S0-ARF-162

Thoracic Surgery

SECOND EDITION

Thoracic Surgery

Edited by

F. GRIFFITH PEARSON, MD
Professor, Division of Thoracic Surgery
Department of Surgery
University of Toronto Faculty of Medicine
Senior Surgeon, Division of Thoracic Surgery
The Toronto General Hospital
Toronto, Ontario, Canada

JOEL D. COOPER, MD
Chief, Division of Cardiothoracic Surgery
Evarts A. Graham Professor of Surgery
Washington University School of Medicine
St. Louis, Missouri

JEAN DESLAURIERS, MD
Professor, Department of Surgery
Laval University Faculty of Medicine
Head, Thoracic Surgery Division
Centre de Pneumologie de l'Hôpital Laval
Ste-Foy, Quebec, Canada

ROBERT J. GINSBERG, MD
Chairman and Professor, Division of Thoracic Surgery
Department of Surgery
University of Toronto Faculty of Medicine
Chief, Division of Thoracic Surgery
The Toronto General Hospital
Toronto, Ontario, Canada

CLEMENT A. HIEBERT, MD
Chairman Emeritus, Department of Surgery
Maine Medical Center
Portland, Maine

G. ALEXANDER PATTERSON, MD
Chief, General Thoracic Surgery
Joseph C. Bancroft Professor of Surgery
Washington University School of Medicine
St. Louis, Missouri

HAROLD C. URSCHEL, JR., MD
Professor, Thoracic and Cardiovascular Surgery
University of Texas Southwestern Medical School
Dallas, Texas

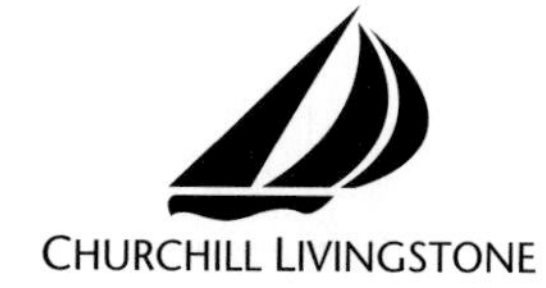

CHURCHILL LIVINGSTONE

An Imprint of Elsevier Science
New York Edinburgh London Philadelphia

CHURCHILL LIVINGSTONE
An Imprint of Elsevier Science

The Curtis Center
Independence Square West
Philadelphia, Pennsylvania 19106

Library of Congress Cataloging-in-Publication Data

Thoracic surgery / [edited by] F. Griffith Pearson . . . [et al.].—2nd ed.

p. cm.

Includes bibliographical references and index.

ISBN 0-443-07595-6

1. Chest—Surgery. I. Pearson, F. Griffith.
[DNLM: 1. Thoracic Surgical Procedures—methods. WF 980 T4865 2001]

RD 536.T458 2002 617.5′4059—dc21

DNLM/DLC 00-057054

Acquisitions Editor: Richard Lampert
Developmental Editor: Melissa Dudlick
Production Manager: Natalie Ware
Manuscript Editor: Veda King
Illustration Specialists: Rita Martello, Walter Verbitski

THORACIC SURGERY ISBN 0-443-07595-6

Printed in the United States of America.

Last digit is the print number: 9 8 7 6 5 4 3 2 1

I thank my wife Hilppa for her patience and ever-present cheerful support. My secretary, Leah Gabriel, was an invaluable resource. Melissa Dudlick, Senior Developmental Editor at WB Saunders, provided a steady stimulus and timely encouragement to our editorial staff during several years of preparation.

F. GRIFFITH PEARSON

To my wife and career-long partner, Janet, whose consistent and unflagging support has made possible all of my professional accomplishments. To my teachers and mentors, especially Griff Pearson, Hermes Grillo, and Ronald Belsey, who have transmitted to me their knowledge, experience, and commitment to the highest standards of clinical care. To my partners and residents over the years for their stimulation and forbearance.

JOEL D. COOPER

This book is dedicated to my wife Debbie and to all the students of Thoracic Surgery.

JEAN DESLAURIERS

My deepest gratitude to Dorrel Granderson for carrying the burden for the second time. To my dear wife, Charlotte, and my children, Karyn, Jordy, and David—thanks for being so patient and understanding during trying times.

ROBERT J. GINSBERG

I wish to thank my secretary, Vicky Bell, for impressive secretarial skills and cheerful assistance. Appreciation also goes to my wife, May Cameron, who, as former head nurse of the thoracic surgical unit at the Toronto General Hospital, had useful insights and suggestions.

CLEMENT A. HIEBERT

I would like to thank my wife Susan—mother, surgeon, scientist, and love of my life. I would also like to acknowledge and thank my four wonderful children—Lachlan, Megan, Brendan, and Caitlan.

G. ALEXANDER PATTERSON

I would like to dedicate my portion of this *Arbeit* to my loving wife Betsey for her understanding of the "time spent away" in thoracic surgery and to my wonderful children—Hal III, Brad, Locke, Amanda, and Susanna—of whom I am extremely proud.

HAROLD C. URSCHEL, JR.

CONTRIBUTORS

Mark S. Allen, MD
Associate Professor of Surgery, Mayo Medical School; Consultant in General Thoracic Surgery, Chair, Division of General Thoracic Surgery, Mayo Clinic, Rochester, Minnesota
Cysts and Duplications in Adults

Scott K. Alpard, MD
Surgical Research Fellow, Division of Cardiothoracic Surgery, University of Texas Medical Branch, Galveston, Texas
Mechanical Ventilatory Assistance

John G. Armstrong, MD, DABR, MRCPI, FFRRCSI
Medical Director, St. Luke's Hospital, Dublin, Ireland
Brachytherapy and Intraoperative Radiotherapy for Non–Small Cell Lung Cancer

Nancy L. Bartlett, MD
Associate Professor of Medicine, Washington University School of Medicine, St. Louis, Missouri
Lymphoma

Gilles Beauchamp, MD
Clinical Professor of Surgery, University of Montreal Faculty of Medicine; Head, Division of Thoracic Surgery, Maisonneuve-Rosemont Hospital, Montreal, Quebec, Canada
Spontaneous Pneumothorax and Pneumomediastinum

Drew C. Bethune, MD, FRCSC
Assistant Professor or Surgery, Dalhousie University Faculty of Medicine; Attending Thoracic Surgeon, Queen Elizabeth II Health Science Centre, Halifax, Nova Scotia, Canada
Acquired Tracheoesophageal Fistula

Akhil Bidani, MD, PhD
Professor of Medicine, Physiology, and Biophysics, University of Texas Medical Branch, Galveston, Texas
Mechanical Ventilatory Assistance

Mark I. Block, MD
Assistant Professor, Division of Cardiothoracic Surgery, Medical University of South Carolina, College of Medicine, Charleston, South Carolina
Thymic Tumors

Philip F. Bongiorno, MD
Senior Resident, Cardiothoracic Surgery, Emory University School of Medicine, Atlanta, Georgia; Attending Surgeon, Section of Cardiothoracic Surgery, Riverside Methodist Hospital, Columbus, Ohio
Blunt Trauma: Chest Wall, Lung, Pleura, Heart, Great Vessels, Thoracic Duct, and Esophagus

Michael Bousamra II, MD
Associate Professor of Surgery, University of Louisville School of Medicine; Director, Lung Transplant Program, and Head of General Thoracic Surgery, University Cardiothoracic Surgical Associates, Jewish Hospital; Attending University of Louisville Hospital, Norton Healthcare Hospitals, and Baptist Hospital East, Louisville, Kentucky
Neurogenic Tumors of the Mediastinum

Arthur D. Boyd, MD
Professor of Surgery, New York University School of Medicine, New York, New York
Thoracic Surgery in the AIDS Patient

Mario Brandolino, MD
Head of Thoracic Surgery Department, Asociaciòn Española, Montevideo, Uruguay
Rare Infections of the Pleural Space

Carl Bredenberg, MD
Professor of Surgery, University of Vermont College of Medicine, Burlington, Vermont; Surgeon-in-Chief, Maine Medical Center, Portland, Maine
Mediastinal Parathyroid Tumors

Robert K. Bright, PhD
Chief, Laboratory of Prostate Biology, Earle A. Chiles Research Institute, Robert W. Franz Cancer Research Center, Providence Portland Medical Center, Portland, Oregon
Non–Small Cell Lung Cancer: Biologic Therapy of Lung Cancer

Joshua H. Burack, MD
Associate Professor of Surgery, State University of New York Health Science Center at Brooklyn; Director, Chest Surgical Service, Kings County Hospital Center, Brooklyn, New York
Pathophysiology and Initial Management of Trauma

Raul Burgos, MD, PhD
Associate Professor, Universidad Autónoma de Madrid; Staff of Cardiovascular Surgery, Clinica Puerta de Hierro, Madrid, Spain
Parasitic Diseases of the Lung and Pleura

Michael Burt, PhD, MD†
Associate Professor, Departments of Surgery and Biochemistry, Cornell University Weill Medical College; Attending Surgeon, Division of Thoracic Surgery, Department of Surgery, Memorial Sloan-Kettering Cancer Center, New York, New York
Rare Primary Malignant Neoplasms

Tada Butler, DO
Department of Family and Community Medicine, University of Arkansas for Medical Sciences, Little Rock, Arkansas

Victor Calvo, MD
Staff Surgeon, La Fe University Hospital, Valencia, Spain
Empyema and Bronchopleural Fistula

Paulo F. Cardoso, MD
Associate Professor of Thoracic Surgery, Department of Surgery, Paulhao Pereira Filho Santa Casa, Porto Allegre, Brazil
Upper Airway Tumors: Primary Tumors

Guy Carrier, MD, CSPQ, FRCP
Associate Professor of Radiology, Department of Radiology, Laval University; Member of Imaging Department, Laval Hospital–University Institute of Cardiology and Pneumology, Quebec, Canada
Diagnostic Procedures for Pleural Diseases

Stephen D. Cassivi, MD
Fellow, Thoracic Surgery, Toronto General Hospital, University of Toronto, Toronto, Ontario, Canada
Surgical Techniques: Videothoracic Transcervical Thymectomy

Alan G. Casson, MB, ChB, MSc, FRCSC, FACS
Professor of Surgery, Dalhousie University Faculty of Medicine; Head, Division of Thoracic Surgery, Queen Elizabeth II Health Science Centre; Head, Surgical Oncology, Cancer Care Nova Scotia, Halifax, Nova Scotia, Canada
Acquired Tracheoesophageal Fistula

Evaristo Castedo, MD
Professor of Surgery, Universidad Autónoma de Madrid; Staff of Cardiovascular Surgery, Clinica Puerta de Hierro, Madrid, Spain
Parasitic Diseases of the Lung and Pleura

Raymond Cloutier, MD, FRCS(C)
Professor of Surgery, Department of Surgery, Laval University Faculty of Medicine; Head of Pediatric Surgery, Centre Hospitalier Univèrsitaire de l'Université Laval, Sainte-Foy, Quebec, Canada
Congenital Eventration and Acquired Elevation of the Diaphragm

†Deceased

Joel D. Cooper, MD
Chief, Division of Cardiovascular Surgery, Evarts A. Graham Professor of Surgery, Washington University School of Medicine, St. Louis, Missouri
Lung Volume Reduction Surgery

Alvin H. Crawford, MD
Professor of Orthopaedics and Pediatrics, University of Cincinnati College of Medicine; Director of Orthopaedic Surgery, Cincinnati Children's Hospital Medical Center, Cincinnati, Ohio
Surgical Techniques for the Chest Wall and Sternum: Thoracoscopic First Rib Resection for Thoracic Outlet Syndrome

R. J. Cusimano, MSc, MD
Associate Professor, University of Toronto Faculty of Medicine; Staff Surgeon, Cardiac Surgery, Toronto General Hospital, Toronto, Ontario, Canada
Anatomy, Physiology and Embryology of the Upper Airway

Pat O. Daily, MD
Medical Director, Cardiovascular and Thoracic Surgery, Sharp Memorial Hospital, San Diego, California
Chronic Pulmonary Embolism

Gail Darling, BSc, MD, FRCS(C), FACS
Associate Professor, Thoracic Surgery, and Program Director, Thoracic Surgery, University of Toronto, Toronto, Ontario Canada
Bacterial Infections of the Lung

Philippe Dartevelle, MD
Professor of Surgery, Paris-Sud University, Paris; Chairman, Department of Thoracic and Vascular Surgery and Heart-Lung Transplantation; Le Plessis Robinson, France
Surgical Techniques: Anterior Approach to Apical Lesions; Resection and Reconstruction of the Superior Vena Cava

Jacob Davtyan, MD
Chief Resident, Section of Cardiothoracic Surgery, Department of Surgery, Emory University School of Medicine, Atlanta, Georgia
Congenital Diaphragmatic Hernias

Marc de Perrot, MD
Fellow, Thoracic Surgery, Toronto General Hospital, University of Toronto, Toronto, Ontario, Canada
Primary Tumors

Denis Desaulniers, MD, FRCS(C)
Clinical Professor, Faculty of Medicine, Laval University; Cardiovascular and Thoracic Surgeon, Laval Hospital, Quebec, Quebec, Canada
Late Sequelae of Thoracic Trauma

Jean Deslauriers, MD, FRCS(C)
Professor of Surgery, Laval University Faculty of Medicine; Head, Thoracic Surgery Division, Centre de Pulmonologie de l'Hôpital Laval, Ste-Foy, Quebec, Canada
Endoscopy: Thoracoscopy for Diagnosis and Staging; Late Complications; Tuberculosis and Atypical Mycobacterial Diseases; Anatomy and Physiology of the Pleural Space; Diagnostic Procedures for Pleural Diseases; Empyema and Bronchopleural Fistula; Fibrothorax and Decortication; Surgical Techniques in the Pleura: Closed Drainage and Suction Systems; Thoracoplasty; Congenital Eventration and Acquired Elevation of the Diaphragm; Diagnostic Strategies in Mediastinal Tumors and Masses; Late Sequelae of Thoracic Trauma

Gregory P. Downey
Director, Division of Respirology; Professor, Department of Medicine, University of Toronto Faculty of Medicine; Staff Physician, The Toronto General Hospital, University Health Networks, Toronto, Ontario, Canada
Bacterial Infections of the Lung

Robert J. Downey, MD
Assistant Professor, Department of Surgery, Weill Medical College of Cornell University; Assistant Attending Surgeon, Division of Thoracic Surgery, Memorial Sloan-Kettering Cancer Center, Department of Surgery, New York, New York
Rare Primary Malignant Neoplasms

Lisa S. Dresner, MD
Associate Professor of Surgery, State University of New York Downstate; Attending Surgeon, King's County Hospital Center, Brooklyn, New York
Pathophysiology and Initial Management of Trauma

John A. Elefteriades, MD
Professor and Chief, Cardiothoracic Surgery, Yale University School of Medicine, Yale–New Haven Hospital, New Haven, Connecticut
The Diaphragm: Phrenic Nerve Pacing

Jeremy J. Erasmus, MBBCh
Associate Professor of Radiology, University of Texas M.D. Anderson Cancer Center, Houston, Texas
Imaging of the Lung

Hao Kenith Fang, MD
Staff Cardiothoracic Surgeon, Good Samaritan Medical Center, Phoenix, Arizona
Unusual Mediastinal Tumors

Ronald Feld, MD
Professor, Department of Medicine, University of Toronto Faculty of Medicine; Staff Physician, Princess Margaret Hospital, University Health Network, Toronto, Ontario, Canada
Small Cell Lung Cancer

Stanley C. Fell, MD
Professor of Cardiothoracic Surgery, Albert Einstein College of Medicine of Yeshiva University; Formerly, Director of Thoracic Surgery, Montefiore Medical Center, Bronx, New York
Mediastinoscopy; Open Lung Biopsy; Surgical Techniques: Segmental Resection; Limited Pulmonary Resection; Anatomy, Embryology, Pathophysiology, and Surgery of the Phrenic Nerve and Diaphragm; Traumatic Diaphragmatic Rupture

Pasquale Ferraro, MD
Assistant Professor, University of Montreal Faculty of Medicine; Thoracic Surgeon and Surgical Director, Lung Transplant Program, Centre Hospitalier de l'Université de Montréal, Montreal, Quebec, Canada
Late Complications

Robert M. Filler, MD
Professor of Surgery and Pediatrics, University of Toronto Faculty of Medicine; Director of Telehealth and External Medical Affairs, The Hospital for Sick Children, Toronto, Ontario, Canada
Benign Conditions: Congenital Anomalies

Matthew J. Fleishman, MD
Radiology Imaging Associates, PC, Denver, Colorado
Imaging of the Diaphragm

Éric Fréchette, MD
Director of Thoracic Surgery, Centre de Pulmonologie de l'Hôpital Laval, Ste-Foy, Quebec, Canada
Congenital Eventration and Acquired Elevation of the Diaphragm

Willard A. Fry, MD
Professor Emeritus of Clinical Surgery, Northwestern University Medical School, Chicago; Former Chief of the Section of Thoracic Surgery, Evanston Hospital, Evanston, Illinois
Surgical Techniques in the Pleura: Open Drainage

Henning A. Gaissert, MD
Assistant Professor of Surgery, Harvard Medical School and Massachusetts General Hospital; Boston, Massachusetts
Endoscopy: Tracheobronchial Stents; Surgical Techniques: Carinal Resection

David S. Gierada, MD
Assistant Professor of Radiology, Chest Radiology Section, Mallinckrodt Institute of Radiology, Washington University School of Medicine, St. Louis, Missouri
Imaging of the Diaphragm

Michelle S. Ginsberg, MD
Assistant Professor of Radiology, Weill Medical College of Cornell University; Director, General Radiology, Assistant Attending, Department of Radiology, Memorial Sloan-Kettering Cancer Center, New York, New York
Imaging of the Lung

Robert J. Ginsberg, MD
Chairman and Professor, Division of Thoracic Surgery, Department of Surgery, University of Toronto Faculty of Medicine; Chief, Division of Thoracic Surgery, The Toronto General Hospital, Toronto, Ontario, Canada
Preoperative Assessment of the Thoracic Surgical Patient: A Surgeon's Viewpoint; Endoscopy: Flexible and Rigid Bronchoscopy; Clinical Features, Diagnosis, and Staging of Lung Cancer; Surgical Management of Non-Small Cell Lung Cancer; Small Cell Lung Cancer; Surgical Techniques: Lobectomy; Superior Sulcus Tumor

Giuseppe Giubilei, MD
Fellow, Thoracic Surgery, Centre de Pneumologie de l'Hôpital Laval, Ste-Foy, Quebec, Canada
Diagnostic Strategies in Mediastinal Tumors and Masses

Lawrence R. Glassman, MD
Assistant Professor of Surgery, New York University School of Medicine; Staff, New York University Hospitals Center and Bellevue Hospital Center.
Thoracic Surgery in the AIDS Patient

Melvyn Goldberg, MD, FRCSC, FACS
Professor, Temple University Medical School; Senior Member and Vice Chairman, Surgical Oncology, Fox Chase Cancer Center, Philadelphia, Pennsylvania
Endoscopy; Laser Therapy; Bullous Disease

Peter Goldstraw, FRCS, FRCS Ed
Consultant Thoracic Surgeon, Royal Brompton Hospital, Sydney Street, London, England
Surgical Techniques: Tracheostomy

Geoffrey M. Graeber, MD
Professor of Surgery and Director of Surgical Research, West Virginia University School of Medicine; Cardiothoracic Surgeon, Monongalia General Hospital, Morgantown, West Virginia
Anatomy and Physiology of the Chest Wall and Sternum; Diagnostic Modalities of the Chest Wall and Sternum; Primary Neoplasms; Surgical Techniques for the Chest Wall and Sternum: Chest Wall Resection; Chest Wall Stabilization; Chest Wall /Soft Tissue Reconstruction; Congenital Diaphragmatic Hernias

Jocelyn Grégoire, MD
Thoracic Surgeon and Consultant, Centre de Pneumologie de l'Hôpital Laval, Ste-Foy; Clinical Instructor, Department of Surgery, Laval University Faculty of Medicine, Quebec City; Quebec, Canada
Surgical Techniques in the Pleura: Closed Drainage and Suction Systems/Thoracoplasty

Hermes C. Grillo, MD
Professor of Surgery, Harvard Medical School; Emeritus Chief of General Thoracic Surgery, Massachusetts General Hospital, Boston, Massachusetts
Benign Conditions: Idiopathic Stenosis; Upper Airway Tumors: Secondary Tumors; Surgical Techniques: Carinal Resections

Ronald F. Grossman, MD
Professor, Department of Medicine, University of Toronto Faculty of Medicine, Toronto; Chief, Department of Medicine, Credit Valley Hospital, Missisauga, Ontario, Canada
Interstitial Lung Disease

Dominique Grunenwald, MD
Professor of Thoracic and Cardiovascular Surgery, University of Paris; Director, Division of Thoracic Surgery, Institut Montsouris, Paris, France
Pulmonary Metastases

Carlos Alberto Guimarães, PhD, MD
Professor, Instituto de Doenças do Tórax da Universidade Federal do Rio de Janeiro; President, Brazilian Society of Thoracic Surgery, Rio de Janeiro, Brazil
Massive Hemoptysis

Patrick J. Gullane, MD, FRCSC, FACS
Professor, Department of Otolaryngology/Surgery, University of Toronto Faculty of Medicine; Otolaryngologist-in-Chief; Director, Head and Neck Program, and Wharton Chair, Head and Neck Surgery, Toronto General Hospital, Toronto, Canada
Anatomy, Physiology, and Embryology of the Larynx; Laryngoscopy

Jeffrey A. Hagen, MD
Associate Professor of Clinical Surgery, Keck School of Medicine, University of Southern California; Chief, Section of Thoracic/Foregut Surgery, LAC/USC Medical Center, Los Angeles, California
Surgery of Myasthenia Gravis

Beverly Hahn, RN
Department of Cardiac Surgery, Christ Hospital, Cincinnati, Ohio
Surgical Techniques for the Chest Wall and Sternum: Thoracoscopic First Rib Resection for Thoracic Outlet Syndrome

David H. Harpole, Jr., MD
Associate Professor of Surgery and Chief of General Thoracic Surgery, Duke University, School of Medicine and Medical Center; Chief of Cardiothoracic Surgery, Durham Veterans Affairs Medical Center, Durham, North Carolina
Bronchial Gland Tumors

Wolfgang Harringer, MD
Assistant Professor of Surgery; Staff Surgeon, Division of Thoracic and Cardiovascular Surgery, Hannover Medical School, Hannover, Germany
Heart-Lung Transplantation

Axel Haverich, MD
Professor of Surgery; Head, Division of Thoracic and Cardiovascular Surgery, Hannover Medical School, Hannover, Germany
Heart-Lung Transplantation

W. Hardy Hendren III, MD
Robert E. Gross, Distinguished Professor of Surgery, Harvard Medical School; Chief of Surgery Emeritus, Children's Hospital; Visiting Surgeon, Massachusetts General Hospital, Boston, Massachusetts
Congenital Deformities of the Chest Wall and Sternum; Cysts and Duplications in Infants and Children

Stephen J. Herman, MD
Associate Professor, Department of Radiology, University of Toronto Faculty of Medicine; Head, Division of Thoracic Imaging, Department of Radiology, The Toronto General Hospital, Toronto, Ontario, Canada
Imaging of the Lung; Imaging of the Mediastinum

Margaret S. Herridge, MD, MSc, MPH, FRCPC
Assistant Professor of Medicine, University of Toronto Faculty of Medicine; Staff Respirologist/Critical Care, Associate Director of Medical-Surgical ICU, University Health Network, Toronto, Ontario, Canada
Bacterial Infections of the Lung

Clement A. Hiebert, MD
Chairman Emeritus, Department of Surgery, Maine Medical Center, Portland, Maine
Laryngeal Nerve Palsy; Mediastinal Parathyroid Tumors

Susan J. Hoover, MD
Clinical Instructor, Department of Surgical Oncology, University of Texas Southwestern Medical Center at Dallas Southwestern Medical School, Dallas, Texas
Infections of the Mediastinum

Tyron Hoover, MD
Pathology Resident, Baylor University Medical Center, Dallas, Texas
Infections of the Mediastinum

David A. Hopkinson, MD
Fellow, Thoracic Surgery, Toronto General Hospital, University of Toronto, Toronto, Ontario, Canada
Benign Conditions: Inflammatory Conditions

Richard I. Inculet, MD, FRCSC
Associate Professor of Surgery, University of Western Ontario Faculty of Medicine; Head, Division of Thoracic Surgery, London Health Sciences Center, London, Ontario, Canada
The Thoracic Duct and Chylothorax

Jonathan C. Irish, MD, MSc, FRCS, FACS
Associate Professor, Department of Otolaryngology, University of Toronto Faculty of Medicine; Staff Surgeon, Department of Surgical Oncology/Otolaryngology, Princess Margaret Hospital, Toronto, Ontario, Canada
Anatomy, Physiology, and Embryology of the Larynx

David R. Jones, MD
Chief Resident, Department of Surgery, West Virginia University School of Medicine; Chief Resident, Ruby Memorial, Morgantown, West Virginia; Chief Resident, Louis A. Johnson Veterans Affairs Medical Center, Clarksburg, West Virginia
Primary Neoplasms

William G. Jones II, MD
Chief, Section of Cardiothoracic Surgery, Methodist Medical Center, Dallas; Attending Cardiothoracic Surgeon, Baylor University Medical Center, Dallas; Doctors Hospital, Dallas; The Medical Center of Mesquite, Mesquite, Texas
Pericardial Disease

Larry R. Kaiser, MD
John Rhea Barton Professor and Chairman, Department of Surgery, University of Pennsylvania School of Medicine, Philadelphia, Pennsylvania
Benign Lung Tumors; Therapeutic Thoracoscopy for Pleural Disease

Riyad Karmy-Jones, MD
Assistant Professor, Thoracic Surgery, University of Washington School of Medicine; Chief, Thoracic Surgery, Harborview Medical Center, University of Washington Medical Center, Division of Cardiothoracic Surgery, Seattle, Washington
Tracheobronchial Trauma

Steven M. Keller, MD
Professor of Cardiothoracic Surgery, Albert Einstein College of Medicine; Chief, Division of Thoracic Surgery, Montefiore Medical Center, Bronx, New York
Surgical Techniques: Mediastinal Lymph Node Dissection

Shaf Keshavjee, MD, MSc, FRCSC, FACS
Associate Professor of Surgery, University of Toronto Faculty of Medicine; Director, Thoracic Surgery Research, and Director, Toronto Lung Transplant Program, The Toronto General Hospital, Toronto, Ontario, Canada
Endoscopy: Flexible and Rigid Bronchoscopy; Benign Conditions: Inflammatory Conditions; Upper Airway Tumors: Primary Tumors; Surgical Techniques: Tracheal Resection; Videothoracoscopic Transcervical Thymectomy

Young T. Kim, MD, PhD
Assistant Professor, Department of Thoracic and Cardiovascular Surgery, Seoul National University College of Medicine; Surgeon, Department of Thoracic and Cardiovascular Surgery; Seoul National University Hospital, Seoul, Korea
Mycotic Infections of the Lung

Thomas J. Kirby, MD, BSc, MBA
Professor of Surgery, Case Western Reserve University School of Medicine; Director of Thoracic Surgery and Lung Transplantation, University Hospitals of Cleveland, Cleveland, Ohio
Endoscopy: Mediastinoscopy; Open Lung Biopsy; Surgical Techniques: Segmental Resection; Limited Pulmonary Resection

Paul A. Kirschner, MD
Professor Emeritus, Cardiothoracic Surgery, Mount Sinai School of Medicine, New York University New York; Consultant, Thoracic Surgery, Veterans Affairs Hospital, Bronx, New York
Anatomy and Surgical Access of the Mediastinum

Paul M. Kirshbom, MD
Fellow in Pediatric Cardiac Surgery, University of Pennsylvania School of Medicine; Instructor of Surgery, Children's Hospital of Philadelphia, Philadelphia, Pennsylvania
Bronchial Gland Tumors

Leslie J. Kohman, MD
Professor of Surgery, State University of New York Medical School, Interim Chair of Surgery, Upstate University Hospital, Syracuse, New York
Biologic Markers of the Mediastinum

Pamela J. Kosco, RN, MPH
Clinical Research Nurse, Memorial Sloan-Kettering Cancer Center, New York, New York
Photodynamic Therapy for Endobronchial Lesions

Dennis Kraus, MD
Associate Clinical Professor, Department of Otorhinolaryngology, Weill Medical College of Cornell University; Staff Surgeon, Division of Head and Neck Surgery, Department of Surgery, Memorial Sloan-Kettering Cancer Center, New York, New York
Laryngeal Nerve Palsy

Florian Lang, Dr Med
Fellow, Academic Staff, University of Lausanne, Faculty of Medicine; Department of Otorhinolaryngology, Head and Neck Surgery, Centre Hospitalier Universitaire Vaudois, Lausanne, Switzerland
Endoscopy: Laser Therapy; Subglottic Resection: Infants and Children; Laryngeal Trauma

Michael P. La Quaglia, MD
Professor of Surgery, Weill Medical College of Cornell University; Chief, Pediatric Surgical Service, Memorial Sloan-Kettering Cancer Center, New York, New York
Congenital Anomalies of the Lung

Robert B. Lee, MD
Associate Professor of Surgery, Clinical Sciences, Division of Cardiothoracic Surgery, University of Mississippi School of Medicine, Jackson, Mississippi
Radionecrosis and Infection of the Chest Wall and Sternum

Stephen Lefrak, MD
Professor of Medicine, Washington University School of Medicine; Director, Lung Volume Reduction Surgery Program; Director, MICU, North Campus; Medical Director, The Jacqueline Maritz Lung Center, Barnes-Jewish Hospital, St. Louis, Missouri
Lung Volume Reduction Surgery

Louis Létourneau, MD, FRCP(C)
Department of Radiology, Centre de Pneumologie, Ste-Foy, Quebec, Canada
Diagnostic Strategies in Mediastinal Tumors and Masses

Dorothea Liebermann-Meffert, Dr Med, FACS
Professor, Technische Universität Munich; Surgeon, Department of Surgery, Chirurgische Klinik und Poliklinik, Klinikum rechts der Isar, Munich, Germany
Laryngeal Nerve Palsy

Jere W. Lord, MD
Chief, Vascular Surgery, Montefiore Hospital, New York, New York
Surgical Techniques for the Chest Wall and Sternum: Surgery of the Clavicle

James D. Luketich, MD
Associate Professor of Surgery, University of Pittsburgh School of Medicine; Chief, Division of Thoracic and Foregut Surgery, Presbyterian University Hospital, Pittsburgh, Pennsylvania
Photodynamic Therapy for Endobronchial Lesions

Paolo Macchiarini, MD, PhD
Professor of Surgery, Hannover Medical School; Chairman, Department of Thoracic and Vascular Surgery, Heidehaus Hospital, Hannover, Germany
Surgical Techniques: Anterior Approach to Apical Lesions; Resection and Reconstruction of the Superior Vena Cava

Susan Mackinnon, MD
Shoenberg Professor and Chief, Division of Plastic and Reconstructive Surgery, Department of Surgery, Washington University School of Medicine, St. Louis, Missouri
Thoracic Outlet Syndromes; Surgical Techniques for the Chest Wall and Sternum: Supraclavicular Approach for Thoracic Outlet Syndrome

Michael A. Maddaus, MD
Associate Professor of Thoracic Surgery, University of Minnesota Medical School–Minneapolis, Minneapolis, Minnesota
Benign Conditions: Postintubation Injury; Tracheomalacia; Subglottic Resection: Adults; Clinical Features, Diagnosis, and Staging of Lung Cancer

Richard A. Malthaner, MD, MSc
Assistant Professor, University of Western Ontario Faculty of Medicine; Staff Surgeon, Division of Thoracic Surgery, London Health Sciences Centre, London, Ontario, Canada
The Thoracic Duct and Chylothorax

Kamal A. Mansour, MD, FACS
Professor of Surgery (Cardiothoracic), Emory University School of Medicine, Atlanta, Georgia
Blunt Trauma: Chest Wall, Lung, Pleura, Heart, Great Vessels, Thoracic Duct, and Esophagus

Nael Martini, MD
Professor of Surgery, Weill Medical College of Cornell University; Attending Thoracic Surgeon, Memorial Sloan-Kettering Cancer Center, New York, New York
Non–Small Cell Lung Cancer: Surgical Management; Surgical Techniques: Lobectomy

Douglas J. Mathisen, MD
Professor of Surgery, Harvard Medical School; Visiting Surgeon and Chief, General Thoracic Surgery, Massachusetts General Hospital, Boston, Massachusetts
Upper Airway Tumors: Secondary Tumors; Surgical Techniques: Carinal Resection

Kenneth L. Mattox, MD
Professor of Surgery, Baylor College of Medicine; Chief of Staff/Chief of Surgery, Ben Taub General Hospital, Houston, Texas
Penetrating Trauma

Carol McGibney, MD, FRCSI, FRCR, FFR(Irel.)
Senior Registrar in Radiation Oncology, St. Luke's Hospital, Dublin, Ireland
Brachytherapy and Intraoperative Radiotherapy for Non–Small Cell Lung Cancer

Karen M. McGinnis, MD
Assistant Professor of Surgery, Beth Israel Medical Center, New York, New York
Biologic Markers of the Mediastinum

Karen M. McRae, MD, CM, FRCPC
Assistant Professor, Department of Anesthesia, University of Toronto Faculty of Medicine; Staff Anesthesiologist, The Toronto General Hospital, Toronto, Ontario, Canada
Anesthesia; Anesthesia for Airway Surgery

Reza John Mehran, MD, CM, FRCSC
Assistant Professor of Surgery, University of Ottawa Faculty of Medicine; Thoracic Surgeon, Ottawa Hospital, Ottawa, Ontario, Canada
Tuberculosis and Atypical Mycobacterial Diseases; Anatomy and Physiology of the Pleural Space; Late Sequelae of Thoracic Trauma

Bryan F. Meyers, MD
Assistant Professor, Division of Cardiothoracic Surgery, Washington University School of Medicine, St. Louis, Missouri
Lung Transplantation; Pericardial Disease

Anthony B. Miller, MB, FRCP
Professor Emeritus, Department of Public Health Sciences, University of Toronto Faculty of Medicine, Toronto, Ontario, Canada; Head, Division of Clinical Epidemiology, Deutsches Krebsforschungszentrum, Heidelberg, Germany
Epidemiology of Lung Cancer

Joseph I. Miller, Jr., MD
Professor of Cardiothoracic Surgery and Chief, General Thoracic Surgery, Emory University School of Medicine, Atlanta, Georgia
Radionecrosis and Infection of the Chest Wall and Sternum; Congenital Diaphragmatic Hernias

Philippe Monnier, Dr Med
Professor, University of Lausanne Faculty of Medicine; Chairman, Department of Otorhinolaryngology, Head and Neck Surgery, Centre Hospitalier Universitaire Vaudois, Lausanne, Switzerland
Endoscopy: Laser Therapy; Subglottic Resection: Infants and Children; Laryngeal Trauma

Clifford Morgan, BM, FRCA
Consultant in Anaesthesia and Critical Care, Royal Brompton Hospital, London, England
Surgical Techniques: Tracheostomy

Sudish C. Murthy, MD, PhD
Staff Surgeon, Division of General Thoracic Surgery, Cleveland Clinic Foundation, Cleveland, Ohio
Thoracic Incisions

John Muscedere, MD, FRCPC
Director, Intensive Care Unit, Hôtel-Dieu Grace Hospital, Windsor, Ontario, Canada
Pulmonary Physiology

Keith S. Naunheim, MD
The Vallee and Melba Willman Professor and Chief of Thoracic Surgery, Saint Louis University School of Medicine; Chief of Thoracic Surgery, John Cochran Veterans Affairs Medical Center, St. Louis, Missouri
Surgical Techniques: Thoracoscopic Mediastinal Surgery

Mitra Niroumand, MD
Associate Physician, Mount Sinai Hospital, Toronto, Ontario, Canada
Interstitial Lung Disease

Denise Ouellette, MD
Associate Clinical Professor, Department of Surgery, University of Montreal Faculty of Medicine; Thoracic Surgeon, Maisonneure-Rosemont Hospital, Montreal, Quebec, Canada
Spontaneous Pneumothorax and Pneumomediastinum

Peter C. Pairolero, MD
Professor, Department of Surgery, Mayo Medical School; Chairman, Department of Surgery, Mayo Clinic and Mayo Foundation, Rochester, Minnesota
Primary Neoplasms

Francisco París, MD
Titular Professor of Surgery, Faculty of Medicine, Valencia University; Head of Thoracic Surgery Service, La Fe University Hospital, Valencia, Spain
Empyema and Bronchopleural Fistula; Fibrothorax and Decortication

Philippe Pasche, Dr Med
Associate Professor, University of Lausanne Faculty of Medicine; Department of Otorhinolaryngology, Head and Neck Surgery, Centre Hospitalier Universitaire Vaudois, Lausanne, Switzerland
Endoscopy: Laser Therapy; Laryngeal Trauma

Harvey I. Pass, MD
Professor of Surgery and Oncology, Wayne State University School of Medicine; Chief, Thoracic Oncology, Karmanos Cancer Institute; Chief, Thoracic Oncology, John Dingell Veterans Hospital, Detroit, Michigan
Non–Small Cell Lung Cancer: Biologic Therapy of Lung Cancer

Helen A. Pass, MD
Staff, William Beaumont Hospital, Royal Oak, Michigan
Non–Small Cell Lung Cancer: Biologic Therapy of Lung Cancer

Ugo Pastorino, MD
Director, Division of Thoracic Surgery, European Institute of Oncology, Milan, Italy
Pulmonary Metastases

Irvin Pathak, MD, FRCSC
Head and Neck Surgeon, Royal Jubilee Hospital, Victoria, British Columbia, Canada
Endoscopy: Laryngoscopy

G. Alexander Patterson, MD, FRCS(C), FACS
Chief, General Thoracic Surgery, Joseph C. Bancroft Professor of Surgery; Head, Section of General Thoracic Surgery, Washington University School of Medicine, St. Louis, Missouri
Endoscopy: Tracheobronchial Stents; Surgical Techniques: Extended Pulmonary Resections; Lung Transplantation; Thoracic Outlet Syndromes; Surgical Techniques for the Chest Wall and Sternum; Supraclavicular Approach for Thoracic Outlet Syndrome

Edward R. Patz, Jr., MD
Professor of Radiology and Pathology, Duke University School of Medicine, Durham, North Carolina
Imaging of the Lung

F. Griffith Pearson, MD
Professor, Division of Thoracic Surgery, Department of Surgery, University of Toronto Faculty of Medicine; Senior Surgeon, Division of Thoracic Surgery, The Toronto General Hospital, Toronto, Ontario, Canada
Anatomy, Physiology, and Embryology of the Upper Airway; Benign Conditions: Postintubation Injury/Tracheomalacia; Upper Airway Tumors: Primary Tumors; Subglottic Resection: Adults; Tracheal Resection

Thomas L. Petty, MD
Professor of Medicine, University of Colorado School of Medicine, Denver; Professor of Medicine, Rush Medical College of Rush University, Chicago; Faculty Consultant, Health One Alliance, Denver, Colorado
Pulmonary Function Testing: A Practical Approach

Andrew F. Pierre, MD, MSc, FRCSC
Chief Resident, Thoracic Surgery, The Toronto General Hospital, University of Toronto, Toronto, Ontario, Canada
Endoscopy: Flexible and Rigid Bronchoscopy

Konstadinos A. Plestis, MD
Assistant Professor, Department of Cardiothoracic Surgery, Jack D. Weiler Hospital of the Albert Einstein College of Medicine, Bronx, New York
Anatomy, Embryology, Pathophysiology, and Surgery of the Phrenic Nerve and Diaphragm

Celeste N. Powers, MD, PhD
Professor, Pathology and Otolaryngology, and Chair, Division of Surgical and Cytopathology, Medical College of Virginia, Virginia Commonwealth University Health Systems; Director, Anatomic Pathology Services, Medical College of Virginia Hospitals, Richmond, Virginia
Biologic Markers of the Mediastinum

Joe B. Putnam, Jr., MD
Professor, Department of Surgery, University of Texas–Houston Medical School and M. D. Anderson Cancer Center, Houston, Texas
Postresection Follow-Up for Non–Small Cell Lung Cancer

Jacquelyn A. Quin, MD
Assistant Professor, Division of Cardiothoracic Surgery, Department of Surgery, Southern Illinois University School of Medicine, Springfield, Illinois
The Diaphragm: Phrenic Nerve Pacing

Alexandre Radu, Dr Med
Research Fellow, University of Lausanne Faculty of Medicine; Department of Otorhinolaryngology, Head and Neck Surgery, Centre Hospitalier Universitaire Vaudois, Lausanne, Switzerland
Laser Therapy

A. C. Ralph-Edwards, MD
Lecturer, University of Toronto Faculty of Medicine; Staff Surgeon, Toronto General Hospital, Toronto, Ontario, Canada
Perioperative Management

Linda M. Razzuk, BA
Premedical Student, University of Texas at Dallas, Dallas, Texas
Infections of the Mediastinum

Maruf A. Razzuk, MD†
Late Professor of Cardiovascular, Thoracic and Vascular Surgery, Baylor University Medical Center, Dallas, Texas
Infections of the Mediastinum

Erino A. Rendina, MD
Associate Professor of Thoracic Surgery; University of Rome "La Sapienza" School of Medicine and Policlinico Umberto I, Rome, Italy
Surgical Techniques: Reconstruction of the Pulmonary Artery

Thomas W. Rice, MD
Head, Section of General Thoracic Surgery, Department of Thoracic and Cardiovascular Surgery, The Cleveland Clinic Foundation, Cleveland, Ohio
Thoracic Incisions; Anatomy of the Lung

Jon H. Ritter, MD
Assistant Professor of Pathology and Immunology, Washington University School of Medicine; Attending Surgical Pathologist, Washington University Medical Center, St. Louis, Missouri
Pathology of Lung Cancer

M. Patricia Rivera, MD
Assistant Professor of Medicine, University of North Carolina–Chapel Hill, Chapel Hill, North Carolina
Pulmonary Infections and the Immunocompromised Host

Francis Robicsek, MD, PhD
Chairman, Department of Cardiovascular and Thoracic Surgery, Carolinas Medical Center; Medical Director, The Carolinas Heart Institute; Clinical Professor of Surgery, University of North Carolina, Charlotte, North Carolina
Complications of Midline Sternotomy; Surgical Techniques for the Chest Wall and Sternum: Combined Exposure of the First Rib: A Modified Approach for the Treatment of Thoracic Outlet Syndrome

Jack A. Roth, MD
Professor of Thoracic and Cardiovascular Surgery and Professor of Molecular and Cellular Oncology, University of Texas Medical School at Houston; Bud Johnson Clinical Distinguished Chair; Chairman, Thoracic and Cardiovascular Surgery; and Director, W. M. Keck Center for Cancer Gene Therapy, The University of Texas M.D. Anderson Cancer Center, Houston, Texas
Biology of Lung Cancer

†Deceased.

Valerie W. Rusch, MD
Professor of Surgery, Cornell University Medical College; Chief, Thoracic Service, Department of Surgery, William G. Cahan Chair of Surgery, Attending Surgeon and Member, Memorial Sloan-Kettering Cancer Center, New York, New York
Pleural Effusion: Benign and Malignant; Mesothelioma and Less Common Pleural Tumors

Alan N. Sandler, MB, ChB
Professor, Department of Anesthesia, University of Toronto Faculty of Medicine; Staff Anesthesiologist, The Toronto General Hospital, Toronto, Ontario, Canada
Anesthesia

Marcel Savary, MD
Honorary Professor, Department of Otolaryngology, Head and Neck Surgery, University of Lausanne Medical School; Centre Hospitaliér Universitaíre Vaudois, Lausanne, Switzerland
Subglottic Resection: Infants and Children

Robert C. Shamberger, MD
Professor of Surgery, Harvard Medical School; Senior Associate in Surgery, Children's Hospital, Boston, Massachusetts
Congenital Deformities of the Chest Wall and Sternum; Cysts and Duplications in Infants and Children

Farid Shamji, MD
Associate Professor, University of Ottawa Faculty of Medicine; Head, Division of Thoracic Surgery, Civic Campus—The Ottawa Hospital, Ottawa, Ontario, Canada
Surgical Techniques: Superior Sulcus Tumor

Frances A. Shepherd, MD, FRCPC
Scott Taylor Chair in Lung Cancer Research, Professor of Medicine, University of Toronto Faculty of Medicine; Senior Staff Physician, Princess Margaret Hospital, Toronto, Ontario, Canada
Chemotherapy for Non–Small Cell Lung Cancer

Thomas W. Shields, MD
Professor Emeritus of Surgery, Northwestern University Medical School, Chicago, Illinois
Mediastinal Thyroid Tumors

Joseph B. Shrager, MD
Assistant Professor of Surgery, University of Pennsylvania School of Medicine; Attending Surgeon, Hospital of the University of Pennsylvania; Director, General Thoracic Surgery, Pennsylvania Hospital, Philadelphia, Pennsylvania
Benign Lung Tumors; Therapeutic Thoracoscopy for Pleural Disease

Cateline Sirois, MD
Resident, Thoracic Surgery, Division of Surgery, Centre de Pneumologie de Laval, Ste-Foy, Quebec, Canada
Thoracoscopy for Diagnosis and Staging

Peter D. Slinger, MD, FRCPC
Professor of Anesthesia, University of Toronto Faculty of Medicine; Staff Anesthesiologist, Toronto General Hospital, Toronto, Ontario, Canada
Anesthesia

Richard M. Slone, MD
Associate Professor of Radiology, Mallinckrodt Institute, Washington University School of Medicine, St. Louis, Missouri
Imaging of the Diaphragm

Arthur S. Slutsky, MD
Professor of Medicine, University of Toronto Faculty of Medicine; Vice-President, Research, St. Michael's Hospital, Toronto, Ontario, Canada
Pulmonary Physiology

Ernesto Soltero, MD
Assistant Professor of Surgery, Division of Cardiothoracic Surgery, Baylor College of Medicine; Acting Chief, Cardiothoracic Surgery, Houston Veteran Affairs Medical Center, Houston, Texas
Penetrating Trauma

Diane E. Stover, MD
Professor of Clinical Medicine, Weill Medical College of Cornell University; Chief of Pulmonary Medicine, Head of General Medicine, Memorial Sloan-Kettering Cancer Center, New York, New York
Pulmonary Infections and the Immunocompromised Host

S. Sundaresan, MD
Associate Professor of Surgery, Northwestern University Medical School; Attending Surgeon, Northwestern Memorial Hospital, Chicago, Illinois
Unusual Mediastinal Tumors

Michael F. Szwerc, MD
Assistant Professor, West Virginia University School of Medicine; Cardiothoracic Surgeon, Monongalia General Hospital, Morgantown, West Virginia
Anatomy and Physiology of the Chest Wall and Sternum

Vicente Tarrazona, MD
Associate Professor of Thoracic Surgery, Department of Surgery, Faculty of Medicine, Valencia University; Head of Thoracic Surgery Unit, Clinic University Hospital, Valencia, Spain
Fibrothorax and Decortication

F. Deaver Thomas, MD
Professor of Radiology and Medicine, State University of New York Medical School; Co-Director of Nuclear Medicine, Department of Radiology, Upstate University Hospital, Syracuse, New York
Biologic Markers of the Mediastinum

Thomas R. J. Todd, MD, FRCSC
Professor of Surgery, University of Toronto Faculty of Medicine, Toronto, Ontario, Canada; Chairman, Department of Surgery, Shaikh Khalifa Medical Center, Abu Dhabi, United Arab Emirates
Perioperative Management; Adult Respiratory Distress Syndrome

Victor F. Trastek, MD
Professor of Surgery, Mayo Medical School, Mayo Clinic Foundation, Rochester, Minnesota; Chairman, Department of Surgery, Mayo Clinic Scottsdale, Scottsdale, Arizona
Mycotic Infections of the Lung

Ryosuke Tsuchiya, MD
Chief, Division of Thoracic Surgery, Department of Surgery, National Cancer Center Hospital, Tokyo, Japan
Bronchoplastic Techniques

Divina M. Tuazon, MD
Senior Fellow, Division of Pulmonary and Critical Care Medicine, University of Texas Medical Branch, Galveston, Texas
Mechanical Ventilatory Assistance

Harold C. Urschel, Jr., MD
Professor, Thoracic and Cardiovascular Surgery, University of Texas Southwestern Medical School; Baylor University Medical Center, Dallas, Texas
General Thoracic Surgery: History and Development; Surgical Techniques: Superior Sulcus Tumor; Thoracic Outlet Syndromes; Surgical Techniques for the Chest Wall and Sternum: Transaxillary Approach with Dorsal Sympathectomy for Thoracic Outlet Syndrome/Recurrent Reoperation Through the Posterior Thoracoplasty Approach with Dorsal Sympathectomy for Thoracic Outlet Syndrome/Surgery of the Clavicle; Infections of The Mediastinum

Éric Vallières, MD, FRCSC
Associate Professor, Thoracic Surgery, University of Washington Medical School and University of Washington Medical Center, Division of Cardiothoracic Surgery, Seattle, Washington
Diagnostic Procedures for Pleural Diseases; Tracheobronchial Trauma

Andrés Varela, MD, PhD
Professor of Surgery, Universidad Autónoma de Madrid; Section Chief of Thoracic Surgery, Clinica Puerta de Hierro, Madrid, Madrid, Spain
Parasitic Diseases of the Lung and Pleura

Federico Venuta, MD
Associate Professor of Thoracic Surgery, University of Rome "La Sapienza" School of Medicine, Policlinico Umberto I, Department of Thoracic Surgery, Rome, Italy
Surgical Techniques: Reconstruction of the Pulmonary Artery

Jorge Nin Vivó, MD
Associate Professor of Anatomy, Faculty of Medicine of Montevideo, Head of Thoracic Surgery Department, Sanatorio Casa de Galicia, Montevideo, Uruguay
Rare Infections of the Pleural Space

Nina D. Wagner, BSN, MSN
Washington University School of Medicine, St. Louis, Missouri
Lymphoma of the Mediastinum

Matthew J. Wall, Jr., MD
Associate Professor, Baylor College of Medicine; Deputy Chief of Surgery, Chief of Cardiothoracic Surgery, Executive Director of Trauma and Critical Care Services, Ben Taub General Hospital, Houston, Texas
Penetrating Trauma

Paul F. Waters, MD, FRCS(C)
Professor of Surgery and Director of Lung Transplant Surgery, Mount Sinai School of Medicine; Chief, Thoracic Surgery, Mount Sinai Medical Center, New York, New York
Surgical Techniques: Pneumonectomy

Tracey L. Weigel, MD
Associate Professor of Surgery, University of Wisconsin Medical School; Head, Section of Thoracic Surgery, University of Wisconsin Hospital and Clinics, Madison, Wisconsin
Photodynamic Therapy for Endobronchial Lesions

Gordon L. Weisbrod, MD, FRCPC
Professor, University of Toronto Faculty of Medicine; Senior Staff Radiologist, University Health Network/ Mount Sinai Hospital, Toronto, Ontario, Canada
Imaging of the Mediastinum

Thomas H. Weisenberger, MD, FACR
Clinical Professor, Department of Radiation Oncology, UCLA School of Medicine, Los Angeles; Medical Director, Cancer Center of Santa Barbara, Santa Barbara, California
Radiotherapy for Non–Small Cell Lung Cancer

Mark R. Wick, MD
Professor of Pathology, University of Virginia School of Medicine; Associate Director of Surgical Pathology, University of Virginia Health System, Charlottesville, Virginia
Pathology of Lung Cancer

Earle W. Wilkins, Jr., MD
Clinical Professor of Surgery, Emeritus, Harvard Medical School; Senior Surgeon, Massachusetts General Hospital, Boston, Massachusetts
General Thoracic Surgery: History and Development

Ian J. Witterick, MD, FRCSC
Assistant Professor, Department of Otolaryngology, University of Toronto Faculty of Medicine, Staff Otolaryngologist, Mount Sinai Hospital; Head of Otolaryngology, Saint Joseph's Health Centre, Toronto, Ontario, Canada
Endoscopy: Laryngoscopy

Randall K. Wolf, MD
Associate Professor, Department of Surgery, Ohio State University School of Medicine; Director of Minimally Invasive Cardiac Surgery and Robotics, Ohio State University Medical Center, Columbus, Ohio
Surgical Techniques for the Chest Wall and Sternum: Thoracoscopic First Rib Resection for Thoracic Outlet Syndrome

Douglas E. Wood, MD
Associate Professor, Thoracic Surgery, University of Washington School of Medicine; Chief, General Thoracic Surgery, Endowed Chair in Lung Cancer Research, University of Washington Medical Center, Seattle, Washington
Tracheobronchial Trauma

Michael G. Wood, MD
Resident in General Surgery, University of Southern California, Keck School of Medicine, Los Angeles, California
Surgery of Myasthenia Gravis

Cameron Wright, MD
Associate Professor of Surgery, Harvard Medical School; Associate Chief, General Thoracic Surgical Unit, Massachusetts General Hospital, Boston, Massachusetts
Germ Cell Tumors of the Mediastinum

Anthony P. C. Yim, DM, FRCS, FACS
Professor and Chief, Division of Cardiothoracic Surgery, The Chinese University of Hong Kong, Prince of Wales Hospital, Hong Kong
Surgical Techniques: Video-Assisted Pulmonary Resections

Maureen Zakowski, MD
Assistant Professor of Pathology, Weill Medical College of Cornell University; Associate Attending Pathologist, Memorial Sloan-Kettering Cancer Center, New York, New York
Rare Primary Malignant Neoplasms

Noe Zamel, MD, FRCPC, FCCP
Professor, Department of Medicine, University of Toronto Faculty of Medicine; Director, Trihospital Pulmonary Function Laboratories, Toronto General, Mt. Sinai and Women's College Hospitals, Toronto, Ontario, Canada
Pulmonary Physiology

Joseph B. Zwischenberger, MD
Professor of Surgery, Medicine, and Radiology; Director, General Thoracic Surgery and ECMO Programs; University of Texas Medical Branch, Division of Cardiothoracic Surgery, Galveston, Texas
Mechanical Ventilatory Assistance

PREFACE

Six years have elapsed since publication of the first editions of *Thoracic Surgery* and *Esophageal Surgery.* In these second editions, all original chapters have been updated and a significant number of new chapters added. Important additions include major advances in the application and acceptance of minimally invasive video-assisted techniques; advances in the technology of imaging with positron emission tomography scanning and ultrasound; the current emphasis on multimodality therapy in the management of many thoracic malignancies (including locally advanced lung and esophageal carcinomas); the expanding field of lung volume reduction surgery and three-field lymphadenectomy for esophageal cancer; and new operative techniques for the management of difficult technical problems, such as resection and reconstruction of the pulmonary artery and superior vena cava.

Otherwise, format and objectives remain the same. Each of the seven medical editors has assumed responsibility for one or more sections in which that particular editor has internationally recognized expertise. Chapter authors were chosen because of their acknowledged expertise in the assigned topic. Content and presentation were designed to create a comprehensive textbook for general reference, with an emphasis on practical guidance for the resident in training and for the established practitioner.

Again, the text has been separated into two volumes in an effort to accommodate the potentially disparate interests of the reader. *Thoracic Surgery* encompasses operative techniques of the airways, lungs, chest wall, and mediastinum. *Esophageal Surgery* will be of interest to general surgeons and gastroenterologists, as well as to thoracic surgeons.

The Department of Surgery at the University of Toronto continues to dominate the background of the editors: Six of the seven current editors hold or have held academic positions in the Division of Thoracic Surgery in Toronto. Many of the individual chapters have been written by graduates of the Toronto General Thoracic Surgery Training Programme.

F. Griffith Pearson

NOTICE

Medicine is an ever-changing field. Standard safety precautions must be followed, but as new research and clinical experience broaden our knowledge, changes in treatment and drug therapy become necessary or appropriate. Readers are advised to check the product information currently provided by the manufacturer of each drug to be administered to verify the recommended dose, the method and duration of administration, and the contraindications. It is the responsibility of the treating physician, relying on experience and knowledge of the patient, to determine dosages and the best treatment for each individual patient. Neither the publisher nor the editor assumes any liability for any injury and/or damage to persons or property arising from this publication.

THE PUBLISHER

CONTENTS

SECTION I

SECTION II

Introduction

CHAPTER 1

General Thoracic Surgery: History and Development

Earle W. Wilkins, Jr.
Harold C. Urschel, Jr.

In his honored speaker's address to the American Association for Thoracic Surgery on the occasion of its 50th annual meeting, the scholarly Leo Eloesser (1970) referred to chest surgery as having "become a purposefully intended and scientifically directed art." That general thoracic surgery is indeed a science complemented by the skilled art of caring for the patient, few would disagree. That it has been purposefully intended may require appraisal and analysis, for which a historical review, seeking common threads of development, is quite admirably suited.

ORIGINS

There is no exact date or specific event that marks the birth of chest surgery. It did not arise de novo in a particular country or in one school of surgery. It appears that after the public demonstration of ether anesthesia by Warren in 1846 and the early understanding of sepsis following Semmelweiss' work in 1847, physicians in a number of countries began to explore the possible application of surgical techniques to the relief of diseases of the thorax. To ascribe priority is surely to pronounce error and invite rebuttal. A series of events and personalities is presented, therefore, only to permit placement of the origins of general thoracic surgery in the context of time and to emphasize the multinational roots of its development.

Czerny of Heidelberg, Germany, a former assistant of the early pioneer of surgery in Vienna, Billroth, performed one of the early resections for carcinoma of the cervical esophagus in 1877. Block of Danzig (now Gdansk, Poland) described his original experimental work in pulmonary resection in rabbits in 1881. Forlanini, professor of medicine in Pavia, introduced the concept of artificial pneumothorax for tuberculous cavities in 1882. De Cérenville of Lausanne, although a professor of clinical medicine and internal pathology, described rib resections for collapsing the lung in 1885. Wheeler of Dublin described a successful resection of a pulsion diverticulum of the pharyngoesophageal junction in 1886. Rehn of Frankfurt am Main in 1897 described the survival of a young man following suture of a stab wound of the right ventricle. Beck of New York advocated visceral pleurectomy in the radical treatment of empyema in 1897. Finally, Jacobaeus of Stockholm introduced the thoracoscope for closed intrapleural pneumonolysis in 1911. Such were examples of the beginnings of thoracic surgery.

INTRAOPERATIVE CONTROL OF RESPIRATION

These pioneering ventures into chest surgery, as innovatively daring as they were, were doomed to limited success until control of respiration in the open chest was achieved. Johann von Mikulicz (1904) of Breslau (now Wroclaw, Poland) initiated research into the development of a differential pressure methodology for control of respiration during surgery. If there was a birth of modern chest surgery, this might be identified as its critical point in time. Eloesser (1965), in an editorial in the *Journal of Thoracic and Cardiovascular Surgery,* suggests that Mikulicz "stumbled on the very birth of modern chest surgery." He was recalling a 1904 scene in Breslau involving Mikulicz's pupil Ferdinand Sauerbruch: ". . . those fiery whitecoats swarming out of the basement into the Silesian twilight heralded the beginnings of controlled respiration."

Sauerbruch developed the negative differential pressure chamber, a complicated system in which the patient and the operating team were closeted in a hermetically sealed space with only the patient's head outside at atmospheric pressure for administration of anesthesia and control of respiration. Meanwhile, Brauer (1904) of Marburg, Germany was developing a positive-pressure method that enclosed only the patient's head, like a diver's helmet according to Borst (1985), for applying anesthesia and positive pressure. Robinson (1910) from the Massachusetts General Hospital in Boston, having worked with both Sauerbruch and Brauer, chose the latter's principle in constructing his own "box," a positive-pressure chamber in which the anesthetist was actually seated with the patient's head enclosed within the chamber.

All these cumbersome methods served as a prelude to the work of Meltzer and Auer of New York (1909) with "continuous respiration without respiratory movements" by means of the intratracheal insufflation of a continuous stream of air and anesthetic vapor. This led ultimately to the intermittent, or phasic, application of positive-pressure respiration and its modern counterpart via the cuffed endotracheal tube. (It should be interjected here that Tuffier of Paris had reported in 1896 his actual development of an intratracheal tube with an inflatable cuff.)

Thus, the development of the methodology of intermittent positive-pressure inflation of the lungs, permitting all the phases of modern intrathoracic surgery, seems to have been "purposefully intended." It constituted what Eloesser called the first milestone in chest surgery.

ANESTHESIA

In addition to the positive-pressure insufflation, another significant advance in thoracic surgical anesthesia was the double-lumen tube, which was developed in England by Robert-Shaw (Wood et al, 1972). This allowed ventilation through one tube, the collapse of the other lung, and easier technical thoracic surgery. In the lateral position, the "down" lung receives most of the blood supply that is shunted in that direction. The Chinese had frequently used this without an endotracheal tube in acupuncture patients who were awake. On opening the chest in the lateral position, the lung collapsed automatically with exposure to positive pressure, and the blood was shunted to the down-side lung. This allowed the same technical advantage of the double-lumen tube in the Western World.

Equally important was the development of the field of endoscopy, which allowed tubes to be used for the diagnosis and treatment of diseases of the larynx, trachea, bronchi, pharynx, esophagus, stomach, and small intestine. Essential to the development of thoracic surgery, endoscopy, anesthesiology, and radiology were all represented in the initial membership of the American Association of Thoracic Surgery.

THE BASIS OF PULMONARY RESECTION

With the ventilatory aspect of anesthesia for the open chest fully achieved, attention slowly turned toward both research and clinical application in pulmonary resection. Brunn (1929) of San Francisco clearly stated the goal of lobectomy: "By this method, the diseased lobe is removed at one stroke, the period of convalescence is diminished, and deformity does not result." The basic challenges in safe pulmonary resection were control of the hilar vessels and closure of the bronchial stump.

Lobectomy

Early efforts at lobectomy involved hilar mass ligature and two-stage resections. Frequently described as ghastly, the staged operation was considered essential because of the fear of bronchial stump blowout. Lilienthal (1922) of New York reported 14 single lobectomies for bronchiectasis with 6 deaths (43%). In this series, he used the presence of adhesions as a guide to staging the lower lobectomy. If the upper lobe were held in an expanded position, he proceeded with single-stage resection; if not, he induced adhesions with gauze abrading of the pleural surfaces and iodoform packing and continued to a two-stage operation. This kind of suppurative lung disease with difficult adhesions and hypertrophy of the bronchial arterial system made early attempts at lobectomy the most hazardous and in large measure may have accounted in this pre-antibiotic era for the high mortality rate.

Despite this early experience of Lilienthal, Eloesser identifies the report of Brunn, including six lobectomies with a single death, as his second milestone in thoracic surgery, stating: "In 1918, Brunn did the first modern closed lobectomy, ligating the vessels, suturing the hilar stump of lung over the severed bronchus, and closing the chest." Brunn used a system of closed chest drainage to maintain expansion of residual lung. Wertheim hysterectomy clamps were used across the lung root pedicle, which was then ligated with double, heavy chromic catgut ties.

Apparently overlooked in these early lobectomies that were done with mass hilar ligature was the report of Davies (1913) of London. In 1912 he had performed a right lower lobectomy for carcinoma in which "the various structures at the pedicle of the lower lobe were ligated separately. . . . The proximal end of the bronchus was stitched over and covered with an adjacent portion of lung." Unfortunately, the patient developed an empyema and died on the eighth day but "at the autopsy, no evidence of leakage from the bronchus could be obtained." It may be assumed that the death of the patient discredited a technique reminiscent of the individual dissection technique developed by Churchill of Boston (1931). In it, Churchill carried out a successful lobectomy for a bronchial adenoma using individual dissection and ligation of vessels and continuous catgut suture of the bronchial stump with coverage by adjacent upper lobe parenchyma.

This work culminated in the classic report of Churchill and Belsey of Bristol, England (1939), working at that time in Churchill's department. In this report, the individual dissection and ligature technique was extended to segmental pulmonary resection. The authors identified the lingula "for descriptive purposes . . . the homologue of the right middle lobe," emphasizing from bronchographic study its frequent (46 of 50 cases) involvement in bronchiectasis. The article concluded with a prophetic sentence: "It is suggested that the bronchopulmonary segment may replace the lobe as the surgical unit of the lung."

Meade (1961) of Ann Arbor, Michigan, in *A History of Thoracic Surgery* insists that Kent of Pittsburgh and Blades of Washington, D.C. (1942) be credited with individual management of vessels and bronchus "for publicizing this technique" in their report on the surgical anatomy of pulmonary lobes.

Pneumonectomy

The concerns facing the pioneers in lobectomy were only magnified when it came to total removal of a lung, not only because of the risk of hemorrhage and the ever-present likelihood of bronchial fistula but also because of the fear of sudden occlusion of a main pulmonary artery. Would a ligature of the pulmonary artery simulate the clinical picture of a massive pulmonary embolus?

The prevention of hemorrhage was facilitated by the introduction by Shenstone and Janes of Toronto (1932) of their lung tourniquet. In this technique, the lung root pedicle was encircled by a snare of heavy cord, which was then tightened, and the lung was cut away leaving a 2-cm cuff of tissue. In their words, "obvious vessels were clamped and ligated and a running suture of chromic catgut was introduced across the pedicle." Graham of St. Louis and Singer (1933) employed the tourniquet in their remarkable and successful one-stage pneumonectomy for carcinoma. Graham was apparently unaware of basic animal experiments, but his anxiety over occlusion of the pulmonary artery was relieved by preliminary tourniquet obliteration of arterial blood flow without apparent change in vital signs. Graham added a complementary thoracoplasty of the third to ninth ribs to reduce the size of the residual pleural space and to minimize the worrisome threat of mediastinal shift. The patient, a physician, survived 30 years until his death at age 78. Graham's pneumonectomy was Eloesser's third milestone in surgery, a courageous accomplishment and a turning point in history.

Archibald of Montreal (1934) reported a successful dissection pneumonectomy performed just 3 months after Graham's feat. Ever after pneumonectomy would be carried out by individual ligation of pulmonary artery and veins. Rienhoff (1933) of Baltimore provided the definitive technique for bronchial closure after pneumonectomy. His technique included "cutting the cartilages at various points, in order to do away with their spring-like action" and suturing "the bronchus with interrupted medium silk sutures." A classic paper by Rienhoff followed in 1942, the result of extensive experimentation with techniques of bronchial closure in dogs, including coverage of the stump with parietal pleura.

Here too, the techniques of hilar dissection and bronchial stump closure seem purposefully intended.

Bronchoplasty

Although it is a significant advance in resection for cancer of the lung, pneumonectomy is a "disease" itself because of morbidity and mortality. Some cases are amenable to resection of the cancer with bronchoplastic preservation of lung tissue after preoperative irradiation. Price-Thomas is given credit for performing bronchoplastic procedures for benign tumors. However, since 1952 Paulson and Urschel have followed over 500 patients undergoing bronchoplastic resection for carcinoma following 3000 cGy of preoperative irradiation that would otherwise have required pneumonectomy. Over the next 50 years, an excellent 5-year survival from 35% to 55% (depending on nodal involvement) has resulted (Paulson, 1971).

Superior Pulmonary Sulcus Carcinoma

Pancoast's tumor, described by radiologists in 1932, was considered unresectable because of its location extending from the lung and involving the lower trunk of the brachial plexus in most cases. Shaw, Paulson, and Urschel, starting from the early 50s, developed a technique of surgical en bloc resection following preoperative irradiation and subsequently used it in over 500 patients. Long-term survival was similar to that of lobectomy for carcinoma, relative to the lymph node stage (Urschel, 2000).

ESOPHAGECTOMY

Early efforts toward esophageal resection were confined to its cervical portion or to extrapleural approaches at the thoracic level. Billroth (1871) had demonstrated in dogs that resection and anastomosis of the cervical esophagus was feasible. His assistant in those animal experiments, Czerny (1877), carried out a partial cervical esophageal resection for carcinoma, as already noted. Meade (1961), the thoracic surgical historian, describes "the first successful intrathoracic resection and anastomosis of the esophagus" by Dobromysslow (1901). A 3- to 4-cm segment was resected, the ends united with two rows of silk sutures, and the anastomosis wrapped with a large posteriorly based skin flap. Although "complete union of the suture line" was demonstrated at 3 weeks, Meade reported that no further follow-up could be discovered. Denk (1913) of Vienna demonstrated in cadavers that the esophagus could be removed by blunt dissection through a subcostal transhiatal approach combined with a cervical dissection. Turner (1933) reported a successful blunt esophagectomy followed by a second-stage completion of an antethoracic skin tube to connect the esophageal and gastric stomas.

The contemporary development of positive-pressure intratracheal anesthesia permitted the direct transthoracic approach to esophageal resection. The pioneering operation was that of Torek (1913) of New York, who carried out a subtotal, left thoracic resection of the esophagus for a squamous carcinoma of the middle third. The 67-year-old woman survived 13 years, fed orally via a rubber tube that connected her cervical esophagostomy and gastrostomy. She refused any attempt at plastic, antethoracic skin tube reconstruction.

Restoration of alimentary continuity following esophagectomy now constituted the principal surgical challenge. In animal experiments, Beck (1905) demonstrated the use of a tube that was of greater curvature than the stomach to replace the lower esophagus. Roux (1907) of Lausanne developed the technique of esophagojejunoplasty for distal esophageal stricture. Kelling (1911) of Dresden devised a technique for use of the colon for esophageal replacement. In his initial case, an isoperistaltic segment of transverse colon was brought up subcutaneously, and its distal end was anastomosed to the stomach at the midsternal level in preparation for ultimate skin-tube connection to the cervical esophagostomy. Kirschner (1920) of Leipzig originated the now standard use of a mobilized stomach to replace the esophagus by dividing the left gastric, left gastroepiploic, and short gastric arteries. He planned an antethoracic, subcutaneous placement of the stomach but never succeeded in using it in a patient with carcinoma.

In light of this burst of both animal experimentation and progressive attempts in humans, it is surprising that the final accomplishment of a successful esophagectomy with an intrathoracic esophagogastric anastomosis did not occur until 1937, when Marshall (1938) of Boston carried out an esophagogastrectomy with re-establishment of continuity by an end-to-side anastomosis. Adams and Phemister (1938) of Chicago followed with a similar successful case, featuring for the first time a two-layer anastomosis using interrupted nonabsorbable sutures, which in this case were linen. Churchill and Sweet (1942) of Boston presented a classic report of 11 resections, emphasizing preservation of gastric blood supply and the meticulous suturing, with two-layer interrupted fine silk, of the anastomosis as the basis for avoiding anastomotic leakage or stricture formation.

Finally, Sweet (1945) and the British surgeon Lewis (1946) extended esophageal resection to any level of carcinoma within the esophagus—Sweet by the strictly left transthoracic, double-rib resection approach and Lewis by the separate laparotomy and right thoracic incisions.

Mahoney and Sherman (1954) of Rochester, New York reintroduced use of the colon to replace the entire thoracic esophagus, utilizing isoperistaltic right colon placed in the anterior mediastinal position. Wilkins (1980) emphasized preference for use of left colon, always following preoperative angiographic mapping of mesenteric blood supply. The colon thus became the accepted alternative choice, after the stomach, for esophageal replacement.

Mark Orringer (1978) of Ann Arbor resurrected and perfected the technique of transhiatal-transcervical esophagectomy without thoracotomy. Once again in the esophagus, a purposefully intended art continued.

GLOBAL FACTORS

Tuberculosis: The White Plague

Delarue (1989) of Toronto apparently coined the term *white plague* in noting that after the conquest of smallpox, tuberculosis remained a worldwide major public health threat. He recorded "little significant change . . . from Hippocratic times to the onset of the twentieth century." Indeed, Robert Koch had discovered the causative bacterial agent, the tubercle bacillus, only in 1882. That was the same year in which Forlanini reported his work with inducing artificial pneumothorax to treat cavitary pulmonary tuberculosis.

Thenceforth, the evolution of forms of therapy for tuberculosis was closely tied to the history of thoracic surgery, in fact defining early surgical techniques. Failure of pneumothorax to provide appropriate cavitary collapse led to the development of extrapleural thoracoplasty. As mentioned earlier, de Cérenville began this work in 1885 with resections of just a few ribs, usually the second and third. Brauer in 1909 related the number of ribs to be resected to the degree of collapse necessary to provide cavity closure. Friedrich (1911) of Marburg described extensive thoracoplasty with removal of portions of ribs 2 through 10. The 3-month mortality, however, was 40%. Brauer then proposed certain modifications: operative staging of the rib resections, subperiosteal rib resection to permit better ultimate stability of the chest wall, and limitation of lengthy rib resections to those underlying the scapula. Wilms (1911) of Basel added removal of the transverse processes posteriorly, and Carter (1932) in the United States added removal of the first rib. The final step in the evolution of extrapleural thoracoplasty was the addition of pulmonary extrafascial apicolysis described by Holst (1933) and Semb (1935), both of Oslo.

The operation of phrenicectomy, like use of pneumoperitoneum to elevate the diaphragm in an effort to promote collapse of lower lobe cavities, enjoyed a transient period of popularity in the 1920s. [*Editor's note*: Probably because it was easily performed.] It never proved effective in cavity closure and was largely abandoned, even before the modern antibiotic era.

The ingenuity of surgeons led to a rash of procedures to modify the standard operation that extrapleural thoracoplasty had become, primarily in an effort to avoid the major chest wall deformity caused by thoracoplasty. The underlying principles of all these were extraparietal pleural dissection to free the lung from the chest wall and placement of substance in the extrapleural space to maintain pulmonary collapse. The variety of substances used included air (the original method), pedicled muscle, fat, and paraffin. A further modification was the subperiosteal stripping of ribs to provide an extraperiosteal space into which materials were introduced, providing a plombage. Popular substances included oil (oleothorax), polyethylene sheets, and Lucite balls. This trend toward plombage was terminated not so much by the onset of the antibiotic era as by the unacceptable rate of complications stemming from foreign body intolerance—tissue reaction, infection, and internal fistulas.

Pulmonary resection for tuberculous cavities dates back to Krönlein (1882) of Zurich but was performed only sporadically and without signal success. Renewed interest followed the work of Churchill and Klopstock (1943), in which lobectomy was selectively carried out in cases not amenable to pneumothorax. However, in a consolidated report of these operations by Meade (1961), the "morbidity ranged from 37% to 70% and mortality rate was 6.2% to 33%."

The era of surgery for tuberculosis culminated after the arrival of antituberculous agent therapy (streptomycin, para-amino-salicylic acid, and isoniazid) in segmental resection with Overholt (Overholt et al, 1950) of Boston and Chamberlain (Chamberlain and Klopstock, 1950) of New York as its principal advocates.

World War I

Two lessons learned from World War I were the management of open chest wounds and the treatment of empyema.

A long held physiologic concept that the mediastinum provided a rigid separation of the lungs was refuted by the deadly experience early in the war with open chest wounds. Meade (1961) quotes the 1917 directive from MacPherson for the Director General of Medical Service, British Armies in France: "An open pneumothorax should be temporarily closed by suture at the earliest opportunity, either in the field ambulance or at the Casualty Clearing Station. If for any reason suturing is impossible, the wound should be packed, and strapped, so as to render it air tight." Only the modern technique of associated tube thoracostomy was missing from that order.

The other physiologic principle evolving from the war stemmed not from war wounding but from epidemic infection. Almost two thirds of deaths in the American army were due to pneumonia and empyema complicating the 1918 influenza epidemic or, tragically, to their treatment early on. Standard protocol had been open drainage of empyema as soon as diagnosed, but in these army cases the infecting organism was often *Streptococcus*. Empyemas were being drained before the lung parenchyma had become adherent to the chest wall, and patients were dying from open pneumothorax. In their work with the Empyema Commission of the U.S. Army, Graham and Bell (1918) concluded (once again to quote Meade): "the principles of treatment of acute empyema are (1) drainage, but with careful avoidance of open pneumothorax during the period of active pneumonia, (2) early sterilization and obliteration of the cavity, and (3) maintenance of the nutrition of the patient." It would take another 25 years and another world war before antibiotics, beginning with penicillin, could be added to the prescription of empyema therapy.

World War II

Whereas the lessons of the first World War dealt with problems of pneumothorax, the principal advance in the handling of chest wounds in World War II involved the management of hemothorax. Contrary to civilian teaching at the time, war experience determined that clotted hemothorax was not uncommon. In spite of clotting, frequent aspiration was possible, or in some cases spontaneous resorption took place. Samson, Burford, Brewer (all later presidents of the American Association for Thoracic Surgery), and Burbank (Samson et al, 1946), in discussing the management of chest wounds in general, introduced the concept of early pulmonary decortication for organizing hemothorax. Their indications for operation included "patients in whom there is at least 50% compression of the lung . . . those in whom aspiration has been unsuccessful and in whom there has been no appreciable pulmonary expansion at the end of 4 to 6 weeks following injury." Although appropriate credit must be given to Eggers (1923) of New York for his work with the radical treatment of empyema, it was this work beginning with Burford's 1943 innovative "decortication in a case of uninfected organizing hemothorax five weeks after injury" that culminated in the modern concept of total pulmonary decortication as expressed in the classic report of Samson and Burford (1947).

The role of the thoracic center, in this case the Army Second Auxiliary Surgical Group's starting of the first Army Thoracic Surgical Center at Bizerte (Tunisia, North Africa), cannot be overstressed in studies on the wet lung syndrome and its treatment with intercostal block, tracheal suction, and repeated bronchoscopy. An abiding principle was that chest wounds in general do not require early thoracotomy.

EVOLUTION OF GENERAL THORACIC SURGERY

Eloesser's fourth milestone in chest surgery was the work of Gibbon (1937, 1954) beginning in 1937 in the development of extracorporeal circulation, which Eloesser characterized as an "idea and its elaboration . . . among the boldest and most successful feats of man's mind." This eventuated in opening the entire field of cardiac surgery, which in turn indirectly supported the distinct specialty of general thoracic surgery. The differences in its evolution in the United States and Canada are worthy of recounting.

United States

It is essential, in understanding the concept of general thoracic surgery as a specialty in its own right, to begin with the early interest in establishing thoracic surgical societies as a means of sharing ideas, techniques of surgery, and patient outcomes. These societies were all established within this century, the first being the New York Thoracic Surgical Society, founded in early 1917. Its prime mover was Meyer, who immediately used this group as a focal point for discussing formation of a national thoracic society. That same year, at the American Medical Association meeting in New York, with the New York society as host to 23 physicians out of some 42 who had published on thoracic subjects, Meyer moved formation of the American Association for Thoracic Surgery (AATS). Its first meeting took place in Chicago in 1918 with Meltzer as president. There were 50 men in the founders' group, which was not limited to thoracic surgeons alone but included interested physicians "*for* thoracic surgery," such as anesthesia, endoscopy, and radiology.

The proceedings of meetings were initially published in 1921 in the newly established *Archives of Surgery.* The *Journal of Thoracic Surgery* became the official organ of the Association in 1931; Graham was its first editor, a position he held until his death in 1957. In a move reflecting the exploding role of cardiac surgery and the burgeoning numbers of papers on cardiovascular surgery, its name was changed in 1959 to the *Journal of Thoracic and Cardiovascular Surgery.*

With a national society and a journal for the publication of its transactions now established, the next issue involved the need for a certifying mechanism and body. In 1937, the AATS appointed a seven-man committee chaired by Eggers to investigate the situation. Only Alexander favored the establishment of a board of thoracic surgery. With only 18 surgeons in the country considering themselves to be thoracic surgeons, the committee advised the AATS that the time was not right for such a board. By 1946, however, particularly with the remarkable thoracic surgical developments during the war, the time was ripe. Another Eggers committee working with the American Board of Surgery (ABS), itself established only in 1937, reported favorably to the AATS this time. So, in 1948 the Board of Thoracic Surgery was created as an affiliate of the ABS. Reflecting the same pressures that beset the Journal, the Board ultimately (1971) became the independent American Board of Thoracic Surgery (ABTS). Although it retained the generic "Thoracic" in its title, the ABTS changed the wording of its certificate to specify accreditation in both thoracic and cardiovascular surgery.

RESIDENCY REVIEW COMMITTEE

Unique in the United States and not present in other countries of the world is the Residency Review Committee (RRC) for each of the subspecialties. The Thoracic Surgery RRC regularly reviews the 90 thoracic training programs for content, educational requirements, and training of the thoracic surgeon. This RRC Accreditation of the Thoracic Surgical training program is totally separate from the certification program as performed by the ABTS. It minimizes "conflict of interest" and also provides the optimal environment for encouraging excellence for thoracic surgeons. After the ABTS was established in 1948, the American Medical Association (AMA) developed the Accreditation Council for Graduate Medical Education (ACGME). It is made up of the American Board of Medical Specialties (ABMS), the American Hospital Association (AHA), the AMA, the American Association for Medical Colleges (AAMC), and the Council for Medical Specialty Societies (CMSS). In addition, it also has representatives from the public and the federal government. This provides a broad base for accreditation of medical specialties. The Residency Review Committee for Thoracic Surgery, under the auspices of the ACGME, is made up of 2 members each from the American College of Surgeons, the AMA and the ABTS. Each of the residencies is reviewed every 5 years at the minimum if the educational techniques are satisfactory. If there is any irregularity, probation, or withdrawals, they are examined more frequently, as often as every year. At the present time, there are slightly over 90 programs, between two and three years in length, for surgeons having completed the requirement for the American Board of Surgery, which is 5 years of general surgery.

The second national thoracic society was established in 1965—the Society of Thoracic Surgeons (STS). This organization permitted an unlimited membership of surgeons who strictly limited their practice to thoracic and cardiovascular surgery and who were accredited by the ABTS. It initiated and promoted its own journal, *The Annals of Thoracic Surgery.*

In his presidential address before the AATS entitled "A Time for Assessment," Paulson (1981) described three stages in the development of thoracic surgery—its establishment, its expansion, and its maturity. Much of the first two of these phases have been discussed earlier in this history. The first successful open heart operation by Gibbon (1953) was the catalyst in the phase of expansion. This took place primarily in the cardiac portion of the specialty, with the development of techniques for coronary bypass, valve replacement, correction of congenital defects, and excision of thoracic aneurysms. In the *maturity* phase, Paulson addressed an imbalance between programs for cardiac surgery and what has come to be termed general thoracic surgery (GTS): "The increase in volume of cardiac surgery has led to a serious imbalance in our educational programs, with subordination of general thoracic surgery to a secondary position in many thoracic surgical training centers." One of the several examples cited was the mean operative experience of ABTS candidates in the period of 1971 to 1980, when only six to nine operations on the esophagus were encountered during an entire training career. This inadequate training experience resulted in either ill-equipped thoracic surgeons or non–board-certified surgeons performing these procedures.

In response to Paulson's recommendations, a Liaison Committee for Thoracic Surgery was established, which involved the Thoracic Surgery Directors Association, the ABTS, the Residency Review Committee, the STS, and the AATS. In a slowly increasing number of training centers, separate GTS programs with their own directors have been set up, collaborating with cardiac surgical programs to meet the ABTS requirements. A general thoracic surgeon finds that he must qualify and be certified in both fields to practice GTS.

Canada

The contrasting development of GTS in Canada was concisely described by Pearson (1990) in his presidential address to the AATS. He cited the combined specialty of thoracic and cardiovascular surgery prevalent in the United States, the United Kingdom, and Europe and then commented that "the evolution of training in thoracic surgery, in Toronto, however, was at variance with this pattern." A separate division of cardiovascular surgery had been created in 1958 with its own "dedicated residency." Thoracic surgery (now GTS) was continued within the two general surgical divisions until 1968, when a separate division of thoracic surgery was established. Pearson described the establishment of separate and autonomous divisions as "chance."

According to Pearson, "thoracic surgery was suffering the neglect of a 'poor relation' in departments of cardiovascular and thoracic surgery throughout the country." In 1976, the Royal College of Physicians and Surgeons of Canada, the one certifying body in Canada, established the Certificate of Special Competence in Thoracic Surgery, which "focused attention on training in thoracic surgery." The Toronto pattern thus had been recognized nationally, and the Certificate of Special Competence had helped enormously along the way in addressing the imbalance between cardiac surgery and GTS. In his expansive history of *Thoracic Surgery in Canada,* Delarue (1989) is quoted: "As a result, there is, at the present time, effective specialty coverage across the length and breadth of this huge country."

Canada, unlike the United States, has achieved a fifth milestone in thoracic surgery, recognition of the specialty of General Thoracic Surgery.

KEY REFERENCES

Borst HG: Hands across the ocean: German-American relations in thoracic surgery. J Thorac Cardiovasc Surg 90:477, 1985.

This was the honored speaker's address before the 1985 annual meeting of the American Association for Thoracic Surgery. Borst, who is professor of surgery in Hannover, Germany, and has experienced medical school and residency training in the United States, is uniquely qualified to trace the beginnings of thoracic surgery in Germany onward to the leadership role of the United States during the dark times in Europe.

Delarue NC: Thoracic Surgery in Canada. Toronto, BC Decker, 1989.

In the words of the subtitle, this is a "a story of people, places, and events, the evolution of a specialty," told in a thoroughly authoritarian style by the late emeritus professor of surgery in the Faculty of Medicine, University of Toronto. It provides the details of the evolution of the specialty of general thoracic surgery in Canada and its credentialing with the Certificate of Special Competence in Thoracic Surgery.

Meade RH: A History of Thoracic Surgery. Springfield, IL, CC Thomas, 1961.

This encyclopedic story of thoracic surgery from earliest times through 1960 is, in the words of Emile Holman in its preface, "less a history and more a textbook giving the development of surgical procedures, embellished by instructive details including results."

Naef AP: The Story of Thoracic Surgery: Milestones and Pioneers. Bern, Hogrefe & Huber, 1990.

A Swiss surgeon's account of the evolution of both general thoracic and cardiovascular surgery, much of it from his own personal experience with the pioneers who created the milestones he has cited.

REFERENCES

Adams WE, Phemister DB: Carcinoma of the lower thoracic esophagus: Report of a successful resection and esophagogastrostomy. J Thorac Surg 7:621, 1938.

Archibald EW: Unilateral pneumonectomy. Ann Surg 100:796, 1934.

Beck C: Demonstrations of specimens illustrating a method of formation of a prethoracic esophagus. IMJ 7:463, 1905.

Beck C: Discussion of Ferguson AH: Thoracoplasty in America and visceral pleurectomy, with report of a case. JAMA 28:58, 1897.

Billroth CAT: Über die Resektion des Ösophagus. Arch Klin Chir 13:65, 1871.

Block MH: Experimentelles zur Lungenresektion. Dtsch Med Wochenschr 7:634, 1881.

Brauer L: Erfahrungen and Überlegungen zur Lungenkollapstherapie: Die ausgedehnte extrapleurale Thorakoplastik. Klin Tuberk 12:49, 1909.

Brauer L: Die Ausschaltung der Pneumothoraxfolgen mit Hilfe des Überdruckverfahrens. Mitt Grenzgeb Med Chir 13:483, 1904.

Brunn H: Surgical principles underlying one-stage lobectomy. Arch Surg 18:490, 1929.

Cérenville ECB de: De l'intervention opératoire dans les maladies du poumon. Rev Med Suisse Rom 5:441, 1885.

Carter BN: A technique for thoracoplasty. Surg Gynecol Obstet 57:353, 1933.

Chamberlain JM, Klopstock R: Further experiences with segmental resection in pulmonary tuberculosis. J Thorac Cardiovasc Surg 20:843, 1950.

Churchill ED, Belsey R: Segmental pneumonectomy in bronchiectasis: Lingula segment of left upper lobe. Ann Surg 109:481, 1939.

Churchill ED, Klopstock R: Lobectomy for pulmonary tuberculosis. Ann Surg 117:641, 1943.

Churchill ED, Sweet RH: Transthoracic resection of tumors of the stomach and esophagus. Ann Surg 115:897, 1942.

Czerny V: Neue Operationen. Zentralbl Chir 4:433, 1877.

Davies HM: Recent advances in the surgery of the lung and pleura. Br J Surg 1:228, 1913.

Denk W: Zur Radikaloperation des Ösophaguskarzinomas. Zentralbl Chir 40:1065, 1913.

Dobromysslow VD: Ein Fall von transpleuraler Ösophagektomie ein Brustabschnitte. Zentralbl Chir 28:1, 1901.

Eggers C: Radical treatment of chronic empyema. Ann Surg 77:327, 1923.

Eloesser L: Milestones in chest surgery. J Thorac Cardiovasc Surg 60:157, 1970.

Eloesser L: Birth of modern chest surgery and von Mikulicz's part in it. J Thorac Cardiovasc Surg 50:757, 1965.

Forlanini C: A contribuzione della terrapie della tisi. Primo caso di tisi pulmonare curato col pneumotorace artificiale. Gaz Osped 68:537, 1882.

Friedrich PL: Statisches und Prinzipielles zur Frage der Rippenresektion ausgedehnten oder beschränkten. Munch Med Wochenschr 58:2041, 1911.

Gibbon JH Jr: The application of a mechanical heart and lung apparatus to cardiac surgery. Minn Med 37:171, 1954.

Gibbon JH Jr: Artificial maintenance of circulation during experimental occlusion of pulmonary artery. Arch Surg 34:1105, 1937.

Graham EA, Bell RD: Open pneumothorax: Its relation to the treatment of acute empyema. Am J Med Sci 156:839, 1918.

Graham EA, Singer JJ: Successful removal of an entire lung for carcinoma of the bronchus. JAMA 101:1371, 1933.

Holst J: Local selective thoracoplasty in pulmonary tuberculosis. Norsk Mag Laegevidensk 94:361, 1933.

Jacobaeus HC: Über Laparo und Thorakoscopie. Beitr Klin Tuberk 25:185, 1912.

Kelling G: Ösophagoplastik mit Hilfe des Querkolon. Zentralbl Chir 38:1209, 1911.

Kent EM, Blades B: Surgical anatomy of the pulmonary lobes. J Thorac Surg 12:18, 1942.

Kirschner MB: Eines neues Verfahren der Ösophagoplastik. Arch Klin Chir 114:606, 1920.

Krönlein RV: Über Lungen-Chirurgie. Berl Klin Wochenschr 8:440, 1882.

Lewis I: The surgical treatment of carcinoma of the oesophagus: With special reference to a new operation for growths of the middle third. Br J Surg 34:18, 1946.

Lilienthal H: Pulmonary resection for bronchiectasis. Ann Surg 75:257, 1922.

Mahoney EB, Sherman CD Jr: Total esophagoplasty using intrathoracic right colon. Surgery 35:937, 1954.

Marshall SF: Carcinoma of the esophagus: Successful resection of lower end of esophagus with reestablishment of esophageal gastric continuity. Surg Clin North Am 18:643, 1938.

Meltzer SJ, Auer J: Continuous respiration without respiratory movements. J Exp Med 11:622, 1909.

Mikulicz J von: Über Operationen in der Brusthöhle mit Hilfe der Sauerbruchschen Kammer. Cited in Eloesser L: Milestones in chest surgery. J Thorac Cardiovasc Surg 60:157, 1970.

Naef AP: Hugh Morriston Davies: First dissection lobectomy in 1912. Ann Thorac Cardiovasc Surg 56:988, 1993.

Orringer MB: Esophagectomy without thoracotomy. J Thorac Cardiovasc Surg 76:643, 1978.

Overholt RH, Woods RM, Ramsay BH: Segmental pulmonary resection: Details of technique and results. J Thorac Cardiovasc Surg 19:207, 1950.

Paulson DL: A time for assessment. J Thorac Cardiovasc Surg 82:163, 1981.

Paulson DL, Urschel HC Jr, McNamara JJ, Shaw RR: Bronchoplastic procedures for bronchogenic carcinoma. J Thorac Cardiovasc Surg 59:38, 1970.

Pearson FG: Adventures in surgery. J Thorac Cardiovasc Surg 100:639, 1990.

Rehn L: Über penetrierende Herzwunden und Herznaht. Arch Klin Chir 55:315, 1897.

Rienhoff WF Jr: Closure of bronchus following total pneumonectomy. Ann Surg 116:481, 1942.

Reinhoff WF Jr: Pneumonectomy: A preliminary report on the operative technique in two successful cases. Johns Hopkins Med J 55:390, 1933.

Robinson S: A positive pressure cabinet for thoracic surgery. Surg Gynecol Obstet 10:287, 1910.

Roux C: L'Esophago-jejuno-gastromie, nouvelle opération pour rétrécissement infranchisable de l'esophage. Semaine Med 27:37, 1907.

Samson PC, Burford TH: Total pulmonary decortication: Its evolution and present concepts of indications and operative technique. J Thorac Cardiovasc Surg 16:127, 1947.

Samson PC, Burford TH, Brewer LA, Burbank B: The management of war wounds of the chest in a base center. J Thorac Cardiovasc Surg 15:1, 1946.

Sauerbruch JF: Über die physiologischen und physikalischen Grundlagen bei intrathorakalen Eingriffen in meiner pneumatischen Operationskammer. Arch Klin Chir 77:977, 1904.

Semb C: Technique of plastic operation of apicolysis. Acta Chir Scand 76:84, 1935.

Shenstone NS, Janes R: Experiences in pulmonary lobectomy. Can J Med 27:138, 1932.

Sweet RH: Surgical management of carcinoma of the mid-thoracic esophagus. N Engl J Med 233:1, 1945.

Torek F: The first successful case of resection of the thoracic portion of the esophagus for carcinoma. Surg Gynecol Obstet 16:614, 1913.

Tuffier T: Régulation de la pression intrabronchique et de la narcose. Compt Rend Soc Biol 3:1086, 1896.

Turner GG: Excision of thoracic oesophagus for carcinoma with construction of extra-thoracic gullet. Lancet 2:1315, 1933.

Urschel HC Jr: Superior pulmonary sulcus tumors. In Skarin AT (ed): Multimodality Treatment of Lung Cancer. New York, Marcel Dekker, 2000.

Wheeler WI: Pharyngocele and dilatation of the pharynx, with existing diverticulum at lower part of pharynx lying posterior to the oesophagus. Dublin J Med Sci 82:349, 1886.

Wilms M: Ein neue Methode zur Verengerung des Thorax bei Lungentuberkulose. Munch Med Wschr 50:777, 1911.

Wilkins EW Jr: Long-segment colon substitution for the esophagus. Ann Surg 192:722, 1980.

Wood RE, Campbell DC, Urschel HC, Jr: Surgical advantages of selective unilateral ventilation. Ann Thorac Surg 14:2, 1972.

CHAPTER **2**

Pulmonary Physiology

John Muscedere
Noe Zamel
Arthur S. Slutsky

An understanding of basic respiratory physiology is important to the diagnosis and treatment of lung disease—this is true whether the clinician is a respiratory physician or thoracic surgeon. In virtually no other organ system is function so closely related to relatively easily measured variables. Respiratory diseases and syndromes can be readily understood if the basic physiology is understood, and indeed, if basic physiology is understood, therapies can be suggested and implemented. Two good examples of this are lung volume reduction surgery for emphysema and ventilator-associated lung injury, both of which are discussed at the end of this chapter, under Applied Pulmonary Physiology.

The comprehension of pulmonary physiology is essential to the provision of excellent care to the thoracic surgical patient. However, the field of pulmonary physiology is extremely vast and rapidly expanding, and due to space constraints this chapter provides only an overview of this area. In this context, only important or classic articles are referenced. References to important review articles on selected topics are provided so that information beyond the scope of this chapter may be readily accessed. The structural basis of pulmonary physiology is discussed first, followed by discussions on the control of breathing, ventilation, diffusion, and pulmonary function studies. The final section on applied pulmonary physiology demonstrates some of the physiologic principles in relation to two common clinical problems: lung volume reduction surgery for emphysema and ventilator-associated lung injury—areas of current clinical and research interest.

RESPIRATORY APPARATUS

Airways

The main purpose of the respiratory system is to deliver oxygen (O_2) and remove carbon dioxide (CO_2) from the bloodstream. In this context, the anatomic structure of the lungs can be viewed as consisting of two regions: (1) the conducting airways, and (2) the gas exchange region.

The conducting airways extend from the nasal passages to the terminal bronchioles. In these airways, gas transport takes place largely by convection—the bulk transport of gas. Distal to the terminal bronchioles, the major gas transport mechanism is diffusion. Because gas exchange does not take place in the conducting airways, the volume of these is given the term *anatomic dead space*. In a normal, upright subject, it is approximately 150 ml (methods to measure this are discussed later in this chapter).

Starting from the trachea, successive branching of the bronchial tree occurs with subsequent narrowing of each individual bronchus. However, because of the increase in the number of airways, the total cross-sectional area increases with each division. As can be seen in Figure 2–1, the total cross-sectional area of the bronchi initially increases slightly and later starts to increase exponentially (West, 1985). Bronchial diameter reaches a minimum of approximately 0.5 to 0.7 mm at the level of the terminal bronchioles and remains constant in spite of subsequent divisions (Bastacky et al, 1983; Horsfeld and Cumming, 1968). It is postulated that the transition from bulk flow to diffusion occurs at this level because the forward velocity of the inspired gas drops dramatically as the cross-sectional area rapidly widens. The average number of divisions or generations of airways from trachea to terminal bronchi is approximately 23, but it may occur in as few as 8 divisions or as many as 25, as idealized in the schematic of Figure 2–2 (Horsfeld and Cumming, 1968).

The primary gas exchange unit of the lung is the acinus. It is the portion of the lung distal to the terminal bronchiole and comprises respiratory bronchioles, alveo-

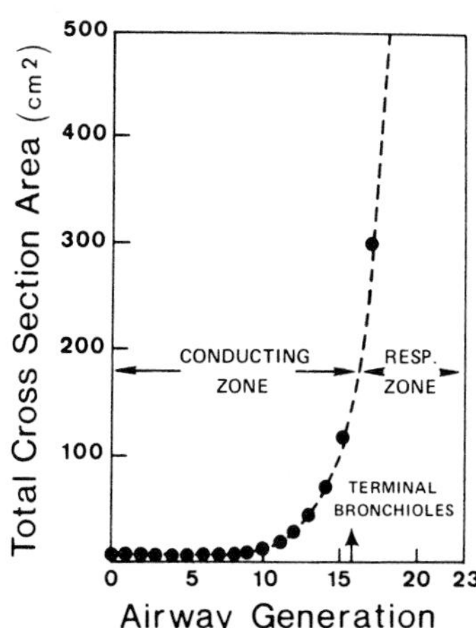

FIGURE 2–1 ■ Cross-sectional area versus airway generation. Note that the total cross-sectional area increases exponentially as the number of airway generations increase. (From West JB: Respiratory Physiology—The Essentials. 3rd ed. Baltimore, Williams & Wilkins, 1985.)

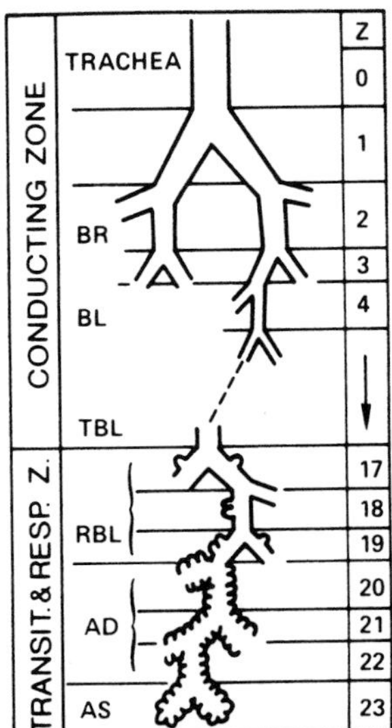

FIGURE 2–2 ■ Diagram of the human bronchial tree. Gas exchange cannot take place prior to division 17, and this volume constitutes the anatomic dead space. (AD, alveolar ducts; AS, alveolar sacs, BL, bronchioli; BR, bronchi; RBL, respiratory bronchioli; TBL, terminal bronchioli; Z, number of airway generations.) (From Weibel ER: Morphometry of the Human Lung. Berlin, Springer-Verlag, 1963.)

lar ducts, alveolar sacs, and alveoli (Fraser et al, 1988). The acini are not completely isolated but are interconnected by small channels known as the pores of Kohn. Also, other poorly demarcated channels are present that may serve the purpose of collateral ventilation (Raskin and Herman, 1975). Although the acinus is the primary gas exchange unit of the lung, it can be further broken down into many interrelated alveoli. The human lung had been thought to contain approximately 300×10^6 alveoli as determined in several studies (Cumming, 1972; Horsfeld and Cumming, 1968). However, a more recent study found that the number of alveoli correlated with body length and ranged from about 200×10^6 to 600×10^6 (Angus and Thurlbeck, 1972). The total alveolar surface area has been found to range from 70 to 100 m^2 (Thurlbeck, 1967; Weibel, 1963).

Pulmonary Circulation

The pulmonary circulation is essential for the lungs to oxygenate and eliminate CO_2. Although the pulmonary circulation receives the entire cardiac output from the right ventricle, in contrast to the systemic circulation, it is very compliant and pressures are quite low, with systolic pressures around 25 mm Hg, diastolic pressures about 8 mm Hg, and mean pressures of approximately 15 mm Hg. It has several unique properties, which makes it ideally suited for the function of gas exchange. These are covered in this section in which we explore its properties and how they relate to lung function as a whole.

As the pulmonary arteries enter the lungs from the hilum, they usually follow the divisions of the bronchi, branching with every bronchial division. However, the number of arterial branches is greater than the number of bronchial branches because the artery undergoes extra divisions, which serve the lung parenchyma. The number of extra branches increases with each additional bronchial branch (Elliot and Reid, 1965). These branches are not usually seen on pulmonary angiography because they tend to arise at very oblique angles, which tends to minimize blood flow under normal conditions.

Once the capillary level is reached, the capillary network becomes very extensive and the total capillary cross-sectional area increases significantly at a rate analogous to the exponential increase in the area of the airways. The capillaries go on to form a large plexus around each alveolus and do not become terminal vessels because they are all interconnected. The capillary network is so extensive that it can be thought of as a continuous sheet of blood enveloping the alveolus (Fung and Sobin, 1968). A red blood cell may pass several alveoli while in the capillary network. Because of this, the residence time of blood in a lung capillary is relatively long (~ 0.5 to 1 second), which under most conditions is sufficient for the blood to become fully equilibrated with alveolar gas. The only situations in which the capillary transit time is thought to be a limiting factor in arterial oxygenation are heavy exercise in low-oxygen atmospheres or in conditions where the alveolar-capillary membrane is abnormal, such as pulmonary fibrosis (Staub, 1963).

Because the capillaries are arranged in extensive, multiply interconnected parallel networks, there is a large degree of reserve. A large number of capillaries can be occluded without an appreciable increase in pulmonary artery pressures. Also, the extensive endothelial surface of the pulmonary capillary network is very well suited for carrying out the metabolic functions of the lung.

To facilitate diffusion, the air-blood barrier may be as thin as 0.5 μm in thickness and at its thinnest there are only three layers (Weibel, 1963). These are the capillary endothelium, fused basement membrane of the endothelial and epithelial layers and the epithelium composed of type I and II pneumocytes (West and Dollery, 1964) (Fig. 2–3).

Pulmonary edema is a common manifestation of derangements in pulmonary physiology. The forces that govern the formation of alveolar fluid are expressed by the Starling equation, which is represented as follows:

$$Qs = Kf\ ((Pc - Pi) - (Op - Oi))$$

where *Qs* is the net flow of fluid across the capillary membrane; *Kf* is the fluid filtration and removal coefficient; *Pc* is the pressure within capillaries; *Pi* is the pressure within the interstitium; *Op* is the plasma oncotic pressure; and *Oi* is the oncotic pressure within the interstitium. This equation forms a conceptual model for relating these forces. The pressure within capillaries and the oncotic pressure within the interstitium tend to draw fluid from the vascular bed into the alveolar spaces. This is counterbalanced by pressure within the interstitium and oncotic pressure within the vasculature, which tend to keep fluid within the capillaries. Pulmonary capillary pressure is less than the oncotic pressure of serum proteins. This tends to draw fluid into the vascular space (Landis and Pappenheimer, 1963). Also, interstitial pressure is subatmospheric (Meyer et al, 1968), and surfac-

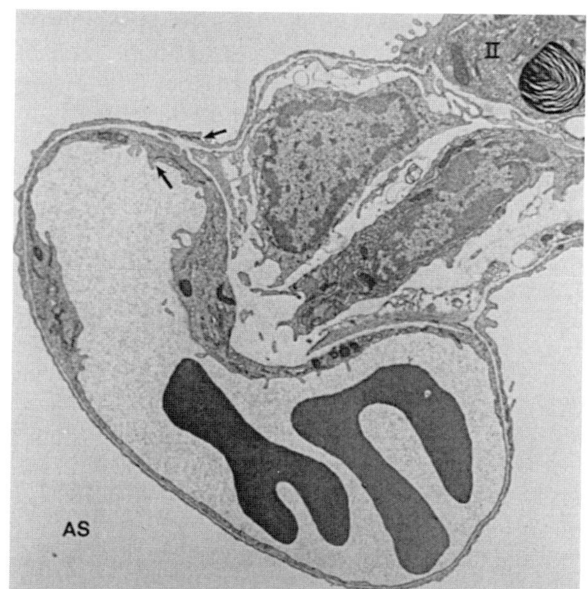

FIGURE 2–3 ■ Alveolar capillary of rat lung. The alveolar space (AS) and intravascular compartment are closely approximated and are separated by the flattened epithelium of a type 1 pneumocyte, fused basement membrane, and nonfenestrated epithelium. (From Schneeberger EE: Structural basis for some permeability properties of the air-blood barrier. Fed Proc 37:2471, 1978.)

tant reduces intra-alveolar surface tension (Prattle, 1965). These favor fluid migration from the air spaces to the interstitium.

However, the net filtration of fluid for a given filtration pressure is governed by the filtration coefficient, which is composed of several protective mechanisms, both active and passive, to prevent alveolar flooding due to the exceedingly thin blood-air barrier within the alveolar spaces. Once fluid arrives in the interstitium, there is efficient lymphatic drainage (Lauweryns, 1965). The final passive guard against alveolar flooding is the barrier of the air-blood interface with the main barrier to permeability residing in the epithelial layer (Schneeberger, 1978).

In addition to passive mechanisms, the lung has active transport pumps to pump fluid from the airways. These are of two types: Na^+,K^+-ATPase pumps, both catecholamine sensitive and insensitive, and molecular water channels (Matthay et al, 1996). These channels are important to the normal function of the lungs but may be even more important in disease states in which alveolar flooding occurs. In disease states, increase in catecholamines may cause upregulation in Na^+,K^+-ATPase, thus increasing alveolar fluid clearance above baseline.

The importance of the integrity of the blood-alveolar interface is seen in disease states in which damage to the epithelial layer and the resultant increase in permeability cause protein-rich, low-pressure pulmonary edema. An example of this is seen with the inhalation of noxious gases, which cause damage to the epithelial layer with a resultant increase in permeability. This is discussed further later in the chapter.

Because lung perfusion is accomplished with relatively low pulmonary artery pressures (mean = 15 mm Hg) and because the lung is approximately 30 cm high in the upright position, the lung is uniquely affected by hydrostatic pressures. That is, perfusion pressures are a sum of the mean pulmonary artery pressure and hydrostatic pressure as measured from the right ventricle (West and Dollery, 1964). This results in large differences in pulmonary blood flow between dependent and nondependent regions of the lung (Ball et al, 1962; Hughes et al, 1968; West and Dollery, 1960) (Fig. 2–4). This gravitational effect can have a marked influence on oxygenation in situations with markedly asymmetric lung injury. In these situations, improvement in oxygenation can occur by placing the patient in a position such that the abnormal lung receives a smaller fraction of the cardiac output ("good side down").

Much of the work on the influence of hydrostatic pressure on lung perfusion has been done by West and colleagues, who have divided the lung into three regions—zones I, II and III—on the basis of perfusion pressure (Ball et al, 1962; Elliot and Reid, 1965; Weibel, 1963; West, 1978) (Fig. 2–5). In zone I, which is found in the apex of the lung (in the upright posture), hydrostatic pressure is greater than perfusion pressure (Glazier et al, 1969) (Fig. 2–6). As a result $P_{alv} > P_{art} > P_{ven}$ where P_{alv} is atmospheric or alveolar pressure, P_{art} is pulmonary artery pressure, and P_{ven} is pulmonary venous pressure. Therefore, under normal conditions in the upright human, no flow occurs in the apex, and ventilation without perfusion occurs.

In zone II conditions, $P_{art} > P_{alv} > P_{ven}$ and flow occurs only when P_{alv} becomes subatmospheric, as occurs during

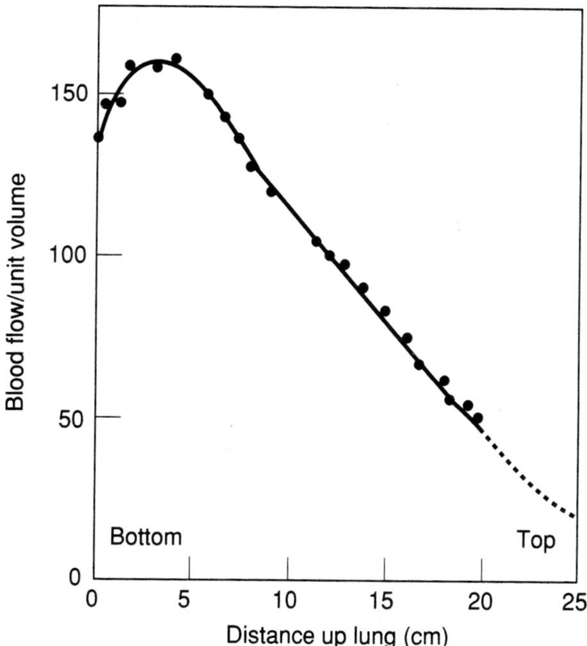

FIGURE 2–4 ■ Perfusion versus blood flow per unit volume of lung in the upright position. The amount of blood flow per lung volume is increased in the bases and reduced in the apex. (Modified from Hughes JMB, Glazier JB, Maloney JE, et al: Effect of lung volumes on the distribution of pulmonary blood flow. Respir Physiol 4:58, 1968.)

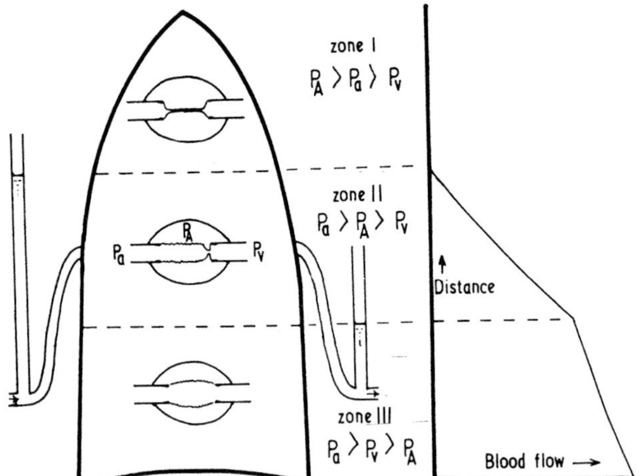

FIGURE 2–5 ■ Three-zone model of lung perfusion. (PA, alveolar pressure; Pa, arterial pressure; Pv, venous pressure.) (From West JB, Dollery CT, Naimark A: Distribution of blood flow in isolated lungs: relation to vascular and alveolar pressures. J Appl Physiol 19:713, 1964.)

inspiration, and flow in this zone ceases during expiration. In zone III, $P_{art} > P_{ven} > P_{alv}$, and therefore perfusion occurs throughout the respiratory cycle. This physiologic concept has a number of clinical implications. For example, when a pulmonary artery catheter is used for hemodynamic measurements, estimation of capillary wedge pressure is based on the assumption that there is a static column of blood between the site of measurement or tip of the catheter and the left atrium. If the pulmonary artery catheter is wedged in a part of the lung that is in zone I, then the pressure transducer will record alveolar pressure rather than left atrial pressure. For accurate readings, the catheter should be wedged in a part of the lung that is in zone III. This is usually the case because the catheter is balloon-tipped and most of the pulmonary blood flow is to zone III; however, if the relationship among P_{art}, P_{ven}, and P_{alv} changes (e.g., addition of high positive end-expiratory pressure (PEEP) acute blood loss, change in position of the patient), then the catheter tip may no longer be in zone III.

Respiratory Mechanics

The mechanical properties of the lung and chest wall are important determinants of function in health and disease. These can be measured and are important clues to the presence of disease. In this section, the mechanics of respiratory function are delineated.

The lungs and the chest wall are elastic structures with inherent recoil and different mechanical properties such that the function of the respiratory system in vivo is determined by the summation of individual characteristics (Fig. 2–7). These properties can be seen by plotting volume versus pressure, as seen Figure 2–8 for each structure individually (Rahn et al, 1946). In this diagram, the static pressure-volume curves of the lungs and relaxed chest wall are shown along with their sum, representing the pressure-volume curve for the total respiratory system. The lungs' resting volume, where the transpulmonary pressure (P_{tp}) is zero, is near residual volume, while the chest wall resting volume where the trans–chest wall pressure is zero is near 80% of total lung capacity (TLC). As the P_{tp} increases with increasing lung volume, the trans–chest wall pressure is positive only over the top 20% of TLC and negative over the lower 80%.

The static functional residual capacity (FRC) is the volume at which the inward recoil of the lungs balances the outward recoil of the chest wall (see Fig. 2–8). A consequence of this is that any alteration in chest wall or lung compliance shifts the FRC. A practical example of this is the increase in FRC due to loss of pulmonary elastic tissue as one ages or in disease states (e.g., emphysema). Also, FRC is reduced in the supine position due to the effect of gravity on outward chest recoil (Sykes et al, 1976). If the FRC is below the volume at which the airways in the most dependent parts of the lung close, atelectasis may result in these regions.

Compliance

Compliance is defined as change in volume divided by change in pressure. Therefore, compliance is the chord

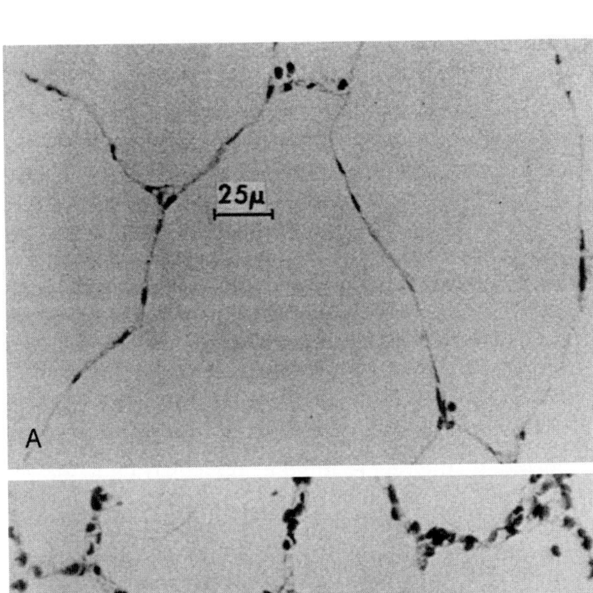

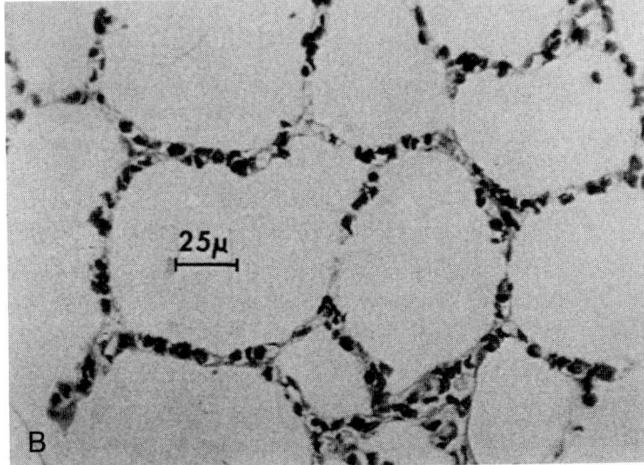

FIGURE 2–6 ■ Rapidly frozen lung specimens taken from the apex, *A*, and basilar, *B*, regions of the lung. Note that the capillaries from the base (zone III conditions) are distended with blood, whereas capillaries in the apex (zone 1) are essentially empty of blood. (From Glazier JB, Hughes JMB, West JB: Measurement of capillary dimensions and blood volume in rapidly frozen lungs. J Appl Physiol 26:65, 1969.)

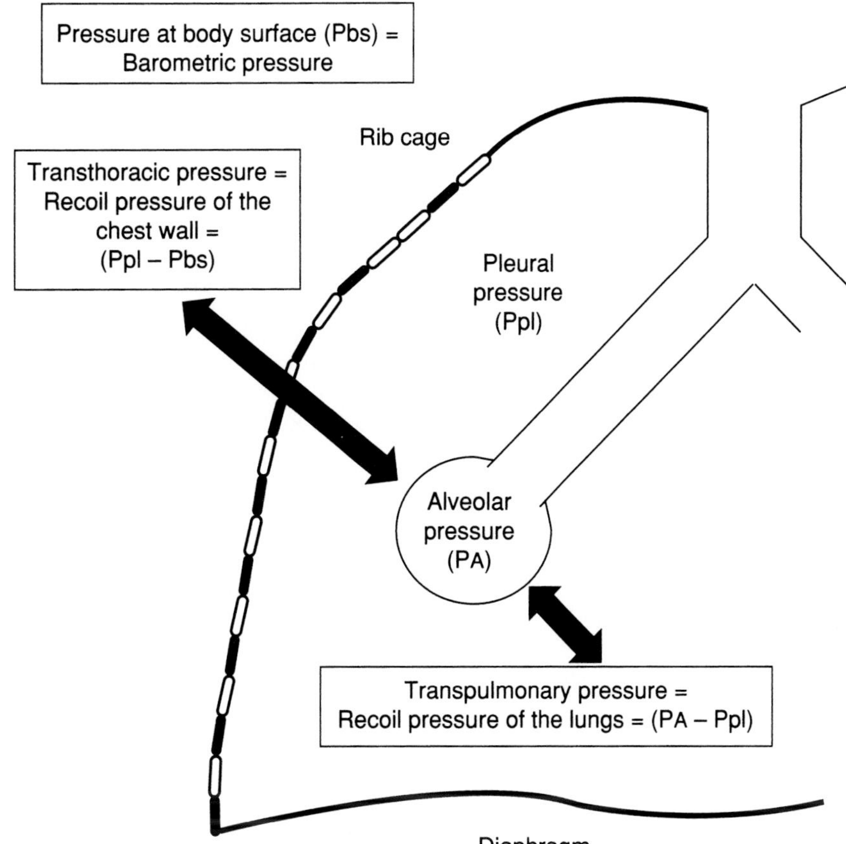

FIGURE 2–7 ■ Schematic diagram illustrating the relationship between the lungs and chest wall.

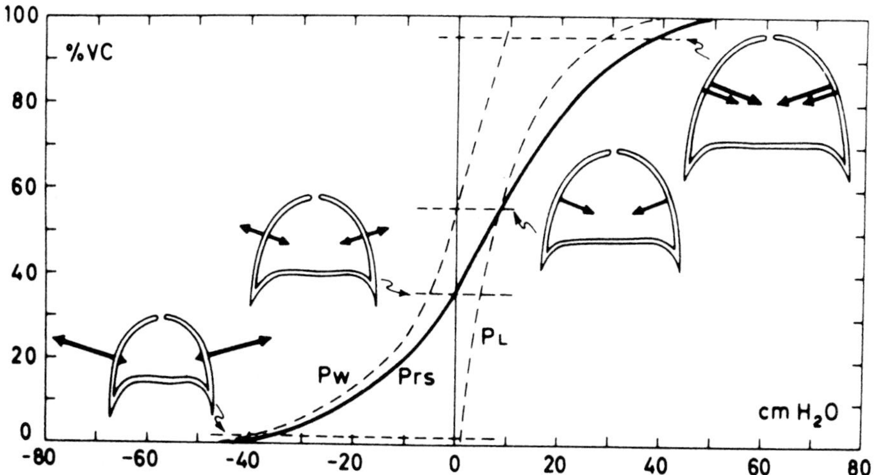

FIGURE 2–8 ■ Pressure-volume curves of the lung (PL), chest wall (Pw) and total respiratory system (Prs). Size of large arrows indicates relative size of recoil forces. Functional residual capacity is reached when outward chest recoil is equal to inward lung recoil. (From Sharp JT, Hammond MD: Pressure-volume relationships. In Crystal RG, West JB [eds]: The Lung: Scientific Foundations. New York, Raven Press, 1991; and from Knowles JH, Hong SK, Rahn H: Possible errors using an esophageal balloon in the determination of pressure-volume characteristics of lung and rib cage. J Appl Physiol 14:525, 1959.)

slope of the pressure-volume curve. It can be determined during static and dynamic conditions. To measure static compliance, equilibration of the respiratory system is allowed to take place, prior to measurement of volume for a given volume. If compliance is measured dynamically, then factors related to distribution of the ventilation may have an influence. As a result, dynamic compliance underestimates static compliance when there is uneven distribution of the ventilation. Lung compliance is directly related to lung volume and decreases with increasing volume, that is, the lung behaves as if it were stiffer as one approaches TLC; the reverse is true with chest wall compliance, which decreases with decreasing volume.

Compliance is analogous to electrical conductance and the compliance of two structures in series is added as follows:

$$\frac{1}{C_T} = \frac{1}{C_1} + \frac{1}{C_2}$$

where C_T is the total compliance and C_1 and C_2 are the individual compliances. As an example, the compliance of chest wall and the lungs is about 0.2 L/cm H_2O each for a total respiratory system compliance of 0.1 L/cm H_2O (Grassino et al, 1991).

Diseases that affect the lung parenchyma directly affect lung compliance. Diseases that lead to a loss of elastic tissue and decreased recoil result in an increase in compliance (e.g., emphysema) with the opposite being true for diseases such as pulmonary fibrosis, as illustrated in Figure 2–9 (Zamel, 1989).

Pressure-Volume Curves

When pressure-volume curves are performed in lungs using air to inflate the lungs, the curves obtained depend on whether the measurements are made during inflation or deflation. This property is common to elastic tissues

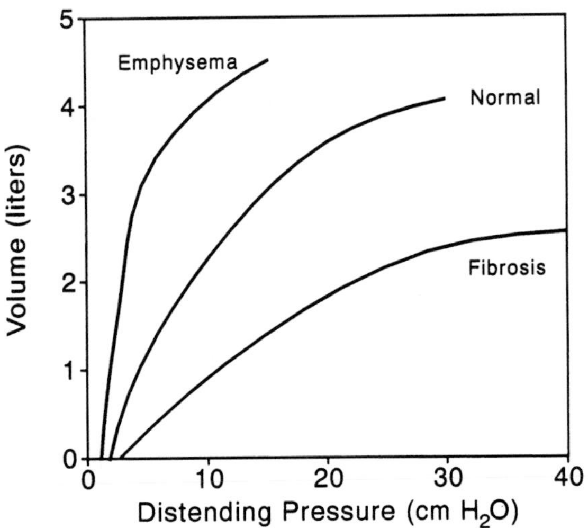

FIGURE 2–9 ■ Static pressure-volume curves for patients with normal lungs, pulmonary fibrosis, and emphysema. Compliance represents the slope of the pressure-volume curve. (Adapted from Murray JF: The Normal Lung. 2nd ed. Philadelphia, WB Saunders, 1986, p. 87.)

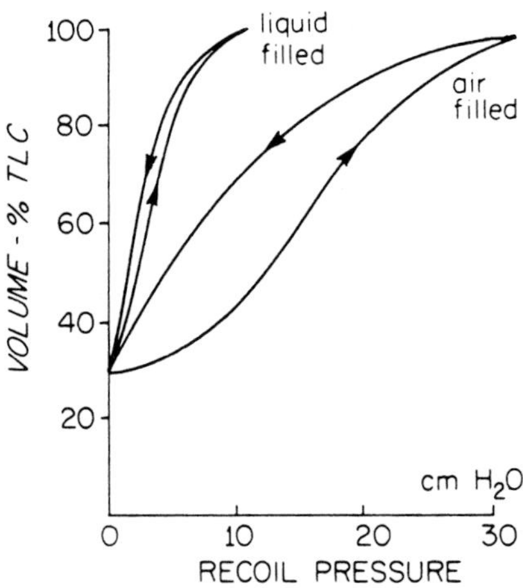

FIGURE 2–10 ■ Static pressure-volume curve of the lung measured during inflation with saline and air. (From Culver BH: Mechanics of ventilation. In Culver BH [ed]: The Respiratory System. Syllabus for Human Biology, Seattle, WA, University of Washington Health Sciences Academic Services, 1990.)

and is called *hysteresis*, which is defined as failure of a system to respond identically to the application and withdrawal of a force, in this case distending pressure (Landowne and Sacy, 1957). However, when the lungs are inflated with liquid, the inflation and deflation loops become virtually identical (i.e., the amount of hysteresis is reduced), as seen in Figure 2–10 (Bachofen et al, 1970; Radford, 1957).

The characteristics of pressure-volume curves of excised lungs are dependent on the amount of lung recoil. Lung recoil is determined by the elasticity of lung parenchyma and surface tension present in the gas-liquid interface. Inflation with liquid abolishes the contribution of surface tension to lung recoil such that the resultant pressure-volume curve is a reflection only of tissue forces and is shifted to the left.

When isolated lungs are deflated to transpulmonary pressures of zero, significant volume remains within the lung. In fact, even if the transpulmonary pressures become negative, little additional volume is removed. This is due to air trapping within alveoli from the closure of small airways and is relatively constant between air- and liquid-filled lungs (Sharp and Hammond, 1991; West, 1985). This is referred to as the closing volume and is approximately 15% of TLC; closing volume increases with age and can be increased with some disease processes (Hoppin et al, 1986). The ex vivo closing volume is the volume at which all the airways are closed, whereas the in vivo closing volume is referred to the lung volume at which the airways in the most dependent parts of the lungs start to close.

Surfactant

Although Von Neergaard, in the 1920s, was the first to suggest that surface tension played a role in lung expansion, it was not until the 1950s that surfactant was isolated and it was recognized that neonatal respiratory distress syndrome was due to surfactant deficiency (Floros, 1990). Since then, surfactant has been shown to have multiple functions and to be crucial for normal lung function.

Surfactant is a heterogeneous mixture of phospholipids and proteins. The composition consists of 80% to 85% phospholipids, 5% to 10%, protein, and 10% neutral lipids, with dipalmitoylphosphatidylcholine as the main surface active agent (Hawgood, 1991; Morton, 1989). The protein components of surfactant are important for its function and are named apoproteins A, B, and C. They appear to be essential to surfactant's secretion, regulation of turnover rate, and distribution into the alveolar liquid layer (Hawgood and Clements, 1990).

The main effect of surfactant is to reduce the surface tension at the interface between air and alveoli, and in doing so it promotes lung stability. Intra-alveolar pressure can be determined by Laplace's law:

$$P = \frac{2T}{r}$$

where *P* is the pressure, *T* is the tension, and *r* is the radius of the alveolus. From this equation, it is evident that for a given surface tension, intra-alveolar pressure will rise as alveolar size falls, and smaller alveoli will tend to empty into larger alveoli, thus initiating a cascade whereby the whole lung becomes unstable. This is where surfactant is critically important. Surfactant reduces surface tension in proportion to the size of the alveolus; the smaller the alveolus, the greater the reduction in surface tension. This is due to compression of the surfactant film as alveolar size falls, whereby overall lung stability is enhanced (Schurch et al, 1976).

Surfactant is important to alveolar fluid handling. Surface tension may be important in determining transvascular water flux. There is experimental evidence that reduction in surfactant activity or an increase in surface tension results in pulmonary edema (Albert et al, 1979; Nieman and Bredenberg, 1985). Surfactant also reduces the work of breathing by increasing pulmonary compliance (Bachofen et al, 1979), functions as an antiadherence agent, and may have immunologic effects such as increasing macrophage recruitment to the lungs (Dobbs, 1989).

Surfactant is synthesized by type II alveolar cells and stored in lamellar bodies (Fig. 2–11). Clearance is accom-

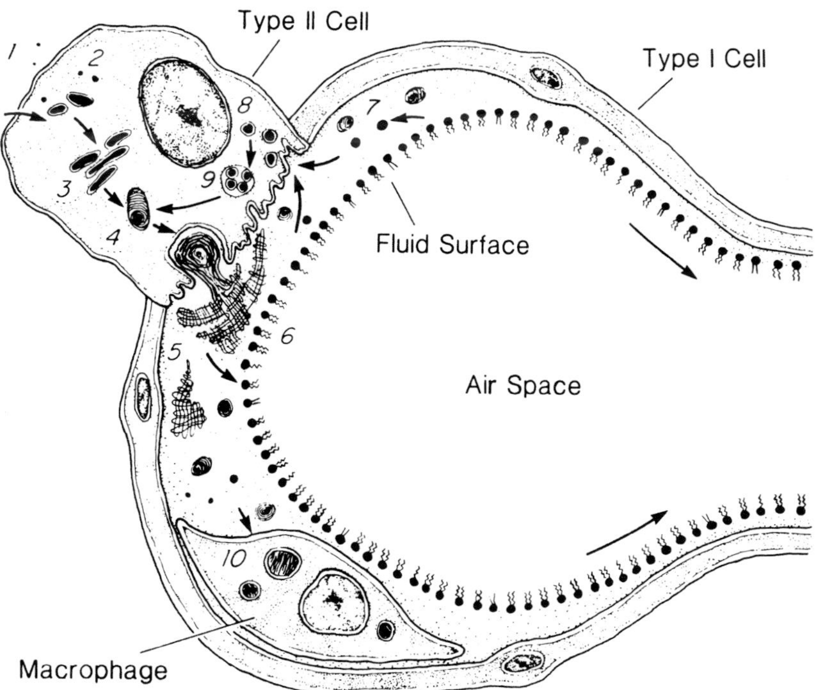

FIGURE 2–11 ■ Schematic diagram of the surfactant system. A single alveolus is shown, with the location and movement of surfactant components depicted. Surfactant components are synthesized from precursors (1) in the endoplasmic reticulum (2) and transported via the Golgi apparatus (3) into lamellar bodies (4), which are the intracellular storage granules for surfactant. After secretion into the liquid that lines the alveolus, the surfactant forms tubular myelin (5), which is thought to generate the surface monolayer (6), which lowers surface tension. Subsequently, surfactant components are taken back into type II cells, possibly in the form of small vesicles (7), apparently by a specific pathway involving endosomes (8) and multivesicular bodies (9) and culminating again in storage of surfactant in lamellar bodies. Some surfactant in the liquid layer is also taken up by alveolar macrophages (10). A single transit of the phospholipid components of surfactant through the alveolar lumen normally takes a few hours. The phospholipids in the lumen are taken back into the type II cell and used approximately 10 times before being degraded. (From Hawgood S, Clements JA: Pulmonary surfactant and its apoproteins. J Clin Invest 86:1, 1990.)

plished by several mechanisms. Reuptake by type II cells, degradation by alveolar macrophages, and clearance up the mucociliary ladder are the most important (Wright, 1990). An example of a disease state arising from disordered surfactant metabolism is alveolar proteinosis, which is characterized by excess surfactant, although it is unclear if it results from increased production or decreased clearance.

CONTROL OF BREATHING

To meet the metabolic demands of the body, the process of respiration has to be tightly controlled such that the delivery of O_2, the removal of Co_2, and the maintenance of pH are ensured. To do this, a central controller, a system of sensors, and a system to effect changes are present. For the respiratory system, the central controller resides in the brain with autonomic control residing in the brain stem, and voluntary control in the cerebrum. The effector system consists of the lungs and the respiratory muscles. The system of sensors is complex and comprises the chemoreceptors in the medulla, the aortic and carotid bodies that respond to changes in pH, P_{CO_2}, and P_{O_2}. Other receptors are the mechanoreceptors in the lungs and chest wall. So that the coordination of breathing such that metabolic demands are met can be understood, each component will be discussed individually.

Receptors

Peripheral Chemoreceptors

The peripheral chemoreceptors are situated within the aortic body and the carotid body, with the carotid body being the more important of the two. They are extremely sensitive to changes in P_{O_2}. Receptor activation and firing starts at a P_{O_2} of 500 mm Hg, and its frequency increases as the P_{O_2} decreases with a marked burst in activity as the P_{O_2} drops below 100 mm Hg (Lahiri et al, 1981) (Fig. 2–12).

These receptors are primarily responsible for the ventilatory response to hypoxia. This is enhanced in the presence of an elevated P_{CO_2}. Overall, approximately 30% of the total ventilatory response to P_{CO_2} is mediated by the carotid bodies (Lugliani et al, 1971). Clinically, this is important in disease states whereby bilateral denervation or destruction of the carotid bodies occurs, as in bilateral carotid endarterectomy, in which the response to hypoxia is abolished and dangerous levels of hypoxemia may occur without compensatory ventilatory responses. There is also evidence that respiratory depression may occur in response to hypoxia without afferent input from the carotid bodies.

Stimulation of the carotid bodies also produces many other effects, such as increased bronchomotor tone, increased catecholamine secretion, and, during sleep, possibly arousal (Phillipson and Sullivan, 1978).

Central Chemoreceptors

The central chemoreceptors consist of a group of cells in the ventrolateral surface of the medulla, approximately 200 to 500 μm below the surface. They respond basically

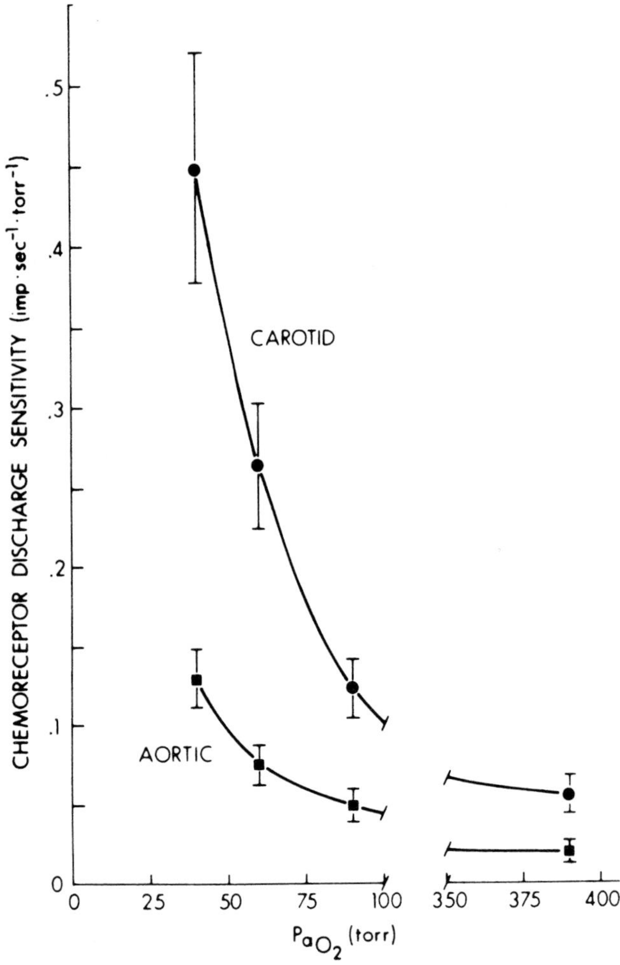

FIGURE 2–12 ■ Response of aortic and carotid body receptors to hypoxia (From Lahiri S, Mokasi A, Mulligan E, Nishino T: Comparison of aortic acid and chemoreceptor responses to hypercapnia and hypoxia. J Appl Physiol 51:55, 1981.)

to hydrogen ion concentrations of the extracellular fluid bathing the cells or cerebrospinal fluid (CSF). An increase in hydrogen ion concentration or decrease in pH causes an increase in ventilation. Because bicarbonate and hydrogen ions do not cross the blood-brain barrier, for changes in CO_2 to effect a change in ventilation, CO_2 must diffuse across the blood-brain barrier and change the pH of the CSF. For full equilibration to take place, a period of hours may be needed. For this reason, the response to metabolic acidosis is less brisk than that for respiratory acidosis because blood hydrogen ion concentration does not directly influence the central chemoreceptors and can only influence them by changing the concentration of bicarbonate in the serum and, secondarily, the plasma CO_2 levels.

Pulmonary Receptors

In the lung, there are three major categories of receptors: pulmonary stretch receptors, irritant receptors, and J receptors.

The pulmonary stretch receptors lie within airway smooth muscle and are activated by lung inflation. The primary effect of activation of these fibers, whose afferent impulses are carried within the vagus, is a slowing of inspiratory frequency owing to an increase in expiratory time (Berger et al, 1977a,b,c). Classically, this is known as the Herring-Breuer reflex. However, this reflex seems to be much more important in some animals and does not seem to be activated for tidal volumes less than about a liter in humans.

Receptors that respond to irritant stimuli are located between airway epithelial cells. They respond to noxious gases, inhaled dust, smoke, cold air, and histamine (Armstrong and Luck, 1974; Sampson and Vidruk, 1975). The afferent impulses are carried within the vagus, and receptor stimulation produces cough, bronchoconstriction, and hyperpnea. They may have a role in asthma because contact with allergen produces histamine release with subsequent activation of the irritant-type receptors.

Type J, or juxtapulmonary-capillary, receptors are present within the wall of the pulmonary capillary. They are believed to be activated by pulmonary congestion or increases in interstitial fluid volume (Paintal, 1973). The afferent impulses are conducted in nonmyelinated fibers in the vagus and result in rapid, shallow breathing. They are thought to play a role in the dyspnea associated with such disease states as left ventricular failure and are not associated with normal respiration.

Other Receptors

Receptors are also located within the nasal passages, pharynx, and upper airways. These are sensitive to various chemical and mechanical stimuli and mediate reflexes such as sneezing, coughing, and laryngeal spasm. They are numerous and beyond the scope of this chapter.

Central Control of Breathing

Respiration is governed by both voluntary and automatic controls, with the cerebral cortex responsible for voluntary control, and the brain stem responsible for automatic breathing. Brainstem control of breathing originates in neurons located within the pons and medulla that are organized into separate groups called the respiratory centers. There are three separate areas: the pneumotaxic center, the apneustic center, and the medullary center, which is divided into an expiratory center and a gasping center (Berger et al, 1977a,b,c; Lumsden, 1923a,b).

The pneumotaxic center is the most caudal of the three and is located in the upper pons. Stimulation of this area appears to inhibit inspiration and cause a switch to expiration. The intensity of the stimulus needed decreases as inspiration progresses (Euler and Trippenbach, 1975). In this way, inspiratory volume is limited, and the respiratory rate is regulated.

The apneustic center lies in the lower pons. It is so named because sectioning of the brain stem above this area results in prolonged inspiratory efforts with occasional expiratory gasps. This has been called *apneustic breathing*. It is a phenomenon that results from prolonged discharge of inspiratory neurons. Various inputs into this area can terminate inspiration by negative feedback.

The medullary center is located in the reticular formation of the medulla and consists of two centers, the dorsal respiratory group and the ventral respiratory group, the dorsal group being responsible for inspiration and the ventral group for expiration. These centers are capable of rhythmically driving the respiratory musculature in the absence of any other input, although the pattern of respiration is abnormal, and gasping predominates. If these centers are destroyed, all automatic respiration ceases (Thurlbeck, 1967). Respiratory rhythm generation is likely within the dorsal respiratory group.

Integration of Breathing Control

The respiratory system has a complex system of sensors and effectors (the lungs and respiratory muscles) with the central nervous system (CNS) to coordinate the response to the stimuli received. Changes in P_{CO_2} or P_{O_2} are the main stimuli that elicit a response. These are usually kept within narrow physiologic ranges. In this section, they are considered separately relative to the reaction they elicit.

Carbon Dioxide

Carbon dioxide elimination is directly related to alveolar ventilation, and as alveolar ventilation increases, the P_{CO_2} falls until a new steady-state level is reached. At any given CO_2 production, the relationship between P_{CO_2} and ventilation is a hyperbolic one (Fig. 2–13) (Berger et al, 1977a,b,c).

For a normal subject, minute ventilation increases linearly with P_{CO_2}. Figure 2–14 plots the ventilatory response to changes in P_{CO_2} and, as can be seen, the degree of response is altered by the subject's P_{O_2}, with greater degrees of hypoxia causing increased ventilation (Nielsen

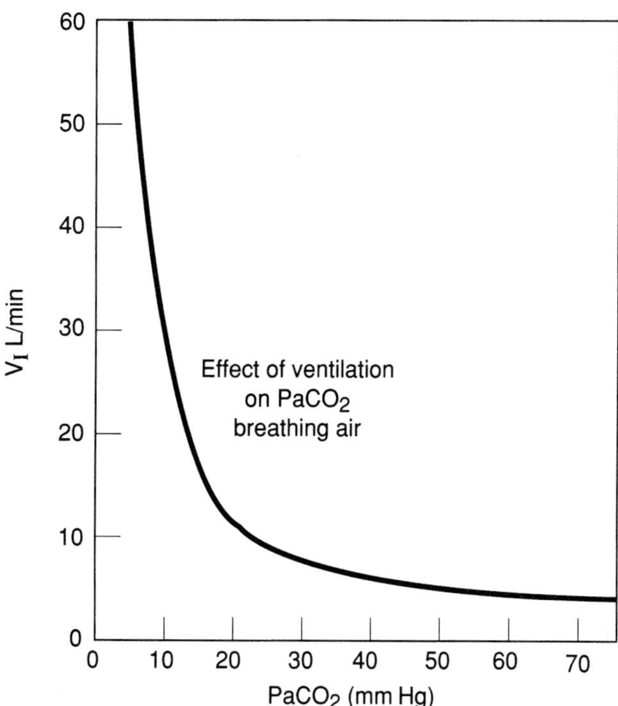

FIGURE 2–13 ■ Effect of ventilation on Pa_{CO_2}.

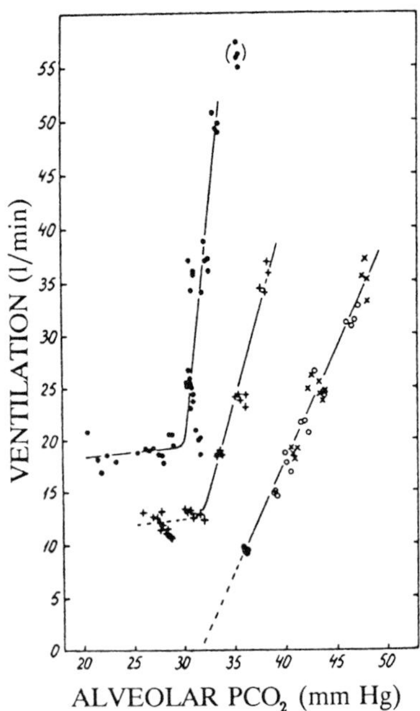

FIGURE 2–14 ■ Ventilatory response to CO_2 at different $Paco_2$ levels. The ventilatory response to CO_2 is enhanced by alveolar hypoxia. (From Nielson M, Smith H: Studies on the regulation of respiration in acute hypoxia. Acta Physiol Scand 24:293, 1951.)

and Smith, 1951). The ventilatory response to hypercapnia is usually measured using the Read technique in which the subject rebreathes from a small bag containing a mixture of CO_2 and O_2 (Read, 1967; Rebuck and Slutsky, 1981). The ventilatory response to CO_2 is quite variable among subjects, but about 80% of subjects have a Pco_2 value between 1 and 4 L/min mm Hg, with women generally having a lower response than men. The ventilatory response to CO_2 diminishes with age, following the use of CNS depressants or an enhancement of cardiovascular fitness.

The response to CO_2 is mainly central, but there is a peripheral contribution. It is estimated that peripheral chemoreceptors contribute 10% to 30% to the response to hypercapnia, but the exact mechanism of this response is not fully known (Rebuck and Woodley, 1975).

Oxygen

The response to hypoxia is mainly a peripheral phenomenon and originates in the carotid bodies, with minimal or no input from the aortic bodies, as manifested by the lack of hypoxic ventilatory drive in patients who have had bilateral carotid body resections (Armstrong and Luck, 1974. Ventilation increases as Po_2 and arterial hemoglobin saturation fall. Ventilation is a hyperbolic function of Pao_2 but is a linear function of arterial hemoglobin saturation (Fig. 2–15) (Rebuck and Slutsky, 1981). The response is variable, but about 80% of healthy subjects have a value between 0.6 and 2.8 L/min/1% fall in Sao_2. (Rebuck and Woodley, 1975). This response is increased in the presence of elevated Pco_2 or decreased pH. The ventilatory response is blunted or reduced in chronic hypoxia (Severinghaus, 1972).

Under normal circumstances, hypoxic ventilatory drive plays a minimal role in the control of respiration. However, in the presence of a chronically elevated Pco_2, the ventilatory response to Pco_2 is reduced. This occurs partly because of the associated metabolic alkalosis in the CSF, which makes the CSF pH much less responsive to changes in Pco_2. In this situation, hypoxic ventilatory drive assumes a prominent role, and the administration of O_2 may depress respiration to dangerous levels (West, 1985).

VENTILATION

Dynamic Aspects of Ventilation

For gas exchange to occur, O_2 must be delivered to the alveoli and CO_2 removed. This is accomplished by bulk transport to the small airways where gas delivery and removal by diffusion become predominant. For gas flow to occur, a pressure gradient must exist between the alveoli and the mouth. The relationship between the pressure gradient from the mouth to the alveoli and net flow is the resistance of the airways. The flow obtained from a given pressure gradient is dependent on whether gas flow is laminar or turbulent. This is determined largely by the Reynold's number (Re), which for flow through a cylindrical tube is given by the equation

$$Re = \frac{vd}{\nu}$$

where v is the velocity of the gas, *d* is the diameter of the cylinder, and ν is the kinematic viscosity (viscosity/density) of the gas flowing in a cylinder. If Re is less than 2100, flow is usually laminar, for Re greater than 4000, flow will be turbulent; and for values of Re between these two values, flow will be transitional

In the lung, flow is turbulent in the larger airways and becomes laminar in small peripheral airways (Netter, 1979). The flow is laminar at the level of the small airways because of their small diameter individually but large cumulative diameter, with the resultant markedly reduced gas velocity. Thus the Reynold's number falls to the critical threshold of 2100. Turbulent gas flow is proportional to gas density and is proportional to the square root of the driving pressure. It is this dependence on gas density that makes the use of gas mixtures such as He-O_2 (mixtures of helium and oxygen) useful in some diseases in which there is upper airway obstruction. (Curtis, 1986; Ta-Shung Lu et al, 1976). Pure helium has a density that is about one-third that of air so that in situations wherein the major pressure drop is related to turbulent flow, a decrease in density will decrease the pressure gradient necessary to generate a given flow rate (Houck et al, 1990).

For laminar flow, flow is proportional to gas viscosity and directly proportional to the driving pressure. In a straight tube or airway, the flow profile is parabolic, with the velocity greatest in the center of the tube and zero at

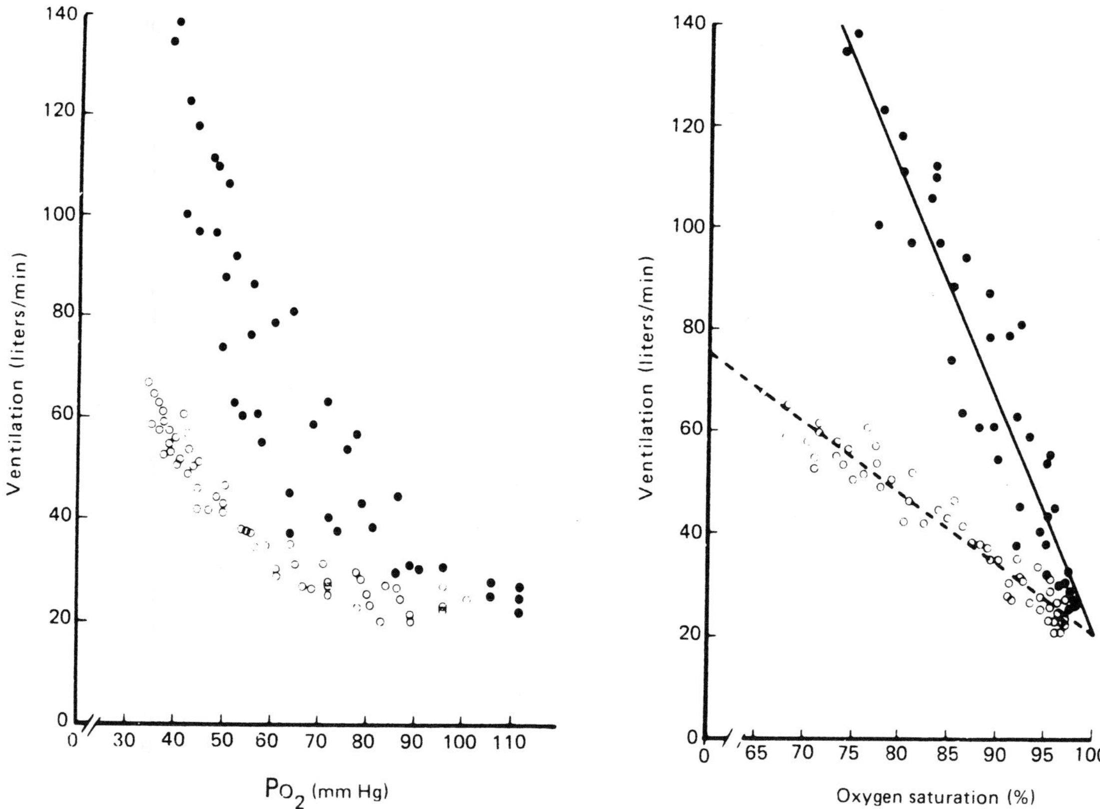

FIGURE 2–15 ■ The ventilatory response to hypoxia in two subjects (*open and closed circles*). Illustrated are a hyperbolic response curve obtained by plotting P_{O_2} and a linear response curve obtained by plotting hemoglobin saturation against ventilation. (From Rebuck AS, Campbell EJM: A clinical method for assessing the ventilatory response to hypoxia. Am Rev Respir Dis 109:345, 1974.)

the wall. Laminar flow can be quantified using Poiseuille's law, which describes the relationship between flow and pressure:

$$V = \frac{\pi r^4 \Delta P}{8 \mu l}$$

where *V* is flow, *r* is the radius of the airway, ΔP is the driving pressure, μ is the gas viscosity, and *l* is the length of the airway.

Because airway resistance (R_{aw}) is the relationship between a pressure gradient and the resultant flow, it is apparent from the previous discussions that in health most of the resistance to flow occurs in the large airways where flow is turbulent and the cumulative airways diameter is relatively small. R_{aw} is also volume dependent owing to the parenchymal recoil applied to the airway walls.

Dead Space

Dead space is defined as the volume of the respiratory apparatus, including the upper airways, which is ventilated but in which gas exchange between the blood and gas phases does not occur. This is arbitrarily divided into anatomic and physiologic dead space. Anatomic dead space is the volume of the conducting airways, which are not specialized for gas exchange. This includes the nasal passages, pharynx, trachea, and airways up to the terminal bronchioles. In the normal individual, the total volume of the anatomic dead space is approximately 150 ml. It also varies with inspiration, posture, and size as the volume of the large airways changes. For normal nonobese individuals in the seated position, the volume of dead space in milliliters approximately equals their body weight in pounds (West, 1985). The most common method of measuring anatomic dead space is Fowler's method (Fowler, 1952). In this method, the subject inhales a single breath of 100% O_2. On expiration, the nitrogen (N_2) concentration is continuously measured at the mouth. The N_2 concentration in the expired gas gradually rises as the 100% O_2 is washed out of the conducting airways by the alveolar gas. It finally plateaus when only alveolar gas is being exhaled. The volume of anatomic dead space is taken as the volume that occurs halfway to the plateau point (Fig. 2–16).

Physiologic dead space is the part of the tidal volume that does not directly participate in gas exchange. Anatomic dead space makes up a portion of physiologic dead space. The rest arises from regions of the lung that have the ability to participate in gas exchange but do so poorly or not at all because of inadequate or no perfusion in relation to the degree of ventilation. Physiologic dead space usually constitutes about 25% to 35% of a normal

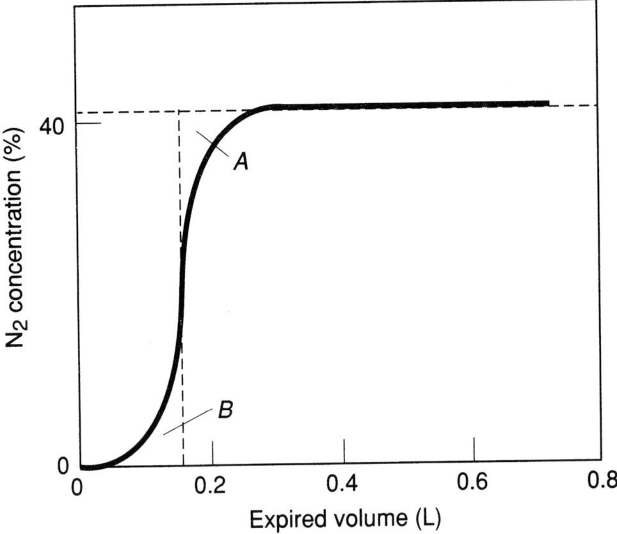

FIGURE 2–16 ■ Fowler's method for determining anatomic dead space. (From Fowler WS: Intrapulmonary distribution of inspired gas. Physiol Rev 32:1, 1952.)

tidal volume (also known as the VD/VT ratio). During exercise, the tidal volume increases, and the VD/DT ratio can fall to as low as 10% to 15%.

Physiologic dead space is usually measured by the Bohr method. This method takes advantage of the fact that inspired air has virtually no CO_2 and that air ventilating perfused lung will equilibrate with the CO_2 within the blood. That is,

$$V_T \times F_{ECO_2} = V_A \times F_{ACO_2}$$

where F_{ECO_2} is the fractional concentration of CO_2 in the mixed expired gas and F_{ACO_2} is the fractional concentration of CO_2 in alveoli. Because $V_T = V_D + V_A$ where V_T is the tidal volume, V_D is the volume of dead space, and V_A is the volume of normally ventilated and perfused alveoli, rearrangement of the above equation produces

$$\frac{V_D}{V_T} = \frac{F_{ACO_2} - F_{ECO_2}}{F_{ACO_2}}$$

Multiplication of the top and bottom by the atmospheric pressure minus the partial pressure of water vapor converts the above to partial pressures:

$$\frac{V_D}{V_T} = \frac{P_{ACO_2} - P_{ECO_2}}{P_{ACO_2}}$$

where P_{ACO_2} is the alveolar partial pressure of CO_2 and P_{ECO_2} is the partial pressure of CO_2 in expired gas. Because P_{ACO_2} is not easy to measure, it is assumed to be equal to P_{ACO_2} and P_{ECO_2} is measured by collecting an expired sample of gas. Physiologic dead space is influenced by a number of factors, including age, body size, duration of inspiration and breath-holding, smoking, and anesthesia.

DIFFUSION

Diffusion is defined as the movement of a gas from an area of high partial pressure to an area of low partial pressure by the process of molecular mixing and not by bulk transfer. The rate of diffusion is determined by the pressure gradient that is driving the diffusion process and the properties of the gas in question and the pressure gradient of the environment through which diffusion takes place.

Gas delivery by bulk transport is effective to the level of the respiratory bronchioles in the lung. At end-inspiration, the fresh gas must mix with the volume of the FRC. Therefore, the mixing of residual alveolar gas and the inspiratory gas is then dependent entirely on diffusion.

Once the inspiratory gas is delivered to the alveolar ducts, oxygen needs to reach the red blood cells in the alveolar capillaries. Oxygen must first diffuse into the alveolar spaces and then sequentially across the alveolocapillary membrane, plasma in the capillaries, the red blood cell membrane, and finally combine with hemoglobin within the red blood cell. The reverse process occurs with CO_2 (West, 1985) (Fig. 2–17).

The rate of diffusion within air is dependent on the molecular weight of the gas whereas diffusion of a gas within a liquid is dependent on the solubility of the gas

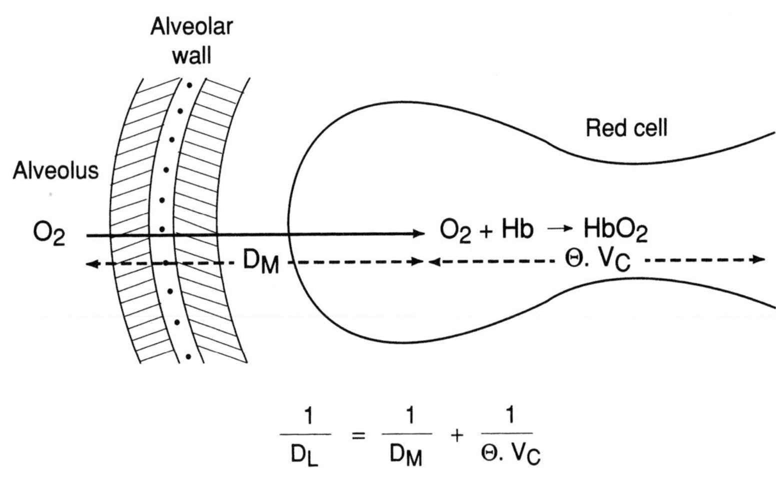

FIGURE 2–17 ■ The components of diffusing capacity. (From West JB: Respiratory Physiology—The Essentials. 3rd ed. Baltimore, Williams & Wilkins, 1985, p. 28.)

in the liquid. CO_2 is heavier than O_2 and it diffuses through air at a slightly slower rate. However because CO_2 is 20 times more soluble than O_2, its rate of diffusion through the red blood cell, plasma, and alveolocapillary membrane is markedly faster than that of O_2.

The process of mixing within the alveolar spaces occurs very quickly, and under normal conditions can be considered to be almost instantaneous; therefore, the rate-limiting step becomes the process of gas transfer from the alveoli to the red blood cell. Because of the greater ease with which CO_2 does this as compared with O_2, pathologic states that impair diffusion affect O_2 transport to a much greater degree. For all intents and purposes, the reserve of CO_2 diffusion is so great that impairments of diffusion, unless extreme, can be considered not to have any effect on CO_2 elimination. This is much different for O_2, however, which, because of its relatively low diffusion reserve, is very sensitive to pathologic processes that impair diffusion.

Under normal circumstances, blood in the alveolar capillary becomes fully oxygenated in the first third of the time spent in the capillary (Fig. 2–18). In states of high cardiac output, the capillary blood time is reduced but the diffusion reserve is still adequate to ensure that the end-capillary blood is fully oxygenated. However, because the diffusion capability is reduced, the time required to fully oxygenate the blood during its course through the capillary becomes progressively longer and finally exceeds the capillary transit time, at which point end-capillary blood will not be fully oxygenated and hypoxia results. In states of high cardiac output, in which the capillary transit time is reduced, hypoxia may be produced. This mechanism likely accounts for the hypoxia seen on exercise in patients with early interstitial lung disease who have normal blood gases at rest. It likely also accounts for a portion of the severe hypoxia seen in hyperdynamic septic patients with lung disease.

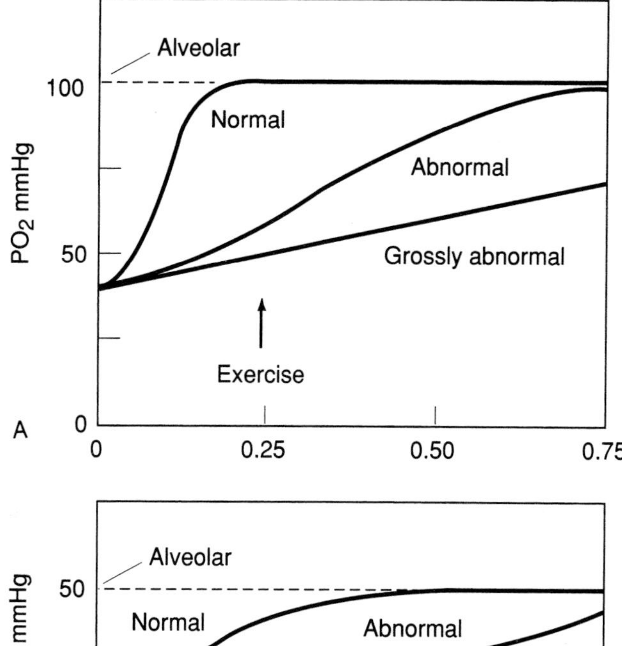

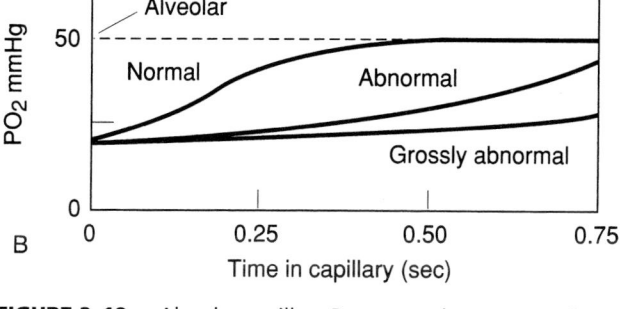

FIGURE 2–18 ■ Alveolar capillary P_{O_2} versus the amount of time spent in the capillary by deoxygenated blood. *A*, Graph is plotted with normal alveolar P_{O_2} levels, and *B*, Graph is plotted with an alveolar P_{O_2} of 50 mm Hg. Both graphs are plotted with normal and abnormal alveolar membranes. Normal capillary transit time is approximately 0.75 second and may be reduced to as little as 0.25 second during exercise or other states of high cardiac output. End-capillary P_{O_2} is a function of transit time, alveolar membrane function, and alveolar P_{O_2}. (From West JB: Respiratory Physiology—The Essentials. 3rd ed. Baltimore, Williams & Wilkins, 1985, p. 28.)

Diffusing Capacity

The measurement of the efficiency of diffusion is termed the *diffusing capacity* (D_L). When the process of diffusion for oxygen is broken down into its individual components, three separate rate-limiting steps are found. The first is the rate of passage of O_2 across the alveolocapillary membrane. The second is the rate of combination of oxygen with hemoglobin on red blood cells. The third element is the driving pressure for the diffusion, which is the difference in pressures between the P_{O_2} in the alveolus and the P_{O_2} in the red blood cell. The equation form for the alveolocapillary membrane becomes

$$\text{Resistance } (R_1) = \frac{1}{D_M}$$

$$D_M = \frac{V}{P_A - P_P} = \text{Conductance} = \frac{1}{\text{Resistance}}$$

where D_M is the diffusing capacity of alveolar-capillary membrane, V is the amount of diffusing gas, P_A is the partial pressure in alveolus, and P_P is the partial pressure in plasma. Similarly, the rate with which a gas combines with the red blood cell (D_B) is proportional to the rate of the reaction and the capillary blood volume present.

$$D_B = \theta V_C = \text{Conductance} = \frac{1}{R_2}$$

$$\text{Resistance } (R_2) = \frac{1}{\theta V_C}$$

where θ is the rate of combination with hemoglobin and V_C is the volume of the capillary in contact with the blood.

Similarly, the total diffusion capacity (D_L) is equal to the inverse of the total resistance to flow (R_L). However, the total resistance is obtained by adding R_1 and R_2. Therefore,

$$R_L = R_1 + R_2$$

and this then becomes

$$\frac{1}{D_L} = \frac{1}{D_M} + \frac{1}{\theta V_C}$$

Measurement of Diffusing Capacity

In practice, the diffusing capacity is measured by using carbon monoxide (CO) as the tracer gas. The advantage of using CO as opposed to oxygen is that it has a very strong affinity for hemoglobin, and under normal circumstances the partial pressure of CO rises only slightly as it diffuses into the capillary. This is in contrast to O_2, which has a moderate affinity for hemoglobin. The capillary partial pressure of O_2 starts to rise after about one third of the blood capillary transit time, thereby reducing the pressure gradient for diffusion. As a result, the transfer of O_2 from the alveolar space to the red blood cell is initially diffusion-limited and later perfusion-limited. Also, CO is readily measured and in low concentrations poses no hazard.

There are two methods in common use for the measurement of diffusing capacity: the single-breath and the steady-state methods. The most common is the single-breath technique, which consists of the rapid inspiration from residual volume of a gas mixture of CO (0.3% to 0.4%), He, O_2, and N_2. The breath is held for 10 seconds, and a sample of alveolar gas is collected on expiration and analyzed for He and CO concentration. The *diffusing capacity* (DLCO) is defined as the volume of CO transferred into the blood per minute per millimeter of mercury of CO partial pressure. It is calculated from the following equation:

$$D_L = \frac{V_I}{t \times P_B} \times \frac{FI_{He}}{FA_{He}} \log_e \left[\frac{FI_{CO}}{FA_{CO}}\right]$$

where V_I is the volume of inspired test gas; t is the time of breath-holding; FI_{CO} is the fraction of inspired CO; FA_{CO} is the fraction of CO in alveolar gas; FI_{He} is the fraction of inspired He; FA_{He} is the fraction of He in alveolar gas; and P_B is the dry atmospheric pressure.

In the steady-state method, the subject breathes a CO gas mixture until alveolar partial pressure of CO (P_{CO}) is constant. Expired gas is then collected and from the volume of expired gas and CO concentration, the uptake of CO can be calculated.

Interpretation

The diffusing capacity can be either elevated or reduced depending on the disease process. The individual components of the equation for diffusing capacity (D_L),

$$\frac{1}{D_L} = \frac{1}{D_M} + \frac{1}{\theta V_C},$$

are useful clues as to the manner in which diseases affect diffusing capacity. D_M depends on the thickness and area of the alveolocapillary membrane, and diseases that affect either one will tend to reduce the diffusing capacity. Examples of such diseases are emphysema and pneumonectomy, whereas those that affect the thickness are interstitial lung disease and pulmonary edema.

Since the θ remains relatively constant, V_C influences the diffusing capacity to a large extent. θV_C is reduced by anemia, pulmonary hypertension, pulmonary embolism and so on; diseases that reduce the amount of hemoglobin or cells in the capillary spaces. Diseases, that increase the amount of blood or hemoglobin within the lung will actually increase the measured diffusing capacity. Examples of this are early mitral stenosis and left-to-right shunt. An extreme example is the elevation of diffusing capacity in pulmonary hemorrhage because of the free hemoglobin within the air spaces. In these situations, the diffusing capacity is a sensitive indicator of recurrent hemorrhage and may be used to follow such diseases as Goodpasture's syndrome.

PULMONARY FUNCTION TESTS

Static Volumes

The volume of the lung can be divided into several compartments. The definitions of these compartments are indicated in Figure 2–19. Total lung capacity (TLC) is the total amount of air within the lungs at maximal inspiration and is equal to the residual volume (RV) plus vital capacity (VC). The VC is the volume obtained when a subject expires from TLC to full expiration and is approximately equal to 70% of the TLC. The volume present within the lung at end-expiration from a normal tidal volume is defined as the FRC. The inspiratory reserve capacity is the volume between TLC and the end-inspiratory volume of normal tidal breathing whereas the expiratory reserve capacity is the volume between residual volume and FRC.

TLC is determined by a combination of inspiratory

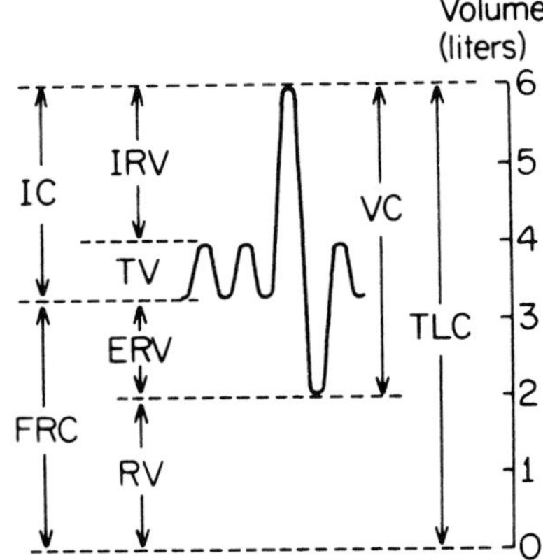

FIGURE 2–19 ■ Divisions of lung volume (ERV, expiratory reserve volume; FRC, functional residual capacity; IC, inspiratory capacity; RV, inspiratory reserve volume; TLC, total lung capacity; TV, tidal volume; VC, vital capacity.) (From Culver BH: Mechanics of ventilation. In Culver BH [ed]: The Respiratory System. Syllabus for Human Biology, Seattle, WA, University of Washington, Health Sciences Academic Services, 1990.)

muscle strength, chest wall recoil, and lung recoil. A decrease in inspiratory muscle strength will decrease TLC, as will increases in either lung or chest wall recoil. RV is determined by expiratory muscle strength, chest wall compliance, and the point at which airway closure takes place. In young people, the RV is greater than that at which airway closure takes place and is mainly dependent on muscle strength. However, with increasing age, airway closure occurs at higher volumes and becomes relatively independent of expiratory muscle strength. As a result RV rises from approximately 25% of TLC at age 20 years to 40% at age 70 years (Fowler, 1952).

As seen previously, FRC is determined by the interplay between lung recoil and chest wall recoil. It may be reduced in states such as obesity and pregnancy and increased in patients with severe chronic obstructive pulmonary disease.

The measurement of these volumes is done by a combination of spirometry and more specialized tests. The tests amenable to measurement with spirometry are the VC, tidal volume, and both the inspiratory capacity and expiratory reserve volume. FRC, TLC, and RV cannot be measured with spirometry.

A common method of measuring static lung volumes is by He dilution, as He is relatively insoluble and is not taken up by the lungs. In this method a known concentration and volume of an He-containing gas is inhaled and allowed to equilibrate with gas in the lung. Subsequently, the He concentration in the exhaled gas is measured. Based on the law of conservation of mass, the volume can be calculated as follows:

$$V_1 \times C_1 = V_2 \times C_2$$

where V_1 is the volume of inhaled gas; C_1 is the concentration of He in the inspired gas; V_2 is the unknown volume to be measured (volume of the lung); and C_2 is the exhaled concentration of He.

The volume measured is a function of the lung volume at which the subject is asked to inhale the He-containing gas. If inhalation commences at the end of a normal tidal volume, then the lung volume measured is the FRC. If inhalation begins at end-expiration, then the lung volume measured is TLC, and RV can be calculated by subtracting VC from TLC.

In practice, there are two methods to measure lung volume by He dilution. They are the single–breath-hold technique, which is usually used to measure TLC (Meneely and Kaltrieder, 1949), and the steady-state method in which equilibrium is achieved over a few minutes. FRC is usually measured by the steady-state method (Ogilivie et al, 1957). A problem with these methods is that they only measure the volume of the air spaces in direct communication with the mouth and may seriously underestimate thoracic gas volume in disease states where there is an airway abnormality or there are noncommunicating pockets of gas, as occurs with bullous lung disease and pneumothorax.

Another method to measure FRC is to use a constant-volume body plethysmograph. This method measures all compressible gas within the thorax. It does this by taking advantage of Boyle's law, which is applicable to constant temperature conditions:

$$PV = \text{Constant}$$

The subject sits in an airtight chamber and pants into a circuit in direct communication with the outside. This produces pressure changes within the chamber that are proportional to the thoracic gas volumes. Because the volume of the chamber is known and the pressure changes are measured, the volume of FRC can be calculated.

The advantage of constant-volume plethysmography is that it measures all gas within the thoracic cavity. However, if changes in abdominal pressure occur, this technique will measure intra-abdominal gas volume as well. Another source of artifact with this technique is the assumption that during a panting maneuver there is equilibration between alveolar and mouth pressure. This may not be the case in severe airway obstruction in which the lack of equilibration may lead to significant overestimation of TLC (Brown and Slutsky, 1984). Also, in patients with severe airway obstruction, there may be large discrepancies between the two methods because the airway obstruction may prevent full equilibration of the He with all the air spaces. In normal individuals, the volumes obtained by He dilution and plesthymography should be nearly identical, and differences greater than 500 ml are considered to be significant and an indicator of air within the thoracic cavity in poor communication with the mouth. To properly interpret lung volumes by plethysmography, a chest radiograph is required to exclude severe bullous disease or pneumothorax.

Flow-Volume Loop

A large amount of information can be obtained using spirometry and examining the relationship between maximal expiratory and inspiratory flow rates and lung volumes. (Hyatt and Black, 1973). Maximal expiratory and inspiratory flow rates are a function of lung volume. Plotting these on a graph produces a flow-volume curve (Fig. 2–20). In practice, the expiratory curve is constructed by having a subject inhale to TLC and then forcefully expire to RV while the inspiratory curve is constructed from the flow rates generated during maximal inspiration from RV to TLC. Typically, the expiratory curve is triangular, with the highest flows near TLC. The inspiratory curve is more symmetric, with highest flows at mid-VC.

If markers of elapsed time are added during expiration, then quantitative measurements of flow with respect to time can be derived. An example is the forced expiratory volume in 1 second, or FEV_1. The forced vital capacity (FVC) is the volume between the RV and TLC. Other measurements, such as maximum flow at 50% and 25% VC ($Vmax_{50}$, $Vmax_{25}$, respectively) can also be derived (see Fig. 2–21). $Vmax_{50}$ and $Vmax_{25}$ are reflective of small airway function and if reduced in comparison with lung volume indicate small airway obstruction (Cosio et al, 1978).

The shape of the flow-volume loop is dependent on

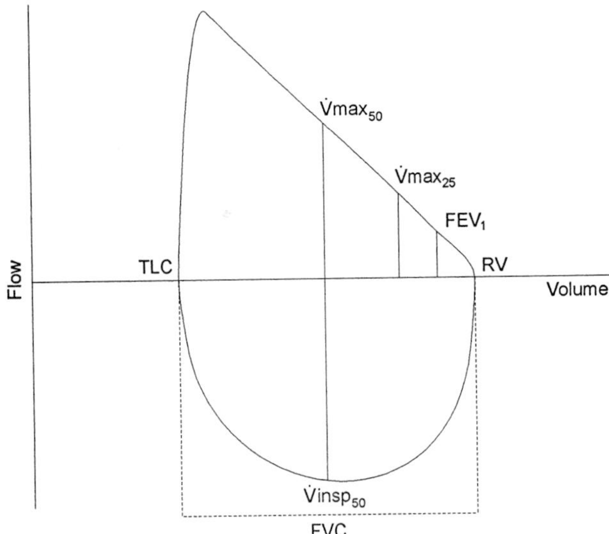

FIGURE 2–20 ■ Idealized diagram of maximal expiratory and inspiratory flow-volume curves. (FEV_1, forced expiratory flow in 1 second; FVC, forced vital capacity; RV, residual volume; TLC, total lung capacity; $\dot{V}insp_{50}$, inspiratory flow at 50% of vital capacity; $\dot{V}\ max_{25}$, flow at 25% of vital capacity; $\dot{V}max_{50}$, flow at 50% of vital capacity.)

the properties of the airways, lung recoil, and lung volume. For this reason it will be altered by disease states that affect any of these. The resultant curves can be divided into three categories and with each there is a corresponding clinical correlate. These are restrictive lung disease, airway obstruction, and upper airway obstruction (Fig. 2–21).

In restrictive lung disease, lung recoil is increased, although total lung volume is reduced. Although absolute flows are reduced because of the low lung volumes, the airways are usually normal. When the measurements of flow are standardized for lung volume, they are increased or normal. An example is the reduction in FEV_1 seen in restrictive lung disease while the FEV_1/FVC (an indicator of lung volume) ratio is increased (Gaensler, 1951). A normal FEV_1/FVC ratio is approximately 70% to 80%. Also, the absolute values of $Vmax_{50}$ and $Vmax_{25}$ are reduced. However, when these are compared with lung volume they are usually appropriately reduced in the absence of airway disease ($Vmax_{50}$ and $Vmax_{25}$ values should be approximately equal to VC and one half the VC in liters, respectively). This illustrates the difficulty in evaluating flow measurements unless they are related to the lung volumes from which they are derived.

In obstructive lung disease, the FEV_1 is reduced, but lung volumes can be increased, and the FVC is much better preserved. Therefore, the FEV_1/FVC ratio is reduced. Although upper airway obstruction can mimic obstructive lung disease, both the inspiratory and expiratory limbs of the flow-volume loop are affected if the obstruction is fixed. This may help distinguish between the two disease processes. A useful measurement of inspiratory flow is the maximum inspiratory flow at 50% VC.

The FEV_1, and all other lung volumes, varies directly with height, inversely with age, and is greater in men than in women. Published tables for all lung volumes are available. Pulmonary function tests are discussed in greater detail in the sections to follow.

If a flow-volume loop is done with minimal effort and then repeated successively with increasing effort until maximal effort is reached, an interesting phenomenon emerges. The peak flow is effort dependent and increases with increasing effort, but 75% to 80% of the expiratory curve turns out to be effort independent (Fig. 2–22). On this portion of the curve, increasing effort will not increase flows. Several theoretical models have been proposed for this phenomenon, but the most simple is the equal pressure point model (Mead et al, 1967). In this model, the effort independence of flow is thought to result from the compression of intrathoracic airways. Increased effort results in the generation of increased positive pleural pressures, which are then transmitted to the intrathoracic airways such that resistance to expiration increases in concert with driving pressure, and flow remains constant.

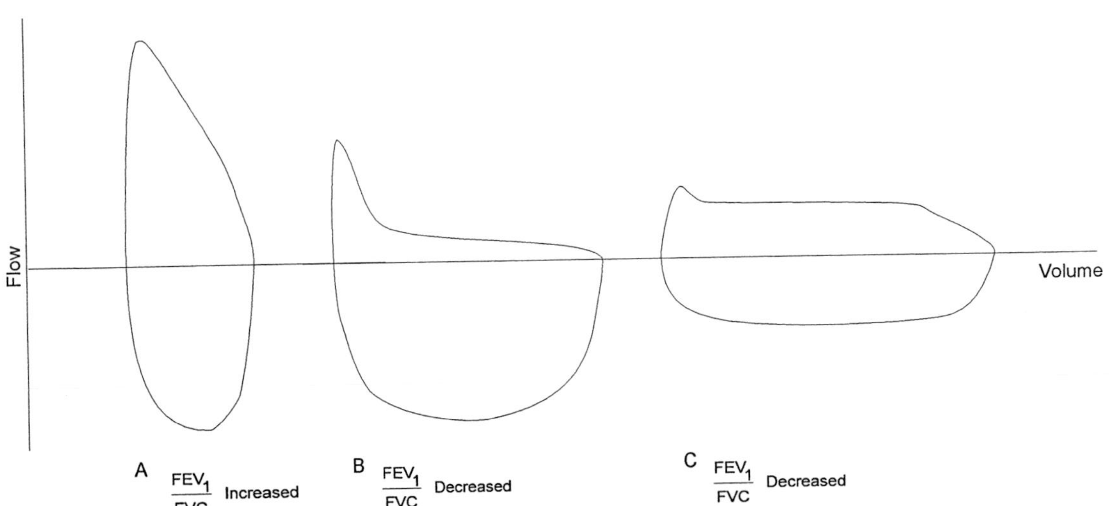

FIGURE 2–21 ■ Representative flow-volume curves of restrictive lung disease, obstructive lung disease, and upper airways obstruction. *A*, Restrictive lung disease; *B*, obstructive lung disease; and *C*, upper airway obstruction.

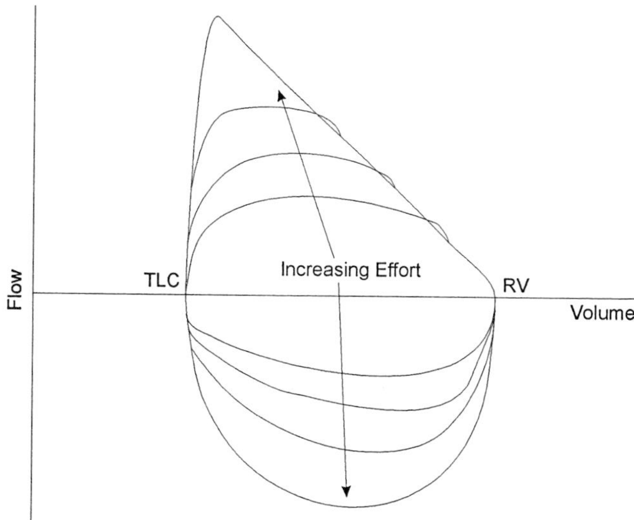

FIGURE 2–22 ■ Effect of effort on the expiratory limb of a flow-volume curve. Note that at low lung volumes, increasing effort causes no increases in maximal flow.

APPLIED PULMONARY PHYSIOLOGY

To gain a better understanding of pulmonary physiology, it is useful to study respiratory diseases and the pathophysiology they produce. The most common manifestation of respiratory disease is altered gas exchange, which is discussed in the following section. Similarly, the concepts of lung volume reduction surgery for emphysema and ventilator-associated lung injury are also reviewed because they can produce important insights into respiratory mechanics and physiology. Additionally, these disease states illustrate the importance of a thorough understanding of pulmonary physiology for the treatment of respiratory disease.

Mechanisms of Altered Gas Exchange

Hypoxia and hypercarbia are common problems faced by clinicians. An understanding of the physiology involved is crucial in dealing with them effectively.

Hypercapnia

Pa_{CO_2} is inversely related to alveolar ventilation and directly related to CO_2 production. This relationship can be expressed as follows:

$$Pa_{CO_2} = K\frac{V_{CO_2}}{V_A}$$

where Pa_{CO_2} is the partial pressure of arterial CO_2; V_{CO_2} is CO_2 production and V_A is alveolar ventilation. The constant *K* has a value of 0.863 mm Hg (Weinberger et al, 1989). Alveolar ventilation can also be expressed in terms of tidal volume (V_T) and dead space (V_D), because

$$V_A = f(V_T - V_D).$$

Therefore, the equation for Pa_{CO_2} becomes

$$Pa_{CO_2} = K\frac{V_{CO_2}}{f(V_T - V_D)}.$$

By looking at the individual terms in the equation, one can readily infer the causes of hypercapnia. CO_2 production is a function of the substrate metabolized for energy and is usually related to the amount of O_2 consumed. This is referred to as the respiratory quotient (RQ) and is expressed as follows:

$$RQ = V_{CO_2} - V_{O_2}$$

where V_{O_2} is O_2 consumption. For carbohydrates, RQ equals 1; for fat, 0.7; and for protein, 0.8; with an average of 0.8 for a typical diet. An increase in CO_2 production does not usually cause hypercapnia, because it can readily be compensated for by increasing alveolar ventilation. However, in individuals who have underlying respiratory compromise, this may not be possible, and increases in CO_2 production may result in significant hypercarbia. An example of this can be found in patients who have respiratory failure secondary to severe chronic obstructive lung disease. In these patients, there may be a role for nutrition supplements high in fat, which have low RQ ratios, such that CO_2 production is minimized in the process of meeting caloric needs.

If CO_2 production is constant, Pa_{CO_2} is inversely proportional to alveolar ventilation. In this case, factors that reduce alveolar ventilation will produce hypercapnia. The causes of alveolar ventilation can be divided into two main groups: central hypoventilation ("won't breathe") or peripheral ("can't breathe"). Central hypoventilation can be caused by a variety of factors, including drugs (e.g., narcotics) and CNS disease. Peripheral hypoventilation can also be caused by a variety of disease processes ranging from airway obstruction, to chest wall disease, to neuromuscular weakness.

From the equation for Pa_{CO_2} in terms of V_{CO_2}, V_T, and V_D, it can also be deduced that as V_D increases in relation to V_T, the denominator falls, and Pa_{CO_2} rises. In other words, the V_D/V_T ratio is important in determining the amount of alveolar ventilation for a given respiratory rate and tidal volume. This may be an important mechanism of hypercapnia in patients with chronic obstructive lung disease who have areas of V/Q mismatch (i.e., increased dead space) but who also tend to have relatively low tidal volumes.

Hypoxia

The causes of arterial hypoxemia can be divided into two broad categories, depending on whether alveolar O_2 levels are normal or reduced. Reduction of alveolar O_2, either focally or diffusely, is a relatively frequent cause of hypoxemia. Alveolar O_2 levels are the result of a balance between the delivery of O_2 and its removal from the alveolus (Hlastala, 1991).[80] Hypoxemia from low alveolar O_2 levels only occurs in situations where delivery of O_2 to the alveolus is reduced relative to the blood flow to that alveolus. This occurs throughout the lung at high altitudes, where the inspired P_{O_2} is low and although hyperventilation is usually present, total O_2 delivery to alveoli is reduced. It also occurs with hypoventilation, because the amount of air and consequently O_2 delivery is reduced. In this situation, if the FIO_2 is increased, it may compensate for the hypoventilation, and hypoxia may be circumvented.

Regional reduction of alveolar O_2 content occurs with ventilation/perfusion (V/Q) mismatch and shunt. In V/Q mismatch, ventilation is inadequate to deliver sufficient amounts of O_2 to fully oxygenate the blood perfusing that alveolus, and shunt is present when there is no ventilation to a perfused alveolus. In V/Q mismatch and shunt, arterial hypoxemia occurs when partially oxygenated blood mixes (in blood vessels downstream from alveolar capillaries) with fully oxygenated blood from regions with normal perfusion and ventilation. An example of hypoxia secondary to V/Q mismatch occurs in obstructive airways disease, in which alveolar ventilation is not uniform and on a regional basis may be inadequate for the amount of perfusion present, while an example of shunt is provided by hypoxia secondary to lobar collapse, as continued perfusion may occur in the absence of ventilation.

Hypoxemia with normal alveolar O_2 levels occurs with abnormalities of diffusion and with very low mixed venous PO_2 ($P\bar{v}O_2$) levels. In these situations, equilibration of alveolar and capillary PO_2 does not occur during the transit time through the alveolar capillaries. In the normal situation, complete equilibration occurs in approximately one third of the capillary transit time, and as a result there is a large degree of reserve present. Abnormalities of diffusion alone in the absence of V/Q mismatch or shunt do not usually cause hypoxemia unless they are present with reduced pulmonary capillary transit times or they are associated with low $P\bar{v}O_2$ (Fraser et al, 1988).[81] An example in which hypoxia is secondary to impaired diffusion and reduced capillary transit time occurs during exercise in patients with pulmonary fibrosis.

A useful method of assessing gas exchange in the lung is to look at the alveolar-arterial PO_2 difference ($PAO_2 - PaO_2$). Under ideal circumstances, alveolar PO_2 (PAO_2) should be equal to PaO_2). The PAO_2 is a function of the inspired O_2 pressure (PIO_2) and the subsequent uptake and replacement of O_2 by CO_2 in the alveolus. As previously stated, the amount of CO_2 exhaled from the lungs for a given O_2 uptake from the lungs is known as the respiratory quotient (RQ). Therefore

$$PAO_2 = PIO_2 - \frac{PaCO_2}{RQ}$$

$P(A-a)O_2$ then is

$$P(A-a)O_2 = PAO_2 - PaO_2$$

Combining these equations gives

$$P(A - A)O_2 = PIO_2 - \frac{PaCO_2}{RQ} - PaCO_2$$

In its full form the equation becomes

$$P(A - a)O_2 = (PB - 47)\,FIO_2 - \frac{PaCO_2}{RQ} - PaO_2$$

where PB is the barometric pressure, 47 mm Hg is the partial pressure of water vapor in fully saturated air, and FIO_2 is the fraction of inspired oxygen. RQ is usually assumed to be approximately 0.8, although this assumption can lead to errors in the calculation, especially in non–steady-state conditions.

If $PAO_2 - PaO_2$ is normal or less than 10, there is unlikely to be any shunt or V/Q mismatch. However, in the presence of V/Q mismatch or shunt, the degree of elevation of $PaO_2 - PaO_2$ does not correlate with the amount of shunt or V/Q mismatch, because then it is also influenced by $P\bar{v}O_2$ and FIO_2. For example, the $PAO_2 - PaO_2$ increases as FIO_2 is increased, although the amount of lung disease remains constant.

The amount of shunt or venous admixture ratio is calculated from the following formula (for its full derivation, see West, 1985, p. 52):

$$\frac{Qs}{Qt} = \frac{Cc'O_2 - CaCO_2}{Cc'O_2 - C\bar{v}O_2}$$

where Qs/Qt is the shunt fraction, $Cc'O_2$ is the O_2 content of end-capillary blood, CaO_2 is the O_2 content of arterial blood, and $C\bar{v}O_2$ is the O_2 content of mixed venous blood (Fig. 2–23).

Lung Volume Reduction Surgery

The interplay between lung dynamics and respiratory muscles is illustrated in the physiologic abnormalities found in patients with emphysema and severe hyperinflation. In emphysema, there is a gradual loss of lung tissue elastic recoil (reduction in driving pressure) combined with airway obstruction such that progressive hyperinflation occurs (Zamel et al, 1976). Pulmonary function studies in emphysema reveal reduction in indices of expiratory flow such as FVC and FEV_1 with hyperinflation as measured by increases in lung volumes such as TLC, FRC, and RV. As hyperinflation occurs, respiratory muscles are placed at a mechanical disadvantage such that progressive respiratory embarrassment occurs. The diaphragm becomes flattened and shortened as the zone of apposition decreases and the diaphragmatic muscle area is reduced leading to significant impairment in func-

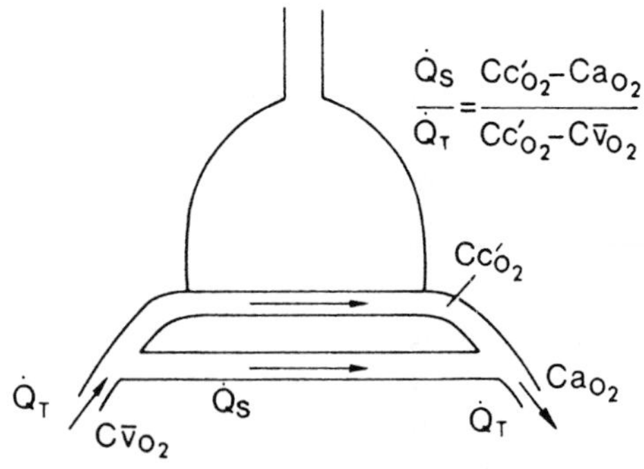

FIGURE 2–23 ■ The influence of shunt on arterial PO_2.

tional muscle strength (Cassart et al, 1997; Similowski et al, 1991). The changes in diaphragmatic function with emphysema are fully covered in the recent reviews of De Troyer (1997) and Ruel and colleagues (1998).

Lung volume surgery as a means of treating emphysema was first carried out in the 1950s and was postulated as a means of improving the physiologic abnormalities observed in patients with severe lung hyperinflation from emphysema (Brantigan and Mueller, 1957). With improvement in surgical techniques and postoperative care, interest in this technique was rekindled in the 1990s (Cooper et al, 1995). Emphysema is amenable to lung volume reduction surgery because hyperinflation is characteristic of the disease along with disease heterogeneity, such that areas that are severely affected and contribute little to lung function can be removed with minimal loss of functional lung tissue but with reduction in hyperinflation. Once the degree of hyperinflation is reduced, respiratory dynamics improve with resultant improvement in function. Improvements in patient functional capacity, in expiratory volume measurements such as FVC and FEV_1, and reduction in lung volumes have been found after lung volume reduction surgery (Date et al, 1998; Gaissert et al, 1996; Meyers et al, 1998). The mechanisms for improvement of lung function have been found to be complex, with the main factor being improvement in lung elastic recoil (Gelb et al, 1996, 1998; Hun et al, 1998). Other contributing factors to the improvement seen after lung volume reduction surgery are an expansion of functional lung tissue, improvement in respiratory muscle function and strength, improvement in the neuromechanical coupling of the diaphragm, and possibly alterations in pulmonary hemodynamics. (Becker et al, 1998; Laghi et al, 1998; Martinez et al, 1997; Wagner, 1998).

Ventilator-Associated Lung Injury

Acute respiratory distress syndrome (ARDS) is a syndrome that clearly demonstrates how derangements in pulmonary physiology cause characteristic clinical syndrome and how a thorough understanding of pulmonary physiology is necessary for the treatment of respiratory patients.

As discussed in previous sections, the prevention of alveolar flooding is an important function of the alveolar capillary blood–air barrier. Alterations in the permeability of this barrier lead to influx of fluid into the alveolus, and if permeability is increased sufficiently, the protective mechanisms in place to ensure that the alveolus remains dry are overwhelmed. This leads to flooding of alveoli by protein-rich fluid, and the syndrome commonly known as ARDS is produced (Petty and Fowler, 1982). Several causes of this are known and include entities such as sepsis, aspiration of gastric contents, multiple trauma, and pancreatitis. Although a diverse group, they all produce disruption of the alveolar-capillary barrier either directly, as occurs in aspiration and inhalation of noxious gases, or indirectly through the effect of mediators on the pulmonary epithelium, as occurs in pancreatitis or sepsis.

The therapy for ARDS is supportive and includes treatment of the underlying cause and mechanical ventilation to correct the resultant gas exchange abnormalities. The goal is to wait until the permeability of the blood-alveolar barrier improves to the point that the mechanisms to keep alveoli dry, as previously discussed, become adequate. However, mortality from ARDS remains high and is usually caused by multisystem organ failure, which occurs during the prolonged period that is required for the ARDS to improve (Krafft et al, 1996). The reasons for this are becoming better defined, and it is likely that ventilator-associated lung injury plays a role (Dreyfuss and Saumon, 1998).

In animal models, high ventilating volumes cause protein-rich pulmonary edema similar to that seen in ARDS (Kolobow et al, 1987; Webb and Tierney, 1974). This results from alveolar overstretch and in part by subsequent disruption of the alveolar epithelium, secondary to breaks in the extremely thin epithelial cell processes (the junctions between cells are extremely strong and are not disrupted as previously suspected). To maintain normal blood gases in the ARDS patient, in previous years mechanical ventilation with very high airway pressures was common and may have worsened the high-permeability pulmonary edema. In addition, it has become apparent that mechanical ventilation at very low lung volumes can also cause marked injury, possibly by the repeated opening and closing of alveolar units. Not only does this pattern of mechanical ventilation cause direct injury, there is evidence that a systemic inflammatory response can occur because of mechanical activation of inflammatory cells recruited to the lung during lung injury (Tremblay et al, 1997). This systemic inflammatory response may lead to the production of mediators, which may produce organ dysfunction and cause multisystem organ failure, which is one of the major determinants of mortality from ARDS (Slutsky and Tremblay, 1998).

It is difficult clinically to ascertain at the bedside whether a particular pattern of ventilation is causing overdistention or whether repeated recruitment or decruitment of lung units is occurring. One approach that has sparked intense interest is the use of the lung or respiratory system pressure-volume curve. The key concepts underlying this approach are that the lower inflection point (LIP) on the inflation limb of the pressure-volume curve represents the start of recruitment and the upper inflection point (UIP) represents the start of overdistention. There are certainly many caveats to this approach: (1) continuing recruitment may occur above the LIP; (2) the UIP may represent the discontinuation of recruitment, rather than the start of overdistention (Hickling, 1998); and (3) a stiff chest wall may markedly alter interpretation of respiratory system pressure-volume curves (Mergoni et al, 1997; Ranieri et al, 1997).

Although controversial, based on this scheme, the best ventilatory strategy for ARDS may be one in which distending pressures are below the upper inflection point and expiratory pressures are above the lower inflection point of a patient's static pressure-volume curve. Typically, in ARDS patients, lung compliance is low, and the pressure-volume curve is shifted to the right. To stay below the upper inflection point, small tidal volumes may need to be used such that alveolar ventilation falls and the Pa_{CO_2} may rise (permissive hypercapnia) (Hickling et al, 1990). In addition, high levels of PEEP may be needed to stay above the lower inflection point. This is dependent on the degree of lung injury present.

In summary, ARDS is a syndrome in which multiple abnormalities of pulmonary physiology are present. The treatment of patients with ARDS requires a thorough understanding of pulmonary physiology and is a good example of the necessity for an intimate knowledge of pulmonary physiology in the treatment of patients with respiratory disorders.

■ REFERENCES

Albert RK, Lakshminarayan S, Hildebrandt WK, Butler J: Increased surface tension favors pulmonary edema formation in anesthetized dogs' lungs. J Clin Invest 63:1015–1016, 1979.

Angus GE, Thurlbeck WM: Number of alveoli in the human lung. J Appl Physiol 32:483, 1972.

Armstrong DJ, Luck JC: A comparative study of irritant and type J receptors in the cat. Respir Physiol 21:47–60, 1974.

Bachofen HP, Gehr P, Weibel ER: Alterations of mechanical properties and morphology in excised rabbit lungs rinsed with a detergent. J Appl Physiol 47:1002–1010, 1979.

Bachofen H, Hildebrandt J, Bachofen M: Pressure-volume curves of air and liquid filled excised lungs—surface tension in situ. J Appl Physiol 29:422–431, 1970.

Ball WC, Stewart PB, Newsham LG S, Bates DV: Regional pulmonary functions studied with xenon-133. J Clin Invest 41:519–531, 1962.

Bastacky J, Hayes TL, Schmidt BV: Lung structure as revealed by microdissection. Am Rev Respir Dis 128:S7–S13, 1983.

Becker MD, Berkmen YM, Austin JH: Lung volumes before and after lung volume reduction surgery. Am J Respir Crit Care Med, 157:1593–1599, 1998.

Berger AJ, Mitchell RA, Severinghaus JW: Regulation of respiration (pt 1). N Engl J Med 297:92–97, 1977a.

Berger AJ, Mitchell RA, Severinghaus JW: Regulation of respiration (pt 2) N Engl J Med 297:139–143, 1977b.

Berger AJ, Mitchell RA, Severinghaus JW: Regulation of breathing (pt 3). N Engl J Med 297:194–201, 1977c.

Brantigan OC and Mueller E: Surgical treatment of pulmonary emphysema. Am Surg 23:789–804, 1957.

Brown R, Slutsky AS: Frequency dependence of plethysmographic measurement of thoracic gas volume. J Appl Physiol 57:1865–1871, 1984.

Cassart M, Pettiwx N, Gevenois PA et al: Effect of chronic hyperinflation on diaphragm length and surface area. Am J Respir Crit Care Med, 156:504–508, 1997.

Cooper JD, Trulock EP, Triantafillou AN: Bilateral pneumonectomy (volume reduction) for chronic obstructive pulmonary diseases. J Thorac Cardiovasc Surg 109:106–119, 1985.

Cosio M, Ghezzo H, Hogg JC: The relationship between structural changes in small airways and pulmonary function. N Engl J Med 298:1277, 1978.

Cumming G: Airway morphology and its consequences. Bull Physiopathol Respir 8:527, 1972.

Curtis JL, Mahlmeister M, Fink JB et al: Helium-oxygen gas therapy. Chest 90:455–457, 1986.

Date H, Goto K, Souda R: Bilateral lung volume reduction surgery via median sternotomy for severe pulmonary emphysema. Ann Thorac Surg 65:939–942, 1998.

De Troyer A: Effect of hyperinflation on the diaphragm. Eur Respir J 10:708–713, 1997.

Dobbs LG: Pulmonary surfactant. Annu Rev Med 40:431–446, 1989.

Dreyfuss D, Saumon G: Ventilator induced lung injury: Lessons learned from experimental studies (state of the art). Am J Respir Crit Care Med 157:294–323, 1998.

Elliot FM, Reid L: Some new facts about the pulmonary artery and its branching pattern. Clin Radiol 16:193–198, 1965.

Floros J: Sixty years of surfactant research. Am J Physiol 2:L238–L240, 1990.

Fowler WS: Intrapulmonary distribution of inspired gas. Physiol Rev 32:1–20, 1952.

Fraser RG, Pare JP, Pare PD et al (eds): Diagnosis of Diseases of the Chest, 3rd ed. Philadelphia, WB Saunders, 1988, p 29.

Freedman S: Mechanics of ventilation. In Brewes RAL, Gibbon GJ, Geddes DM (eds): Respiratory Medicine. London Bailliere Tindall, 1990, pp 114–130.

Fung YC, Sobin SS: Theory of sheet flow in lung alveoli. J Appl Physiol 26:472–478, 1968.

Gaensler EA: Analysis of the ventilatory defect by timed vital capacity measurements. Am Rev Tuberc 64:256, 1951.

Gaissert HA, Trulock EP, Cooper JD et al: Comparison of early functional results after volume reduction or lung transplantation for chronic obstructive pulmonary disease. J Thorac Cardiovasc Surg 111:296–306, 1996.

Gelb AF, Brenner M, McKenna RJ: Serial lung function and elastic recoil 2 years after lung volume reduction surgery for emphysema. Chest 113:1497–1506, 1998.

Gelb AF, Zamel N, Mckenna RJ, Brenner M: Mechanism of short-term improvement in lung function after emphysema reduction. Am J Respir Crit Care Med 154:945–951, 1996.

Glazier JB, Hughes JMB, West JB: Measurement of capillary dimensions and blood volume in rapidly frozen lungs. J Appl Physiol 26:65–76, 1969.

Grassino AE, Roussos C, Macklem PT: Static properties of the chest wall. In Crystal RG, West JB (eds): The Lung: Scientific Foundations, Vol 1. New York, Raven Press 1991; pp 855–867.

Hawgood S: Surfactant: Composition, structure and metabolism. In Crystal RG, West JB (eds): The Lung: Scientific Foundations, Vol 1. New York, Raven Press, pp 247–261, 1991.

Hawgood S, Clements JA: Pulmonary surfactant and its apoproteins. J Clin Invest 86:1–6, 1990.

Hickling KG: The pressure-volume curve is greatly modified by recruitment: A mathematical model of ARDS lungs. Am J Respir Crit Care Med 158:194–202, 1998.

Hickling KG, Henderson SJ, Jackson R: Low mortality associated with low volume pressure limited ventilation with permissive hypercapnea in severe ARDS. Intensive Care Med, 16:372–377, 1990.

Hlastala MI: Ventilation. In Crystal RG, West JB (eds): The Lung: Scientific Foundations. New York, Raven Press, 1991, p 1209.

Hoppin FG, Stothert JC, Greaves IA et al: Lung recoil: Elastic and rheological properties. In Handbook of Physiology. Section 3: The Respiratory System, Vol 3: Fishman AP, Macklem PT, Mead J, Geiger SR (section eds). Bethesda, MD, American Physiological Society, 1986, pp 195–215.

Horsfeld K, Cumming G: Morphology of the bronchial tree in man. J Appl Physiol 24:373, 1968.

Houck JR, Keamy MF, McDonough JM: Effect of helium concentration on experimental upper airway obstruction. Ann Otol Rhinol Laryngol 99:556–561, 1990.

Hughes JMB, Glazier JB, Maloney JE et al: Effect of lung volumes on the distribution of pulmonary blood flow. Respir Physiol 4:58–72, 1968.

Huh J, Brenner M, Chen JC et al: Changes in pulmonary physiology after lung volume reduction surgery in a rabbit model of emphysema. J Thorac Cardiovasc Surg 115:328–335, 1998.

Hyatt RE, Black LE: The flow-volume curve. Am Rev Respir Dis 107:191–199, 1973.

Kolobow TM, Moretti MP, Fumagelli R et al: Severe impairment in lung function induced by high peak airway pressure during mechanical ventilation. Am Rev Respir Dis 135:312–315, 1989.

Kraff P, Fridrich P, Fitzgerald RD et al: The acute respiratory distress syndrome: Definitions, severity and clinical outcome—an analysis of 101 clinical investigations. Intensive Care Med 22:519–529, 1996.

Laghi F, Jubran A, Topeli A et al: Effect of lung volume reduction surgery on neuromechanical coupling of the diaphragm. Am J Respir Crit Care Med 157:475–483, 1998.

Lahiri S, Mokasi A, Mulligan E, Nishino T: Comparison of aortic acid and chemoreceptor responses to hypercapnia and hypoxia. J Appl Physiol 51:55–61, 1981.

Landis EM, Pappenheimer JR: Exchange of substances through capillary walls. In Handbook of Physiology. Section 2: Circulation, Vol 2; Hamilton WF, Dao P (eds): Washington DC, American Physiological Society, 1963, pp. 961–1034.

Landowne M, Sacy WR: Glossary of terms. In Remington JW (ed): Tissue Elasticity. Bethesda, MD, American Physiological Society, 1957, pp. 197–190.

Lauweryns J: The blood and lymphatic microcirculation of the lung. Pathol Annu 6:365–415, 1965.

Lugliani R, Whipp BJ, Seard C, Wasserman K: Effect of bilateral carotid-body resection on ventilatory control at rest and during exercise in man. N Engl J Med 285:1105–1111, 1971.

Lumsden T: Observations on the respiratory centers in the cat. J Physiol (Lond) 57:153–160, 1923a.

Lumsden T: Observations on the respiratory centres. J Physiol (Lond) 57:354–367, 1923b.

Martinez FJ, Montes de Oca M, Whyte RI: Lung volume reduction improves dyspnea, dynamic hyperinflation, and respiratory muscle function. Am J Respir Crit Care Med 155:1984–1990, 1997.

Matthay MA, Folkesson HG, Verkman AS: Salt and water transport across alveolar and distal airway epithelia in the adult lung. Am J Physiol 270:L487–L503, 1996.

Mead J, Turner JM, Macklem PT et al: Significance of the relationship between lung recoil and maximum expiratory effort. J Appl Physiol 22:95–105, 1967.

Meneely GR, Kaltrieder NL: The volume of the lung determined by helium dilution. Description of the method and comparison with other procedures. J Clin Invest 28:129, 1999.

Mergoni M, Martelli A, Volpi A et al: Impact of positive end-expiratory pressure on chest wall and lung pressure-volume curve in acute respiratory failure. Am J Respir Crit Care Med 156:846–854, 1997.

Meyer BJ, Meyer A, Guyton AC: Interstitial fluid pressure versus negative pressure in the lung. Circ Res 22:263–271, 1968.

Meyers BF, Yusen RD, Lefrak SS et al: Outcome of Medicare patients with emphysema selected for, but denied, a lung volume reduction operation. Ann Thorac Surg 66:331–336, 1998.

Morton NS: Pulmonary surfactant: Physiology, pharmacology and clinical uses. Br J Hosp Med 42:52–58, 1989.

Netter FH: The Ciba Collection of Medical Illustrations: Vol 7: The Respiratory System, Summit, NJ, Ciba-Geigy, 1979.

Nielsen M, Smith H: Studies on the regulation of respiration in acute hypoxia. Acta Physiol Scand 24:293, 1951.

Nieman GF, Bredenberg CE: High surface tension pulmonary edema induced by detergent aerosol. J Appl Physiol 58:129–136, 1985.

Ogilvie CM, Forster RE, Blakemore WS, Morton JE: A standardized breath-holding technique for the clinical measurement of diffusing capacity. J Clin Invest 36:1, 1957.

Paintal AS: Vagal sensory receptors and their reflex effects. Physiol Rev 53:159–227, 1973.

Petty TL, Fowler AA: Another look at ARDS. Chest 82:98–104, 1982.

Phillipson EA, Sullivan CE: Arousal: The forgotten response to respiratory stimuli (editorial). Am Rev Respir Dis 118:807, 1976.

Prattle RE: Surface lining of lung alveoli. Physiol Rev 45:48–79, 1965.

Radford EP Jr: Recent studies of mechanical properties of mammalian lungs. In Remington JW (ed): Tissue Elasticity. Bethesda MD, American Physiological Society, 1957, pp. 177–190.

Rahn H, Otis AB, Chadwick LE, Fenn WO: The pressure-volume diagram of thorax and lung. Am J Physiol 146:161, 1946.

Ranieri VM, Brienza N, Santostasi S et al: Impairment of lung and chest wall mechanics in patients with acute respiratory distress syndrome: Role of abdominal distension. Am J Respir Crit Care Med 156:1082–1091, 1997.

Raskin PS, Herman P: Inter-acinar pathways in the human lung. Am Rev Respir Dis 111:489–495, 1975.

Read DJC: A clinical method of assessing the ventilatory response to CO_2. Aust Ann Med 16:20–32, 1967.

Rebuck AS, Slutsky AS: Measurement of the ventilatory response to hypercapnia and hypoxia. In Hornbill TF (ed): Regulation of Breathing, PH. New York, Marcel Dekker pp. 745–772, 1981.

Rebuck AS, Woodley WE: Ventilatory effects of hypoxia and their dependence on P_{CO_2}. J Appl Physiol 38:16–19, 1975.

Ruel M, Deslauriers J, Maltais F: The diaphragm in emphysema. Chest Surg Clin N Am May 8:381–399, 1998.

Sampson SR, Vidruk EH: Properties of irritant receptors in canine lung. Respir Physiol 25:9–22, 1975.

Schneeberger EE: Structural basis for some permeability properties of the air-blood barrier. Fed Proc 37:2471–2478, 1978.

Schurch S, Goerke J, Clements JA: Direct determination of surface tension in the lung. Proc Natl Acad Sci USA 73:4698–4702, 1976.

Severinghaus JW: Hypoxic respiratory drive and its loss during chronic hypoxia. Clin Physiol 2:57–79, 1972.

Sharp JT, Hammond MD: Pressure-volume relationships. In Crystal RG, West JB (eds): The Lung: Scientific Foundations. New York, Raven Press, 1991; pp. 839–854.

Similowski T, Yan S, Gauthier AP et al: Contractile properties of the human diaphragm during chronic hyperinflation. N Engl J Med 325:917–923, 1991.

Slutsky AS, Tremblay LN: Multiple system organ failure. Is mechanical ventilation a contributing factor? Am J Respir Crit Care Med 157:1721–1725, 1998.

Staub NC: Alveolar-arterial oxygen tension gradient due to diffusion. J Appl Physiol 18:673, 1963.

Sykes MK, McNicol MW, Campbell EJM: Respiratory Failure, 2nd ed. Oxford, Blackwell Scientific, 1976.

Ta-Shung Lu, Ohmura A, Wong KC, Hodges MR: Helium-oxygen in treatment of upper airway obstruction. Anesthesiology 678–680, 1976.

Thurlbeck WM: The internal surface of area on non-emphysematous lungs. Am Rev Respir Dis 95:765, 1967.

Tremblay LF, Valenza SP, Ribeiro JL et al: Injurious ventilatory strategies increase cytokines and c-fos m-RNA expression in an isolated rat lung model. J Clin Invest 99:944–952, 1997.

von Euler C, Trippenbach T: Cyclic excitability changes of the inspiratory “off-switch” mechanism. Acta Physiol Scand 93:560–562, 1975.

Wagner PD: Functional consequences of lung volume reduction surgery for COPD. Am Respir Crit Care Med 158:1017–1019, 1998.

Webb HH, Tierney DF: Experimental pulmonary edema due to positive pressure ventilation with high inflation pressures: Protection by positive end-expiratory pressure 110:556–565, 1974.

Weibel ER: Morphometry of the Human Lung. New York, Academic Press, 1963.

Weinberger SE, Schwartzstein RM, Weiss JW: Hypercapnea. N Engl J Med 321:1223, 1989.

West JB: Regional differences in the lung. Chest 74:426–437, 1978.

West JB: Respiratory Physiology—The Essentials, 3rd ed. Baltimore, Williams & Wilkins, 1985.

West JB, Dollery CT: Distribution of blood flow and ventilation-perfusion ratios on the lung measured with radioactive CO_2. J Appl Physiol 15:405–410, 1960.

West JB, Dollery CT: Distribution of blood flow in isolated lungs: Relation to vascular and alveolar pressures. J Appl Physiol 19:713–724, 1964.

Wright JR: Clearance and recycling of pulmonary surfactant. Am J Physiol 259:L1–12, 1990.

Zamel N: Normal lung mechanics. In: Baum GL, Wolinsky E (eds) Textbook of Pulmonary Disease. Boston, Little, Brown, 1989.

Zamel N, Hogg J, Gelb AF: Mechanisms of maximal expiratory flow limitation in clinically unsuspected emphysema and obstruction of the peripheral airways. Am Rev Respir Dis 113:337–345, 1976.

CHAPTER **3**

Pulmonary Function Testing: A Practical Approach

Thomas L. Petty

The value of pulmonary function testing in health and disease is grossly underestimated. In this chapter, a practical approach to the assessment of lung mechanics and gas transfer is presented, which is useful in the diagnosis of pulmonary disease and responses to therapy, in preoperative assessment, and for estimation of the overall prognosis of surgical patients.

HISTORICAL NOTE

John Hutchinson, a surgeon, invented the spirometer and coined the term *vital capacity* (i.e., capacity for life). John Hutchinson was a very precise man. He was a violinist of some reputation. His exacting observations allowed him to learn that vital capacity was directly related to height and inversely related to the age of the patients he studied. In his landmark first paper (Hutchinson, 1846), he cited measurements on 2130 individuals, including deceased patients. John Hutchinson inflated the body of a corpse immediately after death, using a bellows device equipped with a crude endotracheal tube and a valve system. He then allowed the corpse to "exhale" into his spirometer, which accurately measured exhaled volume. Thus he correctly concluded that elastic recoil of the lungs and thorax and open airways were essential for expiratory airflow. He believed that his device would be valuable to the insurance industry of London in predicting premature mortality. Alas, the dogma of the era and the lack of vision of "experts" of the time prevented them from capitalizing on the brilliance of John Hutchinson's predictions. In short, the spirometer was not accepted as a useful medical instrument until many years later. Even today, many physicians and surgeons fail to take advantage of the immense value of simple pulmonary function tests in their daily practice.

Many years later in the landmark Framingham study, (Kannel et al, 1980), it was finally recognized that abnormalities in vital capacity were the best predictors of premature mortality, including deaths from all causes, but especially deaths from heart disease. The reason that the vital capacity is such a powerful indicator of premature morbidity and mortality is because any compromise of ventilatory air space may result from an important heart or lung disease. Therefore, a reduction in vital capacity may be a nonspecific indicator of poor health.

Lung diseases can be classified as obstructive or restrictive, as described later in this chapter. Additionally, pulmonary congestion, cardiomegaly, space–pre-empting intrathoracic malignant or benign lesions, poor physical conditioning, neuromuscular disorders, and marked obesity can all affect the vital capacity. Therefore, it is easy to understand how a simple measurement of expiratory airflow can be the true predictor of the capacity to live (i.e., the vital capacity).

Another surgeon, Gaensler (1951), popularized the concept of the timed vital capacity. The concept of the timed vital capacity or the forced expiratory volume (FEV) over time was first introduced by Tiffeneau in France (1947). In recent years, clinicians have settled on the 1-second vital capacity, or (FEV) in 1 second (FEV_1) as the standard. Other arbitrary times have been used for the FEV such as the FEV in 0.75, 2, or 3 seconds. Recently, the FEV_6 has been designated as a surrogate for the forced vital capacity (FVC), because normal lungs empty in 6 seconds or less. Today, two key spirometric tests have become standard: the FVC or FEV_6 (volume test) and the FEV_1 (flow test). The ratio between the two is another important value. Normally, this ratio is greater than 70%. Therefore, an FEV_1/FVC of 71% is considered to be the lower limit of normal (LLN).

HISTORICAL READINGS

Gaensler EA: Analysis of the ventilatory defect by timed vital capacity. Am Rev Respir Dis 69:256, 1951.

Gilson JC, Hugh-Jones P: The measurement of total lung volume and breathing capacity. Clin Sci 7:185, 1949.

Hutchinson J: On the capacity of the lungs and the respiratory function with a view of establishing a precise and easy method of detecting disease by the spirometer. Med Chir Trans (Lond) 29:137, 1846.

Kannel WB, Lew EA, Hubert HB et al: The value of measuring vital capacity for prognostic purposes. Trans Am Life Insurance Med Dir Am 64:66, 1980.

Leiner GC, Abramowitz S, Small MJ et al: Expiratory peak flow rate. Standard values for normal subjects. Use as a clinical test of ventilatory function. Am Rev Respir Dis 88:644, 1963.

Milic-Emili J, Marazzini L, D'Angelo E: 150 years of blowing: Since John Hutchinson. Can Respir J 4:239–245, 1997.

Ogilvie CM, Forster RE, Blakemore WS et al: A standardized breath holding technique for the clinical measurement of the diffusing capacity of the lung for carbon monoxide. J Clin Invest 36:1, 1957.

Tiffeneau R, Pinelli AF: Air circulant et air captif dans l'exploration de la fonction ventilatrice pulmonaire. Paris Med 133:624–628, 1947.

ORIGINS OF AIRFLOW

Figure 3–1 schematically presents the origins of airflow from the complex respiratory system. After the lungs are fully inflated by a forceful inspiratory effort, the lungs and thorax empty, with a vigorous muscular effort throughout exhalation by force of the elastic recoil of the lungs and the conductance of the airways of the lungs. Conductance is the reciprocal of the airway resistance. Expiratory airflow is a result of the release of stored

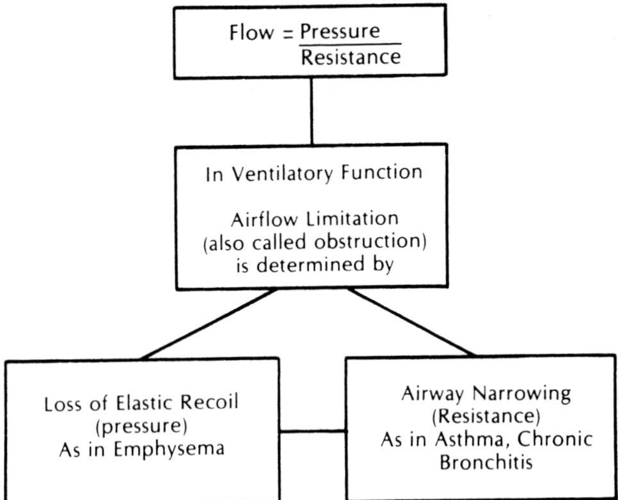

FIGURE 3–1 ■ Origins of airflow. Airflow is a function of alveolar pressure and airways resistance. Expiratory pressure is caused by elastic recoil and muscular effort. Airways resistance is caused by anything that compromises the conducting air passages, such as mucus, bronchospasm, inflammation, mucosal edema, dynamic airways collapse, or combinations. (From Petty TL: Office spirometry. Semin Respir Med 4:184, 1983.)

elastic energy and the fact that airways are normally open. Maximum emptying of the lungs requires a complete forced expiration. The middle stage of expiratory airflow is largely effort-independent and has been termed the *forced expiratory flow between 25% and 75% of the total expiratory flow curve* (FEF_{25-75}) or the maximum midexpiratory flow (MMEF). FEF_{25-75} or MMEF, is not a more sensitive index of airflow; it is only more variable because it is affected by lung volume and, therefore, elastic recoil. This measurement does not have any additional practical value as compared with FEV_1, FVC, and the percentage of predicted airflow (i.e., FEV_1/FVC), and accordingly, both the measurement and term should be abandoned by clinicians. Contrary to previous dogma, it does not measure small airway function any better than the FEV_1 or the FEV_1/FVC ratio.

Not all the air in the lungs can be forcibly inhaled. The FVC is the amount of air that can be exhaled; the residual volume (RV) is the amount of air that cannot be exhaled. The RV and FVC together constitute the total lung capacity (TLC), as seen in Figure 3–2, which conceptualizes the elastic forces of the lung and chest wall as equal but opposite forces at the resting level or functional residual capacity (FRC) *(heavily shaded area between vital capacity and RV).*

Figure 3–3 graphically presents the radiographic features of normal lung emptying. The top of the lung and the diaphragm are outlined with wax pencil. On the left, one can see that the subject has filled his lungs by a forceful inspiratory muscular effort. The diaphragms have descended and the ribs have achieved a horizontal position at full inflation. As seen on the left, the man has now exhaled his FVC within 4 seconds; the FVC was 4.25 L, which is within the normal range. Therefore, some air remains in the top of the lung, which constitutes the RV. This patient's TLC is 5.55 (4.25 FVC + 1.30), which is normal for his sex and height. That the RV is present in the top part of the lung is suggested by studies demonstrating that the upper lobes have less elastic recoil than the lower lobes do (Silvers et al, 1979).

In marked contrast are the inspiratory (left) and expiratory (right) films of a patient with advanced emphysema (Fig. 3–4). Notice the marked hyperinflation. There has been very little lung emptying between the inspiratory and expiratory maneuver. The FVC is 1.25 L, but a huge RV, 6.10 L, remains. Thus, the TLC is 1.25 plus 6.1, or 7.35 L, which is a markedly elevated TLC (140% of normal).

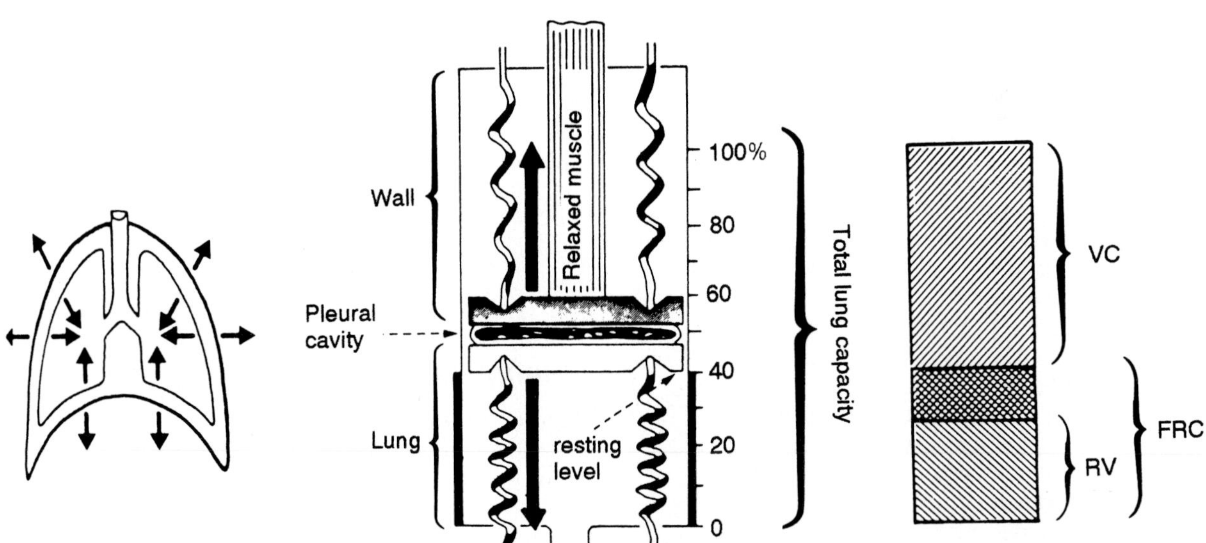

FIGURE 3–2 ■ Balanced opposing elastic forces. Note that the elastic forces of the lung and chest wall are equal but pulling in opposite directions at the resting level or functional residual capacity. (From Cherniack RM: Mechanics of breathing. Semin Respir Med 4:171, 1983).

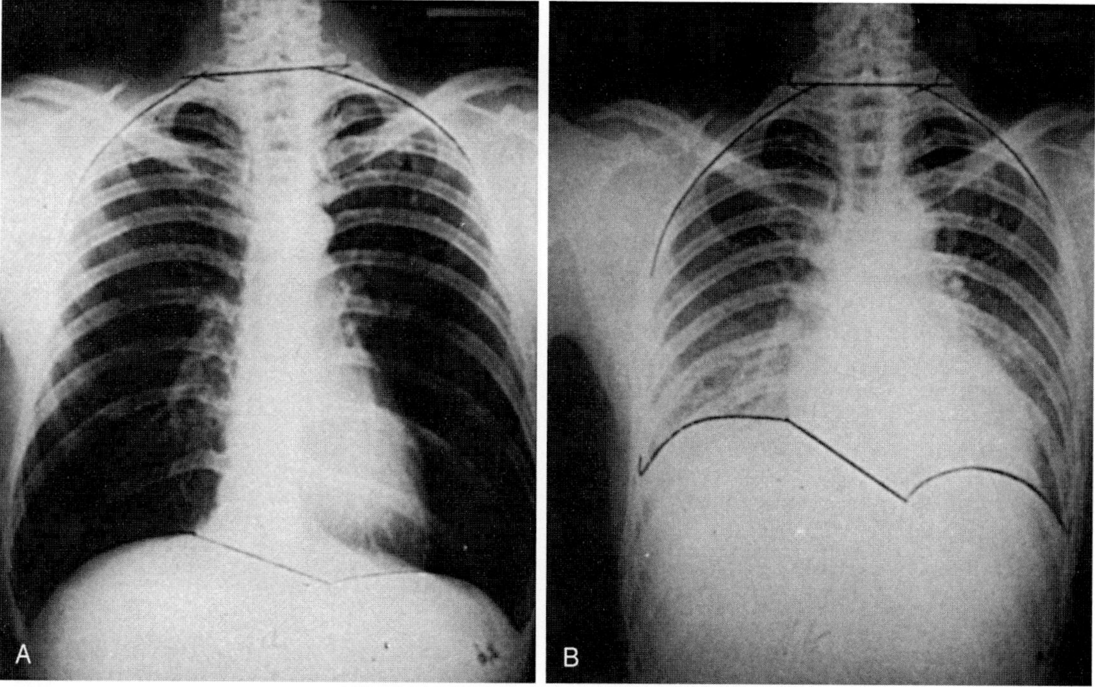

FIGURE 3–3 ■ Normal, *A*, inspiratory and, *B*, expiratory chest radiographs from a young, healthy 24-year-old male volunteer. Note that some air (i.e., the residual volume) remains at the top of the lung following a forced expiration. (From Petty TL: Office spirometry. Semin Respir Med 4:184, 1983.)

Normal expiratory time is 6 seconds or less (Lal et al, 1964). In obstructed breathing states, expiratory time is longer than 6 seconds. This can be easily observed by auscultation over the manubrium using a stopwatch or sweep second hand. A very short expiratory time (e.g., 1 to 2 seconds) strongly suggests increased elastic recoil from pulmonary fibrosis. Therefore, the timing of the expiratory maneuver, as well as the measures of volume and flow, is important and is readily visualized by simple volume over time measurements in classic spirometry. These measurements can also be calculated from flow-volume maneuvers, as illustrated in Figures 3–8 through 3–12.

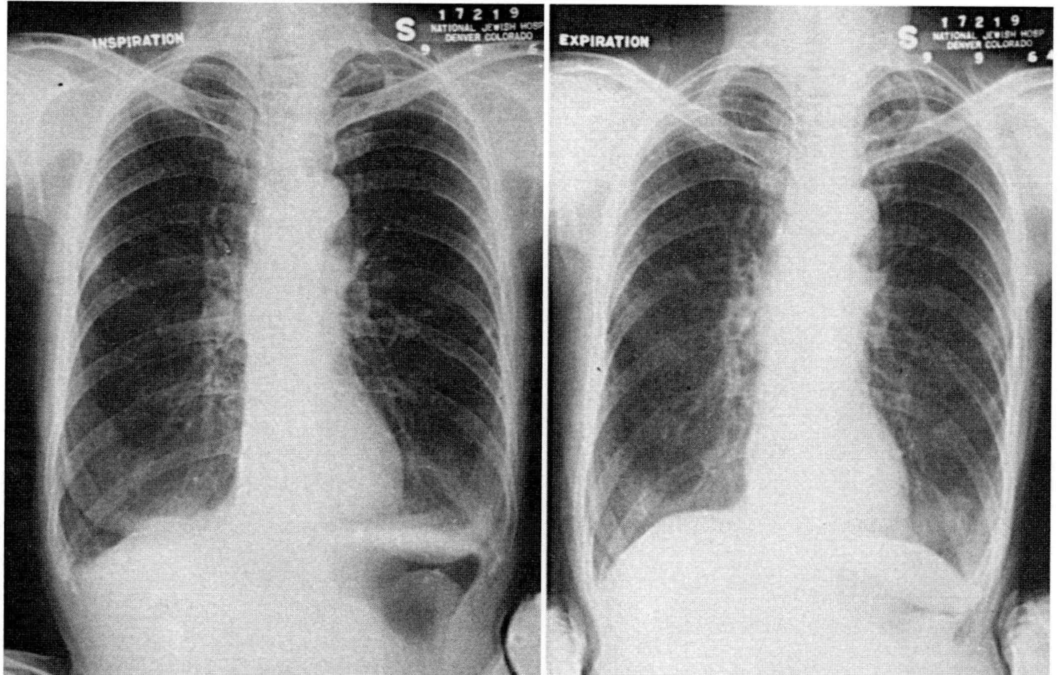

FIGURE 3–4 ■ Inspiratory-expiratory films of a patient with advanced emphysema. Notice that only a small amount of air has been exhaled; this proved to be 1.25 L. The residual volume (i.e., the air remaining in the lung) was 6.10 L. (From Petty TL: Office spirometry. Semin Respir Med 4:184, 1983.)

TESTING METHODS

Spirometry

John Hutchinson's "mysterious machine" was an inverted bell with a water seal. A reproduction of a slight modification of Hutchinson's spirometer is presented in Figure 3–5. Essentially, this same technology was used in the Collins-type instruments, which became the instruments of choice in many pulmonary function laboratories and are still used in some centers today. However, other technologies can accurately measure volume over time; flow transducers, one of which is shown in Figure 3–6, have become the most popular. Also, dry, direct-recording devices are commonly used, as shown in Figure 3–7.

Two methods of expressing the expiratory airflow curve are the volume-over-time curve, which I prefer, and the flow-volume curve, which is somewhat of a fad but also has value. The figures that follow show a comparison of flow-volume and time-volume curves in different situations.

Figure 3–8 presents both the flow-volume and time-volume expiratory airflow curves in a normal person. (The LLN is in parentheses.) Note the rapid emptying of

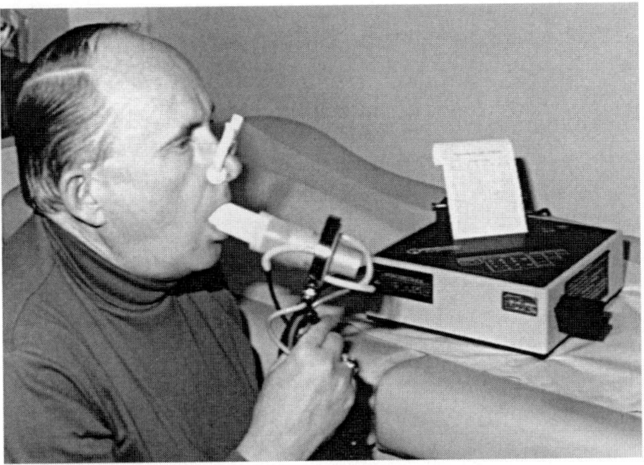

FIGURE 3–6 ■ Flow transducer device, which accurately measures either flow-volume or volume-time curves. Volume is on the vertical and time on the horizontal axis. These devices are popular and convenient. They perform the calculations and give percentages of predicted normal values.

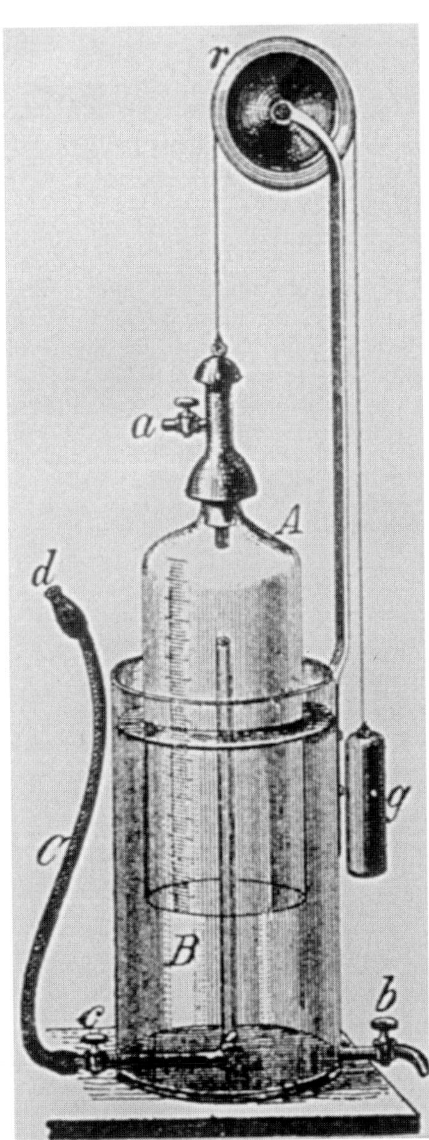

FIGURE 3–5 ■ Reproduction of a slight modification of Hutchinson's original water-sealed spirometer. This device is very similar to the Collins-type spirometers that are still in use and that were the preferred method in the past.

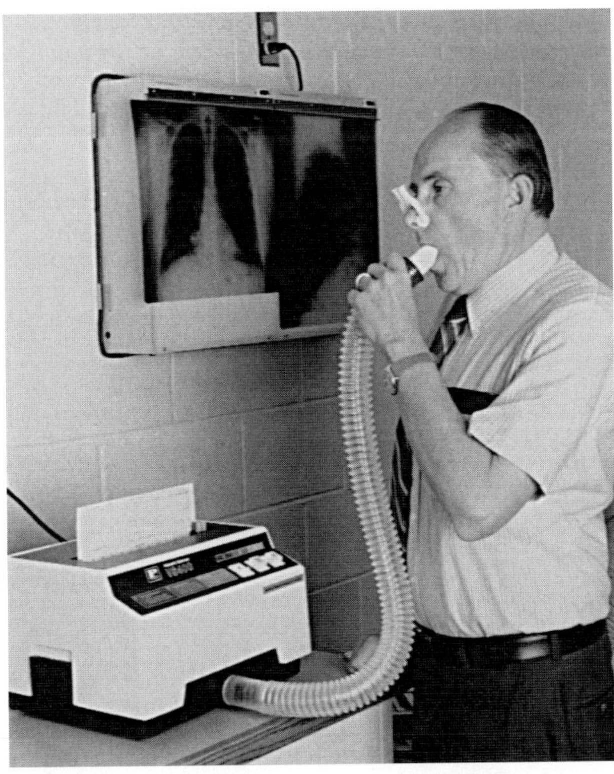

FIGURE 3–7 ■ Example of a simple, dry, direct-recording spirometer suitable for clinic or office use. Many of these spirometers are also used in modern pulmonary function laboratories because their accuracy is equal to or greater than that of more complex spirometers, such as rolling-seal devices (which are not discussed in the text).

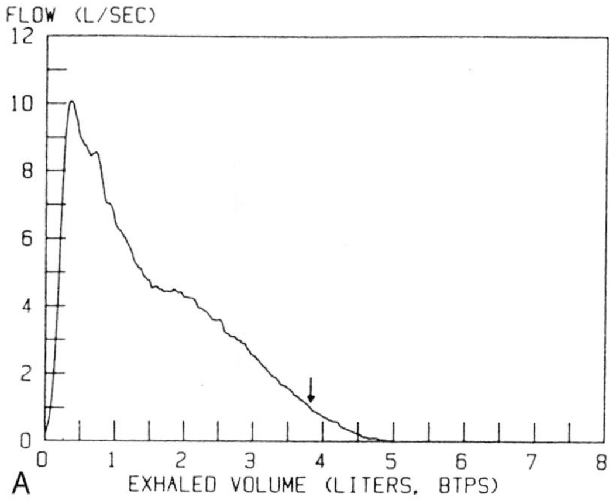

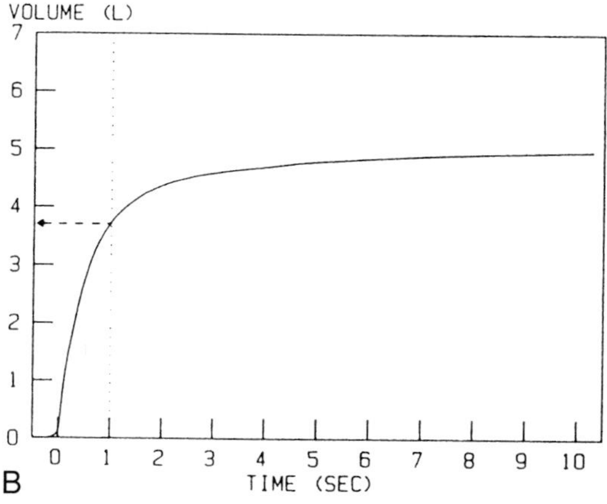

	Result	LLN
FVC	5.00	(3.88)
FEV_1	3.79	(3.12)
$\%FEV_1$	76%	(71%)

FIGURE 3–8 ■ Normal, *A*, flow-volume and, *B*, time-volume curves of a normal individual. LLN indicates lower limit of normal. Notice that the expiratory time can be visualized from the volume-time curve, but the peak flow can only be visualized from the flow-volume curve. Thus, both curves are useful. (From Enright PL, Hyatt PR: Office Spirometry—A Practical Guide to the Selection and Use of Spirometers. Lea & Febiger, Philadelphia, 1987, p. 34.)

the lung with FEV_1 3.79 L as indicated by the arrow on both curves. Figures 3–9 to 3–11 present both the flow-volume and time-volume curves of patients with progressive degrees of obstructive ventilatory disorders. Figure 3–9 shows the pattern of mild airflow obstruction and reveals a concavity of the flow-volume curve. Note that the FVC is above the lower limit of normal, but the FEV_1 (Gaensler, 1951) is below normal. This makes the FEV_1 1% less than the normal 71%. Therefore, there are actually two factors in the low FEV_1 percentage: an increased denominator (volume) and a decreased numerator (flow). Studies in whole, excised, human lungs by my associates and me (Petty et al, 1987) have shown that in the earliest stages of emphysema, TLC increases along with decreased elastic recoil. This is probably the best explanation for the increased FVC and low FEV_1/FVC ratio in the very earliest stages of emphysema.

Figure 3–10 shows the flow-volume and time-volume curves of a patient with moderate air flow obstruction, and Figure 3–11 presents the expiratory airflow curves of a patient with severe airflow obstruction. Finally, Figure 3–12 shows the expiratory flow curves of a patient with moderate airflow *restriction*. Note that, in this case, the expiratory time is shortened, but peak flow is high, owing to excessive elastic recoil from pulmonary fibrosis.

Normal Values

Normal values are based on age, sex, and height (Morris et al, 1971). Younger, taller individuals have better air volume and flow than shorter, older individuals have. Men have slightly higher values than do women. For

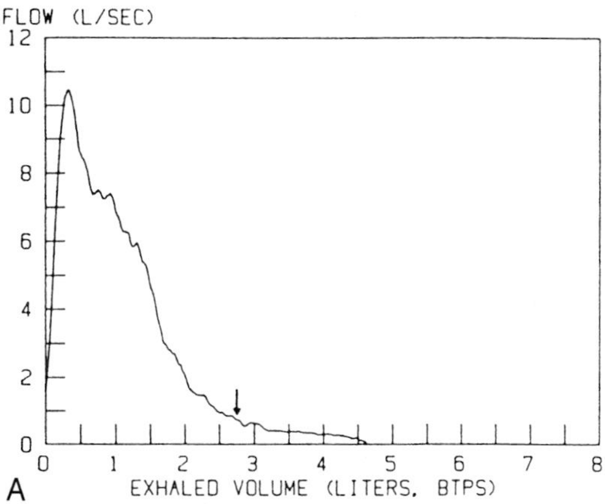

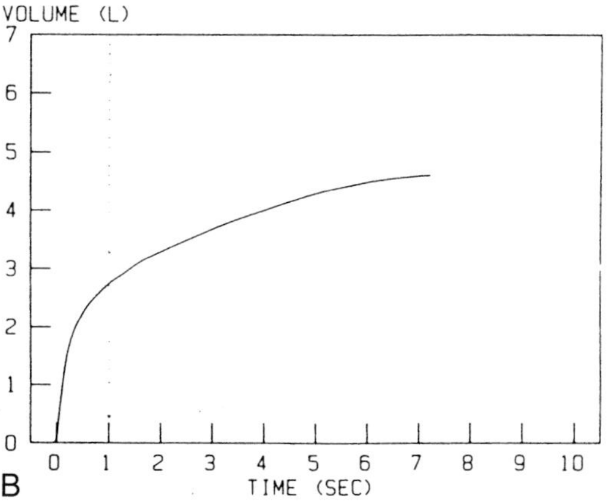

	Result	LLN
FVC	4.60	(3.88)
FEV_1	2.74	(3.12)
$\%FEV_1$	59%	(71%)

FIGURE 3–9 ■ *A*, Flow-volume and, *B*, time-volume curves in a patient with a mild obstructive airflow disorder. (LLN, lower limit of normal.) (From Enright PL, Hyatt PR: Office Spirometry—A Practical Guide to the Selection and Use of Spirometers. Lea & Febiger, Philadelphia, 1987, p. 34.)

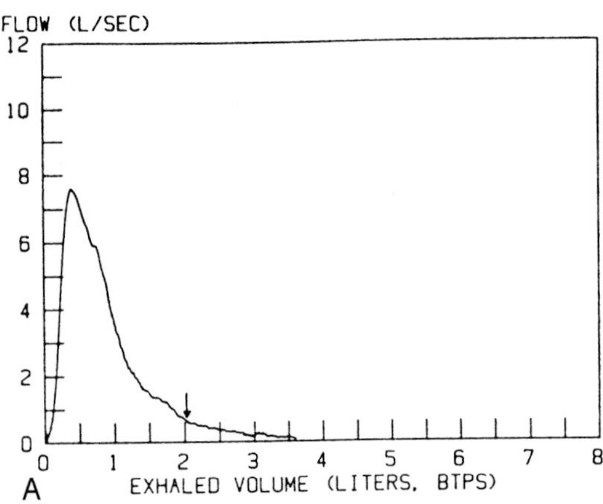

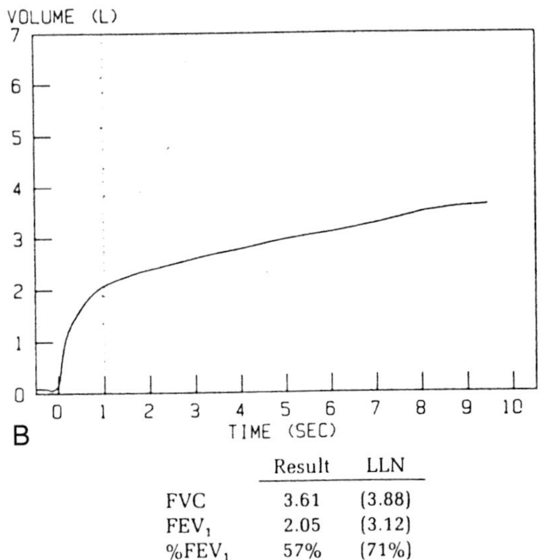

	Result	LLN
FVC	3.61	(3.88)
FEV_1	2.05	(3.12)
$\%FEV_1$	57%	(71%)

FIGURE 3–10 ■ *A*, Flow-volume and, *B*, time-volume curves of a patient with moderate airflow obstruction. (LLN, lower limit of normal.) (From Enright PL, Hyatt PR: Office Spirometry—A Practical Guide to the Selection and Use of Spirometers. Lea & Febiger, Philadelphia, 1987, p. 34.)

some reason, certain ethnic groups, such as blacks, have slightly lower normal values (but most atheletes would deny that this is true) (Rossiter and Weill, 1974).

Figure 3–13 presents normal values for FVC, FEV_1, and the ratio between the two. Using a straightedge to connect age and height helps to determine normal values. A range of 20% is commonly considered normal.

Listed in the box on Ventilatory Disorders are the common disease states that are characterized by obstructive ventilatory defects, airflow disorders in less common disease states, and the common restrictive ventilatory disorders.

Alternatives to Spirometry

There really is no alternative to simple spirometry, but other methods can give insight into abnormalities of airflow and volume. Thus, the experienced clinician can easily estimate ventilatory function. The importance of the expiratory time has already been cited. Additionally, use of a simple peak flowmeter gives a snapshot of flow. Peak flow does not measure the FEV_1, but it tracks FEV_1 accurately in a given individual. Normal values for peak flow have been established (Leiner et al, 1963). Figure 3–14 shows a patient performing the peak flow maneuver.

An important recent development is the advent of simple handheld spirometers that have been produced by industry in response to a new national health care initiative known as the National Lung Health Education Program (NLHEP). The NLHEP aims to identify people who have asymptomatic degrees of airflow obstruction or even undiagnosed restrictive lung diseases by placing spirometers in the hands of all primary care practitioners. This device is illustrated in Figure 3–15. It is really a highly sophisticated device that uses a flow transducer to integrate flow. It has easy input steps for age, sex, height, race, smoking history, and the ambient altitude of testing. The device requires precision within 3%. Additionally, it coaches for better effort, more complete exhalation, and so on. Therefore, it is unlikely that such a spirometer will give falsely low values, because it is virtually impossible to have poor or incomplete efforts within 3% of each other. This spirometer is capable of storing 300 tests. It is used with a stand or docking station, which can con-

VENTILATORY DISORDERS

Common Obstructive Ventilatory Disorders

Asthma
Asthmatic bronchitis
Chronic obstructive bronchitis
Chronic obstructive pulmonary disease*
Cystic fibrosis
Emphysema

Uncommon Obstructive Ventilatory Disorders

Bronchiolitis obliterans (may also show a mild restrictive defect)
Eosinophilic granuloma
Lymphangiomyomatosis
Sarcoidosis (may show a restrictive defect in advanced fibrotic status)

Common Restrictive Ventilatory Disorders

Idiopathic fibrosing alveolitis
Interstitial pneumonitis and fibrosis associated with drug reactions (e.g., to bleomycin) or occupational exposures (e.g., asbestosis)
Fibrotic residue of disseminated granulomas (e.g., tuberculosis, histoplasmosis)
Sarcoidosis
Thoracic deformities
Congestive heart failure

*This is a generic term that combines asthmatic bronchitis, chronic bronchitis, bronchitis, and emphysema. These states commonly overlap.

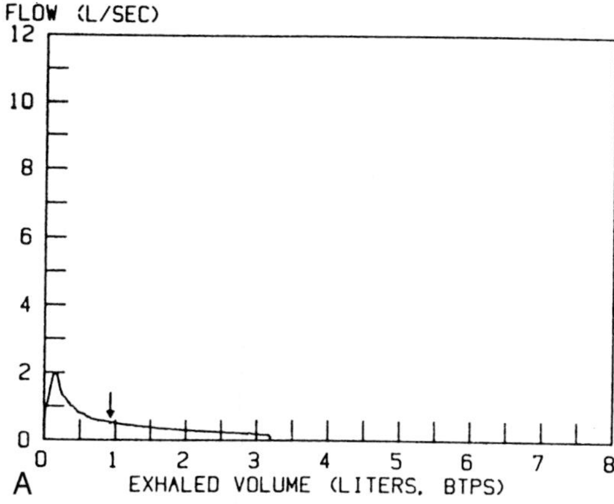

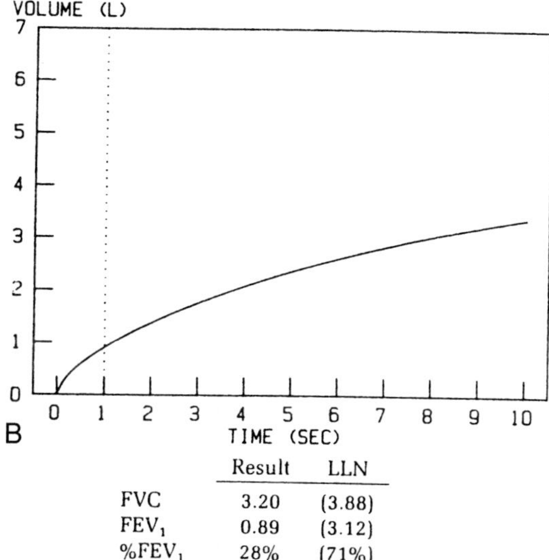

	Result	LLN
FVC	3.20	(3.88)
FEV_1	0.89	(3.12)
$\%FEV_1$	28%	(71%)

FIGURE 3–11 ■ *A,* Flow-volume and *B,* time-volume curves from a patient with advanced airflow obstruction from emphysema. (LLN, lower limit of normal.) From Enright PL, Hyatt PR: Office Spirometry—A Practical Guide to the Selection and Use of Spirometers. Lea & Febiger, Philadelphia, 1987, p. 42.)

nect to a parallel printer. Both volume time and flow volume curves are easily printed for a hard copy in filing. Many other devices are soon to reach the market. Their cost will be $500 or less. They give only two important parameters: FVC, FEV_1, the ratio between the two, and an interpretation of normal in various degrees of obstructive and restrictive ventilatory disorders. It is agreed that such devices will revolutionize the use of spirometry and put it in the hands of all frontline practitioners, as well as specialists.

Other Pulmonary Function Tests

Measurements or estimates of lung volumes are briefly described earlier. These can be accurately estimated from chest radiographs. They can also be measured accurately by the application of Boyle's law through the use of a "body box" (a volume body plethysmograph) (Mead, 1960) or by use of inert gases such as helium or nitrogen (Gilson and Hugh-Jones, 1949) to estimate the FRC, from which the RV can be derived following a forced expiration. The difference between FRC and RV is called the *expiratory reserve volume.* It is only measured to define the RV. TLC can be fairly accurately estimated from full inspiration posteroanterior and lateral chest radiographs. Subtracting the measured FVC from this estimate of TLC gives a fairly accurate estimate of the RV.

Gas Transfer Tests

There are basically two gas transfer tests. One, the diffusion test, measures the simple uptake of carbon monoxide. It measures the integrity of the air-blood interface (Ogilvie et al, 1957). In emphysema, the diffusion test measurement is reduced owing to loss of alveolar walls.

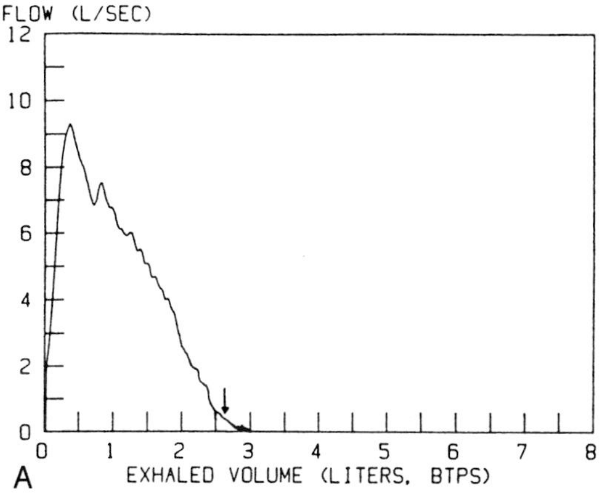

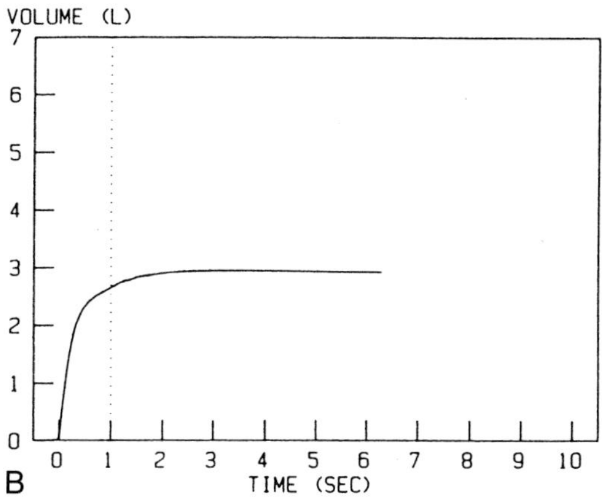

	Result	LLN
FVC	2.97	(3.88)
FEV_1	2.64	(3.12)
$\%FEV_1$	89%	(71%)

FIGURE 3–12 ■ *A,* Flow-volume and, *B,* time-volume curves of a patient with a moderate restrictive ventilatory disorder. Notice that FEV_1 is nearly 90% of FVC; a restrictive disorder is often suggested when this ratio is high. However, normal individuals can often empty most of the lung in 1 second. (LLN, lower limit of normal.) (From Enright PL, Hyatt PR: Office Spirometry—A Practical Guide to the Selection and Use of Spirometers. Lea & Febiger, Philadelphia, 1987, p. 38).

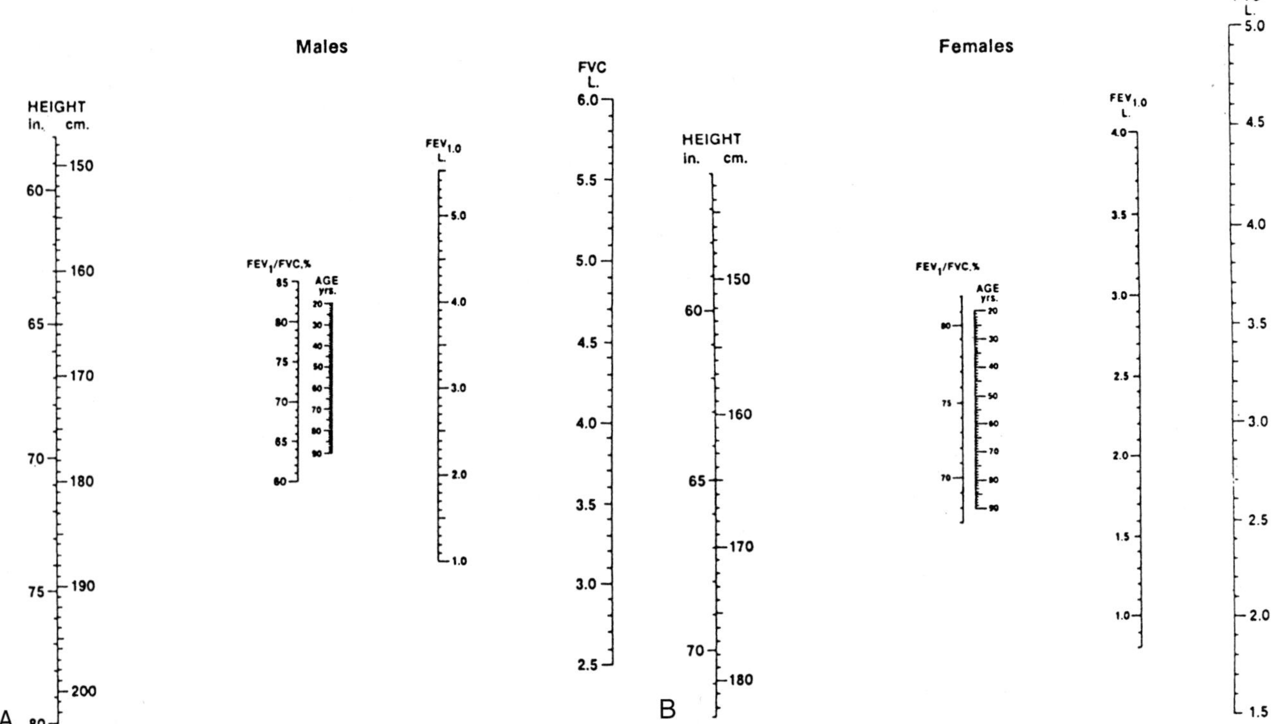

FIGURE 3–13 ■ Nomogram to identify normal spirometry values for, *A*, men and, *B*, women. Place a straight edge to connect age and height to determine normal value. (Adapted from Morris JF, Koski A, Johnson LC: Spirometric standards for healthy nonsmoking adults. Am Rev Respir Dis 103:57, 1971.)

In fibrotic states, it is reduced by a barrier to gas transfer across the air-blood interface. Arterial blood gas determinations can also be used as indicators of gas transfer. The oxygen tension and carbon dioxide tension are also affected by ventilation.

Discussion of the role of arterial blood gases is beyond the scope of this chapter. Basically, oxygen tension, CO_2 tension, and the pH of arterial blood (pHa) are measured. Oxygen saturation is a function of pHa and oxygen tension. Factors that cause hypoxemia are listed below. A useful way of expressing Po_2 as a fraction of alveolar ventilation with shunt factors is presented in the following equation:

$$Po_2 \; \alpha \; (\text{alveolar ventilation/shunt factors})$$

Ventilation-Perfusion Scanning

Fairly accurate estimates of the contribution of each lung or lung region to global lung functions can be made from ventilation-perfusion lung scans. Details of the role of this increasingly popular form of lung imaging are beyond the scope of this chapter, except as commented on below.

> CAUSES OF HYPOXEMIA
>
> Altitude
> Hypoventilation
> Shunt factors
> - Ventilation/perfusion defect
> - Diffusion defect
> - Anatomic shunt

CLINICAL APPLICATIONS OF PULMONARY FUNCTION TESTING

Physicians and surgeons primarily use pulmonary function testing for diagnostic purposes and to guide responses to therapy, such as improvements in airflow or volume with bronchodilators and, when indicated, with the use of corticosteroid drugs. Both internists and surgeons can be guided in estimates of preoperative and postoperative risk by pulmonary function measurements. Many authors have published guidelines regarding the value of pulmonary function measurements to estimate the risk of postoperative complications, but, of course, no single estimate is absolute (Harmon and Lillington, 1979; Stein and Cassara, 1970; Stein et al, 1962; Tisi, 1984). Identification of respiratory insufficiency before surgery can help to reduce postoperative complications by instituting smoking cessation and using bronchoactive drugs (e.g., bronchodilators or corticosteroids) if indicated (Harmon and Lillington, 1979; Stein and Cassara, 1970; Stein et al, 1962; Tisi, 1984).

I firmly believe that any emergency surgery can be performed with relative safety despite severe degrees of respiratory impairment. However, it is important to know the degree of ventilatory impairment to predict the need for postoperative mechanical ventilation and the diffi-

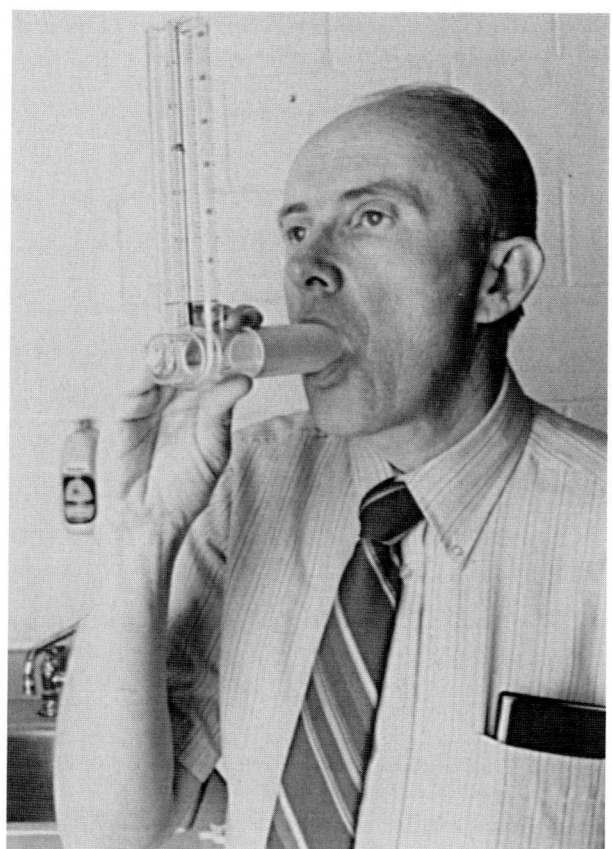

FIGURE 3–14 ■ Popular peak flowmeter, which measures a snap-shot of expiratory airflow. A peak flowmeter does not measure FEV_1 but tracks it in the individual. Conversion formulas exist.

culties in weaning from mechanical ventilation. Nothing is more frustrating than to be consulted for a ventilator-dependent patient in the postoperative period when there are no measurements of pulmonary function prior to major thoracic surgery, including heart transplantation. Often every organ system of the body except the lungs has been measured prior to surgery. One study demonstrated that patients with respiratory impairment in the preoperative period had more postoperative complications and required longer stays in the intensive care unit than did patients with normal pulmonary function. Patients who require valve replacement have a much higher risk of pulmonary complications than do patients who undergo other cardiac procedures (Bevelaqua et al, 1990).

Pulmonary function measurements can also be used as crude but useful indicators of the functional success of resectional surgery for lung cancer and for benign lung disease. The amount of lung to be sacrificed is based on knowledge of the contribution of each of the five lobes. Normally, the right lung accounts for 55% of total lung function, and the left lung accounts for 45%. The right middle lobe and its counterpart, the lingula, on the left, can easily be resected with essentially no compromise in lung function. The large upper and lower lobes simply expand to fill the space previously occupied by these small lobes. Even an upper or lower lobectomy can be tolerated with fairly good postoperative pulmonary function if the remaining lobe or lobes can be expected to expand (i.e., in the absence of fibrosis, bronchial obstruction, and so on). Table 3–1 gives a crude estimate of the lower limits of lung function required with various degrees of lung resection. Of course, however, if a nonfunctional lung is resected, as in cancer, these calculations would be modified. In some cases, thoracic surgery results in actual restoration of lung function, such as with draining of an empyema or decortication. A prospective study showed that fairly accurate estimates of postoperative lung function following resectional surgery can be obtained by estimating the relative contribution of each lung to overall lung function prior to pneumonectomy (Olsen et al, 1974).

LUNG VOLUME REDUCTION SURGERY

The reawakening of interest in the surgical procedure to reduce the lung volume by resecting portions of the lung with predominant emphysema, usually in the upper portion of the lung, will create increased interest in pulmonary function testing for physicians and surgeons in patients with advanced stages of disease. Of course, the purpose of lung volume reduction surgery is to improve ventilatory function by reducing the RV and air trapping through improvement in elastic recoil, which in turn improves airway conductance. The ideal candidate for lung volume reduction surgery is yet to be determined and is the subject of a 17-center trial, known as the National Emphysema Therapy Trial (NETT). It is likely that patients with large lung volume and high RV, but little evidence of intrinsic airways disease (as judged by complex tests of lung function, not covered in this chapter, known as tests of airways resistance), will be ideal candidates. The patient should be free of serious comorbidities such as ischemic heart disease or major organ system insufficiencies. Computed tomography (CT) scans are necessary to assess the regional distribution of emphysema in such patients.

OTHER GLOBAL TESTS OF LUNG FUNCTION

For many years, experienced physicians and surgeons have asked patients about their ability to walk up a few

TABLE 3–1 ■ **Lower Limits of Lung Function Required for Various Degrees of Lung Resection***

	Function Before Surgery	
Degree of Resection	*FEV_1 (L)*	*FVC (L)*
Middle or lingular lobectomy	1.3	2.0
Upper or lower lobectomy	1.5	2.2
Left-sided pneumonectomy	1.8	2.8
Right-sided pneumonectomy	2.0	3.0

*For potential cure of cancer in 6-ft, 55-year-old man.
FEV_1, forced expiratory volume in 1 second; FVC, forced vital capacity.

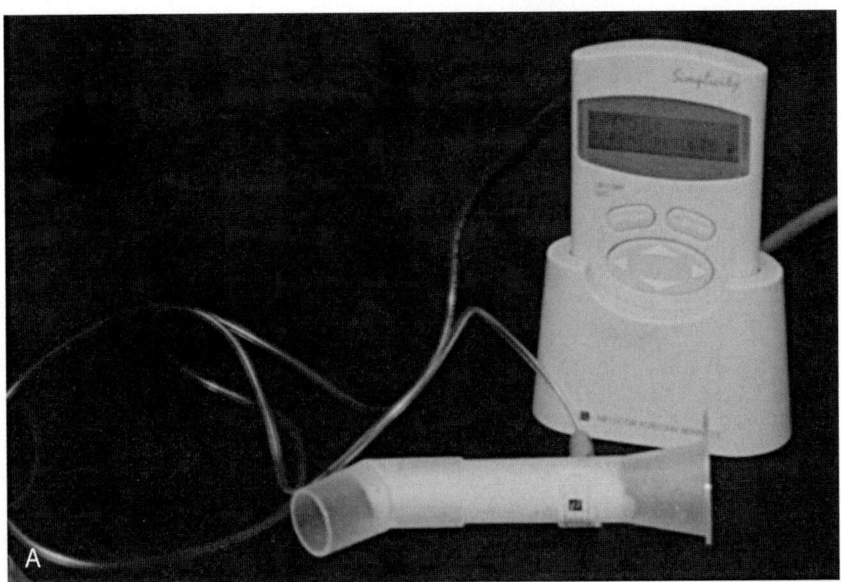

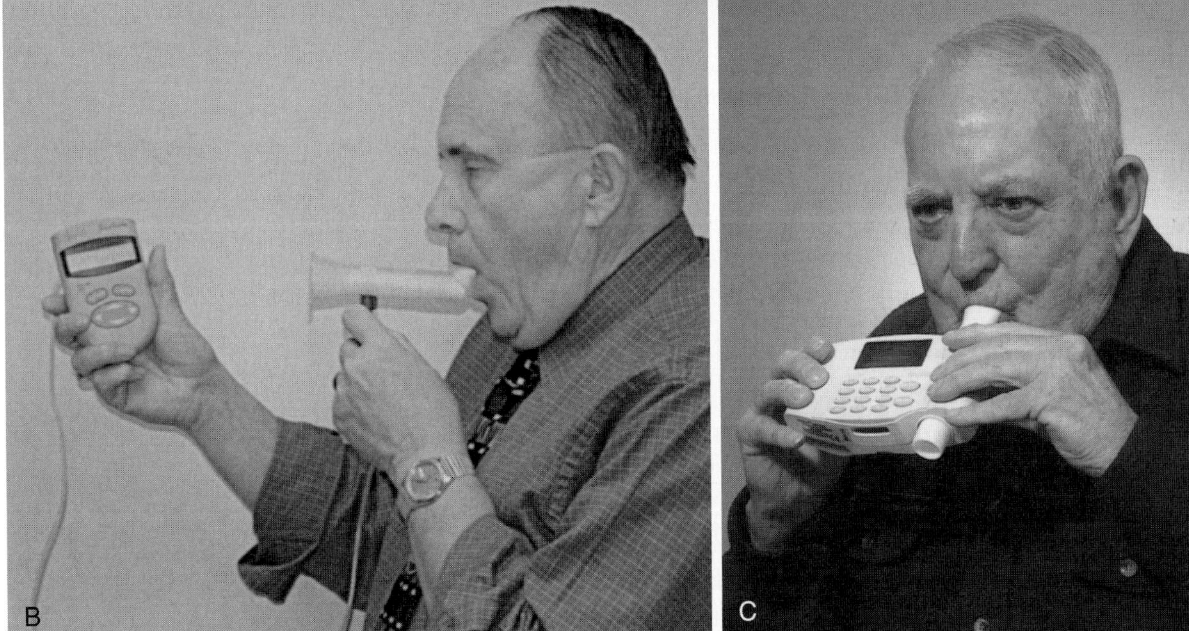

FIGURE 3–15 ■ *A*, A microprocessor spirometer in its stand, with its portable flow transducer. *B*, A technician doing a forced expiratory spirogram, after imputing his age, height, sex, smoking status, race, and the altitude at which the test was performed. This device requires repeatability of FEV_1 and FEV_6 within 200 mL, or 3%, in order to print out results. Thus, it is highly unlikely that it will give falsely low values. *C*, A hand-held device for measuring FEV_1, FVC, and the ratio between the two.

flights of stairs. Many astute clinicians have actually taken corridor and stairwell walks with their patients while assessing respiratory rate, dyspnea, and use of respiratory muscles and feeling the pulse to note tachycardia. The anguished, tachycardic, diaphoretic individual who cannot walkup a half flight of stairs is a poor candidate for any form of surgery!

COMMENTS AND CONTROVERSIES

In this chapter a practical approach to pulmonary function testing is presented and the importance of simple spirometry is emphasized. Dry, direct-recording devices measuring volume (FVC or FEV_6) and flow (FEV_1) are widely used. Only two values, namely the FEV_1 and FVC, and the ratio between the two, are required. New simple handheld spirometers are of great practical value for bedside, clinic, or home measurements of FVC and FEV_1. Lung volume and diffusion tests do not often result in clinical decision-making; these tests are primarily useful in categorizing disease states and for research purposes. As in all medicine and surgery, the values obtained by pulmonary function measurements must be put in the context of the patient, the patient's disease, the dynamics of the disease state, its trends, and the likelihood of improvement with surgical or medical intervention.

■ KEY REFERENCES

Bevelaqua F, Garritan S, Haas F et al: Complications after cardiac operations in patients with severe pulmonary impairment. Ann Thorac Surg 50:602, 1990.

Although patients with severe lung impairment, as identified by abnormal pulmonary function, generally do well after cardiac operations, they have more postoperative pulmonary complications than do patients with no impairment. Patients with restrictive ventilatory disorders have better outcomes than do those with obstructive diseases. Preoperative pulmonary function tests (e.g., spirometry) can alert the surgeon to the possible risk of postoperative complications, but alone these tests do not exclude patients from necessary surgery. Patients with severe pulmonary impairment should be considered for preoperative bronchodilator therapy to maximize pulmonary function prior to surgery. Although the history of pulmonary symptoms is important, it cannot replace spirometry to identify individuals at increased risk of cardiac surgery in the face of chronic obstructive pulmonary disease.

Cooper JD, Trulock EP, Trianta-Fillou AN et al: Bilateral pneumonectomy (volume reduction) for chronic obstructive pulmonary disease. J Thorac Cardiovasc Surg 109:106–116, 1995.

A description of the modified surgical technique to improve the lung's elastic recoil and improve lung function by the resection of regions of emphysematous destruction.

Harmon E, Lillington G: Pulmonary risk factors in surgery. Med Clin North Am 63:1289, 1979.

Pulmonary complications following surgery are common and range from 6% to 60%. The most common complications are atelectasis, pneumonia, pulmonary embolism, and respiratory insufficiency in the immediate postoperative period. Although all patients undergoing general anesthesia and surgery are at risk, those subjected to thoracic and upper abdominal surgery have the greatest chance of developing pulmonary complications.

Postoperative mortality from major surgery in patients over 60 years of age ranged from 10% to 33%, with most deaths owing to respiratory and cardiac causes. Careful fluid management and early mobilization will help mitigate pulmonary complications.

The prediction of surgical risk in thoracic surgery is based on simple spirometric measurements. For example, the mortality following resection for bronchiogenic carcinoma is related to preoperative FEV_1 and age; 40% of patients who had an FEV_1 of less than 2 L and who were older than 60 years of age developed problems.

Kannel WB, Lew EA, Hubert HB et al: The value of measuring vital capacity for prognostic purposes. Trans Am Life Insurance Med Directors Am 64:66, 1980.

A simple test (i.e., the measurement of forced vital capacity) was the best predictor of mortality, including deaths from all causes in this Framingham study. Accordingly, as John Hutchinson, a surgeon, stated, "the vital capacity" is clearly the capacity to live.

Lal S, Ferguson AD, Campbell EJM: Forced expiratory time. A simple test for airways obstruction. BMJ 1:814, 1964.

A simple measurement of expiratory time will help identify patients with airflow obstruction. Normal expiratory time is 6 seconds or less. If the total measured expiratory time is measured with a stopwatch or a sweep second hand while listening to a forced expiration over the manubrium, and this time is significantly longer than 6 seconds, the patient likely has one of the diseases characterized by airflow obstruction.

Morris JF, Koski A, Johnson LC: Spirometric standards for healthy nonsmoking adults. Am Rev Respir Dis 103:57, 1971.

These are important spirometric standards for nonsmoking healthy adults. Normal spirometric values are a function of age, sex, and height. Younger, taller men have higher FVC and FEV_1 than their older, shorter, female counterparts.

Rogers RM, Sciurba FC, Keenan RJ: Lung reduction surgery in chronic obstructive lung disease. Med Clin North Am 80:623–644, 1996.

A state-of-the-art review of the purpose, physiology, and indications for lung volume reduction surgery.

Stein M, Cassara EL: Preoperative pulmonary evaluation and therapy for surgical patients. JAMA 211:787, 1970.

Simple pulmonary function tests using spirometry can help predict patients at poor risk. When patients were treated preoperatively and postoperatively with cessation of smoking, bronchodilator drugs, and inhaled bronchodilators, along with chest physical therapy techniques, a marked reduction in postoperative morbidity and mortality owing to pulmonary complications, was observed. Identifying patients at risk, as strongly indicated by abnormal spirometric tests, and using aggressive therapy should reduce postoperative morbidity and mortality and allow discharge following a shorter hospital stay than would be adequate without this identification or intervention.

■ REFERENCES

Enright PL, Hyatt PR: Office Spirometry: A Practical Guide to the Selection and Use of Spirometers. Philadelphia, Lea & Febiger, 1987.

Gaensler EA: Analysis of the ventilatory defect by timed vital capacity. Am Rev Respir Dis 69:256, 1951.

Gilson JC, Hugh-Jones P: The measurement of total lung volume and breathing capacity. Clin Sci 7:185, 1949.

Hutchison J: On the capacity of the lungs and on the respiratory function with a view of establishing a precise and early method of detecting disease by the spirometer. Med Chir Trans (Lond) 24:137, 1846.

Leiner GC, Abramowitz S, Small MJ et al: Expiratory peak flow rate. Standard values for normal subjects. Use as a clinical test of ventilatory function. Am Rev Respir Dis 88:644, 1963.

Mead J: Volume displacement body plethysmograph for respiratory measurements in human subjects. J Appl Physiol 15:736, 1960.

Ogilvie CM, Forster RE, Blakemore WS et al.: A standardized breath holding technique for the clinical measurement of the diffusing capacity of the lung for carbon monoxide. J Clin Invest 36:1, 1957.

Olsen GN, Block AJ, Tobias JA: Prediction of postpneumonectomy pulmonary function using quantitative macroaggregate lung scanning. Chest 66:13, 1974.

Petty TL, Silvers GW, Stanford RE: Mild emphysema is associated with reduced elastic recoil and increased lung size but not with airflow limitation. Am Rev Respir Dis 136:867, 1987.

Rossiter CE, Weill H: Ethnic differences in lung function: Evidence for proportional differences. Int J Epidemiol 3:55, 1974.

Silvers GW, Petty TL, Stanford RE et al: The elastic properties of lobes of excised human lungs. Am Rev Respir Dis 120:207, 1979.

Stein M, Koota GM, Simon M: Pulmonary evaluation of surgical patients. JAMA 181:765, 1962.

Tisi GM: Evaluating pulmonary function before surgery. J Respir Dis 5:103, 1984.

CHAPTER 4

Preoperative Assessment of the Thoracic Surgical Patient: A Surgeon's Viewpoint

Robert J. Ginsberg

The surgeon is trained to treat patients using invasive modalities. Despite the technical skills acquired, the surgeon is first and foremost a physician and must make use of the deductive skills acquired, not only to determine whether or not a therapeutic intervention is indicated or necessary but also to assess the suitability of the patient to undergo the surgical procedure. This initial assessment must not be delegated to other individuals.

In thoracic surgery, over two thirds of postoperative complications are cardiopulmonary (Deslauriers et al, 1989). In most cases cardiac complications tend to be minor (treatable arrhythmias), whereas pulmonary complications are more morbid and account for most deaths, usually due to respiratory failure.

In the field of general thoracic surgery, more often than not, transthoracic or upper abdominal approaches are used. Because they inhibit postoperative respiratory mechanics, these interventions are associated with high postoperative cardiopulmonary morbidity rates. In most thoracic surgical practices, the predominant illness treated is related to cancer. Our patients most frequently present between the sixth and eighth decades, each decade increasing the risk of postoperative morbidity and mortality (Deslauriers et al, 1989; Ginsberg et al, 1983). Associated cardiopulmonary disease is prevalent in this population.

The necessity for a compulsive attitude toward preoperative evaluation cannot be emphasized enough. Technical misadventures do occur but, with well-trained surgeons, rarely account for the problems seen following thoracic surgical procedures. The majority of postoperative complications and deaths are related to cardiopulmonary events, most of which can be identified and prevented before surgery. Additionally, in pulmonary surgery, the surgeon must ensure that the anticipated resection will allow the patient a reasonable quality of life without chronic respiratory failure.

INITIAL PATIENT ENCOUNTER

The initial patient encounter is by far the most important step in preoperative assessment. Major predictors of postoperative complications include extent of resection, significant cardiopulmonary disease, age, and other comorbid conditions (e.g., diabetes, other systemic illnesses, immune-depressive diseases, drug addiction, obesity, recent weight loss) (Kohlman et al, 1986; Wahi et al, 1989). All these factors must be assessed. The Dripps-American Society of Anesthesiologists classification (Table 4–1) subdivides individuals into five risk categories, which have been correlated with both the morbidity and mortality of operative procedures.

The skills acquired in history-taking, physical examination, and judicious use of laboratory investigation must be honed to perfection. It is a truism that over 75% of the first encounter with the patient should be devoted to accurate history-taking. This initial step not only confirms the diagnosis and determines the indications and the necessity of the potential surgical intervention but also determines the suitability of the patient to undergo such a procedure, the extent of comorbid disease, and the need for further testing. Accurate history-taking can predict 95% of all diagnoses and can predict and, hopefully, thereby prevent most potential postoperative problems. A complete physical examination should never be ignored or delegated to a nonphysician. Use of these tools so painstakingly developed during the medical school apprenticeship in every patient encounter will serve the physician-surgeon well; failure to use them will lead to misdiagnoses, inappropriate treatment, and preventable disasters.

All premorbid conditions must be identified and optimized prior to surgical treatment. Although multivariant analyses have not consistently demonstrated the same adverse prognostic factors, those that seem to be most significant other than intrinsic cardiopulmonary disease

TABLE 4–1 ■ **Dripps–American Society of Anesthesiologists Risk Classification and Associated Estimated Mortality of General Anesthesia**

Class	*Description*	*% Mortality*
1	Normal, healthy	0.08
2	Mild to moderate systemic disease	0.27
3	Severe systemic disease, limited activity	1.8
4	Incapacitating, life-threatening systemic disease	7.8
5	Moribund, 24-hour life expectancy without surgery	9.4

PREOPERATIVE EXERCISE PROGRAM*

This program includes strengthening and flexibility exercises to improve muscle conditioning before surgery.

Arm exercises improve strength and flexibility.

1. Sitting or standing position
2. Place arms out at shoulder level; arms are straight, parallel to floor
3. On breathing in: raise arms above head, touching both palms above head, hold for 2 seconds
4. On breathing out: lower arms slowly, exhale through pursed lips; stop when arms are parallel to floor

Leg exercises improve strength.

1. Sitting position
2. Lift leg off chair, tightening muscles on top of thigh, then extend leg straight, hold for 3 seconds
3. Bend knee and lower slowly, relax then repeat

Repeat 10 times; perform 10 times daily.
Sniff and blow—improve strength of diaphragm

1. Sitting position
2. Sniff twice; hold breath for 2 to 3 seconds
3. Tighten stomach muscles and blow out slowly

Repeat 10 times; perform 10 times daily
Walk 1 mile twice daily, in less than 20 minutes
Climb 2 flights of stairs, quickly, four times daily
Use incentive spirometer for 10 minutes, four times daily
Mobilization—improve mobility and flexibility

1. Sitting position
2. Breathe in, raise arms above head, crossing wrists
3. Breathe out, pursed-lip breathing
   Bend forward touching chest to top of thigh (if possible)
   Lower arms to floor (try to touch fingers to floor)
4. Uncross arms
   Breathe in
   Raise upper body upright
   Stretch arms above head

Cough technique

1. Sitting position
2. Breathe in deeply five times, then
3. Hold breath for 2 seconds
4. Contract abdominal muscles (bearing down)
5. Cough, while maintaining contraction of abdominal muscles
6. Practice this four times daily

*Developed by the MSKCC Thoracic Surgical Service in association with D. Wilson, R.N., R.T. and L. Wall, R.N. and given to patients at their initial encounter.

include recent smoking, recent weight loss greater than 10%, age over 70 years, obesity, and, in cancer surgery, the type and stage of the tumor.

Other factors that may predict a poor outcome from surgical intervention are difficult to classify. It has been my distinct impression that the patient's attitude toward the disease, the desire to have a favorable outcome, and confidence in the doctor are predictive of success. A prospective analysis of quality of life following lung cancer treatment, performed by the Lung Cancer Study Group (Ruckdeschel et al, 1991), confirmed that the patient's attitude toward the disease was the best predictor of long-term survival. Except in emergency life-threatening situations, patients should never be cajoled or forced into accepting surgery. In most cases, this will lead to disastrous results. At times it is best to deny surgical intervention to the patient with a significant negative outlook, especially if other curative options (e.g., radiotherapy for cancer, medical therapy in reflux disease) are available.

PULMONARY ASSESSMENT

Pulmonary complications, especially retained secretions, atelectasis, pneumonia, and respiratory failure, are the most significant problems following thoracic surgical procedures (Deslauriers et al, 1989; Ginsberg et al, 1983). Most patients who are present or former smokers have underlying pulmonary problems, especially chronic obstructive lung disease (COPD) and chronic bronchitis, and most have at least some compromise of pulmonary function.

History

Cardiopulmonary Reserve

A reasonable assessment of cardiopulmonary reserve can be determined by history-taking alone. The dyspnea grade correlates well with pulmonary function testing.

Smoking

A smoking history is relevant. Patients who continue to smoke have a significantly increased risk of postoperative complications, and, whenever possible, surgery should be delayed until smoking has been stopped for a minimum of 1 to 2 weeks, although studies suggest no real benefit until 8 weeks after smoking cessation. The use of the transdermal nicotine patch and newer oral psychotropic agents has made preoperative smoking cessation an achievable goal.

Sputum Production

Daily sputum production, whenever present, should be quantified, and, whenever possible, steps should be taken to decrease this production to minimal levels (cessation of smoking, antibiotics, postural drainage when indicated). If sputum production is present, preoperative sputum cultures may identify a chronic infection owing to a specific organism, which should be treated prior to surgical intervention.

Ability to Cough

The evaluation of the ability of patients to cough by using diaphragmatic and accessory respiratory muscles is an important but often ignored preoperative assessment of real value. Many patients do not know how to produce an effective cough; however, this can be taught preoperatively, so that a more effective cough will be present in the postoperative period. I have found that this type of instruction, together with the use of incentive spirometry, improves postoperative pulmonary toilet.

TABLE 4–2 ■ **Criteria of Pulmonary Function for Lung Resection**

PFT	*Normal*	*Pneumonectomy*	*Lobectomy*	*Wedge or Segment Resection*	*Inoperable*
MVV	>80%	>55%	>40%	>35%	<35%
FEV_1	>2 L	>2 L	>1 L	>0.6 L	<0.6 L
FEV_{25-75}	>2 L	>1.6 L	>0.6 L	>0.6 L	<0.6 L
Stair climbing	>2 flights	2 flights	1 flight	<1 flight	

FEV_1, forced expiratory volume in 1 second; FEV_{25-75}, forced expiratory flow rate from 25% to 75%; MVV, maximal voluntary ventilation (% predicted); PFT, pulmonary function tests. None of these can be considered to be absolute (please see text).
Adapted from Miller JI: Thallium imaging in preoperative evaluation of the pulmonary resection candidate. Ann Thorac Surg 54:249, 1992.

Pulmonary Function Testing

Mountains of literature are available on the value of preoperative pulmonary function testing. The tests range from the simplest medical assessment (e.g., history-taking, physical examination, stairclimbing, and the "match" test) to the most sophisticated exercise testing with calculation of maximal oxygen uptake (Vo_2max) and invasive pulmonary artery pressure (PAP) measurements. All such testing has value (Tables 4–2 and 4–3). It has been well demonstrated that stairclimbing of a fixed height, especially when combined with pulse oximetry, is probably the only cardiopulmonary test required in most patients who otherwise have normal function (Bolton et al, 1987; Ninan, 1997; Olsen et al, 1991; Rao, 1995). However, for various reasons, including medicolegal, preoperative spirometry, estimation of carbon monoxide diffusing capacity (DLCO), and determination of arterial blood gases should be carried out on all patients undergoing thoracic surgical procedures. These relatively simple tests are all that are necessary in most individuals. Abnormalities of these tests, as outlined in Table 4–3, indicate a higher risk of developing postoperative complications. When resection of pulmonary tissue is anticipated, additional pulmonary testing may be of value, including ventilation/perfusion scanning to predict postresection pulmonary capacity, such as predicted postoperative FEV_1 (ppo FEV_1) (Ali et al, 1980; Boysen et al, 1977) and function and exercise testing to determine oxygen saturation after exercise and Vo_2max (Jones, 1975). The latter tests assess general fitness as well as pulmonary function.

TABLE 4–3 ■ **Predictors of Postoperative Mortality and Morbidity**

Test	*Predictive of Increased Morbidity*	*Prohibitive*
Clinical		
Stair climbing	<3 flights (12 m height)	<1 flight
Match test	Failed	
Dyspnea grade	2–4	4
Pulmonary Mechanics		
MVV	<50 L/min	<35% predicted
FEV_1	<50% FVC	<0.6 L
FVC	<50% predicted	<1.0 L
FEV_1/FVC	<60% predicted	<50%
Gas Exchange		
DLCO	<50%	<30%
Po_2 and Sao_2	Desaturation on exercise	Po_2 <45 mm Hg
Pco_2 and actual HCO_3 elevated		Pco_2 >50 mm Hg
$\dot{V}/\dot{Q}$ Scanning Prediction		
FEV_1	<30% predicted	<0.8 L predicted
VC		<1 L predicted
Exercise Testing		
Vo_2max	<20 ml/kg/min	<10 ml/kg/min
PVR		>190 dynes/s/cm^5

DLCO, carbon monoxide diffusion capacity; FEV_1, forced expiratory volume in 1 second; FVC, forced vital capacity; MVV, maximal voluntary ventilation; PVR, pulmonary vascular resistance; VC, vital capacity; Vo_2max, maximal oxygen uptake; $\dot{V}/\dot{Q}$, ventilation/perfusion.
Data from multiple treatises.

The forced expiratory volume in 1 second (FEV_1), which is used by many as the primary predictor of function and resectability, can be misleading in many patients, especially those who are of small stature or who have significant tracheomalacia. The latter patients will have an abnormally low FEV_1, predicted FEV_1, or FEV_1/FVC ratio and on physical examination, forced expiratory maneuvers will cause them to produce an audible, large airway, expiratory wheeze. This malacia can be confirmed by imaging maneuvers (tracheogram, dynamic computed tomography [CT] scan, or ultrasound) or by using fiberoptic bronchoscopy in an awake setting to assess airways collapse by forced expiratory maneuvers. Such patients frequently can tolerate pulmonary resection despite an unusually low FEV_1 even if corrected for body habitus (% predicted FEV_1), especially if appropriate breathing instruction and preoperative control of excessive sputum can be accomplished. Other reasons for a low FEV_1 that can be "ignored" include small body habitus or obstructed airways in diseased areas to be removed. The FEV_1/FVC ratio is a better predictor of postoperative complications, because it assesses the obstructive pulmonary component more accurately. The recent experience with volume reduction surgery for COPD has shown us that FEV_1 cannot be considered an absolute indication of inoperability. We (Korst et al, 1998) have shown that a patient with an extremely low FEV_1 owing to COPD often improves following pulmonary resectional surgery (lobectomy), probably for the same reasons that improvement is seen following volume reduction operations.

Blood Gas Assessment

Arterial blood gas analysis has become an essential preoperative assessment. Occasionally, an unexpected ex-

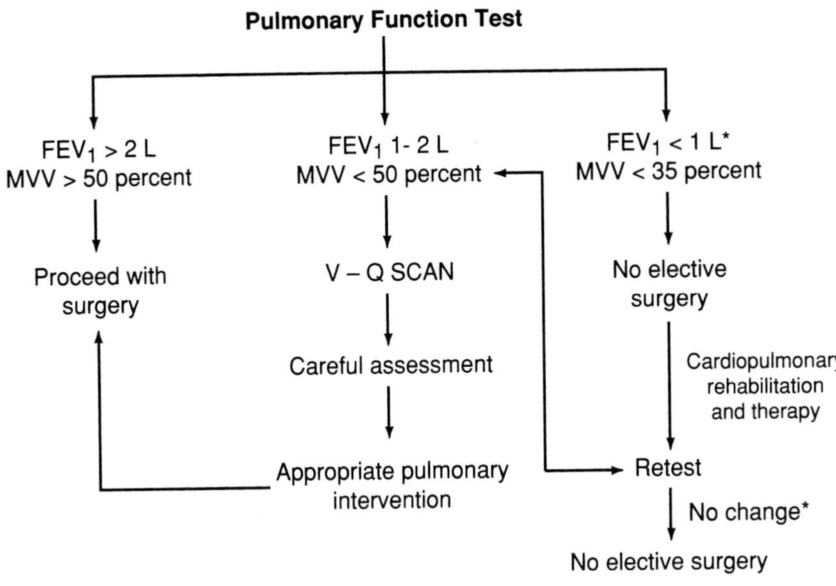

FIGURE 4–1 ■ An algorithm suggesting the schema for evaluating pulmonary function.* The absolute numbers indicated are not absolute and depend on the individual in selected cases, FEV_1 may be as low as 0.6 L/min. (Adapted from Miller JI: Preoperative evaluation. Chest Surg Clin North Am 4:701, 1992.

tremely low preoperative arterial oxygen pressure will indicate that further cardiopulmonary testing is required. Oxygen desaturation on exercise also indicates the need for further investigation. Patients with severe COPD and resting hypercarbia usually have cor pulmonale and can rarely tolerate a pneumonectomy but may be suitable candidates for lesser resections. Additionally, patients who have an elevated bicarbonate as measured by serum electrolytes (not the bicarbonate calculated with blood gas analysis) must be investigated for possible occult carbon dioxide retention and cor pulmonale. Usually, these abnormalities in blood gas analysis are associated with abnormalities seen on DLCO estimation, although the DLCO can vary enormously from laboratory to laboratory.

Ferguson and colleagues (Ferguson 1988, Wang 1999, Wang 1999) have studied DLCO and more recently postoperative predicted DLCO. They have found that the DLCO predicts pulmonary complications and operative mortality. A decreasing DLCO does predict increasing morbidity postoperatively and an absolute ppo DLCO percent less than 50 predicts mortality. This appears to be a better indicator than VO_2max is. In our experience, desaturation on exercise testing correlates with DLCO estimations.

In our own center we have found that the three most important predictors of severe pulmonary complications include: DLCO, FEV_1/FVC ratio, and A-a DO_2 as measured on room air (Melendez, 1998).

The risk of anesthesia and surgical intervention, especially when combined with pulmonary resection, cannot be exactly determined for any individual patient. Guidelines for prediction of high risks and contraindications to pulmonary resection have been suggested by many authors (see Tables 4–2 and 4–3). Although most of these guidelines are relative, in the past it appeared that absolute contraindications to resection included a predicted postoperative FEV_1 of less than 0.8 L, no matter the type of resection, a VO_2max of less than 10 ml/kg/min, and in the case of pneumonectomy, a resting elevated carbon dioxide pressure or cor pulmonale. However, even these criteria on occasion are no longer absolute, especially in dealing with small patients, but they do indicate the need for further investigation and preoperative cardiopulmonary rehabilitation.

Despite all guidelines, the final preoperative pulmonary assessment of the patient depends on the experience of the assessor. There is no formula, no absolute criterion, and, in the case of curable lung cancer, in view of the relative lack of alternative treatments, no absolute contraindication to surgical intervention. One must remember that these parameters predict postoperative morbidity, not mortality, most of which is recoverable, and in the case of lung cancer, treatment of such recoverable morbidity may be acceptable. Moreover, I have been frequently pleasantly surprised at the improvement obtained by prolonged and intensive pulmonary rehabilitation and the smoothness of the postoperative course in patients initially deemed totally inoperable by standard functional assessments. An algorithm suggested by Miller (1992) is a valuable guideline, but even this cannot be considered absolute (Fig. 4–1).

Pulmonary Rehabilitation

Whenever possible, preoperative pulmonary assessment, especially in compromised individuals, should be performed at least 2 weeks prior to anticipated surgery. This allows enough time to correct deficiencies (e.g., by use of antibiotics, bronchodilators when indicated, relief of airway obstructions to reduce infection and so on) and improve function. In some individuals, prolonged preoperative intensive rehabilitation may significantly improve pulmonary function and thus allow surgical intervention that otherwise would have been contraindicated. This should always be attempted before denying patients a curative surgical procedure. In some cases up to 2 months of preoperative therapy, including progressive pulmonary rehabilitation, may be required to optimally prepare the patient for surgery. Even in cancer surgery this delay may

TABLE 4–4 ■ **The New York Heart Association Angina Classification**

Class	*Description*
1	Angina with strenuous exercise
2	Angina with moderate exercise
3	Angina with 1 flight of stairs or 1 to 2 blocks
4	Angina with any activity

be valuable and has not been shown to adversely affect curability.

Preoperative bronchodilator therapy can be extremely useful in improving pulmonary function in selected patients with reactive airways disease. If steroids are to be used, whenever possible the benefit of such therapy should be documented and as low a dose as possible should be used in the perioperative period.

Even in the minimally compromised individual, preoperative cardiopulmonary rehabilitation will have value. A program that we have found to be useful and given to all patients prior to surgery in our institution is outlined in the box titled "Preoperative Exercise Program."

CARDIOVASCULAR ASSESSMENT

The risk of both morbidity and mortality from surgery increases exponentially in patients with significant cardiovascular disease. In the general population, the risk of a postoperative myocardial infarction following general anesthesia is 0.07%. However, this risk increases with a history of previous remote infarction and is significant when a myocardial infarction has occurred within 3 months prior to the expected surgery (Arkins et al, 1964; Steen, 1978). Similar risks have been identified for patients with angina, with an increasing risk for each class of the New York Heart Association Angina Classification (Table 4–4). Similarly, increasing postoperative morbidity and mortality correlate with the New York Heart Association functional class describing dyspnea associated with congestive heart failure. Cardiac predictors of increased risk include hypertension, valvular heart disease, cardiac conduction abnormalities, and preoperative dysrhythmias.

For these reasons, an accurate cardiac history is very important in the preoperative assessment, including documentation of all cardiovascular medications used. A routine electrocardiogram is considered part of the physical examination, as important as auscultation of the heart, measurement of blood pressure, and examination for focal vascular lesions of the carotids, aorta, and femoral vessels.

The overall estimation of cardiac risk has been documented by Goldman (1983), who used nine significant preoperative risk factors and assessed a point value by multivariant risk analysis (Table 4–5). Detsky (1986) added some additional risk factors to the original Goldman index, including angina, pulmonary edema, presence of S3 or jugular venous distention (JVD), and type of operation. It is likely that with modern postoperative care, the risks engendered are much less than originally

DETERMINANTS OF POSTOPERATIVE MORBIDITY AND MORTALITY*

Cardiac disease
Pulmonary disease
Tumor characteristics
  Stage
  Type
General medical conditions
  Diabetes
  Creatinine level
  Hemoglobin level
  Serum albumin level
  Immnosuppressed status
    Steroids
    Chemotherapy
    Other chronic illnesses
  Weight loss >10%
  Age >70
Anticipated surgery
Extent of resection
Additional procedures
Side of pulmonary resection (R > L)
Previous surgery

*Significant cardiopulmonary disease, late tumor stage, and extent of resection appear to be the most significant determinants.

TABLE 4–5 ■ **Goldman Cardiac Risk Index (1983)***

Factors	*Points*
History	
Age >70	5
Myocardial infarction, <6 mo	10
Physical	
Congestive failure	11
Aortic stenosis	3
Electrocardiogram	
Rhythm abnormality	7
PVCs >5/min	7
General	
Po_2 <60 mm Hg, Pco_2 >50 mm Hg, HCO_3 <20 mg/L	3
↑ Creatinine	
Liver disease	
↑ Performance status	
Type of operation	
Intraperitoneal or intrathoracic	3
Emergency	4
Total possible points	53

Class	*Points*	*Severe Morbidity*	*Cardiac Death*
1	0–5	0.7%	0.2%
2	6–12	5%	2%
3	13–25	11%	2%
4	>26	22%	56%

PVCs, premature ventricular contractions.
*With more modern perioperative care, the risks for each class are probably less than those originally predicted.

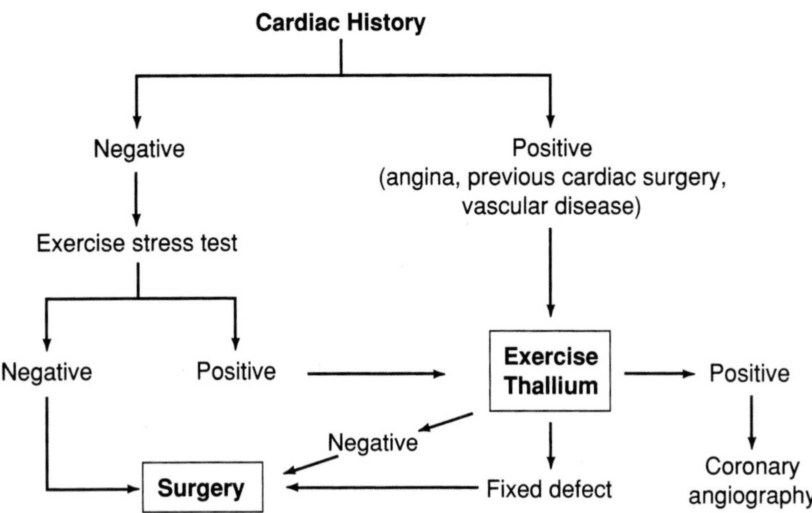

FIGURE 4–2 ■ A suggested algorithm for investigating the cardiac status of all patients over the age of 45 or those with significant risk factors undergoing major thoracic surgery. (Adapted from Miller JI: Preoperative evaluation. Chest Surg Clin North Am 4:701, 1992.)

predicted. Patients in class 3 or 4 according to this risk index require significant preoperative investigation and almost certainly benefit from intensive perioperative monitoring, including the use of intraoperative and postoperative pulmonary artery pressure monitoring. For pulmonary resectional surgery, Epstein and colleagues (1993) have correlated this type of risk index to Vo_2max, which is an estimate of total physical fitness, thus suggesting that Vo_2max is as predictable as other indices already discussed.

Exercise Stress Testing

Much more difficult and germane is the need for preoperative identification of occult coronary artery disease in presumed healthy patients. With increasing frequency, exercise stress tests are being added to routine cardiac assessment for all preoperative thoracic surgical patients older than 45 years of age or with other risk factors. Occult coronary artery disease can be revealed that would indicate the need for more invasive testing, and, when treatable problems are found, they can be corrected before the thoracic operation.

Thallium Imaging

Eagle (1989) identified five clinical predictors for cardiac complications, including age (>70 years), angina pectoris, diabetes, Q waves, and premature ventricular contractions (PVCs) on electrocardiography. With one predictor, there was a 3% risk of cardiac complications; with two or three predictors there was up to a 15% risk. With these statistics plus an abnormal thallium scan, the risk is increased further. More recently, atropine/dobutamine stress echocardiography has been found to satisfactorily replace thallium perfusion scans to identify ischemic events (Poldermans 1995).

For those patients with a positive result on an exercise stress test or a significant history of coronary artery or peripheral vascular disease, exercise thallium testing is indicated. In those patients with no coronary artery disease history, a normal exercise tolerance test result, or a normal thallium test or fixed defect on thallium testing, the risk of surgery, especially in relation to postoperative major cardiac events, is minimal (Lette et al, 1989; Miller, 1992b). The value of preoperative thallium imaging is its ability to identify reversible ischemia with viable myocardium that should be treated prior to thoracotomy. There have been several studies showing a high risk of perioperative cardiac events, including death, for those patients who have untreated, reversible, ischemic defect, in contradistinction to those patients who have fixed defects, in whom the risk of perioperative cardiac events is small (Lette et al, 1990). Miller (1992b) has developed an algorithm for cardiovascular evaluation of patients older than 45 years of age (Fig. 4–2). On the basis of this algorithm, 275 of 2340 patients were selected to undergo thallium imaging. Approximately 50% of these 275 patients had normal thallium imaging; of those with abnormal imaging, 50% had fixed defects. Reversible ischemic changes were identified in approximately 25% of all patients undergoing imaging (1.5% of all patients) and were corrected prior to surgical exploration. The mortality was zero in this group of patients. However, some believe that documented ischemia on stress testing or a significant cardiac or vascular disease history warrants coronary angiography without the need for thallium testing (Jewell, 1985), pointing out the significant false-negative rates of stress testing.

It appears that in the future a more aggressive, proactive approach should be adopted for most patients who have an abnormal exercise tolerance test or history of coronary artery disease, despite a normal electrocardiogram. Whether or not all patients older than 60 years of age should undergo routine thallium imaging despite a normal exercise tolerance test is yet to be determined.

COMORBID DISEASES

It is important to identify comorbid diseases suffered by the patient (e.g., malnutrition, diabetes, peripheral vascular disease, other endocrinopathies) to ensure that these diseases have been optimally controlled and that no further preoperative intervention or treatment is required.

Routine screening of significant electrolytes and blood chemicals will help to identify occult intercurrent disease. When necessary, appropriate consultations with specific specialists may be required for concurrent management of these illnesses. Whenever possible, all such comorbid diseases should be stabilized and treated prior to surgical intervention.

CONCLUSIONS

The preoperative assessment of the thoracic surgical patient is of inestimable value in anticipating and preventing postoperative complications and lessening postoperative morbidity and mortality. The thoracic surgeon need not and should not abrogate the responsibility of this initial assessment, which requires a complete history and physical examination, judicious use of cardiopulmonary testing, and screening for other comorbid diseases. Although many indices and algorithms have been devised to predict postoperative morbidity and mortality, nothing replaces an astute clinician—all of these algorithms and indices must be correlated with the overall clinical assessment of the surgeon. Where indicated, pulmonary rehabilitation, treatment of occult or manifest cardiac disease, and optimization of the treatment of other comorbid disease will decrease the risks associated with major thoracic surgical interventions and hopefully lessen perioperative morbidity and mortality.

COMMENTS AND CONTROVERSIES

I fully agree with Dr. Ginsberg on the importance that should be given to the preoperative evaluation of all patients who are to undergo pulmonary resection. Often these patients are older, and they have significant cardiopulmonary diseases that need to be assessed before surgery.

As discussed by the author, the pulmonary evaluation often starts with a good questionnaire. While taking the clinical history, it is important to realize that many patients will have adjusted their lifestyle and that they may not complain of dyspnea or chest pain simply because they never reach a stage where they become symptomatic. A history of cigarette smoking is easy to record from the patient and, clearly, the postoperative course will be easier if the patient has never smoked or has stopped 2 or 3 months before the operation. Another important feature of the questionnaire is to note the patient's ability to cooperate postoperatively. These issues and others are very important in predicting operative risk and in taking prophylactic measures aimed at reducing morbidity.

No patient should have pulmonary surgery, no matter how limited, without preoperative pulmonary function testing. In many cases, a simple spirometric test will provide enough information to determine that the pulmonary function is normal and that the patient can tolerate pneumonectomy if necessary. The FEV_1 is the most quoted value and many surgeons will not operate on patients with an FEV_1 that is below 0.8 L or on patients in whom the expected postoperative FEV_1 will be 0.8 L or less. I think that, in some cases, an FEV_1 of 0.8 L can be almost normal, particularly if the patient has a small body surface. One should therefore look at the percentage of predicted value rather than at absolute numbers. Similarly, the critical number of 0.8 L is derived from life study analysis done in emphysema patients. These series have shown that once a patient with chronic obstructive lung disease reaches an FEV_1 of 0.8 L, there is a good chance that he will die within the next 5 years of complications of his disease. This, however, does not necessarily apply to patients who will reach a level of 0.8 L because of pulmonary resection, particularly if they stop smoking after surgery. One has therefore to be very careful before turning down a patient for surgery merely on the basis of a predicted negative postoperative period FEV_1 of 0.8 L. As shown by Ginsberg, other tests including D_{LCO} measurements are useful and recognized as good indicators of pulmonary reserve.

In borderline cases, exercise testing with measurements of the V_{O_2}max and arterial P_{O_2} and P_{CO_2} both at rest and during exercise is very useful to help preoperative selection. A P_{CO_2} that rises on minimal exercise is a strong indicator of inadequate reserve and such patients should be looked at very carefully before surgery.

Overall, it is important to understand that no one, single test is predictive of postoperative complications but that patients with poor profiles based on clinical history, spirometric values, or exercise testing are at high risk of morbidity, and, in those cases, the benefits of an operation should be carefully weighed against the risks.

J.D.

■ KEY REFERENCES

Epstein SK, Ealing JL, Daly B, Celli BR: Predicting complications after pulmonary resection: Preoperative exercise testing versus a multifactorial cardiopulmonary risk index. Chest 104:694, 1993.

The author attempts to develop a cardiopulmonary risk index for patients undergoing pulmonary resection demonstrates the value of V_{O_2}max as a single index, which correlates well with a multifactorial index.

Julio ER, Persson AV: Preoperative evaluation of high-risk patients. Surg Clin North Am 65:3, 1985.

Another excellent review of preoperative assessment of the high-risk patient.

Mark JBD (ed): Perioperative cardiopulmonary evaluation and management. Chest 115(Suppl):2, May 1999.

This recent supplement contains many papers discussing perioperative cardiopulmonary evaluation and management and is a worthwhile, up-to-date treatise on the subject.

Miller JI: Preoperative evaluation. Chest Surg Clin North Am 4:701, 1992a.

This outline of a surgeon's approach to preoperative pulmonary and cardiac evaluation of the thoracic surgical patient provides an excellent overview of current practice.

Olsen GN: The evolving role of exercise testing prior to lung resection. Chest 95:218, 1989.

Dr. Olsen, a noted pulmonary physiologist interested in preoperative assessment, here discusses exercise testing including V_{O_2}max assessment.

Smetana GW: Preoperative pulmonary evaluation. N Engl J Med 340:937–944, 1999.

This up-to-date review of preoperative pulmonary evaluation is succinct and worthwhile reading.

Tisi M: Preoperative evaluation of pulmonary function. Am Rev Respir Dis 119:295, 1979.

This excellent review of the early work in preoperative pulmonary function testing is very relevant despite its age.

■ REFERENCES

Ali KM, Mountain CF, Ewer MS et al: Predicting loss of pulmonary function after pulmonary resection for bronchogenic carcinoma. Chest 77:337, 1980.

Arkins R, Smesseart AA, Hicks RG: Mortality and morbidity in surgical patients with coronary artery disease. JAMA 190:485, 1964.

Bolton JWR, Weiman DS, Haynes JL et al: Stairclimbing as an indicator of pulmonary function. Chest 82:783, 1987.

Boysen PG, Block AJ, Olsen GN et al: Prospective evaluation for pneumonectomy using the technetium-99m quantitative perfusion lung scan. Chest 72:422, 1977.

Deslauriers J, Ginsberg RJ, Dubois P et al: Current operative morbidity associated with elective surgical resection for lung cancer. Can J Surg 32:335, 1989.

Detsky AS, Abrams HB, McLaughlin JR et al: Predicting cardiac complications in patients undergoing non-cardiac surgery. J Gen Intern Med 1:211–219, 1986.

Eagle KA, Coley Cm, Newell JB et al: Combining clinical and thallium data optimizes preoperative assessment of cardiac risk before major vascular surgery. Ann Intern Med 110:859–866, 1989.

Epstein SK, Ealing JL, Daly B, Celli BR: Predicting complications after pulmonary resection: Preoperative exercise testing versus a multifactorial cardiopulmonary risk index. Chest 104:694, 1993.

Epstein TA, Tinker AH, Tarhan S: Myocardial re-infarction after anesthesia and surgery. JAMA 339:2566, 1978.

Ferguson MK, Little L, Rizzo L et al: Diffusing capacity predicts morbidity and mortality after pulmonary resection. J Thorac Cardiovasc Surg 96:894–900, 1988.

Ginsberg RJ, Hill LD, Eagan RT et al: Modern 30-day operative mortality for surgical resections in lung cancer. J Thorac Cardiovasc Surg 86:654, 1983.

Goldman L: Cardiac risks and complications of non-cardiac surgery. Ann Surg 198:780, 1983.

Jones NL: Exercise testing in pulmonary evaluation: Rational, methods in normal respiratory response exercise. N Engl J Med 393:541, 1975.

Julio ER, Persson AV: Preoperative evaluation of high-risk patients. Surg Clin North Am 65:3, 1985.

Kohman LJ, Meyer JA, Ikins PM, Oates RP: Random versus predictable risks of mortality after thoractomy for lung cancer. J Thorac Cardiovasc Surg 91:551, 1986.

Korst RJ, Ginsberg RJ, Ailawadi M et al: Lobectomy improves ventilatory function in selected patients with severe COPD. Ann Thorac Surg 66:898–902, 1998.

Lette J, Waters D, Lapointe J: Usefulness of the severity and extent of reversible perfusion defects during thallium-dye dipyridamole imaging for cardiac risk assessment before non-cardiac surgery. Ann J Cardiol 64:276, 1989.

Lette J, Waters D, Lasson DEJ: Postoperative myocardial infarction in cardiac death. Ann Surg 211:84, 1990.

Mark JBD (ed): Perioperative cardiopulmonary evaluation and management. Chest 115(Suppl):2 May 1999.

Melendez JA, Barrera R: Predictive respiratory complication quotient predicts pulmonary complications in thoracic surgical patients. Ann Thorac Surg 66:220–224, 1998.

Miller JI: Preoperative evaluation. Chest Surg Clin North Am 4:701, 1992a.

Miller JI: Thallium imaging in preoperative evaluation of the pulmonary resection candidate. Ann Thorac Surg 54:249, 1992b.

Ninan M, Sommers KE, Landreneau RJ et al: Standardized exercise oximetry predicts postpneumonectomy outcome. Ann Thorac Surg 64:328–332, 1997.

Olsen GN: The evolving role of exercise testing prior to lung resection. Chest 95:218, 1989.

Olsen GN, Bolton JWR, Weunab DS, Hornung CA: Stairclimbing as an exercise test to predict the postoperative complications of lung resection—2 years experience. Chest 99:587, 1991.

Poldermans D, Arnese M, Fioretti PM et al: Improved cardiac risk stratification in major vascular surgery with dobutamine-atropine stress echocardiography. J Am Coll Cardiol 26:648–653, 1995.

Rao V, Todd TRJ, Kuus A et al: Exercise oximetry versus spirometry in the assessment of risk prior to lung resection. Ann Thorac Surg 60:603–609, 1995.

Ruckdeschel J, Piantadori S (for the Lung Cancer Study Group): Quality of life assessment in lung surgery for bronchogenic carcinoma. J Thorac Surg 6:201, 1991.

Smetana GW: Preoperative pulmonary evaluation. N Engl J Med 340:937–944, 1999.

Steen PA, Tinker JH, Tarhan S: Myocardial reinfarction after anesthesia and surgery. JAMA 220:1451, 1978.

Tisi M: Preoperative evaluation of pulmonary function. Am Rev Respir Dis 119:295, 1979.

Wahi R, McMurtrey MJ, DeCaro LF et al: Determinants of perioperative morbidity and mortality after pneumonectomy. Ann Thorac Surg 48:333, 1989.

Wang J, Olak J, Ferguson MK: Diffusing capacity predicts operative mortality but not long-term survival after resection for lung cancer. J Thorac Cardiovasc Surg 117:581–587, 1999.

Wang J, Olak J, Ultman RE, Ferguson MK: Assessment of pulmonary complications after lung resection. Ann Thorac Surg 67:1444–1447, 1999.

CHAPTER **5**

Anesthesia

Karen M. McRae
Peter D. Slinger
Alan N. Sandler

General thoracic surgery encompasses a wide breadth of varied procedures; the authors have had the privilege of practicing anesthesia in an institution in which these procedures are performed with regularity. The practice of thoracic anesthesia requires a firm understanding of pulmonary anatomy and physiology, in addition to technical knowledge and experience. A vast literature describing the care of the patient undergoing thoracotomy for pulmonary resection exists. The bulk of this chapter, which describes the authors' experiences in patient assessment, airway management, lung separation, and the management of perioperative pain, draws on this literature. The chapter ends with a brief overview of some of the particular anesthetic considerations germane to other procedures performed by general thoracic surgeons. Management issues discussed include those related to mediastinal surgery and esophageal surgery, along with a relatively recent endeavor—surgical procedures to improve the quality of life of patients with end-stage lung disease through lung volume reduction and pulmonary transplantation. The anesthetic considerations for airway surgery merit a dedicated chapter (see Chapter 13).

HISTORICAL NOTE

Apparent from the beginning of the provision of anesthesia for thoracic surgery was the challenge of ventilating the open chest. Spontaneous ventilation with an open thorax is hampered by lung collapse, mediastinal and diaphragmatic shift, and paradoxical respiratory movement, all of which hinder operating conditions for all but the simplest procedures. The patient became increasingly hypoxic and hypercapnic, and his desperate respiratory efforts only worsened the situation; thus, the only option was to close the chest. Ferdinand Sauerbruch, a pioneering thoracic surgeon from Breslau, Germany, began to experiment with a negative-pressure chamber to minimize the effect of the pneumothorax. In 1904, he successfully performed chest surgery with the surgical team working inside a chamber held at negative 7 to 8 mm Hg, while the patient's head, and the anesthetist, remained outside. At the same time, his colleague Brauer in Marburg tried a reverse method, "the so-called plus or positive pressure" approach, whereby the patient's head was isolated in a positive-pressure chamber (Sauerbruch, 1908).

Devices for cannulation of the trachea had been described as early as the 18th century by physiologists and physicians interested in the resuscitation of drowning victims and asphyxiated neonates. Until the late 19th century, however, anesthesiologists had not taken an interest in their use (White, 1960). Until 1907, endotracheal anesthesia had been inhalational; patients breathed spontaneously through a mask or a large-bore tube. Barthélemy and Dufour proposed an insufflation method for surgery on the face, whereby a continuous flow of air and chloroform entered the trachea via a catheter advanced to just above the carina (Barthélemy and Dufour, 1907). It was recommended that the catheter not occupy greater than half of the glottis; expired gases escaped through the space between the tube and the trachea. The modest positive airway pressure provided by this technique was soon hailed as the solution to the problem of preventing pulmonary collapse in surgical pneumothorax.

For casualties of the First World War, chest surgery was perfomed using insufflation, or the administration of nitrous oxide and oxygen via a tight-fitting face mask with a continuous positive pressure of approximately 5 mm Hg to promote lung inflation. Intravenous morphine was administered for analgesia. Magill and Rowbotham in Britain, and Guedel and Waters and Flagg in the United States, soon realized that insufflation anesthesia provided inadequate carbon dioxide elimination and offered no protection against pulmonary aspiration.

Following World War I, Ivan W. Magill and Stanley Rowbotham played a prominent role in the development of endotracheal intubation. They gained their expertise working as anesthetists with a British army plastic surgery unit performing early head and neck reconstruction. Rowbotham designed a wide-bore endotracheal tube with an inflatable pharyngeal cuff, but it was Magill's design of a similar endotracheal tube with a tracheal cuff that prevailed. Intubation initially was performed blindly; the anesthesia community's interest in laryngoscopy was not sustained until the 1920s, despite Chevalier Jackson's long-standing use of the laryngoscope for examination of the airway (see Historical Note in Chapter 14).

Guedel and Waters described "a new intratracheal catheter" with an inflatable cuff in 1928 (Guedel et al, 1928), and Magill reported his experience at about the same time (Magill, 1928). Positive-pressure ventilation was now much simplified. The introduction of the tracheal tube was facilitated by the newly popularized laryngoscope. In 1931, separate ventilation of one lung was achieved first by Gale and Waters who used a standard rubber tube molded in hot water to obtain a lateral curve toward the bevel tip (Gale and Waters, 1932). The tube was advanced toward the bronchus until resistance was met. Graham and Singer described the first pneumonectomy using endobronchial anesthesia in 1933.

Ether and cyclopropane were most often used during this era. Cyclopropane was popular in thoracic surgery as a powerful respiratory depressant, making positive-pressure ventilation feasible. The introduction of muscle relaxants into clinical practice in the 1940s greatly facilitated the use of positive-pressure ventilation. Despite the innovation of endobronchial intubation and the use of automatic ventilators for rhythmic ventilation of the lungs as early as the late 1930s, these devices and the personnel skilled in their use were not available outside highly specialized centers. Open chest surgery continued to be performed in spontaneously breathing patients well into the 1950s.

The first era of thoracic surgery was primarily for treatment of infectious disease, tuberculosis, and empyema. Methods to effectively remove secretions and prevent their movement into healthy lung segments were sought. A bronchus blocker placed in the operative lung to contain purulent secretions was first described by Archibald in 1935. The first double lumen tubes were adapted for surgery by Björk and Carlens in 1950, with the same goal. Since that time, advances in anesthetic agents, pain control techniques, and monitoring have led us through the second era defined by surgery for bronchogenic cancer and into the current, third era in which surgery for respiratory failure is successfully performed (Conacher, 1997).

■ *HISTORICAL READINGS*

Archibald EJ: A consideration of the dangers of lobectomy. J Thorac Surg 4:335, 1935.

Barthélemy et Dufour: L'anaesthésie dans la chirurgie de la face. Presse Méd 15:475, 1907.

Björk VO, Carlens E: The prevention of spread during pulmonary resection by the use of a double lumen catheter. J Thorac Surg 20:151, 1950.

Björk VO, Carlens E, Friberg O: Endobronchial anesthesia. Anesthesiology 14:60, 1953.

Flagg PJ: Intratracheal inhalation: Preliminary report of a simplified method of intratracheal anesthesia developed under the supervision of Dr. Chevalier Jackson. Arch Otolaryngol 5:394, 1927.

Gale JW, Waters RM: Closed endobroncheal anesthesia in thoracic surgery: Preliminary report. J Thorac Surg 1:432, 1932.

Graham AE, Singer JJ: Successful removal of the entire lung for carcinoma of the bronchus. JAMA 101:1371, 1933.

Guedel AE, Waters RM: A new intratracheal catheter. Anesth Analg 7:238, 1928.

Guedel AE, Waters RM: Endotracheal anesthesia; a new technic. Ann Otol (St. Louis) 40:1139, 1931.

Magill IW: Endotracheal anaesthesia. Proc Roy Soc Med 22:1, 1928.

Magill IW: Anaesthesia in thoracic surgery with special reference to lobectomy. Proc Roy Soc Med 29:643, 1936.

Rowbotham S, Magill IW: Anaesthetics in plastic surgery of the face and jaws. Proc Roy Soc Med (Section of Anaesthetics) 14:17, 1921.

Sauerbruch EF: Present status of surgery of the thorax. JAMA 51:808, 1908.

White GMJ: Evolution of endotracheal and endobroncheal intubation. Br J Anaesth 32:235, 1960.

PREOPERATIVE ASSESSMENT

Preoperative anesthetic assessment prior to chest surgery is a continually evolving science and art. This section concentrates on preoperative assessment for pulmonary resection surgery in cancer patients. The principles described here apply to all other types of nonmalignant pulmonary resection, and to other chest surgery as well. The major difference in their application is that in patients with malignancy, the risk/benefit ratio of canceling or delaying surgery for each individual patient pending other investigation or therapy is always complicated by the risk of further spread of cancer during any extended interval prior to resection. This is never completely "elective" surgery.

Several general points should be appreciated in the assessment of pulmonary resection patients.

1. *Anesthesiologists are not gatekeepers.* It is rarely the anesthesiologist's function to assess these patients to decide who is or is not an operative candidate. In the majority of situations, the anesthesiologist will be seeing the patient at the end of a referral chain from chest or family physician to surgeon. At each stage, there should have been a discussion of the risks and benefits of the operation. Recent anesthetic and surgical advances have made it so that almost any patient, given a full understanding of the risks and appropriate investigation, can be considered "operable" (Olsen, 1995). The preoperative anesthetic assessment is used first to identify those patients at increased preoperative risk; then that risk assessment is used to stratify perioperative management and focus resources on high-risk patients with the goal of improving their outcome.

2. *Short-term versus long-term survival is currently under study.* Although a massive amount of research has been done on long-term survival (6 months–5 years) following pulmonary resection surgery, there has been a comparatively small volume of research on the short-term (<6 weeks) outcome of these patients. However, this research area is currently very active, and there are several studies that can be used to guide anesthetic management during the immediate perioperative period, when it influences outcome.

3. *Preoperative evaluation comprises two disjoint phases.* Until very recently, preanesthetic management was part of a continuum whereby a patient was admitted preoperatively for testing and the management plan evolved as test results were received. Currently, the reality of practice patterns in anesthesia has changed such that a patient is commonly assessed initially in an outpatient clinic, often not by the members of the anesthesia staff who will actually administer the anesthesia. The actual contact with the responsible anesthesiologist may involve only 10 to 15 minutes prior to induction. It is necessary for the anesthesiologist to organize and standardize the approach to preoperative evaluation for most of these patients into two temporally "disjoint" phases: the initial (clinic) assessment and the final (hallway) assessment. Elements vital to each assessment are described in the following paragraphs.

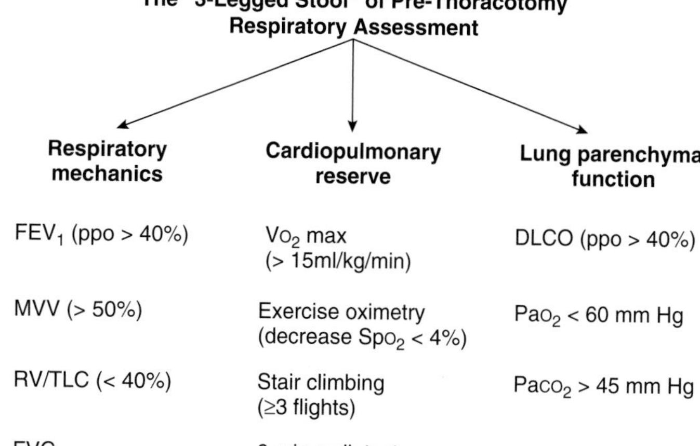

FIGURE 5–1 ■ Three separate but interrelated aspects of respiratory function are used for pre-anesthetic assessment for thoracic surgery. (DLCO, carbon monoxide diffusion; FEV_1, forced expiratory volume in one second; FVC, forced vital capacity; MVV, maximal voluntary ventilation; $Paco_2$, partial pressure of carbon dioxide in arterial blood; Pao_2, partial pressure of oxygen in arterial blood; RV/TLC, residual volume/total lung capacity; Spo_2, pulse oximetry.)

Perioperative Complications

To assess patients for thoracic anesthesia, one must have an understanding of the risks specific to this type of surgery. The major causes of perioperative morbidity and mortality in the thoracic surgical population are respiratory in nature. Surgery and anesthesia alter respiratory function, beginning with the induction of anesthesia and often lasting well into the convalescent period. Atelectasis occurs within minutes of induction, causing reduction in the functional residual capacity (FRC) and lung compliance (Hedensteirna, 1998). Postoperative changes in respiratory function are in part due to the direct effect of the surgical procedure on respiratory muscles (Siafakas et al, 1999). Major respiratory complications of persistent atelectasis, pneumonia, and respiratory failure occur in 15% to 20% of patients and account for the majority of the reported 3% to 4% mortality (Nakahara et al, 1988). It should be appreciated that the thoracic surgical population differs from other adult surgical populations in this respect. For other types of surgery, cardiac and vascular complications are the leading causes of early perioperative morbidity and mortality. Cardiac complications (e.g., arrhythmia, ischemia) occur in 10% to 15% of the thoracic population (Kearney et al, 1994).

Prethoracotomy assessment naturally involves all of the factors in a complete anesthetic assessment: medical history, allergies, medications, condition of upper airway, and so forth. This section focuses on the additional information (beyond that included in a standard anesthetic assessment) needed for management of a pulmonary resection patient.

Assessment of Respiratory Function

Much scientific effort has been spent to try to find a single test of respiratory function that has sufficient sensitivity and specificity to predict outcome for all pulmonary resection patients. It is now clear that no single test will ever accomplish this. There are many factors that determine overall respiratory performance. It is useful to think of respiratory function in three related but somewhat independent areas: respiratory mechanics, gas exchange, and cardiorespiratory interaction. These three factors form the "3-legged stool" of prethoracotomy respiratory assessment (Fig. 5–1).

Respiratory Mechanics

Many tests of respiratory mechanics and volumes show correlation with post-thoracotomy outcome in terms of forced expiratory volume in one second (FEV_1), forced vital capacity (FVC), maximal voluntary ventilation (MVV), residual volume/total lung capacity ratio (RV/TLC), and so forth. It is useful to express these as a percentage of predicted volumes corrected for age, sex, and height (e.g., FEV_1%). Of these, the most valued single test for post-thoracotomy respiratory complications is the predicted postoperative FEV_1 (ppo FEV_1%), which is calculated as

$$\text{ppo } FEV_1\% = \text{preoperative } FEV_1\% \times (1 - \%\text{ functional lung tissue removed}/100)$$

One method of estimating the percentage of functional lung tissue present is based on a calculation of the number of functioning subsegments of the lung removed. Nakahara and associates (1988) found that patients with a ppo FEV_1 greater than 40% had no or minor postresection respiratory complications. Major respiratory complications were seen only in the subgroup with ppo FEV_1 less than 40% (although not all patients in this subgroup developed respiratory complications), and 10 of 10 patients with ppo FEV_1 less than 30% required postoperative mechanical ventilatory support. These key threshold values—30% and 40%—are extremely useful to remember when one is managing these patients. It can be useful just to consider the right upper and middle lobes combined as being approximately equivalent to each of the other three lobes, with the right lung 10% larger than the left. These data of Nakahara are the result of work done in the 1980s. Modern anesthetic management, particularly the use of epidural analgesia, has probably decreased the incidence of complications in the high-risk group (Cerfolio et al, 1996). However, ppo FEV_1 values of 40% and 30% remain useful as reference points for the anesthesiologist. The study by Kearney and colleagues (1994) has confirmed the ppo FEV_1 as the only truly significant independent predictor of complications among a variety of historical, physical, and laboratory tests performed on these patients.

Lung Parenchymal Function

As important to the process of respiration as the mechanical delivery of air to the distal airways is the subsequent ability of the lung to exchange oxygen and carbon dioxide between the pulmonary vascular bed and the alveoli. Traditionally, arterial blood gas data such as $Pao_2 < 60$ mm Hg or $Paco_2 > 45$ mm Hg have been used as cut-off values for pulmonary resection. Cancer resections have now been successfully done, or even combined with volume reduction, in patients who do not meet these criteria (McKenna et al, 1996), although they remain as useful warning indicators. The most useful test of the gas exchange capacity of the lung is the diffusing capacity for carbon monoxide (DLCO). Although the DLCO was initially thought to reflect only diffusion, it actually correlates with the total functioning surface area of the alveolocapillary interface. This simple noninvasive test, which is included with spirometry and plethysmography in most pulmonary function laboratories, is a useful predictor of post-thoracotomy complications. The corrected DLCO can be used to determine a postresection (ppo) value using the same calculation as for the FEV_1. A ppo DLCO less than 40% predicted correlates with both increased respiratory and cardiac complications, and is to a large degree independent of the FEV_1 (Ferguson et al, 1995).

Cardiopulmonary Function

The final and perhaps most important assessment of respiratory function is an assessment of cardiopulmonary interaction. All patients should have some assessment of their cardiopulmonary reserves. The traditional, and still extremely useful, test in ambulatory patients is stair climbing (Olsen et al, 1991). Stair climbing is done at the patient's own pace but without stopping, and is usually documented as a certain number of flights. There is no gold standard for a "flight" but 20 steps at 6 in/step is a frequently used value. The ability to climb 3 flights or more is closely associated with decreased mortality and is somewhat associated with morbidity. Less than 2 flights reflects the performance of those at very high risk.

Formal laboratory exercise testing has become more standardized and thus more valid for the assessment of cardiopulmonary function. Among the many cardiac and respiratory factors tested, the maximal oxygen consumption (VO_2 max) is the most useful predictor of post-thoracotomy outcome. Walsh and co-workers (1994) have shown that in a high-risk group of patients (mean preop $FEV_1 =$ 41% predicted), there was no perioperative mortality if the preoperative Vo_2 max was greater than 15 ml/kg/min. Only 1 of 10 patients with a Vo_2 max greater than 20 ml/kg/min had a respiratory complication. Exercise testing can be modified using bicycle or arm exercises in patients who are not capable of stair climbing.

Complete laboratory exercise testing is labor intensive and expensive. Recently, several alternatives to exercise testing have been demonstrated to have potential as replacement tests for prethoracotomy assessment. The 6-minute walk test (6MWT) shows an excellent correlation with Vo_2 max and requires little or no laboratory equipment. A 6MWT distance of less than 2000 ft correlates with a Vo_2 max of less than 15 ml/kg/min, and also correlates with a fall in oximetry (Spo_2) during exercise. Patients with a decrease in Spo_2 of greater than 4% during exercise (stair climbing 2 or 3 flights or equivalent) are at increased risk of morbidity and mortality (Ninan et al, 1997; Rao et al, 1995). The 6-minute walk test and exercise oximetry may replace the Vo_2 max in the future for assessment of cardiorespiratory function. Both of these tests are still evolving, and for the present, exercise testing will remain the gold standard. Exercise tolerance can be estimated (postresection) based on the amount of functioning lung tissue removed. An estimated ppo Vo_2 max less than 10 ml/kg/min may be one of the few absolute remaining contraindications to pulmonary resection. In a small series reported by Bollinger and associates (1995), mortality was 100% (3/3) in patients with a ppo Vo_2 max less than 10 ml/kg/min.

Ventilation-Perfusion Scintigraphy

Prediction of postresection pulmonary function can be further refined by assessment of the preoperative contribution of the lung or lobe to be resected, using ventilation-perfusion (V/Q) lung scanning. If the lung region to be resected is nonfunctional or is minimally functional, the prediction of postoperative function can be modified accordingly. This is particularly useful in the treatment of pneumonectomy patients and should be considered for any patient who has a ppo FEV_1 less than 40%.

Split-Lung Function Studies

A variety of methods have been described to try to simulate the postoperative respiratory situation by unilateral exclusion of a lung or lobe with an endobronchial tube or blocker, or by pulmonary artery balloon occlusion of a lung or lobe artery. These and other varieties of split-lung function testing have also been combined with exercise to try to assess the tolerance of the cardiorespiratory system to a proposed resection. Although these tests are currently available and are used to guide therapy in certain individual centers, they have not shown sufficient predictive validity for widespread universal adoption in potential lung resection patients. One possible explanation for some predictive failure among these patients may be that lack of a pulmonary hypertensive response to unilateral occlusion may represent a sign of a failing right ventricle, and may be mistakenly interpreted as a good sign of pulmonary vascular reserve. It is conceivable that the future combination of unilateral occlusion studies with echocardiography may be a useful addition to this type of pre-resection investigation.

Combination of Tests to Guide Management

No single test of respiratory function has shown adequate validity as the sole preoperative assessment. Prior to surgery, an estimate of respiratory function in all three areas should be made for each patient. These data can then be

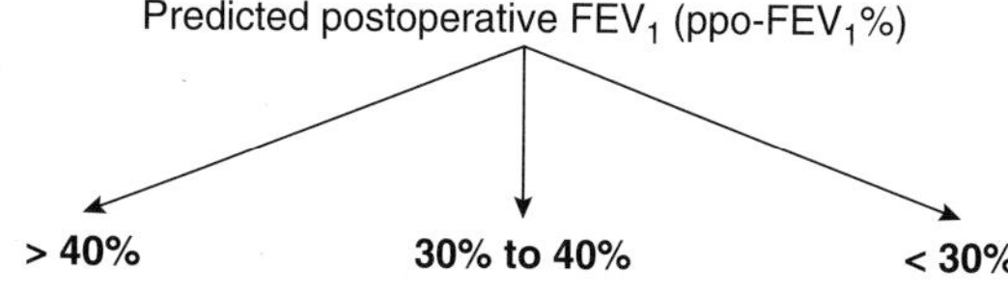

FIGURE 5–2 ■ The preanesthetic assessment is used to guide initial postoperative ventilatory management (see text). (DLCO, carbon monoxide diffusion; FEV_1, forced expiratory volume in one second; V/Q, ventilation/perfusion.)

used to plan intraoperative and postoperative management (Fig. 5–2), as well as to alter these plans when intraoperative surgical factors necessitate that a resection become more extensive than had been foreseen. The management schema outlined in Figure 5–2 is conservative and is based largely on data from the 1980s (Markos et al, 1989). If a patient has a ppo FEV_1 greater than 40%, it should be possible for that patient to be extubated in the operating room at the conclusion of surgery, assuming that the patient is alert, warm, and comfortable ("AWaC"). Patients with a ppo FEV_1 less than 40% usually account for about one fourth of an average thoracic surgical population. If the ppo FEV_1 is greater than 30%, and exercise tolerance and lung parenchymal function exceed the increased risk thresholds, then extubation in the operating room should be possible, depending on the status of associated diseases (see below). Patients in this subgroup who do not meet the minimal criteria for cardiopulmonary and parenchymal function should be considered for staged weaning from mechanical ventilation postoperatively, so that the effect of the increased oxygen consumption of spontaneous ventilation can be assessed. Patients with a ppo FEV_1 of 20% to 30% and favorable predicted cardiorespiratory and parenchymal function can be considered for early extubation if a thoracic epidural analgesia is used (see later). Otherwise, these patients should have a postoperative staged weaning from mechanical ventilation. In the borderline group (ppo FEV_1 30%–40%), the presence of several associated factors and diseases, which should be documented during the preoperative assessment, will enter into the considerations for postoperative management.

Intercurrent Medical Conditions

Age

There does not appear to be any maximum age that is a cut-off to pulmonary resection. For a patient 80 years of age with a stage I lung cancer, the chances of survival to age 85 are better with the tumor resected than without. The operative mortality in a group of patients 80 to 92 years of age was 3%, a very respectable figure, in a series reported by Osaki and colleagues (1994). However, the rate of respiratory complications (40%) was double that expected in a younger population, and the rate of cardiac complications (40%), particularly arrhythmias, was nearly triple that which would be seen in younger patients. Although the mortality resulting from lobectomy among the elderly is acceptable, the mortality from pneumonectomy (22% in patients >70 years), particularly right pneumonectomy, is excessive (Mizushima et al, 1997).

Cardiac Disease

Cardiac complications are the second most common cause of perioperative morbidity and mortality among the thoracic surgical population.

Ischemia. Because the majority of pulmonary resection patients have a smoking history, they already have one risk factor for coronary artery disease (Barry et al, 1989). However, elective pulmonary resection surgery is generally regarded as an "intermediate-risk" procedure in terms of perioperative cardiac ischemia, which is less than that associated with accepted "high-risk" procedures such as major emergency or vascular surgery. The overall documented incidence of post-thoracotomy ischemia is 5%; it peaks on day 2 to 3 postoperatively. This is approximately what would be expected from a similar patient population having major abdominal, orthopedic, or other procedures. The investigation of the patient with cardiac disease as a candidate for noncardiac surgery has been described elsewhere (ACC/AHA, 1996). Beyond the standard history, physical examination, and electrocardiogram, routine screening testing for cardiac disease does not appear to be cost effective for all prethoracotomy patients (Ghent et al, 1994). Noninvasive testing is indicated in patients with major (unstable ischemia, recent infarction, severe valvular disease, significant arrhythmia) or intermediate (stable angina, remote infarction, previous congestive failure, or diabetes) clinical predictors of myocardial risk, as well as in the elderly (Miller, 1992). Therapeutic options to be considered in patients with significant coronary artery disease include optimization of medical therapy and the use of coronary angioplasty or coronary artery bypass, either prior to or at the time of lung resection. Timing of lung resection surgery following a myocardial infarction is always a difficult decision. Based on the data of Rao and co-workers (1983), and generally confirmed by recent clinical practice, limiting the delay to 4 to 6 weeks after myocardial infarction in a medically stable and fully investigated and optimized patient seems acceptable.

Arrhythmia. Dysrhythmia, particularly atrial fibrillation, is a well-recognized complication of all pulmonary resection surgery. Factors known to correlate with an increased incidence of arrhythmia include the amount of lung tissue resected, patient age, the amount of intraoperative blood loss, and the use of intrapericardial dissection. Prophylactic therapy with digoxin has not been shown to prevent these arrhythmias (Ritchie et al, 1992).

Renal Dysfunction

Renal dysfunction following pulmonary resection surgery is associated with a very high incidence of mortality. Golledge and Goldstraw (1994) reported a perioperative mortality of 19% (6/31) in patients who developed any significant elevation of serum creatinine during the post-thoracotomy period, compared with 0% (0/99) in those who did not show any renal dysfunction. The factors that were highly associated ($P < .001$) with an elevated risk of renal impairment are listed in Table 5–1. Other factors that were statistically significant, but less strongly associated with renal impairment, included preoperative hypertension, chemotherapy, ischemic heart disease, and postoperative oliguria (<33 ml/hr). Nonsteroidal anti-inflammatory agents (NSAIDs) were not associated with renal impairment in this series, but are clearly a concern in any thoracotomy patient with an increased risk of renal dysfunction. The high mortality among pneumonectomy patients from either renal failure or postoperative pulmonary edema emphasizes the importance of fluid management in these patients (Slinger, 1995) and the need for close and intensive perioperative monitoring, particularly in those patients taking diuretics or with a history of renal dysfunction.

Chronic Obstructive Pulmonary Disease

The most common concurrent illness in the thoracic surgical population is chronic obstructive pulmonary disease (COPD), which incorporates three disorders—emphysema, peripheral airways disease, and chronic bronchitis. Any individual patient may have one or all of these conditions, but the dominant clinical feature is impairment of expiratory airflow. Historically, patients with a predominantly bronchitic pathology were termed "blue-bloaters." Typically, these patients have excessive sputum production and cough, and are prone to hypoxemia, hypercapnia, and secondary cardiovascular disease. Patients with predominantly emphysematous pathology are the "pink-puffers." They are typically more dyspneic than bronchitics. Asthma, which is considered a separate disease entity involving increased reactivity of the tracheobronchial tree and inflammation, frequently overlaps with COPD such that many COPD patients have a reactive component to their airway obstruction. Assessment of the severity of COPD has traditionally been done on the basis of FEV_1% predicted values. The American Thoracic Society currently categorizes stage I as greater than 50% predicted (this category previously included both "mild" and "moderate" COPD), stage II as 35% to 50%, and stage III as less than 35% (ATS, 1995). Stage I patients should not have significant dyspnea, hypoxemia, or hypercarbia, and other causes should be considered if these are present. Recent advances in our understanding of the pathophysiology of COPD are relevant to perioperative management. These include increased knowledge of the respiratory drive, nocturnal hypoxemia, flow limitation, auto-PEEP (see later), and right ventricular (RV) dysfunction.

TABLE 5–1 ■ Factors Associated with an Increased Risk of Postthoracotomy Renal Impairment

Previous history of renal impairment
Diuretic therapy
Pneumonectomy
Postoperative infection
Blood loss requiring transfusion

Respiratory Drive. Major changes have occurred in our understanding of the control of breathing in COPD patients. Many stage II or III COPD patients have an elevated $Paco_2$ at rest. It is not possible to differentiate these "CO_2 retainers" from nonretainers on the basis of history, physical examination, or spirometric pulmonary function testing. This CO_2 retention seems to be more related to an inability to maintain the increased work of respiration (W_{resp}) required to keep the $Paco_2$ normal in patients with mechanically inefficient pulmonary function; it is not primarily due to an alteration of respiratory control mechanisms. It was previously thought that chronically hypoxemic or hypercapnic patients relied on a hypoxic stimulus for ventilatory drive and became insensitive to $Paco_2$. This explained the clinical observation that COPD patients in incipient respiratory failure could be put into a hypercapnic coma by the administration of a high concentration of oxygen (Fio_2). Actually, only a minor fraction of the increase in $PaCO_2$ in such patients is due to a diminished respiratory drive, as minute ventilation is basically unchanged (Parot et al, 1980). The $Paco_2$ rises because a high Fio_2 causes a relative decrease in alveolar ventilation, as well as an increase in alveolar dead space, by the redistribution of perfusion away from lung areas of relatively normal V/Q matching to areas of very low V/Q ratio. Essentially, the high Fio_2 abolishes hypoxic pulmonary vasoconstriction (HPV) in low-V/Q alveoli. The perfusion then returns to these areas because the previously low alveolar oxygen tension (PAO_2) has been augmented by the increased Fio_2, with no local improvement in ventilation. This new perfusion represents an "intrapulmonary steal" of blood flow from previously well-matched V/Q regions, which thus become relatively overventilated, causing an increased alveolar dead space (V_D). Effective alveolar ventilation falls and $Paco_2$ rises with no change in minute ventilation. This occurs in patients who are mechanically unable to augment their minute ventilation to deal with the rising $Paco_2$. During anesthesia in normal patients, the most common cause of an intraoperative decrease in PaO_2 is an increase in V/Q mismatch, and the most common cause of an elevated $Paco_2$ is inadequate minute ventilation. However, in COPD patients, the rise in $Paco_2$ during administration of a high F_{IO_2} is also due to increased V/Q mismatch (Milic-Emilic and Aubier, 1980).

Nocturnal Hypoxemia. COPD patients desaturate more frequently and severely than do normal patients during sleep (Douglas and Flenley, 1990). This is due to the rapid/shallow breathing pattern that occurs in all patients during REM sleep. In COPD patients breathing air, this causes a significant increase in the respiratory dead space/tidal volume (V_D/V_T) ratio, and a fall in Pa_{O_2} and Pa_{O_2}. This is not the sleep-apnea-hypoventilation syndrome (SAHS). There is no increased incidence of SAHS in COPD. In 8 of 10 COPD patients studied, the oxygen saturation fell to less than 50% at some time during normal sleep, and this was associated with an increase in pulmonary artery pressure. This tendency to desaturate, combined with a postoperative fall in FRC and the use of opioid analgesia, places these patients at high risk for severe postoperative hypoxemia, which occurs during sleep.

Flow Limitation. Severe COPD patients are often flow-limited, even during tidal volume expiration at rest. Flow limitation is present in normal patients only during a forced expiratory maneuver. Flow limitation occurs when an equal pressure point (EPP) develops in the intrathoracic airways during expiration. During quiet expiration in the normal patient, the pressure in the lumen of the airways always exceeds the intrapleural pressure because of the upstream elastic recoil pressure transmitted from the alveoli. The effect of this elastic recoil pressure diminishes as air flows downstream in the airway. With forced expiration, the intrapleural pressure may equal the intraluminal pressure at a certain point—the EPP—which then limits the expiratory flow. Then, any increase in expiratory effort will not produce an increase in flow at that given lung volume (O'Donnell et al, 1987).

Flow limitation occurs particularly in emphysematous patients, who primarily have a problem with loss of lung elastic recoil and have marked dyspnea on exertion. Flow limitation causes dyspnea because of stimulation of mechanoreceptors in the muscles of respiration, the thoracic cage, and the airway distal to the EPP. Any increase in the work of respiration leads to increased dyspnea (Kanek et al, 1985). This variable mechanical compression of airways by overinflated alveoli is the primary cause of the airflow obstruction in emphysema. In patients with a predominantly emphysematous pathology versus those with a bronchitic or asthmatic pathology, the FEV_1 is not as valid an indicator of the severity of disease (Geld et al, 1996). This may explain why emphysematous patients frequently show an improvement in symptoms and plethysmographic respiratory function from beta-agonist bronchodilators without a change in FEV_1.

Auto-PEEP. Patients with severe COPD often breathe in a pattern that interrupts expiration before the alveolar pressure has fallen to atmospheric pressure. This incomplete expiration is due to a combination of factors, including flow-limitation, increased W_{resp}, and increased airway resistance. This interruption leads to an elevation of the end-expiratory lung volume to above the functional residual capacity, even above the already increased FRC due to loss of lung elastic recoil. This positive end-expiratory pressure (PEEP) in the alveoli at rest has been termed auto-PEEP or intrinsic PEEP (Tobin and Lodato, 1989). During spontaneous respiration, the intrapleural pressure must be decreased to a level that counteracts auto-PEEP before inspiratory flow can begin. Thus, COPD patients can have an increased inspiratory load added to their already increased expiratory load. Auto-PEEP becomes even more important during mechanical ventilation. It is directly proportional to tidal volume and inversely proportional to expiratory time (T_e). The presence of auto-PEEP is not detected by the manometer of anesthesia ventilators. It can be measured by end-expiratory flow interruption, a feature available on the newer generation of intensive care ventilators. Auto-PEEP can have significant hemodynamic effects; it has been found to develop in most patients during one-lung anesthesia (Slinger et al, 1998).

Right Ventricular Dysfunction. Right ventricular (RV) dysfunction occurs in up to 50% of COPD patients (Klinger and Hill, 1991). The dysfunctional RV, even when hypertrophied, is poorly tolerant of sudden increases in afterload such as the change from spontaneous to controlled ventilation (Myles et al, 1995). Right ventricular function becomes critical in maintaining cardiac output as the pulmonary artery pressure rises. The RV ejection fraction does not increase with exercise in COPD patients, as it does in normal patients.

Chronic recurrent hypoxemia is the cause of the RV dysfunction and the subsequent progression to cor pulmonale. Patients who have episodic hypoxemia in spite of normal lungs (e.g., Central Alveolar Hypoventilation, SAHS) (MacNee, 1994) develop the same secondary cardiac problems as COPD patients. Cor pulmonale occurs in 40% of adult COPD patients with an FEV_1 less than 1 liter and in 70% with a FEV_1 less than .6l. It is now clear that mortality is primarily related to chronic hypoxemia in COPD patients. The only therapy that has been shown to improve long-term survival and decrease right heart strain in COPD is oxygen. COPD patients who have a resting PaO_2 less than 44 mm Hg should receive supplemental home oxygen, as should those who desaturate less than 55 mm Hg with usual exercise (ATS, 1995). The goal of supplemental oxygen is to maintain a PaO_2 of 60 to 65 mm Hg. Diuretics and phlebotomy (if Hct >55%) decrease the signs and symptoms of RV failure. Compared with chronic bronchitics, emphysematous COPD patients tend to have a decreased cardiac output and a mixed venous oxygen tension while maintaining lower pulmonary artery pressures (Shulman et al, 1984).

Preoperative Therapy of COPD. There are four treatable complications of COPD that must be actively sought and therapy begun at the time of the initial prethoracotomy assessment. These include atelectasis, bronchospasm, chest infection, and pulmonary edema. Atelectasis impairs local lung lymphocyte and macrophage function, thereby predisposing the patient to infection (Nguyen et al, 1991). Pulmonary edema can be very difficult to diagnose by auscultation in the presence of COPD and may present very abnormal radiologic distributions (unilateral, upper lobes, etc.). Bronchial hyperactivity may be a symptom of congestive failure. All COPD patients should receive maximal bronchodilator therapy as guided by their symptoms. Only 20% to 25% of COPD patients respond to corticosteroids. In a patient who is poorly controlled on sympathomimetic and anticholinergic bronchodilators, a trial of corticosteroids may be beneficial (Nisar et al, 1992). It is not clear if corticosteroids are as beneficial in COPD as they are in asthma.

Physiotherapy. Patients with COPD have fewer postoperative pulmonary complications when a perioperative program of intensive chest physiotherapy is followed. Among the different modalities available (e.g., cough and deep breathing, incentive spirometry, PEEP, continuous positive airway pressure [CPAP]), there is no proven superior method (Stock et al, 1985). The important variable is the time spent with the patient and devoted to chest physiotherapy. Family members or nonphysiotherapy hospital staff can easily be trained to perform effective chest physiotherapy. Even in the most severe COPD patient, it is possible to improve exercise tolerance with a physiotherapy program (Niederman et al, 1991). Little improvement is seen before 1 month has passed. Among COPD patients, those with excessive sputum benefit the most from chest physiotherapy.

Pulmonary Rehabilitation. A comprehensive program of pulmonary rehabilitation involving physiotherapy, exercise, nutrition, and education has been shown to consistently improve functional capacity for patients with severe COPD (Kesten, 1997). These programs are usually of several months' duration and are generally not an option in resection for malignancy, although for nonmalignant resection in severe COPD patients, rehabilitation should be considered. The benefits of short-duration rehabilitation programs prior to malignancy resection have not been fully assessed.

Smoking Cessation

Patients having cardiac surgery showed no decrease in incidence of respiratory complications unless smoking was discontinued for longer than 8 weeks before surgery (Warner et al, 1984). Postoperative respiratory complications in patients who stopped for longer than 8 weeks were not frequent (17%), and were not different from those of nonsmokers (11%). The complication rates were higher for those who never stopped (48%) and for those who stopped for less than 8 weeks (56%). Chronic obstructive pulmonary disease was not specifically documented in this study. Carboxyhemoglobin concentrations decrease if smoking is stopped for longer than 12 hours. It is advisable for patients to discontinue smoking for longer than 8 weeks before surgery. The value of shorter periods of abstinence is uncertain. However, complications are decreased in thoracic surgical patients who are not smoking versus those who continue to smoke up until the time of surgery (Dales et al, 1993). It is extremely important for patients to avoid smoking postoperatively. Smoking leads to a prolonged period of tissue hypoxemia. Wound tissue oxygen tension correlates with wound healing and resistance to infection (Jonsson, 1988).

Lung Cancer

At the time of initial assessment, cancer patients should be assessed for the "4 M's" associated with malignancy: mass effects, metabolic abnormalities, metastases, and medications. The use of medications that can exacerbate oxygen-induced pulmonary toxicity such as bleomycin (Ingrassia et al, 1991) and amiodarone (Van Meigham et al, 1994) should be documented.

Postoperative Analgesia

The strategy for postoperative analgesia should be developed and discussed with the patient during the initial preoperative assessment. It is at this time that the risks and benefits of the various forms of post-thoracotomy analgesia should be explained to the patient. Potential contraindications to specific methods of analgesia should be determined, such as coagulation problems, anticoagulant therapy, sepsis, or neurologic disorders. If the patient is to receive prophylactic anticoagulants and the use of epidural analgesia has been selected, then appropriate timing of anticoagulant administration and neuraxial catheter placement needs to be arranged. A common practice is to administer prophylactic anticoagulants after the epidural catheter has been put in place.

Premedication

Premedication should be discussed and ordered at the time of the initial preoperative visit. The most important aspect of preoperative medication is to avoid inadvertent withdrawal of those drugs that are taken for concurrent medical conditions (e.g., bronchodilators, antihypertensives, and β-blockers). For some types of thoracic surgery, such as esophageal reflux surgery, oral antacids and H_2-blockers are routinely ordered preoperatively. Currently, we do not routinely order preoperative sedation or analgesia for pulmonary resection patients. Mild sedation such as an intravenous short-acting benzodiazepine is often given immediately prior to placement of invasive monitoring lines and catheters. In patients with copious secretions, an antisialogogue (such as glycopyrrolate) is useful to facilitate fiberoptic bronchoscopy for positioning of a double-lumen tube or bronchial blocker. To avoid an intramuscular injection, this can be given orally or intravenously immediately after placement of the intravenous catheter. It is common practice to use short-term intravenous antibacterial prophylaxis such as a cephalosporin in thoracic surgical patients. If it is the local practice to administer these drugs prior to admission to the operating room, then they will have to be ordered preoperatively. Consideration for those patients allergic to cephalosporin or penicillin will have to be made at the time of the initial preoperative visit. Recently, our practice has changed from using vancomycin to giving clindamycin to these patients.

TABLE 5–2 ■ Preanesthetic Assessment for Pulmonary Resection

Initial	
ALL PATIENTS	Exercise tolerance, ppoFEV_1%, ? postoperative analgesia, D/C smoking
ppoFEV_1<40%	DLCO, V/Q scan, Vo_2 max
CANCER PATIENTS	The "4 M's": mass effects, metabolic effects, metastases, medications
COPD PATIENTS	Arterial blood gas, physiotherapy, bronchodilators
INCREASED RENAL RISK	Creatinine, BUN
Final	
Review initial assessment and test results. Assess risk of hypoxemia during one-lung ventilation. Assess difficulty of lung isolation: chest radiograph, CT scan.	

BUN, blood urea nitrogen; COPD, chronic obstructive pulmonary disease; CT, computed tomography; DLCO, diffusion capacity for carbon monoxide; ppoFEV_1, predicted postoperative forced expiratory volume in one second; V/Q, ventilation/perfusion.

Final Preoperative Assessment

The final preoperative anesthetic assessment for the majority of thoracic surgical patients is carried out immediately prior to admission of the patient to the operating room. At this time, it is important to review the data from the initial prethoracotomy assessment, as well as the results of tests ordered at that time (Table 5–2). At this time, in addition to routine preanesthetic information, two other specific areas affecting thoracic anesthesia need to be assessed: the potential for difficult lung isolation and the risk of desaturation during one-lung ventilation (Table 5–3).

Difficult Endobronchial Intubation

Anesthesiologists are familiar with the clinical assessment of the upper airway for ease of endotracheal intubation. In a similar fashion, each thoracic surgical patient must be assessed for ease of endobronchial intubation. At the time of the preoperative visit, historical factors or physical findings may lead to suspicion of difficult endobronchial intubation (e.g., previous radiotherapy, infection, or prior pulmonary or airway surgery). In addition, there may be a written bronchoscopy report with a description of anatomic features. However, fiberoptic bronchoscopy is not totally reliable for estimating potential problems with endobronchial tube positioning. The single most useful predictor of difficult endobronchial intubation is the plain chest radiograph (Fig. 5–3).

TABLE 5–3 ■ Factors that Correlate with an Increased Risk of Desaturation During One-Lung Ventilation

- High percentage of ventilation or perfusion to the operative lung on preoperative ventilation-perfusion scan
- Poor Pao_2 during two-lung ventilation, particularly in the lateral position intraoperatively
- Right-sided surgery
- Good preoperative spirometry (FEV_1 or FVC)

FEV_1, forced expiratory volume in 1 second; FVC, forced vital capacity.

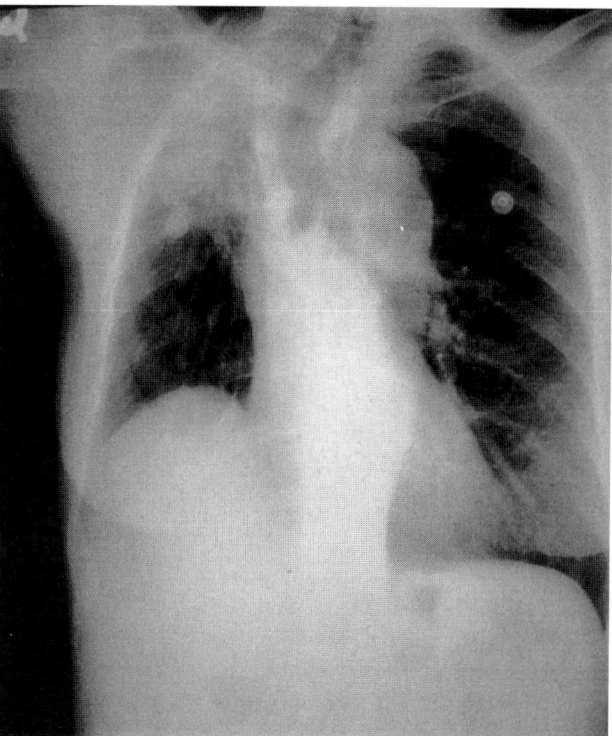

FIGURE 5–3 ■ Preoperative chest radiograph of a 50-year-old female presenting with hemoptysis for a right thoracotomy and possible completion pneumonectomy. The radiologist's report mentions a mass in the right apex and old scarring in the left apex. No verbal or written report can easily describe the obvious potential problem this woman presents for placement of a left-sided, double-lumen endobronchial tube, which can readily be appreciated by examining the actual radiograph.

Endobronchial problems not evident on the plain chest film can sometimes be visualized on the computed tomography (CT) scan. The major factors in successful lower airway management are anticipation and preparation (based on the preoperative assessment).

Prediction of Desaturation During One-Lung Ventilation

In the vast majority of cases, it is possible to predict which patients are most at risk of desaturation during one-lung ventilation (OLV) for thoracic surgery. The factors that correlate with desaturation during OLV are listed in Table 5–3. Identification of those patients most likely to desaturate allows the anesthesiologist and the surgeon to make a more informed decision about the intraoperative use of OLV. In patients at high risk of desaturation, prophylactic measures can be used during OLV to decrease this risk. The most useful prophylactic measure is the use of continuous positive airway pressure (CPAP)—2 to 5 cm H_2O of oxygen to the nonventilated lung (Slinger et al, 1988). Because this tends to make the surgical exposure more difficult, particularly during video-assisted thoracic surgery (VATS), it is worthwhile to identify early those patients who will require CPAP so that it can be instituted at the start of OLV.

The most important predictor of Pao_2 during OLV is the Pao_2 during two-lung ventilation. Although the preoperative Pao_2 correlates with the intraoperative OLV Pao_2, the strongest correlation is with the intraoperative Pao_2 during two-lung ventilation in the lateral position, prior to OLV. The proportion of perfusion or ventilation to the nonoperated lung on preoperative V/Q scans also correlates with the Pao_2 during OLV (Hurford et al, 1987). If the operative lung has little perfusion preoperatively as the result of unilateral disease, the patient is unlikely to desaturate during OLV.

The side of the thoracotomy has an effect on Pao_2 during OLV. Because the left lung is 10% smaller than the right, there is less shunt when the left lung is collapsed. In a series of patients, the mean Pao_2 during left thoracotomy was approximately 70 mm Hg higher than during right thoracotomy (Lewis et al, 1992). The degree of obstructive lung disease correlates in an inverse fashion with Pao_2 during OLV. Other factors being equal, patients with more severe airflow limitation on preoperative spirometry tend to have better Pao_2 during OLV than do patients with normal spirometry. The etiology of this seemingly paradoxical finding is unclear but may be related to the development of auto-PEEP during OLV in obstructed patients (Myles, 1996).

INTRAOPERATIVE MANAGEMENT

Positioning

The majority of thoracic procedures are performed with the patient in the lateral position, most often the lateral decubitus position; however, depending on the surgical technique, a semisupine or semiprone lateral position may be used. These positions have specific implications.

Position Changes

It is awkward to induce anesthesia with the patient in the lateral position. Thus, monitors will be placed and anesthesia will usually be induced in the supine position, then the anesthetized patient will be repositioned for surgery. It is possible to induce anesthesia with the patient in the lateral position, and this may rarely be indicated with unilateral lung diseases, such as bronchiectasis or hemoptysis, until lung isolation can be achieved. However, even these patients will then have to be repositioned, and the diseased lung turned to the nondependent side.

Owing to the loss of venous vascular tone in the anesthetized patient, it is not uncommon to see hypotension when the patient is turned to or from the lateral position. This can occur at the beginning or at the end of the procedure and is more marked in patients who have a degree of intravascular volume depletion and in those with sympathetic blockade from epidural local anesthesia. All lines and monitors will have to be secured during position change and their function reassessed after repositioning. It is useful to make an initial "head-to-toe" survey of the patient after induction and intubation to check oxygenation, ventilation, hemodynamics, lines, monitors, and potential nerve injuries. This survey then must be repeated after repositioning. It is nearly impossible to avoid some movement of a double-lumen tube or bronchial blocker during repositioning (Klein et al, 1998). Certainly, the patient's head, neck, and endobronchial tube should be turned "en bloc" with the patient's thoracolumbar spine. However, the margin of error in positioning endobronchial tubes or blockers is often so narrow that even very small movements can have significant clinical implications. The carina and mediastinum may shift independently with repositioning, and this can lead to distal malplacement of a previously well-positioned tube. Endobronchial tube or blocker position and the adequacy of ventilation must be rechecked by auscultation and fiberoptic bronchoscopy after the patient has been repositioned. Access for additional intravascular lines will be more difficult to attain after the patient has been repositioned. This should be anticipated and all lines placed, whenever possible, with the patient supine.

Neurovascular Complications

There is a specific set of nerve and vascular injuries related to the lateral position that must be understood and appreciated. The brachial plexus is the site of the majority of intraoperative nerve injuries related to the lateral position. These are two varieties: The majority are compression injuries of the brachial plexus of the dependent arm, but there is also significant risk of stretch injury to the brachial plexus of the nondependent arm. The brachial plexus is fixed at two points—proximally by the transverse process of the cervical vertebrae, and distally by the axillary fascia. This two-point fixation, plus the extreme mobility of neighboring skeletal and muscular structures, makes the brachial plexus extremely prone to injury. The patient should be positioned with padding under the dependent thorax to keep the weight of the upper body off the dependent arm brachial plexus. However, this padding will exacerbate the pressure on the brachial plexus if it migrates rostrally into the axilla.

The brachial plexus of the nondependent arm is most at risk if it is suspended from an arm support or "ether screen." Traction on the brachial plexus in these situations is particularly likely to occur if the patient's trunk accidentally slips toward a semiprone or semisupine position after fixation of the nondependent arm. *Vascular* compression of the nondependent arm in this situation is also possible, and it is useful to monitor pulse oximetry in the nondependent hand to observe for this. The arm should not be abducted beyond 90 degrees, and it should not be extended posteriorly beyond the neutral position, nor flexed anteriorly more than 90 degrees.

Anterior flexion of the arm at the shoulder (circumduction) across the chest, or lateral flexion of the neck toward the opposite side can cause a traction injury of the suprascapular nerve. This causes a deep, poorly circumscribed pain in the posterior and lateral aspects of the shoulder and may be responsible for some cases of post-thoracotomy shoulder pain. It is very easy, after the patient has been repositioned in the lateral decubitus position, to cause excessive lateral flexion of the cervical spine because of improper positioning of the patient's head. This malpositioning, which exacerbates brachial plexus traction, can cause a "whiplash" syndrome and can be difficult to appreciate after the surgical drapes have been placed. It is useful to survey the patient from the side of the table immediately after turning, to ensure that the entire vertebral column is aligned properly.

The dependent leg should be slightly flexed, with padding under the knee to protect the peroneal nerve lateral to the proximal head of the fibula. The nondependent leg is placed in a neutral extended position, and padding placed between it and the dependent leg. The dependent leg must be observed for vascular compression. Excessively tight strapping at the hip level can compress the sciatic nerve of the nondependent leg. Other sites particularly prone to neurovascular injury in the lateral position are the dependent ear pinna and eye.

Physiologic Changes in the Lateral Position

Ventilation. Significant changes in ventilation develop between the lungs when the patient is placed in the lateral position. This has been explained by the theory that the lungs move up and down a common compliance curve, with the dependent lung becoming less compliant and the nondependent lung more compliant. However, the reality is more complex (Larsson et al, 1987). The compliance curves of the two lungs are different because of their difference in size. The lateral position, use of anesthesia, paralysis, and opening of the thorax all combine to magnify these differences between the lungs.

The compliance curve (change in volume versus change in pressure) of a lung depends on the balance of two "springs"—the chest wall (normally distending the lung) and the elastic recoil of the lung itself. Any factor that changes the mechanics of either of these springs places the lung on a different compliance curve (Nunn, 1993).

In a healthy, conscious, spontaneously breathing patient, the ventilation of the dependent lung increases by approximately 10% when the patient is turned to the lateral position. Once the patient is anesthetized and paralyzed, the ventilation of the dependent lung then decreases by 15%. Although the distribution of ventilation does not change significantly once the nondependent hemithorax is open, the FRC of this lung tends to increase by approximately 10%. These changes depend on the method used for ventilation in the individual patient. When the chest is open, owing to disruption of the chest wall, both lungs tend to collapse to a minimal lung volume if expiration is prolonged. Thus the end-expiratory volume of each lung is directly a function of the time allowed for expiration. The compliance of the entire respiratory system increases significantly after the nondependent hemithorax is opened (Werner et al, 1984b).

Because of the decrease in FRC and the compliance of the nondependent lung in the lateral position, selective application of PEEP to only this lung improves gas exchange (Bachrendtz and Klingstadt, 1984). However, this is different from the effect of nonselectively applying PEEP to both lungs in the lateral position, where PEEP tends to preferentially go to the most compliant lung regions and to hyperinflate the nondependent lung without causing any improvement in gas exchange (Rehder et al, 1973).

Atelectasis develops in an average of 6% of the lung parenchyma after induction of anesthesia in the supine position. This atelectasis is evenly distributed in the dependent portions of both lungs in the supine position (Klingstedt et al, 1990). Turning the patient to the lateral position results in a slight decrease of total atelectasis to 5% of lung volume, but this is now concentrated totally in the dependent lung.

Perfusion. The teaching has been that turning the patient from the supine to the lateral position will decrease the blood flow of the nondependent lung owing to gravity. This decrease has been assumed to be approximately 10% of the total pulmonary blood flow (Benumof, 1985). However, recent animal work has led to some question about the effect of gravity on pulmonary blood flow distribution (Mure et al, 1998). The distribution of pulmonary blood flow in various positions may be more related to inherent pulmonary vascular anatomic factors than to gravity. The matching of ventilation and perfusion is usually decreased in the lateral compared with the supine position. The pulmonary arteriovenous shunt usually increases from approximately 5% in the supine position to 10% to 15% in the lateral position (Slinger, 1990).

Intraoperative Monitoring

General to All Pulmonary Resections. The majority of these are major operative procedures of moderate duration (2–4 hours); they are performed with the patient in the lateral position with the hemithorax open. Thus, consideration for monitoring and maintenance of body temperature and fluid volume should be given to all of these cases. Monitors are initially placed in the supine position; they have to be rechecked and often repositioned after the patient is turned. It is often very difficult to add additional monitoring, particularly invasive vascular monitoring, after the case is started if complications arise. Thus the risk/benefit ratio often tends to favor overly invasive procedures at the outset. Several intraoperative complications that can occur during all types of surgery are more prone to occur during thoracotomy. The choice of monitoring should be guided by knowledge of the anticipated incidence of specific complications.

Specific to Certain Types of Resection. Some complications are more likely to occur with certain resections—for example, hemorrhage from an extrapleural pneumonectomy, contralateral lung soiling with resection of a cyst or bronchiectasis, or air-leak hypoventilation or tension pneumothorax with a bronchopleural fistula. Monitoring for these specific types of resections is directed in part by the intraoperative complications associated with the underlying surgical disease.

Oxygenation

Significant desaturation (<90%) during one-lung ventilation occurs in approximately 10% of the surgical population in spite of a high FIO_2 (1.0). The significant risk of hypoxemia during one-lung ventilation was one of the major factors that created the demand for on-line monitoring of intraoperative oxygenation. However, for several reasons, pulse oximetry (SpO_2) has not negated the need for direct measurement of arterial PaO_2 via intermittent blood gases in the majority of thoracotomy patients.

First, the PaO_2 value offers a more useful estimate than the SpO_2 of the margin of safety above desaturation. A patient with a two-lung ventilation PaO_2 greater than 400 mm Hg, with an FIO_2 of 1.0 (or an equivalent PaO_2/FIO_2 ratio) is unlikely to desaturate during one-lung ventilation, whereas a patient with a PaO_2 of 200 mm Hg is prone to desaturate during OLV, although both may have SpO_2 values of 99% to 100%. Second, the rapidity of the fall in PaO_2 after the onset of OLV is an indicator of the risk of subsequent desaturation. For this reason, it is useful to measure PaO_2 by arterial blood gases (ABGs) prior to OLV, and 20 minutes after the start of OLV. Third, the delay time for detection of falls in SpO_2 in the supranormal ranges of oxygenation used in thoracic surgery is much longer than for continuous monitoring systems of PaO_2. However, on-line monitoring systems of PaO_2 using optode or similar technology continue to be plagued by problems of reliability and intravascular positioning "wall effect," and are not in widespread clinical use at present. Fourth, there are significant "manufacturer" differences in the accuracy of SpO_2. Although the trends are reliable, before a specific cut-off of SpO_2 value is used as a guideline for treatment of hypoxemia, the accuracy of the oximeter model used should be verified intraoperatively with the ABG measurement. During hypoxemia, SpO_2 sensor malpositioning can cause significant underestimation of saturation (Barker et al, 1993).

Capnometry

It has been shown that the end-tidal CO_2 (PET_{CO2}) is a less reliable indicator of the arterial $PaCO_2$ during one-lung ventilation than during two-lung ventilation, and this $PaCO_2$- PET_{CO2} difference tends to increase during OLV. Although the PET_{CO2} is less directly correlated with alveolar minute ventilation during OLV, because the PET_{CO2} also reflects lung perfusion and cardiac output, it gives an indication of the relative changes in perfusion of the two lungs, independently, during position changes and during OLV. As the patient is turned to the lateral position, the PET_{CO2} of the nondependent lung falls relative to the dependent lung (Werner et al, 1984a), reflecting increased perfusion of the dependent lung and increased dead space of the nondependent lung. However, the fractional excretion of CO_2 is higher from the nondependent lung in most patients owing to the increased fractional ventilation of this lung. Patients with higher fractional excretion of CO_2 from the dependent lung (i.e., better perfusion) during two-lung ventilation tend to have better PaO_2 values during OLV. At the onset of OLV, the PET_{CO2} of the dependent lung usually falls transiently as all the minute ventilation is transferred to this lung. The PET_{CO2} then rises as the fractional perfusion is increased to this dependent lung by collapse and pulmonary vasoconstriction of the nonventilated lung. If there is no correction of minute ventilation, the net result will be both an increased baseline $PaCO_2$ and PET_{CO2} with an increased gradient. However, severe (>5 mm Hg) or prolonged falls in PET_{CO2} can indicate a maldistribution of perfusion between ventilated and nonventilated lungs; these falls may be an early warning of a patient who will subsequently desaturate during OLV.

Invasive Hemodynamic Monitoring

Arterial Line. A significant incidence of transient severe hypotension results from surgical compression of the heart or great vessels during intrathoracic procedures. For this reason, and because of the helpfulness of intermittent ABG sampling, it is useful to have beat-to-beat assessment of systemic blood pressure during the majority of thoracic surgery cases. Exceptions naturally occur during limited procedures such as thoracoscopic resections in younger and healthier patients. For most thoracotomies, a radial artery catheter can be placed in either the dependent or the nondependent arm.

Central Venous Pressures. Central venous pressure (CVP) monitoring and access is a routine procedure for thoracic surgery in many centers. However, it is a common impression that CVP readings with the patient in the lateral position with the chest open are not completely reliable. Certainly, the CVP is a useful monitor postoperatively, particularly in cases for which fluid management is critical (e.g., pneumonectomies). It is our practice to routinely place CVP lines in pneumonectomy patients but not for lesser resections unless there is significant other concurrent illness. For lobectomies that unforseeably become pneumonectomies during the course of the surgery, a CVP catheter is placed at the end of the operation. Our choice, unless there is a contraindication, is to use a high anterior approach to the right internal jugular vein to minimize the risk of pneumothorax for CVP access in all patients. Internal jugular CVP data are not reliable in patients with superior vena cava obstruction.

Pulmonary Artery Catheter. Similar to CVP data, intraoperative pulmonary artery (PA) pressure may be a less accurate indicator of true left heart preload in the lateral position with the chest open than in other clinical situations. This is partly because often it is not known initially if the catheter tip lies in the dependent or the nondependent lung. Also, it is possible that thermodilution cardiac output data may be unreliable if there are significant transient unilateral differences in perfusion between the lungs, as can occur during one-lung ventilation and positive pressure. There is, at present, no consensus on the reliability of thermodilution cardiac output data during OLV. When left-sided PA catheter placement is required, it can be achieved in 50% of patients (versus the usual 10%) by floating the catheter into the PA when the patient is in the right lateral position (Parlow et al, 1992). It is usually possible for the surgeon to confirm the placement of the PA catheter once the chest is open. It is important to remember that a PA catheter ipsilateral to the side of surgery must be withdrawn prior to vascular clamping to avoid transsection. Complications from the use of PA catheters, including arrhythmia, hemorrhage, and pulmonary infarction, are well documented. Also, if a PA catheter lies in the nonventilated lung, it frequently becomes accidentally wedged even without balloon inflation as the lung collapses. The risk/benefit ratio for the routine use of PA catheters for pulmonary resection surgery favors their use only in certain specific cases such as in patients with major coexisting disease (cardiac, renal, etc.) or in those having particularly extensive procedures (e.g., extrapleural pneumonectomy).

Fiberoptic Bronchoscopy

It would be incomplete to discuss monitoring of lung resection candidates without reference to the routine use of fiberoptic bronchoscopy to monitor the position of endobronchial tubes or blockers. Significant malpositioning of left- or right-sided double-lumen tubes, which can lead to desaturation during OLV, is often not detected by auscultation or other traditional methods of confirming tube placement. Positioning of double-lumen tubes or blockers should be confirmed whenever possible after the patient is placed in the surgical position because these tubes or blockers frequently migrate during patient repositioning.

Continuous Spirometry

The recent development of side-stream spirometry has made it possible for inspiratory and expiratory pressure, volume, and flow interactions to be continuously monitored during anesthesia. This monitoring is particularly useful during pulmonary resection surgery. An early indicator of accidental changes in the intraoperative position of a double-lumen tube can be detected on-line by observation of changes in the ventilation pressure-volume loops (Simon et al, 1992). The development of a persistent end-expiratory flow during OLV, which correlates with the development of auto-PEEP, can be seen on the flow-volume loop. Also, the ability to accurately assess changes in inspiratory and expiratory tidal volumes is extremely useful in the assessment and management of pulmonary air leaks.

Transesophageal Echocardiography

The clinical usefulness of transesophageal echocardiography (TEE) for pulmonary resection surgery is currently under investigation. In addition to the well-developed usefulness of TEE as an intraoperative monitor of ischemia and cardiac valvular function, several specific areas of pulmonary resection surgery seem to offer potential applications for TEE.

Right Ventricular Function. TEE has been shown to be capable of monitoring intraoperative changes in right ventricular (RV) function induced by changes in RV afterload (Polart et al, 1994). Thermodilution right ventricular ejection fraction (RVEF) has been used to attempt to predict patients who will not tolerate a major resection. Patients whose RVEF remains greater than 35% with normal pulmonary vascular resistance (PVR) will tolerate a pneumonectomy in spite of pulmonary hypertension and borderline pulmonary function tests (Lewis et al, 1992). Early postoperative changes in right heart function documented by transthoracic echocardiography (TTE) have been shown to be more severe in pneumonectomy patients than in lobectomy patients. TEE may be more useful than thermodilution RVEF for detecting intraoperative changes in RV function (Rafferty, 1993). Thus, intraoperative TEE for major pulmonary resection may offer a more accurate and less invasive method of assessing the effects of pulmonary resection on the right heart.

Pulmonary Flow Redistribution. Because it is possible to measure flow velocities in the pulmonary veins by means of the TEE, it may soon be possible to make useful clinical measurements of the blood flow through each lung independently. This will allow monitoring of physiologic changes in blood flow redistribution during OLV; it also may be useful for guiding therapy such as PEEP to improve oxygenation during OLV.

Reversal of Shunt Patent Foramen Ovale. A rare but documented cause of hypoxemia associated with thoracic surgery is reversal of shunt flow through an undiagnosed patent foramen ovale (PFO) (Diabel et al, 1982). When PEEP (to 15 cm H_2O) was applied during controlled ventilation for nonthoracic surgery, 9% of patients developed a right-to-left intracardiac shunt (Jaffe et al, 1992). TEE should be capable of detecting the potential population of patients who might intraoperatively develop a right-to-left interatrial shunt during OLV for thoracic surgery.

Anesthetic Technique

Essentially, any anesthetic technique that provides safe and stable general anesthesia for major surgery can be, and has been, used for lung resection. There is currently a trend toward the use of combined thoracic epidural and general anesthesia for thoracic surgery: In one recent survey, 10 of 12 Australian hospitals reported that thoracic epidural analgesia (TEA) was the standard method of postoperative pain control. Midthoracic epidurals were used in more than 90% of cases; continuous infusions of local anesthetics and opioids were used in more than 90%, and these were continued for longer than 2 days postoperatively in more than 80% of patients (Cook, 1997). Thoracic epidural analgesia has been suggested to shorten the hospital stay.

Fluid Management

Because of hydrostatic effects, excessive administration of intravenous fluids can cause increased shunting and can subsequently lead to pulmonary edema of the dependent lung (Ray et al, 1974). Because the dependent lung is the lung that must carry on gas exchange during one-lung ventilation, it is best to be as judicious as possible with fluid administration. Intravenous fluids are administered only during lung resection anesthesia to replace volume deficits and for maintenance. No volume is given for theoretical third-space losses during thoracotomy. There is no good evidence that such third-space losses occur during lung resection as they do during abdominal or other types of major surgery.

Temperature

Maintenance of body temperature can be a problem during thoracic surgery because of heat loss from the open hemithorax. This is a particular problem at the extremes of the age spectrum. Most of the body's physiologic functions, including hypoxic pulmonary vasoconstriction (HPV), are inhibited during hypothermia. Increasing the ambient room temperature and using a lower-limb forced-air patient warmer are the best methods for preventing inadvertent intraoperative hypothermia.

Prevention of Bronchospasm

Owing to the high incidence of coexisting reactive airways disease in the thoracic surgical population, it is generally advisable to use an anesthetic technique that decreases bronchial irritability. This is particularly important because the added airway manipulation caused by placement of a double-lumen tube or a bronchial blocker is a potent trigger for bronchoconstriction. The principles of anesthetic management are the same as for any asthmatic patient: Avoid manipulation of the airway in a lightly anesthetized patient, use bronchodilating anesthetics, and avoid drugs that release histamine. For intravenous induction of anesthesia, either propofol or ketamine can be expected to diminish bronchospasm. This benefit is not seen with barbiturate, narcotic, benzodiazepine, or etomidate intravenous induction. For maintenance of anesthesia, propofol or any of the volatile anesthetics will diminish bronchial reactivity. Sevoflurane may be the most potent bronchodilator of the volatile anesthetics (Rooke et al, 1997).

Coronary Artery Disease

Because the lung resection population largely comprises elderly patients and smokers, there is a high coincidence of coronary artery disease. This consideration is a major factor in the choice of anesthetic technique for most thoracic patients. The anesthetic technique should optimize the myocardial oxygen supply/demand ratio by maintaining arterial oxygenation and diastolic blood pressure while avoiding unnecessary increases in cardiac output and heart rate. Thoracic epidural anesthesia/ analgesia may aid in this (Saada et al, 1992).

There are two aspects of anesthetic management that are essentially unique to thoracic surgery—lung separation and management of one-lung anesthesia.

Lung Separation

The three methods of lung separation developed in the 1930s and 1940s still form the basis of modern methods of lung isolation. These include single-lumen endobronchial tubes, double-lumen endobronchial tubes, and bronchial blockers. The second half of this century has seen refinements of the double-lumen tube (DLT) from that of Carlens (1949) to a tube specifically designed for intraoperative use (Robertshaw, 1962), with larger, D-shaped lumina and without a carinal hook. Current disposable polyvinyl chloride DLTs have incorporated high-volume low-pressure tracheal and bronchial cuffs. These recent DLT refinements have two major drawbacks: (1) These tubes now require fiberoptic bronchoscopy for positioning (Slinger, 1989); and (2) a satisfactory right-sided DLT has not yet been designed to deal with the short (average 2 cm) and variable length of the right mainstem bronchus. Recently, there has been a revival of interest in bronchial blockers (BBs) resulting from several factors—design advances such as the Univent tube (Inoue, 1982) and the catheter of Arndt and associates (1999), greater familiarity of anesthesiologists with fiberoptic placement of BBs, and possible cost savings.

Indications for Lung Separation

Because it is impossible to describe one technique as best in all indications for one-lung ventilation (OLV), the various indications are considered separately in the following paragraphs.

Elective Pulmonary Resection, Right-Sided. This is the commonest adult indication for OLV. The first choice is a left DLT (Fig. 5–4). There is a wide margin of safety in the positioning of left DLTs (Benumof, 1987). With blind positioning, the incidence of malposition can exceed 20% but is correctable in virtually all cases by fiberoptic adjustment. A partial resection can proceed to a pneumonectomy, if required, without loss of lung isolation. With a DLT, there is continuous access to the nonventilated lung (NV lung) for suctioning, fiberoptic monitoring of

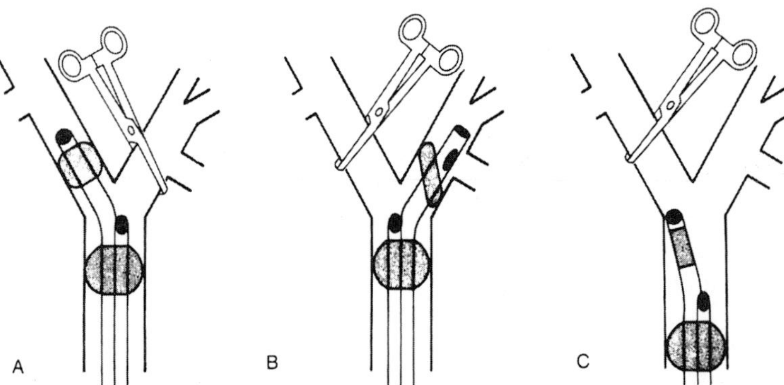

FIGURE 5–4 ■ Use of the left- and right-sided double-lumen endobronchial tubes for left and right lung surgery (as indicated by the *clamp*). *A,* When surgery is performed on the right lung, a left-sided double-lumen tube should be used. *B,* When surgery is performed on the left lung, a right-sided tube can be used. *C,* However, because of the difficulty that may be encountered aligning the ventilating side-slot of a right-sided tube with the right upper lobe bronchial orifice, a left-sided tube can be used and pulled back into the trachea as needed. (From Benumof JL: Anesthesia for Thoracic Surgery. Philadelphia, WB Saunders, 1987.)

position, and continuous positive airway pressure (CPAP), if needed. Possible alternatives include a single-lumen endobronchial tube (EBT) (a standard 7.5-mm, 32-cm-long endotracheal tube [ETT] can be advanced over a fiberoptic bronchoscope [FOB] into the left mainstem bronchus [El Baz et al, 1991]). Or, a Univent tube or BB can be used (the BB can be placed external to, or intraluminally with, an ETT).

Elective Pulmonary Resection, Left-Sided (Not a Pneumonectomy). There is no obvious best choice between a BB and a left DLT. The use of a left DLT for a left thoracotomy is occasionally associated with obstruction of the tracheal lumen by the lateral tracheal wall and subsequent problems with gas exchange in the ventilated lung (V-lung). A right DLT is an alternate choice. Problems with positioning or lung isolation occur much less frequently with right-sided DLTs than was previously thought, when routine FOB placement is used (Campos, 1997).

Left Pneumonectomy. There is no completely satisfactory choice. Any left pulmonary resection may unforeseeably become a pneumonectomy. When a pneumonectomy is foreseen, a right DLT is the best choice. A right DLT permits the surgeon to palpate the left hilum during OLV without interference from a tube or blocker in the left mainstem bronchus. The disposable right DLTs currently available in North America vary greatly in design, depending on the manufacturer (e.g., Mallinckrodt, Rusch, Kendall). The Mallinckrodt design is currently the most reliable. All three designs include a ventilating side-slot in the distal bronchial lumen for right upper lobe ventilation. Positioning this slot can be time consuming. These tubes require relatively high bronchial intracuff pressures (40–50 cm H_2O versus 20–30 cm H_2O for left DLTs). However, this is lower than the range of pressures required by a Univent or by nondisposable DLTs.

Rarely, left lung isolation is impossible in spite of extremely high pressures in the right DLT bronchial cuff. In these cases, a Fogarty catheter can be passed into the left main bronchus after estimation of depth with an FOB. As an alternative, there is no clear preference among a Univent, a left DLT, or another bronchial blocker. These all require intraoperative repositioning, but this usually is not a major problem.

Thoracoscopy. Video-assisted thoracoscopic surgery (VATS) under general anesthesia requires OLV. During open thoracotomy, the lung can be compressed by the surgeon to facilitate collapse prior to inflation of a bronchial blocker. This is not possible during thoracoscopy. The operative lung deflates more easily when the NV lung lumen of a DLT is opened to the atmosphere, than when the 2-mm suction channel of a Univent tube is used. A left DLT is preferred for thoracoscopy of either hemithorax. Spontaneous ventilation without lung isolation is an alternative in some patients (Robinson et al, 1994).

Pulmonary Hemorrhage. Instances of life-threatening pulmonary hemorrhage can occur owing to a wide variety of causes (e.g., aspergillosis, tuberculosis, PA catheter trauma). The primary risk for these patients is asphyxiation, and first-line treatment is lung isolation. There are several problems associated with use of any sort of bronchial blocker in the acute situation: (1) It is often not known which side to occlude; (2) visualization below the vocal cords to aid placement is difficult; and (3) after the blocker is placed, there is no access to the involved lung to monitor bleeding. In patients with pulmonary hypertension, endobronchial blockade can lead to lobar rupture from continued bleeding. A left DLT avoids these problems. Tracheobronchial hemorrhage from blunt chest trauma usually resolves with suctioning; only rarely is lung isolation necessary (Devitt et al, 1991). PA catheter–induced hemorrhage during weaning from cardiopulmonary bypass should be dealt with by resumption of full bypass, bronchoscopy, and lung isolation. Weaning may then proceed without pulmonary resection in some cases (Urschel and Myerowitz, 1993).

Bronchopleural Fistula. This complication involves the triple problem of avoiding tension pneumothorax, ensuring adequate ventilation, and protecting the healthy lung from fluid collection in the involved hemithorax. Management depends on the site of the fistula and the urgency of the clinical situation. For a peripheral bronchopleural fistula in a stable patient, some form of BB such as a Univent tube may be acceptable. For a large central fistula, and in urgent situations, the most rapid and reliable method of securing one-lung isolation and ventilation is a DLT. In life-threatening situations, a DLT can be placed in the awake patient with direct FOB guidance.

Purulent Secretions. For the management of lung abscess and hydatid cysts, lobar or segmental blockade is the ideal. Loss of lung isolation in these cases is not merely a surgical inconvenience, it may be life-threatening. Univent tubes can be used for lobar blockade. A secure technique in these cases is the combined use of a bronchial blocker and a DLT (Otruba and Oxorn, 1992).

Nonpulmonary Thoracic Surgery. Thoracic aortic and esophageal surgery require OLV, as do intrathoracic neurosurgical procedures such as thoracic vertebral resection and sympathectomy. Because there is no risk of ventilated-lung contamination, a left DLT and a BB (Fig. 5–5) are equivalent choices.

Bronchial Surgery. An intrabronchial tumor, bronchial trauma, or a bronchial sleeve resection during lobectomy requires intraluminal access to the ipsilateral mainstem bronchus. Either a single-lumen EBT (Newton et al, 1991) or a DLT in the ventilated lung is preferred.

Unilateral Lung Lavage, Independent Lung Ventilation, and Lung Transplantation. These are all best accomplished with a left DLT.

Upper Airway Abnormalities

It is occasionally necessary to provide OLV in patients who have abnormal upper airways due to previous sur-

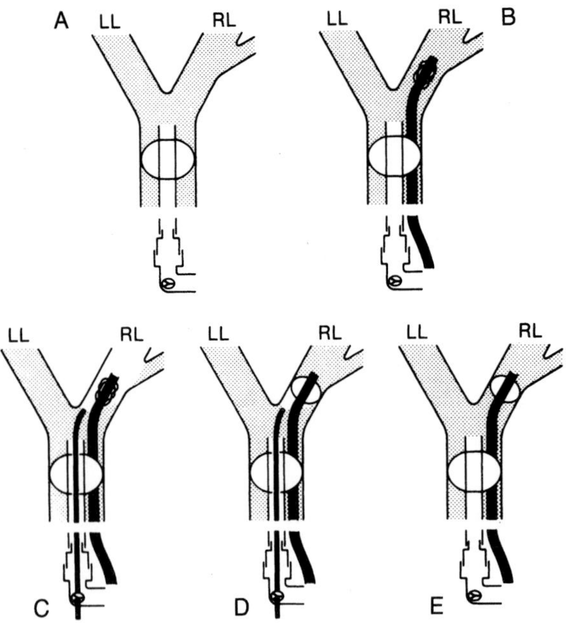

FIGURE 5–5 ■ This figure illustrates the technique of separating the lungs with a single-lumen tube, a fiber-optic bronchoscope, and a bronchial blocker. The sequence of events is as follows. *A,* A single-lumen tube is inserted, and the patient is ventilated. *B,* A bronchial blocker is passed alongside the endotracheal tube. *C,* A fiber-optic bronchoscope is passed through a bronchoscopy connector into the endotracheal tube and used to place the blocker into the desired mainstem bronchus under direct vision; ventilation continues through the endotracheal tube during positioning of the blocker. *D,* The balloon of the bronchial blocker is inflated under direct vision distally in the mainstem bronchus. *E,* The bronchoscope is removed but should remain available to adjust blocker position as needed. (LL, left lung; RL, right lung.) (From Benumof JL: Anesthesia for Thoracic Surgery. Philadelphia, WB Saunders, 1987.)

gery or trauma. The Univent tube may be useful in some of these patients. Smaller DLTs (28 and 26 Fr) are available, but will not permit passage of an FOB of the diameter commonly used to monitor positioning (3.5–4.0 mm). An ETT designed for microlaryngoscopy (5–6 mm internal diameter [ID] and >30 cm in length) can be used as an EBT, with FOB positioning. If the patient's trachea can accept a 7.0-mm ETT, a Fogarty catheter (8/10 Fr venous thrombectomy catheter with a 4-ml balloon) can be passed through the ETT via a fiberoptic bronchoscopy adapter for use as a BB (Larson and Gasior, 1990). If the patient has a tracheostomy, a BB may be used, or a DLT may be inserted through a large tracheal stoma, which occurs when the patient has had a laryngectomy.

Avoiding Airway Trauma

Iatrogenic injury has been estimated to occur in 0.5 to 2 per 1000 cases with DLTs (Massard et al, 1996).

1. The majority of difficult endobronchial intubations can be predicted by viewing the chest radiograph or CT scan.
2. An appropriately sized tube should be used. Too small a tube makes lung isolation difficult. Too large a tube is more likely to cause trauma. Useful guidelines for DLT sizes in adults include the following: females of height less than 1.6 m (63 inch)—35 Fr; females 1.6 m—37 Fr; males of height less than 1.7 m (67 inch)—39 Fr; and males 1.7 m—41 Fr. Tracheobronchial dimensions correlate with height. The average depth at insertion, from the teeth, for a left DLT is 29 cm in an adult; it varies by ±1 cm for each 10 cm of patient height above or below 170 cm (Brodsky et al, 1991).
3. It is prudent to inflate the bronchial cuff or blocker only to the minimum volume required for lung isolation and for the minimum time. This volume is usually less than 3 ml (Slinger and Chripko, 1993). Inflating the bronchial cuff does not stabilize the DLT position when the patient is turned to the lateral position (Desiderio et al, 1997).
4. Nitrous oxide should be used cautiously. Nitrous oxide 70% can increase the bronchial cuff volume from 5 to 16 ml intraoperatively (Peden et al, 1992). The pilot balloon should be periodically assessed during long procedures for signs of elevated pressure.
5. Endobronchial intubation must be done gently and with fiberoptic guidance if resistance is met. A significant number of reports of injury have resulted from patients requiring esophageal surgery in whom the elastic supporting tissue may be weakened and predisposed to rupture from DLT placement.

Other Complications

Malpositioning. Initial malpositioning of DLTs with blind placement can occur in more than 30% of cases (Klein et al, 1998). Verification and adjustment with FOB immediately prior to initiation of OLV is mandatory because these tubes migrate during patient positioning. Malpositioning after the start of OLV due to dislodgment is more of a problem with bronchial blockers than with DLTs.

Airway Resistance. The resistance from a 37 Fr DLT exceeds that of a No. 9 Univent by less than 10% over this range. These flow resistances are both less than those of an 8.0-mm ID ETT, but they exceed those of a 9.0-mm ETT. For short periods of postoperative ventilation and weaning, airflow resistance is not a problem with a DLT.

The three fundamental techniques for lung isolation have not changed over the past 60 years. They include single-lumen endobronchial tubes, double-lumen tubes, and bronchial blockers. The operative team must be comfortable with all three methods of lung isolation to provide adequate lung isolation in the wide variety of patients and clinical situations for which lung separation is now indicated. The **ABC**'s of lung isolation always apply: Know the tracheobronchial **A**natomy, use the fiberoptic **B**ronchoscope, and look at the **C**hest radiograph and CT scan in advance.

Management of One-Lung Ventilation

A unique problem that influences anesthetic management for thoracic surgery is the occurrence of hypoxemia during one-lung ventilation. Reports for the period from 1950 to 1980 describe an incidence of hypoxemia (arterial saturation <90%) of 20% to 25% (Tarhan and Lundborg, 1970). During the 1990s, reports have consistently described an incidence of less than 10% of hypoxemia during one-lung ventilation for thoracic surgery (Hurford and Alfille, 1993). This improvement is most likely due to several factors, including improved lung isolation techniques such as routine fiberoscopy to prevent lobar obstruction from double-lumen tubes, a better understanding of the pathophysiology of one-lung ventilation, and improved anesthetic techniques.

The pathophysiology of one-lung ventilation involves the body's ability to redistribute pulmonary blood flow to the ventilated lung. Several factors can aid or impede this redistribution, and these are under the control of the anesthesiologist to a variable degree.

Intraoperative Position

Most thoracic surgery is performed with the patient in the lateral position, and gravity is thought to increase proportional blood flow to the dependent lung by approximately 10%. In one study, 6 of 8 COPD patients showed an improvement in Pao_2 turning from the supine to the lateral position during OLV (Bardoczky et al, 1998). Recent animal work has cast some doubt on the importance of gravity and position in blood flow distribution (Mure et al, 1998).

Hypoxic Pulmonary Vasoconstriction

This is considered by many authors to be the most important factor governing the redistribution of blood flow during one-lung ventilation. HPV is thought to be able to decrease the blood flow to the nonventilated lung by 50%. The stimulus for HPV is primarily the alveolar oxygen tension (Pao_2), which stimulates precapillary vasoconstriction, redistributing pulmonary blood flow away from hypoxemic lung regions via a pathway involving nitric oxide or cyclooxygenase synthesis inhibition (Lennon and Murray, 1996). The mixed venous Po_2 (Pvo_2) is also a stimulus, although it is considerably weaker than the P_{AO_2}, and the arterial PaO_2 has a biphasic effect on HPV (Marshall et al, 1994).

Surgical trauma to the lung can affect pulmonary blood flow redistribution. Surgery may oppose HPV by release of vasoactive metabolites locally in the lung, or it may cause autonomic effects from trauma to the perihilar plexus. Conversely, surgery can dramatically decrease blood flow to the nonventilated lung by deliberately, or accidentally, mechanically interfering with either the unilateral pulmonary arterial or the venous blood flow.

It is not clear what the mechanical effects of lung collapse are on the pulmonary flow through the nonventilated lung. Some authors have described a local reduction in pulmonary blood flow due to the mechanical effects of collapse. However, this effect may be small and dependent on the experimental preparation because it has not been found in other studies.

Choice of Anesthetic

All of the volatile anesthetics inhibit HPV. This inhibition is dose dependent. Animal studies suggest that this inhibition is also dependent on the agent: Halothane > enflurane > isoflurane. There has been some animal evidence that sevoflurane and desflurane may cause less inhibition. In general, human studies have tended to confirm observations from the animal models, except that no benefit has been shown for sevoflurane or desflurane over isoflurane. Also, no clinical benefit has been shown for total intravenous anesthesia above that seen with the usual clinical concentrations of isoflurane, even though intravenous agents are well documented not to interfere with HPV.

The inability of clinical studies to demonstrate superior oxygenation when vasodilating, volatile anesthetics are avoided during one-lung ventilation (OLV) is not easy to explain. It may be related in part to the fact that the distribution of Pao_2 values in a group of patients during stable OLV is very wide; the standard deviation approaches 100 mm Hg in most studies. Also, the inhibition of HPV by a volatile agent such as isoflurane is only about 20%. This could account for a net difference of only 4% in total shunt during OLV, which is a difference too small to be detected in most clinical studies. In addition, volatile anesthetics cause less inhibition of HPV when delivered to the active site of vasoconstriction via the pulmonary arterial blood than via the alveolus. This pattern is similar to the HPV inhibitory characteristics of oxygen. During established OLV, the volatile agent reaches the hypoxic lung alveoli only via the pulmonary blood. Because the inhibition of HPV is dose dependent, the lower incidence of hypoxemia during OLV in the last decade may be related to the use of lower concentrations of volatile anesthetics. Many of the studies from the 1970s used relatively high doses of halothane.

Cardiac Output

The effects of alterations of cardiac output during OLV are complex. Increasing cardiac output tends to cause increased pulmonary artery pressures and passive dilation of the pulmonary vascular bed, which in turn opposes HPV and has been shown to be associated with increased shunting during OLV. However, in patients with a relatively fixed oxygen consumption, as is seen during stable anesthesia, the effect of an increase in cardiac output is to increase mixed venous oxygen content. Thus, increasing cardiac output during OLV tends to increase both shunt and venous oxygen, which have opposing effects on Pao_2. The net effects of an increase in cardiac output during OLV tend to favor an increase in Pao_2. HPV is decreased by all vasodilators such as nitroglycerin and nitroprusside. In general, vasodilators can be expected to cause a deterioration in Pao_2 during OLV.

Ventilation Strategies

The strategy used to ventilate the ventilated lung during OLV plays an important part in the distribution of pulmonary blood flow between the lungs. It has been the practice of many anesthesiologists to use the same tidal volume during one-lung ventilation as during two-lung ventilation. Although this strategy is adequate for the majority of cases, it is clearly possible to improve gas exchange for selected individual patients by altering the ventilatory variables that are under the control of the anesthesiologist: tidal volume, rate, inspiratory/expiratory ratio, $Paco_2$, peak and plateau airway pressures, and positive end-expiratory pressure.

Respiratory Acid/Base Status. The efficacy of HPV in a hypoxic lung region is increased in the presence of respiratory acidosis and is inhibited by respiratory alkalosis. However, there is no net benefit to gas exchange during OLV from hypoventilation because the respiratory acidosis preferentially increases the pulmonary vascular tone of the well-oxygenated lung, and this opposes any clinically useful pulmonary blood flow redistribution. Overall, the effects of hyperventilation tend to decrease pulmonary pressures.

Positive End-Expiratory Pressure. It is generally accepted that resistance to blood flow through the lung is related to lung volume in a biphasic pattern; it is lowest when the lung is at its functional residual capacity (FRC). As an extension of this, it is theorized that keeping the ventilated lung as close as possible to its normal FRC should favorably encourage pulmonary blood flow to this lung. Several intraoperative factors that are known to alter FRC tend to cause the FRC of the ventilated lung to fall below its normal level; these include lateral position, paralysis, and opening of the nondependent hemithorax, which allows the weight of the mediastinum to compress the dependent lung. Attempts to measure FRC in human patients during OLV have been complicated by the presence of a persistent end-expiratory airflow in most patients. Further investigation has shown that the majority of patients do not actually reach their end-expiratory equilibrium FRC lung volume because of this delayed expiration as they try to exhale a relatively large tidal volume through one lumen of a double-lumen tube. These patients develop an occult positive end-expiratory pressure (auto-PEEP) (Slinger and Hickey, 1998).

Auto-PEEP. Auto-PEEP is most prone to occur in patients with decreased lung elastic recoil, including the elderly and those with emphysema. Auto-PEEP increases as the inspiratory/expiratory (I:E) ratio increases (i.e., as the time of expiration decreases). This auto-PEEP, which averages 4 to 6 cm H_2O in most series of patients studied, opposes factors that tend to diminish dependent-lung FRC during OLV. The effects of applying external PEEP through the ventilator circuit to the lung, in the presence of auto-PEEP, are complex. There tends to be a non-arithmetic additive effect. For most patients with an auto-PEEP of 4 to 6 cm H_2O, the addition of 5 cm external PEEP to the ventilator circuit will result in a net total PEEP to the patient of 7 to 8 cm. Patients with a very low auto-PEEP ($<$2 cm H_2O) will experience a greater increase in total PEEP from a moderate (5 cm H_2O) external PEEP than those with a high level of auto PEEP ($>$10 cm H_2O). Whether the application of PEEP during OLV will improve a patient's gas exchange depends more on the individual's lung mechanics (as demonstrated by the static lung compliance curve) than on the presence or absence of auto-PEEP. If the application of PEEP tends to shift the expiratory equilibration position on the compliance curve toward the lower inflection point (IP) of the curve (i.e., toward the FRC), then external PEEP is of benefit. However, if the application of PEEP raises the equilibration point such that it is farther from the IP, then gas exchange deteriorates. The fall in oxygenation as mean airway pressure is increased is due to the transmission of airway pressure to the pulmonary vasculature and redistribution of blood flow away from the ventilated lung as the airway pressure in the nonventilated hemithorax is atmospheric. Auto-PEEP is difficult to detect and measure using currently available anesthetic ventilators because these ventilators are open to atmosphere during expiration. For auto-PEEP to be detected, the respiratory circuit must be held closed at the end of a normal expiration until an equilibrium appears in the airway pressure. Most current intensive care ventilators can be used to measure auto-PEEP. Many patients show surprisingly high levels of auto-PEEP, often greater than 10 cm H_2O, during OLV using standard ventilatory parameters. Auto-PEEP is dependent on the time of expiration; thus the use of higher I:E ratios or the addition of an end-inspiratory pause tends to increase auto-PEEP.

Tidal Volume. There is without doubt an optimal combination of tidal volume, respiratory rate, I:E ratio, and pressure or volume-controlled ventilation (VCV) for each individual patient during OLV. Traditionally, anesthesiologists have tended to use the same tidal volume for OLV as for two-lung ventilation (e.g., 10 ml/kg). Because of the presumed decrease in FRC with the nondependent thorax open, this was thought to decrease the risk of atelectasis formation in the dependent lung. However, certain individuals have better oxygenation with larger (14 ml/kg) or smaller (8 ml/kg) tidal volumes (Katz et al, 1992). At present, the benefits of alterations in tidal volume are unpredictable. This may be due in part to the interaction of tidal volume with auto-PEEP. The use of 10-ml/kg tidal volumes initially for most patients seems a logical starting point during OLV. Tidal volume should be decreased so that peak airway pressures do not exceed 35 cm H_2O. This corresponds to a plateau airway pressure of approximately 25 cm H_2O. Peak airway pressures exceeding 40 cm H_2O may contribute to hyperinflation damage to the ventilated lung during OLV. Turning the patient to the lateral position increases respiratory dead space and the arterial–to–end-tidal CO_2 tension gradient (a-ET CO_2). This usually requires a 20% increase in minute ventilation to maintain the same $Paco_2$.

Volume-Controlled Versus Pressure–Controlled Ventilation. Traditionally, volume-controlled ventilation has been used in the operating room for all types of surgery. The recent availability of anesthesia ventilators with optional pressure-control modes has made it possible for this form of ventilation to be studied and used during thoracic surgery. In a series of patients, pressure-controlled ventilation resulted in a statistically significant but small improvement in oxygenation (Tugrul et al, 1997). This improvement is most marked (for the same tidal volume) in patients with COPD. Pressure-controlled OLV is very useful in patients with severe obstructive disease such as those undergoing lung volume reduction.

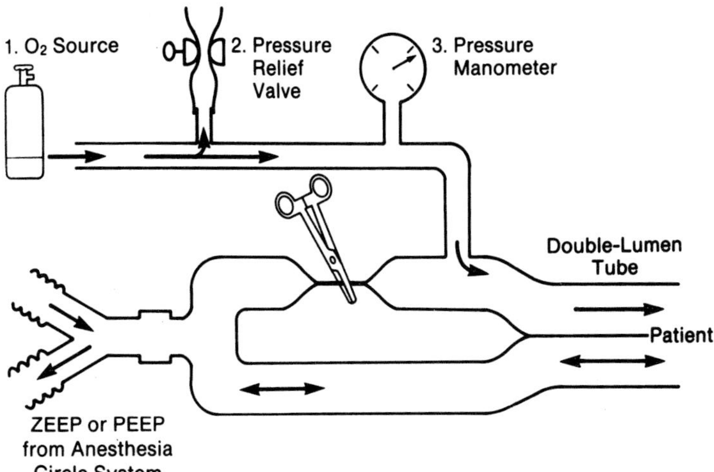

FIGURE 5–6 ■ The three essential components of a nondependent lung continuous positive airway pressure (CPAP) system are (1) an oxygen source, (2) a pressure-relief valve, and (3) a pressure manometer to measure the CPAP. The CPAP is created by the free flow of oxygen into the lung versus the restricted outflow of oxygen from the lung by the pressure-relief valve. (PEEP, positive end-expiratory pressure; ZEEP, zero positive end-expiratory pressure.) (From Benumof JL: Anesthesia for Thoracic Surgery. Philadelphia, WB Saunders, 1987.)

Treatment of Hypoxemia During One-Lung Ventilation

Hypoxemia during one-lung ventilation responds readily to treatment in most cases. Potential therapies are as follows.

Increased FIO_2. The purpose of first-line therapy is normally to increase the FIO_2; this is an option in essentially all patients except those who have received bleomycin or similar therapy that potentiates pulmonary oxygen toxicity.

Continuous Positive Airway Pressure. Continuous positive airway pressure (CPAP) with oxygen to the nonventilated lung is the most useful ventilatory intervention (Capan et al, 1980), apart from augmenting the FIO_2, and has proven to be consistently more reliable at improving oxygenation than other ventilatory maneuvers such as oxygen insufflation to the nonventilated lung, or PEEP to the ventilated lung. There is an important caveat to be observed when CPAP is applied to the nonventilated lung, and that is that CPAP must be applied to a fully inflated lung to be effective. The opening pressure of atelectatic lung regions is greater than 20 cm H_2O; these units will not be recruited by CPAP levels of 5 to 10 cm H_2O. Even a period as short as 5 minutes of collapse prior to CPAP application can have deleterious effects on oxygenation during OLV. When CPAP is properly applied to a fully inflated lung, levels of CPAP as low as 2 to 3 cm H_2O can be used. Because the normal transpulmonary pressure of the lung at FRC is approximately 5 cm H_2O, levels of 5 to 10 cm H_2O CPAP result in a large-volume nonventilated lung, which impedes surgery. Because surgical exposure is the most common indication for one-lung ventilation, it is preferable to use lower levels of CPAP. Owing to lung elastic recoil, this results in a nonventilated lung that is one third to one half of its resting FRC volume; also, during open thoracotomy, it does not interfere with surgical access into the operative hemithorax.

CPAP levels less than 10 cm H_2O do not interfere with hemodynamics. The beneficial effects of low levels of CPAP are primarily due to oxygen uptake from the nonventilated lung and are not due to blood flow diversion to the ventilated lung. CPAP is most effective when oxygen (FIO_2 1.0) is applied to the nonventilated lung. Lower FIO_2 levels of CPAP are of clinical benefit and can be used along with decreased FIO_2 to the ventilated lung in patients at risk of oxygen toxicity.

Numerous anesthetic systems to apply CPAP to the nonventilated lung have been described (Thiagarajah et al, 1984). Essentially all that is required is a CPAP valve and an oxygen source (Fig. 5–6). Ideally the circuit should permit variation of the CPAP level and should include a reservoir bag, to allow easy reinflation of the nonventilated lung, and a manometer, to measure the actual CPAP supplied. Such circuits are commercially available or can be readily constructed from standard anesthetic equipment.

However, CPAP, even when properly administered, is not completely reliable to improve oxygenation during OLV. When the bronchus of the operative lung is obstructed, or is open to the atmosphere (as in a bronchopleural fistula or during endobronchial surgery), CPAP will not improve oxygenation. Also in certain situations, particularly during thoracoscopic surgery in which access to the operative hemithorax is limited, CPAP can interfere with surgery by preventing complete lung collapse.

Positive End-Expiratory Pressure. Positive end-expiratory pressure (PEEP) to the ventilated, dependent lung has often been used to improve oxygenation during one-lung ventilation. During two-lung ventilation in the lateral position, the selective administration of PEEP to the dependent lung can be expected to improve dependent lung mechanics and gas exchange. However, studies of groups of patients consistently show a fall in mean PaO_2 levels when PEEP is applied to the dependent lung during OLV. A small minority (<25%) of patients benefit from PEEP during OLV. Fortunately, these are often the patients with the lowest PaO_2 levels (Cohen and Eisenkraft, 1996).

The unreliability of PEEP for improving PaO_2 during OLV is probably due in part to the interaction of PEEP with auto-PEEP, and in part to the changes that develop in individual lung mechanics during OLV in the lateral position with an open hemithorax. It is possible to identify the subgroup of patients who will benefit from PEEP 5 cm to the ventilated lung during OLV. These are patients with both relatively low $Pa{O_2}$ values during two-lung ventilation in the lateral position (i.e., $Pa{O_2}/F{I}{O_2}$ <360), and with lower than mean auto-PEEP (4 cm H_2O) during OLV.

Tidal volume manipulations benefit certain individuals during OLV, but at present it is not possible to predict which patients, or at what volumes. This is undoubtedly due to complex interaction between the altered lung mechanics and auto-PEEP during OLV. It should be possible with better respiratory monitoring to choose an optimal tidal volume for an individual patient.

Alternative Ventilation Methods. Several alternative methods of one-lung ventilation, all involving partial ventilation of the nonventilated lung, have been described; these improve oxygenation during OLV. These techniques are useful in patients who are particularly at risk of desaturation, such as those who have had previous pulmonary resection of the contralateral lung. These alternatives include the following:

1. *Selective lobar collapse of only the operative lobe in the open hemithorax (Campos, 1997).* This is accomplished by placement of a blocker in the appropriate lobar bronchus of the ipsilateral operative lung.
2. *Differential lung ventilation.* This is done by only partially occluding the lumen of the double-lumen tube to the operative lung (Baraka, 1994).
3. *Intermittent reinflation of the nonventilated lung.* This can be performed by regular re-expansion of the operative lung via an attached CPAP circuit (Malmkvist, 1989).
4. *Two-lung high-frequency positive-pressure ventilation (HFPPV).* The use of very small tidal volume at high rates permits ongoing ventilation of the operative lung with minimal movement of the surgical field (Tsui et al, 1991).
5. *Conventional one-lung ventilation of the nonoperative lung and high-frequency jet ventilation (HFJV) of the operative lung (Godet et al, 1994).* These have both been shown during thoracic surgery to provide superior oxygenation to conventional OLV, or conventional OLV plus CPAP to the nonventilated lung. High-frequency ventilation strategies tend to increase the diameters of the central airways in the operative lung and make pulmonary resection surgically more difficult (Glenski et al, 1986). It seems that these HFV methods are most useful for improving oxygenation during intrathoracic, nonpulmonary surgery such as esophageal or aortic surgery. It has been suggested that avoidance of total intraoperative collapse of the operative lung may improve postoperative pulmonary function and decrease morbidity (Nevin et al, 1987). HFV techniques are also useful because they can be delivered through a catheter in cases involving surgery on the main bronchi, such as sleeve resection (McKinney et al, 1988).

Mechanical Restriction of Pulmonary Blood Flow. It is possible for the surgeon to directly compress or clamp the blood flow to the nonventilated lung. This can be done temporarily in emergency desaturation situations, or definitively in cases of pneumonectomy or lung transplantation. Another technique of mechanical limitation of blood flow to the nonventilated lung is inflation of a pulmonary artery catheter balloon in the main pulmonary artery of the operative lung. The pulmonary artery catheter can be positioned at induction with fluoroscopic guidance, and inflated as needed intraoperatively. This has been shown to be a useful technique for resection of large pulmonary arteriovenous fistulas (Abiad et al, 1995).

Pharmacologic Manipulations. Because patients tend to have a large intrapulmonary shunt (30%–40%) and fixed oxygen consumption during stable one-lung anesthesia, increasing the cardiac output results in a small but clinically useful increase in both $Pv{O_2}$ and $Pa{O_2}$. In a similar sense, eliminating known potent vasodilators such as nitroglycerin and halothane improves oxygenation during OLV.

The use of selective pulmonary vasoactive agents to try to improve oxygenation during thoracotomy has recently been the subject of much interest. The selective administration of the vasodilator prostaglandin E_1 to the ventilated lung (Chen et al, 1996) or a nitric oxide synthase inhibitor (L-NAME) (Freden et al, 1996) to a hypoxic lobe has been shown to result in improved redistribution of pulmonary blood flow in animal models. Selective administration of nitric oxide (NO) alone to the ventilated lung was not shown to be of benefit in humans. The combination of NO (20 ppm) to the nonventilated lung and an intravenous infusion of almitrine, which enhances HPV, has been shown to restore $Pa{O_2}$ values during OLV in humans to essentially the same levels as during two-lung ventilation (Moutafis et al, 1997). It is unlikely that almitrine, which was previously available in North America as a respiratory stimulant, will be reintroduced to this market owing to adverse effects such as hepatic enzyme changes and lactic acidosis. However, the combination of nitric oxide and other pulmonary vasoconstrictors such as phenylephrine has been shown to improve oxygenation in ventilated intensive care unit patients with adult respiratory distress syndrome, and may have applications in OLV.

All treatments outlined as therapy for hypoxemia can be used prophylactically to prevent hypoxemia in patients who are at high risk of desaturation during OLV. These patients can be identified as was previously described in the section on preoperative evaluation, based on data available prior to the onset of OLV. The advantage of *prophylactic* therapy of hypoxemia, in addition to the obvious patient safety benefit, is that maneuvers involving CPAP or alternative ventilation patterns of the operative lung can be instituted at the onset of OLV in a controlled fashion and will not require interruption of surgery and emergent reinflation of the nonventilated lung at a time when it may be extremely disadvantageous.

Ventilation strategies should prioritize the avoidance of hypoxemia and barotrauma over concerns about hypercapnia. Arterial $Pac{O_2}$ of up to 100 mm Hg is well tolerated during OLV for limited periods (Morisaki et al, 1999).

Complex Resections

Bilateral Pulmonary Surgery

Owing to mechanical trauma to the operative lung, the gas exchange in this lung will always be temporarily impaired after one-lung ventilation. Desaturation during bilateral lung procedures is a particular problem during the second period of one-lung ventilation (i.e., during one-lung ventilation of the lung that has already had surgery) (Antognini and Hanowell, 1991). Thus, for bilateral procedures, it is advisable to operate first on the lung that has better gas exchange and less propensity to desaturate during one-lung ventilation. For the majority of patients, this means operating on the right side first.

Bronchopleural Fistula

Whichever surgical procedure is used, there are three specific anesthetic goals in all patients with a bronchopleural fistula. First, healthy lung regions must be protected from soiling by extrapleural fluid from the affected hemithorax. Second, the ventilation technique must avoid development of a tension pneumothorax in the affected hemithorax. And third, the anesthetic technique must ensure adequate alveolar gas exchange in the presence of a low-resistance air leak.

To achieve these three goals, there are two management principles that should be used in essentially all cases. First, a functioning chest drain should be placed prior to the induction of anesthesia and connected to an underwater seal without suction. Second, some method of lung separation should be placed so that the fistula can be isolated as necessary, intraoperatively.

After placement of a chest drain, there are three options for induction of anesthesia. First, a double-lumen tube can be placed in an awake patient with topical anesthesia and its position checked fiberoptically prior to induction. This may be the safest option in some patients because it secures the airway and protects the lung prior to anesthesia and positive-pressure ventilation. However, awake double-lumen intubation is often not simple for either the anesthesiologist or the patient, and most patients can be safely managed using one of the other options. Also, this is often not the best choice in a patient with severely compromised gas exchange because maintaining adequate oxygenation in an already hypoxemic patient can be a problem during awake double-lumen intubation.

The second option for airway management is induction of anesthesia while maintaining spontaneous ventilation until lung isolation is secured. This avoids the risk of tension pneumothorax, and permits favorable matching of ventilation to perfusion. However, a spontaneous ventilation induction may not be desirable if there is a risk of aspiration. Patients with compromised hemodynamics may not tolerate it.

A third option is intravenous induction of general anesthesia and muscle relaxation after meticulous preoxygenation and manual ventilation, using small tidal volumes and low airway pressures until the airway isolation is confirmed. The efficiency of this technique can be improved by using a bronchoscope to guide the double-lumen tube placement during intubation.

The air leak through a bronchopleural fistula is dependent on the pressure gradient between the mean airway pressure at the site of the fistula and the interpleural space. A wide variety of differential methods of ventilation and chest drain management have been used to try to improve the ventilation in patients with bronchopleural fistula both in the operating room and in the intensive care unit. High-frequency ventilation (Bishop et al, 1987), with and without lung or lobar blockade, has been used in certain cases. The lack of agreement on a single best technique for these patients is probably a reflection of the fact that the individual mechanical properties of the air leak vary widely from patient to patient. Similarly, the central-peripheral gradient of mean airway pressures depends on the type of ventilation. High-frequency techniques may permit relatively lower proximal mean airway pressures than does conventional mechanical ventilation, and may be more useful in larger, central air leaks.

Bullae and Blebs

Whenever positive-pressure ventilation is applied to the airway of a patient with a bulla or a bleb, there is risk of rupturing the lesion and causing the development of a tension pneumothorax and bronchopleural fistula. The anesthetic considerations are similar to those for a patient with a bronchopleural fistula, with the exception that it is best not to place a prophylactic chest drain as this may enter the bulla and create a fistula. There is no risk of soiling healthy lung regions with extrapleural fluid, such as exists with fistulas.

For induction of anesthesia, it is usually optimal to maintain spontaneous ventilation until the lung or lobe with the bulla or bleb is isolated. When there is risk of aspiration, or if it is felt that the patient's gas exchange or hemodynamics may not permit spontaneous ventilation for induction, the anesthesiologist must use small tidal volumes and low airway pressures during positive-pressure ventilation until the airway is isolated (Benumof, 1987).

Abscesses, Bronchiectasis, Cysts, Empyema

Chronic infectious lung processes can arise following acute pulmonary infection, or following surgery or trauma. Failure of conservative management with antibotics or closed drainage may lead to the need for surgical intervention. As with bronchopleural fistulas, there is the risk of soiling healthy lung regions with uncontrolled spillage from the lesion. Lung isolation is a primary requirement for anesthesia, and the anesthetic principles and management are similar to those described for fistulas. Also, when an intrathoracic space-occupying lesion is removed, there is the potential for re-expansion pulmonary edema to develop following reinflation of the ipsilateral lung. A slow and gradual reinflation may decrease the severity of this complication (Ray et al, 1984).

MANAGEMENT OF PERIOPERATIVE PAIN

Analgesia during and after thoracic surgery is of particular importance: The classic incision for pulmonary resection, the posterolateral thoracotomy, is reported to be among the most intense clinical pain experiences. The sources of the perceived pain are multiple and depend on the surgical approach; they include the site of the incision, disruption of the ribs and intercostal nerves, inflammation of the chest wall adjacent to the incision, incision or contusion of the pleura and pulmonary parenchyma, and placement of thoracostomy drainage tubes. Additional muscle or joint pain may occur postoperatively, as a result of positioning during surgery. Specifically, ipsilateral shoulder pain is frequently reported after thoracotomy in the lateral decubitus position.

Pain is exacerbated by movement, especially obligatory ventilatory movements, and thus is associated with shallow breathing and inability to cough effectively. Many factors alter pulmonary function and gas exchange after thoracotomy. A restrictive pattern of ventilation is seen after surgery, with significant reductions in forced expiratory volumes for at least 72 hours postoperatively (Craig, 1981). In studies of effort-elicited spirometry, both before and after thoracotomy, expiratory volumes and flow rates measured in the first 24 hours after surgery were between 25% and 67% of preoperative values; increases of 15% to 30% were achieved when a more effective analgesic regimen was used (Sabanathan et al, 1990; Shulman et al, 1984). Hence, effective analgesia allows patients to use an incentive spirometer, to effectively clear secretions, and to participate in chest physiotherapy. Insufficient analgesia is judged to increase the risk of persistent atelectasis and pneumonia, and to hinder early mobilization. Effective pain relief, when integrated with a progressive rehabilitative regimen, is believed to reduce the surgical stress response and organ dysfunction, and to facilitate early oral nutrition and mobilization. Definitive outcome studies are, however, lacking (Kehlet, 1997).

In our practice, a multimodal approach to pain control is adopted; the use of multiple drugs minimizes the side effects of any one. Local anesthetics are used for central neural blockade for major surgery; peripheral nerve blockade and incisional infiltration may be used for smaller incisions. Opioids are used in the neuraxis or systemically. Nonsteroidal anti-inflammatory drugs and acetominophen are used as adjunctive therapy; when delivered consistently, both have an opioid-sparing effect.

Systemic Analgesia

Opioids

Traditional therapy for post-thoracotomy analgesia with systemic opioids (intravenous, intramuscular, subcutaneous) has the significant clinical problem of a narrow therapeutic window. Moderate dose ranges result in adverse effects, including nausea and vomiting, somnolence, and respiratory depression, the latter of which is of particular concern in the context of thoracic surgery. Postoperative pain consists of a constant background pain with acute exacerbation during activity such as cough, deep breathing, and mobilization. Opioids are effective in controlling background pain, but the acute component associated with movement requires plasma levels that might cause sedation at periods of rest. The maintenance of a level of analgesia that does not cause respiratory depression but is adequate to allow mobilization, deep breathing, and coughing is desirable but difficult to achieve with systemic opioids alone. "On demand" intramuscular analgesia has been shown to be ineffective after major surgery. Plasma levels cycle between high peak levels, causing sedation, and ineffective trough levels, causing undue pain. Patient-controlled analgesia (PCA), delivered intravenously, attenuates the peak and trough effects and individualizes analgesia to the patient's requirements. To use PCA effectively, patients need to understand the concept and be physically able to operate the device. The interruption of sleep patterns is inevitable if PCA is in use; plasma levels of opioid become subtherapeutic while the patient is sleeping. The patient must wake up to activate the device. The use of intravenous background infusions of opioid is associated with an increased incidence of respiratory depression. Systemic opioids are generally considered to be the control against which all other treatment modalities are compared, and many studies reflect this (Kavanagh et al, 1994).

Nonsteroidal Anti-Inflammatory Drugs

Nonsteroidal anti-inflammatory drugs (NSAIDs) are frequently used as adjuncts to other forms of analgesia after thoracic surgery; indomethecin has been shown to decrease the opioid requirement by 30% after posterolateral thoracotomy (Pavy et al, 1990). NSAIDs are particularly effective in relief of the pressure and pain at the insertion site of chest tubes, and for the "rubbing" sensation that chest tubes create in the apex or anterior chest wall. Muscle and joint pain related to operative positioning and rib retraction is also relieved. In our practice, all patients who do not have a contraindication to NSAIDs receive perioperative indomethacin (50–100 mg per rectum [PR] q 12 hr) or ketorolac (10–30 mg intravenously [IV] q 6 hr), with dosing dependent on the patient's weight and age. Absolute contraindications include renal insufficiency, peptic ulcer disease with exposure to NSAIDs or recent gastrointestinal hemorrhage, and ongoing surgical bleeding. The low cost of indomethacin results in its frequent use. The duration of NSAID therapy varies between patients, but typically 36 to 48 hours is sufficient, during which period many patients will have had their chest tubes removed. Daily creatinine monitoring is advisable.

NSAIDs act by the reversible inhibition of cyclooxygenase, thereby limiting the production of prostaglandins, prostacyclin, and thromboxane. This has anti-inflammatory benefits but may lead to complications associated with the lack of these eicosanoids. Prostaglandins are involved in gastric protection through the regulation of blood flow to the gastric mucosa, the production of mucus, and the inhibition of gastric acid secretion. Gastrointestinal ulcers in patients taking NSAIDs may be asymptomatic, and are part of a spectrum of diseases that includes erosions and petechiae. Endogenous prostaglandins are important regulators of renal hemodynamics in states of decreased perfusion; in this scenario, NSAIDs can contribute to the development of renal failure. Thromboxane is important for normal platelet function, and platelet aggregation is affected for as long as NSAIDs are present in the circulation (Kruger and McRae, 1999).

These effects are unlikely to cause significant clinical problems with short-term use.

Cyclooxygenase is now known to exist in two isoforms—a constitutive enzyme (COX-1) and an inducible enzyme (COX-2). The eicosanoids produced by COX-2 are suggested to contribute to the inflammatory response, whereas COX-1 is thought to play a role in normal physiologic function. Recently, selective COX-2–inhibiting drugs having an inhibitory effect that is focused on the inflammatory proteins, with a relative sparing of the homeostatic proteins (COX-1), have become available. Meloxicam and celecoxib (Celebrex) are effective anti-inflammatory drugs with fewer gastrointestinal adverse effects, less inhibition of the platelet prostaglandin endoperoxide, and a renal safety profile equivalent to other NSAIDs. Their perioperative use is increasing.

Acetaminophen

Acetaminophen can be a useful adjunct in patients in whom NSAIDs are contraindicated. When it is administered consistently (650 mg q 4 hr per os [PO] or PR), many patients experience considerable relief of muscle and joint pain and chest tube discomfort. Hepatotoxicity is a concern with high doses and prolonged use (>5 g/day for longer than 1 week).

Ketamine

Although it is not widely used in clinical practice, the general anesthetic ketamine in low doses (1 mg/kg intramuscularly [IM]) has been shown to be equivalent to the same dose of meperidine in providing analgesia, but with less respiratory depression (Dich-Nielsen et al, 1992). Laboratory investigation has revealed the role of *N*-methyl-D-aspartate (NMDA) receptor activation in post-injury central sensitization and hyperalgesia, suggesting that ketamine, a noncompetitive NMDA antagonist, may play a role in the treatment of postoperative pain (Kavanagh et al, 1994). Intravenous infusions of ketamine have been used to decrease morphine requirements and may be useful in patients developing spinal cord sensitization. Ketamine will likely be increasingly used as an analgesic adjunct, although the associated psychomimetic effects, particularly hallucinations, will limit the dose range used (Kruger and McRae, 1999).

Blockade of Peripheral Nerves

Local anesthetics may be used to block conduction of the afferent impulse of painful stimuli along intercostal nerves. Single applications of local anesthetic are limited by the duration of action of drug used. To maintain efficacy, repeated injections are required, which are both painful and labor-intensive. Continuous delivery via catheters strategically placed in proximity to nerves supplying the painful area permits prolonged analgesia, but raises concern of local anesthetic toxicity due to systemic drug accumulation.

Recent experimental use of controlled-release bupivacaine in polymer microspheres resulted in analgesia for 48 hours when used for intercostal blocks in an animal model. Longer periods of analgesia resulted when dexamethasone was added to the microspheres. Because of granulomatous reactions found at the sites of injection, the use of bupivacaine-containing microspheres in ongoing clinical trials is currently restricted to wound infiltration (Drager et al, 1998).

Intercostal Blocks

The ventral rami of the twelve thoracic nerves run a lateral course within the groove on the underside of each rib. Intercostal nerve blockade has been used extensively in thoracic surgery. Agents may be delivered percutaneously as a single preoperative treatment, given under direct vision before chest closure, or by postoperative percutaneous injection. The long-acting agent bupivacaine (0.5%) is frequently chosen, with the addition of epinephrine to further prolong its effect. The use of indwelling intercostal catheters is described for infusion or to facilitate repeated injections, but these are not widely used. The main concern with the technique is a high degree of systemic absorption, although clinical studies of patients after thoracic surgery have documented safe plasma levels of local anesthetics. In general, intercostal nerve blockade is effective for supplementing opioid analgesia after thoracotomy pain, but is not adequate as a sole technique.

Extrapleural Paravertebral Blocks

There is renewed interest in the use of unilateral paravertebral neuronal blockade for post-thoracotomy analgesia. The paravertebral space may be located percutaneously and catheterized (Richardson and Lönnqvist, 1998). Alternatively, an extrapleural pocket is made under direct vision, prior to thoracotomy closure; then, a catheter is placed in the most inferior space and directed superiorly (Watson et al, 1999). A local anesthetic bolus through the catheter, when the pleura is intact, spreads over the heads and necks of the ribs above and below the site of injection for at least four dermatomes. Local anesthetic penetrates the intercostal nerves, including the dorsal rami and the sympathetic chain; multilevel intercostal neuronal blockade and unilateral sympathetic blockade are achieved (Richardson and Lönnqvist, 1998). Opioid-sparing effect and improvement in postoperative lung function have been demonstrated using postoperative bupivacaine infusions (Sabanathan et al, 1990). The possibility of systemic bupivacaine toxicity has been investigated because of the high concentrations (0.5%) and volumes (0.1 ml/kg/hr) required for adequate blockade. A steady increase in plasma bupivacaine levels was observed over 5 days of infusion, approaching or exceeding toxic levels on day 4. The free serum bupivacaine levels remained unchanged, however, as the binding protein α_1-acid glycoprotein increased during the postoperative period, providing an explanation for the apparent safety of high concentrations of bupivacaine (Dauphin et al, 1997). Lidocaine has been proposed to be a better choice of drug for extrapleural infusion; a drug with a shorter half-life has less potential for toxicity. Lidocaine (1%) was found to produce equivalent analgesia to bupivacaine

(0.5%) when infused at 0.1 ml/kg/hr in the paravertebral space (Watson et al, 1999).

Extrapleural paravertebral blockade must be distinguished from intrapleural analgesia, whereby local anesthetic is injected into the pleural space. Thirty to forty percent of the local anesthetic is lost if chest tubes are in place. Reports of the efficacy of this technique vary widely (Kruger and McRae, 1999). Objective measures such as improved postoperative pulmonary function or significant opioid-sparing effect are lacking (Kavanagh et al, 1994).

Cryoanalgesia

A cryoprobe may be applied intraoperatively to the posterior aspect of the intercostal nerves at the several interspaces subserving the dermatomal region of the incision. Histologic studies have demonstrated that the resultant nerve injury consists of loss of continuity in the axon with preservation of the endoneurium. Time to recovery of sensation in affected dermatomes depends on the speed of nerve regeneration, in some patients taking as long as 6 months. Although the initial experience with cryoanalgesia was encouraging, later, more definitive studies revealed only minimal efficacy; these studies reported an association between cryoanalgesia and the occurrence of chronic neuralgia (Müeller et al, 1989).

Central Neural Blockade

The mechanisms of action of the delivery of analgesic drugs into the cerebrospinal fluid (intrathecal) and into the epidural space have been extensively reviewed (Cousins and Mather, 1984). There are serious but very infrequent adverse effects, which include spinal cord or nerve trauma, hematoma, and infection or inflammatory reaction associated with introduction of the needle or catheter. Permanent neurologic sequelae are predicted to occur in less than .07% of patients. There is a small risk of headache when puncture of the dura occurs (Giebler, 1997). A single dose of spinal opioid or local anesthetic may be used, particularly for relief of the pain of sternotomy in cardiac surgery. Continuous spinal blockade via an intrathecal catheter is possible, but is not commonly used. The remainder of this discussion addresses continuous epidural analgesia.

Local Anesthetics

Thoracic epidural local anesthetics are administered to create a circumscribed band of dense analgesia in the dermatomal distribution of the thoracic incision. Although epidural local analgesia alone may be effective when given by bolus or by infusion, the sympathectomy created by an extended dense block may cause hypotension and may contribute to excessive fluid loading. Motor block of the limbs occurs with poor catheter placement or excessive dosing. It is our practice to place the epidural catheter into the intervertebral space most closely corresponding to the dermatomal distribution of the incision, and to use a combination of dilute local anesthetic and opioid. Beneficial nonanalgesic effects attributed to the use of epidural local anesthestic include a decrease in the postoperative hypercoagulable state, attenuation of the stress response during surgery, and some cardioprotection due to the blockade of cardiac efferents that induce poststenotic coronary constriction (Kruger and McRae, 1999).

Opioids

Epidural opioid administration has the potential to establish segmental analgesia with little or no contribution from systemic levels of opioid. The lipid solubility of each drug is the primary determinant of its pharmacodynamic profile. Lipophilic drugs such as fentanyl are avidly absorbed by fat; they cross the dura and provide segmental analgesia with rapid onset and short duration of action. The transfer of lipophobic opioids, such as morphine, across the dura is slower, which leads to a slow onset of analgesia. A depot of drug remains in the cerebrospinal fluid for long periods, leading to prolonged analgesia. Morphine, hydromorphone, and meperidine have analgesic effects lasting from 10 to 30 hours, whereas lipophilic agents, such as fentanyl and sufentanil, provide analgesia for approximately 4 hours. Epidural morphine dose requirements are much lower than those for parenteral administration; and intrathecal morphine doses are about one fifth those of epidural morphine, demonstrating a dural transfer fraction of 20% (Kruger and McRae, 1999).

The use of a lipophobic opioid permits analgesic effects far beyond the distribution of local anesthesia. Cephalad flow of cerebrospinal fluid can extend the level of analgesia; as time progresses, a gradient of drug is established from the site of drug delivery. If significant levels reach the medulla, respiratory depression can occur, long after a bolus is administered, or an infusion rate may be increased. Fortunately, delayed respiratory depression is slow in onset and can be readily detected with serial monitoring of respiratory rate and sedation scores, permitting early intervention (deLeon-Casasola et al, 1994). Pruritus and urinary retention are common adverse effects, and both are dose-dependent.

Epidural opioids have been combined with local anesthetics, with the aim of synergistically blocking spinal nociceptive pathways while reducing the dose-related adverse effects of each agent. Investigators have found evidence of such synergism; cerebrospinal fluid levels of sufentanil have been measured to be higher in the presence of bupivacaine, suggesting enhanced availability of the opioid (Hansdóttir et al, 1996). In an animal study, a conformational change of the spinal opioid receptors by bupivacaine was proposed to facilitate morphine-induced antinociception (Tejwani et al, 1992). The use of patient-controlled epidural analgesia (PCEA) for bolus delivery of local anesthetic and opioid-containing solutions allows further tapering of background infusion rates to minimize adverse effects.

An understanding of potential adverse effects and appropriate monitoring permit stabilization of the epidural regimen in a high-intensity unit, as well as continued care on the ward. The safety of neuraxial opioid therapy for routine postoperative care has been established (deLeon-Casasola et al, 1994; Gwirtz et al, 1999). A combination of local anesthetic and opioid is initially used in most patients in our institution; one component may be withdrawn if adverse effects specific to that agent develop.

Pre-emptive Analgesia

The evidence that central nervous system sensitization may increase postoperative pain has recently been reviewed. The hypothesis is that transmission of the noxious afferent input from the incision of the periphery of the central nervous system to the spinal cord induces a prolonged state of central nervous excitability that amplifies subsequent input from the wound, and leads to heightened postoperative pain. By prevention of the transmission of noxious operative input to the spinal cord, a pre-emptive approach can avoid the establishment of central sensitization, resulting in reduced pain, even after the analgesic effects of the pre-emptive agents have worn off (Katz, 2001). The practice of treating pain only after it has been established is being supplanted by a preventative approach. The preincisional administration of systemic analgesic (Katz, 2001), central analgesic (Katz et al, 1992), and peripheral nerve blockade (Richardson and Lönnqvist, 1998), prior to the injury barrage of the incision, is gaining acceptance. The results of clinical studies, however, have proved conflicting. Further research is required to delineate the benefits of pre-emptive analgesia for post-thoracotomy pain. Issues to be determined are the most useful combinations of agents, dosages, timing, and routes of administration, and whether long-term post-thoracotomy chest wall pain can be prevented.

Future Directions

Further advances in perioperative and long-term pain management for thoracic surgery require greater understanding of the mechanisms of the injury incurred by surgery (Benedetti et al, 1998). Reduction in pain is truly a multidisciplinary endeavor. Thoracoscopic surgery, axillary thoracotomy, and muscle-sparing thoracotomy represent an evolution of surgical approach to minimize tissue trauma, resulting in less postoperative pain and less disruption of pulmonary function. Multimodal analgesic regimens represent the current standard of care, but must be tailored to the individual patient, and the procedure performed. The creation of a team of anesthesiologists, surgeons, nurses, and physiotherapists dedicated to thoracic surgery allows hospital staff to acquire expertise from a large number of thoracic patients. Experience with a variety of analgesic techniques is particularly valuable when patients with severely compromised lung function or chronic pain syndromes are cared for.

ANESTHETIC CONSIDERATIONS FOR SPECIFIC THORACIC SURGICAL PROCEDURES

Mediastinoscopy

Paratracheal lymph nodes are sampled during mediastinoscopy through a small suprasternal incision. General anesthesia is almost universally used, with muscle relaxation to prevent coughing, which can produce trauma from the mediastinoscope to surrounding structures. Minimal surgical trespass and the use of short-acting general anesthetic agents have resulted in this procedure being routinely performed on an outpatient basis in our institution, even on patients with significant chronic pulmonary disease. Continuous assessment of right arm perfusion is warranted during manipulation of the mediastinoscope because the innominate artery can be compressed, leading to total cessation of flow to the right upper extremity and right carotid artery. This is particularly important in patients with cerebrovascular disease, in whom transient neurologic deficit has been reported (Ashbaugh, 1970). If the patient's underlying medical condition warrants an arterial line, this should be placed on the right side, with an automatic, noninvasive blood pressure cuff on the left side as a second site for assessing blood pressure. Most patients do not require an arterial line; the pulse oximeter on the right hand, in combination with a second, hand-operated blood pressure cuff ensures continuous flow monitoring on the right and pressure monitoring on both sides.

Torrential hemorrhage may rarely occur from vascular injury at the biopsy site, requiring immediate thoracotomy. Resuscitation fluids administered intravenously in the upper body may spill into the mediastinum. If vascular injury occurs, a lower body intravenous access should be sought (Plummer et al, 1998). Placement of a double-lumen tube may incur significant delay; single-lung ventilation may be achieved with a bronchial blocker, or by advancement of the single-lumen tube into one bronchus. For this reason, the endotracheal tube is left uncut.

Patients are observed in the postanesthetic care unit for signs of stridor or respiratory compromise indicative of vocal cord dysfunction from recurrent laryngeal injury, diaphragmatic dysfunction from phrenic nerve injury, or clinical manifestations of pneumothorax. A chest radiograph is performed prior to discharge.

Mediastinal Mass

Lesions of the mediastinum may be approached via sternotomy or thoracotomy. The anesthetic approach to small lesions does not vary from that of other thoracic procedures. The anesthesiologist is, however, influenced by the presence of a large anterior mediastinal mass (Fig. 5–7). Both complete tracheobronchial obstruction and cardiovascular collapse have occurred with the induction of general anesthesia (Neuman et al, 1984). Positive-pressure ventilation and the use of muscle relaxants contribute to the weight of the mass, thereby compromising vital structures. Under such circumstances, a change to lateral or prone positioning may be life-saving. Rigid bronchoscopy may alternatively bypass the compressed airway. During preoperative assessment, symptoms of concern include positional dyspnea (airway compression) and pre-syncopy during Valsalva's maneuver (pericardial or pulmonary arterial involvement). Superior vena cava obstruction may impair venous return, diminish the utility of upper body intravenous access, and render the upper airway edematous. Among various diagnostic tools,

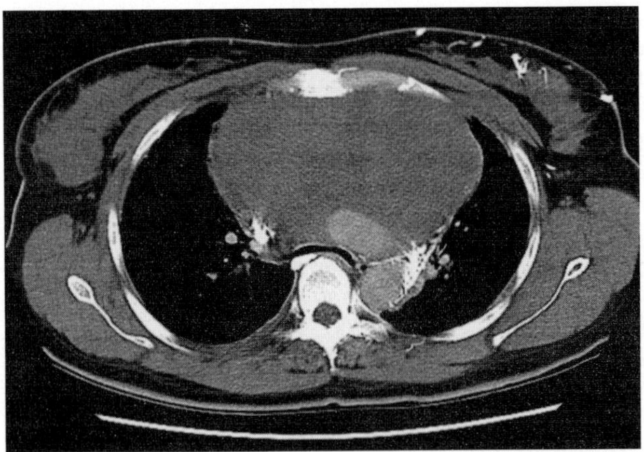

FIGURE 5–7 ■ A computed tomography visualization of severe airway compression at the carinal level by an anterior mediastinal mass.

CT scan, magnetic resonance imaging (MRI), and upright and supine flow-volume loops are useful for the evaluation of compressive airway lesions. Contrast enhancement allows differentiation of vascular involvement.

Surgical intervention is often necessary to ensure an accurate histologic diagnosis; every effort should be made to avoid this high-risk general anesthetic. It may be possible to sample more superficial nodes, or the anterior mass itself, through a small intercostal incision under local anesthesia. Limited preoperative steroid, or radiotherapy, may rapidly decrease the size of the mass, and therefore the risk of general anesthesia; this option should be discussed with the oncology team. If surgery must proceed in a symptomatic patient, awake fiberoptic intubation followed by general anesthesia with spontaneous ventilation has been described (Sibert et al, 1987). A rigid bronchoscope should be immediately available, as well as a stretcher for prone positioning of the patient. Some authors have suggested that all patients in whom imaging reveals more than 50% compression of the airway at the level of the lower trachea or main bronchi should undergo cannulation of their femoral vessels under local anesthesia prior to induction of general anesthesia, in readiness for cardiopulmonary bypass (Goh et al, 1999). A flow chart has been described by Neuman and associates (1984) for the assessment and management of the patient with an anterior mediastinal mass (Fig. 5–8).

Thymectomy for Myasthenia Gravis

Myasthenia gravis is a disease of the neuromuscular junction; affected patients have a decreased number of acetylcholine receptors at the motor endplate. Thymectomy is frequently performed to induce clinical remission. The effects of muscle relaxants are modified by this disease; myasthenic patients are resistant to succinylcholine, so a greater than normal dose is required. The use of succinylcholine is associated with the early onset of phase II block, which can be prolonged. Nondepolarizing muscle relaxants have increased potency and duration, with incomplete antagonism by the intravenous anticholinesterase neostigmine (Baraka et al, 1999). Myasthenic patients

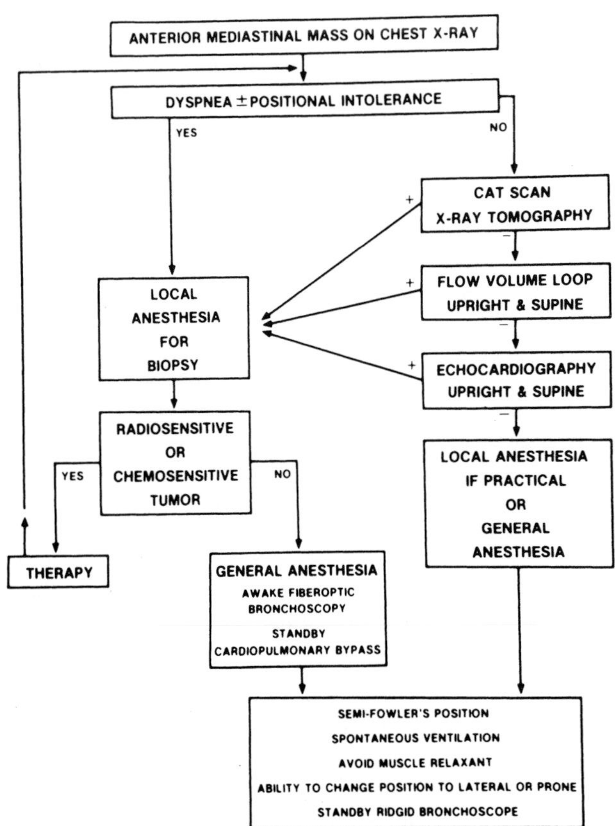

FIGURE 5–8 ■ Flow chart describing the preoperative evaluation of the patient with an anterior mediastinal mass. (−, negative workup; +, positive finding.) (From Neuman G, Weingarten AE, Abramowitz RM et al: The anesthetic management of the patient with an anterior mediastinal mass. Anesthesiology 60:144, 1984.)

are more sensitive to the neuromuscular effects of the halogenated agents and to systemic narcotics. Monitoring for postoperative airway obstruction and hypoventilation is therefore of particular importance.

Thymectomy may be performed via full or partial sternotomy, or a minimally invasive approach via cervicotomy or thoracoscopy may be used. Ideally, the use of neuromuscular relaxation is avoided. Induction of anesthesia with propofol facilitates intubation without the use of muscle relaxants (Scheller et al, 1992). Alternatively, inhalational induction with a halogenated agent such as sevoflurane may be performed. Most patients take pyridostigmine, an oral anticholinesterase, and many patients are on immunosuppressive medication. On the day of surgery, pyridostigmine dosing should be adjusted to ensure coverage of the immediate postoperative period. Some patients require intravenous dosing with neostigmine until they are able to resume oral intake of pyridostigmine.

A scoring system was devised for prediction of the need for prolonged mechanical ventilation after thymectomy via sternotomy. A predictive accuracy of 80% was initially described (Leventhal et al, 1980). Among the criteria that contributed to the predicted need for support were disease duration longer than 6 years, chronic respiratory illness, pyridostigmine dosage greater than 750 mg/day, and vital capacity less than 2.9 liters. When applied to patients undergoing transcervical thymectomy, predictive accuracy fell to 13% (Eisenkraft et al, 1986). Referral for surgery early in the course of the disease and symptom optimization with plasmapheresis, combined with increased use of the transcervical approach, have made the need for postoperative ventilation infrequent.

Esophageal Surgery

Esophageal surgery may be performed for resection of malignant or benign lesions, or for correction of functional abnormality. The potential for esophageal reflux and pulmonary aspiration must be considered at the time of induction, or of emergence from anesthesia, and appropriate antireflux precautions taken. The esophagus may be approached via an abdominal incision (with or without an additional cervical incision) or a lateral thoracotomy, depending on the site of the cancer. Regardless of whether the chest is opened, the diaphragmatic dysfunction that accompanies an upper abdominal incision, combined with trauma to intrathoracic structures, results in a greater degree of respiratory compromise than the extent of the incision would suggest (Siafakas et al, 1999). Pneumonia occurs in as many as 12% of esophagogastrectomy patients (Weissman, 1999).

Fluid management should be liberalized, in contrast to thoracotomy for pulmonary resection, as a significant amount of fluid enters the interstitial space in the abdomen. Volume loading to retain intravascular volume is required; the placement of a central venous catheter is therefore justified, in addition to routine monitors and an arterial line if thoracotomy is performed.

Excellent analgesia is required. Patients benefit from regional analgesia to optimize postoperative pulmonary function, and to facilitate return of spontaneous ventilation. Early extubation after esophagectomy is associated with reduced morbidity and decreased length of stay in high-dependency units. Reductions in hospital stay have been reported when patients receive epidural rather than intravenous morphine (Weissman, 1999). Regional analgesia as part of a multimodal therapy permits good pain control without the use of large doses of parenteral narcotic, which may contribute to postoperative ileus. When the stomach or jejunum is used to replace the esophagus, the neo-esophagus retains a tenuous blood supply; expert management of volume status is required to ensure adequate perfusion of the transplant while providing sufficient analgesia. Increasingly, esophageal procedures are being performed using a laparoscopic approach, thus minimizing tissue trespass, postoperative pain, and pulmonary dysfunction. Laparoscopic upper abdominal surgery, however, is not without respiratory complications, including the occurrence of intraoperative subcutaneous emphysema, pneumothorax, and intravascular carbon dioxide embolism (Wahba et al, 1996).

Lung Volume Reduction

Selected patients with severe, heterogeneous obstructive airway disease may derive benefit from the resection of 20% to 30% of their lung volume. If hyperinflated, poorly perfused areas of the lungs are removed, better ventilation of well-perfused lung may follow, and the benefit of improved pulmonary mechanics may be observed immediately—as early as on emergence from anesthesia. Patients referred for lung volume reduction surgery have extremely reduced FEV_1, often less than 25% of predicted value, and greatly increased residual volume. They are severely dyspneic and frequently oxygen-dependent. When positive-pressure ventilation is initiated, they are prone to dynamic hyperinflation; gas trapping causes increased mean intrathoracic pressure, which can lead to decreased venous return and circulatory compromise. Low peak pressures and increased expiratory time to avoid gas trapping should be used, and extrinsic PEEP should be avoided. Permissive hypercapnia and moderate respiratory acidosis must be tolerated, particularly during one-lung ventilation. Inotropes may be required during positive-pressure ventilation (Conacher, 1997; Triantafillou, 1996).

A double-lumen endotracheal tube is placed in most patients because bilateral volume reduction is usually planned via a thoracoscopic approach. If thoracotomy is required on the first side owing to widespread adhesions, surgery on the second side is postponed. A sternotomy approach may be used in some centers. The prompt return of spontaneous ventilation is paramount. Emphasis is placed on the use of short-acting general anesthetic agents, with minimal residual respiratory depression. A propofol infusion avoids the prolonged emergence from inhaled agents caused by poor V/Q matching. The use of nitrous oxide is avoided because of the potential for enlargement and rupture of noncommunicating bullae. Residual weakness from muscle relaxants is not tolerated. An epidural catheter is placed in all patients, in anticipation of possible thoracotomy, and to optimize analgesia using a multimodal approach. Excellent analgesia is sought to optimize conditions for sustained spontaneous ventilation. At the end of the procedure, the operating table is placed in a sitting position to minimize the weight of the abdominal contents on the diaphragm. When a consistent spontaneous respiratory pattern is observed, the trachea is extubated. Every effort is made to remove the endotracheal tube prior to the onset of coughing, which can significantly increase air leaks from the lung parenchyma. Initially, the patient may require ventilatory assistance with a mask. During recovery from anesthesia, which may be prolonged, constant verbal contact is maintained with the patient. Progressive somnolence is an early sign of hypercapnic respiratory failure. Patients should be nursed in a high-dependency unit in which serial blood gases may be drawn and expert physiotherapy and liberal use of bronchodilator therapy are available. Analgesia is maintained with an epidural infusion of bupivacaine, with or without opioid and systemic NSAIDs.

Lung Transplantation

Anesthetic techniques for pulmonary transplantation vary with the recipient's underlying lung disease, the procedure performed, and regional practices. Care of these patients incorporates principles from both cardiac and thoracic anesthesia. Noninvasive monitors and an arterial line are placed. In our institution, a PA catheter is inserted routinely and is left in place throughout surgery. The PA should be palpated for the presence of the catheter prior to division of the artery; rarely, the catheter must be withdrawn and floated on the other side. We have found that the PA pressure data obtained, even from the operative side, are clinically useful. Transesophageal echocardiography (TEE) is used for establishing a specific diagnosis. Some centers report routine use of TEE during lung transplantation, as well as continuous intra-arterial blood gas analysis. Despite unpredictable end-tidal–to–arterial CO_2 gradients, capnography can be invaluable in monitoring the progress of pulmonary blood flow to a newly reperfused lung, particularly when capnography from each lung is monitored independently.

A variety of induction agents have been described; management of the patient should be guided by underlying disease, airway anatomy, and fasting status. Nitrous oxide is avoided in lung transplantation as it may increase pulmonary vascular resistance, and will expand any gas emboli entrapped in the graft. A narcotic-based anesthetic is given, and provision must be made to ensure amnesia, with a combination of benzodiazepines and propofol infusion.

In Toronto, lung transplantation is performed using cardiopulmonary bypass (CPB) only when indicated. Thirty-three percent of cases require CPB; in 45%, the use of CPB is anticipated for pulmonary hypertension or concomitant cardiac repair; in 55%, CPB is unanticipated and is initiated for hemodynamic instability or inadequate gas exchange. During CPB for cardiac repair, the heart is arrested and the patient is moderately cooled. When lung transplant alone is performed, the heart remains warm and beating. The use of CPB decreases afterload to the right heart, possibly resulting in less right heart dysfunction. There is less hemodynamic instability caused by interruption of venous return by surgical manipulation. Disadvantages in the use of CPB include the obligate infusion of large quantities of crystalloid solution, heparinization with resultant bleeding from raw surfaces, and the occurrence of coagulopathy and fibrinolysis. CPB is associated with activation of neutrophils and platelets, activation of complement, and increased circulating levels of cytokines such as endotoxin, interleukins, and tumor necrosis factor, all of which may contribute to increased reperfusion injury in the allograft. Neurologic deficits and renal dysfunction are common after CPB. The routine use of high-dose steroids in transplantation may attenuate the systemic release of proinflammatory cytokines during transplant procedures using CPB, more so if administered well before initiation of CPB. We therefore administer methylprednisolone 500 to 1000 mg at induction of anesthesia of the recipient, rather than immediately prior to graft reperfusion. The extent to which CPB contributes to morbidity in human lung transplantation is controversial (McRae, 2000a).

During bilateral sequential lung transplantation, initially both lungs are dissected from the chest wall and from the hila. The native lung with the least blood flow on V/Q scan is the first to be removed, followed by engraftment of the first allograft. The allograft is gently reinflated, then ventilated with an FIO_2 of 0.5, PEEP of 5 cm H_2O, and peak airway pressures under 25 cm H_2O. Slow reperfusion of the allograft is accomplished by the removal of the PA clamp over 10 minutes. This modified reperfusion technique promotes vascular recruitment and avoids shear stress injury of high flow reperfusion demonstrated in experimental models. The new allograft is then ventilated with an FIO_2 of 1.0, and removal of the second native lung commences. A period of particular risk of hypoxemia ensues: Ventilation may go preferentially to the compliant allograft, whereas perfusion may be predominantly to the diseased native lung, the vasculature in the allograft being relatively vasoconstricted. Rapid clamping of the native PA improves V/Q mismatch. However, the entire cardiac output is now forced through the allograft, which may amplify pulmonary edema if reperfusion injury has occurred. Separate ventilation of each lung is required in almost all cases, and placement of a left-sided double-lumen tube is preferred.

Ventilation strategy must be adapted to underlying disease. Patients with obstructive airway disease may have hyperinflation and bronchospasm, and are at risk of life-threatening gas trapping with positive-pressure ventilation. Clearance of secretions is important. Patients with pulmonary fibrosis have a reduced gas exchange capability. A small chest cavity often makes surgical manipulation poorly tolerated. High airway pressures, inotropic support, and permissive hypercapnia may be required during one-lung anesthesia so that CPB may be avoided. Patients with vascular disease have near-systemic PA pressures and severe right heart dysfunction with little tolerance for any increase in pulmonary vascular resistance (PVR). Both atelectasis and lung hyperinflation should therefore be avoided. One-lung ventilation is not attempted. All such patients require CPB. The transplanted lung is unique among solid organ transplants in that its primary blood supply, the bronchial circulation, is not surgically re-established. Lung tissue is therefore dependent on collateral flow from the pulmonary circulation to maintain oxygen supply. Thus, when bilateral sequential transplantation is performed using cardiopulmonary bypass, ventilation and perfusion must be provided to the newly reperfused first allograft during engraftment of the second. This is accomplished by reducing the CPB flow to 75% of predicted cardiac output, permitting some ejection of blood into the pulmonary artery (the heart remains warm and beating), and by maintaining ventilation once the allograft is reperfused.

Reperfusion injury is characterized by endothelial dysfunction, increased vascular permeability, and sequestration of neutrophils. Activation of complement occurs. Clinical features include progressive increases in PVR, decreased pulmonary compliance, and impaired gas exchange. Radiographic findings include reticular interstitial infiltrates and air space disease; however, appearance is not related to functional impairment. A spectrum of injury is produced in the transplanted lung, from mild and self-limited dysfunction to fulminant pulmonary edema occurring in the operating room. Injury may be progressive over hours or days. Treatment consists of ventilatory and hemodynamic support and stimulation of cyclic guanosine monophosphate (inhaled nitric oxide) or of cyclic adenosine monophosphate (prostaglandin E_1). In severe pulmonary dysfunction, support with extracorporeal membrane oxygenation (ECMO) has been reported. Nitric oxide (NO) appears to be an important mediator of ischemia-reperfusion injury. Clinically, inhaled NO produces selective pulmonary vasodilatation without systemic hypotension because of avid binding with hemoglobin and a short half-life, making NO an ideal treatment for hypoxia by improved ventilation-perfusion matching. NO may effectively lower PA pressures, thus avoiding the need for CPB during lung transplant procedures. The pulmonary allograft is vulnerable to mechanical and biochemical injury throughout the harvesting, preservation, and engraftment procedures. An understanding of the mechanisms of allograft injury permits the incorporation of strategies for minimizing allograft injury in clinical practice (McRae, 2000b).

■ KEY REFERENCES

Benumof JL: Anesthesia for Thoracic Surgery, 2nd ed. Philadelphia, WB Saunders, 1994.

This single author text is a cohesive review of all aspects of thoracic anesthesia.

Conacher ID: Anaesthesia for the surgery of emphysema. Br J Anaesth 79:530, 1997.

A well-written account of the development of lung volume reduction surgery for patients with end-stage bullous emphysema. The clinical challenges that these patients present and strategies to optimize their ventilation are discussed.

Kavanagh BP, Katz J, Sandler A: Pain control after thoracic surgery; a review of current techniques. Anesthesiology 81:737–759, 1994.

A systematic, critical review of the extensive literature describing analgesic techniques employed for thoracic surgery. The large number of references reviewed reflects the importance of pain management and the variety of approaches to this problem.

Slinger PD: Fiberoptic bronchoscopic positioning of double-lumen tubes. J Cardiothorac Anesth 3:486, 1989.

A clear, concise presentation of a systematic approach to a vital skill in thoracic anesthesia—the placement of double lumen endotracheal tubes using fiberoptic bronchoscopy. Superbly illustrated with line drawings and photographs of the views seen through the bronchoscope, this review allows the reader to recognize correctly positioned and malpositioned double-lumen tubes.

■ REFERENCES

Abiad MG, Cohen E, Krellenstein DL et al: Anesthetic management for resection of a giant pulmonary arterio-venous malformation. J Cardiothorac Vasc Anesth 9:89, 1995.

ACC/AHA American Task Force: Practice guidelines. Anesth Analg 82:854, 1996.

American Thoracic Society: Standards for the diagnosis and care of patients with chronic obstructive pulmonary disease. Am J Respir Crit Care Med 152:S78, 1995.

Antognini SF, Hanowell LH: Intraoperative hypoxemia complicating sequential resection of bilateral pulmonary metastases. Anesthesiology 74:1137, 1991.

Archibald EJ: A consideration of the dangers of lobectomy. J Thorac Surg 4:335, 1935.

Arndt G, Kranner PW, Rusy DA, Love R: Single-lung ventilation in a critically ill patient using a fiberoptically directed wire-guided endobronchial blocker. Anesthesiology 90:1484, 1999.

Ashbaugh DG: Mediastinoscopy. Arch Surg 100:568, 1970.

Bachrendtz S, Klingstadt C: Differential ventilation and selective PEEP during anaesthesia in the lateral decubitus posture. Acta Anaesth Scand 28:252, 1984.

Baraka A: Differential lung ventilation as an alternative to one-lung ventilation during thoracotomy. Anaesthesia 49:881, 1994.

Baraka A, Siddik S, Kawkabani N: Cisatracurium in a myasthenic patient undergoing thymectomy. Can J Anaesth 46:779, 1999.

Bardoczky G, Szegedi L, Capello M et al: Two-lung and one-lung ventilation in COPD patients, the effects of position and F_iO_2. Anesthesiology 89:A1390, 1998.

Barker SS, Hyatt S, Shah NK, Kao J: The effect of sensor malpositioning on pulse oximeter accuracy during hypoxemia. Anesthesiology 79:248, 1993.

Barry J, Mead K, Nadel EC, et al: Effect of smoking on the activity of ischemic heart disease. JAMA 261:398, 1989.

Barthélemy et Dufour: L'anaesthésie dans la chirurgie de la face. Presse Méd 15:475, 1907.

Benedetti F, Vighetti S, Ricco C et al: Neurophysiologic assessment of nerve impairment in posterolateral and muscle-sparing thoracotomy. J Thorac Cardiovasc Surg 115:841, 1998.

Benumof J: One lung ventilation and hypoxic pulmonary vasoconstriction. Anesth Analg 64:821, 1985.

Benumof JL: Sequential one-lung ventilation for bilateral bullectomy. Anesthesiology 67:268, 1987.

Benumof JL: Anesthesia for Thoracic Surgery, 2nd ed. Philadelphia, WB Saunders, 1994.

Benumof JL, Partridge BL, Salvatierra C, Keating J: Margin of safety in positioning modern double-lumen endotracheal tubes. Anesthesiology 67:729, 1987.

Bishop MJ, Benson MS, Sato P, Pierson DJ: Comparison of high frequency jet ventilation with conventional ventilation for bronchopleural fistula. Anesth Analg 66:833, 1987.

Björk VO, Carlens E: The prevention of spread during pulmonary resection by the use of a double lumen catheter. J Thorac Surg 20:151, 1950.

Björk VO, Carlens E, Friberg O: Endobronchial anesthesia. Anesthesiology 14:60, 1953.

Bollinger CT, Wyser C, Roser H et al: Lung scanning and exercise testing for the prediction of postoperative performance in lung resection candidates at increased risk for complications. Chest 108:341, 1995.

Brodsky J, Benumof JL, Ehrenwerth J, Ozaki GT: Depth of placement of left double-lumen endobronchial tubes. Anesth Analg 73:570, 1991.

Campos J, Massa C, Kernstine KH: The incidence of right upper-lobe collapse when comparing a right-sided double-lumen tube versus a modified left double-lumen tube for left-sided thoracic surgery. Anesth Analg 90:535, 2000.

Campos JH: Effects on oxygenation during selective lobar versus total lung collapse with or without continuous positive airway pressure. Anesth Analg 85:583, 1997.

Capan LM, Turndorf H, Patel C et al: Optimization of arterial oxygenation during one-lung anesthesia. Anesth Analg 59:847, 1980.

Carlens E: A new flexible double-lumen catheter for bronchospirometry. J Thorac Surg 18:742, 1949.

Cerfolio RJ, Allen MS, Trastak VF et al: Lung resection in patients with compromised pulmonary function. Ann Thorac Surg 62:348, 1996.

Chen T-L, Ueng TH, Huang C-H et al: Improvement of arterial oxygenation by selective infusion of prostagladin E_1 to the ventilated lung during one-lung ventilation. Acta Anaesthesiol Scand 40:7, 1996.

Cohen E, Eisenkraft SB: Positive end-expiratory pressure during one-lung ventilation improves oxygenation in patients with low arterial oxygen tensions. J Cardiothorac Vasc Anesth 10:578, 1996.

Conacher ID: Anaesthesia for the surgery of emphysema. Br J Anaesth 79:530, 1997.

Cook TM, Riley RH: Analgesia following thoracotomy: A survey of Australian practice. Anaesth Intensive Care 25:520, 1997.

Cousins MJ, Mather LE: Intrathecal and epidural administration of opioids. Anesthesiology 67:427, 1984.

Craig DB: Postoperative recovery of pulmonary function. Anesth Analg 60:46, 1981.

Dales RE, Dionne G, Leech JA, et al: Preoperative prediction of pulmonary complications following thoracic surgery. Chest 104:155, 1993.

Dauphin A, Gupta RN, Young JEM et al: Serum bupivacaine concentrations during continuous extrapleural infusion. Can J Anaesth 44:367, 1997.

deLeon-Casasola OA, Parker B, Lema MJ et al: Postoperative epidural bupivacaine-morphine therapy. Experience with 4227 surgical cancer patients. Anesthesiology 81:368, 1994.

Desiderio DP, Burt M, Kolker AC et al: The effects of endobronchial cuff inflation on double-lumen endobronchial tube movement after lateral decubitus positioning. J Cardiothorac Vasc Anesth 11:595, 1997.

Devitt JH, McLean RF, Koch JP: Anaesthetic management of acute blunt thoracic trauma. Can J Anaesth 38:506, 1991.

Diabel PW, Stutts BS, Jenkins DW et al: Cyanosis following right pneumonectomy. Chest 81:370, 1982.

Dich-Nielsen JO, Svendsen L, Berthelsen P: Intramuscular low-dose ketamine versus pethidine for post-operative pain treatment after thoracic surgery. Acta Anaesthiol Scand 36:583, 1992.

Douglas NJ, Flenley DC: Breathing during sleep in patients with obstructive lung disease. Am Rev Respir Dis 141:1055, 1990.

Drager C, Benziger D, Gao F et al: Prolonged intercostal nerve blockade in sheep using controlled-release of bupivacaine and dexamethasone from polymer microspheres. Anesthesiology 89:969, 1998.

Eisenkraft JB, Papatestas AE, Kahn CH et al: Predicting the need for postoperative mechanical ventilation in myasthenia gravis. Anesthesiology 65:79, 1986.

El Baz N, Faber L, Kittle F, Warren W: Single-lumen tube for two-lung and one-lung ventilation during thoracic surgery. Anesth Analg 72:s64, 1991.

Ferguson MK, Reeder LB, Mich R: Optimizing selection of patients for major lung resection. J Thorac Cardiovasc Surg 109:275, 1995.

Flagg PJ: Intratracheal inhalation: Preliminary report of a simplified method of intratracheal anesthesia developed under the supervision of Dr. Chevalier Jackson. Arch Otolaryngol 5:394, 1927.

Freden F, Berglund JE, Reber A et al: Inhalation of a nitric oxide synthase inhibitor to a hypoxic lung lobe in anaesthetized pigs. Br J Anaesth 77:413, 1996.

Gale JW, Waters RM: Closed endobroncheal anesthesia in thoracic surgery: Preliminary report. J Thorac Surg 1:432, 1932.

Geld AF, Hogg JC, Muller NL: Contribution of emphysema and small airways in COPD. Chest 109:353, 1996.

Ghent WS, Olsen GN, Hornung CA et al: Routinely performed multigated blood pool imaging (MUGA) as a predictor of postoperative complication of lung resection. Chest 105:1454, 1994.

Giebler RM, Scherer RV, Peters J: Incidence of neurological complications related to thoracic epidural catheterization. Anesthesiology 86:55, 1997.

Glenski JA, Crawford M, Reheder K: High-frequency, small volume ventilation during thoracic surgery. Anesthesiology 64:211, 1986.

Godet G, Bertrand M, Rouby JJ, et al: High-frequency jet ventilation vs. continuous positive airway pressure for differential lung ventilation in patients undergoing resection of thoraco-abdominal aneurysms. Acta Anaesthesiol Scand 38:562, 1994.

Goh MH, Liu XY, Goh YS: Anterior mediastinal masses: An anaesthetic challenge. Anaesthesia 54:670, 1999.

Golledge J, Goldstraw P: Renal impairment after thoracotomy: Incidence, risk factors and significance. Ann Thorac Surg 58:524, 1994.

Graham AE, Singer JJ: Successful removal of the entire lung for carcinoma of the bronchus. JAMA 101:1371, 1933.

Guedel AE: Cyclopropane anesthesia. Anesthesiology 1:13, 1940.

Guedel AE, Treweek DN: Ether apnoeas. Curr Res Anesth Analg 13,263, 1934.

Guedel AE, Waters RM: Endotracheal anesthesia; a new technic. Ann Otol (St. Louis) 40:1139, 1931.

Gwirtz KH, Young JV, Byers RS et al: The safety and efficacy of intrathecal opioid analgesia for acute postoperative pain: Seven years' experience with 5969 surgical patients at Indiana University Hospital. Anesth Analg 88:599, 1999.

Hansdóttir V, Woestenborghs R, Nordberg G: The pharmacokinetics of continuous epidural sufentanil and bupivacaine infusion after thoracotomy. Anesth Analg 83:401, 1996.

Hedensteirna G: Gas exchange pathophysiology during anesthesia. Anesthesiol Clin N Am 16:113, 1998.

Hurford WE, Alfille PH: A quality improvement study of placement and complications of double-lumen endobronchial tubes. J Cardiothorac Vasc Anesth 7:517, 1993.

Hurford WE, Kokar AC, Strauss HW: The use of ventilation/perfusion lung scans to predict oxygenation during one-lung anesthesia. Anesthesiology 64:841, 1987.

Ingrassia TS III, Ryu JH, Trasek VF, Rosenow EC III: Oxygen-exacerbated bleomycin pulmonary toxicity. Mayo Clin Proc 66:173, 1991.

Inoue H: New device for one-lung anesthesia: Endotracheal tube with movable blocker. J Thorac Cardiovasc Surg 83:940, 1982.

Jaffe RA, Pinto FS, Schmittger I: Aspects of mechanical ventilation affecting intra-atrial shunt flow during general anesthesia. Anesth Analg 75:484, 1992.

Jonsson K, Hunt TK, Mathes SJ: Oxygen as an isolated variable influences resistance to infection. Ann Surg 208:783, 1988.

Kanek R, Fahey PS, Vanderworf C: Oxygen cost of breathing. Chest 87:126, 1985.

Katz J: Pre-emptive analgesia: Importance of timing. Can J Anaesth 48:105, 2001.

Katz J, Kavanagh BP, Sandler AN et al: Pre-emptive analgesia: Clinical evidence of neuroplasticity contributing to postoperative pain. Anesthesiology 77:439, 1992.

Kavanagh BP, Katz J, Sandler A: Pain control after thoracic surgery; a review of current techniques. Anesthesiology 81:737–759, 1994.

Kearney DJ, Lee TH, Reilly JJ et al: Assessment of operative risk in patients undergoing lung resection. Chest 105:753, 1994.

Kehlet H: Multimodal approach to control postoperative pathophysiology and rehabilitation. Br J Anaesth 78:606, 1997.

Kesten S. Pulmonary rehabilitation and surgery for end-stage lung disease. Clin Chest Med 18:174, 1997.

Klein U, Karzai W, Bloos F et al: Role of fiberoptic bronchoscopy in conjunction with the use of double-lumen tubes for thoracic anesthesia. Anesthesiology 88:346, 1998.

Klinger JR, Hill NS: Right ventricular dysfunction in chronic obstructive pulmonary disease. Chest 99:715, 1991.

Klingstedt C, Hedenstierna G, Lundgust A et al: The influence of body position and differential ventilation on lung dimensions and atelectasis formation in anaesthetized man. Acta Anaesthesiol Scand 34:315, 1990.

Kruger M, McRae K: Pain management in cardiothoracic practice. Surg Clin North Am 79:2, 1999.

Larson CE, Gasior TA: A device for endobronchial blocker placement during one-lung anesthesia. Anesth Analg 71:311, 1990.

Larsson A, Malmkvist G, Warner O: Variations in lung volume and compliance during pulmonary surgery. Br J Anesth 59:585, 1987.

Lennon PE, Murray PA. Attenuated hypoxic pulmonary vasoconstriction during isoflurane anesthesia is abolished by cyclooxygenase inhibition in chronically instrumented dogs. Anesthesiology 84:404, 1996.

Leventhal SR, Orkin FK, Hirsh RA: Predicting postoperative ventilatory need in myasthenia gravis. Anesthesiology 53:26, 1980.

Lewis JW, Serwin JP, Gabriel FS et al: The utility of a double-lumen tube for one-lung ventilation in a variety of non-cardiac thoracic surgical procedures. J Cardiothorac Vasc Anesth 6:705, 1992.

MacNee W: Pathophysiology of cor pulmonale in chronic obstructive pulmonary disease. Am J Respir Crit Care Med 150:833, 1994.

Magill IW: Endotracheal anaesthesia. Proc Roy Soc Med 22:1, 1928.

Magill IW: Anaesthesia in thoracic surgery with special reference to lobectomy. Proc Roy Soc Med 29:643, 1936.

Malmkvist G: Maintenance of oxygenation during one-lung ventilation. Anesth Analg 68:763, 1989.

Markos J, Mullan BP, Hillman DR et al: Preoperative assessment as a predictor of mortality and morbidity after lung resection. Am Rev Respir Dis 139:902, 1989.

Marshall B, Clarke WR, Costarino AT et al: The dose response relationship for hypoxic pulmonary vasoconstriction. Respir Physiol 96:231, 1994.

Massard G, Rouge C, Dabbagh A: Tracheobronchial lacerations after intubation and tracheostomy. Ann Thorac Surg 61:1483, 1996.

McKenna RJ, Fischel RJ, Brenner M, Gelb AF: Combined operations for lung volume reduction surgery and lung cancer. Chest 110:885, 1996.

McKinney M, Coppel DL, Gibbons JR, Cosgrove J: A new technique for sleeve resection and major bronchial resection using twin catheters and high frequency jet ventilation. Anaesthesia 43:25, 1988.

McRae K: Lung transplantation should not be routinely performed with cardiopulmonary bypass. J Cardiothorac Vasc Anesth 14:746, 2000a.

McRae KM: Pulmonary transplantation. Curr Opin Anesthesiol 13:53, 2000b.

Milic-Emilic J, Aubier M: Some recent advances in the study of control of breathing in patients with chronic obstructive lung disease. Anesth Analg 59:865, 1980.

Miller JI: Thallium imaging in preoperative evaluation of the pulmonary resection candidate. Ann Thorac Surg 54:249, 1992.

Mizushima Y, Noto H, Sugiyama S et al: Survival and prognosis after pneumonectomy in the elderly. Ann Thorac Surg 64:193, 1997.

Morisaki H, Serita R, Innami Y et al: Permissive hypercapnia during thoracic anaesthesia. Acta Anaesth Scand 43:845, 1999.

Moutafis M, Liu N, Dalibon N et al: The effects of inhaled nitric oxide and its combination with intravenous almitrene on P_aO_2 during one-lung ventilation in patients undergoing thoracoscopic procedures. Anesth Analg 85:1130, 1997.

Müeller LC, Salzer GM, Ransmayr G et al: Intraoperative cryoanalgesia for postthoracotomy pain relief. Ann Thorac Surg 48:15, 1989.

Mure M, Domino KB, Robertson T et al: Pulmonary blood flow does not redistribute in dogs with reposition from supine to left lateral position. Anesthesiology 89:483, 1998.

Myles P: Auto-PEEP may improve oxygenation during one-lung ventilation. Anesth Analg 83:1131, 1996.

Myles P, Madder H, Morgan EB: Intraoperative cardiac arrest after unrecognized dynamic hyperinflation. Br J Anaesth 74:340, 1995.

Nakahara K, Ohno K, Hashimoto J et al: Prediction of postoperative respiratory failure in patients undergoing lung resection for cancer. Ann Thorac Surg 46:549, 1988.

Neuman GG, Weingarten AE, Abramowitz RM et al: The anesthetic management of the patient with an anterior mediastinal mass. Anesthesiology 60:144, 1984.

Nevin M, Van Besouw JP, Williams CW, Pepper JR: A comparative study of conventional versus high frequency jet ventilation with relation to the incidence of postoperative morbidity in thoracic surgery. Ann Thorac Surg 44:625, 1987.

Newton JR, Grillo HC, Mathisen DJ: Main bronchial sleeve resection with pulmonary conservation. Ann Thorac Surg 52:1272–1275, 1991.

Nguyen DM, Mulder DS, Shennib H: Altered cellular immune function in atelectatic lung. Ann Thorac Surg 151:76, 1991.

Niederman MS, Clemente P, Fein AM et al: Benefits of a multidisciplinary pulmonary rehabilitation program. Chest 99:798, 1991.

Ninan M, Sommers KE, Landranau RJ et al: Standardized exercise oximetry predicts post pneumonectomy outcome. Ann Thorac Surg 64:328, 1997.

Nisar M, Eoris JE, Pearson MG, Calverly PMA: Acute broncho-dilator trials in chronic obstructive pulmonary disease. Am Rev Respir Dis 146:555, 1992.

Nunn JF: Applied Respiratory Physiology, 4th ed. Cambridge, Butterworth Heinmann, 1993, pp 48–52 (Chap 3).

O'Donnell DE, Sami R, Anthonisen NR, Younes M: Effect of dynamic airway compression on breathing pattern and respiratory sensation in severe chronic obstructive pulomonary disease. Am Rev Respir Dis 135:912, 1987.

Olsen GN: Lung cancer resection. Who's inoperable? Chest 108:289, 1995.

Olsen GN, Bolton JW, Weiman DS, Hornung CA: Stair climbing as an exercise test to predict the postoperative complications of lung resection. Two years' experience. Chest 99:587, 1991.

Osaki T, Shirakusa T, Kodate M et al: Surgical treatment of lung cancer in the octogenarian. Ann Thorac Surg 57:188, 1994.

Otruba Z, Oxorn D: Lobar bronchial blockade in bronchopleural fistula. Can J Anaesth 39:176, 1992.

Parlow JL, Milue B, Cervenko FW: Balloon flotation is more important than flow direction in determining the position of flow-directed pulmonary artery catheters. J. Cardiothorac Vasc Anesth 6:202, 1992.

Parot S, Saunier C, Gauthier H et al: Breathing pattern and hypercapnia in patients with obstructive pulmonary disease. Am Rev Respir Dis 121:985, 1980.

Pavy T, Medley C, Murphy DF: Effect of indomethacin on pain relief after thoracotomy. Br J Anaesth 65:624, 1990.

Peden CJ, Galizia EJ, Smith RB: Bronchial trauma secondary to intubation with a PVC double-lumen tube. J Roy Soc Med 85:705, 1992.

Plummer S, Hartley M, Vaughan RS: Anaesthesia for telescopic procedures in the thorax. Br J Anaesth 80:223, 1998.

Polart JI, Visser CA, Everaest JA et al: Doppler evaluation of right ventricular out flow impedence during positive pressure ventilation. J Cardiothorac Vasc Anesth 8:392, 1994.

Rafferty T, LaMantia KR, Davis E et al: Quality assurance for intraoperative transesophageal echocardiography monitoring. Anesth Analg 76:228, 1993.

Rao TKK, Jacob KH, El-Etr AA: Reinfarcation following anesthesia in patients with myocardial infarction. Anesthesiology 59:499, 1983.

Rao V, Todd TRJ, Kuus A et al: Exercise oximetry versus spirometry in the assessment of risk prior to lung resection. Ann Thorac Surg 60:603, 1995.

Ray JF III, Yost L, Moallem S et al: Immobility, hypoxemia and pulmonary arteriovenous shunting. Arch Surg 109:537, 1974.

Ray RJ, Alexander CM, Chen L et al: Influence of the method of re-expansion of atelectatic lung upon the development of pulmonary edema in dogs. Crit Care Med 12:364, 1984.

Rehder K, Wenthe FM, Sesslar AD: Function of each lung during mechanical ventilation with ZEEP and with PEEP in man anesthetized with triopental-meperidine. Anesthesiology 39:597, 1973.

Richardson J, Lönnqvist PA: Thoracic paravertebral block. Br J Anaesth 81:230, 1998.

Ritchie AJ, Bowe P, Gibbons JRP: Prophylactic digitalisation for thoracotomy: A reassessment. Ann Thorac Surg 50:86, 1990.

Ritchie AJ, Danton M, Gibbons JRP: Prophylactic digitalisation in pulmonary surgery. Thorax 47:41, 1992.

Robertshaw FL: Low resistance double-lumen endobronchial tubes. Br J Anaesth 34:576, 1962.

Robinson RJS, Slinger P, Mulder DS et al: Video-assisted thorascopic surgery using a single-lumen tube in spontaneously ventilating anesthetized patients: An alternative anesthetic technique. J Cardiothorac Vasc Anesth 8:693–695, 1994.

Rooke GA, Choi JH, Bishop MS: The effect of isoflurane, halothane, sevoflurane and triopental/nitrous oxide on respirator resistance after tracheal intubation. Anesthesiology 86:1294, 1997.

Rowbotham S, Magill IW: Anaesthetics in plastic surgery of the face and jaws. Proc Roy Soc Med (Section of Anaesthetics) 14:17, 1921.

Saada M, Catoire P, Bonnet F et al: Effect of thoracic epidural anesthesia combined with general anesthesia on segmental wall motion assessed by transesophageal echocardiography. Anesth Analg 75:329, 1992.

Sabanathan S, Mearns AJ, Bickford Smith PJ et al: Efficacy of continuous extrapleural nerve block on post-thoracotomy pain and pulmonary mechanics. Br J Surg 77:221, 1990.

Sauerbruch EF: Present status of surgery of the thorax. JAMA 51:808, 1908.

Scheller MS, Zornow MH, Saidman LJ: Tracheal intubation without the use of muscle relaxants: A technique using propofol and varying doses of alfentanil. Anesth Analg 75:788, 1992.

Shulman M, Sandler AN, Bradley JW et al: Postthoracotomy pain and pulmonary function following epidural and systemic morphine. Anesthesiology 61:569, 1984.

Siafakas NM, Mitrouska I, Bouros D et al: Surgery and the respiratory muscles. Thorax 54:458, 1999.

Sibert K, Biondi JW, Hirsch NP et al: Spomtaneous respiration during thoracotomy in a patient with a mediastinal mass. Anesth Analg 66:904, 1987.

Simon BA, Hurford WE, Alfille PH et al: An aid in the diagnosis of malpositioned double-lumen tubes. Anesthesiology 76:862, 1992.

Slinger P: Fiberoptic bronchoscopic positioning of double-lumen tubes J Cardiothorac Anesth 3:486, 1989.

Slinger P, Chripko D: A clinical comparison of bronchial cuff pressures in three different designs of left double-lumen tubes. Anesth Analg 79:305, 1993.

Slinger P, Hickey D: The infraction between applied PEEP and auto-PEEP during one-lung ventilation. J Cardiothorac Vasc Anesth 12:133, 1998.

Slinger P, McRae K, Winton T et al: Arterial oxygenation during thoracic surgery: A comparison of isoflurane and sevoflurane. Anesth Analg 86:SCA40, 1998.

Slinger P, Triolet W, Wilson J: Improving arterial oxygenation during one-lung ventilation. Anesthesiology 68:291, 1988.

Slinger PD: Anesthesia for lung resection. Can J Anaesth 37:Sxv, 1990.

Slinger PD: Perioperative fluid management for thoracic surgery: The puzzle of post-pneumonectomy pulmonary edema. J Cardiothorac Vasc Anesth 9:442, 1995.

Stock MC, Downs JB, Gauer PK et al: Prevention of postoperative pulmonary complications with CPAP, incentive spirometry and conservative therapy. Chest 87:151, 1985.

Tarhan S, Lundborg RO: Effects of increased expiratory pressure on blood gas tensions and pulmonary shunting during thoracotomy with the use of the Carlens catheter. Can Anaesth Soc J 17:4, 1970.

Tejwani G, Rattan A, McDonald JS: Role of spinal opioid receptors in the antinociceptive interactions between intrathecal morphine and bupivacaine. Anesth Analg 74:726, 1992.

Thiagarajah S, Job C, Rao A: A device for applying CPAP to the non-ventilated upper lung during one-lung ventilation. Anesthesiology 60:254, 1984.

Tobin MJ, Lodato RF: PEEP, auto-PEEP and waterfalls. Chest 96:449, 1989.

Triantafillou AN: Anesthetic management for bilateral volume reduction surgery. Semin Thorac Cardiovac Surg 8:94, 1996.

Tsui SL, Chan CS, Chan ASH et al: A comparison of two lung high frequency positive pressure ventilation and one-lung ventilation plus 5 cm H_2O non-ventilated lung CPAP in patients undergoing anaesthesia for oesophagectomy. Anaesth Intensive Care 19:205, 1991.

Tugrul M, Camci E, Karadeni H et al: Comparison of volume controlled with pressure controlled ventilation during one-lung anesthesia. Br J Anesth 79:306, 1997.

Urschel JD, MyerowitzPD: Catheter-induced pulmonary artery rupture in the setting of cardiopulmonary bypass. Ann Thorac Surg 56(3):585–589, 1993.

Van Miegham W, Collen L, Malysse I et al: Amiodarone and the development of ARDS after lung surgery. Chest 105:1642, 1994.

Wahba RWM, Tessler MJ, Kleinman SJ: Acute ventilatory conplications during laparoscopic upper abdominal surgery. Can J Anaesth 43:77, 1996.

Walsh GL, Morice RC, Putnam JB et al: Resection of lung cancer is justified in high risk patients selected by oxygen consumption. Ann Thorac Surg 58:704, 1994.

Warner MA, Diverti MB, Tinker JH: Preoperative cessation of smoking and pulmonary complications in coronary artery bypass surgery. Anesthesiology 60:383, 1984.

Watson DK, Panian S, Kendall V et al: Pain control after thoracotomy: Bupivacaine versus lidocaine in continuous extrapleural intercostal nerve blockade. Ann Thorac Surg 67:825, 1999.

Weissman C: Pulmonary function after cardiac and thoracic surgery. Anesth Analg 88:1272, 1999.

Weissman C: Pulmonary function after cardiac and thoracic surgery. Curr Opin Anesthesiol 13:47, 2000.

Werner O, Malmkvist G, Beckman A et al: Carbon dioxide elimination from each lung during endobronchial anaesthesia. Effects of posture and pulmonary arterial pressure. Br J Anaesth 56:995, 1984a.

Werner O, Malmkvist G, Beckman A et al: Gas exchange and haemodynamics during thoracotomy. Br J Anaesth 56:1343, 1984b.

White GMJ: Evolution of endotracheal and endobroncheal intubation. Br J Anaesth 32:235, 1960.

CHAPTER **6**

Endoscopy

FLEXIBLE AND RIGID BRONCHOSCOPY

Andrew F. Pierre
Robert J. Ginsberg
Shafique Keshavjee

Flexible Bronchoscopy

Until the 1970s, the airway could only be examined using the rigid bronchoscope. In 1968, Ikeda from Japan introduced the first flexible fiberoptic bronchoscope (Ikeda et al, 1968). Since then it has become an invaluable tool in the diagnosis and management of tracheobronchial and pulmonary diseases. Although the flexible bronchoscope enhances the capabilities of the endoscopist, it does not replace the rigid scope. The rigid bronchoscope is still the optimal instrument for control of airway hemorrhage, the placement of Silastic stents, removal of foreign bodies, and management of airway obstruction. The flexible and rigid bronchoscopes are complementary instruments and should be used as such.

Flexible bronchoscopy has its greatest utility in diagnostic procedures. It is relatively easy to learn to use, it can be used with topical anesthesia and minimal sedation, and serious complications are rare. Specimens may be obtained by direct forceps biopsy, washings, needle biopsies, protected brushings, or transbronchial biopsies—all at relatively low risk to the patient. The flexible scope is an important tool used by thoracic surgeons, pulmonologists, intensivists, anesthesiologists, and otolaryngologists. The flexible bronchoscope may also be used to deliver laser therapy and brachytherapy to the airways.

INDICATIONS

Flexible fiberoptic bronchoscopy is now widely used in the diagnosis and management of inflammatory, infectious, and neoplastic diseases of the lungs. In well-trained hands, the application of the flexible instrument is safe and effective, but experience and sound clinical judgment determine the ultimate indications and utility of flexible bronchoscopy. No list of indications can accurately reflect the changing state of medical technology and capabilities. New instrumentation and techniques will continue to expand the role of flexible bronchoscopy. Also, details of how and when a particular physician decides to perform the procedure for the various indications will depend on several factors related to the disease, the condition of the patient, and the risks and benefits of the procedure in each instance.

All patients should undergo a thorough history and physical examination, and medical problems should be addressed prior to the procedure. A coagulation profile should be obtained if biopsies are planned or the history is suggestive of a coagulopathy. Note in particular that asthma can be triggered and worsened by bronchoscopy—bronchial edema and bronchospasm can result from the procedure. If asthma is adequately treated and controlled, asthmatic patients can be examined safely. Table 6–1 lists the general indications and contraindications for flexible bronchoscopy. Following is a brief discussion of some of the common indications for which a thoracic surgeon might use the flexible bronchoscope.

Pulmonary Lesions or Infiltrates

Indications for flexible bronchoscopy commonly include an abnormal mass or nodule detected on chest radiograph and suspected of being a lung cancer. The exact location of the lesion can be identified, and the mass may be biopsied. The remaining airways are examined carefully for other lesions that might represent metastatic disease or other primaries. Other frequent indications include recurrent pulmonary infiltrates, an unresolving infiltrate, and persistent atelectasis—collapse of a segment, a lobe, or a lung; a mediastinal or hilar mass; or persistent pleural effusions. Bronchoscopy may help in the diagnosis of diffuse parenchymal lung disease when the differential diagnosis includes neoplastic, infectious, or inflammatory lung diseases. Flexible bronchoscopy can be a very useful diagnostic tool in immunocompromised patients with new pulmonary infiltrates. In this population, bronchoalveolar lavage with or without transbronchial lung biopsies frequently helps to define an infectious cause for the new pulmonary infiltrate (Martin et al, 1987). The yield from these procedures is high and has reduced the need for open-lung biopsy in these immunocompromised patients.

Planning a Lung Cancer Operation

Information gathered with the bronchoscopic examination is crucial to the planning of the resection of a lung cancer. The decision to perform a lobectomy, sleeve resection, pneumonectomy, or carinal pneumonectomy will depend on the determination of the exact location of the tumor in the airway and an evaluation of the length of airway involved. For example, a tumor of the right upper lobe extending into the right mainstem bronchus may be resected by pneumonectomy or by a right upper lobe sleeve resection with preservation of the right middle and lower lobes. Information obtained at bronchoscopy is vital to planning this resection and making this decision.

Pulmonary Toilet

The clearing of secretions is very important after a thoracic operation but is especially important following tracheal resections. The flexible scope can be used at the bedside to achieve this goal of pulmonary toilet in the thoracic patient. Topical anesthesia and minimal sedation are required. This technique should be liberally used if patients, for whatever reason, are unable to clear their secretions with chest physiotherapy and more conservative measures.

Endotracheal Intubation and the Intubated Patient

The flexible bronchoscope advanced through a standard single-lumen endotracheal tube can be used for difficult intubations that cannot be obtained by standard techniques. The awake patient is topically anesthetized. The flexible bronchoscope is passed through an endotracheal tube. The bronchoscope is guided into the distal airway, and the endotracheal tube is advanced down the bronchoscope to ensure accurate placement in the trachea. Finally, the position of the endotracheal tube is checked using the scope as it is removed. The patient is then anesthetized and connected to the ventilator.

Following endotracheal intubation with a double-lumen tube, the flexible bronchoscope is used to confirm proper positioning of the bronchial arm and the bronchial balloon. Flexible scopes are also useful for positioning bronchial blockers or Univent tubes for single-lung ventilation.

In the intubated patient, the flexible bronchoscope may be used to evaluate the position and patency of the endotracheal tube, to evaluate hemoptysis, to obtain samples for microbiologic examination, and to clear secretions. These indications commonly arise in the intensive care unit but may also occur in the operating room.

Bronchopleural Fistula

The bronchoscope may help in the diagnosis and management of a bronchopleural fistula. Examination of the bronchial stump may reveal the fistula, and bronchoscopic evaluation can be used to determine if further intervention is required. The scope can be used to help position bronchial blockers or long endotracheal tubes

TABLE 6–1 ■ **American Thoracic Society Guidelines for Flexible Fiberoptic Bronchoscopy**

Diagnostic Uses
To evaluate lung lesions of unknown etiology that appear on the chest x-ray
To assess airway patency
To investigate unexplained hemoptysis, unexplained cough, localized wheeze, or stridor
To search for the origin of suspicious or positive sputum cytology
To investigate the etiology of unexplained paralysis of a vocal cord or hemidiaphragm, superior vena cava syndrome, chylothorax, or unexplained pleural effusion
To evaluate problems associated with endotracheal tubes, such as tracheal damage, airway obstruction, or tube placement
To stage lung cancer preoperatively and subsequently to evaluate, when appropriate, the response to therapy
To obtain material for microbiologic studies in suspected pulmonary infections
To evaluate the airways for suspected bronchial tear or other injury after thoracic trauma
To evaluate a suspected tracheoesophageal fistula
To determine the location and extent of respiratory tract injury after acute inhalation of noxious fumes or aspiration of gastric contents
To obtain material for study from the lungs of patients with diffuse or focal lung diseases
Therapeutic Uses
To remove retained secretions or mucous plugs not mobilized by conventional noninvasive techniques
To remove foreign bodies
To remove abnormal endobronchial tissue or foreign material by use of forceps or laser techniques
To perform difficult intubations
To aid in the delivery of brachytherapy
To aid in the deployment of expandable wire stents
Conditions Involving Increased Risk
Lack of patient cooperation
Recent myocardial infarction or unstable angina
Partial tracheal obstruction
Unstable bronchial asthma
Respiratory insufficiency associated with moderate to severe hypoxemia or any degree of hypercarbia
Uremia and pulmonary hypertension (possible serious hemorrhage after biopsy)
Lung abscess (danger of flooding the airway with purulent material)
Obstruction of the superior vena cava (possibility of bleeding and laryngeal edema)
Debility, advanced age, malnutrition
Unstable cardiac arrhythmia
Respiratory failure requiring mechanical ventilation
Disorders requiring laser therapy, biopsy of lesions obstructing large airways, or multiple transbronchial lung biopsies
The danger of a serious complication is especially high in the following conditions
Malignant arrhythmia
Profound refractory hypoxemia
Severe bleeding diathesis that cannot be corrected when biopsy is anticipated
Contraindications
Absence of consent from the patient or his or her representative
Bronchoscopy by an inexperienced person without direct supervision
Bronchoscopy without adequate facilities and personnel to care for emergencies such as cardiopulmonary arrest, pneumothorax, or bleeding
Inability to adequately oxygenate the patient during the procedure

Adapted with permission from the guidelines for fiberoptic bronchoscopy in adults. Accepted as official position paper by the American Thoracic Society Board of Directors, November 1986; from Sokolowski RW, Burgher LW, Jones FL et al: Guidelines for fiberoptic bronchoscopy in adults. Am Rev Respir Dis. 136:1066, 1987.

for single-lung ventilation if such is required for management of ventilation.

Airway Obstruction

A patient with a persistent lung abscess or pneumonia may have an endobronchial obstruction and should be bronchoscoped. Bronchoscopy in this situation may reveal a foreign body, a tumor, or an extrinsic compression. Occasionally, flexible bronchoscopy can help establish drainage from the affected area of the lung, or a tumor, if present, can be biopsied.

Stridor or localized wheezing may be due to a structural narrowing of the upper airway and trachea and should be evaluated by bronchoscopy. Lesions may include laryngeal abnormalities, vocal cord paralysis, benign and malignant tumors, extrinsic compression, tracheal stricture caused by mucosal pathology, or tracheomalacia. Suspicious lesions can be biopsied. Management will depend on the cause. If tracheal obstruction is suspected, the bronchoscopic examination should be performed in an operating room—where rigid bronchoscopy can be performed first to ensure control of the airway. The flexible bronchoscope can be used through the rigid bronchoscope to examine the distal airway in detail (see the section on Rigid Bronchoscopy).

Bronchial obstruction by tumor is best managed with the rigid bronchoscope, but the flexible scope can aid in many of the maneuvers that are necessary to open the airway. Débridement by laser is slow, but the laser can be used to help achieve hemostasis after manual forceps débridement via the rigid bronchoscope. The airway may then be stented if required (Sonett, 1998). If an expandable metal stent is selected, the stent and delivery device are advanced into the trachea along the rigid scope. The flexible scope is then placed through the rigid scope and used to visualize the stent as it is positioned accurately into the bronchus across the stricture/obstruction. Ventilation is maintained through the side arm of the rigid bronchoscope. Continuous visualization in this fashion ensures that the stent is optimally deployed.

Airway Trauma

Following blunt or penetrating chest trauma, the patient should be bronchoscoped if the lung fails to re-expand after adequate chest tube drainage or if the suspicion of a tracheobronchial injury is high. Such patients may present with high-volume air leaks, persistent pneumothorax, pneumomediastinum, or hemoptysis. Signs and symptoms of a tracheobronchial injury may, however, be subtle in some patients.

Foreign Bodies

The flexible bronchoscope may be used to identify foreign bodies and on occasion may also be used to remove them. However, the rigid bronchoscope is the preferred tool for the removal of foreign bodies, because it facilitates safe and rapid removal and simultaneously provides an excellent airway control for ventilation.

Inhalation Injury

Patients with an inhalation injury should be bronchoscoped to determine the extent of injury. The flexible scope may also be used to facilitate endotracheal intubation of these patients if there is significant airway edema.

Laser Therapy

The flexible bronchoscope facilitates the use of the neodymium:yttrium-aluminum-garnet (Nd:YAG) laser by directing the laser fiber into locations that are difficult to reach with the rigid bronchoscope (Dumon, 1982). This laser may then be used in the management of bronchial obstruction secondary to tumor once distal luminal patency is confirmed. However, the management of bronchial obstruction is best and most safely carried out using a rigid bronchoscope. The flexible scope is used in conjunction with the rigid scope by simply passing it through the lumen of the rigid scope to deliver laser therapy. With this technique, the obstructed airway may be effectively opened using a combination of both manual forceps débridement and laser débridement.

Mediastinal Adenopathy

In certain circumstances, the flexible scope and a Wang needle can be used to perform transbronchial biopsies of mediastinal nodes. However, mediastinal nodes are more commonly sampled by cervical mediastinoscopy.

Lung Transplantation

The flexible bronchoscope is used extensively in the management of the lung transplant patient. Bronchoscopy is an important part of donor assessment and may identify donors who have aspirated, have infections, or have abnormal airway anatomy. The recipient is intubated with a double-lumen endotracheal tube—the position of which is confirmed with the flexible bronchoscope. After completion of the bronchial anastomoses, they are examined endobronchially with the flexible scope, and the distal airways are cleared of blood and secretions. Pulmonary toilet is very important in the postoperative period, and the scope may be used for this purpose at the bedside or in the intensive care unit. Finally, the diagnosis of infection or rejection is heavily dependent on flexible bronchoscopy. The patient undergoes transbronchial lung biopsies under fluoroscopic guidance to diagnose rejection, and bronchoalveolar lavage is used to help diagnose various pulmonary infections in the transplant patient.

EQUIPMENT

The basic setup consists of a flexible fiberoptic bronchoscope, light source, biopsy forceps, and suction (Figs. 6–1 and 6–2). The video bronchoscope has become standard equipment. It provides excellent visualization and is ideal for teaching. Fiberoptic bronchoscopes are classified according to the size (diameter) of their distal ends (Fig. 6–3). Standard adult scopes are 5 to 6 mm in outside diameter with a 2.2- to 2.8-mm working channel. Pediat-

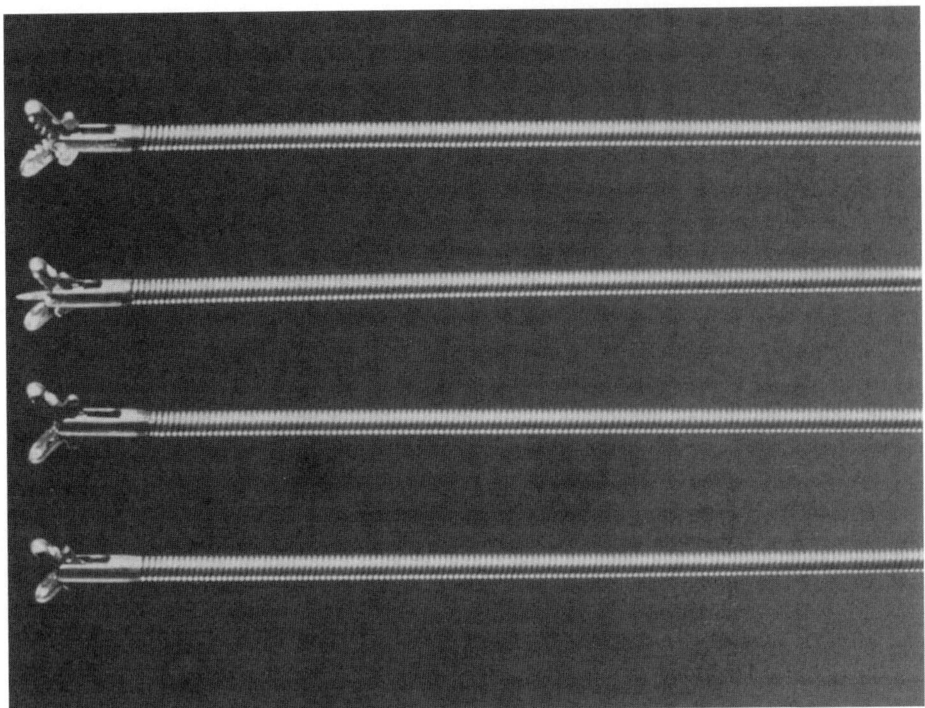

FIGURE 6–1 ■ A selection of flexible biopsy forceps for use through the flexible fiberoptic bronchoscope.

ric scopes are typically 3.5 to 3.6 mm with a smaller (1.2-mm) working channel. With technologic advances, smaller caliber fiberoptic bronchoscopes of high quality are becoming available. Consideration should be given to the intended use of the scope. The suctioning and clearing of secretions is best accomplished through larger scopes with wider working channels, but the ability to reach very distal airways to obtain direct biopsies is greater with smaller scopes. Having two sizes of adult scope and a pediatric scope on hand offers the endoscopist the greatest flexibility.

The endoscopy suite should be equipped with supplemental oxygen, a cardiac monitor, an oxygen saturation monitor, and supplies for cardiopulmonary resuscitation. In addition, the necessary drugs for sedation and topical anesthesia as well as appropriate solutions and containers for cytology, microbiology, and pathology should be present. Table 6–2 lists some of the more common items found in the endoscopy suite. Special equipment such as lasers and brachytherapy are discussed in other chapters of this book; they are not typically involved in the endoscopy suite.

TECHNIQUE

Flexible bronchoscopy can be performed with the surgeon in either the seated or supine position. Patients may be premedicated with intravenous meperidine 25–50 mg and Diazemuls 5–10 mg. The patient gargles with 4% aqueous Xylocaine prior to insertion of the broncho-

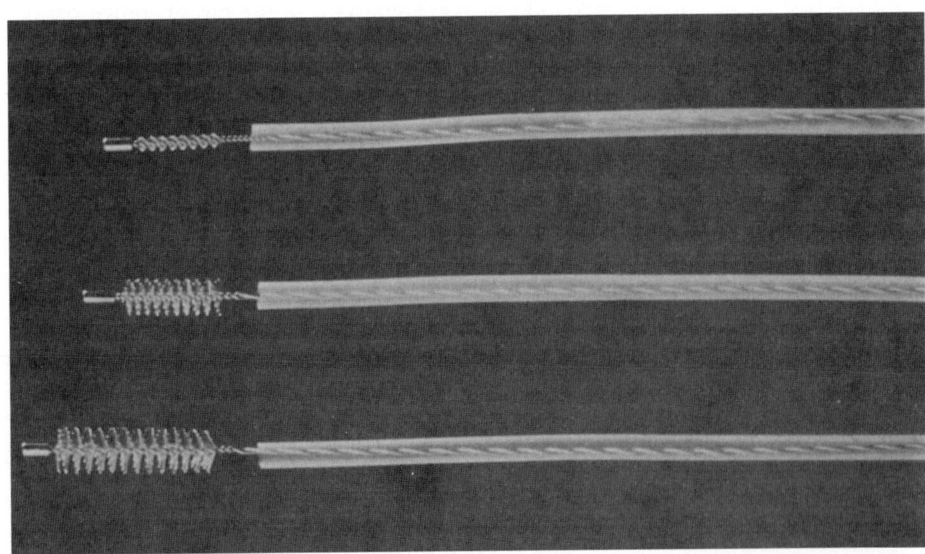

FIGURE 6–2 ■ Bronchial brushes in protective plastic catheter sheaths can be used to obtain protected samples from the distal airways for culture.

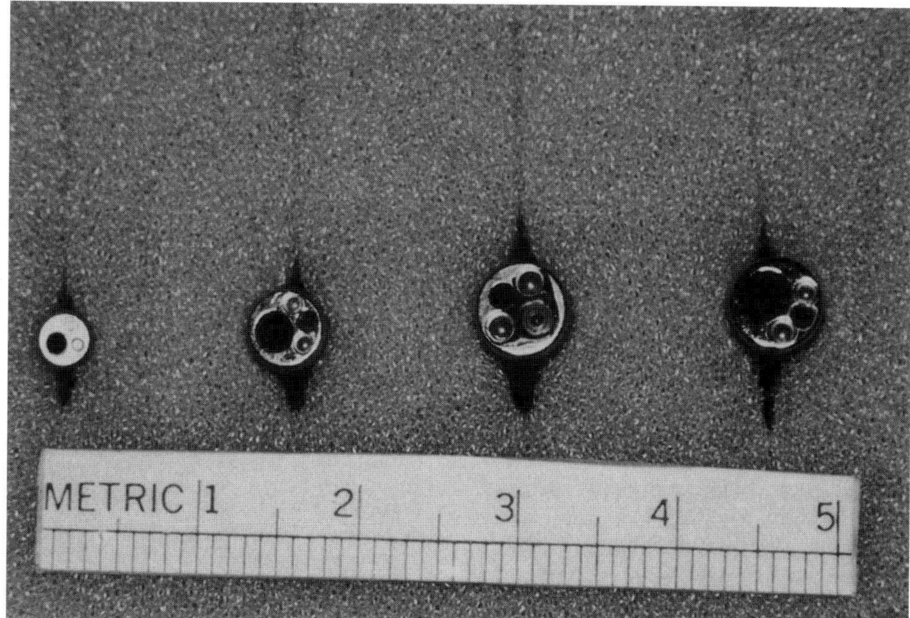

FIGURE 6–3 ■ Distal tips of various size bronchoscopes and their working channels.

scope, and additional topical Xylocaine spray is administered. The scope may be inserted either through the anesthetized naris or orally through a bite-block. In the intubated patient, the scope is inserted through a connector to the endotracheal tube. Xylocaine 2% is then injected through the bronchoscope to anesthetize the hypopharynx, the larynx, the vocal cords, and the tracheobronchial tree in a progressive fashion as the bronchoscope is advanced.

In the very cooperative patient, there is no need for sedation and the procedure can be performed with topical anesthesia alone. However, in the uncooperative patient or in situations in which the airway or respiratory function is compromised, bronchoscopy may be best performed in the operating room with intravenous sedation or under general anesthesia.

The entire tracheobronchial tree, including the vocal cords, should be systematically evaluated at bronchoscopy. Several additional procedures may be carried out after inspection of the airways. These include washings, bronchoalveolar lavage, protected brushings, biopsies, and transbronchial biopsies. Ideally, transbronchial biopsies should be performed with the aid of fluoroscopy to reduce the incidence of pneumothorax. Management of the specimens will depend on the practices of the various laboratories and the practices of the institution involved.

A solution of epinephrine 0.2 to 1 mg in 500 ml normal saline is useful for hemostasis via instillation down the working channel of the bronchoscope when mild to moderate bleeding occurs during bronchoscopy or after a biopsy. Aliquots of 2 to 5 ml are typically used. If in the operating room, the anesthetist should be made aware of the use of this drug as it may affect heart rate and blood pressure.

Refer to later discussions of rigid bronchoscopy, tracheobronchial stents, endoscopic laser therapy, and brachytherapy for more detailed information on the use of flexible bronchoscopy with these techniques and modalities.

TABLE 6–2 ■ **Bronchoscopy Equipment**

Essential
Bronchoscopes
Suction tubing, connectors, wall suction
Biopsy forceps
Syringes (non–Luer-Lok)
Specimen containers
Lidocaine
Pulse oximeter
Cardiac monitor
Oxygen source
Advanced Cardiac Life Support (ACLS) equipment for resuscitation, e.g. endotracheal tubes, medications
Desirable
Cytology brushes
Protected catheter brushes
Video camera and photographic equipment

LIMITATIONS AND COMPLICATIONS

The best visualization is obtained with the larger adult scope and the video camera. Smaller scopes also do not allow for easy clearing of secretions and mucus, and visualization is consequently impaired. Adult scopes usually fit through a No. 7.5 endotracheal tube, but it may be necessary to use a pediatric bronchoscope in smaller endotracheal tubes or in double-lumen endotracheal tubes.

Flexible bronchoscopy performed by experienced endoscopists is a safe procedure. The complications have been well summarized by Pereira and colleagues (1978). The overall mortality in their study was 0.1%. Major complications (respiratory arrest, pneumonia, pneumothorax, and airway obstruction) occurred in 1.7%. Minor complications that included vasovagal reaction, fever, cardiac arrhythmia, nausea/vomiting, and psychotic reactions occurred in 6.5% of patients. Pneumothorax occurred in 5% of transbronchial biopsies. Complications such as pneumothorax are more likely in patients receiving transbronchial lung biopsies, and bleeding is more likely in patients having biopsies of airway lesions. Postbronchoscopy respiratory failure may be anticipated in patients who are already verging on the need for intubation and mechanical ventilation. The relative risks and benefits must always be carefully weighed in each patient who is being considered for a fiberoptic bronchoscopic procedure.

Rigid Bronchoscopy

HISTORICAL NOTE

Bronchoscopy is an invaluable tool for the management of thoracic disease. In addition to being an essential diagnostic modality, it provides direct therapeutic benefits in many situations. Until 1970, the only access to the tracheobronchial tree was provided by the rigid bronchoscope, initially designed by Jackson (Boyd, 1994; Jackson and Jackson, 1950). Although the rigid bronchoscope provided a limited view, the operator could usually visualize the pulmonary segmental orifices of most lobes. However, the rigidity of the instruments limited our ability to obtain biopsy specimens distal to the major bronchi. The development of rigid telescopes with high-quality optics enhanced our ability to examine the subsegmental bronchi and lesions of the central airway in detail.

The introduction of flexible fiberoptic bronchoscopic equipment has enhanced our ability to view the distal segmental bronchi and has simplified the procedure considerably. Both techniques of bronchoscopy—rigid and flexible—have evolved to define their own diagnostic and therapeutic indications. Each system has its strengths and limitations, and the thoracic surgeon should be competent in the use of both modalities to manage the spectrum of thoracic disease that may be confronted. Flexible bronchoscopy is dealt with in detail later in this chapter.

■ *HISTORICAL READINGS*

Boyd AD: Chevalier Jackson: The father of American bronchoesophagoscopy. Ann Thorac Surg 57:502, 1994.

Jackson C, Jackson CL: Bronchoesophagology. Philadelphia, WB Saunders, 1950.

INDICATIONS

Hemoptysis

Although many common respiratory symptoms can be investigated by fiberoptic bronchoscopy, one specific indication for the use of rigid equipment is massive hemoptysis (Wedzicha and Pearson, 1990). A rigid endoscope provides the operator with immediate control of the airway. In addition, it permits the use of large-bore suction equipment to keep the airway clear of blood and clots. Although occlusive balloon catheters or packing (to tamponade bleeding) may be placed in certain circumstances with flexible fiberoptic equipment, they can be positioned with greater control and accuracy under direct vision with the rigid scope, especially when there is significant bleeding that requires efficient suctioning.

INDICATIONS FOR RIGID BRONCHOSCOPY

Massive hemoptysis
Airway obstruction: diagnostic and therapeutic
Foreign body
Tumor: endobronchial, extrinsic compression
Benign stricture
Laser therapy
Endobronchial stenting
Tracheobronchial toilet
Pediatric bronchoscopy
Miscellaneous

Airway Obstruction

In conditions that cause the obstruction of the airway (larynx, trachea, or main bronchi), the use of the rigid bronchoscope is the safest modality for obtaining a diagnosis because it enables secure control of the airway should a problem arise. In many instances, it is both diagnostic and therapeutic.

Foreign Bodies

The need for a rigid bronchoscope for the extraction of foreign bodies is self-evident. In fact, this was the initial indication for which Jackson developed the instrument (Boyd, 1994). With the varied forceps available and the operator working through the scope, a foreign body can be manipulated and extracted directly (Holinder, 1978; Weissberg and Schwartz, 1987).

Malignant Disease

In cases of malignant obstruction, the first priority is the establishment of a safe airway. This is readily achieved with a rigid bronchoscope. Endobronchial tumors may be débrided directly with biopsy forceps, electrocautery, or a laser to establish an improved airway. Such débridement is often impossible with flexible equipment (Hetzel and Smith, 1991). Such cases should be handled in an operating room, where problems with airway control can be readily dealt with if necessary. In cases of obstruction caused by endobronchial pathologic conditions or extrinsic compression, it is safer to keep the patient breathing spontaneously until a secure airway is established.

Once an airway is established, the obstructing lesion can be dilated as the first step. Dilatation may be carried out by the surgeon, first passing the smallest scope that will fit through the stricture and then using sequentially larger scopes for dilatation in a stepwise fashion. Gum-tipped Jackson bougies inserted under direct vision through the bronchoscope can be used in selected cases of tumor obstruction to define the lumen prior to the use of the laser (see later).

Benign Stricture

Rigid bronchoscopy is often the first step in the management of a benign stricture. Tracheal or mainstem bronchial stenoses are often readily dilated with sequential passage of bronchoscopes of increasing diameter. Narrow, tight strictures that will not easily admit the tip of a scope may be initially dilated with gum-tipped Jackson bougies that are passed under direct vision through the bronchoscope. Rigid equipment allows an accurate assessment of the location, caliber, length, and rigidity of the stricture and the status of the distal airway. This detailed examination is essential in the preoperative assessment and planning for airway resection (see Chapter 12).

Laser Therapy

Laser therapy of the airway is dealt with in detail later in this section (see Chapter 14). It is apparent that the use of rigid equipment enhances the surgeon's ability to remove a tumor more rapidly in combination with laser coagulation. The bulk of the endobronchial tumor is directly débrided with large biopsy forceps. The flexible bronchoscope is then passed through the rigid scope to permit use of the Nd:YAG laser to complete the débridement and obtain hemostasis. The CO_2 laser, which cannot be used with a fiberoptic system, mandates the use of rigid equipment. Once again, in cases of airway obstruction, the rigid bronchoscope enables the surgeon to obtain immediate control of the airway safely. The tumor can then be managed by dilatation or débridement prior to the application of the laser. In many such cases, the laser may not be required because gross tumor can be adequately débrided with the biopsy forceps, and bleeding can be controlled with epinephrine solution or electrocautery.

Endobronchial Stents

The placement of endobronchial stents frequently requires the use of the rigid bronchoscope (Cooper et al, 1989). Stents are used in the palliation of obstructing tumors and in stenting the airway for benign stenoses. The indications and techniques for stent placement are described in detail later in this chapter.

Tracheobronchial Toilet

In rare instances, the tracheobronchial toilet of thick secretions cannot be managed adequately with a fiberoptic bronchoscope. Rigid equipment allows the use of larger bore suction equipment and facilitates the removal of such viscid secretions.

Pediatric Bronchoscopy

In children with tiny airways, rigid bronchoscopy is the only option available to inspect the airway because tiny endotracheal tubes will not permit the passage of flexible equipment.

Miscellaneous

Proponents of rigid endoscopy maintain that the assessment of airway invasion by surrounding or extrinsic tumors (e.g., esophageal carcinoma) can be done better with a rigid instrument than with flexible bronchoscopy. The rigidity of the airway is best "felt" with a rigid scope, and the larger biopsy specimens obtained will improve accuracy in the assessment of microscopic submucosal invasion.

METHODS OF ANESTHESIA AND VENTILATION

General Anesthesia

When bronchoscopy is performed under general anesthesia, the patient is supine, usually on an operating table. Intravenous or inhalation general anesthesia, or a combination of both, can be used. The induction is rapid if intravenous agents are used. This is the preferred technique, because it can take 10 to 20 minutes if one "breathes down" the patient with inhalational agents. Once suitable induction has occurred and a muscle relaxant has been administered, the lower jaw should be loose and mobile. This indicates a suitable depth of anesthesia and muscle relaxation for the procedure. The patient should be fully monitored (oxygen saturation, blood pressure, and electrocardiography) throughout the procedure. Additional details on the anesthetic management for rigid bronchoscopy are found in Chapter 5.

Techniques of Ventilation

For rigid bronchoscopic examination, four techniques of ventilation are available: intermittent insufflation, continuous insufflation, Venturi (jet) ventilation, and spontaneous inhalation ventilation.

Intermittent Insufflation

This classic technique of ventilation through the bronchoscope involves intermittent ventilation through either a side port or the proximal end of the bronchoscope to ventilate, oxygenate, and maintain anesthesia. This is carried out simply by the examiner inserting an endotracheal tube, attached to the ventilating system, into either the side port or the open end of the bronchoscope. The endoscopist may have to occlude the upper airway with packing or occlude the nose and mouth by hand if there is a large air leak. This technique is cumbersome and does not allow for continuous viewing through the scope.

Continuous Insufflation

The end of the bronchoscope is fitted with a lens, and a side port is used to ventilate the patient continually while the endoscopist proceeds with the bronchoscopy. This practice provides the advantages of allowing uninterrupted bronchoscopy and using inhalational agents throughout the procedure, thus minimizing the need for intravenous anesthesia. One simply slides the lens open for biopsy sampling or suctioning. This technique is simple and reliable in that it provides relatively continuous viewing and continuous ventilation. The middle bronchoscope in Figure 6–4 is shown fitted with the viewing lens. With the use of rigid telescopes, this ventilation technique provides excellent conditions for continuous, detailed viewing. The lower bronchoscope in Figure 6–4 is shown with the ventilation tubing attached and a Hopkins telescope in place.

Jet Ventilation

The most common form of ventilation used during rigid bronchoscopy is the Venturi technique (Fig. 6–5). This is based on the principle of air entrainment. With a side port or the open proximal end of the scope, a high-pressure (25 to 30 psi) jet of oxygen (delivered at 10 to 20 breaths per minute through an 18-gauge catheter) entrains surrounding ambient air, thus ventilating the patient throughout the procedure. The modified Sanders ventilating system (see Fig. 6–5) and a reducing valve are required (Ehrenwerth and Brull, 1991; Sanders, 1987). With this technique, it is essential that the surgeon wear eye protection because droplets of secretions or blood can be drawn out of the open end of the bronchoscope. Anesthesia is maintained with intravenous agents or muscle relaxants.

Spontaneous Inhalation Ventilation

The technique of spontaneous inhalation ventilation demands a nonapneic patient. Inhalational agents are administered through the side port, and the anesthesia is kept light enough to maintain spontaneous respiration. The major disadvantages are lack of relaxation and exposure of the operator to the anesthetic gases. This technique is useful for the induction of a patient with an obstructive lesion of the airway when the surgeon anticipates that airway control is precarious. With this technique, it is not catastrophic if an airway is not obtained immediately because patients continue to breathe on their own.

Local Anesthesia

Rigid bronchoscopy can be carried out under local anesthesia. However, in most cases, general anesthesia is the usual and preferred technique. The technique of local anesthesia is similar to that used with flexible bronchoscopy (see later) and includes adequate topical anesthesia of the mouth, pharynx, and vocal cords, and intravenous sedation as required. The use of atropine to decrease secretions and inhibit vagal reflexes is helpful. The authors' technique is as follows: administration of a local spray anesthetic to the pharynx and larynx, a transcricoid injection of 2 ml of 1% lidocaine, and premedication with an intravenous narcotic analgesic (e.g., morphine 2 to 5 mg IV). Intravenous sedation with diazepam or midazolam is then titrated to the patient's needs. The need for an adequately sedated and reasonably comfort-

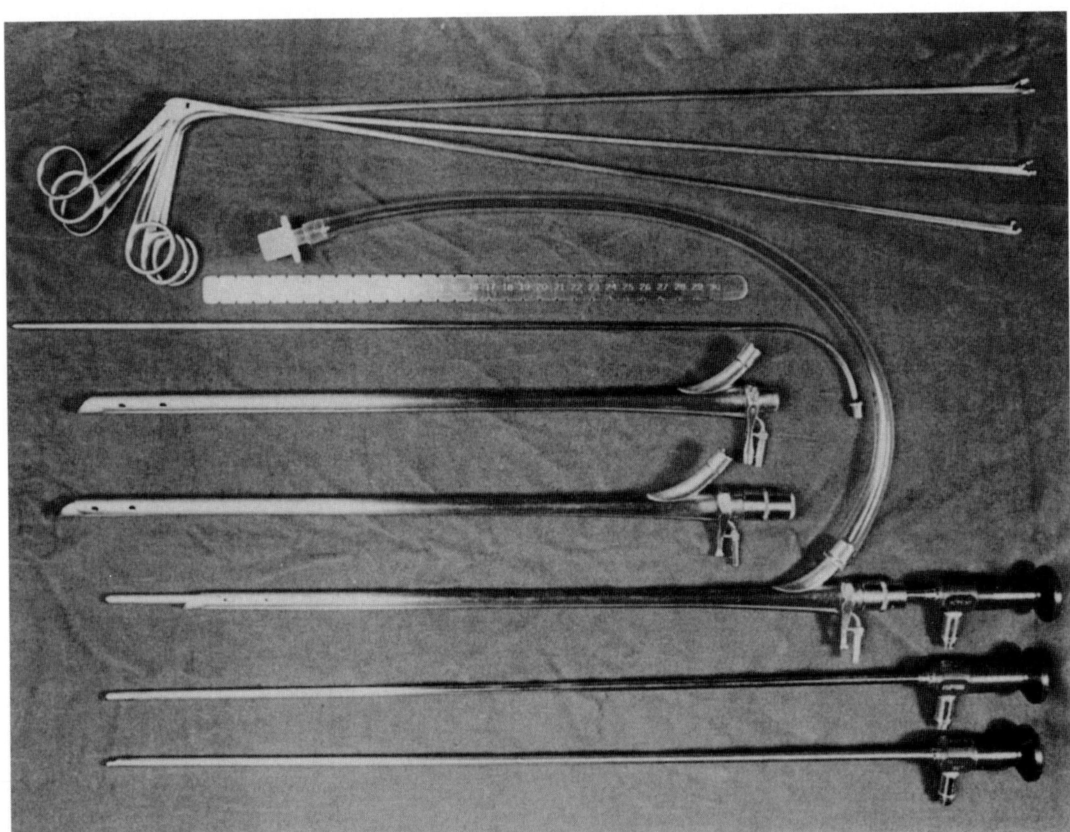

FIGURE 6–4 ■ Basic equipment for rigid bronchoscopy. From *top* to *bottom*: biopsy forceps, ruler, rigid suction cannula, rigid bronchoscopes of varying sizes, and rigid Hopkins telescopes. The *middle bronchoscope* is shown with the viewing lens fitted. The *lower bronchoscope* is illustrated with the ventilation tubing attached to the side port and a 0-degree telescope inserted as it would be during use. The light source and fiberoptic cable are not shown.

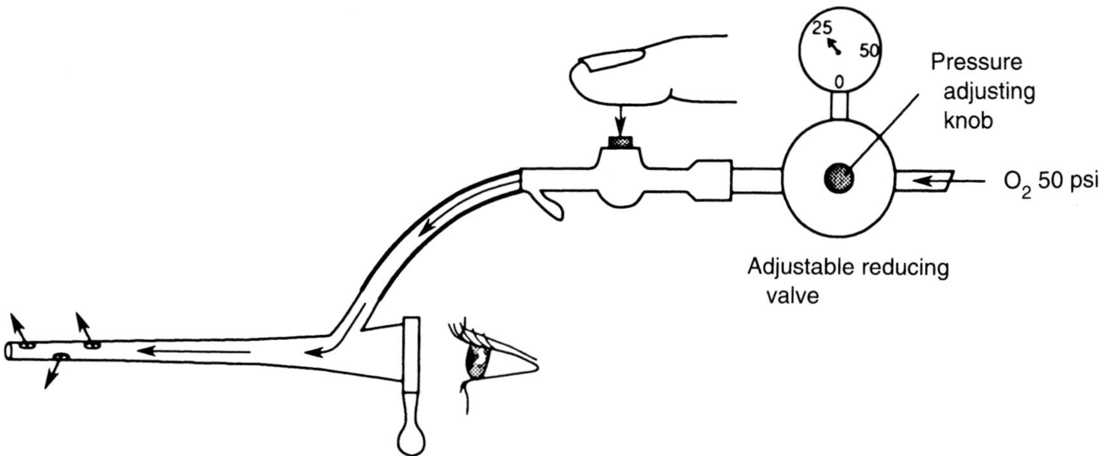

FIGURE 6–5 ■ A schematic illustrating the modified Sanders jet ventilation technique for ventilation through a rigid bronchoscope. The wall oxygen supply at 50 psi is connected to a reducing valve that allows the pressure to be adjusted from 0 to 50 psi. The side port of the bronchoscope is used as the Venturi injector site, and the open end can be used for continuous viewing by the endoscopist. (From Ehrenwerth J, Brull S: Anesthesia for thoracic diagnostic procedures. In Kaplan JA [ed]: Anesthesia, 2nd ed. New York, Churchill Livingstone, 1991.)

able patient cannot be overemphasized because intubation of the airway under local anesthesia requires the patient's cooperation. This can be enhanced with moderate sedation and effective local anesthesia, as described earlier. The procedure may be performed with the patient in a chair (preferably a dental-type chair) or supine on an operating table. If necessary in an emergency, intubation can be carried out on a stretcher or hospital bed. The technique for intubation under local anesthesia is identical to that for general anesthesia (described later).

TECHNIQUE OF RIGID BRONCHOSCOPY

Prior to the induction of anesthesia, the equipment and light source should be checked for proper function. The basic setup includes at least two sizes of bronchoscopes, appropriate suctioning cannulas, a variety of biopsy forceps, and a variety of telescopes (see Fig. 6–4 and Equipment, later).

Care must be taken to protect the patient's eyes, usually with padding and adhesive tape. At all times, the operator must protect the lips and teeth or gums of the patient from injury. A commercial rubber tooth guard is available, but a saline-soaked gauze sponge is adequate. The largest bronchoscope sufficient for the needs of the operator should be chosen. In most instances an 8- or 9-mm (outer diameter) scope is used for men, and a 7- or 8-mm scope is used for women (see Fig. 6–5). Larger-diameter scopes may damage the larynx and may preclude intubation of the smaller distal bronchi. Much smaller equipment is required for infants and children; the selection of the size depends on the size of the child. Scopes as small as 2.5 to 3 mm are required for patients who weigh less than 10 kg.

Placement of the patient's head on a pillow and then extension of the patient's neck so that the chin points vertically (the "sniffing" or "intubating" position) facilitate the introduction of the bronchoscope. With the examiner's thumb always protecting the rigid bronchoscope from injuring the upper teeth, the scope is inserted through one side of the mouth (usually the right side for right-handed operators) or in the midline in edentulous patients. Under direct vision, it is advanced to the posterior median groove of the tongue (Fig. 6–6*A*). The upper teeth must never serve as a fulcrum to lever the bronchoscope into place; the operator's left thumb should bear this pressure and support the scope at all times. The scope is first introduced almost vertically; the proximal end is then brought smoothly downward as the tip follows the contour of the tongue until the instrument is almost horizontal. By gently elevating the tongue and slowly advancing the scope, the operator can identify the epiglottis (see Fig. 6–6*A*). If the epiglottis is not seen (usually because the instrument was advanced too rapidly past it), the scope should be partially withdrawn, and the maneuver should be repeated. The tip of the bronchoscope is insinuated a short distance beyond and posterior to the epiglottis, just far enough to raise it without having it slip off the end of the instrument (see Fig. 6–6*B*). Once the epiglottis is lifted anteriorly with the tip of the bronchoscope, the posterior part of the laryngeal inlet, the arytenoids, and the vocal cords are identified (see Fig. 6–6*B*). Occasionally, external pressure on the larynx by an assistant, to displace it posteriorly, might be required to visualize the cords. In difficult cases, the glottis can be displayed with a laryngoscope held in the left hand, and the bronchoscope is then inserted with the right hand.

Once the glottis is visualized, the bronchoscope is advanced toward the cords (see Fig. 6–6*C*). As the cords are approached, the scope is turned 90 degrees to align the vertical orifice of the glottic chink with the tip of the scope (see Fig. 6–6*D*). The scope is then gently advanced through the larynx into the upper airway. With a gentle twisting motion, the scope is rotated back to the original orientation. No force must be used at this stage. If the examiner advances the scope gently, injuries will not occur. If significant resistance is met, a smaller-sized

Text continued on page 96

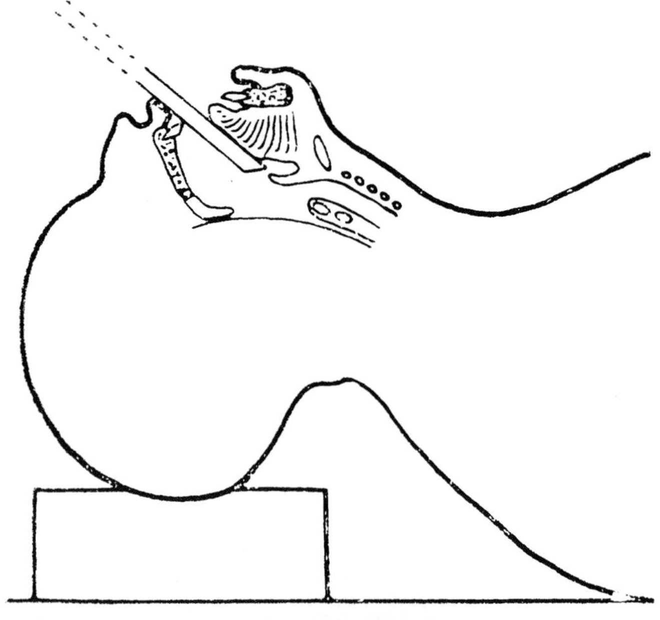

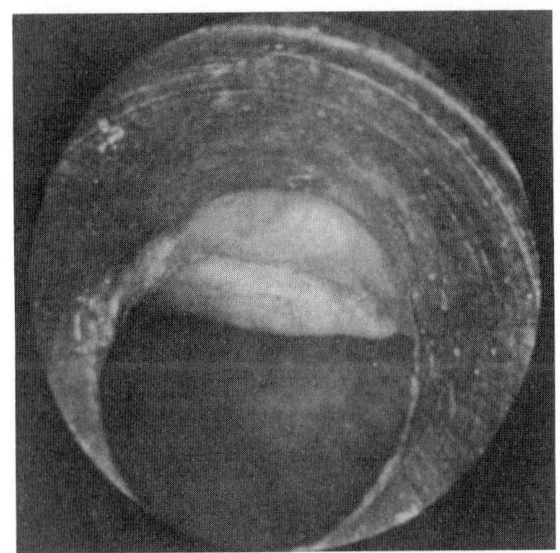

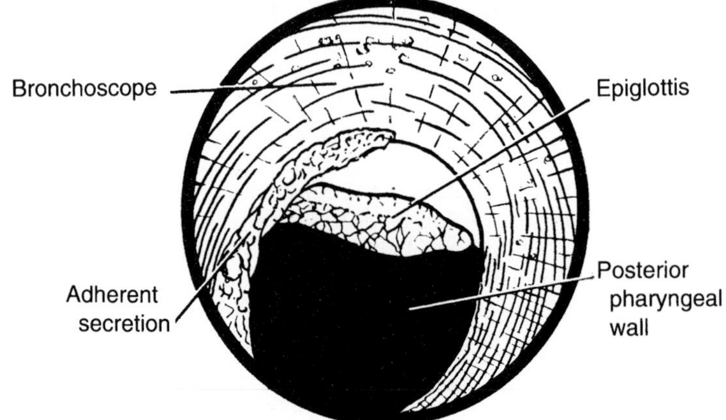

A

FIGURE 6–6 ■ *A*, Visualization of the epiglottis. The tip of the bronchoscope has followed the contour of the tongue toward its root, and the epiglottis has been located and centered in the field of vision.

Illustration continued on opposite page

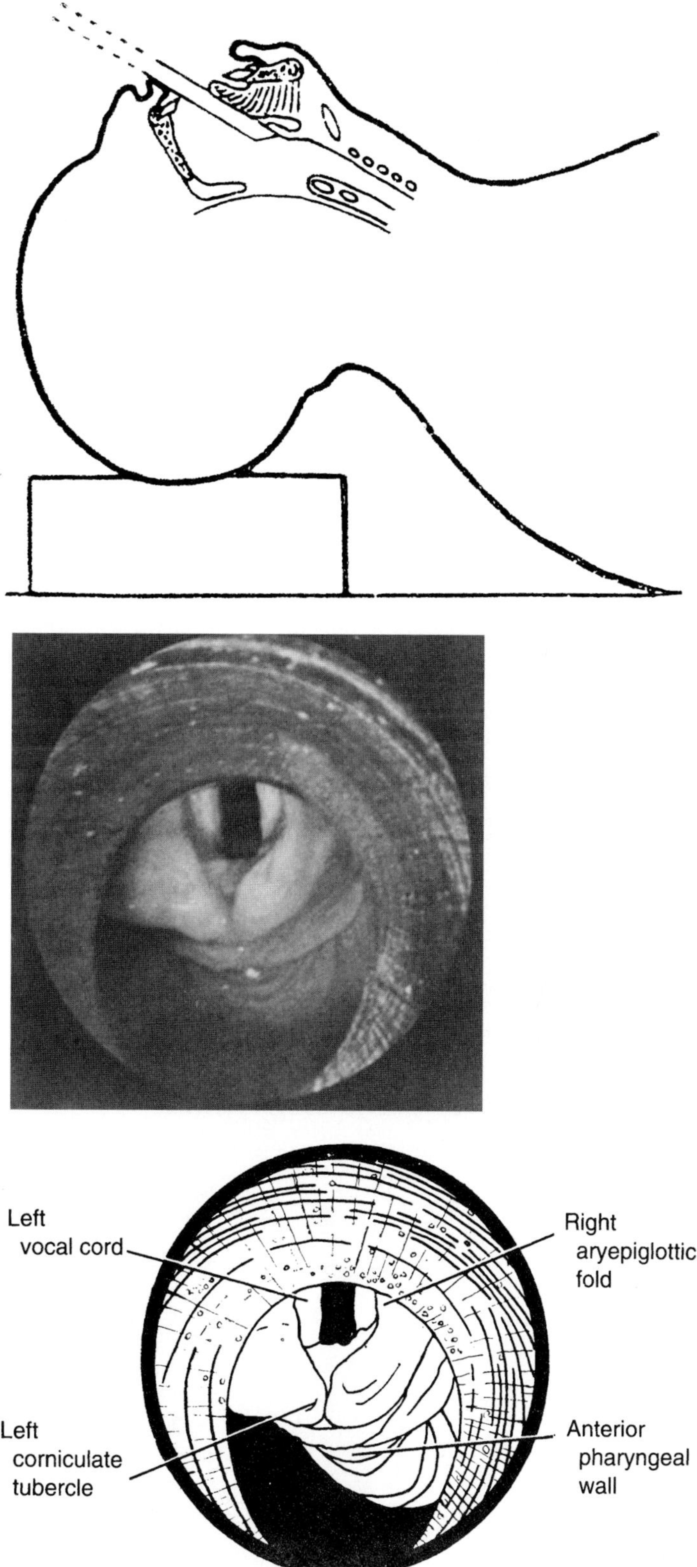

FIGURE 6–6 ■ (*Continued*). *B*, The epiglottis is elevated with the tip of the scope, and the scope is advanced just beyond to demonstrate the glottis. The posterior larynx and vocal cords are clearly visualized.

Illustration continued on following page

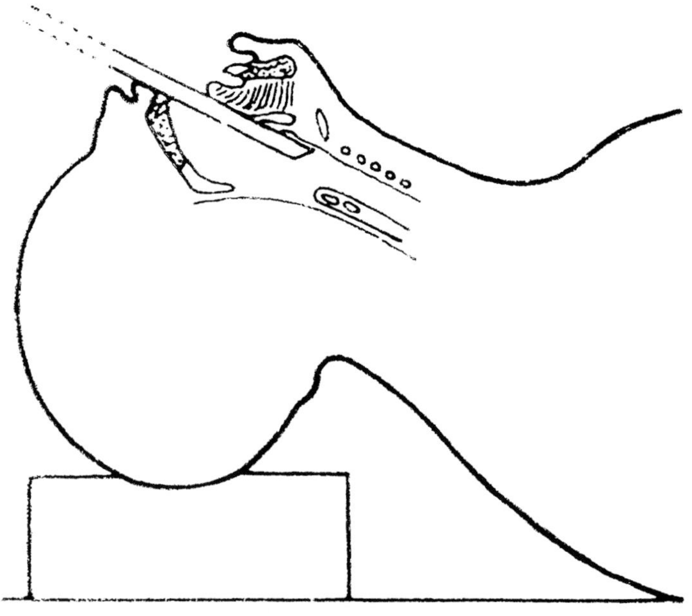

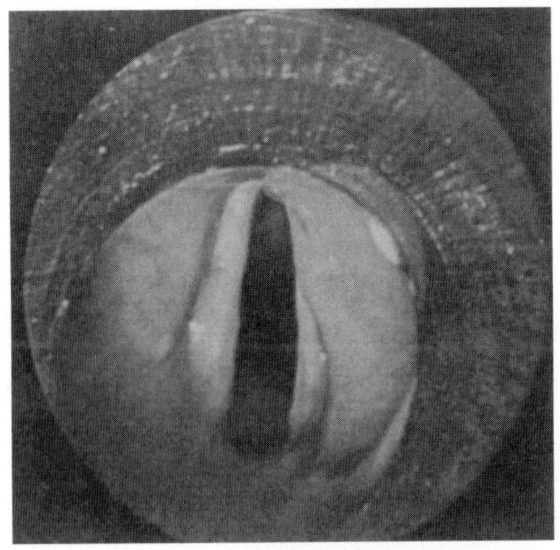

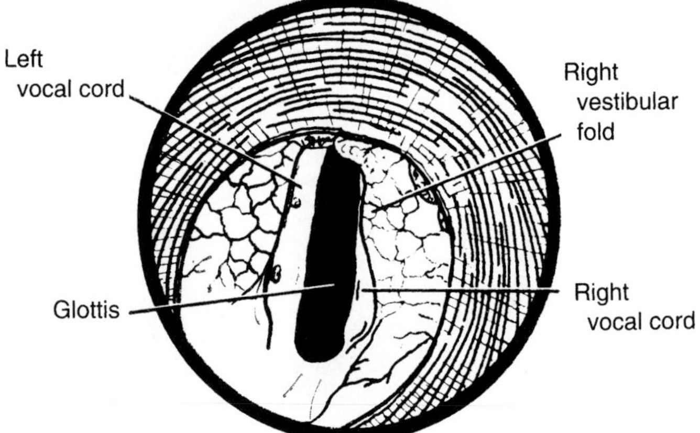

C

FIGURE 6–6 ■ (*Continued*). *C*, The bronchoscope is advanced a little further, and its axis is carefully aligned with that of the glottis and trachea.
Illustration continued on opposite page

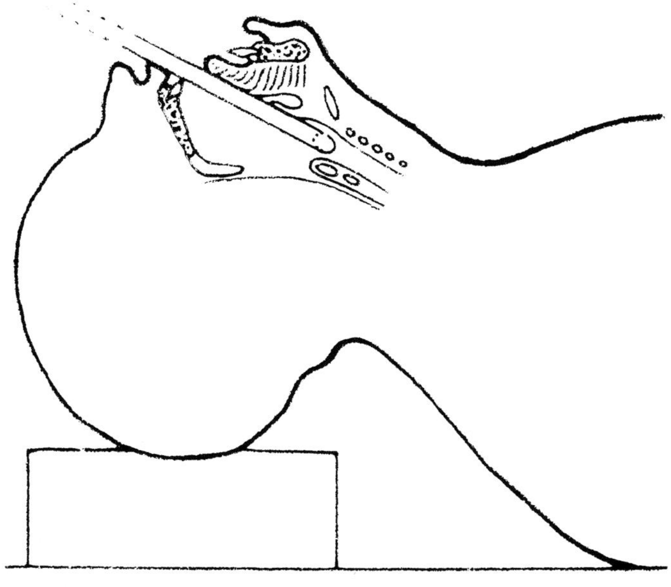

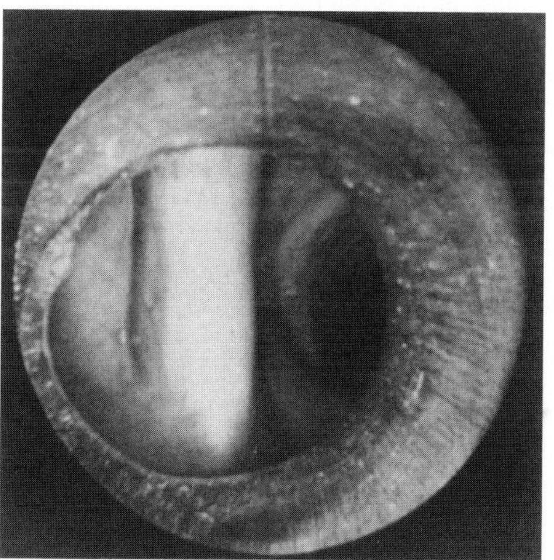

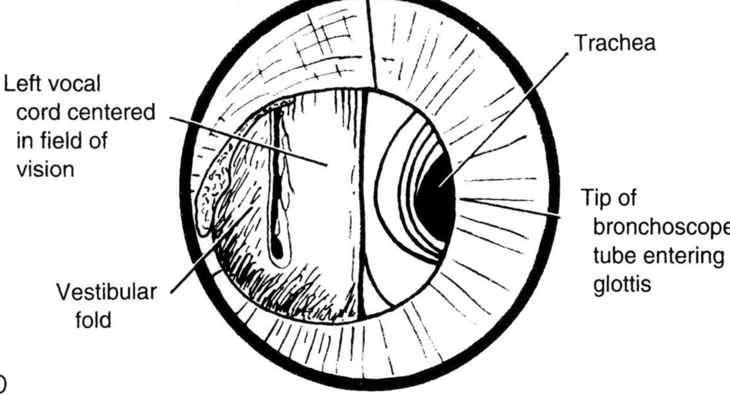

FIGURE 6–6 ■ (*Continued*). *D*, The bronchoscope is turned 90 degrees and gently advanced between the cords into the trachea. The tracheal cartilages are seen in the distance. Once the bronchoscope is in the trachea, it is rotated back to its original orientation for comfortable manipulation, and the pillow behind the patient's head is removed. (From Stradling P: Diagnostic Bronchoscopy: An Introduction, 2nd ed. Baltimore, Williams & Wilkins, 1973.)

bronchoscope should be used. Also, the surgeon should ensure that the lips or pharyngeal tissues are not being inadvertently compressed and injured by the advancing scope.

After intubation, the pillow is removed and the patient's head is extended; care is taken to prevent injury to the cervical spine. The operator is advised to use a mobile stool to sit on and to raise the operating table to a comfortable position before beginning the examination. The scope is then slowly advanced, and the glottis, trachea, and carina are examined. To inspect the left or right side, the patient's head is turned in the opposite direction so that a "straight line" is developed between the oropharynx, the trachea, and the mainstem bronchus to be examined.

To examine the left side, the bronchoscope is placed in the right corner of the mouth, and the patient's head is turned to the right. The scope is gently advanced down the left main bronchus. The lingular and lower lobe bronchi are easily seen. To visualize the segmental and subsegmental bronchi clearly, a telescope (see Fig. 6–4) should be used. A lateral or oblique viewing telescope is required to see the left upper lobe bronchus. The presence of an aortic arch aneurysm is a contraindication to the passing of a rigid instrument down the left mainstem bronchus.

To examine the right bronchial tree, the patient's head is turned to the left, and the bronchoscope is moved to the left corner of the mouth. The right main bronchus and the bronchus intermedius are easily examined. The lower lobe is relatively easily visualized. To examine the middle lobe orifice, the patient's head may have to be extended further to allow the operator an adequate angle to view the anteriorly placed middle lobe orifice. Oblique or lateral viewing telescopes facilitate this task. The lateral viewing telescope is essential to visualize the right upper lobe bronchus and its segmental divisions.

Removal of the rigid bronchoscope should be performed as carefully as its insertion. The opportunity should be taken to examine the entire airway carefully on the way out. This is especially important for the proximal trachea and the subglottic, glottic, and supraglottic areas that may not have been visualized in detail on the way in. Furthermore, if the patient is starting to "lighten" from the anesthetic, this will provide an opportunity to assess the function of the vocal cords.

EQUIPMENT

The performance of rigid bronchoscopy requires several essential pieces of equipment (see Fig. 6–4). Additional components or modifications are available for specialized procedures or are based on operator preference. The basic components are discussed under the categories of bronchoscopes and light sources, suction devices, forceps, and enhanced visualization.

Bronchoscopes

There are a variety of rigid bronchoscopes available; all are variations of the original design by Jackson (Boyd, 1994; Jackson and Jackson, 1950). Several standard rigid bronchoscopes are illustrated in Figure 6–4. The most commonly used sizes in adult practice are in the range of 6 to 9 mm in external diameter and 40 cm in length. For pediatric use, a range of smaller (3- to 6-mm) and shorter scopes are available. A cold halogen light source is connected by a fiberoptic cable to the bronchoscope. The light is transmitted down a fiberoptic fibre bundle along the sidewall of the tube such that the light is emitted from a point just inside the distal tip of the scope.

Suction Devices

One of the major advantages of rigid bronchoscopy is the ability to suction out the airway effectively, especially in cases of massive hemoptysis. An effective (operating room–type) suction source is required. The rigid suction cannula (see Fig. 6–4) must be long enough to protrude from the distal end of the scope that is being used. An insulated suction tube is useful for the application of electrocautery to deal with bleeding after tumor débridement or biopsy.

Forceps

A wide variety of forceps are available for use in varying circumstances. Some of these are illustrated in Figure 6–4. Tissue biopsy forceps are available in several sizes. The large biopsy forceps allow deeper biopsy specimens to be sampled than are generally obtainable with the flexible bronchoscope, but caution must be used to avoid hemorrhage. Aggressive, deep biopsy sampling can remove the full thickness of airway cartilage and lead to troublesome bronchial arterial bleeding. The larger forceps can be used to débride an obstructing tumor or to extract a clot from the airway. A number of forceps are also available that can be used to manipulate, grasp, and extract foreign bodies in the airway. These are stronger than biopsy forceps and more suitably designed for grasping and removing objects.

Enhanced Visualization: Telescopes and Video Display

Rigid Hopkins rod-type telescopes have been developed to examine distal segmental orifices and improve the image (Hopkins, 1976). These solid-rod telescopes produce the best image available, far superior to that seen with fiberoptic equipment. Zero-(forward), 30-, 60-, and 90-degree telescopes are available (see Fig. 6–4). Some telescopes are also equipped with malleable forceps so that biopsy specimens can be taken when this equipment is used. However, in most instances the need to examine segmental and subsegmental orifices is best handled by the insertion of the fiberoptic bronchoscope through the rigid scope to examine the distal structures. Specimens can be taken in the usual fashion with fiberoptic equipment. For this examination, a 7- or 8-mm bronchoscope is necessary to allow passage of the fiberoptic scope, although flexible pediatric bronchoscopes are available for use through smaller tubes.

It can be difficult to teach the fine points of rigid bronchoscopy because of the nature of the examination

(Stradling, 1973). However, cameras are available that mount on the end of the telescope and allow the display of the image on a video monitor. This is of obvious value in the teaching environment and to obtain permanent video or photographic records of the surgeon's observations.

LIMITATIONS AND COMPLICATIONS

There are many potential complications of rigid bronchoscopy, but most can be avoided with careful technique. The major disadvantages of rigid endoscopy include the limitation of view necessitated by the rigid equipment and the need for general anesthesia during this procedure. Because of the rigid nature of the equipment, injury to the upper aerodigestive tract is also a potential complication. The unique complications of rigid endoscopy are injuries to the mouth, pharynx, and upper airway as a result of poor application of the technique. Injuries to the lips, gums, and incisor teeth are avoided with care in the insertion and manipulation of the instrument. Lacerations of the peripharyngeal tissues and injuries to the glottis (e.g., dislocation of the arytenoids) are rare but can occur with forceful manipulation of the scope. A traumatic bronchoscopic examination can result in laryngeal edema, especially in small adults or children, when the bronchoscope may be larger than the laryngeal orifice. Rigid bronchoscopy may be difficult or impossible in patients with certain physical disabilities (e.g., temporomandibular joint fixation or cervical spondylosis) because of the restriction of the opening of the mouth or of the extension of the neck.

Major hemorrhage may occur only when excessive or ill-advised biopsy specimens are taken. The examiner must always remember that the biopsy forceps are large, that bronchial vessels lie in the submucosa, and that certain tumors (e.g., carcinoid) can be highly vascular. If sudden hemorrhage does occur, the main bronchus on the side of bleeding should be intubated with the bronchoscope to diminish spillage into the contralateral lung. Working through the bronchoscope lumen, the surgeon can deal directly with the bleeding site. The topical application of epinephrine solutions (0.2 mg of epinephrine in 500 ml of Ringer's lactate) for vasoconstriction is helpful in some instances. Ventilation of the contralateral lung is maintained through the side ports of the bronchoscope (see Fig. 6–4), which by design will always be in the tracheal lumen. Cauterization, tamponade with epinephrine-soaked gauze, or selective balloon catheterization can be performed through the bronchoscope.

The major anesthetic complication that is seen occurs with the misuse of the Venturi technique. High-pressure jets can produce surgical emphysema, especially if the airway is injured during the procedure. This is extremely rare and is totally avoidable. On occasion, rupture of peripheral pulmonary blebs or bullae can result in a pneumothorax. This complication can occur with any positive–pressure ventilation technique.

SUMMARY

The rigid bronchoscope remains an extremely valuable tool for the diagnosis and management of many thoracic conditions. In certain instances of upper airway obstruction, it may in fact be the only modality that can save a patient's life. It has specific advantages but requires expertise to avoid unnecessary complications. Flexible and rigid bronchoscopy are complementary, rather than mutually exclusive, tools to be used in the diagnosis and therapy of thoracic disease. Although there is some overlap of indications, each modality has its unique indications and limitations, and the thoracic surgeon should be experienced with both techniques to diagnose and treat the spectrum of thoracic disease that may be encountered effectively.

COMMENTS AND CONTROVERSIES

The authors provide a practical summary of the instrumentation, indications, and techniques that are of primary importance to the thoracic surgeon.

Flexible bronchoscopy is very much in the domain of the internist-respirologist, who will frequently refer the lung cancer patient for surgery in accordance with the findings at bronchoscopy. In any patient for whom resection is being considered, it is critically important that the surgeon be familiar with the bronchoscopic findings firsthand, and a repeat endoscopy will frequently be necessary. Such evaluation may be key in the selection of patients for specific techniques such as sleeve resection.

The illustrations demonstrating the pertinent anatomy and technique of rigid bronchoscopy are outstanding and will be very useful for the trainee who is just beginning experience with this procedure. The authors clearly define the indications for rigid bronchoscopy, for which the flexible instrument is inadequate: the management of life-threatening upper-airway obstruction, the control of massive bleeding, and the débridement of obstructing tumors.

F.G.P.

REFERENCES

Boyd AD: Chevalier Jackson: The father of American bronchoesophagoscopy. Ann Thorac Surg 57:502, 1994.

Cooper JD, Pearson FG, Patterson GA et al: Use of silicone stents in the management of airway problems. Ann Thorac Surg 47:371, 1989.

Dumon JF: Treatment of tracheobronchial lesions by laser photoresection. Chest 81:278, 1982.

Ehrenwerth J, Brull S: Anesthesia for thoracic diagnostic procedures. In Kaplan JA (ed): Thoracic Anesthesia, 2nd ed. New York, Churchill Livingstone, 1991.

Hetzel MR, Smith STT: Endoscopic palliation of tracheobronchial malignancies. Thorax 46:225, 1991.

Holinder LD: Use of the open tube bronchoscope in the extraction of foreign bodies. Chest 73:721, 1978.

Hopkins HH: Optical principles of the endoscope. In Berci G (ed): Endoscopy. New York, Appleton-Century-Crofts, 1976.

Ikeda S, Yanain N, Ishikawa S: Flexible bronchofiberscope. Keio J Med 17:1, 1968.

Jackson C, Jackson CL: Bronchoesophagology. Philadelphia, WB Saunders, 1950.

Martin WJ II, Smith TF, Sanderson DR et al: Role of bronchoalveolar lavage in the assessment of opportunistic pulmonary infections: Utility and complications. Mayo Clin Proc 62:549, 1987.

Pereira W Jr, Covenat DM, Snider GL: A prospective cooperative study of complications following flexible fiberoptic bronchoscopy. Chest 73:813, 1978.

Sanders RD: Two ventilating attachments for bronchoscopy. Del Med J 39:170, 1987.

Sonett JR: Endobronchial stents: Primary and adjuvant therapy for endobronchial airway obstruction. Md Med J 47:260, 1998.

Stradling P: Diagnostic Bronchoscopy: An Introduction, 2nd ed. Baltimore, Williams & Wilkins, 1973.

Wedzicha JA, Pearson NC: Management of massive hemoptysis. Respir Med 84:9, 1990.

Weissberg D, Schwartz I: Foreign bodies in the tracheobronchial tree. Chest 91:730, 1987.

MEDIASTINOSCOPY

Thomas J. Kirby
Stanley C. Fell

HISTORICAL NOTE

Cervical mediastinal exploration was originally described by Harken and associates in 1954. Their technique was basically an extension of scalene node biopsy as developed by Daniels (1949) and was used to sample lymph nodes in the superior mediastinum and paratracheal areas. Carlens (1959) and Pearson (1965), using a specially designed mediastinoscope and a suprasternal notch incision, developed and popularized the indications and techniques currently used. Lymph nodes in the aortopulmonary window can be sampled by an anterior mediastinotomy approach, a technique first described by McNeil and Chamberlain (1966). This technique can also be employed on the right side to explore and assess involvement of the anterior mediastinum, right hilum, and superior vena cava. Ginsberg and associates (1987) developed the technique of "extended" cervical mediastinoscopy as an alternative to left anterior mediastinotomy.

■ *HISTORICAL READINGS*

Carlens E: Mediastinoscopy: A method for inspection and tissue biopsy of the superior mediastinum. Chest 36:343, 1959.

Daniels AC: Method of biopsy useful in diagnosing intrathoracic diseases. Dis Chest 16:360, 1949.

Ginsberg RJ, Rice TW, Goldberg M et al: Extended cervical mediastinoscopy: A single staging procedure for bronchogenic carcinoma of the left upper lobe. J Thorac Cardiovasc Surg 94:673, 1987.

Harken DE, Black H, Clauss R, Farrand RE: A single cervical mediastinal exploration for tissue diagnosis of intrathoracic disease. N Engl J Med 251:1041, 1954.

McNeil TM, Chamberlain JM: Diagnostic anterior mediastinoscopy. Ann Thorac Surg 22:260, 1966.

Pearson FG: Mediastinoscopy: A method of biopsy in the superior mediastinum. J Thorac Cardiovasc Surg 49:11, 1965.

INDICATIONS AND DIAGNOSIS

Although mediastinoscopy and mediastinotomy are used primarily in the staging of lung carcinoma, they are also of value in biopsying mediastinal masses and lymph nodes to establish the diagnosis in diseases such as sarcoidosis, lymphoma, and mediastinal tumors. Bronchogenic carcinoma that has metastasized to mediastinal lymph nodes (stage IIIa or IIIb disease) is in most cases not resectable for cure. The results of adjuvant and neoadjuvant radiotherapy or chemotherapy in this group of patients are mixed but for the most part are negative and have not conferred a survival advantage (5-year survival < 10%). Therefore, the importance of establishing involvement of mediastinal lymph nodes with metastatic disease (N2 or N3 disease) prior to thoracotomy is readily apparent. This information will avoid unnecessary thoracotomies in patients with incurable disease (N3 and multistation N2 disease, extracapsular invasion, extension into mediastinal structures [T4 tumors]) and also correctly stage patients who are potential candidates for neoadjuvant trials. Frozen-section results of mediastinal nodes are accurate, allowing the surgeon to proceed immediately to thoracotomy if indicated.

Another staging procedure for assessing the status of mediastinal lymph nodes is transbronchial needle aspiration/biopsy as reported by Wang and associates (1983). This technique is of value in establishing a diagnosis of bronchogenic carcinoma or confirming inoperability in those patients with radiographically unresectable mediastinal lymph node involvement. Otherwise, all patients should be staged with mediastinoscopy or mediastinotomy. These techniques allow accurate assessment of mediastinal lymph node involvement, resulting in an informed and appropriate judgment as to resectability and possible treatment options.

Computed tomography (CT) and magnetic resonance imaging (MRI) are useful screening tests to detect enlargement of mediastinal lymph nodes and direct mediastinal invasion. Although Daly and associates (1984) and Glazer and coworkers (1984) reported sensitivities in the 90% range, Staples and associates (1988) and McLoud and colleagues (1992) reported a sensitivity in the 60% range and a specificity of 50%, defining a lymph node size greater than 1 cm in the short axis as pathologically enlarged. In 1991, one group, reporting on the results from the radiologic oncology group evaluating CT and MR imaging of mediastinal lymph nodes, found a sensitivity of 52% and 48% and a specificity of 69% and 64%, respectively. Compared with the 90% sensitivity and 100% specificity of mediastinoscopy, the relatively poor sensitivity of CT and MRI scanning would, therefore, result in many unnecessary thoracotomies. In a patient with a normal mediastinum by CT scan who is found to have a T1 peripheral carcinoma, mediastinoscopy can be legitimately omitted, but otherwise all patients should be invasively staged. CT scans can also be of value in identifying enlarged mediastinal lymph nodes and mediastinal invasion by tumor. The surgeon is therefore forewarned to pay particular attention to these areas during mediastinoscopy.

There have been many reports on the efficacy of positron emission tomography (PET) scans as a staging modality combined with fluorodeoxyglucose (FDG) to exploit the differences in metabolism between normal and cancerous cells. For a variety of reasons, cancerous cells preferentially trap FDG, thus accounting for the "hot" spots detected by a PET scanner. The overall accuracy of FDG-PET scans in staging the mediastinum is high, easily surpassing that reported for either CT or MRI. Patz and colleagues (1994) reported a sensitivity and specificity for mediastinal lymph nodes staged by PET scanning of 92% and 100%, respectively, compared with 58% and 80% for CT scanning. For combined hilar and mediastinal lymph nodes, the sensitivity and specificity for PET imaging was 83% and 82%, compared with 43% and 85% for CT. Similarly, Sasaki and associates (1996) reported a sensitivity and specificity for PET scan staging of the mediastinum of 76% and 98%, respectively, compared with 65% and 87% for CT scan staging. Al-Sugair and Coleman (1998) give an excellent review of the present application of PET imaging in lung cancer. Overall, there is certainly compelling evidence in the literature that FDG-PET scans are superior to conventional CT/MRI in terms of sensitivity, specificity, and overall accuracy in staging the mediastinum of lung cancer patients. However, the thoracic surgeon is still left with a false-negative rate of 10% to 15%, although this compares favorably with the 8% to 10% false-negative rate reported for mediastinoscopy. PET scanning has the additional advantage over mediastinal biopsy procedures of demonstrating metastatic spread beyond the mediastinum, such as M disease in the liver, lung, adrenal glands, bone, and other sites of hematogenous spread.

Cervical Mediastinoscopy

With a bolster under the patient's shoulders and the neck fully extended, a 3- to 4-cm skin incision is made one fingerbreadth above the suprasternal notch. Dissection is carried down directly in the midline, bluntly separating the strap muscles with the aid of small, right-angle retractors. The thyroid gland is retracted superiorly, with care taken not to avulse the inferior thyroid veins, which can be electrocoagulated or ligated with fine suture to avoid troublesome bleeding. The pretracheal fascia is exposed, opened, and bluntly dissected from the anterior aspect of the trachea by using the index finger. By direct palpation, an attempt is made to identify mediastinal adenopathy, masses, or areas of direct mediastinal invasion. The fascia just inferior and anterior to the innominate artery should be entered to allow the anterior mediastinum and subinnominate space to be assessed. A mediastinoscope can now be introduced along the anterior surface of the trachea (Fig. 6–7). Mediastinal lymph nodes that are accessible to biopsy include the subcarinal (#7), subinnominate (#3a), ipsilateral and contralateral tracheobronchial (#4), and paratracheal (#2) locations. Posterior subcarinal, paraesophageal (#8), and inferior pulmonary ligament (#9) lymph nodes cannot be biopsied through a standard cervical mediastinoscopy or by anterior mediastinotomy.

A metal suction catheter is used as a dissecting instru-

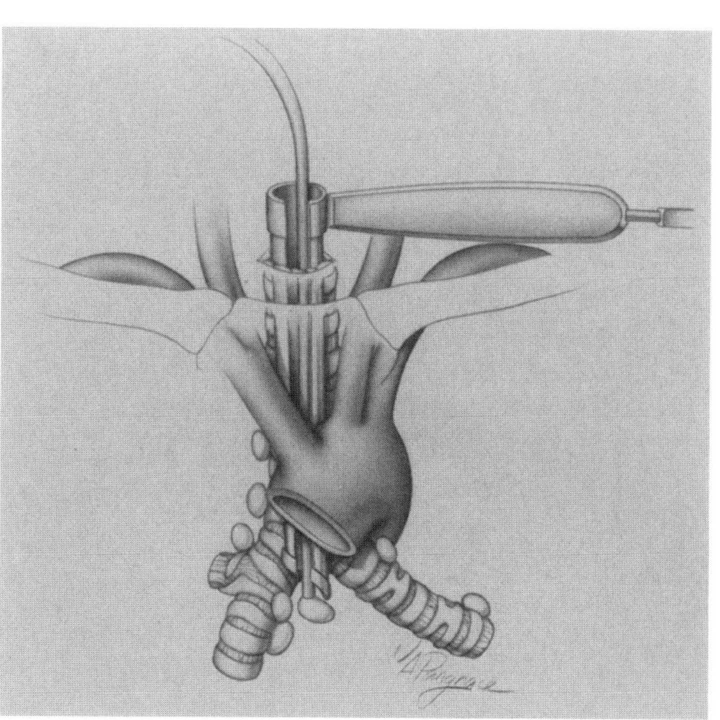

FIGURE 6–7 ■ Cervical mediastinoscopy. A mediastinoscope is introduced through a suprasternal notch incision into the pretracheal space, where samples of paratracheal, tracheobronchial, subcarinal, and subinnominate lymph nodes can be obtained.

ment to further dissect fascial planes and identify lymph nodes and vascular structures. There is usually a firm layer of fascial tissue that has to be opened to gain access to the subcarinal space. If there is any question as to the vascular nature of a structure, it is wise to use a spinal needle mounted on a small syringe to aspirate the structure in question. It is not necessary to remove the entire lymph node to provide representative tissue. Small, bleeding vessels are easily coagulated by using the tip of the suction catheter and touching the proximal end of the catheter with an electrocautery tip. Vascular clips may also be applied through the mediastinoscope. As described by Deslauriers and colleagues (1976), if there is a need to assess the pleural space (e.g., for the presence of an effusion or possible metastatic involvement), the mediastinal pleura just lateral to the trachea can be bluntly broken through, and the mediastinoscope can be introduced to inspect the pleural space and obtain suitable tissue or fluid samples.

Anterior Mediastinotomy

Anterior mediastinotomy was developed by McNeil and Chamberlain (1966) to sample lymph nodes in the subaortic and periaortic regions that are not accessible through cervical mediastinoscopy. Mediastinotomy is classically carried out through the second left intercostal space. The technique can also be employed on the right side to biopsy mediastinal masses and lymph nodes. In the technique as originally described, a vertical parasternal incision removing the second costal cartilage was used. A transverse incision directly over the second intercostal space, which does not remove a costal cartilage, is also effective.

A 3- to 4-cm skin incision is made directly over the second intercostal space just lateral to the sternal border. Dissection is carried down to the pectoralis major, separating its fibers. Electrocautery is used along the superior border of the second costal cartilage to divide the intercostal muscles, with care taken not to injure the internal mammary vessels. An attempt is made to bluntly dissect the mediastinal pleura, with an index finger, down to the aortopulmonary window without entering the pleural space. If the pleural space is entered, a pleural drainage catheter is placed at the end of the procedure, with the anesthesiologist's hand bagging the patient to evacuate all intrapleural air. Unless the underlying lung parenchyma has been injured, one should be able to remove the catheter at the end of the procedure or in the recovery room. If mediastinotomy is being carried out in conjunction with mediastinoscopy, the aortopulmonary window can be bimanually palpated by inserting one index finger through the neck incision and the other through the mediastinotomy incision. This will help in identifying adenopathy or tumor fixation in the area.

A mediastinoscope can now be safely introduced through the incision (Fig. 6–8). Care must be taken not to injure the phrenic or vagus nerves as they pass over the aortic arch. The superior pulmonary vein, aorta, and left main pulmonary artery as it passes under the aortic arch are all at risk of injury. If the proper technique is followed, regional lymph nodes are easily and safely identified and biopsied.

Extended Cervical Mediastinoscopy

Extended cervical mediastinoscopy as described by Ginsberg and associates (1987) can supplant left anterior mediastinotomy and carries the advantage of avoiding a separate incision. Blunt dissection with an index finger is used to open tissue between the innominate and the carotid arteries, superior to the arch of the aorta. A mediastinoscope is then introduced anterior to the aortic arch and between the innominate and carotid arteries

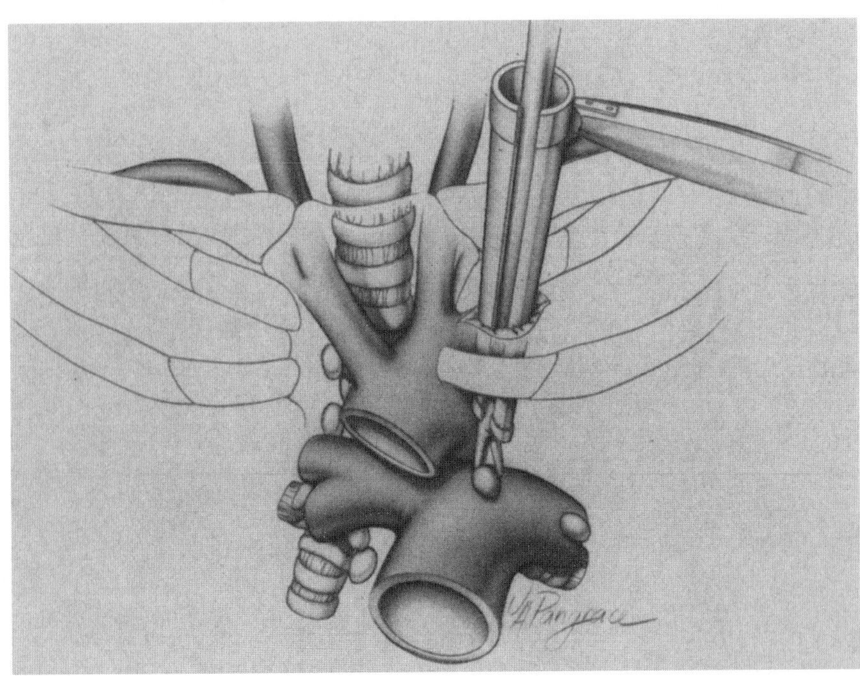

FIGURE 6–8 ■ Anterior mediastinoscopy. A mediastinoscope is introduced through a parasternal incision placed in the second intercostal space. On the left side, this allows periaortic and aortopulmonary window lymph nodes to be sampled.

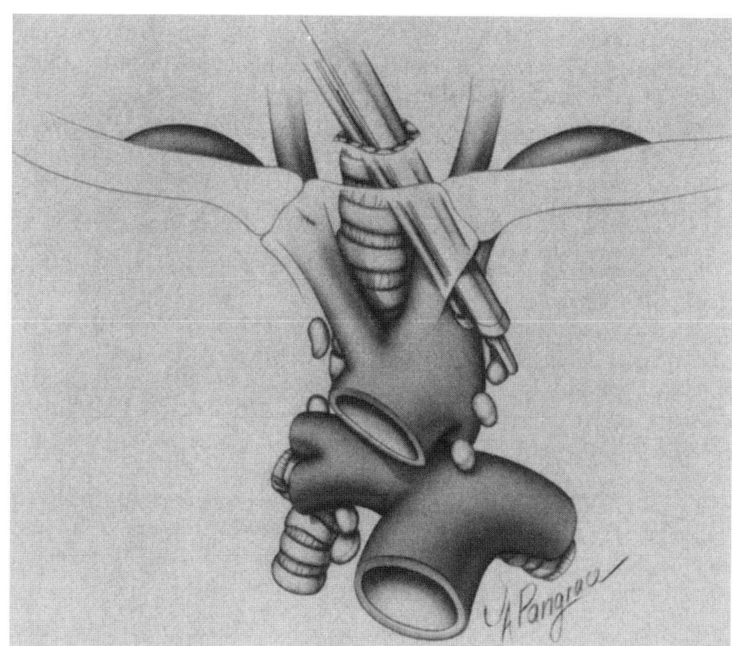

FIGURE 6–9 ■ Extended cervical mediastinoscopy. By the same approach as that for standard cervical mediastinoscopy, a mediastinoscope is introduced over the aortic arch and into the aortopulmonary window.

(Fig. 6–9). The mediastinoscope can then be advanced over the top of the aorta to the aortopulmonary window. In addition to the innominate and carotid arteries, the same nerves and vessels as those in mediastinotomy are at risk of injury.

Scalene Lymph Node Biopsy

The involvement of supraclavicular lymph nodes (stage IIIb disease) is obviously a grave prognostic sign. Enlarged nodes in this area may be simply needle aspirated to confirm involvement, but a negative aspirate does not rule out metastatic disease and will have to be confirmed with an excisional biopsy. Enlarged lymph nodes may be locally excised, or a formal excision of the scalene fat pad may be performed.

A small, 3- to 4-cm incision is placed over the origin of the sternocleidomastoid muscle just above and parallel to the clavicle. Further dissection is carried down between the clavicular and sternal heads, or the entire muscle is retracted medially. This exposes the scalene fat pad, which lies on top of the anterior scalenus muscle, medial to the internal jugular vein (Fig. 6–10). The fat pad is carefully dissected away from the internal jugular vein laterally and the scalenus anterior muscle posteriorly. Care must be taken not to injure the phrenic nerve, which is separated from the operative field by only a thin fascial sheath overlying the scalenus anterior muscle. The transverse cervical artery, which usually enters inferiorly, is divided to allow complete excision of the fat pad, which should contain five or more lymph nodes for pathologic examination.

COMPLICATIONS

In experienced hands, the complications of mediastinoscopy and mediastinotomy are rare (1% to 2%), but the potential for catastrophic complications is apparent. Puhakka (1989) reported on 2021 mediastinoscopies with a complication rate of 2.3% and no associated deaths. Only 10 (0.5%) of these complications were considered major; these were four cases of hemorrhage, three of tracheal rupture, and three of wound infection. Basca and colleagues (1974) reported on 11,623 mediastinoscopies from 15 different series. Bleeding that required operation was noted in 0.1% of cases, with pneumothorax occurring in 0.5% and vocal-cord paralysis in 0.4%. In another series of 1000 cases, Luke and associates (1986) from the University of Toronto reported a 2.3% complication rate. Only three complications were considered major, including two cases of hemorrhage and one of tracheal injury. Minor complications included six pneumothoraces, five wound infections, and nine other complications. There were no reported recurrent nerve injuries.

Major complications during mediastinoscopy are most commonly encountered at either tracheobronchial angle. On the right side, the azygos vein and anterior pulmonary arterial branch to the right upper lobe are at risk of injury. The azygos vein is easily mistaken for an anthracotic lymph node and inadvertently biopsied. Experience and the liberal use of a long aspirating needle prior to biopsy will avoid this complication. Lymph nodes in this area are often directly adherent to branches of the pulmonary artery, which are therefore at risk if deep biopsies are taken or if excessive traction is applied. The apical arterial branch can also be injured if the mediastinoscope is "levered" anteriorly, resulting in a traction injury to the artery. At the left tracheobronchial angle, the left recurrent laryngeal nerve is in close proximity to regional lymph nodes and is easily traumatized if care is not taken. Again, the entire lymph node should not be sampled, because the recurrent laryngeal nerve is usually directly adherent to nodes in this area. Bleeding is best handled with packing placed through the mediastinoscope rather than by electrocautery, which may cause

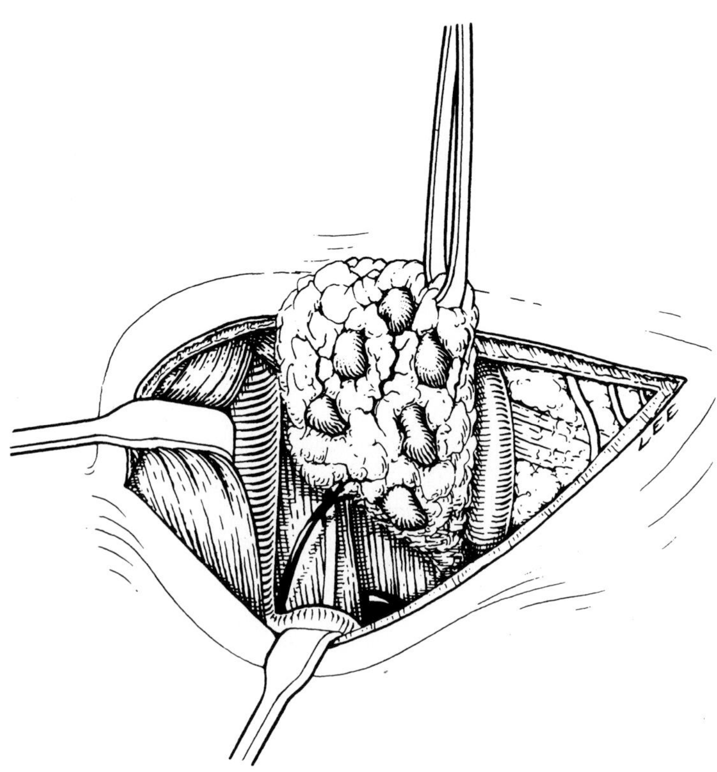

FIGURE 6–10 ■ With the sternocleidomastoid muscle retracted medially, the scalene fat pad is mobilized off the internal jugular vein and the scalenus anterior muscle posteriorly. The phrenic nerve can be seen lying on the scalenus anterior muscle, with the transverse cervical artery entering the fat pad inferiorly.

thermal injury and permanent damage to the recurrent nerve.

In the event of massive bleeding, mediastinal packing will usually control the hemorrhage while blood is obtained and preparations are made for a possible thoracotomy or median sternotomy. Following 10 minutes of gauze tamponade, with the operating room prepared for a major procedure, the gauze packing is gently removed. In many cases, the hemorrhage will have subsided or decreased so that the bleeding site can be identified. In the face of persistent, uncontrollable hemorrhage, the mediastinum should be repacked, and a decision should be made as to whether thoracotomy or median sternotomy would offer the best approach to control hemorrhage in this patient. Median sternotomy is the most versatile incision and allows most injuries to be easily identified and controlled. It also allows the surgeon to expeditiously institute cardiopulmonary bypass to gain control of major vessel injuries. A disadvantage of sternotomy is the greater difficulty in carrying out a definitive pulmonary resection once the hemorrhage is controlled.

Injuries to the esophagus are extremely rare. As the esophagus lies directly posterior to the subcarinal space, most injuries occur during the exploration of this space and the biopsy of subcarinal lymph nodes. This injury is often not recognized at the time of surgery and may be diagnosed postoperatively when the patient develops mediastinitis and an esophagogram is obtained. The detection of cervical or mediastinal air, pneumothorax, or pleural effusion in the early postoperative period should alert the surgeon to the possibility of this complication and lead to further investigation. These injuries are dealt with by the same principles applied to managing other forms of esophageal trauma (see Chapter 68).

Tracheobronchial tree injuries are also rare. They are usually recognized at the time of surgery, when an air leak is encountered. As reported by Puhakka (1989), most of these injuries can be controlled by packing the area with absorbable cellulose gauze (Surgical, Johnson & Johnson, New Brunswick, NJ). If such an injury occurs, it is also prudent to leave a drain in the area. The positive pressure of mechanical ventilation makes even small injuries to the airway appear significant, but once the patient has been extubated and is breathing spontaneously, most of these injuries will close. As reported by Schubach and Landreneau (1992), more extensive injuries can require a direct surgical approach and primary repair.

COMMENTS AND CONTROVERSIES

The authors are both very experienced clinicians and have a long and continuing experience with mediastinoscopy and its variants for histologic evaluation of mediastinal lymph nodes, which can be accessed by these techniques. This updated chapter contains a review of the role and influence of FDG PET scanning, which was not available when the first edition of this text was prepared. It is clear that PET scanning is significantly more sensitive and accurate than CT evaluation and has the added distinct advantage of being instrumental in identifying metastatic disease in sites outside the mediastinum, anywhere that hematogenous disease may appear. As the authors point out, in patients with primary lung cancer, PET scans result in some false-positive reports, which may warrant mediastinoscopy for confirmation, as well as a 10% to 15% incidence of false-negative studies. Although PET scanning has undoubtedly reduced the frequency of mediastinoscopy for the staging of lung cancer, there are many surgeons who continue to regularly employ mediastinoscopy to evaluate most patients because of this small, but potentially important subset of cases with false-negative scans.

F.G.P.

■ KEY REFERENCES

Carlens E: Mediastinoscopy: A method for inspection and tissue biopsy of the superior mediastinum. Chest 36:343, 1959.

The initial report on cervical mediastinoscopy using a suprasternal notch incision as compared with the more cumbersome approach originally reported by Harkens and associates (1949). This technique has withstood the test of time and is still employed today.

Luke WP, Pearson FG, Todd TRJ et al: Prospective evaluation of mediastinoscopy for assessment of carcinoma of the lung. J Thorac Cardiovasc Surg 91:53, 1986.

This report on 1000 mediastinoscopies performed in the staging of lung cancer demonstrates its high level of sensitivity, specificity, and overall accuracy combined with a low operative morbidity.

Pearson FG: Mediastinoscopy: A method of biopsy in the superior mediastinum. J Thorac Cardiovasc Surg 49:11, 1965.

An excellent review of the initial experience of the surgeon responsible for popularizing mediastinoscopy in North America and demonstrating its value in staging bronchogenic carcinoma.

■ REFERENCES

Al-Sugair A, Coleman E: Applications of PET in lung cancer. Semin Nucl Med 28:303, 1998.

Basca S, Czako Z, Vezendi S: The complications of mediastinoscopy. Panminerva Med 16:402, 1974.

Daly BDT Jr, Faling LJ, Pugatch RD et al: Computed tomography: An effective technique for mediastinal staging in lung cancer. J Thorac Cardiovasc Surg 88:486, 1984.

Daniels AC: Method of biopsy useful in diagnosing certain intrathoracic diseases. Dis Chest 16:360, 1949.

Deslauriers J, Beaulieu M, Dufour C et al: Mediastino-pleuroscopy: A new approach to the diagnosis of intra-thoracic diseases. Ann Thorac Surg 22:265, 1976.

Ginsberg RJ, Rice TW, Goldberg M et al: Extended cervical mediastinoscopy: A single staging procedure for bronchogenic carcinoma of the left upper lobe. J Thorac Cardiovasc Surg 94:673, 1987.

Glazer GM, Orringer MB, Gross BH, Quint LE: The mediastinum in non-small cell cancer: CT-surgical correlation. AJR Am J Roentgenol 142:1101, 1984.

Harkens DE, Black H, Clauss R, Farrand RE: A single cervical mediastinal exploration for tissue diagnosis of intrathoracic disease. N Engl J Med 251:1041, 1954.

McLoud TC, Bourgouin PM, Greenberg RW et al: Bronchogenic carcinoma: Analysis of staging in the lymph node mapping and sampling. Radiology 182:319, 1992.

McNeil TM, Chamberlain JM: Diagnostic anterior mediastinotomy. Ann Thorac Surg 2:532, 1966.

Patz EF, Lowe VJ, Goodman PC et al: Thoracic nodal staging with PET imaging with 18-FDG in patients with bronchogenic carcinoma. Chest 108:1617, 1994.

Puhakka H: Complications of mediastinoscopy. J Laryngol Otol 103:312, 1989.

Sasaki M, Ichiya Y, Kuwabara Y et al: The usefulness of FDG-PET for the detection of mediastinal lymph node metastases in patients with non-small cell lung cancer: A comparative study with x-ray CT. Eur J Nucl Med 21:189s, 1996.

Schubach SL, Landreneau RJ: Mediastinoscopic injury to the bronchus: Use of incontinuity bronchial flap repair. Ann Thorac Surg 93:1101, 1992.

Staples CA, Muller NL, Miller RR et al: Mediastinal nodes in bronchogenic carcinoma: Comparison between CT and mediastinoscopy. Radiology 67:367, 1988.

Wang KP, Brower R, Haponik EF, Siegelman S: Flexible transbronchial needle aspiration for staging bronchogenic carcinoma. Chest 84:571, 1983.

THORACOSCOPY FOR DIAGNOSIS AND STAGING

Jean Deslauriers
Cateline Sirois

Video-assisted thoracic surgery (VATS) has now replaced open thoracotomy in the evaluation of many pleuropulmonary disorders. Indeed, in many centers it has become the procedure of choice for the biopsy of diffuse lung disease, indeterminate lung nodules, or pleural infiltrates. Specific advantages of VATS over open thoracotomy include the use of smaller incisions, reduced operative morbidity, and, most importantly, optimal visualization of the entire lung and pleural space.

The role of VATS for pretreatment staging of lung cancer patients is still debated, because accurate staging can be achieved by the use of imaging modalities or less invasive surgical techniques such as cervical mediastinoscopy. VATS appears to be useful to determine if a pleural effusion is due to pleural dissemination or to obstructive pneumonitis or to access lymph nodes in areas that are difficult to reach through standard mediastinoscopy.

In this subchapter, indications, techniques, and complications of thoracoscopy that are used for the diagnosis of pleuropulmonary diseases and staging of lung cancer are reviewed.

HISTORICAL NOTE

In the past, thoracoscopy independent of laparoscopy was a popular diagnostic tool. In 1806, Bozzini (Bloom-

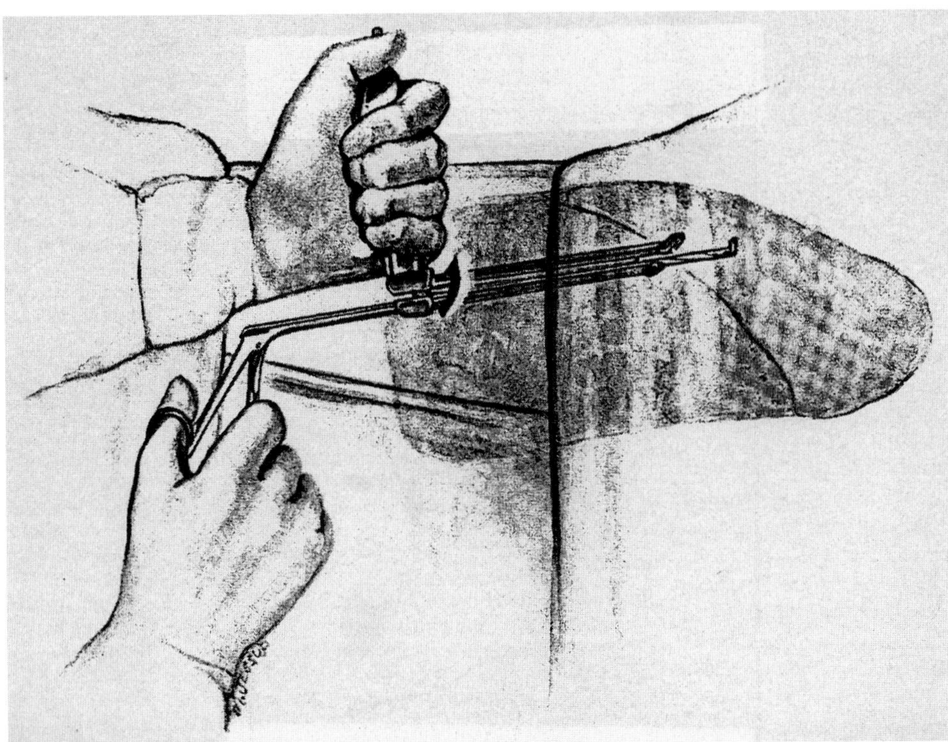

FIGURE 6–11 ■ Use of a fiberoptic mediastinoscope as a thoracoscope. (From Lewis RJ, Kunderman PJ, Sisler GE, Mackenzie JW: Direct diagnostic thoracoscopy. Ann Thorac Surg 21:536, 1976.)

berg, 1978) conceived the first endoscope. This was followed in 1853 by the report of Desormeau, who suggested improvements in the technique (Le Tacon, 1981). Both used a hollow tube lighted by a burning light to visualize the bladder. In 1910, Jacobeus modified the scope and incorporated an Edisonian light. He used a modified cystoscope to cauterize pleural adhesions to facilitate lung collapse in the treatment of tuberculosis (Jacobeus, 1925). Soon after the development of effective antituberculous medications, the use of thoracoscopy started to decline. During those early years, thoracoscopy was also used on occasion and mostly in Europe for the treatment of recurrent malignant pleural effusions and pneumothoraces (Sattler, 1937). In South America, thoracoscopy was used as a method of exploration in penetrating injuries of the thorax (Branco, 1946). Often, physicians avoided the use of thoracoscopy because they feared infection, hemorrhage, and air embolism.

From the early 1960s to 1990, thoracoscopy remained popular in a few centers throughout Europe, the procedure being usually carried out by chest physicians. In his review, Boutin and associates (1981) states that Brandt in Berlin had done over 3000 thoracoscopies under local anesthesia and that 1130 of these cases involved biopsy of diffuse lung diseases or of pulmonary nodules. Only one case of massive hemorrhage was observed, and a positive diagnosis was obtained in 87% of patients. Other significant early contributions were those of Lewis and associates (1976) (Fig. 6–11) and Weisberg and Kaufman (1980). By using a mediastinoscope or a bronchoscope, Lewis and associates studied 40 patients, diagnosing malignant lesions in 21 and finding benign lesions in the others.

In 1981, Maassen from Germany described an improved method of direct thoracoscopy without creating a pneumothorax (Fig. 6–12). Between 1972 and 1979, he performed 1097 pleuropulmonary biopsies and obtained a definitive tissue diagnosis in 86% of cases. Wenderman and associates (1974), who worked with Maassen and adopted his technique, reached a histologically confirmed diagnosis in 87% of 61 patients with diffuse pulmonary disorders. Beaulieu, Deslauriers, and colleagues (1972, 1976) used a cervical mediastinoscopy incision and perforated digitally the mediastinal pleura on either side.

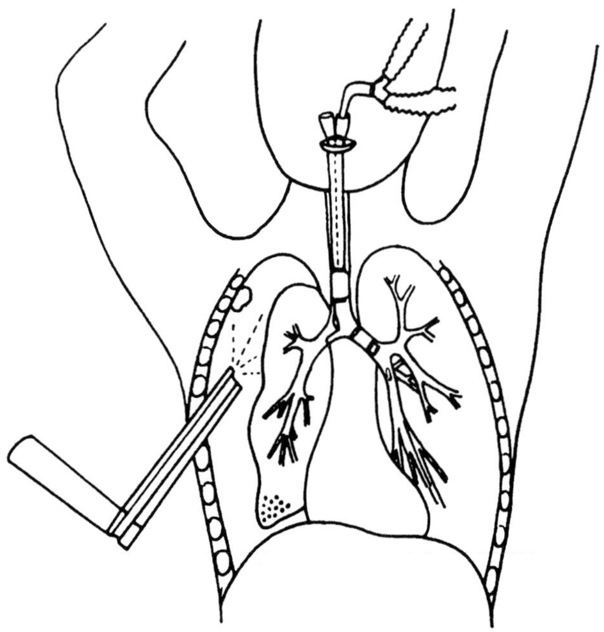

FIGURE 6–12 ■ Technique of direct thoracoscopy as described by Maassen for pleuropulmonary biopsies. (From Maassen W: Thoracoscopie et biopsie pulmonaire sans pneumothorax initial. Poumon-Cœur 37:317, 1981.)

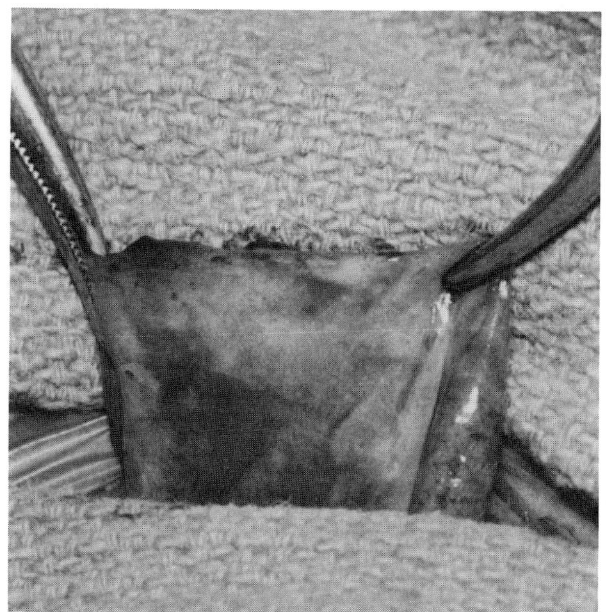

FIGURE 6–13 ■ Operative photograph showing the apex of the lung, which is pulled out through the cervical incision.

They then inserted the mediastinoscope to obtain biopsy material and in some cases were able to pull the lung out through the cervical incision for biopsy (Fig. 6–13). In the latter report, a diagnostic accuracy of 90% was attained in benign pulmonary diseases and of 100% in pleural diseases.

The first significant use of thoracoscopy for the preoperative evaluation of presumed operable lung cancer is credited to le Roux (1968). In a review of 4000 cases of lung cancer seen between 1949 and 1963, he reported 139 thoracoscopies for patients with associated effusions, and, in 82 instances, pleural metastases were found. These patients were not operated on, and 80% of the individuals with gross pleural metastases were dead within 6 months.

Over the years, diagnostic thoracoscopy has been performed in a number of ways. The scope could be a simple mediastinoscope, a flexible bronchoscope, or a rigid thoracoscope with a cold light. Currently, the rigid scope is coupled to a video camera system, which allows the involvement of the whole surgical team in the procedure. Thoracoscopy can be performed under locoregional or general anesthesia, which provides increased liberties for manipulations in the pleural space.

Since 1990, videothoracoscopy has exploded worldwide, and, in 1991, the councils of the American Association for Thoracic Surgery and the Society for Thoracic Surgeons appointed a joint committee to develop standards and guidelines pertaining to therapeutic videothoracoscopy (Miller, 1993). In essence, a clear distinction was established between thoracic surgical procedures being done with video equipment (VATS) and "medical" thoracoscopies primarily used for diagnostic purposes.

■ *HISTORICAL READINGS*

Beaulieu M, Després JP, Lemieux M: Mediastinopleuroscopy: A new technique for the diagnosis of thoracic diseases. Chirurgie 98:355, 1972.

Bloomberg AE: Thoracoscopy in perspective. Surg Gynecol Obstet 147:433, 1978.

Boutin C, Viallat JR, Cargnino P, Farisse P: Indications actuelles de la thoracoscopie. Rev Fr Mal Resp 9:309, 1981.

Branco JMC: Thoracoscopy as a method of exploration in penetrating injuries of the thorax. Dis Chest 12:330, 1946.

Deslauriers J, Beaulieu M, Dufour C et al: Mediastinopleuroscopy: A new approach to the diagnosis of intrathoracic diseases. Ann Thorac Surg 22:265, 1976.

Jacobeus HC: Ueber die Möglichkeit die cystoscopic bei Untersuchung seröses Höhl-lumen anzuwenden. Munch Med Wochenschr 57:2090, 1910.

Jacobeus HC: Die Thorakoscopic und ihre praktische Bedeutung. Ergeb-Ges Med (Berlin) 7:112, 1925.

le Roux BT: Bronchial carcinoma. London, Livingston, 1968.

Le Tacon J: La pneuroscopie. Rappel historique. Poumon-Cœur 37:5, 1981.

Lewis RJ, Kunderman PJ, Sisler GE, MacKenzie JW: Direct diagnostic thoracoscopy. Ann Thorac Surg 21:536, 1976.

Maassen W: Thoracoscopie et biopsie pulmonaire sans pneumothorax initial. Poumon-cœur 37:317, 1981.

Miller JI: The present role and future considerations of video-assisted thoracoscopy in general thoracic surgery. Ann Thorac Surg 56:804, 1993.

Sattler A: The treatment of spontaneous pneumothorax with special reference to thoracoscopy. Beitrin Klinik Tuberkulosis 89:395, 1937.

Weisberg D, Kaufman M: Diagnostic and therapeutic pleuroscopy: Experience with 127 patients. Chest 78:732, 1980.

Wenderman K, Greschuchna D, Maassen W: Results of surgical pleural and pulmonary biopsies. Thorax Chirurgie 22:453, 1974.

BASIC SCIENCE

Thoracoscopy for Undiagnosed Pleural Effusion and Other Pleural Diseases

Any alteration of the fluid transportation system across the pleural space or of the physical and histochemical integrity of the pleural surfaces or of its lymphatic drainage can result in the abnormal accumulation of pleural fluid. Some of the most common etiologic factors associated with abnormal formation and accumulation of pleural fluid are listed in Table 6–3.

Imaging techniques can readily detect effusion but they generally are not very accurate in identifying its etiology. Thoracentesis with biochemical, microbiologic, and cytologic studies is diagnostic in 75% of patients with pleural effusion (Collins and Sahn, 1987), and higher yields can be obtained for diseases that rely less on cytology for their diagnosis such as empyemas, hemothoraces, and chylothoraces. Cytologic analysis, even with repeated examination of large amounts of pleural fluid, is diagnostic in only 60% to 80% of patients with metastatic disease to the pleura (Light, 1983).

The conventional technique of closed pleural biopsy using an Abrams needle provides diagnosis in 38% to 67% of patients with malignancy of the pleura (Canto et al, 1977; Rao et al, 1965) and in 54% to 75% of patients with tuberculous pleuritis (Tomlinson and Sahn, 1987). The mapping of the sites of pleural malignancies shows that most tumors are located in the lower half of the thorax, and in that portion, most are located on the visceral, diaphragmatic, or mediastinal pleura (Canto et al, 1983), none of which are readily accessible to the biopsy needles.

The consequence of the relatively low yield of these investigations is that in about 20% to 25% of patients

TABLE 6–3 ■ **Etiologic Factors Associated with Pleural Effusion**

Pulmonary and pleural infection
Empyema
Mycobacterium tuberculosis
Bacteria
Fungi
Viruses and mycoplasma
Parasitic
Immunologic diseases
Rheumatoid arthritis
Systemic lupus erythematosus
Wegener's granulomatosis
Pleural neoplasms
Bronchogenic carcinoma
Myeloproliferative disorders
Metastatic carcinoma
Mesothelioma
Chest wall tumors
Cardiac disorders
Hemothorax
Chylothorax
Pneumothorax
Abdominal pathology
Pancreatitis
Subphrenic abscess
Malignancy
Renal pathology
Nephrotic syndrome
Hydronephrosis
Dialysis
Glomerulonephritis
Uremiopleuritis
Liver pathology
Miscellaneous
Myxedema
Asbestosis

with pleural effusion, no etiology can be found despite exhaustive and expansive testing (Colt, 1995; Gunnels, 1978; Poe et al, 1984). In a series of 1000 effusions investigated by Boutin and colleagues (1981), 215 defied diagnosis despite repeated pleural fluid analyses and closed pleural biopsies. Of much concern is the 50% of this group that will ultimately show evidence of malignancy. By thoracoscopy, 90% to 100% of the surfaces of both visceral and parietal pleura can be explored, allowing for direct access and biopsy of suspicious areas. Because the biopsy specimens are bigger and obtained from different sites, the yield of what is obtained by percutaneous biopsy is significantly improved (Fig. 6–14).

In 1971, Brandt and Mai reported on 1130 diagnostic thoracoscopies, of which 414 were performed for an undiagnosed pleural effusion. When thoracoscopy was combined with cytologic and bacteriologic studies, only 2.5% of the effusions were still of unknown etiology. In 1991, Wakabayashi reported 315 thoracoscopies performed under general anesthesia with a mortality of 1% and a diagnostic accuracy of 99%. In a collective review of 1500 thoracoscopies from different centers, Menzies and Charbonneau (1991) reported that the diagnostic accuracy of the technique was approximately 90% and morbidity, which included arrhythmias, bleeding, and empyema, was under 3%. In their own series of 102 thoracoscopies performed with the patient under local anesthesia, the diagnostic accuracy was 96%, the sensitivity was 91%, the specificity was 100%, and the negative predictive value was 93%. Major operative complications occurred in 1.9% of cases. Other studies present similar data (Buchhotz et al, 1990; Hucker et al, 1991; Kimura et al, 1990).

Thoracoscopy for Mesothelioma

One of the problems associated with the treatment of malignant mesothelioma is that the diagnosis is often made when the tumor is either unresectable or too extensive to be responsive to any form of therapy. Not unlike other malignancies, it is probable that if the diagnosis were established at an earlier stage, treatment could be more effective and cure rates higher.

Pleural fluid cytology is notoriously unreliable for the diagnosis of mesothelioma, and Legha and Muggia (1977) have shown that it has a diagnostic yield of only 20%. Unless a definite pleural mass is present, percutaneous pleural biopsy is also unreliable. CT scan with contrast media can be of some help (Gore et al, 1998; Maasilta et al, 1991), but the pleural thickening must be within the resolution of the scanner, a situation seldom seen in the early stages of disease. An additional problem with the diagnosis of mesothelioma is that it must be differentiated from metastatic adenocarcinoma, a distinction that is often difficult to establish with the smaller tissue specimens that are obtained by percutaneous techniques. Finally, mesotheliomas have a predilection for costophrenic angles, diaphragm, and mediastinum, all of which are not readily accessible to biopsy needles. In a review of 35 cases of malignant mesotheliomas, Boutin and associates (1979) showed that pleural biopsy by percutaneous technique was conclusive in only 40% of cases, whereas a positive diagnosis was obtained in 94% of cases after thoracoscopy. Sgro and coworkers (1991) also obtained a yield of 85.7% after thoracoscopy in 21 cases of proven mesothelioma. In an interesting study, Grossebner and associates (1999) prospectively analyzed a group of 25 patients in whom mesothelioma was suspected and who had been referred for histologic diagnosis by VATS after failure of other methods. In that series, all patients had a histologic diagnosis made by VATS (mesothelioma: 23; empyema: 2). In addition, patients underwent, during the same procedure, drainage of the effusion, pleurectomy, and lung mobilization; this resulted in significantly fewer hospital admissions and ostensibly improved the quality of life for these patients.

Thoracoscopy for Chest Trauma

Little has been documented about the use of thoracoscopy as an aid to diagnose intrathoracic injuries. In 1946, Branco was the first to describe the use of thoracoscopy in the initial decision-making after penetrating injuries to the chest. In 1981, Sattler reported the use of thoracoscopy in a patient with hemopneumothorax, and more recently, Duzhyi (1991) also described thoracoscopy as the method of choice in the investigation of hemothoraces. In 1992, Feliciano suggested the use of thoracoscopy among other methods in the diagnosis of thoracic inju-

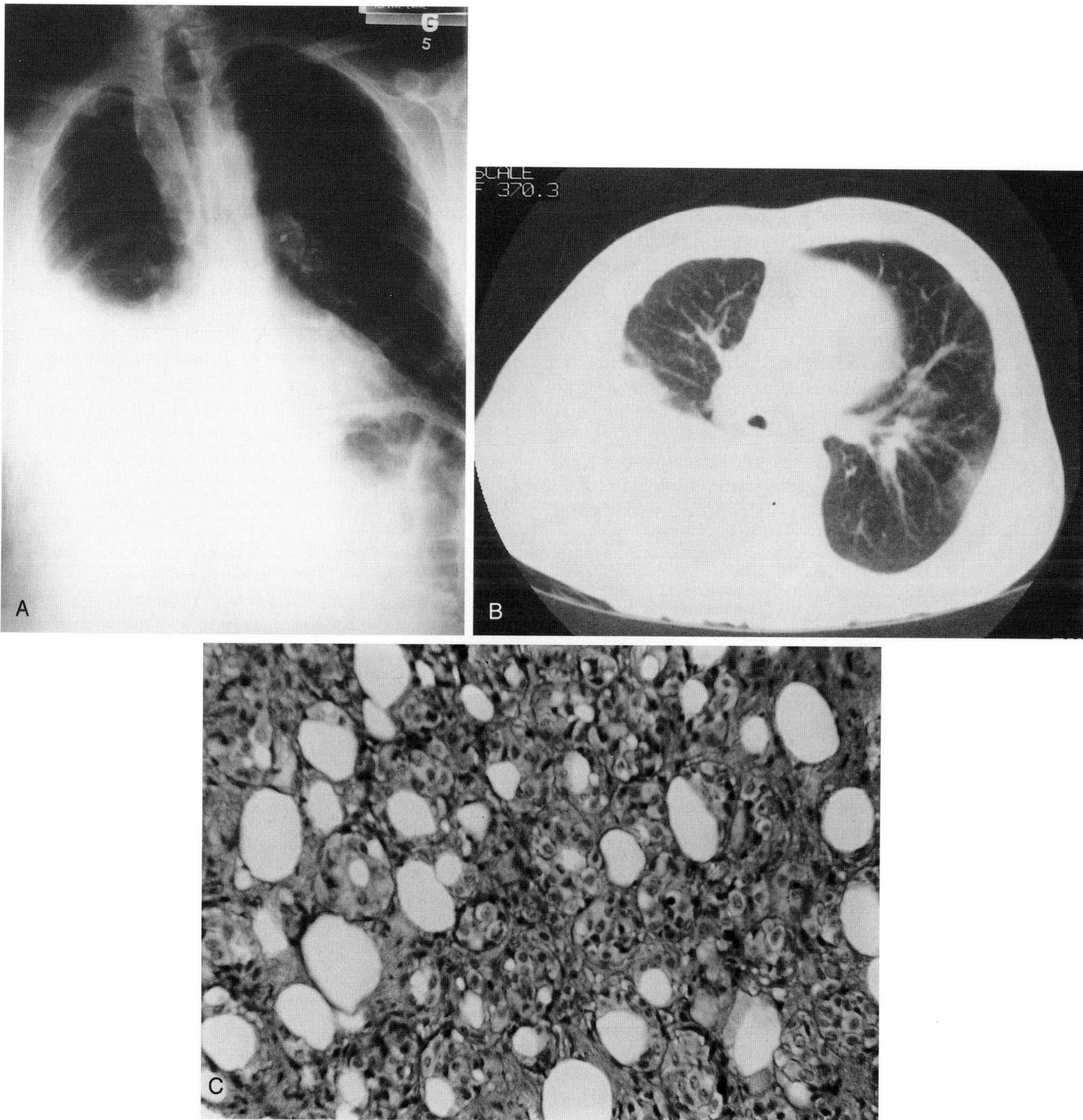

FIGURE 6–14 ■ Standard posteroanterior chest radiograph, *A*, and computed tomography (CT) scan, *B*, of a 56-year-old man with undiagnosed right-sided pleural effusion. Note that on the CT scan there are no pleural nodules or thickening of the parietal pleura. At videothoracoscopy, nodularities located over the lower half of the pleural space were biopsied, and on histology, *C*, these were typical of a malignant, predominantly epithelial mesothelioma.

ries, and 3 years later, Spann and associates (1995) evaluated the role of VATS in the diagnosis of diaphragmatic injuries. Twenty-six patients were enrolled in that study over a 12-month period. Diaphragmatic injuries were documented in 8 patients, and all 8 injuries were identified through videothoracoscopic surgery. The authors concluded that VATS is a safe, expeditious, and accurate method for evaluating the diaphragm in injured patients.

Thoracoscopy for Diffuse Lung Diseases

Thoracoscopic Lung Biopsy for Patients with Acute Respiratory Failure

A number of diagnostic methods are available to determine the nature of pulmonary infiltrates in patients with acute respiratory failure. Although all these methods have merit in certain circumstances, they do not always provide useful information in critically ill patients in whom an accurate diagnosis is essential to the success of treatment. Accordingly, a methodical and structured approach is recommended, with the final diagnosis being made by correlating clinical, bacteriologic, radiologic, and biopsy findings.

Often an adequate clinical history obtained from the referring physician or from relatives and a complete physical examination will narrow the diagnostic possibilities. Similarly, the study of standard chest radiographs or the simple analysis of bronchial secretions or pleural fluid aspirate will help in the assessment of a variety of diffuse pulmonary diseases. Thin-cut CT scanning is also of value in determining the extent of disease and defining anatomic and morphologic patterns that are suggestive of specific diseases.

There is increasing interest in the use of diagnostic bronchoscopy not only because it is readily available and easy to perform but also because it carries a significantly lower morbidity than does open lung biopsy. Conditions such as Wegener's granulomatosis can be found with endobronchial lesions that are easy to access with the bronchoscope. Sputum cultures can identify specific organisms, and when these are negative, bronchial brushings or protected sheath brushing can be carried out. Bronchoalveolar lavage has been shown to be of value in a number of conditions, particularly in identifying *Pneumocystis carinii* or mycobacterial disease in immunosuppressed patients. Transbronchial biopsies can also be valuable to diagnose infected, inflammatory, and malignant lung diseases.

Open lung biopsy has consistently been shown to yield the highest percentage of diagnosis in patients with chronic infiltrative lung disease (Gaensler and Carrington, 1980). In patients with acute respiratory failure, the role of open-lung biopsy is more controversial, and some authors (McKenna et al, 1986; Potter et al, 1985) believe that the findings seldom give specific information about the cause or lead to a change in therapy or better survival rates. In 1988, Warner and colleagues reported a cohort of 80 patients who underwent emergency open-lung biopsy for diffuse pulmonary infiltrates and acute respiratory failure. They noted that a specific etiologic diagnosis was obtained in 66% of patients and that therapy was altered in 70%. Fifteen patients suffered complications possibly related to the biopsy, and only 24 patients (30%) survived hospital discharge. In another series reported by Lachapelle and Morin (1995), a specific diagnosis was made in 21 of 31 patients (68%), and there was a change in diagnosis in 58% (18 of 31 patients). There was, however, no significant difference in survival between patients who received new treatment and those whose therapy was not altered after open-lung biopsy. More recently, Thomas and others (1998) reported the results of open-lung biopsy done at bedside in the intensive care unit. Twenty-six patients underwent biopsy without significant morbidity, and clinical management was changed in 22 (85%) based on biopsy results.

The role of VATS lung biopsy in patients who are on a ventilator with high levels of positive end-expiratory pressure (PEEP) is unclear, because such individuals tolerate very poorly the single-lung ventilation that is necessary to perform the thoracoscopic biopsy. Ferson and Landreneau (1998) also noted that, in these patients, the change from a single-lumen to a double-lumen endotracheal tube may be hazardous. Finally, the application of endo–gastrointestinal anastomosis (endo-GIA) staplers over lung surfaces that are extremely congested and edematous may produce significant tearing of the parenchyma.

Thoracoscopic Lung Biopsy for Interstitial Lung Disease

Because there are several possible etiologies to diffuse lung disease (Table 6–4), a definitive diagnosis is often difficult to obtain, and a surgical lung biopsy is recommended when other less invasive methods have failed. The development of "medical" thoracoscopy and of VATS has allowed minimally invasive methods to be used to establish a diagnosis in these patients.

The evaluation of patients with interstitial lung diseases includes the use of several tests that must be integrated within a structured investigational algorithm. Occasionally, these diseases have characteristic features and

TABLE 6–4 ■ Common Causes of Diffuse Lung Disease

Infection
- Granulomatous disease: tuberculosis, other mycobacterium, fungi
- Nongranulomatous disease: bacteria, virus, mycoplasma

Collagen vascular disease
- Lupus, rheumatoid arthritis, scleroderma, Sjögren's syndrome

Toxicities
- Inhalation disorders
- Drug toxicity, radiation injury
- Contusion

Neoplasms
- Leukemia, lymphoma, bronchoalveolar carcinoma
- Lymphangitic carcinomatosis
- Hematogenous metastasis

Miscellaneous
- Sarcoidosis, Wegener's granulomatosis, idiopathic fibrosis
- Allergic granuloma, eosinophilic granuloma
- Histiocytosis X
- Goodpasture's syndrome
- Interstitial pneumonia: usual, desquamative, bronchiolitis

can be positively diagnosed by clinical examination, sputum analysis, and radiologic features. Many infections, such as tuberculosis, from which mycobacterium tuberculosis can be isolated from the sputum, fall into that category. Unfortunately, most interstitial lung diseases cannot be properly diagnosed or classified without analysis of histologic material.

Fiber optic bronchoscopy combined with brushing, protected specimen brushing (Wimberley et al, 1979), and bronchoalveolar lavage is safe and frequently provides a positive diagnosis particularly in infectious processes such as tuberculosis (Uddenfeldt and Lundgren, 1981) and other mycosis. According to Ferguson (1993), bronchoalveolar lavage is very effective in diagnosing cytomegalovirus infection in transplant patients (Heurlin et al, 1989), and it is the procedure of choice for diagnosing *Pneumocystis carinii* in HIV-infected patients. Bronchoalveolar lavage and transbronchial biopsies (TBBs) are also useful in diagnosing and following patients with uniformly distributed inflammatory disorders such as histiocytosis X (Basset et al, 1977), eosinophilic granuloma, alveolar proteinosis, sarcoidosis (Armstrong et al, 1981), and farmer's lung disease. Indeed, mediastinoscopy with lymph node biopsy is seldom required in the management of sarcoidosis.

In an interesting study, Wall and co-workers (1981) studied 53 patients who underwent transbronchial biopsy for the diagnosis of chronic infiltrative lung diseases. Among these 53 patients, TBB was diagnostic in 20, and the histologic findings in the remaining 33 patients were reported as normal. Open biopsy in these 33 patients resulted in specific diagnoses in 92%, and the authors concluded that TBB diagnoses of interstitial pneumonitis, chronic inflammation, and fibrosis are unreliable. Similar results were obtained by others (Burt et al, 1981; Smith et al, 1977; Wall et al, 1981).

In their classic study published in 1980, Edward Gaensler and his fellow pathologist Charles Carrington reported 502 patients who underwent open lung biopsy. A pathologic diagnosis was established in 92% of these individuals. The mortality rate was 0.3% and the complication rate was 2.5%. In that paper, the authors stressed the importance of avoiding biopsies of the lingula and middle lobe, because these are often the sites of inflammation, scarring, and passive congestion. Subsequently, Flint et al (1995) concluded that a single generous (2 cm or greater diameter) sample obtained from a representative region of the radiographically most involved lobe is sufficient for diagnostic and evaluation purposes. Other authors (Miller et al, 1987; Wetstein, 1986) also select the site of biopsy through a review of the CT scan prior to biopsy and find no evidence that the middle lobe or lingula are inferior sites.

The VATS approach has become the gold standard for elective lung biopsy in patients with diffuse interstitial diseases. The potential advantages of thoracoscopic biopsy over open lung biopsy are its ability to inspect the entire pleural space, the accessibility of different regions of the lung for biopsy (Krasna et al, 1995), and reduced morbidity and postoperative pain (Ferguson, 1993). In one study comparing open versus VATS lung biopsy (Ferson et al, 1993), a significant decrease in hospital stay was noted with thoracoscopic biopsy. In another similar study from the Mayo Clinic (Kadokura et al, 1995), the authors concluded that VATS lung biopsy is an acceptable alternative to open lung biopsy.

Thoracoscopy for Indeterminate Lung Nodules

The solitary pulmonary nodule is a single intrapulmonary spherical lesion that is fairly well circumscribed, is surrounded by normal lung tissue, and measures 3 cm or less. According to Lillington (1991), there are approximately 150,000 new nodules detected each year in the United States, and 40% to 50% of them are malignant, either bronchogenic carcinoma or metastatic nodules, from primaries at other sites (Lillington, 1991; Midthun et al, 1992).

Many noninvasive diagnostic procedures exist for the evaluation of the patient with a solitary pulmonary nodule; these include clinical observation, careful review of standard radiographs and CT scans, and comparison of current films with previous ones to determine the growth of the nodule. If the patient is less than 35 years of age, for instance, and is a nonsmoker, the risk of malignancy is 1% or less (Fraser et al, 1989). By contrast, a nodule of 3 cm or more in diameter is likely to be malignant in over 95% of patients (Westcott, 1988; Zerhouni et al, 1986).

When clinical clues are vague, histologic analysis becomes crucial to assess the indeterminate pulmonary nodule. The yield of fiberoptic bronchoscopy with or without guided biopsies is low, and specific benign diagnoses are seldom established (Cortese and McDougall, 1979; Fletcher and Levin, 1982; Wallace and Deutsch, 1982).

Transthoracic fine needle aspiration (TTNA) done under radiologic guidance has a sensitivity in the range of 70% to 95% in the diagnosis of malignancies (Khouri et al, 1985, 1987; Viggiano et al, 1992), and the diagnostic accuracy of the technique is often proportional to the interest and experience of the operator. With the use of new generations of CT scan, nodules of 5 to 10 mm in diameter can be successfully biopsied (Fig. 6–15).

According to Westcott (1988), 3% to 11% of nodules reported as benign after TTNA will eventually be shown to be malignant when they are resected. The controversy surrounding the role of TTNA is well expressed by Shulkin (1993) in his discussion of a paper by Mack and colleagues on thoracoscopy for the diagnosis of pulmonary nodules (1993). Shulkin states: "A negative biopsy without a specific benign diagnosis provides insufficient evidence of a benign origin for the nodule, and further diagnostic procedures are indicated (Calhoun et al, 1986). In addition, a diagnosis of cancer obtained by TTNA mandates resection anyway. One must therefore question the value of fine-needle aspiration in establishing a diagnosis that avoids the necessity of thoracotomy." It is the authors' view that the diagnostic accuracy of TTNA is currently in the range of 95% and that these results justify its use in most patients with undiagnosed lung nodules. Obviously, the advantages of having this information include proper clinical staging of patients

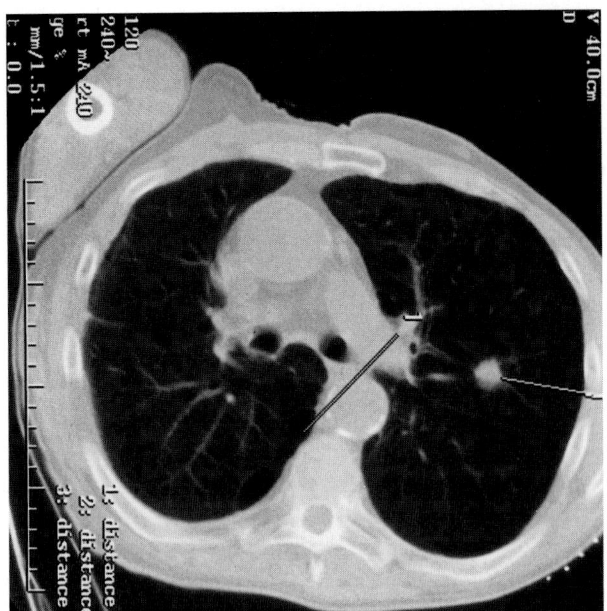

FIGURE 6–15 ■ A computed tomography–guided transthoracic needle aspiration biopsy of a lung nodule.

with lung cancer, proper planning of the resectional procedure, and avoidance of relying on frozen section analysis to make the final decision regarding indication and type of resection.

Several authors (Allen et al, 1993; Decamp et al, 1995; Mack et al, 1993) now recommend thoracoscopic wedge excisions for indeterminate lung nodules not only because it is accurate but also because it avoids undue delays in the treatment of malignancies. Ideal lesions for VATS excision are located in the outer third of the lung or close to an interlobar fissure, and in such cases the accuracy of the technique is approximately 95%. Indeed, Mack and colleagues (1993) state: "If a solitary nodule has been demonstrated to have been present unchanged in size for 2 years, or if there is a benign pattern of calcification present, or if the patient is a non-smoker with no history of malignancy and is less than 30 to 35 years old, then an 'observation only' approach is taken. In most other clinical settings, we proceed with thoracoscopy for diagnosis unless the patient is a prohibitive risk for general anesthesia due to general debilitation or associated cardiac disease." When the nodule is deep into the lung, various intraoperative localization techniques such as methylene blue injection, insertion of a guidewire or ultrasound probes (Shennib, 1993) have been described to facilitate its identification. In one series of 92 patients who underwent VATS resection of lung nodules, the authors (Suzuki et al, 1999) concluded that preoperative marking should be considered when the distance to the nearest pleural surface is more than 5 mm in cases of lung nodules that are 10 mm or less in diameter. In a retrospective analysis comparing CT percutaneous biopsy versus thoracoscopy to diagnose indeterminate pulmonary nodules, Mitruka and colleagues (1995) studied 613 patients with new, noncalcified pulmonary nodules seen over 4½ years. A specific benign or malignant diagnosis was obtained in 96% of patients undergoing VATS biopsy; the authors concluded that "limited accuracy for benign diagnosis with CT requires surgical biopsy for patients with adequate physiologic reserve."

In 1997, Bousamra and Clowry proposed the use of thoracoscopic fine-needle aspiration as an alternative to percutaneous fine-needle aspiration. They reported 8 patients for whom an accurate diagnosis was made within 20 minutes of the biopsy.

Thoracoscopy for Staging Lung Diseases

Staging of Patients with Pneumothoraces

At least two authors (Loddenkemper, 1998; Vanderschueren, 1981) have suggested that patients with spontaneous pneumothoraces should be staged for therapeutic purposes at the time of their pneumothorax. It is to be noted that all proponents of this method are medical specialists rather than surgeons. According to Loddenkemper (1998), "medical thoracoscopy is routinely justified in all patients with spontaneous pneumothorax where tube drainage is indicated, since several advantages are offered: precise assessment of underlying lesions under direct visual control, choice of best (conservative or surgical) treatment measures, direct treatment by coagulation of blebs and bullae, and by severing of adhesions, if necessary, followed by talc poudrage as well as selection of the best location for the chest tube placement." Vanderschueren also suggests the use of thoracoscopy to classify patients in one of four categories, allowing for selection of the most appropriate treatment: stage I: normal lung; stage II: adhesions only; stage III: small blebs; and stage IV: numerous larger bullae. It is the authors' opinion that such procedures are totally unnecessary, particularly in young, healthy individuals with a first episode of primary spontaneous pneumothorax.

Staging of Patients with Lung Cancer

One of the goals of preoperative staging is to recognize local causes of inoperability (irresectable disease). Several authors are now recommending the use of VATS, either as a routine or by indication, to achieve that goal.

Patients with a pleural effusion seen on chest radiograph or CT scanning need further evaluation, and many surgeons recommend the use of VATS exploration if thoracentesis cytology is negative. As suggested by Deslauriers and colleagues (1976), this exploration can be done through the neck at the time of cervical mediastinoscopy or through separate thoracoscopic incisions made over the thoracic cage. If malignant pleuritis or metastatic nodules are found, the tumor should not be resected as le Roux (1968) suggested. The role of VATS to explore the pleura in patients without a pleural effusion on CT scan is more controversial because the chances of finding pleural pathology contraindicating surgical resection are very small. In one series of 154 patients who were submitted to VATS operative staging (Roviaro et al, 1995), seven patients (5%) were found to be unresectable because of pleural dissemination without effusion. Six additional patients were found to be unresectable after VATS exploration because of mediastinal invasion (n = 4), esophageal wall invasion (n = 1), and tumor invasion of the pulmonary artery in the fissure. The significance of pleural effusion in patients with lung cancer is shown in Table 6–5.

In 1997, Asamura and colleagues from the National Cancer Center in Tokyo reported on the results of VATS exploration carried out in 116 patients with histologically/cytologically proven or suspected lung cancer. No pleural effusion was found in 63 patients, whereas in the remaining 53 (46.7%), an effusion was clearly demonstrated on the thoracoscopic images. In most of the patients, the effusion was minimal (<5 ml), but in five individuals, a cytologic examination revealed cancer cells in the effusion. Because of that finding, four of these five patients did not undergo subsequent thoracotomy. It is the authors' opinion that we currently have insufficient data on survival and patterns of recurrences to consider this finding an absolute contraindication to surgical resection.

Very few authors have looked at the role of thoracoscopic exploration to determine local extension of lung cancer and possible unresectability (Weissberg et al, 1981). Indeed, direct parietal extension is not a contraindication to resection, and often thoracoscopy will be unable to differentiate between true parietal extension and dense pleural symphysis secondary to local inflammatory resection. In the series by Roviaro and colleagues (1995), five patients were found to be inoperable because of local invasion, as documented by VATS exploration, but these findings were not confirmed by thoracotomy.

The role of VATS to preoperatively determine the nodal status of patients with presumed operable lung cancer is controversial because mediastinal lymph nodes in the superior mediastinum are accessible to cervical mediastinoscopy (Luke et al, 1986) and those outside the aortic arch to anterior mediastinotomy or extended cervical mediastinoscopy (Ginsberg et al, 1987). According to Goldstraw (1997), "these techniques have been shown to be safe and of proven prognostic significance and to use VATS to access such nodes, in the absence of other indications, seems extravagant." In a prospective study comparing mediastinoscopy with VATS for mediastinal node biopsy, Gossot and coworkers (1996) concluded that the diagnostic yield of mediastinoscopy is comparable to thoracoscopy but that the complication rate and hospital stay of patients undergoing mediastinoscopy are significantly inferior.

In a recent study, Wain (1993) showed that VATS is useful to document visceral pleura invasion and N1 status. Among 11 patients with N1 status, 6 (55%) were identified by VATS. The author concluded that VATS staging data may identify those subpopulations of patients who may benefit from neoadjuvant therapy regimens.

TABLE 6–5 ■ **Significance of Pleural Effusion in Patients with Bronchogenic Carcinoma**

Author (yr)	*No. of Patients*	*Inoperable*	*Operable*
Brinkman (1959)	21	20	1
le Roux (1968)	139	89	50
Decker et al (1978)	73	69	4
Canto et al (1983)	78	70	8
Total	311	248 (80%)	63 (20%)

Thoracoscopy for Diagnosis of Mediastinal Masses

There are few reports that have looked at the role of thoracoscopy for the diagnosis of mediastinal masses. In 1994, Rendina and co-workers from Rome looked at the comparative merits of VATS, mediastinoscopy, and mediastinotomy for mediastinal biopsy. They analyzed 51 patients with mediastinal masses and concluded that mediastinoscopy is indicated in the majority of lesions involving the peritracheal space but that in all other cases, VATS is preferable because it allows removal of large tissue biopsy specimens and even resection with wide surgical exposure and low operative trauma. At least two other series (Kern et al, 1993; Sugarbaker, 1993) have discussed the application of thoracoscopic techniques for the diagnosis of mediastinal masses, mostly those located in the anterior mediastinum. In the series by Kern and colleagues (1993), 22 patients with mediastinal masses were managed by VATS biopsy, and thoracoscopy provided an accurate diagnosis in 19 of the 22 patients (86%) without need for an open diagnostic procedure.

TECHNIQUE

Basic Operation

General endotracheal double-lumen anesthesia is used in all cases, and the patient is positioned for a full posterolateral thoracotomy incision with the surgeon operating from the back of the patient. We use a Storz instrument (Karl Storz GMBH and Co., Mittelstrasse 8, Postfach 230-D-7200, Tullinger, Germany) with an incorporated working channel, and we find that the clarity of the field of vision is improved if the lens tip is covered with a fine layer of anti-fog material (Ultrastop, Sigmapharm, Vienna, Austria). With this extra measure, it is not necessary to warm the scope before introducing it into the pleural space.

One to three trocars are necessary to perform the procedures. The first trocar site, the thoracoscopic trocar, is usually placed in the sixth or seventh intercostal space in the midaxillary line, because in that position and once the lung is collapsed, one has access to well over 75% of the pleural space without any other manipulation. The location of the other one or two trocars is based on the planned procedure and generally in a triangular way to allow for maximum maneuverability. Endo-GIA staplers (Endo-GIA-30, Autosuture; United States Surgical Corp., Newark, CT) are used for lung biopsies. A single chest tube is always left in the pleural space at completion of the procedure. When VATS resection of nodules or wedge biopsies of lung infiltrates are carried out, early chest tube removal (within 90 minutes of the procedure) appears to be a safe and cost-effective practice (Russo et al, 1998).

VATS for Pleural Effusion

If one tries to aspirate the effusate through the working channel of the thoracoscope, the lung will inflate and the lens will often become foggy and covered with blood. It is therefore preferable to have a second trocar (5 mm) usually located in the posterior axillary line in the seventh intercostal space.

Once the cavity is dry, it is fully inspected, and special attention is given to the lower half of the pleural space, particularly the costophrenic angles, which are often not readily visible. Any suspicious-looking pleural lesions or nodules over the lung surface are generously biopsied, and the specimens are sent for pathologic analysis. Part of the specimen has to be sent for electronic microscope analysis, because this examination is essential to differentiate between malignant mesothelioma and metastatic adenocarcinoma. In obvious neoplastic effusion, we terminate the procedure by sprinkling a fine layer of talc powder over the whole lung surface.

VATS for Diffuse Lung Disease and Solitary Lung Nodule

In cases of diffuse lung disease, we perform VATS biopsies according to the techniques described by Kadokura and colleagues (1995), Flint and associates (1995), and Pêgo-Fernandes and coworkers (1998). In every case, the site of biopsy is determined by the extent and location of radiographic abnormalities and by endoscopic visualization of the lung surface. On occasion, palpation of the lung will also help to determine the best site for biopsy. In general, we prefer to biopsy the right lung because it provides more edges due to the extra lobe, and we try to select the biopsy site in an intermediate zone, between the most compromised and apparently normal areas of the lung (Pêgo-Fernandez et al, 1998). We typically take one to three biopsies of the lung to obtain representative tissue, although an interesting study by Flint and coworkers (1995) has shown that a single generous sample (2 cm or greater diameter) obtained from a representative region of the radiographically most involved lobe will be sufficient for diagnostic and evaluative purposes (Fig. 6–16). In that study, 28 patients with idiopathic pulmonary fibrosis were analyzed, and statistically significant differences in histopathologic features were not observed between samples. In a similar study, Chechani and colleagues (1992) evaluated 20 patients in whom a biopsy was done in the most representative region of the lung as documented by radiographs, and a second biopsy was obtained from an adjacent accessible lobe. The same histologic diagnosis was reached for each of the two biopsy samples in all patients, and the authors concluded that when biopsy specimens are obtained from a representative region of the lung, biopsy of other lobes is unnecessary. We always ask the pathologist to do a frozen-section analysis of the specimen to ensure that representative lung tissue has been biopsied.

In cases of lung nodules, trocar placement is based on precise localization of the target by CT scan. If the nodule is not readily seen after adequate lung deflation, instrument or forceps palpation is performed next (Mack, 1993). On occasion, the use of methylene blue on the surface of the lung (Vandoni et al, 1998) or the insertion of a guidewire in the nodule (Mack et al, 1992) will facilitate identification of the site of an occult nodule. As suggested by Mack and associates (1993), all resected nodules are placed inside an endoscopic bag so that no tumor seeding over the trocar sites occurs if the lesion is malignant. Deeper lesions can be thinned out and brought to the surface by using the Nd:YAG laser prior to stapled resection (Landreneau et al, 1992).

VATS for Staging Lung Cancer

According to Roviaro and associates (1995), videothoracoscopic operative staging can entail "avulsion of the pulmonary ligament, and freeing of the pulmonary hilum for easier mobilization of the lung; dissection of the fissure to inspect the integrity of the pulmonary artery; opening the pericardium to examine the possibility of carrying out an intrapericardial ligature of the great vessels in case of suspected infiltration in proximity to their mediastinal origin, and section of the azygos vein to explore mediastinal lymph nodes."

If one is to do VATS operative staging, we recommend the standardized approach described by Wain (1993). Three trocar sites are selected, and the parietal pleura,

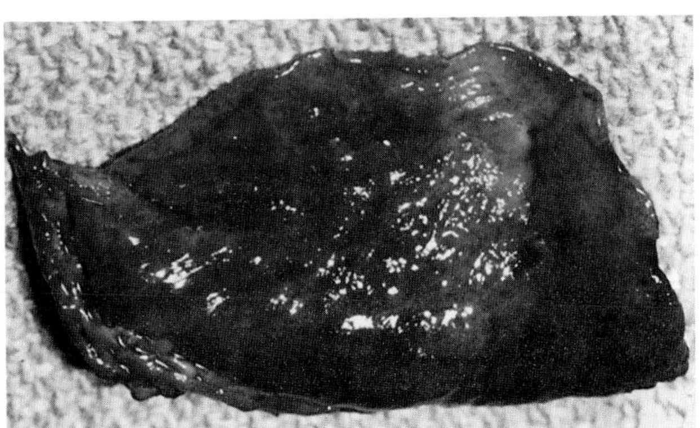

FIGURE 6–16 ■ Specimen of lung biopsy obtained by video-assisted thoracic surgery in a patient with diffuse interstitial disease.

TABLE 6–6 ■ **Comparison of Patients Undergoing VATS Wedge Excision and Patients Undergoing Wedge Excision via Thoracotomy without Prior VATS**

	Thoracoscopy	*Thoracotomy*
Number of patients	64	64
Epidural analgesia	0	49
Mortality	0	0
Complications	4 (6.3%)	6 (9.4%)
Median hospitalization (days, range)	3 (1–10)*	6 (2–13)

*$P < 0.05$.
VATS, video-assisted thoracic surgery.
Adapted from Allen et al: Video-assisted thoracoscopic stapled wedge excision for indeterminate pulmonary nodules. J Thorac Cardiovasc Surg 106:1048, 1993.

Table 6–7 ■ **Comparison of VATS to OLB in Patients with Diffuse Lung Disease**

Author (yr)	*Number of Patients*	*Morbidity (%)*	*Mortality (%)*	*Hospital Stay (days)*	*Diagnostic (%)*
Bensard et al (1993)	VATS 22	4.5	0	2.6 ± 2.2	95
	OLB 21	23.8	4.5	5.7 ± 2.9	100
Ferson et al (1993)	VATS 47	19	6.4	4.9 ± 3.4	100
	OLB 28	50	21.4	12.2 ± 15.2	100
Molin et al (1994)	VATS 16	25	0	4.8 ± 4.0	94
	OLB 21	4.8	4.8	5.0 ± 2.3	95

OLB, open lung biopsy; VATS, video-assisted thoracic surgery.

visceral pleura, lung tumor, hilum, and mediastinum are sequentially explored. Biopsies of nodal tissue are performed using both cup and grasping forceps, and as much nodal tissue as possible is excised. We refer the reader to the excellent article written by Wain (1993) for a complete description of the procedure.

RESULTS

For most series in which VATS was used for diagnosis and staging, minimal operative morbidity and no mortality directly related to the procedure were reported.

Allen and colleagues (1993) presented the results of a comparison between 64 patients who underwent VATS pulmonary wedge excision of lung nodules and 64 patients who underwent wedge excision via thoracotomy without prior VATS (Table 6–6).

In their analysis, postoperative analgesia requirements were less in patients undergoing VATS. These patients could be discharged from the hospital a median of 3 days earlier than patients who had thoracotomy. In the VATS group, complications occurred in 4 patients. These included pneumothorax (n = 2), atrial fibrillation (n = 1), and persistent air leak (n = 1).

In a similar study, Ferson and colleagues (1993) compared open versus thoracoscopic lung biopsy for diffuse infiltration disorders (Table 6–7). Mean duration of chest tube drainage was not significantly different between the two groups, but duration of hospital stay was significantly less for VATS biopsy (4.9 days) than for open biopsy (12.2 days) (P = 0.018). Fourteen of 28 open biopsies resulted in complications compared with 9 of 47 closed biopsies (P = 0.009). In a paper from the Mayo Clinic (Kadokura et al, 1995), complications developed in 11 (15%) of 71 patients in a VATS lung biopsy group compared with 7 (17%) of 42 patients in an open lung biopsy group. It is to be noted that in several series the mortality is significant but that the cause of death is usually a progression of the underlying disease.

The accuracy of VATS to diagnose pleuropulmonary diseases is the same or better than that with open procedures (Zegdi et al, 1998), and a number of series (Bensard et al, 1993; Carnochan et al, 1994; Mouroux et al, 1997) have demonstrated equal success in establishing a pathologic diagnosis with either method (see Table 6–7). According to Miller and colleagues (1992) and Rena and others (1999), this level of accuracy can reach 100% when a wedge excision technique is used for lung biopsy in patients with diffuse pulmonary disease.

CONCLUSION

The development of video-assisted thoracic surgical techniques allows a minimally invasive method to establish a diagnosis in many patients with pleural effusions and diffuse interstitial lung diseases. With the result of these biopsies, treatment strategies will be modified in many patients, and, hopefully, better outcomes will prevail.

The role of VATS for the diagnosis of pulmonary nodules or for the staging of lung cancer remains controversial.

■ *KEY REFERENCES*

Bloomberg AE: Thoracoscopy in perspective. Surg Gynecol Obstet 147:433, 1978.

This is an excellent article that looks at the evolution of thoracoscopy from its beginning until the end of the 1970s.

Ferguson MB: Thoracoscopy for diagnosis of diffuse lung disease. Ann Thorac Surg 56:694, 1993.

The merits and disadvantages of common diagnostic techniques used to pursue a definitive diagnosis of diffuse pulmonary disease are discussed.

Gaensler EA, Carrington CB: Open biopsy for chronic diffuse infiltrative lung disease: Clinical, roentgenographic, and physiological correlations in 502 patients. Ann Thorac Surg 30:411, 1980.

This classic study presents clinical, physiological, roentgenographic, and histologic data concerning 502 patients who had open biopsy for chronic interstitial lung disease.

Mack MJ, Hazelrigg SR, Landreneau RG, Acuff TE: Thoracoscopy for the diagnosis of the indeterminate solitary pulmonary nodule. Ann Thorac Surg 56:825, 1993.

This article provides a clear overview of investigating and managing a patient with a solitary lung nodule.

Shennib H: Intra-operative localization techniques for pulmonary nodules. Ann Thorac Surg 56:745, 1993.

In this article, Shennib describes all methods that can be used for intraoperative localization of nodules to be removed by VATS technique.

Wain JC: Video-assisted thoracoscopy and the staging of lung cancer. Ann Thorac Surg 56:776, 1993.

The author suggests a standardized approach using VATS technique to preoperatively stage lung cancer.

■ *REFERENCES*

Allen MS, Deschamps C, Lee RE et al: Video-assisted thoracoscopic stapled wedge excision for indeterminate pulmonary nodules. J Thorac Cardiovasc Surg 106:1048, 1993.

Armstrong JR, Radke JR, Kuade PA et al: Endoscopic findings in sarcoidosis. Ann Otol 90:339, 1981.

Asamura H, Nakayama H, Kondo H et al: Thoracoscopic evaluation of histologically/cytologically proven or suspected lung cancer: A VATS exploration. Lung Cancer 16:183, 1997.

Basset F, Soler P, Jauraud MC, Bignon J: Ultrastructural examination of broncho-alveolar lavage for diagnosis of pulmonary histiocytosis X. Thorax 32:303, 1977.

Beaulieu M, Després JP, Lemieux M: Mediastino-pleuroscopy: A new technique for the diagnosis of thoracic diseases. Chirurgie 98:355, 1972.

Bensard DD, McIntyre RC Jr, Waring BJ: Comparison of video-thoracoscopic lung biopsy to open lung biopsy in the diagnosis of interstitial lung disease. Chest 103:765, 1993.

Bloomberg AE: Thoracoscopy in perspective. Surg Gynecol Obstet 147:433, 1978.

Bousamra M, Clowry L: Thoracoscopic fine-needle aspiration of solitary pulmonary nodules. Ann Thorac Surg 64:1191, 1997.

Boutin C, Farisse P, Viallat P et al: La thoracoscopie dans le mésothéliome pleural: Intérêt diagnostique, prognostique et thérapeutique. Rev Franç Mal Respir 7:680, 1979.

Boutin C, Viallat JR, Cargnino P et al: Thoracoscopy in malignant pleural effusions. Am Rev Respir Dis 124:588, 1981.

Boutin C, Viallat JR, Cargnino P, Farisse P: Indications actuelles de la thoracoscopie. Rev Fr Mal Resp 9:309, 1981.

Branco JMC: Thoracoscopy as a method of exploration in penetrating injuries of the chest. Dis Chest 12:330, 1946.

Branco JMC: Thoracoscopy as a method of exploration in penetrating injuries of the thorax. Dis Chest 12:330, 1946.

Brandt HJ, Mai J: Differential diagnosis of pleural effusions using thoracoscopy. Pneumologie 145:192, 1971.

Brinkman GL: The significance of pleural effusion complicating otherwise operable bronchogenic carcinoma. Dis Chest 36:152, 1959.

Buchhotz J, Mayer M, Giesekus D: The diagnosis of pleural effusion using thoracoscopy. Zentrabl Chir 115:1565, 1990.

Burt ME, Flye MW, Webber BL et al: Prospective evaluation of aspiration needle, cutting needle, transbronchial and open lung biopsy in patients with pulmonary infiltrates. Ann Thorac Surg 32:146, 1981.

Calhoun P, Feldman PS, Armstrong P et al: The clinical outcome of needle aspiration of the lung when cancer is not diagnosed. Ann Thorac Surg 41:592, 1986.

Cantó A, Blasco E, Casillas M et al: Thoracoscopy in the diagnosis of pleural effusion. Thorax 32:550, 1977.

Cantó A, Rivas J, Saumench J et al: Points to consider when choosing a biopsy method in cases of pleurisy of unknown origin. Chest 84:176, 1983.

Carnochan FM, Walker WS, Cameron EW: Efficacy of video-assisted thoracoscopic lung biopsy: An historical comparison with open lung biopsy. Thorax 49:362, 1994.

Chechani V, Landreneau RJ, Shaikh SS: Open lung biopsy for diffuse infiltrative lung disease. Ann Thorac Surg 54:296, 1992.

Collins TR, Sahn SA: Thoracentesis: Clinical value, complications, technical problems and patient experience. Chest 91:817, 1987.

Colt HG: Thoracoscopy: A prospective study of safety and outcome. Chest 108:324, 1995.

Cortese DA, McDougall JC: Biopsy and brushing of peripheral lung cancer with fluoroscopic guidance. Chest 75:141, 1979.

Decamp MM, Jaklitsch MT, Mentzer SJ et al: The safety and versatility of video-thoracoscopy: A prospective analysis of 895 consecutive cases. J Am Coll Surg 181:113, 1995.

Decker DA, Dines DE, Payne WS et al: The significance of a cytologically negative pleural effusion in bronchogenic carcinoma. Chest 74:640, 1978.

Deslauriers J, Beaulieu M, Dufour C et al: Mediastino-pleuroscopy: A new approach to the diagnosis of intra-thoracic diseases. Ann Thorac Surg 22:265, 1976.

Duzhyi ID: Spontaneous hemopneumothorax. Klin Khir 11:35, 1991.

Feliciano DV: The diagnostic and therapeutic approach to chest trauma. Sem Thorac Cardiovasc Surg 4:156, 1992.

Ferguson MF: Thoracoscopy for diagnosis of diffuse lung disease. Ann Thorac Surg 56:694, 1993.

Ferson PF, Landreneau RJ: Thoracoscopic lung biopsy or open lung biopsy for interstitial lung disease. Chest Surg Clin North Am 8:749, 1998.

Ferson PF, Landreneau RJ, Dowling RD et al: Comparison of open versus thoracoscopic lung biopsy for diffuse infiltrative pulmonary disease. J Thorac Cardiovasc Surg 106:194, 1993.

Fletcher EC, Levin DC: Flexible fiberoptic bronchoscopy and fluoroscopically guided transbronchial biopsy in the management of solitary pulmonary nodules. West J Med 136:477, 1982.

Flint A, Martinez FJ, Young ML et al: Influence of sample number and biopsy site on the histologic diagnosis of diffuse lung disease. Ann Thorac Surg 60:1605, 1995.

Fraser RG, Paré JAP, Paré PD et al: The solitary pulmonary nodule. In Fraser RG, Paré JAP (eds): Diagnosis of disorders of the chest, Vol 2. Philadelphia, WB Saunders, 1989.

Gaensler EA, Carrington CB: Open biopsy for chronic diffuse infiltrative lung disease: Clinical, roentgenographic, and physiological correlations in 502 patients. Ann Thorac Surg 30:411, 1980.

Ginsberg RJ et al: Extended cervical mediastinoscopy: A single staging procedure for bronchogenic carcinoma of the left upper lobe. J Thorac Cardiovasc Surg 94:673, 1987.

Goldstraw P: Surgery: Minimal invasive surgery in lung cancer management. Proceedings of the 1997 World Congress on Lung Cancer, p 18.

Gore RB, Luksza AR, Grunshaw N et al: A new diagnostic schedule for pleural mesothelioma [Abstract]. Thorax 53:19, 1998.

Gossot D, Toledo L, Fritsch S, Celerier M: Mediastinoscopy vs. thoracoscopy for mediastinal biopsy: Results of a prospective nonrandomized study. Chest 110:1328, 1996.

Grossebner MW, Arifi AA, Goddard M, Ritchie AJ: Mesothelioma-VATS biopsy and lung mobilization improves diagnosis and palliation. Eur J Cardiothorac Surg 16:619, 1999.

Gunnels JJ: Perplexing pleural effusion. Chest 74:390, 1978.

Heurlin N, Lonngvist B, Tollemar J, Ehrnet A: Fiberoptic bronchoscopy for diagnosis of opportunistic pulmonary infection after bone marrow transplantation. Scand J Infect Dis 21:359, 1989.

Hucker J, Bhatnaggar NK, Al-Jilaihawi AN, Forrester-Wood CP: Thoracoscopy in the diagnosis and management of recurrent pleural effusions. Ann Thorac Surg 52:1145, 1991.

Jacobeus HC: Die Thorakoscopic und ihre praktische Bedeutung. Ergeb-Ges Med (Berlin) 7:112, 1925.

Jacobeus HC: Über die Möglichkeit die cystoscopic bei Untersuchung seröses Höhl-lumen anzuwenden. Munch Med Wochenschr 57:2090, 1910.

Kadokura M, Colby TV, Myers JL et al: Pathologic comparison of video-assisted thoracic surgical lung biopsy with traditional open lung biopsy. J Thorac Cardiovasc Surg 109:494, 1995.

Kern JA, Daniel TM, Tribble CG et al: Thoracoscopic diagnosis and treatment of mediastinal masses. Ann Thorac Surg 56:92, 1993.

Khouri NF, Meziane MA, Zerhouni EA et al: The solitary pulmonary nodule: Assessment, diagnosis and management. Chest 91:128, 1987.

Khouri NF, Stitik FP, Erozan YS et al: Transthoracic aspiration biopsy of benign and malignant lung lesions. AJR Am J Roentgenol 144:281, 1985.

Kimura M, Nakamura J, Tomizawa S et al: The role of thoracoscopy in pleural biopsy in cases with pleural effusion. Nippon Kyobo Shikkan Gakkai Zasshi 28:882, 1990.

Krasna MJ, White CS, Aisner SC et al: The role of thoracoscopy in the diagnosis of interstitial lung disease. Ann Thorac Surg 59:348, 1995.

Lachapelle KJ, Morin JE: Benefit of open lung biopsy in patients with respiratory failure. Can J Surg 38:316, 1995.

Landreneau RJ, Hazelrigg SR, Ferson PF et al: Thoracoscopic resection of 85 pulmonary lesions. Ann Thorac Surg 54:415, 1992.

le Roux BT: Bronchial carcinoma. London, E and S Livingston, 1968.

Le Tacon J: La pleuroscopie: Rappel historique. Poumon-Coeur 37:5, 1981.

Legha SS, Muggia FM: Pleural mesothelioma: Clinical features and therapeutic implications. Ann Intern Med 87:613, 1977.

Lewis RJ, Kunderman PJ, Sisler GE, MacKenzie JW: Direct diagnostic thoracoscopy. Ann Thorac Surg 21:536, 1976.

Light RW: Pleural diseases. Philadelphia, Lea and Febiger, 1983.

Lillington GA: Management of solitary pulmonary nodules. Dis Mon 37:271, 1991.

Loddenkemper R: Thoracoscopy: State of the art. Eur Respir J 11:213, 1998.

Luke WP, Pearson FG, Todd TRJ et al: Prospective evaluation of mediastinoscopy for assessment of carcinoma of the lung. J Thorac Cardiovasc Surg 91:53, 1986.

Maasilta P, Vehmas T, Kivisaari L et al: Correlations between findings at computed tomography (CT) and at thoracoscopy/thoracotomy/autopsy in pleural mesothelioma. Eur Respir J 4:952, 1991.

Maassen W: Thoracoscopie et biopsie pulmonaire sans pneumothorax initial. Poumon-Cœur 37:317, 1981.

Mack MJ, Gordon MJ, Postma TW et al: Percutaneous localization of pulmonary nodules for thoracoscopic lung resection. Ann Thorac Surg 53:1123, 1992.

Mack MJ, Hazelrigg SR, Landreneau RJ, Acuff TE: Thoracoscopy for the diagnosis of the indeterminate solitary pulmonary nodule. Ann Thorac Surg 56:825, 1993.

McKenna RJ Jr, Campbell A, McMurtrey MJ et al: Diagnosis for interstitial lung disease in patients with acquired immunodeficiency syndrome (AIDS): A prospective comparison of bronchial washing, alveolar lavage, transbronchial lung biopsy, and open-lung biopsy. Ann Thorac Surg 41:318, 1986.

Menzies R, Charbonneau M: Thoracoscopy for the diagnosis of pleural disease. Ann Intern Med 114:271, 1991.

Midthun DE, Swensen SJ, Jett JR: Clinical strategies for solitary pulmonary nodule. Annu Rev Med 43:195, 1992.

Miller D, Allen MS, Trastek VF et al: Video-thoracoscopic wedge excision for diffuse interstitial lung disease. Chest 102(Suppl):169s, 1992.

Miller JI: The present role and future considerations of video-assisted thoracoscopy in general thoracic surgery. Ann Thorac Surg 56:804, 1993.

Miller RR, Nelems B, Muller NL et al: Lingula and right middle lobe biopsy in the assessment of diffuse lung disease. Ann Thorac Surg 44:269, 1987.

Mitruka S, Landreneau RJ, Mack MJ et al: Diagnosing the indeterminate pulmonary nodule: Percutaneous biopsy versus thoracoscopy. Surgery 118:676, 1995.

Molin LJ, Steinberg JB, Lanza LA: VATS increases costs in patients undergoing lung biopsy for interstitial lung disease. Ann Thorac Surg 58:1595, 1994.

Mouroux J, Clary-Meinesz C, Padovani B et al: Efficacy and safety of video-thoracoscopic lung biopsy in the diagnosis of interstitial lung disease. Eur J Cardiothorac Surg 11:22, 1997.

Pêgo-Fernandes PM, Jatine FB, Campos JRM et al: Pulmonary biopsy by video-assisted thoracic surgery: Experience of 76 cases. S Am J Thorac Surg 2:47, 1998.

Poe RH, Israel RH, Utell MJ et al: Sensitivity, specificity, and predictive values of closed pleural biopsy. Arch Intern Med 144:325, 1984.

Potter D, Pass HI, Brower S et al: Prospective randomized study of open lung biopsy versus empirical antibiotic therapy for acute pneumonitis in non-neutropenic cancer patients. Ann Thorac Surg 40:422, 1985.

Rao NV, Jones PO, Greenberg SD et al: Needle biopsy of parietal pleura in 124 cases. Arch Intern Med 115:34, 1965.

Rendina EA, Vinata F, DeGiacomo T et al: Comparative merits of thoracoscopy, mediastinoscopy, and mediastinotomy for mediastinal biopsy. Ann Thorac Surg 57:992, 1994.

Rena O, Casadio C, Leo F et al: Videothoracoscopic lung biopsy in the diagnosis of interstitial lung disease. Eur J Cardiothorac Surg 16:624, 1999.

Roviaro G, Varoli F, Rebuffat C et al: Video-thoracoscopic staging and treatment of lung cancer. Ann Thorac Surg 59:971, 1995.

Russo L, Wiechmann RJ, Magovern JA et al: Early chest tube removal after video-assisted thoracoscopic wedge resection of the lung. Ann Thorac Surg 66:1751, 1998.

Sattler A: La thoracoscopie: Intérêt thérapeutique dans les syndromes pleuro-pulmonaires d'urgence et intérêt diagnostique. Poumon-Cœur 37:265, 1981.

Sattler A: The treatment of spontaneous pneumothorax with special reference to thoracoscopy. Beitr Klin Tuberkulosi 89:395, 1937.

Sgro M, Gorla A, Tacchi G et al: Thoracoscopy in the diagnosis of pleural mesothelioma. Chir Ital 43:95, 1991.

Shennib H: Intraoperative localization techniques for pulmonary nodules. Ann Thorac Surg 56:745, 1993.

Smith CN, Murray GF, Wilcox BR: The role of transbronchial lung biopsy in diffuse pulmonary disease. Ann Thorac Surg 24:54, 1977.

Spann JC, Nwariaku FE, Wait M: Evaluation of video-assisted thoracoscopic surgery in the diagnosis of diaphragmatic injuries. Am J Surg 170:628, 1995.

Sugarbaker DJ: Thoracoscopy in the management of anterior mediastinal masses. Ann Thorac Surg 56:653, 1993.

Suzuki K, Nagai K, Yoshida J et al: Video-assisted thoracoscopic surgery for small indeterminate pulmonary nodules. Chest 115:563, 1999.

Thomas P, Papazian L, Reynaud-Gaubert M et al: Biopsies pulmonaires chirurgicales au lit en réanimation chez les patients ventilés pour un syndrome de détresse respiratoire aiguë. J Chir Thorac Cardiovasc 2:69, 1998.

Tomlinson JK, Sahn SA: Invasive procedures in the diagnosis of pleural disease. Semin Respir Med 9:30, 1987.

Uddenfeldt M, Lundgren R: Flexible bronchoscopy in the diagnosis of pulmonary tuberculosis. Tubercle 62:197, 1981.

Vanderschueren RG: Le talcage pleural dans le pneumothorax spontané. Poumon-Cœur 37:273, 1981.

Vandoni RE, Cutlat JF, Wicky S, Suter M: CT-guided methylene-blue labelling before thoracoscopic resection of pulmonary nodules. Eur J Cardiothorac Surg 14:265, 1998.

Viggiano RW, Swensen SJ, Rosenow EC: Evaluation and management of solitary and multiple pulmonary nodules. Clin Chest Med 13:83, 1992.

Wain JC: Video-assisted thoracoscopy and the staging of lung cancer. Ann Thorac Surg 56:776, 1993.

Wakabayashi A: Expanded applications of diagnostic and therapeutic thoracoscopy. J Thorac Cardiovasc Surg 102:721, 1991.

Wall CP, Gaensler EA, Carrington CB, Hayes JA: Comparison of transbronchial and open biopsies in chronic infiltrative lung diseases. Am Rev Respir Dis 123:280, 1981.

Wallace JM, Deutsch AL: Flexible fiber optic bronchoscopy and percutaneous needle lung aspiration for evaluating the solitary pulmonary nodule. Chest 81:665, 1982.

Warner DO, Warner MA, Divertie MB: Open lung biopsy in patients with diffuse pulmonary infiltrates and acute respiratory failure. Am Rev Respir Dis 137:90, 1988.

Weissberg D, Kaufman M: Diagnostic and therapeutic pleuroscopy: Experience with 127 patients. Chest 78:732, 1980.

Weissberg D, Kaufman M, Schwecher I: Pleuroscopy in clinical evaluation and staging of lung cancer. Poumon-Cœur 37:241, 1981.

Wenderman K, Greschuchna D, Maassen W: Results of surgical pleural and pulmonary biopsies. Thorax Chirurgie 22:453, 1974.

Westcott JL: Percutaneous transthoracic needle biopsy. Radiology 169:593, 1988.

Wetstein L: Sensitivity and specificity of lingula segmental biopsies of the lung. Chest 90:383, 1986.

Wimberely NW, Faling LF, Bartlett JG: A fiberoptic bronchoscopy technique to obtain uncontaminated lower airway secretions for bacterial culture. Am Rev Resp Dis 119:337, 1979.

Zegdi R, Azorin J, Tremblay B et al: Videothoracoscopic lung biopsy in diffuse infiltrative lung diseases: A 5-year surgical experience. Ann Thorac Surg 66:1170, 1998.

Zerhouni EA, Stikik FP, Siegelman SS et al: CT of the pulmonary nodule: A cooperative study. Radiology 160:319, 1986.

CHAPTER 7

Open Lung Biopsy

Thomas J. Kirby
Stanley C. Fell

Open lung biopsy (OLBx), whether by a video-thoracoscopic (VATS) or thoracotomy approach, has proven itself to be an accurate and useful diagnostic technique in the elective setting for patients with undiagnosed lung disease that has failed to be accurately categorized using less invasive approaches, such as transbronchial biopsy and bronchoalveolar lavage. The value of lung biopsy in mechanically ventilated critically ill patients with *undiagnosed* lung disease remains more controversial, as often the pathology of the biopsy reveals nonspecific changes (diffuse alveolar damage). Even when OLBx results in a specific diagnosis and a change in therapy, it is not shown to improve patient survival in most studies. However, the thoracic surgeon is still frequently called on to perform an OLBx, and therefore it is important to have a basic understanding of the disease processes most frequently encountered and of the correct surgical approach in the management of these patients.

PATIENT POSITION

Depending on the surgical approach, there are two options in positioning the patient. For an anterolateral thoracotomy, the patient is placed supine with a roll under the shoulders and hips to rotate the side to be biopsied by 30 degrees (Fig. 7–1). Alternatively, the patient can be placed in a full lateral position, and the chest can be entered through the auscultatory triangle, sparing the latissimus dorsi and the serratus anterior muscles. If exposure is inadequate, it is a simple matter to divide the latissimus (Fig. 7–2). Ruskin and associates (1990) have shown that OLBx can be safely performed in the intensive care unit (ICU), which avoids the logistics of transporting an often critically ill patient for whom adequate ventilation during transportation can be problematic. It is our preference to use an operating room setting whenever possible, because the lighting is better, access to necessary instrumentation is easier, and trained personnel are readily available.

An elective OLBx is probably best approached using VATS as detailed in Chapter 6. In the ventilated, critically ill patient, the purported advantages of VATS vanish. In addition, these patients will not tolerate single lung ventilation, which makes a VATS approach problematic at best.

TECHNIQUE

If an anterolateral thoracotomy approach is selected, a 6- to 8-cm submammary thoracotomy is made, and the chest is entered through the fourth or fifth intercostal space, which enables biopsy specimens to be obtained from both the upper and the lower lobes (see Fig. 7–1). Alternatively, with the patient in the full lateral thoracotomy position, the incision can be placed over the auscultatory triangle, and the chest can be entered by reflecting the latissimus dorsi anteriorly and the trapezius posteriorly (see Fig. 7–2). At least two biopsies from different lobes should be performed to ensure that adequate and representative tissue is obtained. Careful review of the plain chest radiograph and computed tomography (CT) scans will help direct the surgeon to the appropriate areas. Biopsy specimens should be taken from pulmonary parenchyma that appears to be involved by the underlying disease process as well as from areas that by inspection appear relatively normal. This should provide the

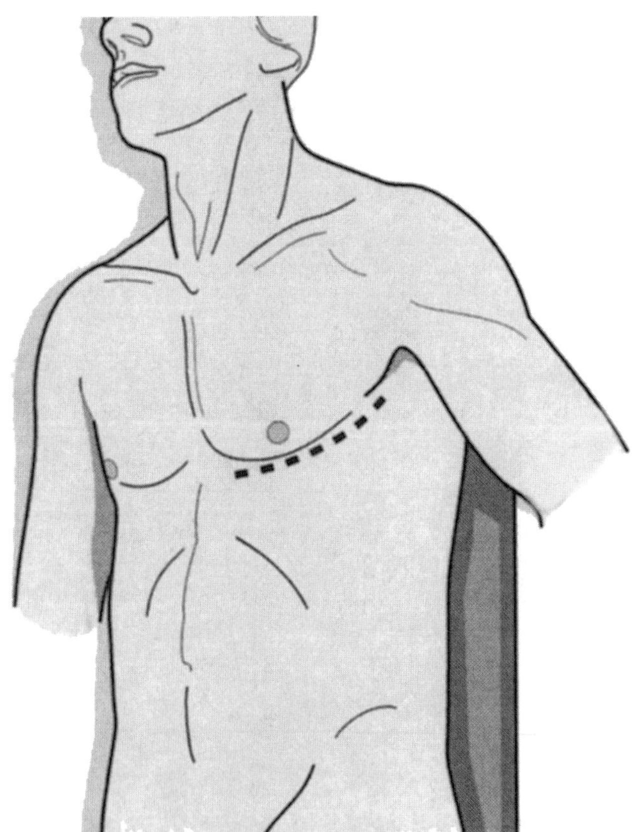

FIGURE 7–1 ■ Positioning for an anterior lateral thoracotomy and open lung biopsy. The patient is placed supine with a roll under the operative side to rotate the chest by 30 degrees.

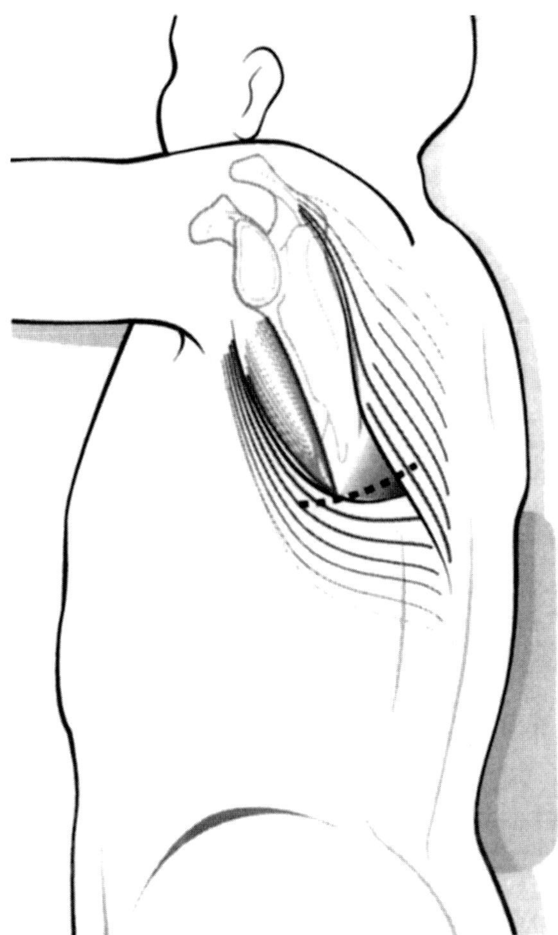

FIGURE 7–2 ■ An alternative approach to an open lung biopsy is a full lateral position, placing the incision over the auscultatory triangle (as illustrated) and entering the chest between the trapezius and latissimus dorsi muscles.

pathologist with representative samples of the disease in various stages of its evolution, increasing the chance for an accurate diagnosis and perhaps aiding in determining the prognosis. Stapling instruments allow biopsies to be expeditiously carried out, providing a secure hemostatic and airtight closure (Figs. 7–3 and 7–4). Prior to the availability of stapling instruments, a lung clamp was simply applied to the outer edge of the lung parenchyma, a specimen was excised, and the cut surface was oversewn (Fig. 7–5).

A frozen section of the biospy specimen should be carried out to ensure that an adequate and diagnostic tissue sample has been obtained as well as to alert the pathologist that special investigations (e.g., electron microscopy, silver staining for pneumocystis) are necessary. It is prudent to avoid biopsying the middle lobe and the lingula, because these pulmonary segments occasionally have microscopic parenchymal fibrosis and vascular changes even in the absence of underlying lung disease. However, it is still possible to obtain diagnostic tissue from these areas as shown by reports from Imoke and colleagues (1983) and Weng and associates (1980). If infection is a preoperative consideration, especially in an immunocompromised patient, a specimen should be sent for appropriate cultures including virus, fungus, tuberculosis, and acid-fast bacillus.

RESULTS

Although there is controversy regarding the value of OLBx in influencing therapy or prognosis, especially in the critically ill patient, there are reports in the literature that support its utility. Nelems and colleagues (1976) reported that the working preoperative diagnosis in patients undergoing OLBx was incorrect 55% of the time but that the diagnostic accuracy of the procedure was 96%. McKenna and associates (1984) reported a 90% accuracy of detecting OLBx, with 71% of patients having their therapy changed as a result. Cheson and colleagues (1985) found that in immunocompromised patients, OLBx led to a definitive diagnosis in 54% and a change of therapy in 38%. Walker and associates (1989) reported on 61 patients who had undergone OLBx, including 22 who were immunocompromised; OLBx gave a specific diagnosis in 13 (59%) and resulted in a change in therapy in 17 (77%). In the 39 nonimmunocompromised patients, a specific diagnosis was only obtained in 8 (21%) and led to a change in therapy in 16 (41%). Warner and colleagues (1988) reported on 80 patients with diffuse pulmonary infiltrates and acute respiratory failure who

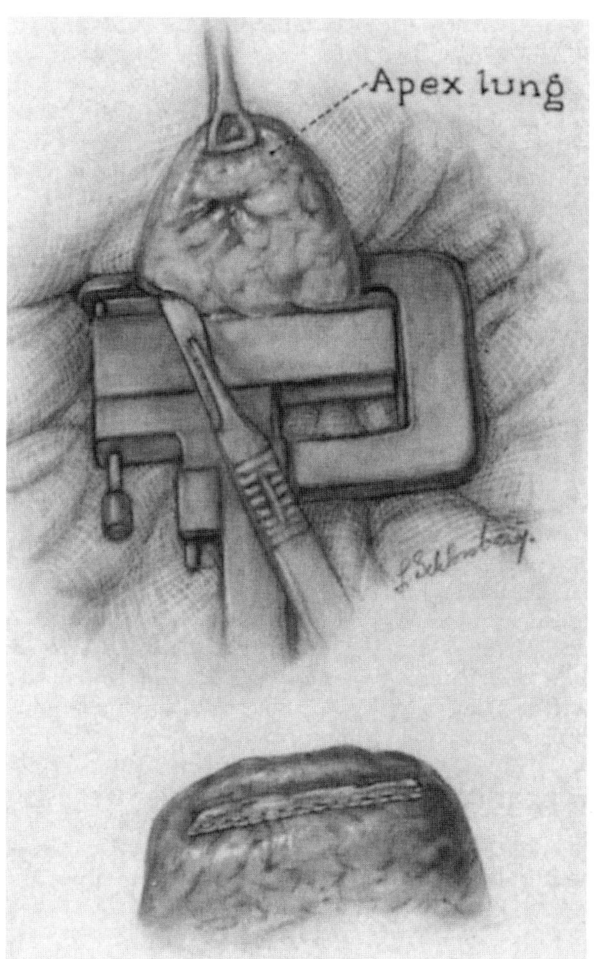

FIGURE 7–3 ■ A linear stapler being used for a wedge biopsy.

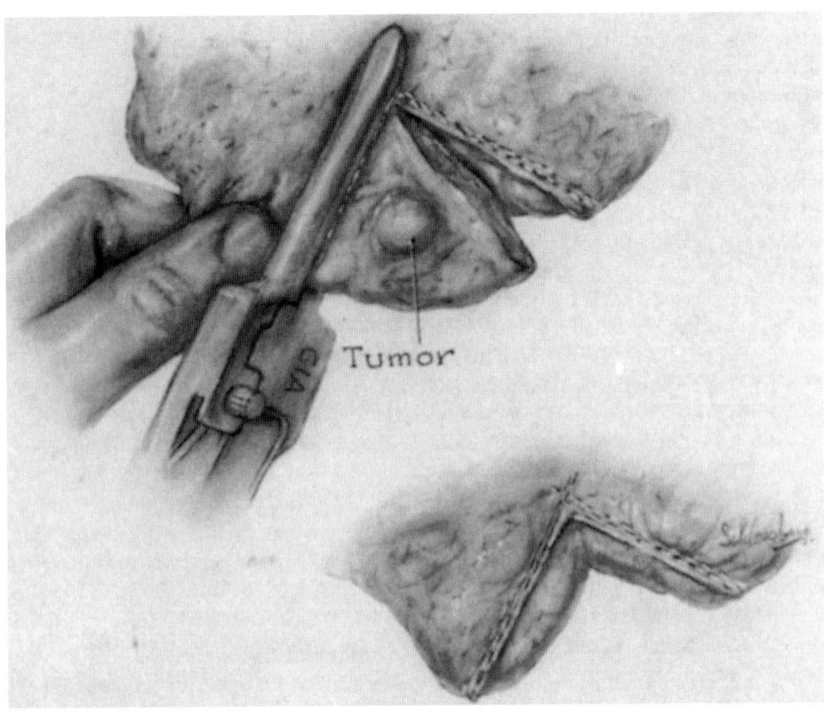

FIGURE 7–4 ■ An alternative method using a linear stapler to obtain an open lung biopsy.

underwent OLBx. OLBx led to a specific diagnosis in 66% and a change in therapy in 70%. However, only 30% of these patients left the hospital, with just 11% surviving for more than 1 year. Survival was best in young patients and in those who did not require preoperative mechanical ventilation. Warner and colleagues (1988) concluded that although OLBx was an accurate diagnostic tool, its utility is limited by the lack of therapy for the underlying disease process.

More recently, Temes and associates (1999) reported on 75 patients undergoing OLBx between 1992 and 1998. They found that the results of lung biopsy lead to beneficial therapeutic changes in 60% of elective, 94% of urgent, and 41% of emergency procedures. The operative mortality for the three groups was 0%, 18%, and 54% respectively. The authors conclude that lung biopsy is appropriate in the elective and urgent settings, but that it is best avoided in critically ill patients. The authors recommend, not unreasonably, that this latter group undergo an empiric course of steroid therapy as this was usually the only therapy that was given to this group based on the finding of OLBx.

Flabouris and Myburgh (1999) reported on 24 mechanically ventilated patients undergoing OLBx. The overall mortality was 8.4%. No patient survived with respiratory failure and organ failures at 2 or more sites.

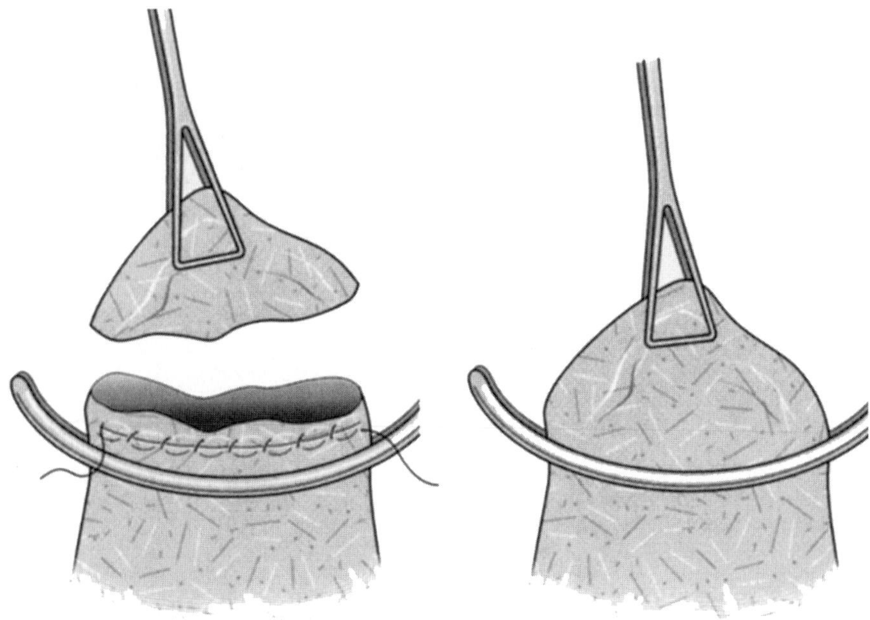

FIGURE 7–5 ■ Prior to the introduction of stapling instruments, noncrushing clamps were used to obtain a lung biopsy, and the cut surface was simply oversewn.

A specific diagnosis was obtained in 46% of cases and alteration in therapy benefited 39% of patients; however, alteration in therapy did not differentiate between survivors.

In patients with hematologic malignancies who developed unexplained pulmonary parenchymal changes, White and colleagues (2000) found that OLBx led to a specific diagnosis in 57% and a change in therapy for 70% of these patients. The authors support the use of OLBx in this setting.

In properly selected cases, OLBx can lead to a specific diagnosis and change in therapy in 50% to 70% of patients. Although in many cases there is no specific therapy for the underlying disease process, the fact that therapy may be added or withheld depending on the correct diagnosis would logically dictate that the procedure offers the best chance for recovery.

The mortality associated with OLBx can be daunting. Saterfield and McLaughlin (1979) reported a 12% mortality, and Nelems and colleagues (1976) reported a 57% mortality. Death is obviously related to the underlying disease process rather than to the operative procedure itself and occurs most frequently with ICU patients who are ventilator-dependent.

■ *KEY REFERENCES*

Temes TR, Joste NE, Qualls CR et al: Lung biopsy: Is it necessary? J Thorac Cardiovasc Surg 118:1097, 1999.

The authors report a retrospective review of 75 immunocompetent patients undergoing lung biopsy between 1992 and 1996. Their results indicate that elective and 'urgent' OLBx is useful in direct therapy but that critically ill patients on ventilators are better off being treated empirically with steroids, because OLBx in this group was associated with a high operative mortality (54%) and rarely resulted in a change in therapy other than immunosuppression.

Teo DC, Ziolo KM, Lange PA et al: The utility of open lung biopsy in the critically ill. Chest 118:169s, 2000.

A current review from a large institution of 125 critically ill patients, 62% of whom were immunosuppressed and the others immunocompetent. The mortality differences between these two groups, 66% versus 42%, respectively, were significant. OLBx led to a specific diagnosis in 68% of immunosuppressed patients, resulting in a change in therapy in 51% and an ultimate overall mortality of 67.5%. The authors conclude that OLBx did not change mortality in critically ill patients with respiratory failure.

Warner DO, Warner MA, Divertie MB: Open lung biopsy in patients with diffuse pulmonary infiltrates and acute respiratory failure. Am Rev Respir Dis 137:90, 1988.

A detailed report on 80 patients with diffuse pulmonary infiltrates and acute respiratory failure. This study shows the accuracy of open lung biopsy in establishing a diagnosis but also points out the limited therapeutic options for most of the underlying disease processes.

Walker WA, Cole HF, Khandekar A et al: Does open lung biopsy affect treatment in patients with diffuse pulmonary infiltrates? J Thorac Cardiovasc Surg 97:534, 1989.

This retrospective review of 61 patients demonstrates the accuracy of open lung biopsy in both immunocompromised and noncompromised patients with diffuse pulmonary infiltrates and how the results of biopsy result in a change in therapy.

■ *REFERENCES*

Cheson BD, Samlowski WE, Tang TT, Spruance SL: Value of open lung biopsy in 87 immunocompromised patients with pulmonary infiltrates. Cancer 55:453, 1985.

Daniels AC: Method of biopsy useful in the diagnosing of certain intrathoracic diseases. Dis Chest 16:360, 1949.

Flabouris A, Myburgh J: The utility of open lung biopsy in patients requiring mechanical ventilation. Chest 115:811, 1999.

Imoke E, Dudgeon DL, Colombana P et al: Open lung biopsy in the immunocompromised pediatric patient. J Pediatr Surg 10:816, 1983.

McKenna RJ Jr, Mountain CF, McMurtrey MJ: Open lung biopsy in immunocompromised patients. Chest 86:671, 1984.

Nelems JM, Cooper JD, Henderson RD et al: Emergency open lung biopsy. Ann Thorac Surg 22:260, 1976.

Ruskin G, Brodman R, Condit D, Karpel J: Prospective evaluation of bedside open lung biopsy [Abstract]. Am Rev Respir Dis 141 (Suppl):A596, 1990.

Saterfield IR Jr, McLaughlin JS: Open lung biopsy in diagnosing pulmonary infiltrates in immunosuppressed patients. Ann Thorac Surg 28:359, 1979.

Weng TR, Levinson H, Wentworth P et al: Open lung biopsy in children. Am Rev Respir Dis 97:673, 1980.

White DA, Wong PW, Downey R: The utility of open lung biopsy in patients with hematologic malignancies. Am J Respir Crit Care Med 161:723, 2000.

CHAPTER **8**

Thoracic Incisions

Sudish C. Murthy

Thomas W. Rice

It is easy for the surgeon . . . to treat in a casual, sometimes cavalier, manner the only visible reminder to the patient of that procedure.

C. Frederick Kittle

The history of thoracic surgery is replete with vivid descriptions of morbid, often gruesome, surgical approaches to the chest (Fig. 8–1, *A* and *B*). The rigidity of the chest wall and the relative lack of mobility of thoracic viscera magnify the importance of a well-conceived incision to facilitate exposure for resectional procedures. A century of experience and technologic advancement has afforded the modern thoracic surgeon the luxury of choosing from a variety of surgical approaches to the chest. However, to successfully utilize this information, the surgeon must be facile with the surgical anatomy of the chest wall and contents, and must understand the advantages and limitations of each incision.

GENERAL CONSIDERATIONS

Regardless of size, the incision should be placed to allow for the best possible exposure of the area that will be the site of the most technically challenging part of the surgery. Consequently, for standard pulmonary resections, incisions should expose the hilum of the lung. Location of the incision must permit rapid extension should circumstances dictate. This mandates a wide sterile prep for most thoracic procedures. Options to widen an existing incision need not be restricted to the linear axis, as counter-incisions or perpendicular incisions can be used for greater surgical exposure. Retractors have been developed to improve exposure from otherwise less-than-adequate incisions (Cooper et al, 1988).

Although thoracotomies can be safely performed in octogenarians (Naunheim et al, 1991), physical condition and body habitus of the patient should be considered when planning the surgical approach. A cachectic, bedridden patient may develop pressure necrosis over a posteriorly placed thoracotomy incision versus a lateral one. Similarly, muscular individuals require much larger subcutaneous dissection if muscle-sparing thoracotomy approaches are considered, and may subsequently be at greater risk for postoperative seroma. Tall individuals with narrow costal flares who require pericardial drainage may be more easily treated from an anterior left minithoracotomy than from a subxiphoid approach. Standard risk factors for wound complications (obesity, diabetes, etc.) should be recognized preoperatively and considered when incisions are planned. Meticulous surgical technique, gentle tissue handling, and excellent hemostasis will minimize local wound problems.

Ancillary services at an institution can greatly impact the surgical plan. If reliable single lung isolation is available, incision size can be drastically reduced and postoperative recovery may be enhanced by epidural analgesia (Lubenow et al, 1994). Preoperative imaging studies are useful to define the pathology and may also help direct the location of the incision (Daly et al, 1991).

Finally, as postoperative survival progressively improves, the long-term sequelae of thoracic incisions must be considered. A muscle-sparing thoracotomy may be less painful and preserve arm function better than the *classic* postero-lateral approach (Ginsberg, 1993; Kittle, 1988), although objective data are insufficient to support this theory (Hazelrigg et al, 1991; Ponn et al, 1992). Post-thoracotomy neuralgia remains a problem without a definitive solution and brachial plexopathy can be a devastating complication of thoracotomy or sternotomy.

With these tenets in mind, the chest can be accessed from anterior, lateral, or posterior (posterolateral) approaches. Combined approaches are commonly utilized. A fundamental understanding of the regional musculoskeletal anatomy is valuable in reconstructing the wound and in predicting postoperative debility that might result.

ANTERIOR CHEST INCISIONS

The musculoskeletal anatomy of the anterior neck, chest and abdomen are represented in Figure 8–2. Important skeletal landmarks include the thyroid cartilage, the suprasternal notch, the sternal angle of Louis, and the xiphoid process. The suprasternal notch lies over the inferior aspect of the second thoracic vertebra (T2), the angle of Louis superimposes onto T4, and the xiphoid approximates T9. When mediastinal structures are projected through the anterior skeleton (Fig. 8–3), the origin of the left innominate vein is beneath the junction of the first right rib and sternum. The top of the aortic arch is posterior to the midportion of the manubrium, and the hila are located deep to the third ribs.

Major anterior muscles include the platysma, sternocleidomastoid (SCM), the pectoralis major, the serratus anterior, and the rectus abdominus. The direction of the muscles should be noted (especially the pectoralis major) to permit muscle-splitting, rather than muscle-dividing incisions if possible. The vascular supply to the pectoralis major is both medial, from internal mammary perforators, and lateral, from the thoracoacromial trunk and

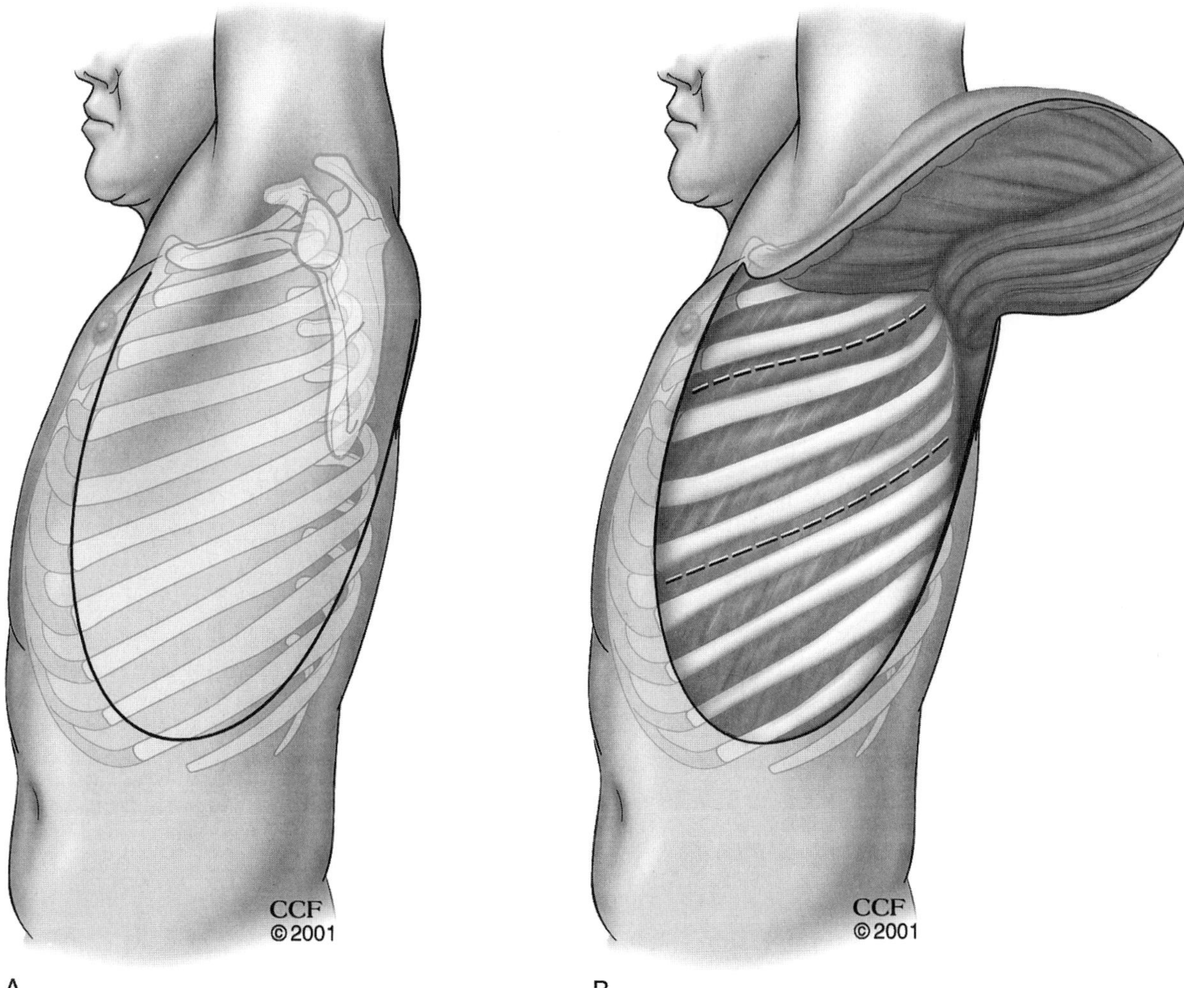

FIGURE 8–1 ■ *A*, Thoracic incision for esophageal resection in 1910. *B*, The scapula was completely mobilized, and the chest was entered at multiple interspaces *(dashed lines)*. (Adapted from Meyer W: Some observations regarding thoracic surgery on human beings. Ann Surg 52:34, 1910; © Cleveland Clinic Foundation, 2001.)

intercostal artery perforators. This becomes relevant when mobilizing the muscle for reconstructive efforts.

Transverse Cervical Incision

The transverse cervical incision is the most common approach to access the thyroid, the cervical trachea, the proximal esophagus, and the superior mediastinum. The surgeon should be familiar with the anatomic relationships of the region (Fig. 8–4*A*). Patients are placed in a supine position on the operating table and arms are tucked at the sides (see Fig. 8–4*B*). Ulnar nerve compression is avoided by appropriate padding, and cervical exposure is augmented by neck hyperextension. For some tracheal procedures, intraoperative neck flexion and extension are necessary and should be permissible. Both surgeon and anesthesiologist should ensure that proper head support is provided prior to the placement of the drapes. Preoperative placement of central venous lines must be done with the operative plan in mind.

The neck is cleansed with alcohol, and a standard iodine-based gel is used to prepare the skin. It is customary to consider the entire neck (to the jaw angle) and the anterior chest as part of the operative field, although after the sterile preparation, these regions may be covered and exposed only if needed. Examination with the patient under anesthesia will help the surgeon identify anatomic landmarks (thyroid cartilage, suprasternal notch, SCM, etc.) prior to commencement of the procedure.

Depending on the patient's anatomy and indication, a standard transverse cervical incision (see Fig. 8–4*C*) is usually made midway between the thyroid cartilage and the suprasternal notch in a convenient skin crease. This location is consistent with the lines of Langer. The knife blade is used to carry the incision through the platysma, which allows for easy identification of this muscle when closing. The incision is easily carried across the SCM or in a cephalad direction toward the mastoid process for additional exposure. Myocutaneous flaps are raised as dissection subadjacent to the platysma is relatively bloodless. In the midline, the strap muscles are then easily identified and bluntly mobilized laterally to expose the thyroid gland.

The cervical trachea is exposed as the thyroid is ele-

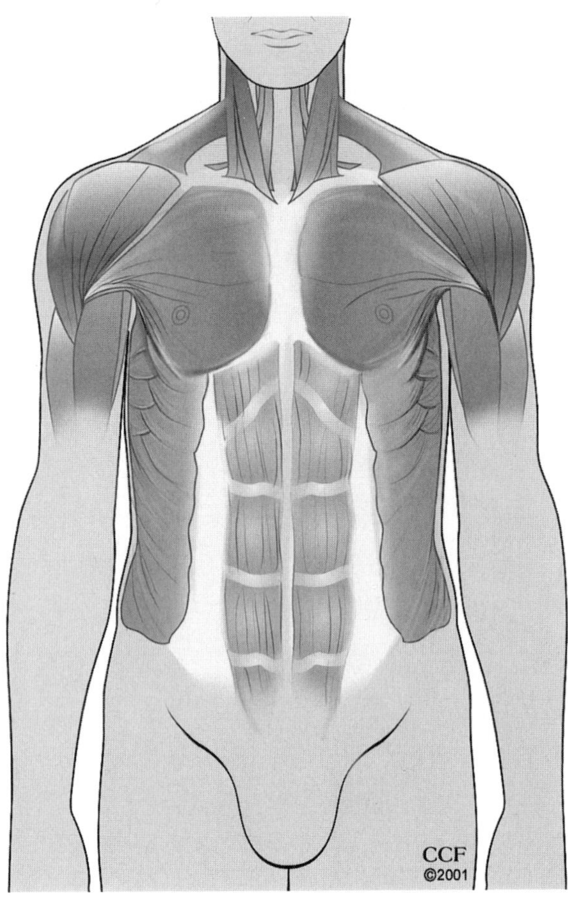

FIGURE 8–2 ■ Musculoskeletal structures encountered with anterior approaches. Important muscle groups include sternocleidomastoid, pectoralis major, serratus anterior, and rectus abdominis. (© Cleveland Clinic Foundation, 2001.)

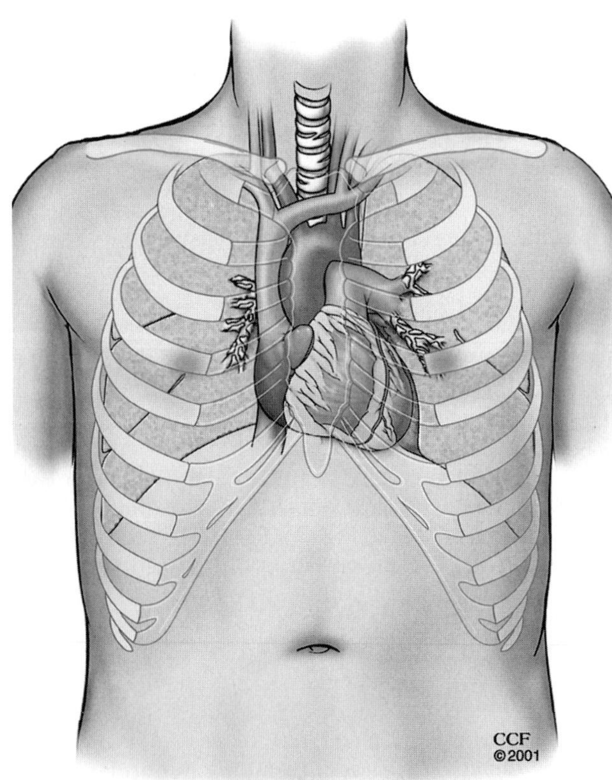

FIGURE 8–3 ■ Anterior projection of major mediastinal structures through the chest wall. (© Cleveland Clinic Foundation, 2001.)

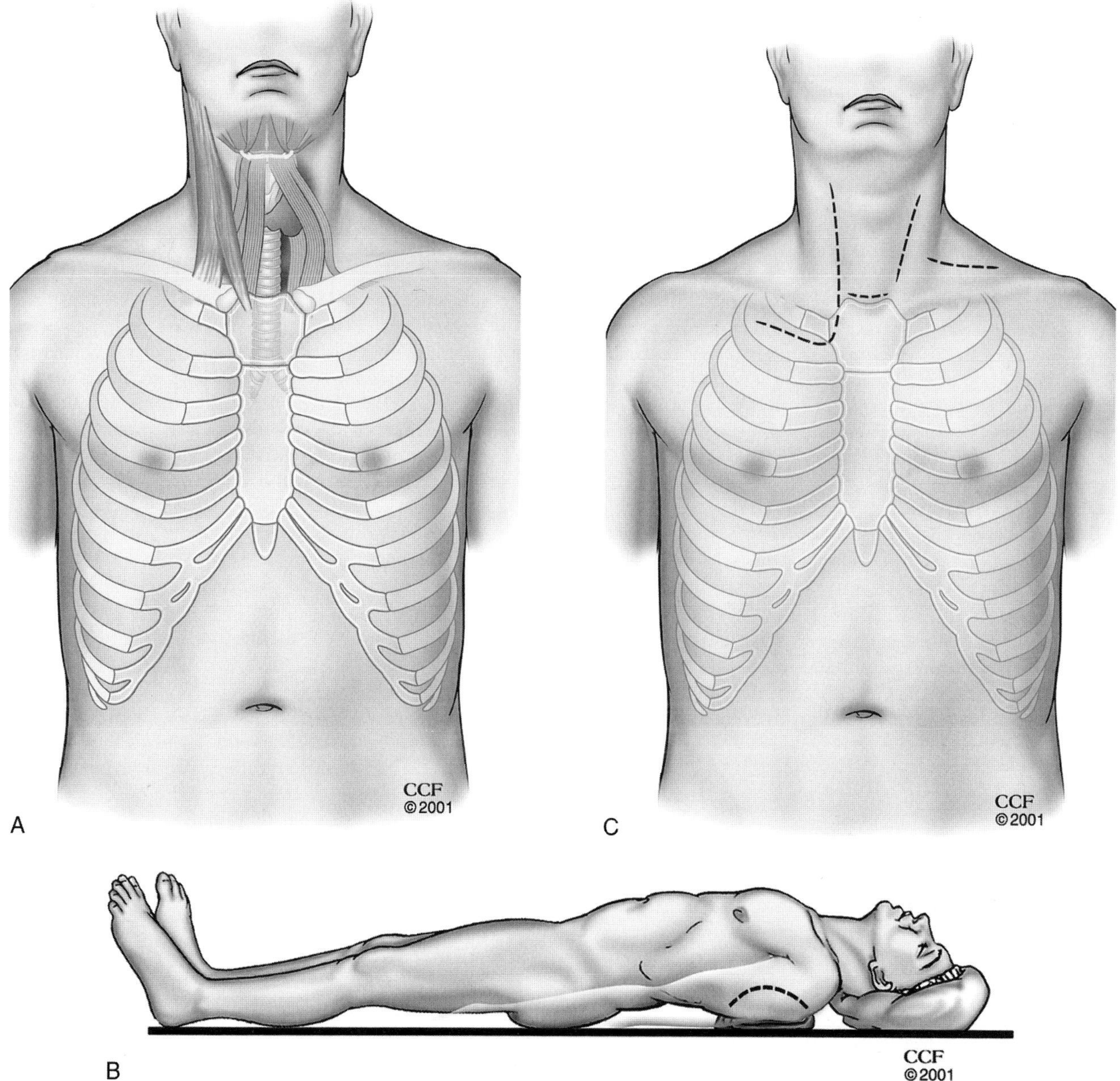

FIGURE 8–4 ■ *A,* Exposure of the neck. With the platysma cut away, the relationship of the deeper cervical muscles should be understood. Exposure to the trachea mandates lateral mobilization of the strap muscles and elevation (or division) of the thyroid isthmus. *B,* Standard position for midline cervical incisions. *C,* Variety of common cervical incisions.

vated superiorly (or the thyroid isthmus divided) and pretracheal (thymic) fat mobilized laterally. This approach is recommended for tracheotomy or tracheal resection (Grillo, 1969). Elevation of the pretracheal fascia permits access to the mediastinum for mediastinoscopy. The transcervical approach to the mediastinum has been used for thymectomy (Cooper et al, 1988) and is occasionally helpful in reoperative parathyroid surgery (Wells and Cooper, 1991) and substernal goiter.

Variations of this incision are frequently used (see Fig. 8–4*C*). With the neck extended and turned to the contralateral side, a transverse incision is started at the lateral border of the SCM and carried laterally across the supraclavicular fossa to facilitate scalene node biopsy. The platysma is incised sharply and the ipsilateral external jugular vein ligated. The SCM can be mobilized medially with cautery to expose the internal jugular vein. The omohyoid muscle courses obliquely in the field and can be mobilized or divided without consequence. The fat pad can then be harvested off the scalene anticus muscle after the phrenic nerve has been identified and preserved. The subclavian artery courses at the inferior aspect of the field, and the thyrocervical trunk can be skeletonized. The left-sided approach may bring the thoracic duct in the field, mandating additional caution when the medial aspect of the fat pad is being mobilized.

The cervical esophagus is exposed with an oblique incision along the anterior border of the SCM (see Fig. 8–4*C*). After the SCM is mobilized laterally, the omohyoid is divided if necessary. To properly mobilize the carotid sheath requires division of the inferior thyroid artery and middle thyroid vein. As the thyroid, trachea, and strap muscles are gently retracted medially and the carotid sheath and SCM moved laterally, the esophagus is approached. Blunt dissection posteriorly along the anterior border of the cervical spine provides the safest route to control the cervical esophagus.

The anterior transcervical approach to superior sulcus tumors (Dart et al, 1979; Dartevelle et al, 1993) permits controlled cervical mobilization for anterior lesions. After appropriate positioning, intersecting incisions are made along the anterior border of the SCM and transversely across to the inferior edge of the medial clavicle (see Fig. 8–4*C*). Much of the dissection is similar to that discussed previously. Notable differences include division of the SCM and the scalenus anticus. After removal of the scalene fat pad, the tumor is carefully assessed. If deemed resectable, the medial half of the clavicle is resected and vascular control is obtained (Fig. 8–5). Division of the scalenus anticus nicely exposes the stellate ganglia for dorsal sympathectomy (Nanson, 1957).

Closure entails repair of divided muscle with interrupted absorbable suture. For large neck procedures, platysma closure should allow a Silastic drain to hold bulb suction. A fine, absorbable, subcuticular suture is used for skin closure. Wound infection is very rare unless a viscus (e.g., esophagus) has been opened or the tissues have been previously irradiated. However, an enlarging hematoma in the neck can rapidly lead to airway compromise. Thus, meticulous hemostasis is required and close postoperative observation is warranted for large neck dissections. Postoperative hoarseness heralds a recurrent nerve injury and ipsilateral diaphragm elevation suggests a phrenic nerve palsy. Familiarity with the surgical anatomy of the region should greatly reduce complications.

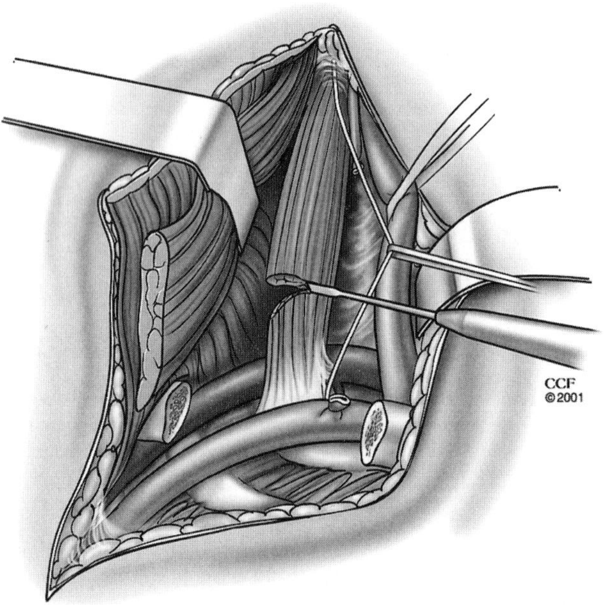

FIGURE 8–5 ■ Anterior transcervical approach to superior sulcus tumors as described by Dartevelle and associates (1993). Schematic represents a right-sided approach. The medial portion of the clavicle *(bottom of the picture)* has been resected. A retractor *(left)* distracts platysma and the cut end of the sternocleidomastoid muscle, exposing the scalene anticus. The phrenic nerve should be mobilized medially to permit safe division of the scalene muscle. (Adapted from Dartevelle FG, Chapelier AR, Macchiarini P, et al: Anterior transcervical-thoracic approach for radical resection of lung tumors invading the thoracic inlet. J Thorac Cardiovasc Surg 105: 1025, 1993; © Cleveland Clinic Foundation, 2001.)

ANTERIOR MEDIASTINOTOMY

The original description of anterior mediastinotomy (McNeil and Chamberlain, 1966) entailed a 6-cm incision along the second intercostal space and removal of the entire cartilaginous portion of the second rib. The internal mammary pedicle was ligated and divided, and the retrosternal extrapleural space was entered by blunt dissection. The procedure was devised to identify patients with unresectable cancer (mediastinal spread) to prevent unnecessary exploratory thoracotomy. Current indications for the procedure are considerably narrower, as accurate radiographic staging and alternative surgical approaches (mediastinoscopy and VATS) have largely supplanted the technique. Occasionally, it is still used for staging patients with left upper lobe bronchogenic cancer. More commonly, anterior mediastinotomy is used to diagnose primary mediastinal masses after percutaneous attempts (e.g., fine-needle aspiration) have failed to provide adequate tissue for complete pathologic analysis.

A preoperative computer tomography scan can help place the incision directly over the pathology, simplifying the procedure. The ipsilateral thorax should be prepped in the event the incision needs to be extended to improve exposure or control hemorrhage. If a mediastinoscope is used to assist in the exposure, seldom is more than a 3-cm incision required. The selected interspace may be widened enough to accommodate the mediastinoscope without rib resection (Fig. 8–6).

The skin incision should be placed directly over the site of the pathology. The pectoralis major muscle can be separated bluntly in the direction of its fibers. To remain in the extrapleural plane, sharp dissection is used to identify the internal mammary pedicle and to distract it laterally. The mediastinum is then entered bluntly, and the mediastinoscope is inserted. If additional space is needed, the medial aspect of the rib cartilage over the internal mammary vascular bundle is removed carefully and sharp dissection is used to expose the vascular pedicle. Rarely will the internal mammary artery need to be sacrificed.

If an intrapleural approach is preferred, the pleural cavity should be entered lateral to the mammary pedicle. When a mediastinoscope is used, lung isolation is generally not needed. The surgeon must be careful not to mistake hilar lymph nodes (N1) for mediastinal lymph nodes (N2), since both may be biopsied through this approach. At the conclusion of the procedure, air is evacuated through a soft catheter left in the pleural space. Suction is applied to the catheter as pectoralis muscle is tightly closed around it with absorbable suture. The catheter is pulled out during a deep breath-hold, and the muscle layer is cinched tight. If a parenchymal lung injury was incurred, a chest tube is warranted.

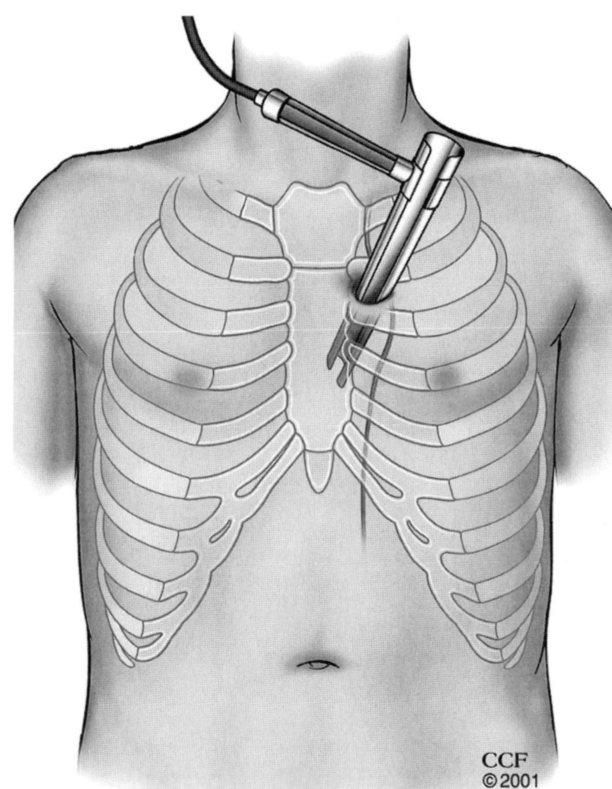

FIGURE 8–6 ■ Modified Chamberlain procedure for access to the superior-anterior mediastinum. A mediastinoscope is used to facilitate exposure and minimize the incision length and morbidity. The scope is inserted medial to the internal mammary pedicle for most applications. (© Cleveland Clinic Foundation, 2001.)

ANTERIOR THORACOTOMY

Anterior thoracotomy has both general thoracic and cardiac surgical applications. It is advantageous in that the patient can remain supine with the expected result of improvement in cardiopulmonary function. The right middle lobe is easily approached anteriorly. Bilateral anterior thoracotomy is gaining popularity for double lung transplantation (Meyers et al, 2000; Pochettino et al, 2000). Moreover, open lung biopsy on critically ill patients can be safely conducted through anterior exposure, as can partial pericardectomy. Similarly, reoperative cardiac surgeries are often approached via anterior thoracotomy (Byrne et al, 2001; Kerr et al, 2001). Because the posterior hilum and the esophagus are poorly exposed, the anterior approach is infrequently used for pulmonary or esophageal resections.

The patient should be placed in a supine position with a paraspinal roll elevating the ipsilateral chest by 20 to 30 degrees (Fig. 8–7, *A* and *B*). A double-lumen endotracheal tube should be placed for lung isolation. Arms are tucked at the sides and elbows are padded. The ipsilateral elbow is elevated if excessive stretch is perceived on the shoulder. After a standard sterile prep and drape, the angle of Louis is identified. This palpable landmark identifies the second rib. For entrance into the chest at interspace 4, an incision is made in the inframammary crease from the sternal edge to the anterior axillary line. The pectoralis major muscle should be divided slightly superior to the skin incision to prevent suture lines from overlapping. Breast tissue is mobilized from the pectoralis fascia with cautery. The cephalad portion of the pectoralis muscle is mobilized medially off the sternum and inferiorly from the ribs until the desired interspace is reached. Internal mammary artery perforators are controlled with cautery or clips.

The ipsilateral lung should be deflated well before the thorax is entered. We do not routinely dissect rib periosteum for a thoracotomy unless the rib is to be resected. Cautery is used to incise the intercostal muscles from the superior aspect of the rib below the interspace. Laterally, serratus muscle is split along the course of its fibers. Slips of pectoralis minor muscle are divided. The pleura is initially entered bluntly to prevent parenchymal injury. Once the lung is collapsed, or retracted, the rest

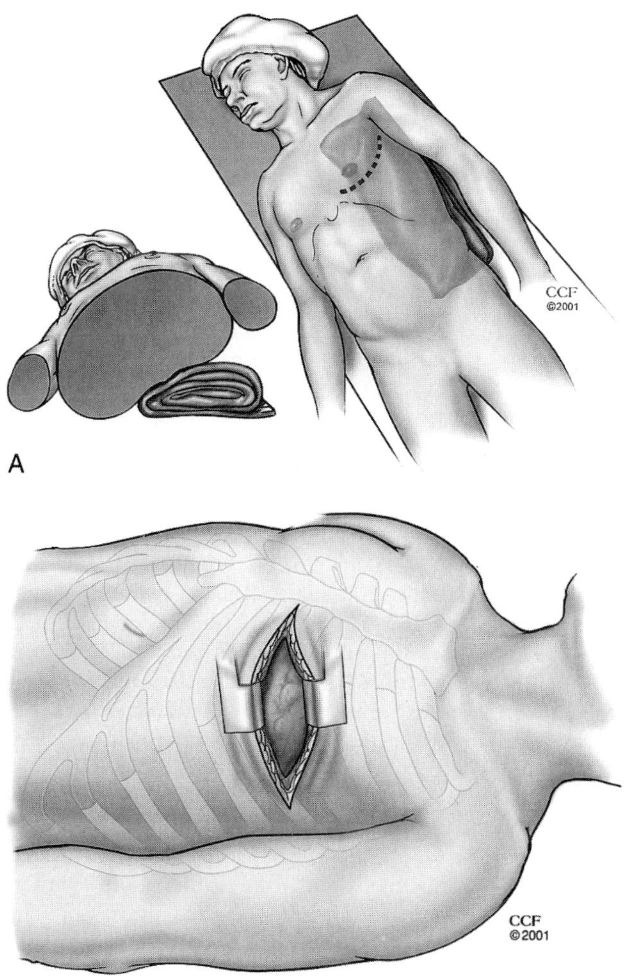

FIGURE 8–7 ■ *A*, Position for anterior thoracotomy. A roll is used to elevate the patient on the ipsilateral side. The ipsilateral arm can be positioned at the side *(as shown)* or elevated across the body. *B*, The pleural cavity is commonly entered at interspace 4. Resection of the sternocostal junction at rib 3 allows sufficient exposure for single lung transplantation *(not shown)*. (© Cleveland Clinic Foundation, 2001.)

of the interspace is opened with cautery. If additional exposure is necessary, the internal mammary pedicle can be divided. This may be facilitated by resecting a small piece of rib cartilage anterior to the bundle. If cephalad exposure is required, the cartilage of the rib above the interspace can be divided. To further increase rib distraction, the intercostal muscles and pleura can be divided posteriorly, well beyond the limits of the incision. Gauze pads are used to cushion the ribs and soft tissues when the rib spreader is applied.

For closure, after chest drains are placed, ribs are reapproximated with heavy gauge (e.g., #2) absorbable suture. We do not routinely drill holes in ribs or tunnel suture subperiosteally to prevent intercostal neuralgia. Rather, sutures are placed to incorporate intercostal muscle from the interspace below to cushion the neurovascular bundle and excessive force is avoided when sutures are tied down. Anteriorly, it is seldom possible to obtain rib-to-rib apposition. Trying to do so predisposes to neurovascular bundle injury. Instead, attention should be paid to meticulous soft tissue closure. The perichondrium should be identified and reapproximated if divided. The medial aspect of the rib is anchored to the sternum with heavy, non-absorbable monofilament suture if necessary. The pectoralis major muscle is repaired with either continuous or interrupted suture technique. Deep dermal tissues and skin are closed with continuous absorbable suture.

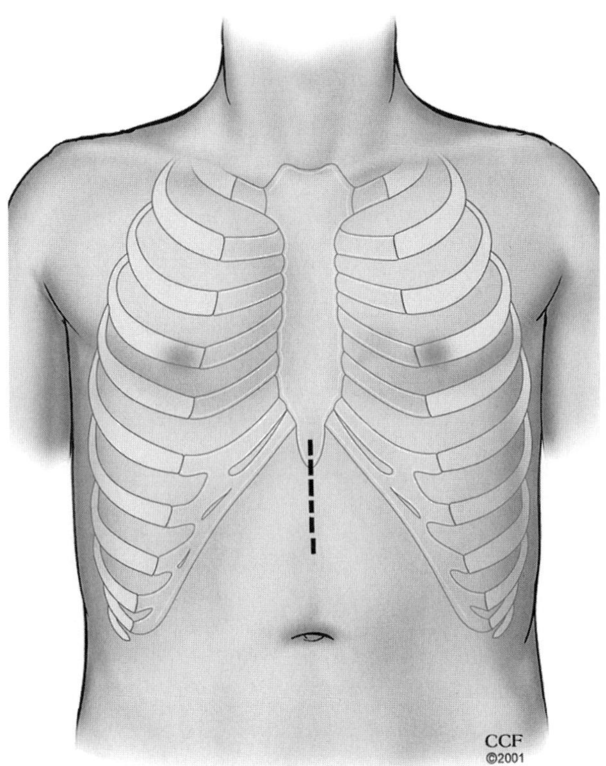

FIGURE 8–8 ■ Location of the incision for a subxiphoid approach to the pericardium. (© Cleveland Clinic Foundation, 2001.)

UPPER MIDLINE

The upper midline abdominal incision has wide application in thoracic surgery. In addition to providing access to the abdominal viscera, the pericardium can be drained, and the gastroesophageal junction can be easily exposed. Moreover, the incision is routinely coupled with other incisions during two- or three-field approaches. Contraindications are few, although a previous laparotomy incision may deter a subxiphoid approach to the pericardium.

Although there remains some disagreement as to the best surgical strategy to manage effusive pericardial disease (Hankins et al, 1980; Larrieu et al, 1986; Piehler et al, 1985), the subxiphoid approach to the pericardium is rapid, effective, and if needed, can be performed without general anesthesia (Stewart, 1974). In obese or tall patients with narrow costal arches, subxiphoid exposure of the pericardium can be difficult (Prager et al, 1982).

Patients with hemodynamically compromising effusive disease (pericardial tamponade) are stabilized medically and percutaneously drained prior to surgery. This should be done the day before; pericardial drains should be left in place. If the pericardium cannot be decompressed, the surgeon must remain with the patient while the patient's abdomen and chest are sterilized and draped prior to anesthesia induction. If the patient is too unstable, the procedure must be done with the patient under local anesthesia and conscious sedation.

The patient is placed supine on the operating table (Fig. 8–8). A roll should be placed behind the lumbar spine so that the patient assumes a lordotic posture. A midline incision is made from the xiphisternal junction to 8 to 10 cm below the tip of the xiphoid. The linea alba is divided, with care being taken to avoid entering the peritoneal cavity. The soft tissue plane behind the xiphoid should be developed bluntly; the xiphoid can be dislocated from the xiphisternal joint after being freed from its fascial and muscular attachments. The diaphragm is depressed posteriorly with a sponge stick, and blunt dissection proceeds superiorly until the pericardium is exposed. The sternum is elevated anteriorly with a hand-held retractor. If a preoperative pericardial catheter was placed, the pericardial space can be filled with 100 to 200 ml of body-temperature, sterile saline to facilitate its identification and permit safe entrance. Once identified, the pericardium is grasped and sharply incised (Fig. 8–9). The space is drained after manual deloculation. A mediastinoscope (Santos et al, 1977) can be used to identify and biopsy pericardial implants. A generous segment of pericardium should be resected (16 to 25 cm^2) to decrease recurrence rate (Larrieu et al, 1986; Piehler et al, 1985; Santos et al, 1977). A chest tube is left in the pericardial space and tunneled out of a separate stab incision for postoperative drainage.

Complications, although rare, can be catastrophic. If the preoperative diagnosis was incorrect and an obliterative pericardial process exists, a coronary artery or ventricle can be lacerated in the surgical attempt to enter the space (Prager et al, 1982). Similarly, for a postcardiotomy, loculated, posterior effusion, a transthoracic approach would be prudent.

Proper reapproximation of the linea alba with heavy suture is necessary to prevent postoperative ventral her-

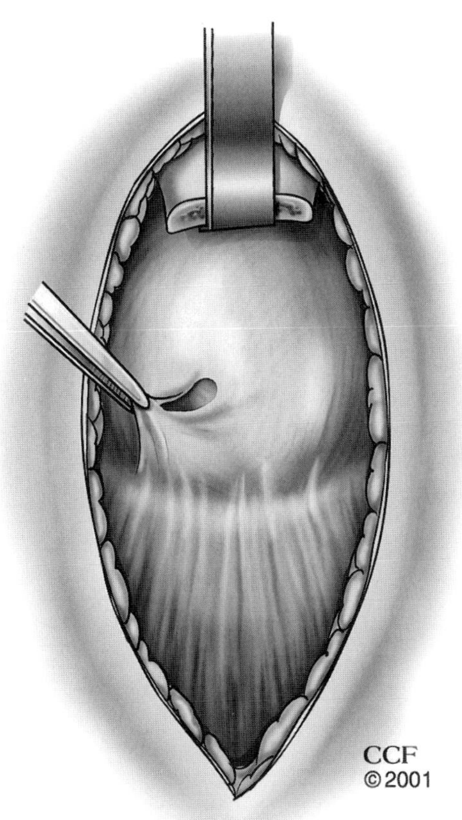

FIGURE 8–9 ■ Subxiphoid pericardial exposure. When the xiphisternum is elevated and the diaphragm depressed, the inferior pericardium is brought into the operative field. The pericardium is then incised sharply to create the window. (© Cleveland Clinic Foundation, 2001.)

nia. Heterotopic ossification is sited as an uncommon late sequela of midline incisions (Reardon et al, 1997). Patients tolerate the incision well and can be mobilized early. Although follow-up echocardiogram is not imperative, it is recommended prior to chest tube removal.

When the upper midline incision is extended down to the umbilicus (Fig. 8–10*A*) and self-retaining retractors are properly placed, the esophageal hiatus can be exposed. After the left lobe of the liver is separated from its ligamentous attachment to the diaphragm and gently tucked beneath the retractor, the hiatus is brought into full view (see Fig. 8–10*B*). Access to the posterior mediastinum can be achieved by vertical division of the diaphragm from the hiatus or through a transverse semicircular incision in the central tendon that spares the hiatus (Thirby et al, 1993). When dividing the diaphragm, attention should be paid to controlling the inferior phrenic vessels and preserving the phrenic nerves. The technique of transhiatal esophagectomy through this approach is described in Chapter 57 of *Esophageal Surgery.*

STERNOTOMY

Median sternotomy was originally described for the management of mediastinal tuberculosis (Milton, 1897). Median sternotomy has since become the most common thoracic incision due to the development of cardiac surgery. By virtue of its midline and anterior location, it has broad applications for noncardiac chest operations as well. The transsternal route is the most direct for thymectomy and other anterior mediastinal tumors. Tracheal (Grillo, 1969; Grillo, 1979) and upper esophageal exposure (Orringer, 1984) is greatly enhanced when cervical incisions are combined with full or partial sternotomy. Median sternotomy can simplify bilateral pulmonary metastasectomy (Regal et al, 1985; Takita et al, 1977) and bilateral lung volume operations (Cooper et al, 1995). Anatomic pulmonary resections can be safely performed through a sternotomy incision (Asaph and Keppel, 1984; Cooper et al, 1978; Urschel and Razzuk, 1986). Transsternal repair of postpneumonectomy bronchopleural fistula has also been reported (Baldwin and Mark, 1985). Sternotomy permits early hilar control for completion pneumonectomy cases and should be considered for uncontrollable hemorrhage that may occur during mediastinoscopy. An additional advantage of sternotomy is the ease of instituting cardiopulmonary bypass from this approach.

The sternotomy incision is performed with the patient supine (Fig. 8–11*A*). Arms should be tucked and elbows padded. Depending on the indication for surgery, the sterile drape may include the entire neck and abdomen. Similarly, the groins may be included if additional access for cardiopulmonary bypass is needed. A double lumen endotracheal tube is preferable for most pulmonary operations except tracheal resection. The standard sternotomy incision is from the suprasternal notch to a point midway between the xiphoid and umbilicus in the midline. The knife is used to carry the incision to the pectoral fascia and linea alba. Cautery can then be applied to control superficial bleeding, score the periosteum, and divide the linea alba. The superior end of the skin incision is retracted in a cephalad manner to expose the top of the manubrium and allow for control of crossing jugular tributaries in the space of Burns. The interclavicular ligament can be divided sharply or with cautery; care must be taken to avoid an anterior coursing innominate artery or vein. Blunt digital dissection is used to open the retrosternal space both superiorly and inferiorly.

Once the sternum is fully exposed, deliberate palpation of the interspaces allows for an accurate assessment of the true midline. If necessary, this can be re-marked with cautery. A reciprocating saw is used to divide the sternum either from top down or bottom up (see Fig. 8–11*B*). Prior to splitting the sternum, the lungs are transiently deflated to prevent unintentional entry into a pleural space. Bleeding is immediately controlled with gauze packing, while periosteal bleeders are selectively cauterized. Marrow bleeding can be controlled by bone wax without significantly increasing infectious complications (Baskett et al, 1999), although biocompatible sealants now exist for this purpose (Kjaergard and Trumbull, 2000).

A choice of sternal spreaders can be used to distract the sternal edges (see Fig. 8–11*C*). Inferior (caudad) placement of retractors seems less frequently associated with rib fracture and brachial plexus injury (Baisden et al, 1984). Sternal edges should be spread only far enough

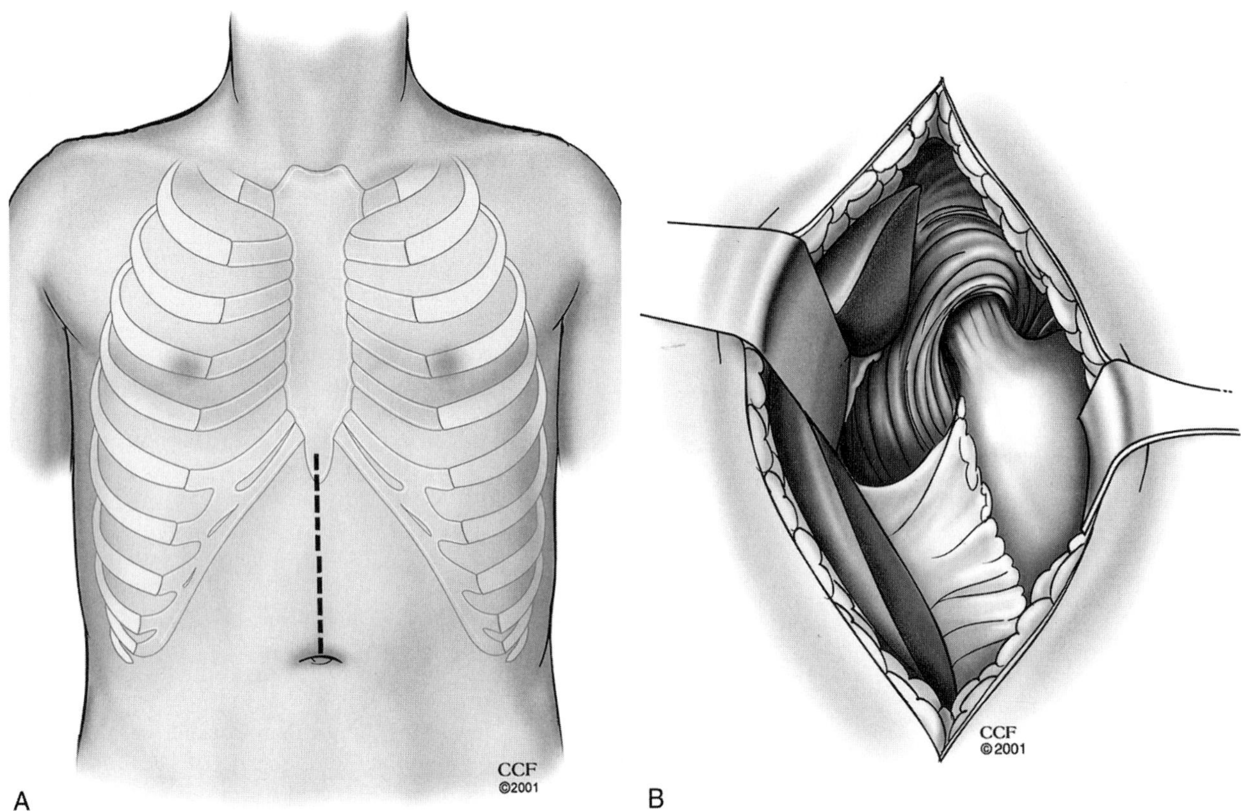

FIGURE 8–10 ■ *A*, Placement of upper midline incision for distal esophageal and diaphragm exposure. *B*, After the left lateral segments of the liver are mobilized toward the midline, the esophageal hiatus is brought into full view. An *upper-hand* retractor greatly improves exposure. (© Cleveland Clinic Foundation, 2001.)

to permit adequate exposure for safe completion of the operation. Anterior diaphragm fibers may prematurely restrict sternal spreading and can be divided. In addition to brachial plexus and rib injury, excessive tension on the innominate vein limits sternal distraction.

Multiple modifications to the skin incision have been made to improve cosmetic results. Common to all is extensive soft tissue mobilization, which allows for complete sternal division. Candidates for skin-sparing operations should be fit and well-nourished, because significant wound healing is required. Steroid use is a relative contraindication.

A limited 10- to 12-cm vertical incision can be made beginning below the angle of Louis. This keeps the scar below the neckline. Subcutaneous flaps are raised laterally off the pectoralis fascia and rectus sheath. Internal mammary perforators are encountered as the flaps are raised. Depending on the size of the incision it may be necessary to undermine the subcutaneous flaps laterally to the midclavicular line. Superiorly, the soft tissue is universally more lax, requiring less dissection for adequate mobilization. Prior to splitting the sternum, the incision should be able to provide exposure from the suprasternal notch to the xiphoid. Because the decreased length of the incision limits the view of operative field, intraoperative repositioning of the sternal retractor is frequently necessary. Subcutaneous drains and compressive dressings should be used postoperatively. A limited "Y" incision has also been described and is similarly performed (Nandi et al, 1979).

The submammary exposure of the sternum is popular for young women (Laks and Hammond, 1980; Martinez-Sanz et al, 1990). Patients are positioned supine with elbows slightly flexed at the patient's side to expose the anterior axillary line (Fig. 8–12). The submammary folds can be marked preoperatively. Beginning just lateral to the nipple, the incision is made in the submammary crease and elevated to a point level with the nipples in the midline. Cautery dissection is used to elevate the breasts and soft tissues, in a triangular fashion, toward both the suprasternal notch and the xiphoid (see Fig. 8–12). The lateral extent of the dissection should not interrupt the lateral perforating branches of the intercostal arteries that perfuse the flap. After completion of the dissection and exposure of the sternum, the superior and inferior flaps are handled gently and retracted with sutures. A standard sternotomy is then performed. When closing, the flaps can be loosely tacked down to the pectoral fascia and closed over vacuum drains. The deep dermis and skin are reapproximated with fine absorbable suture. Compressive dressings are applied to the wound and breast support is provided with an elastic bra.

Wound hematoma and skin necrosis in the central part are observed in 5% to 10% of cases. A horizontal (versus elevated) connecting incision across the sternum has a higher incidence of wound breakdown (de la Riviere et al, 1981). Healing by secondary intention still results in an acceptable cosmetic outcome. Hypertrophic scarring has been noted in 10% to 20% of patients (Deutinger and Domanig, 1992; Martinez-Sanz et al, 1990).

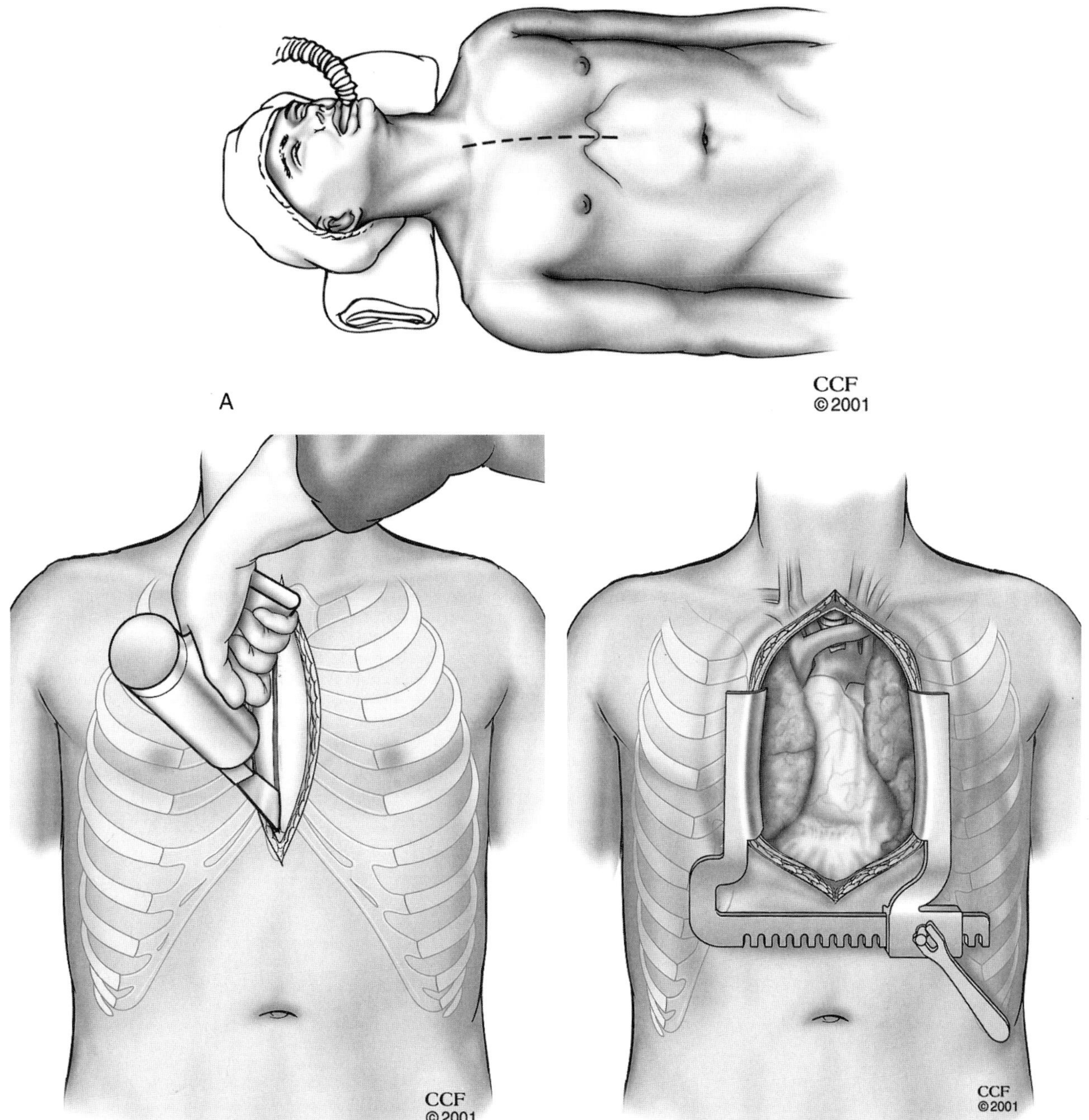

FIGURE 8–11 ■ *A*, Location of incision for median sternotomy. *B*, A sternal saw can be applied either superiorly or inferiorly. It is critical to ensure a midline division of the bone. *C*, The sternal spreader should be applied at the inferior aspect of the incision to reduce the incidence of brachial plexus injury. (© Cleveland Clinic Foundation, 2001.)

Intralesional triamcinolone injection seems effective in these cases (Martinez-Sanz et al, 1990). Decreased areolar sensitivity is reported in 30% of patients (Deutinger and Domanig, 1992). No long-term interference with breast-feeding is reported (Deutinger and Deutinger, 1993).

Regardless of skin incision, rigid reapproximation of the sternum is the single most important factor in preventing sternal dehiscence and deep-seated infection (DiMarco et al, 1989). A variety of strategies have been devised to oppose the sternal edges after sternotomy (DiMarco et al, 1989; Kalush and Bonchek, 1976; Robicsek et al, 1977; Sirivella et al, 1987; Zieren et al, 1993). For uncomplicated cases, a standard stainless steel wire reapproximation is appropriate (Fig. 8–13*A*). Six to seven #6 stainless steel wires should be used. Depending on the patient's size, 2 or 3 wires are placed in the body of the manubrium. The remaining wires are placed parasternally from interspaces 2 through 5. If an osteoporotic or fractured sternum is encountered, the wire-reinforced closure suggested by Robicsek and associates (1977) should be used (see Fig. 8–13*B*). This technique is also useful to help salvage a paramedian sternal split. Mersilene tape, steel bands, and heavy absorbable suture have all been successfully used to close sternotomy incisions.

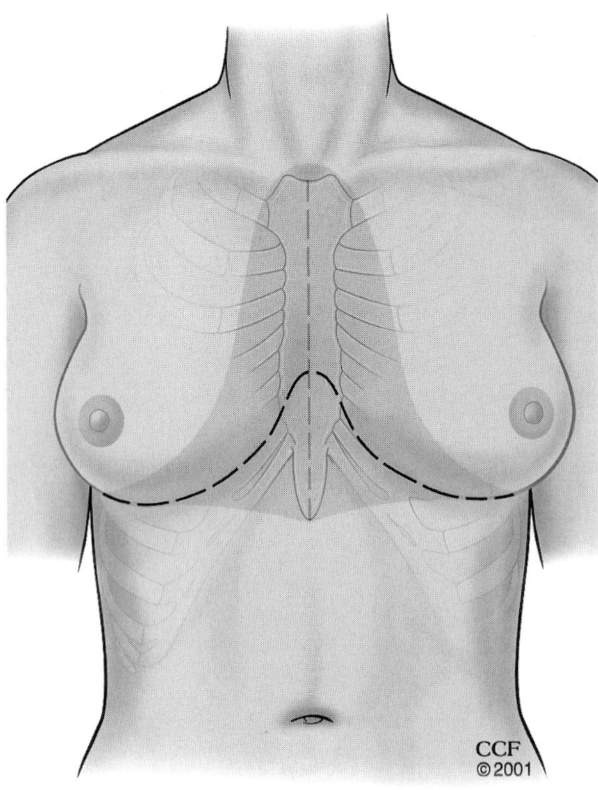

FIGURE 8–12 ■ Submammary incision for sternotomy. Subcutaneous tissue flaps should be raised as depicted by the *shaded areas* in the diagram. The lateral extent of the soft tissue dissection should not be beyond the midclavicular line. (Adapted from Laks H, Hammond GL: A cosmetically acceptable incision for the median sternotomy. J Cardiovasc Surg 79: 146, 1980; © Cleveland Clinic Foundation, 2001.)

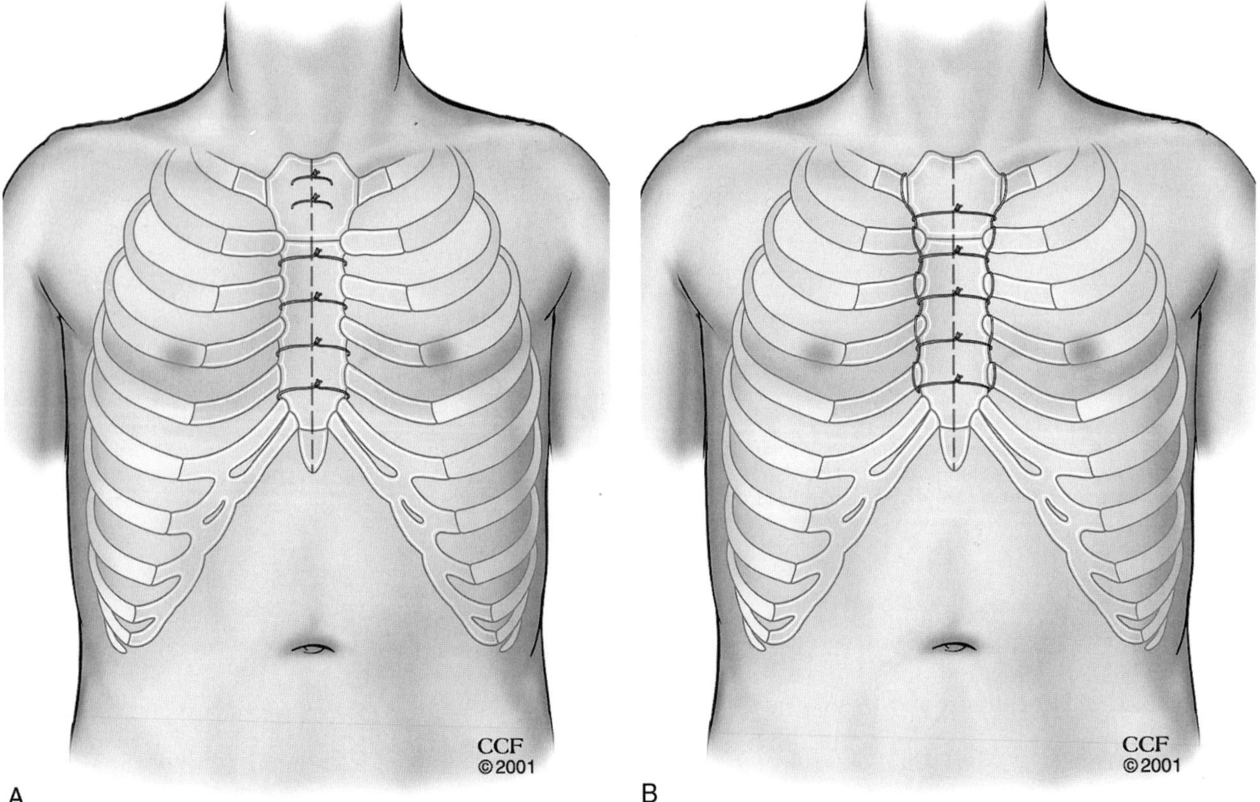

FIGURE 8–13 ■ *A*, Conventional sternal reapproximation with #6 stainless steel. *B*, Sternal closure as proposed by Robicsek. The transverse wires must be placed outside the parasternal weave. (Adapted from Robicsek F, Daugherty HK, Cook JW: The prevention and treatment of sternum separation following open-heart surgery. J Thorac Cardiovasc Surg 73:267, 1977; © Cleveland Clinic Foundation, 2001.)

For patients with preoperative and operative risk factors for sternal wound complications (Demmy et al, 1990; Zacharias and Habib, 1996), the interlocking figure-of-eight closure reported by DiMarco and associates (1989) should be considered.

Although the incidence of mediastinitis following sternotomy is 1% to 2%, the data have been largely derived from cardiac surgical cases. Nonetheless, sternal wound complications do predict a slight long-term survival disadvantage in this population (Stahle et al, 1997). In addition to preoperative patient selection, intraoperative hemostasis and proper sternal closure, early extubation is important in preventing mediastinitis (Demmy et al, 1990). Delayed chest wall complications of median sternotomy include costochondral separation, occult rib fracture, chronic osteomyelitis of the sternum or rib cartilage, sternal non-union, and sternal wire erosion (Weber and Peters, 1986).

PARTIAL STERNOTOMY

Partial sternotomy is a useful adjunct to extend a variety of incisions for additional exposure. It has been combined with a low, collar incision to facilitate tracheal reconstruction (Grillo, 1979), with an oblique cervical incision for upper esophageal (Orringer, 1984) and great vessel exposure, with anterior thoracotomy ("hemi-clamshell"), or with parallel supraclavicular and infraclavicular incisions ("open book incision"). Moreover, when extended in an intercostal space, partial (hemi-) sternotomy can serve as the primary incision for resection of mediastinal malignancy, thymectomy, substernal goiter, or ectopic parathyroid adenoma.

The patient is positioned supine as for a standard sternotomy. The neck should be included in the drape if needed. Flexion and extension of the neck should be possible for tracheal cases. When used as the only incision, an 8 to 10 cm incision can be made beginning at the angle of Louis (Fig. 8–14*A*). Soft tissue flaps are raised as previously described, and the sternum is exposed. A reciprocating saw divides the sternum to the chosen interspace (usually 3 or 4). Given the location of the mass, the saw is used to "T" one side of the sternum towards the mass. A small sternal spreader is used to open the incision. The internal mammary pedicle may need to be divided to improve exposure. Separate lung ventilation is preferable.

After the planned resection is completed, stainless steel wire is used to reapproximate the sternum. An anchoring wire is used to firmly fix the divided bone to the main body of the sternum at the base of the incision (see Fig. 8–14*B*). Suction drains are placed under large subcutaneous flaps.

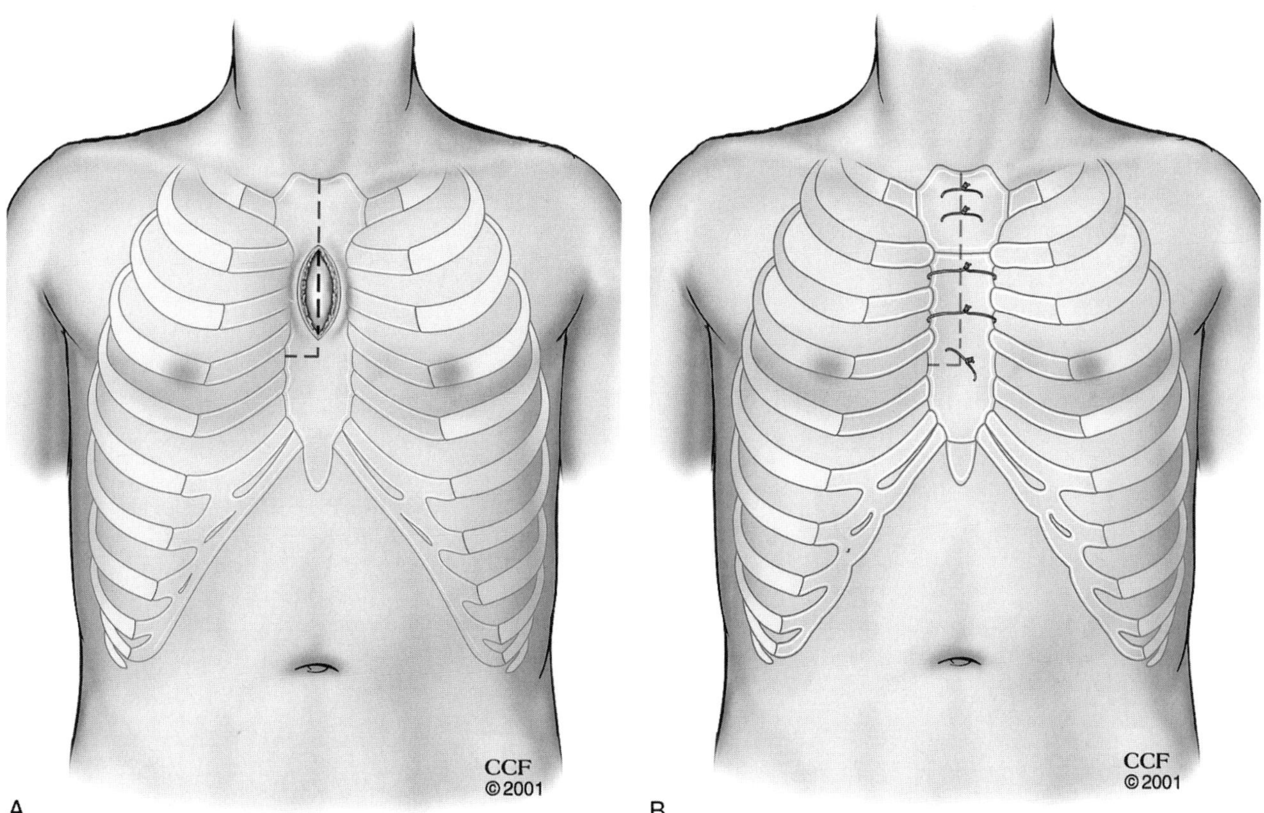

FIGURE 8–14 ■ *A*, Skin incision and position of sternal division for a hemisternotomy. Soft tissue flaps are elevated to expose the upper sternum. The sternum is "T'd" off to the appropriate side. *B*, Wire closure for the partial sternal split is similar to the standard closure with the exception of an inferior anchoring wire placed through the body of the undivided sternum. (© Cleveland Clinic Foundation, 2001.)

THORACOSTERNOTOMY (CLAMSHELL) INCISION

The clamshell incision offers superior exposure of the heart, great vessels, mediastinum, and pulmonary hilum. It has applications in the management of life-threatening traumatic injury, pulmonary metastastectomy (Shimizu et al, 1992) and bilateral sequential double lung transplantation (Kaiser et al, 1991). Rarely, the incision has been used for coronary surgery (Marshall et al, 1988).

After a double lumen endotracheal tube is placed, the patient is positioned supine on the operating table with both arms flexed at the elbows and extended over the face (Fig. 8–15*A*). The patient may be elevated from the table by placement of a roll along the spine and parallel rolls across the scapulae and pelvis. This allows for better exposure should the incision need to be carried more posteriorly. The skin incision is identical to that used for the submammary exposure of the sternum (see Fig. 8–12). Bilateral anterior thoracotomies are performed as previously described; however, rib cartilage is not divided. Interspace 4 is chosen for entrance into the thorax for most cases. Internal mammary pedicles are divided, and suture is ligated. The sternum conjoining the two interspaces is divided with the Gigli saw after the retrosternal space has been dissected bluntly. Bone wax may be applied to the cut ends of the sternum. Rib spreaders are placed bilaterally to open the incision (see Fig. 8–15*B*).

Closure is time consuming. Attention to proper surgical technique is warranted, especially for lung transplant recipients. Over 10% of patients will develop wound complications (Kaiser et al, 1991). In addition to a sturdy thoracotomy closure, the sternum is reapproximated with two interrupted #6 stainless steel wires. Suction drains should be used if large subcutaneous dissections were necessary. Epidural analgesia usually permits early postoperative extubation.

LATERAL CHEST INCISIONS

It is difficult to define the lateral aspect of the chest, yet much is written about anterolateral, posterolateral, and lateral thoracotomies. For the purposes of this discussion, the boundaries of the *lateral* chest stretch from the nipple anteriorly to the scapular tip posteriorly. Incisions contained within these arbitrary boundaries are classified as lateral chest incisions. Because there is a relative paucity of large muscles that span this area (pectoralis major lies anterior and latissimus dorsi lies posterior), most exposures in this location can be done using a muscle-sparing technique. The serratus anterior, the only muscle in the space, runs in a similar direction as the rib interspaces and can be split without difficulty for low thoracotomy approaches. The two most common lateral chest incisions are the "axillary thoracotomy" and the lateral "muscle-sparing" thoracotomy.

AXILLARY THORACOTOMY

Because of the limited exposure of axillary thoracotomy, and the widespread use of video-assisted thoracic surgery (VATS), no longer can sympathectomy (Atkins, 1954), apical bullous disease (Becker and Munro, 1976), or cosmetic concerns (Baeza and Foster, 1976) be considered indications for the approach. The incision has now largely been relegated to a utility incision applicable if problems are encountered in VATS procedures. The transaxillary approach to first rib resection (Roos, 1971) shares the same incision, although the dissection is carried much more superiorly. The axillary thoracotomy provides an approach through the axilla. As the serratus anterior is not part of the axilla, incisions requiring division of this muscle are considered in the lateral thoracotomy section.

Following the induction of general anesthesia (preferably with a double lumen tube), the patient is placed in

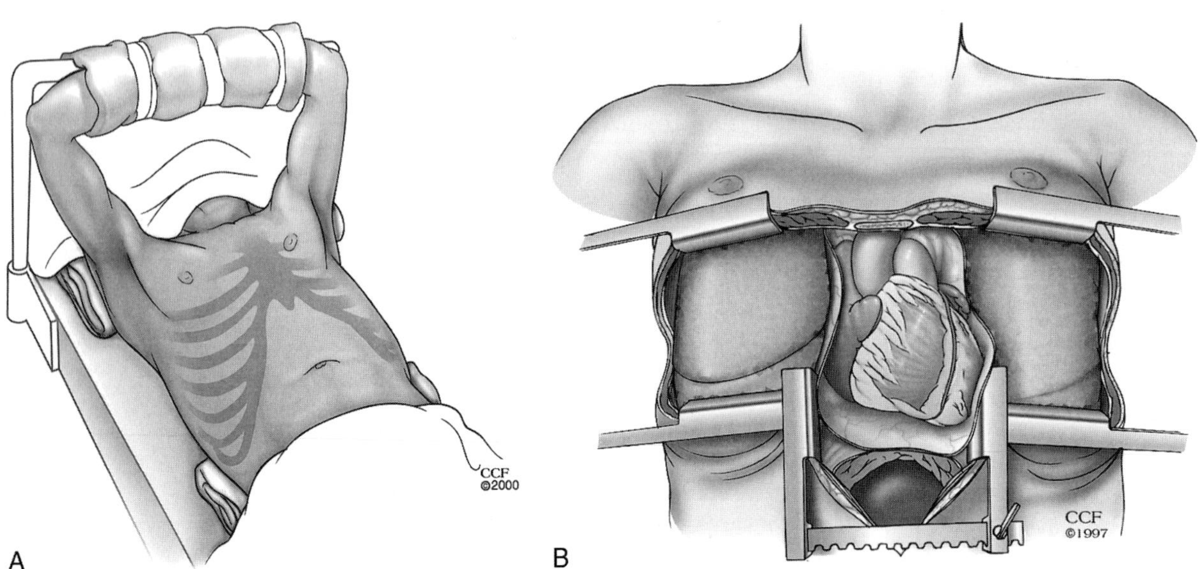

FIGURE 8–15 ■ *A*, Patient position for thoracosternotomy (clamshell) incision. *B*, Excellent exposure is obtained of anterior and middle mediastinal structures. (© Cleveland Clinic Foundation, 2001.)

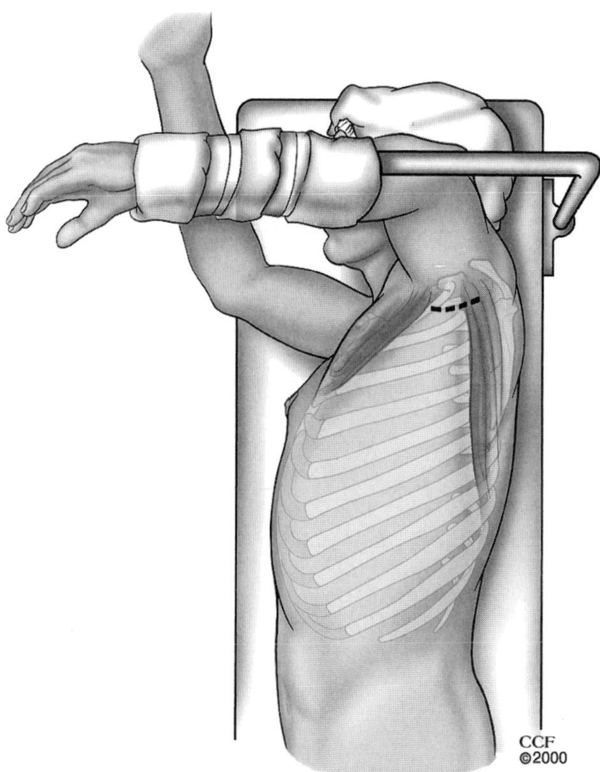

FIGURE 8–16 ■ Patient position and location of the axillary thoracotomy incision. This approach serves as a useful adjunct to video-associated thoracic surgery procedures. (© Cleveland Clinic Foundation, 2001.)

the lateral position on the operating table with the ipsilateral arm flexed and abducted to 90 degrees (Fig. 8–16). A contralateral subaxillary roll is also placed. The entire hemithorax should be included in the sterile field. If the indication is first rib resection, the ipsilateral arm should be included in the sterile preparation. A curvilinear incision is made at the base of the hairline from pectoralis major to latissimus dorsi. After subcutaneous fascia is divided, the axillary fat pad is bluntly dissected superiorly. With the pectoralis major retracted anteriorly and the latissimus dorsi posteriorly, the second intercostal interspace is identified by locating the intercostal brachial nerve. The third interspace is entered anteriorly to the long thoracic nerve by dividing intercostal muscle or resecting the third rib. The long thoracic nerve should be gently mobilized to allow the ribs to be distracted and prevent nerve injury (Massimiano et al, 1988). Intercostal muscles can be divided under both the pectoralis major and the latissimus dorsi muscles to extend the intercostal incision. Superior slips of the serratus anterior muscle may be encountered if the interspace is opened beneath the pectoralis major muscle. These slips can be divided with cautery. Exposure of the first rib through this approach is presented in detail in Chapter 58.

Closure entails rib reapproximation with heavy absorbable suture and repositioning of the axillary fat pad. The superficial fascia should be closed over a suction drain in obese individuals. The skin is closed in the standard fashion.

LATERAL (MUSCLE-SPARING) THORACOTOMY

Muscle-sparing entry of the chest was initially greeted with enthusiasm. There were improvements in postoperative forced expiratory volume in 1 second (FEV_1) and forced vital capacity (FVC) (Lemmer et al, 1990), better shoulder function (Landreneau et al, 1996), and decreased pain (Hazelrigg et al, 1991) compared with the standard muscle-dividing, posterolateral thoracotomy. In addition, involuntary muscular spasm was reported as a late complication of latissimus dorsi division during posterolateral thoracotomy (Kuwabara et al, 1995). These reports have led some to recommend muscle-sparing lateral thoracotomy be used for routine anatomic pulmonary resection (Ginsberg, 1993; Kittle, 1988; Mitchell, 1990). Unfortunately, no controlled studies have documented faster recovery, or better long-term function, when comparing muscle-sparing and muscle-dividing techniques. In fact, Landreneau and colleagues (1996) concluded that the only advantage of muscle-sparing thoracotomy is the preservation of chest wall musculature in the event that rotational muscle flaps would be needed (e.g., bronchopleural fistula closure).

Several variations of the lateral thoracotomy exist. Cosmetically, they differ only in the location of the skin incision (Fig. 8–17). Technically, all involve posterior mobilization of the latissimus dorsi and preservation of the muscle. Serratus anterior is split in the direction of its fibers for more cephalad and anterior chest entry or mobilized anteriorly for lower and more posterior approaches. Functionally, there are slight differences in mediastinal exposure afforded by the various lateral approaches. Some argue that the more anterior approaches should be avoided if extensive chest wall, posterior hilar, or posterior mediastinal involvement exists (Heitmiller and Mathisen, 1989).

The "French" incision (Heitmiller and Mathisen, 1989) is a cosmetic, muscle-sparing anterolateral thoracotomy. The patient is positioned laterally on the operating table and rotated posteriorly 30 to 45 degrees. A deflatable bean bag or cloth rolls are used to fix the patient's position. The axilla is opened as the arm is flexed and abducted 90 degrees. The sterile drape should extend posteriorly to the spine to allow prompt extension of the thoracotomy if needed. The incision is made from the submammary crease (below the nipple) toward a point 1 to 2 cm below the scapular tip. Alternatively, the incision can be carried up toward the axilla in a "lazy-S" manner (Claeys et al, 1995); however, this incision is difficult to extend. The latissimus dorsi is carefully dissected off the serratus anterior and mobilized posteriorly. The long thoracic neurovascular bundle is exposed on the serratus muscle as the latissimus dorsi is dissected. The serratus anterior is divided along its fibers over the chosen interspace (4th or 5th) well anterior to the nerve. The interspace is entered in the standard fashion, and intercostal muscles beyond the operative field are divided to allow maximal spreading of ribs. The interspace can be opened posteriorly down to the costotransverse process articulation, which helps to prevent inadvertent rib fracture when the ribs are separated. A second retractor, placed perpendicular to the rib spreader, is used to distract the latissimus dorsi posteriorly. For closure, ribs are coapted with interrupted heavy (#2) absorbable sutures placed 2 to 3 cm apart. The serratus muscle is repaired with absorbable monofilament or braided suture. The latissimus is restored in its anatomical position with running sutures; the subcutaneous tissue and skin are closed with absorbable running sutures.

If posterior mediastinal exposure is desired, the French incision may be inadequate. A more posterior incision, however, centers the latissimus dorsi in the operative field (see Fig. 8–17). Consequently, more lateral muscle-sparing approaches require that the latissimus be mobilized more completely. As expected, postoperative seroma complicates these approaches.

For the lateral thoracotomy, the patient is placed in a lateral position and the ipsilateral arm positioned in front of the patient (see Fig. 8–17). The patient may be slightly elevated off the operating table, which widens the ipsilateral interspaces. The dependent leg is slightly flexed at the hip and knee; a pillow is placed between legs. A skin incision is extended from the anterior axillary (or midaxillary) line to below the scapular tip. Soft tissue flaps are raised with cautery, and the latissimus muscle is fully mobilized. Like the "French" incision, serratus anterior is usually divided in the direction of its fibers, although the muscle is elevated anteriorly without division to provide exposure through a lower interspace such as the 6th. A closed-suction drain should be tunneled subcutaneously at the conclusion of the procedure.

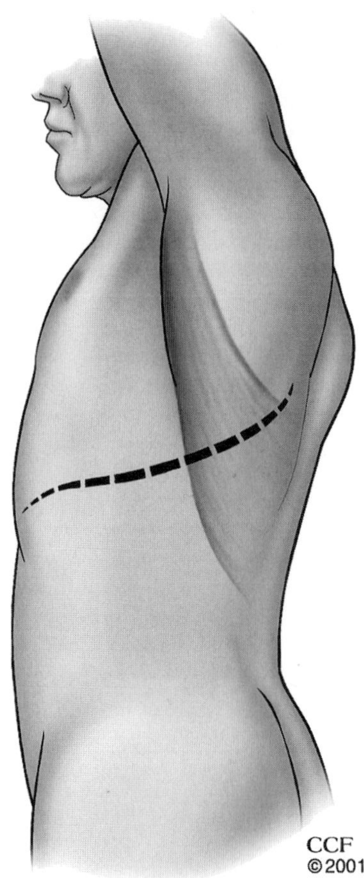

FIGURE 8–18 ■ Standard location of the posterolateral thoracotomy. The incision can be extended posteriorly (and superiorly) to the base of the neck and anteriorly (and inferiorly) to the costal margin. (© Cleveland Clinic Foundation, 2001.)

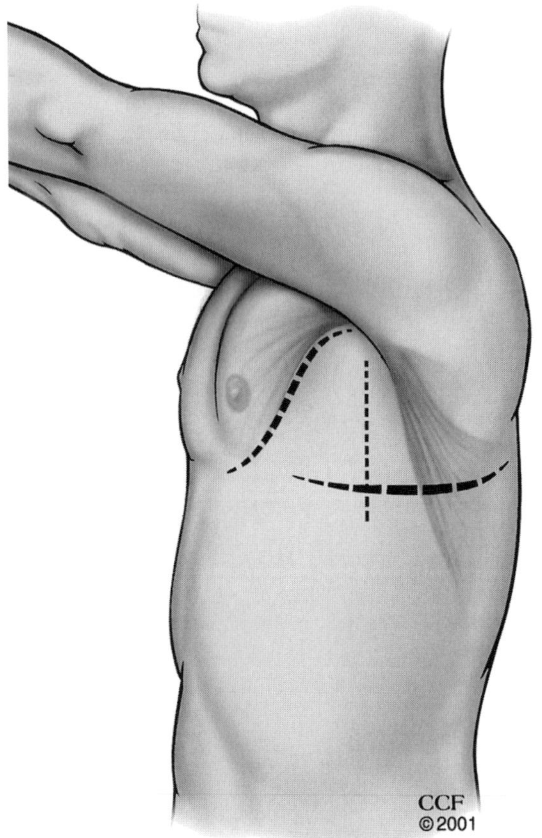

FIGURE 8–17 ■ Common locations of incisions used for lateral thoracotomy. Most of each incision is anterior to the latissimus dorsi allowing for easy posterior mobilization of the muscle. As incisions are placed more posteriorly, muscle-sparing approaches require greater mobilization of the latissimus muscle. (© Cleveland Clnic Foundation, 2001.)

POSTERIOR INCISIONS

Although some consider the *classic* posterolateral thoracotomy (Sweet, 1950) a relic of the past, the utility of this incision cannot be underscored. One might argue that this incision has experienced a renaissance as larger, more complicated pulmonary and esophageal resections have become more common. Current indications include extrapleural pneumonectomy, superior sulcus tumors, tracheal surgery, and resection of advanced malignancy following induction therapy. Often, the serratus anterior can be spared during the thoracotomy, limiting postoperative disability. We routinely employ this approach for single lung transplantation. The posterolateral thoracotomy can also be performed in a muscle-sparing manner (Ashour, 1990). Because the latissimus dorsi is mobilized anteriorly, unlike lateral approaches, the muscle is not stretched against the maximum convexity of the chest. This may result in less muscle stress and quicker recovery (Ashour, 1990).

POSTEROLATERAL THORACOTOMY

The patient is placed in the same position as that described for lateral thoracotomy. The incision is started at the anterior axillary line and continued posteriorly for 2 to 3 cm below the scapular tip. The incision then follows the contour of the posterior border of the scapula superiorly along a line midway between the medial aspect of the scapula and the spine (Fig. 8–18). The dissection is carried down to the latissimus muscle, which is divided with cautery. Vascular pedicles within the muscle are easily identified by associated fatty tissue. The serratus muscle is similarly divided. Division of the serratus slips close to rib insertions ensures that the majority of the muscle will remain innervated. If additional scapular mobility is necessary (e.g., superior sulcus tumor), trapezius and rhomboid muscles can be divided. Ribs are then counted posteriorly, and the appropriate interspace is entered (4th or 5th).

For extended resections, it is occasionally necessary to resect or "shingle" a rib to enhance exposure. For these rare cases, the periosteum is scored longitudinally along the posterior aspect of the rib. A periosteal elevator is used to reflect the periosteum off the rib. Once the intercostal neurovascular bundle is separated from a portion of the underside of the rib, a Doyen raspatory can be used to separate the remaining periosteum over the desired length. The rib is then resected with shears, and the periosteum and pleura are opened to permit access into the pleural cavity.

When a rib is resected, the closure becomes more complicated. If resected properly, the periosteum with attached intercostal muscle can be sewn closed. Otherwise, simply reapproximating the ribs above and below the resection leaves a defect in the chest wall through which the lung may herniate. This defect can be particularly troubling if a pneumonectomy has been performed, as a subcutaneous seroma may result from extravasated pleural fluid. To prevent this complication, slips of muscle can be used to close the defect.

MUSCLE-SPARING POSTEROLATERAL THORACOTOMY

To spare the latissimus dorsi from a posterolateral approach requires anterior mobilization of the muscle. This is achieved by disconnecting the latissimus muscle posteriorly from the thoracolumbar fascia (Fig. 8–19*A*). This incision is used for the majority of our pulmonary resec-

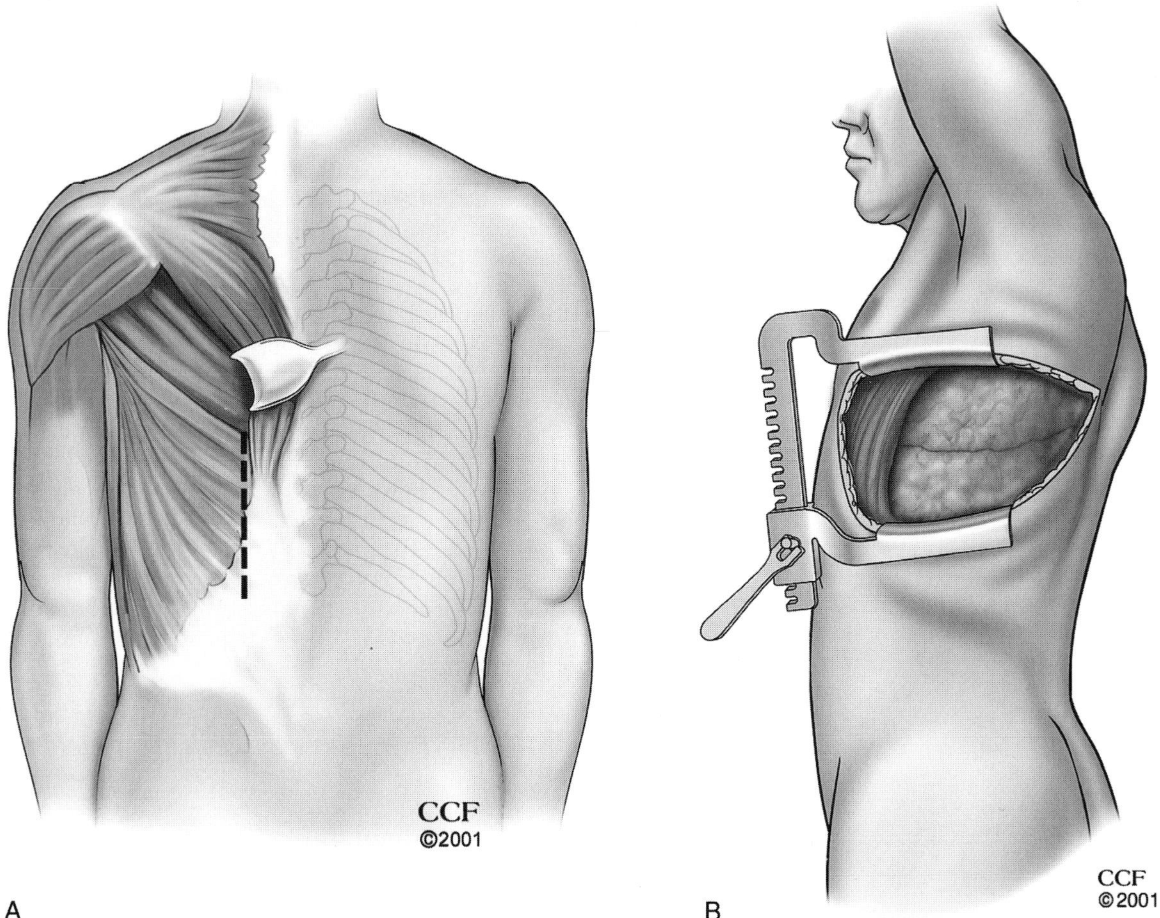

FIGURE 8–19 ■ *A*, For the muscle-sparing posterolateral thoracotomy, the latissimus dorsi is disconnected from the thoracolumbar fascia with cautery *(dashed line)*. *B*, After complete mobilization, both latissimus and serratus muscles can be moved anteriorly and spared. (Adapted from Ashour M: Modified muscle sparing posterolateral thoracotomy. Thorax 45:935, 1990; © Cleveland Clinic Foundation, 2001.)

tions. It offers excellent posterior exposure for complicated hilar dissections and lymphadenectomy. Limited postoperative disability has been encountered with this approach.

After standard posterolateral incision, subcutaneous flaps are raised over the latissimus dorsi superiorly and inferiorly. The plane between the latissimus and trapezius muscles should be developed with cautery. The posterior aspect of the latissimus muscle is then freed from the thoracolumbar fascia with cautery, for 6 to 7 cm. After this maneuver, the latissimus dorsi can easily be reflected anteriorly, exposing the serratus muscle (see Fig. 8–19*B*). After the serratus is moved anteriorly under the latissimus, the interspace is approached and opened.

POSTERIOR THORACOTOMY

Prior to the development of lung isolation, pneumonectomy for suppurative disease was often performed from a posterior approach. This permitted early division of the bronchus and lung collapse. With the bronchus controlled, purulent secretions could not escape from the operated lung and contaminate the contralateral side. Few indications remain for this approach.

The patient is placed in a prone position on a specially designed table that allows anterior access to the chest if necessary (Fig. 8–20). An incision is extended from the anterior axillary line to the base of the neck, midway between the medial edge of the scapula and the spine. Rhomboid, trapezius, latissimus, and serratus muscles are divided. The selected interspace may then be entered.

THORACOABDOMINAL INCISION

The thoracoabdominal incision permits simultaneous dissection in pleural and abdominal cavities. The left-sided approach is particularly attractive to thoracic surgeons. This exposure facilitates esophageal, gastric, splenic, and retroperitoneal surgeries. The closure can be formidable and time consuming. Postoperative recovery has been greatly improved by epidural analgesia.

Left lung isolation is necessary. The patient is placed in a lateral position with the hips rotated posteriorly by an additional 45 degrees (Fig. 8–21). The sterile field should include the left arm and neck if a cervical esophagogastric anastomosis is anticipated. In cases of esophageal malignancy, the abdominal portion of the incision is made first to determine operability. An oblique incision from the midline to the left costal margin is utilized. If the exploration is unremarkable, the incision is continued obliquely across the costal margin and extended upward as a posterolateral thoracotomy incision. Latissimus and serratus muscles are divided, and the chest is entered in either the 6th or 7th interspace. The costal margin is cut sharply. We do not routinely resect a short segment of rib cartilage as advocated by Heitmiller (1988). The exposure is completed by division of the diaphragm. Although the diaphragm can be incised circumferentially, a radial incision can be made if anterior branches of the phrenic nerve are carefully avoided.

The closure must not be looked upon casually as simply the end of a long procedure, but as an entire operation on its own. The diaphragm should be reconstructed with nonabsorbable suture, and the paracostal sutures should be spaced by 2 to 3 cm. The costal margin is repaired with a heavy, absorbable, figure-of-eight suture. This suture should be passed through the diaphragm to buttress the costal margin and prevent herniation. Each muscle layer should be carefully closed with running absorbable suture. Superficial tissues are closed in the standard fashion.

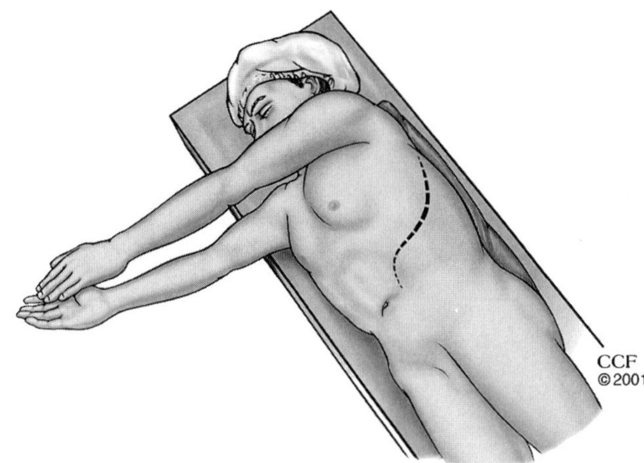

FIGURE 8–21 ■ Incision for thoracoabdominal approach. The patient's hips are rotated back 45 degrees to facilitate the abdominal dissection. (© Cleveland Clinic Foundation, 2001.)

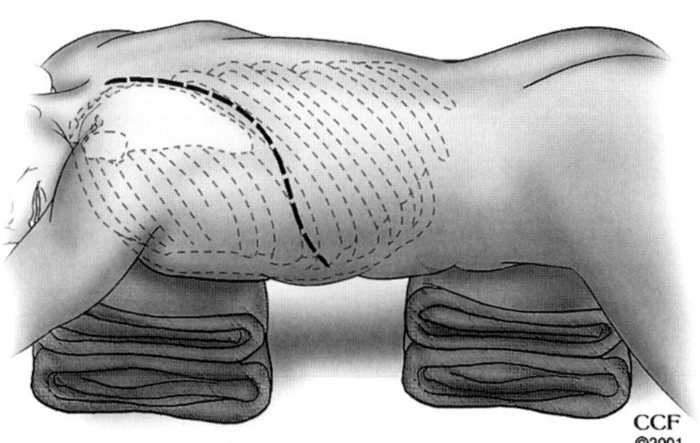

FIGURE 8–20 ■ Location of the posterior thoracotomy incision. With the patient placed prone on the operating table, the posterior thoracotomy incision begins at the base of the neck and is carried inferiorly and anteriorly. The scapula is disconnected from trapezius, rhomboid, and teres muscle groups. (© Cleveland Clinic Foundation, 2001.)

SUMMARY

Since the times of Hippocrates, surgeons have been incising the chest with curative intent. As knowledge has been accumulated and techniques refined, the thoracic surgeon is now armed with a vast array of incisions from which to choose. The difficulty lies in choosing the right one.

■ REFERENCES

Asaph JW, Keppel JF: Midline sternotomy for the treatment of primary pulmonary neoplasms. Ann J Surg 147:589, 1984.

Ashour M: Modified muscle sparing posterolateral thoracotomy. Thorax 45:935, 1990.

Atkins HJB: Sympathectomy by the axillary approach. Lancet 1:538, 1954.

Baeza OR, Foster ED: Vertical axillary thoracotomy: A functional and cosmetically appealing incision. Ann Thorac Surg 22:287, 1976.

Baisden CE, Greenwald LV, Symbas PN: Occult rib fractures and brachial plexus injury following median sternotomy for open-heart operations. Ann Thorac Surg 38:192, 1984.

Baldwin JC, Mark JBD: Treatment of bronchopleural fistula after pneumonectomy. J Thorac Cardiovasc Surg 90:813, 1985.

Baskett RJ, MacDougall CE, Ross DB: Is mediastinitis a preventable complication? A 10-year review. Ann Thorac Surg 67:462, 1999.

Becker RM, Munro DD: Transaxillary minithoracotomy: The optimal approach for certain pulmonary and mediastinal lesions. Ann Thorac Surg 22:254, 1976.

Byrne JG, Aklog L, Adams DH et al: Reoperative CABG using left thoracotomy: a tailored strategy. Ann Thorac Surg 71:196, 2001.

Claeys D, Flamme A, Vanoverbeke H, Muysoms F: Muscle-saving lateral axillary thoracotomy. Acta Chir Belg 95:27, 1995.

Cooper JD, Al-Jilaihawa AN, Pearson, FG et al: An improved technique to facilitate transcervical thymectomy for myasthenia gravis. Ann Thorac Surg 45:242, 1988.

Cooper JD, Nelems JM, Pearson FG: Extended indications for median sternotomy in patients requiring pulmonary resection. Ann Thorac Surg 26:413, 1978.

Cooper JD, Trulock EP, Triantafillou AN et al: Bilateral pneumonectomy (volume reduction) for chronic obstructive pulmonary disease. J Thorac Cardiovasc Surg 109:106, 1995.

Daly BD, Faling LJ, Diehl JT et al: Computed tomography-guided minithoracotomy for the resection of small peripheral pulmonary nodules. Ann Thorac Surg 51:465, 1991.

Dart CH, Braitman HE, Larab S: Supraclavicular thoracotomy for diagnosis of apical lung and superior mediastinal lesions. Ann Thorac Surg 28:90, 1979.

Dartevelle FG, Chapelier AR, Macchiarini P et al: Anterior transcervical-thoracic approach for radical resection of lung tumors invading the thoracic inlet. J Thorac Cardiovasc Surg 105:1025, 1993.

de la Riviere AB, Brom GHM, Brom AG: Horizontal submammary skin incision for median sternotomy. Ann Thorac Surg 32:101, 1981.

Demmy TL, Park SB, Liebler GA et al: Recent experience with major sternal wound complications. Ann Thorac Surg 49:458, 1990.

Deutinger M, Deutinger J: Breast feeding after aesthetic mammary operations and cardiac operations through horizontal submammary skin incision. Surg Gynecol Obstet 176:267, 1993.

Deutinger M, Domanig E: Breast development and areola sensitivity after submammary skin incision for median sternotomy. Ann Thorac Surg 53:1023, 1992.

DiMarco RF Jr, Lee MW, Bekoe S et al: Interlocking figure-of-eight closure of the sternum. Ann Thorac Surg 47:927, 1989.

Ginsberg, RJ: Alternative (muscle-sparing) incisions in thoracic surgery. Ann Thorac Surg 56:752, 1993.

Grillo HC: Surgical approaches to the trachea. Surg Gynecol Obstet 129:347, 1969.

Grillo HC: Surgical treatment of postintubation tracheal injuries. J Thorac Cardiovasc Surg 78:860, 1979.

Hankins JR, Satterfield JR, Aisner J, et al: Pericardial window for malignant pericardial effusion. Ann Thorac Surg 30:465, 1980.

Hazelrigg Sr, Landreneau RJ, Boley TM et al: The effect of muscle-sparing versus standard posterolateral thoracotomy on pulmonary function, muscle strength, and postoperative pain. J Thorac Cardiovasc Surg 101:394, 1991.

Heitmiller RF: The left thoracoabdominal incision. Ann Thorac Surg 46:250, 1988.

Heitmiller RF, Mathisen DJ: French incision. In Grillo HC, Austen WG, Wilkins EW Jr et al (eds): Current Therapy in Cardiothoracic Surgery. Philadelphia, BC Decker, 1989.

Kaiser LR, Pasque MK, Trulock EP et al: Bilateral sequential lung transplantation: The procedure of choice for double-lung replacement. Ann Thorac Surg 52:438, 1991.

Kalush SL, Bonchek LI: Peristernal closure of median sternotomy using stainless steel bands. Ann Thorac Surg 21:172, 1976.

Kerr PC, Ricci M, Abraham R et al: Redo left anterior descending artery grafting via left anterior small thoracotomy: An alternative approach. Ann Thorac Surg 71:384, 2001.

Kittle CF: Which way in? The thoracotomy incision. Ann Thorac Surg 45:234, 1988.

Kjaergard HK, Trumbull HR: Bleeding from the sternal marrow can be stopped using vivostat patient-derived fibrin sealant. Ann Thorac Surg 69:1173, 2000.

Kuwabara S, Fukutake T, Kashata N et al: Associated movement as a sequel to thoracotomy: Aberrant regeneration to the latissimus dorsi muscle. Mov Disord 10:788, 1995.

Laks H, Hammond GL: A cosmetically acceptable incision for the median sternotomy. J Cardiovasc Surg 79:146, 1980.

Landreneau RJ, Pigula F, Luketich JD et al: Acute and chronic morbidity differences between muscle-sparing and standard lateral thoracotomies. J Thorac and Cardiovasc Surg 112:1346, 1996.

Larrieu AJ, Ghosh SC, Ablaza SG et al: Favorable results with the subxiphoid pericardial window technique [Letter]. J Thorac Cardiovasc Surg 91:639, 1986.

Lemmer JH Jr, Gomez MN, Symreng T et al: Limited lateral thoracotomy: Improved postoperative pulmonary function. Arch Surg 125:873, 1990.

Lubenow TR, Faber LP, McCarthy RJ et al: Post-thoracotomy pain management using continuous epidural analgesia in 1,324 patients. Ann Thorac Surg 58:924, 1994.

Marshall WG Jr, Meng RL, Ehrenhaft JL: Coronary artery bypass grafting in patients with a tracheostomy: Use of a bilateral thoracotomy incision. Ann Thorac Surg 46:465, 1988.

Martinez-Sanz R, Fleitas MG, de la Llana R, et al: Submammary median sternotomy. J Cardiovasc Surg 31:578, 1990.

Massimiano P, Ponn, RB, Toole AL: Transaxillary thoracotomy revisited. Ann Thorac Surg 45:559, 1988.

McNeil TM, Chamberlain JM: Diagnostic anterior mediastinotomy. Ann Thorac Surg 2:532, 1966.

Meyer W: Some observations regarding thoracic surgery on human beings. Ann Surg, 52:34,1910.

Meyers BF, Lynch JP, Trulock EP et al: Single versus bilateral lung transplantation for idiopathic pulmonary fibrosis: A ten-year institutional experience. J Thorac Cardiovasc Surg 120:99, 2000.

Mitchell RL: The lateral limited thoracotomy incision: Standard for pulmonary operations. J Thorac Cardiovasc Surg: 99:590, 1990.

Milton H: Mediastinal surgery. Lancet 1:872, 1897.

Morin JE, Long R, Elleker MG, et al: Upper extremity neuropathies following median sternotomy. Ann Thor Surg 34:181, 1982.

Nandi P, Mok CK, Ong GB: Y incision for medial sternotomy. Aust N Z J Surg 49:489, 1979.

Nanson EM. The anterior approach to upper dorsal sympathectomy. Surg Gynecol Obstet 104:118, 1957.

Naunheim KS, Kesler KA, D'Orazio SA, et al. Thoracotomy in octogenarians. Ann Thorac Surg 51:547, 1991.

Orringer MB: Partial median sternotomy: Anterior approach to the upper thoracic esophagus. J Thorac Cardiovasc Surg 87:124, 1984.

Piehler JM, Pluth JR, Schaff HV et al: Surgical management of effusive pericardial disease. J Thorac Cardiovasc Surg 90:506, 1985.

Pochettino A, Kotloff RM, Rosengard BR et al: Bilateral versus single lung transplantation for chronic obstructive pulmonary disease: Intermediate-term results. Ann Thorac Surg 70:1813, 2000.

Ponn RB, Ferneini A, D'Angostino RS et al: Comparison of late pulmonary function after posterolateral and muscle-sparing thoracotomy. Ann Thorac Surg 53:675, 1992.

Prager RL, Wilson CH, Bender HW Jr: The subxiphoid approach to pericardial disease. Ann Thorac Surg 34:6, 1982.

Reardon MJ, Tillou A, Mody DR, Reardon PR: Heterotopic calcification in abdominal wounds. Am J Surg 173:145, 1997.

Regal A, Reese P, Antkowiak J et al: Median sternotomy for metastatic lung lesions in 131 patients. Cancer 55:1334, 1985.

Robicsek F, Daugherty HK, Cook JW: The prevention and treatment of sternum separation following open-heart surgery. J Thorac Cardiovasc Surg 73:267, 1977.

Roos DB: Experience with first rib resection for thoracic outlet syndrome. Ann Surg 173:429, 1971.

Santos GH, Frater RWM: The subxiphoid approach in the treatment of pericardial effusion. Ann Thor Surg 23:467, 1977.

Shimizu N, Ando A, Matsutoni T et al: Transsternal thoracotomy for bilateral pulmonary metastasis. J Surg Oncol 50:105, 1992.

Sirivella S, Zikria EA, Ford WB et al: Improved technique for closure of median sternotomy incisions: Mersilene tapes versus standard wire closure. J Thorac Cardiovasc Surg 94:591, 1987.

Stahle E, Tammelin A, Bergstrom R et al: Sternal wound complications: Incidence, microbiology and risk factors. Euro J Cardiothorac Surg 11:1146, 1997.

Stewart S: Placement of the sutureless epicardial pacemaker lead by the subxiphoid approach. Ann Thorac Surg 18:308, 1974.

Sweet H: Thoracic Incisions. In Sweet H (ed): Thoracic Surgery. Philadelphia, Saunders, pp. 59, 1950.

Takita H, Merrin C, Didolkar MS: The surgical management of multiple lung metastases. Ann Thorac Surg 24:359, 1977.

Thirby RC, Kraemer SJ, Hill LD: Transdiaphragmatic approach to the posterior mediastinum and thoracic esophagus. Arch Surg 128:897, 1993.

Urschel H, Razzuk M: Median sternotomy as the standard approach for pulmonary resection. Ann Thorac Surg 41:130, 1986.

Vander Salm TJ, Cereda JM, Cutler BS: Brachial plexus injury following median sternotomy. J Thorac Cardiovasc Surg 80:447, 1980.

Weber L, Peters RW: Delayed chest wall complications of median sternotomy. South Med J 79:723, 1986.

Wells SA, Cooper JD: Closed mediastinal exploration in patients with persistent hyperparathyroidism. Ann Surg 214:555, 1991.

Zacharias A, Habib RH: Factors predisposing to median sternotomy complications. Chest 110:1173, 1996.

Zieren HU, Muller JM, Zieren J, Pichlmaier H: Closure of partial median sternotomy with absorbable sutures: A practical and safe option. Ann Surg 59:596, 1993.

CHAPTER **9**

Perioperative Management

Thomas R. J. Todd

A. C. Ralph-Edwards

Preoperative preparation and postoperative care have always been important components of thoracic surgical care. For many reasons, their relative importance has grown in recent years. Thoracic procedures have become more complex and are performed on an increasingly elderly population. Neoadjuvant treatment regimens for bronchogenic carcinoma ensure that pulmonary resections will be performed more frequently and that the procedures will be not only complex but also more challenging. The aging of the population has resulted in an increased number of older patients undergoing pulmonary and esophageal resection for malignant disease. In addition, the frequency of immunosuppressive disorders and the reappearance of mycobacterial infections will guarantee the presence of challenging cases of benign disease. These trends and the resulting increase in challenging surgery will demand careful preoperative assessment and rapid recognition and treatment of complications.

HISTORICAL NOTE

When thoracotomy first became feasible, the procedure was conducted without the benefit of readily available blood transfusions and critical care facilities. In addition, knowledge of fluid and electrolyte abnormalities and postoperative fluid shifts was poor. It would take the lessons learned from the Coconut Grove fire in Boston in 1947 and the experience gained from the Korean and Vietnamese conflicts before a thorough understanding of fluid requirements and the effect of resuscitation on pulmonary function was reached. More importantly, the advent of positive pressure ventilation was hastened by a polio epidemic, which largely led to the evolution of modern critical care units.

The technologic developments and the enhanced knowledge of cardiopulmonary physiologic interactions that were the result of this experience have greatly altered our ability to perform thoracic procedures on an increasingly complex patient population. As a result, perioperative management has become a much more involved and important aspect of surgical care.

■ *HISTORICAL READINGS*

Baily CC, Betts RH: Cardiac arrhythmias following pneumonectomy. N Engl J Med 229:356, 1943.

Bettman RB, Tannenbaum WJ: Herniation of the heart through a pericardial incision. Ann Surg 128:1012, 1948.

Cerney CI: The prophylaxis of cardiac arrhythmias complicating pulmonary surgery. J Thorac Surg 34:105, 1957.

Claggett OT, Geraci JE: A procedure for the management of postpneumonectomy empyema. J Thorac Cardiovasc Surg 45:141, 1963.

Eggers C: The treatment of bronchial fistulae. Ann Surg 72:345, 1920.

Goldman L, Caldera DL, Nussbaum SR: Multifactorial index of cardiac risk in noncardiac surgical procedures. N Engl J Med 297:845, 1977.

Shenstone NS: The use of intercostal muscle in the closure of bronchial fistulae. Ann Surg 104:560, 1936.

GENERAL INCIDENCE

The overall perioperative mortality rate is 2.1% to 3.7% for pulmonary resection in most large series (Deslauriers et al, 1989; Ginsberg et al, 1983; Motta and Ratta 1989; Nagasaki et al, 1982; Wahi et al, 1989). The 30-day postoperative mortality rate is 6% to 7.8% for pneumonectomy (right greater than left) and 2% to 2.9% for lobectomy. Harpole and associates (1999) reported mortality rates of 4% for lobectomy and 11.5% for pneumonectomy in a prospective large series of Veterans Affairs patients in the United States. The overall major and minor complication rate of pulmonary resection is high (45.5% to 48%). Complications are noted in 36% to 75% of cases after pneumonectomy and in 41.4% to 50% of cases following lobectomy (Motta and Ratta et al, 1989; Olsen et al, 1991; Wahi et al, 1989). Nonetheless, data would suggest 30-day morbidity rates of 24% for lobectomy and 26% for pneumonectomy (Harpole et al, 1999). DesLauriers and colleagues (1989) report the incidence of major complications or death for lobectomy and pneumonectomy to be 10%. Extended lobectomy or pneumonectomy (on chest wall, tracheal, or pericardial block resection) carries significantly higher risks of death or major complication, at 20% and 17%, respectively. The frequency of bronchial plastic procedures has increased nearly four-fold; 30-day postoperative mortality is 5.5% and 20% for sleeve lobectomy and sleeve pneumonectomy, respectively (Tedder et al, 1992). Of note is the revival of interest in the performance of pulmonary vascular sleeve procedures resections (Rendina et al, 1999). Such are now undertaken with a complication rate that is comparable with standard lobectomy. As a result, patients who are deemed unsuitable for resection on the presumption that a pneumonectomy would seriously impair pulmonary function might be considered for surgical resection. Increased patient age has also been demonstrated to adversely affect outcome: patients under 60 years of age may be expected to have a perioperative mortality rate of 1.3%, those 60 to 69 years old, 4.1%, and those over 70 years old, 7% (Ginsberg et al, 1983). The major causes of death after pulmonary resection include pneumonia and respiratory failure, bronchopleural fistula and empyema, myocardial infarction, and pulmonary embolism (Ginsberg et al, 1983). Ginsberg reported these results from the combined data base of the Lung Cancer Study Group based on their experience since 1977. Data from single institutions suggest that this has not changed significantly since the report by Ginsberg and colleagues (De Perrot et al, 1999; Oliaro et al, 1999; Sioris et al, 1999). Particularly notable is the effect of age on the mortality following pneumonectomy with rates as high as 13.7% reported in patients over 70 years of age (De Perrot et al, 1999).

In this chapter, the principles of perioperative care and the recognition and treatment of selected complications are discussed. Preoperative preparation is discussed in the preceding chapters; only general comments follow here as they relate to the specific complications discussed.

PREOPERATIVE PREPARATION

More than two thirds of the complications occurring in the postoperative period in general thoracic surgical patients are cardiopulmonary in nature. Postoperative respiratory failure, myocardial infarction, and pulmonary embolism may be reduced dramatically by careful patient selection, modification of operative intervention, and use of prophylactic measures to prevent deep venous thrombosis. Strategies for preoperative cardiopulmonary assessment are outlined in Chapters 3 and 4. However, we would stress that careful and systematic evaluation of pulmonary function will lead to identification of a group of patients with poor pulmonary reserve who may benefit from a period of rehabilitation (Filaire et al, 1999). Pulmonary rehabilitation should consist of graded and measurable supervised exercise over 3 to 4 weeks, accompanied by bronchodilator therapy and antibiotics when pathogenic organisms are identified in sputum. Its value in the improvement of exercise tolerance and quality of life in patients with chronic obstructive lung disease has been established (Goldstein et al, 1994). In addition, it appears to be a valuable preoperative adjunct in patients who are undergoing lung volume reduction surgery (Cooper et al, 1995).

Perioperative antibiotic prophylaxis has been demonstrated to reduce the incidence of wound infection from up to 18% to 1% to 5% (Ilves et al, 1981; Krasnik et al, 1991; Wertzel et al, 1992). A single dose of antibiotic with adequate gram-positive and gram-negative coverage is suggested preoperatively and should be continued for no longer than 24 hours postoperatively. Cefuroxime, cefazolin, and penicillin G are all equally effective in reducing wound infections; however, the incidence of empyema and pneumonia is probably unaffected (Ilves et al, 1981; Krasnik et al, 1991; Wertzel et al, 1992). A patient's nutritional status has also been found to correlate with postoperative morbidity. Deslauriers and colleagues (1989) found an 11% increase in major morbidity and death among patients with a greater than 10% weight loss. When assessing patients for pulmonary resection, nutritional status should be considered and measures taken to supplement caloric intake if profound malnutrition is present. Perioperative use of total parenteral nutrition has been shown to benefit only severely malnourished surgical patients in the absence of specific indications for intravenous alimentation (Veterans Affairs Total Parenteral Nutrition Cooperative Study Group, 1991). Nonetheless, the early use of enteral feeding after esophagectomy has been shown to be technically feasible and to be associated with few complications (Braga et al, 2001). In addition, randomized trials suggest that enteral feeding is comparable with TPN in the support of general nutrition—at a fraction of the cost (Braga et al, 2001).

PROPHYLACTIC MEASURES IN THE POSTOPERATIVE PERIOD

Monitoring

Significant improvements have been made in cardiorespiratory monitoring. Both cardiac and pulmonary complications after thoracotomy occur most frequently in the first 2 to 4 days, and this should correspond to the period of most intensive patient monitoring. The goals of monitoring include the provision of information regarding changes in a patient's cardiopulmonary status and the evaluation and appreciation of the results of therapeutic interventions. To provide this level of care, post-thoracotomy patients should be managed in a specialized unit. Ideally, frequent measurements of respiratory rate, heart rate, blood pressure, and arterial oxygen saturation are necessary. Oxygen saturation is readily measured noninvasively. Arterial blood gases should be drawn initially to provide information on postoperative ventilatory status via assessment of carbon dioxide partial pressure ($Paco_2$). Transient elevations of $Paco_2$ may occur secondary to excessive analgesia, failure to adequately reverse anesthesia, and the unmasking of previously unrecognized carbon dioxide retention, which may be seen in the postoperative period as a result of excessive oxygen administration. With carbon dioxide retention, oxygen supplementation should be guided by the saturation recordings from the pulse oximeter to achieve a saturation of no more than 90%. Intra-arterial electrodes that provide continuous oxygen partial pressure (Po_2) and Pco_2 measurements may in part resolve problems of sampling errors and delays in laboratory reporting. Preoperative knowledge of arterial oxygen and carbon dioxide content, combined with physical examination, is critical to direct oxygen therapy and analgesia.

Continuous cardiac rhythm monitoring should also be available, as cardiac arrhythmias are common after thoracotomy. Undiagnosed supraventricular tachycardia may lead to myocardial ischemia or congestive heart failure or may degenerate to a more malignant rhythm. If diagnosed early, the majority of arrhythmias are easily treated. Hypoxia, hypercarbia, anemia, electrolyte abnormalities, and fluid overload are frequently associated inciting abnormalities.

More invasive monitoring is usually reserved for the ventilated patient in whom a widened alveolar-arterial oxygen gradient [$P(A\text{-}a)\ o_2$], hypotension, or both necessitate the availability of frequent arterial blood gas measurements, as well as assessments of cardiac output and oxygen transport. This requires insertion of a Swan-Ganz catheter to obtain cardiac output via thermal dilution, as well as measurements of left ventricular preload (via pulmonary arterial wedge pressure), pulmonary artery pressure, and mixed venous oxygen tension ($P\bar{v}O_2$).

These data permit the calculation of several other parameters, including oxygen transport and left ventricular stroke work. The former is particularly important in determining the optimal level of positive end-expiratory pressure (PEEP) in patients whose PEEP requirements exceed 10 cm H_2O. The optimal PEEP can also be obtained by repeated evaluations of static lung compliance, which is readily estimated by applying a clamp to the expiratory limb of the ventilator tubing at the end of inspiration. The peak airway pressure will fall to the degree determined by the relative contribution of airway resistance and pulmonary compliance to peak area pressure. In the absence of airflow, the plateau pressure obtained following application of the clamp to the expiratory tubing at end-inspiration must be solely due to pulmonary compliance. Some ventilators have an inspiratory hold and, if so, the application of the clamp is unnecessary.

Ventilatory Support

In some patients, continued postoperative ventilation may be desirable as a prophylactic measure. Large-volume fluid resuscitation, hemodynamic instability, myocardial ischemia, prolonged anesthesia, and potential space problems may be more safely managed with a period of elective postoperative mechanical ventilation. This provides time to stabilize the patient and to appreciate the degree of pulmonary parenchymal damage. Short-term positive pressure ventilation in patients undergoing pulmonary decortication or major bullectomy may achieve more complete lung re-expansion, particularly if there is a reduction in pulmonary compliance. The latter is frequently the case for conditions that require decortication, in which the procedure itself leads to excessive extravascular lung water, which will result in stiffer lungs.

Pain Control

Pain following thoracotomy can be severe and often results in an alteration in the pattern of breathing. The patient may generate low tidal volumes, maintaining adequate minute ventilation by an increase in rate. As a result, functional residual capacity will fall and airway closure with attendant atelectasis results. This is compounded by the suppression of cough, which in the presence of augmented secretions in the postoperative period further aggravates airway closure. The result is an impairment in oxygenation owing to the consequent ventilation/perfusion mismatch.

As a result, it is imperative to control pain effectively and early following thoracotomy. There are several options. Narcotic administration has been a mainstay of therapy for decades. The mode of administration has markedly improved from the days of the intramuscular route. Hourly intravenous administration is satisfactory, and the advent of patient-controlled analgesia (PCA) has provided an even greater level of comfort. Adjuvant pain therapy with nonsteroidal compounds is often recommended, whether given orally or as a rectal suppository. In our experience, the latter provides significant improvement in pain control. Epidural administration of opiates takes advantage of the fact that there are specific opiate receptors on the dorsal columns of the spinal cord. A properly functioning epidural catheter permits excellent analgesia with narcotic doses that have few, if any, systemic effects and do not result in impairment of motor function. One must be alert to the possibility of respiratory depression, although this is less likely to occur if the epidural is placed in the lumbar region. In addition, an epidural catheter will usually require the insertion of a urinary catheter. Whether the epidural route offers any therapeutic advantage over PCA remains to be determined and must await randomized clinical trials. An important new area of research currently undergoing clinical trials is that of pre-emptive analgesia, which may increase patient comfort while possibly reducing analgesic requirements (Obata et al, 1999).

Paravertebral thoracic block with bupivacaine has been reported to be superior to epidural routes of administration (Richardson et al, 1999), while at the same time reducing the incidence of complications such as nausea, vomiting, and, especially, hypotension. The latter complication of epidural analgesia is worrisome especially in the pneumonectomy patient who needs increased intravenous fluids.

Oxygen Therapy

Oxygen should only be administered as needed. The availability of cutaneous saturation monitors allows one to titrate the amount required. Given the shape of the oxygen-hemoglobin dissociation curve (Fig. 9–1), the higher the saturation, the greater is the PaO_2 and, hence, the farther away is the patient from the steep portion of the curve. However, one must be mindful of the fact that oxygen administration can have deleterious effects. In a patient with chronic carbon dioxide retention, a hypoxic

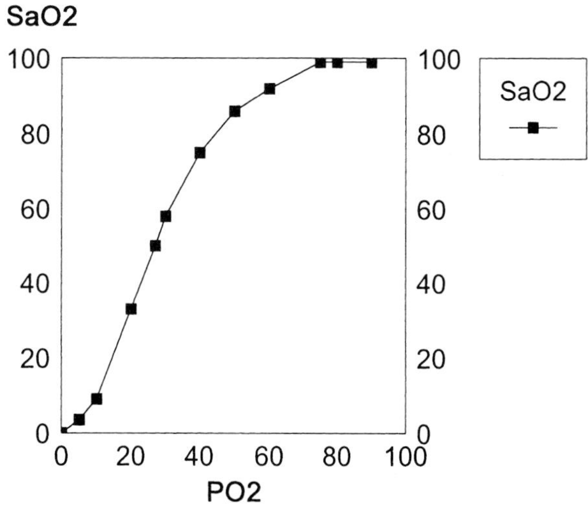

FIGURE 9–1 ■ Oxygen-hemoglobin dissociation curve.

drive to breathing is required, and the elimination of hypoxemia can lead to respiratory depression and further carbon dioxide retention with respiratory acidosis. This emphasizes the need for preoperative blood gas determinations. The presence of an elevated $Paco_2$ in the preoperative period will also be suggested by an abnormally elevated bicarbonate level on serum electrolyte determinations, on which basis the physician should suspect a compensated respiratory acidosis or a primary metabolic alkalosis (often secondary to chronic diuretic therapy). If the $Paco_2$ is elevated preoperatively, desirable oxygen saturations should be 90% or even less. Although the Pao_2 will fall off steeply below this level, the hypoxic drive to breathe will be preserved, and, indeed, these patients tolerate hypoxemia extremely well.

Other complications of excessive oxygen administration include alveolar damage and pulmonary fibrosis in either the ventilated patient (Fox et al, 1981; Sackner et al, 1976) or the patient who has received certain chemotherapeutic agents (Gilson and Sahn, 1985). In addition, excessive oxygen flow may predispose patients to infectious pulmonary complications by drying secretions, inhibiting mucus salivary clearance, and decreasing pulmonary macrophage function.

Intravenous Fluid

Patients undergoing thoracotomy for pulmonary resection should not receive excessive fluid, either in the operating room or postoperatively. Pulmonary surgery is not associated with large postoperative fluid shifts, and intraoperative lung manipulation and collapse not only may impair pulmonary lymphatic drainage in the early postoperative period but also may lead to the increased extravasation of fluid owing to a disruption of the alveolar-capillary membrane. Excessive fluids given perioperatively may result in pulmonary edema, decreased alveolar gas permeability, and decreased pulmonary compliance, which will promote atelectasis and further hypoxia. It is important to remember that epidural analgesia may be associated with increased fluid administration because of induced hypotension. In patients undergoing resection for malignant disease, use of blood products has also been reported to decrease survival and increase the likelihood of recurrence through immunosuppression (Cade et al, 1983; Ziomek et al, 1993). These observations are not, however, universal (Fox et al, 1981). Major gastrointestinal procedures such as esophagectomy require large amounts of perioperative fluid, owing to the increased third-space accumulations that result from such dissections. Such patients should undergo careful monitoring of their fluid status.

MANAGEMENT OF COMPLICATIONS

Pulmonary Insufficiency

Respiratory failure is the major cause of perioperative mortality in patients undergoing pulmonary resection for lung cancer. Postoperative respiratory failure occurs in 0.2% to 2.6% of patients, and there is a 46% to 100% mortality from this complication (Chatila et al, 2000; Deslauriers et al, 1989; Jordan et al, 2000; Nagasaki et al, 1982). Pulmonary complications most frequently occur in the first 2 to 4 days following surgery. As noted, preoperative pulmonary function testing is critical to minimize postoperative pulmonary complications and guide surgical decision making. Determination of the degree of pulmonary impairment and its reversibility will direct preoperative optimization and extent of resection and identify those patients at high risk for life-threatening pulmonary complications after resection (American College of Physicians, 1990). Antibiotics, bronchodilators, cessation of smoking, chest physiotherapy, postural drainage, and exercise may all be employed to enhance pulmonary function preoperatively. Spirometry, arterial blood gas analysis, split perfusion lung scanning, and exercise testing are suggested preoperative investigations in significantly impaired patients. Forced expiratory volume in 1 second (FEV_1) is easily obtained and reproducible. Using this value, the expected postoperative FEV_1 can be determined by the formula

$$\text{Postresection } FEV_1 = \text{preoperative } FEV_1 - X\,(\text{preoperative } FEV_1)$$

where X is the percent perfusion to the proposed area of resection. Regional pulmonary perfusion can be readily obtained preoperatively by quantitative perfusion lung scanning. A predicted postoperative FEV_1 that is less than 0.8 L/min in an adult of average size is associated with significantly increased perioperative morbidity and mortality (Nakahara, et al, 1988). Arterial blood gas analysis is also useful, identifying patients at high risk of respiratory complications postresection. Arterial hypercapnia ($Pco_2 > 45$ mm Hg) is usually considered to be an indicator of significantly increased risk of respiratory failure and death following pulmonary resection, but recent experience with lung volume reduction surgery would cast doubt on this as a reliable indicator. Arterial hypoxemia is also correlated with an increased risk of postoperative complications, although in some patients airway obstruction may cause intrapulmonary shunting, which will be eliminated with resection. In the patient with a main stem bronchial obstruction, hypoxemia may be improved by pneumonectomy.

Because of their failure to either individually or collectively predict morbidity, all these apparent predictors must be assessed in the context of the individual patient. Indeed, we are more concerned with the presence of a preoperatively high Pao_2 (>80 mm Hg) in the presence of impaired pulmonary mechanics. As most patients undergoing pulmonary surgery are heavy smokers and have obstructive lung disease, various degrees of ventilation/perfusion mismatching are usually present. This is particularly the case if pulmonary function testing suggests a marginal FEV_1 or diffusing capacity. Under such circumstances, a Pao_2 above 80 mm Hg can only be achieved if the ventilation/perfusion mismatch has been either eliminated or maximized. In a patient with chronic bronchitis or emphysema, this can occur from destruction or obliteration of portions of the pulmonary capillary bed that have been poorly ventilated. As a result, a high Pao_2 may suggest the early development of pulmonary vascular hypertension. Under such circumstances, preoperative evaluation of pulmonary vascular pressure is advisable.

Preoperative pulmonary assessment as a predictor of postoperative respiratory function has undergone reassessment since the advent of lung volume reduction surgery. As a result absolute values of spirometric parameters may have little relevance if there are areas of hyperinflation and lung destruction that could be rectified through resection. Indeed, there are several anecdotal reports and series of lung volume reduction combined with pulmonary resection undertaken in patients with emphysema and lung cancer (DeMeester et al, 1988; Hayashi et al, 1999; Mentzer et al, 1999; Simone et al, 1999).

Chest physiotherapy has been demonstrated to be effective in preventing postoperative pulmonary complications and should be considered routine postoperative care for patients undergoing thoracotomy (Stiller and Munday, 1992). Patients identified preoperatively with lung diseases or excessive secretions or postoperatively with recurrent laryngeal nerve palsy, phrenic nerve palsy, diaphragmatic reimplantation, or chest-wall resection are at higher risk and should receive more intensive evaluation and treatment. In patients with a history of excessive sputum production, prophylactic minitracheotomy may be advantageous to provide a route for frequent tracheal and bronchial suctioning without flexible bronchoscopy (Au et al, 1989; Nelson, 1992). The development of recurrent laryngeal nerve palsy in the postoperative period may seriously impair the ability to cough and clear secretions. This is particularly a problem following pneumonectomy. When the diagnosis is suggested early, evaluation by laryngoscopy is warranted. If the paralyzed cord is abducted, augmentation should be considered. If one knows that the recurrent nerve has been divided, augmentation with Teflon is appropriate. However, if the paralysis is believed to be temporary, glycerol should be used, as it will be absorbed with time.

Arrhythmias

In 1943, the first recorded cases of cardiac arrhythmias occurring after pulmonary resection were simultaneously reported by Currens and colleagues and Bailey and Betts. The occurrence of cardiac rhythm disturbances is likely related to the magnitude of the operative procedures performed. Cardiac arrhythmias (defined as atrial fibrillation, premature beats, atrial flutter, and ventricular arrhythmias) occurred in 3.1% to 14.3% of patients postlobectomy as compared with 19.4% to 40% for patients after pneumonectomy (Cerney, 1957; Krowka et al, 1987; Motta and Ratto, 1989; Mowrey and Reynolds, 1964; Wahi et al, 1989). The overall rate of postoperative arrhythmia in a large series was 3.2% to 20.8% (Cerney, 1957; Deslauriers et al, 1989; Nagasaki et al, 1982; Von Knorring et al, 1992). In patients undergoing pneumonectomy, arrhythmias were associated with a significantly increased mortality. Of postoperative deaths in patients undergoing pneumonectomy, 81% were preceded by or associated with a tachyarrhythmia (Krowka et al, 1987).

Much speculation exists regarding the causes of postoperative arrhythmias. Most authors consider increased vagal tone, hypoxemia, and intraoperative fluid administration of more than 2 L to be the most important deciding factors. Intraoperative hypotension has also been found to significantly increase the risk of both arrhythmias and myocardial ischemia (Von Knorring et al, 1992). Several series have failed to demonstrate any significant relation between preoperative pulmonary function, surgical indication, or tumor, node, metastasis (TNM) staging of lung cancer and the subsequent development of a tachyarrhythmia. General investigations include serum electrolytes, cardiac enzymes, arterial blood gases, hemoglobin, and electrocardiography (ECG).

Atrial arrhythmias are the most common. Most arrhythmias (96%) occur within the first postoperative week, with a peak incidence at 48 hours (Mowry and Reynolds, 1964; Von Knorring et al, 1992). Atrial fibrillation, atrial flutter, and atrial tachycardia account for most postoperative arrhythmias encountered (42%, 12.5%, and 4%, respectively) (Ritchie et al, 1992). The likelihood of arrhythmia increases with advancing age and previous cardiac history. Ventricular arrhythmias are rare. Prophylaxis of this common complication has received a great deal of attention. Prophylactic digitalization has been suggested for older patients (over 50 years) undergoing pulmonary resection. In several retrospective series, preoperative digitalization was shown to have a variable effect on the incidence of postoperative atrial arrhythmias and mortality (Juler et al, 1969; Shields and Ujiki, 1968). In a prospective randomized series, prophylactic digitalization was found to increase the frequency and severity of postoperative arrhythmias (Ritchie et al, 1992). Most authors do not advocate routine prophylactic digitalization. A prospective randomized trial using flecainide after thoracic operations as prophylaxis for postoperative arrhythmia has demonstrated efficacy with no side effects (Borgeat et al, 1989). These results await further testing in larger trials. Calcium channel blockade has aroused interest. Amar and others (2000) reduced the atrial arrhythmia rate by close to 50% with the use of prophylactic calcium channel blockade.

Therapy for atrial arrhythmias is dependent on correct diagnosis and careful assessment of the patient. Urgency and mode of therapy are dictated by the degree of hemodynamic impairment imposed by the new rhythm. Assessment for congestive heart failure should be made and supplemental oxygen given. Patients who are asymptomatic with a normal blood pressure and new-onset atrial fibrillation are easily treated with intravenous digoxin. Digoxin is the drug of choice in this situation, as it decreases ventricular response rate without impairment of myocardial contractility. The average-size adult should receive 0.5 mg IV, followed by two or three subsequent doses of 0.25 mg given every 6 hours or more rapidly if indicated. Subsequently, a maintenance dose of 0.25 mg PO is given daily; dosage may require adjustment based on renal function. Peak levels of digoxin occur approximately 90 to 120 minutes after intravenous administration; therefore, 1 or 2 hours may be required to obtain an effect. Digoxin levels have little correlation with effects, and adequacy or treatment is best judged by ventricular response rate. Additional doses of digoxin may be required in some cases to bring ventricular response rate below 120 beats/min.

Patients demonstrating evidence of circulatory compromise require more urgent therapy. If hypotension, dizziness, or angina is experienced, verapamil or propranolol may be used in addition to digoxin. Both verapamil (a calcium channel antagonist) and propranolol (a β-blocking agent) produce rapid slowing of ventricular response when administered intravenously. Both should be used in a monitored environment with dosage carefully titrated. Propranolol may be given in 1-mg aliquots every 5 to 8 minutes until the heart rate reaches 120 beats/min or less. Verapamil may be given as 2.5 mg IV as a slow push; the dose may be repeated every 10 to 15 minutes to a maximum of 15 mg. β-Blocking agents should not be used simultaneously with calcium channel blockers because of their possible synergistic negative inotropic and chronotropic effects, which could lead to hypotension or asystole in some patients.

Occasionally patients may experience extreme circulatory compromise with new-onset atrial fibrillation. Patients presenting with profound hypotension, severe angina, and obtundation require emergent treatment. Direct-current cardioversion is a fast and effective mode of treatment for patients in extremis. Following cardioversion, digoxin should be given to reduce the risk of recurrent atrial fibrillation and relative circulatory compromise. Patients who fail to convert to a normal sinus rhythm after the ventricular response rate has been controlled may be treated by chemical cardioversion with propranolol, sotalol, quinidine, or procainamide (Pronestyl). Most patients, however, undergo spontaneous cardioversion after heart rate is controlled with digoxin. Patients with normal sinus rhythm prior to surgery who develop atrial tachyarrhythmias postoperatively are discharged home with digoxin for 6 weeks. This continuation of digoxin is arbitrary.

Postpneumonectomy Empyema

Empyema occurring after pneumonectomy begins as a suppurative contamination of the pneumonectomy space. The incidence of empyema occurring with or without a bronchial fistula has decreased and is now close to 1% (Eckersberger et al, 1990). Empyema may occur early in the postoperative course or may develop years after the procedure. The majority of patients develop empyema within 12 weeks, with 77% having an associated bronchopleural fistula (Shamji et al, 1983). Early empyema may be primary, due to bacterial contamination of the pleural fluid at the time of operation (most common), or secondary, due to contamination from infected residual lung (in the case of lobectomy or wedge resection) or to bronchopleural or esophagopleural fistula (Van Raemdonck et al, 1990). Bronchopleural fistula in this setting is usually a complication of empyema. Empyema occurring months to years after resection is generally considered to arise from hematogenous seeding, but a late fistula should be ruled out.

Staphylococcus is the most frequently occurring pathogen. *Streptococcus* species and gram-negative and anaerobic organisms are also frequently cultured (Shamji et al, 1983). Diagnosis is established by diagnostic thoracocentesis (Papadakis and Wall, 1990). This procedure should be considered whenever patients are febrile, lethargic, or anorexic. Pleural fluid should be aspirated and sent for pH, protein, lactate dehydrogenase (LDH), and glucose determinations; cytology (if a late fistula); and aerobic and anaerobic cultures. Bronchoscopy and esophagography should be performed to rule out a bronchial or esophageal fistula when indicated. Delayed diagnoses may result in sepsis, bronchopleural fistula, pneumonia, or pericarditis.

Therapy consists of early drainage of the pleural space and administration of systemic antibiotics for 48 to 72 hours after drainage has been effected. Eventual obliteration of the space or closure of the draining sinus may be required. In approaching these difficult problems, the algorithm in Figure 9–2 is useful. Tube thoracostomy is essential initial treatment, and bronchoscopy should be performed to ensure that a bronchial fistula has not also developed. If the empyema occurs more than 3 weeks following thoracotomy, one can be assured that sufficient mediastinal fixation has occurred to allow creation of a thoracic window. If, however, the pulmonary resection was performed less than 3 weeks before the tube thoracostomy, a thoracic window should be delayed until the mediastinum has become stabilized. There is some controversy over the fate of the thoracic window. It can represent definitive treatment in high-risk patients with poor functional status. In our opinion, attempts at closure should be delayed for 12 to 24 months to ensure that the risk of recurrence of bronchogenic carcinoma is minimized and to allow the patient time to recover a normal nutritional status. Closure of the window following sterilization of the empyema cavity in the hospital has been reported with variable success (American College of Physicians, 1990; Clagett and Geraci, 1963; Pairoleiro et al, 1991; Shamji et al, 1983; Stafford and Clagett, 1972). Alternatively, thoracoplasty with or without muscle transposition represents a definitive approach to obliteration of the empyema space (Gregoire et al, 1987).

Bronchopleural Fistulas

Bronchopleural fistulas with or without empyema have been identified as a major source of morbidity and mortality in patients undergoing pulmonary resections for malignancy (Deslauriers et al, 1989; Ginsberg et al, 1983; Nagasaki et al, 1982). The incidence of postoperative fistula is approximately 1.6% to 6.2% (Asamura et al, 1992; Motta and Ratto, 1989; Vester et al, 1991; Wahi et al, 1989). Wider resection, residual carcinoma in the bronchial stump, preoperative irradiation, and diabetes have been identified by multivariate analyses to be significant risk factors (Asamura et al, 1992). Most bronchopleural fistulas occur following pneumonectomy (46%), and approximately 75% are right-sided. Radical mediastinal lymphadenectomy also increases the risk of fistula formation because of bronchial devascularization. In patients who have received preoperative radiation, the diagnosis of bronchopleural fistula is made significantly later than in patients who have not had radiotherapy (48 days average versus 18 days) (Vester et al, 1991). Mortality from bronchopleural fistula may be as high as 71% (Asamura et al, 1992). The diagnosis should be suspected

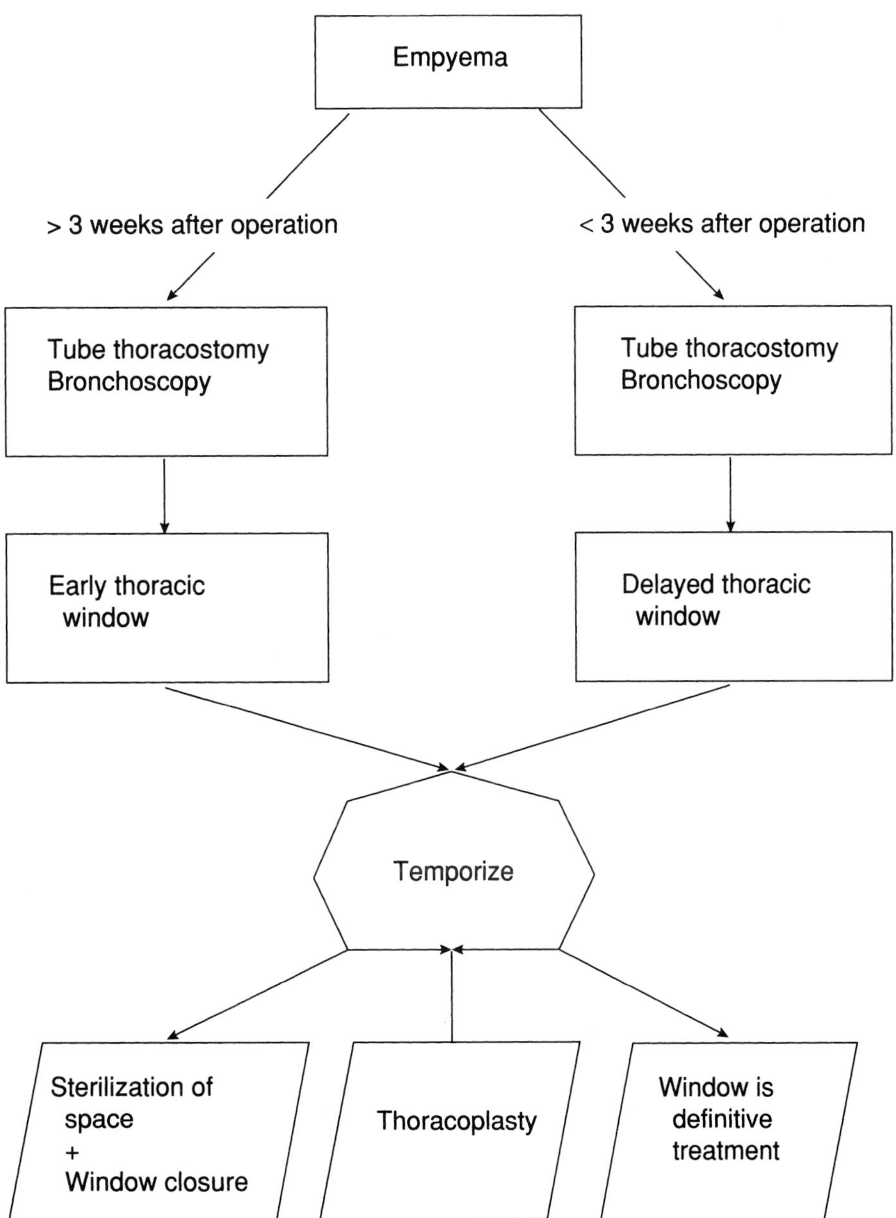

FIGURE 9–2 ■ Suggested algorithm for management of postpneumonectomy empyema.

if there is expectoration of copious amounts of infected material (when fistulas occur late) or serosanguineous fluid (early fistulas); this, however, is often not noted. The clinical scenario of a falling fluid level and a new contralateral infiltrate after pneumonectomy is virtually diagnostic and demands insertion of a chest tube into the space (Fig. 9–3).

The initial therapy for a bronchial stump fistula involves immediate insertion of a chest drain and performance of bronchoscopy to verify the clinical suspicion. Prior to insertion of a thoracostomy tube, the patient should be nursed with the operative side dependent to reduce the incidence of contralateral soiling. Subsequent therapy depends on the time of occurrence of the fistula. Those fistulas that develop within the first week are usually secondary to technical difficulties and are unlikely to be associated with significant pleural infection. Following verification of bronchial stump dehiscence, thoracotomy is recommended in this situation. Reclosure of the bronchial stump is undertaken employing a buttress of pedicled intercostal muscle, pericardium, or omentum. The pleural space should be débrided and lavaged. The role of postoperative irrigation of the pleural space with or without antibiotic solutions—so-called balanced drain age—remains to be determined but empirically would seem to have merit.

Fistulas that occur beyond the 10th postoperative day are usually associated with an empyema. Under such circumstances reoperation is not recommended. Tube thoracostomy and antibiotic coverage for 5 to 7 days are appropriate. If there has been considerable soilage into the contralateral lung, mechanical ventilation may be required. If the fistula is large, high-frequency ventilation may be necessary (Panos et al, 1986). If jet ventilation is unavailable, the fistula can be controlled with either a bronchus blocker or a balloon catheter or by insertion of

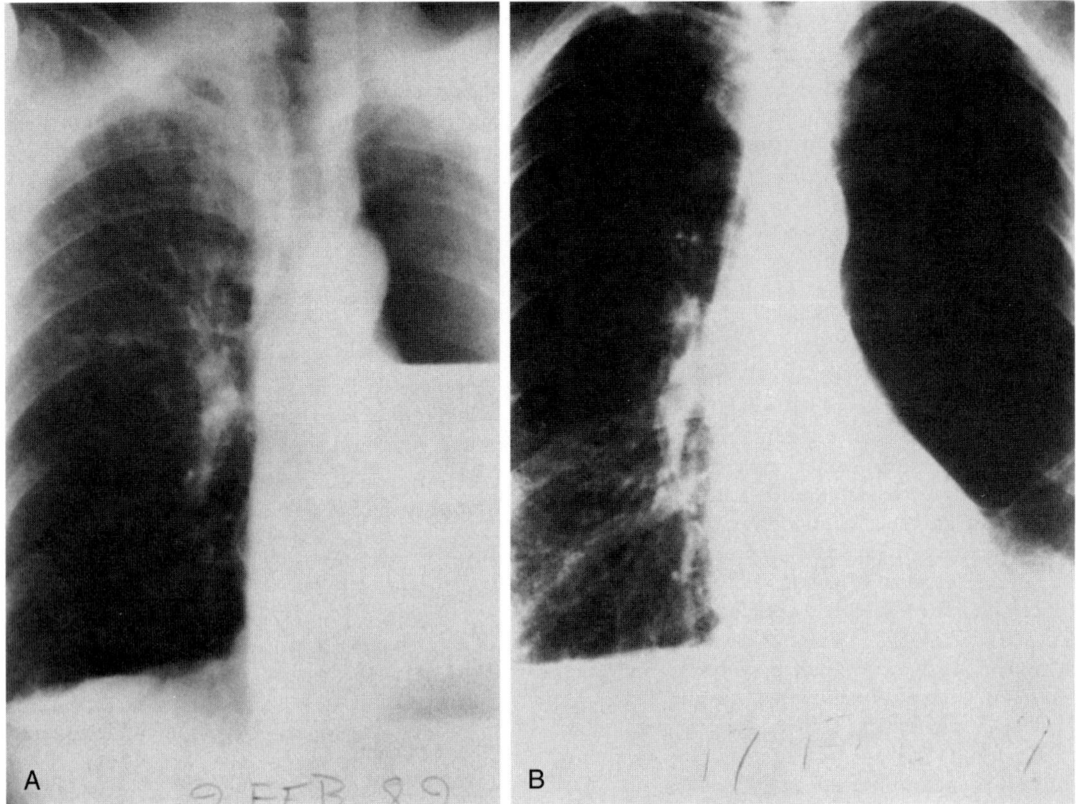

FIGURE 9–3 ■ *A*, Postpneumonectomy chest radiograph at discharge from hospital. *B*, Follow-up chest radiograph demonstrating fallen fluid level.

an uncut endotracheal tube into the contralateral mainstem bronchus. For bronchopleural fistulas that occur following lobectomy, tube thoracostomy may be all that is required. However, following pneumonectomy, a thoracic window is a better option. The window is best created 2 to 3 weeks after the pneumonectomy to ensure that fixation of the mediastinum has occurred. Under these circumstances, closure of the fistula will occur in 30% of cases (Shamji et al, 1983). Fistulas that fail to close can be managed by a thoracoplasty (Gregoire et al, 1987) or by transsternal reamputation of the bronchial stump.

Cardiac Herniation

Cardiac herniation is an infrequently reported complication of intrapericardial pneumonectomy (right more common than left). This complication arises in the immediate postoperative period in patients with residual medium and large (>5 cm) pericardial defects. Onset is sudden and is marked by hypotension, tachycardia, and cyanosis, usually within 24 hours of operation. The mortality rate in cases recognized promptly approaches 50% (Delranija, 1974; Groh and Sunder-Plassmann, 1987). Diagnosis rests on clinical suspicion and critical appraisal of the chest radiograph. Right-sided herniation is unmistakable on chest radiograph, which frequently shows obvious right-sided cardiac subluxation (Fig. 9–4). Left-sided herniation demonstrates a more subtle radiographic change; often, a left shift of the cardiac shadow is seen in conjunction with a rounded opacity in the lower portion of the left hemithorax, representing the strangulated ventricular mass.

Several predisposing factors have been described, including the application of suction to chest tubes, coughing, patient positioning (Bettman and Tannenbaum, 1948), tracheal suctioning, and positive pressure ventilation. Hemodynamic alterations and clinical manifestations vary between right- and left-sided herniation. Right-sided cardiac herniation results in torsion and occlusion of venous inflow via the superior and the inferior vena cava (Delraniya, 1974; Gates et al, 1970; Levin et al, 1971; Takita and Majares, 1970). In addition, the left ventricular outflow tract is distorted and compromised. Left-sided herniation, however, results in constriction of the left ventricle by the sharp edges of the pericardial defect. This results in ischemia, edema, and dysfunction of the herniated myocardium; epicardial vessels may also be lacerated, resulting in bleeding (Glass et al, 1984; Papsin et al, 1993). Electrocardiographic changes may thus frequently accompany left-sided herniation (Yacoub et al, 1968).

Successful management of cardiac herniation requires prompt diagnosis and operation. At operation, the heart must be returned to its normal anatomic position within the pericardial sac, and the pericardial defect must be closed. Numerous methods of obliteration of the right-sided defect have been suggested, including approximation of the epicardium to the pericardium and patching the defect with pleura, fascia, or bovine pericardium. The use of Dacron to close pericardium defects has been

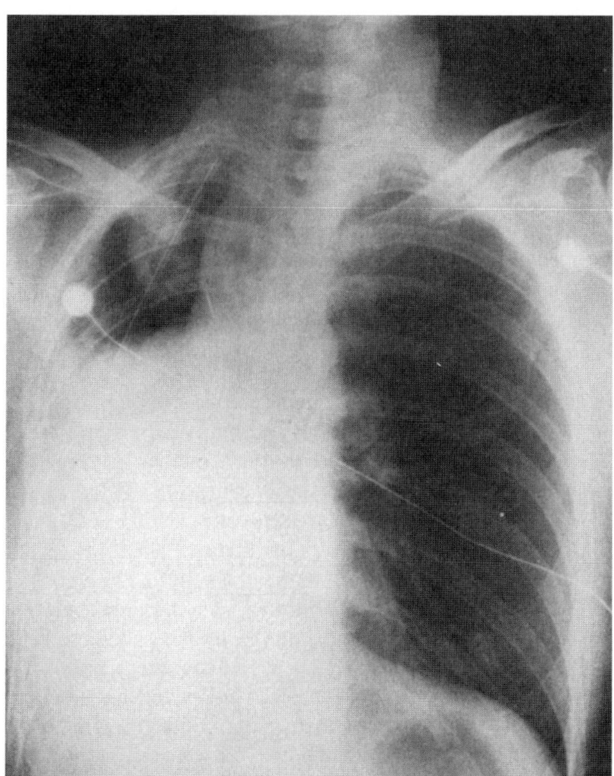

FIGURE 9–4 ■ Chest radiograph after intrapericardial resection of lung tumor demonstrating right-sided cardiac herniation.

associated with septic complications and is not recommended. On the left side, the pericardium may be widely opened to the diaphragm. With this maneuver, the extreme cardiac shift is not eliminated, but cardiac strangulation and infarction are unlikely.

Pulmonary Embolism

Pulmonary embolism occurs in approximately 0.19% to 2.3% of patients undergoing pulmonary resection for malignancy (Asamura et al, 1992; Rogiers et al, 1991a; Tedder et al, 1992). In one series, postoperative pulmonary embolism accounted for 14.3% of early deaths in patients undergoing bronchoplastic procedures (Rogiers et al, 1991b). Most surgical literature concerning perioperative pulmonary embolism and prophylaxis deals with orthopaedic, neurosurgical, and general surgical patients. The reported incidence of symptomatic pulmonary embolism in thoracic surgical patients is low. Once pulmonary embolism is documented, however, the mortality is high (50% to 100%) (Asamura et al, 1992; Tedder et al, 1992; Waller et al, 1993). This observation is likely related to poor cardiopulmonary reserve in this patient population.

Factors predisposing to venous thrombosis are stasis, hypercoagulability, and initimal damage. Most thoracic surgical patients have several risk factors, including advanced age, malignancy, and prolonged duration of general anesthesia (longer than 30 minutes). Some patients may have additional risk factors such as a previous history of deep venous thrombosis (DVT), a known hypercoagulable state, obesity, and heart disease. Thoracic surgical patients constitute a moderate risk group for perioperative thrombotic complications. Patients undergoing surgery without prophylaxis can be expected to have a 10% to 40% risk of calf vein thrombosis, a 2% to 10% incidence of proximal vein thrombosis, and a 0.1% to 0.7% risk of fatal pulmonary embolism (Papadakis and Wall, 1990). Prophylaxis should be considered for most thoracic patients, either with standard heparin administered in a low dose subcutaneously or with low molecular weight heparin. Low-dose heparin is administered subcutaneously, beginning 2 hours prior to surgery and continued every 8 to 12 hours. This regimen has been shown to decrease the incidence of DVT in thoracic surgical patients by approximately 50% (Jackaman et al, 1978). Heparin prophylaxis is associated with an increased risk of bleeding and hematoma formation, but serious complications are minimal (Shirakusa et al, 1990). Low molecular weight heparin has also been shown to be effective in the prevention of thromboembolism in randomized blind trials (Hull et al, 2000; Kakkar et al, 2000).

Diagnosis of DVT and pulmonary embolism is difficult. Physical examination is often misleading, swelling and tenderness are often subtle, and Homan's sign is not accurate. Pulmonary embolism is a complication of DVT; 90% of emboli originate in the deep veins of the lower extremities. Any patient suspected of having DVT should receive a duplex ultrasound scan or venogram. Pulmonary embolism can occur in different forms, depending on the degree of obstruction to blood flow. Small emboli may produce minimal symptoms such as atrial arrhythmias, but, if recurrent, may lead to hypoxia and right-sided cardiac failure. Large emboli often occur with significant hypoxemia and circulatory collapse. The most frequent patient symptoms include chest pain (89%), dyspnea (86%), apprehension (59%), and cough (51%). Dyspnea, cough, fever, and leg cramps are often the first symptoms reported by affected patients. Periodic chest pain and hemoptysis occur more frequently in patients with submissive emboli. Apprehension, syncope, increased pulmonic heart sound, gallop, and murmurs are more frequently present among patients with massive embolism.

Suspected pulmonary embolism mandates urgent investigation and treatment. Arterial blood gas measurements are nonspecific and should not be relied on for diagnosis (Hull et al, 1986). Chest radiograph findings and ECG are useful in the initial investigation to confirm or rule out other important disorders that have a presentation that is similar to that of pulmonary embolism and will be important in the evaluation of subsequent nuclear scans. Patients rarely have findings diagnostic of pulmonary embolism on routine chest radiograph or ECG.

Ventilation/perfusion scans remain the initial investigation of choice for most patients; normal perfusion is associated with a very low incidence of angiographically documented emboli (Miller, 1990). A high-risk scan carries a reliable diagnostic accuracy (Lesser et al, 1992) and should lead to the institution of systemic anticoagulants (Fig. 9–5). A moderate-risk scan presents uncertainty, and if the suspicion of pulmonary embolism is high, a pulmonary angiogram should be obtained. Venti-

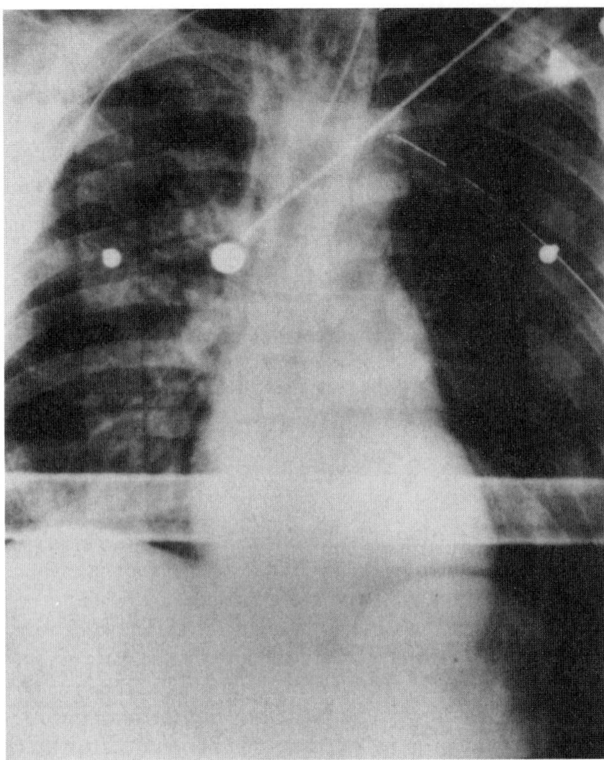

FIGURE 9–5 ■ Chest radiograph of a postoperative patient demonstating pneumomediastinum and pneumopericardium resulting from esophageal perforation.

lated patients and postoperative patients with other pulmonary complications frequently have multiple ventilation defects, rendering ventilation/perfusion scanning in this patient group less useful. Such patients should undergo perfusion scans to direct selective pulmonary angiography. Normally, pulmonary angiography is reserved for the patient with massive pulmonary embolism that requires surgical intervention, the patient with an indeterminant scan, or the patient in whom there is a contraindication to anticoagulation. Documented pulmonary embolism or DVT is treated with specific anticoagulation using heparin. Patients with low risk of anticoagulation-related complications should receive anticoagulants while confirmatory investigations are under way. In those patients who subsequently have a negative ventilation/perfusion scan or angiogram, the heparin therapy may be terminated. Those patients with documented embolism or thrombosis should be anticoagulated with heparin or low molecular weight heparin (Hull et al, 2000) and then converted quickly to warfarin and then continued on oral anticoagulants for 3 to 6 months (Hirsh et al, 2001). Patients allergic to heparin can be anticoagulated with ancrod. Those with contraindications to systemic anticoagulation require surgical prophylaxis against recurrent embolism. Most commonly, a Greenfield filter can be placed radiographically in the inferior vena cava and positioned immediately below the renal veins (Forty et al, 1990).

Tumor Embolism

Massive systemic tumor embolism is a rare but potentially life-threatening complication of pulmonary resection for bronchogenic carcinoma. Embolism occurs most frequently during surgery or in the immediate postoperative period. In most cases, the pulmonary vein is invaded by tumor, and embolization occurs either spontaneously or secondary to surgical manipulation. In 1967, Firor and Pearson reported the first successful removal of a massive tumor embolism situated at the aortic bifurcation. This patient did well after bilateral femoral Fogarty balloon embolectomy but 3 months later died of intracranial and systemic metastasis (Pairolero et al, 1990). Subsequent case reports have stressed the importance of early pulmonary vein ligation prior to manipulation of the lung to prevent gross systemic tumor embolization (Arnold and Pairolero, 1990; Van Raemdonck et al, 1990). Anticipation of the problem preoperatively will likely prevent most embolic phenomena.

Proximal tumors abutting the pulmonary veins or failure to visualize a pulmonary vein during a contrast computed tomography (CT) scan should lead to concern that the tumor is invading the lumen of the vessel or extending into the left atrium. If the problem is unsuspected preoperatively, it may first be recognized on palpation of the vein. Under this circumstance, it is advisable to open the pericardium and apply an atrial clamp beyond the palpable abnormality. A two-dimensional ECG or a transesophageal echocardiogram will further elucidate the situation in such circumstances and alert the surgeon to the possibility of tumor embolism. The lower extremities have been the most frequent site of tumor emboli. Primary bronchogenic carcinoma has been diagnosed in a patient initially presenting with lower limb ischemia secondary to tumor embolism (Peters, 1989). It has been suggested that tumor embolism does not adversely affect prognosis and that outlook is best predicted by TNM staging (Shastri and Spaulding, 1989). Gradual respiratory decompensation secondary to subacute cor pulmonale from microscopic bronchogenic carcinoma embolization has also been well described (Postmus et al, 1989). Massive tumor embolism can be diagnosed by careful physical examination and selective angiography when the latter is deemed necessary. Appropriate initial therapy involves systemic anticoagulation and urgent embolectomy. All extracted embolic material should be sent for pathologic examination.

Lobar Gangrene

Torsion of a remaining lobe following lobectomy or bilobectomy is a rare complication, occurring in approximately 0.2% of surgical patients (Eggers, 1920; Rogiers et al, 1991b). Without prompt diagnosis and treatment, torsion progresses to pulmonary infarction and finally fatal gangrene. The use of a double-lumen endotracheal tube has been implicated in inadvertent intraoperative lobar torsion (Eggers, 1920), but in most cases lobar torsion is believed to occur either because of manipulation at the time of surgery or because of the presence of a complete fissure between the middle lobe and either the upper or the lower lobe. A complete oblique fissure, coupled with the narrow middle lobe hilum, makes the right middle lobe the most frequently involved lobe (Pool and Garlock, 1929). Lobar torsion results in vascular and bronchial obstruction, predisposing the patient to ischemic lung injury. Patients often present with persistently high fever, hemoptysis, and bronchorrhea. Arterial blood gases may be deceptively normal, as the involved lobe may have no perfusion. Typically, serial chest radiographs demonstrate increased volume and density of the involved pulmonary parenchyma. Prominent reticular markings may also be seen secondary to edema from venous obstruction (Wangensteen, 1935). Pleural effusion and abnormal location of bronchovascular markings are less specific associated findings (Eggers, 1920).

Occasionally, a bronchial cutoff is also present. Differentiation from lobar opacification secondary to retained secretions may be difficult. Flexible bronchoscopy, CT scanning, and ventilation/perfusion scanning are adjuncts to diagnosis. Bronchoscopy shows no endobronchial lesion but rather a collapsed bronchus through which the scope may be passed. Removal of the bronchoscope results in prompt reclosure of the affected bronchus. Mucosal erythema and edema may also be evident.

When the diagnosis of lobar torsion is made, immediate operation is mandatory. Repeat thoracotomy is required to untwist the lobe and assess its viability. If diagnosis is early, the involved lobe may yet be viable, and its fixation to the remaining lobe may be sufficient. If ischemic injury is advanced, lobectomy is indicated. Perioperative anesthesia management should include the use of a double-lumen tube. During detorsion, retained secretions or bleeding into the airway may occur; with isolation of the affected lung, soiling of the good lung may be prevented (Shenstone, 1936). Right middle lobe torsion may be prevented in suitable situations (complete fissure with a narrow bronchovascular pedicle) by suturing or stapling the middle lobe to adjacent lung (Gray, 1938; Pool and Garlock, 1929). During the conduct of intrathoracic procedures, care must be taken to avoid unrecognized lobar volvulus.

Esophageal Fistulas

A common cause of esophageal fistulas occurring postoperatively is an anastomotic leak from either an intrathoracic anastomosis or an esophagogastrostomy in the neck. Anastomotic leaks commonly occur within the first 5 to 7 days. Those that are large or are secondary to major necrosis of the gastric tube may occur earlier and in more dramatic fashion. Although commonly occurring with symptoms and signs of sepsis, the intrathoracic anastomotic leak may declare itself with an increasing pleural effusion, supraventricular tachycardia, mediastinal air, and even pneumopericardium and cardiac tamponade (Fig. 9–6). Fistulas into the airway are not common but will usually heal spontaneously if adequate drainage is provided. Esophageal fistulas that occur in the neck usually heal quickly and are of little long-term consequence unless there has been substantial necrosis of the gastric transposition. The latter is suggested by the presence of a foul odor from the mouth and neck and is confirmed by gastroscopy.

Pneumonia

Nosocomial pneumonia usually occurs between the third and seventh day postoperatively. The most common organisms are enteric gram-negative bacilli or those commonly seen colonizing the airways of patients with chronic obstructive lung disease (*Hemophilus influenzae* and *Pneumococcus*). The pathophysiology, diagnosis, and treatment are outlined in detail elsewhere in this book.

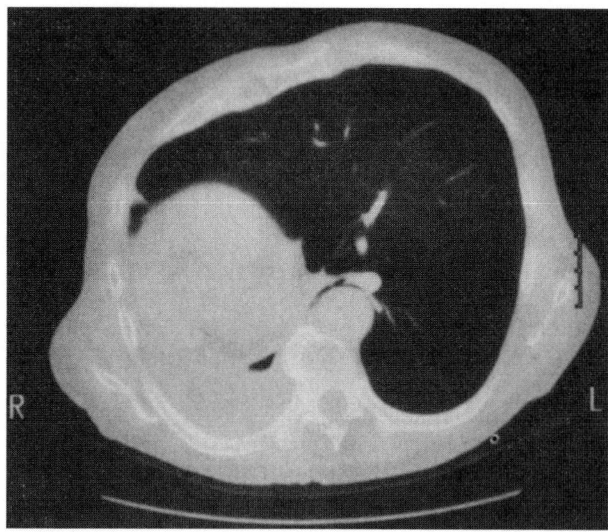

FIGURE 9–6 ■ A computed tomography scan demonstrating extreme mediastinal shift and pulmonary hyperinflation occurring after pneumonectomy.

Postpneumonectomy Syndrome

Airway obstruction may occur following pneumonectomy accompanied by extreme mediastinal shift. This has most commonly been reported following pneumonectomy in children or adolescents. Although originally described following right pneumonectomy (Shepard et al, 1986), it has been observed after left pneumonectomy when there is a right aortic arch (Grillo et al, 1992) or, in two of our cases, in the absence of associated congenital abnormalities. Following a right pneumonectomy, the mediastinum shifts to the right and the heart undergoes a counterclockwise rotation. The left main bronchus is compressed between the aortic arch and the left main pulmonary artery. The abnormality is best seen on CT scanning (Fig. 9–7) and confirmed with bronchoscopy. After a left pneumonectomy, the bronchus intermedius becomes compressed against the thoracic spine (Fig. 9–8) if there is extreme mediastinal shift and clockwise rotation of the heart. Diagnosis is made from a high degree of suspicion. The incidence of the condition is probably considerably greater than reported. It should be considered in any patient with dyspnea following pneumonectomy, particularly when there is significant mediastinal shift.

Surgical correction has involved several elaborate vascular procedures, such as division and bypass of the descending aortic arch. However, most successful corrections have involved mediastinal repositioning, either with autologous tissue (Grillo et al, 1992) or expandable prostheses (Rasch et al, 1990). In our experience (Shamji et al, 1996), the latter has been straightforward and has resulted in reversal of the bronchial obstruction in all four cases attempted. The procedure involves reopening

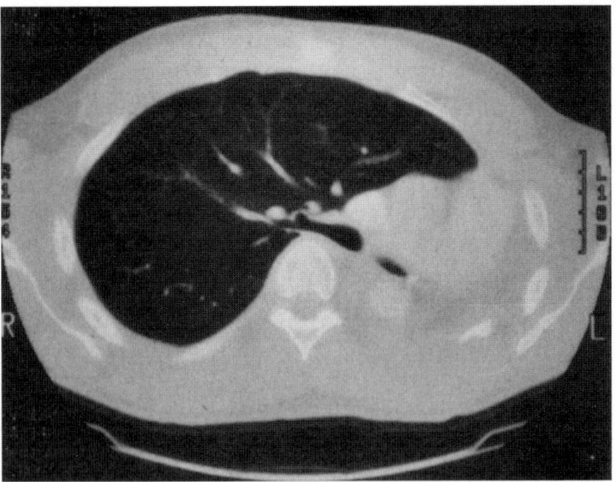

FIGURE 9–7 ■ Obstruction of bronchus intermedius resulting from compression against the thoracic spine.

of the original thoracotomy with division of all adhesions between the parietal pleura and the mediastinal structures. The mediastinum can then be repositioned in the midline, correcting the rotation of the heart. On the right side the correction of the cardiac rotation is facilitated by division of the azygous vein. In our series of four cases, the pericardium was sutured to the anterior chest wall to maintain neutrality and an expandable tissue prosthesis was placed to ensure that no further mediastinal shift would occur. The correction of the airway obstruction is immediate, although bronchomalacia has been reported (Grillo et al, 1992).

Myocardial Ischemia and Infarction

Preoperative assessment of cardiac risk is critical when evaluating potential patients prior to thoracic surgery. Perioperative cardiac complications can be reduced in patients identified as at high risk preoperatively by increased perioperative monitoring, performance of lesser procedures, or medical optimization. Preoperative revascularization using either balloon angioplasty or coronary artery bypass grafting should be considered in appropriate patients with significant coronary artery disease.

Preoperative indicators of increased risk of perioperative cardiac morbidity (myocardial infarction, unstable angina, congestive heart failure, serious dysrhythmia, or cardiac death) include advanced age, history of previous myocardial infarction, congestive heart failure, poorly controlled hypertension, arrhythmias, severe valvular heart disease, angina, and previous coronary artery revascularization.

Age over 70 has been found by Goldman and colleagues (1977) and Detsky and colleagues (1986) to be an independent risk factor for perioperative cardiac events. Age alone may not be as important as the patient's overall physiologic status; however, the leading cause of death in elderly patients undergoing noncardiac surgery is cardiovascular disease.

Patients with a previous myocardial infarction are at greater risk of perioperative myocardial infarction and congestive heart failure as compared with those with no cardiac history. The time interval between surgery and the previous myocardial infarction significantly alters perioperative risk. Within 3 months of an infarction, surgery carries up to a 37% risk of perioperative cardiac morbidity. With time the risk diminishes, remaining constant at approximately 5% after 6 months (Dweyer et al, 1984). Clinical or radiologic evidence of left ventricular failure is associated with a poor prognosis in patients with coronary artery disease. Patients with documented episodes of congestive heart failure may be expected to have a 5-year survival of less than 50% (Multicenter Postinfarction Research Group, 1983).

Hypertension is the most common cardiovascular disease in North America and a major risk factor for the development of atherosclerotic heart disease. Periopera-

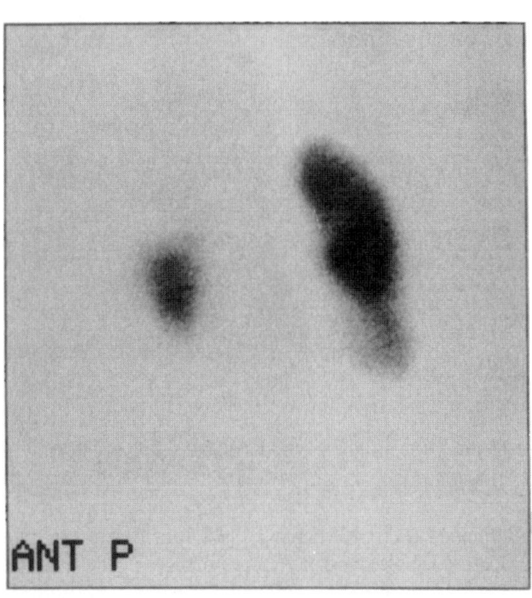

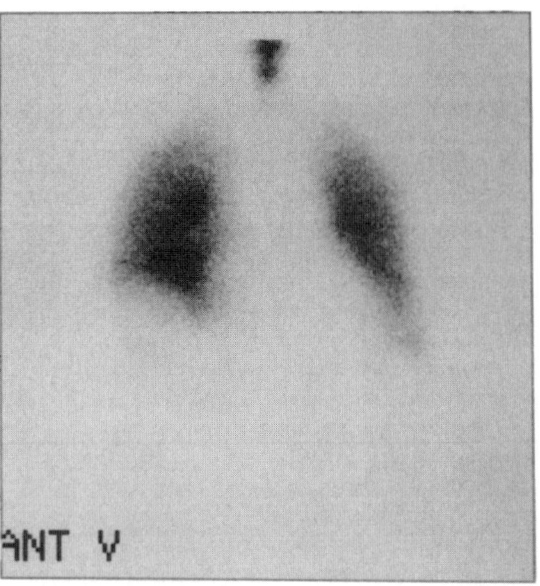

FIGURE 9–8 ■ Ventilation/perfusion scan demonstrating mismatching over the right lung fields.

tive complications are frequent in hypertensive patients who develop either a 50% decrease in intraoperative blood pressure or a 33% or greater decrease for 10 minutes or more as compared with preoperative values (Goldman and Caldera, 1979). Untreated diastolic hypertension greater than 110 mm Hg is also associated with increased frequency of intraoperative hypotension and perioperative myocardial ischemia and renal failure (Martin and Krammerer, 1983; Prys-Roberts et al, 1971).

Arrhythmias are common and benign in normal individuals. In the presence of coronary artery disease or left ventricular dysfunction, however, dysrhythmias may pose considerable risk. In the setting of myocardial ischemia or electrolyte abnormalities, certain arrhythmias may precipitate ventricular fibrillation. Goldman and coworkers (1977) considered a rhythm other than sinus, premature atrial contractions, or more than five premature ventricular contractions per minute on preoperative ECG in patients with known atherosclerotic heart disease to be risk factors for perioperative cardiac morbidity.

Aortic stenosis is associated with left ventricular hypertrophy, subendocardial ischemia, and decreased coronary perfusion pressure. Patients with significant aortic stenosis have dramatically increased risk of perioperative cardiac morbidity.

In ambulatory patients with coronary artery disease, stable angina increases the risk of myocardial infarction and sudden death. The predictive value of stable angina in patients undergoing noncardiac surgery is less clear, however. In thoracic patients, activity level and anginal symptoms may be limited. Class III or IV angina is a significant predictor of cardiac morbidity.

Patients who have had previous coronary artery bypass surgery and have patent grafts are at low risk. In these patients, the risk of surgery is equivalent to that in patients with no documented coronary artery disease for the corresponding age (Foster et al, 1986). No similar data are available relating the risk of surgery in patients who have undergone angioplasty procedures.

Preoperatively, patients with multiple risk factors or symptomatic heart disease should be investigated (Table 9–1). Echocardiography is a noninvasive method for determining left ventricular function and regional wall motion and for estimating pulmonary artery pressure. Dipyridamole-thallium (Persantine) scanning reveals areas of myocardium with restricted perfusion. This test is a highly sensitive predictor of perioperative cardiac events with low specificity (Boucher et al, 1985). In patients with curable pulmonary malignancy and a large reversible defect seen on Persantine-thallium scan, coronary angiography should be pursued. These patients may be candidates for combined or staged revascularization and resection. In patients with amenable significant single-vessel disease, angioplasty may be considered.

Patients undergoing thoracic surgical procedures are frequently at increased cardiac risk; many patients have significant underlying coronary artery disease. Thoracotomy-related supraventricular tachycardia, hypoxia, hypotension, fluid shifts, changes in pulmonary vascular resistance, and medications all may induce myocardial ischemia, which may progress to infarction. Principles of management are prevention and symptomatic care. Those patients who are identified preoperatively as being at increased risk and who are not candidates for revascularization procedures should have management plans carefully considered. Medical treatment or lesser surgical procedures may be appropriate. If these patients are to be treated surgically, preoperative anesthetic assessment should be sought, and patients should be managed postoperatively in an intensive-care setting. Perioperative monitoring with a Swan-Ganz catheter allows more careful fluid management and hemodynamic optimization.

Episodes of myocardial ischemia should be treated promptly with nitrates, calcium channel blockers, β-blockade, and afterload reduction. Predisposing factors (i.e., hypotension, arrhythmia, tachycardia, hypoxia, and anemia) must be treated promptly. Patients with evidence of respiratory failure should be recognized early; those with refractory angina with any degree of respiratory insufficiency may benefit from early intubation and mechanical ventilation. If necessary, patients may be anticoagulated 24 to 48 hours after thoracotomy, and enteric-coated aspirin is indicated in all patients with myocardial ischemia or infarction.

COMMENTS AND CONTROVERSIES

To all surgeons who are involved in the resection or lung parenchyma daily, it is clear that most postoperative complications are preventable. Prophylaxis should start during the preoperative evaluation, and proper selection of patients is one of the most important elements of successful thoracic surgery. Cardiopulmonary function and other significant comorbidities should be carefully evaluated and stabilized before operation. Medical management of chronic obstructive lung disease should be optimized, and the surgeon should never be afraid to ask

TABLE 9–1 ■ **Preoperative Predictors of Perioperative Cardiac Events**

Symptom	*Two-Dimensional Echocardiogram*	*Persantine-Thallium Scan*	*Angiogram*
Atrial arrhythmia	–	–	–
Ventricular arrhythmia	+	–	–
Stable angina	+	+	–
Congestive heart failure	+	–	–
Atypical chest pain	–	+	–
Unstable angina	+	–	+

consultants for their help with either the evaluation or preparation for surgery. Although there are no data on the usefulness of preoperative rehabilitation, it seems clear that for some individuals, 3 to 4 weeks of preoperative rehabilitation is useful to increase their endurance and stamina, and decrease the likelihood of postoperative complications. This rehabilitation, which can be home-based, involves mostly lower-extremity exercises. Objectives are set for each patient, and progress is monitored weekly through telephone or fax transmissions. Patients most likely to benefit from rehabilitation are those with documented abnormalities in gas exchange such as desaturation greater than 4% on exercise or abnormally low $\dot{V}O_2$ *max of* DLCO.

Intraoperatively, several maneuvers can also be done to decrease the incidence of postoperative complications. For instance, one must avoid pneumonectomy if a lesser operation can achieve complete resection of the tumor. The operation should be carried out rapidly so that the anesthetic time is shortened. The surgical technique should be meticulous. Bronchi should be covered when at risk of dehiscence, and potential prolonged air leaks or spaces should be anticipated and prevented by careful oversewing of lung parenchyma and use of either pleural tenting or intraoperative pneumoperitoneum. The amount of time on one-lung anesthesia should be shortened to avoid volutrauma to the opposite lung. The pleural space should be properly drained, and, for most cases, this can be accomplished with a single properly placed chest tube. On opening the chest, one should avoid breaking ribs, because, even with proper pain control, chest expansion will be limited, and efficient coughing will be more difficult.

Optimal pain control is essential during the postoperative period. In most centers, this is accomplished through epidural analgesia. Although this method is generally effective, the patient is often deeply asleep, particularly during the first 12 hours after surgery. Because of that, microaspiration can occur and initiate pulmonary complications. An alternative to epidural analgesia is the technique of intrapleural analgesia, which is reported to have fewer side effects. Sometimes epidural injection will lower the blood pressure and urine output, necessitating boluses of fluid to correct the situation. This may create a hypervolemic status, which could lead to lung edema. The complications of oxygen therapy are well described in this chapter. Undesirable side effects also include stomach distention with nausea and vomiting; dryness of nasopharyngeal airways and mouth; throat irritation; and dependence. In general, patients should be helped with coughing by physiotherapists—even over the weekend.

In general, complications can be anticipated and prevented. For instance, postoperative pneumonia or sputum retention can be diagnosed early. Bedside bronchoscopy should be done as frequently as required. We have found that the use of a minitracheotomy can be very useful to suction secretions in patients who have difficulties in coughing or do not understand the importance of it. If the patient seems to be delirious as is often the case in older individuals, we do not hesitate to involve the psychiatrist early on so that proper medication can be administered.

For patients who have vocal-cord paralysis, we believe that Teflon injection should not be done in the early postoperative period, as it may create laryngeal edema. Indeed, patients often adjust to this situation, and the voice returns to normal at a later date.

J.D.

■ KEY REFERENCES

Claggett OT, Geraci JE: A procedure for the management of postpneumonectomy empyema. J Thorac Cardiovasc Surg 45:141, 1963.

A classic paper describing the difficulties managing postpneumonectomy empyema and the original description of the "Claggett drainage procedure."

DeMeester SR, Patterson GA, Sundaresan RS, Cooper JD: Lobectomy combined with volume reduction for patients with lung cancer and advanced emphysema. J Thorac Cardiovasc Surg 115:681, 1998.

The first series of patients demonstrating that lung-volume reduction surgery improves pulmonary function sufficiently to permit resection for co-existent bronchogenic carcinoma.

Deslauriers J, Ginsberg RJ, Dubois P et al: Current operative morbidity with elective surgical resection for lung cancer. Can J Surg 32:335, 1989.

Experience at two teaching centers over a 6-year period is reported for 1076 consecutive elective pulmonary resections. Frequency of complications and preoperative risk factors are described.

Ginsberg RJ, Hill LD, Eagan RT et al: Modern thirty-day operative mortality for surgical resections in lung cancer. J Thorac Cardiovasc Surg 86:654, 1983.

Report from the lung cancer study group documenting mortality from pulmonary resection for lung cancer. Results from multiple institutions are reported, involving 2200 resections performed over a 3-year period.

Harpole DH, Decamp MM, Daley J et al: Prognostic models of thirty day mortality and morbidity after major pulmonary resection. J Thoracic Cardiovasc Surg 117:969, 1999.

A modern and large multivariate analysis of co-morbidities that identifies risk factors for 30-day mortality and morbidity.

Ilves R, Cooper JD, Todd TRJ, Pearson FG: Prospective, randomized, double-blind study using prophylactic cephalothin for major, elective, general thoracic operations. J Thorac Cardiovasc Surg 81:813, 1981.

One of the earliest well-conducted studies demonstrating a significant reduction in the incidence of postoperative wound infections with the use of prophylactic antibiotics. No reduction in postoperative empyema or pneumonia was seen.

Kakkar VV, Howes J, Sharma V, Kadziola A: A comparative double-blind, randomized trial of a new second generation LMWH (bemiparin) and UFH in the prevention of post-operative venous thromboembolism. The Bemiparin Assessment group. Thromb Haemost 83:523, 2000.

A well-conducted trial demonstrating the efficacy of low molecular weight heparin in the prevention of venothromboembolism.

Tedder M, Anstadt MP, Tedder SD, Lowe JE: Current morbidity, mortality, and survival after bronchoplastic procedures for malignancy. Ann Thorac Surg 54:387, 1992.

A report of 1915 bronchoplastic procedures for carcinoma performed over a 12-year period. Morbidity, mortality, and survival statistics are presented.

■ REFERENCES

Alpard SK, Duarte AG, Bidani A, Zwischenberger JB: Pathogenesis and management of respiratory insufficiency following pulmonary resection. Semin Surg Oncol 18:183, 2000.

Amar D, Roistacher N, Rusch VW et al: Effects of diltiazem prophylaxis on the incidence and clinical outcome of atrial arrhythmias after thoracic surgery. J Thorac Cardiovasc Surg 120:790, 2000.

American College of Physicians: Preoperative pulmonary function testing. Ann Intern Med 112:793, 1990.

Arnold PG, Pairolero PC: Intrathoracic muscle flaps: An account of their use in the management of 100 consecutive patients. Ann Surg 211:656, 1990.

Asamura H, Naruke T, Tsuchiya R et al: Bronchopleural fistulas associated with lung cancer operations: Univariate and multivariate analysis of risk factors, management and outcome. J Thorac Cardiovasc Surg 104:1456, 1992.

Au J, Walker WS, Inglis D, Cameron EW: Percutaneous cricothyroidostomy (minitracheostomy) for bronchial toilet: Results of therapeutic and prophylactic use. Ann Thorac Surg 48:850, 1989.

Bailey CC, Betts RH: Cardiac arrhythmias following pneumonectomy. N Engl J Med 229:356, 1943.

Bettman RB, Tannenbaum WJ: Herniation of the heart through a pericardial incision. Ann Surg 128:1012, 1948.

Borgeat A, Biollaz J, Bayer-Berger M et al: Prevention of arrhythmias by flecainide after noncardiac thoracic surgery. Ann Thorac Surg 48:232, 1989.

Boucher CA, Brewster DC, Darling RC: Determination of cardiac risk by dipyridamole-thallium imaging before peripheral vascular disease. N Engl J Med 312:389, 1985.

Braga M, Gianotti L, Gentilini O et al: Early postoperative enteral nutrition improves gut oxygenation and reduces costs compared with total parenteral nutrition. Crit Care Med 29:242, 2001.

Cade JF, Clegg EA, Westlake GW: Prophylaxis of venous thrombosis after major thoracic surgery. Aust N Z J Surg 53:301, 1983.

Cerney CI: The prophylaxis of cardiac arrhythmias complicating pulmonary surgery. J Thorac Surg 34:105, 1957.

Chatila W, Furukawa S, Criner GJ: Acute respiratory failure after lung volume reduction surgery. Am J Respir Crit Care Med 162:1292, 2000.

Clagett OT, Geraci JE: A procedure for the management of postpneumonectomy empyema. J Thorac Cardiovasc Surg 45:141, 1963.

Cooper JD, Trulove EP, Triantafilzou AN et al: Bilateral pneumonectomy (lung reduction) for chronic obstructive pulmonary disease. J Thorac Cardiovasc Surg 109:106, 1995.

Currens JH, White PD, Churchill ED: Cardiac arrhythmias following thoracic surgery. N Engl J Med 229:360, 1943.

Deiraniya AK: Cardiac herniation following intrapericardial pneumonectomy. Thorax 29:545, 1974.

DeMeester SR, Patterson GA, Sundaresan RS et al: Lobectomy combined with volume reduction for patients with lung cancer and advanced emphysema. Thorac Cardiovasc Surg 90:656, 1998.

De Perrot M, Licker M, Reymond MA et al: Influence of age on operative mortality and long-term survival after lung resection for bronchogenic carcinoma. Eur Respir J 14:419, 1999.

Deslauriers J, Ginsberg RJ, Dubois P et al: Current operative morbidity associated with elective surgical resection for lung cancer. Can J Surg 32:335, 1989.

Detsky AS, Abrams HB, Mclaughlin JR: Predicting cardiac complications in patients undergoing noncardiac surgery. J Gen Intern Med 1:211, 1986.

Dweyer EM, McMaster P, Greenberg H: Nonfatal cardiac events and recurrent infarction in the year after acute myocardial infarction. J Am Coll Cardiol 4:695, 1984.

Eckersberger F, Moritz E, Klepetko W et al: Treatment of postpneumonectomy empyema. Thorac Cardiovasc Surg 38:352, 1990.

Eggers C: The treatment of bronchial fistulae. Ann Surg 72:345, 1920.

Filaire M, Bedu M, Naamee A et al: Prediction of hypoxemia and mechanical ventilation after lung resection for cancer. Ann Thorac Surg 67:1460, 1999.

Firor WB, Pearson FG: Massive systemic tumour embolism during pneumonectomy: Successful removal by means of balloon catheter. Can J Surg 10:200, 1967.

Forty J, Yeatman M, Wells FC: Empyema thoracis: A review of a 4½ year experience of cases requiring surgical treatment. Respir Med 84:147, 1990.

Foster ED, Davis KB, Carpenter JA: Risk of noncardiac operation in patients with defined coronary artery disease: The coronary artery surgery study (CASS) registry experience. Ann Thorac Surg 41:42, 1986.

Fox RB, Shasti DM, Harada N: A novel mechanism for pulmonary oxygen toxicity—phagocyte mediated lung injury. Chest 80 (suppl):35, 1981.

Gates GF, Sette RS, Cope JA: Acute cardiac herniation with incarceration following pneumonectomy. Radiology 94:561, 1970.

Gilson AJ, Sahn SA: Reactivation of bleomycin lung toxicity following oxygen administration: A second response to corticosteroids. Chest 88:304, 1985.

Ginsberg RJ, Hill LD, Eagan RT et al: Modern thirty-day operative mortality for surgical resections in lung cancer. J Thorac Cardiovasc Surg 86:654, 1983.

Glass JD, McQuillen EN, Hardin NJ: Iatrogenic cardiac herniation: Post mortem case. J Trauma 24:632, 1984.

Goldman L, Caldera DL: Risk of general anesthesia and elective operations in hypertensive patients. Anesthesiology 50:285, 1979.

Goldman L, Caldera DL, Nussbaum SR: Multifactorial index of cardiac risk in noncardiac surgical procedures. N Engl J Med 297:845, 1977.

Goldstein RS, Gort EH, Stubbing D et al: Randomized controlled trial of respiratory rehabilitation. Lancet 344:1384, 1994.

Gray HK: The use of pedicle muscle grafts in facilitating obliteration of large, chronic, nontuberculous, pleural empyema cavities. Minn Med 21:608, 1938.

Gregoire R, Deslauriers J, Beaulieu M, Piraux M: Thoracoplasty: Its forgotten role in the management of nontuberculous postpneumonectomy empyema. Can J Surg 30:343, 1987.

Grillo HC, Shepard JO, Mathisen DJ, Kanarek DJ: Postpneumonectomy syndrome: Diagnosis, management, and results. Ann Thorac Surg. 54:638, 1992.

Groh J, Sunder-Plassmann L: Heart dislocation following extensive lung resection with pericardial resection. Anaesthesist 36:184, 1987.

Harpole DH, DeCamp NM, Daley J et al: Prognostic models of thirty-day mortality and morbidity after major pulmonary resection. J Thorac Cardiovasc Surg 117:969, 1999.

Hayashi K, Fukushima K, Sagara Y, Takeshita M: Surgical treatment for patients with lung cancer complicated by severe pulmonary emphysema. Jpn J Thorac Cardiovasc Surg 47:583, 1999.

Hirsh J, Dalen J, Guyatt G: The sixth (2000) ACCP guidelines for antithrombotic therapy for prevention and treatment of thrombosis. American College of Chest Physicians. Chest 119(suppl 1):1S, 2001.

Hull RD, Pineo GF, Francis C et al: Low-molecular-weight heparin prophylaxis using dalteparin extended out-of-hospital versus in-hospital warfarin/out-of-hospital placebo in hip arthroplasty patients: A double-blind, randomized comparison. North American Fragmin Trial Investigators. Arch Intern Med 160:2208, 2000.

Hull RD, Raskob GE, Brant RF et al: Low-molecular-weight heparin versus heparin in the treatment of patients with pulmonary embolism. American-Canadian Thrombosis Study Group. Arch Intern Med 160:229, 2000.

Hull RD, Raskob GE, Hirsh J: The diagnosis of clinically suspected pulmonary embolism. Chest 89:417S, 1986.

Ilves R, Cooper JD, Todd TRJ, Pearson FG: Prospective, randomized, double-blind study using prophylactic cephalothin for major, elective, general thoracic operations. J Thorac Cardiovasc Surg 81:813, 1981.

Jackaman FR, Perry BJ, Siddons H: Deep vein thrombosis after thoracotomy. Thorax 33:761, 1978.

Jordan S, Mitchell JA, Quinlan GJ et al: The pathogenesis of lung injury following pulmonary resection. Eur Respir J 15:790, 2000.

Juler GL, Stemmer EA, Connolly JE: Complications of prophylactic digitalization in thoracic surgical patients. J Thorac Cardiovasc Surg 58:352, 1969.

Kakker VV, Howes J, Sharma V, Kadziola Z: A comparative double-blind, randomized trial of a new second generation LMWH (bemiparin) and UFH in the prevention of post-operative venous thromboembolism. The Bemiparin Assessment group. Thromb Haemost 83:523, 2000.

Krasnik M, Thiis J, Frimodt-Moller N: Antibiotic prophylaxis in noncardiac thoracic surgery: A double-blind study of penicillin vs. cefuroxime. Scand J Thorac Cardiovasc Surg 25:73, 1991.

Krowka MJ, Pairolero PC, Trastek VF et al: Cardiac dysrhythmia following pneumonectomy. Chest 91:490, 1987.

Kutlu CA, Williams EA, Evans TW et al: Acute lung injury and acute respiratory distress syndrome after pulmonary resection. Ann Thorac Surg 69:376, 2000.

Lesser BA, Leeper KV, Stein PD et al: The diagnosis of acute pulmonary embolism in patients with chronic obstructive pulmonary disease. Chest 102:17, 1992.

Levin PD, Faber LP, Carleton RA: Cardiac herniation after pneumonectomy. J Thorac Cardiovasc Surg 61:104, 1971.

Mahon SV, Berry PD, Jackson M: Thoracic epidural infusions for post-thoracotomy pain: A comparison of fentanyl-bupivacaine mixtures versus fentanyl alone. Anaesthesia 544:641, 1999.

Martin DE, Krammerer WS: Hypertensive surgical patient. Surg Clin North Am 63:1017, 1983.

Mentzer SJ, Swanson SJ: Treatment of patients with lung cancer and severe emphysema. Chest (Suppl 6) 116:477S, 1999.

Miller JI: Empyema thoracis (editorial comment). Ann Thorac Surg 50:343, 1990.

Motta G, Ratto GB: Complications of surgery in the treatment of lung cancer: Their relationship with the extent of resection and preoperative respiratory function tests. Acta Chir Belg 89:161, 1989.

Mowry FM, Reynolds EW: Cardiac rhythm disturbances complicating resectional surgery of the lung. Ann Intern Med 61:688, 1964.

Multicenter Postinfarction Research Group: Risk stratification and survival after myocardial infarction. N Engl J Med 309:331, 1983.

Nagasaki F, Flehinger BJ, Martini N: Complications of surgery in the treatment of carcinoma of the lung. Chest 82:25, 1982.

Nakahara K, Ohno K, Hashimoto J: Prediction of postoperative respiratory failure in patients undergoing lung resection for lung cancer. Ann Thorac Surg 46:549, 1988.

Nelson S: Minitracheostomy: The benefits for patient care. Br J Nurs 1:492, 1992.

Obata H, Saito S, Fugita N et al: Epidural block with mepivacaine before surgery reduces long-term post-thoracotomy pain. Can J Anaesth 46:1127, 1999.

Oliaro A, Leo F, Filosso PL et al: Resection for bronchogenic carcinoma in the elderly. J Cardiovasc Surg (Torino) 40:715, 1999.

Olsen GN, Bolton JW, Weiman DS, Hornung CA: Stair climbing as an exercise test to predict the postoperative complications of lung resection: Two years' experience. Chest 99:587, 1991.

Pairolero PC, Arnold PG, Trastek VF et al: Postpneumonectomy empyema: The role of intrathoracic muscle transposition. J Thorac Cardiovas Surg 99:958, 1990.

Pairolero PC, Trastek VF, Allen MS: Empyema and bronchiopleural fistula. Ann Thorac Surg 51:157, 1991.

Panos A, Demajo W, Todd TR: High frequency jet ventilation in the management of bronchopleural fistula (BPF). Chest 89 (suppl):521S, 1986.

Papadakis MA, Wall SD: Failure to recognize late postpneumonectomy empyema. Role of diagnostic thoracentesis. West J Med 153:313, 1990.

Papsin BC, Gorenstein LA, Goldberg M: Delayed myocardial laceration after intrapericardial pneumonectomy. Ann Thorac Surg 55:756, 1993.

Peters RM: Empyema thoracis: Historical perspective (see comments). Ann Thorac Surg 48:306, 1989.

Pool EH, Garlock JH: A treatment of persistent bronchial fistula: An experimental and clinical study. Ann Surg 90:213, 1929.

Postmus PE, Kerstjens JM, de Boer WJ et al: Treatment of postpneumonectomy pleural empyema by open window thoracostomy. Eur Respir J 2:853, 1989.

Prys-Roberts C, Meioche R, Foex P: Studies of anaesthesia in relation to hypertension: Cardiovascular responses of treated and untreated patients. Br J Anaesth 43:122, 1971.

Rasch DK, Grover FL, Schnapf BM et al: Right pneumonectomy syndrome in infancy treated with an expandable prosthesis. Ann Thorac Surg 50:127, 1990.

Rendina EA, Venuta F, De Giacomo T et al: Sleeve resection and prosthetic reconstruction of the pulmonary artery for lung cancer. Ann Thorac Surg 68:995, 1999.

Richardson J, Sabanathan S, Jones J et al: A prospective, randomized comparison of preoperative and continuous balanced epidural or paravertebral bupivacaine on post-thoracotomy pain, pulmonary function and stress responses. Br J Anaesth 83:387, 1999.

Ritchie AJ, Danton M, Gibbons JR: Prophylactic digitalisation in pulmonary surgery. Thorax 47:41, 1992.

Rogiers P, Van Miegham W, Engelaar D, Demedts M: Late-onset postpneumonectomy empyema manifesting as tracheal stenosis with respiratory failure. Respir Med 85:333, 1991a.

Rogiers P, Verschakelen J, Knockaert D, Vanneste S: Occult tuberculous postpneumonectomy space empyema four years after lung resection. Postgrad Med J 67:672, 1991b.

Sackner MA, Landa J, Hirsh J: Pulmonary effects of oxygen breathing—a 6 hour study in normal men. Ann Intern Med 82:40, 1976.

Shamji FM, Deslauriers J, Daniel TM, Matzinger F et al: Post-pneumonectomy syndrome with ipsilateral aortic arch following left pneumonectomy. Ann Thorac Surg 62:1627, 1996.

Shamji FM, Ginsberg RJ, Cooper JD et al: Open window thoracostomy in the management of postpneumonectomy empyema with or without bronchopleural fistula. J Thorac Cardiovasc Surg 86:818, 1983.

Shastri KA, Spaulding MB: Late onset of postpneumonectomy empyema. N Y J Med 89:582, 1989.

Shenstone NS: The use of intercostal muscle in the closure of bronchial fistulae. Ann Surg 104:560, 1936.

Shepard JO, Grillo HC, McLoud TC et al: Right pneumonectomy syndrome: Radiologic findings and CT correlation. Radiology 161:661, 1986.

Shields TW, Ujiki GT: Digitalization for prevention of arrhythmias following pulmonary surgery. Surg Gynecol Obstet 126:743, 1968.

Shirakusa T, Ueda H, Takata S et al: Use of pedicled omental flap in treatment of empyema. Ann Thorac Surg 50:420, 1990.

Simone C, Miller JD, Higgins D: Unilateral lung volume reduction in preparation for contralateral pneumonectomy. Can Respir J 6:102, 1999.

Sinjan EA, Van Schil PE, Ortmanns P et al: Improved ventilatory function after combined operation for pulmonary emphysema and lung cancer. Int Surg 84:185, 1999.

Sirois T, Salo J, Perhoniemi V, Mattila S: Surgery for lung cancer in the elderly. Scand Cardiovasc J 33:222, 1999.

Stafford EG, Clagett OT: Postpneumonectomy empyema: Neomycin instillation and definitive closure. J Thorac Cardiovasc Surg 63:771, 1972.

Stiller KR, Munday RM: Chest physiotherapy for the surgical patient. Br J Surg 79:745, 1992.

Takita H, Majares WS: Herniation of the heart following intrapericardial pneumonectomy: Report of a case and review. J Thorac Cardiovasc Surg 59:443, 1970.

Tedder M, Anstadt MP, Tedder SD, Lowe JE: Current morbidity, mortality, and survival after brochoplastic procedures for malignancy. Ann Thorac Surg 54:387, 1992.

Van Raemdonck D, Kesteman J, Roekaerts F, Jadoul P: Treatment of postpneumonectomy empyema with or without bronchopleural fistula. Acta Chir Belg 90:50, 1990.

Vester SR, Faber LP, Kittle CF et al: Bronchopleural fistula after stapled closure of bronchus. Ann Thorac Surg 52:1253, 1991.

Veterans Affairs Total Parenteral Nutrition Cooperative Study Group: Perioperative total parenteral nutrition in surgical patients. N Engl J Med 325:525, 1991.

Von Knorring J, Lepantalo M, Lindgren L, Lindfors O: Cardiac arrhythmias and myocardial ischemia after thoracotomy for lung cancer. Ann Thorac Surg 53:642, 1992.

Wahi R, McMurtrey MJ, DeCaro LF et al: Determinants of perioperative morbidity and mortality after pneumonectomy. Ann Thorac Surg 48:33, 1989.

Waller DA, Gebitekin C, Saunders MR, Walker DR: Noncardiogenic pulmonary edema complicating lung resection. Ann Thorac Surg 55:140, 1993.

Wangensteen OH: The pedicled muscle flap in the closure of persistent bronchopleural fistula. J Thorac Surg 5:27, 1935.

Wertzel H, Swoboda L, Joos-Wurtomberger A et al: Perioperative antibiotic prophylaxis in general thoracic surgery. Thorac Cardiovasc Surg 40:326, 1992.

Yacoub MH, Williams WG, Ahmad A: Strangulation of the heart following intrapericardial pneumonectomy. Thorax. 23:261, 1968.

Ziomek S, Read RC, Tobler G et al: Thromboembolism in patients undergoing thoracotomy. Ann Thorac Surg 56:223, 1993.

CHAPTER **10**

Mechanical Ventilatory Assistance

Akhil Bidani
Divina M. Tuazon
Scott K. Alpard
Joseph B. Zwischenberger

Ventilatory assistance of the critically ill patient and those requiring short-term ventilatory support (as during surgical procedures) has undergone a tremendous change over the past 3 decades. Attendant on an increased understanding of respiratory pathophysiology and an explosive growth in respiratory care specialists and microprocessor technology, several alternative methods of ventilatory support have been developed in an effort to decrease complications, minimize patient work of breathing, and improve patient outcomes. Because of the bewildering number of options available to the physician, understanding the basic principles, advantages, and disadvantages associated with each choice of ventilatory support is mandatory. In this chapter, we briefly review the goals and indications of ventilatory assistance. This is followed by a discussion of the options and modes of ventilatory assistance and monitoring during ventilatory support. Complications of ventilatory assistance are discussed, as well as approaches to weaning from ventilatory support. We assume the reader is familiar with basic pulmonary physiology.

GOALS OF VENTILATORY ASSISTANCE

The primary goal of mechanical ventilatory support is to provide adequate pulmonary gas exchange. The need for mechanical ventilatory support may be manifested by primary CO_2 retention (ventilatory failure), inadequate arterial oxygenation (oxygenation failure), or a combination of both. Secondary goals of mechanical ventilatory assistance are: (1) support of fatigued ventilatory muscles and provision of lung rest; (2) avoidance of complications associated with positive-pressure ventilation; and (3) promotion of lung healing by minimizing ventilator-associated lung injury through restoration of alveolar patency and improved ventilation-perfusion ($\dot{V}/\dot{Q}$) relationships, thereby obviating the need for high concentrations of supplemental oxygen, which may induce a secondary oxidant-induced lung injury. The need for and type of mechanical ventilatory support in a particular patient depends on the mechanism (Fig. 10–1), severity, and expected duration of the respiratory failure. Additionally, a history of cardiopulmonary problems and the specific clinical objectives of the individual patient are important in determining the type and level of mechanical ventilatory support. Ventilatory support for acute respiratory failure has been viewed largely as supportive but is becoming increasingly recognized as appropriate management for the patient-ventilator system with a positive effect on patient outcome. The overall goals of mechanical ventilatory assistance are summarized in Table 10–1 (AARC, 1992; Hinson and Marini, 1992; Pierson, 1983; Tobin, 1994; Tobin and Danzker, 1988; Vanderwarf, 1999).

The spontaneously breathing individual has an intact ventilatory control system, including feedback from peripheral and central chemoreceptors and mechanoreceptors from the lung and chest wall. These provide input to the central integrator-controller, which generates neural output at an appropriate frequency to signal inspiratory effort and generate negative intrathoracic pressure that allows inspiratory flow into the lungs. Exhalation occurs when the ventilatory control system signals relaxation of the inspiratory muscles (with or without active exhalation of the expiratory muscles). The relative amounts of time spent during inspiration and expiration are determined by the magnitude of the respiratory drive and interactions among stimuli received from other receptors.

TABLE 10–1 ■ **Goals of Mechanical Ventilatory Assistance**

Improvement in pulmonary gas exchange
Reverse hypoxemia (optimize $\dot{V}/\dot{Q}$)
Reverse acute respiratory acidosis
Relieve respiratory distress
Decrease work of breathing
Reverse respiratory muscle fatigue
Alter pressure-volume relationship
Prevent and reverse alveolar atelectasis
Improve pulmonary/thoracic compliance
Avoid further lung injury
Avoid complications

$\dot{V}/\dot{Q}$, ventilation-perfusion ratio.

Adapted from Tobin MT: Mechanical ventilation. N Engl J Med 330:1056, 1994. Reprinted, by permission, from the New England Journal of Medicine.

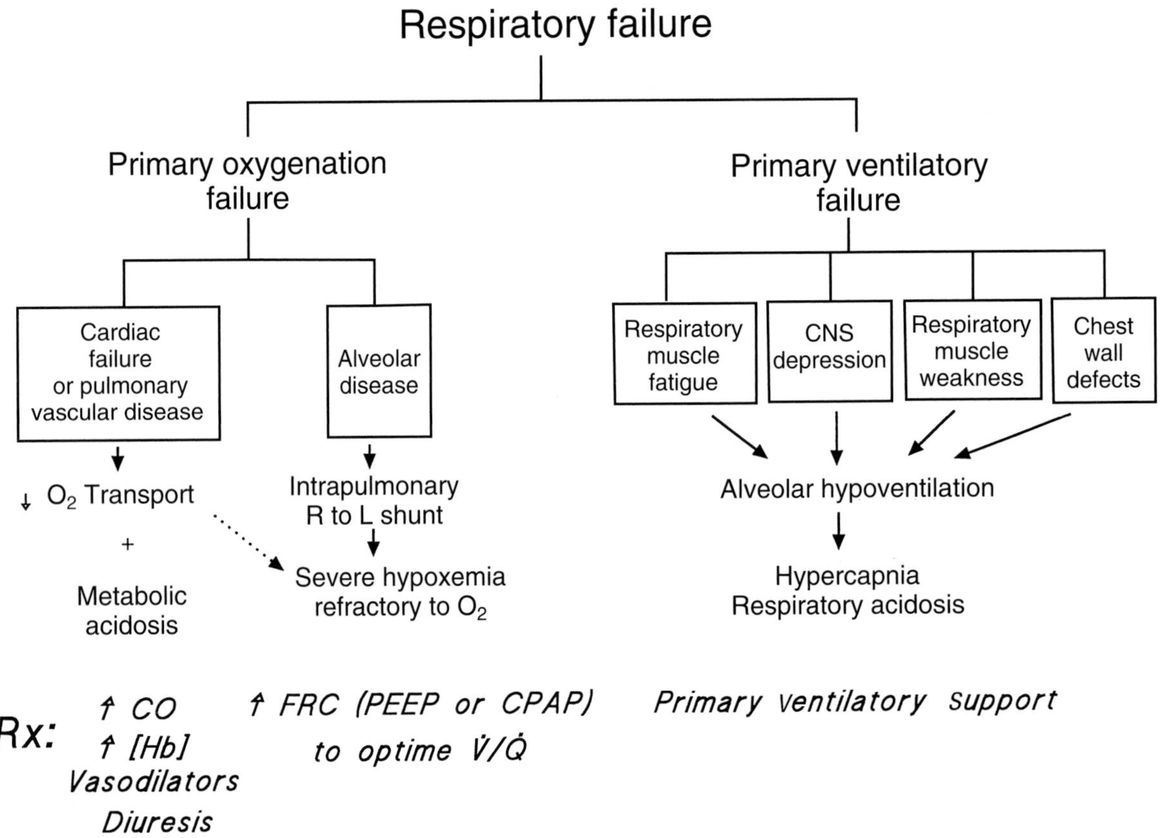

FIGURE 10–1 ■ Modalities of respiratory failure. (CPAP, continuous positive airway pressure; PEEP, positive end-expiratory pressure.)

In contrast, in the patient receiving ventilatory support, the vital role of feedback to the ventilatory control system is supplanted by the open-loop, physician-dependent ventilatory settings of different aspects of the "supported breath," among which are the tidal volume (VT), respiratory rate, magnitude and time course of inspiratory flow, and the inspiration-expiration ratio (I/E ratio). In a lung with heterogeneous distribution of "disease," application of positive pressure at the airway opening may cause either alveolar recruitment or alveolar overdistention (Fig. 10–2). Recruitment of collapsed alveoli should improve static lung compliance, decrease shunt fraction, and have minimal effect on cardiac output (Bartlett, 1996). The "normal" regions of the lung, which have the best regional compliance, are most vulnerable to alveolar overdistention, with resulting increase in pulmonary vascular resistance, decrease in cardiac output, and increased dead-space ventilation. Thus, positive-pressure ventilation can have both beneficial and detrimental effects on the diseased lung. Consequently, inappropriate "ventilator settings and management" can create numerous pulmonary and extrapulmonary problems and complications.

INDICATIONS FOR VENTILATORY ASSISTANCE

Ventilatory assistance is a life-saving intervention that allows maintenance of adequate gas exchange during acute conditions. By improving gas exchange and relieving respiratory distress, ventilatory support can help the patient overcome an episode of acute lung injury, and provide opportunity for the lungs to heal. Although frequently life-saving, ventilatory assistance is also associated with numerous complications. Accordingly, ventilator settings require repeated adjustment to minimize the risk of such complications, and every effort should be made to wean the patient from ventilatory assistance at the earliest time. When executed judiciously, ventilatory assistance can come close to replacing the normal functions of the lungs and chest bellows, and can support gas exchange and lung inflation in a reasonably normal fashion.

Inadequate Alveolar Ventilation

The adequacy of alveolar ventilation is reflected by the arterial blood P_{CO_2} (Pa_{CO_2}). An elevated Pa_{CO_2} indicates alveolar hypoventilation (see Fig. 10–1). When alveolar hypoventilation occurs rapidly enough to produce a significant respiratory acidosis, acute ventilatory failure is present. On the other hand, long-standing or slowly developing alveolar hypoventilation will manifest as a chronic compensated respiratory acidosis (chronic ventilatory failure) that can be well tolerated and in and of itself does not necessitate ventilatory assistance, unless the patient's mental status declines. When CO_2 retention develops slowly, how far must the arterial pH (pHa) fall to justify the institution of ventilatory assistance? There

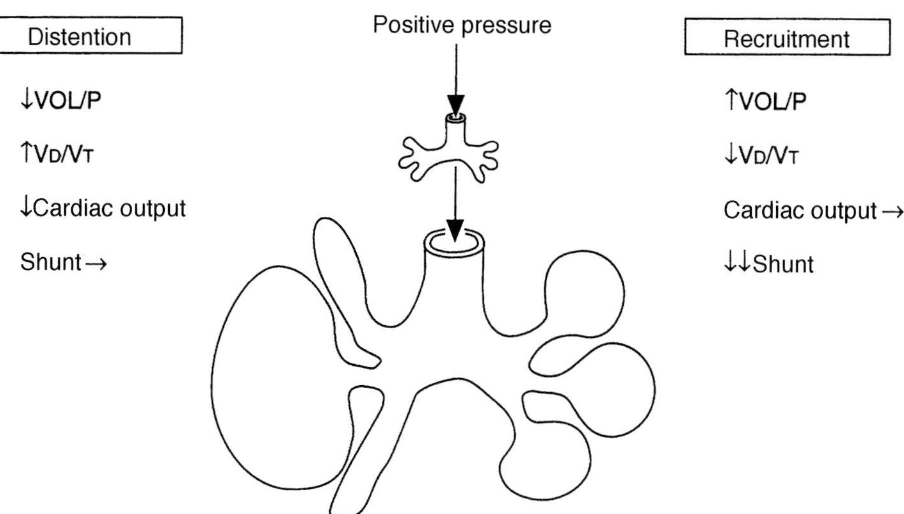

FIGURE 10–2 ■ Positive airway pressure may result in either alveolar recruitment or alveolar overdistention. Alveolar recruitment opens up collapsed alveoli resulting in increased static compliance, decreased intrapulmonary shunt, and no decrement in cardiac output. Alveolar overdistention can increase pulmonary vascular resistance, decrease cardiac output, and increase dead-space ventilation. (From Bartlett RH: Respiratory physiology and pathophysiology. In Bartlett RH [ed]: Critical Care Physiology. Boston, Little, Brown, 1996.)

is no definite answer to this question, but a pHa of less than 7.30 may be an appropriate cut-off value. This is based, in part, on a study by Zwillich and associates (1974) that indicated higher morbidity and mortality in patients with a pHa of less than 7.30. Although pHa is a more accurate indicator of acute ventilatory failure than is Pa_{CO_2}, trends in Pa_{CO_2} and pHa may be equally important. Worsening acute respiratory acidosis over minutes or hours, particularly in the face of intensive therapy, should be an indication for ventilatory assistance, irrespective of the actual value of pHa. Patients with alveolar hypoventilation and respiratory acidosis should be in a monitored environment so that ventilatory assistance can be provided emergently prior to hemodynamic compromise.

Diminished or Unstable Ventilatory Drive

Diminished ventilatory drive in relation to metabolic needs is manifested by a decreased respiratory rate or even apnea. It is an independent indication for ventilatory assistance if its cause cannot immediately be reversed. Although hypoxic or hypercapnic drive cannot be readily measured at the bedside, the finding of respiratory acidosis in the absence of airway or neuromuscular disease suggests that one or both of these may be impaired (see Fig. 10–1). Additionally, a risk exists for sudden apnea or life-threatening hypoventilation in the initial hours following closed-head injury, drug overdose, or massive cerebrovascular accident. Therefore, ventilatory support can be appropriate in such circumstances, even in the absence of hypercapnia.

Severe Hypoxemia

Hypoxemia of mild to moderate severity can usually be managed by the administration of supplemental oxygen via a face mask. With more severe hypoxemia, usually secondary to right-to-left shunting of blood flow, very severe $\dot{V}/\dot{Q}$ mismatching, or markedly reduced mixed venous P_{O_2} (see Fig. 10–1), it may be difficult to restore arterial P_{O_2} to 60 mm Hg with supplemental oxygen via a face mask. Mechanical ventilatory assistance in these patients improves oxygenation by at least three mechanisms: (1) delivery of a high fractional inspired O_2 to the airway; (2) decreased work of breathing; and (3) use of positive end-expiratory pressure (PEEP), which allows recruitment of collapsed alveolar units, thereby improving $\dot{V}/\dot{Q}$ matching. The severity of hypoxemia, although not specific to the need for ventilatory assistance, may serve as a reasonable index of the severity of the patient's illness. The severity of hypoxemia can be assessed by several calculated indices. Among these are the Pa_{O_2}/F_{IO_2} ratio and the a/A ratio (Pa_{O_2}/PA_{O_2}). A patient with a Pa_{O_2} of 90 mm Hg while breathing 30% F_{IO_2} would have a Pa_{O_2}/F_{IO_2} of 300. However, none of these quantitative measures of hypoxemia has been prospectively evaluated as an independent criterion for the institution of ventilatory assistance (Tobin, 1994).

Inadequate Lung Expansion

Inadequate lung expansion during acute illness may lead to the development of atelectasis or pneumonia, even if alveolar ventilation is adequate as assessed by Pa_{CO_2}. Inadequate lung expansion may occur during general anesthesia, after upper abdominal surgery, following trauma, or in the setting of acute restrictive pulmonary disease. Spontaneous vital capacity (VC) is probably the most practical method of assessment. Rapid shallow breathing, as commonly assessed by the ratio of spontaneous respiratory rate to spontaneous VT during assessment for weaning (see later), is also a good indicator of inadequate pulmonary expansion (Tobin and Yang, 1990).

Inadequate Ventilatory Muscle Function

Inadequate ventilatory muscle function can lead to inadequate lung expansion, loss of lung compliance, atelectasis, and pneumonia. When severe, this may lead to inadequate alveolar ventilation. Maximum voluntary ventilation is a useful measure of ventilatory muscle function, although VC and maximum inspiratory pressure

(PImax) are more readily assessed. Sequential determinations of these functions can be extremely helpful in following the progression of ventilatory muscle weakness in acute neuromuscular disorders such as Guillain-Barré syndrome. In this setting, it is prudent to initiate ventilatory assistance when the VC falls to 10 to 15 ml/kg, or the PImax falls to 20 to 25 cm H_2O, rather than waiting for acute respiratory acidosis to develop (Tobin, 1994).

Excessive Work of Breathing

Excessive work of breathing is manifested by rapid shallow breathing. A respiratory rate in the mid-30s per minute or higher in an acutely ill patient suggests that the work of breathing may exceed that which can be sustained by the patient (Tobin, 1994). Although otherwise healthy individuals can maintain a minute ventilation ($\dot{V}E$) twice that of normal indefinitely, when resting ventilation required to maintain a normal $Paco_2$ exceeds 10 to 15 L/min in the setting of severe acute illness or underlying pulmonary disease, acute respiratory acidosis or inadequate lung expansion is likely to develop. The $\dot{V}E$ required to maintain a normal $Paco_2$ is determined by CO_2 production, which reflects metabolic needs, and dead-space ventilation, and is an index of the efficiency of ventilation. Although these factors are rarely measured directly in patients who are not already intubated, consideration should be given to factors that might be expected to increase one or both of them in the acutely ill patient.

DETERMINANTS OF VENTILATOR-INITIATED BREATH

Ventilatory modes are defined by inspiratory events or phase variables (ACCP, 1993; Bersten and Oh, 1997; Chatburn, 1994; Hubmayr, 1994; Pierson, 1999; Pilbeam, 1997; Sassoon, 1992). The physical principles underlying the different breath types and ventilatory modes are discussed in the following paragraphs.

Breath Duration and Type

Each breath is composed of four phases: (1) inspiratory phase; (2) change from inspiration to expiration; (3) expiratory phase; and (4) change from expiration to inspiration. In order to appreciate the differences among these alternative breaths and phases of each breath, one must understand the concepts of control variables and phase variables. A *control variable* is the variable that the ventilator manipulates to initiate inspiration. Specific control variables are pressure, volume, flow, and time. *Phase variables* are used to initiate some phase of each ventilatory cycle. Specifically, these are trigger, limit, and cycle. The trigger variable causes inspiration to begin. The limit variable is the pressure, flow, or volume target that cannot be exceeded during inspiration. When the limit variable (i.e., the target) is reached, inspiration is terminated. The cycle variable is the pressure, volume, flow, or time that terminates inspiration. The various modes of mechanical ventilation refer to different patterns of control variables and phase variables. Depending on the distribution of the workload between the patient and the ventilator, four clinically different breath types can be provided during mechanical ventilation: (1) mandatory; (2) assisted; (3) supported; and (4) spontaneous.

A *mandatory breath* is triggered, limited, and cycled off by the machine, which does all the ventilatory work. An *assisted breath* is triggered by the patient, and limited and cycled off by the machine. The patient does the work of initiating the breath only, while the ventilator does the rest. A *supported breath* is triggered by the patient, limited by the ventilator, and cycled off by the patient. The patient does the work of initiating the breath and then interacts with the ventilator to perform a variable amount of the remaining work. A *spontaneous breath* is triggered, limited, and cycled off by the patient, who performs all of the ventilatory work.

Initiation (Trigger). A ventilator breath may be initiated by the machine (machine-triggered, controlled breath) or by the patient (patient-triggered, assisted breath). In a controlled breath, inspiration is triggered at a time set by the ventilator, regardless of the patient's effort and respiratory cycle. In an assisted breath, inspiration is triggered when the patient generates a negative airway pressure below a preset threshold (usually -2 cm H_2O), called the "sensitivity." The ventilator rate is dependent on the patient rate, unless efforts are too feeble to reach the sensitivity threshold.

Limit (Target). The limit, or target, for each breath defines the primary ventilator mode and is either a preset VT, or preset airway pressure. In the volume-limited mode, the ventilator delivers a set flow for a set time, until the preset VT is achieved. The peak airway pressure that results is variable and depends on the peak flow rate, tubing and airway resistance, and lung and chest wall compliance. In the pressure-limited mode, the ventilator delivers a variable (often decelerating) flow to maintain the preset airway pressure limit. The VT that results is variable, and depends on the peak flow rate, tubing and airway resistance, and lung and chest wall compliance. In the case of pressure-supported ventilation (PSV), the VT also depends on patient effort.

Cycle Off. The phase variable used by the ventilator to cycle from inspiration to expiration defines the cycle off function. This can be VT, airway pressure, elapsed time, or inspiratory flow rate. The breath may be cycled off to expiration as soon as the preset VT or airway pressure has been achieved (volume-cycled, pressure-cycled). The inspiratory time can be prolonged by the addition of a phase of zero flow, called an "inspiratory pause," and the breath cycles off once the predetermined time has elapsed (time-cycled), as in pressure-controlled ventilation (PCV). The breath may cycle off to expiration when the patient's inspiratory flow rate declines to about 25% of the peak flow rate (flow-cycled), as in PSV.

OPTIONS IN VENTILATORY ASSISTANCE

Invasive Versus Noninvasive Ventilatory Assistance

Ventilatory assistance may be provided invasively, that is, via an artificial airway (invasive ventilatory assistance

[IVA]) or via the use of tight-fitting nasal or facial masks (noninvasive positive-pressure ventilatory assistance [NIPPVA]). Because of the unique aspects of non-invasive ventilatory assistance (NIVA), we reserve discussion of this option to the end of this chapter.

Negative Versus Positive Pressure

To accomplish ventilation, a pressure difference must be phasically applied across the lung. This pressure gradient may be generated by negative pressure in the pleural space or by positive pressure applied to the airway opening, or a combination of both (Pierson, 1999). In recent years, powerful negative pressure units have become available that allow phasic tidal pressure swings and are capable of increasing resting lung volume by sustaining a negative pressure gradient, as well as vibrating the chest wall and air column to improve gas exchange and secretion clearance (Levine et al, 1990). If perfected, such devices could see increased use in the intensive care unit (ICU) setting. For now, most ventilatory assistance is provided via positive pressure ventilators.

Pressure Versus Volume-Targeted Ventilation

The fundamental difference between pressure and volume-targeted ventilation is implicit in their names: pressure-targeted modes guarantee pressure at the expense of allowing variable V_T, whereas volume-targeted modes guarantee flow (and consequently the volume provided to the circuit in the allowed inspiratory time) at the expense of allowing airway pressure to vary with changes in airway impedance (AARC, 1992). In a well-monitored patient, pressure-targeted and volume-targeted modes can be used with virtually identical effects. If pressure control is used, the targeted inspiratory pressure (above PEEP) and the inspiratory time must be selected (usually with consideration of the desired V_T). If volume-cycled ventilation is used, one may select (depending on the ventilator) either V_T and flow delivery pattern (waveform and peak flow) or flow delivery pattern and minimum $\dot{V}_E$.

Volume-targeted modes provide a preset volume unless a specified pressure limit is exceeded. Major advantages with volume-targeted ventilation are the capacity to deliver a fixed V_T (except in the presence of a gas leak), the flexibility of flow and volume adjustments, and adequate power to ventilate difficult patients (Hess and Kacmarek, 1996; Pierson, 1999). All ventilators currently used for continuous support in adults offer volume cycling as a primary option. Despite its advantages for acute care, it should be noted that volume cycling also suffers from some important disadvantages. Volume-cycled modes cannot ventilate effectively and consistently unless the airway is well sealed. Furthermore, once the inspiratory flow rate is set, the inflation time of the machine is fixed and remains unresponsive to the patient's native cycling rhythm. Perhaps most important, excessive alveolar pressure may be required to deliver the desired V_T with changes in the patient's airway resistance or lung compliance (C_L). With volume-targeted modes, if the patient's lungs get stiffer, the V_T and overall ventilation stay the same while the airway pressures go up, increasing the likelihood of ventilator-induced lung injury, overt barotrauma, and compromised cardiac function. With pressure-targeted modes, if the overall compliance of the system decreases (say, with the onset of pulmonary edema), peak airway pressure would stay the same while the delivered V_T would decrease, thus worsening respiratory acidosis, atelectasis, and gas exchange.

MODES OF VENTILATORY ASSISTANCE

A classification of common ventilator modes (AARC, 1995; Del Valle and Hecker, 1995; Hubmayr, 1994; MacIntyre, 1988; Marini, 1993; Nahum and Marini, 1996; Pierson, 1999; Sassoon et al, 1990; Sassoon, 1991; Tobin and Danzker, 1988) is provided in Table 10–2. These are divided into volume-targeted and pressure-targeted modes (Figs. 10–3 and 10–4).

Volume-Targeted Modes

Volume-Controlled Ventilation (VCV) or Controlled Mechanical Ventilation (CMV). All breaths are initiated at a set time (machine-triggered, controlled breaths) and delivered with a preset flow pattern to achieve a set V_T (volume-limited). The ventilator cycles off to expiration once the V_T has been delivered (volume-cycled), unless an inspiratory pause is added for a predetermined time

TABLE 10–2 ■ **Modes of Mechanical Ventilation**

Ventilatory Mode	*Breath Type*	*Initiation*	*Cycle off*
Volume-Targeted			
Volume-controlled ventilation	Mandatory	Time	Volume, time
Volume-assisted ventilation	Assisted	Patient	Volume, time
Volume assist-control ventilation	Assisted/mandatory	Patient/time	Volume, time
Intermittent mandatory ventilation	Spontaneous/mandatory	Time	Volume, time
Synchronized intermittent mandatory ventilation	Spontaneous/mandatory	Patient/time	Volume, time
Pressure-Targeted			
Pressure support ventilation	Supported	Patient	Flow
Pressure control ventilation	Mandatory	Time	Time
Pressure assist-control ventilation	Assisted/mandatory	Patient/time	Time

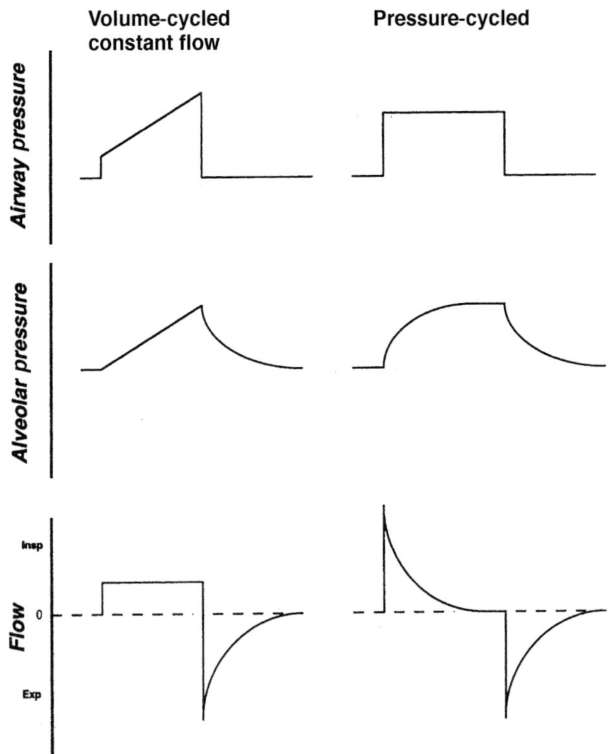

FIGURE 10–3 ■ Idealized airway pressure, alveolar pressure, and flow tracings during volume-cycled ventilation (with constant inspiratory flow) and pressure-cycled ventilation. (From Marcy TW, Marini JJ: Control mode ventilation and assist/control ventilation. In Stock MC, Perel A [eds]: Mechanical Ventilatory Support. Philadelphia, Lippincott Williams & Wilkins, 1997.)

(time-cycled). V̇E is determined solely by the ventilator. The airway pressure alarm limit is usually set at 60 cm H_2O. If this pressure is exceeded, which could occur with coughing, bucking, bronchospasm, or stiff lungs, an alarm sounds and the ventilator cycles to expiration without delivering the entire preset VT. VCV is useful in patients who are anesthetized, heavily sedated, paralyzed, or who have severe neuromuscular disorders. This mode completely eliminates the patient's work of breathing.

Volume-Assisted Ventilation (VAV) or Assisted Mechanical Ventilation (AMV). The ventilator delivers a breath when the patient triggers the machine by a spontaneous inspiratory effort, or automatically if the patient fails to make such an effort within a preselected time frame. One sets VT, the backup rate, the sensitivity, and the inspiratory flow rate (IFR). Although VT is set in this mode, the volume delivered to the patient may be markedly decreased in patients with abnormal pulmonary mechanics owing to volume compression in the ventilator tubing (2 to 4 ml may be "lost" for each 1 cm H_2O of airway pressure). All breaths are initiated by patient inspiratory effort above threshold (patient-triggered, assisted breaths). When a breath is triggered, the full preset VT is delivered, that is, the patient cannot breathe spontaneously between machine breaths. The V̇E is determined by the product of the machine-delivered VT and the patient's respiratory rate. Patient work of breathing is greater than with VCV, but is still largely provided by the ventilator. VAV mandates spontaneous ventilation and is contraindicated in patients with heavy sedation, muscle relaxation, or in patients who are too weak to initiate a breath. This mode is dangerous during central hyperventilation. Patients who are very anxious can trigger the ventilator too frequently, leading to an extremely high V̇E with associated acute respiratory alkalosis and arrhythmias.

Volume Assist-Controlled Ventilation (VACV). This mode is also referred to as ACV (Pierson, 1999). VACV is a combination of VAV and VCV. A minimum controlled ventilator rate is set, but patient-triggered breaths are allowed if the spontaneous rate exceeds the controlled rate. This mode can thereby prevent hypoventilation but, like VAV, will exacerbate hyperventilation. Sensitivity to inspiratory effort can be adjusted to require a small or large negative pressure deflection, below the set level of end-expiratory pressure needed to initiate the machine's inspiratory phase. Alternatively, many of the latest-generation machines can be flow-triggered, initiating a cycle when a flow deficit is sensed in the expiratory limb of the circuit relative to the inspiratory limb during the exhalation period. Both may be effective. As a safety mechanism, a "backup rate" is set, so that if the patient does not initiate a breath within the number of seconds dictated by that frequency, a machine cycle is initiated automatically (Marcy and Marini, 1997).

Intermittent Mandatory Ventilation (IMV). The patient receives periodic positive-pressure breaths from the ventilator at a preset volume and rate, but spontaneous breathing is also permitted—unlike the situation with VACV (Sassoon et al, 1994). Spontaneous breathing is usually achieved through the use of a demand valve, which can result in a considerable increase in the work of breathing. This mode is essentially VCV imposed on spontaneous ventilation. At an operator-set frequency (the IMV rate) the ventilator provides a positive-pressure breath to the patient regardless of the phase of the patient's cycle. It is identical to a VCV breath (machine-triggered, volume-limited, volume- or time-cycled). However, an additional circuit provides a continuous gas flow that allows the patient to breathe spontaneously between machine breaths. The total V̇E is the sum of machine V̇E and patient V̇E. The underlying premise of IMV has been that the degree of respiratory muscle rest is proportional to the number of breaths received from the ventilator. However, recent studies show that patients may have difficulty in adapting to the intermittent nature of ventilatory assistance (Tobin, 1994). Instead, respiratory center output appears to be preprogrammed, and it does not adjust to breath-to-breath changes in inspiratory load, which occurs during IMV. Consequently, IMV can contribute to the development of respiratory muscle fatigue (Brochard, 1994; Tobin, 1994).

Synchronous IMV (SIMV). This mode is a modification of IMV in which the patient is allowed to trigger the IMV breath in a manner analogous to VAV (Sassoon et al, 1994). However, if the patient does not breathe within

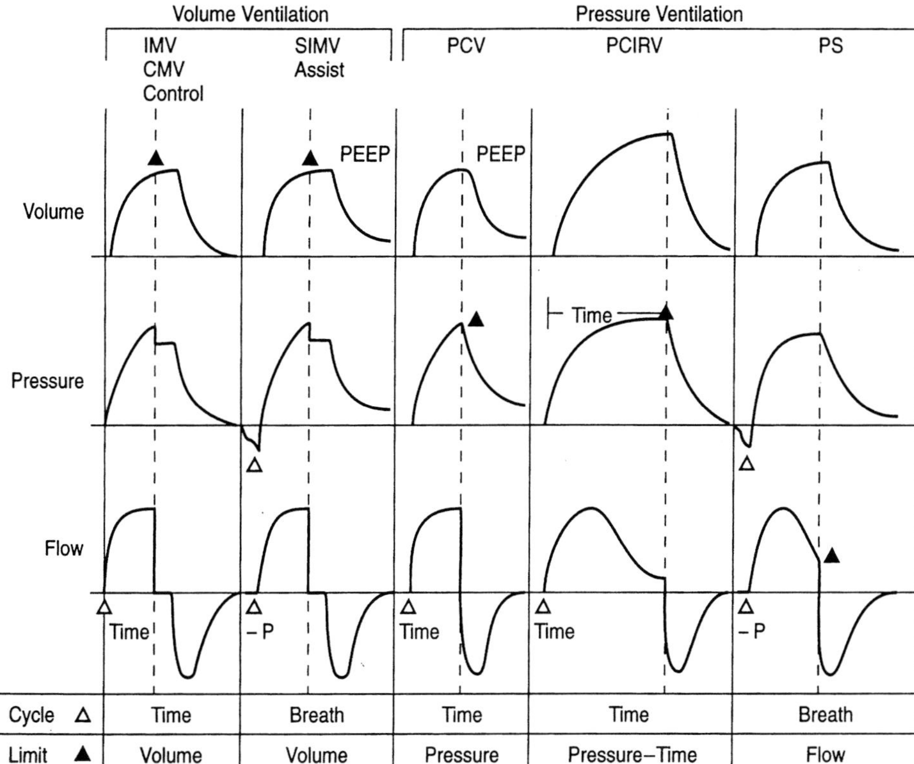

FIGURE 10–4 ■ Patterns of airflow, airway pressure, and lung volume during mechanical ventilation. Gas flow is initiated (cycle △) by either patient effort *(−P)* or set time cycle. Inspiratory flow ceases (limit ▲) when a pre-set volume, pressure, or flow is achieved. (CMV, continuous mechanical ventilation; IMV, intermittent mandatory ventilation; PCIRV, pressure-controlled inverted-ratio ventilation; PCV, premature ventricular contraction; PEEP, positive end-expiratory pressures; PS, pressure support.) (From Bartlett RH: Respiratory physiology and pathophysiology. In Bartlett RH [ed]: Critical Care Physiology. Boston, Little, Brown, 1996.)

an allotted "window" (i.e., 6 seconds if the IMV rate is set at 10 breaths/min), the ventilator delivers a VCV breath. Thus, SIMV may be thought of as VACV superimposed on spontaneous ventilation.

Comparison Between Volume-Targeted Modes

Since the introduction of SIMV to adult ventilation 20 years ago, a debate has raged over whether SIMV or VACV is "better." If the ventilator rate is set high enough that all the patient's ventilation needs are met, and the patient is not dyspneic, then VACV and SIMV are essentially equivalent. The ventilator provides *full ventilatory support* (i.e., it supplies all the energy required to ventilate the lungs). The difference occurs when the patient wants more ventilation than the ventilator provides, either by the backup rate in the VACV mode, or by the "mandatory" rate in the SIMV mode. In VACV, the patient can increase the ventilator's output by triggering breaths more frequently than the set backup rate. Depending on the set triggering sensitivity, the IFR, and other factors, the patient is required to do a variable amount of work to get this extra ventilation. Under ideal circumstances, the patient gives a little "tug," the additional breath is delivered immediately and fast enough to satisfy the patient, and little work is done over and above full ventilatory support. Unfortunately, this is often not the case, and adjusting VACV to maximize patient comfort with continuous triggering is a challenge. With SIMV, when the patient wants more ventilation than that provided by the set volume of mandatory breaths, the patient must take unassisted spontaneous breaths through the ventilator circuit. Because this may require substantial effort, the spontaneous breaths taken by patients on SIMV tend to be small in comparison with the mandatory breaths. A fundamental hypothesis underlying SIMV is that patients *should* do some breathing work to maintain ventilatory muscle tone. After 20 years of experience and dozens of studies, this hypothesis remains unproven, and we still do not know whether it is better for patients' ventilatory muscles to be exercised or rested during mechanical ventilation (Tobin, 1994). However, putting the SIMV hypothesis into full effect means that the mandatory rate should be low so that the patient contributes a substantial portion of the total $\dot{V}_E$. Because initiating spontaneous breaths and breathing through the circuits of some ventilators can be uncomfortable, a number of techniques have been introduced to reduce the effort. These include continuous flow, flow-by, and inspiratory pressure support (see later).

Pressure-Targeted Modes

Pressure-Supported Ventilation (PSV). This mode allows the physician to set a level of pressure to boost each breath (Brochard, 1994). The machine attempts to maintain airway pressure at a preset level until the patient's inspiratory flow rate decreases below a certain threshold value, such as 25% of the peak flow. V_T is determined by the preset level of pressure support, patient effort, and pulmonary mechanics. This mode is a unique, patient-triggered, pressure-limited, flow-cycled mode that can allow close tracking of the patient's ventilatory effort and very precise decremental withdrawal of ventilatory support of the work of breathing. It provides the greatest patient-ventilator interaction of any of the conventionally used ventilatory modes. Once initiated, there is a rapid flow of fresh gas until the airway pressure limit (above baseline PEEP) is achieved. Thereafter, the inspiratory flow adjusts via microprocessor circuitry to keep the airway pressure constant. The patient can continue to inhale actively and increase the delivered VT above that provided by the ventilator alone. When the patient's inspiratory flow rate declines to 25% of the peak flow rate, the ventilator cycles off into expiration. The actual VT delivered for a given level of PSV depends on patient effort, airway resistance, and chest wall and lung compliance.

Advantages of Pressure-Supported Ventilation. PSV combines the power of the machine and that of the patient, providing assistance that ranges from no support at all to fully powered ventilation, depending on the machine-developed pressure relative to patient effort. Because the depth, length, and flow profile of the breath are influenced by the patient, well-adjusted PSV tends to be relatively comfortable for the patient. PSV has its widest application as a weaning mode (Brochard, 1994). Pressure support is also valuable in offsetting the resistive work required to breathe spontaneously through an endotracheal (ET) tube, as during continuous positive airway pressure (CPAP) or SIMV. The pressure support level should be adjusted to maintain an adequate VT at an acceptable frequency (<30 breaths/min). In theory, PSV can provide sufficient power for the entire work of breathing if set to meet or exceed the average inspiratory pressure requirement (Brochard, 1994; Pierson, 1999).

Problems with Pressure-Supported Ventilation. PSV requires the ventilatory cycle to be patient-initiated and cannot adjust itself to changes in the ease of chest inflation. Therefore, PSV is not an ideal mode for patients with unstable ventilatory drive or highly variable thoracic impedance (e.g., bronchospasm, copious secretions, or changing auto-PEEP). Furthermore, because the ability of most ventilator systems to provide a true square-wave of airway pressure tends to deteriorate as ventilatory demands increase, VT resulting from PSV tends to be frequency-dependent. It needs to be emphasized that pressure support is a spontaneous breathing mode: if the patient does not breathe, nothing happens. Pressure support is often combined with SIMV during partial ventilatory support, so that each spontaneous breath receives a positive-pressure assist (Brochard, 1994; Pierson, 1999).

Pressure-Controlled Ventilation. Pressure-controlled is a machine-triggered, pressure-limited, and time-cycled mode intended for patients with acute respiratory failure, severe hypoxemia, and poor lung compliance (Marini, 1994). Immediately after initiation of the breath, fresh gas flow rapidly achieves the preset pressure limit above baseline PEEP. For example, PCV of 25 cm H_2O added to 10 cm H_2O PEEP achieves a peak airway pressure of 35 cm H_2O. Thereafter, flow decelerates to zero with an inspiratory pause that sustains airway pressure at the limit for the defined inspiratory time, when it cycles off. This allows precise definition of inspiratory and expiratory ratios. In PCV, maximal pressure is controlled, but VT is a complex function of applied pressure and its rate of approach to target pressure, available inspiratory time, and the impedance to breathing (compliance, inspiratory and expiratory resistance, and auto-PEEP). Prolongation of inspiratory time such that the I/E ratio is greater than 1:1 is known as pressure-controlled inverse ratio ventilation (PC-IRV) (Marini, 1994).

Advantages of Pressure-Controlled Ventilation. Limiting peak airway pressure may decrease the risk of volutrauma or barotrauma. Precise control of IFR, inspiratory time, and mean airway pressure (Paw) allows IRV, which enhances alveolar inflation, recruitment, and oxygenation, and may decrease the supplemental oxygen requirements. High-flow capacity, pressure-targeted ventilation compensates well for small air leaks and is therefore quite appropriate for use with leaking or uncuffed ET tubes, as in neonatal or pediatric patients. Because of its virtual "unlimited" ability to deliver flow and its decelerating flow profile, pressure-targeted ventilation is also an appropriate choice for spontaneously breathing patients with high inspiratory flow demand, which usually peaks early in the ventilatory cycle. Decelerating flow profiles also tend to improve the distribution of ventilation in a lung with heterogeneous mechanical properties (widely varying time constants) (Marini, 1994; Nahum and Marini, 1996). Apart from their application in limiting the lung's exposure to high airway pressure and barotrauma, pressure-targeted modes can also be helpful in adult patients in whom the airway cannot be completely sealed (e.g., bronchopleural fistula).

Disadvantages of Pressure-Controlled Ventilation. (1) PCV and PC-IRV evoke patient discomfort, and heavy sedation is usually required. (2) Increased Paw may impair cardiac filling, although transmission of high airway pressures to the vasculature may be attenuated by lung stiffness. (3) Inverse I/E ratio may result in inadequate expiratory time, air trapping, breath "stacking," and the development of auto-PEEP (intrinsic PEEP). This in turn may lead to hypercapnia.

Combined Modes

In certain situations it is desirable to adjust midinspiratory flow in response to changing patient needs, or alternatively, to restrict maximal cycling pressure but ensure delivery of a specified VT. As a result of advances in computer microprocessor technology, this has led to "combination modes" (Pierson, 1999).

Pressure-Regulated Volume Control. This mode satisfies a target VT with the least cycling pressure within the predetermined inspiratory time (AARC, 1995). Inflation pressure is continuously regulated in response to changes in inflation impedance so as to satisfy the preset VT. If a satisfactory VT is achieved by spontaneous patient effort, no ventilatory assistance is provided.

Volume Support. In this mode, the flow-cycled pressure support is adjusted (up or down) to achieve the primary target (VE) while guaranteeing a minimum VT (Hess and Kacmarek, 1996). When breathing frequency declines, the $\dot{V}E$ may increase by as much as 50% over a baseline minimum to satisfy the target $\dot{V}E$.

Volume-Assured Pressure Support. In this mode, a fixed level of pressure support is supplemented by gas from a backup source if the PSV is insufficient to meet a target VT (Kacmarek and Hess 1994; Pierson, 1999).

High-Frequency Ventilation

High-frequency ventilation (HFV), 150 to 300 breaths/min, delivers respiratory tidal volumes (1 to 3 ml/kg) averaging significantly less than anatomic dead space. Because of the reduced tidal volumes, peak inspiratory pressures (PIPs) during HFV are less than those in conventional ventilation. High-frequency oscillatory ventilation (HFOV) uses a reciprocating piston, diaphragm, or bellows to generate a sinusoidal respiratory waveform during the breathing cycle. Several randomized studies in neonates have demonstrated a decreased incidence of barotrauma, bronchopulmonary dysplasia (BPD), and decreased need for extracorporeal membrane oxygenation (ECMO) (Clark et al, 1994). Improvements in oxygenation can be attributed to the static inflation (up to 30 cm H_2O). High-frequency jet ventilation (HFJV) consists of the intermittent delivery of gas through a small-bore cannula within the airway in short bursts. Rates are commonly 100 to 200 breaths/min and the expiratory phase of the cycle is entirely passive, dependent on chest wall and lung compliance. The primary use is as a rescue therapy in adults with acute respiratory failure–related hypoxemia in the face of high PEEP or a significant air leak.

VENTILATOR SETTINGS

The initial ventilator settings are estimated on the basis of the patient's size and clinical condition and are generally altered after obtaining arterial blood gases or other laboratory information (Hubmayr, 1994; Kacmarek, 1992; Nahum and Marini, 1996; Pierson, 1999; Tobin and Danzker, 1988; Wood and Hall, 1993). Depending on the stability of the patient's clinical state, the settings should be assessed repeatedly and may require adjustment.

Fractional Inspired Oxygen Concentration

Initially, FIO_2 should be set deliberately on the high side, with later adjustment guided by pulse oximetry or blood gases. Immediately after intubation, for example, it is generally prudent to administer pure oxygen until adequate arterial oxygenation has been confirmed. Many predictive equations have been created to aid in the selection of a satisfactory FIO_2, but none is sufficiently accurate to substitute for a trial-and-error approach (Tobin, 1994). The risk of oxygen toxicity is minimized by using the lowest FIO_2 with which satisfactory arterial oxygenation is achieved. The usual goal is a PaO_2 of approximately 60 mm Hg or an arterial oxygen saturation (SaO_2) of 90%, as higher values do not substantially enhance tissue oxygenation. The response to a change in FIO_2 depends on the underlying pathophysiology, because right-to-left shunts do not respond as well to increased FIO_2 as do hypoventilation or $\dot{V}/\dot{Q}$ mismatch (Nelson, 1993). Exposure to an FIO_2 of 100% for up to 24 hours probably does not pose a significant clinical risk, although prolonged exposure to this concentration is clearly toxic (Durbin and Wallace, 1993; Jenkinson, 1993). An FIO_2 of 0.5 is generally considered safe for several weeks if necessary in the management of hypoxemia. For FIO_2 values between 0.5 and 1.0, the duration of safe exposure before the onset of toxicity is unknown, but there is more to fear from severe hypoxemia in critically ill patients than from the potential threat of oxygen toxicity.

Tidal Volume

It had been customary to use tidal volumes that are two to three times higher than normal during mechanical ventilation (10 to 15 ml/kg) (Marini, 1993; Marini and Kelsen, 1992). This approach has been challenged by convincing data in experimental animals showing that alveolar overdistention can produce pulmonary epithelial, endothelial, and basement membrane injuries that are associated with increased microvascular permeability and lung rupture (Dreyfuss et al, 1988; Kacmarek and Chiche, 1998; Parker et al, 1993; Tsuno et al, 1990). Although data are incomplete, there is a growing tendency to use lower tidal volumes, namely, 5 to 7 ml/kg, particularly in acute respiratory distress syndrome (ARDS). Ideally, one would wish to titrate delivered volume based on monitoring of alveolar volume, but this is not feasible. A reasonable substitute is to monitor peak alveolar pressure (Palv), which can be estimated from the plateau in airway pressure; this is measured by briefly occluding the ventilatory circuit at end-inspiration in a relaxed patient. The plateau pressure (P_{plat}) should be maintained at less than 35 cm H_2O (Gattinoni et al, 1994; Marini and Kelsen, 1992). As additional experimental data become available, it is possible that an even lower P_{plat} will be considered a desirable target (Brochard et al, 1998; Hudson, 1998; Kacmarek and Chiche, 1998). The associated reduction in delivered volume can result in an increase in $PaCO_2$; this strategy is called "permissive hypercapnia" or "controlled hypoventilation" (Bidani et al, 1994; Hickling et al, 1994; Tuxen, 1994). When titrating VT, it is important to focus on pHa rather than $PaCO_2$. If pHa decreases below 7.20, one could administer alkaline solutions, such as bicarbonate, but this is of unproven benefit and a subject of controversy (Bidani and DuBose, 1995; Tuxen, 1994). Several uncontrolled studies suggest that controlled hypoventilation results in a lower mortality than does conventional mechanical ventilation in patients with acute severe asthma who require ventilator support (Darioli and Perret, 1984). In recent studies Amato and colleagues (1995, 1998) have reported improved survival in ARDS patients using a "lung-protective" strategy (VT of 6 to 8 ml/kg and adequate PEEP to ensure alveolar recruitment) compared with ARDS patients managed using traditional ventilator management.

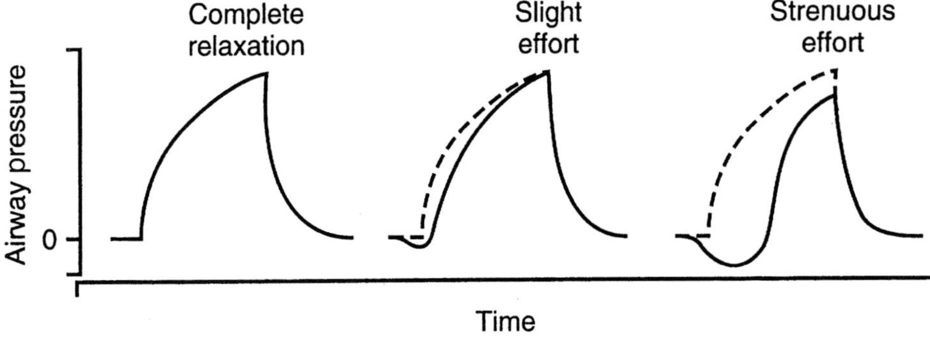

FIGURE 10–5 ■ Airway pressure waveforms during assist-control ventilation (VACV). With no patient effort, a convex inspiratory pattern is present, but with increasing patient inspiratory effort and inadequate inspiratory airflow, a concave pressure waveform is noted. (From Tobin MT: Mechanical ventilation. N Engl J Med 330:1056, 1994.)

Ventilatory Rate

Selection of the ventilatory rate depends on the mode of ventilatory support (Hubmayr, 1994). With VACV, the backup rate should be approximately 4 breaths/min less than the patient's spontaneous rate. This ensures that the ventilatory will supply an adequate volume should the patient have a sudden decrease in respiratory center output. Another reason for this approach is that a substantial difference between the machine backup rate and the patient's spontaneous rate promotes breathing patterns with inverse I/E time ratios, which can be very uncomfortable (Hubmayr, 1994). With IMV, the ventilator rate is usually set at a high initial value (15 to 20 breaths/min) and then reduced in accordance with the patient's tolerance. With PSV, the ventilatory rate is not set.

Sensitivity Setting

Most ventilators are triggered by a change in airway pressure, and sensitivity is usually set at −1 to −2 cm H_2O. However, with poorly responsive demand valves, the actual pressure generated by the patient may be considerably greater (Sassoon, 1992). If the trigger setting is too sensitive, autocycling and severe respiratory alkalosis can occur. Flow triggering is available on some ventilators; this appears to involve less patient work than pressure triggering does (Kacmarek and Hess, 1994). Some patients, especially those with chronic obstructive pulmonary disease (COPD) and a high $\dot{V}_E$, develop gas trapping and have a positive Palv at end-expiration. This auto-PEEP makes ventilator triggering more difficult because the patient needs to generate a negative pressure equal in magnitude to the level of auto-PEEP in addition to the set sensitivity (Hubmayr, 1994). This is one of the factors that may account for the observation of a patient who is unable to trigger the ventilator despite making obvious respiratory efforts (Tobin, 1994).

Inspiratory Flow Rate

Depending on the specific machine, the IFR may be independently adjusted, or is determined by alteration of the V_T, ventilator rate, and the I/E ratio. Generally, an IFR of approximately 60 L/min achieves optimal gas exchange. However, an IFR of 100 L/min is preferred in patients with COPD, probably because the resulting reduction in the I/E ratio, with associated prolongation of expiration, allows regions of air trapping to empty more completely (Connors et al, 1981; Tobin, 1994). If the flow rate is insufficient to meet a patient's ventilatory demands, the patient will pull against his or her own pulmonary impedance and that of the ventilator, with consequent increase in the work of breathing (Tobin, 1994). Examining the contour of the airway pressure waveform is helpful when adjusting the flow rate and trigger sensitivity (Sassoon, 1991). Ideally, the waveform should demonstrate a smooth rise and convex appearance during inspiration. In contrast, a prolonged negative phase with excessive scalloping of the tracing signifies unsatisfactory sensitivity and flow settings (Fig. 10–5) (Marcy and Marini, 1997; Marini et al, 1985; Sassoon, 1991).

Positive End-Expiratory Pressure

No other area of ventilatory management has aroused as much controversy as PEEP, and there is still no consensus on its use (Albert, 1985; Hudson et al, 1988; Kacmarek and Pierson, 1988; Romano, 1985; Rossi and Ranieri, 1994). Some consider PEEP to have no application other than to ameliorate life-threatening hypoxemia and decrease exposure to a potentially toxic F_{IO_2}. In this view, one strives for a satisfactory arterial Pa_{O_2} with the lowest level of PEEP (Albert, 1985; Horton and Cheney, 1975; Suter et al, 1975). Others have been enthusiastic about liberal application of PEEP in most cases of respiratory insufficiency. It had been postulated that early use of PEEP may modify the natural course of acute lung injury or ARDS, and may prevent its development, but this has not been demonstrated in patients at risk for developing ARDS (Pepe et al, 1984). Clearly, PEEP may have both beneficial and detrimental effects based on the clinical setting (Table 10–3). In patients with ARDS, PEEP usually produces a significant improvement in Pa_{O_2}. This is primarily due to a reduction in intrapulmonary shunt as a result of alveolar recruitment of atelectatic regions, and by redistribution of lung water from the alveoli to the perivascular interstitial space (Malo et al, 1984). Provided this improvement in Pa_{O_2} is not offset by a fall in cardiac output, supplemental oxygen requirements can be reduced. This is the major therapeutic effect of PEEP (see Fig. 10–2) (Pepe et al, 1984). The addition of PEEP also influences lung mechanics. Patients with acute lung injury commonly have a decreased end-expiratory lung volume, and, therefore, tidal breathing occurs on the low

TABLE 10–3 ■ **Beneficial and Detrimental Effects of Positive End-Expiratory Pressure**

Beneficial Effects	*Detrimental Effects*
Alveolar recruitment	Alveolar overdistention (barotrauma)
Vascular derecruitment	Depression of cardiac output
Improvement of Pa_{O_2}	Increased intracranial pressure (with high levels of PEEP)
Protection against ventilator-induced lung injury	Decreased renal and portal blood flow (related to decreased cardiac output)
Reduction of inspiratory workload	May increase inspiratory work of breathing
	Worsened hypoxemia (unilateral lung disease)

Pa_{O_2}, partial pressure of arterial oxygen; PEEP, positive end-expiratory pressure.

flat portion of the pressure-volume curve. By shifting tidal breathing to a more compliant portion of the curve, PEEP can decrease the work of breathing, and may prevent phasic alveolar recruitment or derecruitment (Marini, 1993; Marini et al, 1985). In patients with air flow limitation and auto-PEEP who have difficulty in triggering the ventilator, the addition of external PEEP (to a level not exceeding the level of auto-PEEP) can help to counteract this problem, because alveolar pressure needs to be decreased only below the level of external PEEP rather than below zero to trigger the ventilator (Tobin and Lodato, 1989). In addition to the injury induced by high inflation pressures, mechanical ventilation at a low end-expiratory lung volume aggravates lung injury in experimental animals, and probably in humans, owing to shear stresses associated with repeated closing and opening of lung units (Muscedere et al, 1994; Rossi and Ranieri, 1994). There is still some debate as to the level of PEEP required to splint the lung open, but it is most likely 2 cm H_2O above the lower inflexion point, Pflex, on the pressure-volume curve of the respiratory system (Fig. 10–6) (Rossi and Ranieri, 1994).

Institution of PEEP should be done in a systematic manner, with small stepwise increments of 3 to 5 cm H_2O, with evaluation of the response to each change (Rossi and Ranieri, 1994). Several alternative approaches have been suggested to determine the optimal level of PEEP, but none has been shown to be clearly superior (Pepe et al, 1984). The best PEEP is achieved when the FI_{O_2} can be reduced to an acceptable level without compromising tissue oxygen delivery. A methodical approach also is required when PEEP is being reduced or discontinued. Abrupt cessation may produce hypoxemia that takes hours or days to reverse or requires reinstitution of PEEP at a higher level than that used before its suspension (Tobin, 1994; Rossi and Ranieri, 1994).

Patient Positioning

Many diseases affect the lung in a nonhomogeneous manner (Gattinoni et al, 1994; Tobin, 1994). Consequently patient positioning (supine versus prone) can have significant effects on arterial oxygenation (Albert et al, 1987; Flatten et al, 1998). The prone position improves oxygenation in approximately 50% of patients with ARDS (Gattinoni et al, 1994), allowing reduction of FI_{O_2} and PEEP. The likelihood of response to prone positioning is generally higher early in the course of ARDS, and patients may derive benefit only hours after repositioning has occurred. Although the hemodynamic parameters tend to remain unchanged, hypotension, desaturation, and cardiac arrhythmias may occur in the transition from the supine to the prone position. There are unresolved questions about the precise mechanism for improvement in gas exchange in the prone position in patients with ARDS. Animal data obtained by Albert and colleagues (Albert et al, 1987; Lamm et al, 1994) suggest that there is improved perfusion to nondependent regions in the prone position compared with that in the supine position. In a canine model of oleic acid–induced lung injury, the Pa_{O_2} improved from 140 ± 112 mm Hg (FI_{O_2} = 1.0) in the supine position to 453 ± 54 mm Hg in the prone position. Pa_{CO_2} and pHa were unaffected by the position change. Regional $\dot{V}/\dot{Q}$ analysis indicated that the increased Pa_{O_2} was a result of improved dorsal lung ventilation in the prone position, without significant decrease in ventral lung ventilation, while regional perfusion was not markedly altered by the positional change.

COMPLICATIONS OF VENTILATORY ASSISTANCE

A host of complications and other adverse events can occur while patients are receiving ventilatory assistance (Benson and Pierson, 1988; Cullen and Caldera, 1979; Gammon et al, 1995; Pepe and Marini, 1982; Pierson, 1990; Pinsky, 1990; Strieter and Lynch, 1988; Zimmermann et al, 1982). In many instances, the complications are due as much to the underlying illness, its severity, and the intensive care environment as to the mechanical ventilation itself.

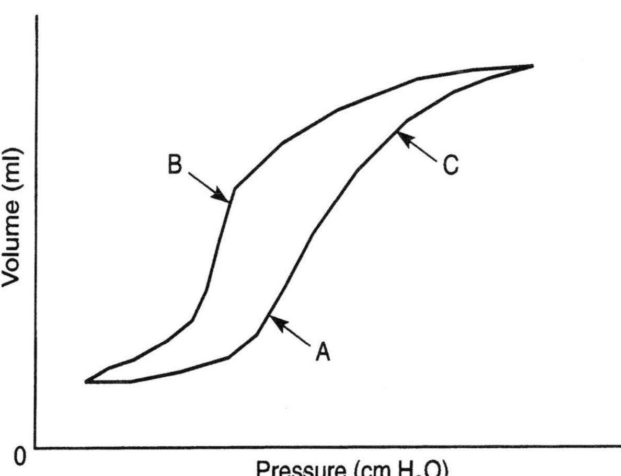

FIGURE 10–6 ■ Schematic representation of pressure-volume curve of a patient with acute respiratory distress syndrome. Point A represents recruitment of collapsed alveoli during *inspiration.* Point C represents alveolar overdistention during *inspiration.* Point B represents corresponding alveolar derecruitment during *expiration.*

Ventilation-Perfusion Mismatch

Positive-pressure ventilation often results in worsening of $\dot{V}/\dot{Q}$ mismatch and may result in impairment of oxygen uptake in the lung (Pierson, 1999). Gravitational forces favor perfusion to the dependent lung zones, but gas delivered by positive-pressure ventilation follows the path of least resistance, so that ventilation is greatest in the nondependent zones (Pierson, 1999). During spontaneous breathing the diaphragm actively ventilates dependent lung zones, but with paralysis and heavy sedation the diaphragm is passively pushed cephalad by the abdominal viscera into the dependent lung zones, further impairing ventilation of these regions (Tobin, 1994).

Impairment of Alveolar Ventilation

High airway pressures (particularly in the presence of hypovolemia) may result in dynamic compression of perfused pulmonary capillaries and thereby convert functioning alveolar-capillary units to physiologic dead space. If $\dot{V}_E$ is fixed, that is, if the patient cannot increase the respiratory rate because of sedation, alveolar ventilation may decrease due to the increased dead space fraction. Therefore, during positive-pressure ventilatory support, intravascular volume needs to be carefully assessed and repleted. Otherwise, increased alveolar dead space can increase the ventilatory requirement, which, if not met, may lead to the development of hypercapnia and respiratory acidosis.

Circulatory Impairment

Increased intrathoracic pressure decreases venous return, cardiac output, and renal blood flow (Pierson, 1990; Strieter and Lynch, 1988; Zimmermann et al, 1982). Measured intravascular pressure (central venous pressure [CVP], pulmonary artery occlusion pressure [PAOP]) and cardiac preload appear to increase, but the effective transmural pressure declines because of the increased intrapleural pressure (Ppl). Circulatory effects are directly proportional to the elevation of intrathoracic pressure, and are exacerbated by hypovolemia (Harken et al, 1974). The adverse circulatory effects of mechanical ventilation are fewer in stiff, noncompliant lungs, which attenuate the transmission of intra-alveolar pressure to the intravascular space. Mean intrathoracic pressures tend to be lower with partial than with full ventilatory support, and the more the patient breathes spontaneously, the less the tendency will be to compromise cardiac output. On the other hand, patients who actively fight the ventilator may experience severe circulatory compromise regardless of ventilator mode. PEEP greater than 10 cm H_2O may compress the pulmonary capillary bed, increase right ventricular afterload and pressure, shift the intraventricular septum, and impede left ventricular filling (Bishop et al, 1991; Jardin et al, 1981; Zimmermann et al, 1982).

Renal and Hepatic Dysfunction

Reductions in portal flow have been associated with the use of PEEP in patients receiving ventilatory assistance, which can potentially lead to hepatic dysfunction (Bennett and Vender, 1997; Pierson, 1990; Strieter and Lynch, 1988). Reductions in renal blood flow have been documented in patients receiving mechanical ventilation and PEEP, particularly in the setting of prolonged respiratory failure (Doherty and Sladen, 1989). It is not clear whether these changes are due primarily to changes in cardiac output (owing to the cardiac effects of positive-pressure ventilation and PEEP).

Intracranial Pressure

ICP may increase, but because cerebrospinal fluid pressure rises equally in the closed cranium, the distending pressure across the brain should not increase (Pierson, 1990). The rise in ICP may be minimized in the head-up position. High intrathoracic pressure may impede venous return from the head and may increase ICP and exacerbate neurologic injury. Increased ICP, again mainly when PEEP is used, can occur as a result of pressure on vertebral and jugular venous systems, and this can impair cerebral perfusion in patients with head injury, causing loss of cerebral autoregulation.

Gastric Distention

Patients receiving mechanical ventilation, particularly those with low lung and chest wall compliance, may develop gastric or intestinal distention with air (Strieter and Lynch, 1988). The mechanism is believed to be due to an air leak around the cuff of the ET tube that can overcome the resistance of the lower esophageal sphincter. This problem can be alleviated by passage of a small-bore nasogastric tube.

Acid-Base Problems

Acid-base disturbances related to suboptimal ventilator adjustment can be clinically important. Prominent among these is acute respiratory alkalosis, usually in patients with underlying chronic ventilatory insufficiency (compensated CO_2 retention). Failure to appreciate a patient's elevated baseline Pa_{CO_2}, and management that results in a "normal" Pa_{CO_2} of 40 mm Hg in such patients, can acutely produce a dangerous, posthypercapnic metabolic alkalosis (often with pHa >7.55) that can cause cardiac arrhythmias and later result in an inability to wean (Pierson, 1999).

Air Trapping, Dynamic Hyperinflation, and Auto-PEEP

Understanding the phenomenon of air trapping, dynamic hyperinflation, and auto-PEEP is central to avoiding complications, performing accurate hemodynamic monitoring, and preventing unnecessary patient discomfort (Benson and Pierson, 1988; Lodato and Tobin, 1991; Pepe and Marini, 1982; Tobin, 1990). In the presence of expiratory air flow obstruction (e.g., in COPD or asthma), or when $\dot{V}_E$ exceeds 15 to 20 L/min, exhalation of a delivered mechanical breath may not be complete by the time the next breath is given (Leatherman, 1996). When this happens, both overall lung volume and *alveolar* pressure remain increased at end-expiration, resulting in the same physiologic effects as with excessive externally applied PEEP (e.g., hyperinflation and decreased cardiac output). Auto-PEEP is common, occurring to some degree in one third or more of all patients with acute respiratory failure, and is physiologically important in perhaps half of these cases (Pepe and Marini, 1982; Pierson, 1999). Auto-PEEP cannot be read from the ventilator's airway pressure manometer during routine operation, and one of several special maneuvers must be performed to detect it. The usual method is via an end-expiratory pause (Fig. 10–7). This permits brief equalization of pressures, from alveolus to central airways, to inspiratory circuit, and allows auto-PEEP to be read on the pressure manometer (see Fig. 10–7). Auto-PEEP cannot conveniently be measured in all clinical circumstances (e.g., patient actively exhaling or continuously triggering in the VACV mode). To reduce auto-PEEP, overall expiratory time must be increased to permit more complete exhalation. Airway obstruction (by bronchospasm or secretions) should be treated aggressively. Two other maneuvers to increase expiratory time, regardless of the ventilator mode, are to increase inspiratory flow rate (e.g., to 80 L/min) and to use a low-compressible-volume ventilator circuit (Tobin, 1994).

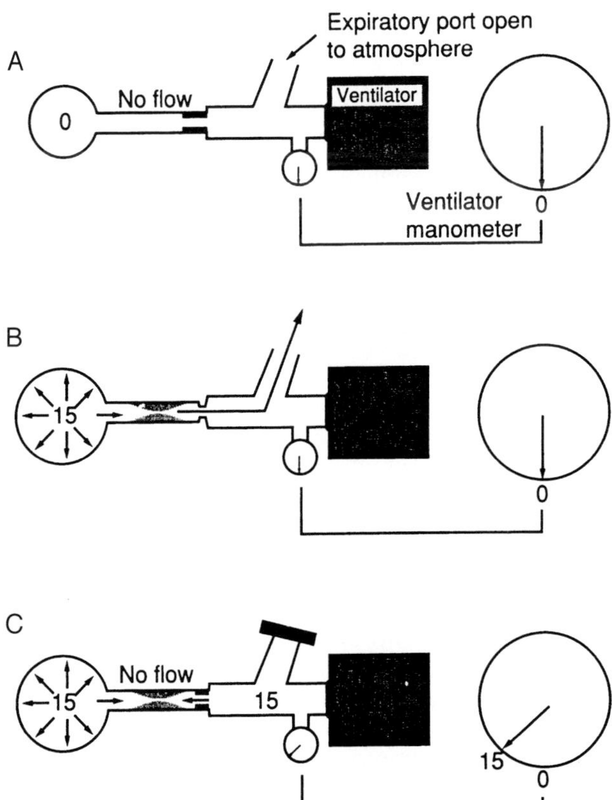

FIGURE 10–7 ■ Relationship among alveolar, central airway, and ventilator circuit pressure under *A*, normal conditions; *B*, in the presence of a severe dynamic airway obstruction, with the expiratory port open; and *C*, in the presence of severe dynamic airflow obstruction, with the expiratory port occluded. Self-controlled positive end-expiratory pressure (auto-PEEP) is identified by creating an end-expiratory hold, allowing alveolar, central, and ventilatory pressure to equilibrate. Note that during expiratory hold, following equilibration, auto-PEEP is read on the system manometer. (From Pepe PE, Marini JJ: Occult positive end-expiratory pressure in mechanically ventilated patients with airflow obstruction: The auto-PEEP effect. Am Rev Respir Dis 126:166, 1982.)

TABLE 10–4 ■ **Steps for Reducing Dynamic Hyperinflation and Self-Controlled Positive End-Expiratory Pressure**

Eliminate unnecessary ventilation
- Wean patient completely if possible
- Minimize number of large-volume ventilator breaths
- Correct overventilation and respiratory alkalosis by decreasing rate or tidal volume or both
- If auto-PEEP impairs cardiac function, allow Pa_{CO_2} to rise above normal

Decrease expiratory airflow obstruction
- Treat bronchospasm aggressively with bronchodilators, steroids, etc., as needed
- Keep airways free of secretions
- Replace small-diameter endotracheal tube with larger one

Maximize expiratory portion of ventilatory cycle
- Increase peak inspiratory flow rate to 70–100 L/min
- Replace standard, corrugated ventilator circuit with low-compressible-volume tubing

Auto = PEEP, self-controlled positive end-expiratory pressure; Pa_{CO_2}, partial pressure of arterial carbon dioxide.

Adapted from Pierson DJ: Invasive mechanical ventilation. In Albert RK, Spiro SG, Jett JR (eds): Comprehensive Respiratory Medicine. London, Mosby, 1999, pp 11.1–11.20.

Another consequence of auto-PEEP is that the patient must develop a greater negative pleural (alveolar) pressure to overcome the auto-PEEP with every breath to create a negative pressure at the proximal airway and thus initiate inspiratory air flow pressure to trigger the ventilator. This greatly increases the patient's work of breathing and may be an important cause of "fighting the ventilator." If the auto-PEEP cannot be eliminated, externally applied PEEP may reduce the muscular effort the patient must exert to trigger the ventilator; the Ppl must now be reduced to just below the external PEEP level rather than to below ambient pressure to trigger a breath. In this setting external PEEP should not increase lung volume and overall PEEP. This can be monitored using PIP. If the latter is not increased when external PEEP is added, overall lung volume has not been increased. A logical approach to evaluate and reduce dynamic hyperinflation and auto-PEEP is provided in Table 10–4.

Barotrauma

The term *barotrauma* currently applies both to extra-alveolar air (classic barotrauma) and parenchymal lung damage that may be caused by ventilatory support (Pierson 1988, 1998). The main clinical forms of barotrauma encountered during ventilatory support are pneumothorax, pneumomediastinum, and subcutaneous emphysema (Fig. 10–8). In adults, only the first of these is potentially life-threatening. Air embolism, also life-threatening, occurs during mechanical ventilation, but is uncommon. These forms of barotrauma generally result from alveolar rupture into the interstitium of an adjacent bronchovas-

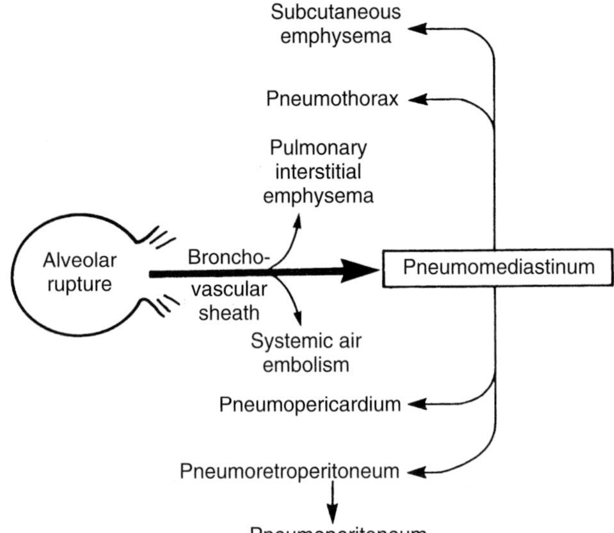

FIGURE 10–8 ■ Pathogenesis of the various clinical manifestations of extra-alveolar air following alveolar rupture during mechanical ventilation. (From Pierson DJ: Complications associated with mechanical ventilation. Crit Care Clin 6:711, 1990.)

cular sheath, with subsequent dissection to the mediastinum and elsewhere, rather than from direct alveolar rupture into the pleural space. Pneumothorax can result from direct puncture of the visceral pleura during central line placement or other procedures. Barotrauma is more likely to occur in the presence of local pulmonary hyperinflation, which may develop in obstructive lung disease, a unilateral or localized process such as lobar pneumonia or atelectasis, or when a "diffuse" acute pathologic process is unevenly distributed, as is typical in ARDS. It is also more common when tidal volumes greater than 12 ml/kg or high levels of PEEP are used (Pierson, 1988). No controlled study has shown that barotrauma is more frequent with the use of volume-targeted rather than pressure-targeted ventilation (Gammon et al, 1995). Chest tube insertion for pneumothorax occurring during mechanical ventilation is sometimes followed by a persistent air leak (bronchopleural fistula), particularly in ARDS. The leak may reach several hundred milliliters per breath and can be associated with moderately severe hypercapnia. Much anecdotal literature exists on novel methods for decreasing a bronchopleural air leak. However, such measures are seldom effective in clinical practice, and it is unlikely that they affect the clinical course (Pierson, 1998). The leak will virtually always resolve without specific measures if the underlying pulmonary process resolves, and it will persist despite all measures as long as the lung disease does not improve.

Volutrauma (Ventilator-Induced Lung Injury)

Over the past decade, there has been a re-evaluation of the paradigm of maintaining normocapnia in mechanically ventilated patients. Considerable animal and human data suggest that conventional tidal volumes of 10 to 15 ml/kg may be associated with alveolar overdistention leading to "volutrauma" or ventilator-induced lung injury (VILI) that might either initiate or further exacerbate acute lung injury. Traditional ventilatory support for respiratory failure has utilized volume-controlled mechanical ventilation using supraphysiologic tidal volumes (10 to 15 ml/kg) because of the observation that high lung volumes minimize atelectasis and prevent deterioration in oxygenation in patients undergoing anesthesia (Bendixen et al, 1963). This strategy often required high airway pressures to deliver these volumes and maintain normocapnia in patients with severe lung injury. In fact, the original description of ARDS included high inspiratory ventilator pressures as part of the definition (Ashbaugh et al, 1967). Webb and Tierney (1974) were the first investigators to recognize the possibility of ventilator-induced parenchymal lung injury as separate from the previously recognized forms of barotrauma. Rats ventilated at high airway pressures (45 cm H_2O) developed alveolar edema, hypoxemia, and decreased C_L, with death occurring within 1 hour. They theorized that the interstitial edema may be due to pulmonary interdependence and that the alveolar edema may be from depletion or inactivation of surfactant. Dreyfuss and colleagues (1988) likewise showed that application of high-inflation-pressure ventilation in rats resulted in a high permeability edema of the lung after only 20 minutes, and resulted in histologic findings similar to those seen in human ARDS.

To discern whether high Palv or alveolar overdistention was the likely causative factor in the observed pulmonary edema, Dreyfuss and coworkers (1988) subjected rats to five ventilatory modes: (1) control group (low-pressure–low-volume positive-pressure ventilation), (2) high-pressure–high-volume group, (3) high-pressure–low-volume group achieved by thoracoabdominal strapping, (4) low-pressure–high-volume group achieved by iron lung ventilation, and (5) high-pressure–high-volume group with 10 cm H_2O PEEP added. No significant difference between the control and the high-pressure–low-volume group was seen; however, the lungs from the groups ventilated with high volumes developed severe high-permeability edema, regardless of whether positive or negative pressure was the generating force. This study strongly suggested that alveolar overdistention was more important in ventilator-associated lung injury than was high Palv. Hernandez and colleagues (1989) similarly found that chest wall restriction limited high airway pressure–induced lung injury in immature rabbits, using capillary filtration coefficient (K_{fc}) as the marker of lung injury. Tsuno and colleagues (1990) analyzed the histopathologic changes in baby pig lungs after mechanical ventilation at high peak airway pressures. After ventilation at a PIP of 40 cm H_2O for 22 ± 11 hours, one group of pigs was sacrificed and the lungs examined. Alveolar hemorrhage, alveolar neutrophil infiltration, alveolar macrophage and type II pneumocyte proliferation, interstitial congestion and thickening, interstitial lymphocyte infiltration, emphysematous change, and hyaline membrane formation were noted. Similar histopathologic changes appear in the early stages of ARDS (Bachofen and Weibel, 1982; Croce et al, 1999; Tomashefski, 1990). Another group of pigs were continued on mechanical ventilation for an additional 3 to 6 days using conventional ventilatory parameters (V_T = 15 ml/kg; PIP = 30 cm H_2O; $Pa{CO_2}$ = 40 mm Hg) and then sacrificed for analysis. This group had the changes noted earlier coupled with prominent organized alveolar exudate, consistent with changes seen in the late stages of ARDS (Bachofen and Weibel, 1982; Tomashefski, 1990). A control group ventilated at PIP of 18 cm H_2O showed no histopathologic change in the lung (Dreyfuss et al, 1988). These studies suggest a clear association between alveolar overdistention and lung injury, similar to that seen in ARDS. However, the exact mechanism of the injury remains unclear (Dreyfuss and Saumon, 1992).

The degree to which conclusions can be extrapolated from animal studies to humans is unknown. Rouby and associates (1993) have demonstrated that these microscopic changes associated with mechanical ventilation can be observed in postmortem examinations. When air space enlargement (alveolar overdistention or intraparenchymal pseudocysts) was used to define barotrauma in 30 patients (20 with ARDS, 6 with pneumonia, and 4 with pulmonary contusion), the more severe abnormalities were associated with higher positive air pressure (PAP) (56 ± 18 cm H_2O versus 44 ± 10 cm H_2O), more days exposed to an F_{IO_2} higher than 0.6 (8.6 ± 9.4 days versus 1.9 ± 2 days), and greater weight loss (6.3 ± 9.2 kg versus 0.75 ± 5.8 kg).

Therefore, there are compelling data to re-evaluate the traditional use of "normal" tidal volumes of 12 ml/kg, and to consider tidal volumes in the range of 6 to 8 ml/kg in most patients with acute respiratory failure or ARDS (Bidani et al, 1994; Bone, 1993; Marini and Kelsen, 1992). It is of interest that Ranieri and colleagues (1999) reported that a variety of inflammatory cytokines remained elevated in the bronchoalveolar lavage fluid of patients with ARDS receiving "conventional" mechanical ventilation but progressively declined in patients receiving a lung-protective mechanical ventilation strategy. Studies by Amato and associates (1995, 1998) have reported improved survival in ARDS patients using a lung-protective strategy. Even more recently, in a National Institutes of Health (NIH)–supported ARDS network trial, comparing a V_T of 6 ml/kg with a V_T of 12 ml/kg, the study was terminated because of significant survival benefit in the low V_T group (Hudson, 1999).

Nosocomial Pneumonia

Nosocomial pneumonia is common in ventilated patients (Craven and Stieger, 1989; Pierson, 1990). If proper techniques for airway suctioning, aerosol administration, and tubing changes are used, pneumonia seldom results from contaminated equipment. Instead, it reflects the vulnerability of critically ill patients to their own oropharyngeal and gut organisms and to infection spread by inadequate handwashing and other physical contact. Prophylactic antimicrobial agents administered systemically appear to be ineffective in preventing pneumonia, and can promote the development of infection with resistant organisms (Pierson, 1999). Newer techniques using a combination of topical oropharyngeal agents and systemic antibiotics have gained popularity, especially in Europe, but have not yet been sufficiently validated to warrant widespread use.

Airway Problems

Complications can occur during intubation (e.g., trauma, right mainstem bronchus intubation, hypoxia), while the tube is in place (e.g., laryngeal injury, tracheal injury, hemorrhage, infection), at the time of extubation (e.g., laryngospasm, aspiration), or subsequently (e.g., hoarseness, laryngeal stenosis, tracheal stenosis) (Heffner, 1990). Right mainstem bronchial intubation can result in overdistention of the right lung, with alveolar rupture and tension pneumothorax, as well as left lung atelectasis. The distal tip of most tracheal tubes can be identified radiographically, and it should lie at least 4 cm above the carina, because neck flexion can advance the tube tip distally by as much as 4 cm in some adult patients. Radiographic or endoscopic confirmation of tube placement following intubation is more reliable than physical examination. Should patients be intubated nasally or orally? Some clinicians avoid nasotracheal intubation altogether because of the risk of sinusitis and otitis. Others use the nasotracheal route whenever possible, especially in patients who are alert, because of the perception that it results in less discomfort (Heffner, 1990). Intracuff pressures should be monitored and kept in the range of 25 to 30 cm H_2O. Studies have shown that pressures exceeding 30 cm H_2O are associated with an increased likelihood of mucosal necrosis and subsequent tracheal stenosis. Lower pressures, however, may be insufficient to prevent aspiration of oropharyngeal secretions around the cuff (Heffner, 1990).

Prolonged Muscle Weakness

Prolonged muscle weakness following the use of muscle relaxants such as vecuronium is a recently appreciated syndrome that can substantially increase a patient's requirement for ICU care. It was initially reported in patients with status asthmaticus who were treated with sedation and paralysis, in conjunction with high doses of corticosteroids (Hansen-Flaschen et al, 1993; Shapiro et al, 1993). Myopathy, elevation of serum creatine phosphokinase, or both also occur in patients with other diagnoses who receive muscle relaxants during ventilatory support (Hansen-Falaschen et al, 1993; Segredo et al, 1992).

Deteriorating Oxygenation in the Ventilated Patient

Deteriorating oxygenation during mechanical ventilation, a common reason for fighting the ventilator, should initiate a systematic search for specific mechanisms and therapy rather than simply an increase in F_{IO_2}, or the level of PEEP. Possible causes of worsening oxygenation fall into several categories (Glauser et al, 1988). The problem could be with the ventilator and its circuitry. The patient's primary disease process (e.g., pneumonia, ARDS) could be worsening, or a new medical problem may have appeared. Examples of the latter include pneumothorax, acute lobar atelectasis, pulmonary edema from fluid overload, nosocomial pneumonia or sepsis, aspiration of gastric contents, retained secretions, and bronchospasm. A fall in cardiac output can also cause worsening oxygenation in a patient with a significant intrapulmonary right-to-left shunt. Interventions and procedures can also lead to a decline in oxygenation. Examples include the effects of airway suctioning, chest physiotherapy, or even changes in body position, especially in patients with heterogeneously distributed pulmonary disorders. Bronchoscopy, thoracentesis, and hemodialysis can also result in a decline in oxygenation (Glauser et al, 1988). A number of drugs administered to patients undergoing mechanical ventilation can interfere with arterial oxygenation. Among these are vasodilators (which can increase right-to-left shunt), β-blockers (which can depress cardiac output and induce bronchospasm), and bronchodilators (which can alter $\dot{V}/\dot{Q}$ ratios).

NONINVASIVE POSITIVE-PRESSURE VENTILATORY ASSISTANCE

Sullivan and colleagues (1981) proposed the use of nasal CPAP for the treatment of obstructive sleep apnea. Mask CPAP therapy for obstructive sleep apnea was the springboard to the development of NIPPVA for patients with chronic ventilatory failure. The techniques of CPAP and NIPPVA are, of course, different despite the fact that similar face masks or nasal masks can be used for both. During CPAP, patients continue to breathe spontaneously at their own rate and depth, whereas during NIPPVA $\dot{V}_E$ is augmented with gas flow, which is determined predominately by the ventilator. NIPPVA was first applied to patients with neuromuscular disorders and chest wall disease, but has recently been extended to subgroups of patients with COPD (Hill, 1993, 1999).

The mechanism underlying the use of NIPPVA is the same as for invasive positive-pressure ventilatory assistance (IPPVA). Positive pressure is applied intermittently via the airways, increasing transpulmonary pressure and inflating the lungs. Exhalation is achieved by passive lung recoil. The success of NIPPVA is dependent on the patient's ability to cooperate and synchronize breathing with the ventilator, and users of NIPPVA cannot be heavily sedated or paralyzed in order to gain synchrony. In addition, the patient's upper airway must permit air flow into the lungs. Although this is usually readily achieved in the conscious, cooperative patient, it may be problematic in uncooperative, obtunded, or sleeping patients.

Meduri and associates (1989) were the first to report the use of NIPPVA to avoid ET intubation in patients with acute respiratory failure. Brochard and colleagues (1990) subsequently used face mask NIPPVA to treat 13 patients with acute exacerbations of COPD, only one of whom required ET intubation, compared with 11 of 13 historically matched controls. This study generated considerable enthusiasm, particularly because NIPPVA-treated patients also required less time on the ventilator and in the ICU, suggesting that NIPPVA might reduce ventilator-associated morbidity and costs. Numerous studies examining the efficacy of NIPPVA in various forms of acute respiratory failure have subsequently been published (Hill, 1999). Roughly, half of the published studies have used pressure-limited techniques and the other half volume-controlled ventilatory modes via nasal or oronasal masks. Success rates (defined as the ability of patients to tolerate NIPPVA and avoid intubation) have been similar among most studies using either ventilator mode, ranging from roughly two thirds to three fourths of entered patients. In a direct comparison of the two modes, Vitacca and colleagues (1993) found similar success rates, but higher comfort ratings and lower complication rates among patients using the pressure support mode.

Despite the lack of randomized, controlled trials, published studies strongly support the conclusion that NIPPVA successfully avoids intubation in the majority of selected patients (mainly COPD patients), with most series reporting success rates of 60% to 80% (Hill, 1999). Among randomized, controlled trials, Kramer and coworkers (1995) showed a reduction in the percentage of patients needing intubation from 73% in controls to 26% in the NIPPVA group, and, in a subgroup with COPD, a reduction from 67% in controls to 9%. In a study of patients with COPD exacerbations, Brochard and associates (1995) found an almost identical reduction in intubation rates, from 74% in controls to 24% in NIPPVA-treated patients. Therefore, evidence from controlled studies supports the use of NIPPVA to avoid intubation. This conclusion applies mainly to patients with acute exacerbations of COPD.

Studies examining the efficacy of NIPPVA in patients with acute respiratory failure due to causes other than COPD have too few patients to allow firm conclusions, but several observations can be made: (1) Patients with acute deterioration owing to restrictive thoracic disease do well, as long as there is no associated problem with excessive secretions or swallowing dysfunction (Meduri et al, 1991). (2) Patients with hypoxemic respiratory failure, but without hypercapnia (e.g., that caused by severe pneumonia or ARDS), do less well (Wysocki et al, 1995). (3) Other subgroups of patients with acute respiratory failure that may benefit from NIPPVA include postoperative patients who deteriorate following extubation and those with acute respiratory failure who decline intubation (Benhamou et al, 1992). Acute asthma, exacerbations of cystic fibrosis, and cardiogenic pulmonary edema may also be managed successfully, but more studies are needed to define the role of NIPPVA in these latter forms of acute respiratory failure (Hill, 1999; Lapinsky et al, 1994; Piper et al, 1992).

Patient selection is crucial in the use of NIPPVA in acute respiratory failure (Table 10–5) (Hill, 1993, 1999; Meyer and Hill, 1994). In addition to those requiring immediate intubation, patients with compromised upper airway function should be excluded (Hill, 1999). This includes those at risk for aspiration due to swallowing dysfunction and those unable to clear secretions due to excessive production or impaired cough. Patients with unstable medical conditions such as hypotensive shock, uncontrolled arrhythmias, acute cardiac ischemia, or uncontrolled gastrointestinal bleeding should be managed using IVPPVA. Patients with anatomic abnormalities or injuries that interfere with interface fitting are poor candi-

TABLE 10-5 ■ Characteristics of Patients Successfully Treated with Noninvasive Positive Pressure Ventilation

Cooperative patient
Intact neurologic function
Able to coordinate breathing with ventilator
Moderate to moderately high (but not very high) severity of illness
Intact dentition
Able to control oral and pulmonary secretions
Moderate hypercapnia
Moderate respiratory acidosis (pH > 7.20)

Adapted from Hill NS: Noninvasive mechanical ventilation. In Albert RK, Spiro SG, Jett JR (eds): Comprehensive Respiratory Medicine. London, Mosby, 1999, pp 12.1–12.10.

dates. Additionally, uncooperative, agitated patients who are continually removing the mask cannot benefit from NIPPVA. The cause and potential reversibility of the acute respiratory deterioration are also important considerations in patient selection. It is again emphasized that patients with acute deterioration of COPD appear to be good candidates. In this regard, NIPPVA may be viewed as a "crutch" that assists the patient through a critical interval, allowing time for other therapies such as bronchodilators, steroids, or diuretics to act. Therefore, patients with status asthmaticus or acute pulmonary edema may also be good candidates, although the role of NIPPVA in these latter conditions has not been fully evaluated. More severe forms of respiratory failure that require prolonged periods of ventilatory support, such as severe status asthmaticus, complicated pneumonia, or ARDS, should be managed using IPPVA.

Methods

A well-fitting and comfortable interface is crucial to the success of NIPPVA (Hill, 1999). Nasal masks or oronasal face masks are suitable. Success rates of studies using different masks are comparable; mask selection depends mainly on practitioner and patient preference. Nasal masks have the advantage of leaving the mouth uncovered, allowing speech and eating during use, and perhaps enhancing patient tolerance. However, air leaking through the mouth is common during nasal ventilation, a problem that may be alleviated by switching to oronasal masks. Air leaks can also occur with the oronasal mask if there is an inadequate seal over the chin. Because oronasal masks interfere with speech and eating during use, they may be less well tolerated than nasal masks. Whichever interface is selected, an optimal fit is most important (Hill, 1999).

Ventilator Selection

Several different ventilators have been used in studies on NIPPVA in either pressure-limited or volume-limited modes. Standard critical care ventilators may be adapted to deliver NIPPVA in either the pressure support or volume control modes, and portable pressure support devices such as the BiPAP S/T (Respironics, Inc., Murrysville, PA) or Quantum (Healthdyne, Marietta, GA) have seen increasing use in the acute setting (Confalonieri et al, 1994; Kramer et al, 1995). These ventilators are compact, highly portable, and cost less than standard critical care ventilators. They cycle between higher inspiratory positive airway pressure (IPAP) and lower expiratory positive airway pressure (EPAP) settings as determined by a sensitive flow-triggering or time-cycling, closely resembling pressure support modes on standard ventilators. However, these devices deliver lower maximal pressures (20 to 30 cm H_2O), and have less sophisticated alarms than do standard critical care ventilators, and should be limited to less critically ill patients in closely monitored settings.

Settings

Low initial pressures facilitate patient acceptance of NIPPVA. Typical starting pressure support settings are 4 to 10 cm H_2O and PEEP of 2 to 4 cm H_2O (8 to 12 cm H_2O for IPAP and 2 to 4 cm H_2O for EPAP). For volume ventilation, initial tidal volumes range from 10 to 15 ml/kg. The ventilator is set in the VAV or VACV mode to allow patient triggering. An oxygen cannula is connected directly to the mask or entrained into the tubing, with inspiratory flow titrated to maintain the desired oxygen saturation. The patient is then coached to relax and let the device assist breathing. As patients adapt, the IPAP, or VT, is gradually increased as tolerated to achieve a small reduction in $Pa{CO_2}$ (5 to 10 mm Hg). EPAP can be increased if oxygenation remains inadequate (Hill, 1999). Successfully managed patients usually rapidly synchronize their breathing with the device and demonstrate a reduction in respiratory rate, heart rate, and $Pa{CO_2}$ within the first few hours of initiation (Meduri et al, 1991; Soo Hoo et al, 1994).

Problems

In properly selected patients, NIPPVA is safe and well tolerated, and most of the relatively few complications are interface related. Approximately 10% to 25% of patients fail to tolerate the interface despite adjustments in strap tension, repositioning, and trials of different sizes and types of mask. Some air leaking through the mouth (with nasal masks) or around the mask is inevitable. Pressure support–type devices compensate for air leaks by maintaining inspiratory airflow during leaking; tidal volumes on volume-limited ventilators may be increased to compensate. To reduce air leak through the mouth, patients are coached to keep the mouth shut, chin straps are used, or an oronasal mask may be tried. Pneumothoraces and painful gastric dilatation are unusual, probably because inflation pressures are low compared with those used with invasive ventilation. Lack of patient cooperation interferes with efficacy and may be ameliorated by judicious use of sedation, such as low doses of benzodiazepines. Unremitting agitation should be considered an indication for intubation. Aspiration is a reported complication (Meduri et al, 1991), but unusual in patients with swallowing dysfunction. Those patients who have problems clearing secretions are excluded.

TABLE 10–6 ■ **Comparison of ECMO, $ECCO_2R$, $AVCO_2R$, and Total Artificial Lung**

Parameter	*ECMO*	*$ECCO_2R$*	*$AVCO_2R$*	*Total Artificial Lung*
Setting	Respiratory/cardiac failure	Respiratory failure	Respiratory failure (investigational)	Respiratory failure (experimental)
Location	Extrathoracic	Extrathoracic	Extrathoracic	Extrathoracic
Type of support	VA (cardiac) VV (respiratory)	VV (respiratory) (CO_2)	AV (respiratory) (CO_2)	PA–PA or PA–LA
Blood flow	High (70–80% CO)	Medium (30% CO)	Low (10%–15% CO)	Total (100%)
Ventilatory support	Pressure-controlled ± high PEEP 10–12 breaths/min	High PEEP 2–4 breaths/min High F_{IO_2}	Volume-controlled (algorithm-driven)	None necessary
Average length of extracorporeal support	Days–weeks	Days–weeks	Days–weeks	Days
Complications	Bleeding Organ failure	Bleeding	Bleeding	Bleeding

AV, arteriovenous; $AVCO_2R$, arteriovenous carbon dioxide removal; PEEP, positive end-expiratory pressure; CO, cardiac output; ECMO, extracorporeal membrane oxygenation; $ECCO_2R$, extracorporeal carbon dioxide removal; F_{IO_2}, fraction of inspired oxygen; PA-LA, pulmonary artery-to-left artery; PAP, pulmonary artery pressure; PA-PA, pulmonary artery-to-pulmonary artery; VA, venoarterial; VV, venovenous.

Adapted from Alpard SK, Zwischenberger JB: Extracorporeal gas exchange. Respir Care Clin 4:711, 1998.

In summary, use of NIPPVA to treat patients with acute respiratory failure has increased substantially in recent years (Hill, 1993, 1999; Meyer and Hill, 1994; Rocker et al, 1999). This has been related to advances in noninvasive interfaces (nasal masks) and ventilator modes (pressure support). In the acute setting, evidence now supports the use of NIPPVA for acute deterioration of COPD, respiratory insufficiency after postoperative extubation, and acute respiratory failure in patients who decline intubation. Indications in patients with respiratory failure due to conditions other than COPD have not been fully established, but anecdotal experience suggests that selected patients with acute asthma, acute pulmonary edema, restrictive lung disease, and pneumonia may also benefit. Application of appropriate selection criteria appears to be important, because neither patients with mild deterioration nor those with severe deterioration who need immediate intubation are likely to benefit. In this regard, it is worthwhile to note that in the study of Brochard and colleagues (1995), only 30% of all patients with COPD admitted during the study period met the criteria for enrollment in that study. Patients with inability to protect the upper airway, excessive airway secretions, other unstable medical conditions, and inability to cooperate should be excluded.

ALTERNATIVE MEANS OF RESPIRATORY SUPPORT

The use of oxygenator technology to accomplish partial or total gas exchange (O_2 or CO_2), with or without cardiac support, is based on the premise that "lung rest" facilitates repair and avoids the barotrauma or volutrauma of ventilator management (Alpard and Zwischenberger, 1998; Bartlett, 1990; Kolobow, 1988; Lewandowski et al, 1992; Pesenti et al, 1997; Slutsky, 1985; Zwischenberger et al, 1999). The basic technique involves a permeable membrane gas exchanger, either extracorporeal or intracorporeal, with or without use of a pump. Large vessel cannulation is typically needed in patients with extracorporeal support. Depending on the design and application of the technology, the circuit orientation can be venovenous; venoarterial, as with ECMO; or arteriovenous, as with arteriovenous CO_2 removal ($AVCO_2R$). Various extracorporeal techniques are compared in Table 10–6.

ECMO, a modification of cardiopulmonary bypass, decreases the mortality of neonatal respiratory distress syndrome and is capable of total gas exchange. Infants with a predicted mortality of 90% have been treated with ECMO, and a nationwide experience of over 15,000 patients shows a greater than 80% survival (Bartlett, 1997). Adult ECMO has also demonstrated improved survival in selected patients (Kolla et al, 1997; Lewandowski et al, 1997). The Extracorporeal Life Support Organization database on all adults with severe respiratory failure demonstrates a cumulative short-term survival rate of 47% (Tracy et al, 1995).

Gattinoni and associates (1978) and Kolobow and coworkers (1978) introduced the use of extracorporeal CO_2 removal ($ECCO_2R$) in both animals and humans, where the focus was on CO_2 removal to facilitate a reduction in ventilatory support. CO_2 removal was accomplished via extracorporeal circulation through the membrane lung, while oxygenation was maintained by simple diffusion or "apneic oxygenation" as O_2 was supplied via constant flow to alveoli maintained with PEEP. Gattinoni and colleagues (1986) demonstrated a decrease in mortality in patients managed with $ECCO_2R$ and low-frequency, pressure-limited ventilation. Morris and colleagues (1994), however, compared conventional ventilation with pressure-controlled inverse ratio ventilation, with or without $ECCO_2R$ in 40 ARDS patients. No significant difference in survival was found between the two groups, with rates of 42% and 33%, respectively. Of note, the majority of patients were hypercapnic on randomization, and although mean peak airway pressures were significantly lower in the new therapy group, they remained elevated (57.8 versus 49.5 cm H_2O). The improvement in survival seen with current techniques of venovenous and venoarterial ECMO and $ECCO_2R$ has since been duplicated at various centers worldwide, with an overall survival rate of 46% in patients thought to have a 90% mortality risk (Lewandowski et al, 1997).

As an alternative to the complexities of extracorporeal devices, Mortensen and Berry (1989) proposed the use of an intravenous gas exchange device in patients with acute respiratory failure. The IVOX intravenacaval gas exchange device developed by Cardiopulmonics, Inc. (Salt Lake City, UT) consists of multiple hollow fibers that are positioned under fluoroscopy into the vena cava via a surgical venotomy in the common femoral vein. Oxygen is drawn through the lumen of each hollow fiber at subatmospheric pressure to prevent gas embolism, and gas exchange with free-flowing venous blood takes place across the fiber wall. Available in sizes 7 to 10 (membrane surface area = 0.21 to 0.52 m^2), it was anticipated that IVOX would result in clinically significant improvement in gas exchange with fewer complications than those associated with extracorporeal circuits. Clinical studies have demonstrated transfer rates for O_2 and CO_2 of 40 to 70 ml/min, or approximately 25% to 30% of metabolic demand (Conrad et al, 1994). Based on measurements of CO_2 transfer by different sizes of IVOX in a sheep model, Tao and colleagues (1996) have calculated that the membrane surface area required to excrete 150 ml/min CO_2 with a vena cava blood flow of 4 L/min at normocapnia ($Pa{CO_2}$ = 40 mm Hg) is approximately 1.8 m^2, considerably greater than the largest (size 10) IVOX (0.52 m^2). High levels of hypercapnia ($Pa{CO_2}$ = 100 mm Hg) can reduce the required surface area by 80% to 0.49 m^2 (Bidani et al, 1996). Permissive hypercapnia and active blood mixing have been incorporated in other intracorporeal devices, such as the intravenous membrane oxygenator designed by the University of Pittsburgh group (Federspiel et al, 1997).

$AVCO_2R$ is achieved with a simple percutaneous arteriovenous shunt that eliminates a substantial portion of ECMO-related components, reducing the extent of exposure to foreign surfaces and eliminating the pump. The procedure involves cannulation of the femoral artery and vein, with a membrane oxygenator interposed in the circuit (Awad et al, 1991; Brunston et al, 1996, 1997; Young et al, 1992). Blood flows spontaneously through the oxygenator because of the pressure gradient between the artery and vein. The circuit is essentially identical to that used for continuous arteriovenous hemofiltration. The difference is in the use of a gas exchange device (membrane oxygenator) in place of a hemofilter, and a larger vascular cannula (~ No. 17 French) to accommodate substantially greater blood flows. Using a mathematical model, it has been estimated that shunt flows of 10% to 15% of the cardiac output can support total CO_2 removal at levels of $Pa{CO_2}$ that are physiologically tolerable (Conrad et al, 1998). In a sheep model of smoke inhalation injury, $AVCO_2R$ facilitated significant reductions in ventilator settings without compromising systemic $Pa{O_2}$ or $Pa{CO_2}$, while removing 96% of CO_2 metabolic production. Following a feasibility trial, $AVCO_2R$ is undergoing initial clinical trials (Zwischenberger et al, 1999).

MONITORING OF PATIENTS RECEIVING VENTILATORY ASSISTANCE

Patients receiving ventilatory assistance are vulnerable to the development of several complications or may suffer deterioration of the underlying illness (Tobin, 1990). Both of these problems are reflected in several dependent variables of airway mechanics and gas exchange. Close monitoring of airway mechanics and gas exchange is necessary to evaluate the physiologic state of the patient and the need and nature of interventions to deal with either inadequate gas exchange or abnormalities in airway mechanics (Rossi et al, 1998). Secondarily, these measurements provide insight into the pathophysiology of the patient's illness.

Basic Concepts in Airway Mechanics

Under static conditions in intubated, completely relaxed patients, airway pressure is equal to the elastic recoil pressure of the respiratory system (lung plus chest wall) (Alex and Tobin, 1999; Hess and Kacmarek, 1996; it is important to recognize that the chest wall includes the rib cage and the diaphragm). The pressure required to inflate the lung by a certain volume (ΔV) corresponds to the change in transpulmonary pressure (ΔP_L = Palv − Ppl), where Palv is alveolar pressure and Ppl is intrapleural pressure. *Lung compliance* (C_L), the inverse of lung elastance (E_L), is defined as the pressure required to cause a unit change in lung volume ($C_L = \Delta V/\Delta P_L$). Under passive conditions, the pressure required to simultaneously distend the chest wall by the same ΔV is determined by the average change in "intrathoracic pressure" ($\approx \Delta P_L$). The compliance of the relaxed chest wall is derived by ($C_W = \Delta V/\Delta Ppl$). The lung and chest wall are arranged in series, and thus the pressure required to distend the respiratory system (lung plus chest wall) may be expressed in terms of an overall elastance of the respiratory system ($E_{RS} = E_L + E_{CW}$). Expressed in terms of the compliance of the respiratory system (C_{RS}), $1/C_{RS} = 1/C_L + 1/C_{CW}$ or $C_{RS} = (C_L)(C_W)/(C_L + C_W)$. Thus, changes in the chest wall can have an independent and significant effect on the compliance of the respiratory system. The lung and chest wall display different pressure-volume relationships (Alex and Tobin, 1999). The overall pressure-volume relationship of the overall respiratory system is sigmoid in shape (see Fig. 10–6), and overall compliance (C_{RS}) is greatest during the mid-volume change. At both extremes of lung volumes, C_{RS} is low because either the pressure-volume curve of the lung becomes flat as the lung gets fully inflated, or the pressure-volume curve of the chest wall becomes flat as the thoracic volume is reduced. High lung volumes can occur during mechanical ventilation as a result of large tidal volumes, dynamic hyperinflation, or inappropriately high levels of PEEP. At low lung volumes, reduced C_{RS} may be secondary to obesity or abdominal distention (Table 10–7) (Hess and Kacmarek, 1996).

The slope of the pressure-volume curve of the respira-

TABLE 10–7 ■ **Causes of Decreased Compliance and Increased Airway Resistance in Patients Receiving Ventilatory Assistance**

Decreased Compliance	*Increased Airway Resistance*
Pneumothorax	Bronchospasm
Mainstem intubation	Airway secretions
Pulmonary edema	Small endotracheal tube
Large pleural effusion	Bronchial edema
Obesity	
Ascites	
Abdominal distention	
Pulmonary consolidation	
Acute lung injury	
Chest wall deformity	

tory system may be altered by abnormalities in either the lung or the chest wall (Tobin, 1990). Elastic recoil of the lung is decreased in emphysema (increased CL), while lung recoil is increased with pulmonary edema or interstitial fibrosis (decreased CL). Increased stiffness of the chest wall (decreased CCW) can be seen in patients with kyphoscoliosis, obesity, or massive ascites (see Table 10–7). CL also depends on the number of alveolar units available to accept the VT. As the chest expands, the number of recruited alveolar units tends to increase, increasing CRS. The reverse phenomenon, derecruitment, occurs during tidal lung deflation, producing hysteresis of the static pressure-volume curve of the respiratory system (see Fig. 10–6).

Typical airway pressure waveforms during mechanical ventilation are shown in Figures 10–3 and 10–4. With volume-targeted ventilation, airway pressure increases during the inspiratory phase as the VT is delivered. The time course of the airway pressure change depends on the inspiratory flow pattern. If a constant flow pattern is chosen, there will be a linear increase in airway pressure during inspiration. With a decelerating inspiratory flow pattern, the inspiratory pressure waveform will be convex. The PIP varies directly with inspiratory airway resistance, end-inspiratory flow, VT, PEEP, and CRS. Depending on the inspiratory flow waveform, PIP may not occur at end-inspiration (Alex and Tobin, 1999; Tobin, 1990).

An end-inspiratory pause of 0.5 to 2.0 seconds allows equilibration between proximal airway pressure and Palv (Alex and Tobin, 1999). During the end-inspiratory pause, there is no flow, and a pressure plateau develops as proximal airway pressure equilibrates with Palv. The proximal airway pressure during the inspiratory pressure is referred to as plateau pressure (P_{plat}) and represents peak Palv (Fig. 10–9). The difference between PIP and peak Palv is due to the inspiratory resistance of the respiratory system (airway resistance plus ET tube resistance) and the difference between peak Palv and total PEEP is due to the elastic properties of the respiratory system (i.e., CL + CCW).

During pressure-targeted ventilation, PIP and peak Palv may be equal (Hess and Kacmarek, 1996). This is due to the flow waveform that occurs during this mode of ventilation (see Fig. 10–3). With pressure-targeted ventilation, inspiratory flow decreases during inspiration and is often followed by a period of zero flow at end-inspiration. During this period of no flow, proximal airway pressure should be equal to peak Palv (see Fig. 10–9). Based on the previously mentioned considerations, PIP should be lower during pressure-targeted ventilation than during volume-targeted ventilation. With volume-targeted ventilation, PIP will be greater than peak Palv owing to the presence of end-inspiratory flow. With pressure-targeted ventilation, PIP will equal Palv if end-inspiratory flow is zero. With all factors held constant (e.g., VT, lung impedance, PEEP), peak Palv is identical for volume-targeted and pressure-targeted ventilation.

Static Compliance. The difference between P_{plat} and total PEEP ($[PEEP]_{tot}$) is determined by the combined static compliance of the lung and chest wall (Alex and Tobin, 1999; Hess and Kacmarek, 1996). The static compliance can be calculated from $C_{RS} = V_T/(P_{plat} - [PEEP]_{tot})$, where $(PEEP)_{tot}$ includes any auto-PEEP that is present. The VT is the actual VT delivered to the patient and should be corrected for the effects of volume compressed in the circuit. The P_{plat} should be determined from an end-inspiratory pause in a relaxed or sedated patient (i.e.,

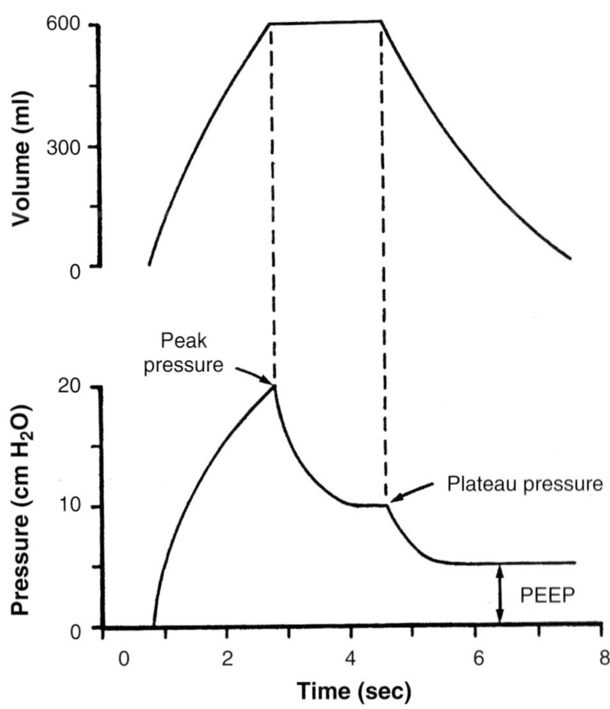

FIGURE 10–9 ■ Relationship between tidal volume and airway pressure in a patient receiving mechanical ventilation. The inspiratory plateau in the volume tracing is achieved by using "inspiratory hold" or by occluding the expiratory port long enough (1 to 2 seconds) to allow the airway pressure to reach a constant value. This pressure is referred to as the "plateau pressure" and represents the elastic recoil pressure of the total respiratory system at end-inflation volume. (PEEP, positive end-expiratory pressure.) (From Tobin MJ, Danzker DR: Ventilatory support: Who, when, and how? In Miller TA [ed]: Physiological Basis of Modern Surgical Care. St. Louis, Mosby–Year Book, 1988.)

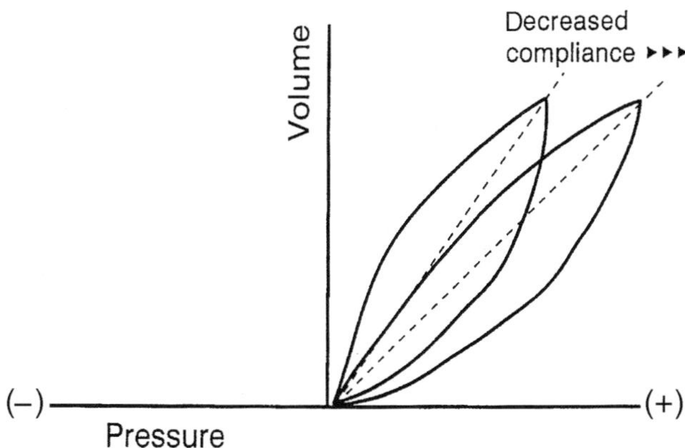

FIGURE 10–10 ■ Pressure-volume loop during passive mechanical ventilation. The slope of the line connecting the points of zero flow at the beginning of inspiration to point-of-zero flow at the beginning of expiration represents the lung plus chest wall compliance. A shift of the pressure-volume loop to the right represents a decrease in compliance. (From Hess DR, Kacmarek RM [eds]: Essentials of Mechanical Ventilation. New York, McGraw-Hill, 1996.)

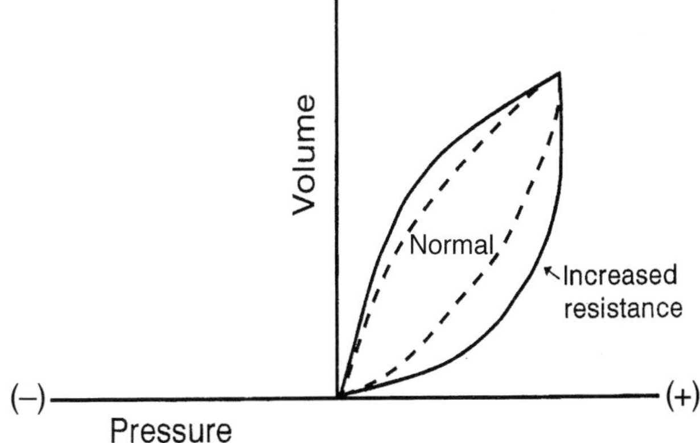

FIGURE 10–11 ■ The area under the dynamic pressure-volume loop is a measure of the resistive work. An increase in airway resistance causes an increase in the area within the pressure-volume loop. (From Hess DR, Kacmarek RM [eds]: Essentials of Mechanical Ventilation. New York, McGraw-Hill, 1996.)

the patient should not have any active inspiratory effort) that is long enough to produce equilibration between proximal airway pressure and Palv (Tobin, 1990). Alterations in overall CRS result in changes in the slope of the pressure-volume curve (Fig. 10–10).

Airway Resistance. The difference between PIP and P_{plat} is determined by inspiratory resistance and end-inspiratory flow (Hess and Kacmarek, 1996). During constant-flow volume-targeted ventilation, inspiratory resistance (RI) can be approximated by $RI = (PIP - P_{plat})/\dot{V}I$, where $\dot{V}I$ is the inspiratory flow. Expiratory resistance may be approximated by $RE = (P_{plat} - [PEEP]_{tot})/\dot{V}Emax$, where $\dot{V}Emax$ is the peak expiratory flow. RI is typically smaller than RE because of the increased airway diameter during inspiration, and the added impedance of the ET tube. Some causes of increased airway resistance are listed in Table 10–7. During mechanical ventilation, the resistance of the ET tube (Ret) in series with the RRS is implicitly included in the measured overall resistance (Rtot) (during both inspiration and expiration), such that RRS = Rtot − Ret (MacIntyre and Gropper, 1995; Marini, 1998). The effect of increased airway resistance on the pressure-volume curve is shown in Figure 10–11.

Mean Airway Pressure. Many of the beneficial and deleterious effects of mechanical ventilation are a function of Paw. Factors affecting Paw are PIP, PEEP, the I/E ratio, respiratory rate, and the inspiratory pressure waveform. Increments in inspiratory time cause an increase in Paw, whereas an increase in the expiratory time reduces Paw (Hess and Kacmarek, 1996).

Waveform Analysis—Flow-Volume and Pressure-Volume Loops. It is important to understand the difference between pressure versus time and flow waveforms versus time, as seen on graphic readouts (see Figs. 10–3 and 10–4) during mechanical ventilation and pressure versus volume, and flow versus volume loops for mechanically ventilated breaths (Figs. 10–10, 10–11, 10–12, and 10–13) (Bardoczky and d'Hollander, 1992; Henning et al, 1977; Rahoof and Khan, 1998; Waugh et al, 1999). The presence of a lower inflection point on the pressure versus volume curve (see Fig. 10–6) in the early stages of inspiration implies alveolar recruitment and may be used to guide the use of PEEP. The presence of an upper deflection point may help to recognize alveolar overdistention (see Fig. 10–6). Changes in the slope of the line

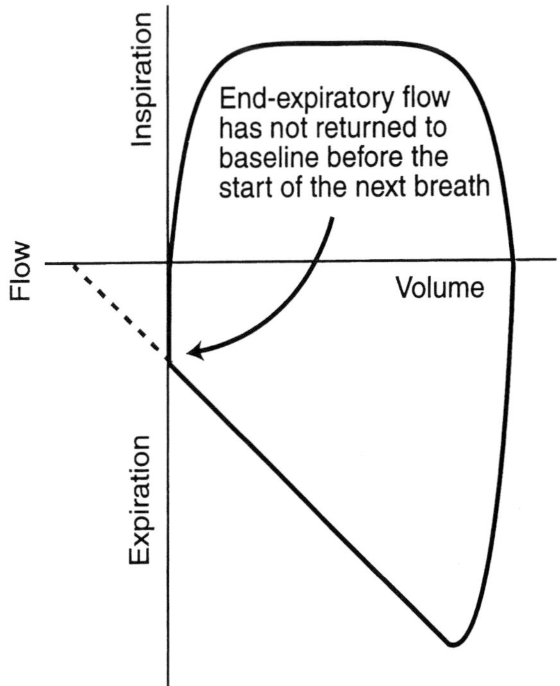

FIGURE 10–12 ■ Recognition of air-trapping and self-controlled end-expiratory pressure (auto-PEEP) from the flow-volume loop during mechanical ventilation. In the presence of auto-PEEP, expiratory flow does not reach zero prior to the initiation of inspiratory flow. (From Waugh JB, Deshpande VM, Harwood RJ: Rapid Interpretation of Ventilator Waveforms. Englewood Cliffs, NJ, Prentice Hall, 1999.)

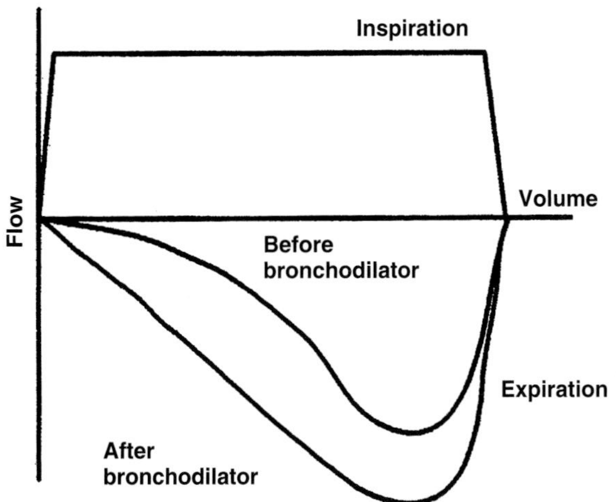

FIGURE 10–13 ■ Idealized flow-volume loop during mechanical ventilation, before and after bronchodilator administration. Inspiratory flow is limited because of the fixed endotracheal tube resistance. Before bronchodilator, the expiratory flow versus exhaled-volume loop is biphasic or "scooped" owing to increased expiratory airflow resistance. Following bronchodilator administration, there is an increment in the peak expiratory flow as well as straightening of the expiratory flow loop, indicating improvement in expiratory airflow obstruction.

connecting points of zero flow on the pressure-volume loop can provide a visual clue to a change in the overall respiratory system static compliance (see Fig. 10–12). The area under the dynamic pressure-volume loop provides information on airway resistance (see Fig. 10–13). Flow versus volume loops may be used to detect expiratory or inspiratory air flow obstruction, assess quantitative response to bronchodilators, and detect the presence of auto-PEEP (see Figs. 10–12 and 10–13). On most ventilators additional monitoring packages are available that combine information obtained from an esophageal catheter (for estimation of Ppl) and produce breath-by-breath information on several aspects of respiratory mechanics, including the work of breathing, the pressure-time product, dynamic compliance, mean airway resistance, and other measures of pulmonary mechanics.

Gas Exchange Indices

Arterial Oxygenation. The PaO_2/PAO_2 ratio is relatively stable with changes in inspired oxygen concentration and the level of alveolar ventilation, and is the preferred method for following the efficacy of arterial oxygenation in mechanically ventilated subjects (Nelson, 1993; Wood and Hall, 1993). PAO_2 is estimated using the ideal alveolar gas equation ($PAO_2 = [PB + P_{plat} - P_{AH_2O}] \times FIO_2 - PACO_2/RQ$). Generally, PB, the barometric pressure, is assumed to be 760 mm Hg; the P_{plat} is ignored; the water vapor pressure (P_{AH_2O}) is assumed to be 47 mm Hg; and the respiratory quotient (RQ) is assumed to be 0.8. Alternatively, the P/F ratio (PaO_2/FIO_2) may be used, because it is easier to calculate than the PaO_2/PAO_2 ratio. The PAO_2/FIO_2 ratio is affected by changes in $PaCO_2$ but appears to correlate well with the extent of pulmonary shunt.

Oxygen Delivery Index (ODI). The ODI is calculated as ODI = (CI) ($[O_2]a$), where CI is cardiac index and $[O_2]a$ is the arterial oxygen content.

Oxygen Utilization Coefficient (OUC). The OUC, also called the O_2 extraction ratio, is calculated as OUC = (VO_2)/(CO $[O_2]a$). OUC may be estimated from SaO_2 (via pulse oximetry) and SvO_2 (mixed venous blood oxyhemoglobin saturation via mixed venous blood oximetry): OUC = $(SaO_2 - SvO_2)/SaO_2$. This index quantitates the oxygen consumption (VO_2) relative to the peripheral oxygen delivery. OUC greater than 0.35 indicates that an excessively high oxygen extraction is required to satisfy the patient's metabolic needs (Nelson, 1993).

Mixed Venous Oxyhemoglobin Saturation. SvO_2 reflects the relative balance between VO_2 and peripheral oxygen delivery (DO_2 = (CO) ($[O_2]a$). It is calculated as $SvO_2 = 1 - (VO_2/DO_2)$. The four primary determinants of SvO_2 are SaO_2, hemoglobin concentration ([Hb]), cardiac output, and VO_2. SvO_2 is a sensitive but nonspecific indicator of the imbalance between VO_2 and DO_2. It is affected more by low-extraction, high-flow tissues (such as the kidney) than by high-extraction, low-flow vascular beds (such as the myocardium).

Intrapulmonary Shunt. The intrapulmonary shunt fraction (Qs/Qt) is estimated from a simplified two-compartment model in which part of the blood reaching the left side of the circulation is completely oxygenated by passage through ventilated lung units that are perfused (i.e., with $\dot{V}/\dot{Q} = 1$), and part of the blood is mixed venous blood that passes from the right side of the circulation to the left without exposure to ventilated alveoli (i.e., with $\dot{V}/\dot{Q} = 0$). It is estimated from the equation $Qs/Qt = ([O_2]c - [O_2]a)/([O_2]c - [O_2]v)$ (Nelson, 1993). Blood oxygen content is estimated from the general equation $[O_2] = 1.34$ [Hb] SO_2. This calculation ignores the concentration of physically dissolved oxygen. End-capillary oxyhemoglobin saturation $(ScO)_2$ is assumed to be 100%. SAO_2 is measured while the patient is transiently switched to 90% FIO_2. Contrary to previous practice, 100% FIO_2 is avoided as it tends to promote absorption atelectasis in very low $\dot{V}/\dot{Q}$ ratios ($\dot{V}/\dot{Q} < 0.01$). The Qs/Qt is the gold standard for clinical assessment of lung oxygenation function. Unfortunately, it is an invasive measurement as it requires determination of SvO_2, necessitating placement of a Swan-Ganz catheter.

Ventilation-Perfusion Index. The ventilation-perfusion index (VQI) (Nelson, 1993) is an approximation of Qs/Qt that can be performed on a continuous basis using combined arterial and mixed venous oximetry and is calculated as VQI = $(1 - SaO_2)/(1 - SvO_2)$. The VQI reflects Qs/Qt when arterial saturation is reduced. In the presence of high intrapulmonary shunts, when SaO_2 is less than 1, the VQI reasonably approximates Qs/Qt (Nelson, 1993).

Dead Space Ventilation. VD/VT is that fraction of the $\dot{V}E$ that does not participate in alveolar gas exchange and is a measure of the efficiency of ventilation (Nelson, 1993).

It may be estimated from the Bohr equation $V_D/V_T = (Pa_{CO_2} - Pe_{CO_2})/Pa_{CO_2}$, based on the Pa_{CO_2} and mixed expired P_{CO_2} (Pe_{CO_2}). The collection of expired gas to estimate Pe_{CO_2} can be laborious and requires meticulous attention to detail.

PRACTICAL GUIDELINES FOR VENTILATOR MANAGEMENT

Regardless of the specific issues associated with each of the following settings, the following general principles are important when providing ventilatory assistance (Pierson, 1995):

- Limit peak Palv to less than 35 cm H_2O
- Watch for and avoid the development of auto-PEEP
- Use low levels of pressure support (e.g., 5 to 8 cm H_2O) during periods of spontaneous breathing, with or without CPAP
- Use the lowest F_{IO_2} necessary to maintain Pa_{O_2} of 60 mm Hg

A summary of recommended ventilator settings are provided in Table 10–8. Some details of disease-specific ventilatory management are discussed in the following paragraphs.

"Routine" Ventilatory Assistance

Many patients who require a period of invasive mechanical ventilation have relatively normal underlying lung function. What may be referred to as "routine" ventilatory assistance is encountered most frequently in the postoperative period or in the setting of short-term loss of spontaneous ventilation, such as with a drug overdose. In such settings, a volume-targeted mode such as VACV is simplest and most reliable, and usually requires fewer adjustments than does pressure-targeted ventilation. One can add 5 cm H_2O of PEEP to counteract the modest drop in functional residual capacity (FRC) that may occur with ET intubation, although this is probably unnecessary in most patients (Pierson, 1999).

Chronic Obstructive Pulmonary Disease

Whether an upper respiratory infection, increased bronchospasm, inspissated secretions, fluid overload, or other cause is responsible, decompensation in patients with COPD is primarily caused by increased work of breathing (Schmidt and Hall, 1989). Signs of ventilatory muscle fatigue and weakness (rapid shallow breathing, use of accessory muscles, abdominal paradox) are usually present (Tobin, 1994). Because these patients may have underlying CO_2 retention, pHa, rather than the absolute P_{CO_2} value, should be used to diagnose and gauge the severity of acute respiratory failure (Leatherman, 1996; Pierson, 1999). The majority (80% to 90%) of episodes can be managed without intubation and mechanical ventilation, and this should be a primary goal. Overoxygena-

TABLE 10–8 ■ Recommended Ventilatory Settings

Short-term ventilatory support in patients with normal lungs
- Mode: SIMV or VACV
- Tidal volume: 10–12 ml/kg
- Initial rate: 10–15 breaths/min, adjusted to maintain Pa_{CO_2} of 35–45 mm Hg
- PEEP: 5 cm H_2O (optional)
- F_{IO_2}: 0.30–0.50 (as required to maintain $Pa_{O_2} > 70$ mm Hg)

Short-term ventilatory support in acute respiratory failure
- SIMV or VACV
- Tidal volume: 10–12 ml/kg (except in obstructive lung disease; see below)
- Initial rate: 10–15 breaths/min adjusted to maintain Pa_{CO_2} of 35–45 mm Hg
- PEEP: 10–12 cm H_2O; adjust as necessary
- F_{IO_2}: as necessary to keep Pa_{O_2} in the range of 60–80 mm Hg

Acute lung injury/ARDS
- SIMV or VACV or PCV
- Tidal volume: 5–8 ml/kg, plateau pressure < 35 cm H_2O
- Rate: 15–25 breaths/min, limited by development of auto-PEEP
- PEEP: in most instances, 10–15 cm H_2O (based on pressure-volume curve)
- Sedate patient to prevent "fighting the ventilator" or increased respiratory rates over those set (to minimize auto-PEEP)
- Mean airway pressure: mild injury, 15–20 cm H_2O; moderate injury, 20–25 cm H_2O; severe injury, 25–30 cm H_2O
- F_{IO_2}: as low as possible to maintain $Pa_{O_2} > 50$ mm Hg in severe injury
- Permissive hypercapnia: allow Pa_{CO_2} to increase into the 60–100 mm Hg range, if necessary, to maintain plateau pressure < 35 cm H_2O

Acute respiratory failure in obstructive lung disease
- SIMV rather than VACV (to avoid hyperinflation)
- Tidal volume: 7–10 ml/kg
- Initial rate: 6–8 breaths/min
- Pressure support: 5–8 cm H_2O (to minimize work of breathing during spontaneous breaths)
- Peak inspiratory flow rate: 60–90 L/min
- PEEP: adjust to about 80% of measured auto-PEEP level (or ≤ 5 cm H_2O)
- F_{IO_2}: sufficient to maintain $Pa_{O_2} > 60$ mm Hg
- Sedation as necessary to ensure that patient rests during the first 24 hr

Acute neuromuscular disease
- SIMV (with sufficient mandatory rate to prevent hypercapnia) or VACV
- Tidal volume: 10–12 ml/kg
- Rate: 10–15 breaths/min or more
- Peak inspiratory flow adjusted to patient comfort
- PEEP: 5 cm H_2O
- F_{IO_2}: sufficient to keep $Pa_{O_2} > 60$ mm Hg (generally 0.21–0.40)

Intracranial hypertension
- Rate > 15 breaths/min to keep Pa_{CO_2} of 25–30 mm Hg
- PEEP: avoid (may raise intracranial pressure), unless needed for hypoxemia; if PEEP is necessary, raise head of bed to counteract increased hydrostatic pressure
- Sedation to prevent patients from coughing violently or "fighting the ventilator"
- Avoid "routine" chest physical therapy

F_{IO_2}, fraction of inspired oxygen; Pa_{CO_2}, partial pressure of arterial carbon dioxide; Pa_{O_2}, partial pressure of arterial oxygen; PCV, pressure control ventilation; PEEP, positive end-expiratory pressure; SIMV, synchronized intermittent mandatory ventilation; VACV, volume assist-control ventilation.

Adapted from Pierson DJ: Invasive mechanical ventilation. In Albert RK, Spiro SG, Jeff JR (eds): Comprehensive Respiratory Medicine. London, Mosby, p 11.1–11.20.

tion should be avoided, with the patient's hypoxemia being treated initially with 1 to 2 L/min of nasal oxygen (or 24% to 28% Ventumask), with incremental increases until the PaO_2 is greater than 50 mm Hg but below 60 to 65 mm Hg. Acute severe hypoxemia (PaO_2 < 50 mm Hg) should always be treated, and the great majority of patients will not develop clinically significant acute respiratory acidosis as long as the PaO_2 is not raised initially above about 65 mm Hg. Patients with COPD are at increased risk for circulatory impairment and barotrauma when subjected to invasive mechanical ventilation. The most common problem is pulmonary hyperinflation, which patients who suffer obstructive lung disease typically have at baseline, and which worsens during times of acute exacerbation. The three main goals of invasive mechanical ventilation in patients who have acutely exacerbated COPD are to: (1) rest the ventilatory muscles, (2) avoid further dynamic hyperinflation, and (3) avoid overventilation and acute alkalemia. Resting the ventilatory muscles may be achieved either by providing full ventilatory support using volume-targeted ventilation (with either VACV or SIMV, so that the patient makes no respiratory effort), or by providing partial ventilatory support using PSV, such that tachypnea and respiratory distress are relieved. Tidal volumes in the range of 5 to 8 ml/kg and rapid inspiratory flow (e.g., 80 to 100 L/min) are preferred to maximize expiratory time and avoid air trapping.

This is one of the two clinical settings in which permissive hypercapnia is appropriate, the other being acute lung injury or ARDS, as discussed later. When the degree of air flow limitation is severe, it may not be possible to provide a sufficient $\dot{V}_E$ (i.e., respiratory rate × V_T) to reduce the $PaCO_2$ enough to produce a near-normal pH without a resultant worsening hyperinflation. In obstructive lung disease, PEEP serves a different function than it does in acute lung injury. The purpose here is not to increase lung volume (which is already excessive), but to decrease the muscular effort required to trigger the ventilator during weaning or to breathe spontaneously in the presence of dynamic hyperinflation and auto-PEEP.

Mechanical Ventilation of Patients with Severe Asthma

The most important factor in the decision to intubate a patient with asthma is not any absolute numeric value of PaO_2, respiratory rate, or pulsus paradoxus, but is based on an overall clinical assessment of the degree of respiratory distress, hemodynamics, and the patient's mental status. A patient with marked hypercapnia on presentation, but who is not in extremis, may respond rapidly to aggressive medical therapy with or without noninvasive ventilation, and may not need intubation. Conversely, a patient with less hypercapnia but with a deteriorating mental status despite full medical therapy may require intubation. The mechanical ventilation of patients with severe asthma continues to be associated with a high morbidity (hypotension, 23%; pulmonary barotrauma, 12%) and mortality (overall, 12%; Tuxen, 1996). Hypotension and barotrauma are almost exclusively confined to patients who have been mechanically ventilated. It is now clear that much of this morbidity, and 20% to 35% of the mortality, is probably due to unrecognized or undertreated dynamic pulmonary hyperinflation (DHI), with auto-PEEP arising during mechanical ventilation.

DHI occurs during mechanical ventilation because airflow obstruction leads to inspired volume being incompletely exhaled prior to the arrival of each new breath (Tuxen, 1996). DHI continues until an equilibrium point is reached whereby the increased lung volume results in a sufficient increase in the elastic recoil pressure and reduction in small airway resistance to enable exhaled volume to equal inhaled volume. The primary determinants of this equilibrium point are the severity of airflow obstruction, the V_T, and the expiratory time (a function of both the respiratory rate and the inspiratory flow rate $\dot{V}_I$).

Current recommendations for mechanical ventilation include sedation, with or without transient initial paralysis, hypoventilation using an initial V_T of 6 to 8 ml/kg, a respiratory rate of 10 to 12 breaths/min, and $\dot{V}_I$ of 80 to 100 L/min. Ventilation should then be adjusted based on DHI and not $PaCO_2$. If the DHI is excessive, the respiratory rate should be reduced. If the DHI is not excessive, then the rate can be increased. PCV with a suitable I/E ratio is a reasonable alternative. Uncommonly, patients with exceptionally severe asthma may develop excessive DHI despite moderate hypoventilation. Any unexplained hypotension, apparent cardiac tamponade, or electromechanical dissociation occurring during mechanical ventilation of a patient with airflow obstruction should first be given an apnea test (discontinuation of mechanical ventilation) before any other delaying or potentially harmful diagnostic or therapeutic procedures are attempted (Tuxen, 1994).

Acute Lung Injury and Acute Respiratory Distress Syndrome

Patients with ARDS present great challenges for effective mechanical ventilation. These patients have decreased pulmonary compliance, increased airways resistance, and increased dead space. The approach to mechanical ventilation for patients with ARDS has changed as our understanding of ARDS has evolved (Bone, 1993; Hinson and Marini, 1992; Koleff and Schuster, 1995; Matthay, 1996; Pierson, 1995; Schuster, 1995). Previously, ARDS was viewed as a homogeneous disease in which alveolar compliance was uniformly decreased. The goal of mechanical ventilation was to deliver a normal V_T to each individual alveolus during inspiration and to prevent collapse of the alveolus during expiration. Therefore, the approach was to use tidal volumes appropriate for normal patients (12 ml/kg) and to use PEEP to recruit collapsed alveoli and maintain alveolar expansion during expiration (Fig. 10–14). Because patients with ARDS have extremely low compliance at these tidal volumes, this approach resulted in extremely high PIPs (60 to 100 cm H_2O). Additionally, because dead space is markedly increased in ARDS, high respiratory rates were required and patients frequently developed intrinsic PEEP (auto-PEEP or dynamic hyperinflation due to inadequate time for exhalation of the inspired volume) in addition to the applied PEEP.

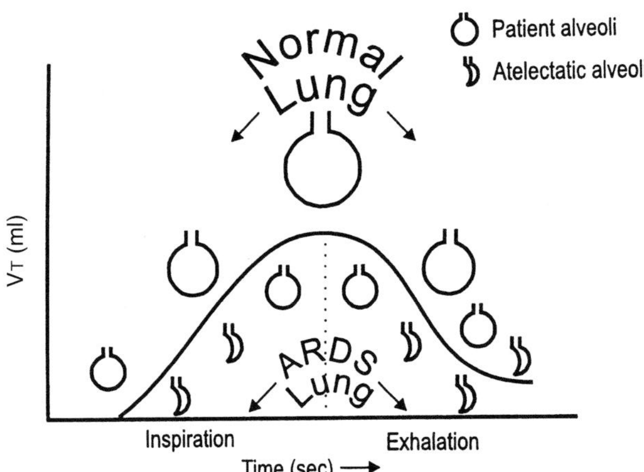

FIGURE 10–14 ■ In acute respiratory distress syndrome (ARDS), alveoli may collapse during early to mid-exhalation and may open only during mid-inspiration to late inspiration. Appropriate use of positive end-expiratory pressure (PEEP) may prevent the phasic opening and closing of alveoli during the ventilatory cycle, thus attenuating ventilator-induced lung injury and also improving arterial oxygenation. (From Rahoof S, Khan FA: Mechanical Ventilation Manual. Philadelphia, American College of Physicians, 1998.)

The approach to mechanical ventilation of ARDS has been altered by the development of two concepts: heterogeneity of lung injury in ARDS and the recognition of ventilator-induced lung injury (volutrauma). Although chest radiographs may show a homogeneous increase in lung density in ARDS, computed tomography (CT) scans of the chest demonstrate marked variability in density from region to region. $\dot{V}/\dot{Q}$ distributions, measured by the multiple inert gas elimination technique, demonstrate the entire range from shunt, to normal, to dead-space units. Histologic examination demonstrates marked variability in injury among adjacent lung areas. The diminished compliance of the lung in ARDS is therefore primarily explained by a reduced number of normal alveoli rather than by a normal number of poorly compliant alveoli. Accordingly, Gattinoni and colleagues (1987, 1988, 1994) have popularized the "baby lung" concept whereby the patient with ARDS is considered to have a severely diminished volume of normal lung with no effective ventilation in the remainder of the lung. Appropriate ventilation would therefore use tidal volumes appropriate to a baby-sized rather than to an adult-sized lung. The recognition of heterogeneity of lung units has additional implications for mechanical ventilation in ARDS. Each lung unit can be considered to have its own resistance and compliance so that the time constants for inflation of lung units may vary. Although the maximal possible inflation of a lung unit is determined by the PIP and the compliance of that unit, the actual inflation is also dependent on the duration of the PIP and the time constant of the lung unit. Lung units with normal compliance but increased resistance will be underinflated if high airway pressure is maintained for only a brief period of time.

Based on a better understanding of lung mechanics and recognition of the heterogeneity of parenchymal involvement in different phase of ARDS, new lung-protective strategies of ventilator management have evolved (Hickling, 1990; Marini, 1993; Pierson, 1995). The overall goal is to support gas exchange at an acceptable level while avoiding ventilator-induced lung injury. These principles are best illustrated on a pressure-volume curve corresponding to an ARDS patient shown in Figure 10–6. Static CL increases as recruitable areas of atelectasis open (at the lower inflection point, *A*). At higher inflation pressures, compliance decreases as overdistention of individual lung units occurs (at the upper inflection point, *C*). It is believed (Marini, 1993) that lung injury can occur when the patient's lungs are inflated at volumes both below the lower inflection point and above the upper inflection point. Point *B* represents alveolar derecruitment during expiration. Thus, the optimal ventilation strategy seeks to carry out the ventilation between points *A* and *C* on the curve (see Fig. 10–6). This means that a certain minimum level of PEEP is required to avoid alveolar derecruitment at point *B*, but that the VT must be kept small so that the end-inspiratory P_{plat} does not exceed that at the upper inflection point (Marini and Kelsen, 1992; Pierson, 1995). It has been suggested that the upper and lower inflection points be determined for each patient by constructing a pressure-volume curve. However, studies indicate that in most patients, ventilation will stay between points *A* and *C* using 8 to 15 cm of PEEP, and a VT of 5 to 8 ml/kg (Marini and Kelsen, 1992; Pierson, 1995). In addition, because an alveolar distending pressure of 30 to 35 cm H_2O is the injury threshold in most animal studies, efforts should be made to keep P_{plat} less than 30 to 35 cm H_2O.

These concepts have led to the application of PC-IRV in ARDS. During PCV, the peak airway pressure is maintained throughout the duration of inspiration, allowing inflation of all lung units to a degree dependent primarily on compliance. Thus, lung units that are not inflated during conventional VCV may be inflated during PCV, a process called "alveolar recruitment." These recruited lung units are then maintained open by the addition of an appropriate level of PEEP. The combination of a low level of PEEP and a moderate but constant level of inspiratory pressure during PCV results in an elevated Paw at a lower peak pressure than occurs during VCV. However, significant controversy exists regarding whether PCV (usually with IRV) actually produces any additional benefit over VCV. Multiple studies have documented that for a similar VT, PCV results in a lower peak airway pressure than does VCV. However, recent data suggest that the higher peak airway pressure with VCV versus PCV may be an artifact related to the site of measurement. Due to the resistance of the ET tube, the high flow rates used with VCV in patients with ARDS result in a significant pressure gradient between the proximal and distal ends of the ET tube. The difference between peak and plateau pressures during VCV in ARDS may be due to this gradient, rather than to redistribution of ventilation during the inspiratory pause (Pierson, 1999; Tobin, 1994). Lessard and colleagues (1994) noted that increased mean airway pressures with PC-IRV actually worsened oxygenation compared with volume or PCV at a similar level of PEEP. At present, it is difficult to determine whether PCV, with or without IRV, provides advantages over conventional VCV. Many studies did not compare the different modes at similar levels of VT, $(PEEP)_{tot}$, and Paw. Additionally, some studies suggest that the beneficial effects of PC-IRV may not occur for several hours, so that the demonstration of equivalent short-term effects may be misleading. Use of PC-IRV must weigh the potential benefits (decreased lung injury, improved gas exchange) against the potential hazards (decreased VT, decreased CO). In general, the use of PC-IRV requires deep sedation, with or without paralysis of the patient; frequent evaluation of intrinsic PEEP, VT, and Paw; and invasive hemodynamic monitoring to determine any adverse affects of increased Paw and intrinsic PEEP.

In managing patients who have severe ARDS, one may have to accept "permissive hypoxemia" as well as permissive hypercapnia. Although the goal is to maintain Pa_{O_2} in the normal range, this may not be attainable in some patients without the use of potentially injurious levels of PEEP. A Pa_{O_2} of 50 to 55 mm Hg (oxygen saturation as measured by pulse oximetry [Sp_{O_2}] of 85% to 90%) is usually well tolerated if hemoglobin concentration and cardiac function are adequate. Appropriate sedation is usually required when pursuing the lung-protective ventilatory strategy in ARDS.

Unilateral and Asymmetric Lung Disease

Patients who have lobar pneumonia, lobar or whole-lung atelectasis, or other markedly asymmetric pulmonary involvement present a special problem for ventilatory assistance, particularly in the presence of severe hypoxemia. Such patients illustrate why PEEP should not automatically be applied as treatment for hypoxemic respiratory failure. CRS is much higher in relatively normal areas of the lung than in areas of consolidation or collapse. As a result, application of PEEP can preferentially expand these more normal areas of the lung, yet not produce the desired effect in the diseased lung. Distention of normal lung regions can raise pulmonary vascular resistance sufficiently and divert blood to the abnormal areas. Accordingly, applying PEEP can worsen rather than improve arterial oxygenation in such instances (see Table 10–3) (Pierson, 1995).

Neuromuscular Disease

The most commonly encountered acute neuromuscular diseases are high cervical spinal cord injury and acute inflammatory polyneuropathy (e.g., Guillain-Barré syndrome). Ventilatory drive is intact but patients lack sufficient neuromuscular function to maintain normal CO_2 removal, lung inflation, airway protection, and secretion clearance. Development of frank respiratory acidosis is a late sign, and ventilatory assistance should be instituted when VC falls below about 10 ml/kg, or maximum inspiratory force falls to less than 20 cm H_2O, without waiting for CO_2 retention to develop. Patients who have acute neuromuscular disease or cervical spinal cord injury, where lung function is relatively normal, may benefit from ventilator management at higher than usual tidal volumes and flows. Such patients may experience dyspnea at tidal volumes of 10 to 12 ml/kg, which improves when larger volumes (12 to 16 ml/kg) are used. Similarly, such patients typically prefer faster inspiratory flows (e.g., 80 to 100 L/min). Such settings often result in a mild-to-moderate respiratory alkalosis, which is usually well tolerated. Many patients who have traumatic quadriplegia or other acute neuromuscular disorder experience recurrent atelectasis, which can cause more severe hypoxemia than is usually seen with lobar collapse in other clinical settings. Ventilation with larger than usual tidal volumes, with or without the addition of low-level PEEP, is important in such patients to prevent recurrence. Frequent changes in posture may also be beneficial.

Acute Brain Injury

Patients who have closed head injury or other acute brain insult may lose the normal autoregulation of cerebral perfusion pressure. In such patients anything that decreases mean arterial pressure or raises CVP must be avoided. Therefore, PEEP is used cautiously, if at all, in patients who have acute brain injury, because the raised intrathoracic pressure can be transmitted via the vertebral veins to the central nervous system. Maneuvers that induce coughing and thus raise ICP, such as tracheal suctioning, are avoided whenever possible. For many years, deliberate hyperventilation to Pa_{CO_2} levels of 25 to 30 mm Hg was an integral part of ventilator management in patients who had acute brain injury. Firm data in support of this practice are lacking (Pierson, 1995, 1999).

Flail Chest

Several studies demonstrate that the clinical course and outcome of flail chest injury are determined mainly by the underlying pulmonary injury rather than the flail segment. Patients who sustain multiple rib fractures without associated lung contusion or pneumonia generally recover uneventfully, whereas flail chest in the setting of acute lung injury typically follows the course of that illness, with little additional morbidity related to the chest wall instability. Ventilator management of patients with a flail chest is therefore the same as for the underlying pulmonary injury. Attention must be given to pain control. Often one can use full ventilatory support until the patient is ready for weaning. Intercostal nerve blocks or administration of epidural narcotics can greatly aid in pain control and ventilator weaning in such patients.

WEANING FROM VENTILATORY ASSISTANCE

Discontinuation of mechanical ventilation is usually not a problem in patients requiring short-term ventilator support, but it may be difficult in patients recovering from an episode of acute respiratory failure (Hall and Wood, 1987; MacIntyre and Stock, 1990; Tobin, 1994; Yang and Tobin, 1991). Weaning such patients from the ventilator can be a major clinical challenge. The initiation of weaning from ventilatory support requires careful timing. If delayed unnecessarily, the patient remains at risk of ventilator-associated complications. If performed prematurely, severe cardiopulmonary decompensation may occur and further delay extubation. Before attempting to wean the patient from the ventilator, the patient's pulmonary function should be stable or improving and there should be no evidence of hemodynamic instability. If extubation is anticipated, clinical evaluation of the patient's ability to protect the upper airway and to cough needs to be verified.

When ventilatory support has been required for 1 to 2 weeks or longer, factors in addition to the respiratory status of the patient become increasingly important (Pierson, 1999). These nonrespiratory factors emphasize that prolonged acute respiratory failure is typically associated with multisystem dysfunction, resulting in a variety of abnormalities that can interfere with weaning. The patient's overall medical condition is an important determinant. Such patients often remain unstable, requiring frequent ventilator changes, which precludes the possibility of totally spontaneous ventilation. In prolonged acute illness, weaning depends on the balance between ventilatory demand and patient capability. Frequently, weaning must be deferred because the $\dot{V}E$ required to keep the $PaCO_2$ in the normal range is too high (e.g., 16 to 18 L/min instead of the expected 10 L/min). In such cases, at least one of two possible physiologic derangements may be present: hypermetabolism (increased CO_2 production) or inefficient ventilation (increased dead-space ventilation, VD/VT). Causes of hypermetabolism include fever, sepsis, excessive skeletal muscle activity (e.g., shivering, seizures, or agitation), or overzealous caloric supplementation, especially with carbohydrate calories. Inefficient ventilation is a hallmark of severe obstructive lung disease and is also a characteristic feature of late ARDS. Bedside measurement of both CO_2 production and VD/VT may be helpful in identifying the cause or causes of excessive $\dot{V}E$ requirement. Elevated CO_2 production may be due to fever, thyrotoxicosis, excessive parenteral nutrition, or a generalized catabolic state (Pierson, 1999). Elevated dead space ventilation (manifested as increased VD/VT), may be due to hypovolemia, excessive airway pressures, or pulmonary vascular disease (Pierson, 1999).

Drugs can interfere with weaning, either by suppressing ventilatory drive or by compromising ventilatory muscle function (Pierson, 1999). All sedatives, tranquilizers, and hypnotics depress ventilatory drive, albeit to varying degrees. Muscle relaxants such as vecuronium and pancuronium, often used as adjuncts in ventilatory management, can cause muscle weakness and prolong weaning in two ways: Clearance of these agents may be prolonged for days in the presence of renal insufficiency; a recently described myopathy, most often seen with concurrent systemic administration of corticosteroids, can produce muscle weakness that lasts for many weeks (Hansen-Flaschen et al, 1993). Aminoglycoside antibiotics can produce neuromuscular paralysis, although this is rarely seen today.

Predicting Weaning Outcome

Several of the indices used to predict the outcome of a weaning trial are listed in Table 10–9.

Gas Exchange. Discontinuation of ventilator support is not advisable in a patient with persistent hypoxemia, for example, with a PaO_2 less than 55 mm Hg and FIO_2 of at least 0.40. A number of indices derived from arterial blood gas (ABG) measurements have been proposed as predictors of weaning outcome, but have not been shown to be consistently helpful (Tobin and Alex, 1994; Tobin and Yang, 1990). Additionally, none of the ABG criteria listed in Table 10–9 have been subjected to prospective investigation.

TABLE 10–9 ■ Variables Used to Predict Weaning Outcome

Gas Exchange
$PaO_2 > 60$ mm Hg with $FIO_2 < 0.35$
$PaO_2/FIO_2 > 200$
Ventilatory Pump
Vital capacity >10–15 ml/kg body weight
Maximum inspiratory pressure < −30 cm H_2O
Minute ventilation <10 L/min
Maximum voluntary ventilation greater than twice resting minute ventilation
Normal rib cage abdominal motion
CROP index >13 ml/breaths/min (see text)
Ventilatory endurance index (Jabour) <4/min
Frequency-to-tidal volume ratio (*f*/VT) <100 breaths/min/L

FIO_2, fraction of inspired oxygen; PaO_2, partial pressure of arterial oxygen.

Adapted from Tobin MJ, Yang K: Weaning from mechanical ventilation. Crit Care Clin 6:725, 1990.

Maximum Inspiratory Pressure. PImax provides a global assessment of the strength of all the inspiratory muscles and is one of the standard measurements used to predict weaning outcome. In a classic study, Sahn and Lakshminarayan (1973) found that a PImax value of −30 cm H_2O or less predicted successful weaning, whereas a PImax value higher than −20 cm H_2O predicted weaning failure. However, in a subsequent prospective study conducted in patients with ARDS (20 patients), left-sided heart failure (20 patients), and neuromuscular disease (7 patients), Tahvanainen and associates (1983) found that a PImax criterion of −30 cm H_2O was false negative in 100% of patients and false positive in 26%. Subsequent studies have also found that PImax has limited power in predicting weaning outcome, especially in those patients receiving prolonged mechanical ventilation (Fiastro et al, 1988; Tobin, 1994).

Vital Capacity. VC is the largest volume of gas that a patient is able to exhale after a maximal inspiration. A value of VC of 10 ml/kg has been suggested as being essential to sustain spontaneous ventilation, suggesting that a VC of greater than 10 to 15 ml/kg could predict weaning success (Tobin and Alex, 1994). However, Tahvanainen and associates (1983) found that a VC of greater than 10 ml/kg was false positive in 18% of patients and false negative in 50%. Similarly, Milbern and colleagues (1978), in a prospective study of 33 postoperative patients, found that a VC of 15 ml/kg was false positive in 15% of patients and false negative in 63%.

Thoracic Compliance. A decrease in static thoracic compliance is associated with disorders of the thoracic cage, or a reduction in the number of functioning lung units (pneumonia, pneumothorax, pulmonary edema, etc.). Total static thoracic compliance of the respiratory system has been suggested as a useful predictor of weaning outcome (Tobin and Alex, 1994). A successful weaning outcome is considered unlikely in patients with an effective thoracic compliance of less than 25 ml/cm H_2O, because the associated increase in the work of breathing would make it difficult to sustain the level of ventilation necessary for adequate gas exchange (Tobin and Alex, 1994; Tobin and Yang, 1990). An associated index, called the "effective dynamic compliance," obtained by dividing VT by the difference in peak airway pressure and $(PEEP)_{tot}$, has also been proposed as being useful to assess the overall impedance of the respiratory system (Tobin and Alex, 1994). Despite the attractiveness and potential usefulness of static thoracic compliance and effective dynamic compliance, there have been few studies that evaluate their role in predicting weaning outcome.

Minute Ventilation and Maximum Voluntary Ventilation. The relationship between $\dot{V}E$ and $PaCO_2$ provides a good indication of the demands placed on the respiratory system. A high $\dot{V}E$ in the presence of hypercapnia indicates the presence of either increased CO_2 production or a high VD/VT. Maximum voluntary ventilation (MVV) is the volume of air that can be inhaled or exhaled with maximum effort over 1 minute. A $\dot{V}E$ of less than 10 L/min is the conventional index of a successful weaning outcome (Tobin and Alex, 1994). In a study by Sahn and Lashminarayan (1973), all patients who had a $\dot{V}E$ of less than 10 L/min, and the ability to double this value (during an MVV maneuver), were weaned successfully, whereas 71% of those who did not meet both criteria required continued ventilatory support. However, Tahvanainen and colleagues (1983), using the criterion of less than 10 L/min, failed to wean 11% of favorable patients (false positives), and observed false-negative results in 25%. The ability to double $\dot{V}E$ during an MVV maneuver was false positive in 5% of patients and false negative in 76% of patients. Other investigators have also reported a high rate of false-negative and false-positive results using the $\dot{V}E$ and MVV criterion (Tobin, 1994).

Airway Occlusion Pressure. Airway occlusion pressure is proportional to the respiratory drive and is a well-accepted way of estimating weaning probability. *Airway occlusion pressure* is defined as the airway pressure generated at 0.1 second ($P_{0.1}$) after initiating an inspiratory effort against an occluded airway. In healthy subjects, $P_{0.1}$ is generally 2 cm H_2O (Tobin and Alex, 1994). Herrera and coworkers (1985) first suggested that measurements of $P_{0.1}$ might be useful in predicting the outcome of a weaning trial. These investigators obtained 52 measurements in 20 patients requiring ventilatory support for acute respiratory failure (due to COPD in 11 patients, and to other causes in 9 patients). All of their patients had $P_{0.1}$ greater than 2 cm H_2O. In 78% of instances, weaning was successful when the $P_{0.1}$ was equal to or less than 4.2 cm H_2O. In a subsequent study, Sasson and colleagues (1987) obtained $P_{0.1}$ measurements within 5 minutes of discontinuing ventilatory support in 12 patients with COPD who met "standard" weaning criteria (PImax ≤ -20 cm H_2O, and VC $\geq$ 10 ml/kg). These investigators found that all patients failed the weaning trial when the $P_{0.1}$ was greater than 6 cm H_2O, whereas all 7 patients who were successfully weaned had a $P_{0.1}$ of less than 6 cm H_2O (Sasson et al, 1987). Using the data reported by Herrera and colleagues (1985), Sassoon and associates (1987) and subsequently by Montgomery and coworkers (1987), Tobin and Yang (1990) estimated that the application of $P_{0.1}$ equal to or less than 4.2 cm H_2O as a predictor of weaning success was associated with a 44% false-positive rate and a 50% false-negative rate. A $P_{0.1}$ of less than 6 cm H_2O was associated with a 46% false-positive rate and a 33% false-negative rate. Clearly, more prospective data are necessary to evaluate the usefulness of airway occlusion pressure to predict successful weaning outcomes.

Rib Cage and Abdominal Motion. The chest wall has two compartments, the rib cage and the abdomen, and assessment of their relative motion can help in the detection of respiratory dysfunction and distress. Asynchronous and paradoxic motion of the rib cage and abdomen can be assessed by an index called the maximum compartmental amplitude-to-VT ratio, which relates the total extension of both the rib cage and abdomen to VT; a high value suggests that weaning is unlikely to be successful (Tobin et al, 1986, 1987). An increase in the breath-to-breath variation of the compartmental contribution to VT also appeared to predict weaning failure (Tobin et al, 1987).

Rapid Shallow Breathing. Patients who fail a weaning trial develop an immediate increase in respiratory frequency (*f*) and a decrease in VT following discontinuation of ventilator support (Tobin and Alex, 1994). In a study by Yang and Tobin (1991), measurements of *f* and VT were combined as an index of rapid shallow breathing—the *f*/VT ratio. In an initial "training data set" obtained in 36 patients, the authors found that an *f*/VT value of 105 breaths/min/L best differentiated patients who were successfully weaned from those in whom weaning failed. The predictive power of this value was then assessed in 64 patients who constituted the "prospective-validation data set" (Yang and Tobin, 1991). The positive and negative predictive values were 0.78 and 0.95, respectively, which were the highest values noted for any of the predictive indices in the study.

Integrative Indices. Weaning failure is commonly multifactorial in origin, and therefore it is not surprising that an index that assesses a single function may be unreliable. Accordingly, an index that integrates a number of physiologic functions would be expected to have greater predictive accuracy. Such an index is the CROP index (Yang and Tobin, 1991), which incorporates a measure of pulmonary gas exchange and an assessment of the demands placed on the respiratory system and the capacity of the respiratory muscles to handle them:

$$\text{CROP Index} = \frac{(C_{dyn})(\text{PImax})(PaO_2/PAO_2)}{\text{Respiratory rate}}$$

where C_{dyn} is dynamic compliance, and PaO_2/PAO_2 is the arterial-alveolar ratio and a measure of gas exchange. Successful weaning is reliably suggested by a CROP index greater than 13, whereas difficult weaning frequently occurs with a CROP index between 11 and 13, and unsuccessful weaning attempts occur with a CROP index of less than 11. When examined prospectively, this index had positive and negative predictive values of 0.71 and 0.70, respectively (Yang and Tobin, 1991).

Another integrative index of *ventilatory endurance* and gas exchange was developed by Jabour and colleagues (1991). This index uses the pressure-time index (PTI), an estimate of the efficiency of gas exchange (the $\dot{V}E$ needed to bring $PaCO_2$ to 40 mm Hg, or $\dot{V}E40$), and VT during spontaneous breathing (sb): Integrative index = PTI × ($\dot{V}E40/(VT)sb$). The investigators found that this index had a positive predictive value of 0.96 and a negative predictive value of 0.95. However, assessment was performed on a post hoc basis, and they did not examine accuracy prospectively.

Methods of Weaning

A list of techniques used for weaning is provided in Table 10–10.

TABLE 10–10 ■ **Different Strategies Used in Weaning Following Short-Term Ventilatory Support**

Strategy	*Rationale and Technique*
T-piece	Abrupt reloading of ventilatory muscles, using a brief trial of spontaneous ventilation to demonstrate that the patient can breathe without assistance once predictive variables suggest that it will be successful; the patient is disconnected from the ventilator and a high flow of warmed, humidified, oxygen-enriched air is provided during trial
Intermittent mandatory ventilation (IMV)	Gradual reloading of ventilatory muscles as tolerated by patient until all ventilator-provided breaths are discontinued; a volume-targeted technique in which the number of mandatory breaths is progressively decreased, with the adequacy of the patient's efforts assessed by comfort, breathing pattern, and arterial blood gas values; the patient remains connected to the ventilator until weaning is complete
Pressure support	Gradual reloading of ventilatory muscles as tolerated by patient until all positive pressure inspiratory assistance is discontinued; a pressure-targeted technique in which the patient is switched to spontaneous breathing with positive pressure inspiratory assist, and the inspiratory pressure level is progressively decreased as tolerated; the patient remains connected to the ventilator until weaning is complete

Adapted from Pierson DJ: Invasive mechanical ventilation. In Albert RK, Spiro SG, Jett JR (eds): Comprehensive Respiratory Medicine. London, Mosby, 1999, pp 11.1–11.20.

Abrupt Discontinuation. Patients who require brief periods of ventilatory assistance can resume spontaneous respiration with little difficulty. For example, many patients undergoing uncomplicated cardiac surgery can be extubated within a few hours of surgery (Prakash, 1982). Patients should be carefully observed for tachypnea, signs of respiratory distress, and abnormalities in the breathing pattern while breathing spontaneously, without ventilatory support, before extubation.

Gradual T Tube Weaning. To assess a patient's ability to sustain spontaneous ventilation, the patient can be disconnected from the ventilator and receive supplemental oxygen through a T tube system (Tobin and Alex, 1994). During such a trial, the patient's clinical status is monitored closely. Some physicians have used relatively brief trials of spontaneous breathing (~ 5 minutes) interposed with periods of mechanical ventilation of increasing duration. Other physicians proceed directly from high levels of ventilator assistance to a spontaneous breathing trial. If the patient does not develop signs of intolerance, extubation is performed without any further weaning maneuvers.

Intermittent Mandatory Ventilation. IMV was the first alternative approach to T tube trials (Tobin and Alex, 1994). It involves a gradual reduction in the amount of support being provided by the ventilator and a progressive increase in the amount of respiratory work being performed by the patient. When used for weaning, the IMV rate is usually reduced in steps of 1 to 3 breaths/min, and an arterial blood gas sample is obtained after about 30 minutes. With application of IMV, patient effort is thought to be reduced in proportion to the number of breaths delivered by the ventilator. Recent evidence, however, suggests that this is not correct. Rather, as the synchronized IMV rate is decreased, inspiratory work and pressure-time product increase progressively, both for spontaneous breaths and for assisted breaths (Marini et al, 1988). This is largely due to the inability of the respiratory center output to adapt to intermittent support, as demonstrated in a recent study using electromyograms of the diaphragm and sternomastoid muscles (Imsand et al, 1994).

Pressure Support Ventilation. PSV augments a spontaneous breath with a fixed amount of positive pressure and is commonly used to counteract the work of breathing imposed by ET tubes and ventilator circuits (Brochard, 1994). Theoretically, this should help with weaning, because a patient who is comfortable at the level of PSV that compensates for increased work should be able to sustain ventilation following extubation. However, the resistance posed by an ET tube varies with the diameter and flow rates, and even when these values are constant, resistance will vary as a result of tube deformation and adherent secretions. Indeed, Brochard and associates (1991) demonstrated that the level of PSV necessary to eliminate imposed work varied considerably (3 to 14 cm H_2O) from patient to patient. Likewise, Nathan and colleagues (1993) could not define a level of PSV that predicted respiratory work following extubation. These studies (Brochard et al, 1991; Nathan et al, 1993) suggest that the use of PSV to predict a patient's ability to sustain ventilation following extubation may be misleading.

Relative Efficacy of Weaning Techniques. Three early studies compared the efficacy of IMV versus trials of spontaneous breathing and noted little or no difference between them (Tobin and Alex, 1994). These studies had the problems of retrospective design, inappropriate study populations, and poorly standardized protocols. In addition, most were conducted before the widespread use of PSV. In a recent, rigorously controlled study, Brochard and associates (1994) found that weaning time was significantly shorter with PSV (5.7 ± 3.7 days) than with IMV (9.9 ± 8.2 days) or trials of spontaneous breathing (8.5 ± 8.3 days). In contrast, using a similar experimental design, Esteban and colleagues (1995) found that a once-daily trial of spontaneous breathing led to extubation about three times more quickly than did IMV, and about twice as quickly as PSV. No differences were noted in the rate of successful weaning between a once-daily trial of spontaneous breathing and intermittent trials of spontaneous breathing (attempted at least twice a day). Nor were differences noted between IMV and PSV. The reason for the different outcomes in these two studies is likely explained by the constrained manner in which IMV and trials of spontaneous breathing were used in the study of Brochard and associates (1994). During application of IMV, patients had to tolerate a ventilator rate of 4 breaths/min or less for at least 24 hours before extubation. In contrast, Esteban and colleagues (1995) extubated patients as soon as they tolerated a ventilator rate of 5 breaths/min for 2 hours. For the trials of spontaneous breathing in the study of Brochard and associates (1994), physicians could request up to three separate trials over a 24-hour period, each lasting for 2 hours, before deciding to extubate a patient. Esteban and colleagues (1995) extubated patients in the once-daily trials of spontaneous breathing, as soon as this was tolerated for 2 hours. Some findings in these two studies are complementary: both demonstrate that the pace of weaning depends on the manner in which the technique is applied. When IMV and trials of spontaneous breathing are used in a constrained manner, weaning is delayed compared with PSV. When a spontaneous breathing trial is used once a day, weaning appears to be expedited.

In summary, most patients can be easily weaned from mechanical ventilation, but a troublesome minority have considerable difficulty (Tobin and Alex, 1994). The major determinants of weaning outcome include the adequacy of pulmonary gas exchange, respiratory muscle function, and psychological problems. Many of the physiologic indices that have been used to predict weaning outcome are frequently inaccurate. Of those available, the f/V_T ratio appears to be the most reliable. A number of techniques can be used for weaning. Of these, a once-daily trial of spontaneous breathing may be the most useful.

COMMENTS AND CONTROVERSIES

The management of thoracic surgical patients, in the ICU and on ventilators for respiratory assistance, is often a shared responsibility between the surgeon, the surgeon's house staff, and intensivists who may work primarily, or full time, in the ICU. The lines of responsibility remain blurred on many occasions, even though the unit may be designated as "closed" and presumably is the primary responsibility of personnel in the ICU. In my opinion, it is a major loss of important, often rapidly changing, educational experience for both operating surgeon and resident if aspects of supervision and ongoing patient care are entirely entrusted to the incumbent ICU staff. It is admittedly difficult for the surgeon to remain abreast of frequent new developments and management techniques in this volatile field, but the effort to do so is almost certainly rewarded with benefit to surgeon, surgical students, and most important, patients.

Drs. Bidani, Tuazon, Alpard, and Zwischenberger provide a thorough review of all pertinent aspects relating to mechanical ventilation in surgical patients: indications, methods, and complications are all presented with an effort to impart practical, applicable, current information. Although most of us will not remember many of the tortuous formulas expressed in the vocabulary of the respiratory physiologist and intensivist, each section provides clearly expressed, practical, summary information and recommendations, often in clearly illustrated tabular form. This chapter has been prepared for thoracic surgeons, under the direction of a thoracic surgeon (Dr. Zwischenberger) who has an internationally recognized expertise as a clinician, investigator, and educator in this field.

F. G. P.

REFERENCES

AARC: Consensus Conference on the Essentials of Mechanical Ventilation. Respir Care 37:999, 1992.

AARC, American Association for Respiratory Care Consensus Group: Assessing innovations in mechanical ventilatory support. Respir Care Clin N Am 40:926, 1995.

ACCP: American College of Chest Physicians Consensus Conference on Mechnical Ventilation. Chest 104:1833, 1993.

Albert RK: Least PEEP: Primum non nocere. Chest 87:2, 1985.

Albert RK, Leasa D, Sanderson M et al: The prone position improves arterial oxygenation and reduces shunt in oleic acid–induced acute lung injury. Am Rev Respir Dis 135:628, 1987.

Alex CG, Tobin MJ: Assessment of pulmonary function in critically ill patients. In Shoemaker WC, Ayres SM, Grenvik A et al (eds): Textbook of Critical Care, 4th ed. Philadelphia, WB Saunders, 1999, pp 1222–1232.

Alpard SK, Zwischenberger JB: Extracorporeal gas exchange. Respir Care Clin 4:711, 1998.

Amato MB, Barbas CS, Medeiros DM et al: Beneficial effects of the "open lung approach" with low distending pressures in acute respiratory distress syndrome. A prospective randomized study on mechanical ventilation. Am J Respir Crit Care Med 152:1835, 1995.

Amato MB, Barbas CS, Medeiros DM et al: Effect of a protective-ventilation strategy on mortality in the acute respiratory distress syndrome. N Engl J Med 338:347, 1998.

Ashbaugh DG, Bigelow DB, Petty TL, Levine BL: Acute respiratory distress syndrome in adults. Lancet 2:319, 1967.

Awad JA, Deslauriers J, Major D et al: Prolonged pumpless arteriovenous perfusion for carbon dioxide extraction. Ann Thorac Surg 51:534, 1991.

Bachofen M, Weibel ER: Structural alterations of lung parenchyma in the adult respiratory distress syndrome. Clin Chest Med 3:35, 1982.

Bardoczky G, d'Hollander A: Continuous monitoring of the flow-volume loops and compliance during anesthesia. J Clin Monit Comput 8:251, 1992.

Bartlett RH: Extracorporeal life support for cardiopulmonary failure. Curr Probl Surg 27:621, 1990.

Bartlett RH: Respiratory physiology and pathophysiology. In Bartlett RH: Critical Care Physiology. Boston, Little, Brown, 1996, pp 48–100.

Bartlett RH: Extracorporeal life support registry report. ASAIO J 43:104, 1997.

Bendixen HH, Hedley-Whyte J, Laver MB: Impaired oxygenation in surgical patients during general anesthesia with controlled ventilation: a concept of atelectasis. N Engl J Med 269:991, 1963.

Benhamou D, Girault C, Faure C et al: Nasal mask ventilation in acute respiratory failure. Chest 102:912, 1992.

Bennett HB, Vender JS: Positive-pressure ventilation: Renal, hepatic and gastrointestinal function. In Stock MC, Perel A (eds): Mechanical Ventilatory Support. Philadelphia, Lippincott Williams & Wilkins, 1997, pp 75–85.

Benson MS, Pierson DJ: Auto-PEEP during mechanical ventilation of adults. Respir Care Clin N Am 33:557, 1988.

Bersten AD, Oh TE: Ventilators and resuscitators. In Oh TE (ed): Intensive Care Manual, 4th ed. Oxford, Butterworth-Heinemann, 1997, pp 256–265.

Bidani A, DuBose TD: Acid-base regulation: Cellular and whole body. In Arieff AI, DeFronzo RA (eds): Fluid, Electrolyte, and Acid Base Disorders, 2nd ed. New York, Churchill Livingstone, 1995, pp 69–103.

Bidani A, Tzouanakis AE, Cardenas VJ JR et al: Permissive hypercapnia in acute respiratory failure. JAMA 272:957, 1994.

Bidani A, Zwischenberger JB, Cardenas V: Intracorporeal gas exchange: Current status and future development. Intensive Care Med 22:91, 1996.

Bishop MH, Jorgens J, Shoemaker WC et al: The relationship between ARDS, pulmonary infiltration, fluid balance, and hemodynamics in critically ill surgical patients. Am Surg 57:785, 1991.

Bone R: The ARDS lung: New insights from computed tomography. JAMA 269:2134, 1993.

Brochard L: Pressure support ventilation. In Tobin MJ (ed): Principles and Practice of Mechanical Ventilation. New York, McGraw-Hill, 1994, pp 239–257.

Brochard L, Isabey D, Piquet J et al: Reversal of acute exacerbations of chronic obstructive lung disease by inspiratory assistance with a face mask. N Engl J Med 323:1525, 1990.

Brochard L, Rua F, Lorino H et al: Inspiratory pressure support compensates for the additional work of breathing caused by the endotracheal tube. Anesthesiology 75:739, 1991.

Brochard L, Rauss A, Benito S et al: Comparison of three methods of gradual withdrawal from ventilatory support during weaning from mechanical ventilation. Am J Respir Crit Care Med 150:896, 1994.

Brochard L, Mancebo J, Wysocki M et al: Noninvasive ventilation for acute exacerbations of chronic obstructive pulmonary disease. N Engl J Med 333:817, 1995.

Brochard L, Roudot-Thoraval F, Roupie E et al: Tidal volume reduction for prevention of ventilator-induced lung injury in acute respiratory distress syndrome. Am J Respir Crit Care Med 158:1831, 1998.

Brunston RL Jr, Tao W, Bidani A et al: Determination of low blood flow limits for arteriovenous carbon dioxide removal ($AVCO_2R$). ASAIO J 42:M845, 1996.

Brunston RL Jr, Zwischenberger JB, Tao W et al: Total arteriovenous carbon dioxide removal ($AVCO_2R$): Simplifying extracorporeal support for severe respiratory failure. Ann Thorac Surg 64:1599, 1997.

Chatburn RL: Classification of mechanical ventilation. In Tobin MJ (ed): Principles and Practice of Mechanical Ventilation. New York, McGraw-Hill, 1994, pp 37–64.

Clark RH, Yoder BA, Sell MS: Prospective, randomized comparison of high frequency oscillation and conventional ventilation in candidates for extracorporeal oxygenation. J Pediatr 124:447, 1994.

Confalonieri M, Aiolfi S, Gandola L et al: Severe exacerbations of chronic obstructive pulmonary disease treated with BiPAP by nasal mask. Respiration 61:312, 1994.

Connors AF, McCaffree DR, Gray BA: Effect of inspiratory flow rate on gas exchange during mechanical ventilation. Am Rev Respir Dis 124:537, 1981.

Conrad SA, Bagley A, Bagley B et al: Major findings from the clinical trials of the intravascular oxygenator. Artif Organs 18:846, 1994.

Conrad SA, Brown EG, Grier LR et al: Arteriovenous extracorporeal carbon dioxide removal ($AVCO_2R$): A mathematical model and experimental evaluation. ASAIO J 44:267, 1998.

Craven DE, Stieger R: Pathogenesis and prevention of nosocomial pneumonia in the mechanically ventilated patient. Respir Care Clin N Am 34:85, 1989.

Croce MA, Fabian TC, Davis KA et al: Early and late acute respiratory distress syndrome: Two distinct clinical entities. J Trauma 46:361, 1999.

Cullen DJ, Caldera DL: The incidence of ventilator-induced pulmonary barotrauma in critically ill patients. Anesthesiology 50:185, 1979.

Darioli R, Perret C: Mechanical controlled hypoventilation in status asthmaticus. Am Rev Respir Dis 129:385, 1984.

Del Valle RM, Hecker RB: A review of ventilatory modalities used in the intensive care unit. Am J Anesthesiol 12:23, 1995.

Doherty D, Sladen RN: Effects of positive airway pressure on renal function. Probl Respir Care 2:369, 1989.

Dreyfuss D, Saumon G: Barotrauma is volutrauma, but which volume is the one responsible? Intensive Care Med 18:139, 1992.

Dreyfuss D, Soler P, Basset G et al: High inflation pressure pulmonary edema: Respective effects of high airway pressure, high tidal volume, and positive end-expiratory pressure. Am Rev Respir Dis 137:1159, 1988.

Durbin CG, Wallace KK: Oxygen toxicity in the critically ill patient. Respir Care Clin N Am 38:739, 1993.

Esteban A, Frutos F, Tobin MJ et al: A comparison of four methods of weaning patients from mechanical ventilation. N Engl J Med 332:345, 1995.

Federspiel WJ, Hout MS, Hewitt TJ et al: Development of a low flow resistance intravenous oxygenator. ASAIO J 43:M725, 1997.

Fiastro JF, Habib MP, Shon BY et al: Comparison of standard weaning parameters and mechanical work of breathing in mechanically ventilated patients. Chest 94:232, 1988.

Flatten H, Aardal S, Hevroy O: Improved oxygenation using the prone position in patients with ARDS. Acta Anaesthesiol Scand 42:329, 1998.

Gammon RB, Shin MS, Groves RH Jr et al: Clinical risk factors for pulmonary barotrauma: A multivariate analysis. Am J Respir Crit Care Med 152:1235, 1995.

Gattinoni L, Kolobow T, Tomlinson T et al: Low frequency positive pressure ventilation with extracorporeal CO_2 removal (LFPPV-$ECCO_2R$): An experimental study. Anesth Analg 57:470, 1978.

Gattinoni L, Pesenti A, Mascheroni D et al: Low frequency positive pressure ventilation with extracorporeal CO_2 removal in severe acute respiratory failure. JAMA 256:881, 1986.

Gattinoni L, Pesenti A, Avalli L et al: Pressure-volume curve of total respiratory system in acute respiratory failure. Computed tomographic scan study. Am Rev Respir Dis 136:730, 1987.

Gattinoni L, Pesenti A, Bombino M et al: Relationships between lung computed tomographic density, gas exchange and PEEP in acute respiratory failure. Anesthesiology 69:824–832, 1988.

Gattinoni L, Bombino M, Pelosi P et al: Lung structure and function in different stages of severe adult respiratory distress syndrome. JAMA 271:1772, 1994.

Glauser FL, Polatty RC, Sessler CN: Worsening oxygenation in the mechanically ventilated patient: Causes, mechanisms, and early detection. Am Rev Respir Dis 138:458, 1988.

Hall JB, Wood LDH: Liberation of the patient from mechanical ventilation. JAMA 257:1621, 1987.

Hansen-Flaschen H, Cowen I, Raps EC: Neuromuscular blockade in the ICU: More than we bargained for? Am Rev Respir Dis 147: 234, 1993.

Harken AH, Brennan MF, Smith B et al: The hemodynamic response to positive end-expiratory pressure in hypovolemic patients. Surgery 74:786, 1974.

Heffner JE: Airway management in the critically ill patient. Crit Care Clin 6:533, 1990.

Henning R, Shuhin H, Weil M: The measurement of the work of breathing for the clinical assessment of ventilator dependence. Crit Care Med 5:264, 1977.

Herrera M, Blasco J, Venegas J et al: Mouth occlusion pressure ($P_{0.1}$) in acute respiratory failure. Intensive Care Med 11:134, 1985.

Hernandez LA, Peevy KJ, Moise AA, Parker JC: Chest wall restriction limits high airway pressure–induced lung injury in young rabbits. J Appl Physiol 66:2364, 1989.
Hess DR, Kacmarek RM: Basic pulmonary mechanics during mechanical ventilation. In Hess DR, Kacmarek RM (eds): Essentials of Mechanical Ventilation. New York, McGraw-Hill, 1996, pp 171–176.
Hickling KG: Ventilatory management of ARDS: Can it affect the outcome? Intensive Care Med 16:219, 1990.
Hickling KG, Walsh J, Henderson S et al: Low mortality rate in adult respiratory distress syndrome using low-volume, pressure-limited ventilation with permissive hypercapnia: A prospective study. Crit Care Med 22:1568, 1994.
Hill NS: Noninvasive ventilation: Does it work, for whom, and how? Am Rev Respir Dis 147:1030, 1993.
Hill NS: Noninvasive mechanical ventilation. In Albert RK, Spiro SG, Jett JR (eds): Comprehensive Respiratory Medicine. London, Mosby, 1999, pp 12.1–12.10.
Hinson JR, Marini JJ: Principles of mechanical ventilator use in respiratory failure. Annu Rev Med 43:341, 1992.
Horton WG, Cheney FW: Variability of effect of positive end-expiratory pressure. Arch Surg 110:395, 1975.
Hubmayr RD: Setting the ventilator. In Tobin MJ (ed): Principles and Practice of Mechanical Ventilation. New York, McGraw-Hill, 1994, pp 191–206.
Hudson LD: Protective ventilation for patients with acute respiratory distress syndrome. N Engl J Med 338:385, 1998.
Hudson LD: Progress in understanding ventilator-induced lung injury. JAMA 282:77, 1999.
Hudson LD, Weaver LJ, Haisch CE et al: Positive end-expiratory pressure: Reduction and withdrawal. Respir Care Clin N Am 33:613, 1988.
Imsand C, Fiehl F, Perret C et al: Regulation of inspiratory neuromuscular output during synchronized intermittent mechanical ventilation. Anesthesiology 80:13, 1994.
Jabour ER, Rabil DM, Truwit JD et al: Evaluation of a new weaning index based on ventilatory endurance and the efficiency of gas exchange. Am Rev Respir Dis 144:531, 1991.
Jardin F, Forest JC, Boisante L et al: Influence of positive end-expiratory pressure on left ventricular performance. N Engl J Med 304:387, 1981.
Jenkinson SG: Oxygen toxicity. New Horiz 1:504, 1993.
Kacmarek RM: Management of the patient-mechanical ventilator system. In Pierson DJ, Kacmarek RM (eds): Foundations of Respiratory Care. New York, Churchill Livingstone, 1992, pp 973–997.
Kacmarek RM, Chiche JD: Lung protective ventilatory strategies for ARDS—the data are convincing! Respir Care Clin N Am 43:724, 1998.
Kacmarek RM, Hess DR: Basic principles of ventilator machinery. In Tobin MJ (ed): Principles and Practice of Mechanical Ventilation. New York, McGraw-Hill, 1994, pp 65–110.
Kacmarek RM, Pierson DJ: Positive end-expiratory pressure (PEEP). Respir Care Clin N Am 33:456, 1988.
Koleff MH, Schuster DP: The acute respiratory distress syndrome. N Engl J Med 332:27, 1995.
Kolla S, Awad SS, Rich PB et al: Extracorporeal life support for 100 adult patients with severe respiratory failure. Ann Surg 226:544, 1997.
Kolobow T: An update on adult extracorporeal membrane oxygenation–extracorporeal CO_2 removal. Am Soc Artif Intern Organs Trans 34:1004, 1988.
Kolobow T, Gattinoni L, Tomlinson T et al: An alternative to breathing. J Thorac Cardiovasc Surg 75:261, 1978.
Kramer N, Meyer P, Meharg J et al: Randomized, prospective trial of noninvasive positive pressure ventilation in acute respiratory failure. Am J Respir Crit Care Med 151:563, 1995.
Lamm WJE, Graham MM, Albert RK: Mechanism by which the prone position improves oxygenation in acute lung injury. Am J Respir Crit Care Med 150:184, 1994.
Lapinsky SE, Mount DNB, Mackey D et al: Management of acute respiratory failure due to pulmonary edema with nasal positive pressure support. Chest 105:229, 1994.
Leatherman JW: Mechanical ventilation in obstructive lung disease. Clin Chest Med 17:577, 1996.
Lessard MR, Guerot E, Lorino H et al: Effects of pressure-controlled ventilation with different I:E ratios versus volume-controlled ventilation on respiratory mechanics, gas exchange, and hemodynamics in patients with adult respiratory distress syndrome. Anesthesiology 80:983, 1994.
Levine S, Levy S, Henson D: Negative-pressure ventilation. Crit Care Clin 6:505, 1990.
Lewandowski K, Slama K, Falke KJ: Approaches to improve survival in severe ARDS. In Vincent JL (ed): Update of Intensive Care and Emergency Medicine. Berlin, Springer-Verlag, 1992, pp 372–383.
Lewandowski K, Rossaint R, Pappert D et al: High survival rate in 122 ARDS patients managed according to a clinical algorithm including extracorporeal membrane oxygenation. Intensive Care Med 23:819, 1997.
Lodato RF, Tobin MJ: Estimation of auto-PEEP. Chest 99:520, 1991.
MacIntyre NR: New forms of mechanical ventilation in the adult. Clin Chest Med 9:47, 1988.
MacIntyre NR, Gropper C: Monitoring ventilatory function II: Respiratory system mechanics and muscle function. In Levine RL, Fromm RE (eds): Critical Care Monitoring. St Louis, Mosby–Year Book, 1995, pp 179–190.
MacIntyre NR, Stock CM: Weaning mechanical ventilatory support. In Kirby RR, Banner MJ, Downs JB (eds): Clinical Applications of Ventilatory Support. New York, Churchill Livingstone, 1990, pp 263–276.
Malo J, Ah I, Wood LDH: How does positive end-expiratory pressure reduce intrapulmonary shunt in canine pulmonary edema? J Appl Physiol 57:1002, 1984.
Marcy TW, Marini JJ: Control mode ventilation and assist/control ventilation. In Stock MC, Perel A (eds): Mechanical Ventilatory Support. Philadelphia, Lippincott Williams & Wilkins, 1997, pp 89–109.
Marini JJ: Patient-ventilator interaction: Rational strategies for acute ventilatory management. Respir Care 38:482, 1993.
Marini JJ: Pressure-controlled ventilation. In Tobin MJ (ed): Principles and Practice of Mechanical Ventilation. New York, McGraw-Hill, 1994, pp 305–318.
Marini JJ: Pulmonary mechanics in critical care. In Dantzker DR, Scharf SM (eds): Cardiopulmonary Critical Care, 3rd ed. Philadelphia, WB Saunders, 1998, pp 223–244.
Marini JJ, Kelsen SG: Retargeting ventilatory objectives in adult respiratory distress syndrome: New treatment prospects—persistent questions. Am Rev Respir Dis 146:2, 1992.
Marini JJ, Capps JS, Culver BH: The inspiratory work of breathing during assisted mechanical ventilation. Chest 87:612, 1985.
Marini JJ, Smith TC, Lamb VJ: External work output and force generation during synchronized intermittent mechanical ventilation: Effect of machine assistance on breathing effort. Am Rev Respir Dis 138:1169, 1988.
Matthay MA: The acute respiratory distress syndrome. N Engl J Med 334:1469, 1996.
Meduri GU, Conoscenti CC, Menashe P et al: Noninvasive face mask ventilation patients with acute respiratory failure. Chest 95:865, 1989.
Meduri GU, Abou-Shala N, Fox RC et al: Noninvasive face mask mechanical ventilation in patients with acute hypercapnic respiratory failure. Chest 100:445, 1991.
Meyer P, Hill NS: Noninvasive positive pressure ventilation to treat respiratory failure. Ann Intern Med 120:760, 1994.
Milbern SM, Downs JB, Jumper LC et al: Evaluation of criteria for discontinuing mechanical ventilation support. Arch Surg 113:1441, 1978.
Montgomery AB, Holle RHO, Neagley SR et al: Prediction of successful ventilatory weaning using airway occlusion pressure and hypercapnic challenge. Chest 91:496, 1987.
Morris A, Wallace CJ, Menlove RL et al: Randomized clinical trial of pressure-controlled inverse ratio ventilation and extracorporeal CO_2 removal for adult respiratory distress syndrome. Am J Respir Crit Care Med 149:295, 1994.
Mortensen JD, Berry G: Conceptual and design features of a practical, clinically effective intravenous mechanical blood oxygen/carbon dioxide exchange device (IVOX). Int J Artif Organs 12:384, 1989.
Muscedere IG, Mullen IBM, Gan K et al: Tidal ventilation at low airway pressures can augment lung injury. Am J Respir Crit Care Med 149:1327, 1994.
Nahum A, Marini JJ: Recent advances in mechanical ventilation. Clin Chest Med 17:355, 1996.
Nathan SD, Ishaaya AM, Koerner SK et al: Prediction of minimal

pressure support during weaning from mechanical ventilation. Chest 103:1215, 1993.

Nelson LD: Assessment of oxygenation: Oxygenation indices. Respir Care Clin N Am 38:631, 1993.

Parker JC, Hernandez LA, Peevy KJ: Mechanisms of ventilator-induced lung injury. Crit Care Med 21:131, 1993.

Pepe PE, Marini JJ: Occult positive end-expiratory pressure in mechanically ventilated patients with airflow obstruction: The auto-PEEP effect. Am Rev Respir Dis 126:166, 1982.

Pepe PE, Hudson LD, Carrico CI: Early application of positive end-expiratory pressure in patients at risk of adult respiratory distress syndrome. N Engl J Med 311:281, 1984.

Pesenti A, Bombino M, Marcolin R et al: Extracorporeal techniques to support ventilation. In Stock MC, Perel A (eds): Mechanical Ventilatory Support. Philadelphia, Lippincott Williams & Wilkins, 1997, pp 233–245.

Pierson DJ: Indications for mechanical ventilation in acute respiratory failure. Respir Care Clin N Am 28:570, 1983.

Pierson DJ: Alveolar rupture during mechanical ventilation: Role of PEEP, peak airway pressure, and distending volume. Respir Care Clin N Am 33:472, 1988.

Pierson DJ: Complications associated with mechanical ventilation. Crit Care Clin 6:711, 1990.

Pierson DJ: Ventilator management of ARDS: Emerging Concepts. Crit Care Alert 2:68–72, 1995.

Pierson DJ: Barotrauma and bronchopleural fistula. In Tobin MJ (ed): Principles and Practice of Intensive Care Monitoring. New York, McGraw-Hill, 1998, pp 857–890.

Pierson DJ: Invasive mechanical ventilation. In Albert RK, Spiro SG, Jett JR (eds): Comprehensive Respiratory Medicine. London, Mosby, 1999, pp 11.1–11.20.

Pilbeam SP: Physical characteristics of mechanical ventilators. In Respiratory Care, 4th ed. Philadelphia, JB Lippincott, 1997, pp 643–690.

Pinsky MR: Effects of mechanical ventilation on the cardiovascular system. Crit Care Clin 6:663, 1990.

Piper AJ, Parker S, Torzillo PJ et al: Nocturnal nasal IPPV stabilized patients with cystic fibrosis and hypercapnic respiratory failure. Chest 102:846, 1992.

Prakash O, Meij S, Van Der Borden B: Spontaneous ventilation test vs intermittent mandatory ventilation: An approach to weaning after coronary bypass surgery. Chest 811:403, 1982.

Rahoof S, Khan FA: Mechanical Ventilation Manual. Philadelphia, American College of Physicians, 1998, p 94.

Ranieri VM, Suter PM, Tortorella C et al: Effect of mechanical ventilation on inflammatory mediators in patients with acute respiratory distress syndrome—a randomized controlled trial. JAMA 282:54, 1999.

Rocker GM, Mackenzie MG, Williams B et al: Noninvasive positive pressure ventilation: Successful outcome in patients with acute lung injury/ARDS. Chest 115:173, 1999.

Romano E: Best PEEP: A still unsolved problem. Chest 87:551, 1985.

Rossi A, Ranieri VM: Positive end-expiratory pressure. In Tobin MJ (ed): Principles and Practice of Mechanical Ventilation. New York, McGraw-Hill, 1994, pp 259–304.

Rossi A, Polese G, Milic-Emili J: Monitoring respiratory mechanics in ventilator-dependent patients. In Tobin MJ (ed): Principles and Practice of Intensive Care Monitoring. New York, McGraw-Hill, 1998, pp 553–596.

Rouby JJ, Lherm T, Lassale ME et al: Histologic aspects of pulmonary barotrauma in critically ill patients with acute respiratory failure. Intensive Care Med 19:383, 1993.

Sahn SA, Lakshminarayan S: Bedside criteria for discontinuation of mechanical ventilation. Chest 63:1002, 1973.

Sassoon CSH: Positive pressure ventilation: Alternate modes. Chest 100:1421, 1991.

Sassoon CSH: Mechanical ventilator design and function: The trigger variable. Respir Care Clin N Am 37:1056, 1992.

Sassoon CSH, Te TT, Mahute CK et al: Airway occlusion pressure: An important indicator for successful weaning in patients with chronic obstructive pulmonary disease. Am Rev Respir Dis 135:107, 1987.

Sassoon CSH, Mahutte CK, Light RW: Ventilator modes: Old and new. Crit Care Clin 6:605, 1990.

Sassoon CS, Del Rosano N, Fei R et al: Influence of pressure- and flow-triggered synchronous intermittent mandatory ventilation on inspiratory muscle work. Crit Care Med 22:1933, 1994.

Schmidt GA, Hall JB: Acute on chronic respiratory failure: Assessment and management of patients with COPD in the emergent setting. JAMA 261:3444, 1989.

Schuster DP: What is acute lung injury? What is ARDS? Chest 107:1721, 1995.

Segredo V, Caldwell JE, Matthay MA et al: Persistent paralysis in critically ill patients after long-term administration of vecuronium. N Engl J Med 327:524, 1992.

Shapiro JM, Condos R, Cole RP: Myopathy in status asthmaticus: Relation to neuromuscular blockade and corticosteroid administration. Intensive Care Med 8:144, 1993.

Slutsky AS: Nonconventional methods of ventilation. Am Rev Respir Dis 138:175, 1985.

Soo Hoo GW, Silverio S, Williams J: Nasal mechanical ventilation for hypercapnic respiratory failure in chronic obstructive pulmonary disease: Determinants of success and failure. Crit Care Med 22:1253, 1994.

Strieter RM, Lynch JP: Complications in the ventilated patient. Clin Chest Med 9:127, 1988.

Sullivan CE, Issa FG, Berthon-Jones M et al: Reversal of obstructive sleep apnea by continuous positive airway pressure applied through the nares. Lancet 1:862, 1981.

Suter PM, Fairley HB, Isenberg MD: Optimum endexpiratory pressure in patients with acute pulmonary failure. N Engl J Med 292:284, 1975.

Tahvanainen J, Salenpera M, Nikki P: Extubation criteria after weaning from intermittent mandatory ventilatory and continuous positive airway pressure. Crit Care Med 11:702, 1983.

Tao W, Bidani A, Cardenas VJ et al: Strategies to maximize CO_2 transfer of an intravenacaval gas exchange device (IVOX). ASAIO J 41:M567, 1996.

Tobin MJ: Mechanical ventilation. N Engl J Med 330:1056, 1994.

Tobin MJ: Respiratory monitoring during mechanical ventilation. Crit Care Clin 6:679, 1990.

Tobin MJ, Alex CA: Discontinuation of mechanical ventilation. In Tobin MJ (ed): Principles and Practice of Mechanical Ventilation. New York, McGraw-Hill, 1994, pp 1177–1206.

Tobin MJ, Danzker DR: Ventilatory support: Who, when, and how? In Miller TA (ed): Physiological Basis of Modern Surgical Care. St Louis, Mosby–Year Book, 1988, pp 565–588.

Tobin MJ, Lodato RF: PEEP, auto-PEEP, and waterfalls. Chest 96:449, 1989.

Tobin MJ, Perez W, Guenther SM et al: Does ribcage abdominal paradox signify respiratory muscle fatigue? J Appl Physiol 63:851, 1987.

Tobin MJ, Perez W, Guenther SM et al: The pattern of breathing during successful and unsuccessful trials of weaning from mechanical ventilation. Am Rev Respir Dis 134:1111, 1986.

Tobin MJ, Yang K: Weaning from mechanical ventilation. Crit Care Clin 6:725, 1990.

Tomashefski JF Jr: Pulmonary pathology of the adult respiratory distress syndrome. Clin Chest Med 11:593, 1990.

Tracy TF, Delosh T, Stolar: The registry of the Extracorporeal Life Support Organization. In Zwischenberger JB, Bartlett RH (eds): ECMO: Extracorporeal cardiopulmonary support in critical care. Ann Arbor, MI, Extracorporeal Life Support Organization, 1995, pp 251–260.

Tsuno K, Prato P, Kolobow T: Acute lung injury from mechanical ventilation at moderately high airway pressures. J Appl Physiol 69:956, 1990.

Tuxen DV: Permissive hypercapnia. In Tobin MJ (ed): Principles and Practice of Mechanical Ventilation. New York, McGraw-Hill, 1994, pp 371–392.

Tuxen DV: Mechanical ventilation in severe asthma. In Evans T, Hinds C (eds): Recent Advances in Critical Care Medicine, vol 4. London, Churchill-Livingstone, 1996, pp 165–189.

Vanderwarf C: Mechanical ventilation. In Fink JB, Hunt GE (eds): Clinical Practice in Respiratory Care. Philadelphia, Lippincott Williams & Wilkins, 1999, pp 405–436.

Vitacca M, Rubini F, Fogho K et al: Non-invasive modalities of positive pressure ventilation improved the outcome of acute exacerbations in COLD patients. Intensive Care Med 19:450, 1993.

Waugh JB, Deshpande VM, Harwood RJ: Rapid Interpretation of Ventilator Waveforms. Englewood Cliffs, NJ, Prentice Hall, 1999, p 85.

Webb HH, Tierney DF: Experimental pulmonary edema due to intermittent positive pressure ventilation with high inflation pressures:

Protection by positive end-expiratory pressure. Am Rev Respir Dis 110:556, 1974.

Wood LDH, Hall JB: A mechanistic approach to providing adequate oxygenation in acute hypoxemic respiratory failure. Respir Care Clin N Am 38:784, 1993.

Wysocki M, Tric L, Wolff MA et al: Noninvasive pressure support ventilation in patients with acute respiratory failure: A randomized comparison with conventional therapy. Chest 107:761, 1995.

Yang K, Tobin M: A prospective study of indexes predicting the outcome of trials of weaning from mechanical ventilation. N Engl J Med 324:1445, 1991.

Young JD, Dorrington KL, Blake GJ et al: Femoral arteriovenous extracorporeal carbon dioxide elimination using low blood flow. Crit Care Med 20:805, 1992.

Zimmerman GA, Morris AH, Cengiz M: Cardiovascular alterations in the adult respiratory distress syndrome. Am J Med 73:25, 1982.

Zwillich CW, Pierson DJ, Creagh CE et al: Complications of assisted ventilation: A prospective study of 354 consecutive episodes. Am J Med 57:161, 1974.

Zwischenberger JB, Conrad, Alpard SA et al: Percutaneous extracorporeal arteriovenous CO_2 removal for severe respiratory failure. Ann Thorac Surg 68:181, 1999.

CHAPTER **11**

Late Complications

Jean Deslauriers
Pasquale Ferraro

When patients are discharged from the hospital after pulmonary resections, they are still at risk of developing late complications related to their operations. These are uncommon events that, for the most part, become apparent during the first year of follow-up. Although late complications are seldom life threatening, delayed diagnosis or mismanagement often leads to chronicity and prolonged disability.

HISTORICAL NOTE

Although the first successful resection for lung cancer was in 1932, complications following partial lung resections for pulmonary disease prior to this were common. The first successful anatomic resection depended on solving technical problems leading to major complications.

Very early on, problems related to the bronchial closure had been identified. Kummel (1911) performed a pneumonectomy, clamping the pedicle and leaving the clamps in situ since individual ligation was unknown at the time. The patient died of complications after only 6 days. In 1912, Davies performed the first lobectomy for lung cancer. Prior to this, the only resections were very primitive operations that included exteriorization of the tumor, suturing the visceral and parietal pleura together, and ultimately cauterizing the eviscerated mass (Pean, 1895). Following Brunn's 1929 description of intercostal drainage and underwater seal, lobectomy became a distinct possibility. But, unfortunately, empyema and bronchopleural fistula continued to be major problems. Prevention of these complications due to technical problems awaited the development of individual ligation, pioneered by the efforts of Hinz (1923), Churchill (1933), Rienhoff (1933), and Churchill and Belsey (1939).

It was not until these techniques had been developed that patients survived long enough to be followed and the late complications of pulmonary resection slowly became evident.

■ *HISTORICAL READINGS*

Brunn HB: Surgical principles underlying one-stage lobectomy. Arch Surg. 18:490, 1929.

Churchill ED: The surgical treatment of carcinoma of the lung. J Thorac Surg 2:254, 1933.

Churchill E, Belsey HR: Segmental pneumonectomy in bronchiectasis. Ann Surg 109:481, 1939.

Davies HM: Recent advances in the surgery of the lung and pleura. Br J Surg 1:228, 1913–1914.

Hinz R: Totale extirpation der linken lunge wegen bronchial carcinoma. Arch Klin Chir 124:104, 1923.

Kummel H: Proceedings of the 40th Congress, Berlin, April 19–22, 1911. Verh Dtsch Ges Chir 40:147, 1911.

Pean J: Chirurgie des poumons. Discussion Ranc Chir Proc Verh Paris 9:72m, 1895.

Rienhoff WF: Pneumonectomy. A Preliminary report of operative technique in two successful cases. Bull Johns Hopkins Hosp 53:390, 1933.

INFECTIONS AND SPACE COMPLICATIONS

Persistent Spaces After Lobectomy or Lesser Resections

Persistent pleural air spaces following lobectomies or lesser resections are common, and for many years, they were thought to lead inevitably to infection if left untreated (Rainer and Newby, 1967; Kirsh et al, 1975). Consequently, numerous intraoperative and postoperative prophylactic measures, such as tailoring thoracoplasty, pleural tent, pneumoperitoneum, phrenoplasty, and high postoperative intrapleural suction, were designed to prevent such spaces from occurring (Kirsh et al, 1975).

In 1959, Shields et al published a classic article on the fate of persistent pleural air spaces following resection for pulmonary tuberculosis. A review of 584 pulmonary resections revealed an incidence of 128 (21.9%) persistent pleural air spaces postoperatively. Of these spaces, 86 (67.1%) were asymptomatic, and 42 (32.9%) were symptomatic. The asymptomatic spaces were benign with respect to the patient's course; the symptomatic spaces were hazardous and accounted for complications of varying severity in all 42 patients, with eventual death of 3. It was concluded that prophylaxis with careful dissection in the intersegmental or interlobar plane and closure of any major leaks at the time of stripping was the best management.

In 1966, Barker and co-workers questioned the then-accepted concept that all postresectional thoracic spaces represented frank bronchial leaks that required active surgical intervention. It was assumed that bronchopleural fistulas constituted a prelude to empyemas, and hence active prophylaxis and therapy of these spaces should be initiated early. In this series, 730 partial lung resections were performed for pulmonary tuberculosis, and 86 patients had postresection spaces (Table 11–1). Fifteen patients had persistent spaces for longer than 4 weeks after their operations, and of these, 5 closed spontaneously within 1 year. Only two patients had evidence of a major pleuropulmonary communication, and in both cases, long-term follow-up did not turn up important complications. In a similar study, Silver and associates (1966)

TABLE 11–1 ■ **Fate of 86 Postresection Spaces**

Fate	*No. Patients (%)*
Spontaneous obliteration	76 (88)
Less than 4 wk	71
4 wk to 1 yr	5
Persistent for 1–10 yr	10 (11)
Uninfected	8
With bronchopleural fistula	2

From Barker WL, Langston HT, Naffah P: Post-resectional thoracic spaces. Ann Thorac Surg 2:299, 1966.

concluded that most postresectional residual spaces resolve without complications or major surgical intervention.

Normally, the space after lobectomy or lesser resection is obliterated by the shift of adjacent dynamic structures, such as the heart, mediastinum, and diaphragm; the approximation of ribs with internal bulging of the intercostal muscles; the hyperinflation of the remaining lung; and the intrapleural accumulation of blood and serum in recesses and fissures. This obliteration is facilitated by the negative intrapleural pressure, the lack of air leakage from the lung or bronchus, and the unimpaired expansibility of the lung.

Risk factors for the development of persistent spaces are the inability of the lung to fill the hemithorax, such as occurs in patients with underlying fibrosis or the presence of a bronchopleural fistula either at the alveolar or the bronchial level. On the basis of their studies, Barker and co-workers (1966) classified persistent postresection spaces as benign or malignant. A benign space is characterized as one that is small and getting smaller on serial radiographs, is thin walled, and has no or minimal and decreasing fluid. It occurs in a patient who has no fever or leucocytosis and who has no major symptoms (Fig. 11–1). Most of these spaces have no bronchial or alveolar communications and have an intraspace pressure that is negative and disappears without therapy over a period of weeks or months (Fig. 11–2).

In contradistinction to patients with benign spaces, patients with malignant spaces have fever and leucocytosis, and they are generally ill (Barker et al, 1966). These spaces are large and getting larger, have a thick wall, and contain fluid in increasing amounts. These infected spaces are usually obvious during the early postoperative period, but sometimes they are only diagnosed at the time of the first or second postoperative visit (Fig. 11–3). Clinically, these patients present with a failure to thrive, purulent bronchorrhea with or without hemoptysis, unresolving chest pain, and sometimes spiking temperature.

After lung cancer surgery, most residual air spaces are not infected and should be observed until their complete resolution. Investigation by thoracentesis or other procedures is not indicated and may in fact be contraindicated because of the risks of infecting a previously sterile space. These recommendations apply to all asymptomatic spaces whether they have an air fluid or not and whether they persist for only a few weeks postoperatively or for years. However, if the patient develops systemic or local symptoms of infection or if the space is enlarging, appropriate therapy should be instituted promptly.

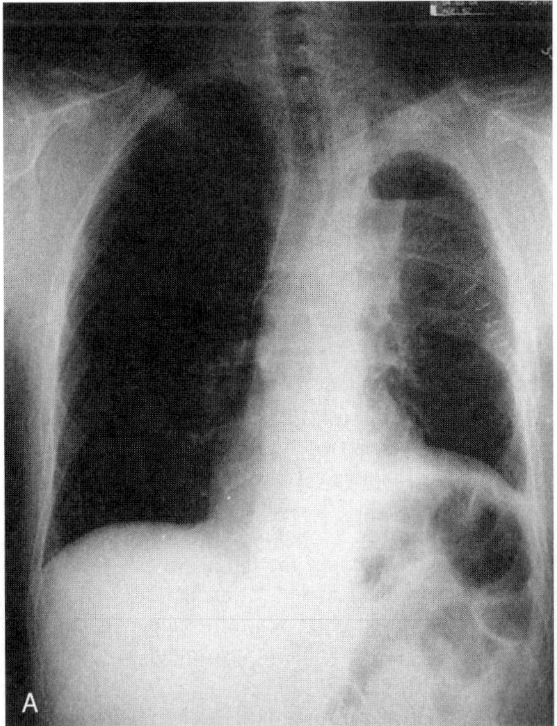

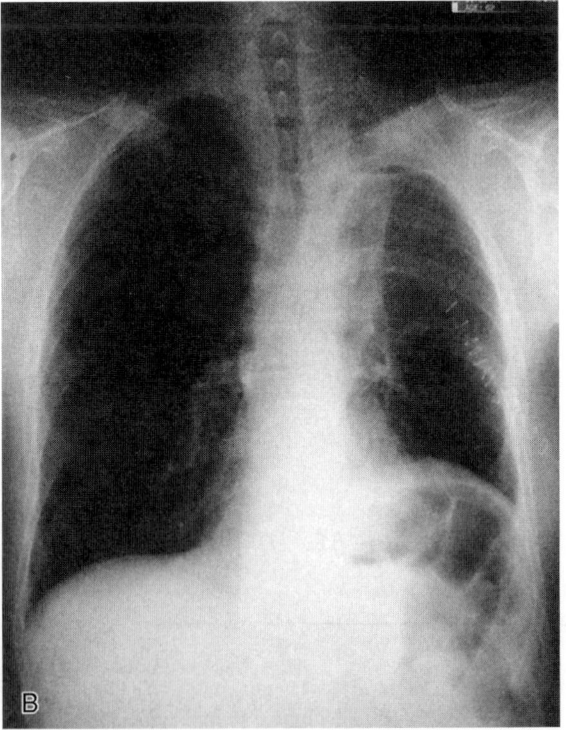

FIGURE 11–1 ■ Asymptomatic benign space following left upper lobectomy. *A*, Early postoperative chest radiograph showing a thin-walled air space located anteriorly and at the apex. *B*, Near-complete disappearance of the space 10 days postoperatively.

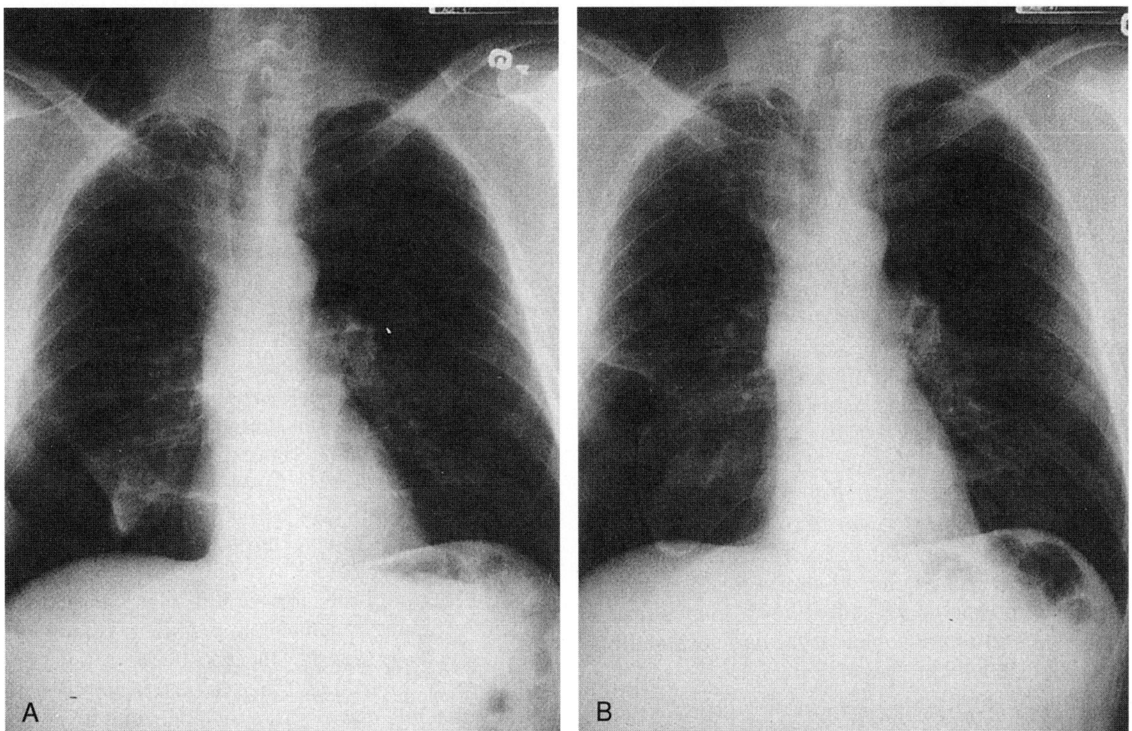

FIGURE 11–2 ■ Asymptomatic benign space following right lower lobectomy. *A,* Postoperative posteroanterior chest radiograph taken 3 weeks postoperatively and showing a large basal space. *B,* Four weeks later, the space is smaller, and the patient has remained asymptomatic.

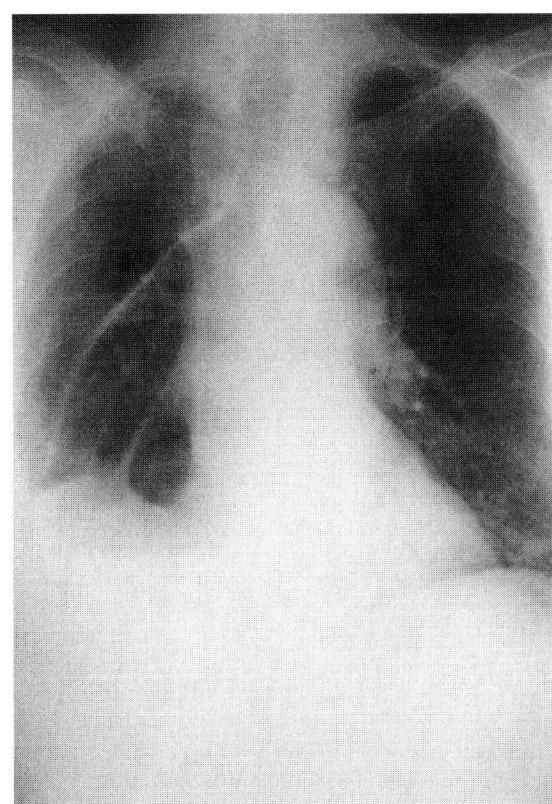

FIGURE 11–3 ■ Symptomatic space following lower and middle lobectomy. Posteroanterior chest radiograph showing a large thick-walled air space with multiple air-fluid levels diagnosed 5 months postoperatively.

Late Empyema and Bronchopleural Fistula

Definition and Incidence

Although late empyemas and bronchopleural fistulas may occur separately, they generally are associated with one another and thus are discussed together in this chapter.

Late-onset postpneumonectomy empyema has been arbitrarily defined by Kerr (1977) as an empyema occurring 3 months after surgery in a patient with an uneventful postoperative course. The overall incidence of postoperative empyemas is between 2% and 13% after pneumonectomy (Leroux et al, 1986) and less than 1% after lobectomy. The exact incidence of late-onset empyemas, however, is unknown, although it is likely to represent a rare complication.

In their original article on open drainage and irrigation for postpneumonectomy empyemas, Clagett and Geraci (1963) make one of the first references to the occurrence of late empyema. In a series also from the Mayo Clinic (Pairolero, et al, 1990), the interval between pneumonectomy and the diagnosis of subsequent empyema ranged from 1 week to 33 years (median, 4 weeks). The complication was apparent within 4 months of pneumonectomy in 32 patients (71%) and later than 4 months in 13 patients (29%). In three patients, the empyema developed after 5 years (10.5, 13, and 33 years). In the Toronto series (Shamji et al, 1983), the complication was apparent within 12 weeks of the operation in 23 cases (74.2%) and after 3 months in the remaining 8 individuals (25.8%).

The overall incidence of postresectional bronchopleural fistula is 1% to 3% (Boyd and Spencer, 1972; Vester et al, 1991; Williams and Lewis, 1976), but precise data on the occurrence of late fistulas is lacking because most occur in association with empyemas. Steiger and Wilson (1984) reported six cases of late fistulas in a series of 11 patients, and Vester and co-workers (1991) described 14 late cases from a series of 35 patients with postoperative fistulas. The latter group also showed that in patients who received preoperative irradiation, a significantly longer time (average, 48 days) elapsed before the diagnosis of bronchopleural fistula than in the other patients (average, 18 days). Asamura and associates (1992) presented 13 patients with late fistulas among 52 patients with bronchopleural fistulas developing after pulmonary resection.

Pathophysiology

The exact pathophysiology of late-onset empyema is not completely understood. As suggested by Witz and Roeslin (1981), two possibilities exist. In most cases, the empyema results from a bronchopleural or an esophagopleural fistula with contamination of the postpneumonectomy space. In Kerr's series (1977), fistulas (two bronchial and two esophageal) were found in four of nine patients presenting with empyemas 8 months to 13 years after pneumonectomies. The second possible mechanism of infection involves the contamination of the pleural cavity during the initial surgery. Microorganisms may lodge in small pockets or loculations of fluid and lie dormant for months or years before producing an empyema. Although plausible, this hypothesis cannot be verified with any certainty.

PATHOGENESIS OF LATE POSTRESECTION EMPYEMAS

- Secondary to late bronchopleural or esophagopleural fistula
- Contamination of the space during the initial surgery
- Seeding through the hematogenous route
- Direct spread through the esophageal hiatus or diaphragm

In theory, seeding of the postpneumonectomy space may also occur by the hematogenous route, as is the case with bacterial endocarditis. This mechanism is supported by a number of authors. In five cases of late-onset empyema (Kerr, 1977), patients had signs of infection in the contralateral lung, and pneumococcal and streptococcal agents were isolated from the empyema. In 1983, Model (1983) described a case of empyema occurring 10 years after pneumonectomy in a patient receiving therapy for pneumonia. Bellamy and associates (1991) also reported three cases of late empyema (7, 10, and 30 months after resection) with organisms of blood-borne origin. The bacteria isolated were *Pasteurella multocida, Campylobacter fetus,* and various anaerobes in the third patient. Rogiers and colleagues (1991b) described a case of empyema 4 years after pulmonary resection for carcinoma in which *Mycobacterium tuberculosis* was cultured. In all these reports, the authors concluded that the pleural space had been contaminated by blood-borne agents because no evidence of bronchial or esophageal fistulas could be found. A final theory was proposed by Holden and co-workers (1972) in the discussion of a case of late postpneumonectomy empyema occurring in a patient soon after appendiceal peritonitis. The same *Bacteroides* species were isolated in the cultures of the empyema and of the intra-abdominal contents. In this case, spread probably occurred through the esophageal hiatus or the diaphragm.

Although the exact pathogenesis of late bronchopleural fistulas is unknown, different hypotheses exist. In the early postoperative period, bronchopleural fistulas are secondary to technical errors in bronchial stump closure. Intermediate fistulas, such as those seen 8 to 10 days after resection, result from a failure in the healing process. Extensive dissection around the bronchus may damage its blood supply and lead to ischemia and impaired healing. Other factors may also be involved. In a multivariate analysis of risk factors in 1360 patients, Asamura and investigators (1992) showed that wider resections, such as pneumonectomies, residual carcinoma, preoperative irradiation, and diabetes, significantly increased the risk of postoperative bronchopleural fistulas. Late-occurring bronchopleural fistulas are generally believed to be caused by an underlying empyema because the presence of an infectious process in the pleural cavity impairs healing and may lead to the breakdown of the stump. Other possible factors are the presence of an occult bronchopleural fistula, which was undetected early postoperatively; the presence of residual cancer at the bronchial margin (Soorae and Stevenson, 1979); and a long stump (Lynn, 1958), which can lead to infection and dehiscence.

Clinical Features and Diagnosis

The clinical features associated with late-onset empyemas vary greatly and often are nonspecific. Patients may be asymptomatic; may show mild symptoms of pulmonary sepsis with fever, productive cough, and dyspnea; or may present with severe toxemia. If undetected, the empyema may rupture into the bronchus, flooding the contralateral lung and causing respiratory distress. Factors such as the size of the empyema, the bacterial agent involved, the presence of an underlying bronchopleural fistula, and the patient's general condition usually determine the extent of the symptoms.

In Kerr's (1977) report, five of nine patients presented with an empyema necessitatis (Fig. 11–4). In Stafford and Clagett's (1972) series of 18 cases of postpneumonectomy empyema, 10 patients had late-onset empyemas (6 weeks to 26 years after surgery). The diagnosis was overlooked in these cases, and 6 of 10 patients presented with an empyema necessitatis. In one other case of late empyema (Rogiers, et al, 1991a), the patient presented with respiratory failure secondary to tracheal compression by the empyema, and he was quickly relieved of his symptoms by thoracentesis.

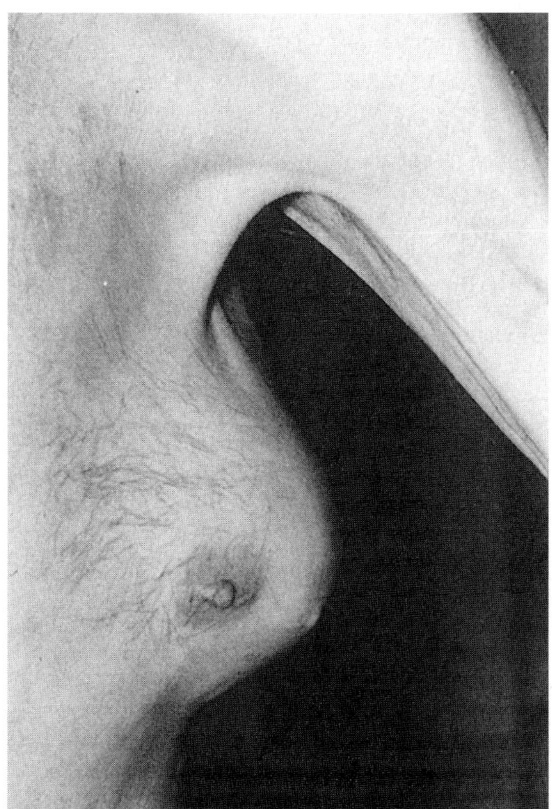

FIGURE 11–4 ■ A patient presenting with an empyema necessitatis secondary to a postpneumonectomy empyema.

Late bronchopleural fistulas may present with signs and symptoms of an empyema, or affected patients may develop sudden dyspnea, subcutaneous emphysema, and contralateral deviation of the trachea. Expectoration of purulent material associated with these symptoms is virtually diagnostic of the complication. Khargi and others (1993) also showed that, in rare cases, bleeding can occur from the pulmonary artery stump in patients with a postpneumonectomy bronchopleural fistula.

The diagnosis of late-onset empyema may be difficult and is usually delayed (Kerr, 1977; Rogiers et al, 1991a). The history and physical examination are often unrewarding unless signs of a bronchopleural fistula are present. A standard chest radiograph alone, however, may lead to the diagnosis. The physician must specifically look for a fall in the fluid level (more than 1.5 cm) or a new fluid level, the presence of loculated intrapleural gas, or a mediastinal shift to the nonoperated side (Friedman and Hellekant, 1977). Also recommended in the workup are chest computed tomography (CT) scans and bronchoscopy, which are useful to exclude associated or recurrent carcinomas. This workup also documents the presence or absence of a bronchopleural fistula and evaluates the pleural cavity in regard to its size and the exact site of the empyema. A diagnosis of empyema must always be confirmed by thoracentesis with appropriate cultures and biochemical and cytologic examinations being carried out on the aspirated fluid or pus. A suspected bronchopleural fistula may be demonstrated by the use of a xenon gas ventilation-isotope scan (Lowe and Siddiqui, 1984; Moote, et al, 1987). Although seldom required, bronchography with Lipiodol instillation in the bronchial stump and methylene blue injection into the pleural space with subsequent appearance of colored sputum may be valuable.

Management

The management of late empyemas or bronchopleural fistulas is similar to that of these complications occurring early during the postoperative period. Initially, it includes control of respiration, tube thoracostomy, appropriate systemic antibiotics, and nutritional support (Erola, et al, 1988; Grégoire, et al, 1987; Pairolero, et al, 1992). Although open window thoracostomy may only be necessary in selected cases refractory to closed chest drainage, some authors (Goldstraw, 1979; Lemmer et al, 1985; Stafford and Clagett, 1972; Virkkula and Kostiainen, 1970) recommend open pleural drainage in all patients.

Long-term management is individualized and varies according to the success of the initial measures, the patient's condition, the presence of an associated bronchopleural fistula, and the surgeon's experience. The objectives are sterilization of the space, closure of the fistula, and obliteration of the remaining pleural cavity (Allen et al, 1992). A Clagett procedure may be sufficient for a late empyema without a bronchopleural fistula (Bellamy et al, 1991; Kerr, 1977). If unsuccessful, an intrathoracic muscle transposition (Erola et al, 1988; Miller et al, 1984; Pairolero et al, 1990) or a space-reducing thoracoplasty (Grégoire et al, 1987; Hopkins et al, 1985) may be required. The management of an empyema associated with a bronchopleural fistula requires open chest drainage. Persistent fistulas necessitate the use of a muscle transposition and/or thoracoplasty procedure. If basic surgical principles are respected and if there is no recurrent carcinoma, the results are generally satisfactory, with success rates of 70% to 90%.

Persistent Spaces After Pneumonectomy

Pathogenesis and Clinical Features

Christiansen and associates (1965) studied the chest radiographs of 60 pneumonectomized patients and calculated that filling of the pleural space is a phenomenon that requires 3 weeks to 7 months to take place. They suggested that the pleural space fills progressively with serosanguineous fluid and plasma and that the gradual organization of the fluid completely obliterates the hemithorax. In 1969, Suarez and co-workers reviewed autopsy protocols in 37 cases in which pneumonectomy had been performed at the Mayo Clinic (average time between pneumonectomy and death, 46.7 months). Of the patients studied, 10 had specific evidence of total obliteration, and 27 exhibited some degree of residual space. The amount and character of the fluid found in such spaces were not related to the postoperative interval.

As in obliteration of the postlobectomy space, obliteration of the postpneumonectomy space is aided by the shift of adjacent mediastinal structures, elevation of the diaphragm, approximation of the ribs with internal bulging of the intercostal muscles, intrapleural collection of blood and serum, and negative intrapleural pressure. In a study by Suarez and associates (1969), most cases of complete obliteration demonstrated an extensive shift of the mediastinal structures and a diaphragmatic leaf located at or above the fourth rib posteriorly.

Not unlike what can be observed after partial resection, some patients without a demonstrable fistula never fill their postpneumonectomy spaces; other empty their spaces during the early period of follow-up. This syndrome is called "postpneumonectomy pneumothorax" or persistent space after pneumonectomy.

All these patients have a microscopic fistula, which is often impossible to document, either because it is too small or because it is only intermittently patent. Classically, these individuals are asymptomatic. However, on the chest radiograph (Fig. 11–5), the fluid level in the pneumonectomy space is lower than it was previously, and the mediastinum has shifted contralaterally toward the remaining lung. In these cases, the pleural fluid is probably reabsorbed by the parietal pleura because of pressure changes from negative to atmospheric in the space.

Management

When the patient with this complication is asymptomatic, management should be conservative, and approximately 75% of such patients either reaccumulate pleural fluid (Fig. 11–6) or maintain an empty space without further complications. The patient should be told about the problem and be instructed to watch for signs and symptoms of empyema or bronchopleural fistula. If a fistula is identified or an empyema develops, the management should be the same as previously described.

Late Esophagopleural Fistula

The occurrence of an esophagopleural fistula following pneumonectomy is an uncommon event, and in early reports (Dumont and DeGraef, 1961; Takaro et al, 1960) most were seen after pulmonary resections done for tuberculosis or suppurative diseases. The diagnosis of an esophagopleural fistula may be difficult and overlooked; patient management still represents an important challenge for the thoracic surgeon.

Incidence and Pathogenesis

The incidence of postpneumonectomy esophagopleural fistula is estimated to be 0.4% to 0.6% by Takaro and co-workers (1960); Evans (1972); and more recently, Shama and Odell (1985). Although these fistulas were thought to occur more frequently after surgery for tuberculosis, this may not be the case. The incidence in Takaro and co-workers' series (1960) of 934 resections for tuberculosis was similar to that of Evans (1972) who reported on 1389 pneumonectomies done for carcinomas. Thus, the large number of esophagopleural fistulas reported after tuberculosis surgery probably only reflects the greater prevalence of the disease at the time.

Following pneumonectomy, esophagopleural fistulas occur predominantly on the right side (75% to 88% of all cases) (Engelman et al, 1970; Takaro et al, 1960) because, on that side, the esophagus lies close to the hilum and carinal nodes. In the left hemithorax, the aorta is interposed between the esophagus and pleural cavity and therefore protects against the development of esophagopleural fistulas. The most common sites of fistula formation are the carinal and subcarinal regions (Benjamin et al, 1969; Dumont and DeGraef, 1961; Takaro et al, 1960). As described by Dumont and DeGraef (1961), the blood supply to the esophagus in these locations is segmental and often deficient, thus creating an area of vulnerability.

The pathophysiology of esophagopleural fistula formation is multifactorial and may vary depending on the onset of the fistula. In Takaro and co-workers' (1960) review of 33 cases, the esophagopleural fistula developed within 3 months of surgery in 16 patients. In the remaining 17 patients, the fistula occurred from 3 months to 6 years after the pneumonectomy. Shama and Odell (1985) reported three cases of early-onset esophagopleural fistula and four cases of fistulas occurring 3 years, 6 years, 17 years, and 25 years postoperatively.

Most authors agree that, in cases of early esophagopleural fistulas (less than 3 months), direct trauma and devascularization of the esophagus are responsible for the development of the fistula (Benjamin et al, 1969; Dumont and DeGraef, 1961; Engelman et al, 1970; Shama and Odell, 1985; Takaro et al, 1960). Other possible etiologic factors include the presence of caseating lymph nodes adherent to the esophageal wall or direct inflammatory

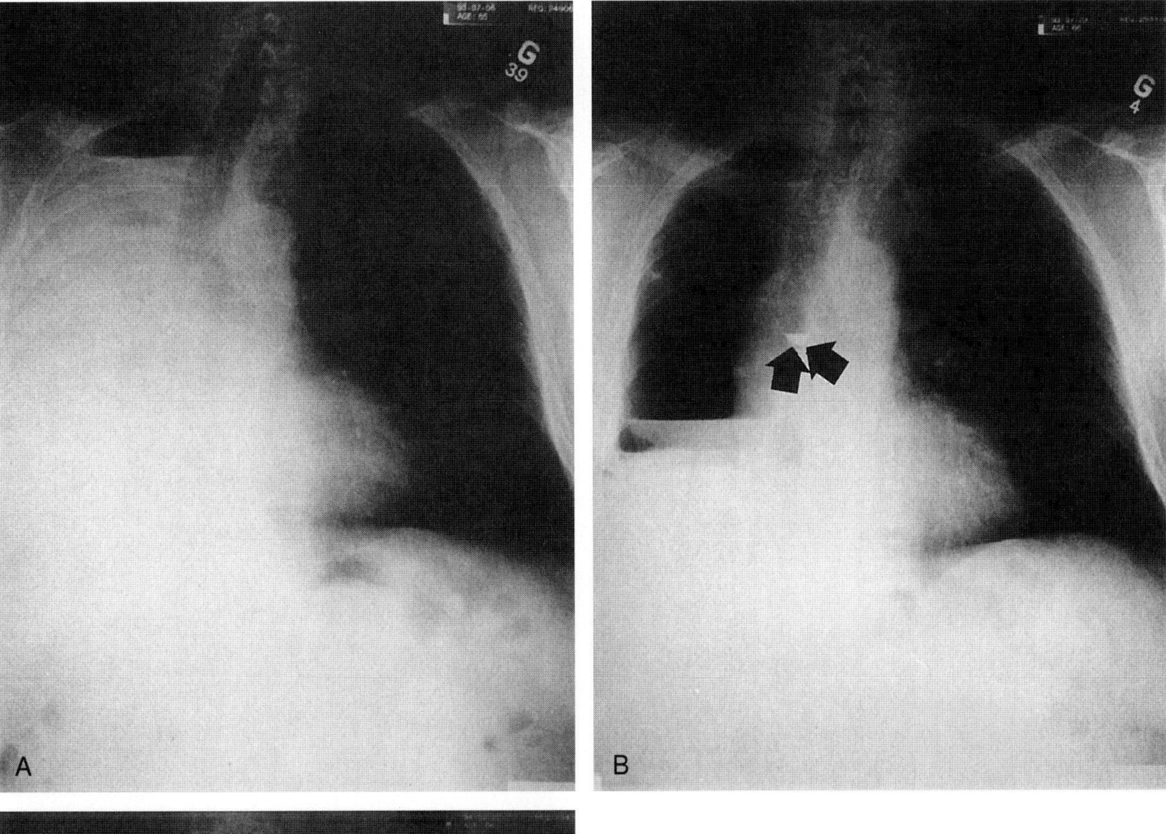

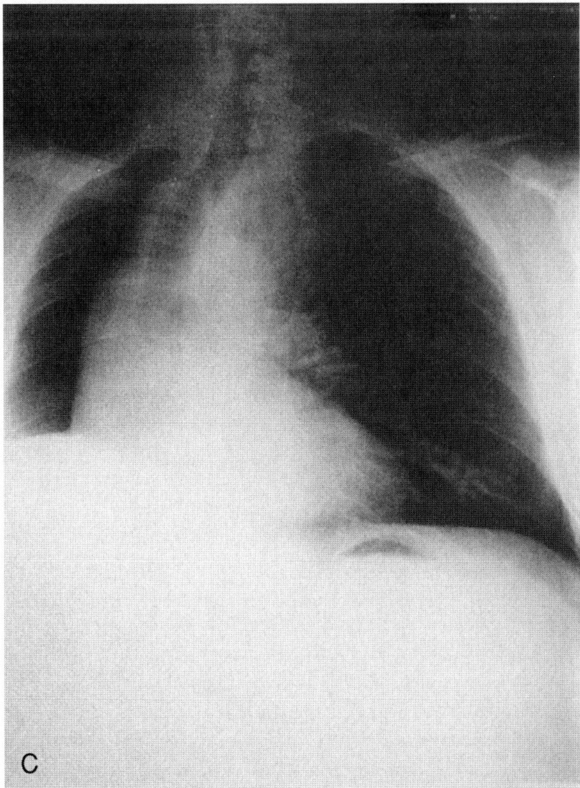

FIGURE 11–5 ■ Persistent space after pneumonectomy. Posteroanterior chest radiographs taken *A,* 2 weeks; *B,* 1 month; and *C,* 6 months after right pneumonectomy. The patient is completely asymptomatic and being followed conservatively. Several bronchoscopies have failed to demonstrate a bronchopleural fistula. Note that Lipiodol instillation in the bronchus does not show a fistula (*arrows, B*) and that the mediastinum has remained shifted toward the operated side.

involvement of the esophagus by a suppurative process. These conditions make the pulmonary resection more difficult and increase substantially the risk of inadvertent injury to the esophagus.

In contrast to early esophagopleural fistulas, the pathogenesis of late-onset fistulas remains unclear. Takaro (1960) and Benjamin (1969) and their co-workers suggested that a chronic infectious process, such as an empyema, a periesophageal abscess, or a peribronchial abscess, may rupture into the esophagus and create a

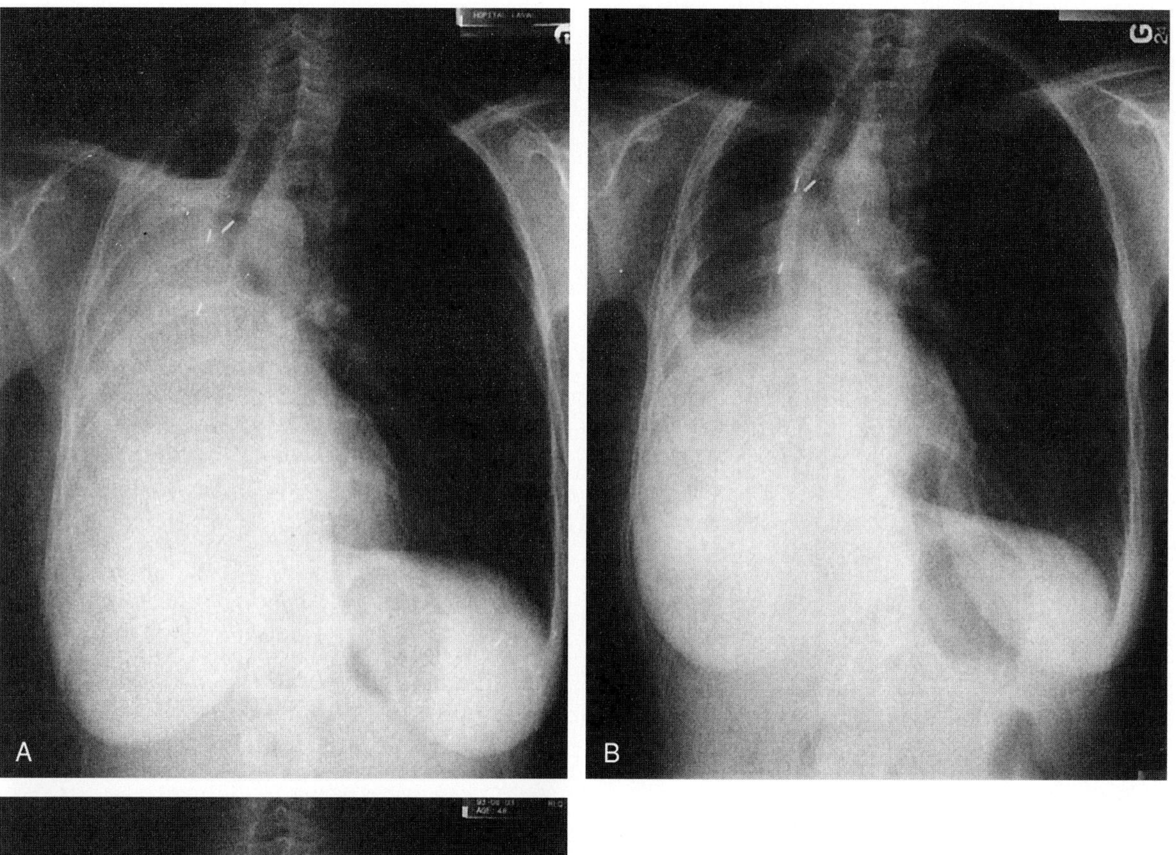

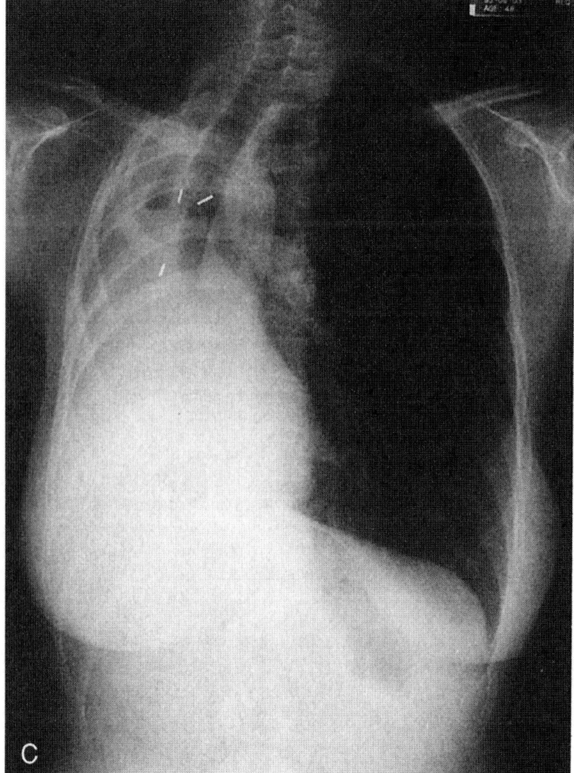

FIGURE 11–6 ■ Persistent space after pneumonectomy. Posteroanterior chest radiograph taken *A,* 4 weeks; *B,* 8 weeks; and *C,* 6 months after pneumonectomy. Note that the pleural fluid decreased initially in the space but later reaccumulated. No bronchopleural fistula was ever demonstrated.

fistula. In a report on three patients and a review of 49 collected cases from the literature, Van den Bosch and associates (1980) stated that an infectious process may be responsible for late-onset esophagopleural fistula. Evans (1972) found that a bronchopleural fistula was present in seven of eight patients with an esophagopleural fistula, and all patients presented an empyema for a period of 1 to 22 months prior to the diagnosis of the esophagopleural fistula.

In 1961, Dumont and DeGraef (1961) suggested that a mechanical process, such as traction on the esophageal wall, creates an inflammatory reaction, which leads to the formation of a fistula between the esophageal lumen and pleural cavity. According to this hypothesis, the empyema is the result and not the cause of the fistula.

Symes and co-workers (1972) proposed a different mechanism to explain the pathogenesis of esophagopleural fistulas. They presented the case of a 62-year-old man in whom a left pneumonectomy had been performed for a bronchogenic carcinoma. Sixteen months later, the patient developed an esophagopleural fistula that was attributed to recurrent lung carcinoma because there were no signs of empyema or bronchopleural fistula. Esophagopleural fistula may thus occur as a result of recurrent local disease.

Clinical Features and Diagnosis

Early diagnosis of an esophagopleural fistula is essential to reduce the rates of patient morbidity and mortality. The clinical features are often those of an empyema or bronchopleural fistula, but the diagnosis of an esophagopleural fistula must be considered when a suspected bronchopleural fistula has been ruled out. These patients may present with varying degrees of toxicity, fever, dyspnea, chest pain, and possible subcutaneous emphysema. On occasion, however, they present with malnutrition, weight loss, and fatigue, a clinical picture that may be difficult to distinguish from that of a locally recurrent or disseminated carcinoma. On thoracentesis, the finding of food particles or gastric juices confirms the diagnosis. The presence of desquamated epidermoid cells in the pleural fluid is pathognomonic, as reported by Eriksen (1964).

The diagnostic workup must include standard chest radiographs, CT scan, and a bronchoscopy to eliminate recurrent disease and the commonly associated bronchopleural fistula. A contrast esophagogram (Fig. 11–7) and esophagoscopy establish the diagnosis, locate the site of the fistula, and help estimate its size. In selected cases, ingestion of methylene blue or the helium test (Van den Bosch et al, 1980) may also be useful.

Management

Although a variety of procedures exist, the management of esophagopleural fistulas must be individualized, and both the patient's condition and the specific characteristics of the fistula must be considered. In Takaro and coworkers' (1960) series, 8 patients were treated by direct repair of the fistula (1 death); 4 patients, by gastric or colonic interposition (4 deaths); 10 patients, by chest wall surgery, including drainage and Schede thoracoplasty (2 deaths); and 10 patients, by conservative measures (9 deaths). Overall, 21% of patients were cured, and a mortality rate of 49% was reported. These authors concluded that therapy of these fistulas is complicated and unsatisfactory.

Successful management of patients must include adequate nutritional support and effective therapy of the associated empyema. Sethi and Takaro (1978) and Van den Bosch and associates (1980) recommend total parenteral nutrition; others, such as Shama and Odell (1985) and Faber and co-workers (1990), advocate enteral feeding. Closed or open pleural drainage with irrigation is required to treat the empyema (Benjamin et al, 1969;

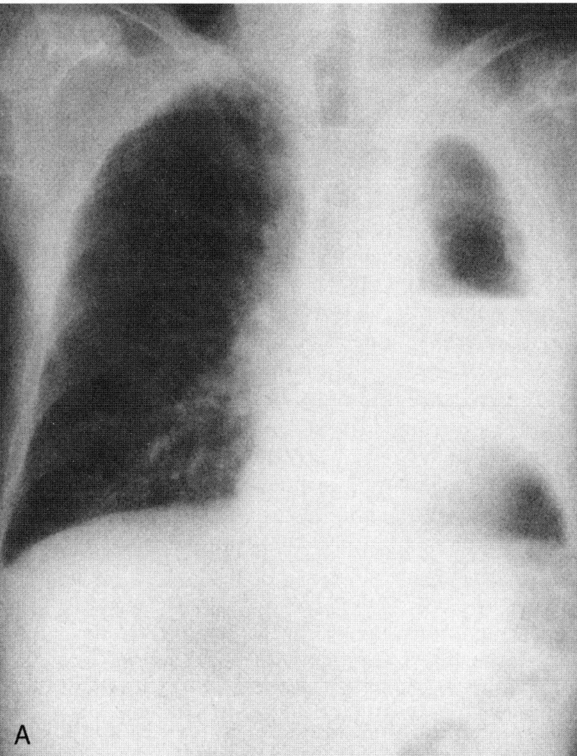

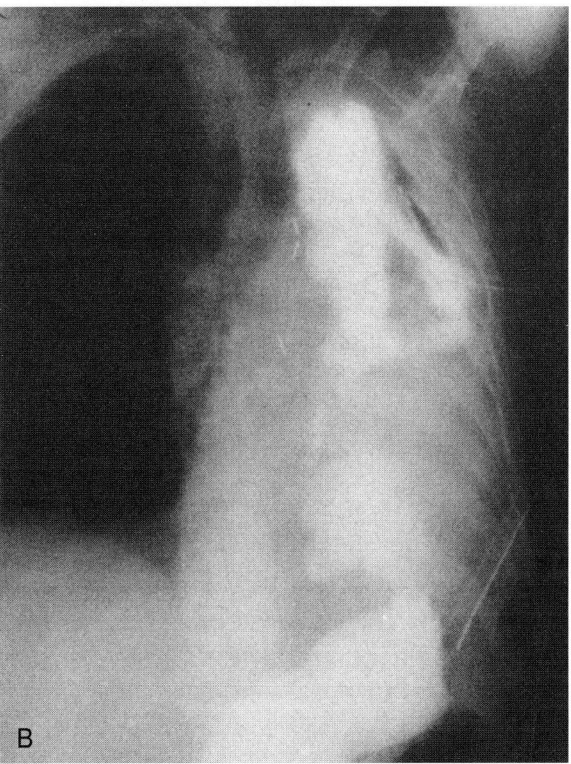

FIGURE 11–7 ■ Esophagopleural fistula. *A,* Posteroanterior chest radiograph showing a fluid level in a left pneumonectomy space 3 months following incomplete resection of lung cancer followed by radiation. *B,* Contrast esophagogram established the diagnosis of a late esophagopleural fistula.

Dumont and DeGraef, 1961; Shama and Odell, 1985; Takaro et al, 1960). After the infectious process is under control and the patient is stable, attention can be turned to the fistula.

Complicated reconstructions, such as gastric or colonic interposition, are not suitable in these frail patients. We agree with those who recommend direct primary repair of the fistula reinforced with pleura, omentum, or a pedicled chest wall or intercostal muscle flap (Benjamin et al, 1969; Efthimidis et al, 1974; Engelman, et al, 1970; Mud et al, 1987; Richardson et al, 1976). An 86% success rate is reported with this procedure from a literature review (Sethi and Takaro, 1978). A space-reducing thoracoplasty may be added if the postpneumonectomy space is large and shows signs of residual infection (Evans, 1972; Richardson et al, 1976).

Shama and Odell (1985) offer an interesting alternative to the therapy of these fistulas. Although the procedure is condemned by Evans (1972) and Sethi and Takaro (1978), Shama and Odell recommend open drainage of the empyema and prolonged nasogastric feeding. After the fistula has healed, attempts are made at sterilizing the cavity by irrigation. These authors successfully treated five of seven patients in this fashion and believe that treating the empyema is the key to the problem and that the fistula heals by itself after the empyema is under control. This approach is valid and justified in elderly patients who cannot tolerate more extensive procedures.

When the esophagopleural fistula is secondary to recurrent carcinoma, only palliative therapy can be offered. As reported by Symes and co-workers (1972), an endoluminal esophageal prosthesis may occlude the fistula and alleviate the patient's symptoms.

LATE BRONCHIAL COMPLICATIONS OTHER THAN FISTULA

Bronchial Stump Suture Granulomas

Granulations at the bronchial suture line are almost always caused by the use of highly reactive suture material, such as silk or Tevdek. In a report from Stanford (Baumgartner and Mark, 1981), all eight patients with bronchial margin granulations had their bronchi closed with Tevdek, which is a multifilament plastic nonabsorbable suture material. The median time between the resection and the development of respiratory symptoms was 18 months (8 to 57 months).

Scott and co-workers (1975, 1976) addressed the problem of healing of the bronchial stump when different methods of closure were used. They compared closure and inflammatory reactions when silk, chromic catgut, and stainless steel staples were used for bronchial closure in experimental animals. They concluded that, compared to silk and nylon, the onset of the exudative reaction is delayed and at all times minimal with staples. Because most surgeons currently use staple closure for bronchi, granulation tissue is now seldom seen as a complication of surgery. When it occurs, it is almost always caused by relative ischemia or impaired healing of the bronchus.

Patients with bronchial stump suture granulomas nearly always complain of a dry irritative cough. This symptom may be intermittent and relieved by the spontaneous expectoration of granulation tissue or suture material. Hemoptysis is not uncommon but is seldom of a life-threatening nature.

The diagnosis of bronchial stump suture granulomas can be made at bronchoscopy by which both granulations and suture material can be seen. A local inflammatory reaction can also be seen. Bronchoscopy is also useful to rule out the presence of locally recurrent carcinoma.

Management consists of removing all exposed sutures with the flexible or rigid bronchoscope, and in Baumgartner and associates' (1981) series, immediate and sustained relief was obtained in seven of eight patients.

Long Stump Syndrome

Lynn (1958) was one of the first surgeons to recognize that one of the most important sources of breakdown of the bronchus stump was the failure to observe high division of the bronchus. He made the following observation: "If the bronchus is not divided almost flush with the trachea during pneumonectomy or as close to the parent bronchus as possible during segmental resection or lobectomy, then a stump for the accumulation of secretions is left. This is the greatest source of postoperative infection, delayed healing and breakdown."

Long stump syndromes are uncommon and mostly seen after left pneumonectomy (Fig. 11–8) or middle and lower lobectomies. The clinical presentation is usually that of recurring infection, chronic purulent bronchorrhea, and hemoptysis. At bronchoscopy, the stump is markedly inflamed, and suture granulomas are often present.

The management can be conservative, with respiratory hygiene, postural physiotherapy, and antibiotics or, when necessary, granulomas can be removed by bronchoscopy. Occasionally, the stump has to be reresected.

Anastomotic Strictures After Sleeve Resection

The incidence of granuloma formation at the anastomosis after sleeve resection has been reduced to virtually 0% with the use of absorbable sutures. Nevertheless, if they should occur and be symptomatic with stridor, hemoptysis, or recurrent pneumonia, granulomas can be removed, sometimes with the adjacent sutures, through the bronchoscope.

Late anastomotic strictures are caused by an interrupted blood supply or anastomotic dehiscence with secondary healing and stricture formation. In most reported series, the incidence of this complication ranges from 2% to 5%. Therapy consists of repeated dilatations and removal of granulation tissue, reresection, and anastomosis or completion pneumonectomy. In a recent series of 142 patients who underwent sleeve resection for lung cancer (Mehran et al, 1994), 4 patients had a late complication at the site of the bronchial anastomosis. Among these, two had granulation tissue that was successfully removed with a bronchoscope, and two had a fibrous stricture that was dilated in one but necessitated completion pneumonectomy in the other. Tsang and Goldstraw (1989)

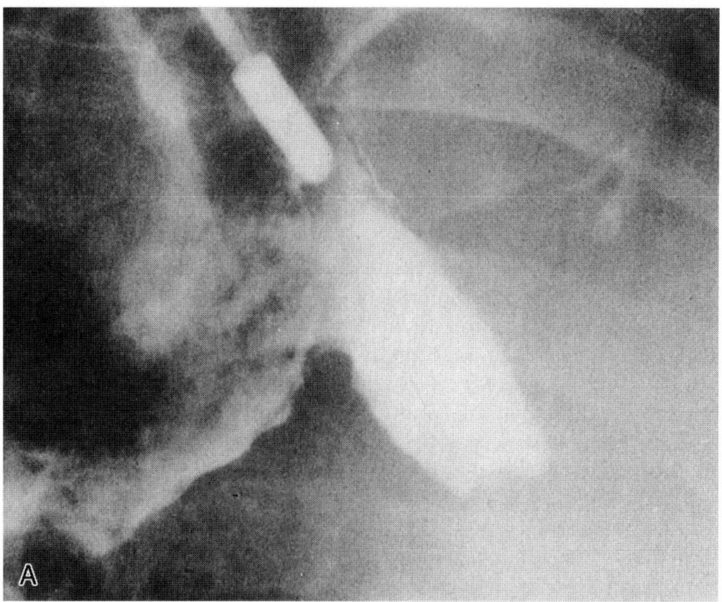

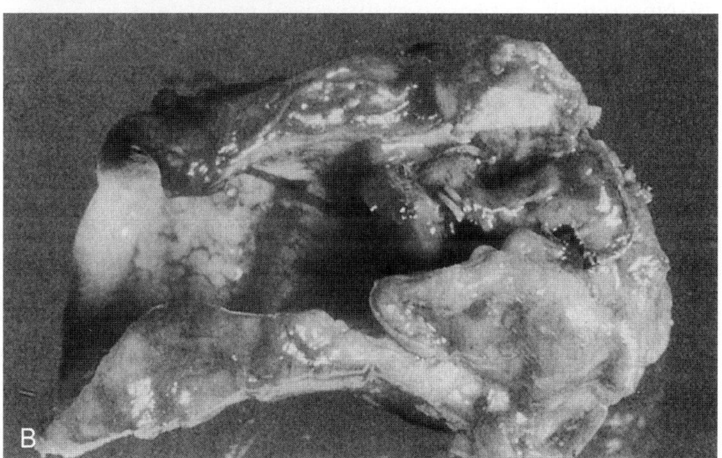

FIGURE 11–8 ■ Long stump syndrome. *A,* Bronchogram showing a long stump after left pneumonectomy. This patient was symptomatic and underwent reresection through a median sternotomy. *B,* The resected specimen showing large amounts of granulation tissue in the stump.

showed that endobronchial stenting with a Silastic prosthesis may also be a valid option in the therapy of this complication.

POST-THORACOTOMY CHEST PAIN

Definitions and Incidence

The concepts of post-thoracotomy pain and of its management are complex and fascinating. Over the years, great advances have been made in the therapy of pain in the early postoperative period with developments in preemptive analgesia, postoperative maintenance therapy, and patient-controlled analgesia. Unfortunately, compared with early post-thoracotomy pain, much less is known about chronic pain, which is an unnecessary source of anxiety and discomfort for a patient who has undergone a thoracotomy and curative resection for a malignancy. Generally, surgeons find the therapy of these pain syndromes frustrating because the results are often unsatisfactory.

Post-thoracotomy pain is important because it is usually more severe and of longer duration than pain following other surgical procedures (Conacher, 1990); Loan and Morrison, 1967). The post-thoracotomy pain syndrome refers to pain in the area of the surgical incision that lingers beyond the expected postoperative course (Jackson, 1993). The International Association for the Study of Pain (1986) defines this syndrome as pain that recurs or persists along a thoracotomy scar at least 2 months following the surgical procedure. Other authors, such as Sutton (1993), consider post-thoracotomy pain chronic only if it lasts for more than 6 months postoperatively and is unrelated to the underlying pathologic condition.

Following thoracotomy, mild chest pain without repercussions on daily life is common, with an incidence of 44% to 54% as reported by Kalso (1992) and Dajczman and their co-workers (1991). The presence of severe disabling chronic pain is, however, less common, with an estimated incidence of 5% (Conacher, 1992; Sutton, 1993). It is often described as a sensation of continuous burning or aching in the scar with a dysesthetic or lancinating component extending beyond the immediate area of the incision (Jackson, 1993). Patients may complain of a dull or stabbing pain, numbness, or hyperesthesia or of secondary features, such as frozen shoulder or back pain. Conacher (1992) describes post-thoracotomy pain syndrome more specifically as a post-thoracotomy neuralgia, which is a benign pain condition unrelated to the underlying pathologic condition.

Pathophysiology and Clinical Features

The exact cause of chronic post-thoracotomy pain is unknown. Following surgery, nociceptive stimuli arise from the skin incision, damaged costovertebral structures, fractured or excised ribs, and parietal pleura. These injuries cause direct mechanical and thermal damage to nerve endings and sensitization of primary afferent nociceptors (Sabanathan et al, 1993). The stimuli from the chest wall structures and pleura are conducted to the central nervous system by the intercostal nerves, those from the diaphragmatic pleura by the phrenic nerve, and those from the lung and mediastinum by the vagus nerve (Conacher, 1990). Although these events are important in the development of acute post-thoracotomy pain, their role in chronic pain is unclear. Furthermore, psychological factors affecting the patient's personality and emotional status may also influence the occurrence and severity of chronic pain (Jackson, 1993; Loan and Morrison, 1967).

Different causes of chronic post-thoracotomy pain have been described, and it is important to distinguish pain as the "symptom" from pain as the "disease" (Jackson, 1993). In the presence of recurrent carcinoma, infectious process, or fractured ribs, pain results from an identifiable source, which is the symptom of an underlying problem. In a study by Kanner and associates (1982), a recurrent cancer or infectious complication was found in 29 of 32 patients evaluated for persistent post-thoracotomy pain. Thus, all patients presenting with chronic chest pain must be thoroughly evaluated by clinical history, complete physical examination, and a workup that includes a chest radiograph, a CT scan (or magnetic resonance imaging), and a bone scan. If the cause of pain is identified, it can be appropriately treated.

When no cause is found, the chronic pain should be dealt with as a disease process. These forms of post-thoracotomy pain syndrome are considered benign and are either neurogenic or musculoskeletal in origin. A number of phenomena are associated with post-thoracotomy neurogenic pain. The pain may first result from entrapment of nerve fibers in the scar tissue (intercostal neuralgia). In these patients, light touch produces intense radiating pain, accompanied by a burning sensation if a reflex sympathetic dystrophy is associated. The relief of pain with injection of a local anesthetic is virtually diagnostic of this condition. Another cause of neurogenic pain is a neuroma. A palpable mass in the wound, the loss of pinprick sensation over the skin, and pain on palpation lead to this diagnosis. Third, sympathetic dystrophy presents as a burning pain associated with hyperpathia, decreased skin temperature, and increased sweating (Ramamurthy, 1986).

Benign musculoskeletal post-thoracotomy pain syndromes are less common than pain of neurogenic origin. As discussed previously, recurrent tumor and metastatic disease must first be ruled out, and associated conditions, such as shoulder bursitis or tendinitis, must also be looked for. Unrecognized rib fractures at the time of thoracotomy may be involved in the production of pain. Section of the richly innovated chest wall muscles produces extensive soft tissue injury and inflammation, which may also generate musculoskeletal pain syndromes through a variety of chemical mediators (Conacher, 1990).

It has been shown that muscle-sparing thoracotomy incisions are associated with less pain in the early postoperative period Hazelrigg et al, 1991; Lemmer et al, 1990. Their impact on chronic chest pain, however, is unknown. A specific type of musculoskeletal post-thoracotomy pain, known as myofascial pain syndrome, has been described (Jackson, 1993). Patients have trigger points or localized areas in thoracic muscles, such as the serratus anterior or latissimus dorsi, which produce pain that is referred to distant sites when palpated.

How does the severity of early postoperative pain correlate with the development of chronic chest pain? In Kalso and associates[2] (1992) study, patients who had persistent pain had significantly more pain during the first postoperative week compared with those without chronic pain. However, no difference was found in the amounts of opioids given or in the nurses' comments when comparing the patients. It seems that patients with persistent pain are inclined to remember more pain. As shown by Eich and others (1985), memory about the intensity of past physical pain depends on the intensity of present pain.

Management

The management of patients with post-thoracotomy pain syndrome is difficult and benefits from a multidisciplinary approach. A hospital pain "team" can play a key role in developing an appropriate therapeutic plan. In a review of 73 cases of post-thoracotomy neuralgia (more than 3 months' duration), Conacher (1992) found that more than 70% of patients received three or more different therapeutic modalities. These included analgesics (narcotics or nonsteroidal anti-inflammatory drugs [NSAIDs]); local anesthetics or local steroids; transcutaneous electric nerve stimulation (TENS); cryotherapy; surgical or chemical neurolysis; and acupuncture. Despite the great number and variety of therapies, no patients admitted to being relieved of all symptoms.

It has been shown that peripheral nerve injuries may produce central changes in the dorsal root ganglia and that, after such central processes are established, pain may persist independent of peripheral stimulation (Melzack and Loeber, 1978). This hypothesis may explain why local therapy of post-thoracotomy pain syndrome is often frustrating and unsuccessful.

When dealing with benign neurogenic or musculoskeletal chronic chest pain, local measures may nonetheless be valuable. They represent first-line therapy. Intercostal neuralgias or nerve entrapment are initially treated with intercostal nerve blocks using a local anesthetic (e.g., bupivacaine) with or without steroids. A thoracic epidural infusion or paravertebral blocks may be useful. Kirvela and Antila (1992) reported on the use of paravertebral nerve blocks in 32 patients with chronic chest pain. Although 58% of patients were relieved, only 8% were relieved for more than 4 months.

Cryoanalgesia has also been recommended for neuralgia. First described by Lloyd and co-workers (1976), cryoanalgesia uses extreme cold (−75°C) to cause temporary disruption of nerve conduction and thus alleviate pain. A number of recent reports, however, have condemned its use (Berrisford and Sabanathan, 1990; Conacher, 1986; Orr et al, 1981; Roxburgh et al, 1987). In Conacher's (1986) study on cryotherapy for post-thoracotomy neuralgia, 21% of patients showed no improvement, and 29% were actually worse after therapy.

When a neuroma is found or suspected, a small amount (less than 1 mL) of anesthetic may be infused into it. If the pain is relieved, the procedure is repeated with a neurolytic phenol solution (Jackson, 1993). Wound exploration and surgical excision are also possible but carry the risk of creating further damage. The presence of a sympathetic dystrophy requires paravertebral sympathetic blocks, nerve root blocks, or an epidural infusion (Ramamurthy, 1986).

The therapeutic options for musculoskeletal chronic chest pain include physical therapy to strengthen muscle tone and improve shoulder mobilization. Heat massages and ultrasound may also be valuable (Jackson, 1993), and NSAIDs may be added to the physical therapy. The use of TENS is also recommended, especially in the presence of myofascial pain syndrome. Oral and systemic medication (narcotics, NSAIDs, and tricyclic antidepressants) and different neuroablative techniques are available and important adjuncts to the local therapeutic measures described.

In all cases of post-thoracotomy pain syndrome, it is essential and important foremost to exclude the presence of recurrent cancer, metastatic disease, or an infectious complication. The patient must then be reassured as to the benign nature of the problem. Understanding the underlying pathophysiology and obtaining a working diagnosis are crucial to provide adequate and successful patient management. Although they often only offer temporary relief, local therapeutic measures continue to represent the mainstay of therapy for chronic chest pain.

LATE PHYSIOLOGIC COMPLICATIONS

Postpneumonectomy Syndrome

Definitions and Incidence

The postpneumonectomy syndrome is caused by airway obstruction, which is itself secondary to the extreme mediastinal shift and rotation after pneumonectomy. In this situation, the mainstem bronchus becomes compressed between the spine and aorta posteriorly and the pulmonary artery anteriorly. This syndrome mainly occurs in younger patients in whom the bronchus is softer and more compressible. It has been described almost exclusively after right pneumonectomy (Grillo et al, 1992).

The exact incidence of the postpneumonectomy syndrome is unknown, although Jansen and co-workers (1992) reported only 1 case among 640 patients who had undergone pneumonectomies (incidence of 0.2%). This low incidence likely reflects the older age of the patients undergoing pneumonectomy for lung cancer.

Pathogenesis

In a classic review, Grillo and associates (1992) reported on 11 patients with the postpneumonectomy syndrome and concluded that the airway obstruction clearly results from mediastinal displacement.

After right pneumonectomy, the mediastinum moves counterclockwise to the right and posteriorly (Shepard et al, 1986). The realignment of intrathoracic structures results in tracheal displacement to the right and compression of the left main bronchus, and sometimes the distal trachea, as it angles beneath the aorta and is flattened against the vertebral column or against the descending aorta (Grillo et al, 1992) (Fig. 11–9). Szarnicki and colleagues (1978) also showed the same findings in a child in whom the lower trachea was compressed by the arch of the aorta after right pneumonectomy.

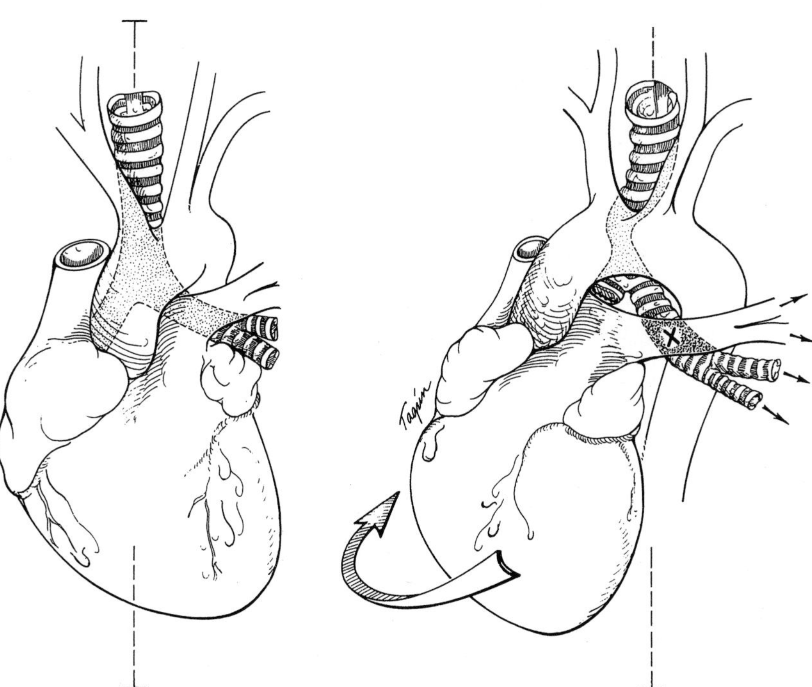

FIGURE 11–9 ■ Postpneumonectomy syndrome after right pneumonectomy with left-sided arch. This diagram shows that the trachea and carina are displaced to the right with left main bronchus compression between the left pulmonary artery and descending aorta or against the spine. The *dashed vertical line* indicates the midline. (From Grillo HC, Shepard JAO, Mathisen DJ, Kanorck DJ: Post-pneumonectomy syndrome: Diagnosis, management, and results. Ann Thorac Surg 54:638, 1992.)

Although Grillo (1992) and others (Quillin and Shakleford, 1991) reported the same syndrome after left pneumonectomy, all these patients had a right-sided aortic arch. In Quillin and Shakleford's case, the right-sided descending aorta and ligamentum arteriosum played a central role in the bronchial obstruction. In the cases that occurred after left pneumonectomy, Grillo and colleagues (1992) showed that, because the right main bronchus is so much shorter than the left, it is not uncommon to find that the right upper lobe bronchus and the bronchus intermedius are also compressed against the vertebral column.

These observations may not be entirely true, because we now have seen four cases of postpneumonectomy syndrome occurring after left pneumonectomy and a normally located left-sided aortic arch (Daniel and co-workers, personal communication, 1994) (Fig. 11–10). In these cases, the right main bronchus, right upper lobe bronchus, and right bronchus intermedius are stretched,

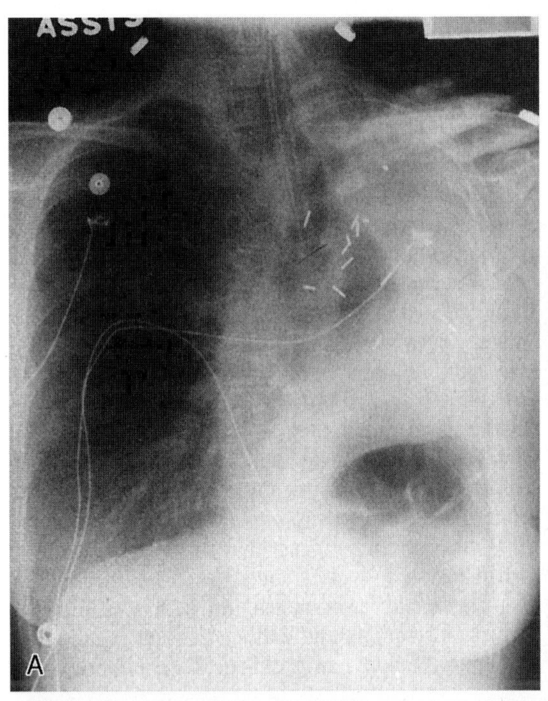

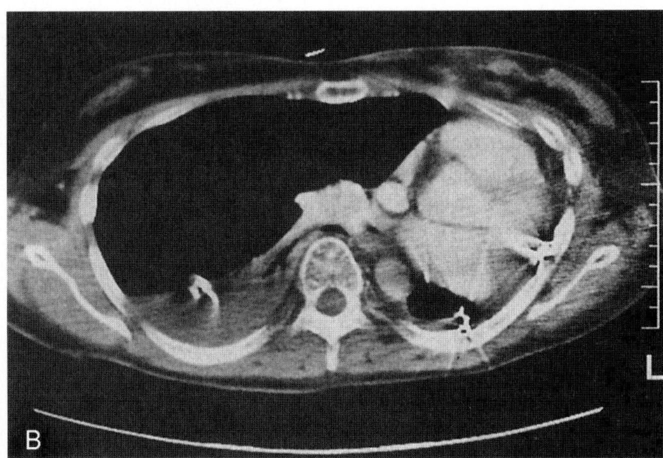

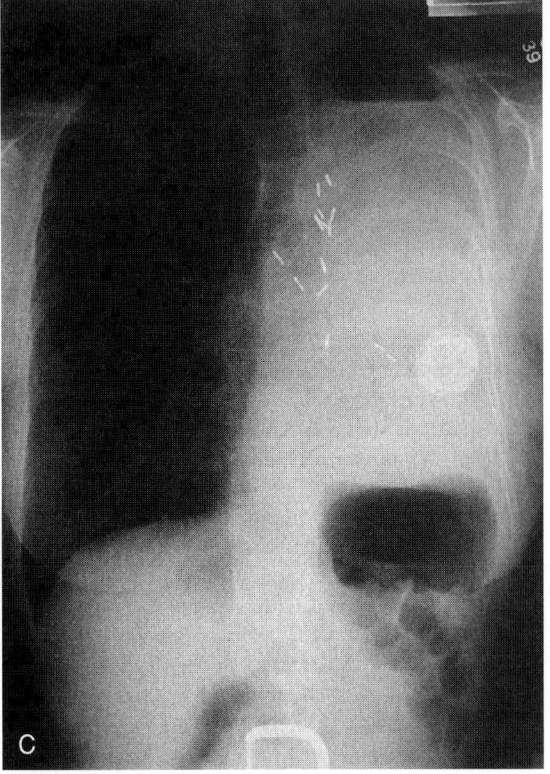

FIGURE 11–10 ■ Postpneumonectomy syndrome after left pneumonectomy and left-sided arch. *A,* Standard chest radiograph taken 1 year after left pneumonectomy and showing extreme mediastinal shift. There is an infiltrate in the right lower lung, and the patient had to be intubated. *B,* Scan showing the mediastinal shift and severe narrowing of the right main bronchus. *C,* The mediastinum has been repositioned in a central position by the insertion of a Silastic expander. The patient has remained well 2 years after the insertion of the prosthesis.

tented, and compressed between the spine posteriorly and the pulmonary artery anteriorly.

Rusch and colleagues (1990) and others (Powell et al, 1979) showed that these syndromes are more likely to develop in infants and young children, presumably because of increased mobility of the mediastinum, increased elasticity and compliance of the remaining lung (which allows overdistention), and greater compressibility of the trachea and bronchi (which have less cartilaginous support).

Clinical Features and Diagnosis

Patients can present with an acute onset of dyspnea and airway obstruction, or they can present with a more insidious onset of symptoms, such as repeated bouts of pulmonary infection, persistent cough, and stridor. The interval between the pneumonectomy and the onset of symptoms is variable, and in Grillo and colleagues' (1992) series, it ranged from 5 months to 17 years. Shepard and associates (1986) also presented the case of one patient who developed the syndrome 37 years after pneumonectomy. In many patients, the symptoms are well tolerated until a critical point of airway obstruction is reached, which brings about acute respiratory failure.

The diagnosis of postpneumonectomy syndrome is based on a high index of suspicion and a methodical multimodality investigation in which CT scanning and bronchoscopic examination are the most important. Conventional radiographic examination always show extreme posterior mediastinal displacement, anterior lung herniation, and stretching of the remaining main bronchus over the spine. CT of the chest is essential to demonstrate the rotation of the heart and great vessels and the exact site and extent of bronchial obstruction against the spine (Grillo et al, 1992). Confirmation of bronchial narrowing can finally be obtained by bronchoscopy which can also demonstrate the presence or absence of bronchomalacia.

Management

Surgical therapy of the postpneumonectomy syndrome is directed toward correcting the tracheobronchial compression and diminishing the extreme mediastinal shift and rotation (Riveron et al, 1990). Relieving the obstruction by way of lysis of adhesions (Wasserman et al, 1979); suspension of the mediastinum, pericardium, and pulmonary artery to the anterior chest wall (Adams et al, 1972); division of the aortic arch with placement of a Dacron prosthesis (Szarnicki et al, 1978); and phrenectomy have all been reported, but they have had variable and unpredictable results.

Using the concept that Lucite balls can prevent overexpansion of the remaining lung after pneumonectomy (Johnson et al, 1949), Silastic breast implants (Wasserman et al, 1979), and more recently tissue expanders, such as those used by plastic surgeons, have been successfully used to reposition and maintain the mediastinum toward the midline. These prostheses are inserted in the pleural space and filled with the necessary amount of fluid to replace the mediastinum to the midline, a motion that can be monitored by measuring the central venous pressure. The operation is fairly simple, and the improvement is often immediate and dramatic.

One of the problems associated with the correction of this syndrome is the presence of bronchomalacia in the involved bronchus. In these patients, simple mediastinal replacement and fixation by filler material seems to be insufficient, and Grillo and associates (1992) proposed the placement of bronchial stents, which are either internal or specially constructed T tubes.

Late Respiratory Failure

As pneumonectomy became the standard of care for the therapy of bronchogenic carcinoma in the 1940s, attention was drawn to the functional changes in the remaining lung, and pulmonary insufficiency was recognized as a potential late complication. Gaensler and colleagues (1955) in an early report on 460 patients found dyspnea with severe or total disability postoperatively in 7.8% of patients. This group also recognized respiratory failure as an important cause of late death. A number of studies on respiratory and circulatory alterations following pulmonary resection appeared thereafter in the literature (Burrows et al, 1960; De Graff et al, 1965; Gorlin et al, 1957; Harrison et al, 1958).

How do we explain the occurrence of respiratory insufficiency several months or years after a pneumonectomy? It is well known that several structural and physiologic changes develop in the remaining lung parenchyma. Experimental studies in animals subjected to pneumonectomy have shown overdistention and emphysematous changes in the contralateral lung. The lung also has histologic evidence of hyperplasia with fragmentation of the alveoli and loss of elastic tissue (Longaire and Johansmann, 1940). Harrison and associates. (1958) believed that these changes could cause an increase in airway resistance with abnormal alveolar gas mixing and arterial oxygen desaturation, eventually leading to late pulmonary failure. The destructive changes in the alveolar walls following surgery were termed "compensatory emphysema" by Phillips and co-workers (1941), but other authors did not demonstrate such changes in the remaining lung after pneumonectomy (Birath et al, 1947; Burrows et al, 1960; Jones et al, 1960).

A number of hypotheses concerning hemodynamic and circulatory alterations have also been proposed. In a patient who has undergone pneumonectomy, the blood flow through the remaining lung is substantially increased, but the total capillary bed available for gas exchange remains unchanged. When the oxygen requirements and pulmonary blood flow increase on exertion, the capillary bed cannot accommodate the demand, and this may result in pulmonary hypertension and arterial oxygen desaturation (Harrison et al, 1958). Burrows and co-workers (1960) also suggested that exercise may have an active vasomotor effect on the lung, thus creating pulmonary artery hypertension, which could in turn lead to progressive pulmonary failure. In a study of postpneumonectomy patients, De Graff and associates (1965) found a reduction in maximal oxygen intake on exercise, and neither a reduced ventilation nor a lower diffusing capacity was responsible for the changes. These authors believed a decrease in cardiac output was the limiting factor.

In these early reports, the investigational methods were few, and thus a correlation between structural and physiologic changes and clinical outcome could not be demonstrated. The more recent development of dynamic respiratory studies and of sophisticated hemodynamic monitoring apparatuses has provided a wealth of information. Boushy and others (1971), in a study of 62 patients who had undergone preoperative and postoperative pulmonary function tests, found that changes in exercise tolerance after resection were not related to morphologic emphysema or bronchitis in the remaining lung. Lobectomies were shown to have little effect on exercise capacity and late respiratory failure (Berend et al, 1980; Vejlsted and Halkier, 1982). After surgery, there are generally no alterations in the distribution of ventilation or the diffusing capacity, and modifications in pulmonary function simply reflect changes in pulmonary volumes.

Van Meighem and Demedts (1989) reported on cardiopulmonary function following lung resections for carcinoma. They found a decrease in vital capacity (15% for lobectomies and 35% to 40% for pneumonectomies) and a decrease in static lung compliance (increase in elastic recoil pressures and transdiaphragmatic pressures). At rest, patients had normal pulmonary artery pressures and vascular resistances; during exercise, an increase in pulmonary artery pressure and an absence of the physiologic decrease in pulmonary vascular resistance were noted. In postpneumonectomy patients, these authors suggest that there may be a relative increase in vasoactive substances, such as angiotensin II, leading to systemic vasoconstriction with a secondary decrease in stroke volume and cardiac output. These vascular and pulmonary hemodynamic changes alter pulmonary function and may in theory predispose to late pulmonary failure.

Mossberg and co-workers (1976) studied working capacity and exercise limitation in pneumonectomized patients. They found a reduction in ventilatory function (increase in static pulmonary volumes and decrease in dynamic volumes), a decrease in diffusing capacity, impaired gas exchange, a low stroke volume, and an elevated left atrial pressure and pulmonary artery pressure during exercise, all of which contributed to a lower working capacity. In a more recent comprehensive study, Pelletier and colleagues (1990) reported a 25% decrease in maximal working capacity following pneumonectomy. Dyspnea increased significantly for a given workload after pneumonectomy, whereas no significant change was found following lobectomy. In this report, the reduction in forced expiratory volume could explain only 30% of the change in the working capacity. A number of other mechanisms, such as the characteristics of the respiratory muscles and different hemodynamic parameters, are thus probably also involved.

Late respiratory failure following pulmonary resection is an important cause of patient morbidity and death, and its pathophysiology is complex, multifactorial, and not completely understood. Hemodynamic and ventilatory factors and parenchymal structural changes are involved. A thorough preoperative evaluation is therefore required in all patients with a limited pulmonary reserve, especially if they are 70 years of age or older.

COMMENTS AND CONTROVERSIES

As can be seen from this review, late complications of pulmonary surgery are rare events, but when they occur, they usually are difficult to diagnose and treat. They should be distinguished from recurrent carcinoma, and it is not unusual for patients to be told that they are terminally ill with tumor when the problem is a postpneumonectomy empyema or a postpneumonectomy syndrome.

It is for these reasons that we recommend a close follow-up for at least the first 2 years after the operation. All patients should be seen and have a chest radiograph 1 month postoperatively and again every 3 months for the following 2 years. In our unit, each patient is also given a pamphlet that lists and explains symptoms, such as fever, chest pain, and purulent sputum, that may be indicative of a pending late complication.

J. D.
P. F.

Late-appearing empyema following lobectomy or pneumonectomy can be a daunting problem. The initial management by tube thoracostomy and ultimately open drainage is a standard technique. In most instances, open window thoracostomy is required to effect better mechanical débridement. My associates and I prefer repeated daily packing of saline or hypochlorite-impregnated gauze. Ultimately, tailoring thoracoplasty or muscle transposition may be necessary to close the space. However, we have found that repeated packing, especially with situations less than pneumonectomy in the lower regions of the chest, can close the space by progressive fibrosis and contraction.

In late-appearing fistulas, we firmly believe in the initial strategy of tube thoracostomy and closed chest drainage. Following this, open thoracotomy is performed once it is determined that the patient can ventilate with an open chest wound as determined by releasing the thoracostomy tube from its underwater position. Open-window thoracostomy is often successful in closing the fistula and cleaning the contaminated space. We prefer a large window (2 to 3 ribs, 6- to 7-cm length being removed) and repeated packing of the cavity to effect mechanical debridement. In a significant number of such patients, the fistulas close. Once open-window thoracostomy is performed, the patient can be treated as an outpatient.

For persisting fistulas, a variety of approaches have been suggested, including ipsilateral thoracotomy and direct closure using a vascularized flap of transposed muscle (intercostal, chest wall, rectus abdominis) or a vascularized pedicle of omentum. If a fistula is not present, attempts at sterilization of a persisting cavity (the Clagett procedure) can be very successful if particular attention is directed toward mechanical débridement of the cavity and replacement of the empyema wall with healthy granulation tissue before sterilization.

Anastomotic strictures following sleeve resections can occasionally be treated by laser resection if the stricture is extremely short. This is best done using a carbon dioxide laser, incising the stricture radially in quadrants over 4 or 5 sessions.

I have found, on occasion, that post-thoracotomy pain is caused by cross-union of ribs inadvertently fractured at thoracotomy. This malunion can be identified by specific rib radiographs or tomograms. Surgical removal of the cross-union and freeing of the entrapped nerve can relieve the problem. Prevention of late post-thoracotomy pain may be related to amelioration of the early post-thoracotomy pain, which appears to be almost inevitable. A recent development is the use of "pre-emptive analgesia," which appears to be extremely effective in diminishing early postoperative pain. This includes preoperative institution of analgesia by percutaneous paravertebral block or epidural analgesia.

The postpneumonectomy syndrome has only recently been described. The procedure of choice appears to be repositioning of the mediastinum. On occasion, this has been sucessfully treated by intrabronchial insertion of expandable metallic stents. However, results based on late follow-up of such stents are unavailable.

The occurrence of late respiratory failure, especially following right pneumonectomy, is a disappointing result. This whole area remains a challenge, in being able not only to predict this complication but also to prevent its occurrence and manage it once it is manifest. We require more reports on its incidence, especially following pneumonectomy, and more reports on very long-term follow-up of pulmonary function in resected patients. This is an area worth further study.

R. J. G.

■ KEY REFERENCES

Gaensler EA, Cugell DW, Lindgren I et al: The role of pulmonary insufficiency in mortality and invalidism following surgery for pulmonary tuberculosis. J Thorac Surg 29:163, 1955.

Classic analysis of pulmonary function after pneumonectomy by a physiologist-surgeon.

Grillo HC, Shepard JAO, Mathisen DJ, Kanorek DJ: Post-pneumonectomy syndrome. Diagnosis, management, and results. Ann Thorac Surg 54:638, 1992.

Best article on the postpneumonectomy syndrome, with clear descriptions and pathogenesis, pathophysiology, and principles of management.

Lynn RB: The bronchial stump. J Thorac Surg 36:70, 1958.

A good overview of the principles involved in bronchial stump closure and healing.

Pairolero P, Arnold PG, Trastek VF et al: Post-pneumonectomy empyema—the role of intrathoracic muscle transposition. J Thorac Cardiovasc Surg 99:958, 1990.

The results of a large series of early and late postpneumonectomy empyemas treated by muscle filling of the space.

Shama DM, Odell JA: Esophageal fistula after pneumonectomy for inflammatory disease. J Thorac Cardiovasc Surg 89:77, 1985.

Discussion of the pathophysiology and principles of management of patients with esophagopleural fistula.

Shields TW, Lees WMM, Fox RT, Salazar G: Persistent pleural air space following resection for pulmonary tuberculosis. J Thorac Cardiovasc Surg 38:523, 1959.

Excellent review of the incidence and rate of postresectional spaces. Provides guidelines as to the strategy of management.

■ REFERENCES

Infectious and Space Complications

Allen MS, Deschamps C, Trastek VF, Pairolero PC: Bronchopleural fistula. Chest Surg Clin North Am 2:823, 1992.

Asamura M, Naruke T, Tsuchiya R et al: Bronchopleural fistulas associated with lung cancer operations. J Thorac Cardiovasc Surg 104:1456, 1992.

Barker WL, Langston HT, Naffah P: Post-resectional thoracic spaces. Ann Thorac Surg 2:299, 1966.

Bellamy J, Saada J, Dang QD: Pyothorax tardifs d'origine hématogène après pneumonectomie. Ann Chir 45:182, 1991.

Benjamin I, Olsen AM, Ellis FH: Esophagopleural fistula. A rare post-pneumonectomy complication. Ann Thorac Surg 7:139, 1969.

Boyd AD, Spencer FC: Bronchopleural fistulas. How often should they occur? Ann Thorac Surg 13:195, 1972.

Brunn HB: Surgical principles underlying one-stage lobectomy. Arch Surg 18:490, 1929.

Christiansen KH, Morgan SW, Karich AF, Takaro T: Pleural space following pneumonectomy. Ann Thorac Surg 1:298, 1965.

Churchill ED: The surgical treatment of carcinoma of the lung. J Thorac Surg 2:254, 1933.

Churchill E, Belsey HR: Segmental pneumonectomy in bronchiectasis. Ann Surg 109:481, 1939.

Clagett OT, Geraci JE: A procedure for the management of postpneumonectomy empyema. J Thorac Cardiovasc Surg 45:141, 1963.

Davies HM: Recent advances in the surgery of the lung and pleura. Br J Surg 1:228, 1913–1914.

Dumont A, De Graef J: La fistule esophagopleurale, complication tardive de la pneumonectomie. Lyon Chir 57:481, 1961.

Efthimiadis M, Xanthakis D, Primikyrios N et al: Late esophagopleural fistula after pneumonectomy for bronchial carcinoma. Chest 65:579, 1974.

Engelman RM, Spencer FC, Berg P: Post-pneumonectomy esophageal fistula. Successful one-stage repair. J Thorac Cardiovasc Surg 59:871, 1970.

Eriksen KR: Esophagopleural fistula diagnosed by microscopic examination of pleural fluid. Acta Chir Scand 128:771, 1964.

Erola S, Virkkula L, Varstela E: Treatment of post-pneumonectomy empyema and associated bronchopleural fistula. Scand J Thorac Cardiovasc Surg 22:235, 1988.

Evans JP: Post-pneumonectomy oesophageal fistula. Thorax 27:674, 1972.

Faber C, Kartheuser A, Buche M et al: Fistules oesophago-respiratoires traitées par suture primaire. A propos de deux observations de fistule oeso-pleurales et de deux observations de fistules oeso-bronchiques. Ann Chir 44:290, 1990.

Friedman PJ, Hellekant CAG: Radiologic recognition of bronchopleural fistula. Radiology 124:289, 1977.

Goldstraw P: Treatment of post-pneumonectomy empyema: The case of fenestration. Thorax 34:740, 1979.

Grégoire R, Deslauriers J, Beaulieu M, Piraux M: Thoracoplasty: Its forgotten role in the management of non-tuberculous postpneumonectomy empyema. Can J Surg 30:343, 1987.

Hinz R: Totale extirpation der linken lunge wegen bronchial carcinoma. Arch Klin Chir 124:104, 1923.

Holden MP, Wooler GH: Pus somewhere, pus nowhere else, pus above the diaphragm: Post-pneumonectomy empyema necessitatis. Am J Surg 124:669, 1972.

Hopkins RA, Ungerleider RM, Staub EW et al: The modern use of thoracoplasty. Ann Thorac 40:181, 1985.

Kerr WF: Late onset post-pneumonectomy empyema. Thorax 32:149, 1977.

Khargi K, Duurkens VAM, Knaepen PJ, de la Rivière AB: Hemorrhage due to inflammatory erosion of the pulmonary artery stump in post-pneumonectomy bronchopleural fistula. Ann Thorac Surg 56:357, 1993.

Kirsh MM, Rotman H, Behrendt DM et al: Complications of pulmonary resection. Ann Thorac Surg 20:215, 1975.

Kummel H: Proceedings of the 40th Congress, Berlin, April 19–22, 1911. Verh Dtsch Ges Chir 40:147, 1911.

Lemmer HJ, Botham MJ, Orringer MB: Modern management of adult thoracic empyema. J Thorac Cardiovasc Surg 90:849, 1985.
Leroux BT, Mohlala ML, Odell JA, Whitton FD: Suppurative disease of the lung and pleural space. Part I: Empyema thoracis and lung abscess. Curr Probl Surg 23:1, 1986.
Lowe RE, Siddiqui AR: Scintimaging of bronchopleural fistula: A simple method of diagnosis. Clin Nucl Med 9:10, 1984.
Miller JI, Mansour KA, Nahai F et al: Single stage complete muscle flap closure of the post-pneumonectomy empyema space: A new method and possible solution to a disturbing complication. Ann Thorac Surg 38:227, 1984.
Model D: Occult empyema presenting ten years after pneumonectomy. Lancet 22:192, 1983.
Moote D, Ehrlich L, Martin RH: Post-pneumonectomy bronchopleural fistula imaged by ventilation lung scanning. Medicine 12:337, 1987.
Mud HJ, Van Houten H, Slingerland R et al: A modified pectoralis muscle flap for closure of post-pneumonectomy esophagopleural fistula: Technique and results. Ann Thorac Surg 43:359, 1987.
Pairolero P, Deschamps C, Allen MS, Trastek MS: Postoperative empyema. Chest Surg Clin North Am 2:813, 1992.
Pean J: Chirurgie des poumons. Discussion Ranc Chir Proc Verh Paris 9:72m, 1895.
Rainer WG, Newby JP: Prevention of residual space problems after pulmonary resection. Am J Surg 114:744, 1967.
Richardson JD, Campbell D, Trinkle JK: Esophagopleural fistula after pneumonectomy. Chest 69:795, 1976.
Reinhoff WF: Pneumonectomy. A preliminary report of operative technique in two successful cases. Bull Johns Hopkins Hosp 53:390, 1933.
Rogiers PH, Van Mieghem W, Engelaar D, Demedts M: Late onset post-pneumonectomy empyema manifesting as tracheal stenosis with respiratory failure. Respir Med 85:333, 1991a.
Rogiers PH, Verschakelen J, Knockaert D, Vanneste S: Occult tuberculous post-pneumonectomy space empyema four years after lung resection. Postgrad Med J 67:672, 1991b.
Sethi GK, Takaro T: Esophagopleural fistula following pulmonary resection. Ann Thorac Surg 25:74, 1978.
Shamji FM, Ginsberg RJ, Cooper JD et al: Open window thoracostomy in the management of post-pneumonectomy empyema with or without bronchopleural fistula. J Thorac Cardiovasc Surg 86:818, 1983.
Silver AN, Epinas EE, Byron FX: The fate of the post-resection space. Ann Thorac Surg 2:311, 1966.
Soorae AS, Stevenson HM: Survival with residual tumor on the bronchial margin after resection for bronchogenic carcinoma. J Thorac Cardiovasc Surg 78:175, 1979.
Stafford EG, Clagett OT: Post-pneumonectomy empyema. Neomycin instillation and definitive closure. J Thorac Cardiovasc Surg 63:771, 1972.
Steiger Z, Wilson RF: Management of bronchopleural fistulas. Surg Gynecol Obstet 158:267, 1984.
Suarez J, Clagett OT, Brown AL: The post-pneumonectomy space: Factors influencing its obliteration. J Thorac Cardiovasc Surg 57:539, 1969.
Symes JM, Page AJF, Flavell G: Esophagopleural fistula: A late complication after pneumonectomy. J Thorac Cardiovasc Surg 63:783, 1972.
Takaro T, Walkup HE, Okano T: Esophagopleural fistula as a complication of thoracic surgery. A collective review. J Thorac Cardiovasc Surg 40:179, 1960.
Van den Bosch JMM, Swierenga J, Gelissen HJ, Laros CD: Post-pneumonectomy oesophagopleural fistula. Thorax 35:865, 1980.
Vester SR, Faber LP, Kittle CF et al: Bronchopleural fistula after stapled closure of bronchus. Ann Thorac Surg 52:1253, 1991
Virkkula L, Kostiainen S: Post-pneumonectomy empyema in pulmonary carcinoma patients. Scand J Thorac Cardiovasc Surg 4:267, 1970.
Williams NS, Lewis CT: Bronchopleural fistula: A review of 86 cases. Br J Surg 63:520, 1976.
Witz JP, Roeslin N: Les empyèmes et fistules bronchiques après pneumonectomie. Résultat d'une enquête à propos de 444 observations. Ann Chir 35:669, 1981.

Late Bronchial Stump Complications Other Than Fistulas

Baumgartner WA, Mark JBD: Bronchoscopic diagnosis and treatment of bronchial stump suture granulomas. J Thorac Cardiovasc Surg 81:553, 1981.
Lynn RB: The bronchus stump. J Thorac Surg 36:70, 1958
Mehran RJ, Deslauriers J, Piraux M et al: Survival related to nodal status after sleeve resection for lung cancer. J Thorac Cardiovasc Surg 107:576, 1994.
Scott RN, Faraci RP, Goodman DG et al: The role of inflammation in bronchial stump healing. Ann Surg 181:4, 1975.
Scott RN, Faraci RP, Hough A, Chrétien PB: Bronchial stump closure techniques following pneumonectomy. A serial comparative study. Ann Surg 184:205, 1976.
Tsang V, Goldstraw PL: Endobronchial stenting for anastomotic stenosis after sleeve resection. Ann Thorac Surg 48:568, 1989.

Post-Thoracotomy Chest Pain

Berrisford RG, Sabanathan SS: Cryoanalgesia for post-thoracotomy pain (Letter). Ann Thorac Surg 49:509, 1990.
Conacher ID: Therapists and therapies for post-thoracotomy neuralgia. Pain 48:409, 1992.
Conacher ID: Pain relief after thoracotomy. Br J Anaesth 65:806, 1990.
Conacher ID: Percutaneous cryotherapy for post-thoracotomy neuralgia. Pain 25:227, 1986.
Dajczman E, Gordon A, Krelsman M, Wolkove N: Long term post-thoracotomy pain. Chest 99:270, 1991.
Eich E, Reeves JL, Jaeger B, Graff-Radford SB: Memory for pain: Relation between past and present pain intensity. Pain 23:375, 1985.
Hazelrigg S, Landreneau RJ, Boley TM et al: The effect of muscle sparing versus standard posterolateral thoracotomy on pulmonary function, muscle strength and postoperative pain. J Thorac Cardiovasc Surg 101:394, 1991.
International Association for Study of Pain: Post-thoracotomy pain syndrome (XVII-14), classification of chronic pain. Pain 3 (Suppl):S138, 1986.
Jackson KE: Postthoracotomy pain syndromes. In Gravlee GP, Rauck RI (eds): Pain Management in Cardiothoracic Surgery. Philadelphia, JB Lippincott, 1993.
Kalso E, Perttunen K, Kaasinen S: Pain after thoracic surgery. Acta Anaesthesiol Scand 36:96, 1992.
Kanner RM, Martin N, Foley KM: Nature and incidence of post-thoracotomy pain (Abstract). Proc Am Soc Clin Oncol 2:152, 1982.
Kirvela O, Antila M: Thoracic paravertebral block in chronic post-operative pain. Reg Anesth 17:348, 1992.
Lemmer J, Gromez MN, Symreng T et al: Limited lateral thoracotomy improved postoperative pulmonary function. Arch Surg 125:873, 1990.
Lloyd JW, Barnard JDW, Glynn CJ: Cryoanalgesia, a new approach to pain relief. Lancet 2:932, 1976.
Loan WB, Morrison TD: The incidence and severity of postoperative pain. Br J Anaesth 39:695, 1967.
Melzack R, Loeber JD: Phantom body pain in paraplegics: Evidence for a central pattern generating mechanism for pain. Pain 4:195, 1978.
Orr JA, Keeman DJ, Dundee NN: Improved pain relief after thoracotomy: Use of cryopcrobe and morphine infusion. BMJ 283:945, 1981.
Ramamurthy S: Thoracic and low back pain. In Raj P (ed): Practical Management of Pain. Chicago, Year Book Medical Publishers, 1986, p 464.
Roxburgh JC, Markland CG, Ross BA, Kerr WF: Role of cryanalgesia in the control of pain after thoracotomy. Thorax 42:292, 1987.
Sabanathan S, Richardson T, Mearns AJ: Management of pain in thoracic surgery. Br J Hosp Med 50:114, 1993.
Sutton BA: Post-operative management and the provision of pain relief. In Gothard JWW (ed): Anaesthesia for Thoracic Surgery. Oxford, England, Blackwell Scientific Publications, 1993, p 122.

Late Physiologic Complications

Adams HD, Junod FL, Aberdeen E, Johnson J: Severe airway obstruction caused by mediastinal displacement after right pneumonectomy in a child: Case report. J Thorac Cardiovasc Surg 63:534, 1972.
Berend N, Woolcock AJ, Marlin GE: Effects of lobectomy on lung function. Thorax 35:145, 1980.
Birath G, Crafoord G, Rudstron P: Pulmonary function after pneumonectomy and lobectomy. J Thorac Surg 16:492, 1947.
Boushy SF, Billig DM, North LB, Helgason AH: Clinical course related to pre-operative and post-operative pulmonary function in patients with bronchogenic carcinoma. Chest 59:383, 1971.

Burrows B, Harrison RW, Adams WE et al: The post-pneumonectomy state. Clinical and physiologic observations in thirty-six cases. Am J Med 28:281, 1960.

De Graff AC, Taylor HF, Ord JW et al: Exercise limitation following extensive pulmonary resection. J Clin Invest 44:1514, 1965.

Gorlin R, Knowles JH, Storey FS: Effects of thoracotomy on pulmonary function. J Thorac Surg 34:242, 1957.

Harrison RN, Adams WE, Long ET et al: The clinical significance of cor pulmonale in the reduction of cardiopulmonary reserve following extensive pulmonary resection. J Thorac Surg 36:352, 1958.

Jansen JP, de la Rivière AB, Carpentier-Alting MP et al: Post-pneumonectomy syndrome in adulthood. Surgical correction using an expandable prosthesis. Chest 101:11, 1992.

Johnson J, Kirby CK, Lazatin CS, Cooke JA: The clinical use of a prosthesis to prevent overdistention of the remaining lung following pneumonectomy. J Thorac Surg 18:164, 1949.

Jones JJ, Robinson JL, Meyer BW, Motley HL: Primary carcinoma of the lung. A follow-up study including pulmonary function studies of long-term survivors. J Thorac Cardiovasc Surg 39:144, 1960.

Longaire JJ, Johansmann R: An experimental study of the fate of the remaining lung following total pneumonectomy. J Thorac Surg 10:131, 1940.

Mossberg B, Bjök VO, Holmgren A: Working capacity and cardiopulmonary function after extensive lung resections. Scand J Thorac Cardiovasc Surg 10:247, 1976.

Pelletier C, Lapointe L, Leblanc P: Effects of lung resection on pulmonary function and exercise capacity. Thorax 45:497, 1990.

Phillips FJ, Adams WE, Hrdina LS: Physiologic adjustment in sublethal reduction of lung capacity in dogs. Surgery 9:25, 1941.

Powell RW, Luck SR, Raffensperger JG: Pneumonectomy in infants and children: The use of a prosthesis to prevent mediastinal shift and its complications. J Pediatr Surg 14:231, 1979.

Quillin SP, Shakleford GD: Post-pneumonectomy syndrome after left lung resection. Radiology 179:100, 1991.

Rasch DK, Grover FL, Schnapf BM: Right pneumonectomy syndrome in infancy treated with an expandable prosthesis. Ann Thorac Surg 50:127, 1990.

Riveron FA, Adams C, Lewis JW et al: Silastic prosthesis plombage for right post-pneumonectomy syndrome. Ann Thorac Surg 50:465, 1990.

Shepard JA, Grillo HC, McLoud TC et al: Right pneumonectomy syndrome: Radiologic findings and CT correlation. Radiology 161:661, 1986.

Szarnicki R, Maurseth K, de Leval M, Stark J: Tracheal compression by the aortic arch following right pneumonectomy in infancy. Ann Thorac Surg 25:231, 1978.

Van Mieghem W, Demedts M: Cardiopulmonary function after lobectomy or pneumonectomy for pulmonary neoplasm. Respir Med 83:199, 1989.

Vejlsted H, Halkier E: Pre- and post-operative lung function after pulmonary resection. Scand J Thorac Cardiovasc Surg 16:87, 1982.

Wasserman K, Jamplis RW, Lash H et al: Post-pneumonectomy syndrome: Surgical correction using Silastic implants. Chest 75:78, 1979.

Larynx and Upper Airway

CHAPTER 12

Anatomy, Physiology, and Embryology

ANATOMY, PHYSIOLOGY, AND EMBRYOLOGY OF THE LARYNX

Jonathan C. Irish
Patrick J. Gullane

PHYSIOLOGY

The larynx plays an important role in the production of speech and sound as well as a protector of the airway during swallowing. In their role as a digestive tract conduit, the structures cranial to the cricopharyngeus muscle play a role in three of the four phases of the normal swallow. The first two phases of swallowing, the oral and oral preparatory phases, are voluntary, whereas the third and fourth phases, the pharyngeal and esophageal phases, are involuntary (Mandelstam and Lieber, 1970). During the involuntary phase of swallowing, coordinated activity between the swallowing center, mediated in the reticular formation of the brain stem, and the adjacent respiratory center is critical for respiration to cease during the initiation of the swallow (Miller, 1972). In addition to the brief cessation of respiration and the coordinated neuromuscular activity of the pharyngoesophageal complex for propulsion of the food bolus, airway protection during the swallow is also performed by the sphincteric actions of the larynx. Laryngeal closure is achieved when the epiglottis covers the laryngeal introitus, the ventricular folds (false vocal folds) close, and the true vocal folds adduct (Ardran and Kemp, 1967).

During the normal swallow, the larynx is elevated and moves anteriorly under the base of the tongue, allowing the passive closure of the epiglottis over the laryngeal aperture (Fink and Demarest, 1978). Anterior movement of the larynx away from the esophagus also "stretches" the cricopharyngeus muscle, allowing the food bolus to pass through the upper esophageal sphincter.

Speech production is an obvious function of the larynx. The current theory of speech production, the myoelastic theory, suggests that the larynx is pivotal (Van den Berg, 1958). This theory recognizes that the larynx is a pliable, elastic, muscular organ, with the ability to generate closure with vocal cord adduction and the ability to finely tune speech by alteration of the mass and tension of the vocal folds. The ability to generate glottic closure enables subglottic pressure to build up until it is greater than the glottic closing pressure, allowing escape of air. This periodic opening and closing of the glottis causes compression and rarefaction of air, resulting in the physical phenomenon of sound. The frequency of vocal cord opening corresponds to the frequency of the sound produced. Fine tuning of the sound is secondary to finer alterations in the intrinsic muscles of the larynx, allowing variation of vocal-fold mass (greater mass, lower frequency) and vocal-fold tension (increased tension, higher frequency). Vocal-cord pathology such as a polyp results in a "raspy" voice often lower in frequency (secondary to increased mass) and diplophonic in quality.

Effort-induced approximation of the false and true vocal folds is critical for producing the "tussive squeeze" and "bechic blast" that are necessary for normal cough production (Adrian et al, 1953). This function also allows performance of Valsalva maneuvers, which are essential for lifting heavy objects and for normal defecation. Failure to generate effort-induced approximation of the glottis, as in recurrent laryngeal-nerve paralysis, can result in aspiration, with the situation further aggravated by the inability of the patient to produce an effective cough, often resulting in pneumonia. Medialization of the paralyzed cord by Teflon augmentation or medialization thyroplasty can restore this ability.

EMBRYOLOGY

At approximately the 26th day of embryonic development, the endodermally lined rudiment of the respiratory tree develops as the median laryngotracheal groove (Fig. 12–1*A*). This groove develops in the caudal end of the ventral wall of the pharynx, and over the course of the fourth week of development, it deepens and elongates to form a diverticulum. The edges of the tube fuse, forming a septum, and thus providing a functional and anatomic separation of the pharyngoesophageal complex from the laryngotracheal complex. The fusion commences caudally and extends cranially, excluding the slitlike opening into the pharynx. Failure of fusion during this period of embryonic development may result in a posterior laryngeal cleft, while failure of caudal septal fusion is the presumed etiologic basis of a congenital tracheoesophageal fistula. The endodermally lined tube gives rise to the mucosal epithelium and glandular elements of the larynx, trachea, and bronchi, and the splanchnic mesenchyme, into which the diverticulum grows, gives rise to the supporting connective tissue, cartilage, nonstriated muscle, and vasculature of the laryngotracheal complex.

In the fourth week of development, the primitive larynx is bounded cranially by the hypobranchial eminence (formed by the third and fourth arches) and bounded laterally by the folds of the sixth branchial arch. By the sixth week of embryonic development, mesenchymal proliferation occurs on both sides of the laryngotracheal groove, forming the arytenoid swellings (see Fig. 12–1*B*). With this proliferation, the laryngeal aperture changes from a vertical slit or cleft shape to a T shape. During the second month of prenatal development, the arytenoid swelling differentiates into the arytenoid and corniculate cartilages as derivatives of the sixth branchial arch. At this time, the aryepiglottic folds develop, joining the arytenoids to the epiglottis, which has developed from the hypobranchial eminence (see Fig. 12–1*C*). During this time, the laryngotracheal lumen is obstructed by an epithelial plug and by mucosa-mucosa adherence, which undergoes recanalization during the third month of prenatal life. Failure of recanalization has been proposed as an etiology of congenital glottic and subglottic stenosis.

The thyroid cartilage develops from the fourth branchial arch with the fusion of two lateral plates, each with two chondrification centers. The cricoid cartilage and tracheal cartilages develop from the sixth branchial arch during the sixth week of embryologic development.

The development of each branchial arch is accompanied by that of an accompanying arch nerve and artery. The artery from the third arch ultimately forms the proximal part of the common carotid artery and the internal carotid artery. The superior laryngeal nerve and subclavian artery are the nerve and artery of the fourth arch, and the recurrent laryngeal nerve and ligamentum arteriosum are the neurovascular structures of the sixth branchial arch.

DESCRIPTIVE ANATOMY

The larynx in men is opposite the third to sixth cervical vertebrae, whereas in women and children it lies in a more cranial position. Although there is little difference in the size of the laryngeal aperture between boys and girls before puberty, after puberty the anteroposterior diameter of the larynx increases dramatically in males to 36 mm compared with 26 mm in females.

Laryngeal Cartilages

The rigid framework of the larynx is provided by nine cartilages (Fig. 12–2). The thyroid, cricoid, and epiglottic cartilages are unpaired, and the arytenoid, corniculate, and cuneiform cartilages are paired.

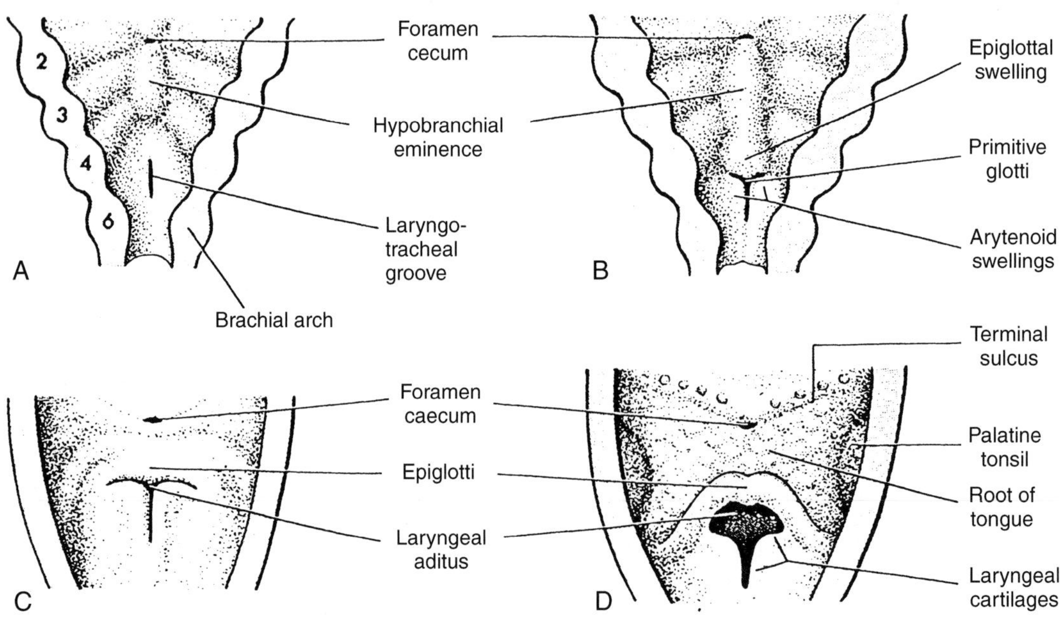

FIGURE 12–1 ■ Successive stages of development of the larynx at *A*, 4 weeks; *B*, at 5 weeks; *C*, at 6 weeks; and *D*, at 10 weeks. (From Moore K: The Developing Human, 2nd ed. Philadelphia, WB Saunders, 1977.)

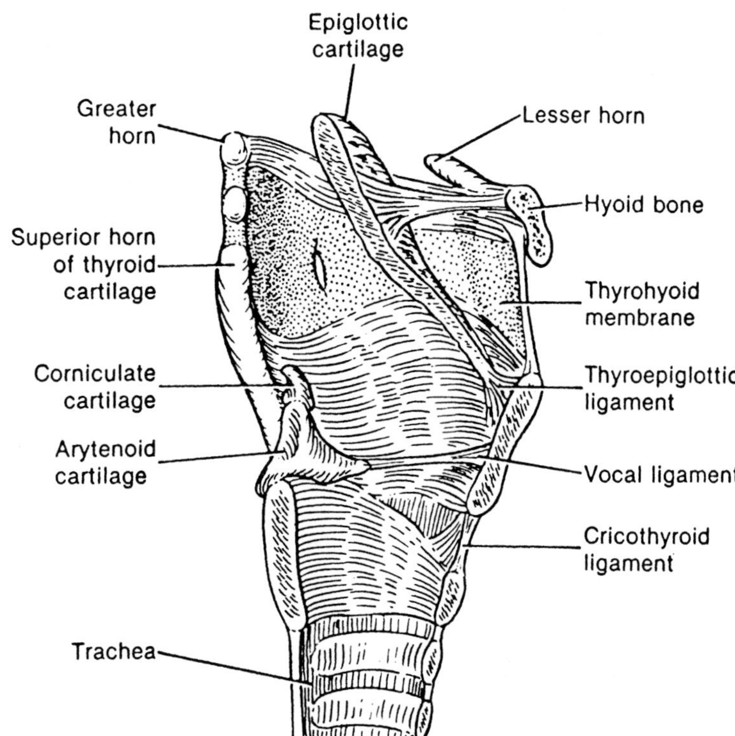

FIGURE 12–2 ■ The laryngeal bones and cartilages in sagittal section. (From Cummings C et al [eds]: Otolaryngology, Head and Neck Surgery. St. Louis, CV Mosby, 1986.)

Thyroid Cartilage

The longest and largest of the laryngeal cartilages is the thyroid cartilage, which consists of two laminae fusing in the midline with a 90-degree angle in men and a 120-degree angle in women. From the posterior border of the thyroid cartilage, two slender processes extend superiorly and inferiorly, forming the superior and inferior cornua, respectively. A facet on the medial surface of the inferior cornu marks the cricothyroid joint and allows the thyroid cartilage to tilt or glide anteriorly or posteriorly on the cricoid cartilage. The superior border of the thyroid cartilage is attached to the hyoid bone by the thyrohyoid membrane. The inferior attachment to the cricoid is provided by the cricothyroid membrane, which attaches to the inner aspect of the medial portion of the inferior border of the thyroid cartilage. The external surface of the thyroid laminae is marked by an oblique line curving downward and forward from the superior cornu. This line marks the attachment for the inferior constrictor muscle of the pharynx and for the sternothyroid and thyrohyoid muscles.

Cricoid Cartilage

The signet ring–shaped cricoid cartilage is the only complete cartilaginous ring in the air passage. The posterior lamina is deep and thick, and the anterior arch is narrow. The cricoid is attached to the thyroid cartilage by the cricothyroid ligament. At the junction of the lamina and the arch is a facet that articulates with the inferior cornu of the thyroid. The other important joints of the cricoid are the paired cricoarytenoid joints, which are synovial joints that allow rotation and glide of the arytenoids on the sloping shoulders of the cricoid lamina. As with any synovial joint, arthritic processes such as rheumatoid arthritis may cause inflammation and ultimately ankylosis of the cricoarytenoid joint.

Arytenoid Cartilages

The paired arytenoid cartilages are shaped like irregular, three-sided pyramids. The three points of the pyramid are the superiorly projecting apex, the anteriorly projecting vocal process attaching to the vocal ligament, and the laterally projecting muscular process to which the lateral and posterior cricoarytenoid muscles attach. The base of the arytenoid is concave, providing an articulating relationship with the gently sloping shoulders of the cricoid lamina.

Corniculate and Cuneiform Cartilages

The corniculate cartilages are conical nodules of elastic fibrocartilage attached to the apices of the arytenoid cartilages. The cuneiform cartilages are elongated pieces of fibrocartilage lying in the aryepiglottic folds. The function of these small cartilages is not clear, but they may provide increased structure and prevent collapse of the aryepiglottic folds into the laryngeal inlet.

Epiglottis

The epiglottis is a thin sheet of elastic fibrocartilage shaped like a leaf. In neonates and infants, the epiglottis is omega-shaped, forming a long, floppy, deeply grooved structure, while in adults it has a gradually curving semi-elliptical shape. The epiglottis is attached to the thyroid cartilage anteriorly by the thyroepiglottic ligament. The epiglottis forms the anterior wall of the laryngeal inlet, and laterally its margins are continuous with the aryepiglottic folds forming the lateral walls of the inlet. Anteriorly, the epiglottis is attached to the hyoid bone by the hyoepiglottic ligament, thereby dividing the epiglottis into an infrahyoid and a suprahyoid segment. The mucous membrane covering the epiglottis is continuous with that of the posterior tongue. Three folds of mucous membrane are reflected onto the pharyngeal part of the tongue and onto the lateral walls of the pharynx, forming a median glossoepiglottic fold and two lateral glossoepiglottic folds. Between each of the lateral folds and the median fold are depressions called the epiglottic valleculae.

The corniculate, cuneiform, and arytenoid apices are composed of elastic fibrocartilage with little tendency to calcify. The thyroid, cricoid, and the greatest part of the arytenoid cartilages are composed of hyaline cartilage and can begin calcification in early adulthood, which can mimic the appearance of a foreign body on lateral soft tissue radiographs.

Ligaments

The extrinsic ligaments of the larynx, including the thyrohyoid ligament, the cricotracheal ligament, and the hyoepiglottic ligament were previously discussed. The intrinsic ligaments are divided into two major groups by the laryngeal vestibule. Superior to the vestibule is the quadrangular membrane, the free inferior margins of which constitute the ventricular ligament, which is covered by mucous membrane forming the false cords or vestibular folds.

The second network of ligaments is positioned inferior to the laryngeal ventricle and consists of the vocal ligament and conus elasticus. The vocal ligament runs anteriorly from the junction of the laminae of the thyroid cartilage to its posterior attachment with the vocal processes of the arytenoid. The vocal ligament forms the superior free edge of the conus elasticus. The conus spreads like a draped tent from the vocal ligament to its attachment to the cricoid cartilage. The vocal ligament forms the fibrous core of the true vocal cord. The ligament and fibrous layers of the larynx can play critical roles as barriers in the prevention of tumor spread. Breach of tumor across these anatomic barriers into the paraglottic and pre-epiglottic spaces portends poor patient outcome and survival.

Interior of the Larynx

The cavity of the larynx extends from the pharynx at the laryngeal inlet called the rima glottis to the trachea beginning at the lower border of the cricoid cartilage. The larynx is divided into three parts by the vestibular and vocal folds. Above the vestibular folds, the cavity of the larynx is called the vestibule. Between the vestibular and vocal folds lies the ventricle, which arises through a narrow horizontal slit laterally. Extending superiorly from the anterior part of the ventricle is a pouchlike structure called the saccule, which ascends between the ventricular folds and the inner surface of the thyroid cartilage (Fig. 12–3).

The high density of mucous glands in the ventricle and saccule has led to the belief that they play a particularly important role in lubrication of the larynx and therefore are important in voice production. The ventricle is separated from the subglottis by the vocal folds, which are two folds of mucous membrane that closely adhere to the underlying vocal ligaments, consisting of the free, upper, thickened margins of the conus elasticus. Lateral to the vocal ligament lies the vocalis muscle, which by contraction and stretching plays an integral role in the determination of voice quality. The subglottic space extends from the vocal folds to the lower border of the cricoid cartilage, where the trachea begins.

Laryngeal Musculature

The muscles of the larynx are divided into intrinsic and extrinsic groups.

Extrinsic Musculature

The extrinsic muscles move the larynx as a whole and originate outside the larynx. These muscles are further subdivided into depressors of the larynx (omohyoid, sternohyoid, and sternothyroid) and elevators of the larynx

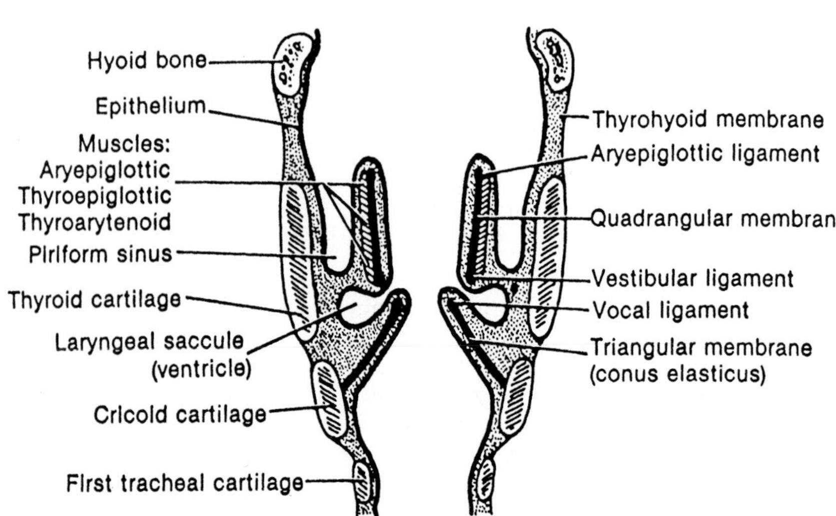

FIGURE 12–3 ■ Schematic drawing of a coronal section of the larynx demonstrating the supporting ligaments and membranes. (From Cummings C et al [eds]: Otolaryngology, Head and Neck Surgery. St. Louis, CV Mosby, 1986.)

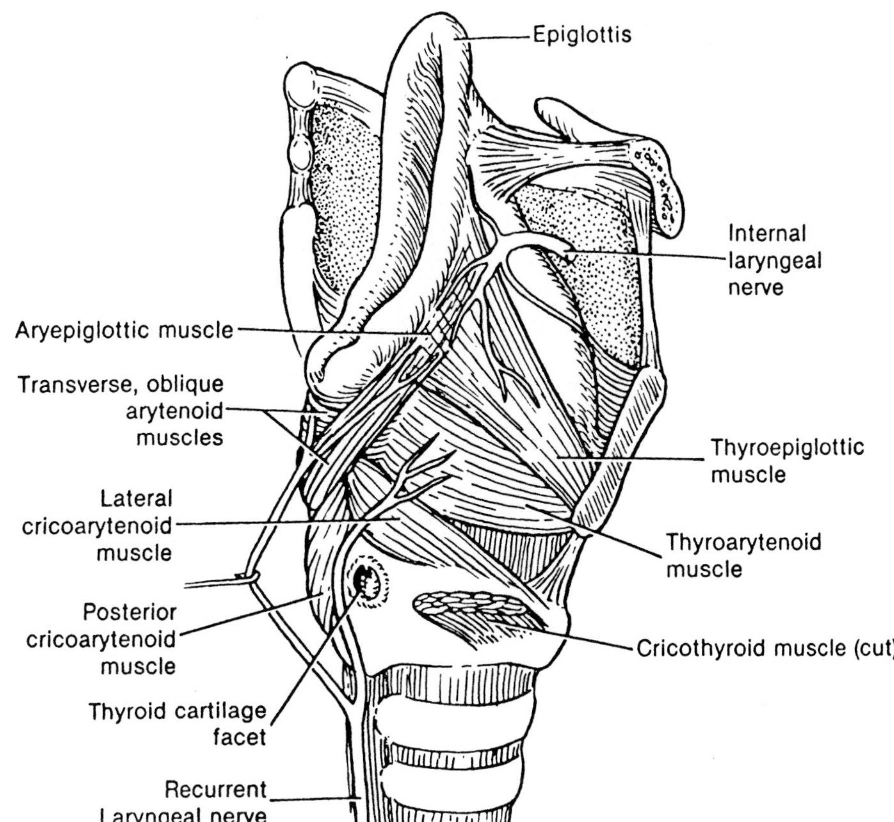

FIGURE 12–4 ■ Lateral view of laryngeal muscles and nerves. (From Cummings C et al [eds]: Otolaryngology, Head and Neck Surgery. St. Louis, CV Mosby, 1986.)

(stylohyoid, digastric, mylohyoid, geniohyoid, stylopharyngeus, and thyrohyoid). Except for the thyrohyoid muscle, which elevates the larynx but draws the hyoid and thyroid cartilages together, all the elevators elevate both the hyoid and the larynx as a unit.

Intrinsic Musculature

The intrinsic muscles (Fig. 12–4) are concerned with movements of the laryngeal parts and have both their origin and insertion within the larynx. The prime function of these muscles is to make alterations in vocal cord length and tension and to change the size and shape of the rima glottis. The intrinsic muscles of the larynx are best subdivided into three groups.

The first group of muscles consists of those that open and close the glottis. The posterior cricoarytenoid muscles are the primary abductors of the vocal cords, and the lateral cricoarytenoid muscles are the primary adductors of the vocal cords. The interarytenoid muscles include the transverse and the oblique arytenoid muscles, both of which act as adductors of the vocal cords by approximation of the arytenoids. Some of the fibers of the oblique arytenoid muscle continue as the aryepiglottic muscle, which ensures that the epiglottis is drawn inferiorly simultaneously with vocal-cord adduction. This action of laryngeal inlet closure plays an important role in the normal swallow.

The second group of intrinsic laryngeal muscles comprises those that control the tension of the vocal ligaments. The main tensor of the vocal folds is the cricothyroid muscle. This muscle arises on the cricoid cartilage and inserts into the anterior aspect of the inferior margins of the thyroid cartilage. Therefore, contraction of this muscle tilts the thyroid cartilage anteriorly on the cricoid, increasing the distance between the thyroid and the arytenoid cartilages, thus elongating the vocal ligaments and increasing vocal pitch. The main relaxors of the vocal folds are the thyroarytenoid muscles, which arise from the posterior surface of the thyroid cartilage and insert on the anterolateral surfaces of the arytenoid cartilages. The vocalis muscle is part of the thyroarytenoid muscle.

The final group of intrinsic muscles are those whose primary function is to alter the shape of the laryngeal inlet. The thyroepiglottic muscle is formed from the superior fibers of the thyroarytenoid muscles and functions to widen the laryngeal inlet. The aryepiglottic muscle is formed from fibers of the oblique arytenoid muscles and closes the inlet.

Blood Supply

The blood supply of the larynx is derived from the superior thyroid artery through its superior laryngeal and cricothyroid branches and from the inferior thyroid artery through its inferior laryngeal branch (Fig. 12–5).

The superior thyroid artery, which arises from the external carotid artery and passes deep to the thyrohyoid muscle, piercing the thyrohyoid membrane with the internal branch of the superior laryngeal nerve, supplies the internal surface of the larynx. The inferior thyroid artery arises from the thyrocervical trunk of the first part of the subclavian artery and gives rise to the inferior

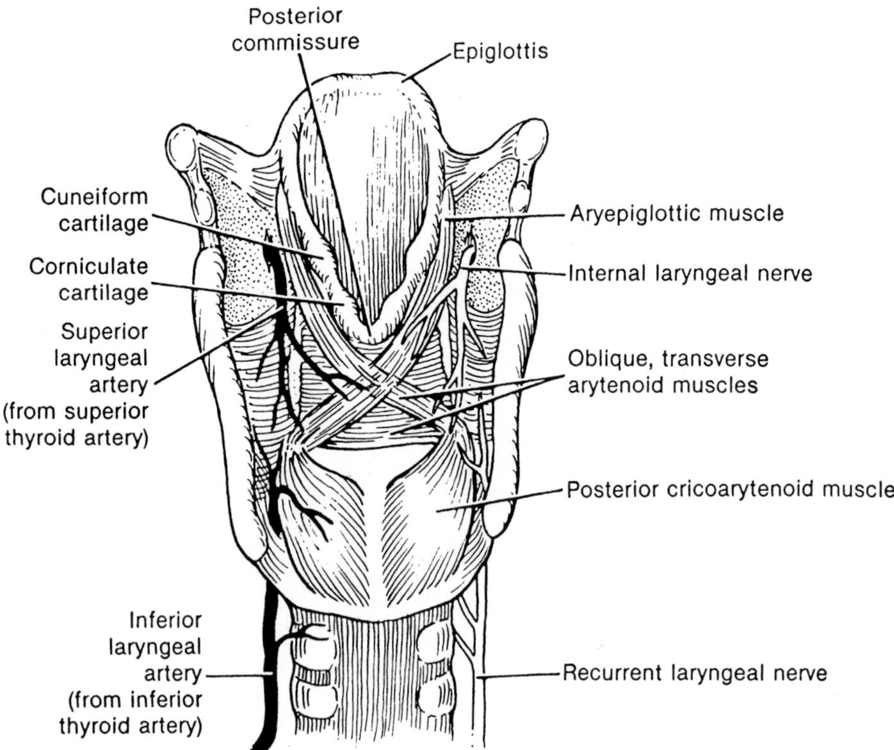

FIGURE 12–5 ■ Posterior view of the larynx demonstrating intrinsic muscles, nerves, and vascular supply. (From Cummings C et al [eds]: Otolaryngology, Head and Neck Surgery. St. Louis, CV Mosby, 1986.)

laryngeal branch at the level of the lower border of the thyroid gland. The artery, which enters the larynx and runs along with the recurrent laryngeal nerve beneath the lower border of the inferior constrictor, supplies the inferior internal larynx.

The veins leaving the larynx accompany the arteries, with the superior vessels entering the internal jugular vein by way of the superior thyroid vein and the inferior veins draining into the brachiocephalic vein through the inferior thyroid vein. Additional venous drainage is through the middle thyroid vein into the internal jugular vein.

Lymphatics

Lymphatic drainage of the larynx occurs by way of two main pedicles. Superior to the vocal folds, the lymphatic circulation accompanies the superior laryngeal artery through the thyrohyoid membrane. The superior pedicle ultimately drains into the superior deep cervical lymph nodes. Inferior to the vocal folds, the lymphatics drain to the inferior deep cervical lymph nodes via the prelaryngeal, pretracheal, and paratracheal lymph nodes.

Innervation

The innervation of the larynx is provided by the vagus nerve by way of the superior and recurrent laryngeal branches (see Fig. 12–5). The motor innervation arises within the nucleus ambiguus, while the parasympathetic supply arises from the dorsal motor nucleus of the vagus (Yoshida et al, 1982).

The superior laryngeal nerve divides within the carotid sheath into two terminal branches, the internal laryngeal nerve (sensory and autonomic) and the external laryngeal nerve (motor). The internal laryngeal nerve pierces the thyrohyoid membrane with the superior laryngeal artery, supplying sensation (including stretch receptor and proprioceptive information) to the larynx superior to the vocal folds. The external laryngeal nerve accompanies the superior thyroid artery descending posterior to the sternothyroid muscle, supplying motor innervation to the cricothyroid muscle.

The recurrent laryngeal nerve on the right loops under the right subclavian artery and ascends in the tracheoesophageal groove. On the left, the nerve passes under the aortic arch and ligamentum arteriosum to reach the tracheoesophageal groove. On both sides, the nerve accompanies the laryngeal branch of the inferior thyroid artery and passes deep to the inferior constrictor muscle behind the cricothyroid joint. The motor supply innervates all the intrinsic laryngeal musculature except the cricothyroid muscle, while the sensory branch supplies the laryngeal mucosa inferior to the vocal folds.

The extrinsic muscles of the larynx receive their motor innervation from the ansa cervicalis derived from cervical roots C1, C2, and C3.

■ *KEY REFERENCES*

Basmajian JV: Grant's Method of Anatomy, 10th ed. Baltimore, Williams & Wilkins, 1980.

A traditional text, but remains highly regarded as concise, with simple, easily reproducible line drawings.

Fink BR, Demarest RI: Laryngeal Biomechanics. Cambridge, MA, Cambridge University Press, 1978.

Good, detailed review of the physiologic detail of laryngeal function.

Hollinshead WH: Anatomy for Surgeons: The Head and Neck, 2nd ed. Hagerstown, MD, Harper & Row, 1968.

Clinically applied anatomy of the head and neck, with excellent accompanying text.

Moore KL: The Developing Human: Clinically Oriented Embryology, 3rd ed. Philadelphia, WB Saunders, 1982.

Development of the larynx, esophagus, and related structures of the upper aerodigestive tract is fully described and illustrated with clinical relevance.

REFERENCES

Adrian GM, Kemp FH, Manen L: Closure of the larynx. Br J Radiol 26:497, 1953.

Ardran J, Kemp F: The mechanism of the larynx. II. The epiglottis and closure of the larynx. Br J Radiol 40:372, 1967.

Graney DO: Larynx/hypopharynx anatomy. In Cummings C et al (eds): Otolaryngology: Head and Neck Surgery. St. Louis, CV Mosby, 1986.

Mandelstam P, Lieber A: Cineradiographic evaluation of the esophagus in normal adults. Gastroenterology 58:32, 1970.

Miller A: Characteristics of the swallowing reflex, induced by peripheral nerve and brain stem stimulation. Exp Neurol 34:210, 1972.

Van den Berg J: Myoelastic-aerodynamic theory of voice production. J Speech Hear Res 1:227, 1958.

Yoshida Y, Miyazaki T, Hirano M et al: Arrangement of motoneurons innervating the intrinsic laryngeal muscles of cats as demonstrated by horseradish peroxidase. Acta Otolaryngol (Stockh) 94:329, 1982.

ANATOMY, PHYSIOLOGY, AND EMBRYOLOGY OF THE UPPER AIRWAY

R. J. Cusimano
F. Griffith Pearson

EMBRYOLOGY

Trachea

The development of the respiratory system begins at 4 weeks of gestation with the development of an endodermal bud growing into the splanchnic mesenchyme. The endodermal components become the epithelium and glands, while the mesenchyme becomes cartilage, connective tissue, and muscular components (Moore, 1977; Salassa et al, 1977). Growth occurs in both length and circumference. Longitudinal growth occurs first by the laying down of new cellular elements followed by a lengthening of the cartilage, intervening connective tissue, and muscle. Circumferential growth of the trachea is uniform, unlike the growth and lengthening of bones, which grow at each end. Burrington (1978) found, in examinations of both animal and human material, that increases in the circumference of the trachea occur by the simultaneous process of uniform growth of the convex side of the trachea and remodeling by resorption along the concave surface. In this manner, the whole cartilage grows as a unit. Interestingly, while the growth at each segment is uniform, the different levels grow to different extents so that the trachea is funnel shaped, being larger at the larynx than at the carina (Wailoo and Emery, 1982). This funnel shape is especially evident in the antenatal period and in the youngest babies and children. Because of the uniform, almost radial growth along the surface of each tracheal ring, incisions made in a vertical direction can be expected to have little influence on the final cross-sectional area of a growing trachea.

Tracheal Glands

Tracheal glands develop from the endodermal layer of the developing embryo, development generally occurring after that of the cartilage, between 10 and 25 weeks' gestation. Thereafter, there is no further increase in the number of new glands (Reid, 1976). Glandular development after this stage occurs by an increase in the acinar components, thus increasing the mass but not the number of glands. After birth, the density of glands gradually decreases. Thus, while there are 7.3 glands per square millimeter at birth, by 8 years of age the density has decreased to 2.3. The adult trachea generally contains less than one gland per square millimeter (Tos, 1970).

Cilia

The cilia of the trachea develop within the first half of gestation, and by 24 weeks their development is complete (Galliard et al, 1989). There is constant differentiation from columnar undifferentiated epithelium through primitive ciliated cells to the final form.

Blood Supply

During prenatal life, the blood supply of the trachea is segmental. Thus, multiple pairs of arteries arise in segmental fashion from the aorta to supply both trachea and esophagus. With time, the segmental distribution disappears, and branches that originate from the thyroid artery and aorta (via bronchial vessels) become the major sources of blood supply (Reid, 1976).

ANATOMY

Trachea

Length

The trachea is a cartilaginous and membranous tube that connects the larynx with the bronchi. It is continuous with the larynx at the level of the cricoid cartilage. The upper trachea is normally found at the level of the sixth or seventh cervical vertebra, and the lower end lies at the fourth or fifth thoracic vertebra. On full inspiration, the distal end of the trachea may descend to the level of the sixth vertebra. In the adult resting state, the total length of the trachea is 10 to 11 cm, with approximately 5 cm lying superior to the suprasternal notch.

The noncartilaginous portions of the trachea between rings are elastic and allow lengthening or shortening of the trachea during respiration (or neck flexion or extension). Thoracic surgeons use this knowledge in the management of tracheal resections. It is desirable to minimize anastomotic tension by maintaining neck flexion after segmental tracheal resections. Surgeons commonly suture the chin to the skin of the manubrium to prevent neck extension during the first postoperative week.

Projected anteriorly, the tracheal bifurcation, or carina, lies at the level of the manubriosternal junction, or the second inner end of the costal cartilage. In children, the carina lies at the level of the third costal cartilage (Nagaishi, 1972; Williams and Warwick, 1981). The trachea runs in the median plane, and the carina is usually slightly to the right of the midline.

Shape

The cross-sectional shape of the trachea is determined by the horseshoe-shaped cartilage anteriorly and the membranous portion posteriorly. The most common cross-sectional configuration of the trachea is elliptical (larger transverse than anteroposterior diameter, 33% of cases). A C shape (equal transverse and anteroposterior diameters) is found in 26% of cases, and the U-shaped trachea accounts for 21%. A triangular, cross-sectional shape occurs in less than 10% of the population, and a circular variant accounts for less than 1% of cases (Meta and Myat, 1984). Asymmetric shapes are found, and males and females differ not only in the size of the tracheas but also in the most common shape. Meta and Myat reported that the U-shaped trachea was the most common variant in adult men, and an elliptical shape was most common in adult women. Tracheal shape also changes as the individual grows and during the different phases of a respiratory cycle (Kawakami et al, 1991).

The adult trachea has an almost constant dimension for its entire length, but the pediatric trachea does not. Wailoo and Emery (1982) studied humans from 28 weeks of gestation to 4 years of age and found that the trachea was a funnel-shaped structure that is larger at the larynx than at the carina. This was most pronounced in the prenatal and neonatal stages. With growth, the difference in size between larynx and carina decreased until it was negligible, creating a cylindrical rather than a funnel-shaped trachea. There is generally no difference between the dimensions in young children; however, after the age of 14, the size of the female trachea tends to remain constant, and the male trachea continues to enlarge (but not lengthen), even after somatic growth ceases (Griscom and Wohl, 1986).

Tracheal Rings

There are between 16 and 20 horseshoe-shaped tracheal rings, which are composed of hyaline cartilage. There is variation in size and shape, and the average ring in an adult is approximately 4 mm wide and 1 mm thick. Some rings are fused over variable circumferential distances, and there is a great variability among individuals in this respect. Although the cartilaginous rings are resilient and compliant in childhood and early adulthood, they tend to calcify with age. Calcification may occur earlier when certain lung diseases are present. This is thought to occur through the chelation of calcium by the acid glycoprotein of the cartilage (Reid, 1976). Each cartilage is enveloped by perichondrium, which is continuous with a sheet of dense connective tissue made up primarily of collagen with some elastin. The collagen and elastin are diagonally apposed, allowing both for changes in diameter of the airway and for some elastic recoil when the distending stress is removed. The connective tissue is continuous with the posterior or membranous trachea. This gradual calcification and resultant loss of compliance with age has clinical implications: blunt trauma may be better tolerated by the young patient because of higher compliance compared with the elderly. During tracheal resections, mobilization of a compliant trachea may allow a greater extent of resection without the anastomotic tension that is possible in the elderly patient with a rigid, calcified upper airway.

Membranous Trachea

The membranous trachea consists of an enveloping fibrous sheath, smooth muscle, epithelium, and glands. The smooth muscle component consists mostly of transverse fibers with some vertical elements external to the transverse layer. The cartilaginous part of the trachea also contains small amounts of muscle (Håkansson et al, 1976). It is the soft, distensible, membranous trachea that allows most of the moment-to-moment change in size of the tracheal lumen.

Glands

The luminal surface of the trachea consists of pseudostratified, columnar cells, some goblet cells, and many glandular openings. The glands are situated in the membranous trachea and in the intercartilaginous components of the cartilaginous trachea. They are layered in the submucosa, with ducts extending through the mucosa and opening into the lumen. Glands are distributed in three layers: the first layer lies immediately below the mucosa; deep to this lies the transverse muscle layer, which contains the greatest concentration of glands; and a third deep layer lies on the fibrous sheath with a flattened, platelike distribution. External to the fibrous sheath and perichondrium of the trachea is an envelope of fascia, which blends with the surrounding muscle.

External to the enveloping fascia there is no glandular tissue.

Blood Supply

Macroscopic. The blood supplies of the trachea and esophagus are similar and closely linked. That of the trachea is segmental prenatally; however, there are primarily two sources after birth. The cervical trachea receives its arterial blood supply from the inferior thyroid artery and its branches. There is a rich anastomotic connection between the ascending branches of the bronchial vessels and the descending branches of the inferior thyroid vessels. As their name implies, the bronchial vessels also supply the bronchi themselves. Figure 12–6 demonstrates the rich anastomotic network of the trachea and the major origins from the inferior thyroid and bronchial vessels.

Miura and Grillo (1966) studied the blood supply of the cervical trachea and found that the inferior thyroid artery gives rise to branches that not only serve the esophagus but also the trachea. They found that a variable number of vessels pass to the trachea on the way to the thyroid gland. Typically there are three parathyroid branches, with one of the three dominant, most commonly the inferior one. Occasionally, a vessel arises directly from the subclavian artery, usually on the right side. When this occurs, two rather than three prethyroid branches of the inferior thyroid artery are present. These branches, regardless of origin, anastomose with the bronchial vessels and also provide blood supply to the esophagus (Fig. 12–7). The superior thyroid artery has anastomotic connections with the inferior thyroid artery and thus supplies the trachea (and esophagus) only indirectly.

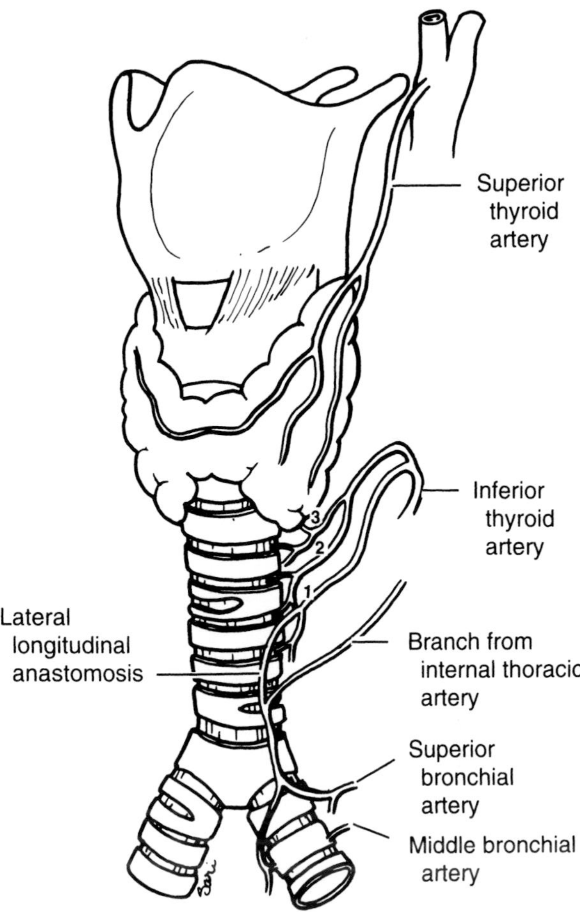

FIGURE 12–7 ■ Left anterior view of the blood supply of the trachea. A most important supply to the cervical trachea arises from the three branches of the inferior thyroid artery, one of which is usually dominant. There is an occasional branch derived from the subclavian artery. The superior thyroid artery only provides contributions through its anastomoses with the inferior thyroid artery. (From Salassa JR, Pearson BW, Payne WS: Gross and microscopical blood supply of the trachea. Ann Thorac Surg 24:100, 1977.)

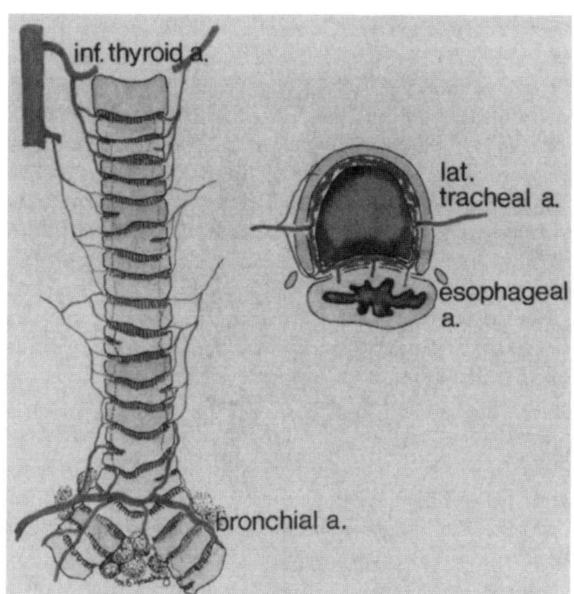

FIGURE 12–6 ■ The important components of the tracheal circulation. Substantial contributions are provided by the inferior thyroid vessels above and the bronchial vessels below. These vessels anastomose with one another and, along with additional contributions from the aorta and other great vessels, form a lateral arcade, which then supplies the rich submucosal plexus through vessels passing between the cartilages anterior to the tracheal esophageal grooves. These lateral tracheal vessels supply the trachea in segmental fashion.

From the work of Cauldwell and colleagues (1948) and Salassa and associates (1977), it is known that the bronchial vessels are also a major source of blood to the trachea. There may be some variation in the origin and number of bronchial vessels, both between species (McLaughlin, 1983) and between individuals, but the most common arrangement (40% of cases) is to have two left and one right bronchial vessel originating directly from the aorta. Approximately 50% of such bronchial arteries arise at the level of the sixth thoracic vertebra, whereas a smaller number (35%) arise at the level of the fifth vertebra. Occasionally there is only one left bronchial vessel (20% of cases), and occasionally there are two right vessels (20%). Two thirds of all right lungs are supplied by a single bronchial vessel, whereas only one third of all left lungs are singly supplied (Cauldwell et al, 1948).

The trachea is also supplied by branches that originate from the subclavian artery, the internal mammary artery, or the brachiocephalic (innominate) artery (Fig. 12–8). The bronchial vessels usually arise from the aorta (the right from the lateral or posterolateral part and the left from the anterior surface or the convex surface of the aortic arch), but they can and frequently do originate from a common trunk with an intercostal artery. This is found more commonly on the right side. More recently, Schreinemakers and colleagues (1990) and Couraud and associates (1992) studied the tracheal and bronchial vasculature in humans to better evaluate the role of the bronchial circulation in human lung transplantation. Their findings confirmed the observations of Cauldwell and associates and Salassa and colleagues. They also documented the importance of the right first intercostal artery, noting that many bronchial trunks arise from the *right* but not the left first intercostal artery. Cauldwell and co-workers (1948) found that 90% of the intercostobronchial arteries arose from the right first intercostal artery and only 6% arose from the left (Fig. 12–9). The esophagus is supplied by twigs from these vessels as they supply the trachea. A knowledge of the anatomy of the bronchial arteries has allowed some surgeons to incorporate a bronchial artery anastomosis into the lung transplant operation. There appears to be early improvement in the mucosal circulation of the donor airway and theoretical benefits for tracheal healing (Couraud et al, 1992; Daly et al, 1993; Laks et al, 1991).

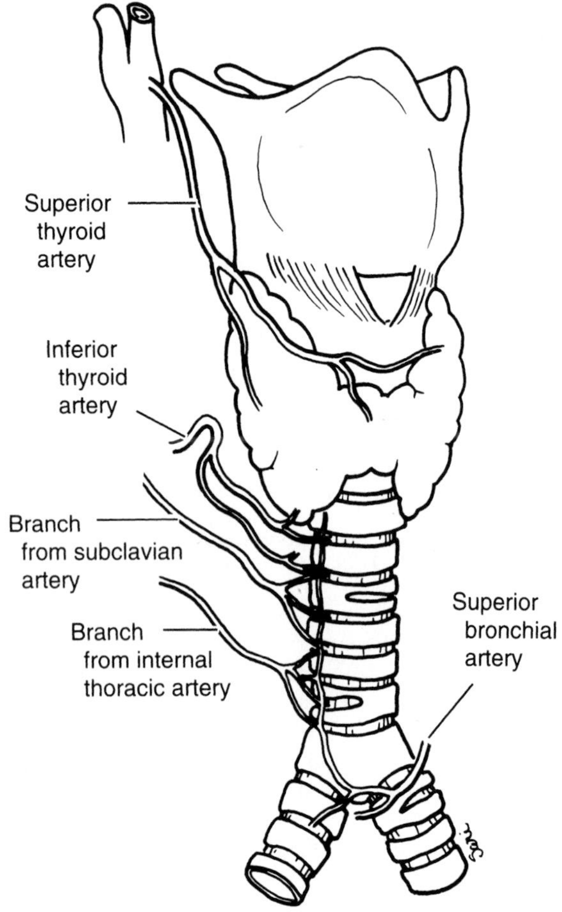

FIGURE 12–8 ■ Right anterior view of the tracheal blood supply, demonstrating alternate mechanisms of supply. In this diagram, arterial branches arise from the innominate artery, a supreme intercostal artery, and the internal thoracic or vertebral artery. Such vessels usually anastomose with the lateral longitudinal arcade, which is supplied inferiorly through the bronchial circulation originating directly from the aorta or from intercostal vessels. The first intercostal artery on the right side is commonly the most important contributor to the tracheal circulation. (From Salassa JR, Pearson BW, Payne WS: Gross and microscopical blood supply of the trachea. Ann Thorac Surg 24:100, 1977.)

Microcirculation. Once the arteries reach the tracheoesophageal groove, they divide into primary tracheal and primary esophageal branches. Tracheal vessels enter the trachea in its lateral wall 0.7 to 1.5 cm anterior to the tracheoesophageal groove. After entering the trachea, lateral longitudinal and transverse intercartilaginous arteries are formed that connect the superior to the inferior vessels and supply blood in a circumferential manner to the trachea (Fig. 12–10). The lateral longitudinal arteries may be large—up to 1 to 2 mm in diameter—and form an important anastomotic connection for the entire trachea. To safely preserve blood supply, mobilization of long segments of trachea, especially along the posterolateral aspects, should be minimized during tracheal surgery. Bleeding from these vessels can be brisk and alarming in the case of accidental laceration, as may occasionally occur during lymph node biopsy in the paratracheal or subcarinal space.

Throughout the length of the trachea is an extensive submucosal plexus, fed by transverse intercartilaginous arteries, each of which penetrates the soft tissue space between the cartilaginous rings and runs anteriorly. As they reach the midline, they dive more deeply and terminate in the submucosal plexus. Conversely, there is *no* blood supply external to the cartilages. Thus, the cartilages receive their nutrient supply from the submucosal arterial plexus. It is therefore understandable that the tracheal rings may be damaged by ischemic injury due to overinflation of endotracheal tube cuffs.

The membranous trachea is not supplied by the transverse intercartilaginous arteries. Small twigs from these vessels pass posteriorly, but they tend to stop at the cartilage-membrane junction. The membranous portion is supplied by secondary tracheal twigs, which arise from primary esophageal branches of the tracheoesophageal arteries. These secondary tracheal twigs enter the membranous portion of the trachea and feed the submucosal plexus of the posterior wall of the trachea. These secondary arteries are well developed and form longitudinal arcades that span several segments.

Carina

The most inferior portion of the trachea, the bifurcation, is called the carina. It normally lies slightly to the right of the midline and is at the level of the fourth or fifth vertebra posteriorly and the sternomanubrial junction anteriorly. In normal individuals the left mainstem bronchus lies under the aortic arch, and for this reason, the carina, proximal left mainstem bronchus, and distal

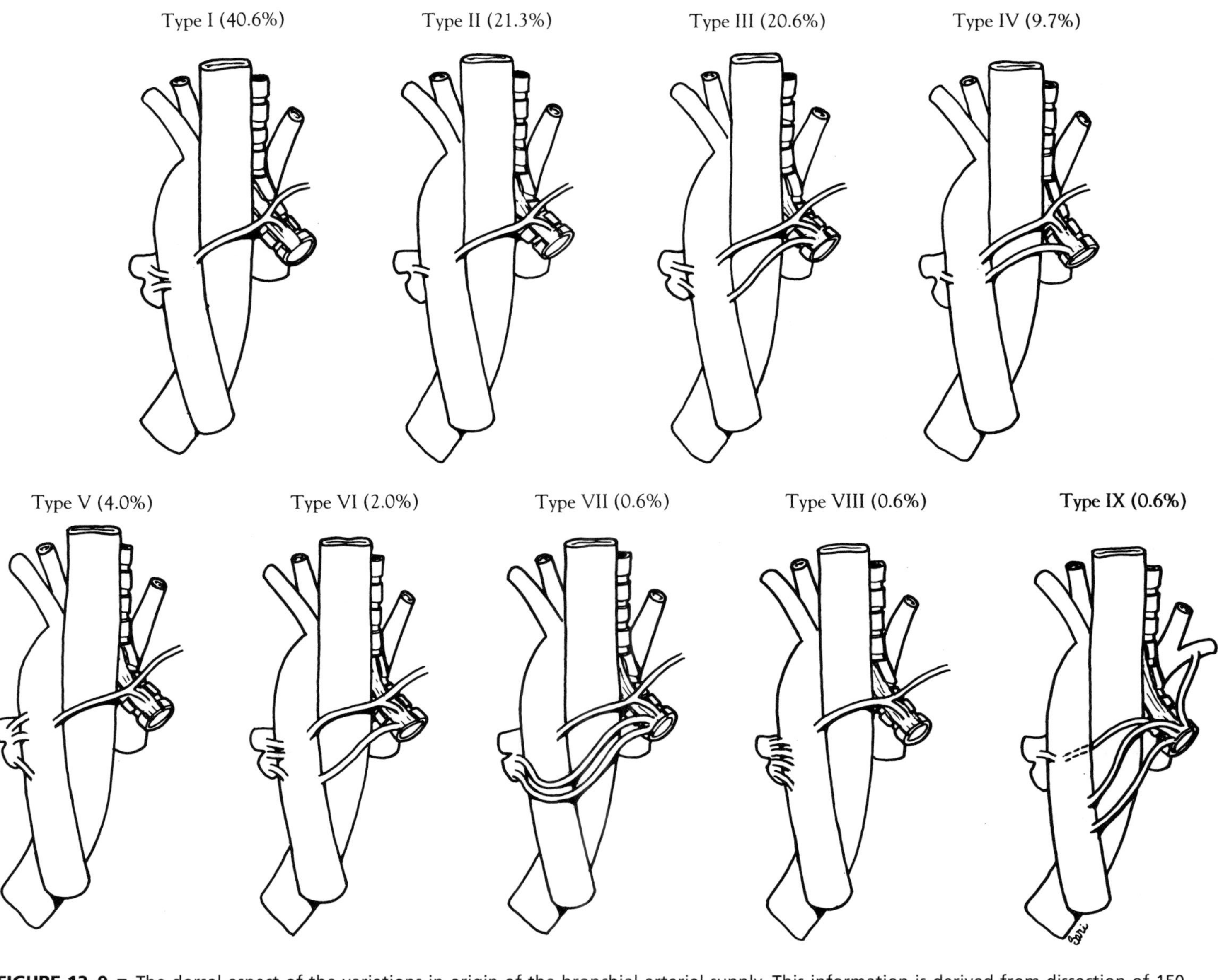

FIGURE 12–9 ■ The dorsal aspect of the variations in origin of the bronchial arterial supply. This information is derived from dissection of 150 cadavers and classified on the basis of the origin, number, and course of the vessels. (From Cauldwell EW, Siekert RG, Linninger RE, Anson BJ: The bronchial arteries, an anatomic study of 150 human cadavers. Surg Gynecol Obstet 86:395, 1948.)

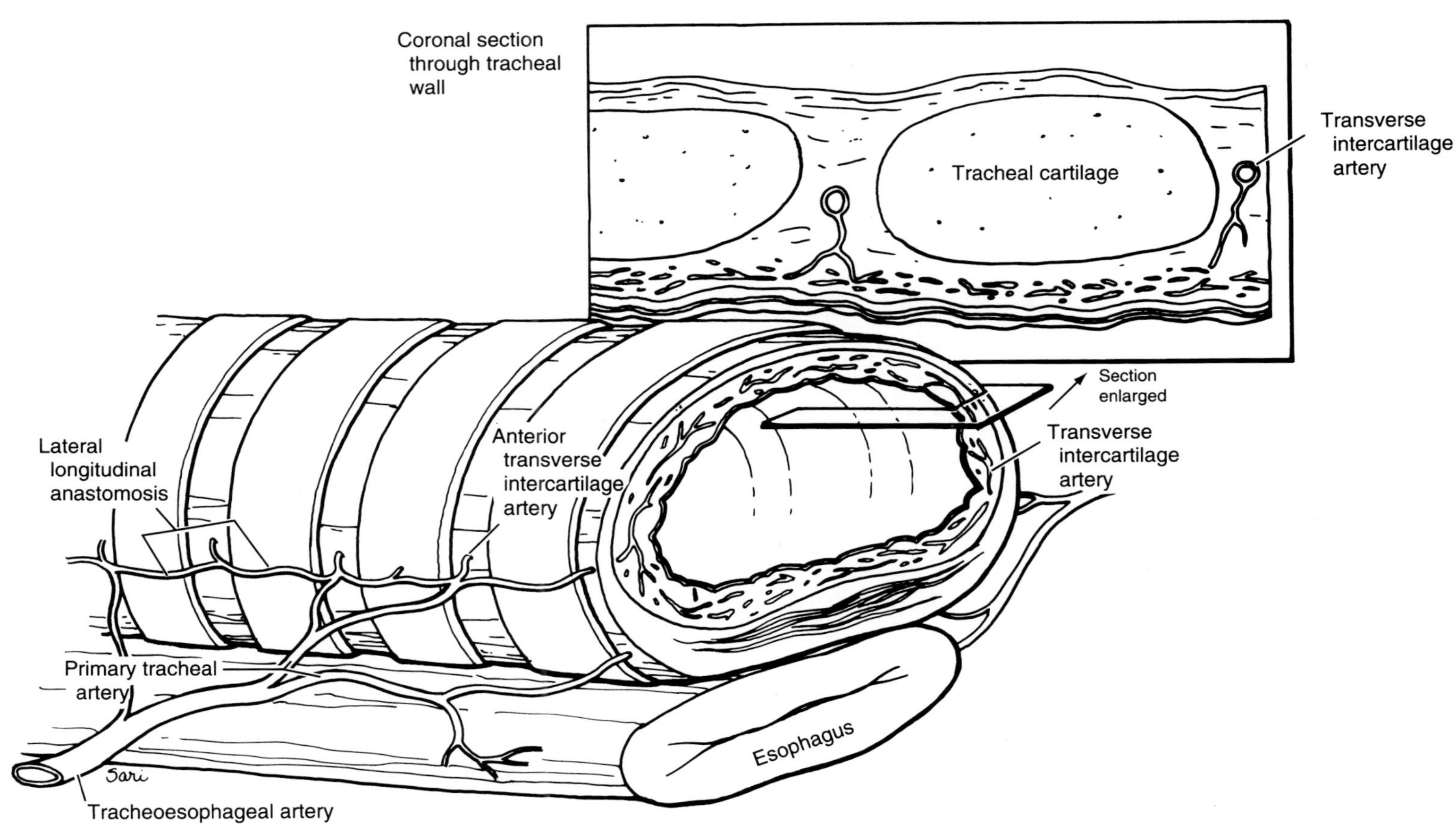

FIGURE 12–10 ■ Microcirculation of the trachea and esophagus. There is a rich submucosal plexus but no similar plexus of vessels on the external surface. Tracheal cartilage is nourished entirely from the submucosal circulation. (From Salassa JR, Pearson BW, Payne WS: Gross and microscopical blood supply of the trachea. Ann Thorac Surg 24:100, 1977.)

trachea are difficult to access through a left thoracotomy. Exposure is excellent through a high (fourth interspace) right thoracotomy. The angle between the two mainstem bronchi varies among individuals and is generally greater in children than in adults (Kubota et al, 1986). The configuration of the cartilages at the carina is quite variable. Occasionally a tracheal ring arising from the right or left mainstem bronchus extends under the crotch of the carina. Most often, however, there is a symmetric contribution from each side, with or without fusion at the carinal bifurcation (Vanpeperstraete, 1973). The blood supply at the carina is very robust and comes primarily from bronchial vessels, which branch to supply both the trachea and the bronchi. There is an abundance of lymph nodes in the crotch of the carina, which drain each side of the tracheobronchial tree and the lungs.

PHYSIOLOGY

There are three aspects of tracheal physiology that warrant discussion: changes in airway size, ciliary clearance, and humidification of tracheobronchial secretions.

Airway Size

Alterations in tracheal diameter and length occur with each respiration. During inspiration, both the length and the diameter increase in size, which facilitates airflow. The airway resistance is decreased (it is inversely related to the fourth power of the radius), as is the muscular work to move air. It is this capacity to change radius that accounts for different lung volumes in individuals with similar tracheal areas. Tracheal area is related more to gender (males having larger tracheas than females despite equivalent total lung capacities) than it is to lung volume (Martin et al, 1987). The length of the trachea can increase by one vertebral size on full inspiration, which allows for the descent of the diaphragm during inspiration.

Ciliary Action

The epithelium of the trachea consists of pseudostratified ciliated columnar epithelium with interspersed goblet cells. Ciliary action gently wafts debris proximally from more distal airways, and the mucoid material is then either expectorated or swallowed. This occurs by a rhythmic contraction of the cilia at a rate of 160 to 1500 times per minute and moves debris at a rate of about 16 mm/min (Paparella and Shumrick, 1980). Hypoxia as well as hyperoxia can decrease the beat frequency of these cilia. While it is said that cigarette smoking also decreases the frequency and thus the clearance, some find this not to be the case (Konietzko et al, 1981). The average beat frequency is similar regardless of the primary disease process (Konietzko et al, 1981). A rise in temperature causes an increase in beat frequency. The metabolic rate of the tracheal mucosa is quite high owing to the ciliary and glandular function. In fact, the oxygen consumption of the tracheal mucosa exceeds that of both the liver and the beating heart (Widdicombe, 1993).

Tracheobronchial Secretions

Tracheobronchial secretions consist of the output of the mucous glands under vagal and parasympathetic drug stimulation and of the goblet cells under the influence of local irritants. The sympathetic nervous system plays no known role in the production of these secretions. The total volume of the secretions is difficult to measure but under normal circumstances varies from 10 to 100 ml/day. The mucous layer forms a coat on the surface of the airway, which not only moistens the inspired air but also may limit evaporation from the trachea and bronchi. This mucous coat, which is about 5 μm in thickness, also carries foreign debris out of the airway. These secretions contain immunoglobulins, lysozymes, and other bacteriostatic and bacteriocidal components; they are 95% composed of water, with carbohydrates, proteins, and lipids making up most of the remaining 5% (Yeager, 1971). Output from the goblet cells is strongly stimulated by local irritants.

■ *KEY REFERENCES*

Cauldwell EW, Siekert RG, Linninger RE, Anson BJ: The bronchial arteries: An anatomic study of 150 human cadavers. Surg Gynecol Obstet 86:395, 1948.

The most comprehensive study of the tracheal and bronchial circulations. All subsequent studies have confirmed the findings in this report.

Salassa JR, Pearson BW, Payne WS: Gross and microscopical blood supply of the trachea. Ann Thorac Surg 24:100, 1977.

A study of the tracheal blood supply that is pertinent to surgery of the trachea, particularly circumferential resection and reconstruction by primary anastomosis. The report was written by an anatomist and two Mayo Clinic surgeons.

■ *REFERENCES*

Burrington JD: Tracheal growth and healing. J Thorac Cardiovasc Surg 76:453, 1978.

Couraud L, Baudet E, Martigne C et al: Bronchial revascularization in double lung transplantation: A series of 8 patients. Ann Thorac Surg 53:88, 1992.

Daly RC, Tadjkarimi S, Khaghani A et al: Successful double-lung transplantation with direct bronchial artery revascularization. Ann Thorac Surg 56:885, 1993.

Galliard DA, Lallement AV, Petit AF, Puchelle ES: In vivo ciliogenesis in human fetal tracheal epithelium. Am J Anat 185:415, 1989.

Griscom NT, Wohl ME: Dimensions of the growing trachea related to age and gender. AJR Am J Roentgenol 146:233, 1986.

Håkansson CH, Mercke U, Sonesson B, Toremalm NG: Functional anatomy of the musculature of the trachea. Acta Morphol Neerl Scand 14:291, 1976.

Kawakami Y, Nishimura M, Kusaka H: Tracheal dimensions at full inflation and deflation in adolescent twins. J Appl Physiol 70:1781, 1991.

Konietzko N, Nakhosteen JA, Mizera W et al: Ciliary beat frequency of biopsy samples taken from normal persons and patients with various lung diseases. Chest 80(Suppl):855, 1981.

Kubota Y, Toyoda Y, Nagata N et al: Tracheo-bronchial angles in infants and children. Anesthesiology 64:374, 1986.

Laks H, Louie HW, Haas GS et al: New technique of vascularization of the trachea and bronchus for lung transplantation. J Heart Lung Transplant 10:280, 1991.

Martin R, Castile RG, Fredberg JJ et al: Airway size is related to sex but not lung size in normal adults. J Appl Physiol 63:2042, 1987.

McLaughlin RF: Bronchial artery distribution in various mammals and in humans. Am Rev Respir Dis 128:S57, 1983.

Meta S, Myat HM: The cross-sectional shape and circumference of the human trachea. Ann R Coll Surg Engl 66:3568, 1984.

Miura T, Grillo JC: The contribution of the inferior thyroid artery to the blood supply of the human trachea. Surg Gynecol Obstet 123:99, 1966.

Moore K: The Developing Human, 2nd ed. Philadelphia, WB Saunders, 1977.

Nagaishi C: Functional Anatomy and Histology of the Lung. Baltimore, University Park Press, 1972.

Paparella MM, Shumrick DA: Otolaryngology, 2nd ed. Philadelphia, WB Saunders, 1980.

Reid L: Visceral cartilage. J Anat 122:349, 1976.

Schreinemakers HHJ, Weder W, Miyoshi S et al: Direct revascularization of bronchial arteries for lung transplantation: An anatomical study. Ann Thorac Surg 49:44, 1990.

Tos M: Anatomy of the tracheal mucous glands in man. Arch Otolaryngol Head Neck Surg 92:132, 1970.

Vanpeperstraete F: The cartilaginous skeleton of the bronchial tree. Adv Anat Embryol Cell Biol 48:1, 1973.

Wailoo MP, Emery JL: Normal growth and development of the trachea. Thorax 37:584, 1982.

Widdicombe J: New perspectives on basic mechanisms in lung disease 4: Why are the airways so vascular? Thorax 48:290, 1993.

Williams PL, Warwick R: Gray's Anatomy, 33rd ed. Edinburgh, Churchill Livingstone, 1981.

Yeager H: Tracheobronchial secretions. Am J Med 50:493, 1971.

CHAPTER **13**

Anesthesia for Airway Surgery

Karen M. McRae

The Shared Airway

Surgery of the upper airway requires diagnostic or therapeutic manipulation of the respiratory tree despite ongoing ventilation. Review of historical literature reveals that the anatomic and physiologic challenges posed by the earliest surgeries are the same ones that we face today. Whether internal or external access to the conducting airway is required, anesthesiologist and surgeon, who must work together closely, share the airway.

The anesthetic technique is determined by the chosen mode of ventilation. Anesthetic agents with rapid onset and short duration have now become available, permitting a deep plane of general anesthesia with prompt recovery and resumption of spontaneous ventilation necessary to successful extubation of patients with compromised airway anatomy. Clinicians have responded to the challenge of ventilating the patient undergoing airway surgery with a wide variety of innovative techniques. In this chapter, an overview of both short-acting anesthetic agents and of ventilation modalities is presented, followed by the applications described for each type of airway procedure.

HISTORICAL NOTE

Early in his career, Chevalier Jackson (1905), a practitioner of endoscopy from the beginning of the 20th century, wrote:

> Tracheoscopy and bronchoscopy by mouth may be done under cocaine if the patient is stolid. In sensitive men, and in women and children, deep, relaxing, general anesthesia will always be required, and thus must be supplemented with cocaine locally . . . Chloroform anesthesia, with the patient in the recumbent position, the head hanging over the end of the table . . . offers so many advantages that (the writer) does not feel inclined to try any other.

The hazards of general anesthesia were recognized. With an experience accumulated of thousands of cases, Jackson's opinion of the merits of various anesthetic techniques during bronchoscopy and laryngoscopy had been significantly altered, as revealed in his book, *Bronchoesophagology* (Jackson and Jackson, 1950).

> General anesthesia is rarely justified in children, and not often in adults. The various kinds of inhalation anesthetics are inconvenient and many of them dangerous because they are explosive* . . . Sodium pentothal given intravenously has been found satisfactory but for safety it requires an anesthetist with technical skill and experience in its use.

Jackson recognized the importance of correct patient positioning for successful endoscopy. He suggested that "the muscular tension exerted by some patients in assuming and holding a faulty position is almost as much of a hindrance as to peroral endoscopy as is the faulty position itself."

Rapid insertion of the laryngoscope by a well-rehearsed team was recommended. Chevalier Jackson performed endoscopy primarily for purposes of diagnosis, dilatation of stenoses, and removal of foreign bodies. These examinations were necessarily brief.

Although many early endoscopists advocated the use of topical anesthesia, review of their regimen revealed considerable reliance on systemic premedication before topicalization of the airway. The use of an intramuscular opioid agent (most often morphine) and an anticholinergic agent (scopolamine or atropine), with dose adjustment for patient age and size, was suggested to precede the application of topical anesthesia with allowance for sufficient time for its effect. The addition of nembutal was recommended in patients with "a tendency to sensitivity to local anesthetic drugs," and barbiturates were known to reduce the manifestations of local anesthetic toxicity. Of available local anesthetics, cocaine was often used, as were pontocaine and larocaine (Jackson and McReynolds, 1940; Putney, 1939).

As bronchoscopic procedures of increased duration and complexity were performed, the attendant risks were described. "Debris in the respiratory tract of an unconscious patient without an adequate cough reflex may lead to his death by asphyxia" (Churchill-Davidson, 1952). In 1954, MacIntosh, the Nuffield Professor of Anaesthetics at Oxford University, wrote:

> At many centers abroad topical analgesia is used as a routine, but has taken a heavy toll. Its application is often left to a junior assistant armed with a barber's spray having a large reservoir of cocaine or a methocaine solution. . . . Death from 'idiosyncrasy' to the local analgesia is only too frequent.

Intravenous (IV) pentothal induction of general anesthesia and brief neuromuscular blockade with succinylcholine, with intermittent mask ventilation during which a directed application of nebulized cocaine to the airway structures, was recommended (MacIntosh, 1947). Once topicalization was complete, spontaneous ventilation was allowed to resume and bronchoscopy was performed in the anesthetized airway as the barbiturate was metabolized (MacIntosh, 1954).

A method of *positive-pressure ventilation* during bron-

*Ether, widely used in the first half of the 20th century, is highly explosive.

choscopy was first suggested by Muendnich and Hoflehner in 1953, and a simple modification of the standard bronchoscope was described soon thereafter (Safar, 1958). The ventilating bronchoscope allowed prolonged examination in the apneic patient. The newly introduced inhalational agent halothane was described for bronchoscopic examination in spontaneously breathing children in 1959; more rapid recovery was observed than when ether or IV barbiturates were used (Brown, 1959). In Brown's report, the children were allowed to breathe spontaneously despite the attachment of an anesthetic delivery circuit. The author warned that if a muscle relaxant was used, cyanosis could rapidly occur.

The advent of arterial blood gas (ABG) analysis introduced new evidence to the debate of the relative merits of topical versus general anesthesia and spontaneous versus controlled ventilation. Patients managed by topical anesthesia were not infrequently hypoxic and hypercapnic before bronchoscopy, a result of the respiratory depression from premedicants. Ventilation tended to improve with the stimulation of the procedure. Patients managed with general anesthesia and spontaneously breathing inhalational agents were well oxygenated but tended to experience hypercapnia during bronchoscopy (Carnes and Fabian, 1961). Patients in whom ventilation was controlled with positive pressure via a ventilating bronchoscope with a wide side arm exhibited high arterial oxygen tension and could easily be hyperventilated (Schoenstadt et al, 1965).

Sanders (1967) first devised a method to deliver jet ventilation via a rigid bronchoscope that permitted positive-pressure ventilation in the absence of a gas tight system. With this technique, high-pressure gas source is connected to a narrow cannula, positioned at the inlet of the bronchoscope; gas boluses are delivered by means of a hand-operated switch. In the lumen of the bronchoscope, the high-velocity stream of gas encounters stationary gas, and friction causes the quiescent gas to decelerate the moving stream; in turn the moving gas accelerates the quiescent gas. Each jet bolus therefore entrains ambient air, substantially augmenting the volume of the bolus and diluting the oxygen fraction of the jet. Widely, but incorrectly, attributed to the *Venturi principle*, this is in fact an illustration of *Newton's law of motion* (Hunsaker, 1994; Ihra and Aloy, 2000).

Sanders' innovation inspired a proliferation of techniques utilizing gases at high flows for ventilation during bronchoscopy. Placement of an injector that exactly fitted the side arm of a bronchoscope permitted delivery of larger breath volumes with lower driving pressures than with a jet catheter held within the inlet or side port (Carden et al, 1973).

Gillick (1974) described a ventilation catheter that could be independently passed into the trachea, through which gas boluses could be injected. The catheter tended to position itself in the anterior commisure of the larynx as the bronchoscope was subsequently inserted. The original catheter described was a nasogastric sump tube with a reinforcing wire threaded down the narrow lumen to maintain catheter position with each bolus injection. The diameter of the ventilation port was larger than jet catheters (5 mm) and permitted high gas flows with lower driving pressures. Both the injection bronchoscope and the inflation-catheter techniques resulted in less entrainment of ambient air. When oxygen was used, high arterial oxygen tensions could be achieved. These systems could be adapted to deliver air or nitrous oxide mixtures.

With a spectrum of ventilation techniques available, prolonged examination and incision of laryngeal and intrabronchial structures were possible. Fiberoptic bronchoscopy was introduced into clinical practice in 1968 and offered access to more peripheral airway lesions. In the early 1970s, laser resection of airway structures was introduced, further expanding therapeutic options.

■ *HISTORICAL READINGS*

Brown D: Halothane-oxygen anaesthesia for bronchoscopy. Anaesthesia 14:135, 1959.

Carden E, Burns WW, McDevitt NB et al: A comparison of Venturi and side-arm ventilation in anaesthesia for bronchoscopy. Can Anaesth Soc J 20:569, 1973.

Carnes MA, Fabian LW: Anesthesia for bronchoscopy and bronchography. Anesth Analg 40:567, 1961.

Churchill-Davidson HC: Anaesthesia for bronchoscopy. Anaesthesia 7:237, 1952.

Gillick JS: The inflation-catheter technique for ventilation during bronchoscopy. Anesthesiology 40:503, 1974.

Jackson C: Foreign bodies in the trachea, bronchi and oesophagus—the aid of oesophagoscopy, bronchoscopy, and magnetism in their extraction. Laryngoscope 4:257, 1905.

Jackson C, Jackson CL: Bronchoesophagology. Philadelphia, WB Saunders, 1950.

Jackson CL, McReynolds GS: Anesthesia for peroral endoscopy. Ann Otol Rhinol Laryngol 49:1048, 1940.

MacIntosh RR: Anaesthesia for bronchoscopy. Anaesthesia 9:77, 1954.

MacIntosh RR: Technique of laryngeal anaesthesia. Lancet 2:54, 1947.

Muendnich K, Hoflehner G: Die Narkose-Beatmungs-bronchoscopie. Anaesthetist 21:121, 1953.

Putney FJ: Anesthesia for peroral endoscopy. Laryngoscope 49:55, 1939.

Safar P: Ventilating bronchoscope. Anesthesiology 19:406, 1958.

Sanders RD: Two ventilating attachments for bronchoscopes. Del Med J 39:170, 1967.

Schoenstadt DA, Doneker TG, Arnold HS et al: A re-examination of the ventilating bronchoscope. J Thorac Cardiovasc Surg 49:525, 1965.

ANESTHETIC AGENTS

Whereas a wide spectrum of anesthetic agents have been used for airway surgery, several short-acting drugs have become available in the last decade that have transformed the anesthesiologist's ability to provide profound general anesthesia for short procedures with rapid recovery. This advance has permitted many laryngoscopic and bronchoscopic procedures to be scheduled on an outpatient basis. The rapid return of airway reflexes, muscle strength, and an alert, conscious state is particularly important in patients with severely compromised respiratory function and residual airway obstruction for resumption of effective spontaneous ventilation. The use of short-acting agents during longer airway procedures (e.g., reconstruction) facilitates prompt extubation.

The ideal volatile anesthetic agent would have very low solubility in blood, allowing rapid equilibration between delivered alveolar concentration and the site of effect—the central nervous system (CNS). This facilitates prompt induction of anesthesia, titration of drug during the maintenance period, and rapid emergence and recovery.

Two new volatile anesthetic agents with low blood solubility were introduced into clinical practice in the early 1990s: *desflurane* and *sevoflurane*. Sevoflurane has the advantage of being pleasant-smelling and nonirritating to the airways and thus is most suitable for the inhalation induction required in some airway procedures (Smith et al, 1996).

The IV anesthetic *propofol* is almost insoluble in aqueous solutions, making it necessary for it to be solubilized in a lecithin preparation. High lipid solubility contributes to a rapid onset of unconsciousness with its administration. Recovery from the effects of propofol is due to rapid metabolism. The drug has no active metabolites. Unlike barbiturates, propofol is associated with little postoperative sedation and nausea. This drug was key to the popularization of total IV anesthesia in the 1980s (Sebel and Lowdon, 1989).

The ultra-short-acting opioid *remifentanil* possesses a rapid onset of action and half-life elimination time of only 3 to 5 minutes by mechanisms of redistribution and ester hydrolysis. It is unique among opioids, in that a steady-state infusion wears off in predictable fashion, independent of the infusion's duration (Bürkle et al, 1996).

Alfentanil also has rapid onset and is short-acting. It is eliminated by rapid redistribution and hepatic metabolism. Small bolus doses (10 μg/kg) wear off rapidly (15 minutes). The elimination half-time, however, tends to increase with the duration of the infusion.

Fentanyl, an opioid of intermediate duration, is also commonly used for bronchoscopy. A dose of 2 μg/kg generally lasts less than an hour.

Opiates are particularly useful for attenuating the stress response to airway instrumentation. Remifentanil is increasingly used for patients with tenuous respiratory status for stressful procedures with minimal postoperative pain and in my practice is the drug of choice as an adjunct to a general anesthetic for patients with cardiovascular or respiratory disease who are undergoing laryngoscopy or bronchoscopy. An infusion of 0.5 μg/kg/min is started during preoxygenation. A maintenance infusion of 0.2 μg/kg/min is used in younger patients, 0.1 μg/kg/min for older patients.

Beta-adrenergic blockade may also be used to attenuate tachycardia and hypertension during airway manipulation. *Esmolol* is an IV β_1 receptor antagonist with an ester group incorporated into its structure; this allows rapid degradation by erythrocyte esterases, with a resultant half-life of about 9 minutes. Esmolol is β_1 cardioselective, having little effect on bronchial tone, and is advantageous in patients with reactive airway disease. A bolus dose of 500 μg/kg may be followed by an infusion of 100 to 300 μg/kg if prolonged effect is required.

Muscle relaxants are classified according to their ability to depolarize the neuromuscular junction. *Succinylcholine* is a depolarizing muscle relaxant in clinical use since the 1940s. Rapid, profound relaxation is achieved within 1 minute of administration of 1.5 mg/kg, ideal for rapid intubation. The drug wears off within minutes by diffusion from the neuromuscular junction. These characteristics make it the ideal drug for short procedures in which profound muscle relaxation is necessary but in which rapid recovery is required. An intubating dose may be followed by an infusion, titrated to effect. A succinylcholine infusion can be turned off and on (e.g., for assessment of vocal cord function). Extended infusion is not recommended, since a phase II response (a prolonged and unpredictable neuromuscular blockade) may occur. Succinylcholine has some unfortunate side effects; myalgias are common, transient increase in serum potassium levels can be clinically significant in the hyperkalemic patient, and a malignant hyperthermia reaction occurs infrequently in the susceptible individual.

The ideal short-acting, nondepolarizing agent has yet to be developed; *rocuronium* has a rapid onset but is of intermediate duration. *Mivacurium* is considered to be short-acting; it has a slower onset and offset than succinylcholine and an inconsistent time to maximum blockade. In this author's experience, mivacurium does not reliably provide the profound blockade required for stimulating procedures, such as rigid bronchoscopy. The same is said of the new rapid-onset, short-acting, nondepolarizing relaxant *rapacuronium* (Goulden and Hunter, 1999).

MODES OF VENTILATION: JET VENTILATION

Surgical intervention in the airway presents unique ventilation difficulties. Clinicians have devised creative solutions for the challenges presented by airway surgery, and there has been a proliferation of airway devices and ventilation techniques described. *Jet ventilation* releases high gas flow through a small orifice, permitting ventilation of the open airway via laryngoscopes and bronchoscopes, with minimal obstruction of the surgical field. The use of long catheters of small caliber permits ventilation of the distal airways. *High-frequency* techniques optimize lung recruitment while avoiding high peak pressure and cause minimal movement of the surgical field. Each technique has been successfully used in series of patients. A summary of these reports is presented in Tables 13–1 and 13–2. Many of the devices described in these reports are specific to the institution in which they are used; most important, when adopting a ventilation technique that exposes the patient's airway to high gas flows or pressures, the practitioner must be aware of potential complications.

Low-frequency jet ventilation (LFJV) is accomplished by the release of gas under high pressure (50–60 psi) through an orifice (~1 mm), as described by Sanders (1967). A pressure regulator is required to maintain constant flow, and a hand-held on-off valve is released intermittently; jet pulses are delivered at a rate of 10 to 20 per minute. Physiologic tidal volumes are generated, and chest movement is clearly visible. The resultant motion of airway structures during LFJV usually necessitates intermittent periods of apnea, when resection is required. Distinct advantages of this approach are its simplicity and lack of specialized equipment.

Initially developed for ventilation of patients with acute lung injury in the intensive care unit, *high-frequency ventilation* (HFV) techniques, including *high-frequency jet ventilation* (HFJV), *high-frequency positive pres-*

TABLE 13–1 ■ **Characteristics of Modes of Ventilation During Airway Surgery**

	Can Ventilate Open Airway	*Immobility of Operative Field*	*Specialized Equipment Required*	*Airway Pressure Monitoring*	*Potential for Barotrauma*	*Gas Entrainment During Ventilation*	*Airway Gas Composition and Monitoring*
Intermittent positive-pressure ventilation	No	No	No, routine anesthetic machine	Pressure depends on ventilator settings, reliable	Minor	No	Stable and accurate
Low-frequency jet ventilation	Yes	No	Simple gas injector only	Intermittently high, difficult	Yes, high	Yes	Variable and difficult
High-frequency jet ventilation	Yes	Yes	Yes, specialized ventilator	Can be high*; difficult, especially around jet nozzle	Yes	Yes, degree of entrainment is application-dependent (see Table 13–2)	Variable and difficult
High-frequency positive-pressure ventilation	Yes	Yes	Yes, specialized ventilator	Low peak, mean, transpulmonary pressure; difficult	Yes	Minor	Stable and accurate
High-frequency oscillation	Yes	No	Yes, specialized ventilator	High mean pressure; difficult	Yes	No	Stable and accurate

*Gas trapping and hyperinflation common.
Adapted from McRae K: Anesthesia for airway surgery. Anesthesiol Clin North Am 19:498, 2001.

sure ventilation (HFPPV), and *high-frequency oscillation* (HFO) were introduced in the 1970s and 1980s.

The mechanical effects of the use of high frequencies are crucial to understanding the mechanisms of gas transfer in HFV. Increasing respiratory rates (and volumes) decrease pulmonary emptying time, moderate gas trapping occurs, and the lung is held in a distended state. Peripheral airway pressures are continuously positive with all high-frequency techniques, with low mean and peak pressures achieved (Carlon et al, 1981; Glenski et al, 1986; Howland et al, 1987; Sjostrand, 1980). This is analogous to maintenance of lung volume with high positive end-expiratory pressure (PEEP) without the need to impose large tidal volume excursion to remove carbon dioxide (CO_2).

Elimination of CO_2 in HFV has been extensively studied and is probably a result of bulk convection created by even small tidal volumes and by molecular diffusion (a decreasing gradient of CO_2 from the alveoli to the conducting airways) enhanced by the turbulence created by convective flow (*Taylor dispersion*) (Froese and Bryan, 1987). These mechanisms permit effective removal of CO_2 despite the use of tidal volumes less than the lung's dead space. Lung distention promotes alveolar recruitment, increased functional residual capacity (FRC), and decreased areas of low ventilation-perfusion ($\dot{V}/\dot{Q}$), enhancing oxygenation. HFV has been extensively applied to airway surgery (see Table 13–2). An obvious advantage is the lower peak airway pressures generated with HFV, compared with conventional *intermittent positive-pressure ventilation* (IPPV), permitting diminishing air leak. The use of low tidal volumes at high respiratory rates offers the advantage of minimal movement of the operative field. Interruption of ventilation may not be required during resection.

HFJV resembles its low-frequency counterpart (LFJV), in that gas is delivered from a high-pressure gas source via a stiff, small-bore catheter positioned in the airway. Rather than a hand-held switch, the jet stream is cut by a high-frequency pneumatic or electronically controlled flow interrupter. As the high-velocity gas jet enters the airway, additional gas is entrained at the jet nozzle, contributing to the delivered tidal volumes, which remain small in comparison to conventional ventilation (Carlon et al, 1981). Variables that can be regulated during HFJV include (1) driving pressure, (2) frequency, and (3) inspiratory time, usually set at 20% to 30% of the cycle. Ventilation rates span 100 to 400 breaths/min, tidal volumes delivered are 2 to 5 ml/kg. Increased driving pressure and inspiratory time can result in impedance in expiratory gas flow, gas trapping, development of auto-PEEP, and impaired CO_2 elimination (Beamer et al, 1984).

HFJV has been used with success to support gas exchange in experimental conducting airway disruption; the driving pressure of the gas and size of the jet nozzle have been shown to be crucial. When a constant driving pressure was used, an increase in nozzle size was required to maintain gas exchange with increasing air leak; however, a larger nozzle used with a smaller air leak resulted in lung overdistention and systemic hypotension (Carlon et al, 1983).

HFPPV of small tidal volumes (3–5 ml/kg at 60–100 breaths/min) may be delivered by means of a conventional ventilator of low internal volume and negligible internal compliance; known volumes and gas mixtures are delivered. Initially, HFPPV was applied via an insufflation catheter placed at the tip of an endotracheal tube. An injection catheter with multiple side holes was recommended both to increase turbulence, thereby reducing injection jet effect, and to minimize entrainment. Later, a pneumatic valve system was devised that permitted HFPPV through a side port of an open ventilator circuit. External PEEP may be added.

Delivered volume using the pneumatic valve is dimin-

TABLE 13–2 ■ **Jet Ventilation and High-Frequency Ventilation in Airway Surgery**

Ventilation Mode	*Anesthetic Application*	*Reports/Technique Used*	*Reference*	*Advantages*	*Disadvantages*
Low-frequency jet ventilation 10–20 breaths/min, tidal volumes variable (in range of conventional ventilation)			For all applications	Simple apparatus	Difficulty in monitoring gas composition and airway pressure, significant movement of surgical field
	Suspension-laryngoscopy	Supraglottic; catheter down axis of laryngoscope	Spoerel & Greenway, 1973	Chest movement clearly visible, glottis unobstructed	Ventilation decreased by catheter malalignment, movement of vocal cords, intermittent apnea required
	For laser resection	Ventilating laryngoscope	Shikowitz et al, 1991	No combustible airway devices during laser therapy	Movement of vocal cords, intermittent apnea required
	Rigid bronchoscopy	Through lumen of rigid bronchoscope using hand-held injector with narrow orifice (~1 mm)	Sanders, 1967	Chest movement visible	Tracheal gas composition variable Aspiration of blood and debris into trachea
		High-pressure injector fitting on side arm	Carden, 1974	Less gas entrainment than in Sanders technique	As above
		12–18 French nasogastric tube used as endotracheal inflation catheter, based on patient's weight	Gillick, 1974	Less gas entrainment than in Sanders technique	As above
	For laser resection	Hand-held injector, by way of bronchoscope	Duckett et al, 1985; Perera & Mallon, 1987; Vourc'h, 1980, 1983	No combustible devices in airway during laser therapy	Apnea required for resection
		Using a low-frequency automated jet ventilator by way of the bronchoscope	Conacher et al, 1998	Operator's hands are free	As above
	Tracheal reconstruction			Simplicity of equipment, both catheters and gas injectors	Movement of surgical field, intermittent apnea required for resection Aspiration of blood and debris into distal lumen

Table continued on following page

TABLE 13–2 ■ **Jet Ventilation and High-Frequency Ventilation in Airway Surgery** *Continued*

Ventilation Mode	*Anesthetic Application*	*Reports/Technique Used*	*Reference*	*Advantages*	*Disadvantages*
		8 French suction catheter advanced through endotracheal tube across defect into distal trachea	Lee & English, 1974		
		5-mm endotracheal tube advanced into distal trachea, mainstem bronchus across defect	Baraka, 1977; Baraka et al, 1986	As above	As above
		Nasogastric tube advanced through single-lumen endotracheal tube, single or bilateral bronchial catheters	McClish et al, 1985	Larger catheters; lower driving pressure causes less entrainment of room air and debris	As above
		Ventilation by way of T tube, 2-mm catheter advanced into extraluminal limb of T tube	Baraka et al, 1982	As above	As above
High-frequency jet ventilation 100–400 breaths/min 1.7–6.6 Hz 2–5 ml/kg breath volume			For all applications	Immobility of operative field	Gas trapping and hyperinflation common Difficulty monitoring gas composition and airway pressure
	Fiberoptic bronchoscopy	By way of 2-mm suction port of bronchoscope	Sivarajan et al, 1995	Can ventilate while viewing airway	Experimental*
	Fiberoptic bronchoscopy, operative	Nasotracheal insertion of 14 French nylon catheter into trachea	Hautmann et al, 2000		Catheter must be removed during stent placement
	Suspension laryngoscopy	Supraglottic, ventilating laryngoscope	Bacher et al, 2000a&b; Ihra et al, 1999	Glottis unobstructed	Vocal cord movement seen Ventilation decreased by malalignment of bronchoscope Unclear how much entrainment

		Subglottic; 3.5–4.0-mm catheter in trachea	Babinski et al, 1980	Minimal entrainment of gas and debris	Tube present in glottis
	For laser resection	Subglottic; laser-resistant 2.7-mm catheter in trachea	Brooker et al, 1998	Minimal entrainment of smoke, gas, and debris	Ventilation catheter in glottis during laser pulses; potential for combustion
	Rigid bronchoscopy for laser resection	Ventilation through rigid bronchoscope during resection of tracheal/bronchial stenosis	Vourc'h, 1983b	Minimal movement operative field	Inadequate ventilation during bronchial resection adequate for tracheal ventilation
	Tracheal resection			Elimination of endotracheal tube from field, narrow ventilation minimally obstructive Can ventilate throughout resection Continuous gas flow from trachea	Jet effect may displace catheter
	High tracheal resection	Jet catheter through laryngeal mask airway, across defect	Adelsmayr et al, 1998	Laryngeal mask airway permits mobilization of high lesion	As above
	Tracheal, sleeve resection	14 French jet catheter through endotracheal tube, across defect	Magnusson et al, 1997; Watanabe, 1988	As above	As above
	Carinal resection	Two 12 and 14 French jet catheters through endotracheal tube, into bilateral bronchi	Perera, 1993	Oxygenation maintained in patient with limited reserve	As above
High-frequency positive-pressure ventilation 60–100 breaths/min 1–1.7 Hz 3–5 ml/kg breath volume			For all applications	Immobility of operative field Minimal gas entrainment	Specialized ventilator required Difficulty monitoring airway pressure
	Fiberoptic bronchoscopy	High-frequency positive-pressure ventilation via endotracheal tube	Flatau et al, 1982	Peak airway pressures significantly less than during conventional positive-pressure ventilation	As above
	Suspension laryngoscopy	Ventilation catheter in trachea, multiple side holes at tip	Eriksson & Sjostrand, 1980	Continuous positive airway pressure, flow directed out of glottis, minimal entrainment, stable gas mixture	As above

Table continued on following page

TABLE 13–2 ■ **Jet Ventilation and High-Frequency Ventilation in Airway Surgery** *Continued*

Ventilation Mode	*Anesthetic Application*	*Reports/Technique Used*	*Reference*	*Advantages*	*Disadvantages*
	Rigid bronchoscopy	By way of bronchoscope side arm, pneumatic valve effect	Eriksson & Sjostrand, 1980	Lower peak airway pressures than low-frequency jet ventilation, IPPV, continuous positive airway pressure, minimal entrainment, stable gas mixture	As above
	Endobronchial laser resection	Long ventilation catheter in contralateral bronchus	Medici et al, 1999	Protection of nonaffected lung	As above
	Tracheal resection				
	High tracheal resection	2-mm catheter by way of Montgomery T tube	El-Baz et al, 1982a	Able to ventilate throughout resection. Elimination of endotracheal tube from field, narrow catheters minimally obstructive	Successful ventilation under both topical and general anesthesia
	Midtracheal stenosis	5-mm catheter advanced through endotracheal tube	Eriksson et al, 1975	As above	
	Carinal resection, sleeve pneumonectomy	2-mm catheter advanced through trachea into bronchus to be anastomosed	El-Baz et al, 1982b	As above	

	Tracheal, carinal resections	Sterile catheter placed into open distal airway across surgical field during reconstruction	Young-Beyer & Wilson, 1988	Catheter easily placed by surgeons	
High-frequency oscillation					
60-3000 breaths/min 1-50 Hz 1–3 ml/kg breath volume	Rigid bronchoscopy	Delivered externally by way of body cuirass	Natalini et al, 2000	Bronchoscope free of ventilatory attachments	Specialized ventilator required
	Airway surgery, around hilum	Piston pump oscillator ventilating through single	Glenski et al, 1986	Attempted ventilation throughout resection	Hypercapnia common, 10% of patients hypoxic, required change of ventilation pattern Suboptimal conditions due to movement of the airways, not recommended Specialized ventilator required Difficulty monitoring airway pressure

*Experimental application; not recommended by author.
Adapted from McRae K: Anesthesia for airway surgery. Anesthesiol Clin North Am 19:499, 2001.

ished by some degree of escape of inspired gas through the expiratory limb. Ventilation nomograms for laryngoscopic and bronchoscopic HFPPV have been developed for different brands of bronchoscopes and insufflation catheters of various sizes. Upper airway examination and surgery currently constitute the primary applications of this ventilation technique. Little hemodynamic derangement has been described (Sjostrand, 1980).

HFO is a mode of ventilation that uses very high frequencies (up to 50 Hz) and very small tidal volumes (as little as 1 ml/kg). A reciprocating piston-type pump is used to oscillate gas in a sinusoidal pattern via an endotracheal tube. Fresh gas is entrained from an ancillary circuit located between the patient and oscillator.

HFO is dependent on active injection and withdrawal of gas from a lung suspended in inflation by continuous positive airway pressure (CPAP), and CO_2 removal is dependent on stroke amplitude and oscillator frequency. Clinical studies of HFO show higher mean airway pressures than with conventional mechanical ventilation, yet little hemodynamic compromise. There is renewed interest in HFO in critical care, a field in which it is considered a promising but experimental mode of ventilation for patients with adult and infant respiratory distress syndrome (Krishnan and Brower, 2000).

Disadvantages of high-frequency techniques include a requirement for specialized ventilator equipment and technical difficulty in monitoring ventilation parameters. The variable positioning of ventilation catheters during airway surgery likely precludes the use of optimal sites for airway pressure monitoring. Peripheral airway pressures may be markedly different from pressures in the large airways as a result of gas trapping inherent to the use of high respiratory rates, short expiratory times, and expiratory flow limitation. Delivered breath volumes are nearly impossible to quantify with an open airway, and serial ABG analysis is essential to detect hypoventilation. For longer procedures, humidification of gases must be provided in order to avoid drying of the airway mucosa and desiccation of secretions; this is particularly difficult when jet techniques are used.

All modes of HFV require that the delivery circuit have minimal compliance. Review of the HFV literature is notable for the variation in devices described in different clinical reports. Many ventilators and breathing circuits, having been built in a hospital laboratory, are specific to an institution. The systematic characterization of operating conditions is often lacking. Many devices are in fact hybrids, superimposing a high-frequency mode on conventional IPPV or displaying features of two forms of HFV (Froese and Bryan, 1987). To further confuse matters, innovative clinicians have combined both LFJV and HFV during one lung ventilation for bronchoplasty with IPPV of the contralateral lung, usually to minimize shunting during an operative procedure (Benumof, 1994).

There is inherent risk in the use of high-flow, high-pressure gas pulses in the airway and even more so when delivered at rapid rates. Catheter position and alignment within the tracheobronchial tree must be known at all times and is made more difficult by manipulation of the airway during surgery. Free egress of expired gas and adequate expiratory time must be maintained in order to avoid inadvertent hyperinflation. Whereas CPAP is expected in HFV and is beneficial in maintaining lung recruitment, the use of higher ventilation rates and higher volumes may result in occult PEEP (Howland et al, 1987). The resulting lung hyperinflation can lead to impedance of venous return and hemodynamic compromise, particularly if the chest is closed.

Barotrauma and volotrauma in the form of pneumothorax, pneumomediastinum, and subcutaneous emphysema have been reported with all forms of HFV and with LFJV. The use of distal airway pressure monitoring as well as automatic shutoff mechanisms to prevent further gas flow into the lungs in the event of high airway pressure is advocated (Froese and Bryan, 1987).

Although there are many reports of the adaptation of volatile agent vaporizers for use with HFV (Baraka et al, 1986; Eriksson et al, 1975; Gillick, 1974), this is unnecessary because current practice offers ideal total IV anesthetic regimens. The use of newer, short-acting volatile agents that involve the high flows required of HFV would be wasteful and costly.

Anesthesia for Endoscopic Surgery of the Airway

The surgeon and anesthesiologist should review all available knowledge of the patient's airway pathology. Depending on the urgency of the procedure, pulmonary function tests, particularly the flow-volume loop (Fig. 13–1), chest x-ray and computed tomography (CT) or magnetic resonance imaging (MRI) delineating the airway may be available. Patients should be examined for evidence of airway obstruction, the use of accessory muscles, or stridor. In adult patients, stridor is a sign of significant airway obstruction; and the tracheal diameter is usually 6 mm or less (Young-Beyer and Wilson, 1988). A clear plan of the procedure should be made. The surgical team, adjunct airway equipment, and surgical instruments must be present at the time of induction of anesthesia, particularly when difficult mask ventilation or intubation is anticipated.

Patient Positioning and Monitoring

The procedure is performed with the patient supine on a bed, usually in an operating room. Patients with respiratory compromise may breathe more effectively in a sitting position, and the bed should be adjustable to this position during induction of anesthesia and emergence. The bed should have an adjustable headpiece, permitting flexion and extension of the neck. The availability of equipment for airway management and resuscitation must be ensured before any form of bronchoscopy. If rigid bronchoscopy or suspension laryngoscopy is to be performed, appropriate ventilation devices to be used should be operational before the procedure is begun.

Reliable IV access must be secured. Noninvasive monitoring with a continuous electrocardiogram (ECG), pulse oximetry, and blood pressure cuff is required. When general anesthesia is induced, exhaled gas should be ana-

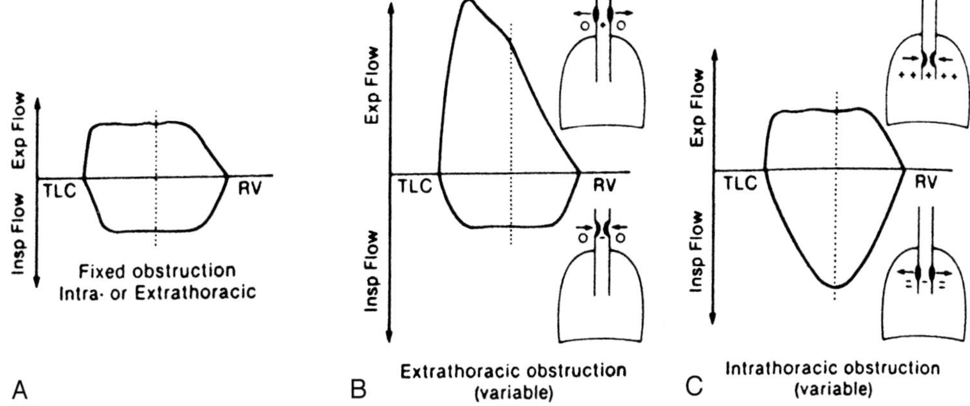

FIGURE 13–1 ■ Maximum inspiratory and expiratory flow-volume loops may detect airway pathology in fixed obstruction of the intrathoracic or extrathoracic trachea, *A*, extrathoracic variable obstruction, *B*, and intrathoracic variable obstruction, *C*. The schematic represents the relative pressure generated within and outside the trachea during the maneuver. (RV, residual volume; TLC, total lung capacity.) (From Benumof JL: Anesthesia for Thoracic Surgery, 2nd ed. Philadelphia, WB Saunders, 1995.)

lyzed for oxygen, CO_2 fraction, and anesthetic agents. Arterial cannulation is indicated for blood pressure measurement in patients in whom hemodynamic instability is anticipated or in those with respiratory compromise sufficient to warrant serial ABG analysis during or after the procedure. When rigid bronchoscopy is performed emergently to relieve airway obstruction, invasive monitoring may have to be secured after ventilation is established, airway management being the priority.

Before airway examination, the patient's eyes should be shielded from mechanical injury, contamination by washing fluids, and unpleasant stimulation from bright lights. When general anesthesia is used, the eyes should be taped shut. When the patient is sedated, the eyes may be covered with a soft towel. When rigid endoscopy is performed, scrupulous attention is paid to the protection of patient's teeth; a tooth guard may be used. Patients should be warned in advance of the potential for dental trauma, and any prior damage should be documented.

Fiberoptic Bronchoscopy

Patient Characteristics and Physiologic Effects

The flexible fiberoptic bronchoscope permits examination and biopsy of peripheral airway lesions. The patient's cervical spine remains in an anatomic position; significant pressure on airway structures is not required. There is less neurohumoral stress response than when rigid bronchoscopy is used. Nonetheless, myocardial ischemia may occur, particularly in older patients (Matot et al, 1997). Fiberoptic bronchoscopy is commonly performed using conscious sedation and application of topical anesthetic to the airway, both of which may contribute to a patient's inability to protect the airway from aspiration of stomach contents should regurgitation occur. All patients should therefore fast before all elective airway procedures. The flexible bronchoscope may be introduced via the nasal or oral route.

Fiberoptic bronchoscopy is not without deleterious physiologic effects. Matsushima and colleagues (1984) showed that sedated, spontaneously breathing patients had decreased forced expiratory volume (FEV_1) and increased FRC during flexible bronchoscopy and decreased arterial oxygen tension after the procedure. These investigations suggested that the changes in pulmonary mechanics were caused by the loss of 10% to 15% of the airway cross-section from the presence of the bronchoscope in the trachea.

The application of suction in the airway can predispose to atelectasis and increased work of breathing. Bronchospasm can be provoked by airway manipulation and compounded by bronchial edema. Supplemental oxygen should be applied and the patient should be recovered and weaned from oxygen during monitoring of peripheral oxygen saturation. Patients should be assessed clinically for signs of hypoventilation, and ABG analysis should be performed if indicated.

Anesthetic Techniques

Topical Anesthesia with Conscious Sedation

Benzodiazepines (midazolam, 0.05 mg/kg IV, lorazepam 1–2 mg SL) and parenteral opioids (fentanyl, 1–2 g/kg, demerol 0.5–1.0 mg/kg) are frequently used by endoscopists for conscious sedation for bronchoscopy, with the dose adjusted for the patient's age and physiologic condition. More infrequently, a low dose of ketamine (0.2–0.4 mg/kg) is used, but excessive salivation and hallucinations may occur. A sedative dose of propofol (50 μg/kg/min) is commonly administered by anesthesiologists when providing conscious sedation during airway examination.

Many practitioners advocate the use of an anticholinergic drug to minimize airway secretions. Glycopyrrolate has the advantage over atropine of not crossing the blood-brain barrier; hence, there is less tendency for confusion, particularly in older adults. Both drugs have comparable antisialogogic and hemodynamic effects and may be administered by the intramuscular (IM) or IV route (Gronnebech et al, 1993). The routine use of anticholinergic drugs has been questioned in one randomized study showing no benefit over placebo in the performance of flexible bronchoscopy (Cowl et al, 2000).

Local anesthetics may be applied to the airway through a number of techniques, with the purpose of blunting laryngeal and cough reflexes. Many procedures, including airway stent placement, may be accomplished using thorough topicalization alone (Coolen et al, 1994). Topical drug application may be accomplished by the use of an atomizer to direct spray to the mucosa of the larynx and trachea. Local anesthetic agents may be nebulized by means of oxygen flow of less than 6 L per minute. A spray of 30- to 60-μm droplets is produced that, when inhaled, is deposited in the airway to the trachea. Anesthesia of the trachea may be accomplished with a transtracheal injection or direct spray of local anesthetic via the suction port of the bronchoscope under direct vision. Airway topicalization may be supplemented with discrete nerve blocks. A multitude of nerves supply the nasopharynx and oropharynx (Sanchez et al, 1996). Typically, the glossopharyngeal and superior laryngeal nerves are blocked with the transoral or percutaneous approach.

Lidocaine is the most common choice of local anesthetic for bronchoscopy. Cocaine, benzocaine, and tetracaine are also used. Vigilant observation of the patient for signs of local anesthetic toxicity is essential; signs and symptoms of neuroexcitation (dizziness, restlessness, visual and auditory disturbances) precede seizure, coma, and cardiovascular collapse.

Treatment consists of cardiovascular and respiratory support until the local anesthetic diffuses from the sodium channels in cardiac and neural tissue. Systemic absorption of local anesthetic from the oropharyngeal mucosa is slow, but rapid absorption can take place in the conducting airways and alveoli. During airway topicalization, a considerable amount of local anesthetic may be swallowed; in the acidic environment of the stomach, absorption is reduced. It may be difficult to estimate the dose the patient has absorbed.

The maximum recommended doses of topical lidocaine is 5 mg/kg. My choice is to use lidocaine for topicalization of the oropharynx, whereas cocaine is used to anesthetize the nasopharynx when nasal intubation is required. Cocaine is applied with pledgets to the nasopharyngeal mucosa and is particularly useful for vasoconstriction of the nasal mucosa and prevention of epistaxis. The maximum recommended dose is 2 mg/kg.

General Anesthesia

Fiberoptic bronchoscopy is frequently performed in intubated patients under general anesthesia, particularly when combined with another procedure, such as mediastinoscopy or esophagoscopy. The flexible bronchoscope is introduced into the endotracheal tube via a swivel connector.

Most patients require assisted ventilation during prolonged flexible bronchoscopy via an endotracheal tube under general anesthesia. Placement of a 5.7-mm fiberoptic bronchoscope into an 8.0-mm endotracheal tube results in a reduction of cross-sectional area of more than 50%, increasing airway resistance manyfold. Although the authors of one study preferred the use of HFPPV over conventional ventilation, citing lower peak airway pressures and higher systemic arterial pressures with similar alveolar ventilation and oxygenation, seldom is this clinically necessary (Flatau et al, 1982). A large series of interventional fiberoptic bronchoscopy procedures was described using HFJV delivered via a 14-gauge intratracheal catheter. General anesthesia was used in only 82% of cases; the rest of the procedures were performed using airway topicalization. Moderate hypercapnia was common but not deleterious. The use of this technique for airway dilatation and expandable stent placement was thought to be a viable alternative to the use of the rigid bronchoscope (Hautmann et al, 2000).

Endotracheal intubation is not a requirement for flexible bronchoscopy with general anesthesia; masks specifically adapted to this purpose, with the inclusion of an endoscopy port, are available. This technique is most often used in small children in whom an endotracheal tube is of insufficient caliber to admit a bronchoscope. The *laryngeal mask airway* (LMA), first described in 1983, is increasingly used in the management of difficult airway problems. An elliptical inflatable mask is connected to a diagonally cut clear plastic airway. The mask is seated in the hypopharynx after induction of general anesthesia (Fig. 13–2), and neuromuscular blockade is rarely required (Brain, 1983). Propofol as a general anesthetic is particularly well suited to the insertion of the laryngeal mask, since airway reflexes are better suppressed than by barbiturates or inhalational agents. Spontaneous ventilation may be rapidly re-established. Inspection of the supraglottic, glottic, and infraglottic structures can be accomplished by insertion of a fiberoptic bronchoscope through the mask. Vocal cord function may be assessed in this way because neuromuscular relaxation is

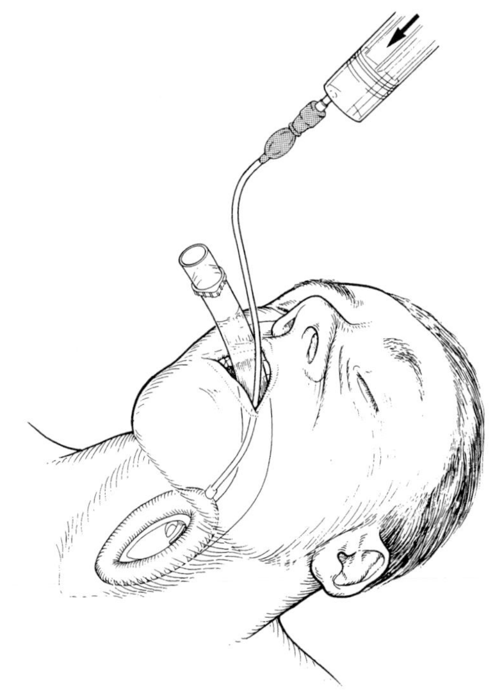

FIGURE 13–2 ■ Correct position of the laryngeal mask airway (LMA). (From Brain AI: The Laryngeal Mask Airway, instruction manual.)

not required. The larger diameter of the laryngeal mask airway permits bronchoscopy with little increase in airway resistance. Bronchoscopy is successfully performed during spontaneous ventilation (Ferson et al, 1997), CPAP (Brimacombe and Dunbar-Reid, 1996), and conventional IPPV (Dich-Nielsen and Nagel, 1993). The laryngeal mask airway offers no protection against pulmonary aspiration, however, and the patient may experience laryngospasm.

Rigid Bronchoscopy

Patient Characteristics and Physiologic Effects

The rigid bronchoscope is used for diagnostic purposes and is the instrument of choice for therapeutic interventions such as the dilatation of tracheal stenoses, resection of airway tumors, removal of foreign bodies, and control of bleeding. Airway stents or Montgomery T tubes may be placed for a variety of malacic and compressive airway pathologic processes (Cooper et al, 1989). Instrumentation of the upper respiratory tract results in a significant sympathoadrenal stress response (Tomori and Widdicombe, 1969). Increases in heart rate and both systemic pressure and pulmonary artery pressure (PAP) are seen and may be prolonged. Myocardial oxygen consumption rises, and dysrhythmias may occur. Patients presenting for rigid bronchoscopy frequently have lung cancer; many are elderly smokers with attendant risks of peripheral and coronary artery disease. The incidence of myocardial ischemia during and after rigid bronchoscopy may be as high as 10% to 15% (Hill et al, 1991).

The optimal patient head position to facilitate access to the trachea, for both rigid bronchoscopy and endotracheal intubation, probably varies from patient to patient. The first description of the "sniffing position" to facilitate rigid bronchoscopy is attributed to Chevalier Jackson (Jackson, 1913). Anterior flexion of the lower cervical spine and cervico-occipital extension is achieved by placement of a pillow under the supine patient's head. The conventional rationale that the alignment of three anatomic axes (oral, laryngeal, and pharyngeal) is achieved has been questioned by anatomic studies, which suggest that glottic visualization may be successful with simple head extension (Adnet et al, 2001) (Fig. 13–3). In my observations of many rigid bronchoscopies, I have noted that the bronchoscope at times can be easily inserted in the trachea with the patient's head in the sniffing position. More often, however, the glottis is located in the sniffing position, the pillow is then removed, and the neck is further extended for cannulation of the trachea.

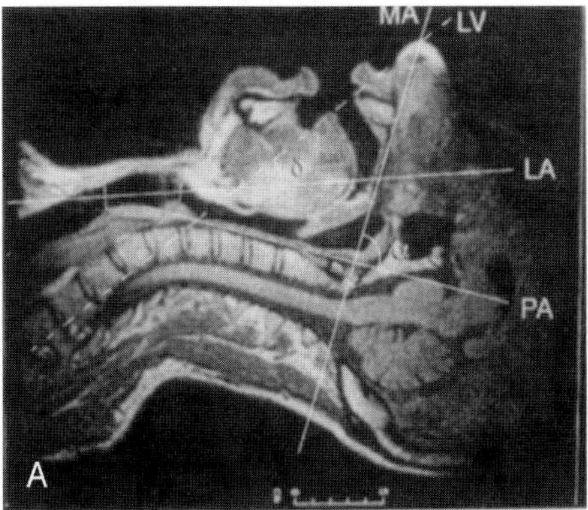

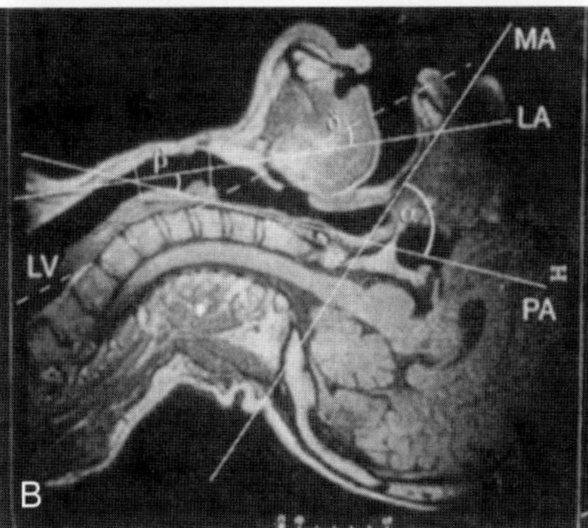

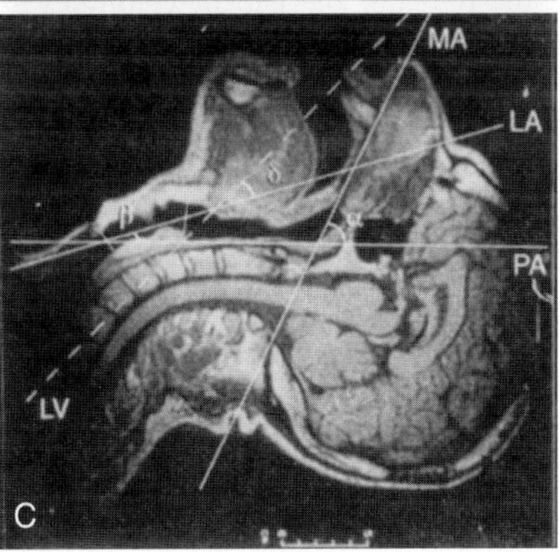

FIGURE 13–3 ■ Magnetic resonance images of three anatomic axes (mouth axis [MA], pharyngeal axis [PA], laryngeal axis [LA] and the line of vision [LV]) in three head positions: *A*, neutral, *B*, head extension, and *C*, the "sniffing position." (From Adnet F, Borron SW, Dumas JL et al: Study of the "sniffing position" by magnetic resonance imaging. Anesthesiology 94:83, 2001.)

Extensive cervical fusion or ankylosing spondylitis may preclude adequate positioning. Preoperatively, symptoms of cervical spine pathology should prompt a lateral neck radiograph in flexion and extension, as should a history of congenital or acquired disease that predisposes patients to cervical spine instability. Down syndrome and certain forms of dwarfism can cause hypoplasia of the odontoid process of C2 or laxity of the atlantoaxial ligament (Auden, 1999; Rehl, 1998).

Patients with rheumatoid arthritis may develop atlantoaxial (C1–C2) subluxation from the inflammatory erosion of the joints and ligaments that stabilize the odontoid. Atlantoaxial subluxation can result from neck flexion, extension, and rotation, depending on the distribution of joint destruction; less frequently, subaxial (below C2) subluxation may occur. In the worst-case scenario, acute subluxation may result in spinal cord and vertebral artery compression, causing quadriparesis or sudden death.

Cervical involvement in rheumatoid arthritis is common (affecting up to 86% of patients with long-standing disease) and may occur in the absence of signs or symptoms. A comprehensive review of the anatomic basis of rheumatoid cervical joint disease has been described by MacArthur and Kleinman (1993).

Anesthetic and Ventilation Techniques

Rigid bronchoscopy in an awake patient receiving local anesthesia alone is almost unheard of in modern practice. General anesthesia should provide an unconscious state, muscular relaxation, abolition of respiratory tract reflexes, and rapid recovery. The anatomy of the patient's airway influences the choice of induction technique. When the upper airway anatomy is essentially normal, an IV induction agent is given with a dose of neuromuscular relaxant and the ability to ventilate by mask is ensured.

In our practice, propofol is used almost exclusively for induction of anesthesia. The choice of neuromuscular relaxant is influenced by the duration of the procedure; when rapid or intermittent return of spontaneous ventilation is required, succinylcholine is given as a bolus, followed by an infusion titrated to effect. For longer procedures, one of the intermediate-acting muscle relaxants (rocuronium or vecuronium) is used. Direct laryngoscopy may be performed in order to spray the vocal cords with lidocaine, and this may reduce the incidence of laryngospasm on emergence. Formal topicalization of the oropharynx and trachea may further blunt the stress response. The rigid bronchoscope may then be inserted.

In the setting of airway compromise secondary to stricture, obstruction, or compression, an inhalation induction may be chosen; if insertion of the bronchoscope proves to be difficult, the patient continues to breathe spontaneously. The application of 100% oxygen by a tight-fitting mask results in an increased oxygen fraction (FIO_2) in FRC as nitrogen is washed out, providing an oxygen reserve if airway obstruction occurs. Preoxygenation is followed by inhalation induction with a volatile anesthetic in 100% oxygen via a slowly increasing concentration.

Sevoflurane is particularly well suited to this application. The patient continues to breathe spontaneously but may require some assistance. Gentle positive airway pressure may stent open collapsed airways and increase tidal volume. Depending on the minute ventilation and the induction agent used, an inhalation induction may require well over 20 minutes. When a deep plane of anesthesia is achieved, a local anesthetic may be applied to the upper airway before instrumentation. When airway patency is ensured by placement of the bronchoscope and successful ventilation, a muscle relaxant may be used. After surgical intervention the patient's airway patency is hopefully much improved.

Alternatively, even in the presence of significant airway obstruction, an IV induction may be chosen if it is thought that an airway can be rapidly established with a rigid bronchoscope. This approach depends on the immediate presence of an experienced bronchoscopist.

After preoxygenation, propofol is titrated to unconsciousness and IV succinylcholine is then given to allow rapid insertion of the bronchoscope. This approach may be required when a patient with imminent airway obstruction cannot tolerate inhalation induction. If the bronchoscope cannot be inserted, ventilation may be difficult and the risk of hypoxia or death is present. The decision to use this approach should be made by surgeon and anesthesiologist together. The patient and family should be informed of the risk if possible.

The choice of agent for maintenance of anesthesia depends on the ventilation technique during rigid bronchoscopy. The development of LFJV into the open rigid bronchoscope is outlined in the Historical Notes earlier. Alternatively, conventional anesthetic circuits may be connected to the side arm of the bronchoscope, which is wedged between the patient's vocal cords. When the aperture window is closed, positive pressure may be generated within the circuit. When side-arm ventilation is used, volatile anesthetic agents may be combined with nitrous oxide. Halothane, enflurane, and isoflurane have been used for many years. In a recent study of endoscopy in children, Meretoja and associates (1996) compared the use of sevoflurane–nitrous oxide and halothane–nitrous oxide. Children receiving sevoflurane experienced more rapid physiologic and psychomotor recovery, with fewer arrhythmias noted. It was concluded that sevoflurane is a superior anesthetic for this application. Gas leakage through the larynx about the bronchoscope can be reduced by the application of gentle pressure on the patient's throat; however, some contamination of the operating room environment is inevitable. High gas flows are required during side-arm ventilation, which consumes large quantities of anesthetic gases.

Continuous IV anesthesia is almost exclusively used in the author's practice, using propofol 50 to 250 μg/kg/min. Both side arm and LFJV are used. IV maintenance of anesthesia is most commonly used during jet ventilation techniques. The safety of IV anesthesia for rigid bronchoscopy has been established (Perrin et al, 1992). From the early days of rigid bronchoscopy, there has been discussion of the need for muscle relaxants and positive-pressure ventilation (PPV) versus the maintenance of spontaneous breathing (Kovacs, 1957). The debate continues to this day: One randomized study suggested that controlled negative pressure ventilation in paralyzed patients reduced the need for opioids and shortened recovery time compared with spontaneous assisted ventilation (Natalini et al, 1998).

In my opinion, the most compelling argument for the use of muscle relaxants is the facilitation of ventilation by whatever means. In particular, the use of jet ventilation and HFV is made safer when the patient cannot cough and the chest wall is compliant. Jet ventilation under any circumstance requires caution because barotrauma and pneumothorax are significant risks. An increase in volume flow through the jet generates a proportional rise in inflation pressure: A reduction of the cross-sectional area of the bronchoscope, with the jet left unchanged, produces an exponential increase in inflation pressure (Spoerel and Grant, 1971). LFJV ventilation should therefore be suspended when other instruments are placed within the bronchoscope. Because of the movement of airway structures when IPPV via the side arm or LFJV is used, patients are frequently hyperventilated with high oxygen fractions. The surgeon operates during periods of apnea. When high flow oxygen is applied to the bronchoscope side arm, some diffusion respiration occurs, during which moderate hypercapnia is well tolerated.

HFV has been adapted for use through the rigid bronchoscope. Small tidal volumes delivered at high frequency have the advantage of maintaining a relatively motionless field; HFV can be maintained throughout the procedure. The side arm of the Storz bronchoscope has a configuration that lends itself to the delivery of HFPPV using the pneumatic valve principle. Ventilation nomograms have been developed and were used extensively in one center (Borg et al, 1980). FRC was increased in contrast to awake, spontaneous ventilation (Eriksson and Sjostrand, 1980).

In one study of rigid bronchoscopy in patients with tracheal stenosis, HFJV was compared with LFJV (Vourc'h et al, 1983b). Operating conditions were deemed better with HFJV; however, gas exchange, which was stable with LFJV, deteriorated with use of the highest frequencies of HFJV.

Ironically, the use of a technique considered redundant in 1967 by Sanders—external ventilation using a body cuirass—has been combined with the HFO principle to create a new ventilation modality that has been applied in anesthetized, paralyzed patients undergoing rigid bronchoscopy. Of patients ventilated in this manner, 9% required interruption of the procedure for manual ventilation due to hypoxemia (Natalini et al, 2000). Negative-pressure ventilation techniques are not a common practice but are being investigated. The advantage to their use is that there are no ventilation attachments on the bronchoscope (Natalini et al, 1998, 2000).

After removal of the bronchoscope, patients may be reintubated with an endotracheal tube, or the airway can be maintained with a mask or laryngeal mask airway during emergence.

Attempts to attenuate the sympathoadrenal stress response to bronchoscopy have included the use of topical and IV lidocaine, α-adrenergic and β-adrenergic blockade, and the use of vasodilators—all with limited success. IV opiates, prior to induction with pentothal, suppress the hypertensive response and the increase in the rate-pressure product. Unfortunately, the doses of opiate required (fentanyl, 6 μg/kg or alfentanil 18 μg/kg) also produce prolonged respiratory depression, making this approach of limited utility for short procedures (Wark et al, 1986).

Induction of general anesthesia with propofol has since been shown to provide hemodynamic stability during bronchoscopy. The addition of alfentanil, 18 μg/kg, does not attenuate the stress response further (Hill et al, 1991). The ultra-short-acting narcotic remifentanil and the β-blocker esmolol are frequently used in our practice to control hypertension and tachycardia. Outcome studies of the use of these agents during bronchoscopy have yet to appear. Preoperative oral dosing of the α-blocking agent clonidine (300 μg) may attenuate tachycardia and hypertension during rigid bronchoscopy, but it is not widely used, probably because of concern that the sedating effects of clonidine might delay emergence and fitness for hospital discharge (Matot et al, 2000).

Suspension Laryngoscopy

Patient Characteristics and Physiologic Effects

Considerations for suspension laryngoscopy are similar to those for rigid bronchoscopy. Additionally, there may be obstructing or friable lesions in the patient's mouth or pharynx.

Anesthetic and Ventilation Techniques

Operative laryngoscopy can be performed around a small endotracheal tube; however, obstruction of the surgical field is inevitable. The open end of the suspension laryngoscope above the glottis precludes conventional positive-pressure ventilation. The high-flow ventilation techniques first proposed for rigid bronchoscopy have been applied extensively in microlaryngoscopic procedures; the use of jet ventilation improves visibility and access to the operative field. The patient may undergo an inhalational or IV induction. Supraglottic LFJV is accomplished by a Sanders injector connected to a small catheter (0.9–1.1 mm), aligned along the axis of the suspension laryngoscope (Spoerel and Greenway, 1973).

Gas entrainment results in significantly greater volumes delivered, as much as a 20-fold increase of the jet volume. Delivery of gas is critically dependent on alignment of the gas jet catheter along the axis of the glottic opening. As much as 50% of ventilated volume may be lost by poor catheter placement (Hunsaker, 1994). Ventilating laryngoscopes with built-in ventilation channels were devised soon thereafter (Oulton and Donald, 1971), most recently to accommodate multifrequency jet ventilation (Bacher et al, 2000b; Ihra et al, 1999). When supraglottic jet ventilation is used, blood and debris may be entrained into the trachea. Tracheal pressure and gas composition are difficult to monitor.

Subglottic jet ventilation is preferred by some; a long catheter of small diameter (2.5–4.0 mm) is inserted into the tracheal inlet, independent of the laryngoscope. Jet ventilation of a flexible tube in this position tends to cause whipping of the catheter in the trachea. Various means have been used to stabilize intratracheal ventilation tubes (Gillick, 1976). Long, narrow endotracheal tubes with a full-sized inflatable cuff were devised (Carden and Crutchfield, 1973) but can be difficult to insert, particularly in the presence of laryngeal pathology (El-Naggar et al, 1974). Complete egress of air must be carefully monitored with a cuffed tube to avoid overinflation of the lungs. Small-diameter subglottic tubes are not easily used to assist conventional ventilation of the wakening patient (Gillick, 1976) but continued HFV may be possible (Babinski et al, 1980). Ventilation catheters can be left in the glottis during emergence to retain access to the airway should the patient experience respiratory distress and need to be reanesthetized.

Most recently, a subglottic catheter was designed with a basket on its tip to prevent contact of the jet nozzle with the tracheal mucosa. A second lumen, which ends proximal to the jet nozzle, permits aspiration of airway gas for analysis (Brooker et al, 1998; Hunsaker, 1994). With intratracheal jet ventilation techniques, entrainment of gas and debris is decreased, permitting better prediction of the intratracheal oxygen fraction (Bacher et al, 2000a; Gillick, 1976).

HFV techniques result in improved oxygenation, probably by preservation of lung volumes by CPAP. Laryngoscopic HFPPV is delivered via an intratracheal insufflation catheter with multiple side holes at its tip; a continuous gas flow is directed through the larynx (Borg et al, 1980). When HFJV is applied via subglottic catheter, debris adhering to the larynx moves slowly in an oral direction (Baer, 2000). The continuous gas flow from HFV is proposed to remove smoke, debris, and blood from the airway, particularly when subglottic ventilation is used (Evans et al, 1994). The effect of CPAP to prevent entrainment, when HFV is delivered by a supraglottic route, remains unclear.

Combined frequency jet ventilation (simultaneous application of LFJV and HFJV) during laryngeal surgery has now been shown to result in better gas exchange than monofrequent LFJV or HFJV, particularly when supraglottic delivery is used (Bacher et al, 2000a, 2000b). Of particular interest is the calculation of the degree of gas entrainment by measurement of the oxygen fraction delivered by the ventilator and the resulting oxygen fraction in the trachea for each mode of ventilation:

- ~ 10% of ventilated gas entrained during subglottic LFJV
- ~ 8.5% during subglottic combined-frequency ventilation
- ~ 55% during supraglottic combined-frequency ventilation

Gas entrainment presumably reflects the potential contamination of the airway by entrainment of blood and debris.

The accuracy of airway pressure monitoring during supraglottic or subglottic jet ventilation remains the subject of considerable concern. A stable pressure signal cannot be picked up near a jet nozzle; it is likely that pressure catheters positioned well into the trachea are required (Bacher et al, 2000b; Baer, 2000; Ihra and Aloy, 2000). Continuous monitoring of gas composition and end-tidal carbon dioxide remains problematic, and accuracy is dependent on the configuration of the ventilation device, gas sampling site, and respiratory pattern (Bacher et al, 2000b; Baer et al, 1995). ABG analysis remains the "gold standard" for the adequacy of ventilation.

During direct laryngoscopy, maintenance of anesthesia with an IV technique is most commonly used. Profound neuromuscular blockade is used to avoid coughing during high-flow ventilation; doses of relaxants for blockade of the larynx and diaphragm must be larger than doses needed for other skeletal muscles. The laryngeal muscles, therefore, recover more quickly than the forearm, a traditional monitoring site. The use of muscle relaxants and monitoring of the resulting blockade have been systematically studied during direct laryngoscopy. Baer (1984) advocated the use of continuous monitoring of the airway pressure curve to reflect recovery of laryngeal muscle function in order to avoid patient injury from barotrauma.

Succinylcholine produces a more intense block in laryngeal muscles in a shorter time compared with nondepolarizing vecuronium, rocuronium, mivacurium, and rapacuronium (Goulden and Hunter, 1999). In a recent cost analysis (Puura et al, 1999), succinylcholine infusion had the most rapid onset, was associated with the least time spent waiting for the return of neuromuscular function, and incurred the lowest expense of relaxant regimens studied for use during endolaryngeal procedures. Of nondepolarizing drugs, the short-acting agent mivacurium caused the least delay and, despite the apparent high cost of the drug, was more economical than any of the relaxants of intermediate duration. Atracurium, vecuronium, and rocuronium each cost more because of the prolonged recovery time.

Endotracheal Laser Surgery

Suspension Laryngoscopy or Bronchoscopy

Laser resection may be used in patients with benign pharyngeal, tracheal, or bronchial strictures or for palliation of airway tumors. In our institution, the CO_2 laser is used primarily for glottic airway lesions during suspension laryngoscopy. The neodymium-yttrium-aluminum-garnet (Nd-YAG) laser is used for tracheal and bronchial diseases. Numerous reviews of laser safety are available (Dumon et al, 1984; Shapshay and Beamis, 1986). Eye protection for the patient and surgical team is essential.

Limitation of combustible material and gas mixtures in the airway during the application of laser pulses is fundamental. Oxygen and nitrous oxide are combustible, and the use of an air-oxygen gas mixture with limitation of oxygen fraction to less that 30% is suggested (Baer et al, 1995). For laser use during direct laryngoscopy, rubber endotracheal tubes wrapped with reflective metal foil have been used. To provide laser resistance, the cuff is filled with water rather than air. Wrapped endotracheal tubes are of relatively large diameter and limit exposure of the larynx. Small-diameter, laser-resistant, cuffed endotracheal tubes (silicone-, foil-, and fluoroplastic-wrapped, metal) and subglottic ventilation catheters (fluoroplastic, metal) are commercially available for delivery of both conventional and HFV. Only metallic devices are truly incombustible. The risk of ignition of laser-resistant tubes is much greater with the Nd-YAG laser (Sosis, 1996).

The Nd-YAG laser is conducted through a fiberoptic filament, which enables access to peripheral airway lesions. Many surgeons have adopted a combination of rigid and fiberoptic bronchoscopy (Conacher et al, 1998; Medici et al, 1999). The use of a rigid bronchoscope permits mechanical débridement and rapid response in the case of hemorrhage, which can be a lethal complication (Dumon et al, 1984). The flexible bronchoscope, inserted through the rigid scope, allows access to peripheral lesions. The laser filament is inserted through the suction port of the flexible bronchoscope, and the resection can thus be viewed (Fig. 13–4). Ventilation is delivered via the side arm of the bronchoscope; conventional side-arm ventilation, LFJV, and high-frequency techniques have been described. Insertion of flexible fiberoptic bronchoscope via the laryngeal mask airway can facilitate Nd-YAG laser resection of obstructive tumors of the subglottis (Jameson et al, 2000), high trachea (Divatia et al, 1994), and carina (Slinger et al, 1992).

The technique of anesthetic induction is based on the degree and site of airway obstruction. The use of neuromuscular blockade is essential during laser pulses because misdirection of the beam can cause serious injury. Patients who undergo resection of tumor are usually

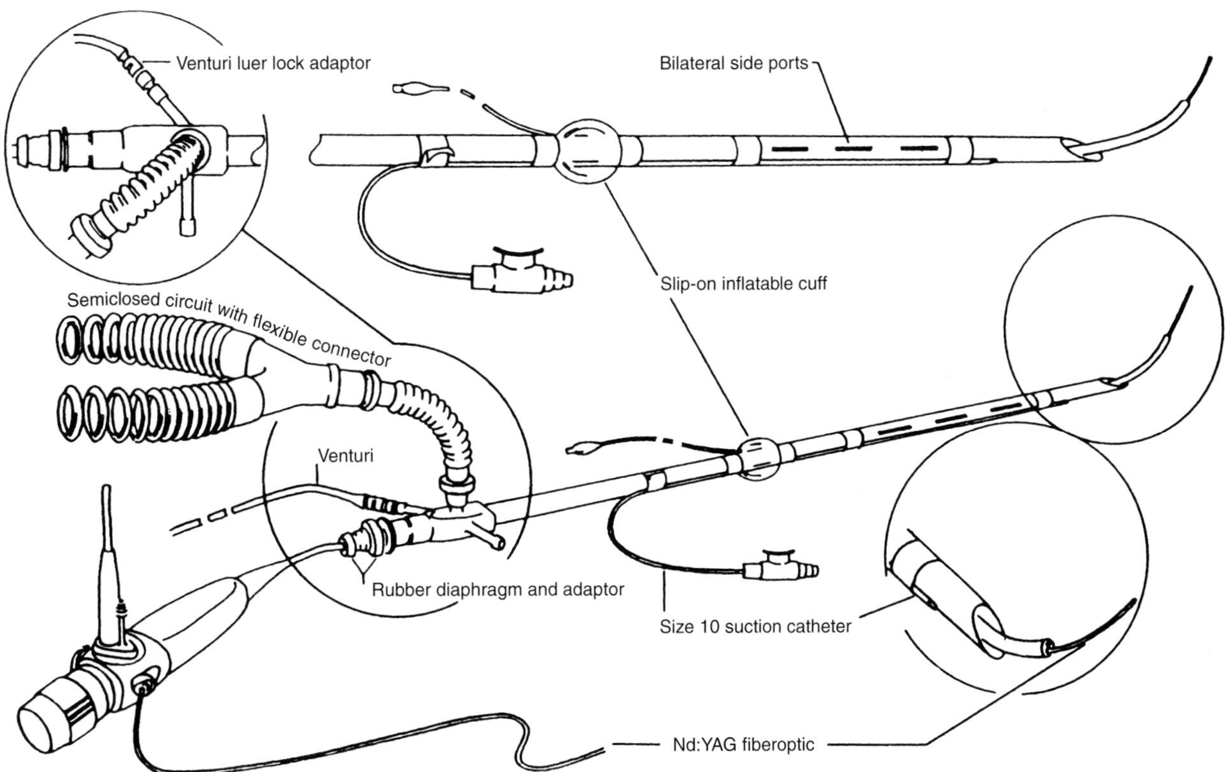

FIGURE 13–4 ■ Apparatus for laser resection by combined use of fiberoptic and rigid bronchoscopes. (From Perera ER, Mallon JS: General anaesthetic management for laser resection of central airway lesions in 85 procedures. Can J Anaesth 34:383, 1987.)

in a palliative phase of treatment, and many are debilitated with significant respiratory compromise.

A major source of morbidity is hypoxemia, both from airway obstruction and postoperatively from retained secretions, blood, and tumor debris. In the past, anesthetic induced respiratory depression was cited as a significant contributing factor to hypoxemia (Dumon et al, 1984); the use of short-acting general anesthetic agents is indicated to optimize return of spontaneous ventilation and recovery of airway function. An arterial line for sequential ABG analysis is indicated in all but the simplest resections and may be particularly useful during the postoperative phase. Improvement of respiratory status is expected after resection of major obstructing lesions (Conacher et al, 1998).

Retrospective reviews of anesthetic technique during laser airway resection comparing the use of inhalational anesthesia with conventional IPPV via side arm of the bronchoscope, versus total IV anesthesia with LFJV, have produced conflicting recommendations. Duckett and associates (1985) found increased periods of hypercapnia with side arm ventilation, whereas Perera and Mallon (1987) reported fewer. The increase in postoperative respiratory complications, including delayed extubation, postextubation stridor, and reintubation in patients receiving IV anesthesia, can be attributed to the use of a now redundant barbiturate technique (Perera and Mallon, 1987).

Vourc'h (1983) recommended the use of LFJV via the rigid bronchoscope during resection of endobronchial lesions and the use of HFJV when the bronchoscope remained within the trachea. In a report of laser resection of endobronchial tumors, prevention of soiling of the nonoperative lung was attributed to the use of HFPPV via a multiport endobronchial catheter, independent of the rigid bronchoscope (Medici et al, 1999). HFPPV through side holes generates an upward stream, which may prevent aspiration of smoke and debris and clear the field of laser smoke. In all series, periods of desaturation and hypercapnia were common, emphasizing the need for vigilance during these procedures.

Removal of Foreign Bodies

Patients who present with a foreign body in the airway are often young children or adults with a decreased ability to reason because of intoxication or psychiatric illness. The patient may be acutely dyspneic and uncomfortable. In many cases the patient has recently eaten, and aspiration of stomach contents during the procedure is a significant concern. Spontaneous ventilation should be maintained until the foreign body is removed. Positive pressure may induce a ball-valve effect or might dislodge the object distally, into a less accessible part the airway tree, or proximally, causing complete airway obstruction. These patients present a significant dilemma to the anesthesiologist, in that an inhalational induction is required in a patient who has a full stomach and thus an increased risk of aspiration. One survey of pediatric anesthesiologists revealed that most would perform an inhalation induction without the application of cricoid pressure (Kain et al, 1994).

Anesthesia for Tracheal Resection and Reconstruction

TRACHEOSTOMY

Tracheostomy is the most common incision of the airway. The anesthetic management of the patient greatly depends on the clinical circumstances of the procedure. Chevalier Jackson (1950) wrote

> Tracheostomy is too often postponed until it becomes an emergency, and often a desperate emergency. The patient is often exhausted in his fight for air, the respiratory centers are so fatigued by the prolonged high carbon dioxide tension that respiratory movements are ceasing. After they stop, the heart muscle may quit for want of its oxygen supply; at best it will continue functioning but three minutes. The patient's appearance is ghastly . . . a general anesthetic would be promptly fatal.

Emergency tracheostomy is required in patients with rapidly expanding laryngotracheal tumors, epiglottitis, hemorrhage from recent cervical surgery, submandibular cellulitis (Ludwig's angina), or trauma obstructing the airway. Awake, fiberoptic intubation after topical application of a local anesthetic agent to the airway may prove impossible or may result in further airway compromise.

Tracheostomy is performed with the patient awake and with the use of a local anesthetic by the surgeon. The patient is kept in a sitting position, with assisted delivery of 100% oxygen by mask to optimize failing gas exchange. A patient in extremis often has little recollection of the procedure. Hypercapnia probably contributes to a decreased level of consciousness.

After the airway has been surgically established and ventilation resumes, the patient may be given an amnesic drug. When tracheostomy is performed with the patient awake and prior to the occurrence of critical airway obstruction, reassurance and cautious sedation may be provided to the patient. Anxiolytic drugs should be supplemented with the judicious use of an analgesic drug, usually an IV opiate. Cautious sedation may improve gas exchange in an anxious patient; a quieter breathing pattern produces less turbulent flow in the airway, thereby decreasing resistance.

Tracheostomy may be performed after the induction of general anaesthesia and placement of an endotracheal tube. Depending on the difficulty presented by the patient's airway anatomy, intubation may have been accomplished (1) with the patient awake after airway topicalization by a flexible fiberoptic bronchoscope or via direct laryngoscopy, (2) after inhalation induction with a volatile agent, or (3) after IV induction using muscle relaxants. Elective tracheotomy is routinely performed before laryngectomy and major head and neck resection and reconstruction.

Tracheostomy is commonly performed in patients with anticipated prolonged weaning from mechanical ventilation to optimize pulmonary toilet and to decrease airway resistance and dead space. A tracheotomy tube is more comfortable than an orotracheal tube. A variety of anesthetic techniques can be used, with or without the use of muscle relaxants. When neck dissection is performed and the surgeon is ready to incise the trachea, the endotracheal tube cuff is deflated to decrease the risk of rupture.

After tracheal incision, the endotracheal tube is withdrawn under direct vision and the tracheotomy tube is inserted. Because of the need for short periods of apnea with the airway open, performance of tracheostomy on patients dependent on maximal ventilator settings or very high PEEP is not recommended. Usually, a cuffed tracheotomy tube is placed, secured with sutures or tied about the patient's neck. Positive-pressure ventilation may be resumed or, if the patient's pulmonary status permits, spontaneous ventilation may be possible after emergence from anesthesia. At the time of induction of subsequent anesthetic agents, the breathing circuit easily connects to the tracheotomy tube. Ventilatory management of the patient when a Montgomery T tube has been placed via a tracheotomy is discussed later in this chapter.

HISTORICAL NOTE

From the very beginning of tracheal surgery, the greatest challenge facing the anesthesiologist has been how to ventilate the patient adequately before and during airway resection. Collaboration between anesthesia and surgical colleagues was required.

Early reports of tracheal tumor resection by Belsey (1950) described reconstruction of the trachea after the surgeon advanced the intratracheal tube beyond the tracheal defect. A wire coil was constructed over the cuff of the intratracheal tube. A free graft of fascia covered the wire skeleton, and the intratracheal tube was withdrawn.

In 1957, Barclay and colleagues reported on the carinal resection of a low tracheal tumor with the use of cross-field intubation and ventilation of the left bronchus while the right mainstem bronchus was sutured to the remaining trachea (Fig. 13–5). Ventilation was then resumed via the tracheal tube, and left bronchial anastomosis was performed.

In 1963, Grillo and coworkers described the performance of a similar procedure under critical circumstances in which tracheal obstruction had progressed to severe dyspnea and pulmonary hyperinflation. During cross-field ventilation of the left lung, the right pulmonary artery was clamped so that the unventilated lung was not perfused. Elimination of shunt maintained "the best possible tissue oxygenation," permitting an unhurried reconstruction. "The operative requirement for complete anesthetic control during all phases of tracheal surgery is met by the technic of transitory physiologic pneumonectomy" (Grillo, 1963).

Geffin and associates reported the anesthetic management of Grillo's first 31 cases to undergo tracheal resection and reconstruction (Geffin et al, 1969). The problems of anesthetic induction and control of the airway were fully described. Prolonged incision and complex reconstruction of the airway in patients with even more compromise of pulmonary function have demanded further innovation on the part of anesthesiologists and surgeons. A spectrum of ventilation strategies have been used, not only to maintain ventilation but to optimize

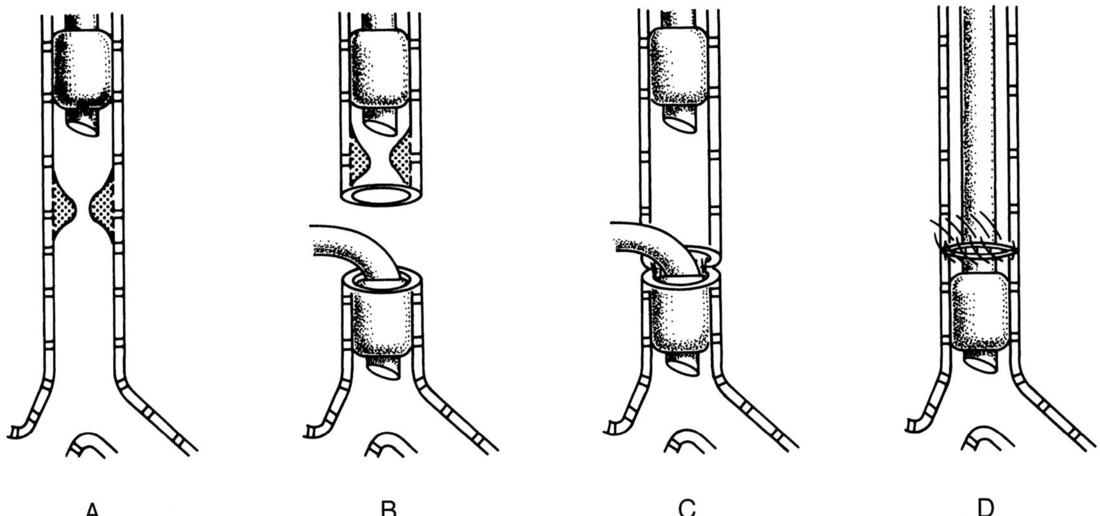

FIGURE 13–5 ■ Airway management for resection of a high tracheal lesion using intermittent positive-pressure ventilation. *A*, Initial intubation above the lesion. *B*, A sterile cross-field endotracheal tube is placed distal to the lesion once the airway has been incised. *C*, Suturing of the posterior wall of the anastomosis. *D*, The cross-field endotracheal tube is removed, the original tube is advanced across the anastomosis, and the anterior repair is completed. (From Benumof ER: Anesthesia for Thoracic Surgery, 2nd ed. Philadelphia, WB Saunders, 1995.)

operating conditions. Evidence of the success of this evolving collaboration lies in the large series of successful procedures reported.

■ *HISTORICAL READINGS*

Barclay RS, McSwan N, Welsh TH: Tracheal reconstruction without the use of grafts. Thorax 12:177, 1957.

Belsey R: Resection and reconstruction of the intrathoracic trachea. Br J Surg 38:200, 1950.

Geffin B, Bland J, Grillo HC: Anesthetic management of tracheal resection and reconstruction. Anesth Analg 48:884, 1969.

Grillo HC, Bendixen HH, Gephart T: Resection of the carina and lower trachea. Ann Surg 158:889, 1963.

TRACHEAL RESECTION

Preoperative Assessment

A complete radiologic assessment should define the tracheal lesion. Preoperatively, surgeons and anesthesiologists should be familiar with findings from the chest radiograph and other modalities. A CT scan of the neck and thorax is usually available. Increasingly, three-dimensional (3D) images are being constructed from helical CT data. Pulmonary function tests, including spirometry and flow-volumes loops, should be performed unless the patient is at risk of imminent airway obstruction (see Fig. 13–1).

The surgical approach to tracheal resection depends on the site and extent of the lesion. A cervical incision may be made with relatively little tissue trespass, extension into the thorax via sternotomy, or full posterolateral right thoracotomy if access to midtracheal and carinal lesions is required (Grillo, 1969).

When thoracotomy is planned, provision should be made for effective postoperative analgesia. The use of regional analgesia is ideal when a short-acting general anesthetic is used to optimize prompt extubation. Manipulation of airway and mediastinal structures intraoperatively may provoke significant stress response or arrhythmias. A preoperative electrocardiogram (ECG) should be obtained in all patients to assess cardiac rhythm. Patients over 40 years of age with symptoms or significant risk factors for coronary artery disease should undergo echocardiography, persantine thallium stress testing, and coronary angiography if indicated. Risk stratification is then possible, with institution of antianginal medication when appropriate.

Cardiac assessment is recommended when carinal resection with pneumonectomy is anticipated (Dartevelle and Macchiarini, 1996). If hemodynamically significant coronary artery lesions are identified, the decision to proceed with surgery should be made on a case-by-case basis. The use of perioperative β-blockade confers survival benefit in patients at high risk for coronary artery disease (Palda and Detsky, 1997). No data, however, exist that are specific to thoracic surgical patients, in whom obstructive pulmonary disease may preclude the use of β-blockers.

Identification and treatment of reversible pulmonary disease are warranted. Airway stenting may permit a period of medical optimization of the patient (Licker et al, 1997). Smoking cessation is vital. Postoperative mechanical ventilation is undesirable; the presence of an endotracheal tube may predispose new suture lines to ischemia, necrosis, and dehiscence. Severe respiratory compromise caused by parenchymal lung disease or neuromuscular disorder is a serious concern and may preclude tracheal resection (Pinsonneault et al, 1999).

Patient Monitoring

For continuous blood pressure monitoring, an arterial catheter should be placed, usually in the left radial artery.

The innominate artery lies anterior to the trachea; compression or division of this vessel renders inaccurate arterial measurement in the right arm. Arterial cannulation also provides immediate access for ABG analysis, which is essential during complex resections or in the event of postoperative respiratory distress. Central venous or pulmonary artery catheterization should be used as indicated by the patient's cardiopulmonary status. Avoidance of the area of incision must be considered in their placement; a jugular, subclavian, or antecubital approach may be used. A urinary catheter is usually placed. The patient's temperature is monitored and maintained. In the unusual case of cervical exenteration, in which elective division of the innominate artery is contemplated, electroencephalographic monitoring has been recommended (Grillo and Mathisen, 1990).

Anesthesia and Ventilation Techniques

Careful questioning of the patient may reveal a position-dependent increase in airway obstruction, particularly intolerance to lying supine. Induction of anesthesia may be performed with the patient sitting. Any difficulty encountered at previous intubation or bronchoscopy should be communicated to the team. A clear, coordinated plan is required. In many cases, induction of anethesia is followed by rigid bronchoscopy for dilatation of tracheal stenosis or by débridement of tumor prior to placement of an orotracheal tube.

A variety of anesthetic regimens have been used, including inhalational induction with volatile anesthetics and IV induction agents with and without the use of neuromuscular relaxants (Pinsonneault et al, 1999). In the setting of airway compromise, careful preoxygenation, followed by inhalation induction with a volatile anesthetic in 100% oxygen using a slowly increasing concentration, is recommended. When a deep plane of anesthesia is achieved, a local anesthetic (often lidocaine) is applied to the vocal cords and upper airway before instrumentation.

If the tracheal anatomy has already been fully defined and rigid bronchoscopy is not required, awake intubation of the trachea is an option. The patient receives sedation, and a topical anesthetic is applied to the airway. The patient is intubated with a small orotracheal tube, preferably under the guidance of fiberoptic bronchoscope. Once the ability to deliver positive-pressure ventilation is confirmed, the patient may then receive a general anesthetic.

The ideal endotracheal tube for tracheal reconstruction is a long, flexible, reinforced tube with a short, low-pressure, high-volume cuff and with a short segment beyond the cuff. These features allow manipulation of the tube without kinking and ventilation of both lungs through a short tracheal stump without encroachment on the operative site (Hannallah, 1995).

With the tracheal obstruction bypassed and positive-pressure ventilation now possible, a dose of muscle relaxant is usually given and ventilation is provided during the period of open airway. A spectrum of ventilation techniques are described next.

Distal Tracheal Intubation, Intermittent Positive-Pressure Ventilation

Early reports of tracheal tumor resection described reconstruction of the trachea after an intratracheal tube was advanced by the surgeon beyond the tracheal defect (Belsey, 1950). Advancement of the orotracheal tube across the surgical field into the distal trachea or bronchus is an option now seldom used, because a full-sized endotracheal tube obstructs access to the surgical field. An exception is the patient with airway trauma and tracheoesophageal fistula, in whom a defect in the trachea exists prior to the induction of anesthesia (see later).

The use of "cross-field" intubation and ventilation of the distal airway was first described for the resection of a low tracheal tumor (Barclay et al, 1957). Geffin and colleagues (1969) fully described the variations of cross-field ventilation to be used for high and low tracheal lesions. An orotracheal tube is placed above the lesion. As the airway is divided, the surgeon advances a second, sterile endotracheal tube across the field into the distal trachea (see Fig. 13–5).

In our institution, when subglottic resection is performed, a reinforced endotracheal tube is inserted in the distal trachea, is passed under the sterile drapes lateral to the patient's face, and is connected to the anaesthetic circuit. Lower tracheal resection may necessitate the use of a second, sterile anaesthetic circuit originating from the surgical field.

After reanastomosis of the posterior trachea, the distal tube is withdrawn and the orotracheal tube is advanced and used for ventilation. Lower tracheal and carinal resection require some modification of the technique (Figs. 13–6 and 13–7). The distal tube is advanced into the left mainstem bronchus below the lesion. The resected trachea and the right mainstem bronchus are anastomosed, the orotracheal tube is advanced across the suture line, and one-lung ventilation of the right lung is accomplished while the left mainstem bronchus is anastomosed to the side of the trachea. The orotracheal tube is then withdrawn above both suture lines until extubation.

This technique necessitates intermittent periods of apnea as surgeons withdraw the distal tracheal tube for better exposure and placement of sutures. Increased oxygen concentration is used when ventilating (>70%) in order to delay desaturation. Periods of moderate hypercapnia are inevitable. Independent distal cannulation of both bronchi has been described. A variety of endotracheal tubes of different sizes should be available for distal cannulation (Theman et al, 1976).

Jet Ventilation and High-Frequency Ventilation

LFJV with intermittent apnea was first described for tracheal resection in the 1970s (Ellis et al, 1976; Lee and English, 1974). A variation of this technique is still favored by some groups (McClish et al, 1985). The use of a narrow, long catheter permits ventilation of the distal airway using a device well away from the surgical field, and the small diameter is unlikely to obstruct surgical access to the airway. The ultimate catheter position varies with the procedure performed. A high tracheal stenosis may not admit a regular-sized endotracheal tube. Jet ven-

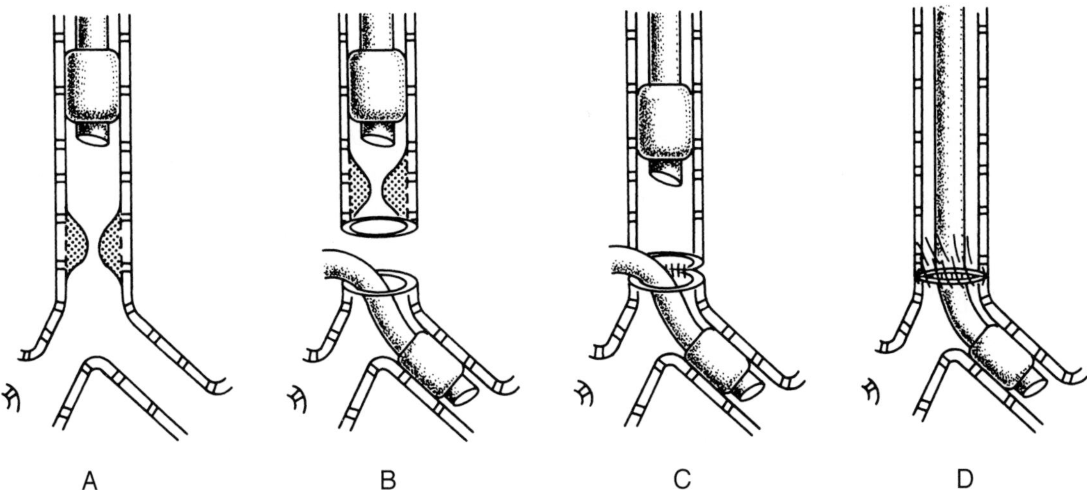

FIGURE 13–6 ■ Airway management for resection of a low tracheal lesion using intermittent positive-pressure ventilation. *A,* Initial intubation above the lesion. *B,* A sterile cross-field left endobronchial tube is placed distal to the lesion once the airway has been incised. *C,* Suturing of the posterior wall of the anastomosis. *D,* The cross-field endobronchial tube is removed, the original tube is advanced across the anastomosis into an endobronchial position, the anterior repair is completed. Geffin's original representation included snaring of the right pulmonary artery during *B* and *C* to diminish shunt during one-lung ventilation. (From Benumof ER: Anesthesia for Thoracic Surgery, 2nd ed. Philadelphia, WB Saunders, 1995.)

tilation via a long small orotracheal tube has been used throughout such resections (Baraka, 1977; Baraka et al, 1986). More often, an orotracheal tube is placed above the tracheal lesion and the narrow ventilation catheter is advanced into the distal airway after incision of the trachea. Distal LFJV of both lungs is used during tracheal resection (Ellis et al, 1976; Lee and English, 1974).

The use of independent, simultaneous catheter ventilation of each bronchus has been described in carinal resection (Clarkson and Davies, 1978). Unpredictable tidal volumes are generated using LFJV; however, they are sufficiently large to cause movement of the surgical field. Intermittent apnea is usually required. When high driving pressure (50–60 psi) is used through a narrow catheter, a high flow jet is produced (up to 100 L/min), entraining air, blood, and debris from the field into the distal airway. Blood may spray from the surgical field. When larger ventilation catheters are used, high flows can be maintained with lower driving pressure and air entrainment is reduced, permitting less dilution of the oxygen jet as demonstrated by the high arterial oxygen tensions that can be achieved. Longer periods of apnea are therefore possible (McClish et al, 1985).

HFV has been assessed in the setting of airway resec-

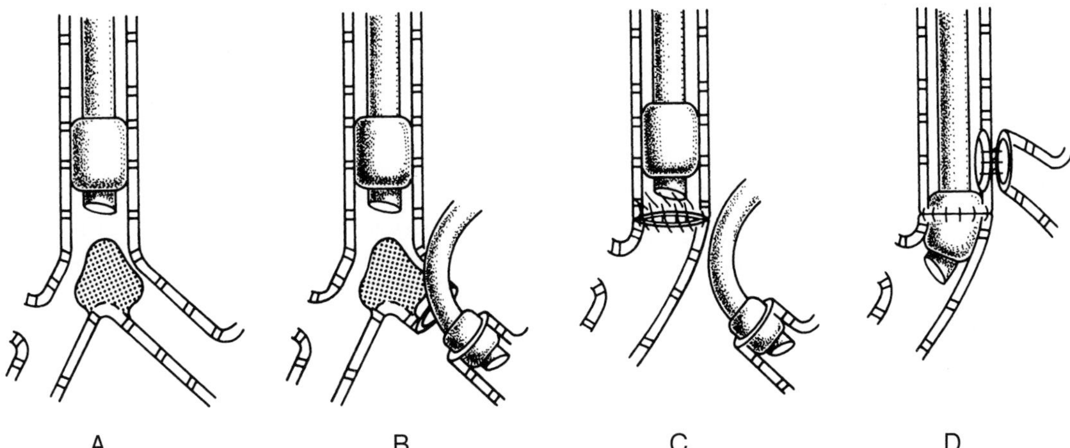

FIGURE 13–7 ■ Airway management for resection of a carinal lesion using intermittent positive-pressure ventilation. *A,* Initial intubation above the lesion. *B,* A sterile cross-field left endobronchial tube is placed after the left mainstem bronchus has been incised. *C,* The trachea is anastomosed to the unventilated right main bronchus. *D,* The cross-field endobronchial tube is removed, the original tube is advanced across the anastomosis into a right endobronchial position during anastomosis of the left mainstem bronchus to the trachea. Geffin's original representation included snaring of the right pulmonary artery during *B* and *C* to diminish shunt during one-lung ventilation. (From Benumof ER: Anesthesia for Thoracic Surgery, 2nd ed. Philadelphia, WB Saunders, 1995.)

tion. An obvious advantage is the lower peak airway pressures generated with HFV, compared with conventional IPPV, which permits ventilation with an open airway without a large air leak. The use of low tidal volumes at high respiratory rates offers the advantage of minimal movement of the operative field, and interruption of ventilation is not required during many procedures.

In the intensive care unit, *HFJV* is delivered via a narrow ventilating catheter advanced through an orotracheal tube. The optimal position of the catheter tip is the subject of considerable debate (Froese and Bryan, 1987). During airway surgery, a narrow ventilating catheter may be advanced across a stenosis or surgically created defect; the catheter position is therefore further influenced by the nature of the procedure. The catheter is positioned in the distal trachea for resection of a stenotic tracheal segment (Magnusson et al, 1997) and in the distal bronchus for sleeve resection (Watanabe et al, 1988). Bilateral bronchial catheters have been reported in carinal resection when desaturation occurred during HFJV of one lung (Perera, 1993).

All reports emphasize that ventilator frequency and driving pressure must be adjusted to the patient's respiratory compliance and the proportion of lung segments being ventilated. Although bilateral bronchial ventilation has been recommended for patients with decreased pulmonary reserve, improved oxygenation may be achieved using minimal driving pressure on the operative lung, minimizing lung inflation and impairment of surgical field (Perera et al, 1993).

Eriksson and colleagues (1975) first described tracheal resection via *HFPPV*, with gas delivery using the pneumatic valve principle during bronchoscopic examination of the lesion and via a 5-mm diameter insufflation catheter threaded into the distal trachea during resection and anastomosis. An injection catheter with multiple side holes was recommended to increase turbulence, thereby reducing injection jet effect.

El-Baz and coauthors (1982a) described the use of HFPPV during complex tracheal reconstruction using a 2-mm insufflation catheter via a Montgomery T tube. HFPPV via the same type of catheter inserted down the endotracheal tube and across the resected airway during sleeve resection and carinal resection was further reported (El Baz et al, 1981, 1982b). Excellent surgical conditions, with minimal motion of the field, and uninterrupted access to the circumference of the anastomosis were described. Continuous outflow of gas through the open bronchus was felt to minimize soiling with blood. Placement of a sterile ventilation catheter in the distal airway across the surgical field has also been used to deliver HFPPV (Young-Beyer and Wilson, 1988).

Only one report of the use of *HFO* during airway resection was found. Changes of large airway diameter were observed during HFO using relatively large tidal volumes and low frequency for this technique (1.6 ml/kg at 3 Hz). No comment was made on the adequacy of gas exchange during attempted airway resection. HFO is dependent on active injection and withdrawal of gas from a lung suspended in inflation by CPAP. It is unlikely that this strategy can be maintained in the presence of a proximal airway opening. HFO is therefore unsuited to surgery of the conducting airways but has been used successfully in peripheral lung resection (Glenski et al, 1986).

Extraordinary Ventilation Strategies

Extracorporeal Circulation

Cardiopulmonary bypass (CPB) without circulatory arrest was first used for resection of a carinal tumor in 1959 (Woods et al, 1961), followed by reports of small series in both adults (Neville, 1965) and children (Louhimo, 1987). Then as now, systemic anticoagulation required for CPB may introduce formidable problems, notably intrapulmonary hemorrhage (Geffin et al, 1969).

Today CPB is considered only under specific circumstances:

1. Tracheoplasty of long segments in small children in whom small airway caliber precludes other options (Benca et al, 1988).
2. Combined cardiac and pulmonary procedures (Ernst et al, 1999).
3. Repair of complex tracheobronchial injuries (Symbas et al, 1992).
4. When tracheal occlusion is imminent by a lesion that is unlikely to be bypassed by tracheotomy or rigid bronchoscopy (Wilson et al, 1984).

The practice of having a perfusionist and CPB pump at hand during elective complex airway resections can thus be justified. Extracorporeal membrane oxygenation (ECHO) has been successfully used to support small children throughout the preoperative period (Angel et al, 2000).

Hyperbaric Oxygenation

The use of hyperbaric oxygenation may supplement differential lung ventilation by conventional and HFV modes when these methods fail in the repair of a large tracheal tear (Ratzenhofer-Komenda et al, 2000). Hyperbaric conditions enhance oxygen delivery via increased oxygen dissolved in the plasma. This approach requires the performance of surgery within a hyperbaric chamber with compression of the entire surgical team and must be considered experimental.

Spontaneous Ventilation

A departure from the use of general anesthesia with neuromuscular relaxation involves case reports of a small number of patients allowed to breathe spontaneously throughout tracheal resection (Vyas et al, 1983) and tracheoesophageal (TE) fistula repair (Joynt et al, 1996; Pittoni et al, 1993). IV anesthesia was provided to these patients with endotracheal oxygen insufflation. Some aspiration of blood and debris from the surgical field was noted. The reported patients were well oxygenated and stable despite moderate respiratory acidosis; however, it is unlikely that patients with significant limitation of pulmonary reserve would tolerate this approach.

Reconstruction of the Airway

When the airway is open, the surgeon is able to manipulate the endotracheal tube; to easily retrieve the distal tip, the surgeon may affix a suture to the Murphy eye. The endotracheal tube may be replaced during the procedure should it be damaged; after removal of the proximal connector, the tube with pilot balloon is passed retrograde through the trachea into the oropharynx, where it is retrieved by the anesthesiologist. During airway reconstruction, the use of long, uncut polyvinyl chloride endotracheal tubes is recommended to permit positioning distal to surgical anastomoses. When the airway is closed, conventional positive-pressure ventilation through the orotracheal tube is resumed.

A Montgomery T tube may be left in the trachea, in which case the surgeon fits a small (usually 6.0-mm) endotracheal tube into the proximal limb. This press fit permits positive-pressure ventilation until emergence, when the endotracheal tube is removed by steady traction while the surgeon maintains the position of the T tube with a clamp on the cervical arm. Head flexion delivers the cervical trachea into the mediastinum. When surgery significantly shortens the trachea, a guardian stitch is placed after skin closure, between the skin of the chin and the anterior chest (Fig. 13–8). Patients should be warned that the head will be flexed at the time of emergence, and all efforts should be made to maintain the flexed position during the postoperative period to avoid traction on the new repair.

Tracheal Procedures with Specific Anesthetic Considerations

Airway Trauma

Injury to the conducting airways may be the result of blunt or penetrating trauma, often other injuries are present. In rare instances, the membranous trachea may be injured during airway instrumentation, particularly during double-lumen tube placement, becoming apparent immediately after extubation. Whereas small tears may be managed conservatively, urgent repair is required when significant clinical manifestations, such as hemoptysis, dyspnea, and pneumomediastinum occur or if bronchoscopic examination reveals gaping of the edges of the tear during respiratory flow. Repair may be possible transtracheally via an extended cervicotomy, or thoracotomy may be required (Mussi et al, 2000). Unlike the situation with other tracheal surgery, the patient has a defect in the major conducting airways prior to the induction of anesthesia. Preoperative assessment must be limited by the urgency of the procedure. Pulmonary function testing with spirometry is contraindicated because positive airway pressure increases subcutaneous emphysema.

Intubation of the patient for surgery is best accomplished under bronchoscopic guidance while the patient is breathing spontaneously, either awake with upper airway topicalization or after inhalation induction. When a transtracheal approach is used, the surgeon makes an anterior tracheotomy and passes a small endotracheal tube distally to be used intermittently for ventilation. The repair is performed during periods of apnea, when the tube is withdrawn.

Tracheoesophageal Fistula

Congenital TE fistula is recognized in the neonatal period. Adults may acquire such a lesion from trauma, neoplasia, or radiotherapy. In cases of TE fistula, contamination of the airway with gastric contents and preexisting pulmonary injury may have occurred. Positive-pressure ventilation is avoided because gastric insufflation may

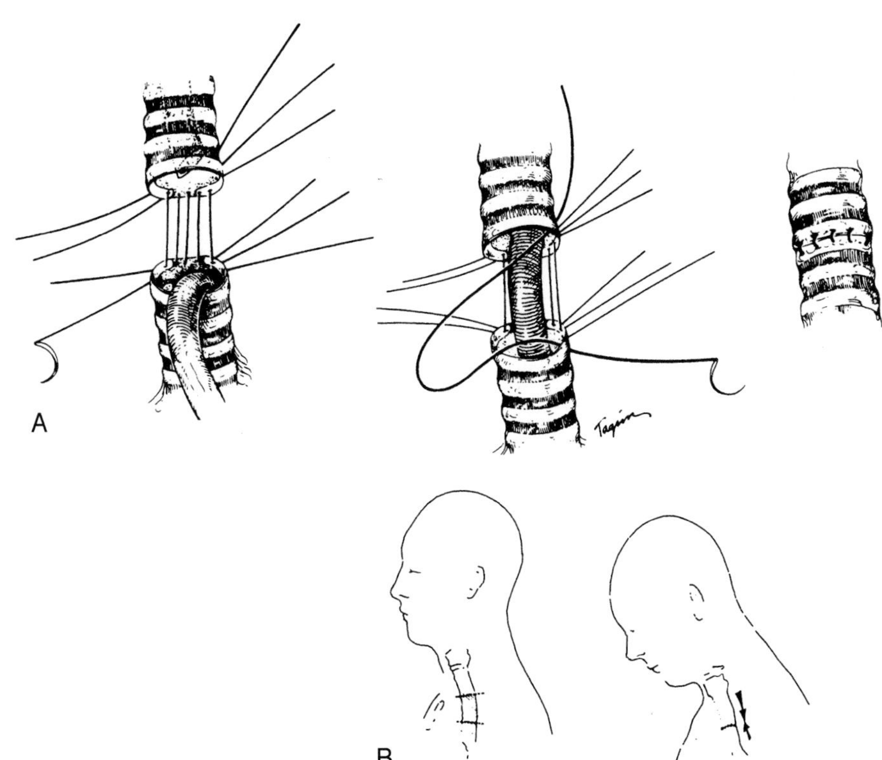

FIGURE 13–8 ■ Head flexion delivers the cervical trachea into the mediastinum to facilitate re-approximation of the edges of the trachea. A guardian stitch is placed after skin closure, between the skin of the chin and the anterior chest. (From Grillo HC: Congenital lesions, neoplasms and injuries to the chest. In Sabiston DC, Spencer FC [eds]: Gibbon's Surgery of the Chest. Philadelphia, WB Saunders, 1976.)

result in increased intrathoracic pressure, difficult ventilation, and impaired venous return (Salem et al, 1973).

Placement of an endotracheal tube beyond the fistula while maintaining spontaneous ventilation is recommended. A novel variation of this strategy was described in an adult who presented for resection of a large carinal TE fistula. To isolate each lung independently, two 5.0-mm microlaryngoscopy endotracheal tubes were placed sequentially in each bronchus following inhalation induction of anesthesia using sevoflurane. Conventional IPPV was then initiated (Au et al, 1999).

EMERGENCE AFTER AIRWAY SURGERY

The resumption of sustained spontaneous ventilation is essential. Prompt extubation is sought after airway reconstruction to avoid positive pressure or endotracheal tube cuff trauma to the new anastomosis, which might predispose to ischemia and dehiscence. Most patients breathe more comfortably in a sitting position, which helps to remove the weight of abdominal contents from the diaphragm and increases functional lung capacity. The oropharynx is thoroughly suctioned, neuromuscular blockade is fully reversed, and the patient is extubated when awake and able to maintain patency of the upper airway and to mobilize secretions.

The author's practice is to use an infusion of *propofol* for the final stages of the procedure, which permits rapid emergence to a wakeful state without agitation. This is important to avoid abrupt neck extension with possible anastomotic traction injury in the case of tracheal resection. Maintenance of normothermia is important because shivering increases oxygen consumption, which is particularly problematic if the airway is compromised. Humidification of inhaled gases minimizes the inspissation of dried airway secretions.

The laryngeal mask airway is being used for an increasing variety of airway procedures (Adelsmayr et al, 1998; Divatia et al, 1994), and for non-airway surgery in patients with airway disease and for non-airway surgery in patients with airway compromise (Rothschild and Kavee, 1997). Emergence with the laryngeal mask airway in place provokes minimal airway irritation and coughing, and patients often atraumatically remove the laryngeal mask airway themselves.

Reintubation after tracheal reconstruction may be difficult; the patient's neck is positioned in extreme flexion, the airway may be edematous and bloody, and there is potential for mechanical injury to the new anastomosis. If required, endotracheal tube positioning is best accomplished under direct vision with a fiberoptic bronchoscope. When an airway stent is left in place, the trachea should not be intubated blindly from above.

Telescoping of a small endotracheal tube into the stent may be possible using a bronchoscope. This technique should be applied with great care when a self-expanding metal stent has been placed for airway stenosis; it takes several hours for the stents to expand completely. Insertion of an endotracheal tube may distort or dislodge the stent, especially if the balloon cuff becomes snagged. The laryngeal mask airway may be positioned above the stented airway, particularly if a short period of ventilatory assistance is required, or to facilitate emergence from anesthesia.

The airway with a Montgomery T tube can be ventilated in several ways. The side arm protruding via a cervical tracheal stoma can accommodate an endotracheal tube connector (a 4.0- to 6.0-mm endotracheal tube), permitting connection to standard ventilation circuits. If positive pressure is required, the open upper limb must be obstructed to prevent loss of airway gas. The patient's mouth and nose may be manually held shut, packing may be placed in the pharynx, or an embolectomy catheter (Fogarty No. 14) may be directed into the upper limb of the T tube via the side arm of the stent and the balloon inflated (Lane et al, 1981). LFJV may also be initiated via the side arm (Baraka et al, 1982).

IMMEDIATE POSTOPERATIVE COMPLICATIONS

In all surgical patients, residual anesthetics, analgesics, and neuromuscular blockade may contribute to hypoventilation, atelectasis, and poor mobilization of secretions, leading to postoperative respiratory compromise. Additional pulmonary complications may be a direct result of surgery to the airway. Airway obstruction should be suspected if the patient is in respiratory distress, particularly if stridor is evident. Before emergence, the tracheobronchial tree should be examined and any residual blood in the airway should be carefully removed. Despite this, bleeding may be ongoing or old clot may be mobilized from the lung periphery. Airway caliber may be further compromised by edema.

Steroids are used empirically. Controlled studies of their use in airway surgery are entirely lacking. Dexamethasone is frequently chosen for its long duration of action; however, several hours may be required after dosing (4–10 mg IV) for edema to subside.

For many years, racemic epinephrine, a β_2 and α-mucosal vasoconstrictor (0.5 ml of 2.25% nebulized with 2 ml saline) has been advocated for treatment of postintubation edema and is used in our institution after airway surgery if required. The racemic form (an equal mixture of the D- and L-isomers of epinephrine) is increasingly unavailable in many countries, and the use of a similar dose of the more common 1% L-epinephrine is proposed to be equally effective (Nutman et al, 1994). Helium and oxygen mixtures, provided by a rebreathing face mask, may permit increased ventilation in patients with a narrowed conducting airway and is useful as a supportive measure while definitive therapy is pursued. Breathing with airway obstruction may be viewed as breathing through an orifice, which implies turbulent flow. Under turbulent conditions, gas flow varies with inverse square root of density. The low density of helium permits a 1.5-fold increase in relative flow of the commercially available heliox (70% helium/30% oxygen) over air and oxygen mixtures (Doyle and O'Grady, 1995). The high helium fraction required to significantly reduce the work of breathing through an orifice precludes the high oxygen fraction desirable if there is coexisting compromise in parenchymal gas exchange. When airway compromise is refractory to medical therapy, reintubation may be required.

Pulmonary parenchymal injury may occur; in a review of cases of pulmonary edema associated with airway obstruction after surgery, more than 20% of cases were in adults being treated for airway tumor (Lang et al, 1990). Spontaneous inspiratory efforts against an obstructed upper airway result in marked negative intrapleural and transpulmonary pressures, causing edema formation, usually within minutes. Laryngospasm is a frequent precursor. Bronchoscopic findings include pink frothy secretions and punctate hemorrhagic lesions throughout the tracheobronchial tree (Koch et al, 1996). Treatment is supportive and includes reestablishment of airway patency, oxygen supplementation, and diuresis; 85% of patients require reintubation, usually of short duration (Lang et al, 1990).

Pulmonary aspiration of acidic stomach contents is a particular concern during and after airway surgery, a point at which the trachea is not protected by an endotracheal tube, such as rigid bronchoscopy. When aspiration occurs, it is frequently at the time of airway manipulation (Tasch and Stoelting, 1996). Some patient groups are at increased risk (e.g., patients undergoing emergency procedures, probably because of an unfasted state). Lung transplant recipients, frequent candidates for dilatation and stenting of allograft anastomoses, are susceptible to gastric dysmotility and reflux (Berkowitz et al, 1995). Aspiration may occur after completion of the airway procedure; patients with newly placed T tubes may have difficulty closing the glottis. Laryngeal dysfunction is common after thyrohyoid and suprahyoid release procedures during tracheal resection (Grillo et al, 1995).

Despite an impressive array of antacids, gastric acid secretion blockers, antiemetics, and gastric prokinetic agents, such chemoprophylaxis remains unproven in the prevention of the secondary lung injury of acid aspiration. Once aspiration has occurred, treatment is supportive: bronchoscopy for removal of particulate matter and ventilation with PEEP. Mortality remains ~5%.

■ KEY REFERENCES

Geffin B, Bland J, Grillo HC: Anesthetic management of tracheal resection and reconstruction. Anesth Analg 48:884, 1969.

This paper, presented at the International Anesthesia Research Society in March 1969, elegantly presents the techniques of upper and lower airway management developed during a pivotal period of the development of tracheal reconstruction at the Massachusetts General Hospital. The discussion generated by the paper reveals the increasing appreciation of the etiologic mechanism of postintubation stenoses and the clinical dilemmas presented by these injuries.

Pinsonneault C, Fortier J, Donati F: Tracheal resection and reconstruction. Can J Anaesth 46:439, 1999.

This review of both the surgical and anesthesia literature of the last 30 years emphasizes shared airway management. A variety of anesthetic drug regimens are reported according to regional practices.

■ REFERENCES

Adelsmayr E, Keller C, Erd G et al: The laryngeal mask and high-frequency jet ventilation for resection of high tracheal stenosis. Anesth Analg 86:907, 1998.

Adnet F, Borron SW, Dumas JL et al: Study of the "sniffing position" by magnetic resonance imaging. Anesthesiology 94:83, 2001.

Angel C, Murillo C, Zwischenberger J et al: Perioperative extracorporeal membrane oxygenation for tracheal reconstruction in congenital tracheal stenosis. Pediatr Surg Int 16:98, 2000.

Au CL, White SA, Grant RP: A novel intubation technique for tracheoesophageal fistula in adults. Can J Anaesth 46:688, 1999.

Auden SM: Cervical spine instability and dwarfism: Fiberoptic intubations for all. Anesthesiology 91:580, 1999.

Babinski M, Smith RB, Klain M: High-frequency jet ventilation for laryngoscopy. Anesthesiology 52:178, 1980.

Bacher A, Lang T, Weber J et al: Respiratory efficacy of subglottic low-frequency, subglottic combined-frequency, and supraglottic combined-frequency jet ventilation during microlaryngeal procedures. Anesth Analg 91:1506, 2000a.

Bacher A, Pichler K, Aloy A: Supraglottic combined frequency jet ventilation versus subglottic monofrequent jet ventilation in patients undergoing microlaryngeal surgery. Anesth Analg 90:460, 2000b.

Baer G: Complications and technical aspects of jet ventilation for endolaryngeal procedures. Acta Anaesth Scand 44:1273, 2000.

Baer GA: Laryngeal muscle recovery after suxamethonium. Anaesthesia 39:143, 1984.

Baer G, Paloheimo M, Rahnasto J et al: End-tidal oxygen concentration and pulse oximetry for monitoring oxygenation during intratracheal jet ventilation. J Clin Monit 11:373, 1995.

Baraka A: Oxygen-jet ventilation during tracheal reconstruction in patients with tracheal stenosis. Anesth Analg 56:429, 1977.

Baraka A, Mansour R, Jaoude CA et al: Entrainment of oxygen and halothane during jet ventilation in patients undergoing excision of tracheal and bronchial tumors. Anesth Analg 65:191, 1986.

Baraka A, Muallem M, Noueihid R et al: Oxygen jet ventilation of patients with tracheal T-tube. Anesth Analg 61:622, 1982.

Barclay RS, McSwan N, Welsh TH: Tracheal reconstruction without the use of grafts. Thorax 12:177, 1957.

Beamer WC, Prough DS, Royster RL et al: High-frequency jet ventilation produces auto-PEEP. Crit Care Med 12:734, 1984.

Belsey R: Resection and reconstruction of the intrathoracic trachea. Br J Surg 38:200, 1950.

Benca JF, Hickey PR, Dornbusch JN et al: Ventilatory management assisted by cardiopulmonary bypass for distal tracheal reconstruction in a neonate. Anesthesiology 68:270, 1988.

Benumof JL: Anesthesia for Thoracic Surgery, 2nd ed. Philadelphia, WB Saunders, 1994, pp 534–535.

Berkowitz N, Schulman LL, McGregor C, Markowitz D: Gastroparesis after lung transplantation. Chest 108:1602, 1995.

Borg U, Eriksson I, Sjöstrand U: High-frequency positive-pressure ventilation (HFPPV): A review based upon its use during bronchoscopy and for laryngoscopy and microlaryngeal surgery under general anesthesia. Anesth Analg 59:594, 1980.

Brain AIJ: The laryngeal mask: A new concept in airway management. Br J Anaesth 55:801, 1983.

Brimacombe J, Dunbar-Reid K: The effect of introducing fiberoptic bronchoscopes on gas flow in laryngeal masks and tracheal tubes. Anaesthesia 51:923, 1996.

Brooker CR, Hunsaker DH, Zimmerman AA et al: A new anesthetic system for microlaryngeal surgery. Otolaryngol Head Neck Surg 118:55, 1998.

Brown D: Halothane-oxygen anaesthesia for bronchoscopy. Anaesthesia 14:135, 1959.

Bürkle H, Dunbar S, van Aken H: Remifentanil: A new, short-acting, μ-opioid. Anesth Analg 83:646, 1996.

Carden E, Burns WW, McDevitt NB et al: A comparison of Venturi and side-arm ventilation in anaesthesia for bronchoscopy. Can Anaesth Soc J 20:569, 1974.

Carden E, Crutchfield W: Anesthesia for microsurgery of the larynx. Can Anaesth Soc J 20:378, 1973.

Carlon GC, Griffin J, Ray C et al: High frequency jet ventilation in experimental airway disruption. Crit Care Med 11:353, 1983.

Carlon GC, Kahn RC, Howland WS et al: Clinical experience with high frequency ventilation. Crit Care Med 9:1, 1981.

Carlon GC, Ray C, Klain M: High-frequency positive-pressure ventilation in management of a patient with bronchopleural fistula. Anesthesiology 52:160, 1980.

Carnes MA, Fabian LW: Anesthesia for bronchoscopy and bronchography. Anesth Analg 40:567, 1961.

Churchill-Davidson HC: Anaesthesia for bronchoscopy. Anaesthesia 7:237, 1952.

Clarkson WB, Davies JR: Anaesthesia for carinal resection. Anaesthesia 33:815, 1978.

Conacher ID, Paes LL, McMahon CC et al: Anesthetic management of laser surgery for central airway obstruction: A 12-year case series. J Cardiothorac Vasc Anesth 12:153, 1998.

Coolen D, Slabbynck H, Galdersmans D et al: Insertion of a self-expandable metal stent using topical anaesthesia and a fiberoptic bronchoscope: A comfortable way to offer palliation. Thorax 49:87, 1994.

Cooper JD, Pearson FG, Patterson GA et al: Use of silicone stents in the management of airway problems. Ann Thorac Surg 47:371, 1989.

Cowl CT, Prakash UB, Kruger BR: The role of anticholinergics in bronchoscopy: A randomized clinical trial. Chest 118:188, 2000.

Dartevelle P, Macchiarini P: Carinal resection for bronchogenic cancer. Semin Thorac Cardiovasc Surg 8:414, 1996.

Dexter TJ: The laryngeal mask airway: A method to improve visualisation of the trachea and larynx during fiberoptic assisted percutaneous tracheostomy. Anaesth Intensive Care 22:35, 1994.

Dich-Nielsen JO, Nagel P: Fiberoptic bronchoscopy via the laryngeal mask. Acta Anaesthesiol Scand 37:17, 1993.

Divatia JV, Sareen R, Upadhye SM et al: Anaesthetic management of tracheal surgery using the laryngeal mask airway. Anaesth Intensive Care 22:69, 1994.

Doyle DJ, O'Grady KF: Physics and the airway: Essentials for the clinician. Anesthesiol Clin North Am 13:277, 1995.

Duckett JE, McDonnell TJ, Unger M et al: General anaesthesia for Nd:YAG laser resection of obstructing endobronchial tumours using the rigid bronchoscope. Can Anaesth Soc J 32:67, 1985.

Dumon JF, Shapshay S, Bourcereau J et al: Principles for safety in application of neodymium-YAG laser in bronchology. Chest 86:163, 1984.

Ellis RH, Hinds CJ, Gadd LT: Management of anaesthesia during tracheal resection. Anaesthesia 31:1076, 1976.

El-Baz N, El-Ganzouri A, Gottschalk W et al: One-lung high frequency positive pressure ventilation for sleeve pneumonectomy: An alternative technique. Anesth Analg 60:683, 1981.

El-Baz N, Holinger L, El-Ganzouri A: High-frequency positive-pressure ventilation for tracheal reconstruction supported by tracheal T-tube. Anesth Analg 61:796, 1982a.

El-Baz N, Jensik R, Penfield Faber L et al: One-lung high-frequency ventilation for tracheoplasty and bronchoplasty: A new technique. Ann Thorac Surg 34:564, 1982b.

El-Naggar M, Keh E, Stemmers A et al: Jet ventilation for microlaryngeal procedures: A further simplified technic. Anesth Analg 53:797, 1974.

Eriksson I, Sjostrand U: Effect of high-frequency positive-pressure ventilation (HFPPV) and general anesthesia on intrapulmonary gas distribution in patients undergoing diagnostic bronchoscopy. Anesth Analg 59:585, 1980.

Eriksson I, Nilsson LG, Nordstrom S: High-frequency positive-pressure ventilation during transthoracic resection of tracheal stenosis and during preoperative bronchoscopic examination. Acta Anaesthesiol Scand 19:113, 1975.

Ernst M, Koller M, Grobholtz et al: Both atrial resection and superior vena cava replacement in sleeve pneumonectomy for advanced lung cancer. Eur J Cardiothorac Surg 15:530, 1999.

Evans KL, Keene MH, Bristow ASE: High-frequency jet ventilation—a review of its role in laryngology. J Laryngol Otol 108:23, 1994.

Ferson DZ, Nesbitt JC, Nesbitt K et al: The laryngeal mask airway: A new standard for airway evaluation in thoracic surgery. Ann Thorac Surg 63:768, 1997.

Flatau E, Lewinsohn G, Konichezky S et al: Mechanical ventilation in fiberoptic-bronchoscopy: Comparison between high frequency positive pressure ventilation and normal frequency positive pressure ventilation. Crit Care Med 10:733, 1982.

Froese AS, Bryan AC: High frequency ventilation. Am Rev Respir Dis 135:1363, 1987.

Geffin B, Bland J, Grillo HC: Anesthetic management of tracheal resection and reconstruction. Anesth Analg 48:884, 1969.

Giesecke AH, Gerbershagen HU, Dortman C et al: Comparison of the ventilating and injection bronchoscopes. Anesthesiology 38:298, 1973.

Gillick JS: The inflation-catheter technique for ventilation during bronchoscopy. Anesthesiology 40:503, 1974.

Gillick JS: The inflation-catheter technique of ventilation during laryngoscopy. Can Anaesth Soc J 23:534, 1976.

Glenski JA, Crawford M, Rehder K: High-frequency, small-volume ventilation during thoracic surgery. Anesthesiology 64:211, 1986.

Goulden MR, Hunter JM: Rapacuronium (Org 9487): Do we have a replacement for succinylcholine? Br J Anaesth 82:490, 1999.

Grillo HC: Surgical approaches to the trachea. Surg Gynecol Obstet 129:347, 1969.

Grillo HC, Bendixen HH, Gephart T: Resection of the carina and lower trachea. Ann Surg 158:889, 1963.

Grillo HC, Donahue DM, Mathisen DJ et al: Postintubation tracheal stenosis: Treatment and results. J Thorac Cardiovasc Surg 109:486, 1995.

Grillo HC, Mathisen DJ: Cervical exenteration. Ann Thorac Surg 49:401, 1990.

Gronnebech H, Johansson G, Smedebol M et al: Glycopyrrolate versus atropine during anaesthesia for laryngoscopy and bronchoscopy. Acta Anesthesiol Scand 37:454, 1993.

Hannallah MS: The optimal breathing tube for tracheal resection and reconstruction. Anesthesiology 83:419, 1995.

Hautmann H, Gamarra F, Henke M, et al: High-frequency jet ventilation in interventional fiberoptic bronchoscopy. Anesth Analg 90:1436, 2000.

Hill AJ, Feneck RO, Underwood SM et al: The haemodynamic effects of bronchoscopy: Comparison of propofol and thiopentone with and without alfentanil pretreatment. Anaesthesia 46:266, 1991.

Howland WS, Carlon GC, Goldiner PL et al: High-frequency jet ventilation during thoracic surgical procedures. Anesthesiology 67:1009, 1987.

Hunsaker DH: Anesthesia for microlaryngeal surgery: The case for subglottic jet ventilation. Laryngoscope 104:1, 1994.

Ihra G, Aloy A: On the use of Venturi's principle to describe entrainment during jet ventilation. J Clin Anesth 12:417, 2000.

Ihra G, Hieber C, Schabernig C et al: Supralaryngeal tubeless combined high-frequency jet ventilation for laser surgery of the larynx and the trachea. Br J Anaesth 83:940, 1999.

Jackson C: Foreign bodies in the trachea, bronchi and oesophagus—the aid of oesophagoscopy, bronchoscopy, and magnetism in their extraction. Laryngoscope 4:257, 1905.

Jackson C: The technique of insertion of intratracheal insufflation tubes. Surg Gynecol Obstet 17:507, 1913.

Jackson C, Jackson CL: Bronchoesophagology. Philadelphia, WB Saunders, 1950.

Jackson CL, McReynolds GS: Anesthesia for peroral endoscopy. Ann Otol Rhinol Laryngol 49:1048, 1940.

Jameson JJ, Moses RD, Vellayappan U et al: Use of the laryngeal mask airway for laser treatment of the subglottis. Otolaryngol Head Neck Surg 123:101, 2000.

Joynt GM, Chui PT, Mainland P et al: Total intravenous anesthesia and endotracheal oxygen insufflation for repair of tracheoesophageal fistula in an adult. Anesth Analg 82:661, 1996.

Kain ZN, O'Connor EZ, Berde CB: Management of tracheobronchoscopy and esophagoscopy for foreign body in children: A survey study. J Clin Anesth 6:28, 1994.

Klein U, Karzai W, Gottschall R et al: Respiratory gas monitoring during high-frequency jet ventilation for tracheal resection using a double lumen jet catheter. Anesth Analg 88:224, 1999.

Koch SM, Abramson DC, Ford M et al: Bronchoscopic findings in post-obstructive pulmonary oedema. Can J Anaesth 43:73, 1996.

Kovacs S: Method of ventilation during bronchoscopy. Anesthesiology 18:335, 1957.

Krishnan JA, Brower RG: High-frequency ventilation for acute lung injury and ARDS. Chest 118:795, 2000.

Lane GA, Steude G, Pashley NRT: Anesthesia for a patient with a tracheal T-tube stent. Anesth Analg 60:218, 1981.

Lang SA, Duncan PG, Shepard DAE et al: Pulmonary oedema associated with airway obstruction. Can J Anaesth 37:201, 1990.

Lee P, English ICW: Management of anesthesia during tracheal resection. Anaesthesia 29:305, 1974.

Licker M, Schweizer A, Nicolet G et al: Anesthesia of a patient with an obstructing tracheal mass: A new way to manage the airway. Acta Anaesthesiol Scand 41:34, 1997.

Louhimo I, Leijala M: Cardiopulmonary bypass in tracheal surgery in infants and small children. Prog Pediatr Surg 21:98, 1987.

MacArthur A, Kleinman S: Rheumatoid cervical joint disease: A challenge to the anaesthetist. Can J Anaesth 40:154, 1993.

MacIntosh RR: Anaesthesia for bronchoscopy. Anaesthesia 9:77, 1954.
MacIntosh RR: Technique of laryngeal anaesthesia. Lancet 2:54, 1947.
Magnusson L, Lang FJW, Monnier P et al: Anaesthesia for tracheal resection: Report of 17 cases. Can J Anaesth 44:1282, 1997.
Matot I, Kramer MR, Glantz L et al: Myocardial ischemia in sedated patients undergoing fiberoptic bronchoscopy. Chest 112:1454, 1997.
Matot I, Sichel JY, Yofe V et al: The effect of clonidine premedication on hemodynamic responses to microlaryngoscopy and rigid bronchoscopy. Anesth Analg 91:828, 2000.
Matsushima Y, Jones RL, King EG, et al: Alterations in pulmonary mechanics and gas exchange during routine fiberoptic bronchoscopy. Chest 86:184, 1984.
McClish A, Deslauriers J, Beaulieu M et al: High-flow catheter ventilation during major tracheobronchial reconstruction. J Thorac Cardiovasc Surg 89:508, 1985.
Medici G, Mallios C, Custers WT et al: Anesthesia for endobronchial laser surgery: A modified technique. Anesth Analg 88:298, 1999.
Meretoja OA, Taivainen T, Raiha L et al: Sevoflurane–nitrous oxide or halothane–nitrous oxide for paediatric bronchoscopy and gastroscopy. Br J Anaesth 76:767, 1996.
Muendnich K, Hoflehner G: Die Narkose-Beatmungs-bronchoscopie. Anaesthetist 21:121, 1953.
Mussi A, Ambrogi MC, Menconi G et al: Surgical approaches to membranous tracheal wall lacerations. J Thorac Cardiovasc Surg 120:115, 2000.
Natalini G, Cavaliere S, Seramondi V et al: Negative pressure ventilation vs. external high-frequency oscillation during rigid bronchoscopy. Chest 118:18, 2000.
Natalini G, Vitacca M, Cavaliere S et al: Negative pressure ventilation vs. spontaneous assisted ventilation during rigid bronchoscopy. Acta Anaesthesiol Scand 42:1063, 1998.
Neville WE, Thomason RD, Peacock H, Colby C: Cardiopulmonary bypass during non-cardiac surgery. Arch Surg 92:516, 1966.
Nutman J, Brooks LJ, Deakins KM et al: Racemic versus L-epinephrine aerosol in the treatment of postextubation laryngeal edema: Results from a prospective, randomized, double-blind study. Crit Care Med 22:1591, 1994.
Oulton JL, Donald DM: A ventilating laryngoscope. Anesthesiology 35:540, 1971.
Palda VA, Detsky AS: Perioperative assessment and management of risk from coronary artery disease. Ann Intern Med 127:313, 1997.
Perera ER, Mallon JS: General anaesthetic management for laser resection of central airway lesions in 85 procedures. Can J Anaesth 34:383, 1987.
Perera ER, Vidic DM, Zivot J: Carinal resection with two high-frequency jet ventilation delivery systems. Can J Anaesth 40:59, 1993.
Perrin G, Colt HG, Martin C, et al: Safety of interventional rigid bronchoscopy using intravenous anesthesia and spontaneous assisted ventilation. Chest 102:1526, 1992.
Pinsonneault C, Fortier J, Donati F: Tracheal resection and reconstruction. Can J Anaesth 46:439, 1999.
Pittoni G, Davia G, Tottoletto F: Spontaneous ventilation and epidural anesthesia in a patient with a large tracheoesophageal fistula and esophageal cancer undergoing colonic interposition. Anesthesiology 79:855, 1993.
Puura AI, Rorarius MGF, Manninen P et al: The cost of intense neuromuscular block for anesthesia during endolaryngeal procedures due to waiting time. Anesth Analg 88;1335, 1999.
Putney FJ: Anesthesia for peroral endoscopy. Laryngoscope 49:55, 1939.
Ratzenhofer-Komenda B, Offner A, Kaltenbock F et al: Differential lung ventilation and emergency hyperbaric oxygenation for repair of a tracheal tear. Can J Anaesth 47:169, 2000.
Rehl G: Massive pyramidal tract signs after endotracheal intubation: A case report of spondyloepiphyseal dysplasia congenita. Anesthesiology 89:1262, 1998.
Rothschild MA, Kavee EH: The modified laryngeal mask airway: Four head and neck procedures in two children with mild subglottic stenosis. Int J Pediatr Otolaryngol 41:163, 1997.
Safar P: Ventilating bronchoscope. Anesthesiology 19:406, 1958.
Salem MR, Wong AY, Lin YH et al: Prevention of gastric distension during anesthesia for newborns with tracheoesophageal fistulas. Anesthesiology 38:82, 1973.
Sanchez A, Trivedi NS, Morrison DE: Preparation of the patient for awake intubation. In Benumof JL (ed): Airway Management: Principles and Practice. St. Louis, Mosby–Year Book, 1996, pp 159–182.
Sanders RD: Two ventilating attachments for bronchoscopes. Del Med J 39:170, 1967.
Schoenstadt DA, Doneker TG, Arnold HS et al: A re-examination of the ventilating bronchoscope. J Thorac Cardiovasc Surg 49:525, 1965.
Sebel PS, Lowdon JD: Propofol: A new intravenous anesthetic. Anesthesiology 71:260, 1989.
Shapshay SM, Beamis JF: Safety precautions for bronchoscopic Nd-YAG laser surgery. Otolaryngol Head Neck Surg 94:175, 1986.
Shikowitz M, Abramson AL, Liberatore L: Endolaryngeal jet ventilation: A ten-year review. Laryngoscope 101:455, 1991.
Sivarajan M, Stoler E, Kil HK et al: Jet ventilation using fiberoptic bronchoscopes. Anesth Analg 80:384, 1995.
Sjostrand U: High-frequency positive-pressure ventilation: A review. Crit Care Med 8:345, 1980.
Slinger P, Robinson R, Shennib H et al: Alternative technique for laser resection of a carinal obstruction. J Cardiothorac Vasc Anesth 6:749, 1992.
Smith I, Nathanson M, White PF: Sevoflurane: A long awaited anaesthetic. Br J Anaesth 76:435, 1996.
Sosis MB: Anesthesia for laser airway surgery. In Benumof JL (ed): Airway Management: Principles and Practice. St. Louis, Mosby, 1996.
Spoerel WE, Grant PA: Ventilation during bronchoscopy. Can Anaesth Soc J 18:178, 1971.
Spoerel WE, Greenway RE: Technique of ventilation during endolaryngeal surgery under general anaesthesia. Can Anaesth Soc J 20:369, 1973.
Symbas PN, Justicz AG, Ricketts RR: Rupture of the airways from blunt trauma: Treatment of complex injuries. Ann Thorac Surg 54:177, 1992.
Tasch MD, Stoelting RK: Aspiration prevention, prophylaxis, and treatment. In Benumof JL (ed): Airway Management: Principles and Practice. St. Louis, Mosby–Year Book, 1996, pp 183–201.
Theman TE, Kerr JH, Nelems JM et al: Carinal resection: A report of two cases and a description of the anesthetic technique. J Thorac Cardiovasc Surg 71:314, 1976.
Tomori Z, Widdicombe JG: Muscular, bronchomotor and cardiovascular reflexes elicited by mechanical stimulation of the respiratory tract. J Physiol 200:25, 1969.
Vourc'h G, Fischler M, Michon et al: High frequency jet ventilation v. manual jet ventilation during bronchoscopy in patients with tracheo-bronchial stenosis. Br J Anaesth 55:969, 1983.
Vourc'h G, Fischler M, Michon et al: Manual jet ventilation v. high frequency ventilation during laser resection of tracheo-bronchial stenosis. Br J Anaesth 55:973, 1983.
Vourc'h G, Tannieres ML, Toty L et al: Anaesthetic management of tracheal surgery using the neodynium:yttrium-aluminum-garnet laser. Br J Anaesth 52:993, 1980.
Vyas AB, Lyons SM, Dundee JW: Continuous intravenous anaesthesia with Althsin for resection of tracheal stenosis. Anaesthesia 38:132, 1983.
Wark K, Lyons J, Feneck O: The haemodynamic effects of bronchoscopy: The effect of pretreatment with fentanyl and alfentanil. Anaesthesia 41:162, 1986.
Warner MA, Warner MA, Weber JG: Clinical significance of pulmonary aspiration during the perioperative period. Anesthesiology 78:58, 1993.
Watanabe Y, Murakami S, Iwa T et al: The clinical value of high-frequency jet ventilation in major airway reconstructive surgery. Scand Thorac Cardiovasc Surg 22:227, 1988.
Wilson RF, Steiger Z, Jacobs J et al: Temporary partial cardiopulmonary bypass during emergency operative management of near total tracheal occlusion. Anesthesiology 61:103, 1984.
Woods FM, Neptune WF, Palatchi A: Resection of the carina and main-stem bronchi with the use of extracorporeal circulation. Engl J Med 264:493, 1961.
Young-Beyer P, Wilson RS: Anesthetic management for tracheal resection and reconstruction. J Cardiothorac Anesth 2:821, 1988.

CHAPTER **14**

Endoscopy

LARYNGOSCOPY

Ian J. Witterick
Patrick J. Gullane
Irvin Pathak

Laryngoscopy is an important part in the examination of the upper aerodigestive tract to (1) identify benign and malignant disease, (2) evaluate vocal cord mobility, and (3) assess laryngeal trauma and stenosis. Direct laryngoscopy implies that the larynx is seen in a direct line from the examiner's eye to the area of interest. It usually requires a hollow metal scope to be placed through the mouth to the area of interest. Indirect laryngoscopy involves various devices, including mirrors and fiberoptic scopes (flexible or rigid), to direct an image of the larynx and pharynx to the examiner's eye.

INDIRECT LARYNGOSCOPY

Indications

Indirect laryngoscopy is a routine part of the examination of the head and neck. It is particularly important in patients with a history of smoking and alcohol abuse because of the known risk of upper aerodigestive tract malignancies associated with these habits. It is advisable to perform indirect laryngoscopy in any patient who complains of dysphagia, odynophagia, or hoarseness for greater than 2 to 3 weeks. It can also be used with appropriate instrumentation to sample lesions in the larynx, remove foreign bodies, and augment the vocal cords with temporary (Gelfoam, glycerin) or permanent (Teflon) materials.

When indirect laryngoscopy is properly performed in a cooperative patient, a good view of the base of tongue, the vallecula, the supraglottic and glottic larynx, and the posterior pharyngeal wall can be obtained. It may be difficult to assess the pyriform sinuses, the laryngeal surface of the epiglottis, and the subglottis fully. The postcricoid area cannot usually be fully visualized. The one contraindication to indirect laryngoscopy is a suspected case of supraglottitis or epiglottitis in a child. Traction on the tongue and insertion of a laryngeal mirror may precipitate an acute airway obstruction. If the diagnosis is in question, it may be possible to examine these patients with a flexible scope inserted transnasally. Alternatively, the patient can be taken to the operating room for inhalational induction, direct laryngoscopy, and intubation.

Instruments

The larynx may be examined indirectly with a mirror or flexible or rigid fiberoptic scopes. The mirror has stood the test of time and is adequate for the examination of most patients. Good illumination is required. Either a head mirror and appropriate light source or a head light with its own built-in light source is used. Flexible and rigid scopes have revolutionized the examination of the larynx and pharynx. The flexible scope in particular is superior in patients who are difficult to examine with a mirror or rigid scope because of gagging or an overhanging epiglottis. The flexible scope does not trigger the pharyngeal gag reflex and can be manipulated posterior to the epiglottis.

Rigid scopes come in a variety of designs, but basically they are similar to a 90-degree periscope (Fig. 14–1). The light is conducted along fiberoptic cables out of the end of the instrument and directed at the target. Some scopes have built-in zoom lenses, which magnify the larynx and give an excellent view of vocal cord pathologic conditions. Rigid scopes may be ineffective in patients with a prominent gag reflex or in those in whom the epiglottis is displaced posteriorly.

Flexible laryngoscopes are similar to bronchoscopes except they are shorter, have a smaller diameter, and usually do not come equipped with suction (Fig. 14–2). A lever mechanism manipulates the end forward or backward but not from side to side. Therefore, orientation of the end of the scope is important before insertion. Transnasal insertion usually does not trigger the pharyngeal gag reflex. Flexible bronchoscopes can be substi-

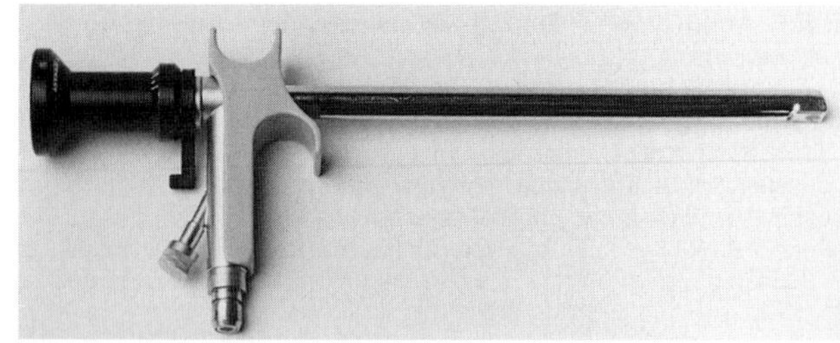

FIGURE 14–1 ■ Rigid fiberoptic scope for examination of the pharynx and larynx.

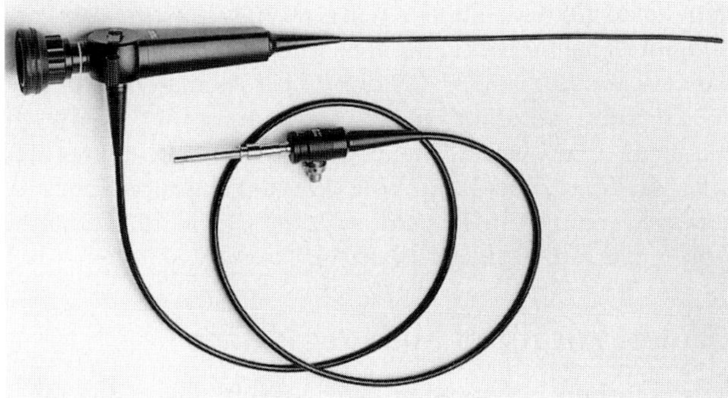

FIGURE 14–2 ■ Flexible fiberoptic scope for examination of the pharynx and larynx.

tuted, but the diameter of some may be too large to fit comfortably through the nose. Pediatric bronchoscopes are of similar caliber but are more difficult to manipulate because of added length. They do not give as wide or as bright a view as does a flexible laryngoscope.

Another advantage of the fiberoptic systems is the ability to connect them to camera and video devices. High-quality still and motion pictures can be produced for documentation, discussion with colleagues, or teaching. A strobe light can be connected to slow laryngeal vocal cord vibrations perceptively and allow an assessment of subtle laryngeal pathologic conditions (Sodersten and Lindestad, 1992).

Anesthesia

Most patients can be examined without anesthesia. If the patient has a prominent gag reflex, the anterior tonsillar pillars, base of tongue, and posterior oropharyngeal wall can be sprayed with a topical anesthetic (e.g., 10% lidocaine spray). Having the patient gargle with a topical anesthetic (e.g., 2% to 5% lidocaine) is also effective. Rarely is a superior laryngeal nerve block required (subcutaneous infiltration of a local anesthetic 1 cm anterior to the superior thyroid cornua and 1 cm superior to the thyroid cartilage). When a flexible laryngoscope is passed transnasally, the procedure is much more comfortable for the patient if topical anesthesia is used. Topical cocaine (4%) is particularly effective because it decongests and anesthetizes at the same time. Attention to the maximum dose of the anesthetic per kilogram of weight must be observed, particularly in children and in patients with cardiac disease.

Technique

Mirror

Laryngeal mirrors are readily available and inexpensive, but they require some practice to be used effectively. The examiner and patient are seated comfortably at eye level (Fig. 14–3). A head mirror or head light is used to focus light on the soft palate and the posterior pharyngeal wall. The mirror is warmed with hot water, heated beads, or a flame to prevent the patient's respirations from fogging the mirror during the examination. To avoid burning the patient, the temperature should be tested on the examiner's hand before the instrument is inserted. Alternatively, defogging solution may be used. If the examiner is right handed, the left hand is used to hold the protruded tongue with a folded gauze. If the examiner needs both hands free, the patient may be asked to hold out his or her own tongue. The right hand directs the mirror towards the posterior oropharyngeal wall and angles it so that a view of the base of tongue, vallecula, hypopharynx, and larynx is obtained. It is helpful to have the patient pant, and it is often necessary to touch and elevate the soft palate to gain an adequate view. The patient attempts to vocalize "eee" so that vocal cord mobility may be assessed and also to rotate the larynx anteriorly for improved visualization. The larynx and pharynx should be examined in a systematic fashion, which may require several trials.

It is important to remember that, with a mirror, the anterior and posterior relationships of the larynx are reversed but right and left remain the same when the examiner looks at the reflected image. An easy way to understand this is to draw two labeled vocal cords on a piece of paper and position them so that the anterior commissure is facing the examiner (i.e., the patient is facing the examiner). When the mirror is held over the paper, it will be noted how the right and left cords remain on the same side, but the anterior and posterior dimensions are reversed. This reversal makes instrumentation of the larynx with a mirror confusing. An advantage of both the rigid and the flexible telescopes is that there is no reversal, and a true image of the larynx is obtained.

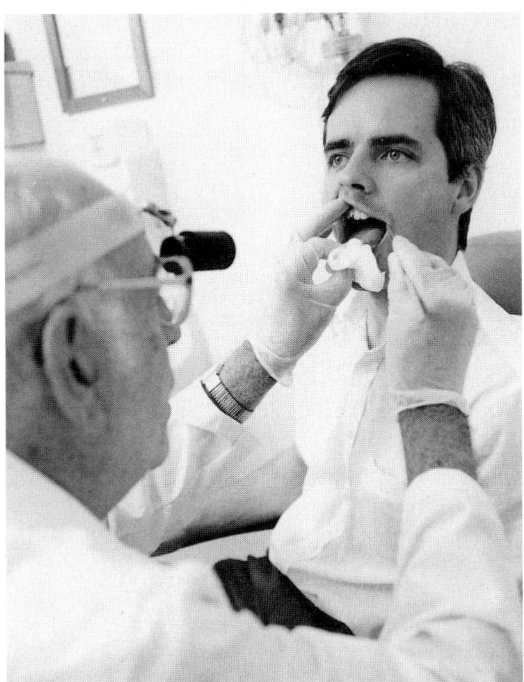

FIGURE 14–3 ■ Indirect mirror laryngoscopy. Note the examiner's hand retracting the tongue with a folded gauze while the right hand positions the mirror.

Rigid Telescope

Examination with the rigid scope is similar to that with the mirror. The protruded tongue is held with one hand while the telescope is inserted through the mouth toward the posterior oropharyngeal wall. It often touches the wall. The telescope can be rotated to view the entire larynx and pharynx while the patient pants or attempts to vocalize "eee." If the telescope is equipped with a zoom lens, particular areas can be examined with magnification.

Flexible Telescope

The patient is asked if one nasal passage is more patent, or preferably patency is assessed by anterior rhinoscopy. After topical anesthesia is administered, the scope is directed along the floor of the nose adjacent to the inferior turbinate or between the inferior and middle turbinates. In the nasopharynx, the scope is directed posterior to the soft palate, and a panoramic view of the base of tongue, larynx and pharynx is obtained. The scope is then directed towards areas of interest for a closer examination in a systematic fashion. The subglottis and trachea can be examined in a systematic fashion. The access to difficult-to-examine areas is superb, although the illumination and clarity may not always be as good as those with a mirror or rigid scope (Fig. 14–4).

DIRECT LARYNGOSCOPY

Indications

Direct laryngoscopy is the preferred technique for the detailed evaluation of laryngeal tumors, stenosis, and trauma (Benjamin, 1990, 1993; Kleinsasser, 1991). The extent of any disease process can be precisely characterized, and appropriate biopsies can be taken. Areas that are not amenable to examination with indirect methods can be evaluated, such as the laryngeal ventricles, the subglottis, the postcricoid area, and the pyriform sinuses. The vocal cords and arytenoid processes may be palpated to ascertain whether vocal cord immobility is due to paralysis or ankylosis. The vocal cords may be augmented with Gelfoam, fat, or Teflon. Laryngeal lesions may be removed using either cold microlaryngeal instrumentation or various types of lasers.

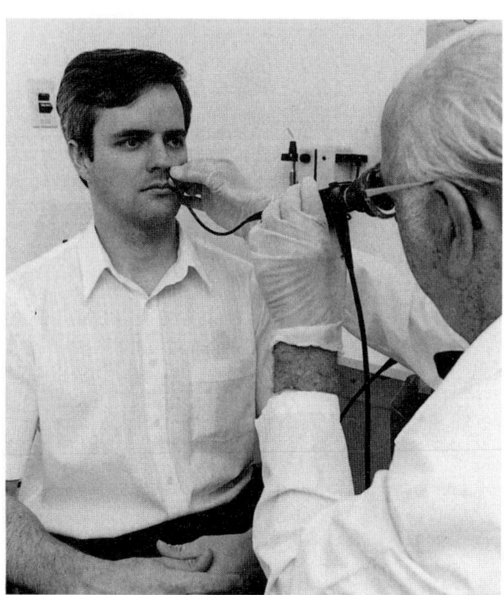

FIGURE 14–4 ■ Flexible laryngoscopy.

Contraindications and Precautions

It is inappropriate to administer general anesthesia when the patient has a laryngeal obstruction (e.g., neoplasm, foreign body, or edema). When the pharyngeal tone is lost, a marginal airway may advance to total obstruction. There are several options in this situation, including awake intubation (often with the aid of a flexible bronchoscope [Roberts, 1991]) and tracheotomy under local anesthesia. Unfavorable patient anatomy may create impossible or dangerous situations for direct laryngoscopy. Examples include ankylosing spondylitis, rheumatoid arthritis, and cervical spine fractures or dislocation. Other anatomic features that may make laryngoscopy difficult include a small mandible, trismus, long central incisors, a short neck, or the inability to extend the neck. Other examples of possible instances of difficult laryngoscopic intubation include measurements of mouth opening (interincisal gap), thyromental distance, length of mandibular ramus, atlanto-occipital extension, and the assessments of oropharyngeal view. This last assessment is graded according to the Mallampati classification as modified by Samsoon and Young: grade 1—good) visualization of the soft palate and tonsillar pillars; grade 2—pillars obscured by the soft palate but posterior oropharyngeal wall visible; grade 3—soft palate and base of uvula visible; and grade 4—soft palate not visible. Although these measures may be somewhat helpful, they are not foolproof as interobserver reliability is often poor (Karkouti et al, 1996).

Preoperative Preparation

The patient is placed in the supine position on a head support that raises the head approximately 10 cm above the operating room table. This flexes the neck onto the chest and places the patient in the Boyce or "sniffing" position, which is the optimal endoscopic position for visualization of the larynx. Secretions can be minimized if the patient is given a drying agent preoperatively, such as atropine or glycopyrrolate.

Anesthesia

Direct laryngoscopy can be performed under local or general anesthesia. General anesthesia is preferred for patient comfort and muscular relaxation. Local anesthesia is used in circumstances in which vocal cord mobility or assessment of the voice is important (e.g., Teflon augmentation).

Ventilation may be carried out with or without the use of an endotracheal tube during direct laryngoscopy. Techniques of ventilation using an endotracheal tube may be divided into large-tube or small-tube techniques. With the large-tube technique, a standard 7 to 9 French endotracheal tube is used. This presents a significant obstruction to the surgeon's view, especially of the posterior commissure. This can be overcome to some extent by moving the tube into the anterior glottis. The small-tube technique involves the use of an endotracheal tube ranging from 5 to 6 mm inside diameter. The primary difficulty with this tube arises if adequate time is not given for expiration, resulting in raised intrathoracic pressure and possible hypotension, pneumothorax, or pneumomediastinum. In most cases, positive-pressure ventilation may be provided for up to 1 hour with a small tube. In most cases, the tube lies posterior to the laryngoscope and is taped to the face of the patient or held by the anesthetist at the left oral commissure so that it can be removed from the path of entry of the laryngoscope through the right side of the oropharynx. Care must also be taken with the use of lasers so that the tube is not inadvertently punctured, which may initiate an endotracheal tube fire. This risk can be reduced by the use of a "laser" tube, placing wet cottonoids around the tube to act as a heat sink and using blue dye in the endotracheal tube cuff to warn of laser puncture.

Nonintubation techniques in current use entail some form of jet ventilation. This involves the entrainment of room air by a jet stream of gas based on the principles elucidated by Bernoulli and Venturi. This, in essence, means that the faster moving stream of gas gives up some of its velocity to the slowly moving room air such that the entrained room air is dragged into the moving stream. Jet ventilation may be divided into supraglottic, subglottic, transtracheal, or high-frequency ventilation techniques. Supraglottic jet ventilation is the most common method in use but has some disadvantages, including soiling of the trachea with blood and debris, inefficient ventilation due to turbulence, and gastric distension. Subglottic ventilation does not have these problems but does carry with it an increased risk of barotrauma. Transtracheal jet ventilation is rarely used. High-frequency jet ventilation uses respiratory rates at 1 Hz and at relatively low volumes. This enhances diffusion and interregional mixing within the lungs and may have a place in patients with chronic obstructive pulmonary disease, poor compliance, or obesity (Hunsaker, 1994; Shikowitz et al, 1991).

Protection of Teeth

The patient's upper dentition is at risk for damage during direct laryngoscopy. It is important to note dental work and loose teeth prior to the procedure and to point these out to the patient. Gauze or a prefabricated plastic dental guard are most useful to prevent dental abrasion. A guard may help to distribute pressure, but does not allow the upper teeth to be used as a fulcrum during exposure of the larynx in a difficult patient. In patients who require frequent endoscopies or those with precarious dentition, a customized acrylic or plastic plate of the upper dentition is useful to reduce dental trauma. It is much easier to position the scope in patients who do not have teeth or who have large gaps in their upper teeth.

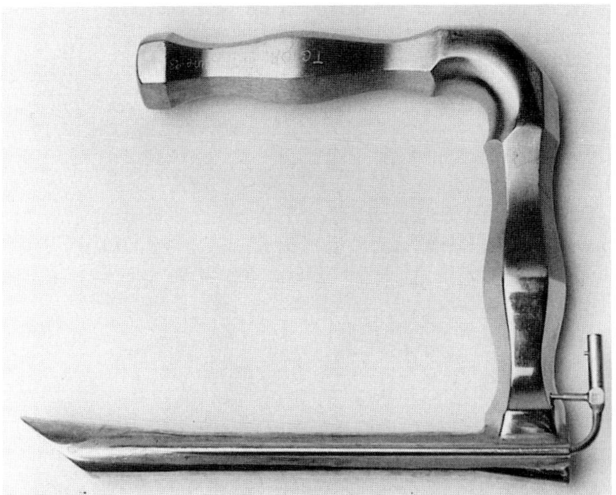

FIGURE 14–5 ■ Anterior commissure scope.

Instruments

There are many laryngoscopes that can be used to carry out direct laryngoscopy. To examine the entire larynx, the Holinger anterior commissure laryngoscope is excellent because its hourglass shape allows it to reach most sites (Figs. 14–5 and 14–6). Unfortunately, the panoramic view is lost and each site must be sequentially examined. Furthermore, binocular visualization is not possible. For delicate laryngeal surgery, it is preferable to select the widest scope that can be inserted to expose the anterior commisure.

A variety of shapes and sizes of laryngoscopes is required to meet the needs of the entire spectrum of patients (see Fig. 14–6). The Dedo laryngoscope is a good standard laryngoscope because it allows for a panoramic view of the endolarynx, and it can be used in most patients. The Lindholm laryngoscope (Fig. 14–7) is designed so that its anterior aspect sits in the vallecula. This allows for visualization of both the supraglottis and the glottis. For further access to the supraglottis, a bivalve

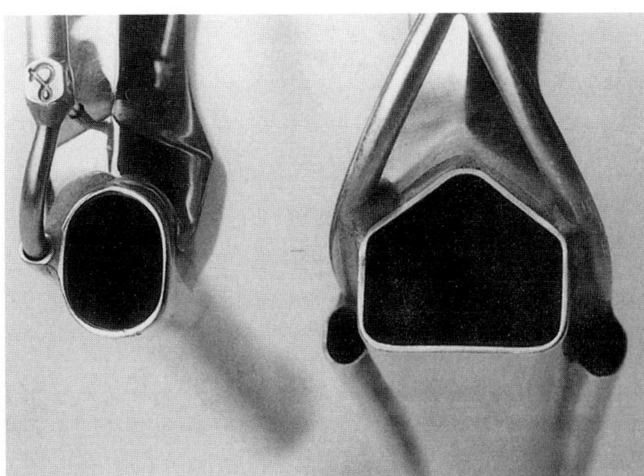

FIGURE 14–6 ■ Two examples to illustrate the different luminal sizes of direct laryngoscopes: anterior commissure scope (*left*) and Dedo scope (*right*).

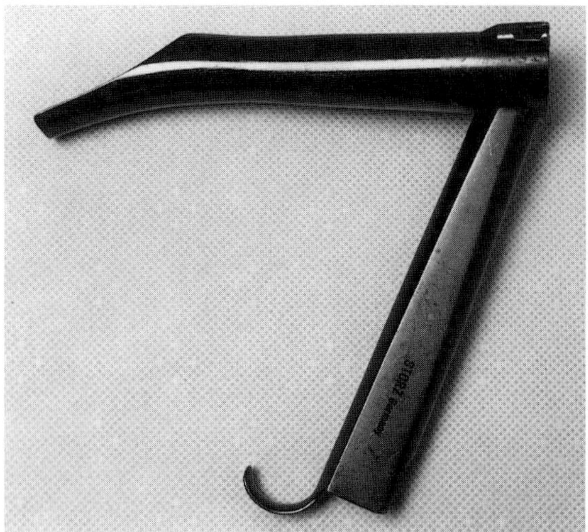

FIGURE 14–7 ■ Lindholm laryngoscope.

laryngoscope may be used (Zeitels and Vaughn, 1990). The Weerda laryngoscope is a bivalve scope that has two adjustable blades, allowing the diameter of the scope to be enlarged after insertion into the larynx. The subglottis is an area that can be difficult to access with a conventional laryngoscope. A subglottoscope with an elongated tube and a diameter that is large enough to allow binocular visualization is available for this purpose (Ossoff et al, 1991). Laryngoscopes have one or two ports for fiberoptic light carriers. The Kanto-Berci video microlaryngoscope (Fig. 14–8) has a port for the insertion of a rigid telescope for both illumination and magnification. Ports may also be present to allow for jet ventilation or smoke evacuation. The use of these ports for jet ventilation is less efficient than holding the jet in the middle of the laryngoscope lumen that allows for more efficient entrainment of room air.

The laryngoscope may be held with one hand, or alternatively may be suspended to allow both hands to be used. Two commonly used suspension devices are the Lewy and Boston systems. The Lewy suspension device is light, easy to attach and detach, and provides excellent stabilization of the laryngoscope within the larynx (Fig. 14–9). The Lewy system may exert unacceptable pressure on the upper dentition when exposure of the larynx is difficult. The Boston suspension system is favored in these patients as it allows proper positioning of the head and neck, minimizing pressure on the maxillary teeth (Fig. 14–10). This system does take longer time to set up and position accurately. Magnification of the larynx can be accomplished with an operating microscope (Fig. 14–11). The axis of the microscope is aligned with the axis of the scope. A 400-mm objective lens has a focal length that is long enough to allow instrumentation of the larynx without the instrument hitting the microscope. It is usually not possible to get binocular vision through

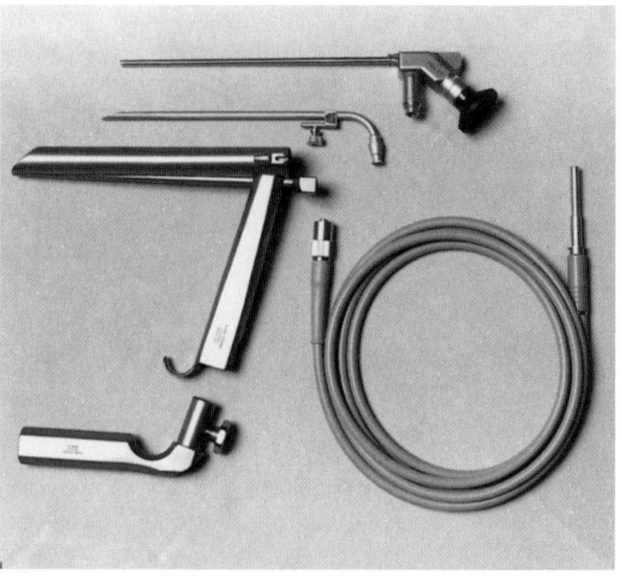

FIGURE 14–8 ■ Kantor-Berci video microlaryngoscope.

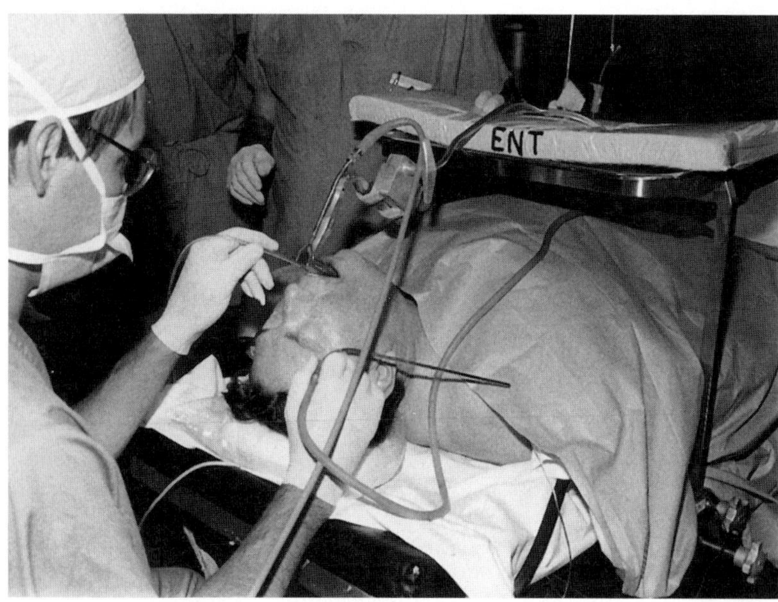

FIGURE 14–9 ■ Lewy suspension system with jet Venturi. This system is placed on a Mayo stand over the patient's upper chest and attached to the laryngoscope.

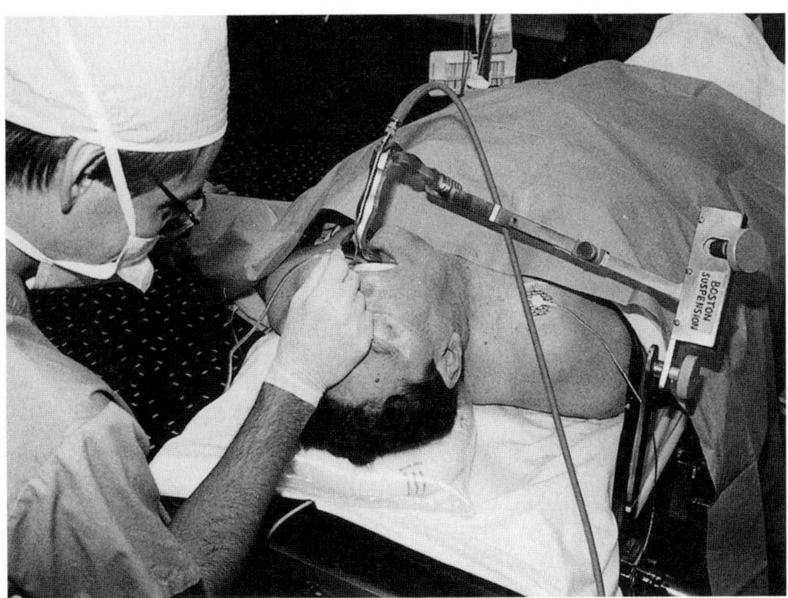

FIGURE 14–10 ■ Boston suspension system. To avoid excessive pressure on the maxillary dentition, the teeth are not used as a fulcrum with this system.

narrow scopes, and hence there is a need for the widest scope possible that will expose the area of interest. For microlaryngeal surgery, a support stand such as a Mayo stand may be placed at the head to rest one's elbows. An alternative to the use of a microscope is a rigid fiberoptic telescope that can be inserted through the suspended laryngoscope to examine the larynx in detail. These are available in various angles from 0 to 90 degrees.

The epithelium of the vocal cords can be characterized further through the use of contact endoscopy. Contact endoscopy involves the staining of the vocal cords with methylene blue followed by visualization with a contact endoscope. This allows the examination of cellular detail of the vocal cord epithelium (Andrea et al, 1995).

Lasers can be used for select purposes in the larynx, such as excision of laryngeal cancer or papillomata. The most common method is to use a carbon laser by attaching a micromanipulator to the operating microscope. The surgeon aims the laser with a joy stick. The carbon dioxide laser is invisible so that a coaxial red helium-neon beam is required for aiming. This allows for ablation or excision of the lesion.

Technique

The airway must be stable, and the patient must be relaxed. This is best provided through close collaboration between surgeon and anesthesiologist. It is again stressed that general anesthesia should not be administered if there is concern regarding the patency of the airway. In most cases, induction is carried out with an intravenous agent after preoxygenation. The procedure is carried out with neuromuscular paralysis to allow easy insertion of the laryngoscope. Anesthesia is maintained with volatile agents such as nitrous oxide, halothane, or enflurane. Propofol is an intravenous agent that can provide com-

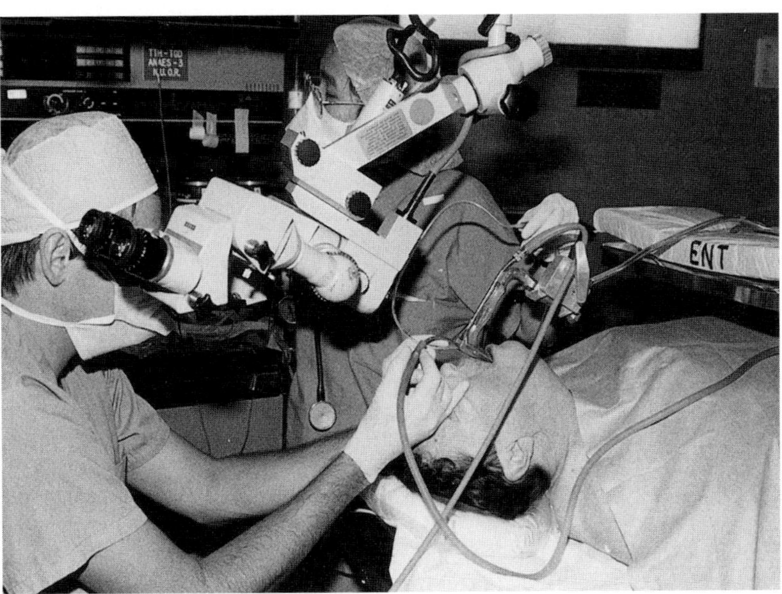

FIGURE 14–11 ■ Direct microlaryngoscopy.

plete anesthesia by itself. The eyes are taped shut to prevent corneal abrasion. Ventilation is achieved by intubation or jet ventilation as discussed earlier. The surgeon sits at the head of the table and introduces the laryngoscope with his or her left hand, through the patient's mouth to the epiglottis. It is important not to crush the lips or tongue during manipulation of the laryngoscope. The tip of the laryngoscope is passed under the epiglottis, which is displaced anteriorly. The scope is advanced to the laryngeal inlet as far as necessary to expose the internal surface of the larynx. The scope can be suspended at this point or held in the hand to examine various parts of the larynx systematically, including the true and false vocal cords, anterior and posterior commissures, ventricles, subglottis, epiglottis, pyriform sinus, vallecula, and postcricoid area. It is often necessary to push on the thyroid or cricoid cartilage externally to bring structures into view through the scope. Fine dissecting instruments are required for microsurgery of the larynx.

Local anesthesia is commonly applied topically to the larynx at the conclusion of laryngoscopy to prevent postoperative laryngospasm. Most patients have minimal pain after the procedure and can return to a normal diet. The patient's voice may be hoarse after the procedure, depending on the amount of instrumentation. He or she should be instructed to speak softly for short periods and to avoid whispering, shouting, or long conversations.

■ *KEY REFERENCES*

Benjamin B: Diagnostic Laryngology: Adults and Children. p. 1. WB Saunders, Philadelphia, 1990

This atlas of laryngology will assist the reader in the differential diagnosis and correct interpretation of various laryngeal abnormalities in both adults and chidren.

Kleinsasser O: Microlaryngoscopy and Endolaryngeal Microsurgery: Techniques and Typical Findings. 3rd Ed. p. 1. Mosby Year Book, St. Louis, 1991

This is a beautifully illustrated book of typical findings seen with direct laryngoscopy. It will give the reader an appreciation of the variety of laryngeal pathologic conditions examined under the operating microscope.

■ *REFERENCES*

Andrea M, Dias O, Santos A: Contact endoscopy during microlaryngeal surgery: A new technique for endoscopic examination of the larynx. Ann Otol Rhinol Laryngol 104:333, 1995.

Benjamin B: Prolonged intubation injuries of the larynx: Endoscopic diagnosis, classification and treatment. Ann Otol Rhinol Laryngol 160(Suppl):1, 1993.

Bourgain JL, McGee K, Cosset MF et al: Carbon dioxide monitoring during high frequency jet ventilation for direct laryngoscopy. Br J Anaesth 64:327, 1990.

Hunsaker D: Anesthesia for microlaryngeal surgery: The case for subglottic jet ventilation. Laryngoscope 104:1, 1994.

Karkouti K, Rose D, Ferris L et al: Interobserver reliability of ten tests used for predicting difficult tracheal intubation. Can J Anaesth 43:554, 1996.

Ossoff R, Duncavage I, and Dere H: Microsubglottiscopy: An expansion of operative microlaryngoscopy. Otolaryngol Head Neck Surg 104:842, 1991.

Roberts JT: Preparing to use the flexible fiberoptic laryngoscope. J Clin Anesth 3:64, 1991.

Shikowitz M, Abramson A, Liberatore L: Endolaryngeal jet ventilation: A 10-year review. Laryngoscope 101:455, 1991.

Sodersten M, Lindestad PA: A comparison of vocal fold closure in rigid telescopic and flexible fiberoptic laryngostroboscopy. Acta Otolaryngol (Stockh) 112:144, 1992.

Zeitels S, Vaughn C: The adjustable supraglottiscope. Otolaryngol Head Neck Surg 103:487, 1990.

LASER THERAPY

Philippe Pasche
Alexandre Radu
Florian Lang
Melvyn Goldberg
Philippe Monnier

HISTORICAL NOTE

Although the principles of light-amplification–stimulated emission of electromagnetic radiations (LASERS) have been known since the beginning of the century (Einstein, 1917), the first laser (a ruby laser) was not developed until 1960. Since the mid-1960s, ruby lasers in ophthalmology have pioneered the use of lasers in medicine. Subsequently, new sources for emitting in ultraviolet, visible, and infrared light have appeared on the market. These include the excimer lasers, krypton laser, argon laser, potassium-titanyl-phosphate laser (KTP), dye lasers, the neodymium:yttrium-aluminum-garnet (Nd:YAG) laser, the erbium and holmium lasers, and the carbon-dioxide (CO_2) laser.

The first applications of laser technology for use in bronchology date from the 1970s; Strong and Jako (1972) used the CO_2 laser for removing benign tumors, specifically tracheobronchial papillomas. In 1976, Laforet reported the first application of this laser for treating malignant obstructive lesions of the trachea and the bronchi. Later, the indications for employing the CO_2 laser were expanded to include benign tracheal stenoses. At the end of the 1970s, the Nd:YAG laser was introduced in France by Toty (1979) and Dumon (1982) and in Japan by Oho (1983) for the palliative treatment of inoperable tracheobronchial tumors. In the United States, these techniques were developed by Shapshay (1997) and Brutinel (1987) in the beginning of the 1980s. Due to its physical properties, the Nd:YAG laser remains the laser of choice for the removal of obstructive tumors in the tracheobronchial tree. Due to its physical properties, the KTP laser, which is strongly absorbed by pigments in tissues (hemoglobin, melanin), is becoming increasingly popular for the treatment of some highly vascularized tumors (hemangiomas) and intrabronchial metastasis of melanomas.

Another laser application in bronchoesophagology is represented by photodynamic therapy with the goal of curing superficial cancers (in situ and microinvasive carcinomas). Palliative photodynamic therapy for inoperable bronchial cancers has limited indications, owing to potential complications (hemorrhages and fistulas) and the risk of cutaneous photosensitization to the sun (Smith et al, 1993).

■ *HISTORICAL READINGS*

Brutinel WM, Cortese DA, McDougall JC et al: A two-year experience with neodymium-YAG laser in endobronchial obstruction. Chest 91:159, 1987.

Dumon JF, Reboud E, Garbe L et al: Treatment of tracheobronchial lesions by laser photoresection. Chest 81:278, 1982.

Einstein A: On the quantum theory of radiation. Physikal Z 18:121, 1917.

Laforet KG, Berger RL, Vaughn CW: Carcinoma obstructing the trachea: Treatment by laser resection. N Engl J Med 214:941, 1976.

Oho K, Ogawa I, Amemiya R et al: Indication for endoscopic Nd:YAG laser surgery in the trachea and bronchus. Endoscopy 15:302, 1983.

Shapshay S: Endoscopic treatment of subglottic and tracheal stenosis by radial laser incision and dilatation. Ann Otol Rhinol Laryngol 99:661, 1987.

Smith SGT, Bedwell J, MacRobert AJ et al: Experimental studies to assess the potential of photodynamic therapy for the treatment of bronchial carcinomas. Thorax 48:474, 1993.

Strong MS, Jako JG: Laser surgery in the larynx: Early clinical experience with continuous CO_2 laser. Ann Otol Rhinol Laryngol 81:791, 1972.

Toty L, Personne C, Hertzog P et al: Utilisation d'un faisceau laser (YAG) à conducteur souple, pour le traitement endoscopique de certaines lésions trachéobronchiques. Rev Fr Mal Respir 7:57, 1979.

PROPERTIES OF LASERS

Each laser has its own particular properties based on its wavelength (Table 14–1). Although they have very different configurations, all lasers are composed of three fundamental elements:

1. An active substance (lasing medium), either atoms or molecules, which are excited by an energy source and emit photons of a concisely defined wavelength. The choice of the medium (e.g., gas, crystal, or dye) defines the wavelength of the laser and therefore its properties.
2. The energy source that excites the active substance; this is the pumping source.
3. The optical resonator, which is formed by two mirrors, separated by a cylindrical cavity in which the active substance is found.

We differentiate the following lasers: crystal solids lasers (ruby, 696 nm; KTP, 532 nm; Nd:YAG, 1064 nm), gas lasers (HeNe, 632.8 nm; CO_2, 10,600 nm; argon, 488 and 514 nm; krypton, 407 nm), dye lasers (variable wavelength depending on the dye), and semiconductor lasers.

Effects on Tissue

The effects of laser beams on tissue are primarily dependent on the type of laser used (wavelength of the laser) and the type of tissue under consideration (optical properties of biologic tissues). When a laser comes in contact with a tissue, four phenomena, of varying degrees, can be produced:

1. Reflection: partially seen on the surface of biologic tissues.
2. Transmission: total or partial (e.g., the total transmission of the argon laser through water and glass, through the cornea and the vitreous body of the eye, and through the urinary bladder filled with saline; the same is true to a lesser degree for the Nd:YAG laser).
3. Absorption: Based on the wavelength and the biologic tissue composition, a laser beam may be absorbed to a greater or lesser degree (e.g., strong absorption of the CO_2 laser by saline, strong absorption of the argon and the KTP lasers by hemoglobin and melanin pigments).
4. Diffusion into the adjacent tissue: coherence and collimation properties of the laser beams are partially lost in relation to the wavelength and the type of tissue considered. The energy concentration is lost due to its diffusion in the tissue. The heat flows into the adjacent tissue and causes thermal damage (e.g., strong diffusion of the Nd:YAG laser in biologic tissues).

TABLE 14–1 ■ **Characteristics of Lasers in Clinical Use**

Variable	*CO_2*	*Nd:YAG*	*Argon/KTP*	*Argon-Tunable Dye*
Wavelength (nm)	10.600	1.060	500/532	630
Power (W)	40	100	5–20	2
Transmission system	Mirrors	Fiberoptic	Fiberoptic	Fiberoptic
Absorption in tissues	High	Low	Selective	Selective for photodynamic therapy
Coagulation effect	Low	High	Medium	None
Cutting effect	High	Low	Low	None
Penetration	1 mm	10–15 mm	5 mm	8–10 mm

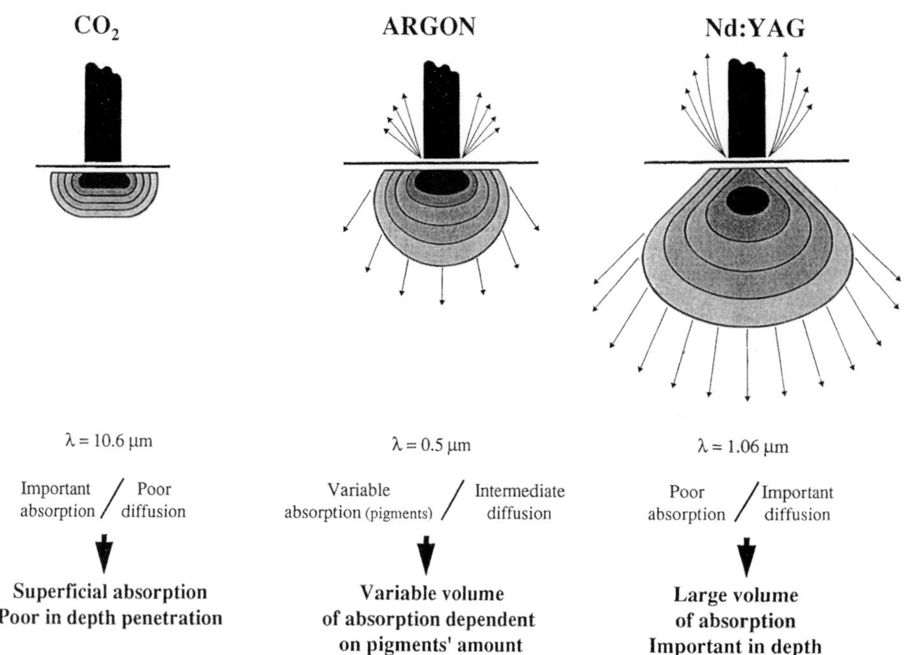

FIGURE 14–12 ■ Comparison of the effect on tissue with carbon dioxide, argon, and neodymium:yttrium lasers.

Thermal Effect

In prevailing use, it is the thermal effect of the laser beam that is exploited. Laser energy, absorbed by the tissue, is converted into heat. According to the temperature reached, various tissue effects are observed: coagulation (blanching of the lesion), protein denaturation (gray coloring of the lesion), carbonization (black coloring of the lesion), and vaporization (tissue volatilization) (Fig. 14–12).

Other than the types of laser and tissue characteristics, two other important parameters aid in the control of the laser effects on tissue: the power density (concentration of energy per surface unit expressed in watt/cm^2) and the exposure time. The power density increases when the spot size is reduced. The energy delivered to the tissue can be expressed by the formula:

$$\text{delivered energy (joules)} = \text{power density (watt/cm}^2) \times \text{exposure time (sec)}.$$

Photochemical Effect

In general, a pump laser (argon, KTP, Nd:YAG) is required to excite the dye, the wavelength of which depends on its type. Dye lasers are basically used in bronchology for photodynamic therapy of early cancers (in situ carcinoma and microinvasive carcinoma), which do not infiltrate beyond the cartilage and do not cause lymph node metastases (Monnier, 1991). The effect is not thermal but photochemical. The principle is such that a photosensitizer, usually from the porphyrin group, is injected intravenously several hours or days before therapeutic endoscopy. Its preferential retention in cancer cells leads to destruction of the tumor by a photochemical effect caused by weak irradiation (0.1 W) by a dye laser. The wavelength is selected according to the peak absorption of the photosensitizer and the desired tissue penetration. Most porphyrins have strong fluorescent properties, and these same substances can therefore be used equally well for the photodetection of early cancers that may still be invisible by traditional endoscopic methods (photodiagnostic imaging).

ENDOSCOPIC ANATOMY

When using a laser in the airways, accurate knowledge of the anatomic configuration of the surrounding structures is essential to avoid potential complications, especially vascular damage.

The first third of the trachea is positioned close, anteriorly and laterally, to the thyroid gland and, posteriorly, to the esophagus; no major vessels are in direct contact with the trachea at this level. The second third of the trachea is mainly surrounded by vascular structures (Fig. 14–13*A*). Anteriorly, the trachea is crossed by the innominate artery and the left innominate vein; on left side, the trachea is close to the left carotid artery and posteriorly to the esophagus. At the level of the carina, the aortic arch runs over the left anterolateral wall of the trachea (see Fig. 14–13*B*). The left mainstem bronchus is surrounded by vessels, and the laser must be handled with great precaution in this area: the anterior wall is crossed by the left pulmonary artery and the posterior wall by the descending aorta (see Fig. 14–13*C*). On the right, the azygos vein runs around the proximal right mainstem bronchus, which is crossed underneath by the right pulmonary artery on its anterior wall. Further down, the left mainstem bronchus is surrounded by the pulmonary vein anteriorly and by the pulmonary artery on the external wall (see Fig. 14–13*D*). The anterior wall of the distal right mainstem bronchus is crossed by the right pulmonary artery (see Fig. 14–13*E*). In the left and right lower lobes, the pulmonary artery stays on the external wall of

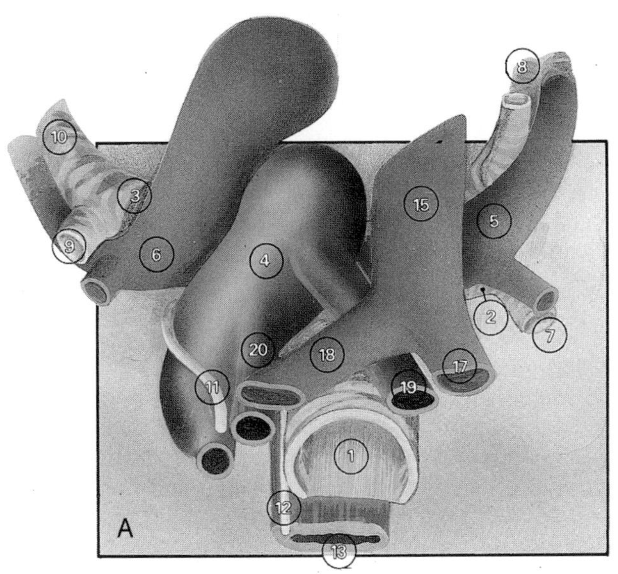

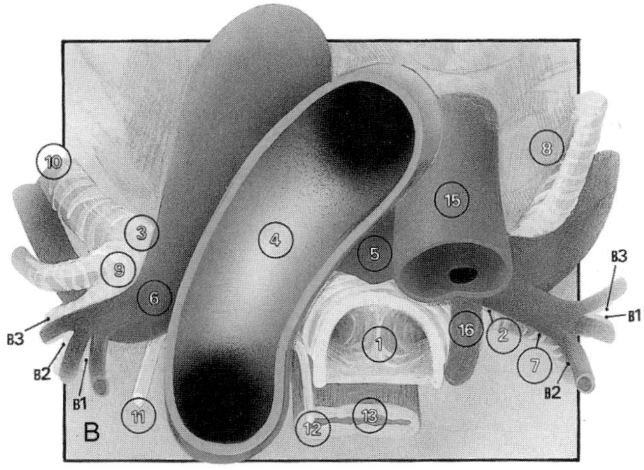

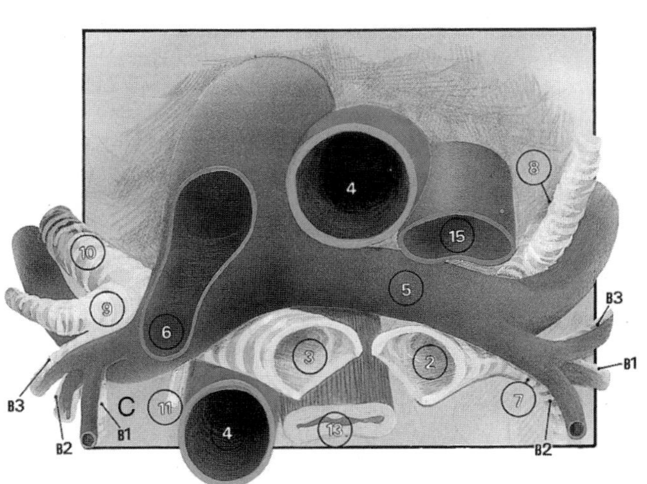

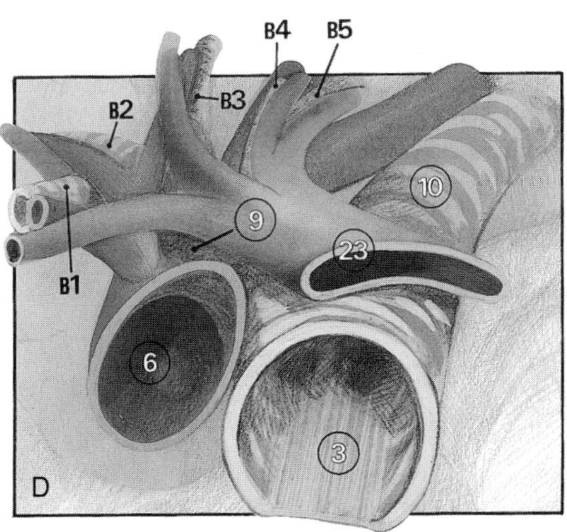

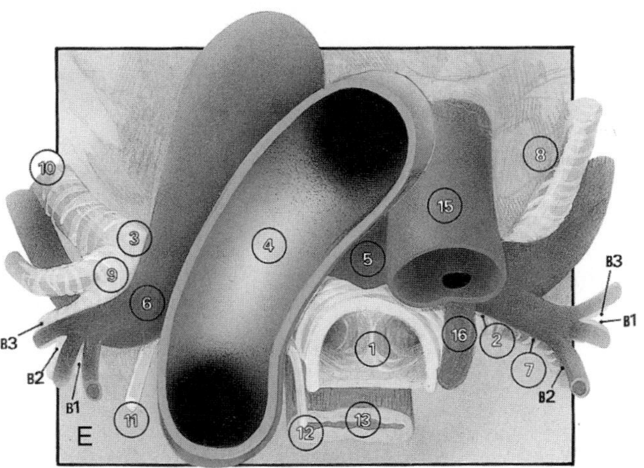

FIGURE 14–13 ■ Endoscopic anatomy of the trachea and the bronchi. *A*, Above the aortic arch. *B*, Right mainstem bronchus. *C*, At the aortic arch level. *D*, Below the carina. *E*, Left mainstem bronchus. *1*, trachea; *2*, right mainstem bronchus; *3*, left mainstem bronchus; *4*, aorta; *5*, right pulmonary artery; *6*, left pulmonary artery; *7*, right upper lobe bronchus; *8*, truncus intermedius; *9*, left upper-lobe bronchus; *10*, left lower-lobe bronchus; *11*, vagus nerve; *12*, recurrent nervus; *13*, esophagus; *15*, superior vena cava; *16*, azygos vein; *17*, right innominate vein; *18*, left innominate vein; *19*, innominate artery; *20*, left carotid artery; *21*, right upper pulmonary vein; *23*, left upper pulmonary vein. (From Dumon JF: Personal slides.)

the bronchus, the pulmonary vein is situated on the internal wall, and the branches of these vessels are on the posterior wall. The risk of vascular damage during laser therapy is much higher distally because the pulmonary vasculature is more closely related to the lobar bronchi than to the mainstem bronchi; furthermore, the wall of the airway is much thinner distally and has incomplete cartilaginous rings.

THERMAL LASERS

Carbon Dioxide Laser

The CO_2 laser is a gas laser that emits light with a wavelength of 10,600 nm. The spot size varies in diameter from 0.16 to 2 mm, as a function of the focal distance and the transmission systems (microspot, guide). The beam is strongly absorbed by water and by all biologic tissues with a composition, of 90% water. Absorption is totally independent of the presence of hemoglobin or melanin. All of the beam's energy contributes to the vaporization of certain tissue volume by instantaneous dessication without heat dispersion by conduction. These properties make it a precise scalpel that ensures hemostasis of all vessels with a caliber less than 0.5 mm. Thus, the tissue neighboring a zone that is excised by a CO_2 laser remains intact. This causes a weak inflammatory reaction and a diminution of fibrous scarring reactions. If energy delivery is restricted to a series of high-intensity pulses (superpulse or ultrapulse technology), the efficiency of vaporization is optimal, and thermal damage through conduction is reduced to a minimum. This thermal damage can be reduced by: (1) using a pulsed wave, rather than a continuous-wave mode; (2) using a high energy level during a short-duration pulse; (3) avoiding carbonization at the impact site by using a high-power density and by wiping away debris. The new generation of CO_2 lasers, capable of operation with a duty cycle of 1:3 (ultrapulse laser) produce higher peak powers (up to 500 watts) during a very short time (1000 msec), maintaining the peak throughout the entire pulse. This results in a significantly greater pulse energy and allows a clean, bloodless, and char-free tissue ablation with minimal thermal damage to the adjacent tissue. A major inconvenience of the CO_2 laser is that the beam is transmittable only in a straight line, necessitating the use of articulating arms and mirrors as intermediaries.

The improvement of adding hand-regulated accessories to the rigid bronchoscope has facilitated its use in the trachea and in the mainstem bronchi, but its capabilities are practically excluded at the level of the distal airway routes (lobar and segmental bronchi), despite the development of semiflexible guides that can convey the beam through the biopsy channel of the fibroscope. Nevertheless, the angulation provided by these guides is inferior to those of the fiberoptic used with Nd:YAG, argon, and KTP lasers. Direct laryngoscopy with an operating microscope coupled with the CO_2 laser provides excellent access to the larynx and the subglottic space. The binocular vision and the microprecision of the system allow the removal of tissue in the supraglottic, the glottic, and the subglottic regions, preserving the adjacent structures such as the vocal ligaments and the subglottic and tracheal cartilages. Lesions most successfully treated in this way include small glottic cancers, glottis synechia and webs, papillomas of the glottis, subglottic hemangiomas, and tracheal webs.

Methodology

Because a rigid bronchoscope or laryngoscopic exposure must be used, patients are placed under general anesthesia. There are now many options for ventilating the patient, depending on the preference of the surgical/anesthesiology team, the nature of the lesion and the age of the patient. When using a laryngoscopic exposure with the microscope, the patient is curarized. The ventilation is delivered either through an endotracheal protected tube made with laser resistant material, or it is administered with high-frequency jet ventilation by an injection system through the glottis or by a transtracheal catheter introduced percutaneously. In children and newborn babies, endoscopic treatment can present difficult problems related to the small dimension of the upper airway. The jet ventilation goes through thin injection systems and procures the following advantages: a clear vision of the operative field, a good respiratory gas exchange, an elimination of the risk of ignition of an endotracheal tube by the laser, decreased risks of broncho-aspiration of blood and debris, and the possibility to provide oxygen or mechanical ventilation in the postoperative period (Depierraz et al, 1994). The technique of successive apneas consists of alternatively ventilating the patient with a conventional endotracheal tube between the laser work. The patient is monitored by pulse oxymetry and is reintubated before oxygen saturation drops. Another option is Venturi ventilation with the Venturi catheter placed through the laryngoscope and above the vocal cords at all times.

When using a rigid bronchoscope, the method of ventilation may vary from spontaneous to controlled jet ventilation with a Sanders injector at conventional frequencies or jet ventilation with appropriate equipment at high frequencies. With jet ventilation, total intravenous anesthesia is necessary. The patient's eyes are protected

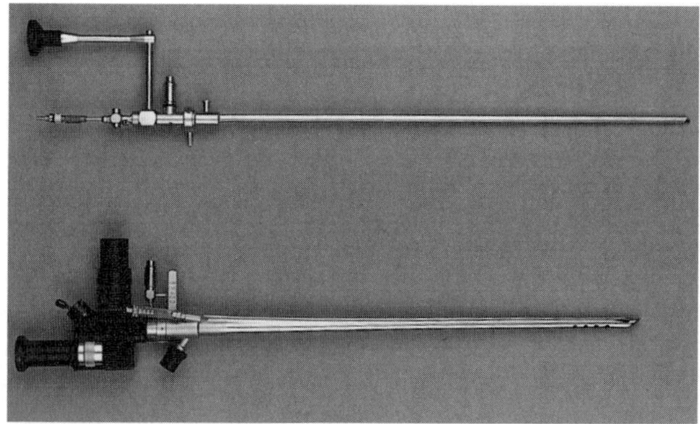

FIGURE 14–14 ■ Bronchoscopes for CO_2 laser. *Top*, Exelite guide (Coherent, Inc., Santa Clara, CA, USA) adapted on a bronchoscope whose optical element is mounted in a bayonnet shape; *Bottom*, Bronchoscope with a CO_2 laser coupler (Karl Storz, Berlin). A micromanipulator allows the laser beam to be oriented through the bronchoscope.

with moist gauze, and all personnel in the operating theater must wear protective goggles.

Once adequate ventilation has been established, the laser port is connected to the ventilating bronchoscope by means of a coupler (Fig. 14–14), and the laser beam can be fired directly down the bronchoscope into the area of pathology. The oxygen concentration during the laser procedure is kept below 30% to minimize intraoperative combustion and fire. Potential sources of combustion, such as unprotected polyvinyl chloride tubes, cotton pledgets, and carbonized tissue should be avoided. Because of the risk of combustion, nitrogen protoxide should be avoided.

Advantages and Disadvantages

The CO_2 laser is a precise cutting instrument, and it affords hemostasis only to the microcirculation. There is little perioperative edema next to the focal point of the beam, and excellent healing ability exists in the adjacent tissue. The new ultrapulse CO_2 laser minimizes the thermal effect to the surrounding tissue and the formation of scar tissue. It is the ideal laser for the treatment of benign pathologies of the larynx and tracheobronchial tree where protection of the underlying tissues (vocal ligament and cartilaginous framework) is essential. Tracheotomy can be avoided in most cases. The necessity of using a rigid system for treating laryngeal and subglottic pathologies with the CO_2 laser is not a disadvantage, as this affords excellent stability for precise work with the operating microscope in suspension laryngoscopy.

Unfortunately, the hemostasis of vessels that are greater than 0.5 mm is poor with the CO_2 laser. Furthermore, this instrument requires a cumbersome delivery system of articulated arms with several built-in prisms for the transmission of the light beam. This is necessary because the extremely long wavelength of the CO_2 laser cannot be transmitted through flexible fibers. Thus, general anesthesia with rigid endoscopy is required. However, the development of laser couplers with micromanipulators that are adaptable to a rigid endoscope allows the treatment of lesions located in the trachea and the mainstem bronchi. However, more distal lesions are not accessible to rigid endoscopy and are best treated with a flexible endoscope and a KTP or Nd:YAG laser. Because of its poor coagulation effect, the CO_2, laser has been replaced by the Nd:YAG laser for the de-obstruction of malignant tumors of the airways.

Nd:YAG Laser

The Nd:YAG is a crystal solid-state laser emitting at 1064 nm, with a minimum diameter spot size of 0.6 mm. In contrast to the CO_2 laser, the Nd:YAG laser is poorly absorbed by water. A large part of its energy is diffused by conduction in the tissue; thus, a high power is necessary to achieve a vaporization effect. With respect to the mucous membranes, underlying tissue injury is approximately 600 times more prominent than with the CO_2 laser and reaches a depth of several millimeters. With this laser, more edema and greater inflammatory reaction are seen than with the CO_2 laser. The Nd:YAG laser thus lends itself less well to precise tissue resection than does the CO_2 laser, but its coagulation and vaporization effects are excellent. Its beam is transmitted by a Teflon-coated flexible quartz fiber with a diameter of 1.8 or 2.2 mm, which can easily be introduced into a rigid or flexible endoscope and oriented in any angle.

Because of its effects of coagulation and capability of vaporizing large amounts of tissue, the Nd:YAG laser is indicated in bronchology to remove tumoral obstructions, but it should not be used for the treatment of benign strictures.

Methodology

The goal of bronchoscopic debulking of tumors using the Nd:YAG laser is to improve respiratory function or to diminish the risk of bronchopneumonia. This implies functional lung parenchyma and preserved vascularization by the pulmonary arteries and veins beyond the obstruction. The preoperative assessment involves a history, physical examination, recent chest radiograph or computed tomography (CT) scan, and routine blood tests, including arterial blood gases. On occasion, a ventilation/perfusion scan is helpful in identifying an occluded pulmonary artery to the involved lung that might preclude an attempt to reopen the airway. An atelectasis of longer than 3 weeks has little chance to be reventilated after de-obstruction of the bronchus because of chronic bronchopneumonia. The need for perfect cooperation between the surgeon and the anesthetist cannot be overstated. For both, the airway is a shared facility, and discussion is essential before the procedure commences and throughout its course. A bronchoscopy under local anesthesia is often useful to confirm the value of de-obstruction, especially if the patient is referred. The method that should be used to apply laser treatment in bronchology (fiberoptic mode in local anesthesia versus rigid mode in general anesthesia) is a subject of controversy (Chan, 1990); uncontrolled and dreadful complications including death from massive hemorrhage have been reported with the flexible bronchoscope.

Based on safety considerations for the patient and the time required for the procedure, we strongly recommend the use of a rigid endoscope under general anesthesia. Its efficacy is clearly superior to that of bronchofibroscopy used under local anesthesia. Bronchofibroscopes do not allow the rapid and efficient control of potential major complications (hemorrhage and hypoxia) in high-risk patients, who represent most the patients treated for palliative tumoral de-obstruction. This view is supported by most centers that have extensive experience treating this pathology (Beamis, 1991; Brutinel et al, 1987; Cavalièr, 2000; Dumon, 1982; Edell et al, 1993). The rigid bronchoscope allows control of the ventilation during the entire procedure and ensures a good visualization of the surgical field because of the easy cleaning of the telescope without retracting the rigid tube. Nevertheless, for selected indications, it is possible to use a bronchofibroscope with local anesthesia for the removal of small benign tumors and of granulation tissue following surgery (Personne, 1990). This type of therapeutic endoscopy in local anesthesia should, however, take place in a set-up that is equipped with facilities for general anesthesia in case uncontrollable hemorrhage should occur

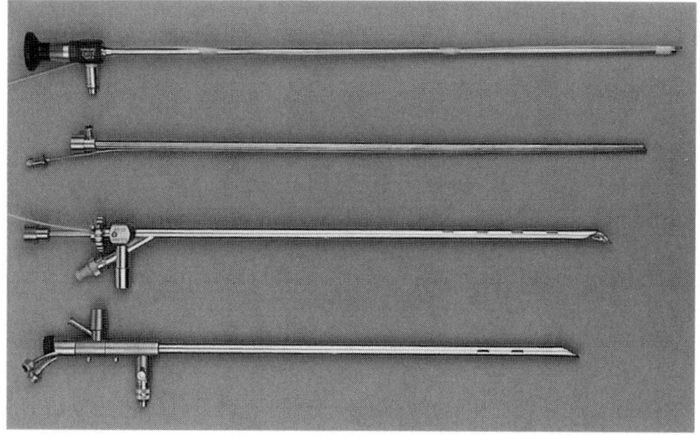

FIGURE 14–15 ■ Bronchoscope for neodymium:yttrium aluminum-garnet laser. *Top,* The laser fiber is attached with adhesive strips directly to the optic. An external canal has been added to the intermediary guide of the bronchoscope to allow the passage of the fiber. *Second from bottom,* An intermediary guide with a canal for the laser fiber, which can be oriented up to 45 degrees at the tip of the bronchoscope, is adaptable with the universal bronchoscope; *Bottom,* Laser bronchoscope by Shapsay with two or three channels for the laser fiber, the aspiration of secretion, and the aspiration of smoke. (*Bottom two,* Karl Storz, Berlin).

during the procedure. With the aim of mastering all situations, the endoscopist must be instructed in bronchofibroscopy as well as in the handling of the rigid instrumentation (Kvale, 1990). Many specific laser bronchoscopes have been developed, but a standard ventilating bronchoscope is most often used (Fig. 14–15). Different techniques of ventilation are adaptable to the bronchoscope, such as intermittent or continuous insufflation or Venturi (jet) ventilation at conventional or high frequencies (see the chapter on rigid bronchoscopy). We prefer the Venturi ventilation for the following reasons: high-frequency jet ventilation in an open circuit has the advantage of keeping the patient well ventilated during the various endoscopic maneuvers, such as changing or cleaning the optic, aspiration of the secretion and blood, and tamponade with cotton swabs soaked in adrenaline. Inconveniences include the drying out of the bronchial mucosa and the risks associated with barometric trauma (e.g., pneumothorax, pneumomediastinum, gastric distention). These complications have diminished since the introduction of monitoring the end-respiratory pressure, which permits interruption of the procedure in cases of poor expiration and excessive alveolar pressure. The smoke produced by the vaporization is immediately removed and does not disturb the surgeon's vision.

During the entire procedure, the patient must be monitored. Close attention must be paid to the electrocardiogram, the transcutaneous oxygen saturation, the expired carbon dioxide, and arterial tension. The fraction of inspired oxygen (FIO_2) should be less than 30% to prevent the risk of combustion or fire. Because nitrogen protoxide is just as good a combustor as oxygen, its use should be avoided during laser endoscopic surgery. Anesthesia is maintained by intravenous agents. Choice of anesthesia is left to the anesthetist's judgment based on the patient's condition. When the oxygen saturation falls, the laser is stopped, and the patient is again ventilated through a closed circuit with 100% FIO_2.

The removal of the obstruction starts with coagulation some distance away from the lesion (blanching of the tumor), with a low power setting (30 to 35 W, for 3 to 5 sec). The aim is to reduce the perioperative bleeding as much as possible. The vaporization effect occurs by placing the fiber closer to the lesion with a higher power setting (40 to 50 W), in the continuous emission mode (2 to 3 sec) or with intermittent shots of 0.8 to 1.4 seconds. This depends on the effect desired or the proximity of vascular structures neighboring the lesion. When used in a continuous mode, the laser is waved over the surface of the tumor with a laser beam parallel to the tracheobronchial wall. The lesion is then removed with the beveled tip of the bronchoscope and cored out until the tip of the instrument is passed beyond the obstruction. Pieces of the tumor are extracted with the biopsy forceps (Fig. 14–16); blood and secretions are aspirated using a large caliber suction device, and hemostasis is obtained with cotton swabs soaked in adrenaline or by repeated washings with a cool saline solution.

The external shaft of the rigid bronchoscope also plays a significant role in ensuring hemostasis because it compresses the bleeding surface of the tumoral stenosis. Complete vaporization and hemostasis of the tumor is then achieved in a retrograde fashion by lasering tumor debris and bleeding sources from a distance with the Nd:YAG laser. This also offers the distinct advantage of enabling visualization of the bronchial lumen throughout the laser work, thus minimizing the risk of perforation of vascular structures and of the bronchial wall. In cases of massive hemorrhage, the main bronchus is totally packed with a re-absorbable hemostatic compress (Surgicel) or an inflatable balloon (Fogarty catheter), and the open-tube bronchoscope is introduced into the healthy main bronchus to ensure ventilation of the contralateral lung and to suck out blood clots. Afterwards, the bleeding area covered with the re-absorbable compress is vaporized with the laser to ensure that the hemostasis and

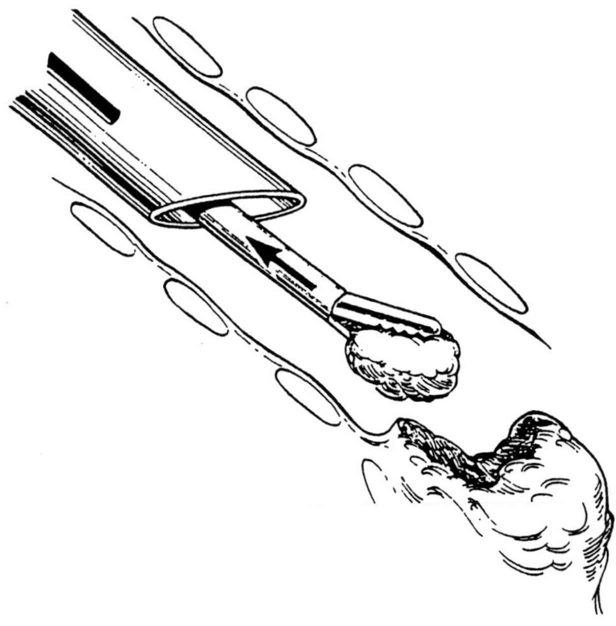

FIGURE 14–16 ■ After photocoagulation with the neodymium:yttrium-aluminum-garnet laser, the tumor can be removed by physical débridement using large biopsy forceps through the ventilating bronchoscope.

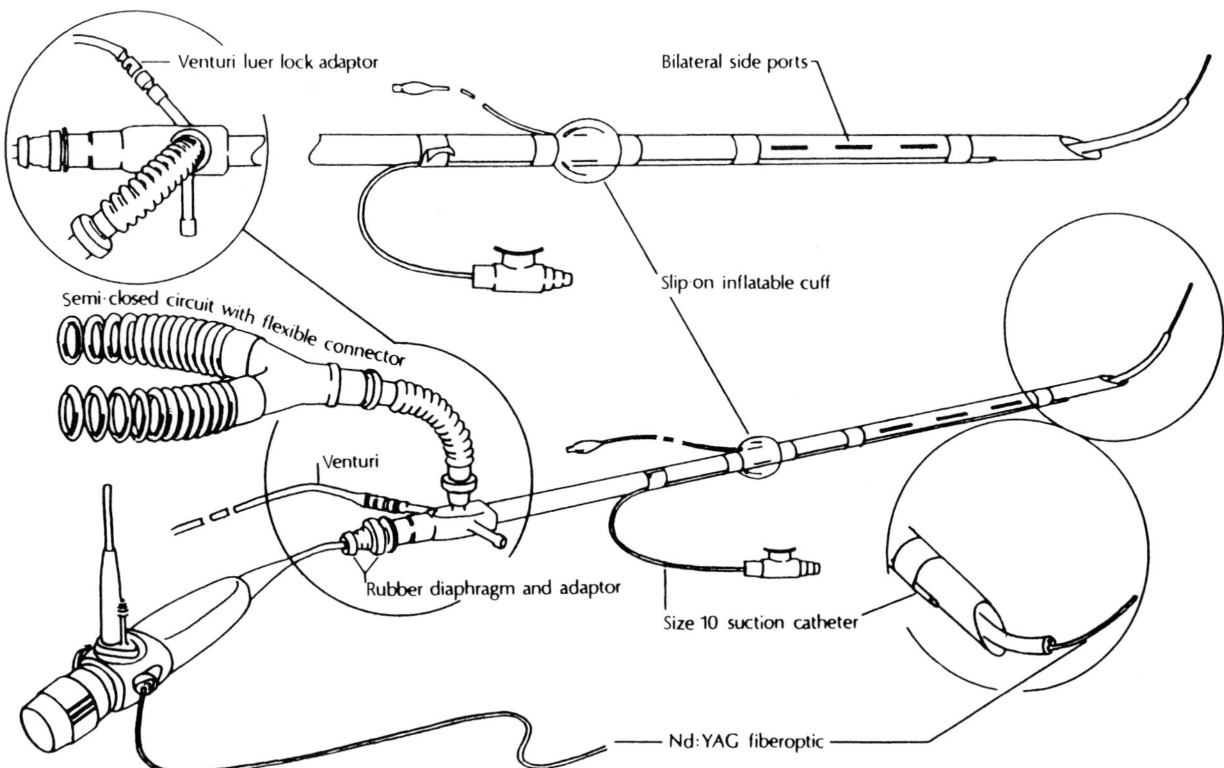

FIGURE 14–17 ■ A technique illustrated by Perera demonstrating the bronchoscopy/anesthesia technique for laser resection of airway lesions (From Perera ER, Mallon JS: General anesthetic management for laser resection of central airway lesion in 85 procedures. Can J Anaesth 34:383, 1987.)

the debris are gently aspirated. When hemostasis has been achieved with a Fogarty catheter, the balloon is slowly deflated under direct visualization after 3 to 5 minutes. If the hemostasis is not satisfactory or the risk of recurrence appears too high, then the catheter with the balloon inflated is kept in place for 24 to 48 hours. The removal is done under general anesthesia or local anesthesia with all of the facilities for general anesthesia available if needed.

By attaching a ventilator to the side port of the bronchoscope and occluding its open end, the anesthesia system can be converted to a conventional closed ventilation system. A flexible bronchoscope can then be passed through a grommet occluding the open end of the bronchoscope, and a laser fiber can be passed through the channel of the fiberoptic bronchoscope and positioned under the direct vision of the operator in the area to be treated (Fig. 14–17).

Laser treatment of distal obstructive malignant lesions is not effective in improving ventilation. For that reason, this method is essentially used for treatment of the distal airway for obstructive pneumonitis and recurrent hemoptysis. It is used occasionally to vaporize the tumoral bed and to clean the distal airway at the end of the intervention (Fig. 14–18). Another application is the treatment of peripheral benign lesions, such as papillomas or hemangiomas, that are not accessible with the CO_2 laser.

To maintain the effects of treatment as long as possible and to avoid multiple hospitalizations, the laser treatment is usually followed by the immediate insertion of an endobronchial prosthesis (see later). Prophylactic antibiotic therapy is advisable. The patient is extubated, if the oxygen saturation so permits, or reintubated with an endotracheal tube. After laser obstruction removal, maintenance of bronchial permeability depends on the diameter of the bronchus and the speed of tumor growth.

The postoperative period in high-risk patients is especially critical. They require strict cardiorespiratory moni-

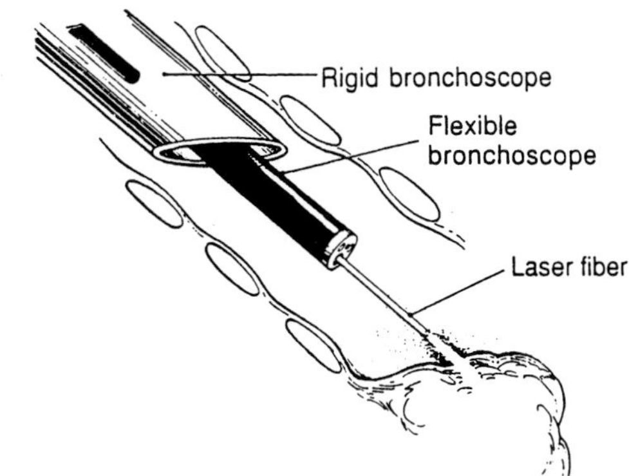

FIGURE 14–18 ■ Laser therapy with bronchofibroscope. For distal lesions of the airways, laser therapy is performed by direct observation of the laser through the fiberoptic bronchoscope, which is passed initially through the rigid endoscope. If suctioning is required during therapy, then the flexible bronchoscope can be removed, and ventilation can be converted to a jet system. Débridement can then occur simply through the rigid bronchoscope.

toring in the recovery room. The most frequent complications are hypoxia, followed by respiratory depression owing to anesthetic agents (Hanowell, 1991), obstruction of a bronchus by blood clots or secretions, or cardiovascular complications. In the days following the intervention, bronchofibroscopies for cleaning purposes under local anesthesia are sometimes necessary to evacuate a mucus or fibrin plug. Respiratory physiotherapy is also helpful over a span of several days.

Advantages

The Nd:YAG laser has characteristics that produce excellent vaporization of large tumor masses with good coagulation properties. Safe and effective ablation can be performed much more quickly than with the CO_2 laser. It is strongly recommended that a rigid open tube bronchoscope be used for the palliative treatment of obstructing inoperable bronchial cancer (Brutinel et al, 1987; Dumon, 1987). However, the flexible bronchoscope introduced through the rigid instrument may be used in selected cases for the treatment of benign, well-circumscribed tumors of lobar or segmental bronchi. However, the risk of bronchial and vascular perforations with massive hemorrhage must not be underestimated.

KTP and Argon Lasers

The KTP (532 nm, spot size 0.15-mm diameter) corresponds to an Nd:YAG laser coupled to a crystal, which doubles the wavelength of the Nd:YAG from 1064 to 532 nm. The laser can be used either in the Nd:YAG mode or in the KTP mode.

The argon laser (488 and 514 nm, spot size 0.15 mm diameter) has a wavelength close to that of the KTP laser, and, based on this, it also has similar effects on tissue. Nevertheless, the absorption peak in hemoglobin is somewhat lower than that of the KTP laser. Its tissue penetration depth is difficult to predict, and it is extremely dependent on the degree of tissue vascularization and pigmentation. The use of these two lasers requires accurate knowledge of tissue interactions with each organ and each lesion of interest. For the mucous membranes, tissue damage is approximately 10 times greater than that caused by the CO_2 laser (i.e., approximately 1 to 2 mm). The beams of the argon and KTP lasers are transmitted through a flexible fiber. With a lower power setting, it has a coagulating effect, and with a higher power setting, a vaporization effect.

The KTP laser has not been widely used in bronchology owing to its physical properties as discussed and owing to its purchase cost, which is comparable with the combined cost of a CO_2 and an Nd:YAG laser. However, combined Nd:YAG/KTP laser machines are becoming commercially available and will likely modify some of the indications in bronchology. In comparison with the CO_2 laser, the KTP laser can also be used with a bronchofibroscope. In bronchology, the argon laser is especially useful in photodynamic therapy at 514 nm or as a pump laser on a dye-emitting laser in the red at 630 nm.

COMPLICATIONS OF THERMAL LASER THERAPY

Hypoxemia

The risk of intraoperative and postoperative hypoxemia is high in those patients whose oxygen saturation at ambient air pressure is already low owing to their underlying bronchopulmonary illness. This risk is accentuated by the impossibility of using the laser with 100% FIO_2 ventilation, based on danger of tracheal fire. Blood gas level is monitored during the whole procedure, and the endoscopist and anesthesiologist team should anticipate the hypoxemia. It can occur rapidly, depending on the localization of the obstruction. An obstruction at the level of the trachea, of the carina, or of the two mainstem bronchi constitutes a high risk for hypoxemia. Airway patency can be rapidly re-established by passing the bronchoscope beyond the obstructive tumor and changing the jet ventilation to a close ventilation circuit with 100% oxygen. Secretions, blood clots, and necrotic debris accumulated beyond the obstruction are aspirated, and the lungs are washed with a saline solution. Severe hypoxemia may occur following severe hemorrhage or bronchial collapse by loss of cartilaginous support from extensive tumoral destruction or repetitive vaporizations (Maire, 1989). Endoprostheses can be used to avoid this complication (Cavalière, 1996; Colt, 1991; Edell, 1993; Monnier, 1996; Sonett, 1995). Postoperatively, in the recovery room, pooling of secretions and blood may compromise the airway, and the patient may benefit from flexible bronchoscopy to evacuate the secretions. On occasion, the patency of the mainstem bronchus is improved by the laser treatment, but the patient remains hypoxemic, owing to a dead space effect resulting from a nonperfused but ventilated lung.

Hemorrhage

Based on a large series of studies published by experienced surgeons, the risk of fatal hemorrhage during laser de-obstruction is relatively rare. Nevertheless, it represents a grave danger because it leads to severe hypoxemia with risk of death. Brutinel and colleagues (1987), Beamis (1991), and Cavalière and coworkers (1996), respectively, reported 5.6%, 0.5%, and 0.7% intraoperative and immediate postoperative hemorrhages. Knowledge of the anatomy of the pulmonary vasculature and its relationship to the airway is essential to prevent dramatic hemorrhage. If a massive tracheal hemorrhage occurs, then the rigid bronchoscope is passed through the bleeding area, and the hemorrhage is controlled by tamponade with the bronchoscope and with gauze soaked in adrenaline. After the re-establishment of the ventilation, the de-obstruction is performed in a retrograde manner. With massive bronchial hemorrhage, the bronchoscope is immediately introduced in the healthy main bronchus, which is cleared by blood aspiration. After a ventilation phase with 100% oxygen, the hemorrhage is treated (in order of importance) by coagulation, tamponade with the tip of the bronchoscope, or by obstruction of the bronchus with reabsorbable compress or an inflatable balloon (Fogarty catheter).

Perforations and Fistulas

Perforations of the bronchial tree may be complicated by pneumothorax, pneumomediastinum, mediastinal fistula, tracheo-broncho-esophageal fistula, and massive or fatal hemorrhage. Fistula can occur in cases of excessive thermal damage or in the presence of large necrotic tumors, mainly on the posterior wall of the trachea and the left mainstem bronchus where the cartilaginous framework is absent. When isolated lesions are identified bronchoscopically in these particular locations, esophagoscopy must be performed to rule out a primary malignancy in the esophagus with anterior penetration into the posterior wall of the airway. One can avoid these complications by strictly vaporizing the posterior wall with weak laser power and with tangential laser beam application.

Pneumothorax

Pneumothorax without perforation is a rare complication of barotrauma associated with both jet and conventional positive-pressure ventilation. It does happen on occasion, and once recognized it should be treated simply by chest tube drainage. Brutinel and colleagues (1987) and Cavalière and coworkers (1996) report 0.5% and 0.3% of pneumothoraces, respectively.

Endobronchial Spill

Occasionally, when an obstructing malignancy has been removed, the airway and lung beyond contain purulent material owing to obstruction and accumulation or to acute endobronchial drainage of a parenchymal abscess cavity. Care must be taken to avoid spillage to the contralateral lung, both during the operation and immediately postoperatively.

Fire

Fire in the area during laser therapy can always be avoided with proper care. The target of the laser beam should always be visible to the operator, and nothing, such as a suction catheter or normal tissues, should inadvertently be fired upon. The tip of the laser fiber should be at least 5 mm beyond the end of the flexible bronchoscope. If it is retracted into the bronchoscope, then the tip of the bronchoscope will be severely damaged. The FIO_2 during therapy should always remain less than 30%.

General Complications

Various cardiovascular complications (rhythm disturbances, infarcts, cardiac arrests, pericarditis, pulmonary edema) and cerebral gas emboli should also be mentioned (Golish, 1992; Ross, 1988).

In spite of all of these potential complications in high-risk patients, the mortality rate is less than 2% (Brutinel et al, 1987; Cavalière et al, 1996; Dumon, 1982).

CLINICAL APPLICATIONS OF THE THERMAL LASER IN AIRWAY OBSTRUCTION

Endoscopic Treatment of Papillomatosis and Benign Tumors

Papillomatosis and benign tumors of the larynx and of the tracheobronchial tree are good indications for endoscopic laser treatment. For most cases, the CO_2 laser is the laser of choice. It has minimal scatter and deep coagulation effect, and it, therefore, preserves the adjacent tissue from thermal damage. It offers the possibility of a total resection, and if there is recurrence, the endoscopic treatment does not preclude a later surgical resection, if indicated. Tumors in the peripheral bronchi that are not accessible with a rigid endoscope are treated with the KTP or Nd:YAG lasers. The fiber is passed through the canal of a bronchofibroscope. The danger of the procedure is related to absorption into tissue, strongly dependent on pigment for the KTP laser, with the risk of perforation and hemorrhage.

Recurrent respiratory papillomatosis (juvenile or adult) is the most frequent benign lesion treated with the CO_2 laser. The larynx is the principal site involved, but isolated tracheal and bronchial papillomas occur, mostly in adults (Fig. 14–19). Although the CO_2 laser does not reduce the frequency of recurrence, it allows a complete

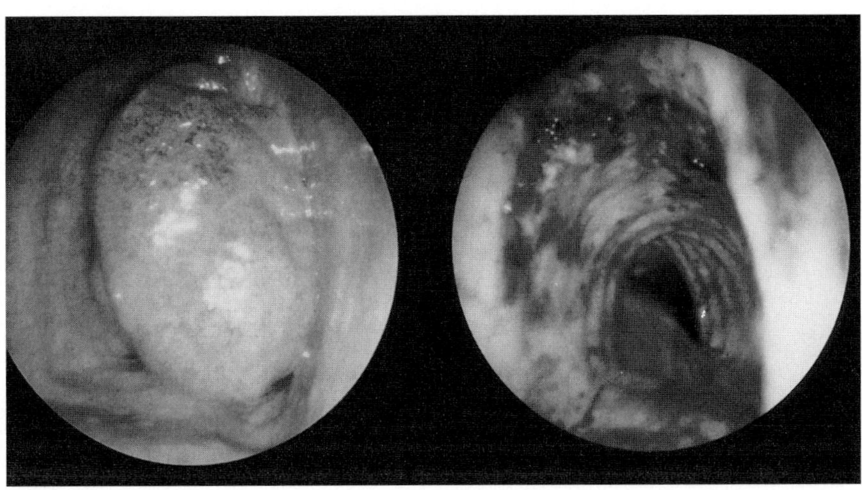

FIGURE 14–19 ■ Papilloma implanted in the anterior wall of the proximal trachea resected with the CO_2 laser coupled to a bronchoscope.

removal of the lesion with minimal hemorrhage. It is important to avoid any source of hemorrhage in the operative field because it diminishes the quality of the resection and increases the diffusion of the heat into the surrounding tissues. Because papillomatosis is a pathology that is strictly limited to the mucosa, the underlying tissues must be preserved. When extensive papillomatosis causes an obstruction of the airways, laser debulking is indicated to avoid a tracheotomy. Total removal is, therefore, not possible without damage to the adjacent structures. For these cases, to reduce volume and the recurrence of the papillomas, the laser treatment is often associated with interferon administration or with concomitant local injection of antiviral agents (cidofovir). The combination of these treatments leads to a complete eradication of the illness in some cases.

Subglottic hemangioma can be treated by resection with the CO_2 laser coupled with a laser bronchoscope or in suspension laryngoscopy with a micromanipulator coupled to the microscope. Hemangioma involving the near total or total circumference is removed in two sessions to avoid a circular stenosis. The CO_2 laser is also indicated for the removal of other benign tumors such as lipomas, chondromas, leiomyomas, hamartomas, and other pathologies such as Wegener granulomatosis and histiocytomas. The KTP laser, owing to its absorption peak in hemoglobin, is indicated for the treatment of well-vascularized tumors. Amyloidosis can be a difficult problem to treat owing to its infiltration into the cartilaginous wall and its spread all along the tracheobronchial tree. Total excision is generally not possible, and the only goal of the treatment is to restore the patency of the airways.

Endoscopic Treatment for Tracheobronchial Cicatricial Stenoses

The management of cicatricial stenoses of the airway is a difficult therapeutic problem. They are often associated with laryngeal lesions and are most frequently located at the subglottic and superior tracheal regions (sequelae of intubation, tracheotomy, or trauma). Pretherapeutic endoscopic assessment must be carried out in a rigorous manner (see chapter on subglottic resection in children). It comprises a functional examination of the vocal cords and a laryngotracheoscopy ranging at least from the epiglottis to the carina. This examination should provide the following information: (1) mobility of the vocal cords, (2) exact location of the lesion (distance in centimeters and the number of normal tracheal rings between the level of the glottis and the superior pole of the stenosis on one side; distance between the inferior pole of the stenosis and the carina on the other); and (3) the length and the diameter of the lesion (Monnier et al, 1998).

Based on the type of stenosis encountered, various therapeutic surgical or endoscopic modalities exist. Because of the development of therapeutic bronchoscopy with the CO_2 laser, certain endoscopic therapies have become possible. In all cases of cicatricial stenosis, the risk of aggravating the initial situation exists; it is thus necessary to respect the indications rigorously and to know when to propose surgical resection before "attempting" laser therapy as a first step (Mudry and Monnier, 1994; Simpson et al, 1982).

Indications

Indications for endoscopic laser therapy include the following:

1. A thin, scarred diaphragm that is less than 1 cm in length without cartilaginous collapse or localized tracheal malacia (Fig. 14–20*A*, *B*): preferentially, ultrapulsed CO_2 laser with a microlite spot is used to avoid heat diffusion into the surrounding tissue. Circular vaporization should be avoided, and, based on the technique proposed by Shapsay (1987), we prefer to carry out radial incisions of the stenosis with the laser beam and then gently dilate the stricture with Savary-Gilliard dilators. This will maintain intact mucosal bridges in the area of the stenosis and afford better re-epithelialization. Vaporization of the perichondrium and cartilage should be avoided, as this may lead to serious deformations of the framework, which could make further therapy necessary.
2. Failures from previous surgery that require further intervention: with this type of indication, it is difficult to provide guidelines concerning the techniques to be used. The most conservative therapy possible is indicated to

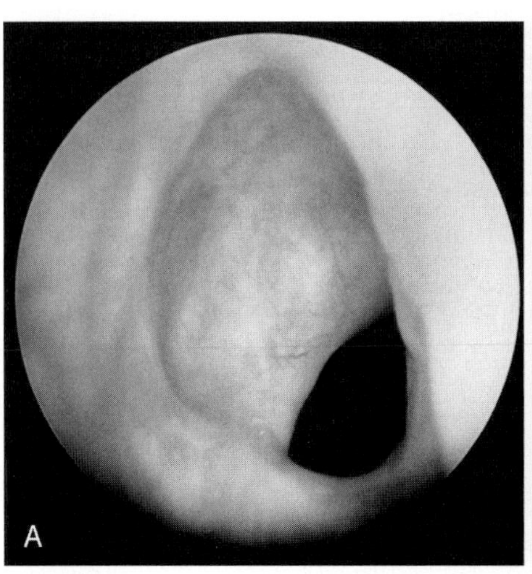

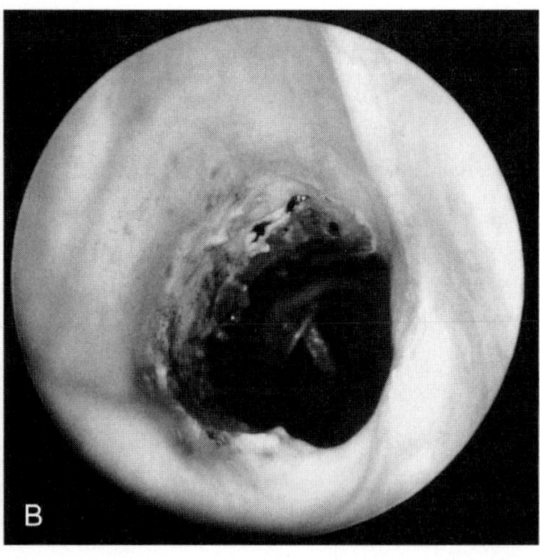

FIGURE 14–20 ■ *A*, Thin scarred diaphragm less than 1 cm situated in the subglottis. *B*, After resection with CO_2 laser coupled with an operating microscope.

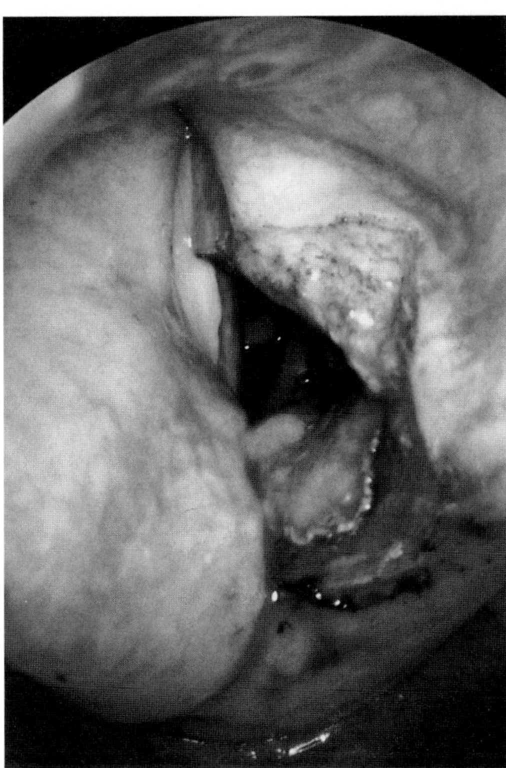

FIGURE 14–21 ■ Left CO_2 laser arytenoidectomy for bilateral vocal cord paralysis after extensive thyroid surgery. An internal mucosal flap is elevated to cover the excision area.

avoid further aggravation of the situation. In the face of such restrictive situations, it may be necessary to refrain from any attempt at endoscopic therapy and to rely on endoluminal stenting.

3. Postoperative inflammatory granulations at the level of a surgical anastomosis, at the level of a suprastomal spur in a tracheotomized patient, or at the level of the tip of the cannula. The CO_2 laser remains the best laser for vaporization of granulations.

4. Bronchial anastomostic stenosis after lung transplantation: airway stenosis or malacia after lung transplantation occurs in about 10% of the patients, and treatment is required if they are symptomatic (Bolot et al, 1998; Sonett et al, 1995). Short diaphragm-like stenoses without malacia are treated with CO_2 laser and dilatation. Cartilage necrosis that is due to ischemic injury during the immediate postoperative period is complicated by bronchomalacia and fibrotic lesion. In these cases, laser treatment must be combined with stent implantation.

5. Symptomatic bilateral vocal cord paralysis can be treated by CO_2 laser arytenoidectomy with an operating microscope in suspension laryngoscopy (Fig. 14–21).

Perioperative Adjuvant Therapies

The efficacy of perioperative adjuvant therapies such as corticosteriods (systemic or intralesional) and antibiotics remains controversial. Corticosteroids are administered with the hope of reducing postoperative edema and later formation of scar tissue. However, they may delay epithelialization and inhibit effective epithelial healing with the risk of infection. Actually, there is no consensus on the proper use and benefit of corticosteroids. Because infections delay the healing process and favor the formation of scar tissue, prophylactic and postoperative administration of antibiotics is generally advocated. Regarding corticosteroids, no data have defined the real effect of antibiotics on the outcome. The authors routinely administer systemic antibiotics and local application of ointment containing an antibiotic and a corticosteroid (Diprogenta, Essex Chemie). This approach has had excellent results for prevention of inflammatory granulations.

Contraindications

Contraindications to endoscopic laser therapy include destruction of the cartilaginous framework, tracheomalacia, stenosis longer than 1 cm, and total stenosis. If the indications and contraindications for endoscopic therapy (discussed) are ignored, irreversible damage may ensue from repeated laser therapy. At the end of the 20th century, it was the trend of certain endoscopists to combine laser therapy with an endotracheal stent placement as a first treatment modality in all cicatricial stenoses of the airway. This attitude must be severely condemned. The best chance for the patient lies in the initial treatment; therefore, a recommendation for surgery must be carefully considered. No endoscopic treatment will ever achieve the quality of results obtained by a segmental resection of the trachea with end-to-end anastomosis. Additionally, stenting of the airway always carries the risk of aggravating the initial condition by inducing granulation tissue and, eventually, stenosis at both ends of the tracheal prosthesis.

From 1973 to 1998, the authors treated 84 laryngotracheal stenoses by endoscopic means. According to Cotton's classification (Cotton, 1984), 20% of the stenoses were grade I, 35% grade II, 44% grade III, and none was grade IV. Thirteen percent of the patients had received multiple surgeries previously and had no further open surgical alternatives. Twenty-four percent had a tracheostomy, 25% presented with a dyspnea at rest, and 51% complained of exertional dyspnea. Endoscopic treatment consisted of CO_2 or Nd:YAG laser treatment with contact sapphire, dilatation, or stenting. With a mean follow-up of 2 years, 80% of the patients recovered an airway size that averaged 50% to 100% of the normal lumen. Decannulation was possible in 70% of the tracheostomized cases (14/20). After treatment, 46% practice sports freely, 43% complain of exertional dyspnea, 4% have a dyspnea at rest, and 7% are still tracheostomy-dependent. Compared with other groups (Metha et al, 1993; Ossof et al, 1985; Shapsay, 1987), these results are fairly good but are clearly inferior to those achieved by surgical resection (Monnier et al, 1998).

Palliative Endoscopic Therapy for Tracheobronchial Cancer

Indications

To eliminate unnecessary surgical risks, it is important to choose those patients capable of being helped by removal of obstruction by laser treatment. One must ensure that

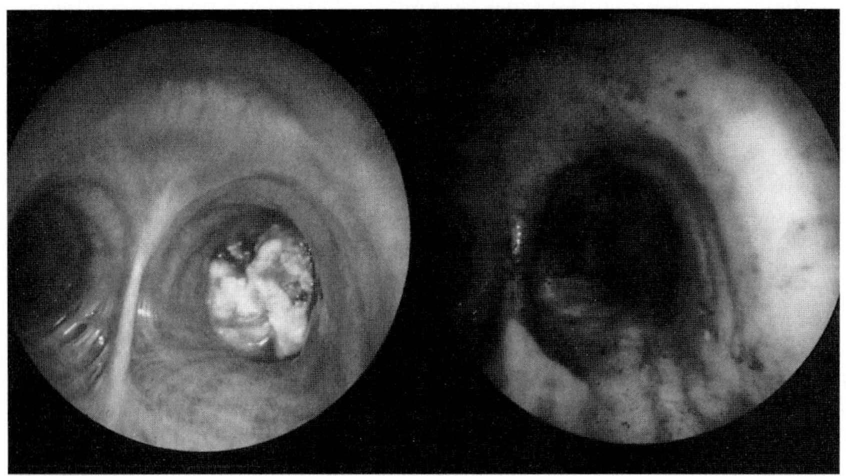

FIGURE 14–22 ■ Obstruction of the right mainstem bronchus from an epidermoid carcinoma and recanalization of the bronchial lumen after neodymium:yttrium-aluminum-garnet laser debulking.

the patient can indeed benefit from the intervention. The primary indication is restoration of the airway patency to reduce dyspnea. Drainage of an obstructive pneumonia and hemostasis of a hemorrhagic tumor are rarer indications. Our eligibility criteria include the following:

1. The tumor should basically be exophytic if therapy is to be by laser alone (Fig. 14–22). However, this condition is less strict with the possibility of stenting the airways (Cavaliere et al, 1996; Monnier et al, 1996). If mixed (extrinsic and intrinsic) compression is present, a lumen that is large enough to allow the introduction of a prosthesis is created by the laser, which acts on the intrinsic compression to restore a sufficient lumen.
2. If possible, a lumen should always be present to reduce the risk of creating a perforation of the bronchus or of the large vessels. In inoperable cases, preventive vaporization of the tumor is recommended before it completely obstructs the lumen, even if it is producing no symptoms, or if these symptoms are minor (Dierkesmann, 1990).
3. In the bronchi, the length of the tumor should not exceed 4 cm (Edell and Shapsay, 1994).
4. Because the therapeutic effect increases with the more proximal site of the obstruction, the best indications for therapy are obstructions at the level of the trachea and mainstem bronchi. At the periphery (lobar and segmental bronchi), the only valuable indications are hemostasis and drainage of an obstructive bronchopneumonia. However, in segmental bronchi the risk of vascular perforation is extremely high, owing to the partial obstruction of the bronchial wall by the tumor. In fact, laser indications are almost restricted to benign lesions at this level.
5. The pulmonary parenchyma beyond the obstruction must still be functional. An atelectasis of more than 3 weeks' duration has little chance of re-expanding after the reopening of the obstructed bronchus.

Results

Dumon and associates (1982), using a specially constructed rigid bronchoscope for laser endoscopy, performed 1500 procedures in 817 patients. The immediate results after reopening of the main airway obstructions (trachea, right and left mainstem bronchi) were excellent in 75%, fair in 15%, and poor in 10% of cases. As laser treatments addressed more distal obstructions, the efficacy of the procedure was directly reduced. Dumon's group also performed laser endoscopy on 122 benign lesions, achieving good results in 90 of these patients with a 1-year follow-up. Hayata and colleagues (1989) and Unger (1985) demonstrated that Nd:YAG therapy was effective in improving ventilation by both objective and subjective assessments in 78% and 77% of patients, respectively. Therapy was most effective in patients who had proximal tracheobronchial lesions, integrity of the cartilaginous wall, healthy parenchyma distal to the lesion, benign lesions, and partial obstructions.

Miller (1989) has compared CO_2 with Nd:YAG laser endoscopy for obstructing lesions in 89 patients with 102 procedures performed. This study demonstrated good to excellent results in 81% of those treated by CO_2 laser and 91.5% in those treated by Nd:YAG laser. The Nd:YAG therapy was easier to use and involved a shorter anesthesia time and a shorter time in the operating room. It was less expensive overall.

Cavalière and coworkers (1996) reported 13 years of experience with endoscopic treatment of malignant airway obstruction, including laser therapy, brachytherapy, and stenting, in more than 2000 patients. Good results were obtained in 93% of patients with bronchogenic carcinoma. Extrinsic compression, extensive infiltration of the airways, and voluminous extraluminal infiltration were poor prognostic factors. More peripheral location of lesions was associated with a less favorable outcome. The best results were obtained for tumors located in the trachea, the mainstem bronchi, and the truncus intermedius (>90% of good results). Less favorable results were obtained for tumors situated in the right upper lobe with good results in only 49% of cases.

An improvement of pulmonary function has been seen in a similar percentage of patients in another series (George et al, 1990; Mohsenifar et al, 1988) with better results for proximal lesions. For most patients, the quality of life was considerably improved and death by asphyxiation was avoided (Daddi et al, 1998; Stanopoulos et al, 1993). For ethical reasons, there is no way of determining if the survival of patients is prolonged because randomized studies in patients with dyspnea cannot be undertaken. Endobronchial laser therapy is usually the final attempt after other treatments have been unsuccessful. However, the influence of this procedure on survival and the circumstances of death remain unclear, although survival is not the main goal of a palliative treatment. The interval between treatment and relapse averages 2 to 3 months (Clarke et al, 1994; Hetzel, 1995). Patients who are treated for relief of hemoptysis tend to have a recurrence of their symptoms within 30 days of the treatment. Patients treated for dyspnea or cough tend to have a recurrence of symptoms later, approximately 60 to 90 days after treatment (Clarke et al, 1994).

The optimal combination of treatment modalities (laser alone, laser with external beam radiation or brachytherapy, laser with endobronchial stents) is also not defined. Macha and colleagues (1994) evaluated the survival and the pattern of failure in patients treated with laser compared with patients treated with radiotherapy: the incidence of terminal hemorrhage was four times higher in patients treated with laser (34.5%), but survival was similar in the two groups. This suggests that survival time is not shortened by laser therapy but corresponds to that expected in patients with submucosal tumors treated with external radiotherapy and reflects different patterns of tumor growth with respect to mucosal destruction. When full recanalization was achieved, the survival was prolonged by 4 months. The median survival was 12 months.

A combination of endobronchial brachytherapy and laser de-obstruction has been used in patients with endobronchial disease to prevent the regrowth of the tumor and to provide good palliation of the symptoms for the duration of survival (Cavalière et al, 1996). Brachytherapy may not bring any benefit to those patients who present with severe dyspnea, because the survival duration is very short (Ordanel, 1997). For patients with higher expectations for survival, the use of laser treatment as an adjunct to endobrachytherapy is controversial, because of the risk of fatal hemorrhage (Macha et al, 1994). Suh and coworkers (1994) reported a series of 37 patients treated with brachytherapy with or without laser resection. Both groups had good to excellent palliation of symptoms. Catheter placement was easier following laser resection in patients with exophytic endobronchial lesions. Median survival rate was also higher, although this may have been related to selection criteria. Hemorrhage occurred in 33% of laser-treated patients and in 25% of non–laser-treated patients; however, the difference was not statistically significant. Lesions located in the upper lobe bronchus had a greater risk for fatal hemorrhage. Survival was improved in both groups of patients receiving external beam boost as an adjunct. Ordanel (1997) reports a 20% actuarial risk of fatal hemoptysis at 2 years in patients treated with laser and brachytherapy, and Macha and associates (1995) reported a 21% rate of fatal hemorrhage in patients treated exclusively with endobrachytherapy. Based on the literature, it seems that prior laser resection increases the risk of hemoptysis, but the reason may be related more to patient selection and the pattern of growth of the tumor rather than to the treatment itself. There is a suggestion that laser de-obstruction in adjunct to external or internal radiotherapy may provide longer symptom relief in selected patients than does external or internal radiotherapy alone (Jain et al, 1985; Joyner et al, 1985; Maire and Monnier, 1989).

Failure of treatment—mostly related to incomplete deobstruction, extrinsic compression, endobronchial tumoral regrowth or fistula—has stimulated the development of endobronchial prostheses (see later). Numerous stents are available with a good immediate palliative effect (Cavalière et al, 1996; Dumont, 1982; Freitag, 2000; Lam, 1996; Monnier et al, 1996). If their indications are clear in extrinsic compressions, in loss of cartilage support after laser de-obstruction, and in fistulas, their role has to be defined when they are used preventively to avoid the regrowth of the tumor or in association with external or internal radiotherapy.

The relief of symptoms and enhanced quality of life are the principal goals of palliative treatment. From this point of view, these different therapeutic options should be used separately or in association and adapted for each case considering the previous treatments and the clinical status. Assessment of long-term results is more difficult to evaluate because survival is not the principal goal of palliative treatment.

CONCLUSION

The role of interventional bronchoscopy has expanded with the advent of lasers. Our experience has shown that the use of the rigid endoscope can effectively treat lesions, and when both safety measures and indications are respected, low mortality and morbidity rates are observed. For inoperable tumors, tracheal or bronchial prosthesis is becoming a very useful adjunct to laser removal of obstructions. Nevertheless, progress remains to be made in the development of new prostheses that are better tolerated and instrumentation that facilitates easy insertion and removal of prostheses. Endoscopic treatment of benign stenoses should be reserved for selected cases. In many situations, surgery remains the treatment of choice. As we do not yet know the long-term outcomes of prostheses, these should only be used as the last choice in cases of benign pathology, when no other treatment can be proposed. In this context, newly designed resorbable prosthesis could be a solution for the future.

PHOTOCHEMICAL LASER THERAPY

Definition and Benefits

Since 1982, photodynamic therapy (PDT) has emerged as a promising technique for the treatment of various cancers, including those of the tracheobronchial tree. Its principle consists of administration of a photosensitizer, which is preferentially retained in neoplastic cells, followed by activation of the dye by visible light of a specific wavelength, usually emitted by a laser. The combination of the photosensitizing drug and the light induces a photochemical process with formation of singlet oxygen and other oxygen radicals, leading to the localized destruction of the targeted tumor. The benefits of PDT render this procedure very attractive. Photodynamic therapy is minimally invasive, nonmutilating, and causes few side effects. This relatively new therapeutic modality also has the distinct advantage that it can be repeated multiple times because neither resistance nor cumulative toxicity have yet been observed. Photodynamic therapy has the potential to be used in association with other procedures as it involves a different curative process. Although a controversial issue with PDT, the relative affinity of the photosensitizer for the pathologic cells allows a somewhat selective necrosis of the tumor with preservation of normal tissue. This property, together with the excellent healing, renders PDT more attractive than other thermal techniques, such as laser or electrocautery, for the cure of early, superficial bronchial cancers.

Methodology

Hematoporphyrin derivative (HpD), a complex mixture of porphyrins, was the first photosensitizer tested in clinical studies. Its application in treatment of malignancies of the lung was first reported by Hayata and associates in 1982. A more purified form of HpD, dihematoporphyrin ester (DHE), which is also known as Photofrin II, was subsequently synthesized. In clinical trials, the dyes are injected intravenously at doses of 2.5 to 5 mg/kg of body weight for HpD and 1 to 2.5 mg/kg for Photofrin II. Both compounds are activated with monochromatic light of 630 nm wavelength for about 20 to 30 minutes. Illumination usually takes place 48 or 72 hours after the administration of the drugs. At that time, the difference in the concentration of the dye between tumoral and healthy tissue is believed to be at its peak. However, despite good clinical results, the first-generation photosensitizers suffer from some significant drawbacks: lack of clearly defined chemical composition; relatively low phototoxicity requiring high drug and light doses; and long-term skin photosensitization. Moreover, the wavelength (630 nm) normally used to activate HpD and Photofrin II is not optimal in terms of light penetration in tissues.

Hence, several new second-generation photosensitizers have been developed and introduced in preclinical and clinical trials. Among them, tetra (*m*-hydroxyphenyl) chlorin (mTHPC) has been evaluated in the treatment of early tumors with promising results. The mTHPC shows distinct advantages compared with the first-generation photosensitizers in terms of chemical purity, phototoxicity, and duration of skin photosensitization. It is usually activated at 652 nm, resulting in deeper tissue penetration of light of at least 1 cm. Most clinical protocols for mTHPC-PDT propose a standard drug dose of 0.15 mg/kg administered intravenously 4 days before illumination with an exposure time that is usually less than 2 minutes. Although other dyes, such as benzoporphyrin derivative (BPD), are currently being investigated in PDT trials for lung cancer, clinical results have not yet been published in the medical literature.

Photodynamic therapy can be performed either under local anesthesia using the flexible fiberoptic bronchoscope or under general anesthesia with the manipulation of a rigid bronchoscope. However, endoscopists prefer to perform PDT under general anesthesia to have an optimal view of the setting. Moreover, during general anesthesia the cough reflex is abolished and breathing movements are reduced, thus allowing a more accurate illumination of the tumoral field.

Accurate dose and intensity of light as well as availability of adequate optical devices are necessary to obtain optimal destruction of the lesions. The light dose, expressed in joules per centimeter squared (J/cm^2), and the irradiance, expressed in milliwatts per centimeter squared (mW/cm^2), vary with each photosensitizer. They are sometimes correlated to the relative fluorescence signal of the illuminated area, but usually they are chosen empirically. Endoscopic delivery of the light into the tracheobronchial tree requires an optical quartz fiber coupled to a laser light source. The fiber is inserted through the biopsy channel of a rigid or flexible bronchoscope, and its tip is connected to a light delivery system and guided to the site of the tumor. The most frequently used light source for PDT in the bronchi is the argon ion laser pumping a tunable dye laser. The laser containing the dye allows the use of a broad spectrum of emission wavelengths according to the absorption characteristics of the various dyes. This laser system has the disadvantage, however, of being very heavy and expensive. More convenient laser light sources in terms of cost and ease of handling, such as semiconductor laser diodes, have been developed and have been progressively introduced in PDT. They are designed at different but fixed wavelengths.

Because selectivity of the photosensitizers for the neoplastic tissues is still a debatable issue, especially in early cancers, homogeneous and total illumination of the tumor is mandatory to achieve complete eradication. Various light distributors have been designed with the goal of optimally matching the light delivery with the complex geometry of the tracheobronchial tree and tumors. The devices are optimized for delivering accurate light intensity to the tumor with minimal losses. Illumination is carried out by either a microlens fiber tip, in cases of a small circumscript lesion, or a cylindrical diffusor of well-defined length and with a window adjusted to the extension of the tumor. Further advances in laser technology and improvements in light delivery systems and dosimetry will render PDT more accessible and efficient.

Indication

The conventional treatment for the cure of lung cancer is surgical resection with or without radiotherapy or chemotherapy. However, in some cases, tumors are discovered at an advanced stage where even radical surgery cannot achieve complete eradication of the lesion, and only palliative treatments can be proposed. In a few cases, superficial tumors are detected at an early stage, especially during follow-up endoscopies in patients treated for a previous malignancy and who are at high risk for the development of multiple primary lesions. These latter patients are often in poor general condition owing to previous radical procedures directed to the initial tumor, or they have limited cardiac and pulmonary function. In these carefully selected cases, an effective and minimally invasive method may be taken into account as an alternative to surgery for the treatment of early lung cancers.

In the tracheobronchial tree, PDT alone has been applied as an experimental treatment in early superficial malignancies with a curative intent and in invasive carcinomas as a palliative treatment. Photodynamic therapy has also been performed as an additional local treatment prior to external radiation or surgery to limit the extent of resection. However, the limited tissue penetration by activated light in this procedure precludes complete eradication of large obstructing airway lesions. Moreover, the use of PDT to palliate advanced lesions has shown only moderate advantages compared with other methods such as thermal YAG laser vaporization with endobronchial stenting and brachytherapy. Although PDT temporarily reduces the volume of bulky and invasive tumors and thus maintains the patency of the airway, its benefit is limited by severe potential complications, such as hemorrhage, bronchopleural fistula, and airway compromise that are related to the procedure. The only possible indication for the use of PDT as a palliative treatment in invasive lung tumors might be for lesions located in the upper and lower lobes where stenting is difficult to perform.

The main interest in using PDT is the treatment of early cancers, which are those defined as either in situ (i.e., intraepithelial with no invasion of the basement membrane) or microinvasive (i.e., with no invasion beyond the cartilage or bronchial muscular layer). PDT has been successfully used for early malignancies in the bronchi, especially in sites where surgery is contraindicated. These superficial tumors are radiographically occult and can be considered as local lesions with almost no risk of developing lymph node metastasis. Sputum cytology and thorough endoscopic examination as part of a systematic screening program allow detection and localization of early lung cancers (most of these tumors do not cause any symptoms). However, accurate localization and delimitation of the lesion, which sometimes might even be occult, rely on the endoscopist's skills, and in many cases success is difficult to achieve. Hence, the search for new imaging technologies that would improve detection and localization of early cancers is mandatory. Recent development of fluoroscopic devices based on the tumor autofluorescence characteristics would, in combination with PDT, likely increase the chances of a cure for early lung cancers and consequently improve long-term survival in a high-risk population.

Results

Several studies have confirmed the efficacy of PDT for the treatment of in situ and microinvasive squamous cell carcinomas of the tracheobronchial tree.

Kato (1998) reported on 95 patients with 116 superficial early-stage lung cancers using HpD and Photofrin II. Complete response was achieved in 77 patients (81.1%) and partial remission was obtained in 18 cases. Recurrence occurred in 12 (15.6%) among 77 patients with complete response. Response was related to the size of the tumor, with those less than 2 cm in length obtaining almost 100% complete remission. Seventy-two patients were free of disease 2 to 195 months after treatment. Eighteen patients with partial remission were treated by other therapies, primarily surgery. The overall 5-year survival rate for all patients treated by PDT, predicted according to Kaplan-Meier analysis, was 68.4%, but raised to 94.8% when death due to other diseases was excluded.

Cortese and associates (1997) studied a group of 21 patients with 23 early-stage squamous cell carcinomas of the lung treated by HpD-PDT. The patients were eligible for surgery but were offered PDT as an alternative to resection. A complete response was noted in 15 patients (71%) after an initial PDT session, and 11 of them were still disease-free 1 year after treatment. Two of these 11 patients developed a second primary lung cancer, and they subsequently underwent surgical resection. Therefore, 9 of the original 21 patients (43%) were spared a surgical procedure with a mean follow-up of 68 months. The authors concluded with 95% confidence that at least 22% of patients with early stage squamous cell lung carcinoma who are treated with PDT can be spared surgical resection.

Grosjean and colleagues (1996) reported on 16 early squamous cell carcinomas of the bronchi in 13 patients treated with mTHPC-PDT alone. Twelve lesions were considered in situ and 4 were microinvasive. Eleven of the 12 in situ carcinomas (92%) and 2 of the 4 microinvasive tumors (50%) had a complete response. In all but 2 lesions, complete remission was achieved after only one session of PDT. All of the eradicated malignancies showed no recurrence after a follow-up ranging from 4 to 61 months. The only major complication encountered after the procedure in a single case was a complete bronchial stenosis.

Several factors have been pointed out for failures of PDT, even in patients with early lung cancers. Tumor understaging is one factor because precise assessment of depth of tumor infiltration as well as ability to visualize the distal margin is difficult to estimate with the available technology in some cases. Another reason that may account for an incomplete response in some treatments is that tumors are likely to be only partially included in the illumination field. The complex geometry of some lesions expanding from a spur into different adjacent segmental divisions may be responsible for inadequate light delivery and probably plays a role in the nonsterilization of the tumors. Finally, insufficient light dose that is due to interpatient variability in the dye concentration at the time of PDT might account for the incomplete eradication of some lesions. Adjusting the light dose to the dye fluorescence signal measured prior to irradiation could help to minimize the risk of undertreating the lesions.

Complications

The most common complication of PDT, which is related to the procedure itself and not specifically to the treatment in the lungs, is skin photosensitization. The prolonged retention of the dye in the skin depends on the type of photosensitizer administered. Skin burns can occur up to 2 months after HpD or Photofrin II and 1 month after mTHPC injection. Cutaneous reactions can, however, be minimized if exposure to sunlight or to other sources of bright light are strictly avoided until the complete clearance of the dye. Another complication encountered is bronchial stenosis, which is believed to be caused by the lack of drug selectivity for the tumoral tissue. Because PDT is seldom used for treatment of large and bulky lesions, complications such as fistulas, hemorrhage, or airway obstruction caused by edema and fibrinous plugs are very rare. In the latter cases, bronchoscopy is usually carried out 2 days after PDT to remove the necrotic tissue and, thus, to prevent obstructive pneumonia or respiratory distress. Other, less serious complications such as ulcerating bronchitis, fever, pleural effusion, allergic reactions, or mild and transient liver dysfunction have been reported.

Discussion

Photodynamic therapy can be considered a useful alternative to standard procedures. Pulmonary function can be preserved and mortality and morbidity can be minimized in some very selected patients with early lung cancers. This technique, which is well tolerated and allows a rapid recovery, does not preclude the use of possibly more aggressive treatments in cases of failure. Other therapeutic modalities, such as YAG laser, stenting, and brachytherapy have limited the role of PDT in the palliation of bulky and obstructive tumors in the tracheobronchial tree. However, PDT has been confirmed as an effective endobronchial treatment for early cancers. Complete remission can be achieved for radiographically occult lesions, which should appear superficial with an entire visualization at bronchoscopy and be less than 2 cm in diameter. In addition, the use of optimal light dosimetry with adequate light diffusers renders PDT safer. However, PDT is still an experimental procedure, and the number of research groups using this technique is relatively limited. More prospective studies, such as those of Cortese and associates (1997), would be necessary to assess the real benefit of PDT for early lung carcinomas in comparison with surgery. Moreover, further improvement in imaging technology, such as endoscopic ultrasonography with higher resolution miniprobes, to better detect and assess tumor extension in early cancers, as well as availability of new photosensitizers with increased selectivity and limited skin photosensitization are indispensable for wider acceptance of PDT in the field of early lung cancer. In addition, optimization of light dosimetry and development of less expensive and more compact light delivery systems will render PDT more accessible and attractive.

SUMMARY

Laser bronchoscopy for inoperable malignant obstruction of the airway is considered an effective palliative treatment. Accumulated experience has defined the most valuable indications and appropriate methodologies in use. Airway stenting is routinely recommended as an adjunctive measure to laser recanalization of obstructing tumors. However, the role and benefits of brachytherapy are still being debated in terms of duration of palliation of symptoms and quality of life rather than in terms of survival.

Laser treatment is best done with rigid bronchoscopy under general anesthesia for safety reasons, speed of resection, and comfort for the patient. Exophytic lesions of the trachea and mainstem bronchi are most amenable to laser bronchoscopy, and the improvement in symptoms correlates best with the improved patency of large airways. In most patients, the major portion of the endobronchial debulking procedure can be performed quickly and safely by physically coring out the exophytic tumor mass with the rigid end of the bronchoscope. Total recanalization results in an increase in survival compared with unsuccessful recanalization. As an adjunctive treatment, insertion of autoexpandable or semirigid silicone prostheses allows airway patency to be restored in cases of extrinsic compression associated with endoluminal tumor or of a collapse of the bronchial wall after repeated laser de-obstructions. The efficacy of stenting in preventing tumoral endoluminal regrowth of the tumor is controversial because prostheses tend to be occluded by secretions. Some data (Macha et al, 1995; Ordanel, 1997) suggest that endoluminal brachytherapy combined with laser and stenting or as a single treatment modality if the airway is already patent, improve the quality of the palliation, even if hemorrhage seems to be more frequent. Ideally, the best combination of these different modalities would be to evaluate them in randomized studies, but this is not acceptable for ethical reasons. Therefore, the endoscopist should manage all of these various palliative therapies to choose the best treatment, based on experience and the patient's condition.

The main interest in using photodynamic therapy remains the treatment of early cancers. There is no advantage for its use in the palliative treatment of obstructing lesions, except perhaps in fairly distal lesions of the lobar bronchi where Nd:YAG laser treatments are dangerous.

Treatment of cicatricial stenoses of the airways with the CO_2 laser should be performed with rigorous adherence to the indications. The endoscopist should know the indications for surgical resection before attempting laser therapy as a first measure because of the risk of aggravating the initial condition.

COMMENTS AND CONTROVERSIES

Other than the use of photochemical excitation, laser endoscopy is a palliative technique employing yet another form of thermal destruction. Other methods to relieve airway obstructions include the simple "coring-out" technique best described by Mathisen—endoscopic electrocautery and endoscopic cryotherapy. However, with increasing experience, Nd:YAG laser coagulation appears to be the preferred approach when thermal destruction of obstructing lesions is required. Over the years, with experience, its safety and efficacy have been improved, and, as the authors describe, the indications for its use and its limitations are now well enunciated.

In the very proximal airway, the CO_2 laser continues to be valuable because of its precision. Beyond the mainstem bronchi, the value of thermal coagulation for obstructing lesions becomes less and less apparent.

All practicing thoracic surgeons should include these

modalities in their armamentarium, because, frequently, this technique is useful following a coring-out of a large, obstructing tumor.

To avoid repetitive endoscopic procedures, we prefer to combine this approach with more definite local treatments such as endobronchial brachytherapy or external-beam radiotherapy. As well, when appropriate, stents have been used with increasing frequency, especially the covered stents, which help to avoid ingrowth of tumor.

Because of the increasing availability and use of photodynamic therapy in the treatment of lung cancer, a separate chapter has been added to discuss this modality (see Chapter 32).

R. J. G.

■ KEY REFERENCES

Cavalière S, Dumon JF: Laser Bronchoscopy. In Bolliger CT, Mathur PN (ed): Interventional Bronchoscopy: Progress in Respiratory Research, Vol 30, Basel, S Karger, 2000.

Excellent chapter on laser bronchoscopy with extensive description of the technique. This book covers all the topics on interventional bronchoscopy.

Cavalière S, Venuta F, Foccoli P, et al: Endoscopic treatment of malignant airway obstructions in 2,008 patients. Chest 110:1536, 1996.

A report of a 13-year experience with endoscopic treatment of malignant obstructions by Nd:YAG laser, stents, and brachytherapy. The indications and the complications of each treatment modality are discussed.

Cortese DA, Edell ES, Kinsey JH: Photodynamic therapy for early stage squamous cell carcinoma of the lung. Mayo Clin Proc 72:595, 1997.

A prospective study assessing the benefit of photodynamic therapy for early lung carcinomas in comparison with surgery.

Dougherty TJ, Gomer CJ, Henderson BW et al: Photodynamic therapy. J Natl Cancer Inst 90:889, 1998.

A complete review discussing all of the important issues related to photodynamic therapy.

Edell E, Shapsay S: Laser Bronchoscopy. In Prakash U (ed): Bronchoscopy. New York, Raven, 1994.

This book is an excellent review of diagnostic and interventional bronchoscopy, and it contains many illustrations.

Hetzel MR (ed): Outcome, morbidity and mortality of Nd-Yag laser photoresection: Minimally Invasive Techniques in Thoracic Medicine and Surgery. London, Chapman & Hall, 1995, pp 137–146.

A review of 21 reported series by centers experienced in using these techniques.

Macha HN, Becker KO, Kemmer HP: Pattern of failure and survival in endobronchial laser resection. Chest 105:1668, 1994.

A prospective series that evaluates the influence of laser resection on survival and the pattern of failure.

■ REFERENCES

Beamis JF, Vergos K, Rebeiz EE et al: Endoscopic laser therapy for obstructing tracheobronchial lesions. Ann Otol Rhinol Laryngol 100:413, 1991.

Brutinel WM, Cortese DA, McDougall JC et al: A two-year experience with neodymium-YAG laser in endobronchial obstruction. Chest 91:159, 1987.

Bolot G, Poupart M, Pignat J-C et al: Self-expanding metal stent for the management of bronchial stenoses and bronchomalacia after lung transplantation. Laryngoscope 108:1230, 1998.

Cavalière S, Foccoli P, Farina PL: Nd:YAG laser bronchoscopy: A five-year experience with 1396 applications in 1000 patients. Chest 94:15, 1988.

Chan AL, Tharratt RS, Siefkin AD et al: Nd:YAG laser bronchoscopy: Rigid or fiberoptic mode? Chest 98:271, 1990.

Clarke CP, Ball DL, Sephton R: Follow-up of patients having Nd-YAG laser resection of bronchostenotic lesion. J Bronchol 1:19, 1994.

Colt HG, Dumon JF: Lasers et endoprothèses en bronchopneumologie. Rev Pneumol Clin 47:65, 1991.

Cotton RT: Pediatric laryngotracheal stenosis. J Pediatr Surg 19:699, 1984.

Daddi G, Puma F, Avenia N et al: Resection with curative intent after endoscopic treatment of airway obstruction. Ann Thorac Surg 65:203, 1998.

Depierraz B, Ravussin P, Brossard E et al: Percutaneous transtracheal jet ventilation for paediatric endoscopic laser treatment of laryngeal and subglottic lesion. Can J Anaesth 41:1200, 1994.

Dhingra JK, Perrault DF Jr, McMillan K et al: Early diagnosis of upper aerodigestive tract cancer by autofluorescence. Arch Otolaryngol Head Neck Surg 122:1181, 1996.

Dierkesmann R: Indication and results of endobronchial laser therapy. Lung 168(Suppl 1):1095, 1990.

Dougherty TJ, Kaufman JE, Goldfarb A et al: Photoradiation therapy for the treatment of malignant tumors. Cancer Res 38:2628, 1978.

Dumon JF, Reboud E, Garbe L et al: Treatment of tracheobronchial lesions by laser photoresection. Chest 81:278, 1982.

Edell ES, Cortese DA, McDougall JC: Ancillary therapies in the management of lung cancer: Photodynamic therapy, laser therapy, and endobronchial prosthetic devices. Mayo Clin Proc 68:685, 1993.

Freitag L: Tracheobronchial stents. In Bolliger CT, Mathur PN: Interventional Bronchoscopy: Progress in Respiratory Research, Vol 30. Basel, S Karger, 2000.

Furuse K, Fukuoka M, Kato H et al: A prospective phase II study on photodynamic therapy with Photofrin II for centrally located early-stage lung cancer. J Clin Oncol 11:1852, 1993.

George PJM, Clarke G, Tolfree S et al: Changes in regional ventilation and perfusion of the lung after endoscopic laser treatment. Thorax 45:248, 253, 1990.

Golish JA, Pena CM, Mehta AC: Massive air embolism complicating Nd:YAG laser endobronchial photoresection. Las Surg Med 12:338, 1992.

Grosjean P, Savary J-F, Wagnières G et al: Tetra (m-hydroxyphenyl) chlorine clinical photodynamic therapy of early bronchial and oesophageal cancers. Lasers Med Sci 11:227, 1996.

Hanowell LH, Martin WR, Savelle JE, Foppiano LE: Complications of general anesthesia for Nd:YAG laser resection of endobronchial tumors. Chest 99:72, 1991.

Hayata Y, Kato H, Furuse K et al: Photodynamic therapy of 168 early stage cancers of the lung and esophagus. Lasers Med Sci 11:255, 1996.

Hetzel MR, Smith SGT: Endoscopic palliation of tracheobronchial malignancies. Thorax 46:325, 1991.

Hetzel MR, Nixon C, Edmondstone WM et al: Laser therapy in 100 tracheobronchial tumors. Thorax 40:341, 1985.

Jain PR, Dedhia HV, Lapp NL et al: Nd:YAG laser followed by radiation for treatment of malignant airway lesions. Lasers Surg Med 5:47, 1985.

Joyner LR, Maran AG, Sarama R et al: Neodymium-YAG laser treatment of intrabronchial lesions. Chest 87:418, 1985.

Kato H: Photodynamic therapy for lung cancer: A review of 19 years experience. J Photochem Photobiol B 42:96, 1998.

Kvale P: Training in laser bronchoscopy and proposals for credentialing. Chest 97:983, 1990.

Laforet KG, Berger RL, Vaughn CW: Carcinoma obstructing the trachea: Treatment by laser resection. N Engl J Med 214:941, 1976.

Lam S: Bronchoscopic, photodynamic, and laser diagnosis and therapy of lung neoplasms. Curr Opin Pulm Med 2:271, 1996.

Lam S, Muller NL, Miller RR et al: Predicting the response of obstructive endobronchial tumors to photodynamic therapy. Cancer 58:2298, 1986.

Lipson RL, Baldes EJ, Olsen AM: The use of a derivative of hematoporphyrin in tumor detection. J Natl Cancer Inst 26:1, 1961.

Macha HN, Becker KO, Kemmer HP: Pattern of failure and survival in endobronchial laser resection: A matched pair study. Chest 105:1668, 1994.

Macha HN, Wahlers B, Reichle C, von Zwehl D: Endobronchial radiation therapy for obstructing malignancies: Ten years experience with iridium-192 high-dose radiation brachytherapy afterloading technique in 365 patients. Lung 173:271, 1995.

Maire R, Monnier PH: Le laser-YAG dans le traitement endoscopique palliatif du cancer trachéo-bronchique: indications, modalités et résultats. ORL, Aktuelle Probleme der Otorhinolaryngologie 12:146, 1989.

Metha AC, Harris RJ, De Boer GE: Endoscopic management of benign airway stenosis. Clin Chest Med 16:401, 1995.

Metha AC, Lee FY, Cordaso EM et al: Concentric tracheal and subglottic stenosis. Chest 104:674, 1993.

Miller JI: Comparison of Nd:YAG and CO_2 laser bronchoscopy in the management of tracheobronchial lesions. In Martini N (ed): International Trends in General Thoracic Surgery, Vol 5: Thoracic Surgery: Frontiers and Uncommon Neoplasms. St. Louis, CV Mosby, 1989.

Mohsenifar Z, Jasper AC, Koerner SK: Physiologic assessment of lung function in patients undergoing laser photoresection of tracheobronchial tumors. Chest 93:65, 1988.

Monnier P, Fontolliet C, Wagnieres G et al: Further appraisal of PDI and PDT of early squamous cell carcinomas of the pharynx, esophagus and bronchi. In Spinelli P, Dal Fante M, Marchesini R (eds): Photodynamic Therapy and Biomedical Lasers. Excerpta Medica, International Congress Series 1992. pp 7–14.

Monnier PH, Fontolliet CH, Wagnieres G et al: The possibilities and limitations of the endoscopic and photodynamic treatments of early squamous cell cancer of the upper aero-digestive tract, bronchi and oesophagus. Acta Endoscopica 21:641, 1991.

Monnier P, Lang F, Savary M: Partial cricotracheal resection for severe pediatric subglottic stenosis: Update of the Lausanne experience. Ann Otol Rhinol Laryngol 107:961, 1998.

Monnier P, Mudry A, Stanzal F, Haeussinger K et al: The use of the covered wallstent for the palliative treatments of inoperable tracheobronchial cancers. Chest 110:1161, 1996.

Mudry A, Monnier P: Les sténoses cicatricielles glotto-sous-glottiques: place du traitement endoscopique. ORL Aktuelle Probleme der Otorhinolaryngologie 17:137, 1994.

Oho K, Ogawa I, Amemiya R et al: Indication for endoscopic Nd:YAG laser surgery in the trachea and bronchus. Endoscopy 15:302, 1983.

Ono R, Ikeda S, Suemasu K: Hematoporphyrin derivative photodynamic therapy in roentgenographically occult carcinoma of the tracheobronchial tree. Cancer 69:1696, 1992.

Ornadel D, Duchesne G, Wall P et al: Defining the roles of high dose rate endobronchial brachytherapy and laser resection for recurrent bronchial malignancy. Lung Cancer 16:203, 1997.

Ossof RH, Tucker GF, Duncacage JA et al: Efficacy of bronchoscopic carbon dioxide laser surgery for benign strictures of the trachea. Laryngoscope 95:1220, 1985.

Personne C, Colchen A, Bonnette P et al: Laser in bronchology: Methods of application. Lung 168(Suppl):1085, 1990.

Ross D, Mohsenifar Z, Koerner SK: Survival characteristics after Neodymium:YAG laser photoresection in advanced stage lung cancer. Chest 98:581, 1990.

Ross DJ, Mohsenifar Z, Potkin RT, Roston WL et al: Pathogenesis of cerebral air embolism during neodymium:YAG laser photoresection. Chest 94:660, 1988.

Schuitmaker JJ, Baas P, Van Leengoed HLLM et al: Photodynamic therapy: A promising new modality for the treatment of cancer. J Photochem Photobiol B 34:3, 1996.

Shapshay S: Endoscopic treatment of subglottic and tracheal stenosis by radial laser incision and dilatation. Ann Otol Rhinol Laryngol 96:661, 1987.

Simpson GT, Strong MS, Healy GB et al: Predictive factors of success or failure in the endoscopic management of laryngeal and tracheal stenosis. Ann Otol Rhinol Laryngol 91:384, 1982.

Smith SGT, Bedwell J, MacRobert AJ et al: Experimental studies to assess the potential of photodynamic therapy for the treatment of bronchial carcinomas. Thorax 48:474, 1993.

Sonett JR, Keenan RJ, Ferson PF et al: Endobronchial management of benign, malignant, and lung transplantation airways stenoses. Ann Thorac Surg 59:1417, 1995.

Stanopoulos IT, Beamis JF, Martinez FJ et al: Laser bronchoscopy in respiratory failure from malignant airway obstruction. Crit Care Med 21:386, 1993.

Stewart F, Baas P, Star W: What does photodynamic therapy have to offer radiation oncologists (or their cancer patients)? Radiother Oncol 48:233, 1998.

Strong MS, Jako JG: Laser surgery in the larynx: Early clinical experience with continuous CO_2 laser. Ann Otol Rhinol Laryngol 81:791, 1972.

Suh JH, Dass KK, Pagliaccio L et al: Endobronchial radiation therapy with or without Neodymium:yttrium-aluminum-garnet laser resection for managing malignant airway obstruction. Cancer 73:2583, 1994.

Sutedja TG, Schreurs AJ, Vandearschueren RG, et al: Bronchoscopic therapy in patients with intraluminal typical bronchial carcinoid. Chest 107:556, 1995.

Sutedja TG, Postmus PE: Photodynamic therapy in lung cancer: A review. J Photochem Photobiol B 36:199, 1996.

Toty L, Personne C, Hertzog P et al: Utilisation d'un faisceau laser (YAG) à conducteur souple, pour le traitement endoscopique de certaines lésions trachéobronchiques. Rev Fr Mal Respir 7:57, 1979.

Unger M: Neodymium:YAG laser therapy for malignant and benign endobronchial lesion. Clin Chest Med 6:277, 1985.

Van den Bergh H: On the evolution of some endoscopic light delivery systems for photodynamic therapy. Endoscopy 30:392, 1998.

Wagner I, Ayache D, Denoyelle F, Garabedian EN: Traitement par broncholaser CO_2 des sténoses trachéobronchiques acquises chez des enfants porteurs d'une dysplasie bronchopulmonaire. Arch Pédiatr 3:1079, 1996.

TRACHEOBRONCHIAL STENTS

Henning A. Gaissert

G. Alexander Patterson

The purpose of tracheobronchial stents is to maintain airway patency through strictures that are not amenable to resection and reconstruction. Unlike tracheostomy tubes, these stents permit translaryngeal airflow, thus providing a humidified airway and preservation of the voice. Stents have been used successfully in a variety of benign and malignant strictures of the trachea and mainstem bronchi. They are placed under bronchoscopic control and may reside in the airway lumen for extended periods of time. Most experience has been gained with

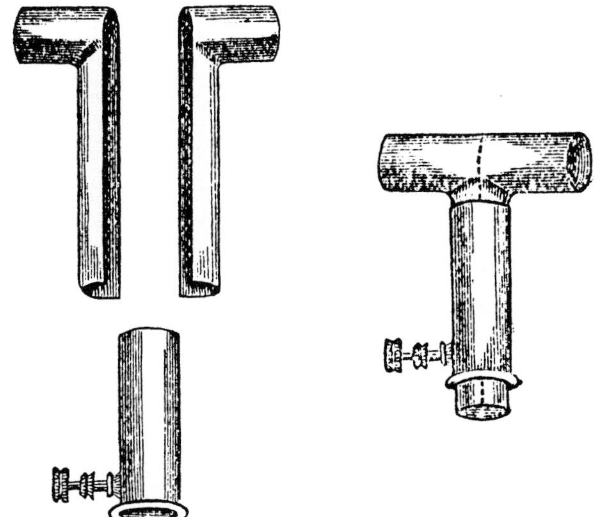

FIGURE 14–23 ■ Bond's tracheal T tube. (From Bond CJ: Note on the treatment of tracheal stenosis by a new T shaped tracheotomy tube. Lancet 1:539, 1891.)

tubes made of silicone rubber. Wire mesh tubes have been introduced in recent years; however, long-term experience with their use is limited.

HISTORICAL NOTE

The concept of stenting for the treatment of airway disease probably originated toward the end of the 19th century, although tracheostomy tubes have been known for much longer. In 1872, Trendelenburg of Berlin reported the use of a metal coil spring covered with rubber tubing to stent a stenosis of the cervical trachea in a young woman. The T-shaped tracheotomy tube depicted in Figure 14–23 was described in a brief case report by the surgeon Bond in 1891. This metal cannula was made for a tracheal stricture caused by a suicidal knife wound. It consisted of two halves that were separately introduced into the trachea and held together by a metal collar fixed with a screw over an external side arm. The side arm was closed to allow the patient to breathe and talk naturally.

Montgomery used a similar device made of rigid acrylic in 1964 and later modified this tube using flexible silicone rubber (Montgomery, 1965). Subsequent reports emphasized the safety and success of T tubes in the treatment of subglottic stenosis (Montgomery, 1968), in the palliation of malignant strictures, as a temporizing therapy prior to definitive tracheal resection, and for salvage of the airway after failed reconstruction (Cooper et al, 1981). Tracheobronchial Y stents and straight endobronchial stents have been developed as permanent palliative devices. Such stents have been invaluable in the management of airway complications following lung transplantation.

The purpose of the original Montgomery tube was the definitive treatment of strictures in the cervical trachea. It has been repeatedly demonstrated that the inert Silastic material allows airway epithelium to resurface a granulating stricture. However, current experience suggests that most tracheal strictures will not respond to transient stenting alone and require additional reconstructive procedures because of the concurrent loss of stabilizing cartilage.

■ *HISTORICAL READINGS*

Bond CJ: Note on the treatment of tracheal stenosis by a new T-shaped tracheotomy tube. Lancet 1:539, 1891.

Montgomery WW: T-tube tracheal stent. Arch Otolaryngol 82:320, 1965.

Trendelenburg F: Beitraege zu den Operationen an den Luftwegen. Langenbecks Arch Chir 13:335, 1872.

INDICATIONS

Airway stents are used for benign and malignant strictures that require repeated dilatation and are unsuitable for surgical reconstruction. The general condition of the patient may preclude safe resection because of the presence of prohibitive perioperative risk factors, the likelihood of postoperative ventilator dependence or the use of high-dose steroid medication. The stricture may have anatomic characteristics that indicate the need for stenting, such as extensive length or poor quality of the remaining airway. The presence of active tracheobronchial inflammation may call for a delay of reconstructive procedures to allow accurate estimation of the true length of involved airway at a later date.

Tracheal lesions most commonly in need of stenting are produced by the effects of long-term mechanical ventilatory support. Strictures at the site of the endotracheal tube cuff, a previous tracheostomy site, or in the subglottic space may require stenting prior or subsequent to resection. Such postintubation strictures and inflammatory strictures that occur as a result of burn injury were among the most common indications for T tube insertion in the Massachusetts General Hospital experience (Table 14–2). The palliation of malignant obstruction by either an intrinsic endoluminal tumor or an extrinsic tumor compression is an additional important indication.

TABLE 14–2 ■ **Diagnosis in 140 Patients Undergoing T Tube Placement at Massachusetts General Hospital**

Diagnosis	Number
Postintubation stenosis	86
Burn	13
Malignant airway tumor	12
Radiation stenosis	4
Relapsing polychondritis	4
Tracheomalacia	4
Vascular malformation	3
Sarcoidosis	2
Trauma	2
Necrotizing tracheitis	2
Mucopolysaccharidosis	2
Postpneumonectomy syndrome	2
Tracheobronchomegaly (Mounier-Kuhn)	1
Tuberculosis	1
Idiopathic stenosis	1
Tracheopathia osteoplastica	1

From Gaissert HA, Grillo HC, Mathisen DJ, Wain JC: Temporary and permanent restoration of airway continuity with the tracheal T-tube. J Thorac Cardiovasc Surg 107:600, 1994.

Isolated bronchial stenosis that is not amenable to surgical resection or dilatation is rare. The emergence of lung transplantation as an accepted treatment of end-stage lung disease has been accompanied by complications at the airway anastomosis. The incidence of such complications is high after en bloc, double-lung transplantation involving a single tracheal anastomosis without bronchial revascularization. The incidence of airway complications has been reduced dramatically by improved allograft preservation, superior immunosuppression, and the introduction of bilateral bronchial anastomoses (Patterson et al, 1990). However, ischemia at the bronchial suture line remains an important cause of delayed anastomotic healing in approximately 19% of patients and results in stricture development in 6% of patients (Cooper et al, 1994).

STENT TYPES

An airway stent should not interfere with usual daily activities and should be easily placed and replaced in the event of dislodgment. The properties expected from an airway stent are restoration of a sufficient luminal diameter, undisturbed passage of air through the larynx to provide for humidification of inspired air and phonation, minimal interference with clearance of secretions, a simple cleaning procedure (if at all necessary), and uncomplicated removal once it becomes obstructed or is no longer needed.

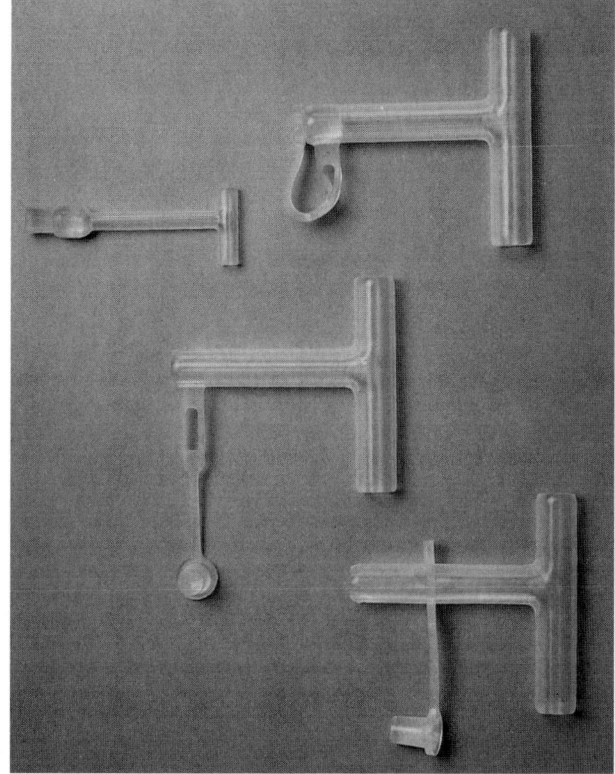

FIGURE 14–24 ■ Silicone tracheal T tube. (Courtesy of Hood Laboratories, Pembroke, MA.)

Tracheal T Tube

The largest and longest clinical experience in the treatment of tracheal strictures has been gained with the silicone T tube. These tubes are generally well tolerated and reliable. Once inserted, they function for long periods, in some patients for many years, without causing further damage to the tracheal wall.

The T tube is a hollow cylinder made of medical-grade silicone rubber that is closed with a plug (Fig. 14–24). The tube is produced in sizes from 4.5 to 16 mm outer diameter (Hood Laboratories, Pembroke, MA). Sizes 4.5 to 9 are generally used for infants and children, 10 to 14 for adult women, and 12 to 16 for men. The upper and lower limbs of the tube are manufactured in various lengths and can be custom-made to meet individual specification. Additional modifications of the T tube, with and without the side arm, are used to stent unilateral main bronchial strictures.

TY Tube

The therapy of benign and malignant strictures with diffuse involvement of the trachea and main bronchi or local obstruction at the carina is challenging. Westaby and colleagues (1982) described a modified T tube by the addition of a Y-shaped extension for intubation of both main bronchi. TY tubes contain a bifurcated extension to fit into carina and both main bronchial lumina (Fig. 14–25). Accurate placement of this tube is particularly important to achieve a correct fit for the two angulations at the stoma and the carina. TY tubes are therefore usually custom-made for an individual patient. Because of their length and two points of fixation, these tubes may cause granulations in the area where the edge of the tube is in contact with the wall of the smaller-caliber main bronchus. However, successful long-term intubation has been performed in many children and adults.

Y Stent

The bifurcated Y tubes have been particularly useful in patients without tracheal stomas who have tracheal or proximal main bronchial strictures. Tracheal, carinal, or proximal bronchial compression by tumor can be effectively palliated by such stents. Various left main bronchial limb lengths are available (Fig. 14–26).

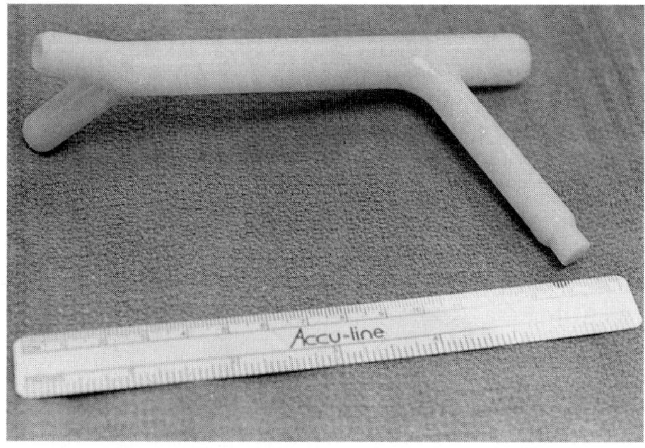

FIGURE 14–25 ■ TY tube.

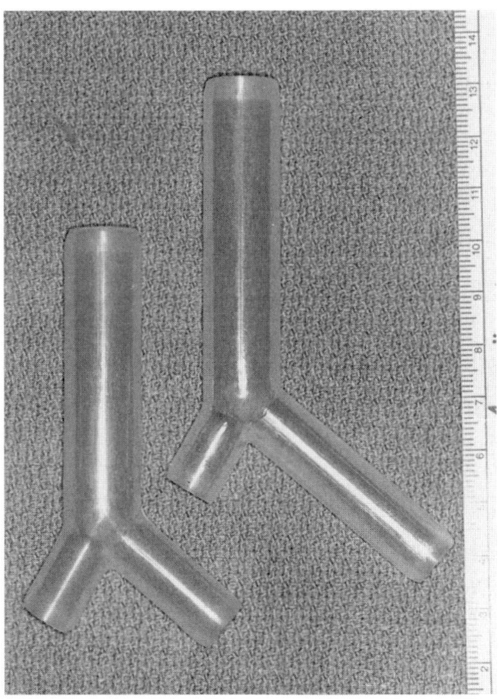

FIGURE 14–26 ■ Y stent.

Bronchial Stent

Straight silicone endobronchial stents are available with outer diameters from 6 to 10 mm or as customized tubes (Hood Laboratories, Pembroke, MA) (Fig. 14–27). These tubes are flanged on both ends to prevent dislodgment

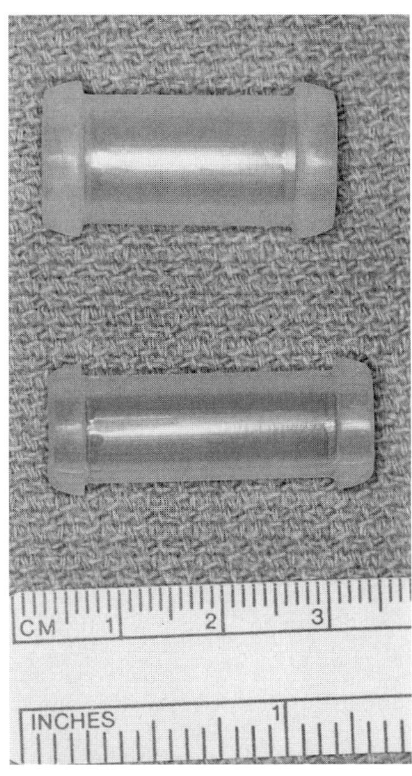

FIGURE 14–27 ■ Bronchial stent with flange.

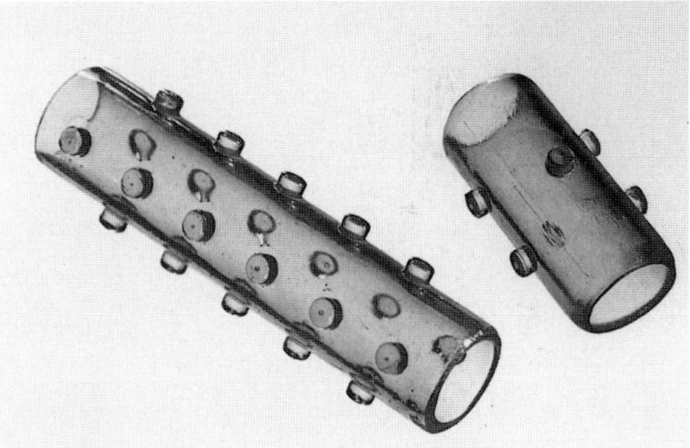

FIGURE 14–28 ■ Dumon studded endobronchial stent. (Courtesy of Bryan Corp., Woburn, MA.)

and have remained in place for extended periods. The selection of a correct stent size and length is critically important. The tube must be long enough to enable its flanges to anchor the tube within the stricture, short enough to avoid compromise of a lobar bronchus distally or the trachea proximally, and of satisfactory diameter to maintain airway caliber. In our early experience, we fashioned bronchial stents from the sidearm of a T tube. This is still used on occasion to create an elliptical distal flange, which will seat nicely at the point of bronchial bifurcation.

Dumon (1990) introduced a Silastic stent for use specifically in the trachea and bronchus (Fig. 14–28). Four rows of studs oriented at 90-degree angles on the external surface are intended to prevent dislodgment (Bryan, Woburn, MA). He reported on 118 stents placed in 66 patients, of whom 38 had malignant disease (Dumon, 1990). Eleven patients had more than one stent placed simultaneously. Cannular migration occurred in 12 instances. Relief of obstructive symptoms was achieved in all but two patients. Overall tolerance appears to be similar to that with other silicone tubes.

Wire Stent

Self-expanding wire-mesh stents of the Gianturco or Wallstent type were introduced to palliate strictures of the biliary tree. In the United States, approval by the Food and Drug Administration has been granted recently for use in the treatment of airway disease. The Gianturco stent (Cook Co., Bloomington, IN) is a stainless steel wire that is shaped into a cylindrical zig-zag formation of 5 to 10 turns and discharged from a cartridge. The Wallstent (Schneider Co., Minneapolis, MN) consists of woven filaments of alloy steel released from an introducer catheter (Fig. 14–29). The Microvasive stent (Boston Scientific, Watertown, MA) is an open-ended cylindrical mesh constructed from a single strand of wire and configured into circumferential interwoven loops (Fig. 14–30). This stent is deployed from a delivery catheter by release of a crocheted suture.

The uncovered wire stents with open interstices may ride across a bronchial orifice without disturbing aeration. A plastic-covered version prevents ingrowth of gran-

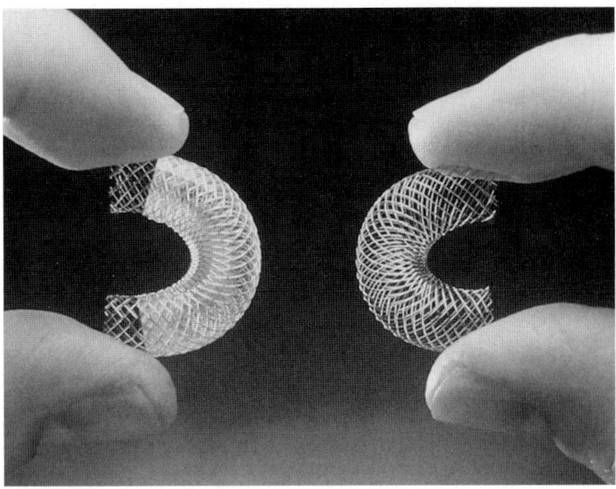

FIGURE 14–29 ■ Wallstent tracheobronchial endoprosthesis with (*left*) and without (*right*) plastic cover. (Courtesy of Boston Scientific, Waltham, MA.)

ulations and incorporation into the wall of the airway. Covered stents are useful for palliation of malignant fistulas between respiratory tract and esophagus. These fistulas usually require concomitant insertion of stents into esophagus and airway (Fig. 14–31). Once inserted, all wire stents expand to a predetermined diameter, and exposed wire is gradually embedded by overgrowth of epithelium. The wire is difficult, if not impossible, to remove at this point, which is desirable in some patients to facilitate natural mucociliary clearance and inconsequential in others with limited survival. However, careful consideration should precede the use of any wire stent in benign disease.

INSERTION TECHNIQUE

All patients who are under consideration for placement of a tracheobronchial stent undergo a complete examination of their airway. Endoscopic evaluation of the airway must be performed in an anesthetized, spontaneously breathing patient. Muscular paralysis, while advantageous for vigorous dilatation and stent placement, must not be instituted until a detailed examination is completed and the surgeon is certain an airway can be subsequently maintained. Optimal assessment of the lower airway anatomy is obtained with flexible bronchoscopy. Assessment of fixation, precise measurements, and satisfactory dilatation is best achieved by rigid bronchoscopic equipment. The patency and function of the larynx should be ascertained with a laryngoscopic examination, particularly if the stent replaces a tracheostomy. The condition of the vocal cords, the size of the subglottic space, and the proximity of the stricture to the larynx should be visualized. The distance from vocal cords to carina and tracheal stoma, and from the upper and lower extent of the stricture to these reference points, is recorded. The required stent dimensions and the need for a custom-designed tube are determined.

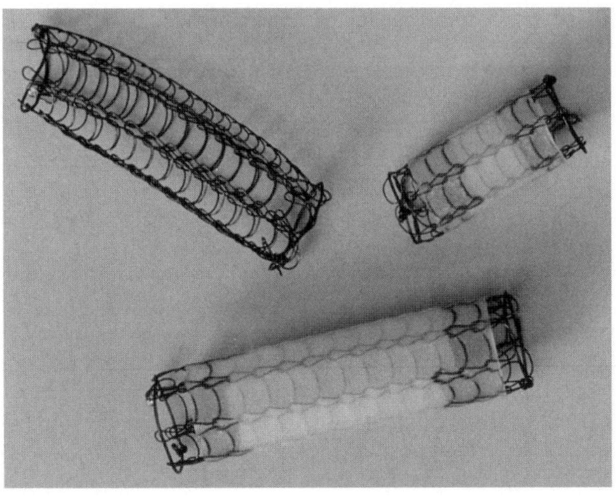

FIGURE 14–30 ■ Microvasive stent in covered and uncovered versions. (Courtesy of Boston Scientific, Waltham, MA.)

Dilatation

Rigid endoscopy should be used exclusively for dilatation of airway strictures. The Holinger bronchoscope is suitable to dilate tracheal and bronchial strictures with a preserved, recognizable lumen. This endoscope has a round lip, which, for this purpose, is insinuated into the stricture and advanced in a corkscrew motion. The dilatation is started with a small, pediatric-size instrument and continued with larger sizes. A particularly tight stricture can be initially stretched using peripheral vascular angioplasty catheters of various sizes inflated under direct bronchoscopic vision. Gum-tipped Jackson esophageal dilators are used when there is uncertainty about the course of the lumen. They are also helpful in the dilatation of laryngeal and subglottic strictures. Hegar dilators are well suited for tracheal dilatation through a stoma. Dilatation to a diameter that is at least as big as the external diameter of the intended stent is advisable unless the stent is self-expanding.

Ventilation

Jet ventilation is employed using Venturi ventilation through the rigid bronchoscope for most routine dilatations and stent placements. Intraoperative ventilation through a T tube is provided by the operator by fitting the side arm with a suitable 15-mm endotracheal tube adapter and ventilating with high tidal volumes to compensate for escape of gases through the upper limb. Alternatively, intermittent ventilation through the stoma can be used.

T Tube Insertion

T tubes may be inserted through the tracheal stoma or, mounted on a rigid bronchoscope, through the mouth. A tracheal stoma is created at the time of T tube insertion, if it is not previously present. Standard insertion through the stoma is satisfactory for most patients; the latter technique provides control of the airway during the entire procedure and is therefore preferred for unstable patients with critical stenosis or limited pulmonary reserve.

Correct seating of the stent in the airway is critical for success. In particular, pressure of the edge of the tube on

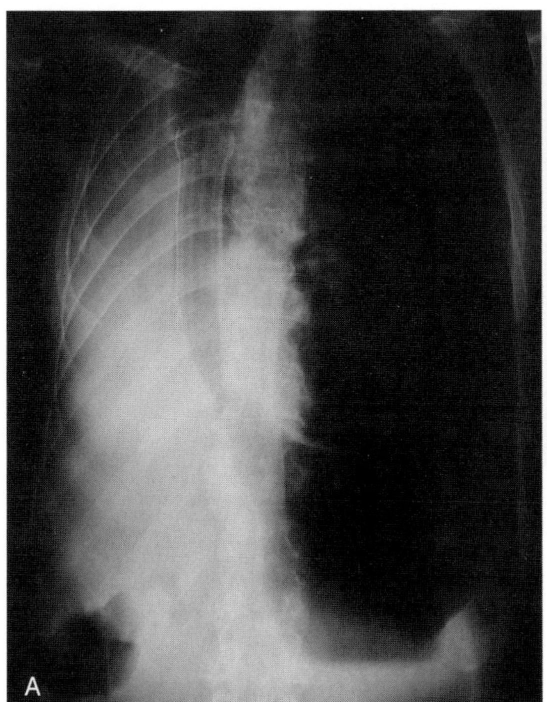

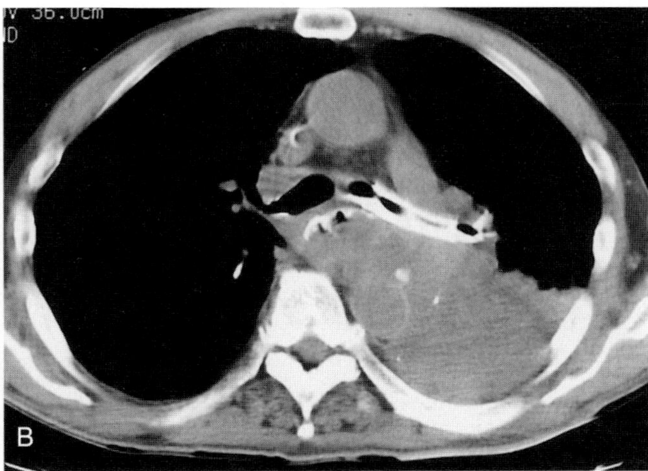

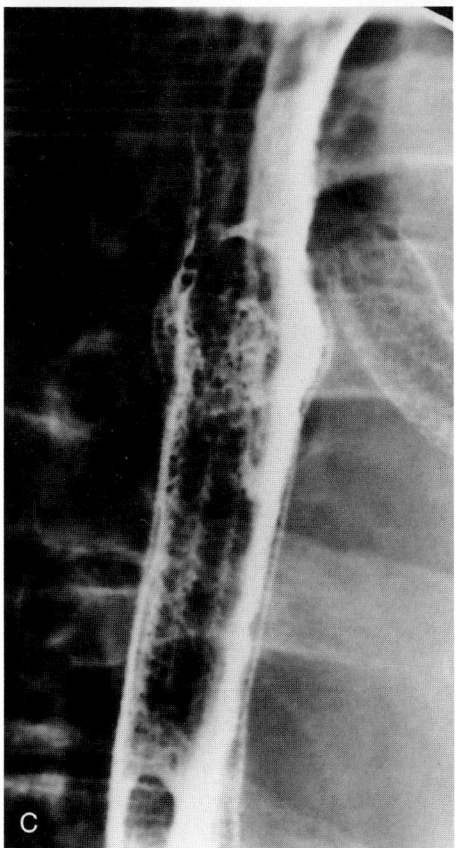

FIGURE 14–31 ■ Endoluminal stenting of esophagus and left mainstem bronchus for malignant esophagorespiratory fistula. *A*, Nodal recurrence after right pneumonectomy for lung cancer. The patient survived for 4 months after stent insertion. *B* and *C*, Unresectable carcinoma of the esophagus. *B*, A computed tomography scan demonstrates spill of esophageal contrast into the airway and a poorly fitted metal stent in the left main bronchus. *C*, A barium swallow after replacement of the bronchial stent and insertion of a new esophageal stent shows occlusion of the fistula. This patient survived for 1 month. Both patients tolerated a soft solid diet.

the mucosal surface must be avoided to prevent granulations. For the same reason, the tube should terminate well below the cords or it should be placed through the true vocal cords. Trimming of the cannula is performed in the operating room with a scalpel blade, and edges are rounded with sterilized sandpaper. To achieve a perfect fit, the tube may have to be repeatedly reinserted and trimmed.

Insertion Through the Stoma

For standard insertion of a T tube, the lower limb of the tube is introduced into the tracheal stoma and advanced

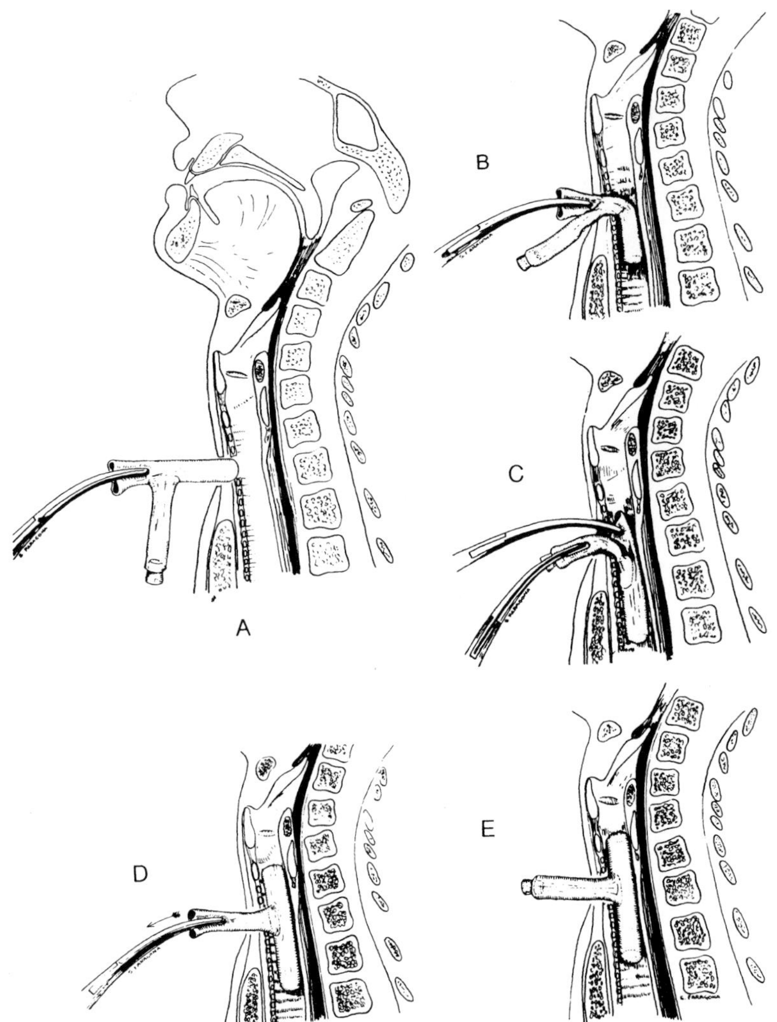

FIGURE 14–32 ■ *A* to *E*, T tube insertion through the stoma. See explanation in the text. (From Landa L: The tracheal tube: In tracheal surgery. In Grillo HC, Eschapasse H (eds): International Trends in General Thoracic Surgery, Vol 2. Philadelphia, WB Saunders, 1987.)

towards the carina (Fig. 14–32*A*). The upper limb is grasped with a Kelly clamp and gently pushed downwards until the entire length of the T tube is inside the tracheal lumen (Fig. 14–32*B* and *C*). At this point, the first Kelly clamp is detached while a second clamp is used to pull on the side arm to straighten the cannula inside the trachea (Fig. 14–32*D*). This maneuver is difficult to perform if the tip of the tube has to be guided through a stricture above the stoma.

For modified insertion through the stoma using a bronchoscope, a long umbilical tape is passed through both the side arm and the upper limb of a T tube and guided into the stoma, where it is grasped with a rigid bronchoscope (Fig. 14–33*A*). The tube is then inserted into the trachea (Fig. 14–33*B* and *C*). Traction is then exerted on the oral string while the side arm tape is kept steady (Fig. 14–33*D*).

Peroral Insertion

To place a T tube through the mouth, a well-lubricated endotracheal tube is passed over a rigid bronchoscope. The silicone cannula is mounted on the tip of the bronchoscope, and the entire assembly is advanced into the airway. When the stent is in the proposed position, it is pushed off with the endotracheal tube while the bronchoscope is withdrawn. A heavy gauge suture fixed to the side arm and previously passed perorally through the stoma is then grasped to properly guide the side arm through the stoma. The position of the tube is inspected with a fiberoptic bronchoscope.

An alternative peroral method was described by Cooper and colleagues (1989). A Pilling bronchoscope is fitted with a balloon. When this is inflated, it will firmly hold a T tube in place for insertion (Fig. 14–34). The advantage of this technique is that direct vision of the airway and ventilation are maintained throughout placement.

STENTING A GLOTTIC AIRWAY

In strictures that extend to the vocal cords, in the presence of active mucosal inflammation that involves the glottic or subglottic larynx, or in the immediate postoperative period after a high subglottic anastomosis, the laryngeal airway is often obstructed. Placement of the upper end of a T tube immediately below the cords results in granulations beneath the cords and increased obstruction. In this circumstance, the tube is positioned above the

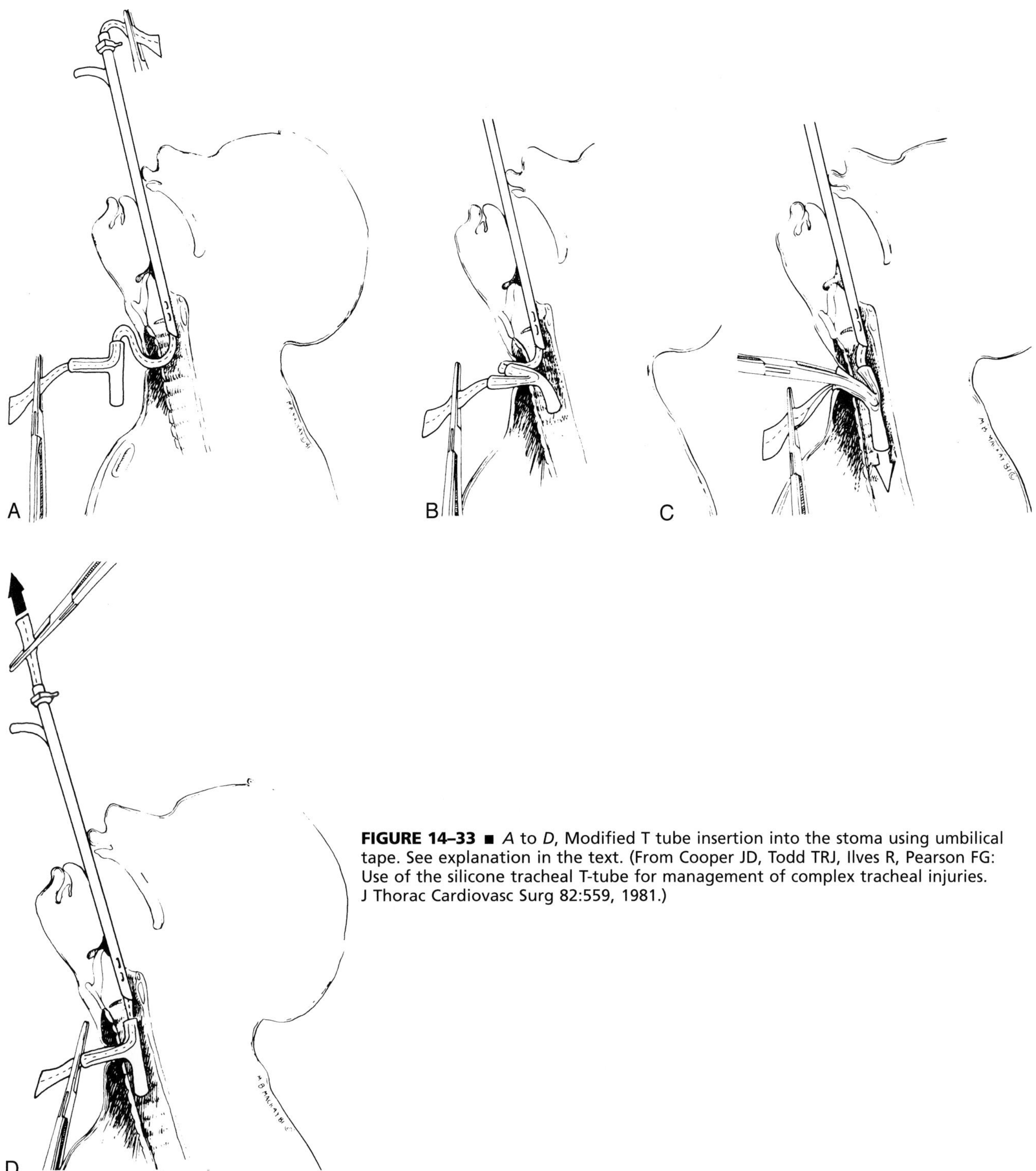

FIGURE 14–33 ■ *A* to *D*, Modified T tube insertion into the stoma using umbilical tape. See explanation in the text. (From Cooper JD, Todd TRJ, Ilves R, Pearson FG: Use of the silicone tracheal T-tube for management of complex tracheal injuries. J Thorac Cardiovasc Surg 82:559, 1981.)

true vocal cords to terminate below the false cords as proposed by Cooper and coworkers (1981). Aspiration is prevented by approximation of the false cords and epiglottic closure, and any contact with the undersurface of the epiglottis must be prevented. Patients can talk with a whispered voice, which usually improves over time. A supraglottic tube may remain in place for periods lasting from months to more than 1 year, without deterioration of vocal cord function. This use of the T tube has particular application in the treatment of inflammatory strictures that are related to inhalation injury (Gaissert et al, 1993).

TY Tube Insertion

Insertion of the TY tube is accomplished through the tracheal stoma using two ureteral catheters or small-caliber, gum-tipped bougies in both mainstem bronchi as guides. The cannula is then advanced over the catheters

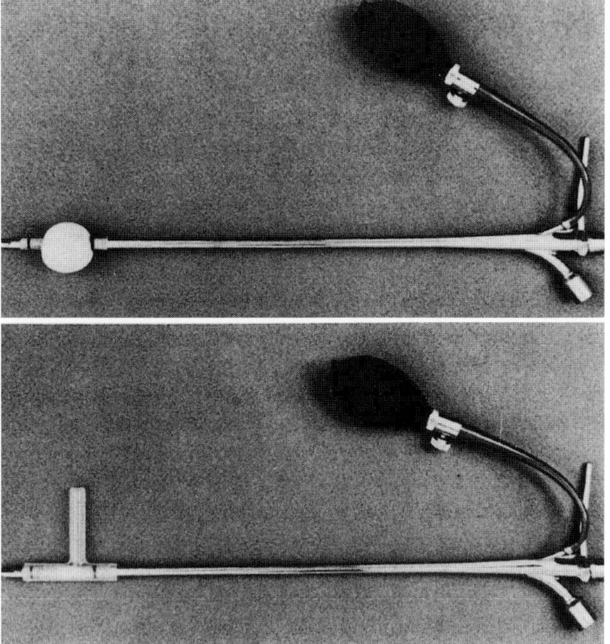

FIGURE 14–34 ■ Pilling bronchoscope adapted for peroral insertion of tracheal T tube. The inflatable balloon at the tip of the bronchoscope secures the T tube during insertion. A heavy silk tie is passed through the stoma and attached to the side arm. After translaryngeal insertion of the bronchoscope, the balloon is released, and traction on the silk tie guides the horizontal limb through the stoma. (From Cooper JD, Pearson FG, Patterson GA et al: Use of silicone stents in the management of airway problems. Ann Thorac Surg 47:371, 1989.)

towards the carina, and its upper limb is inserted into the cervical trachea with the standard or modified technique. Proper seating of the tube is ascertained with a flexible bronchoscope.

Y Stent Insertion

In patients without tracheal stoma, Y tubes are placed as shown in Figure 14–35. The right limb is inverted into the tracheal limb. A rigid bronchoscope, premounted with an 8.5 or 9 mm endotracheal tube, is advanced through the left limb of the Y tube. The bronchoscope is passed to the desired location in the left main bronchus and then withdrawn; the stent is left in place. Through the rigid scope, now in the tracheal portion of the stent, a biopsy forceps is used to place the invaginated right limb out into the right main bronchus. The previously described technique for insertion of TY tubes using catheters or bougies as guides may also be used, but it is more tedious.

Bronchial Stent Insertion

In our experience, the Hood stent was used for bronchial stent insertion. The technique is similar to that described for Y tubes. This method is straightforward for proximal right main bronchial strictures and satisfactory for proximal left main bronchial strictures. However, positioning of stents is difficult in small-caliber, distal, left main bronchial strictures. In lowering a 5-mm or smaller bronchoscope to pass into the distal bronchus, the surgeon's vision is obstructed by the bend in the instrument. In this circumstance, the stent should be mounted on a rigid 0-degree telescope.

T Tube in Children

T tube placement in children is more difficult than that in adults. Of 21 patients under the age of 20 years reported in one study, T tubes were tolerated in all 11 patients older than 10 years, but failed in one half of the children who were younger than 10 years (Gaissert et al, 1994). Most failures were due to obstruction at the subglottic end of the tube. Although the success rate is lower than that in adults, T tube stenting is an important part of the management of airway disease in children, because it allows postponement of reconstruction until the airway has completed its growth and the chances for success are greatest.

Postoperative Care

After T tube insertion, the side arm is plugged when the patient has recovered from anesthesia. Transient laryngeal edema may cause temporary obstruction of the airway, which usually improves within the first two days. If occlusion of the side arm is not tolerated, the side arm is left open. Adjustments in length or position of the tube in the operating room may be necessary. A short course of parenteral steroids may, on occasion, improve the local swelling.

In the first postoperative week, constant humidification of inspired air is important to keep secretions moist and prevent crusting. This is particularly important for T tubes with open side arms and small-caliber bronchial stents. Humidity is administered with a tracheostomy

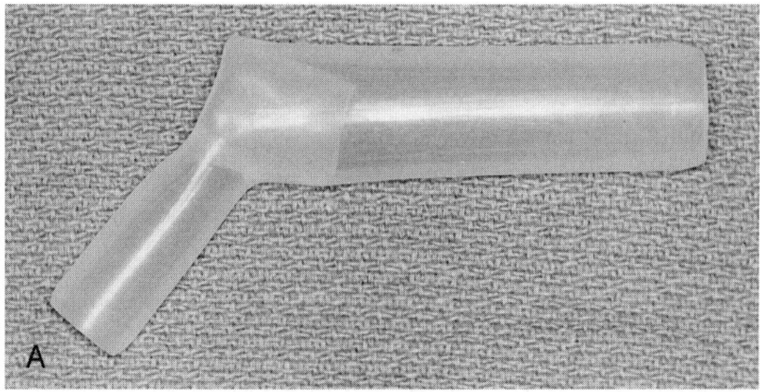

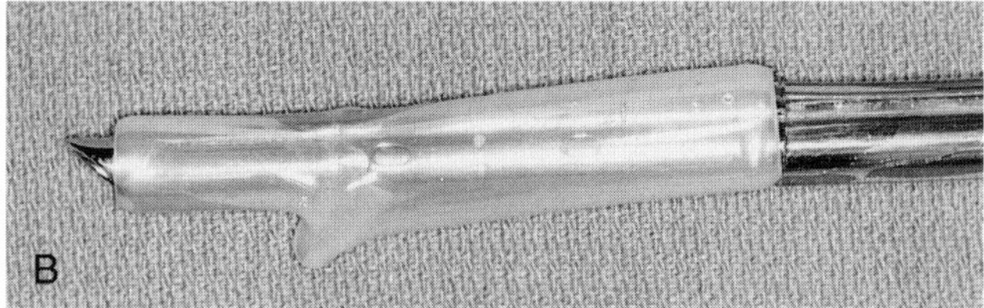

FIGURE 14–35 ■ Insertion of bronchial stent. *A*, Y stent with inverted right bronchial arm. *B*, Bronchial stent and endotracheal tube, used as a pusher, both fitted over bronchoscope.

mask while the side arm is unplugged and with a face mask when it is closed. For T tubes, sterile saline solution is instilled three times daily and the T tube is suctioned through the side arm. After the first week, humidification is discontinued. Daily inhalations with *N*-acetylcysteine are continued for bronchial stents and in some patients with T tubes. The patient is taught to clean and suction the T tube independently before discharge from the hospital.

Wire Stent Insertion

Wire stents may be inserted in the awake, sedated patient or under general anesthesia. In the awake patient, fiberoptic bronchoscopy is used for visualization and dilatation of the stricture. A fluoroscopy unit should be available if deployment of the stent is not observed directly through the bronchoscope. The anatomic limits of the stricture are then outlined with external radiopaque markers.

The selected stent length should cover the total length of the tumor and extend into normal mucosa, and the stent diameter should approximate the normal airway lumen or be slightly larger. The delivery catheter is advanced into the airway and the stricture is centered between the radiopaque markers on the catheter. The stent is then released from the deployment device. The stent position can be corrected with the help of a grasping or biopsy forceps during bronchoscopy. Overgrowth of epithelium may occur as early as 2 weeks after insertion, and any shift in position is difficult thereafter.

Pitfalls

T Tube

A T tube fails for three reasons. Anatomic obstruction occurs when the tube is wedged against the wall of the airway or when contact with the sidewall causes granulations. Most commonly, the point of obstruction is in the subglottic space or, in TY tubes, in the bronchus. The tip of the T tube must be tailored to avoid contact with the conus elasticus or the vocal cords during normal laryngeal excursion or cough. If the subglottic space is markedly narrowed, the T tube may have to be placed above the vocal cords. Dried secretions may occlude the lumen. This occurs when the side arm is left open for extended periods of time without humidification or when the patient does not clean the tube. Aspiration may ensue when the T tube interferes with epiglottic descent and glottic closure during swallowing. However, prior episodes of aspiration, masked by a tracheostomy, may only become apparent after T tube insertion. These problems typically occur immediately, or within the first 2 months after tube placement. Often they resolve spontaneously, or can be corrected, and T tube stenting should, therefore, not be prematurely abandoned without further effort at placement. When the T tube is positioned with the upper end above the vocal cords in an effort to restore translaryngeal airflow and voice, insertion may not be tolerated in as many as 20% of patients (Gaissert et al, 1994).

Bronchial Stents

Because bronchial stents are not anchored to the airway like T tubes, they are prone to movement. Overdilatation of a stricture prior to stent placement or the use of a small, loose stent may prevent the tight fit at the waist of the stenosis that is required to hold the stent in place. In addition, the distal tip of the stent sits just proximal to the lobar carina. Inaccurate placement leads easily to obstruction of a lobar orifice. The stent may be placed too distal, if two segmental orifices are mistaken for the lobar carina.

Wire Stents

Wire stents are poorly tolerated in inflammatory strictures. Gianturco stents are associated with a high rate of migration and wire fracture. Erosion of adjacent pulmonary vascular structures with fatal hemorrhage has been reported (Nashef et al, 1992). Tracheal suction catheters may become lodged in wire struts or may dislocate the stent. Nasotracheal suctioning should, therefore, be performed with caution.

RESULTS

Reports by Cooper and associates (1981, 1989) and Gaissert and colleagues (1994) examine the wide spectrum of airway problems encountered with the T tube in a large number of patients with long follow-up periods. Table 14–3 shows the duration of intubation in 112 patients after successful T tube placement. Patients accept the T tube despite the presence of an unattractive silicone side arm in the neck. This side arm may even be shortened and buried under the skin as described by Keszler (1987). Complications necessitating stent removal occur typically within the first 2 months. Once a silicone tube remains beyond this period of time, long-term stenting is usually well tolerated.

Patients typically feel immediate relief of airway obstruction after stent insertion. Gelb and others (1992) documented significant improvement of forced expiratory volume in one second and maximum expiratory flow rates in 15 patients with tracheal, Y and bronchial, stents. Post-transplant strictures may stabilize after prolonged intubation. In our experience, most stents are only temporarily required. The anastomotic site should, therefore, be inspected 6 to 12 months after insertion to determine

TABLE 14–3 ■ **Duration of T Tube Intubation in 112 Patients**

Duration of Intubation	*No.*
Less than 1 month	5
1 to 3 months	12
3 to 12 months	46
1 to 5 years	37
Longer than 5 years	12

From Gaissert HA, Grillo HC, Mathisen DJ, Wain JC: Temporary and permanent restoration of airway continuity with the tracheal T-tube. J Thorac Cardiovasc Surg 107:600, 1994.

whether bronchial patency can be maintained without the stent.

The growing experience with the technology of self-expanding metal stents in biliary and endovascular applications has led to improved airway stents. The primary indication for wire stents remain strictures in patients with limited life expectancy. Wilson and associates (1996) reported on 56 patients with unresectable cancer and life-threatening airway obstruction or collapse of one lung. Seventy-seven percent of patients showed symptomatic improvement. The authors provide spirometric data and dyspnea scores for some of their patients. Bolot and colleagues (1998) used the Gianturco stent for 23 bronchial strictures in 18 patients after lung transplantation.

COMMENTS AND CONTROVERSIES

Surgical reconstruction is the primary and preferred treatment of a tracheal or bronchial stricture, because resection removes the obstruction, is followed by excellent long-term results, and rids the patient from the nuisance of tubes. Under certain circumstances, an operation is not advised, and a tracheobronchial stent may offer excellent palliation. We prefer silicone cannulas such as the T tube or bronchial stent, because they are nonreactive, well tolerated, and easily removable.

The wire stents offer advantages, such as the ease of insertion and their self-expanding property. However, the incorporation of wire into the wall of the airway must be considered irreversible. In the authors' opinion, their use should, therefore, be restricted to patients with limited life expectancy.

H. A. G.
G. A. P.

KEY REFERENCES

Cooper JD, Pearson FG, Patterson GA et al: Use of silicone stents in the management of airway problems. Ann Thorac Surg 47:371, 1989.

This is a detailed description of the indications for tracheobronchial stents and the techniques of their placement.

Gaissert HA, Grillo HC, Mathisen DJ, Wain JC: Temporary and permanent restoration of airway continuity with the tracheal T-tube. J Thorac Cardiovasc Surg 107:600, 1994.

This is a summary of the extensive Massachusetts General Hospital experience with the tracheal T tube.

Montgomery WW: Manual care of the Montgomery silicone tracheal T-tube. Ann Otol Rhinol Laryngol 73 (Suppl.):1, 1980.

This is a concise guide for inpatient and outpatient care of the tracheal T tube—written by its inventor.

REFERENCES

Bond CJ: Note on the treatment of tracheal stenosis by a new T-shaped tracheotomy tube. Lancet 1:539, 1891.

Bolot G, Poupart M, Pignat JC et al: Self-expanding metal stents for the management of bronchial stenosis and bronchomalacia after lung transplantation. Laryngoscope 108:1230, 1998.

Cooper JD, Patterson GA, Trulock EP: Results of single and bilateral lung transplantation in 131 consecutive recipients. J Thorac Cardiovasc Surg 107:460, 1994.

Cooper JD, Pearson FG, Patterson GA et al: Use of silicone stents in the management of airway problems. Ann Thorac Surg 47:371, 1989.

Cooper JD, Todd TRJ, Ilves R, Pearson FG: Use of the silicone tracheal T-tube for the management of complex tracheal injuries. J Thorac Cardiovasc Surg 82:559, 1981.

Dumon JF: A dedicated tracheobronchial stent. Chest 97:328, 1990.

Gaissert HA, Grillo HC, Mathisen DJ, Wain JC: Temporary and permanent restoration of airway continuity with the tracheal T-tube. J Thorac Cardiovasc Surg 107:600, 1994.

Gaissert HA, Lofgren RH, Grillo HC: Upper airway compromise after inhalation injury: Complex strictures of larynx and trachea and their management. Ann Surg 218:672, 1993.

Gelb AF, Zamel N, Colchen A et al: Physiologic studies of tracheobronchial stents in airway obstruction. Am Rev Respir Dis 146:1088, 1992.

Keszler P: The tracheal T-tube: For indwelling intubation as an alternative management method. In Grillo HC, Eschapasse H (eds): International Trends in General Thoracic Surgery, Vol 2. Philadelphia, WB Saunders, 1987.

Landa L: The tracheal T tube: In tracheal surgery. In Grillo HC, Eschapasse H (eds): International Trends in General Thoracic Surgery, Vol 2. Philadelphia, WB Saunders, 1987.

Montgomery WW: The surgical management of supraglottic and subglottic stenosis. Ann Otol 77:534, 1968.

Montgomery WW: T-tube tracheal stent. Arch Otolaryngol 82:320, 1965.

Nashef SA, Dromer C, Velly JF et al: Expanding wire stents in benign tracheobronchial disease: Indications and complications. Ann Thorac Surg 54:937, 1992.

Patterson GA, Todd TR, Cooper JD et al: Airway complications after double lung transplantation. J Thorac Cardiovasc Surg 99:14, 1990.

Trendelenburg F: Beitraege zu den Operationen an den Luftwegen. Langenbeck Arch Chir 13:335, 1872.

Wallace MJ, Charnsangavej C, Ogawa K et al. Tracheobronchial tree: Expandable metallic stents used in experimental and clinical applications. Radiology 158:309, 1986.

Westaby S, Jackson JW, Pearson FG: A bifurcated silicone rubber stent for relief of tracheobronchial obstruction. J Thorac Cardiovasc Surg 83:414, 1982.

Wilson GE, Walshaw MJ, Hind CRK: Treatment of large airway obstruction in lung cancer using expandable metal stents inserted under direct vision via the fiberoptic bronchoscope. Thorax 51:248, 1996.

CHAPTER **15**

Benign Conditions

CONGENITAL ANOMALIES

Robert M. Filler

The two most common congenital anomalies of the trachea are tracheomalacia and tracheal stenosis. Tracheomalacia is decreased rigidity of the trachea caused by a structural abnormality of its wall. In childhood, this arises from faulty development of the trachea, whereas in adults, it is usually secondary to obstructive lung disease. This anomaly is most commonly present in children who are born with esophageal atresia and tracheal esophageal fistula, but it is also associated with lesions that apply external pressure to the trachea, such as a double aortic arch or a paratracheal tumor (Baxter et al, 1963). Tracheomalacia may also occur as an isolated event. Congenital tracheal stenosis, which may involve all or a portion of the length of the trachea, is almost always secondary to a developmental defect in which the pars membranacea of the trachea is deficient, and the wall consists of complete or almost complete cartilaginous rings.

In the following discussion of the clinical syndromes associated with these abnormalities, special focus is on diagnosis and management.

Tracheomalacia

HISTORICAL NOTE

In 1948, Gross and Neuhauser described a condition in which the trachea was compressed by "an anomalous innominate artery," for which suspension of the innominate artery gave relief. In the subsequent years, the existence of the so-called innominate artery syndrome was questioned by many because anatomic dissections and angiographic findings failed to corroborate the presence of an anomalous innominate artery. In 1969, Mustard and associates reported 285 cases of symptomatic tracheal compression by the innominate artery, 39 of which were treated surgically. These authors believed that tracheal compression was due to mediastinal crowding and that suspension of the innominate artery provided more space in the mediastinum. Many of the children in the series of Mustard and associates had been born with esophageal atresia. Subsequent reports suggest that the innominate artery syndrome is identical to what we now call tracheomalacia. In 1969, Benjamin and others demonstrated that an abnormally soft trachea (tracheomalacia) rather than aortic root anomalies was responsible for tracheal obstruction, at least in those children who also had been born with esophageal atresia. In 1976, Filler and colleagues described life-threatening anoxic spells caused by tracheomalacia after repair of esophageal atresia and indicated that displacement of the aorta anteriorly to the undersurface of the trachea (aortopexy) could be curative. Further experience in a variety of pediatric centers has now indicated that aortopexy will alleviate the symptoms associated with severe tracheomalacia, and a definite anatomic abnormality has been identified (DeLorimier et al, 1990; Heimansohn et al, 1991; Kiely et al, 1987; Schwartz and Filler, 1980; Wailoo and Emery, 1979.

HISTORICAL READINGS

Benjamin B, Cohen D, Glasson M: Tracheomalacia in association with congenital tracheoesophageal fistula. Surgery 79:504, 1969.

DeLorimier A, Harrison M, Hardy K et al: Tracheobronchial obstructions in infants and children. Ann Surg 212:277, 1990.

Filler RM, Rossello PJ, Lebowitz RL: Life-threatening anoxic spells caused by tracheal compression after repair of esophageal atresia: Correction by surgery. J Pediatr Surg 11:739, 1976.

Gross KE, Neuhauser EB: Compression of the trachea by an anomalous innominate artery: An operation for its relief. Am J Dis Child 75:570, 1948.

Heimansohn D, Kesler K, Turrentine M: Anterior pericardial tracheoplasty for congenital tracheal stenosis. J Thorac Cardiovasc Surg 102:710, 1991.

Kiely EM, Spitz L, Brereton R: Management of tracheomalacia by aortopexy. Pediatr Surg Int 2:13, 1987.

Mustard WT, Bayliss CE, Fearon B et al: Tracheal compression by the innominate artery in children. Ann Thorac Surg 8:312, 1969.

Schwartz MZ, Filler RM: Tracheal compression as a cause of apnea following repair of tracheoesophageal fistula: Treatment by aortopexy. J Pediatr Surg 15:842, 1980.

Wailoo MP, Emery JL: The trachea in children with tracheoesophageal fistula. Histopathology 3:329, 1979.

BASIC SCIENCE

The variations in the size of the tracheal lumen depends on the rigidity of its wall and the difference between the intraluminal and extraluminal forces that act on it. Because of these relationships, the lumen of the normal, somewhat flexible, intrathoracic trachea increases during inspiration and decreases during expiration in response to a decrease and then an increase in intrathoracic pressure. In the patient with an abnormally soft trachea, the changes in tracheal caliber caused by ventilation are magnified, so that in the most severe cases, complete collapse of the trachea may occur, even during unlabored expiration. When higher intrathoracic pressures are gen-

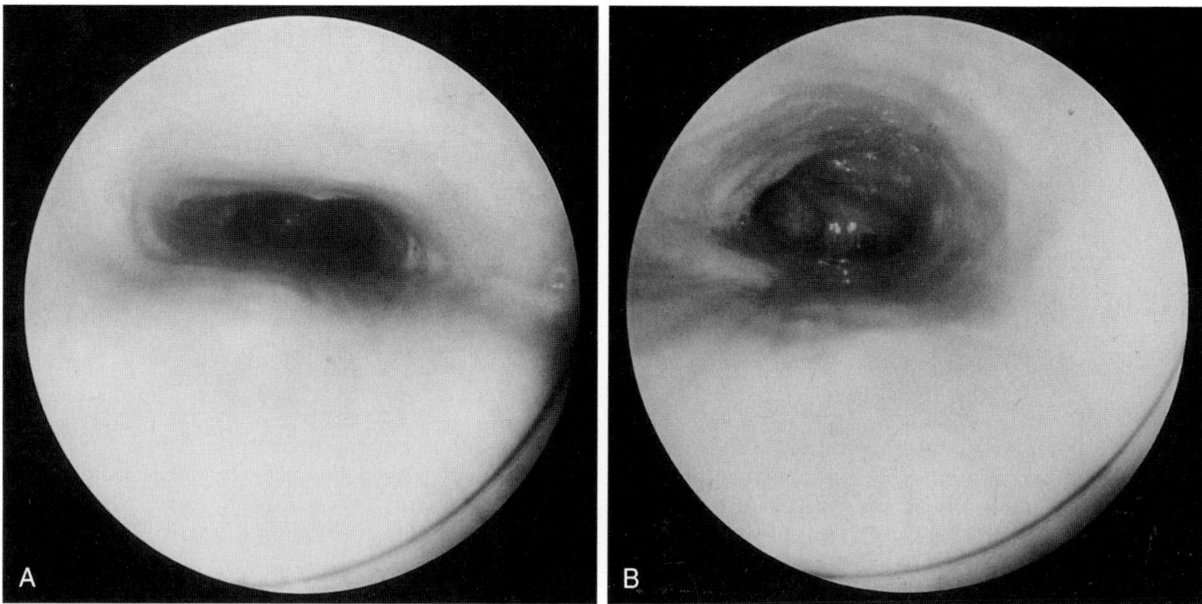

FIGURE 15–1 ■ An endoscopic view of the trachea above the carina in a spontaneously breathing 3-month-old child with tracheomalacia. *A,* Before aortopexy. Note the elliptical, narrowed lumen and the bulging of the elongated membranous trachea posteriorly. *B,* After aortopexy. The incomplete cartilaginous rings can be appreciated in the anterior wall of the trachea, whose lumen is now wider during the phases of respiration and during coughing.

erated, as during a cough or in clinical situations in which lung compliance is reduced, obstruction to the outflow of air is even greater. Because inspiratory efforts cause the trachea to enlarge, obstruction to air inflow does not occur in tracheomalacia. Tracheomalacia in the cervical trachea rarely produces airway obstruction during quiet or forceful respiration because the pressures inside and outside the cervical trachea are equal (i.e., atmospheric) when the glottis is open. The dynamics of airway collapse have been discussed in detail by Wittenborg and coworkers (1969).

In addition to changes in airway size that occur in response to variations in intrathoracic pressure, changes can occur from compression of an abnormally soft trachea by adjacent intrathoracic structures, especially the esophagus, posteriorly, and the ascending aorta and aortic arch and its branches, anteriorly. The size and position of the aorta are relatively constant, but esophageal diameter is increased by swallowing, gastroesophageal reflux, and the presence of obstructive lesions of the lower esophagus. As a result, patients with tracheomalacia often have their most severe symptoms during or shortly after eating, when the esophagus is most distended.

A variety of structural abnormalities can produce tracheomalacia; however, the most common type encountered in childhood is found in children also born with esophageal atresia. The structural defect was first described by Wailoo and Emery (1979), who studied an unselected sequential series of tracheas obtained from 53 deceased infants and children born with esophageal atresia and tracheoesophageal fistula (TEF). Their evaluations showed that in 75% of these cases, there was a segment of trachea in which cartilaginous rings were fragmented or had an elliptical rather than a C shape. The membranous portion of this segment of the trachea was extremely wide and floppy, so that even minor forces acting on the trachea would cause apposition of its anterior and posterior walls. These pathologic findings correspond precisely to those seen at bronchoscopy in children with symptomatic tracheomalacia (Fig. 15–1).

Several causes have been postulated for the association between tracheomalacia and esophageal atresia. Because the trachea and the esophagus are derived from the foregut, a faulty division of the foregut, which is the presumed cause of esophageal atresia, can be expected also to affect the adjacent trachea. Evidence to support this possibility can be found in Wailoo and Emery's (1979) studies, in which esophageal muscle was often present in the membranous trachea at the site of the other tracheal abnormalities. This finding suggests that when the foregut divides, the esophagus receives too little (atresia) and the trachea receives too much (tracheomalacia). Davies and Cywes (1978) surmised that the dilated esophagus above the site of atresia may compress the fetal trachea and prevent its normal development. They also suggested that abnormal tracheal development could be due to the loss of intratracheal pressure in the fetus through a TEF, because the fluid that normally fills the embryonic airway may provide the mechanism of internal support for the growing trachea.

Tracheomalacia sometimes becomes apparent only after surgery for lesions that mechanically compress the trachea, such as a vascular ring or a tumor. While it is possible that trauma during surgery contributes to postoperative tracheomalacia, it is more likely that long-term compression of the trachea is responsible for abnormal tracheal development. Other developmental defects of cartilage and complete absence of tracheal cartilage are much less common causes of tracheomalacia (Cox and Shaw, 1965; Johner and Szanto, 1970).

DIAGNOSIS

Clinical Features

The symptoms of tracheomalacia are due to airway obstruction during expiration. Most children have a typical barking cough, which is probably due to vibration of the opposing anterior and posterior tracheal walls (Benjamin et al, 1969). Recurrent pneumonia is common in these patients, presumably because airway collapse during coughing prevents effective clearance of airway secretions. In some children, airway obstruction during normal ventilation is so severe that airway intubation is necessary, and in others the diagnosis of tracheomalacia is not really appreciated until the airway cannot be extubated after a surgical procedure such as repair of esophageal atresia or a vascular ring. The most serious symptom, and the one that is the most frequent reason for surgery, is a life-threatening "dying spell." Spells, which often do not appear until 2 or 3 months of age, are characterized by cyanosis that rapidly progresses to apnea, bradycardia, and, if uninterrupted, even cardiac arrest. Characteristically, spells occur during feeding or within 5 to 10 minutes of a meal. Benjamin and associates (1969) and Mustard coworkers (1969) suggested that the spells are due to a vagal reflex that arises from the tracheal wall when the trachea collapses.

Our experience, however, suggests another mechanism. Transcutaneous oxygen pressure ($tcPO_2$) monitoring during feedings in a small group of infants with spells associated with tracheomalacia showed a progressive fall in $tcPO_2$ during uninterrupted bottle feeding, with bradycardia developing as $tcPO_2$ fell; $tcPO_2$ and heart rate returned to normal as soon as the feeding was interrupted. We theorize that the spell is secondary to progressive hypoxia, which occurs because the lumen of the malacic trachea is compressed by an esophagus filled with milk. Because esophageal dilatation is extremely common in children after repair of esophageal atresia because of poor esophageal peristalsis, esophageal stricture, or gastroesophageal reflux, it is not surprising that spells related to feeding are extremely common in this subset of tracheomalacia patients. Because similar-type spells can be due to cardiac or neurologic causes, complete evaluation of the child's neurologic and cardiac status is also necessary in these cases.

Natural History

Symptoms that are due to tracheomalacia tend to improve with time, presumably because the trachea becomes more rigid with growth. In patients with the most severe symptoms, such as dying spells, one cannot delay treatment to see how much improvement occurs with time. However, for those with mild or even intermediate symptoms, such as recurrent pneumonia, a wait-and-see attitude is sometimes justified.

Differential Diagnosis

Symptoms of tracheomalacia can be caused by a variety of conditions. However, in the setting in which they occur, the primary diagnoses that must also be considered are gastroesophageal reflux, esophageal stricture, recurrent tracheoesophageal fistula, and neurologic and cardiac conditions that could cause anoxic syncopal attacks.

Investigative Techniques

The diagnosis of tracheomalacia should be suspected on the basis of a clinical history of apneic spells, recurrent pneumonia, or inability to extubate the airway because of expiratory obstruction, especially in children with a history of esophageal atresia, vascular ring, or a previous mass around the trachea. Investigations to confirm the diagnosis are relatively straightforward. A narrowing of the air-filled trachea can be noted on the lateral view of a plain chest radiograph in almost all children with tracheomalacia whose airways are not intubated. A better evaluation of tracheal dynamics is obtained radiographically with the image intensifier by continuous visualization of the trachea during several respiratory cycles. At the same time, the esophagus should be filled with radiocontrast material so that the relationship between esophageal size and tracheal diameter can be appreciated. The radiocontrast study is also needed to determine if gastroesophageal reflux, esophageal stricture, recurrent tracheoesophageal fistula, or poor esophageal motility is present. Typical radiographic findings in tracheomalacia are shown in Figure 15–2.

Bronchoscopy provides a definitive diagnosis in these cases (see Fig. 15–1). General anesthesia is usually necessary for bronchoscopy, but the child must be breathing spontaneously, and not paralyzed, for proper evaluation of the trachea. In the symptomatic case, the tracheal lumen has an eliptical shape. Anterior vascular pulsations are usually evident, and the membranous portion of the trachea is usually enlarged and bulging into the lumen, more on the left than on the right. The cartilaginous tracheal rings may appear to be discontinuous. Anterior and posterior collapse of the lumen occurs during expiration, and in severe cases, complete airway occlusion is noted when a cough is stimulated. Because of the need for general anesthesia, bronchoscopy is usually the last test to be performed in suspected cases of tracheomalacia. In general, one should be prepared to proceed with definitive surgery at the time of bronchoscopy if the diagnosis of severe tracheomalacia is confirmed.

MANAGEMENT

Principles

Many children with minor degrees of airway collapse do not require specific therapy. The abnormally soft trachea tends to become more rigid with continued growth and development, and symptoms can be expected to improve in the first 1 or 2 years of life.

Symptoms that are life-threatening or are likely to represent a significant health hazard require surgical intervention. The major indications for surgery are noted in Table 15–1. We believe that a single dying spell due to tracheomalacia is an indication for surgery. Likewise, there appears to be little justification for delaying surgical correction for the child who requires a tracheostomy or

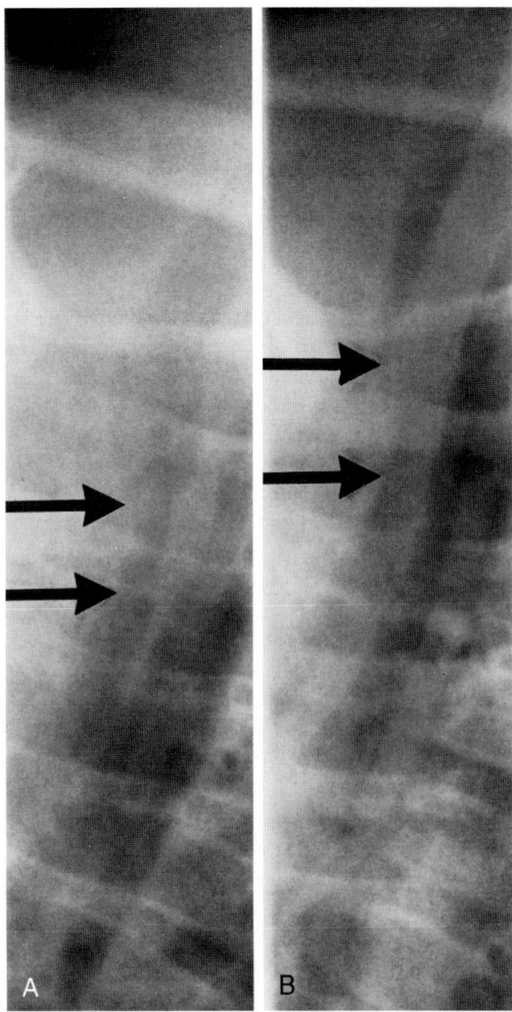

FIGURE 15–2 ■ Lateral chest films in a 2-month-old child with tracheomalacia. Note the tracheal air shadow. *A,* During inspiration, a slight indentation related to the aorta is seen on the anterior wall of the trachea (*between arrows*). *B,* During expiration, the tracheal air shadow disappears in this same region (*between arrows*) as the trachea collapses.

an endotracheal tube to keep the airway patent. Sometimes it is difficult to decide how many episodes of pneumonia are acceptable before advising surgery. Certainly, more than three documented episodes in a year would seem excessive, especially if a severe anatomic abnormality is seen at bronchoscopy.

TABLE 15–1 ■ **Tracheomalacia Treated by Aortopexy 1978–1991**

Primary Indication for Aortopexy (a)	*No. of Patients (n = 46)*	*Outcome*	
		Success	*Failure*
Dying spells	33	32	1 (b)
Airway intubation needed			
Nasotracheal	5	5	
Tracheostomy	4	2	2 (c)
Recurrent pneumonia	4	3	1

a, 5 patients also had splint: b, Dead of undetermined cause: c, Tracheostomy eventually removed.

Surgical Therapy

Tracheomalacia can be treated by several surgical techniques. A tracheostomy will provide an internal tracheal splint and has been used by some in the hope that improvement would accompany growth (Shapiro and Martin, 1981). Wiseman and associates (1985) successfully treated tracheomalacia and bronchomalacia with airway intubation and continuous positive airway pressure (CPAP) for 14 weeks. This duration of CPAP is probably not sufficient for most infants with airway collapse, because significant spontaneous improvement in tracheomalacia is unlikely before 1 or 2 years of age. Johnston and others (1980) used a free-rib graft as a splint for the trachea in two children in whom a tracheostomy tube failed to stabilize the malacic segment. Our experience indicates that aortic suspension is an effective and safe method of therapy for most tracheomalacia patients. Stenting of the malacic segment with a balloon expandable stent has been shown to be a less invasive option than aortopexy (Filler, 1998).

Aortopexy

Our original decision to use aortopexy (Fig. 15–3) for tracheomalacia was based on the favorable reports of Gross and Neuhauser (1948) and Mustard and coworkers (1969) in treating what they called the innominate artery compression syndrome. Many of their patients undoubtedly had what we are now calling tracheomalacia. The rationale for the procedure is that the trachea will be pulled anteriorly when the aorta is suspended from the sternum if the connective tissue between the two is not disturbed. This translocation will change the configuration of the cross section of the malacic trachea from an ellipse to a circle and prevent apposition of its anterior and posterior walls. In addition, anterior displacement of the trachea will minimize airway compression by the esophagus.

Anesthesia for aortopexy is planned to permit intraoperative endoscopic examination of the affected portion of the airway and immediate assessment of the adequacy of repair. For this purpose, anesthetic gases are delivered through a ventilating bronchoscope with a telescope attachment. Although the telescope takes up a portion of the lumen of the bronchoscope and resistance to airflow is increased, the anesthetist can still maintain satisfactory ventilation.

A left anterior thoracotomy through the third interspace is used to gain access to the anterior mediastinum for aortopexy. The left lobe of the thymus is excised to expose the aorta and its first branches and to create a space to translocate these vessels. The tissue plane between the aorta and trachea is not dissected, because it is this attachment that pulls the trachea forward when the aorta is suspended from the sternum. Three or four 3–0 nonabsorbable vascular sutures are placed into the adventitia and a portion of the media at three locations—namely, the ascending aorta, the origin of the

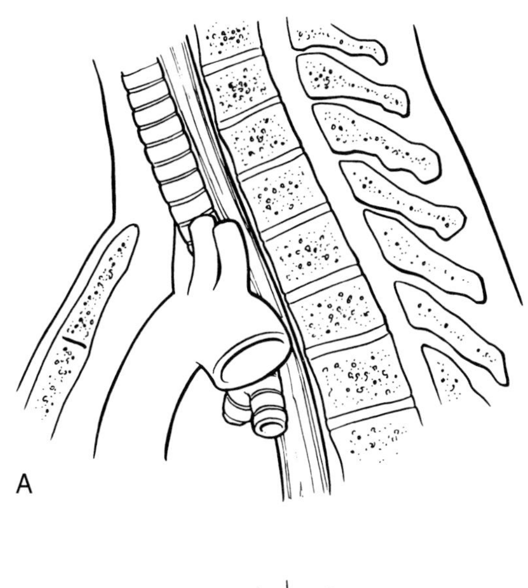

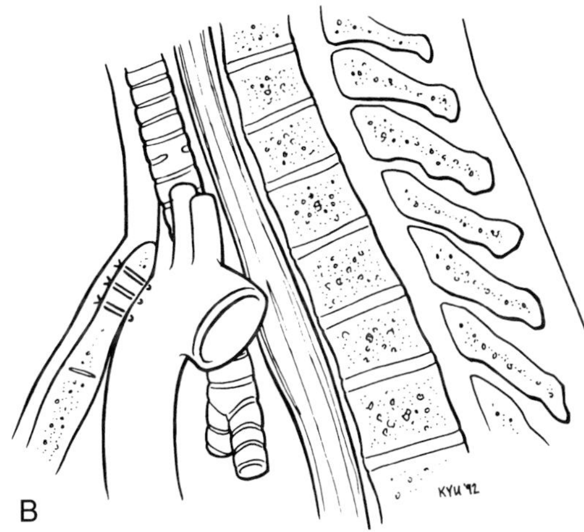

FIGURE 15–3 ■ Mediastinal anatomy in tracheomalacia and the effect on aortopexy. *A,* A sagittal view of the chest showing the relationships between the aorta, the trachea, and the esophagus. The malacic trachea can be compressed by the adjacent aorta, but when the esophagus is empty or the child is not coughing, there is usually no appreciable airway obstruction. However, when the esophagus dilates (during swallowing or reflux), the trachea collapses between it and the aorta. Respiratory symptoms and apneic spells occur at this time. *B,* The operative procedure pulls the aorta anteriorly and displaces the anterior wall of the trachea as well. The filled esophagus no longer causes critical airway narrowing.

right innominate artery, and the aortic arch just beyond the origin of the innominate artery. A subcutaneous pocket is created anterior to the upper sternum, and both ends of the vascular sutures are passed through the entire thickness of the sternum into this pocket. The sutures are pulled up simultaneously, and they are tied sequentially after bronchoscopic observation indicates a satisfactory improvement in the tracheal configuration. If the correction is not satisfactory, one or two additional sutures may be of help; otherwise, insertion of a tracheal stent will be necessary.

In patients with a tracheostomy tube in place prior to surgery, we have removed it and replaced it with a nasotracheal tube 1 week before aortopexy. This allows the stoma to close, which minimizes the possibility of bacterial contamination of the wound at the time of aortopexy. This step is especially important if a prosthetic splint is implanted.

Perioperative Care

Management of the child after surgery is relatively simple. The airway is extubated immediately in most patients. Antibiotics are not used, and analgesics are needed for 1 to 3 days postoperatively. Physiotherapy to ensure adequate coughing and ventilation is necessary, but endotracheal suctioning is almost never needed.

Results of Aortopexy

From 1978 to 1991, 46 children had aortopexy for tracheomalacia at our institution (Filler et al, 1982). A splint was also applied to the external circumference of the trachea in 3 of these cases. Tracheomalacia was associated with esophageal atresia in 34 children and was an isolated finding in 12. The major indications for surgery and outcomes of treatment are listed in Table 15–1. This treatment was judged a complete success in 42 children. Aortopexy was considered a "Failure" if the major indication for surgery was not completely eliminated. Of the four "Failures" noted in Table 15–1, one died at home 6 months after aortopexy of unknown cause; two with tracheostomies could not be decannulated for more than 1 month after aortopexy; and one had additional episodes of pneumonia.

Aortopexy has been well tolerated, and operative complications in our hands and those of others have been minimal. Evaluation of the aortic suspension by postoperative echocardiogram in a limited number of patients indicates that the aorta remains attached to the sternum for at least a year following surgery. Although this is theoretically a problem, there have been no reports of long-term vascular complications from aortopexy.

Treatment of tracheomalacia by aortopexy has been the subject of several reports by other authors, and their results are similar to our own. Kiely and associates (1987) reported on 25 aortopexies in 22 children with associated esophageal anomalies, mostly esophageal atresia and tracheoesophageal fistulas. Excellent results were obtained in 17 children, with only one long-term failure. Of interest is that symptoms worsened after aortopexy in two of children, both of whom had recurrent tracheoesophageal fistula and severe gastroesophageal reflux. Division of the fistula and fundoplication in each case proved to be curative.

Tracheal Stents

In the early 1990s, we began inserting stents into the airway endoscopically as an adjunct to other surgical measures to treat selected cases of airway malacia and stenosis. The Palmaz stainless steel balloon inflatable stent has been used exclusively by us since 1992. This stent was designed for use in the vascular system, but it is well suited to the small airway because it is relatively nonreactive and its mesh-like characteristic in the expanded state allows it to be placed across the mouth of a branch airway without obstructing it. It is readily available in sizes that are useful for the small and large airways of the infant and child. Palmaz stents can be inserted through a rigid bronchoscope or endotracheal tube using videoradiography to follow the movement of the bronchoscope and to ensure the proper placement of the stent. The technical details of stent insertion and removal have been published (Filler et al, 1998).

Stenting for tracheomalacia was first used by us in a child who was born with esophageal atresia and tetralogy of Fallot. Aortopexy was not a treatment option for tracheomalacia in this case, because a dilated aorta was already in juxtaposition to the undersurface of the sternum. The successful outcome of stenting in this child led us to consider the stenting option for all cases of tracheomalacia.

Guidelines for stenting of subsequent patients were based on this initial experience, work done in our animal laboratory (Fraga et al, 1997), and the knowledge of the natural history of tracheomalacia. The indications for stenting were identical to those used for aortopexy. Except for the first case, bronchoscopy was not performed after stenting in the absence of symptoms until planned stent removal 1 year post insertion. We presumed that the tracheal wall would no longer collapse at this time. From 1993 to 1998, tracheomalacia was treated with a Palmaz stent in eight infants. The favorable outcomes are noted in Table 15–2. The bronchoscopic appearance of a stent in its expanded state in the trachea and the accompanying chest radiograph are seen in Figure 15–4*A*, *B*, and *C*. The only troublesome complication of stenting has been the formation of granulation tissue over the stent, which occurred in 4 of 8 children. This was manifested by noisy breathing with some evidence of inspiratory airway obstruction. The granulation tissue was scraped away at bronchoscopy in all, but symptomatic recurrences required stent removal at 4 and 5 months after stenting in two children, respectively. Despite earlier than planned removal, symptoms that led to stenting never recurred in these children, suggesting that stenting for less than 1 year might be satisfactory. All 8 children

TABLE 15–2 ■ **Tracheomalacia Treated by Stenting 1993–1998**

Primary Indication for Stent	*No. of Patients (n = 8)*	*Outcome*	
		Success	*Failure*
Dying spells	4	4(a)	
Inability to extubate	3	3	
Recurrent pneumonia	1	1	

a, Stents removed earlier than planned in 2 children.

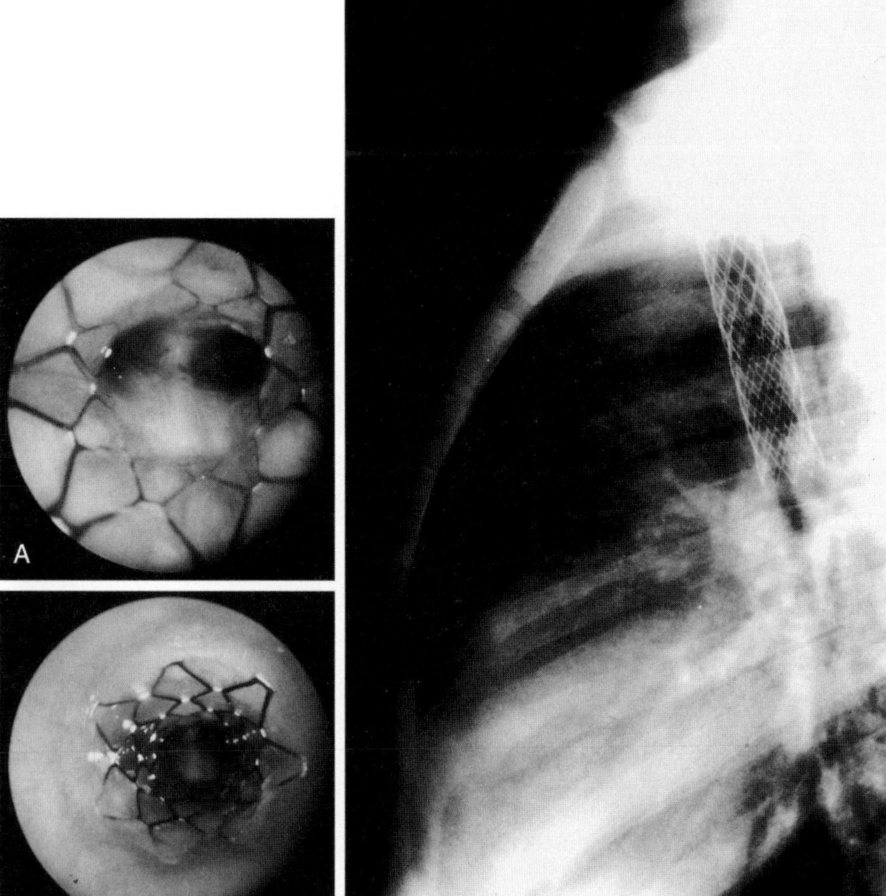

FIGURE 15–4 ■ *A,* This 3-month-old was born with esophageal atresia and tracheoesophageal fistula. Because of dying spells and confirmed tracheomalacia, two overlapping Palmaz stents were inserted in the trachea. The illustration shows the expanded stent just above the carina. *B,* This illustration was taken at the proximal end of the stent. *C,* Post-stenting lateral chest radiograph.

are well, and all stents have been removed. Because stenting is less invasive than aortopexy, and the outcomes are comparable, stenting is now our procedure of choice for infants and children with tracheomalacia. Additional details of stenting have been published (Filler, 1998).

A variety of indwelling stents are now available, although except for the one described by Vinograd and colleagues (1994), none have been designed with the airway in mind. For the infant and small child, a balloon expandable stent such as the Palmaz stent appears to be preferable to a spring stent such as the Gianturco stent, which expands to a size that is larger than the tracheal diameter. Such stents exert continuous pressure on the airway wall until the spring is completely expanded, thus increasing the risk of late perforation. The final diameter of the Palmaz stent can be selected by the operator at the time of insertion. Vinograd and associates (1994) described a novel airway coiled ribbon stent made of nitinal, a nickel-titanium alloy, which expands when heated and contracts when cooled. It is inserted (and removed) in its small cold state and expands to a preselected diameter at body temperature. The ability to decrease the stent size with simple cooling may make its removal easier than the removal of the Palmaz stent.

Splinting Operations

Collapsing airways have been stabilized by the application of a variety of "splints" about the external circumference of the trachea. Herzog and associates (1968) described the use of a free autologous rib graft to stent the adult trachea. Johnston and coworkers (1980) applied the same technique in two children, but long-term results have not been published. Rainer and others (1968) first used prosthetic splinting in 23 adults with tracheomalacia caused by severe chronic obstructive lung disease. In their cases, the widened membranous trachea was plicated and covered with a Dacron-reinforced Silastic prosthesis. Several years ago we implanted a Silastic-reinforced Marlex mesh device in five children with tracheomalacia. The device has not adversely affected tracheal growth in animals or in long-term clinical follow-up of these and other children (Filler et al, 1982; Murphy et al, 1983; Vinograd et al, 1987). Our indication for the application of an airway splint in tracheomalacia was long-segment tracheal collapse or collapse that could not be corrected by aortopexy. With the availability of intraluminal stents, which can be implanted less invasively, splinting no longer appears to be indicated in the management of tracheomalacia in the small child.

COMMENTS AND CONTROVERSIES

One of the frequent clinical decisions to be faced is how to deal with the severely symptomatic child who is found to have both tracheomalacia and gastroesophageal reflux. This complex of abnormalities occurs frequently in the group of children born with esophageal atresia. The reflux of gastric contents into the esophagus may actually cause tracheal collapse if a dilated esophagus, filled in retrograde fashion, impinges on a flaccid trachea. In our series, 14 of the 35 children who had esophageal atresia were diagnosed as having reflux before surgery for tracheomalacia. Five of these had undergone an antireflux procedure elsewhere because of the belief that gastroesophageal reflux was responsible for the life-threatening respiratory symptoms, and three others required a fundoplication after aortopexy. Four additional children who developed gastroesophageal reflux after aortopexy also needed fundoplication, although not for respiratory symptoms.

In those children who are found to have gastroesophageal reflux during evaluation for tracheomalacia or vice versa, if the major symptom is a dying spell or recurrent pneumonia and if radiography and bronchoscopy show complete or near-complete closure of the trachea on swallowing and coughing, we and others (Kiely et al, 1987) would elect to proceed with aortopexy rather than fundoplication as the initial step in surgical management.

For aortopexy, the aorta can be approached through a left or right anterior thoracotomy or a sternal split. We have found the left-sided approach to be the easiest, although this is not always possible because of a previous surgical procedure. With sternotomy, the effect of the aortic suspension cannot be determined until the sternum is closed; if the desired change in tracheal shape is not achieved, the sternum must be reopened. In contrast, closure of an anterior thoracotomy does not change the spatial relationships of the structures affected by aortopexy.

To reduce the possibility of aortic tear from the deep sutures that we use to suspend the aorta, some surgeons prefer to attach a patch of synthetic material to the adventitia of the aorta with many superficial sutures and then to sew the synthetic fabric to the undersurface of the sternum. Because we have had no complications from sutures placed through a partial thickness of the aortic wall, this additional step seems unnecessary. The bleeding that sometimes occurs when the aortic suture is placed indicates that the lumen has been entered. If this occurs, the suture is removed, and gentle pressure is applied to the needle hole. When bleeding stops, a new suture can be placed.

The use of stents in the airway is so new that one cannot be dogmatic about their use at this time. Aortopexy has been the standard treatment for tracheomalacia in many institutions for the past 2 decades, and it is the gold standard against which one must compare new treatments. Stents are easily implanted with minimally invasive techniques. However, one must be cautious about removal, especially if granulations that form on it have been removed with a laser. We reported a death at the time of stent removal in such a child whose stent was placed elsewhere. The stent was "welded" into the tracheal wall by the laser treatment, making it impossible to remove, even at autopsy. To date we have been very impressed with the outcomes of stenting for tracheomalacia and recommend it as a better procedure than aortopexy. However, important questions remain: What are the long-term effects of stenting? Will the trachea grow normally? How long is stenting necessary? How safe is removal? What can be done to make removal easier? How much practice does one need to be competent?

R. M. F.

Tracheal Stenosis

HISTORICAL NOTE

Wolman (1941) reported 11 cases of congenital tracheal stenosis, including one of his own, that had been documented since 1832. One child with dyspnea for the first 7 years of life improved after tracheostomy, but all others died. Benjamin and colleagues (1981) reviewed 21 cases of congenital tracheal stenosis seen in Sydney, Australia, between 1971 and 1980. Despite nine deaths in that series, the authors emphasized that 12 of the 21 patients survived after mostly conservative treatment (excepting one pneumonectomy and one tracheopexy), and they concluded "there appears to be little place for surgical resection of the stenosis . . . . " Case reports of successful segmental resection of tracheal stenosis in babies started to appear in the 1980s (Harrison et al, 1980; Healy et al, 1988; Mansfield, 1980; Mattingly et al, 1981; Minato et al, 1986; Nakayama et al, 1982; Weber et al, 1982). Aggressive surgical treatment of symptomatic lesions is now the accepted standard, although methods of tracheoplasty have varied at different surgical centers.

■ *HISTORICAL READINGS*

Benjamin B, Pitkin J, Cohen D: Congenital tracheal stenosis. Ann Otol Rhinol Laryngol 90:364, 1981.

Harrison MR, Heldt GP, Brasch RC et al: Resection of distal tracheal stenosis in a baby with agenesis of the lung. J Pediatr Surg 15:938, 1980.

Healy GB, Schuster SR, Jonas RA et al: Correction of segmental tracheal stenosis in children. Ann Otol Rhinol Laryngol 97:444, 1988.

Mansfield PB: Tracheal resection in infancy. J Pediatr Surg 15:79, 1980.

Mattingly WT Jr, Belin RP, Todd EP: Surgical repair of congenital tracheal stenosis in an infant. J Thorac Cardiovasc Surg 81:738, 1981.

Minato N, Itoh K, Ohkawa Y et al: Surgical treatment of congenital distal tracheal stenosis involving the carina. Ann Thorac Surg 42:326, 1986.

Nakayama DK, Harrison MR, DeLorimier AA et al: Reconstructive surgery for obstructing lesions of the intrathoracic trachea in infants and small children. J Pediatr Surg 17:854, 1982.

Weber TR, Eigen H, Scott PH et al: Resection of congenital tracheal stenosis involving the carina. J Thorac Cardiovasc Surg 84:200, 1982.

Wolman IJ: Congenital stenosis of the trachea. Am J Dis Child 61:1263, 1941.

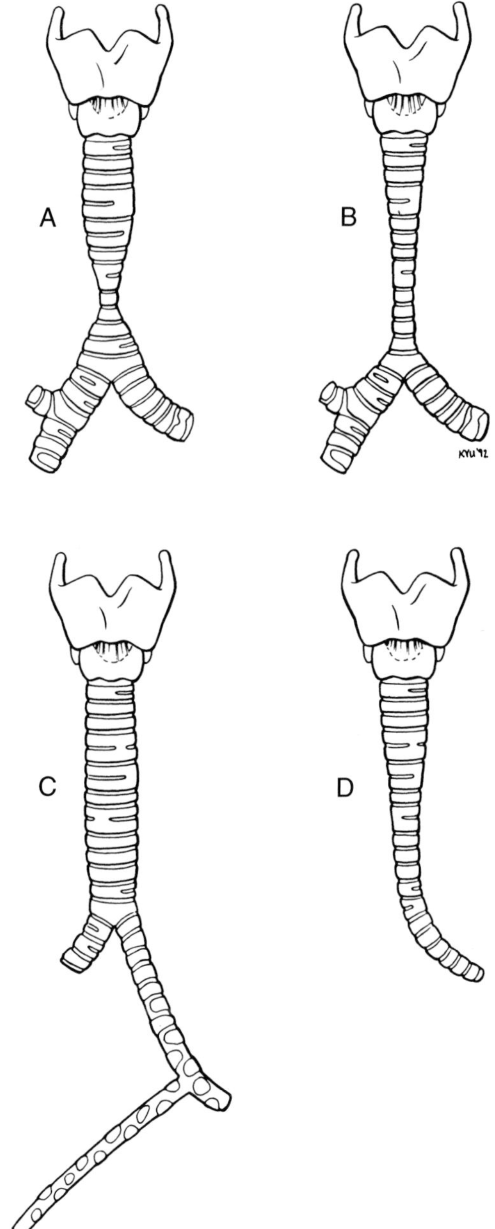

FIGURE 15–5 ■ Types of congenital tracheal stenosis commonly encountered. *A,* Short segment. *B,* Long, funnel-like narrowing. The carina and the upper bronchi can be involved. *C,* Abnormal branching of the bronchi. In this example, the two lower lobes on the right are supplied by a bronchus originating on the left. Major stenosis of this type usually begins at the carina and extends distally, often on both right and left sides. *D,* Tracheal stenosis is associated with pulmonary agenesis on the right.

BASIC SCIENCE

With rare exception, congenital tracheal stenosis is caused by absence of all or most of the membranous portion of the affected tracheal segment. From their review of the literature, Cantrell and Guild (1964) described three basic anatomic patterns: generalized tracheal hypoplasia, funnel-like stenosis, and segmental stenosis. These stenoses are often associated with other anomalies of the tracheobronchial tree, the most common of which are pulmonary artery sling; aberrant right middle and lower lobe bronchi arising from the left mainstem bronchus; and unilateral pulmonary agenesis or hypoplasia (Fig. 15–5). The so-called pulmonary artery sling represents an aberrant left pulmonary artery, which arises from the right pulmonary artery and passes behind the trachea to the left lung (Fig. 15–6). In children with congenital tracheal stenosis, a pulmonary artery sling coexists in about 50% of the cases. Similarly, among children in whom a sling is identified, about 50% also have congenital tracheal stenosis. The severity and type of tracheal stenosis is independent of the presence of the vascular sling. Berdon and associates (1984) coined the term *ring-sling syndrome* for those cases in which a pulmonary artery sling coexists with complete cartilaginous O tracheal rings. The surgeon must be aware of this

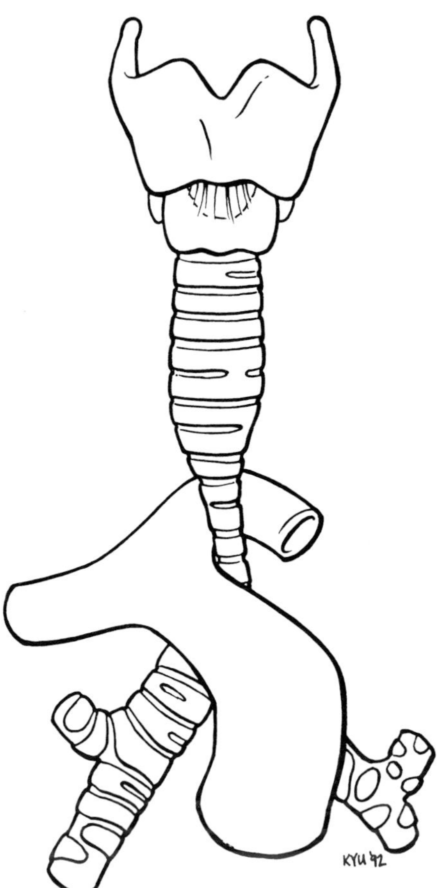

FIGURE 15–6 ■ Tracheal stenosis is associated with aberrant left pulmonary artery (sling) in 50% of cases. Repair of the sling will not correct the intrinsic tracheal problem.

association, for, in these cases, repair of the vascular anomaly alone will not eliminate intrinsic airway obstruction.

DIAGNOSIS

Clinical Features

Clinical features associated with congenital tracheal stenosis are listed in Table 15–3 (Loeff et al, 1988b). Most commonly, children present in the first few months of life because of stridor or pneumonia.

Natural History

The length and degree of narrowing varies significantly between cases. Children without life-threatening symptoms may grow and develop normally, although a degree of airway obstruction and stridor may be obvious during exercise, when ventilation increases. It appears that in some cases the airway diameter can increase with growth even in the absence of a membranous trachea (Benjamin et al, 1981). However, in children with severe stridor owing to tracheal stenosis, death can be expected in hours or days.

Differential Diagnosis

In young infants who present with stridor due to airway obstruction, the differential diagnosis includes congenital tracheal stenosis; complete vascular ring, including double aortic arch; subglottic hemangioma; and more rarely, unusual pharyngeal and paratracheal tumors, cysts, and infections.

Investigative Techniques

High-contrast radiographs plus fluoroscopy in two projections will give fairly accurate information about an infant's airway. Barium swallow is useful in children with airway obstruction to see if a vascular ring or pulmonary artery sling is present. In addition, paratracheal or esophageal masses can be identified by the impression that they make on the esophageal lumen. However, additional information is usually necessary to make an accurate anatomic diagnosis and to plan appropriate therapy.

Tracheobronchography

In the past, we relied primarily on tracheobronchography for the most accurate evaluation of children with congenital tracheal stenosis. When performed properly, this technique will clearly outline the degree and extent of narrowing and will delineate anomalies of airway branching. It will allow the surgeon to decide whether or not surgery will help and what procedure might be best suited for the specific anatomic abnormality.

The major problem with tracheobronchography is that the injection of contrast material into a severely narrowed airway may convert a partial obstruction into a complete one, either by plugging the narrowed lumen with contrast

TABLE 15–3 ■ **Clinical Features in 22 Cases of Congenital Tracheal Stenosis**

Characteristics	*No. of Patients*
Total number of patients	22
Boys	13
Girls	9
Age of onset of symptoms	
0–3 months	18
4–12 months	4
Presenting symptoms	
Stridor	18
Recurrent pneumonia	10
Cyanosis	7
Wheezing	2
Respiratory arrest	2
Associated anomalies	
Vascular ring or sling	11
Hypoplastic aortic arch	2
Other aberrant vessels	4
Osteocartilaginous	9
Cardiac	8
Gastrointestinal	4
Renal	3
TEF = EA, H-type TEF	2

EA, esophageal atresia; TEF, tracheoesophageal fistula.
Data from Loeff DS, Filler RM, Vinograd I et al.: Congenital tracheal stenosis: A review of 22 patients from 1965 to 1987. J Pediatr Surg 23:744, 1988b.

agent or by inciting an inflammatory reaction within its wall. If tracheobronchography is attempted, fluoroscopic control is essential. Minimal quantities of contrast material should be used, and contrast must be carefully aspirated after the study. An operating room must be ready to accept the infant for urgent surgical repair should condition deteriorate. Because other diagnostic procedures have largely replaced tracheobronchography, radiocontrast agents designed specifically for airway use are no longer being manufactured. As a result, small quantities of water-soluble, non-ionic radiocontrast agents are now used but their safety has not yet been completely established.

Computed Tomography

Spiral computed tomography (CT) scanning with three-dimensional reconstruction is now our procedure of choice to evaluate the airway in cases of congenital tracheal stenosis. This technique can detect a pulmonary artery sling, abnormal tracheobronchial branching, aortic arch anomalies, and most of the rarer causes of tracheal obstruction. The display of the length and degree of airway narrowing is appropriate for surgical decision making. An example is shown in Figure 15–7.

Magnetic Resonance Imaging

We have had no significant experience with magnetic resonance imaging (MRI) in these cases. Because many infants with severe congenital tracheal stenosis have a precarious airway or require ventilatory support, MRI with the techniques used in most centers may be hazardous.

Bronchoscopy

Bronchoscopy is useful to resolve any doubt concerning the diagnosis of congenital tracheal stenosis and to confirm the site and degree of stenosis at the upper end of the narrowed trachea. However, when tracheal obstruction is severe, even the smallest bronchoscope or telescope will not pass into the narrowed segment, and the total length of stenosis and the presence of abnormal airway branching may not be obvious endoscopically. If bronchoscopy is attempted, the surgeon must be prepared to proceed immediately with surgical repair, because trauma to the narrowed tracheal wall may precipitate total airway obstruction.

Cardiac Evaluation

Cardiac catheterization is not necessary to determine whether a pulmonary artery sling is present if a CT scan with injection of radiocontrast material has been obtained. However, in those children with associated heart defects, complete cardiac evaluation, including echocardiogram and heart catheterization, may be indicated.

MANAGEMENT

Principles

The obvious goal of surgery is to eliminate airway narrowing without compromising future growth of the tracheobronchial tree. In the small infant and child, procedures to accomplish this end are not without significant risks, and sophisticated surgical judgment is required to reach a satisfactory conclusion. The decision to proceed with operative correction depends on the magnitude of ventilatory embarrassment and on the surgeon's experience in the use of available corrective procedures, knowledge of what such an operation can be expected to achieve, and complete understanding of the mortality and morbidity associated with the corrective operation. For example, we would usually advise surgery for the child with moderate respiratory obstruction with a short ste-

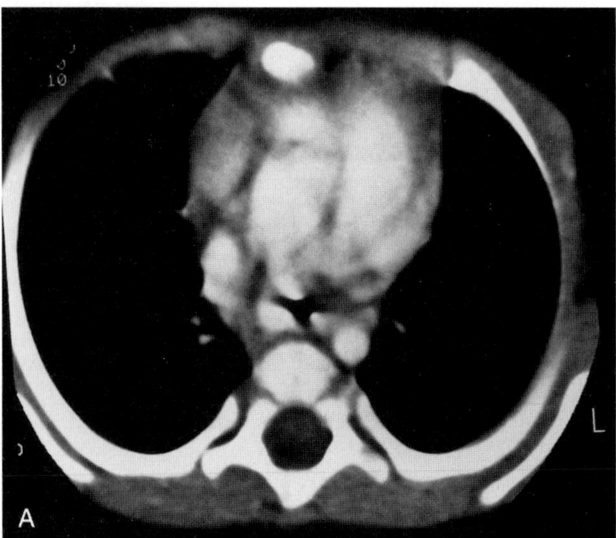

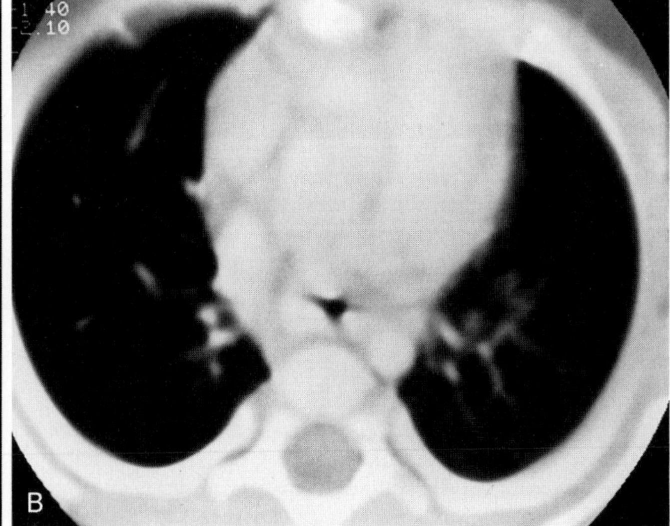

FIGURE 15–7 ■ A computed tomography scan of a 7-month-old child with tracheal stenosis that involves 2.5 cm. of distal trachea but not carina. Stenosis is associated with aberrant left pulmonary artery (sling). *A,* A mediastinal window is cut just above the carina. The contrast-filled aberrant pulmonary artery can be seen behind the tracheal air shadow. *B,* The tracheal window gives a more accurate measurement of the size of the tracheal lumen, which in this case measures 2.5 mm.

notic segment manageable by resection. However, in the child with identical symptoms caused by long-segment stenosis, a nonoperative approach might be chosen initially, because the risk and morbidity of tracheoplasty is so much greater. Postponement to a later date when the child is larger might improve outcome. Help in making this decision can be obtained by measuring the diameter of the airway lumen on a CT scan with proper window and comparing it with predicted normals (Griscom and Wohl, 1986). Loeff and associates (1988b) published a graph showing the relationship between airway diameter and body length in normal infants and children. By comparison, in 13 patients who died with severe tracheal stenosis, the airway was consistently less than 50% of normal. In the small infant, this translates to a tracheal diameter of 2 to 2.5 mm. Conversely, these data suggest that if the airway diameter is significantly greater than 50% of normal, imminent death is unlikely, and the decision for repair can be deferred safely.

Operative Technique

Operations to correct tracheal stenosis fall into three categories: dilatation, resection and anastomosis, and tracheoplasty.

Balloon Dilatation

Although there has been little clinical experience to date, a few reports suggest that balloon dilatation may have a place in the treatment of congenital tracheal stenosis (Bagwell et al, 1991; Messineo et al, 1992b). We have used balloon dilatation on many occasions to treat tracheal strictures that develop after tracheal resection, tracheoplasty, and tracheal intubation injuries. Equipment developed for balloon angioplasty is well suited for the small trachea. Radiographic control is useful to ensure that the balloon is in proper position and that the airway is not overdistended to the point of rupture. Dilatation as a primary treatment for congenital stenosis awaits further experience. Certainly, in the neonate or premature infant, it may be the only procedure that can be performed.

Resection and Anastomosis

Segmental resection of stenotic lesions less than five rings in length with end-to-end anastomosis is accepted by most tracheal surgeons as the treatment of choice. My group and others (DeLorimier et al, 1990; Grillo and Zannini, 1984) have had success with resection of 50% of the tracheal length (up to nine rings). The techniques of resection enunciated by Grillo and Mathisen (1988) have been adopted by most surgeons performing these operations. The trachea can be exposed anteriorly through the neck, by sternotomy, or through a right posterior lateral thoracotomy. The anterior or posterior surface of the trachea can be exposed along its entire length, but care should be taken to preserve the lateral tracheal blood supply. Initial circumferential tracheal dissection should be limited to 1 to 2 cm above and below the narrowed area to preserve the tracheal blood supply. Any posterolateral dissection must be on the tracheal wall to avoid recurrent nerve injury. Both ends of the stenosis should be resected to normal-diameter trachea.

For tracheal anastomosis, four to five sutures are placed in the posterior trachea with knots on the outside and are not tied until all are in place. Ventilation is maintained through a separate anesthesia circuit connected to the distal trachea. After the posterior sutures are tied, a translaryngeal endotracheal tube is advanced across the anastomosis, and the anterior row of sutures is placed. When the distal stenosis extends to the carina, it is easier to perform the operation with cardiopulmonary bypass rather than to have ventilation tubes providing a precarious airway in the operative field. Absorbable suture material should be used to minimize formation of intraluminal granulation tissue after surgery. Polyglycolic acid, polydioxanone, and polyglactin all seem adequate (Friedman et al, 1990). Traction sutures placed in the medial and lateral trachea on either side of and at least 1 cm proximal and distal to the anastomosis may be tied together after completion of the anastomosis to relieve tension on the suture line. Head-restraining sutures between the chin and the chest wall or a prosthetic brace to keep the neck flexed postoperatively can be helpful to reduce anastomotic tension when long segments of trachea are removed. My colleagues and I have had no experience with laryngeal release procedures for severe length problems (Dedo and Fishman, 1969; Montgomery, 1974).

Tracheoplasty

Tracheoplasty is reserved for long-segment tracheal stenosis, which cannot be treated by resection and end-to-end anastomosis. The basic technique, which is similar in all tracheoplasties described, is illustrated in Figure 15–8.

The stenotic section of the trachea is incised in the anterior midline (or posterior midline if a posterior lateral approach is used) to one ring beyond the narrowing, which often means extension into the upper end of a bronchus. An interposition graft is then sutured to the edges of the open trachea to enlarge the lumen. A variety of grafts have been employed, including tantalum (Loeff et al, 1988a), esophagus (Ein et al, 1982), dura (Lobe et al, 1987), cartilage (Kimura et al, 1982; Lobe et al, 1987; Kamata et al, 1997), pericardium (Idriss et al, 1984; Heimansohn et al, 1991), periosteum (Cohen et al, 1986), and cadaveric tracheal allografts (Elliot et al, 1996).

In the literature, pericardium and costal cartilage have been used most frequently. We have had experience with all types of grafts, and, unfortunately, none has been ideal. The pericardial graft is taken from the anterior pericardium, and its size is designed to enlarge the trachea 1.5-fold. It is sewn to the edge of the trachea with a continuous stitch of absorbable 5–0 or 6–0 sutures. The pericardial patch should be sutured to the undersurface of the aorta and mediastinal structures to prevent collapse until the graft becomes stiff, presumably by fibrosis. In addition, after surgery the trachea is kept intubated with a nasotracheal tube for 10 to 14 days. Heimansohn and colleagues (1991) recommend that children be kept pharmacologically paralyzed and sedated until the pericardium adheres to mediastinal structures.

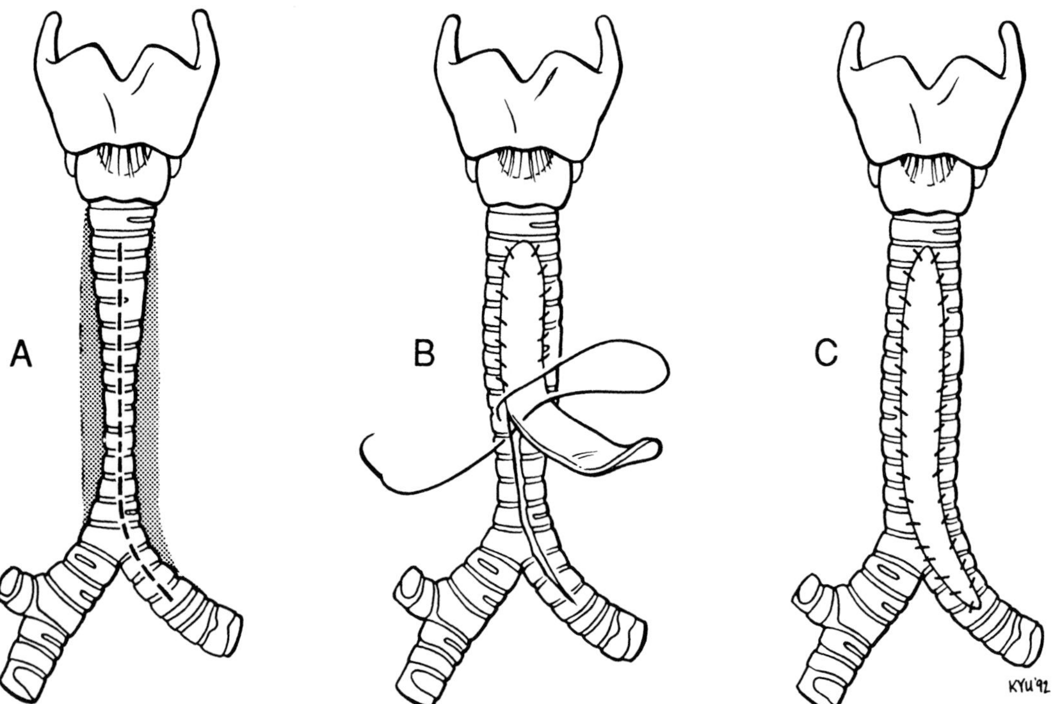

FIGURE 15–8 ■ General technique of tracheoplasty. *A,* The stenotic segment of trachea is opened longitudinally to an airway of normal diameter superiorly and inferiorly. *B,* Tissue selected for grafting is sutured to the defect with running or interrupted sutures of absorbable material. *C,* Completed tracheoplasty.

When cartilage is inserted as a graft, its rigidity precludes the need to fix it to other mediastinal structures. Also, intubation and paralysis beyond 1 or 2 days after surgery are often not necessary. However, later complications may require prolonged endotracheal intubation. We have found that sufficient length of cartilage can be obtained from the costal margin by subperichondrial resection. The thickness of the cartilage can be reduced by scraping it with a scalpel, leaving the side facing the lumen slightly concave. Continuous or interrupted sutures of 5–0 to 6–0 absorbable material pass easily through the cartilage of the young child so that implantation is not a problem. The goal is to use a piece of cartilage that will maximize the size of the lumen.

Periosteum for a tracheal graft is obtained by making a longitudinal incision over the anterior aspect of the tibia. A graft that starts below the tibial tubercle and extends to just above the ankle is adequate to cover the longest tracheal defects. A graft 7 to 10 mm wide can be obtained. Tibial periosteum in the infant is thick and has a leathery quality, which makes for easy handling and suturing. The outermost surface of periosteum should face the lumen. The graft is best obtained prior to thoracotomy and cardiopulmonary bypass if that is to be used, so that it is available when needed and at a time when the child is not heparinized. Hemostasis should be complete by the time heparin is given for cardiopulmonary bypass. Animal and clinical experience with free grafts of periosteum show that bone will grow from the graft, which becomes rigid within 2 weeks (Cohen et al, 1986).

When the esophagus is used to cover the tracheal defect, the trachea is opened in the posterior midline. The intact anterior wall of the esophagus is sutured to the edges of the defect to eliminate air leak (Ein et al, 1982).

In 1989, Tsang and colleagues described a slide tracheoplasty for tracheal stenosis, which obviates the need for a graft. This tracheoplasty was used in two children, ages 10 months and 3 months. Each had a funnel-type stenosis of the trachea not involving the carina. The trachea was divided at the midpoint of the stenosis. Both segments of the trachea were opened longitudinally and spatulated, the upper segment posteriorly and the lower segment anteriorly. The open segments were slid on top of one another and sutured in place. This tracheoplasty shortens the trachea and uses living tracheal tissue for coverage. One child was well 12 months later. Grillo (1994) reported 3 successful outcomes in 3 children, and Dayan and colleagues (1997) had 1 success in the 2 children treated.

A critical issue in tracheoplasty is the maintenance of ventilation during the operation. We believe, as do others (Bando et al, 1996; Idriss et al, 1984; Heimansohn et al, 1991), that cardiopulmonary bypass is the most reliable and safest method to ensure adequate oxygenation and still allow excellent exposure of the entire trachea and upper bronchi. Through a sternotomy incision, we have used right atrial and aortic cannulas for bypass. The catheters can be fixed in place and kept out of the surgeon's way even in the smallest infant. We have not found a need to use the femoral artery for arterial inflow. Cardiopulmonary bypass also allows easy rerouting of an aberrant left pulmonary artery and the repair of other cardiac defects that may be present (Yamaguchi et al,

1990). With the trachea open during bypass, it is helpful to place balloon catheters through an endotracheal tube into each bronchus to prevent accumulation of blood in the lower airways. Excessive bleeding at the cut edges of the trachea caused by heparinization has not been troublesome during or after bypass.

Formerly we used fibrin glue at the junction of the graft and trachea to minimize the possibility of an air leak at the completion of tracheoplasty. However, in several children who needed a second operation, we believed that excessive fibrous tissue at the graft site might have been due in part to use of the fibrin. Because small air leaks around the graft close spontaneously in a few minutes when airway pressures are not excessive, fibrin glue does not seem to be needed.

The adequacy of tracheoplasty can be judged by the pressures required for lung expansion and the rapidity of lung collapse during expiration. When the extracorporeal circuit is turned off, arterial and venous bypass cannulas should be left in place until one is certain that adequate ventilation can be achieved through an endotracheal tube with reasonable airway pressures.

Airway stenting is important after tracheoplasty, not only to ensure adequate ventilation and airway toilet following surgery but also to provide temporary rigidity to an airway that might collapse following tracheoplasty, especially when a nonrigid tissue such as pericardium is used to cover the tracheal defect. Standard endotracheal tubes suffice in most cases, but when the bronchi must be stented, this presents an enormous problem in the small child. We have tried to intubate one bronchus and leave an opening at the carina for ventilation of the other, but this has invariably failed. Similarly, the development of Y-shaped stents for small children has been unsuccessful because the small lumen of these stents plug frequently, and the distal ends cannot be prevented from occluding upper lobe bronchi. We believe that this contributes to the poor long-term results of tracheoplasty in infants and children with stenosis extending well into one or both bronchi. However, the insertion of a Palmaz stent into the bronchus at the time of tracheoplasty might solve this problem.

Postoperative Care

The major problem following tracheoplasty is maintenance of a patent airway. In the first 2 weeks after surgery, airway secretions are usually the major cause of airway obstruction. Usually these can be handled easily with suctioning, especially when an endotracheal tube has been left in place. Suction catheters must be used with care, because the delicate, narrow airway of the infant can be traumatized easily by these catheters, especially because the distal end of the tracheoplasty is usually beyond the end of the tracheoplasty is usually beyond the end of the endotracheal tube.

In the next several weeks to months after surgery, three more difficult-to-treat problems causing airway obstruction may arise; these are formation of granulation tissue, airway collapse, and airway stricture.

Despite all precautions to minimize formation of granulation tissue, such as the use of low-reactive absorbable suture material and the avoidance of airway trauma by suction catheters, the healing of the tracheal repair is often associated with the formation of granulation tissue at suture lines and on the surface of grafts. Even a ring of granulation tissue that is 1 to 2 mm thick in the lumen of a small infant's airway can result in significant obstruction, in contrast to a ring of equal thickness in an adult. Its presence is signaled by airway obstruction, usually in the region of the carina and bronchial orifices. The granulations can be identified by bronchoscopy and can be removed by suction or foreign-body forceps. Rarely, excision with a laser can be helpful. However, if a metallic stent is in the lumen, laser therapy should be avoided because it tends to weld the device to the wall of the airway. Because the trauma of granulation tissue removal (by whatever method) often begets more granulations, this complication can be extremely troublesome. The need for repeated endoscopic procedures is to be expected. Granulation tissue formation ceases only when the grafted tissues or sutures are completely epithelialized. Because any manipulation of a healing tracheoplasty tends to produce granulation tissue, we remove such tissues only when they cause significant airway obstruction, not prophylactically.

Intrathoracic airway collapse causing airway obstruction tends to occur at a grafted area of the trachea when the graft has little or no rigidity. Pericardium is a flexible tissue, which allows airway collapse at least until it becomes more rigid by ingrowth of fibrous tissue. Therefore, when pericardium is used, the graft should be sutured to other mediastinal structures, and the grafted area should be stented with an endotracheal tube for approximately 2 weeks (Heimansohn et al, 1991). Providing high end-expiratory pressures with a ventilator may help keep the airway open until the graft becomes rigid. Using the wall of the esophagus for tracheoplasty can also be associated with significant tracheal collapse. The muscular esophageal wall ordinarily does not become rigid after surgery, and long-term airway intubation can be anticipated postoperatively with this type of repair. Free periosteal grafts tend to become rigid in 1 to 2 weeks, at which time calcium can be seen radiographically (Cohen et al, 1986).

In our experience, stricture at the tracheoplasty site as a complication of the tracheoplasty procedure occurs commonly, regardless of the tissue used for grafting. Usually the stricture develops in the distal trachea and carina just beyond the tip of the endotracheal tube stent. This complication is often blamed on faulty blood supply or a lack of stenting. It seems likely that trauma from suction catheters is also at least a part of the problem. Our first approach to treating strictures has been balloon dilatation. By using balloons designed for angioplasty, satisfactory dilatation can be achieved, at least temporarily. The need for repeat dilatation is the rule. With epithelialization of the graft, the intervals between dilatations increases; however, dilatations over many weeks are usually necessary. We have also resorted to surgical resection of the stricture with end-to-end anastomosis or regrafting using cardiopulmonary bypass. Despite many frustrations and long hospitalizations, some infants can be salvaged after apparent initial failure.

In 1988, my colleagues and I reported the use of a coiled stainless steel stent, which could be inserted endoscopically, to treat recurrent tracheoplasty strictures (Loeff et al, 1988a). This type of stent was not successful over the long term because granulation tissue formed through and over the coils and obstructed the airway. Subsequently, we and others (Domschke et al, 1990; Dumon, 1990; Filler et al, 1998; Santoro et al, 1993) have treated strictures by inserting expandable metal stents (Palmaz stents) into the trachea and bronchi through a bronchoscope or endotracheal tube with radiographic control, as noted in the section on Tracheomalacia. Although granulation tissue still tends to be a problem with these stents, we have been able to cope with the problem by repeated bronchoscopic removal. To date, we have inserted one to four Palmaz stents in the trachea or bronchi in 5 children with unremitting stricture following airway surgery.

Results

Because congenital tracheal stenosis is relatively rare, the number of cases in the largest series ranges from 5 to 18 (Andrews et al, 1994; Bando et al, 1996; DeLorimier et al, 1990; Dunham et al, 1994; Heimansohn et al, 1991; Idriss et al, 1984; Loeff et al, 1988b). The children treated in these reports had varying lengths of tracheal stenosis, and the degree of narrowing in each case was not similar. In addition, follow-up was often inadequate for judging the long-term results, which is especially important because laboratory and clinical experience suggest that tracheoplasty may reduce subsequent tracheal growth (Dykes et al, 1990). Because of the small numbers and these other variables, one cannot draw clear-cut conclusions as to the best method of repair. Nevertheless, some generalizations seem warranted. When resection of the narrowed segment and end-to-end anastomosis are possible, survival is the rule by methods currently available in most centers. No current method will correct all the variants of congenital tracheal stenosis. When severe stenosis extends into one or both bronchi, the results from all types of tracheoplasty are poor.

Most tracheoplasty experience has been with cartilage and pericardial grafts. Given the limitations in evaluating surgical results, encouraging results have been reported, especially with pericardium. In the series of Heimansohn and colleagues (1991), seven of eight patients survived, and Dunham and others (1994) had 15 of 18 long-term survivors in a series initiated by Idriss and associates (1984).

Our experience and that of others indicates that success in the treatment of tracheal stenosis requires diligent monitoring of ventilation and recognition and treatment of granulation tissue and scarring, which is secondary to the healing process, especially in the smallest patients.

COMMENTS AND CONTROVERSIES

Our experience and that of others indicates that there is still much to be accomplished in treating congenital tracheal stenosis.

As noted throughout this section on congenital tracheal stenosis, the primary issues involved in its treatment include indications for surgery; type of operation to be selected; graft selection when tracheoplasty is performed; the value of dilatation as primary treatment; and the exclusive use of cardiopulmonary bypass for extensive tracheoplasties. Except perhaps for the last issue, defensible recommendations await further laboratory and clinical experience.

Our experience with intraluminal stents in selected cases indicates that this is an important area for further fruitful exploration. Questions still to be answered include long-term effects of stents on tracheal growth; the necessity and the techniques for removal at a later date; ideal prosthetic material; ideal size and shape of the stent; and the value of implanting stents at the time of initial tracheoplasty.

Replacement of narrowed segments of trachea and bronchi with allografts of appropriate size has been explored in our laboratory, and a few clinical trials have been reported (Elliot, 1996). Using a pig model, we have replaced airway segments with free, nonvascularized, fresh and cryopreserved tracheal allografts and cryopreserved cartilage. Transplanted cartilage is replaced with fibrous tissue, and its growth is less than that of the normal adjacent trachea. However, the luminal surface of the grafts becomes epithelialized and the airway size appears to be adequate. In addition, the ability to use cryopreserved tissue would allow us to store tracheas and cartilage for later use (Messineo, 1992a).

R. M. F.

■ KEY REFERENCES

Filler F, Forte V, Chait P: Tracheobronchial stenting for the treatment of airway obstruction. J Pediatr Surg 33:304, 1998.

The technique and results of stenting with balloon expandable stents in selected cases of airway are noted.

Filler RM, Messineo A, Vinograd I: Severe tracheomalacia associated with esophageal atresia: Results of surgical treatment. J Pediatr Surg 27:1136, 1992.

This study reviews a 15-year experience with the surgical treatment of tracheomalacia in 32 children. Indications for surgery, types of operative procedures, and their techniques are reviewed.

Grillo HC: Slide tracheoplasty for long-segment congenital tracheal stenosis. Ann Thorac Surg 58:619, 1994.

This clear description of the technique of slide tracheoplasty should be useful to those planning to perform this innovative operation.

Heimansohn DA, Kesler KA, Turrentine MW et al: Anterior pericardial tracheoplasty for congenital tracheal stenosis. J Thorac Cardiovasc Surg 102:710, 1991.

This paper clearly outlines the technique of tracheoplasty using a pericardial patch. The authors indicate the value of cardiopulmonary bypass for the procedure and outline the details of postoperative care, including paralysis and ventilation. The surgical approach used in this paper can be applied equally well to tracheoplasties when tissue other than pericardium is used. These authors report their experience with eight cases with very good results.

■ REFERENCES

Bagwell C, Talbert J, Tepas J: Balloon dilatation of long-segment tracheal stenosis. J Pediatr Surg 26:153, 1991.

Bando K, Turrentine M, Sun K et al: Anterior pericardial tracheoplasty for congenital tracheal stenosis: Intermediate to long-term outcomes. Ann Thorac Surg 62:981, 1996.
Baxter JD, Dunbar JS: Tracheomalacia. Ann Otol Rhinol Larnygol 72:1013, 1963.
Benjamin B, Cohen D, Glasson M: Tracheomalacia in association with congenital tracheoesophageal fistula. Surgery 79:504, 1969.
Benjamin B, Pitkin J, Cohen D: Congenital tracheal stenosis. Ann Otol Rhinol Laryngol 90:364, 1981.
Berdon WE, Baker DH, Wung JT et al: Complete cartilage-ring tracheal stenosis associated with anomalous left pulmonary artery: The ring-sling complex. Radiology 152:57, 1984.
Blair GK, Filler RM, Cohen R: Treatment of tracheomalacia: 8 years' experience. J Pediatr Surg 21:781, 1986.
Campbell AH, Young IF: Tracheobronchial collapse, a variant of obstructive respiratory disease. Br J Dis Chest 57:174, 1963.
Cantrell JR, Guild HG: Congenital stenosis of the trachea. Am J Surg 108:297, 1964.
Cogbill TH, Moore FA, Accurso FJ et al: Primary tracheomalacia. Ann Thorac Surg 35:538, 1983.
Cohen RC, Filler RM, Konuma K et al: A new model of tracheal stenosis and its repair using free periosteal grafts. J Thorac Cardiovasc Surg 92:296, 1986.
Cox WL Jr, Shaw RR: Congenital chondromalacia of the trachea. J Thorac Cardiovasc Surg 49:1033, 1965.
Davies MR, Cywes S: The flaccid trachea and tracheoesophageal congenital anomalies. J Pediatr Surg 13:363, 1978.
Dedo HH, Fishman NH: Laryngeal release and sleeve resection for tracheal stenosis. Ann Otol Rhinol Laryngol 78:285, 1969.
DeLorimier A, Harrison M, Hardy K et al: Tracheobronchial obstructions in infants and children. Ann Surg 212:277, 1990.
Domschke W, Foers EC, Matek W et al: Self-expanding mesh stent for esophageal cancer stenosis. Endoscopy 22:134, 1990.
Dumon J: A dedicated tracheobronchial stent. Chest 97:328, 1990.
Dunham ME, Holinger LD, Backer CL et al: Management of severe congenital tracheal stenosis. Ann Otol Rhinol Laryngol 103:351, 1994.
Dykes EH, Bahoric A, Smith C et al: Reduced tracheal growth after reconstruction with pericardium. J Pediatr Surg 25:25, 1990.
Ein SH, Friedberg J, Williams WG et al: Tracheoplasty: A new operation for complete congenital tracheal stenosis. J Pediatr Surg 17:872, 1982.
Elliott MJ, Haw MP, Jacobs JP et al: Tracheal reconstruction in children using cadaveric homograft trachea. Eur J Cardiothorac Surg 10:707, 1996.
Fallis J, Filler RM, Lemoine G: Pediatric Thoracic Surgery. New York, Elsevier Science, 1991
Filler RM, Buck JR, Bahoric A et al: Treatment of segmental tracheomalacia and bronchomalacia by implantation of an airway splint. J Pediatr Surg 17:597, 1982.
Filler RM, Forte V, Chait P: Tracheobronchial stenting for the treatment of airway obstruction. J Pediatr Surg 33:304, 1998.
Filler RM, Rossello PJ, Lebowitz RL: Life-threatening anoxic spells caused by tracheal compression after repair of esophageal atresia: Correction by surgery. J Pediatr Surg 11:739, 1976.
Fraga JC, Filler RM, Forte V et al: Experimental use of Palmaz metallic stent in normal and operated trachea in cats. Revista HCPA 17:109, 1997.
Friedman E, Perez-Atayde A, Silvera M et al: Growth of tracheal anastomoses in lambs. J Thorac Cardiovasc Surg 100:188, 1990.
Grillo HC: Slide tracheoplasty for long-segment congenital tracheal stenosis. Ann Thorac Surg 58:613, 1994.
Grillo HC, Mathisen DJ: Surgical management of tracheal strictures. Surg Clin North Am 68:511, 1988.
Grillo HC, Zannini P: Management of obstructive tracheal disease in children. J Pediatr Surg 19:414, 1984.
Griscom NT, Wohl ME: Dimensions of the growing trachea related to age and gender. AJR 146:233, 1986.
Gross RE, Neuhauser EB: Compression of the trachea by an anomalous innominate artery: An operation for its relief. Am J Dis Child 75:570, 1948.
Harrison MR, Heldt GP, Brasch RC et al: Resection of distal tracheal stenosis in a baby with agenesis of the lung. J Pediatr Surg 15:938, 1980.
Healy GB, Schuster SR, Jonas RA et al: Correction of segmental tracheal stenosis in children. Ann Otol Rhinol Laryngol 97:444, 1988.
Heimansohn D, Kesler K, Turrentine M: Anterior pericardial tracheoplasty for congenital tracheal stenosis. J Thorac Cardiovasc Surg 102:710, 1991.
Herzog H, Keller R, Maurer W et al: Distribution of bronchial resistance in obstructive pulmonary diseases and in dogs with artificially induced tracheal collapse. Respiration 25:381, 1968.
Idriss F, DeLeon SY, Ilbawi MN et al: Tracheoplasty with pericardial patch for extensive tracheal stenosis in infants and children. J Thorac Cardiovasc Surg 88:527, 1984.
Johner CH, Szanto PA: Polychondritis in a newborn presenting as tracheomalacia. Ann Otol Rhinol Laryogol 79:1114, 1970.
Johnston MR, Loeber N, Hillyer P et al: External stent for repair of secondary tracheomalacia. Ann Thorac Surg 30:291, 1980.
Kamata S, Usui N, Ishikawa S et al: Experience in tracheobronchial reconstruction with a costal cartilage graft for congenital tracheal stenosis. J Pediatr Surg 32:54, 1997.
Kiely EM, Spitz L, Brereton R: Management of tracheomalacia by aortopexy. Pediatr Surg Int 2:13, 1987.
Kimura K, Mukohara M, Tsugawa C et al: Tracheoplasty for congenital stenosis of the entire trachea. J Pediatr Surg 17:869, 1982.
Lobe TE, Hayden CK, Nicolas D, Richardson CJ: Successful management of congenital tracheal stenosis in infancy. J Pediatr Surg 22:1137, 1987.
Loeff DS, Filler RM, Gorestein A et al: A new intratracheal stent for tracheobronchial reconstruction. J Pediatr Surg 23:1173, 1988a.
Loeff DS, Filler RM, Vinograd I et al: Congenital tracheal stenosis: Review of 22 patients from 1965 to 1987. J Pediatr Surg 23:744, 1988b.
Mansfield PB: Tracheal resection in infancy. J Pediatr Surg 15:79, 1980.
Mattingly WT Jr, Belin RP, Todd EP: Surgical repair of congenital tracheal stenosis in an infant. J Thorac Cardiovasc Surg 81:738, 1981.
Messineo A, Filler RM, Bahoric A et al: Repair of long tracheal defects with cryopreserved cartilaginous allografts. J Pediatr Surg 27:1131, 1992a.
Messineo A, Forte V, Joseph T et al: The balloon posterior tracheal split: A technique for managing tracheal stenosis in the premature infant. J Pediatr Surg 27:1142, 1992b.
Minato N, Itoh K, Ohkawa Y et al: Surgical treatment of congenital distal tracheal stenosis involving the carina. Ann Thorac Surg 42:326, 1986.
Montgomery WW: Suprahyoid release for tracheal stenosis. Arch Otolaryngol Head Neck Surg 99:225, 1974.
Murphy P, Filler RM, Muraji T et al: Effect of prosthetic airway splint on the growing trachea. J Pediatr Surg 18:872, 1983.
Mustard WT, Bayliss CE, Fearon B et al: Tracheal compression by the innominate artery in children. Ann Thorac Surg 8:312, 1969.
Nakayama DK, Harrison MR, DeLorimier AA et al: Reconstructive surgery for obstructing lesions of the intrathoracic trachea in infants and small children. J Pediatr Surg 17:854, 1982.
Rainer WG, Newby JP, Kelble DL: Long-term results of tracheal support surgery for emphysema. Chest 53:765, 1968.
Schwartz MZ, Filler RM: Tracheal compression as a cause of apnea following repair of tracheoesophageal fistula: Treatment by aortopexy. J Pediatr Surg 15:842, 1980.
Shapiro RS, Martin WM: Long custom-made plastic tracheostomy tube in severe tracheomalacia. Laryngoscope 91:355, 1981.
Tsang V, Murday A, Gillbe C et al: Slide tracheoplasty for congenital funnel-shaped tracheal stenosis. Ann Thorac Surg 48:632, 1989.
Vinograd I, Filler RM, Bahoric A: Long-term functional results of prosthetic airway splinting in tracheomalacia and bronchomalacia. J Pediatr Surg 22:38, 1987.
Vinograd I, Filler RM, England SJ et al: Tracheomalacia: An experimental animal model for a new surgical approach. J Surg Res 42:597, 1987.
Vinograd I, Klin B, Brosh T et al: A new intratracheal stent made from nitinol, an alloy with "shape memory effect." J Thorac Cardiovasc Surg 1107:1255, 1994.
Wailoo MP, Emery JL: The trachea in children with tracheoesophageal fistula. Histopathology 3:329, 1979.
Weber TR, Eigen H, Scott PH et al: Resection of congenital tracheal stenosis involving the carina. J Thorac Cardiovasc Surg 84:200, 1982.
Wiseman NE, Duncan PG, Cameron CB: Management of tracheobron-

chomalacia with continuous positive airway pressure. J Pediatr Surg 20:489, 1985.
Wittenborg MM, Gyepes MT, Crocker D: Tracheal dynamics in infants with respiratory distress, stridor and collapsing trachea. Radiology 88:653, 1969.
Wolman IJ: Congenital stenosis of the trachea. Am J Dis Child 61:1263, 1941.
Yamaguchi M, Yoshihiro O, Hosokawa Y et al: Concomitant repair of congenital tracheal stenosis and complex cardiac anomaly in small children. J Thorac Cardiovasc Surg 100:181, 1990.

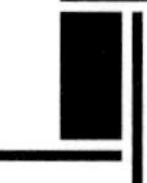

POSTINTUBATION INJURY

Michael A. Maddaus
F. Griffith Pearson

Postintubation injury is the most common cause of benign, stenotic lesions of the upper airway. Such injury may be produced by either translaryngeal intubation or tracheostomy.

After tracheostomy, stenotic lesions may be the result of injury at the level of the tracheostoma or at the level of the inflatable cuff. Full-thickness erosion of the tracheal wall occasionally results in tracheoinnominate artery fistula or tracheoesophageal fistula.

Translaryngeal intubation may result in damage to the glottis, the subglottic segment, or the trachea itself. It usually follows periods of prolonged intubation with a translaryngeal cuffed tube, in an intensive care setting, for the support of ventilation. The laryngeal injury most commonly occurs in the posterior interarytenoid area and restricts abduction of the vocal cords. Significant subglottic lesions usually result in circumferential stenosis.

HISTORICAL NOTE

Postintubation injury is a rare complication of tracheostomy with an uncuffed tube. It only became a significant problem with the advent of mechanical ventilatory support using cuffed endotracheal tubes. Trendelenburg reported on the use of a cuffed tracheostomy tube in 1871 (Trendelenburg, 1871). But the use of cuffed tubes did not become widespread until the introduction of mechanical ventilators and cuffed tracheostomy tubes during the 1952 epidemic of poliomyelitis in Europe (Lassen, 1956). During the early 1960s, postintubation tracheal stenosis was increasingly recognized as a frequent, life-threatening complication of assisted ventilation with cuffed tubes. A prospective study initiated in 1967 identified a 17.5% incidence of functionally significant tracheal stenosis in 153 surviving patients who had undergone mechanical ventilation with cuffed tracheostomy tubes (Pearson, Goldberg, and daSilva, 1968; Pearson and Andrews, 1971). In that study, most of the postintubation strictures occurred either at the stoma or under the inflatable cuff; the most severe lesions were seen at the cuff level.

Subsequent investigation focused on the mechanisms of injury. It soon became apparent that the greatest damage occurred because of pressure ischemia under the small-volume, noncompliant inflatable cuffs that were used during those early years. In 1969, Cooper and Grillo showed that mucosal ulceration with exposure of underlying cartilage occurred within as few as 48 hours of cuff inflation. Inflation pressures of up to 100 mm Hg were necessary to obtain an airtight seal with these low-volume cuffs (Webb, 1973). Such high pressures deformed the wall of the trachea until the tracheal contour matched that of the balloon.

Having identified the pathophysiology of these injuries, Grillo and associates (1971) then developed a large-volume, low-pressure cuff—a prototype for the cuff design in current use on tracheostomy and endotracheal tubes. This large-volume floppy cuff has a resting diameter of about 3 cm. Inflation with 2 to 6 ml of air usually fills the trachea, allows the cuff to conform to the normal tracheal shape, and provides an airtight seal. Most important, cuff inflation pressures are in the same range as the peak airway pressures generated during mechanical ventilation.

These early experiences took place during a time when translaryngeal intubation was maintained for relatively brief periods preceeding tracheostomy. During the 1970s, however, translaryngeal intubation was rarely maintained beyond 48 to 72 hours. But since then, the ongoing trend has been to maintain patients with longer and longer periods of nasotracheal or orotracheal intubation. Although the incidence of post-tracheostomy stenosis is now markedly reduced, longer periods of translaryngeal intubation (often for 2 or 3 weeks) have increased the incidence of post-intubation stenosis at the level of the glottis and subglottic segment.

■ *HISTORICAL REFERENCES*

Andrews MJ, Pearson FG: The incidence and pathogenesis of tracheal injury following cuffed tube tracheostomy with assisted ventilation: An analysis of a two year prospective study. Ann Surg 173:249, 1971.
Cooper JD, Grillo HC: Experimental production and prevention of

injury due to cuffed tracheal tubes. Surg Gynecol Obstet 129:1235, 1969.

Grillo HC, Cooper JD, Geffin B et al: A low pressure cuff for tracheostomy tubes to minimize tracheal injury: A comparative clinical trial. J Thorac Cardiovasc Surg 62:898, 1971.

Lassen HCA: Management of life-threatening poliomyelitis. E and S Livingstone, London, 1956.

Trendelenburg F: Beitrage zu den Operationen an den Luftwegen. Arch Klin Chir 12:112, 1871.

Webb WR, Ozdemir IA, Ikins PM et al: Surgical management of tracheal stenosis. Ann Surg 179:819, 1973.

BASIC SCIENCE

Anatomy

The trachea extends from the inferior cricoid margin to the carina, averages between 10 and 13 cm in length, and contains between 18 and 22 cartilaginous rings (about 2 rings per cm of length). The average internal diameter of the trachea is 2.3 cm. Tracheal blood supply arises from the inferior thyroid arteries above and from the bronchial circulation below. Anastomotic branches of these vessels enter the trachea at its posterolateral margin and are segmental in their distribution. In view of this segmental distribution, the tracheal circulation may be impaired if circumferential mobilization is extended beyond 1 to 2 cm (Fig. 15–9).

The anatomy and relationships of the recurrent laryngeal nerves at the level of the larynx and upper airway is illustrated in Figure 15–10. A knowledge of this anatomy is essential during any circumferential resection of the trachea or adjacent cricoid cartilage. These nerves ascend in the tracheoesophageal groove—they pass deep to the inferior border of the cricothyroid muscle, posterior to the cricothyroid articulations. Only above this level do the nerves enter the laryngeal musculature. Thus, it is possible to preserve the recurrent nerves when operating in the region of the posterior cricoid cartilage, as long as the posterior perichondrium or a thin shell of posterior cricoid plate is maintained intact.

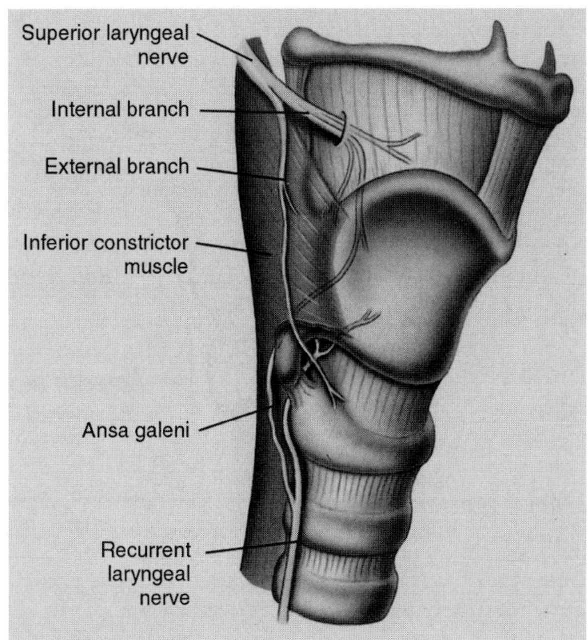

FIGURE 15–10 ■ This diagram illustrates the course and anatomic relationships of the recurrent laryngeal nerves at the upper trachea and cricoid levels.

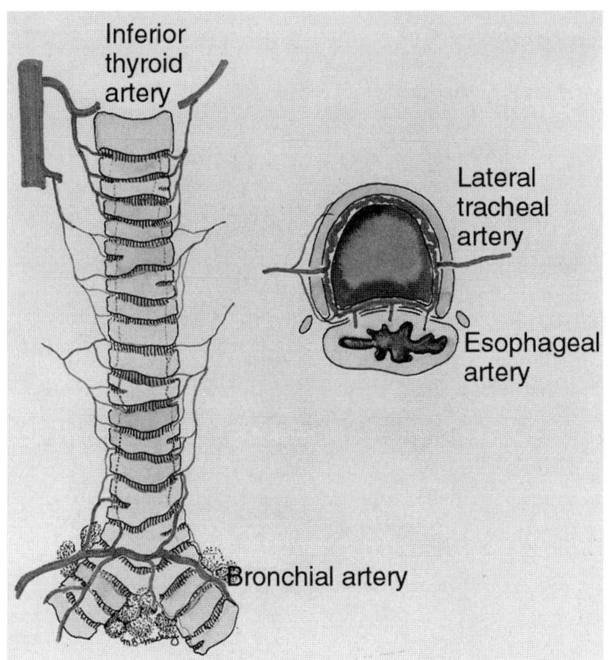

FIGURE 15–9 ■ This diagram illustrates the important features of tracheal circulation. The most robust contributions to this circulation arise from the inferior thyroid arteries above, and the bronchial arteries below. These vessels anastomose in an arcade lying along the posterolateral margins of the trachea. They feed the submucosal plexus by intercartilagenous branches, which are segmental in distribution.

The anatomy of the larynx and upper airway is provided in detail in Chapter 12. But to provide a clear understanding of postintubation injury at the level of the larynx and subglottis, some details of anatomy warrant emphasis. The larynx has three key cartilaginous components that provide skeletal support for the airway and vocal function: thyroid cartilage, cricoid cartilage, and paired arytenoid cartilages. The thyroid cartilage is the outer protective cover for the entire larynx; it articulates inferiorly with cricoid cartilage at the cricothyroid joints (Fig. 15–11). The cricoid cartilage is the first full ring of the upper airway; it has an anterior arch that is similar in height to a normal tracheal ring. This arch expands into a broadly based posterior plate or rostrum. Both the inner and the outer aspects of the cricoid cartilage are covered with a stout perichondrial layer, which may be an important feature during segmental resection and primary reconstruction at the subglottic level.

The paired arytenoid cartilages rest on the superior surface of the posterior cricoid plate; they articulate with the cricoid cartilage at the cricoarytenoid joints. The vocal ligaments or cords arise behind, from the vocal processes of the arytenoid cartilages, and attach anteriorly to the thyroid cartilage (see Fig. 15–11). The action of vocal muscles on the arytenoid cartilages produces changes in both position and tension of the vocal cords. These changes are responsible for important aspects of

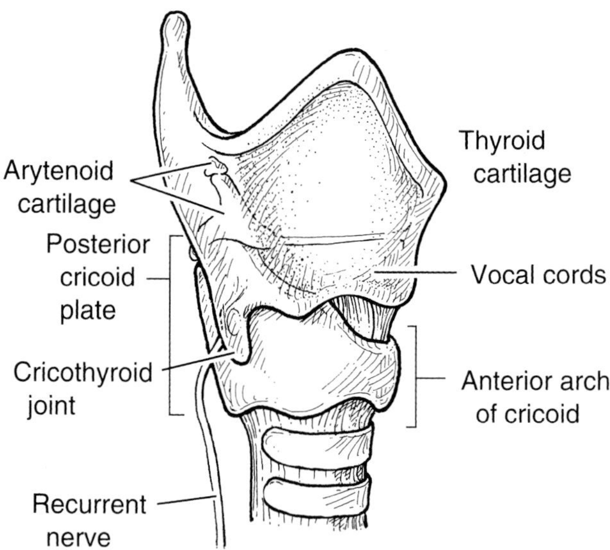

FIGURE 15–11 ■ This diagram illustrates the thyroid, cricoid, and arytenoid cartilages and their relationships.

the normal range of vocal function and require full mobility of the cricoarytenoid articulations. The subglottic larynx begins immediately below the vocal folds; it extends to the inferior margin of the cricoid cartilage and the interface with the first tracheal ring. The subglottic space is the narrowest part of the upper airway aside from the larynx. The subglottis has an internal diameter between 1.5 and 2 cm. It is surrounded throughout by the cricoid cartilage, which provides rigid structural support for both the subglottic and the laryngeal apertures.

Pathophysiology

The mechanisms by which translaryngeal intubation or tracheostomy produce airway injury are diverse: the injury may be secondary to the inflated cuff, to the rigid walls of the endotracheal tube, or to the site where a tracheostomy or cricothyroidotomy was created.

Cuff Level Injury

Various degrees of injury under the inflatable cuff are the most frequent complication after either endotracheal intubation or tracheostomy. These injuries occur despite the widespread use of high-volume, low-pressure floppy cuffs. Normal capillary perfusion pressure is no more than 20 to 30 mm Hg; hyperinflation of the cuff may lead to circumferential mucosal ischemia and ulceration. Schmidt and others (1979) demonstrated that mucosal injury occurred within as little as 4 hours after overinflation of a floppy cuff. When mucosal ulceration occurs, the underlying tracheal cartilage is exposed and may become devitalized and disappear. After extubation, healing usually occurs with the formation of a firm fibrous scar, which results in varying degrees of stenosis (Fig. 15–12*A* and *B*). Circumferential injury and cicatrix produce the most extreme degrees of obstruction. On occasion, relatively little collagen is laid down in an area of destruction, which results in a malacic segment. Full-thickness erosion of the anterior wall of the mediastinal

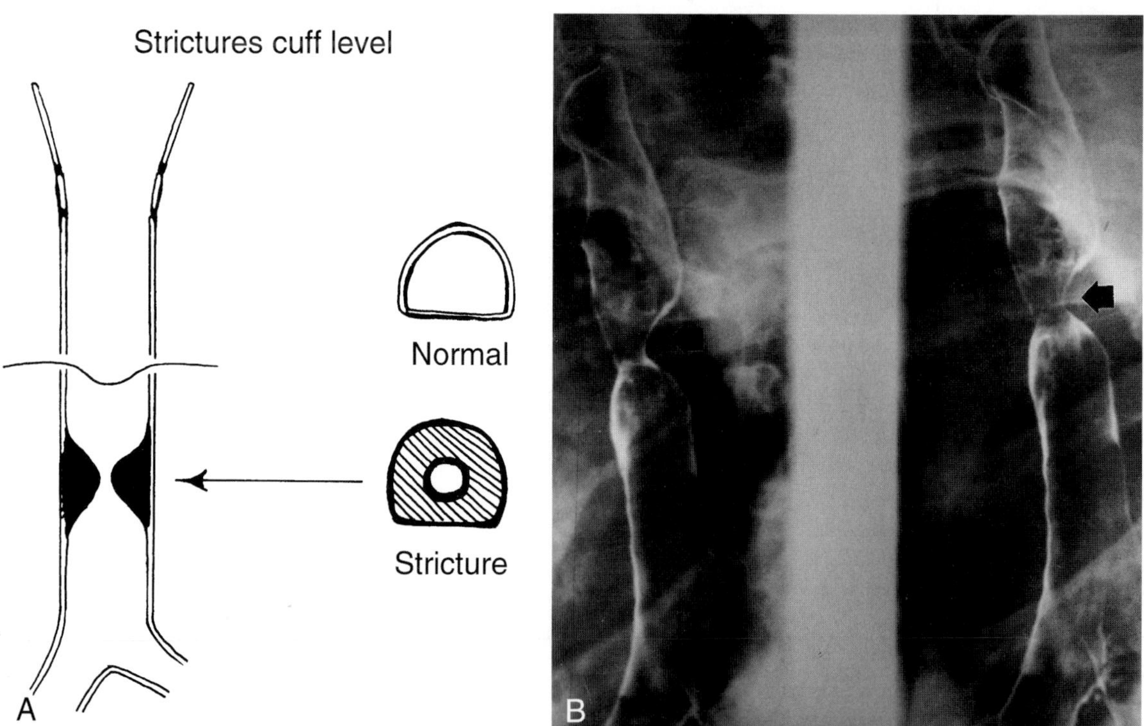

FIGURE 15–12 ■ *A,* This diagram illustrates a typical concentric, fibrous stricture caused by injury under the inflatable cuff. These lesions are usually short (no more than 2 to 3 cm). *B,* A contrast tracheogram illustrating a relatively tight cuff stricture (*black arrow*).

trachea may result in a tracheoinnominate artery fistula. Destruction of the posterior membranous trachea may lead to a tracheoesophageal communication.

To minimize cuff-related injury, cuff pressure should be maintained below 20 mm Hg whenever possible. Alternatively, the cuff may be inflated to a level that provides an air-tight system. Repeated checks are needed to ensure that minimal inflation is maintained. In some cases, if the peak airway pressures are unduly high, maintaining a small leak around the cuff may be desirable to avoid hyperinflation injury.

Stomal Injury

Stomal stenosis was clearly identified as a complication of cuffed tracheostomy tubes in a prospective study by Pearson (1968; 1971). In that early study, functionally significant stomal stenosis occurred in 12% of surviving patients who had undergone mechanical ventilation with cuffed tracheostomy tubes. The incidence of stomal stenosis increased significantly with the use of larger-diameter tracheostomy tubes. The smallest possible tube that is satisfactory for ventilation and tracheal toilet is recommended for either translaryngeal intubation or tracheostomy. Factors promoting stenosis include pressure and leverage on the stomal margins because of fixation of the ventilator attachments, and pooling of infected secretions above the inflated tracheostomy cuff. After extubation, the stomal margins fall together, with some degree of anterolateral scarring and loss of luminal diameter in every patient (Fig. 15–13*A*). In functionally significant lesions, the defect is usually triangular, with preservation of the posterior membranous airway (Fig. 15–13*B* and *C*).

On occasion, airway obstruction may be due to soft inflammatory granulations that develop at the margins of the stoma or adjacent to areas of ulceration under the inflatable cuff. These granulations may result in airway obstruction after decannulation, but are usually easily managed by endoscopic removal. To prevent stomal stenosis, the tracheostomy tube should be introduced at the level of the second or third rings; the least amount of cartilage should be removed that still permits introduction of the tube. The smallest possible tracheostomy tube that still provides a satisfactory airway is recommended. Ventilator connections that result in leverage and pressure at the stoma margins, with tubing supports and swivel connectors, will reduce lateral pressure at the stoma.

Glottic and Subglottic Injury

After translaryngeal intubation, the most common site of injury is the larynx or subglottis. This area is the narrowest part of the upper airway, and the subglottic segment is circumferentially encased with unyielding cricoid cartilage. At the level of the glottis and vocal cords, endolaryngeal tubes most commonly damage the posterior structures with ulceration of the interarytenoid mucosa. This damage may be followed by the development of a fibrous, posterior glottic stenosis. The most severe of these posterior injuries may involve one or both cricoarytenoid joints. The usual result is limited abduction of one or both vocal cords.

Subglottic stenosis is more commonly due to circumferential injury resulting in a concentric stricture, rather than to an isolated posterior injury. Occasionally, anterior commissure stenosis is produced at the glottic level.

It is very likely that some degree of mucosal injury occurs in most patients undergoing translaryngeal intubation for more than a few days. But after recovery, most have reasonably normal function. One prospective study, by Whited (1984), demonstrated a relationship between the incidence of posterior commissure stenosis and the length of time the patient was intubated: stenosis occurred in 12% of patients intubated for longer than 11 days. Colice and associates (1989) and Kastanos and colleagues (1983) reported a high incidence of acute injury (mucosal ulceration), but did not find a clear correlation between the length of intubation and the degree of significant, permanent injury.

Subglottic injury may occur when the tracheostomy is incorrectly placed through the first tracheal or anterior cricoid ring. It may also occur after cricothyroidotomy. In each of these circumstances, the anterior cricoid arch may be lost with variable degrees of injury of the posterior cricoid plate.

Postintubation Stenosis

CLINICAL PRESENTATION

Symptoms usually appear within 1 to 6 weeks after extubation. This delay in onset is due to the ongoing development and maturation of scar tissue at the site of airway damage. Both Andrews (1971) and Couraud (1987) noted that 80% of patients develop symptoms within 3 months of extubation. Less commonly, symptoms may be evident immediately after extubation. Very rarely, symptoms may be delayed for up to several years (Couraud, 1987).

Dyspnea on exertion is the primary symptom in all patients with clinically significant obstruction. Depending on the degree of stenosis, dyspnea ranges from a mild limitation of breathing during heavy exertion to marked shortness of breath even during minimal activity such as speaking. In most patients, narrowing of the lumen to less than 50% of its normal cross-sectional area results in dyspnea only with significant exertion. Narrowing of the lumen to less than 25% of its normal cross-sectional area will usually produce dyspnea and stridor at rest; such patients may be at risk of asphyxia from an inability to clear secretions.

Stridor is classically accentuated during inspiration. However, if the obstructive lesion is in the mediastinal trachea (where intrathoracic pressure increases with exhalation against an obstruction), or if there is associated tracheomalacia, the stridor may be predominantly expiratory. Frequent, but often overlooked, symptoms of severe airway narrowing are a characteristic brassy cough and difficulty raising secretions.

Not infrequently these symptoms lead to a misdiagnosis of asthma or bronchitis. Because of the respiratory

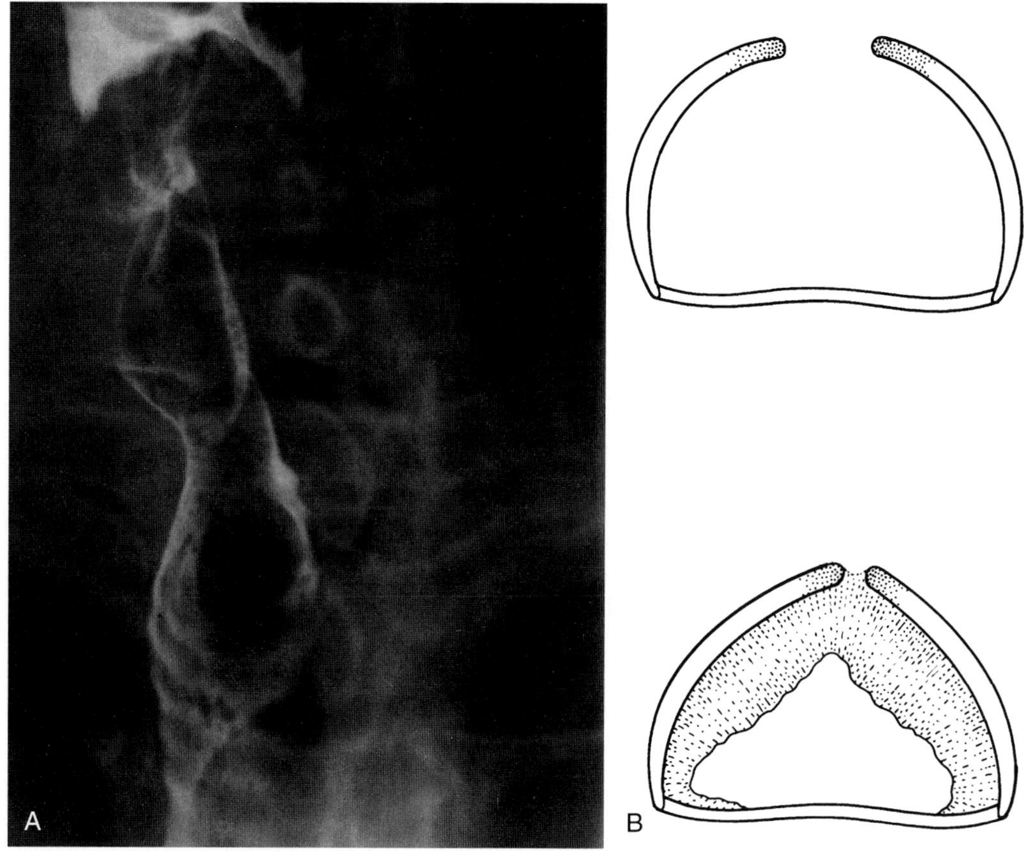

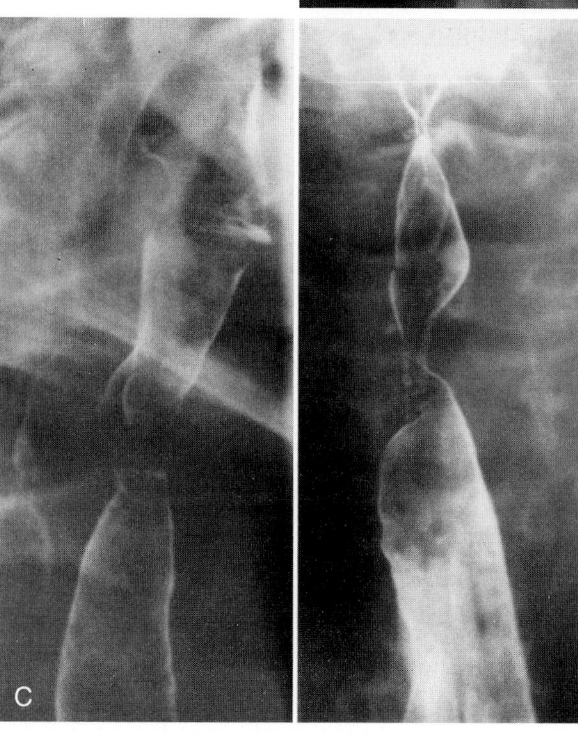

FIGURE 15–13 ■ *A,* A contrast tracheogram showing the typical anterolateral defect at the stomal level after tracheostomy. This relatively mild lesion was asymptomatic. *B,* This diagram illustrates the mechanism of stomal stenosis. A variable segment of cartilage is lost anteriorly (*top*); with healing, the remaining margins fall together and form scar tissue in the anterolateral parts of the trachea. The membranous trachea is relatively preserved, and a triangular stenosis results. *C,* A contrast tracheogram illustrating a severe stomal stenosis.

disorder that initiated the need for assisted ventilation, symptoms can understandably be attributed to manifestations of the original respiratory illness. The correct diagnosis is frequently delayed.

Symptom severity usually correlates with the degree of stenosis. If the lumen is greater than 5 mm (in adults), symptoms may be subtle and diagnosis difficult. Such patients may accept a modest loss of exercise tolerance without seeking help. In patients whose pulmonary function is already impaired (e.g., those with chronic obstructive pulmonary disease), a lesser reduction in airway diameter may result in more severe symptoms. Stridor is present only when the diameter of the airway is reduced to 4 or 5 mm; it may be noticeable only with exertion or during forcible inspiration and exhalation.

Changes in vocal function occur with lesions involving the glottis. Patients with postintubation laryngeal injury and stenosis have variable degrees of hoarseness and loss of vocal power. Rarely, recurrent nerve injury occurs as a complication of tracheostomy and may be the cause of hoarseness.

RADIOLOGY

Radiologic evaluation begins with plain posteroanterior and lateral chest radiographs. These radiographs provide information about the status of the lungs; on occasion, a narrowing in the airway may be obvious. Laryngeal stenosis and subglottic stenosis are rarely defined on plain chest radiograph. Stomal stenosis in the cervical airway is sometimes evident on plain film—at a level above the manubrium. The mediastinal airway is rarely defined accurately on plain chest films. Tomograms (anterior-posterior and lateral) of the larynx, trachea, and main bronchi are useful, providing reasonably precise information about the location, length, and extent of the stenosis. Familiarity and expertise with tomography has declined due to the increasing use of computed tomography (CT). CT provides accurate information about the location, length, and extent of narrowing. CT also demonstrates changes in the tracheal wall and adjacent soft tissues (information not provided by tomography or plain chest films). However, CT has lacked the ability to provide sagittal images comparable in accuracy to those of tomography. The recent development of helical (or spiral) CT using thin cuts (1–3 mm) with multiplanar reconstruction provides outstanding cross-sectional and sagittal images. Using this technique, Whyte and others (1995) found a sensitivity, specificity, and accuracy of 93%, 100%, and 94% compared with bronchoscopy. Helical CT with thin cuts and multiplanar reconstruction may be particularly useful in evaluating lesions involving both the larynx and the subglottis. Dynamic MRI can provide functional information about areas of potential malacia. A more detailed evaluation of radiology is provided in Chapter 21.

BRONCHOSCOPY

Bronchoscopy is a mainstay of evaluation. Much can be learned from flexible endoscopy under topical anaesthesia. With the patient breathing spontaneously and able to vocalize, an assessment can be made of vocal cord function and the more distal airway dynamics during inspiration, expiration, forced expiration, and coughing. Segments of tracheomalacia may only be evident at such an examination. However, the examiner has no control over a critically obstructed airway when using a flexible bronchoscope. Unlike a rigid scope, a flexible scope cannot be used to maintain the airway. Nor is the suction satisfactory in the face of abundant or tenacious secretions lying distal to a point of obstruction.

At some point in the evaluation of all patients with functionally significant stenosis, rigid bronchoscopy—conducted in an operating room, preferably under general anesthesia—is desirable. With the patient awake, vocal cord function and areas of malacia may be assessed with the rigid bronchoscope as well. It is possible to identify the exact anatomic location and diameter of the stenosis (including its position relative to the larynx above and the carina below) and to assess the rigidity of the stenosed segment. During either rigid or flexible bronchoscopy, it is important to evaluate the status of the mucosa adjacent to the proximal and distal margins of the damaged segment. Most importantly, a tight and disabling stricture may be dilated at the time of rigid bronchoscopy: dilatation may be initiated by passing gum-tipped bougies through the scope, then passing progressively larger-diameter bronchoscopes fully through the stenosis until a safe and adequate airway has been obtained. Dilatation allows safe and satisfactory relief of obstruction in almost all patients, for days or weeks. It also permits a more leisurely approach to planning subsequent care.

TREATMENT

Emergency Care

On occasion, patients with severe stenosis and disabling, life-threatening obstruction require emergency intervention. Treatment is initiated with humidified oxygen or a mixture of helium and oxygen (heliox). It also includes measures to reduce the inflammatory or edematous component of the obstruction (e.g., nebulized racemic epinephrine inhalation, intravenous steroid [a 500-mg bolus of Solu-Medrol], or steroid-containing [Beclovent] inhalation). These measures can be undertaken while preparing for emergency bronchoscopy in the operating room. Rigid bronchoscopy, with general anaesthesia, is preferable. The techniques of anesthesia are detailed in Chapter 5. In patients with postintubation strictures, it is almost always possible to obtain airway control using a rigid bronchoscope. Indeed, Couraud (1987) has found it unnecessary to do emergency tracheostomies in these patients. If possible, every effort should be made to avoid tracheostomy: it will only complicate the pathology and may make subsequent surgery more difficult. In that rare instance when tracheostomy is deemed unavoidable, the tube should be introduced through an area of damaged trachea, so that the extent of any subsequent resection is not increased. Emergency resection has no role in these patients.

Elective Care

The options in elective care for patients with subglottic or tracheal stenosis include interval dilation, laser resection, internal stents, staged plastic reconstructions, circumferential resection and primary anastomosis, and permanent tracheostomy.

Dilatation

Dilatation is useful to establish a safe airway at the onset of treatment. Additional interval dilatation may be useful in maintaining the airway while acute inflammatory features of the original injury resolve and mature. Except for very short strictures (less than 0.5 cm long), dilatation alone is rarely, if ever, successful in restoring an adequate airway. In the occasional patient who is reluctant to undergo resection, repeated elective dilatations may maintain a safe level of airway patency. The need for repeated, and often increasingly frequent, dilatations usually convinces the patient of the need for surgical resection.

Laser Resection

Laser resection has been popularized in recent years for managing many airway lesions. For benign strictures, however, its benefit is almost always temporary. Only very short strictures are amenable to definitive management by laser resection. Such strictures are usually weblike lesions in which a four-quadrant laser incision may be successful (Fig. 15–14). In the subglottic region, laser resection is generally contraindicated because of the potential for damaging the underlying cricoid cartilage.

Internal Stents

A stent is useful in the following circumstances: (1) as a temporary measure to avoid the need for repeated dilatations while waiting for inflammation to subside or while waiting for the patient's general condition to improve before definitive surgical resection and (2) as an alternative to permanent tracheostomy in patients who are not candidates for resection and primary anastomosis.

Of the variety of stents available, a silicone T tube (Montgomery T tube) is most commonly used in the trachea. A Silastic T tube has the distinct advantage over open tracheostomy of maintaining both adequate humidification of the airway and normal speech. In cases of subglottic stenosis, the proximal arm of the T tube must be positioned with the open end lying just above the level of the vocal cords. In this position, the tube is remarkably well tolerated. Although the vocal cords are unable to function, patients are able to produce a "hypopharyngeal voice," which is sufficient for reasonable communication. Although aspiration is common initially, it usually resolves completely within a few days or weeks. Aspiration may be a more difficult problem for some elderly patients or for patients with other pathologic defects or complications.

Three other stent options exist. The Gianturco Z stent (Cook Inc., Bloomington, IN, USA) is a stainless steel monofilament self-expanding stent. Its use is not recommend for tracheal or subglottic stenoses due to the potential for tracheal erosion from the high radial force exerted by the stent. The Wallstent (Schneider Inc., Minneapolis, MN, USA), a recently popularized self-expanding wire mesh stent, exerts less radial force than the Gianturco stent, is available in larger sizes to fit the trachea, and is available with a silicone covering that will prevent ingrowth of tissue. In patients with tracheal stenoses or malacia, the Wallstent is an alternative to the Montgomery T tube. Its advantages are its stability within the airway, no external components, and the ability of the airway to epithelialize over the nonsilicone-covered stents. Disadvantages include the inability to use these stents for lesions near the vocal cords, and the significant difficulty of removal by rigid bronchoscopy. Although experience is very limited, stents made of nitinol (a

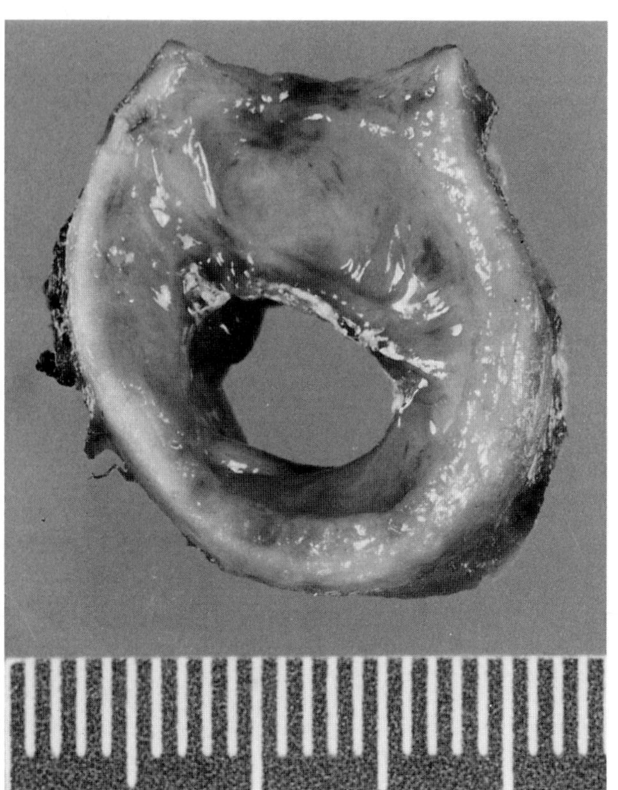

FIGURE 15–14 ■ Photograph of a resected, short, postintubation stricture at the cuff level. This stricture was less than 5 mm long, was resected in 1969 before endobronchial lasers were available, and would be suitable for laser management today.

titanium alloy that has a temperature dependent "shape memory effect") (Vinograd et al, 1994) may be of value in select patients with tracheal and subglottic stenoses and tracheomalacia (DeRowe et al, 1998; Tsugawa et al, 1997).

Staged Plastic Reconstruction

Staged plastic reconstruction, popularized by otolaryngologists, is most widely used to manage subglottic strictures. Most procedures involve vertical division of the anterior and posterior walls of the subglottic space (cricoid cartilage) and placement of some type of autogenous tissue graft between the divided ends of the cartilage. These steps are designed to achieve permanent enlargement of the subglottic airway. Grafts have been obtained from many sources, including free segments of bone or cartilage, as well as composite pedicled grafts. As recently as 1991, McCaffrey reported on the use of costal cartilage grafts placed in anterior vertical incisions in the thyroid and cricoid cartilages. Of 21 patients with isolated subglottic stenosis, 16 (76%) had a satisfactory postoperative airway. Five patients (24%) could not be extubated.

Segmental Resection and Primary Anastomosis

Most functionally significant postintubation strictures are best managed by segmental resection and reconstruction with primary anastomosis. Most postintubation injuries involve relatively short segments (1 to 4 cm). They can be reliably managed by circumferential resection and end-to-end anastomosis, without resorting to special techniques of airway mobilization at the upper and lower ends of the trachea. On occasion, longer segments are damaged; it is usually possible to resect about half the length of the adult trachea if supraglottic and infracarinal mobilization techniques are also used.

Details of operative technique (including indications, perioperative management, complications, and results) are provided in Chapter 9.

Several principles for successful reconstruction by primary anastomosis warrant emphasis:

1. Accurate, preoperative identification of the precise level and length of the lesion to be excised is critical. Doing so is particularly important in the case of benign strictures. This information determines the operative exposure and anticipates the mobilizing procedures. Preoperative tomograms and CT scans, combined with the findings at bronchoscopy, are most useful.
2. The tracheal margins at the level of the anastomosis should be as healthy as possible. When appropriate, acute mucosal inflammation should be allowed to subside before resection, and the excision should include all significantly diseased tissue. Both preoperative and postoperative tracheostomy should be avoided if possible, because an open tracheostomy inevitably results in some degree of chronic inflammatory change.
3. It is essential to preserve the tracheal circulation and to avoid undue tension at the anastomosis. These surgical platitudes are, nevertheless, critical for obtaining a healthy, healing suture line. With the mobilization required for resection, it is important to preserve the segmental blood supply, which enters the trachea through a series of small, posterolateral branches. Once the lesion has been resected, the remaining tracheal ends should not be mobilized circumferentially for more than about 1 cm.

Grillo (1979) clearly defined these contraindications to resection:

1. Continued need for, or high likelihood of, future ventilatory support;
2. Medical inability to withstand operation (rarely a contraindication if the resection is manageable through a cervical incision);
3. Tracheal lesions requiring resection of lengths that cannot be technically reconstructed by primary anastomosis; and
4. Anticipation of a future tracheostomy and presence of certain neurologic diseases associated with repeated aspiration. Relative contraindications include the use of high-dose steroids at the time of surgery and a history of prior radical local irradiation in the field of the resection.

RESULTS OF RESECTION AND PRIMARY ANASTOMOSIS

In general, the results of resection and reconstruction by primary anastomosis for benign tracheal stenoses are excellent. We reported on 34 patients with benign postintubation strictures (Andrews and Pearson, 1973). In that series, there was 1 operative death, and results were unsatisfactory, but not fatal, for 3 other patients; results were good to excellent for the remaining 30 patients. In that early period, 7 patients developed restenosis requiring reoperation and resection, 5 of whom ultimately obtained a good result. Grillo reported on resection and primary anastomosis in 208 patients with postintubation strictures (1979): 185 of those lesions were produced by cuffed tracheostomy tubes. Between 2 and 7 cm of trachea were resected. Overall results were good in 168 patients and satisfactory in 21; treatment failed in only 9 patients (4%). Both of these early reports—Andrews and Pearson (1973) and Grillo (1979)—concerned patients with postintubation strictures involving the trachea; only an occasional lesion extended above the lower border of the cricoid cartilage.

Similarly, the results of resection and primary anastomosis in patients with subglottic stenosis are excellent. Using the technique of partial cricoid resection, preservation of recurrent nerves, and primary thyrotracheal anastomosis (Pearson, 1975), we reported on 38 patients with isolated, benign subglottic stenosis (Maddaus and Pearson, 1992). Our series had no operative mortality; all 38 patients were decannulated. Restenosis occurred in 2 patients—we successfully managed them by re-resection in 1 patient and by dilatation and laser ablation of anastomotic granulation tissue in the other. Ultimately, therefore, all 38 patients had satisfactory results. In that same article (Maddaus and Pearson, 1992), we reported on 16 patients with combined laryngeal and subglottic lesions managed by synchronous subglottic resection combined with laryngeal reconstruction. The care of these 16 patients was in collaboration with our otolaryngology department. Of the 16 patients, 15 were decannulated and maintained a satisfactory glottic and subglottic airway.

The technique of partial cricotracheal resection with primary anastomosis has also been applied successfully to children with subglottic stenosis (see Chapter 19).

Grillo (1992) reported on 80 patients with subglottic stenosis managed by segmental resection and primary thyrotracheal anastomosis. He used his own modified technique for subglottic resection and reconstruction. Of these 80 patients, 50 had postintubation injuries. There was 1 operative death. All 49 survivors improved; most had good to excellent results. None required long-term tracheostomy. Couraud (1988) reported on a large number of postintubation injuries involving either subglottis alone or subglottis with concomitant laryngeal injury. Results were good to excellent in 95% of the patients; all were extubated.

Patients with recurrent stenosis after resection and primary anastomosis are a particular challenge. Donahue and colleagues (1997) at Massachusetts General Hospital reported on 75 patients who underwent reoperations for restenosis of the trachea; 16 of these patients came from a group of 32 with unsuccessful primary repair (out of 450 patients who underwent primary resections and reconstructions at that institution). The cause of the restenosis was often difficult to determine. In about 50% of the patients, the cause was felt to be secondary to excessive anastomotic tension and tracheal devascularization. Granulations were also felt to play a role, particularly in anastomoses performed with permanent (as opposed to absorbable) sutures.

Clinically, postoperative restenosis became symptomatic within 1 to 2 weeks after the original operation. Donahue and colleagues emphasize the following points in caring for this complex group of patients:

1. Initial management should be conservative. Reoperation should be delayed until inflammation and fibrosis subside, typically 4 to 6 months. During this time, 50% of Donahue's patients were cared for by either observation or repetitive dilatation. The remaining patients had airway obstruction that was unmanageable by dilatation and were managed by either a T tube (preferred) or tracheostomy placed through the most damaged or stenotic portion of the airway.
2. Most reoperations can be accomplished through an anterior cervical collar incision (73/75). In 18 patients, a partial upper sternotomy was added for additional exposure.
3. Avoiding anastomotic tension is critical. Donahue used a laryngeal release in 19 patients (15 suprahyoid, 4 thyrohyoid). A suprahyoid release is preferred because it results in less laryngeal dysfunction and aspiration).

The major complication rate in Donahue's series was 39%. Anastomotic granulations (most secondary to permanent suture use) occurred in 15 patients and significant dysphagia in 4. Both of these complications could be minimized by using absorbable sutures and avoiding thyrohyoid laryngeal release. There were two postoperative deaths (2.6%). Yet, the overall outcome of reoperative tracheal resection in Donahue's series was good (normal activity and good voice) in 59 patients (78.6%) and satisfactory (dyspnea on exertion and an adequate voice) in 10 (13.3%). Reoperation failed (need for permanent tracheostomy or T tube) in 4 (5.3%) patients. Donahue emphasized that the selection of patients for reoperation is governed primarily by the surgeon's judgment of the degree of anastomotic tension that re-resection would create. Patients considered to be at risk for excessive anastomotic tension are best treated with a permanent T tube or other endotracheal stent.

Tracheoinnominate Artery Fistula

HISTORICAL NOTE

The first report of massive hemorrhage caused by a tracheoinnominate artery fistula (TIF) after tracheostomy was by Korte in 1897. The patient, a 5-year-old girl with diphtheria, died of exsanguinating hemorrhage. In 1924, Schlaepfer reviewed the literature regarding 115 patients with TIF; the incidence of TIF was 0.5% to 4.5% after tracheostomy. Couraud (1966) reported detailed pathologic observations in 6 patients: 4 had fistulas due to circumferential tracheal erosion by the cuff, extending through the anterior wall into the innominate artery. The anterior wall of the trachea was adherent to the artery, and hemorrhage occurred directly into the airway through a fistula measuring between 0.5 and 3.0 mm in diameter. In the other 2 patients, erosion occurred at the inferior border of the tracheal stoma because of pressure necrosis of the arterial wall against the undersurface of the tracheostomy tube. Of the 6 patients, 2 had a premonitory hemorrhage of bright red blood, at 8 and 124 days, respectively, after tracheostomy.

■ *HISTORICAL REFERENCES*

Couraud L, Favarel-Garrigues JC, Chevais G et al: Cataclysmic creation of the tracheal hemorrhage following tracheostomy: Anatomical etiological and therapeutical consideration. Ann Chir Thor Car 5:772, 1966.

Korte W: Uber einige seltenere nach krankheiten nach der tracheotomie wegen diphtheritis. Arch Klin Chir 24:238, 1897.

Schlaepfer K: Fatal hemorrhage following tracheotomy for laryngeal diphtheria. JAMA 82:1581, 1924.

TIF is a rare, but frequently lethal, complication of intubation or tracheostomy. Nelems and others reviewed the literature in 1988. Of 175 reported patients, only 24 survived (86% mortality rate).

Figure 15–15 illustrates the mechanisms of postintubation TIF. The most common cause is due to too at low placement of the tracheal stoma—such placement allows the cannula to abut and erode the innominate artery. This mechanism of fistula formation is preventable by placing the stoma at the level of the second or third tracheal ring. The innominate artery normally lies at the level of the fifth or sixth tracheal ring behind the manubrium. In children and young adults, however, it may lie in the neck above the sternal notch. In such patients, mobilization of the arterial wall adjacent to the stoma must be

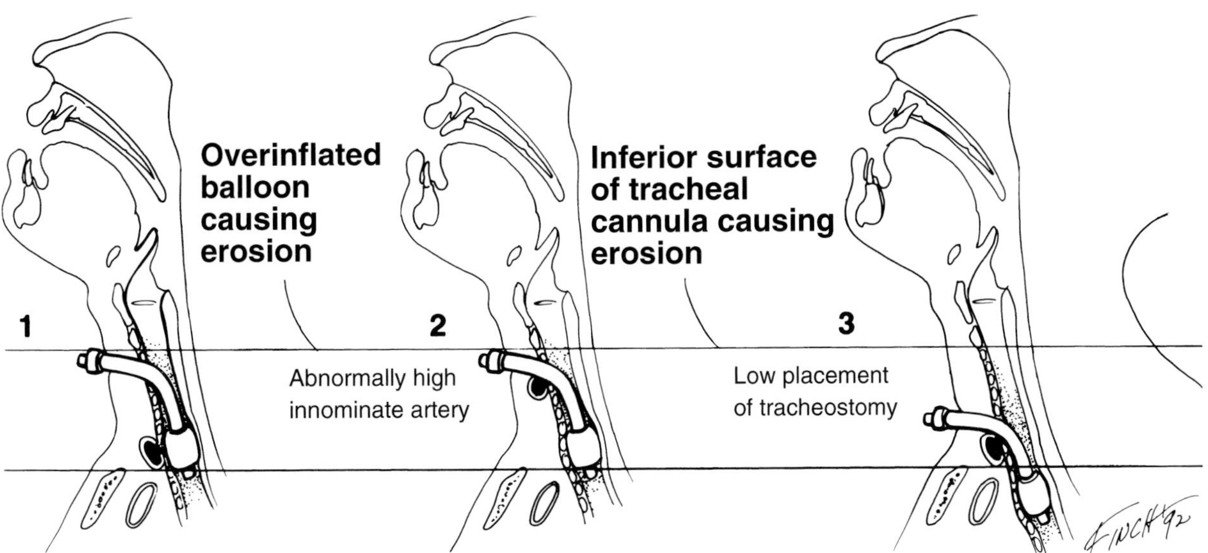

FIGURE 15–15 ■ This diagram illustrates the mechanisms of tracheoinnominate artery fistula. The fistula may occur from erosion of the anterior wall under the inflatable cuff or at the level of the stoma because of pressure from the tracheostomy tube itself. In the latter case, the innominate artery courses above the manubrium in the neck, or the tracheal stoma is created at too low a level.

avoided, and the stoma must be placed to avoid possible contact and erosion.

Other causes of TIF include tracheal wall necrosis that is due to cuff hyperinflation, which results in erosion of the anterior tracheal wall into the innominate artery. A normally placed tracheostomy may occasionally erode the adjacent distal tracheal cartilage and ultimately abut the innominate artery, with subsequent fistula formation.

TIF can complicate tracheal resection, extended laryngectomy, and prosthetic tracheal reconstruction. Arterial fistula after tracheal resection was reported by Grillo (1979) in 0.5%, and by Deslauriers (1975) in 3.0% of tracheal reconstructions with end-to-end anastomoses. These fistulas result from erosion of the arterial wall by the contiguous tracheal anastomosis and suture material. Grillo (1979) recommends protecting any tracheal anastomosis that lies near the innominate artery and uses local tissue such as surrounding fat, thymus, or strap muscle. Nelems (1987) described fistula formation after extended laryngectomy in 2 patients who required extensive tracheal resection for distal tracheal spread of a laryngeal tumor. After dehiscence of the cutaneous tracheostomy stoma because of undue tension, the innominate artery was exposed and eroded by the laryngectomy tube.

CLINICAL FEATURES

TIF presents with massive bleeding. Jones (1976) noted that 72% of patients bled within 21 days after tracheostomy. Premonitory hemorrhage—often significant, but not life-threatening—may precede massive bleeding. Premonitory bleeding can manifest as bleeding around the tracheostomy tube (often falsely attributed to the tracheostomy wound), bleeding through the tracheostomy tube (often falsely attributed to tracheal suctioning or tracheitis), or bleeding through the mouth or nose (often ignored). It is critical to recognize that bleeding from any of the above sites may represent a TIF.

MANAGEMENT

In all patients with a tracheostomy and with possible premonitory bleeding, flexible bronchoscopy is advised to define the cause. If the findings suggest arterial injury, the neck incision is reopened, and the wound is explored in the operating room. Before exploration, an endotracheal tube is placed with the tip above the tracheostomy. With the airway thus controlled, the tracheostomy tube is partially withdrawn and the neck incision is reopened to fully assess the tracheostomy site. If no fistula is found, the wound is closed, and the tracheostomy is replaced. If a fistula is found, it is managed by resecting the damaged arterial segment, with subsequent closure of the divided ends. Repair of the defect in the arterial wall is contraindicated—the repair site subsequently breaks down resulting in recurrent bleeding.

In patients with massive bleeding—which is the usual scenario—care involves three simultaneous priorities: control of the airway, control of bleeding, and resuscitation. Initially, the tracheostomy balloon is hyperinflated in an effort to compress the artery anteriorly (Fig. 15–16). If hyperinflation is successful, an assistant is assigned to hold the tracheostomy tube securely in position. Simultaneously, an endotracheal tube is passed, with the tip placed just above the tracheostomy site to ensure control of the airway. If hyperinflation is unsuccessful, the tracheostomy wound is widely opened, and the innominate artery is compressed anteriorly against the manubrium with a finger (see Fig. 15–16). A rigid bronchoscope can also be used to compress the hyperinflated tracheostomy balloon against the innominate artery and the sternum for control of bleeding (Cooper, 1987) (see Fig. 15–16). Blood can then be cleared from the distal tracheobronchial

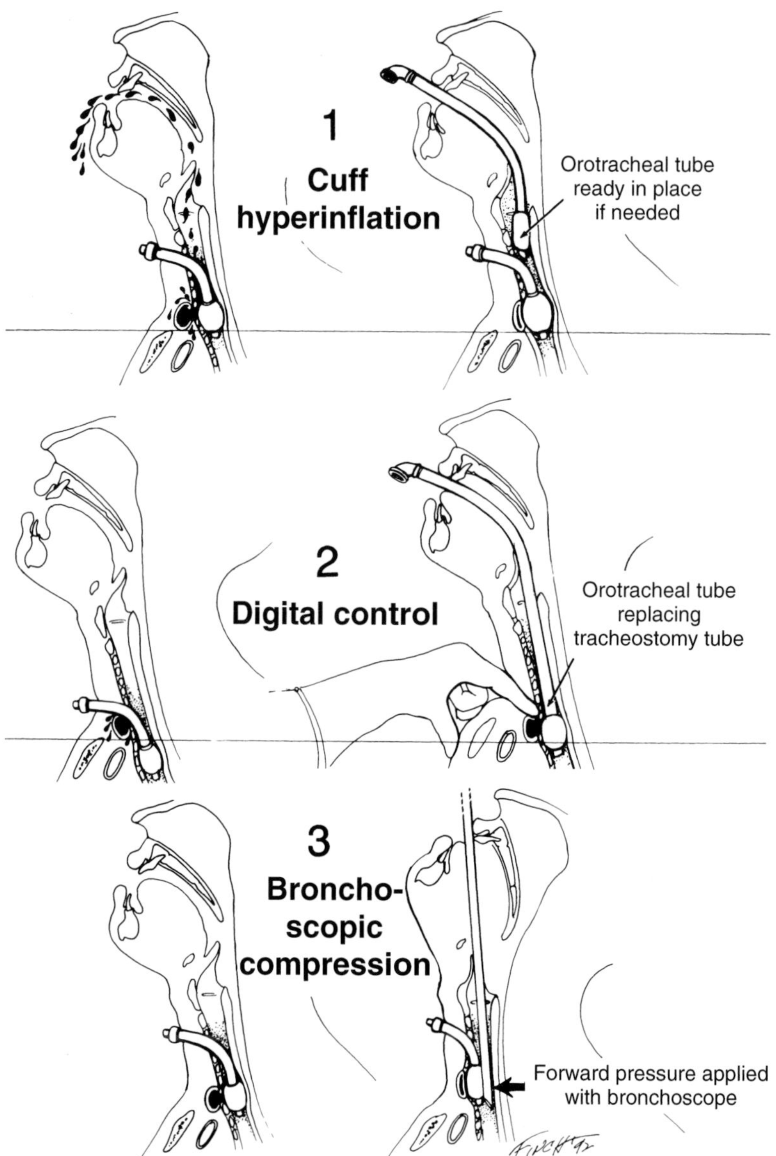

FIGURE 15–16 ■ This diagram illustrates the steps in the emergency management of tracheoinnominate artery fistula.

tree, and the patient can be ventilated. Jet ventilation may be preferable in this situation, if available.

With the airway secure and the bleeding controlled, the patient is cross-matched, sedated if necessary, and, if not already there, transported to the operating room. Under general anesthesia, the entire neck and chest are prepared and draped. The incision for fistula repair extends the tracheostomy incision combined with a partial upper sternotomy with extension into the right third or fourth intercostal space (Cooper, 1977; Nelems, 1988). Full sternotomy adds a higher risk of infection from the contaminated tracheostomy site. After the thymus is cleared and the innominate vein is retracted, proximal and distal control of the innominate artery is obtained. The artery is dissected free from the trachea, and the fistula is resected. It may be necessary to resect the innominate artery at its point of origin from the aorta. The suture line may be flush with the aortic wall. Arterial wall repair is contraindicated. Jones (1976) reported only a 18% survival rate after repair. Deslauriers (1975) also noted that repair almost inevitably fails, even when bolstered with autogenous tissue.

The controversy about vascular reconstruction is still unresolved, although anecdotal reports strongly suggest that bypass to the right carotid system is unnecessary. Most authors, therefore, advise resection of the innominate artery without vascular bypass.

If the operative field is grossly infected, the tracheal defect may be packed open to await secondary closure with granulation tissue. If the operative field is clean, the defect may be closed primarily and covered with soft tissue. The airway is managed by translaryngeal intubation, with the balloon cuff positioned below the tracheal wall defect.

Tracheoesophageal Fistula

Tracheoesophageal fistula (TEF) results from destruction of the posterior membraneous trachea, which most commonly occurs after prolonged mechanical ventilation, particularly in simultaneous association with nasogastric intubation.

HISTORICAL NOTE

Before 1960, the most common cause of benign TEF was granulomatous mediastinal infection or trauma. In the early 1960s, Flege (1967) reported on TEF due to injury by cuffed endotracheal tubes. By 1973, Thomas had amassed 46 cases of benign postintubation TEF, documenting that cuffed tube intubation was the leading cause. A variety of methods have been used to manage these fistulas. Early attempts at direct repair were made by Braithwaite (1961), Flege (1967), and Thomas (1973), all with some success. In 1976, Grillo noted that these fistulas were frequently associated with a damaged and stenosed tracheal segment at the same level as the fistula. He described a single-stage technique for simultaneous closure of the esophageal defect, circumferential tracheal resection, and primary tracheal anastomosis, performed through an anterior cervical approach.

■ *HISTORICAL READINGS*

Braithwaite FC: Closure of a tracheo-esophageal fistula. Br J Plast Surg 14:138, 1961.

Flege JB Jr: Tracheoesophageal fistula caused by cuffed tracheostomy tube. Ann Surg 166:153, 1967.

Grillo HC, Moncure AC, McEnany MT: Repair of inflammatory tracheoesophageal fistula. Ann Thorac Surg 22:112, 1976.

CLINICAL PRESENTATION

Tracheoesophageal fistulas occur predominantly in patients who require prolonged mechanical ventilation combined with nasogastric intubation. Cuff inflation compresses the membranous trachea and anterior esophageal wall against the nasogastric tube, leading to full-thickness necrosis and fistula formation. Many patients have a concurrent circumferential injury to the tracheal wall at cuff level.

A TEF may be heralded by a marked increase in tracheal secretions with the characteristics of saliva. Patients on oral nutrition may cough when swallowing liquids; particular foods may appear in the tracheal aspirate. Patients with reflux may have repeated aspiration of gastric juice through the fistula and into the tracheobronchial tree. Gross gastric distention due to "ventilation" of the esophagus and stomach through the fistula occurs if the cuff is positioned above the fistula.

Confirmation of the suspected diagnosis is generally simple. Tracheoesophageal fistulas are usually sizeable. They are easy to visualize by removing the tracheostomy tube and identifying the TEF directly through the stoma. Alternatively, the tracheostomy tube can be pulled back, and a flexible bronchoscope can be inserted through the tracheostomy to visualize the defect. Esophagoscopy, with the tracheostomy cuff inflated, allows visualization of the fistula, which is typically located on the anterior wall of the esophagus 1 to 2 cm below the tracheostomy stoma. Contrast studies are usually unnecessary. The large size of the fistula allows direct visualization in nearly all patients.

Grillo (Mathisen, 1991) eloquently described his extensive experience with nonmalignant TEF. The initial dilemma is whether or not to repair the fistula while the patient still requires assisted ventilation. The few reported attempts to achieve closure in this circumstance have been failures. With a documented tracheoesophageal fistula in a patient who still requires ventilation, Grillo recommends the following steps: Remove the nasogastric tube. Ensure that the tracheostomy has a low pressure cuff that is not overinflated, and attempt to place the cuff below the fistula. If absolutely necessary, keep the cuff at the level of the fistula. Establish a gastrostomy (to prevent gastroesophageal reflux) and a feeding jejunostomy. Manage salivary secretions by frequent suctioning. In the rare patient who appears disabled because of aspiration of salivary secretions, a tube pharyngostomy or cervical esophagostomy may be necessary. The patient is weaned as tolerated from ventilator support. Esophageal diversion is only used if disabling and life-threatening aspiration continues, despite the above measures, or if supracarinal fistula cannot be controlled with the cuffed tube.

Once the patient is off the ventilator, a single-stage repair is performed. Because many fistulas involve simultaneous circumferential tracheal injuries, repair often requires a segmental tracheal resection and reanastomosis, along with repair of the esophageal defect.

Figure 15–17 illustrates placement of a collar incision over the tracheostomy stoma. Because many of these fistulas are at a level below the manubrium, partial upper sternotomy may be necessary.

With small fistulas and lesser degrees of tracheal damage, repair consists of identifying and dividing the fistula, closing the tracheal defect with interrupted 4–0 Vicryl sutures, and closing the esophageal defect in two layers. A pedicle of strap muscle is interposed between the esophageal and the tracheal suture line to prevent recurrence (Fig. 15–18).

In patients with extensive or circumferential tracheal damage, the fistula is identified and divided, the damaged trachea is resected, and a primary tracheal anastomosis is performed. The esophageal defect is closed in two layers (Fig. 15–19), and strap muscle is interposed between the two suture lines. If a tracheostomy is required for postoperative airway management, it is placed, if possible, at least two tracheal rings below the tracheal anastomosis.

Grillo (1991) reported on 38 patients with nonmalignant TEF in whom 41 operations were performed. In 9 patients with smaller fistulas and a normal trachea, simple division and closure of the fistula was performed. Twenty-nine patients underwent tracheal resection and esophageal repair. There were 3 recurrent fistulas: 2 were managed by re-resection and 1 healed spontaneously with simple drainage. Of the 34 surviving patients, 33 were capable of normal oral intake. Five patients required esophageal dilatation because of narrowing at the level of the esophageal fistula repair. Thus, in most patients, a single-stage repair can be performed with a low rate of

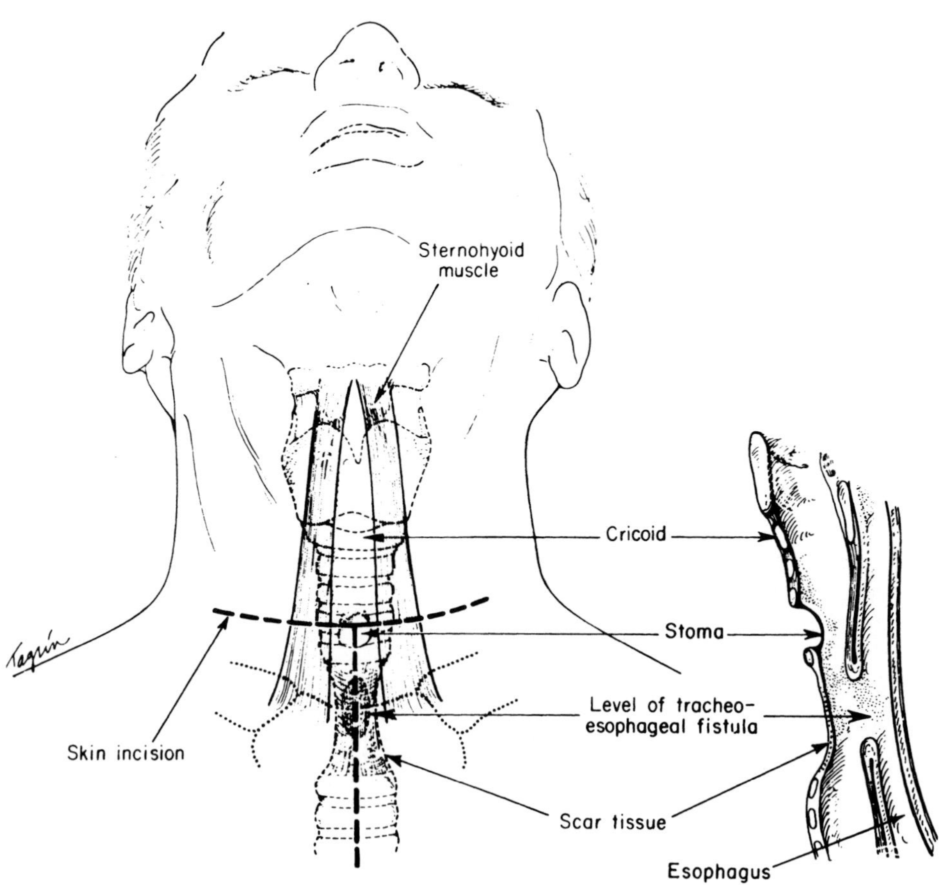

FIGURE 15–17 ■ This diagram illustrates the position of a cervical incision, centered over the tracheostomy stoma with a vertical extension for partial upper sternotomy, in the management of postintubation tracheoesophageal fistula.

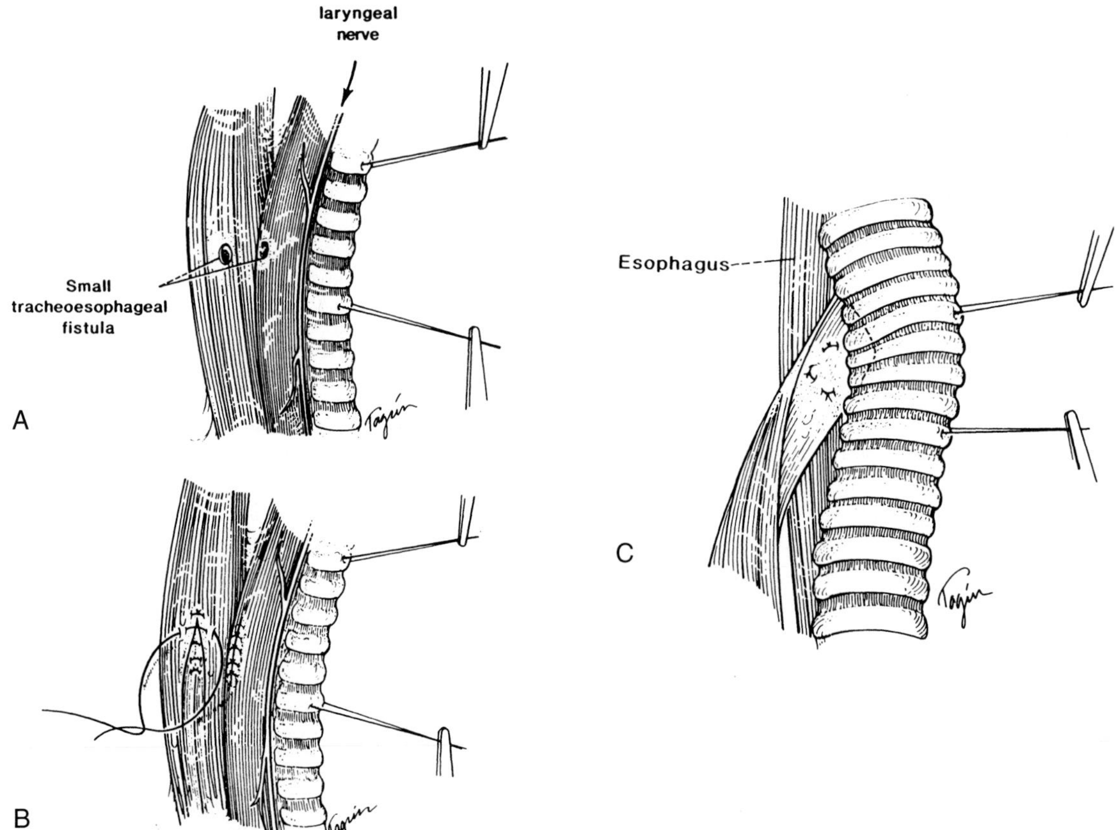

FIGURE 15–18 ■ This diagram illustrates repair of a small tracheoesophageal fistula without significant tracheal injury. The fistula is closed on both tracheal and esophageal sides (*B*), and a pedicle flap of strap muscle is interposed between the esophagus and the trachea at the level of the suture lines (*C*).

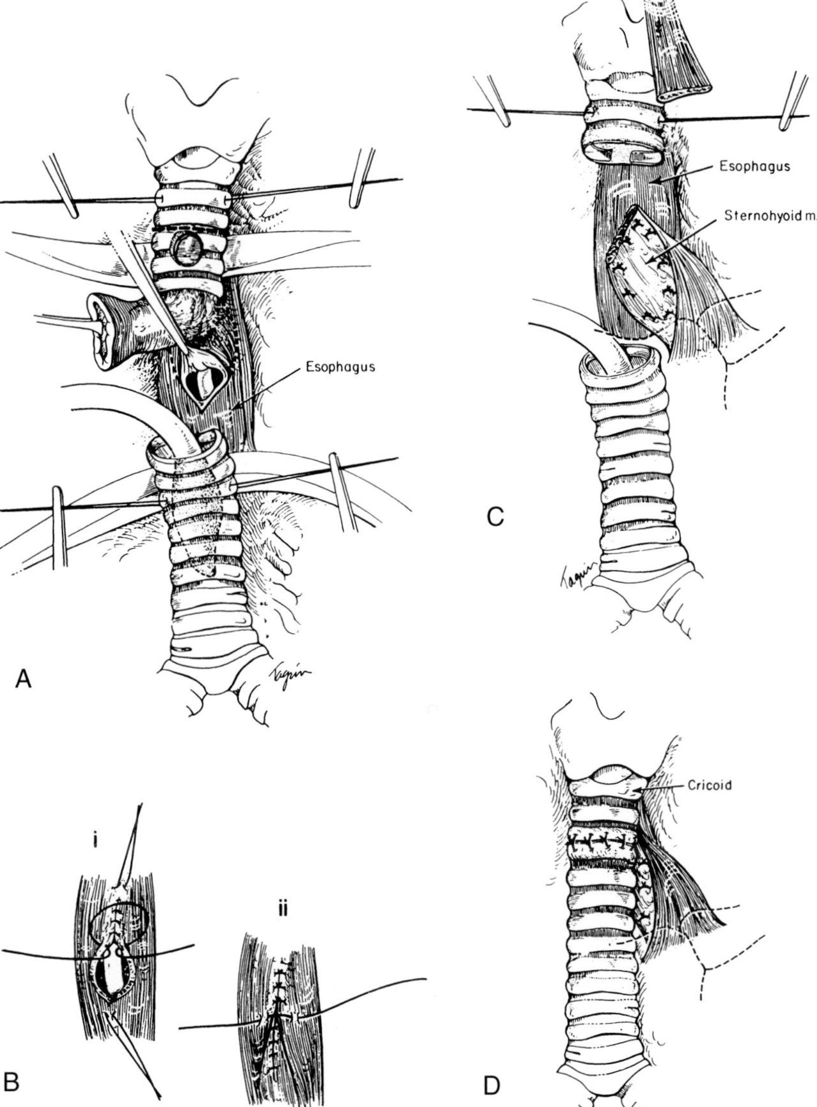

FIGURE 15–19 ■ This diagram illustrates the steps for closure in a tracheoesophageal fistula in which extensive tracheal damage requires a concomitant tracheal resection. The fistula is divided, and the trachea is transected below the level of the tracheal injury (*A*). The tracheal side of the fistula is closed with a single layer of interrupted absorbable sutures, and the esophageal side of the defect is closed in two layers (*B*). The damaged tracheal segment is removed, usually including the tracheostomy stoma, and a pedicled flap cuff sternohyoid muscle is sutured in place over the esophageal closure (*C*). The tracheal anastomosis is then completed (*D*).

recurrence and with good prospects of restoring normal oral alimentation.

■ KEY REFERENCES

Cooper JD: Complications of tracheostomy: Pathogenesis, treatment, and prevention. International Trends in General Thoracic Surgery, Vol 2. Philadelphia, WB Saunders, 1987.

This comprehensive review of postintubation injury caused by tracheostomy provides a clear exposition of pathogenesis and recognition. It also includes important statements about injury prevention in the current era.

Couraud L, Hafez A: Acquired and non-neoplastic subglottic stenoses. In International Trends in General Thoracic Surgery, Vol. 2. Philadelphia, WB Saunders, 1987.

This is a comprehensive report of a large, carefully documented experience with laryngotracheal injury. It catalogs Couraud's experience beginning in the early 1960s, which parallels the evolution in management of subglottic stenosis: from simple dilatation, through staged plastic reconstruction, and ultimately to techniques for circumferential resection and primary anastomosis.

Mathisen DJ, Grillo HC, Wain JC et al: Management of acquired nonmalignant tracheoesophageal fistula. Ann Thor Surg 52:759, 1991.

This is a detailed review of the largest reported experience with postintubation tracheosophageal fistula in the world. It details pathogenesis, diagnosis, and patient care, with an emphasis on the importance of identifying and documenting significant associated tracheal injury.

■ REFERENCES

Andrews MJ, Pearson FG: An analysis of 59 cases of tracheal stenosis following tracheostomy with cuffed tube and assisted ventilation, with special reference to diagnosis and treatment. Br J Sur 60:208, 1973.

Andrews MJ, Pearson FG: Incidence and pathogenesis of tracheal injury following cuffed tube tracheostomy. Ann Thorac Surg 12:359, 1971.

Braithwaite FC: Closure of a tracheo-esophageal fistula. Br J Plast Surg 14:138, 1961.

Colice GL, Stukel TA, Dain B: Laryngeal complications of prolonged intubation. Chest 96:877, 1989.

Cooper JD: Complications of tracheostomy: Pathogenesis, treatment, and prevention. In International Trends in General Thoracic Surgery, Vol 2. WB Saunders, Philadelphia, 1987.

Cooper JD, Grillo HC: The evolution of tracheal injury due to ventilatory assistance through cuffed tubes: A pathologic study. Ann Surg 169:334, 1969.

Cooper JD, Grillo HC: Experimental production and prevention of injury due to cuffed tracheal tube. Surg Gynecol Obstet 129:1235, 1969.
Couraud L, Brichon PY, Velly JF: The surgical treatment of inflammatory and fibrous laryngotracheal stenosis. Eur J Cardiothorac Surg 2:410, 1988.
Couraud L, Hafez A: Acquired and non-neoplastic subglottic stenoses. In International Trends in General Thoracic Surgery, Vol. 2. W.B. Saunders Co., 1987.
DeRowe A, Finkelstein Y, Ophir D: Self-expanding and self-retaining spiral coil stent for the treatment of severe subglottic stenosis in adults: Initial clinical experience. Otolaryngol Head Neck Surg 118:249, 1998.
Deslauriers J, Ginsberg RJ, Nelems JM, Pearson FG: Innominate artery rupture: A major complication of tracheal surgery. Ann Thorac Surg 20:671, 1975.
Donahue DM, Grillo HC, Wain JC et al: Reoperative tracheal resection and reconstruction for unsuccessful repair of postintubation stenosis. J Thorac Cardiovasc Surg 114:934, 1997.
Donnelly WH: Histopathology of endotracheal intubation: An autopsy study of 99 cases. Arch Pathol Lab Med 88:511, 1969.
Flege JB Jr: Tracheoesophageal fistula caused by cuffed tracheostomy tube. Ann Surg 166:153, 1967.
Gerwat J, Bryce DP: The management of subglottic laryngeal stenosis by resection and direct anastomosis. Laryngoscope 84:940, 1974.
Grillo HC: Surgical treatment of post-intubation tracheal injuries. J Thorac Cardiovasc Surg 78:860, 1979.
Grillo HC, Cooper JD, Geffin B et al: A low pressure cuff for tracheostomy tubes to minimize tracheal injury: A comparative clinical trial. J Thorac Cardiovasc Surg 62:898, 1971.
Grillo HC, Mathisen DJ, Wain JC: Laryngotracheal resection and reconstruction for subglottic stenosis. Ann Thorac Surg 53:54, 1992.
Grillo HC, Moncure AC, McEnany MT: Repair of inflammatory tracheoesophageal fistula. Ann Thorac Surg 22:112, 1976.
Grillo HC, Zannini P, Michelassi F: Complications of tracheal reconstruction. J Thorac Cardiovasc Surg 91:322, 1986.
Jones JW, Reynolds M, Hewitt RL et al: Tracheoinnominate artery erosion: Successful surgical management of a devastating complication. Ann Surg 184:194, 1976.
Kastanos N, Estpoa Miro R, Marin Perez A et al: Laryngotracheal injury due to endotracheal intubation: Incidence, evolution, and predisposing factors. A retrospective long-term study. Crit Care Med 11:362, 1981.
Lassen HCA: Management of life-threatening poliomyelitis. London, E and S Livingstone, 1956.
Maddaus MA, Toth JL, Gullane PJ, Pearson FG: Subglottic tracheal resection and synchronous laryngeal reconstruction. J Thoracic Cardiovasc Surg 104:1443, 1992.
Mathisen DJ, Grillo HC, Wain JC et al: Management of acquired nonmalignant tracheoesophageal fistula. Ann Thor Surg 52:759, 1991.
McCaffrey TV: Management of subglottic stenosis in the adult. Ann Otol Rhinol Laryngol 100:90, 1991.
Montogomery WW: Suprahyoid release for tracheal anastomosis. Arch Otolaryngol 99:255, 1974.
Mulliken JB, Grillo HC: The limits of tracheal resection with primary anastomosis. J Thorac Cardiovasc Surg 55:418, 1968.
Nelems B: Tracheoarterial fistula. In Grillo HC, Eschapasse H (eds): International Trends in General Thoracic Surgery, Vol 2. Philadelphia, WB Saunders, 1987.
Ogura JH, Powers WE: Functional restitution of traumatic stenosis of the larynx and pharynx. Laryngoscope 74:1081, 1964.
Pearson FG: A prospective study of tracheal injury complicating tracheostomy with a cuffed tube. Ann Otol Rhinol Laryngol 77:867, 1968.
Pearson FG, Andrews MJ: Detection and management of tracheal stenosis following cuffed tube tracheostomy. Ann Thorac Surg 12:359, 1971.
Pearson FG: Primary tracheal anastomosis after resection of the cricoid cartilage with preservation of recurrent laryngeal nerves. J Thorac Cardiovasc Surg 70:806, 1975.
Pearson FG, Brito-Filomen L, Cooper JD: Experience with partial cricoid resection and thyrotracheal anastomosis. Ann Otol Rhinol Laryngol 95:582, 1986.
Schmidt WA, Schaap RN, Mortensen JD: Immediate mucosal effects of short-term, soft-cuff, endotracheal intubation. Arch Pathol Lab Med 103:516, 1979.
Stern Y, Walner D, Gerber M, Cotton R: Partial cricotracheal resection with primary anastomosis in the pediatric age group. Ann Otol Rhinol Laryngol 106:891, 1997.
Streitz JM, Shapshay SM: Airway injury after tracheostomy and endotracheal intubation. Surg Clin North America 71:1211, 1991.
Thomas AN: Management of tracheoesophageal fistula caused by cuffed tracheal tubes. Am J Surg 124:181, 1972.
Trendelenburg F: Beitrage zu den Operationen an den Luftwegen. Arch Klin Chir 12:112, 1871.
Tsugawa C, Nishijima E, Murahi T et al: A shape memory airway stent for tracheobronchomalacia in children: An experimental and clinical study. J Ped Surg 32:50, 1997.
Tucker HM: The Larynx. New York, Thieme, 1987.
Vinograd I, Klin B, Brosh T et al: A new intratracheal stent made from nitinol, an alloy with "shape memory effect." J Thorac Cardiovasc Surg 107:1255, 1994.
Webb WR, Ozdenin IA, Ikins PM et al: Surgical management of tracheal stenosis. Ann Surg 179:819, 1973.
Whited RE: A study of endotracheal tube injury to the subglottis. Laryngoscope 95:1216, 1985.

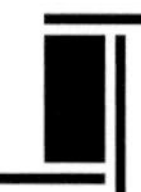

IDIOPATHIC STENOSIS

Hermes C. Grillo

A lower laryngeal and upper tracheal circumferential fibrous stenosis that is of idiopathic origin is occasionally seen. Although such patients are characterized principally by the fact that they have no known cause for the stenosis, the lesions also share typical features of location, configuration, clinical evolution, and specific pathology.

HISTORICAL NOTE

Brandenburg (1972) described three cases of idiopathic subglottic stenosis seen over 10 years, two of which were complicated by retro-orbital pseudotumor. Several other case reports have appeared (Havas et al, 1984; Jazbi et al, 1977; Mikaelian 1974). Grillo (1982), Grillo and others (1992), and Maddaus and colleagues (1992) noted a number of these patients in reports on single-stage laryngotracheal resection and reconstruction. In 1993, Grillo and others reported 49 patients with this entity, provided a detailed picture of the pathology, and described the natural history, surgical management, and results of treatment.

■ HISTORICAL READINGS

Brandenburg JH: Idiopathic subglottic stenosis. Trans Am Acad Ophthalmol Otolaryogol 76:1402, 1972.

Grillo HC: Primary reconstruction of airway after resection of subglottic laryngeal and upper tracheal stenosis. Ann Thorac Surg 33:3, 1982.

Grillo HC, Mathisen DJ, Wain JC: Laryngotracheal resection and reconstruction for subglottic stenosis. Ann Thorac Surg 53:54, 1992.

Havas T, Dodd M, Weldon B et al: A case report of subglottic stenosis. Aust N Z J Surg 54:291, 1984.

Jazbi B, Goodwin C, Tackett D, Faulkner S: Idiopathic subglottic stenosis. Ann Otol Rhinol Laryngol 86:644, 1977.

Maddaus MA, Toth JLR, Gullane PJ, Pearson FG: Subglottic tracheal resection and synchronous laryngeal reconstruction. J Thorac Cardiovasc Surg 104:144, 1992.

Mikaelian DO: Idiopathic subglottic stenosis in an adult. J Laryngol Otol 88:467, 1974.

BASIC SCIENCE

Idiopathic stenosis is a circumferential fibrotic stenosis, which begins at varying distances from the vocal cords, usually in the subglottic larynx but occasionally in the upper trachea only, and extends into the upper trachea. The tissue is dense and fibrous, although mucosal bleeding occurs easily on instrumentation. In a few patients, more florid granulation tissue or even ulceration is present, but this is unusual. The proximal end of the stricture begins subtly somewhere below the vocal cords, but its inferior border in the trachea is usually quite sharp. The usual length of stenosis measures between 2 and 3 cm with a range of 1.5 to 5 cm. Trachea distal to the lesion is normal. The effective lumen may be as narrow as 2 mm but more frequently ranges from 5 to 7 mm.

Dense, white, fibrous tissue replaces the lamina propria of the trachea. No calcification or ossification is encountered. Fibrosis is of the keloidal type, with thick bundles of eosinophilic collagen separated by sparse fibroblasts (Fig. 15–20). Some patients have areas of spindle cell proliferation with regimentation of nuclei, but such cellular regions represent a minority of the affected area. Mucous glands may be entrapped by fibrosis and become dilated. Lymphocytes are modest in number and sometimes are almost lacking. A few histiocytes associated with lymphocytes are embedded in the cellular fibrosis.

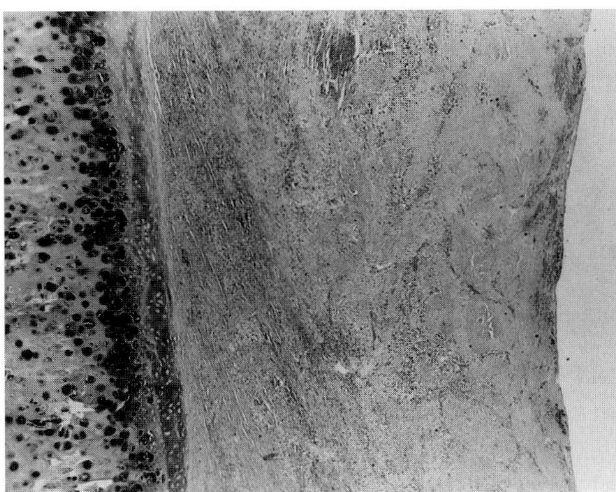

FIGURE 15–20 ■ Histopathology of idiopathic tracheal stenosis. Dense fibrosis of the keloidal type replaces the lamina propria of the mucosa. The epithelium (*right*) has squamous metaplasia. The inner perichondrium (*left*) is normal (× 30). (From Grillo HC, Mark EJ, Mathisen DJ, Wain JC: Idiopathic laryngotracheal stenosis and its management. Ann Thorac Surg 56:80, 1993.)

The surface epithelium usually shows squamous metaplasia (see Fig. 15–20), sometimes with granulation tissue noted. Cartilaginous rings remain intact or in some cases show slight loss of basophilic chondroitin sulfate from chondrocytes along the inner perichondrium. Little, if any, destruction of cartilage is seen, and no pus, eosinophiles, plasma cells, polychondritis, granulomas, vasculitis, granulomatosis of the Wegener type, amyloid, organisms, or foreign particles are seen. Cultures for bacteria, mycobacteria, and fungi have been repeatedly negative. Antineutrophil cytoplasmic antibody (ANCA) tests have been negative in all but one patient with poorly defined periarteritis.

Koufman (1991) postulated silent gastroesophageal reflux as a cause, but this is not borne out in two large series (Dedo et al, 2001; Grillo et al, 1993).

DIAGNOSIS

Clinical Features

Of 49 patients seen by Grillo and others (1993), 46 were women ranging in age from 18 to 80 years, with most in their 30s to 60s. Symptoms were initially dyspnea on effort, progressing to dyspnea at rest, noisy breathing, wheezing, or stridor. The duration of symptoms before evaluation varied from 4 months to 15 years, with most patients reporting symptoms of 1 to 3 years duration. None had been intubated for ventilation. A few had had brief anesthesia, with or without intubation, probably unrelated to their pathology. None had had bacterial tracheitis, tuberculosis, histoplasmosis, diphtheria, scleroma, or other specific tracheal infections. None had suffered external trauma to the trachea, inhalation burns, or irradiation. The age of onset, relative brevity of symptom duration, and pathologic findings ruled out congenital lesions. Sarcoid, relapsing polychondritis, Wegener's granulomatosis, and amyloid disease were not present. Two patients had vague arthralgia, and polyarteritis was suspected in one. The remaining 46 had no systemic symptoms or illnesses previously, concurrently, or subsequently.

Natural History

Most patients had had symptoms for 1 to 3 years prior to their clinical recognition, but in others the symptoms could be traced back for as long as 15 years. Initially, and continuing in many cases, the therapy was dilatation. Stenosis then recurred with its original or even greater tightness over varying periods, sometimes weeks and sometimes years. Lesions have never regressed spontaneously over long periods of follow-up. In only 2 of the 49 patients was there evidence of extension of stenosis into more distal areas of the trachea following initial resection.

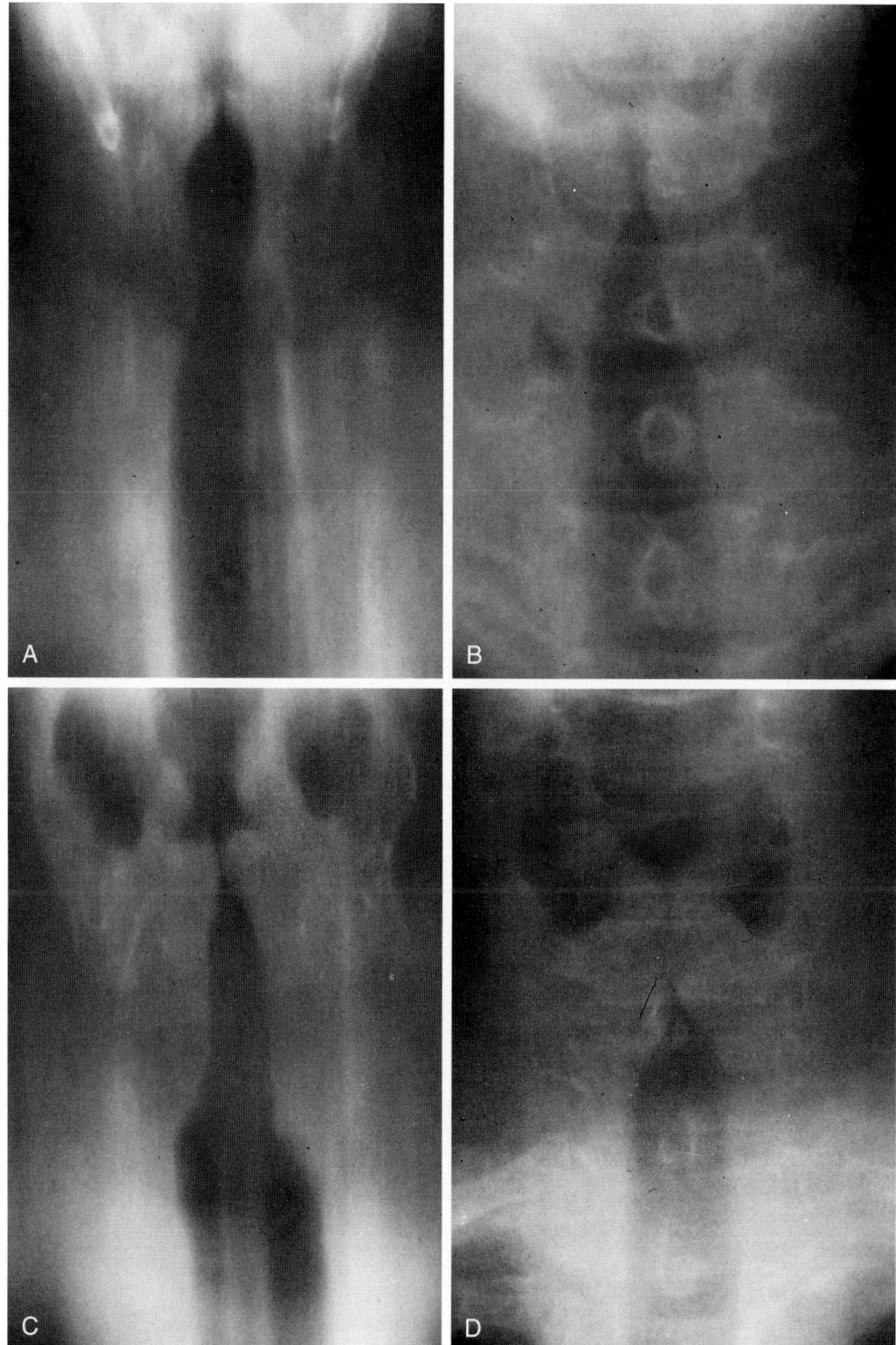

FIGURE 15–21 ■ Radiographs of the larynx and upper trachea in idiopathic laryngotracheal stenosis. *A,* Tomographic cut showing false and true vocal cords and a narrowed but still adequate immediate subglottic space, with maximal narrowing in the lower subglottic larynx and uppermost trachea. The distal trachea is normal in diameter. *B,* Postoperative radiograph using a copper filter for clarity. A nearly normal subglottic configuration has been attained. *C,* The subglottic narrowing here is more severe and commences immediately below the vocal cords. *D,* Postoperative view. (From Grillo HC, Mark EJ, Mathisen DJ, Wain JC: Idiopathic laryngotracheal stenosis and its management. Ann Thorac Surg 56:80, 1993.)

As noted, no signs of disease elsewhere or of systemic illness appeared. No association with gastroesophageal reflux was found.

Differential Diagnosis

Idiopathic stenosis is a diagnosis made initially by its typical clinical characteristics and by exclusion of any other etiology. These conditions have been noted in previous paragraphs. The pathology of a resected specimen is typical and rules out the diagnoses of polychondritis, Wegener's granulomatosis, and other entities.

Investigative Techniques

Simple radiologic techniques (Momose and MacMillan, 1978) demonstrate the location and extent of the lesion very well (Fig. 15–21). These may be supplemented with tomograms. Crisp, linear images such as these are generally of more use than CT scans, which provide cross-sectional images. Linear pictures show where the lesion begins and ends and its severity, as well as the amount of subglottic space remaining for reconstruction. Flow-volume loops demonstrate extrathoracic fixed obstruction as might be expected (Fig. 15–22). Direct endoscopy usually demonstrates normal vocal cord function with subglottic stenosis, as described (Fig. 15–23). The proximity and severity of the process in relation to the undersurface of the vocal cords are of greatest importance in determining the ease with which surgical correction may be done with a reasonable chance of success.

MANAGEMENT

Principles

Because of the unknown nature of the disease process and uncertainty about its future progression, patients were approached conservatively. Therapy consisted of dilatation at intervals, as necessary for relief of severe symptoms. The period of relief obtained varied greatly. Surgical resection and reconstruction have been increasingly performed, as favorable results were obtained. When the disease involves the larynx, as is often the case, techniques are used that provide correction in a single stage.

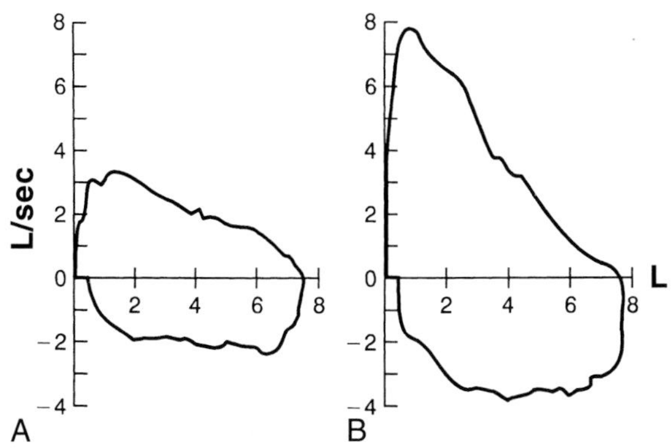

FIGURE 15–22 ■ *A,* Preoperative and *B,* postoperative flow-volume loops in idiopathic stenosis. Measurements were made at a 3-year interval. Forced expiratory volume in 1 second rose from 2.7 to 3 L, and peak expiratory flow rate from 4 to 7.7 L/sec. Surgery corrected the marked reduction in inspiratory flow. (From Grillo HC, Mark EJ, Mathisen DJ, Wain JC: Idiopathic laryngotracheal stenosis and its management. Ann Thorac Surg 56:80, 1993.)

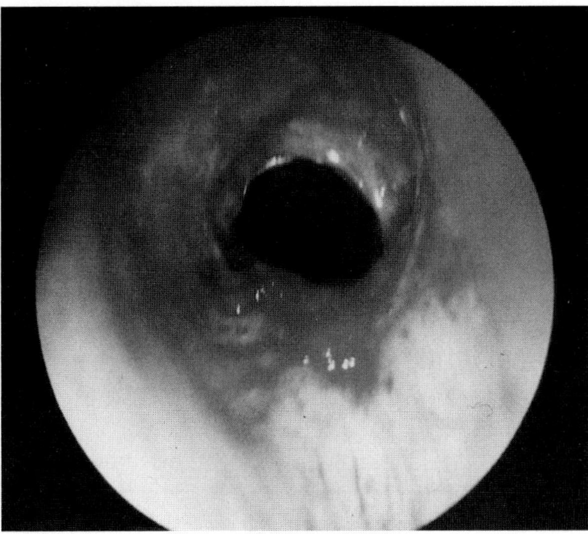

FIGURE 15–23 ■ Bronchoscopic view of typical subglottic stenosis. Lesions are concentric, although sometimes eccentric. Mucosal vascularity, but no granulation tissue, is present. (From Grillo HC, Mark EJ, Mathisen DJ, Wain JC: Idiopathic laryngotracheal stenosis and its management. Ann Thorac Surg 56:80, 1993.)

Operative Technique

Dilatation

Dilatation is performed under general anesthesia, administered by an inhalation technique without respiratory paralysis. The subglottic larynx is visualized with use of a rigid ventilating bronchoscope, through which small Jackson bougies are introduced to initiate dilatation. When lumen of adequate size is achieved, Jackson-type rigid bronchoscopes are passed serially, appropriate sizes from the range of 3.5-, 4-, 5-, and 6-mm bronchoscopes being selected. If dilatation is to be therapeutic, adult-sized rigid bronchoscopes may also be used to obtain satisfactory diameter, but these should not be so large that severe damage is caused. I prefer not to use a laser in these maneuvers for fear of creating more damage, which may interfere with future surgical repair. A tracheostomy is never performed, because such would complicate surgical repair. However, if a tracheostomy is already in place, anesthesia is delivered through the tracheostomy tube, and the dilatation becomes a simpler process.

Surgical Correction

When idiopathic stenosis involves only the upper trachea or extends only to the lower margin of cricoid cartilage, standard segmental circumferential resection is performed with end-to-end anastomosis. This usually requires anastomosis of the trachea to the inferior margin of the cricoid cartilage. However, when stenosis involves the

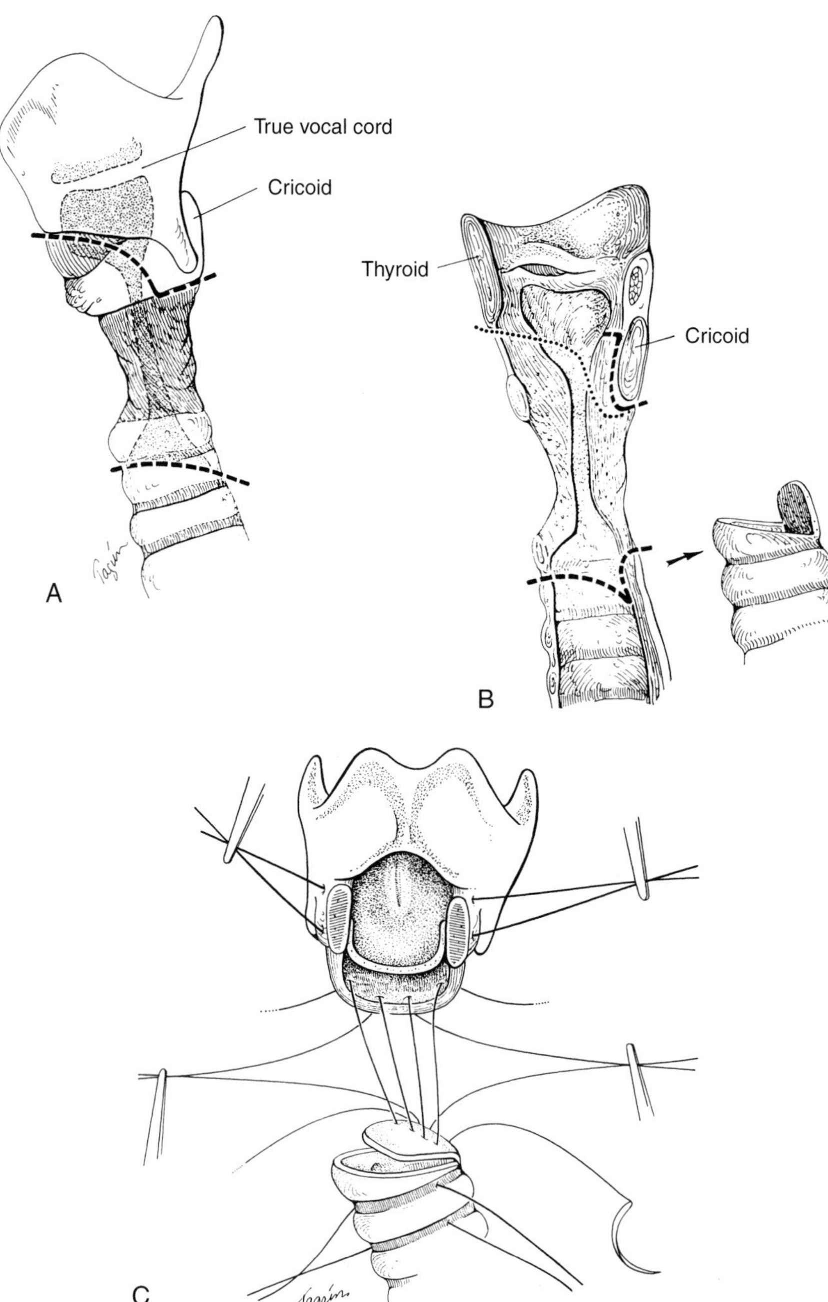

FIGURE 15–24 ■ Technique of laryngotracheal resection and reconstruction. *A,* External lines of division of the larynx and trachea are indicated by *dashed lines.* The anterior cricoid arch is removed. *B,* When the subglottic intralaryngeal stenosis is circumferential, scar tissue is removed from the front of the posterior cricoid lamina, baring the cartilage, as shown. The residual posterior cricoid lamina protects the recurrent laryngeal nerves. Distally, the trachea is beveled over the length of one cartilage, as shown, to fit the anterolateral subglottic defect that has been created. A broad-based flap of membranous tracheal wall is fashioned to resurface the bared cricoid plate. *C,* The posterior flap is fixed to the lower margin of the cricoid plate with four extraluminal sutures (4–0 Tevdek). The lateral traction sutures (2–0 Vicryl) are also shown in the larynx proximally and in the trachea distally. (*Figure continues.*)

subglottic larynx, as is most often the case, resection must be modified to preserve the posterior skeleton of the larynx with the entry point of the two recurrent laryngeal nerves (Grillo, 1982; Grillo et al, 1992). In these cases, the anteroinferior portion of the larynx below the glottic commissure is resected, including the anterior portion of the circumferential stenosis. An arcuate line of incision transects the midpoint of the lateral laminae of the cricoid cartilage and sweeps up in a curve that goes beneath the inferior margin of the thyroid cartilage in the midline anteriorly (Fig. 15–24*A*). The posterior portion of circumferential stenosis that remains is resected from the anterior surface of the posterior cricoid plate, baring the cartilage. The proximal line of resection may be almost at the arytenoid cartilages. The distal normal trachea is beveled for use in the reconstruction (see Fig. 15–24*B*). The first good cartilage below the stricture is salvaged and is cut backward in a sloping line toward its posterior ends on either side so that a "prow" is created of this single cartilage. This slides into the similarly shaped defect in the inferior part of the anterior laryngeal wall. Posteriorly, a broad-based flap of membranous wall is fashioned, which serves to resurface the bared posterior cricoid plate.

Lateral traction sutures (2–0 Vicryl) are placed in lateral midpoints of the trachea on either side below the line of anastomosis and proximally in the lateral laryngeal wall at the junction of the thyroid cartilage and remaining cricoid plates. Anastomosis is commenced with 4–0 Vicryl sutures, which are placed from the posterior mucosa

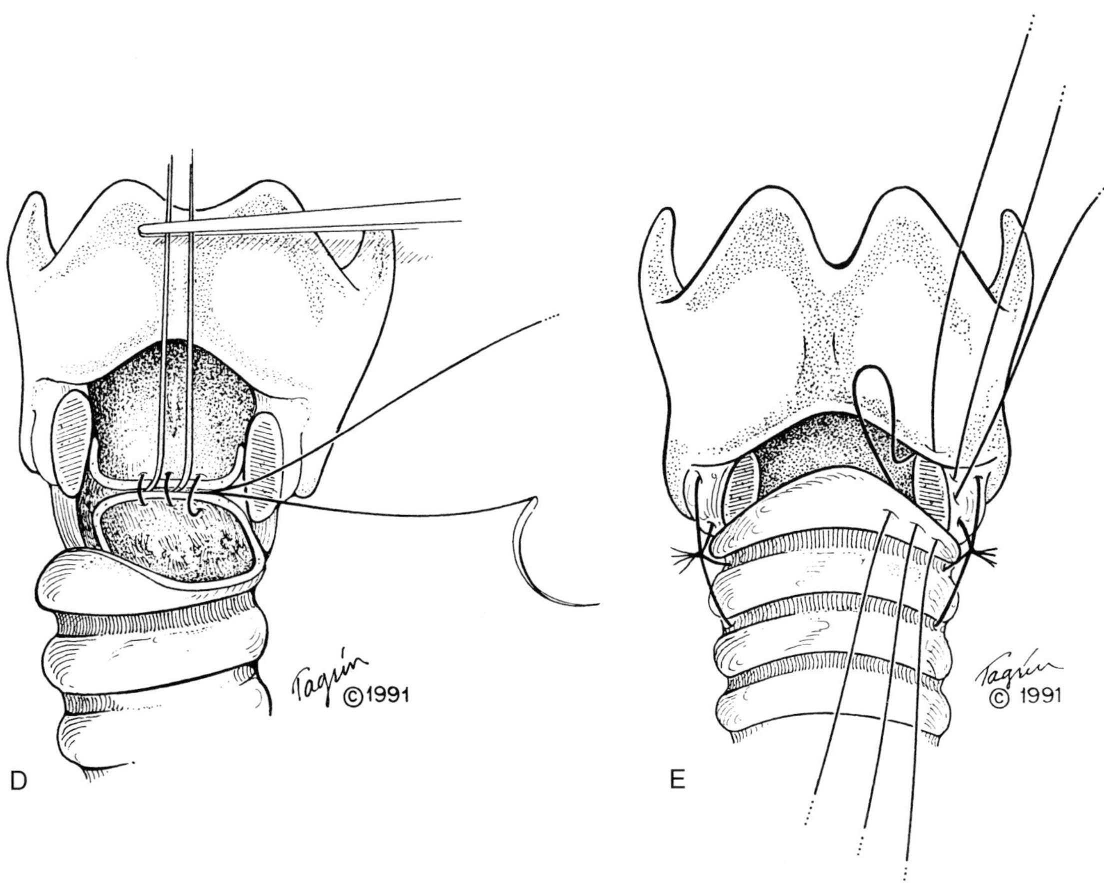

FIGURE 15–24 ■ (*Continued.*) *D,* Posterior mucosal anastomotic sutures (4–0 Vicryl) are placed with knots to lie behind the mucosa. Traction sutures are omitted in this diagram for simplicity. *E,* After placement of all the posterior and posterolateral anastomotic sutures as far anteriorly as the lateral stay sutures, the patient's neck is flexed, and the stay sutures, external fixing Tevdek sutures, and posterior mucosal sutures are tied, in that order. The anterior and anterolateral anastomotic sutures are then placed and finally tied serially. (*A* and *B* from Grillo HC: Primary reconstruction of airway after resection of subglottic laryngeal and upper tracheal stenosis. Ann Thorac Surg 33:3, 1983. *C* through *E* from Grillo HC, Mathisen DJ, Wain JC: Laryngotracheal resection and reconstruction for subglottic stenosis. Ann Thorac Surg 53:54, 1992.)

of the larynx to the membranous wall flap, with knots inverted from the lumen (see Fig. 15–24*C*). The sutures are placed but not tied. Four nonabsorbable sutures (4–0 Tevdek) are placed in a line across the back of the base of this flap to the inferior margin of the posterior cricoid plate to fix the flap against the cartilage (Fig. 15–24*D*). These are clipped to the drapes, two on each side.

Sutures lateral to the midline traction sutures on either side are placed through the cartilage of the larynx and the trachea, along with one or two sutures anterior to the location of the traction sutures. The traction sutures are then approximated, with cervical flexion, to relieve tension on the anastomosis. The sutures are tied in the following order: (1) posterior Tevdek approximating sutures; (2) posterior mucosal flap sutures; (3) anastomotic sutures posterior to the lateral traction sutures. The remaining anterior anastomotic sutures are then placed, and the anastomosis is completed (Fig. 15–24*E*). The anterior flap of cartilage from the trachea that is used to fill in the defect in the larynx is fashioned from a single ring to avoid floppiness.

Of the 35 patients who underwent single-stage resection and reconstruction, 32 achieved good or excellent results in terms of respiration and voice. Two needed annual dilatations. Six were treated by proximal tracheal resection with cricotracheal anastomosis. The other 29 patients with involvement of the subglottic larynx in varying degrees of severity were managed by laryngotracheal resection as described. In 7 of the 29, a posterior flap was not necessary because of the location of the posterior portion of the stenosis, which could be removed by simple resection. In the others, a flap was necessary to resurface the posterior plate of the cricoid cartilage. Concomitant temporary tracheostomies for 2 to 4 weeks were necessary in 3 of 22 undergoing laryngotracheal resection and reconstruction with a posterior stenotic component. In only one was suprahyoid laryngeal release necessary. The approach for all was through a cervical incision.

Perioperative Care

In all laryngotracheal anastomoses in which a normal subglottic airway is not present even at the final point of anastomosis, patients must be observed closely following surgery for signs of airway obstruction. If progressive glottic or subglottic edema occurs postoperatively, the patient should be intubated promptly with a small-bore, uncuffed, endotracheal tube. After several days, a trial of tube removal is made. If the airway is inadequate, a small tracheostomy tube is inserted very carefully in the now sealed tissue planes at a preselected point inferior to the anastomotic line. The anastomosis itself is protected at the original operation with thyroid isthmus or other tissue, and if the innominate artery is close to the area of potential tracheostomy, a strap muscle is sutured down to the trachea over the innominate artery to protect it. Using this technique, we have had no difficulties involving arterial injury in these resections or others of this type. In the series of 35 patients who underwent operation for idiopathic stenosis, no late intubations or tracheostomies were necessary.

Results

Of the 49 patients seen with this diagnosis (Grillo et al, 1993), 35 underwent surgical resection. The reasons for nonresectional therapy in 9 of the other 14 patients were severe stenosis close to the vocal cords, which prohibited reconstruction, in four patients; an excessive length of involvement, prohibiting anastomosis, in one; ease of conservative management in three; and demonstrated mucosal ulcerations in one. The other five patients were seen in consultation but underwent therapy elsewhere.

Of the 35 patients who underwent single-stage resection and reconstruction, 32 achieved good or excellent results in terms of respiration and voice. Two needed annual dilatations, and in one, failure demanded permanent tracheostomy. Of 26 patients followed for 1 to 15 years, 10 attained excellent results with respect to both airway and voice, and 22 had good results. A patient with a good result was considered to be one who is left with a slight change in vocal characteristics such as weakness in ability to project the voice or inability to sing as well as preoperatively. Minimal dyspnea on major exertion was also so categorized. Two patients had fair results, meaning either vocal hoarseness or an intermittently weak voice and low exercise tolerance owing to limited airway diameter, which limited activity. Failure occurred in one patient previously operated on elsewhere. Patients with good or excellent results have not required further dilatations or other therapy of any type.

In contrast to the curative surgical management described, Dedo and Catten (2001) treated 50 patients with multiple endoscopic laser submucosal resection. The treatment was regarded as palliative, requiring indefinite repetition.

■ *KEY REFERENCE*

Grillo HC, Mark EJ, Mathisen DJ, Wain JC: Idiopathic laryngotracheal stenosis and its management. Ann Thorac Surg 56:80, 1993.

Clinical characteristics, diagnosis, pathology, management, and results in idiopathic laryngotracheal stenosis are described as studied in 49 patients, 35 of whom were treated surgically. This appears to be the first definitive study of this topic.

■ *REFERENCES*

Brandenburg JH: Idiopathic subglottic stenosis. Trans Am Acad Ophthalmol Otolaryngol 76:1402, 1972.

Dedo HH, Catten MD: Idiopathic progressive subglottic stenosis: Findings and treatment in 52 patients. Ann Otol Rhinol Laryngol 110:305, 2001.

Grillo HC: Primary reconstruction of airway after resection of subglottic laryngeal and upper tracheal stenosis. Ann Thorac Surg 33:3, 1982.

Grillo HC, Mathisen DJ, Wain JC: Laryngotracheal resection and reconstruction for subglottic stenosis. Ann Thorac Surg 53:54, 1992.

Havas T, Dodd M, Weldon B et al: A case report of subglottic stenosis. Aust N Z J Surg 54:291, 1984.

Jazbi B, Goodwin C, Tackett D, Faulkner S: Idiopathic subglottic stenosis. Ann Otol Rhinol Laryngol 86:644, 1979.

Koufman JA: The otolaryngologic manifestations of gastroesophageal reflux disease (GERD). Laryngoscope 101(Suppl 53):1, 1991.

Maddaus MA, Toth JLR, Gullane PJ, Pearson FG: Subglottic tracheal resection and synchronous laryngeal reconstruction. J Thorac Cardiovasc Surg 104:1443, 1992.

Mikaelian DO: Idiopathic subglottic stenosis in an adult. J Laryngol Otol 88:467, 1974.

Momose K, MacMillan AS Jr: Roentgenologic investigations of the larynx and trachea. Radiol Clin North Am 16:321, 1978.

TRACHEOMALACIA

Michael A. Maddaus
F. Griffith Pearson

In most individuals, the trachea and the main bronchi are pliant, elastic structures that undergo significant changes in length during extension of the neck and with each inspiration. Shortening occurs during neck flexion, expiration, and coughing. During the phases of respiration, a concomitant, relatively diffuse change occurs in the diameter of the tracheal lumen. During forced expiration or coughing, the tracheal cartilages are compressed, and the diameter of the lateral walls of the cartilaginous rings is reduced. In addition, some forward displacement, or "herniation," of the posterior, membranous wall usually occurs. Tracheomalacia is defined as a pathologic exaggeration of these changes. It may result in functionally significant interference with airflow and impaired clearance of tracheobronchial secretions. On occasion, extreme degrees of malacic collapse may result in cough syncope.

HISTORICAL NOTE

In 1954, Herzog of Switzerland was the first to describe a syndrome of "expiratory stenosis of the trachea and mainstem bronchi"; this syndrome is now identified as tracheomalacia secondary to emphysema. Herzog defined the condition as "an alteration of the elastic fibers of unknown etiology, always associated with chronic inflammation." He noted that it is found primarily in "men over the age of 50 with chronic bronchitis." Herzog and Nissen (1954) described the first clinical attempts at surgical treatment of this condition by stabilizing the membranous trachea with thin bone grafts. Rainer (1965) reported his clinical experience with his own technique of stabilization of the membranous trachea: in the region of the malacic segment, he sutured a thin plate of silicone rubber (covered with Marlex mesh) over the plicated membranous trachea, then fixed it to the free margins of the tracheal cartilages. He observed both subjective and objective improvement in some patients.

■ *HISTORICAL READINGS*

Herzog H, Nissen R: Ershlaffung und exspiratorische Invagination des membranosen Teils der intrachorakalen Luftrohre und der Hauptbronchien als Urasche der asphyktischen Anfalle beim Asthma bronchiale und bei der chronischen asthmoiden Bronchitis des Lungenemphysems. Schweiz med Wchnschr, 84:217, 1954.

Rainer WG, Hutchinson D, Newby JP et al: Major airway collapsibility in the pathogenesis of obstructive emphysema. J Thorac Cardiovasc Surg 46:559, 1963.

Rainer WG, Feilder EM, Kelble L: Surgical technique of major airway support for pulmonary emphysema. Am J Surg 110:788, 1965.

ETIOLOGY

Congenital

Congenital anomalies include:

1. Rare, segmental cartilaginous defects (more commonly of the main bronchi);
2. Congenital vascular rings and anomalous innominate artery;
3. The syndrome of tracheobronchomegaly (also known as tracheal diverticulosis, and the Mounier-Kuhn syndrome).

The Mounier-Kuhn syndrome is a diffuse dilatation of the tracheobronchial tree; it may involve the airway from the larynx to the subsegmental bronchi (Johnson and Green, 1965, Mounier-Kuhn, 1932). In 1973, Bateson reviewed 55 reported cases and noted the following: The syndrome occurs primarily in males and usually causes bouts of coughing, purulent sputum, or pneumonia during the third and fourth decades. Chest radiograph is often diagnostic, typically revealing a striking enlargement of the trachea and bronchi. Bronchoscopy typically reveals redundant semicircular folds of mucous membrane and saccular pouches (hence, the name "tracheal diverticulosis").

The cause of the Mounier-Kuhn syndrome is unknown. A decrease in the number of airway elastic fibers has been reported. The syndrome may be associated with the Ehlers-Danlos syndrome and other connective tissue disorders (Aaby, 1966; Ayres, 1981). The trachea and bronchi—abnormally compliant because of atrophic changes in the cartilage—collapse easily with coughing or forced expiration (Al-Mallah, 1968; Katz, 1962). Fluoroscopy demonstrates a striking airway dilatation during inspiration, and collapse occurs during expiration or cough. Pooling of secretions occurs in the trachea and main bronchi (Johnson, 1965).

Acquired

Post-traumatic

Segmental areas of tracheomalacia may occur after any injury that results in loss of cartilage. The most common cause is postintubation injury at the stomal or cuff sites. Postintubation tracheomalacia is more frequent in the early phase of injury, in association with acute inflammation. In most patients, the "softening" disappears as the scar matures and as inflammation subsides. Most postintubation injuries heal by dense scar formation and stenosis. In some cases (most notably with administration of high dose steroids), scar formation is minimal, and malacia rather than fibrous stenosis occurs.

Emphysema and Chronic Bronchitis

Most patients with advanced emphysema and chronic bronchitis have some degree of malacia affecting part, or all, of the trachea and main bronchi. The cause appears related to a decrease in the amount of cartilage (Maisel, 1968; Thurlbeck, 1974). On occasion, the degree of malacia results in functional air flow impairment and inability to raise secretions across the malacic segment. In such patients, the changes in airway diameter that normally occur with changes in intrathoracic pressure are pathologically exaggerated.

Saber-sheath trachea is characterized by marked coronal narrowing of the trachea—to less than two thirds that of the sagittal diameter. The coronal narrowing, usually easily identified on a posterior-anterior chest radiography involves only the intrathoracic trachea and ends abruptly above the level of the thoracic inlet. The cause is unknown. Because it is invariably associated with significant chronic obstructive pulmonary disease, the deformity may be due to chronic compression by the overinflated lungs. Saber-sheath narrowing appears to be a fixed abnormality without a tendency to malacia and collapse, likely due to the extensive tracheal calcification seen in most cases (Greene, 1975).

Chronic External Compression

This condition is most commonly caused by compression of the upper mediastinal trachea by a benign mediastinal goiter. On occasion, other mediastinal lesions that are contiguous with the trachea (e.g., teratoma, thymoma, bronchogenic cyst) may induce an area of segmental tracheomalacia. Segmental malacia of a main bronchus may occur after pneumonectomy if the carinal airway is markedly displaced and, if a main bronchus is compressed, by the underlying thoracic spine.

Relapsing Polychondritis

This systemic disease affects cartilage in several areas of the body, including the cartilage of the ear, nose, larynx, and tracheobronchial tree. An autoimmune connective tissue disease, it is thought to be secondary to production of autoantibodies to cartilage (Ebringer, 1981; Foidart, 1978). Occasionally, it is associated with other systemic connective tissue disorders such as systemic lupus erythematosus. Pathologically, a tracheal chondritis is initially seen (most often demonstrated by nasal biopsy). The disease is characterized by an infiltration of lymphocytes and plasma cells; with time, the destroyed cartilage is replaced by fibrous tissue. A diffuse disease, relapsing polychondritis may involve different segments of the airway to varying degrees. Dolan, in 1966, noted that the involved segments may demonstrate either a fixed obstruction or a variable malacic obstruction. Relapsing polychondritis usually occurs in the third or fourth decade, with equal incidence in males and females. As noted by McAdam, 1976, the tracheobronchial tree is involved in over 50% of patients; in severe cases, airway symptoms can be disabling. Respiratory involvement is the leading cause of death from this disease (Hughes, 1972).

DIAGNOSIS

Symptoms are related to collapse of the airway and occur with increases in intrathoracic pressure. They include expiratory wheezing or stridor, particularly with exertion; a barking cough; and an inability to clear secretions. Physical examination may reveal an audible wheeze, or stridor with forced expiration. Auscultation over the suprasternal notch during forced expiration or cough may disclose a sharp, loud knock early in expiration. Postintubation malacia in the cervical trachea may be palpable on physical examination.

Pulmonary function studies show a break in the expiratory phase of the spirogram (Campbell, 1965; Gandevia, 1963). The break in the expiratory curve to a flat plateau is assumed to represent the moment of large airway collapse after dead space air has been exhaled. It is at this point in the cycle that a sharp knock may be heard with a stethoscope placed over the upper sternum.

IMAGING

Plain posterior-anterior and lateral chest radiographs, tracheal tomograms, and computer tomography (CT) scans may show no abnormality: these studies provide only static images of the airways. However, they do show some changes in specific types of tracheomalacia. In the Mounier-Kuhn syndrome, the diagnosis is immediately apparent on a plain chest radiograph, which shows an overall increase in the caliber of the trachea and bronchi, as well as a unique, corrugated, diverticular airway appearance. With Saber-sheath trachea, the coronal diameter of the trachea is markedly reduced on a posterior-anterior chest radiograph, whereas the sagittal diameter, seen in the lateral film, is increased (normally, the two diameters are roughly equal). Any mediastinal mass compressing the trachea, such as a benign goiter, may be evident on a plain chest radiograph.

If the diagnosis is not apparent on static images, *cine studies* of the trachea and main bronchi, with or without contrast, will dynamically display the airways and provide critical diagnostic information. Cine studies demonstrate the presence of airway collapse and the anatomic levels involved. The lateral projection is an essential component, particularly in patients with malacia due to emphysema and bronchitis (Fig. 15–25).

Bronchoscopy, another important diagnostic modality, may be done with either rigid or flexible instruments. It should be done under local anesthesia, allowing observation of the airway during spontaneous respiration, deep breathing, forced expiration, and cough. Abnormal collapse of the airway is typically identified during expiration, especially with forced expiration and cough. In cases of malacia that is associated with emphysema, the membranous trachea is widened and redundant and may lack the normal longitudinal folds. During expiration, anterior displacement of the redundant membranous trachea is pronounced, resulting in a semilunar or "new moon" configuration of the airway lumen. In some cases, the airway closes completely at certain points in the cycle, as the redundant membranous trachea becomes apposed to the inner surface of the cartilaginous rings. These changes may be diffuse or segmental in distribution, although they commonly involve the origins of the main bronchi.

The dynamic changes seen on cineradiography, or at bronchoscopy, may be dramatically demonstrated at the time of surgery. If the malacia is due to emphysema, gross widening of the posterior tracheal wall is evident, and abnormal softening of the cartilages is readily palpable. With the patient breathing spontaneously, expiration will produce invagination of the membranous wall in that part of the malacic airway beyond the endotracheal tube. Stimulation of cough by carinal irritation will produce abrupt collapse and forward herniation of the posterior wall, even in the open thorax.

MANAGEMENT

Postintubation Malacia

Post-intubation tracheomalacia results in defects that are usually similar to the more common post-intubation fibrous strictures. Some degree of malacia is often observed during the early phase of postintubation injury, in association with acute inflammation. In most patients, this softening disappears as the inflammation subsides and the scar matures. High-dose steroids undoubtedly interfere with the formation of normal scar tissue and predispose to malacia rather than cicatricial stenosis.

At bronchoscopy, malacic segments can be easily dilated, because the luminal circumference is often normal. A rigid bronchoscope may be easily advanced through

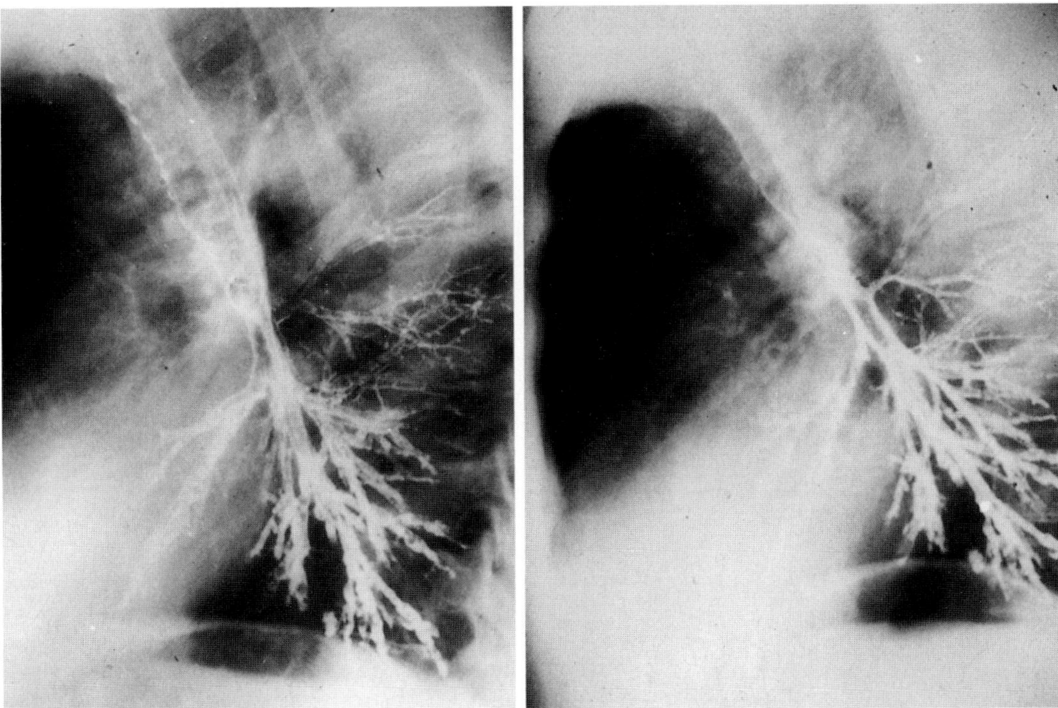

FIGURE 15–25 ■ Contrast tracheogram illustrating pronounced narrowing of the trachea during cough, in a patient with chronic bronchitis and emphysema.

the collapsed segment. Obviously, such dilatation is of no therapeutic benefit. Disabling postintubation malacia is usually best managed by segmental resection and primary anastomosis. Otolaryngologists have reported successful alternative techniques, such as ceramic ring reinforcement of the malacic segment (Amedee, 1992). In our opinion, such techniques are unwarranted because of the need to implant foreign material, particularly given the demonstrated safety and effectiveness of resection and primary repair. In those rare instances when an operation is deemed impossible, internal stenting with either a silicone Montgomery T tube or a wire mesh stent (Wallstent, Schneider Inc., Minneapolis, MN, USA) may provide a safe and satisfactory airway.

Emphysema and Chronic Bronchitis

A number of surgical techniques may provide external support of the trachea and main bronchi in selected patients with functionally disabling malacia secondary to emphysema and chronic bronchitis.

Herzog and Nissen, in 1954, were the first to describe a technique of external support using either autologous or homologous arches, or rings of bone. Rainer, in 1965, reported on 12 patients in whom a slab of specially prepared silicone and Marlex mesh was secured to a membranous wall of the trachea, with reefing of the redundant membranous component. In some patients with significant cartilaginous malacia, polypropylene rings were added anterolaterally. Exposure was obtained in all cases through a right posterolateral thoracotomy through the bed of the fifth rib. Four late deaths (3 to 11 months postoperatively) occurred: three were due to unrelated disease and one was due to erosion of the prosthesis into the airway, resulting in a fatal, distal pneumonia. Of the eight longer-term survivors, four significantly improved clinically, and all eight saw quantitative improvement in pulmonary function tests. In 1968, Rainer reported on 19 patients, 3 of whom died from complications of esophageal and aortic erosion by the prosthesis.

Urschel (personal communication) has amassed experience with about 40 patients, and in all but 2, the malacia was secondary to emphysema and bronchitis. One of those 2 had congenital Mounier-Kuhn syndrome; the other had a "giant trachea" of no known etiology. Urschel used a modification of the posterior Marlex mesh support developed by Rainer (Fig. 15–26). His experience has yet to be critically assessed with long-term evaluation. He did note severe and fatal complications owing to erosion of the airway or adjacent organs, and infection. There were, however, excellent immediate and long-term results.

An alternative technique, described by Hanawa in 1990, involves stabilization of the membranous wall using Marlex mesh with lyophilized human dura. The support is secured by bonding with fibrin glue. Hanawa used this technique in one patient with emphysematous tracheomalacia. The patient's cough syncope and airway collapse disappeared completely after surgery.

Dunn and colleagues, in a 1990 case report, emphasized an important feature of the pathology of tracheomalacia secondary to emphysema. Preoperative cine studies and bronchoscopy in one patient showed evidence of collapse of a segment of trachea above the aortic arch; the patient underwent thoracotomy, with the intention of

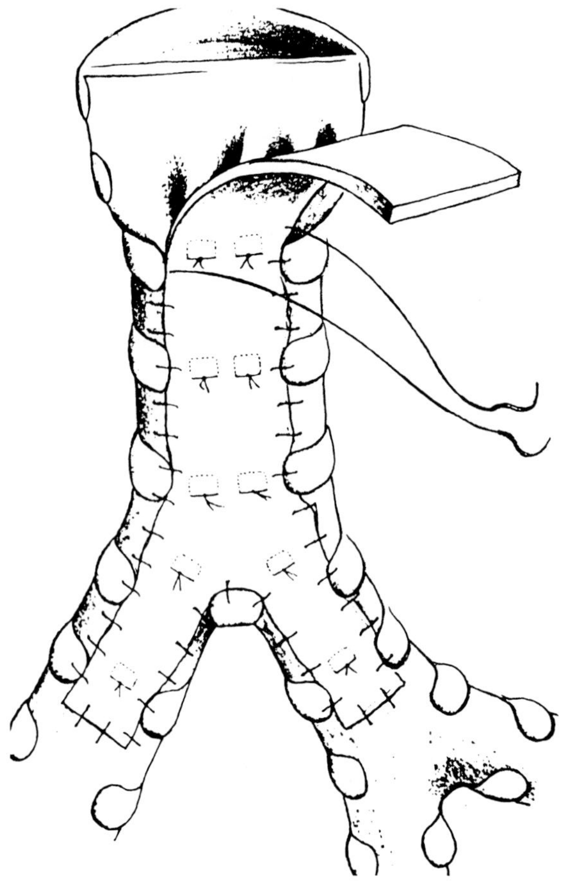

FIGURE 15–26 ■ This diagram illustrates Urschel's modification of Rainer's technique of tracheal stabilization. Urschel uses a silicone and Marlex plate to "reef" and stabilize the membranous part of the trachea and main bronchi.

resection with primary anastomosis. However, at surgery, the defect in cartilaginous support was found to extend from the thoracic inlet to the carina and major bronchi. The reason for the discrepancy between the preoperative assessment and the operative findings was that collapse occurred predominantly at the weakest site of the tracheal wall: resection and repair may then be followed by collapse of the adjacent segment.

Finally, internal stenting with either a silicone Montgomery T tube, a wire mesh stent (Wallstent, Schneider Inc., Minneapolis, MN, USA), or nitinol stent may be of value (see Postintubation Injury earlier in this chapter). Any of these stents can be ordered or custom-made to fit various size airways.

Chronic Compression

It is not possible to evaluate the extent of malacia in a patient with tracheal compression due to a mediastinal goiter before the enlarged gland has been resected and the pressure relieved. In most of these cases, the compressed segment of trachea is abnormally soft, but presents no airway problem after extubation. Most cases are manageable without a period of postoperative airway support. However, if breathing and coughing are critically impaired after extubation, an indwelling T tube offers an immediate solution; it can almost always be removed within a few weeks or months. A T tube is unquestionably superior to a conventional open tracheotomy. Other reported options include application, for external support, of a Marlex mesh wrap (Meurala, 1982) or of artificial rings of Gore-Tex and stainless steel wire (Geelhoed, 1988). Depending on the length of the involved segment, resection with primary anastomosis may occasionally be used.

In cases of relapsing polychondritis, with either diffuse or segmental malacic segments, some type of internal stent may provide good palliation.

SUMMARY

In summary, surgical experience is limited with respect to this type of diffuse malacic change. Undoubtedly, many patients may benefit from the available techniques, but the indications for selection have yet to be clearly defined. More sophisticated tests of airway dynamics are needed to better delineate indications for surgery. In some patients, internal stenting with silicone rubber tubes (T tubes, TY tubes, or Y tubes) or with a wire mesh stent may be a better alternative to external surgical stenting.

■ *KEY REFERENCES*

Rainer WG, Hutchinson D, Newby JP et al: Major airway collapsibility in the pathogenesis of obstructive emphysema. J Thorac Cardiovasc Surg 46:559, 1963.

This report clearly defines the pathophysiology of the most common form of tracheomalacia, one that is secondary to obstructive emphysema.

Rainer WG, Newby JP, Kelble DL: Long-term results of tracheal support surgery for emphysema. Dis Chest 53:765, 1968.

This is the first paper reporting longer-term follow-up in patients with tracheomalacia secondary to emphysema who have undergone surgical stabilization of the redundant membranous trachea. The authors also define details of surgical technique that might still be applied today.

■ *REFERENCES*

Aaby GV, Blake HA: Tracheobronchomegaly. Ann Thorac Surg 2:64, 1966.

Al-Mallah Z, Quantock OP: Tracheobronchomegaly. Thorax 23:230, 1968.

Amedee RG, Mann WJ, Lyons GD: Tracheomalacia repair using ceramic rings. Otolaryngol Head Neck Surg 106:270, 1992.

Ayres J, Rees J, Cochrane GM et al: Hemoptysis and non-organic upper airway obstruction in a patient with previously undiagnosed Ehlers-Danlos syndrome. Br J Dis Chest 75:309, 1981.

Bateson EM, Woo-Ming M: Tracheobronchomegaly. Clin Radiol 24:354, 1973.

Campbell AH, Gaulks LW: Expiratory air-flow pattern in tracheobronchial collapse in emphysema. Am Rev Resp Dis 92:781, 1965.

Dolan DL, Lemmon GB, Teitelbaum SL: Relapsing polychondritis: Analytical literature review and studies on pathogenesis. Am J Med 41:285, 1966.

Dunn WF, Hubmayr RD, Pairolero PC et al: The assessment of major airway function in a ventilator-dependent patient with tracheomalacia. Chest 97:939, 1990.

Ebringer R, Rook G, Swana GT et al: Auto-antibodies to cartilage and type II collagen in relapsing polychondritis and other rheumatic diseases. Ann Rheum Dis 40:473, 1981.

Foidart JM, Abe S, Martin GR et al: Antibodies to type II collagen in relapsing polychondritis. N Engl J Med 299:1203, 1978.

Gandevia B: The spirogram of gross expiratory tracheobronchial collapse in emphysema. Quart J Med 32:23, 1963.
Geelhoed GW: Tracheomalacia from compressing goiter: Management after thyroidectomy. Surgery 104:1100, 1988.
Greene R, Lechner GL: Saber-sheath trachea: A clinical and functional study of marked coronal narrowing of the intrathoracic trachea. Radiology 115:265, 1975.
Hanawa T, Ikeda S, Funatsu T et al: Development of a new surgical procedure for repairing tracheobronchomalacia. J Thorac Cardiovasc Surg 100:587, 1990.
Herzog H, Nissen R: Ershlaffung und exspiratorische Invagination des membranosen Teils der intrachorakalen Luftrohre und der Hauptbronchien als Urasche der asphyktischen Anfalle beim Asthma bronchiale und bei der chronischen asthmoiden Bronchitis des Lungenemphysems. Schweiz med Wchnschr 84:217 1954.
Hughes RAC, Berry CL, Seifert M et al: Relapsing polychondritis: Three cases with a clinicopathological study and literature review. Quart J Med 41:363, 1972.
Johnson RF, Green RA: Tracheobronchomegaly: Report of five cases and demonstration of a familial occurrence. Am Rev Resp Dis 91:35, 1965.
Katz I, LeVine M, Herman P: Tracheobronchomegaly: The Mounier-Kuhn syndrome. AJR Am J Roentgenol 88:1084, 1962.
Maisel JC, Silvers GW, Mitchell RS et al: Bronchial atrophy and dynamic expiratory collapse. Am Rev Respir Dis 98:988, 1968.
McAdam LP, O'Hanlan A, Bluestone R et al: Relapsing polychondritis: Prospective study of 23 patients and a review of the literature. Medicine 55:193, 1976.
Meurala H, Halttunen P, Standertskjold-Nordenstam C-G, Keskitalo E: Surgical support of collapsing intrathoracic tracheomalacia after thyroidectomy. Acta Chir Scand 148:127, 1982.
Mounier-Kuhn P: Dilatation de la trachee: Constations radiographiques et bronchoscopiques (Tracheal dilatation: Roentgenographic and bronchographic findings). Lyon Med 150:106, 1932.
Rainer WG, Feiler EM, Kelble DL: Surgical technic of major airway support for pulmonary emphysema. Am J Surg 110:788, 1965.
Rainer WG, Hutchinson D, Newby JP et al: Major airway collapsibility in the pathogenesis of obstructive emphysema. J Thorac Cardiovasc Surg 46:559, 1963.
Rainer WG, Newby JP, Kelble DL: Long term results of tracheal support surgery for emphysema. Dis Chest 53:765, 1968.
Thurlbeck WM, Pun R, Toth J et al: Bronchial cartilage in chronic obstructive lung disease. Am Rev Respir Dis 109:73, 1974.

INFLAMMATORY CONDITIONS

David N. Hopkinson
Shaf Keshavjee

Of relevance to thoracic surgeons are a few relatively uncommon inflammatory/infectious conditions and anatomic abnormalities, which may occur with symptoms of upper airway obstruction, or which may develop subsequent to the diagnosis of the primary systemic condition. If the tracheal lumen is compromised by any of these disorders, the spirometry and flow-volume loops demonstrate typical changes, with a disproportionate reduction in peak expiratory flow rate (PEFR) as compared with that of the first-second forced expiratory volume (FEV_1). Forced vital capacity (FVC) is usually unaltered. Fixed obstruction causes a reduction of both inspiratory and expiratory airflow. A dynamic obstruction in the extrathoracic airway has maximal effect on inspiration, whereas a dynamic lesion in the intrathoracic is manifest on expiration. An analysis of the flow-volume loops assists in determining the location and nature of the obstruction, and whether they are fixed or dynamic (Miller, 1973).

This chapter deals mainly with the involvement of the trachea by Wegener's granulomatosis, and still rarer conditions that cause tracheal narrowing, including tracheobronchopathia osteochondroplastica, tuberculosis, relapsing polychondritis, amyloidosis, "sabre-sheath" trachea, mediastinal fibrosis, and tracheobronchomegaly.

The diagnosis has often been made radiologically and occasionally by blood tests by the time the patient presents to the thoracic surgeon. Bronchoscopy and confirmatory biopsy may be required. Therefore, the role of the surgeon is often in securing patency of the upper airway with rigid bronchoscopy and dilatation and by tracheotomy in the most severe forms of these conditions. Occasionally, curative resection is indicated.

Wegener's Granulomatosis

HISTORICAL NOTE

In 1936, Wegener, in Breslau, described a syndrome in three patients, in whom necrotizing granulomata were found in the upper and lower respiratory tract. By 1954, an additional seven patients had been described, and consequently the definite criteria for the diagnosis of the disease were established (see later).

INCIDENCE

Wegener's granulomatosis is rare, with an incidence of two cases per million. It can occur at any age, with a peak in the 4th or 5th decade. The mean age is around 40 and almost any age above infancy may be affected, with no gender predilection. Most patients are Caucasian.

ETIOLOGY

The etiology of Wegener's granulomatosis remains unknown, and although the disease resembles an infectious process, no causative agent has been isolated.

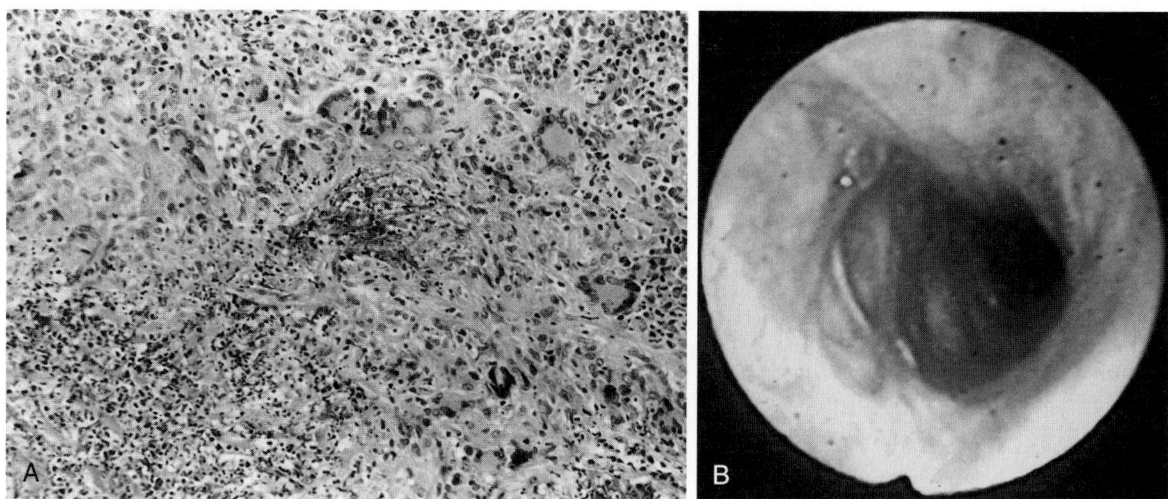

FIGURE 15–27 ■ Wegener's granulomatosis. Note the presence of giant cells and granulomata.

SYMPTOMS

Initial upper respiratory tract symptoms are common. Rhinorrhea, sinusitis, and ulceration of nasal membranes are early features, accompanied later by persistent cough and hemoptysis. Generalized features include fever, malaise, arthralgia, and night sweats. Hematuria and ocular symptoms may be present. Any of these symptoms may be present in isolation, or in combination with others, and there is often a delay in diagnosis. In the presence of tracheal granulomata (Fig. 15–27), symptoms of upper airway obstruction may be present, although it is rare for this to be the presenting feature (2%). Tracheal stenosis has been shown to be a feature in 16% of patients at sometime during the course of the disease (Hoffman et al, 1992).

DIAGNOSIS

The American College of Rheumatology has defined diagnostic criteria for Wegener's granulomatosis as follows: (1) Abnormal urinary sediment, red-cell casts or greater than five red cells per high power field; (2) nodular cavities on plain chest radiograph; (3) oral ulcers or nasal discharge; and (4) granulomatous inflammation on tissue biopsy. Two or more of these 4 features are highly suggestive of the diagnosis (Leavitt et al, 1990).

There are no specific laboratory tests. There may be anemia, leukocytosis, and elevated erythrocyte sedimentation rate (ESR). Chest radiography may demonstrate parenchymal infiltrates. Nodules up to 10 cm in diameter occur, and central necrosis may give the appearance of cavitating lesions (Yoshikawa et al, 1986). There is a strong positive correlation with the presence of antineutrophilic cytoplasmic antibody (ANCA). The ANCA level appears to correlate with disease activity (Specks et al, 1989).

Because of the frequency of nasal involvement, the otolaryngologist plays an important role in the early diagnosis and treatment of Wegener's granulomatosis. (McDonald and DeRemme, 1983). Biopsy of the nose and paranasal sinuses reveals typical perivascular inflammation, giant cells, and granulomata (Fraser and Paré, 1995). The subglottis and upper trachea involved and lend themselves to CT imaging, which will define the site, level, and submucosal extent of tracheal involvement (Stein et al, 1986). The differential diagnosis includes carcinoma, lymphoma and tuberculosis.

TREATMENT

Treatment of the systemic manifestations involves corticosteroids, which invoke a variable response, together with cyclophosphamide (Arauz and Fonseca, 1982; Hoffman et al, 1992). Management of specific subglottic and tracheal involvement depends on the extent of the disease. Unfortunately, in many cases it is rarely sufficiently localized to permit resection with a primary anastomosis, and the imaging often serves to define the most appropriate level for tracheotomy (Stein et al, 1986). In some instances, this becomes permanent, although a few patients may be decannulated (Arauz and Fonseca, 1982).

Historically, there has been concern about the wisdom of surgical intervention during concurrent immunosuppressive therapy and the possible recurrence of disease at the tracheal anastomosis (McDonald et al, 1982). However, if it can be demonstrated by serial ANCA assay that the disease is in remission, then in the presence of an isolated tracheal lesion (usually subglottic), surgery should be considered. A report of a series of five such selected cases demonstrated the feasible option of surgical resection with primary thyrotracheal anastomosis (see Chapter 14). Clinical remission had been achieved using cyclophosphamide and prednisone. There was no postoperative morbidity despite concurrent cytotoxic and steroid therapy in some cases (Herridge et al, 1996).

Tracheobronchopathia Osteochondroplastica

ETIOLOGY

This rare condition, affecting predominantly men over 50 years of age, is characterized by the development of

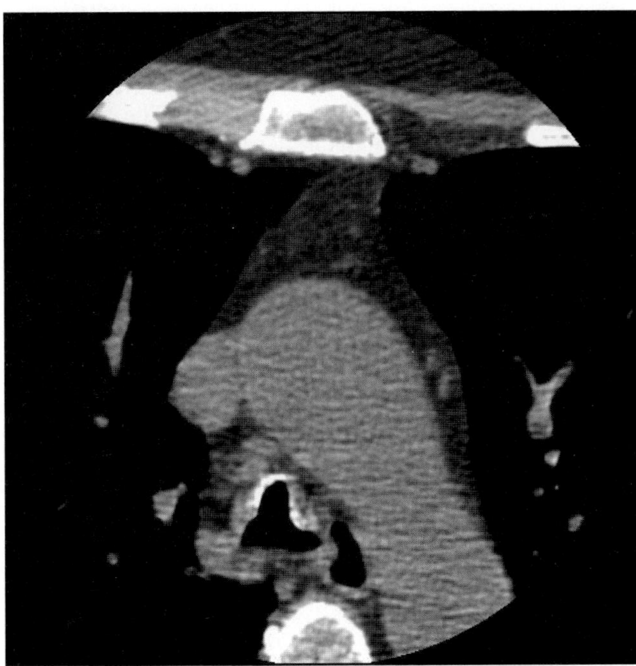

FIGURE 15–28 ■ Tracheopathia osteochondroplastica: computer tomographic appearance.

spicules or nodules of cartilage and bone in the submucosa of the trachea and bronchi (Baird and McCartney, 1966). Histologically, these lesions, which usually arise in continuity with the cartilaginous elements of the upper airway, may contain bone and marrow. The condition has been linked with amyloidosis (Sakula, 1968) and is thought, by some, to be a late complication of this chronic condition in which dystrophic calcification of any organ affected may occur (Clee et al, 1983). However, although amyloidosis can involve the entire circumference of the trachea, tracheopathia does not. It has also been reported in association with *Mycobacterium avium-intracellulare* (Baugnee, 1995). The diagnosis is often made only at post-mortem.

SYMPTOMS

Clinical features of tracheobrachopathia osteochondroplastica include a gradual onset of exertional dyspnea owing to airway obstruction, and hemoptysis caused by mucosal ulceration (Clee, 1983).

DIAGNOSIS

Flow-volume loops show typical obstructive features for this condition and are used to monitor disease progression (Neinhuis, 1990). Diagnosis is made by CT, which easily defines the sites of irregular calcification (Fig. 15–28). Distally, involvement may become more circumferential. Bronchoscopy reveals the irregular, hard, nodules that protrude into the tracheal lumen (Fig. 15–29).

TREATMENT

Dilatation and removal of part, or some of the bone spicules may be possible using a rigid bronchoscope. Other methods described include cryotherapy, laser excision, and external beam irradiation (Neinhuis et al, 1990). Rarely does the condition progress beyond mild to moderate airflow limitation.

Relapsing Polychondritis

ETIOLOGY

Relapsing polychondritis is a systemic disease that may affect any cartilage-containing structure (Dolan et al, 1966). It affects both sexes equally, unless there is airway involvement, in which case females are affected predominantly. It is associated with systemic lupus erythematosus

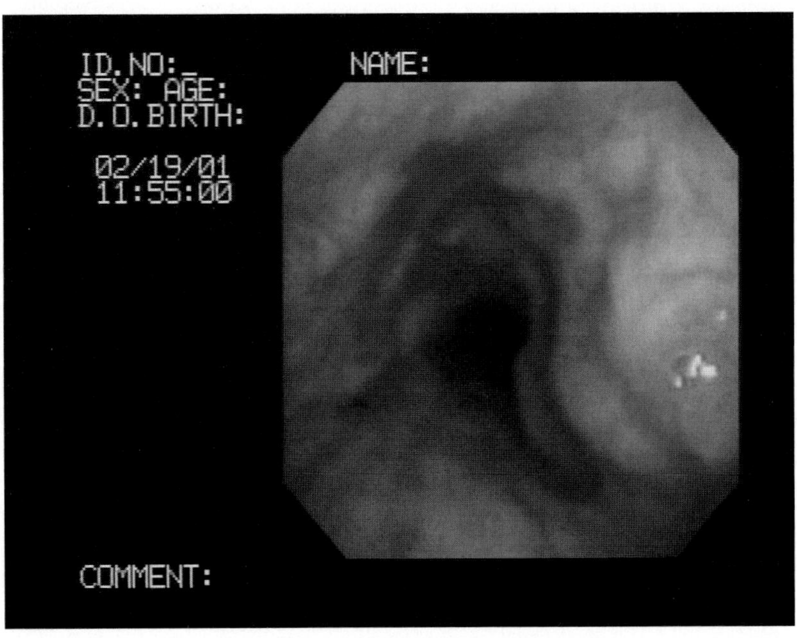

FIGURE 15–29 ■ Tracheopathia osteochondroplastica: bronchoscopic appearance.

and Wegener's granulomatosis, and, therefore, it is generally thought to be an autoimmune disease (Fraser and Paré, 1995). It is characterized by symmetrical narrowing of the upper airways (typically the subglottic region) giving rise to a fixed upper-airway obstruction. However, it may affect any part of the trachea or main bronchi down to the segmental orifices.

DIAGNOSIS

Diagnosis of the generalized disorder is by demonstration of recurrent inflammation of at least three cartilaginous sites. Usually, these are the nasal septum and the aural helix, although occasionally a tracheal biopsy is required. Biopsy demonstrates perivascular infiltration of plasma cells and lymphocytes. Auto-antibodies to cartilage have been demonstrated in a high proportion of patients (Foidart et al, 1978). Tracheal lesions take up Gallium-67, which may serve to localize the disease and assess ongoing disease activity (Dupont et al, 1983). Inspiratory flow rates are reduced less than expiratory flow rates, which is typical of intrathoracic large airway obstruction.

Bronchoscopy is useful in determining the nature and extent of the disease. It should be remembered that deaths have occurred during this procedure. Bronchoscopy may reveal severe inflammation of the tracheobronchial tree or collapse of the airways. These may open on introduction of the bronchoscope, but collapse on withdrawal.

TREATMENT

Medical management involves use of corticosteroids, which may attenuate progression of the tracheal narrowing. Pulsed high-dose steroids are given in acute exacerbations of chondritis at any site. Immunosuppressive agents such as methotrexate, azathioprine, and cyclosporine are used with variable efficacy in an attempt to lower the doses of prednisone required for maintenance therapy (Trentham and Le, 1998). Tracheal cartilage may collapse suddenly, requiring emergency tracheotomy. The Montgomery T tube (Neville, 1990) and metallic stents have been used (Dunne and Sabanathan, 1994). Tracheotomy alone, in the presence of extensive disease, is of no value without the addition of positive pressure ventilation. Dynamic obstruction secondary to collapse of the upper airway may be amenable to splinting techniques. Localized disease may be treated by supporting the posterior membranous wall (Herzog, 1987). A variety of materials have been used in this and other disorders causing tracheal collapse, including dura mater, pericardium, and GoreTex mesh (Halttunen, 1981). In extensive disease, external splintage through a right thoracotomy has been described, applying tissue adhesive or sutures to stabilize the soft, redundant posterior membranous trachea (Eng, 1989).

"Sabre-sheath" trachea

Normally, the sagittal diameter of the trachea is slightly greater than the coronal diameter. In this rare condition, which affects mostly males, the coronal diameter of the intrathoracic portion is reduced by more than 50%. The narrow section typically extends proximally from the carina along the entire thoracic trachea. The subglottic portion is unaffected. Tracheal calcification commonly occurs, rendering the condition easily detectable on posteroanterior and lateral radiographs (Green and Lechner, 1945).

Tracheobronchomegaly

Tracheobronchomegaly condition predominantly affects men in their 4th or 5th decade. Cystic dilatation of the tracheo bronchial tree may occur anywhere from the larynx to the periphery of the lung. It is characterized by markedly increased compliance of the trachea, abnormal flaccidity, and the propensity to collapse during forced expiration. Diverticula-like protrusions of intercartilaginous tissue extend outwards. A tracheal diameter greater than 3 cm (up to 5 cm) is typical and usually confirms the diagnosis. Although the clinical features are similar to the syndrome of tracheomalacia (due to any cause), it represents a distinct disease entity.

Granulomatous Conditions

TUBERCULOSIS

Focal involvement of the trachea by *Mycobacterium tuberculosis* may arise as a primary focus within the mucosa of the trachea, or by direct extension of infection from a contiguous lymph node. A primary focus within the lung parenchyma may also invade the tracheal wall. Rarely, the proximal airways may be involved due to hematogenous miliary tuberculosis via the bronchial arteries. Tracheal tuberculosis is usually associated with parenchymal disease, but active tracheobronchial infection may persist in a chronic form after the pulmonary disease has healed (Fraser and Paré, 1995). In early infection, the mucosa appears irregular and edematous. Later, ulcers and fibrotic stenosis may be evident, requiring dilatation stent placement or resection. Biopsy demonstrates typical inserting granulomatous inflammation.

AMYLOIDOSIS

Other chronic inflammatory conditions such as sarcoidosis and amyloidosis may cause diffuse narrowing. Amyloidosis appears as smooth, greyish-yellow sessile tumors. Intermittent bronchoscopic resection is the usual mode of treatment (Fleming, 1980), although the use of carbon-dioxide laser photoresection has been described (Breuer 1985). Following this modality, subglottic edema may ensue requiring temporary tracheotomy.

SCLEROMA

Scleroma typically affects the paranasal sinuses and is caused by chronic granulomatous infection with *Klebsiella rhinoscleromatis*. Tracheal involvement occurs in approximately 5% of cases and is characterized by either diffuse symmetric narrowing or nodular masses (Choplin et al, 1983). This is usually a late complication of a chronic disease process.

FIBROSING MEDIASTINITIS

Mediastinal granuloma and fibrosis are chronic forms of mediastinitis that can occasionally give rise to extrinsic compression of the lower trachea. In granuloma, the pathology is confined to lymph nodes that exhibit capsular fibrosis. With fibrosis, the reaction infiltrates the entire mediastinum. Infection with tuberculosis or histoplasmosis is thought to be the cause of most cases, and tracheal or bronchial compression is reported in up to 50% of cases (Goodwin, 1972). Stenting of the lower trachea may be required when the airway lumen has been compromised either by progressive stenosis or direct lymph node erosion.

MISCELLANEOUS

Ankylosis of the cricoarytenoid joint may occur in longstanding rheumatoid arthritis (Kandora et al, 1985). Intratracheal thymus has been documented as a rare cause of tracheal obstruction (Martin and McAllister, 1987).

SUMMARY

The thoracic surgeon should be aware of these challenging conditions, which require diagnosis and consideration of palliative forms of therapy such as tracheotomy and stent placement. However, in experienced hands, surgery may cure localized tracheal lesions and vascular anomalies, with good results.

■ *REFERENCES*

Arauz JC, Fonseca R: Wegener's granulomatosis appearing initially in the trachea. Ann Otol Rhinol Laryngol 91:593, 1982.

Akyol MU, Martin AA, Dhurandhar N, Miller RH: Tracheobronchopathia osteochondroplastica: A case report and review of the literature. Ear Nose Throat J 72:347, 1993.

Baird RD, McCartney JW: Tracheobronchopathia osteoplastica. Thorax 21:321, 1966.

Baugnee PE, Delaunois LM: *Mycobacterium avium-intracellulare* associated with tracheobronchoplastica osteochondroplastica. Eur Respir J 8:180, 1995.

Breuer R, Simpson GT, Robinow A et al: Tracheobronchial amyloidosis: Treatment by carbon-dioxide laser photoresection. Thorax 40:870, 1985.

Choplin RH, Wehunt WD, Theros EG et al: Diffuse lesions of the trachea. Semin Roentgenol 18:38, 1983.

Clee MD, Anderson JM, Johnston RN et al: Clinical aspects of tracheobronchopathia osteochondroplastica. Br J Dis Chest 77:308, 1983.

Dolan DC, Lemmon GB, Treitelbaum SC: Relapsing polychondritis: Analytical literature review and studies on pathogenesis. Am J Med 41:285, 1966.

Dunne JA, Sabanathan S: Use of metallic stents in relapsing polychondritis. Chest 105:864, 1994.

Dupont A, Bossuyt A, Sommers G et al: Relapsing polychondritis: Gallium-67 uptake in recurrent lung lesions. J Nucl Med Allied Sci 27:57, 1983.

Eng J, Sabanathan S: Tissue adhesive in bronchial closure. Ann Thorac Surg 48:683, 1989.

Eng J, Sabanathan S: Airway complications in relapsing polychondritis. Ann Thorac Surg 51:686, 1991.

Fleming AFS, Fairfax AJ, Arnold AG, Lane DJ: Treatment of endobronchial amyloidosis by intermittent bronchoscopic resection. Br J Dis Chest 74:183, 1980.

Foidart JM, Abe S, Martin GR et al: Antibodies to type II collagen in relapsing polychondritis. N Engl J Med 299:1203, 1978.

Fraser RS, Paré JAP: Diseases of the airways. In Fraser RS, Paré JAP, Fraser RG, Paré PD (eds): Synopsis of diseases of the chest. 3rd ed. Philadelphia, WB Saunders, 1995.

Goodwin RA, Nickell JA, Des Prez RM: Mediastinal fibrosis complicating healed primary histoplasmosis and tuberculosis. Medicine 51:227, 1972.

Greene R, Lechner GL: "Sabre-sheath trachea": Clinical and functional study of marked coronal narrowing of the intrathoracic trachea. Radiology 115:265–269, 1975.

Herridge MS, Pearson FG, Downey GP: Subglottic stenosis complicating Wegener's granulomatosis: Surgical repair as a viable treatment option. J Thorac Cardiovasc Surg 111:961, 1996.

Herzog H, Heitz M, Keller R, Graedel E: Surgical therapy for expiratory collapse of the trachea and large bronchi. In Grillo HC, Eschapsse H (eds): International Trends in General Thoracic Surgery, Vol 2. Philadelphia, W.B. Saunders, 1987.

Hoffman GS, Ken GS, Leavitt RY et al: Wegener's granulomatosis: An analysis of 158 patients. Ann Intern Med 116:488, 1992.

Kandora TF, Gilmore IM, Sorber JA et al: Cricoarytenoid arthritis presenting as a respiratory arrest. Am Emerg Med 14:700, 1985.

Leavitt RY, Fauchi AS, Bloch DA et al: The American College of Rheumatologists 1990 criteria for the classification of Wegener's granulomatosis. Arthritis Rheum 33:1101, 1990.

McDonald TJ, DeRemee RA: Wegener's granulomatosis. Laryngoscope 93:220, 1983.

McDonald TJ, Neel HB, DeRemee RA: Wegener's granulomatosis of the subglottis and upper portion of the trachea. Ann Otol Rhinol Laryngol 91:588, 1982.

Maayan C, Mogle P, Tal A et al: Prolonged wheezing and tracheal compression caused by aberrant right subclavian artery. Thorax 36:793, 1981.

Martin KW, McAllister WH: Intratracheal thymus: A rare cause of airway obstruction. AJR Am J Roentgenol 149:1217, 1987.

Miller RD, Hyatt RE: Evaluation of obstructing lesions of the trachea and larynx by flow volume loops. Am Rev Resp Dis 108:475, 1973.

Nienhuis DM, Prakash UB, Edell ES: Tracheobronchopathia osteochondroplastica. Ann Otol Rhinol Laryngol 99:689, 1990.

Sakula A: Tracheobronchopathia osteoblastica: Its relationship to primary tracheobronchial amyloidosis. Thorax 23:105, 1968.

Specks U, Wheatley CL, McDonald TJ et al: Anticytoplasmic auto antibodies in the diagnosis and follow-up of Wegener's granulomatosis. Mayo Clinic Proc 64:28, 1989.

Stein MG, Gamsu G, Webb WR, Stulbarg MS: Computed tomography of diffuse tracheal stenosis in Wegener granulomatosis. J Comput Assist Tomogr 10:868, 1986.

Trentham DE, Le CH: Relapsing polychondritis. Ann Intern Med 129:114, 1998.

Yoshikawa Y, Watanabe T: Pulmonary lesions in Wegeners granulomatosis: A clinicopathologic study of 22 autopsy cases. Hum Pathol 17:401, 1986.

CHAPTER **16**

Laryngeal Nerve Palsy

Clement A. Hiebert
Dorothea Liebermann-Meffert
Dennis H. Kraus

The larynx is wired to the brain by four nerves, the lower two of which, the right and left recurrent laryngeal nerves (RLNs), lie in corridors alongside the trachea, esophagus, and great vessels, corridors defined by Liebermann-Meffert and colleagues in 1999. In contrast to these gross conduits for air, food, and blood, the recurrent nerves are inconspicuous strings, easily mistaken for connective tissue and exposed to invasion by cancer, stretching by an aneurysm, or crushing by a surgical instrument. It is an unwelcome fact that most laryngeal nerve trauma occurs in the operating room (Table 16–1).

The purpose of this chapter is to review the asymmetric anatomy and function of the laryngeal nerves, draw attention to the consequences of their being disabled, and look at what may be done when the circuits are interrupted.

HISTORICAL NOTE

Although Hippocrates recognized the clinical symptoms of hoarseness and dysphagia, the historian Major (1954) credits Marinos, an anatomist in AD 100, with identifying the inferior nerves to the larynx and the 2nd-century surgeon Galen with proving their function. Major tells how Galen returned to Pergamon after 11 years of anatomic study in Alexandria and shortly thereafter was appointed surgeon at the gladiatorial amphitheater, a natural venue for studying cross-sectional neck anatomy. It was an era when dissection of a human cadaver was reckoned an unholy act. Galen purportedly demonstrated that dividing the laryngeal nerves in a laboratory pig destroyed the animal's ability to squeal. By tracing the parent nerve, that is, the vagus, to the brain, he disproved the philosophically agreeable, but archaic, dogma that speech emanates from the heart.

Except for observations of wounds produced by swords and spears, surgeons had little opportunity to study cadavers until the Renaissance ushered in an enlightened attitude toward dissecting the human body. Even so, the 1700 years between Galen and the 19th century saw little in the way of new or useful information until operations on the thyroid gland and cervical esophagus reintroduced the surgeon to the subject of laryngeal nerve injury.

According to Major, the earliest observation of a nonrecurrent laryngeal nerve was made in a cadaver by Stedman (1823). One hundred years later, Pemberton and Beaver (1932) recognized the implications for a surgeon operating in the neck or thoracic inlet.

In 1833, Hooper observed the complementary role of the external branch of the superior laryngeal nerve in raising the pitch of a singer's voice. Years later, Terracol (1931) confirmed the cricothyroid muscle as an essential cord adductor.

Using optical magnification, Liebermann-Meffert and colleagues (1999) have reported on 34 postmortem studies showing overlapping innervation of all but one of the laryngeal muscles, new information that may explain the variable consequences of single nerve injury.

■ *HISTORICAL READINGS*

Leibermann-Meffert DMI, Walbrun BW, Hiebert CA, Siewert JR: Recurrent and superior laryngeal nerves: A new look with implications for the esophageal surgeon. Ann Thorac Surg 67:217–223, 1999.

Major RH: A History of Medicine, Vol 1. Springfield, IL, Charles C Thomas, 1954, pp 191, 220.

TABLE 16–1 ■ **Incidence (%) of the Causes of Vocal Cord Paralysis in Various Series Reported**

	Hagan (N = 100)	*Maisel and Ogura (N = 181)*	*Titche (N = 134)*	*Parnell and Brandenburg (N = 100)*	*Average*
Neoplastic	23	20	38	35	29
Traumatic	9	23	11	12	14
Surgical	35	23	11	28	24
CNS disease	13	8	16	7	11
Inflammatory	10	6	20	6	10.5
Toxic	5	—	—	2	1.5
Idiopathic	5	20	4	10	10

Modified from Montgomery WW. Surgery of the Upper Respiratory System, Vol. 2, 2nd ed. Malvern, PA. Lea & Febiger, 1989, p 607.

Pemberton J, Beaver MG: Anomaly of the right recurrent laryngeal nerve. Surg Gynecol Obstet 54:594, 1932.

Stedman GW: A singular distribution of some of the nerves and arteries of the neck and the top of the thorax. Edinb Med Surg J 19:564, 1823; (cited in Henry JF, Audifrett J, Denizot A, Plan M: The nonrecurrent inferior laryngeal nerve: Review of 33 cases, including two on the left side. Surgery 104:6, 1988)

LARYNGEAL NERVE FUNCTION

The key functions of the laryngeal nerves are the following:

- Opening the cords for breathing
- Sealing the airway for swallowing
- Approximating the cords for phonation

The first two functions are critical to survival, in contrast to phonation, an embellishment for speaking, humming, singing, laughing, crying, and saying "Aaaah" in the doctor's office. Breathing and swallowing keep us going, but the ability to speak and to sing makes life worthwhile. Figure 16–1 lists the essential and ornamental uses of the vocal cords in various positions. Most of these functions are voluntary. An exception is the act of swallowing, which abruptly closes the glottis and cancels both phonation and breathing. It is impossible to speak and to swallow at the same time.

Speech rides on expiration, with one exception—the *gasp.* Triggered by astonishment, fear, pain, or delight, the gasp is a vocalized exclamation point formed by *inspiring* through drawn cords. The pitch and length of the gasp reveal both the character and intensity of what may be joy or alarm. Opening that perfect present, for example, might evoke an appreciative gasp of delight, in contrast to a long inhaled wail appropriate to discovering a corpse in the bedroom closet. Gasping is part of everyday communication in the Scottish Highlands and Down East Maine where "ayuh," uttered rapidly *on inspiration,* is a curious shibboleth meaning "yes."

ANATOMY

Recurrent Laryngeal Nerve Anatomy

Each RLN arises from the ipsilateral vagus, which, in turn, springs from the medulla oblongata to become, at the start, the longest and broadest of all the cranial nerves (Fig. 16–2).

On the *left* side, the RLN is given off close to the ligamentum arteriosum whence it loops front to back around the aorta before ascending to the neck under cover of loose connective tissue. The left RLN is longer and lies measurably closer to the esophageal wall than the nerve on the right (Liebermann-Meffert et al, 1999).

The *right* RLN arises at the level of the first portion of the subclavian artery around which it loops to ascend on a somewhat more diagonal line than its opposite number. The asymmetric course of the RLNs is of interest to esophageal surgeons, who generally choose the left thoracic inlet as the avenue for transposing stomach or colon to the neck. The RLN is less in the way. Additionally, the cervical esophagus veers slightly to the left (see Chapter 2, *Esophageal Surgery* 2nd ed, Fig. 1–7) making the construction of an anastomosis from that side easier for a right-handed surgeon.

At the level of the thyroid gland the nerve's slack and sinuous course straightens, and 2 or 3 cm before each RLN enters the larynx it crosses loops of the inferior thyroid artery, which may be anterior, posterior, or on both sides of the nerve. Precise dissection, clamping, and ligation of vessels is required. In half of human dissec-

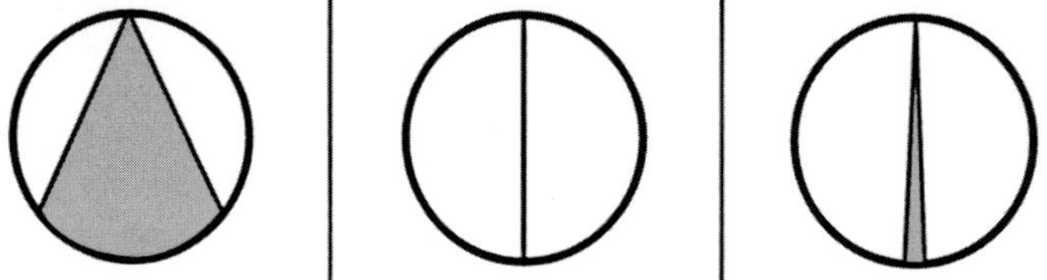

Cord Position	Abducted (open)	Adducted (sealed)	Adducted (loosely)
Primary Use	Breathing	Airway protection while swallowing Coughing	Speaking Singing Humming
But also for:	Huffing Whispering Gargling Whistling Blowing out a candle Sniffing a rose	Straining to initiate urination or defecation Parturition	Laughing Crying Clearing phlegm Groaning Moaning Shouting Gasping

FIGURE 16–1 ■ Overview of laryngeal functions.

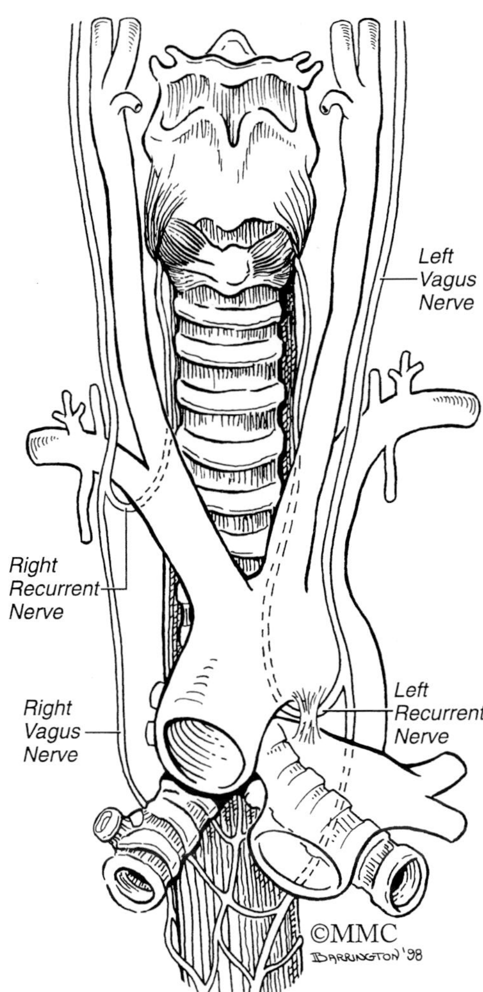

FIGURE 16–2 ■ Anatomy of the right and left recurrent laryngeal nerves. Tracheal and esophageal branches are not shown.

tions of this area, Liebermann-Meffert and colleagues (1999) found short RLN twigs that penetrated the deep surface of the thyroid gland. The significance of these small nerves is not known.

Before each recurrent nerve enters the larynx, it sends 8 to 14 short branches into the *lateral* wall of the esophagus and trachea. These branches are visible during operations on the upper sphincter, especially if one chooses a lateral approach, uses optical loupes, and gently draws the RLN away from the tracheoesophageal groove. The parent nerve dives into the laryngopharynx at the lateral caudal margin of the cricopharyngeus. On entering the larynx, the terminal branches of the RLN lie firmly rooted between the thin mucosa and its backing of cartilage and bone. It has occurred to at least one of us (CAH) that local pressure from an indwelling tube in the airway or pharynx, however well-positioned, may explain idiopathic postintubation laryngeal nerve paresis.

A new finding by Liebermann-Meffert and colleagues (1999) is the overlapping innervation of the laryngeal muscles by terminal twigs of both recurrent and superior laryngeal nerves with the exceptions that the posterior cricoarytenoid muscle appears to be innervated by the RLN alone and the cricothyroideus muscle receives only fibers from the superior laryngeal nerve (SLN).

Nonrecurrent Laryngeal Nerve

Of special anatomic concern to surgeons is the nonrecurrent laryngeal nerve (Fig. 16–3), an uncommon but important anomaly associated with a right subclavian artery that arises from the left side of the aortic arch distal to the origin of the left subclavian artery. The developing recurrent nerve, having no vessel around which to loop, passes directly from the vagus to the larynx. The investigation of dysphagia lusoria with contrast studies of the aortic arch and esophagus makes the diagnosis. In a review of 6307 operations on the thyroid or parathyroid glands, Henry (1988) found 33 instances of nonrecurrent inferior laryngeal nerves, 31 of which were on the right side. The two patients with a left nonrecurrent nerve had situs inversus and a right-sided arch.

Superior Laryngeal Nerves

Using magnified dissection techniques, Liebermann-Meffert and colleagues (1999) traced the SLN from its bifur-

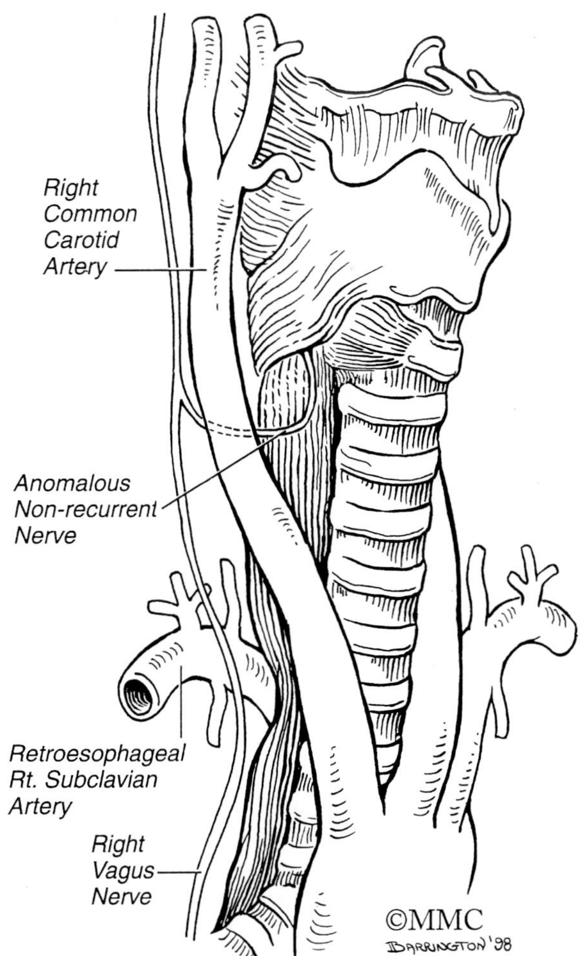

FIGURE 16–3 ■ Anatomy of the nonrecurrent nerve. Note the esophageal compression by the anomalous retroesophageal right subclavian artery.

cation into internal and external divisions above and behind the crotch of the carotid arteries. The external branch innervated the cricothyroid muscle while the internal branch pierced the thyroid membrane, split into three divisions, and sent branches to the aryepiglotticus, arytenoideus transversus, arytenoideus obliquus, and cricoarytenoideus lateralis.

The upper laryngeal nerves are subject to injury during wide dissection of the superior pole vessels during thyroidectomy. Unless involved with cancer, the SLNs can usually be avoided by precise isolation of the pole vessels before clamping or ligating them. In contrast to the RLNs, the SLNs are rarely encountered by the thoracic surgeon.

CAUSES OF RECURRENT NERVE PALSY

Natural Causes

Among the natural causes of RLN paralysis are invasion by primary or metastatic cancer of the lung, trachea, esophagus, or thyroid gland. Dayal (1981) noted that the left nerve is twice as frequently involved as the right, a not surprising discovery given its longer course and proximity to hilar lymph nodes. Less frequently, an aortic aneurysm or dilated left atrium may disable the nerve. Other nonmalignant causes of laryngeal nerve dysfunction include alcoholism, lead poisoning, and radiation. Dayal alleges that one third of all cases of vocal cord paralysis are idiopathic.

Iatrogenic Causes

Surgical damage to the RLNs is said to occur in 0.05% to 37% of operations in the neck or upper thorax (Orringer and Orringer, 1983). Injury at times may be unavoidable, especially when one is operating for cancer and requires wide margins. An incomplete listing of operations with inherent risk for RLN damage would include the following.

- Transhiatal esophagectomy
- Thyroidectomy
- Parathyroid exploration
- Correction of Zenker's diverticulum
- Carotid artery surgery
- Pleural pneumonectomy
- Right upper lobectomy
- First rib resection
- Aortic arch surgery
- Carotid body resection
- Nerve sheath tumor resection
- Radical neck dissection
- Tracheal resection
- Patent ductus arteriosus correction
- Pancoast's tumor resection
- Mediastinal tumor resection

SELECTED POINTS ON AVOIDING OPERATIVE INJURY

Transhiatal Esophagectomy

Transhiatal esophagectomy exposes the left recurrent nerve to neuropraxis from traction or avulsion during blunt dissection in the region of the aortic arch. Orringer and Orringer (1983) recommend keeping the index and third fingers of each hand closely applied to the anterior and posterior aspects of the esophagus.

A second area of RLN vulnerability is in the neck, where the nerve lies more or less parallel to the trachea and in front of and somewhat lateral to the esophagus. Medial retraction of the trachea with a self-retaining retractor can cause pressure damage to the nerve and ostensibly did so in 38% of Orringer and Orringer's (1983) first series of patients undergoing transhiatal esophagectomy. The authors later eschewed use of a self-retaining retractor and by 1991 had reduced the incidence of RLN palsy to 2.5%. Our recommendation is to expose and identify the nerve and to position the retractor(s) with the left nerve in view.

The right recurrent nerve is vulnerable during encirclement of the cervical esophagus with a rubber drain or tube such as routinely used for traction. The far side of the esophagus is not visible, and if the right-angled clamp or Semb dissector drifts from the outer esophageal muscle layer it can inadvertently capture the right laryngeal nerve. A No. 46 French bougie passed through the mouth may help to define the far unseen edge of the esophagus.

Liebermann-Meffert and colleagues (1999) note that transsecting the esophagus close to the pharynx exposes the RLNs and branches to the esophagus and trachea to injury and suggest that an anastomosis is more safely constructed given 2.5 cm or more of proximal esophagus.

Other Procedures

Operations about the cervical trachea inevitably carry a risk for disrupting the RLNs. Pearson (personal communication, 1999) and Grillo (1983) agree that the safest approach when operating for benign disease is to keep the dissection close to the trachea and to reduce the current to the lowest hemostatically useful level.

Visualization of the recurrent nerves makes sense when contemplating wider resections for malignant tracheal tumors or in operations for tumors of the thyroid gland or esophagus that have invaded the trachea. When paresis of a single vocal cord already exists, it is in the patient's interest to identify and preserve the functioning nerve, at least until it is clear that the tumor is otherwise nonresectable.

In contrast to operations on the larynx or cervical trachea, when the patient is likely to have been alerted to the possibility of laryngeal dysfunction, awakening to speech and swallowing problems following procedures unrelated to the larynx can be difficult for the physician to explain and for the patient to understand. Better that the surgeon discuss the possibility with the patient beforehand.

Searching for parathyroid glands, especially aberrant ones, inevitably puts the nerves at risk. The special circumstance of a right-sided parathyroid tumor presenting as a mediastinal shadow may be more safely approached through the neck.

Idiopathic Postoperative Paresis

Using human specimens and optically magnified dissection technique, Liebermann-Meffert and colleagues

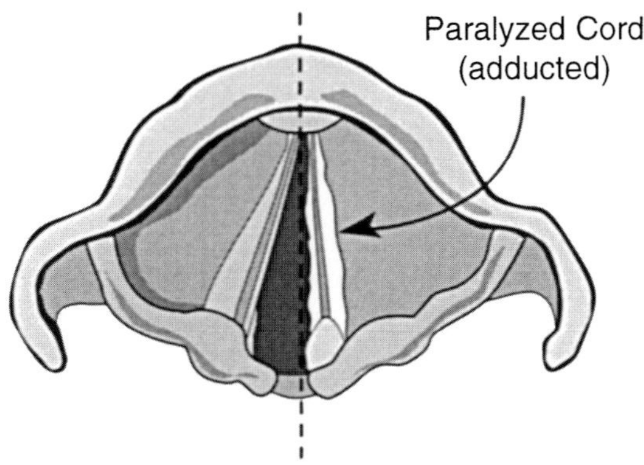

FIGURE 16–4 ■ Paralyzed cord (adducted position).

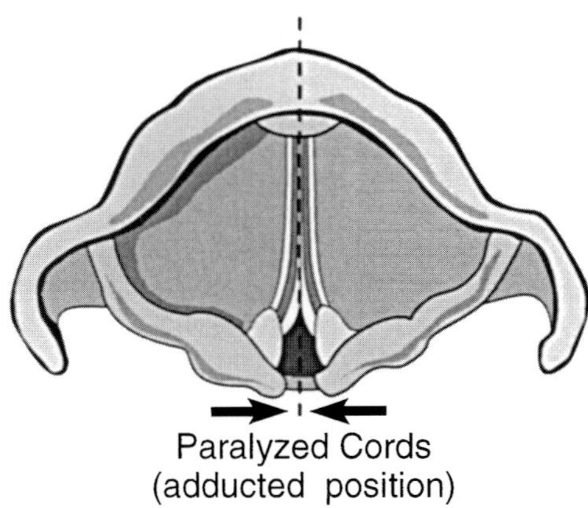

FIGURE 16–6 ■ Paralyzed cords (adducted position).

(1999) have shown that the terminal branches of the RLNs lie essentially unprotected beneath the thin mucosa of the pharynx and larynx. The question of occult pressure injury from an adjacent endotracheal tube is noted. The same reasoning would seem to apply to electing an endoscopic approach for Zenker's diverticulum. When intubated patients undergoing operations remote from the neck have postoperative dysphagia, dysphonia, and aspiration, such symptoms are likely to be viewed as idiopathic RLN palsy. Given the anatomic information now available, it at least seems possible that the culprit is an indwelling airway tube positioned against an uncushioned laryngeal nerve. The matter remains speculative, pending further study.

DIAGNOSIS

Clinical Features of Recurrent Nerve Injury

The most conspicuous evidence of unilateral nerve failure is change in the pitch, force, and timbre of phonation, but the spectrum of symptoms varies from near-normal speech to hoarseness, breathlessness, choking, and aspiration. Montgomery (1989) catalogs three objective variables: (1) unilaterality or bilaterality of recurrent nerve failure, (2) position of the cords, and (3) compensatory movement of the functioning cord.

The default position of a paralyzed vocal cord is determined by the sum of the vector forces acting on that cord. This resultant varies. Some examples follow.

Unilateral paralysis with cord adducted. Unilateral paralysis with the cord in the position of adduction (Fig. 16–4) impairs pitch in singing, but the speaking voice and airway may be close to normal. No treatment is required.

Unilateral paralysis with cord abducted. Unilateral paralysis of the RLN and the cord in the position of abduction (Fig. 16–5) results in breathy hoarseness or aphonia, depending on the degree of abduction. The afflicted individual is unable to cough or laugh. Aspiration, especially of liquids, is the rule. In time, the normal cord may swing across the midline and partially close the chink, but given no improvement within 6 months to 1 year, either injection of the immobile cord or a phonoplastic operation may be performed to enhance cord approximation (see Management).

Bilateral paralysis with cords adducted. Bilateral RLN paralysis with the cords adducted (Fig. 16–6) places the patient in constant danger of obstruction and almost always requires a permanent tracheostomy. Without such a vent the patient must suffer inspiratory stridor and the possibility of unheralded asphyxiation.

Bilateral paralysis with cords abducted. Bilateral paralysis with the cords abducted (Fig. 16–7) leaves the patient without a voice. Coughing is ineffective. Aspiration of

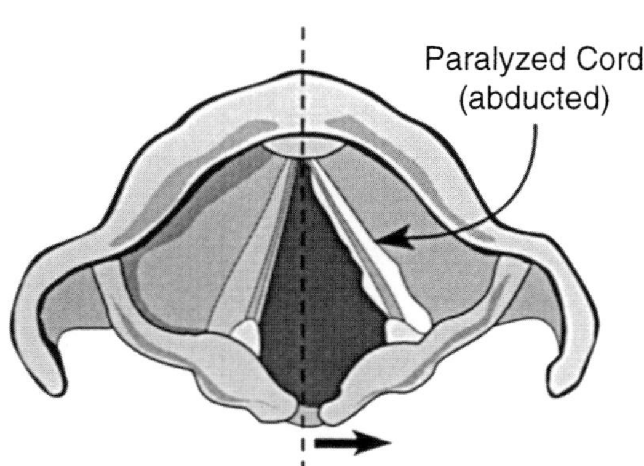

FIGURE 16–5 ■ Paralyzed cord (abducted position).

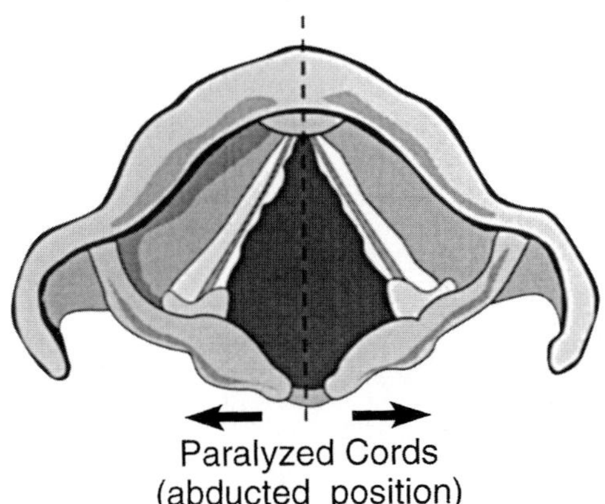

FIGURE 16–7 ■ Paralyzed cords (abducted position).

saliva and food is severe, and tracheostomy with a cuffed tube may be required as a temporizing measure. For the long term, Montgomery (1989) suggests either laryngectomy and tracheostomy or Habal and Murray's (1972) operation of sealing the larynx permanently with a flap of epiglottis.

There is a human side to the loss of recurrent nerve function that is not conveyed by anatomic descriptions. Explanation is less awkward for the surgeon when nerves succumb to natural events, such as invasion by a tumor; then we tell the patient, "You have a paralyzed vocal cord." When the nerve may have been cut with the scalpel or Bovie knife, a less incriminating euphemism emerges: "hoarseness," we say. The patient could tell us more if we took the time to ask: aspiration results when reflexes that normally shunt air to the trachea and food to the pharynx fail. With time the patient learns to swallow without aspirating by pressing the chin against the chest. Coughing is ineffective, as are lesser efforts to clear the throat. A Valsalva maneuver is impossible. Singing, laughing, and raising the voice, let alone shouting, are compromised. Force and timbre of the voice may improve as the working cord moves across the midline, but toward evening fatigue sets in.

MANAGEMENT

In deciding which patients require surgical rehabilitation for vocal cord paralysis, there are several factors to be considered. Is the RLN bruised, severed, or merely shaken up (Fig. 16–8)? Will the nerve recover on its own? Has there been previous operative or radiation treatment for a head or neck cancer? What is the overall prognosis for the patient? Unoperated patients or patients with a nonresectable intrathoracic malignancy who present with vocal cord paralysis will almost never regain nerve function. Other patients in whom "curative" left upper lobectomy, pneumonectomy, or cervical esophagectomy has been performed, and in whom the proximal vagus nerve, RLN, or both have been skeletonized but left anatomically intact, may have return of function up to 1 year from the time of the operation, according to Woo and colleagues (1991).

Hoarseness, taken alone, is only a relative indication for early surgical treatment, an exception being the individual who is professionally dependent on oral communication. Multiple symptoms are a different matter. Dysphagia, aspiration, and inability to generate a proper cough generally argue for early correction. When return of cord function is in doubt, laryngeal electromyography (EMG) may help to identify surgical candidates.

Temporary Dysfunction

When spontaneous return of laryngeal function is anticipated, temporizing procedures are often useful. The majority of these are based on adding bulk to the paralyzed vocal cord so as to advance its free edge toward the midline. A variety of fillers are available, including Gelfoam, fat, collagen, and glycerin.

Fat and collagen tend to migrate or resorb. Therefore, in the setting of expected return of function. to inject Gelfoam into the substance of the deficient cord. This procedure is performed in the operating room using topical anesthesia and intravenous sedation. Gelfoam powder is converted to a paste with sterile saline and then loaded into a Bruening injector; it resembles a caulking gun. Utilizing an anterior commissure laryngoscope, the para-

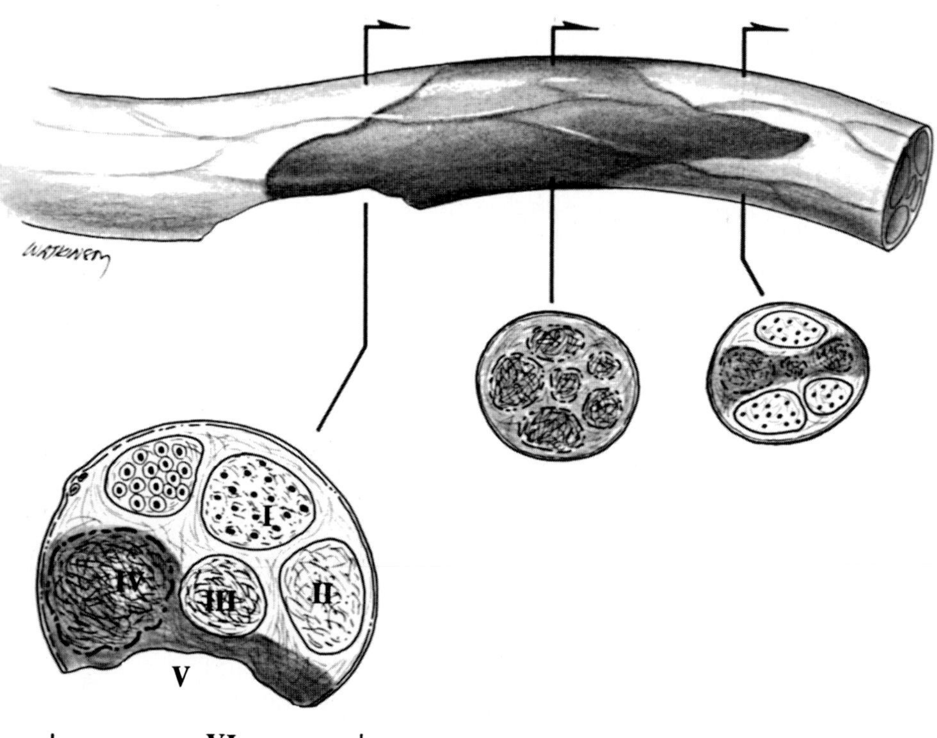

FIGURE 16–8 ■ Mackinnon's sixth-degree injury, a situation where fibers and fascicles are variably injured. The likelihood of spontaneous recovery is certain with first- and second-degree injuries and nil with fourth- and fifth-degree injuries.

lyzed vocal cord is identified and the false vocal cord is retracted laterally. The needle is then positioned in the substance of the vocal fold, and the Gelfoam is injected (Fig. 16–9). An attempt is made to overcorrect slightly, anticipating possible resorption of the Gelfoam paste over 4 to 8 weeks. Patients usually receive steroids for a short period to prevent or minimize airway obstruction.

More permanent cord enhancement may be achieved using a custom-cut wedge of silicone to nudge the disabled cord toward the midline (Figs. 16–10, 16–11, and 16–12). This open technique is especially useful for patients for whom laryngeal electromyelography is unavailable and the return of vocal function is uncertain. Patients are informed of the possibility of subtle voice changes due to scarring, as well as the need to remove the implant should there be a spontaneous return of vocal cord function.

Permanent Dysfunction

For the patient with a permanent vocal cord paralysis either from deliberately or inadvertently sacrificing a laryngeal nerve during, say, a cancer operation, there are various options. Mackinnon and Dellon (1988) suggest an epineural repair when the ends will come together (Fig. 16–13) and insertion of a short graft taken from a cervical sensory nerve when they will not. Recovery of the voice following end-to-end repair has been reported, but the skeptic will note the extremely variable response of patients to unilateral vocal cord paralysis. Compensation by the contralateral cord is a factor, and spontaneous recovery of a less than completely damaged RLN may occur over 6 to 9 months.

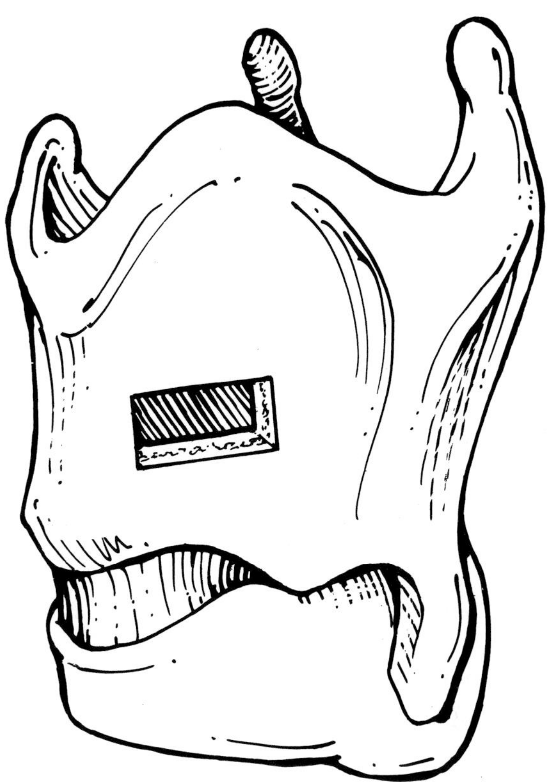

FIGURE 16–10 ■ Preparation of thyroid cartilage for silicone wedge insertion.

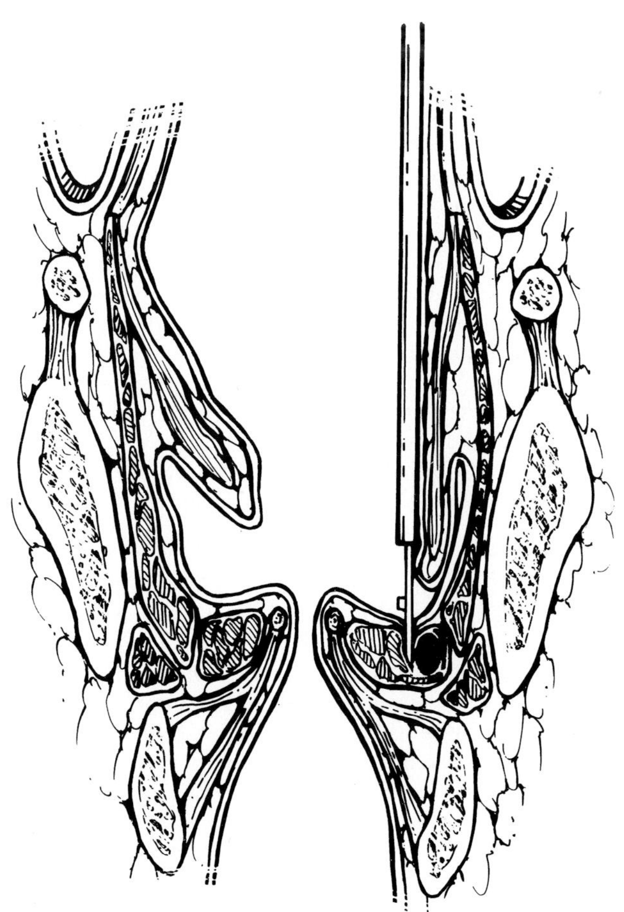

FIGURE 16–9 ■ Technique of Gelfoam injection to advance the functional free edge of a denervated cord toward the midline.

The situation may be urgent following operations requiring placement of a double-lumen endotracheal tube for one-lung ventilation. Patients may initially have good vocal cord function, owing to edema from intubation trauma, and this edema may effectively medialize the paralyzed vocal cord. After the initial 48 to 72 postoperative hours, however, the edema resolves and the patient experiences increasing hoarseness, aspiration, pulmonary congestion, and an ineffective cough. The situation may require repeated bronchoscopy for clearing secretions and consideration of urgent permanent medialization. "Medialization" refers to improving speech, swallowing, and breathing functions by moving the paralyzed cord to a medial position.

A number of techniques are available for permanent medialization. As noted earlier, neither fat nor collagen injections reliably remain in the paralyzed vocal cord, and over the years the standard treatment was cord augmentation with Teflon. But Teflon proved to have its own shortcomings, the most significant of which was the development of a chronic granuloma. Teflon technique, furthermore, proved a challenge to teach because once injected the material cannot be withdrawn.

During the last two decades, Teflon injection has

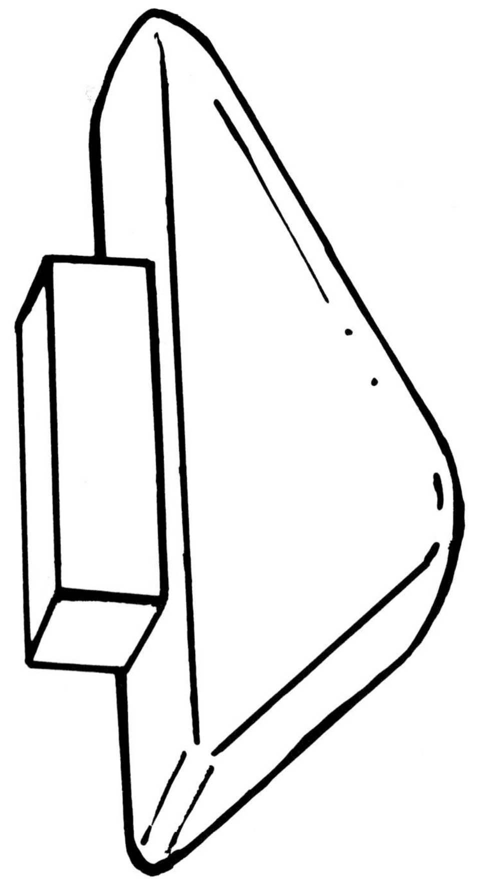

FIGURE 16–11 ■ Enlarged view of silicone wedge.

largely been replaced by open medialization, described by Meurman (1952), modified by Isshiki and colleagues (1974), and tested by others, including Kraus and coworkers (1999). This transcutaneous procedure is performed under local and topical anesthesia and consists of positioning a hand-crafted Silastic implant in a pocket on

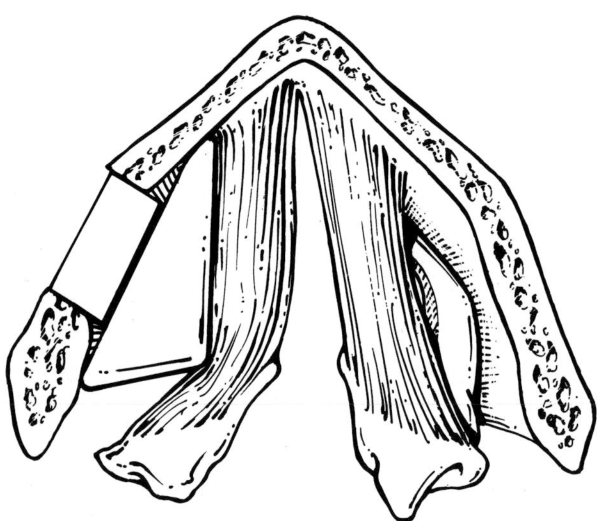

FIGURE 16–12 ■ Cutaway view of the partially medialized cord.

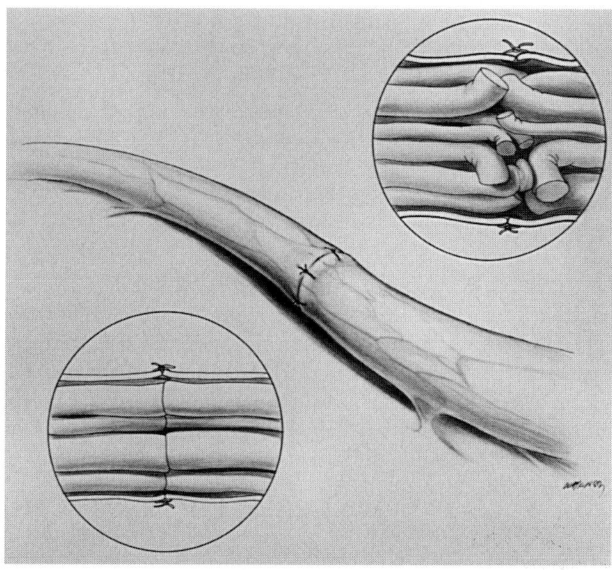

FIGURE 16–13 ■ Repaired nerve. The surgeon's expectation *(lower left)* is contrasted with the all too frequent result *(upper right).* Accurate alignment of sensory and motor neurons is elusive. (From Mackinnon SE: Upper extremity nerve injuries: Primary repair and reconstruction. In Cohen ML [ed]: Mastery of Surgery—Plastic Surgery. Boston, Little, Brown, 1992.)

the deep surface of the thyroid cartilage; this implant partially displaces the paralyzed cord toward the midline. Kraus and colleagues have noted satisfactory or excellent results in 57 of 63 patients with RLN palsy attributed to intrathoracic malignancy.

The major shortcoming of Silastic medialization is the residual triangular gap in the posterior commissure at the level of the arytenoid cartilage. Isshiki and colleagues (1978) and Netterville and associates (1993) recommend adding another suture to close the chink, a maneuver that improves phonation, breathing, and swallowing without aspiration. Kraus and associates (1999) agree.

The incidence of bleeding, infection, implant extrusion, and airway obstruction is approximately 1% each. Infection has decreased with the use of perioperative antibiotics, and transient airway edema has been reduced since the introduction of intravenous steroids. Nevertheless, long-term survival of these patients is not very likely. Palliation remains the goal.

The patient with *bilateral* vocal cord paralysis constitutes a different problem. If the vocal cords meet in the midline, patients may be able to generate good voice and, in some instances, swallow agreeably. The lurking lifelong threat, however, is sudden compromise of the airway. Traditionally these patients have been treated with a permanent tracheostomy. Ventilation improvement is dramatic, but accumulating secretions sentence survivors to living an arm's length away from a suction device.

If the patient has adequate respiration, and functional return of at least one cord is anticipated, a laser arytenoidectomy to widen the posterior commissure may be elected. Enthusiasm for doing this, however, is tempered by the knowledge that these patients will continue to have difficulty sealing the airway during swallowing.

CONCLUSIONS AND RECOMMENDATIONS

As with other functions of the human body that are taken for granted, the larynx, that quintessential instrument of human connectedness, attracts the physician's attention only when it breaks down. The laryngeal nerves cross the domains of thoracic, vascular, esophageal, and general thoracic surgeons and are easily injured. They tend to quit when squeezed by an aneurysm, invaded by cancer, or pinched by a forceps. It is a sobering fact that most RLN failure is iatrogenic. Knowing the fine anatomy of the nerves, the details of diagnosis, and techniques to restore laryngeal function is important, but the best approach is prevention. Based on a successful operative experience of deliberately exposing the RLN over 600 times, one of us (CAH) offers the following prescription:

- It is better to learn the anatomy of the laryngeal nerves in the dissecting room than in the operating room.
- Use a headlamp and optical loupes.
- Beware of grasping or cutting any filamentous structure until the recurrent nerve has been identified. (There are a few exceptions, notably in tracheal surgery and mediastinoscopy.)
- Even after identifying the nerve, remember that its meandering course may catch the inattentive operator unaware.
- Be gentle with retraction and sparing with the cautery.
- When possible, construct an esophagogastrostomy at least 2.5 cm away from the pharyngoesophageal junction.
- Alert the patient beforehand of the possibility of nerve damage, and note that the conditions for which the thoracic surgeon usually operates, if uncorrected, also place the respiratory, swallowing, and speech functions at risk.

COMMENTS AND CONTROVERSIES

Recurrent laryngeal nerve palsies can be devastating for the patient as well as the surgeon. Many of the common symptoms attributed to this dysfunction include hoarseness, which is sometimes debilitating, inability to cough and clear secretions, and aspiration, especially of liquids. Less recognized is the inability to modulate the expiratory phase of breathing, which results in loss of intrinsic positive end-expiratory pressure, early airway collapse during the expiratory phase, atelectasis, and pneumonia. The patient often experiences significant shortness of breath because of this. All of these complications can be devastating, especially in the face of a recently reconstructed esophagogastric anastomosis or pneumonectomy. For this reason, at Memorial Sloan-Kettering we have taken a very aggressive approach in the early recognition and management of postoperative RLN palsy. Once it is recognized, if symptomatic, we advocate early correction, usually within 48 hours of the primary surgery. If, on the other hand, the patient's contralateral vocal cord is compensating, no correction is necessary. The authors have described the various methods of correction in detail.

In bilateral vocal cord palsies, immediate tracheostomy is not always necessary. However, the patient must be observed extremely closely and when episodes of recurrent stridor are evident, tracheostomy is required to protect the airway. In such cases, a vented tracheostomy will allow for speech and, ultimately, a small T tube can be employed, keeping the T portion occluded to be opened at night during sleeping hours and whenever an episode of stridor begins.

In many of these cases, the palsy is not permanent and up to 1 year is required for recovery of function.

As stated, prevention is the key to success, as this requires gentle dissection, avoidance of significant retraction when performing surgery around the cervical esophagus and trachea, and avoidance of unipolar cautery in the region of the recurrent nerves.

R.J.G.

KEY REFERENCES

Liebermann-Meffert DMI, Walbrun BW, Hiebert CA, Siewert JR: Recurrent and superior laryngeal nerves: A new look with implications for the esophageal surgeon. Ann Thorac Surg 67:217–223, 1999.

A painstaking anatomic study of the laryngeal nerves. Among the findings are overlapping innervation of the RLN with the SLN and a plausible explanation of idiopathic vocal cord paralysis.

Mackinnon SE, Dellon AL: Surgery of the Peripheral Nerve. New York, Thieme, 1988.

A thorough, scholarly, and beautifully illustrated examination of nerve injury and repair.

Montgomery WW: Laryngeal paralysis. In Surgery of the Upper Respiratory System, Vol 2, 2nd ed. Malvern, PA, Lea & Febiger, 1989, p 607.

An excellent overview covering all aspects of laryngeal paralysis.

Rice DH: Laryngeal reinnervation. Laryngoscope 92:1049, 1982.

A useful review of the multitude of procedures attempted to improve the lot of patients with vocal cord paralysis, with discussion and suggestions for further research.

REFERENCES

Dayal DS: Clinical Otolaryngology. Philadelphia, Lippincott, 1981.

Grillo HC: Congenital lesions, neoplasms, and injuries of the trachea. In Sabiston DC, Spencer FC (eds): Gibbon's Surgery of the Chest, Vol 1. 4th ed. Philadelphia, WB Saunders, 1983.

Habal MB, Murray JE: Surgical treatment of life-endangering chronic aspiration pneumonia. Use of an epiglottic flap to the arytenoids. Plast Reconstr Surg 49:305, 1972.

Henry JF: Nonrecurring recurrent laryngeal nerve. Surgery 104:977, 1988.

Isshiki N, Morita H, Okamura H et al: Thyroplasty as a new phonosurgical technique. Acta Otolaryngol (Stockh) 78:451–457, 1974.

Isshiki N, Tanabe M, Sawanda M: Arytenoid adduction for unilateral vocal cord paralysis. Arch Otolaryngol 104:555–558, 1978.

Kraus DH, Ali MK, Ginsberg RJ et al: Vocal cord medialization for unilateral vocal cord paralysis associated with intrathoracic malignancies. J Thorac Cardiovasc Surg 111:334–341, 1996.

Kraus DH, Orlikoff RF, Risk SS, Rosenberg DB: Arytenoid adduction as an adjunct to type I thyroplasty for unilateral vocal cord paralysis. Head Neck 21:52–59, 1999.

Liebermann-Meffert DMI, Walbrun BW, Hiebert CA, Siewert JR: Recurrent and superior laryngeal nerves: A new look with implications for the esophageal surgeon. Ann Thorac Surg 67:217–223, 1999.

Mackinnon SE: Upper extremity nerve injuries: Primary repair and reconstruction. In Cohen ML (ed): Mastery of Surgery—Plastic Surgery. Boston, Little, Brown, 1992.

Mackinnon SE, Dellon A: Surgery of the Peripheral Nerve. New York, Thieme, 1988, p 35.

Major RH: A History of Medicine, Vol 1. Springfield, IL, Charles C Thomas, 1954, pp 191, 220.

Meurman Y: Operative mediofixation of the vocal cord in complete unilateral paralysis. Arch Otolaryngol (Stockh) 55:544–553, 1952.

Montgomery WW: Laryngeal paralysis. In Surgery of the Upper Respiratory System, Vol 2, 2nd ed. Malvern, PA, Lea & Febiger, 1989, p 607.

Netterville JL, Stone RE, Luken ES, et al: Silastic medialization and arytenoid adduction: The Vanderbilt experience. Ann Otol Rhinol Laryngol 102:413–424, 1993.

Orringer MB, Orringer JS: Esophagectomy without thoracotomy: A dangerous operation? J Thorac Cardiovasc Surg 85:72, 1983.

Pemberton J, Beaver MG: Anomaly of the right recurrent laryngeal nerve. Surg Gynecol Obstet 54:594, 1932.

Rice DH: Laryngeal reinnervation. Laryngoscope 92:1049, 1982.

Stedman GW: A singular distribution of some of the nerves and arteries of the neck and the top of the thorax. Edinb Med Surg J 19:564, 1823; cited in Henry JF, Audifrett J, Denizot A, Plan M: The nonrecurrent inferior laryngeal nerve: Review of 33 cases, including two on the left side. Surgery 104:6, 1988.

Woo P, Colton R, Brewer D, Casper J: Functional staging for vocal cord paralysis. Otolaryngol Head Neck Surg 105:440–448, 1991.

CHAPTER 17

Acquired Tracheoesophageal Fistula

Alan G. Casson

Drew C. Bethune

DEFINITION

An acquired communication (i.e., fistula) between the trachea and esophagus is an uncommon lesion, which may be classified by etiology, anatomic site of communication, or mode of onset (acute, subacute, chronic). In current clinical practice, malignancy, prolonged tracheal intubation, and trauma are the most frequent predisposing factors for acquired tracheoesophageal fistula. Management may be challenging, to control not only the underlying disease but also the life-threatening pulmonary complications associated with this condition.

This chapter does not address congenital tracheoesophageal fistula, which is discussed in detail in Chapter 8, *Esophageal Surgery,* 2nd ed.

HISTORICAL NOTE

Trauma, granulomatous infections of the mediastinum, and malignancy were considered to be the most frequent predisposing factors for acquired tracheoesophageal fistula until the late 1950s and early 1960s (Coleman, 1957; Wychulis and Ellis, 1966). With increasing use of mechanical ventilation, the importance of prolonged tracheal intubation, particularly related to cuff inflation pressures, was appreciated throughout the next decade (Bargh and Slawson, 1965; Cooper and Grillo, 1969; Flege, 1967; Thomas, 1972, 1973). Early surgical attempts to close the fistula, using various operative strategies, were generally unsuccessful, until Grillo and colleagues (1976) reported their initial, successful experience with a single-stage repair, performed after patients were weaned from the ventilator.

■ *HISTORICAL READINGS*

Bargh W, Slawson KB: Experience with an artificial ventilation unit. Br J Anaesth 37:574, 1965.

Coleman FP: Acquired nonmalignant esophagorespiratory fistula. Am J Surg 93:321, 1957.

Cooper JD, Grillo HC: The evolution of tracheal injury due to ventilatory assistance through cuffed tubes: A pathologic study. Ann Surg 169:334, 1969.

Flege JB: Tracheoesophageal fistula caused by cuffed tracheostomy tube. Ann Thorac Surg 166:153, 1967.

Grillo HC, Moncure AC, McEnany MT: Repair of inflammatory tracheoesophageal fistula. Ann Thorac Surg 22:113, 1976.

Thomas AN: Management of tracheoesophageal fistula caused by cuffed tracheal tubes. Am J Surg 124:181, 1972.

Thomas AN: The diagnosis and treatment of tracheoesophageal fistula caused by cuffed tracheal tubes. J Thorac Cardiovasc Surg 65:612, 1973.

Wychulis AR, Ellis FH: Acquired non-malignant esophagotracheobronchial fistula. JAMA 196:117, 1966.

BASIC SCIENCE

Etiology

Acquired tracheoesophageal fistula has a diverse etiology. In current clinical practice, it is most frequently a consequence of malignancy, including direct invasion by esophageal, lung, or thyroid tumors (Dartevelle and Macchiarini, 1996; Green et al, 1983); mediastinal non-Hodgkin's and Hodgkin's lymphomas (Ling and Bushunow, 1996; Orvidas et al, 1994; Small et al, 1995); prolonged ventilation (Cherveniakov et al, 1996; Couraud et al, 1996; Dartevelle and Macchiarini, 1996; Mathisen et al, 1991); penetrating and blunt thoracic trauma (Reed et al, 1995; Sebastian and Wolfe, 1997; Weber et al, 1996; Weiman et al, 1995, 1996); and iatrogenic injury, following esophageal resection (Bartels et al, 1998; Houben, 1998), laryngectomy (Buchanan et al, 1995), esophageal dilatation for caustic injury (Cherveniakov et al, 1996; Mutaf et al, 1995), tracheal intubation for inhalation injury (Tan et al, 1993), esophageal stenting (Schowengerdt, 1999), and bronchial artery infusion therapy (Yiengpruksawan et al, 1984). Although chemotherapy (Jougon and Couraud, 1998) and chemoradiotherapy (Kinsman et al, 1996) for mediastinal lymphomas have been implicated as etiologic factors, this has recently been disputed (Raijman et al, 1997).

A variety of mediastinal infections and granulomatous processes are still associated with the development of acquired tracheoesophageal fistula, including tuberculosis (Shah et al, 1994); mediastinal actinomycosis (Dux et al, 1994); herpes esophagitis (Cirillo et al, 1993); Wegener's granulomatosis (Conces et al, 1995); acquired immunodeficiency syndrome (Chow et al, 1992; Temes et al, 1995); dual infection with *Candida albicans* and cytomegalovirus (Rusconi et al, 1994); and *Staphylococcus aureus* neck abscess (Ahmad and Lee, 1999). Esophageal foreign bodies (Rahbar and Farha, 1978; Tucker et al, 1994) and Zenker's diverticulum (Senders and Babin, 1983) have also been implicated.

Pathophysiology

In a landmark study, Cooper and Grillo (1969) reported the evolution of tracheoesophageal fistulas developing in patients requiring prolonged mechanical ventilation for respiratory failure. Direct pressure necrosis by high-pressure cuffs of endotracheal or tracheostomy tubes resulted in microscopic ulceration of the tracheal mucosa within 3 to 5 days. This progressed to deeper, confluent ulceration exposing the tracheal cartilage. Whereas healing resulted in circumferential stricture formation or tracheomalacia (if cartilaginous support is lost), persistent inflammation and infection resulted in fragmentation of cartilage and ulceration. Full-thickness inflammation of the posterior membranous trachea resulted in perforation into the adjacent esophagus, which remained compressed against the vertebral bodies. The presence of a rigid nasogastric tube appeared to provide a fixed point for ulceration. Other contributing factors included diabetes mellitus, steroid use, hypotension, and excessive movement of the endotracheal or tracheostomy tube.

The pathophysiology of acquired tracheoesophageal fistula associated with other etiologic factors varies: transmural invasion of the esophageal wall in herpes infection, vasculitis associated with cytomegalovirus infection, necrosis of the tracheal and esophageal walls following bronchial artery infusion, and direct tumor invasion have all been proposed.

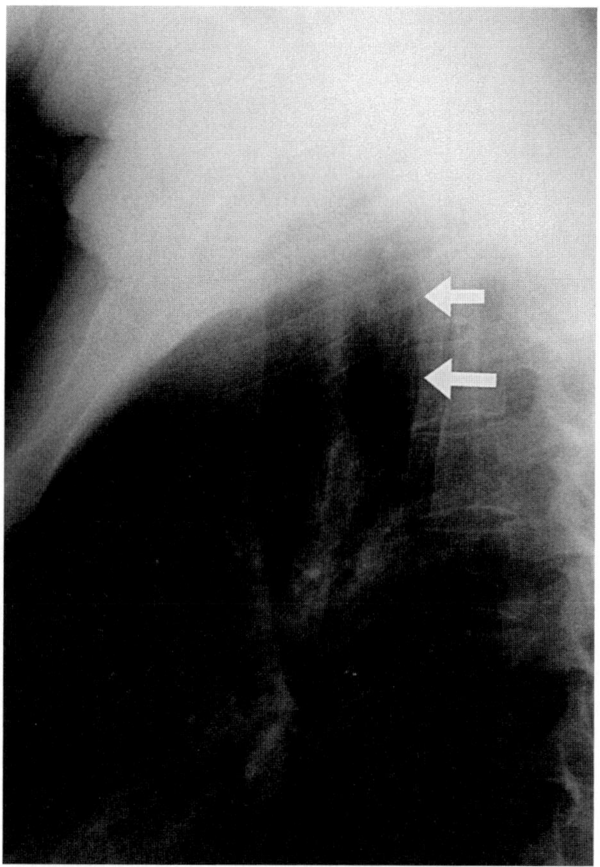

FIGURE 17–1 ■ Lateral chest radiograph illustrating a prominent, dilated, air-filled esophagus *(arrows)* posterior to the trachea. The patient was subsequently diagnosed with a malignant tracheoesophageal fistula. (Courtesy of H. Henteleff MD.)

DIAGNOSIS

Clinical Features

Because symptoms and signs of a tracheoesophageal fistula may vary widely depending on the etiology and clinical setting, a high index of suspicion for this diagnosis should be maintained. The clinical presentation will range from symptoms and signs directly attributable to the fistula, to complications (principally pulmonary) arising from the fistula and from the underlying disease.

In patients who can swallow, persistent and often violent coughing, especially with liquids, is highly suggestive of a communication between the esophagus and airway. Patients may expectorate sputum mixed with food, particulate matter, or colored dye if given orally. Chest pain and hemoptysis are infrequent.

However, for most patients requiring mechanical ventilation, suctioning of gastric contents from the airway, often associated with sudden gastric distention, are virtually diagnostic for a tracheoesophageal fistula.

Natural History

Spontaneous closure of an acquired tracheoesophageal fistula is infrequent, although this has been reported for small, linear fistulas of traumatic origin (Couraud et al, 1996).

In acute tracheoesophageal fistula, usually post-traumatic, mediastinitis and abscess formation may occur. However, in the majority of patients, the tracheoesophageal fistula has evolved relatively slowly, with the development of fibrous adhesions between the esophageal wall and membranous trachea, protecting the mediastinum from contamination. The degree of pulmonary contamination initially depends on the size and location of the fistula, as well as the position of the patient. Overflow of esophageal, oral, or gastric contents across the fistula into the tracheobronchial tree results in various pulmonary sequelae, including bronchial obstruction, pneumonia, respiratory distress, and adult respiratory distress syndrome (ARDS), which are inevitably fatal if untreated. Long-term prognosis is also dependent on the underlying disease and the extent of nutritional depletion.

Differential Diagnosis

It is important to differentiate direct communication (i.e., fistula) from indirect contamination (i.e., aspiration) of the airway, which may result from anatomic or functional esophageal obstructions. These include benign and malignant esophageal strictures, primary and secondary motor disorders of the esophageal body, neurogenic or myogenic cricopharyngeal disorders, and other functional diseases, including achalasia and gastroesophageal reflux disease.

Investigative Techniques

Radiologic Techniques

A plain chest radiograph may initially be normal, but will subsequently demonstrate the spectrum of pulmonary complications attributable to the fistula (i.e., pulmonary infiltrates, pneumonia, ARDS). Occasionally, other nonspecific, and subtle, findings may suggest the diagnosis; for example, air within the dilated esophagus (Fig. 17–1). Although computed tomography (CT) has been reported to be diagnostic (Berkmen and Auh, 1985; Lee et al, 1996), this study is more useful for the investigation and staging of underlying disease.

The diagnosis of a tracheoesophageal fistula may be made (sometimes inadvertently) at the time of contrast esophagography (Fig. 17–2*A*). In this situation, dilute barium is preferred to hyperosmolar, water-soluble contrast agents, which may result in clinically significant aspiration pneumonitis (see Fig. 17–2*B*). The barium esophagogram will also provide useful information about the extent of esophageal obstruction.

Endoscopy

Endoscopic examination of the upper aerodigestive tract is the most useful technique to diagnose a tracheoesophageal fistula, to evaluate associated disease, and to exclude foreign bodies. Bronchoscopy and esophagoscopy may be performed using rigid or flexible instrumentation and under general or local anesthesia, as determined by the clinical setting.

Bronchoscopy is the most useful examination to directly visualize the location and extent of the fistula. Biopsies of the posterior membranous trachea adjacent to the fistula should be taken to obtain a histologic diagnosis if malignancy is suspected. The entire trachea should be examined for associated mucosal ulceration, stricture, or tracheomalacia, including the tracheostoma if present. The distal tracheobronchial tree should also be visualized, and secretions should be suctioned and sent for culture to identify microorganisms as a guide to systemic antibiotic therapy.

A large fistula may also be visualized directly and biopsied by esophagoscopy. However, this technique is less accurate in evaluating smaller fistulas, which may remain hidden in folds of esophageal mucosa. Esophagogastroscopy is essential to evaluate the extent of associated esophageal disease, especially if esophageal stenting is planned.

MANAGEMENT

Principles of Management

Few individuals, or centers, have an extensive experience with the management of acquired tracheoesophageal fistulas, as they have a varied etiology and are relatively uncommon. Two large series reported surgical experience with only 38 patients (Mathisen et al, 1991) and 41 patients (Gudovsky et al, 1993) over 20 years.

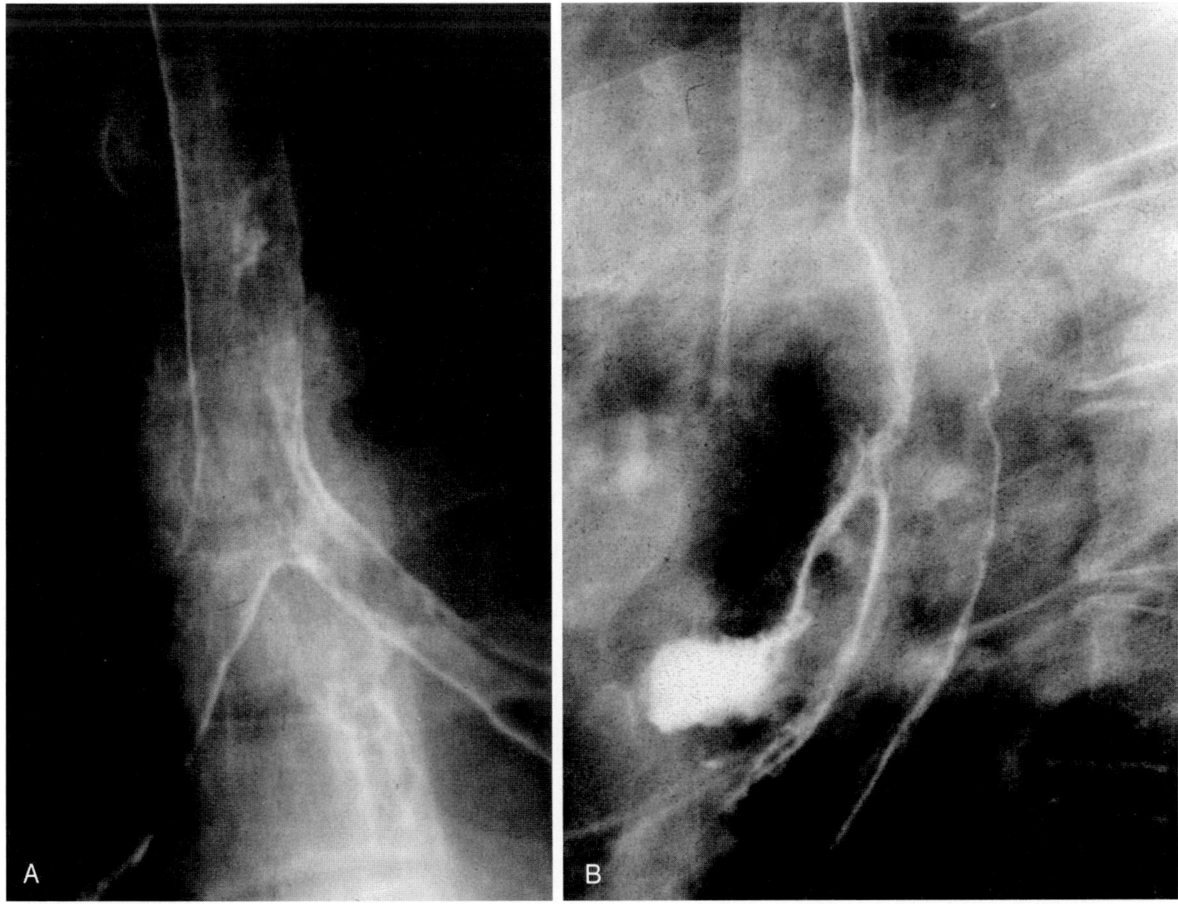

FIGURE 17–2 ■ Posteroanterior, *A*, and oblique, *B*, projections taken during a single-contrast barium swallow. Barium is seen in the tracheobronchial tree as well as in the esophagus, confirming a tracheoesophageal fistula. The esophagus, distal to the fistula, is partially obstructed by tumor.

Prevention of this complication by use of low-pressure, high-volume cuffed tracheostomy and endotracheal tubes is obviously important. Although newer designs of cuffed tubes have been introduced over the past 2 decades, it is important that the volume of air introduced into the cuff is monitored and does not exceed the minimum necessary to produce a seal. Additionally, concurrent use of rigid nasogastric tubes should be avoided.

Management of an established fistula depends on several factors, including the location of the fistula, its etiology, the degree of pulmonary contamination and need for ongoing respiratory support, and the general physiologic or performance status of the patient. The principal goal of management is to prevent soilage of the respiratory tree.

For the majority of patients with incurable malignancy, stenting (esophageal, tracheal, or both) is widely used to minimize pulmonary contamination and restore swallowing. In highly selected patients, esophageal diversion or bypass to exclude the fistula will achieve these goals. For occasional patients with advanced malignancy, no further treatment may be entirely appropriate.

Surgical repair is the only "curative" treatment and is applicable for patients with benign disease. The goals of surgery are to close the fistula, to prevent a recurrence, and to treat any underlying disease (if possible). Various surgical approaches are described in the following sections. However, the timing of surgery is a matter of considerable judgment. In general, a conservative approach is adopted until the patient is weaned from the ventilator. During this time, several maneuvers are initiated: when feasible, the cuffed tube is positioned below the fistula to reduce pulmonary contamination; any indwelling nasogastric tube is removed and a gastrostomy is placed to decompress the stomach to reduce gastroesophageal reflux; a feeding jejunostomy is placed for enteral nutrition; and pulmonary sepsis is treated aggressively with physiotherapy, positioning, bronchoscopy, and antibiotics. Very occasionally, esophageal diversion, comprising end-cervical esophagostomy, ligation of the cardia, decompressive gastrostomy, and feeding jejunostomy, may be required (Couraud et al, 1996; Hilgenberg and Grillo, 1983; Utley et al, 1978). In current practice this is rarely necessary if the preceding maneuvers are initiated promptly and effectively, but may be appropriate for selected patients with a distal fistula (Mathisen et al, 1991).

After pulmonary sepsis is controlled and the patient is weaned from the ventilator, a single-stage repair is performed. Attempts to repair tracheoesophageal fistulas while patients are still ventilated are reported (Thomas, 1973) but are generally unsuccessful as most patients have ongoing pulmonary sepsis, predisposing to poor healing, mediastinal infection, and bleeding.

Although healing of tracheoesophageal fistulas is reported occasionally after endoscopic electrocautery (Couraud et al, 1996), application of tissue glue or sealant (Bartels et al, 1998; Goh et al, 1994), and chemoradiotherapy (Ahmad et al, 1998), such techniques are not generally used in current clinical practice.

Operative Approaches

Anesthetic Considerations

Anesthetic techniques applicable to tracheal surgery are described in detail elsewhere. The airway may be controlled by orotracheal intubation distal to the fistula or by using a sterile armored tube placed directly into the distal trachea or bronchus across the operative field. High-frequency jet ventilation is useful for stenotic segments or for distal lesions. Use of short-acting anesthetic agents and muscle relaxants permits spontaneous ventilation during induction and throughout the procedure, and facilitates early extubation.

Incisions and Exposure

Exposure of the tracheoesophageal fistula may be obtained using a low transverse collar incision, incorporating the tracheostome, or using a left lateral incision anterior to the sternomastoid. If further exposure of the distal trachea is required, either incision may be extended as a partial upper midline sternotomy. A right posterolateral thoracotomy through the fourth interspace provides excellent exposure of the esophagus, distal trachea, and carina.

Identification of the fistula may require extensive dissection in view of local inflammation. The ipsilateral recurrent laryngeal nerve and the posterior membranous trachea, especially inferior to the fistula, are most at risk during the dissection. Careful placement of a small bougie in the esophagus may assist the dissection.

Direct Closure

A small fistula may be divided and the edges of the tract débrided. The membranous trachea is closed primarily using a single layer of interrupted absorbable sutures, placed carefully without tension. The esophageal wall should be closed longitudinally in two layers. The strap muscles (sternothyroid, sternohyoid, sternocleidomastoid) are mobilized to interpose between the suture lines to prevent a recurrence.

Tracheal Resection

A larger tracheal defect, especially associated with stenosis, will require tracheal resection, as described elsewhere. Extensive tracheal devascularization should be avoided, and care should be taken to avoid and preserve the recurrent laryngeal nerves. Transsection of the trachea provides satisfactory exposure of the fistula, and a segmental resection is performed. The primary tracheal anastomosis is performed with carefully placed interrupted absorbable sutures, without tension. Additional mobilization of the trachea (preserving the lateral vascular pedicles) or a laryngeal release may be required to reduce anastomotic tension. As described earlier, the esophageal defect is closed in two layers, and strap muscles are interposed between the suture lines to prevent recurrence.

A tracheostomy is rarely necessary, but if required, should be placed at least two rings distal to the anastomosis. Alternatively, a Silastic tracheal T tube may be used.

Esophageal Diversion

Several techniques of esophageal diversion or bypass are reported, with the aim of preventing contamination of the tracheobronchial tree and restoration of swallowing

(Burt, 1996; Meunier et al, 1998). However, these procedures are generally associated with high morbidity and mortality, and are limited to the following uncommon situations: as an alternative to stenting in good-performance patients with malignant tracheoesophageal fistulas, prior to the development of significant pulmonary sepsis; for patients with fistulas involving the distal trachea or carina; and for ventilated patients with ongoing tracheobronchial contamination despite placement of a decompressive gastrostomy, and so on.

An end-cervical esophagostomy will effectively divert salivary secretions, but reconstruction of the upper gastrointestinal tract, using stomach, colon, or free jejunal interposition, will be required as a second-stage procedure. Reflux of gastric contents may be reduced using a decompressive gastrostomy and positioning, but absolute exclusion of the esophagus requires ligation or stapling of the esophagus at the esophagogastric junction (Couraud et al, 1996; Urschel et al, 1974). This may lead to distention (or rupture) of the distal blind esophageal pouch if the fistula remains in continuity with the airway in a ventilated patient. This can be avoided by occlusion or ligation of the esophagus distal to the fistula, or alternatively, decompression of the distal esophageal pouch may be achieved with a Roux-en-Y jejunal loop.

Stenting

Intubation and stenting of an obstructing esophageal tumor, occluding the associated fistula, will prevent ongoing airway contamination, and restore swallowing. This palliative approach is appropriate for the majority of patients with advanced esophageal malignancy, who may achieve a quite satisfactory quality of life.

The endoesophageal prosthesis must be placed with care to minimize morbidity, and should be impermeable to tumor growth. Although many conventional esophageal stents are available, improved occlusion of the fistula is seen with stents incorporating an expandable foam cuff. The development of self-expanding covered stents, placed endoscopically or radiologically, has proved increasingly useful (Ell et al, 1995; Good et al, 1997; Han et al, 1996; Kozarek et al, 1996; Raijman, 1998; Wong and Goldstraw, 1995).

Palliation of a malignant tracheoesophageal fistula may also be achieved using airway stents alone (Albes et al, 1994; Kawashima et al, 1996) or by a combination of airway and esophageal stents (Freitag et al, 1996; Witt et al, 1996).

Early and Late Results

Based on the experience of a limited number of physicians and centers, it appears as though the optimal strategy to manage an acquired (benign) tracheoesophageal fistula is to perform a single-stage repair after the patient is weaned from mechanical ventilation. Mortality rates below 12% (Couraud et al, 1996; Dartevelle and Macchiarini, 1996; Mathisen et al, 1991) are anticipated, in contrast to mortality rates of 29% (Couraud et al, 1996) to 36% (Meunier et al, 1998) in a comparable series of patients undergoing esophageal bypass. Recurrence rates after primary closure of the fistula approximate 8% (Dartevelle and Macchiarini, 1996; Mathisen et al, 1991).

For malignant tracheoesophageal fistula, the long-term prognosis often depends on tumor histology and stage. Initial reports of palliative esophageal stenting using modern techniques suggest this may be performed safely, but to date little consideration has been given to quality of life.

COMMENTS AND CONTROVERSIES

Casson and Bethune provide a clear and concise review of a problem that is frequently complex, because each patient may present with unique problems. One of the most difficult situations is the patient who has a tracheoesophageal fistula that continues to contaminate the airway with gastroesophageal secretions for whom continued assisted ventilation with a cuffed endotracheal tube is essential. Any attempt to surgically close the fistula with the continued requirement for intubation and ventilatory support is almost certain to fail. The endotracheal tube, with its inflated cuff, continues to traumatize and interfere with the vascularity of the region of repair. In this circumstance, esophageal exclusion by the firing of a double layer of staples across the distal end of the esophagus will prevent the potentially lethal continuation of airway contamination with gastric content. Distal esophageal stapling is a relatively simple operative procedure, and today may well be done using a laparoscopic or thoracoscopic approach. A double layer of staples, without division of the esophagus, does not devascularize any part of the esophageal wall, and the esophageal lumen will reopen, spontaneously and completely, within a few months. This maneuver will provide many weeks of airway protection, allowing delay of definitive repair, awaiting the time when the patient is no longer ventilator dependent. Experience with this management sequence is most clearly defined in a recent publication by Couraud (Couraud, 1996).

The use of self-expanding wire stents may provide prompt palliation for selected malignant fistulae. An occasional patient with a malignant fistula may be selected for bypass.

F.G.P.
A.G.C.

KEY REFERENCES

Couraud L, Ballester MJ, Delaisement C: Acquired tracheoesophageal fistula and its management. Semin Thorac Cardiovasc Surg 8:392, 1996.

Dartevelle P, Macchiarini P: The management of acquired tracheoesophageal fistula. Chest Surg Clin N Am 6:819, 1996.

Mathisen DJ, Grillo HC, Wain JC, Hilgenberg AD: Management of acquired nonmalignant tracheoesophageal fistula. Ann Thorac Surg 52:759, 1991.

REFERENCES

Ahmad HF, Hussain MA, Grant CE, Wadleigh RG: Closure of tracheoesophageal fistulas with chemotherapy and radiotherapy. Am J Clin Oncol 21:177, 1998.

Ahmad I, Lee WC: Methicillin-resistant *Staphylococcus aureus* neck infections resulting in a delayed abscess and a tracheoesophageal fistula. ORL J Otorhinolaryngol Relat Spec 61:45, 1999.

Albes JM, Prokop M, Gebel M et al: Bifurcate tracheal stent with a foam cuff for tracheo-esophageal fistula. J Thorac Cardiovasc Surg 42:367, 1994.

Bargh W, Slawson KB: Experience with an artificial ventilation unit. Br J Anaesth 37:574, 1965.

Bartels HE, Stein HJ, Siewert JR: Respiratory management and outcome of non-malignant tracheo-bronchial fistula following esophagectomy. Dis Esophagus 11:125, 1998.

Berkmen YM, Auh YH: CT diagnosis of acquired tracheoesophageal fistula in adults. J Comput Assist Tomogr 9:302, 1985.

Buchanan CC, Vaughan RS, Verdi I et al: Right upper lobectomy in a patient with an iatrogenic tracheo-oesophageal fistula after laryngectomy. Br J Anaesth 74:461, 1995.

Burt M: Management of malignant esophagorespiratory fistula. Chest Surg Clin N Am 6:765, 1996.

Cherveniakov A, Tzekov C, Grigov GE, Cherveniakov P: Acquired benign esophago-airway fistulas. Eur J Cardiothorac Surg 10:713, 1996.

Chow CC, Kotlyarov EV, Fantry GT et al: Ga-67 citrate in diagnosing tracheosophageal fistula in a patient with AIDS. Clin Nucl Med 17:103, 1992.

Cirillo NW, Lyon DT, Schuller AM: Tracheoesophageal fistula complicating herpes esophagitis in AIDS. Am J Gastroenterol 88:587, 1993.

Coleman FP: Acquired nonmalignant esophagorespiratory fistula. Am J Surg 93:321, 1957.

Conces DJ, Kesler KA, Datzman et al: Tracheoesophageal fistula due to Wegener granulomatosis. J Thorac Imaging 10:126, 1995.

Cooper JO, Grillo HC: The evolution of tracheal injury due to ventilatory assistance through cuffed tubes: A pathologic study. Am Surg 169:334, 1969.

Couraud L, Ballester MJ, Delaisement C: Acquired tracheoesophageal fistula and its management. Semin Thorac Cardiovasc Surg 8:392, 1996.

Dartevelle P, Macchiarini P: The management of acquired tracheoesophageal fistula. Chest Surg Clin N Am 6:819, 1996.

Dux M, Gehling U, Schmitteckert H et al: Mediastinal actinomycosis with formation of an esophagotracheal fistula. Radiologie 34:537, 1994.

Ell C, May A, Hahn EG: Gianturco Z-stents in the palliative treatment of malignant esophageal obstruction and esophagotracheal fistulas. Endoscopy 27:495, 1995.

Flege JB: Tracheoesophageal fistula caused by cuffed tracheostomy tube. Ann Thorac Surg 166:153, 1967.

Freitag L, Tekolf E, Steveling H et al: Management of malignant esophagotracheal fistulas with airway stenting and double stenting. Chest 110:1155, 1996.

Goh PM, Kum CK, Toh EH: Endoscopic patch closure of malignant esophagotracheal fistula using Histoacryl glue. Surg Endosc 8:1434, 1994.

Good S, Asch M, Jaffer N, Casson AG: Radiologic placement of metallic esophageal stents. Can Assoc Radiol J 48:340, 1997.

Green RP, Biller HF, Sicular A et al: Cervical tracheoesophageal fistula. Laryngoscope 93:364, 1983.

Grillo HC, Moncure AC, McEnany MT: Repair of inflammatory tracheoesophageal fistula. Ann Thorac Surg 22:113, 1976.

Gudovsky LM, Koroleva NS, Biryukov YB et al: Tracheoesophageal fistulas. Ann Thorac Surg 55:868, 1993.

Han YM, Song HY, Lee JM et al: Esophagorespiratory fistulae due to esophageal carcinoma: Palliation with a covered Gianturco stent. Radiology 199:65, 1996.

Hilgenberg AD, Grillo HC: Acquired nonmalignant tracheoesophageal fistula. J Thorac Cardiovasc Surg 85:492, 1983.

Houben CH: Tracheobronchial lesions following esophagectomy: Prevalence, predisposing factors and outcome. Br J Surg 85:1015, 1998.

Jougon J, Couraud L: Esophageal patching for an unsuturable tracheoesophageal fistula. Eur J Cardiothorac Surg 14:431, 1998.

Kawashima O, Yoshida I, Ishikawa S et al: Use of an intratracheal silicone prosthesis (Dumon type) for the treatment of tracheoesophageal fistula due to advanced lung cancer. Surg Today 26:915, 1996.

Kinsman KJ, DeGregorio BT, Katon RM et al: Prior radiation and chemotherapy increase the risk of life-threatening complications after insertion of metallic stents for esophagogastric malignancy. Gastrointest Endosc 43:196, 1996.

Kozarek RA, Raltz S, Brugge WR et al: Prospective multicenter trial of esophageal Z-stent placement for malignant dysphagia and tracheoesophageal fistula. Gastrointest Endosc 44:562, 1996.

Lee S, Mergo PJ, Ros PR: The leaking esophagus: CT patterns of esophageal rupture, perforation and fistulization. Crit Rev Diagn Imaging 37:461, 1996.

Ling D, Bushunow P: Tracheoesophageal fistula in a patient with recurrent Hodgkin's disease. Chest 109:850, 1996.

Mathisen DJ, Grillo HC, Wain JC, Hilgenberg AD: Management of acquired nonmalignant tracheoesophageal fistula. Ann Thorac Surg 52:759, 1991.

Meunier B, Stasik C, Raoul JL et al: Gastric bypass for malignant esophagotracheal fistula: A series of 21 cases. Eur J Cardiothorac Surg 13:184, 1998.

Mutaf O, Avanoglu A, Mevsim A et al: Management of tracheoesophageal fistula as a complication of esophageal dilations in caustic esophageal burns. J Pediatr Surg 30:823, 1995.

Orvidas LJ, McCaffrey TV, Lewis JE et al: Lymphoma involving the esophagus. Ann Otol Rhinol Laryngol 103:843, 1994.

Rahbar A, Farha SJ: Acquired tracheoesophageal fistula. J Pediatr Surg 13:375, 1978.

Raijman I: Endoscopic management of esophagorespiratory fistulas: Expanding our options with expandable stents. Am J Gastroenterol 93:496, 1998.

Raijman I, Siddique I, Lynch P: Does chemoradiation therapy increase the incidence of complications with self-expanding coated stents in the management of malignant esophageal stricture? Am J Gastroenterol 92:2192, 1997.

Reed WJ, Doyle SE, Aprahamian C: Tracheoesophageal fistula after blunt chest trauma. Ann Thorac Surg 59:1251, 1995.

Rusconi S, Meroni L, Galli M: Tracheoesophageal fistula in an HIV-1-positive man due to dual infection of Candida albicans and cytomegalovirus. Chest 106:284, 1994.

Schowengerdt CG: Tracheoesophageal fistula caused by a self-expanding esophageal stent. Ann Thorac Surg 67:830, 1999.

Sebastian MW, Wolfe WG: Traumatic thoracic fistulas. Chest Surg Clin N Am 7:385, 1997.

Senders CW, Babin RW: Management of benign fistulae between Zenker's diverticulum and the trachea. Ann Otol Rhinol Laryngol 92:349, 1983.

Shah CP, Yeolekar ME, Pardiwala FK: Acquired tracheoesophageal fistula. J Postgrad Med 40:83, 1994.

Small D, Caplan S, Sheiner N et al: Tracheoesophageal fistula as the initial presentation of Hodgkin's disease. South Med J 88:664, 1995.

Tan KK, Lee JK, Tan I et al: Acquired tracheoesophageal fistula following tracheal intubation in a burned patient. Burns 19:360, 1993.

Temes RT, Wong RS, Davis M et al: Esophago-airway fistula in AIDS. Ann Thorac Surg 60:440, 1995.

Thomas AN: The diagnosis and treatment of tracheoesophageal fistula caused by cuffed tracheal tubes. J Thorac Cardiovasc Surg 65:612, 1973.

Thomas AN: Management of tracheoesophageal fistula caused by cuffed tracheal tubes. Am J Surg 124:181, 1972.

Tucker JG, Kim HH, Lucas GW: Esophageal perforation caused by coin ingestion. South Med J 87:269, 1994.

Urschel HC, Razzuk MA, Wood RE et al: Improved management of esophageal perforation: Exclusion and diversion in continuity. Ann Surg 179:587, 1974.

Utley JR, Dillon ML, Todd EP et al: Giant tracheoesophageal fistula. J Thorac Cardiovasc Surg 75:373, 1978.

Weber SM, Schurr MJ, Pellett JR: Delayed presentation of a tracheoesophageal fistula after blunt chest trauma. Ann Thorac Surg 62:1850, 1996.

Weiman DS, Walker WA, Brosnan KM et al: Noniatrogenic esophageal trauma. Ann Thorac Surg 59:849, 1995.

Weiman DS, Pate JW, Walker WA et al: Combined gunshot injuries of the trachea and esophagus. World J Surg 20:1099, 1996.

Witt C, Ortner M, Ewert R et al: Multiple fistulas and tracheobronchial stenoses require extensive stenting of the central airways and esophagus in squamous cell carcinoma. Endoscopy 28:381, 1996.

Wong K, Goldstraw P: Role of covered esophageal stents in malignant esophagorespiratory fistula. Ann Thorac Surg 60:199, 1995.

Wychulis AR, Ellis FH: Acquired non-malignant esophagotracheobronchial fistula. JAMA 196:117, 1966.

Yiengpruksawan A, Watanabe G, Ono Y et al: Tracheoesophageal fistula as a result of bronchial artery infusion therapy. Int Surg 69:351, 1984.

CHAPTER **18**

Upper Airway Tumors

PRIMARY TUMORS

Shaf Keshavjee
Marc de Perrot
Paulo Cardoso
F. Griffith Pearson

Primary tumors of the trachea are rare with an incidence of less than 0.2 per 100,000 persons per year and a prevalence of 1 per 15,000 autopsies. The great majority of primary tumors in adults are malignant, whereas in children most are benign. Squamous cell carcinoma and adenoid cystic carcinoma are the most frequent histologic types encountered in the adult population; other tumors account for only occasional case reports. Over the last 40 years, considerable improvement has been made in tracheal resection, and surgery has become the treatment of choice for most primary tracheal tumors. However, because of the rarity of these tumors, only a few centers throughout the world have reported significant experience with their surgical management.

This chapter does not discuss laryngeal neoplasms. Tumors involving the main carina are considered in Chapter 19, and secondary neoplasms of the upper airway are dealt with later in this chapter.

HISTORICAL NOTE

Prior to the 1960s, tracheal resection was limited by the assumption that no more than three or four tracheal rings (up to 3 cm) could be resected circumferentially and reconstructed by primary anastomosis (Barclay et al, 1957). During these early years, there were numerous reports of experimental and clinical efforts to replace segments of the resected trachea with a variety of prosthetic materials, both solid and porous. Belsey (1946) was the first to resect an adenoid cystic carcinoma of the thoracic trachea and to report reconstruction of the human trachea using fascia lata reinforced with stainless steel wire. Beall and associates (1963) reported on experimental and clinical experience with a porous prosthesis of heavy Marlex mesh, and our group subsequently reported our preliminary clinical experience with this same prosthesis (Pearson et al, 1968). In the early 1970s, Neville and colleagues (1972) also developed the use of a solid silicone prosthesis for both tracheal and carinal replacement.

Between 1960 and 1970, significant technical advances resulted from increased experience with postintubation tracheal injury secondary to cuffed endotracheal tubes and mechanical ventilation. Techniques of mobilization were developed (Grillo et al, 1964) that made it possible to resect up to half the length of the adult trachea and achieve reconstruction by primary end-to-end anastomosis. Furthermore, techniques were developed for circumferential resection and primary reconstruction at both the subglottic (Pearson et al, 1975) and carinal (Grillo, 1982) levels.

■ *HISTORICAL READINGS*

Barclay RS, McSwan N, Welsh TM: Tracheal reconstruction without the use of grafts. Thorax 12:177, 1957.

Beall AC Jr, Harrington OB, Greenberg SD et al: Circumferential replacement of thoracic trachea with Marlex mesh. JAMA 183:1082, 1963.

Belsey R: Stainless steel wire suture technique in thoracic surgery. Thorax 1:39, 1946.

Grillo HC: Carinal reconstruction. Ann Thorac Surg 34:356, 1982.

Grillo HC, Dignan EF, Miura T: Extensive resection and reconstruction of mediastinal trachea without prosthesis or graft: An anatomical study in man. J Thorac Cardiovasc Surg 48:741, 1964.

Neville WE, Hamouda F, Andersen J, Dwan FM: Replacement of the intrathoracic trachea and both stem bronchi with a molded Silastic prosthesis. J Thorac Cardiovasc Surg 63:569, 1972.

Pearson FG, Cooper JD, Nelems JM, Van Nostrand AW: Primary tracheal anastomosis after resection of the cricoid cartilage with preservation of recurrent laryngeal nerves. J Thorac Cardiovasc Surg 70:806, 1975.

Pearson FG, Henderson RD, Gross AE et al: The reconstruction of circumferential tracheal defects with a porous prosthesis: An experimental and clinical study using heavy Marlex mesh. J Thorac Cardiovasc Surg 55:605, 1968.

BASIC SCIENCE: PATHOLOGY

Benign Tracheal Neoplasms

Benign tumors of the trachea may arise from any component of the tracheal wall and account for 90% of primary neoplasms in children. Conversely, less than 10% of primary neoplasms in the adult trachea are benign.

Papillomas are the most common neoplasms in the pediatric population and are usually multifocal, with diffuse involvement of the larynx, trachea, and more rarely, the bronchial tree and lung. A viral etiology has been well

TABLE 18–1 ■ **Primary Tumors of the Trachea and Carina: Reported Series of Resected Cases**

Authors	*Span of Study*	*Number of Cases Reported*	*Number of Cases Resected*	*Adenoid Cystic Carcinoma No. (%)*	*Squamous Cell Carcinoma No. (%)*
Pearson et al (1984)	1963–1983	44	39	28 (64)	9 (20)
Grillo and Mathisen (1990)	1962–1989	198	132	80 (40)	70 (36)
Regnard et al (1996)	1970–1993	208	208	65 (31)	94 (45)
Perelman et al (1996)	1963–1995	144	102	66 (46)	21 (15)
Refaely and Weissberg (1997)	1975–1994	22	22	13 (59)	5 (23)

established and involves primarily human papillomavirus (HPV) 6 and 11. The virus is most likely transmitted vertically from vaginal condylomas in the mother; no cases of horizontal transmission to siblings and other family members have been reported (Sun et al, 2000). Patients with HPV 11 have been reported to have a more aggressive course and to be at increased risk of malignant transformation into squamous cell carcinoma (Rabah et al, 2001). Although juvenile papillomatosis almost always regresses after puberty, endoscopic ablation of symptomatic lesions is often required during childhood. In some instances, improvement has been reported with interferon therapy (Goepfert et al, 1982).

Another tumor of epithelial origin is the neuroendocrine carcinoid neoplasm (Briselli et al, 1978; Perelman and Koroleva, 1987). As has been reported for neuroendocrine carcinoma of the bronchial tree, some of these tumors can be listed in the benign category, whereas others undoubtedly behave more aggressively with histologic evidence of direct local invasion into contiguous structures. Carcinoid tumors may appear hypervascular at bronchoscopic and histologic examination and, thus, may occasionally be confused with glomus tumor, which is a benign vascular lesion also reported in the trachea (Lange et al, 2000; Menaissy et al, 2000).

Tumors of mesenchymal origin include chondroma, neurilemmoma, schwannoma, fibroma, and lipoma (Grillo and Mathisen, 1990; Pearson et al, 1984; Perelman and Koroleva, 1987). Of these, chondroma is the most frequent and is commonly located in the upper trachea at the cricoid level (Neis et al, 1989). It is often difficult or impossible for the pathologist to distinguish between a benign chondroma and a low-grade chondrosarcoma on the basis of histology. In addition, benign chondroma may potentially degenerate into malignant chondrosarcoma over time (Salminen et al, 1990). Rarer mesenchymal tumors include leiomyoma, hemangioma, myoblastoma, and benign epithelial polyp (Grillo, 1978; Perelman and Koroleva, 1987; Xu et al, 1987).

Malignant Tracheal Neoplasms

More than 90% of primary tumors of the trachea and carina in the adult population are malignant. The most common types are squamous cell carcinoma and adenoid cystic carcinoma, which account for approximately two thirds of primary tracheal malignancies. The proportion of squamous cell carcinomas usually predominates in surveys of primary tracheal tumors, but these tumors are often diagnosed at an advanced stage and are not amenable to resection (Gelder and Hetzel, 1993; Manninen et al, 1991; Yang et al, 1997). Therefore, the proportion of adenoid cystic carcinomas is often higher in surgical series (Grillo and Mathisen, 1990; Pearson et al, 1984; Perelman et al, 1996; Refaely and Weissberg, 1997). Five large series of surgical resection of primary tumors of the trachea and carina have been reported over the last 20 years (Table 18–1). These series included a total of 616 cases, of which 41% were adenoid cystic carcinoma and 32% squamous cell carcinoma; 503 underwent resection and reconstruction of the trachea. The pathology and clinical features of squamous cell carcinoma and adenoid cystic carcinoma are described later in some detail.

Adenoid Cystic Carcinoma

Adenoid cystic carcinoma was first described by Billroth in 1859 and for many years was called "cylindroma." The gross appearance of the tumor may suggest benignity in that the overlying tracheal mucosa is frequently intact (Fig. 18–1) and the progression of these tumors is often exceedingly slow. It is apparent, however, that these are malignant neoplasms with universal evidence of local

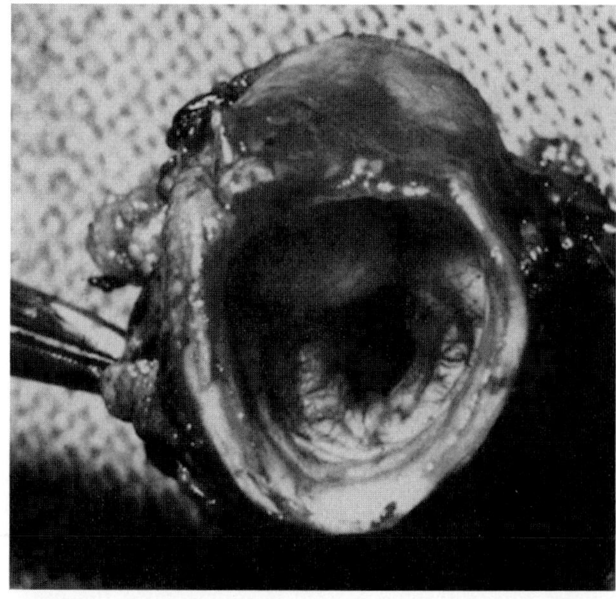

FIGURE 18–1 ■ Photograph illustrating the gross appearence of a freshly resected specimen of adenoid cystic carcinoma, such as might be seen at bronchoscopy. The overlying mucosa is intact, and the gross margins of the tumor appear circumscribed.

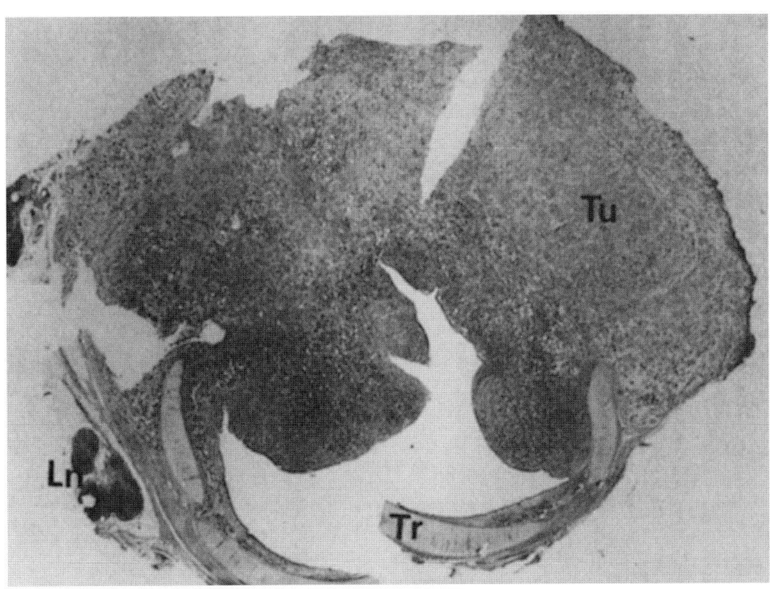

FIGURE 18–2 ■ A whole-mount histologic section of a resected specimen of adenoid cystic carcinoma. The tumor extends through the full thickness of the tracheal wall, and there is as much gross tumor lying outside the lumen as within. (Ln, lymph node; Tr, tracheal cartilage; Tu, tumor.)

invasion on histologic examination. Indeed, these tumors are nearly always found to extend beyond the visible and palpable confines of the gross lesion at the time of surgery. Microscopic spread occurs both circumferentially and longitudinally in the tracheal wall, particularly in the submucosal plane and on the external surface of the trachea in the perineural lymphatic spaces. The gross and microscopic features of this tumor are illustrated in Figures 18–1 to 18–4. Because of the microscopic extension of the tumor, frozen section evaluation of resection margins is of critical importance at the time of resection if a complete and potentially curative operation is the objective. However, one should not forget that these tumors are extremely slow growing, and complete resection should not compromise safety by creating excessive anastomotic tension.

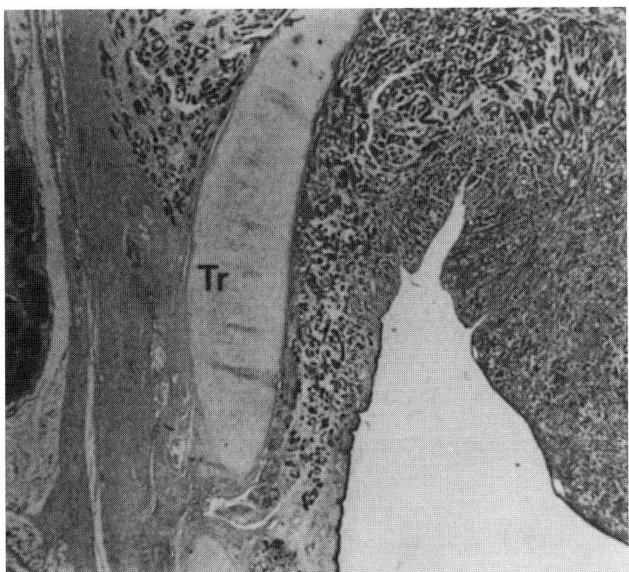

FIGURE 18–3 ■ Photomicrograph illustrating the extensive submucosal spread of adenoid cystic carcinoma. The spread occurs both longitudinally and circumferentially and is neither visible nor palpable to the operating surgeon. The overlying mucosa is intact. Only intraoperative frozen section assessment will identify such involvement. (Tr, tracheal cartilage.)

Metastases to regional lymph nodes are reported in approximately 13% of patients. Hematogenous metastases occur most commonly in the lungs (76%), but there may be occasional spread to the liver, brain, or bone (Maziak et al, 1996; Pearson et al, 1974). The natural history of this tumor, even in untreated cases, is often that of a slow and insidious progression. Local recurrences have been observed by one of us (F.G.P.) more than 25 years following a presumably complete resection (Figs. 18–5 to 18–9). Pulmonary metastases are frequently asymptomatic when first identified on plain chest films and may remain so for long periods (years) in some patients (Pearson et al, 1974). Hence, asymptomatic pulmonary metastasis is not necessarily a contraindication to resection of the primary tumor in selected cases (Maziak et al, 1996; Regnard et al, 1996).

Adenoid cystic carcinoma occurs with equal frequency in men and women and in all age groups from the teens through the nineties. There is no relationship to cigarette smoking.

Squamous Cell Carcinoma

Squamous cell carcinoma occurs predominantly in men (3:1 male/female ratio), and has an age distribution similar to that of squamous cell carcinoma of the lung, with a predominance in the sixth and seventh decades. The great majority of patients presenting with squamous cell tumors of the trachea are smokers, and up to 40% of them may present with a previous history, a concurrent finding, or a later occurrence of squamous cell carcinoma in another location along the respiratory tract (Grillo and Mathisen, 1990; Hadju et al, 1970; Li et al, 1990).

The gross appearance of these tumors is similar to that of squamous cancer of the bronchus in any other location. They are almost always ulcerated lesions, and hemoptysis is a common presenting symptom. Unfortu-

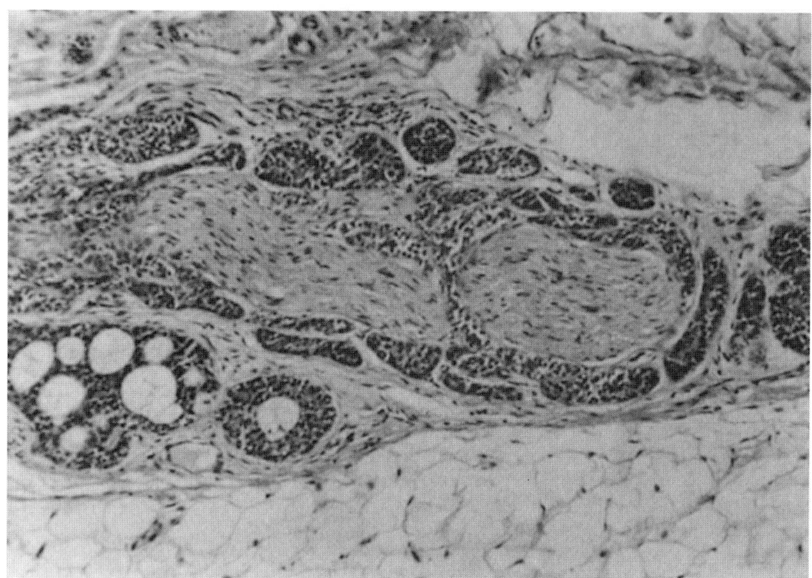

FIGURE 18–4 ■ Photomicrograph illustrating adenoid cystic carcinoma, spreading longitudinally on the outer surface of the trachea, in the perineural lymphatics. This type of microscopic spread is invisible and produces no gross abnormality in the appearance of the external tracheal wall.

nately, the incidence of regional lymph node metastasis is high, and the tumor is frequently locally advanced and unresectable at the time of presentation. Hematogenous spread is similar to that of bronchogenic carcinoma.

Other Primary Malignancies

The remaining primary malignancies are rare and include adenocarcinoma, small cell carcinoma, chondrosarcoma, leiomyosarcoma, carcinosarcoma, spindle cell sarcoma, synovial cell sarcoma, and melanoma (Grillo and Mathisen, 1990; Pearson et al, 1984; Sykes et al, 1997). Mucoepidermoid carcinoma and mixed adenosquamous tumors may also arise from the tracheal or carinal epithelium (Grillo and Mathisen, 1990). Primary tracheal non-Hodgkin's lymphoma and plasmacytoma have also been reported in some cases (Fidias et al, 1996; Grillo, 1978; Hadju et al, 1970; Kairalla et al, 1988; Neis et al, 1989).

DIAGNOSIS AND CLINICAL FEATURES

Signs and Symptoms

The clinical presentation of tracheal tumors may reflect upper airway obstruction (dyspnea, wheezing, and stridor), mucosal irritation and ulceration (cough and he-

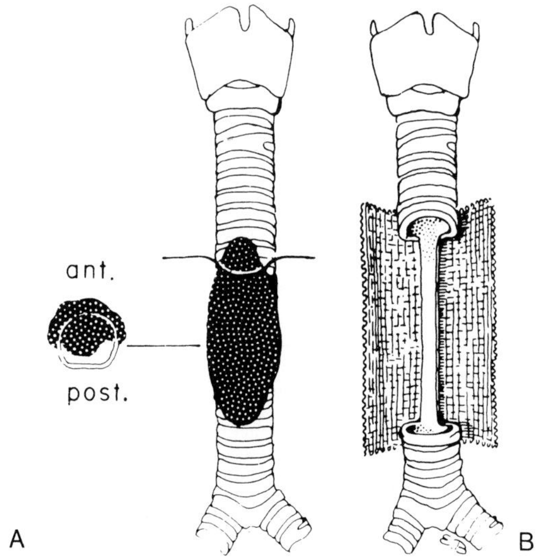

ant.

post.

A B

FIGURE 18–5 ■ *A,* Diagram illustrating a tumor in the upper mediastinal trachea in a 15-year-old girl. This patient had a 2-year history of a condition diagnosed as "asthma and chronic bronchitis." The tumor was an adenoid cystic carcinoma. *B,* This tumor was resected in 1963 in the first case in which the author (F.G.P.) used a cylinder of heavy-duty Marlex mesh for replacement. A 6.5-cm segment was resected, and a strip of membranous trachea was preserved as a potential source for early epithelization of the internal surface of the prosthesis.

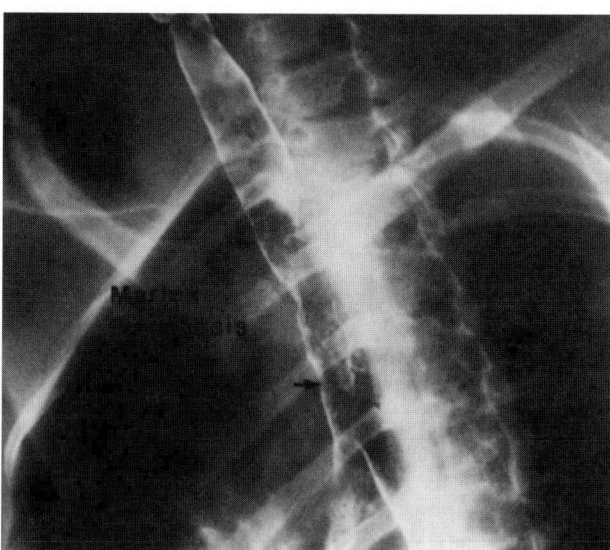

FIGURE 18–6 ■ A contrast tracheogram from the same patient shown in Figure 18–5. This tracheogram was taken 4 years after prosthetic replacement, and the patient maintained an excellent airway until that time. During the following year she developed slowly progressive narrowing at the upper end of the prosthesis, with associated dyspnea. *Arrows* indicate ends of Marlex prosthesis.

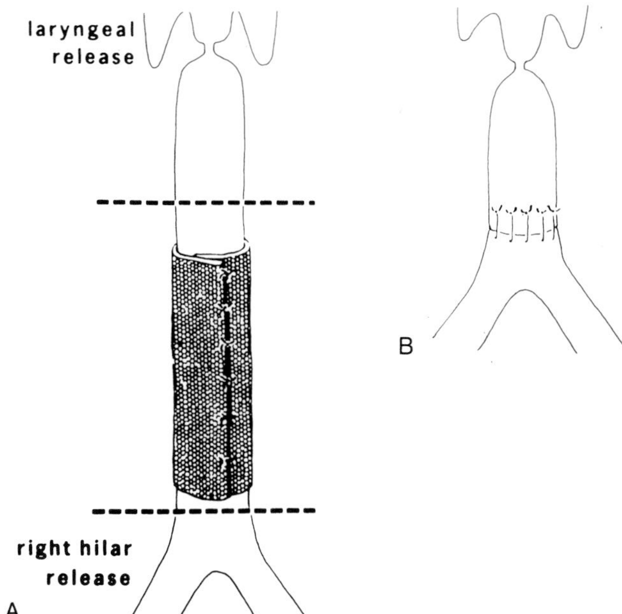

FIGURE 18–7 ■ The same patient shown in Figures 18–5 and 18–6. The diagram illustrates the operative procedure performed in 1968, 5 years after the initial prosthetic replacement. The entire prosthesis was resected. *A*, By using a suprathyroid release procedure above and a right intrapericardial release below, it was possible to achieve a successful primary anastomosis, *B*.

moptysis), or direct invasion and involvement of contiguous structures (recurrent nerve palsy, dysphagia), or such tumors may be the result of distant metastasis. Upper airway obstruction is characterized by dyspnea, stridor, wheezing, and cough. Because these symptoms are commonly encountered in respiratory dysfunction, many patients with tracheal tumors are treated for "asthma" or "chronic bronchitis" for long periods prior to receiving the correct diagnosis. Furthermore, many of these tumors do grow very slowly (benign tumors, adenoid cystic carcinoma, carcinoid tumors, mucoepidermoid carcinoma), and symptoms of obstruction may continue for months or even years without development of life-threatening airway impairment.

It is understandable that the correct diagnosis of primary tracheal tumor is frequently delayed because these neoplasms are so uncommon that they are rarely, if ever, encountered by most physicians. When symptoms of cough, wheezing, and dyspnea are investigated with plain chest films, there may be no apparent abnormality in the mediastinum or tracheal air column. If abnormalities do exist in the plain chest film, they are often subtle and easily overlooked.

Radiology

Plain chest films, anteroposterior and lateral tomograms, and contrast tracheograms are all valuable modalities for imaging tracheal tumors. However, tracheal masses can be identified on chest radiographs in only approximately half of cases (Li et al, 1990). Computed tomography (CT) provides the most informative evaluation, with delineation of both the intraluminal and the extraluminal extent of tumor and relatively accurate evaluation of the relationship of tumor to adjacent structures. CT is recommended in all cases for staging and for directing management (Morency et al, 1989). Three-dimensional reconstructions of the entire airway can be obtained routinely with helical CT scanners. These images provide invaluable anatomic information to the surgeon regarding extent of airway involvement and potential for resection and reconstruction. Therefore, as a rule, contrast tracheograms are not used anymore. A contrast esophagogram, however, identifies esophageal involvement and may be obtained as part of the CT scan or as a separate study.

Magnetic resonance imaging (MRI) has not proved superior to CT in the detection and evaluation of mediastinal masses, although MRI can occasionally be of benefit when vascular and cardiac invasion are questioned. There have been few studies comparing MRI and CT for endobronchial tumors. Although MRI has the advantage of providing coronal and sagittal planes, CT usually shows tumor extension and anatomic details more precisely than does MRI (Aberle et al, 1991; Naidich, 1990). Cur-

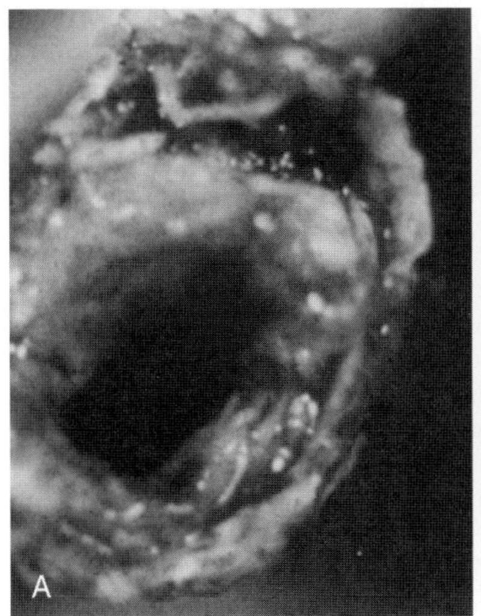

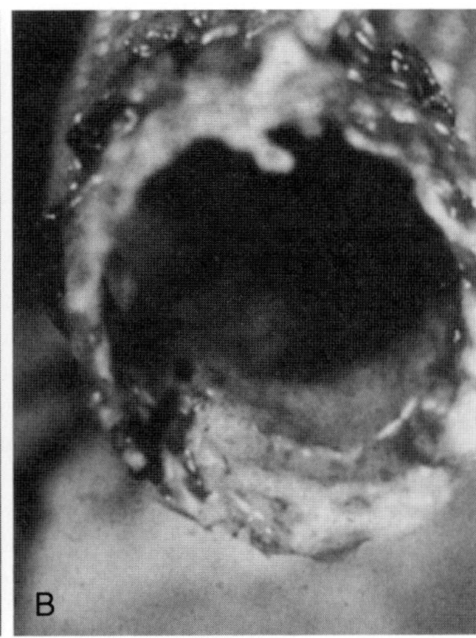

FIGURE 18–8 ■ Photograph of same patient as that in Figures 18–5 to 18–7 showing the gross appearance of the resected prosthesis. *A*, There was concentric stenosis due to fibrosis and granulations at the upper end. *B*, The lower end was epithelized and widely patent.

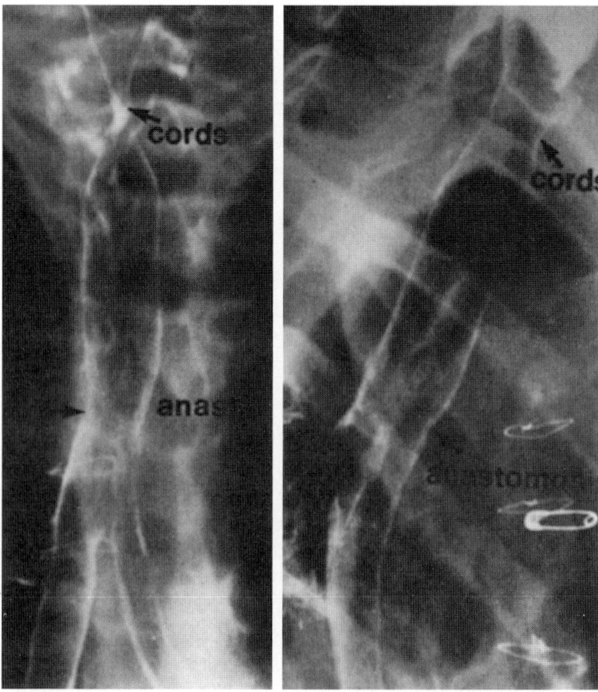

FIGURE 18–9 ■ A contrast tracheogram in the same patient shown in Figures 18–5 to 18–8, obtained 1 year following resection and primary reconstruction. A widely patent airway was obtained, and the degree of tracheal shortening is apparent. This patient survived for an additional 24 years before succumbing to airway obstruction from a local recurrence in the distal remaining trachea. This recurrence did not become clinically evident until 1989, 26 years following the first operation with prosthetic reconstruction. (Cords, *upper arrows*; anastomosis, *lower arrows*.)

rently, there is no clear advantage of MRI over CT imaging in the evaluation of primary tracheal tumors.

Pulmonary Function Studies

Pulmonary function tests may alert the physician to the possibility of upper airway obstruction and may help the physician to make a correct diagnosis. An obstructive pattern combined with a lack of response to bronchodilator medication may suggest a fixed upper airway obstruction. Flow-volume loops may clearly indicate upper airway obstruction, with plateauing of the inspiratory or expiratory phase depending on the location of the tumor in relation to the mediastinum. In most cases, both limbs of the flow-volume loop are flattened (Fig. 18–10). Gelb and associates (1988) have addressed the problem of interpreting false-negative results. Fredberg and colleagues (1980) have described a technique for measuring upper airway diameters by acoustic reflection directed at the patient's mouth; these "tracheal echograms" provide relatively accurate quantitative measurements of airway diameter and reveal the precise level of obstruction relative to the vocal cords. This technique also identifies areas of lesser obstruction that would not be picked up in the flow-volume curves.

Endoscopy

Bronchoscopy is essential in all cases and provides the simplest and most reliable approach for biopsy and tissue diagnosis. The extent of intraluminal involvement is ascertained, and precise measurements define the margins of the tumor and the relationship to the carina, cricoid, and vocal cords. This information is essential for planning the operative approach and the details of surgical resection. Biopsies taken at and beyond the margins of visible tumor may detect microscopic extension of disease and can further facilitate judgment concerning the necessary extent of resection.

In patients with significant upper airway obstruction or massive hemoptysis, the flexible bronchoscope is ineffective. These are potentially life-threatening conditions that require rigid bronchoscopy to provide adequate control of the airway. In most cases, the bronchoscope can be advanced beyond the tumor to provide access for ventilation. The tracheal lumen may be enlarged by endoscopic removal of tumor using biopsy forceps, coagulation, or laser resection (see Chapter 6). Whenever possible, tracheotomy is to be avoided because it may complicate any subsequent resection and reconstruction.

MANAGEMENT

We again emphasize that most primary tracheal tumors are malignant, are usually locally advanced at the time of symptomatic presentation and diagnosis, and are frequently at a stage that precludes a complete resection. However, careful assessment is required to ensure that the patient has the opportunity for a curative resection if at all possible. Both curative and palliative approaches are presented in the following paragraphs.

Tracheal Resection and Primary Reconstruction

With few exceptions such as primary tracheal lymphoma and small cell carcinoma of the trachea that may be treated primarily with chemoradiation therapy, surgical resection and primary reconstruction of the trachea is the best therapy for all neoplasms that can be completely resected. It is assumed that all malignant tumors extend through and beyond the tracheal wall, which makes endoscopic resection (including laser resection) inevitably

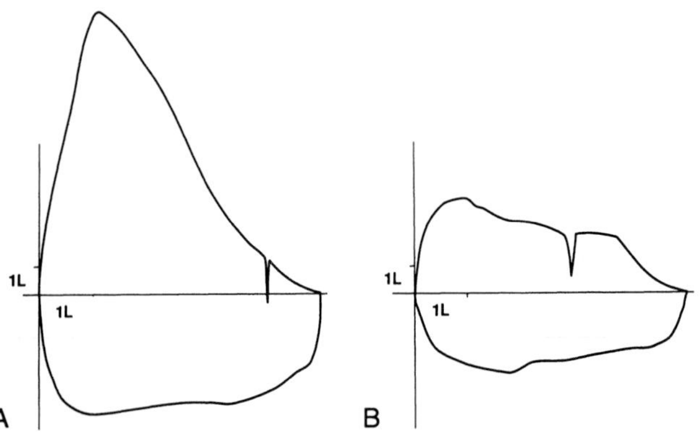

FIGURE 18–10 ■ A flow-volume loop illustrating the typical flattening of both inspiratory and expiratory curves associated with a fixed obstruction in the trachea due to neoplasm. *A*, Normal. *B*, Tracheal obstruction.

incomplete, and therefore inadequate, in otherwise operable patients.

A cervical collar incision provides adequate access for most tumors confined to the cervical and upper mediastinal trachea. The mediastinal trachea is well exposed throughout its length via a median sternotomy, although a right posterolateral thoracotomy may provide preferable exposure for selected tumors that involve the distal trachea and require a concomitant carinal resection (Grillo and Mathisen, 1990; Pearson et al, 1984). The technique of resection for a tumor of the mediastinal trachea is illustrated in Figures 18–11 to 18–14. An extended resection is necessary for the management of many of these tracheal neoplasms. With few exceptions, it is usually possible to remove approximately half the length of the adult trachea and achieve reconstruction by primary anastomosis. Such extended resections require mobilization of the anterior and anterolateral aspects of the trachea from top to bottom and may necessitate the addition of release procedures at the upper and lower ends of the trachea. The operative details describing these procedures are provided in Chapter 19. An illustrative case of a patient requiring extended resection for adenoid cystic carcinoma is depicted in Figures 18–15 through 18–17.

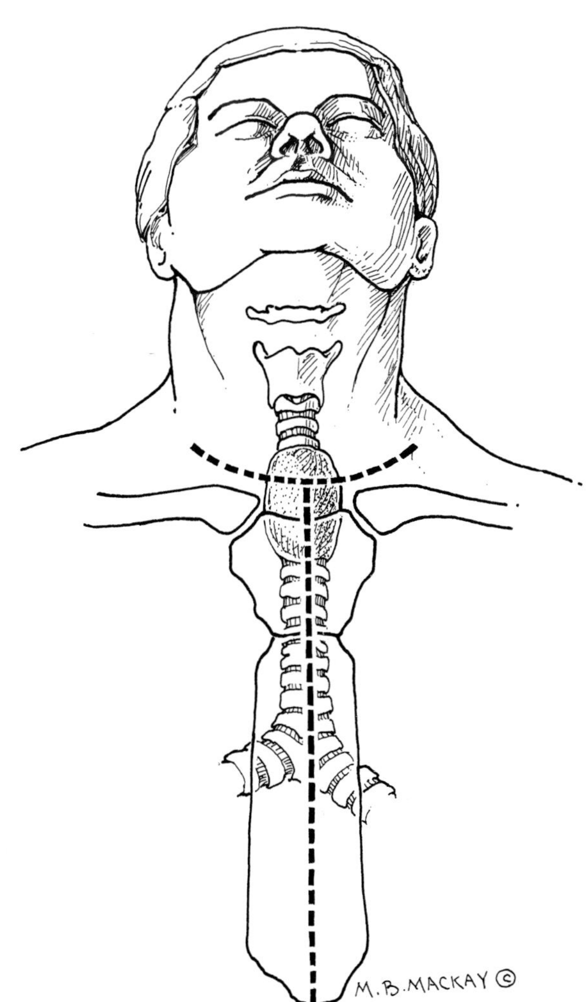

FIGURE 18–11 ■ Diagram illustrating the incision most commonly used for tracheal tumors that extend to the mediastinal trachea: a generous collar incision and a full median sternotomy.

A difficult problem for the surgeon in many of these operations relates to the extent of resection that should be undertaken. Until the airway has been divided and frozen section of the resection margins performed, it is impossible to judge the extent of resection required to remove the tumor. It may be necessary to accept microscopic disease at one or both margins rather than to extend the resection beyond the limits of safety. This decision must be made at a time when the airway has already been divided, the tumor resected, and there is no option other than reconstruction. Microscopic tumor at the resection margin does not appear to impair healing, and long-term survival may still be possible, particularly in patients with adenoid cystic tumors (Grillo and Mathisen, 1990; Pearson et al, 1984).

There are technical problems that complicate resection at the upper and lower ends of the trachea. The various approaches to carinal resection are well described by Grillo and Mathisen (1990). In selected cases, neoplasms involving the subglottic airway may be managed by circumferential resection of the distal cricoid with preservation of the larynx and vocal function (Pearson et al, 1986).

Role of Radiotherapy

Improvement in surgical techniques and anesthesiology over the last four decades has led surgery to be the treatment of choice for primary tracheal neoplasms. However, because of the narrow resection margins and the radiosensitivity of adenoid cystic carcinoma and squamous cell carcinoma, adjuvant radiotherapy is usually combined with surgery even if the resection margins are free of tumors and no lymph node metastasis is detected. A dosage of 50 Gy or higher is generally recommended.

Radiation therapy alone may occasionally be associated with early good response, but local recurrence is almost uniform. No one has reportedly survived for longer than 10 years following radiotherapy alone (Grillo, 1993). Grillo and Mathisen (1990) reported that surgery provided at least a triple survival time for squamous cell carcinoma and adenoid cystic carcinoma when compared with radiation only. In Toronto, only 3 of 32 patients with adenoid cystic carcinoma of the trachea treated by primary resection developed a local recurrence, whereas 5 of 6 patients treated by radiation alone presented with recurrence in the trachea (Maziak et al, 1996).

Results of Resection and Primary Reconstruction

Complications

The operative mortality reported in five recent major publications dealing with resection and reconstruction of the trachea for primary tracheal tumors ranged between 5% and 15% (Table 18–2). Lethal complications included anastomotic dehiscence, pneumonia and respiratory failure, pulmonary embolism, and tracheoinnominate artery fistula. A majority of these lethal complications occurred after resection-reconstruction of the carina and may have

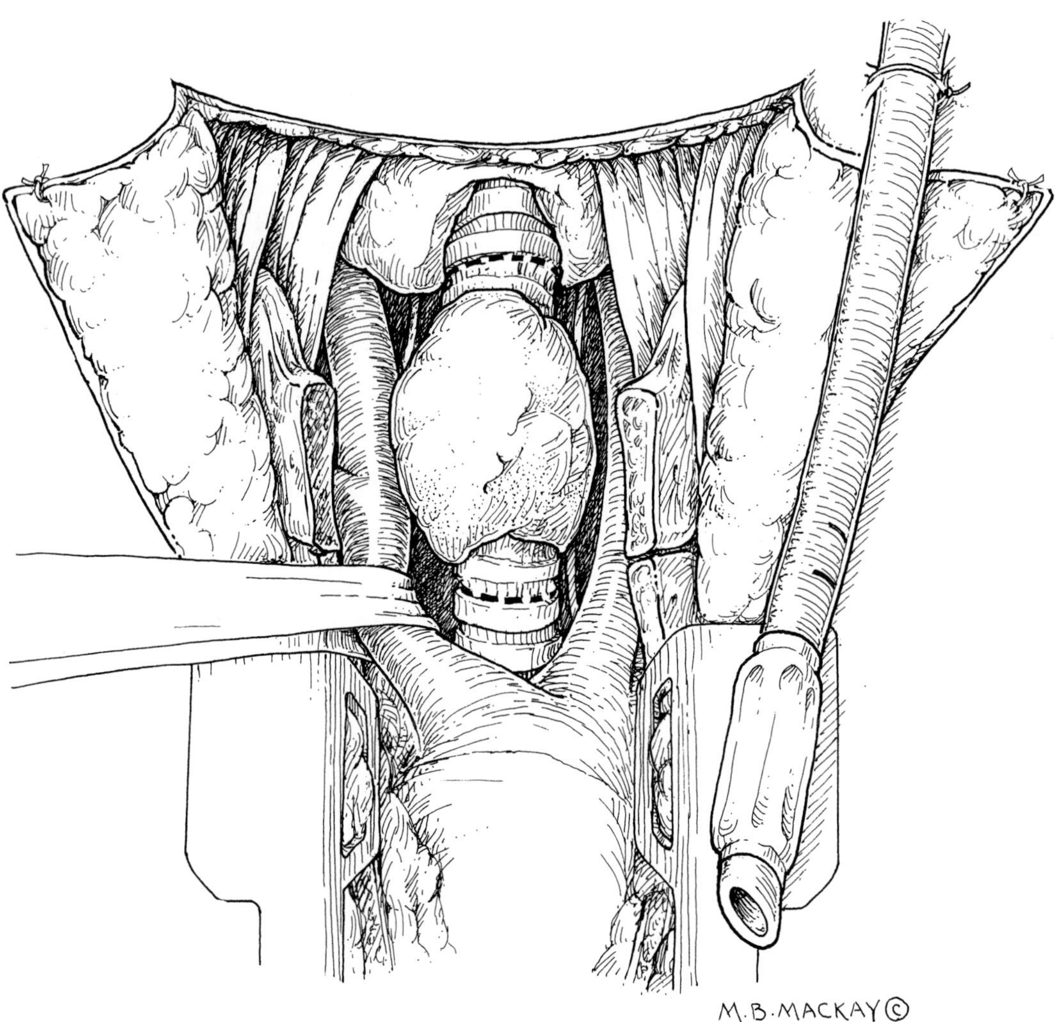

FIGURE 18–12 ■ The intraoperative appearance following retraction of the sternal margins, reflection of the strap muscles above, and exposure of the trachea from the thyroid isthmus above to the top of the aortic arch below. In this patient the resection can be achieved with this exposure. The proposed resection margins are illustrated with dotted lines. For more distal resections, it may be necessary to open the pericardium vertically front and back, with lateral retraction of the ascending aorta to the patient's left and the superior vena cava to the patient's right. This will expose the entire mediastinal trachea, the carina, and the origin of both main bronchi.

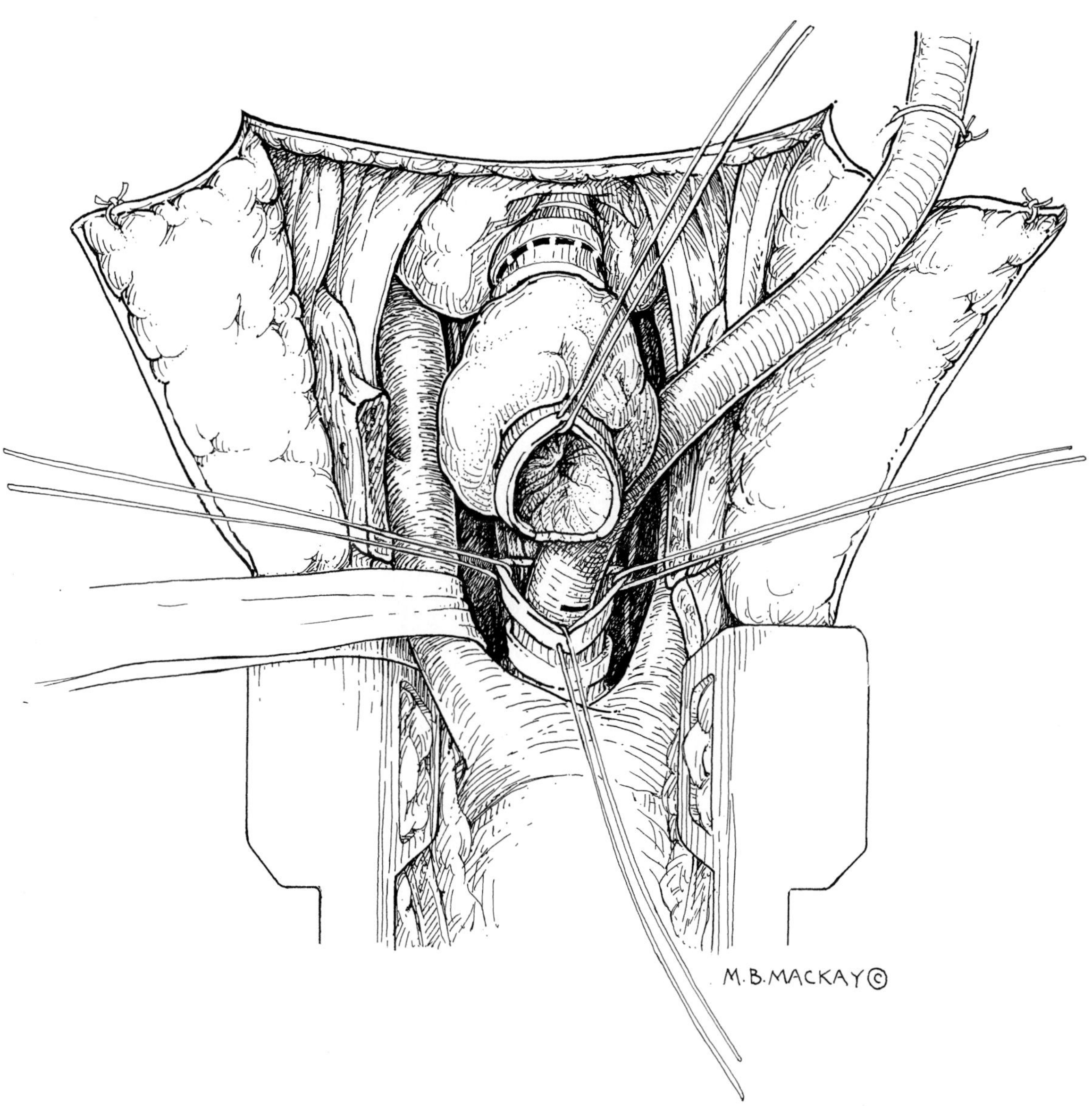

FIGURE 18–13 ■ The airway has been divided 1 cm beyond the gross distal margin of the tumor. Three stay sutures are used to stabilize the distal tracheal stump, which has been intubated with an armored endotracheal tube for ventilation. At this point, a circumferential ring is taken from the distal trachea and submitted to pathology for frozen section assessment.

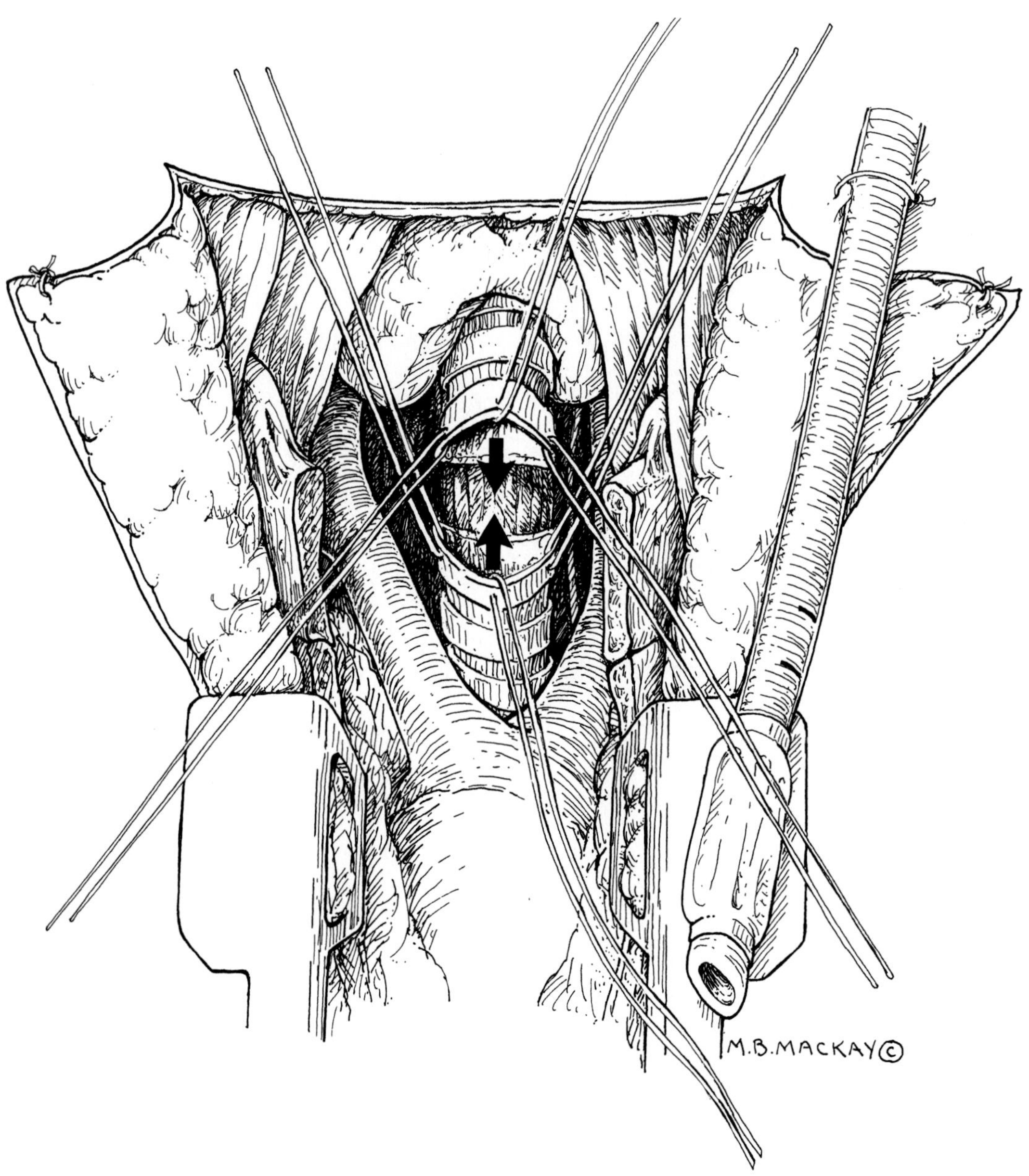

FIGURE 18–14 ■ The tumor has been resected, the divided tracheal ends have been evaluated by frozen section assessment, and each end has been stabilized with three stay sutures in preparation for primary anastomosis. Details of anastomotic technique can be found in Chapter 19.

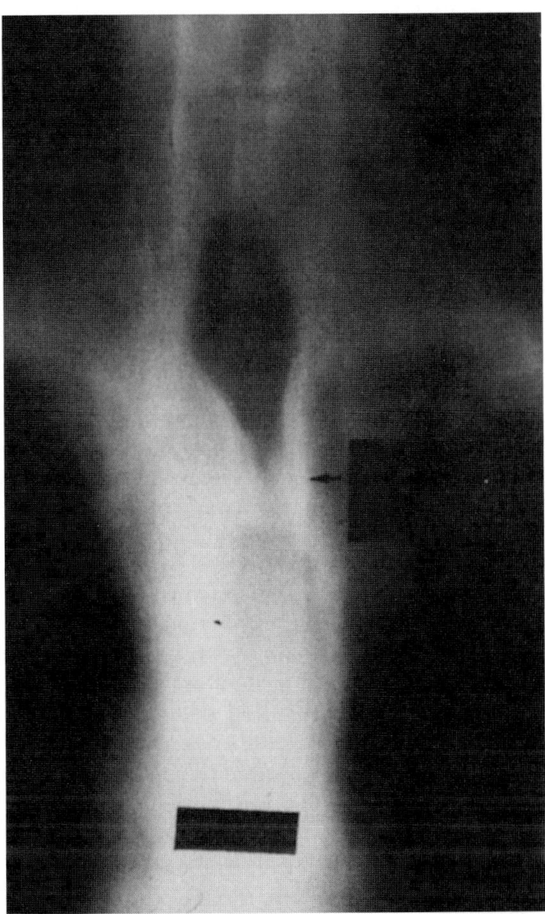

FIGURE 18–15 ■ Contrast tracheogram illustrating a large, lobulated filling defect in the mediastinal trachea. This was due to an adenoid cystic carcinoma in a 58-year-old patient with a 1-year history of slowly progressing wheezing and dyspnea.

been due to excessive tension at the anastomotic sites (Grillo and Mathisen, 1990; Pearson et al, 1984; Perelman et al, 1996).

Nonlethal complications ranged between 20% and 40% and included anastomotic leakage, pneumonia, recurrent nerve palsy (usually transient), aspiration with deglutition following superior release procedures, and late stenosis at the anastomosis. These late strictures were the result of either dehiscence or ischemia at the anastomotic margins and were successfully managed by dilatation, laser therapy, or reoperation (Grillo and Mathisen, 1990; Pearson et al, 1984; Regnard et al, 1996). In a multi-institutional series of 208 patients, Regnard and his colleagues (1996) observed four significant risk factors of postoperative complications: (1) the length of resection (the longer the tracheal resection, the higher the morbidity), (2) the need for laryngeal release, (3) the type of surgical procedure (laryngotracheal or carinal resection having a higher risk than standard tracheal resection), and (4) the histologic type (the postoperative mortality was higher among patients with squamous cell carcinoma than with other tumors). Older age of the patient, positive margins at resection, and lymph node involvement did not significantly increase the postoperative complication rate.

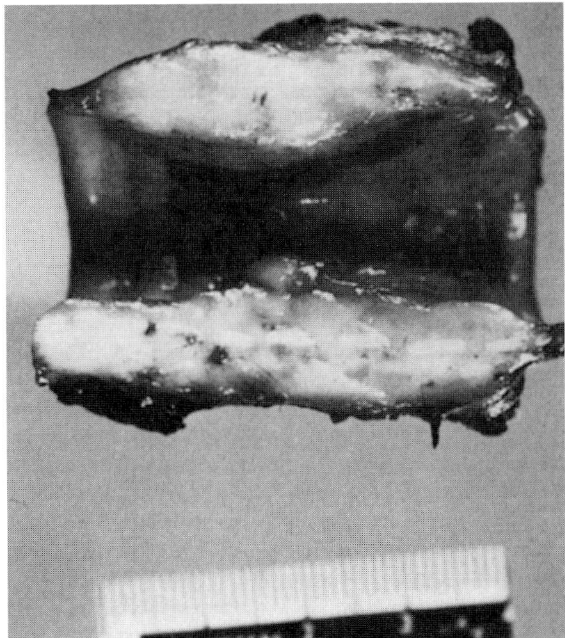

FIGURE 18–16 ■ The gross apperance of the freshly resected specimen. In this longitudinal cross section of the airway, it is evident that 10 tracheal rings have been removed. Including separately submitted resection margins, this represented removal of more than half of the trachea, a length of 8 cm. A diffusely infiltrating adenoid cystic tumor is seen invading the full circumference of the resected segment.

Survival

Long-term survival is excellent in patients with adenoid cystic carcinoma and ranges between 50% and 57% at 10 years (Table 18–3). Survival was better for patients with complete resection margins and negative regional lymph nodes than for those with incomplete resections or positive lymph nodes. However, because of the slow progression of the disease and the small number of patients, the difference never reached statistical significance (Grillo and Mathisen, 1990; Maziak et al, 1996; Regnard et al, 1996). Metastasis occurred after a mean interval of 100 months from the initial diagnosis of the primary tumor and remained asymptomatic for long periods (Maziak et al, 1996). Because there is no evidence that chemotherapy

TABLE 18–2 ■ **Resection and Anastomosis for Primary Tracheal Tumors: Operative Mortality***

Authors	*No. Cases Resected*	*Operative Mortality*	
		No.	*%*
Pearson et al (1984)	33	2	6.1
Grillo and Mathisen (1990)	132	7	5.3
Regnard et al (1996)	208	22	10.5
Perelman et al (1996)	97	14	14.4
Refaely and Weissberg (1997)	22	1	4.5

*Tracheas reconstructed with prosthetic material were excluded.

TABLE 18–3 ■ **Five and 10-Year Survival Following Surgical Resection of Adenoid Cystic Carcinoma of the Trachea**

Authors	*No. Cases Resected*	*Follow-up (yrs)*	*Survival (%)*	
			5-year	*10-year*
Grillo and Mathisen (1990)	60	26	72	53
Regnard et al (1996)	65	23	73	57
Maziak et al (1996)	32	32	79	51
Perelman and Koroleva (1987)	56	20	66	56
Prommegger and Salzer (1998)	14	26	79	57
Azar et al (1998)	5	25	75	50

is useful in the management of these metastases, they should not be treated unless they are symptomatic.

Survival following resection for squamous cell carcinoma is less favorable, and the reported experience is smaller. Perelman and Koroleva (1987) reported a 15% 5-year survival in 20 patients. Grillo and Mathisen (1990) reported 14 of 41 patients alive and free of disease between 3 and 15 years after resection. If it is assumed that these represent ultimate 5-year survivors, the projected survival rate is as high as 35%. Pearson and co-workers (1984) reported four of nine patients living and clinically free of disease at 6, 16, 21, and 56 months after operation. Two patients died at 6 and 46 months, respectively, with recurrent cancer.

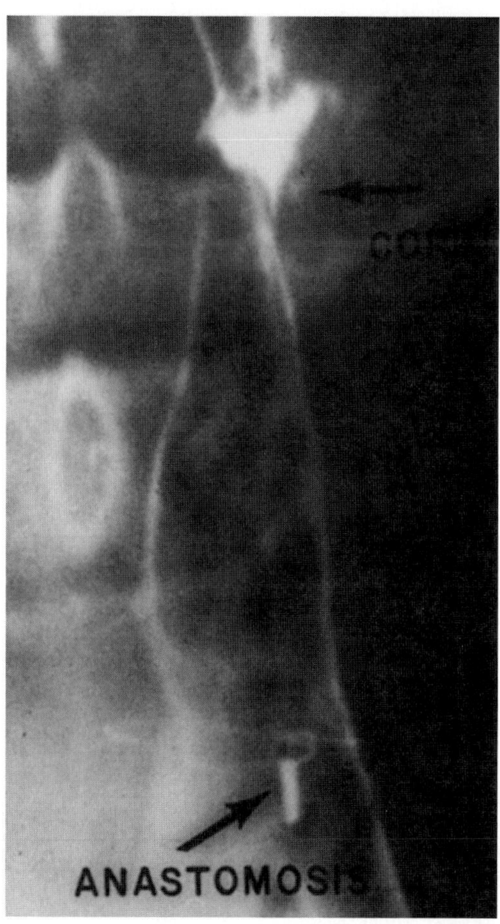

FIGURE 18–17 ■ A contrast tracheogram in the same patient shown in Figures 18–15 and 18–16, obtained 1 year after resection. There is a widely patent airway, and a marked degree of tracheal shortening.

Miscellaneous Reports

Heitmiller and associates (1989) reported their experience with resection for mucoepidermoid tumors of the tracheobronchial tree. Of 18 patients, 3 with primary tracheal tumors were seen during a 41-year period at the Massachusetts General Hospital. These authors confirmed that mucoepidermoid carcinoma presents with different grades of malignancy. All patients who underwent complete resection for well-differentiated, low-grade tumors were long-term survivors, whereas patients with high-grade tumors died within 2 years of resection.

Daniel and colleagues (1980) reported on a single case of granular cell myoblastoma of the trachea managed by resection; this was part of a literature review identifying management and outcome in 44 patients with this type of tumor. There were no instances of tumor recurrence in patients managed by surgical resection. In cases managed by bronchoscopic removal, however, the recurrence rate was 54%. The obvious recommendation was that surgical resection is the treatment of choice.

Fidias and co-workers (1996) reported on a case of primary tracheal non-Hodgkin's lymphoma and reviewed five other cases reported in the literature. The authors concluded that primary tracheal or tracheobronchial non-Hodgkin's lymphoma should be treated like any other stage I extranodal lymphoma with limited chemotherapy followed by radiation therapy. Surgery should be reserved as a salvage therapy for resistant disease or tracheomalacia.

Shankar and associates (1990) reported on four patients in whom the primary tracheal malignancy was initially managed by resection using the neodymium: yttrium-aluminum-garnet (Nd:YAG) laser to open an obstructed airway. In these cases, 2 months elapsed before elective tracheal resection was performed, presumably in order to avoid impaired healing, which might occur secondary to thermal damage created by the laser. There were no anastomotic complications in these four patients, and good long-term results were reported.

Terz and colleagues (1980) reported an unusual experience with 21 patients managed by tracheal resection and reconstruction of the airway with mediastinal tracheostomy. The tracheostomy tube was brought out through a bipedicled flap of soft tissue and skin. A mediastinal lymphadenectomy was performed in all 21 patients, and simultaneous neck dissections were done in 9 patients. Of the 21 patients, 8 (38%) died during their hospital stay as a result of rupture of a major vessel, mediastinitis, or pulmonary insufficiency. Three patients (14%) were long-term survivors. The authors justifiably concluded their report with a statement of caution about the application of this approach.

Resection and Prosthetic Replacement

Belsey (1950) was the first to describe prosthetic replacement of a circumferential tracheal defect in a patient. He fashioned a tubular prosthesis from autogenous fascia lata reinforced with a coil of stainless steel wire. During the next decade, there were anecdotal reports of clinical reconstructions using a variety of solid tubes, which included substances such as glass, stainless steel, and tantalum. Both solid and porous materials were used. A porous substance used for tracheal replacement has the presumed advantage of becoming infiltrated with host granulation tissue, which may penetrate to the endoluminal surface and create a base for subsequent epithelization. Bucher and co-workers (1951) were the first to report on the use of a porous stainless steel wire mesh prosthesis. In 1960, Usher and Ochsner reported laboratory studies with a porous prosthesis of "heavy-duty" Marlex mesh, and in 1963, Beall and associates reported its application in two patients.

Pearson and colleagues initiated laboratory studies with the same Marlex prosthesis in 1962 and reported results along with a preliminary report of replacement in two patients (Pearson et al, 1968). They subsequently reported experience in seven patients with a cylinder of heavy Marlex mesh for replacement of extensive circumferential defects (Pearson et al, 1984). In three of the seven patients, an excellent functional airway was obtained for 2, 5, and 7.5 years, respectively (one of these patients is shown in Figures 18–5 to 18–9). There were, however, four deaths related to the prosthesis; carinal dehiscence occurred in one case and tracheoinnominate artery fistula in the other three. The vascular fistulas all occurred within 3 weeks of operation.

The last patient in this series was operated on in 1972 for recurrent adenoid cystic carcinoma following a prior extended resection. At the second operation, the surgery required esophageal replacement, laryngectomy, and removal of the entire trachea to the level of the carina (Fig. 18–18). The airway was reconstructed with a cylinder of heavy Marlex mesh, which was anastomosed distally at the carina and sutured to the skin proximally as a terminal stoma in the suprasternal notch. The innominate artery was deliberately resected in this patient to avoid tracheoinnominate artery fistula. The patient, a 65-year-old man, lived for 7½ years with a satisfactory airway and subsequently died of unrelated disease at age 72.

Neville was the first to report on the clinical use of a solid silicone rubber tube for tracheal replacement (Neville et al, 1972). Neville and co-workers subsequently accumulated significant experience and reported on 35 patients managed by reconstruction with a tube of solid, silicone rubber (Neville et al, 1990). A straight prosthesis was used for tracheal replacement in 27 patients (20 with postintubation strictures and 7 with neoplasms), and a bifurcation stent was used for carinal replacement in 8 patients, all with neoplastic disease. A Dacron-reinforced sewing ring was devised at each end of the prosthesis to secure better fixation at the proximal and distal margins. Cardiopulmonary bypass was recommended and was used in a majority of these cases.

It was observed that the silicone replacement was

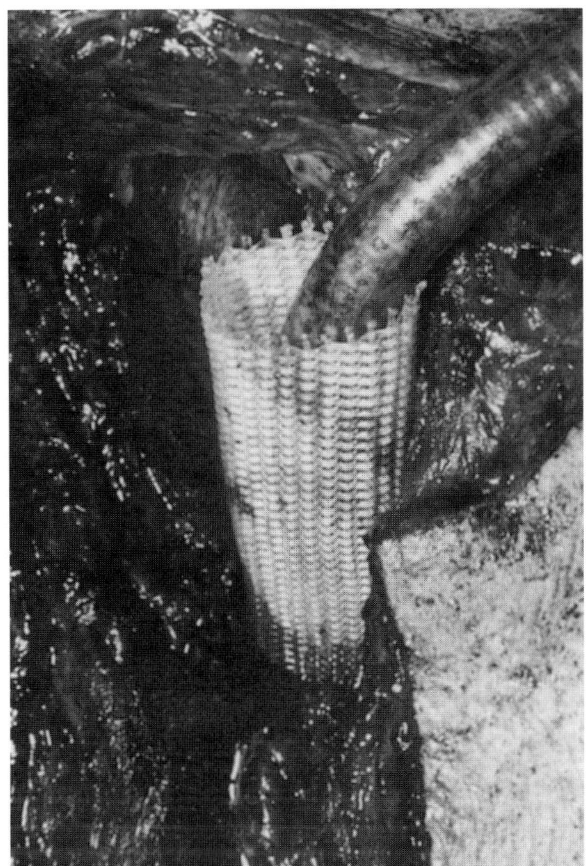

FIGURE 18–18 ■ Intraoperative photograph illustrating replacement of the entire remaining upper airway with a cylindrical prosthesis of heavy Marlex mesh. At operation, the larynx and entire trachea were removed through a cervical incision, median sternotomy, and laparotomy, and the mediastinal trachea was replaced with the Marlex prosthesis. The distal end has been sutured to the main carina, and the upper end has been intubated for intraoperative ventilation. The upper end was brought out as a terminal stoma through the skin of the suprasternal notch. The overlying innominate artery was resected, and the involved thoracic esophagus was replaced with stomach.

never intimately incorporated into the host tissues but remained in an encapsulated pocket of connective tissue, similar to the envelope that surrounds a silicone breast implant. Granulation tissue developed unpredictably at the interface between the native trachea or bronchus and the prosthesis. The inner surface never became epithelized. Complications included obstruction due to granulation tissue, dehiscence requiring reoperation, erosion of the innominate artery, and retention of secretions. It is impossible to precisely quantitate the incidence of complications in their reports. It is also clear that a majority of the 20 patients with postintubation strictures could have been managed by circumferential resection and primary anastomosis; it is exceptional for postintubation injuries to involve an extent of airway that precludes primary reconstruction. Neville and associates are the only surgeons to have recommended widespread application of cardiopulmonary bypass for tracheal replacement surgery in adults.

Subsequent to the report of Neville and associates in

1972, Toomes and colleagues (1985) published experience with nine patients who were operated on between 1979 and 1984 with use of the Neville prosthesis. Eight of these nine patients were operated on for locally advanced malignancy, and the remaining patient had relapsing polychondritis. Resection and reconstruction required the use of a straight Neville prosthesis in five cases and a bifurcation prosthesis in four. Circumferential segments between 6 and 9 cm in length were resected, and resections of this extent may indeed require prosthetic replacement. None of the nine patients required cardiopulmonary bypass for the procedure. Five of these patients died of complications of the prosthesis and operation—two of cardiorespiratory insufficiency, two of tracheoinnominate artery erosion (15 days and 10 months post surgery, respectively), and one of dehiscence. Toomes and coworkers concluded that the morbidity and mortality with this method of tracheal replacement were unacceptable.

The need for prosthetic reconstruction of the airway appears very limited at present. With use of currently available techniques, the majority of resectable lesions can be reconstructed by primary anastomosis with autologous tissues. In those rare cases in which prosthetic replacement is considered, one of us (F.G.P.) would recommend using a porous material and would select heavy duty Marlex mesh as the best available. The prosthesis should be enveloped with a pedicle graft of omentum. Because soft tissue interposition does not provide dependable protection to the innominate artery, resection of the overlying segment of the innominate artery at the time of operation is recommended. If a prosthesis is used, the shortest possible length of cylinder should be employed. If, for example, 80% of the trachea is resected, it is not necessary to use a prosthesis representing the full length of the missing segment. With the use of known techniques of mobilization, the ends of the airway can be approximated, and a prosthesis that may be less than half the length of the normal airway can be inserted without anastomotic tension. The shorter the prosthesis, the less formidable the problem of obtaining endoluminal epithelial cover and avoiding late stenosis.

It must be emphasized that since the first tracheal allotransplantation, which was performed in a human in 1979 (Rose et al, 1979), considerable advances have been made in tracheal allograft transplantation. Cadaveric trachea may be either freeze-dried and radiated (cryopreservation), or chemically stored (chemical preservation), in order to decrease its allogenicity before implantation (Herberhold et al, 1999; Kunachak et al, 2000). Although clinical experience is increasing, application has been limited primarily to children with long-segment congenital tracheal stenosis or recurrent tracheal stenosis in whom previous surgical therapy has failed (Jacobs et al, 1999; Kunachak et al, 2000). The role of tracheal homografting in the management of tracheal disease is not yet established, but this technique may hold future potential for application in patients who require airway resection beyond the current limits of extended resection and reconstruction.

Endoscopic Débridement

Endoscopic procedures are mainly used for palliative therapy of malignant neoplasms. As with any form of upper airway obstruction, it may be possible to secure an improved and safer airway by using a rigid bronchoscope and removing the endoluminal neoplasm with biopsy forceps, suction, or electrocoagulation. Since its first description in the early 1970s by Strong and associates (1973), laser resection has become increasingly popular and is often combined with other bronchoscopic techniques. Endoscopic laser resection with routine bronchoscopic follow-up may occasionally be an acceptable approach to the management of benign pedunculated tumors with no demonstrable extratracheal component (Perelman et al, 1996; Rusch and Schmidt, 1994). Techniques of laser bronchoscopy are described in Chapter 14.

Internal Stents

Some form of internal stent may be used to secure a patent airway in patients with otherwise unmanageable neoplasms. Such therapy is obviously palliative. The options include silicone tubes of various configuration (T, Y, and TY tubes) and internal, self-expanding covered wire stents such as Gianturco and Wall stents and UltraFlex-Microvasive stents. A detailed description of the indications and techniques for the employment of tracheobronchial stents is provided in Chapter 14. Some features of the expandable wire stents are clearly advantageous—no external limb, wider diameters with a more effective internal diameter, and ease of insertion. Incorporation of these stents into the airway may be difficult to reverse. The use of an uncovered wire stent is contraindicated in patients with neoplasms because the tumor will grow through the interstices of the mesh.

COMMENTS AND CONTROVERSIES

Most primary neoplasms of the trachea are malignant, and adenoid cystic carcinoma and squamous cell carcinoma are by far the most common histologic types. Using currently available techniques of mobilization and "release," the surgeon can safely resect long, circumferential segments and can achieve primary reconstruction without the need for a prosthesis in the majority of operable patients. As experience with carinal resection improves, innovations in the techniques of reconstruction have advanced our capability to manage tumors at this level. Cervical collar incision, with a full median sternotomy, is our incision of choice in most patients requiring a concomitant carinal resection for a primary tracheal tumor.

Worthwhile survival can be obtained in patients with adenoid cystic carcinoma, squamous cell carcinoma, and other primary malignant tumors of the trachea as long as a complete and potentially curative resection is done. In the majority of patients with adenoid cystic tumors, even an incomplete resection may be compatible with long periods of symptom-free palliation. Most adenoid cystic carcinomas are radiosensitive, and adjuvant radiation is recommended in all resected tumors of this cell type. Radical radiation therapy is the treatment of choice in patients with unresectable adenoid cystic carcinoma and often results in significant regression of the tumor and palliation, which may endure for several years. Pulmo-

nary metastases occur in about one third of patients with adenoid cystic carcinoma. When first seen, the metastases are often asymptomatic, progress slowly, and may remain symptom-free for many years. In selected patients, therefore, the presence of asymptomatic, synchronous pulmonary metastases is not necessarily a contraindication to resection of an obstructing primary adenoid cystic carcinoma.

Safe and reliable methods of prosthetic replacement remain elusive. The experience of one of us (F.G.P.) with heavy duty Marlex mesh was unsatisfactory owing to an unacceptable operative mortality. The relatively favorable clinical experience reported by Neville and associates with a solid, silicone rubber prosthesis has not been reproduced by others. We emphasize again that the need for prosthetic reconstruction is very limited. With the use of currently available techniques, the majority of resectable lesions can be reconstructed by primary anastomosis with autologous tissue.

Although there is some encouraging work using tracheal homograft in humans, experience remains limited mainly to children with long-segment congenital tracheal stenosis or recurrent tracheal stenosis in whom previous surgical therapy has failed.

S. K.
M. de P.
F. G. P.

■ KEY REFERENCES

Grillo HC, Mathisen DJ: Primary tracheal tumors: Treatment and results. Ann Thorac Surg 49:69, 1990.

This is a detailed review and analysis of the largest reported series of primary tracheal tumors, in which 132 cases were managed by resection, with an operative mortality of 5%.

Pearson FG, Todd TRJ, Cooper JD: Experience with primary neoplasms of the trachea and carina. J Thorac Cardiovasc Surg 88:511, 1984.

This report includes an analysis of the unique pathology and natural history of 44 patients with primary tracheal tumors. A description of the transpericardial approach to the mediastinal trachea and carina is provided.

■ REFERENCES

Aberle DR, Brown K, Young DA et al: Imaging techniques in the evaluation of tracheobronchial neoplasms. Chest 99:211, 1991.

Azar T, Abdul-Karim FW, Tucker HM: Adenoid cystic carcinoma of the trachea. Laryngoscope 108:1297, 1998.

Barclay RS, McSwan N, Welsh TM: Tracheal reconstruction without the use of grafts. Thorax 12:177,1957.

Beall AC Jr, Harrington OB, Greenberg SD et al: Circumferential replacement of thoracic trachea with Marlex mesh. JAMA 183:1082, 1963.

Belsey R: Stainless steel wire suture technique in thoracic surgery. Thorax 1:39, 1946.

Belsey R: Resection and reconstruction of the intrathoracic trachea. Br J Surg 38:200, 1950.

Briselli M, Mark EJ, Grillo HC: Tracheal carcinoids. Cancer 42:2870, 1978.

Bucher RM, Burnett WE, Rosemond GP: Experimental reconstruction of tracheal and bronchial defects with stainless steel wire mesh. J Thoracic Surg 21:572, 1951.

Daniel TM, Smith RH, Faunce HF, Sylves VM: Transbronchoscopic versus surgical resection of tracheobronchial granular cell myoblastomas. Suggested approach based on follow up of all treated cases. J Thorac Cardiovasc Surg 80:898, 1980.

Fidias P, Wright C, Harris NL et al: Primary tracheal non-Hodgkin's lymphoma. A case report and review of the literature. Cancer 77:2332, 1996.

Fredberg JJ, Wohl MEB, Glass GM, Dorkin HL: Airway area by acoustic reflections measured at the mouth. J Appl Physiol 48:749, 1980.

Gelb AF, Tashkin DP, Epstein JD et al: Diagnosis and Nd:YAG laser treatment of unsuspected malignant tracheal obstruction. Chest 94:767, 1988.

Gelder CM, Hetzel MR: Primary tracheal tumours: A national survey. Thorax 48:688, 1993.

Goepfert H, Sessions RB, Gutterman JV et al: Leukocyte interferon in patients with juvenile laryngeal papillomatosis. Ann Otol Rhinol Laryngol 91:431, 1982.

Grillo HC: Tracheal tumors: Surgical management. Ann Thorac Surg 26:112, 1978.

Grillo HC: Carinal reconstruction. Ann Thorac Surg 34:356, 1982.

Grillo HC: Primary tracheal tumors. Thorax 48:681, 1993.

Grillo HC, Dignan EF, Miura T: Extensive resection and reconstruction of mediastinal trachea without prosthesis or graft: An anatomical study in man. J Thorac Cardiovasc Surg 48:741, 1964.

Grillo HC, Mathisen DJ: Primary tracheal tumors: Treatment and results. Ann Thorac Surg 49:69, 1990.

Hadju SI, Huvos AG, Goodner JT et al: Carcinoma of the trachea: Clinicopathologic study of 41 cases. Cancer 25:1448, 1970.

Heitmiller RF, Mathisen DJ, Ferry JA et al: Mucoepidermoid lung tumors. Ann Thorac Surg 47:394, 1989.

Herberhold C, Stein M, Bierhoff E, Kost S: Tracheal reconstruction with preserved tracheal homograft—new aspects. Laryngorhinootologie 78:54, 1999.

Jacobs JP, Quintessenza JA, Andrews T et al: Tracheal allograft reconstruction: The total North American and worldwide pediatric experiences. Ann Thorac Surg 68:1043, 1999.

Kairalla RA, Carvalho CRR, Parada AA et al: Solitary plasmacytoma of the trachea treated by loop resection and laser therapy. Thorax 43:1011, 1988.

Kunachak S, Kulapaditharom B, Vajaradul Y, Rochanawutanon M: Cryopreserved, irradiated tracheal homograft transplantation for laryngotracheal reconstruction in human beings. Otolaryngol Head Neck Surg 911:122, 2000.

Lange TH, Magee MJ, Boley TM et al: Tracheobronchial glomus tumor. Ann Thorac Surg 70:292, 2000.

Li W, Ellerbroek NA, Libshitz HI: Primary malignant tumors of the trachea. A radiologic and clinical study. Cancer 66:894, 1990.

Manninen MP, Antila PJ, Pukander JS, Karma PH: Occurrence of tracheal carcinoma in Finland. Acta Otolaryngol 111:1162, 1991.

Maziak DE, Todd TRJ, Keshavjee SH et al: Adenoid cystic carcinoma of the airway: Thirty-two-year experience. J Thorac Cardiovasc Surg 112:1522, 1996.

Menaissy YM, Gal AA, Mansour KA: Glomus tumor of the trachea. Ann Thorac Surg 70:295, 2000.

Morency G, Chalaoui J, Samson L, Sylvestre J: Malignant neoplasms of the trachea. J Can Assoc Radiol 40:198, 1989.

Naidich DP: CT/MR correlation in the evaluation of tracheobronchial neoplasia. Radiol Clin North Am 28:555, 1990.

Neis PR, McMahon MF, Norris CW: Cartilaginous tumors of the trachea and larynx. Ann Otol Laryngol 98:31, 1989.

Neville WE, Bolanowski PJP, Kotia GG: Clinical experience with the silicone tracheal prosthesis. J Thorac Cardiovasc Surg 99:604, 1990.

Neville WE, Hamouda F, Andersen J, Dwan FM: Replacement of the intrathoracic trachea and both stem bronchi with a molded Silastic prosthesis. J Thorac Cardiovasc Surg 63:569, 1972.

Pearson FG, Brito Flomeno LT, Cooper JD: Experience with partial cricoid resection and thyrotracheal anastomosis. Ann Otol Rhinol Laryngol 95:582, 1986.

Pearson FG, Cooper JD, Nelems JM, Van Nostrand AW: Primary tracheal anastomosis after resection of the cricoid cartilage with preservation of recurrent laryngeal nerves. J Thorac Cardiovasc Surg 70:806, 1975.

Pearson FG, Henderson RD, Gross E et al: The reconstruction of circumferential tracheal defects with a porous prosthesis: An experimental and clinical study using heavy Marlex mesh. J Thorac Cardiovasc Surg 55:605, 1968.

Pearson FG, Thompson DW, Weissberg D et al: Adenoid cystic carcinoma of the trachea. Ann Thorac Surg 18:16, 1974.

Pearson FG, Todd TRJ, Cooper JD: Experience with primary neoplasms of the trachea and carina. J Thorac Cardiovasc Surg 88:511, 1984.

Perelman MI, Koroleva N, Birjukov J, Goudovsky L: Primary tracheal tumors. Semin Thorac Cardiovasc Surg 8:400, 1996.
Perelman Ml, Koroleva NS: Primary tumors of the trachea. In Grillo HC (ed): International Trends in General Thoracic Surgery, Vol 2. Philadelphia, WB Saunders, 1987, p 91.
Prommegger R, Salzer GM: Long-term results of surgery for adenoid cystic carcinoma of the trachea and bronchi. Eur J Surg Oncol 24:440, 1998.
Rabah R, Lancaster WD, Thomas R, Gregoire L: Human papillomavirus-11–associated recurrent respiratory papillomatosis is more aggressive than human papillomavirus-6–associated disease. Pediatr Dev Pathol 3:68, 2001.
Refaely Y, Weissberg D: Surgical management of tracheal tumors. Ann Thorac Surg 64:1429, 1997.
Regnard JF, Fourquier P, Levasseur P: Results and prognostic factors in resections of primary tracheal tumors: A multicenter retrospective study. J Thorac Cardiovasc Surg 111:808, 1996.
Rose KG, Sesterhenn K, Wustrow F: Tracheal allotransplantation in man. Lancet 1:433, 1979.
Rusch VW, Schmidt RA: Tracheal schwannoma: Management by endoscopic laser resection. Thorax 49:85, 1994.
Salminen US, Haltunen P, Taskinen E, Mattila S: Recurrence and malignant transformation of endotracheal chondroma. Ann Thorac Surg 49:830, 1990.
Shankar S, George PJ, Hetzel MR, Goldstraw P: Elective resection of tumors of the trachea and main carina after endoscopic laser therapy. Thorax 45:493, 1990.
Strong MS, Jako GJ, Polanyi T, Wallace RA: Laser surgery in the aerodigestive tract. Am J Surg 126:529, 1973.
Sun JD, Weatherly RA, Koopmann CF, Carey TE: Mucosal swabs detect HPV in laryngeal papillomatosis patients but not family members. Int J Pediatr Otorhinolaryngol 53:95, 2000.
Sykes AT, Rokkas CK, Kajdacsy-Balla A, Haasler GB: Primary tracheal synovial cell sarcoma: A first report. J Thorac Cardiovasc Surg 114:678, 1997.
Terz JJ, Wagman LD, King RE et al: Results of extended resection of tumors involving the cervical part of the trachea. Surg Gynecol Obstet 151:491, 1980.
Toomes H, Mickisch G, Bogt-Moykopf I: Experiences with prosthetic reconstruction of the trachea and bifurcation. Thorax 40:32, 1985.
Usher FC, Ochsner JL: Marlex mesh: A new polyethylene mesh for replacing tissue defects. Surg Forum 10:319, 1960.
Xu L-T, Sun Z-F, Li Z-J et al: Clinical and pathological characteristics in patients with tracheobronchial tumor. Report of 50 patients. Ann Thorac Surg 43:276, 1987.
Yang KY, Chen YM, Huang MH, Perng RP: Revisit of primary malignant neoplasms of the trachea: Clinical characteristics and survival analysis. Jpn J Clin Oncol 27:305, 1997.

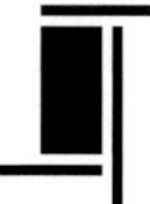

SECONDARY TUMORS

Hermes C. Grillo
Douglas J. Mathisen

Secondary tumors most often involve the trachea or carina by direct invasion from the adjacent organ of origin—larynx, thyroid, lung, or esophagus. The two categories of secondary tumors involving trachea and carina that are most appropriately treated surgically are carcinoma of the thyroid and bronchogenic carcinoma.

This chapter section is divided into three parts: (1) thyroid cancer invading the airway; (2) bronchogenic carcinoma involving the carina; and (3) other secondary tumors involving the airway.

Thyroid Cancer

HISTORICAL NOTE

Resection of the larynx and upper trachea has been performed for many years for both well- and poorly differentiated invasive carcinoma of the thyroid (Frazell and Foote, 1958; Hendrick, 1963), sometimes with surprisingly long-term palliation or apparent cure. Patients are few in number who have well-differentiated carcinoma involving the trachea or adjacent larynx in limited enough fashion to be resectable with the involved airway and yet permit primary reconstruction. The techniques of airway reconstruction that have evolved over the past 30 years have been applied only slowly to these cases. Ishihara and associates (1978) reported on 11 such patients. In the Western Hemisphere, Grillo reported an initial case in 1965, and with Zannini (1986) described 19 patients who underwent resection for papillary or mixed papillary and follicular carcinoma of the thyroid, as well as 3 who underwent this surgery for undifferentiated carcinoma. In 16, primary reconstruction was performed, and for the other 6, therapy was en bloc cervicomediastinal resection with end tracheostomy. Of the 16 having airway reconstruction, 15 had good surgical results with speech preservation. Eight patients were alive without disease at up to 9 years, and only 2 developed airway recurrence. By 1991, Ishihara had performed 60 resections for thyroid cancer invading the airway. Maeda and associates (1989) recorded 151 patients in Japan with tracheoplasty for thyroid cancer (26.7% of all tracheoplasties in Japan). Grillo and colleagues (1992) described 34 patients at Massachusetts General Hospital who underwent resection for thyroid cancer invading the airway of 52 who presented with such involvement.

■ *HISTORICAL READINGS*

Grillo HC, Zannini P: Resectional management of airway invasion by thyroid carcinoma. Ann Thorac Surg 42:287, 1986.
Ishihara T, Kobayashi K, Kikuchi K et al: Surgical treatment of advanced thyroid carcinoma invading the trachea. J Thorac Cardiovasc Surg 102:717, 1991.

BASIC SCIENCE

Well-differentiated thyroid carcinoma usually runs an indolent course, frequently with long-term survival (Beahrs et al, 1981). Airway invasion, however, is directly responsible for many late deaths due to thyroid cancer and is a source of profound morbidity due to airway hemorrhage and suffocation (Silliphant et al, 1964). Thyroid cancer that invades the airway early usually does so by direct involvement of the airway closest to the tumor; this occurs in 1% to 6.5% of patients (Lawson et al, 1977). Tsumori and co-workers (1985) reported that 50% of papillary and follicular carcinomas that invaded the airway showed poor differentiation, as compared with 11.4% of noninvasive thyroid cancers of the same histology. Invasion also tends to be seen in older patients, in whom papillary and follicular thyroid cancers are more aggressive, although the spectrum is broad. Nomori and associates (1990) found that the nuclear area of tumor cells was significantly greater in cases with tracheal invasion than in those without. Both Tsumori and colleagues and Nomori and co-workers noted that the tumors had sometimes become less well differentiated than they were originally.

The prognosis of thyroid cancers invading the airway appears to correlate with the site and depth of invasion (Tsumori et al, 1987). Shin and associates (1993) classified papillary thyroid cancer invading the trachea as follows: stage 0, tumor confined to the thyroid gland; stage I, extension through the capsule to abut the perichondrium but without cartilaginous erosion or intercartilaginous invasion; stage II, destruction of cartilage or intercartilaginous invasion; stage III, extension into the lamina propria of the tracheal mucosa; stage IV, extension through the tracheal mucosa. Clinical results correlated well with these stages, in general confirming the observations of Tsumori and colleagues (1987).

Because of the location of the thyroid gland, the subglottic larynx may also be invaded. The corresponding recurrent laryngeal nerve is often paralyzed, paretic, or encircled by tumor. Adjacent esophagus or cricopharyngeus may be involved. The tumor may penetrate into any depth of the airway. Recurrent tumors are too often permitted to grow to large sizes even though they frequently respond little to radioactive iodine therapy (RaI) or external radiotherapy. Poorly differentiated tumors in their initial presentation may involve the larynx to such a degree that its salvage is not possible. Invasion may include the pharynx and esophagus as well.

DIAGNOSIS

The patient with differentiated thyroid carcinoma involving the airway may present with classical signs of airway involvement, mainly hemoptysis and sometimes dyspnea on exertion or wheezing. More often, airway involvement is not symptomatic because the tumor has not yet penetrated the mucous membrane or projected any distance into the lumen. A firm mass that is not freely movable over the airway may be palpable. All too often, tracheal and laryngeal involvement is detected only at thyroidectomy. Under these circumstances, the thyroid surgeon, often unskilled in techniques of airway resection and reconstruction, will "shave off" the tumor from the airway wall.

In addition to the usual diagnostic approach to thyroid cancer (thyroid function studies, thyroid scan, and needle biopsy), flexible bronchoscopy is advisable in every patient. CT scanning should include the chest to search for pulmonary metastases. MRI is also useful in defining these lesions. The neck should be imaged by means of thin-section CT scans, which are most likely to identify involvement of the tracheal wall or intrusion into the lumen. Linear radiographic studies of the trachea, including filtered views and crisp tomography, are of great use in determining the extent of gross involvement of the larynx and trachea and also the relative proportion of uninvolved airway, which is important to the surgeon considering resection and reconstruction (Fig. 18–19). Fluoroscopy of the larynx adds information about function of the vocal cords to that obtained by direct laryngoscopy. A barium swallow may define the bulk of the tumor and detect involvement of the proximal esophagus.

In some cases considered for cervical exenteration, arch angiography may detect involvement of mediastinal vessels and may be useful for studying cerebral blood supply in the event that mediastinal tracheotomy should become necessary and require prophylactic division of the brachiocephalic artery. Bone scan is performed to search for skeletal metastases.

MANAGEMENT

Principles

The purposes of resection of thyroid cancer invading the airway are (1) to attempt to achieve cure by accomplishing complete resection of the tumor; (2) to provide prolonged palliation by relief or prevention of airway obstruction in patients with slowly progressive neoplasms; and (3) to prevent death by asphyxiation or hemorrhage. Resection and reconstruction of involved airway as part of the complete local excision of thyroid cancer, particularly as an initial procedure, accomplishes the primary goals of conventional thyroid cancer surgery. It does not represent a radical extension of surgery for thyroid cancer. Where resection and reconstruction of the airway can effect complete removal of the disease, it is illogical simply to shave off a cancer, leaving the local tumor to recur in the airway. This is done all too frequently, however, because a surgeon performing thyroidectomy may not be competent to perform airway surgery. Hence, it is important that efforts be made to attempt to diagnose such involvement in advance of surgical exploration so that the patient can be referred for needed care. The alternative is to refer a patient for resection of the airway immediately after discovery of such involvement in the operating theater.

Follow-up results suggest strongly that patients in whom either of these alternatives has been followed are the two groups in whom the best long-term results and even cure may be expected (Grillo et al, 1992). Late removal of recurrent tumor obstructing the airway, occurring sometimes years after the initial tumor has been

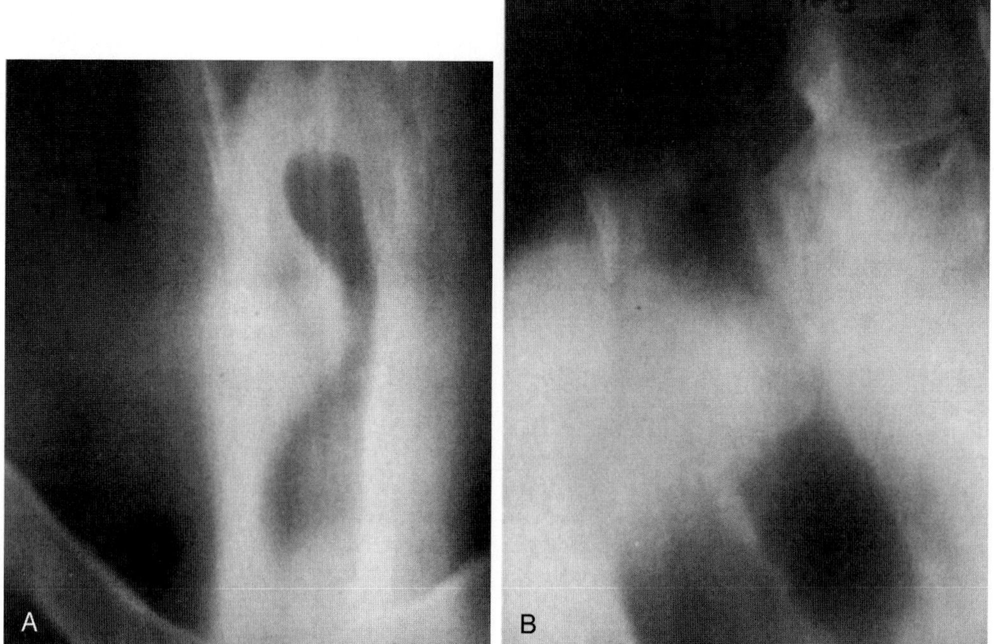

FIGURE 18–19 ■ Tomograms of mixed papillary and follicular carcinoma invading the subglottic larynx and upper trachea. *A,* Anterior view: tumor is seen protruding on the right invading the subglottic larynx just below the conus elasticus. The alae of the thyroid cartilage may be seen just above the tumor mass on the right. *B,* Lateral view: the calcified thyroid cartilage is seen just above the mass. (From Grillo HC, Zannini P: Resectional management of airway invasion by thyroid carcinoma. Ann Thorac Surg 42:287, 1986.)

shaved off the trachea, is effective palliation but not often curative. Remote metastases have often occurred by this time. The finding of pulmonary metastases from slowly progressive differentiated carcinoma of the thyroid is not an absolute contraindication to therapy of the airway disease, however. Almost uniformly, localized involvement of the airway by carcinoma of the thyroid involves only one recurrent laryngeal nerve. Thus, a still functional larynx can be preserved by conserving the nerve on the opposite side.

Radical techniques of cervical or cervicomediastinal exenteration, on the other hand, should be applied very selectively. Such radical technique appears justifiable when the tumor is localized but involves larynx too extensively for salvage, and sometimes the pharynx and esophagus as well. This occurs more commonly with aggressive, poorly differentiated carcinoma. A second situation justifying radical technique is massive recurrence of differentiated carcinoma, often over years and usually after unsuccessful treatment with RaI and external radiotherapy. Such patients may be miserable, with poorly functioning tracheostomies accompanied by local bleeding, loss of voice, and inability to swallow food or even saliva. Cervical pain further aggravates their condition. In such patients, radical excision may offer palliation even if pulmonary metastases are present.

Operative Technique

Resection and Reconstruction

Careful endoscopic examination requires a rigid instrument with a Storz-Hopkins magnifying telescope rather than a flexible bronchoscope, so that precise information can be obtained about the gross extent of involvement proximally and distally. Measurements are made of the extent of grossly uninvolved trachea that will be available for reconstruction. The same general guiding principles of extent of resection that apply in surgery for primary tracheal tumors (Grillo and Mathisen, 1990b) also apply here. Because resection often extends proximally to include a portion of the subglottic larynx on one side, the distal trachea must be divided in an irregular, bayonet-like pattern so that the two ends of the airway can be slid together for reconstruction (Grillo and Zannini, 1986). This requires a longer resection than simply the distance from the inferior border of the cricoid cartilage to a point just distal to the tumor. This length must be considered in planning the reconstruction.

Approach comes almost uniformly through a low collar incision, elevating flaps well up onto the larynx as necessary and extending to the sternal notch below. If the tumor is recurrent or invasive, strap muscles or residual tissue overlying the tumor is excised en bloc. The limits of tumor are defined by dissection before irrevocable steps are taken. This includes superior and inferior definition of the extent of tumor, lateral definition of the carotid arteries and internal jugular veins, and later in the dissection, the extent, if any, of involvement of the upper esophagus and cricopharyngeus. Because such involvement is proximal, at the level where the thyroid gland is most closely adjacent to the trachea, upper sternal division has not been required.

There are three principal patterns by which the trachea has been resected for invasive differentiated thyroid carcinoma (Grillo and Zannini, 1986) (Fig. 18–20). The first consists of sleeve resection, performed when the trachea alone is involved. The superior margin is usually at the inferior border of the cricoid cartilage. In a second situation, in which the tumor involves the cricoid on one side, the line of proximal division may be beveled to transect the larynx above the point of involvement, including part of the cricoid cartilage on one side. Because the recurrent laryngeal nerve on that side is almost uniformly involved by tumor in such a case, no additional avoidable functional loss is incurred by deliberate division of the paralyzed nerve as it enters the larynx posteriorly on that side.

More complicated is the third situation, in which the tumor creeps up higher into the larynx on one side, so that a straight beveled line of resection is not feasible (Fig. 18–21). In such a case, we prefer to commence division beneath the cricoid cartilage on the uninvolved side and to angle the incision upward anteriorly, staying away from the gross border of the tumor; we then curve the incision to divide the larynx beneath the paralyzed vocal cord, carrying it down in a curve to leave a margin of uninvolved tissue around the tumor, and finally dropping vertically or obliquely in the posterior part of the laryngeal wall. Each resection is necessarily individualized (Fig. 18–22). Frozen sections are obtained at the points nearest the tumor, preferably sampled from tissue that remains in the patient rather than from the resected specimen. This is definitive for the surgeon and pathologist, eliminating any question about the location of cancer cells. If tumor is still present, the surgeon may take additional tissue, remembering, however, that reconstruction is the goal. The trachea distal to the tumor is trimmed to fit the irregular lateral defect that has been created in the larynx.

Microscopically positive margins may have to be accepted occasionally if this is necessary to salvage a functional larynx. With well-differentiated carcinoma, often characterized by slow clinical progression, this seems preferable to laryngectomy. External radiation is administered after healing, provided that prohibitive doses have not been given in the past. Laryngectomy can be performed later should tumor recur locally in the larynx.

Reconstruction is accomplished with 4–0 Vicryl sutures, all sutures being placed prior to being tied (Grillo, 1988). Lateral traction sutures are employed to take tension off the anastomosis while it is being accomplished. Ventilation is managed across the operative field in the usual manner in a methodical and unhurried fashion. With very extensive resection, suprahyoid laryngeal release (Montgomery, 1974) may be employed, although this has rarely been necessary in these cases. Even with the known occurrence of microscopic foci of papillary carcinoma elsewhere in an involved gland, we have not considered it necessary to remove the opposite lobe of thyroid in all cases; a second clinically significant cancer on the opposite side is rare. This conservative approach further ensures that damage will not be done to the opposite and uninvolved recurrent laryngeal nerve. Total thyroidectomy is performed if indicated.

If reconstruction is particularly high or if the laryngeal airway seems to be tenuous because of edema, protective tracheostomy is advised. The anastomosis is covered with available adjacent tissue (muscle). The brachiocephalic

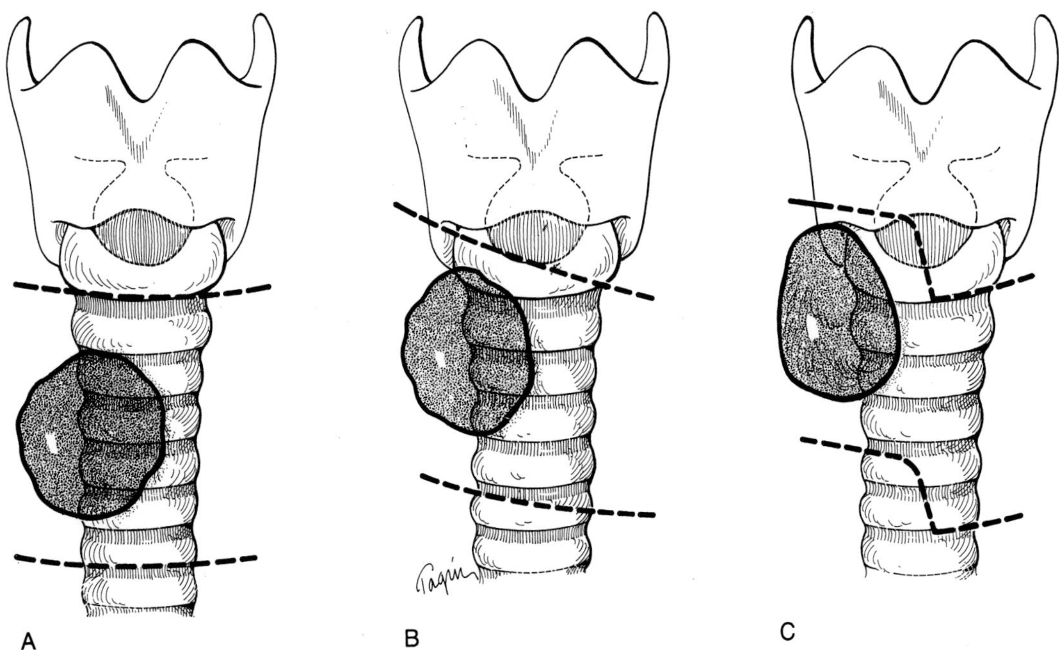

FIGURE 18–20 ■ Types of resection of upper airway for thyroid carcinoma. *A,* Sleeve resection of trachea. *B,* A portion of the lower cricoid is beveled to remove an additional margin above the tumor. The recurrent laryngeal nerve may or may not be involved in such a case. *C,* Tailored line of resection to obtain a margin around the tumor with deeper and more proximal invasion of the cricoid cartilage. The recurrent laryngeal nerve in such a case is almost uniformly paralyzed prior to resection. (From Grillo HC, Zannini P: Resectional management of airway invasion by thyroid carcinoma. Ann Thorac Surg 42:287, 1986.)

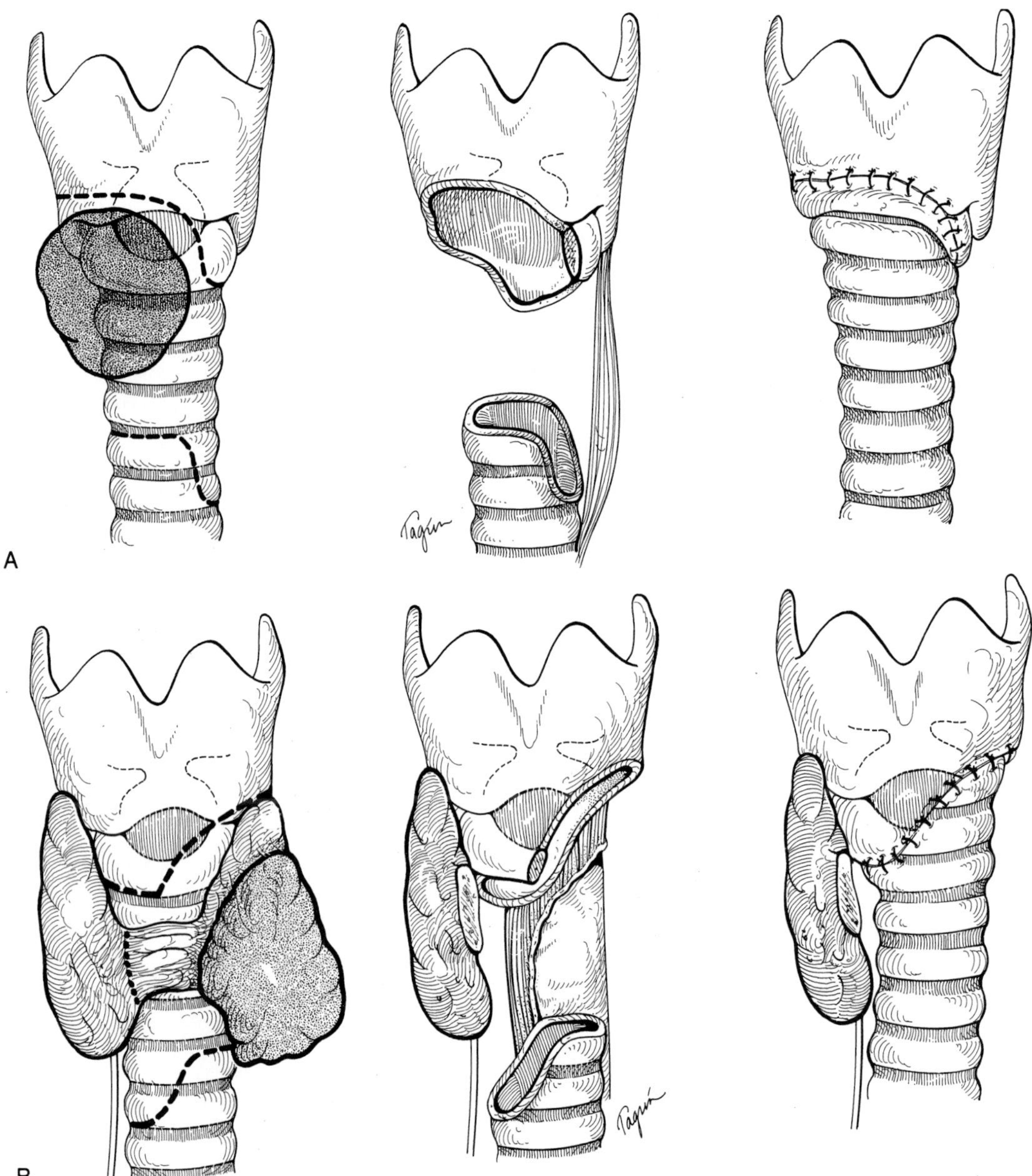

FIGURE 18–21 ■ Examples of complex resections. *A*, Resection of mixed papillary and follicular carcinoma for recurrence 2 years after total thyroidectomy. The left recurrent laryngeal nerve was preserved anatomically and functionally. *B*, Mixed papillary and follicular carcinoma, not previously treated, managed by resection of part of the larynx, trachea, and anterolateral muscular wall of the esophagus. (From Grillo HC, Zannini P: Resectional management of airway invasion by thyroid carcinoma. Ann Thorac Surg 42:287, 1986.)

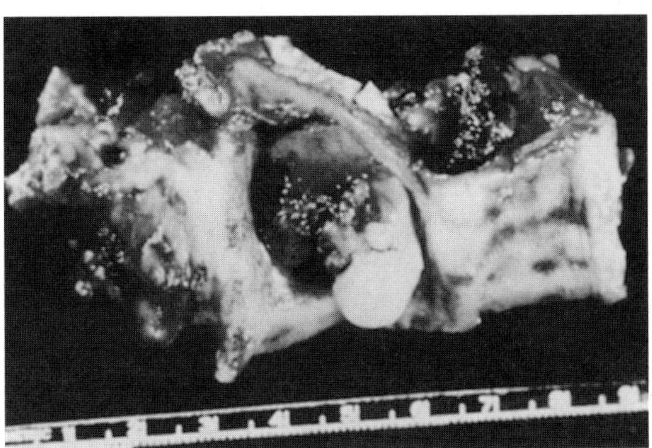

FIGURE 18–22 ■ Follicular carcinoma recurrent 4 years after total thyroidectomy, which in turn was preceded by right hemithyroidectomy 2 years earlier. The proximal resection line includes a beveled portion of the cricoid cartilage. The right recurrent laryngeal nerve was paralyzed preoperatively. The patient died almost 7 years following this resection from mediastinal metastases. (From Grillo HC: Congenital lesions, neoplasms and injuries of the trachea. In Sabiston DC Jr, Spencer FC [eds]: Gibbon's Surgery of the Chest, 5th ed. Philadelphia, WB Saunders, 1983.)

artery is protected by suturing strap muscle or other available tissue over the artery against the trachea in order to prevent potential erosion of the artery by a low-placed tracheostomy tube (in a shortened trachea). A small tracheostomy tube is inserted into the resulting triangular space 1.5 to 2 cm distal to the anastomosis.

If it is uncertain whether the airway might be edematous postoperatively, or if there is concern about the short distance available for placement of a tracheostomy tube adjacent to the anastomosis, the anastomosis and brachiocephalic artery are walled off as described, and a single, silk, marking suture is placed on the tracheal wall at the point where a tracheostomy may later be placed (Grillo, 1982b). The patient is awakened and the airway examined with a flexible bronchoscope. If there is any question about adequacy of the glottis because of edema, an uncuffed small-bore nasotracheal tube is placed. After 5 days, this is removed in the operating room and the airway again examined. If it is adequate, the patient is observed closely for another period of days. If it does not appear adequate, tracheotomy is performed in the premarked spot without interfering with the now-sealed suture lines. The tracheostomy is removed when glottic edema subsides. Decadron, as well as racemic epinephrine, is administered perioperatively and immediately postoperatively in most patients.

When the outer esophageal wall is involved, we have removed the full thickness of the muscularis, leaving an intact mucosa. In other patients, we have removed the full thickness of the esophageal wall, closing the esophagus in linear fashion with two layers of interrupted 4–0 silk sutures in the manner described by Sweet (1950). A thus-narrowed esophagus remains an adequate conduit for saliva and for initial liquid feedings. It usually dilates spontaneously later without the need even for mechanical dilatation, which may, however, occasionally be needed. A pedicled strap muscle or other tissue is placed between an esophageal suture line and the airway anastomosis to prevent fistulization.

The surgery is precise and demanding, but functional results are excellent. The patient will initially have a hoarse voice if one recurrent laryngeal nerve has been sacrificed. Often, this is largely self-corrected over 6 to 12 months. If at the end of that time, the voice remains inadequate, the vocal cord may be stiffened by a variety of procedures such as Teflon injection. Because so many patients improve spontaneously, such procedures are deferred for 1 year. The airway is usually wholly satisfactory.

Cervical Exenteration

There is limited application for the drastic approach of cervical exenteration to airway involvement by thyroid cancer. However, exenteration can be a remarkably effective palliative measure for a patient who is facing strangulation by tumor, usually recurrent, or less commonly, for the patient who is faced with a primary carcinoma of rapid local growth that is still resectable (Fig. 18–23). Rarely, resection may be curative.

If the pharynx and esophagus are also involved, our technique of resection consists of blocking out all tissue from above the hyoid bone, including the lower pharynx, and from carotid sheath to carotid sheath laterally to the upper mediastinum below (Grillo and Mathisen, 1990a). The vertebral spine forms the floor of the dissection. A long, horizontal incision along the top of the clavicles is used. If tumor extends low on the trachea, a mediastinal tracheostomy is performed, with removal of the heads of the clavicles and the first two costal cartilages and division of the sternum at the level of the second interspace. The feasibility of resection is determined initially by dividing the sternum horizontally through the second interspace and vertically through the manubrium. If resection is safely possible, the bony plaque is removed.

The trachea is divided well below the tumor but is not mobilized except on its anterior surface, with careful preservation of the lateral blood supply. A second, inferior horizontal incision beneath the mammary crease allows a bipedicled cutaneous flap to fall into the mediastinum for stomal anastomosis without tension. The inferior deficit in skin is closed with a skin graft (Fig. 18–24). In the case of a very low mediastinal tracheostomy (within 2 to 3 cm of the carina)—rarely necessary for thyroid cancer, even for recurrent disease—the brachiocephalic artery may be electively divided after it is first occluded and the electroencephalographic monitors, which are placed in all such cases, are checked. Esophageal continuity is established with stomach or left colon.

The omentum is also advanced substernally in such cases, particularly if the patient has received heavy irradiation, as many have. The omentum covers major mediastinal vessels, buttresses the neo-esophageal anastomosis, and surrounds the trachea just beneath its anastomosis to the skin (Mathisen et al, 1988). Postoperative separation of the anastomosis in the vicinity of the innominate artery, due to irradiation or tension, thus does not necessarily produce a disastrous vascular fistula. Cervicomediastinal exenteration is a lengthy and complex procedure that demands rigorous indications and considerable experience.

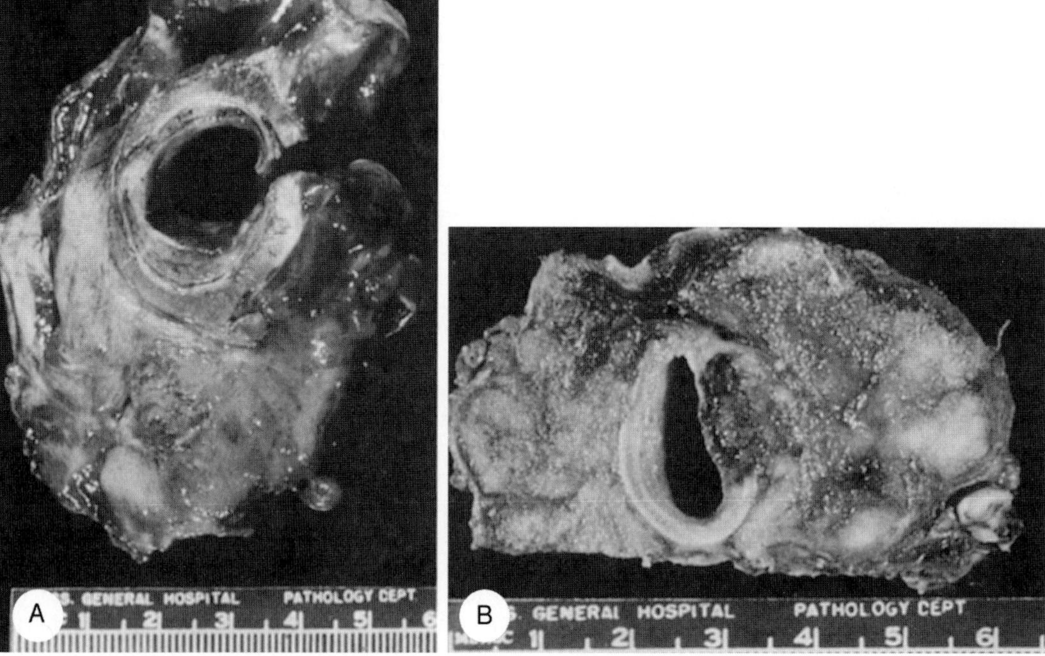

FIGURE 18–23 ■ *A,* Squamous cell carcinoma of the thyroid, which required resection of larynx, trachea, and esophagus. *B,* Papillary carcinoma, which required tracheal resection, neck dissection, and removal of the anterolateral wall of the esophagus. (From Grillo HC, Zannini P: Resectional management of airway invasion by thyroid carcinoma. Ann Thorac Surg 42:287, 1986.)

Early Results

Of 52 patients with thyroid cancer invading the airway seen between 1964 and 1991, resection was not performed in 18 because of either distant disease, extensive local disease, or the desire to preserve laryngeal function in cases where only an operation including laryngectomy would have been adequate (Grillo et al, 1992). The other 34 patients underwent resectional therapy; 27 of these had reconstruction of the airway and 7 had exenteration with end tracheostomies. The distribution was even between males and females, and their ages ranged from 17 to 79 years, with a mean of 61. Among the patients who had the reconstructive procedure, 16 had papillary carcinoma, 5 had follicular carcinoma, 4 carcinoma of mixed histology, and 2 poorly differentiated carcinoma. The cancers of those undergoing resection without reconstruction comprised three papillary, one follicular, and three of more aggressive histology. Of those who had reconstruction, 15 had unilateral recurrent laryngeal nerve paralysis, but 11 of these had had prior surgery. Only 9 of the 27 patients undergoing reconstruction had had no prior therapy or ^{131}I radiotherapy only. The other 18 had undergone resection, including hemithyroidectomy and subtotal thyroidectomy. Neck dissections had been performed in some. Five of the patients were referred immediately after the surgeon identified tracheal invasion, but 13 others were referred at the time of recurrence, the original tumor having been shaved off the trachea. The interval between initial surgical treatment and airway resection ranged from 1 to 47 years. A number had undergone ^{131}I therapy, chemotherapy, and external irradiation. Some had tracheostomies. Only three of those undergoing exenteration had had no prior therapy; the other four had had thyroidectomy, ^{131}I therapy, and external irradiation.

Ten patients underwent tracheal sleeve resection, six had partial oblique resection of the cricoid cartilage with a laryngotracheal anastomosis, and ten underwent complex resection with individually designed lines of resection through the larynx to accomplish maximal tumor removal but preservation of laryngeal function. In three patients, a complementary tracheotomy was performed because the immediate adequacy of the airway at the conclusion of the surgery was in question. Laryngeal release was not required. Of the 27, 15 showed lymph node metastases, and in 13, positive resection margins were accepted in order to salvage the larynx. Eight patients received radioactive iodine therapy, and seven received external radiation.

Two deaths occurred in this group of 27 patients. The first was the result of failure of anastomotic healing in a patient who had undergone 7800 cGy of irradiation 6 years prior to reconstruction, following incomplete resection of cancer. This resection was attempted prior to the time when omental augmentation was used for irradiated airways. A second patient died from respiratory arrest due to airway obstruction; a temporary tracheostomy would have obviated this occurrence. One patient suffered right vocal cord paralysis not present preoperatively and not the result of elective resection of a recurrent laryngeal nerve. Mild dysphagia in three patients resolved, with one patient requiring dilatation.

Late Results

In the reconstruction group, 11 of the 25 survivors of surgery died of cancer from 3 months to 10¼ years

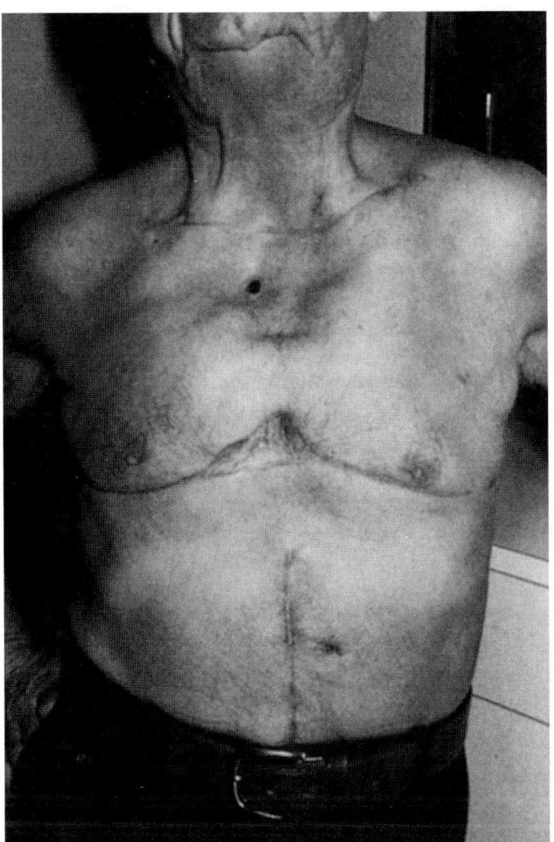

FIGURE 18–24 ■ Postoperative status of patient whose specimen is shown in Figure 18–23*A*. The mediastinal tracheostomy may be seen in a depressed portion of the chest wall, where the upper part of the sternum, the heads of the clavicles, and the first two cartilages have been removed. A skin graft covers the relaxing incision, which permitted the flap to drop into the mediastinum.

following reconstruction (Fig. 18–25). Two patients with undifferentiated thyroid cancer died from distant metastases within 6 months of resection. Cancer of the airway recurred in only two patients in the group, which indicates the accomplishment of one of the primary goals of surgery, obviation of death by airway obstruction. The average duration of survival among these 11 patients was 3 years and 7 months. The usual cause of death was metastatic disease in the mediastinum, lungs, or brain. One patient died of leukemia, which was possibly related to earlier ^{131}I therapy. Of the 13 surviving patients, 12 were without evidence of cancer at the time of follow-up (1 month to 14½ years following airway surgery); the other patient had pulmonary metastases. The average survival of the 13 patients was 5 years and 9 months at the time of follow-up. In two patients, local nodal recurrences had been excised at varying intervals following the initial airway resection.

Of the 13 surviving patients, 9 had undergone airway resection as part of the initial surgical treatment or had been referred immediately after a surgeon found evidence of tracheal invasion at thyroidectomy (see Fig. 18–25). Of 17 patients eligible for 5-year follow-up, 10 were alive at 5 years and 9 at 10 years. Of 11 survivors with positive microscopic margins, 3 were alive without evidence of disease up to 6 years after resection. Six of the others died of thyroid cancer, one died of leukemia, and one was alive with pulmonary metastases. The six who died of thyroid cancer lived from 3 months to more than 10 years following resection.

It is also worth noting that seven patients had evidence of pulmonary metastasis at the time of airway resection performed to achieve palliation. The metastases were known to be slowly enlarging. While two of these died within 1 year of the airway procedure (with undifferentiated carcinoma), the average survival for the whole group was 4.2 years, and the patient surviving the longest was still alive for longer than 10½ years following surgery.

In the nonreconstruction group who underwent radical resection, one patient with sarcoma died of metastases 2 years and 7 months following resection, one with squamous carcinoma died 7 years and 4 months after resection, three died of other diseases without evidence of recurrence, and one remained alive 3 years later but had developed asymptomatic pulmonary metastases.

COMMENTS AND CONTROVERSIES

Although differentiated carcinoma that invades the airway appears often to be aggressive in character, many tumors run an indolent course, with potential for long-term survival. Complete resection of the local disease, including involved airway, appears to be the best therapy, providing potential for cure when it is done as part of the initial therapy, and for prolonged palliation when it is done for late recurrent disease. External irradiation, radioactive iodine, and chemotherapy have often not proved to be effective agents for management of such residual disease. Various techniques of coring out the airway, either mechanically or by laser, provide temporary palliation but should otherwise be applied only when resection is not possible. Even when cure is not achieved, prolonged palliation is often obtained by resection, and devastating airway complications are avoided.

For these reasons, bronchoscopy and careful CT examination should be part of the preoperative investigation of all patients with thyroid carcinoma. Either the preoperative discovery of invasion or its finding at thyroidectomy should dictate prompt referral to a center where appropriate airway reconstruction can be performed. Every effort should be made to save the larynx. In a highly selected group of patients, radical resection, including laryngectomy in patients with no hope of laryngeal salvage, is indicated. Even the presence of slowly growing pulmonary metastases is not a contraindication for resection because this is compatible with prolonged survival.

H. C. G.
D. J. M.

Bronchogenic Carcinoma

HISTORICAL NOTE

Techniques of carinal resection and reconstruction (Grillo, 1982a) have been applied frequently for bronchogenic carcinoma. Mathey and co-workers (1966) and Jensik and associates (1972) were among the earliest to

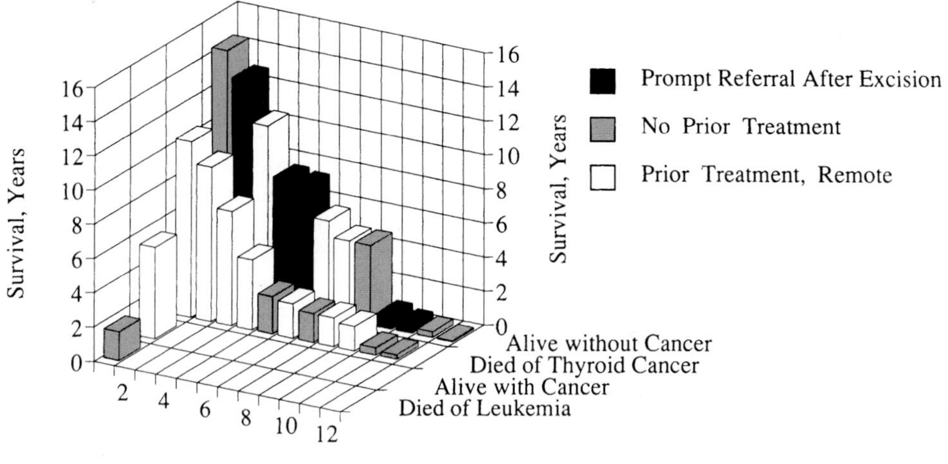

FIGURE 18–25 ■ Performance of 25 survivors in the reconstructed group. Long-term palliation achieved in some patients who died of thyroid cancer is to be noted. Also striking is the number of patients alive without cancer who had undergone resection either primarily or following prompt referral upon discovery of airway invasion. (From Grillo HC, Suen HC, Mathisen DJ, Wain JC: Resectional management of thyroid carcinoma invading the airway. Ann Thorac Surg 54:3, 1992.)

practice sleeve pneumonectomy for bronchogenic carcinoma. Indeed, classification of bronchogenic cancer invading the carina into stage IV was dictated largely by the rarity of technical expertise for such resections. Even main bronchial invasion has been classified as stage IIIB. Since the late 1970s, carinal resection for bronchogenic carcinoma has been reported in North America by Deslauriers and colleagues (1978), Jensik and co-workers (1982), and Mathisen and Grillo (1991); in Europe by Dartevelle and associates (1988) and Perelman and Koroleva (1980); and in Japan by Ishihara and colleagues (1977) and Naruke and co-workers (1982), among others. Excessive mortality has attended extension of surgery to this group of patients. Mathisen and Grillo (1991) called attention to the alarming occurrence of acute postoperative adult respiratory distress syndrome (ARDS) in these patients.

■ *HISTORICAL READINGS*

Jensik RJ, Faber P, Milloy FJ, Goldin MD: Tracheal sleeve pneumonectomy for advanced carcinoma of the lung. Surg Gynecol Obstet 134:231, 1972.

Mathey J, Binet JP, Galey JJ et al: Tracheal and tracheobronchial resection. J Thorac Cardiovasc Surg 51:1, 1966.

BASIC SCIENCE

When bronchogenic carcinoma invades the trachea directly from parenchymal contiguity, the disease is usually so extensive that segmental resection of the trachea is precluded. On the other hand, when bronchogenic carcinoma is centered in the proximal main bronchus or involves the carina, it should be considered for resection. The disease must be localized enough so that resection of the involved carina will not result in reconstruction under tension. The generally safe limit of such resection in right carinal pneumonectomy is approximately 4 cm between the distal end of the trachea and the left main bronchus. With carinal resection alone, which preserves the right lung, resection may be somewhat more extensive because of the greater possibility for mobilization of the right lung unhindered by the aortic arch. This applies also to the rare left carinal pneumonectomy for bronchogenic carcinoma.

Considerations regarding lymph node involvement are the same as for any other resection of carcinoma of the lung. N3 disease is out of bounds, and N2 disease would be resected only as part of a protocol approach with adjunctive therapy. Because of the extensiveness of the operation and the still high mortality, it is important that one search exhaustively for remote metastases prior to performing resection.

Carcinoma involving the right upper lobe at its origin may easily extend up the short length of the right main bronchus to involve the carina. On the left side, the bronchus is considerably longer, and carcinoma of the left upper lobe, which is less common than that of the right upper lobe, is not likely to extend to the carina. In all series, the number of right carinal pneumonectomies for bronchogenic carcinoma is far greater than the rare left-sided resection.

Of 37 patients undergoing carinal resection for bronchogenic carcinoma, 26 had squamous carcinoma, 9 adenocarcinoma, 1 large cell carcinoma, and 1 adenosquamous carcinoma (Mathisen and Grillo, 1991).

Particularly in right carinal pneumonectomy, significant interruption of tracheobronchial lymphatics necessarily occurs even when no effort is made to perform radical lymphadenectomy of the subcarinal, precarinal, and right paratracheal lymph nodes.

DIAGNOSIS

Involvement of the carina by bronchogenic carcinoma must be assessed with great care by conventional imaging, which includes CT scanning of the chest and upper abdomen. Crisp carinal tomograms are useful for demonstrating the gross extent of the lesion both within and outside of the lumen of the trachea, and equally importantly, for making clear the relative proportion of airway that may be uninvolved by tumor (Fig. 18–26). This is confirmed intraluminally by bronchoscopy. Even when flexible bronchoscopy has been performed for preliminary assessment, we prefer to carry out rigid bronchoscopy with Storz-Hopkins magnifying telescopes under general anesthesia for precise definition at the time of resection. The lengths of airway that are and are not involved are determined by differences with a rigid bronchoscope; the level of carina, the proximal extent of gross tumor, and the inferior border of the cricoid cartilage are noted successively. Particular attention is paid to extent of involvement of the opposite main bronchus. Extension of tumor down the opposite main bronchus for any distance, particularly down the left side when the tumor is predominantly on the right, may severely compromise or make impossible the approximation of the airway without tension. Mediastinoscopy is important for assessment of lymph node involvement to supplement information from the CT scan. Mediastinoscopy is preferably performed concurrently with the planned resection so that tissue planes and definition between scar and tumor are not obscured.

All patients who are being considered for carinal resection in connection with bronchogenic carcinoma must be evaluated by pulmonary function studies and quantitative ventilation-perfusion scans to determine what pulmonary function will be present postoperatively. In a few patients in whom pneumonectomy would not have been tolerated and whose tumor was localized, it was possible to perform carinal resection and right upper lobectomy with reimplantation of the middle and lower lobes or the lower lobe. Exploration was necessary before a final decision could be made about resectability.

MANAGEMENT

Principles

The patient must have disease that is not so extensive locally that the resulting resection will run a high risk of technical failure due to tension at the anastomosis. Lymph node involvement must be carefully analyzed, and an appropriate decision must be made according to the surgeon's policy for the management of involved mediastinal lymph nodes. Distant metastases must be ruled out. The patient's functional limitations for resection must be defined. It must be made clear to the patient that the risk of carinal resection is presently greater than that of total pneumonectomy.

Operative technique is discussed in Chapter 14.

Early Results

Among 37 patients (age range, 29 to 70; mean, 53 years), some had had prior pneumonectomy, others, thoracotomy and biopsy. Mediastinoscopy was negative in all but three, who were entered into a protocol for therapy of N2 disease with neoadjuvant chemotherapy and radiotherapy. Right carinal pneumonectomy was performed in 21 patients, lymph node dissection in 7, partial lateral resection of superior vena cava in 3, and partial resection of muscular wall of the esophagus in 1. Seven patients underwent carinal resection with preservation of all pulmonary parenchyma, and seven underwent right upper lobectomy and carinal resection with salvage and reimplantation of middle and lower lobes. In two patients with recurrent bronchial stump cancer, one on the right and one on the left, resection of the involved airway was performed through the right chest. Because both had received 4400 cGy of radiation 3 years previously, the anastomoses were wrapped with omentum.

In 17 patients, there were no complications. Many in this population with a history of smoking required fre-

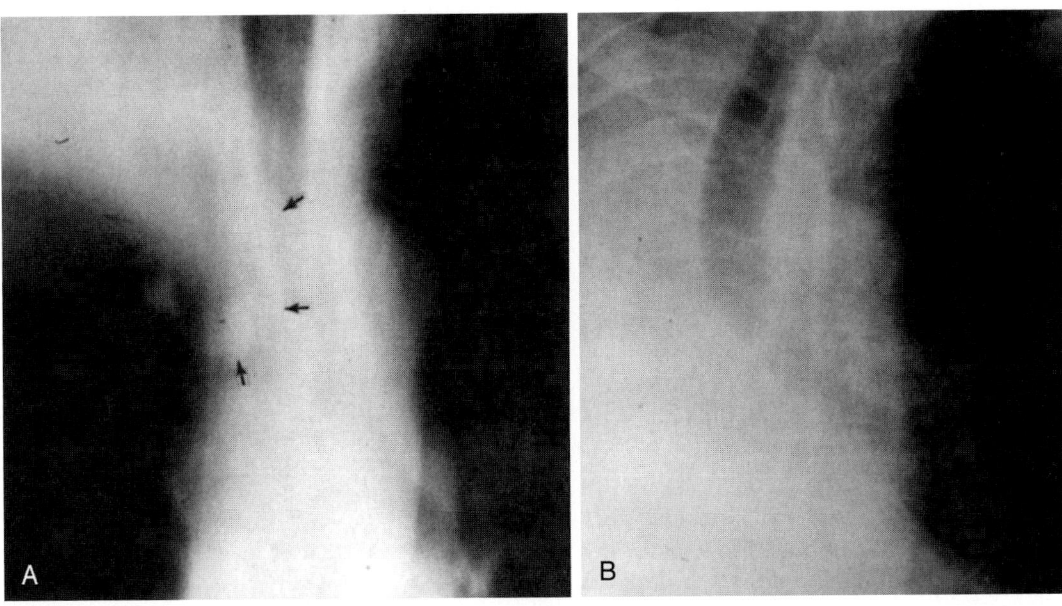

FIGURE 18–26 ■ *A,* Preoperative tomogram demonstrating a large cell carcinoma invading the carina and lower trachea *(arrows). B,* Postoperative image. The patient achieved a 5-year survival.

quent postoperative chest physiotherapy and flexible bronchoscopy to clear secretions. Six developed atelectasis, five developed pneumonia, and nine had postoperative atrial fibrillation. The ominous complication of pulmonary infiltration and respiratory failure occurred in three (8%), and all died despite vigorous therapy. Bacteriologic findings were unimpressive. Seven patients developed anastomotic problems, which in two consisted of stenosis of the right main bronchial anastomosis with the side of the trachea, and in one involved the bronchus intermedius. Two stenoses were repaired successfully surgically and others were managed conservatively by dilatation or laser therapy. Three patients died ultimately of anastomotic complications, principally separation: In one of them, much more than 4 cm of trachea had been resected after prior resection 9 years earlier; one required prolonged mechanical ventilation, and separation followed; and the third died during endoscopic manipulation of an occluded reimplanted right lower lobe bronchus. Three patients had left vocal cord dysfunction, presumably due to injury to the left recurrent nerve; in two, the problem resolved spontaneously, but one required vocal cord injection with Teflon. Early postoperative mortality was 8%, but delayed mortality was nearly 11%. The late deaths were due to anastomotic complications related to either tension or ischemia. The overall mortality rate was therefore 18.9%.

Mortality rates of 29% and 27% were reported, respectively, by Jensik and colleagues (1982) and by Deslauriers and co-workers (1985). The series of Dartevelle and associates (1988) showed mortality reduced to 11%. A significant number of early postoperative deaths following right carinal pneumonectomy are due to a particularly aggressive and rapidly moving ARDS-like syndrome. The operation may go smoothly, after which the patient may be extubated early and appear to be in fine condition for 24 hours. At 36 to 48 hours, a diffuse infiltrate appears in the remaining lung (Fig. 18–27). This progresses relentlessly to complete "whiteout" of the lung, and ultimately to death. At postmortem, the lung is wet and heavy, and nonspecific bacteria, if any, are cultured. A postmortem diagnosis of bronchopneumonia does not appear to be supported. This syndrome also follows conventional right pneumonectomy, but rarely. Peters and colleagues (1987) describe this sequence as postpneumonectomy pulmonary edema, attributing it most likely to perioperative intravenous fluid overload. In reviewing our case data, we have not found a correlation between the amount of perioperative fluid administered and the occurrence of this dreaded complication. Nonetheless, we manage these patients with minimum fluid administration.

Lymphatic interruption and barotrauma have also been hypothesized as causes. Nitric oxide treatment seemed to reduce the previously high mortality (Mathisen et al, 1998). Reduced incidence of this dire complication may be due to adjustment of intraoperative airway ventilatory pressure and tidal volumes to avoid barotrauma to the lung.

Late Results

Our series produced five absolute 5-year survivors (5 to 10 years), nine patients alive between 1½ and 3½ years without evidence of disease, and two dead of other causes at 2½ years.

Five patients were alive without disease less than 1 year after surgery. Eight patients died of recurrent disease between 1 and 3½ years after operation. Actuarial survival is 19%. This compares with a 5-year actuarial survival of 15% in the series of Jensik and co-workers (1982), 23% in the series of both Deslauriers and associates (1985) and Dartevelle and colleagues (1988), and 20% by Roviaro and co-workers (1994). In 1996, Dartevelle estimated a 5-year survival rate over 40%. The patients of Jensik and associates (1982) were not staged with respect to mediastinal lymph node metastases.

Recent review of 60 carinal resections for broncho-

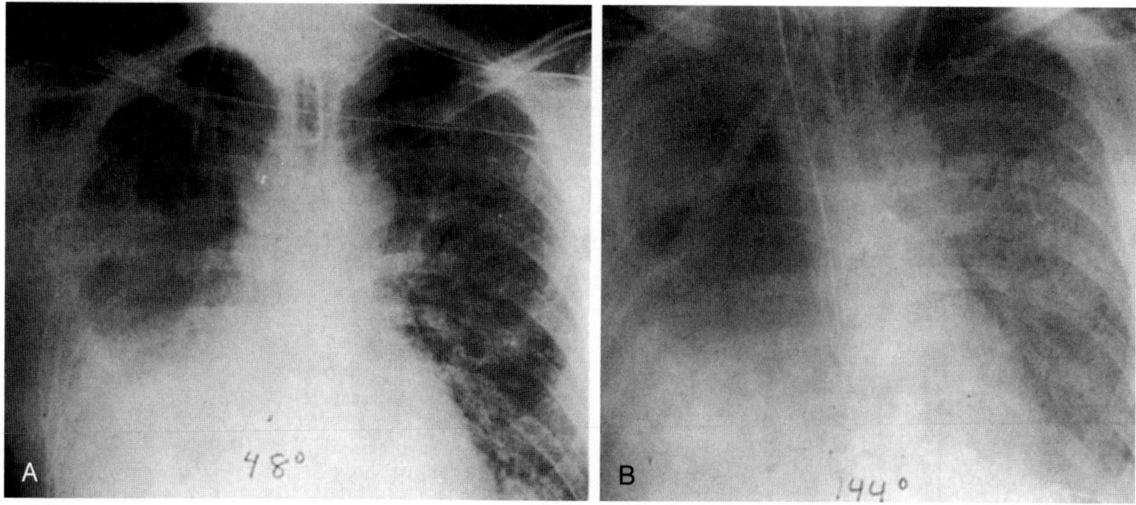

FIGURE 18–27 ■ Postpneumonectomy pulmonary edema. Following an uneventful right carinal pneumonectomy, this patient developed a "ground glass" infiltrate in his left lung at approximately 26 hours. *A,* Pulmonary infiltrate at 48 hours. *B,* Progression of adult respiratory distress syndrome at 6 days. Death followed despite maximum therapy.

genic carcinoma (Mitchell, 2001) shows a drop in operative mortality from 20% to 10%, 5-year survival of all patients at 42%, and strong influence of lymph node involvement on survival: N0 51%, N1 32%, N2/N3 12%.

COMMENTS AND CONTROVERSIES

With the development of carinal surgery, carinal pneumonectomy or carinal resection with various types of reconstruction has become feasible with growing safety. The techniques are applicable to bronchogenic carcinoma that involves the carina and that would otherwise be potentially curable. Involvement of the main bronchus or carina, therefore, should not by itself exclude surgical consideration, even if currently classified as stage IIIB or IV. Such patients must be very carefully appraised for extent of local and distant disease and for anatomic feasibility of safe resection. With careful attention to selection of patients, surgical technique, and perioperative management, complications from the surgery itself decrease steadily. The ominous exception is postpneumonectomy pulmonary edema, or ARDS. Its cause remains uncertain, as do, therefore, methods for prevention and treatment. A 5-year survival rate between 20% and 25% may be anticipated if patients with N2 disease are excluded. The N0 patients should probably be reclassified into stage IIIA.

H. C. G.
D. J. M.

Other Tumors

Recurrence of squamous carcinoma of the larynx at the tracheal stoma after laryngectomy has been approached by radical resection (Sisson et al, 1962). This has usually followed either postoperative irradiation that failed to prevent recurrence or failed radiation therapy for recurrence. Such resection frequently requires radical excision, including adjacent cervical tissues and esophagus. Reconstruction is performed much as described for cervical exenteration for extensive thyroid carcinoma. Because of cutaneous involvement by recurrent tumor and irradiation, it is frequently necessary to rotate unirradiated myocutaneous flaps to cover the lower neck and upper mediastinum and to establish a low mediastinal tracheostomy.

All too often, however, cancer recurs soon after resection (Krespi et al, 1985). Lymphatics are probably permeated with cancer paratracheally for some distance distally. Justification for such extensive surgery is therefore questionable.

Cervicomediastinal exenteration has also been performed for other secondary tumors invading the trachea, including postcricoidal squamous carcinoma of the esophagus that involves the larynx and upper trachea, so that laryngeal salvage is impossible (see Chapter 60). Adenoid cystic carcinoma may also invade the larynx in an unsalvageable manner, as well as the upper portion of the trachea and less often the wall of the esophagus.

Generally, resection of the trachea for direct involvement by esophageal carcinoma other than the postcricoidal type is not advised. The extent of involvement is usually so great that curative resection is unlikely. Tracheoesophageal fistula due to esophageal carcinoma is an extreme example. In a rare patient following preoperative neoadjuvant therapy, if the only point of apparent nonresectability is a short segment of trachea, it has seemed worthwhile to resect this segment and perform direct tracheotracheal anastomosis. One must be particularly cautious in such cases because the blood supply of the trachea may well be damaged by the extensive dissection performed for removal of the esophagus. Through a large part of the body of the trachea, segmental arteries provide an anterior branch to the trachea and a posterior one to the esophagus. If combined resection is performed, advancement of the omentum is advisable. This is brought up with the stomach, which is used to reconstruct the esophagus. Extension of radical esophageal resection to include tracheal segmental resection in any programmatic way is not advised.

KEY REFERENCES

Dartevelle PG, Khalife J, Chepelier A et al: Tracheal sleeve pneumonectomy for bronchogenic carcinoma: Report of 55 cases. Ann Thorac Surg 46:68, 1988.

In 55 tracheal sleeve pneumonectomy patients, mortality was 10.9%, the lowest recorded. Actuarial survival was 23% at 5 years and correlated with node involvement.

Deslauriers J: Involvement of the main carina. In Delarue NC, Eschapasse H (eds): Lung Cancer. International Trends in General Thoracic Surgery, Vol 1. Philadelphia, WB Saunders, 1985, p 139.

In 27 patients, a 23% 5-year survival was obtained, but operative mortality was 27%. The authors identify the cause of death as infection but describe what may well be "postpneumonectomy pulmonary edema" (ARDS).

Grillo HC, Suen HC, Mathisen DJ, Wain JC: Resectional management of thyroid carcinoma invading the airway. Ann Thorac Surg 54:3, 1992.

The principles of application of airway resection for invading thyroid carcinoma are stated on the basis of 34 resections, including 27 with reconstruction. Results and long-term follow-up are detailed.

Ishihara T, Kobayashi K, Kikuchi K et al: Surgical treatment of advanced thyroid carcinoma invading the trachea. J Thorac Cardiovasc Surg 102:717, 1991.

In 60 patients, thyroid cancer invading the trachea was removed, resulting in 5- and 10-year survival rates for complete resection of 78% and for incomplete resection of 44% and 24%, respectively.

Jensik RJ, Faber JP, Kittle CF et al: Survival in patients undergoing tracheal sleeve pneumonectomy for bronchogenic carcinoma. J Thorac Cardiovasc Surg 84:489, 1982.

This is the first large series of such patients, listing 34, with a 15% 5-year survival but 29% mortality. The high mortality clearly differentiated the magnitude of the procedure from standard pneumonectomy.

Mathisen DJ, Grillo HC: Carinal resection for bronchogenic carcinoma. J Thorac Cardiovasc Surg 102:16, 1991.

Of the 37 patients in this series, 8% suffered early death, principally due to respiratory distress syndrome of a characteristic type. Late operative deaths were due to anastomotic complications. Actuarial 5-year survival was 19%.

REFERENCES

Abbruzzini P: Trattamento chirurgico delle fistole del broncho principale consecutive a pneumonectomia per tubercolosi. Chir Torac 14:165, 1961.

Beahrs OH, Kiernan PD, Hubert JP Jr: Cancer of the Head and Neck. New York, Churchill Livingstone, 1981.

Dartevelle P, Macchiarini P: Carinal pneumonectomy for bronchogenic carcinoma. Semin Thorac Cardiovasc Surg 8:414, 1996.

Dartevelle PG, Khalife J, Chepelier A et al: Tracheal sleeve pneumonectomy for bronchogenic carcinoma: Report of 55 cases. Ann Thorac Surg 46:68, 1988.

Deslauriers J: Involvement of the main carina. In Delarue NC, Eschapasse H (eds): Lung Cancer. International Trends in General Thoracic Surgery, Vol 1. Philadelphia, WB Saunders, 1985, p 139.

Deslauriers J, Beaulieu M, Benazera A, McClish A: Sleeve pneumonectomy for bronchogenic carcinoma. Ann Thorac Surg 28:465, 1978.

Frazell EL, Foote FW Jr: Papillary cancer of the thyroid: A review of 25 years of experience. Cancer 11:895, 1958.

Friedman M, Danielzadeh JA, Caldarelli DD: Treatment of patients with carcinoma of the thyroid invading the airway. Arch Otolaryngol Head Neck Surg 120:1377, 1994.

Grillo HC: Circumferential resection and reconstruction of mediastinal and cervical trachea. Ann Surg 162:374, 1965.

Grillo HC: Carinal resection. Ann Thorac Surg 34:356, 1982a.

Grillo HC: Primary reconstruction of airway after resection of subglottic and upper tracheal stenosis. Ann Thorac Surg 33:3, 1982b.

Grillo HC: Congenital lesions, neoplasms and injuries of the trachea. In Sabiston DC Jr, Spencer FC (eds): Gibbon's Surgery of the Chest, 5th ed. Philadelphia, WB Saunders, 1983, p 335.

Grillo HC: Atlas of General Thoracic Surgery. Philadelphia, WB Saunders, 1988.

Grillo HC, Mathisen DJ: Cervical exenteration. Ann Thorac Surg 49:401, 1990a.

Grillo HC, Mathisen DJ: Primary tracheal tumors: Treatment and results. Ann Thorac Surg 49:69, 1990b.

Grillo HC, Suen HC, Mathisen DJ, Wain JC: Resectional management of thyroid carcinoma invading the airway. Ann Thorac Surg 54:3, 1992.

Grillo HC, Zannini P: Resectional management of airway invasion by thyroid carcinoma. Ann Thorac Surg 42:287, 1986.

Hendrick JW: An extended operation for thyroid carcinoma. Surg Gynecol Obstet 116:183, 1963.

Ishihara T, Ikeda T, Inoue H, Fukai S: Resection of cancer of the lung and carina. J Thorac Cardiovasc Surg 73:936, 1977.

Ishihara T, Kikuchi K, Ikeda T et al: Resection of thyroid carcinoma infiltrating the trachea. Thorax 33:378, 1978.

Ishihara T, Kobayashi K, Kikuchi K et al: Surgical treatment of advanced thyroid carcinoma invading the trachea. J Thorac Cardiovasc Surg 102:717, 1991.

Jensik RJ, Faber JP, Kittle CF et al: Survival in patients undergoing tracheal sleeve pneumonectomy for bronchogenic carcinoma. J Thorac Cardiovasc Surg 84:489, 1982.

Jensik RJ, Faber P, Milloy FJ, Goldin MD: Tracheal sleeve pneumonectomy for advanced carcinoma of the lung. Surg Gynecol Obstet 134:231, 1972.

Krespi YP, Wurster CF, Sisson GA: Immediate reconstruction after total laryngopharyngoesophagectomy and mediastinal dissection. Laryngoscope 95:156, 1985.

Lawson W, Som MP, Biller HF: Papillary carcinoma of the thyroid invading the upper air passages. Ann Otol Rhinol Laryngol 86:751, 1977.

Maeda M, Nakamoto K, Ohta M et al: Statistical survey of tracheobronchoplasty in Japan. J Thorac Cardiovasc Surg 97:402, 1989.

Mathey J, Binet JP, Galey JJ et al: Tracheal and tracheobronchial resections; technique and results in 20 cases. J Thorac Cardiovasc Surg 51:1, 1966.

Mathisen DJ, Grillo HC: Carinal resection for bronchogenic carcinoma. J Thorac Cardiovasc Surg 102:16, 1991.

Mathisen DJ, Grillo HC, Vlahakes GJ, Daggett WM: The omentum in the management of complicated cardiothoracic problems. J Thorac Cardiovasc Surg 95:677, 1988.

Mathisen DJ, Kuo EY, Hahn C et al: Inhaled nitric oxide for adult respiratory distress syndrome following pulmonary resection. Ann Thorac Surg 65:1894–1902, 1998.

Mitchell JD, Mathisen DJ, Wright CD et al: Resection for bronchogenic carcinoma involving the carina: Long-term results and effect of nodal status on outcome. J Thorac Cardiovasc Surg 121:465, 2001.

Montgomery WW: Suprahyoid release for tracheal stenosis. Arch Otolaryngol Head Neck Surg 99:255, 1974.

Naruke T, Yoneyama T, Ogata T et al: Bronchoplastic procedures for lung carcinoma. J Thorac Cardiovasc Surg 84:489, 1982.

Nishida T, Nakao K, Hamaji M: Differentiated thyroid carcinoma with airway extension: Indication for tracheal resection based on the extent of cancer invasion. J Thorac Cardiovasc Surg 114:84, 1997.

Nomori H, Kobayaski K, Ishihara T et al: Thyroid carcinoma infiltrating the trachea: Clinical histologic, and morphometric analyses. J Surg Oncol 44:78, 1990.

Perelman MI, Koroleva NS: Surgery of the trachea. World J Surg 4:583, 1980.

Perelman MI, Koroleva NS: Primary tumors of the trachea. In Grillo HC, Eschapasse H (eds): International Trends in General Thoracic Surgery Major Challenges for the Thoracic Surgeon, Vol 2. Philadelphia, WB Saunders, 1987.

Peters RM: Postpneumonectomy pulmonary edema. In Grillo HC, Eschapasse H (eds): International Trends in General Thoracic Surgery: Major Challenges for the Thoracic Surgeon, Vol 2. Philadelphia, WB Saunders, 1987.

Roviaro GC, Varioli F, Rebuffat C et al: Tracheal sleeve pneumonectomy for bronchogenic carcinoma. J Thorac Cardiovasc Surg 107:13, 1994.

Shin DH, Mark EJ, Suen HC, Grillo HC: Pathological staging of papillary carcinoma of the thyroid with airway invasion based upon the anatomic manner of extension to the trachea. Hum Pathol 24:866, 1993.

Sillphant WM, Klinck GH, Levitin MS: Thyroid carcinoma and death: A clinicopathological study of 193 autopsies. Cancer 17:513, 1964.

Sisson GA, Straehley CJ Jr, Johnson NE: Mediastinal dissection for recurrent cancer after laryngectomy. Laryngoscope 72:1064, 1962.

Sweet RH: Thoracic Surgery. Philadelphia, WB Saunders, 1950.

Tsuchiya R, Goya T, Naruke T, Suemasu K: Resection of tracheal carina for lung cancer. J Thorac Cardiovasc Surg 99:779, 1990.

Tsumori T, Nakao K, Miyata M et al: Clinicopathologic study of thyroid carcinoma infiltrating the trachea. Cancer 56:2843, 1985.

Tsumori T, Nakao K, Miyata M et al: Clinicopathologic study on the mode and degree of invasion of the trachea by thyroid carcinoma. Nippon Geka Gakkai Zasshi 88:600, 1987.

Waller DA, Gebitekin C, Saunders NR, Walker DR: Noncardiac pulmonary edema complicating lung resection. Ann Thorac Surg 55:140, 1993.

CHAPTER **19**

Surgical Techniques

TRACHEOSTOMY

Peter Goldstraw

Clifford Morgan

HISTORICAL NOTE

The term tracheostomy (Greek: *tracheo* + *stomoun*) will be used throughout this chapter as it describes the purpose of this operation, that is, making an opening into the trachea (Sebastian, 1999). This operation is rooted in antiquity (Goodall, 1934); the literature relevant to the modern surgeon began with the work of Jackson early in the 20th century (Jackson, 1937). The operation became more widely utilized with the need for prolonged ventilatory assistance and the technical refinements that made this possible (Cooper, 1987; Gothard, 1993).

HISTORICAL READINGS

Goodall EW: The story of tracheotomy. Br J Child Dis 31:167, 1934.

Jackson C, Jackson CL: The larynx and its disorders. Philadelphia, WB Saunders, 1937.

INDICATIONS

A *permanent* end-tracheostomy is required if laryngectomy has been performed. The technique and indications for this operation are not covered in this chapter because they belong to the realm of head and neck surgery, but the thoracic surgeon may become involved if extended resection requires esophageal reconstruction or the creation of an anterior mediastinal tracheostomy (Orringer, 1992).

A *temporary* side-tracheostomy may be advisable for one or more of the following indications:

1. **To facilitate the maintenance or weaning from prolonged positive-pressure ventilation.** The increasing skills of the intensivist and the wider availability of intensive care units (ICUs) has made this by far the most common indication for tracheostomy. Prolonged intermittent positive-pressure ventilation (IPPV) is commonplace in the treatment of respiratory failure, whether following trauma or surgery for severe lung disease or as part of the management of multiple organ failure. As the period of orotracheal or nasotracheal intubation lengthens, there is increased concern regarding the possibility of consequent laryngeal injury. Unfortunately, there is no consensus as to the appropriate time to perform tracheostomy in these circumstances. Laryngeal damage may be initiated within the first day after intubation (Weymuller, 1998), but the incidence of granuloma, voice impairment, and chronic stenosis increases as the period of intubation lengthens (Whited, 1983). Improvements in the management and supervision of orotracheal and nasotracheal tubes in the ICU, coupled with frequent inspection of the larynx for early signs of damage, has allowed longer periods of ventilation without tracheostomy. However, if the patient's prognosis suggests that weaning from ventilation is likely to become an issue at some stage, most intensivists would recommend tracheostomy after 7 to 10 days of IPPV.

Other factors are clearly important in this decision (Watson, 1983). Some patients with severe respiratory failure are so critically dependent on a pattern of lung volume recruitment ventilation that even a brief interruption may result in prolonged deterioration in blood oxygenation. It is neither advisable nor necessary to perform tracheostomy under those circumstances unless there is a coincidental critical airway management issue that also has to be dealt with. It is unwise to perform tracheostomy during a period in which there is real or potential hemodynamic instability. This is particularly so if the patient has to be moved from the ICU to an operating room for the procedure but may also be relevant to ICU bedside procedures if the patient is dependent on multiple drugs or devices. The presence of any coagulopathy is a relative contraindication to tracheostomy. There are common circumstances in which clotting factors or platelets are deficient or dysfunctional, and anticoagulants may have been administered for prophylaxis against thromboembolic complications. It is usually wise to delay tracheostomy in the presence of sepsis or the systemic inflammatory response syndrome (SIRS). Bacteremia associated with tracheostomy, particularly percutaneous tracheostomy (Teoh, 1997), may cause or exacerbate a sepsis syndrome or the new tracheostomy wound may be colonized by pre-existing systemic sepsis. Once infected, the tracheostoma may then itself become a troublesome secondary site of nosocomial infection. The timing and indication for tracheostomy, and the choice of technique, must be made on an individual patient basis.

Once established, the tracheostomy is much more comfortable for the patient than either orotracheal or nasotracheal intubation, and it allows less analgesia or sedation. Weaning from prolonged IPPV is facilitated by tracheostomy in that it protects the airway from aspiration, allows tracheobronchial toilet, reduces dead space, and allows IPPV support to be given intermittently as needed.

2. **In the relief of acute or anticipated upper airway obstruction.** Since the decline of diphtheria, relief of upper airway obstruction is an uncommon indication for tracheostomy, but it may be required for trauma or laryngeal edema. Prophylactic tracheostomy undertaken prior to certain complex maxillofacial operations such as intubation would prove difficult, perhaps fatally so, if airway obstruction occurred postoperatively.

3. **To protect the airway from laryngeal incompetence such as aspiration of gastric contents and swallowed material.** This is rarely, of itself, the reason for tracheostomy, but it is an additional advantage of a cuffed endotracheal tube if tracheostomy is used to facilitate prolonged IPPV. Inevitably, such patients experience uncoordinated swallowing as a result of both muscle wasting and the mechanical effects of tracheostomy. The problem may be exacerbated by neurologic injury.

4. **To allow tracheobronchial toilet**—when cough is ineffective or soiling is excessive.

5. **To allow long-term, intermittent ventilatory support**—often on a domiciliary basis. This may require positive pressure ventilation or merely the ability to bypass the upper airway, as seen in patients with obstructive sleep apnea.

TECHNIQUE

A temporary tracheostomy may be performed using either an open technique or a percutaneous puncture.

Open tracheostomy has changed little since the days of Jackson. If the appropriate conditions can be provided in the ICU, the patient can be spared the disruption of transportation to the operating room. A firm bed is needed; this can be a problem because most long-term IPPV patients are now nursed on soft mattresses to protect pressure areas. Diathermy, suction, adequate assistance, and a good light are essential. We have found a headlight useful, which is something that Jackson also recommended. The operation is now routinely performed under general anesthesia. After induction, rigid bronchoscopy is performed to check the larynx and trachea for any damage resulting from intubation, to exclude any cause of airway obstruction, and to undertake bronchial toilet. It is our practice to leave the bronchoscope in place throughout the operation, maintaining gas exchange using the Sanders injector (Feneck, 1987). This allows bronchoscopic assistance in positioning the tracheostomy incision and in tube placement. Most tracheostomies are performed by surgeons who are unfamiliar with bronchoscopy. However, in most situations, the intensivist or anesthetist should be able to provide some endoscopic guidance using a fiberoptic bronchoscope inserted through the endotracheal tube.

The patient is positioned supine with the neck extended using a sandbag under the shoulders. A 3-cm transverse incision is placed midway between the thyroid cartilage and the suprasternal notch. The tissues are dissected vertically in the midline until the trachea is identified. The pretracheal fascia is incised vertically, and the thyroid isthmus is reflected superiorly to expose the trachea. It is rare to find the isthmus so intrusive as to require division, but, if necessary, it can be divided with the diathermy or with transfixion.

It is advisable to pause at this point and to check the equipment once more. A range of tracheostomy tubes should be available in appropriate sizes. The cuff is inflated, checked for leaks, fully deflated once more, and lubricated. The anesthetist should check the connections to ensure that they fit the tracheostomy tube and ventilator. The suction should be connected and functioning. A pointed blade, a tracheal hook retractor, and a Trousseau tracheal dilator should all be available.

There is continued debate as to the best tracheostomy incision. Patients undergoing tracheostomy are nursed in an intensive care setting such that early acute displacement should be rare, and patients should have a patent larynx, which permits easy oral intubation should displacement occur. There is, therefore, little indication for the flap tracheostomy that was popularized by Bjork (Bjork, 1960). We have seen several strictures associated with this type of tracheotomy, although the role of tracheal incision in the genesis of stricture is debated, and there are those who would maintain that the flap tracheostomy is associated with a lower incidence of stricture (Lulenski, 1975). We recommend a vertical incision through tracheal rings 2 to 4, a method that is universally recommended in pediatric practice (Albert, 1998).

The trachea is elevated and fixed using the hook retractor on the cricoid. A needle is inserted at the proposed site of tracheotomy, and the bronchoscopist directs the surgeon to the midline at the correct level. The tracheal incision is started with the pointed blade. If the operation is performed with an endotracheal tube in place, the tube is usually ruptured at this point. This should not hinder ventilation unless pulmonary compliance is very poor. Nevertheless, it is important to proceed smoothly and without delay. The tracheal incision is extended through rings 2 to 4 until the retractor can allow sufficient distraction to admit the tracheostomy tube and its trocar. It is surprisingly easy to place the tracheostomy tube into the mediastinum, anterior to the trachea. Bronchoscopic confirmation that the tube is correctly placed within the distal trachea is reassuring. The trocar is removed, the cuff is inflated, and ventilation is undertaken through the tracheostomy tube. Once this is safely achieved, the bronchoscope or orotracheal tube can be removed. These steps are frequently performed in a slightly hurried fashion. Hence, once ventilation is stable, the cuff should be deflated and refilled with the minimum amount of air required to produce a seal at the lowest cuff pressure. The skin is then sutured loosely around the tube.

The surgeon's final responsibility is to secure the tube to prevent displacement. The sandbag should be removed before doing this to ensure that the neck is in a neutral position. We prefer to have the flaps of the tracheostomy tube sutured to the skin until the tube is changed after approximately 1 week. At this time, ties are more comfortable, and a track is available if displacement occurs.

Cricothyroidostomy has been advocated at various times. It can be accomplished speedily and, therefore, remains popular when emergency relief is required for laryngeal or upper airway obstruction. Cricothyroidostomy as an elective procedure was abandoned after being decried by Jackson (Jackson, 1921), who confused matters somewhat by linking it with high tracheostomy. One should remember that in Jackson's era, tracheostomy was done under local anesthesia, often under less than optimal conditions. Properly performed, cricothyroidostomy has a very low complication rate (Brantigan, 1976). It is particularly attractive as an alternative to tracheostomy after median sternotomy, because the incision is better suited, and there is theoretically less risk of sternal contamination and wound infection. This advantage no longer pertains because of the insurgence of widespread use of percutaneous tracheostomy (see later). The risks of laryngeal stenosis after cricothyroidostomy are greater if there has been prior endotracheal intubation, the largest group in whom tracheostomy is now necessary (Burkey, 1991). Grillo, whose opinion on all airway matters must be respected, has pointed out that stenosis after cricothyroidostomy might be infrequent but may result in subglottic stenosis, a notoriously difficult problem to correct surgically (Grillo, 1995a). For these reasons, we do not recommend the operation on an elective basis.

Percutaneous minitracheostomy is enormously valuable in the management of sputum retention after surgery (Hopkinson, 1984). It requires a special disposable pack marketed for this purpose. It is readily performed in the ward bed under local anesthetic. The neck is extended over a pillow, and the trachea is fixed between the thumb and the forefingers of the left hand while the pretracheal tissues are infiltrated with local anesthetic. It is helpful to puncture the cricothyroid membrane and inject a little local anesthesia into the trachea to suppress the cough response. A vertical incision is performed through the skin and into the cricothyroid membrane, using the pointed, guarded knife provided. Bleeding is unlikely because the veins lie laterally, but if bleeding does occur, it is best to stop, control the bleeding with a few minutes of compression, and then try again a few millimeters to one side. Once the membrane has been punctured, the blunt guidewire is inserted into the trachea, and the tube is passed over it using the Seldinger technique. We find it useful to have a small, curved hemostat available in case the cricothyroid membrane is calcified. Passage of the guidewire is facilitated by gentle dilatation using the hemostat. Suction should be available to remove blood from the airway and provide immediate clearance of retained secretions. The tube is held in place by adjustable straps that are comfortable and fit all neck sizes.

Percutaneous Tracheostomy

In the past, tracheostomy for intensive care patients implied a surgical procedure performed by surgeons and often in an operating-room environment. There were variations on the theme. In some cases the operation was performed at the bedside in the ICU, thus avoiding the need for disruptive transfers of critically ill patients to and from the operating room. The major motivation for self sufficiency in tracheostomy was the perceived delays and disruption of an ICU care program that resulted from dependency on visiting surgeons, whether or not the procedure was ultimately performed at the bedside or in an operating room. Another possible motivating factor was the perception that ICU specialists probably have a consistently lower threshold for initiating tracheostomy than do the attending surgical staff or the surgeons who are specifically consulted to perform the procedure. It has been suggested that the introduction of an alternative to open surgical tracheostomy increased the frequency of the use of tracheostomy over and above any changes in workload or case mix (Simpson, 1999).

The most widely practiced alternative to open tracheostomy is the technique of progressive dilatation over a percutaneously inserted guidewire, first described by Ciaglia in 1985. There have been modifications and refinements of this technique subsequently, most notably the awareness that endoscopic guidance by fiberoptic bronchoscopy (Marelli, 1990) or using the rigid bronchoscope (Brimacombe, 1995) is essential to the safe execution of this operation.

The perceived advantages of percutaneous tracheostomy over open surgical tracheostomy include:

- Self sufficiency of the ICU medical staff
- Less disruption of patient care
- Superior cosmetic result for the patient
- Lower cost in the operating room compared with tracheostomy
- Avoidance of some of the risks associated with open tracheostomy (e.g., stoma adjacent to recent median sternotomy incision)

The Ciaglia Technique

The surgeon must be familiar with the method and must be capable of dealing with the potential complications of bleeding and airway disruption. The likelihood of conditions requiring conversion to open tracheostomy is arguable. This only occurred in 2 patients in one reported series of 35 patients undergoing percutaneous dilatational tracheostomy (Carillo, 1997). Some may contend that such a situation mandates the presence of a surgeon who is capable of performing tracheostomy or that the surgeon should perform the percutaneous procedure. However, in actual practice, the need for conversion to open tracheostomy is exceptionally rare and not generally an immediate necessity. In the event of failure of the percutaneous technique, it is usually best to retreat and secure the airway by endotracheal intubation rather than proceeding directly to surgical tracheostomy. The pragmatic approach is to have readily available surgical equipment and expertise but to assume in most cases that they will not be needed.

Contraindications to the percutaneous technique include:

Absolute:

- In emergency situations—in which cricothyroidostomy or surgical tracheostomy is to be preferred.
- Where neck manipulation is contraindicated—for example, suspected or known cervical spine injury.

Relative:

- Hemodynamic instability.
- Severe pulmonary failure in which the need for high airway pressures must be maintained constantly.
- Significantly enlarged thyroid gland.
- Coagulopathy.
- Recent neck surgery.
- Pediatric patients.

The procedure is not suitable for a lone surgeon. It requires a skilled team working together to minimize potential complications. The team must include:

- The operator.
- Someone to look after the conventional airway until tracheostomy is achieved and to restore the airway if the percutaneous procedure is not successful.
- Someone to provide endoscopic observation of the procedure, using either the fiberoptic bronchoscope inserted via the endotracheal tube or a rigid bronchoscope.
- Someone to monitor the patient's general condition throughout the procedure while those more directly involved are somewhat focused on the airway.

Obviously there are many potential variations on the above theme and the possibility that one person may be responsible for more than one of the duties. Proprietary single use kits are available, which provide almost all of the equipment needed for the procedure. Standard tracheostomy tubes are perfectly adequate, but specially designed tracheostomy tubes adapted for percutaneous insertion are available.

The patient is prepared and draped as for open tracheostomy with the neck fully extended and stabilized in this position by a pillow or sandbag. The head of the bed is elevated by 30 to 40 degrees to reduce venous pressure.

General anesthesia is required, as the procedure is quite stimulating. Neuromuscular blocking drugs are usually used, which allows control of respiration. The inspired oxygen concentration is often increased temporarily because of the brief interruption of normal ventilation during the procedure. It may also be advisable to increase the mean and end-expiratory pressures of the ventilator profile to maintain lung volume recruitment with the partially open airway. The detailed requirements of ventilatory management will be specific to each individual patient. Local anesthesia with topical infiltration of a suitable agent is very helpful, and the addition of epinephrine aids short-term hemostasis. Some surgeons also instill local anesthetic into the trachea at the time of first tracheal puncture to suppress airway reactivity. Inspection and palpation identify anatomical landmarks. The aim is to enter the trachea between the first and second or between the second and third tracheal cartilages. A vertical incision is made in the midline, 1 to 1.5 cm inferiorly from the level of the cricoid cartilage. At this stage, the endotracheal tube must be withdrawn several centimeters to avoid impaling it at the time of tracheal puncture. The kit includes a catheter-over-needle, which is inserted in the midline and angled slightly inferiorly into the trachea. The free aspiration of air will indicate that the needle is in the trachea; its correct position in the midline and between the appropriate tracheal cartilages is confirmed endoscopically. The needle is removed, and the catheter is advanced into the trachea.

The J-ended guidewire supplied in the set is introduced through the catheter and passed several centimeters into the trachea. The catheter is then removed. The tip of the wire should remain above the carina. It is very important to maintain the position of the wire relative to the trachea throughout the rest of the procedure if injury to the posterior tracheal wall is to be avoided. Initial dilatation is done using a short dilator over the wire. The dilator is introduced with a slight twisting motion while the guidewire is anchored by the operator's other hand (or by an assistant). A slight "give," or "pop," is felt as the tip of this dilator enters the trachea; this event is confirmed visually by endoscopy. This dilator is removed while maintaining the position of the guidewire. The next step is to advance the guiding catheter over the guidewire. This reinforces the assembly to allow the more substantial subsequent dilatations. There is an arrow on the proximal end of the guiding catheter to indicate the direction of insertion. There is a bulbous "safety ridge" near the distal end to indicate the correct insertion depth. With the safety ridge positioned at the level of the skin, the proximal end of the guiding catheter should be aligned with a solder mark on the guidewire. This ensures that the guidewire is anchored at the correct depth during the subsequent passage of dilators. Graduated dilators of increasing size are passed over the guidewire/catheter assembly. Insertion of the smallest of the dilators is often the most difficult step in the procedure, because the increase in diameter is greatest during this maneuver. Maintaining the guidewire at the optimal depth is crucial in preventing damage to the posterior tracheal wall. Firm pressure in the direction of the carina and a slight twisting motion is required. Endoscopic monitoring is helpful at this point. A fine, curved hemostat may be useful at this stage; it can be used in a spreading motion to follow the wire and dissect along the track. The dilatation procedure is continued until the stoma is slightly greater than the diameter of the desired tracheostomy tube.

The chosen tracheostomy tube is threaded onto the appropriate size dilator. This requires generous lubrication so that the largest possible dilator is used for the tube. The tracheostomy tube balloon must be totally deflated, and the outside of the tube must be thoroughly lubricated to facilitate insertion over the guidewire/catheter assembly. There may be significant resistance to insertion (more than that encountered with a substantially larger dilator) because of the shoulder between the shaft of the dilator and the leading edge of the tracheostomy tube. If too much resistance is encountered, it may be necessary to repeat dilatation with the largest size dilator or to use further blunt dissection with the hemostat. Endoscopic control at this stage is helpful to confirm correct placement and alignment, but this may be difficult as the force for passage required may compress the trachea and obscure the view.

As soon as the tracheostomy tube has been inserted, the dilator on which it was loaded and the guidewire/catheter assembly are removed. Correct placement and alignment of the tube are confirmed endoscopically, first from above and then through the lumen of the tracheostomy tube. Tracheal toilet to remove blood is performed as necessary. The ventilator circuit is attached to the tracheostomy tube, and adequate inflation of the cuff is confirmed. The tracheostomy tube is then secured in place by sutures, ties, or both.

Bleeding into the trachea may have occurred but almost always stops when the superficial source of the bleeding is tamponaded by the tracheostomy tube. The patient may require further tracheal suction or endoscopic toilet to remove operative blood from the trachea and proximal bronchi.

The Impact of Percutaneous Tracheostomy

The Ciaglia technique was first described in 1985, but within 10 years it had become well established in most large ICUs. A postal survey in the United Kingdom (Cooper, 1998) confirmed that percutaneous tracheostomy was used by over 78% of respondents (76% response rate) and that the Ciaglia technique was the one most commonly used. Interestingly, only 31.3% of respondents claimed to routinely use fiberoptic endoscopy during the procedure. Several studies reporting the short-term complications and long-term follow-up have found results comparable with or superior to traditional open tracheostomy (Ciaglia, 1992; Walz, 1998). Operating time is shorter and costs are lower when compared with procedures that require the use of an operating room (McHenry, 1999). However, there are those who challenge this economic assessment when comparing percutaneous tracheostomy with open tracheostomy at the bedside performed by experienced surgical intensivists (Porter, 1999). In this study, there was no economic advantage for the percutaneous technique when compared with bedside open tracheostomy and no technical problems with the latter when compared with contemporaneous patients who were undergoing open tracheostomy in the operating room.

Simpson and colleagues (Simpson, 1999) showed an apparent increase in the proportion of ICU patients who were subjected to tracheostomy by any technique following the introduction of the percutaneous technique. This may significantly increase the total number of tracheostomy complications observed overall. This factor needs to be considered when assessing the true impact of percutaneous tracheostomy.

The loss of surgical experience with open tracheostomy is a concern, as there are occasions when the percutaneous technique is either not available or not appropriate, especially in an emergency situation in which speed may be of the essence.

The influence of the learning curve is well recognized in percutaneous tracheostomy, particularly because those who usually perform it are not surgeons. There is no substitute for practical experience; however, training using an animal or cadaveric model can be valuable (Gardiner, 1998; Trottier, 1999). These models have been used to study the most significant and worrying complication of percutaneous dilatational tracheostomy—damage or perforation of the posterior tracheal wall. In one study (Trottier, 1999), 7 of 24 (29%) patients sustained complications of percutaneous dilatational tracheostomy, 3 of which (12.5%) were posterior wall perforations that were associated with tension pneumothorax. These workers studied this injury in swine and cadaveric models, and the mechanism of injury was thought to be related to improper stabilization of the guiding catheter resulting in its withdrawal into the dilating catheter.

Alternative Techniques

Other methods based on the percutaneous dilatational technique have been described, such as tracheostomy by guidewire dilating forceps (GWDF) (van Heerbeek, 1999). This technique has the additional attraction of being quicker because there is a single-stage dilatation and tube insertion process. Early results appear to be comparable with those reported using the Ciaglia technique (Ambesh, 1998; Leonard, 1999) but there is less experience with the newer technique. There may be a more significant learning curve associated with the GWDF technique, which could result in an increased complication rate compared with that of the Ciaglia method (Powell, 1998).

TRACHEOSTOMY TUBES

Clinical and experimental studies of postintubation and post-tracheostomy stenosis have incriminated cuff design (Andrews, 1971; Cooper, 1969). All such tubes have large-volume, floppy cuffs that seal the airway against aspiration and loss of positive ventilation pressure by molding to the ovoid shape of the airway at low pressure rather than distorting the airway to fit a spherical balloon. In most circumstances, standard tracheostomy tubes are adequate, but there is a wide range of tubes for specific functional or anatomical situations. If the anatomy of the neck is distorted by obesity, previous surgery, or kyphoscoliosis, the alignment of the tracheostomy may cause the distal lumen to impact on the posterior tracheal wall. The resultant injury is exacerbated by the trauma of repeated suction and may cause ulceration and even penetration. In such cases, the use of a tracheostomy tube with a hinged flange may allow better orientation. Some patterns of tracheostomy tubes have a moveable flange that can be fixed at skin level once the distal orifice of the tube has been positioned optimally under endoscopic control. Flexible, armored tubes are versatile and will adjust in shape to fit most difficult anatomical situations. However, in extreme situations, the manufacturers of tracheostomy tubes can provide a custom-built tube specifically for any individual patient.

Fenestrated tubes are useful in the weaning of some patients from ventilator dependence. These tubes have single or multiple openings on the upper wall of the tube at its "elbow," which are occluded by an inner tube during IPPV. When the cuff is deflated, the inner tube is removed, and the outer stoma of the tracheostomy tube is occluded, the patient can temporarily regain laryngeal function, allowing phonation and encouraging morale. Simply reversing these steps allows further periods of ventilatory support whenever necessary. A similar situation can be achieved in many patients by replacing the standard tracheostomy tube with a similar but smaller size. Once the cuff is deflated, there is sufficient space for the patient to breathe and phonate around the outside of the tube. Another pattern of tracheostomy tube facilitates speech by the insufflation of air or oxygen through a small channel that enters the trachea above the cuff and below the larynx. In practice, it is difficult for the patient to learn to speak with this method. The channel does, however, allow aspiration of any pooled secretions from above the tracheostomy cuff. This may help prevent colonization of the lungs with pharyngeal and gut-derived organisms.

TRACHEOSTOMY CARE

Early displacement of the tracheostomy tube may occur when the patient is being moved for nursing care or physiotherapy. It is important that everyone involved in the care of the patient is aware of this possibility. The complication should be suspected if ventilation becomes unsatisfactory or airway pressure rises. If displacement is suspected, management will depend on a number of factors. What is the immediacy of the situation? Is any difficulty anticipated with oral intubation? What expertise is immediately available? If there is time and bronchoscopy facilities are available, the fiberoptic instrument can be inserted through the tracheostomy tube to check its position. This also allows the clearance of any obstructing secretions. If satisfactory placement of the tube cannot be confirmed, and if oral intubation is straightforward in this patient, it is best to relieve the immediate problem by inserting an orotracheal tube and removing the tracheostomy tube. The tracheostomy tube can then be replaced surgically, later, under controlled circumstances. If oral intubation is not possible, or if it is extremely difficult, one would hope that a Bjork flap had been performed!

Humidification and warming of the inspired air is necessary. This is provided routinely through the ventilator circuit, but once IPPV is discontinued, it should be continued through a separate humidifier. There are a number of compact devices that fit the tracheostomy tube and humidify inspired air by recycling exhaled moisture.

Coughing is difficult in the absence of laryngeal function. Suction should be undertaken as frequently as necessary by the nursing staff. Physiotherapy helps propel sputum to the central airways from where it can be removed by suction.

Stenosis at the stoma may be related to excessive angulation and tube erosion (Grillo, 1995a). The tracheostomy tube and its attachments to the ventilator should, therefore, be fixed into adjustable clamps to prevent undue movement or pressure.

The tracheostomy tube should be changed periodically. The ideal period between tube changes will depend on individual patient characteristics. From a practical ward management perspective, it is probably best to have a standard policy for changing the tube every week, earlier if crusting forms.

EXTUBATION

Laryngeal function should be checked once continuous IPPV is no longer required, which will allow the cuff to be deflated during the periods off the ventilator. Clinical observation and careful inspection of the tracheal aspirate is usually sufficient to exclude aspiration. That which is swallowed should vary in consistency during the assessment period.

In adults, once prolonged unassisted ventilation has been accomplished without the patient tiring, the tracheostomy tube is removed. The tract remains patent for a few days, usually allowing re-insertion of the tube if the decision to extubate proves incorrect. During this time, the stoma can be intermittently occluded by digital pressure to allow coughing and speech. An occlusive dressing will become sodden. Dry dressings with light adhesive tape are all that is necessary as long as the patient is properly instructed.

In children, cuffed tubes are used less often, and most pediatric intensivists would progressively reduce the size of the tube over several days before extubation (Watson, 1983). If, in a small child, the tracheostomy has been in place for a long period, bronchoscopy is recommended prior to decannulation (Albert, 1998).

If it is thought that sputum clearance might be a continued problem after extubation, a minitracheostomy tube can be inserted before the tract closes.

COMPLICATIONS

The complications of tracheostomy are largely common to all methods. The management of such complications will be covered in detail elsewhere; however, some complications warrant comment and emphasis.

Bleeding may be due to a coagulopathy or a local vascular injury and may be predictive of an impending innominate artery erosion. The coagulation status of all patients should be checked prior to tracheostomy, especially those who have been seriously ill in the ICU for prolonged periods. Most bleeding associated with tracheostomy is minor and originates from small vessels close to the skin. Local venous damage may complicate the percutaneous techniques, but this is less likely if the incision remains in the midline, and the tracheostomy tube usually controls such venous bleeding. However, if the venous pressure is elevated, control by an open operation is preferable. Arterial bleeding 1 to 3 weeks after tracheostomy raises the possibility of impending arterial erosion. Tracheoinnominate artery erosion occurs in approximately 0.6% of tracheostomies. This complication may be due to a tracheostomy below the fourth tracheal ring, a high position of the innominate artery such that the posterior surface of the tube erodes the artery, or excessive movement of the tracheostomy tube resulting in erosion at the tip of the cannula; or it may be the result of high cuff pressure causing erosion of the anterior tracheal wall (Jones, 1976). A premonitory bleed occurs in one third to one half of all such cases (Jones, 1976; Nelems, 1987). Although this possibility must be investigated urgently, it is often difficult to identify the site of arterial damage, and all one can do is to be prepared for subsequent events. Emergency management may salvage only 14% of these cases (Nelems, 1987). As with most complications, prevention is preferable!

Bacteremia may occur as a result of tracheostomy. In one study, 11 positive blood cultures were found in 106 patients (10.4%) undergoing percutaneous dilatational tracheostomy compared with 7 (6.6%) of 106 patients with the "same patient characteristics" managed by open tracheostomy (Teoh, 1997). *Staphylococcus* species, usually *S. epidermidis,* was the most common organism found in the blood of both groups.

The airway maneuvers involved during tracheostomy, by any technique, may exacerbate *raised intracranial pressure.* Theoretically, this is least likely to occur during open tracheostomy, but even with open operation there will be a brief interruption of normal ventilation, which may cause elevation of the arterial partial pressure of carbon dioxide or a transient fall in oxygen saturation. Either change may result in a significant elevation in intracranial pressure in at-risk patients. When doing a percutaneous tracheostomy, the additional physical stimulation and compression of the neck may produce an even more significant rise of intracranial pressure. However, this does not seem to create a major problem provided that intracranial pressure is monitored (Carillo, 1997).

Tracheoesophageal fistula can occur following open or percutaneous tracheostomy. The timing, however, is different. When associated with open operation, the fistula develops late, owing to erosion of the posterior tracheal wall. The fistula becomes apparent when gastric dilatation occurs or if the tracheal aspirate becomes voluminous or contains aspirated feed. The presence of a nasogastric tube has been implicated (Grillo, 1987). Following the percutaneous operation, the fistula may occur acutely due to penetration of the posterior tracheal wall during insertion of the dilator or tube. Unfortunately, recognition may be delayed. This complication is not completely avoided by bronchoscopic guidance, if this is performed using the fiberoptic instrument. We have studied this problem by monitoring percutaneous tracheostomy using the rigid bronchoscope. The guidewire migrates progressively distally to become impacted in the bronchial tree. The pressure that is required to insert the larger bougies and the tube mounted upon them compresses the tracheal lumen and the guidewire concertinas. Using the fiberoptic bronchoscope, one cannot see the bougie penetrating the posterior wall. The rigid instrument can hold the anterior wall forward during this maneuver. Laceration of the posterior wall is not uncommon, but complete penetration and fistulation is fortunately rare. The suction-aspiration of fresh blood soon after tracheostomy is suggestive of posterior wall laceration and merits bronchoscopy, using the flexible instrument through the tracheostomy tube. The injury may be missed, however, if the tracheostomy tube covers the area of the laceration. If the tracheostomy has been done recently, it is probably unwise to remove it, and suspected injury is treated expectantly.

Stenosis occurs following all techniques of tracheostomy. This is a complex issue on which it is difficult to obtain comparative data. Most patients will have had a period of endotracheal intubation prior to tracheostomy. Upper airway problems arising after such treatment may be erroneously attributed to the tracheostomy procedure. Although endoscopy will help distinguish lesions at the level of the vocal cords, tracheostomy is undertaken through a segment of airway that may have been traumatized by prior intubation (Santos, 1989). Most tracheostomy procedures are undertaken in ICU patients with severe, life-threatening problems. As many as 60% of such patients will not survive to qualify for long-term complications (Friman, 1976). In as many as 50% of the survivors, the recovery is slow and incomplete, such that they fail to reach a level of activity sufficient to reveal the airway problem (Law, 1997). There is the possibility that by studying only those who live for a period after decannulation we will underestimate the true incidence of the complication.

Stenosis may occur at the level of the stoma, at the cuff level, or at both sites (Grillo, 1995b). The method of tracheostomy can only have an impact on lesions at the level of the stoma, and even here there will be confounding factors such as the nursing care of the tracheostomy tube. The reported incidence of any complication must reflect the diligence with which it is sought. Some reports have only recorded those cases in which stenosis after tracheostomy was severe enough to cause stridor (Toursarkissian, 1994), whereas others have systematically evaluated airway cross-sectional anatomy using lung function test, radiology, and endoscopic studies (Andrews, 1971; Friman, 1976; Law, 1997). In one, large recent study (Walz, 1998), only one out of 106 long-term survivors developed clinically significant tracheal stenosis, but 46 (43.4%) had a subclinical stenosis of at least 10% of the cross-sectional area of the trachea.

Generally, the reported incidence of stenosis with open techniques is somewhat higher than that so far reported with percutaneous tracheostomy (Worthley, 1992). One prospective, randomized trial has suggested that the overall incidence of complications is lower with the percutaneous technique (Hazard, 1991). Surgeons may respond by stating that the incidence of complications reflects the level of surgical skill and contend that more serious complications are more common after percutaneous operation. This debate is somewhat sterile, as most tracheostomies are done on intensive care patients who require prolonged IPPV and will be managed by a percutaneous procedure. Some surgeons may be pleased that their operating lists are no longer disrupted by the need for such "housekeeping operations."

A persisting stoma may have to be closed surgically. This is a simple surgical procedure. The stomal margins are mobilized, and fibrous tissue is approximated to close the tracheal defect. If this is not possible, soft tissue cover is sufficient. A persistent stoma is usually associated with a long-standing tracheostomy and epithelialization of the tract. One should be on guard, however, for the occasional case in which the persistent stoma is associated with a proximal stenosis of the larynx.

COMMENTS AND CONTROVERSIES

This chapter provides an excellent overview of current indications, practices, and techniques of tracheostomy, and reflects the combined opinions and perspectives of two experienced, pragmatic clinicians working in separate specialties within the same hospital: Peter Goldstraw, an internationally prominent thoracic surgeon, and Clifford Morgan—anesthetist, intensivist, and current director of a very active ICU.

They emphasize the role and importance of percutaneous tracheostomy, and of mini-tracheostomy, in current practice. Indeed, percutaneous tracheostomy is often the elective procedure of choice for many ICU patients today, with the recognition that there are some clear contraindications to its use in selected cases. With experience, whether the procedure is done by a surgeon or by an intensivist, the percutaneous operation is simpler, and less expensive in both time and money, than the traditional open procedure. It can be done in the ICU without moving the patient, under local anesthesia if desired; it is usually completed more quickly; and it has the same or even a lower incidence of complications. "Experience" is the key word. Patient selection and attention to technical precautions and details are critical to satisfactory outcomes; these important details are clearly stated and well summarized by the authors.

The use of mini-tracheostomy to maintain a clear airway in the early postoperative period, in selected patients, is also well presented. The authors frequently use the mini-procedure in their practice at the Royal Brompton Hospital. Unfortunately, this relatively simple operation is much underutilized in many thoracic surgical centers throughout the world. Although the authors make brief comment about each of the serious complications of tracheostomy—TE fistula, tracheo-innominate artery fistula, and tracheal stenosis—these problems are described in much greater detail in accompanying chapters in this section on Upper Airway Surgery.

F. G. P.

■ REFERENCES

Albert D, Leighton S: Stridor and airway management. In Cummings CW, Fredrickson JM, Harker LE et al (eds): Paediatric Otolaryngology, Head and Neck Surgery. St Louis, Mosby, 1998.

Ambesh SP, Kaushik S: Percutaneous dilational tracheostomy: The Ciaglia method versus the Rapitrach method. Anes Analg 87:556, 1998.

Andrews MJ: The incidence and pathogenesis of tracheal injury following tracheostomy with cuffed tube and assisted ventilation: An analysis of a 3-year prospective study. Br J Surg 58:749, 1971.

Bjork VO: Partial resection of the only remaining lung with the aid of respiratory treatment. J Thorac Cardiovasc Surg 39:179, 1960.

Brantigan CO, Grow JB: Cricothyroidotomy: Elective use in respiratory problems requiring tracheotomy. J Thorac Cardiovasc Surg 71:71, 1976.

Brimacombe J, Clarke G: Rigid bronchoscope: A possible new option for percutaneous dilational tracheostomy. Anesthesiology 83:646, 1995.

Burkey B, Esclamado R, Morganroth M: The role of cricothyroidotomy in airway management. Clin Chest Med 12:561, 1991.

Carrillo EH, Spain DA, Bumpous JM et al: Percutaneous dilational tracheostomy for airway control. Am J Surg 174:469, 1997.

Ciaglia P, Firsching R, Syniec C: Elective percutaneous dilational tracheostomy: A new simple bedside procedure—preliminary report. Chest 87:715, 1985.

Ciaglia P, Graniero KD: Percutaneous dilational tracheostomy: Results and long-term follow-up. Chest. 101:464, 1992.

Cooper JD, Grillo HC: Experimental production and prevention of injury due to cuffed tracheal tubes. Surg Gynaecol Obstet 129:1235, 1969.

Cooper JD: Complications of tracheostomy: Pathogenesis, treatment and prevention. In Grillo HC, Eschapasse H (eds): International Trends in General Thoracic Surgery: Major Challenges. Philadelphia, WB Saunders, 1987.

Cooper RM: Use and safety of percutaneous tracheostomy in intensive care. A report of a postal survey of ICU practice. Anaesthesia 53:1209, 1998.

Feneck R: Anaesthesia for diagnostic thoracic surgical procedures. In Gothard JWW (ed): Clinical Anaesthesiology: Thoracic Anaesthesia. London, Bailliere Tindall, 1987.

Friman L, Hedenstierna G, Schildt B: Stenosis following tracheostomy: A quantitative study of long term results. Anaesthesia 31:479, 1976.

Gardiner Q, White PS, Carson D et al: Technique training: Endoscopic percutaneous tracheostomy. Br J Anaesth 81:401, 1998.

Goodall EW: The story of tracheotomy. Br J Child Dis 31:167, 1934.

Gothard JWW: Anaesthesia for Thoracic Surgery, ed 2. London, Blackwell, 1993.

Grillo HC: Postintubation tracheo-esophageal fistula. In Grillo HC, Eschapasse H (eds): International Trends in General Thoracic Surgery: Major Challenges. Philadelphia, WB Saunders, 1987.

Grillo HC: Congenital lesions, neoplasms, inflammation, infections, injuries, and other lesions of the trachea. In Sabiston DC, Spencer FC (eds): Surgery of the Chest, 6 ed. Philadelphia, WB Saunders, 1995a.

Grillo HC, Donahue DM, Mathisen DJ et al: Postintubation tracheal stenosis: Treatment and results. J Thorac Cardiovasc Surg 109:486, 1995b.

Hazard P, Jones C, Benitone J: Comparative clinical trial of standard operative tracheostomy with percutaneous tracheostomy. Crit Care Med 19:1018, 1991.

Hopkinson RB, Matthews HR: Treatment of sputum retention by minitracheotomy. Br J Surg 71:147, 1984.

Jackson C: High tracheotomy and other errors the chief causes of chronic laryngeal stenosis. Surg Gynaecol Obstet 32:392, 1921.

Jackson C, Jackson CL: The Larynx and its Disorders. Philadelphia, WB Saunders, 1937, pp 455–494.

Jones JW, Reynolds M, Hewitt RL et al: Tracheo-innominate artery erosion: Successful surgical management of a devastating complication. Ann Surg 184:194, 1976.

Law RC, Carney AS, Manara AR: Long-term outcome after percutaneous dilational tracheostomy: Endoscopic and spirometry findings. Anaesthesia 52:51, 1997.

Leonard RC, Lewis RH, Singh B et al: Late outcome from percutaneous tracheostomy using the Portex kit. Chest 115:1070, 1999.

Lulenski GC, Batsakis JG: Tracheal incision as a contributing factor to tracheal stenosis: An experimental study. Ann Otol 84:781, 1975.

Marelli D, Paul A, Manolidis S et al. Endoscopic guided percutaneous tracheostomy: Early results of a consecutive trial. J Trauma 30:433, 1990.

McHenry CR, Raeburn CD, Lange RL et al: Percutaneous tracheostomy: A cost-effective alternative to standard open tracheostomy. Am Surg 65: 92, 1999.

Nelems B: Tracheoarterial fistula. In Grillo HC, Eschapasse H (eds): International Trends in General Thoracic Surgery: Major Challenges. Philadelphia, WB Saunders, 1987.

Orringer MB: Anterior mediastinal tracheostomy with and without cervical exenteration. Ann Thorac Surg 54:628, 1992.

Porter JM, Ivatury RR: Preferred route of tracheostomy—percutaneous versus open at the bedside: A randomized, prospective study in the surgical ICU. Am Surg 65:142, 1999.

Powell DM, Price PD, Forrest LA: Review of percutaneous tracheostomy. Laryngoscope 1998; 108: 170, 1998.

Santos PM, Afrassiabi A, Weymuller EA Jr: Prospective studies evaluating the standard endotracheal tube and a prototype endotracheal tube. Ann Otol Rhinol Laryngol 98:935, 1989.

Sebastian A: A Dictionary of the History of Medicine. New York, Parthenon, 1999, p 722.

Simpson TP, Day CJ, Jewkes CF et al: The impact of percutaneous tracheostomy on intensive care unit practice and training. Anaesthesia 54:186, 1999.

Teoh N, Parr MJ, Finfer SR: Bacteraemia following percutaneous dilational tracheostomy. Anaesth Intensive Care 25:354, 1997.

Toursarkissian, B, Zweng TN, Kearney PA et al: Percutaneous dilational tracheostomy: Report of 141 cases. Ann Thorac Surg 57:862, 1994.

Trottier SJ, Hazard PB, Sakabu SA et al: Posterior tracheal wall perforation during percutaneous dilational tracheostomy: An investigation into its mechanism and prevention. Chest 115:1229, 1999.

van Heerbeek N, Fikkers BG, van den Hoogen FJ et al: The guidewire

dilating forceps technique of percutaneous tracheostomy. Am J Surg 177: 311, 1999.
Walz MK, Peitgen K, Thurauf N et al: Percutaneous dilational tracheostomy: Early results and long-term outcome of 326 critically ill patients. Intensive Care Med 24:685, 1998.
Watson CB: A survey of intubation practices in critical care medicine. Ear Nose Throat J 62:494, 1983.
Weymuller EA Jr: Acute airway management. In Cummings CW, Fredrickson JM, Harker LE et al (eds): Otolaryngology, Head and Neck Surgery, 3 ed. St Louis, Mosby, 1998.
Whited RE: Posterior commissure stenosis post long-term intubation. Laryngoscope 93:1314, 1983.
Worthley LIG, Holt A: Percutaneous tracheostomy. Intensive Care World 9:187, 1992.

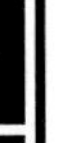

SUBGLOTTIC RESECTION: ADULTS

Michael A. Maddaus
F. Griffith Pearson

The subglottic airway extends from the inferior margin of the vocal cords above to the lower border of the cricoid cartilage below. Resection of the subglottic airway is complicated by the following factors:

1. It is in close proximity to the vocal cords.
2. Complete transection of the subglottic airway at any level above the cricothyroid joints will divide the recurrent laryngeal nerves.
3. The posterior rim of the upper border of the cricoid cartilage supports the arytenoid cartilages, which play a critical role in vocal function.

The technique of subglottic resection, which is described in detail later, allows transverse division of the airway up to the level of the inferior border of the vocal cords without transection of intact recurrent laryngeal nerves. At the level of the inferior border of the posterior cricoid plate, the recurrent nerves pass behind the cricoid cartilage. On each side, the nerve passes behind the cricothyroid articulation and continues a vertical ascent to the superior border of the cricoid cartilage, at which point it passes forward to supply the glottic muscles. As long as the tissues lying behind the cricoid cartilage are undisturbed, both recurrent laryngeal nerves can be predictably preserved.

HISTORICAL NOTE

Ogura and Powers (1964) were the first to describe a segmental resection of the cricoid cartilage with primary thyrotracheal anastomosis. They reported on seven patients with subglottic obstruction secondary to blunt trauma. In all these patients, however, the recurrent laryngeal nerves were avulsed and paralyzed on both sides as a result of the original trauma. In 1974, Gerwat and Bryce described a technique of partial cricoid resection using an oblique line of transection of the subglottic airway (Fig. 19–1), which removed the anterior cricoid arch but preserved the posterior cricoid cartilage and recurrent nerves above the level of the cricothyroid joints. With this technique, however, the level of resection of the posterior subglottic airway was limited.

In 1975, Pearson and colleagues described a technique of transverse resection of the subglottic airway at any

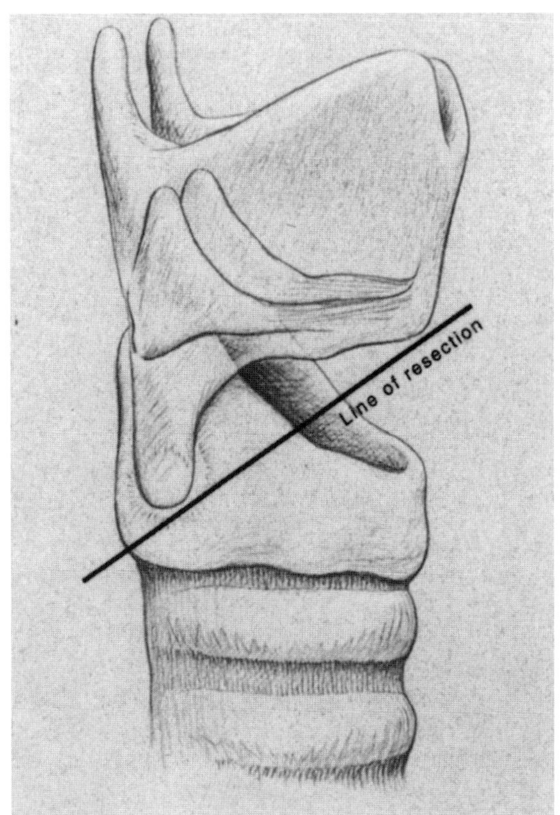

FIGURE 19–1 ■ Diagram illustrating lateral view of the larynx and the upper airway. The line of resection begins at the inferior border of the thyroid cartilage anteriorly and passes below the cricothyroid joint behind. This line of resection allows preservation of the recurrent laryngeal nerves and was the technique of partial cricoid resection described by Gerwat and Bryce (1974).

level below the vocal cords, with preservation of intact recurrent laryngeal nerves. This was accomplished by maintaining a posterior shell of cricoid cartilage. A primary thyrotracheal anastomosis was performed within 1 cm or less of the inferior margin of the vocal cords. This is the technique that we describe in detail in the section, Operative Technique.

■ HISTORICAL READINGS

Gerwat J, Bryce DP: The management of subglottic laryngeal stenosis by resection and direct anastomosis. Laryngoscope 84:940, 1974.

Ogura JH, Powers WE: Functional restitution of traumatic stenosis of the larynx and pharynx. Laryngoscope 74:1081, 1964.

Pearson FG, Cooper JD, Nelems JM et al: Primary tracheal anastomosis after resection of the cricoid cartilage with preservation of recurrent laryngeal nerves. J Thorac Cardiovasc Surg 70:806, 1975.

ANATOMY

A clear knowledge of the anatomy of the region is essential to an understanding of this operative technique. The anatomy of the larynx and upper airway is described in detail in Chapter 12. Some features warrant emphasis (Fig. 19–2). The cricoid cartilage is the first full ring of the upper airway, has an anterior arch similar in height to a normal tracheal ring, and expands into a broad posterior plate or rostrum. Both the inner and outer aspects of the cricoid cartilage are covered with a stout perichondrial layer, which may be freed from the underlying cartilage during certain stages of the operation. Paired arytenoid cartilages rest on the superior border of the posterior cricoid plate and articulate at the cricoarytenoid joints. The vocal cords are attached posteriorly to the vocal processes of the arytenoid cartilages and attach anteriorly to the thyroid cartilage. The subglottic larynx begins immediately below the vocal folds and extends to the inferior margin of the cricoid cartilage. The subglottic space is the narrowest part of the upper airway aside from the larynx. The subglottis has an internal diameter that is between 1.5 and 2 cm in adults and is completely surrounded by the cricoid cartilage.

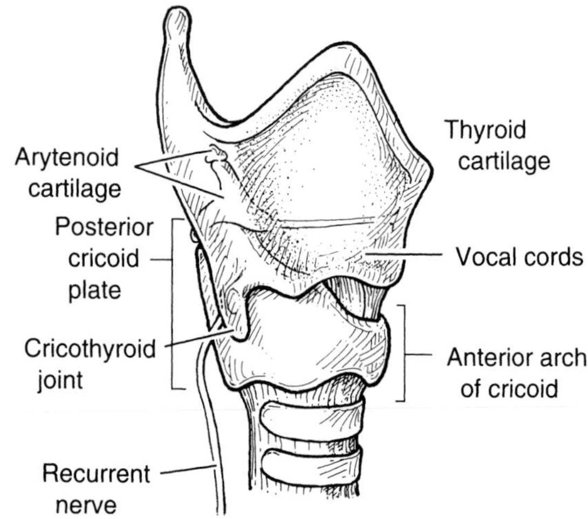

FIGURE 19–2 ■ Diagrammatic illustration, lateral view, showing the pertinent anatomy of the larynx and the subglottic and upper tracheal airways.

ANESTHETIC TECHNIQUE

When necessary, the stenosis is dilated prior to operation. With the patient asleep, gum-tipped esophageal bougies are directed through a conventional intubating laryngoscope. This is the least traumatic technique for dilatation of the subglottic region. Following passage of a 34 French (F) gum-tipped bougie, the anesthetist should easily pass a No. 6 or 6.5 endotracheal tube. If the intubation is difficult owing to a tight stenosis, an uncuffed tube may be preferable, because an air seal will be secured at the level of the stricture. A rigid bronchoscope can be used as the dilating instrument, but this procedure is more traumatic than that using the tapered bougies.

Once the distal airway is divided, an armored endotracheal tube is introduced through the distal trachea, and the proximal end of the tube is passed at the side of the cheek and under the drapes to the anesthetist (Fig. 19–3A).

INDICATIONS

Postintubation injury remains the most common cause of subglottic stenosis that is amenable to resection and primary reconstruction (Fig. 19–4). The injury follows translaryngeal intubation, with or without a subsequent tracheotomy. A high tracheotomy or cricothyroidotomy may result in injury within the cricoid ring, even in the absence of prior translaryngeal intubation. Other causes of benign stenosis are blunt trauma with cricotracheal disruption, idiopathic subglottic stenosis, inhalation injury owing to thermal or chemical burns, and rare miscellaneous conditions such as primary amyloidosis.

On occasion, neoplasms of the upper airway may be amenable to subglottic resection with sparing of the larynx and voice. To date we have used this approach in 13 patients: adenoid cystic carcinoma—4, squamous cell carcinoma—2, mucoepidermoid carcinoma—2, neurofibroma—2, thyroid carcinoma—2 and chondrosarcoma—1. It should be emphasized, however, that a majority of primary malignancies involving the subglottic airway will be best managed by a resection that includes a laryngectomy.

Monnier and Savary (1993) were the first to demonstrate the successful application of this operation in infants and children suffering from obstruction due to postintubation stenosis or congenital subglottic stenosis. In this second edition, Monnier has described his modified technique and results in detail (see Chapter 22). They have shown that such resections do not interfere with the normal growth and development of the larynx and subglottis in long-term follow-up.

MANAGEMENT

Operative Technique

Subglottic Resection

The neck is fully extended, with some type of bolster placed behind the scapulae. Exposure is obtained with a generous collar incision, which is located at a level that will best expose the pathology in the upper airway. Sub-

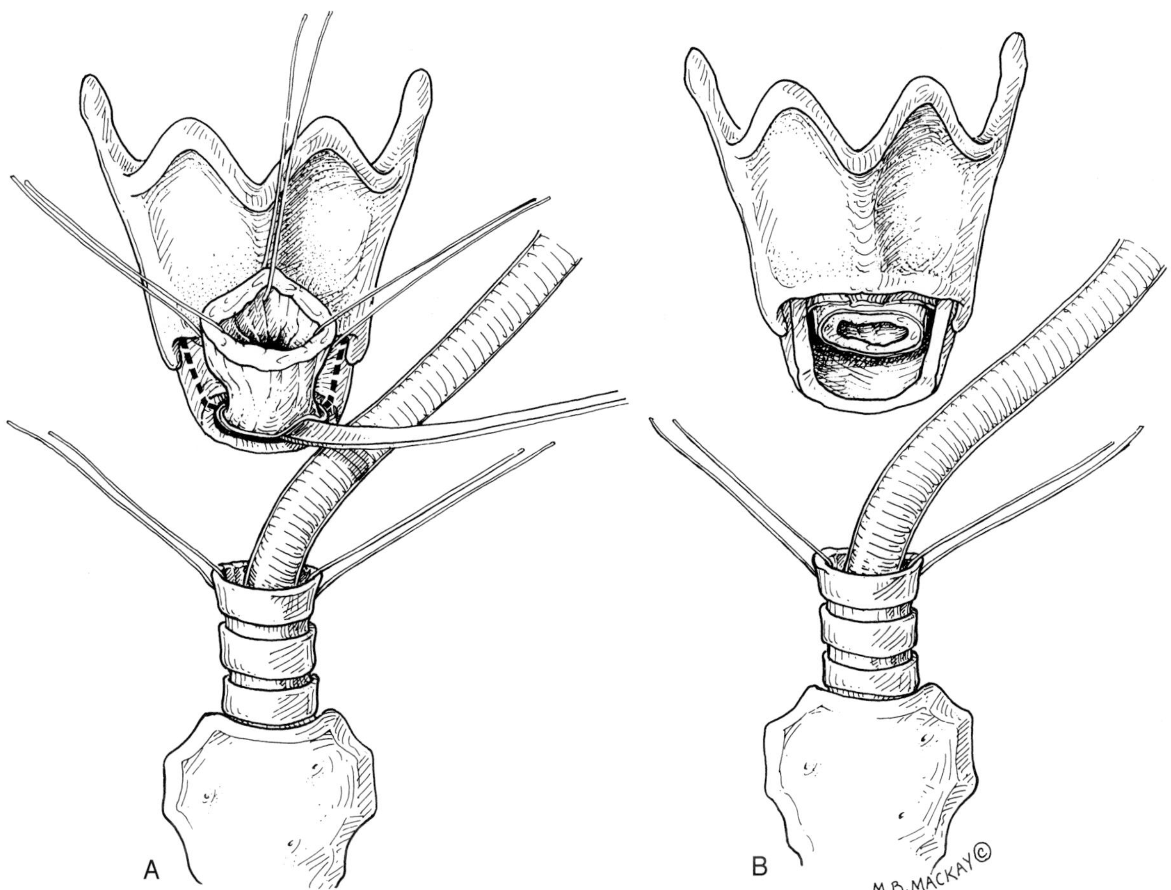

FIGURE 19–3 ■ *A*, The airway has been divided just beyond the stenotic lesion, and the distal trachea has been intubated with the armored endotracheal tube. Stay sutures have been placed in the divided tracheal ends. The anterior and lateral components of the cricoid cartilage have been removed, and it is now possible to develop the subperichondrial plane in front of the posterior cricoid plate. This is usually done with a small orthopedic elevator. This avascular plane can be developed posteriorly and laterally to a level just below the arytenoid cartilages and vocal folds. *B*, The soft tissue airway is now divided above the lesion, through an area of healthy mucosa in the subglottic region. This line of division may lie within a few millimeters of the inferior margins of the vocal cords. A posterior shell of the remaining cricoid cartilage is exposed and protects the posteriorly situated recurrent nerves.

platysmal skin flaps are developed to provide exposure from the thyroid notch above to the suprasternal notch below. The strap muscles are reflected from the midline to expose the anterior aspect of the thyroid and cricoid cartilages and the adjacent cervical trachea (Fig. 19–5). In these cases the pathology lies within the cricoid ring and commonly extends to the adjacent cervical trachea. The lines of resection for this isolated subglottic lesion are illustrated in Figure 19–6.

The upper trachea in the region of the diseased segment is freed circumferentially to the level of the inferior border of the cricoid ring. Dissection is maintained immediately against the outer surface of the airway, which protects the recurrent laryngeal nerves posterolaterally. In patients with benign lesions, no attempt is made to identify the recurrent nerves, which are frequently obscured by peritracheal scar. When operating for neoplasm, however, it may be necessary to identify one or the other recurrent laryngeal nerve to determine the extent of neoplastic involvement. If the nerve is infiltrated by tumor, it may have to be sacrificed and resected.

Once the inferior border of the cricoid cartilage has been identified, the exposed perichondrium is incised with a scalpel or by cautery. In most patients it is possible to free the perichondrium from the underlying cartilage by using a small orthopedic elevator (Fig. 19–7). The entire circumference of the inferior border of the cricoid cartilage is exposed under the perichondrium, and the entire anterolateral ring of the cricoid cartilage is then freed from its perichondrial cover (Fig. 19–8). The exposed anterior and lateral aspects of the cricoid arch are then removed, usually in piecemeal fashion, with small rongeurs (Fig. 19–9).

The trachea is then transected at the distal end of the lesion, and the distal airway is intubated with an armored endotracheal tube (see Fig. 19–3*A*). Stay sutures are placed in the divided tracheal ends, above and below. It is now possible to develop the subperichondrial plane in front of the posterior cricoid plate. Once again, by using an orthopedic elevator, this avascular plane can be freed almost to the inferior margins of the cricoarytenoid joints (see Fig. 19–3*A*). The airway is then divided above the stenosis, through healthy mucosa in the subglottic region (see Fig. 19–3*B*). This line of division may lie within a

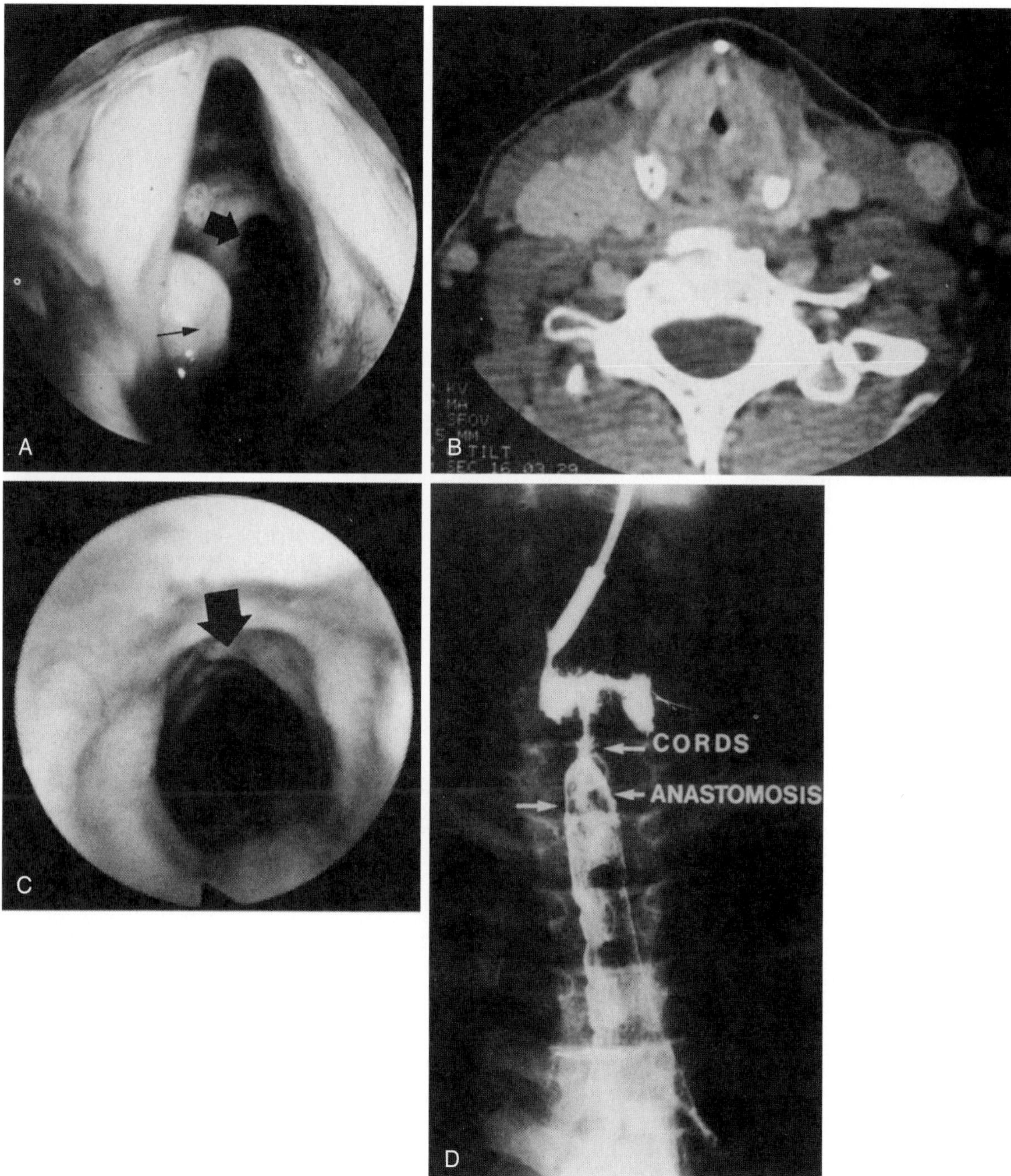

FIGURE 19–4 ■ *A*, Postintubation injury. There is a polypoid granulation projecting from the posterior third of the left vocal cord *(small arrow)*. In the subglottic area, a concentric stenosis is just visible *(large arrow)*. *B*, A computed tomography scan (1.5-mm–interval cut) at the subglottic level showing a severe stenosis with marked circumferential submucosal thickening (scar). (Same patient as in *A*.) *C*, Photograph obtained 1 year after subglottic resection and reconstruction by primary thyrotracheal anastomosis. The subglottic airway is healthy throughout, with a complete mucosal covering and normal airway diameters. The thin line of scar that identifies the anastomosis is almost invisible *(arrow)*. (Same patient as in *A* and *B*.) *D*, Contrast tracheogram obtained 1 year after operation in the same patient. The anastomosis is widely patent and lies within 1 cm of the inferior aspect of the vocal cords.

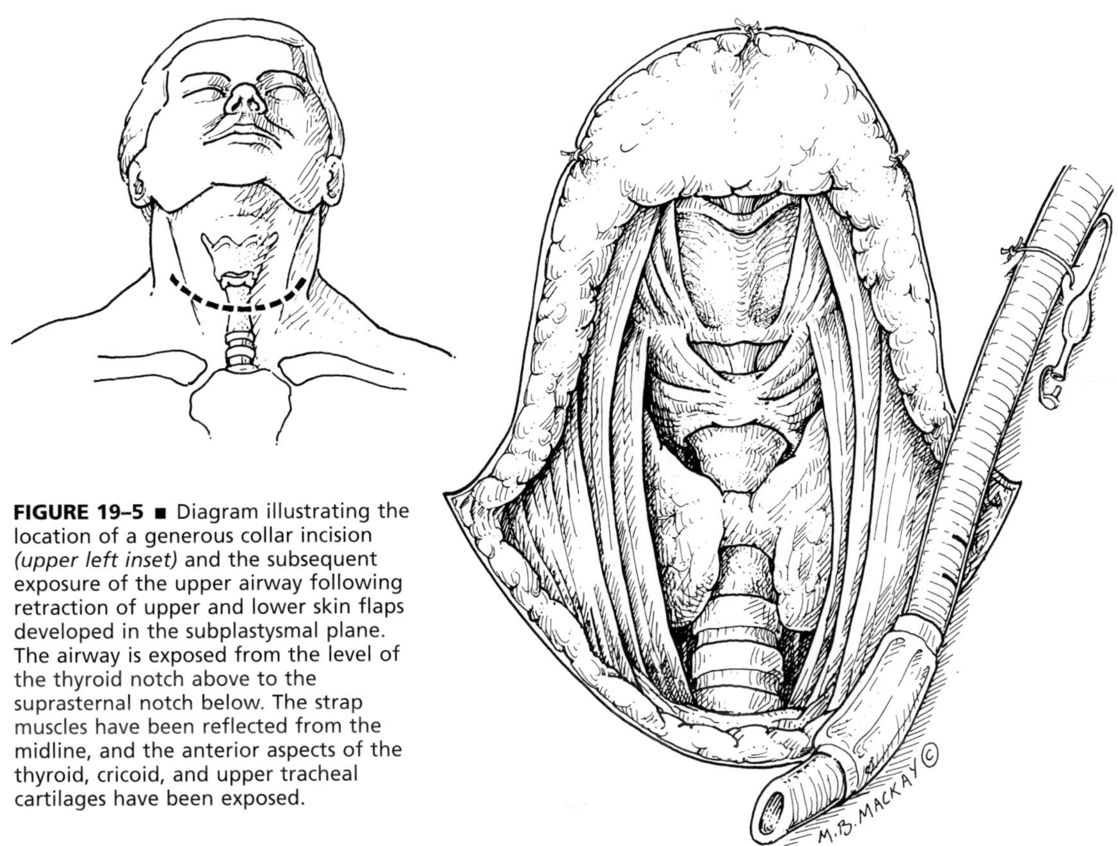

FIGURE 19–5 ■ Diagram illustrating the location of a generous collar incision *(upper left inset)* and the subsequent exposure of the upper airway following retraction of upper and lower skin flaps developed in the subplastysmal plane. The airway is exposed from the level of the thyroid notch above to the suprasternal notch below. The strap muscles have been reflected from the midline, and the anterior aspects of the thyroid, cricoid, and upper tracheal cartilages have been exposed.

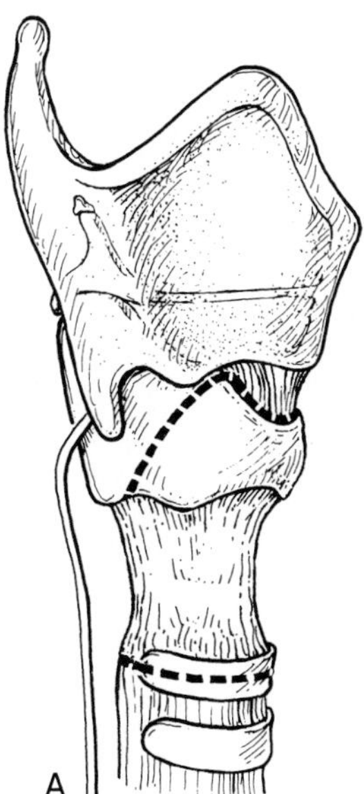

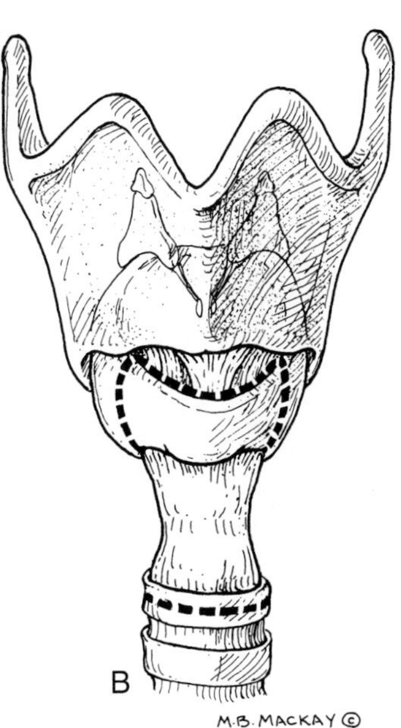

FIGURE 19–6 ■ Lateral *(A)* and anteroposterior *(B)* projections showing the resection margins for a benign postintubation stenosis, which involves the subglottic airway, within the cricoid ring, as well as the proximal cervical trachea.

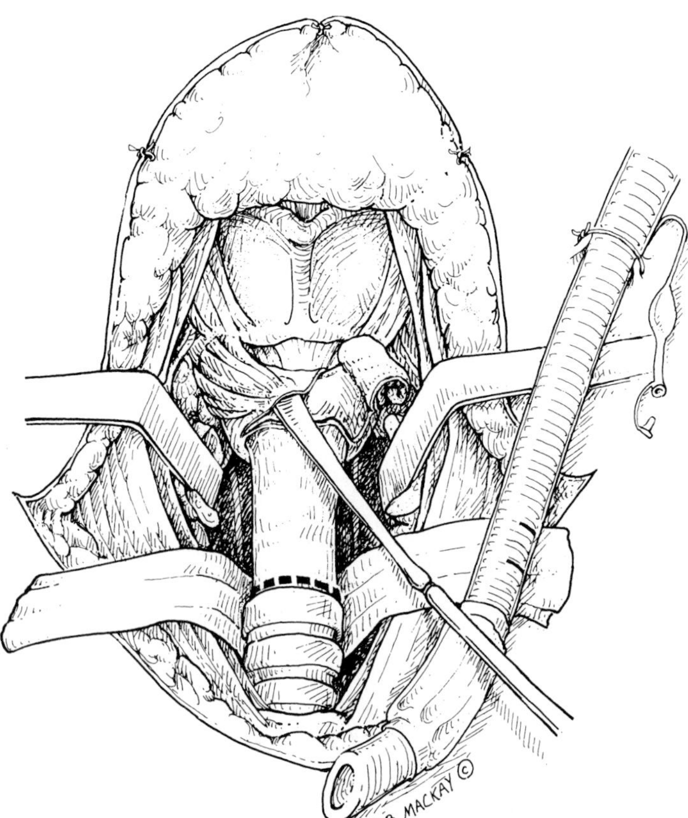

FIGURE 19–7 ■ Diagram illustrating technique of subperichondrial exposure of the anterior and lateral aspects of the cricoid cartilage. The perichondrium has been incised along the inferior border of the arch and is being freed from the underlying cartilage by means of a small orthopedic elevator. The damaged and stenotic lesion extends for several centimeters below the cricoid and has been mobilized circumferentially. The distal airway will be divided at the level of the *dotted line*, and an armored orotracheal tube has been secured along the left side of the neck for intubation of the distal airway following transection.

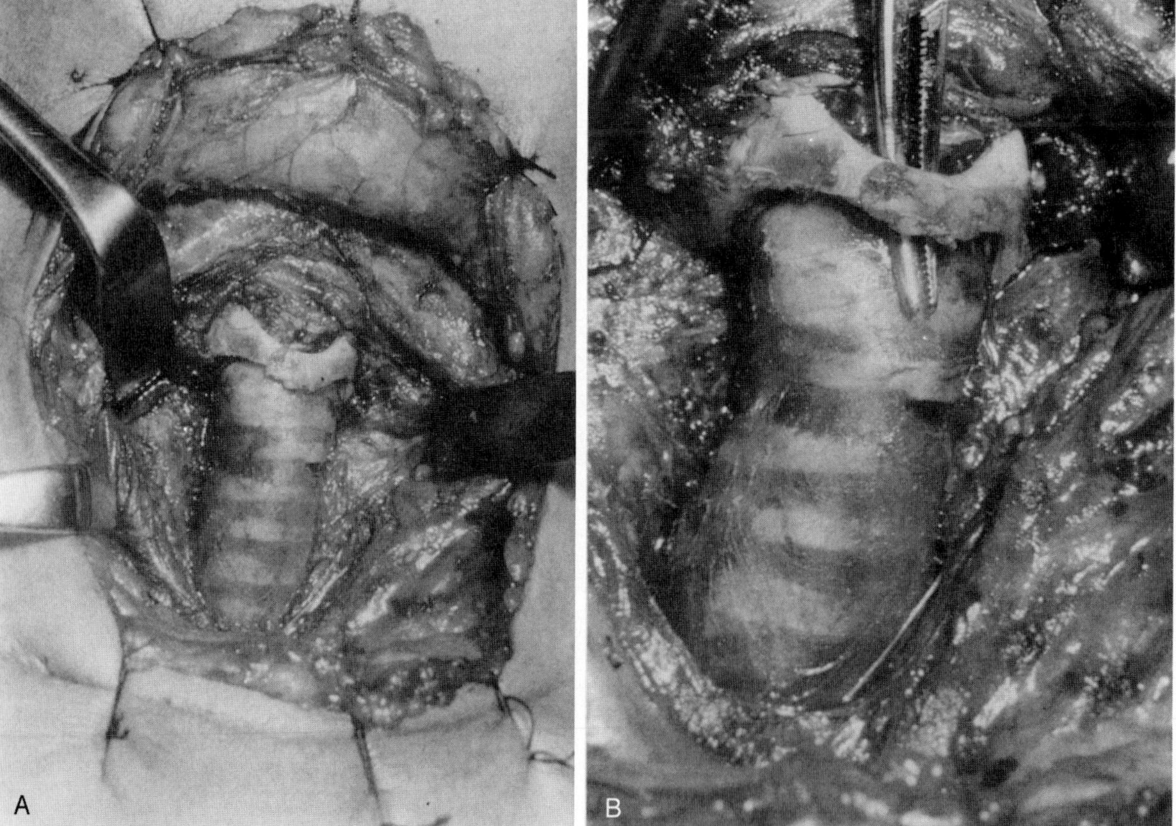

FIGURE 19–8 ■ *A*, Operative photograph illustrating the anterior cricoid cartilage after it has been freed completely of its perichondrial cover. *B*, The tip of a hemostat has been passed behind the anterior cricoid arch, demonstrating the circumferential mobilization.

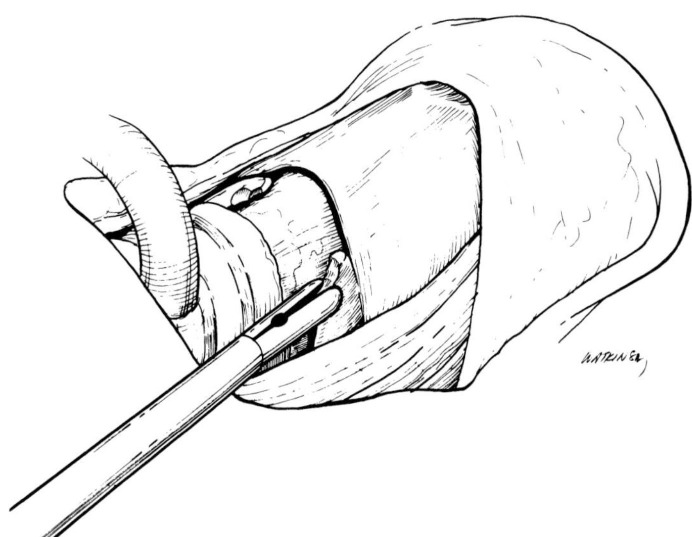

FIGURE 19–9 ■ Diagram illustrating removal of the exposed anterior and lateral aspects of the cricoid arch using a small rongeur.

few millimeters of the inferior margins of the vocal folds. The posterior shell of the remaining cricoid cartilage is exposed and protects the posteriorly situated recurrent laryngeal nerves.

If the external, posterior aspect of the cricoid plate is freed subperichondrially, the posterior cartilage may also be removed up to the level of the proposed anastomosis. This may be necessary in patients with a damaged or chronically infected posterior cricoid cartilage. The remaining subglottic airway now consists of a stout tube of perichondrium with underlying mucosa and submucosa. There will inevitably be a discrepancy in luminal diameter between the subglottic airway (smaller) and the cut end of the distal trachea. It is usually desirable to plicate the membranous component of the distal trachea to accommodate these differences in diameter (Fig. 19–10*A*).

An end-to-end thyrotracheal anastomosis is performed using interrupted sutures (see Fig. 19–10*B*). Our preference is to use 35-gauge stainless steel wire on the posterior wall with knots tied on the inside. The lateral and anterior part of the anastomosis is completed with interrupted sutures of 3–0 or 4–0 Vicryl, with knots tied on the outside.

Subglottic Resection and Synchronous Laryngeal Reconstruction

Synchronous laryngotracheal injury is commonly seen following prolonged translaryngeal intubation (Maddaus et al, 1992). The most common glottic injury is a posterior interarytenoid stenosis, which restricts abduction of the vocal cords. These combined injuries are best managed collaboratively with the otolaryngologist. A review of our group's experience with postintubation glottic injury was reported by Pearson and Gullane (1995).

The lines of incision and transection for a synchronous combined procedure are illustrated in Figure 19–11. The technique of mobilization of the cervical trachea and cricoid is similar to that used for resection of isolated subglottic stenosis (Fig 19–12). In these cases, however, the thyroid cartilage is divided in the midline anteriorly (Fig. 19–13*A*). When the margins of the laryngofissure are retracted laterally, the vocal cords and upper subglottic region are exposed. (In Figure 19–3*B*, the subglottic pathology is resected, but the interarytenoid scar remains—see *dotted line*.)

When the interarytenoid scar is excised, a posterior mucosal defect is created, which extends to the upper margins of interarytenoid mucosa (Fig. 19–14*A*). This

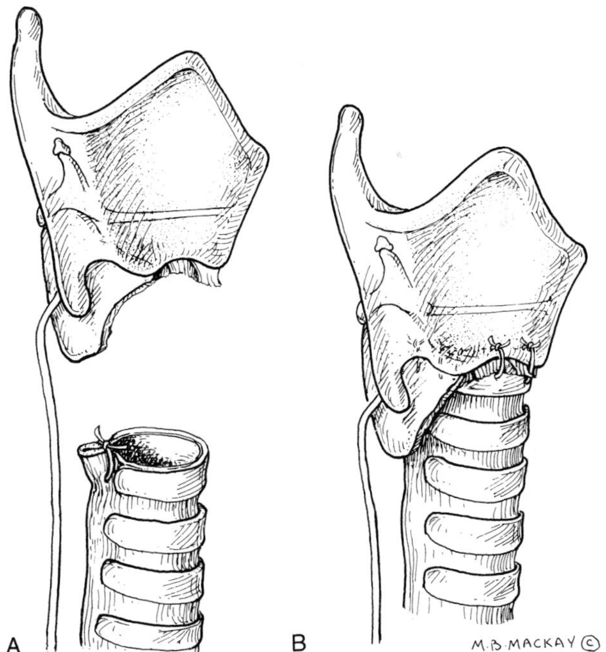

FIGURE 19–10 ■ *A*, Diagram illustrating the technique of plication of the membranous trachea to match the luminal diameters of the tracheal and subglottic airways at the level of anastomosis. This also restores a complete cartilaginous ring in the subglottic larynx. *B*, Diagram illustrating an end-to-end thyrotracheal anastomosis. This anastomosis is begun posteriorly using interrupted sutures of fine-gauge (35 French) stainless steel wire, with the knots tied inside. The lateral and anterior margins of the anastomosis are then closed by interrupted sutures of 3–0 or 4–0 Vicryl with the knots tied on the outside.

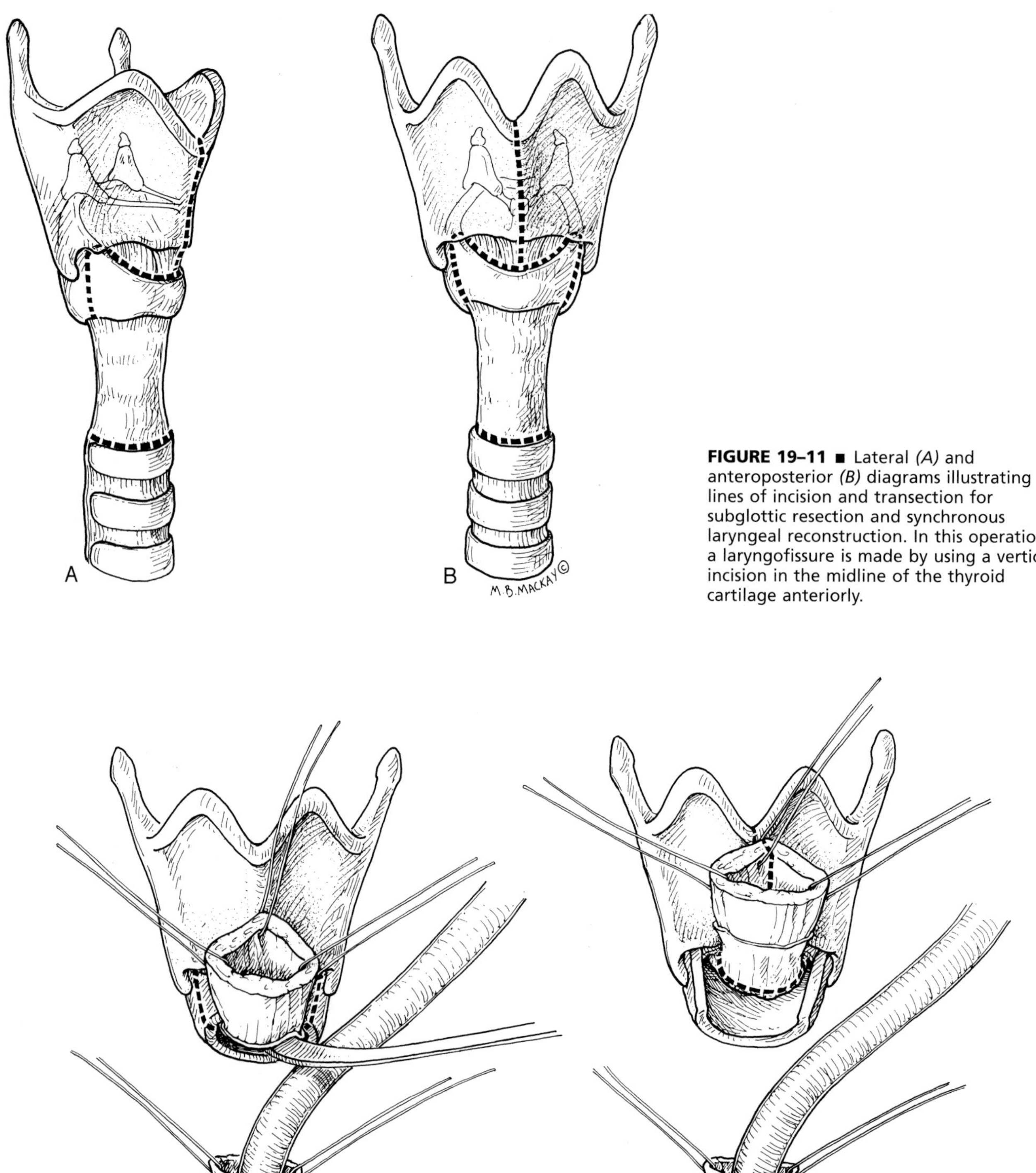

FIGURE 19–11 ■ Lateral *(A)* and anteroposterior *(B)* diagrams illustrating the lines of incision and transection for subglottic resection and synchronous laryngeal reconstruction. In this operation, a laryngofissure is made by using a vertical incision in the midline of the thyroid cartilage anteriorly.

FIGURE 19–12 ■ *A*, Diagram illustrating mobilization and resection of the subglottic defect. The cricoid arch has been freed subperichondrially and resected, and the trachea has been divided below the lesion and intubated for ventilation. The avascular, subperichondrial plane in front of the posterior cricoid plate is being developed with a small orthopedic elevator. *B*, The stenotic lesion in the subglottic airway has been freed posteriorly to a level above the pathology.

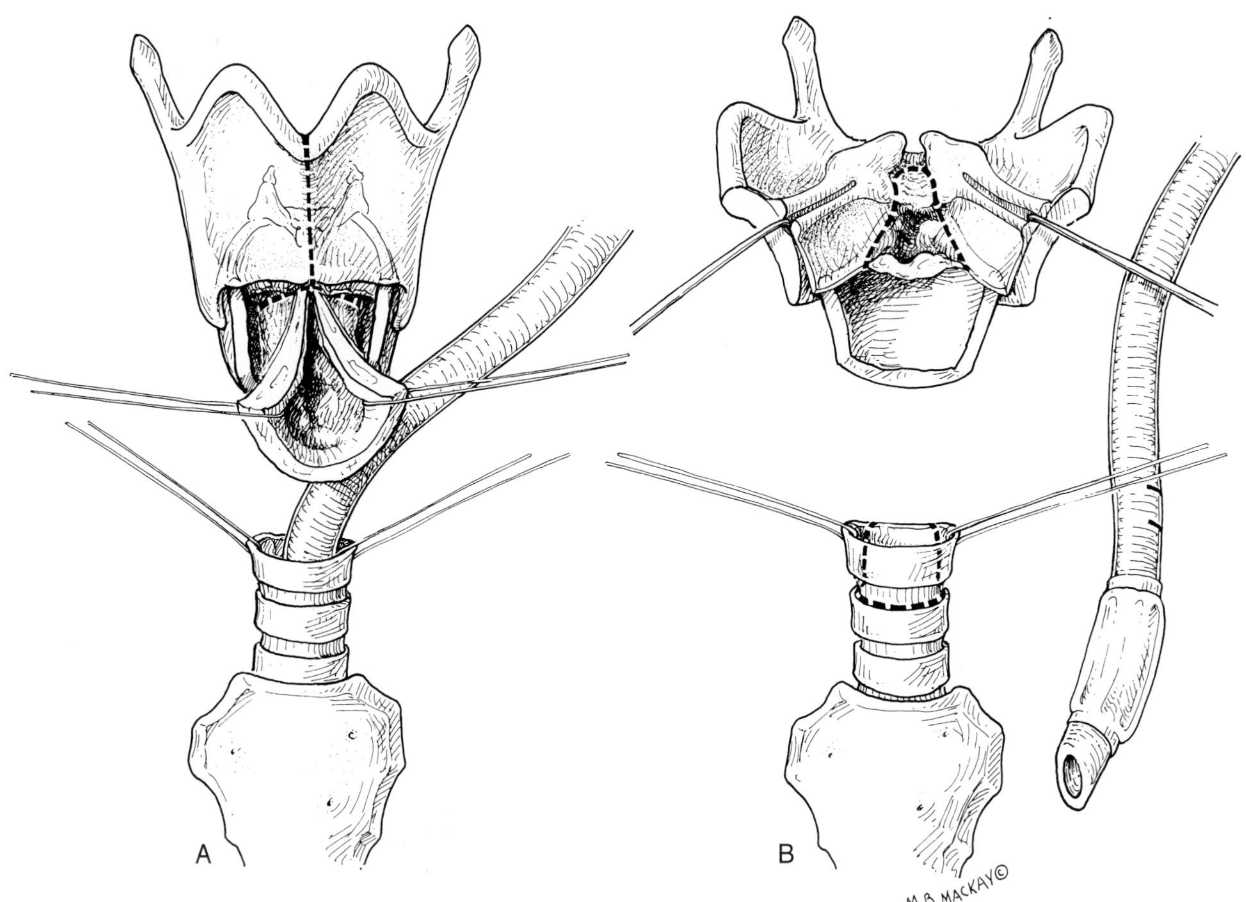

FIGURE 19–13 ■ *A*, Diagram illustrating the diseased and stenotic airway, which has been opened anteriorly in the midline to the level of the thyroid cartilage. The subglottic airway will be transected above the pathology *(transverse dotted line)* and the larynx exposed by a laryngofissure. *B*, The laryngofissure has been completed and the diseased subglottic segment resected. The margins of the thyroid cartilage are separated with small retracting hooks, which are positioned at the anterior ends of the vocal cords in the diagram. Following resection of the subglottic stenosis, a broad plate of inferior cricoid cartilage is exposed. There is still a dense interarytenoid scar, which will be excised within the margins of the *upper dotted line*. A posterior pedicled flap of membranous trachea will be fashioned from the distal cut margin of the airway *(lower dotted line)* and will be used to resurface the interarytenoid defect.

defect will be resurfaced by using a pedicled flap of membranous trachea fashioned from the distal tracheal margins (see Fig. 19–14*B*). To create this vascularized pedicle of membranous trachea, it is necessary to resect one or two of the anterolateral cartilaginous rings. The mucosal flap is then secured with interrupted sutures of fine-gauge stainless steel wire, as illustrated in Figure 19–14. Figures 19–15 to 19–19 are operative photographs illustrating laryngofissure, excision of interarytenoid scar, and preparation of a pedicled flap of posteromembranous distal trachea, which will be used to resurface the posterior glottic defect. The remainder of the thyrotracheal anastomosis is completed with interrupted 3–0 or 4–0 Vicryl sutures. The laryngofissure is closed anteriorly with interrupted 3–0 or 4–0 Vicryl sutures (Fig. 19–20). When the subglottic anastomosis lies within a few millimeters of the vocal cords, there is an unpredictable risk of postoperative glottic edema. This problem is managed by placement of a small distal tracheostomy tube or placement of a silicone Montgomery T tube, with the upper limb of the T tube lying 0.5 to 1 cm above the vocal cords, as illustrated in Figure 19–20. Depending on the status of the airway at the margins of this high anastomosis, the T tube may be left in position for intervals varying from a few weeks to 3 or more months.

The incision is closed as described previously. A stout suture of 5–0 Tevdek secures the skin of the chin to the skin of the chest to maintain neck flexion during the first postoperative week.

Postoperative Management

If a Montgomery T tube is placed, the cervical arm should be closed or corked, so that breathing occurs through the nose and mouth and the normal mechanisms for humidification of the airway are preserved. If the cervical arm of the T tube is not closed, and the patient is allowed to breathe through the cervical stoma, there is a serious risk of life-threatening airway obstruction. The tracheal arm of the T tube can become plugged with desiccated secretions owing to failure of adequate humidification. The Montgomery T tube has no inner cannula, and such obstruction may only be relieved by the immediate removal of the T tube. If a small distal tracheostomy is placed, this, too, may be corked if the patient can breathe

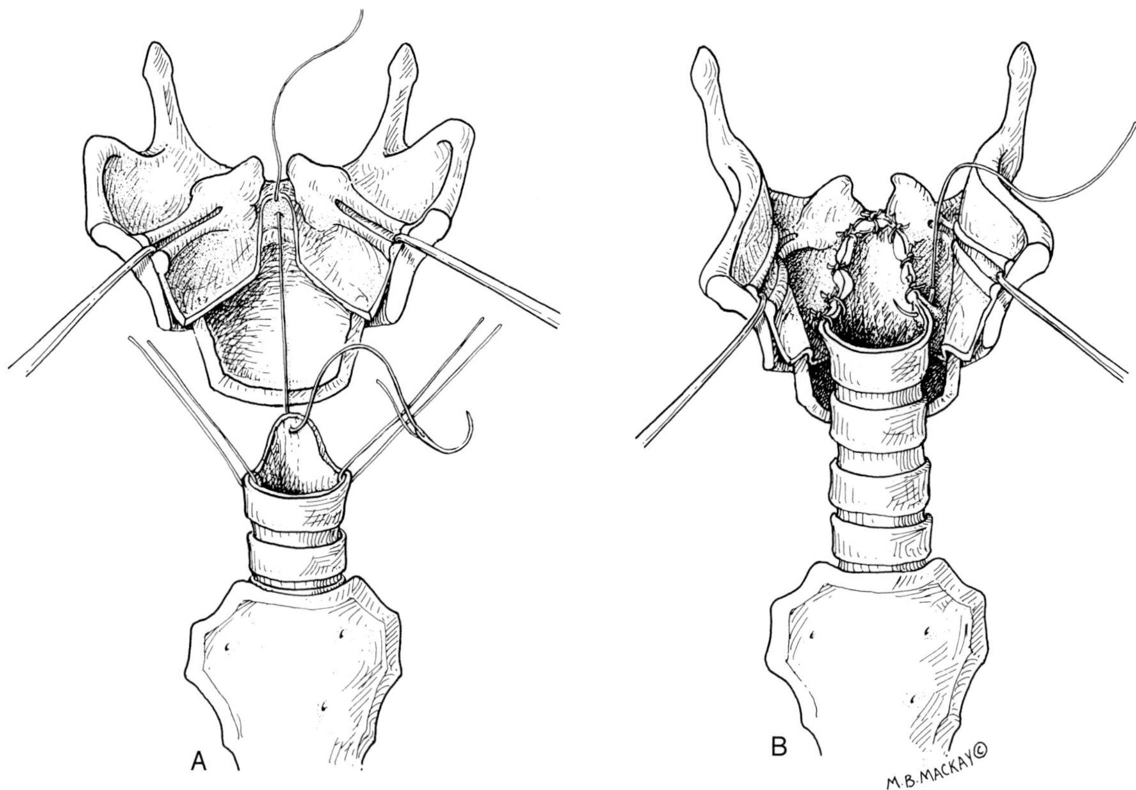

FIGURE 19–14 ■ *A*, The posterior mucosal flap has been developed at the distal resection margin, and the first of a series of interrupted sutures is placed to secure the flap in the interarytenoid defect. *B*, The completed closure of the posterior defect is illustrated. We prefer fine-gauge stainless steel wire for this part of the anastomosis, with the knots tied on the inside.

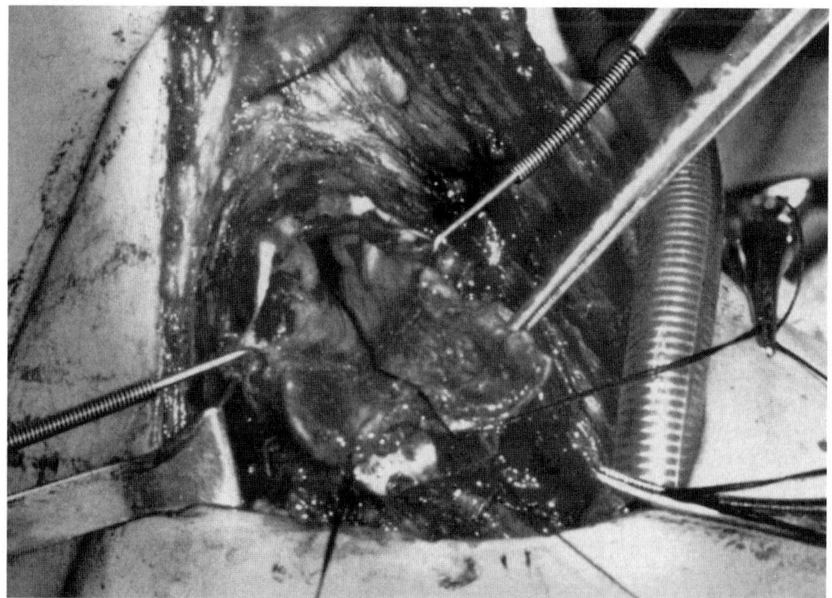

FIGURE 19–15 ■ Operative photograph showing the larynx and subglottic areas following resection of the anterior cricoid arch and laryngofissure. Fine hook retractors are being used to spread the anterior margins of the thyroid cartilage. In the photograph, the vocal cords lie about 5 mm superior to the position of the hook retractors. The ulcerated, thickened, and stenosed subglottic segment begins immediately below these small retractors and extends posteriorly into the interarytenoid mucosa.

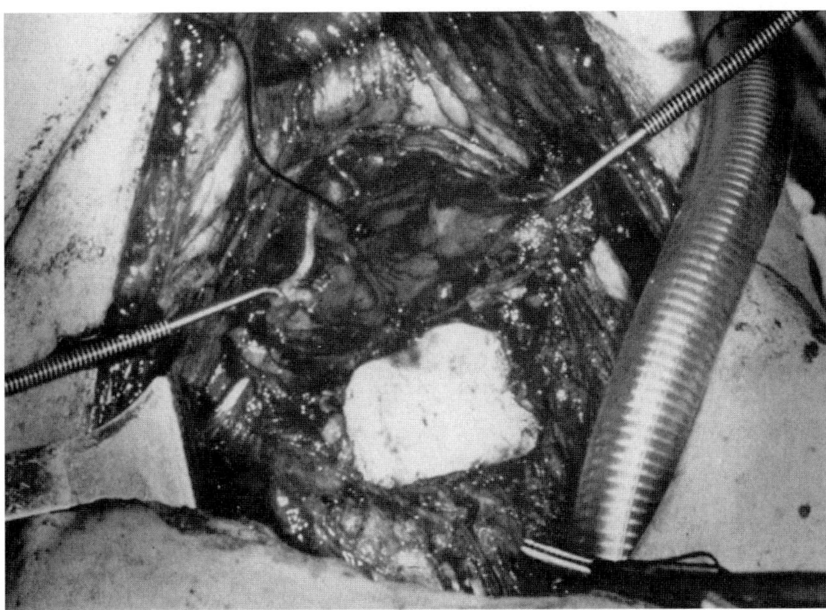

FIGURE 19–16 ■ Photograph of the same patient shown in Figure 19–14, following resection of the stenosed subglottic segment and interarytenoid scar. A broad plate of posterior cricoid cartilage is exposed below. The fine hook retractors lie just below the inferior margin of the vocal folds.

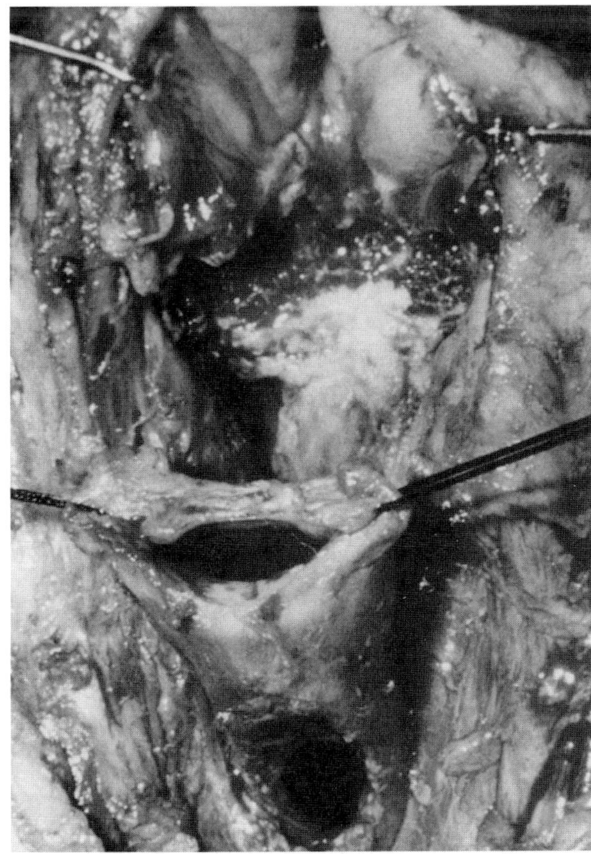

FIGURE 19–17 ■ The distal airway has been stabilized with two posterolateral stay sutures. At the *bottom* of the photograph, the stoma of a prior tracheostomy is seen. The uppermost cartilaginous rings of the distal airway will be resected to develop a vascularized posterior mucosal flap.

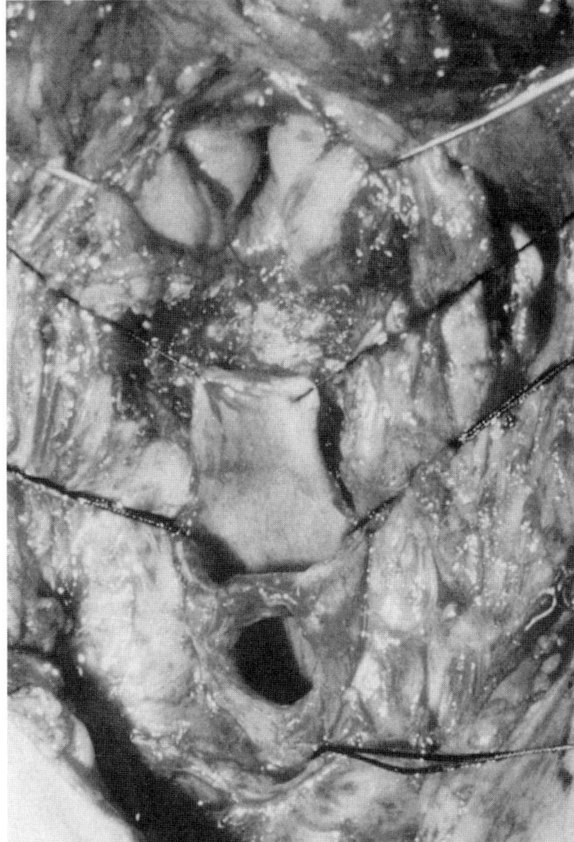

FIGURE 19–18 ■ The anterolateral margins of the distal airway have been trimmed back, with preservation of a pedicle of posterior membranous trachea. The pedicled flap has been stabilized with two fine stay sutures. The old tracheostomy stoma now lies within a few millimeters of the tracheal margin. Just above the mucosal flap, a bare area of cricoid is seen, and above this the mucosal surface of the airway lies immediately below the vocal cords.

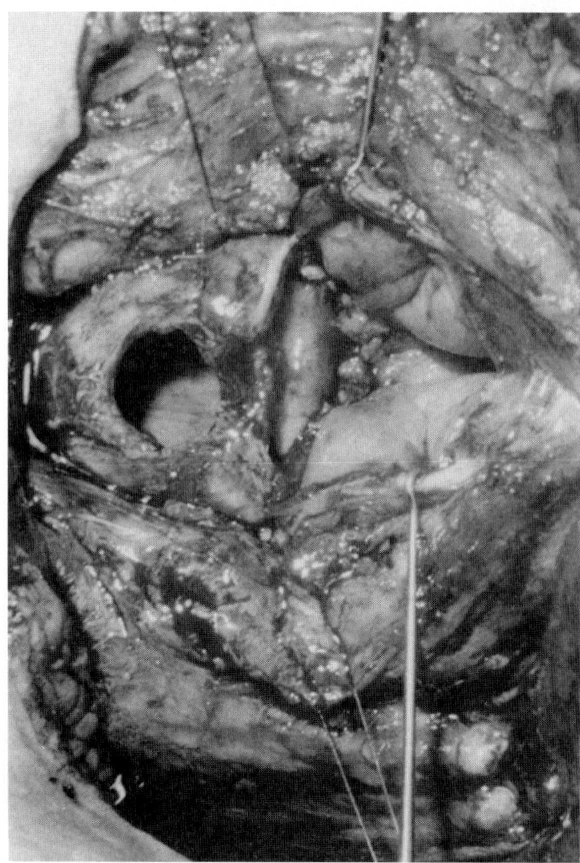

FIGURE 19–19 ■ The distal airway has been elevated in preparation for the anastomosis. The posterior flap is now lying just below the mucosal defect between the arytenoid cartilages. This pedicle will be secured in place with interrupted sutures of fine gauge (35 French) stainless steel wire with the knots tied inside.

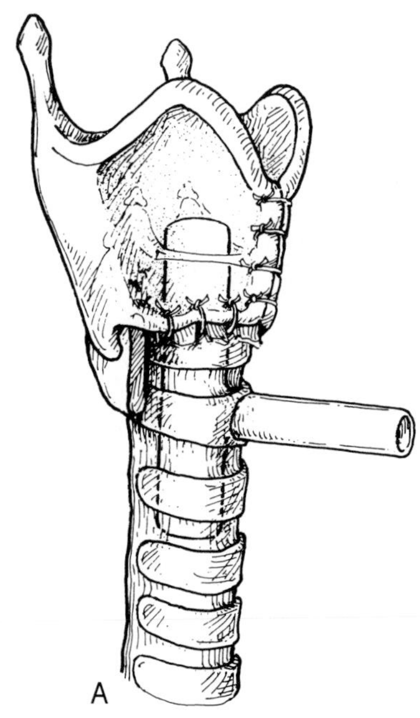

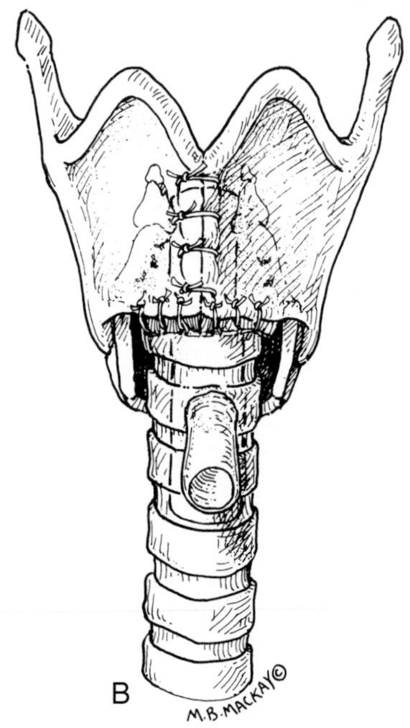

FIGURE 19–20 ■ Lateral *(A)* and anteroposterior *(B)* diagrams illustrating the completed thyrotracheal anastomosis and closure of the laryngofissure. A silicone T tube has been placed with the proximal limb lying 0.5 cm above the vocal cords.

adequately around it. If not, it is important to provide adequate humidification with a tracheostomy mask during the early postoperative period.

The chin suture is removed at the end of 1 week. It is recommended that the anastomosis be examined by flexible bronchoscopy at that time. If the margins are well vascularized and healing cleanly, it is almost certain that a satisfactory result will be obtained, and it is safe to discharge the patient.

COMPLICATIONS AND RESULTS

The complications and results of subglottic and laryngotracheal resection in adults are reported in publications by Pearson and colleagues (1975, 1986, 1996), Maddaus and co-workers (1992), Couraud and others (1987, 1996), Grillo (1982, 1992), Donahue (1997), Zannini (1999) and Macchiarini (2001). Summary information from these reports may be found in Chapter 15.

Since the original publication by Monnier and Savary (1993) reporting experience in infants and children, there has been a slow but increasingly enthusiastic endorsement of their single-stage technique of partial cricoid resection and laryngotracheal reconstruction in the pediatric age group: Stern (1997), Vollrath (1999), and Monnier and co-workers' updated experience in 1999 (Monnier et al, 1999).

■ *KEY REFERENCES*

Monnier P, Savary M: Partial cricoid resection with primary tracheal anastomosis for subglottic stenosis in infants and children. Laryngoscope 103:1273, 1993.

These authors are the first in the world to report a successful experience with subglottic resection in infants and children. The indications for operation and the details of technique in this age group are clearly outlined.

Pearson FG, Cooper JD, Nelems JM et al: Primary tracheal anastomosis after resection of the cricoid cartilage with preservation of recurrent laryngeal nerves. J Thorac Cardiovasc Surg 70:806, 1975.

The operative technique of partial cricoid resection, preservation of recurrent laryngeal nerves, and primary thyrotracheal anastomosis is described in detail in this original report. The description includes anatomic diagrams, intraoperative photographs, and photographs of cadaver dissections illustrating pertinent details of anatomy in this region.

■ *REFERENCES*

Couraud L, Hafez A: Acquired and non-neoplastic subglottic stenoses. In Grillo HC, Eschapasse H (eds): International Trends in General Thoracic Surgery: Major Challenges, Vol 2. Philadelphia, WB Saunders, 1987.

Couraud L, Jougon JB, Velly JF: Surgical treatment of nontumoral stenosis of the upper airway. Ann Thorac Surg 60: 250, 1995.

Couraud L, Jougon JB, Ballesteer M: Techniques of management of subglottic stenosis with glottic and supraglottic problems. Chest Surg Clin North Am 6:791, 1996.

Donahue DM, Grillo HC, Wain JC et al: Reoperative tracheal resection and reconstruction for unsuccessful repair of postintubation stenosis. J Thorac Cardiovasc Surg 114:934, 1997.

Gerwat J, Bryce DP: The management of subglottic laryngeal stenosis by resection and direct anastomosis. Laryngoscope 84:940, 1974.

Grillo HC, Mathisen DJ, Wain JC: Laryngotracheal resection and reconstruction for subglottic stenosis. Ann Thorac Surg 53:54, 1992.

Grillo HC: Primary reconstruction of airway after resection of subglottic and upper tracheal stenosis. Ann Thorac Surg 33:3, 1982.

Macchiarini P, Verhoye J, Chapelier A et al: Partial cricoidectomy with primary thyrotracheal anastomosis for postintubation subglottic stenosis. J Thorac Cardiovasc Surg 121: 68, 2001.

Maddaus MA, Toth JL, Gullane PJ, Pearson FG: Subglottic tracheal resection and synchronous laryngeal reconstruction. J Thorac Cardiovasc Surg 104:1443, 1992.

Monnier P, Lang F, Savary M: Partial cricoid resection for severe pediatric subglottic stenosis: Update of the Lausanne experience. Ann Otol Rhinol Laryngol 107: 961, 1998.

Monnier P, Lang F, Savary M: Cricotracheal resection for pediatric subglottic stenosis. Int J Pediatr Otorhinolaryngol 49:283, 1999.

Ogura JH, Powers WE: Functional restitution of traumatic stenosis of the larynx and pharynx. Laryngoscope 74:1081, 1964.

Pearson FG, Brito-Filomen L, Cooper JD: Experience with partial cricoid resection and thyrotracheal anastomosis. Ann Otol Rhinol Laryngol 95:582, 1986.

Pearson FG, Gullane P: Subglottic resection with primary tracheal anastomosis: Including synchronous laryngotracheal reconstructions. Semin Thorac Cardiovasc Surg 8:381, 1996.

Pearson FG: Technique of management of subglottic stenosis. Chest Surg Clin North Am 6:683, 1996.

Stern Y, Gerber ME, Walner DL et al: Partial cricotracheal resection with primary anastomosis in the pediatric age group. Ann Otol Rhinol Laryngol 106:891, 1997.

Vollrath M, Freihorst J, von der Hardt H: Surgery of acquired laryngotracheal stenosis in childhood: Experiences from 1988 to 1998. II. The cricotracheal resection [German]. HNO 47:611, 1999.

Zannini P, Melloni G, Carretta A: Laryngotracheal resection and reconstruction by Grillo's technique for postintubation stenosis. Minerva Chir 54:107, 1999.

SUBGLOTTIC RESECTION: INFANTS AND CHILDREN

Philippe Monnier
Florian Lang
Marcel Savary

The principle of subglottic resection in infants and children is basically identical to that described for adults, but because a child's airway is smaller the postoperative management is more challenging. Furthermore, pediatric subglottic stenosis (SGS) is often associated with posterior glottic stenosis, and sometimes laryngeal and mediastinal malformations significantly add to the therapeutic challenge. However, the worst situations seen in this group of pathologies always result (1) from previous failed laryngotracheal reconstructions (LTRs) that can distort the laryngeal framework; (2) from inappropriate overuse of the laser; and (3) from misplacement of the tracheostoma that unecessarily damages the normal trachea. Needless to say, the best chance for the patient lies in the first operation. This implies that the surgeon in charge of this problem is fully trained in pediatric upper airway endoscopy and laryngotracheal surgery, because inappropriate initial management of SGS may lead to permanent, intractable sequelae.

HISTORICAL NOTE

In 1953, Conley reported the first successful cricotracheal resection in a patient operated on for a chondroma of the cricoid cartilage. Almost 10 years later, Shaw and colleagues (1961) and then Ogura and Powers (1964) revisited this technique for the correction of traumatic stenosis of the larynx and trachea. However, cricotracheal resection only gained wider acceptance in the mid-1970s, thanks to the reports of larger series published by Gerwat and Bryce (1974) and Pearson and colleagues (1975). These authors were the first to perform a partial cricotracheal resection (PCTR) with preservation of both recurrent laryngeal nerves (RLNs). Since then, PCTR has become the treatment of choice for the cure of SGS in adults (Couraud et al, 1985; Grillo et al, 1992; Pearson et al, 1986).

Ranne and associates (1991) are credited with the first report of a series of seven PCTRs performed in children with recurrent subglottic stenosis. Decannulation was accomplished 3 to 12 weeks following operation in all cases. However, this short-lived experience never stimulated the medical community and, for several reasons including the lack of training in tracheal surgery, otolaryngologists and pediatric surgeons have been reluctant to use PCTR in infants and children. The main allegations have included the risk of injury to the RLNs, the possible dehiscence of the anastomosis, and the interference with the normal growth of the larynx.

Although Savary's pioneering work with PCTR in pediatric cases dates back to the late 1970s, this surgical procedure only emerged as a superior alternative to LTR for the cure of severe SGS in infants and children after the first report of the authors' experience in 15 cases with an update in 1998 on 31 cases (Monnier et al, 1993). In 1997, the department of pediatric otolaryngology in Cincinnati (Stern et al, 1997) adhered to this technique in selected indications and reported results from 16 additional pediatric cases. Overall, decannulation for severe SGS was achieved after PCTR in 111 (92.5%) of the 120 pediatric cases published in the literature at the turn of the 20th century (Monnier et al, 2001; Rutter et al, 2001; Triglia et al, 2000; Vollrath et al, 1999).

■ *HISTORICAL READINGS*

Conley JJ: Reconstruction of the subglottic air passage. Ann Otol Rhinol Laryngol 62:477, 1953.

Gerwat J, Bryce DP: The management of subglottic laryngeal stenosis by resection and direct anastomosis. Laryngoscope 84:940, 1974.

Monnier P, Savary M, Chapuis G: Partial cricoid resection with primary tracheal anastomosis for subglottic stenosis in infants and children. Laryngoscope 103:1273, 1993.

Pearson FG, Cooper JD, Nelems JM et al: Primary tracheal anastomosis after resection of the cricoid cartilage with preservation of recurrent laryngeal nerves. J Thorac Cardiovasc Surg 70:806, 1975.

Ranne RD, Lindley S, Holder TM et al: Relief of subglottic stenosis by anterior cricoid resection: An operation for the difficult case. J Pediatr Surg 26:255, 1991.

BASIC SCIENCE

Etiology and Pathophysiology

In the pediatric age group, SGS is acquired after prolonged intubation in most cases (Weymuller, 1988). In newborns, however, congenital SGS represents the third most common laryngeal anomaly after laryngomalacia and bilateral vocal fold paralysis. According to Holinger (1980), congenital SGS is classified into cartilaginous and soft tissue stenoses. It is present when the lumen of the cricoid region measures less than 4 mm in diameter in a full-term infant or 3 mm in a premature infant. The cartilaginous type results from a failure of complete recanalization of the laryngeal lumen after the eighth week of gestation. The cricoid may be normal in shape but too small for the infant's size or it may show different abnormalities comprising a general thickening of the cricoid ring, a large anterior or posterior lamina, or an elliptical shape. Sometimes, a trapped first tracheal ring is responsible for the small size of the subglottis.

The membranous form of congenital SGS is due to a thickening of the submucosa with an increase in fibrous connective tissue and hyperplasia and dilatation of the mucous glands. In contrast to the cartilaginous type, it is soft to palpation and generally circumferential.

In approximately 50% of cases, a congenital SGS is associated with mediastinal malformations including cardiovascular, tracheobronchial, or esophageal anomalies (Morimitsu, 1981). For the thoracic surgeon and the anesthetist, this implies that any mediastinal malformation warrants a pretherapy bronchoesophagoscopy to rule out a minor asymptomatic congenital SGS. This will avoid the disastrous consequence of a failed extubation leading to SGS after an elective cardiac or esophageal surgery in a newborn child who has been intubated with a normal-sized endotracheal (ET) tube for its age, but which is obviously too large for the size of its subglottic airway. The trauma induced to the subglottic airway will result in the typical combined (congenital and acquired) subglottic stenosis.

Since McDonald and Stocks (1965) introduced long-term intubation for the management of neonates requiring prolonged ventilatory support, SGS has become a well-recognized entity in pediatric intensive care units (ICUs). Improving the stiffness and biocompatibility of ET tubes as well as the nursing conditions in the ICU has led to a gradual decrease in the incidence of SGS resulting from elective intubation in full-term or premature infants. Injuries leading to SGS in infants and children are more likely to occur after traumatic intubations for resuscitation, after intubation for severe cranial injuries, when laryngoscopy is difficult because of anatomic problems, or when a mild congenital subglottic stenosis has been overlooked. Any systemic condition that diminishes capillary perfusion (e.g. shock, anemia) or that increases the susceptibility to infection (e.g., diabetes, immunosuppression) will aggravate the subglottic damage caused by the indwelling ET tube (Komorn et al, 1973).

At the acute stage, hyperemia and edema of the vocal folds, ulcerated troughs at the medial surface of the arytenoids with flanges of granulation tissue, and swelling or ulceration of the subglottic mucosa may all explain the reasons for failed extubation (Benjamin, 1993). Before planning a tracheotomy, a conservative treatment should always be attempted to avoid the development of cicatricial stenosis of the larynx and subglottis. In suspension microlaryngoscopy, endolaryngeal granulation tissue is gently removed with a biopsy forceps, and the child is reintubated with a one-size-smaller tube (soft Portex ET tube). An endolaryngeal plug of a corticosteroid-gentamicin ointment is then applied around the tube to the endolarynx and subglottis and systemic antibiotics and corticosteroids are given for 5 to 7 days. A tentative extubation is made 2 to 4 days later. If a tracheotomy is deemed unavoidable at this stage, it should be placed as close as possible to the subglottis to avoid any further damage to the normal trachea. Whenever possible, the larynx should not remain unstented, because acute lesions of intubation will evolve into contracting scars leading to subglottic stenosis or posterior glottic stenosis.

DIAGNOSIS

Infants and children with mild to moderate (<60% reduction in luminal size) SGS may become symptomatic only during upper respiratory tract infection. They present with an inspiratory stridor, dyspnea, and marked suprasternal and intercostal retractions. Recurrent or prolonged episodes of croup indicate possible SGS and warrant an endoscopic evaluation.

In cicatricial stenosis, the endoscopic evaluation of the larynx and trachea gives all information required for the preoperative workup. Vocal-fold mobility is assessed by transnasal fibroscopy with mask ventilation in deep halothane anesthesia and spontaneous ventilation. This examination also gives information on the patency of the nose, the choanae, and the nasopharynx (Fig. 19–21). Differentiating vocal-fold immobility owing to a neurogenic cause from an interarytenoid fibrous adhesion is done by carefully inspecting the posterior commissure of the larynx using a 30-degree, angled telescope and by direct palpation of the arytenoid cartilages during suspension microlaryngoscopy. A fixed arytenoid raises the sus-

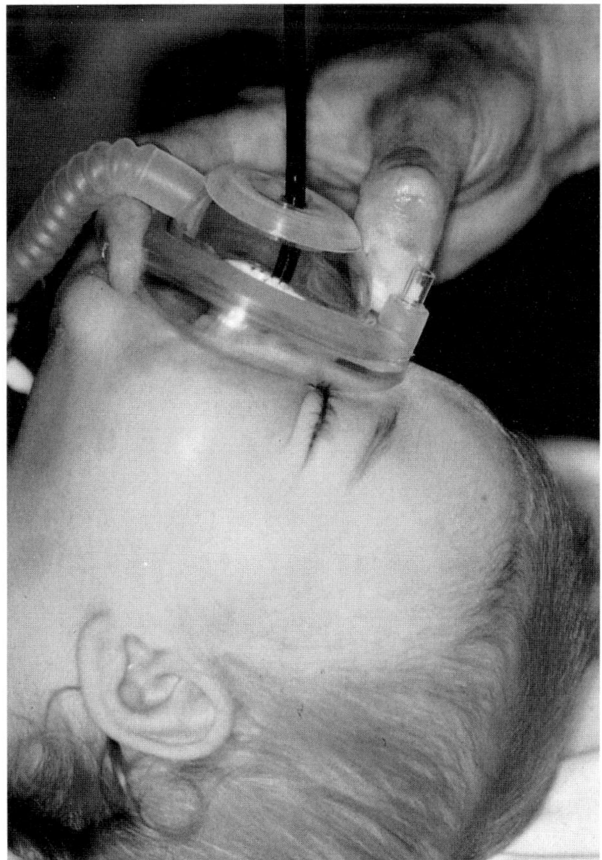

FIGURE 19–21 ■ Transnasal laryngotracheal fibroscopy with mask ventilation. In small children, this technique allows a thorough evaluation of vocal fold mobility and tracheal dynamics in spontaneous ventilation.

picion of a fibrous ankylosis of the joint, but in the most difficult cases, this diagnosis is only safely made during open surgery.

Location, extention, and degree of stenosis are assessed using a bare magnifying telescope and the intubation laryngoscope while the patient is under general anesthesia and fully relaxed (Fig. 19–22). The exact location of the stenosis with respect to the vocal folds, the tracheostoma, and the carina are given in millimeters and according to the number of residual normal tracheal rings above and below the tracheostoma. The degree of the stenosis is measured by passing telescopes, endotracheal tubes, or bougies of different sizes through the stricture (Fig. 19–23). In the pediatric community, the Myer-Cotton (1994) airway grading system is routinely used. This system classifies SGS in four grades (I: 0% to 50% obstruction; II: 51% to 70% obstruction; III: 71% to 90% obstruction; IV: 100% obstruction) and helps predict the rate of success after LTRs, because the less severe grades (I and II) have a far better outcome than the most severe grades (III and IV), which correspond to a total or subtotal obstruction.

For PCTR, this grading system is not useful as a predictor of success or failure, because the stenotic segment is fully resected. The endoscopy report should also mention the presence of any localized tracheomalacia as well as a possible infection of the airway. A bacteriologic smear is routinely taken. Finally, in the presence of a congenital subglottic stenosis, a bronchoesophagoscopy is performed to rule out a mediastinal malformation (e.g., tracheoesophageal fistula, tracheobronchial anomalies, extrinsic vascular compression of the airway).

If a precise description and measurements of the stenosis are obtained from the endoscopy, radiographs add little to the preoperative workup. However, lateral soft tissue and anteroposterior high kilovoltage radiographs are useful in documenting the length of the segment to be resected in cases of complete stenosis of the airway.

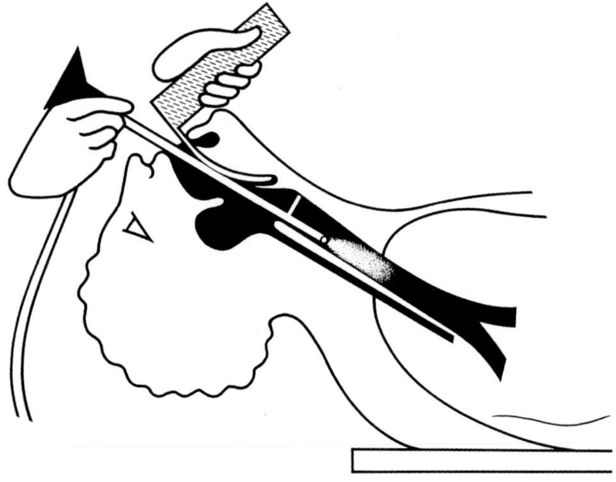

FIGURE 19–22 ■ Direct laryngotracheoscopy with a 0-degree bare telescope. The larynx is exposed with an intubation laryngoscope. The 0-degree bare telescope is used to assess the location, extension, and size of the stenosis. Examination down to the carina is possible without mucosal trauma and risk of worsening a dyspneic, nontracheotomized child.

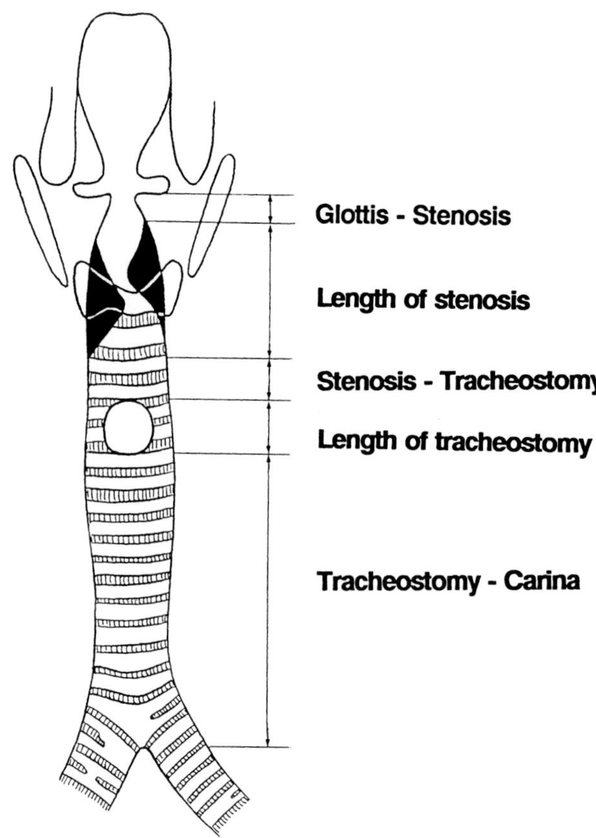

FIGURE 19–23 ■ Endoscopy report for subglottic stenosis. Precise measurements with reference to the vocal folds, tracheostoma, and carina should be given in all cases, including the number of residual normal tracheal rings. A precise surgical strategy is made at that time, taking all parameters into account: vocal fold mobility, extension and degree of stenosis, location of tracheostoma, length of residual normal trachea, and segments of tracheomalacia.

When a malformation of the mediastinum is suspected, computed tomography or magnetic resonance imaging are the exams of choice (Volg et al, 1990).

Finally, if a single-stage operation is planned, pulmonary function tests and neurologic evaluation should be considered, especially in children with malformations or previous long-term intubation for neonatal dyspnea of different etiologies. Gastroesophageal reflux disease should be systematically ruled out or actively treated if present.

MANAGEMENT

Indications

PCTR is the procedure of choice for the treatment of severe SGS (>70% luminal obstruction) of congenital or acquired etiology, but it is generally advisable to wait until the child reaches 10 kg of body weight before surgery is undertaken. The latter is performed as a single-stage operation without the need for a tracheotomy when there is no glottic involvement such as posterior glottic stenosis (with or without cricoarytenoid ankylosis), anterior laryngeal web extending into the subglottis, or diffuse endolaryngeal scarring and distortion of the laryngeal framework resulting from failed LTRs. When an SGS is combined with a posterior glottic stenosis, PCTR is then supplemented with a posterior cricoid split and costal cartilage graft that need stenting and maintenance of the tracheostoma until a complete healing of the subglottic area is obtained.

Anesthetic Technique

Jet Ventilation for Nontracheotomized Children

In nontracheotomized children, the induction of anesthesia is done by mask ventilation with halothane, followed by fentanyl and vecuronium. The stenosis is dilated with tapered bougies, and the child is intubated with the largest nasotracheal tube that will pass the stenosis. As the stenosis will be resected, the trauma induced to the subglottis by dilatations has no adverse consequence on the final outcome. Anesthesia maintenance is achieved with propofol, fentanyl, and vecuronium as needed. Once the cricothyroid membrane is incised, the ET tube is withdrawn, and its tip is securely fixed with a Mersilene thread. A 10-French and 400-mm long catheter (external diameter: 3.3 mm) is passed through the tube and placed distally into the trachea by the surgeon. Once the jet catheter is correctly placed, the ET tube is further withdrawn out of the operation field.

Resection of the stenosis is then performed under excellent visual control, because the jet catheter may easily be displaced out of the operation field. The stenotic segment is resected, and after the posterior anastomosis is completed, all sutures for the lateral and anterior anastomosis are placed. Just before the sutures are tied, the distal trachea is rinsed with saline to moisten the mucosa and clean blood and secretions from it, and the ET tube is pushed down into the trachea over the jet catheter, using the leading Mersilene thread. The jet catheter is withdrawn and normal ventilation is ensured through the ET tube repositioned beyond the anastomosis. All sutures are then tied with the knots on the outside (Magnusson et al, 1997).

Conventional Ventilation System in Tracheotomized Children

This setup is used in tracheotomized children whose tracheostomas will be resected during the same procedure. Two sets of ventilation tubes are prepared before draping the patient; one on the thorax for ventilation through the tracheostoma, another at the head of the patient for ventilation through a nasotracheal tube at the end of the operation. The whole dissection and resection of the stenosis is done while the patient is ventilated through the tracheostoma. The sutures of the posterior anastomosis and two lateral cricotracheal stitches are placed and tied while the child is still ventilated through the tracheal stump. Then, either a jet catheter or a nasotracheal tube is pushed beyond the posterior anastomosis into the distal trachea, and the rest of the lateral and anterior sutures are placed with the knots tied on the outside.

Operative Technique

Purely Subglottic Stenosis

The procedure is performed with the neck fully extended. A collar incision is usually made at the level of the second tracheal ring. In tracheotomized child, a horizontal crescent-shape excision of the skin is made around the stoma. The subplatysmal skin flaps are elevated, and the strap muscles are separated from the midline to provide exposure from the hyoid bone to the suprasternal notch. The isthmus of the thyroid gland is transected in the midline. The trachea is dissected anteriorly and laterally without identification of the RLNs by staying in close contact with the underlying cartilaginous rings. The vascular supply coming laterally from the tracheoesophageal grooves should always be carefully preserved, especially in extensive mobilization of the distal trachea.

At the level of the cricoid arch, a vertical midline incision is made, and the cricothyroid muscles are sharply dissected off of the underlying cartilage until the cricothyroid joint is identified bilaterally. After stay sutures are placed to the distal normal tracheal wall, the inferior resection line is made first at the lower end of the stenosis or at the level of the tracheostoma, if the latter is to be resected during the same surgical procedure. This allows a view of the stenosis from below and affords a good distal airway for ventilation. The membranous trachea is then dissected and separated from the anterior wall of the esophagus over a distance that corresponds to the height of the cricoid plate (Fig. 19–24).

Unnecessary extensive separation of the trachea from the esophagus should be avoided. The advancement of the distal tracheal stump upward is achieved by freeing

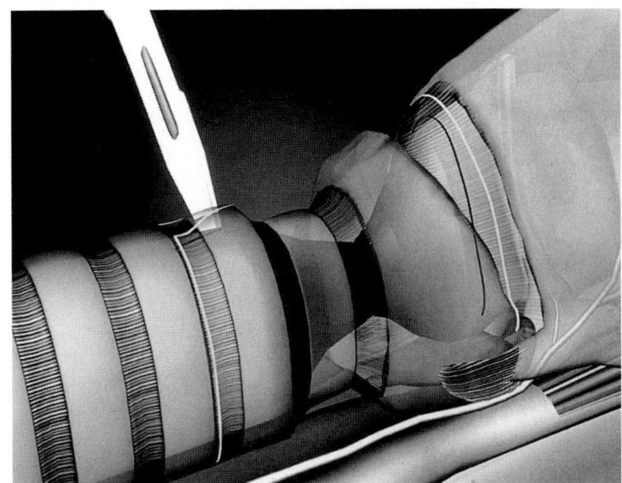

FIGURE 19–24 ■ Resection lines for subglottic stenosis (lateral view). After careful preparation and mobilization of the trachea and larynx, the superior resection line is made at the inferior margin of the thyroid cartilage. The inferior resection line is carried out one ring below the first normal tracheal ring to harvest an anterior pedicled wedge of cartilage that will be used to enlarge the subglottic lumen (see Fig. 19–25). The lateral resection line is made just anterior to the cricothyroid joint on both sides. The recurrent laryngeal nerve is shown here for anatomical purposes only; it is deliberately not identified during the surgery (see text for details).

the cartilaginous rings from the mediastinal structures anteriorly and laterally only. Due to its elasticity, the esophagus will shorten spontaneously without anterior bulging.

The superior incision is started at the inferior margin of the thyroid cartilage in front and is passed laterally just anterior to the cricothyroid joints. This results in the complete resection of the anterior cricoid arch, while avoiding injury to the recurrent laryngeal nerves that run posteriorly to the joint. In the subglottis, the uppermost incision of the posterior mucosa is made just below the cricoarytenoid joints, and the submucosal fibrosis constituting the posterior aspect of the subglottic stenosis is fully resected, thus exposing the cricoid plate completely.

As the luminal diameter of the distal airway is always much larger than that of the proximal subglottic resection line, the first normal tracheal ring used for the anastomosis must be adapted to the size of the subglottic lumen. In children, the difference in diameter between the subglottic space and the tracheal stump is even more pronounced than it is in adults. Any attempt at reducing the caliber of the trachea should be avoided. Instead, one should enlarge the subglottic lumen as much as possible without compromising voice quality. This is best achieved by widening the cricoid plate posteriorly and laterally with a diamond burr and by performing an inferior midline thyrotomy up to the level of the anterior commissure of the larynx, without transecting it (Fig. 19–25).

Because the thyroid cartilage is usually soft and pliable in infants and children, the inferior margins of both thyroid alae are easily spread apart. In this way, the subglottic lumen is enlarged considerably, while the anterior commissure is kept intact, thus preserving a good voice. The triangular defect is filled in with a mucosa-

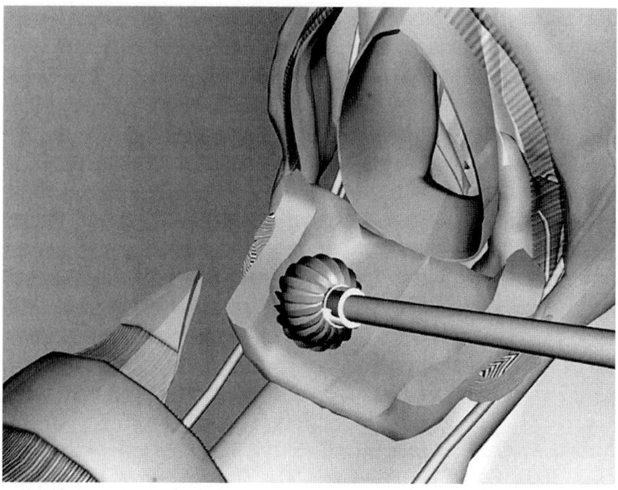

FIGURE 19–25 ■ Oblique view of the subglottis after resection of the stenotic segment. After resection of the anterior arch of the cricoid, the fibrous tissue constituting the posterior aspect of the stenosis is fully resected. The uppermost posterior section of the mucosa passes immediately below the cricoarytenoid joints. The denuded cricoid plate is then flattened down with a diamond burr. This will allow a better adaptation of the tracheal stump to the subglottis. The cartilaginous wedge of anterior trachea will be used to enlarge the subglottic lumen.

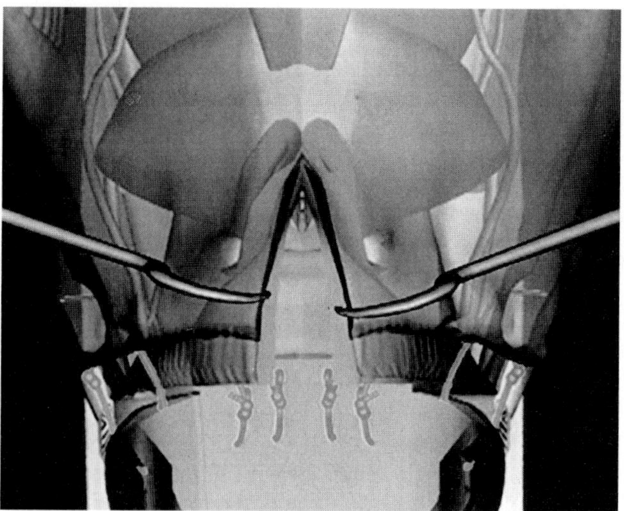

FIGURE 19–26 ■ Partial inferior midline thyrotomy (frontal view). An inferior midline thyrotomy is carried out up to the anterior commissure of the vocal folds, without transecting it. This corresponds to half the distance from the thyroid notch to the inferior margin of the thyroid cartilage. The thyroid alae are easily spread apart in children to increase the subglottic lumen. The wedge of cartilage pedicled to the first normal tracheal ring is used to fill in the subglottic defect resulting from the inferior midline thyrotomy. 6–0 or 5–0 Vicryl sutures are used for the posterior anastomosis with the knots tied inside the lumen.

lined cartilaginous wedge that is obtained from the first normal tracheal ring below the resected stricture (see Fig. 19–24). This requires an additional resection of the lateral portion of the first normal tracheal ring used for the anastomosis. The denuded cricoid plate is covered with the membranous trachea after its upward mobilization (Fig. 19–26).

Interrupted Vicryl sutures (6–0 or 5–0 in children) are used for the posterior anastomosis, with the knots tied inside the lumen. The disadvantage of having a few sutures tied inside the lumen posteriorly is largely compensated for by the optimal approximation of the mucosa that is difficult to obtain with the knots tied outside the lumen (see Fig. 19–26). Fibrin glue is used to secure the membranous trachea to the cricoid plate. Depending on the child's age, 4–0 or 3–0 Vicryl sutures are used for the anterior and lateral anastomosis. The first stitch is passed through the posterolateral aspect of the first normal tracheal ring and through the cricoid plate laterally. It should emerge in a subperichondrial plane from the outer surface of the cricoid plate to avoid any lesion to the recurrent laryngeal nerves. This stitch is extremely important and should be placed as meticulously as possible to bring the mucosa of the subglottis in close contact with the mucosa of the trachea (Fig. 19–27). The thyrotracheal anastomosis is completed by placing the Vicryl sutures between the tracheal ring and the thyroid cartilage anteriorly, with the knots tied on the outside. A tension-releasing suture is also placed between the third or fourth tracheal ring laterally and the border of the cricoid plate (Figs. 19–27 and 19–28).

Various techniques of tracheal and supralaryngeal release may be used to diminish the tension on the suture

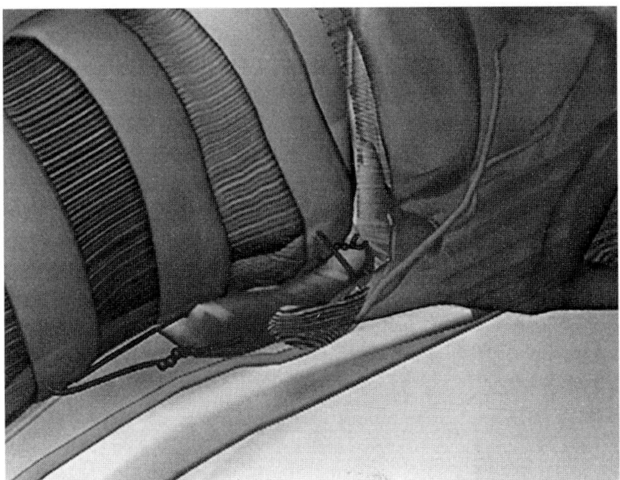

FIGURE 19–27 ■ Thyrotracheal anastomosis (lateral view). The first posterolateral stitch is passed between the first tracheal ring and the cricoid plate. The stitch should emerge in a subperichondrial plane from the outer surface of the cricoid plate to avoid any lesion to the recurrent laryngeal nerves. A second stitch, placed between the third tracheal ring and the inferior border of the cricoid plate, is used to release the tension at the site of the anastomosis.

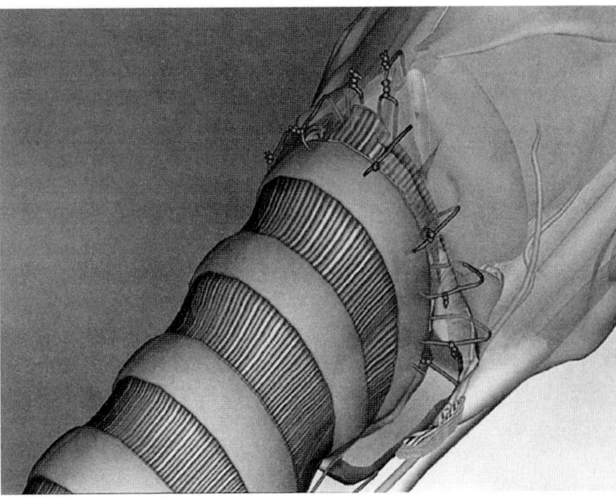

FIGURE 19–28 ■ Completion of thyrotracheal anastomosis (oblique view). Except for the most posterior suture, which is placed between the trachea and the cricoid plate, all lateral and anterior stitches are passed between the tracheal ring and the thyroid cartilage. The adaptation of the large tracheal ring to the narrower subglottic space is facilitated by the enlargement of the subglottic lumen with a partial inferior midline thyrotomy. The triangular defect is then filled in with the cartilaginous wedge pedicled to the tracheal ring used for the anastomosis.

line. This depends on the length of the tracheal segment to be resected and on the individual anatomy. Usually, the advancement of the distal tracheal stump upward is much easier in children than it is in adults. If necessary, a laryngeal release will suffice; hilar mobilization, sometimes used in adults, should remain as an exception in children.

At the end of the procedure, the neck is maintained in a flexed position. Sutures placed from the chin to the chest are never used to limit the extension of the neck during the postoperative period, although this measure has been recommended by different authors (Fig. 19–29).

Subglottic Stenosis Combined with Glottic Pathologies

Initially used for purely subglottic stenosis, partial cricotracheal resection with primary thyrotracheal anastomosis has proved to be also very efficient for the cure of

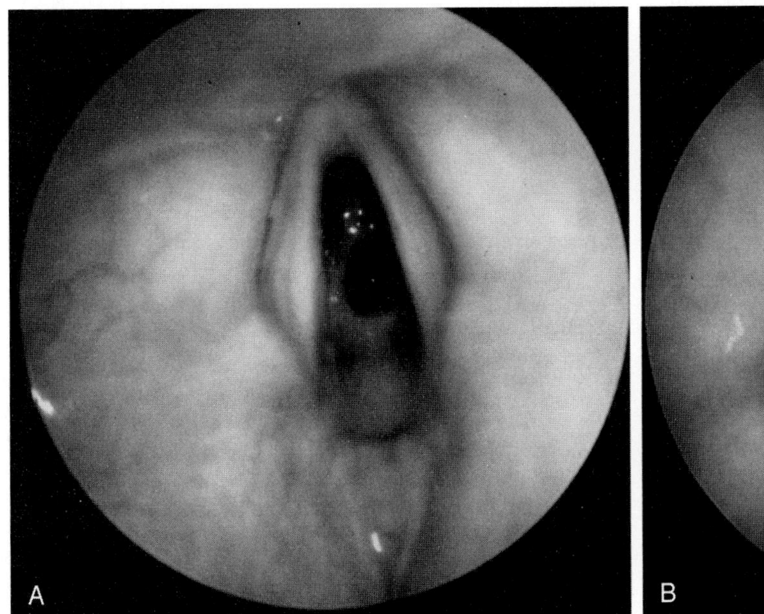

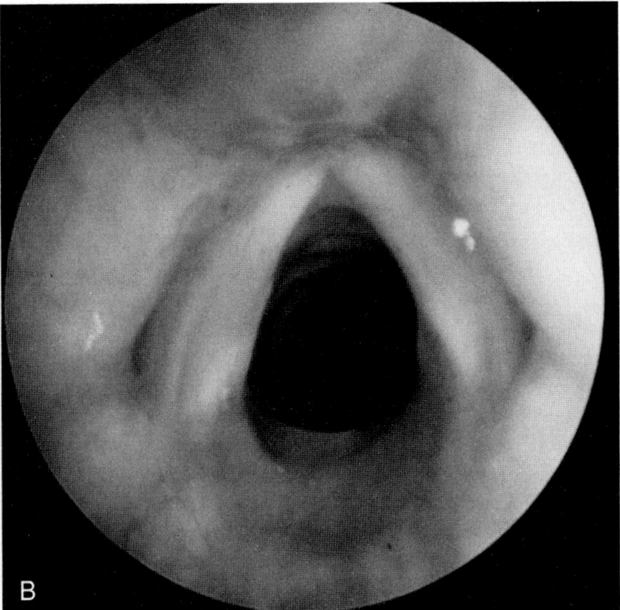

FIGURE 19–29 ■ Endoscopic views of a grade III subglottic stenosis prior to and after partial cricotracheal resection. *A*, Subtotal obstruction of the subglottis resulting from prolonged intubation in a 2.5-year-old child. *B*, Postoperative view showing a large and patent lumen. Note the integrity of the vocal folds, ensuring a normal voice.

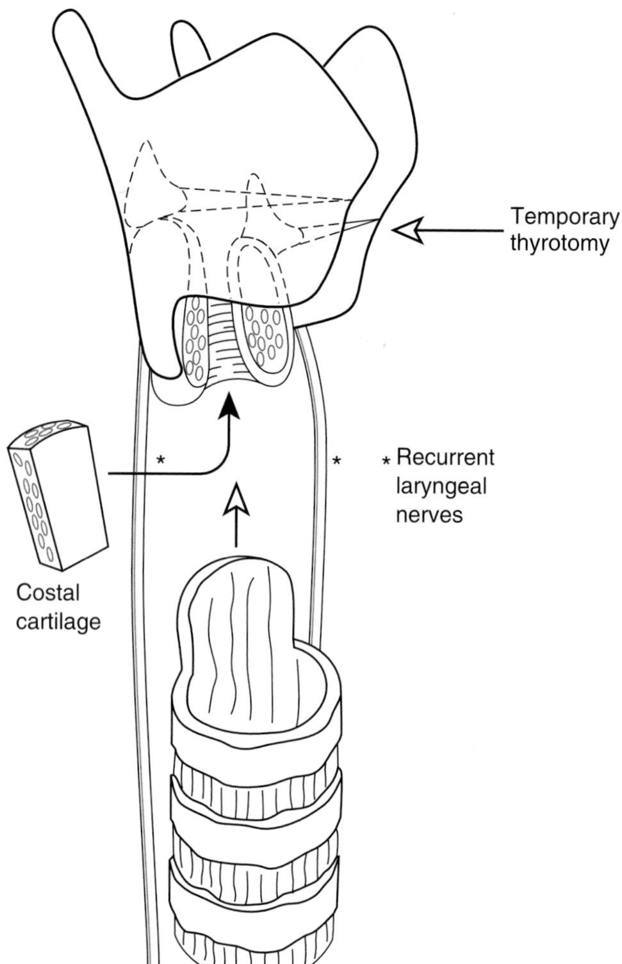

FIGURE 19–30 ■ Cricotracheal resection with posterior cricoid split and costal cartilage graft for the cure of combined subglottic and posterior glottic stenosis. Partial cricotracheal resection (PCTR) is performed according to the conventional technique. A pedicled flap of membranous trachea is obtained by removing two more rings of the tracheal stump distally. A posterior midline incision of the cricoid plate is made through a temporary thyrotomy, and a costal cartilage graft is interposed between the two parts of the posterior cricoid *(black arrow)*. The trachea is advanced upward *(open arrow)*, and its membranous portion is sutured to the mucosa of the posterior commissure of the larynx. The lateral and anterior anastomosis is completed as in conventional PCTR. A full mucosalized anastomosis is obtained in this way. A laryngeal stent is used for 3 to 4 weeks if the tracheostoma site remains in place. Stenting with a nasotracheal tube for 1 week proved sufficient in the two cases treated thus far without tracheostomy.

combined subglottic and glottic pathologies (posterior glottic stenosis, anterior web extending into the subglottis, combined glottic and supraglottic scarring, and distortion of the larynx after failed LTR). The surgical procedure is then modified as follows: A complete laryngofissure is created, and the posterior cricoid plate is divided in the midline up to the transverse interarytenoid muscle. If the latter is embedded in scar tissue, it is transected without injuring the underlying pharyngeal mucosa. The two parts of the posterior cricoid are then sufficiently distracted to allow the correct positioning of the costal cartilage harvested from the seventh or eighth rib. The graft must be flush with the cricoid plate, with the perichondrium facing the lumen. Lateral flanges of perichondrium help stabilize the graft that is fixed in place with 4.0 Vicryl sutures (Fig. 19–30).

By resecting two more rings of the tracheal stump distally, a pedicle flap of membranous trachea is created. The trachea is then advanced upward, and its membranous portion is sutured with 5.0 or 6.0 Vicryl sutures to the mucosa of the posterior commissure of the larynx. The lateral and anterior anastomosis is completed as in conventional PCTR using 4.0 or 3.0 Vicryl sutures. A fully mucosalized anastomosis is thus obtained. The closure of the laryngofissure over a nasotracheal tube or a stent is performed meticulously by placing a 3.0 Vicryl suture exactly at the level of the vocal cords to restore a sharp anterior commissure (Fig. 19–31).

The cartilaginous wedge pedicled to the tracheal ring that is used for the anastomosis is inserted between the alae of the thyroid cartilage inferiorly to enlarge the subglottic lumen without compromizing voice quality. Next, the isthmus of the thyroid gland is resutured in the midline, over the anastomosis, to optimize the vascular supply.

POSTOPERATIVE CARE

After surgery, nontracheotomized children stay under close supervision in the ICU until extubation is achieved. Broad spectrum antibiotics and antireflux medication are given to all patients for a minimum of 10 days or until a mucosalized anastomosis is obtained. Corticosteroids are started only on the day prior to extubation and continued for the following days, if necessary.

Depending on the child's age, a first control endoscopy is performed at 5, 7, or 10 days postoperatively. If there is only mild to moderate edema of the vocal folds and subglottis, the child is tentatively extubated. In the case of significant edema, the child is reintubated with a one-size-smaller tube, and a plug of corticosteroid-gentamicin ointment is applied to the endolarynx. The next tentative extubation is planned for 2 days later. Additional endoscopic controls are routinely performed at 3 weeks and 3 months. The final result may then be optimized at three months by gentle bougienage with Savary-Gilliard dilators.

MATERIAL AND RESULTS

From August 1978 to December 2000, 58 infants and children underwent PCTRs for severe (Cotton's grade III or IV) SGS at our institution. In 18 (31%) of the 58 patients, the SGS was combined with a posterior glottic stenosis that necessitated the removal of a cicatricial interarytenoid adhesion in 11 patients and a combined PCTR with a posterior costal cartilage graft in 7 patients, four of whom had a bilateral cricoarytenoid ankylosis.

The operation was performed before age 1 in 9 children, before age 3 in another 19 children, and before age 13 in the rest of the patients. In 7 patients, the resection included only the anterior arch of the cricoid and in the remaining 51 patients it included a segment of trachea (1 to 8 rings) to remove the tracheostoma during the same surgical procedure. A laryngeal release was done in 5 patients.

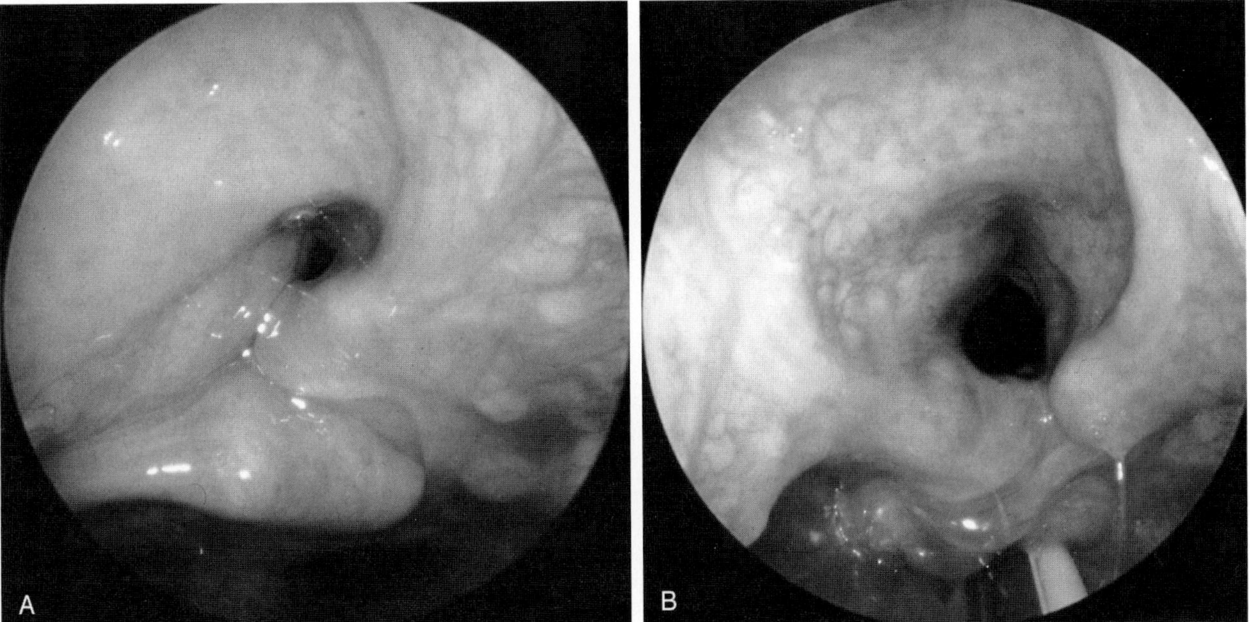

FIGURE 19–31 ■ Endoscopic views of a failed laryngotracheoplasty prior to and after partial cricotracheal resection (PCTR) combined with posterior costal cartilage graft. *A*, Preoperative view showing a distorted larynx with overlapping aryepiglottic folds and grade III combined glottic and subglottic stenosis, resulting from failed laryngotracheal reconstruction. *B*, Postoperative view showing the restoration of a patent airway after PCTR combined with a posterior cricoid split and costal cartilage graft. The tracheostoma was resected at the time of surgery and stenting was ensured with a nasotracheal Portex tube for 10 days only.

Postoperatively, a normal lumen was formed in 42 patients, a better than grade I stenosis (80%-size lumens) in 15 patients, and a complete restenosis in one patient. This last patient, a 13-year-old boy, had a remarkable tendency to form keloid skin scars. Forty-four (76%) of the 58 patients engage in sports freely without exertional dyspnea. Nine patients live normally, but present a slight stridor with some dyspnea while exercising. One patient is still tracheotomy dependent. Three children still await decannulation and 1 infant died of a massive broncho-aspiration 2 months after PCTR. Postoperative follow-up is longer than 10 years in 12 patients, 5 to 10 years in 13 patients, 1 to 5 years in 28 patients and less than 1 year in 5 patients. Eight patients have reached adulthood, and their laryngotracheal development is normal.

COMPLICATIONS

Although we had no case with a lesion of the RLNs, we have to report one complete failure in a grade IV glotto-subglottic stenosis. Another 5 month-old child with multiple malformations successfully underwent a PCTR but died 6 weeks after the operation from a massive broncho aspiration, and a 13-year-old girl sustained an ischemia of the upper thoracic medulla with subsequent paraplegia resulting from a thrombosis of the anterior spinal artery. This event was related to a previous severe neck trauma and not to the surgery itself. These complications should indicate the importance of comorbidity factors including multiple malformations, neurologic disabilities, previous head and neck trauma, and pulmonary condition resulting from prematurity or duration of tracheotomy.

Minor complications included anterior subglottic granulations in 2 patients, a partial dehiscence of the anastomosis in another 3 patients, and a tracheostoma leak in one patient. After vaporization of the granulation with the carbon dioxide laser in 3 patients, and after an open revision in 4 (7%) patients, an excellent final result was obtained in all patients.

DISCUSSION

This series of 58 consecutive PCTRs for severe SGS in pediatric patients compares most favorably with LTRs still performed in most centers for the same indications (Cotton et al, 1989; Hartley et al, 2000). Even in experienced pediatric otolaryngologic departments, the decannulation rate for grade III and IV SGS is only approximately 60% after a single-stage LTR in children (Cotton et al, 1995); (Narcy et al, 1990). Stern (1997) and then Vollrath (1999), Triglia (2000), and Rutter (2001) used PCTR in selected patients and reported good results in 62 patients overall, with a decannulation rate of 90% for severe (grade III and IV) subglottic stenosis.

Of the three main potential complications of the surgery, injury to the RLNs should not be a problem if the principles of the operation are carefully respected (Monnier et al, 1998). The concern of interference with normal laryngotracheal growth is now obsolete; all 12 patients followed for more than 10 years show a normal development of their laryngotracheal airway, including 8 patients who have reached adulthood. Partial dehiscence of the anastomosis only represents a potential complication if an extensive tracheal resection is needed. A laryngeal release procedure or a hilar mobilization should help solve the problem in most instances. However, the most difficult situations always result from failed previous LTRs and from misplacement of the stoma at the time of the tracheotomy. A better education of the medical community should help minimize undue tracheal damage by placing the tracheotomy through the stenosis in tracheal strictures and as close as possible to the subglottis (through the first tracheal ring) in laryngo-subglottic stenosis. Furthermore, pediatric surgeons and otolaryngologists should carefully learn the technique of PCTR in infants and children to achieve better results than with LTRs.

The unresolved issues are related to SGS combined with vocal-fold immobility. Posterior glottic stenosis without cricoarytenoid ankylosis may be treated with PCTR and resection of the interarytenoid fibrous adhesion or possibly with a posterior cricoid split and costal cartilage graft. A pedicle flap of membranous trachea is then used to cover the denuded cricoid plate or cartilage graft (see Fig. 19–30).

In the case of bilateral cricoarytenoid ankylosis combined with SGS, the end result will always represent a trade-off between airway patency and quality of voice. A staged operation is often necessary to reach the best result by performing a vocal-fold lateralization procedure. The risk of bronchoaspiration in these “frozen” larynges should, however, not be underestimated.

CONCLUSION

In pediatric severe SGS, PCTR with primary thyrotracheal anastomosis represents a real breakthrough in the surgical armamentarium to resolve this difficult problem.

Similar and generally good results may be expected if the surgery is performed meticulously with magnifying glasses. The use of a steady normal tracheal ring for the anastomosis and the placement of stitches in a submucosal plane to obtain a full mucosalized anastomosis in the subglottic area are of the utmost importance.

Problems still exist when the SGS is associated with extensive tracheal damage or with a bilateral cricoarytenoid ankylosis. For the latter, PCTR can be combined with a posterior costal cartilage graft (according to Rethi) covered by a flap of membranous trachea, or with a vocal-fold lateralization procedure in a second stage.

■ *KEY REFERENCES*

Benjamin B: Prolonged intubation injuries of the larynx: Endoscopic diagnosis, classification and treatment. Ann Otol Rhinol Laryngol 160S:1, 1993.

A comprehensive description of the pathophysiology and morphology of acute lesions of intubation and their evolution into fibrocicatricial sequelae leading to impairment of laryngeal function and subglottic stenosis.

Cotton RT, Myer CM, O'Connor DM, Smith ME: Pediatric laryngotracheal reconstruction with cartilage grafts and endotracheal tube stenting: The single-stage approach. Laryngoscope 105:818, 1995.

A report of the largest world experience on single-stage laryngotracheal reconstruction for pediatric subglottic stenosis with detailed information on postoperative results obtained for different degrees of subglottic stenosis.

Monnier PH, Lang F, Savary M: Partial cricotracheal resection for severe pediatric subglottic stenosis: Update of the Lausanne experience. Ann Otol Rhinol Laryngol 107:961, 1998.

An update of the author's experience on 31 cases of partial cricotracheal resection for the cure of severe subglottic stenosis in infants and children. Detailed information on operative technique, postoperative care, results, and complications is given for all cases that were followed very closely.

Pearson FG, Brito-Filomeno L, Cooper JD: Experience with partial cricoid resection and thyrotracheal anastomosis. Ann Otol Rhinol Laryngol 95:582, 1986.

A report of a series of 28 partial cricotracheal resections for subglottic stenosis in adults, with a follow-up longer than 5 years in half of the patients. Twenty-six widely patent anastomoses were formed after surgery, and in two patients, a partial restenosis occurred that resulted in some limitations in exercise tolerance.

■ *REFERENCES*

Cotton RT, Gray SD, Miller RP: Update of the Cincinnati experience in laryngotracheal reconstruction. Laryngoscope 99:1111, 1989.

Couraud L, Hafez A, Velly JF: Current reconstructive management of subglottic stenosis of the larynx with reference to sixty consecutively treated cases. J Thorac Cardiovasc Surg 33:263, 1985.

Grillo HC, Mathisen DJ, Wain JC: Laryngotracheal resection and reconstruction for subglottic stenosis. Ann Thorac Surg 53:54, 1992.

Hartley BEJ, Cotton RT: Paediatric airway stenosis: Laryngotracheal reconstruction or cricotracheal resection? Clin Otolaryngol 25:342, 2000.

Holinger LD: Etiology of stridor in the neonate, infant and child. Ann Otol Rhinol Laryngol 89:397, 1980.

Komorn RM, Smith CP, Erwin JR: Acute laryngeal injury with short-term endotracheal anesthesia. Laryngoscope 83:683, 1973.

Magnusson L, Lang F, Monnier Ph, Ravussin P: Anaesthesia for tracheal resection: Report of 17 cases. Can J Anaesth 44:1282, 1997.

McDonald IH, Stocks JG: Prolonged nasotracheal intubation: A review of its development in a paediatric hospital. Br J Anaesth 37:161, 1965.

Monnier P, Lang F, Savary M: Partial cricotracheal resection for severe pediatric subglottic stenosis: Update of the Lausanne experience. Ann Otol Rhinol Laryngol 107:961, 1998.

Monnier P, Lang F, Savary M: Traitement des sténoses sous-glottiques de l'enfant par résection crico-trachéale: Expérience lausannoise dans 58 cas. Ann Otolaryngol Chir Cervicofac (in press), 2001.

Morimitsu T, Matsumoto I, Okada S et al: Congenital cricoid stenosis. Laryngoscope 91:1356, 1981.

Myer CM, O'Connor DM, Cotton RT: Proposed grading system for subglottic stenosis based on endotracheal tube sizes. Ann Otol Rhinol Laryngol 103:319, 1994.

Narcy P, Contencin P, Fligny I: Surgical treatment for laryngotracheal stenosis in the pediatric patient. Arch Otolaryngol Head Neck Surg 116:1047, 1990.

Ogura JH, Powers HE: Functional restitution of traumatic stenosis of the larynx and pharynx. Laryngoscope 84:1081, 1964.

Rethi A: An operation for cicatricial stenosis of the larynx. J Laryngol Otol 70:283, 1956.

Rutter MJ, Hartley BEJ, Cotton RT: Cricotracheal resection in children. Arch Otolaryngol Head Neck Surg 127:289, 2001.

Shaw R, Paulsen DL, Kee JL: Traumatic tracheal rupture. J Thorac Cardiovasc Surg 42:281, 1961.

Stern Y, Gerber ME, Walner DL, Cotton RT: Partial cricotracheal resection with primary anastomosis in the pediatric age group. Ann Otol Rhinol Laryngol 106:891, 1997.

Triglia JM, Nicollas R, Roman S, Pech C: La résection crico-trachéale chez l'enfant. Indications, technique, résultats. Ann Otolaryngol Chir Cervicofac 117:155, 2000.

Volg TH, Wilimzig C, Bilaniuk LT: MR imaging in pediatric airway obstruction. J Comput Assist Tomogr 14:182, 1990.

Vollrath M, Freihorst J, von der Hardt H: Die Chirurgie der erworbenen laryngotrachealen Stenosen im Kindes-alter-Erfahrungen und Ergebnisse Von 1988–1998. Teil II: Die cricotracheale Resection. HNO 47:611, 1999.

Weymuller EA Jr: Laryngeal injury from prolonged endotracheal intubation. Laryngoscope 455:98, 1988.

TRACHEAL RESECTION

Shaf Keshavjee
F. Griffith Pearson

HISTORICAL NOTE

Prior to 1960, reports of segmental tracheal resection and reconstruction by primary anastomosis were rare and anecdotal. At most, it was assumed that no more than two or three tracheal rings (3 cm) could be resected and restored by primary anastomoses. With the advent of mechanical ventilation and the increasing use of cuffed endotracheal tubes, a spate of postintubation tracheal injuries were reported in North America and Europe. The management of these injuries provided a major stimulus to the development of new techniques of resection and reconstruction. Grillo (1970) described techniques of mobilization of the anterolateral aspects of the trachea and elevation of the main carina by an intrapericardial release of the right pulmonary hilum, and he also highlighted the importance of neck flexion in minimizing tension on a primary anastomosis. By using these maneuvers, it became possible to resect 4- to 5-cm long segments of the adult trachea and to obtain predictable healing by primary anastomosis.

The addition of the superior laryngeal release operation (Dedo and Fishman, 1969) and the technique of suprahyoid release (Montgomery, 1974) increased the capability of extended tracheal resection and primary reconstruction. By using these superior release procedures, it is usually possible to remove approximately half the length of the adult trachea and reconstitute the airway by end-to-end anastomosis. During the same decade, techniques were developed for resection of the carina, below, and the subglottic airway, within the cricoid ring. The techniques of subglottic and carinal resection are detailed in separate parts of this chapter, by Maddaus and Pearson and by Mathisen and Grillo, respectively.

■ *HISTORICAL READINGS*

Dedo HH, Fishman NH: Laryngeal release and sleeve resection for tracheal stenosis. Ann Otol Rhinol Laryngol 78:285, 1969.

Grillo HC: Surgery of the trachea. In Ravitch MM (ed): Current Problems in Surgery. Chicago, Year Book Medical Publishers, 1970.

Montgomery WW: Suprahyoid release for tracheal stenosis. Arch Otolaryngol 99:255, 1974.

INDICATIONS

Among the indications for tracheal resection and reconstruction are postintubation strictures (including upper airway burns), idiopathic stenosis, benign and malignant neoplasms, some congenital anomalies, and rare conditions such as selected cases of tracheomalacia. The incidence, pathogenesis, and principles of management of these conditions are discussed in Chapter 15. At present, postintubation stricture is the most common indication for resection. These lesions are frequently no more than a few centimeters in length and rarely require special mobilization techniques for management. In contrast, a majority of tracheal neoplasms are malignant and locally extensive at the time of symptomatic presentation, and they frequently require extended resection using many or all of the available maneuvers to achieve a satisfactory primary reconstruction.

MANAGEMENT

Preoperative Assessment

Preoperative assessment includes history and physical examination, a combination of imaging modalities, and bronchoscopy. From the information obtained by imaging and endoscopy, it is possible to obtain a precise evaluation of the nature, location, and extent of the lesion prior to resection. This information determines the operative exposure and mobilizing procedures that are anticipated. Details of preoperative evaluation are provided in the section on postintubation injury by Maddaus and Pearson in Chapter 15.

Risk Factors

It is important to identify several significant risk factors: (1) the presence of ongoing inflammation or infection, (2) diabetes, (3) previous radiation in the operative field, (4) therapy with high-dose steroids, and (5) age.

Particularly in patients with postintubation injury, it is desirable to delay resection and reconstruction until active inflammatory changes beyond the margins of the stricture subside. Early in the evolution of such injury, these changes are common, and time is required simply to allow the process to mature and for the adjacent inflammatory changes to settle. On occasion, the resolution of inflammation is expedited by removing an indwelling tracheostomy tube and maintaining the airway by interval dilatation if necessary. Alternatively, in selected cases, the tracheostomy tube may be replaced with a T tube, which provides a well humidified and closed airway and is less irritating to the tracheal mucosa than is an open tracheostomy tube (Cooper, et al., 1989; Montgomery, 1968; Pearson, 1983).

Radical radiotherapy (dosage of 400 cGy or greater) creates a significant risk to airway healing (Mathisen et al, 1988; Tsubota et al, 1975). Unless some form of additional protection is provided, the anastomosis frequently fails in an irradiated field, with dehiscence, progressive necrosis, and further destruction of the remaining airway. At first, Grillo refrained from operating on these patients because of the anticipated high morbidity and mortality. He was the first to recommend use of a vascularized pedicle to support healing at the anastomosis and, with Mathisen (1988), reported on a group of successful cases that were managed with the addition of a pedicled graft of omentum. The effects of irradiation on tracheal healing were documented in an animal study by Tsubota and colleagues (1975).

Diabetics have a known propensity for impaired healing and a reduced tolerance to contamination and infection. Needless to say, all airway surgery is relatively contaminated with oropharyngeal pathogens. Similarly, administration of steroids (especially in high dosage) appears to impede healing and increase the risk of infection. Whenever possible, patients should be weaned from steroid medication preoperatively. In diabetics or patients requiring perioperative high-dose steroids, it may be desirable to support the anastomosis with some form of vascularized pedicle, such as omentum, muscle flap, pericardium, or thymus.

Age is a variable risk factor owing to loss of upper airway elasticity in older patients, which may limit the extent of segmental resection that can be reconstructed by primary anastomosis.

Anesthesia

The management of anesthesia for tracheal resection is challenging and requires close cooperation between the anesthesiologist and the surgical team. The induction must be carefully planned, and the surgeon should be present and available to secure the airway with a rigid bronchoscope whenever necessary. A rigid bronchoscope can be used to dilate a stenotic airway when necessary to accommodate the appropriate-sized endotracheal tube.

A detailed description of the anesthetic techniques for tracheal resection is provided by McCrae and Slinger in Chapter 13. Some important steps in management are repeated here for emphasis: the airway is usually transected on the distal side of the lesion, and the distal trachea is intubated with a cuffed, armored, endotracheal tube. In all operations done through a cervical incision, the proximal end of the armored tube can be passed under the surgical drape alongside the upper neck and jaw, directly to the anesthetic connections at the patient's head. When the operative field requires either a sternotomy or a thoracotomy, it is usually necessary to use a set of sterile anesthetic connections, extending from the armored tube across the operative field and under the drapes to the anesthetist. The armored tube is intermittently withdrawn and reinserted during the conduct of the tracheal anastomosis.

Jet ventilation offers an alternative technique and has the advantage of permitting continuous operation without intermittent withdrawal and reinsertion of the endotracheal tube. Familiarity with the technique of jet ventilation is essential in avoiding forceful insufflation, barotrauma, or air embolism. Jet ventilation is preferred in those circumstances in which an airway that cannot be easily or reliably intubated must be ventilated, such as the bronchus intermedius or the distal left main bronchus. Oxygen saturation and carbon dioxide tension should be recorded throughout the procedure.

In most cases, it is desirable to have the patient resume spontaneous respiration and awaken as quickly as possible following termination of surgery. The sooner the orotracheal tube is removed, the better, because the cuffed tube may impair circulation at the anastomosis as long as it remains inflated in the upper airway.

Operative Technique

The patient is placed in the supine position. An inflatable bag is positioned transversely beneath the scapulae so that reversible hyperextension of the neck is easily obtained. A generous collar incision usually provides ample exposure (Fig. 19–32) for lesions involving the upper one half to two thirds of the trachea. Occasionally, extension to a sternotomy may be required. Lesions in the distal one third of the trachea are commonly approached with a right posterolateral thoracotomy through the fourth intercostal space.

An alternate approach to the mediastinal trachea is through a full median sternotomy. This exposure has several distinct advantages over a right posterolateral thoracotomy in selected cases. A median sternotomy should be selected in situations (usually involving neoplasms) in which there is the possibility of extension to a carinal or more distal resection. This is particularly useful in cases of malignancy involving the carina, in which the extent of involvement of the left main bronchus cannot be assessed with certainty preoperatively. In some cases, extensive involvement of the left main bronchus precludes anastomosis, necessitating a left pneumonectomy, which is possible through a median sternotomy. To obtain exposure of the distal trachea, carina, and both main bronchi through a median sternotomy, it is necessary to divide the pericardium both anteriorly and posteriorly, using vertical incisions extending from the innominate artery above to the right main pulmonary artery below. The ascending aorta and superior vena cava are freed intrapericardially and then retracted laterally. Once the posterior pericardium is divided, the carina and main bronchi are clearly displayed and accessible. Through this midline exposure, bilateral intrapericardial releases can be performed, and a cervical incision may be added if a suprathryoid or suprahyoid laryngeal release is required. Thus, exposure from the hyoid bone to the carina can be obtained through a median sternotomy combined with a cervical incision.

The technique for circumferential resection of short tracheal segments is relatively straightforward. Several important principles should again be emphasized:

1. Accurate preoperative identification of the precise level and length of the lesion to be resected is necessary.
2. Resection should be performed through healthy trachea. Reconstruction with inflamed tissue will prejudice the success of a primary anastomosis.
3. To preserve circulation, the airway should not be circumferentially mobilized for more than 1 cm beyond the resection margin. The anterior and anterolateral aspects of the trachea from the cricoid to the carina can be mobilized without compromising the circulation that

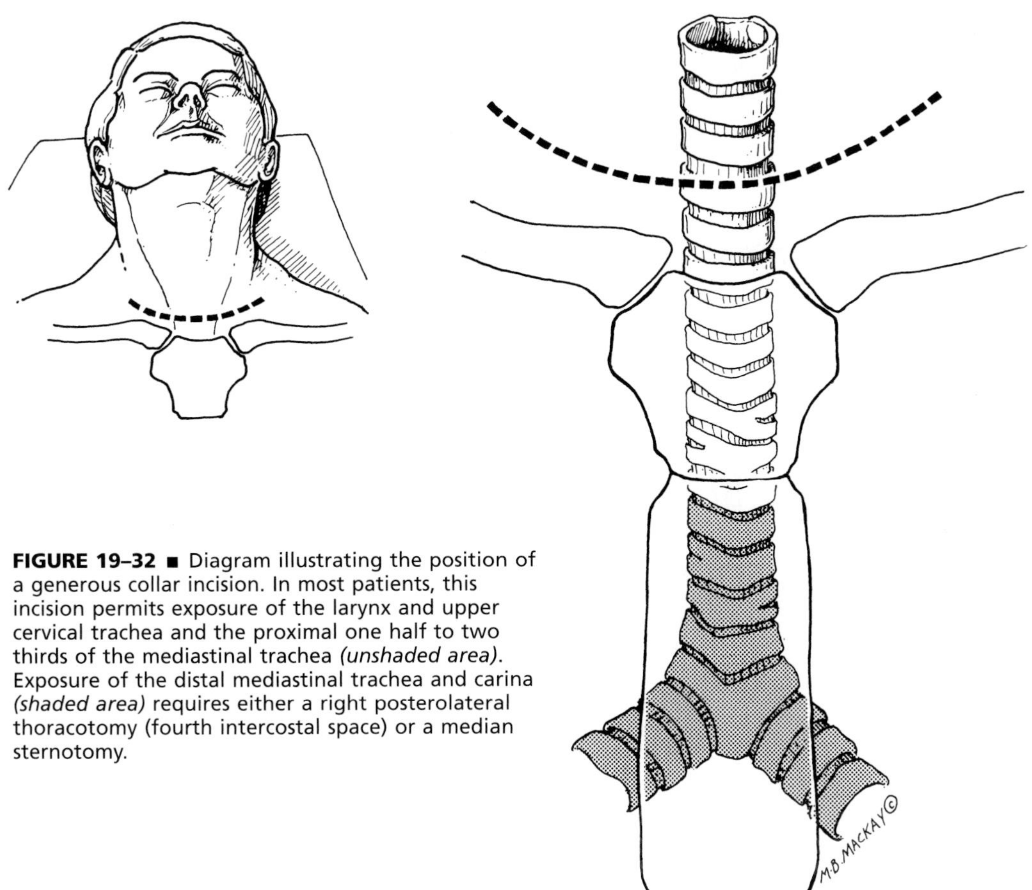

FIGURE 19–32 ■ Diagram illustrating the position of a generous collar incision. In most patients, this incision permits exposure of the larynx and upper cervical trachea and the proximal one half to two thirds of the mediastinal trachea *(unshaded area)*. Exposure of the distal mediastinal trachea and carina *(shaded area)* requires either a right posterolateral thoracotomy (fourth intercostal space) or a median sternotomy.

enters posterolaterally. This mobilization often improves the mobility of the distal trachea and decreases tension on the anastomosis. The membranous trachea can be mobilized posteriorly in the midline in circumstances in which there is a desperate need for additional length. This maneuver is rarely necessary, and it is usually not performed because it will diminish some of the blood supply provided by esophageal collaterals.

4. Tension at the anastomosis should be avoided.

Resection of the Trachea

The airway between the hyoid bone above the trachea and the junction between the middle and lower thirds of the mediastinal trachea is usually accessible through a generous collar incision (see Fig. 19–32). Resection within these boundaries rarely requires a median sternotomy except in patients with a very short neck, those with a dorsal kyphosis, or some older patients with a rigid, inelastic trachea.

Skin flaps are elevated in the plane deep to the platysma and are developed to expose the airway from the inferior border of the thyroid cartilage to the suprasternal notch. The strap muscles are separated in the midline to expose the anterior tracheal wall (Fig. 19–33). The thyroid isthmus is divided between suture ligatures if necessary for exposure. With the neck in full extension, the upper mediastinal trachea is elevated into the operative field and the area to be resected is identified. In the case of benign stricture, the tracheal wall is often deformed, may be enveloped by fibrous tissue, and can be densely adherent to adjacent structures (see Fig. 19–33). Occasionally, the area to be resected is not readily apparent, and the external aspect of the trachea looks normal. In such cases the location of the lesion can be determined from the measurements obtained at preoperative (or intraoperative) bronchoscopy. These predetermined distances can be confirmed by using a sterile ruler intraoperatively, with the lower border of thyroid cartilage, cricoid cartilage, or main carina as an identifiable external landmark. If there is still doubt about the location of the lesional margins, their position can be confirmed with flexible bronchoscopy: the combination of the site of the bronchoscope light seen in the operative field and a transtracheally positioned needle viewed through the bronchoscope will accurately localize the position for the initial incision in the airway.

In benign disease, the strictured segment is mobilized circumferentially by sharp dissection, which is maintained as close to the tracheal wall as possible, particularly at the tracheoesophageal angles in which the recurrent laryngeal nerves run. No effort is made to identify the nerves in these cases. In resection for malignant disease, however, the recurrent nerves should be clearly defined above and below the tumor. A decision can then be made as to whether the nerve has to be sacrificed to achieve complete resection. Circumferential mobilization should not extend more than 1 cm above and below the segment to be resected (Fig. 19–34).

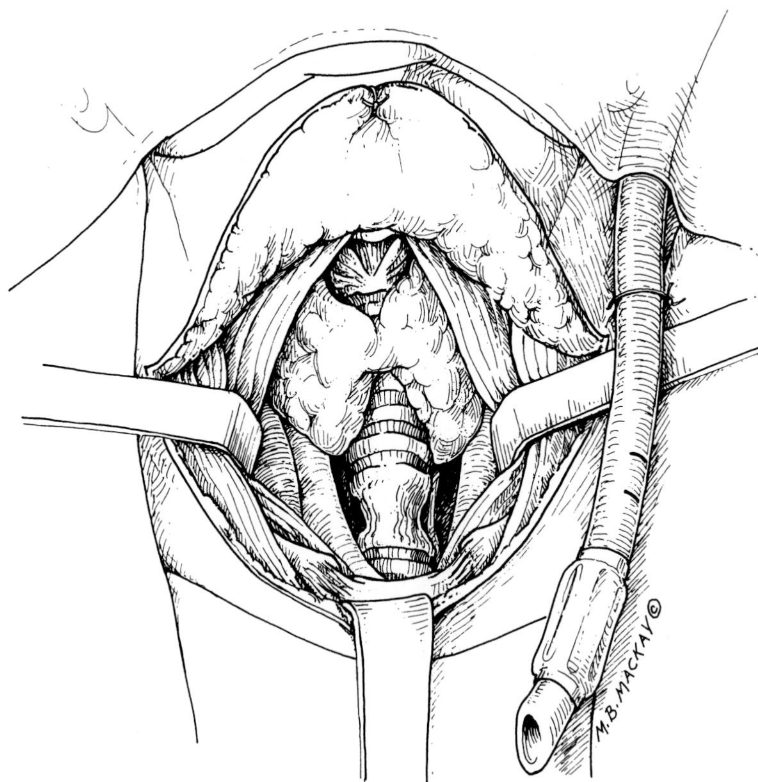

FIGURE 19–33 ■ Subplatysmal skin flaps have been developed to allow exposure of the airway from the suprasternal notch below to the thyroid notch above. The soft tissues are divided vertically in the midline from the thyroid cartilage to the suprasternal notch, with lateral mobilization and retraction of the strap muscles. This exposes the anterior wall of the larynx and trachea with the overlying thyroid isthmus in the region of the cricoid cartilage. A short area of circumferential scarring is depicted in the airway just above the suprasternal notch. Exposure of this segment has been facilitated by hyperextension of the neck and a bolster between the shoulders. An endotracheal tube has been positioned on the left side of the neck prior to division of the airway at the lower border of the stricture.

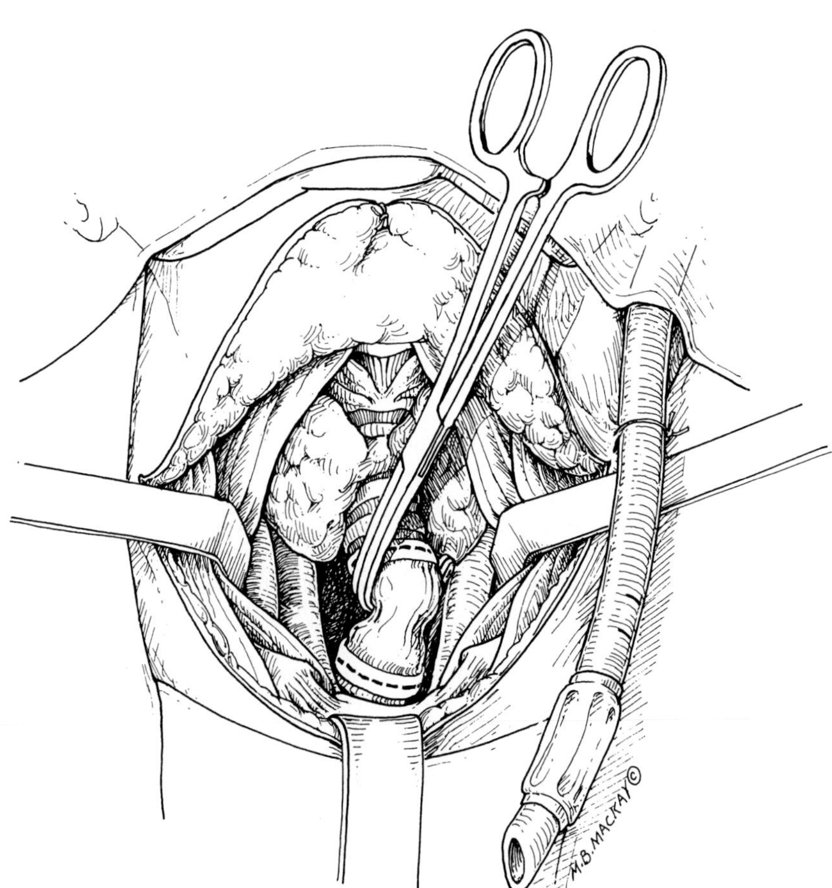

FIGURE 19–34 ■ In this diagrammatic representation of a benign postintubation stricture, the lesion has been mobilized circumferentially by maintaining sharp dissection immediately against the tracheal wall. The normal trachea on each side of the lesion is mobilized circumferentially for no more than 1 cm to preserve a good circulation at the subsequent tracheal margins *(dotted line)*.

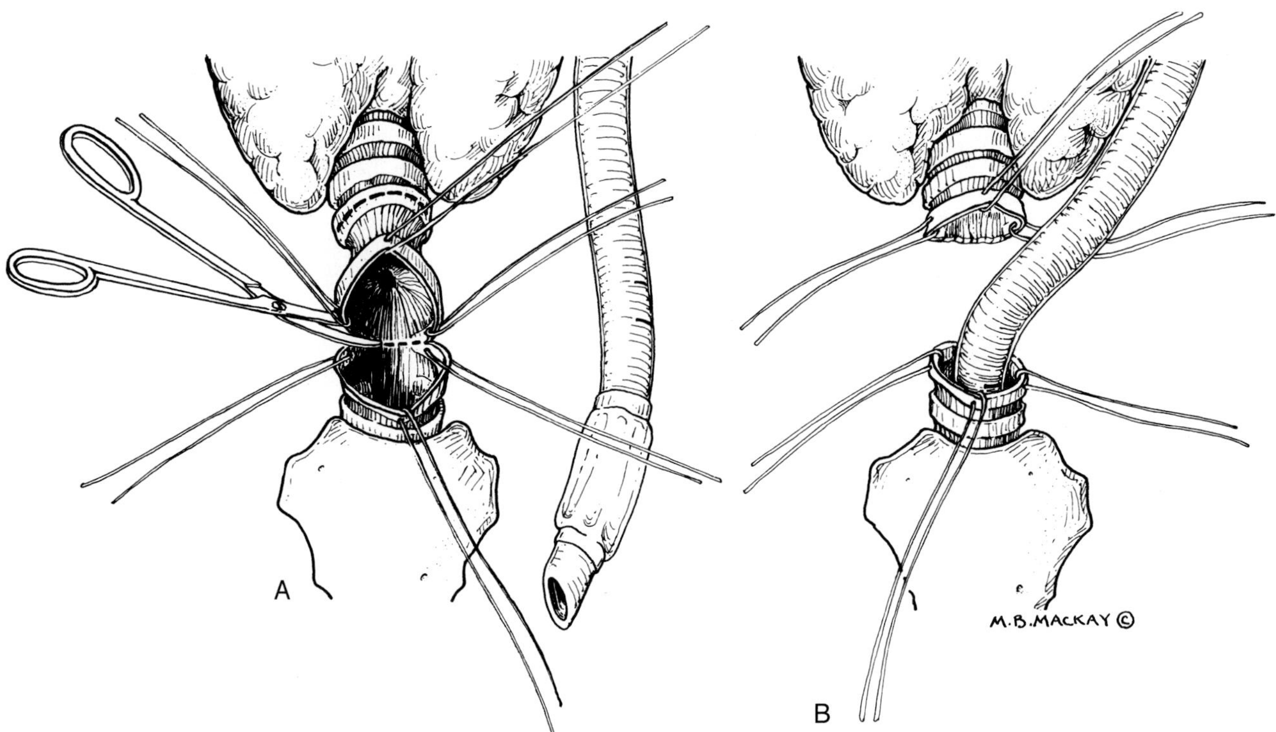

FIGURE 19–35 ■ *A*, The airway is divided distally just beyond the stricture. Stay sutures have been placed in the midline anteriorly and posterolaterally at the junction between tracheal cartilage and membranous trachea. *B*, With the airway completely divided, the distal end is intubated with an armored tube, which has been secured laterally to the skin of the neck and passed alongside the jaw and under the drapes to the anesthetic connections at the head of the operating table.

The airway is divided transversely through healthy trachea immediately below the segment to be resected. This incision is placed conservatively, with the surgeon choosing to divide the trachea through abnormal tissue if in doubt, because a more distal resection is always possible. Following incision of the cartilaginous wall anteriorly and laterally, 2–0 Vicryl stay sutures are placed in the midline anteriorly and also on each side at the junction between the cartilaginous and the membranous trachea, approximately one ring away from the divided edge (Fig. 19–35*A*). Traction on these sutures will accurately display the normal shapes and diameters of the tracheal lumen and membranous tracheal wall, which otherwise may be deformed and contracted. These stay sutures also prevent retraction of the distal tracheal stump into the mediastinum once the trachea is completely transected.

Following division of the trachea, the oral endotracheal tube is pulled back into the proximal airway, and the distal trachea is intubated with a flexible, cuffed, armored endotracheal tube (see Fig. 19–35*B*). The trachea is then divided above the lesion through healthy airway, and similar stay sutures are placed to display the upper tracheal margin. In the case of malignant disease, frozen section evaluation of the tracheal margins is an essential requirement.

Prior to performance of the anastomosis, the inflatable bag beneath the scapulae is deflated and the neck is flexed to shorten the distance between the tracheal ends. The anastomosis is begun by placing a row of interrupted sutures in the posterior membranous trachea (Fig. 19–36*A*). These sutures are placed at 2- to 3-mm intervals, taking approximately a 3-mm bite of trachea on each side of the tracheal margin. The endotracheal tube is intermittently removed and replaced, as required, in order to place the sutures. The entire posterior row is placed before any sutures are tied (see Fig. 19–36*B*). Our preference is to use fine (35-gauge) stainless steel wire with knots tied on the inside. This technique permits precise approximation of the posterior tracheal wall under direct vision. By means of appropriate traction on the stay sutures, all tension is removed from the tracheal ends while the posterior sutures are being tied. Once the sutures in the membranous trachea have been tied, the distal airway is extubated, and the original orotracheal tube is carefully advanced across the anastomosis into the distal airway. The anastomosis is then completed by using similarly placed, interrupted sutures of 4–0 Vicryl in the anterolateral cartilaginous wall, with the knots tied on the outside (Fig. 19–37).

In an alternative technique, practiced by Grillo (1970), the anastomosis is performed by using interrupted 4–0 Vicryl sutures only. All sutures are placed without tying, starting in the middle of the membranous trachea and progressing around each side to the front. The tracheal ends are then approximated, and the stay sutures of 2–0 Vicryl are tied to ablate tension when the 4–0 Vicryl sutures are tied. The 4–0 Vicryl sutures are tied sequentially, with knots on the outside, beginning in the midline anteriorly and working around the back on both sides.

Tension on the completed anastomosis should be minimal, and secure apposition should be possible with use

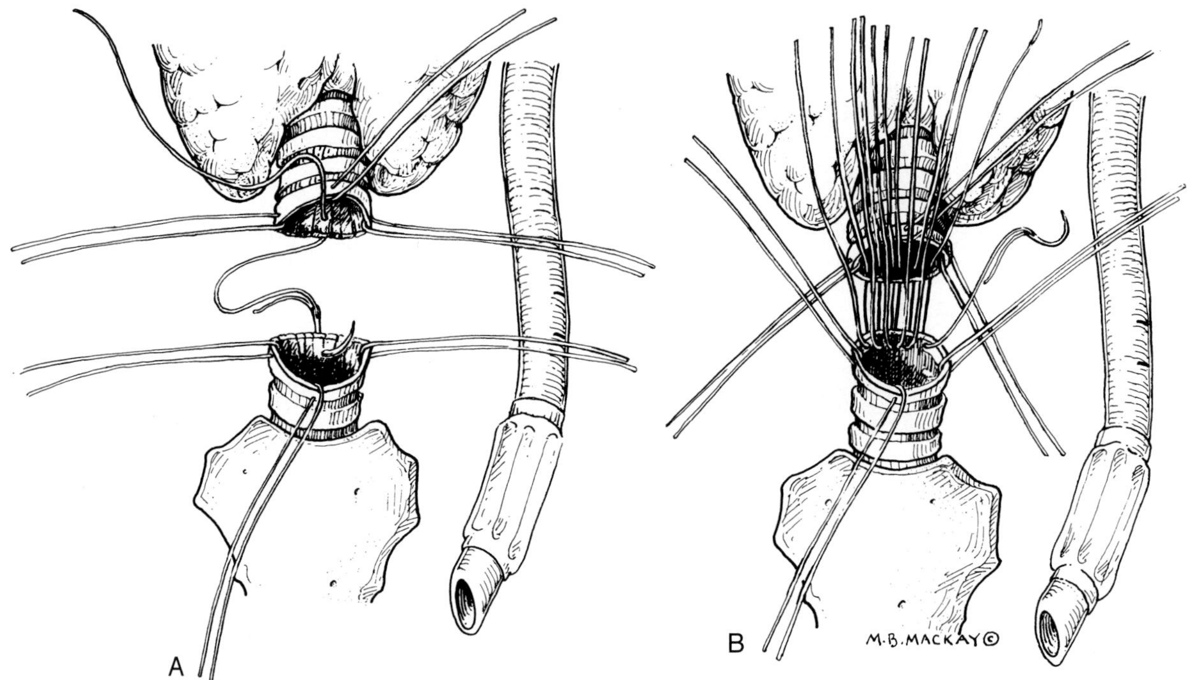

FIGURE 19–36 ■ *A*, The stricture has been resected, stay sutures placed in the proximal tracheal margin, and the posterior layer of anastomotic sutures begun. Reasonably deep 3- to 4-mm bites are taken in the tracheal wall on each side. *B*, Interrupted sutures are placed across the entire posterior wall of the anastomosis without being tied. An absorbable suture such as 3–0 or 4–0 Vicryl may be used for this part of the anastomosis. We prefer fine (35-gauge) stainless steel wire for this part of the anastomosis with the knots tied on the inside.

of relatively fine suture material. Unfortunately, there is no practical method to quantitate tension at the anastomosis, and this evaluation must be learned through experience.

After completion of the anastomosis, its integrity can be checked by manual ventilation of the patient to 20 to 30 cm H_2O with the cuff deflated. The thyroid gland or the strap muscles are approximated in the midline to buttress the anastomosis. A drain is placed alongside the trachea and brought out through a separate stab wound.

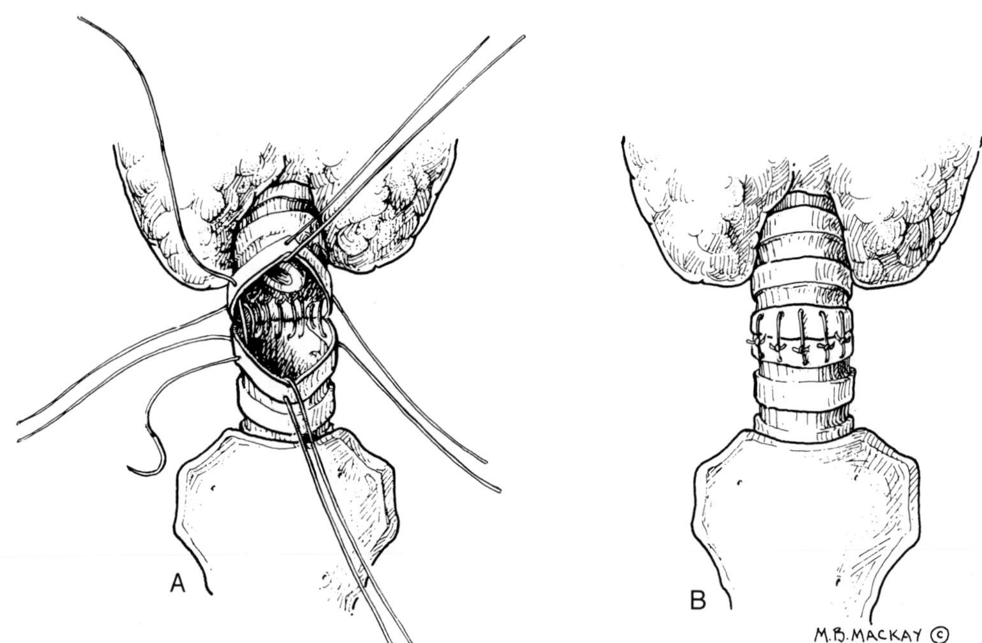

FIGURE 19–37 ■ *A*, Sutures on the posterior wall have been tied. At this point the orotracheal tube (lying just proximal to the anastomosis) is advanced across the anastomosis into the distal trachea. *B*, The anastomosis is completed.

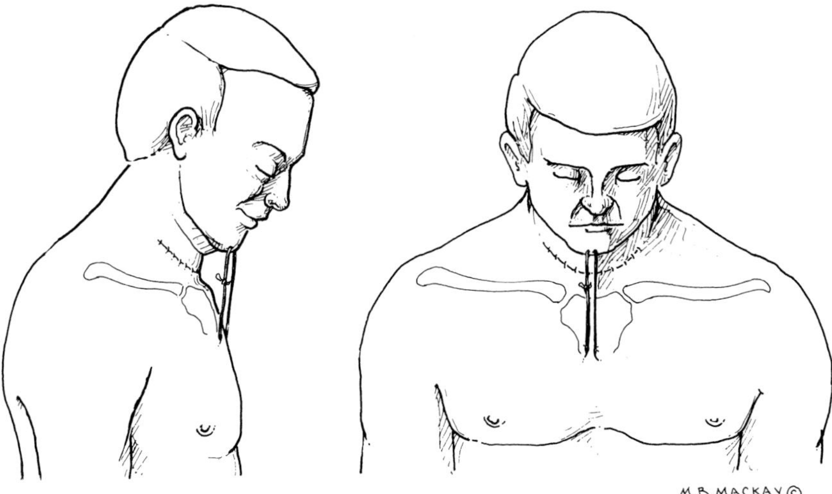

FIGURE 19–38 ■ At the end of the operation and before the patient is awake, a stout suture (#5 Tevdek) is secured as shown in the diagrams, between the skin of the point of the chin and the midline of the chest over the manubrium. This maintains neck flexion for the first postoperative week.

It is essential to maintain neck flexion during the postoperative period. This is simply and effectively achieved by securing a stout suture between the skin of the chin and the skin of the anterior chest (Fig. 19–38). This suture is left in place for 7 days to protect the tracheal anastomosis. It is surprisingly well tolerated by the patient.

It is desirable to extubate the patient in the operating room. If patency of the airway is equivocal—a situation usually due to acute edema—a distal No. 4 or 5 uncuffed tracheostomy tube is placed prior to closure. Alternatively, if the airway obstruction is minor or expected to be short-lived, translaryngeal intubation with a small, uncuffed tube may suffice. In those cases in which there is concern about the viability of the anastomosis, a silicone Montgomery T tube can be used to stent the anastomosis. This not only protects and maintains continuity of the airway but may prevent or diminish stricture development during the healing phase.

Mobilization and Release Procedures

If attempts to approximate the ends of the divided airway suggest that undue tension would result, there are several mobilization and release procedures that can be used to resolve the problem. These include neck flexion, which has its maximal effect in the cervical trachea but still reduces some tension in resections involving the lower trachea. Digital dissection of the trachea along the anterior, pretracheal "mediastinoscopy plane" is a useful technique that will provide additional mobility. The suprahyoid and suprathryoid laryngeal release procedures and the intrapericardial hilar releases are mobilization techniques that reduce anastomotic tension by elevation of the carina.

Suprathyrold Laryngeal Release

The suprathryoid laryngeal release operation, described by Dedo and Fishman in 1969, permits resection of an additional 2 to 3 cm of trachea by "dropping" the larynx and reducing tension at the anastomosis. To perform this procedure, the upper skin flap of the cervical incision is extended to the level of the hyoid bone. The sternohyoid strap muscles are retracted laterally, and the thyrohyoid muscles on each side are freed and divided transversely (Fig. 19–39, *dotted lines*). This exposes the thyrohyoid membrane and a centrally placed thyrohyoid ligament. The membrane and ligament are divided anteriorly and laterally between the superior cornua of the thyroid cartilage (Fig. 19–40*A*). The tips of the superior cornua are amputated, with care taken to avoid injury to the superior laryngeal nerves and their accompanying vessels, which are usually readily identified on each side (see Fig. 19–40*B*).

After division of the thyrohyoid membrane and ligament, the submucosa of the anterior pharyngeal wall is exposed. It is easily recognized by the rich submucosal plexus of vessels that it possesses. Thus, all the anterior and lateral soft-tissue attachments lying between the inferior border of the hyoid bone and the superior border of the thyroid cartilage, except for the underlying mucous membrane, have been divided. It is now possible to drop the larynx at least 2 to 3 cm inferior to its original position (see Fig. 19–40*B*). This operation may be complicated by transient postoperative supraglottic edema and is frequently associated with uncoordinated swallowing and with aspiration. Although these problems are usually transient, troublesome or disabling aspiration may be more prolonged and pronounced in elderly patients and in patients with reduced mobility of the larynx owing to previous surgery or radiation effects.

Suprahyoid Laryngeal Release

The suprahyoid release, originated by Montgomery in 1968, results in a laryngeal drop of similar magnitude to that achieved with the suprathyroid release. It has the reported advantage, however, of causing a diminished incidence and severity of incoordinate swallowing.

To perform this procedure, the upper skin flap is extended to the suprahyoid region. Alternatively, this operation may be performed through a separate transverse incision, which is centered over the hyoid bone. The muscular attachments (mylohyoid, geniohyoid, and genioglossus muscles) on the central two thirds of the superior aspect of the hyoid bone are completely tran-

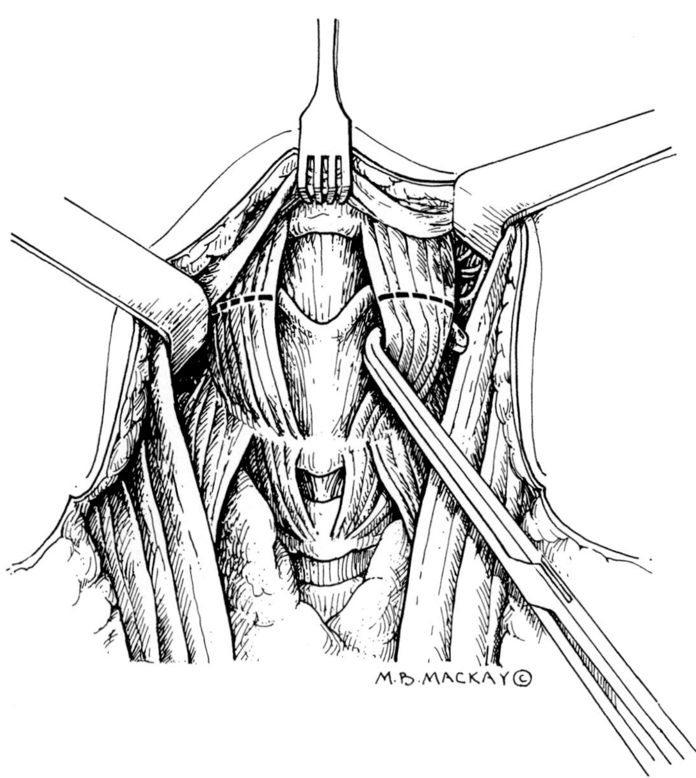

FIGURE 19–39 ■ Diagram illustrating the suprathyroid laryngeal release: the sternohyoid strap muscles have been retracted laterally, the thyrohyoid muscles on each side have been freed circumferentially, and the *dotted line* identifies the point of division of the thyrohyoid muscles.

sected to expose the pre-epiglottic space (Fig. 19–41*A*). The lesser cornua of the hyoid bone are transected, and the body of the hyoid bone is then divided just anterior to the tendinous attachments of the digastric muscles on each side. This separates the body of the hyoid from the greater horns and allows the larynx to drop for 2 to 3 cm (see Fig. 19–41*B*).

Intrapericardial Pulmonary Hilar Release

A right hilar release (Fig. 19–42) allows elevation of the carina or distal trachea for approximately 2 cm. To begin, the inferior pulmonary ligament is divided. Intrapericardial mobilization of the right pulmonary hilus is then accomplished by circumferential division of the pericardium and its reflections a few millimeters beyond the

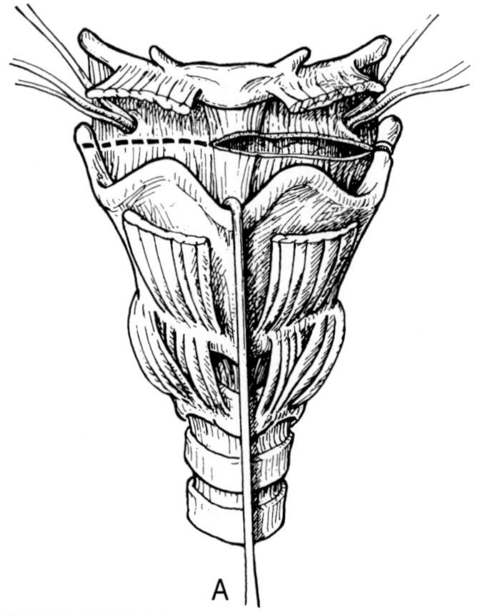

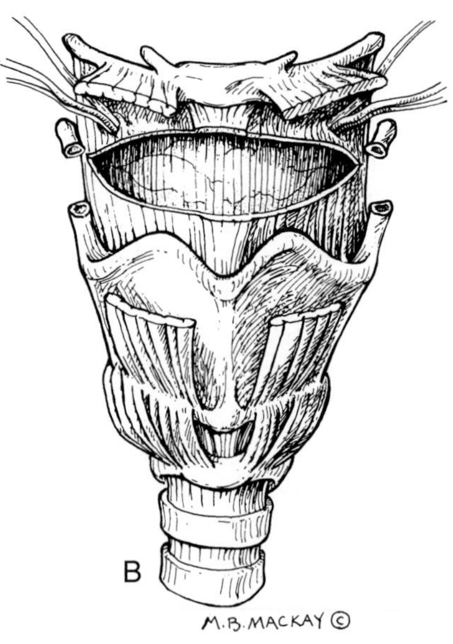

FIGURE 19–40 ■ *A*, Following division of the thyrohyoid muscles, the thyrohyoid membrane and a centrally placed thyrohyoid ligament are displayed. *B*, The thyrohyoid membrane and ligament are divided anteriorly and laterally between the superior cornua of the thyroid cartilage. The tips of the superior cornua are amputated, with care taken to avoid injury to the superior laryngeal nerves and vessels. It is now possible to "drop" the larynx at least 2 to 3 cm inferior to its original position.

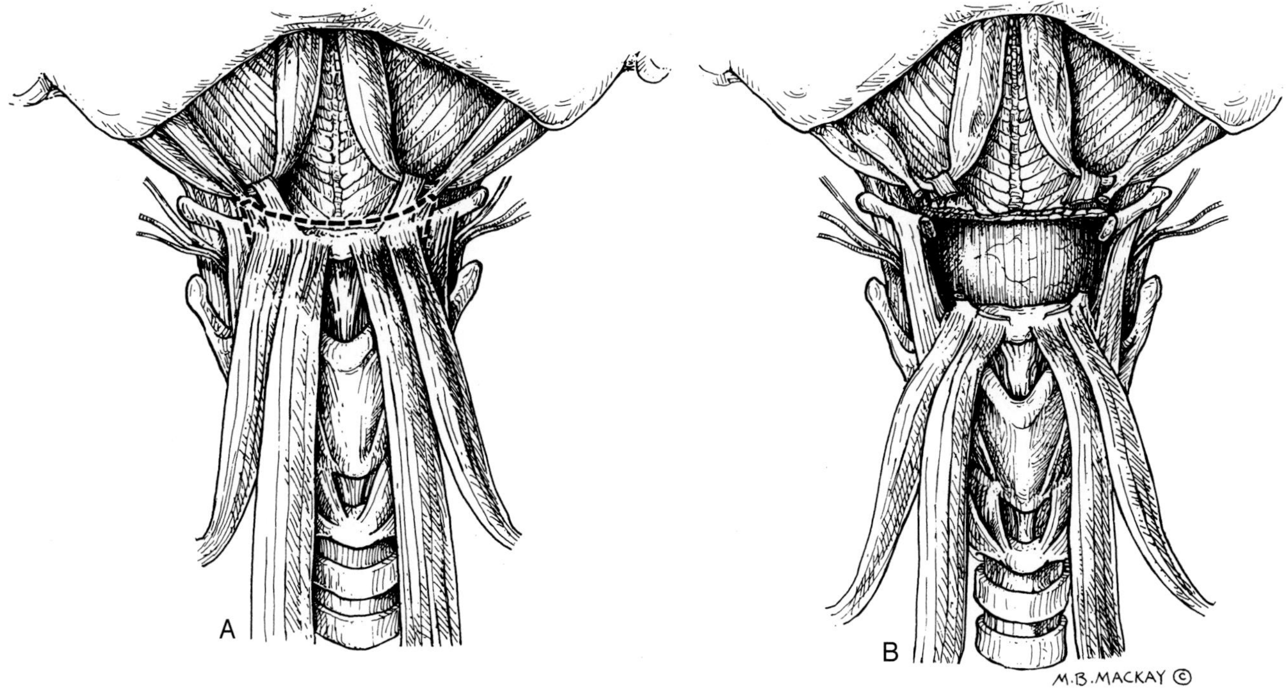

FIGURE 19–41 ■ *A*, Diagram illustrating the suprahyoid laryngeal release: Muscular attachments on the central two thirds of the upper margin of the hyoid bone are transected *(dotted line)* to expose the pre-epiglottic space. The lesser cornua of the hyoid bone are amputated, and the body of the hyoid bone is divided just anterior to the tendinous attachments of the digastric muscles on each side. *B*, This procedure separates the body of the hyoid from the greater horns and allows the larynx to "drop" 2 to 3 cm.

pericardial reflection on the superior and inferior pulmonary veins and the right pulmonary artery. The pericardium is divided close to the hilar reflection, and the right pulmonary artery is freed to its origin. In freeing the origin of the right main bronchus, care is taken to preserve the bronchial arterial circulation. To complete the release on the right side, the intrapericardial septum, which joins the lateral aspect of the atrium and inferior vena cava to the pericardium, is divided from the level of the inferior pulmonary vein to the diaphragm. There is no such septum on the left side.

A hilar release on the left side does not yield as much additional length as is obtained on the right. On the left side, the aortic arch restricts upward movement of the left main bronchus. The mobilization procedure is similar to that described for the right side, except that there is no intrapericardial septum to divide, and the ductus arteriosus must be divided to allow the hilum to shift upwards. The left main bronchus is freed, but care is taken to preserve its systemic bronchial blood supply.

Complications

The potential early and late complications of tracheal resection are listed later.

Mild to moderate airway obstruction can be treated with heliox (80% helium, 20% oxygen), racemic epinephrine inhalational therapy, and bolus administration of steroid (500 mg Solu-Medrol) as necessary. One or two such doses of steroid do not appear to significantly impair tracheal healing. Severe airway obstruction should be anticipated and treated intraoperatively with a distal tracheotomy under carefully controlled conditions, preferably with use of a flexible bronchoscope.

Minor air leaks at suture holes usually seal spontaneously and promptly. Larger leaks, if noticed at surgery, should be closed, usually by buttressing the leak site with vascularized tissue. If postoperative subcutaneous emphysema develops, the incision may have to be partially opened to achieve decompression. Pneumothorax is another potential postoperative complication and should be ruled out by an early postoperative chest radiograph.

POTENTIAL COMPLICATIONS OF TRACHEAL RESECTION

Early

Airway obstruction—edema
Air leak, subcutaneous emphysema
Recurrent laryngeal nerve injury—transient, permanent
Aspiration, dyscoordinate swallowing
Anastomotic dehiscence
Bleeding
Infection, abscess

Late

Restenosis, failure of healing
Suture-line granuloma
Tracheoesophageal fistula
Trachea-innominate artery fistula

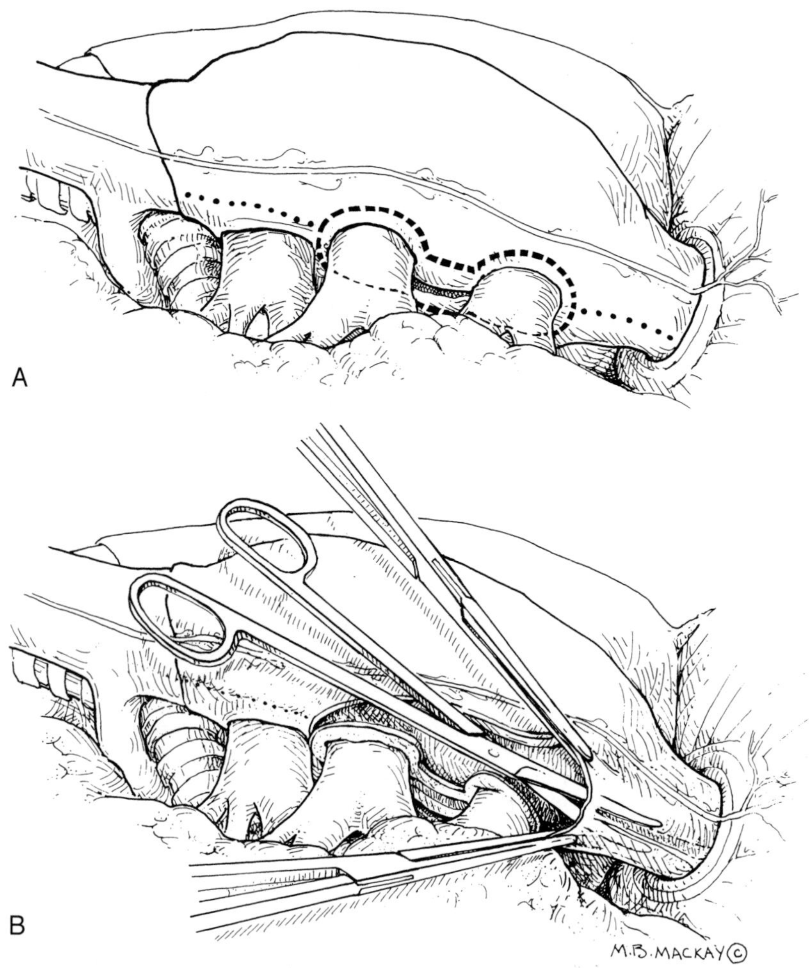

FIGURE 19–42 ■ *A*, Diagram illustrating the technique of right hilar pulmonary release. The *dotted lines* indicate the line of incision of the pericardium, a few millimeters outside the pericardial reflections on the pulmonary veins. The *upper dotted line* indicates the extension of the incision anterior to the right main pulmonary artery and bronchus, which gives exposure for circumferential mobilization of these two structures, which lie outside the free pericardial space. The *lower dotted line* indicates the location of the fibrous pericardial septum, which lies between the pericardium and the inferior vena cava, and separates the pericardial space on the right side into anterior and posterior compartments. *B*, The pericardium has been opened circumferentially around the pulmonary veins. The fibrous septum between the pericardium and the inferior vena cava is being divided from the lower border of the inferior pulmonary vein to the diaphragm. This allows the right side of the heart (right and left atria), the pulmonary artery, and the right main bronchus and carina to be elevated in a cephalad direction by several centimeters.

Permanent *inadvertent* injury to the recurrent laryngeal nerve is not common if the operative principles described above are followed. Transient dysfunction may be seen, however, and is presumably the result of reversible injury owing to traction or mobilization.

Patients are started on clear fluids on the first postoperative day and are usually quickly advanced to a full diet. Following a laryngeal release procedure, however, patients may experience considerable difficulty with swallowing and aspiration.

Incoordinate swallowing and aspiration are usually most troublesome with liquids and less of a problem with solid food. In most patients, the disability is transient and short-lived and results in a minor delay of a full recovery. Longer-term and disabling problems with aspiration are more often seen in the elderly patient or in cases in which laryngeal mobility is impaired by prior neck surgery or cervical irradiation.

A bronchoscopic examination should be performed postoperatively to evaluate healing of the anastomosis in all patients. This is usually done prior to discharge from the hospital about 1 week after surgery, or sooner if there is concern about the integrity of the anastomosis. If a dehiscence involving more than one third of the circumference of the airway is encountered, a Montgomery T tube stent should be placed. Smaller areas of separation usually heal without stricture formation but warrant follow-up with repeated bronchoscopic examination. Bleeding is an uncommon complication of tracheal surgery.

Infections occur infrequently relative to the amount of contamination that accompanies all tracheal surgery. Prophylactic antibiotics are given immediately before surgery, and one or two doses are given postoperatively. The course of antibiotics may be extended in patients with residual sepsis or risk factors such as diabetes or steroid therapy. If the patient does develop a wound infection, or is suspected of having a deep infection, the wound should be widely opened to provide immediate drainage. An undrained abscess may abut and necrose the tracheal anastomosis and drain internally.

Re-stenosis is a delayed complication, which is usually manifested within 4 to 6 weeks of surgery. Therapy consists of dilatation (repeated if necessary) and re-resection in selected cases. Grillo has reported experience with reoperation following unsuccessful repair for postintubation tracheal stenosis (Donahue, 1997). Where re-resection is not possible, insertion of a permanent stent may be the only option. Suture-line granulomas are uncommon with the use of absorbable suture or stainless steel suture. If they do occur, the granulomatous tissue can be removed through the rigid bronchoscope with biopsy forceps. Granulation tissue can also be treated with a silver nitrate stick or a judiciously applied laser.

Another potential late complication is fistulization between the tracheal anastomosis and the esophagus or the innominate artery. The management of these conditions is discussed elsewhere in this chapter. These complications can be avoided in most cases. During dissection of the trachea, the innominate artery should not be unduly mobilized if denuded. If the artery lies near the completed anastomosis, it can be protected with a muscular or omental pedicle. Similarly, if an esophageal repair is part of the tracheal operation, a buttress of vascularized tissue (usually strap muscle) should be interposed between the esophagus and the trachea at the level of anastomosis or repair.

■ *KEY REFERENCES*

Donahue DM, Grillo HC, Wain JC et al: Reoperative tracheal resection and reconstruction for unsuccessful repair of postintubation stenosis. J Thorac Cardiovasc Surg 114:934, 1997.

The only paper that describes a significant and detailed experience with reoperation for failure following resection for postintubation stenosis. Seventy-five patients were reoperated between 1966 and 1997. Complication rates were higher than they were for first-time resections and were most pronounced in the 19 patients requiring a laryngeal release at the time of reoperation. The authors clearly demonstrate, however, that a successful outcome can be obtained in most such cases.

Grillo HC: Surgery of the trachea. In Ravitch MM (ed): Current Problems in Surgery. Chicago, Year Book Medical Publishers, 1970.

A comprehensive review of the advances in surgical techniques for tracheal resection that occurred prior to 1970. The basic principles pertaining to segmental resection were established and have changed little since this publication.

Pearson FG: Advances in Tracheal Surgery. Chicago, Year Book Medical Publishers, 1983.

A review of advances in tracheal surgery following Grillo's landmark publication in 1970. Among these advances are improved techniques for segmental resection, including the carina below and the subglottis above, and the use of median sternotomy for selected cases of segmental resection.

■ *REFERENCES*

Cooper JD, Pearson FG, Patterson CA et al: Use of silicone stents in the management of airway problems. Ann Thorac Surg 47:371, 1989.

Dedo HH, Fishman NH: Laryngeal release and sleeve resection for tracheal stenosis. Ann Otol Rhinol Laryngol 78:285, 1969.

Mathisen DJ, Grillo HC, Vlahakes GJ, Daggett WM: The omentum in the management of complicated cardiothoracic problems. J Thorac Cardiovasc Surg 95:677, 1988.

Montgomery WW: The surgical management of supraglottic and subglottic stenosis. Ann Otol Rhinol Laryngol 77:534, 1968.

Tsubota N, Simpson WJ, Van Nostrand AWP, Pearson FG: The effects of pre-operative irradiation on primary tracheal anastomosis. Ann Thorac Surg 20:152, 1975.

CARINAL RESECTION

Douglas J. Mathisen
Hermes C. Grillo
Henning A. Gaissert

The intrathoracic portion of the trachea is the last unpaired organ of the body to fall to the surgeon, and the successful solution of the problem of its reconstruction may mark the end of the "expansionist" epoch in the development of surgery.

—Ronald H. R. Belsey
Bristol, England
1946

In 1946, Belsey could not have predicted the challenges of organ transplantation to the thoracic surgeon, but his admonition regarding resection and reconstruction of the intrathoracic trachea remains true even today. Techniques for resection and reconstruction of the trachea and carina are available, but they are not widely accepted and practiced. Unique perioperative complications, high operative mortality rates, technical challenges, and evolution of the understanding of the limits of resection are but a few of the hurdles remaining. Until these hurdles are cleared, experience with carinal resection remains limited to only few institutions around the world.

Successful resection and reconstruction of the carina initially faced four major challenges: preoperative evaluation of the extent of disease, technique of surgery, anesthetic management, and postoperative care. The techniques for reconstruction and anesthesia have been established but need continued refinement to improve current results. Postoperative care needs further refinement to reduce the complications and improve the operative mortality rates, thereby improving the chances for long-term survival.

HISTORICAL NOTE

Early surgical efforts involved lateral or wedge resections of the airway. Prosthetic materials were used because of the uncertainty of airway healing and because of concern about the extent of resection of the airway that would allow safe reconstruction. Belsey's initial report (1946) of intrathoracic tracheal resection described reconstruction with prosthetic material after lateral resection of the distal airway, including the carina, in one patient. Juvenelle and Citret in 1951 were among the earliest to report experimental results of carinal resection in dogs. The first report of complicated carinal resection and reconstruction in humans was in 1957 by Barclay and associates. They reported successful resection of the carina for a cylindroma, with end-to-end reconstruction between the trachea and the right mainstem bronchus and implantation of the left mainstem bronchus into the side of the bronchus intermedius. Grillo and colleagues in 1963 and Grillo in 1982 described carinal resection and reconstruction. Grillo presented a comprehensive approach to carinal reconstruction based on experience with 36 cases. Other significant reports of carinal resection and reconstruction included those by Mathey and others (1966), Eschapasse (1974), and Perelman (1976). Jensik and coworkers (1972) reported 17 patients undergoing tracheal sleeve pneumonectomy for lung cancer. Results, mostly for lung cancer, reported operative mortality ranging from 10.9% to 29% (Dartevelle and Chapelier, 1988; Deslauriers, 1985; Jensik et al, 1982; Mathisen and Grillo, 1991; Perelman and Koroleva, 1980; Tsuchiya et al, 1990).

■ *HISTORICAL READINGS*

Barclay RS, McSwan N, Welsh TM: Tracheal resection without the use of grafts. Thorax 12:177, 1957.

Belsey R: Resection and reconstruction of the intrathoracic trachea. Br J Surg 38:200, 1946.

Dartevelle PG, Chapelier A: Tracheal sleeve pneumonectomy for bronchogenic carcinoma: A report of 55 cases. Ann Thorac Surg 46:68, 1988.

Deslauriers J: Involvement of the main carina. In Delarue NC, Eschapasse H (eds): International Trends in General Thoracic Surgery, Vol 1. Philadelphia, WB Saunders, 1985.

Eschapasse H: Les tumeurs tracheales primitives: Traitement chirurgical. Rev Fr Mal Respir 2:425,1974.

Grillo HC: Carinal resection. Ann Thorac Surg 34:356, 1982.

Grillo HC, Bendixen HH, Gephart T: Resection of the carina and lower trachea. Ann Surg 158:889, 1963.

Jensik RJ, Faber JP, Kittle CF et al: Survival in patients undergoing tracheal sleeve pneumonectomy for bronchogenic carcinoma. J Thorac Cardiovasc Surg 84:489, 1982.

Jensik RJ, Faber LP, Milloy FJ, Goldin MD: Tracheal sleeve pneumonectomy for advanced carcinoma of the lung. Surg Gynecol Obstet 134:232, 1972.

Juvenelle A, Citret C: Transplantation de la bronche souche et résection de la bifurcation tracheale. J Chir (Paris) 67:666, 1951.

Mathey J, Binet JP, Galey JJ et al: Tracheal tracheobronchial resection. J Thorac Cardiovasc Surg 51:1, 1966.

Mathisen DJ, Grillo HC: Carinal resection for bronchogenic carcinoma. J Thorac Cardiovasc Surg 102:16, 1991.

Mathisen DJ, Grillo HC: Endoscopic relief of malignant airway obstruction. Ann Thorac Surg 48:469, 1989.

Mathisen DJ, Grillo HC, Vlahakes GJ, Daggett WM: The omentum in the management of complicated cardiothoracic problems. J Thorac Cardiovasc Surg 95:677, 1988.

Perelman M: Surgery of the Trachea. Moscow, Moscow Mir, 1976.

Perelman M, Koroleva N: Surgery of the trachea. World J Surg 4:583, 1980.

Tsuchiya R, Goya T, Naruke T, Suemasu K: Resection of tracheal carina for lung cancer. J Thorac Cardiovasc Surg 99:941, 1990.

PREOPERATIVE EVALUATION

The risks of surgery demand careful preoperative assessment of each patient. Computed tomography (CT), magnetic resonance imaging (MRI), and plain linear tomography are all helpful in assessing the extent of disease and the involvement of the airway. Conventional tomography has been particularly helpful in determining the extent of airway involvement and defining the carina radiologically, regardless of the etiology of the problem. All patients with lung cancer should undergo routine radiologic evaluation for metastatic disease. Spiral CT scans and virtual bronchoscopy are increasingly more useful in imaging the central airways.

Patients should be carefully screened from a general medical point of view, and each patient should be particularly screened for coronary disease. Stress thallium studies and echocardiography are used when indicated. Most importantly, all patients should be evaluated to be certain they will have adequate pulmonary function to tolerate such operations and such pulmonary resection as may be indicated. Smoking must stop and medical regimens must be optimized for underlying chronic obstructive lung disease. Chronic bronchitis should be treated vigorously. All steroids should be discontinued prior to the time of surgery. Arterial blood gases, spirometry, and quantitative ventilation/perfusion scans have become routine. Diffusion capacity, maximum oxygen uptake, and exercise testing are also useful in assessing high-risk patients. Predicted postoperative forced expiratory volume in 1 second should be at least 800 ml/sec, but this figure is only a guideline in the context of the patient's size and general medical condition.

Preoperative radiation for lung cancer is advocated by some authors but is probably associated with a higher incidence of complications (Jensik et al, 1982). Preoperative radiation should not exceed 4000 cGy and is generally given over a period of 3 to 4 weeks. An additional interval of 3 to 4 weeks is allowed for the acute inflammatory effects of radiation to subside. Radiation in excess of 5000 cGy given 1 year or more prior to planned resection should be viewed as a relative contraindication. If circumstances dictate carinal resection, omentum should be wrapped around the anastomosis to aid healing and to buttress the anastomosis (Mathisen et al, 1988). Chronic steroid dependency also precludes safe carinal resection.

ANESTHESIA

Anesthetic management is an important consideration in patients undergoing carinal resection. If an obstructing tumor exists, an adequate airway must be provided to allow safe conduct of anesthesia. This can be accomplished at the time of planned resection by rigid bronchoscopes and biopsy forceps or by laser (Mathisen and Grillo, 1989; Shapshay et al, 1985). The risk of bleeding is minimal with either technique. If postobstructive pneumonia is present, it may be desirable to relieve the obstruction and to treat the pneumonia prior to proceeding to carinal resection. In the face of severe obstruction, preliminary "coring out" of the airway may provide time for any necessary study, medical therapy, or weaning from steroids.

The anesthetic technique of choice in our institution

has been a deep Ethrane anesthesia that avoids long-acting muscle relaxants and narcotics (Wilson, 1988).

This technique allows spontaneous ventilation by the patient, which is especially important in difficult airway situations, and it facilitates extubation at the end of the procedure.

The choice of endotracheal tube is also important. Double-lumen tubes are generally not useful for carinal resection. Abbott (1950) initially recommended the use of a long tube advanced through the divided end of the trachea into the remaining mainstem bronchus. Grillo and associates (1963) advocated intubation of the left mainstem bronchus across the operative field, with sterile tubing passed off to the anesthesiologist. El-Baz and colleagues (1982) later advocated high-frequency ventilation, which has become the preferred method of airway management for some.

Our preferred method of airway management is with an extra-long oral endotracheal tube initially. This can be directed into the opposite bronchus if collapse of the operated lung is desired, or a bronchial blocker can be used. Once the carina has been resected, the opposite bronchus (usually the left mainstem) is intubated with a sterile, flexible Tovell tube. Sterile connecting tubing is passed to the anesthesiologist. The tube can be removed for brief periods to allow precise placement of sutures. When the anastomosis is ready to be approximated, the original long oral endotracheal tube is advanced from above across the anastomosis into the mainstem bronchus. Previously placed stay and anastomotic sutures are then tied. Special circumstances occasionally arise that require bifid catheters for selective high-frequency ventilation of upper and lower lobes or, rarely, two separate anesthesia machines and small Tovell tubes to accomplish the same effect. Cardiopulmonary bypass is almost never required for carinal resection. In the extraordinarily complex situation in which bypass might seem useful, the risk of parenchymal hemorrhage negates its use.

Any surgical team performing carinal resection must be equipped and familiar with all the techniques of airway management to ensure safe conduct of the operation. Complete control of ventilation and oxygenation must be maintained continuously.

Operative Technique

Bronchoscopy

Careful bronchoscopic evaluation to determine the extent of involvement and the adequacy of the remaining airway is invaluable. The distal trachea, carina, and mainstem bronchi should be carefully inspected for signs of involvement. We find that more precise assessment is possible with rigid ventilating bronchoscopes and Storz-Hopkins telescopes than with flexible fiberoptic instruments. It is always difficult to know the maximum amount of airway that can be removed to allow safe, tension-free anastomosis; this varies from patient to patient. For the most common carinal resection, namely right carinal pneumonectomy, the length of distal trachea, carina, and left mainstem bronchus resection should not exceed 4 cm in most patients. Length in excess of 4 cm will produce excessive anastomotic tension and predisposes to separation or stenosis. This does not apply to anastomosis of right main bronchus to trachea.

Mediastinoscopy

All patients with lung cancer should undergo mediastinoscopy to evaluate mediastinal nodes and the degree of extraluminal tumor involvement. The presence of positive mediastinal nodes should preclude resection in most patients with primary carinal tumors because these are first-level nodes for such tumors in lung cancer cases. The management of N2 nodes should follow the surgeon's protocol for such a stage. To avoid fibrosis, which would limit mobility of the airway, and to eliminate intraoperative confusion between scar and tumor, it is preferable to perform mediastinoscopy at the time of planned resection. Dissection of the pretracheal plane increases mobility of the airway in patients without lung cancer as well, although the plane is easily dissected intrathoracically. Blunt dissection of the carina at mediastinoscopy may facilitate dissection of this area at the time of thoracotomy and may be useful in separating the left recurrent nerve from the left lateral wall of the trachea.

Incisions

The most common incision to gain access to the carina for carinal resection or right carinal pneumonectomy or to the stump of either mainstem bronchus and the carina is a right posterolateral thoracotomy. Median sternotomy is adequate for limited carinal resection; this is carried out transpericardially between the superior vena cava and the ascending aorta laterally and the innominate vein and the pulmonary artery superiorly and inferiorly. These structures need to be fully mobilized to give adequate exposure. The pericardium is opened anteriorly and posteriorly.

Left carinal pneumonectomy poses difficult exposure problems. Limited resection of the carina can be done through a left thoracotomy but requires mobilization of the aorta to gain access to the carina. Tapes can then be passed around the distal trachea and right mainstem bronchus to facilitate exposure (Newton et al, 1991) (Fig. 19–43). Cervical flexion to devolve the lower trachea is essential to the exposure. More extensive involvement of the carina, distal trachea, or right mainstem bronchus precludes this approach. Bilateral, submammary, transsternal (clamshell) thoracotomy has been the most useful approach under these conditions. Access is adequate but should be used only for the fittest of patients. Median sternotomy also has a limited role in a few lesions involving the left mainstem and carina. Left hilar mobilization, if required, is difficult or impossible through sternotomy in many patients, because excessive traction on the heart is required.

Release Maneuvers

One of the most important reasons for technical failure following carinal resection is excessive anastomotic tension. Surgeons performing carinal resection should be very familiar with the available maneuvers to reduce anastomotic tension. The simplest maneuver, as with

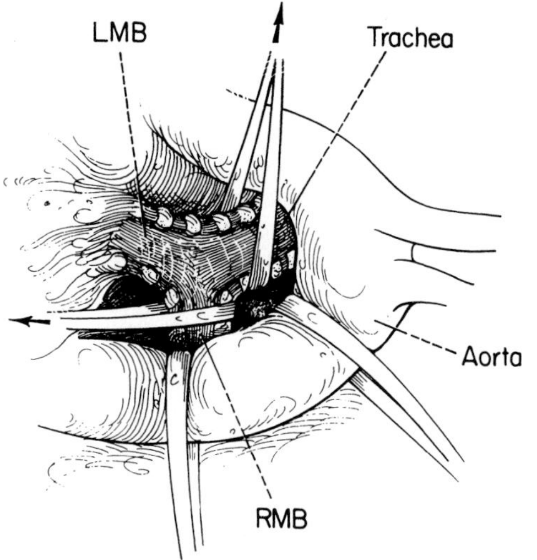

FIGURE 19–43 ■ Exposure for left carinal resection through left thoracotomy. The aortic arch is mobilized and retracted. Tapes are passed around the distal trachea and right main bronchus (RMB) and retracted to bring the carina into the operative field.

tracheal resection, is flexion of the neck. This allows devolvement of the trachea into the mediastinum and should be done in all cases just prior to approximation of the airway. Mobilization of the anterior pretracheal plane, avoiding injury to the lateral blood supply to the trachea, increases the mobility of the airway and should be done in all patients, often by mediastinoscopy. Dissection of the left mainstem bronchus in a similar fashion, avoiding its lateral blood supply, will slightly increase the mobility of the distal airway as well. A stitch between the chin and chest, placed at the completion of the operation, holds the patient's head in flexion, avoiding excessive tension in the early postoperative period. The stitch is cut on the seventh postoperative day. Laryngeal release for carinal reconstruction has not been helpful in gaining additional length and has been abandoned in most cases.

For carinal resection involving anastomosis of the trachea to right mainstem bronchus, division of the inferior pulmonary ligament and mobilization of the right hilum are important. A U-shaped incision in the pericardium below the inferior pulmonary vein will allow the hilar structures and bronchus to advance (Fig. 19–44). Additional length may be obtained by completely incising the pericardium around the hilar vessels. It is best to preserve a posteriorly based pedicle of tissue that includes bronchial vessels and lymphatics whenever complete incision of the pericardium is performed.

Special mention should be made of those resections involving only the carina. Attempting to "recreate" a carina by joining the left and right mainstem bronchi will not allow much, if any, cephalad advancement of the neocarina, because in such an instance, length can be obtained largely by devolvement of the trachea from above. The left main bronchus remains tethered by the aortic arch.

SURGICAL TECHNIQUE

Because of the narrow margin between success and failure, precise surgical technique is required. Careful, gentle handling of the tissues is crucial; every attempt should be made to avoid trauma to the bronchial mucosa. Sharp, single, clean transection lines are imperative. The blood supply to the trachea is predominantly segmental, and every effort should be made to avoid interruption. Lateral dissection proximal and distal to the proposed lines of transection should be limited to 1 to 2 cm. Size discrepancy usually exists between the proximal and the distal ends of the airway, and no attempt should be made to

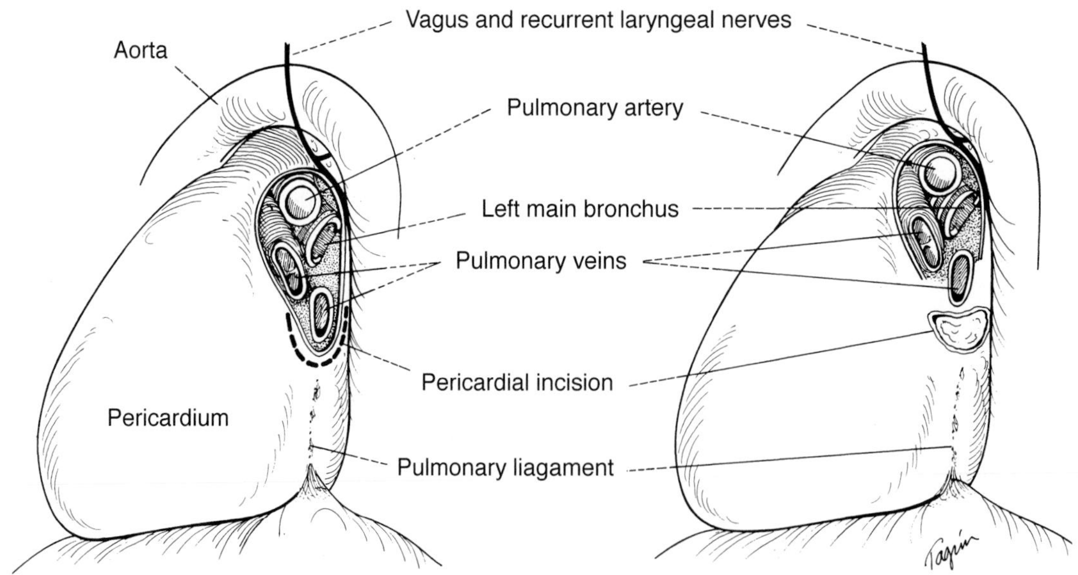

FIGURE 19–44 ■ The left-sided intrapericardial hilar release technique showing the U-shaped pericardial incision, which allows 1 to 2 cm of upward hilar mobility to facilitate the creation of a tension-free anastomosis.

alter either end; narrowing the proximal end or creating a V in the distal end is unnecessary. All airway anastomoses should be covered by local vascularized tissues. This may add to the blood supply but, most importantly, separates these suture lines from nearby vascular structures and suture lines. Pleural flaps, pericardial fat pads, pedicled intercostal muscle flaps, and even omentum can be used. The principles apply to all the reconstructive procedures discussed later.

The goal of surgery should be a tension-free anastomosis with clear surgical margins. Because of the limits of safe resection, a balance must be struck between the desire for clear margins and the ability to safely reconstruct the airway. Clear margins are most desirable for invasive carcinoma. Failure to achieve clear margins, even with postoperative radiotherapy, will invariably lead to recurrence in squamous carcinoma, but this does not appear to be equally true for adenoid cystic carcinoma, in which microscopically positive margins seem to be successfully managed with postoperative radiotherapy.

MODES OF RECONSTRUCTION

A variety of techniques for reconstruction of the carina have been proposed and used (Fig. 19–45). In practice, the applicability of each technique is determined by the required extent of resection of various parts of the carina. The first reconstructive technique described in the next paragraph applies when no pulmonary tissue is resected, and the other techniques are used after varying amounts of pulmonary resection have been performed.

The simplest technique is the approximation of the medial walls of the right and left main bronchi to one another to fashion a new carina with the trachea. This

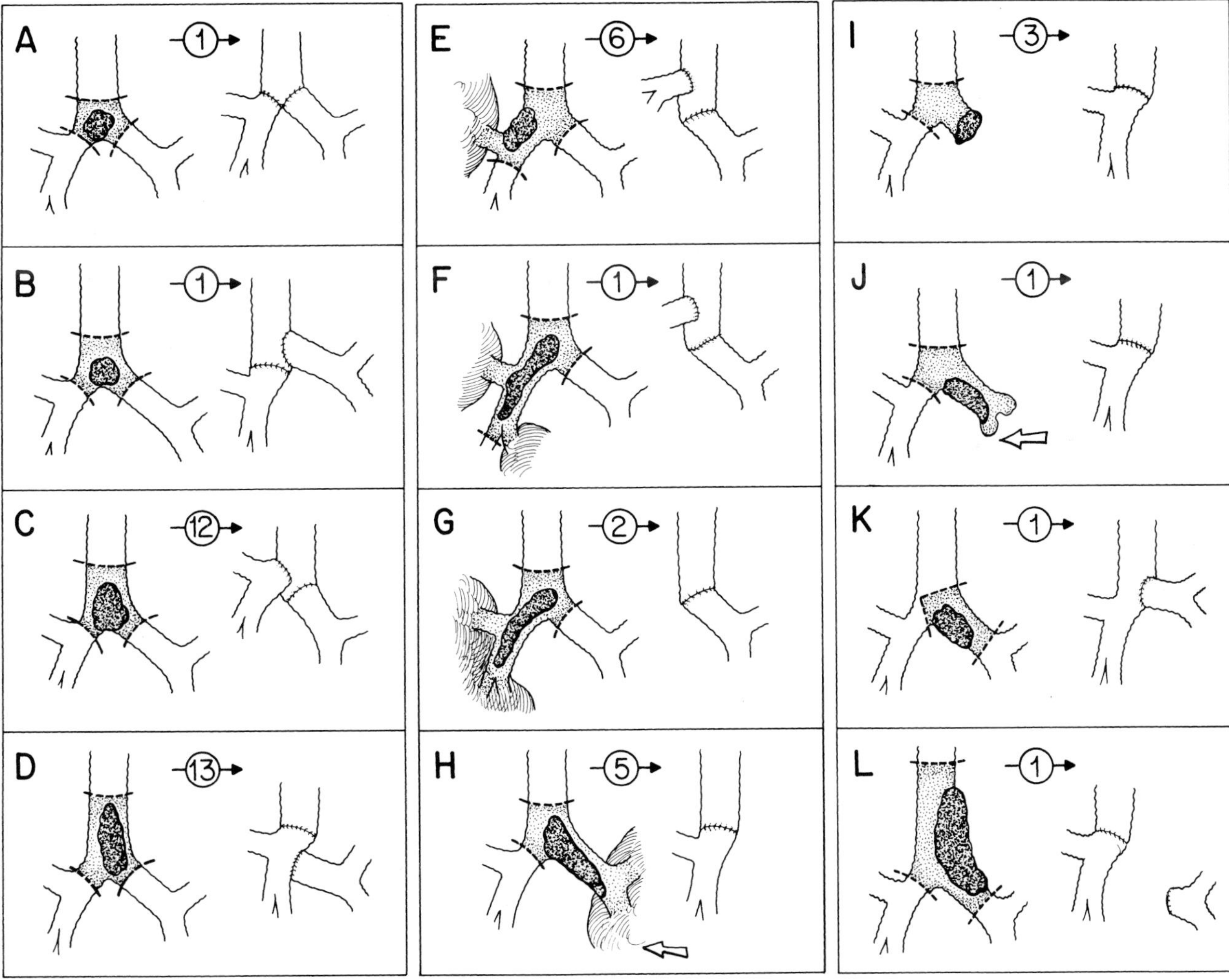

FIGURE 19–45 ■ Modes of carinal resection and reconstruction that have been used for tracheal and carinal tumors. *Circled number* is number of patients. *Open arrows* indicate side of approach when not conventionally right-sided. *A*, Limited resection permits carinal restitution. *B*, Technique used in initial carinal resection; technique in *A* would now be used. *C*, More extensive resection. *D*, Greater length of trachea (technique of Barclay and co-workers [1957]). *E*, Involvement of right main bronchus and right upper lobe bronchus, requiring right upper lobectomy. *F*, Middle lobe also removed; right lower lobe bronchus may be anastomosed to left main bronchus. *G*, Right carinal pneumonectomy. *H*, Left carinal pneumonectomy. *I*, Resection of carina after previous left pneumonectomy. *J*, Resection of carina with extra long stump. *K*, Wedge removal of left main bronchus from the right. *L*, Tracheocarinal resection with long segment of left main bronchus, and exclusion of remaining left lung from the right; left pneumonectomy also through bilateral thoracotomy.

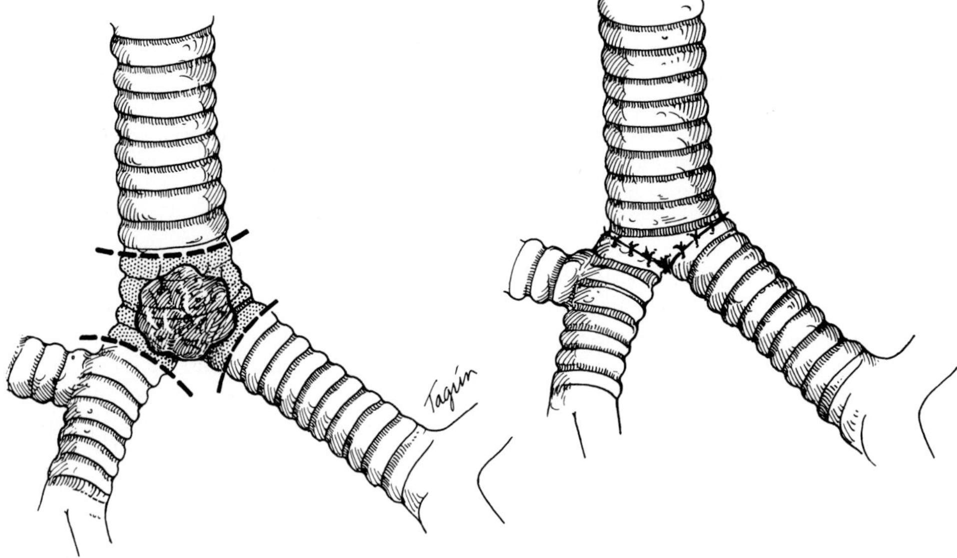

FIGURE 19–46 ■ Resection with restitution of newly created carina. This technique is applicable only for small, centrally placed tumors.

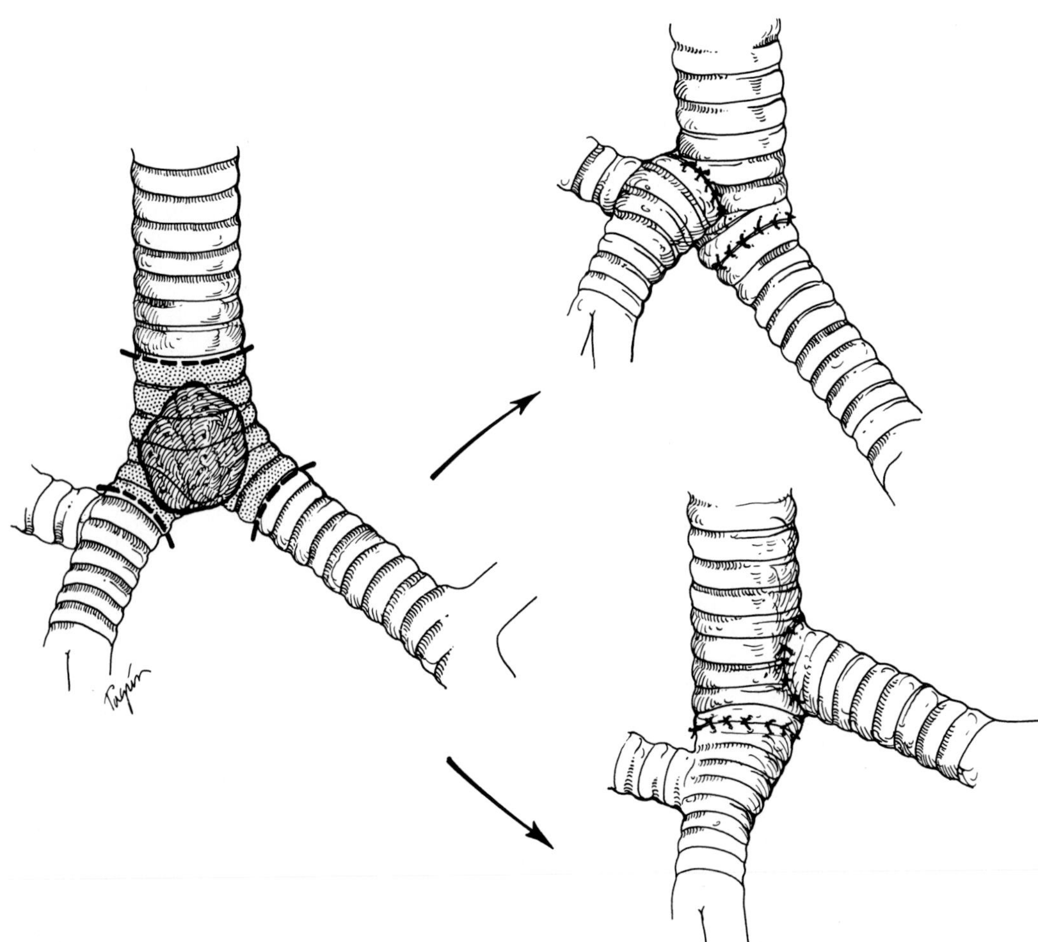

FIGURE 19–47 ■ Carinal reconstruction after resection, with the trachea anastomosed end-to-end to either the left or the right main bronchus and the other bronchus placed into the lateral wall of the trachea above the first anastomosis. The diagram at *upper right* shows the more commonly used technique.

technique is applicable only in cases of very small tumors that require limited resection of the trachea and bronchi (Fig. 19–46). Suturing the two bronchi together restricts the mobilization of the newly created carina. The left main bronchus has very little mobility, even if its anterior surface has been bluntly dissected; it is held in position by the aortic arch. Closure of the gap must, therefore, be accomplished by bringing the trachea down to the new carina.

When the tumor is more extensive, requiring a larger portion of trachea to be resected, end-to-end plus end-to-side tracheobronchial anastomosis is the method of choice (Fig. 19–47). The possibility of approximation after resection is determined, with the patient's neck flexed, by drawing together lateral traction sutures that have been placed in the trachea and bronchi. In some cases it is easier to approximate the trachea to the left main bronchus than to the right main bronchus. The tube across the operative field may be intermittently removed, if necessary, during placement of the sutures. It is preferable to place all the anastomotic sutures prior to drawing the lateral traction sutures together and then to tie each of the anastomotic sutures in sequence. In this anastomosis, most of the length is gained by bringing the proximal trachea down to the end of the left main bronchus. After completion of this anastomosis, the endotracheal tube is passed into the left main bronchus, and the right main bronchus is elevated and anastomosed to the side of the trachea. The opening is ovoid and is placed in the cartilaginous wall to provide more rigidity. Rarely, it is easier to anastomose the trachea to the right main bronchus and to implant the left main bronchus into the left lateral wall of the trachea. Access for this anastomosis is not as easy.

When a greater length of trachea must be removed, the distance between the relatively immobile left main bronchus and the stump of the trachea is too great to be spanned by bringing the trachea down. Under these circumstances, the right lung is mobilized, the right main bronchus is brought up for direct end-to-end anastomosis to the trachea, and the left main bronchus is implanted across the mediastinum into the side of the bronchus intermedius (Fig. 19–48). A "reverse" procedure can be done but is rarely required (see Fig. 19–48).

If the lesion involves the carina and the right main bronchus to the right upper lobe bronchus, the problem is more complex. The lower trachea and carina, plus the right main bronchus and upper lobe, are resected. The bronchus intermedius is transected below the takeoff of the upper lobe bronchus; the trachea and left main bronchus are anastomosed; and after mobilization of the right hilum intrapericardially, the bronchus intermedius is elevated and implanted in the lateral wall of the trachea, about 1 cm above the previously described anastomosis (Fig. 19–49). This may lead to excessive anastomotic tension, dictating implantation of the bronchus intermedius into the left main bronchus or sacrifice of the residual right lung, if feasible.

The most common resection of the carina involves the entire right lung and carina (Fig. 19–50) because of the

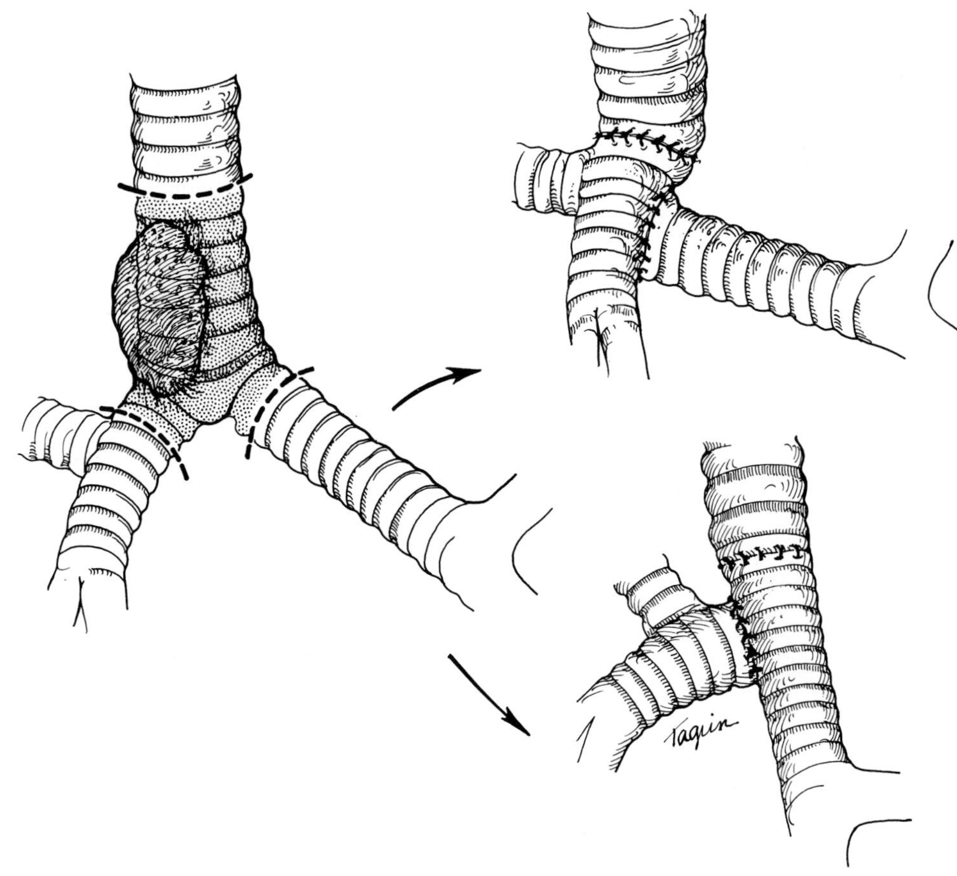

FIGURE 19–48 ■ More extensive tracheal resection, with advancement of the right main bronchus to the end of the trachea and implantation of the left main bronchus into the bronchus intermedius *(upper right)*. The reverse procedure *(lower right)* is rarely applicable, because the left main bronchus is very fixed.

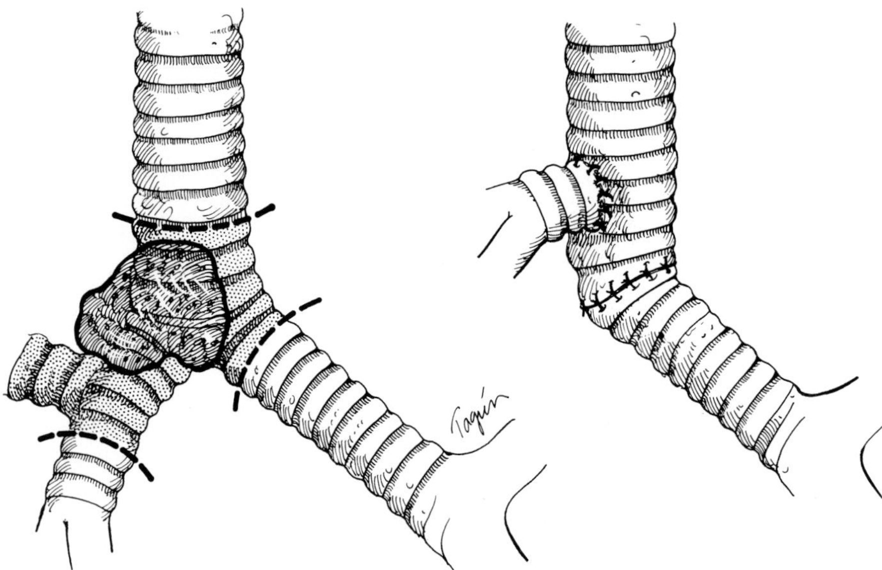

FIGURE 19–49 ■ Carina resection with right upper lobectomy. With mobilization, the bronchus intermedius is advanced to the side of the trachea and implanted above the anastomosis of the trachea and the left main bronchus.

frequency of bronchogenic carcinoma relative to other primary carinal neoplasms. Anastomosis is between the distal trachea and the left mainstem bronchus. The procedure is performed for tumors of the right lung that involve the carina and require pneumonectomy. The hilar structures are carefully dissected as for right pneumonectomy. The azygous vein is divided, and the distal trachea and left mainstem bronchus are encircled with tape.

Once it has been determined that resection is feasible, vascular structures are divided as for right pneumonectomy. Sterile tubing is passed from the operative field to the anesthesiologist to allow ventilation of the left lung across the operative field. Two midlateral traction sutures are placed proximally on the trachea and distally on the left mainstem bronchus. These sutures are 2–0 Vicryl and are placed full thickness and vertically 4 mm from the point of transection. The airway is then divided, and the oral endotracheal tube is pulled out of the way into the proximal trachea. The left mainstem bronchus is intubated with a sterile Tovell tube. Frozen section specimens are taken from the proximal and distal margins. With cervical flexion, the traction sutures are used to approximate the two ends tentatively to ensure that the airway can be reconstructed. A balance must be struck between the extent of resection for margin and the ability to reconstruct the airway. The pretracheal plane should have been dissected at mediastinoscopy, but if not, it can be done at this time. To improve mobility, the left mainstem can be dissected anteriorly, avoiding the lateral blood supply.

Once clear frozen-section margins have been confirmed, individual anastomotic sutures of 4–0 Vicryl are placed. The sutures are placed so the knots are on the outside 3 to 4 mm from the cut edge of the airway. The first suture is placed in the 6 o'clock position of airway as seen from the operative field. Individual sutures for the anastomosis are completed, the operating table is leveled, the patient's head is maximally flexed, the original oral tube is advanced carefully from above, and the traction sutures are drawn together and tied. The individ-

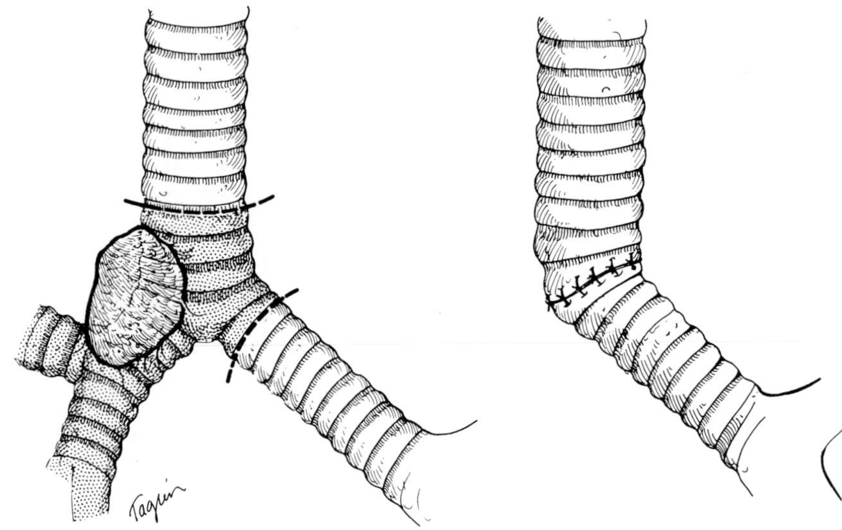

FIGURE 19–50 ■ Lung cancer involving carina. In this situation the right lung is involved. The right lung and carina are resected, and the trachea is anastomosed to the left main bronchus.

ual sutures are tied in the reverse order of that in which they were placed, so that the last suture to be tied is the first stitch in the 6 o'clock position.

Occasionally the oral endotracheal tube pushes against the left mainstem, distracting it and preventing approximation with the trachea. If this occurs, the tube is withdrawn and a high-frequency ventilation catheter is passed through the oral endotracheal tube across the anastomosis and into the left mainstem bronchus. High-frequency ventilation is terminated when the anastomosis is completed. The anastomosis is inspected through the oral endotracheal tube with a flexible bronchoscope. The anastomosis is checked to be certain it is airtight by flooding the operative field with saline and sustaining a breath at 30 or 40 cm H_2O. A superiorly based pericardial fat pad or a pleural flap is elevated and passed circumferentially around the anastomosis and secured to the airway with fine interrupted sutures. The pleural space is irrigated copiously, and a chest tube is placed to be managed as for a pneumonectomy.

When tumor involves the lower trachea and a large part of the left main bronchus, the problem becomes very difficult. When the left main bronchus is divided close to the bifurcation into the upper and lower lobes from beneath the aorta and the trachea cannot be brought down to that point, there is no way to advance the residual left main bronchus to a resected trachea. Perelman and Koroleva (1980) have managed this problem by stapling the left main bronchus distal to the tumor and reanastomosing the trachea to the right main bronchus. In 10 patients, they noted no difficulty with shunting or infection in the left lung; however, massive vascular shunting through the nonaerated left lung may occur, requiring left pneumonectomy. These authors now recommend ligation of the left pulmonary artery also. Bilateral anterolateral thoracotomy can be performed for tracheal resection, left pneumonectomy, and anastomosis of the trachea to the right main bronchus; however, such procedures produce major physiologic stresses.

In patients with involvement of most of the left main bronchus and very limited involvement of the carina, pneumonectomy and carinal resection can be performed from the left hemithorax. With flexion of the neck and with tapes placed around the lower trachea and the right main bronchus, it is possible to draw the airway up beneath the aortic arch and to place appropriate traction sutures, excise the carina, and anastomose the trachea to the right main bronchus. Exposure is difficult, and fortunately this approach is rarely required. Bilateral submammary transsternal thoracotomy, another approach giving better access, is suitable only for the fittest of patients. Prolonged mechanical ventilation can be anticipated.

Tumor recurrence in the stump following left pneumonectomy may require resection of the carina (Fig. 19–51). Resection is performed through the right chest, and ventilation is maintained in the right lung, working with the lung gently retracted and incompletely collapsed. High-frequency ventilation may be of value, and a great deal of understanding, patience, and cooperation must exist between the surgeon and the anesthesiologist. Recurrence in the stump following right pneumonectomy can be approached through the right chest. Dissection is difficult and mobility is reduced because of the associated fibrosis, but the procedure is applicable for selected patients.

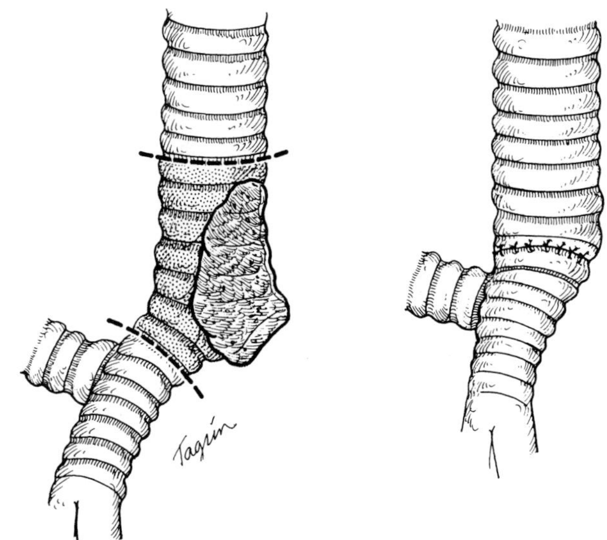

FIGURE 19–51 ■ Carinal resection after prior pneumonectomy. Except for one patient who had an abnormally long residual left main bronchial stump, these procedures were carried out through the right hemithorax.

Staged resections of the carina have been abandoned because of the excessive mortality and morbidity associated with these procedures. There is no uniformly dependable prosthesis for tracheal or carinal replacement.

POSTOPERATIVE CARE

Postoperative care begins in the operating room. The anesthesiologist must be constantly vigilant to clear secretions and blood from the airway in an aseptic manner. Fluids must be minimized to avoid fluid overload and subsequent pulmonary edema. It is always best to perform bronchoscopy at the completion of the procedure to remove any retained secretions and inspect the anastomosis.

Early postoperative management requires great attention to detail and dedication on the part of all involved. Adequate pain control is paramount and has been greatly facilitated by epidural analgesia, patient-controlled analgesia, and intercostal nerve blocks. Vigorous chest physiotherapy should be instituted early and often. Nasotracheal suction or direct aspiration with a flexible bronchoscope should be performed whenever needed. Minitracheotomy through the cricothyroid membrane with a small (4 French) cannula has greatly aided pulmonary toilet in some patients (Wain et al, 1990). Sputum cultures should be monitored daily and antibiotics adjusted accordingly.

Fluid and electrolyte management are crucial in the early postoperative period. A problem resembling the adult respiratory distress syndrome (ARDS) is the leading cause of early mortality in some series (Mathisen and Grillo, 1991). The etiology is still uncertain, with barotrauma, fluid overload, lymphatic dysfunction, or an inflammatory response from surgery being postulated. Early presentation has been with hypoxia, tachypnea, and a "ground glass" appearance on radiography of the remaining lung. It usually presents 36 to 72 hours postoperatively. Measures to treat it include intubation, diuresis, fluid restriction, broad-spectrum antibiotics, and frequent suctioning. The use of inhaled nitric oxide has shown promise in a small number of patients treated for post-pneumonectomy ARDS (Mathisen, 1998). Therapy must be instituted early along with other supportive measures. Radiographic and clinical response has been dramatic. Patients must be monitored for side effects, but to date few if any have been identified. ARDS has been fatal often despite all these measures.

Atrial arrhythmias are common, just as in patients undergoing conventional pneumonectomy. Digoxin and calcium channel blockers are indicated. (β-Blockers should be used with caution in this group of patients because of the limitations of pulmonary reserve.)

Patients should undergo bronchoscopy at about 1 week postoperatively to check the adequacy of healing. Any sign of early ischemia or necrosis must be followed very closely. Bronchopleural fistula must be treated with drainage and antibiotic coverage. If dehiscence and anastomotic separation occur, internal stenting is necessary with a long, custom-made Silastic T tube or a tracheostomy tube. Initial management may require a carefully placed long endotracheal tube. It may be necessary in these extreme situations to buttress the anastomosis with pedicled intercostal muscle or omentum. Delayed stenosis should be managed with dilatations or stenting. Re-resection is possible in some patients, but a sufficient period should elapse to allow resolution of inflammation and fibrosis. Anastomotic complications represent the leading cause of delayed mortality in most series.

There are many challenges in performing carinal resection. It remains a relatively uncommon surgical procedure, but experience is increasing. With this increased experience has come decreased operative mortality. Our own personal experience has seen the operative mortality reduced from 20% to 10% in the last half of our series (Mitchell, 1999). Others have reported no operative mortality in a small series (Roviaro, 1994). A better understanding of the safe limits of resection has undoubtedly contributed to the reduced mortality from anastomotic complications. The encouraging experience with nitric oxide for post-pneumonectomy ARDS may hold promise for this devastating complication following carinal resection. Reported survival rates for bronchogenic cancer involving the carina exceed 40% (Dartevelle, 1996; Mitchell, 2001). With operative mortality rates falling below 10% and survival rates improving, carinal resection remains an important surgical option in specific cases.

COMMENTS AND CONTROVERSIES

Grillo and Mathisen have accumulated and reported in detail the most extensive experience in the world with the difficult technical problem of carinal resection. The critical details of operative technique are clearly presented and illustrated, and include the practical features of perioperative care.

The only opinion with which I disagree is their perception that median sternotomy has "a limited role in some lesions involving the left mainstem and carina." I believe that median sternotomy may afford better access than thoracotomy in a significant number of appropriately selected cases. We reported our experience with median sternotomy for carinal resection for primary tumors of the trachea and carina in 1984 (Pearson, 1984). Median sternotomy was used in 7 of the 13 carinal resections and has since been utilized in more than half of the subsequent cases. Exposure of the carina and main bronchi through a median sternotomy requires a transpericardial approach. The anterior pericardium is divided vertically to permit mobilization of the aortic arch, which is then retracted laterally to the left. The superior vena cava is displaced laterally and to the right. The right main pulmonary artery is freed circumferentially and displaced inferiorly. The posterior pericardium is then divided vertically, and the entire mediastinal trachea and carina are clearly exposed and accessible. This technique of operative exposure has several distinct advantages over a right posterolateral thoracotomy in selected cases.

1. Any pulmonary resection is possible through a median sternotomy. Five of thirteen patients undergoing carinal resection required excision of the right main bronchus and right upper lobe. Two additional patients required a concomitant left pneumonectomy.

2. A cervical collar incision combined with a median sternotomy provides easy access for a superior laryngeal or suprahyoid release procedure, when required.

3. Median sternotomy also affords access for both a right and a left pulmonary hilar release (see Chapter 22).

Using this exposure, we performed a carinal resection on a 52-year-old male patient that included a 4-cm circumferential segment of distal trachea and 2.5 cm of the left main bronchus, followed by successful primary reconstruction. Mobilization included bilateral pulmonary hilar releases.

F. G. P.

REFERENCE

Pearson FG, Todd TRJ, Cooper JD: Experience with primary neoplasms of the trachea and carina. J Thorac Cardiovasc Surg 88:511, 1984.

KEY REFERENCES

Dartevelle PG, Chapelier A: Tracheal sleeve pneumonectomy for bronchogenic carcinoma: A report of 55 cases. Ann Thorac Surg 46:68, 1988.

This is a report of the largest series available on sleeve pneumonectomy for bronchogenic carcinoma. The results are excellent, with a very low operative mortality reported—10.9%.

Grillo HC: Carinal resection. Ann Thorac Surg 34:356, 1982.

This report describes a variety of techniques suitable for carinal resection. Detailed information on the different techniques is provided. Many etiologies other than lung cancer that require carinal resection and reconstruction are also included.

Jensik RJ, Faber LP, Milloy FJ, Goldin MD: Tracheal sleeve pneumonectomy for advanced carcinoma of the lung. Surg Gynecol Obstet 134:232, 1972.

This is a report of the first series of any significant number of patients undergoing sleeve pneumonectomy for carcinoma of the lung. The authors describe in detail their results, their techniques, complications, mortality, and long-term results.

Mathisen DJ, Grillo HC: Carinal resection for bronchogenic carcinoma. J Thorac Cardiovasc Surg 102:16, 1991.

This contemporary report of the authors' experience with carinal resection for bronchogenic carcinoma includes techniques other than sleeve pneumonectomy. This represents one of the few series to include procedures of re-creation of the carina and carinal resection plus right upper lobectomy for cancer.

Mitchell JD, Mathisen DJ, Wright CD et al: Clinical experience with carinal resection. J Thorac Cardiovasc Surg 117:39, 1999.

Mitchell JD, Mathisen DJ, Wright CD et al: Resection for bronchogenic carcinoma involving the carina: Long-term results and effect of nodal status on outcome. J Thorac Cardiovasc Surg 121:465, 2001.

Wilson RS: Tracheal resection. In Marshall BE, Longnecker DE, Fairley HB (eds): Anesthesia for Thoracic Procedures. Boston, Blackwell, 1988.

This is an excellent reference on anesthetic techniques for thoracic procedures in general and for carinal resections in particular. Several techniques are described, all of which should be well known to those working in the area of carinal resection and reconstruction.

■ *REFERENCES*

Abbott OA: Experiences with the surgical resection of the human carina, tracheal wall, and contralateral bronchial wall in cases of right total pneumonectomy. J Thorac Cardiovasc Surg 19:906, 1950.

Barclay RS, McSwan N, Welsh TM: Tracheal resection without the use of grafts. Thorax 12: 177, 1957.

Belsey R: Resection and reconstruction of the intrathoracic trachea. Br J Surg 38:200, 1946.

Dartevelle P, Macchiarini P: Carinal pneumonectomy for bronchogenic carcinoma. Semin Thorac Cardiovasc Surg 8:414, 1996.

Deslauriers J: Involvement of the main carina. In Delarue NC, Eschapasse H (eds): International Trends in General Thoracic Surgery, Vol 1. Philadelphia, WB Saunders, 1985.

El-Baz J, Jensik R, Faber LP, Faro RS: One-lung high-frequency ventilation of tracheoplasty and bronchoplasty: A new technique. Ann Thorac Surg 34:564, 1982.

Eschapasse H: Les tumeurs tracheales primitives. Traitement chirurgical. Rev Fr Mal Respir 2:425, 1974.

Grillo HC, Bendixen HH, Gephart T: Resection of the carina and lower trachea. Ann Surg 158:889, 1963.

Jensik RJ, Faber JP, Kittle CF et al: Survival in patients undergoing tracheal sleeve pneumonectomy for bronchogenic carcinoma. J Thorac Cardiovasc Surg 84:489, 1982.

Juvenelle A, Citret C: Transplantation de la bronche souche et résection de la bifurcation tracheale. J Chir (Paris) 67:666, 1951.

Mathey J, Binet JP, Galey JJ et al.: Tracheal tracheobronchial resection. J Thorac Cardiovasc Surg 51:1, 1966.

Mathisen DJ, Grillo HC: Endoscopic relief of malignant airway obstruction. Ann Thorac Surg 48:469, 1989.

Mathisen DJ, Grillo HC, Vlahakes GJ, Daggett WM: The omentum in the management of complicated cardiothoracic problems. J Thorac Cardiovasc Surg 95:677, 1988.

Mathisen DJ, Kuo EY, Hahn C et al: Inhaled nitric oxide for ARDS following pulmonary resection. Ann Thorac Surg 65:1894, 1998.

Newton JR Grillo HC, Mathisen DJ: Main bronchial sleeve resection with pulmonary conservation. Ann Thorac Surg 52:1272, 1991.

Perelman MI: Surgery of the trachea. Moscow, Moscow Mir 1976.

Perelman M, Koroleva N: Surgery of the trachea. World J Surg 4:583, 1980.

Roviaro GC, Varoli F, Rebuffat C et al: Tracheal sleeve pneumonectomy for bronchogenic carcinoma. J Thorac Cardiovasc Surg 107:13, 1994.

Shapshay SM, Dumon JF, Beamis JF: Endoscopic treatment of tracheobronchial malignancy: Experience with the Nd:YAG and CO_2 lasers in 506 operations. Otolaryngol Head Neck Surg 93:205, 1985.

Tsuchiya R, Goya T, Naruke T, Suemasu K: Resection of tracheal carina for lung cancer. J Thorac Cardiovasc Surg 99:941, 1990.

Wain JC, Wilson DJ, Mathisen DJ: Clinical experience with minitracheostomy. Ann Thorac Surg 49:881, 1990.

Lung

CHAPTER 20

Anatomy of the Lung

Thomas W. Rice

HISTORICAL NOTE

Graham and Singer (1933) reported the first successful pneumonectomy for therapy for bronchogenic carcinoma. The left pneumonectomy was performed by mass ligation of the pulmonary hilum. Although it was not the first pulmonary resection, this landmark procedure marked the beginning of modern thoracic surgery. Mass ligation became a curiosity, however, and careful identification and precise control of the individual structures of the pulmonary hilum, lobes, and segments was soon considered standard procedure. Recognition and preservation of the pulmonary arterial supply, the pulmonary venous drainage, and the bronchial anatomy permit conservation of the parenchyma. This is the cornerstone of pulmonary surgery.

HISTORICAL READING

Graham EA, Singer JJ: Successful removal of an entire lung for carcinoma of the bronchus. JAMA 101:1371, 1933.

BRONCHOPULMONARY SEGMENT

The anatomic and surgical unit of the lung is the bronchopulmonary segment. A review of pulmonary embryology is helpful for understanding this pulmonary element and the congenital abnormalities of the lung bud (i.e., congenital lobar emphysema, cystic adenomatoid malformation, pulmonary sequestration, and bronchogenic cyst. The lung develops from a foregut bud with continual branching of the principal structures. The lung bud is first seen in the embryo at 3 weeks. In the fourth week, the branching begins with the growth of the right and left main bronchi. Further development is asymmetric, principally because of the absorption of the left eparterial bud. Rapid growth of the airway by terminal branching ensues. By the 17th week, 70% of the airway has been formed. The alveoli appear between 20 and 24 weeks in utero.

The pulmonary vascular plexus and venous drainage originate from the splanchnic plexus, which is carried with the developing lung buds. The pulmonary arteries arise from the sixth aortic arch as bilateral buds. These grow into the lung and connect with the developing pulmonary plexus. On the right, absorption of the dorsal sixth aortic arch bud allows the potential separation of the pulmonary from the systemic vasculature. On the left, persistence and growth of the dorsal bud and its connection to the ventral bud form the fetal and neonatal communication between the pulmonary and systemic vascular circuits—the ductus arteriosus.

The repetitive branching of the airway and vasculature allows the evolution of independent lung units. Bronchopulmonary segments are subdivisions of the lung that function as individual units because they possess their own bronchus, pulmonary arterial supply, and venous drainage. Each segment may be individually removed without disturbing the function of adjacent segments if the bronchovascular anatomy is appreciated and precisely controlled. The bronchial anatomy of the segment is most constant. The pulmonary artery accompanies the bronchus but has a more variable pattern. The pulmonary veins do not accompany the artery and bronchus in the center of the bronchopulmonary segment but run in the intersegmental planes. Pulmonary veins drain adjacent segments and mark the boundaries of this anatomic unit (Fig. 20–1). Ramsey (1949) emphasized the importance of the venous drainage pattern of the bronchopulmonary segments. Appreciation of the venous drainage is crucial in the identification of the segment and the successful completion of a segmental or lobar resection.

The right lung, which is the larger of the two lungs, has three lobes: upper, middle, and lower. The right major fissure runs obliquely along the lateral surface of the lung from a superior and posterior position to an inferior and anterior position. The major fissure separates the lower lobe from the upper and middle lobes. The minor fissure, which is less well developed, runs horizontally to separate the upper lobe from the middle lobe. The right lung is composed of 10 segments (Fig. 20–2). The upper lobe has three segments: apical, posterior, and anterior. The middle lobe has two segments: lateral and medial. The lower lobe has five segments: superior, medial basal, anterior basal, lateral basal, and posterior basal.

The left lung has two lobes: upper and lower. The

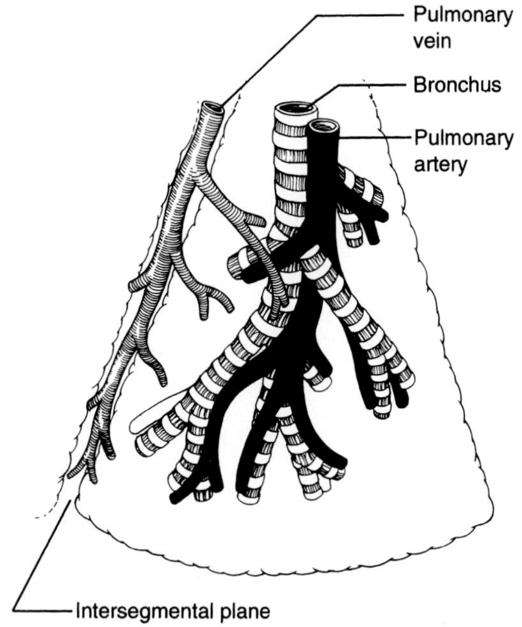

FIGURE 20–1 ■ The bronchopulmonary segment.

lingula, which is the anatomic equivalent of the middle lobe, is part of the left upper lobe. The left major fissure runs obliquely along the lateral surface of the lung from a superior and posterior position to an inferior and anterior position. The major fissure separates the upper lobe from the lower lobe. The left lung is composed of eight segments (see Fig. 20–2). The upper lobe has four segments: apical posterior, anterior, superior (lingular), and inferior (lingular). The lower lobe has four segments: superior, anteromedial basal, lateral basal, and posterior basal. Fewer segments exist in the left lung because of sharing of the segmental bronchi by subsegmental bronchopulmonary units, which in the right lung are segments. The apical and posterior segments of the right upper lobe correspond to one segment in the left upper lobe where these two subsegments share a common segmental bronchus (apical posterior). Similarly, the anterior basal and medial basal subsegments of the left lower lobe share the common anteromedial basal segmental bronchus. This variation is of greatest interest at bronchoscopy. At surgery, these subsegments can be dissected; this may be useful in surgery of the left upper lobe but is generally not advantageous in the left lower lobe.

Anomalies of lobation are usually the result of too few or too many fissures. Absences or incomplete development of the major or minor fissures cause fusion of adjacent lobes. Accessory fissures correspond to the planes of division between bronchopulmonary segments and account for many of the previously reported accessory lobes. The cardiac lobe is the medial basal segment of the lower lobe, which is demarcated by an intersegmental fissure. Similarly, the superior segment in the lower lobe and the lingula in the upper lobe can be separated by an accessory fissure. Accessory lobes are seen in two cases. If no bronchial communication exists,

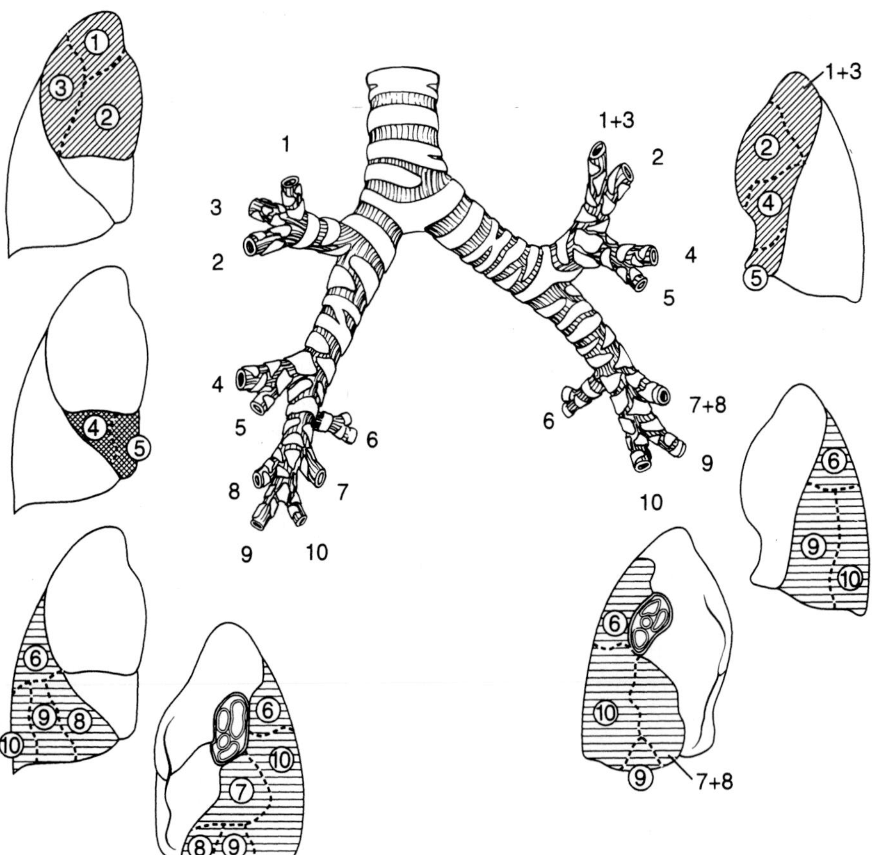

FIGURE 20–2 ■ The lobes and segments of the lung. Right upper lobe segments: 1, apical; 2, anterior; 3, posterior. Right middle lobe segments: 4, lateral; 5, medial. Right lower lobe segments: 6, superior; 7, medial basal; 8, anterior basal; 9, lateral basal; 10, posterior basal. Left upper lobe segments: 1 and 3, apical posterior; 2, anterior; 4, superior (lingular); 5, inferior (lingular). Left lower lobe segments: 6, superior; 7 and 8, anteromedial basal; 9, lateral basal; 10, posterior basal.

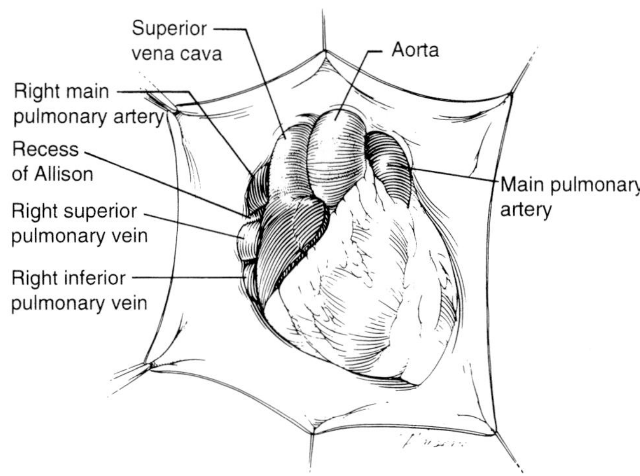

FIGURE 20–3 ■ The right intrapericardial anatomy.

these accessory lobes are really extralobar sequestrations. Rarely, an accessory lobe has a bronchial connection; this is seen in the tracheal lobe. This lobe is the apical segment of the right upper lobe with a tracheal origin of the segmental bronchus. Agenesis or aplasia of the lung results from maldevelopment of the lung bud.

INTRAPERICARDIAL ANATOMY

The control of the pulmonary vessels within the pericardium was first advocated by Allison (1946) and further refined by Healey and Gibbon (1950). The ability to control the pulmonary vasculature within the pericardium is crucial for lung transplantation, for the resection of central tumors and tumors with hilar invasion, and for the management of distal vascular problems in which proximal control is required. The serous pericardium reflects onto the pulmonary vessels, as they originate within or enter the fibrous pericardial sac and must be divided to mobilize these vessels. The lack of complete pericardial investage sometimes obscures the vessel and may make identification and mobilization difficult.

The pulmonary trunk arises from the infundibulum of the right ventricle and, at its origin, overlies the aorta. It then passes to the left and rises superiorly and posteriorly for about 4 to 6 cm. It is contained in the serous pericardium with the aorta. In this position, it lies between the right and left atria. Below the aortic arch, it bifurcates into the right and left main pulmonary arteries.

The right main pulmonary artery (Fig. 20–3) arises from the main pulmonary artery to pass transversely posterior to the aorta and superior vena cava. More than three fourths of its length is within the pericardial sac. Behind the aorta and superior vena cava, this artery constitutes the superior border of the transverse sinus. It is covered by serous pericardium for more than three fourths of its circumference. Its posterior surface is directly applied to the fibrous pericardium and is not covered by serous pericardium. The pulmonary artery may be safely controlled in this location by retracting the aorta medially and the superior vena cava laterally. After the right pulmonary artery is mobilized, it may be retracted, and division of the posterior fibrous pericardium provides transpericardial access to the trachea and main bronchi. As the right pulmonary artery passes from behind the vena cava, it exits the pericardial sac. In this position, it forms the superior border of the postcaval recess of Allison. The medial border is the superior vena cava; the inferior border is the superior pulmonary vein; and the lateral border is the pericardial sac. In about 5% of patients, there is no postcaval recess. The right pulmonary artery exits the pericardial sac when it is still in the retrocaval position.

The right superior pulmonary vein enters the pericardium and is covered by serous pericardium for more than two thirds of its circumference. It immediately drains into the left atrium. The right inferior pulmonary vein is covered by serous pericardium over only one third of its circumference, and total lack of this covering in half of patients with lung disease makes it appear that the right inferior pulmonary vein has no intrapericardial component. Mobilization of the inferior pulmonary vein's short, stubby, pericardial attachments and division of the frenulum of pericardium that runs to the inferior vena cava provide additional mobility of the hilum. This maneuver is sometimes required during intrathoracic tracheobronchial resections for the relief of tension at the airway anastomosis. The vein then drains into the left atrium. On the right, a common pulmonary vein is found in about 3% of patients. The junction between the right and left atria lies just anterior to the termination of the right pulmonary veins. Additional pulmonary venous length may be obtained by dissection within the (developing) intra-atrial groove.

The left pulmonary artery (Fig. 20–4) arises from the main pulmonary artery and passes inferiorly and posteriorly before exiting the pericardium from under the aortic arch. As it leaves the pericardial sac, half of its circumference is covered by serous pericardium; this

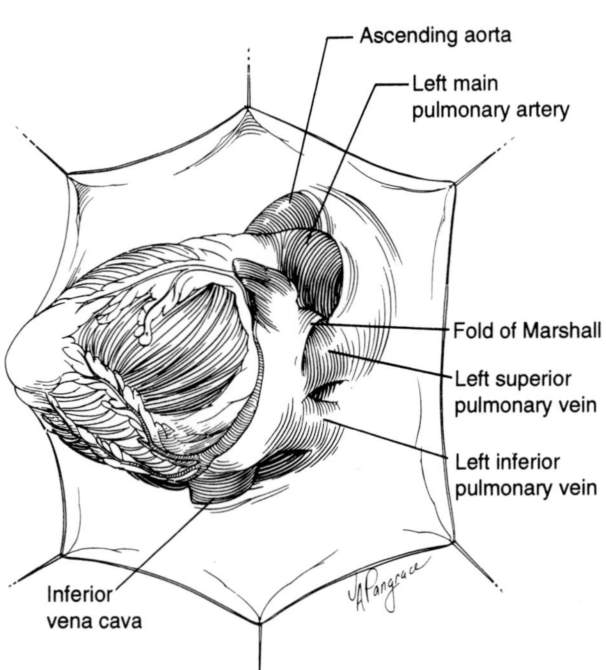

FIGURE 20–4 ■ The left intrapericardial anatomy.

must be divided to control the pulmonary artery at this point. The left pulmonary recess is bordered by the left main pulmonary artery superiorly, the left superior pulmonary vein inferiorly, and the fibrous pericardium laterally. The medial border is the fold of Marshall, which contains the remnant of the left superior vena cava. This is patent in less than 1% of patients and may be divided to provide improved intrapericardial access to the left main pulmonary artery and left superior pulmonary vein.

The left superior pulmonary vein enters the pericardium to be covered by serous pericardium on two thirds of its circumference. Immediately below and inferior to this is the left inferior pulmonary vein. This vein is the most distinct and free of all the pulmonary vessels, with 90% of its circumference covered by serous pericardium. Unlike the pulmonary veins on the right, about 25% of patients have a common left pulmonary vein within the pericardium.

Anomalies of the pulmonary arteries and pulmonary veins may be classified as abnormalities of number or of site of origin or termination. Aberrations of the main pulmonary artery are typically accompanied by anomalies of the heart and great vessels. Main pulmonary artery anomalies are uncommon and consist of agenesis, hypoplasia, or abnormal origin and cause vascular rings that result in airway and esophageal compression. Accessory pulmonary arteries may arise from the aorta or its branches. This is usually seen in pulmonary sequestrations or pulmonary atresia with ventricular septal defect, but it may occur without associated disease. Anomalies of pulmonary veins are more common. An abnormal number of veins is seen most frequently as a common left pulmonary vein or as separate veins that drain the upper, middle, and lower lobes on the right. Anomalous pulmonary venous drainage can be partial or complete. The veins typically drain into the superior vena cava, right atrium, coronary sinus, inferior vena cava, persistent left vena cava, or systemic veins.

HILUM

The principal structures passing to and from the lung at the mediastinal border are the bronchus, the pulmonary artery, and the superior and inferior pulmonary veins, which constitute the pulmonary hilum. The lung is fixed centrally by the hilum and the inferior pulmonary ligament. The inferior pulmonary ligament is the reflection of the inferior mediastinal parietal pleura onto the lung, where it envelops the inferior pulmonary vein. On both sides, the hilum is subtended by a vascular arch: on the right by the azygos vein and on the left by the aortic arch. The hilum is bordered by nerves and systemic vessels: the phrenic nerve and its vascular bundle anteriorly and the vagus nerve and bronchial vessels posteriorly.

The right main bronchus is the most superior and posterior of the right hilar structures and passes into the hilum after exiting the mediastinum below the azygos vein (Fig. 20–5). The right pulmonary artery exits the pericardium behind the superior vena cava and enters the hilum. In the right hilum, the right pulmonary artery lies inferiorly and anteriorly to the bronchus, partially

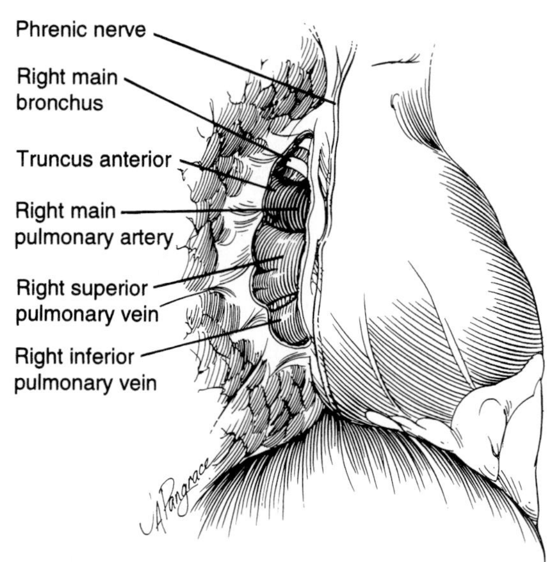

FIGURE 20–5 ■ The right hilar anatomy, anterior view.

obscuring the bronchus. The truncus anterior, the first branch of the right pulmonary artery, originates from the pulmonary artery before it enters the lung. The superior pulmonary vein passes from the pulmonary parenchyma to lie anterior to the pulmonary artery and slightly below the truncus anterior branch of the right pulmonary artery. Here, it overlaps and obscures the intraparenchymal continuation of the pulmonary artery, the pars intralobares. The superior pulmonary vein receives four component branches. Three branches drain the upper lobe, and three are superficial. The most superior is the apical anterior vein; just below this is the inferior vein, which drains the inferior surface of the anterior segment. Entering the vein deep from the pulmonary parenchyma and from its posterior aspect is the posterior vein, which principally drains the posterior segment of the right upper lobe. The most inferior venous tributary is the middle lobe vein. The inferior pulmonary vein lies posterior and inferior to the superior pulmonary vein. It comprises two tributaries: the superior and common basal branches. Lying anterior to the hilum on the superior vena cava and pericardium is the right phrenic nerve.

The posterior right hilum (Fig. 20–6) is bordered superiorly by the azygos vein. The short membranous portion of the right main bronchus passes from under the arch of the azygos vein to terminate as the right upper lobe bronchus and the bronchus intermedius. Lying inferior and posterior to the bronchus intermedius is the inferior pulmonary vein. The superior branch of the inferior pulmonary vein, which drains the superior segment of the right lower lobe, is best identified posteriorly. The esophagus and right vagus nerve lie immediately posterior to the right hilum. Lying behind these structures is the azygos vein, which arches over the right main bronchus just above the origin of the right upper lobe. The most constant position of the thoracic duct in the thoracic cavity is inferior to the right hilum (Fig. 20–7). Here, in its supradiaphragmatic location, it can be found between the azygos vein and aorta, bordered anteriorly by the esophagus and posteriorly by the vertebral column.

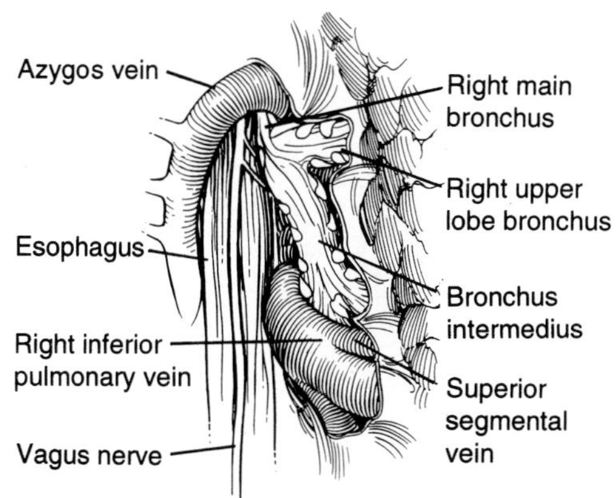

FIGURE 20–6 ■ The right hilar anatomy, posterior view.

The left main bronchus is 4 to 6 cm long and passes under the aortic arch to lie posteriorly in the hilum. Unlike the right side, where the bronchus remains the most posterior structure, on entering the lung on the left, the left main bronchus is sandwiched between the superior pulmonary vein anteriorly, the pulmonary artery superiorly and posteriorly, and the inferior pulmonary vein inferiorly.

The left pulmonary artery (Fig. 20–8) is the most anterior superior structure in the left pulmonary hilum. The ligamentum arteriosum is found as the pulmonary artery exits the pericardium. This is the remnant of the ductus arteriosus, which connects the aortic arch to the left pulmonary artery in utero. At this point, the left recurrent laryngeal nerve loops around the aorta at the lateral margin of the ligamentum arteriosum (Fig. 20–9). The pulmonary artery leaves the pericardium and passes over the left main bronchus. The first branch of the artery, the truncus anterior, which supplies the anterior segment of the left upper lobe, originates before the pulmonary artery passes around the left upper lobe bronchus to enter the left lung posteriorly. The superior pulmonary vein lies anterior and inferior to the pulmonary artery and is composed of three draining veins: apical posterior, anterior, and lingular. The inferior pulmonary vein lies inferior and posterior to the superior pulmonary vein and is found at the apex of the pulmonary ligament.

The posterior left hilum (Fig. 20–10) consists of the pulmonary artery superiorly, the left main bronchus, and the inferior pulmonary vein inferiorly. The esophagus and left vagus nerve lie immediately posterior to the left pulmonary hilum. The descending thoracic aorta lies behind these structures.

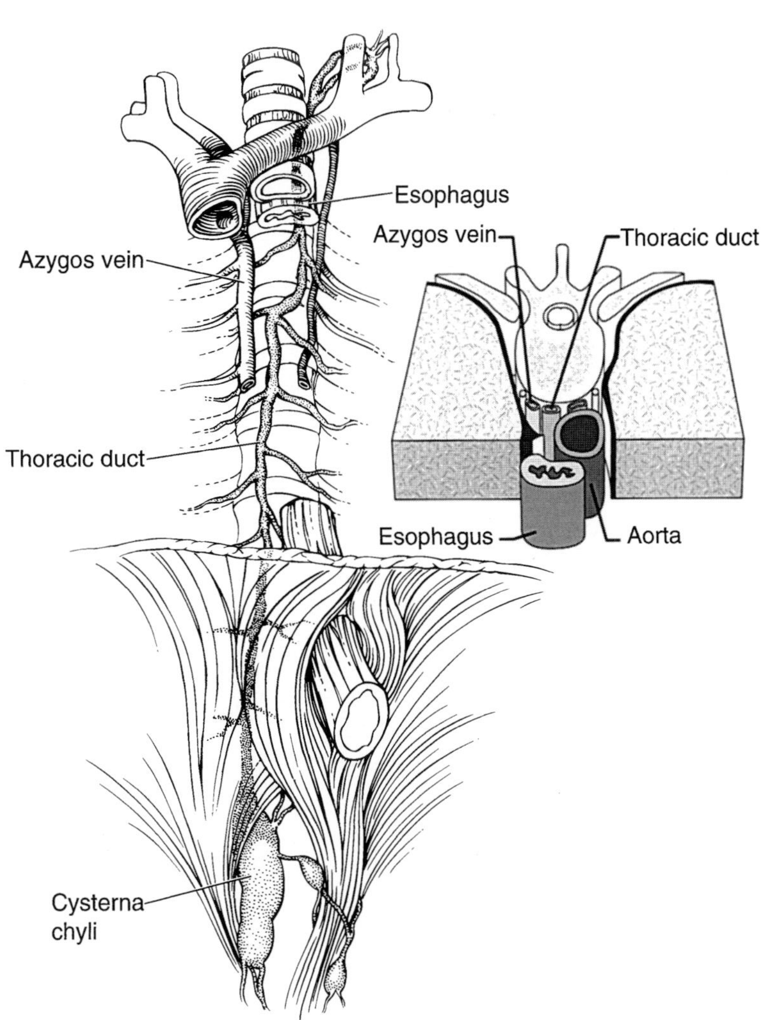

FIGURE 20–7 ■ The course and relationship of the thoracic duct.

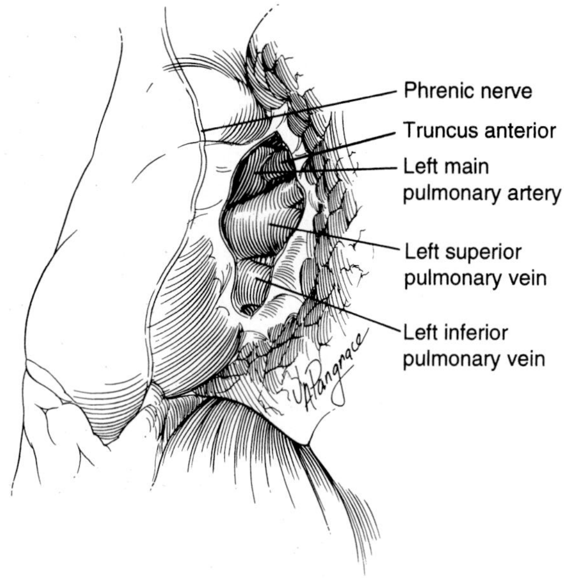

FIGURE 20–8 ■ The left hilar anatomy, anterior view.

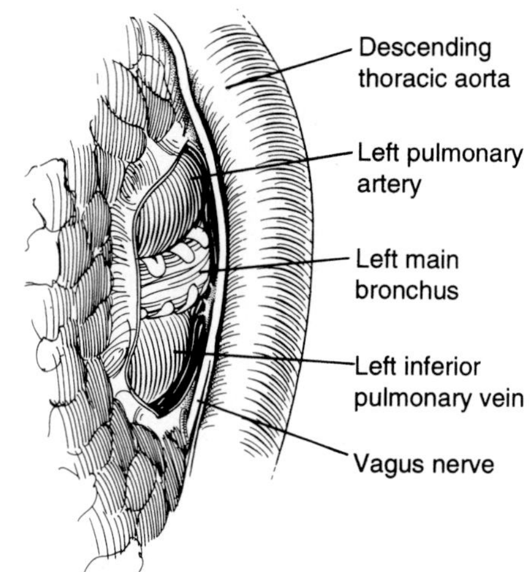

FIGURE 20–10 ■ The left hilar anatomy, posterior view.

RIGHT UPPER LOBE

The right upper lobe bronchus (previously called the *eparterial bronchus*) arises from the lateral wall of the right main bronchus immediately after the origin of the right main bronchus from the trachea. The bronchus passes at right angles to the right main bronchus and bronchus intermedius to enter the right upper lobe. The anomalies of the right upper lobe bronchus have been outlined by le Roux (1962). The origin of the right upper lobe bronchus is anomalous in 3% of patients. The most common bronchial anomaly of the right upper lobe is the origin of the apical segmental bronchus from the trachea (tracheal bronchus) or right main bronchus, which is reported in 1.4% of patients. Absence of a true right upper lobe bronchus with immediate division into the segmental bronchi is seen in 1.1% of patients. The entire right upper lobe bronchus may originate from the trachea in 0.5% of patients.

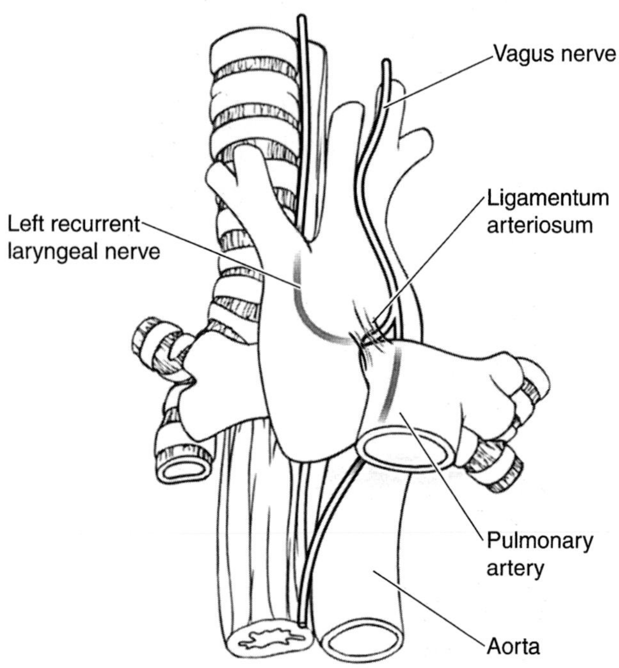

FIGURE 20–9 ■ The course and relationship of the left vagus and left recurrent laryngeal nerves.

The pulmonary arterial supply of the right upper lobe arises from two main branches: the truncus anterior branch, which originates in the hilum, and the ascending branches, which originate within the pulmonary parenchyma. The variations of the pulmonary artery anatomy of the right upper lobe are well outlined by Milloy and colleagues (1963). The truncus anterior is the first and largest branch of the right pulmonary artery. It usually bifurcates after traveling for about 1 cm. In 3.6% of patients, the anterior trunk is split, and two small branches arise separately from the main pulmonary artery. Rarely, the anterior trunk has three branches. The truncus anterior is found in all patients. In 10% of patients, the truncus anterior is the only arterial supply of the right upper lobe.

The ascending branches of the right upper lobe originate from the pulmonary artery after it enters the pulmonary parenchyma. These branches ascend to enter the inferior surface of the right upper lobe. In 90% of patients, there is an ascending arterial contribution. In 60% of patients, there is one branch; in 29%, two branches; and in 1%, three ascending branches. The ascending artery may be a posterior ascending branch that supplies the posterior segment of the right upper lobe. This is the most common ascending artery and is seen in 88% of patients with ascending arteries. This artery arises from the lateral and posterior aspect of the pulmonary artery, opposite the middle lobe branch, and it lies anterior to the junction of the inferior margin of the upper lobe bronchus and the bronchus intermedius. In 12% of patients, this artery originates from a common trunk with the superior segmental artery. The anterior ascending artery is seen in 25% of patients and supplies a portion of the anterior segment of the right upper lobe. It arises from the lateral aspect of the pulmonary artery opposite the middle lobe branch. Ninety-nine percent of these arterial branches are single, and only 1% arise from a common trunk with the middle lobe artery.

The superior pulmonary vein drains both the upper and middle lobes. It is crucial during a right upper lobectomy to identify and preserve the middle lobe vein. The venous drainage of the upper lobe is variable but usually consists of three venous tributaries: the apical anterior, the inferior, and the posterior veins.

The azygous lobe is the major anomaly in the segmentation of the right upper lobe, and it is seen in less than 1% of patients. It is not a supernumerary lobe but instead is a segregated portion of the right upper lobe. As such, it does not have an individual or anomalous bronchovascular supply. The azygous lobe is associated with the azygos vein, which has a long, dangling mesentery; this accessory lobe is formed medial to the pleural septation of the azygos vein.

RIGHT MIDDLE LOBE

The bronchus intermedius is the continuing right bronchus after the origin of the right upper lobe. It is 2 to 4 cm long and terminates at the origin of the middle and lower lobe bronchi. The middle lobe bronchus is on average 1.8 cm long. Generally, the bronchus bifurcates to form the two segmental bronchi; rarely (in 3% of patients), a bifurcate bronchus is seen (Boyden and Hamre, 1951).

An analysis of 225 specimens by Wragg and associates (1968) demonstrated that the pulmonary arterial supply of the middle lobe is from one artery in 46.5% of patients. It usually arises as the first branch of the pars intralobares after the origin of the truncus anterior. It originates from the anterior and medial surface of the pulmonary artery at the level of the ascending branch of the upper lobe. More commonly (in 51.5% of patients), the middle lobe is supplied by two arteries. This second artery arises, in 48.5% of patients, from the pulmonary artery at the level of and opposite to the branch to the superior segment of the right lower lobe. This second branch arises from the ascending branch of the right upper lobe in 0.5% of patients and from a common trunk with a basal segmental artery in 2.5% of patients. Rarely (in 2% of patients), three branches supply the middle lobe.

The middle lobe vein joins the upper lobe vein to form the superior pulmonary vein. Lindskrog and associates (1949) demonstrated that in most patients (64%), the two segmental veins join to form the middle lobe vein. In 36% of patients, the two segmental veins terminate separately at the superior pulmonary vein.

RIGHT LOWER LOBE

The segmental bronchi of the right lower lobe arise with the middle lobe bronchus at the termination of the bronchus intermedius. The superior segmental bronchus originates from the posterior and lateral aspect of the bronchus intermedius, usually opposite or slightly above the middle lobe bronchus. In 6% of patients, the superior segmental bronchus arises as two separate orifices that are 6 to 10 mm apart (Ferry and Boyden, 1951). Below these are the four basal segmental bronchi of the right lower lobe. Usually, the medial basal segmental bronchus is the most proximal basal branch. The anterior basal bronchus is next, and then a common stem for the lateral basal and posterior basal bronchi is usually seen. The middle lobe bronchus must be protected during right lower lobectomy. The abrupt termination of the bronchus intermedius into the middle lobe bronchus and superior and basal segmental bronchi makes compromise of the middle bronchial lobe bronchus a distinct possibility if the lower lobe segmental bronchi are taken en masse. Identification of all three bronchi and separate control of the superior segmental and basal segmental bronchi minimize this complication.

Wragg and associates (1968) provided the largest modern description of the arterial supply of the right lower lobe. In 78% of patients, the superior segment of the right lower lobe is supplied by a single arterial branch. Two branches to the superior segment are seen in 21% of patients. Rarely (in less than 1% of patients), three branches to this segment are found. Branches to the segment may be displaced in their origin or arise as common trunks, either from the ascending branch of the upper lobe or from the basal segmental arteries of the lower lobe. Twelve percent to 14% of arterial branches to the superior segment may arise from a common branch with the ascending branch of the upper lobe. In 6% of patients, the superior segmental artery may arise from a basal segmental artery. The basal segmental arterial supply is variable, but generally this artery, which lies posterolateral to the bronchus, sends branches to the anterior basal and medial basal segments. The pulmonary artery then terminates by division into the lateral basal and posterior basal segmental arteries.

The inferior pulmonary vein usually consists of two segmental tributaries: the superior and the common basal veins. Generally, the common basal vein is composed of two major veins: the superior basal vein (which drains the medial basal, anterior basal, and lateral basal segments) and the inferior basal vein (which usually drains the lateral basal and posterior basal segments). One third of patients may have three and four branches of the common basal vein. Rarely, venous drainage is received from the posterior segment of the right upper lobe or from the middle lobe.

LEFT UPPER LOBE

The left main bronchus, which is 4 to 6 cm long, passes at an oblique angle under the aortic arch and bifurcates to form the upper and lower lobe bronchi. The left upper lobe bronchus, which originates much lower than does the right upper lobe bronchus, bifurcates almost immediately, forming the lingular orifice and the common bronchus to the anterior and apical posterior segments.

The pulmonary arterial supply of the left upper lobe is the most variable of all lobes. In an analysis of 300 specimens, Milloy and colleagues (1968) provided the most complete description of the left upper lobe arterial supply. The number of branches varies from one to eight. In 46% of patients, three branches supply the left upper lobe, and in 36%, four branches are found. The arterial branches arise as two groups: the truncus anterior and the posterior arterial branches, which originate in the fissure along the inner curve of the pulmonary artery.

The truncus anterior is large, short, and partially hidden by the superior pulmonary vein. It is the origin of a hidden deep branch to the anterior or lingular segments in one fourth of patients and is frequently invaded by large left upper lobe tumors. All these factors make mobilization of the truncus anterior hazardous and lead surgeons to refer to the truncus anterior as the "artery of sorrow." In less than 1% of patients, the truncus anterior is the only arterial supply of the left upper lobe. In about 70% of patients, two branches of the anterior trunk are present and, in near-equal proportions, one or three branches. In most patients, the apical posterior and anterior segments are supplied by this branch (62.3%). In 8% of patients, the anterior and lingular segments are supplied by this branch. In 15.6% of patients, three branches of this artery supply all segments of the left upper lobe. In 13.9% of patients, only one branch is seen, supplying variably the apical posterior or anterior segments.

The remaining blood supply of the left upper lobe comes from the posterior segmental arteries. These arteries arise along the inner curve of the pulmonary artery, in the fissure as it wraps around the left upper lobe bronchus. These vessels pass into the posterior aspect of the left upper lobe. There may be zero to five posterior artery branches. In 65% of patients, no common trunks are seen. In 35% of patients, however, common trunks of these posterior branches are found. In 5% of patients, there is only one posterior branch to the left upper lobe; in 46%, two; in 36%, three; in 12%, four; and in 1%, five posterior branches. The segmental arterial supply to the left upper lobe is variable, with anterior and lingular segments receiving one to three branches. The apical posterior segment may receive as many as four separate branches.

The venous drainage of the left upper lobe is similarly divergent. The superior pulmonary vein may receive two major branches, three major branches, or a number of radiating veins. Generally, it is the terminus of the anterior, apical posterior, and lingular veins; however, these veins may have multiple branches. Because the vein lies anterior to the pulmonary artery, all except its deep branches may be appreciated in the anterior dissection of the hilum.

LEFT LOWER LOBE

The lower lobe bronchus arises with the upper lobe bronchus at the termination of the left main bronchus. The first segmental branch, the superior segmental bronchus, originates posteriorly and laterally. In less than 1% of patients, it has a bifurcate origin. About 1 to 2 cm beyond this, the common basal trunk is found. In 80% of patients, it immediately bifurcates; in the remainder, it branches into the three segmental bronchi (Pitel and Boyden, 1953).

The arterial supply of the left lower lobe is derived solely from arteries arising in the fissure. The superior segment of the lower lobe is supplied by a single artery in 72% of patients (Wragg et al, 1968). In 26% of patients, two superior segmental arteries are found. In 2% of patients, three arteries supply the superior segment. These arteries usually arise directly from the pulmonary artery; however, in less than 3% of patients, one may originate from a common trunk with a posterior artery of the left upper lobe. In as many as 12% of patients, a common trunk with a basal segmental artery is found. The frequency of a shared trunk with a basal segmental artery is similar for the superior segments of both the right and left lower lobes. A common trunk with an upper lobe artery is seen more commonly on the right.

The basal segmental artery is the termination of the left pulmonary artery after the origin of the superior segmental and lingular branches. In about half of patients, the artery bifurcates to supply the anteromedial segment and the combination of the posterior and lateral segments. In the remaining patients, the branching varies and ranges from two to four segmental branches.

The venous drainage of the left lower lobe is similar to that of the right lower lobe. The inferior pulmonary vein receives two major branches: the superior segmental and the common basal veins.

FISSURES

The relationship of the bronchovascular structures of the lobes and segments is best appreciated by describing their relationship during control of the fissures.

Right Major Fissure

The pulmonary artery may be palpated at the confluence of the major and minor fissures (Fig. 20–11). Dissection of the pulmonary parenchyma permits the pulmonary artery to be identified in its interlobar position. The posterior branch of the superior pulmonary vein commonly runs in this interlobar plane and may overlay and obscure the pulmonary artery. In addition, an interlobar lymph node (R11), commonly referred to as the *sump node*, is found overlying the pulmonary artery. After identification of the pars intralobares, the branches of the pulmonary artery in this area may be mobilized. They are identified as follows: anteriorly, the superior branch of the middle lobe; posteriorly and superiorly, the posterior ascending branch of the right upper lobe; posteriorly and inferiorly, the superior segmental arterial branch of the right lower lobe; and inferiorly, the bifurcating termination of the pulmonary artery supplying the basal segments. Dissection in the notch between the posterior ascending and superior segmental arterial branches allows the identification of a posterior interlobar lymph node (R11; see Fig. 20–11*A*).

Next, the hilum is approached posteriorly, and the angle between the inferior margin of the right upper lobe bronchus and the bronchus intermedius is dissected (see Fig. 20–11*B*). In this notch between the bronchi, the posterior aspect of the posterior interlobar lymph node is seen. The posterior superior portion of the major fissure may be controlled if the posterior interlobar lymph node is mobilized and the posterior dissection around the bronchi is then connected to the posterior

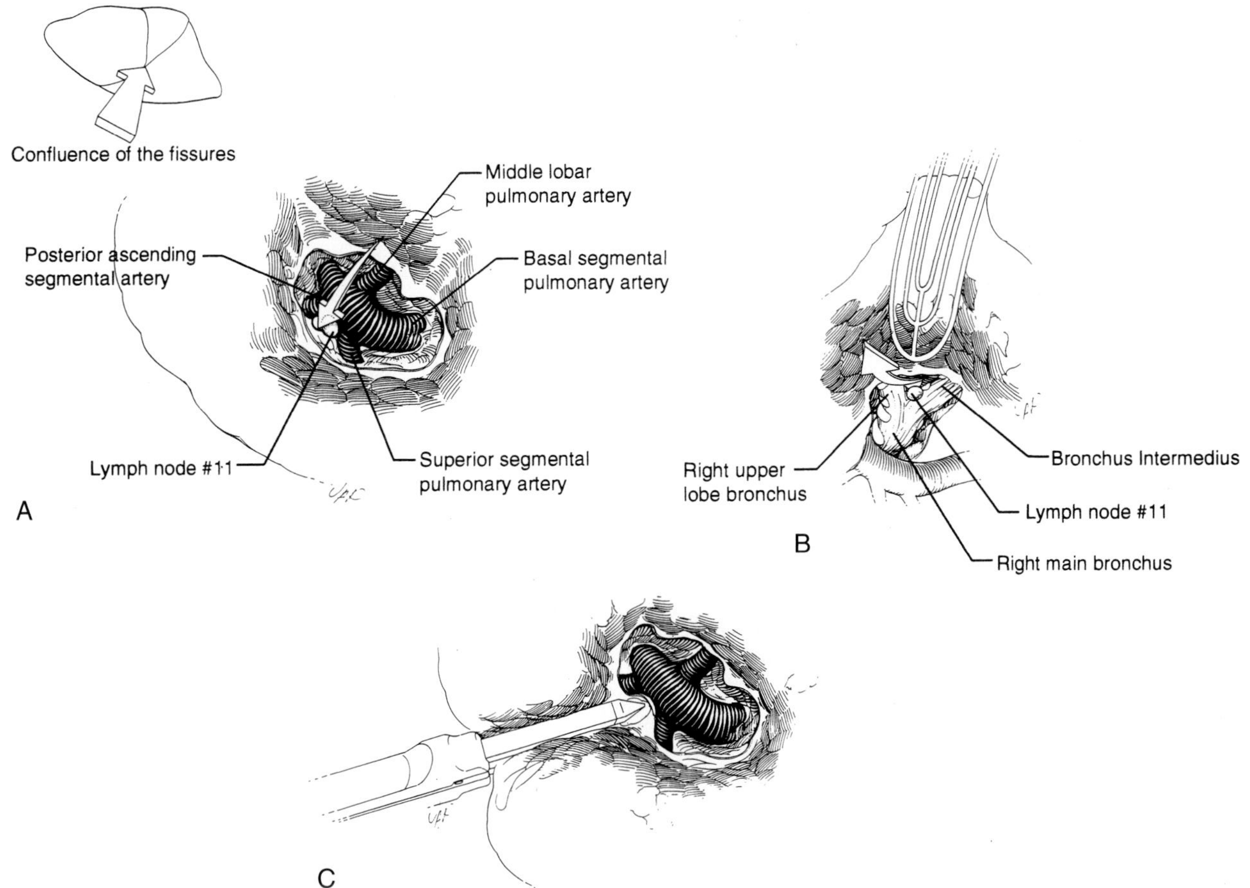

FIGURE 20–11 ■ The posterior superior dissection of the right major fissure. *A,* Dissection at the confluence of the fissures allows identification of the pars intralobares of the pulmonary artery and its major branches. The dissection is carried out between the posterior ascending segmental artery and the superior segmental artery. *B,* The posterior hilar dissection is carried out between the inferior margin of the right upper lobe bronchus and the bronchus intermedius. *C,* The posterior superior portion of the right major fissure is completed by connecting the dissections of both the pulmonary artery *(A)* and the bronchus *(B).*

and lateral pulmonary arterial dissection in the fissure (see Fig. 20–11*C*).

Return to the confluence of the fissures allows control of the anterior inferior portion of the right major fissure (Fig. 20–12*A*). Dissection in the notch between the inferior pulmonary artery branch of the middle lobe and the adjacent basal segmental artery reveals the bronchi deep to these arteries. An anterior interlobar lymph node (R11) is found lying in the notch between the middle lobe and the basal segmental bronchi.

Next, the hilum is approached anteriorly, and the space between the superior and inferior pulmonary veins is cleared (see Fig. 20–12*B*). Dissection in this notch allows the identification of the middle lobe and basal segmental bronchi and the anterior surface of the previously identified anterior interlobar lymph node. The anterior inferior portion of the major fissure may be controlled if the anterior interlobar lymph node is mobilized and the anterior dissection around the pulmonary veins is connected to the anterior and lateral pulmonary arterial dissection in the fissure (see Fig. 20–12*C*).

Right Minor Fissure (Horizontal Fissure)

The horizontal fissure is usually incomplete (poorly developed). Generally, it is the last structure controlled in a middle or upper lobectomy; however, management of this fissure may be necessary as an early step in these surgical procedures. Again, the control of this fissure commences with a dissection at the confluence of the fissures. The pars intralobares of the pulmonary artery is identified in the fissure. The superior arterial branch of the middle lobe is identified anteriorly. In about one fourth of patients, the anterior ascending branch of the right upper lobe is found at this level, lying opposite the highest middle lobe branch (Fig. 20–13*A*).

Next, the hilum is approached anteriorly, and the space between the middle lobe vein and the inferior segment vein of the upper lobe is dissected (see Fig. 20–13*B*). Care must be taken during dissection not to damage the posterior vein branch, which joins the upper lobe vein from deep within the pulmonary parenchyma. The minor fissure may be controlled if the anterior dissection around the superior pulmonary vein is connected to the lateral pulmonary arterial dissection in the fissure (see Fig. 20–13*C*).

Left Major Fissure

The pulmonary artery may be palpated in the midportion of the major fissure (Fig. 20–14). Dissection of the pul-

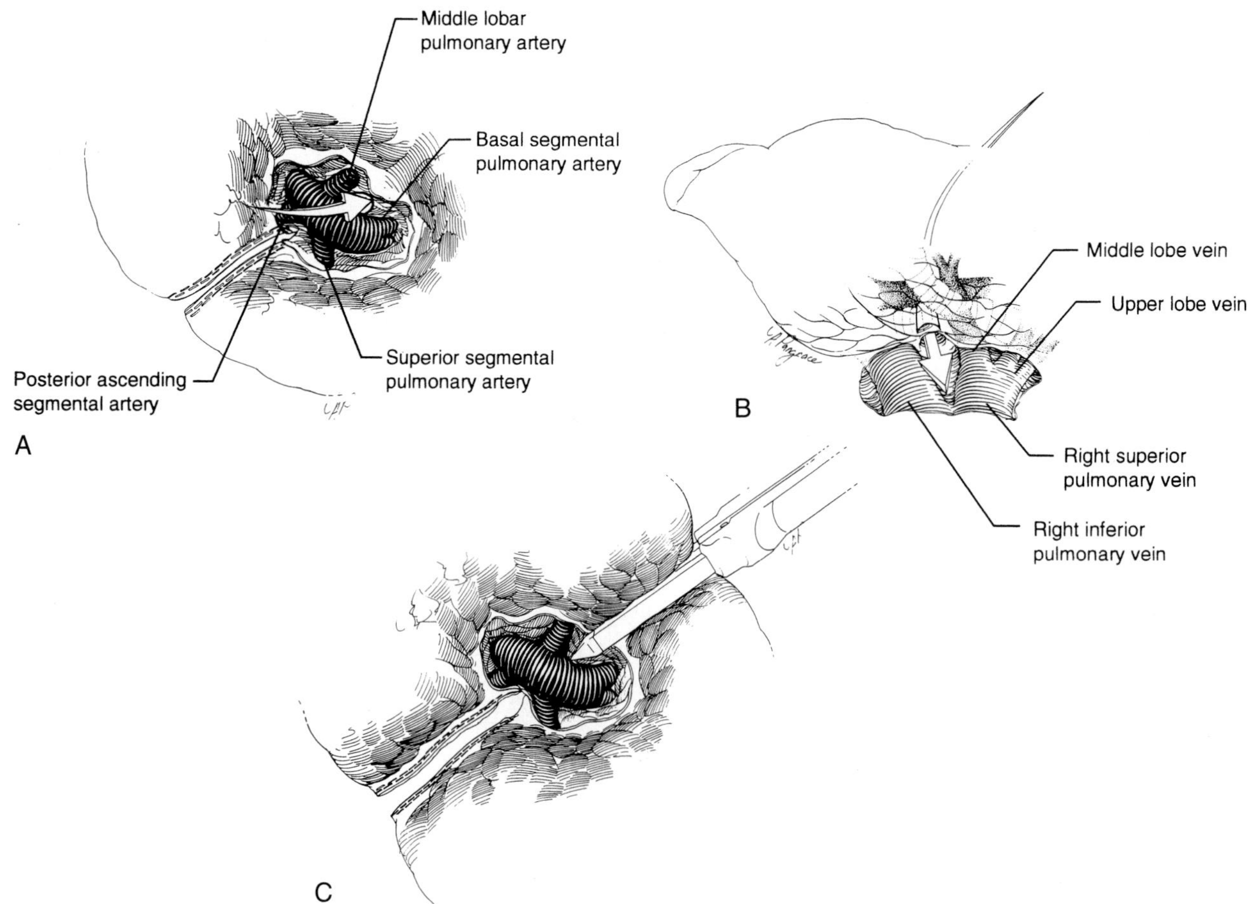

FIGURE 20–12 ■ The anterior inferior dissection of the right major fissure. *A*, Dissection at the confluence of the fissures allows identification of the pars intralobares and its branches in the fissure. The dissection is carried out between the inferior middle lobe artery and the basal segmental artery. *B*, The anterior hilar dissection is carried out between the superior and inferior pulmonary veins. *C*, The anterior inferior portion of the right major fissure is completed by connecting the dissection of both the pulmonary artery *(A)* and the pulmonary veins *(B)*.

monary parenchyma permits the pulmonary artery to be identified in its interlobar position. An interlobar lymph node (L11), the left sump node, is found overlying the pulmonary artery. The branches of the pulmonary artery may now be mobilized: anteriorly, the posterior branches of the upper lobe supplying the apical posterior and lingular segments; posteriorly, the superior segmental artery; and inferiorly, the basal segmental arteries (see Fig. 20–14*A*).

Next, the hilum is approached posteriorly, and the main pulmonary artery is mobilized as it enters the pulmonary parenchyma (see Fig. 20–14*B*). Dissection allows the posterior surface of the superior segmental artery to be defined. The posterior superior portion of the major fissure may be controlled if the posterior dissection of the pulmonary artery at the hilum is connected in the plane of the pulmonary artery to the lateral pulmonary arterial dissection in the fissure (see Fig. 20–14*C*). Care is taken to dissect in the plane above the pulmonary arterial adventitia and between the posterior branches to the upper lobe and the superior segmental branch to the lower lobe.

Return to the fissure allows control of the anterior inferior portion of the left major fissure. Dissection in the notch between the lingular segmental artery branch and the adjacent basal segmental artery reveals the bronchi deep to these arteries. An anterior interlobar lymph node (L11) is found lying in the notch between the lingular and basal segmental bronchi (Fig. 20–15*A*).

Next, the hilum is approached anteriorly, and the space between the superior and inferior pulmonary veins is cleared (see Fig. 20–15*B*). Dissection in this notch allows identification of the lingular and basal segmental bronchi and the anterior surface of the previously identified anterior interlobar lymph node. The anterior inferior portion of the major fissure may be controlled if the anterior interlobar lymph node is mobilized and the anterior dissection around the pulmonary veins is connected to the anterior and lateral pulmonary arterial dissection in the fissure (see Fig. 20–15*C*).

PULMONARY LYMPHATICS

Narake and colleagues (1978) were the first to propose a mapping system for the regional lymph nodes of the lung. This refined map is now a mainstay in the staging of primary bronchogenic carcinomas (Fig. 20–16) (Mountain and Dressler, 1997). The regional lymph

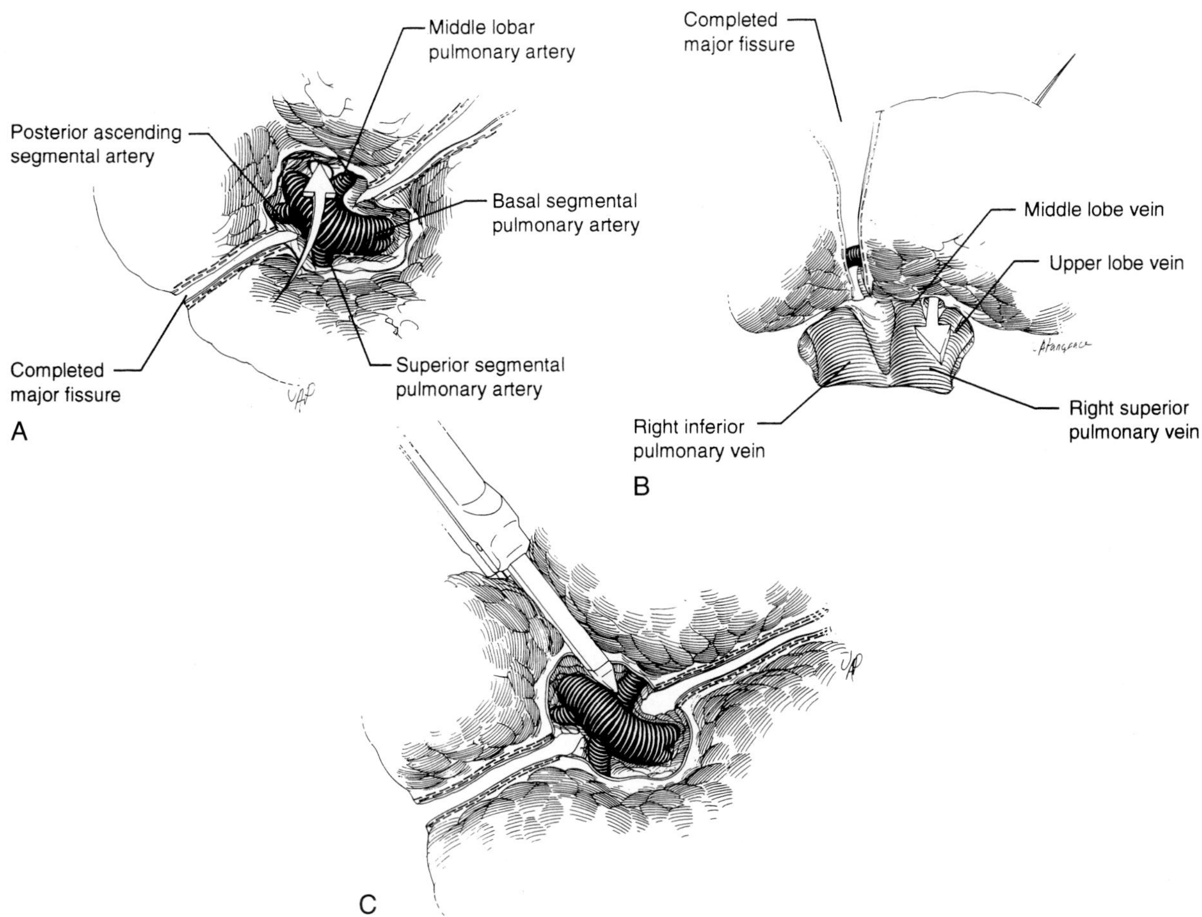

FIGURE 20–13 ■ The dissection of the minor (horizontal) fissure. *A*, Dissection at the confluence of the fissures allows identification of the pars intralobares and the branches to the middle lobe. *B*, The anterior hilar dissection is carried out between the middle lobe vein and the inferior segmental vein of the upper lobe. *C*, The minor fissure is completed by connecting the dissections of both the pulmonary artery *(A)* and the pulmonary veins *(B)*.

nodes of the lung are arranged into 1 of 14 lymph node stations. Lymph nodes 1 through 9 are mediastinal lymph nodes. Metastases to mediastinal lymph nodes represent N2 or N3 disease (in the tumor, nodes, and metastasis [TNM] staging system), depending on whether the metastases are ipsilateral (N2) or contralateral (N3). Hilar lymph nodes are designated as station 10. Lymph nodes 11 through 14 are intrapulmonary lymph nodes. Metastases to lymph nodes 10 through 14 are termed stage N1 disease. If no lymph node metastases are found, the regional lymph node status is stage N0. Supraclavicular lymph nodes are not included in this map, but metastases to regional lymph nodes on either side of the neck are classified as N3 disease.

The highest mediastinal node is a pretracheal node, sometimes called the *Delphian lymph node*. It is frequently involved with thyroid carcinoma but is infrequently a site of metastasis in primary lung cancer. It is encountered at the beginning of mediastinoscopy during the identification of the pretracheal plane. Lymph nodes 2, 4, and 7 are found around the trachea and are easily assessed at mediastinoscopy. These are the right and left paratracheal (2R and 2L), the right and left tracheobronchial angle (4R and 4L), and the subcarinal (7) lymph nodes. These nodes may also be identified at thoracotomy, but sampling of 2L and 4L may be difficult because they are obscured by the aortic arch.

Not obtainable by standard cervical mediastinoscopy are lymph nodes in the prevascular (3a), retrotracheal (3p), subaortic (5), and para-aortic (6) spaces. These may be obtained by anterior mediastinotomy (the Chamberlain procedure), thoracoscopy, or thoracotomy. Extended cervical mediastinoscopy has been used to access lymph node stations 5 and 6 (Ginsberg et al, 1987). The paraesophageal (8) and inferior pulmonary ligament (9) lymph nodes can be sampled by thoracoscopy or dissected at thoracotomy. Hilar lymph nodes (10) may be obtained by mediastinotomy, thoracoscopy, or thoracotomy.

Interlobar lymph nodes (11) are found in the fissures, surrounding the pulmonary arteries or bronchi. Lobar (12), segmental (13), and subsegmental (14) lymph nodes can be reliably sampled only at thoracotomy.

The classic drainage pathway of the pulmonary lymphatics is from subpleural lymphatic vessels along lymphatic channels that are associated with the pulmonary veins to reach larger channels that run with the arteries and bronchi. These deeper lymphatic channels drain into segmental, lobar, interlobar, hilar, and mediastinal nodes. Riquet and coworkers (1989) demonstrated segmental

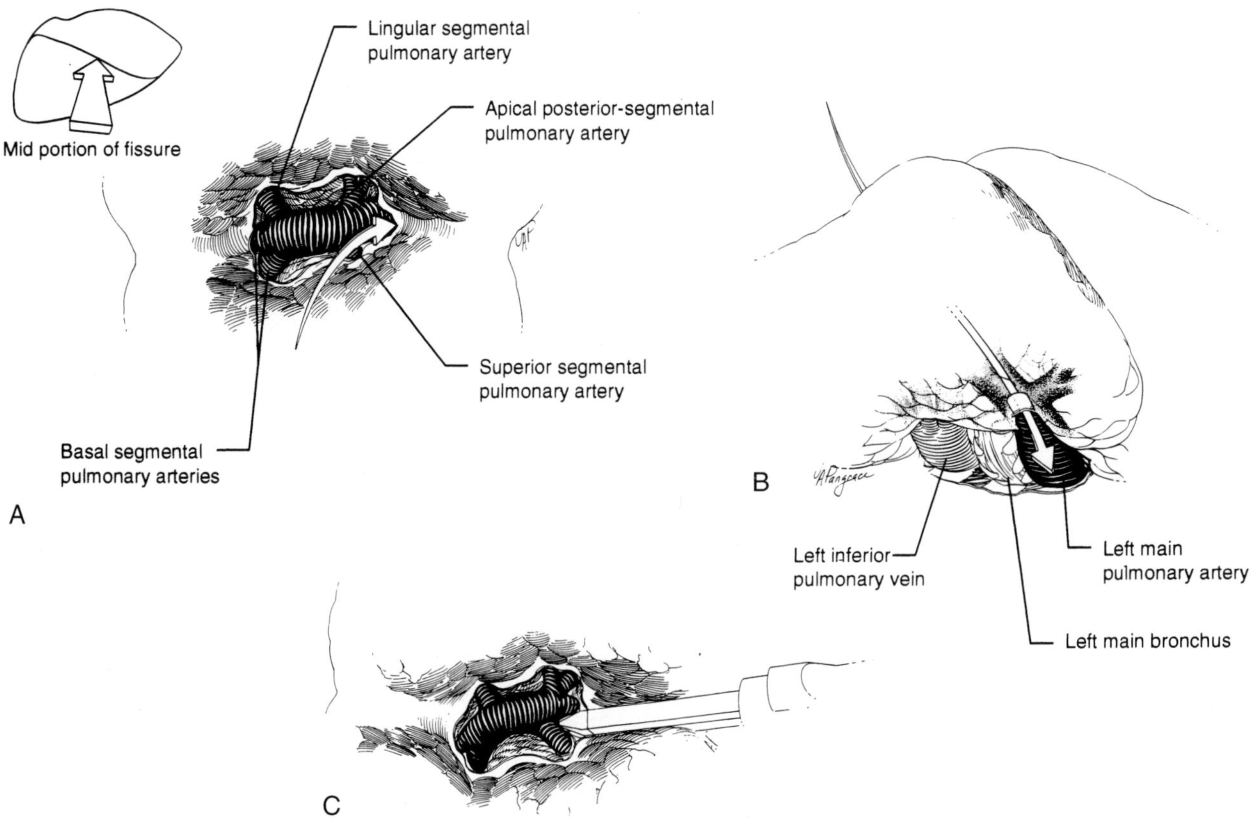

FIGURE 20–14 ■ The posterior superior dissection of the left major fissure. *A*, Dissection in the midportion of the left major fissure allows the pulmonary artery in its interlobar position and the branches of the pulmonary artery to be identified. *B*, The posterior hilar dissection of the pulmonary artery allows identification of the branches to the upper and lower lobes. *C*, The posterior superior portion of the left major fissure is developed by connecting the pulmonary arterial dissection in the fissure *(A)* to the posterior hilar arterial dissection *(B)*.

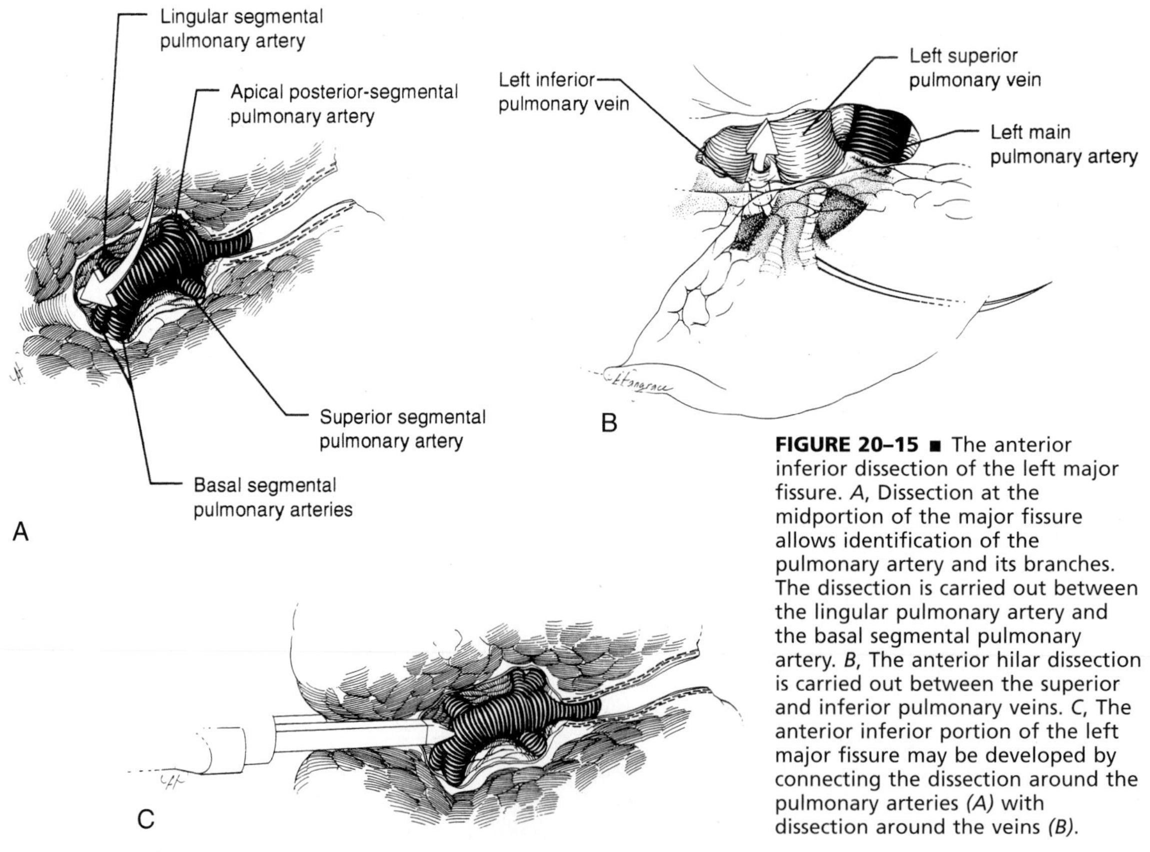

FIGURE 20–15 ■ The anterior inferior dissection of the left major fissure. *A*, Dissection at the midportion of the major fissure allows identification of the pulmonary artery and its branches. The dissection is carried out between the lingular pulmonary artery and the basal segmental pulmonary artery. *B*, The anterior hilar dissection is carried out between the superior and inferior pulmonary veins. *C*, The anterior inferior portion of the left major fissure may be developed by connecting the dissection around the pulmonary arteries *(A)* with dissection around the veins *(B)*.

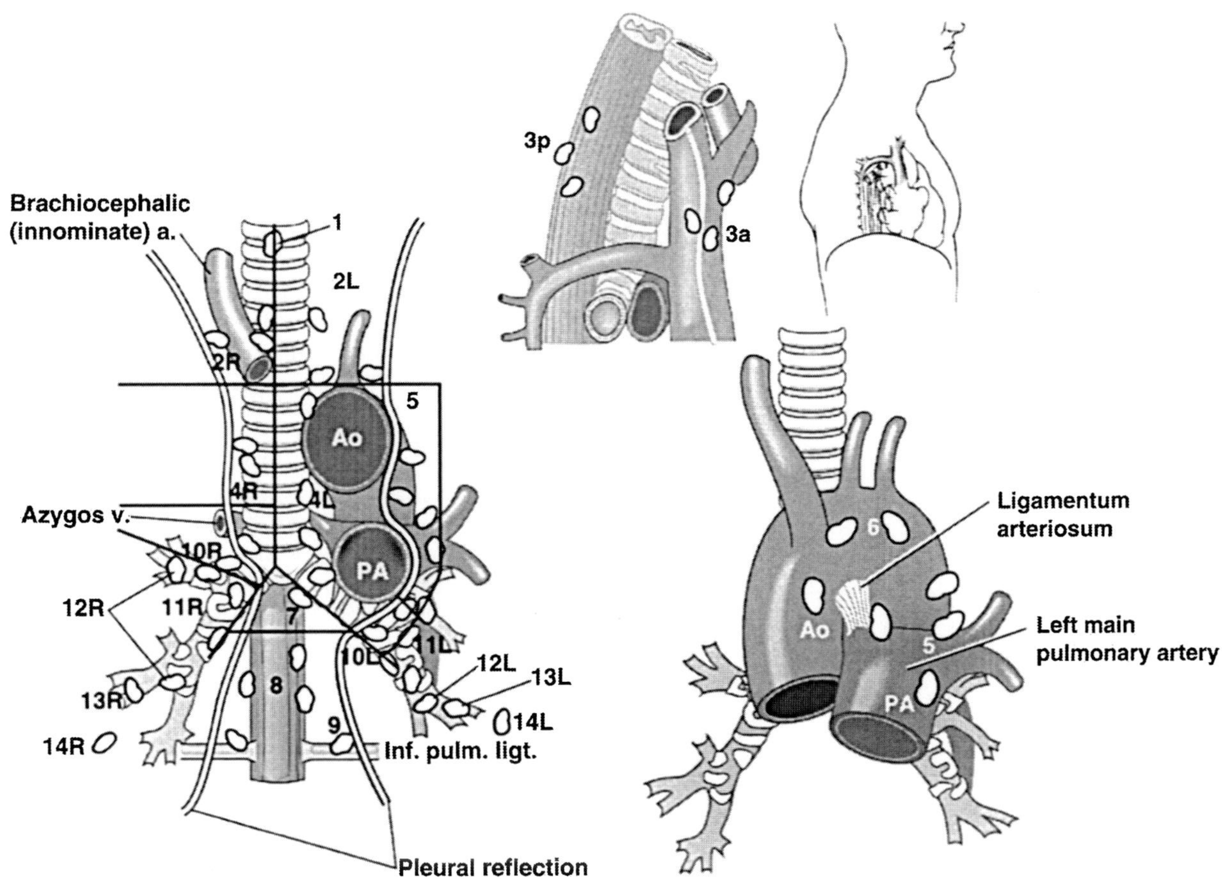

FIGURE 20–16 ■ Regional lymph nodes: 1, highest mediastinal; 2R, right paratracheal; 2L, left paratreacheal; 3a, prevascular; 3p, retrotracheal; 4R, right tracheobronchial; 4L, left tracheobronchial; 5, aortopulmonary; 6, para-aortic; 7, subcarinal; 8, paraesophageal; 9, pulmonary ligament; 10R, right hilar; 10L, left hilar; 11L, interlobar; 12L, lobar; 13L, segmental; 14L, subsegmental. (a., artery; Ao, aorta; Inf. pulm. ligt., inferior pulmonary ligament; PA, pulmonary artery; v., vein.)

drainage of subpleural lymphatic channels in 90.5% of patients. In 9.5% of patients, the drainage is intersegmental. In 77.8% of right-sided studies, intrapulmonary drainage was demonstrated; however, 22.2% of patients had direct drainage to mediastinal lymph nodes, bypassing the classic drainage pattern. This was slightly more common on the left. Twenty-five percent of studies show direct mediastinal drainage that circumvents the classic intrapulmonary pathway.

The drainage of the parenchymal lymphatic channels to mediastinal lymph nodes is generally ipsilateral and directed toward the trachea. Anomalies of drainage are more likely to be found on the left. The left lower lobe lymphatic vessels may drain through the subcarinal lymphatic channels to the right-sided mediastinal nodes in up to one third of patients. Drainage, however, appears to be predominantly left sided. Baker and associates (1967) demonstrated, in live human subjects, drainage of left lower lobe lymphatic channels to left scalene nodes in eight of nine patients, but to right-sided scalene nodes in only three of nine. The left upper lobe has dual drainage, with lymph flowing from lobar, interlobar, and hilar nodes to subcarinal, left tracheobronchial, and paratracheal lymph nodes. The alternate pathway is to the subaortic, periaortic, and anterior mediastinal nodes. In patients with left upper lobe tumors and N2 disease, one third have metastases that are confined to the classic pathway, one third have metastases that are confined to the alternate pathway by the subaortic window, and one third have metastases to both chains.

In patients with bronchogenic carcinoma and positive mediastinoscopy, Funatsu and colleagues (1992) found the greatest incidence of contralateral mediastinal metastases in left lung and lower lobe tumors. Spread to contralateral mediastinal nodes (N3 disease) was found in 50% of left lower lobe tumors and in 35% of left upper lobe tumors. For right lung tumors with positive mediastinoscopy, 42% of right lower lobe tumors, 18% of right upper lobe tumors, and none of the middle lobe tumors had metastases to contralateral mediastinal nodes, despite the fact that middle lobe tumors often drain to subcarinal lymph nodes as their first mediastinal nodal station.

BRONCHIAL CIRCULATION

Most bronchial arteries arise from the anterolateral aspect of the aorta or its branches within 2 to 3 cm of the origin of the left subclavian artery (Fig. 20–17). About 20% of origins are either higher or lower. Usually, the arteries to the right and left lungs arise separately; however, common trunks may be found in 25% of patients. Origin from the intercostal arteries is uncommon on the left but

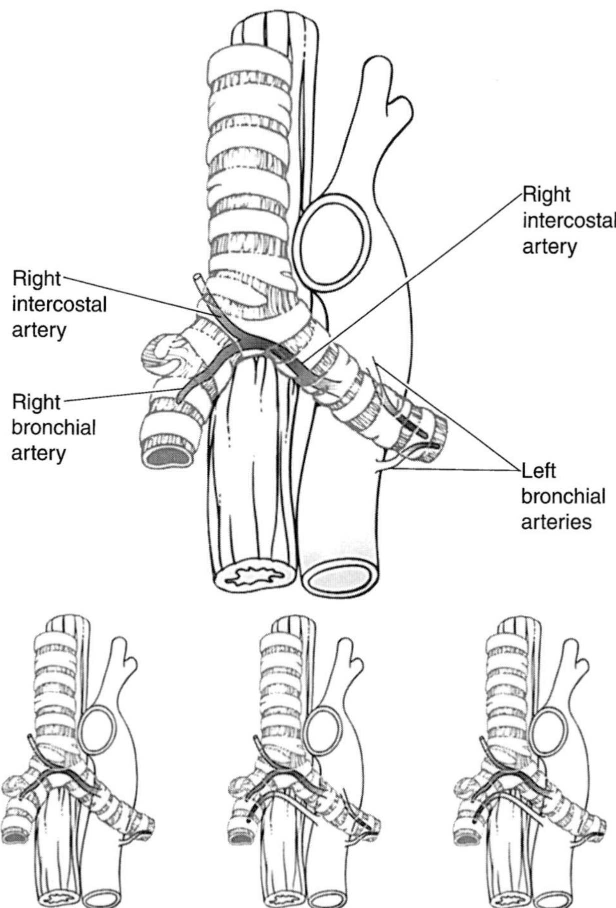

FIGURE 20–17 ■ The bronchial arterial anatomy is variable. The most frequent bronchial arterial supply is one right artery arising from an intercostal artery and two left arteries with separate aortic origins. The inset *(bottom)* demonstrates the next three most common bronchial arterial arrangements.

common on the right. Liebow (1965) and Cauldwell and associates (1948), in two large autopsy series, found an intercostal origin for a right bronchial artery in 43% to 89% of specimens. There are two arteries to each lung in 20% to 30% of patients. The most common distribution of the bronchial arteries is three bronchial arteries; dual supply to the left is more common. There are two left arteries and one right artery in 20% to 40% of patients, and two right arteries and one left artery in 10% to 16% of patients. There may be one artery to each lung in 10% to 21% of patients.

Before reaching the airway, the bronchial arteries give off esophageal branches. These, along with direct branches from the aorta, account for a significant portion of the midthoracic esophageal blood supply. The arteries then pass posteriorly to the airway to lie on the membranous portion of the mainstem bronchi. They divide to supply lobar and segmental branches. There is a rich anastomosis with the pulmonary artery. These anastomoses are important for the initial blood supply of the airway after bronchoplastic resections and pulmonary transplantation.

Most of the venous drainage from the bronchial arteries passes into the pulmonary venous system. Marchand and coworkers (1950) pointed out, however, that a second group of veins forms a venous network around the first two or three divisions of the bronchi that drain a small portion of bronchial arterial blood into the azygous system on the right or the hemiazygos on the left.

PULMONARY NERVES

The vagus nerves and the sympathetic plexus send branches to the lungs. In the hilum, they form a poorly developed anterior plexus around the main pulmonary arteries and a well-developed posterior plexus around the bronchi. The nerves then pass into the pulmonary parenchyma, where they divide into the periarterial plexus or the peribronchial plexus. The periarterial plexus contains only nonmyelinated fibers; both myelinated and nonmyelinated fibers are found around the bronchus. Bronchoplastic procedures, lung transplantation, and sometimes hilar dissections result in denervation of the lung. The loss of neural control of the bronchial glands and the smooth muscle of the bronchi and arteries is of minimal clinical importance. Loss of the cough reflex as a result of this denervation can be critical.

COMMENTS AND CONTROVERSIES

The importance of a detailed knowledge of the physical anatomy of the thorax cannot be underestimated in the training and practice of a general thoracic surgeon. For surgeons in training, this chapter should be read and reread. Intimate knowledge of the anatomy of the fissures, the recesses of the pericardium, and the relationships of the lobes and vascular structures of the mediastinum allows the thoracic surgeon complete command in the operating room, despite the intricacies of the surgery. Detailed knowledge of lymphatic drainage, including the anatomy of the thoracic duct, is important in the staging of lung cancer and the avoidance of thoracic duct catastrophes.

After obtaining this knowledge, before embarking on an unusual or new surgical procedure, it has been our practice to reinforce this knowledge by spending time in the postmortem room, dissecting the area of concern on cadavers, before embarking on a new adventure.

Dr. Rice's chapter provides a basis for knowledge of the surgical anatomy and of the practical applications in performing pulmonary resections and reconstructions.

R.J.G.

■ KEY REFERENCES

Milloy FJ, Wragg LE, Anson BJ: The pulmonary arterial supply to the right upper lobe of the lung based upon a study of 300 laboratory and surgical specimens. Surg Gynecol Obstet 116:34, 1963.

A large, modern study using current terminology describes the variations in the pulmonary arterial supply of the right upper lobe. This is the first in a series of three articles that describe the lobar pulmonary artery supply.

Milloy FJ, Wragg LE, Anson BJ: The pulmonary artery supply to the upper lobe of the left lung. Surg Gynecol Obstet 126:811, 1968.

The second in the series, this article outlines the variations in the pulmonary arterial supply of the left upper lobe.

Wragg LE, Milloy FJ, Anson BJ: Surgical aspects of the pulmonary artery supply to the middle lobe and lower lobes of the lungs. Surg Gynecol Obstet 127:531, 1968.

The last of this series, this large, modern study describes the variations in the pulmonary arterial supply of the middle and lower lobes.

■ REFERENCES

Allison PR: Intrapericardial approach to the lung root in the treatment of bronchial carcinoma by dissection pneumonectomy. J Thorac Cardiovasc Surg 15:99, 1946.

Baker NK, Hill N, Ewy GH, Marable S: Pulmonary lymphatic drainage. J Thorac Cardiovasc Surg 54:695, 1967.

Boyden EA, Hamre CJ: An analysis of variations in the bronchovascular patterns of the middle lobe in fifty dissected and twenty injected lungs. J Thorac Cardiovasc Surg 21:172, 1951.

Cauldwell EW, Siekert RG, Lininger RE, Anson BJ: The bronchial arteries: An anatomic study of 150 human cadavers. Surg Gynecol Obstet 86:395, 1948.

Ferry RM Jr, Boyden EA: Variations in the bronchovascular patterns of the right lower lobe of fifty lungs. J Thorac Cardiovasc Surg 22:188, 1951.

Funatsu T, Yoshito M, Hatakenaka R et al: The role of mediastinoscopic biopsy in preoperative assessment of lung cancer. J Thorac Cardiovasc Surg 104:1688, 1992.

Ginsberg RJ, Rice TW, Goldberg M et al: Extended cervical mediastinoscopy: A single staging procedure for bronchogenic carcinoma of the left upper lobe. J Thorac Cardiovasc Surg 94:673, 1987.

Graham EA, Singer JJ: Successful removal of an entire lung for carcinoma of the bronchus. JAMA 101:1371, 1933.

Healey JE Jr, Gibbon JM: Intrapericardial anatomy in relation to pneumonectomy for pulmonary carcinoma. J Thorac Cardiovasc Surg 19:864, 1950.

le Roux BT: Anatomical abnormalities of the right upper bronchus. J Thorac Cardiovasc Surg 44:225, 1962.

Liebow AA: Patterns of origin and distribution of the major bronchial arteries in man. Am J Anat 117:19, 1965.

Lindskrog GE, Liebow AA, Hales MR: Bilobectomy: Surgical and anatomic considerations in resection of right middle and lower lobes through the intermediate bronchus. J Thorac Cardiovasc Surg 18:616, 1949.

Marchand P, Gilroy JC, Wilson VH: An anatomical study of the bronchial vascular system and its variations in disease. Thorax 5:207, 1950.

Milloy FJ, Wragg LE, Anson BJ: The pulmonary arterial supply to the right upper lobe of the lung based upon a study of 300 laboratory and surgical specimens. Surg Gynecol Obstet 116:34,1963.

Milloy FJ, Wragg LE, Anson BJ: The pulmonary artery supply to the upper lobe of the left lung. Surg Gynecol Obstet 126:811, 1968.

Mountain CF, Dressler CM: Regional lymph node classification for lung cancer staging. Chest 111:1718, 1997.

Narake T, Suemasu K, Ishikawa S: Lymph node mapping and curability at various levels of metastasis in resected lung cancer. J Thorac Cardiovasc Surg 76:832, 1978.

Pitel M, Boyden EA: Variations in the bronchovascular patterns of the left lower lobe of fifty lungs. J Thorac Cardiovasc Surg 26:633, 1953.

Ramsey BH: The anatomic guide to the intersegmental plane. Surgery 25:533, 1949.

Riquet M, Hidden G, Debesse B: Direct lymphatic drainage of lung segments to the mediastinal nodes. J Thorac Cardiovasc Surg 97:623, 1989.

Wragg LE, Milloy FJ, Anson BJ: Surgical aspects of the pulmonary artery supply to the middle lobe and lower lobes of the lungs. Surg Gynecol Obstet 127:531, 1968.

CHAPTER **21**

Imaging of the Lung

Michelle S. Ginsberg
Jeremy J. Erasmus
Edward R. Patz, Jr.
Stephen J. Herman

HISTORICAL NOTE

Shortly after the discovery of x-rays in November 1895, their use in recognizing thoracic disease quickly became apparent (Eisenberg, 1991). As early as May 1896, descriptions of both film and fluoroscopic findings in diseases of the lungs and heart were published. It became evident that chest radiography could detect some diseases much earlier than had previously been possible; for example, in 1897 Dr. Williams of Boston noted that pulmonary tuberculosis could be detected earlier by chest radiography than by any other method. The diagnosis of bronchogenic carcinoma was similarly improved.

The development of computed tomography (CT) in the 1970s improved the detection of diseases of both the lungs and the mediastinum. Additionally, it led to a better understanding of many of the poorly understood patterns of disease as seen on the plain chest radiograph. High-resolution CT (HRCT) further improved our ability to image lung diseases. CT made two major evolutionary leaps during the 1990s. The first of these occurred early in that decade with the introduction of spiral or helical volumetric CT scanners, creating new applications that could not have been attempted before, such as CT angiography (CTA) and virtual bronchoscopy. The second leap occurred mid-decade with the introduction of dual detector row spiral CT, followed by the introduction of the multidetector CT (MDCT), with four detector rows. The major advantages are improved volume coverage and longitudinal spatial resolution.

Magnetic resonance imaging (MRI), developed in the 1980s, has been of great use in the diagnosis of cardiovascular disorders. Recent advances in the MR coils and pulse sequence technology have increased its applications to include vascular anatomy, cardiac anatomy, myocardial perfusion, and myocardial wall motion. The superior soft tissue resolution of MRI has helped in the evaluation of chest wall and mediastinal invasion by tumors.

The most exciting new technology is that of positron emission tomography (PET) imaging, which is still evolving and is not universally available at this writing, even in advanced countries.

■ *HISTORICAL REFERENCE*

Eisenberg RL: Radiology: An Illustrated History. St. Louis, Mosby–Year Book, 1991.

NONINVASIVE PLAIN RADIOGRAPHY

Air Space Versus Interstitial Disease

Pulmonary parenchymal diseases can be subdivided radiologically and pathologically into air space and interstitial categories (Fig. 21–1). With air space disease, the pathologic process is the result of increased amounts of water-dense material located predominantly within alveolar air spaces. Interstitial disease is manifested by increased water-dense material located predominantly within the pulmonary interstitial tissues, which include the alveolar walls, interlobular septa, subpleural spaces, and bronchovascular bundles (Heitzman, 1984).

Air space disease is manifested radiologically by the appearance of small (5 to 10 mm in diameter), fluffy, ill-defined nodular densities that tend to coalesce when adjacent to each other (Fig. 21–2). Each of these individual opacities is known as an "acinar shadow." Although there is no universal agreement, it is believed that these opacities represent a single pulmonary acinus filled with a water-dense material (Ziskind et al, 1963). In many air space diseases, the bronchi in the affected lung remain air filled and can be seen as tapering, branching, lucent structures within the diseased area (Fleischner, 1948). These lucencies are known as "air bronchograms" (Felson, 1973), a highly indicative (but not absolute because they can be seen rarely with interstitial disease) finding that air space disease is involved. The individual acinar shadows coalesce to form larger and larger areas of opacification, which are somewhat ill defined and irregular in outline. Depending on the cause, these areas of opacification are distributed either in a patchy distribution in the lungs or more focally in one region. With some causes, (e.g., pneumococcal pneumonia) there may be rapid spread of the disease centrifugally with time. Such spread is usually limited by a pleural surface (i.e., the process appears to stop at a pleural fissure).

Interstitial diseases manifest radiologically in a nodular pattern, a reticular pattern, or a combined, reticulonodular pattern. Interstitial nodules are tiny (2 to 3 mm in diameter), multiple, discrete, round densities that are usually easily distinguished from air space nodules in that they are smaller and remain discrete where they appear to be adjacent to one another (Fig. 21–3). Reticu-

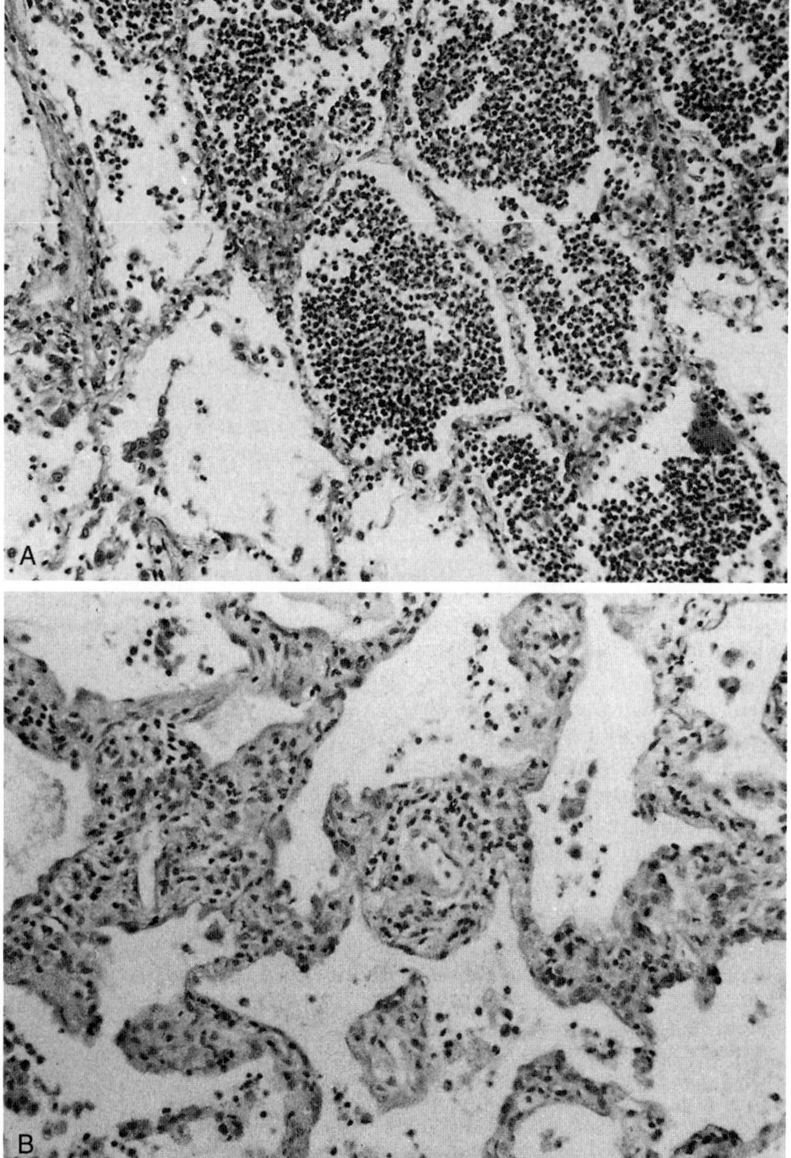

FIGURE 21–1 ■ Microscopic pathologic specimens. *A*, Air space disease. In this patient with bronchopneumonia, innumerable polymorphonuclear cells fill the air spaces; the alveolar walls are intact. *B*, Interstitial disease. In this patient with fibrosing alveolitis, the air spaces are relatively free of disease; there is marked thickening of the pulmonary interstitium.

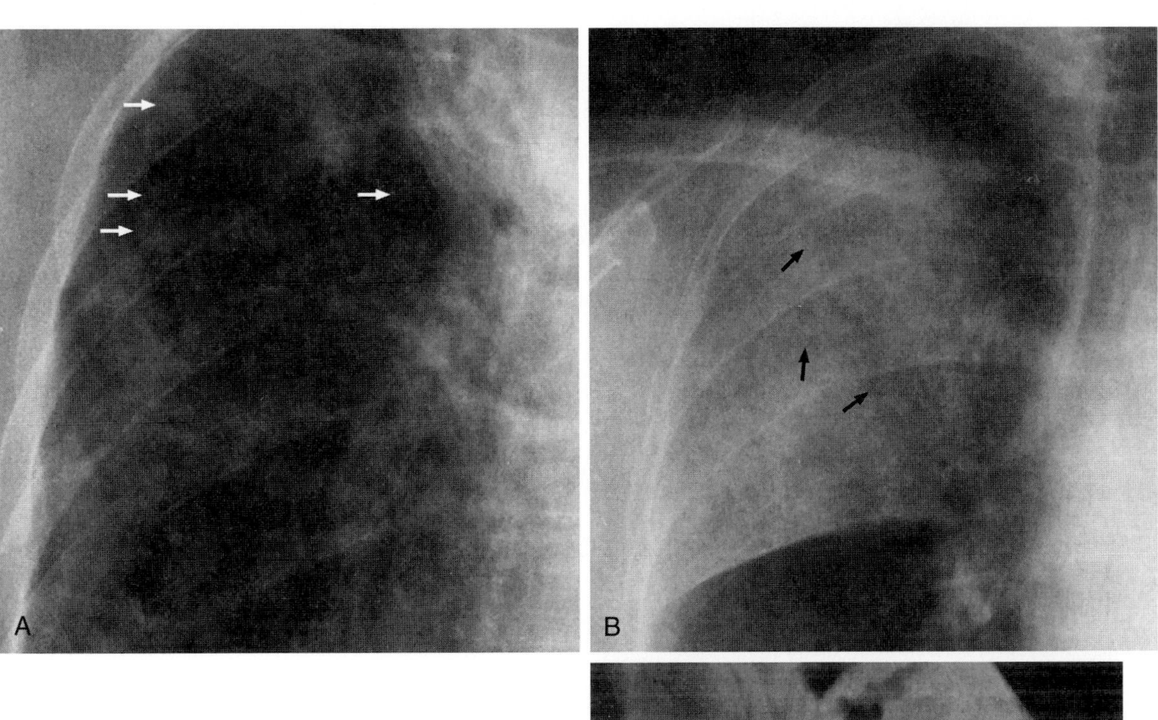

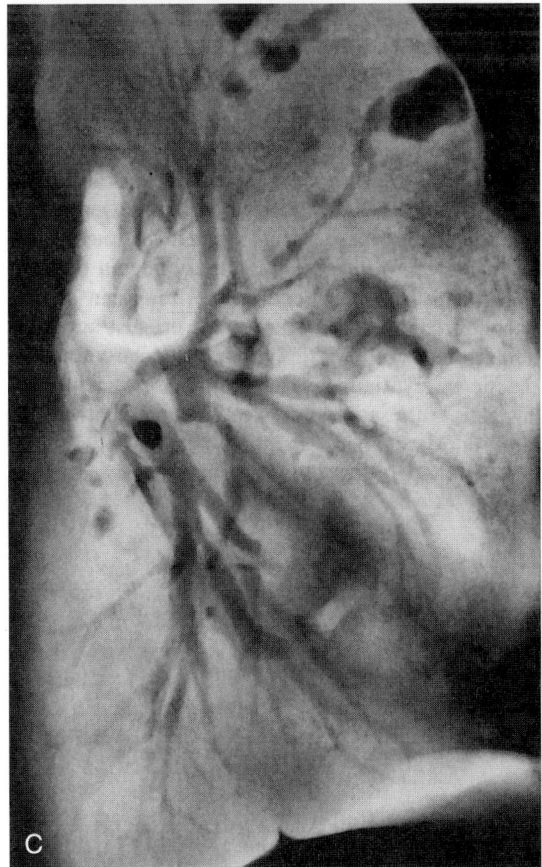

FIGURE 21–2 ■ Air space disease. *A*, Acinar shadows *(arrows)* are noted on this close-up view of the right middle and upper lung of this 33-year-old man with active tuberculosis. *B*, Right upper-lobe pneumonia. The consolidation in the right upper lobe is being contained by the minor fissure. Faint air bronchograms are noted within the consolidated lung *(arrows)*. *C*, Radiograph of lung specimen removed at autopsy. The lungs are totally consolidated and air filled within the consolidated lung, producing air bronchograms.

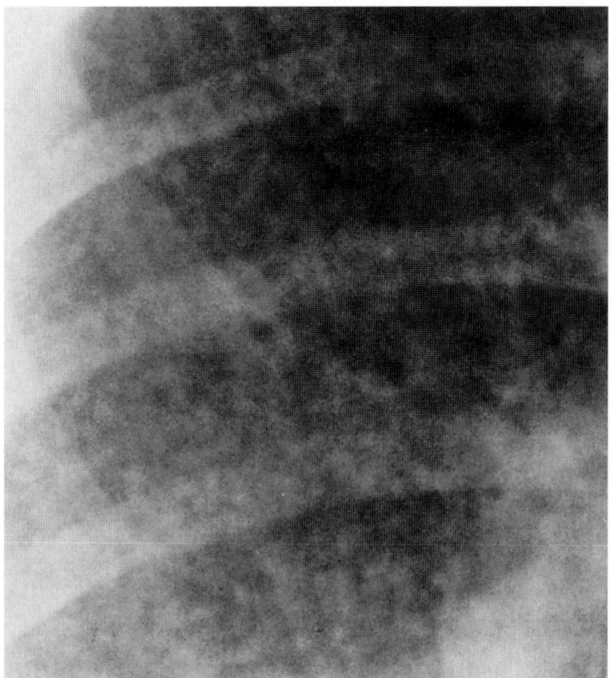

FIGURE 21–3 ■ Interstitial nodules. Close-up view of posteroanterior chest radiograph of a 16-year-old girl with sarcoidosis. Note the innumerable, well-defined nodular densities each measuring 1 to 2 mm in diameter.

lar densities are a network of lines that are thin (1 to 2 mm in width) and well defined. This network can be either fine (in which case the black spaces between the linear densities are small and the linear densities themselves are thin) or coarse (in which case the black spaces are larger, up to 1 cm or more in diameter, with thicker, white linear margins) (Fig. 21–4). When the interstitial process involves an interlobular septum, the so-called Kerley B lines appear. These appear as thin (about 0.5 to 1 mm thick), linear densities about 1 cm in length that meet the pleural surface at right angles. Although they are often considered to indicate pulmonary edema (which is a common cause of their occurrence), they can be caused by any condition in which a water-dense process accumulates in the interlobular septi (e.g., heart failure or lymphangitic spread of carcinoma). Disease in the interstitium that accompanies bronchovascular bundles causes these structures to be somewhat prominent and more poorly defined.

Lobar Collapse

Lobar collapse is extremely important to recognize because it may be missed clinically but may be the result of potentially treatable diseases, such as bronchogenic carcinoma or an aspirated foreign body. Lobar collapse can be recognized by direct and indirect signs (Fraser et al, 1988; Fig. 21–5).

The main direct signs of lobar collapse are opacity of the lobe and evidence of loss of volume of the lobe. Another direct sign, displacement of a pleural fissure, represents the margin of a lobe itself and indicates that one of the lobes has lost volume. Additional direct signs include displacement of blood vessels and major bronchi.

With the loss of volume in lobar collapse, a number of compensatory mechanisms come into play. These form the so-called indirect signs and include: elevation of the ipsilateral hemidiaphragm (most prominent when a lower lobe is collapsed), hilar displacement, mediastinal shift, and compensatory hyperinflation. The part of the mediastinum that shifts is usually that which is closest to the collapsed lobe. For example, with upper lobe collapse, tracheal shift is the main finding; with lower lobe collapse, there is a shift of the heart. Compensatory hyperinflation is noted in the lung closest to the collapsed lobe. For example, with left lower lobe collapse, the left upper lobe appears relatively hyperlucent compared with the right lung. This is because it has expanded into the space formerly occupied by the left lower lobe and its vessels, and the parenchyma are now more spread out than they were previously. A collapsed lobe is generally of increased density because of the relative lack of air within it. Occasionally the ribs adjacent to the collapsed lobe are more crowded than are the corresponding ribs on the contralateral side, although this is not the most prevalent sign of collapse.

Patterns of collapse of each of the five pulmonary lobes and combinations of lobes have been described in detail elsewhere (Fraser et al, 1988; Proto and Thomas, 1980; Robbins and Hale, 1945a to 1945f; Robbins et al, 1945). Examples of these are shown in the accompanying figures (see Fig. 21–5).

The causes of atelectasis have been divided into four main types: resorptive (obstructive), passive (relaxation), adhesive, and cicatrization (Fraser et al, 1988). Resorptive or obstructive atelectasis occurs when the normal communication between the trachea and alveoli is lost; this form is discussed later. Passive or relaxation atelectasis occurs when a space-occupying lesion, most often a pneumothorax or pleural effusion, "compresses" adjacent lung (in fact, the lung is not truly compressed by these processes but rather is allowed to return to its resting size by the local loss of "negative" pleural pressure). Adhesive atelectasis refers to situations in which increased surface tension in the alveoli, probably caused by loss of surfactant, causes the alveoli to collapse (e.g., acute radiation-induced pneumonitis). Cicatrization atelectasis occurs secondary to pulmonary fibrosis, which may be local or general.

It is most important to distinguish resorptive atelectasis from the other three forms because the bronchial obstruction must be recognized and treated. Generally, this is not a problem because obstructive atelectasis is the only form that tends to involve an entire lobe or segment of lung. Rarely, some cicatrizing diseases, such as tuberculosis, can involve an entire lobe and leave it scarred and atelectatic, but this is not difficult to distinguish from an obstructive collapse (Fig. 21–6). Additionally, by their nature the other three forms should contain air bronchograms. In contrast, all air distal to an obstructing airway lesion is absorbed, and usually air bronchograms are not seen with resorptive atelectasis. However, air bronchograms by themselves should not be used to determine if the cause of a lobar collapse is airway ob-

Text continued on page 451

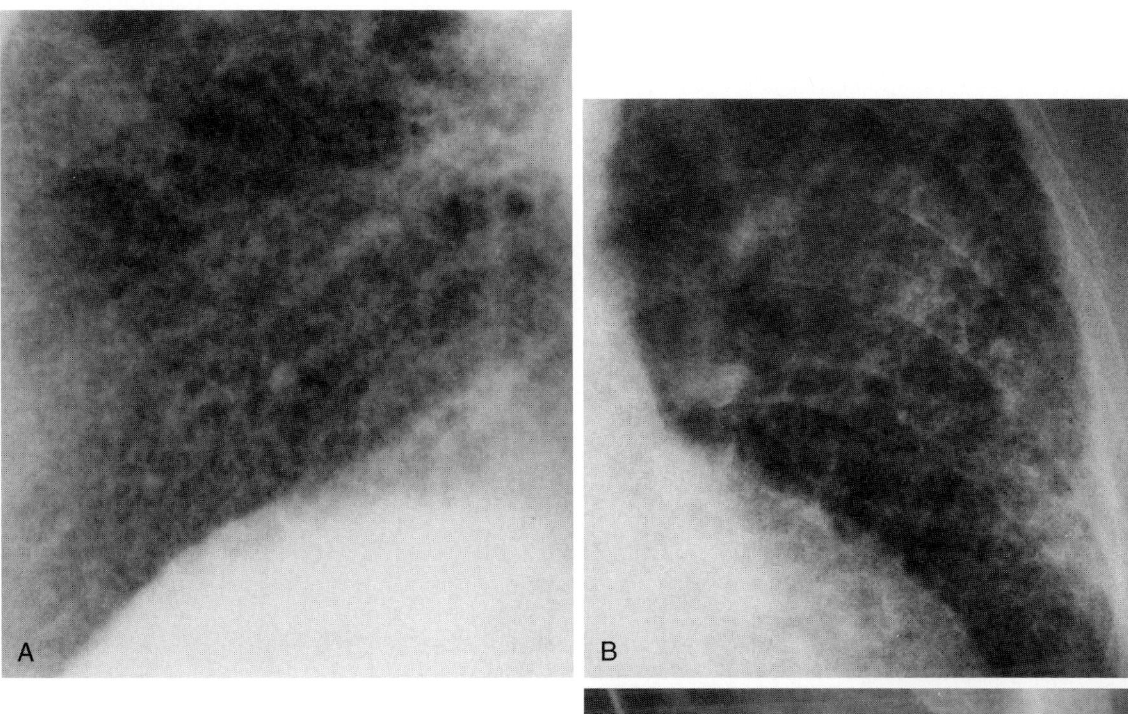

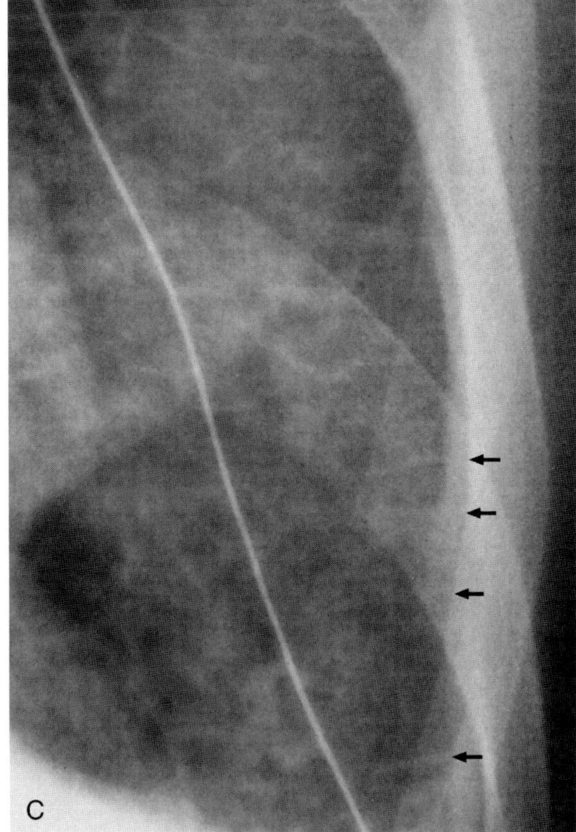

FIGURE 21–4 ■ Reticular interstitial disease. *A*, Fine reticular disease. Close-up view of right lung base of 59-year-old woman with fibrosing alveolitis. *B*, Close-up view of left midlung reveals a coarse reticular pattern in this 62-year-old man with farmer's lung. *C*, Close-up view of posteroanterior chest radiograph of a patient with pulmonary edema. Kerley B lines *(arrows)* are short, straight, thin lines running perpendicular to and abutting the pleural surface.

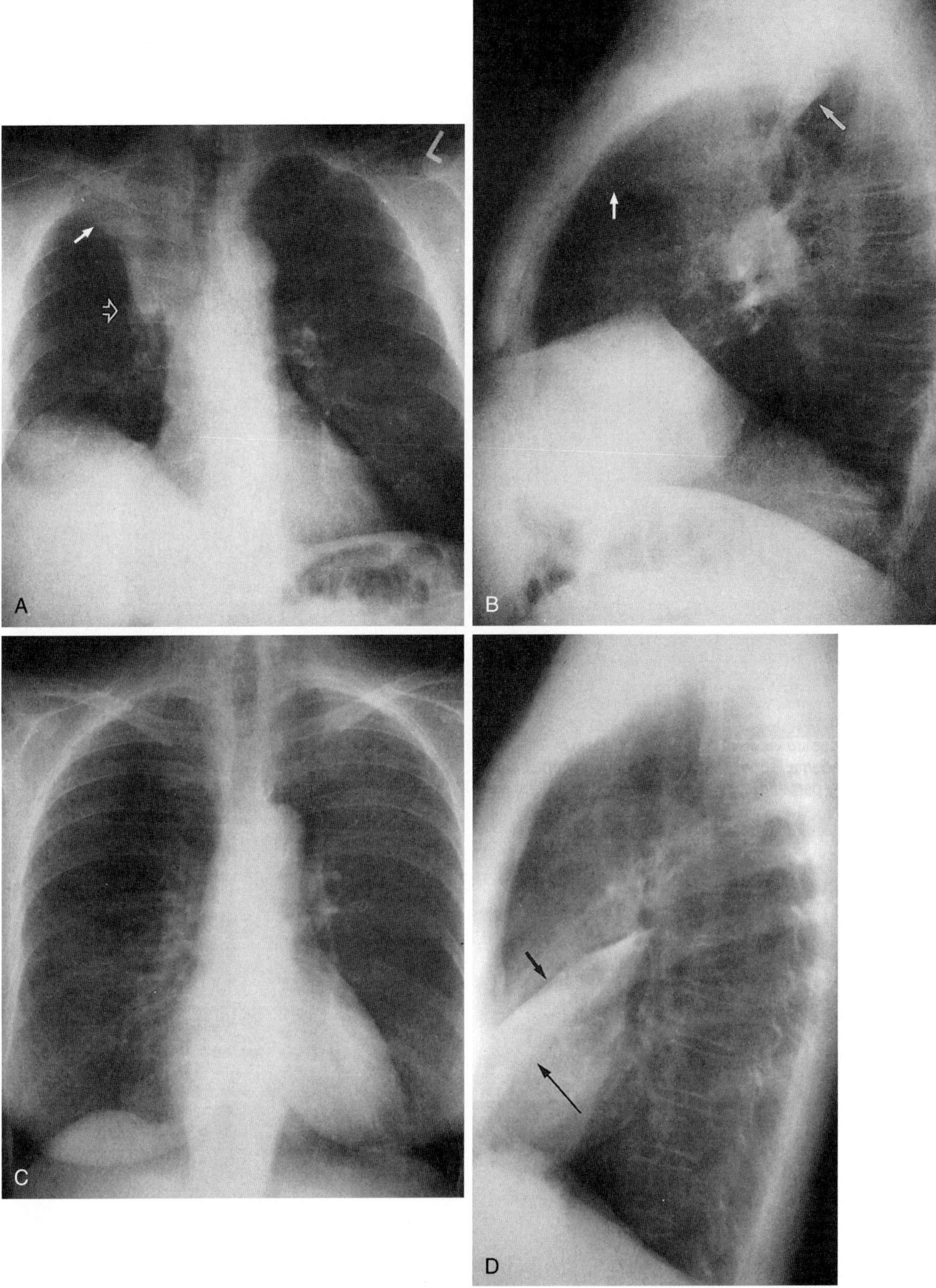

FIGURE 21–5 ■ *A* and *B*, Right upper-lobe collapse. The minor fissure is displaced superiorly on the posteroanterior and lateral views *(small arrows)*; the superior aspect of the major fissure is displaced anteriorly on the lateral view *(large arrows)*. There is elevation of the right hilum and right hemidiaphragm and displacement of the trachea to the right. Note the presence of a central convexity in the region of the hilum *(open arrows)*, the Golden S sign. *C* and *D*, Right middle-lobe collapse. On the posteroanterior view, there is loss of visualization of the right heart border (silhouette sign), with a slight increase in the density of the right base medially. On the lateral view, there is displacement of the minor fissure inferiorly *(short arrow)* and the inferior aspect of the major fissure anterosuperiorly *(long arrow)*. Because of the relatively small size of the middle lobe, indirect compensatory signs are not present.

Illustration continued on opposite page

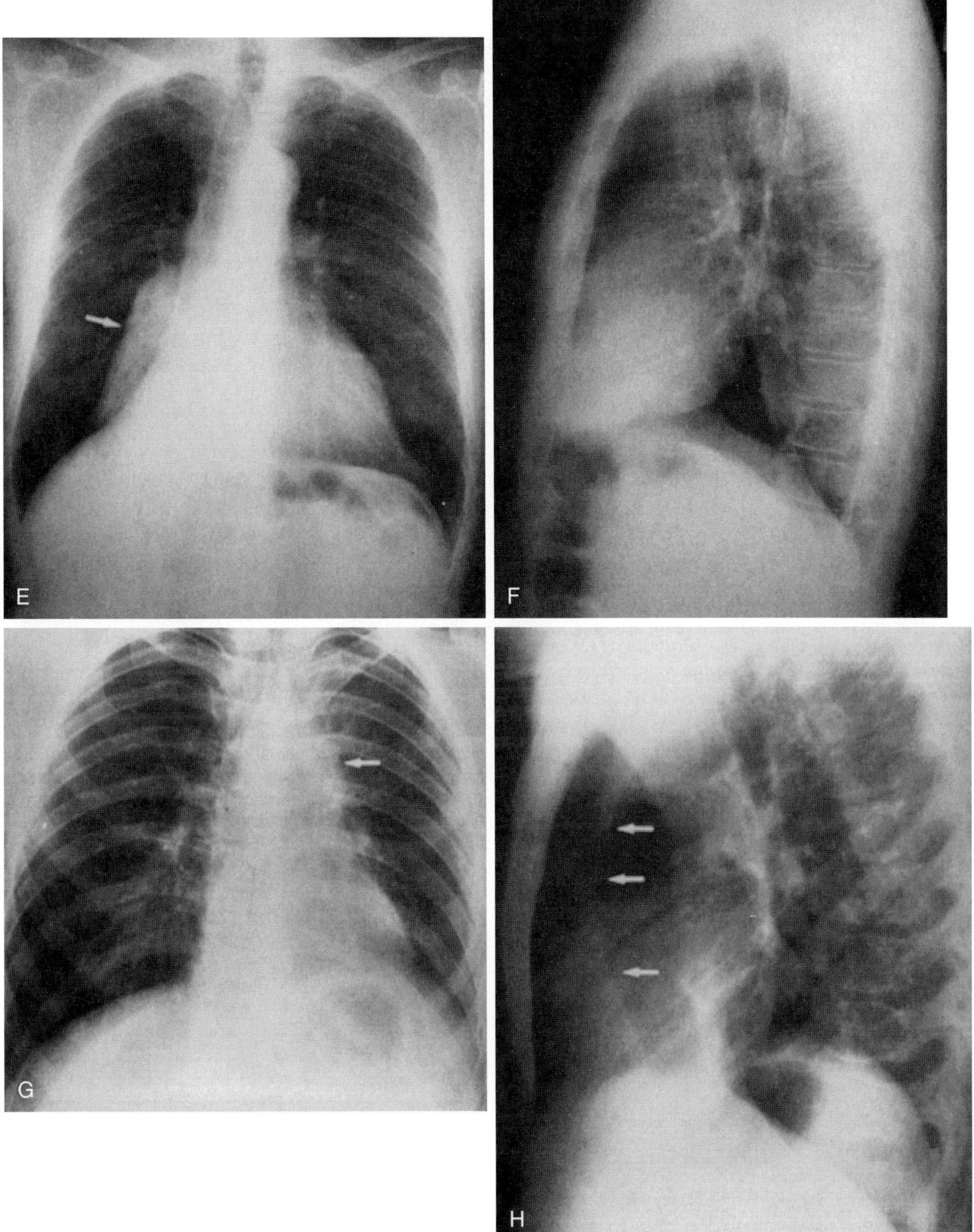

FIGURE 21–5 ■ *(Continued) E* and *F*, Right lower-lobe collapse. The major fissure is displaced inferomedially *(arrow)*. Indirect signs include relative hyperlucency of the right lung, especially the right middle lobe (compare with corresponding locations on the left), inferior displacement of the right hilum, shift of the trachea to the right, and slight elevation of the right hemidiaphragm, especially medially. On the lateral view, note that the density of the thoracic spine decreases from the upper to the midthoracic spine but then increases inferiorly because of the overlying airless lobe. *G* and *H*, Left upper-lobe collapse. On the lateral view, there is displacement of the left major fissure anteriorly with increased density of the collapsed lobe anterior to it. On the posteroanterior view, there is elevation of the left hemidiaphragm, elevation of the left hilum *(arrow)*, shift of the trachea and the heart to the left, and a generalized increase in the density of the left hemithorax.

Illustration continued on following page

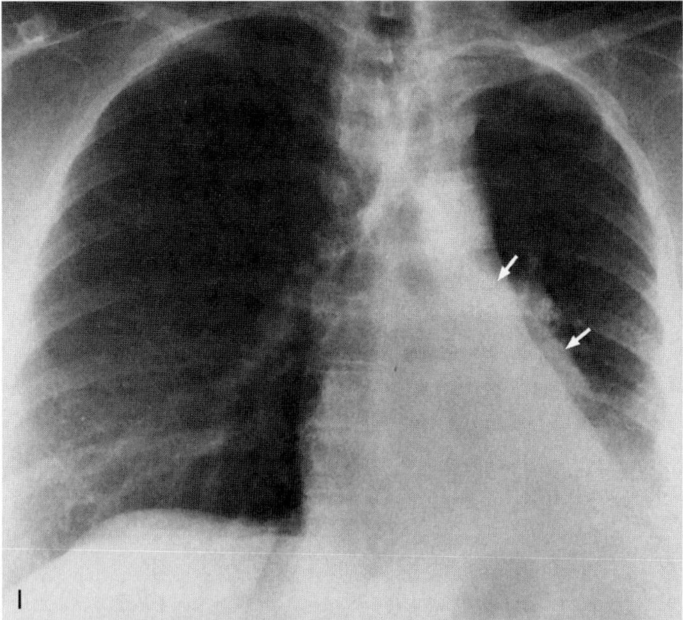

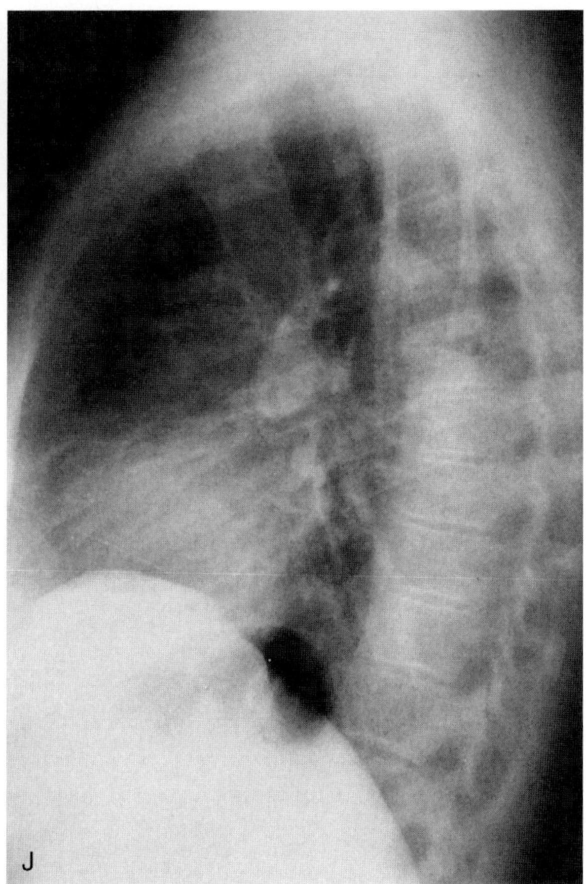

FIGURE 21–5 ■ *(Continued) I* and *J*, Left lower-lobe collapse. The inferomedially displaced left major fissure is seen *(arrows)* just lateral to the left cardiac margin. Additionally, there is increased inferior displacement of the left hilum and elevation of the left hemidiaphragm. On the lateral views, note the increase in the density of the lower thoracic spine compared with that of the upper spine. Note also the loss of visualization of the left hemidiaphragm as a result of the now airless left lower lobe.

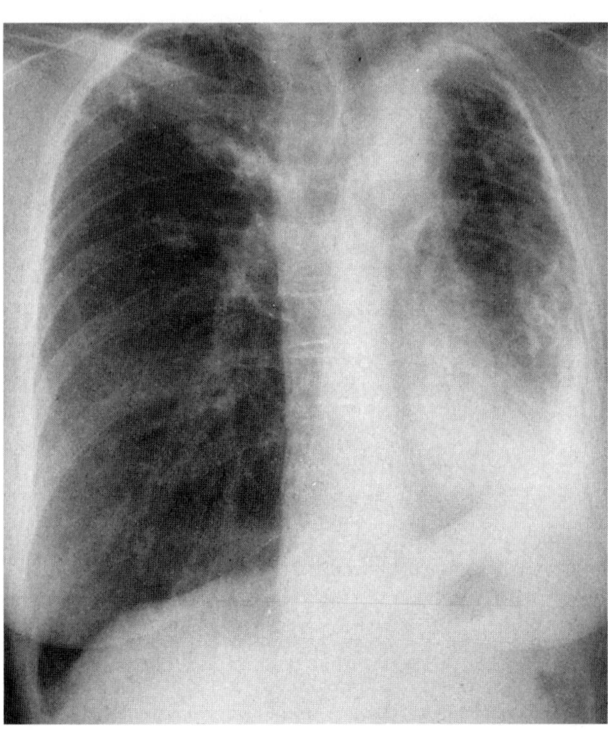

FIGURE 21–6 ■ This elderly woman with known tuberculosis from many years earlier has significant bilateral, upper-lobe atelectasis, especially on the left. The type of atelectasis demonstrated in this patient does not indicate an endobronchial tumor.

struction (Woodring, 1988). Two other radiographic signs, central bronchial narrowing or cutoff and the so-called Golden S sign, are accurate in determining if the atelectasis is the result of an obstructing tumor or not (Woodring, 1988). The latter refers to the presence of a central convexity at the hilum, the convexity being the margin of the central tumor itself (Golden, 1925; see Fig. 21–5*A*).

A somewhat unique form of parenchymal collapse known as "round atelectasis" exhibits some well-described, characteristic features (Schneider et al, 1980). It appears as a pleural-based, well-defined, round or oval opacity, usually occurring in the lung base posteriorly, with adjacent pleural thickening and curving pulmonary vessels sweeping into it (Fig. 21–7). These features are better seen on CT (see Computed Tomography).

Pulmonary Nodules and Masses

When a pulmonary nodule or mass is seen, the main consideration is whether the lesion is benign or malignant. A number of signs suggest one or the other. One that suggests malignancy is the presence of poorly defined margins, especially if there is spiculation forming so-called corona radiata (Fig. 21–8). The latter refers to short linear opacities extending from the margin of the mass into the adjacent lung. Although formerly believed to be a definite indication of malignancy (and known as corona maligna), corona radiata have been recognized in some benign diseases. However, they are definitely highly suggestive of malignancy. Malignant nodules tend to be lobulated in contour and generally do not contain calcium. The rare malignant nodule that does contain calcium is usually larger than 2 cm, and, when present, the calcium is most often eccentrically located. If old films are available, any increase in the size of the mass makes it suspicious for a malignancy. Additionally, malignancy should be suspected when there are associated signs, such as lymphadenopathy, bone destruction, or pleural effusion. Cavitation of the mass does not help in making the distinction; however, the thickness of its wall does (Woodring et al, 1980; Woodring and Fried, 1983). If the maximum wall thickness is 4 mm or less, the mass is most likely benign. If the thickness is greater than 1.5 cm, the mass is likely to be malignant; otherwise, the mass must be considered indeterminate.

Signs that the nodule or mass is benign include well-defined margins and a smooth contour, although both features are also seen with metastases. However, the most important signs that a nodule is benign include calcification and growth rate. There are certain patterns of calcification that are pathognomonic of benign disease (Fig. 21–9). If the nodule contains a central nidus of calcification, diffuse calcification, or lamellated (ring-like) calcification, then granulomatous disease is almost certain. So-called popcorn calcification (i.e., lumps of calcium seen throughout the mass) indicates that the mass is probably a benign hamartoma. If old films are available, then the growth rate of the nodule can be estimated. By measuring its diameter on both studies and calculating its volume, the doubling time of the nodule can be determined. If the doubling time is 7 days or less, or 465 days or greater, then benign disease is almost certain (Nathan et al, 1962). Of note, primary lung tumors that are 1 cm or less in diameter are usually not visible on plain chest radiographs; therefore, it is not possible to calculate an accurate growth rate for small nodules developing in areas that were previously normal.

Pragmatically, a nodule that either exhibits a benign calcific pattern or exhibits no growth over a 2-year period may be considered benign; otherwise, it must be considered suspicious for malignancy. It must be noted that occasionally some tumors, especially bronchoalveolar cell carcinoma, exhibit no growth over 2 years. This possibility must always be kept in mind.

Line Shadows

Linear densities are a common finding in the lungs and can be the result of a number of different causes, the most common of which are scarring, subsegmental (discoid or plate) atelectasis, and Kerley B lines (described earlier) (Fig. 21–10). Any parenchymal process that heals with the development of scar tissue can leave behind permanent, thin, linear opacities that can run in any direction and remain visible for the rest of the patient's life. Subsegmental atelectasis appears as a linear density up to about 1 cm in diameter and many centimeters in length. Its pathogenesis is poorly understood (Westcott and Cole, 1985).

Other causes of line shadows include mucoid impaction (dilated, mucus-filled bronchi caused by bronchial obstruction or thick, inspissated mucus), bronchial wall thickening (which can cause the appearance of parallel lines, so-called tram tracks, or thickening of the circular shadow of a bronchus seen end on), and the walls of bullae. Of course, an extrathoracic cause, such as a skinfold, clothing, or a bed sheet, must always be kept in mind.

Increased Radiolucency

There are many causes of increased radiolucency of the lungs. These can be categorized into four main groups: artifactual, extrapulmonary, decreased perfusion, and increased aeration. Artifactual lucency occurs when the film is obtained with the patient rotated to one side, with the side to which the patient is rotated being more radiolucent. A relative lack of overlying soft tissues (e.g., mastectomy) causes ipsilateral lucency. One of many possible causes of decreased perfusion (e.g., pulmonary embolism [PE], arterial obstruction by tumor, or congenital pulmonary arterial agenesis) can cause focal lucency. Relative hyperinflation of a portion of the lung is a significant cause that must be recognized because it can be the result of bronchial obstruction; however, compensatory hyperinflation (e.g., atelectasis or resection of another lobe) and the presence of emphysema or a bulla are more common causes. A film obtained during expiration can often be helpful in assessing hyperlucent lung; if it is the result of a bronchial obstruction, the hyperlucency is accentuated on the expiratory film (Fig. 21–11).

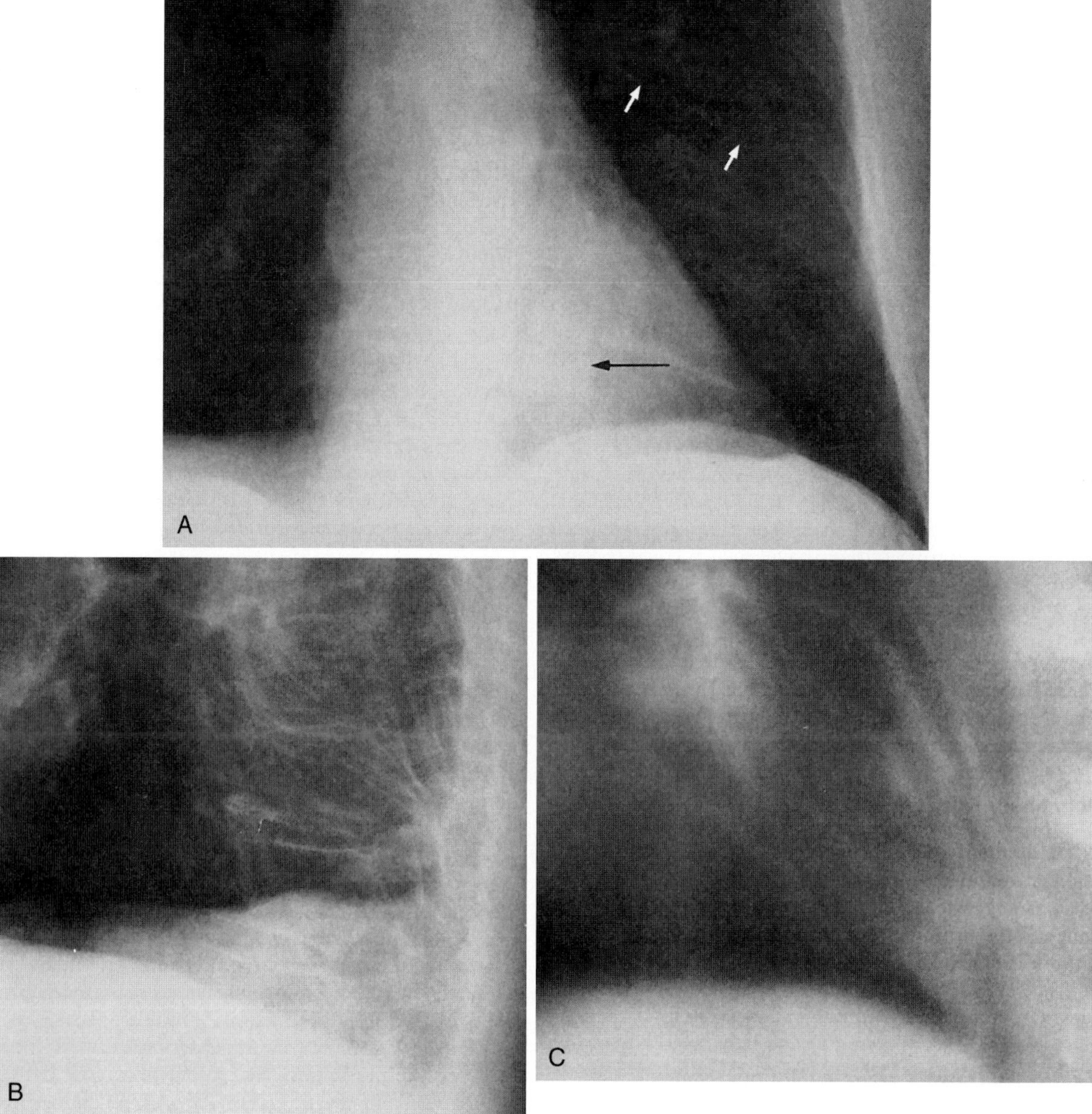

FIGURE 21–7 ■ Round atelectasis. *A*, Close-up view of a posteroanterior chest radiograph reveals a nodular density measuring 2 cm in diameter in the left lower lobe *(black arrow)*. Note the mild, left lower-lobe volume loss, as evidenced by the slightly inferiorly displaced left major fissure *(white arrows)*. *B*, On the lateral view, linear densities are seen extending posteriorly toward the thickened pleura. *C*, Plain tomogram. This study clearly reveals curving vessels sweeping into the nodular density in the left lower lobe. There is adjacent pleural thickening (note that the lung is separated from the posterior rib by a water-dense band).

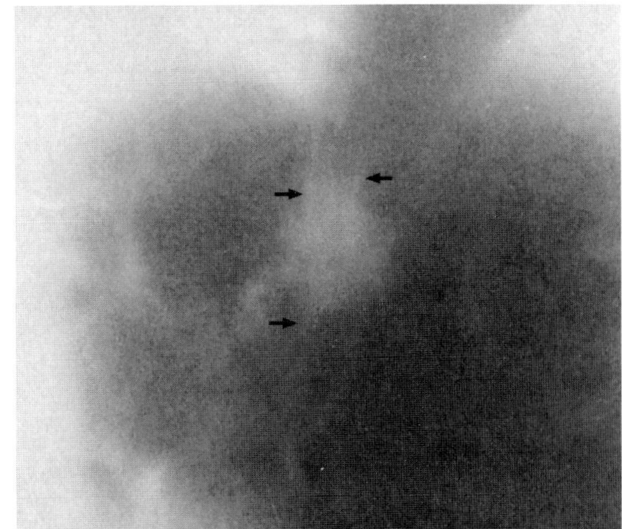

FIGURE 21–8 ■ Bronchogenic carcinoma in a 60-year-old man. This somewhat ill-defined nodule has prominent spiculated margins. Specifically, there are linear opacities extending from the surface of the nodule into the adjacent lung, so-called corona radiata *(arrows)*.

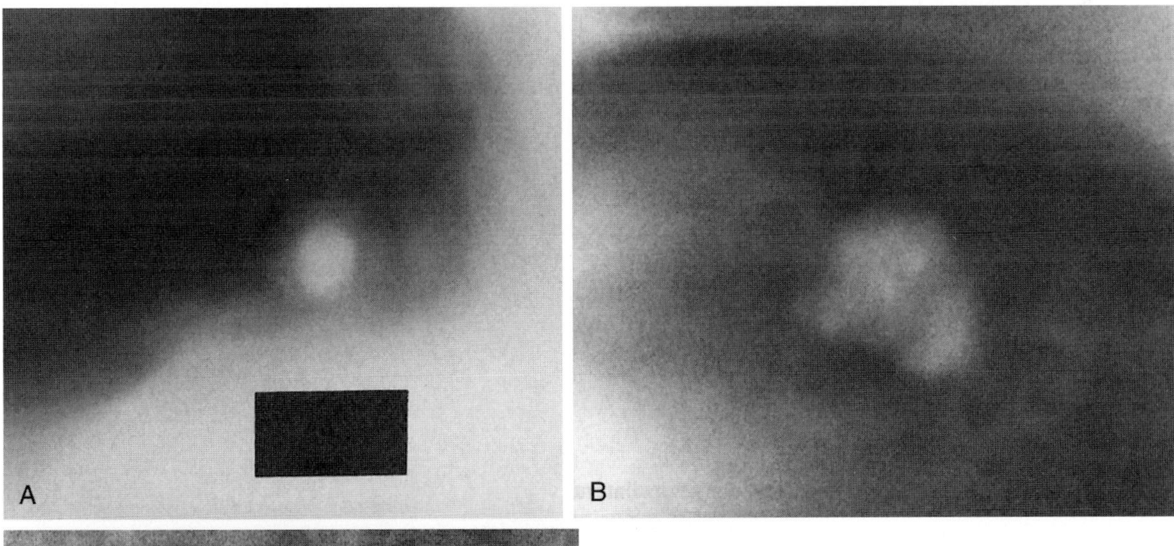

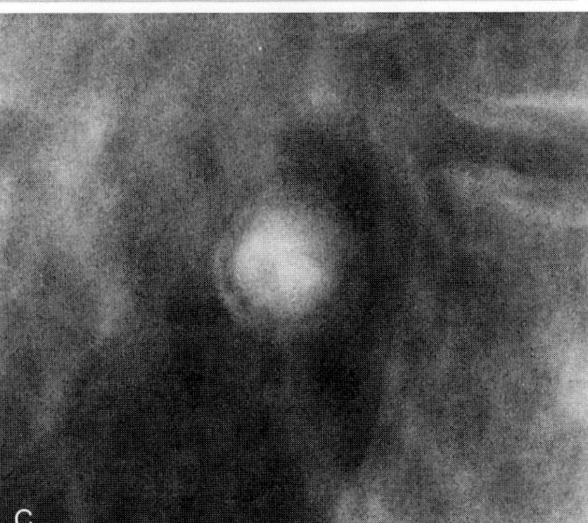

FIGURE 21–9 ■ Patterns of calcification in benign nodules *A*, Close-up view of a tomogram of a smooth, well-defined nodule with dense central calcification. *B*, Popcorn calcification in a presumed pulmonary hamartoma. *C*, Close-up view of a nodule containing a large, central nidus of calcification and peripheral, lamellated calcification.

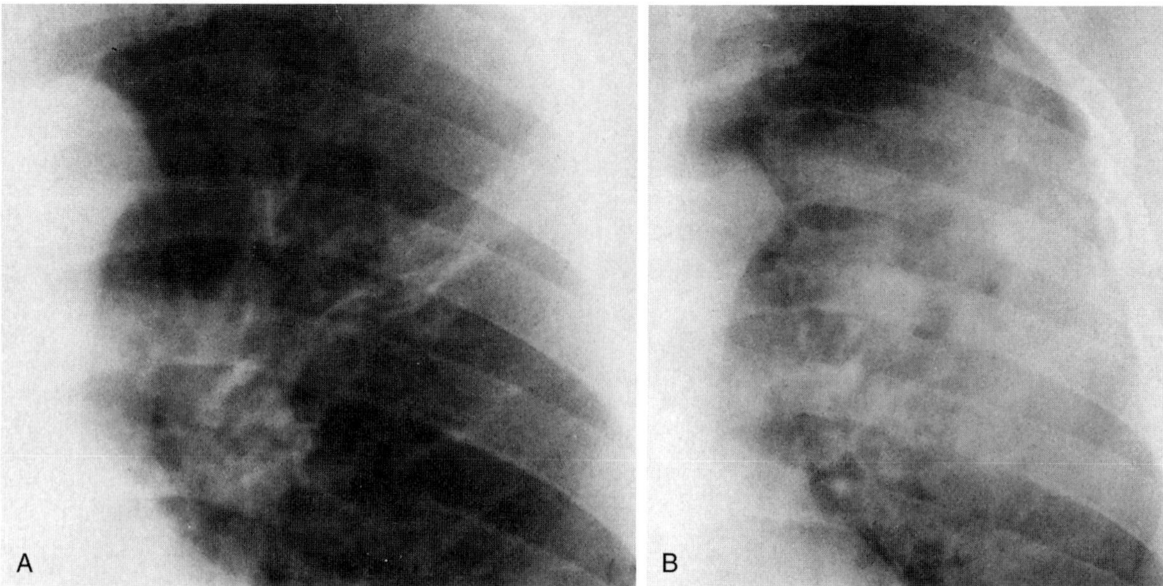

FIGURE 21–10 ■ *A*, Linear densities in the left perihilar region are typical of both pulmonary fibrosis and subsegmental atelectasis. *B*, One year earlier, this patient had a necrotizing pneumonia in this region and was left with permanent linear scarring.

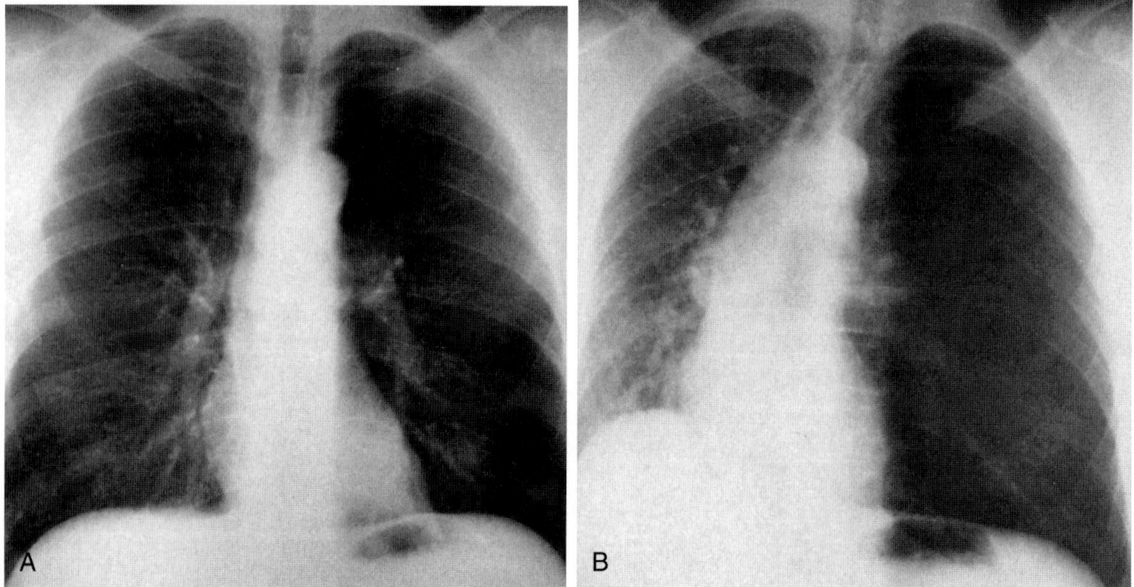

FIGURE 21–11 ■ *A*, Inspiration posteroanterior chest radiograph reveals mild hyperlucency of the left hemithorax. *B*, Expiration view reveals marked hyperlucency of the left lung with significant shift of the mediastinum to the right. These findings suggest bronchial obstruction. At bronchoscopy, this 49-year-old man was found to have a bronchogenic carcinoma that completely occluded the left mainstem bronchus.

Pulmonary Versus Extrapulmonary Disease

When an opacity is seen in the periphery of the lung, the clinician must determine if it is a pulmonary lesion extending to the pleura or if it actually represents an extrapulmonary lesion that is bulging into the lung. It is not always possible to be certain which of these is the correct situation; however, a number of signs can be helpful (Fig. 21–12). If the opacity forms acute angles with the chest wall, then most likely it is of pulmonary origin. If the angles are obtuse, then it more often represents an extrapulmonary lesion. Extrapulmonary lesions tend to be uniform in density (although pulmonary lesions may be so as well); however, if an air bronchogram is seen within the lesion then it is definitely pulmonary in origin. A pulmonary lesion may have well- or ill-defined margins, but an extrapulmonary lesion has extremely well-defined margins (as a result of the overlying visceral pleura), and these margins are convex toward the lung (Fig. 21–13).

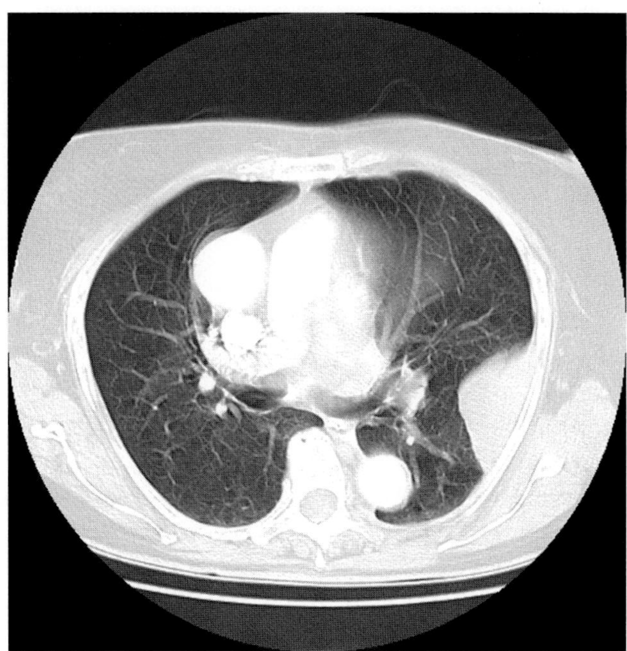

FIGURE 21–13 ■ Lymphomatous mass (in a 75-year-old woman) with obtuse angles characteristic of a pleural-based lesion.

EXTRA VIEWS

Although CT use has surpassed that of additional plain film views for the evaluation of vague opacities, there remain several projections that are still useful. Oblique views can be obtained if a density is not clearly parenchymal or osseous. It may demonstrate that the lesion lies in an overlying rib on both oblique projections and, therefore, represents a rib lesion (e.g., bone island) and not a parenchymal one. Nipple markers can be obtained to mark a nipple or a skin lesion that may mimic a parenchymal nodule. A lordotic view is a form of oblique view in which the beam is angled 15 to 20 degrees craniad. It is rarely used but is intended to demonstrate the lung apices free from superimposed shadows of the clavicle and first rib. It is useful in distinguishing pulmonary shadows from incidental osteochondromas or bony irregularities of the costochondral junctions. Frequently, however, patients still require a CT scan for confirmation.

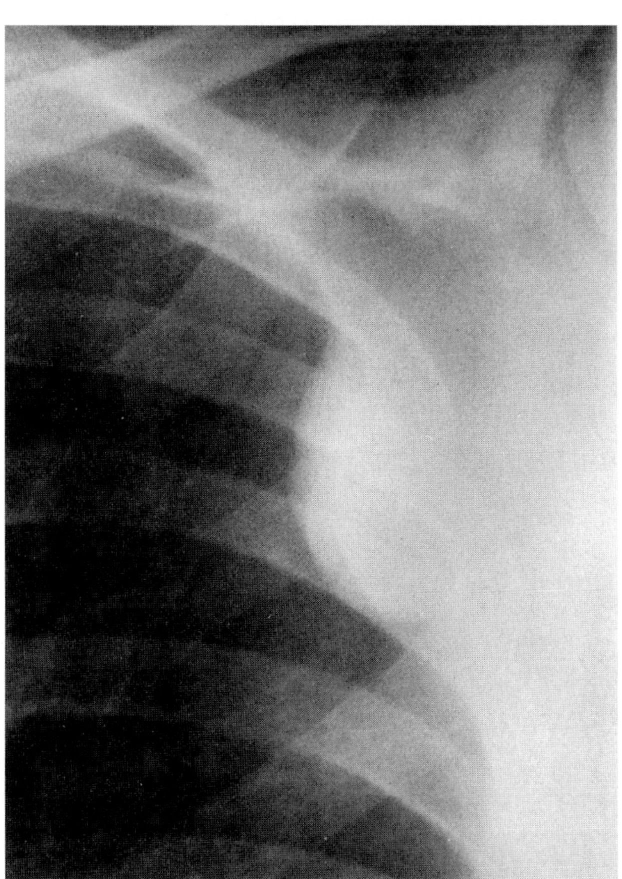

FIGURE 21–12 ■ Intercostal lipoma. Note the typical characteristics of this extrapulmonary lesion, which is protruding into the thorax. It is well defined and makes obtuse angles where it contacts the chest wall. Additionally, it is homogeneous in density and convex toward the lung.

DIGITAL CHEST RADIOGRAPHY

Digital technology has begun to replace conventional films at many institutions. It has become apparent that digital image acquisition, transmission, display, and storage have advantages in chest radiography. This system uses conventional radiographic equipment and a reusable photostimulable phosphor plate that can store an electronic latent image when exposed to x-rays. The phosphor plate is a large-area detector housed in a "filmless" cassette that traps electrons in direct proportion to the x-ray energy beam. The latent image is processed using a low-energy (red) laser beam, resulting in the emission of a blue light that is collected and converted to an electronic signal with an optically coupled photomultiplier tube. The output signal is digitized, scaled, manipulated, and translated into a gray scale image that mimics the characteristics of screen-film detectors. In the digital environment, image manipulation and postprocessing algo-

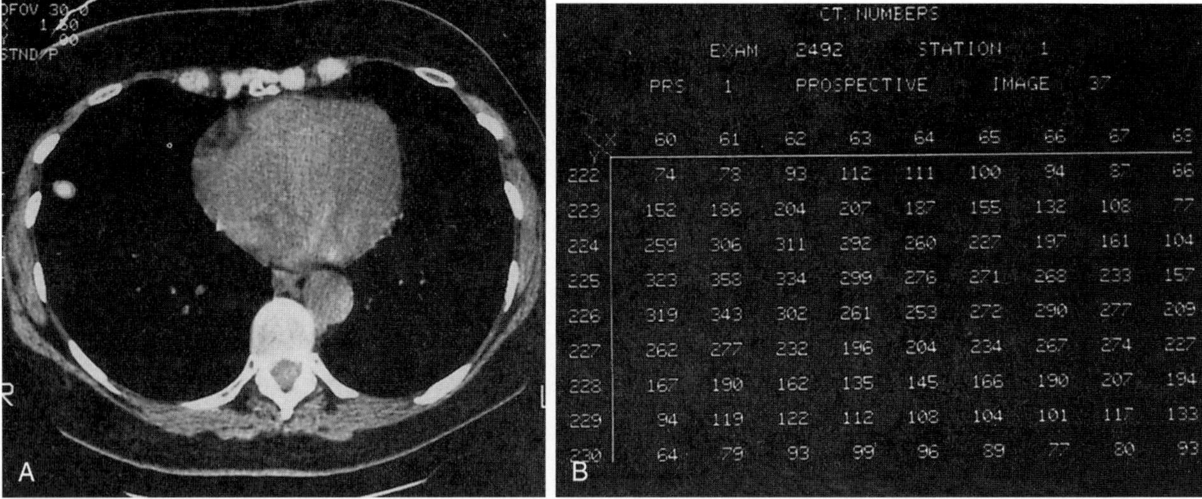

CT NUMBERS

EXAM 2492 STATION 1

PRS 1 PROSPECTIVE IMAGE 37

Y \ X	60	61	62	63	64	65	66	67	68
222	74	78	93	112	111	100	94	87	66
223	152	186	204	207	187	155	132	108	77
224	259	306	311	292	260	227	197	161	104
225	323	358	334	299	276	271	268	233	157
226	319	343	302	261	253	272	290	277	209
227	262	277	232	196	204	234	267	274	227
228	167	190	162	135	145	166	190	207	194
229	94	119	122	112	108	104	101	117	133
230	64	79	93	99	96	89	77	80	93

FIGURE 21–14 ■ *A*, Old granulomatous disease. Thin-section computed tomography scan through the lower lung reveals a nodule in the right lower lobe measuring 1 cm in diameter and containing a dense calcified central nidus. *B*, Computer readout of the density (in Hounsfield units [H]) of each of the pixels in the central part of this nodule. Note that many of these pixels have values greater than 200 H, indicating calcification.

rithms can overcome errors in exposure to produce an image within the gray-scale range that is appropriate for the chest. This ability to retrieve an image of diagnostic quality from a suboptimal exposure has led to the increasing implementation of such systems, particularly for portable chest radiography. These images may be displayed on laser-printed film or video monitors, transferred to remote sites for viewing, or archived for later reference (Ravin, 1997).

COMPUTED TOMOGRAPHY

Solitary Pulmonary Nodule

When a solitary pulmonary nodule (SPN) is identified on two views on a chest radiograph, a CT of the chest is performed with intravenous contrast for evaluation in staging of presumed bronchogenic carcinoma. If, however, there is a question as to whether a small nodule is calcified, the nodule is localized on the CT topogram, and multiple, thin (1 to 1.5 mm), contiguous sections are imaged through the nodule to further characterize it. By this method, an accurate picture of the internal characteristics of the nodule can be obtained without any effects of partial volume averaging. That is, because the thickness of tissue being imaged is such that no lung is included with the nodule, the CT numbers obtained are not affected by the air in the adjacent lung. An idea of the amount and distribution of calcium (and fat) in the nodule is thus determined. The resultant image is viewed in the standard fashion and as a matrix of numbers (Fig. 21–14). Generally, densities of 200 Hounsfield units (H) or greater are said to reflect calcium; numbers in the −40 to −120 H range indicate fat. Thin-section, CT densitometry, with or without the use of a phantom, facilitates the ability to detect calcification that cannot be identified on chest radiographs. The technique of CT densitometry was first introduced in 1980 by Siegelman and colleagues. Use of the phantom technique has largely fallen out of favor, due to substantial variability in Hounsfield unit readings between examinations and between CT scanners. However, CT densitometry is widely used to determine the amount of calcium or fat in a nodule.

If calcium is seen in the nodule, then the pattern of calcification is examined. Certain "benign" types of calcifications indicate a specific benign type of diagnosis such as granuloma or hamartoma (Fig. 21–15). Eccentric, scattered, or amorphous calcifications in nodules do not confirm benignity. Tumors occasionally arising around pre-existing calcific scars at times engulf a previous granuloma. In such cases, the calcification is most likely to be eccentric. Another explanation for eccentric calcification is reactivation of an old granulomatous process. In either case, the presence of a mass with eccentric calcification warrants further diagnostic evaluation. In the case of multiple pulmonary nodules, it must be em-

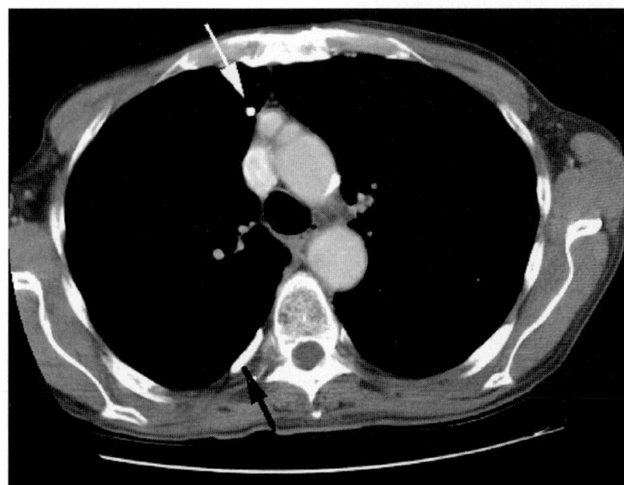

FIGURE 21–15 ■ Small calcified granuloma in the right upper lobe *(white arrow)*. Note also calcified pleural plaque in the right thorax posteriorly *(black arrow)*.

phasized that patients may have calcified granulomas and also develop carcinomas. Therefore, the presence of calcium in one nodule is meaningless with regard to the evaluation of a second nodule. The detection of minimal calcification in a mass must be cautiously interpreted. Microscopic calcifications in primary lung tumors and metastatic tumors, particular from mucin-producing adenocarcinoma and certainly from primary bone tumors, are not rare (Fig. 21–16). Calcification from metastases of osteosarcoma may be readily detected by conventional radiographs, but the microscopic calcification seen in primary lung tumor is rarely detected by conventional radiography. Detection of minimal calcification by thin-section CT or CT with a reference phantom may lead to an incorrect diagnosis of a benign process.

CT can also make a specific benign diagnosis when fat is identified within a pulmonary nodule, indicating a hamartoma (Fig. 21–17). If no calcium or fat is seen within the nodule, then it is considered suspicious for malignancy.

If a lesion can be demonstrated to be new or enlarging, or confirmation of stability over a 2-year period is not possible because no prior chest radiographs exist, an SPN must be considered to be indeterminate and very likely malignant. The following criteria are recommended for avoiding the potential pitfalls of thin-section CT: (1) Benign calcification should extend over 10% of the cross-section area of the nodule; and (2) The calcification must have a symmetric pattern of deposition, for example, diffuse, laminated, or central nidus.

Once a noncalcified nodule has been confirmed, radiographic features, including the borders and texture of the lesion, should be characterized. The borders may be smooth, lobular, ill defined, or spiculated. Although the

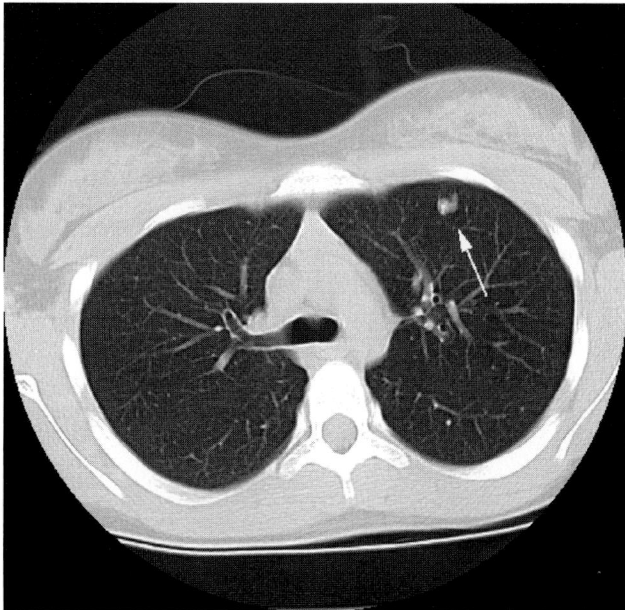

FIGURE 21–16 ■ Sixteen-year-old girl with osteosarcoma of distal femur diagnosed 3 years earlier. Computed tomography scan shows 1 × 0.8 cm partly calcified pulmonary nodule *(arrow)* in left upper lobe. Histopathologic examination of wedge resection specimen showed osteogenic sarcoma.

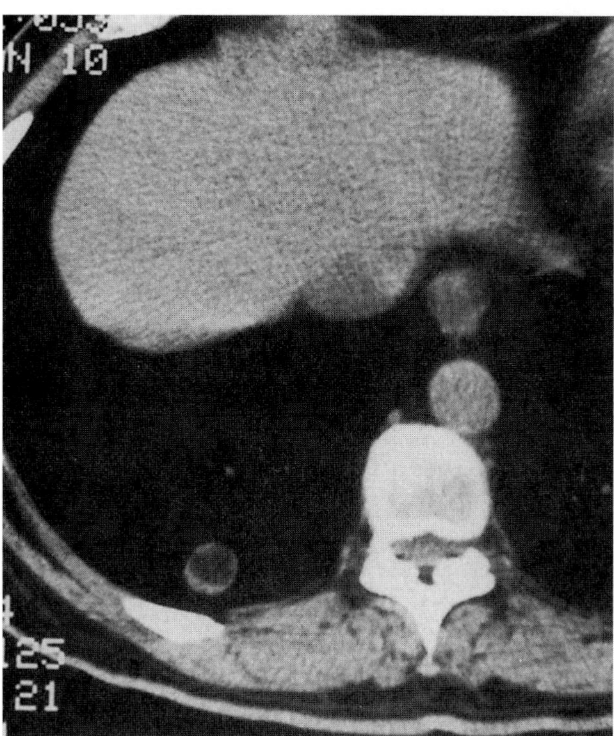

FIGURE 21–17 ■ Pulmonary hamartoma. Thin-section computed tomography scan shows a nodule in the right lower lobe, which is composed almost entirely of fat.

border characteristics are valuable, they are rarely reliable for making a definitive diagnosis. As a primary carcinoma of the lung grows, it continues to invade the surrounding parenchyma. The mass not only enlarges but may become irregular, more spiculated, and possibly even ill defined. Although the border characteristics may not be diagnostic on a single study, on serial studies they may be virtually diagnostic. However, although a smooth border is not typical of primary lung carcinoma, this appearance should not be used to exclude the diagnosis. Well-differentiated adenocarcinomas and squamous cell tumors may present as well-circumscribed, solitary nodules. In contrast, a sharply circumscribed nodule is the expected appearance for a solitary metastasis. Of note, a bronchial carcinoid, which most frequently occurs in the proximal bronchi, may also arise from more peripheral bronchi and present as a solitary nodule.

There is no single diagnostic technique that can determine with 100% accuracy that a nodule is benign or malignant. Many new emerging technologies are being investigated to improve our ability to make this distinction. Using the hypothesis that malignant nodules enhance substantially more than benign nodules, it has been demonstrated that malignant neoplasms enhanced statistically significantly more than granulomas and benign neoplasms by at least 20 H or more (Swensen et al, 1996). Another study demonstrated significantly higher peak heights of enhancement between malignant and inflammatory nodules versus benign nodules. However, no statistically significant difference in the peak height was found between malignant and inflammatory nodules (Zhang et al, 1997). Studies have also evaluated contrast

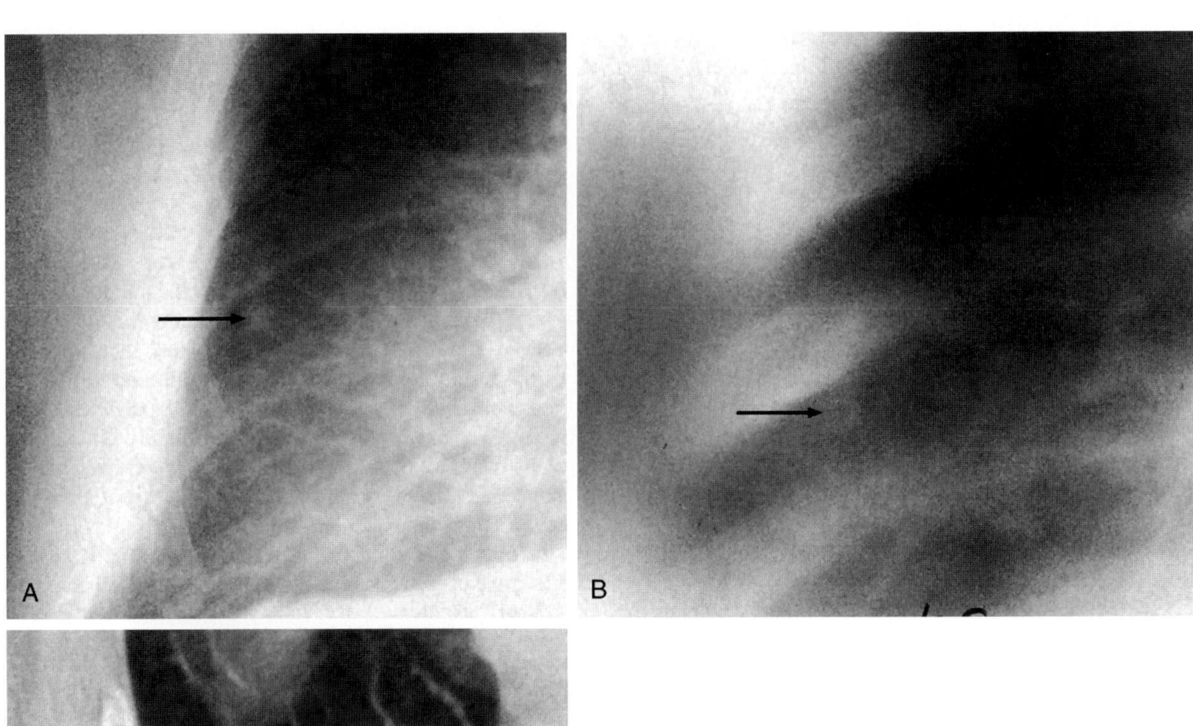

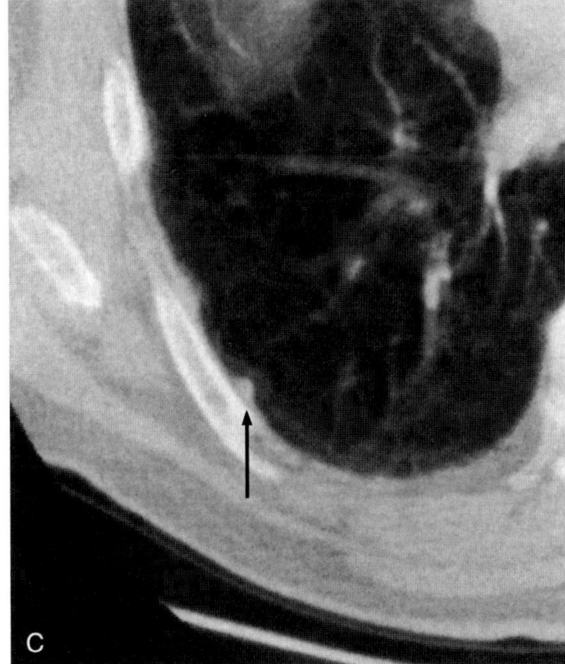

FIGURE 21–18 ■ "Pulmonary" nodule. *A,* Close-up view of a posteroanterior chest radiograph reveals a nodular density *(arrow)*, measuring 8 mm in diameter and projecting over the lateral aspect of the right midchest. *B,* Plain tomogram. This study confirms the presence of this nodule but cannot determine its exact location. Because the nodule is in focus with the adjacent rib, we can state that the nodule lies in a peripheral location. *C,* Computed tomography scan. This study reveals that the nodular density represents a focal area of pleural thickening rather than a true *(arrow)* pulmonary nodule.

enhancement patterns of nodules with dynamic contrast-enhanced MRI and have tried to differentiate between benign and malignant nodules. This has been less successful in part because small nodules, particularly those 1 cm or less, are not reliably identified on MRI. PET scanning is becoming a common technique for the evaluation of SPN; this is discussed in more detail in the PET section.

Evaluation of the SPN with repeated CT scans to depict growth of the nodule has also been investigated. Preliminary experience with early repeat CT suggested that a single repeat CT scan obtained within 30 days after the first scan can depict growth even in tumors as small as 5 mm in diameter. This technique is not available for routine clinical use because it requires software implementation that is not available at most centers (Yankelevitz et al, 1999).

Other Focal Lesions

CT is useful in determining if a suspicious nodule seen on the plain radiograph lies within the lung or not (Fig. 21–18). For example, lesions such as bone islands, costochondral junctions, tortuous mediastinal vessels, and focal areas of pleural thickening can all be clearly distinguished from true pulmonary nodules by CT.

Pulmonary hamartomas can often be diagnosed as such by CT densitometry by finding a well-defined nodule containing fat (−40 to −120 H) with or without calcium. In one large study of 47 patients with this lesion (Siegelman et al, 1986b), fat without calcium was found in 18 patients, fat with calcium in 10 patients, and calcium alone in 2 patients.

Round atelectasis is a unique form of chronic atelectasis that resembles a mass. The mechanism that leads to the formation of round atelectasis is uncertain. One suggestion is that a pleural effusion occurs initially and causes elevation and compression atelectasis of the adjacent lower lobe (Hanke, 1980). The atelectatic lung may adhere to the parietal pleural and to the major fissure. As the pleural effusion clears, the atelectatic lung folds in on itself, leading to the condition of round atelectasis, sometimes referred to as "rounded" atelectasis.

CT demonstrates vessels and bronchi coursing into a region of round atelectasis, thereby proving the true nature of what might otherwise be considered a nonspecific pulmonary mass by chest radiography. In certain instances, these curving vessels form the so-called comet-tail sign. Other CT features of round atelectasis include a rounded, pleural-based mass; adjacent pleural thickening; an ill-defined margin medially where it contacts the incoming vessels; and the frequent presence of air bronchograms within it (Doyle et al, 1984; McHugh et al, 1989). Lesions demonstrating classic features of round atelectasis can be conservatively managed with serial CT scans. Newly diagnosed lesions should be followed up at 3, 6, 12, and 24 months to ensure stability of the lesion for a minimum of 2 years (Kuhlman, 1997). Lesions with an atypical appearance may require needle biopsy or thoracoscopic sampling for definitive diagnosis. However, the biopsy results should be interpreted cautiously because samples of areas of rounded atelectasis sometimes demonstrate misleading findings.

CT is useful in demonstrating arteriovenous malformations (AVMs) as the cause of a pulmonary nodule (Fig. 21–19). The feeding artery and draining vein are usually clearly visualized. The presence of large vessels entering a nodule should strongly suggest a diagnosis of AVM (Fig. 21–20). It is imperative to rule out the possibility of AVM prior to either transbronchial or percutaneous biopsy.

Sequestrations can usually be definitively diagnosed with helical CT following a bolus injection of intravenous contrast because the vascular supply can be determined as primarily from the pulmonary artery (i.e., AVM) or the aorta (i.e., sequestration). If the lesion opacifies in phase with the pulmonary artery or vein, it is supplied by the pulmonary artery; if its peak opacification coincides with or immediately follows peak aortic enhancement, then its vascular supply is primarily systemic. Pulmonary venous drainage may be demonstrable with an intralobar sequestration, whereas systemic venous drainage may be seen in an extralobar sequestration, a lesion that usually does not require surgical resection. MRI may also be used to define and characterize the size and course of anomalous feeding vessels.

Lung Cancer Staging

The role of CT in the initial staging of patients with bronchogenic carcinoma is controversial. It has been used in assessing the tumor (T), node (N), and metastasis (M) aspects of the disease (TNM staging), but the following discussion is limited to only the N and T factors.

The CT technique that is most often used includes 7-mm–thick, contiguous images from the thoracic apex into the upper abdomen, including the liver and adrenal glands. Intravenous contrast material aids in detecting hepatic lesions and in assessing hila and the mediastinum in problematic situations. Additional 2- to 3-mm–thick images through the hilar regions are also helpful. The nodes may be round or oblong on the CT transverse images, and some interpreters measure the long axis of the nodes. Others measure the short axis. There is no definite consensus as to which is superior. Nodes tend to be oblong in the superoinferior direction, but this is difficult to assess on CT scanning. For example, if a lymph node in the right paratracheal region is seen on two contiguous images, it cannot be ascertained if this actually represents one oblong node or two separate nodes lying one above the other. Therefore, lymph node size as measured by CT may not be equal to the size measured pathologically. In addition, there are some specific pitfalls that are well known in the assessment of mediastinal nodes. For example, one must be careful not to interpret the top of the left pulmonary artery as an anteroposterior window node. Similarly, the transverse sinus of the pericardium, located just posterior to the ascending aorta and just above the right pulmonary artery, must not be mistaken for a lymph node.

N Factor

A number of studies were performed on normal patients to determine the upper limits of normal for each of the

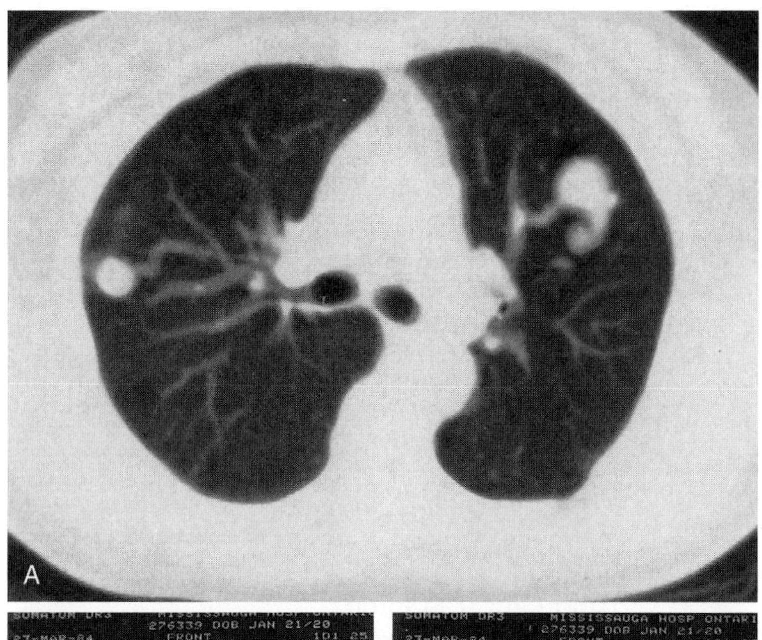

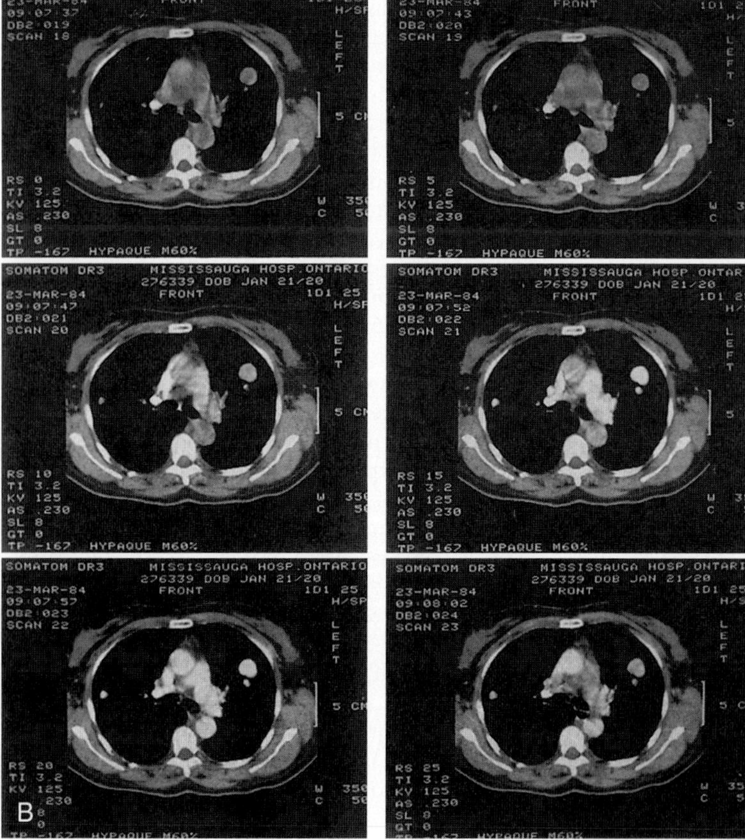

FIGURE 21–19 ■ A 64-year-old woman with known Rendu-Osler-Weber disease. *A*, CT scan. Bilateral upper lobe pulmonary nodules are noted, along with dilated feeding vessels. *B*, Six images from a dynamic scan through the same level. The pulmonary nodules pick up contrast as soon as it is seen in the left pulmonary artery *(third image)*. Maximum opacification is present on the fourth image, and by the sixth image, the density of the nodules has returned almost to baseline.

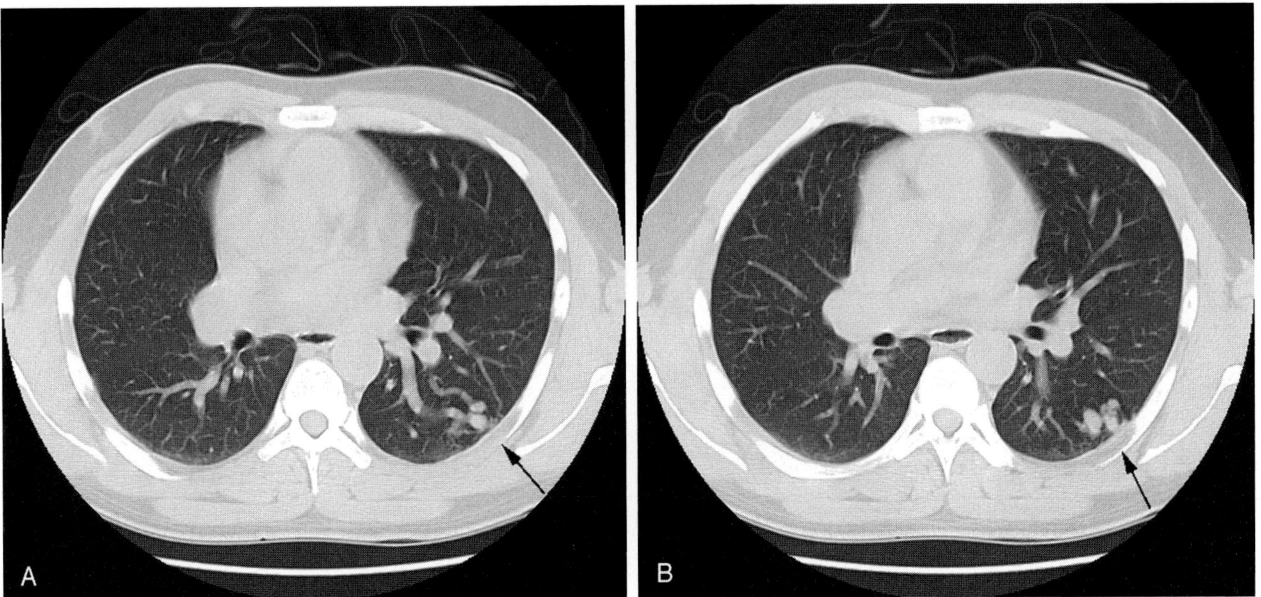

FIGURE 21–20 ■ *A* and *B*, 30-year-old man with juvenile polyposis status following colectomy. Cluster of nodules *(arrow)* is seen in the superior segment of the left lower lobe with a draining vein and arterial supply representing an arteriovenous malformation.

American Thoracic Society nodal stations (Genereux et al, 1984; Glazer et al, 1985b; Kiyono et al, 1988; Quint et al, 1986). The largest nodes are generally found in the right tracheobronchial angle region (station 10R) and in the subcarinal region (7). In practice, the upper limit of normal is considered to be 1 cm; this size is used whether the long or short axis is measured.

A large number of studies looked at the ability of CT to detect mediastinal nodal disease. These were summarized in several reviews (Aronchick, 1990; Libshitz, 1990; Webb, 1987). Using 1 cm as the criterion for abnormality, from these studies a range of sensitivities of 29% to 95% is found, with a range of specificities from 46% to 94% (Libshitz, 1990). The published studies differ greatly in a number of details, including the prevalence of granulomatous disease, prevalence of metastatic disease, relative proportion of each T stage, prospective versus retrospective CT technique, and, very importantly, the extent of nodal dissection (Freedman, 1992). In those studies in which complete nodal dissection is the therapy of choice, relatively lower sensitivities were noted (Freedman, 1992; McLoud et al, 1992; Webb et al, 1991) as would be expected. If a normal-sized node is not resected (e.g., as might occur if it is not palpable during thoracotomy), then the result is called a "true negative" by CT; however, this would be a "false negative" if a complete nodal dissection had been performed and the node were found to contain a tumor.

In clinical practice, two specific questions arise in analyzing the patient. These are: (1) What is the clinical significance of having one or more nodes greater than 1 cm in diameter? and (2) What is the clinical significance if all nodes are less than 1 cm in size?

Nodes between 1 and 2 cm in diameter have a 25% to 30% chance of harboring a tumor; nodes greater than 2 cm in diameter have a 70% to 75% chance of harboring a tumor (Libshitz, 1990) (Fig. 21–21). Therefore, even patients with nodes larger than 2 cm in diameter have a 25% to 30% chance of having no tumor within these lymph nodes. Thus, nodal enlargement alone on CT scanning does not make a patient's condition inoperable; biopsy proof is required.

In patients with no enlarged lymph nodes, the chance of mediastinal involvement is generally in the 3% to 16% range (Gross et al, 1988; McKenna et al, 1985b; Whittlesey, 1988) (Fig. 21–22). In fact, little correlation between the presence of mediastinal nodal metastases and nodal size has been demonstrated. Metastases may be found in 21% of normal nodes (Arita et al, 1995), and up to 40% of enlarged nodes in some series are not cancerous (Arita et al, 1996). Some interpret these figures to mean that the patient can undergo thoracotomy directly (Whittlesey, 1988); others believe that mediastinoscopy is still necessary (Patterson et al, 1987). The issue must be individualized to the particular institution, and there must be good communication between the surgeon and the radiologist as to what is and is not thought to be significant.

The finding of normal-sized, mediastinal nodes by CT does not imply that the patient is free of metastatic disease. In fact, such patients have a 25% chance of having stage Ml disease (Sider et al, 1988).

A number of questions still remain unanswered. For example, there is some evidence that CT scanning accuracy can be improved by using different nodal sizes in different stations. As stated earlier, superior mediastinal nodes are normally smaller than are pericarinal nodes. Average normal 2R nodes measure 3 mm in diameter; average normal 10R nodes measure 7 mm. If one assumes that the presence of tumor enlarges the lymph node diameter by 5 mm, then a 2R node becomes 8 mm in size and will still be called normal, using 1 cm as the

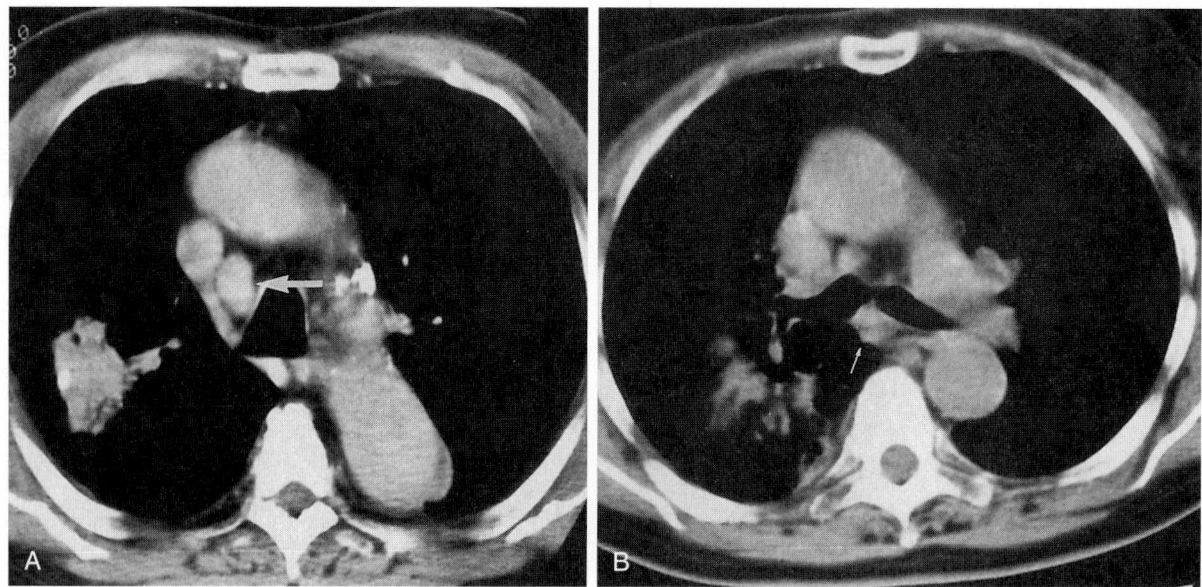

FIGURE 21–21 ■ *A*, Computed tomography scan in this 74-year-old man reveals a right upper-lobe bronchogenic carcinoma with an enlarged lymph node in the right tracheal bronchial angle region *(arrow)*. Pathologic examination revealed malignant cells in this nodule, which has been removed at mediastinoscopy. *B*, In this 70-year-old woman with a right upper lobe, bronchogenic carcinoma, an enlarged node measuring 1.7 × 1.3 cm in size is seen in the posterior subcarinal region *(arrow)*. This node was found to be free of tumor at thoracotomy.

cutoff. A 10R node becomes 12 mm in size and is considered positive. From this analysis, we might predict that the sensitivity for the 2R nodal station would be low but the specificity would be high. This is exactly what was found. For example, in one study (Staples et al, 1988) the sensitivity in the 2R region was found to be 0.22; the specificity was 0.98. This is in contrast to the observed 10R sensitivity and specificity of 0.63 and 0.73, respectively.

Similarly, cell type may play a role in affecting the CT accuracy. False-negative nodal disease appears more likely with adenocarcinoma than with squamous cell carcinoma (Staples et al, 1988). Additionally, the location of the primary tumor is believed by some to be a factor, although this is also controversial. Although some reports have demonstrated that the sensitivity of CT scanning is higher for central than for peripheral tumors (Staples et al, 1988), the opposite was found to be the case in a meta-analysis study (Dales et al, 1990).

MRI and CT have been shown to have comparable accuracy in the evaluation of mediastinal lymph-node metastases. This is an expected finding because both techniques rely predominately on size criteria for determining nodal status. There are, however, potential advantages and disadvantages of MRI when compared with CT. An advantage of MRI relates to its multiplanar imaging capabilities, which may be helpful in assessing lymph nodes in areas that are difficult to assess in the

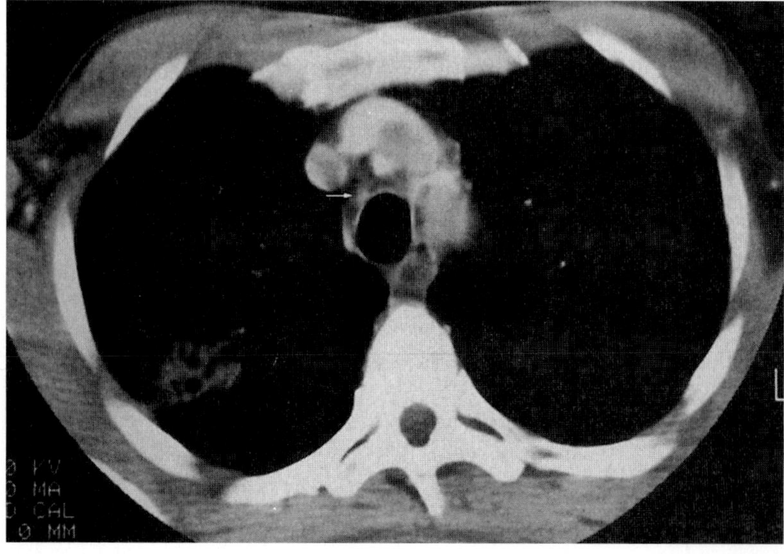

FIGURE 21–22 ■ Computed tomography scan of high paratracheal region in this 53-year-old man will a right upper-lobe, bronchogenic carcinoma. A tiny 2R node, measuring about 2 mm in diameter *(arrow)*, was found to contain tumor at mediastinoscopy.

axial plane, particularly the aortopulmonary window and subcarinal region. A second possible advantage relates to the ease of distinguishing lymph nodes from blood vessels on MRI. Although this distinction is usually readily apparent on CT images, difficulties infrequently arise in patients with contraindications to intravenous contrast. Thus, MRI may be helpful as a problem-solving tool for inconclusive CT cases. There is a disadvantage to MRI because calcification within lymph nodes may be overlooked. Thus, an enlarged calcified lymph node from prior granulomatous infection may be misdiagnosed as metastatic disease. An exciting area of investigation is physiologic MRI of the lymph nodes with iron oxide. This technique is based on the principle that differing cell types demonstrate varying degrees of iron-oxide uptake. Thus, normal and metastatic lymph nodes can be differentiated by their signal characteristics. This is currently being evaluated in clinical trials.

PET scanning has recently emerged as another modality to stage lung cancer and is discussed in a separate section. A recent meta-analysis comparing PET and CT for the demonstration of mediastinal nodal metastases in patients with non–small cell lung cancer indicated PET as superior to CT for mediastinal staging (Dwamena 1999).

It appears that the use of CT scanning (versus mediastinoscopy) in evaluating patients with mediastinal nodal disease varies from institution to institution, and it is important that the radiologist and the surgeon discuss each case individually. Although it is invasive and requires a general anesthetic, mediastinoscopy has a better sensitivity and specificity than does CT scanning, MRI, or PET. Additionally, it must be stressed that the clinician must prove the presence of metastatic disease in enlarged nodes and not deem the patient's condition inoperable by cross-sectional imaging alone.

T Factor

Although a large number of studies have investigated mediastinal nodal disease, few have examined chest wall and mediastinal invasion by the primary tumor. The surgeon may want to know if the chest wall is involved prior to thoracotomy because of the increased morbidity and mortality rates associated with chest wall resection (Patterson et al, 1982) compared with the general situation (Ginsberg et al, 1983). Additionally, it affects the surgical approach because the surgeon does not want to make the thoracotomy incision at the level of chest wall invasion, and the prognosis for a patient with N1 or N2 disease and chest wall involvement is poor (Patterson et al, 1982; Piehler et al, 1982).

Generally speaking, CT performs poorly in the assessment of chest wall involvement in most cases (Glazer et al, 1985a; Pennes et al, 1985). Many different CT signs were examined, including the length of contact of the tumor with the chest wall, the angles that were made at the point of contact, and the presence of asymmetry of the chest wall soft tissues adjacent to the tumor. None of these signs was reliable. Highly predictive signs of chest wall invasion are definite rib destruction and the presence of a large, soft tissue mass in the adjacent chest wall (Glazer et al, 1985a; Pennes et al, 1985; Fig. 21–23). If there is no evidence of pleural thickening, the chest wall is not involved (Glazer et al, 1985a; Pennes et al, 1985). MRI is better than CT scanning in assessing chest wall involvement. However, this does not mean that CT plays no role. For example, it may demonstrate clearly that a mass that appears contiguous with the chest wall on the plain chest radiograph is actually separate from it.

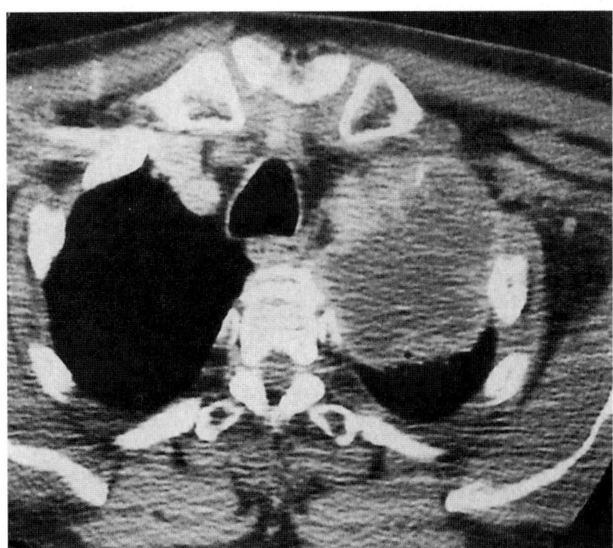

FIGURE 21–23 ■ Computed tomography scan in this 78-year-old man with a left upper-lobe, bronchogenic carcinoma reveals that the tumor is extending directly into the chest wall, almost completely destroying the left first rib.

Similar to chest wall involvement, CT assessment of mediastinal invasion is poor (Glazer et al, 1989b; Scott et al, 1988; Webb et al, 1991). Most investigators used the findings of gross interdigitation of the tumor with mediastinal fat or encasement of mediastinal structures as indications of mediastinal invasion (Figs. 21–24 and

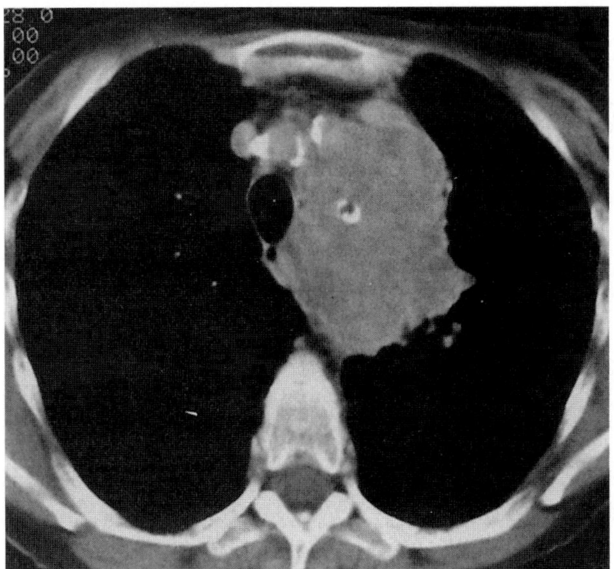

FIGURE 21–24 ■ This left upper-lobe carcinoma has extended directly into the mediastinum where it can be seen to be surrounding the calcified left subclavian artery completely.

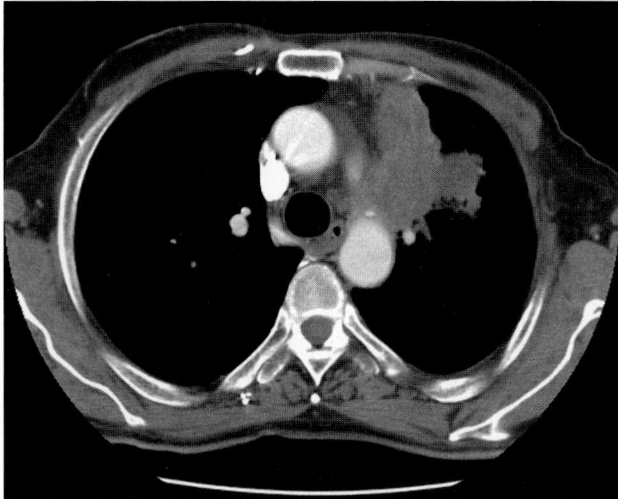

FIGURE 21–25 ■ Large, left upper lobe, squamous cell cancer. Loss of fat plane between the mass and mediastinum suggests invasion of the mediastinum.

21–25). However, even these signs were shown to lack sensitivity and to be poor predictors of mediastinal invasion (Herman et al, 1991b). Other criteria were also studied in this regard, including the angle that the tumor makes with the mediastinum, the length of contact, whether vessels are indented by the tumor, whether there is bronchial wall thickening, the presence or absence of a fat plane between the mass and the mediastinal structures, and the degree of contact with the aorta (Fig. 21–26). Using these criteria, sensitivity was found to range from 53% to 84% and specificity from 57% to 94% (Baron et al, 1982; Martini et al, 1985; Kameda et al, 1988; Rendina et al, 1987; Webb et al, 1991; Wursten and Vock, 1987). Importantly, the positive predictive value is in the 64% to 84% range (Baron et al, 1982; Wursten and Vock, 1987), and, therefore, the clinician must not assume that a tumor is inoperable from CT criteria alone.

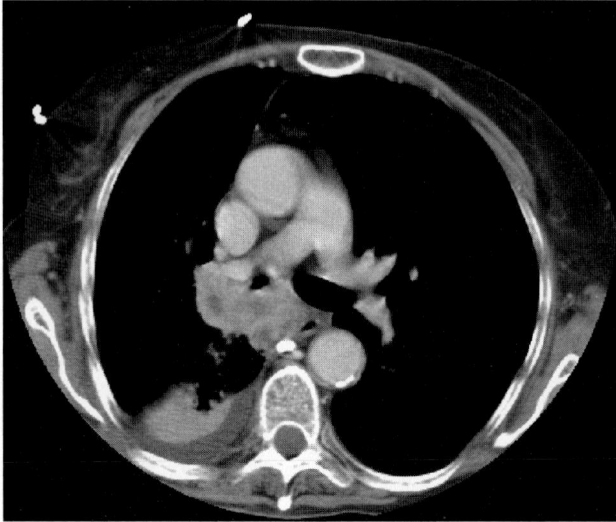

FIGURE 21–26 ■ Squamous cell carcinoma invading the right mainstem bronchus and bronchus intermedius with extension to the right main pulmonary artery. Resultant partial collapse of right lower lobe. Note mediastinal shift to the right owing to the volume loss. A small pleural effusion is also present.

CONCLUSIONS

Although CT scanning provides excellent visualization of the mediastinum, it is not accurate enough to allow the clinician to deem a patient's condition inoperable by CT criteria alone. This applies to both the presence of nodal involvement and mediastinal invasion. Other means of detecting involvement with certainty must be used. That is, enlarged lymph nodes require histologic proof of metastatic involvement. Similar proof of direct mediastinal invasion may be necessary, although not uncommonly, certain clinical features are sufficient. For example, tumor surrounding the superior vena cava in the presence of clinical superior vena caval syndrome or a tumor in the aortopulmonary window in the presence of a left vocal cord paralysis is good evidence of direct mediastinal invasion.

Some other uses of CT in patients with bronchogenic carcinoma include its use as a guide to the radiotherapist, its ability to detect recurrent disease in patients who have had a pneumonectomy (Glazer et al, 1984a; Peters et al, 1983), and its ability to distinguish recurrent tumor from radiation fibrosis (Bourgouin et al, 1987).

Central Airway Disease

Bronchoscopy is superior to CT scanning in determining if an airway lesion is endobronchial, submucosal, or extrabronchial (Naidich et al, 1990). Although an unequivocal filling defect within an airway is highly suggestive of endobronchial disease (Fig. 21–27), the CT finding of narrowing cannot be definitive in distinguishing among these three (Fig. 21–28). However, CT scanning is much better for detecting the extent of extrabronchial disease than is bronchoscopy and, therefore, can be useful in guiding the bronchoscopist to the site of a transbronchial needle biopsy (Fig. 21–29). In addition, by demonstrating the extent of peribronchial tumor, CT scanning was shown to be useful in predicting which patients will benefit from photodynamic therapy by virtue of harboring early T1 tumors (Zwirewich et al, 1988).

A number of studies have been performed that compared CT and fiberoptic bronchoscopy in the detection of abnormalities of the central airways. In one large study (Naidich et al, 1987) using 1.5- and 10-mm thick sections and bronchoscopy as the procedure of choice, CT had a sensitivity of 90% and a specificity of 92%; all malignant lesions were accurately visualized. In another study (Mayr et al, 1989), the use of contiguous 4-mm-thick sections was found to yield a sensitivity and specificity of 100%.

If a specific airway is closely associated with a pulmonary mass, forming the so-called positive bronchus sign, it has been shown that a transbronchial biopsy is more likely to have a positive yield (Naidich et al, 1988). In this study, the yield from transbronchial biopsy was 60% in patients with this sign but only 30% in those without it. In another study of 33 patients with proven bronchogenic carcinoma (Gaeta et al, 1991), transbronchial bi-

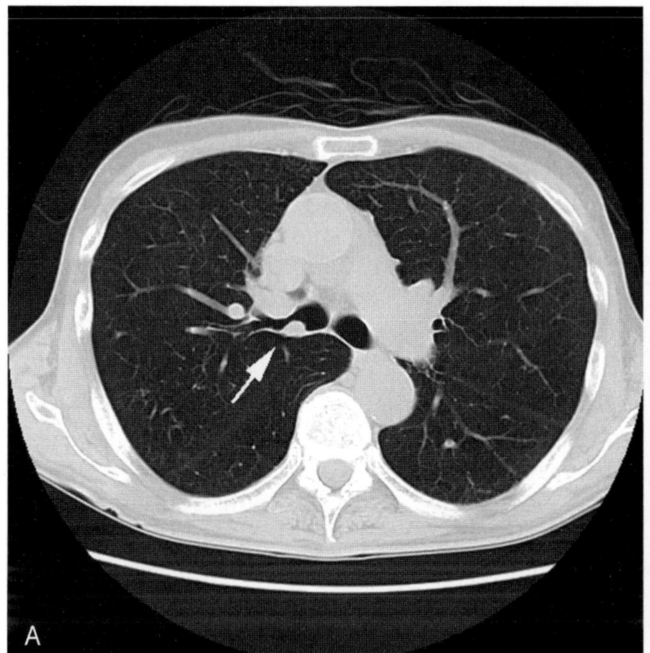

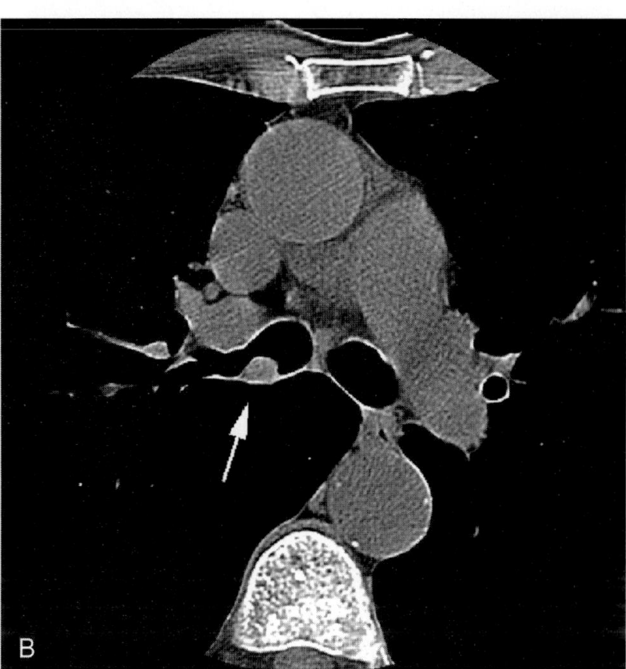

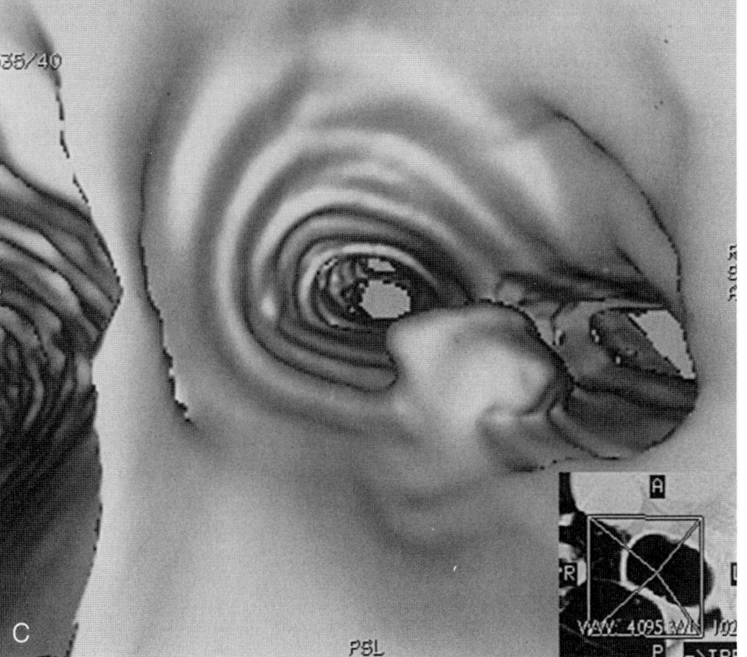

FIGURE 21–27 ■ *A*, Computed tomography scan of a 75-year-old with rectal cancer demonstrates a 7 × 10 mm polypoid lesion in the right mainstem bronchus *(arrow)*. *B*, Follow-up 3-mm prone images exclude mucus by demonstrating the lesion's adherence to the posterior wall. Biopsy of this lesion demonstrated a carcinoid. *C*, Virtual bronchoscopic rendering of the lesion in the right mainstem bronchus. The bronchus intermedius and right upper-lobe bronchus are seen distal to the lesion.

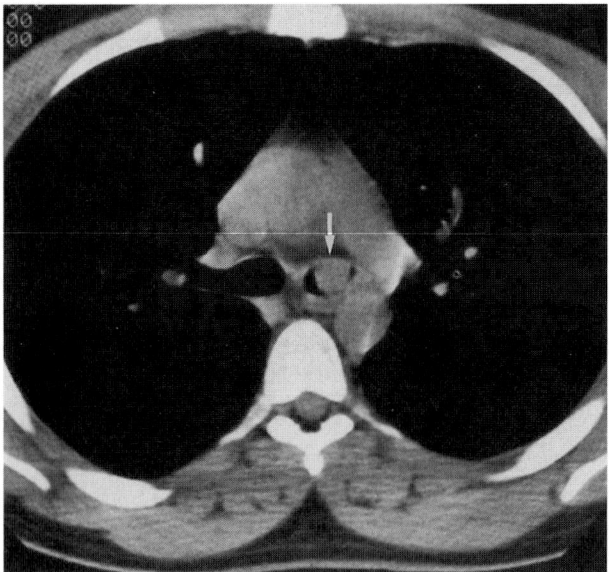

FIGURE 21–28 ■ Computed tomography scan of a 20-year-old man with a mucoepidermoid tumor in the left mainstem bronchus *(arrow)*. The presence of soft tissue within an airway, as exemplified by this case, is highly suggestive of endobronchial tumor.

opsy and brushing revealed tumor in 13 of 22 (59%) patients with the sign but only 2 of 11 (18%) without it. If the sign was present in a fourth-order bronchus, then there was a 90% success rate at bronchoscopy, compared with a 33% success rate when the sign was present in fifth through seventh-order bronchi.

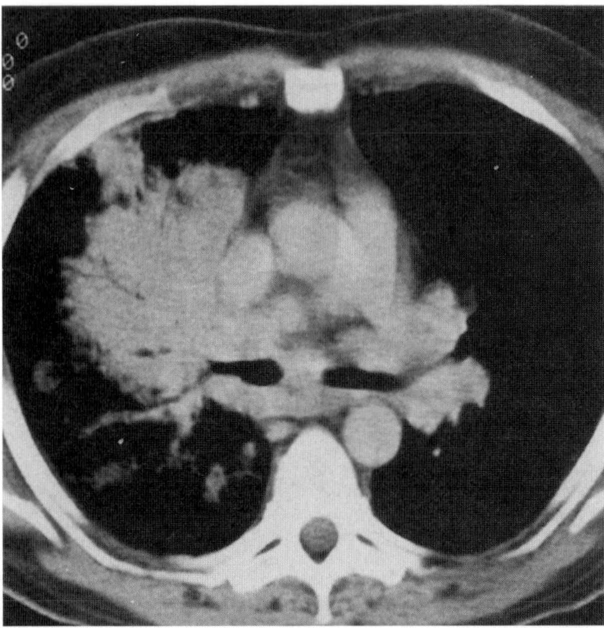

FIGURE 21–29 ■ Bronchoscopy in this 51-year-old man with bronchogenic carcinoma revealed a splayed carina and occlusion of one segmental branch of the right upper lobe by extrinsic compression. The right upper-lobe bronchus itself is normal. The computed tomography scan in this patient reveals extensive tumor surrounding the right upper-lobe airways and the right mainstem bronchus itself.

CT has been shown to be very useful in evaluating patients with hemoptysis (Naidich et al, 1990) (Fig. 21–30). In this study of 58 patients investigated by plain radiography, CT, and fiberoptic bronchoscopy, airway abnormalities were detected at CT in 28 patients (48%). Eighteen of these patients had central airway problems (including all such lesions detected by bronchoscopy), and 10 had bronchiectasis. All 24 patients ultimately proven to have malignant disease had abnormal CT scan results (17 had a central airway abnormality, and 21 had a mass lesion).

Lobar Collapse

CT was shown to be useful in assessing patients with lobar collapse (Naidich et al, 1983a, 1983b). It may demonstrate evidence of a central bronchial abnormality or hilar mass that is causing a bronchial obstruction when no such mass is evident on the plain radiograph (Woodring, 1988; Figs. 21–31 and 21–32). Occasionally, a small hilar mass can be simulated by lobar vessels. If this is considered a possibility, images through this region must be obtained following a bolus of intravenous contrast material.

A characteristic finding of central bronchial obstruction on CT, which cannot be seen by chest radiography, is the presence of so-called mucus bronchograms (Woodring, 1988; Fig. 21–33). In this situation, dilated bronchi filled with low-density material can be seen within the collapsed lobe. This finding suggests a central obstructing lesion (Glazer et al, 1989a). Similarly, the absence of air bronchograms on CT suggests, but not definitely, the presence of obstruction; in one study (Woodring, 1988) it was associated with obstruction 89% of the time. In 34% of those with air bronchograms, a central obstruction was present (Woodring, 1988).

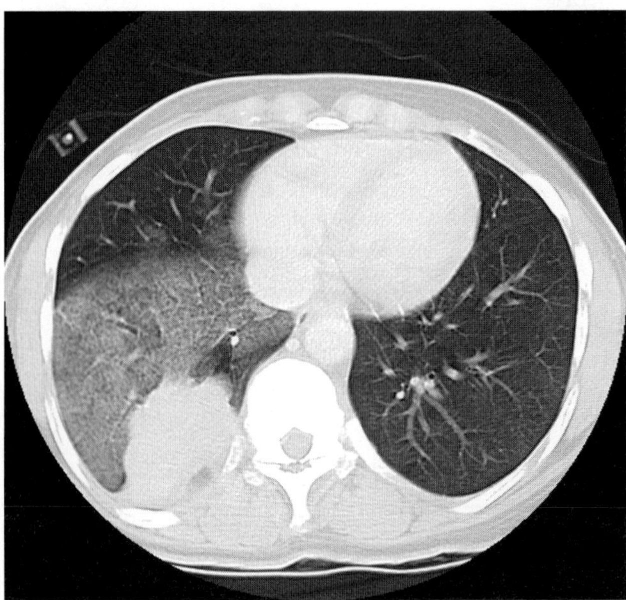

FIGURE 21–30 ■ Forty-five-year-old woman with known right lower-lobe adenocarcinoma presented with hemoptysis. New ground-glass opacity adjacent to the mass is consistent with hemorrhage.

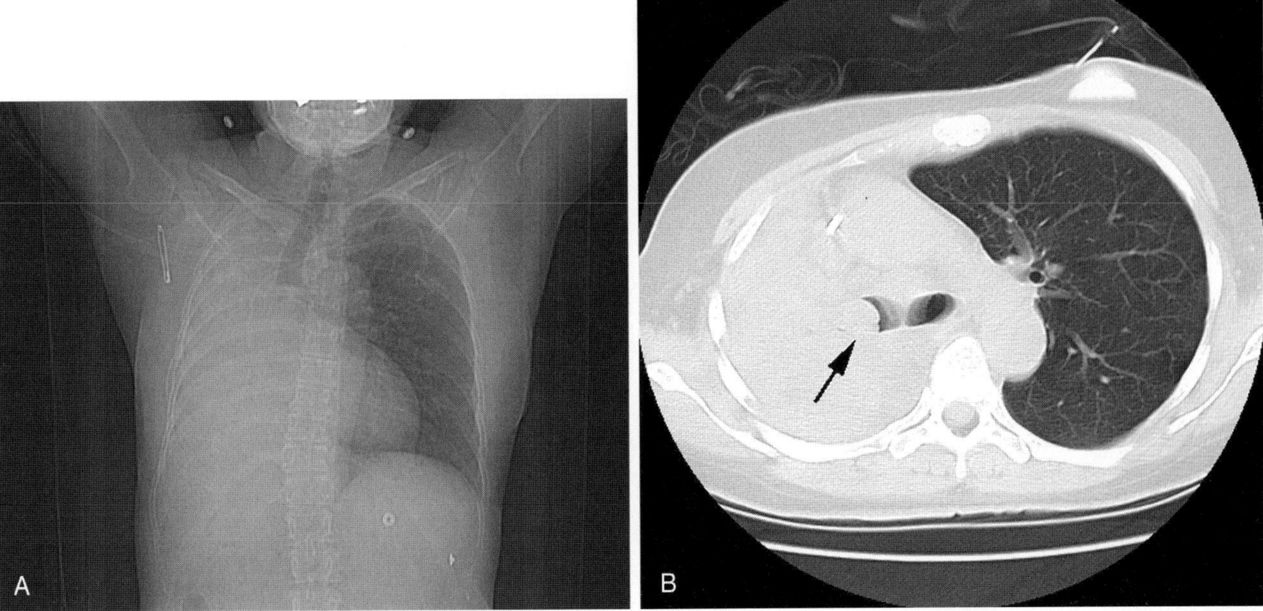

FIGURE 21–31 ■ *A*, Computed tomography scout topogram demonstrates complete opacification of the right hemithorax and volume loss. Cutoff of the right mainstem bronchus suggests an underlying mass with complete collapse of right lung as well as a pleural effusion. *B*, Obstructing mass in the right mainstem bronchus *(arrow)*.

Bronchiectasis

Bronchiectasis is defined as irreversible, abnormal dilatation of one or more bronchi. Thin-section CT of the chest has replaced bronchography as the technique for diagnosis of bronchiectasis because of its demonstrated accuracy and relative noninvasiveness. In the early years of CT scanning, controversy existed regarding the accuracy of CT in the diagnosis of bronchiectasis. On a segment-by-segment basis, the sensitivity of CT compared with that of bronchography was found to be low, in the 63% to 66% range (Cooke et al, 1987; Silverman and Godwin, 1987). Cystic bronchiectasis was clearly seen, but varicose and cylindrical bronchiectases were more difficult to detect (Muller et al, 1984). However, with the advent of HRCT (utilizing 1- and 1.5-mm sections obtained every 10 mm), even cylindrical bronchiectasis can be accurately assessed. CT is considered to be the procedure of choice for imaging this condition (Muller, 1991), having replaced contrast bronchography.

Bronchiectasis is classified on CT as cylindrical, vari-

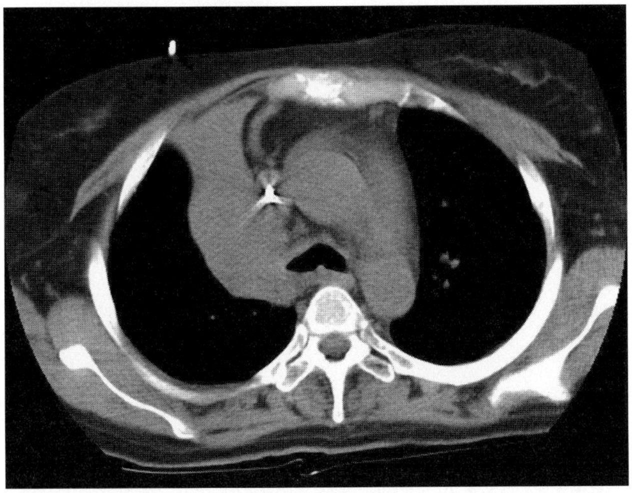

FIGURE 21–32 ■ Forty-three-year-old woman with aplastic anemia and graft-versus-host disease presented with a cough following bone marrow transplant. Bronchoscopy revealed a mucus plug causing the right upper lobe collapse.

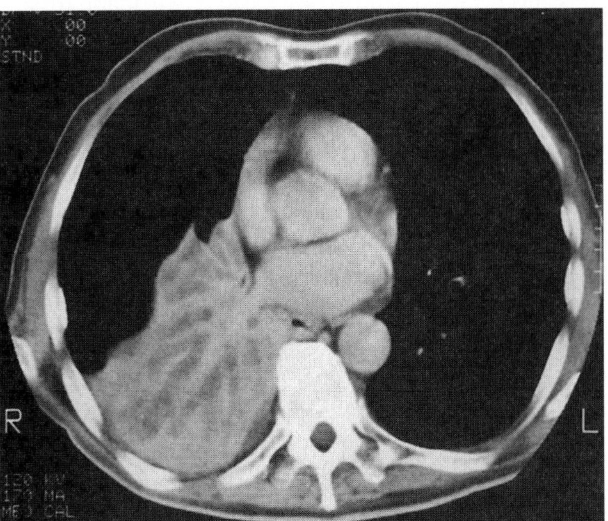

FIGURE 21–33 ■ This 74-year-old man had a bronchogenic carcinoma causing complete obstruction of the bronchus intermedius and complete collapse of the right middle and lower lobes. The computed tomography scan reveals dilated bronchi filled with relatively low-density bronchial secretions (mucus bronchograms).

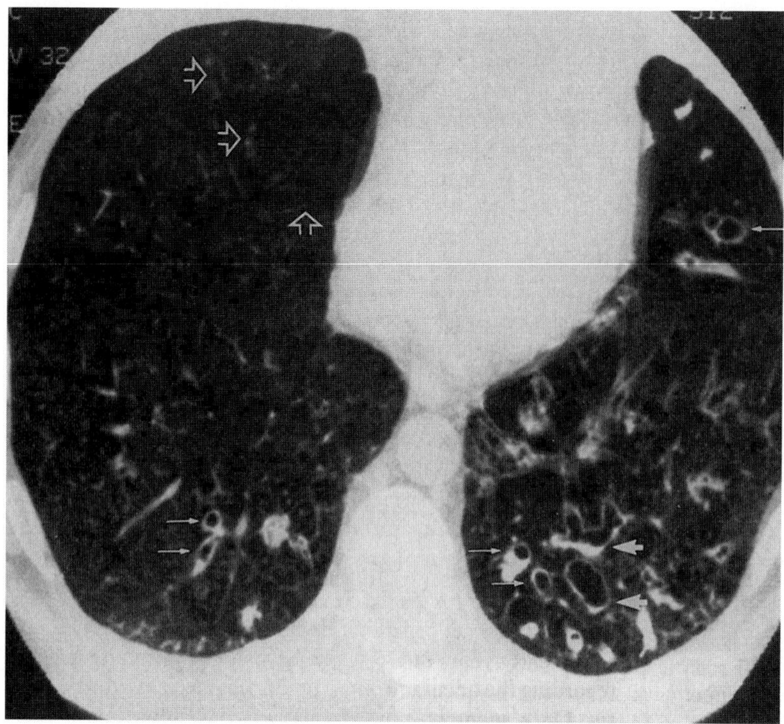

FIGURE 21–34 ■ Bronchiectasis. This high-resolution computed tomography image reveals moderately severe cystic bronchiectasis in the left lower lobe, with small amounts of fluid present in some of the cysts *(short solid arrows)*. Cylindrical bronchiectasis is seen in both lower lobes and in the lingula *(long narrow arrows)*. Note also the emphysema in the right middle lobe *(open arrows)*.

cose, or cystic. Cylindrical bronchiectasis is diagnosed when lack of bronchial tapering or smooth bronchial dilatation occurs, with the internal bronchial diameter being greater than that of the accompanying pulmonary artery. Varicose bronchiectasis is the diagnosis when an irregular or beaded dilatation of the bronchus occurs. Cystic bronchiectasis is diagnosed when strings or clusters of cysts are evident. Cystic bronchiectasis and varicose bronchiectasis imply more bronchial destruction than cylindrical bronchiectasis and might be expected to be associated with more severe clinical symptoms. Bronchiectasis is diagnosed with HRCT when abnormally dilated, thick-walled airways are seen (Figs. 21–34 and 21–35). Normally, bronchi are visualized only in the inner and middle thirds of the lung with HRCT. With bronchiectasis, because of the dilatation of the airways and thickening of their walls, bronchi can be seen more peripherally. A length of an abnormal bronchus will be seen if it is running in the transverse plane. When oblique or vertical, the abnormal bronchus appears to be oval or round in configuration, respectively. Because bronchi are accompanied by branches of the pulmonary artery, a signet ring appearance is frequently seen when these abnormal airways are observed sagittally. Varicose bronchiectasis can be recognized by the beaded appearance of the bronchial wall. With cystic bronchiectasis, there are several, large, air-containing spaces, with water-dense walls, which may contain air-fluid levels. The cysts frequently are arranged linearly, which can be noted either directly on a single transverse image or more indirectly by analyzing contiguous images. CT findings commonly associated with bronchiectasis include bronchial wall thickening, mucoid impaction, atelectasis, and decreased lung attenuation assumed to represent air trapping.

Several interpretative errors can occur on CT scans. One common error is to mistake the same "dots" that are due to bronchiectasis and mucous plugging of small airways for true nodules or tiny cavities. Bronchiectasis, particularly milder forms of the disease, is much harder to appreciate and easily overlooked on conventional CT

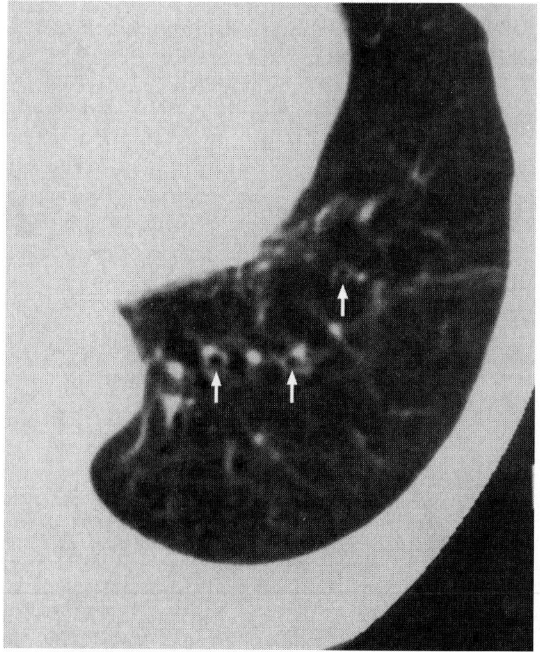

FIGURE 21–35 ■ Bronchiectasis. Close-up view of high-resolution computed tomography scan of the left lower lobe. Note that the bronchi *(arrows)* are larger than their accompanying pulmonary artery, indicating mild cylindrical bronchiectasis.

or spiral scans using standard-slice collimation—7 to 10 mm. Sensitivity for detecting bronchiectasis is much improved by utilizing the HRCT technique. Grenier and colleagues reported a sensitivity of 96% and a specificity of 93% in detecting bronchiectasis compared with bronchography using 1.5 collimation HRCT at 10-mm intervals. False-positive readings of bronchiectasis also occur, usually when motion artifact, often in the paracardiac zone of the lung, creates "double-vessels" images that resemble the tram-tracking of bronchiectasis.

HRCT is, therefore, very useful in the evaluation of patients with suspected bronchiectasis. It may clearly demonstrate disease in several locations, obviating surgery in most instances. It has emerged as the imaging modality of choice for evaluating bronchiectasis; HRCT has all but eliminated the use of bronchography. It must be emphasized that, despite the excellent sensitivity of HRCT, bronchiectasis may be focal and exceedingly subtle on HRCT scans.

Diffuse Lung Disease

Much literature has been devoted to the assessment of diffuse lung disease by CT scanning. A number of excellent reviews (Genereux, 1989; Klein and Gamsu, 1989; Muller et al, 1990a; Muller et al, 1990b; Muller, 1991;) and an entire book (Webb et al, 1996) are available for the interested reader. In this section, a few highlights are summarized.

Both standard CT scanning and HRCT (especially) have been shown to be very useful in evaluating patients with diffuse lung disease (Fig. 21–36). These techniques

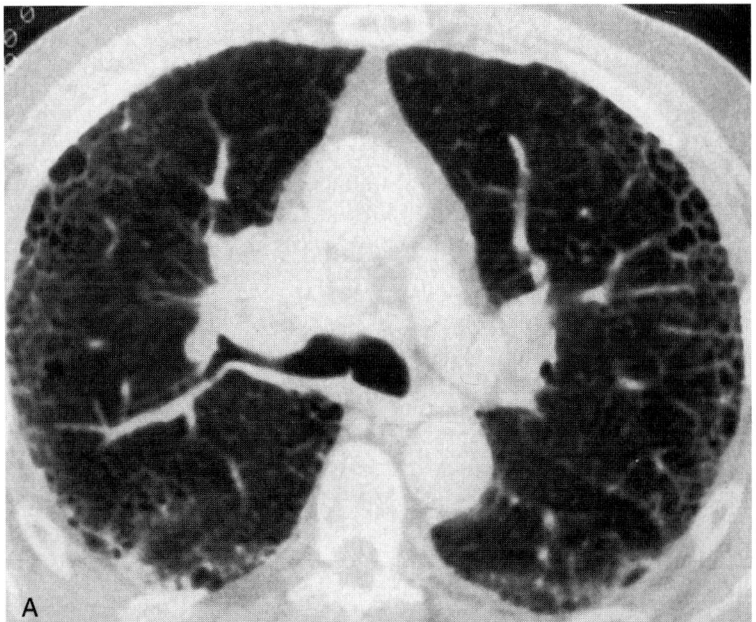

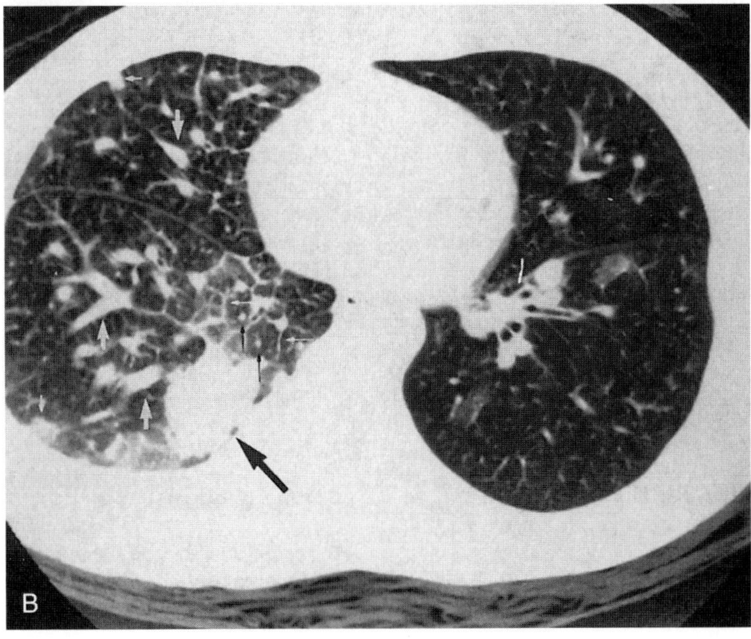

FIGURE 21–36 ■ *A*, Fibrosing alveolitis. This high-resolution computed tomography scan reveals reticular interstitial disease, with cyst formation, in a characteristic peripheral distribution. The patient also has a right upper lobe, bronchogenic carcinoma, which extends into the mediastinum. *B*, Lymphangitic carcinomatosis. High-resolution computed tomography scan from a 36-year-old man with a right lower-lobe adenocarcinoma *(large black arrow)*. In the right base, there are prominent bronchovascular bundles *(wide white arrows)*, nodules *(short white arrows)*, and polygonal shadows with irregular walls *(long white arrows)* and a central dot *(small black arrows)*.

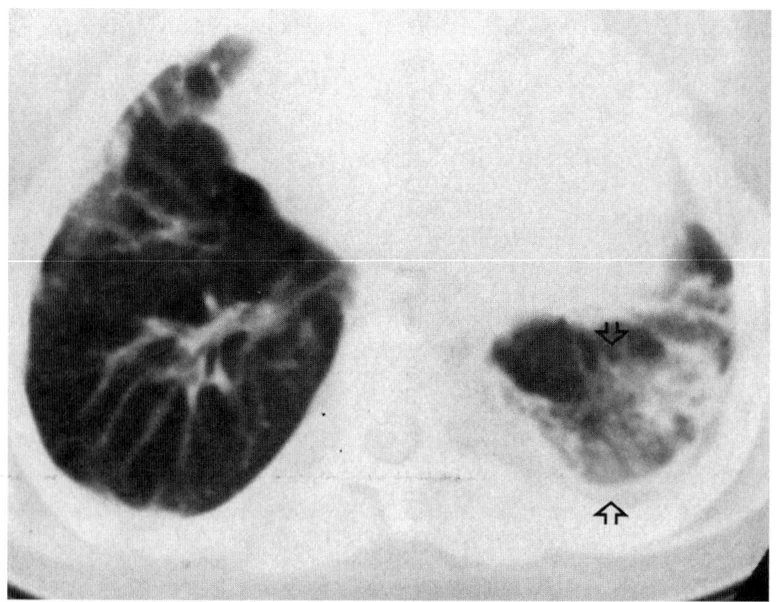

FIGURE 21–37 ■ The presence of the air space disease in the left lower lobe *(between arrows)* suggests active disease in this patient with biopsy-proven fibrosing alveolitis. Areas such as this are more likely to yield active disease than are more peripheral areas of reticular disease, which generally represent scarring (as shown in Fig. 21–36*A*).

are helpful in revealing definite abnormalities in cases in which the chest radiograph is normal; this has been reported for a number of conditions, including fibrosing alveolitis (Strickland and Strickland, 1988), sarcoidosis (Brauner et al, 1989), asbestosis (Aberle et al, 1988), and lymphangitic carcinomatosis (Stein et al, 1987). Therefore, HRCT should be performed in patients with clinical or pulmonary function evidence of diffuse lung disease and abnormal chest radiograph. Even when a definite diagnosis cannot be made by CT, it may still be helpful by suggesting both the most appropriate type of biopsy that should be performed and the optimal location for the biopsy.

Besides the ability to detect disease in the presence of a normal chest radiograph, CT (and HRCT) scanning have been shown to allow the clinician to be much more specific in diagnosing the patient's disease (Grenier et al, 1991; Mathieson et al, 1989). Additionally, this diagnosis can be made with much more confidence (Grenier et al, 1991; Mathieson et al, 1989). Even if a specific diagnosis cannot be made, the techniques have been shown to be excellent for determining whether the patient needs a transbronchial or open lung biopsy (Mathieson et al, 1989). The former is suggested when there is evidence of peribronchial disease, which is the case with diseases such as sarcoidosis or lymphangitic carcinoma. When the lung disease is seen to be more peripheral within the parenchyma, an open lung or video-assisted thoracoscopic biopsy is more likely necessary. CT has also been shown to be useful in directing the surgeon to the optimal site for the lung biopsy (Fig. 21–37). Not only are abnormal areas clearly seen but also regions suggesting the presence of active disease can be detected. This was shown in patients with fibrosing alveolitis (Muller et al, 1987) in whom "ground glass" densities, as opposed to more reticular densities, have been shown to be associated more likely with active disease, as opposed to residual fibrosis. If a biopsy is obtained from the region of fibrosis, then it might be impossible to determine the cause of the original process. However, if a biopsy can be obtained from the more active areas, then characteristic pathologic lesions are frequently seen that allow a more specific diagnosis to be made (Miller et al, 1987).

Metastatic Disease

CT is currently the procedure of choice for the detection of pulmonary metastatic disease in patients with a known extrathoracic primary tumor (Davis, 1991). CT has been shown to be much more sensitive than radiography in this regard (Heaston et al, 1983; Vanel et al, 1984) because it detects both smaller and more nodules (Fig. 21–38). However, more nodules are found by thoracot-

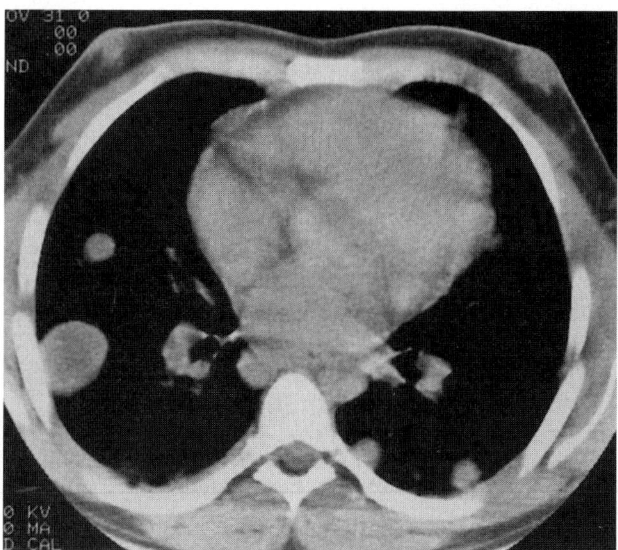

FIGURE 21–38 ■ Computed tomography scan of 22-year-old man with metastatic choriocarcinoma of the testis. There are several pulmonary nodules of varying size bilaterally. Note the gynecomastia; this patient's β-human chorionic gonadotropin level was greater than 300,000 units.

omy (Schaner et al, 1978). Unfortunately, not all of the nodules that are detected turn out to be metastases but are instead the result of other conditions, such as old granulomatous disease, intrapulmonary lymph nodes, or areas of fibrosis (Peuchot and Libshitz, 1987; Fig. 21–39). The false-positive rate depends on a number of factors, including the site of the primary tumor, the patient's age, and whether prior therapy was given. For example, sarcomas are more likely to metastasize to the lungs than are carcinomas; therefore, pulmonary nodules in a patient with the former are more likely to be metastases than are those in a patient with a carcinoma (Peuchot and Libshitz, 1987). Similarly, younger patients are less likely to have previous granulomatous disease; their nodules are therefore more likely to be caused by metastatic disease (Putnam et al, 1984; Wellner and Putnam, 1986). A patient being investigated after treatment may have so-called sterile metastases, residual areas of scar tissue where viable tumor had originally been; these can be confused with true metastases on CT (Hidalgo et al, 1983).

In a study comparing the features of metastatic and benign nodules (Gross et al, 1985), the former were found to be more numerous, larger, and more rounded. The presence of calcium was associated with benign disease. Other features that suggest that a nodule is a metastasis are the presence of a feeding vessel into the center of the nodule (Milne and Zarhouni, 1987), beaded adjacent interlobular septi (Ren et al, 1989), and possibly a zone of hyperlucency distal to the nodule (Naidich et al, 1991). We reviewed the etiology of 426 pulmonary nodules resected at video-assisted thoracic surgery (VATS) and found that in patients with a known malignancy, nodules that were 5 mm or smaller were more likely to be benign (58% of 275 resected pulmonary nodules), whereas pulmonary nodules greater than 5 mm, but smaller than or equal to 1 cm, were more likely to be malignant (69% of 149 resected nodules). Multiple nodules were more likely to be malignant than a single nodule in patients with a known malignancy (Ginsberg et al, 1999).

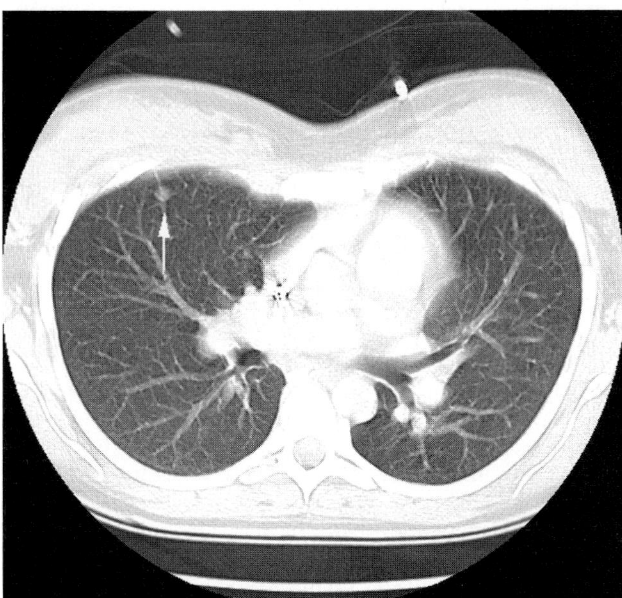

FIGURE 21–39 ■ Twenty-one-year-old woman with Ewing's sarcoma. Computed tomography scan demonstrated three subcentimeter nodules that at resection were all benign. Nodule in the right middle lobe represented a benign lymph node *(arrow)*.

In practice it can be difficult to be certain whether the multiple pulmonary nodules demonstrated by CT in a patient with a known primary tumor represent metastases or not, and the probability is subjectively assigned based on the aforementioned factors. If the nodules are large enough, a sample can be taken from one of them by transthoracic needle biopsy (TNB) of the lung (see Transthoracic Needle Biopsy). However, they are often too small for this to be possible. In these cases, a clinical decision must be made either to obtain tissue by open lung biopsy or VATS or to repeat the CT in 1 to 2 months, with the assumption that metastases are likely to enlarge.

Lung Abscess Versus Empyema

It is important to be able to distinguish between a lung abscess and empyema because patient management differs, depending on which condition is present. Generally, lung abscesses tend to be spherical, with thick, irregular, lobulated walls, and they cause little compression of the adjacent lung. Empyemas tend to be oblong; have smooth, thin walls; and may cause compression of adjacent lung.

Although lung abscess and empyema frequently can be differentiated on the chest radiograph, CT has been shown to be excellent at distinguishing between them (Figs. 21–40 and 21–41). Lung abscesses have thick, irregular walls; the walls of empyemas tend to be uniformly thin and smooth (Baber et al, 1980; Pugatch et al, 1978; Stark et al, 1983). These latter walls, which are better assessed if the study is performed after the injection of contrast, represent the separated visceral and parietal pleura. Their visibility forms the so-called split pleura sign, an excellent sign of an empyema (Stark et al, 1983). Compression of the adjacent lung is much more commonly seen with empyema, as would be expected. If the entire lesion is considered three-dimensionally, then lung abscesses tend to be spherical. Empyemas are oblong, either in an anteroposterior, lateral, or craniocaudal direction. Another helpful but less definite feature is the fact that lung abscesses tend to form acute angles with the chest wall or mediastinum; empyemas tend to form obtuse angles.

Pulmonary Embolism

Recent advances in CT have enabled this technique to be applied to the diagnosis of PE. The technique for performing pulmonary CTA using a helical scanner employs thinner (2.5 mm) collimation. Scans are performed in a caudal to cranial direction acquiring a volume from the inferior pulmonary veins to the aortic arch within a breath-hold. Faster contrast injection rates are used. CTA using helical or electron-beam CT has been suggested as a study that may have both high sensitivity and high

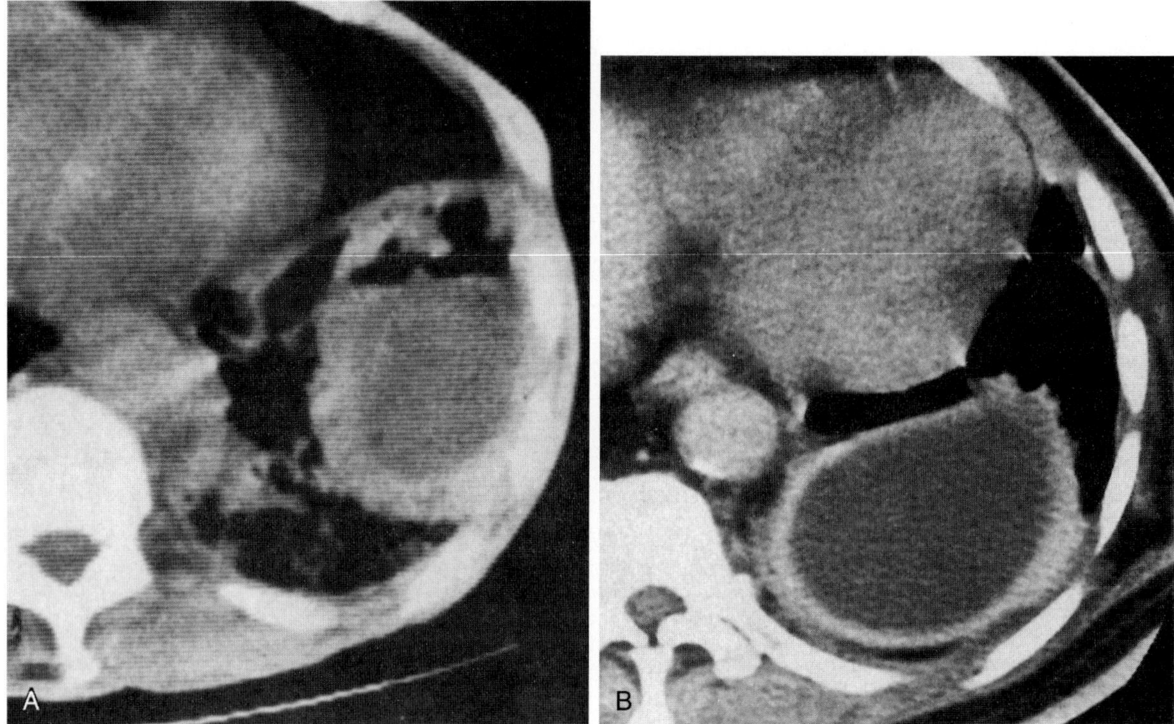

FIGURE 21–40 ■ *A*, Close-up view of computed tomography scan of a patient with a left lower-lobe abscess. The walls of this abscess are thick and irregular. The mass is spherical (confirmed by synthesis of multiple adjacent images, not shown). The abscess makes acute angles with the chest wall. Lung windows (not shown) did not show adjacent atelectases. *B*, Empyema. The walls of this left lower lobe lesion are thin and smooth. Its shape is only slightly oblong on this view, but examination on several other images reveals that it was oblong in a craniocaudal direction. Although it is making acute angles with the chest wall, the other features are highly indicative of empyema.

specificity for the diagnosis of acute PE (Fig. 21–42). In 1992, Remy-Jardin and colleagues published a prospective comparison of helical CT and pulmonary arteriography in which they reported a sensitivity of 100% and a specificity of 96% for the helical diagnosis of PE. In a 1996 study, the same authors performed a larger investigation of helical CT and reported a sensitivity of 91% and a specificity of 78%. The authors of two other prospective studies (Goodman et al, 1995; Teigen et al, 1995) compared CT with arteriographic correlation and reported a sensitivity of 63% and 65% and a specificity of 89% and 97%. Despite the wide range of reported sensitivities, the clinical use of CT for the diagnosis of PE has been growing. The initial diagnostic study in patients suspected of having PE often is ventilation-perfusion (VQ) scintigraphy. However, CTA has been increasingly performed as the initial diagnostic study. This is especially the case in patients who have numerous pulmonary abnormalities on their chest radiographs and are more likely to have an indeterminate VQ study. Additional imaging is indicated in those patients with indeterminate VQ scans and those with discrepancies between the results of the VQ study and those of clinical assessment. Pulmonary angiography may then be needed to help confirm or exclude PE. Even if available, however, pulmonary angiography is generally underused because it is invasive and expensive. A major advantage of CT over conventional angiography is that CT, in addition to revealing intraluminal filling defects, allows concurrent evaluation of the lung parenchyma and pleural space.

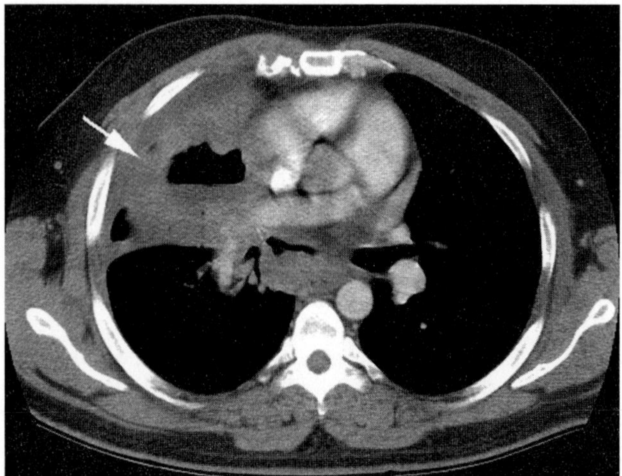

FIGURE 21–41 ■ Thirty-six-year old with lymphoma and necrotizing pneumonia in the right upper and right middle lobes developed an abscess with air fluid level *(arrow)* necessitating percutaneous catheter drainage.

Interest has focused on the development of a reliable, accurate, and readily available technique for diagnosing PE. MRI and magnetic resonance angiography (MRA) have also been used. The use of faster magnetic resonance hardware combined with dynamic gadolinium enhancement has made it possible to perform high-resolution angiography during a single, suspended breath. A prelim-

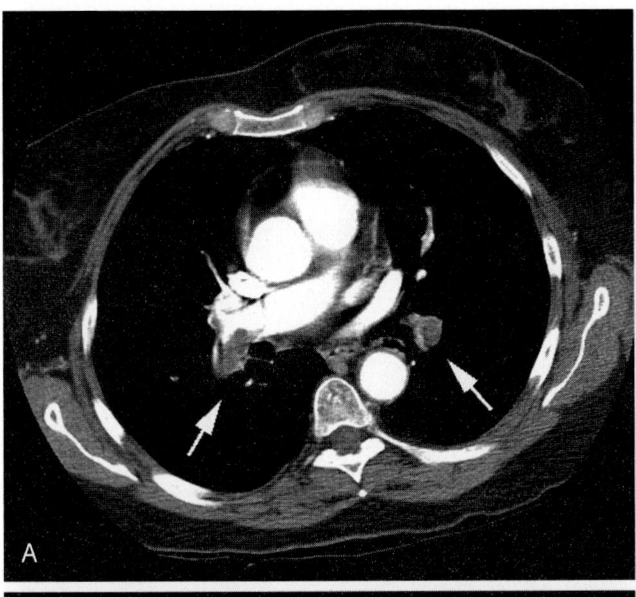

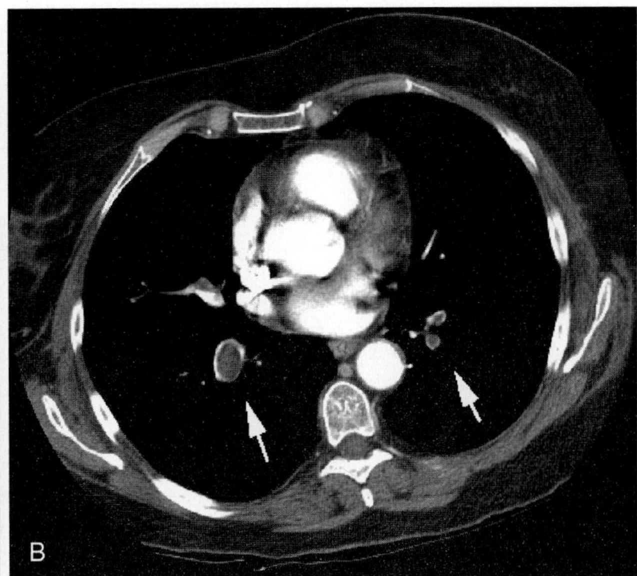

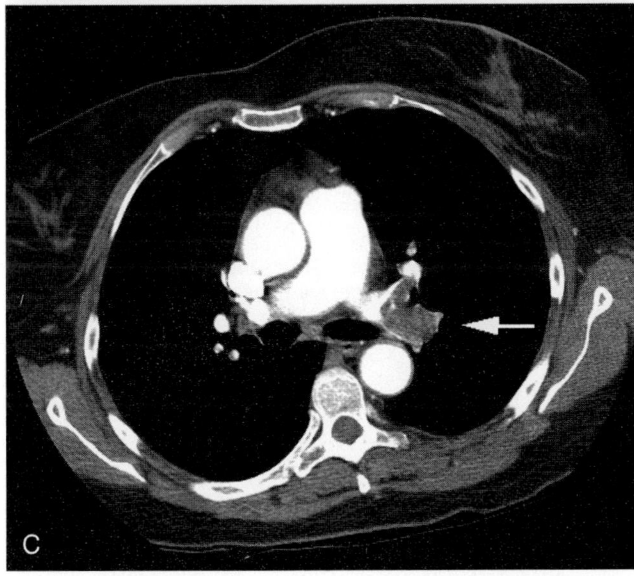

FIGURE 21–42 ■ Sixty-four-year-old woman with breast cancer and known deep vein thrombosis. *A*, Computed tomography scan demonstrating large thrombus in the right main pulmonary artery *(arrow)* and left lower-lobe pulmonary artery *(arrows)*. *B*, Several pulmonary emboli in lower-lobe segmental branches *(arrows)*. *C*, Large thrombus in the left main pulmonary artery.

inary study (Meaney et al, 1997) performed standard pulmonary angiography and MRA in 30 patients suspected of having PE. MRA detected all 5 of 5 lobar and 16 of 17 segmental angiographically proven emboli. However, none of the patients had subsegmental emboli.

Subsegmental vessels can indeed be imaged with MRA, but the accuracy of MRA for the detection of subsegmental clot is less impressive. A recent study evaluated MRA versus conventional angiography in 36 patients (Gupta et al, 1999). Of 19 acute pulmonary emboli depicted on angiography, 6 were missed by MRA. Four of these were subsegmental. MRA has a high sensitivity and specificity for central, lobar, and segmental vessels but has limitations that are similar to those with CT in its ability to detect subsegmental clots (Maki et al, 1999). MRA has the advantage of not requiring iodinated contrast material in patients with marginal renal function. The high cost and lower availability of MRA compared with CTA have made it less prevalent as the initial imaging study for the evaluation of PEs.

New Computed Tomography Techniques

The introduction of helical (spiral) CT has significantly changed the use of CT. Helical scanners employ slip-ring technology to acquire data continuously as the patient is translated through the gantry. With the patient translating inside the rotating gantry, the path of the x-ray source describes a spiral, or helix, with its focus along a line passing through the rotational isocenter perpendicular to the plane of rotation. Because there are no interscan delays, the rate of coverage along this line is equal to the table speed. Thus, in the same amount of time, spiral scanners can acquire a volume of CT data four to nine times larger than the conventional scanner of the 1980s. This is of particular advantage in scanning the chest. An increase in the number of sections that may be acquired per breath-hold greatly increases the detection rate of small pulmonary nodules by eliminating respiratory misregistration (Kalender et al, 1994; Remy-Jardin et al, 1993). Helical CT also allows reconstruction of the ac-

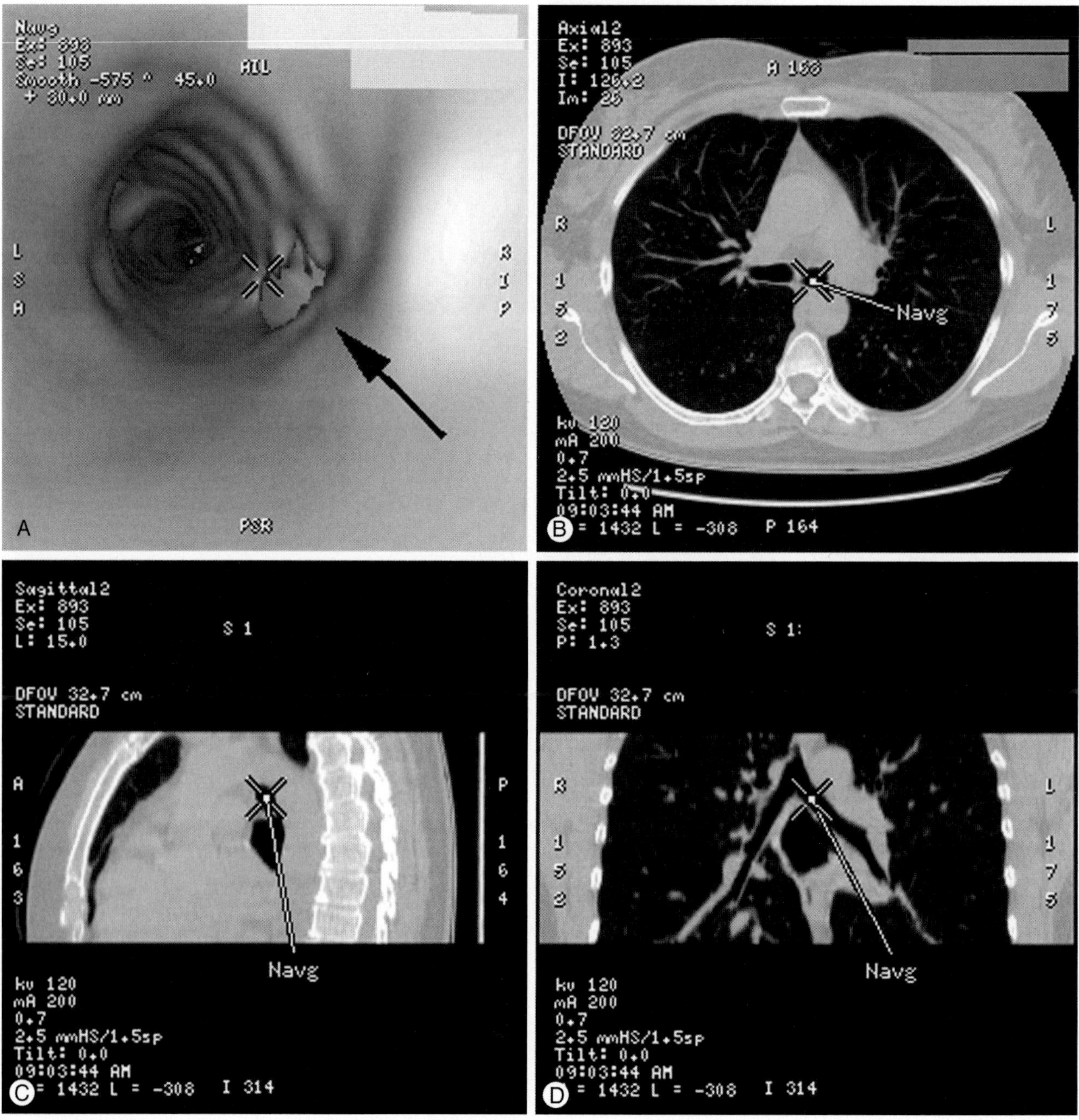

FIGURE 21–43 ■ *A,* Subcarinal mediastinal air cyst shown to communicate with the left mainstem bronchus *(arrow)* on virtual bronchoscopy. Thin-section axial section did not reveal this communication. *B,* Axial; *C,* sagittal (reformatted); and *D,* coronal (reformatted) images are shown as reference guide to the corresponding navigational site on virtual bronchoscopy.

quired helical CT data set in overlapping sections, further improving the detection of subcentimeter nodules (Urban et al, 1993). Moreover, helical CT typically utilizes thinner image sections (e.g., 5 to 7 mm) than does conventional CT, resulting in sharper images with less partial-volume averaging effects.

At many facilities, radiologists are now interpreting CT studies on workstations rather than on radiographic film. Scrolling through helical CT images on a computer workstation in a sequential "ciné" mode has distinct technical and perceptual advantages, significantly increasing the detection rate of pulmonary nodules 5 mm in diameter or smaller compared with film-based viewing; no significant advantage has been demonstrated for lesions larger than 5 mm (Tillich et al, 1997).

The improved resolution that is offered by helical CT has led to the clinical use of three-dimensional reconstruction techniques, such as virtual bronchoscopy (VB). Preliminary data have shown that 90% of bronchi (up to third-order) measurable on multiplanar CT reformation are also measurable on VB (Summers et al, 1996). VB offers the advantage of being able to visualize areas beyond even high-grade stenosis. However, it is still not possible to detect very small lesions with VB. Preliminary observations suggest that VB simulations accurately represent major endobronchial anatomic findings (Vining et al, 1996). This new representation of helical CT data might be helpful for postoperative follow-up examination, such as after stent implantation, and can be carried out without additional risk to the patient (Fleiter et al, 1997). It does require special fiberoptic bronchoscopy knowledge of the radiologist and experience with three-dimensional reconstruction and is therefore only available at certain institutions (Fig. 21–43).

MAGNETIC RESONANCE IMAGING

MRI has limited use in the investigation of pulmonary parenchymal problems because of the inherent magnetic properties of the lung. The lung produces little MR signal. The emergence of newer generation MR scanners with high performance gradient systems is changing the role of MR imaging of the lung. State-of-the-art MR capabilities now include functional imaging such as perfusion and ventilation, which will open a scope for assessing regional pulmonary functions of the lung (Hatabu et al, 1999a).

There are a number of aspects of bronchogenic carcinoma in which MRI plays a definite role. It is the primary imaging modality for local staging of superior sulcus (Pancoast) tumors. This peripheral lung carcinoma at the apex of the lung frequently invades the pleura, spine, and chest wall, including the brachial plexus and the subclavian vessels. MR imaging is superior to CT in evaluating the extent of this tumor because of its multiplanar imaging capabilities and better tissue contrast (Heelan et al, 1989; Manfredi et al, 1996) (Fig. 21–44). Vessel involvement may not be determined unless actual disruption of blood flow is demonstrated. Therefore, distinguishing simple abutment from invasion of the vessel wall remains a problem (Freundlich et al, 1996). MRI may be better than CT in the diagnosis of

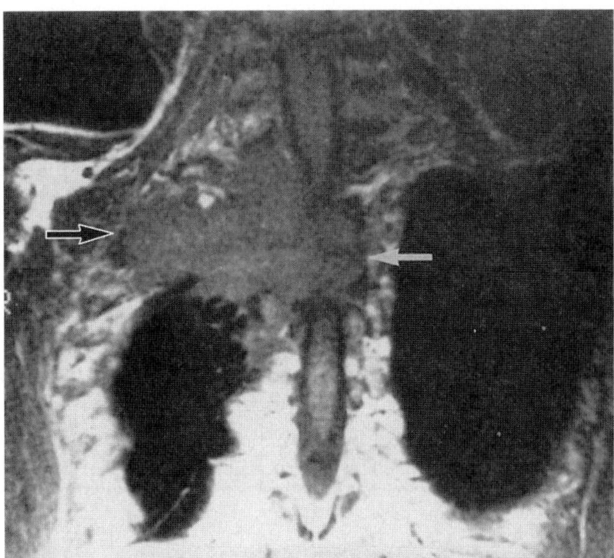

FIGURE 21–44 ■ T_1-weighted image in the coronal plane of a 66-year-old man with a right upper-lobe Pancoast's tumor. Note the extension of this tumor into the chest wall *(black arrow)* and spinal canal *(white arrows).*

mediastinal invasion by the primary tumor (Kameda et al, 1988; Webb et al, 1991). The thin layer of extrapleural fat may be better shown on MRI than on CT. Tumor invasion into the chest wall must cross this fat plane, and discontinuity of the fat line may be evident (Padovani et al, 1993).

In practice, MRI should be regarded as a primary imaging method in cases of central lung tumors in patients who cannot receive iodinated contrast for CT and as a secondary problem-solving method in cases in which CT proves inconclusive with regard to tumor involvement of major mediastinal structures.

MRI is no different than CT scanning in detecting mediastinal nodal involvement with bronchogenic carcinoma (Musset et al, 1986; Poon et al, 1987; Webb et al, 1985; Webb et al, 1991). MRI and CT demonstrate similar accuracy in detecting mediastinal lymph node metastasis, with a sensitivity of approximately 65% and a specificity of approximately 72%, but lesser values have been reported (Gdeedo et al, 1997). Unfortunately, MRI cannot identify lymph-node metastasis based solely on T_1 and T_2 relaxation times. In practice, therefore, MRI uses size criteria, as does CT. In this regard, CT scanning is probably better than MRI because of its increased spatial resolution for identifying relationships with bronchi and fissures. Similarly, because MRI cannot detect calcification, it may misrepresent calcified nodes as malignant when CT would have correctly identified them as benign.

MRI can be used to distinguish between central tumor and adjacent atelectasis with T_1-weighted images after injection of gadolinium contrast media (Ho and Prince, 1998). CT is able to do this at least as well if a bolus of contrast material is administered (Tobler et al, 1987). MRI has been shown to be accurate in distinguishing obstructive from nonobstructive atelectasis by differences in the signal pattern of the collapsed lung (Herold et al, 1991).

MRI can demonstrate tumor necrosis after radiation therapy. Gadolinium-enhanced imaging improves the detection of viable tumor and necrosis. Some studies suggest T_2-weighted images may be helpful in differentiating recurrent tumor from fibrosis. However, it can be difficult to differentiate tumor from an inflammatory response, a common sequela following irradiation (Glazer et al, 1985c; Lee and Glazer, 1990).

The interested reader is invited to refer to reviews on the uses of MRI in the assessment of mediastinal and vascular diseases, a discussion beyond the scope of this chapter (Edelman et al, 1996; Hatabu et al, 1999b). It has been shown to be useful in cardiac, paracardiac, and aortic disease and in the evaluation of patients with posterior mediastinal masses and residual masses following treatment of lymphoma.

NUCLEAR IMAGING

Ventilation/Perfusion Scanning

A perfusion lung scan, as its name implies, produces an image of the distribution of pulmonary blood flow throughout both lungs (Fig. 21–45). While in the supine position (to minimize the effects of gravity), the patient is given an intravenous injection of macroaggregated albumin, which has been radiolabeled with technetium (^{99m}Tc). This material is composed of particles of such a size (5 to 100 μm) that they become trapped in the pulmonary capillaries. The amount given (1 to 4 $\times$ 10^5 particles) is such that less than 1 in 1000 capillaries, in normal lungs, become obstructed (Melter and Guiberteau, 1991). A gamma camera is placed over the patient's chest, and an image reflecting pulmonary blood flow is obtained from six to eight directions.

A ventilation scan is used in a corresponding manner to obtain images reflecting the distribution of airflow to the lungs (see Fig. 21–45). A number of different radioactive gases are available for this purpose. Some (e.g., ^{133}Xe) are inhaled by the patient in the sitting position while a gamma camera records the distribution of the radioactivity. Multiple images are obtained during the washin, equilibrium, and washout phases of the test. Areas of abnormal ventilation, including air trapping, are therefore recorded. A different technique involves the use of radioactive aerosols, the most common one being nebulized diethyltriaminepentaacetic acid (^{99m}Tc-DTPA). This mixture is inhaled, and the gas is deposited in the lungs, again in a distribution reflecting alveolar ventilation. The advantage of this technique is that multiple images can be obtained from different directions, and these are chosen to correspond to those obtained during the perfusion scan. In this way, pairs of images reflecting both ventilation and perfusion are obtained in multiple directions, allowing accurate comparison of these two aspects of pulmonary function in each lung region.

Two large prospective trials (Hull et al, 1985; The PIOPED Investigators, 1990) helped to define the role of VQ scanning in the evaluation of patients with suspected PE (Fig. 21–46). A discussion of this topic is a chapter unto itself, and only a summary is presented here. Most investigators believe that a normal perfusion scan rules out PE with enough certainty that no further consideration need be given to this diagnosis, and another cause for the patient's problems must be sought. In general, a high-probability VQ pattern is specific enough that therapy may be given without further testing. However, if there is a contraindication to anticoagulation, then CTA or pulmonary angiography should be performed to increase the certainty of the diagnosis. Additionally, because emboli may take years to resolve, a high-probability scan may reflect old embolic disease. In the PIOPED study (The PIOPED Investigators, 1990), the positive predictive value of a high probability scan was 91% in those without a history of prior PEs, but it fell to 74% in those with a prior history.

The clinical situation of a low- or intermediate-probability scan is much more controversial (Juni and Alavi, 1991). In this circumstance, the clinician must always keep in mind that PEs result, almost always, from deep venous thrombosis in the leg or pelvic veins. Therefore, attention must be paid to this primary disease. The finding of venous thrombosis necessitates anticoagulation. However, if the results of these two studies are negative and the clinical suspicion remains high, additional imaging may be necessary. One study (Ferretti et al, 1997) found that CTA allowed accurate diagnosis of acute PE in patients suspected of having acute PE, with an intermediate probability VQ scan and normal duplex ultrasound of the legs.

The VQ scan is also used in preoperative assessment as a means of calculating the amount of functioning lung that will be removed by the proposed resection and has value especially in assessing higher-risk patients for pneumonectomy. The preoperative VQ scan can accurately predict how much the lung or lobe to be resected contributes to overall total lung function (Ryo, 1990). A preoperative VQ scan can accurately predict the 3- and 6-months' postoperative percentage of vital capacity, forced vital capacity, and forced expiratory volume in 1 second in patients who will undergo pulmonary resection for lung cancer (Imaeda et al, 1995).

Gallium Scanning

Both inflammatory and neoplastic tissues take up and concentrate ^{67}Ga citrate. It can therefore be used to locate abscesses and assess diffuse inflammatory conditions in the lungs; additionally, it has been used in the staging of patients with lymphoma. One disadvantage of ^{67}Ga is that imaging cannot take place until about 48 hours following its administration.

This radiopharmaceutical agent is useful in detecting otherwise hidden abscesses, although, if a specific site is suspected of harboring an abscess by clinical criteria, it is better to perform a CT of the region rather than ^{67}Ga imaging. A number of conditions are associated with diffuse pulmonary uptake of ^{67}Ga. These include pneumonia from *Pneumocystis carinii*, active sarcoidosis, active idiopathic pulmonary fibrosis, miliary tuberculosis, bleomycin toxicity, acute radiation pneumonitis, and lymphangitic carcinoma (Melter and Guiberteau, 1991).

^{67}Ga single-photon emission CT has been shown to improve significantly both the sensitivity and specificity

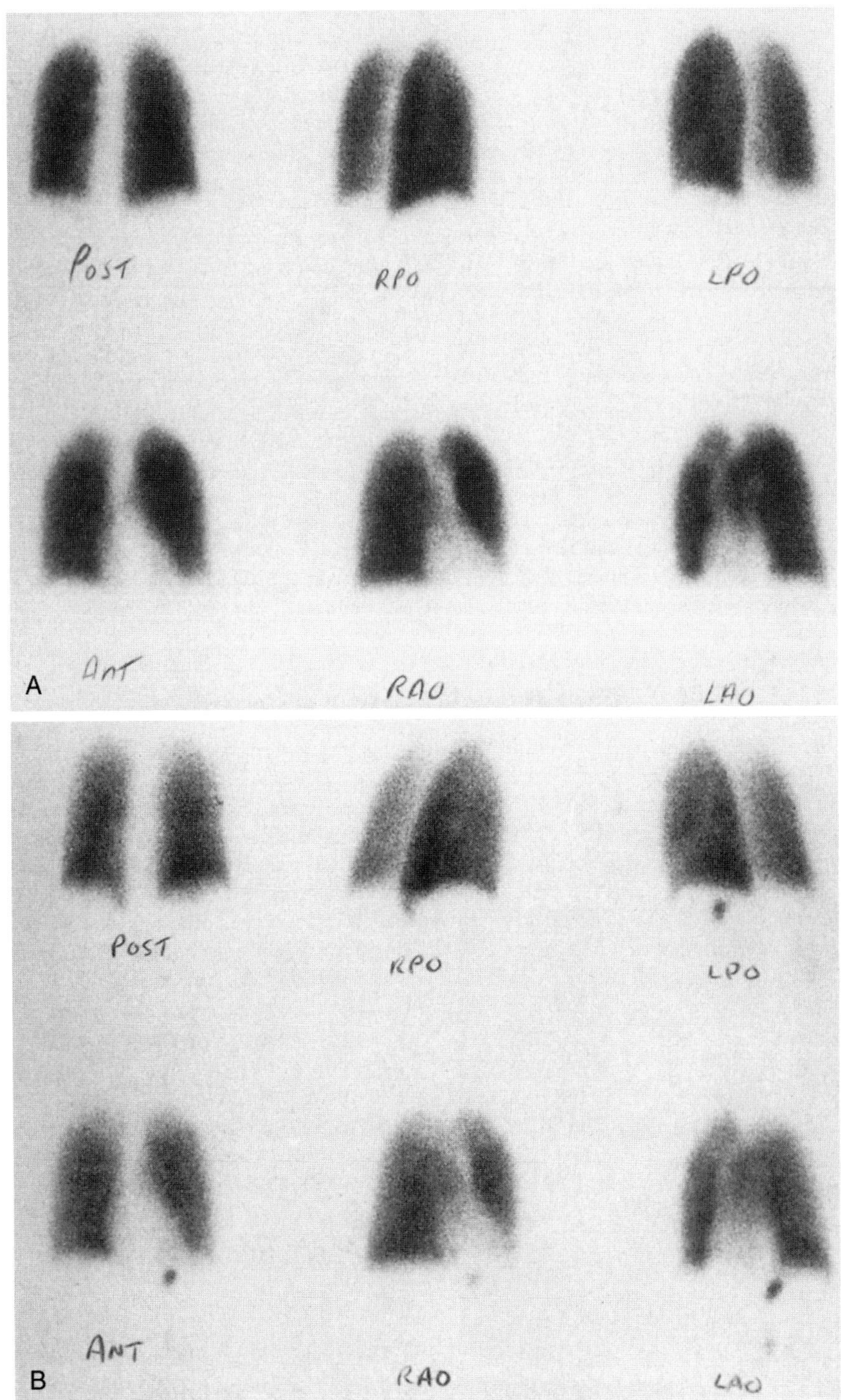

FIGURE 21–45 ■ Normal V/Q scan. *A*, Perfusion scan. *B*, Ventilation scan. There is homogeneous distribution of radioactivity throughout the lungs on both studies. (Courtesy of K. Yip, MD.)

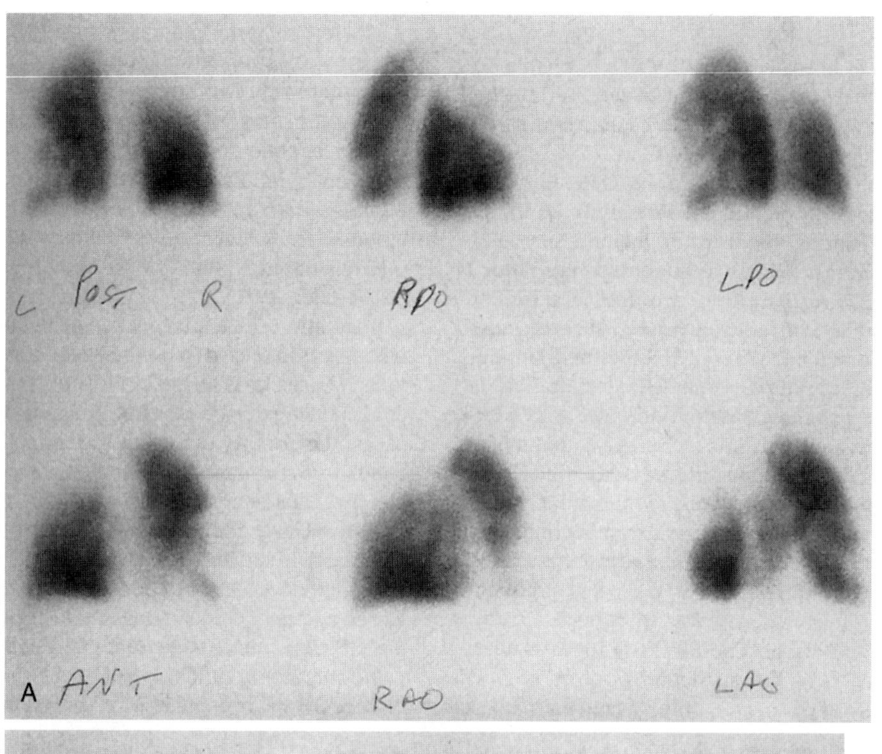

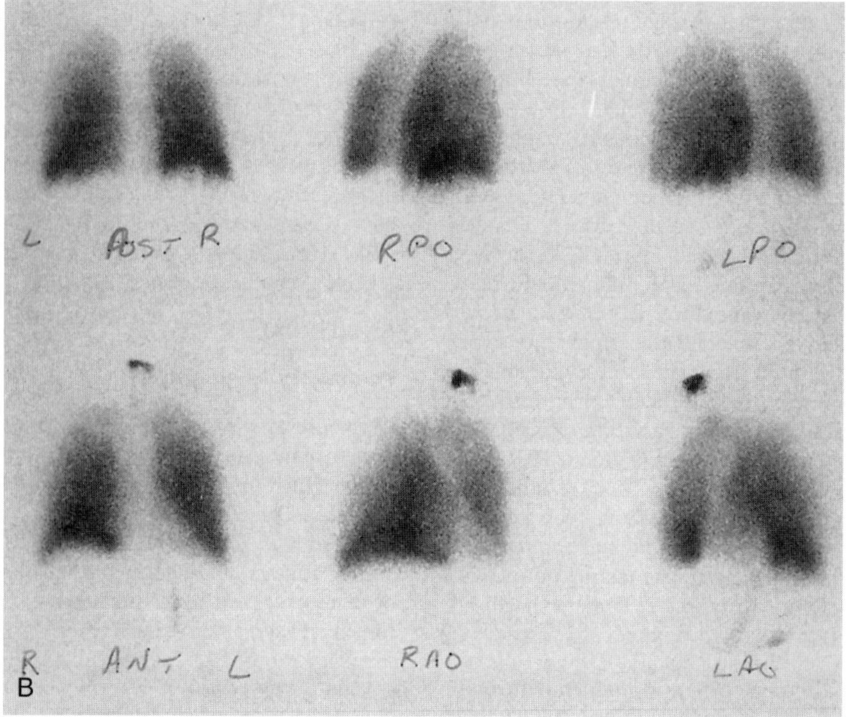

FIGURE 21–46 ■ VQ scan of pulmonary emboli. *A*, Perfusion scan. *B*, Ventilation scan. There is no flow to the entire right upper lobe, the anteromedial basal segment of the left lower lobe, or the lingula. Ventilation to these regions, and to the rest of both lungs, is normal. These multiple large areas of V/Q mismatch are highly predictive of pulmonary emboli. (Courtesy of K. Yip, MD.)

over ^{67}Ga planar imaging in the staging of patients with lymphoma (Front et al, 1990; Tumeh et al, 1987). Additionally, ^{67}Ga scanning appears to be better than CT for predicting the outcome of these patients (Front et al, 1992). Following treatment for lymphoma, patients are commonly left with a so-called residual mass on CT. It is impossible to know whether such a mass represents residual tumor requiring further treatment or is just scar tissue requiring observation only. ^{67}Ga scanning (Front et al, 1990) and MRI (described earlier) were shown to be useful in determining whether such residual mass represents a residual tumor.

POSITRON EMISSION TOMOGRAPHY IMAGING IN LUNG CANCER

PET has become an important imaging modality in the evaluation of the cancer patient. PET provides physiologic information that supplements conventional radiologic imaging of both cardiac and intrathoracic (pulmonary, hila, mediastinal) abnormalities. Although several PET agents are currently available, 18F-2-deoxy-D-glucose (FDG) is the most commonly used radionuclide for tumor imaging in the thorax. FDG, a D-glucose analog labeled with a positron-emitting ^{18}F, is preferentially absorbed by tumor cells because of their increased glucose metabolism. Once inside the cell, FDG initially proceeds through the glycolytic pathway, accelerated by increased levels of the enzyme hexokinase. This enzyme phosphorylates FDG, although FDG-6-phosphate (FDG-6-P) cannot be further metabolized, and thus the imaging agent becomes trapped within the cell. It is this increased uptake, trapping, and accumulation of FDG by tumor cells that theoretically permits differentiation between benign and malignant tissue (Hatanaka, 1974; Nolop, 1987; Patz, 1994; Wahl, 1991).

Positron Emission Tomography Fundamentals

Positrons are emitted from unstable nuclei and travel only a few millimeters before they are annihilated with an electron. This interaction results in the production of two 511 KeV gamma rays that travel in opposite (~180 degrees) directions. These photons are simultaneously captured by crystal detectors, and the result of the coincident detection is used to reconstruct a cross-sectional image. Spatial resolution is determined by the geometry of the single or multiple ring array gantry and the aperture utilized. Correction for surrounding tissue attenuation permits accurate radionuclide measurement and quantitation of the photons. Clinically useful biologic or physiologic evaluation can be obtained by binding the positron-emitter isotopes to metabolic substrates such as glucose (FDG) and amino acids (methylmethionine C 11).

Techniques

Because elevated serum glucose levels can decrease cellular FDG uptake, patients are required to fast for several hours before PET imaging (Langen, 1993; Lindholm, 1993). FDG is injected intravenously and transmission scans using a rotating ^{68}Ge pin source are performed to locate the area of interest. Multiple emission images (field of view 15 cm, resolution 5 mm) are then obtained approximately 30 to 60 minutes after injection of FDG. Results are displayed in axial, sagittal, and coronal projections on standard workstation monitors. A new acquisition and processing method has been utilized to generate whole-body images (Lewis, 1994; Rege, 1993; Valk, 1995). This technique consists of a series of overlapping transaxial images from which two-dimensional projection and tomographic coronal and sagittal images are generated (DeGrado, 1994; Lewis, 1994; Rege, 1993; Valk, 1995).

Increased glucose metabolism can be assessed visually on PET images by comparing the activity of the lesion with the background activity or by semiquantitative analysis using calculated standardized uptake ratios (SUR) according to the following formula:

$$\text{SUR} = \frac{\text{Mean ROI activity (mCi/ml)}}{\text{injected dose (mCi)/body weight (kg)}}$$

An SUR less than 2.5 is generally considered to be indicative of a benign lesion (Lowe, 1994; Patz, 1993).

As the indications and demand for PET imaging have increased over the past several years, development of FDG imaging on a variety of modified gamma cameras has taken place (Coleman, 1999; Shreve, 1998; Tatsumi, 1999; Zimmy, 1999). These alternatives are less expensive but do not have the same performance characteristics as the dedicated PET scanner. Several studies have shown that gamma camera imaging has lower resolution compared with PET scanners, particularly for lesions that are less than 1.5 cm in diameter (Shreve, 1998; Tatsumi, 1999; Zimmy, 1999). In one study, only 55% of tumors identified by PET were identified on a gamma camera system (Shreve, 1998), and in another study an inappropriate therapeutic decision would have been made in 29% of patients (Lonneux, 1998). Although modified gamma cameras may provide information about larger lesions and tumor staging, they cannot yet replace dedicated FDG-PET scanning in most oncology patients.

FDG-PET Indications

FDG-PET of thoracic abnormalities is clinically useful in differentiating benign and malignant focal pulmonary abnormalities, staging lung cancer, and evaluating patients after treatment of lung cancer.

Focal Pulmonary Abnormalities

Lung cancer is a major health problem and the leading cause of cancer-related deaths in the United States (Osteen, 1990). Prognosis depends on a number of factors including stage at presentation, histology, performance status, and treatment (Boring, 1993). Between 20% and 30% of patients with lung cancer present with a solitary pulmonary opacity. Early detection and confirmation that these lesions are primary lung malignancies is important (Viggiano, 1992). Unfortunately, lung cancer and benign pulmonary abnormalities can have similar morphologic features, and many lesions remain indeterminate after standard evaluation with chest radiographs, CT, or MRI. Depending on the clinical history and likelihood of malignancy, indeterminate focal pulmonary lesions can then be either observed, biopsied (transthoracic needle aspiration [TNA] or transbronchial needle aspiration), or resected. A nondiagnostic TNA or bronchoscopic biopsy is not uncommon if the lesion is benign (Berquist, 1980). Furthermore, because the decision to resect an indeterminate nodule is usually subjective (depending on the perceived probability that the nodule is malignant), up to 60% of resected nodules are benign (Edwards, 1962; Lillington, 1982; Lillington, 1993). The unnecessary cost and morbidity of resecting these lesions can be reduced by FDG-PET imaging. FDG-PET is accurate in differentiating benign from malignant lesions as small as 10 mm with an overall sensitivity, specificity, and accuracy of 96%, 88%, and 94%, respectively, in the detection of malignancy (Conti, 1996; Gupta, 1992; Gupta, 1996; Hübner, 1996; Patz, 1993; Scott, 1994) (Fig. 21–47). FDG-PET is clinically useful in directing clinical management of a solitary focal pulmonary opacity for several reasons:

1. The probability of malignancy with a positive FDG-PET study is high (90% if the patient is more than 60 years old), and focal pulmonary opacities with increased FDG uptake should be considered malignant. False-positive studies have, however, been reported with infectious and inflammatory processes such as active tuberculosis, histoplasmosis, and rheumatoid nodules (Dewan, 1993; Kubota, 1990; Patz, 1993; Quint, 1995; Strauss, 1991).
2. The probability of malignancy is low (less than 5%) with a negative study (Dewan, 1997; Gupta, 1996), and focal pulmonary opacities with low FDG uptake can be followed radiologically. Rarely, false-negative studies can occur with pulmonary malignancies (carcinoid tumors and bronchioloalveolar carcinoma can have lower FDG uptake than expected for malignant tumors) (Erasmus, 1998; Higashi, 1997; Lowe, 1998). Additionally, small (<10 mm) lung cancers can be falsely negative due to limitations in spatial resolution and paucity of tumor cells within the lesion (Lowe, 1998).

PET imaging is currently used as a complementary study to thoracic CT. Decision-analysis models indicate that the use of CT and FDG-PET imaging for evaluating focal pulmonary lesions is the most cost-effective and useful strategy in determining patient management over a large pretest likelihood (12% to 69%) of having a malignant nodule (Gambhir, 1998). With a low (up to 12%) or high (>90%) pretest likelihood of malignancy, the most cost-effective strategies are observation and resection, respectively (Gambhir, 1998). In the management of a focal pulmonary lesion within the pretest likelihood of 1% to 7%, an estimated 15% fewer patients will undergo resection if FDG-PET imaging is included in the assessment.

Although FDG-PET imaging is more expensive than other imaging modalities, its high accuracy and minimal risk make it cost effective in the evaluation of focal pulmonary opacities. It has been estimated that the combination of FDG-PET and CT to evaluate a focal pulmonary lesion in the pretest likelihood of 1% to 7% range will save $1192 per patient ($62.7 million annually) in medical treatment costs compared with the use of CT alone (Gambhir, 1998). Currently, the limited availability and expense of PET imaging has restricted its widespread application.

Staging Lung Cancer

Once the diagnosis of lung cancer has been established, accurate staging becomes essential for therapeutic decisions and prognostic information. The TNM staging system for non–small cell cancer provides a standardized

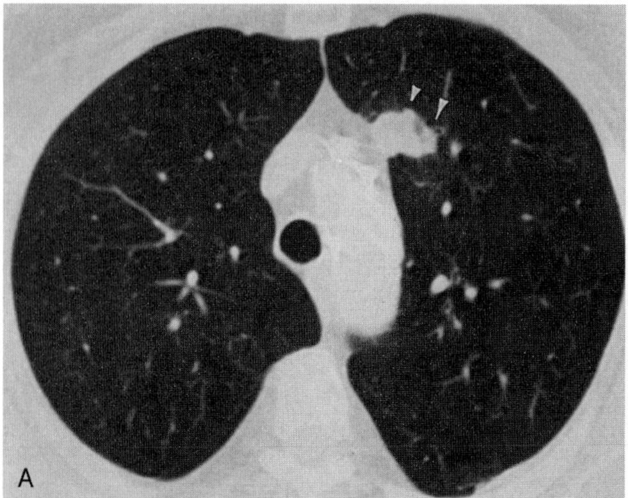

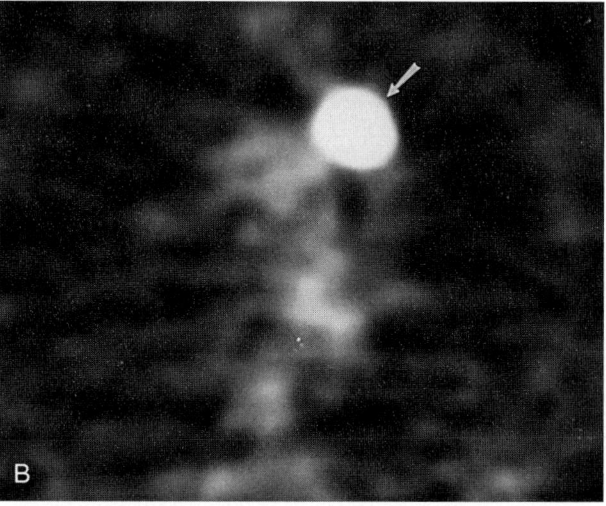

FIGURE 21–47 ■ Seventy-seven-year-old asymptomatic woman with solitary pulmonary nodule detected on routine radiograph (not shown). *A*, Axial chest computed tomography scan confirmed a nodule in the left upper lobe *(arrowheads)*. There was no intrathoracic lymphadenopathy. *B*, Axial positron emission tomography scan image showed increased fluorodeoxyglucose uptake in the left upper lobe nodule *(arrow)*. Hilar and mediastinal activity was normal. Transthoracic needle aspiration biopsy confirmed non–small cell lung cancer.

description of the anatomic extent of disease and is used to differentiate stage I to IIIa (potentially resectable) from stage IIIb to IV (nonresectable) (Epstein, 1986; Friedman, 1988; Mann, 1988; Mountain, 1986; Mountain, 1988; Stitik, 1990; Stitik, 1994; Templeton, 1990). The use of imaging in determining clinical staging (cstage) is not clearly delineated, although chest radiographs, CT, and occasionally MRI are often performed and used together with clinical information and invasive procedures to differentiate patients with resectable disease from those with nonresectable disease (Broderick, 1997; Chen, 1997; Quint, 1995; Shaffer, 1997; Stitik, 1990; Templeton, 1990).

Despite extensive preoperative evaluation, patients who are considered surgical candidates according to their cstage can have lesions that are unresectable at surgery (Kadvi, 1991). With the addition of FDG-PET, the accuracy of clinical staging has improved, and it has been suggested that this strategy is more cost-effective than conventional imaging alone (Gambhir, 1996; Kutlu, 1998). In several studies, as many as 18% of patients who are considered to have resectable malignancy will have more advanced disease demonstrated by PET and will be nonresectable (Lewis, 1994; Weder, 1998).

Primary Tumor (T)

CT is usually used in the evaluation of the primary tumor to determine the size, anatomic location, and extent of local invasion (T status) (Mountain, 1997). In comparison, the poorer spatial resolution of PET precludes accurate anatomic assessment of T status; that is, it is often not possible to determine whether the lesion is completely surrounded by lung parenchyma (T_1) or invading adjacent structures including the pleura, chest wall, diaphragm, and mediastinum (T_2 to T_4). PET assessment of T status consequently differs from conventional anatomic imaging in that most PET studies are interpreted as positive or negative for malignancy. Because PET is usually used in combination with CT, anatomic and physiologic information is obtained that can be used to stage the primary tumor. It is unclear whether the lack of anatomic detail of PET, when used alone, has clinical significance.

Nodal Disease

CT and MRI are often used to evaluate the hilar and mediastinal lymph nodes. Size is usually the only criterion used to distinguish normal and abnormal nodes because morphology of lymph nodes (shape and definition) and T_1/T_2 signal characteristics are usually not useful (Quint, 1995). A short axis nodal diameter of 1 cm is often used as the upper limit of normal, although metastatic disease can be found in normal-sized nodes, and enlarged nodes may be reactive (Glazer, 1985; Glazer, 1988). If mediastinal nodes are larger than 1 cm in diameter, the accuracy of CT and MRI for mediastinal nodal metastases is 56% to 82% and 50% to 82%, respectively (Klein, 1991; Martini, 1985; Musset, 1986; Staples, 1988; Webb, 1988; Webb, 1991). Although CT and MRI can accurately demonstrate hilar and mediastinal nodes, the specificity is too low to be more than an adjunct to invasive (mediastinoscopy, bronchoscopy) sampling (McLoud, 1992). The limitations of chest radiographs and CT/MRI, which depend on morphologic and anatomic findings, may be overcome by metabolic changes in tumor cells. In several studies, FDG-PET consistently has been shown to be more accurate than CT in determining nodal status (81% to 100% and 52% to 85%, respectively) (Guhlmann, 1997; Gupta, 1992; Patz, 1993; Patz, 1995; Sazon, 1996; Steinert, 1997; Vansteenkiste, 1998; Wahl, 1994). FDG-PET is more sensitive and specific than CT in detecting metastatic disease in normal-sized nodes and in the differentiation of enlarged benign nodes from enlarged nodal metastases (Boiselle, 1998; Guhlmann, 1997; Kutlu, 1998; Steinert, 1997; Wahl, 1994; Vansteenkiste, 1997; Vansteenkiste, 1998). PET has been reported to correctly increase or decrease the nodal staging as determined by CT in 21% of presurgical patients (Valk, 1995) (Fig. 21–48). The combined use of CT and FDG-PET to stage intrathoracic nodal metastases is clinically useful and cost effective (Gambhir, 1996). It reduces the probability that a patient with unresectable mediastinal nodal metastases will undergo an attempt at curative resection and has been shown to save $1154 per patient and give a small increase in life expectancy (Gambhir, 1996) (Fig. 21–49).

Invasive nodal sampling will be required until noninvasive imaging can reliably improve its specificity to greater than 90% (Malenka, 1991; Valk, 1995). This is the value required for noninvasive imaging to have the same predicted outcome as invasive staging of the mediastinum. FDG-PET and CT assessment of mediastinal nodal metastases has a higher negative predictive value (92% to 100%) than mediastinoscopy and could reduce the need for invasive staging (Steinert, 1997; Valk, 1995; Vansteenkiste, 1997; Vansteenkiste, 1998; Wahl, 1994). It has been suggested that invasive mediastinal staging could be omitted when the PET study is normal. Although PET has a high positive predictive value, false-positive results can occur with infection, active inflammation, hyperplasia, sarcoidosis, and anthracotic nodes (Guhlmann, 1997; Lewis, 1994; Valk, 1995). Invasive mediastinal staging, consequently, should still be performed if there is increased nodal uptake in the mediastinum to prevent denying a patient a potentially curative resection. It has been estimated that the use of this strategy in the staging of mediastinal nodes would dramatically reduce invasive mediastinal staging (Vansteenkiste, 1997; Vansteenkiste, 1998).

Metastatic Disease

The occurrence of distant metastatic disease at presentation ranges from 11% to 36% (Matthews, 1976; Quint, 1996). Common sites of metastases are the liver, adrenal glands, bones, and brain (Klein, 1991; Quint, 1996). Staging performed on the basis of symptomatology, abnormal laboratory indices, and conventional radiologic imaging will incorrectly stage some patients with M_1 disease for curative resection (accuracy of 49.3%, positive predictive value of 36%, and negative predictive value of 86.8%) (Quinn, 1986; Salvatierra, 1990; Weder, 1998). Routine radiologic evaluation for occult metastases in the absence of clinical or laboratory findings is controversial

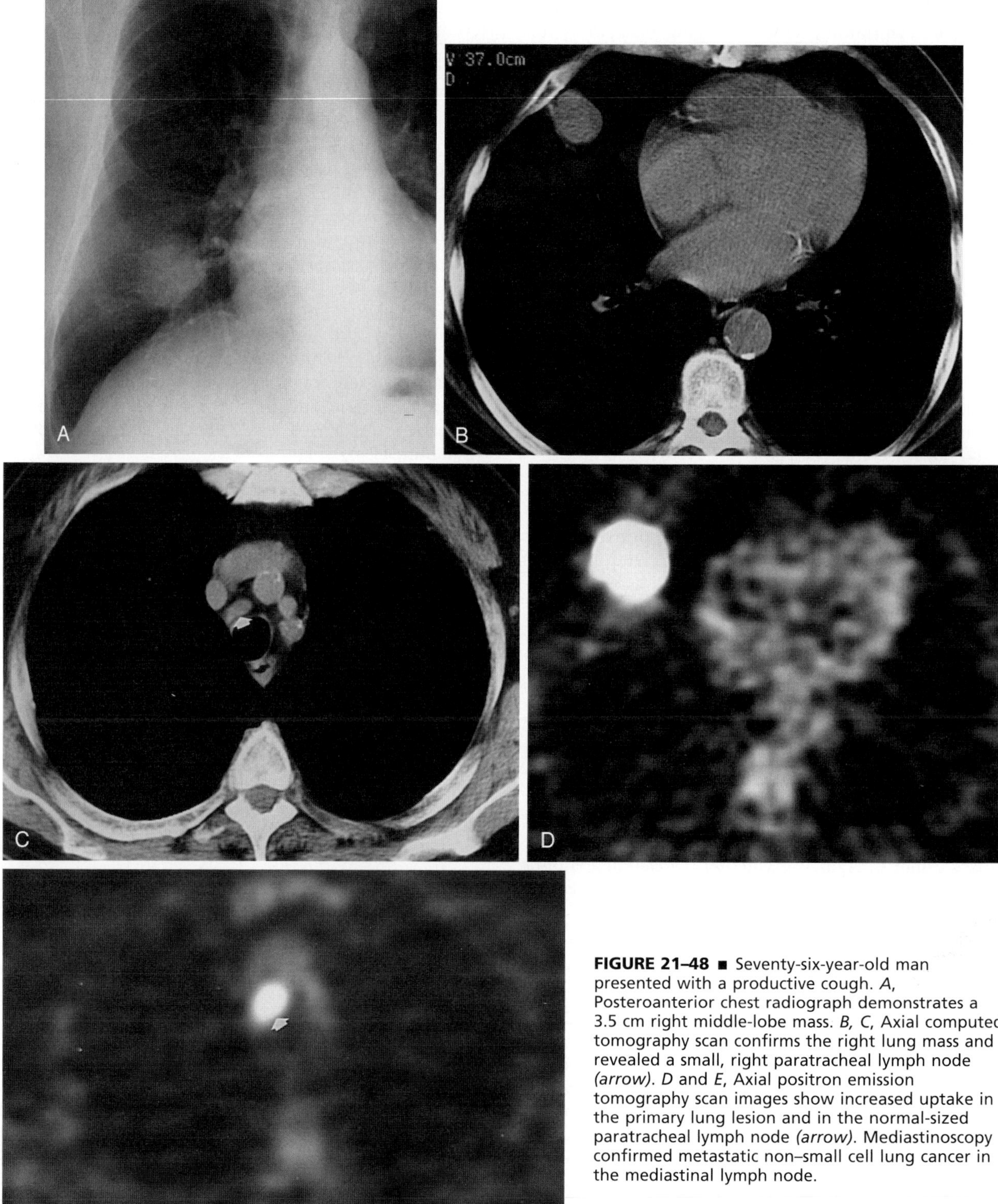

FIGURE 21–48 ■ Seventy-six-year-old man presented with a productive cough. *A*, Posteroanterior chest radiograph demonstrates a 3.5 cm right middle-lobe mass. *B, C,* Axial computed tomography scan confirms the right lung mass and revealed a small, right paratracheal lymph node *(arrow)*. *D* and *E*, Axial positron emission tomography scan images show increased uptake in the primary lung lesion and in the normal-sized paratracheal lymph node *(arrow)*. Mediastinoscopy confirmed metastatic non–small cell lung cancer in the mediastinal lymph node.

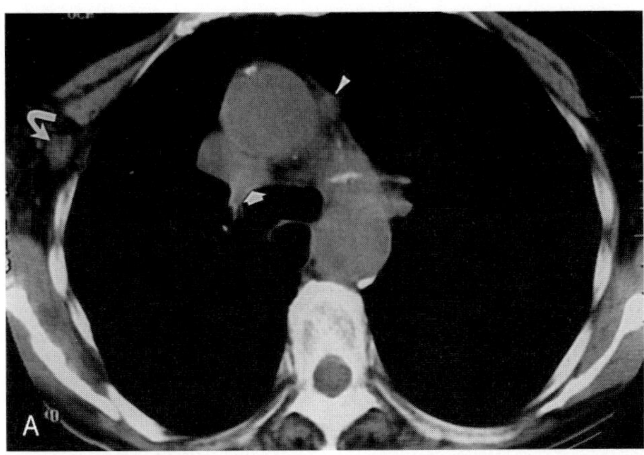

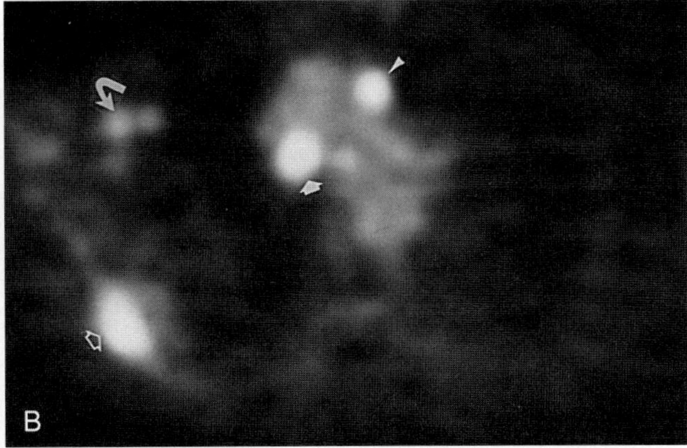

FIGURE 21–49 ■ Seventy-year-old woman with non–small cell lung cancer. *A*, Computed tomography scan shows enlarged right paratracheal lymph node *(arrow)* and small prevascular lymph node *(arrowhead)*. Note the small right axillary lymph node *(curved arrow)*. *B*, Axial positron emission tomography scan demonstrates increased activity in both mediastinal nodal stations consistent with nodal metastases. There is increased fluorodeoxyglucose uptake in right axillary nodes *(curved arrows)* and right scapula *(open arrow)* suggestive of metastatic disease. Biopsy of right scapula confirmed metastasis.

and not clearly defined (Klein, 1991; Little, 1990; Stitik, 1990; Templeton, 1990). Whole-body PET imaging has the capability to stage intrathoracic and extrathoracic disease in a single study and has a higher specificity than does CT in the detection of metastases in the liver, adrenals, and extrathoracic lymph nodes (Erasmus, 1997; Hustinx, 1998; Lewis, 1994; Rege, 1993; Valk, 1995; Weder, 1998). FDG-PET has been shown to detect occult extrathoracic metastases in 11% to 14% of patients selected for curative resection and alters management in as many as 40% of cases (Lewis, 1994; Valk, 1995; Weder, 1998). Additionally, once an unsuspected extrathoracic lesion is found on PET images, metastases should be highly suspected because there are few false-positive results (Fig. 21–50).

Approximately 10% of patients with lung cancer have an adrenal mass at presentation (Klein, 1991; Oliver, 1984; Sandler 1982). Nonfunctioning cortical adenomas occur as an incidental finding in 3% to 5% of the population, and in the absence of extrathoracic metastases an adrenal mass is more likely to be an incidental or benign finding (Klein, 1991; Oliver, 1984). CT and MRI features favoring malignancy include large size (>3 cm in diameter), poorly defined margins, irregular enhancing rim, invasion of adjacent structures, low attenuation values (<10 H), and high signal intensity on T_2-weighted sequences (Dunnick, 1990; Lee, 1991; McNicholas, 1995; Mitchell, 1992; Reinig, 1986). Unfortunately, after extensive, noninvasive evaluation, some adrenal lesions remain radiologically indeterminate and patients proceed to biopsy. Even percutaneous biopsy, however, although accurate (83% to 100%), can produce false-negative results (Bernardino, 1988; Pagani, 1983). FDG-PET imaging is an accurate, noninvasive way to differentiate benign from metastatic adrenal masses in patients with lung cancer (Erasmus, 1997) (Fig. 21–51). Because of the high sensitivity for detecting metastatic adrenal disease, patients with non–small cell lung carcinoma should be considered for curative surgical resection if FDG uptake is normal in an adrenal mass. Those patients with small cell lung carcinoma and an adrenal mass with normal FDG uptake should be treated as though they have limited stage disease. The specificity for malignancy is not optimal (≤80%), however, and patients with an isolated adrenal lesion and increased activity on the FDG-PET study should have a biopsy in an attempt to confirm metastatic disease before surgical resection.

Because conventional radiologic screening (radiographs, radionuclide technetium isotope medronate methylene diphosphonate [^{99}Tc-MDP]) for occult skeletal metastases has a low specificity, evaluation for metastases is usually performed only if the patient has focal bone pain or elevated serum alkaline phosphatase (Little, 1990; Quinn, 1986; Salvatierra, 1990). FDG-PET imaging has been shown to have fewer false-positive studies than radionuclide ^{99}Tc-MDP in patients with lung cancer who are being evaluated for skeletal metastases (Bury, 1998). Furthermore, in a recent study evaluating the detection of extrathoracic metastases in lung cancer using whole-body PET, skeletal metastases were detected in 13% of the patients, approximately 75% of whom were asymptomatic (Weder,1998) (Fig. 21–52).

Isolated metastases to the central nervous system (CNS) have been reported to be a rare occurrence in patients with non–small cell lung cancer and, when present, are frequently associated with an abnormal neurologic examination (Hooper, 1984; Klein, 1991). Although asymptomatic CNS metastases occur in 2.7% to 9.6% of patients with non–small cell lung cancer, routine CT or MRI of the CNS is controversial (Hooper, 1984; Mintz, 1984; Quinn, 1986; Salvatierra, 1990). Although whole-body FDG-PET can detect occult CNS metastases, the accuracy of PET, although unknown, is almost certainly lower.

Recurrent Disease

Response to therapy is continually reassessed using chest radiographs, CT, or MRI. Distinguishing persistent or recurrent lung cancer and metastatic pleural or mediastinal disease from post-treatment fibrosis, benign pleural thickening, and hyperplastic nodes presents a problem in

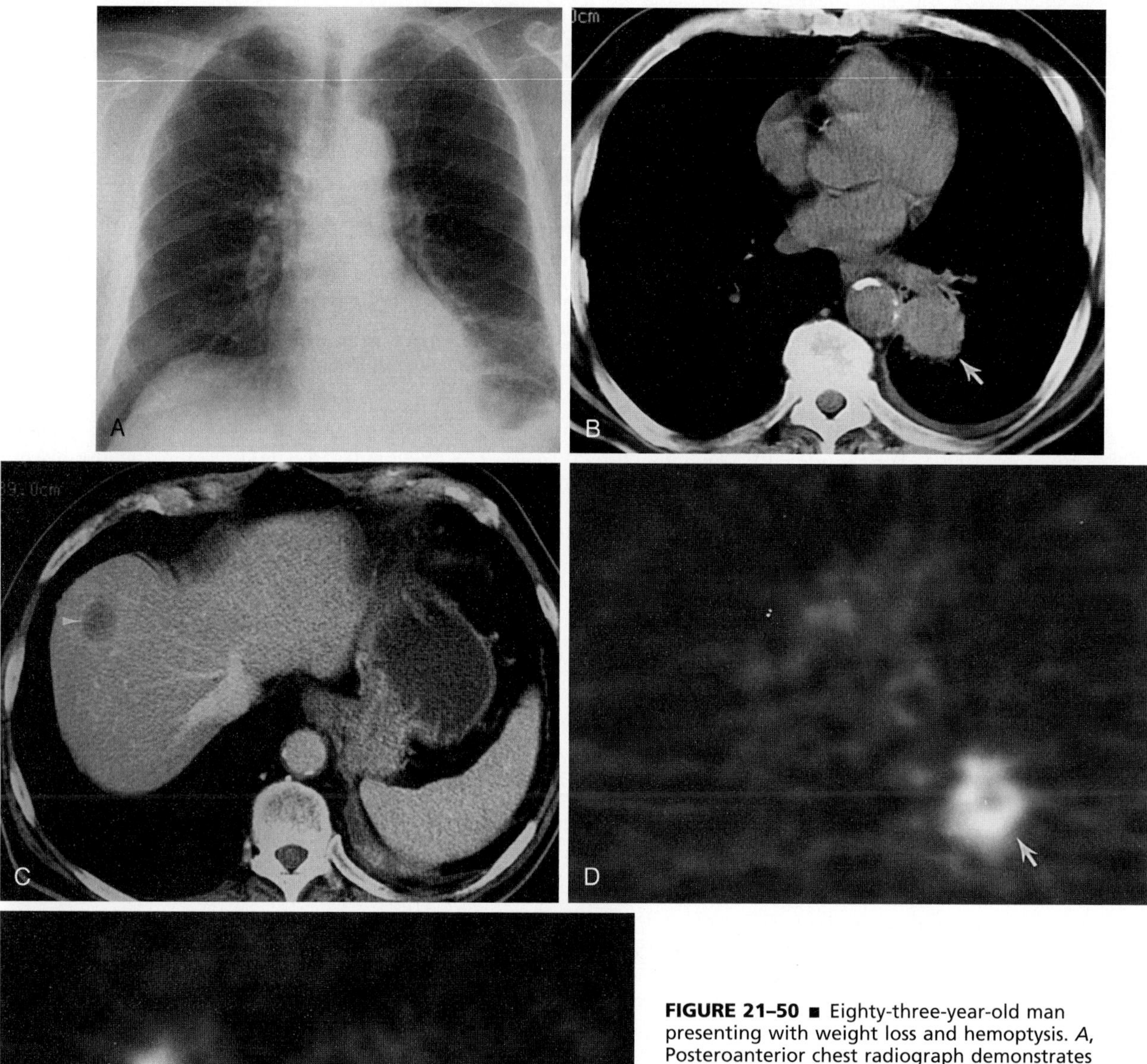

FIGURE 21–50 ■ Eighty-three-year-old man presenting with weight loss and hemoptysis. *A*, Posteroanterior chest radiograph demonstrates homogeneous opacity in the retrocardiac region suggestive of left lower-lobe atelectasis. *B* and *C*, Computed tomography scan confirms a nodular 3.5-cm left lower-lobe mass *(arrow)* and a low-attenuation lesion in the liver *(arrowhead)*. *D* and *E*, Axial positron emission tomography images show increased uptake in the primary lung lesion and in the liver lesion. Biopsy of lung and liver lesion confirmed non–small cell lung cancer (*V*, vertebral body).

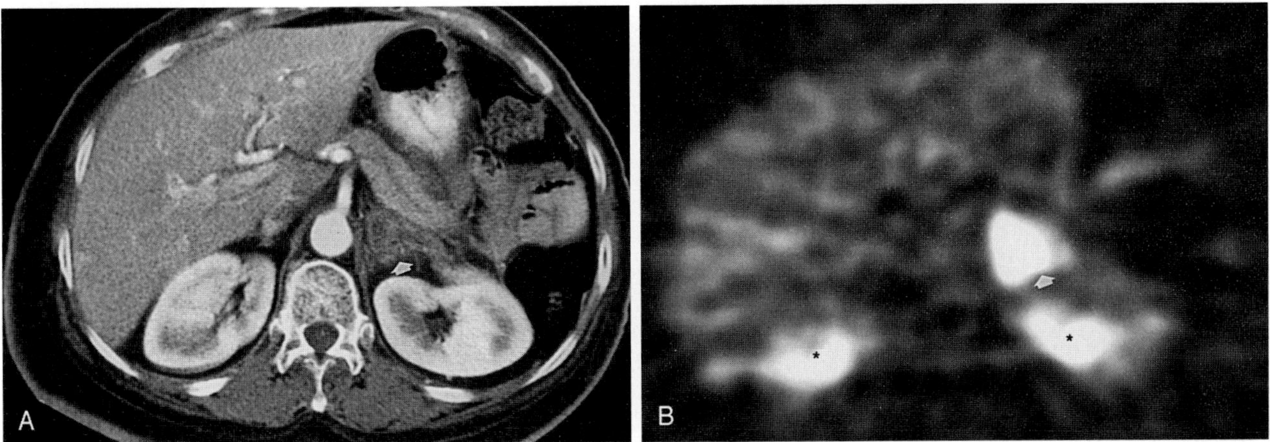

FIGURE 21–51 ■ Fifty-five-year-old woman with non–small cell lung cancer. *A*, Computed tomography axial images shows a 2-cm left adrenal mass *(arrow)*. *B*, Axial positron emission tomography image shows marked fluorodeoxyglucose uptake in the left adrenal mass. Percutaneous biopsy confirmed metastatic disease. Note the normal fluorodeoxyglucose activity in the renal collecting systems (*).

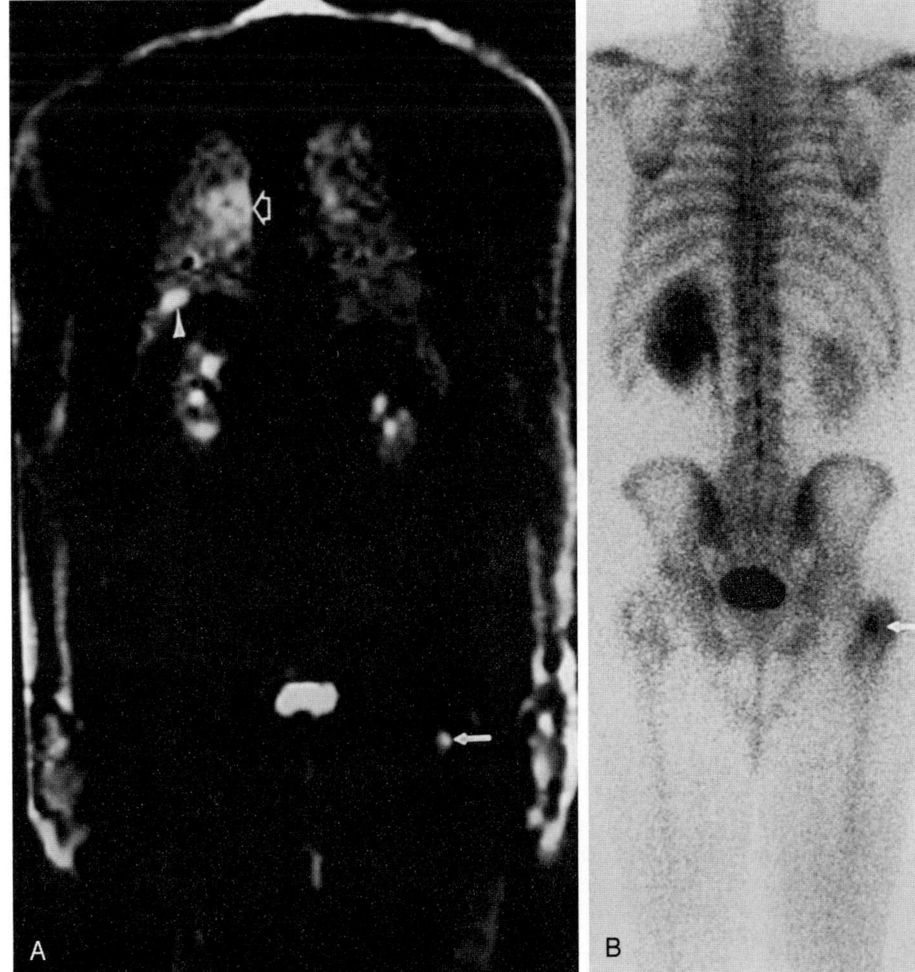

FIGURE 21–52 ■ Sixty-nine-year-old woman with non–small cell lung cancer and left hip pain. *A*, Coronal, whole-body, fluorodeoxy-glucose–positron emission tomography images show hypermetabolism suspicious for metastases in the right lower lobe mass *(arrowhead)*, right hilum *(open arrow)*, and left femur *(arrow)*. *B*, ^{99m}Tc labeled methylene diphosphonate (MDP) bone scan *(anterior projection)* shows uptake in proximal left femur consistent with osseous metastasis.

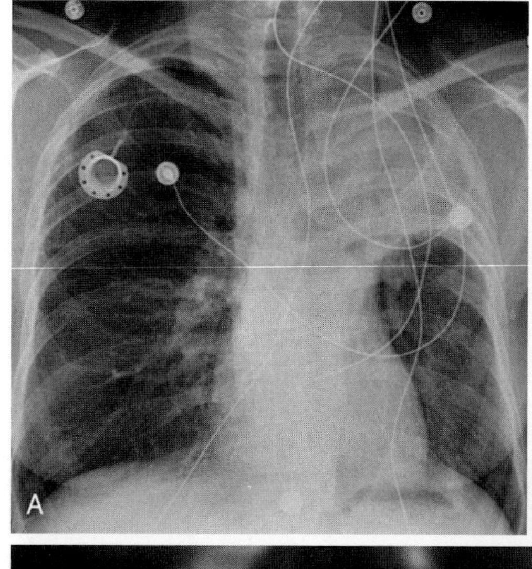

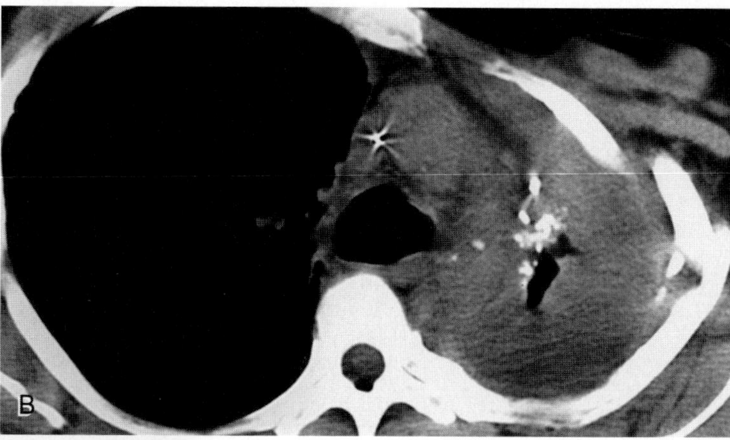

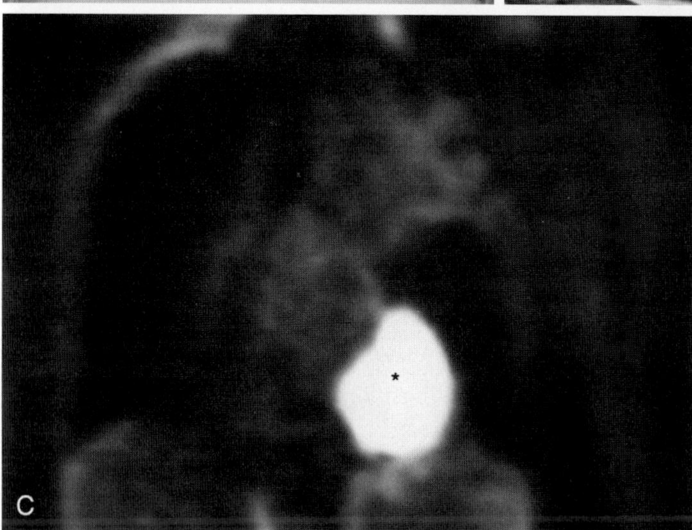

FIGURE 21–53 ■ Forty-seven-year-old woman with history of non–small cell lung cancer undergoing evaluation for possible aortic valve prosthesis replacement. *A*, Posteroanterior chest radiograph demonstrates surgical and radiation changes in the left upper lobe. *B*, Computed tomography scan confirms the nonspecific left apical opacity. *C*, Coronal positron emission tomography image reveals no significant uptake in the left hemithorax, and follow-up radiographs were stable without evidence of recurrent disease. Note the normal left ventricular activity (*).

the management of patients with lung cancer (Frank, 1995). Biopsies or sequential follow-up studies have traditionally been used to make this distinction. PET imaging may have an important role in guiding patient care after treatment because it is more accurate than conventional studies in detecting recurrent tumor (accuracy of 78% to 98%, and sensitivity and specificity of 97% to 100% and 62% to 100%, respectively) (Conti, 1996; Frank, 1995; Hübner, 1995; Ichiya, 1991; Inoue, 1995; Kim, 1992; Kubota, 1992; Patz, 1994) (Fig. 21–53). False-positive studies can be caused by post-treatment inflammatory changes and, therefore, it is recommended that PET studies are not obtained until 4 to 5 months after irradiation (Frank, 1995).

Monitoring patients using serial FDG-PET studies can detect local recurrence before conventional imaging and thus allow earlier treatment. Relying on patient symptomatology to determine local recurrence can delay diagnosis, although the effect on survival and prognosis needs to be determined (Frank, 1995).

Prognostic Potential and Therapeutic Response

Preliminary studies suggest a possible role for PET as a prognostic marker. Patients with significant increased FDG uptake in the primary lesion have a worse survival rate relative to those with modest FDG activity (Ahuja, 1998). This fact may have a role in treatment planning as well as in assessing the response to therapy (Abe, 1990; Kiffer, 1998; Knopp, 1994; Kubota, 1992; Munley, 1999). A decrease in FDG uptake after therapy suggests improved survival directly related to the magnitude of diminished activity (Abe, 1990; Smith, 1998). FDG uptake has been reported to return to normal in patients with a complete response but remains elevated in those with only a partial response. This appears to correlate with disease-free periods, which are significantly longer in patients with decreases in uptake relative to those patients in whom FDG uptake remains high (Abe, 1990).

Summary

PET has become an invaluable tool in the evaluation and management of thoracic abnormalities. It is more accurate than CT or MRI in characterizing indeterminate focal abnormal pulmonary opacities, staging lung cancer, and assessing the therapeutic response following treatment. Whole-body study PET imaging in lung cancer also appears to be the most cost-effective, efficient way to noninvasively evaluate these patients. When more studies are performed, the full clinical utility of this imaging modality will be determined.

INVASIVE IMAGING

Pulmonary Angiography

Although pulmonary angiography is the gold standard in the diagnosis of PE (Fig. 21–54), it is rarely used. Other indications include the investigation of congenital lesions (e.g., pulmonary AVMs), acquired vascular abnormalities (e.g., pulmonary arterial or venous obstruction from mediastinitis), involvement of central vessels by bronchogenic carcinoma (rarely used for this reason since the advent of CT), and, again rarely, the investigation of hemoptysis.

The advent of CTA and MRA have virtually replaced the use of pulmonary angiography for the detection of PE (see the PE section for further discussion). The impression that pulmonary angiography is an invasive and expensive test associated with significant complications has led to its underuse as well (Goodman, 1984; Newman, 1989). In fact, the morbidity and mortality rates of the procedure are quite low, with reported mortality rates being about 0.1% to 0.2% (Goodman, 1984; Mills et al, 1980; Perlmutt et al, 1987) and morbidity of significance rates of about 1.5% to 3% percent (Goodman, 1984; Mills et al, 1980).

The exact sensitivity of pulmonary angiography is unknown, but it is certainly not 100%. In part, this is caused by interobserver interpretation differences (The PIOPED Investigators, 1990) and in part by the occasional finding of emboli at autopsy following a negative angiogram (Cheery et al, 1981). However, for practical purposes, a negative study, when properly performed, essentially rules out clinically significant PEs (Cheery et al, 1981; Novelline et al, 1978). The specificity is believed to be high (Goodman, 1984).

Bronchial Arteriography

Bronchial arteriography is performed for the diagnosis of severe hemoptysis (Johnsrude et al, 1987; Remy-Jardin

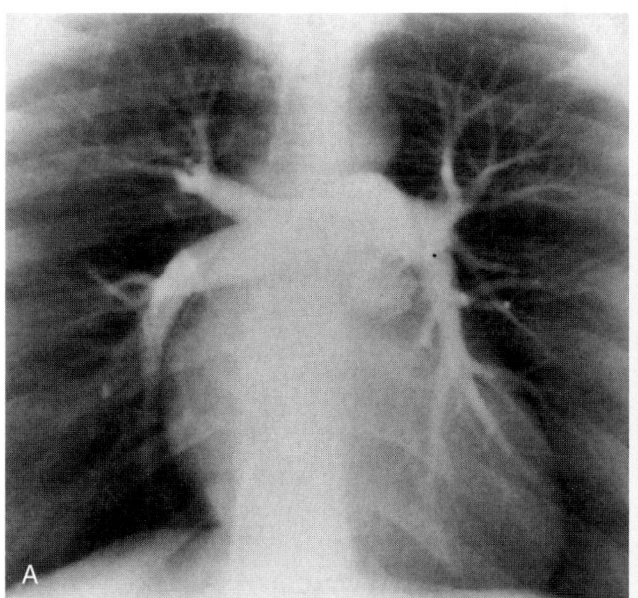

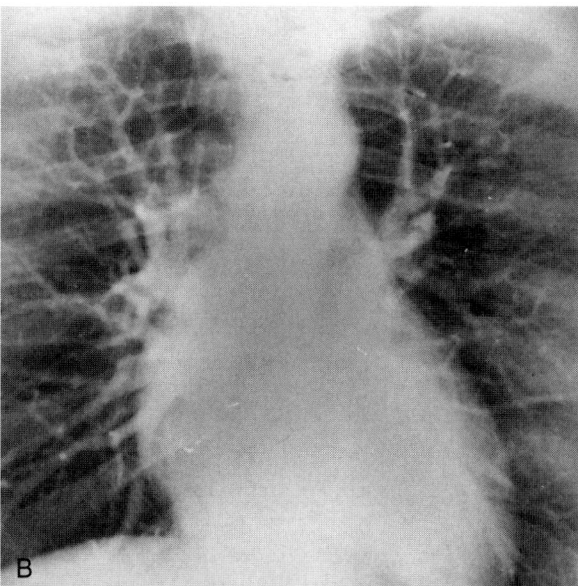

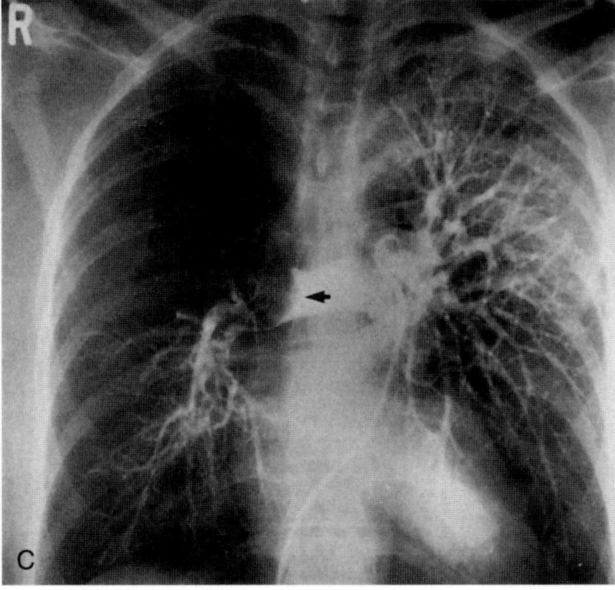

FIGURE 21–54 ■ Pulmonary arteriogram. *A*, Normal arterial phase. Contrast has been injected through a catheter with its tip just into the left main pulmonary artery. *B*, Normal venous phase. *C*, Pulmonary embolism. A large filling defect *(arrows)* representing a large, obstructing pulmonary embolism is seen in the distal right main pulmonary artery. Note the paucity of flow to the right upper lung (compare with the left side).

and Remy, 1991). The procedure involves selective placement of a catheter into a bronchial artery followed by the injection of contrast material (Fig. 21–55).

When performing bronchial arteriography, it must be kept in mind that an intercostal, or some other nonbronchial, arterial source may be contributing to the hemoptysis, especially when the patient has associated pleural inflammatory disease. If the bleeding is found to be the result of a bronchial arterial cause, then it can often be controlled by therapeutic embolization, using one of a number of different materials, including polyvinyl alcohol (Ivalon) microparticles or absorbable gelatin sponge (Gelfoam) (see Fig. 21–55*B*). The main problem that must be avoided is inadvertent obstruction of the anterior spinal artery, which may lead to transverse myelitis. Refer to the chapter on massive hemoptysis in this text.

Aortography

Although aortography has many uses in the investigation of various pathologic processes involving the aorta, the main indication in the context of this chapter is for the diagnosis of bronchopulmonary sequestration (Fig. 21–56). MRI and CTA have recently obviated the need for a more invasive procedure such as aortography. If the feeding arteries and draining veins are adequately demonstrated on one of these studies, no further evaluation is needed. However, in case of doubt, aortography should be performed for surgical planning (Hang et al, 1996). In this case, a catheter is placed within the lower thoracic aorta, and contrast is injected. The finding of an anomalous vessel (or vessels) feeding an abnormal portion of the lung is diagnostic of sequestration. This anomalous vessel must not be confused with a hypertrophied

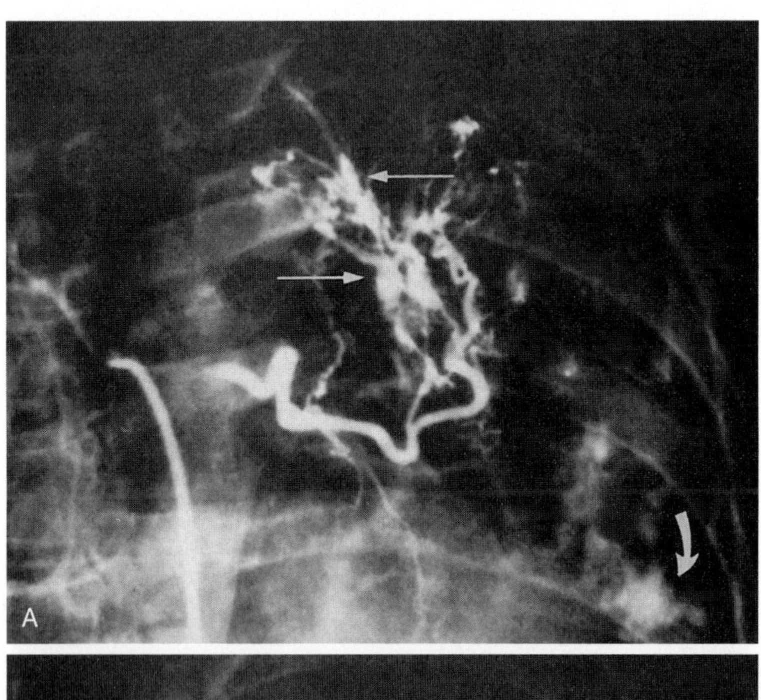

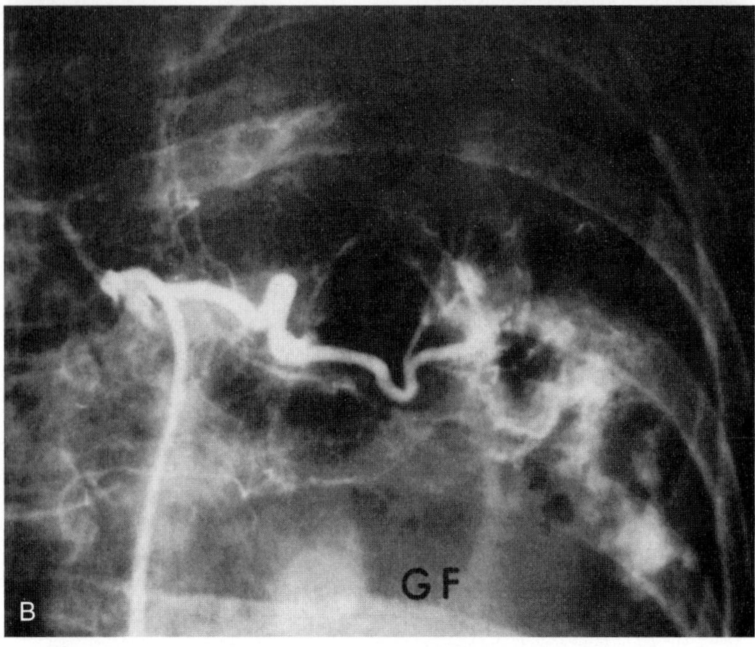

FIGURE 21–55 ■ *A*, Bronchial arteriogram in a patient with previous tuberculosis and recurrent hemoptysis. Arteriography reveals multiple dilated abnormal vessels *(straight arrows)*. *B*, Following the injection of absorbable gelatin sponge, there is no flow to these abnormal vessels. The calcific density (*curved arrow* in *A*) is related to the previous tuberculous infection. (Courtesy of K. Sniderman, MD.)

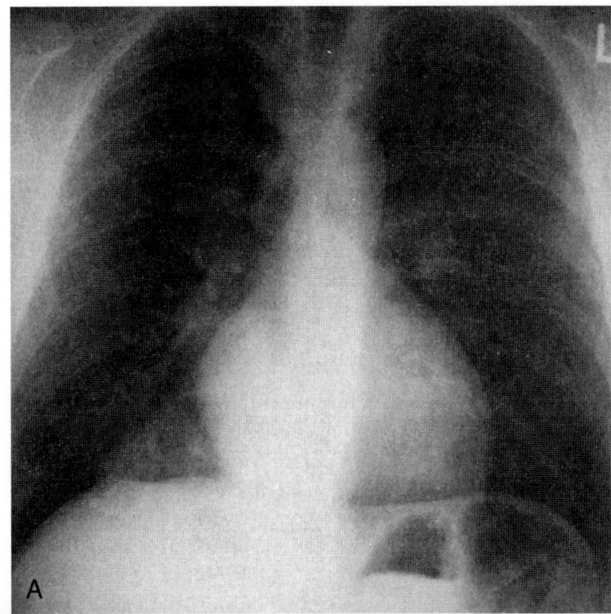

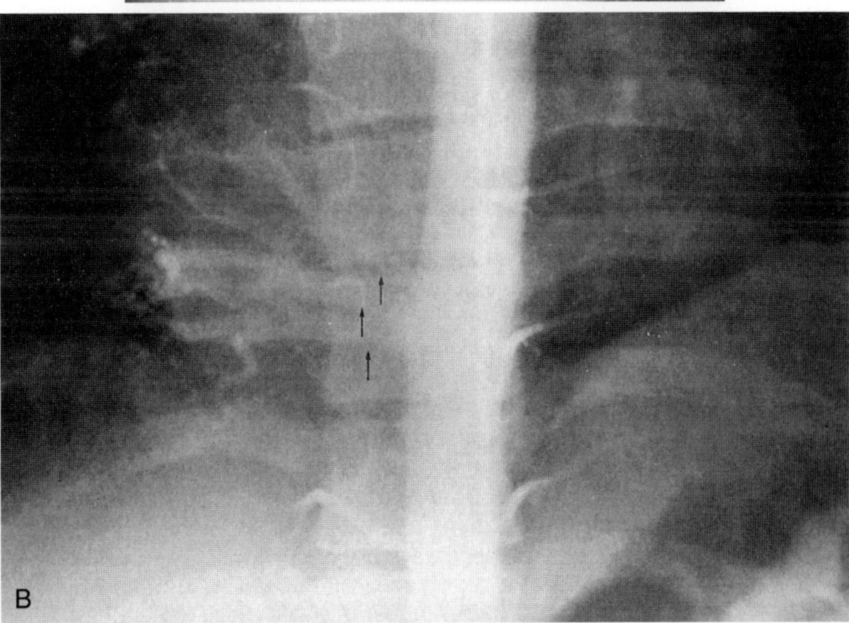

FIGURE 21–56 ■ Bronchopulmonary sequestration. *A*, Posteroanterior chest radiograph. This 27-year-old had a history of recurrent fever, chills, and dry cough. The radiograph reveals an ill-defined mass in the medial aspect of the right lower lobe. *B*, Aortogram reveals three anomalous vessels *(arrows)* feeding this bronchopulmonary sequestration.

inferior phrenic or intercostal artery, which may be feeding a noncongenital chronic inflammatory pulmonary process. Additionally, it must be kept in mind that the finding of an anomalous vessel alone is not diagnostic of sequestration; systemic supply to a normal portion of lung is a well-described phenomenon.

The aortic injection may be followed by selective catheterization of the anomalous vessel. In this way, both the number of anomalous vessels (by the aortogram) and their venous drainage (by the selective studies) can be determined. Intralobar sequestrations generally have pulmonary venous drainage; extralobar ones usually have systemic drainage, most often into the inferior vena cava or hepatic veins.

TRANSTHORACIC NEEDLE BIOPSY

Although TNB of the lung was first performed more than 100 years ago, the technique did not achieve widespread popularity until the 1960s, when Nordenstrom (1966) introduced thin needles (18 to 20 gauge) along with biplanar fluoroscopic guidance and improved cytologic methods (Fig. 21–57). Although cytologic examination continues to be the principal pathologic method of assessment, newer coaxial cutting needles may now acquire core biopsy tissue fragments that are large enough for histologic examination (Lucidarme, 1998). In addition, although fluoroscopic guidance is used in most instances, CT guidance allows the radiologist to assess more difficult pulmonary lesions (vanSonnenberg et al, 1988). Also, it is now possible to obtain diagnostic material from hilar, mediastinal, and pleural lesions by using either fluoroscopic or CT guidance (Weisbrod, 1987; Wernecke et al, 1989; Westcott, 1987).

TNB has become widely accepted as a safe and accurate method for establishing the diagnosis of pulmonary nodules and masses. It can also be used in the diagnosis

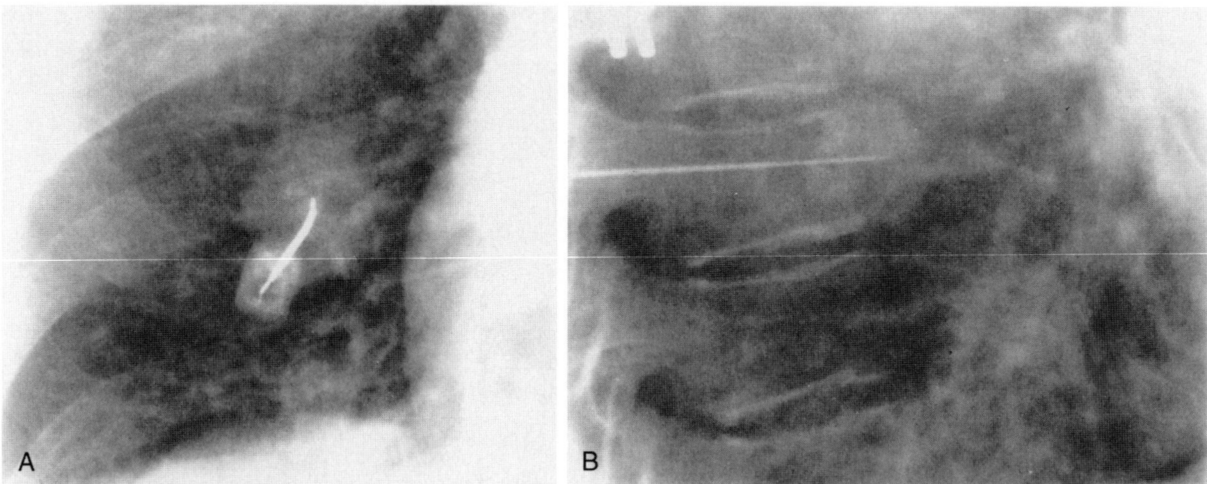

FIGURE 21–57 ■ Transthoracic needle biopsy. *A*, Frontal and *B*, lateral views reveal the tip of the needle within the central portion of the pulmonary nodule, an optimal position for sampling a lesion such as this.

of many intrathoracic pathologic processes, including pleural, rib, hilar, or mediastinal masses; or undiagnosed pulmonary infiltrates, especially when neoplasia or infection are considered possible (Perlmutt et al, 1989; Weisbrod, 1990; Westcott, 1988).

The value of TNB has been questioned because the patient will need to undergo thoracotomy whether malignancy is found or not. However, many surgeons use TNB in such cases for a number of reasons. Knowing that a patient has definite bronchogenic carcinoma prior to thoracotomy allows better planning of operating room time, reduces the need for intraoperative quick sections of the nodule, and allows the patient and family to be better informed of what to expect from the operation. In addition, TNB can make a definite benign diagnosis on occasion or may find small cell carcinoma (which can be reliably diagnosed), both of which may obviate thoracotomy. Furthermore, it has been shown that TNB can shorten both the time from admission to diagnosis and the length of hospital stay and reduce the number of thoracotomies and the hospitalization costs (Gobien et al, 1983).

Absolute contraindications to the procedure include patients with uncorrected bleeding disorders; uncooperative patients, including those with intractable coughing; and patients with suspected hydatid cysts. Relative contraindications include severe emphysema and significant pulmonary arterial hypertension.

Patients undergoing TNB do not require premedication. After informed consent is obtained, the patient is placed on the fluoroscopic table, and the opacity to be sampled is localized. The skin is washed with antiseptic solution, and a local anesthetic is instilled, with particular attention to the skin and subpleural regions. An attempt is made to avoid pleural transgression with the local anesthetic needle. The biopsy needle is then slowly advanced into the lesion, using frequent fluoroscopic assessment of its course.

Needles may be of the aspirating or cutting variety, in addition to biopsy ones. Techniques include both the single-pass technique, in which several needles are passed through the pleural surface either one at a time or in tandem, or the coaxial method, in which a 19G introducer needle is advanced through the chest wall into the lung with its tip placed at the edge of the nodule. Subsequential 22G needles are placed through it. With this technique, there is only one pleural puncture, theoretically reducing the risk of pneumothorax. Fine-needle aspiration requires finalizing preparation, preferably with an on-site cytopathologist on hand during the procedure to deem the specimen adequate before the biopsy is terminated. In cases in which cytopathology is not available, 18G core needle biopsy with histologic specimens can be obtained; biopsy guns are particularly useful for this evaluation.

Following the procedure, patients are closely watched for the development of a pneumothorax. Vital signs are taken every 15 minutes for 1 hour and then every 30 minutes until the first chest radiograph. This is obtained routinely at 4 hours with inpatients and at 2 hours with outpatients. In a series of 2421 TNBs, pneumothorax occurred in 34.1%, and chest tubes were required in 7.8% of the biopsies (Weisbrod, 1990). A more recent study in a smaller series had pneumothorax as a complication in 44.6% (54 of 121 procedures) with a chest tube required in 14.9%. If a chest tube is required, it generally becomes apparent within the first hour following the procedure, often within the first few minutes (Perlmutt et al, 1986).

Hemoptysis occasionally occurs following the procedure, almost always within the first few minutes, and is usually self-limited. Such hemorrhage may manifest as self-limited hemoptysis or increased attenuation around a nodule. However, fatalities caused by massive hemorrhage have been reported (Berquist et al, 1980); in these cases, bronchial blockers must be placed immediately. The theoretical possibility of spread of the tumor along the needle track is extremely unlikely with the use of small-gauge needles; it is limited to case reports (Muller et al, 1986).

The sensitivity of TNB in diagnosing malignancy has been reported to range from 64% to 97% (Weisbrod, 1990). The correlation between the cytologic and final histologic diagnosis of cell type has been good. The diagnostic accuracy of TNB is significantly less accurate for small pulmonary nodules than for large nodules; however, the complication rates for both are low (Huanqi et al, 1996). The use of CT has made it possible to perform biopsies on small nodules and other lesions that were previously invisible or unapproachable with fluoroscopic guidance. In a series by Westcott and colleagues, CT guidance was used for approximately 90% of the biopsies on 64 small pulmonary nodules, less than 15 mm. Pneumothorax occurred in 27%; chest tube placement was necessary in only 4%.

TNBs can also be useful in the diagnosis of mediastinal lymphadenopathy. Protopatas and colleagues (1996) performed biopsies in the hilum or mediastinum in 111 patients with suspected neoplasms. TNB can be used as a useful alternative to mediastinoscopy. It is safe in these regions, with pneumothorax and chest tube insertion rates of 19.2% and 4.8%, respectively (Weisbrod, 1987). Because the pleura is frequently not transgressed in many of these cases, these rates are actually lower than those found with pulmonary biopsies. When these biopsies are interpreted cytologically, immunohistochemical analysis is important, especially in distinguishing lymphoma from thymoma (Herman et al, 1991a). Although the accuracy is high in the diagnosis of metastatic disease and germ cell tumors, it is lower with thymoma, lymphoma, and neurogenic tumors (Herman et al, 1991a; Weisbrod, 1987).

There are limitations to using TNB to stage lung cancer. One limitation is that lymph node sampling is incomplete. Lymph nodes less than 1.5 cm are not usually sampled; therefore, cancer-containing, normal-size lymph nodes will not be detected. Also, there is a potential for occasional false-positive results. Additionally, a negative biopsy result does not absolutely rule out lymph node involvement with malignancy. At our institution, it is generally not performed. Our patients usually undergo mediastinoscopy before surgery.

TNB has been shown to have significant value in the diagnosis of pulmonary infections, with clinically useful information being found in 81% of those with suspected infection and with a specific organism being found in 76% of those in whom infection was ultimately diagnosed (Conces et al, 1989). However, because fiberoptic bronchoscopy has a very high diagnostic yield and a lower chance of causing pneumothorax, TNB should probably be used only in those patients in whom bronchoscopic results are negative.

Besides infection, other specific benign diagnoses that can be identified include hamartoma and pulmonary infarction (Westcott, 1988). When a proven benign condition is ultimately shown to be present, TNB makes a specific diagnosis in 11.7% to 68% of cases (Perlmutt et al, 1989). In the absence of a specific benign diagnosis, the procedure should be repeated at least once. The reliability of a nonmalignant result depends to a large degree on the radiologist performing the biopsy and the cytopathologist interpreting the specimen. However, if the clinician still suspects malignancy after a negative biopsy result (e.g., lesion is new or enlarging or has spiculated margins), then a video-assisted thoracic biopsy or an open biopsy should be performed. If the clinician is less suspicious, then regular follow-up CT scans must still be performed to be certain that the lesion is stable or becoming smaller. In one study (Calhoun et al, 1986) of 116 patients with nonmalignant nonspecific benign diagnoses after TNB, 33% were subsequently found to have a malignant process.

COMMENTS AND CONTROVERSIES

Because of the importance of imaging in the practice of thoracic surgery, this expanded chapter has been provided. As editors, it is our belief that thoracic surgeons must be as accomplished as radiologists in interpreting chest radiographs and CT and MRI scans. The importance of a continuing dialogue between surgeons and radiologists cannot be overemphasized. This is best accomplished by personal review of the radiographic films with the radiologist rather than by depending on reading their reports. The value of the thoracic surgeon attending weekly pathologic-radiologic conferences to maintain these skills cannot be overemphasized.

There is no doubt that the field of imaging has accelerated faster than any other clinically applied area of medicine. In the future we can look forward to further advances in functional imaging (e.g., MRI), computerized three-dimensional imaging, refinements in noninvasive angiography, computerized transmission of imaging materials, and radionuclide scanning.

This chapter, written by radiologists specializing in the field of thoracic imaging, provides a basis for understanding the expanding field of pulmonary imaging. However, the thoracic surgical trainee or practitioner is well advised to read thoroughly the textbooks identified by the authors in the annotated references. Unfortunately, not all thoracic surgeons have the advantage of an expert chest radiographer in their own institution. Therefore, the surgeon must be as well (or better) versed in the imaging of the thorax as are general radiologists.

R.J.G.

KEY REFERENCES

Armstrong P, Wilson AG, Dee P, Hansell DM: Imaging of Diseases of the Chest, 3rd ed. St. Louis, Mosby–Year Book, 2000.

This is an excellent, up-to-date textbook designed for radiologists, chest physicians, and thoracic surgeons. Although it stresses plain chest radiograph interpretation, it also fully integrates other newer imaging modalities such as CT, MRI, and nuclear medicine.

Felson B: Chest Roentgenology. Philadelphia, WB Saunders, 1973.

This book is a classic and is mandatory reading for any serious student of chest radiology. Although lacking in some up-to-date details of specific thoracic diseases, it contains a wealth of information regarding plain film image interpretation, both of the lung and of the nonpulmonary thoracic structures.

Fraser RG, Pare JAP, Pare PD et al: Diagnosis of Diseases of the Chest, 3rd ed. Vol 1–4. Philadelphia, WB Saunders, 1988–1991.

This four-volume set is encyclopedic in scope and contains the answer to virtually any question that could be asked dealing with chest disease, whether regarding the cause, epidemiology, pathologic conditions, clinical manifestations, pulmonary function, or imaging. Therapeutics are not covered. In addition to this information, it contains tables of differential diagnoses based on radiographic patterns and more than 20,000 references dealing with thoracic diseases.

Heitzman ER: The Lung: Radiologic-Pathologic Correlations, 2nd ed. St. Louis, Mosby–Year Book, 1984.

This book provides an explanation of all major radiographic signs of disease by demonstrating their genesis based on pathologic correlations, both gross and microscopic. By reading the book, the clinician gains a thorough understanding of the pathologic and radiologic signs of pulmonary diseases; it is mandatory reading for radiology residents.

McLoud TC: Thoracic Radiology: The Requisites. St. Louis, Mosby, Inc., 1998.

This is a basic text in thoracic radiology. It is extensively supplemented by tables and boxes that summarize key information presented in the text. Each chapter is outlined in detail at the beginning. It is a concise overview of many topics; however, it is not intended as a comprehensive text.

Naidich DP, Zerhouni EA, Siegelman SS: Computed Tomography and Magnetic Resonance Imaging of the Thorax, 2nd ed. New York, Raven Press, 1991.

This is a superb book that thoroughly covers what its title suggests. In addition to providing a discussion of the imaging findings in all important thoracic diseases, it presents this information in a practical manner so that it is useful in day-to-day practice.

Reed JC: Chest Radiology Plain Film Patterns and Differential Diagnosis, 4th ed. St. Louis, Mosby–Year Book, 1997.

A unique format with 24 chapters that open with unidentified radiographs followed by a series of questions designed to help identify the pattern of disease presented. The answers are a discussion with a step-by-step approach to eliminating inappropriate diagnoses and arriving at the correct one.

■ REFERENCES

Abe Y, Matsuzawa T, Fujiwara T et al: Clinical assessment of therapeutic effects on cancer using ^{18}F-2-fluoro-2-deoxy-D-glucose and positron emission tomography: Preliminary study of lung cancer. Int J Radiat Oncol Biol Phys 19:1005–1010, 1990.

Aberle DR, Gamsu G, Ray CS, Feuerstein IM: Asbestos-related pleural and parenchymal fibrosis: Detection with high-resolution CT. Radiology 166:729, 1988.

Ahuja V, Coleman RE, Herndon J, Patz EF Jr: The prognostic significance of fluorodeoxyglucose positron emission tomography imaging for patients with non–small cell lung carcinoma. Cancer 83:918–924, 1998.

Arita T, Kuramitsu T, Kawamura M et al: Bronchogenic carcinoma: Incidence of metastases to normal sized lymph nodes. Thorax 50:1267, 1995.

Arita T, Matsumoto T, Kuramitsu T et al: Is it possible to differentiate malignant mediastinal nodes from benign nodes by size? Reevaluation by CT, transesophageal echocardiography, and nodal specimen. Chest 110:1004, 1996.

Armstrong P, Wilson AG, Dee P, Hansell DM: Imaging of Diseases of the Chest, 2nd ed. St. Louis, Mosby–Year Book, 1995.

Aronchick JM: CT of mediastinal lymph nodes in patients with non–small cell lung carcinoma. Radiol Clin North Am 28:573, 1990.

Baber CE, Hedlung LW, Oddson TA, Putman CE: Differentiating empyemas and peripheral pulmonary abscesses. Radiology 135:755, 1980.

Baron RL, Levitt RG, Sagel SS: Computed tomography in the preoperative evaluation of bronchogenic carcinoma. Radiology 145:727, 1982.

Bergin CJ, Glover GM, Pauly J: Magnetic resonance imaging of lung parenchyma. J Thorac Imag 8:12, 1993.

Bernardino ME: Management of the asymptomatic patient with a unilateral adrenal mass. Radiology 166:121–123, 1988.

Bernardino ME, Walther MM, Phillips VM et al: CT-guided adrenal biopsy: Accuracy, safety, and indications. AJR Am J Roentgenol 144:67–69, 1985.

Berquist TH, Bailey PB, Cortese DA, Miller WE: Transthoracic needle biopsy accuracy and complications in relation to location and type of lesion. Mayo Clin Proc 55:475, 1980.

Boiselle PM, Patz EF Jr, Vining DJ et al: Imaging of mediastinal lymph nodes: CT, MR, and FDG PET. Radiographics 18(5):1061–1069, 1998.

Boring CC, Squires TS, Tong T: Cancer statistics, 1993. CA Cancer J Clin 43:7–23, 1993.

Bourgouin P, Cousineau G, Lemire P et al: Differentiation of radiation-induced fibrosis from recurrent pulmonary neoplasm by CT. J Can Assoc Radiol 38:23, 1987.

Brauner MW, Grenier P, Mompoint D et al: Pulmonary sarcoidosis: Evaluation with high-resolution CT. Radiology 172:467, 1989.

Broderick LS, Tarver RD, Conces DJ Jr: Imaging of lung cancer: Old and new. Semin Oncol 24:411–418, 1997.

Bury T, Barreto A, Daenen F et al: Fluorine-18 deoxyglucose positron emission tomography for the detection of bone metastases in patients with non–small cell lung cancer. Eur J Nucl Med 25(9):1244–1247, 1998.

Calhoun P, Feldman PS, Armstrong P et al: The clinical outcome of needle aspirations of the lung when cancer is not diagnosed. Ann Thorac Surg 41:592, 1986.

Cartier Y, Kavanagh PV, Johkoh T et al: Bronchiectasis: Accuracy of high-resolution CT in the differentiation of specific diseases. AJR Am J Roentgenol 173:47, 1998.

Case TA, Durney CH, Ailion DC et al: A mathematical model of diamagnetic line broadening in lung tissue and similar heterogeneous systems: Calculations and measurements. J Magn Reson 73:304, 1987.

Cheely R, McCartney WH, Perry JR et al: The role of noninvasive tests versus pulmonary angiography in the diagnosis of pulmonary embolism. Am J Med 70:17, 1981.

Chen MYM, Chiles C, Choplin RH, Aquino SL: Bronchogenic carcinoma: A survey of CT protocols for staging disease. Acad Radiol 4:687–692, 1997.

Cirimelli KM, Colletti PM, Beck S: Metastatic choriocarcinoma simulating an arteriovenous malformation on chest radiography and dynamic CT. J Comput Assist Tomogr 12:317, 1988.

Cleman RE, Laymon CM, Turkington TG: FDG imaging of lung nodules: A phantom study comparing SPECT, camera-based PET, and dedicated PET. Radiology. 210(3):823–828, 1999.

Coche EE, Müller NL, Kim K et al: Acute pulmonary embolism: Ancillary findings at spiral CT. Radiology 207:753, 1998.

Conces DJ Jr, Clark SA, Tarver RD, Schwenk GR: Transthoracic aspiration needle biopsy: Small value in the diagnosis of pulmonary infections. AJR Am J Roentgenol 152:31, 1989.

Conti PS, Lilien DL, Hawley K et al: PET and [^{18}F]-FDG in oncology: A clinical update. Nucl Med Biol 23:717–735, 1996.

Cooke JC, Currie DC, Morgan AD et al: Role of computed tomography in diagnosis of bronchiectasis. Thorax 42:272, 1987.

Cox JE, Chiles C, McManus CM et al: Transthoracic needle aspiration biopsy: Variables that affect risk of pneumothorax. Radiology 212:165, 1999.

Cutillo AG, Ganesan K, Ailion DC et al: Alveolar air-tissue interface and nuclear magnetic resonance behavior of lung. J Appl Physiol 70:2145, 1991.

Dales RE, Stark RM, Raman S: Computed tomography to stage lung cancer. Approaching a controversy using meta-analysis. Am Rev Respir Dis 141:1096, 1990.

Davis SD: CT evaluation for pulmonary metastases in patients with extrathoracic malignancy. Radiology 180:1, 1991.

Davis SD, Zirn JR, Govoni AF, Yankelevitz DF: Peripheral carcinoid tumor of the lung: CT diagnosis. AJR Am J Roentgenol 155:1185, 1990.

de Geer G, Gamsu G, Cann C, Webb WR: Evaluation of a chest phantom for CT nodule densitometry. AJR Am J Roentgenol 147:21, 1986.

DeGrado TR, Turkington TG, Williams JJ et al: Performance characteristics of a whole-body PET scanner. J Nucl Med 35:1398–1406, 1994.

Dewan NA, Gupta NC, Redepenning LS et al: Diagnostic efficacy of PET-FDG imaging in solitary pulmonary nodules. Chest 104:997–1002, 1993.

Dewan NA, Shehan CJ, Reeb SD et al: Likelihood of malignancy in a solitary pulmonary nodule. Chest 112:416–422, 1997.

Doyle TC, Lawler GA: CT features of rounded atelectasis of the lung. AJR Am J Roentgenol 143:225, 1984.

Drucker EA, Rivitz SM, Shepard JO et al: Acute pulmonary embolism: Assessment of helical CT for diagnosis. Radiology 209:235, 1998.

Dunnick NR: Adrenal imaging: Current status. AJR Am J Roentgenol 154:927–936, 1990.

Dwamena BA, Sonnad SS, Angobaldo JO, Wahl RL: Metastases from non–small cell lung cancer: Mediastinal staging in the 1990s: Meta-analytic comparison of PET and CT. Radiology 213:530, 1999.

Edelman RR, Hesselink JR, Zlatkin MB: Clinical Magnetic Resonance Imaging, Vol 2, 2nd ed. Philadelphia, WB Saunders, 1996.

Edelman RR, Wielopolski P, Schmitt F: Echo-planar MR imaging. Radiology 192:600, 1994.

Edwards WM, Cox RS Jr, Garland LH: The solitary nodule (coin lesion) of the lung: An analysis of 52 consecutive cases treated by thoracotomy and a study of preoperative diagnostic accuracy. AJR Am J Roentgenol 88:1020–1042, 1962.

Eisenberg RL: Radiology: An Illustrated History. St. Louis, Mosby–Year Book, 1991.

Epstein DM, Stephenson LW, Gefter WB et al: Value of CT in the preoperative assessment of lung cancer: A survey of thoracic surgeons. Radiology 161:423–427, 1986.

Erasmus JJ, McAdams HP, Patz EF Jr et al: Evaluation of primary pulmonary carcinoid tumors using FDG-PET. AJR Am J Roentgenol 170:1369–1373, 1998.

Erasmus JJ, Patz EF, McAdams HP et al: Evaluation of adrenal masses in patients with bronchogenic carcinoma by using 18F-fluorodeoxyglucose positron emission tomography. AJR Am J Roentgenol 168:1357–1360, 1997.

Felson B: Chest Roentgenology. Philadelphia, WB Saunders, 1973.

Ferretti GR, Bosson JL, Buffaz PD et al: Acute pulmonary embolism: Role of helical CT in 164 patients with intermediate probability at ventilation-perfusion scintigraphy and normal results at duplex US of the legs. Radiology 205:453, 1997.

Fleischner FG: The visible bronchial tree: A roentgen sign in pneumonic and other pulmonary consolidations. Radiology 50:184,1948.

Fleiter T, Merkle EM, Aschoff AJ et al: Comparison of real-time virtual fiberoptic bronchoscopy in patients with bronchial carcinoma: Opportunities and limitations. AJR Am J Roentgenol 169:1591, 1997.

Frank A, Lefkowitz D, Jaeger S et al: Decision logic for retreatment of asymptomatic lung cancer recurrence based on positron emission tomography findings. Int J Radiat Oncol Biol Phys 32:1495–1512, 1995.

Fraser RG, Pare JAP, Pare PD et al: Diagnosis of Diseases of the Chest, Vol 1, 3rd ed. Philadelphia, WB Saunders, 1988.

Freedman P: Editorial. Radiology 182:307, 1992.

Freundlich IM, Chasen MH, Varma DGK: Magnetic resonance imaging of pulmonary apical tumors. J Thorac Imaging 11(3):210, 1996.

Friedman PJ: Lung cancer: Update on staging classifications. AJR Am J Roentgenol 150:261–264, 1988.

Front D, Ben-Haim S, Israel O et al: Lymphoma: Predictive value of Ga-67 scintigraphy after treatment. Radiology 182:359, 1992.

Front D, Israel O, Epelbaum R et al: Ga-67 SPECT before and after treatment of lymphoma. Radiology 175:515, 1990.

Gaeta M, Pandolfo I, Volta S: Bronchus sign on CT in peripheral carcinoma of the lung: Value in predicting results of transbronchial biopsy. AJR Am J Roentgenol 157:1181, 1991.

Gambhir SS, Hoh CK, Phelps ME et al: Decision tree sensitivity analysis for cost-effectiveness of FDG-PET in the staging and management of non–small-cell lung carcinoma. J Nucl Med 37:1428–1436, 1996.

Gambhir SS, Shepherd JE, Shah BD et al: Analytical decision model for the cost-effective management of solitary pulmonary nodules. J Clin Oncol 16:2113–2125, 1998.

Garg K, Sieler H, Welsh CH et al: Clinical validity of helical CT being interpreted as negative for pulmonary embolism: Implications for patient treatment. AJR Am J Roentgenol 172:1627, 1999.

Garg K, Welsh CH, Feyerabend AJ et al: Pulmonary embolism: Diagnosis with spiral CT and ventilation-perfusion scanning: Correlation with pulmonary angiographic results or clinical outcome. Radiology 208:201, 1998.

Gdeedo A, Van Schil P, Corthouts B et al: Comparison of imaging TNM [(i)TNM] and pathological TNM [pTNM] in staging of bronchogenic carcinoma. Eur J Cardiothorac Surg 12:224, 1997.

Genereux GP: The Fleischner Lecture: Computed tomography of diffuse pulmonary disease. J Thorac Imaging 4:50, 1989.

Genereux GP, Howie JL: Normal mediastinal lymph node size and number: CT and anatomic study. AJR Am J Roentgenol 142:1095, 1984.

Ginsberg MS, Griff SK, Go BD et al: Pulmonary nodules resected at video-assisted thoracoscopic surgery: Etiology in 426 patients. Radiology 213:277, 1999.

Ginsberg RJ, Hill LD, Eagan RT et al: Modern 30 day operative mortality for surgical resections in lung cancer. J Thorac Cardiovasc Surg 86:654, 1983.

Glazer GM, Gross BH, Aisen AM et al: Imaging of the pulmonary hilum: A prospective comparative study in patients with lung cancer. AJR Am J Roentgenol 145:245–248, 1985a.

Glazer GM, Gross BH, Quint LE et al: Normal mediastinal lymph nodes: Number and size according to American Thoracic Society mapping. AJR Am J Roentgenol 144:261, 1985b.

Glazer GM, Orringer MB, Chenevert TL et al: Mediastinal lymph nodes: Relaxation time/pathologic correlation and implications in staging of lung cancer with MR imaging. Radiology 168:429–431, 1988.

Glazer HS, Anderson DJ, Sagel SS: Bronchial impaction in lobar collapse: CT demonstration and pathologic correlation. AJR Am J Roentgenol 153:485, 1989a.

Glazer HS, Aronberg DJ, Sagel SS, Emami B: Utility of CT in detecting postpneumonectomy carcinoma recurrence. AJR Am J Roentgenol 142:487, 1984a.

Glazer HS, Duncan-Meyer J, Aronberg DJ et al: Pleural and chest wall invasion in bronchogenic carcinoma: CT evaluation. Radiology 157:191, 1985a.

Glazer HS, Kaiser LR, Anderson DJ et al: Indeterminate mediastinal invasion in bronchogenic carcinoma: CT evaluation. Radiology 173:37, 1989b.

Glazer HS, Lee JK, Levitt RG et al: Radiation fibrosis: Differentiation from recurrent tumor by MR imaging. Radiology 156:721, 1985c.

Gobien RP, Bouchard EA, Gobien BS et al: Thin needle aspiration biopsy of thoracic lesions: Impact on hospital charges and patterns of patient care. Radiology 148:65, 1983.

Godwin JD, Speckman JM, Fram EK et al: Distinguishing benign from malignant pulmonary nodules by computed tomography. Radiology 144:349, 1982.

Golden R: The effect of bronchostenosis upon the roentgen-ray shadows in carcinoma of the bronchus. AJR Am J Roentgenol 13:21, 1925.

Goodman LR: CT of acute pulmonary emboli: Where does it fit? Radiographics 17:1037, 1997.

Goodman LR, Curtin JJ, Mewissen MW et al: Detection of pulmonary embolism in patients with unresolved clinical and scintigraphic diagnosis: Helical CT versus angiography. AJR Am J Roentgenol 164: 1369, 1995.

Goodman LR, Lipchik RJ: Diagnosis of acute pulmonary embolism: Time for a new approach. Radiology 199:25, 1996.

Goodman PC: Pulmonary angiography. Clin Chest Med 5:465, 1984.

Grenier P, Maurice F, Musset D et al: Bronchiectasis: Assessment by thin-section CT. Radiology 161:95, 1986.

Grenier P, Valeyre D, Cluzel P et al: Chronic diffuse interstitial lung disease: Diagnostic value of chest radiography and high-resolution CT. Radiology 179:123, 1991.

Gross BH, Glazer GM, Bookstein FL: Multiple pulmonary nodules detected by computed tomography: Diagnostic implications. J Comput Assist Tomogr 9:880, 1985.

Gross BH, Glazer GM, Orringer MB et al: Bronchogenic carcinoma metastatic to normal-sized lymph nodes: Frequency and significance. Radiology 166:71, 1988.

Gückel C, Schnabel K, Deimling M, Steinbrich W: Solitary pulmonary nodules: MR evaluation of enhancement patterns with contrast-enhanced dynamic snapshot gradient-echo imaging. Radiology 200:681, 1996.

Guhlmann A, Storck M, Kotzerke J et al: Lymph node staging in non-small cell lung cancer: Evaluation by [18F]FDG positron emission tomography (PET). Thorax 52:438–441, 1997.

Gupta A, Frazer CK, Ferguson JM et al: Acute pulmonary embolism: Diagnosis with MR angiography. Radiology 210:353, 1999.

Gupta NC, Frank AR, Dewan NA et al: Solitary pulmonary nodules: Detection of malignancy with PET with 2-[F-18]-fluoro-2-deoxy-D-glucose. Radiology 184:441–444, 1992.

Gupta NC, Maloof J, Gunel E: Probability of malignancy in solitary pulmonary nodules using fluorine-18-FDG and PET. J Nucl Med 37:943–948, 1996.

Halbsguth A, Schulze W, Ungeheur E, Hoer PW: Pitfall in the Cl diagnosis of pulmonary arteriovenous malformation. J Comput Assist Tomogr 7:710, 1983.

Hang JD, Guo QY, Chen CX, Chen LY: Imaging approach to the diagnosis of pulmonary sequestration. Acta Radiol 37(6):883, 1996.

Hanke R, Kretzschmar R: Round atelectasis. Semin Roentgenol 15:174, 1980.

Hatabu H: MR pulmonary angiography and perfusion imaging: Recent advances. Semin Ultrasound CT MR 18:349, 1997.

Hatabu H, Chen Q, Levin DL et al: Ventilation-perfusion MR imaging of the lung. Magn Reson Imaging Clin North Am 7(2):379, 1999a.

Hatabu H, Stock KW, Sher S et al: Magnetic resonance imaging of the thorax. Clin Chest Med 20 (4):775, 1999b.

Hatanaka M: Transport of sugars in tumor cell membranes. Biochim Biophys Acta 355:77–104, 1974.

Heaston DK, Putman CE, Rodan BA et al: Solitary pulmonary metastases in high-risk melanoma patients: A prospective comparison of conventional and computed tomography. AJR Am J Roentgenol 141:169, 1983.

Heelan RT, Demas BE, Caravelli JF et al: Superior sulcus tumors: CT and MR imaging. Radiology 170:637, 1989.

Herman SJ, Holub RV, Weisbrod GL, Chamberlain DW: Anterior mediastinal masses: Utility of transthoracic needle biopsy. Radiology 180:167, 1991a.

Herman SJ, Winton T, Weisbrod GL et al: Mediastinal invasion by bronchogenic carcinoma: CT signs. Radiology 190:841, 1994.

Herold CJ, Kuhiman JE, Zerhouni EA: Pulmonary atelectasis: Signal patterns with MR imaging. Radiology 178:715, 1991.

Hidalgo H, Korobkin M, Kinney TR et al: The problem of benign pulmonary nodules in children receiving cytotoxic chemotherapy. AJR Am J Roentgenol 140:21, 1983.

Higashi K, Seki H, Taniguchi M et al: Bronchioloalveolar carcinoma: False-negative results on FDG-PET. J Nucl Med 38:79, 1997.

Ho VB, Prince MR: Thoracic MR aortography: Imaging techniques and strategies. Radiographics 18:287, 1998.

Hooper RG, Tenholder MF, Underwood GH et al: Computed tomographic scanning of the brain in initial staging of bronchogenic carcinoma. Chest 85:774–776, 1984.

Huanqi L, Boiselle PM, Shepard JAO et al: Diagnostic accuracy and safety of CT-guided percutaneous needle aspiration biopsy of the lung: Comparison of small and large pulmonary nodules. AJR Am J Roentgenol 167:105, 1996.

Hübner KF, Buonocore E, Gould HR et al: Differentiating benign from malignant lung lesions using "quantitative" parameters of FDG PET images. Clin Nucl Med 21:941–949, 1996.

Hübner KF, Buonocore E, Singh SK et al: Characterization of chest masses by FDG positron emission tomography. Clin Nucl Med 20:293–298, 1995.

Hull RD, Hirsh J, Carter CJ et al: Diagnostic value of ventilation-perfusion lung scanning in patients with suspected pulmonary embolism. Chest 88:819, 1985.

Hustinx R, Paulus P, Jacquet N et al: Clinical evaluation of whole-body 18F-fluorodeoxyglucose positron emission tomography in the detection of liver metastases. Ann Oncol 9:397–401, 1998.

Huston J III, Muhm JR: Solitary pulmonary nodules: Evaluation with a CT reference phantom. Radiology 170:653, 1989.

Huston J III, Muhm JR: Solitary pulmonary opacities: Plain tomography. Radiology 163:481, 1987.

Ichiya Y, Kuwabara Y, Otsuka M: Assessment of response to cancer therapy using fluorine-18-fluorodeoxyglucose and positron emission tomography. J Nucl Med 32:1655–1660, 1991.

Im JG, Gamsu G, Gordon D et al: CT densitometry of pulmonary nodules in a frozen human thorax. AJR Am J Roentgenol 150:61, 1988.

Imaeda T, Kanematsu M, Asada S et al: Prediction of pulmonary function after resection of primary lung cancer: Utility of inhalation-perfusion SPECT imaging. Clin Nuc Med 20(9):729, 1995.

Inoue T, Kim E, Komaki R et al: Detecting recurrent or residual lung cancer with FDG-PET. J Nucl Med 36:788–793, 1995.

Joharjy IA, Bashi SA, Adbullah AK: Value of medium-thickness CT in the diagnosis of bronchiectasis. AJR Am J Roentgenol 149:1133, 1987.

Johnsrude IS, Jackson DC, Dunnick NR: A Practical Approach to Angiography, 2nd ed. Boston, Little, Brown, 1987.

Jones FA, Wiedemann HP, O'Donovan PB, Stoller JK: Computerized tomographic densitometry of the solitary pulmonary nodule using a nodule phantom. Chest 96:779, 1989.

Juni JE, Alavi A: Lung scanning in the diagnosis of pulmonary embolism: The emperor redressed. Semin Nucl Med 21:281, 1991.

Kadvi MA, Dussek JE: Survival and prognosis following resection of primary non small cell bronchogenic carcinoma. Eur J Cardiothorac Surg 5:132–136, 1991.

Kalender WA, Polacin A, Suss C: A comparison of conventional and spiral CT: An experimental study on the detection of spherical lesions. J Comput Assist Tomogr 18:167, 1994.

Kauczor HU, Ebert M, Kreitner KF et al: Imaging of the lungs using 3He MRI: Preliminary clinical experience in 18 patients with and without lung disease. J Magn Reson Imaging 3:538, 1997.

Kazerooni EA, Lim FT, Mikhail A, Martinez FJ: Risk of pneumothorax in CT-guided transthoracic needle aspiration biopsy of the lung. Radiology 193:371, 1996.

Khan A, Herman PG, Vorwerk P et al: Solitary pulmonary nodules: Comparison of classification with standard, thin-section, and reference phantom CT. Radiology 179:477, 1991.

Khouri NF, Meziane MA, Zerhouni EA et al: The solitary pulmonary nodule: Assessment, diagnosis, management. Chest 91:128, 1987.

Kiffer JD, Berlangieri SU, Scott AM et al: The contribution of ^{18}F-fluoro-2-deoxy-glucose positron emission tomographic imaging to radiotherapy planning in lung cancer. Lung Cancer 19:167–177, 1998.

Kim EE, Chung S, Haynie TP: Differentiation of residual or recurrent tumors from posttreatment changes with F-18-FDG PET. Radiographics 12:269–279, 1992.

Kim K, Müller NL, Mayo JR: Clinically suspected pulmonary embolism: Utility of spiral CT. Radiology 210:693, 1999.

Kiyono K, Sone S, Sakai F et al: The number and size of normal mediastinal lymph nodes: A postmortem study. AJR Am J Roentgenol 150:771, 1988.

Klein J, Gamsu G: High resolution computed tomography of diffuse lung disease. Invest Radiol 24:805, 1989.

Klein JS, Webb WR: The radiologic staging of lung cancer. J Thorac Imaging 7:29–47, 1991.

Knopp MV, Bischoff H, Rimac A et al: Clinical utility of positron emission tomography with FDG for chemotherapy response monitoring—A correlative study of patients with small cell lung cancer. J Nucl Med 35:75, 1994.

Kubota K, Matsuzawa T, Fujiwara T et al: Differential diagnosis of lung tumor with positron emission tomography: A prospective study. J Nucl Med 31:1927–1933, 1990.

Kubota K, Yamada S, Ishiwata K et al: Positron emission tomography for treatment evaluation and recurrence detection compared with CT in long-term follow-up cases of lung cancer. Clin Nucl Med 17:877–881, 1992.

Kuhlman JE: Complex diseases of the pleural space: The 10 questions most frequently asked of the radiologist: New approaches to their answers with CT and MR imaging. Radiographics 17:1043, 1997.

Kutlu CA, Pastorino U, Maisey M, Goldstraw P: Selective use of PET scan in the preoperative staging of NSCLC. Lung Cancer 21:177–184, 1998.

Langen KJ, Braun U, Kops ER et al: The influence of plasma glucose levels on fluorine-18-fluorodeoxyglucose uptake in bronchial carcinomas. J Nucl Med 34:355, 1993.

Lee JKT, Glazer HS: Controversy in the MR imaging appearance of fibrosis. Radiology 177:21, 1990.

Lee JKT, Sagel SS, Stanley RJ, Heiken JP: Computed Tomography with MRI Correlation, Vol 1. Philadelphia, Lippincott-Raven, 1998.

Lee MJ, Hahn PF, Papanicolaou N et al: Benign and malignant adrenal masses: CT distinction with attenuation coefficients, size, and observer analysis. Radiology 179:415–418, 1991.

Lewis P, Griffin S, Marsden P et al: Whole-body ^{18}F-fluorodeoxyglucose positron emission tomography in preoperative evaluation of lung cancer. Lancet 344:1265–1266, 1994.

Libshitz HI: Computed tomography in bronchogenic carcinoma. Semin Roentgenol 25:64, 1990.

Libshitz HI, Jing BS, Wallace S, Logothetis CJ: Sterilized metastases: A diagnostic and therapeutic dilemma. AJR Am J Roentgenol 140:15, 1983.

Light JP, Oster WF: Clinical and pathological reactions to the bronchographic agent Dionosil aqueous. AJR Am J Roentgenol 98:468, 1966.

Lillington GA: Pulmonary nodules: Solitary and multiple. Clin Chest Med 3:361–367, 1982.

Lillington GA, Caskey CI: Evaluation and management of solitary multiple pulmonary nodules. Clin Chest Med 14:111–119, 1993.

Lindholm P, Minn H, Leskinen-Kallio S et al: Influence of the blood glucose concentration on FDG uptake in cancer—A PET study. J Nucl Med 34:1, 1993.

Little AG, Stitik FP: Clinical staging of patients with non–small cell lung cancer. Chest 97:1431–1438, 1990.

Lonneux M, Dleval D, Bausart R et al: Can dual-headed 18F-FDG SPET imaging reliably supersede PET in clinical oncology? A comparative study in lung and gastrointestinal tract cancer. Nucl Med Commun 19:1047–1054, 1998.

Lowe VJ, Fletcher JW, Gobar L et al: Prospective investigation of PET in lung nodules (PIOPILN). J Clin Oncol 16:1075–1084, 1998.

Lowe VJ, Hoffman JM, DeLong DM et al: Semiquantitative and visual analysis of FDG-PET images in pulmonary abnormalities. J Nucl Med 35:1771–1776, 1994.

Lucidarme O, Howarth N, Finet JF, Grenier PA: Intrapulmonary lesions: Percutaneous automated biopsy with a detachable, 18-gauge, coaxial cutting needle. Radiology 207:759, 1998.

Lynch DA, Newell J, Hale V et al: Correlation of CT findings with clinical evaluations in 261 patients with symptomatic bronchiectasis. AJR Am J Roentgenol 173:53, 1999.

Mahoney MC, Shipley RT, Corcoran HL, Dickson BA: CT demonstration of calcification in carcinoma of the lung. AJR Am J Roentgenol 154:255, 1990.

Mai VM, Knight-Scott J, Berr SS: Improved visualization of the human lung in 1H MRI using multiple inversion recovery for simultaneous suppression of signal contributions from fat and muscle. Magn Reson Med 41:866, 1999.

Maki DD, Gefter WB, Alavi A: Recent advances in pulmonary imaging. Chest 116:1388, 1999.

Malenka DJ, Colice GL, Beck JR: Does the mediastinum of patients with non-small cell lung cancer require histologic staging? Am Rev Respir Dis 144:1134–1139, 1991.

Manfredi R, Pirronti T, Bonomo L et al: Accuracy of computed tomography and magnetic resonance imaging in staging bronchogenic carcinoma. MAGMA 4:257, 1996.

Mann H, Karwande SV: The new proposed international staging system for lung cancer. Semin Ultrasound CT MR 9:34–39, 1988.

Martini N, Heelan R, Westcott J et al: Comparative merits of conventional, computed tomographic, and magnetic resonance imaging in assessing mediastinal involvement in surgically confirmed lung carcinoma. J Thorac Cardiovasc Surg 90:639–648, 1985.

Mathieson JR, Mayo JR, Staples CA, Muller NL: Chronic diffuse infiltrative lung disease: Comparison of diagnostic accuracy of CT and chest radiography. Radiology 171:111, 1989.

Matthews MJ: Problems in morphology and behavior of bronchopulmonary malignant disease. In Israel L, Chahinian AL (eds): Lung cancer: Natural History, Prognosis, and Therapy. New York, Academic Press, 1976, pp 23–62.

Mayo JR, Remy-Jardin M, Müller NL et al: Pulmonary embolism: prospective comparison of spiral CT with ventilation-perfusion scintigraphy. Radiology 205:447, 1997.

Mayr B, Ingrisch H, Haussinger K et al: Tumors of the bronchi: Role of evaluation with CT. Radiology 172:647, 1989.

McHugh K, Blaquiere RM: CT features of rounded atelectasis. AJR Am J Roentgenol 153:257, 1989.

McKenna RJ Jr, Libshitz HI, Mountain CT: Roentgenographic evaluation of mediastinal nodes for preoperative assessment in lung cancer. Chest 88:206, 1985.

McLoud TC: Thoracic Radiology: The Requisites. St. Louis, Mosby, Inc., 1998.

McLoud TC, Bourgouin PM, Greenberg RW et al: Bronchogenic carcinoma: Analysis of staging in the mediastinum with CT by correlative lymph node mapping and sampling. Radiology 182:319–323, 1992.

McNicholas MM, Lee MJ, Mayo-Smith WW et al: An imaging algorithm for the differential diagnosis of adrenal adenomas and metastases. AJR Am J Roentgenol 165:1453–1459, 1995.

Meaney JFM, Weg JG, Chenevert TL et al: Diagnosis of pulmonary embolism with magnetic resonance angiography. N Engl J Med 336:1422, 1997.

Metter FA, Guiberteau MJ: Essentials of Nuclear Medicine Imaging, 3rd ed. Philadelphia, WB Saunders, 1991.

Miller RR, Nelems B, Muller NL et al: Lingular and right middle lobe biopsy in the assessment of diffuse lung disease. Ann Thorac Surg 44:269, 1987.

Milne ENC, Zerhouni EA: Blood supply of pulmonary metastases. J Thorac Imaging 2:15, 1987.

Mintz BJ, Tuhrim S, Alexander S et al: Intracranial metastases in the initial staging of bronchogenic carcinoma. Chest 86:850–853, 1984.

Mitchell DG, Crovello M, Matteucci T et al: Benign adrenocortical masses: Diagnosis with chemical shift MR imaging. Radiology 185:345–351, 1992.

Mountain CF: A new international staging system for lung cancer. Chest 89(Suppl):225S–233S, 1986.

Mountain CF: Prognostic implications of international staging system for lung cancer. Semin Oncol 15:236–245, 1988.

Mountain CF: Revisions in the international system for staging lung cancer. Chest 111:1710–1717, 1997.

Muller NL: Clinical value of high-resolution CT in chronic diffuse lung disease. AJR Am J Roentgenol 157:1163, 1991.

Muller NL, Bergin CJ, Miller RR, Ostrow DN: Seeding of malignant cells into the needle track after lung and pleural biopsy. J Can Assoc Radiol 37: 192, 1986.

Muller NL, Bergin CJ, Ostrow DN, Nichols DM: Role of computed tomography in the recognition of bronchiectasis. AJR Am J Roentgenol 143:971, 1984.

Muller NL, Miller RR: Computed tomography of chronic diffuse infiltrative lung disease, Part 1. Am Rev Respir Dis 142:1206, 1990a.

Muller NL, Miller RR: Computed tomography of chronic diffuse infiltrative lung disease, Part 2. Am Rev Respir Dis 142:1440, 1990b.

Muller NL, Staples CA, Miller RR et al: Disease activity in idiopathic pulmonary fibrosis: CT and pathologic correlation. Radiology 165:731, 1987.

Munden RF, Pugatch RD, Liptay MJ et al: Small pulmonary lesions detected at CT: Clinical importance. Radiology 202:105, 1997.

Munley MT, Marks LB, Scarfone C et al: Multimodality nuclear medicine imaging in three-dimensional radiation treatment planning for lung cancer: Challenges and prospects. Lung Cancer 23:105–114, 1999.

Munro NC, Cooke JC, Currie DC et al: Comparison of thin section computed tomography with bronchography for identifying bronchiectatic segments in patients with chronic sputum production. Thorax 45:135, 1990.

Musset D, Grenier P, Carette MF et al: Primary lung cancer staging: Prospective comparative study of MR imaging with CT. Radiology 160:607–611, 1986.

Naidich DP, Funt S, Ettenger NA, Arranda C: Hemoptysis: CT bronchoscopic correlations in 58 cases. Radiology 177:357, 1990.

Naidich DP, Lee JJ, Garay SM et al: Comparison of CT and fiberoptic bronchoscopy in the evaluation of bronchial disease. AJR Am J Roentgenol 148:1, 1987.

Naidich DP, McCauley DI, Khouri NF et al: Computed tomography of lobar collapse. I: Endobronchial obstruction. J Comput Assist Tomogr 7:745, 1983a.

Naidich DP, McCauley DI, Khouri NF et al: Computed tomography of lobar collapse. II: Collapse in the absence of endobronchial obstruction. J Comput Assist Tomogr 7:758, 1983b.

Naidich DP, Sussman R, Kutcher WL et al: Solitary pulmonary nodules: CT-bronchoscopic correlation. Chest 93:595, 1988.

Naidich DP, Zerhouni EA, Siegelman SS: Computed Tomography and Magnetic Resonance Imaging of the Thorax, 2nd ed. New York, Raven Press, 1991.

Nathan MH, Collins VP, Adams RA: Differentiation of benign and malignant pulmonary nodules by growth rate. Radiology 79:221, 1962.

Newman GE: Pulmonary angiography in pulmonary embolic disease. J Thorac Imaging 4:28, 1989.

Nolop KB, Rhodes CG, Brudin LH: Glucose utilization in vivo by human pulmonary neoplasm. Cancer 60:2682–2689, 1987.

Nordenstrom B: New technique for transthoracic biopsy of lung changes. Br J Radiol 38:550, 1965.

Novelline RA, Baltarowich OH, Athanasoulis CA et al: The clinical course of patients with suspected pulmonary embolism and a negative pulmonary arteriogram. Radiology 126:561, 1978.

Oliver TW Jr, Bernardino ME, Miller JI et al: Isolated adrenal masses in non–small-cell bronchogenic carcinoma. Radiology 153:217–218, 1984.

Osteen RT: Cancer Manual, 8th ed. Boston, American Cancer Society, 1990, pp 1–576.

Padovani B, Mouroux J, Seksik L et al: Chest wall invasion by bronchogenic carcinoma: Evaluation with MR imaging. Radiology 187:33–38, 1993.

Pagani JJ: Normal adrenal glands in small cell lung carcinoma: CT-guided biopsy. AJR Am J Roentgenol 140:949–951, 1983.

Patterson GA, Ginsberg RJ, Poon PY et al: A prospective evaluation of magnetic resonance imaging, computed tomography, and mediastinoscopy in the preoperative assessment of mediastinal node status in bronchogenic carcinoma. J Thorac Cardiovasc Surg 94:679, 1987.

Patterson GA, Ilves R, Ginsberg RJ et al: The value of adjuvant radiotherapy in pulmonary and chest wall resection for bronchogenic carcinoma. Ann Thorac Surg 34:692, 1982.

Patz EF Jr, Lowe VJ, Hoffman JM et al: Focal pulmonary abnormalities: Evaluation with F-18 fluorodeoxyglucose PET scanning. Radiology 188:487–490, 1993.

Patz EF Jr, Lowe VJ, Hoffman JM et al: Persistent or recurrent bronchogenic carcinoma: Detection with PET and 2-[F-18]-2-deoxy-D-glucose. Radiology 191:379–382, 1994.

Patz EF Jr, Goodman PC: Positron emission tomography imaging of the thorax. Radiol Clin North Am 32:811–823, 1994.

Patz EF Jr, Lowe VJ, Goodman PC, Herndon J: Thoracic nodal staging with positron emission tomography (PET) and ^{18}-F-2 fluoro-2-deoxy-D-glucose in patients with bronchogenic carcinoma. Chest 108:1617–1621, 1995.

Pennes DR, Glazer GM, Wimbish KJ et al: Chest wall invasion by lung cancer: Limitations of CT evaluation. AJR Am J Roentgenol 144:507, 1985.

Perlmutt LM, Braun SD, Newman GE et al: Timing of chest film follow-up after transthoracic needle aspiration. AJR Am J Roentgenol 146: 1049, 1986.

Perlmutt LM, Johnston WW, Dunnick NR: Percutaneous transthoracic needle aspiration: A review. AJR Am J Roentgenol 152:451, 1989.

Peters JC, Desai KK: CT demonstration of postpneumonectomy tumor recurrence. AJR Am J Roentgenol 141:259, 1983.

Peuchot M, Libshitz HI: Pulmonary metastatic disease: Radiologic-surgical correlation. Radiology 164:719, 1987.

Piehler JM, Pairolero PC, Weiland LH et al: Bronchogenic carcinoma with chest wall invasion: Factors affecting survival following en bloc resection. Ann Thorac Surg 34:684, 1982.

Poon PY, Bronskill MJ, Henkelman RM et al: Mediastinal lymph node metastases from bronchogenic carcinoma: Detection with MR imaging and CT. Radiology 162:651, 1987.

Prokop M, Debatin JF: MRI contrast media: New developments and trends: CTA vs. MRA. Eur Radiol 5:299, 1997.

Proto AV, Thomas SR: Body computed tomography: Pulmonary nodules studied by computed tomography. Radiology 156:149, 1985.

Proto AV, Tocino I: Radiographic manifestations of lobar collapse. Semin Roentgen 15:117, 1980.

Protopapas Z, Westcott JL: Transthoracic needle biopsy of mediastinal lymph nodes for staging lung and other cancers. Radiology 199:489, 1996.

Pugatch RD, Faling LJ, Robbins AH, Snider GL: Differentiation of pleural and pulmonary lesions using computed tomography. J Comput Assist Tomogr 2:601, 1978.

Putnam JB, Roth JA, Wesley MN et al: Analysis of prognostic factors in patients undergoing resection of pulmonary metastases from soft tissue sarcomas. J Thorac Cardiovasc Surg 87:260, 1984.

Quinn DL, Ostrow LB, Porter DK et al: Staging of non–small cell bronchogenic carcinoma. Chest 89:270–275, 1986.

Quint LE, Francis IR, Wahl RL et al: Preoperative staging of non–small-cell carcinoma of the lung: Imaging methods. AJR Am J Roentgenol 164:1349–1359, 1995.

Quint LE, Glazer GM, Orringer MB et al: Mediastinal lymph node detection and sizing at CT and autopsy. AJR Am J Roetngenol 147:469, 1986.

Quint LE, Tummala S, Brisson LJ et al: Distribution of distant metastases from newly diagnosed non–small cell lung cancer. Ann Thorac Surg 62:246–250, 1996.

Ravin CE, Chotas HG: Chest radiography. Radiology 204:593, 1997.

Reed JC: Chest Radiology Plain Film Patterns and Differential Diagnosis, 4th ed. St. Louis, Mosby–Year Book, 1997.

Rege SD, Hoh CK, Glaspy JA: Imaging of pulmonary mass lesions with whole-body positron emission tomography and fluoro-deoxyglucose. Cancer 72:82–90, 1993.

Reinig JW, Doppman JL, Dwyer AJ et al: Adrenal masses differentiated by MR. Radiology 158:81–84, 1986.

Remy-Jardin M, Remy J: Embolization for the treatment of hemoptysis. In Kadir S (ed): Current Practice of Interventional Radiology. Philadelphia, BC Decker, 1991.

Remy-Jardin M, Remy J, Deschildre F et al: Diagnosis of pulmonary embolism with spiral CT: Comparison with pulmonary arteriography and scintigraphy. Radiology 200:699, 1996.

Remy-Jardin M, Remy J, Giraud F, Marquette CH: Pulmonary nodules: Detection with thick spiral CT versus conventional CT. Radiology 187:513, 1993.

Remy-Jardin M, Remy J, Wattinne L, Giraud F: Central pulmonary thromboembolism: Diagnosis with spiral volumetric CT with the single-breath-hold technique: Comparison with pulmonary angiography. Radiology 185:38, 1992.

Ren H, Kuhiman JE, Hruban RH et al: Computed tomography of inflation-fixed lungs: The beaded septum sign of pulmonary metastasis. J Comput Assist Tomogr 13:411, 1989.

Rendina EA, Bognolo DA, Mineo TC et al: Computed tomography for the evaluation of intrathoracic invasion by lung cancer. J Thorac Cardiovasc Surg 94:57, 1987.

Robbins LL, Hale CH: The roentgen appearance of lobar and segmental collapse of the lung: Preliminary report. Radiology 44:107, 1945a.

Robbins LL, Hale CH: The roentgen appearance of lobar and segmental collapse of the lung. II: The normal chest as it pertains to collapse. Radiology 44:543, 1945b.

Robbins LL, Hale CH: The roentgen appearance of lobar and segmental collapse of the lung. III: Collapse of an entire lung or the major part thereof. Radiology 45:23, 1945c.

Robbins LL, Hale CH: The roentgen appearance of lobar and segmental collapse of the lung. IV: Collapse of the lower lobes. Radiology 45: 120, 1945d.

Robbins LL, Hale CH: The roentgen appearance of lobar and segmental collapse of the lung. V: Collapse of the right middle lobe. Radiology 45:260, 1945e.

Robbins LL, Hale CH: The roentgen appearance of lobar and segmental collapse of the lung. VI: Collapse of the upper lobes. Radiology 45:347, 1945f.

Robbins LL, Hale CH, Merrill OK: The roentgen appearance of lobar and segmental collapse of the lung. I: Technique of examination. Radiology 44:471, 1945.

Ryo UY: Prediction of postoperative loss of lung function in patients with malignant lung mass. Radiol Clin North Am 28(3):657, 1990.

Sakai S, Murayama S, Murakami J et al: Bronchogenic carcinoma invasion of the chest wall: Evaluation with dynamic ciné MRI during breathing. J Comput Assist Tomogr 4:595, 1997.

Salvatierra A, Baamonde C, Llamas JM et al: Extrathoracic staging of bronchogenic carcinoma. Chest 97:1052–1058, 1990.

Sandler MA, Pearlberg JL, Madrazo BL et al: Computed tomographic evaluation of the adrenal gland in the preoperative assessment of bronchogenic carcinoma. Radiology 145:733–736, 1982.

Sazon DAD, Santago SM, Hoo GWS et al: Fluorodeoxyglucose-positron emission tomography in the detection and staging of lung cancer. Am J Respir Crit Care Med 153:417–421, 1996.

Schaner KG, Chang AK, Doppman JL et al: Comparison of computed and conventional whole lung tomography in detection of pulmonary nodules: A prospective radiologic-pathologic study. AJR Am J Roentgenol 131:51, 1978.

Schneider HJ, Felson B, Gonzalez LL: Rounded atelectasis. AJR Am J Roentgenol 134:225, 1980.

Schwartz LH, Ginsberg MS, Burt ME et al: MRI as an alternative to CT-guided biopsy of adrenal masses in patients with lung cancer. Ann Thorac Surg 65:193, 1998.

Scott IR, Muller NL, Miller RR et al: Resectable stage III lung cancer: CT, surgical and pathologic correlation. Radiology 166:75, 1988.

Scott WJ, Schwabe JL, Gupta NC et al: Positron emission tomography of lung tumors and mediastinal lymph nodes using [18F] fluorodeoxyglucose. Ann Thorac Surg 58:698–703, 1994.

Shaffer K: Imaging and medical staging of lung cancer. Hematol Oncol Clin North Am 11:197–213, 1997.

Shreve PD, Stevenson RS, Deters EC et al: Oncologic diagnosis with 2-[fluorine-18]fluoro-2-deoxy-D-glucose imaging: Dual-head coincidence gamma camera versus positron emission tomographic scanner. Radiology 207:431–437, 1998.

Sider L, Horejs D: Frequency of extrathoracic metastases from bronchogenic carcinoma in patients with normal-sized hilar and mediastinal lymph nodes on CT. AJR Am J Roentgenol 151:893, 1988.

Siegelman SS, Khouri NF, Leo FP et al: Solitary pulmonary nodules: CT assessment. Radiology 160:307, 1986.

Siegelman SS, Khouri NF, Scott WW Jr et al: Pulmonary hamartoma: CT findings. Radiology 160:313, 1986b.

Siegelman SS, Zerhouni EA, Leo FP et al: CT of the solitary pulmonary nodule. AJR Am J Roentgenol 135:1, 1980.

Silverman PM, Godwin JD: CT/bronchographic correlations in bronchiectasis. J Comput Assist Tomogr 11:52, 1987.

Smith TAD: FDG uptake, tumour characteristics and response to therapy: A review. Nucl Med Commun 19:97–105, 1998.

Staples CA, Müller NL, Miller RR et al: Mediastinal nodes in bronchogenic carcinoma: Comparison between CT and mediastinoscopy. Radiology 167:367–372, 1988.

Stark DD, Ferderle MP, Goodman PC et al: Differentiating lung abscess and empyema: Radiography and computed tomography. AJR Am J Roentgenol 141:163, 1983.

Stein MG, Mayo J, Muller N et al: Pulmonary lymphangitic spread of carcinoma: Appearance on CT scans. Radiology 162:371, 1987.

Steinert H et al: Non–small cell lung cancer: Nodal staging with FDG PET versus CT with correlative lymph node mapping and sampling. Radiology 202:441–446, 1997.

Stevens GM, Jackman RJ: Outpatient needle biopsy of the lung: Its safety and utility. Radiology 151:301, 1984.

Stitik FP: Staging of lung cancer. Radiol Clin North Am 28:619–630, 1990.

Stitik FP: The new staging of lung cancer. Radiol Clin North Am 32:635–647, 1994.

Strauss LG, Conti PS: The applications of PET in clinical oncology. J Nucl Med 32:623–648, 1991.

Strickland B, Strickland NH: The value of high definition, narrow section computed tomography in fibrosing alveolitis. Clin Radiol 39:589, 1988.

Sumners RM, Feng DH, Holland SM, Sneller MC, Shelhamer JH: Virtual bronchoscopy: Segmentation method for real-time display. Radiology 200:857, 1996.

Sumners RM, Selbie WS, Malley JD et al: Polypoid lesions of airways: Early experience with computer-assisted detection by using virtual bronchoscopy and surface curvature. Radiology 208:331, 1998.

Swensen SJ, Brown LR, Colby TV et al: Lung nodule enhancement at CT: Prospective findings. Radiology 201:447, 1996.

Swensen SJ, Harms GF, Morin RL, Myers JL: CT evaluation of solitary pulmonary nodules: Value of 185-H reference phantom. AJR Am J Roentgenol 156:925, 1991.

Tatsumi M, Yutani K, Watanabe Y et al: Feasibility of fluorodeoxyglucose dual-head gamma camera coincidence imaging in evaluation of lung cancer: Comparison with FDG-PET. J Nucl Med 40:566–573, 1999.

Teigen CL, Maus TP, Sheedy PF et al: Pulmonary embolism: Diagnosis with contrast enhanced electron-beam CT and comparison with pulmonary angiography. Radiology 194:313, 1995.

Templeton PA, Caskey CI, Zerhouni EA: Current uses of CT and MR imaging in the staging of lung cancer. Radiol Clin North Am 28:631–646, 1990.

The PIOPED Investigators: Value of the ventilation/perfusion scan in acute pulmonary embolism: Results of the Prospective Investigation of Pulmonary Embolism Diagnosis (PIOPED). JAMA 263:2753, 1990.

Tillich M, Kammerhuber F, Reittner P et al: Detection of pulmonary nodules with helical CT: Comparison of ciné and film-based viewing. AJR Am J Roentgenol 169:1611, 1997.

Tolly TL, Feldmeier JE, Czarnecki D: Air embolism complicating percutaneous lung biopsy. AJR Am J Roentgenol 150:555, 1988.

Tumeh SS, Rosenthal DS, Kaplan WD et al: Lymphoma: Evaluation with Ga-67 SPECT. Radiology 164:111, 1987.

Urban BA, Fishman EK, Kuhlman JE et al: Detection of focal hepatic lesions with spiral CT: Comparison of 4- and 8-mm interscan spacing. AJR Am J Roentgenol 160:783, 1993.

Valk PE, Pounds TR, Hopkins DM et al: Staging non–small cell lung cancer by whole-body positron emission tomographic imaging. Ann Thorac Surg 60:1573–1582, 1995.

Vanel D, Henry-Amar M, Lumbroso J et al: Pulmonary evaluation of patients with osteosarcoma: Roles of standard radiography, tomography, CT, scintigraphy, and tomoscintigraphy. AJR Am J Roentgenol 143:519, 1984.

vanSonnenberg E, Casola G, Ho M et al: Difficult thoracic lesions: CT-guided biopsy experience in 150 cases. Radiology 167:457, 1988.

Vansteenkiste JF, Stroobants SG, De Leyn PR et al: Lymph node staging in non-small-cell lung cancer with FDG-PET scan: A prospective study on 690 lymph node stations from 68 patients. J Clin Oncol 16:2142–2149, 1998b.

Vansteenkiste JF, Stroobants SG, De Lelyn PR et al: Mediastinal lymph node staging with FDG-PET scan in patients with potentially operable non-small cell lung cancer. Chest 112:1480–1486, 1997a.

Viggiano RW, Swensen SJ, Rosenow III EC: Evaluation and management of solitary and multiple pulmonary nodules. Clin Chest Med 13:83–95, 1992.

Vining DJ, Liu K, Choplin RH, Haponik EF: Virtual bronchoscopy: Relationships of virtual reality endobronchial simulations to actual bronchoscopic findings. Chest 109:549, 1996.

Wahl RL, Hutchins CD, Buchsbaum DJ et al: ^{18}F-2-deoxy-2-fluoro-D-glucose uptake into human tumor xenografts: Feasibility studies for cancer imaging with positron emission tomography. Cancer 67:1544–1550, 1991.

Wahl RL, Quint LE, Greenough RL et al: Staging of mediastinal non-small cell lung cancer with FDG PET, CT, and fusion images: Preliminary prospective evaluation. Radiology 191:371–377, 1994.

Ward HB, Pliego M, Diefenthal HC, Humphrey EW: The impact of phantom CT scanning on surgery for the solitary pulmonary nodule. Surgery 106:734, 1989.

Webb WR: MR imaging in the evaluation and staging of lung cancer. Semin Ultrasound CT MRI 9:53–66, 1988.

Webb WR: Plain radiography and computed tomography in the staging of bronchogenic carcinoma: A practical approach. J Thorac Imaging 2:57, 1987.

Webb WR: Radiologic evaluation of the solitary pulmonary nodule. AJR Am J Roentgenol 154:701, 1990.

Webb WR, Gatsonis C, Zerhouni EA et al: CT and MR imaging in staging non-small cell bronchogenic carcinoma: Report of the Radiologic Diagnostic Oncology Group. Radiology 178:705–713, 1991.

Webb WR, Jensen BG, Sollitto R et al: Bronchogenic carcinoma: Staging with MR compared with staging with CT and surgery. Radiology 156:117, 1985.

Webb WR, Muller NL, Naidich DP: High-Resolution CT of the Lung. Philadelphia, Lippincott-Raven, 1996.

Weder W, Schmid RA, Bruchhaus H et al: Detection of extrathoracic metastases by positron emission tomography in lung cancer. Ann Thorac Surg 66:886–893, 1998.

Weisbrod GL: Percutaneous fine-needle aspiration biopsy of the mediastinum. Clin Chest Med 8:27, 1987.

Weisbrod GL: Transthoracic percutaneous lung biopsy. Radiol Clin North Am 28:647, 1990.

Wellner LJ, Putnam CE: Imaging of occult pulmonary metastases: State of the art. CA Cancer J Clin 36:48, 1986.

Wernecke K, Vassallo P, Peters PE, von Bassewitz DB: Mediastinal tumors: Biopsy under US guidance. Radiology 172:473, 1989.

Westcott JL: Percutaneous transthoracic needle biopsy. Radiology 169:593, 1988.

Westcott JL: Transthoracic needle biopsy of the hilum and mediastinum. J Thorac Imaging 2:41, 1987.

Westcott JL, Cole C: Plate atelectasis. Radiology 155:1, 1985.

Westcott JL, Rao N, Colley DP: Transthoracic needle biopsy of small pulmonary nodules. Radiology 202:97, 1997.

Whittlesey D: Prospective computed tomographic scanning in the staging of bronchogenic cancer. J Thorac Cardiovasc Surg 95:876, 1988.

Woodring JH: Determining the cause of pulmonary atelectasis: A comparison of plain radiography and CT. AJR Am J Roentgenol 150:757, 1988.

Woodring JH, Fried AM: Significance of wall thickness in solitary cavities of the lung: a follow-up study. AJR Am J Roentgenol 140:473, 1983.

Woodring JH, Fried AM, Chuang VP: Solitary cavities of the lung: Diagnostic implications of cavity wall thickness. AJR Am J Roentgenol 135:1269, 1980.

Wursten HU, Vock P: Mediastinal infiltration of lung carcinoma (T4N0-1): The positive predictive value of computed tomography. Thorac Cardiovasc Surg 35:355, 1987.

Yankelevitz DF, Davis SD, Chiarella DA, Henschke CI: Pitfalls in CT-guided transthoracic needle biopsy of pulmonary nodules. Radiographics 16:1073, 1996.

Yankelevitz DF, Gupta R, Zhao B, Henschke CI: Small pulmonary nodules: Evaluation with repeat CT: Preliminary experience. Radiology 212:561, 1996.

Zerhouni EA, Boukadoum M, Siddiky MA et al: A standard phantom for quantitative analysis of pulmonary nodules by computed tomography. Radiology 149:767, 1983.

Zerhouni EA, Spivey JF, Morgan RH et al: Factors influencing quantitative CT measurements of solitary pulmonary nodules. J Comput Assist Tomogr 6:1075, 1982.

Zerhouni EA, Stitik FP, Siegelman SS et al: CT of the pulmonary nodule: A cooperative study. Radiology 160:319, 1986.

Zhang M, Kono M: Solitary pulmonary nodules: Evaluation of blood flow patterns with dynamic CT. Radiology 205:471, 1997.

Zimmy M, Kaiser HJ, Cremerius U et al: F-18-FDG positron imaging in oncological patients: Gamma camera coincidence detection versus dedicated PET. Nuklearmedizin 38:108–114, 1999.

Ziskind MM, Weill H, Rayzant AR: The recognition and significance of acinus-filling processes of the lung. Am Rev Respir Dis 87:551, 1963.

Zwirewich CV, Muller NL, Lam SCT: Photodynamic laser therapy to alleviate complete bronchial obstruction: Comparison of CT and bronchoscopy to predict outcome. AJR Am J Roentgenol 151:897, 1988.

CHAPTER **22**

Congenital Anomalies of the Lung

Michael P. La Quaglia

Congenital anomalies of the lung are closely related abnormalities that arise during an early stage of embryonic foregut maturation. Therefore, they have been referred to as "lung-bud anomalies" or "congenital bronchopulmonary foregut abnormalities." They may be detected during the early neonatal period by acute symptoms of increased intrathoracic pressure or, rarely, with congestive heart failure (CHF). Less severe problems can be associated with milder forms of these developmental abnormalities, which result in partial obstruction of secondary bronchi. Congenital pulmonary anomalies may be asymptomatic until later in childhood or early adulthood when they can appear on radiographs as radio-opaque areas within normal pulmonary tissue or recurrent pulmonary infection. Eventually localized bronchiectasis may become evident. These congenital bronchopulmonary anomalies include congenital lobar emphysema, bronchogenic cysts, cystic adenomatoid malformation, or pulmonary sequestration. Because the development of the pulmonary circulation is an intimate component of lung development, pulmonary arteriovenous malformations (AVMs) are considered in this context.

HISTORICAL NOTE

Congenital lobar emphysema was described by Nelson in 1932, and the pathologic features, in particular the deficiency of bronchial cartilage, were defined by Overstreet in 1939. Gross and Lewis (1945) performed a successful lobectomy for this condition in 1945, and the term *congenital lobar emphysema* was first used in 1951 (Lewis et al, 1951).

The initial description of bronchogenic cysts of the mediastinum was by Meyer (1859) in 1859, and the first English language description was by Blackader and Evans (1911) in 1911. The first successful resection was performed in 1948 by Maier (1948). At the time of a report of a series by Eraklis and colleagues in 1969, consisting of 10 patients, only 25 previous cases had been described in the literature.

Congenital cystic adenomatoid malformation of the lung was first recognized as a distinct entity by Ch'in and Tang in 1949.

Huber, in 1777, described an aberrant artery arising from the aorta and supplying a normal right lower lobe. In separate studies in 1861, Rokitansky and Rektorzik described cases of what is now called extralobar pulmonary sequestration. Pryce, in 1946, originated the term pulmonary sequestration and defined the anatomy.

The first lucid description of an abnormal connection between an artery and vein is attributed to Hunter (1757), who described a traumatic AVM in 1757 (Young, 1988). Hunter made the first clinical correlation between a palpable thrill and this lesion. Osler (1901) described a syndrome of hereditary telangiectasias of the skin and mucous membranes in 1901. He also noted that it had first been reported by Rendu in 1896. A report by Parkes Weber (1907) followed. The disease, which is now called Rendu-Osler-Weber syndrome, or hereditary hemorrhagic telangiectasia, is inherited as a mendelian dominant gene and is characterized by numerous spider angiomas of the skin and mucous membranes along with the development of AVMs of the liver and lungs. Arteriographic embolization of AVMs was first applied to spinal cord lesions and subsequently adapted for use in visceral and pulmonary locations (Djindjian et al, 1973).

HISTORICAL READINGS

Blackader AD, Evans DJ: A case of mediastinal cyst producing compression of the trachea, ending fatally in an infant of nine months. Arch Pediatr 28:194, 1911.

Ch'in KY, Tang MY: Congenital adenomatoid malformation of one lobe of a lung with general anasarca. Arch Pathol 48:221, 1949.

Djindjian R, Cophignon J, Theron J et al: Embolization by superselective arteriography from the femoral route in neuroradiology. Review of 60 cases: I. Technique, indications, complications. Neuroradiology 6:20, 1973.

Erakis AJ, Griscom NT, McGovern JB: Bronchogenic cysts of the mediastinum in infancy. N Engl J Med 281:1150, 1969.

Gross RE, Lewis JE: Defect of the anterior mediastinum. Surg Gynecol Obstet 80:549, 1945.

Huber JJ: Observationes aliquot de arteria singulari pulmoni concessa. Acta Helvet 8:85, 1777.

Hunter W: The history of an aneurysm of the aorta with some remarks on aneurysms in general. Obs Soc Phys (Lond) 1:323, 1757.

Lewis JE Jr: Pulmonary and bronchial malformations. In Holder T, Ashcraft KE (eds): Pediatric Surgery. Philadelphia, WB Saunders, 1980.

Maier HC: Bronchogenic cysts of the mediastinum. Ann Surg 127:476, 1948.

Meyer H: åber angeborene blasige Missbildung der Lungen nebst einigen Bemerkungen uber Cyanose aus Lungenleiden. Arch Pathol Anat 16:78, 1859.

Nelson RL: Congenital cystic disease of the lung. J Pediatr 1:233, 1932.

Osler W: On a family form of recurring epistaxis associated with multiple telangiectases of skin and mucous membrane. Bull Johns Hopkins Hosp 12:333, 1901.

Overstreet RM: Emphysema of a portion of the lung in the early months of life. Am J Dis Child 57:861, 1939.

Parkes Weber F: Multiple hereditary developmental angiomata of the skin and mucous membranes associated with recurring hemorrhages. Lancet 2:160, 1907.

Pryce DM: Lower accessory pulmonary artery with intralobar sequestration of lung: A report of seven cases. J Pathol Bacteriol 48:457, 1946.

Rektorzik E: Ueber accessorischen Lungenlappen. Woch Z Aerzte 17:4, 1861.

Rendu M: Epistaxis répétées chez un sujet porteur de petite angiomes cutanes et muqueux. Bull Soc Med Hôp (Paris) 13:731, 1896.

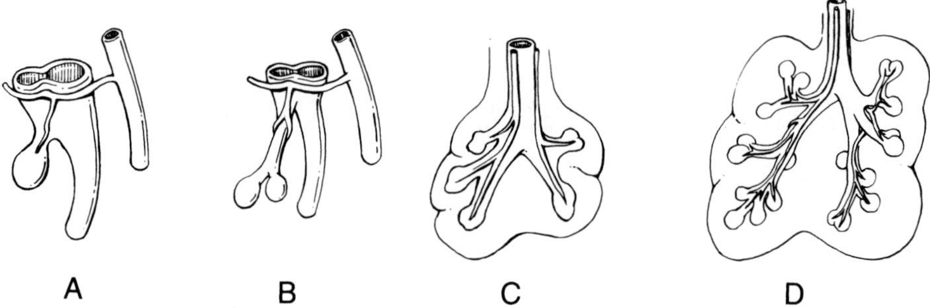

FIGURE 22–1 ■ The progression of events in normal lung development. *A*, Outpouching from the pharyngeal part of the primitive foregut has occurred. Branches from the aorta are also beginning their ingrowth. *B*, The primitive anlagen of the right and left lungs have formed. *C* and *D*, The subsequent subdivision of the lung forms the alveoli with their attendant vascular supply.

Robertson R, James ES: Congenital lobar emphysema. Pediatrics 8:795, 1951.

Rokitansky C: Lehrbuch der pathologischen Anatomie, 3rd ed. Vienna, 1861.

Young AK: Arteriovenous malformations. In Mulliken JS, Young AE (eds): Vascular Birthmarks (Hemangiomas and Malformations). Philadelphia, WB Saunders, 1988.

BASIC SCIENCE

Pulmonary Embryology

The steps in the development of the respiratory system from the primitive foregut are depicted in Figure 22–1. The respiratory tract is represented by a groove in the ventral wall of the foregut at the fourth week of gestation (Gray and Skandalakis, 1972; Langman, 1969; Sorokin, 1965; Willis, 1962). The groove itself will become a portion of the pharynx and the retrotracheal portion of the esophagus. However, the pulmonary groove soon forms a diverticulum with an elongated slit-like opening into the pharyngoesophageal part of the foregut (see Fig. 22–1*A*). The length of the slit is gradually reduced by posteroanterior ingrowth and fusion of its lateral lips, thus forming a partition that separates the trachea from the upper esophagus. Finally, only the upper end remains patent as the definitive laryngeal orifice. This mechanism forms a basis for understanding the various forms of esophageal atresia and tracheoesophageal fistulas.

During the second month of gestation, the pulmonary diverticulum grows rapidly downward and forms the larynx, trachea, bronchi, and lungs. The pharyngeal diverticulum, or bud, elongates, and its tip swells, finally dividing to form the precursors of the primary bronchus of each lung (see Fig. 22–l*B*). These lung buds elongate, swell, and subdivide, as do their descendants, until a large, interbranching network of tubules is formed. This constitutes the early bronchial tree (see Figs. 22–l*C* and *D*).

Branching is not strictly dichotomous; the left primary bronchus forms a more obtuse angle with the trachea compared with the right. As the epithelium pushes out from the pharyngeal floor, it is accompanied by mesenchyme that originated beneath the laryngotracheal groove (Ham and Baldwin, 1941). This mesenchyme gradually condenses around the tracheobronchial tree and differentiates into cartilage, adventitial connective tissue, blood vessels, and lymphatic channels. The lung of a young fetus resembles an exocrine gland with numerous ducts ending in sac-shaped expansions that lie embedded in connective tissue. They lack a rich blood supply at this point but, in the second phase of lung development, the major blood vessels enlarge and the number of capillaries increases until the lung becomes the most highly vascularized organ in the body.

Alveolar formation is related to growth of the vasculature and is first observed in human fetuses at 18 weeks' gestation when angiogenesis is firmly under way in the mesenchyme (Loosli and Potter, 1951). Capillaries grow into the cuboidal endodermal lining (although unproved, it is generally accepted that the lining of the lung arises from endoderm), and the loops push into the lumen of the airway. The interface of alveolar and endothelial cells is depicted in Figure 22–2. The capillaries become more abundant as gestation proceeds, they are separated from the endothelium by the basement membrane, and the lining epithelium is stretched over. The bodies of the cells are tucked into spaces between the capillary loops, becoming type I cells, while some of the fetal cuboidal epithelium differentiates into cytosome containing cubical or polygonal cells. These become the alveolar, or type II, cells.

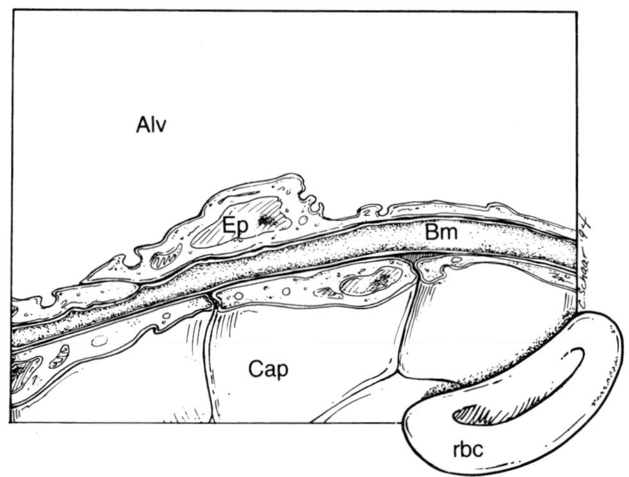

FIGURE 22–2 ■ Alveolar and endothelial cells lie near each other in the developing lung.

The modification of the epithelium of the terminal air sacs into type I or II cells occurs during the 24th to 28th weeks of gestation. Because type II cells produce surfactant and do not develop before the 24th to 28th week, fetuses cannot survive the extrauterine environment if they are born at an earlier gestational age. Terminal budding continues to produce new alveolar regions. At birth, five or six generations of respiratory bronchioles are present. In humans, the number of alveoli continues to increase up to the eighth year of life, and adults usually have two generations of respiratory bronchioles (Engel, 1953). The dimensions of the pulmonary zones and segments may expand until the age of 40 years. Premature birth has no effect on subsequent lung development.

The blood vessels of the lung are derived from two sources: the plexiform network of vessels developing in the pulmonary mesenchyme and the heart. Like bronchi, the vessels may vary in their course based on the selection of channels from the pre-existing mesenchymal network.

This background on pulmonary embryology may help the reader visualize the mechanisms by which the following congenital anomalies arise.

Incidence of Various Malformations

Vogt-Moykopf and colleagues (1992) did a survey of 59 hospitals that were performing thoracic surgery, 14 of which supplied data. Of the 1347 anomalies diagnosed, 1343 were treated surgically, and 5 patients died within the first 30 postoperative days (0.3%). In a retrospective study of 6350 thoracotomies over a 10-year period (1978 to 1988), 198 pulmonary anomalies were identified (Vogt-Moykopf et al, 1993). Table 22–1 illustrates the relative prevalence of the anomalies described.

Congenital Lobar Emphysema

BASIC SCIENCE

Etiology

Congenital lobar emphysema is defined as a postnatal overdistention of one or more lobes of a histologically normal lung (Berlinger et al, 1987; Haller et al, 1979; Lacquet and Lacquet, 1977; Michelson, 1977; Monin et al, 1979). Usually the upper and middle lobes are affected. In most patients, the process is confined to a single lobe. The cause of lobar emphysema may vary, depending on the clinical situation, but the common mechanism of action must involve a ball-valve obstruction of a lobar or segmental bronchus. This allows distal air trapping with resultant hyperinflation, causing additional bronchial obstruction. An estimated 50% of cases of congenital lobar emphysema are associated with decreased bronchial cartilage. Bronchoscopic observation in one 3-year-old patient showed evidence of dynamic airway collapse on expiration, suggesting that lung hyperinflation was secondary to bronchomalacia (Doull et al, 1996). In the acquired form of lobar emphysema, seen in infants with bronchopulmonary dysplasia, the obstruction may be caused by endobronchial granulation tissue. Another cause of bronchial obstruction in both the congenital and acquired form is absence or weakening of the supporting tracheal or bronchial cartilages. This allows the bronchus to collapse with expiration and results in progressive air trapping. In congenital lobar emphysema, cartilaginous malformation can result from absent or inadequate migration of mesenchyme into the endodermal pharyngeal pouch during the 18th week of gestation or improper differentiation of mesenchyme into cartilaginous and fibrous supporting structures.

Extrinsic bronchial obstruction may also play a role in some cases of congenital lobar emphysema. There are many reports of associated cardiac anomalies in infants with this lung anomaly (Borg et al, 1975; Gordon and Dempsey, 1990; Keller, 1983; Roguin et al, 1980). In one study, seven infants who were autopsied were shown to have developed lobar emphysema because of a check valve mechanism created by compression of the bronchi by a distended pulmonary artery (Isogima et al, 1978). All had clinical evidence of a severe left-to-right shunt prior to death. In the same report, eight additional infants, also with left-to-right shunts and concurrent severe lobar emphysema, showed resolution of the emphysema after correction of the cardiac lesion. The authors concluded that resection of the emphysematous lobe should be avoided in favor of repair of the congenital heart defect in this subset of patients. In another report, three patients with patent ductus arteriosus and respiratory failure were described (Toran et al, 1989). Dilatation of the pulmonary arteries led to bronchial compression, which resulted in lobar emphysema. In this report, the

TABLE 22–1 ■ **Major Developmental Anomalies of the Lung**

Anomaly	*Prevalence*	*Associated Anomalies*
Congenital lobar emphysema	Not uncommon	Bronchogenic cyst, PDH, tetralogy of Fallot, ventricular septal defect
Bronchogenic cyst	Uncommon	Abnormalities of the pulmonary artery
Cystic adenomatoid malformation	Rare	No significant association
Pulmonary sequestration	Not uncommon	No significant association
Pulmonary arteriovenous malformation	Rare	Rendu-Osler-Weber syndrome*
Congenital pulmonary hypoplasia or aplasia	Complete is extremely rare; unilateral is not uncommon	Microphthalmia, Potter's syndrome

*Fifteen percent of patients with Rendu-Osler-Weber syndrome have pulmonary arteriovenous malformations.

authors considered those with left-sided lobar emphysema to be a special group for whom extrinsic compression was the principal pathophysiologic factor. In addition to patent ductus arteriosus, double aortic arch, tetralogy of Fallot, ventricular septal defect, and congenital absence of the pulmonic valve have also been associated with lobar emphysema. Hasse and colleagues (1975) reported on six patients with congenital lobar emphysema, three of whom had associated patent ductus arteriosus, with one of these also manifesting a double aortic arch. Two of the three with congenital cardiovascular anomalies responded to division of the obstructing vascular anomaly without the need for a lobectomy. It is estimated that congenital heart defects may be present in 20% of patients with lobar emphysema. Correction of the cardiac anomaly without a pulmonary lobectomy is recommended.

Rarely, this condition may arise because of a polyalveolar lobe (Tapper et al, 1980). This entity is defined as a threefold to fivefold increase in alveolar number, as determined by microscopic point counting of random lung sections. The airways and arteries are normal for age in number, size, and structure. Air may enter alveoli by collateral channels but have no way to get out, resulting in lobar emphysema. The therapy is similar to that for other forms of the disease. Congenital lobar emphysema has also been associated with pectus excavatum, right-sided aortic arch, bilateral diaphragmatic eventration, and mediastinal bronchogenic cyst (Engel et al, 1984; Fukumoto et al, 1991; Gille et al, 1979). Successful therapy of bilateral lobar emphysema has also been described (Ekkelkamp and Vos, 1987). There are a number of reports in the literature of the development of lobar emphysema in dogs and cats that is usually associated with malformations of the bronchial cartilages (Hoover et al, 1992; La Rue et al, 1990; Orima et al, 1992; Voorhout et al, 1986).

DIAGNOSIS

Clinical Features

Congenital lobar emphysema most commonly affects newborns and small infants who have varying degrees of respiratory distress. One half of the cases are seen in the first 4 weeks of life, and most are diagnosed before the sixth month of life. Less frequently seen are patients with this disorder who are older than 1 year at presentation and rare cases of presentation in adulthood. Respiratory distress may be severe, with an infant in the first hours or days manifesting dyspnea, tachypnea, cyanosis, wheezing, coughing, thoracic or epigastric retractions, and nasal flare. The respiratory distress may be severe enough to require endotracheal intubation and urgent surgical intervention within the first 6 hours after birth (Canty, 1977; Keith, 1977; Senyuz et al, 1989; Warner et al, 1982). Later symptoms can include failure to thrive, faintness, psychomotor retardation, malformation of the thorax, and recurrent pulmonary infection (Al-Salem et al, 1990).

On physical examination, the chest wall on the involved side is more prominent but has decreased respiratory excursion. Breath sounds are paradoxically decreased over the affected lobe; the apical pulse is shifted away from the side of involvement. The diaphragm may also be depressed on the ipsilateral side. Congenital lobar emphysema can be mimicked by bronchogenic cysts (Okur et al, 1996; Williams et al, 1996).

Imaging and Other Diagnostic Studies

The plain chest radiograph is the best initial diagnostic tool. Typical findings include overinflation of a pulmonary lobe with mediastinal shift to the contralateral side (Fig. 22–3). The lobes most commonly affected are the left upper lobe (43%), right upper lobe (20%), and the right middle lobe (32%) (Man et al, 1983). Bilateral involvement may occur in 20% of cases; solitary disease of a lower lobe is rare. Because of air trapping, the mediastinal shift can increase on expiration. In addition, the affected lobes may herniate across the mediastinum. The findings on chest radiography may be confused with those of atelectasis with compensatory emphysema, congenital cyst, postpneumonic pneumatocele, pneumothorax, infectious obstructive emphysema, pulmonary interstitial emphysema, unilateral hyperlucent lung (Swyer-James syndrome, Macleod's syndrome), congenital cystic adenomatoid malformation, pneumomediastinum, and diaphragmatic hernia.

Computed tomography (CT) is a useful adjunct in the diagnosis of congenital lobar emphysema (Markowitz et al, 1989; Pardes et al, 1983). Mediastinal masses, especially bronchogenic cysts, bronchial anatomy down to the segmental level, and, occasionally, pulmonary artery slings can all be detected by CT. If the patient's condition allows it, CT of the chest should be performed soon

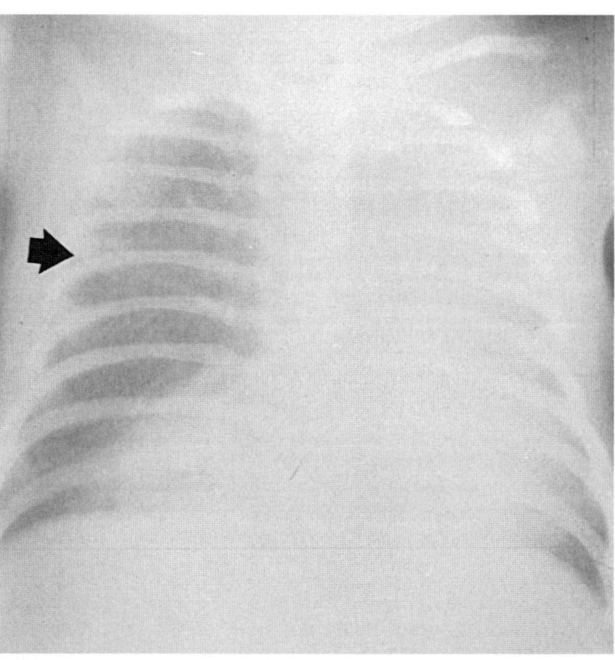

FIGURE 22–3 ■ A plain chest radiograph of a newborn with congenital lobar emphysema. Hyperexpansion and mediastinal shift with contralateral atelectasis are noted.

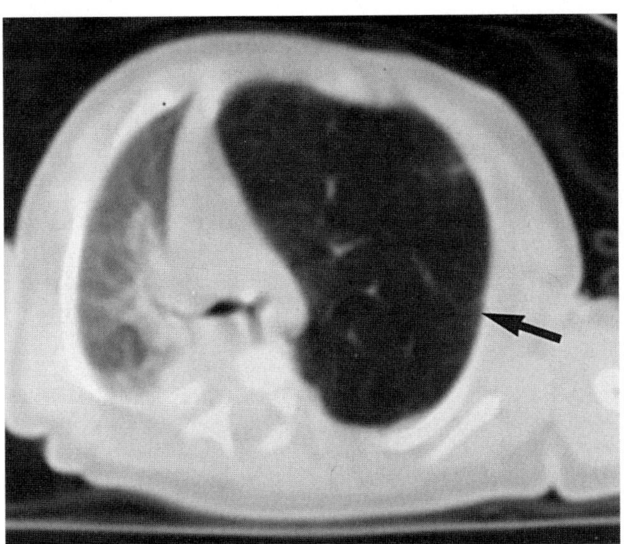

FIGURE 22–4 ■ A computed tomography scan of an infant with congenital lobar emphysema. This clearly demonstrates the hyperexpansion and mediastinal shift associated with this lesion.

after plain chest radiographs have raised a suspicion of congenital lobar emphysema (Fig. 22–4).

Bronchography is contraindicated. Because the bronchial tree is already severely compromised, intrabronchial administration of contrast agents may severely worsen the patient's clinical status.

Ventilation scintigraphy with a submicronic (0.2 to 0.8 μm in diameter) radioaerosol can show unventilated pulmonary segments and provide confirmatory data in patients suspected of having congenital lobar emphysema on chest radiographs (Loewy et al, 1987). In this technique, the child breathes radioactive (^{99m}Tc-sulfur colloid) aerosol through an anesthesia bag for 2 minutes followed by imaging. Children with murmurs, cyanosis, or other clinical findings that suggest congenital heart disease may require cardiac catheterization in a facility equipped to perform this and to undertake the repair of any cardiac anomalies.

Diagnostic bronchoscopy should be performed when there is a question of bronchial compression by vascular structures. Bronchoscopy can determine the sites of compression and might aid in planning future therapy. Fiberoptic bronchoscopy performed through a short endotracheal tube is suitable for this diagnostic procedure. Bronchoscopy has also shown evidence of tracheal stenosis in some of these patients (Doull et al, 1996).

MANAGEMENT

Therapy

The therapy for isolated congenital lobar emphysema is the prompt resection of the involved lobe (Hailer et al, 1979; Hill et al, 1988; Michelson, 1977; Vogt-Moykopf et al, 1992). In anesthesia management, the underlying air-trapping obstruction must be considered, and high ventilatory pressure should be avoided (Cote, 1978; Goto et al, 1987). In patients with congenital heart disease that causes a right-to-left shunt, a full preoperative cardiac evaluation is required. Repair of the heart defect might result in the relief of the lobar emphysema and should be given precedence, although some of these patients might also eventually require a lobectomy (Isojima et al, 1978). Similar conclusions hold for patients with congenital vascular anomalies that cause lobar emphysema by vascular compression of the bronchus. Division of the compressing ductus arteriosus or vascular ring may obviate the need for lobectomy and should be done first. If irreversible, bronchomalacia was induced by the vascular compression, lobectomy may ultimately be required.

The reported mortality rate associated with the surgical correction of congenital lobar emphysema is 10% to 28% and depends on the frequency of associated anomalies (Knoop et al, 1984; Urban et al, 1975). Complete clinical recovery should be expected for children without congenital heart defects. Long-term follow-up demonstrates that the development and physical performance in these patients is roughly equivalent to those of normal controls. The pulmonary volumes are about 90% of predicted, suggesting compensatory growth of the remaining lung tissue (Frenckner and Freychuss, 1982).

There is a subset of patients with congenital lobar emphysema but without serious or life-threatening symptoms who may not require surgical intervention. In a retrospective study, Kennedy and colleagues (1991) performed serial chest radiographs (N = 12) and follow-up ventilation/perfusion (V/Q) scans (N = 6) on 12 children who were treated without surgery. In all 12 patients, improvement in symptoms was accompanied by improved lung appearance on plain chest radiographs. In the six that underwent V/Q scans, an increase in ventilation was more marked than was the improvement in perfusion. The indications for surgical intervention depend on the acuity of presenting symptoms. Usually, urgent thoracotomy with lobectomy must be performed, but, as noted above, some patients may require only observation if symptoms are less acute.

Occasionally, bronchoscopic stenting of a bronchomalacic lobar bronchus will reduce air trapping and allow for a more controlled resection (Phillipos et al, 1998). There are reports of a series of patients whose congenital lobar emphysema was treated using stapled lung volume reduction surgery.

Bronchogenic Cysts

BASIC SCIENCE

Pathophysiology

Bronchogenic cysts originate before the bronchi are formed and may be either mediastinal or intrapulmonary. In children, most bronchogenic cysts are located in the mediastinum (65%), with the rest located intraparenchymally (27%) and in the inferior pulmonary ligament (8%) (DiLorenzo et al, 1989). The mediastinal lesions can be close to the carina, mainstem bronchi, trachea, esophagus, or pericardium. Eraklis and colleagues (1969) noted that obstructing carinal lesions that produced severe symptoms were difficult to locate until the mediastinal

TABLE 22–2 ■ **Bronchogenic Cysts**

Author (Year)	*No. of Patients*	*Ages*	*Symptoms*	*Size (cm)*	*Therapy*	*Follow-Up*
Opsahl and Berman (1962)	1	20 days	Dyspnea, cough	3	Resection	Alive and well
Eraklis et al (1969)	10	Birth, 2 days, 6 mo, 6 mo, 23 mo, 1.5 yr	Dyspnea and respiratory distress in younger patients	2, 2, 3, 3.5, 4, 4	Resection in eight	Three dead, two untreated, seven alive and well
Pokorny (1974)	11	Three before 5 mo, eight after 2 yr	Stridor, three with mild respiratory symptoms, five incidental	—	—	—
Canty et al (1975)	2	Birth, 10 days	Airway obstruction	—	Unroofing	Two alive and well
Haller et al (1975)	2	1 day, 6 weeks	Tachypnea, cyanosis	4, —	Resection	Two alive and well
Bower and Kiesewetter (1977)	6	Three < 1 yr, 3 yr, 6 yr, 10 yr	The three patients < 1 yr had respiratory symptoms	—	Resection	Six alive and well
Snyder (1985)	23	Range from 1 week to 14 yr	Younger patients present with pneumonia, stridor, cough	—	Resection	—
St. Georges et al (1991)	86	Range from 16 to 19 yr	Chest pain, cough, dyspnea, fever	—	Resection	All alive and well

pleura had been divided and retracted anteriorly. Bronchogenic cysts constitute 10% to 15% of all mediastinal masses and occur in 1 of 40,000 to 1 of 68,000 admissions.

Etiology

The precise embryologic steps leading to the development of a bronchogenic cyst are unknown. It is clear from the previous discussion of normal lung development that the respiratory system develops by outpouching of the primitive foregut. Clinical differentiation between mediastinal bronchogenic cysts and esophageal duplication cysts can be very difficult because of this development from the primitive foregut (Nobuhara et al, 1997). Most hypotheses regarding the development of bronchogenic cysts (and also cystic duplications of the esophagus) invoke a process of abortive pouching out and pinching off of a primitive lung bud from the foregut (Balquet, 1984; Letanche et al, 1984). Because of its foregut origin, a bronchogenic cyst may be lined by ciliated columnar (respiratory) or squamous epithelium. Both linings have mucous bronchial glands, which cause the cyst to fill under pressure. This causes pressure on surrounding structures, particularly the membranous trachea or bronchi, and may lead to severe respiratory obstruction. Bronchogenic cysts may also contain focal intramural areas of hyaline cartilage or smooth muscle (Coselli et al, 1987). They are most often found near the carina in the middle part of the mediastinum. The process of abnormal budding leads to centrally located cysts if they occur early in gestation; later occurrences may give rise to peripheral intraparenchymal lesions that may retain a bronchial communication to the airway.

DIAGNOSIS

Clinical Features

Bronchogenic cysts of the mediastinum can occur from infancy to late adulthood. Different presenting symptoms are observed in each group (Buckner et al, 1989; Cartmill and Hughes, 1989; DiLorenzo et al, 1989; Feketi et al, 1988; Koskas et al, 1992). Most newborns present with life-threatening respiratory distress and require urgent intervention (Bower and Kiesewetter, 1977; Haller et al, 1979). Older children and adults have milder symptoms or are diagnosed because of the incidental finding of a mediastinal mass or evidence of bronchial obstruction on imaging studies. This is illustrated in Table 22–2, in which the age range and presenting symptoms are cross-tabulated. In the report by St. Georges and colleagues (1991), which deals with patients older than 16 years of age at diagnosis, cysts are categorized as mediastinal or pulmonary. There were 66 patients in the mediastinal group, of whom 44 (66%) were symptomatic. The most common presenting complaints were chest pain, cough dyspnea, fever, purulent sputum, anorexia, and dysphagia. Also, patients with mediastinal lesions were more likely to have severe symptoms. Of the 22 patients with intrapulmonary cysts, 18 were symptomatic. These most commonly presented with cough, fever, dyspnea, and purulent sputum. In both sets, hemoptysis was uncommon.

Bronchogenic cysts that cause airway obstruction have also been reported in the cervical area (Canty and Hendren, 1975; Cohen et al, 1985; Park and Buford, 1955). These usually occur in infants and are associated with acute respiratory symptoms. Transdiaphragmatic bronchogenic cysts and a cyst presenting as a supraclavicular mass have also been reported (Amendola et al, 1982; Dubois et al, 1981). There is a report of a fatal air embolus occurring in an adult with a giant intrapulmonary bronchogenic cyst (Zaugg et al, 1998).

Cysts in children younger than 1 year of age, especially newborns, usually cause severe airway obstruction with dyspnea, tachypnea, retractions, flaring, and air trapping with distal emphysema. In this age group, the lesion is almost always mediastinal. Bronchogenic cysts diagnosed later in childhood or in adulthood usually do not cause severe respiratory distress. Chest pain, cough, fever, and purulent sputum are more frequently observed. Up to 37% of older patients may also be asymptomatic (Cioffi et al, 1998).

Imaging and Other Diagnostic Studies

Plain chest radiographs are the standard initial study for myriad intrathoracic conditions. DiLorenzo and colleagues (1989), in describing 26 children with bronchogenic cysts, reported that plain chest radiographs were accurately diagnostic in 20 (77%). Suen and colleagues (1993), reporting on 42 patients ranging in age from 8 to 62 years (mean age, 34.8 years), noted that the diagnostic accuracy of plain chest radiographs was 88%. Bronchogenic cysts most commonly appeared as homogeneous water density shadows. Two of their patients had air-fluid levels, and both of these lesions were intrapulmonary. In the five patients not diagnosed by plain chest radiographs, all lesions were in a subcarinal position. Plain chest radiographs alone can accurately diagnose 80% to 90% of cases, and they are useful in initial screening (Figs. 22–5 and 22–6).

Experience with CT supports this imaging modality as the best study for diagnosing bronchogenic cysts. CT scans correctly identified the lesions in 100% of patients from the two studies discussed previously. The findings included a round, well-circumscribed, unilocular, or multilocular mass with a density ranging from that of water (0 to 20 Hounsfield units [H]) to as high as 91 H. Occasionally, an intrapulmonary bronchogenic cyst is air filled, implying bronchial communication (Figs. 22–7 and 22–8).

There is less experience with magnetic resonance imaging (MRI). Suen and colleagues (1993) reported that six of their patients underwent MRI, with definite findings noted in five. In one patient, CT was required to differentiate the cystic contents from fat. Most bronchogenic cysts (five of six) imaged using this modality showed high signal intensity on both T_1- and T_2-weighted images.

Ultrasound has rarely been performed for this lesion. In two cases reported by Suen and colleagues (1993), an anechoic lesion was identified. There are significant technical problems with routine thoracic ultrasound. Barium swallow was diagnostic in only two of six lesions in one report.

Bronchoscopy performed as part of the diagnostic workup for a bronchogenic cyst usually reveals extrinsic bronchial compression. Occasionally, there is evidence

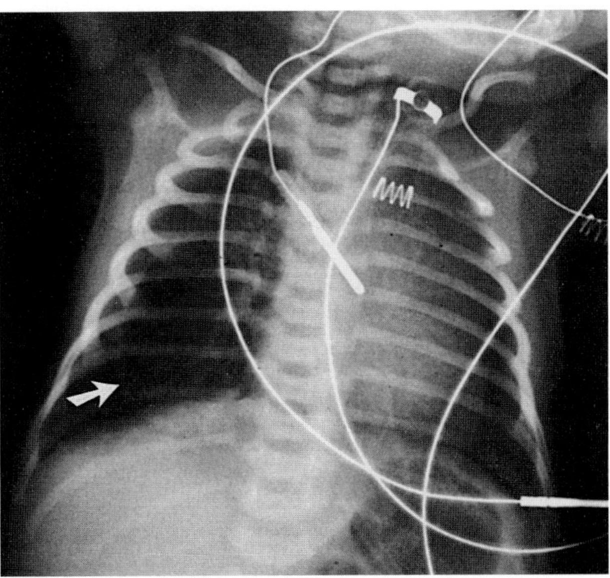

FIGURE 22–6 ■ A plain chest radiograph demonstrating an intralobar bronchogenic cyst with bronchial communication.

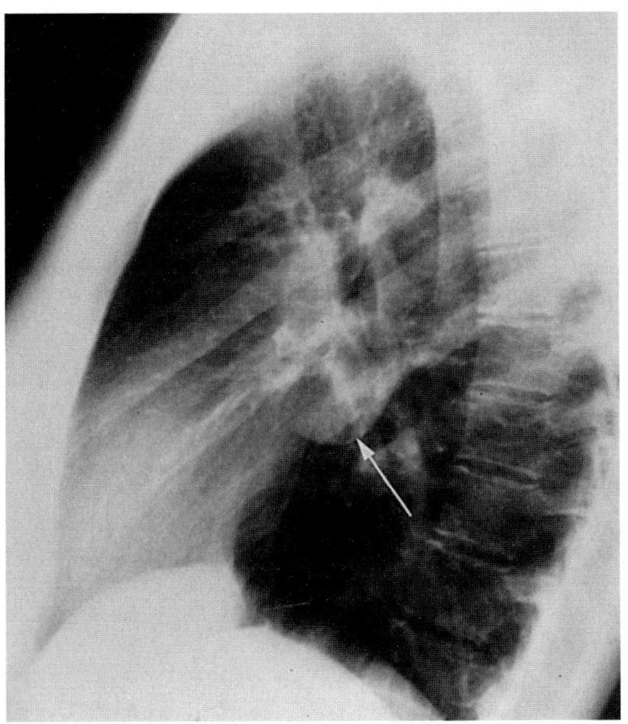

FIGURE 22–5 ■ A lateral chest radiograph demonstrating a mediastinal bronchogenic cyst.

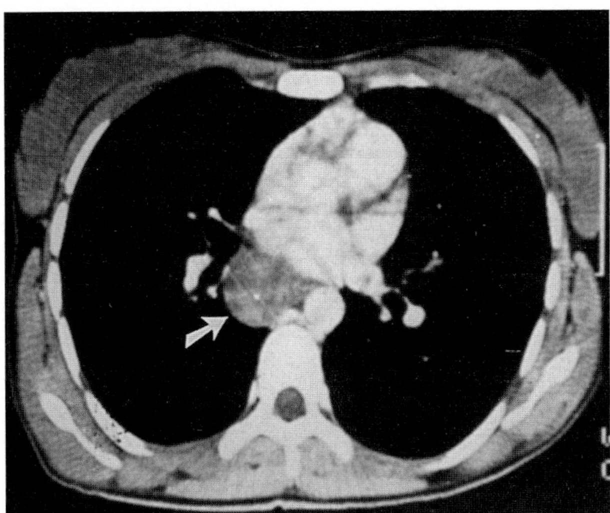

FIGURE 22–7 ■ Computed tomography scan of the mediastinal bronchogenic cyst seen in Figure 22–5.

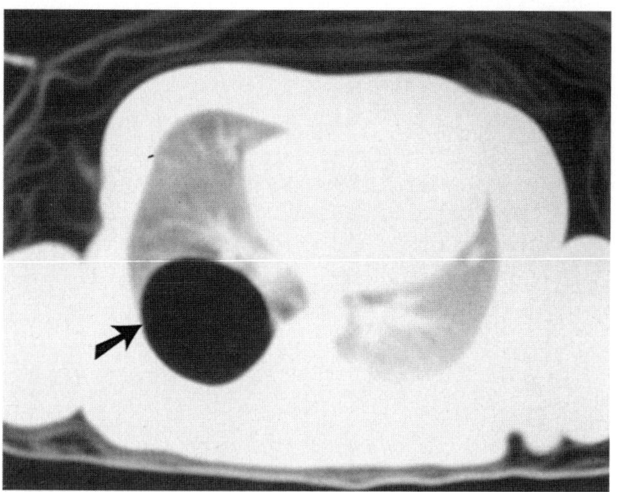

FIGURE 22–8 ■ Computed tomography scan of the intralobar bronchogenic cyst seen in Figure 22–6.

of a fistulous communication between the cyst and the bronchial tree. This may appear as either a fistulous tract or the drainage of mucopurulent material into the bronchus. Reported bronchoscopic abnormalities varied from 1 of 4 (25%) to 9 of 26 (35%) patients in two reported series (DiLorenzo et al, 1989; Suen et al, 1993).

In summary, patients with clinical findings suggesting bronchogenic cyst require a screening plain chest radiograph followed by axial CT of the chest. These studies should confirm the lesion and identify its anatomic location in almost 100% of patients. Bronchoscopy is not routinely indicated but will show evidence of external compression, cysts, or bronchial fistulas in approximately one third of patients.

MANAGEMENT

Therapy

Bronchogenic cysts are usually treated by thoracotomy and excision of the cyst (Balquet, 1984; Eraklis et al, 1969; Opsahl and Berman, 1962; Suen et al, 1993). The anatomic location can be precisely determined using the plain chest radiograph and imaging studies. The cyst is usually approached by a posterolateral thoracotomy. Subcarinal lesions are normally approached from the right side. Exposure is facilitated by the placement of a double-lumen endotracheal tube and ipsilateral collapse of the lung. In younger patients, a bronchial blocker can be used. The objective of the surgery is complete cyst removal, if feasible. This may be impossible or entail inordinate danger to the patient if the cyst has adhered to the membranous portion of the trachea or mainstem bronchi or if the cyst is inflamed. In these cases, opening the cyst and removing the mucous lining layer may be performed. Because removal of the inner layer prevents cyst distention with mucus secretions, the resultant airway compression is relieved. It is preferable to remove the cyst entirely if possible because rare cases of malignant degeneration have been reported.

Adults with bronchogenic cysts may be asymptomatic or have minimal complaints. Ginsberg and Kirby (1989) suggested that small, asymptomatic bronchogenic cysts in adult patients can be followed with serial chest radiographs, although larger or enlarging cysts should be removed. Several authors have also suggested that cyst aspiration, cyst wall biopsy, and possible removal of the cyst or intralesional instillation of a sclerosant (e.g., tetracycline) could be accomplished mediastinoscopically (Carlens, 1959; Ginsberg et al, 1972; Pursel et al, 1966). Finally, Lewis and colleagues (1992) reported on two cases of mediastinal bronchogenic cysts in adults (31 and 40 years old) who underwent thoracoscopic drainage and wall resection. A laser was used to ablate one of the cysts completely. The thoracoscopic approach has become more common recently (Cioffi et al, 1998; Cuypers et al, 1996; Koizumi et al, 1998; Yim et al, 1996). Complete resection is preferable to cyst aspiration because it allows removal or ablation of the entire lesion, preventing the possibility of malignant degeneration. Intrapulmonary cysts can usually be extirpated by lesser resections—for example, segmentectomy or wedge excision.

Cystic Adenomatoid Malformation

BASIC SCIENCE

Pathophysiology

This condition is characterized by overgrowth of bronchioles. Defining histologic criteria include increased terminal respiratory structures appearing as cysts lined by cuboidal or pseudostratified columnar epithelium, an increase of elastic tissue within cyst walls along with polypoid mucosa, an absence of cartilage in the cyst wall, lining mucous cells, and no inflammatory process (Bale, 1979; Olson and Mendelsohn, 1978). Cystic adenomatoid malformation may occur as three distinct histologic subtypes. Type I is the most common (55%) and consists of large cystic spaces within a single pulmonary lobe. Type II (40% of cases) is composed of numerous small cysts measuring 1 to 10 mm in diameter. Type III is a solid mass without cysts consisting of adenomatoid hyperplasia or bronchial structures (Miller et al, 1980; Rosado-de-Christenson and Stocker, 1991; Stocker et al, 1977). In a large institutional series (34 cases) reported by Mentzer and colleagues (1992), the malformation was unilateral in all cases and involved the left and right lungs with equal frequency. The majority (67%) were classified as Stocker type I cystic adenomatoid malformations; 24% were type II and 9% were type III. Most patients were treated by lobectomy or segmental-wedge resection, and only one patient in this series required pneumonectomy. Both rhabdomyosarcoma and bronchoalveolar carcinoma have been reported in previously undiagnosed congenital cystic adenomatoid malformations of the lung (d'Agostino et al, 1997; Kaslovsky et al, 1997).

Etiology

In a study using postmortem bronchography or serial microscopic section of lungs in four patients with congenital cystic adenomatoid malformation, Moerman and colleagues (1992) showed segmental bronchial absence or atresia to be present in each. These observations provide evidence that the primary defect in this condition is bronchial atresia. The morphologic subtype of congenital cystic adenomatoid malformation is thought to be dependent on the type of secondary dysplastic lung growth beyond the atretic segment. The exact cause of the bronchial atresia may be heterogeneous. Possible mechanisms include primary disruption in cell growth or interruption of the fetal bronchial circulation. The simultaneous occurrence of congenital cystic adenomatoid malformation with pulmonary sequestration and polyalveolar lobe has been reported (Wagenvoort et al, 1991; Yogasakaran and Sudhaman, 1991; Zangwill and Stocker, 1993). There is also a report of twins in which one fetus had a cystic adenomatoid malformation and the other was normal (Rebarber and Mohan, 1992).

Recently, Boglino and colleagues (1992) reported that cystic adenomatoid malformations from six patients showed significant reactivity with antibodies to the neuropeptide neurotensin. This neuropeptide and others are thought to play a role in immune reactivity, especially the cytolytic activity of activated macrophages. Normal lung from the same patients was much less reactive. These data suggest that in utero infection is a possible cause of cystic adenomatoid malformation. In another pathophysiologic review, it was concluded that congenital cystic adenomatoid malformation was characterized by increased cell proliferation and decreased apoptosis (Cass et al, 1998).

DIAGNOSIS

Fetal Diagnosis

During the last decade, there has been significant progress in fetal diagnosis based on improvements in fetal ultrasound (Boulot et al, 1991; Deacon et al, 1990; Heydanus et al, 1993; Morris et al, 1991; Sherer et al, 1992; Taguchi et al, 1993). Congenital cystic adenomatoid malformation is one such pulmonary process in which prenatal diagnosis is readily accomplished. Furthermore, it is now appreciated that a large fetal lung mass can cause mediastinal shift, pulmonary hypoplasia, polyhydramnios, and cardiovascular compromise, which leads to fetal hydrops and death (Adzick et al, 1993; Heij et al, 1990; Walker and Cudmore, 1990). The overall prognosis is dependent on the size of the mass and the extent of the secondary physiologic derangements caused by mediastinal compression. Additionally, the Fetal Treatment Center at the University of California at San Francisco has reported three cases of congenital cystic adenomatoid malformation that decreased in size during pregnancy, with one of the lesions regressing almost entirely (Adzick et al, 1993). Other groups have reported the same findings more recently (Golaszewski et al, 1998). The prenatal diagnosis of congenital cystic adenomatoid malformation is a clinical reality that has an impact on therapeutic alternatives.

Clinical Features

As is the case with bronchogenic cysts, congenital cystic adenomatoid malformations are found in newborns and infants with tachypnea, cyanosis, retractions, and respiratory distress. Most patients present in the first month of life with acute respiratory symptoms. Air trapping may occur in cystic areas of the anomaly and result in a clinical and radiographic picture that is reminiscent of lobar emphysema. The cystic distention may rarely result in rupture, causing a pneumothorax or tension pneumothorax (Bentur et al, 1991; Hilpert and Pretorius, 1990; Kleinman et al, 1982). Older children usually complain of cough and fever or have recurrent respiratory infections. They may be asymptomatic and their condition incidentally diagnosed on plain chest radiographs. Because air trapping with resultant mediastinal compression is the operative pathophysiologic mechanism, the condition of the patient may deteriorate rapidly when he or she is intubated and placed on positive-pressure ventilation. The clinician must be aware of this possibility and be prepared to perform thoracotomy and resection rapidly.

Imaging and Diagnostic Studies

As noted previously, ultrasound is instrumental in diagnosing cystic adenomatoid malformation in a fetus as early as the 20th week of gestation (Morcos and Lobb, 1986; Nugent et al, 1989; Scholz and Kuhnt, 1990). Simultaneous assessment for polyhydramnios and fetal hydrops can also be performed and is valuable to determine the prognostic risk. Some cystic adenomatoid malformations may also undergo spontaneous regression; therefore, serial ultrasound is helpful during follow-up and in planning either fetal or neonatal intervention. More recently, rapid intrauterine MRI has become a useful tool for fetal diagnosis (Hubbard et al, 1998).

After birth, patients often have respiratory distress, and plain chest radiographs are again the most important initial diagnostic study (Fig. 22–9). It is important to realize that congenital cystic adenomatoid malformation

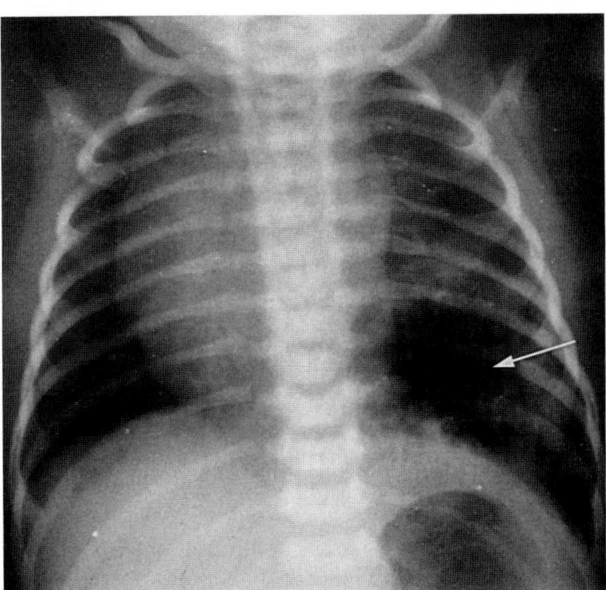

FIGURE 22–9 ■ A plain chest radiograph demonstrating a congenital cyst adenomatoid malformation.

has been confused with congenital diaphragmatic hernia (foramen of Bochdalek), congenital lobar emphysema, bronchogenic cyst, and pneumothorax. The findings observed on plain chest radiographs include single or multiple large cysts, multiple small cysts of uniform size, and solid-appearing masses. Masses are typically intrapulmonary and contain scattered radiolucent areas. Some cysts within the malformation may contain air-fluid levels. In addition, a mediastinal shift away from the lesion is observed when the lesion is expanding because of air trapping. This also implies a bronchial communication. Cystic adenomatoid malformations that cause chronic symptoms (infection or cough) later in life do not usually communicate with the bronchus. Unlike lobar emphysema, most cystic adenomatoid malformations are observed in the lower lobes.

After plain chest radiographs have revealed a unilateral multilocular density in one hemithorax, the next step diagnostically is the introduction of a small amount of water-soluble contrast material through a nasogastric tube to verify that the intestinal tract lies below the diaphragm and thus differentiate cystic adenomatoid malformation from diaphragmatic hernia. The radiographic appearance of bowel loops in the thorax can be confused with the appearance of cystic adenomatoid malformations. No further imaging studies are required after ruling out a foramen of Bochdalek hernia. If additional information is required, CT of the chest may be helpful (Fig. 22–10).

MANAGEMENT

Therapy

Therapy may be divided into prenatal and postnatal categories. Because prenatal diagnosis and assessment of prognostic risk are both feasible with advanced technology, it is reasonable to consider prenatal intervention. Pioneering work in fetal therapy for this lesion was performed at the Fetal Treatment Center of the University of California at San Francisco (Adzick et al, 1993, 1985; Adzick and Harrison, 1993; Harrison et al, 1990). After first establishing a clinical protocol that allowed fetal operative intervention in humans, this group was able to report on their experience in nine cases of fetal intervention for cystic adenomatoid malformation. In six of these cases, resection of the massively enlarged lobe was performed; the other three underwent thoracoamniotic shunt. Four patients who underwent in utero resection were alive 6 to 21 months after birth. The authors note that ultrasound-guided percutaneous drainage results in only a temporary reduction in the size of the cyst, and reaccumulation with recurrent mediastinal compression occurs within 24 to 48 hours after thoracentesis. Other centers have reported their experience with antenatal intervention for congenital cystic adenomatoid malformation (Clark et al, 1987; Dumez et al, 1993; Nicolaides et al, 1987). In a large retrospective review of 175 fetal lung lesions from the Center for Fetal Diagnosis and Treatment at the Children's Hospital of Philadelphia, there were 134 fetuses with congenital cystic adenomatoid malformations (Adzick et al, 1998). Of these, 14 were terminated through elective abortion, 101 were managed expectantly, 13 underwent fetal surgery, and six had placement of a thoracoamniotic shunt. All those with congenital cystic adenomatoid malformations that were not associated with nonimmune hydrops survived. Of 25 with large congenital cystic adenomatoid malformations that had associated hydrops and were managed expectantly, all fetuses died before or shortly after birth. Fetal surgical resection was performed between 21 and 29 weeks of gestation in 13 hydropic fetuses, and eight were able to continue gestation with subsequent hydrops resolution and neonatal survival. Six fetuses with large solitary cysts underwent thoracoamniotic shunting, and five survived. Because fetal surgery requires extensive scientific and clinical experience, it is appropriate for patients with prenatally diagnosed congenital cystic adenomatoid malformations to be referred to centers experienced with the myriad details of antenatal diagnosis and therapy.

Congenital cystic adenomatoid malformations that are detected postnatally are treated by posterolateral thoracotomy and resection of the involved lung tissue (Hailer et al, 1979; Nishibayashi et al, 1981; Ribet et al, 1990; Wesley et al, 1986; Wolf et al, 1980). Usually, an entire lobe is replaced by the adenomatous process, and lobectomy is required. In cases that are diagnosed prenatally but exhibit intrauterine regression, only a small residual is found at thoracotomy, and a more limited resection is possible. Furthermore, in some patients intrauterine regression of the cystic adenomatoid malformation may progress to a point at which no surgical intervention is required (Adzick et al, 1985; Fine et al, 1988; Hatjis and Wall, 1992; Saltzman et al, 1988). When doing exploratory surgery on these patients, it should be realized that the normal anatomic structures may be absent or grossly distorted. The best approach is a slow, careful, serial ligation of the vessels to the involved lobe followed by bronchial division. The results of surgical resection in postnatal disease are good, with resolution of the respiratory distress in most patients.

Atkinson and colleagues (1992) reported on three patients who developed pulmonary hypertension after postnatal resection of congenital cystic adenomatoid malformations. All three did predictably well for a short period after the thoracotomy but required extracorporeal mem-

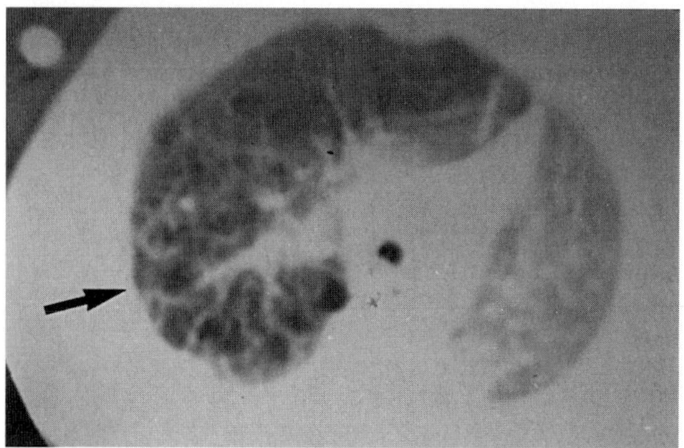

FIGURE 22–10 ■ Computed tomography scan of a cystic adenomatoid malformation.

brane oxygenator support for 66 to 112 hours for the subsequent development of pulmonary hypertension with hypoxemia and acidosis. All patients had the type I histologic subtype. The authors noted that in one patient, histologic examination of the resected lung tissue showed marked smooth muscle thickening in a pulmonary arteriole. This was in contrast to the previously reported findings of normal pulmonary vasculature in all three histologic subtypes of cystic adenomatoid malformation.

Pulmonary Sequestration

BASIC SCIENCE

Pathophysiology

Pulmonary sequestrations are masses of nonfunctioning pulmonary tissue that lack a normal communication with the tracheobronchial tree (Gottrup and Lund, 1978; Sieber, 1986; Stocker and Kagan-Hallet, 1979). They may occur within the substance of the lung (intralobar) or originate in an extralobar location. They normally receive their arterial blood supply directly from the thoracic or abdominal aorta or from intercostal branches (Ferris et al, 1983; Stocker, 1989). Sequestrations are differentiated from accessory pulmonary lobes, which are separated from the normal lung by pleural investments but maintain a normal communication with the trachea, bronchi, or foregut. Accessory pulmonary lobes are extralobar. The incidence of pulmonary sequestration is greater in male patients, by a ratio of 3:1 (Louie et al, 1993).

Embryology

It is thought that pulmonary sequestrations arise as accessory lung buds, which then migrate with the developing esophagus. This may account for the variable blood supply and occasional foregut communications observed with these lesions. Some have speculated that intralobar sequestrations may be acquired rather than congenital (Buntain et al, 1977; Carter, 1969; Iwai et al, 1973; Stocker and Malczak, 1984). Autopsy studies reveal inflammatory changes within intralobar sequestrations in support of this concept. However, Nicolette and colleagues (1993), in examining four surgical specimens, were able to demonstrate progression from no inflammatory changes in a 3-week-old infant to severe bronchiectasis and marked acute and chronic inflammation in a patient operated on at 6 years of age (Holder and Langston, 1986). This progression of inflammatory changes supports a congenital cause for these intralobar sequestrations. Congenital cystic adenomatoid malformations (type II) have been observed within extralobar pulmonary sequestrations, suggesting similar etiologic factors (Nicolette et al, 1993; Yogasakaran and Sudhaman, 1991). Other variations include a case of a bilateral sequestration with a bridging tunnel (horseshoe sequestration) (Zangwill and Stocker, 1993), pericardial sequestrations (Cerruti et al, 1993; Levi et al, 1990), and an association with congenital bronchoesophageal fistulas (Akin et al, 1991). In this latter case, the communication between the sequestration and the esophagus was identified by esophagogram and illustrated the possibility that pulmonary sequestrations can have abnormal communications with the foregut. Some of these foregut communications have been shown to contain pancreatic tissue (Evers et al, 1990). Sixty to ninety percent of sequestrations are located in the left posteroinferior thorax close to the diaphragm and lower lobe. The posterobasal segment of the left lower lobe is a common site for intralobar sequestrations, but intralobar lesions have also been identified in the upper lobes and rarely in the middle lobe or bilaterally. There have also been reports of sequestrations occurring below the diaphragm (Black and Welch, 1986; Lager et al, 1991; Sargent et al, 1992; Shih et al, 1990; Stern et al, 1990; Tilson and Touloukian, 1976).

The blood supply to pulmonary sequestrations is systemic and consists of one large branch or many small branches from the thoracic aorta. The systemic arterial supply may be large enough to cause a severe left-to-right shunt, with resultant CHF or hemoptysis (Brus et al, 1993; Levine et al, 1992; Matzinger et al, 1992). Aneurysmal degeneration has been reported in the abnormal sequestration vasculature. A rupture with hemothorax may occur, or the vessels may fistulize to the pulmonary artery (Hayakawa et al, 1991). The venous drainage from a pulmonary sequestration may be through the pulmonary or azygos veins.

Extralobar sequestrations have the consistency of liver and do not contain air spaces; intralobar lesions may contain air spaces but have no normal communication with the normal tracheobronchial tree. Infected sequestrations can demonstrate air-fluid levels, implying communication to the tracheobronchial tree, probably caused by erosion and fistulization. There is a report of a sequestration containing a fungal mycetoma (Koyama et al, 1992). Chronic inflammation in a sequestration may result in malignant change, as evidenced by a report of mesothelioma (Uppal et al, 1993), or it may result in the development of hundreds of neuroendocrine tumorlets in a chronically scarred intralobar sequestration (Paksoy et al, 1992).

DIAGNOSIS

Clinical Features

Feeding difficulties, failure to thrive, dyspnea, cyanosis, and other signs of respiratory distress are frequent clinical findings in these patients (Pelosi et al, 1992; Piccione and Burt, 1990). In older patients the sequestration may be asymptomatic and observed as an incidental finding on chest radiographs (Grove et al, 1990). Older patients may also present with symptoms of chronic pulmonary infection or even bronchiectasis. Rarely, patients may have a continuous murmur that radiates to the back. With aneurysmal degeneration of the systemic feeding artery to the sequestration with subsequent thrombosis or rupture, hemoptysis or hemothorax may result. Because a sequestration is a form of systemic-pulmonary shunt some patients may present with CHF (Fabre et al, 1998). If the sequestration arises below the diaphragm, it may appear as an abdominal mass, usually in the suprarenal area. Some of these suprarenal sequestrations may spontaneously involute (Daneman, et al, 1997). There have been reports of simultaneous, bilateral pulmonary sequestrations (Jeanfaivre et al, 1997).

Imaging and Diagnostic Studies

Antenatal ultrasound diagnosis has been reported. However, Dolkart and colleagues (1992) noted that the definitive identification of pulmonary sequestrations is only made in 35% of cases, based on the typical ultrasonographic finding of a fetal mass (thoracic or sometimes infradiaphragmatic [Sugio et al, 1992]). When these lesions were noted with fetal hydrops, stillbirth or neonatal death was universal. Fetal hydrops was observed in 35% of cases. Associated findings included polyhydramnios, fetal pleural effusions, mediastinal shifts, and pulmonary hypoplasia. Preterm labor was also more frequently observed in the face of this in utero diagnosis.

Matzinger and colleagues (1992) reported finding a hyperechoic mass in the right upper quadrant of a fetus at 20 and 33 weeks' gestation. This was thought to be a neuroblastoma but on exploration was found to be an infradiaphragmatic pulmonary sequestration. Others have reported that fetal pulmonary sequestrations are echogenic on ultrasound but may have small hypoechoic areas.

After birth, the usual initial imaging study is a plain chest radiograph (Fig. 22–11). In the case of extralobar sequestrations, the lung tissue has no connection with the bronchial tree and, therefore, has the consistency of liver. This appears as a mass, usually between the lower lobe and the diaphragm, on plain chest films. Intralobar sequestrations may resemble a mass. Sometimes intralobar lesions contain air secondary to abnormal connections with the tracheobronchial tree, and the radiographic picture is cystic. Rarely, both intralobar and extralobar sequestrations have been observed in the same patient (Dolkart et al, 1992). Aortography with a demonstration of the abnormal systemic feeding vessel to the sequestration has been used as a confirmatory procedure (Fig. 22–12). Duplex Doppler ultrasound has demonstrated the anomalous aortic branches without the morbidity of aortography (general anesthesia and risk of arterial injury or thrombosis) (Eisenberg et al, 1992; Kim et al, 1993). Abdominal vessels cannot be seen on plain radiographs, and CT or MRI images should be obtained to provide adequate anatomic detail. CT scans and magnetic resonance angiography (MRA) may allow visualization of the arterial inflow and give information similar to that provided by contrast aortography (Hemanz-Schulman et al, 1991; Kauczor et al, 1992) (Figs. 22–13 and 22–14). In most cases, a plain chest radiograph followed by Doppler ultrasound and CT or MRI to demonstrate systemic feeding vessels provides adequate diagnostic and anatomic information for surgery in the case of thoracic sequestrations. More detailed imaging studies are required when an infradiaphragmatic lesion is suspected.

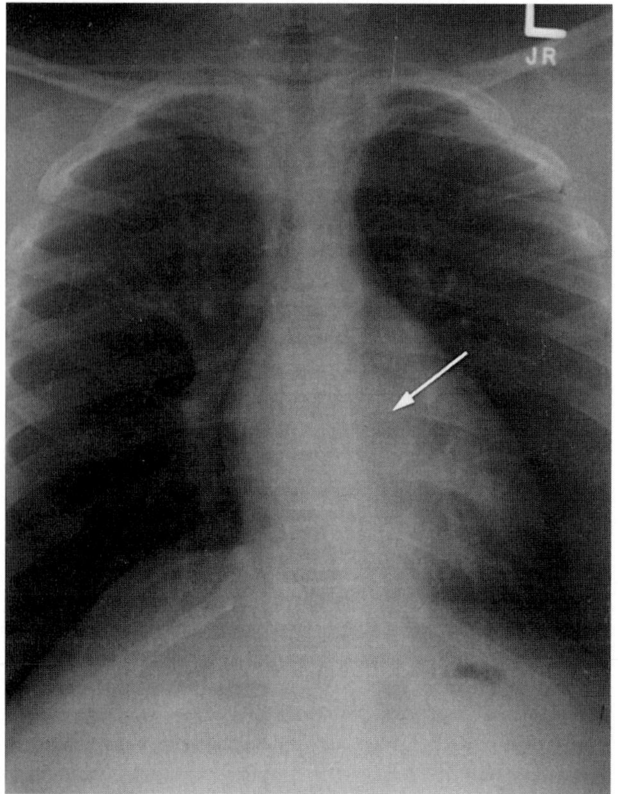

FIGURE 22–11 ■ Plain chest radiograph of a left posterior pulmonary sequestration.

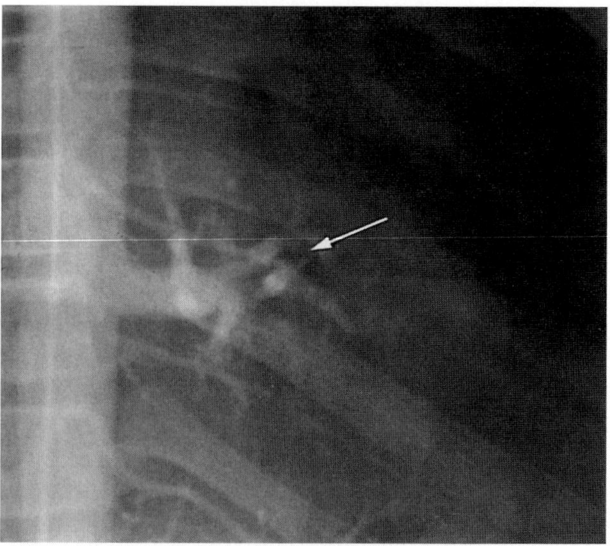

FIGURE 22–12 ■ Aortography of the same patient whose sequestration is depicted in Figures 22–13 and 22–14. This shows a large feeding vessel *(arrow)* derived from the lower thoracic aorta with what appear to be four major subdivisions.

MANAGEMENT

Therapy

The therapy of pulmonary sequestrations is resection, with the specific approach dependent on the location of the lesion. Lower interspace posterolateral thoracotomy is performed for thoracic lesions. Retroperitoneal or abdominal sequestrations may require a laparotomy or even a thoracoabdominal approach. In general, it is preferable

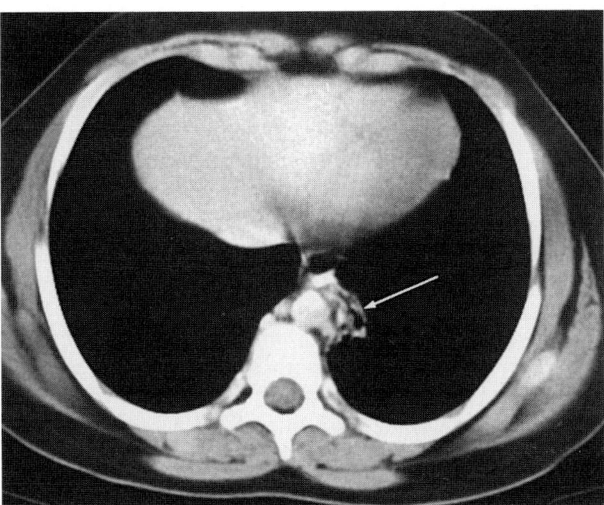

FIGURE 22–13 ■ Computed tomography scan of a left posterior pulmonary sequestration. The arterial blood supply derived from the thoracic aorta is visible.

to identify and ligate the arterial supply to the sequestration as the initial maneuver in the resection (Fig. 22–15). Serious hemorrhage may occur if these feeders are not identified and ligated. Care must be taken to identify and isolate vessels of abdominal origin. Resection can usually be performed without major morbidity and is curative. Intralobar lesions almost always require lobectomy. Extralobar sequestrations that are invested with a separate layer of visceral pleura are simply resected. It is possible to remove selected pulmonary sequestrations using a videothoracoscopic approach; there has been one report of a successful outcome in a six-month old infant (Mezzetti et al, 1996). Arterial embolization of the systemic blood supply has also been used to treat pulmonary sequestrations (Park et al, 1998).

In one large review, 26 cases of pulmonary sequestration occurring from 1959–1997 were reported (Halkic et al, 1998). Nineteen of the 26 (73%) were intralobar. In the seven extralobar cases the localization was basal in five (71%) and between the upper and lower lobe in two (21%). Lobectomy was performed in 46% and was the most common treatment. Segmental resections were done 30% of the time and bilobectomies were performed in 4%. There was no mortality and postoperative morbidity was low. Finally, the prenatal diagnosis of pulmonary sequestration is becoming more frequent. In an analysis of 10 patients who were diagnosed between the 20th and 33rd week of gestation, an absolute or relative regression in the size of the mass was noted in five (50%) (Becmeur et al, 1998). The systemic arterial blood supply was identified by Doppler ultrasound in four patients. Two fetal interventions were required. One fetus required three paracenteses of ascites and amniotic fluid, which then allowed a term delivery. The second fetus developed a hydrothorax that was treated with a pleuroamniotic shunt. All ten patients underwent surgery after birth with no mortality.

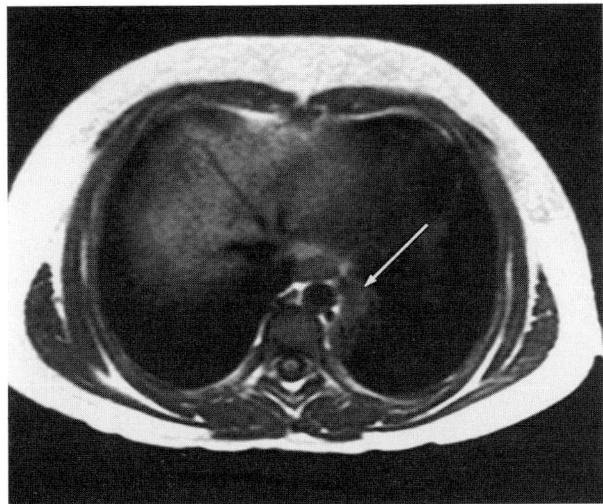

FIGURE 22–14 ■ Magnetic resonance imaging scan of the same pulmonary sequestration imaged in Figure 22–13. Again, the systemic blood supply is evident.

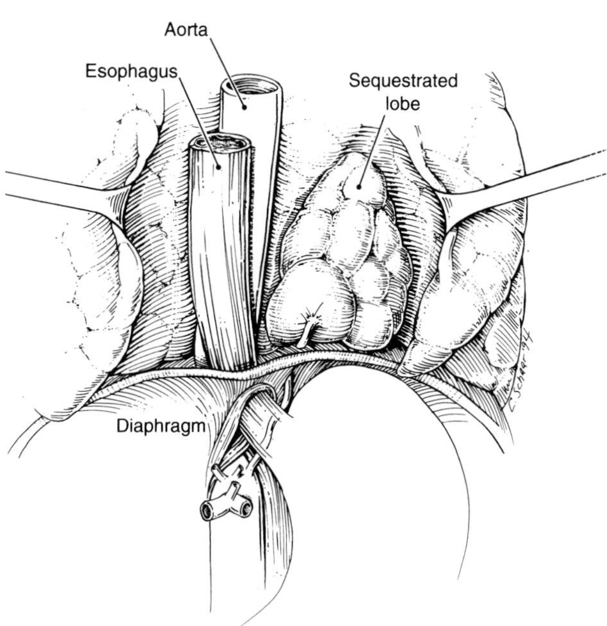

FIGURE 22–15 ■ An illustration of a left posterior pulmonary sequestration showing the systemic arterial supply arising from below the diaphragm. Major hemorrhage can result from a failure to recognize this anomaly and inadvertent division of these vessels during resection.

Congenital Pulmonary Vascular Malformations

BASIC SCIENCE

Pathophysiology

These lesions are characterized by an unusual communication between abnormal pulmonary arteries and pulmonary veins, which results in greater or lesser degrees of right-to-left shunting.

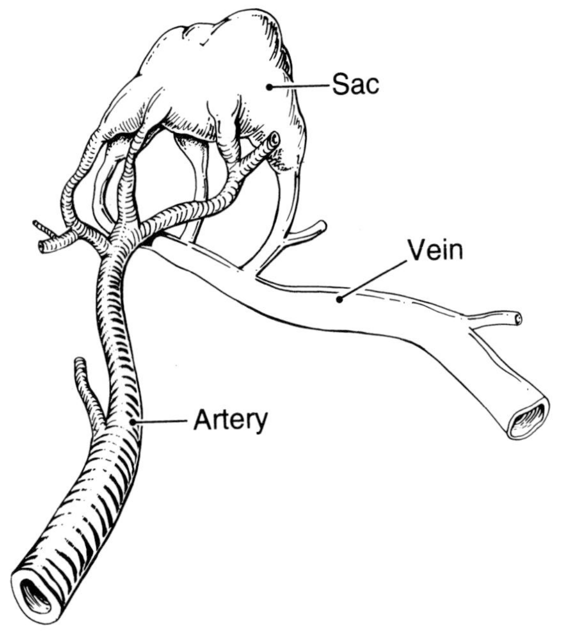

FIGURE 22–16 ■ An illustration depicting the anatomic lesion in arteriovenous malformations. The sac-like malformation is thin walled and easily ruptured or torn with resultant severe hemorrhage.

Embryology

As noted previously, the ingrowth of mesenchyme into the foregut pharyngeal pouch brings with it the capacity for the development of the pulmonary vasculature. During blood vessel development, primitive arteriovenous connections form to initiate the flow of blood. Subsequent vascular remodeling results in normal vessel development. AVMs result from unknown stimuli during the stage of arteriovenous communication in the retiform plexus. The large friable sac that results can be the source of serious hemorrhage (Fig. 22–16).

DIAGNOSIS

Clinical Features

Patients with pulmonary AVMs may present with the Rendu-Osler-Weber syndrome (cutaneous and mucosal spider angiomas) (57%), hemoptysis, dyspnea on exertion (67%), CHF, or a major neurologic event, such as a stroke or intracerebral abscess (33%) (Djindjian et al, 1973; Maruyama et al, 1989; Puskas et al, 1993). The degree of CHF is dependent on the size of the right-to-left shunt (Ribet and Denimal, 1991; Whyte et al, 1992). A continuous murmur may be heard over the involved hemithorax. Because a thrombus may develop in the abnormal vessels constituting these lesions, some patients may have evidence of systemic emboli, especially stroke, brain abscess, or multiple distant abscesses. There is also a reported association between multiple pulmonary AVMs and polysplenia (Papagiannis et al, 1993). Dyspnea may also be a prominent symptom.

Imaging and Diagnostic Studies

Plain chest radiographs show a solid mass in the lung, and it may be difficult to differentiate an AVM from a lung tumor. In one reported case, an AVM closely simulated a bronchogenic carcinoma on plain chest radiographs, but no lesion was palpable at thoracotomy. The diagnosis was only made postoperatively (Kilgore and Chasen, 1983). In the past, pulmonary arteriograms have been diagnostic and also present the opportunity for therapeutic embolization. More recently, MRI has been able to differentiate vascular malformations (hemangiomas or venous and AVMs) with a high degree of accuracy (Gutierrez et al, 1984; Dinsmore et al, 1990; Webb et al, 1984). MRI with the addition of MRA is an adequate confirmatory test and gives good information concerning feeding vessels, multiple lesions, and anatomic localization. Other imaging modalities that have been used for the evaluation of pulmonary AVMs include CT with contrast and contrast (agitated saline) echocardiograms (Barzilai et al, 1991; Remy et al, 1992).

MANAGEMENT

Therapy

The therapy for symptomatic congenital pulmonary AVMs previously consisted of surgical resection when feasible. This is useful for localized and large lesions. There has been a trend, however, to treat these lesions using angiographic embolization (Hartnell et al, 1990; Hughes and Allison, 1990; Jackson et al, 1990; Najarian et al, 1998). An assortment of balloons, springs, coils, and thrombogenic materials has been used with good initial success. Because embolization avoids the morbidity of thoracotomy and, at least in short-term follow-up, is effective in reducing the right-to-left shunt and ameliorating the symptoms of heart failure, it is now considered first-line therapy (Goergen and Sacharias, 1992; Pennington et al, 1992) (Figs. 22–17 and 22–18). A pulmonary AVM is depicted in Figure 22–17, and its successful

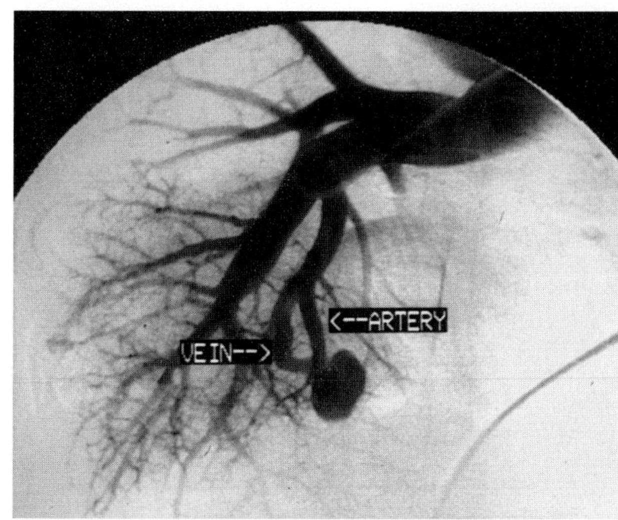

FIGURE 22–17 ■ A pulmonary arteriogram demonstrating an arteriovenous malformation.

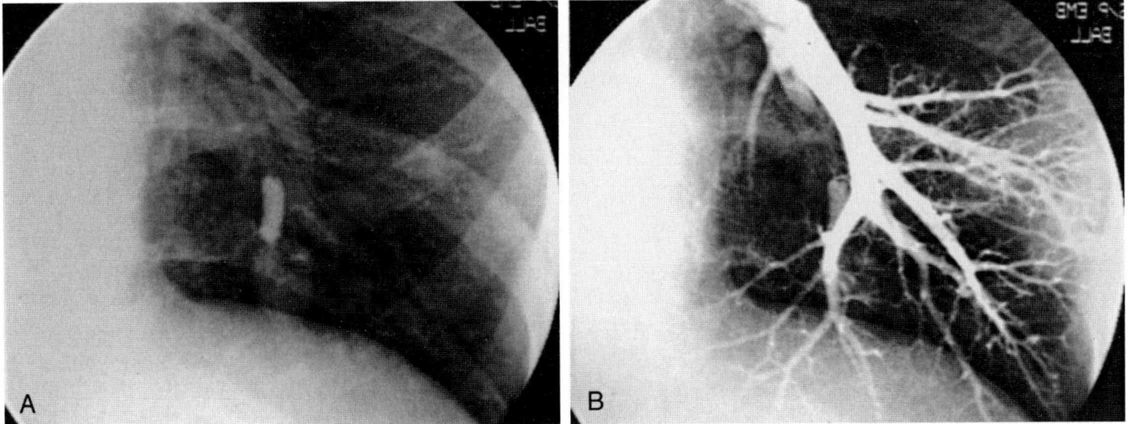

FIGURE 22–18 ■ *A*, A plain chest radiograph showing a detachable intravascular balloon positioned in the large feeding vessel to the arteriovenous malformation (AVM) depicted in Figure 22–17. *B*, Successful obliteration of the AVM following detachment of the intravascular balloon. Assorted other devices (e.g., springs, Gelfoam) are now commonly used for this purpose.

therapy by embolization is shown in Figure 22–18. Surgery should be reserved for localized lesions that have recurred or not responded to embolic therapy. In very large malformations, the combination of embolization followed by surgical removal may be advantageous in preventing infection in a large mass of infarcted lung tissue.

Lung Aplasia and Hypoplasia

BASIC SCIENCE

Pathophysiology

Pulmonary tissue may fail to develop totally or partially, giving rise to pulmonary aplasia or hypoplasia (Boxer et al, 1978; Campanella and Odell, 1987; Chilvers et al, 1990; Goergen and Sacharias, 1992; Gwinn et al, 1976; Hofner et al, 1979; Maltz and Nadas, 1968; Oran et al, 1979; Oyamada et al, 1953; Sbokos and McMillan, 1977; Shenoy et al, 1979). An entire lung on one side may be missing, or one or more lobes may be absent. Uncommonly, agenesis of both lungs may also occur (Claireaux and Ferreira, 1958; Kaya and Dilmen, 1989; Ostor et al, 1978). There is a reported association between bilateral pulmonary agenesis and microphthalmia (Toriello et al, 1985).

Embryology

Potter's syndrome, which consists of bilateral renal agenesis associated with a typical appearance of the facies and pulmonary hypoplasia, suggests a connection between renal and pulmonary development (Gale and Stocker, 1987; Hislop et al, 1979; Loendersloot et al, 1978; Nakamura et al, 1985; Ray et al, 1975; Stechele and Straub, 1978; Spear et al, 1987; Tinaztepe et al, 1983). It is postulated that fetal lung development is controlled in utero by the kidneys, possibly through the secretion of growth factors. Brinsmead and colleagues (1980), in a study on nephrectomized fetal lambs, showed that the fetal serum concentrations of placental lactogen and somatomedins were higher in the anephric animals (Greene et al, 1986). It has been theorized that the kidney plays a role in the clearance of these hormones in the fetus. It is speculated that the pulmonary growth retardation after fetal nephrectomy may be the result of increased binding of somatomedins by serum proteins or inhibition of somatomedin action by unidentified serum factors. Similarly, somatomedin-like receptor activity was greater in nephrectomized animals. These observations indicate that there is a feedback loop between the fetal lung and kidney, a theory that has been under intense investigation, because renal maldevelopment is usually associated with pulmonary dysgenesis.

In other experiments of this nature, complete tracheal or laryngeal obstruction has been associated with pulmonary hyperplasia (Brinsmead et al, 1980; Scurry et al, 1989). However, fetuses with incomplete tracheal or laryngeal obstruction (stenosis) usually develop pulmonary aplasia or hypoplasia (Harrison et al, 1980; Konoshi et al, 1986; Voland et al, 1986; Wigglesworth et al, 1987). For unknown reasons, complete fetal airway obstruction stimulates lung growth, but incomplete obstruction suppresses it. There is also a strong reported association of pulmonary dysgenesis with tracheoesophageal fistula and esophageal atresia (Benson et al, 1985; Black and Welch, 1986; Brereton and Rickwood, 1983; DeBuse and Morris, 1973; Ein et al, 1989; Knowles et al, 1988; McCormick and Kuhns, 1979; Takayanagi et al, 1987). Pulmonary aplasia has also been associated with the absence of the phrenic nerve on the ipsilateral side (Hoffman et al, 1989). Cardiac, vertebral, diaphragmatic, and rib anomalies have also been reported in conjunction with pulmonary dysgenesis (Chavaiittamrong et al, 1980; Courtney and MacKinnon, 1990; Gaziel et al, 1983; Goldstein and Reid, 1980; Sbokos and McMillan, 1977; Toriello and Bauserman, 1985; Wigglesworth et al, 1987), as have Fryn's syndrome, the scimitar syndrome, and omphalocele (Osborne et al, 1989; Vasquez Sanchez et al, 1986).

A number of reports have cited the existence of cytogenetic abnormalities in patients with lung agenesis or hypoplasia (Hatanaka et al, 1984; Hood et al, 1990; Say et al, 1980; Schober et al, 1983). At present, however, there is no known specific genetic defect associated with aplasia or hypoplasia of the lung.

DIAGNOSIS

Clinical Features

Bilateral pulmonary agenesis, or severe hypoplasia, results in stillbirth or rapid death of the newborn. Other patients with severe hypoplasia may present with respiratory distress. Hemoptysis resulting from pulmonary artery hypertension has also been reported (Cogswell and Singh, 1986; Hubsch et al, 1987; Lopez-Majano, 1985; Mehta et al, 1987; Pflueger et al, 1984). Patients with slight degrees of hypoplasia or with aplasia of a single lobe may be asymptomatic and the condition identified incidentally. Other patients may have coughing, wheezing, or pulmonary infection. The symptoms also depend on the extent and type of concomitant anomalies.

MANAGEMENT

Therapy

No therapy may be required for asymptomatic patients, and those with severe or bilateral dysplasia may not survive long enough for intervention to take place. In patients with severe symptoms who can be stabilized, pulmonary transplantation may offer hope of long-term survival.

Miscellaneous Lesions

Given the complexity of lung development, myriad other categories of congenital lesions can be imaged. Fortunately, other congenital pulmonary anomalies are even more uncommon than those discussed. There have been various reports of lymphangiomas or simple congenital cysts. With regard to the latter, there is controversy over whether they actually constitute a category separate from bronchogenic cyst. The clinician must assess the lesion and direct therapy based on the severity of symptoms.

COMMENTS AND CONTROVERSIES

The role of fetal surgery and the use of endoscopic techniques in the treatment of congenital pulmonary anomalies remain controversial. Great strides have been made in antenatal diagnosis and intervention, but precise indications have not been elucidated for all lesions. Also, long-term follow-up to judge the results of therapy is not available. Finally, the cost of fetal intervention has not been weighed against its potential benefits. In the present climate of fiscal responsibility in medicine, these issues will have to be addressed. Nevertheless, this is a frontier of surgery and should be explored. It must be emphasized that fetal intervention is complicated and there are inherent risks, not only to the fetus but also to the healthy mother. This type of surgery should be undertaken only in centers that have a record of excellence in both the technical and scientific aspects of prenatal intervention, so that valid conclusions regarding toxicity and efficacy can be obtained.

As more procedures are successfully performed with the use of endoscopic techniques, it is logical to expect that pulmonary anomalies will be treated videothoracoscopically under certain circumstances.

M.P.L.Q.

The exciting developments occurring in antenatal diagnosis and fetal surgery reside within the province of pediatric surgeons. In large tertiary referral centers, where pediatric cardiothoracic surgery is a burgeoning subspecialty, cardiothoracic surgeons almost certainly will be exploring this new field. Most cardiothoracic surgeons encounter congenital anomalies when they appear in the young adult. This is especially true of pulmonary sequestration, bronchogenic cysts, and AV malformations.

Unlike Dr. La Quaglia, I have always preferred to treat even intralobar pulmonary sequestration by segmentectomy and have accomplished this quite successfully, thereby preserving the rest of the otherwise normal lower lobe. Bronchogenic cysts can develop late complications as documented by St. Georges et al (1991). A significant number of these patients, even when watched closely, will develop major complications, including airway obstruction. For this reason, especially with the advent of simpler approaches such as video-assisted thoracoscopy, most bronchogenic cysts should be excised to avoid the complications of late rapid enlargement. This is especially true of mediastinal cysts, which can cause life-threatening airway compression.

With increasing expertise by interventional radiologists, embolization has become the treatment of choice in all centers for pulmonary AVMs. However, there is a steep learning curve associated with this technique, and it probably should be used only by those with significant expertise in angiographic embolization of these malformations.

R.J.G.

REFERENCES

Adzick NS, Harrison MR: Management of the fetus with a cystic adenomatoid malformation. World J Surg 17:342, 1993.

Adzick NS, Harrison MR, Flake AW et al: Fetal surgery for cystic adenomatoid malformation of the lung. J Pediatr Surg 28:806, 1993.

Adzick NS, Harrison MR, Glick PL et al: Fetal cystic adenomatoid malformation. J Pediatr Surg 20:483, 1985.

Adzick NS, Harrison MR, Crombleholme TM et al: Fetal lung lesions: Management and outcome. Am J Obstet Gynecol 179:884, 1998.

Ahn CM, Kim HJ, Cho HK et al: A case of intrapericardial extralobar pulmonary sequestration: First case in Korea. Korean J Intern Med 6:85, 1991.

Al-Salem AH, Adu-Gyamfi Y, Grant CS: Congenital lobar emphysema. Can J Anaesth 37:377, 1990.

Amendola MA, Shirazi KK, Brooks J et al: Transdiaphragmatic bronchopulmonary foregut anomaly: "Dumbbell bronchogenic cyst." Am J Radiol 138:1165, 1982.

Atkinson JB, Ford KG, Kitagawa H et al: Persistent pulmonary hypertension complicating cystic adenomatoid malformation in neonates. J Pediatr Surg 27:54, 1992.

Ayme S, Julian C, Gambarelli D et al: Fryn's syndrome: Report on 8 new cases. Clin Genet 35:191, 1989.

Bale PM: Congenital cystic malformation of the lung. A form of congenital bronchiolar (adenomatoid) malformation. Am J Clin Pathol 71:411, 1979.

Balquet P: Bronchogenic cysts compressing the trachea and main bronchus. Chir Pediatr 24:270, 1984.

Barzilai B, Waggoner AD, Spessert C et al: Two-dimensional contrast echocardiography in the detection and follow-up of congenital pulmonary arteriovenous malformations. Am J Cardiol 68:1507, 1991.

Becmeur F, Horta-Geraud P, Donato L, Sauvage P: Pulmonary sequestrations: prenatal ultrasound diagnosis, treatment, and outcome. J Pediatr Surg 33:492, 1998.

Benson JE, Olsen MM, Fletcher BD: A spectrum of bronchopulmonary anomalies associated with tracheoesophageal malformations. Pediatr Radiol 15:377, 1985.

Bentur L, Canny G, Thorner P et al: Spontaneous pneumothorax in cystic adenomatoid malformation. Unusual clinical and histologic features. Chest 99: 1292, 1991.

Berlinger NT, Porto DP, Thompson TR: Infantile lobar emphysema. Ann Otol Rhinol Laryngol 96:106, 1987.

Black MD, Bass J, Martin DJ, Carpenter BF: Intraabdominal pulmonary sequestration. J Pediatr Surg 26:1381, 1991.

Black PR, Welch KJ: Pulmonary agenesis (aplasia), esophageal atresia, and tracheoesophageal fistula: A different treatment strategy. J Pediatr Surg 21:936, 1986.

Blackader AD, Evans DJ: A case of mediastinal cyst producing compression of the trachea, ending fatally in an infant of nine months. Arch Pediatr 28:194, 1911.

Blott M, Nicolaides K, Greenough A: Postnatal respiratory function after chronic drainage of fetal pulmonary cyst. Am J Obstet Gynecol 159:858, 1988.

Boglino C, Inserra A, Serventi P et al: Neurotensin localization in adenomatoid cystic malformation versus normal lung: Preliminary report of six consecutive cases. J Pediatr Surg 27:57, 1992.

Borg SA, Young LW, Roghair GD: Congenital avalvular pulmonary artery and infantile lobar emphysema. A diagnostic correlation. AJR Am J Roentgenol 125:412, 1975.

Boulot P, Pages A, Deschamps F et al: Early prenatal diagnosis of congenital cystic adenomatoid malformation of the lung (Stocker's type I): A case report. Eur J Obstet Gynecol Reprod Biol 41:159, 1991.

Bower RJ, Kiesewetter WB: Mediastinal masses in infants and children. Arch Surg 112:1003, 1977.

Boxer RA, Hayes CJ, Hordof AJ, Mellins RB: Agenesis of the left lung and total anomalous pulmonary venous connection. Hemodynamic studies before and after complete surgical correction. Chest 74:106, 1978.

Brereton RJ, Rickwood AM: Esophageal atresia with pulmonary genesis. J Pediatr Surg 18:618, 1983.

Brinsmead MW, Waters MJ, Thorburn GD et al: Increase in placental lactogen and somatomedins after nephrectomy. J Dev Physiol 2:205, 1980.

Brus F, Nikkels PG, van Loon AJ, Okken A: Non-immune hydrops fetalis and bilateral pulmonary hypoplasia in newborn infant with extralobar pulmonary sequestration. Acta Paediatr 82:416, 1993.

Buckner CB, Walker CW, Shah HR, Fitzrandolph RL: Bronchogenic cysts. Am Fam Physician 40:167, 1989.

Buntain WL, Woolley MM, Mahour GH et al: Pulmonary sequestration in children: A twenty-five year experience. Surgery 81:413, 1977.

Campanella C, Odell JA: Unilateral pulmonary agenesis: A report of 4 cases. South Afr Med J 71:785, 1987.

Canty TG: Congenital lobar emphysema resulting from a bronchial sling around a normal right main pulmonary artery. J Thorac Cardiovasc Surg 74:126, 1977.

Canty TG, Hendren WH: Upper airway obstruction from foregut cysts of the hypopharynx. J Pediatr Surg 10:807, 1975.

Carlens E: Mediastinoscopy: A method for inspection and tissue biopsy in the superior mediastinum. Dis Chest 36:343, 1959.

Carter R: Pulmonary sequestration: Collective review. Ann Thorac Surg 7:68, 1969.

Cartmill JA, Hughes CF: Bronchogenic cysts: A persistent dilemma. Aust NZJ Surg 59:253, 1989.

Cass DL, Quinn TM, Yang EY et al: Increased cell proliferation and decreased apoptosis characterize congenital cystic adenomatoid malformation of the lung. J Pediatr Surg 33:1043, 1998.

Cerruti MM, Marmolejos F, Cacciarelli T: Bilateral intralobar pulmonary sequestration with horseshoe lung. Ann Thorac Surg 55:509, 1993.

Chavaiittamrong B, Podhipleux P, Pongpipat D: Agenesis of the left lung associated with vertebral anomalies, fusion of rib and sacralization: report of a case. J Med Assoc Thai 63:46, 1980.

Chilvers ER, Whyte MK, Jackson JE et al: Effect of percutaneous transcatheter embolization on pulmonary function, right-to-left shunt, and arterial oxygenation in patients with pulmonary arteriovenous malformations. Am Rev Respir Dis 142:420, 1990.

Ch'in KY, Tang MY: Congenital adenomatoid malformation of one lobe of a lung with general anasarca. Arch Pathol Lab Med 48:221, 1949.

Cioffi U, Bonavina L, De Simone M et al: Presentation and surgical management of bronchogenic esophageal duplication cysts in adults. Chest 113:1492, 1998.

Claireaux AK, Ferreira HP: Bilateral pulmonary agenesis. Arch Dis Child 33:364, 1958.

Clark SL, Vitale DJ, Minton SD et al: Successful fetal therapy for cystic adenomatoid malformation associated with second-trimester hydrops. Am J Obstet Gynecol 157:294, 1987.

Cogswell TL, Singh S: Agenesis of the left pulmonary artery as a cause of hemoptysis. Angiology 37:154, 1986.

Cohen SR, Thompson JW, Brennan LP: Foregut cysts presenting as neck masses. A report on three children. Ann Otol Rhinol Laryngol 94:433, 1985.

Coselli MP, de Ipolyi P, Bloss RS et al: Bronchogenic cysts above and below the diaphragm: Report of eight cases. Ann Thorac Surg 44:491, 1987.

Cote CJ: The anesthetic management of congenital lobar emphysema. Anesthesiology 49:296, 1978.

Courtney SP, MacKinnon AK: Pulmonary agenesis associated with fourteen other congenital abnormalities. Br J Clin Pract 44:291, 1990.

Cuypers P, De Leyn P, Cappelle L et al: Bronchogenic cysts: a review of 20 cases. Eur J Cardiothorac Surg 10:393, 1996.

D'Agostino S, Bonoldi E, Dante S et al: Embryonal rhabdomyosarcoma of the lung arising in a cystic adenomatoid malformation. J Pediatr Surg 32:1381, 1997.

Daneman A, Baunin C, Lobo E et al: Disappearing suprarenal masses in fetuses and infants. Pediatr Radiol 27:675, 1997.

Deacon CS, Smart PJ, Rimmer S: The antenatal diagnosis of congenital cystic adenomatoid malformation of the lung. Br J Radiol 63:968, 1990.

DeBuse PJ, Morris G: Bilateral pulmonary agenesis, oesophageal atresia, and the first arch syndrome. Thorax 28:526, 1973.

Di Lorenzo M, Collin PP, Vaillancourt R, Duranceau A: Bronchogenic cysts. J Pediatr Surg 24:988, 1989.

Dinsmore BJ, Gefter WB, Hatabu H, Kressel HY: Pulmonary arteriovenous malformations: Diagnosis by gradient-refocused MR imaging. J Comp Assist Tomogr 14:918, 1990.

Djindjian R, Cophignon J, Theron J et al: Embolization by superselective arteriography from the femoral route in neuroradiology. Review of 60 cases: I. Technique, indications, complications. Neuroradiology 6:20, 1973.

Dolkart LA, Reimers FT, Helmuth WV et al: Antenatal diagnosis of pulmonary sequestration: A review. Obstet Gynecol Surv 47:515, 1992.

Doull IJ, Connett GJ, Warner JO: Bronchoscopic appearance of congenital lobar emphysema. Pediatr Pulmonol 21:195, 1996.

Doyle AJ: Demonstration of blood supply to pulmonary sequestration by MR angiography. AJR Am J Roentgenol 158:989, 1992.

Dubois P, Belanger R, Wellington JL: Bronchogenic cyst presenting as a supraclavicular mass. Can J Surg 24:530, 1981.

Dumez Y, Mandelbrot N, Radunovic N et al: Prenatal management of congenital cystic adenomatoid malformation of the lung. J Pediatr Surg 28:36, 1993.

Ein SH, Shandling B, Wesson D, Filler RM: Esophageal atresia with distal tracheoesophageal fistula: Associated anomalies and prognosis in the 1980s. J Pediatr Surg 24:1055, 1989.

Eisenberg P, Cohen HL, Coren C: Color Doppler in pulmonary sequestration diagnosis. J Ultrasound Med 11:175, 1992.

Ekkelkamp S, Vos A: Successful surgical treatment of a newborn with bilateral congenital lobar emphysema. J Pediatr Surg 22:1001, 1987.

Engel S: The structure of the respiratory tissue in the newly-born. Acta Anat (Baser) 19:353, 1953.

Engle WA, Lemons JA, Weber TR, Cohen MD: Congenital lobar emphysema due to a bronchogenic cyst. Am J Perinatol 1:196, 1984.

Eraklis AJ, Griscom NT, McGovern JB: Bronchogenic cysts of the mediastinum in infancy. N Engl J Med 281:1150, 1969.

Evers WB, Vissers R, van Noord JA: Pulmonary sequestration with congenital broncho-oesophageal fistula. Eur Respir J 3:1067, 1990.

Fabre OH, Porte HL, Godart FR et al: Long-term cardiovascular consequences of undiagnosed intrapulmonary sequestration. Ann Thorac Surg 65:1144, 1998.

Fekete F, Rongere C, Foulon JP, Molas G: Bronchogenic esophageal cysts in the adult. Four cases. Presse Med 17:851, 1988.

Ferris EJ, Smith PL, Mirza FH et al: Intralobar pulmonary sequestration: Value of aortography and pulmonary arteriography. Cardiovasc Intervent Radiol 4:17, 1981.

Fine C, Adzick NS, Doubilet PM: Decreasing size of a congenital cystic adenomatoid malformation in utero. J Ultrasound Med 7:405, 1988.

Frenckner B, Freychuss U: Pulmonary function after lobectomy for congenital lobar emphysema and congenital cystic adenomatoid malformation: A follow-up study. Scand J Thorac Cardiovasc Surg 16:293, 1982.

Fukomoto K, Matsuzaki Y, Yoshioka M et al: Congenital bronchomalacia of the left main bronchus combined with lobar emphysema, pectus excavatum and right aortic arch: A case report. Nippon Kyobu Geka Gakkai Zasshi 39:943, 1991.

Gale DH, Stocker JT: Cloacal dysgenesis with urethral, vaginal outlet, and anal agenesis and functioning internal genitourinary excretion. Pediatr Pathol 7:457, 1987.

Gaziel Y, Hoek BB, van Niekerk CH: Agenesis of the right lung associated with hypoplasia of the fourth right rib. A case report. S Afr Med J 64:871, 1983.

Gille P, Aubert D, Menget A, Thura JP: Bilateral congenital eventration of the diaphragm with giant lobar emphysema. Chir Pediatr 20:359, 1979.

Ginsberg RJ, Atkins RW, Paulson DL: A bronchogenic cyst successfully treated by mediastinoscopy. Ann Thorac Surg 13:266, 1972.

Ginsberg RJ, Kirby TJ: Bronchogenic cysts. In Grillo HC, Austin WG, Wilkins EW Jr et al (eds): Current Therapy in Cardiothoracic Surgery. Toronto, BC Decker, 1989.

Goergen SK, Sacharias NR: Pulmonary arteriovenous malformations: Pathology, clinical features and treatment with balloon and coil occlusion. Australas Radiol 36:222, 1992.

Golaszewski T, Bettelheim D, Eppel W et al: Cystic adenomatoid malformation of the lung: Prenatal diagnosis, prognostic factors and fetal outcome. Gynecol Obstet Invest 46:241, 1998.

Goldstein JD, Reid LM: Pulmonary hypoplasia resulting from phrenic nerve agenesis and diaphragmatic amyoplasia. J Pediatr 97:282, 1980.

Gordon I, Dempsey JE: Infantile lobar emphysema in association with congenital heart disease. Clin Radiol 41:48, 1990.

Goto H, Boozalis ST, Benson KT, Arakawa K: High-frequency jet ventilation for resection of congenital lobar emphysema. Anesth Analg 66:684, 1987.

Gottrup F, Lund C: Intralobar pulmonary sequestration. A report of 12 cases. Scand J Respir Dis 59:21, 1978.

Gray, Skandalakis: Embryology for Surgeons. Philadelphia, WB Saunders, 1972.

Greene RA, Bloch MJ, Huff DS, Iozzo RV: MURCS association with additional congenital anomalies. Hum Pathol 17:88, 1986.

Gross RE, Lewis JE: Defect of the anterior mediastinum. Surg Gynecol Obstet 80:549, 1945.

Grove MK, Goodwin CD, Nanagas VN: Extralobar pulmonary sequestration. Cleve Clin J Med 57:88, 1990.

Gutierrez FR, Glazer HS, Levitt RG, Moran JF: NMR imaging of pulmonary arteriovenous fistulae. J Comput Assist Tomogr 8:750, 1984.

Gwinn JL, Lee FA, Davachi F, Rothberg M: Radiological case of the month. Agenesis of the left lung. Am J Dis Child 130:1121, 1976.

Halkic N, Cuenoud PF, Corthesy ME et al: Pulmonary sequestration: A review of 26 cases. Eur J Cardiothorac Surg 14:127, 1998.

Haller JA Jr, Golladay ES, Pickard LR et al: Surgical management of lung bud anomalies: Lobar emphysema, bronchogenic cyst, cystic adenomatoid malformation, and intralobar pulmonary sequestration. Ann Thorac Surg 28:33, 1979.

Haller JA Jr, Shermeta DW, Donahoo JS, White JJ: Life-threatening respiratory distress from mediastinal masses in infants. Ann Thorac Surg 19:364, 1975.

Ham AW, Baldwin KW: A histological study of the development of the lung, with particular reference to the nature of alveoli. Anat Rec 81:363, 1941.

Harrison MR, Adzick NS, Jennings RW et al: Antenatal intervention for congenital cystic adenomatoid malformation. Lancet 336:965, 1990.

Harrison MR, Heldt GP, Brasch RC et al: Resection of distal tracheal stenosis in a baby with agenesis of the lung. J Pediatr Surg 15:938, 1980.

Hartnell GG, Jackson JE, Allsion DJ: Coil embolization of pulmonary arteriovenous malformations. Cardiovasc Intervent Radiol 13: 347, 1990.

Hasse J, Lincoln JC, Paneth M: Differentiated surgical therapy in congenital lobar emphysema. Thoraxchir Vask Chir 23:250, 1975.

Hatanaka K, Ozaki M, Suzuki M et al: Trisomy 16ql3qter in an infant from a t(ll;l6)(q25;ql3) translocation-carrier father. Hum Genet 65:311, 1984.

Hatjis CG, Wall P: Type II congenital cystic adenomatoid malformation of the lung with a mediastinal shift. A case report. J Reprod Med 37:753, 1992.

Hayakawa K, Soga T, Hamamoto K et al: Massive hemoptysis from a pulmonary sequestration controlled by embolization of aberrant pulmonary arteries: Case report. Cardiovasc Intervent Radiol 14:345, 1991.

Heij HA, Ekkelkamp S, Vos A: Diagnosis of congenital cystic adenomatoid malformation of the lung in newborn infants and children. Thorax 45:122, 1990.

Hernanz-Schulman M, Stein SM, Neblett WW et al: Pulmonary sequestration: Diagnosis with color Doppler sonography and a new theory of associated hydrothorax. Radiology 180:817, 1991.

Heydanus R, Stewart PA, Wladimiroff JW, Los FJ: Prenatal diagnosis of congenital cystic adenomatoid lung malformation: A report of seven cases. Prenat Diagn 13:65, 1993.

Hill RC, Mantese V, Spock A, Wolfe WG: Management of an unusual case of congenital lobar emphysema. Pediatr Pulmonol 5:252, 1988.

Hilpert PL, Pretorius DH: The thorax. In Nyberg DA, Mahony BS, Pretorius DH (eds): Diagnostic Ultrasound of Fetal Anomalies. Chicago, Year Book Medical Publishers, 1990.

Hislop A, Hey E, Reid L: The lungs in bilateral renal agenesis and dysplasia. Arch Dis Child 54:32, 1979.

Hoffman MA, Superina R, Wesson DE: Unilateral pulmonary agenesis with esophageal atresia and distal tracheoesophageal fistula: Report of two cases. J Pediatr Surg 24:1084, 1989.

Hofner W, Bardach G, Ferlitsch A, Kotscher E: Diagnosis of combined malformation of the lung and pulmonary vessels. Rontgenblatter 32:384, 1979.

Holder PD, Langston C: Intralobar pulmonary sequestration. Pediatr Pulmonol 2:147, 1986.

Hood OJ, Hartwell EA, Shattuck KE, Rosenberg HS: Multiple congenital anomalies associated with a 47,XXX chromosome constitution. Am J Med Genet 36:73, 1990.

Hoover JP, Henry GA, Panciera RJ: Bronchial cartilage dysplasia with multifocal lobar bullous emphysema and lung torsions in a pup. J Am Vet Med Assoc 201:599, 1992.

Hubbard AM, Crombleholme TM: Anomalies and malformations affecting the fetal/neonatal chest. Semin Roentgenol 33:117, 1998.

Huber JJ: Observationes aliquot de arteria singulari pulmoni concessa. Acta Helv 8:85, 1777.

Hubsch P, Pichler W, Lang I, Mlczoch J: Isolated agenesis of the right pulmonary artery with late manifestation of pulmonary artery hypertension. Rontgenblatter 40:23, 1987.

Hughes JM, Allison DJ: Pulmonary arteriovenous malformations: the radiologist replaces the surgeon. Clin Radiol 41:297, 1990.

Hunter W: The history of an aneurysm of the aorta with some remarks on aneurysms in general. Obstet Soc Phys (London) 1:323, 1757.

Isojima A, Yuasa H, Kusagawa M et al: Surgical treatment of infantile lobar emphysema in cardiovascular disease with left-to-right shunts. Jpn J Surg 8:57, 1978.

Iwai K, Shindo G, Hajikano H et al: Intralobar sequestration with special reference to developmental pathology. Am Rev Respir Dis 107:911, 1973.

Jackson JE, Whyte MK, Allison DJ, Hughes JM: Coil embolization of pulmonary arteriovenous malformations. Cor Vasa 32:191, 1990.

Jeanfaivre T, Afi M, L'hoste P, Tuchais E: Simultaneous discovery of bilateral intralobar and extralobar pulmonary sequestrations. Ann Thorac Surg 63:1171, 1997.

Kaslovsky RA, Purdy S, Dangman BC et al: Bronchoalveolar carcinoma in a child with congenital cystic adenomatoid malformation. Chest 112:548, 1997.

Kauczor HU, Knopp MV, Branscheid D, Semmler W: Pulmonary sequestration: Diagnosis based on MR angiographic findings. AJR Am J Roentgenol 159:429, 1992.

Kaya IS, Dilmen U: Agenesis of the lung. Eur Respir J 2:690, 1989.

Keith HH: Congenital lobar emphysema. Pediatr Ann 6:36, 1977.

Keller MS: Congenital lobar emphysema with tracheal bronchus. Can Assoc Radiol J 34:306, 1983.

Kennedy CD, Habibi P, Matthew DJ, Gordon I: Lobar emphysema: long-term imaging follow-up. Radiology 180:189, 1991.

Kilgore TL, Chasen MH: Pulmonary arteriovenous fistula simulating a vanishing tumor. South Med J 76:884, 1983.

Kim HJ, Kim JH, Chung SK et al.: Coexistent intralobar and extralobar pulmonary sequestration: Imaging findings. AJR Am J Roentgenol 160:1199, 1993.

Kleinman CS, Donnerstein RL, DeVore GR et al: Fetal echocardiography for evaluation of in utero congestive heart failure: A technique for study of nonimmune hydrops. N Engl J Med 306:568, 1982.

Knoop U, Gharib M, Ewerback H, Ebel KD: Monatsschr Kinderheilkd 132:780, 1984.

Knowles S, Thomas RM, Lindenbaum RH et al: Pulmonary agenesis as part of the VACTERL sequence. Arch Dis Child 63:723, 1988.

Koizumi K, Tanaka S, Haraguchi S et al: Thoracoscopic enucleation of a submucosal bronchogenic cyst of the esophagus: Report of two cases. Surg Today 28:446, 1998.

Kolls JK, Kiernan MP, Ascuitto RJ et al: Intralobar pulmonary sequestration presenting as congestive heart failure in a neonate. Chest 102:974, 1992.

Konoshi H, Nakamura H, Mizukami Y et al: A case of pulmonary genesis associated with congenital tracheal stenosis and aberrant left pulmonary artery. Rinsho Hoshasen 31:741, 1986.

Koskas M, Tournier G, Baculard A et al: Bronchogenic cysts in the carina. Rev Mal Respir 9:509, 1992.

Koyama A, Sasou K, Nakao H et al: Pulmonary intralobar sequestration accompanied by aneurysm of an anomalous arterial supply. Intern Med 31:946, 1992.

Lacquet LK, Lacquet AM: Congenital lobar emphysema. Prog Pediatr Surg 10:307, 1977.

Lager DJ, Kuper KA, Haake GK: Subdiaphragmatic extralobar pulmonary sequestration. Arch Pathol Lab Med 115:536, 1991.

Langman J: Medical Embryology. Baltimore, Williams & Wilkins, 1969.

LaRue MJ, Garlick DS, Lamb CR, O'Callaghan MW: Bronchial dysgenesis and lobar emphysema in the adult cat. J Am Vet Med Assoc 197:886, 1990.

Letanche G, Boyer J, Guibert B et al: Bronchogenic cysts and their atypical localizations. A case of pleurodiaphragmatic cyst. Rev Pneumol Clin 40:191, 1984.

Levi A, Findler M, Dolfin T et al: Intrapericardial extralobar pulmonary sequestration in a neonate. Chest 98:1014, 1990.

Levine MM, Nudel DB, Gootman N et al: Pulmonary sequestration causing congestive heart failure in infancy. Ann Thorac Surg 34:581, 1982.

Lewis JE Jr: Pulmonary and bronchial malformations. In Ashcraft KW, Holder TM (eds): Pediatric Surgery. Philadelphia, WB Saunders, 1992.

Lewis RJ, Caccavale RJ, Sisler GE: Imaged thoracoscopic surgery: A new thoracic technique for resection of mediastinal cysts. Ann Thorac Surg 53:318, 1992.

Loendersloot EW, Verjaal M, Leschot NJ: Bilateral renal agenesis (Potter's syndrome) in two consecutive infants. Eur J Obstet Gynecol Reprod Biol 8:137, 1978.

Loewy J, O'Brodovich H. Coates G: Ventilation scintigraphy with submicronic radioaerosol as an adjunct in the diagnosis of congenital lobar emphysema. J Nucl Med 28:1213, 1987.

Loosli CG, Potter EL: The prenatal development of the human lung. Anat Rec 109:320, 1951.

Lopez-Majano V: Hemoptysis and pulmonary artery agenesis: case report. Eur J Nucl Med 11:91, 1985.

Louie HW, Martin SM, Mulder DG: Pulmonary sequestration: 17-year experience at UCLA. Am Surg 59:801, 1993.

Maier HC: Bronchogenic cysts of the mediastinum. Ann Surg 127:476, 1948.

Maltz DL, Nadas AS: Agenesis of the lung. Presentation of eight new cases and review of the literature. Pediatrics 42:175, 1968.

Man DW, Hamdy MH, Hendry GM et al: Congenital lobar emphysema: Problems in diagnosis and management. Arch Dis Child 58:709, 1983.

Markowitz RI, Mercurio MR, Vahjen GA et al: Congenital lobar emphysema. The roles of CT and scan. Clin Pediatr 28:19, 1989.

Maruyama J, Watanabe M, Onodera S et al: A case of Rendu-Osler-Weber disease with cerebral hemangioma, multiple pulmonary arteriovenous fistulas and hepatic arteriovenous fistula. Jpn J Med 28:651, 1989.

Mashiach R, Hod M, Friedman S et al: Antenatal ultrasound diagnosis of congenital cystic adenomatoid malformation of the lung: spontaneous resolution in utero. J Clin Ultrasound 21:453, 1993.

Matzinger MA, Matzinger FR, Matzinger KE, Black MD: Antenatal and postnatal findings in intra-abdominal pulmonary sequestration. Can Assoc Radiol J 43:212, 1992.

McCormick TL, Kuhns LR: Tracheal compression by a normal aorta associated with right lung agenesis. Radiology 130:659, 1979.

Mehta AC, Livingston DR, Kawalek W et al: Pulmonary artery agenesis presenting as massive hemoptysis: A case report. Angiology 38:67, 1987.

Mentzer SJ, Filler RM, Phillips J: Limited pulmonary resections for congenital cystic adenomatoid malformation of the lung. J Pediatr Surg 27:1410, 1992.

Meyer H: Über angeborene blasige Missbildung der Lungen nebst einigen Bemerkungen uber Cyanose aus Lungenleiden. Arch Pathol Anat 16:78, 1859.

Mezzetti M, Dell'Agnola CA, Bedoni M et al: Video-assisted thoracoscopic resection of pulmonary sequestration in an infant. Ann Thorac Surg 61:1836, 1996.

Michelson E: Clinical spectrum of infantile lobar emphysema. Ann Thorac Surg 24:182, 1977.

Miller RK, Sieber WK, Yunis EJ: Congenital adenomatoid malformation of the lung. A report of 17 cases and review of the literature. In Sommers SC, Rosen PP (eds): Pathology Annual: Part I. East Norwalk, CT, Appleton-Century-Crofts, 1980.

Moerman P, Fryns JP, Vandenberghe K et al: Pathogenesis of congenital cystic adenomatoid malformation of the lung. Histopathology 21:315, 1992.

Monin P, Didier F, Vert P et al: Giant lobar emphysema-neonatal diagnosis. Pediatr Radiol 8:259, 1979.

Morcos SF, Lobb MO: The antenatal diagnosis by ultrasonography of type III congenital cystic adenomatoid malformation of the lung. Case report. Br J Obstet Gynaecol 93:1002, 1986.

Morris E, Constantine G, McHugo J: Cystic adenomatoid malformation of the lung: An obstetric and ultrasound perspective. Eur J Obstet Gynecol Reprod Biol 40:11, 1991.

Najarian KE, Morris CS: Arterial embolization in the chest. J Thorac Imaging 13:93, 1998.

Nakamura Y, Funatsu Y, Yamamoto I et al: Potter's syndrome associated with renal agenesis or dysplasia. Morphological and biochemical study of the lung. Arch Pathol Lab Med 109:441, 1985.

Nelson RL: Congenital cystic disease of the lung. J Pediatr 1:233, 1932.

Nicolaides KH, Blott M, Greenough A: Chronic drainage of fetal pulmonary cyst. Lancet 1:618, 1987.

Nicolette LA, Kosloske AM, Bartow SA, Murphy S: Intralobar pulmonary sequestration: A clinical and pathological spectrum. J Pediatr Surg 28:802, 1993.

Nishibayashi SW, Andrassy RJ, Wooley MM: Congenital cystic adenomatoid malformation: A 30-year experience. J Pediatr Surg 16:704, 1981.

Nobuhara KK, Gorski YC, La Quaglia MP, Shamberger RC: Bronchogenic cysts and esophageal duplications: Common origins and treatment. J Pediatr Surg 32:1408, 1997.

Nugent CE, Hayashi RH, Rubin J: Prenatal treatment of type I congenital cystic adenomatoid malformation by intrauterine fetal thoracentesis. J Clin Ultrasound 17:675, 1989.

Okur H, Kucukaydin M, Ozturk A et al: Giant bronchogenic cyst presenting as a lobar emphysema in a newborn. Ann Thorac Surg 62:276, 1996.

Olson JL, Mendelsohn G: Congenital cystic adenomatoid malformation of the lung. Arch Pathol Lab Med 102:248, 1978.

Opsahl T, Berman EJ: Bronchiogenic mediastinal cysts in infants: Case report and review of the literature. Pediatrics 40:372, 1967.

Oran O, Caglar M, Kale G, Kanra G: Unilateral pulmonary agenesis-presentation of two new cases. Turk J Pediatr 21:16, 1979.

Orima H, Fujita M, Aoki S et al: A case of lobar emphysema in a dog. J Vet Med Sci 54:797, 1992.

Osborne J, Masel J, McCredie J: A spectrum of skeletal anomalies associated with pulmonary agenesis: Possible neural crest injury. Pediatr Radiol 19:425, 1989.

Osler W: On a family form of recurring epistaxis associated with multiple telangiectases of skin and mucous membrane. Bull Johns Hopkins Hosp 12:333, 1901.

Ostor AG, Stillwell R, Fortune DW: Bilateral pulmonary agenesis. Pathology 10:243, 1978.

Overstreet RM: Emphysema of a portion of the lung in the early months of life. Am J Dis Child 57:861, 1939.

Oyamada A, Gasul BM, Holinger PH: Agenesis of the lung. Report of a case with review of all previously reported cases. Am J Dis Child 85:182, 1953.

Paksoy N, Demircan A, Altiner M, Artvinli M: Localized fibrous mesothelioma arising in an intralobar pulmonary sequestration. Thorax 47:837, 1992.

Papagiannis J, Kanter RJ, Effman EL et al: Polysplenia with pulmonary arteriovenous malformations. Pediatr Cardiol 14:127, 1993.

Pardes JG, Auh YH, Blomquist K et al: CT diagnosis of congenital lobar emphysema. J Comput Assist Tomogr 7:1095, 1983.

Park OK, Buford CH: Bronchogenic cyst of neck and superior mediastinum. Ann Surg 142:130, 1955.

Park ST, Yoon CH, Sung KB, et al: Pulmonary sequestration in a newborn infant: Treatment with arterial embolization. J Vasc Interv Radiol 9:648, 1998.

Parkes Weber F: Multiple hereditary developmental angiomata of the skin and mucous membranes associated with recurring haemorrhages. Lancet 2:160, 1907.

Pelosi G, Zancanaro C, Sbabo L et al: Development of innumerable neuroendocrine tumorlets in a pulmonary lobe scarred by intralobar sequestration: Immunohistochemical and ultrastructural study of an unusual case. Arch Pathol Lab Med 116:1167, 1992.

Pennington DW, Gold WM, Gordon RL et al: Treatment of pulmonary arteriovenous malformations by therapeutic embolization. Am Rev Respir Dis 145:1047, 1992.

Pflueger SM, Scott CI Jr, Moore CM: Trisomy 7 and Potter's syndrome. Clin Genet 25:543, 1984.

Phillipos EZ, Liebskal K: Flexible bronchoscopy in the management of congenital lobar emphysema in the neonate. Can Respir J 5:219, 1998.

Piccione W Jr, Burt ME: Pulmonary sequestration in the neonate. Chest 97:244, 1990.

Pryce DM: Lower accessory pulmonary artery with intralobar sequestration of lung. A report of seven cases. J Pathol 48:457, 1946.

Pursel SE, Hershey EA, Day JC, Barrett RJ: An approach to cystic lesions of the mediastinum via the mediastinoscope. Ann Thorac Surg 2:752, 1966.

Puskas JD, Allen MS, Moncure AC et al: Pulmonary arteriovenous malformations: Therapeutic options. Ann Thorac Surg 56:253, 1993.

Ray D, Hrudayanath P, Pulimood BM: Pulmonary agenesis associated with crossed renal ectopia. Indian J Chest Dis Allied Sci 17:90, 1975.

Rebarber A, Mohan R: Prenatal diagnosis of cystic adenomatoid malformation of one fetus in a twin pregnancy: an unusual presentation. J Ultrasound Med 11:305, 1992.

Rektorzik E: Ueber accessorischen Lungenlappen. Wochenschr Z Aerzte 17:4, 1861.

Remy J, Remy-Jardin M, Wattinne L, Deffontaines C: Pulmonary arteriovenous malformations: Evaluation with CT of the chest before and after treatment. Radiology 182:809, 1992.

Rendu M: Epistaxis répétées chez un sujet porteur de petite angiomes cutanes et muqueux. Bull Soc Med Hôp (Paris) 13:731, 1896.

Ribet M, Denimal F: Pulmonary arteriovenous malformations. Chirurgie 117:533, 1991.

Ribet M, Pruvot FR, Dubos JP et al: Congenital cystic adenomatoid malformation of the lung. Eur J Cardiothorac Surg 4:403, 1990.

Robertson R, James ES: Congenital lobar emphysema. Pediatrics 8:795, 1951.

Roguin N, Peleg N, Lemer J et al: The value of cardiac catheterization and cineangiography in infantile lobar emphysema. Pediatr Radiol 10:71, 1980.

Rokitansky C: Lehrbuch der pathologischen Anatomie, 3rd ed. Vienna, 1861.

Rosado-de-Christenson ML, Stocker JT: Congenital cystic adenomatoid malformation. Radiographics 11:865, 1991.

Saltzman DH, Adzick NS, Benacerraf BR: Fetal cystic adenomatoid malformation of the lung: Apparent improvement in utero. Obstet Gynecol 71:1000, 1988.

Sargent MA, Liu PC, Smith CR, Daneman A: Infradiaphragmatic pulmonary sequestration. Can Assoc Radiol J 43:208, 1992.

Say B, Carpenter NJ, Giacoia G, Jegathesan S: Agenesis of the lung associated with chromosome abnormality (46,XX, 2p+). J Med Genet 17:477, 1980.

Sbokos CG, McMillan IKR: Agenesis of the lung. Br J Dis Chest 71:183, 1977.

Schober PH, Muller WD, Behmel A et al: Pulmonary agenesis in partial trisomy 2p and 21q. Klin Padiatr 195:291, 1983.

Scholz P, Kuhat C: Congenital cystic malformation of the lung in a fetus. Zentralbl Gynakol 112:289, 1990.

Scurry JP, Adamson TM, Cussen LJ: Fetal lung growth in laryngeal atresia and tracheal agenesis. Aust Paediatr J 25:47, 1989.

Senyuz OF, Danismend N, Erdogan E et al: Congenital lobar emphysema: A report of 5 cases. Jpn J Surg 19:764, 1989.

Shah VK, Marar UK, Gandhi MJ et al: Agenesis of lung with pulmonary hypertension. J Assoc Physicians India 34:819, 1986.

Shenoy SS, Culver GJ, Pirson HS: Agenesis of lung in an adult. AJR Am J Roentgenol 133:755, 1979.

Sherer DM, Abramowicz JS, Metlay LA et al: Nonimmune fetal hydrops caused by bilateral type III congenital cystic adenomatoid malformation of the lung at 17 weeks gestation. Am J Obstet Gynecol 167:503, 1992.

Shih SL, Lin JC, Chen BF et al: Extralobar pulmonary sequestration of the left retroperitoneum. Australas Radiol 34:356, 1990.

Sieber WK: Lung cysts, sequestration, and bronchopulmonary dysplasia. In Welch KJ, Randolph JG, Ravitch MM et al (eds): Pediatric Surgery. Chicago, Year Book Medical Publishers, 1986.

Sorokin S: Recent work on developing lungs. In DeHaan RL, Ursprung H (eds): Organogenesis. New York, Holt, Rinehart and Winston, 1965.

Spear GS, Yetur P, Beyerlein RA: Bilateral pulmonary agenesis and microphthalmia. Am J Med Genet Suppl 3:379, 1987.

Stechele U, Straub E: Potter-syndrome. Klio Padiatr 190:139, 1978.

Stern E, Brill PW, Winchester P, Kosovsky P: Imaging of prenatally detected intra-abdominal extralobar pulmonary sequestration. Clin Imaging 14:152, 1990.

St. Georges R, Deslauriers J, Duranceau A et al: Clinical spectrum of bronchogenic cysts of the mediastinum and lung in the adult. Ann Thorac Surg 52:6, 1991.

Stocker JT: Pediatric Pulmonary Disease. New York, Hemisphere, 1989.

Stocker JT, Kagan-Hallet K: Extralobar pulmonary sequestration: analysis of 15 cases. Am J Clin Pathol 72:917, 1979.

Stocker JT, Madewell JE, Drake RM: Congenital cystic adenomatoid malformation of the lung. Classification and morphologic spectrum. Hum Pathol 8:155, 1977.

Stocker JT, Malczak HT: A study of pulmonary ligament arteries: Relationship to intralobar pulmonary sequestration. Chest 86:611, 1984.

Suen HC, Mathisen DJ, Grillo HC et al: Surgical management and radiological characteristics of bronchogenic cysts. Ann Thorac Surg 55:476, 1993.

Sugio K, Kaneko S, Yokoyama H et al: Pulmonary sequestration in older children and in adults. Int Surg 77:102, 1992.

Taguchi M, Shimizu K, Ozaki Y et al: Prenatal diagnosis of congenital cystic adenomatoid malformation of the lung. Fetal Diagn Ther 8:114, 1993.

Takayanagi K, Grochowska E, Abu-el Nas S: Pulmonary agenesis with esophageal atresia and tracheoesophageal fistula. J Pediatr Surg 22:125, 1987.

Tapper D, Schuster S, McBride J et al: Polyalveolar lobe: Anatomic and physiologic parameters and their relationship to congenital lobar emphysema. J Pediatr Surg 15:931, 1980.

Tilson DD, Touloukian RJ: Mediastinal enteric sequestration with aberrant pancreas. A forme fruste of the intralobar sequestration. Ann Surg 176:669, 1976.

Tinaztepe K, Balci S, Tinaztepe B, Dagli E: Potter's syndrome: Bilateral renal agenesis (a report of two cases emphasizing associated malformations). Turk J Pediatr 25:179, 1983.

Toran N, Ruiz de Miguel C, Reig J, Garcia-Bonafe M: Lobar emphysema associated with patent ductus arteriosus and pulmonary obstructive vascular disease. Pediatr Pathol 9:163, 1989.

Toriello HV, Bauserman SC: Bilateral pulmonary agenesis: Association with the hydrolethalus syndrome and review of the literature from a developmental field perspective. Am J Med Genet 21:93, 1985.

Toriello HV, Higgins JV, Jones AS, Radecki LL: Pulmonary and diaphragmatic agenesis: Report of affected sibs. Am J Med Genet 21:87, 1985.

Uppal MS, Kohman LJ, Katzenstein AL: Mycetoma within an intralobar sequestration: Evidence supporting acquired origin for this pulmonary anomaly. Chest 103:1627, 1993.

Urban AK, Stark J, Waterston DJ: Congenital lobar emphysema. Thoraxchir Vask Chir 23:255, 1975.

Vasquez Sanchez J, Diaz de la Vega V, Lupi Herrera E et al: Scimitar syndrome. Arch Inst Cardiol Mex 56:157, 1986.

Vogt-Moykopf I, Rau B, Branscheid D: Surgery for congenital malformations of the lung. Ann Chir 46:141, 1992.

Vogt-Moykopf I, Rau B, Branscheid D: Surgery for congenital malformations of the lung. Ann Radiol 36:145, 1993.

Voland JR, Benirschke K, Saunders B: Congenital tracheal stenosis with associated cardiopulmonary anomalies. Pediatr Pulmonol 2:247, 1986.

Voorhout G, Goedegebuure SA, Nap RC: Congenital lobar emphysema caused by aplasia of bronchial cartilage in a Pekingese puppy. Vet Pathol 23:83, 1986.

Wagenvoort CA, Zondervan PE: Polyalveolar lobe and congenital cystic adenomatoid malformation type II: Are they related? Pediatr Pathol 11:311, 1991.

Walker J, Cudmore RE: Respiratory problems and cystic adenomatoid malformation of the lung. Arch Dis Child 65:649, 1990.

Warner JO, Rubin S, Heard BE: Congenital lobar emphysema: A case with bronchial atresia and abnormal bronchial cartilages. Br J Dis Chest 76:177, 1982.

Webb WR, Gamsu G, Golden JA, Crooks LE: Nuclear magnetic resonance of pulmonary arteriovenous fistula: Effects of flow. J Comput Assist Tomogr 8:155, 1984.

Wesley JR, Heidelberger KP, DiPrieto MA et al: Diagnosis and management of congenital cystic disease of the lung in children. J Pediatr Surg 21:202, 1986.

Whyte MK, Peters AM, Hughes JM et al: Quantification of right to left shunt at rest and during exercise in patients with pulmonary arteriovenous malformations. Thorax 47:790, 1992.

Wigglesworth JS, Desai R, Hislop AA: Fetal lung growth in congenital laryngeal atresia. Pediatr Pathol 7:515, 1987.

Williams S, Burton EM, Day S et al: Combined sequestration, bronchogenic cyst, and dysgenetic lung simulating congenital lobar emphysema. South Med J 89:1220, 1996.

Willis RA: The Borderland of Embryology and Pathology. Washington, DC, Butterworths, 1962.

Wolf SA, Hertzler JH, Phillipart AI: Cystic adenomatoid dysplasia of the lung. Pediatr Surg 15:925, 1980.

Yim AP, Lam HC, Ho JK: Thoracoscopic lobectomy for an infected intrapulmonary bronchogenic cyst. Surg Endosc 10:439, 1996.

Yogasakaran BS, Sudhaman DA: Congenital cystic adenomatoid malformation of the lung in combination with a pulmonary sequestration. J Cardiovasc Vasc Anesth 5:368, 1991.

Young AK: Arteriovenous malformations. In Mulliken JB, Young AE (eds): Vascular Birthmarks (Hemangiomas and Malformations). Philadelphia, WB Saunders, 1988.

Zangwill BC, Stocker JT: Congenital cystic adenomatoid malformation within an extralobar pulmonary sequestration. Pediatr Pathol 13:309, 1993.

Zaugg M, Kaplan V, Widmer U et al: Fatal air embolism in an airplane passenger with a giant intrapulmonary bronchogenic cyst. Am J Respir Crit Care Med 157:1686, 1998.

CHAPTER **23**

Infections

BACTERIAL INFECTIONS OF THE LUNG

Gail Darling

Gregory P. Downey

Margaret S. Herridge

Lower respiratory tract infections, including pneumonia and its complications, are of substantial importance to the thoracic surgeon. From a historical perspective, suppurative diseases of the lung, such as empyema, lung abcess, and bronchiectasis, provided a major impetus for the development of thoracic surgery as a specialty and, until as recently as 40 years ago, represented the major focus of practice. Currently, lower respiratory tract infections represent the principal cause of mortality globally and, in North America, the major cause of death due to infectious diseases. Lower respiratory tract infections may lead to suppurative complications requiring surgical intervention or may complicate the postoperative course of thoracic surgical patients. Since the advent of antibiotics, the spectrum and clinical course of pneumonia have changed radically. The purpose of this chapter is to provide a practical review of this field with specific recommendations for diagnosis and treatment of lower respiratory tract infections.

PNEUMONIA

Despite the advent of potent antibiotics and effective vaccines, pneumonia remains a common and potentially fatal illness. Although the exact incidence is difficult to ascertain, in North America pneumonia represents the sixth most common cause of death and the most common cause of death from infectious diseases (Bruchhaus et al, 1998; Garibaldi, 1985). There are approximately 4 million cases of community-acquired pneumonia annually, of which approximately 20% will result in hospitalization. Although mortality in the outpatient setting is low (1% to 5%), it approaches 25% in hospitalized patients and may be even higher in those requiring admission to an intensive care unit. Current recommendations for the treatment of pneumonia focus on the presence or absence of comorbid conditions, the severity of illness, and whether treatment is to be given on an outpatient or inpatient basis (Mandell et al, 2000; Mandell, 1999; Niederman et al, 1993).

Definition

Pneumonia is defined as an infection of the lower respiratory tract that involves the secondary lobules of the lung: the respiratory bronchioles, alveolar ducts, and alveoli. It usually presents with a constellation of symptoms and signs that include fever, cough with or without sputum production, dyspnea, and chest pain in association with abnormal findings on physical examination of the chest and parenchymal infiltrates on the chest radiograph. It is to be distinguished from acute bronchitis which, although it can have a similar clinical presentation, represents infection of the tracheobronchial tree without parenchymal involvement as determined radiographically.

Epidemiologic Classification of Pneumonia

Because of dramatic changes in the epidemiology and treatment of pneumonia, traditional classification schemes and diagnostic approaches are obsolete (Cassiere, 1998a; Lynch et al, 1998; Marrie, 1998a, 1998b). During the initial evaluation of patients with suspected pneumonia, the microbial pathogen is rarely known, making the initial choice of antibiotic therapy empiric. However, the use of a diagnostic algorithm and taxonomy based on epidemiologic evidence and the clinical characteristics of patients provides a rational process for the selection of antibiotics. According to this algorithm (Table 23–1), pneumonia is currently divided into community-acquired and hospital-acquired (nosocomial) pneumonias, rather than typical versus atypical pneumonias as in previous practice (Sarosi, 1999). Two additional important categories of pneumonia include aspiration pneumonia and pneumonia in the immunocompromised host.

Community-acquired pneumonia occurs in patients who have not recently (within 14 days) been hospitalized in an acute or chronic care facility including nursing homes and is usually due to bacteria or viral pathogens. These pneumonias are further subdivided based on the mode of presentation and characteristics of the host. Pneumonia is increasingly common in older patients and in those with other comorbid conditions including chronic obstructive pulmonary disease (COPD), congestive heart failure (CHF), diabetes mellitus, renal insufficiency, and chronic liver disease. This has important implications for the nature of the infecting organisms,

TABLE 23–1 ■ **Classification of Types of Pneumonia**

Type of Pneumonia	*Subclassification*
Community-acquired pneumonia	Age <60, no other illness Age >60 or coexisting illness Severe or rapidly progressing pneumonia Pneumonia in nursing home residents
Nosocomial pneumonia	Ventilator-associated pneumonia Non–ventilator-associated pneumonia
Aspiration pneumonia	Infectious pneumonia Chemical pneumonitis
Pneumonia in the immunocompromised host	HIV/AIDS Chemotherapy for neoplastic diseases Organ or bone marrow transplant Diabetes Other immunocompromised states (e.g., hypogammaglobulinemia, neutrophil deficiencies, cellular)

initial treatment recommendations, and ultimately the prognosis (Fine et al, 1996, 1997, 1999).

Nosocomial pneumonia is defined as pneumonia occurring 48 to 72 hours after admission to a hospital. This type of pneumonia commonly reflects some type of compromise in host defense mechanisms and although the cause is usually bacterial (often due to gram-negative bacilli), fungal infection is also observed.

Aspiration pneumonia can be further divided into chemical pneumonitis resulting from aspiration of gastric contents and bacterial aspiration pneumonia.

Pneumonia in the immunocompromised host can be subdivided further based on the nature of the immunocompromised state (e.g., associated with human immunodeficiency virus (HIV) infection, chemotherapy, or organ transplantation).

Community-Acquired Pneumonia

Pathogenesis

Bacterial pneumonia is most commonly the result of bronchogenic spread of infection following microaspiration of infected oropharyngeal secretions. An important consideration is that the oropharyngeal flora changes after 48 to 72 hours of hospitalization and is one factor that accounts for differences in bacteriology between community-acquired and nosocomial pneumonia. Although aspiration of oropharyngeal secretions is common, occurring in 50% of normal subjects during sleep and in up to 70% of subjects with impaired consciousness (Huxley et al, 1978), the host defenses of the lung such as mucociliary clearance are usually able to clear potential pathogenic organisms and prevent parenchymal infection. However, under the appropriate conditions, including impaired host defenses (smoking, malnutrition, impaired cough), large bacterial load, or a virulent pathogen, these infectious particles are able to reach the terminal airways and alveoli where infection is initiated. The anatomic distribution of the resultant pneumonia is variable. Although not completely understood, factors that predispose to a multifocal distribution of pneumonia include the characteristics of the infecting organism and the host, including pre-existing COPD; concomitant viral tracheobronchitis, which impairs mucociliary clearance; and, aspiration of macroscopic particulate matter. Organisms such as *Streptococcus pyogenes*, virulent gram-negative bacteria, or anaerobic bacteria, are often associated with multifocal pneumonia.

Infectious agents can also reach the lower respiratory tract by direct inhalation. This route is common for the respiratory viruses *Mycoplasma pneumoniae, Chlamydia pneumoniae, Legionella* species, *Mycobacterium tuberculosis*, and certain fungi such as *Histoplasma capsulatum*. Less frequently, bacteria, such as *Staphylococcus aureus* and gram-negative enteric bacilli, can infect the lung hematogenously via the pulmonary and bronchial arteries, which may be secondary to intravascular infections such as septic thrombophlebitis or right-sided endocarditis.

Host Defense Mechanisms

The epithelial surface of the respiratory tract is a barrier between the host and the environment. That the lung is routinely exposed to potential pathogens yet maintains its sterility is a testimony to the effectiveness of the defenses of the respiratory system. These defenses include the aerodynamic filtration provided by the upper airway, the cough reflex, mucociliary clearance, phagocytic cells of the innate immune system (neutrophils and macrophages), endogenous antimicrobial products of the epithelial cells (e.g., defensins), and specific humoral (mucosal IgA and IgG) and cellular (lymphocytes) immunity (Reynolds, 1999). These defenses can become compromised at many levels. The upper airway filtration system can be bypassed by intubation or tracheostomy. Indeed, these represent important risk factors for nosocomial pneumonia (see later). Diminished ability to cough and clear secretions may be due to respiratory muscle weakness (severe COPD, prolonged steroid treatment, malnutrition), decreased level of consciousness, or severe incisional chest wall pain. Mechanical impedance to the clearance of secretions may be due to an endobronchial tumor or foreign body, including stents and T tubes. Mucociliary clearance can be impaired by recent cigarette smoking (up to 1 month prior to operation), inhalational anesthetics, alcoholism, COPD, cystic fibrosis, or ciliary dysmotility syndromes. The immune system can also be compromised by malnutrition, alcoholism, renal or hepatic failure, hypoxia, chemotherapy or radiation therapy, and congenital or acquired immunoglobulin deficiencies. These factors must be recognized and corrected, if possible, for effective treatment of pneumonia.

Microbiology

Community-acquired pneumonia can be caused by a wide variety of bacterial, viral, and fungal pathogens (Table 23–2). A definitive microbiologic diagnosis is made in only approximately 50% of cases, despite diag-

TABLE 23–2 ■ **Bacteriology of Community-Acquired Pneumonia**

Patients Without Comorbidity and Age <60	*Patients with Comorbidity or Age >60*	*Hospitalized Patients with Community-Acquired Pneumonia*	*Severely Ill Hospitalized Patients with Community-Acquired Pneumonia*
S. pneumoniae	*S. pneumoniae*	*S. pneumoniae*	*S. pneumoniae*
M. pneumoniae	Respiratory viruses	*H. influenzae*	*Legionella* species
Respiratory viruses	*H. influenzae*	Polymicrobial (including anaerobic bacteria)	Aerobic gram-negative bacilli
C. pneumoniae	Aerobic gram-negative bacilli	Aerobic gram-negative bacilli	*M. pneumoniae*
H. influenzae	*S. aureus*	*Legionella* species	Respiratory viruses
Legionella species	*M. catarrhalis*	*S. aureus*	*H. influenzae*
S. aureus		*C. pneumoniae*	*M. tuberculosis*
M. tuberculosis	*M. tuberculosis*	Respiratory viruses	Endemic fungi
Endemic fungi	Endemic fungi	*M. pneumonia*	
Aerobic gram-negative bacilli		*M. catarrhalis*	
		M. tuberculosis	
		Endemic fungi	

nostic efforts (Bates et al, 1992). Bacterial pathogens responsible for pneumonia have traditionally been divided into "typical" organisms, including *Streptococcus pneumoniae. Haemophilus influenzae, S. aureus, Pseudomonas aeruginosa, Klebsiella pneumoniae*, and "atypical" organisms, including *Legionella* species, *M. pneumoniae*, and *C. pneumoniae*. Although this scheme is useful in the epidemiologic classification of pneumonias, it is important to note that *the clinical syndrome associated with the different pathogens cannot be reliably distinguished on clinical or radiographic grounds* (Fang, 1990).

Pneumonia Caused by *S. pneumoniae* as a Paradigm for Bacterial Pneumonia

S. pneumoniae (pneumococcus) remains the most common cause of community-acquired pneumonia and is responsible for between 5% and 20% of cases. However, evidence suggests that many culture-negative cases of pneumonia are in fact caused by *S. pneumoniae*: sputum cultures are negative in about one half of cases with pneumococcal bacteremia (Barrett-Connor, 1971); invasive techniques to obtain uncontaminated lower respiratory tract secretions (transtracheal and transthoracic aspiration) have identified *S. pneumoniae* in a high percentage of cases (Bartlett and Mundy, 1995); and about two thirds of bacteremic pneumonias are attributable to *S. pneumoniae* (Fine et al, 1996). Risk factors for pneumococcal pneumonia include advanced age, alcoholism, cigarette smoking, dementia, malnutrition, infection with HIV, and the presence of chronic illness (e.g., congestive heart failure, chronic renal failure). Patients who have undergone splenectomy have an increased risk for pneumococcal bacteremia and overwhelming sepsis because the spleen is the primary site of clearance of the organism.

The clinical features of this pneumonia are fever, cough, and production of purulent sputum. Radiographically, infiltrates associated with *S. pneumoniae* can range from a classic lobar distribution to patchy bilateral infiltrates. Small parapneumonic effusions are commonly present but empyema is uncommon (1% to 2% of cases). Bacteremia occurs in 20% to 30% of cases, and extrapulmonary infections include sinusitis, otitis media, meningitis, and endocarditis.

Until recently, penicillin has been the recommended treatment for *S. pneumoniae*. However, the increasing incidence of penicillin-resistant organisms has become a worldwide problem (Low, 1998). In areas where penicillin resistance is high, alternative antibiotics, including second-generation cephalosporins such as cephuroxime and macrolides such as clarithromycin or azithromycin, should be considered.

Other Bacterial Pneumonias. Infections with other bacteria, including *H. influenzae, S. aureus, Moraxella catarrhalis*, and other gram-negative bacteria such as *P. aeruginosa* and *K. pneumoniae* account for between 3% and 10% of cases of community-acquired pneumonia (Bartlett and Mundy, 1995). Pneumonia caused by *S. aureus* is seen most commonly in the elderly and in patients recovering from influenza. This is usually a rapidly progressing pneumonia involving the formation of pneumatoceles and abcesses that are associated with a high mortality rate. Pneumonia caused by *S. pyogenes* (group A streptococcus) is usually a rapidly progressing infection associated with empyema formation. Anaerobic organisms of oropharyngeal origin (*Bacteroides* species, *Fusobacterium*) are the most common cause of "aspiration pneumonia" and are associated with necrotizing pneumonia, abcess formation, and empyema. The role of anaerobic organisms in the syndrome of community-acquired pneumonia is uncertain, in large part because routine culture techniques are not suitable for their culture. However, several studies have suggested that anaerobic organisms may account for up to 30% of pneumonias (Bartlett and Mundy, 1995).

Atypical organisms, including *M. pneumoniae, Legionella* species, and *C. pneumoniae*, are frequently seen in community-acquired pneumonia in younger adults (File et al, 1998).

Pneumonia due to *M. pneumoniae* is the second most common cause of pneumonia (after *S. pneumoniae*) in North America as well as in other parts of the world (Marrie et al, 1996). However, it is likely that the incidence may be higher than reported because undoubtably many mild cases go unreported. *M. pneumoniae* is transmitted from person to person by infected respiratory droplets, and the incubation period varies from 1 to 3 weeks. The incidence of infection is highest in children of school age, in military recruits, and in college students. There are no clinical features—symptoms, physical findings, or radiographic appearances—that can reliably distinguish pneumonia due to *Mycoplasma* species from community-acquired pneumonias of bacterial origin. Moreover, the culture of *M. pneumoniae* is difficult, so a definitive diagnosis depends on serologic testing.

Pneumonia Caused by Mycoplasma *Species.* The clinical presentation of pneumonia caused by *Mycoplasma* species is usually gradual, involving headache, malaise, chills (but not rigors), low-grade fever, sore throat, rhinorrhea, ear pain, and cough, which is often intractable (Lieberman, 1996). Wheezing and dyspnea may occur, and infection due to *M. pneumoniae* has been associated with exacerbations of asthma (Kraft et al, 1998). (The abnormalities found on physical examination of the chest are often minimal, although crackles and wheezes may be present. Extrapulmonary involvement may include skin rash, arthritis, evidence of hemolysis, and involvement of the central nervous system (aseptic meningitis, peripheral neurophathy, cranial nerve palsies). Radiographic abnormalities that have been described commonly include pulmonary infiltrates in a peribronchial distribution, nodular infiltrates, areas of plate-like atelectasis, and hilar adenopathy. Pleural effusions can occur in up to one quarter of cases. Laboratory abnormalities include anemia, which may be hemolytic and associated with a positive Coombs test due to cold agglutinins. The latter are not specific for *M. pneumoniae* and may be seen with other infections such as the Epstein-Barr virus. The white blood cell count is usually normal. Definitive serologic diagnosis requires demonstration of a 4-fold or greater rise (or a single titer greater than 1:32) in IgM or IgG, which is measured by a complement fixation test. Other tests are available, including enzyme-linked immunosorbent assay (ELISA), antigen detection (antigen-capture enzyme immunoassay), and polymerase chain reaction (PCR) detection of genomic DNA (Ramirez et al, 1996).

Pneumonia Caused by Legionella *Species.* Pneumonia due to the *Legionella* species (*Legionella pneumophila*), first identified in 1976 during an outbreak of pneumonia at a convention of the American Legion in Philadelphia (Fraser et al, 1977), is a relatively common cause of both community-acquired and hospital-acquired pneumonia. Symptoms of pneumonia (chills, fever, cough, dyspnea, chest pain) are the predominant clinical manifestation of infection with *Legionella* species but nonpulmonary manifestations such as gastrointestinal symptoms (diarrhea, nausea, vomiting, and abdominal pain), myalgias, arthralgias, lethargy, and neurologic abnormalities (headache, decreased level of consciousness) are common. Fever is usually present and can be higher than 40°C, and bradycardia relative to the temperature elevation is common, especially in elderly patients. Crackles and signs of consolidation are commonly noted on physical examination of the chest. Nonpulmonary findings on physical examination include various rashes and neuropathies.

A variety of laboratory abnormalities are observed in patients with pneumonia caused by *Legionella* species, including leukocytosis, hematuria, renal and hepatic dysfunction, thrombocytopenia, hyponatremia, and coagulopathy. Although there are no characteristic radiographic abnormalities, the most common pattern is a patchy unilobar infiltrate that progresses to consolidation. Other patterns can be present, including diffuse bilateral interstitial infiltrates. Pleural effusions are common.

Clues to diagnosis of infection by *Legionella* species include the presence of gastrointestinal symptoms, the gram stain of respiratory secretions showing many neutrophils but few organisms, hyponatremia, and failure to respond to β-lactam antibiotics.

Pneumonia Caused by Chlamydia *Species. Chlamydia* species (*C. pneumoniae*, *C. psittaci*) are obligate intracellular parasites whose role in the pathogenesis of pneumonia became apparent during the 1990s. Estimates using serologic techniques have put the incidence of infection with *C. pneumoniae* as high as 10% to 20% in patients with community-acquired pneumonia who did not require hospitalization (Chirgwin et al, 1991; Marrie et al, 1996). There have also been associations of chlamydial infections with coronary artery disease (Thom et al, 1992) and asthma (Emre et al, 1995).

There are no distinguishing clinical features of pneumonia with *C. pneumoniae*, although gradual onset of symptoms, pharyngitis, hoarseness, and sinusitis have been commonly reported. As with other atypical pneumonias, the white blood cell count tends to be normal. The chest radiograph commonly demonstrates one or a few areas of patchy consolidation. Extrapulmonary manifestations of *C. pneumoniae* include meningoencephalitis, Guillain-Barré syndrome, arthritis, and myocarditis. The diagnosis of *C. pneumoniae* infection can be difficult to establish because most laboratories do not have the capability to culture the organism. Techniques that are useful include nasopharyngeal swabs (not sputum culture), serologic testing, antigen detection, and PCR.

Clinical Evaluation of Patients with Community-Acquired Pneumonia

During the initial evaluation of a patient with suspected pneumonia, there are several immediate priorities (Fig. 23–1). The highest priority is given to cardiopulmonary stabilization, including treatment of acute respiratory failure if present. Early institution of antibiotic therapy is essential to effective treatment. Broad-spectrum antibiotics chosen according to the clinical situation should be initiated promptly. Ideally, sputum and blood cultures should be obtained prior to the institution of antibiotics, but *antibiotic therapy should not be delayed* if the patient is unable to provide a sputum sample. The next decisions are whether hospitalization is required and whether intensive care monitoring is indicated.

Patients with community-acquired pneumonia usually come to medical attention based on the development of

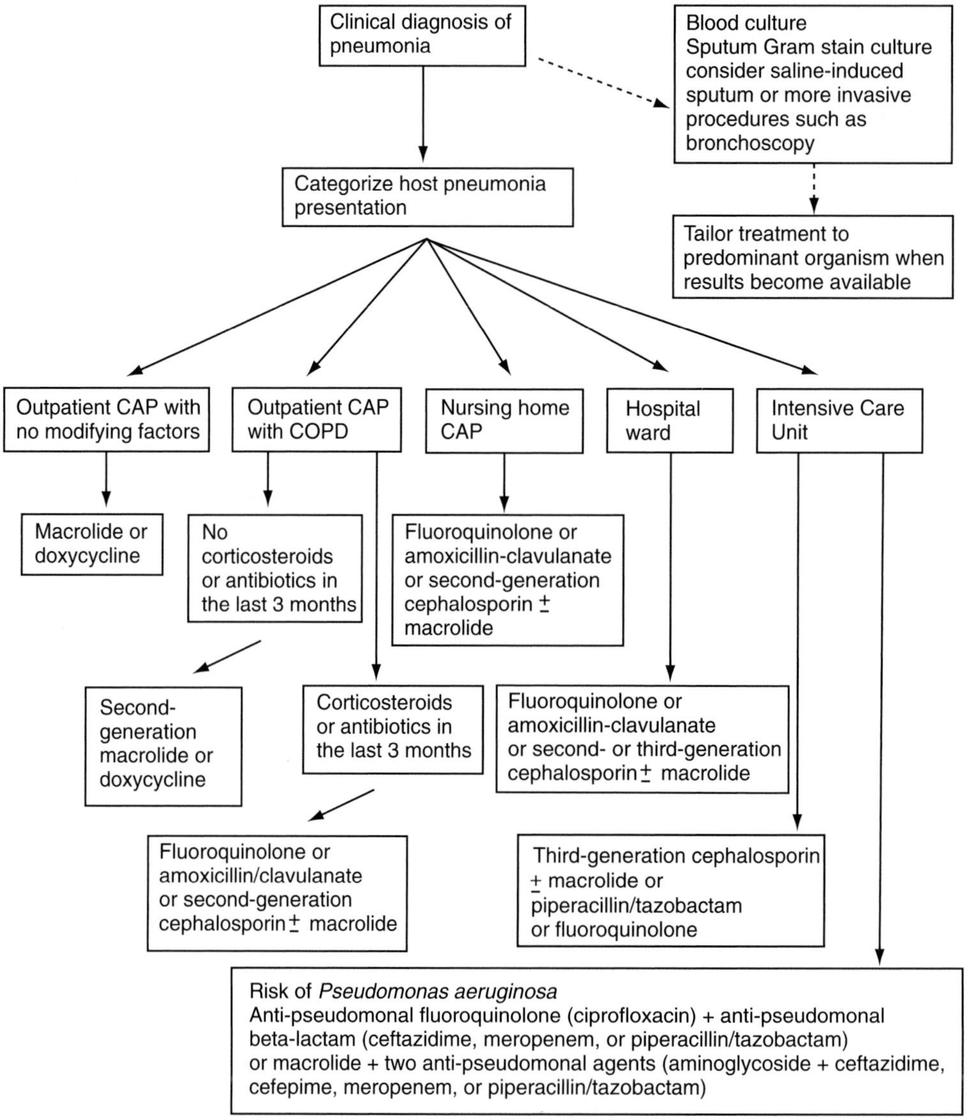

Clinical diagnosis of pneumonia

Blood culture
Sputum Gram stain culture
consider saline-induced sputum or more invasive procedures such as bronchoscopy

Tailor treatment to predominant organism when results become available

Categorize host pneumonia presentation

Outpatient CAP with no modifying factors

Outpatient CAP with COPD

Nursing home CAP

Hospital ward

Intensive Care Unit

Macrolide or doxycycline

No corticosteroids or antibiotics in the last 3 months

Fluoroquinolone or amoxicillin-clavulanate or second-generation cephalosporin ± macrolide

Second-generation macrolide or doxycycline

Corticosteroids or antibiotics in the last 3 months

Fluoroquinolone or amoxicillin-clavulanate or second- or third-generation cephalosporin ± macrolide

Fluoroquinolone or amoxicillin/clavulanate or second-generation cephalosporin ± macrolide

Third-generation cephalosporin ± macrolide or piperacillin/tazobactam or fluoroquinolone

Risk of *Pseudomonas aeruginosa*
Anti-pseudomonal fluoroquinolone (ciprofloxacin) + anti-pseudomonal beta-lactam (ceftazidime, meropenem, or piperacillin/tazobactam) or macrolide + two anti-pseudomonal agents (aminoglycoside + ceftazidime, cefepime, meropenem, or piperacillin/tazobactam)

FIGURE 23–1 ■ Flow chart for patients with community-acquired pneumonia (CAP). COPD, chronic obstructive pulmonary disease.

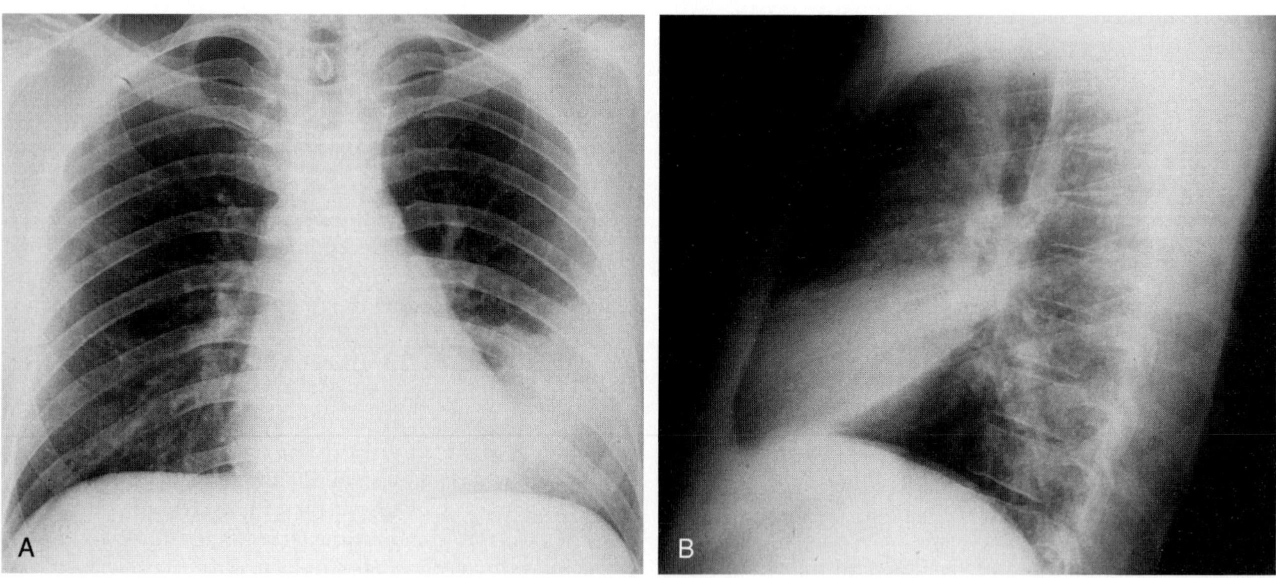

FIGURE 23–2 ■ Posteroanterior *(A)* and lateral *(B)* chest radiograph illustrating lobar consolidation in the lingula owing to mycoplasma.

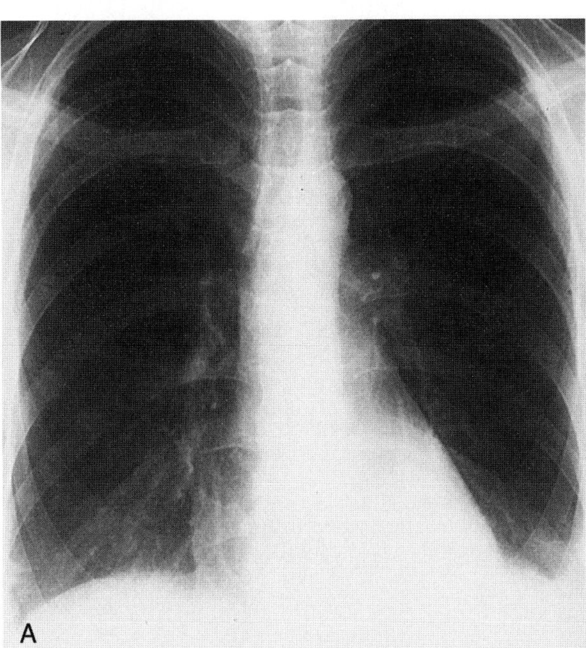

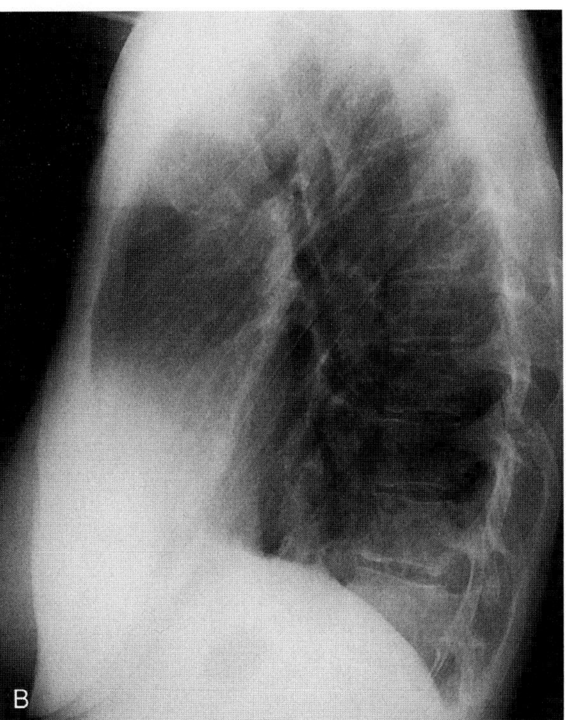

FIGURE 23–3 ■ Posteroanterior *(A)* and lateral *(B)* chest radiograph illustrating bronchopneumonia in the posterior basal segment of the left lower lobe owing to *Haemophilus influenzae.*

symptoms that include fever or hypothermia, rigors, sweats, cough, with or without sputum production, alteration of the color of respiratory tract secretion, chest discomfort, or dyspnea (Metlay et al, 1997). Nonrespiratory symptoms such as headache, abdominal pain, anorexia, nausea, myalgias, arthralgias, or mental confusion may be present in 10% to 30% of patients. Nonspecific symptoms are common in elderly patients.

Abnormalities on physical examination may include the presence of fever (80%), tachypnea (45% to 70%), and tachycardia. Examination of the chest reveals the presence of crackles or wheeze in most patients or, less commonly (30% to 40% of patients), signs of consolidation. As many of the symptoms and signs of pneumonia are nonspecific, it is essential that a chest radiograph be obtained for the proper diagnosis and management of pneumonia.

The majority of patients have leukocytosis that ranges from 15 to 30 $\times$ 10^8/L, often with an increased percentage of immature cells (left shift) which indicates mobilization of the bone marrow reserves in response to the infection. The presence of leukopenia (white blood cell count $< 3 \times 10^8$/L) carries a poor prognosis.

Radiographic Evaluation. The presence of a pulmonary infiltrate on a chest radiograph, when the clinical and microbiologic features are compatible, represents the gold standard for the diagnosis of pneumonia, although the radiographic picture may lag behind the clinical presentation. In concert with other clinical information, the radiographic picture can favor one or several causative agents (Tenholder et al, 1998). Possible radiographic patterns include lobar or segmental consolidation (Fig. 23–2); patchy bronchopneumonia (Fig. 23–3); nodules (large, small, miliary) (Fig. 23–4); and interstitial process (Fig. 23–5). Lobar or segmental consolidation is commonly seen with pneumococcal or *H. influenzae* pneumonia but can also be associated with pneumonias due to *Legionella* or *Mycoplasma* species. Pneumonia associated with large

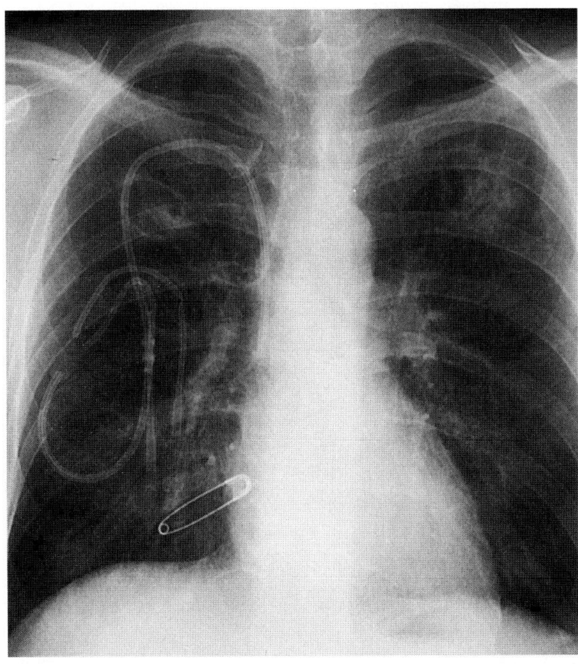

FIGURE 23–4 ■ Nodular infiltrates with cavitation in the upper lobes on the posteroanterior chest radiograph of a patient with pneumonia caused by *Enterobacter cloacae.*

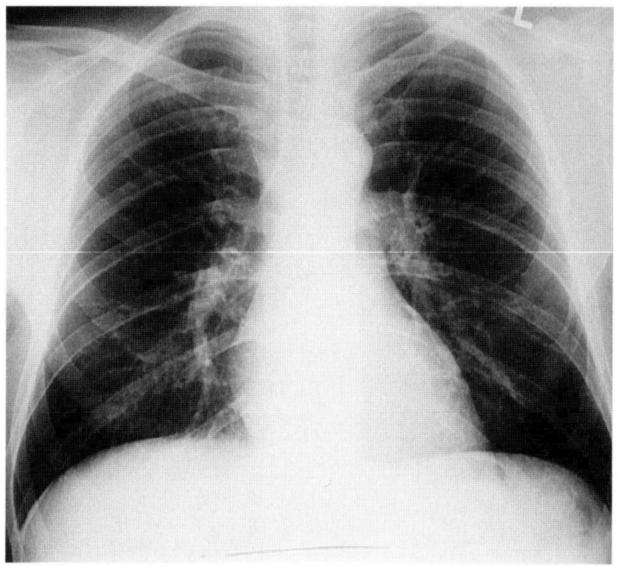

FIGURE 23–5 ■ Interstitial infiltrates illustrated on the posteroanterior chest radiograph of a patient with cytomegalovirus pneumonia.

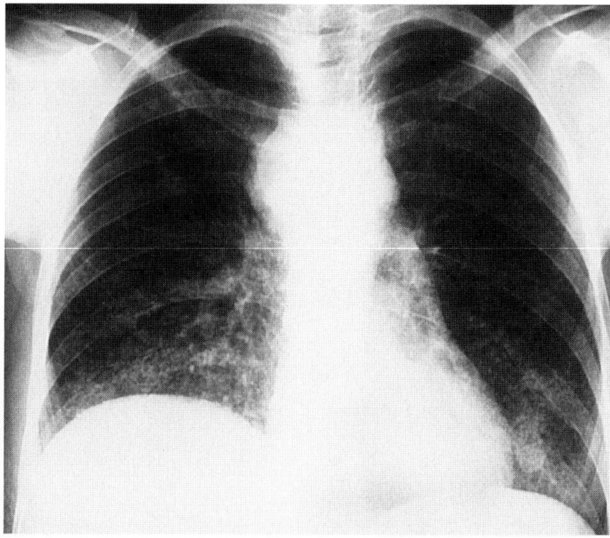

FIGURE 23–7 ■ Posteroanterior chest radiograph illustrating the typical miliary pattern of tuberculosis. Also note the prominent right paratracheal lymphadenopathy.

nodules raises the possibility of infection with *S. aureus* (Fig. 23–6) or gram-negative organisms such as *P. aeruginosa*, especially with hematogenous spread due to endocarditis or an infected vascular access catheter. Fungal pneumonias can be associated with nodules that commonly cavitate. A miliary pattern (1- to 2-mm nodules the size of millet seeds (Fig. 23–7) is highly suggestive of mycobacterial (*M. tuberculosis)* or fungal infection. An intersitital pattern (Fig. 23–8) is associated with infection by virus or *Mycoplasma* or *Chlamydia* species but can also be seen with bacterial pneumonias, including *S. pyogenes*. Pleural effusions may be associated with pneumonias due to many infectious agents but effusions that are large and appear early in the course of pneumonias are often associated with *S. pyogenes* pneumonia and anaerobic pneumonias.

Sputum Examination. The determination of the microbiologic cause of a pneumonia is difficult and, despite best efforts, is successful in only about one half of cases (Bates et al, 1992). The utility of sputum examination in establishing the microbiologic source of pneumonia is controversial, and current guidelines de-emphasize this procedure (Plouffe et al, 1998). However, examination of sputum, especially of sputum induced by inhalation of hypertonic saline and examined using special stains, can be helpful in the identification of *M. tuberculosis* and *Pneumocystis* and *Legionella* species. A Gram stain of

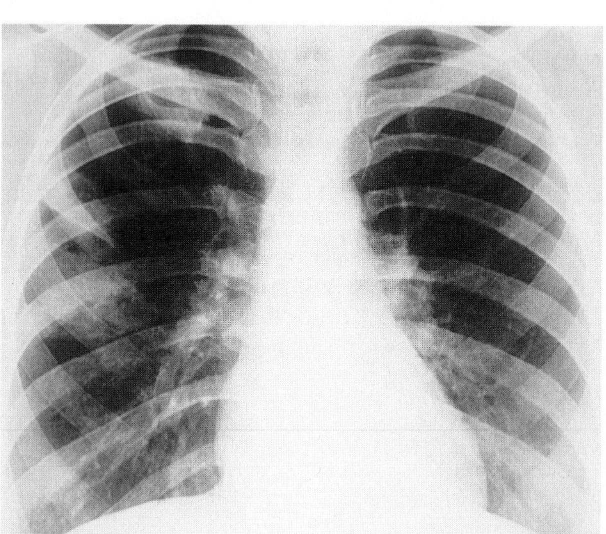

FIGURE 23–6 ■ Posteroanterior chest radiograph illustrating cavitating large nodules in the right upper lobe in a patient with *Staphylococcus aureus* pneumonia.

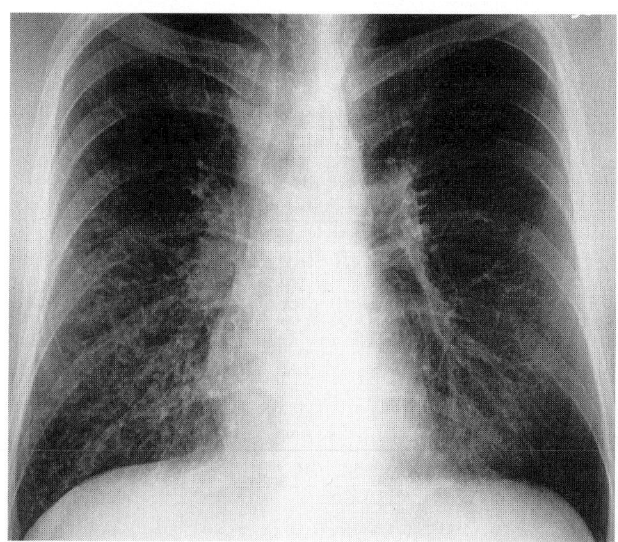

FIGURE 23–8 ■ Posteroanterior chest radiograph illustrating an interstitial pattern in a patient with *Mycoplasma* pneumonia. This pattern is one of several radiographic patterns seen with *Mycoplasma* (see Fig. 23–2).

expectorated induced sputum is helpful if an adequate sample is obtained and if there is a predominant organism. Several factors may contribute to the unreliability of sputum examination, including delays in reaching the laboratory, operator variation in staining techniques, the fact that one third of patients are not able to produce a sputum specimen, and the fact that up to one quarter of patients have received antibiotics prior to the collection of the sputum specimen. However, when performed by experienced laboratory personnel, Gram stain of sputum has been shown to be valuable in the prediction of common types of bacterial pneumonia (Fine et al, 1991). Moreover, what is absent on the Gram stain (e.g., neutrophils or gram-negative bacilli) is often important in making decisions about initial antibiotic choices. *Collection of a sputum specimen should not delay initiation of antibiotic therapy.*

Sputum cultures are helpful if there is a pure growth of a pathogen, of *M. tuberculosis*, of *Legionella* species, or of endemic fungi. Cultures are also useful if resistant organisms are identified.

Invasive Diagnostic Testing. Attempts to obtain uncontaminated lower respiratory secretions by means of invasive measures that include transtracheal aspiration, transbronchial protected specimen brush (PSB), and bronchoalveolar lavage (BAL) are not commonly performed in the setting of community-acquired pneumonia (Mares and Wilkes, 1998). However, if an accurate diagnosis is essential in an extremely ill patient, bronchoscopy and PSB or BAL should be considered. Transtracheal aspiration is associated with significant morbidity and is not frequently used.

If a pleural effusion is present, pleural fluid cultures are highly specific for the causative agent of the underlying pneumonia.

Serologic and Other Blood Testing. Serologic studies are required to establish the cause of atypical pneumonias, including those caused by *Mycoplasma, Legionella*, and *Chlamydia* species. Because the results of these tests are often delayed as long as several weeks, clinical decisions regarding therapy must be made long before the test results are available. However, there are certain exceptions. For example, the findings of *Legionella* antigen or a *Chlamydia* antigen in serum or urine may sometimes be rapidly available and therefore of use in determining or tailoring therapy.

Blood cultures should be obtained from any patient sick enough to warrant hospitalization even though only 10% to 20% of patients will be bacteremic.

Molecular Medicine and Diagnostic Testing. Rapid developments in the field of molecular medicine have had a strong impact on diagnostic testing, including that for pneumonia. Methods of detecting specific pathogens in respiratory secretions (e.g., sputum or the results of BAL) using sensitive immunofluorescent techniques are currently available. As an example, the direct fluorescent antigen (DFA) test for *Legionella* species is used commonly. The use of the PCR for the detection of mycobacterial, *Chlamydia*, and *Legionella* DNA is also becoming possible and it has a rapid turnaround time. However, large studies are needed to validate these techniques before their use becomes widespread.

Therapy for Patients with Community-Acquired Pneumonia

At the time of initial evaluation of patients with suspected pneumonia, a specific microbiologic diagnosis can rarely be made because neither the clinical presentation nor the commonly used diagnostic tests (sputum Gram stain, chest radiograph) are sensitive or specific enough to identify the pathogenic microorganism; therefore antibiotic therapy must be chosen empirically. Eventually, days or weeks later, a specific diagnosis may be made. This information is often more useful for epidemiologic purposes than for initial clinical decision making. Empiric therapy is based on the setting in which the infection was acquired and the clinical characteristics of the patient (see Table 23–1). Initial guidelines for the treatment of community-acquired pneumonia focused on the presence or absence of comorbid conditions, the severity of illness, and whether treatment was to be given on an outpatient or inpatient basis (Farber, 1999; Mandell, 1999; Niederman et al, 1993; Woodhead, 1998; Wunderlink, 1998). However, several developments have transpired since the publication of these guidelines. First, recent epidemiologic studies have provided a basis for more accurate risk prediction and decisions about hospital admission (Auble et al, 1998; Fine et al, 1997). Second, the prevalence of antibiotic resistance in common lower respiratory pathogens has increased the necessity of re-evaluating the choice of antimicrobial agents (Cunha and Shea, 1998). Third, a myriad of antibiotics, including new macrolides and quinolones, are now available; they have improved activity and pharmacokinetic properties such as enhanced oral bioavailability. Finally, the availability of home intravenous antibiotic programs and home nursing care has greatly reduced the need for and duration of hospitalization (Mandell et al, 2000).

Choice of Antibiotic Therapy for Community-Acquired Pneumonia. The general approach to the treatment of community-acquired pneumonia is to categorize patients according to whether they can be treated as outpatients, are nursing-home residents, or require hospitalization. Patients with risk factors associated with a poor prognosis should be hospitalized (Table 23–3). It is to be noted that bacterial pneumonia after recent influenza infection can be life-threatening, particularly in elderly patients (Louria et al, 1959; Schwartzmann et al, 1971). In the majority of patients with community-acquired pneumonia, no pathogen has been identified. Thus, in most instances, the physician initiates empiric antibiotics on the basis of epidemiologic data. If the causative pathogen is identified (either initially or at a later time), the antibiotic spectrum should be directed specifically against this organism. When no pathogen is discovered, broad-spectrum empiric antibiotics are continued (Bernstein, 1999). Table 23–4 outlines an approach to the initial antibiotic therapy for patients, based on the most recent guidelines (Mandell et al, 2000). It is to be emphasized that these

TABLE 23–3 ■ **Risk Factors Associated with Poor Outcome in Community-Acquired Pneumonia**

Coexisting Conditions	Laboratory Abnormalities
Age >60	Leukocytosis $>30 \times 10^9$/L
COPD	Leukopenia $<4 \times 10^9$/L or absolute neutrophil count $<1 \times 10^9$/L
Bronchiectasis	Urea >7 mM/L (20 mg/dl)
Chronic renal failiure	Hemoglobin <90 g/L
Congestive heart failure	Hypoxemia: Pa_{O_2} <60 mm Hg
Chronic liver disease	Hypercapnea: Pa_{CO_2} >50 mm Hg
Alcoholism	Metabolic acidosis
Malnutrition	Coagulopathy (increased partial thromboplastin time, decreased platelet count, or presence of fibrin split products)
Previous splenectomy	Multilobular or rapidly progressive radiography infiltrates
Recent hospitalization (<1 yr)	Presence of a pleural effusion
Physiologic Abnormalities	**Atypical Presenting Features**
Respiratory rate >30 breaths/min	Confusion
Hypotension	Predominantly nonrespiratory complaints
Systolic blood pressure <90	Absence of fever
Diastolic blood pressure <60 mm Hg	
Temperature >38.3°C or <36.5°C	
Tachycardia >120 bpm	

COPD, chronic obstructive pulmonary disease.

guidelines should be used as a guide rather than as an inflexible set of rules. Individual patient factors, such as the presence of comorbid illness, the severity of illness, local microbiologic information (hospital resistance patterns and so forth), and response to initial therapy, should be considered in making the final decision.

For outpatients with no comorbid illness who are 60 years of age or younger, initial treatment with a macrolide (erythromycin, clarithromycin, or azithromycin) or doxycycline should suffice to cover common bacterial (*S. pneumoniae*) and atypical pathogens (*M. pneumoniae, C. pneumoniae*). Erythromycin is often poorly tolerated whereas the newer macrolides are substantially more expensive. Patients with COPD who have not received antibiotics or oral glucocorticoids in the past 3 months have an increased risk of infection with *H. influenzae, M. catarrhalis*, and enteric gram-negative rods, so treatment with a newer (respiratory) quinolone such as levofloxacin or sparfloxacin is recommended. Alternative treatment strategies for these patients include amoxicillin-clavulanate or a second-generation cephalosporin (cefuroxime, cefpodoxime, or cefprozil), usually with the addition of a macrolide. For patients who are older than 60 or who have comorbid illness, broader spectrum antibiotics are recommended. For patients with suspected aspiration in an outpatient setting, amoxicillin-clavulanate, clinda-

TABLE 23–4 ■ **Empiric Antimicrobial Selection for Adults with Community-Acquired Pneumonia**

Patient	*Medications*
Outpatient without modifying factors	1st choice: macrolide (erythromycin, clarithromycin, or azithromycin) 2nd choice: doxycycline
Outpatient with modifying factors	
COPD (no recent antibiotic or steroids)	Same as outpatient without modifying factors
COPD (recent antibiotic or PO steroids)	1st choice: respiratory quinolone (levofloxacin, sparfloxacin) 2nd choice: amoxicillin/clavulanate ± macrolide or second generation cephalosporin ± macrolide
Suspected aspiration	1st choice: amoxicillin/clavulanate or clindamycin 2nd choice: respiratory quinolone with enhanced activity against anaerobes (clinafloxacin or moxifloxacin)
Nursing home resident residing in a nursing home	1st choice: respiratory quinolone (levofloxacin, sparfloxacin) or amoxicillin/clavulanate 2nd choice: second-generation cephalosporin plus macrolide
Nursing home resident in hospital	Identical to treatment of other hospitalized patients
Hospitalized patient on medical ward	1st choice: respiratory quinolone (levofloxacin, sparfloxacin) 2nd choice: dual therapy with second- or third-generation cephalosporin plus macrolide
Hospitalized patient in intensive care unit	1st choice: dual therapy with respiratory quinolone (levofloxacin,) plus β-lactamase (cefotaxime, ceftriaxone, ceftazidime, piperacillin-tazobactam, imipenem, meropenem, aztreonam) or dual therapy of respiratory quinolone + aminoglycoside (gentamicin, tobramycin, amikacin) 2nd choice: triple therapy with β-lactamase plus aminoglycoside plus macrolide

mycin, or a newer quinolone with activity against anaerobic oropharyngeal bacteria, such as levofloxacin or sparfloxacin, is recommended. Residents of nursing homes who have pneumonia should be evaluated with the same prediction rules for hospitalization as patients with community-acquired pneumonia. For patients who do not require hospitalization, a newer quinolone (levofloxacin or sparfloxacin) or amoxicillin-clavulanate with or without a macrolide is recommended. An alternative choice would be a second-generation cephalosporin with or without a macrolide.

Patients with community-acquired pneumonia who require hospitalization can be subdivided into those who can be managed on a general medical ward and those who require cardioventilatory support in an intensive care unit. For the former, the focus of treatment is on several pathogens including *S. pneumoniae* (with the potential to be bacteremic), *H. influenzae*, enteric gram-negative bacilli, and severe infection by *Legionella* or *Chlamydia* species. Recommendations for the treatment of patients on a general medical ward include a respiratory quinolone (levofloxacin, sparfloxacin) or a second- (cefuroxime) or third- (cefotaxime, ceftriaxone, ceftazidime, or cefepime) generation cephalosporin plus a macrolide. If aspiration is suspected, a respiratory quinolone with activity against anaerobes, such as clinafloxacin or moxifloxacin, should be considered. For patients requiring intensive care support, treatment is directed against the more resistant gram-negative bacilli, including *P. aeruginosa*, and the multiresistant gram-negative bacilli (which may be acquired nosocomially subsequent to admission to the intensive care unit). For these patients, dual therapy with a respiratory quinolone plus either a β-lactamase (cefotaxime, ceftriaxone, ceftazidime, piperacillin-tazobactam, carbapenem, or aztreonam) or an aminoglycoside (gentamicin, tobramycin, or amikacin) is recommended. Alternatively, triple therapy with a β-lactamase plus an aminoglycoside and a macrolide can be considered. Once the causative agent has been identified, the initial (empiric) therapy can be narrowed and directed at the specific pathogens.

Special Considerations. Treatment with β-lactamase antibiotics such as penicillins and cephalosporins is effective for infections caused by sensitive pyogenic organisms such as *S. pneumonia*, but these agents are not effective in treating organisms such as *M. pneumoniae, C. pneumoniae*, and *Legionella* species. First-generation macrolides such as erythromycin are effective against these three organisms as well as *S. pneumoniae* but not against *H. influenzae*, and they are often poorly tolerated because of gastrointestinal side effects. In outpatients in whom these organisms are a possibility (e.g., smokers), monotherapy with a second-generation macrolide, such as clarithromycin or azithromycin, or a quinolone such as levofloxacin is possible. Interactions between macrolides and other drugs, including anticoagulants, theophylline, antiarrhythmics, and immunosuppressive agents (cyclosporin, tacrolimus), must be taken into consideration when prescribing these agents.

Duration of Antibiotic Therapy. The optimum duration of parenteral therapy, the timing of conversion from intravenous to oral therapy, and the duration of oral therapy are important variables for which there are no firm answers (Cassiere, 1998b). The presence of coexisting illness, the severity of the pneumonia, the nature of the infecting organism, the subsequent hospital course, the presence of bacteremia, and the presence of complications are all factors that should be considered in making decisions about the route and duration of antibiotic therapy. In general, bacterial infections such as *S. pneumoniae* and *H. influenzae* should be treated for 7 to 10 days. Infection due to *M. pneumoniae* and *C. pneumoniae* should be treated for 10 to 14 days. The duration of treatment of infection due to *Legionella* species should be 14 days in immunocompetent patients and up to 21 days in immunocompromised patients.

Shorter courses of therapy for pneumonia may be possible in certain cases. Newer macrolides such as azithromycin have a much longer serum (11–14 hours) and tissue half-life than most other antibiotics, which allows the shortening of therapy (equivalent to the "area under the curve"). A cautionary note should be added, however, because at the doses currently approved, azithromycin does not achieve high serum levels and should not be used in cases in which bacteremia is known or suspected. The optimal duration of antibiotic therapy is uncertain, and additional studies are needed to address this important issue.

The decision regarding the timing of the switch from parenteral to oral therapy should be made based on considerations concerning both the patient and the pharmacologic characteristics of the antibiotic. The patient must be able to take medication orally (have an adequate level of consciousness or a feeding tube) and must have a functioning gastrointestinal tract. With respect to the antibiotic, the primary issue is whether oral administration is able to achieve adequate serum and tissue levels. For certain antibiotics including chloramphenicol, trimethoprim-sulfamethoxazole, doxycycline, and fluoroquinolones such as ciprofloxacin and levofloxacin, oral administration achieves levels comparable to those reached by means of the intravenous route (Cunha, 1991). With other agents, in which bioavailability by means of the oral route is not as good, the switch from parenteral to oral therapy should occur after the patient has been stabilized and is improving on parenteral therapy so higher tissue levels are no longer required. Practically, this means after 3 to 6 days of parenteral therapy, when the clinical condition of the patient has stabilized and fever has subsided (Cassiere 1998b; and Paladino, 1991).

Assessment of the Initial Response to Therapy. Most patients with community-acquired pneumonia respond to initial empiric therapy in 48 to 72 hours with resolution of fever and normalization of the white blood cell count. Abnormalities on physical examination such as crackles may persist for longer than 1 week in 40% of patients.

Radiographic Clearance of Pneumonia. A difficult but not uncommon problem in pneumonia patients is slow recovery and delayed resolution of radiographically observable infiltrates. Factors that impact negatively on pneumonia resolution include advanced age and the presence of serious comorbid illnesses such as diabetes mellitus, renal disease, or COPD. In addition, certain properties of the infecting agent (e.g., intrinsic virulence) may interact with host factors and advanced age to delay resolution of pneumonia. For example, 50% of patients with pneumococcal pneumonia have radiographic clearing at 5 weeks, and the majority clear within 2 to 3 months. Recent data demonstrate that radiographic resolution is most strongly influenced by the number of lobes involved and the age of the patient. Radiographic clearance decreases by 20% per decade after age 20, and patients with multilobar infiltrates take longer to clear than those with unilobar disease. If the patient has either no identifiable factors associated with prolonged resolution of pneumonia or the repeat chest radiograph at 1 month shows no appreciable change, further diagnostic testing is indicated.

Failure to Respond Adequately to Initial Therapy. Several questions arise when a patient does not respond as expected to the initial therapy. Is the antibiotic therapy appropriate and adequate? Is the infection caused by an unusual organism? A careful re-evaluation of the history, including country of origin, travel, and unusual exposures, is important under these circumstances. Organisms to be considered in patients with persistent clinical and radiographic features include viral infections, *M. tuberculosis*; fungi such as *Histoplasma* species, *Blastomyces* species, and *Coccidioides* species; and parasites such as *Pneumocystis carinii* and *Paragonimus* species. Is it an infective process or something unrelated, such as CHF, pulmonary embolus, pulmonary hemorrhage, eosinophilic pneumonia, or vasculitis? Has a nosocomial infection developed such as antibiotic-induced colitis, or is there a complication of the pneumonia?

Complications of Pneumonia. Complications of pneumonia include empyema, lung abscess, bacteremia or septicemia, and extrapulmonary sites of infection, including otitis media, sinusitis, endocarditis, pericarditis, brain abscess, and meningitis. These complications should be considered in patients who respond inadequately to antibiotics. The early identification and treatment of parapneumonic effusions is essential to prevent the need for operative drainage procedures.

ACUTE BRONCHITIS (TRACHEOBRONCHITIS)

Acute inflammation involving the mucosa of the trachea and bronchi is extremely common and of diverse etiology. Irritants such as constituents of the smoke of tobacco and cannabis, gases such as ammonia, trace elements such as vanadium and cadmium, air pollutants such as sulfur dioxide and nitrogen dioxide as well as industrial byproducts, including cotton and bagasse, can induce acute inflammation of the trachea and bronchi. The most common cause of acute tracheobronchitis is infection due to viruses, *Mycoplasma* species, bacteria, or parasites. Viruses known to be associated with acute tracheobronchitis include respiratory syncytial viruses, rhinoviruses, echo viruses, parainfluenza viruses types 1, 2, and 3, Coxsackie viruses, influenza viruses, adenoviruses, herpes viruses, and corona viruses. The syndromes caused by these viruses are virtually inseparable, although some reasonable estimations of the likelihood of a particular agent can be made on the basis of the season of the year and the age of the patient.

With respect to bacterial bronchitis, the most common organisms include *H. influenzae*, *S. pneumoniae*, and *M. catarrhalis*. Other, less common causes include *Bordetella pertussis*, which is surprisingly common, even in adults, *Legionella* species, *M. pneumoniae,* and *C. pneumoniae*. Less common, but especially likely in patients who have resided or vacationed in tropical climates, are parasites such as those of the *Strongyloides* and *Ascaris* species as well as *Syngamus laryngeus*, which can be associated with acute tracheobronchitis.

The clinical syndrome of acute tracheobronchitis is similar to that of pneumonia except that the chest radiograph is negative and there is production of mucoid or purulent sputum, frequently in association with a low-grade fever. Other symptoms may include small amounts of hemoptysis and substernal pain that is often of a burning quality and accentuated on inspiration. Dyspnea is usually not a significant component of acute tracheobronchitis except in the presence of underlying disease such as COPD (see later), in patients with asthma, or in very young children. In particular, tracheobronchitis may precipitate an asthma attack, which should be treated specifically. Some patients are left with a nonspecific bronchial hyper-reactivity syndrome characterized by a persistent nonproductive cough.

A Gram stain of the sputum usually shows a predominance of mononuclear cells in viral tracheobronchitis (except in adenoviruses), whereas in infections by bacteria and *Mycoplasma* species, there is a striking prodominance of neutrophilic polymorphonuclear leukocytes.

The treatment of acute tracheobronchitis depends on the clinical setting in which it is observed, the appearance of the sputum (including the Gram stain) and findings on physical examination of the chest. In young, previously well patients, most episodes of acute bronchitis are caused by respiratory viruses. In smokers, *H. influenzae* is more common; in elderly patients with comorbidities, bacterial infection should be considered. If there is significant production of purulent sputum that has a neutrophilic predominance on Gram stain, it is suggestive of a bacterial source, and antibiotic administration is appropriate. Reasonable antibiotics would include amoxicillin with clavulanic acid, doxycycline, trimethoprim, sulfamethoxazole, a second-generation macrolide such as clarithromycin or azithromycin or, if resistant organisms are suspected, a quinolone such as ciprofloxacin. The use of humidified air, the maintenance of oral hydration and, in the presence of wheezing, bronchodilator therapy are appropriate. In general, acute tracheobronchitis is not a life-threatening disease except in the presence of underlying disorders such as asthma or COPD or in young children in whom it may precipitate respiratory failure. In cases in which acute tracheobronchitis is recurrent, the possibilities of a tracheoesophageal fistula in infants or gastroesophageal reflux with aspiration in adults should be considered and appropriate diagnostic evaluation conducted.

EXACERBATION OF CHRONIC OBSTRUCTIVE PULMONARY DISEASE

COPD refers to a group of disorders that most commonly coexist, including chronic bronchitis, emphysema, and small-airways disease (Ferguson, 1998; Rennard, 1998; Senior and Anthonisen, 1998). These disorders are characterized by limitation of airflow (obstruction) that is due in large part to smoking-related damage to the airways and lung parenchyma. As opposed to asthma, in which airways obstruction is mainly reversible, in COPD the obstruction is largely irreversible. Familiarity with these entities and their treatment is important for the thoracic surgeon because the presence of COPD can complicate the pre- and postoperative course of many thoracic surgical patients.

Acute exacerbations of COPD, also termed acute exacerbations of chronic bronchitis, are common, especially during the winter months. The symptoms of an acute exacerbation include an increase in dyspnea, wheeze, cough, and sputum production, many of which may be present but to a lesser extent in their baseline state. There are many potential causes for an exacerbation of COPD that include viral and bacterial infection, cigarette smoke, environmental (air) pollution, allergies, drug toxicity, and coexisting medical illness such as CHF or pulmonary embolism. Indeed, several of these predisposing factors may coexist.

The most appropriate therapy for such exacerbations, especially the benefits of antibiotic therapy, have been the subject of intense debate for more than 30 years (Grossman, 1998). Among the problems are the heterogeneous nature of the patients, the small sample size, and the lack of appropriate controls for many studies. Most current guidelines recommend a multifaceted approach to therapy that includes the use of bronchodilators, systemic glucocorticoids, antibiotics, measures to enhance sputum production, and attention to coexisting medical conditions.

Inhaled bronchodilators are an important component of the initial therapy. Current guidelines recommend the use of inhaled ipratropium bromide (Atrovent), in part because it is an effective bronchodilator and also because of its relative lack of toxicity. Inhaled β_2 agonists such as salbutamol, terbutaline, and metaproterenol are also effective bronchodilators but carry risks for toxicity, including tachycardia, cardiac arrhythmias, and hypokalemia. Systemic glucocorticoids are an important component of therapy for an acute exacerbation of COPD. Evidence has suggested that a 3-day course of intravenous methylprednisolone (Solu-Medrol, 125 mg intravenous [IV] qid) followed by completion of a 2-week course of tapering prednisone is of maximal benefit (Niewoehner et al, 1999). However, it should be noted that the use of parenteral glucocorticoids is associated with increased complication, including gastrointestinal bleeding.

Despite many studies, the role of bacterial infection and antimicrobial therapy in the treatment of acute exacerbations of COPD remains controversial (Grossman, 1998; Wilson, 1998). It must be remembered that up to one half of exacerbations are either viral or noninfectious in nature. However, current recommendations are that severe exacerbations be treated with antibiotics. The major bacterial pathogens isolated during exacerbations of COPD include *H. influenzae*, *M. catarrhalis*, and *S. pneumoniae*. There is no single antibiotic that is clearly superior in the treatment of these exacerbations. Reasonable choices would include amoxicillin-clavulanate, doxycycline, trimethoprim-sulfamethoxazole, a second-generation cephalosporin such as cefuroxime axetil, ciprofloxacin, or azithromycin. As patients who have been on recent antibiotic therapy or on systemic corticosteroids have a higher incidence of resistant gram-negative bacilli, antibiotic therapy should be directed against these agents.

Perhaps most important is the attention to details in these patients who may have multiple medical problems contributing to or complicating the exacerbation.

NOSOCOMIAL PNEUMONIA

Nosocomial pneumonia is the second most common nosocomial infection after nosocomial urinary tract infection, and it has the highest fatality rate of all nosocomial infections (Mandell and Campbell, 1998). Crude mortality rates of up to 70% have been reported, and attributable mortality rates have been reported to be in the 33% to 50% range (Kollef, 1999). Mortality increases if mechanical ventilation is required. The pathogenesis is related to the microaspiration or silent aspiration of oropharyngeal flora. Normal individuals aspirate small amounts of oropharyngeal secretions during sleep. There are no untoward consequences because the flora in healthy individuals is composed of relatively benign commensal organisms (Kollef, 1999). However, with illness or trauma requiring hospitalization, oropharyngeal flora shifts to include gram-negative bacilli because of the relative loss of oropharyngeal cell surface fibronectin (Kollef, 1999). Although gram-negative organisms may predominate, in up to 50% of cases, more than one pathogen may be discovered, and in approximately half of those cases, no etiologic agent can be isolated (Kollef, 1999).

Many factors can predispose patients to aspiration, but in many cases of nosocomial pneumonia, particularly in the postoperative patient, no aspiration is identified. Microaspiration undoubtably occurs, but what tips the balance such that infection results? Surgery may cause impaired host cell–mediated immunity. Endotracheal intubation causes increased mucus production and impaired mucociliary clearance and bypasses the normal protective barrier of the glottis. Painful incisions may result in decreased tidal volumes, atelectasis, decreased functional residual capacity and impaired ability to cough and clear secretions (Mayhall, 1997; McEachern and Campbell, 1998).

With increased duration of hospitalization, the flora of the orophaynx changes and becomes dominated by gram-negative bacteria. Why this occurs is not clear but the source of these bacteria is the gastrointestinal tract. Treatment is usually broad-spectrum antibiotics but with increased gram-negative coverage (Baughman et al, 1999).

Ventilator-Associated Pneumonia

Ventilator-associated pneumonia (VAP) refers to nosocomial bacterial pneumonia that has developed in patients receiving mechanical ventilation (Chastre and Fagon, 1994). VAP that occurs in the initial 48 to 72 hours after tracheal intubation usually results from aspiration complicating the intubation process and is due to antibiotic-sensitive bacteria (*S. aureus*, *H. influenzae*, and *S. pneumoniae*). VAP occurring after this period (late-onset VAP) is commonly caused by antibiotic-resistant organisms, including oxacillin-resistant *S. aureus*, *P. aeruginosa Acinetobacter* species, and *Enterobacter* species. The risk of VAP increases with the duration of intubation and may reach 68% in those ventilated for more than 30 days (Langer et al, 1989). The main risk factors of VAP are the need for reintubation and gastric aspiration (Torres et al, 1990). Other risk factors include old age, thoracic or upper abdominal surgery, malnutrition, obesity, chronic lung disease, and concurrent antibiotic use (Haley et al, 1981; Hanson et al, 1992).

Diagnosis and Treatment of Ventilator-Associated Pneumonia

The role of fiberoptic bronchoscopy employing either the PSB or BAL to retrieve lower respiratory tract secretions in the initial evaluation of suspected VAP remains controversial (American Thoracic Society, 1996, Niederman et al, 1994). PSB is highly specific but has a high false-negative rate (DeCastro et al, 1991; Moser et al, 1982). BAL is highly sensitive but not specific (Chastre et al, 1988; Kirkpatrick and Bass, 1989). Its advocates argue that many noninfectious processes can produce a clinical picture indistinguishable from VAP, and knowledge of a specific cause of a VAP allows the physician to narrow the spectrum of antibiotic coverage, thus reducing the selection pressure for antimicrobial resistance and cost of therapy. Others argue that without knowledge of whom should be tested, of the frequency of testing, or of the accuracy of the results, this procedure should be abandoned. To date, no studies have demonstrated that these interventions have altered patient outcome. BAL or PSB may be useful in a patient with diffuse infiltrates when pneumonia is suspected, when a patient fails to respond to clinically appropriate treatment, or when a patient develops signs of new infection while on therapy.

The value of blind sampling techniques and quantitative culture of tracheal aspirates is uncertain because both areas suffer from poor study design and the results are inconclusive (Mandell and Campbell, 1998).

Treatment of VAP consists of general supportive care and the administration of broad-spectrum antibiotics. Canadian and American guidelines for empiric antibiotic coverage of VAP have been published; they stratify treatment recommendations by clinical severity (American Thoracic Society, 1996, Mandell et al, 1993). The choice of antibiotics should be influenced by the rapidity of onset of the pneumonic process, the severity of the illness from a cardiorespiratory perspective, the immunocompetence of the patient, and the known characteristics of the indigenous microbial flora. A reasonable combination would be an aminoglycoside or a third-generation cephalosporin plus clindamycin. Monotherapy with a fluoronated quinolone such as ciprofloxacin, third-generation cephalosporin, imipenem, or meropenem may be appropriate. However in the setting of the intensive care unit, antipseudomonal coverage must be considered and double coverage is usually prudent.

PNEUMONIA IN THE IMMUNOCOMPROMISED HOST

Approach to the Diagnosis of Pulmonary Infection in the Recipient of a Solid-Organ Transplant

Susceptibility to different infections occurs at different time points in the post-transplant clinical course in solid organ recipients. The post-transplant course for all organ transplant patients can be divided into three time periods: the first month after transplant, the period 1 to 6 months after transplant, and the late period, more than 6 months after transplant. When considered in conjunction with various radiographic patterns, a valuable differential diagnosis can be associated with each time point (Table 23–5) (Fishman and Rubin, 1998; Rubin, 1994).

Two major causes of pneumonia in the first month after transplantation are (1) the recurrence of an incompletely treated pneumonia that was present prior to transplantation and (2) infection due to aspiration of nosocomial flora as a result of postoperative vomiting (Fishman and Rubin, 1998). Extensive lung injury and prolonged intubation in the lung transplant recipient lead to an early increased risk of postoperative bacterial pneumonia. Despite this being the period of highest daily dose of immunosuppression, opportunistic infections are not prominent in the first month. This underscores the importance of sustained exposure to immunosuppressive therapy as the major determinant of susceptibility to opportunistic pathogens (Rubin, 1994).

Cytomegalovirus (CMV) and other immunomodulating viruses are the predominant opportunistic infections that occur between 1 and 6 months after transplantation. CMV exerts its effects by directly causing pneumonia; can contribute to graft-versus-host disease (GVHD) and lead to an increased need for immunosuppression and an escalation in the risk for opportunistic infection, and can increase the likelihood of pulmonary infections, including *Aspergillus* species, *Pneumocystis carinii* pneumonia (PCP), and *Nocardia asteroides*. The risk of active disease is greatest in the seronegative solid organ recipient of an organ from a seropositive donor. Also, in the absence of specific prophylaxis, pulmonary infections due to PCP and *Aspergillus* and *Nocardia* species are common.

Beyond 6 months post-transplantation, patients with good graft function will have more modest immunosuppression and are susceptible to community-acquired respiratory syncytial virus infection (RSV) and influenza as well as pneumococcal pneumonia. Patients with poorer graft function and those who require more aggressive

TABLE 23–5 ■ **Differential Diagnosis of Fever and Pulmonary Infiltrates in Organ Transplant Recipients**

	Rate of Progression of Illness	
Radiographic Pattern	*Acute (<24 hr)*	*Subacute-Chronic (dy-wk)*
Consolidation	Pulmonary edema Pulmonary hemorrhage Bacterial pneumonia Thromboembolism	Fungal Nocardial Tuberculous Viral *Pneumocystis carinii* pneumonia Drug-related
Peribronchovascular	Pulmonary edema	Viral *Pneumocystis carinii* pneumonia Fungal Nocardial Tuberculous Tumor (post-transplant lymphoproliferative disorder)
Nodular infiltrate	Bacterial pneumonia Pulmonary edema	Fungal Nocardial Tuberculous *Pneumocystis carinii* pneumonia

immunosuppression are at high risk for infection with *Cryptococcus neoformans*, PCP, *N. asteroides* and *Aspergillus* species.

The principles for diagnosis in organ transplant recipients are very similar to those for neutropenic and bone marrow transplant patients. The cornerstone of diagnosis is BAL with or without transbronchial biopsy. Several centers strongly advocate the routine inclusion of transbronchial biopsies in patients with diffuse pulmonary involvement because of the increased diagnostic yield in PCP and cryptococcal infection (Rosenow, 1990). Thoracoscopic biopsy has come into wider use in patients with peripheral or pleural-based processes because it provides a better specimen for culture and pathologic assessment and has less associated morbidity and mortality than open-lung biopsy (Rubin, 1994). Percutaneous needle biopsy is the procedure of choice for invasive diagnosis of focal pulmonary processes; open lung biopsy should be reserved for patients with rapid clinical deterioration and those who have central radiographic findings not amenable to thoracoscopic biopsy (Rubin, 1994).

ASPIRATION PNEUMONIA

The term *aspiration* may refer to one of three aspiration syndromes: gastric acid aspiration, bacterial pneumonia secondary to aspiration of oropharyngeal secretions, or aspiration of a foreign body causing airway obstruction. This section discusses only gastric acid aspiration syndrome and pneumonia due to aspiration of oropharyngeal secretions.

Acid Aspiration Syndrome

Acute lung injury secondary to gastric acid aspiration was first described by Mendelsohn in association with parturition (Mendelsohn, 1946). Aspiration remains a cause of maternal morbidity in the modern era and is a concern during any general anesthesia. In the recent literature, the incidence of aspiration associated with elective anesthesia is very low—0.00002% (Mellin-Olsen et al, 1996) to 0.0003% (Warner et al, 1993)—but it increases for emergency procedures to 0.001%. Aspiration occurred in 3.5% of patients intubated in the emergency room, as reported by Thibodeau and colleagues (1997). Even so, sequelae were rare. In the pediatric population, the incidence is 0.10% for elective general surgery (Borland et al, 1998).

Historically, gastric acid aspiration was associated with a 50% to 60% mortality rate. The severity of the injury is related to the pH and amount of gastric acid aspirated (Greenfield et al, 1989; James et al, 1984; Teabout, 1952; Wynne, 1982; Wynne et al, 1981). Aspiration of volumes greater than 50 ml with a pH less than 2.5 results in a significant and potentially life-threatening lung injury. The presence of particulate matter in addition to acid is especially damaging (Knight et al, 1993).

Neutralization of acid or reduction in acid production by using sodium citrate, H_2 antagonists, or proton pump inhibitors has become standard in the anesthetic management of the high-risk patient. This may be responsible for the decrease in morbidity and mortality currently reported in association with aspiration on intubation. Current mortality rates for aspiration on induction of anesthesia are approximately zero to 5% (Mellin-Olsen et al, 1996; Warner et al, 1993).

Diagnosis

In the situation of an unwitnessed aspiration, the diagnosis may be difficult to prove. There are four situations in which aspiration is more likely to occur: (1) loss of airway-protective reflexes, as in general anesthesia; (2) structural and functional abnormalities of the esophagus and pharynx; (3) gastroesophageal reflux; and (4) postoperative acute gastric dilatation. A patient with minimal symptoms and no sequelae may go undiagnosed, but more commonly, the patient will present with respiratory distress and hypoxia. A chest radiograph may show air space disease localized to a single (most commonly, the superior segment of the right lower lobe) or multiple dependent areas of the lung or there may be bilateral diffuse infiltrates. Bronchoscopy may reveal particulate debris, gastric fluid, or bile. In a situation in which there are no obvious findings, a BAL may be helpful if lipid-laden macrophages are detected.

Pathophysiology

Aspiration of acid results in a biphasic pattern of injury. The initial phase is the result of direct tissue injury by acid. The second phase results from neutrophil activation and a systemic inflammatory response. (Knight et al, 1992). There may be a third phase if secondary bacterial infection occurs. Acid aspiration causes immediate damage to the ciliated respiratory epithelium and the alveolar lining cells, resulting in a significant loss in pulmonary defenses. A volume of 25 to 50 ml may be dispersed throughout the lungs in less than a minute (Dal Santo, 1986; Hamelberg and Bosomworth, 1964). The acid alone destroys preformed surfactant, and damage to the alveolar lining cells results in loss of surfactant production. Destruction of the alveolar capillary barrier and basement membrane, mediated by reactive oxygen species and elastase, results in increased capillary permeability (Goldman et al, 1992b). The protein-rich alveolar fluid that results from the increase in capillary permeability inactivates any remaining surfactant, but also neutralizes any gastric acid. A cascade of neutrophil-mediated injury may then occur (Goldman et al, 1993). Neutrophil migration mediated by intercellular adhesion molecule-1 (ICAM-1) (Nagase et al, 1996) followed by thromboxane-dependent sequestration of neutrophils and subsequent activation (mediated by TNFα, IL8, and complement) leads to both a local and a systemic inflammatory response which may result in diffuse lung injury, acute respiratory distress syndrome (ARDS), or multiorgan failure (Goldman et al, 1990).

The patient may succumb from refractory respiratory failure within days, or the chemical pneumonitis may resolve quickly without significant sequelae. However, progression to ARDS (Fig. 23–9) and multiorgan failure may occur. A secondary bacterial pneumonia may further compromise the damaged lungs (Folkesson et al, 1995; Goldman et al, 1990, 1992a, 1992b, 1993; Weiser et al, 1997; Yamada et al, 1997).

Treatment

Once acid aspiration has occurred, the treatment is supportive. There is no role for steroids or prophylactic antibiotics. (Buchman et al, 1984; Gates et al, 1983; Glauser et al, 1979; Murray, 1979; Sukumaran et al, 1980; Wynne et al, 1979). Bronchoscopy should be performed, particularly in the setting of a witnessed aspiration, to suction out the airways and remove particulate debris. Small-volume aspiration may cause asthma-like symptoms that will respond to aerosolized bronchodilators. Although adrenergic brochodilators are most commonly used, anticholinergic bronchodilators may be useful, as there is evidence that the bronchospasm is vagally mediated (Boyle et al, 1985).

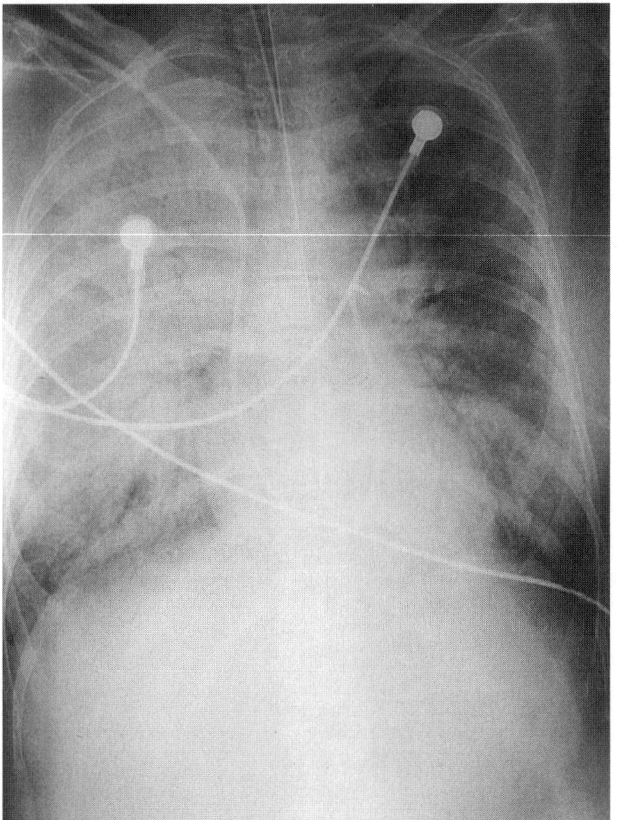

FIGURE 23–9 ■ Chest radiograph showing adult respiratory distress syndrome from massive gastric acid aspiration. The patient is intubated and has a balloon flotation catheter in place.

Adequate oxygenation must be maintained but if mechanical ventilation is required, care must be taken to avoid further lung injury by avoiding hyperoxia (Nader-Djalal et al, 1997, 1998) and barotrauma. Experimental work in animals suggests that exogenous surfactant may be helpful in acid aspiration syndrome but there is no clinical data from humans to support this (Eijking et al, 1993; Zucker et al, 1992).

Vigilance in detecting and aggressively treating any secondary bacterial pneumonias is essential. The ultimate choice of antimicrobial treatment, if infection supervenes, is determined by the clinical setting in which the aspiration occurred.

Bacterial Aspiration Pneumonia

Even normal subjects aspirate small volumes during sleep (Gleeson et al, 1997; Huxley et al, 1978); therefore, in order for pneumonia to occur there must be a breakdown in host defenses or the volume of bacterial inoculum of the aspiration must be large or particularly virulent. Most commonly, a depressed level of consciousness leads to loss of protective airway reflexes and allows a more significant volume of aspiration to occur. This may be due to general anesthesia, sedatives or analgesics, drug overdose, trauma to the central nervous system, infection, or stroke.

Structural or functional abnormalities of the larynx, pharynx, or esophagus may also predispose to aspiration. Recurrent laryngeal nerve paralysis or neuromuscular disease affecting the pharynx impairs the ability to protect the airway; esophageal disease such as achalasia, Zenker's diverticulum, malignant obstruction, or reflux may overwhelm intact defenses with large quantities of aspirated material (Belsey, 1960). As noted earlier, acid aspiration results in injury to the tracheobronchial tree and the lung itself, which in turn impairs host defenses and predisposes the patient to secondary bacterial pneumonia. Smoke or other noxious gas inhalation injuries may cause a similar breakdown in host defenses.

Aspiration pneumonia is a significant cause of morbidity and mortality in intubated patients and in patients recovering from stroke. A great deal of effort has been directed toward preventing aspiration pneumonia in intubated patients, including subglottic drainage, semirecumbent positioning, nasojejunal enteral feeding, and acid suppression as well as antibiotic strategies (Stoutenbeek and van Saene, 1997; Mahul et al, 1992; Orozco-Levi et al, 1995; Torres et al, 1992). Although some improvement has been noted by some authors, none of these strategies has been completely effective in preventing microaspiration. Similarly, there appears to be no difference in effect between a surgically placed feeding gastrostomy versus jejunostomy (Fox et al, 1995) or in nasojejunal or nasogastric feeds versus surgically placed or percutaneous feeding tubes (Kadakia et al, 1992; Strong et al, 1992). Perhaps most effective is semirecumbent positioning and the monitoring of gastric residuals, which should be kept at less than 30% of the hourly rate for continuous feeds. Because aspiration of oropharyngeal secretions is a major source of nosocomial pneumonia, and colonization of the stomach due to acid-suppressing regimens has been implicated in gram-negative pneumonia, The Canadian Critical Care Trials Group has compared sucralfate with ranitidine for ulcer prophylaxis to prevent bacterial overgrowth in the stomach, but this strategy showed no benefit in reducing nosocomial pneumonia (Cook et al, 1998).

Diagnosis and Treatment

The diagnosis of aspiration pneumonia is based on clinical suspicion in the appropriate clinical setting, associated with the typical radiologic findings of air-space disease in dependent areas of the lung, most commonly the superior segment of the right lower lobe and the posterior segment of the right upper lobe, particularly if more than one area is involved.

In a setting in which aspiration due to swallowing dysfunction is suspected, video fluoroscopy is the gold standard to assess function and detect silent aspiration. Although documentation of aspiration does not prove the cause of pneumonia, increased severity of aspiration on videofluoroscopy has been found to be associated with increased risk of pneumonia (Martin et al, 1994; Schmidt et al, 1994). Collins and Bakheit (1997) reported the use of pulse oximetry during swallowing assessment to detect aspiration in dysphagic stroke patients and found a reliability of 81.5%. Zaidi and colleages (1996) found similar results. The addition of methylene blue to tube feeds has not been proven to be reliable in detecting aspiration whereas testing of tracheal aspirates with glucose oxidase strips has had mixed success (Kingston et al, 1991; Kinsey et al, 1994; Potts et al, 1993). The finding of lipid-laden macrophages on bronchoalveolar lavage is associated with aspiration. Adams and colleagues (1997) have reported that a lipid-laden macrophage index of >100 has a sensitivity of 94%, a negative predictive value of 98%, a specificity of 89%, and a positive predictive value of 71%.

In the setting of a bacterial aspiration pneumonia, as opposed to gastric acid aspiration, treatment with antibiotics is appropriate. In a nonhospitalized population, coverage against gram-positive organisms and oral anaerobes is required. The choice of antibiotics may include penicillin or clindamycin (Jacobson et al, 1997, Mier et al, 1993). Ticarcillin-clavulanate has also been found to be effective in treating penicillin-resistant anaerobes. Ceftriaxone and metronidazole are not as effective (Brook, 1996). In hospitalized patients, antibiotics must also be effective against gram-negative organisms (see Table 23–4).

LUNG ABSCESS

Definition

A lung abscess is a localized collection of pus contained in a cavity that is formed by the destruction of pulmonary parenchyma. This excludes infected bullae and cysts in which infection develops within a pre-existing space. Nonetheless, the diagnosis and management of these conditions have some features in common with a true lung abscess. Although most often solitary, multiple abscesses may occur secondary to a primary bacteremia or in immunosuppressed patients. If present for more than 6 weeks an abscess is considered chronic.

Lung abscesses may be further classified, based on cause, into primary or secondary. Primary lung abscesses occur as a result of necrotizing pulmonary infections, including those occurring in immunosuppressed hosts, or due to aspiration of either gastrointestinal contents or oropharyngeal secretions (Table 23–6). Secondary lung abscesses occur as a complication of bacteremia or bronchial obstruction, as an extension of adjacent suppurative infections such as subphrenic or hepatic abscesses, or as infection of a lung destroyed by infarction or tumor.

Historical Note

The monograph on lung abscess written by Brock and colleagues in 1942 described the clinical features of lung abscess and proposed that the pathogenesis of lung abscess is aspiration of infected oropharyngeal secretions. This theory was based on the observation that most abscesses occur in the posterior segment of the right upper lobe and the superior segment of the right lower lobe, the axillary segments, so called because of their proximity to the lateral chest wall. The orifices of these segments are directly in line with the upper respiratory tract when the patient is recumbent. Brock's hypothesis

TABLE 23–6 ■ **Etiologic Classification of Lung Abscesses**

PRIMARY
Aspiration
Impaired level of consciousness (general anesthesia, drugs or alcohol, stroke, etc.)
Poor oral hygiene (gingivodental sepsis)
Esophageal disease (achalasia, Zenker's diverticulum, GERD)
Necrotizing pneumonia
Virulent organisms (*S. aureus*, *K. pneumoniae*, Friedländer's bacillus)
Fungi
Tuberculosis
Immunodeficiency
Immunosuppression for organ transplantation
Steroid therapy
Cancer chemotherapy
Diabetes
Malnutrition
SECONDARY
Bronchial obstruction
Cavitating lesions (neoplasm, infarct)
Direct extension (amebiasis, subphrenic abscess)
Hematogenous
CONGENITAL OR ACQUIRED CYSTS
Hydatid, tuberculosis, bronchogenic cyst, bullae

GERD, gastroesophageal reflux disease.

is supported by the finding that 75% of all lung abscesses occur in these segments and in the superior segment of the left lower lobe (Bernhard et al, 1963; Shafron and Tate, 1968).

Hippocrates is credited with the first description of the treatment of a lung abscess—percutaneous drainage of the abscess, an approach that is enjoying a resurgence in popularity. The importance of pleural symphysis having occurred prior to the performance of any drainage procedure became appreciated in the late 19th century. It was recognized that in the absence of pleural symphysis, percutaneous drainage of a lung abscess may result in a pyopneumothorax, which was commonly fatal. In 1947, Monaldi reported a two-stage procedure in which pleural symphysis was induced by performing a short rib resection and inserting a piece of gauze to act as an irritant; after 4 to 7 days, drainage could be safely accomplished as a second stage, once pleural symphysis had occurred (Monaldi, 1947). Current techniques for percutaneous drainage utilize the principle of pleural symphysis using computed tomography (CT) scanning or ultrasound as a guide to minimize the amount of lung parenchyma traversed and to localize sites where pleural symphysis has most likely occurred.

After the development of antibiotics, first the sulphonamides in 1938 and then penicillin in 1941, the incidence of lung abscess diminished with effective therapy for primary pneumonias. Cancer chemotherapy, immunosuppression for transplantation or autoimmune diseases, and infections such as HIV (Furman et al, 1996) have resulted in an increase in lung abscesses due to unusual or opportunistic organisms.

Pathophysiology

Aspiration of infected oropharyngeal secretions is the most common cause of primary lung abscess. Gingivodental sepsis is associated with an increased risk of pneumonia and abscess because it increases the bacterial load of the aspirated oropharyngeal secretions. The risk of aspiration is increased by conditions of impaired consciousness or suppressed cough reflex, including general anesthesia, intravenous sedation, ingestion of alcohol or other drugs, seizure or coma resulting from any cause. Neurologic diseases acting centrally, such as a stroke, or locally, such as amyotrophic lateral sclerosis, may impair swallowing and increase the risk of aspiration. Esophageal diseases, including gastroesophageal reflux, diverticula (especially Zenker's diverticulum), achalasia or other motility disorders, strictures, and esophageal cancer causing either obstruction or fistulization into the trachea are also associated with an increased risk of aspiration.

Although aspiration has long been considered the principal cause of primary lung abscess, a report by Pohlson and colleagues (1985) suggested that the pattern of occurrence of lung abscess was changing; they found that 40% of cases of abscess were due to a necrotizing pneumonia caused by a virulent organism such as *S. pyogenes*, *K. pneumoniae*, or *S. aureus*. In an immunosuppressed host, pneumonia and lung abscess may be caused by the usual pathogens as well as by opportunistic organisms. Secondary lung abscess is most often caused by an obstructing bronchial carcinoma or, rarely, an aspirated foreign body or extrinsic compression of the bronchus by lymphadenopathy. Secondary infections of cavitating necrotic lung cancers or other cavitating lesions due to pulmonary infarction, tuberculosis, or other granulomatous diseases are also considered lung abscesses. Infected cysts or bullae are not true abscesses but present in a similar fashion. Lung abscesses may also occur secondary to extension of adjacent infection in the liver or subphrenic space penetrating across the diaphragm. Bacteremia causing multiple small lung abscesses may mimic metastases and are associated with infected indwelling vascular access catheters, intravenous drug use, or endocarditis.

Microbiology

Bacteria isolated from lung abscesses reflect the underlying pathophysiology. In community-acquired pneumonia, the bacteria are predominantly gram-positive; in hospital-acquired pneumonia, they are 60% to 70% gram-negative. Immunosuppressed patients may develop infections due to the usual pathogens as well as to less virulent and opportunistic organisms such as *Salmonella* species, *Legionella* species, *P. carinii*, atypical mycobacterium, and fungi (Naidich et al, 1991; Pohlsan et al, 1985).

A primary lung abscess resulting from pneumonia may be due to α- and β-hemolytic streptococcus, *S. aureus*, *S. pneumoniae*, *K. pneumoniae*, *Streptococcus viridans*, and *H. influenzae*. In nosocomial pneumonias, gram-negative bacteria predominate including *K. pneumoniae*, *H. influenzae*, and other species, such as *Proteus* species, *P. aeruginosa*, *Escherichia coli*, *Enterobacter cloacae*, and *Eikenella corrodens*.

In lung abscess due to aspiration, mixed flora are often present and anaerobes play an important role. Aerobic gram-positive cocci and facultative gram-negative bacilli have been most commonly cultured, including *S. aureus*, *S. pyogenes*, *K. pneumoniae*, *E. coli*, and *Pseudomonas* species (Bartlett et al, 1974; Frieden et al, 1991; Kaye et al, 1990). However with improved anaerobic culture techniques and invasive sampling techniques, a predominance of anaerobic bacteria such as species of the *Bacteroides*, *Peptococcus*, *Peptostreptococcus*, *Fusobacterium*, *Veillonella*, and *Clostridium* genera have been reported in abscess aspirates (Bartlett et al, 1974; Henriquez et al, 1991; Lee et al, 1991).

An average of 2.1 to 3.25 isolates per patient have been cultured from samples obtained by percutaneous aspiration of lung abscesses (Grinan et al, 1990; Hammond et al, 1995; Yang et al, 1991), and 58% to 66% of isolates contain anaerobes.

Clinical Presentation

The typical presentation may include cough, fever, chills, malaise, fatigue, weight loss, pleuritic chest pain, dyspnea and, less commonly, hemoptysis, but the onset may be insidious, and chronicity, weight loss, and malaise may predominate.

Putrid sputum, although uncommon early in the course of the illness, occurs in 40% to 75% of patients once cavitation occurs (Wiedemann and Rice, 1995). Production of large quantities of foul sputum, once communication with the bronchial tree has occurred, may lead to infection of the noninvolved lung and respiratory failure. Hemoptysis may occur and varies from blood-streaked sputum to life-threatening hemorrhage. Sudden onset of septic shock and respiratory failure may result from rupture of the abscess into the pleural space and subsequent pyopneumothorax. The mortality rate of those with lung abscess in the preantibiotic era was 56% to 60% but has decreased to 5% to 10% except in the presence of immunosuppression, where rates have increased to 9% to 28% (Bernhard et al, 1963; Chidi and Mendelsohn, 1974; Delarue et al, 1980; Fox et al, 1954; Hagan and Hardy, 1983; Mori et al, 1993; Pohlson et al, 1985).

Physical findings may be minimal but are most commonly consistent with those of pneumonia. In a chronic abscess, clubbing and cachexia may be the predominant findings.

A careful history should be obtained, focusing not just on the symptoms of the infection and its complications, but also on the possible predisposing factors and looking for causes of impaired consciousness, for neurologic and esophageal conditions, and for causes of bronchial obstruction.

Diagnosis

The diagnosis is suspected based on the clinical presentation. Once an abscess is suspected, a chest radiograph may demonstrate a cavitating lesion with an air-fluid level. There is usually an air-fluid level on both the posteroanterior (PA) and lateral views, and the wall of the abscess is relatively thin (Swensen et al, 1991). However, in some patients, a slowly resolving infiltrate may be all that is seen on the plain radiograph. As pointed out by Boon and colleagues (1996), this is a problem particularly in mechanically ventilated patients in the intensive care unit who are examined only by portable chest radiograph machines. In these situations, a CT scan is invaluable for demonstrating a cavitating lesion. A CT scan is also useful to clarify the diagnosis when a plain radiograph is not diagnostic, to help rule out endobronchial obstruction, to more accurately assess the thickness of the walls of the cavity, and to look for an associated mass or other pathology, including other small abscesses.

A cavitating carcinoma is not infrequently mistaken for a lung abscess. The lack of fever and leukocytosis suggests a noninfectious cause, but if the tumor is infected, the clinical presentations of the two are indistinguishable. The failure of the abscess to resolve with appropriate management or the finding of a thick, irregular wall or a mass associated with the abscess suggests an underlying malignancy.

A loculated or interlobar empyema may be mistaken for a lung abscess, but CT findings will clearly differentiate the two in most cases. A loculated empyema has smooth borders. If in the fissure, it has a lenticular shape; if adjacent to the chest wall, it forms an obtuse angle with the chest wall. A split pleura sign may be present and an air-fluid level is uncommon.

Infected cysts or bullae present with the same clinical picture as a lung abscesses, and their management is similar. They are easily distinguished by CT scanning, which shows a smooth, thin-walled cavity with little surrounding inflammation. A parasitic cyst may be associated with peripheral eosinophilia.

Less common differential diagnoses include other cavitating lesions such as tuberculosis, fungal infections, actinomycosis, bronchiectasis, and noninfectious inflammatory conditions such as Wegener's granulomatosis.

Additional investigations include a complete blood count with differential white cell count, sputum culture, blood cultures, and a bronchoscopy. A bronchoscopy is essential to rule out endobronchial obstruction, usually due to tumor but occasionally due to the presence of a foreign body. During bronchoscopy, cultures may be obtained by means of BAL, but if the patient has been on systemic antibiotics for more than 24 hours, bronchoscopic cultures are commonly sterile. PSB appears to offer no additional benefit over BAL. Bronchoscopy may be used to establish drainage of the abscess but sudden drainage of a giant abscess can be hazardous, causing flooding of the tracheobronchial tree, disseminating infection, and possibly causing asphyxia. Transtracheal aspiration has been reported to yield more accurate culture data but is not well tolerated by most patients. Alternatively, samples for culture can be obtained by means of fine-needle aspiration (FNA) using ultrasound or CT guidance. This technique is usually well tolerated by patients, obtains samples uncontaminated by upper respiratory tract flora, allows for more reliable anaerobic culture, and may be accompanied by therapeutic percutaneous drainage of the abscess (Grinan et al, 1990; van Sonnenberg et al, 1991; Yang et al, 1991). Yang and colleagues (1991) reported a 94% success rate in obtaining a culture of pathogens using FNA as compared to an 11% rate using sputum culture and a 3% rate using BAL. There was a low rate of pneumothorax (6%), and none of those patients required a chest tube. Grinan and coworkers (1990) reported similarly encouraging results, with 82% positive cultures and 14% pneumothorax. It is important to note that in 43% of patients, antibiotics were changed as a result of an FNA. This procedure is also useful in identifying unusual organisms.

Management

The mainstay of treatment is systemic antibiotics. The choice of antibiotic depends on the clinical situation. Intravenous antibiotics should be administered until the patient is no longer toxic (1–2 weeks). The antibiotics may then be changed to an oral regimen of equal efficacy and continued for a prolonged course of 4 to 8 weeks (Weiss and Cherniack, 1974). High-dose penicillin (up to 20 million units per day) is effective for most abscesses and historically has been the drug of choice. However, recent studies have demonstrated the superiority of clindamycin (600 mg IV every 6 hours) primarily because of penicillin-resistant *Bacteroides* species (Bartlett et al, 1974; Guidiol et al, 1990; Levison et al, 1983). Metronidazole alone is insufficient, presumably because of the presence of aerobic and microaerophilic streptococci, resulting in only 50% response rates (Perlino, 1981), but in nosocomial infections, a third-generation cephalosporin and metronidazole may be an appropriate choice.

Supportive therapies include nutritional support and treatment of predisposing factors. Chest physiotherapy and possibly bronchoscopy to facilitate bronchial toilet are often recommended, but most abscesses communicate with the bronchial tree and patients drain spontaneously. Because of the risk of flooding the contralateral lung with infected secretions, bronchoscopy is best reserved for diagnostic purposes.

Most lung abscesses (85% to 90%) respond within 2 weeks to medical management and resolve radiographically over 2 to 5 months (Wiedemann and Rice, 1995). The lack of clinical response to medical therapy within 2 weeks suggests the need for invasive culture techniques (FNA) to ensure that antibiotic coverage is appropriate; bronchoscopy if not already performed, to rule out endobronchial obstruction; re-evaluation of the diagnosis; and possible external drainage or surgical resection.

Indications for intervention include failure of medical therapy, abscess under tension, abscess increasing in size while on appropriate antibiotics, contralateral lung contamination, abscess larger than 4 to 6 cm in diameter, rising fluid level, persistent ventilator dependency, necrotizing infection with multiple abscesses, hemoptysis, rupture into the pleural space with pyopneumothorax, and inability to exclude a cavitating carcinoma.

External drainage may be accomplished by means of tube thoracostomy, percutaneous drainage using CT or ultrasound guidance, or surgical cavernostomy. First performed by Hippocrates, percutaneous drainage of lung abscess has gained popularity in the past 10 to 15 years. The exact timing of and indications for percutaneous drainage require the judgment of the treating physician or surgeon. Based on expanding experience and success, early drainage has been practiced with increasing frequency (Fig. 23–10). The effectiveness of percutaneous drainage is high, with cure rates of 73% to 100% (Lambiase et al, 1992; Rice et al, 1987; van Sonnenberg et al, 1991; Weidemann and Rice, 1995; Yellin et al, 1985). The major concerns are the risk of empyema, hemorrhage, pneumothorax, and bronchopleural fistula. The rate of complications is lower with radiologically placed drainage tubes (Mengoli, 1985; Weidemann and Rice, 1995). Overall morbidity is low (zero to 21%) as is mortality (zero to 9%), with most deaths occurring in critically ill patients (Rice et al, 1987).

The technique for percutaneous drainage of a lung abscess utilizes either CT or ultrasound to localize the abscess and determine the optimal location for tube placement in order to take advantage of pleural symphysis or at least minimize the amount of lung traversed by the catheter (Klein et al, 1995). The patient is positioned so that the abscess is in a dependent position so as to minimize the chance of soilage of the contralateral lung. Using either a Seldinger or a trocar technique, the abscess is localized, punctured, and then drained using a No. 12 French (or larger) catheter, aspirating manually as much of the abscess contents as possible, and then irrigating the cavity with saline. The drainage catheter is attached to a standard chest drainage system with −20 cm of water suction.

The choice between tube thoracostomy and radiologically placed catheter drainage depends on the treating physician's preference and the availability of interventional radiology. Radiologic techniques appear to be equally efficacious and have a lower incidence of complications as well as the advantage of allowing localization of the optimal site for tube placement. However, an unstable patient may be better served by a chest tube that is placed expeditiously while at the bedside than by being transported to the radiology department. Surgical cavernostomy may be useful when tube drainage is unsuccessful, particularly in the situation of a necrotizing pneumonia with multiple loculated abscesses, but it may be associated with a higher incidence of bronchopleural fistula.

Surgical resection is required in less than 10% of cases of lung abscess (Weidemann and Rice, 1995). The most common indication for surgery is the suspicion of, or inability to rule out, a cavitating lung cancer. Lack of response to antibiotics as seen on radiology, absense of fever and leukocytosis, and a thick-walled cavity may be clues to an underlying malignancy.

Massive hemoptysis or rupture into the pleural space with resulting pyopneumothorax are indications for emergency surgery. Hemoptysis occurs in 11% to 15% of cases of lung abscess; of these 20% to 50% include massive hemoptysis (Thoms et al, 1972). Medical management of massive hemoptysis in this setting is associated with a 70% mortality rate (Garzon, 1972). Bronchial artery embolization may be an alternative to emergency surgery and may be useful for stabilizing the patient and allowing the contralateral lung to recover so that surgery may take place in a controlled setting. In the presence of

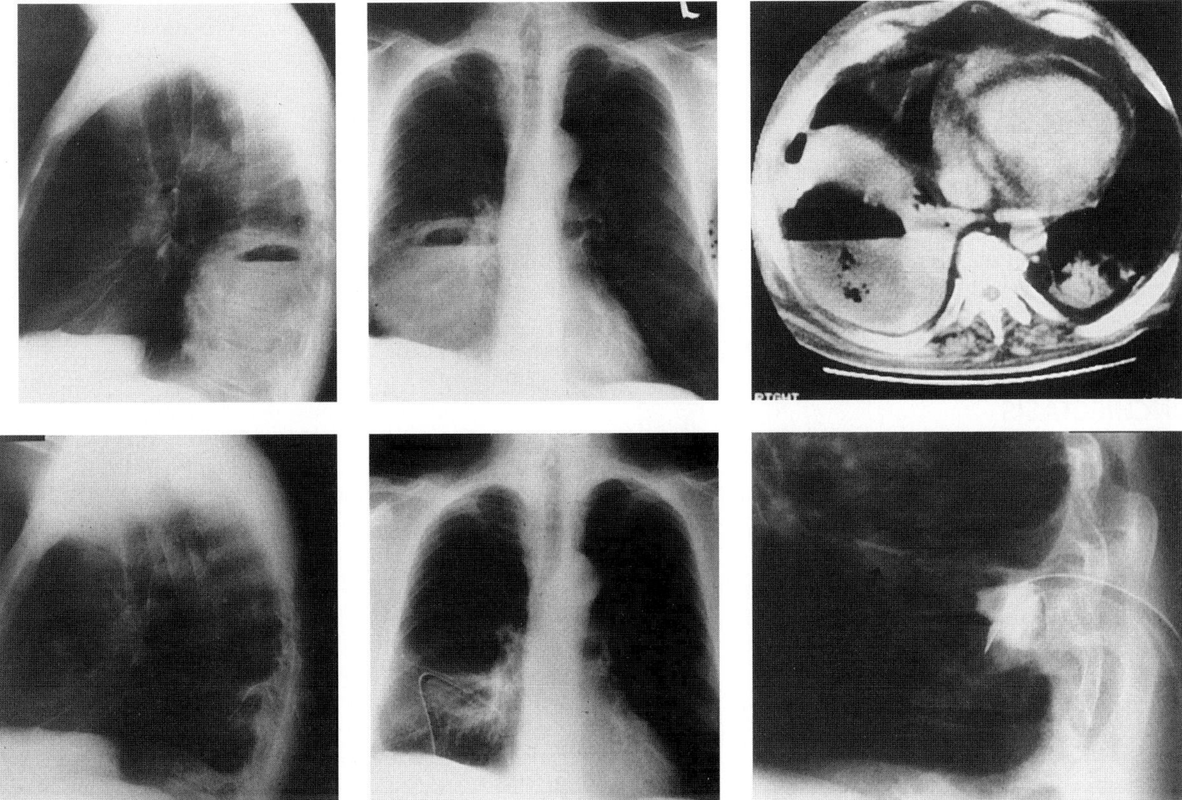

FIGURE 23–10 ■ Lateral and posteroanterior views and computed tomography (CT) scan of a large acute lung abscess *(upper panels)*. Resolution of the CT scan with simple percutaneous drainage followed by the chest tube insertion using the percutaneous tract *(lower panels)*.

a destructive infection, rebleeding is highly probable and resection, once the patient is stabilized, is recommended, assuming the patient can tolerate a pulmonary resection from the perspective of cardiopulmonary reserve. Lobectomy is the preferred resection for both bleeding and pyopneumothorax. A Monaldi procedure or other rib resection procedures may be performed for drainage of a pyopneumothorax if the patient is unstable or cannot tolerate resection. For drainage of an uncomplicated lung abscess, the Monaldi procedure has largely been superseded by percutaneous radiologic techniques.

The most important intraoperative consideration is protection of the contralateral lung, whatever the indication for surgery. The use of a double-lumen tube, a bronchial blocker, or contralateral mainstem intubation minimizes contamination of the dependent lung during surgery. Particularly in the presence of massive hemoptysis, rapid control of the airway is essential. Early clamping of the involved bronchus and minimal manipulation of the involved lobe also help to minimize spillage. Unfortunately, these are usually challenging resections because of the increased vascularity and lymphadenopathy secondary to the infection, making access and control of the hilum difficult.

Results

In the preantibiotic era, the mortality rate in cases of lung abscess was 30% to 50%. In the modern era, the mortality is 5% to 20%, with 75% to 88% of patients cured with medical therapy alone. Surgical treatment has a 90% success rate, with a mortality rate of 1% to 13% (Delarue et al, 1980; Mengoli, 1985; Rice et al, 1987). With the increase in the number of immunosuppressed patients, the incidence of lung abscess is rising and with it, the mortality rate, reported to be 28% in this patient population. The success rate with percutaneous drainage varies from 73% to 100% with no mortality.

SUMMARY

The incidence of lung abscess is again rising with increasing numbers of immunosuppressed patients. The most common cause of lung abscess is aspiration of infected oropharyngeal secretions, followed by necrotizing primary pneumonias. Bacteremia may result in multiple abscesses. Most abscesses contain mixed flora of anaerobes with either gram-positive cocci (if community-acquired) or gram-negative bacilli (if nosocomial). In immunosuppressed patients, unusual or opportunistic infections must be considered. In the assessment of the patient with a lung abscess, predisposing factors such as esophageal or neurologic problems must be ruled out. The differential diagnosis of cavitating lung lesions must be addressed, particularly if the abscess fails to respond to appropriate therapy. The primary treatment is intravenous antibiotics. Percutaneous techniques (FNA) for obtaining culture material have proven to be useful in establishing a microbiologic diagnosis and guiding appropriate antibiotic choice. External drainage using percutaneous radiologic techniques have also proven to be useful and safe and are preferred over surgical drainage. The indications for surgical intervention have changed and include inability to rule out cancer, massive hemoptysis, and rupture into the pleural space. Radiologic drainage techniques are preferred for giant abscesses or abscesses that fail to resolve or are increasing in size. The mortality rate among patients with lung abscesses has diminished dramatically since the preantibiotic era but is higher in immunosuppressed patients.

BRONCHIECTASIS

Definition

Bronchiectasis is defined as an abnormal and permanent dilatation of bronchi. The condition, which may be either localized or diffuse, is caused by destruction of the elastic and muscular components of the bronchial walls (Barker, 1995; Ip and Lam, 1996; Mysliwiec and Pina, 1999). Although this definition is based on pathologic examination, a clinical diagnosis is often suggested in a patient with chronic or recurrent pulmonary infections in association with significant amounts of sputum production. The latter can vary from a few tablespoons to several cups of sputum per day (Nicotra, 1994).

Etiology

The cause of bronchiectasis can be congenital or acquired. Bronchiectasis due to congenital causes is more likely to be diffuse, whereas if caused by infection it is more likely to be localized. Postinfectious bronchiectasis tends to affect the upper lobes if secondary to tuberculosis and the lower lobes if due to other bacterial or viral pathogens.

It should be remembered, however, that bronchiectasis is the consequence of the inflammation and destruction of the bronchial wall, which is the result of infection. In the past, bronchiectasis in childhood was commonly a complication of measles or pertussis. These are now relatively less common causes in North America because of effective immunization practice. At present, the predominant childhood viral infections associated with the development of bronchiectasis include adenoviruses and influenza viruses. Bacterial infections, especially those with potentially necrotizing organisms such as *S. aureus*, *K. pneumoniae*, *H. influenzae*, and anaerobes are important causes of bronchiectasis when there is a delay in the antibiotic treatment. Bronchiectasis has also become more prominent in patients with HIV infection, as well as in the lung transplant population with chronic obliterative bronchiolitis. Although relatively uncommon in North America, tuberculosis remains a significant cause of bronchiectasis in underdeveloped countries due to the necrotizing effect of the mycobacterium on the pulmonary parenchyma and associated airways. In addition, mediastinal lymphadenopathy can cause extrinsic compression of airways with obstruction, and endobronchial involvement can cause bronchostenosis, resulting in compromised drainage and, eventually, bronchiectasis.

Bronchial obstruction caused by extrinsic compression of a bronchus and endobronchial compression related to neoplasia are potential causes of bronchiectasis. Malignant tumors are unusual causes of bronchiectasis, usually because of the rapidity of progression of their clinical course. However, more slowly growing tumors such as carcinoids can be associated with bronchiectasis. Foreign-body aspiration with endobronchial obstruction is an important and potentially reversible cause of bronchiectasis, especially in children. An antecedent history of a predisposing event (e.g., seizure, loss of consciousness, dental procedure) should be sought.

Congenital impairment of host defense mechanisms is another important cause of bronchiectasis. Generalized impairment of lung defenses occurs with immunoglobulin deficiencies including panhypogammaglobulinemia, IgG subclass deficiency, and selective IgA deficiency (Takaro et al, 1977). Cystic fibrosis is an important cause of bronchiectasis that tends to involve primarily the upper lobes. It is important to remember that some of the milder mutations of cystic fibrosis can be associated with late-onset (age 40–50) bronchiectasis in patients with few or no other manifestations of the disease, such as in males with congenital bilateral absence of the vas deferens.

Ciliary dysmotility syndromes are another congenital cause of bronchiectasis. Numerous defects are included in this classification, including structural abnormalities of the dynein arms, radial spokes, and other components of the microtubules (Eliasson et al, 1977; Santamaria et al, 1999; Sturgess et al, 1986). In these syndromes, the cilia are dyskinetic, and their propulsive action is diminished, leading to impairment of clearance of secretions, bacterial colonization and, eventually, infection. The clinical manifestations of this disorder include recurrent upper and lower respiratory infections, including sinusitis, otitis media, bronchiectasis, and immotile sperm. When associated with situs inversus, it is called Kartagener's syndrome (Kinney and DeLuca, 1991). Less common congenital abnormalities of bronchial cartilage and connective tissues may also be associated with bronchiectasis.

Noninfectious causes of bronchiectasis include inhalation of toxic gases such as ammonia and aspiration of gastric contents, which result in severe and destructive inflammatory responses in the airways. Immune disorders such as allergic bronchopulmonary aspergillosis in which an immune response *to Aspergillus* organisms that have colonized the airway in association with asthma can lead to proximal cylindrical bronchiectasis (Cockrill and Hales, 1999). Bronchiectasis can also occur in other presumed immunologic diseases, including ulcerative colitis, rheumatoid arthritis, and Sjögren's syndrome. α-Antitrypsin deficiency, in which early onset and severe pan-acinar emphysema is the usual manifestation, may also be accompanied by bronchiectasis (Longstreth et al, 1975).

Pathology

The original pathologic classification of bronchiectasis by Reid (1986) included three principal types: cylindrical, varicose, and saccular (cystic). In cylindrical bronchiectasis, which is often associated with tuberculosis, the bronchi are uniformly dilated until the dilatation ends abruptly at the junction of smaller airways, where there is obstruction by secretions. In varicose bronchiectasis, the affected bronchi have an irregular or beaded pattern of dilatation resembling varicose veins. In saccular or cystic bronchiectasis, which is the most common form to occur after obstruction or infection, the bronchi are usually in a state of dilatation and have the appearance of a balloon at the periphery, ending in blind sacs without obvious bronchial structures distal to the areas of dilatation. The bronchial dilatation associated with bronchiectasis is associated with inflammatory changes in the walls of medium-sized airways that lead to the destruction of normal structural components of the wall, including cartilage, muscle, and elastic tissue, which are replaced by fibrous tissue. The dilated airways are commonly filled with pools of thick, purulent material, and more distal airways are often occluded by secretions or obliterated by fibrous tissue. There are associated features, including bronchial and peribronchial inflammation, fibrosis, ulceration of the bronchial wall, squamous metaplasia, and mucous gland hyperplasia. The parenchyma that is supplied by the affected airways is commonly abnormal, with varying amounts of fibrosis, emphysema, pneumonia, and atelectasis. The end result of this inflammation is enhanced vascularity of the bronchial wall with associated enlargement of the bronchial arteries and abnormal anastomosis between bronchial and pulmonary arterial circulations. This is extremely important as these anastomotic lesions are often the source of massive hemoptysis requiring urgent angiographic or surgical intervention.

Clinical Manifestations

Patients typically present with recurrent or persistent cough with purulent sputum production. As the disease progresses, hemoptysis becomes frequent and may be life threatening. The bleeding is due to inflamed and friable airway mucosa, and as the disease progresses, massive bleeding can result from erosions of the hypertrophied bronchial arteries. However, it is important to note that in many cases, patients with bronchiectasis may be asymptomatic or have a nonproductive cough ("dry bronchiectasis"). These patients often have involvement of the upper lobes.

Patients often have associated airways hyper-reactivity with wheezing and response to an inhaled bronchodilator. However, many patients have associated small-airways disease that contributes to symptomatology but may not be responsive to bronchodilators.

Radiographic and Laboratory Findings

The chest radiograph, although not very sensitive, may reveal evidence of bronchiectasis. In patients with mild disease, the chest radiograph may be normal, but in patients with saccular bronchiectasis, prominent cystic spaces (see Fig. 23–10), often with air-fluid levels, are visible. Areas of bronchial wall thickening ("tram tracks") (Fig. 23–11) or ring shadows may be apparent on closer inspection. Areas of the lung subserved by these airways may demonstrate decreased aeration and atelectasis or pulmonary infiltrates.

Before the advent of CT scanning, bronchography was the standard procedure for the diagnosis of bronchiectasis and for delineating the areas of involvement. This procedure involved the installation of a radiopaque iodinated lipid material through a catheter or bronchoscope (Fig. 23–12). This technique, however, has been supplanted by CT, which provides an excellent view of dilated airways in cross-section images (Fig. 23–13). The use of high-resolution CT scanning in which the images are on the order of 1 mm in thickness has improved sensitivity for the detection of bronchiectasis (Fig. 23–14) and is currently the gold standard for diagnosis (Hansell, 1998; Smith and Flower, 1996).

The sputum culture of patients with bronchiectasis is often positive for bacterial pathogens such as *S. pneumo-*

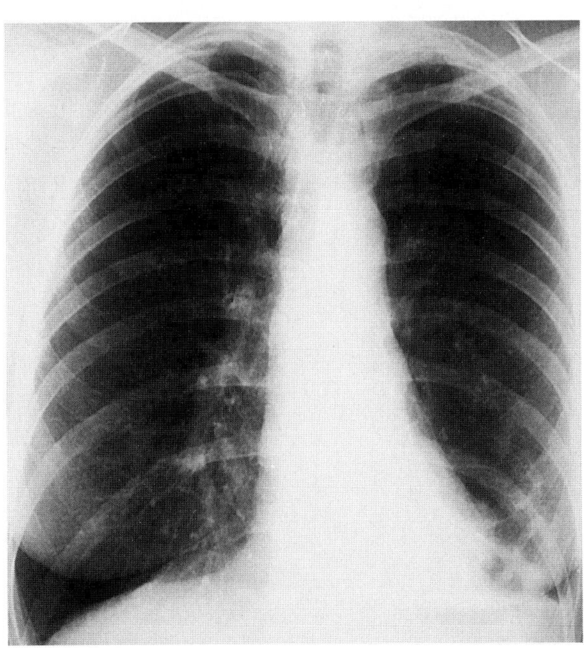

FIGURE 23–11 ■ Posteroanterior chest radiograph illustrating cystic bronchiectasis in the left lower lobe.

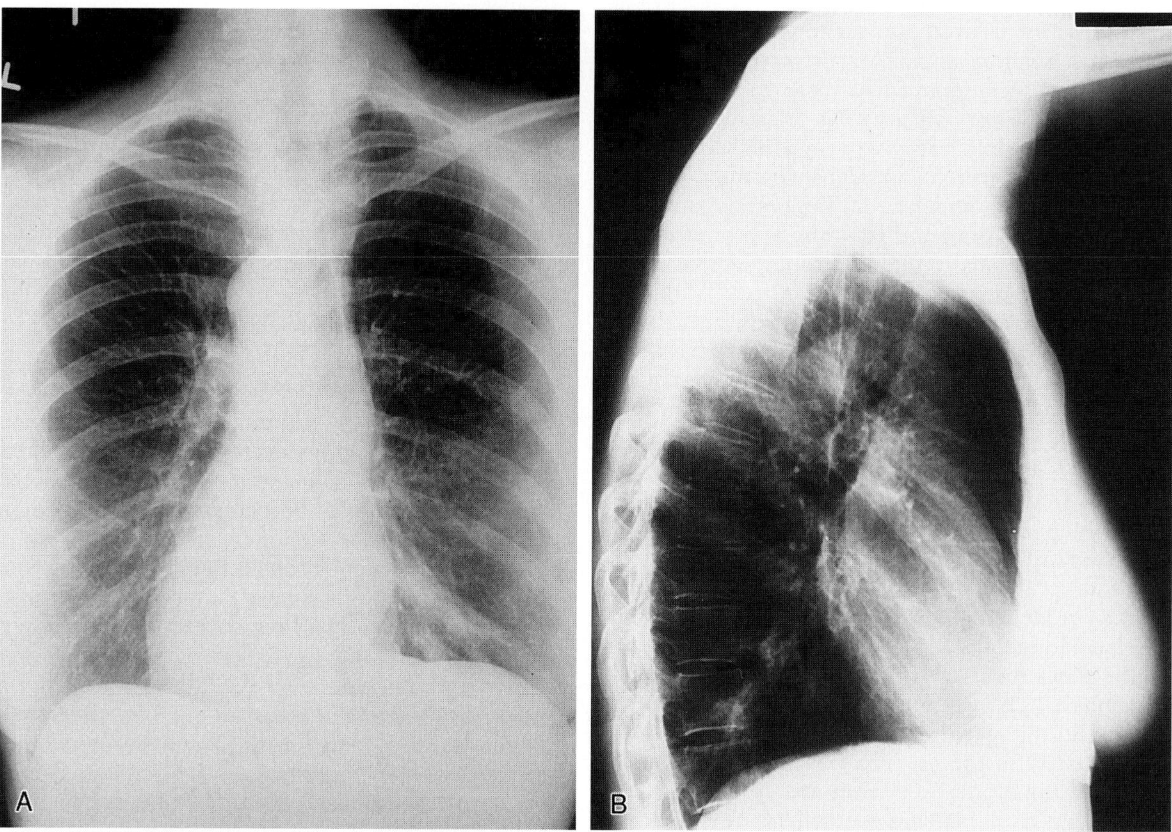

FIGURE 23–12 ■ Posteroanterior (*A*) and lateral (*B*) radiograph illustrating bronchiectasis with bronchial-wall thickening.

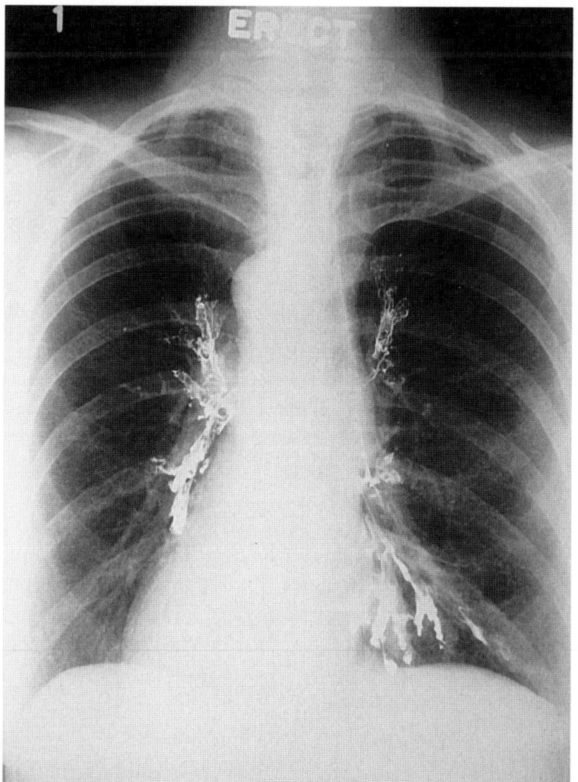

FIGURE 23–13 ■ Bronchogram illustrating varicose bronchiectasis.

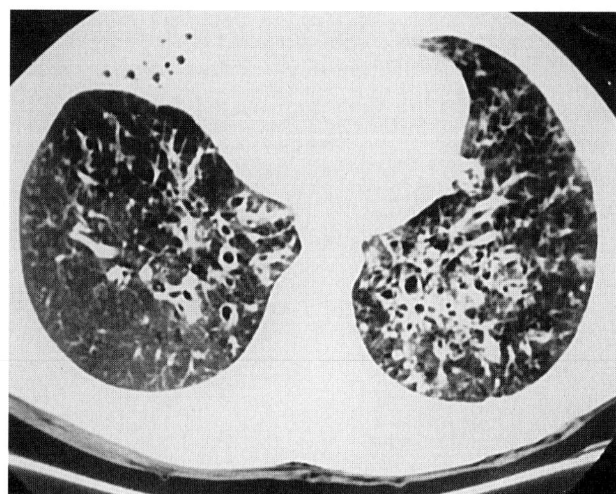

FIGURE 23–14 ■ High resolution computed tomography scan illustrating dilated airways in diffuse bronchiectasis.

niae, *H. influenzae*, and *P. aeruginosa*. In fact, the presence of mucoid *P. aeruginosa* in sputum cultures is so highly associated with bronchiectasis that its presence should alert the physician to consider this possibility, even in the absence of other findings (Nicotra et al, 1995). It is common to find the lung colonized with nontuberculous mycobacteria such as *Mycobacterium avium* complex which can lead to additional problems. Fungal colonization with organisms such as those of the *Aspergillus* genus can also create problems and can also give rise to the syndrome of allergic bronchopulmonary aspergillosis with superimposed asthma.

Treatment

The treatment of bronchiectasis initially should be directed at the elimination of a reversible underlying cause, improved clearance of tracheal and bronchial secretions, control of infection, and reversal of airflow limitation with bronchodilators. Appropriate treatment of an underlying cause, for example, an endobronchial tumor or a foreign body, is obvious. Patients with hypogammaglobulinemia should be treated with intravenous gammaglobulin replacement on a life-long basis (Quartier et al, 1999). Patients with tuberculosis obviously should receive a full course of antituberculous therapy, and patients with allergic bronchopulmonary aspergillosis should be treated with corticosteroids plus monitoring of serum IgE levels, which reflect the underlying eosinophilic inflammatory response in the airways.

In the past, chest physiotherapy with vibration, percussion, and, especially, postural drainage was the cornerstone of therapy. In this era of broad-spectrum antibiotics, these principles are often forgotten, but to the detriment of the patient. Courses of antibiotics for acute exacerbations should be broad-spectrum and directed at underlying culture and sensitivity results. It is often preferable to give a 2 to 3 week course of intravenous antibiotics followed by oral antibiotic therapy, which will result in a more long-lasting remission. Mucolytic agents such as N-acetyl cysteine (Mucomyst) or recombinant DNAase may be of use in patients with cystic fibrosis, but its benefit in patients with bronchiectasis in the absence of cystic fibrosis has never been demonstrated.

Bronchodilators are useful to improve the effects of obstruction and facilitate the clearance of secretions, especially in patients with demonstrable reversible airflow limitation.

Surgical Considerations

In the past, surgical therapy was the foundation of treatment for patients with focal bronchiectasis. In this era of effective antibiotic therapy and supportive treatment, surgery has become much less common (Dogan et al, 1989; Sanderson et al, 1974). However, it is important to recognize that patients with refractory symptoms despite excellent medical management may benefit substantially from resection of a localized bronchiectatic segment or lobe. Before considering resection, an uncorrectable predisposing factor (e.g., ciliary dysmotility) should be excluded because multifocal disease is always present. A thorough evaluation of the chest CT scan should be undertaken prior to making a final decision about resection to ensure that there is no multifocal involvement (which is often subtle). The surgical approach should be planned to spare as much normal parenchyma as possible. Patients with end-stage lung disease resulting from bronchiectasis might be candidates for bilateral lung transplantation.

Surgical intervention is often considered in patients with massive hemoptysis that originates from hypertrophied bronchial arteries. However, it is essential to recognize that surgical resection should be considered only in a patient with sufficient pulmonary reserve. Embolization of bronchial arteries in cases of massive hemoptysis is a viable alternative but may be associated with re-bleeding. In patients with massive hemoptysis in whom pulmonary reserve is limited and who therefore could not withstand a resection, embolization is often the only practical consideration.

SUMMARY

Despite the advent of newer and more potent antibiotics, bacterial infections of the respiratory tract remain an important cause of morbidity and mortality. The ability of the medical profession to treat critical illnesses and immunosuppressive diseases with life-supporting therapies and potent new drugs has resulted in an increase in these infections, which are often due to unusual or opportunistic organisms. This increasing complexity of illness is associated with increases in mortality.

Treatment of community-acquired pneumonia is based on epidemiologic principles, as the infecting organism is rarely known at the time of presentation. These principles classify pneumonia into community-acquired and hospital-acquired. The earlier classification of pneumonia as typical or atypical is obsolete and not clinically useful because the clinical syndrome associated with the various pathogens cannot be reliably distinguished on clinical or radiographic grounds. Prompt institution of antibiotic therapy is key to the successful treatment of pneumonia and should never be delayed while waiting for a sputum sample to be obtained, much less cultured. Sputum cultures are often negative or nondiagnostic, but this does not indicate the absence of infection.

Community-acquired pneumonia is commonly caused by gram-positive and atypical organisms, whereas nosocomial pneumonia is commonly caused by gram-negative organisms and occasionally by fungi. VAP is a subcategory of nosocomial pneumonia, so treatment should be aimed at gram-negative organisms, particularly *Pseudomonas* species.

Another category, aspiration pneumonia, has caused some confusion as it comprises three syndromes: chemical gastric acid pneumonitis, bacterial-aspiration pneumonia, and foreign-body aspiration. Although antibiotics have no role in chemical-aspiration pneumonitis, they are critical in bacterial-aspiration pneumonia and in the bacterial pneumonia that may complicate chemical-aspiration pneumonitis.

Treatment of a COPD exacerbation is controversial but current guidelines recommend combination therapy including antibiotics, inhaled bronchodilators, and systemic corticosteroids. Also, comorbidities should be addressed, as they are often important coprecipitants.

Lung abscess may complicate a necrotizing pneumonia or aspiration syndrome. The mainstay of treatment is systemic, prolonged antibiotic therapy. In some cases external drainage of a lung abscess may be required or, rarely, surgical resection. Radiologic techniques for managing complications such as massive hemoptysis associated with bronchiectasis or lung abscess or primary drainage of a lung abscess that fails to respond to treatment have become the standard of care in many centers and have facilitated the care of these problems such that patients can be stabilized prior to surgery and many avoid surgery altogether.

Bacterial infections remain important in the practice of thoracic surgery as a major source of morbidity and, occasionally, of mortality, but the role of surgery in the management of these problems is usually limited to the treatment of complications.

COMMENTS AND CONTROVERSIES

The role of surgeons in the management of chronic bacterial infections of the lung has certainly changed over the past few decades in most areas of North America and other first-world countries. The incidence of bronchiectasis has diminished and, with modern antibiotic therapy, it is relatively rare that surgical resection is required. In less highly developed countries, surgical resection for bronchiectasis remains much more common. With the introduction of effective methods of percutaneous drainage and antibiotic therapy, lung abscess as a surgical problem has also decreased dramatically. Replacing these problems is the very high incidence of nosocomial infections that can occur within hospitals and that plague thoracic surgeons. With the age of our population increasing, many more elderly patients do undergo major surgical resections. These same patients may have occult aspiration as a result of reflux disease, impaired nutrition, or impaired defense mechanisms leading to postoperative pulmonary infarctions. As well, patients who present with suspected tumors may have community-acquired infections requiring treatment. All of these pulmonary infections require therapy, and often the surgeon plays an important role in their management. For this reason, the authors have detailed the management of both community-acquired and nosocomial infections. Whenever possible, as outlined in the chapter, monotherapy is preferable so as to avoid the problems of superinfection so often seen in intensive care units.

Although these infectious conditions rarely require major surgical intervention, surgeons continue to play an important role in their therapy. In many cases, such as reflux disease, obstructed bronchi, and so forth, following initial treatment, the underlying cause of the pulmonary infection must be investigated and ultimately dealt with.

R. J. G.

REFERENCES

Adams R, Ruffin R, Campbell D: The value of the lipid-laden macrophage index in the assessment of aspiration pneumonia. Aust N Z J Med 27: 550, 1997.

American Thoracic Society: Hospital-acquired pneumonia in adults: Diagnosis, assessment of severity, initial antimicrobial therapy and preventative strategies. Am J Respir Crit Care Med 153:1711, 1996.

Auble TE, Yealy DM, Fine MJ: Assessing prognosis and selecting an initial site of care for adults with community-acquired pneumonia. Infect Dis Clin North Am 12:741, 1998.

Barker AF: Bronchiectasis. Semin Thorac Cardiovasc Surg 7: 112, 1995.

Barrett-Connor E: The value of sputum culture in the diagnosis of pneumococcal pneumonia. Am Rev Respr Dis 103:845, 1971.

Bartlett JG, Gorbach SL, Tally FP et al: Bacteriology and treatment of primary lung abscess. Am Rev Respir Dis 109:510, 1974.

Bartlett JG, Mundy LM: Community-acquired pneumonia. N Engl J Med 333:1618, 1995.

Bates JH, Campbell GD, Barr AL et al: Microbial etiology of acute pneumonia in hospitalized patients. Chest 101:1005, 1992.

Baughman RP, Conrado CE: Diagnosis of lower respiratory tract infections: What we have and what would be nice. Chest 113:219S, 1998.

Baughman RP, Tapson V, McIvor A, et al: The diagnosis and treatment challenges in nosocomial pneumonia. Diagn Microbiol Infect Dis 33:131, 1999.

Belsey R: The pulmonary complications of oesophageal disease. Br J Dis Chest 54:342, 1960.

Bernhard WF, Malcolm JA, Wylie RH: Lung abscess: A study of 148 cases due to aspiration. Dis Chest 43:620, 1963.

Bernstein JM: Treatment of community-acquired pneumonia—IDSA guidelines. Infectious Diseases Society of America (In-process citation). Chest 115:9S, 1999.

Boon ES, Grupa N, Langenberg CJ et al: Concealed lung abscess in critically ill, mechanically ventilated patients. Neth J Med 48:100, 1996.

Borland LM, Sereika SM, Woelfel SK et al: Pulmonary aspiration in pediatric patients during general anesthesia: Incidence and outcome. J Clin Anesth 10:95: 1998.

Boyle JT, Tuchamn DN, Altshulter SM et al: Mechanisms for the association of gastroesophageal reflux and bronchospasm. Am Rev Respir Dis 121:S16, 1985.

Brock RC, Hodgkiss F, Jones HO: Bronchial embolism and posture in relation to lung abscess. Guy's Hosp Rep 91:131, 1942.

Brook I. Treatment of aspiration or tracheostomy-associated pneumonia in neurologically impaired children: Effect of antimicrobials effective against anaerobic bacteria. Int J Pediatr Otorhinolaryngol 35:171, 1996.

Bruchhaus JD, McEachern R, Campbell GD Jr: Hospital-acquired pneumonia: Recent advances in diagnosis, microbiology and treatment. Curr Opin Pulm Med 4: 180, 1998.

Buchman SR, Sugarman JH, Tatum JL et al: Failure of methylprednisolone, ibuprofen or prostacyclin to reduce HCl-induced pulmonary albumin leak in dogs. Surgery 92:163, 1984.

Cassiere HA, Niederman MS: Community-acquired pneumonia. Dis Mon 44:613, 1998a.

Cassiere HA, Fein AM: Duration and route of antibiotic therapy in community-acquired pneumonia: Switch and step-down therapy. Semin Respir Infect 13:36, 1998b.

Chastre J, Fagon JY: Invasive diagnostic testing should be routinely used to manage ventilated patients with suspected pneumonia. Am J Respir Crit Care Med 150:570, 1994.

Chastre J, Fagon JY, Soles P et al: Diagnosis of nosocomial bacterial pneumonia in intubated patients undergoing ventilation: Comparison of the usefulness of BAL and PSB. Am J Med 85:498, 1988.

Chidi CC, Mendelsohn HJ: Lung abscess: A study of the result of treatment based on 90 consecutive cases. J Thorac Cardiovasc Surg 68:168, 1974.

Chirgwin K, Roblin PM, Gelling M et al: Infection with *Chlamydia pneumoniae*. in Brooklyn. J Infect Dis 163:757, 1991.

Cockrill BA, Hales CA: Allergic bronchopulmonary aspergillosis. Annu Rev Med 50:303, 1999.

Collins MJ, Bakheit AM: Does pulse oximetry reliably detect aspiration in dysphagic stroke patients? Stroke 28:1773, 1997.

Cook D, Guyatt G, Marshall J et al: A comparison of sucralfate and ranitidine for the prevention of upper gastrointestinal bleeding in patients requiring mechanical ventilation. N Engl J Med 338:791, 1998.

Cunha BA: Antibiotic pharmacokinetic considerations in pulmonary infections. Semin Respir Infect 6:168, 1991.

Cunha BA, Shea KW: Emergence of antimicrobial resistance in community-acquired pulmonary pathogens. Semin Respir Infect 13:43, 1998.

Dal Santo G: Acid aspiration: Pathophysiological aspects, prevention and therapy. Int Anesth Clin 24:31, 1986.

DeCastro FR, Violan JS, Capuz BL et al: Reliability of the bronchoscopic protected specimen brush in the diagnosis of pneumonia in mechanically ventilated patients. Crit Care Med 19:171, 1991.

Delarue NC, Pearson FG, Nelems JM et al: Lung abscess: Surgical implications. Can J Surg 23:297, 1980.

Dogan R, Alp M, Kaya S et al: Surgical treatment of bronchiectasis: A collective review of 487 cases. Thorac Cardiovasc Surg 37:183, 1989.

Eijking EP, Gommers D, So KL et al: Prevention of respiratory failure after hydrochloric acid aspiration by intratracheal surfactant instillation in rats. Anesth Analg 76:472, 1993.

Eliasson RM, Mossberg B, Camner P et al: The immotile cilia syndrome: A congenital ciliary abnormality as an etiologic factor in chronic airway infections and male sterility. N Engl J Med 297:1, 1977.

Emre U, Sokolovskaya N, Roblin PM, et al: Detection of anti-*Chlamydia pneumoniae* IgE in children with reactive airway disease. J Infect Dis 172:265, 1995.

Fang GD, Fine M, Orloff J et al: New and emerging etiologies for community-acquired pneumonia with implications for therapy. A prospective multicenter study of 359 cases. Med 69:307, 1990.

Farber MO: Managing community-acquired pneumonia: Factors to consider in outpatient care. Postgrad Med 105:106, 1999.

Ferguson GT: Management of COPD: Early identification and active intervention are crucial. Postgrad Med 103:129, 1998.

File TM Jr, Tan JS, Plouffe JF: The role of atypical pathogens: *Mycoplasma pneumoniae*, *Chlamydia pneumoniae*, and *Legionella pneumophila* in respiratory infection. Infect Dis Clin North Am 12:569, 1998.

Fine MJ, Orloff JJ, Rihs JD et al: Evaluation of housestaff physicians' preparation and interpretation of sputum Gram stains for community-acquired pneumonia [see comments]. J Gen Intern Med 6:189, 1991.

Fine MJ, Smith MA, Carson CA et al: Prognosis and outcomes of patients with community-acquired pneumonia. A meta-analysis. JAMA 275:134, 1996.

Fine MJ, Hough LJ, Medsger AR et al: The hospital admission decision for patients with community-acquired pneumonia: Results from the pneumonia Patient Outcomes Research Team cohort study [see comments]. Arch Intern Med 157:36, 1997.

Fine MJ, Stone RA, Singer DE, et al: Processes and outcomes of care for patients with community-acquired pneumonia: Results from the Pneumonia Patient Outcomes Research Team (PORT) cohort study. Arch Intern Med 59:970, 1999.

Fishman JA, Rubin RH: Infection in Organ-Transplant Recipients. N Engl J Med 338:1741, 1998.

Folkesson HG, Matthay MA, Hebert CA, Broaddus VC: Acid aspiration–induced lung injury in rabbits is mediated by interleukin-8–dependent mechanisms. J Clin Invest 96:107, 1995.

Fox JR, Hughes CA, Sutcliff WD: Nonputrid lung abscess. J Thorac Surg 27:255, 1954.

Fox KA, Mularski RA, Sarfati MR et al: Aspiration pneumonia following surgically placed feeding tubes. Am J Surg 170:564, 1995.

Fraser DW, Tsai TR, Orenstein W et al: Legionnaires' disease: Description of an epidemic of pneumonia. N Engl J Med 297:1189, 1977.

Frieden TR, Biebuyck J, Hierholzer WJ: Lung abscess with group A beta-hemolytic streptococcus: Case report and review. Arch Int Med 151:1655, 1991.

Furman AC, Jacobs J, Sepkowitz KA: Lung abscess in patients with AIDS. Clin Infect Dis 22:81, 1996.

Garibaldi RA: Epidemiology of community-acquired respiratory tract infections in adults: Incidence, etiology, and impact. Am J Med 78:32, 1985.

Garzon AA: Life-threatening hemoptysis in primary lung abscess. Ann Thorac Surg 14:357, 1972.

Gates S, Huang T, Cheney FW: Effects of methylprednisolone on resolution of acid aspiration pneumonitis. Arch Surg 118:1262, 1983.

Glauser FL, Millen JE, Falls R: Increased alveolar epithelial permeability with acid aspiration. The effects of high-dose steroids. Am Rev Respir Dis 120:1119, 1979.

Gleason PP, Kapoor WN, Stone RA et al: Medical outcomes and antimicrobial costs with the use of the American Thoracic Society guidelines for outpatients with community-acquired pneumonia. JAMA 278:32, 1997.

Gleeson K, Eggli DF, Maxwell SL: Quantitative aspiration during sleep in normal subjects. Chest 111:1266, 1997.

Goldman G, Welbourn R, Kobzik L et al: Tumor necrosis factor-alpha mediates acid aspiration–induced systemic organ injury. Ann Surg 212:513, 1990.

Goldman G, Welbourn R, Kobzik L et al: Synergism between leukotriene B4 and thromboxane A2 in mediating acid-aspiration injury. Surgery 111:55, 1992a.

Goldman G, Welbourn R, Kobzik L et al: Reactive oxygen species and elastase mediate lung permeability after acid aspiration. J Applied Physiol 73:571, 1992b.

Goldman G, Welbourn R, Klausner JM et al: Leukocytes mediate acid aspiration–induced multiorgan edema. Surgery 114:13, 1993.

Greenfield LJ, Singleton RP, McCaffree DR et al: Pulmonary effects of experimental graded aspiration of hydrochloric acid. Ann Surg 170:74, 1989.

Grinan NP, Lucena FM, Romera JV et al: Yield of percutaneous needle lung aspiration in lung abscess. Chest 97:69, 1990.

Grossman RF: The value of antibiotics and the outcomes of antibiotic therapy in exacerbations of COPD. Chest 113(4 suppl): 249S, 1998.

Guidiol F, Manresa MD, Pallares R et al: Clindamycin vs penicillin for anaerobic lung infections. Arch Int Med 150:2525, 1990.

Hagan JL, Hardy JD: Lung abscess revisited: A survey of 184 cases. Ann Surg 197:755, 1983.

Haley RW, Hooten TM, Culver D et al: Nosocomial pneumonia in US hospitals 1975–1976: Estimated frequency by selected characteristics of patients. Am J Med 70:947, 1981.

Hamelburg W, Bosomworth PP: Aspiration pneumonitis: Experimental studies and clinical observations. Anesth Analg 43:669, 1964.

Hammond JM, Potgieter PD, Hanslo D et al: The etiology and antimicrobial susceptibility patterns of microorganisms in acute community-acquired lung abscess. Chest 108:937, 1995.

Hansell DM. Bronchiectasis. Radiol Clin North Am 36:107, 1998.

Hanson LC, Weber DJ, Rutala WA: Risk factors for nosocomial pneumonia in the elderly. Am J Med 92:161, 1992.

Henriquez AH, Mendoza J, Gonzalez PC: Quantitative culture of bronchoalveolar lavage from patients with anaerobic lung abscesses. J Infect Dis 164:414, 1991.

Huxley EJ, Viroslav J, Gray WR, Pierce AK: Pharyngeal aspiration in normal adults and patients with depressed consciousness. Am J Med 64:564, 1978.

Ip MS, Lam WK: Bronchiectasis and related disorders. Respirology 1:107, 1996.

Jacobson SJ, Griffiths K, Diamond S et al: A randomized controlled trial of penicillin vs clindamycin for the treatment of aspiration pneumonia in children. Arch Pediatr Adolesn Med 151:701, 1997.

James CF, Modell JH, Gibbs CP et al: Pulmonary aspiration: Effects of volume and pH in the rat. Anesth Analg 63:665, 1984.

Kadakia SC, Sullivan HO, Starnes E: Percutaneous endoscopic gastrostomy or jejunostomy and the incidence of aspiration in 79 patients. Am J Surg 164:114, 1992.

Kaye MG, Fox MJ, Bartlett JG et al: The clinical spectrum of *Staphylococcus aureus* pulmonary infection. Chest 97:788, 1990.

Kingston GW, Phang PT, Leathley MJ: Increased incidence of nosocomial pneumonia in mechanically ventilated patients with subclinical aspiration. Am J Surg 161:589, 1991.

Kinney TB, DeLuca SA. Kartagener's syndrome. Am Fam Physician 44:133, 1991.

Kinsey GC, Murray MJ, Swensen SJ, Miles JM: Glucose content of tracheal aspirates: Implication for the detection of tube-feeding aspiration. Crit Care Med 22: 1557, 1994.

Kirkpatrick MB, Bass JB: Quantitative bacterial cultures of BAL fluids and protected brush catheter specimens from normal subjects. Am Rev Respir Dis 139:546, 1989.

Klein JS, Schultz S, Heffner JE: Interventional radiology of the chest: Image-guided percutaneous drainage of pleural effusion, lung abscess and pneumothorax. AJR Am J Roentgenol 164:581, 1995.

Knight PR, Druskovich G, Tait AR, Johnson KJ: The role of neutrophils, oxidants and proteases in the pathogeneisis of acid pulmonary injury. Anesthesiology 77:772, 1992.

Knight PR, Rutter T, Tait AR et al: Pathogenesis of gastric particulate lung injury: A comparison and interaction with acidic pneumonitis. Anesth Analg 77:754, 1993.

Kollef MH: The prevention of ventilator-associated pneumonia. N Engl J Med 340:627, 1999.

Kraft M, Cassell GH, Henson JE et al: Detection of *Mycoplasma pneumoniae* in the airways of adults with chronic asthma. Am J Respir Crit Care Med 158:998, 1998.

Lambiase RE, Deyoe L, Cronan JJ et al: Percutaneous drainage of 335 consecutive abscesses: Results of primary darinage with 1 year follow-up. Radiology 184:167, 1992.

Langer M, Mosconi P, Cigada M et al: Long-term respiratory support and risk of pneumonia in critically ill patients. Am Rev Respir Dis 140:302, 1989.

Lee SK, Morris RF, Cramer B: Percutaneous needle aspiration of neonatal lung abscesses. Pediatr Radiol 21:254, 1991.

le Roux BT, Mohlala ML, Odell JA, Whitton ID: Suppurative diseases of the lung and pleural space. II: Bronchiectasis. Curr Probl Surg 23:93, 1986.

Levison ME, Mangurra CT, Lorber B et al: Clindamycin compared with penicillin for the treatment of anaerobic lung abscess. Ann Intern Med 98:466, 1983.

Lieberman D, Schlaeffer F, Lieberman D et al: *Mycoplasma pneumoniae* community-acquired pneumonia: A review of 101 hospitalized adult patients. Respiration 63:261, 1996.

Longstreth GF, Weitzman SA, Browning RJ et al: Bronchiectasis and homozygous alpha-1-antitrypsin deficiency. Chest 67:233, 1975.

Louria DB, Blumenfeld HL, Ellis JT et al: Studies on the influenza in the pandemic of 1957–58. II: Pulmonary complications of influenzae. J Clin Invest 38:213, 1959.

Low DE: Resistance issues and treatment implications: *Pneumococcus, Staphylococcus aureus*, and gram-negative rods. Infect Dis Clin North Am 12:613, 1998.

Lynch JP III, Martinez FJ: Community-acquired pneumonia. Curr Opin Pulm Med 4:162, 1998.

Mahul P, Auboyer C, Jospe R et al: Prevention of nosocomial pneumonia in intubated patients: Respective role of mechanical subglottic secretions drainage and stress ulcer prophylaxis. Int Care Med 18:20, 1992.

Mandell LA: Antibiotic therapy for community-acquired pneumonia. Clin Chest Med 20:589, 1999.

Mandell LA, Campbell GD: Nosocomial pneumonia Guidelines: An International Perspective. Chest 113:188S, 1998.

Mandell LA, Marrie TJ, Grossman RF, et al: Summary of Canadian guidelines for the management of community-acquired pneumonia; an evidence-based update by the Canadian Infectious Disease Society and the Canadian Thoracic Society. Can Resp J 7:371, 2000.

Mandell LA, Marrie TJ, Niederman MS et al: Initial antimicrobial treatment of hospital-acquired pneumonia in adults: A conference report. Can J Infect Dis 4:317, 1993.

Mares DC, Wilkes DS: Bronchoscopy in the diagnosis of respiratory infections. Curr Opin Pulm Med 4:123, 1998.

Marrie TJ, Peeling RW, Fine MJ et al: Ambulatory patients with community-acquired pneumonia: The frequency of atypical agents and clinical course. Am J Med 101:508, 1996.

Marrie TJ: Community-acquired pneumonia: Epidemiology, etiology, treatment. Infect Dis Clin North Am 12:723, 1998a.

Marrie TJ: Epidemiology of mild pneumonia. Semin Respir Infect 13:3, 1998b.

Martin BJ, Corlew MM, Wood H et al: The association of swallowing dysfunction and aspiration pneumonia. Dysphagia 9:1, 1994.

Mayhall CG: Nosocomial pneumonia: Diagnosis and Prevention. Infect Dis Clin North Am 11:427, 1997.

McEachern R, Campbell GD Jr: Hospital-acquired pneumonia: Epidemiology, etiology, and treatment. Infect Dis Clin North Am 12:761, 1998.

Mellin-Olsen J, Fasting S, Gisvold SE: Routine preoperative gastric emptying is seldom indicated: A study of 85,594 anaesthetics with special focus on aspiration pneumonia. Acta Anaesth Scan 40:1184, 1996.

Mendelsohn CL: Aspiration of stomach contents into the lungs during obstetric anesthesia. Am J Obstet Gynecol 52:191, 1946.

Mengoli L: Giant lung abscess treated by tube thoracostomy. J Thorac Cardiovasc Surg 90:186, 1985.

Metlay JP, Kapoor WN, Fine MJ: Does this patient have community-acquired pneumonia? Diagnosing pneumonia by history and physical examination [see comments]. JAMA 278:1440, 1997.

Mier L, Dreyfuss D, Darchy B et al: Is penicillin G an adequate initial treatment for aspiration pneumonia? A prospective evaluation using a protected specimen brush and quantitative cultures. Int Care Med 19:279, 1993.

Monaldi V: Endocavitary aspiration: Its practical applications. Tubercle 28:223, 1947.

Mori T, Ebe T, Takahashi M et al: Lung abscess: Analysis of 66 cases from 1979 to 1991. Int Med 32:278, 1993.

Moser KM, Maurer J, Jassi L et al: Sensitivity, specificity and risk of diagnositic procedure in a clinical model of *Streptococcus pneumoniae* pneumonia. Am Rev Respir Dis 125:436, 1982.

Murray HW: Antimicrobial therapy in pulmonary aspiration. Am J Med 66:188, 1979.

Mysliwiec V, Pina JS: Bronchiectasis: The "other" obstructive lung disease. Postgrad Med 106:123, 1999.

Nader-Djalal N, Knight PR, Davidson BA, Johnson K: Hyperoxia exacerbates microvascular lung injury following acid aspiration. Chest 112:1607, 1997.

Nader-Djalal N, Knight PR, Thusu K et al: Reactive oxygen species contribute to oxygen-related lung injury after acid aspiration. Anesth Analg 87:127, 1998.

Nagase T, Ohga E, Sudo E et al: Intercellular adhesion molecule-1 mediates acid aspiration–induced lung injury. Am J Resp Crit Care Med 154:504, 1996.

Naidich DP, McGuinness G: Pulmonary manifestations of AIDS: CT and radiographic correlations. Radiol Clin North Am 29:999, 1991.

Nicotra MB: Bronchiectasis. Semin Respir Infect 9:31, 1994.

Nicotra MB, Rivera M, Dale AM et al: Clinical, pathophysiologic, and microbiologic characterization of bronchiectasis in an aging cohort [see comments]. Chest 108:955, 1995.

Niederman MS, Bass JB Jr, Campbell GD et al: Guidelines for the initial management of adults with community-acquired pneumonia: Diagnosis, assessment of severity, and initial antimicrobial therapy. Am Rev Respir Dis 148:1418, 1993.

Niederman MS, Torres A, Summer W: Invasive diagnostic testing is not needed routinely to manage suspected ventilator-acquired pneumonia. Am J Respir Crit Care Med 150:565, 1994.

Niewoehner DE, Erbland ML, Deupree RH et al: Effect of systemic glucocorticoids on exacerbations of chronic obstructive pulmonary disease: Department of Veterans Affairs Cooperative Study Group [see comments]. N Engl J Med 340:1941, 1999.

Orozco-Levi M, Torres A, Ferrer M et al: Semirecumbent position protects from pulmonary aspiration but not completely from gastroesophageal reflux in mechanically ventilated patients. Am J Resp Crit Care Med 152:1387, 1995.

Paladino JA, Sperry HE, Backes JM et al: Clinical and economic evaluation of oral ciprofloxacin after an abbreviated course of intravenous antibiotics. Am J Med 91:462, 1991.

Perlino CA: Metronidazole vs clindamycin treatment of anaerobic pulmonary infection. Arch Intern Med 141:1424, 1981.

Plouffe JF, McNally C, File TM Jr et al: Value of noninvasive studies in community-acquired pneumonia. Infect Dis Clin North Am 12:689, 1998.

Pohlson EC, McNamara JJ, Char C et al: Lung abscess: A changing pattern of disease. Am J Surg 150:97, 1985.

Potts RG, Zaroukian MH, Guerrero PA et al: comparison of blue dye visualization and glucose oxidase test strip methods for detecting pulmonary aspiration of enteral feedings in intubated adults. Chest 103:117, 1993.

Quartier P, Debre M, Deblic J et al: Early and prolonged intravenous immunoglobulin replacement therapy in childhood agammaglobulinemia: a retrospective survey of 31 patients. J Pediatr 134:589, 1999.

Ramirez JA, Ahkee S, Tolentino A et al: Diagnosis of *Legionella pneumophila*, *Mycoplasma pneumoniae*, or *Chlamydia pneumoniae* lower respiratory infection using the polymerase chain reaction on a single throat swab specimen. Diagn Microbiol Infect Dis 24:7, 1996.

Reid LM: The pathology of obstructive and Inflammatory airway diseases. Eur J Respir Dis Suppl 147:26, 1986.

Rennard SI: COPD: Overview of definitions, epidemiology, and factors influencing its development. Chest 113(4 suppl):235S, 1998.

Reynolds HY: Defense mechanisms against infections. Curr Opin Pulm Med 5:136, 1999.

Rice TW, Ginsberg RJ, Todd TRJ: Tube drainage of lung abscess. Ann Thor Surg 44:356, 1987.

Rosenow EC III: Diffuse pulmonary infiltrates in the immunocompromised host. Clin Chest Med 11:55, 1990.

Rubin RH: Infection in the organ transplant recipient. In Rubin RH,

Young LS (eds): Clinical Approach to Infection in the Compromised Host, 3d ed. New York, Plenum, 1994, p 629.

Sanderson JM, Kennedy MC, Johnson MF, Manley DC: Bronchiectasis: Results of surgical and conservative management: A review of 393 cases. Thorax 29:407, 1974.

Santamaria F, de Santi MM, Grillo G et al: Ciliary motility at light microscopy: A screening technique for ciliary defects (In process citation). Acta Paediatr 88:853, 1999.

Sarosi GA: "Atypical pneumonia": Why this term may be better left unsaid. Postgrad Med 105:131, 1999.

Schmidt J, Holas M, Halvorson K, Reding M: Videofluoroscopic evidence of aspiration predicts pneumonia and death but not dehydration following stroke. Dysphagla 9:7, 1994.

Schwartzmann SW, Adler JL, Sullivan RJ et al: Bacterial pneumonia during the Hong Kong influenza epidemic of 1968–1969: Experience in a city-county hospital. Arch Intern Med 127:1037, 1971.

Senior RM, Anthonisen NR: Chronic obstructive pulmonary disease (COPD). Am J Respir Crit Care Med 157:S139, 1998.

Shafron RD, Tate F: Lung abscesses: A five-year evaluation. Dis Chest 53:12, 1968.

Smith IE, Flower CD: Review article: Imaging in bronchiectasis: Br J Radiol 69:589, 1996.

Stoutenbeek CP, van Saene HK: Nonantibiotic measures in the prevention of ventilator-associated pneumonia. Sem Resp Infections 12:294, 1997.

Strong RM, Condon SC, Solinger MR et al: Equal aspiration rates from postpylorus and intragastric-placed small-bore nasoenteric feeing tubes: A randomized, prospective study. JPEN J Parenter Enteral Nutr 16:59, 1992.

Sturgess JM, Thompson MW, Czegledy-Nagy E, Turner JA: Genetic aspects of immotile cilia syndrome. Am J Med Genet 25:149, 1986.

Sukumaran M, Granada MJ, Berger HW et al: Evaluation of corticosteroid treatment in aspiration of gastric contents: A controlled clinical trial. Mt Sinai J Med 47:335, 1980.

Swensen SJ, Peters SG, LeRoy AJ et al: Radiology in the intensive care unit. Mayo Clin Proc 66:396, 1991.

Takaro T, Scott SM, Bridgman AH et al: Suppurative diseases of the lungs, pleura and pericardium. Curr Probl Surg 14:9, 1977.

Teabout JR II: Aspiration of gastric contents: An experimental study. Am J Pathol 28:51, 1952.

Tenholder MF, Greene LM, Thomas AM: The role of radiology in pulmonary infectious disease. Curr Opin Pulm Med 4:142, 1998.

Thibodeau LG, Verdile VP, Bartfield JM: Incidence of aspiration after urgent intubation. Am J Emerg Med 15:562, 1997.

Thom DH, Grayston JT, Siscovick DS et al: Association of prior infection with *Chlamydia pneumoniae* and angiographically demonstrated coronary artery disease. JAMA 268:68, 1992.

Thoms NW, Wilson RF, Puro HE et al: Life-threatening hemoptysis in primary lung abscess. Ann Thor Surg 14:347, 1972.

Torres A, Aznar B, Gatell JM et al: Incidence, risks and prognosis of nosocomial pneumonia in mechanically ventilated patients. Am Rev Respir Dis 142:523, 1990.

Torres A, Serra-Battles J, Ros E et al: Pulmonary aspiration of gastric contents in patients receiving mechanical ventilation: The effect of body position. Ann Int Med 116:540, 1992.

van Sonnenberg E, D'Agostino HB, Casola G et al: Lung abscess: CT-guided drainage. Radiology 178:347, 1991.

Warner MA, Warner ME, Weber JG: Clinical significance of pulmonary aspiration during the perioperative period. Anesthesiology 78:56, 1993.

Weiser MR, Pechet TT, Williams JP et al: Experimental murine acid aspiration injury is mediated by neutrophils and the alternative complement pathway. J Appl Physiol 83:1090, 1997.

Weiss W, Cherniack NS: Acute nonspecific lung abscess: A controlled study comparing orally and parenterally administered penicilin G. Chest 66:348, 1974.

Wiedemann HP, Rice TW: Lung abscess and empyema. Sem Thor Cardiovasc Surg 7:119, 1995.

Wilson R: The role of infection in COPD. Chest 113(4 suppl):242S, 1998.

Woodhead M: Management of pneumonia in the outpatient setting. Semin Respir Infect 13:8, 1998.

Wunderlink RG: Clinical practice guidelines for the management of pneumonia—do they work? New Horiz 6:75, 1998.

Wynne JW: Aspiration pneumonitis: Correlation of experimental models with clinical disease. Clin Chest Med 3:25, 1982.

Wynne JW, Ramphal R, Hood CI: Tracheal mucosal damage after aspiration: A scanning electron microscope study. Am Rev Respir Dis 124:728, 1981.

Wynne JW, Reynolds JC, Hood IC et al: Steroid therapy for pneumonitis induced in rabbits by aspiration of foodstuff. Anesthesiology 51:11, 1979.

Yamada H, Kudoh I, Nishizawa H et al: Complement partially mediates acid aspiration–induced remote organ injury in the rat. Acta Anaesth Scand 41:713, 1997.

Yang PC, Luh KT, Lee YC et al: Lung abscesses: US examination and US-guided transthoracic aspiration. Radiology 180:171, 1991.

Yellin A, Yellin EO, Lieberman Y: Percutaneous tube drainage: The treatment of choice for refractory lung abscess. Ann Thor Surg 39:265, 1985.

Zaidi NH, Smith HA, King SC et al: Oxygen desaturation on swallowing as a potential marker of aspiration in acute stroke. Age Aging 24:267, 1996.

Zucker AR, Holm BA, Crawford GP et al: PEEP is necessary for exogenous surfactant to reduce pulmonary edema in canine aspiration pneumonitis. J App Physiol 73:679, 1992.

TUBERCULOSIS AND ATYPICAL MYCOBACTERIAL DISEASES

Reza John Mehran

Jean Deslauriers

There is no more dangerous disease than pulmonary phthisis, and no other is so common . . . it destroys a very great part of the human race.

Antoine Portal, Paris, 1832

Pulmonary mycobacterial diseases are pathologic processes in which the lung is infected with mycobacterial organisms. Tuberculosis is caused by *Mycobacterium tuberculosis* but species of *Mycobacteria* other than *tuberculosis* can produce similar pathologic changes. The infection involves mainly the lungs, where the result of cell-mediated immunity is characterized by granuloma formation.

Approximately 8 million new cases of tuberculosis are still reported worldwide every year, and they result in 3 million deaths. A significant number of these cases are related to the emergence of the HIV syndrome, which results in greater risks of transmission as well as increased host susceptibility and drug resistance to treatment. Currently, more than two thirds of reported cases of tuberculosis occur in nonwhite population groups, and risk factors other than HIV include substance abuse, low social status, illegal immigration, residence in correctional and nursing home facilities, and noncompliant behavior toward treatment.

The study of tuberculosis is a fascinating travel through the history of medicine and surgery since the dawn of civilization. At the beginning of the 20th century, tuberculosis was indeed the foremost single cause of death among adults and at that time, a system of sanatoriums that emphasized bed rest and nutrition was created to help fight the disease. It was in those institutions that cavity closure by means of surgical modalities, such as phrenic nerve crush, thoracoplasty, and plombage, were found to be of value in controlling the infection. In the United States as well as throughout Europe, these developments paralleled very closely those of thoracic surgery as a surgical speciality.

In this chapter, the authors review the pertinent aspects of the surgical treatment of mycobacterial diseases as they apply to the practice of thoracic surgery at the beginning of the 21st century.

HISTORICAL NOTES

In the Paleolithic period (the stone age), human species were essentially living in herds and did not have domesticated animals. Tuberculosis and other infectious diseases may have occurred sporadically, but they probably did not occur in epidemic form. In the Neolithic period (10,000–7000 BC), humans apparently shifted from food gathering to food producing. Primitive settlements were developed and animals were raised and maintained. Because a social network of more than 180 to 440 persons is required for tuberculosis infection to become endemic in a community, the disease probably became endemic among animals long before it affected humans.

Epidemic transmission began with increasing population density, and it slowly spread as members of large European communities traveled worldwide (Diamond, 1992). Because of its enormous ravages, tuberculosis became known as the Great White Plague throughout feudal Europe (Dubos and Dubos, 1952). In the late 18th century, 40% of deaths in London were thought to be due to tuberculosis. Among Native Americans, there is almost no evidence of tuberculosis prior to the European migration.

From the time of Hippocrates (Table 23–7), tuberculosis was known as *phthisis*, a term derived from the Greek language and meaning decaying. The swollen glands of

TABLE 23–7 ■ **Milestones in the Evolution of the Description of Tuberculosis**

Event	*Date*	*Comment*
Pott's disease in the Neolithic age	5000 BC	
Clay tablets from the library of Assyrian King Assurbanipal	668–626 BC	Earliest description of tuberculosis
Hippocrates, Greece	460–375 BC	Phthisis described in the second book of *De Morbis*
Galen, Greece	129–200	Contagiousness of tuberculosis
King's Evil	Middle Ages	The magic touch of the hands of the kings of France on scrofula
The Great White Plague	1600s	Spread of tuberculosis throughout Europe
Franciscus Delaboe Sylvius, Holland	1679	Tubercle; line of beads; pathologic description of tuberculosis adenopathy
James Carson, England	1819	Idea of pneumothorax in the treatment of tuberculosis; animal model
J. Hastings and R. Storks, England	1844	Cavernostomy
William Morton, Boston	1846	Discovery of anesthesia
Herman Brehner, Germany	1859	Notion of rest in sanatorium for the treatment of tuberculosis
Carlo Forlanini, Italy	1882	First artificial pneumothorax
Robert Koch, Germany	1882	Identification of tubercle bacilli
Edouard Bernard de Cerenville, Switzerland	1885	Description of thoracoplasty
Marin Theodore Tuffier, France	1891	Apicolysis
E. Delorme, France	1894	Pulmonary decortication
Wilhelm Conrad Roentgen, Germany	1895	Discovery of radiography
H. Schlange, Germany	1907	Extrapleural plombage
Hans Christian Jacobeus, Sweden	1912	Thoracoscopy for parietal pneumolysis
A. Bernou	1922	Oleothorax
H. Lilienthal, U.S.	1933	Pneumonectomy
S. Freedlander, U.S.	1935	Lobectomy
Selman Waksman, U.S.	1944	Streptomycin, isolated from soil saprophytes; Nobel prize in 1952
E.H. Robitzek and I.J. Selikoff, U.S.	1952	First clinical trial proving the efficacy of isoniazid, discovered by V. Clarin in 1945, France
Worldwide	1980s	Resurgence of resistant strains of tuberculosis and renewed interest in surgery as a treatment modality

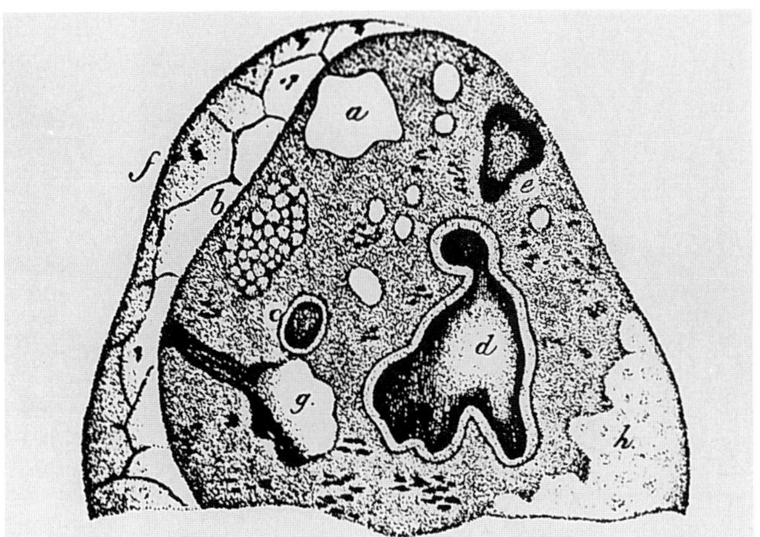

FIGURE 23–15 ■ Laënnec's illustration of different forms of tuberculous matter with (a) immature or crude tubercles; (b) yellow groups of incipient tubercles, still grey and semitransparent externally; (c) small cartilaginous cysts emptied of tuberculous contents; (d) tuberculous excavation entirely empty and lined by two membranes, the exterior semicartilaginous and the interior soft—a bronchial tube opens into this excavation; (e) small, empty, tuberculous excavation, not lined by any membrane; (f) surface of the lung; (g) tubercle partly softened and evacuated; (h) incipient tuberculous infiltration of the pulmonary tissue. (From Comroe JH Jr: T.B. or not T.B.? I. The cause of tuberculosis. Am Rev Respir Dis 117:138, 1978.)

the neck were known as *scrofula* and *king's evil.* Ever since the reign of Clovis (5th century), the kings of France were believed to have received a healing power from God, and this power started the ceremony of the Touch to cure the swollen glands of the neck. Tuberculosis of the skin was termed *lupus vulgaris* and that of the spine *Pott's disease*, a term derived from the name of Percivall Pott, an 18th century British surgeon. Indeed, the vertebral fusion and deformity of the spine that characterize Pott's disease have enabled historians to establish the existence of tuberculosis in mummies dating from 2000 to 4000 BC.

In the early 17th century, tuberculosis was also known as consumption (from the Latin word *consumere*, meaning to eat up, to devour), asthenia, *tabes* (meaning decline), bronchitis, inflammation of the lungs, lactic fever, and gastric fever. Until the late 19th century, however, these terms were also used when referring to other diseases of the lungs, such as cancer, lung abscesses, and silicosis. At that time, tuberculosis struck hardest among young men and women, condemning many of them to early death.

The theory of contagion was described in 1546 by a Florentine physician named Hieronymus Fracastorius. That discovery led not only to increased efforts to find the cause of disease but also to the spread of "magical thinking" throughout Europe. Examples of this thinking include the story of a physician who became "consumptive" because he was in the habit of "tasting" the sputum of his patients and the practice of treating tuberculosis with human milk. As early as 1699, Italy and later Spain developed restrictive quarantine laws, which were not without consequence to the misery of many, including Frédéric Chopin who was denied hospitality on the Island of Majorca. At that time, the sanitation rules of Majorca were very strict and everything touched by phthisic patients had to be burned, a burden no hotel wanted to assume. In 1650, the Medical Faculty of Paris expressed some doubts about the contagiousness of phthisis, and this concept soon spread all over northern Europe, where some physicians believed that heredity had more to do with the spread of the disease than did contagion.

In 1679, Franciscus Delaboe Sylvius, a Dutch iatrochemist, described in his work *Opera Medica* the characteristic lung nodules associated with tuberculosis and called them *tubercula*, or *small knots*. The first credible theory that tuberculosis might be due to infectious organisms (the germ theory) was put forth in 1722 by Benjamin Martel of London. He proposed that tuberculosis was caused by animaliculae (small animals) that could be transmitted from a consumptive lung. In 1821, René Théophile Hyacinthe Laënnec, a French physician, was the first to group tuberculosis in all of its forms into a single disease, and it became known as the totalitarum theory of Laënnec. The following paragraph is from Comroe (1978), who commented on the work of Laënnec:

> By careful examination of tuberculous patients during life and complete study of the lungs (Fig. 23–15) of the unfortunate patients who came to the autopsy room (which was the early fate of most of them), he determined that the characteristic lesion of "consumption" in all of the organs and tissues that it attacked was the tubercle; that tubercles may break down in lungs and form cavities but that the latter may be sealed over by a new membrane and in effect healed; and that the existence of cavities can be detected using a stethoscope during the life of a patient, by a new physical sign, pectoriloquism (transmission of the patient's voice through a cavity in the lungs and the chest wall to a stethoscope on the chest).

In 1839, Johann Lucas Schönlein, professor of medicine in Zurich, suggested using the term *tuberculosis* for all manifestations of phthisis because the tubercle was the fundamental anatomic basis of the disease. The first convincing evidence that tuberculosis was an infectious disease was provided in 1868 by Jean-Antoine Villemin, who performed experiments on rabbits and was able to reproduce the disease by injecting infectious sputum and caseum material into healthy animals.

In 1882, Robert Koch made a presentation at the Berlin physiologic society that forever changed the thinking about tuberculosis as an infectious disease. He described the tuberculous bacillus, an organism known to

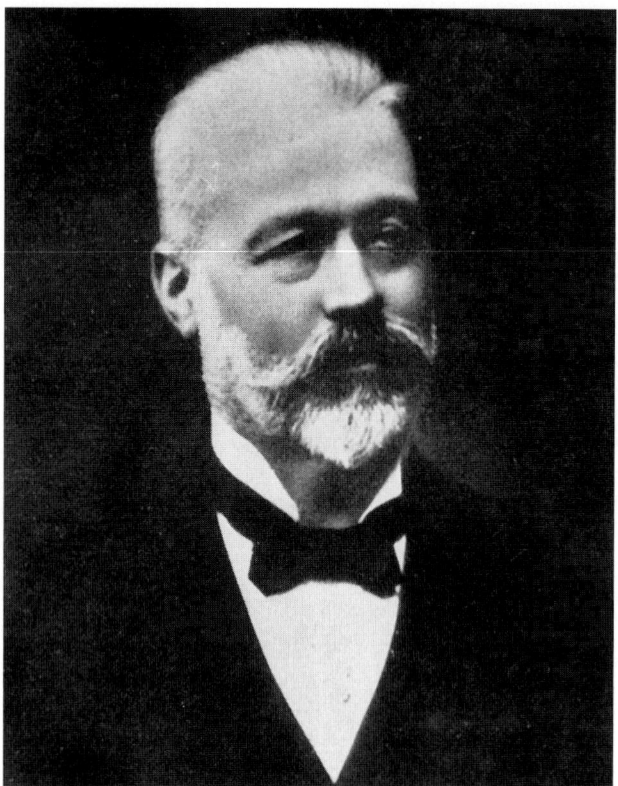

FIGURE 23–16 ■ Carlo Forlanini (1847–1918), Pavia, Italy. (From Alexander J: The collapse therapy of pulmonary tuberculosis. Springfield, Charles C. Thomas, 1937.)

this day as the Koch bacillus, and convincingly demonstrated it to be the cause of disease. He also established the principles of its bacteriology by specifying that it was necessary to isolate the bacteria from the body, to grow them in pure culture, and to administrate the isolate to animals to reproduce the same morbid condition (Koch's principles) (Koch, 1882). Soon after his discovery, Koch introduced a secret vaccine for the treatment of tuberculosis, but unfortunately, the vaccine was made of virulent bacteria and patients became actively infected after the vaccination. Koch was severely criticized for not revealing the content of his vaccine (Dubos and Dubos, 1952).

Albert Calmette was a French physician who was appointed in 1895 to the directorship of the newly founded Pasteur Institute in Lille, France. With the help of Camille Guérin, a veterinarian, they produced a vaccine of boiled, completely attenuated cultures of *Mycobacterium bovis*. Even if the efficacy of the bacille Calmette-Guérin (BCG) vaccine is still largely unknown, it is now used worldwide (Centers for Disease Control, 1991).

Rest resulted in the cure of some patients, but not all of those afflicted with tuberculosis were so lucky. Indeed, the mortality of patients admitted to New York State sanatoriums between the years 1908 and 1914 was 69% for those with advanced disease, 23% for those with moderately advanced disease, and 13% for those with minimal disease (Alling and Bosworth, 1960).

The history of operation for pulmonary tuberculosis is nowhere better summarized than in John Alexander's *The Collapse Therapy of Pulmonary Tuberculosis* (1937). The original idea of accelerating the healing of tuberculous cavities by facilitating their collapse dates back to the end of the 18th century. After having observed a favorable evolution of tuberculous lesions in patients with spontaneous pneumothoraces, Forlanini, in 1894, (Fig. 23–16), thought that adequate treatment of active tuberculosis could be supplemented by the creation and maintenance of intrapleural pneumothoraces. This concept led to the reporting of good results a full 2 years before the actual discovery of radiography.

The principle involved in therapy of tuberculosis by means of artificial pneumothoraces was the promotion of immobilization and collapse of the cavity by suppressing the effects of lung elasticity. By freeing pleural adhesions with a thoracoscope, in 1925, Jacobeus (Fig. 23–17) reemphasized the importance of this technique and he was able to widen its indications. The procedure was done with two incisions, one for the thoracoscope and one for a galvanocautery. It was a long operation, often done in several sittings. Because lung tissue was commonly contained within the adhesion, Eloesser and Brown in 1924 suggested that these adhesions be divided extrapleurally in order to avoid tearing the lung (Fig. 23–18) (Fey et al, 1955). The technique was, however, not without its problems, and accidental lung perforation could lead to bronchopleural fistulas and empyema. The collapse had to be maintained for a period of 4 years after a good result had been obtained and this could be done only in a sanatorium.

Phrenicectomy (Stuertz, 1912) was also advocated to reduce respiratory movements by way of diaphragmatic

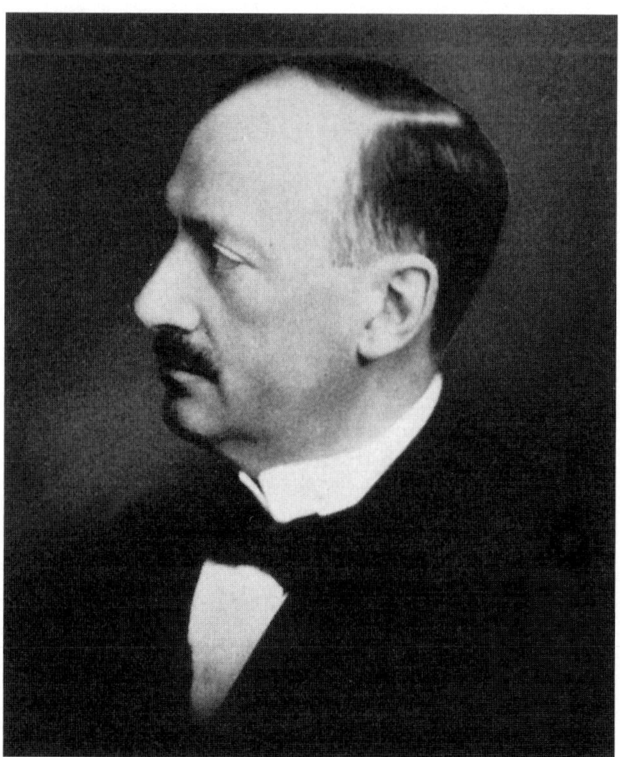

FIGURE 23–17 ■ Hans Christian Jacobeus, Stockholm, Sweden. (From Alexander J: The collapse therapy of pulmonary tuberculosis. Springfield Charles C. Thomas, 1937.)

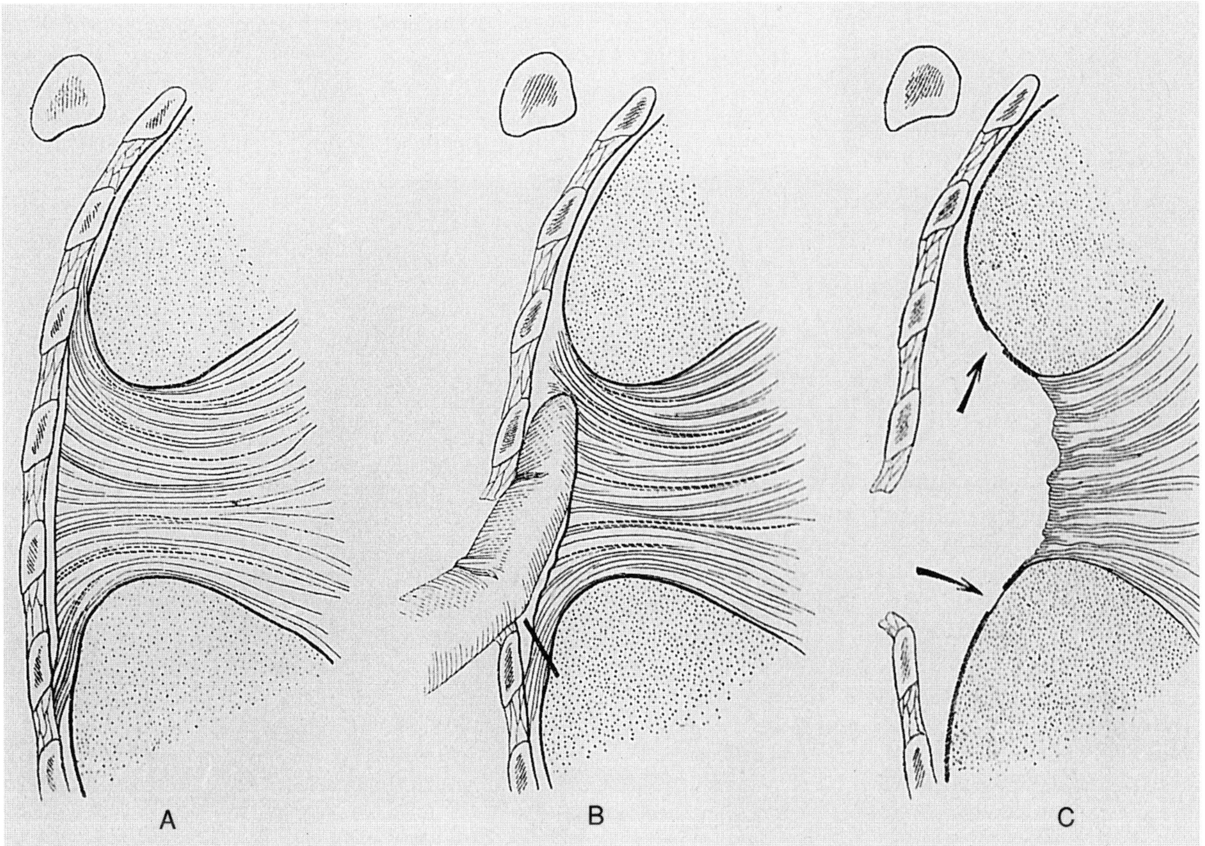

FIGURE 23–18 ■ Technique for open division of adhesions. *A*, Large insertion of the adhesion, *B*, mobilization and division in the endofascia plan, and *C*, division of the adhesion around its base (*arrows*). (From Fey B et al: Traité de technique chirurgicale. Paris, Masson et Cie Éditeurs, Librairies de l'Académle de Médecine, 1955.)

paralysis. The procedure became rapidly popular because it was considered a small operation with no major sequelae (Fey et al, 1955). Unfortunately, phrenicectomy immobilized mostly the lower lobes, whereas the lesions were usually located in the upper lobes. Often the phrenic nerve had collaterals, and it was necessary to divide the subclavian nerve or tear the nerve for a certain distance (Fig. 23–19) in order to ensure that no collateralization or regeneration would occur. The phrenic nerve could also be destroyed by alcoholization carried out by injecting 2 ml of alcohol until the nerve "turned white." While this procedure was being performed, gauze was put around the nerve so that the brachial plexus would not be injured. Often scalenotomy was done to increase the benefits of phrenicectomy by immobilizing the first two ribs. It was done at the same time as phrenicectomy and through the same incision. Other procedures used to increase the collapse of the lung included the creation of a pneumoperitoneum (Vajda, 1933) or intercostal neurotomy (open division or alcoholization). In 1993, Andreas Naef commented on the physicians who performed these operations: "These procedures were conceived and performed by physicians, often themselves former tuberculosis patients who tried to break away from the frustrating passivity of 'bed rest'. Some of these medical men were highly skillful and monopolized the field before surgeons could get into the act—a lesson to be remembered today."

At about the same time, surgical collapse of underlying pulmonary cavities was obtained by rib resection, an operation called thoracoplasty. In 1885, a Lausanne physician named Édouard de Cerenville (Fig. 23–20) described a technique in which short segments of two or more ribs were resected in order to collapse the chest

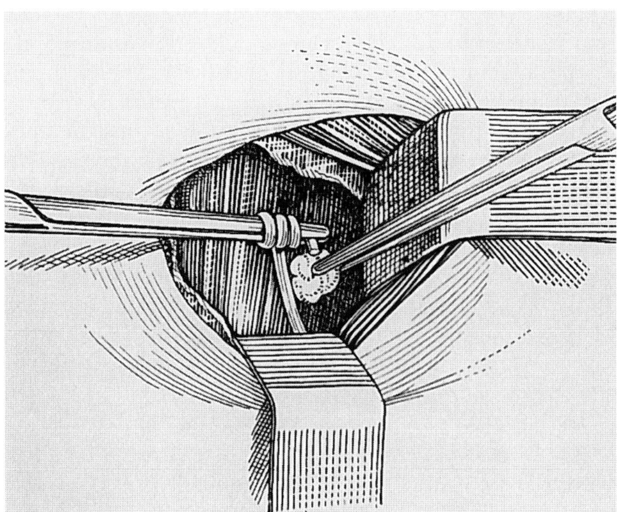

FIGURE 23–19 ■ Technique of tearing the phrenic nerve by rolling it around a clamp. (From Fey B et al: Traité de technique chirurgicale. Paris, Masson et Cie Éditeurs, Librairies de l'Académe de Médecine, 1955.)

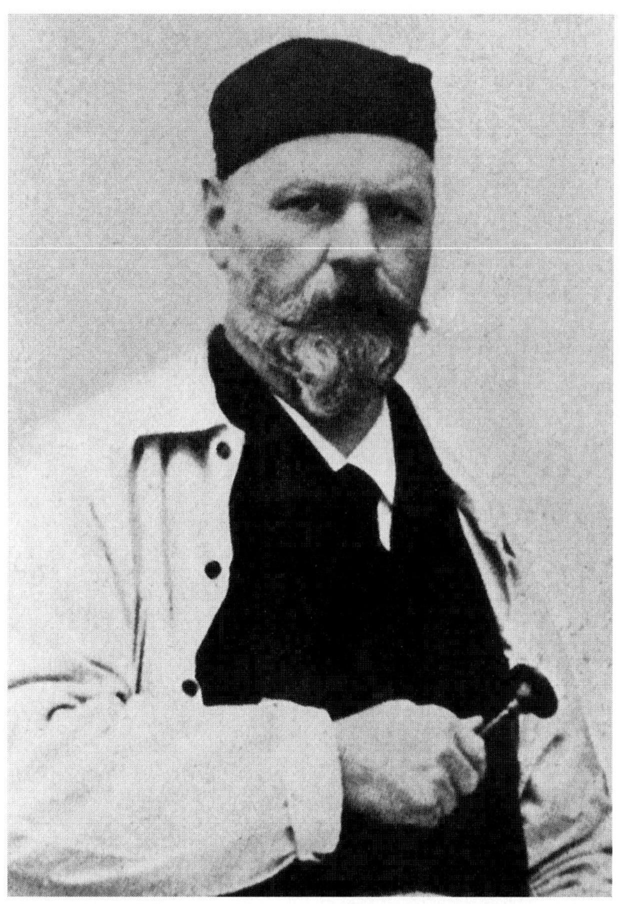

FIGURE 23–20 ■ Édouard Bernard de Cerenville (1843–1915), Lausanne, Switzerland. (From Alexander J: The collapse therapy of pulmonary tuberculosis. Springfield, IL, Charles C Thomas, 1937.)

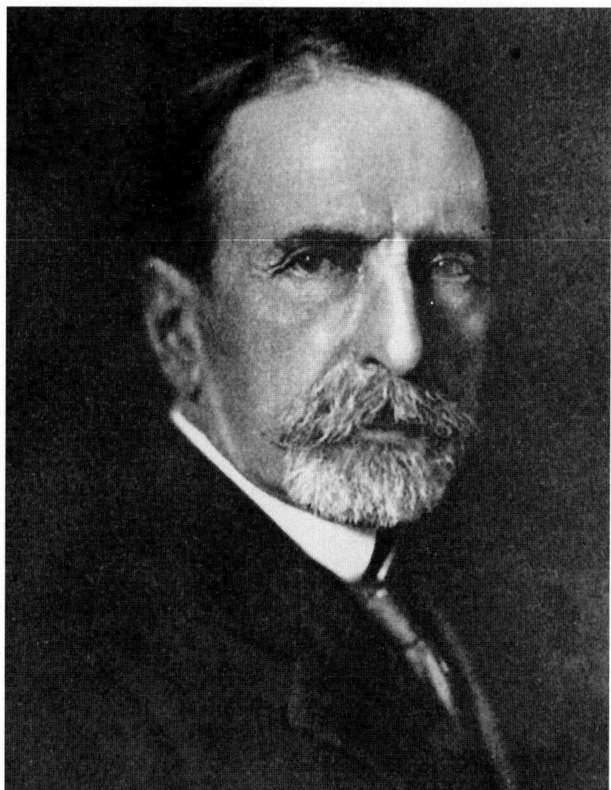

FIGURE 23–21 ■ Théodore Tuffier (1857–1929), Paris, France. (From Alexander J: The collapse therapy of pulmonary tuberculosis. Springfield, IL, Charles C Thomas, 1937.)

wall over areas of apical cavitary tuberculosis. The concept used in this operation was to promote "scar" retraction of tuberculous cavities—that is, to promote retraction of the lung and subsequent scarring by secondary healing. The thoracoplasty described by Schede in 1890 was an operation that included not only multiple rib resections but also the removal of the periosteum, intercostal muscles and nerves, and parietal pleura.

In 1926, Tuffier (Fig. 23–21) was able to free the apex of the lung by using a procedure he called *apicolysis*. This could be done extrapleurally or extrafascially (outside the endothoracic fascia) in such a way as to create a space, which he filled with fatty tissues taken from the patient. This concept became the basis for future procedures such as the extrapleural plombage collapse therapy, obtained by filling the space with slightly heated paraffin (oleothorax) or lucite balls. Each of these techniques had its advantages and disadvantages (Table 23–8).

Collapse therapy for tuberculosis was rendered obsolete by surgical resection. This change of procedure was received with much skepticism and when Freedlander had the courage to present an unsuccessful case of lobectomy for tuberculosis at the 1935 meeting of the American Association for Thoracic Surgery, he was congratulated by Coryllos and Eloesser but criticized by Alexander (Náef, 1993), who favored thoracoplasty in all but a few exceptional situations. Pulmonary resection was very dangerous in sputum-positive patients because bronchial closure seldom healed, and the resulting postoperative tuberculous or mixed tuberculous and pyogenic empyemas usually resulted in death (Meyer, 1991).

The outcome for patients with tuberculosis changed dramatically in November 1944, when a 21-year-old woman with advanced pulmonary tuberculosis received the first injection of streptomycin, which was isolated by Selman Waksman from a soil yeast called *Streptomyces griseus*. Equally or even more dramatic were the results of the first use of isoniazid, reported in a clinical trial by Robitzek and Selikoff (1952). Soon, many of the sanatori-

TABLE 23–8 ■ **Collapsotherapy**

Procedure	*Advantages*	*Disadvantages*
Thoracoplasty	Good patient tolerance if <6 ribs are resected	Definitive collapsus Deformities of the thorax Often done in 2 or 3 stages
Extrapleural pneumothorax	Reversible	Maintenance of pneumothorax
	No deformity Advantageous in extensive lesions	Infection of the space
Extramusculoperiosteal plombage	Same as extrapleural pneumothorax	Infection Late complications

ums around the world became deserted, although one can reflect on how the sanatoriums actually helped patients; a stress-free lifestyle lived in the open air are combined with good hygiene and nutrition are still acknowledged as being beneficial to the treatment of many diseases.

■ *HISTORICAL READINGS*

Alexander J: The Collapse Therapy of Pulmonary Tuberculosis. Springfield, IL, Charles C Thomas, 1937.

Alling DW, Bosworth EB: The after-history of pulmonary tuberculosis. VI. The first fifteen years following diagnosis. Am Rev Respir Dis 81:839, 1960.

Centers for Disease Control. Case Curriculum on Tuberculosis. Atlanta, GA, Centers for Disease Control, 1991.

Comroe JH Jr: T.B. or not T.B. 1. The cause of tuberculosis. Am Rev Respir Dis 117:137, 1978.

de Cerenville EB: De l'intervention dans les maladies du poumon [French]. Rev Med Suisse Normande 5:441, 1885.

Diamond JM: The arrow of disease. Discover 13:64, 1992.

Dubos R, Dubos J: The White Plague. Boston, Little Brown, 1952.

Fey B, Morocquot P, Oberlin S et al: Traité de technique chirurgicale, Vol IV, 2nd ed [French]. Paris, Librairies de l'Académie de Médecine, 1955.

Forlanini C: Primi tentativi di pneumothorax artificiale della tisi pulmonare [Italian]. Gazzetta Medicale di Torino 45:381, 1894.

Jacobeus HC: Die thorakoscopic und ihre praktische bedeutung [German]. Ergebges Med (Berlin) 7:112, 1925.

Koch R: Die aetiologie der tuberkulose. Berlin Klin Wochenschr 19:221, 1882.

Laënnec RTH: De l'auscultation médiate ou traité du diagnostic des maladies des poumons et du cœur [French]. Paris, Brosson et Chaudé, 1819; Forbes J: A treatise on the diseases of the chest [trans]. London, T and C Underwood, 1821.

Meyer JA: Tuberculosis, the Adirondacks, and coming of age for thoracic surgery. Ann Thorac Surg 52:881, 1991.

Naef AP: The 1900 tuberculosis epidemic—Starting point of modern thoracic surgery. Ann Thorac Surg 55:1375, 1993.

Pepper W: A system of practical medicine by American authors, Vol 3. Philadelphia, Lea Brothers, 1885.

Robitzek EH, Selikoff IJ: Hydrazine derivatives of isonicotinic acid (Rimifon, Marsilid) in the treatment of active progressive caseous-pneumonic tuberculosis. A preliminary report. Am Rev Tuberc 65:402, 1952.

Schede M: Die behandlung der empyeme [German]. Verh Long Innere Med Wiesbaden 9:41, 1890.

Stuertz A: Experimenteller beitrag zur "zserchfellbewegung nach einseitiger phrecus *durchtrennung*" [German]. Dtsch Med Wochenschr 38:897, 1912.

Tuffier T: Du décollement pariétal en chirurgie pulmonaire [French]. Arch Med Chir App Respir 1:32, 1926.

Vajda L: Ob das pneumoperitoneum in der kollapsetherapie der beiderseitigen lungentuberkulose angewandt werden kenn? [German]. Ztschr Tuberk 67:371, 1933.

BASIC SCIENCE

Microbiology

Most *Mycobacterium* species are soil and water saprophytes capable of degrading organic material into forms usable by other organisms. These bacteria have characteristics that are close to some yeasts; hence the term *mycobacteria*. Their most precisely defining characteristic, however, is the property of acid-fastness—that is, the ability to withstand decolorization by an acid-alcohol mixture after being stained with such stains as Ziehl-Neelsen (Fig. 23–22) or auramine 0 (Barksdale and Kim, 1977). In addition to being acid-fast, *Mycobacterium* species are primarily intracellular parasites, have slow rates of growth, are obligate aerobes and, in normal hosts, induce a granulomatous response. A classification of the most common *Mycobacterium* species is given in Table 23–9.

The tuberculosis complex includes *Mycobacterium tuberculosis (MTB)*, which is the agent of nearly all tuberculosis in humans; *M. bovis*, which occurs infrequently because milk is pasteurized; and *M. africanum*, a cause of disease in Africa.

The DNA structures of *MTB* and *M. bovis* are so similar that it has been suggested that *MTB*, which appears to be a more highly evolved species, is the result of a mutation of *M. bovis*. According to Manchester (1984), this muta-

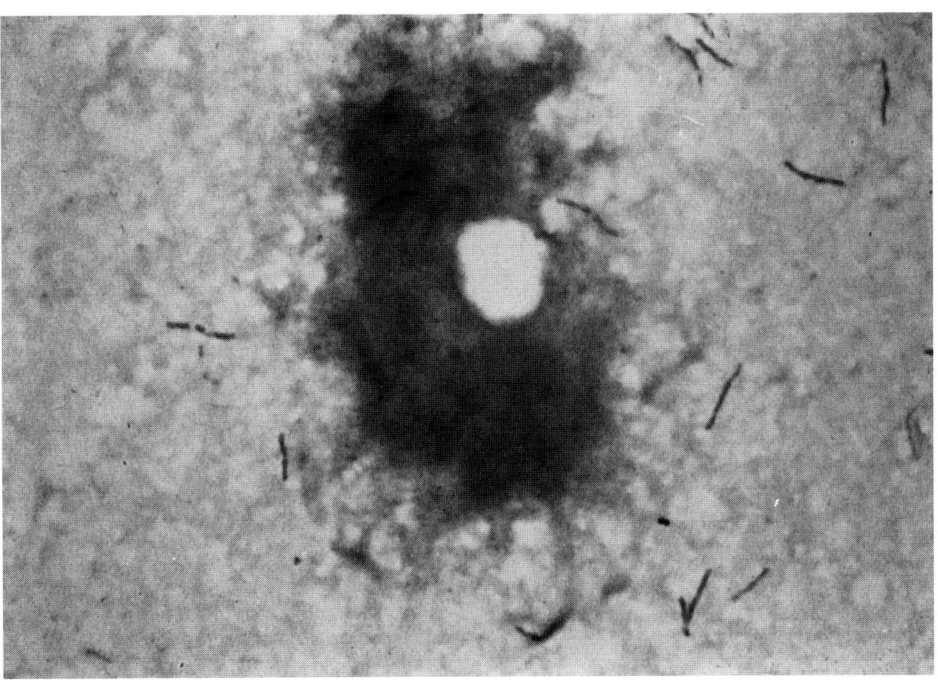

FIGURE 23–22 ■ Acid-fast tuberculous bacilli. The bacteria form a curved rod that measures approximately 0.3 to 0.6 μm.

TABLE 23–9 ■ **Species of *Mycobacterium***

Tuberculosis complex
M. tuberculosis (MTB)
M. bovis
M. africanum
Mycobacteria other than tubercle bacilli (MOTT): Slow-Growing Organisms
M. avium complex
M. kansasii
M. scrofulaceum
M. ulcerans
M. xenopi
M. szulgai
M. simiae
M. haemophilum
M. genovense
Mycobacteria other than tubercle bacilli (MOTT): Fast-Growing Organisms
M. fortuitum
M. chelonei

From Wolinsky E: Nontuberculous mycobacteria and associated diseases. Am Rev Resp Dis 119:107, 1979.

tion may have occurred once humans started to live in larger groups and to domesticate cattle, sometime between 8000 and 4000 BC. *MTB* is an aerophilic organism, as opposed to the micro-aerophilic nature of *M. bovis*, which is why the preponderance of *MTB* infections occur in the lungs.

Transmission and Pathogenesis

The transmission of *MTB* and *M. africanum* usually occurs by way of an airborne or aerosol route, whereas the transmission of *M. bovis* to humans usually occurs by way of the gastrointestinal tract, with cattle being the intermediate host. Bronchial air flow favors the deposition of inhaled bacilli in the basal segment of the lower lobes and the anterior segment of the upper lobes, areas known as the primary infection segments. In 1989, Dannenberg described the three stages of primary infection. In the first stage, scavenger nonactivated alveolar macrophages ingest the tubercle bacilli. During that stage, bacilli multiplication is inhibited or they are destroyed, depending on their virulence and macrophage microbiocidal activity. Infected macrophages release chemotactic factors that attract additional macrophages. The second stage, the symbiotic stage, occurs from day 7 to day 21. During that time, the bacteria continue to grow in macrophages, and monocytes migrate to the site of infection. The patient is often asymptomatic, and chest radiographs may be entirely normal or show only small areas of pneumonitis. The third stage, which occurs after 3 weeks, is characterized by the onset of cell-mediated immunity and delayed hypersensitivity. Alveolar macrophages demonstrate an increased ability to destroy the bacilli and, as a result, there is no longer an increase in the number of organisms. There is an increase in macrophage death, which results in the formation of a granuloma, the characteristic pathologic finding in tuberculosis. Tuberculous granulomas are characterized by the accumulation of blood-derived macrophages; epithelioid cells, which are the degenerating macrophages; and multinucleated giant cells, which are fused macrophages with nuclei around the periphery (Langhan's cells). T lymphocytes are also found around the periphery of the granuloma.

Macrophage death causes central caseation. *Caseum*, the Latin word for *cheese*, is cellular debris of the consistency of soft cheese; in such an environment, low oxygen tension inhibits both macrophage function and bacillary growth. Around the caseum are activated and nonactivated macrophages. A Ghon focus is a single small lesion in the lung, typically located at the apex of the upper lobes or in the upper part of the lower lobes. Although Anton Ghon (Ober, 1983) was not the first to describe the primary pulmonary lesion, he was the first to provide a detailed description of active pulmonary tuberculosis based on autopsy findings. A Ghon complex, or Ranke complex, is a combination of a lung lesion and a calcified hilar node. A Ghon complex is often the only remaining evidence of the primary infection.

During the fourth stage of infection, reactivated tuberculosis, hydrolytic enzymes liquefy the caseum, transforming it into an excellent medium for the growth of *Mycobacterium* species. Once the bronchial structures are involved, the liquefied material is easily expectorated. Bloodstream seeding also occurs during this stage.

Typically, but not exclusively, reactivation tuberculosis starts in the apical or posterior segments of one or both of the upper lobes. These sites, referred to as Simon's foci, are believed to be seeded during the early bacteremia of primary infection. It is likely that reactivation occurs because of the relatively higher partial oxygen tension in the upper portions of the lung, *MTB* being an obligate aerobe that reproduces most successfully in a high-oxygen environment. In HIV infection, the macrophages and T lymphocytes that normally control primary infection are disabled; this results in the greater susceptibility to and virulence of tuberculosis in that group of patients.

Exposure to a patient with active tuberculosis results in infection in approximately one third of individuals who do not have HIV (Grzybowski et al, 1975). Of these, 3% to 5% develop active tuberculosis within 1 year, and an additional 3% to 5% reactivate at a later date. There is convincing evidence that in most adults, tuberculosis occurs as a result of the reactivation of organisms that were seeded during primary infection (Stead, 1967).

Epidemiology

Crowding in European cities and the occurrence of the Industrial Revolution in Europe provided the environmental conditions necessary for an endemic disease to become epidemic. Currently, about 1.7 billion people, or about one third of the world's population, are or have been infected with *MTB* (Kochi, 1991). In 1990, 8 million new cases of tuberculosis were documented, and 95% of them occurred in the developing countries of the western Pacific and Southeast Asia. During that year, 2.9 million people died of the disease, making tuberculosis a huge socioeconomic burden on both industrial and developing countries. In industrial countries, most cases occur in the elderly population, whereas in developing countries,

80% of cases occur in the under-60 age group, resulting in a significant impact on productivity.

Since 1984, more than 20,000 cases have been reported annually in the United States. These cases are seen predominantly in geographic areas and demographic groups that include large numbers of people with AIDS as well as foreign-born persons who have emigrated from regions such as Asia, Africa, and Latin America in which rates of occurrence are high. Other high-risk groups include patients in close contact with others who are known to have tuberculosis; people with medical conditions such as silicosis, diabetes, immunosuppression, intestinal bypass, and malignancy; low-income individuals who have poor medical resources; alcohol and intravenous drug abusers; and persons institutionalized in correctional and nursing home facilities.

In North America, multiple-drug–resistant tuberculosis (MDRTB) is a problem that has emerged in several major urban centers. In a study done in New York City, for instance, 33% of patients with positive cultures had isolates resistant to one or more antituberculous drugs (Frieden et al, 1993), and the strongest predictor of drug resistance was a previous history of antituberculous therapy. Other risk factors for MDRTB identified in that study were HIV infection and intravenous drug abuse.

Screening for Tuberculosis Infection

The objective of screening for tuberculosis in countries such as Canada and the United States, where administration of the bacille Calmette-Guérin (BCG) vaccine is not universal, is the identification of infected people who could benefit from preventive therapy. The Mantoux single subdermal injection of 0.1 ml purified protein derivative (PPD) containing 5 tuberculin units is the favored method. At 48 hours, an erythematous reaction 5 mm or larger is considered positive in individuals who have been in close contact with persons known to be infected, those with suspicious chest radiographs, and HIV patients. A 10 mm reaction is positive for people without those risk factors. A 15 mm reaction is classified as positive in all other persons. Positive tuberculin reactions in BCG-vaccinated persons usually indicate infection with *MTB*, but this is unpredictable. Mycobacteria other than tubercle bacilli (MOTT) react to other specific PPD skin tests such as the PPD-B which is used for the screening of *M. avium* (Battey's bacillus).

Clinical Presentation

The clinical presentation of a patient infected with tuberculosis is determined by the site of primary infection, the stage of disease, and the magnitude of cell-type immunity response mounted by the host to resist the infection. Current experience indicates that in 80% to 90% of cases of tuberculosis occurring in patients without HIV, the disease involves the lungs. In most of these patients, involution and healing occur and a dormant phase, which can last a lifetime, follows in 85% to 90% of those infected. During this dormant phase, the only evidence of infection with *MTB* may be a positive skin test to tuberculin or a Ghon complex seen on a chest radiograph. Reactivation will occur in 10% to 15% of infected persons, with half reactivating within the first 2 years after primary infection. In North America, reactivation classically occurs in middle-aged adults, and in 80% of cases, it involves the lungs. Reactivation at extrapulmonary sites, such as lymph nodes, pleura, or the musculoskeletal system, occurs in 20% of patients without AIDS but in 50% of patients who are HIV-positive (Winn and Prechter, 1994).

During the first weeks after contamination, pulmonary tuberculosis is often asymptomatic because the host's immune reaction is minimal. Indeed, systemic symptoms of low-grade fever, malaise, and weight loss are often so gradual that they are largely unnoticed. Cough due to the accumulation of secretions is most commonly seen when cavitation occurs and, in general, the amount of sputum increases with progressive pulmonary excavation. Hemoptysis is often caused by complications such as bronchiectasis, erosion into vascular malformations associated with cavitation (Rasmussen's aneurysms), or aspergillosis. Pleural or chest wall pain occurs with pleural involvement; dyspnea is common during acute febrile periods. Acute dyspnea may also result from a spontaneous pneumothorax or a rapidly developing pleural effusion.

Extrapulmonary tuberculosis is secondary to hematogenous or lymphatic spread of pulmonary lesions, and virtually any organ can become infected. Swallowed secretions can result in the infection of the gastrointestinal tract. In a retrospective review of 104 patients with thoracic tuberculosis, Lardinois and colleagues (1997) showed that 69.2% of patients presented with an infection of the pulmonary parenchyma, 20.2% presented with pleural tuberculosis, 2.9% with tuberculosis of the chest wall, 7.7% with mediastinal tuberculosis, and 3.8% with bronchial stenosis. Other extrapulmonary sites of interest to the thoracic surgeon are the larynx (Almeyda et al, 1997); the pericardium, where tuberculosis may cause constrictive pericarditis (Gregory et al, 1998); and the pleural space (Campos-Rodriguez et al, 1997).

TREATMENT

Medical Treatment

The recommendation of the Centers for Disease Control for initial therapy for people with active tuberculosis is a 6-month regimen consisting of isoniazid, rifampin, and pyrazinamide given for 2 months, followed by isoniazid and rifampin given for 4 months, in patients with susceptible organisms who are compliant with treatment (Centers For Disease Control, 1991). With this regimen, close to 90% of patients will have bacteriologically negative sputum at the end of the 6-month period. In patients suspected of having resistant organisms, alternative drugs such as ethambutol or streptomycin can also be started until drug sensitivities are obtained.

Indications for Surgical Treatment

With the advent of effective antituberculous medication, the role of surgery in the management of tuberculosis

TABLE 23–10 ■ Treatment of Tuberculosis: Indications for Surgery

Complications resulting from previous surgery
  Delayed complications of plombage
  Complications of insufficient surgery
Failure of medical therapy
  Progressive disease, lung destruction, and left bronchus syndrome
  Lung gangrene
  Drug resistance
  Aspergillosis complicating treatment
Surgery for diagnosis
  Pulmonary lesions of unknown cause
  Mediastinal adenopathy of unknown cause
Complications of scarring
  Massive hemoptysis
  Cavernoma
  Lung cancer
  Tracheo- or bronchoesophageal fistula
  Bronchiectasis
  Extrinsic airway obstruction by tuberculous lymph nodes
  Endobronchial tuberculosis and bronchostenosis
  Middle lobe syndrome
Extrapulmonary thoracic disease
  Tuberculosis of the heart and great vessels
  Vascular malformations
  Constrictive pericarditis
  Cold abscesses and osteomyelitis of the chest wall
  Pott's disease
Pleural tuberculosis
  Pleural effusion
  Bronchopleural fistula
Infections with *Mycobacteria* other than tubercle bacilli (MOTT)

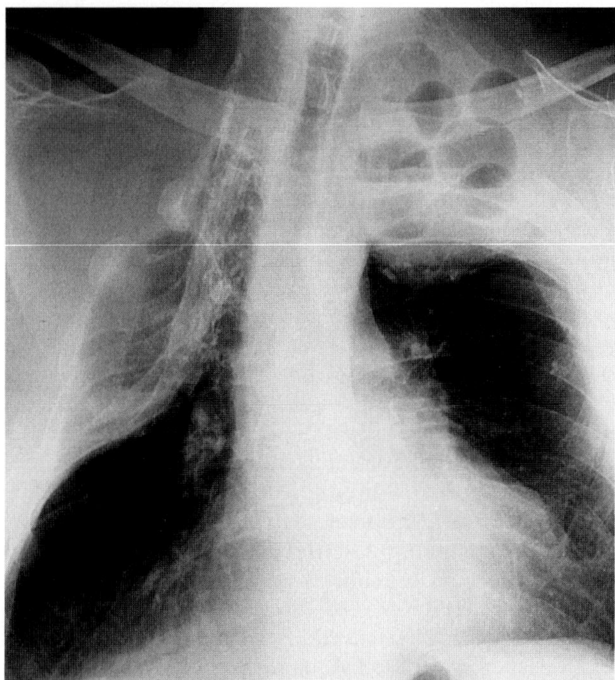

FIGURE 23–23 ■ Posteroanterior chest radiograph of a 74-year-old man who presented with an unrelated upper respiratory tract infection. He had previously been treated for tuberculosis by thoracoplasty on the right and plombage with lucite balls on the left.

has greatly diminished and is now reserved mainly for the treatment of complications of the disease. Indications for surgery differ slightly depending on geographic location. The most common surgical indication in the United States, for example, is multiple-drug–resistant tuberculosis with destroyed lung and persistent cavitary disease. By contrast, the majority of operations in Canada and Europe are performed for complications of therapy or late sequelae of previously cured tuberculosis.

The indications for surgery for *MTB* can be grouped into seven main categories (Table 23–10): (1) complications resulting from previous surgery, (2) failure of medical therapy, (3) diagnosis, (4) complications of scarring, (5) extrapulmonary thoracic disease, (6) pleural tuberculosis, and (7) infection by MOTT.

Complications Resulting from Previous Surgery

Delayed Complications of Plombage. Enthusiasm for the surgical treatment of tuberculosis by thoracoplasty began at the end of the 19th century and was greatest at the time of John Alexander's publication in the early part of the 20th century. During those years, a large number of patients were treated with thoracoplasty and plombage, and many of them were still alive in the latter part of the century but were suffering from late complications of these procedures.

Although various materials, such as rubber bags and sheeting, paraffin packs, Polystan sponges, and fiberglass, were used for plombage, lucite balls (Fig. 23–23) were universally preferred. These spheres were made of translucent methyl methacrylate with diameters of about 2.5 cm. Despite an increasing number of delayed complications (Table 23–11) and the abandonment of the procedure at Duke University in 1948, plombage procedures with lucite balls remained in vogue for many more years because it could be performed in one stage, could be done on sick patients, and was associated with less physical deformity than was thoracoplasty.

Initially performed extrapleurally, the procedure was regularly complicated by erosion into the lung. Because of this complication, the procedure was later performed extraperiosteally, where a thick layer of tissue between the foreign material used in the plombage and the lung itself could prevent erosion. Because of its final appearance, the procedure became known as the birdcage operation.

Unfortunately, lucite balls tended to migrate, either in the mediastinum, where they compressed mediastinal structures, or under the skin, which was more common because of the low resistance to migration offered by the devitalized ribs. Migration in the mediastinum could lead

TABLE 23–11 ■ Common Late Complications of Plombage

Super infection	Malignant changes
Migration of foreign material	Expanding hematomas
Erosion of adjacent organs	

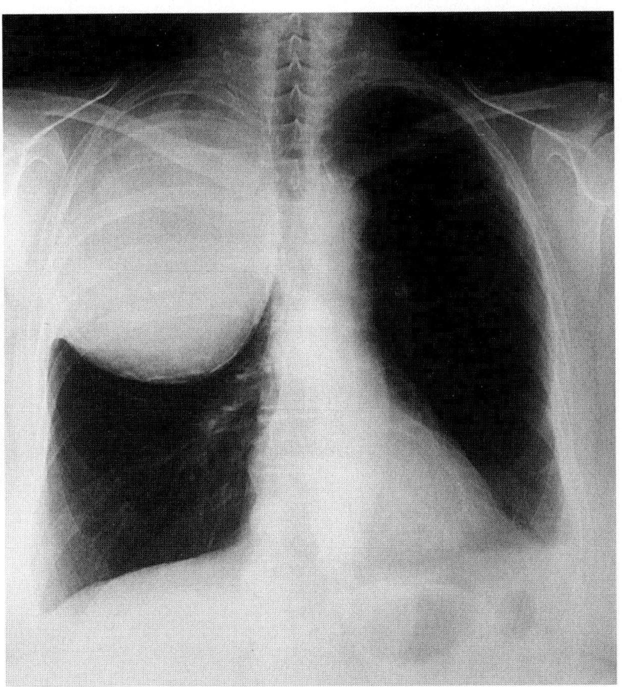

FIGURE 23–24 ■ Posteroanterior chest radiograph of an asymptomatic 62-year-old man treated 30 years previously with paraffin plombage. Note the large collection, which is sometimes called a "paraffinoma."

to erosion of the esophagus, sometimes including passage of the balls into the esophagus, causing small bowel obstruction (Horowitz et al, 1992; Tate, 1980). Erosion of the aorta or subclavian artery occurred with ball migration into immediate para-aortic locations. Severe hemoptysis was reported after erosion of intercostal arteries (Massard et al, 1997), and obstruction of the vena cava has also been documented (Skinner and Sinclair, 1992). Cephalad migration with impingement on the branches of the brachial plexus often caused chest wall pain.

Oleothorax utilized a wax-based, malleable material made of paraffin, bismuth, and mineral oil to induce pulmonary collapse. After insertion, the material became surrounded by a calcified membrane (Fig. 23–24), which could break after trauma or other abnormal contusion of the chest wall. The oil or the wax could then migrate toward the skin, causing a pleurocutaneous fistula (Kirshenbaum et al, 1995) or toward the mediastinum, causing a bronchopleural fistula (Iuchi et al, 1984; Tsou et al, 1978).

A patients can also experience septic complications of the plombage space. Because of increased intracavitary tension, the first sign of infection is commonly an acute swelling of the collapsed space which can in turn initiate migration of the foreign bodies used for the plombage. A surgeon, unaware of the underlying condition, may incise and drain what is assumed to be a subcutaneous abscess. Late empyema can develop years after artificial pneumothorax (Massard et al, 1995) or longstanding oleothorax (Tsou et al, 1978), and *Aspergillus* species, anaerobes, *Haemophilus influenzae*, *Staphylococcus aureus*, *Klebsiella* species, *Streptococcus pneumoniae*, and even *MTB* (Harris et al, 1996) have been isolated from the site of a plombage-cutaneous fistula. Treatment of an infected plombage space or of migration of plombage material consists in the removal of the foreign bodies, empyemectomy, lung resection, and thoracoplasty with or without the use of muscle transposition to fill the residual space (Stobernack et al, 1997; Thomas et al, 1995; Vigneswaran and Ramasastry, 1996). Intraoperative fluoroscopy may be necessary to ascertain that all foreign material has been removed. Often, the lucite balls have been inserted within a bag or have been attached to a string, which makes their removal easier.

Tension pleural effusions can occur 20 or more years after therapeutic pneumothoraces. They usually present with a sudden increase in dyspnea, and chest radiographs may show increased opacity with mediastinal shift (Neff and Buchanan, 1975). Patients with chronic residual spaces after treatment for tuberculosis can also present with effusions yielding fluid that has the appearance of lymph. Although cholesterol concentrations can be over 150 mg/dl, no chylomicrons are found—hence the term *pseudochylothorax* described these effusions (Campos-Rodriguez et al, 1997).

A number of patients, reported on primarily in the Japanese literature, have presented with rapidly growing chest wall or intrathoracic tumors. This condition has been described as occurring after thoracoplasty performed because of tuberculosis as well as after lung and chest wall resection carried out for other pathologic conditions. Such a lesion, called chronic expanding hematoma, is made of non-neoplastic reactive tissue consisting of blood surrounded by dense fibrous tissue. Other terms for this unusual entity include old ancient hematoma, Masson's pseudoangiosarcoma, and papillary endothelial hyperplasia (Duarte et al, 1999; Hanagiri et al, 1997). The hematoma presents as a new, expanding lesion on the chest wall or thoracic cavity years after the initial procedure, and it is often difficult to differentiate it from a relatively more common malignant vascular neoplasm such as an angiosarcoma. The cause of this pseudotumor is unclear but reaction to a foreign body has been suggested by Fukai et al (1990).

Another unusual problem associated with the long-term presence of foreign bodies is the development of a malignancy. Whether the malignancy is caused by the chemical structure of the implanted material or by associated chronic inflammation resulting from the implantation is still debated. In addition, primary extraskeletal chondrosarcoma (Thompson and Entin, 1969); malignant fibrous histiocytoma (Fauquert et al, 1989; Takanami et al, 1994); liposarcoma (Ojika et al, 1997); and type B non-Hodgkin's lymphoma (Borrelly et al, 1996; Molinie et al, 1996) have been documented in plombage space years after the initial procedure.

In view of the severity of some of these late complications, it is probably safe to recommend ablation of plombage material, even in asymptomatic patients.

Complications of Insufficient Surgery. The most important surgical principle of pulmonary resectional surgery for tuberculosis is to remove all gross disease while leaving enough tissue for adequate pulmonary function. Another important principle is to undertake lung resection only in patients with converted sputum. Unfortunately, antituberculous medications do not always sterilize necrotic or scarred lesions, and *MBT* can remain active (Klingensmith and Beckley, 1963). Whether microscopic active disease should be allowed to remain, especially in patients with resistant *MBT* in order to preserve pulmonary function or whether the resection should be extended to encompass all disease is still a matter of controversy.

It is not unusual to encounter patients presenting with complications such as bronchopleural fistulas that are clearly related to persistent or reactivated disease (Halezeroglu et al, 1997) or recurrences in the pleural space, where effusions, containing mixed bacteria and mycobacteria have been reported in a number of series, particularly in patients with active disease at the time of surgery (Rizzi et al, 1997).

Other sites of postoperative recurrence that may require surgical reintervention include the pericardium and lymph nodes. Tuberculous pericarditis is estimated to occur in 1% to 2% of cases of pulmonary tuberculosis, and most patients present with symptoms of constrictive pericarditis (Cacoub et al, 1991; Nataf et al, 1993). Despite adequate medical treatment, some patients may require pericardial resection to relieve the symptoms of tamponade. Because complete pericardial resection is usually not possible, the procedure leaves foci of active disease, which can be associated with late complications, such as chronic sinus tracts or mediastinal abscesses (Gregory et al, 1998).

Incomplete resection of tuberculous adenitis in the neck can also lead to the formation of sinus tracts to the skin. When biopsy of these nodes is necessary for diagnostic purposes, complete excision followed by adequate long-term medical therapy is recommended so as to avoid this problem.

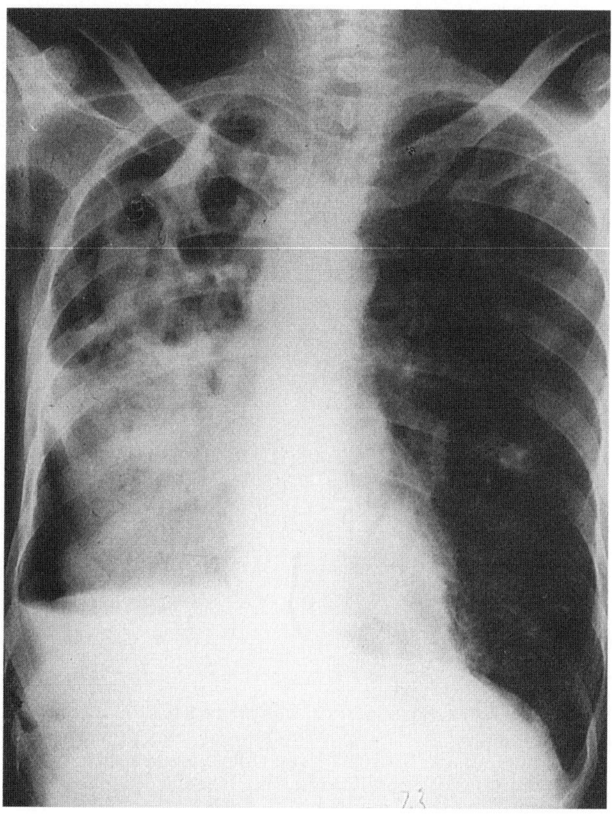

FIGURE 23–25 ■ Posteroanterior chest radiograph of a 46-year-old man with a destroyed right lung; there are disseminated cavities throughout the entire lung field.

Failure of Medical Therapy

Progressive Disease, Lung Destruction, and Left Bronchus Syndrome. Unilateral total lung destruction is a well-recognized complication of tuberculosis. Late presentation, errors in diagnosis, poor compliance, or insufficient treatment account for the largest number of patients presenting with this condition, which is characterized by extensive disease that includes fibrosis, widespread cavitation, and bronchiectasis. In a review of 1600 cases of pulmonary tuberculosis, Ashour et al (1990) found that post-tuberculous lung destruction occurred in 1% of patients. Characteristically, these individuals had had tuberculosis for many years and presented with huge cavitary complexes involving one of the hemithoraces (Fig. 23–25). In the series by Bobrowitz and colleagues (1974), of 18 patients whose lungs had been destroyed secondary to tuberculosis, the most disabling symptom was shortness of breath due to functional exclusion, although hemoptysis was an important complication too and was the cause of death in three patients.

Post-tuberculous lung destruction occurs more commonly on the left side (Fig. 23–26) than on the right (Ashour et al, 1990), a finding thought to result from the anatomy of the left main stem bronchus, which is longer and narrower than the right and therefore more prone to extrinsic compression as it courses beneath the aorta; this is referred to by Ashour and colleagues as left bronchus syndrome. In such cases, pneumonectomy may be indicated for hemoptysis, chronic bacterial superimposed infection, or simply to provide symptomatic relief.

In a series of 118 consecutive patients who underwent pneumonectomy for destroyed lung (tuberculosis: n = 43) between 1986 and 1996, Halezeroglu and colleagues (1997) reported that the combined morbidity and mortality rate of the operation was significantly higher in patients with preoperative empyema ($P < .003$); tuberculosis ($P < .03$); and right pneumonectomy ($P < .03$). The authors concluded that extrapleural dissection, buttressing the bronchial stump, and postoperative irrigation of the cavity could help decrease the rate of postoperative complications.

Lung Gangrene. Lung gangrene is a rare form of parenchymal destruction that has a rapid and virulent clinical course. Initially, the radiographic features show pulmonary consolidation soon followed by extensive necrosis with cavitation. The necrotic tissue can present as a mass within the cavity and can simulate a mycetoma.

Acute pulmonary gangrene is usually caused by bacteria such as *Klebsiella pneumoniae*, *S. pneumoniae*, and *H. influenzae*, but in a review of 22 cases, Khan and colleagues (1980) were able to document that 4 of the cases were related to *MBT*. Vascular thrombosis and arteritis

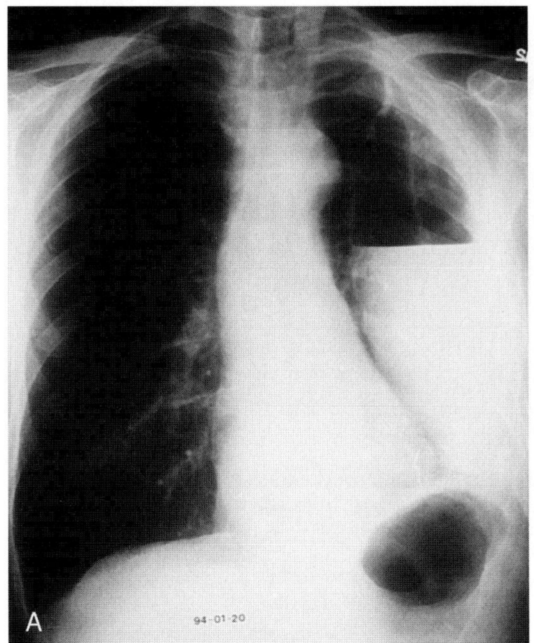

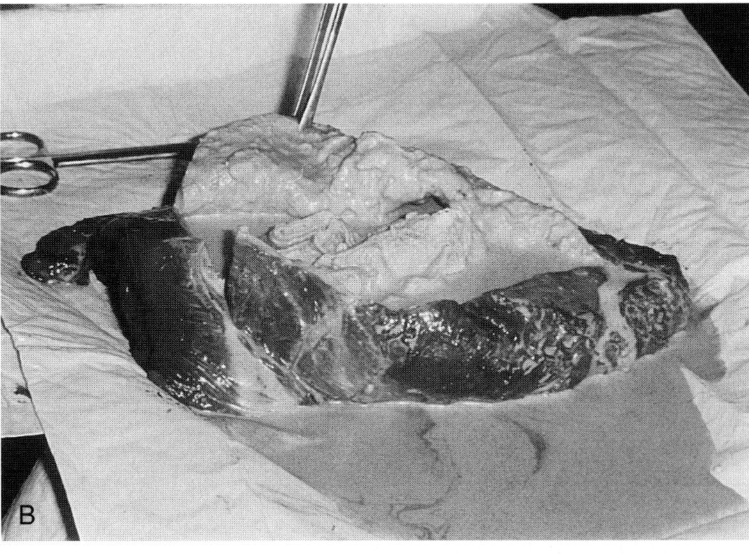

FIGURE 23–26 ■ *A*, Posteroanterior chest radiograph of an elderly man with a left destroyed lung, bronchopleural fistula, and empyema. In a case such as this, it is difficult to differentiate between a truly destroyed lung and a tuberculous empyema with relatively expandable underlying lung. In 1975, Brezler and Abeles suggested that thoracoscopy could be helpful in establishing the distinction because in destroyed lung, large bronchial openings might be visible. *B*, Thick pus (mixed bacterial and tuberculous) contained within the space.

were found in three of these four patients and, according to the authors, this vascular complication was the likely cause of pulmonary gangrene. In such cases, indications for surgery must be individualized; patients not responding to medical therapy and those progressing to the formation of an abscess are likely to benefit from pulmonary resection. Because all cases harbor active infection, prophylactic measures should be taken to prevent the formation of bronchopleural fistulas and empyema. The incision, for instance, must be designed to allow for preservation of the latissimus dorsi or the serratus anterior, which can be used as a vascularized, pediculed tissue flap.

Drug Resistance. Despite aggressive prophylactic education, tighter control of the care of tuberculosis patients, and the commitment of additional resources to tuberculosis control programs, compliance with medical therapy has always been difficult to enforce. The more recent problem of MDRTB, which is on the rise throughout the world, is particularly prevalent in countries that cannot afford increasing costs of treatment. In the United States, resistant organisms cause approximately 7% of cases of tuberculosis but in some cities, resistant organisms may cause 12% to 56% of cases (Goble, 1986).

MDRTB, which is defined as resistance to two or more drugs, including isoniazid and rifampin, is a major challenge because relapse rates as high as 44% have been reported with medical therapy alone (Goble et al, 1988). Although drug resistance is usually due to inadequate prior medical therapy or to secondary resistance, some reports have identified a number of patients with de novo drug resistance.

According to Pomerantz and colleagues (1991), the addition of surgery to medical treatment may improve the outcome in as many as 90% of these patients. The presence of MDRTB is therefore an indication for surgery if the disease is localized and if the patient can tolerate surgery (Iseman et al, 1990; Treasure and Seaworth, 1995). The presence of MDRTB is associated with significantly higher operative morbidity than that found in patients with nonresistant disease (Reed et al, 1989). This increased morbidity is related to positivity of sputum at the time of surgery (up to 50% of patients), previous thoracotomy, previous chest radiation, polymicrobial contamination, and poor nutritional status (Pomerantz and Brown, 1997).

The association of MDRTB with HIV is a major health problem. In 1992, Busillo and associates reported a mortality of 62% in 24 patients with HIV who were infected with MDRTB. Management of these patients is very difficult because of the large number of drugs required, each of which has its own toxicity. Although its use has not yet been clearly documented, it is possible that surgery may have a role to play in this subset of patients.

The medical treatment of active tuberculosis should begin empirically with the use of three, four, or even five first-line drugs, including at least two drugs to which the mycobacteria are sensitive, because resistance can develop if a single agent is being used. The drugs and their dosage are then readjusted after drug-specific sensitivities are obtained.

Sputum conversion in patients with sensitive organisms should take place within 3 months of the beginning of treatment. Failure to convert sputum after that length of time is highly suspicious for the presence of a resistant strain (Iseman and Goble, 1988). Once drug resistance has been established, administering medical therapy alone has been associated with mortality rates as high as 50% (Madsen and Iseman, 1994).

When surgery is combined with postoperative chemotherapy, cure rates of up to 90% have been achieved (Kir et al, 1997; Pomerantz and Brown, 1997). In a series of 99 patients with MDRTB, Iseman and coworkers (1990) used three criteria to select patients who would benefit from surgery: (1) patients with drug resistance and high probability of failure; (2) patients with localized disease amenable to resection; and (3) patients with enough drug reactivity to allow healing of infected bronchial stumps. In this group of patients, sputum negativity was obtained in 25 of 27 survivors.

The optimal duration of preoperative and postoperative chemotherapy is still debated, but negative cultures at the time of surgery clearly decrease operative morbidity and mortality (Pomerantz et al, 1991). For this reason, prior medical treatment of at least 3 to 6 months is recommended (van Leuven et al, 1997). At the time of surgery, the extent of resection should be based on both the amount of lung involved and the preoperative functional status; whenever possible, all cavitary lesions and areas of destroyed lung should be removed. Whether residual tissue can act as a nidus for relapse is controversial. In 1997, van Leuven and colleagues showed that higher percentages of nonconversion and failure of surgical therapy occurred when lobectomies or segmentectomies were performed than occurred when penumonectomies were performed. Other factors thought to increase the likelihood of relapse after lung resection are the postoperative occurrence of bronchopleural fistulas and infected spaces (Blackwood and Andrews, 1967). To prevent these complications, Pomerantz and Brown (1997) recommended routine use of muscle and omental plombage to cover bronchial stumps and fill the pleural space. In their series, they reported only one fistula after 62 pneumonectomies. When pneumonectomy is necessary, an extrapleural approach eliminates the possibility of contamination of the residual thoracic space.

Surgery decreases the pool of viable bacteria but seldom does it eradicate it completely. Therefore, drug therapy must be continued postoperatively. Some authors advocate treatment for a period as long as 3 years postoperatively (Iseman et al, 1990), but this seems long and impractical. In 1997, van Leuven and colleagues proposed a tailored approach that takes into account the amount of residual disease, the sputum status at the time of operation, the microbiology of the resected specimen, and the initial indication for surgery when determining the length of postoperative drug therapy. In their series, the average length of postoperative drug therapy was about 8 months. In all cases, adequate long-term follow-up is necessary to document relapses that occur while still on treatment and reinfections that occur once the treatment has been completed.

Aspergillosis Complicating Treatment. Aspergillosis is an infectious disease caused by various *Aspergillus* species, the most common being *Aspergillus fumigatus.* This fungus grows as a saprophyte in patients with structural lung damage and colonizes cavities secondary to tuberculosis, lung cysts, lung abscesses, bronchiectasis, neoplasms, and sarcoidosis. Other types of aspergillosis involving the lung include allergic bronchopulmonary aspergillosis, which is seen in atopic patients, and invasive aspergillosis, which occurs in immunodeficient patients (Fraser, 1993).

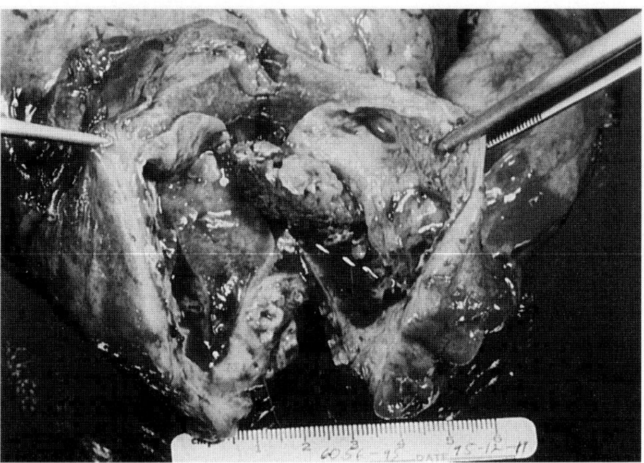

FIGURE 23–27 ■ Resected specimen showing a typical aspergilloma within a pre-existing tuberculous cavity. The fungus ball is made of fungi, necrotic debris, inflammatory cells, and red blood cells.

When aspergillosis infects a lung cavity, necrotic tissue loosens and forms a mass of hyphae tangled with inflammatory and red blood cells (Fig. 23–27). It appears on chest radiographs as a dense ball capped by a slim meniscus of air within the cavity (a fungus ball, or mycetoma). The most common clinical presentation of aspergilloma is hemoptysis, which in some series occurs in up to 91% of patients (Chen et al, 1997). Massive hemoptysis, which is the result of vascular erosion by the fungus or is secondary to the production of endotoxins with hemolytic properties (Pennington, 1980), is associated with mortality rates varying from 25% to 100% (Karas et al, 1976; Solit et al, 1971).

Medical therapy for aspergillomas that involves antifungal agents is usually ineffective, but cavernoscopic evacuation of aspergillomas followed by repeated intracavitary instillation of antifungal agents has been used successfully as an alternative method of palliation in patients in whom surgery is a great risk (Subba et al, 1984). Bronchial artery embolization can also be used to gain time until further therapy can be initiated (Remy et al, 1977) but ultimately, surgical resection offers the best chance for cure. Operative mortality rates are in the range of 5% to 7% (Adeyemo et al, 1984; Al-Majed et al, Butz et al, 1985), and the complications of resection are low, especially if the patient does not have active tuberculosis at the time of operation.

For Diagnosis

Pulmonary Lesion of Unknown Cause. The various clinical presentations of pulmonary tuberculosis represent different manifestations of the host's reaction to the infection. At one end of the spectrum, there is a simple granuloma known as tuberculoma, whereas at the other end, there is cavitation with or without pulmonary destruction. Lymph node involvement may result in bronchial invasion with secondary stenosis or distal bronchiectasis.

On standard chest radiographs, tuberculomas present as pulmonary nodules. Overall, they represent 14% of all solitary pulmonary nodules and 25% of all granulomas (Steele, 1964). They are usually located at the periphery of the lung, immediately beneath the pleura. On cut section they appear as concentric rings of lamellar layers with some degree of caseation not always visible to the naked eye. Unfortunately, no single microscopic feature can differentiate tuberculomas from other granulomatous lesions of the lung, and the diagnosis has to be confirmed by Ziehl-Neelsen staining, culture, or other fluorescent or immunoperoxidative techniques.

Because most patients have no documented history of tuberculosis, the diagnosis of tuberculoma is often made after resection of a solitary nodule of unknown cause (Lai et al, 1996). On chest radiograph, the differential diagnosis between a tuberculous granuloma and lung cancer is not always clear, and there is great variation among individuals in the interpretation of radiographic signs, even among chest specialists (Tokuda et al, 1990). Most radiologic signs are of low specificity for predicting malignancy and, in addition, the site of the lesion has no real predictive value (Ramos-Martinez et al, 1998). In recent years, several authors have shown that contrast computed tomography (CT) scanning with incremental dynamic studies, using 20 Hounsfield units as a threshold, appears to be a good indicator of malignancy (Potente et al, 1997; Yamashita et al, 1995). The CT halo sign is a low attenuation zone around a pulmonary nodule, which is usually seen with aspergillomas but has also been reported with tuberculomas (Gaeta et al, 1992). The discovery on thin-section CT of a bronchus leading into the lesion, also called the positive CT bronchus sign, is more often seen with malignant lesions (Russi et al, 1992), whereas ring or central curvilinear enhancement due to central caseation has been reported in 75% of tuberculomas (Murayama et al, 1995).

In an interesting study carried out in an area endemic for tuberculosis, Lai and associates (1996) found that transbronchial needle aspirations and brushings were diagnostic in 55% of patients with tuberculomas and 70% of patients with malignancies. Of the tuberculomas, 45% yielded positive cultures, and rates were even higher when lesions were large. When transthoracic needle biopsy is used, a specific diagnosis of benign disease is definitely helpful, but a report that suggests only nonspecific cellular elements should prompt repeat biopsy or excisional biopsy (Steen-Hansen and Thommesen, 1988).

Pulmonary mucoceles are the result of chronic airway obstruction that can be caused by broncholithiasis, strictures, and tuberculomas. Mucoceles often present as solitary masses that are indistinguishable from malignancies on radiographs (Miyoshi et al, 1996). Although CT scanning may provide more information about the content of the cyst, surgical resection is often necessary to establish the diagnosis.

Mediastinal Adenopathy of Unknown Cause. Tuberculosis of the lymph nodes is one of the most common presentations of extrapulmonary tuberculosis. Although most commonly found in the cervical region, tuberculous lymphadenitis can also involve mediastinal lymph nodes (Fig. 23–28). Typically, patients have few or no systemic symptoms, but radiologic evidence of slowly enlarging mediastinal adenopathy may be found, and it can be

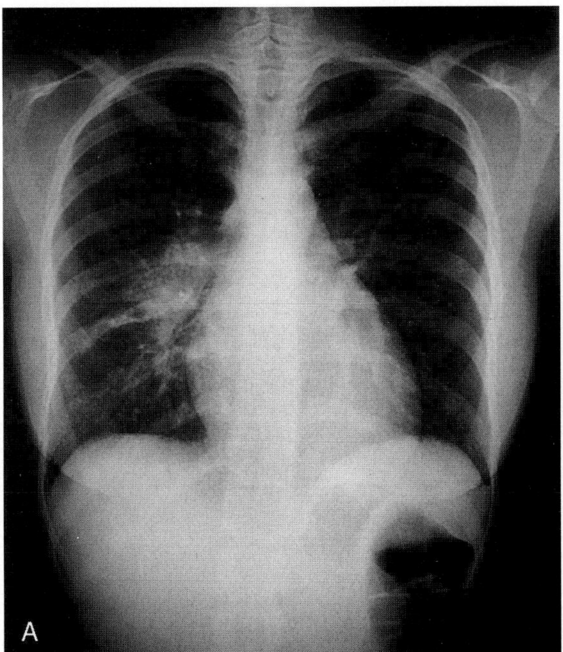

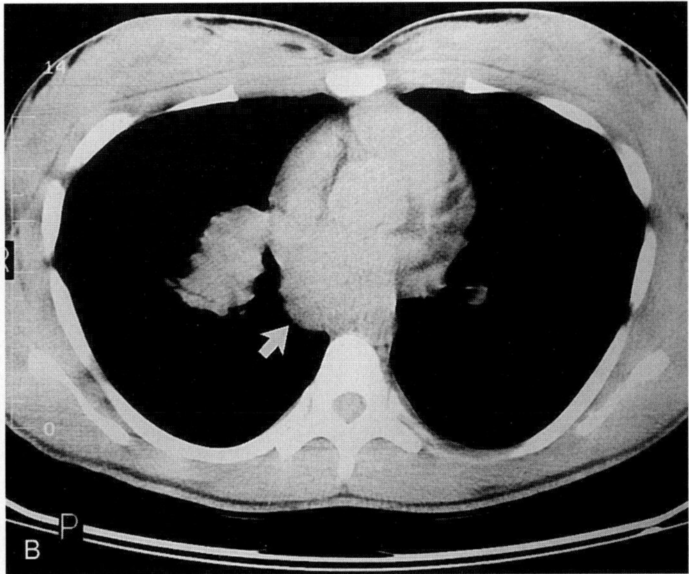

FIGURE 23–28 ■ Posteroanterior chest radiograph (*A*) and computed tomography scan (*B*) of a 19-year-old female with nonspecific upper respiratory tract symptoms. Note the enlarged lymph nodes mostly visible in the subcarinal space (*arrows*). Thoracoscopic biopsy showed caseous granulomatosis, which smeared positive for acid-fast bacilli.

difficult to differentiate from other causes of mediastinal node enlargement. Because most patients do not have active pulmonary disease at the time of presentation, positive diagnosis is based on the isolation of mycobacteria in lymph nodes. Fine-needle aspiration is safe and has a sensitivity of about 80% and very good specificity (Sloane, 1995). Cervical mediastinoscopy and transtracheal and thoracoscopic biopsies are alternative methods that can be used to obtain tissue for diagnosis. Surgical removal of the nodes is indicated only in patients with complications resulting from the adenopathy.

Patients with mediastinal tuberculous lymphadenitis should be treated with isoniazid and rifampin for at least 6 months, with an initial 2-month course of pyrazinamide (McCarthy and Rudd, 1989).

Complications of Scarring

Massive Hemoptysis. The majority of patients with hemoptysis and active tuberculosis (Fig. 23–29) bleed because of systemic bronchial circulation, which becomes abundant around the infected sites. In addition, the incorporation of pulmonary vessels into the wall of tuberculous cavities causes small dilations of these vessels, which are referred to as Rasmussen's aneurysms (Rasmussen and Moore, 1968). These aneurysms have been found to be present in 4% of autopsies of patients with tuberculosis (Auerbach, 1939). Bleeding from tuberculous lesions is usually the result of bronchial ulcerations into bronchial arteries or into Rasmussen's aneurysms. Occasionally, bleeding can be secondary to necrosis of small branches of pulmonary veins, erosion of old, calcified nodes through a bronchus (broncholith), or acute tuberculous ulcerations of the bronchial mucosa.

Cavernoma. One of the main indications for surgery in the golden days of tuberculosis was a large pulmonary cavern, which was the result of limited pulmonary destruction and was a walled-off portion of acutely infected parenchyma often located at pulmonary apices. The wall of a cavern is made of granulation tissue encircled by a layer of fibrous tissue in which Rassmussen's aneurysms can be found. Caverns are often the site of reactivation and can be associated with such complications as bleeding and formation of aspergillomas. Whenever possible, large caverns should be resected, but unfortunately, such lesions commonly occur in debilitated patients with severe underlying lung disease in whom major resection is not possible. In these patients, thoracoplasty combined with muscle plombage may be useful to collapse the cavern. Another option for management is a cavernostomy or cavernoplasty known as speleoplasty. This technique involves sterilization of the cavern by drug instillation, followed by its opening and the closure of visible bronchi. The cavity is then obliterated with stitches or muscle plombage (Perelman and Strelzov, 1997; Wu et al, 1996).

Lung Cancer. The association of lung cancer and tuberculosis has been reported with sufficient frequency to suggest that there is more than a coincidental connection. The linkage could occur by way of two different pathways. First, tuberculosis can be reactivated by bronchogenic carcinoma (Snider and Placik, 1969), either locally by means of the erosion of encapsulated caseous foci or systemically by means of the debilitation associated with the malignancy. The second possible link is the development of malignancies in areas of healed tuberculosis. In 1991, Dacosta and Kinare reported 29 cases of tuberculo-

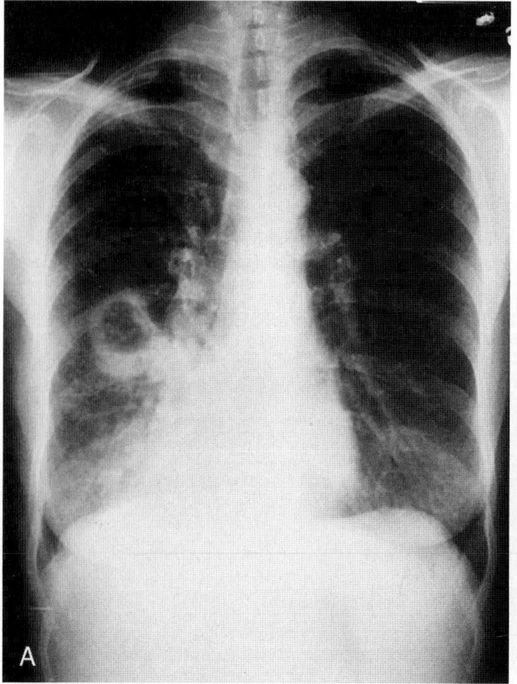

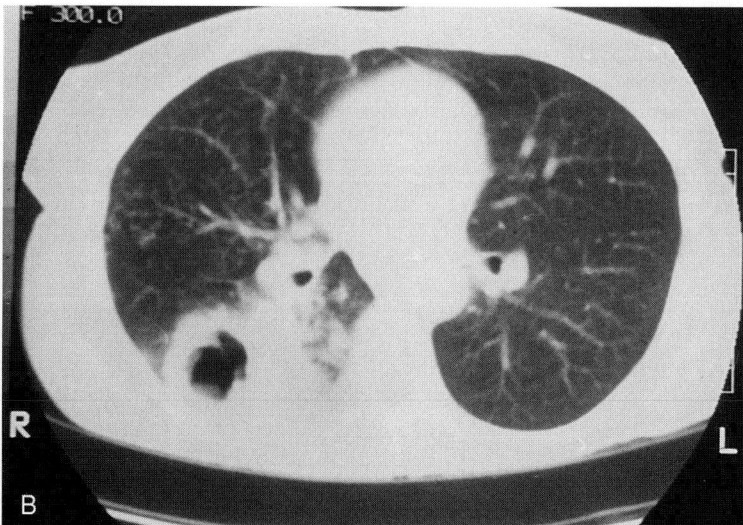

FIGURE 23–29 ■ Posteroanterior chest radiograph (*A*) and computed tomography scan (*B*) of a 30-year-old woman who presented with massive hemoptysis owing to active cavitary tuberculosis in the right lower lobe.

sis associated with 221 cases of mostly undifferentiated carcinomas, and adenocarcinomas of the lung. The typical presentation was that of a lung cancer's developing at the site of a parenchymal scar that had been stable for many years. In another study of 124 patients with coexisting bronchogenic carcinoma and pulmonary tuberculosis, Snider and Placik (1969) found that tuberculosis preceded the discovery of carcinoma in 56% of patients, and in 44% of cases, the two conditions were synchronous and were documented within 6 months of each other. The association of carcinoma with scarring is thought to be due to the poor clearance of carcinogens in scar areas or to the hyperplasia and metaplasia associated with healing and to the production of growth-factor–like substances. Tuberculosis is not the only source of scarring, and virtually any pathologic condition that produces scars within the lung can be associated with malignancy. For instance, malignancies have been described at sites of traumatic scarring associated with explosive shrapnels, bullet wounds, or knife injuries (Chauduri, 1973), and in association with silicosis (Galietti et al, 1989), fibrosing alveolitis end-stage lung disease (Meyer and Liebow, 1965), and scleroderma (Twersky et al, 1976).

The recovery of acid-fast bacilli in suspected cases of bronchogenic carcinoma should never delay diagnostic procedures aimed at confirming the cancer. Similarly, patients with a known history of tuberculosis should be followed regularly to detect not only recurrences of the disease but also the development of scar carcinomas.

Tracheo- or Bronchoesophageal Fistulas. Although the majority of acquired nonmalignant tracheoesophageal fistulas result from complications of mechanical ventilation (Mathisen et al, 1991), they can occasionally be associated with mediastinal granulomatosis. In those cases, the fistulas are produced by the continuous pressure on and scarring of infected mediastinal nodes located between the trachea and esophagus. The anatomic locations of fistulas are variable; they have been reported at the levels of the trachea, right main stem bronchus, left main stem bronchus, and right lower lobe bronchus (Spalding et al, 1978).

Unless surgery is urgently required, a trial of medical therapy seems to be a reasonable first-line approach because some of these fistulas may heal with medical therapy alone (Conjalka et al, 1980). Patients with significant associated esophageal or bronchial stenosis and patients in whom the diagnosis of malignancy cannot be excluded might require surgery (Spalding et al, 1978). Correction requires closure of the esophageal defect, segmental resection of the trachea, and tissue interposition (Macchiarini et al, 1993).

Bronchiectasis. The true incidence of bronchiectasis associated with tuberculosis is unknown but it can be the cause of recurrent and sometimes massive hemoptysis as well as chronic infection (Curtis, 1957). Bronchiectasis is caused by fibrosis and destruction of the lung, which causes retraction and dilation of the bronchi (Curtis, 1957), or is secondary to bronchial obstruction and includes postobstruction bacterial colonization. The bronchial obstruction itself results from bronchial stenosis due to fibrosis or extrinsic compression by cavernomas or enlarged lymph nodes (Rosenzweig and Stead, 1966).

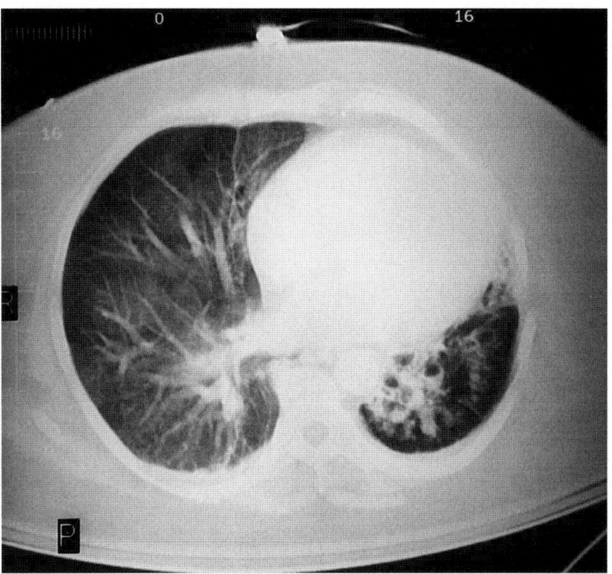

FIGURE 23–30 ■ A computed tomography scan of a 51-year-old woman previously treated for tuberculosis and referred for massive hemoptysis. Note the bronchiectasis in the apical segment of the left lower lobe.

Bronchiectasis associated with tuberculosis is most often found in the spontaneously well-drained apical and posterior segments of the upper lobes (dry bronchiectasis), and in these cases, the clinical presentation is most commonly in the form of hemoptysis. Unless the hemoptysis is massive, patients should be considered for surgery only after a long trial of medical therapy. If the hemoptysis is recurring despite adequate medical management, surgical resection should be considered, particularly if the bronchiectasis is localized and if resection is likely to result in complete removal of the disease (Fig. 23–30).

Extrinsic Obstruction by Tuberculous Lymph Nodes. Enlarged tuberculous nodes can occasionally compromise the lumen of airways. Although mediastinal adenopathy can be found in about 50% of patients requiring admission for complications of pulmonary tuberculosis, in only 2% do they cause airway compression severe enough to require surgical intervention (Worthington et al, 1993). In extreme cases the nodes can actually unload caseum into the bronchial lumen, resulting in sudden respiratory deterioration and even death. Children are particularly prone to mediastinal lymph node compression, probably because of their as yet poorly developed cartilaginous structures. More rarely, calcified lymph nodes (broncholiths) erode into airways and cause bleeding and obstruction.

Extrinsic airway obstruction is usually responsive to medical therapy, primarily to corticosteroids. In the rare cases in which the obstruction becomes clinically significant, surgical decompression may be necessary. The operation is carried out through a right thoracotomy and consists of incision and aspiration or curettage of nodal contents. Excision of the entire lymph node is usually not recommended so as to avoid iatrogenic lacerations of the airways (Worthington et al, 1993). As some of these lymph nodes may contain a liquefied core, endobronchial débridement and drainage is sometimes possible (Schwartz et al, 1988).

Endobronchial Tuberculosis and Bronchostenosis. Endobronchial tuberculosis is seen in 10% to 37% of patients with pulmonary tuberculosis (Hsu et al, 1997) and if untreated, it eventually leads to bronchostenosis (Hoheisel et al, 1994). The stenosis results from local infection and subsequent scarring. Because the lower and middle lobes are more commonly affected than the upper lobes, it is possible that gravity plays an important role in the pathogenesis of this complication. Clinically, patients present with cough, bronchorrhea, and shortness of breath on exertion, with typical collapse or consolidation seen on chest radiographs (Fig. 23–31). The diagnosis of post-tuberculous bronchostenosis is made by bronchoscopic examination and bronchial biopsy. Sputum analysis and smears are notoriously unreliable in the majority of these patients, even in the early stages of disease.

Once cicatricial bronchostenosis is well established, medical management has little to offer unless the patient has evidence of active tuberculosis (Kim et al, 1993). Surgical treatment should be based on the general status of the patient and the location of the stenosis. Balloon dilation, metallic stenting, laser vaporization, and bronchoplastic resection have been accomplished with good results (Hsu et al, 1997; Kato et al, 1993; Sawada et al, 1993; Tong and Van Hasselt, 1993; Watanabe et al, 1997). In order to prevent relapses or restenosis, continuous antituberculous chemotherapy should be given for 9 to 12 months postoperatively.

Middle Lobe Syndrome. Isolated atelectasis of the middle lobe is known as middle lobe syndrome. Although originally described as occurring only in the middle lobe, the process can involve the lingula as well. The syndrome is due to extrinsic nodal compression of the bronchus of lingula or middle lobe, which results in postobstructive

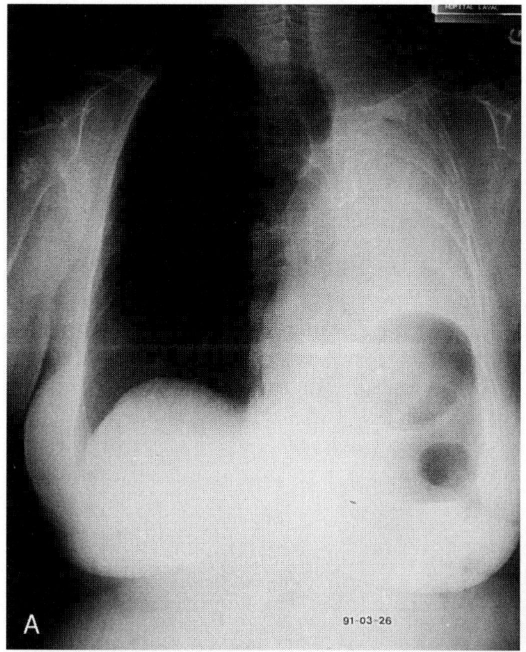

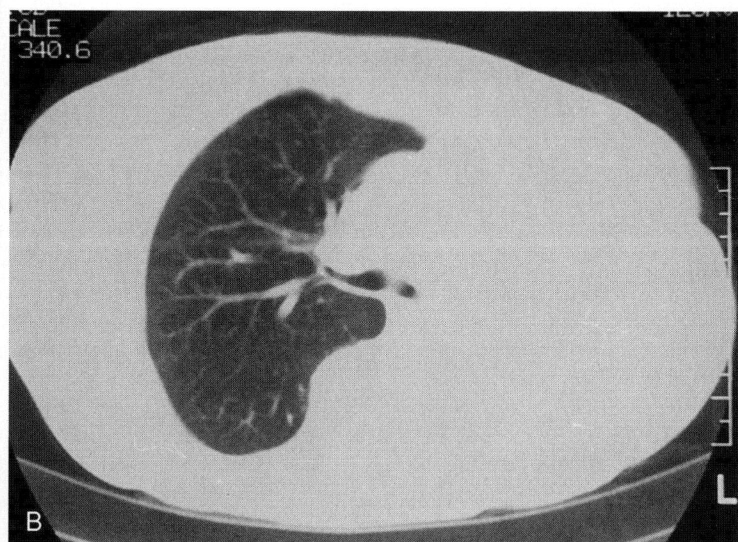

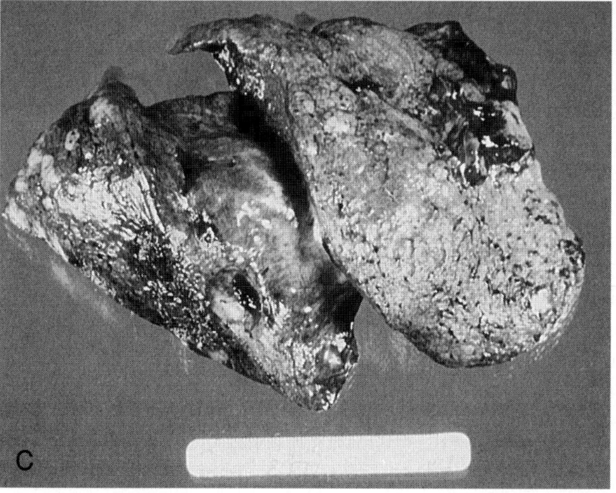

FIGURE 23–31 ■ Posteroanterior chest radiograph (*A*) and computed tomography scan (*B*) of an 80-year-old woman with distal left mainstem bronchus complete obstruction. Both the radiograph and the scan show complete atelectasis of the left lung. At operation, the lung (*C*) was found to be completely consolidated and had to be removed.

atelectasis and chronic pneumonitis. Although this process could conceivably occur anyplace in the lung, the middle lobe and lingula are particularly susceptible because of the long and narrow bronchus and the absence of collateral ventilation in patients with complete fissures (Pomerantz et al, 1996). The predominant symptoms are recurrent infection and atelectatic middle lobe on chest radiograph, with or without hilar lymph adenopathies. Bronchoscopy often shows a tight stenosis of the middle lobe bronchus (Lindskog and Spear, 1955).

In patients with middle lobe syndrome, it is important to rule out endobronchial obstruction by a malignant neoplasm, which could produce the same radiologic appearance. Once the diagnosis of benign disease has been established clearly, patients should be screened for tuberculosis, and symptomatic patients fit for surgery should undergo pulmonary resection. In an interesting series of 229 patients infected with mycobacterial organisms, Pomerantz and colleagues (1996) found 13 cases of middle lobe syndrome. Curiously, the authors noted that all patients involved were slender females with various combinations of skeletal abnormalities. All were treated by resection of the involved lobe or segments, and only two patients experienced postoperative reactivation of tuberculosis requiring additional antibiotic therapy. All patients were symptomatically improved following surgery.

Extrapulmonary Thoracic Disease

Tuberculosis of the Heart and Great Vessels. Tuberculosis extends to the heart and great vessels by way of direct spread from the lung or mediastinal lymph nodes or by means of bloodstream dissemination (Rawls et al, 1968). In 1935, Horn and Saphir classified myocardial tuberculosis into three main categories: miliary, nodular, and infiltrating. The most common clinical presentations are those of bleeding due to the rupture of tuberculomas or tuberculous abscesses, obstruction of the inflow or outflow tracts by tuberculomas, and conduction disturbances (Chang et al, 1999; Rawls et al, 1968).

Commonly, however, patients with cardiac tuberculosis present with nonspecific symptoms of weight loss, asthenia, dyspnea, and cardiac dysrythmias. They nearly always have evidence of concomitant active tuberculosis, so any patient presenting with active tuberculosis and cardiac arrhythmias should be evaluated for cardiac tuberculosis. The treatment of cardiac tuberculosis involves antituberculous medication unless mechanical consequences ensue. In such cases, surgical therapy should aim at resolving the mechanical complication rather than at full resection of the disease. Postoperatively, all patients should be started on antituberculous medication so as to treat residual disease as well as to avoid recurrences.

Vascular Malformations. Tuberculous involvement of the great vessels is caused primarily by the invasion of the wall of the vessel by adjacent tuberculous processes or, occasionally, by direct implantation of circulating mycobacteria (Efremidis et al, 1976). The result is either compression and stenosis of the involved segments of the vessel, with vascular insufficiency, or aneurysmal dilation with the risk of rupture. Because of its mediastinal location, the pulmonary artery is particularly prone to compression by surrounding lymph nodes. In 1996, Cohen and colleagues reported the case of a 35-year-old woman with symptoms similar to those of pulmonary embolism who was found to have near complete obstruction of the right pulmonary artery due to tuberculous lymphadenitis. The diagnosis was made by the recovery of acid-fast bacilli in the resected specimen. Efremidis and coworkers (1976) also reported the case of a 60-year-old woman with a rapidly expanding sacular aneurysm of the aortic arch but with no clinical evidence of ongoing tuberculosis. The diagnosis was made by the recovery of acid-fast bacilli in the resected aneurysmal wall. In 1988, Masjedi and associates reported a rare case of a bronchoaortic fistula that presented with massive hemoptysis. Bronchoscopy showed a brown vegetative mass protruding into the left mainstem bronchus 2 to 3 cm below the carina, and postmortem examination revealed the cause of the fistula to be mediastinal granulomatous disease.

A number of other extrapulmonary vascular malformations due to tuberculosis can also occur within the chest. They present with abnormal communications between chest wall systemic vessels and pulmonary artery circulation as a result of chronic scarring of the interposing tuberculous lung. Cohen and colleagues (1975) described such communications between the internal thoracic artery and the pulmonary artery branches of the left upper lobe in a 25-year-old asymptomatic man who presented with a continuous murmur over the left precordium. Ando and associates (1996) reported the case of a 77-year-old woman with active tuberculosis and a continuous-flow murmur over the left anterior chest wall. Cardiac catheterization and subclavian arteriography revealed abnormal communication between the subclavian and pulmonary arteries. Untreated pulmonary systemic shunts due to tuberculosis can result in pulmonary hypertension, heart failure, and possible rupture. Medical therapy should always supplement surgical resection.

Constrictive Pericarditis. Tuberculous pericarditis occurs in 1% to 4% of patients with tuberculosis (Heurich et al, 1995), and it is a common cause of pericardial effusion in patients with AIDS. The evolution of tuberculous pericarditis classically occurs in four stages. The fibrinous, stage (stage I) is characterized by deposition of fibrin and a granulomatous reaction within the pericardium and pleural space. This is followed by an effusion (stage II) with a predominance of lymphocytes; over time, the effusion resolves and the pericardium thickens (stage III). At that stage, there is dense deposition of scar tissue and calcifications within the pericardium. The organization of this fibrous tissue eventually leads to myocardial constriction (stage IV). Clinically, the symptoms are those of a chronic nonspecific illness associated with the signs and symptoms of restrictive pericardial disease. Dyspnea, chest pain, and pedal edema are common (Heurich et al, 1995). Electrocardiography is usually nonspecific, whereas chest radiographs may show some evidence of cardiomegaly. Tuberculin skin tests are unreliable, especially in patients with AIDS (Quale et al, 1987; Shafer et al, 1991). Echocardiography is extremely valuable in assessing the size of the effusion and the status of the underlying myocardium but is less useful in evaluating the thickness of the pericardial sac, a finding that is essential for the diagnosis of constrictive pericarditis. A thoracic CT scan with contrast is a better examination, and it has eliminated the need for cardiac catheterization (Suchet and Horwitz, 1992).

A positive diagnosis of pericardial tuberculosis can be made only by the identification of mycobacterium in the pericardial fluid or by direct visualization of the stigmata of the infection on the pericardium itself. Measurement of adenosine deaminase and carcinoembryonic antigen levels in the pericardial fluid can be useful in differentiating an effusion secondary to tuberculosis from one associated with malignancy or acute viral pericarditis. Adenosine deaminase is elevated in the pericardial fluid of a patient with tuberculosis, whereas the carcinoembryonic antigen is significantly higher in a patient with a malignancy (Koh et al, 1997).

Surgical procedures are generally indicated for patients with cardiac tamponade, patients with progressive pericardial effusion who are on appropriate medical therapy, and patients with constrictive pericarditis (Quale et al, 1987). In patients with suspected effusive tuberculous pericarditis, it is recommended that a pericardial window be performed; this not only allows for the rapid evacuation of the fluid but also provides a large specimen for analysis. The subxyphoid, left anterior thoracotomy, or left thoracoscopic approaches are safe and effective. Patients with thick pericardium are prone to develop severe constrictive pericarditis, so in that circumstance, early pericardiectomy has been advocated. Patients with constrictive pericarditis should be considered for surgery when they have evidence of calcifications or show no clinical improvement after 4 to 6 weeks of antituberculous medication (Strang, 1984). The surgical approach can be a median sternotomy or a left anterolateral thoracotomy, and the pericardium is excised from phrenic nerve to phrenic nerve, with decortication of the diaphragm and the anterolateral surfaces of the heart. The procedure is generally well tolerated and the majority of patients do not require cardiopulmonary bypass (Arsan et al, 1994; Trotter et al, 1996). In a series reported by Heurich and colleagues (1995), complete resolution of cardiac symptoms occurred in 94% of patients.

Cold Abscesses and Osteomyelitis of the Chest Wall. *MTB* can spread to the chest wall directly from a contiguous infected lung or through lymphatic dissemination (Faure et al, 1998). The clinical presentation may mimic that of a pyogenic abscess, although most patients have active pulmonary tuberculosis or a history of prior tuberculosis at the time of presentation (Kelley and Micozzi, 1984). Tuberculous abscesses occur more frequently in the parasternal area (Fig. 23–32) and over the shaft of the ribs. Because most of these abscesses are asymptomatic, with the contents under no tension, and the skin overlying the abscess usually of normal appearance, the term *cold abscess* has been used to describe them. Often the lesions are accompanied by destructive changes in the underlying bone or cartilage. In the absence of pleuropulmonary tuberculosis, the diagnosis is difficult to

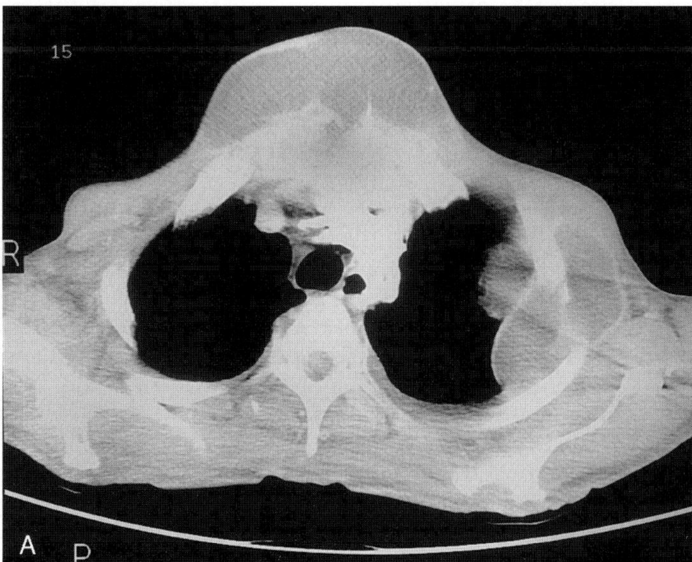

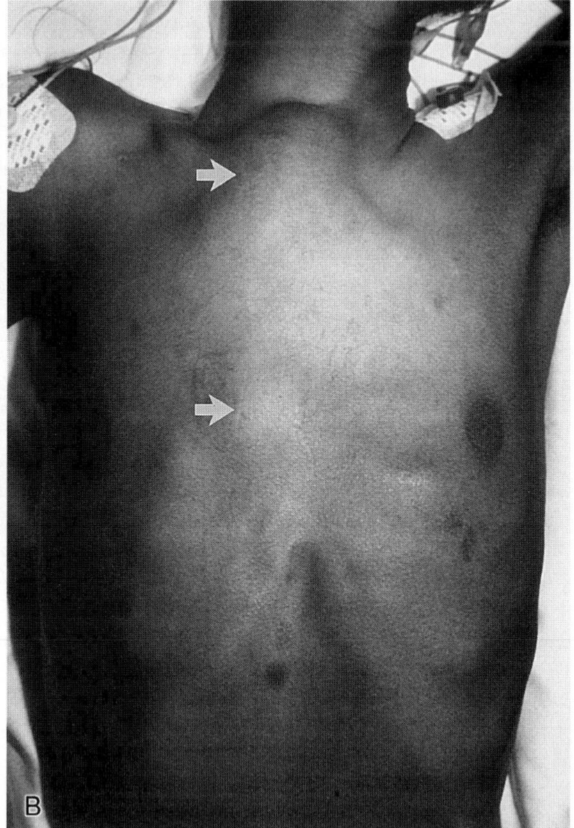

FIGURE 23–32 ■ *A*, A computed tomography scan of a 29-year-old man with active pulmonary tuberculosis and a fluctuating lesion of the anterior chest wall. *B*, Photograph showing large anterior chest wall abscesses *(arrows)* that, at surgery, extended to the underlying sternum and ribs. The patient had a good response to débridement and medical therapy.

establish, as needle aspirates are diagnostic in only 22% to 28% of patients (Faure et al, 1998; Hsu et al, 1995). However, the combination of rib destruction and an extrapleural soft tissue mass in Asian or African immigrants makes the diagnosis of tuberculosis very likely (Brown, 1980). CT characterizes these cold abscesses as low-density collections, often with enhancing rings and occasional calcifications (Adler et al, 1993).

Chest wall abscesses should be treated with a combination of medical and surgical therapies. If a lesion continues to develop or fails to show regression with medical treatment, surgical débridement, including resection of the necrotic ribs, cartilages, and visible adenopathies, is necessary. The authors usually leave the skin incision open, but some surgeons prefer to close it so as to avoid the formation of sinus tracts. Chemotherapy after surgery should be continued for 6 to 9 months. Using this regimen, the only recurrences reported have been in patients who failed to comply with chemotherapy after surgery (Faure et al, 1998; Hsu et al, 1995).

Pott's Disease. Tuberculosis of the spine, also known as Pott's disease, occurs in approximately 1% of patients with tuberculosis (Davidson and Horowitz, 1970). It is characteristically a chronic and slowly progressive disease as compared to pyogenic osteomyelitis, which has a more acute course. The presentation of spinal tuberculosis is nonspecific and most patients have back pain with varying degrees of neurologic impairment. Neurologic complications are more common when the disease involves the thoracic spine.

Clinicians encountering destructive spinal disease must have a high degree of suspicion for a diagnosis of tuberculosis. Indeed, none of the available diagnostic modalities is very specific or sensitive. In a study of 19 patients with Pott's disease, Omari and coworkers (1989) found a positive tuberculin skin test in 18, but only 42% of patients had abnormal chest radiographs. In a similar study involving 20 patients, Rezai and associates (1995) found a positive tuberculin skin test in 19 patients, and 65% showed evidence of concomittant pulmonary tuberculosis. Currently, CT scanning and magnetic resonance imaging (MRI) are important diagnostic tools for assessing the side and degree of vertebral involvement. Some of the typical CT findings are vertebral body destruction, space narrowing, and psoas or paraspinous abscesses (Omari et al, 1989). CT-guided biopsy can also be used in most patients; it reveals acid-fast bacilli or granulomatous disease in 50% to 75% of cases (Omari et al, 1989; Rezai et al, 1995).

Treatment of Pott's disease without neurologic complications can be medical or surgical. However, operative débridement results in faster recovery and less spinal deformity (Rezai et al, 1995). Pott's disease with neurologic deficit is best treated by radical surgery, and in these patients the urgency of the condition allows little time to pinpoint the diagnosis, which is often established postoperatively. Early operative treatment minimizes neurologic deterioration and spinal deformity and allows for earlier ambulation (Omari et al, 1989; Rezai et al, 1995). The indications for surgery are given in Table 23–12.

Spinal tuberculosis is best approached through a thoracotomy; a thoracic surgeon is often called upon to perform the opening of the chest and exposure of the vertebral bodies. The side on which the thoracotomy is performed is determined by the side on which there is maximal bony involvement or spinal cord compression. The disks above and below the affected vertebral bodies are resected along with the posterior longitudinal ligament in order to drain any epidural abscess. Autologous iliac crest bone grafting is then performed. Anterior or posterior instrumentation is usually reserved for patients in whom more than one vertebral body is to be resected and in whom the thoracolumbar spine is involved. In order to avoid relapses, all patients should be managed postoperatively with external bracing as well as antituberculous medication for periods of 6 to 9 months.

TABLE 23–12 ■ Criteria for Surgical Management of Pott's Disease

Neurologic deficit	Noncompliance with medication
Spinal instability or deformity	Nondiagnostic biopsy
Unresponsiveness to medical therapy	

From Rezai AR, Lee M, Cooper PR et al: Modern management of spinal tuberculosis. Neurosurgery 36:87, 1995.

Pleural Tuberculosis

Pleural Effusion. Involvement of the pleura (Fig. 23–33) is a common extrapulmonary manifestation of pulmonary tuberculosis. Pleural tuberculosis is caused by the presence of *MTB* in the pleural space and is thought to be secondary to the rupture of a caseous pulmonary lesion. The amount of pleural effusion present is determined by the interaction between the bacilli antigen and sensitized CD4T lymphocytes. The result of this interaction is a delayed hypersensitivity reaction, which produces an increase in capillary permeability. There is also an accumulation of helper T cells potentiating the inflammatory reaction (Ellner et al, 1988).

Pleural effusions can appear at any time during the natural course of tuberculosis and can be associated with both primary and reactivation diseases. Typically, patients present with symptoms of pleural involvement, including pleuritic chest pain, fever, dyspnea or, rarely, chest wall masses and pleurocutaneous sinus tracks. The effusion commonly appears in the absence of radiographic or clinical evidence of pulmonary tuberculosis. Although tuberculous pleural effusions can regress spontaneously, active pulmonary tuberculosis develops in 30% to 50% of such patients, indicating the importance of diagnosing and treating these effusions early (Sahn, 1988).

Up to one third of patients may not demonstrate positive tuberculin skin tests at the time of presentation, a phenomenon explained by the preferential sequestration of antigen-specific CD4 T cells in the pleural space and by the presence of suppressor cells in the blood (Ellner et al, 1988). Unless anergic, most patients eventually convert, usually 6 to 8 weeks later. The pleural fluid of tuberculous effusions is clear and citrus in color and is an exudate. Pleural fluid protein and lactate dehydrogenase are elevated, whereas the pH is less than 7.4 and

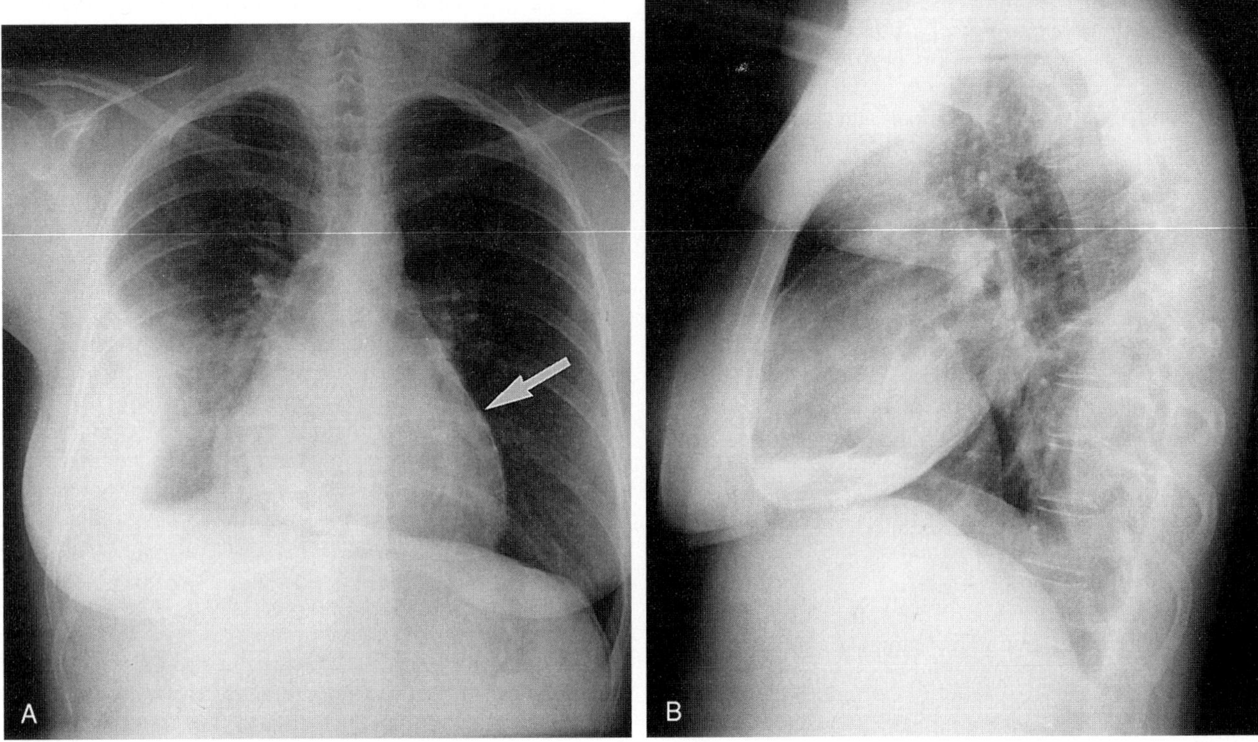

FIGURE 23–33 ■ Posteroanterior (*A*) and (*B*) chest radiographs of a 30-year-old woman with a loculated right pleural tuberculous empyema. Note the pericardial calcifications *(arrow)* indicating concomitant pericardial involvement.

the glucose contents are in the range of 60 mg/dl. The total cell count is usually fewer than 6000 cells/μl, the cell population being made predominantly of T lymphocytes, with an absence of mesothelial cells (Antony, 1987). The ratio of pleural fluid to serum inadenosine deaminase is a new marker that has been found to be above 1.5 in 85.7% of tuberculous effusions (Valdes et al, 1993). The concentration of cholesterol increases in chronic tuberculous effusions and in some cases the pleural fluid may even have a milky appearance (pseudochylothorax).

Pleural fluid cultures are not sensitive; they may yield MBT in only 50% of cases (Antony, 1987). The diagnosis must therefore be confirmed by pleural biopsy, which can yield MBT or granulomas in 75% to 80% of patients. If bedside pleural biopsy fails to provide a diagnosis, diagnostic thoracoscopy should be carried out (Suzuki et al, 1993). With open biopsy, granulomas can be found in up to 60% of cases, but this finding is not pathognomonic of tuberculosis because granulomas can also be found in other pathologic conditions, such as sarcoidosis, rhumatoid arthritis, and fungal infections. Pleural biopsies can be complemented by internal mammary lymph node biopsy. Using this technique, Villegas and colleagues (1970) were able to confirm a diagnosis in 62.5% of cases of tuberculous pleural effusion.

Surgical drainage of the pleural space should be performed only in patients who have large effusions. The management of pleural tuberculosis is otherwise mainly medical. Treatment with two drugs for a period of 9 months is recommended, although more recently, successful treatment courses of 6 months, using isoniazid and rifampin, have been reported (Dutt et al, 1992). Drugs must be adjusted to the sensitivity of the organism, and treatment should be prolonged in cases of drug resistance and in HIV patients.

As a result of lung trapping, failure of pulmonary expansion after adequate medical therapy can occur in up to 50% of patients (Barbas et al, 1991). If this situation develops, intervention is indicated in young patients and in patients with significant pulmonary restriction (Fig. 23–34). Another possible complication of tuberculous pleurisy that requires surgical management is bacterial contamination of the pleural space. In this condition, tube thoracostomy with negative suction should be used first, but if lung expansion cannot be obtained, open decortication or empyemectomy may become necessary.

Bronchopleural Fistula. A bronchopleural fistula is a rare complication of pulmonary tuberculosis. It results from the opening of a pulmonary cavitation into the pleural space or from the erosion of a pleural empyema into the lung. The clinical picture is variable; some patients have an air-fluid level that is found incidentally on a chest radiograph, whereas others present with life-threatening tension pneumothoraces. The most common clinical presentation, however, is in the form of a slowly progressive emaciating disease that can eventually lead to the demise of the patient if left untreated. In a study reported by Donath and Khan (1984), 7 of 13 patients with bronchopleural fistulas had prior evidence of pleural disease in the form of fibrothoraces. All patients had histories of tuberculosis and none had been compliant with their medications. These findings underline the importance of

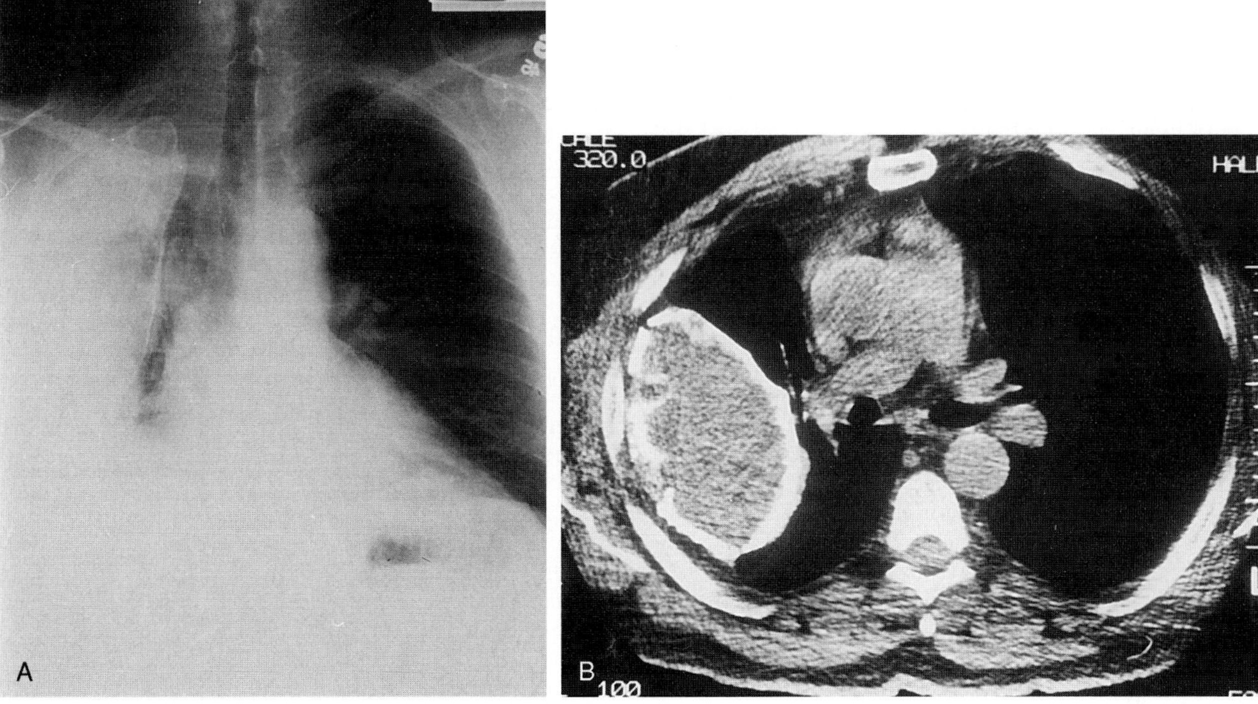

FIGURE 23–34 ■ Posteroanterior chest radiograph (*A*) and computer tomography scan (*B*) of a 60-year-old man with post-tuberculous fibrothorax.

early and adequate treatment of pleural tuberculosis as well as the importance of pleural scarring in the etiology of bronchopleural fistulas.

The initial management of tuberculous bronchopleural fistulas consists of tube drainage and antibiotic therapy. Although tube thoracostomy has been used on a permanent basis (Donath and Khan, 1984), it is generally a temporary measure that allows rapid resolution of sepsis and optimal preparation of patients for more definitive therapy. In elderly patients with chronic sepsis and in patients with AIDS, open drainage by way of a thoracic window is an alternative.

Once drainage of the pleural cavity has been established, sepsis is under control, and tuberculosis is adequately treated medically, low-risk patients can be offered permanent repair of the fistula. Preparation for this can take 3 to 6 months, as patients with ongoing active tuberculosis at the time of surgery have higher risks for surgical complications in the form of pleural empyema and dehiscence of the repair. The objective of surgery is to close the fistula and obtain full lung re-expansion through decortication alone or by filling the pleural cavity with muscle or omentum flaps. Pulmonary resection should be reserved for patients in whom the underlying lung has been seriously damaged and is beyond salvage. Because patients undergoing pulmonary resection, especially pneumonectomy, are at high risk for bronchial dehiscence, the bronchial stump should always be reinforced with viable vascularized autografts. If the pleural space has been contaminated during pneumonectomy, Miller and associates (1975) suggest the use of balanced drainage for 2 to 3 weeks, followed by the establishment of a continuous irrigation system with antibiotics for another 2 weeks. Tubes are removed once the cavity is sterile.

Infections with Mycobacteria Other than Tubercle Bacilli

In North America, MOTT infections are more common than *MTB* infections, and this is particularly true in patients affected by AIDS. The most common organs involved by atypical mycobacteria are the lungs, cervical lymph nodes, soft tissues, bones, and joints. These infections share with *MTB* a number of clinical and bacteriologic similarities, and they often are indistinguishable from one another. Unfortunately, most nontuberculous mycobacteria are resistant to usual antituberculous therapies.

MOTT infections are also known as nontuberculous mycobacterial disease (NTM), yellow bacillus (*M. kansasii*), Battey bacillus (*M. avium*), anonymous mycobacteria, Lady Windermere syndrome (*M. avium*), and MAC (*M. avium* and *M. intracellulare* complex). Many atypical mycobacteria are human saprophytes but some can produce clinical infections. The MOTT, most commonly associated with lung disease are *M. avium-intracellulare*, *M. kansasii*, and *M. abscessus*. On occasion, *M. fortuitum* has also been found to cause sternal osteomyelitis and contamination of porcine valves (Robicsek et al, 1978). *M. kansasii* are the most common atypical mycobacteria in the central United States, whereas MAC is the most common in the southern and southeastern United States. In some laboratories, MAC is even more common than *MTB* and has become the most common mycobacterial species (Nelson et al, 1998). Some atypical mycobacteria can be normal inhabitants of the airway, so clinically significant disease is diagnosed by evidence of lung lesions on radiographs and by repeated isolation of the organisms from bronchial secretions (Bailey, 1983).

MAC typically produces a fibrocavitary disease of the upper lobes in white males who tend to be alcoholic and in smokers with underlying chronic obstructive pulmonary disease. It can also affect patients with few or no risk factors and it has shown a predilection for the lingula and middle lobe in nonsmoking females, a clinical condition known as Lady Windermere syndrome (Reich and Johnson, 1992). At the present time, the most effective drug therapy is the combination of clarithromycin with rifabutin or rifampin and ethambutol until the patient is culture-negative for 1 year. For the first 2 to 4 months, streptomycin should be added to the regimen if there is extensive disease such as cavitary lesions. In a significant number of patients, sterile sputum is the outcome of this regimen, but the main drawback of medical management remains drug toxicity and treatment compliance.

Surgical resection is indicated for localized disease; by combining surgery with medical therapy, sputum conversion can be achieved in 88% to 94% of patients, with relapse rates of less than 6% (Moran et al, 1983; Nelson et al, 1998; Shiraishi et al, 1998). Sputum conversion seems to be more permanent after surgery. In an interesting study, Moran and colleagues (1983) documented that 90% of their patients who were sputum-negative at the time of operation had positive cultures or smears from resected lung tissue. It is possible that the resection of these foci of persistent disease may lead to better long-term outcome when compared to medical therapy alone. The length of postoperative medical therapy is not standardized, although drugs should be given for at least 1 year.

Patients infected with *M. kansasii* are typically in their 50s; risk factors for this disease include cigarette abuse, pneumoconiosis, HIV infection, and living in the midwestern United States. This infection is medically easier to treat than MAC, so surgery is seldom indicated.

Infection by *M. abscessus* has a clinical presentation different from that of infection by other MOTT. It tends to affect white females and present radiographically as a diffuse, patchy interstitial disease difficult to diferentiate from scarring or fibrosis. *M. abscessus* pneumonia has a progressive and slow course that can cause death if left untreated. Because *M. abscessus* is resistant to antituberculous medication, medical therapy alone is usually not successful, and surgery should be considered if the disease is localized and the patient can tolerate surgery.

Outcome of Surgical Treatment

The surgical experience accumulated over the past 40 years indicates that the role of surgery in the treatment of tuberculosis is unquestionable (Table 23–13). With proper indications for surgery, sputum-conversion rates as high as 95% can be obtained (Rieder, 1996). Because the same results can be expected in patients harboring sensitive organisms who comply with treatment, surgery should always be considered an adjunct to proper medical therapy. In established cases of tuberculosis, no patients should be operated upon without proper antibiotic coverage of at least 3 months' duration, and surgeries should always be followed by complete courses of therapy, the lengths of which are dictated by the resistance of the organisms and the susceptibilities of the hosts. In patients with normal immune systems, postoperative medical treatment should include at least two drugs (isoniazid and rifampin) for 6 months. In immunocompromised patients such as those with HIV in whom multiple-drug–resistant tuberculosis is prevalent, postoperative treatments should be carried out for periods of 9 to 12 months, or longer in cases of true resistance (Iseman et al, 1990).

The role of surgery is to remove the burden of mycobacteria in actively infected patients or to treat debilitating consequences due to the ongoing scarring process that characterizes the healing of tuberculosis. It is indeed very difficult to sterilize cavernomas or destroyed lungs, probably because the disease is too far advanced or medications are unable to penetrate the lesions. When such permanent anatomic changes occur, medical treatment alone has a high failure rate and the addition of surgery to remove nidus of active tuberculosis may improve the cure rate of the disease (Mouroux et al, 1996).

Proper preoperative evaluation and optimization of the patient's status are essential, and unless there is an emergency such as a massive hemoptysis, time must be taken to sterilize the sputum of all patients prior to surgery. The nutritional status of the patient should be addressed, as many of these patients present with advanced states of malnutrition due to months of chronic debilitating disease. The feasibility of resection should be evaluated, and attention should be given to the cardiorespiratory status as it is in any patient who is to have pulmonary resection. A CT scan should be provided to all patients to determine the extent of the disease, predict operative difficulties, and assess the status of the contralateral lung.

Bronchoscopy should always be performed to document possible tuberculous endobronchial disease and to determine the extent of resection likely to be necessary. If a bronchial closure encompasses an area involved by tuberculous bronchitis, it will be associated with a significantly higher risk of dehiscence and formation of a bronchopleural fistula (Pomerantz, 1993). During surgery, double-lumen endotracheal tubes should be used not only to deflate the lung but also to avoid contamination of the contralateral lung by pus and debris produced by the manipulation of the resected lung. In patients with chronic pulmonary tuberculosis, pleural adhesions are common and a network of systemic-to-pulmonary neovascularization often involves these adhesions. The presence of these adhesions makes the dissection of the lung tedious and prone to a significant amount of blood loss. Lymph nodes involved by granulomatosis are often adherent to the surrounding vessels, making their skeletonization around the hilum more dangerous. In such cases, the dissection must be extended more proximally so as to encompass as much disease as possible.

When pneumonectomy is required, care must be taken not to contaminate the pleural space. If the risks of contamination are high, pneumonectomy should be per-

TABLE 23–13 ■ **Review of Worldwide Experiences in Performing Surgery for Tuberculosis**

Author, Year, Location	*Patients (No.)*	*Indication for Surgery*	*Morbidity (%)*	*Mortality (%)*	*Outcome*	*Comments*
Cole and Alley: 1955, U.S.	513	Tuberculoma to destroyed lung	34	6.4	85% conversion	32.5% had no medical therapy prior to surgery; 20.6% had septic complications; only 4% of patients had antibiotherapy prior to surgery. All patients with BPF had positive TB cultures in the bronchial resection margin.
Dagher et al: 1959, U.S.	207	Surgery for moderately advanced and advanced TB	27	4.8	NA	
Floyd et al: 1959, U.S.	430	Surgery for TB, not specified	18.8	2.3	NA	BPF in 10.5% of cases (28% of pneumonectomies); 11% had positive cultures.
Neptune et al: 1970, U.S.	186	Cavity 56%, tuberculoma 13%, drug resistance 9.7%, empyema 4.8%, ? carcinoma 3.7%, removal of plombage 9%	8	1.3	0.5% reactivation due to early discontinuation of drugs	Collapse therapy in 20%; 12.3% of patients were on steroids.
Delarue et al: 1975, Canada	146	Cavity 32%, positive sputum 30%, resistance 24.6%, empyema 1.3%	49	9	NA	BPF in 20%
Das and David: 1975, India	805	Cavities, tuberculoma, lung destruction, positive sputum, drug resistance, bronchiectasis, bronchostenosis	12.8	2.8	2.6% reactivation	BPF in 3.1%; all patients had at least 6 mo of preoperative chemotherapy.
Moran et al: 1983, U.S.	37	Localized disease (MOTT) with failure of medical therapy	NA	0		All were MAC; 67% were sputum-negative at the time of surgery.
Reed et al: 1989, U.S.	24	Hemoptysis 58%, drug resistance 21%, ? neoplasia 12.5%, bronchiectasis 8%	46 (major 16.7%)	0	2 reactivations in the contralateral lung	12.5% had MOTT; 12.5% had BPF/empyema.
Whyte et al: 1989, U.K.	31	Destroyed lung, hemoptysis, cavity, BPF/empyema	16	0	NA	In patients suspected of carcinoma, 16% had a history of TB and 12% had been exposed to TB. Only one patient was on preoperative chemotherapy. 10% had carcinoma. All complications occurred in patients with active TB.
Treasure and Seaworth: 1995, U.S.	59	MDRTB 32%, BPF 20%, destroyed lung 12%, solitary nodule 12%, hemoptysis 8%, cavity 7%, trapped lung, empyema	20.3	0	89% cure rate in MDRTB	Pneumonectomy with muscle flaps in 23%; BRF in 3% of patients
Rizzi et al: 1995, Italy	206	? Cancer 24%, cavity 22%, bronchiectasis 16%, hemoptysis 16%, progression 8.5%, lung destruction 8%, BPF 3%	29.1	3	86.2% conversion	Tuberculoma and pleural TB were excluded from the study. Association with scar cancer existed in 33% and with mycetoma in 45%. 1.4% had MOTT. 38.8% had positive sputum at surgery. Higher morbidity occurred in patients with positive sputum.
Wu et al: 1996, China	107	Cavity 35.5%, aspergilloma 25%, destroyed lung 18.7%, tuberculoma 13%, empyema 3.7%, tracheobrochial stenosis 3.7%	16.8	1.8	96% conversion	6.5% BRF; muscle flaps used with cavernostomy in 6.5%.

Table continued on following page

TABLE 23–13 ■ **Review of Worldwide Experiences in Performing Surgery for Tuberculosis** *Continued*

Author, Year, Location	*Patients (No.)*	*Indication for Surgery*	*Morbidity (%)*	*Mortality (%)*	*Outcome*	*Comments*
Mouroux et al: 1996, France	59	Group I, 42%: Solitary nodule, pulmonary lesion/infiltrate, pleural effusion;	4	4	Favorable in all	Classic 6-mo postoperative medical treatment: 4 drugs for 2 mo, 2 drugs for 4 mo
		Group II, 30.5%: Cavity, destroyed lung, chronic loculated pleural effusion;	16.6	5.5	Favorable in all	9 to 12 mo medical treatment: 4-drug treatment for 3 to 6 mo followed by 2 drugs 3 to 6 mo later, depending on sputum status
		Group III, 27%: Pyothorax, bronchiectasis, aspergilloma, fistulized nodes	31.2	12.5	Favorable in all	Classic 6-mo treatment if the cultures of the specimen were positive; 4-mo empiric treatment with 2 drugs if the cultures were negative.
Perelman and Strelzov: 1997, Russia	502	Cavernous TB 39%, tuberculoma 32%, pleuritis/empyema 26%, mediastinal adenopathy 13%, focal TB 2.8%, caseous pneumonia 0.8%	20	2	6.6% reactivation, 82.7% conversion	50% had positive sputum; no HIV. Most complications were associated with pleural TB.
Halezeroglu et al: 1997, Turkey	118	Destroyed lung 100%, active TB 43%	11.9	5.9	NA	Increased rate of BPF and mortality if empyema, active TB, and right pneumonectomy were present.
Kir et al: 1997, Turkey	27	Destroyed lung 18.5%, cavitary disease 81.5%	NA	0	3.7% relapse	All MDRTB in HIV-negative patients. All patients were on antibiotherapy prior to surgery. Good nutritional status in all patients. All patients had negative preoperative cultures. BPF in 7.4% due to extensive bronchial dissection.
van Leuven et al: 1997, South Africa	62	Failure of conversion 39%, high risk of relapse 22%, drug resistance 21%, relapse 18%	23	1.6	75% conversion with surgery alone, 80% relapse free	All MDRTB
Pomerantz and Brown: 1997, U.S.	130	Hemoptysis, bronchial stenosis, BPF, cavitary lesions, destroyed lung	12.3	2.3	90% cure rate	All MDRTB. 50% sputum-positive at the time of surgery; 37% muscle flap; 2.3% BPF
Nelson et al: 1998, U.S.	28	Cavitary disease in MAC 100%	32	7	93% conversion rate at 3 months, 3.6% relapse	Poor nutritional status; 50% culture-negative at the time of surgery. Most common complication was prolonged air leak, which was treated by thoracoplasty. BPF in 3.6% was treated with omentopexy. Drug therapy was continued for 3 to 12 mo postoperatively.
Shiraishi et al: 1998, Japan	33	Localized MAC 100%	15+	0	94% conversion, 6% relapse	55% sputum-positive at the time of surgery; 15% had thoracoplasty for residual space; BPF in 3%

TB, tuberculosis; BPF, bronchopleural fistula; MOTT, mycobacteria other than tubercle bacilli; MAC, *Mycobacterium avium* complex disease; MDRTB, multiple drug–resistant tuberculosis.

formed in an extrapleural fashion. On occasion, thoracoplasty may be a useful adjunct to reduce the size of the pleural cavity occupied by a small lung or to treat bronchopleural fistulas (Delarue et al, 1975).

Proper chest drainage is essential after any kind of surgery for tuberculosis. Large tubes with side holes must be used to avoid the accumulation of clots in the pleural cavity, which can result in lung entrapment, empyema, or even disseminated intravascular coagulation (Rocco et al, 1994). Bronchopleural fistula is a serious complication of surgery for tuberculosis, but in most recent series the incidence has been less than 10%. The type of closure (sutures vs. stapler) does not appear to be a risk factor (Kir et al, 1997), but active tuberculosis and active ongoing suprainfection by gram-negative bacteria are significant risk factors for this complication (Pomerantz et al, 1991). Pulmonary resection should therefore always be complemented by covering the bronchial stump with vascularized pedicled flaps such as intercostal muscle, latissimus dorsi, or omentum. Patients with bronchopleural fistulas should be first treated with tube thoracostomy, and the surgeon's urge to close the fistula should be restrained until sputum and pleural cultures have tested negative.

If the objective of surgical treatment is sputum conversion and maintenance of that conversion, complete resection of the focus of disease along with proper antibiotic therapy are essential. Unfortunately, the rate of relapse is high in patients with sputum positivity at the time of surgery, in patients who develop postoperative bronchopleural fistulas or empyemas, in patients with positive smear or cultures of the resected specimen (Blackwood and Andrews, 1967), in patients with multiple-drug–resistant tuberculosis (Goble et al, 1993), and in patients with inadequate medical therapy (Mahmoudi and Iseman, 1993). There is also a higher percentage of nonconversion with lobectomy and segmentectomy as compared to pneumonectomy, suggesting that a more radical procedure may be more effective than a smaller resection (van Leuven et al, 1997).

CONCLUSION

Successful treatment of tuberculosis depends on prompt diagnosis and proper medical therapy. The increase in the number of new tuberculosis cases and the number of patients with multiple-drug–resistant tuberculosis is related at least in part to pitfalls in the primary care of patients. In a study of 35 patients, Mahmoudi and Iseman (1993) detected errors in management in 28. These errors led to prolonged hospital stays, to the development of sclerotic pulmonary lesions, and to increased costs. When patients fail medical therapy or are at high risk to do so, surgery remains an efficacious tool in the management of this difficult problem.

Acknowledgement

The authors thank Dr. André Crépeau, senior thoracic surgeon, for his bibliography and Dr. Ian Hammond, chief of radiology at Ottawa General Hospital, for some of the radiographs used to illustrate this chapter.

COMMENTS AND CONTROVERSIES

With the advent of effective chemotherapy and early diagnosis, the role of surgery in tuberculosis has decreased. However, because of the high incidence of the disease in developing countries like India, a significant number of our patients do require surgical intervention. One of the main indications in our clinic for surgery is massive hemoptysis. This can occur at any stage of the disease. It may be the first symptom to occur during the treatment of the active phase of disease or it may occur as a result of healed scars. We still perform staged thoracoplasties for patients unsuitable for resection because of extensive endobronchial diseases for MDRTB and for tubercular empyema with bronchopleural fistula.

R. S.

The role of the thoracic surgeon in managing pulmonary tuberculosis has decreased remarkably since the advent of effective antimicrobial agents. Table 23–7 describes the evolution of thoracic surgical treatments over the past 150 years. Indeed, the foundations and development of thoracic surgery lie in the management of infectious diseases such as tuberculosis and empyema. The recent resurgence of resistant forms of tuberculosis, especially in the immunocompromised host, makes this infection a common presentation to thoracic surgeons for diagnosis and for management of its complications. This is especially true in third-world countries. I've asked Dr. Rajan Santosham to comment on the practice in India, where tuberculosis is prevalent. He mentions the common necessity of surgery for the treatment of hemoptysis. This is discussed in Chapter 27 in relation to tuberculosis. The reader is also referred to further discussions of tuberculosis in the immunocompromised host and in the AIDS patient (Chapter 23).

R. J. G.

KEY REFERENCES

Rizzi A, Rocco G, Robustellini M et al: Results of surgical management of tuberculosis: Experience in 206 patients undergoing operation. Ann Thorac Surg 59:896, 1995.

This article shows that aggressive surgical treatment of MDRTB is warranted to achieve eradication of the disease.

Pomerantz M: Surgery for tuberculosis. Chest Surg Clin North Am 3:723, 1993.

This is an excellent review of current indications for surgery of tuberculosis.

Mouroux J, Maalouf J, Padovani B et al: Surgical management of pleuropulmonary tuberculosis. J Thorac Cardiovasc Surg 111:662, 1996.

This article evaluates the role of surgery for diagnostic and therapeutic purposes in the management of pleuropulmonary tuberculosis.

Iseman MD, Madsen L, Gable M, Pomerantz M: Surgical intervention in the treatment of pulmonary disease caused by drug-resistant mycobacterium tuberculosis. Am Rev Respir Dis 141:623, 1990.

This review shows that resectional surgery benefits selected patients with MDRTB.

Perelman MI, Strelzov VP: Surgery for pulmonary tuberculosis. World J Surg 21:457, 1997.

The authors report one of the largest recent experiences with surgery for tuberculosis.

REFERENCES

Adeyemo AO, Odelowo EO, Makanjuola DI: Management of pulmonary aspergilloma in the presence of active tuberculosis. Thorax 39:862, 1984.

Adler BD, Padley SP, Muller NL: Tuberculosis of the chest wall: CT findings. J Comput Assist Tomogr 17:27, 1993.
Alexander J: The Collapse Therapy of Pulmonary Tuberculosis. Springfield, IL, Charles C Thomas, 1937.
Alling DW, Bosworth EB: The after-history of pulmonary tuberculosis. VI. The first fifteen years following diagnosis. Am Rev Respir Dis 81:839, 1960.
Al-Majed SA, Ashour M, el-Kassimi FA et al: Management of post-tuberculous complex aspergilloma of the lung: Pole of surgical resection. Thorax 45:846, 1990.
Almeyda J, Tolley NS, Ghufoor K, Mochoulis G: Subglottic stenosis secondary to tuberculosis. Int J Clin Pract 51:402, 1997.
Ando M, Onizuka O, Kawano M et al: Pulmonary and endobronchial tuberculosis with subclavian artery-pulmonary shunts. Nippon Kyobu Shikkan Gakkai Zasshi 34:374, 1996.
Antony VB: Pleural tuberculosis. Sem Respir Med 9:54, 1987.
Arsan S, Mercan S, Sarigul A et al: Long-term experience with pericardiectomy: Analysis of 105 consecutive patients. Thorac Cardiovasc Surg 42:340, 1994.
Ashour M, Pandya L, Mezraqui A et al: Unilateral post-tuberculous lung destruction: The left bronchus syndrome. Thorax 45:210, 1990.
Auerbach O: Pathology and pathogenesis of pulmonary arterial aneurysm in tuberculous cavities. Am Rev Tuber 39:99, 1939.
Bailey WC: Treatment of atypical mycobacterial disease. Chest 84:625, 1983.
Barbas CS, Cukier A, de Varvalho CR et al: The relationship between pleural fluid findings and the development of pleural thickening in patients with pleural tuberculosis. Chest 100:1264, 1991.
Barksdale L, Kim KS: Mycobacterium. Bacteriol Rev 41:217, 1977.
Blackwood JM, Andrews NC: Analysis of recurrent tuberculosis after resection. Dis Chest 52:768, 1967.
Bobrowitz ID, Rodescu D, Marcus H, Abeles H: The destroyed tuberculous lung. Scand J Resp Dis 55:82, 1974.
Borrelly J, Sebbag H, Vignaud JM: False empyema after artificial pneumothorax. An original entity: type B non-Hodgkin malignant lymphoma Ann Chir 50:405, 1996.
Brown TS: Tuberculosis of the ribs. Clin Radiol 31:681, 1980.
Busillo CP, Lessnau KD, Sanjana V et al: Multidrug-resistant mycobacterium tuberculosis in patients with human immunodeficiency virus infection. Chest 102:797, 1992.
Butz RO, Zvetina JR, Leininger BJ: Ten-year experience with mycetomas in patients with pulmonary tuberculosis. Chest 87:356, 1985.
Cacoub P, Wechsler B, Chapelon C et al: Chronic constrictive pericarditis: 27 cases. Presse Med 20:2185, 1991.
Campos-Rodriguez F, Alfageme-Michavila I, Hernandez-Borge J et al: Pseudochylothorax: Review of 5 cases. Arch Bronconeumol 33:422, 1997.
Centers for Disease Control: Core Curriculum on Tuberculosis. Atlanta, GA, Centers for Disease Control, 1991.
Chang BC, Ha JW, Kin JT et al: Intracardiac tuberculoma. Ann Thorac Surg 67:226, 1999.
Chauduri MR: Primary pulmonary scar carcinoma. Indian J Med Res 61:858, 1973.
Chen JC, Chang YL, Luh SP et al: Surgical treatment for pulmonary aspergilloma: A 28-year experience. Thorax 52:810, 1997.
Cohen AS, Beaconsfield T, Al-Kutoubi A et al: Pulmonary artery reconstruction for tuberculosis. Ann Thorac Surg 61:1257, 1996.
Cohen EM, Loew DE, Messer JV: Internal mammary arteriovenous malformation with communication to the pulmonary vessels. Am J Cardiol 35:103, 1975.
Cole FH, Alley FH: An analysis of pulmonary resection in 513 cases of tuberculosis. Surg Gynecol Obstet: 413, 1955.
Comroe JH Jr: T.B. or not T.B. 1. The cause of tuberculosis. Am Rev Respir Dis 117:137, 1978.
Conjalka MS, Usselman J, Hassidim K, Freedman S: Successful medical treatment of a tuberculosis B-E fistula. Mt Sinai J Med 47:283, 1980.
Curtis JK: The significance of bronchiectasis associated with pulmonary tuberculosis. Am J Med 22:894, 1957.
Dacosta NA, Kinare SG: Association of lung carcinoma and tuberculosis. J Postgrad Med 37:185, 1991.
Dagher IK, Simeone FA, Neville WE et al: A review of the complications of resection in the treatment of pulmonary tuberculosis. Surg Gynecol Obstet :61, 1959.
Dannenberg AM Jr: Immune mechanisms in the pathogenesis of pulmonary tuberculosis. Rev Infect Dis 11:S369, 1989.
Das PB, David JG: Role of surgery in the treatment of pulmonary tuberculosis. Car J Surg 18:512, 1975.
Davidson PT, Horowitz I: Skeletal tuberculosis: A review, with patient presentation and discussion. Am J Med 48:77, 1970.
de Cerenville EB: De l'intervention dans les maladies du poumon [French]. Rev Med Suisse Normande 5:441, 1885.
Delarue N, Pearson FG, Henderson RD et al: Experience with surgical salvage in pulmonary tuberculosis: Application to general thoracic surgery. Can J Surg 18:519, 1975.
Diamond JM: The arrow of disease. Discover 13:64, 1992.
Donath J, Khan FA: Tuberculous and post-tuberculous bronchopleural fistula: Ten-year clinical experience. Chest 86:697, 1984.
Duarte IG, Chang HJ, Kennedy JC, Miller JI Jr: Papillary endothelial hyperplasia presenting as a chest wall neoplasm. Ann Thorac Surg 67:238, 1999.
Dubos R, Dubos J: The White Plague, Boston, Little Brown, 1952.
Dutt AK, Moers D, Stead WW: Tuberculous pleural effusion: 6-month therapy with isoniazid and rifampin. Am Rev Respir Dis 145:1429, 1992.
Efremidis SC, Lakshamanan S, Hsu JT: Tuberculous aortitis: A rare cause of mycotic aneurysm of the aorta. Am J Roentgenol 127:859, 1976.
Ellner JJ, Barnes PF, Wailis RS et al: The immunology of tuberculous pleurisy. Semin Resp Infect 3:335, 1988.
Fauquert P, Saraux A, Guillermit MN et al: Histiocytome fibreux malin thoracique: A propos d'un cas survenant après pneumothorax thérapeutique avec plombage par billes [French]. Semin Hop Paris 65:2181, 1989.
Faure E, Souilamas R, Riquet M et al: Cold abscess of the chest wall: A surgical entity? Ann Thorac Surg 66:1174, 1998.
Fey B, Morocquot P, Oberlin S et al: Traité de Technique Chirurgicale [French], Vol IV, 2nd ed. Paris, Masson, 1955.
Floyd RD, Hollister WF, Sealy WC: Complications in 430 consecutive pulmonary resections for tuberculosis. Surg Gynecol Obstet Oct: 467, 1959.
Forlanini C: Primi tentativi di pneumothorax artificiale della tisi pulmonare [Italian]. Gaz Med Torino 45:381, 1894.
Fraser RS: Pulmonary aspergillosis: Pathologic and pathogenic features. Pathol Annu 28:231, 1993.
Frieden TR, Sterling T, Pablos-Mendez A et al: The emergence of drug-resistant tuberculosis in New York City. N Engl J Med 328:521, 1993.
Fukai I, Sano M, Niwa H et al: Giant chest wall tumor resulting from tissue reaction to foreign bodies. Ann Thorac Surg 50:754, 1990.
Gaeta M, Volta S, Stroscio S et al: CT "halo sign" in pulmonary tuberculoma. J Comput Assist Tomogr 16:827, 1992.
Galietti F, Giorgis GE, Oliaro A et al: Lung diseases associated with silicosis: Study of 618 cases. Minerva Med 80:987, 1989.
Goble M, Hersburg CR, Waite D et al: Treament of isoniazid- and rifampin-resistant tuberculosis. Am Rev Respir Dis 137:24, 1988.
Goble M, Iseman MD, Madsen LA et al: Treatment of 171 patients with pulmonary tuberculosis resistant to isoniazid and rifampin. N Engl J Med 328:527, 1993.
Goble M: Drug-resistant tuberculosis. Semin Resp Infect 1:220, 1986.
Gregory AK, Connery CP, Anagnostopoulos CE: A late complication of tuberculous pericarditis after partial pericardial resection. Ann Thorac Surg 65:542, 1998.
Grzybowski S, Barnett GD, Styblo K: Contacts of cases of active pulmonary tuberculosis. Bull Int Union Tuberc 50:90, 1975.
Halezeroglu S, Keles M, Uysal A et al: Factors affecting postoperative morbidity and mortality in destroyed lung. Ann Thorac Surg 64:1635, 1997.
Hanagiri T, Muranaka H, Hashimoto M et al: Chronic expanding hematoma in the chest. Ann Thorac Surg 64:559, 1997.
Harris A, Burge S, Williams S, Desai S: Cutaneous tuberculous abscess: A management problem. Br J Dermatol 135:457, 1996.
Heurich AE, Quale JM, Burack JH: Pericardial tuberculosis. In Rom WN, Garay S (eds): Tuberculosis. Boston, Little Brown, 1995, p 531.
Hoheisel G, Chan BK, Chan CH et al: Endobronchial tuberculosis: Diagnostic features and therapeutic outcome. Respir Med 88:593, 1994.
Horn H, Saphir O: The involvement of the myocardium in tuberculosis: A review of the literature and report of 3 cases. Am Rev Tuberc 32:492, 1935.
Horowitz MD, Otero M, Thurer RJ, Bolooki H: Late complications of plombage. Ann Thorac Surg 53:803, 1992.

Hsu HS, Hsu WH, Huang BS, Huang MH: Surgical treatment of endobronchial tuberculosis. Scand Cardiovasc J 31:79, 1997.

Hsu HS, Wang LS, Wu YC et al: Management of primary chest wall tuberculosis. Scand J Thorac Cardiovasc Surg 29:119, 1995.

Ip MS, So SY, Lam WK, Mok CK: Endobronchial tuberculosis revisited. Chest 89:727, 1986.

Iseman MD, Goble M: Treatment of tuberculosis. Adv Intern Med 33:253, 1988.

Iseman MD, Madsen L, Goble M, Pomerantz M: Surgical Intervention in the treatment of pulmonary disease caused by drug-resistant *Mycobacterium tuberculosis*. Am Rev Respir Dis 141:623, 1990.

Iuchi K, Ri T, Nakamura K et al: A case of bronchopleural fistula with expectoration of wax after extraperiosteal paraffin plombage 11 years earlier [Japanese]. Rinsho Kyobu Geka 4:745, 1984.

Jacobeus HC: Die thorakoscopic und ihre praktische bedentung [German]. Ergebges Med (Berlin) 7:112, 1925.

Karas A, Hankins JR, Attar S et al: Pulmonary aspergillosis: An analysis of 41 patients. Ann Thorac Surg 22:1, 1976.

Kato R, Kakizaki T, Hangai N et al: Bronchoplastic procedures for tuberculous bronchial stenosis. J Thorac Cardiovasc Surg 106:1118, 1993.

Kelley MA, Micozzi MS: Rib lesions in chronic pulmonary tuberculosis. Am J Phys Anthropol 65:381, 1984.

Khan FA, Rehman M, Marcus P, Azueta V: Pulmonary gangrene occurring as a complication of pulmonary tuberculosis. Chest 77:76, 1980.

Kim YH, Kim HT, Lee KS et al: Serial fiberoptic bronchoscopic observations of endobronchial tuberculosis before and early after antituberculous chemotherapy. Chest 103:673, 1993.

Kir A, Tahaoglu K, Okur E, Hatipoglu T: Role of surgery in multi-drug-resistant tuberculosis: Results of 27 cases. Eur J Cardiothorac Surg 12:531, 1997.

Kirshenbaum KJ, Burke RC, Kirshenbaum MD, Cavallino RP: Pleurocutaneous fistula as a complication of oleothorax: CT findings in three patients. Clin Imaging 19:125, 1995.

Klingensmith WE, Beckley W: Resectional surgery in pulmonary tuberculosis: Its bacteriologic basis. J Thorac Cardiovasc Surg 45:146, 1963.

Koch R. Die aetiologie der tuberculosis [German]. Berlin Klin Wochenschr 19:221, 1882.

Kochi A: The global tuberculosis situation and the new control strategy of the World Health Organization. Tubercle 72:1, 1991.

Koh KK, In HH, Lee KH et al: New scoring system using tumor markers in diagnosing patients with moderate pericardial effusions. Int J Cardiol 61:5, 1997.

Laënnec RTH: De l'auscultation médiate ou traité du diagnostic des maladies des poumons et du cœur [French]. Paris, Brosson et Chaudé, 1819. Forbes J: A treatise on the diseases of the chest [trans.]. London, T and C Underwood, 1821.

Lai RS, Lee SS, Ting YM et al: Diagnostic value of transbronchial lung biopsy under fluoroscopic guidance in solitary pulmonary nodule in an endemic area of tuberculosis. Respir Med 90:139, 1996.

Lardinois D, Furrer M, Mouton W et al: Surgical aspects of mycobacterioses: Evolution during the last 20 Years. Schweiz Med Wochenschr 127: 1961, 1997.

Lindskog GE, Spear HC: Middle-lobe syndrome. N Engl J Med 253:489, 1955.

Macchiarini P, Delamare N, Beuzeboc P et al: Tracheoesophagel fistula caused by mycobacterial tuberculosis adenopathy. Ann Thorac Surg 55:1561, 1993.

Madsen LA, Iseman MD: Management of drug-resistant tuberculosis. Chest Surg Clin North Am 3:715, 1994.

Mahmoudi A, Iseman MD: Pitfalls in the care of patients with tuberculosis: Common errors and their association with the acquisition of drug resistance. JAMA 270:65, 1993.

Manchester K: Tuberculosis and leprosy in antiquity: An interpretation. Med Hist 28:162, 1984.

Masjedi MR, Davoodian P, Forouzesh M, Abttahi SJ: Broncho-aortic fistula secondary to pulmonary tuberculosis. Chest 94:199, 1988.

Massard G, Rouge C, Wihlm JM et al: Decortication is a valuable option for late empyema after collapse therapy. Ann Thorac Surg 60:888, 1995.

Massard G, Thomas P, Barsotti P et al: Long-term complications of extraperiosteal plombage. Ann Thorac Surg 64:220, 1997.

Mathisen DJ, Grillo HC, Wain JC, Hilgenberg AD: Management of acquired nonmalignant tracheoesophageal fistula. Ann Thorac Surg 52:759, 1991.

McCarthy OR, Rudd RM: Six months' chemotherapy for lymph node tuberculosis. Respir Med 83:425, 1989.

Meyer EC, Liebow AA: Relationship of interstitial pneumonia, honeycombing and atypical epithelial proliferation to cancer of the lung. Cancer 18:322, 1965.

Meyer JA: Tuberculosis, the Adirondacks, and coming of age for thoracic surgery. Ann Thorac Surg 52:881, 1991.

Miller JI, Flemming WH, Hatcher CR Jr: Balanced drainage of the contaminated postpneumonectomy space. Ann Thorac Surg 19:585, 1975.

Miyoshi K, Matsui J, Gangi J, Shinoura S: A case of endobronchial tuberculosis with peripheral mucoid impaction showing a solitary pulmonary nodular shadow. Kyobu Geka 49:1119, 1996.

Molinie V, Pouchot J, Navratil E et al: Primary Epstein-Barr virus-related non-Hodgkin's lymphoma of the pleural cavity following long-standing tuberculous empyema. Arch Pathol Lab Med 120:288, 1996.

Moran JF, Alexander LG, Staub EW et al: Long-term results of pulmonary resection for atypical mycobacterial disease. Ann Thorac Surg 35:597, 1983.

Mouroux J, Maalouf J, Padovani B et al: Surgical management of pleuropulmonary tuberculosis. J Thorac Cardiovasc Surg 111:662, 1996.

Murayama S, Murakami J, Hashimoto S et al: Noncalcified pulmonary tuberculomas: CT enhancement patterns with histological correlation. J Thorac Imaging 10:91, 1995.

Náef AP: The 1900 tuberculosis epidemic—starting point of modern thoracic surgery. Ann Thorac Surg 55:1375, 1993.

Nataf P, Cacoub P, Dorent R et al: Results of subtotal pericardiectomy for constrictive pericarditis. Eur J Cardiothorac Surg 7:252, 1993.

Neff TA, Buchanan BD: Tension pleural effusion: A delayed complication of pneumothorax therapy in tuberculosis. Am Rev Respir Dis 111:543, 1975.

Nelson KG, Griffith DE, Brown BA, Wallace RJ Jr: Results of operation in the mycobacterium avium-intracellulare lung disease. Ann Thorac Surg 66:325, 1998.

Neptune WB, Kim S, Bookwalter J: Current surgical management of pulmonary tuberculosis. J Thorac Cardiovasc Surg 60:384, 1970.

Ober WB: Ghon but not forgotten: Anton Ghon and his complex. Pathol Annu 18:79, 1983.

Ojika T, Mukohyama N, Tsuzuki T, Kohketsu H: A case of liposarcoma associated with chronic tuberculous empyema. Kyobu Geka 50:345, 1997.

Omari B, Robertson JM, Nelson RJ, Chiu LC: Pott's disease: A resurgent challenge to the thoracic surgeon. Chest 95:145, 1989.

Pennington JE: Aspergillus lung disease. Med Clin North Am 64:475, 1980.

Pepper W: A system of practical medicine by American authors, Vol 3. Philadelphia, Lea Brothers, 1885.

Perelman MI, Strelzov VP: Surgery for pulmonary tuberculosis. World J Surg 21:457, 1997.

Pomerantz M, Brown JM: Surgery in the treatment of multidrug-resistant tuberculosis. Clin Chest Med 18:123, 1997.

Pomerantz M, Denton JR, Huitt GA et al: Resection of the right middle lobe and lingula for mycobacterial infection. Ann Thorac Surg 62:990, 1996.

Pomerantz M, Madsen L, Goble M, Iseman M: Surgical management of resistant mycobacterial tuberculosis and other mycobacterial pulmonary infections. Ann Thorac Surg 52:1108, 1991.

Pomerantz M: Surgery for tuberculosis. Chest Surg Clin North Am 4:723, 1993.

Potente G, Iacari V, Caimi M: The challenge of solitary pulmonary nodules: HRCT evaluation. Comput Med Imaging Graph 21:39, 1997.

Quale JM, Lipschik GY, Heurich AE: Management of tuberculous pericarditis. Ann Thorac Surg 43:653, 1987.

Ramos-Martinez A, Martin-Jimenez T, Portero Navio JL et al: Solitary pulmonary nodule: Application of Bayes theorem in prediction of malignancy [Spanish]. Arch Bronconeumol 34:4, 1998.

Rasmussen V, Moore WD: Hemoptysis, especially when fatal, in its anatomical and clinical aspects (trans). Edin Med J 14:385, 1968.

Rawls WJ, Shuford WH, Logan WD et al: Right ventricular outflow tract obstruction produced by a myocardial abscess in a patient with tuberculosis. Am J Cardiol 21:738, 1968.

Reed CE, Parker EF, Crawford FA Jr: Surgical resection for complications of pulmonary tuberculosis. Ann Thorac Surg 48:165, 1989.

Reich JM, Johnson RE: *Mycobacterium avium* complex pulmonary disease presenting an isolated lingular or middle lobe pattern. Chest 101:1605, 1992.

Remy J, Arnaud A, Fardou H et al: Treatment of hemoptysis by embolization of bronchial arteries. Radiology 122:33, 1977.

Rezai AR, Lee M, Cooper PR et al: Modern management of spinal tuberculosis. Neurosurgery 36:87, 1995.

Rizzi A, Rocco G, Robustellini M et al: Results of surgical management of tuberculosis: Experience in 206 patients undergoing operation. Ann Thorac Surg 59:896, 1995.

Rizzi A, Rocco G, Robustellini M et al: Modern morbidity following pulmonary resection for postprimary tuberculosis. World J Surg 21:488, 1997.

Robicsek F, Daugherty KH, Cook JW et al: *Mycobacterium fortuitum* epidemics after open-heart surgery. J Thorac Cardiovasc Surg 75:91, 1978.

Robitzek EH, Selikoff IJ: Hydrazine derivatives of isonicotinic acid (Rimifon, Marsilid) in the treatment of active progressive caseous-pneumonic tuberculosis: A preliminary report. Am Rev Tuberc 65:402, 1952.

Rocco G, Rizzi A, Robustellini M et al: About the surgical treatment of pulmonary mycetoma. Ann Thorac Surg 57:260, 1994.

Rosenzweig DY, Stead WW: The role of tuberculosis and other forms of bronchopulmonary necrosis in the pathogenesis of bronchiectasis. Am Rev Resp Dis 93:769, 1966.

Russi EG, Gaeta M, Pergolizzi S et al: Contribution of computerized tomography to the diagnosis of patients with non-calcified solitary pulmonary nodule, without known neoplasm [Italian]. Radiol Med (Torino) 83:243, 1992.

Sahn SA: State of the art: The pleura. Am Rev Respir Dis 138:184, 1988.

Sawada S, Fujiwara Y, Furui S et al: Treatment of tuberculous bronchial stenosis with expandable metallic stents. Acta Radiol 34:263, 1993.

Schede M: Die behandlung der enpyema [German]. Verh Long Innere Med Wiesbaden 9:41, 1890.

Schwartz MS, Kahlstrom EJ, Hawkins DB: Airway obstruction secondary to tuberculosis lymph node erosion into the trachea: Drainage via bronchoscopy. Otolaryngol Head Neck Surg 99:604, 1988.

Shafer RW, Kim DS, Weiss JP et al: Extrapulmonary tuberculosis in patients with human immunodeficiency virus infection. Medicine 70:384, 1991.

Shiraishi Y, Fukushima K, Komatsu H, Kurashima A: Early pulmonary resection for localized *Mycobacterium avium* complex disease. Ann Thorac Surg 66:183, 1998.

Skinner JS, Sinclair DJ: Fatal mediastinal compression as a late complication of surgical plombage. Thorax 47:321, 1992.

Sloane MF: Mycobacterial lymphadenitis. In Rom WN, Garay S (eds): Tuberculosis. Boston, Little Brown, 1995, p 580.

Snider GL, Placik B: The relationship between pulmonary tuberculosis and bronchogenic carcinoma: A topographic study. Am Rev Resp Dis 99:229, 1969.

Solit RW, McKeown JJ Jr, Smullens S, Fraimow W: The surgical implications of intracavitary mycetomas (fungus ball). J Thorac Cardiovasc Surg 62:411, 1971.

Spalding AR, Burney DP, Richie RE: Acquired benign bronchoesophageal fistulas in the adult. Ann Thorac Surg 28:378, 1978.

Stead WW: Pathogenesis of a first episode of chronic pulmonary tuberculosis in man: Recrudescence of residuals of the primary infection or exogenous reinfection? Am Rev Respir Dis 95:729, 1967.

Steele JD: The Solitary Pulmonary Nodule. Springfield, IL, Charles C Thomas, 1964.

Steen-Hansen E, Thommesen P: Clinical management of the benign cytological report in patients with solitary pulmonary nodules. Rontgenblatter 41:458, 1988.

Stobernack A, Achatzy R, Engelmann C: Spätkomplikationen nach extrapleuraler pneumolyse wegan lungentuberkulose [German]. Chirurg 68:921, 1997.

Strang JI: Tuberculous pericarditis in Transkei. Clin Cardiol 7:667, 1984.

Stuertz A: Experimenteller Beitrag Zur "Zserchfellbewegung nach einselitiger Phrecus durchtrennung" [German]. Dtsch Med Wochensdr 38:897, 1912.

Subba Rao RS, Curzon PG, Muers MF, Watson DA: Cavernoscopic evacuation of aspergilloma: A alternative method of palliation for hemoptysis in high-risk patients. Thorax 39:394, 1984.

Suchet IB, Horwitz TA: CT in tuberculous constrictive pericarditis. J Comput Assist Tomogr 16:391, 1992.

Suzuki H, Tanaka K, Tonozuka H et al: Clinical study of tuberculous pleuritis, diagnosed by thoracoscopy using flexible fiberoptic bronchoscope. Nippon Kyobu Shikkan Gakkai Zasshi 31:139, 1993.

Takanami I, Imamura T, Morota N, Kodaira S: Malignant fibrous histiocytoma of the chest wall developing after pleuropneumonectomy performed for tuberculous pyothorax: Report of an unusual case. J Thorac Cardiovasc Surg 108:395, 1994.

Tate CF 3rd: Intestinal obstruction in a 55-year-old man with previous thoracic surgery (extrapleural plombage). JAMA 243:1077, 1980.

Thomas GE, Chandrasekhar B, Grannis FW Jr: Surgical treatment of complications 45 years after extraperiosteal pneumonolysis and plombage using acrylic resin balls for cavitary pulmonary tuberculosis. Chest 108:1163, 1995.

Thompson JR, Entin SD: Primary extraskeletal chondrosarcoma: Report of a case arising in conjunction with extrapleural lucite ball plombage. Cancer 23:936, 1969.

Tokuda H, Aoki M, Isoe K et al: The efficacy of x-ray signs for differential diagnosis of small lung cancer and tuberculoma. Committee for Lung Cancer Mass Screening, JATA. Kekkaku 65:13, 1990.

Tong MC, van Hasselt CA: Tuberculous tracheobronchial strictures: Clinicopathological features and management with the bronchoscopic carbon dioxide laser. Eur Arch Otorhinolaryngol 250:110, 1993.

Treasure RL, Seaworth BJ: Current role of surgery in *Mycobacterium tuberculosis*. Ann Thorac Surg 59:1405, 1995.

Trotter MC, Chung KC, Ochsner JL, McFadden PM: Pericardiectomy for pericardial constriction. Am Surg 62:304, 1996.

Tsou E, Yeager H Jr, Katz S: Late bronchopleural fistula and *Hemophilus influenzae* empyema complicating longstanding oleothorax: Report of two cases. Chest 74:5, 1978.

Tuffier T: Du décollement pariétal en chirurgie pulmonaire [French]. Arch Med Chir App Respir 1:32, 1926.

Twersky J, Twersky N, Lehr C: Scleroderma and carcinoma of the lung. Clin Radiol 27:203, 1976.

Vajda L: Ob das Pneumoperitoneum in der Kollapsetherapic der beiderseitigen Lungentuberkulose Angewandt Werden Kenn [German]? Ztschr Tuberk 67:371, 1933.

Valdes L, San Jose E, Alvares D et al: Diagnosis of tuberculous pleurisy using the biologic parameters adenosine deaminase, lysozyme and interferon gamma. Chest 103:458, 1993.

van Leuven M, De Groot M, Shean KP et al: Pulmonary resection as an adjunct in the treatment of multiple drug-resistant tuberculosis. Ann Thorac Surg 63:1368, 1997.

Vigneswaran WT, Ramasastry SS: Paraffin plombage of the chest revisited. Ann Thorac Surg 62:1837, 1996.

Villegas AH, Naveiro JJ, Tedin DV, Cueto DG: The diagnostic value of internal mammary lymph node biopsy in nonpurulent pleural effusion: Experience in 60 cases. Chest 58:345, 1970.

Watanabe Y, Murakami S, Oda M et al: Treatment of bronchial stricture due to endobronchial tuberculosis. World J Surg 21:480, 1997.

Whyte RI, Deegan SP, Kaplan DK et al: Recent surgical experience for pulmonary tuberculosis. Resp Med 83:357, 1989.

Winn RE, Prechter GC: Pulmonary tuberculosis. In Hoeprich PD, Jordan MC, Ronald AR (eds): Infectious Diseases. Philadelphia, JB Lippincott, 1994, p 447.

Wolinsky E: Nontuberculous mycobacteria and associated diseases. Am Rev Resp Dis 119:107, 1979.

Worthington MG, Brink JG, Odell JA et al: Surgical relief of acute airway obstruction due to primary tuberculosis. Ann Thorac Surg 56:1054, 1993.

Wu MH, Lin MY, Tseng YL, Lai WW: Results of surgical treatment of 107 patients with complications of pulmonary tuberculosis. Respirology 1:283, 1996.

Yamashita K, Matsunobe S, Tsuda T et al: Solitary pulmonary nodule: Preliminary study of evaluation with incremental dynamic CT. Radiology 194:399, 1995.

MYCOTIC INFECTIONS OF THE LUNG

Young T. Kim
Victor F. Trastek

Fungal infection of the lung results from inhalation of an infectious agent. In cases of systemic fungal infection remote from the lung, the portal of entry with rare exceptions is the airway. In all probability, asymptomatic or mild pulmonary infection occurs and clears spontaneously in such patients.

In earlier years these infections were most commonly due to primary pathogens, such as *Histoplasma capsulatum, Coccidioides immitis, Blastomyces dermatitidis, Sporothrix schenckii*, and *Paracoccidioides brasiliensis*. These were thought to arise de novo, and it was only after the development of more sophisticated knowledge of the immune system that it was recognized that some of these earlier cases presented in immunocompromised individuals. In recent years a large number of cases have been caused by secondary or opportunistic pathogens, such as *Cryptococcus neoformans, Torulopsis glabrata*, and species of *Candida, Mucor*, and *Aspergillus* (Medoff and Kobayashi, 1980).

The major fungi that produce pulmonary manifestations were first described nearly a century ago. Better understanding of these conditions began to accumulate with the development of satisfactory antituberculous drugs and the emergence of resectional surgery for the therapy of tuberculosis in the early 1950s. As resectional therapy came into common use, it became apparent that some of the patients whose conditions were diagnosed as tuberculosis on the basis of chest radiographic findings were indeed suffering from deep-seated fungal infections, particularly chronic cavitary histoplasmosis (Furcolow and Brasher, 1956).

Major impetus to rational therapy for pulmonary fungal infections came with the isolation of amphotericin B from a soil actinomycete, which provided for the first time an effective antifungal agent to be used in primary therapy of most of the major fungal diseases or as adjunctive support to surgical therapy in the management of fungal infection (Gold et al, 1955–1956).

Clear understanding of the nature of fungal infections in humans included the knowledge that during primary fungal infections millions of people have sustained subclinical infections with modification of skin test or serologic findings but with little evidence that clinical infection ever existed or will ever develop. Many more patients show slight evidence of clinical disease, which clears rapidly and has no long-lasting effects. Serious fungal infection thus represents the small tip of a large iceberg. In addition, it is now recognized that some of the most difficult and rapidly advancing fungal infections are those caused by secondary or opportunistic pathogens in immunocompromised patients; this is found in an increasingly lethal pattern. The enlarging pool of these patients has been defined through the widespread use of corticosteroids to treat many conditions, of immunosuppressive agents after organ transplantation, of the use of chemotherapy to treat neoplasms, and of the discovery and description in the 1980s of AIDS. The old concept of pathogenic and nonpathogenic fungi is no longer clear (Van Trigt, 1990).

HISTORICAL NOTE

In this time of increasing knowledge and awareness of pulmonary fungal infection, it is interesting to trace the early discovery and understanding that progressed at a snail's pace in most instances. Histoplasmosis serves as an example. The first two cases were discovered in two young adult laborers from Martinique who died within 6 months of their arrival to work on the Panama Canal (Darling, 1906). Eight months later Darling found a third case in a 55-year-old Chinese worker who had lived in Panama for 15 years but had lived and worked in the Canal Zone for only 6 months. Although Darling remained in Panama until 1915, he attributed the fact that he could not find another case to the sanitation efforts of Colonel William E. Gorgas. Not until 15,000 autopsies had been performed (autopsy rate, 80%) and 45 years had passed was another case found in Panama (Draheim et al, 1951), although a later article (Zimmerman, 1954) reported another Panamanian case that occurred in 1931 and was found in the autopsy files in 1954. The first clinical case recognized in the United States was reported from Minnesota (Riley and Watson, 1926).

Darling had incorrectly identified the offending organism as a protozoan. The first accurate determination that it was indeed a fungus came from cultures of a clinical case (DeMonbreum, 1934).

In a 1951 survey, 138 cases of histoplasmosis were found in the literature, 65 of them pulmonary. Two additional cases of pulmonary parenchymal involvement confined to a lobe were treated by lobectomy, apparently the earliest example of pulmonary resection for this condition (Hodgson et al, 1951).

At about this time improved antituberculous drugs were developed, and resectional surgery for tuberculosis was extended. A number of solitary nodules from lung that had been designated as tuberculomas on the basis of their granulomatous appearance on microscopic examination were restudied with the then-new periodic acid–Schiff stain (Klingman and Mescon, 1950) and were confirmed to be due to *H. capsulatum*. The organism was also identified in hilar nodes (Puckett, 1953).

Surgical resection of chronic cavitary progressive disease developed after the observation that this condition was a problem in tuberculosis sanatoriums, either because it had been misdiagnosed and treated as tuberculosis or because it was coexisting as acid-fast infection (Furculow and Brasher, 1956).

Other manifestations of infection by *H. capsulatum* soon came to light, and surgical therapy was proposed for the diagnosis or therapy of the complications of this disease such as superior vena caval obstruction and for prophylactic resection of mediastinal granuloma, in the hope of averting caval obstruction, mediastinal fibrosis, bronchial obstruction, or esophageal involvement.

With the development of immunosuppression resulting from modern therapeutic methods and the description of AIDS by Gottlieb and colleagues (1981), a number of fungal infections, including histoplasmosis, have played a prominent role as determinants of survival in this group of seriously ill patients, and the role of the surgeon in obtaining tissue for prompt diagnosis and therapy has been accentuated in those cases that defy less invasive diagnostic procedures (Trachiotis et al, 1992).

Although histoplasmosis was described in 1906, only sporadic cases were documented during the next 30 years, and the impression was that it was a uniformly fatal disease. The true picture of a disease that affected large numbers of people, most of them in a benign manner, emerged as skin and serologic testing became available. A rather effective albeit toxic antifungal agent (amphotericin B) was discovered by Gold and colleagues (1955–1956). A number of series assessed surgical therapy of chronic progressive (cavitary) histoplasmosis. With refinement of the antifungal agent and careful studies, the role of surgery in this condition has diminished, but there remain surgical roles in the diagnosis and therapy of certain complications of histoplasmosis.

The evaluation of these changes spans nearly a century and closely parallels discoveries in the other major fungal infections. Blastomycosis in the cutaneous form was described as a protozoan infection at the turn of the past century (Gilchrist, 1894). The systemic form was reported a few years later based on a fatal case (Walker and Montgomery, 1902). Coccidioidomycosis was first described in Buenos Aires (Wernicke, 1892). This author also incorrectly identified the organism found in the tumors as a protozoan. *Sporotrichum schenckii* was named for its discoverer (Schenck, 1898) and later redesignated *Sporothrix schenckii*. Stoddard and Cutter (1916) described the pathologic and clinical features of cryptococcosis in humans. It was called torulosis. Sluyter was the first to describe aspergillosis (Sluyter, 1847). French pigeon handlers and hair manipulators were observed to suffer from this infection toward the end of the 19th century (Takaro, 1969). Sporadic cases of pulmonary mucormycosis were reported from Germany after the initial report by Furbringer (1876). Central nervous system and orbital cases were reported in the United States in 1943, but the first case of pulmonary mucormycosis in this country occurred in San Antonio in 1947 (Baker and Severance, 1948). Baker (1956) subsequently reported five more pulmonary cases and added three more cases from the literature. In his analysis he grouped the earlier German cases separately because the fungal hyphae were different from those seen in the later U.S. cases and concluded that, although they appeared acceptable as instances of mucormycosis, they were probably due to other forms of Phycomycetes.

Factors that certainly contributed to improved knowledge of pulmonary fungal infections include greatly improved anatomic knowledge of the lung which facilitated surgical resection; the availability of adjunctive streptomycin, which allowed surgical resection of tuberculosis and thus advanced the knowledge and practice of pulmonary surgery; and improved staining and culture methods that defined the cause of pathologic pulmonary conditions more accurately. All these developments occurred between 1940 and 1950.

■ *HISTORICAL READINGS*

Gold W, Stout HA, Pagano JF, Donovich R: Amphotericins A & B, antifungal antibiotics produced by a streptomycete. I. In vitro studies. Antibiot Annu 3:579, 1955–1956.

Hodgson CH, Weed LA, Clagett OT: Pulmonary histoplasmosis. JAMA 145:807, 1951.

Klingman AM, Mescon H: The periodic acid–Schiff stain for the demonstration of fungi in animal tissues. J Bacteriol 60:415, 1950.

Melick DW: Excisional surgery in pulmonary coccidioidomycosis. J Thorac Cardiovasc Surg 20:66, 1950.

Takaro T: Mycotic infections of interest to thoracic surgeons. Ann Thorac Surg 3:72, 1967.

DIAGNOSIS

Patients who have mycotic lung infections present with a wide spectrum of clinical manifestations, from the asymptomatic patient to the immunosuppressed patient with an opportunistic, life-threatening fungal infection.

In the present era, taking a careful history is important in regard to the possibility of fungal infection. Malnourished, debilitated, or diabetic patients; those who are receiving intensive antibiotic therapy; those with blood dyscrasias; and those with Hodgkin's disease have shown increased incidence of fungal infections. Although pulmonary or meningeal cryptococcosis has been most commonly associated with AIDS, all of the major fungal infections are now found to infect patients who have this syndrome (Ampel et al, 1989; Chechani et al, 1989; Chuck and Sande, 1989; Clark et al, 1990; McKinsey et al, 1989). In addition, it has long been recognized that patients with the pulmonary manifestations of tuberculosis, sarcoidosis, and lung cancer have commonly acquired pulmonary fungal infections.

The geographic nature of the three major pulmonary fungal diseases (histoplasmosis, coccidioidomycosis, and blastomycosis) has been well defined (Takaro, 1967). A geographic history may be useful in patients with new symptoms who have recently traveled to an endemic area. Histoplasmosis occurs most commonly in the states that border the Missouri, Ohio, and Mississippi River valleys. Blastomycosis is most common in the southeastern states. Coccidioidomycosis is found in California, Nevada, Arizona, New Mexico, and Texas in the lower Sonoran life zone.

When the patient presents with upper or lower respiratory symptoms of fever, cough, sputum production, hemoptysis, or pleuritic pain, a chest radiograph is commonly obtained. In most instances it will offer some indication of pulmonary, mediastinal, or pleural involvement.

It is to be emphasized that a firm diagnosis of fungal infection is made only after the demonstration of the presence of the organism in body exudates or tissues. Growth in culture is preferred, but recognition in smear, fresh mounts, or tissue sections sometimes is sufficient (Buechner et al, 1973). Specific immunologic changes in host response may provide a strong indication of the diagnosis and may often lead to therapy before actual isolation of the organism can be achieved (Seabury, et al, 1971).

Once a pulmonary site is identified, specific diagnostic methods can be applied. Sputum retrieval is best accomplished by the induction of sputum production with warm aerosol treatments. Single sputum obtained in this manner should be promptly submitted to the laboratory. Twenty-four-hour sputum collections are of no value because of overgrowth by bacteria and saprophytic yeasts. A minimum of six induced sputum specimens obtained on successive mornings is recommended (Seabury et al, 1971).

Bronchial washings or brushings may be useful, but in most instances sputum specimens are more reliable. Prompt delivery to the laboratory must again be emphasized if growth of fungi is to be successful. Bronchoalveolar lavage (BAL) of a bronchus that serves the involved area of the lung holds promise. Malabonga (1991) notes that lavage plus bronchial washings have a combined sensitivity on the smear equal to that of transbronchial biopsy and superior to that of transbronchial biopsy on the fungal culture in a small series of patients with AIDS and cryptococcal disease. Although open lung biopsy was previously the procedure of choice to identify pulmonary processes with certainty, the improvement of transbronchial techniques for diagnosis and the addition of transthoracic needle biopsy or radiographic insertion of a pigtail catheter into an abscess cavity or effusion in most cases will suffice to make the diagnosis with less risk to the patient.

Bonfils-Roberts and colleagues (1990) outlined the precipitous drop in the use of open lung biopsy in seriously ill patients with AIDS and noted that in only 1 of 66 cases was a successful therapeutic change initiated based on open lung biopsy findings. In this group 22 patients with severe respiratory failure died within 1 month, 3 during operation. Only 3 of the 66 had fungal infections.

Other diagnostic procedures include sampling of lymph nodes by scalene node biopsy or by mediastinoscopy for examination and culture, direct needle biopsy of an involved area of the lung, and the analysis of prostatic secretions. Between 10% and 15% of patients with blastomycosis have involvement of the genitourinary tract, and prostatic secretions contain the organism (Seabury et al, 1971). In patients with AIDS and cryptococcal meningitis who have relapses after apparent successful primary therapy, recurrent infection can most often be diagnosed in urine obtained after prostatic massage (Larsen et al, 1989). Of 12 patients with urine cultures positive for *C. immitis*, fractional urine samples helped identify the prostate as the site of infection in 4 (Peterson et al, 1976). The authors stress the importance of including a rectal examination with the collection of prostatic secretions for culture. The epididymis and the upper urinary tract were also involved. Most patients were immunosuppressed. Spinal fluid analysis has been especially useful in meningitis induced by *Cryptococcus, Coccidioides,* and, more rarely, *Histoplasma* species.

Occasionally blood, bone marrow, joint fluid, skin biopsy specimens that include ulcerative lesions or draining sinus tracts, and biopsy samples of mucous membranes may lead to the diagnosis in extrapulmonary mycotic infections.

Although the search for the causative agent in tissues or secretions continues, serologic or immunologic tests may be an aid to diagnosis, and skin tests may be useful in epidemiologic studies. Skin tests, as a rule, should not be used for diagnosis because (1) their value is limited, (2) cross-reactions occur in histoplasmosis, coccidioidomycosis, and blastomycosis, (3) a positive skin test result indicates that infection has occurred sometime in the past but does not clarify the present clinical situation, (4) the skin test is of no use in early disease because positivity develops only after several weeks, and (5) the skin test elevates the level of serologic titers and interferes with their use in the establishment of a diagnosis or in the interpretation of disease progress by changing serologic titers. This interference may seriously affect the ability of the clinician to assess the progress or lack thereof of the therapy and can produce far more confusion than enlightenment.

Culturing of Clinical Specimens

Once clinical specimens have been obtained and promptly delivered to the laboratory, the growth of the culture is the responsibility of the laboratory, but a basic knowledge of the useful media enhances the possibility that the physician will reach a correct diagnosis. The basic culture media are Sabouraud's dextrose agar, brain-heart infusion agar, and Sabouraud's heart infusion agar. These may be prepared with plain blood or with 5% sheep blood. The sheep blood preparation is useful for tissue, bone marrow, or cerebrospinal fluid culture. All these media can be prepared with inhibitory agents, such as chloramphenicol or cycloheximide, and inhibitory agar is most effective for the culture of any specimen that may be contaminated with bacteria or saprophytic fungi, the rapid overgrowth of which may prevent the growth of the true pathogen. Examples of such specimens are sputum, bronchial washings, nose and nasal sinus, skin, and mucous membranes. Spinal fluid does not require inhibitory media because it is rarely contaminated (Sarosi et al, 1985). Prior to taking the culture, the laboratory will apply techniques such as the selection of purulent parts of a specimen, homogenization, filtration, or centrifugation to concentrate the suspected organism and enhance the likelihood of producing a successful culture. Useful culture methods for specific fungal infections are indicated in the sections on specific diseases. In general, fungi grow slowly in culture, and cultures must be kept for a minimum of 30 days before the results are reported to be negative (Sarosi et al, 1985). Some fungi may require up to 8 weeks for specific isolation and identification (Seabury et al, 1971).

Serologic Diagnosis of Fungal Infections

The two types of serologic tests that are useful in the diagnosis of myocotic disease detect specific antibodies against fungal antigens or specific circulating fungal antigens (Sarosi et al, 1985). Antibody testing is the most common. IgM antibodies detected by a tube precipitin test appear early after infection and usually are not detectable after 6 months. Their presence suggests recent infection. IgG antibodies appear somewhat later, peak at 6 to 12 weeks, and may be present for months or years. These are usually found by performing a complement fixation test. Immunodiffusion tests also detect serum antibodies, usually of the types detected by IgG antibodies. Immunodiffusion is much easier to perform than complement fixation but is less sensitive (Sarosi et al, 1985). Other serologic tests that detect fungal antibodies include counterimmunoelectrophoresis, enzyme-linked immunosorbent assay, passive hemagglutination assay, latex agglutination, and radioimmunoassay (Penn et al, 1983).

Single-specimen serologic testing is much less effective than serial examinations that allow the physician to follow the titers. Titers vary among laboratories and within the same laboratory. When serial testing is desired, part of a specimen should be analyzed for screening and the remainder frozen, to be sent in along with later specimens for simultaneous analysis. In general, serial examinations with intervals of fewer than 3 weeks are not useful (Seabury et al, 1971).

Direct detection of specific circulating fungal antigens indicates the presence of a fungus and that the infection is active. Detection of cryptococcal polysaccharide capsular antigen by the latex agglutination test is the best example of antigen determination and the most important serologic test in the diagnosis of cryptococcosis (Penn et al, 1983). The most useful serologic tests in specific fungal infections are outlined in the sections that describe each disease.

INDIVIDUAL FUNGAL INFECTIONS

Much knowledge about fungal disease was gleaned during an era in medicine and surgery when methods of diagnosis were inadequate. Although the physician must be ever vigilant in the handling of specimens from transbronchial biopsies, bronchial washings, percutaneous lung biopsies, and routine sputum or induced sputum specimens, the availability of these methods has sharply reduced the need for surgical therapy in cases of fungal infections, with a few notable exceptions. A discussion of individual fungal infections highlights the current knowledge of these conditions. The individual drugs used in their management are shown in Table 23–14.

Although it is difficult to establish the frequency of occurrence of fungal infections because of the large numbers of subclinical cases, a reasonable estimate can be made.

Pulmonary mycosis can present a challenge to the general thoracic surgeon. Although the role of the surgery is commonly one of diagnosis, many interesting and difficult therapeutic situations can arise. Because fungal infection of the lung presents with various spectrums of illness, the approach to the treatment of pulmonary mycosis should be individualized.

Histoplasmosis

Histoplasmosis is a fungal infection caused by the dimorphous fungus *Histoplasma capsulatum*, which exists in mycelial form in the soil and in yeast form at body temperature. In the United States, this disease is endemic to the Midwest and Mississippi River Valley (Buechner et al, 1970).

Although millions of people have been infected with this fungus, relatively few show signs of the disease. Occasionally, particularly in immunocompromised hosts, the infection becomes systemic and more virulent. Acute forms of the disease present as primary or disseminated pulmonary histoplasmosis, and chronic forms present as pulmonary granuloma (histoplasmoma), chronic cavitary histoplasmosis, mediastinal granuloma, fibrosing mediastinitis, or broncholithiasis.

History

The first case of human infection by *H. capsulatum* was described by Samuel Darling in 1905 based on an autopsy specimen from a Martinique native who had died of disseminated histoplasmosis (Darling, 1906). The organism received its name because he erroneously thought it was a protozoan, as it was found in histiocytes with capsule. Later studies demonstrated that it was a fungus that did not have a capsule (DeMonbreum, 1934; Ribi and Salvin, 1956). The first case in the United States was reported in 1926 (Riley and Watson), and the first report of the disease in a living patient, an infant with disseminated histoplasmosis, was made in 1934 (Dodd and Tompkins).

A dramatic shift in the understanding of the disease occurred in the 1940s when the histoplasmin skin test was developed. During World War II, many healthy young men and women were rejected for service in the armed forces because of calcification seen on the routine chest radiograph, as they were thought to be evidence of healed miliary tuberculosis. However, extensive skin-testing surveys for histoplasmosis proved that infection by *H. capsulatum* was the most common cause of pulmonary calcification in the United States (Chase, 1970). These reports changed the perception of histoplasmosis, once considered a fatal disseminated disease; it became clear that it was a common and usually self-limited infection in endemic areas.

The arrival of amphotericin B in the 1950s provided highly effective therapy for patients requiring treatment. In the 1980s, new oral therapy for histoplasmosis first appeared in the form of azole compounds. The appearance of acquired immune deficiency syndrome (AIDS)

TABLE 23–14 ■ **Antifungal Agents in Fungal Infections**

Fungal Disease	*Presentation*	*Drug Choice*	*Alternative*	*Possibly Effective (Insufficient Data)*
Aspergillosis	Invasive	AMB (+flucytosine?)	—	Itraconazole
	ICH	AMB (+flucytosine?)	—	Itraconazole
Blastomycosis	Usual case	Observe for progression	AMB if further progression	Itraconazole
	Severe, meningeal, GU, ventilator-dependent, ICH	AMB		—
Candidiasis	Oral, esophageal	Fluconazole	AMB, oral ketoconazole	—
	Deep seated	AMB (+flucytosine?)	—	Fluconazole
Coccidioidomycosis	Acute pulmonary	None	—	—
	Acute pulmonary +ICH	AMB	—	Fluconazole, itraconazole
	Disseminated	Ketoconazole (AMB if progresses)	—	Fluconazole, itraconazole
	Meningeal	AMB (IV and intrathecal)	—	Fluconazole, itraconazole
	AIDS			
	Initial	AMB (IV and intrathecal)	—	Fluconazole, itraconazole
	Maintenance	AMB	—	
Cryptococcosis	Pulmonary	None	AMB	—
	Pulmonary progression	AMB + flucytosine	—	—
	Disseminated	AMB (+ flucytosine?)	—	—
	Meningeal	AMB + flucytosine	—	Fluconazole, itraconazole
	AIDS			
	Meningeal	AMB (+flucytosine?)*	—	Fluconazole, itraconazole
	Acute maintenance	Fluconazole	AMB	Itraconazole
Histoplasmosis	Acute pulmonary	None	AMB, is progressive	—
	Pneumonia, ventilator dependent, ICH	AMB	—	—
	Chronic pulmonary	Ketoconazole	AMB	Itraconazole
	AIDS			
	Initial	AMB	—	Itraconazole
	Maintenance	AMB	Ketoconazole	Itraconazole
Mucormycosis	Rhinocerebral	AMB + surgery	—	—
	Pulmonary	AMB + early surgery	—	—
	Disseminated	AMB	—	—
Paracoccidioidomycosis	Stable patient	Ketoconazole	Itraconazole	—
	Unstable patient	AMB (with or without sulfadiazine)	—	—
Sporotrichosis	Lymphocutaneous	Potassium iodide	—	Itraconazole, fluconazole
	Pulmonary	AMB	Ketoconazole	Itraconazole

ICH, immunocompromised host; AMB, amphotericin B; GU, genitourinary; IV, intravenous.
*Sarosi (1990) noted that most patients with cryptococcosis and AIDS present with marginal bone marrow reserves and are likely to incur severe myelosuppression from the use of flucytosine.

and the increased number of immunocompromised hosts provided the background for further understanding of the disease and its therapy.

Epidemiology

The incidence of histoplasmin sensitivity in the United States population is about 22%. However, the skin test is positive in up to 80% of the population of the Ohio and Mississippi River Valleys of the central United States. It is thought that 500,000 new cases of histoplasmosis develop each year in the United States. Endemic areas usually have a warm, humid climate and a large migratory bird population.

The yeast phase of *H. capsulatum* that exists in the body tissue is thought not to be contagious. There is no evidence of human-to-human or animal-to-human spread except in unusual routes such as direct inoculation during surgery or autopsy. The infectious particles are microspores from the mycelial phase. Casual exposure to a small number of airborne spores usually results in an asymptomatic or minimally symptomatic infection that is self-limited. However, heavier exposure may result in symptomatic illness. In urban areas, people can be infected by exposure to dust from major construction, including road building and urban renewal (Wheat et al, 1981).

Pathophysiology

Histoplasmosis affects primarily the respiratory system. Inhaled spores or mycelial fragments can lodge in an alveolus or interstitial space where they germinate into the yeast form, causing a localized or patchy pneumonitis (Procknow et al, 1960). Fungemia and subsequent hematogeneous dissemination from the lungs to the other tissues can occur during the first 2 weeks of infection (Fojtasek et al, 1993; Paya et al, 1987). About 10 to 14 days after the inoculation, the cellular immune response develops, mediated initially by polymorphonuclear leukocytes and later by lymphocytes and mononuclear phagocytes. The organism reproduces within macrophages and subsequently spreads via lymphatics to mediastinal lymph nodes and then throughout the reticuloendothelial system (Fojtasek et al, 1993; Goodwin and Des Prez, 1978). Immune thymus-derived lymphocytes and activated macrophages assume fungicidal properties (Allendoerfer et al, 1997). Therefore, in the immunocompromised host, progressive illness such as hematogenous dissemination involving extrapulmonary tissue may follow (Wheat et al, 1982). As cellular immunity develops, an intense inflammatory reaction occurs that produces varying degrees of caseation necrosis at the site of involvement. The histoplasmin serum antibody to *H. capsulatum* appears 4 to 6 months after inoculation and skin tests then become positive. Eventually, the lesion heals by fibrous encapsulation and subsequent calcification. It is common for the lung to develop a scar, which presents clinically as an indeterminate nodule. The surrounding lymph nodes drain the infected area, causing lymphadenopathy or mediastinal granuloma in either a calcified or an uncalcified form. Further sclerosis caused by the progression of this process is possibly due to the subsequent rupture of the node and the spread of the caseating material, which causes an intense immunogenic response. Therefore, this infection causes a spectrum of problems. An uncalcified, indeterminate mass in the lung or mediastinum may require invasive surgical diagnostic procedures to rule out carcinoma. Other problems may occur, including erosion or compression of surrounding mediastinal structures, such as the esophagus, trachea, pulmonary artery and vein, pericardium, and superior vena cava (Fig. 23–35).

Clinical Features

Presenting signs and symptoms are dependent upon the inoculum size and host factors that include immune status, previous exposure, and the presence of chronic lung disease.

Acute Pulmonary Histoplasmosis. After low-level exposure, less than 5% of exposed individuals develop symptomatic disease. However, following heavy exposure, most patients develop symptomatic infection. The most common symptoms include flu-like pulmonary illness with fever, chills, headache, joint and muscle pains, nonproductive cough, and central or pleuritic chest pain (Wheat et al, 1981). Radiographs of the chest may be normal or may show enlarged hilar or mediastinal lymph nodes, with or without small parenchymal patch infiltrates. Most patients improve in a few weeks (Brodsky et al, 1973) but some may suffer fatigue for several months (Wheat et al, 1981). After more intensive exposure, patients may develop respiratory insufficiency with diffuse pulmonary involvement.

Histoplasmoma. As the pulmonary infiltrates from the acute pulmonary histoplasmosis heal, they may consolidate into a solitary nodule known as histoplasmoma. Histoplasmoma is usually found as asymptomatic coin-shaped lesions on routine chest radiographs. In rare instances, progressive enlargement may occur at a rate of 1 to 2 mm per year to produce a 3- to 4-cm mass over 10 to 20 years (Deschamps et al, 1993). Most granulomas eventually become calcified. Central calcification and concentric calcific laminations are pathognomonic of benign disease (Goodwin and Des Prez, 1978). When noncalcified, however, these lesions may be impossible to differentiate from neoplasm (Connell and Muhm, 1976). In this situation, appropriate diagnostic evaluation should be undertaken, including a chest scan by computed tomography (CT) with contrast or by magnetic resonance imaging (MRI) and, at times, surgical excision. Antifungal therapy is not required.

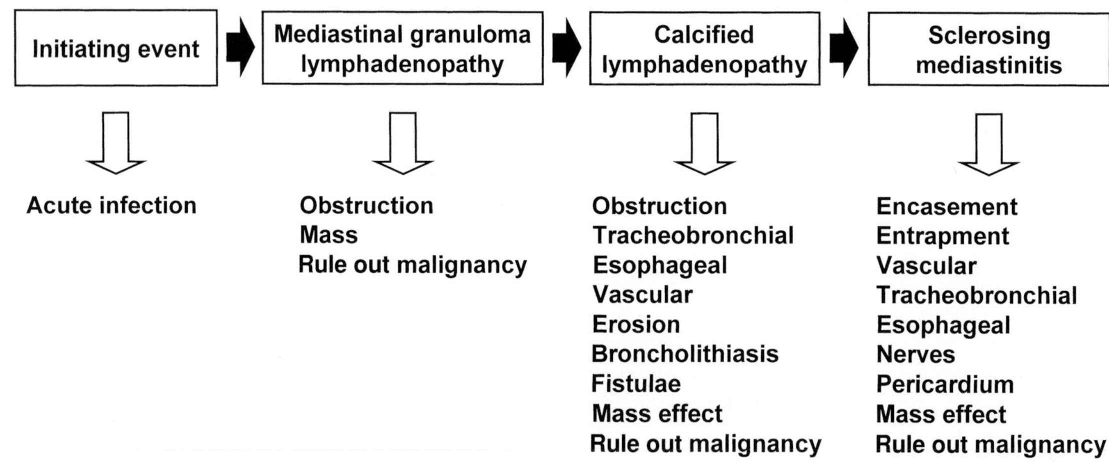

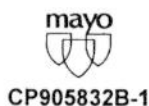

FIGURE 23–35 ■ Spectrum of clinical problems caused by *Histoplasmosis capsulatum*. (Courtesy of the Mayo Clinic.)

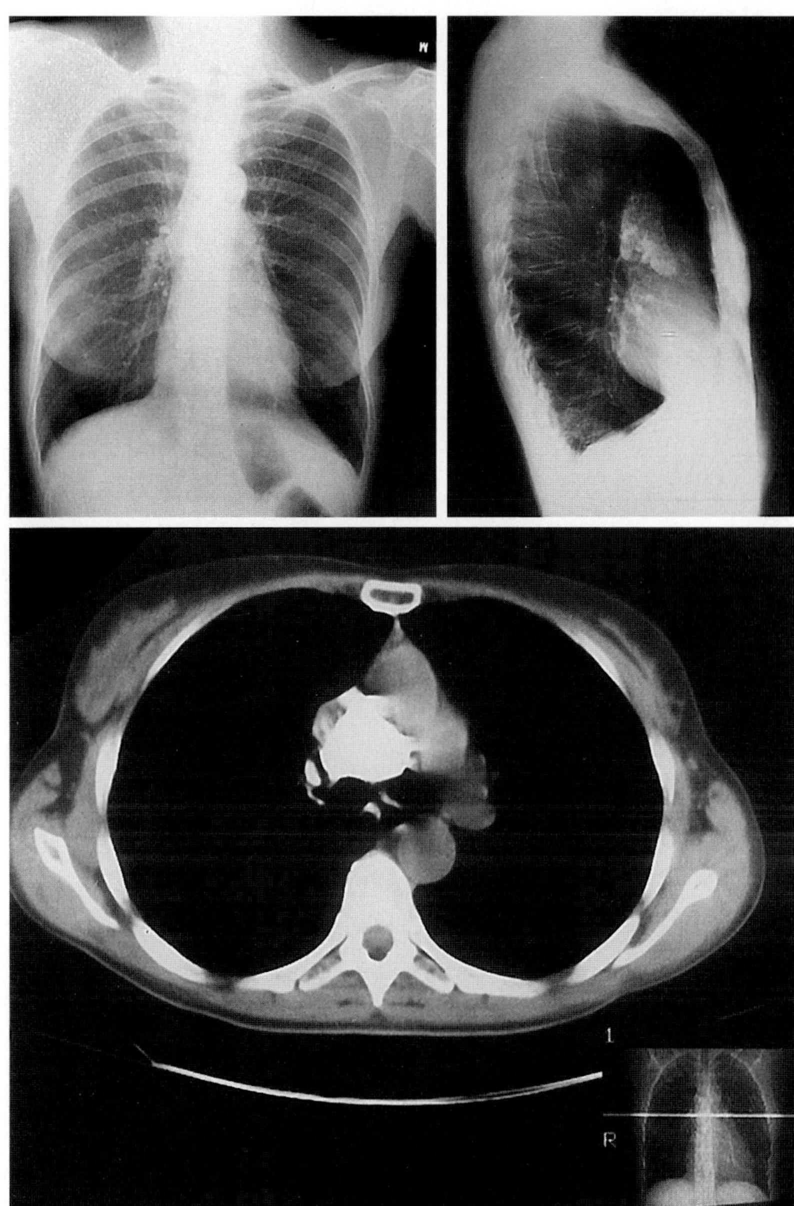

FIGURE 23–36 ■ Mediastinal granuloma in a 45-year-old female. Note calcified, enlarged lymph node in right paratracheal area.

Mediastinal Granuloma and Fibrosing Mediastinitis. Fusion of caseous mediastinal lymph nodes can result in a single large mass that becomes encapsulated (Goodwin and Des Prez, 1978). Histoplasmosis has been implicated as the most common cause of mediastinal granuloma. The granuloma usually develops in the right paratracheal and hilar area (Strimlan et al, 1975) (Fig. 23–36). When noncalcified, the mass is indeterminate, and a tissue diagnosis is required to exclude malignancy (Garrett and Roper, 1986). Depending on the location and suspected diagnosis, various diagnostic methods, such as mediastinoscopy, mediastinotomy, thoracoscopy, or thoracotomy, may be used to obtain tissue (Ferguson et al, 1987; Trastek et al, 1986; Trastek, 1987). With progressive increase in the size of the mediastinal mass, obstructive syndromes may result from compression of the superior vena cava, tracheobronchial tree, or pulmonary artery (Dines et al, 1979; Garrett and Roper, 1986; Schowengerdt et al, 1969; Wieder et al, 1982). Rarely, mediastinal masses or nodes may impinge on the esophagus causing dysphagia (Savides et al, 1995). Caseating lymph nodes have also been reported to rupture in the esophagus (Fig. 23–37), airway, and mediastinum (Coss et al, 1987; Schneider and Reid, 1975; Schowengerdt et al, 1969). These syndromes represent active inflammation of the mediastinal lymph nodes and usually improve slowly. Although about 40% of the patients with mediastinal granuloma are asymptomatic (Dines et al, 1979; Sakulsky et al, 1967; Strimlan et al, 1975), the remainder have cough, dyspnea, pain in the chest, fever, wheezing, dysphagia, and hemoptysis.

Fibrosing mediastinitis is a late stage of mediastinal granuloma that is caused by histoplasmosis. After the infection of the histoplasmosis, the mediastinal granulomas may rupture, spreading their caseous material into the mediastinum where an intense inflammatory reaction develops. As the resultant inflammation heals, variable amounts of collagen are deposited, resulting in dense

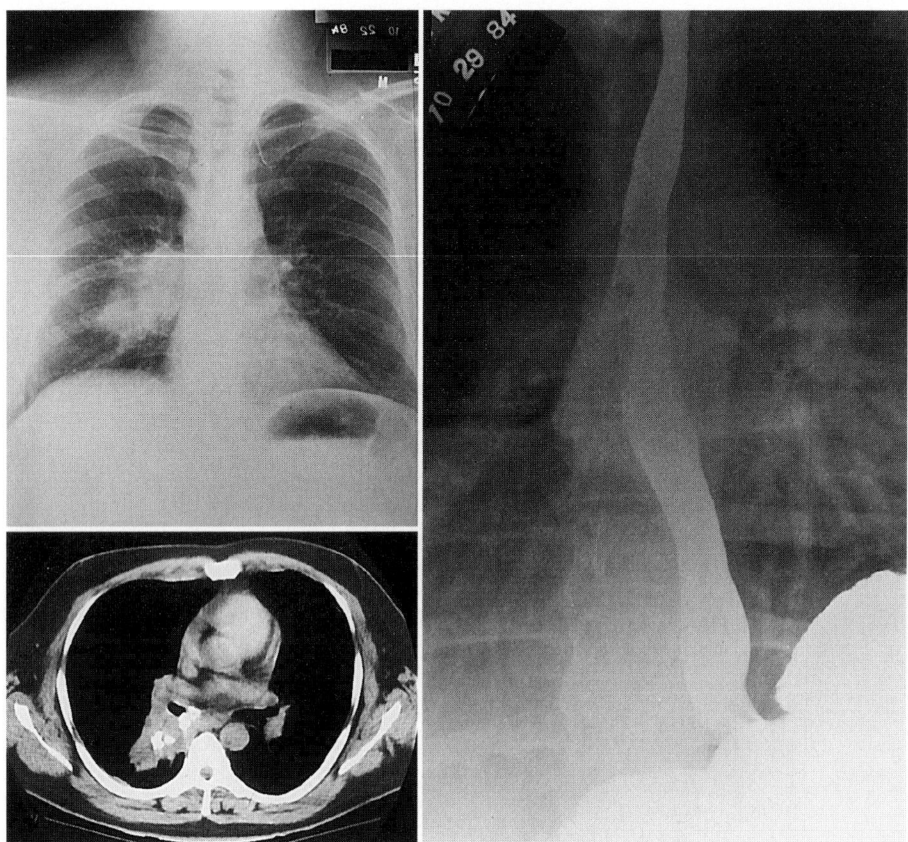

FIGURE 23–37 ■ Mediastinal granuloma eroding the esophagus in a 63-year-old female patient.

fibrosis that encases mediastinal structures. This process is thought to be a tissue response to the fungal antigen rather than distortion by mass effect as occurs in mediastinal granuloma (Goodwin et al, 1972). Signs and symptoms are determined by the extent of the fibrosis and subsequent structure compression. Fibrosing mediastinitis can affect all mediastinal structures, and it is the most common cause of benign obstruction of the superior vena cava (Mahajan et al, 1975). Fibrosis may also exhibit obstruction of the airways, pulmonary arteries and veins, and esophagus (Garrett and Roper, 1986; Loyd et al, 1988; Schowengerdt et al, 1969). Fibrosis also may invade the thoracic duct, recurrent laryngeal nerve, or, in rare cases, the atrium (Garrett and Roper, 1986; Schowengerdt et al, 1969). Recurrent and often serious hemoptysis may result from parenchymal damage caused by airway obstruction and vascular compromise (Loyd et al, 1988). Chest radiographs are commonly negative but may show superior mediastinal widening, paratracheal mass, and calcification resulting from healed infection (Dines et al, 1979). Many times, a CT scan delineates the extent of the fibrosis and identifies the structures involved (Shin and Ho, 1984). Ventilation-perfusion lung scans may show reduced blood flow in patients with pulmonary artery or vein obstruction (Fig. 23–38). The clinical course of mediastinal granuloma with fibrosing mediastinitis is benign but can be slowly progressive (Miller and Sullivan, 1973).

Fungal stains of tissues are positive in over half of cases, but cultures are usually negative (Garrett and Roper, 1986; Loyd et al, 1988), which supports the hypothesis that fibrosing mediastinitis is an excessive scarring reaction to past infection. Serologic tests are positive in two thirds of cases (Loyd et al, 1988). Strongly positive skin test reactivity to histoplasmin, as evidence of prior histoplasmosis, can be demonstrated in most cases (Garrett and Roper, 1986).

Broncholithiasis. The pathogenesis of broncholithiasis is thought to be related to the tissue's late response to healing granulomatous pulmonary infections. When the lymph nodes and pulmonary granulomas calcify over time, they may cause pressure atrophy of the bronchial wall with subsequent erosion and migration of the lymph node into the bronchus, forming broncholithiasis (Trastek et al, 1985) (Fig. 23–39). Histoplasmosis is one of the most common causes of broncholithiasis in North America (Bhagavan et al, 1971), whereas tuberculosis is the major cause in Europe (Dixon et al, 1984). Patients usually present with cough, hemoptysis, and dyspnea. Sometimes patients experience expectorating rock-like particles of tissue (see Fig. 23–39). Life-threatening complications such as massive hemoptysis or bronchoesophageal fistula may develop (Trastek et al, 1985). The diagnosis of broncholithiasis may be difficult and is most commonly based upon symptoms, radiographic findings, and bronchoscopic findings. A chest radiograph may show hilar or mediastinal calcification, and a bronchoscopy can often reveal an image of the stone. Because neoplasm must always be suspected, biopsy with bronchial brushing for cytologic examination should always be performed during bronchoscopy. Organisms may be demonstrated by fungal stains in the calcified nodes, but cultures are usually negative. Thus, antifungal therapy

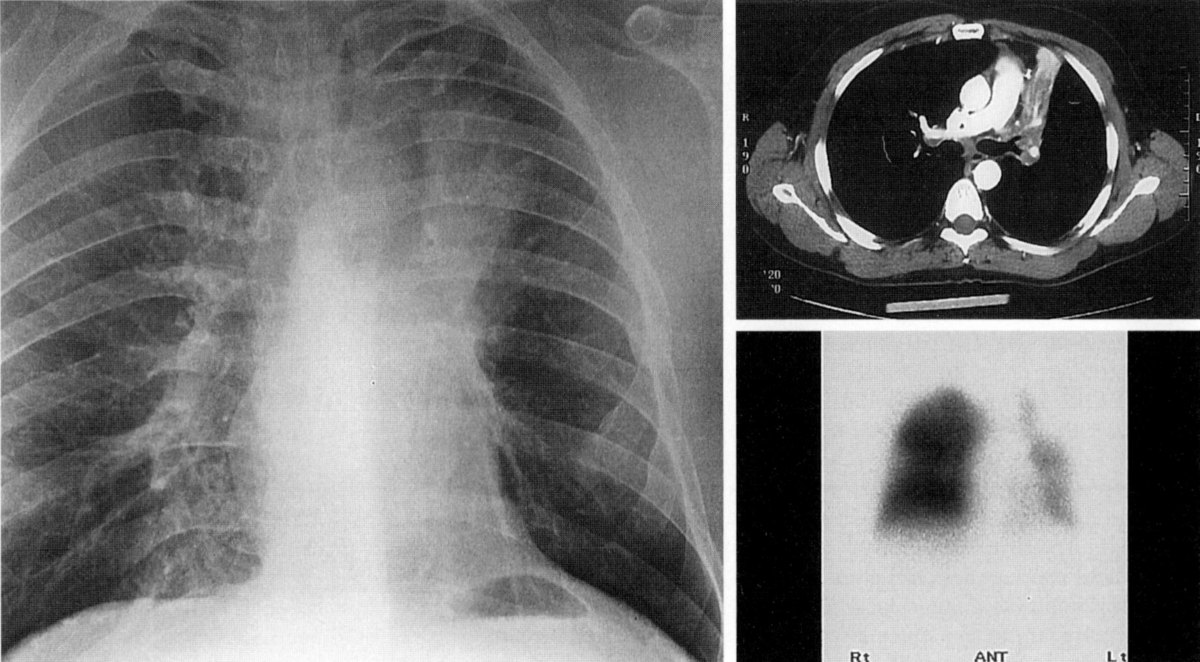

FIGURE 23–38 ■ A 37-year-old male patient with mediastinal fibrosis. This computed tomography scan shows collapse of the left upper lobe with occlusion of the left upper lobe bronchus. The left pulmonary artery is encased by the fibrotic change of the mediastinum. A perfusion scan demonstrates reduced blood flow to the left lung.

would not be expected to be effective. In patients with serious complications, surgical therapy is required.

Pericarditis and Rheumatologic Symptoms. Pericarditis may occur as an immunologic reaction to histoplasmosis in the adjacent mediastinal lymph nodes (Wheat et al, 1983). A history of acute pulmonary histoplasmosis can be recognized. Pericardial fluid is usually sterile, which suggests an inflammatory reaction rather than an infection of the pericardium. The pericardial effusion resolves in response to anti-inflammatory medications without antifungal therapy. Patients with large effusions causing hemodynamic compromise may require drainage of the pericardial fluid or may need corticosteroid therapy if the patient is not immunocompromised or has no evidence of disseminated histoplasmosis. Constrictive pericarditis is an occasional late sequela of this syndrome.

Rheumatologic symptoms can occur in less than 10% of patients with acute histoplasmosis. The symptoms include arthralgia, arthritis, and erythema nodosum (Rosenthal et al, 1983). The symptoms usually resolve spontaneously or in response to treatment with nonsteroidal anti-inflammatory agents (Wheat, 1989).

Adult Respiratory Distress Syndrome. Severe acute infections may occur following heavy exposure. Severe dysp-

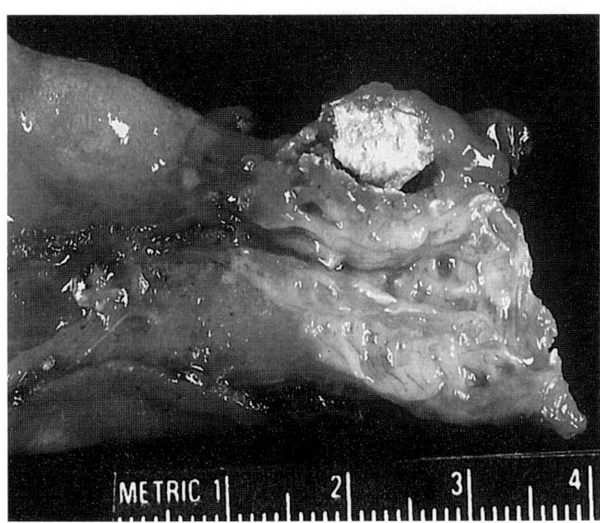

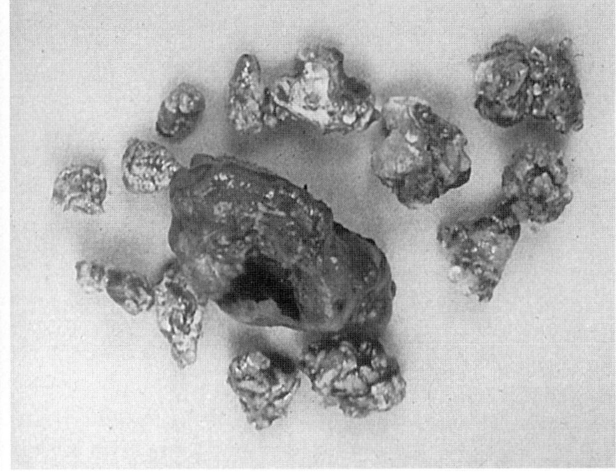

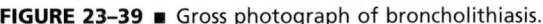

FIGURE 23–39 ■ Gross photograph of broncholithiasis.

nea, fever, and cough develop within 2 weeks of exposure; they are associated with the observance of diffuse nodular infiltrates on a radiograph of the chest. Such a patient may become markedly hypoxemic and show a clinical pattern of adult respiratory distress syndrome but will respond rapidly to amphotericin B in combination with glucocorticoid steroid therapy.

Chronic Cavitary Histoplasmosis. Chronic cavitary histoplasmosis occurs in about 10% of patients who present with symptomatic histoplasmosis. The majority of these patients have abnormal lung tissue such as chronic obstructive pulmonary disease (COPD) (Goodwin and Des Prez, 1978). The symptoms and the findings on radiographs of the chest resemble those of pulmonary tuberculosis. The typical radiographic pattern is repeating episodes of patch consolidation followed by cavitation, scarring, and partial resolution, which leads to a progressive loss of lung tissue. Patients present symptoms of COPD, such as dyspnea and cough, as well as those of chronic infections, such as fever, night sweats, weight loss, and chronic pulmonary histoplasmosis. These symptoms may progress into cavitary enlargement and new cavity formation, may spread to other areas of the lungs, and may form bronchopleural fistulas (Rubin et al, 1959). As concurrent neoplastic or other infectious diseases can coexist in chronic pulmonary histoplasmosis, steps should be taken to exclude cancer if the patient does not respond to treatment.

Disseminated Histoplasmosis. Progressive disseminated histoplasmosis may result from exogenous infection or reinfection or from reactivation of dormant foci. Although progressive disseminated histoplasmosis occasionally develops in immunocompetent patients, most cases occur in patients with depressed T cell function such as those with Hodgkin's disease and other lymphoreticular malignancies, those receiving immunosuppressive therapy, and those undergoing organ transplantation. Human immunodeficiency virus (HIV)–infected patients have the highest risk. So if patients have unexplained progressive disseminated histoplasmosis, serologic tests for anti-HIV antibodies are indicated. Symptoms of progressive disseminated histoplasmosis are nonspecific and include low-grade fever, weight loss, and malaise. The chest radiograph may be normal or diffuse abnormal. Physical examination may reveal hepatomegaly, splenomegaly, or lymphadenopathy. Extreme cases may present with overwhelming infection manifested by shock, respiratory distress, hepatic and renal failure, obtundation, and disseminated intravascular coagulation (Wheat et al, 1990).

Diagnosis

The diagnosis of acute-phase histoplasmosis can be made by means of a smear, a culture, direct biopsy of tissue, or serology. Fungal staining of tissue sections or Write staining of peripheral blood smears may be helpful for rapid diagnosis (Fig. 23–40). Serologic tests have been used to make presumptive diagnoses in patients from endemic areas with typical symptoms. As less than 5% of residents of endemic areas are seropositive by complement fixation, background seropositivity is not a limiting factor of this test (Wheat et al, 1982b). A complement fixation test using yeast and mycelial antigens is more sensitive than an immunodiffusion test (Wheat et al, 1982b). A serum complement fixation titer of 1:32 or more or a 4-fold rise in titer during illness is considered diagnostic (Goodwin et al, 1981). Although the histoplasmin skin test has been a valuable epidemiologic tool, the strong likelihood of positive skin reactions in endemic areas invalidates the test as a diagnostic procedure (American Thoracic Society, 1988). Skin-test reactivity persists for years after recovery from histoplasmosis. Skin tests may be falsely

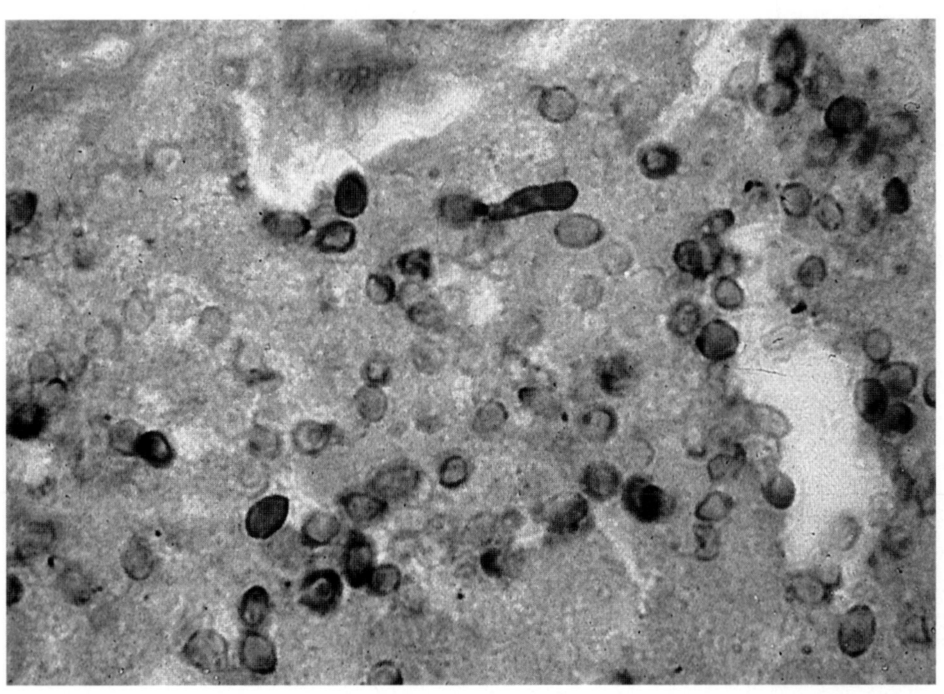

FIGURE 23–40 ■ Mediastinal lymph node biopsy specimen demonstrating *Histoplasmosis capsulatum*. (Silver methenamine; original magnification ×100.)

negative in up to 20% of patients with chronic pulmonary histoplasmosis and in more than 50% with disseminated histoplasmosis. More recently, a method of detecting a glycoprotein antigen in the blood or urine has been developed; it offers rapid diagnosis in patients with severe manifestations of histoplasmosis (Wheat et al, 1986). A definitive diagnosis of histoplasmosis is made by isolation of *H. capsulatum* in clinical specimens, but it may be difficult to demonstrate the organism because of the long incubation time necessary for culture or because of an inadequate specimen. Cultures are positive in 85% of patients with disseminated histoplasmosis, with the highest yield coming from the bone marrow (Wheat, 1997). In patients with diffuse interstitial or miliary infiltrates, the organism may be cultured from the sputum, alveolar lavage specimen, or lung tissue in up to 70% of cases (Sathapatayavongs et al, 1983; Smith and Utz, 1972; Wheat et al, 1992).

Patients with self-limited, acute pulmonary histoplasmosis, mediastinal granuloma, pericarditis, and rheumatologic manifestations demonstrate positive culture rates of only 10%. As a consequence, only a screening radiograph in an asymptomatic patient may uncover an indeterminate solitary pulmonary nodule or a right paratracheal or hilar mass. Other evaluations may include a CT scan with contrast, bronchoscopy, upper gastrointestinal endoscopy, MRI, or echocardiography aimed at the area involved. However, when histoplasmosis presents as a solitary pulmonary nodule, bronchoscopy and noninvasive testing are rarely positive (Prechter and Prakash, 1989). Needle aspiration of these nodules can occasionally isolate the organism, but more often the tissue specimen is inadequate for diagnosis, and a larger tissue sample is required (Conces et al, 1987). Identifying histoplasmosis as the cause of mediastinal granuloma and fibrosing mediastinitis is difficult because special stains and cultures of mediastinal tissues are often negative (Dines et al, 1979; Mathisen and Grillo, 1992). Unfortunately, most patients are in a more chronic phase in which it can be very difficult if not impossible to make this diagnosis retrospectively, even with serologic testing. Failure to document the organism, however, does not exclude *H. capsulatum* as the causative agent.

Treatment

Acute Pulmonary Histoplasmosis. Antifungal therapy is unnecessary in most cases of acute pulmonary histoplasmosis, even when symptoms are present. Patients recover spontaneously in a few weeks following low-level exposure. After more extensive exposure, however, patients may remain symptomatic for a longer time or may present with potentially lethal infection. If patients show moderately severe symptoms that are not improving after 2 to 4 weeks of observation, antifungal therapy may be helpful, especially in immunocompromised hosts. In immunocompetent patients, the treatment of choice is amphotericin B at a cumulative total dose of 500 to 1000 mg. Patients usually respond within 1 to 2 weeks, and no further therapy is needed. In patients who are immunocompromised, the same initially intensive therapy employing amphotericin B should be administered until clinical stabilization has been achieved, that is followed by oral therapy employing 400 mg itraconazole daily. Oral therapy is usually continued until the immunosuppressed state is no longer present; however, it should be continued for life in patients with severe immunosuppression, including all patients coinfected with HIV. Patients with extensive acute pulmonary histoplasmosis who are dyspneic and hypoxic should be treated with antifungal therapy (Kataria et al, 1981; Wynne and Olsen, 1974). If patients remain untreated, the recovery may be slow or the outcome may be fatal (Prior et al, Rubin et al, 1959). In severely ill patients, corticosteroids are also reported to be helpful (Kataria et al, 1981; Wynne and Olsen, 1974).

Histoplasmoma. When an abnormal shadow is seen on a chest radiograph or CT scan in an asymptomatic patient, surgical intervention may be needed to rule out malignancy. Indications for surgical intervention include (1) need to diagnose an acute process with open lung or nodal biopsy and (2) need to rule out carcinoma in a patient presenting with an uncalcified mass in the lung or mediastinum. It is recommended that a limited approach—video-assisted thoracoscopic surgery or limited thoracotomy—be used for local excision to achieve a diagnosis.

Mediastinal Granuloma and Fibrosing Mediastinitis. Many times, a mediastinal granuloma may present as an indeterminate mass producing no symptoms. The excision of this mass is necessary in order to establish a diagnosis. If the diagnosis is not a question, medical therapy may be considered in a patient with symptoms. Several papers have reported successful therapy with amphotericin B in a patient with tracheal obstruction (Greenwood and Holland, 1972) or esophageal fistulas or abscesses (Coss et al, 1987; Jenkins et al, 1976). A trial of itraconazole or ketoconazole is suggested in a patient with symptomatic airway obstruction (Greenwood and Holland, 1972). If a patient remains symptomatic despite medical therapy, surgical excision may be considered. Although complete excision is possible (Dines et al, 1979), an intense inflammatory reaction often increases the risk of injury to adjacent structures. Not infrequently the fibrocalcific reaction is so extensive that the dissection of the hilar structures is difficult. Meticulous dissection is warranted to avoid massive hemorrhage from pulmonary vessels and to avoid injury to the esophagus or bronchial tree. By achieving proximal and distal control of pulmonary vessels ahead of time, catastrophic bleeding can be prevented. Placing a nasogastric tube in the esophagus allows the esophagus to be identified easily during the dissection. The goal of surgery is to remove the calcified granuloma; en bloc resection is not necessary (Fig. 23–41). Unroofing the mass by evacuating the caseous debris is helpful (Garrett and Roper, 1986). To avoid injury to the adjacent structure, the wall of the granuloma may be left intact. The injury sites can be reinforced after repair by using muscle flap or pericardial tissues. Between 1939 and 1975, 10 patients were treated at the Mayo Clinic for esophageal involvement by mediastinal granuloma. The number rep-

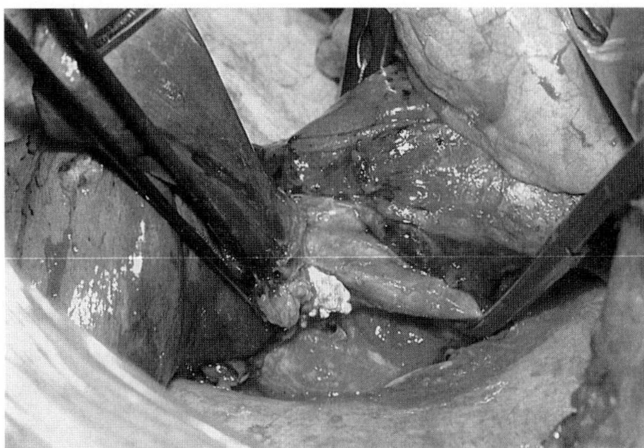

FIGURE 23–41 ■ Removal of calcified granuloma. The goal of the surgery is to remove the calcified granuloma. En bloc resection is not necessary.

resents 10.5% of the total number of mediastinal granulomas seen during that period. One case was complicated by the presence of a fistula; four patients underwent surgical resection or repair, and all experienced relief of their symptoms (Fig. 23–42).

Controversy persists as to the prophylactic role of surgery in asymptomatic patients with large mediastinal granulomas (Mathisen and Grillo, 1992). Resection of enlarged mediastinal lymph nodes has been recommended to prevent progression to fibrosing mediastinitis (Dines et al, 1979). However, aggressive medical or surgical intervention is usually not recommended for asymptomatic patients because the progression of granulomatous mediastinitis to fibrosing mediastinitis has not been documented and there is no prospective study available to justify the debulking of disease in the hope of preventing subsequent fibrosis or compression (Greenwood and Holland, 1972).

If superior vena cava obstruction becomes symptomatic, reconstruction using spiral vein grafts has been successful at the authors' institution (Gloviczki et al, 1992; Parish et al, 1981) (Fig. 23–43). A Gore-Tex graft can be used when the saphenous vein is not available. The long-term durability of the spiral vein graft has been excellent: 14 of 16 grafts are still patent after as long as 23 years of follow-up (Doty, 1982; Doty et al, 1999). Although the early patency rate is 92% in Gore-Tex grafts, the long-term patency rate is inferior to that of saphenous vein graft (62% in 24 months) (Dartevelle et al, 1987). Intraluminal stenting of the superior vena cava has been advocated as a method of relieving these symptoms that is simpler and results in less morbidity.

Palliation of dyspnea and hemoptysis has also been achieved by performing appropriate lobectomy in selected patients who experience focal pulmonary venous obstruction (Dye et al, 1977). In most cases, however, diffuse or central involvement of the pulmonary vessels makes surgical release of the involved structures technically impossible (Garrett and Roper, 1986). Severe stenosis of the tracheobronchial tree presents a similar challenge to the surgeon. Mathison and Grillo suggested that the careful use of bronchoplastic procedures and lung resection would provide relief of symptoms in most pa-

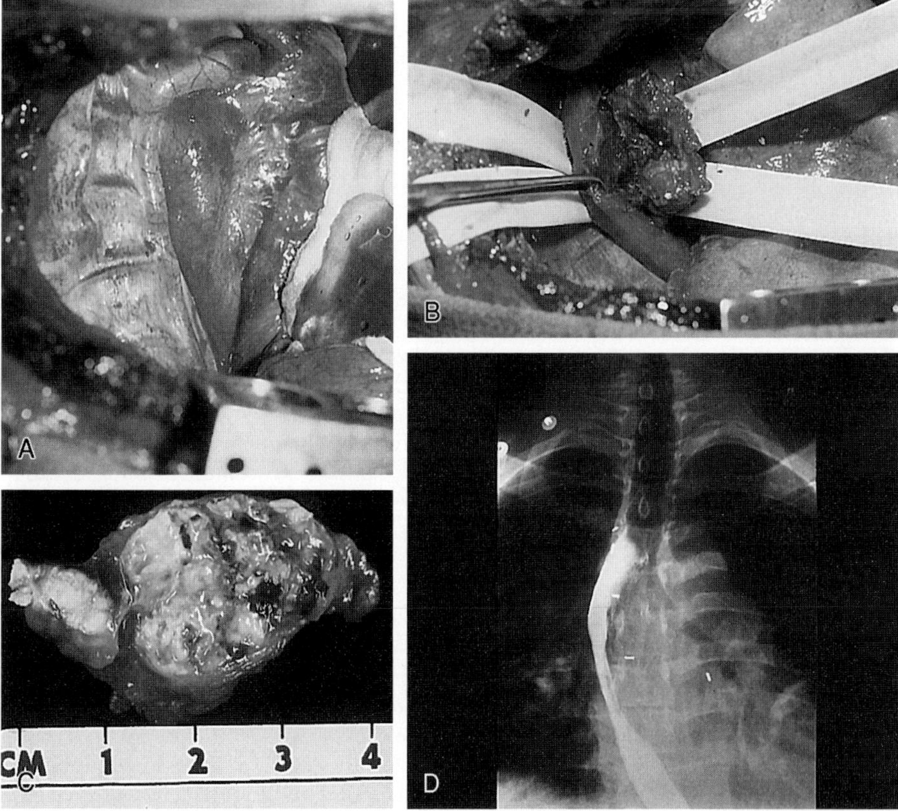

FIGURE 23–42 ■ Operative findings (*A* and *B*), gross specimen (*C*), and postoperative esophagogram (*D*) of mediastinal granuloma invading the esophagus.

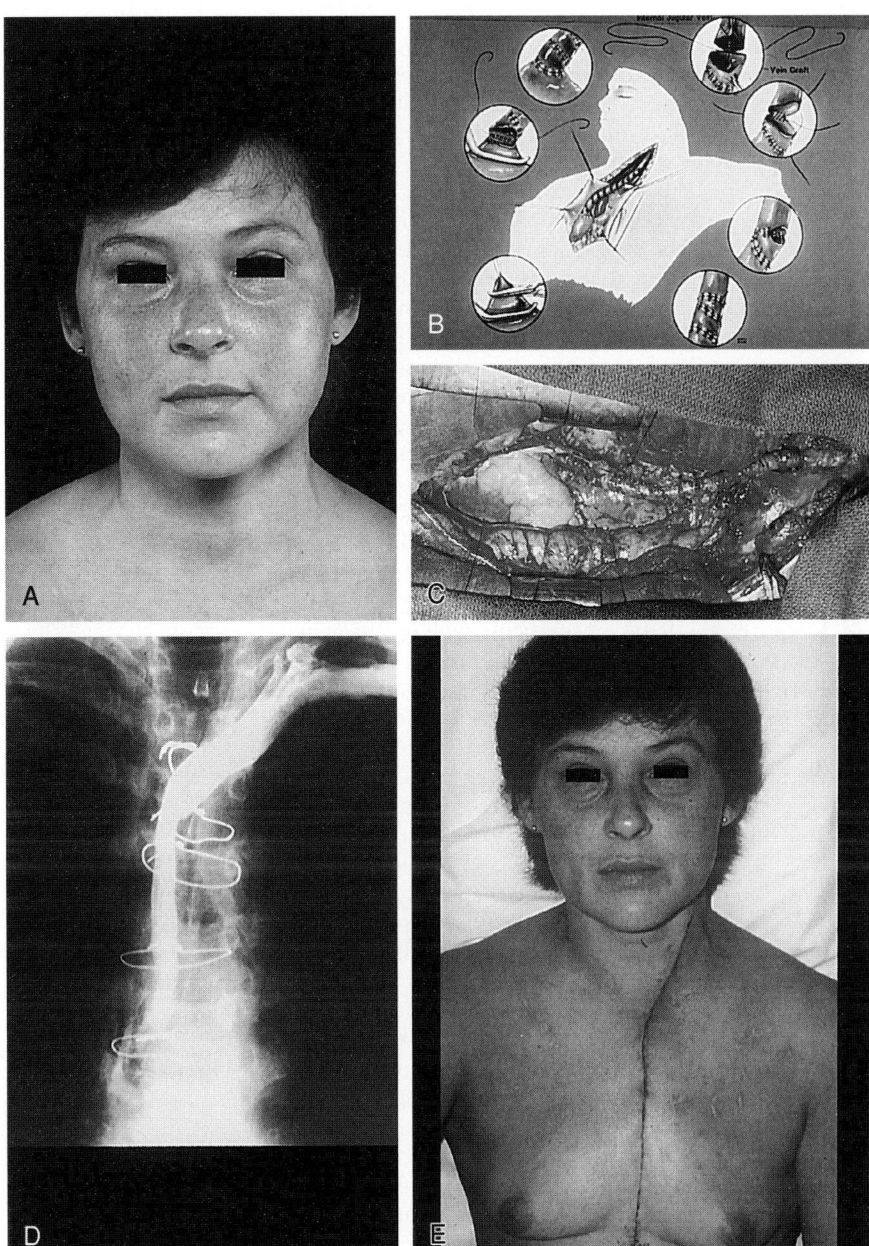

FIGURE 23–43 ■ Superior vena cava obstruction. Note markedly swollen face before operation (*A*) was relieved after the operation (*E*). Operative procedure (*B*), operative photography (*C*), and postoperative angiogram (*D*).

tients. However, mortality rates remain significant—approximately 25% (Mathisen and Grillo, 1992).

It has been frequently stated that neither antifungal nor anti-inflammatory treatment ameliorates the outcome of fibrosing mediastinitis (Goodwin et al, 1972; Loyd et al, 1988), but some have reported responses to antifungal therapy (Urschel et al, 1990). A short-term trial (3 months) of antifungal treatment seems reasonable, especially if complement fixation titers and sedimentation rates are elevated. If follow-up CT scans and clinical evaluation show evidence of response, treatment should be continued for at least 1 year. Itraconazole appears to be the most appropriate treatment. The use of corticosteroids seems inappropriate, however. These patients often experience bacterial superinfections (Loyd et al, 1988), which should be treated with antibiotics. A CT scan should be repeated yearly to mark the progression of the fibrosis and assess indications for surgery.

Broncholithiasis. Surgical removal by means of bronchoscopy or thoracotomy has been recommended as the definitive treatment for broncholithiasis. Surgical indications for broncholithiasis include intractable cough, persistent or massive hemoptysis, suppurative lung disease, bronchiectasis or bronchostenosis, bronchoesophageal or aortotracheal fistula, and uncertainty about the diagnosis. To preserve adequate pulmonary function, surgical removal should be as conservative as possible (Trastek et al, 1985). Bronchoplastic procedures or bronchotomy should be utilized if technically feasible.

At the Mayo Clinic, between 1969 and 1984, 52 patients were diagnosed with broncholithiasis. Almost all (97%) showed symptoms; 40 underwent surgery. Of these 40, all experienced relief of symptoms, and the mortality rate was reasonable (2.5%). The other 12 patients underwent endoscopic removal first, and 8 of them required surgery either immediately after the procedure or later.

Pericarditis and Pneumatologic Symptoms. Pericarditis and rheumatologic manifestations are caused by the inflammatory response to the infection; patients with symptoms respond to anti-inflammatory therapy, but antifungal therapy is not recommended.

Chronic Cavitary Histoplasmosis. Chronic pulmonary histoplasmosis is the most common form of histoplasmosis for which antifungal therapy is prescribed. In many patients, ketoconazole therapy, 400 to 800 mg daily for 6 to 12 months, is effective (National Institute of Allergy and Infections Diseases, 1985). If patients relapse after the treatment is stopped, re-treatment is required, with additional ketoconazole or with another oral agent such as itraconazole (Quinones et al, 1989). Itraconazole can also be used as an initial therapy, with a dose of 400 mg per day for 6 to 12 months (Dismukes et al, 1992). For patients who could take itraconazole or ketoconazole, fluconazole (200–400 mg daily) is not recommended, as it was reported to be less effective (64% response) (McKinsey et al, 1996). For patients who fail to respond or have repeated relapses after oral azole drug therapy, amphotericin B is indicated. The minimal total cumulative dose of 35 mg/kg is administered during a 16- to 20-week period. However, even after this regimen, relapses can occur, primarily as a result of defects in the hosts, such as structural abnormalities in the lungs or depressed immunity, rather than of the development of drug resistance.

Although in the past, several papers have reported surgical resection for chronic cavitary histoplasmosis, surgery is rarely indicated now because of the availability of effective antifungal therapies. Also, surgical resection is frequently contraindicated, as the respiratory reserve is usually diminished in these types of patients. Although severe hemoptysis may be an indication for emergency resection of cavitary lesions, bronchial artery embolization should be considered first.

Disseminated Histoplasmosis. The development of antifungal therapy has reduced the mortality rate in cases of disseminated histoplasmosis to less than 25% (Reddy et al, 1970; Sathapatayavongs et al, 1983), as compared to a rate of 80% if no treatment is given (Rubin et al, 1959). Amphotericin B is the drug of choice for progressive disseminated histoplasmosis; a cumulative dose of 40 mg/kg is usually recommended. Relapse is rare unless the patient has AIDS, in which case relapse is almost universal after discontinuing amphotericin B. It is now recommended that after the induction therapy of 500 to 1000 mg of amphotericin B, AIDS patients with disseminated histoplasmosis should be given 400 mg of itraconazole daily for life to prevent relapse (Wheat et al, 1993).

Aspergillosis

Aspergillus is a ubiquitous fungal genus that comprises more than 350 recognized species, of which *A. fumigatus*, *A. flavus*, and *A. niger* are the most common disease-causing species. The conidia (spores) released from the conidiophores of Aspergillus species are small in diameter (2.5–3.0 μm) and are easily inhaled. Consequently, the lung is the most common site of infection. Clinical manifestations include three types: a localized form, aspergilloma, which is generally considered to be an opportunistic infection in individuals with underlying lung disease; an allergic form, which represents a complex immunologic reaction of the host to a relatively innocuous exposure to a noninvasive *Aspergillus* species; and a disseminated form, which develops in immunosuppressed patients. Surgical interventions occur under two circumstances. The first is the occasional open lung biopsy for invasive aspergillosis in an immunocompromised patient, and the second is resection for complications of aspergilloma.

History

The *Aspergillus* genus was first identified in 1729 by priest and botanist Micheli, who chose the name *Aspergillus* because of the similarity in appearance of these spore-bearing heads and the brush (aspergillum) that Micheli, as a priest, used to sprinkle holy water (Hinson et al, 1952). The first human infection was described by Bennett in 1842 in a patient with tuberculosis. In 1847, Sluyter described a patient who had died of a chest illness and was found to have a fungal mass in a lung cavity. The fungus was originally reported as *mucor* but later was recognized as an *Aspergillus* species. Virchow, in 1856, reported the first four cases of this disease with pathologic evidence on autopsy, and subsequent reports verified the existence of this entity as a definitive clinical problem.

Epidemiology

Aspergillus species are ubiquitous saprophytes that are widely distributed in nature (Fig. 23–44). They exist in soil, decaying vegetation, roting wood, fur, swimming pool water, flour, human hair, ordinary foods, hospital wards, and as a common contaminant in bacteriology laboratories. of the approximately 350 species of *Aspergillus* that have been identified (Conen et al, 1962), human infection is most commonly produced by *A. fumigatus*. Other species reported to be pathogenic to humans include *A. flavus, A. niger, A. terreus, A. nidulans, A. caneus, A. sulphureus, A. glaucus, A. oryzai, and A. sycowi*. Aspergillosis is found in all races. It is more common in adults than in children and in males than in females (Sochocky, 1972).

The number of spores of *Aspergillus* species in the air increases during the autumn and winter. The incidence of aspergillosis in humans has increased, and it is now the third most common systemic fungal infection requiring hospitalization in the United States (Pennington, 1993).

Classification

The manifestation of aspergillosis varies in severity from saprophytism to fulminant, fatal infection, depending on the quantity of the inhaled spore and the physical condition of the patient (Sochocky, 1972). In 1952, Hinson and colleagues classified pulmonary aspergillosis into three types: the noninvasive bronchial allergic form, invasive aspergillosis, and saprophytic aspergilloma. The non-

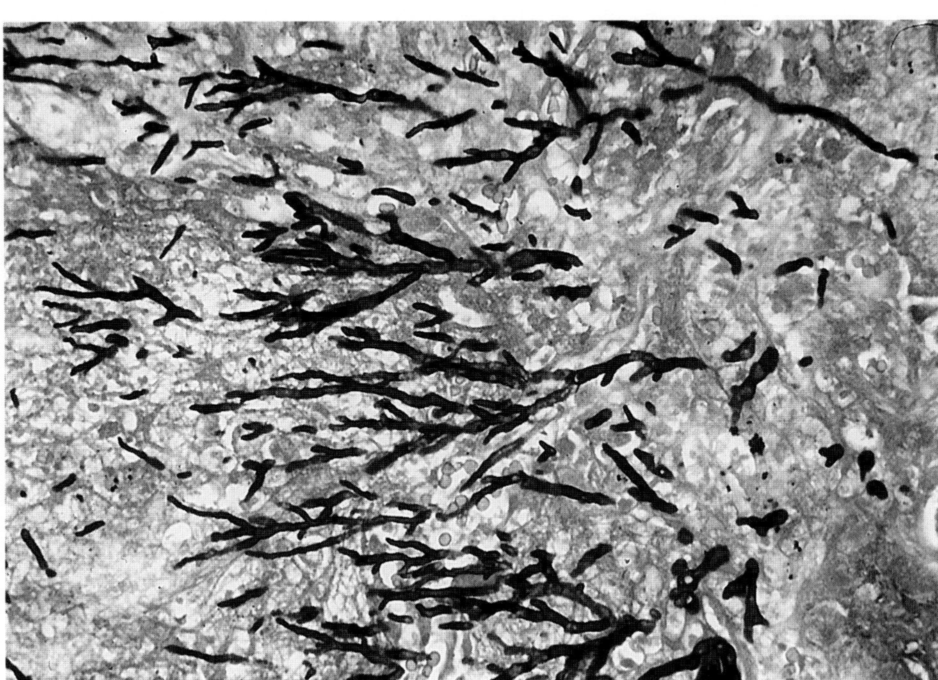

FIGURE 23–44 ■ *Aspergillus fumigatus* showing dichotomous branching pattern and prominent septation.

invasive allergic form results in respiratory symptoms owing to an immunologic reaction to the fungus in the tracheobronchial tree. This form of aspergillosis causes productive cough, fever, episodic wheezing, fleeting pulmonary infiltrates, eosinophilia, and elevated IgE antibodies to *Aspergillus* species. Unless severe bronchiectasis results, allergic aspergillosis is not a condition that requires surgery and is beyond the scope of this chapter. Often associated with this condition are areas of mucoid impaction that may simulate tumors; they usually clear after a course of steroids.

Invasive aspergillosis occurs almost exclusively in immunocompromised hosts. It arises in necrotizing bronchopneumonia and invades the lung parenchyma and pulmonary vessels. This leads to thrombosis and hemorrhagic infarction. Lysis of the infarcted lung results in the development of a mycotic lung sequestrum that may appear radiographically to be a cavity (Suen et al, 1993).

Saprophytic disease is caused by the colonizing of the pre-existing cavities of the lung. This leads to the formation of a tangled mass of hyphae, blood elements, and debris in the cavity that is called a mycetoma, a fungus ball or, most commonly, an aspergilloma. This saprophytic form is the most common manifestation of pulmonary aspergillosis.

It is noteworthy, however, that considerable clinical overlap among these three syndromes may occur. Patients with mycetoma may develop an allergic bronchopulmonary aspergillosis component of the disease (Ein et al, 1979). Likewise, rapidly invasive pneumonia may suddenly arrest and manifest as a mycetoma (Lipinski et al, 1978). Furthermore, a chronic mycetoma may suddenly break down and become a rapidly invasive pulmonary infection (Rosenberg et al, 1982).

Aspergilloma. A mycetoma is a ball of mycelia lying free in a pulmonary cavity that communicates with the bronchial tree. It is regarded as a saprophytic manifestation of a fungus growing in a preformed and poorly drained lung space. An aspergilloma may be discovered incidentally at autopsy or by routine radiographic examination. An important clinical point regarding aspergilloma is to determine whether it is a clinically significant lesion that requires therapy.

Incidence and Predisposing Factors

The incidence of aspergilloma in the general population is unknown. Various diseases that create cavitary lung lesions can be predisposing factors for aspergilloma. The most common antecedent to the development of an aspergilloma is tuberculosis. Among patients with pulmonary tuberculosis who had open negative cavitary lesions larger than 2.5 cm, 11% were found to have aspergilloma (British Tuberculosis Association, 1968). Fougner and Gjonr (1958) first reported the association between sarcoidosis and aspergilloma. Aspergilloma has also been noted to be associated with the sequelae of pulmonary infarction, histoplasmosis, pneumoconiosis, ankylosing spondylitis, congenital heart disease, healed abscess cavities, radiation fibrosis, bullous emphysema, pneumothorax, cavitary bronchogenic carcinoma, bronchiectasis, alveolar proteinosis, postlobectomy bronchial stump, blastomycosis, cryptococcosis, echinococcus cyst, allergic bronchopulmonary aspergillosis, invasive aspergillosis in immunocompromised hosts, and congenital pulmonary cysts. Systemic diseases such as myeloproliferative disease, diabetes, chronic steroid therapy, and other immunosuppressed conditions may increase susceptibility to aspergilloma formation.

Pathogenesis

The natural history of an aspergilloma is highly variable. In the initial stage, the sporulating conidiophores grow

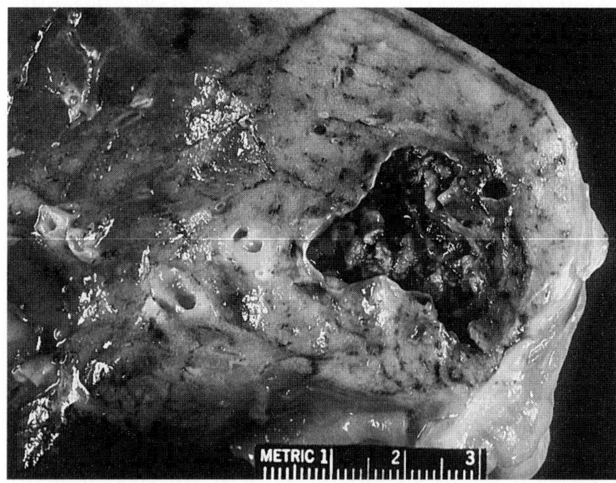

FIGURE 23–45 ■ Gross specimen of aspergilloma.

on the wall of a cavity. Although mycelia frequently grow into the walls of the cavity the fungus does not generally invade surrounding lung parenchyma or spread via the blood (Varkey and Rose, 1976). The growing mycelia subsequently peel off the wall and form a fungus ball (Fig. 23–45). Necrotic lung tissue is colonized by the fungus, which forms vegetative-type, viable hyphae. In its fully developed stage, the fungus both grows and dies in the cavity. Subsequently, the mycetoma is composed of both living and dead fungus. The growing fungus forms one or more brownish balls as mycelia and debris are shed. The epithelial lining of the cavity is rarely maintained and gets larger as the result of the growth of mycelia and the inflammatory reaction caused by the mycotoxin. Fibrotic scarring develops following the formation of granulation tissue. The fungus grows in a partially filled cavity, causing the mycetoma to grow over a period of time. Such lesions may remain stable, increase in size, or spontaneously resolve without treatment. The eventual course of the fungus ball is apparently determined by the predominance of living or dead organisms. If local conditions favor death, the fungus ball usually liquefies and is expectorated in sputum. Less commonly, the mycetoma remains as a calcification of a residual mass of dead fungi.

In 1960, Belcher and Pulmmer classified the aspergilloma into simple and complex types. Simple aspergillomas develop in isolated, thin-walled cysts lined by ciliated epithelium, and the surrounding lung is normal (Fig. 23–46). The formation of the cysts precedes the formation of the fungus ball. Simple aspergillomas sometimes reach considerable size. Complex aspergillomas de-

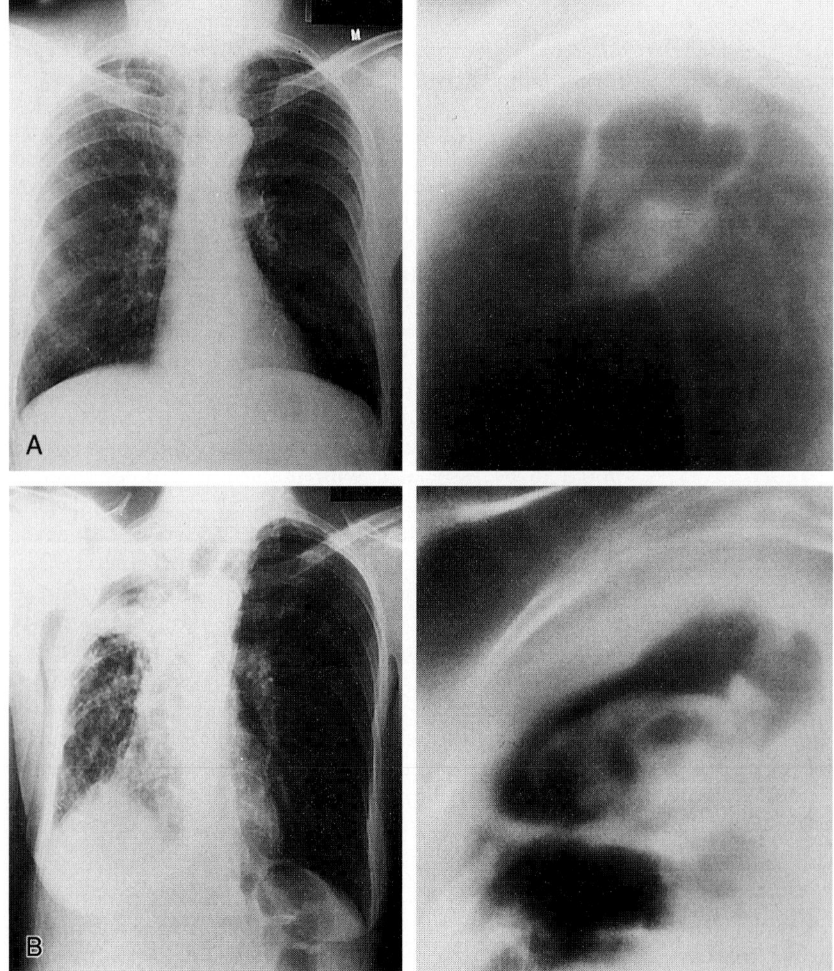

FIGURE 23–46 ■ Chest radiograph of simple aspergilloma (*A*) and a complex aspergilloma (*B*). Simple aspergilloma shows a characteristic round, dense opacity occupying the cavity surrounded partially by a crescent of air. Note the severely destroyed underlying right lung in complex aspergilloma.

velop in cavities formed by gross disease in the surrounding lung tissue, such as chronic tuberculosis, chronic lung abscess, advanced sarcoidosis, or bronchiectasis (see Fig. 23–46). A significant number of patients with complex aspergillomas are also immunosuppressed, and fungal septa may be observed to be invading lung parenchyma. Complex aspergillomas cause more severe symptoms and postoperative complications.

Clinical Features

Patients with aspergilloma may exist without clinical symptoms, and the lesions may remain stable for years. Sometimes the diagnosis is made on routine chest radiography. The most common symptom associated with an aspergilloma is hemoptysis. The severity may vary from infrequent, small episodes of blood-tinged sputum to massive and fatal hemorrhage. Less common symptoms include chronic cough with sputum, clubbing, malaise, weight loss, and reactive airway disease. Fever may suggest a superimposed bacterial infection resulting from bronchial obstruction. Slowly progressive dyspnea resulting from thickening of the pleura over the cavity may occur rarely. The underlying pulmonary condition is an important factor in determining the outcome because most deaths are due to chronic respiratory failure or pneumonia (Suen et al, 1993).

Diagnosis

In many instances, an aspergilloma lesion is found incidentally during routine chest radiography. In other cases, the diagnosis may be made during evaluation of hemoptysis. A characteristic radiographic sign of aspergilloma is a round, dense opacity occupying some or most of the cavity and surrounded partially by a crescent of air (Monod's sign), mostly in the upper lung (Deve, 1938; Pesle and Monod, 1954). Conventional tomography or CT scans help to define the fungus ball within the cavity. If the fungus ball has completely filled the cavity, the air space may not be observed on the radiograph of the chest. The apical portion of the upper lobe or the superior segment of the lower lobe is usually involved by aspergilloma, reflecting the association with pulmonary tuberculosis and sarcoidosis. In patients predisposed by allergic bronchopulmonary aspergillosis, however, the mid lung is commonly involved. Other radiologic findings include irregular calcific densities within the cavity, pleural thickening overlying the cavity, bronchiectasis in the region of the aspergilloma, and an extra area of patch infiltrate and lobar shrinkage contiguous to the cavity (Johnson, 1977; Levin, 1956; Libshitz et al, 1974; Pimentel, 1966).

Direct examination of the sputum using polarizing light microscopy in patients with hemoptysis may reveal the birefringent calcium oxalate crystals that are commonly found in pulmonary aspergillosis. Sputum cultures frequently yield the fungus. Culture confirmation of the fungus in sputum depends on whether the fungus ball consists of viable or dead fungus and also on the patency of the bronchus leading from the aspergilloma (Kahanpaa, 1972). Positive culture rates had been reported to be between 55% and 100% of patients with positive skin tests (Israel and Ostrow, 1969; Krakowka et al, 1978; McCarthy and Pepys, 1973). However, a single positive sputum culture has little specificity because of the ubiquitous nature of *Aspergillus* species (Garvey et al, 1977). If the cavity does not communicate with the bronchial tree, a sputum culture may be falsely negative (Saab and Almond, 1974). BAL may significantly increase the likelihood of isolating the fungus and is thought to be more meaningful than sputum culture (Genoe et al, 1972; George et al, 1978; Karas et al, 1976). Bronchoscopy is also indicated to localize hemoptysis. When the cavity is located in the peripheral area of the lung, percutaneous transthoracic needle aspiration may be diagnostically useful. Direct staining of the aspirate with methenamine silver can confirm the diagnosis (Henderson et al, 1975).

Serologic testing is helpful in situations in which the cultures are negative. A serum-precipitating antibody test is both sensitive and specific in the setting of a radiologically suspicious lesion (British Tuberculosis Association, 1968; American College of Chest Physicians, 1973; Pennington, 1993). Skin testing with the antigen to the *Aspergillus* species is positive in 22% of patients and is less helpful in the evaluation of patients with aspergilloma (American College of Chest Physicians, 1973). If pleural aspergillosis is suspected, pleural biopsy may also be useful. In patients with massive hemoptysis, the diagnosis is often made after surgical resection.

Treatment

Because the natural history of aspergilloma is highly variable, the treatment plan should be individualized for each patient. An asymptomatic aspergilloma usually does not require treatment unless the patient presents with a mass of unknown cause. Although a few cases of aspergilloma have resolved spontaneously (Jewkes et al, 1983; Varkey and Rose, 1976), most cases persist and many patients develop hemoptysis. The incidence of hemoptysis has been reported to be between 50% and 80% (Levin, 1956; McCarthy and Pepys, 1973). According to the report of Karas and colleagues 8 of 23 patients had a life-threatening hemorrhage during the period of 1 year. Approximately 4% of the patients died of hemoptysis and 5% of the patients required surgical resection (Karas et al, 1976). The risk of massive hemoptysis is not related to the size or duration of the aspergilloma, the type of underlying disorder, or the presence of a previous major or minor episode of hemoptysis. Once hemoptysis has occurred, the possibility of fatal hemorrhage was reported to increase as much as 30% (Garvey et al, 1978), and the risk of death from massive hemoptysis has been estimated to occur in 5% to 28% of patients (Faulkner et al, 1978; Karas et al, 1976). Massive hemoptysis can occur in both simple and complex aspergillomas.

In general, if a patient presents with mild non–life-threatening hemoptysis, the initial treatment can be medical management, including bed rest in a semisitting position, oxygenation, humidification, cough suppressants, postural drainage, and oral or parenteral antibiotics. Such a patient should be followed closely for evidence of rebleeding. In a case of more severe hemoptysis, a bronchoscopy should be performed to confirm the focus of the bleeding, which is usually evident radiologically. Cold saline lavage often stops the bleeding temporarily. Bronchial artery embolization can arrest bleeding in most cases. However, hemoptysis recurs in more than 50% of cases, probably because of extensive collaterals (Suen et al, 1993). If the bleeding is massive, tamponade of the bleeding's focus with properly placed balloons may be required to control an acute episode. Double-lumen endotracheal tubes may be necessary to protect the contralateral lung from aspiration of blood. Thoracotomy and resection should be performed if the patient can tolerate the procedure. Systemic antifungal agents are not effective for aspergilloma (al-Majed et al, 1990; Garvey et al, 1977; Israel and Ostrow, 1969; Kilman et al, 1969; Massard et al, 1992). Direct endobronchial or intracavitary instillations of various antifungal agents have been tried. Hargis and colleagues (1980) treated 6 patients who had symptomatic pulmonary aspergilloma with a percutaneous instillation of intracavitary amphotericin B. Five patients received the full course of treatment; one patient did not tolerate the therapy and had systemic reactions. Four of the fully treated patients improved, and the other failed to respond. This experience is encouraging and suggests a nonsurgical alternative for poor surgical candidates. However, others have reported profound bronchospasm and advised considerable caution when attempting such local instillations (Pennington, 1993).

The choice of surgical management of aspergilloma is based on the balance between the risk involved with the disease and the risk involved with surgery. In a case of simple aspergilloma, the risk, for hemoptysis is present and the surgical risk is minimal; therefore, resection is indicated. In a case of complex aspergilloma, because of the higher surgical risk, resection should be recommended only in low-risk patients. In high-risk patients, secondary procedures such as cavernostomy with muscle flap transposition may be used. It would also be reasonable to consider intracavitary instillation of antifungal agents (Giron et al, 1998) or bronchial embolization for this group of patients. In a comparison study of medical and resectional therapy, Jewkes and colleagues (1983) found a similar 5-year survival rate in patients with minor or no hemoptysis who had undergone medical therapy (65%) versus resectional therapy (75%). However, for patients with recurrent frank hemoptysis or a single major bleed, the 5-year survival rate was 41% in the medical and 84% in the resectional treatment group, suggesting the necessity of resectional therapy in this group of patients. In general, indications for surgical treatment include (1) recurrent gross hemoptysis, (2) life-threatening hemoptysis, (3) chronic cough with systemic symptoms, (4) progressive infiltrate around the mycetoma, and (5) the presence of a mass of unknown cause.

The goal of surgery should be a limited resection that encompasses all diseased tissue. Operations of complex aspergillomas are often technically challenging because of the dense fibrosis around the cavity, the obliteration of pleural space and fissures, the enlarged and tortuous bronchial arteries, and the diseased pulmonary parenchyma surrounding the lesion. The inflammatory fibrosis of the pulmonary parenchyma and pleura may make the remaining lungs unable to expand fully and fill the pleural space after the resection. Efforts to obliterate any postresectional residual space should be made. Various techniques, including a pleural tent, pneumoperitoneum, decortication, muscle flap, omental transposition or, in rare conditions, thoracoplasty, should be considered after the resection (al-Zeerah and Jeyasingham, 1989; Daly et al, 1986; Massard et al, 1992). It may also be helpful to reinforce the bronchial stump with healthy tissue to prevent bronchopleural fistula.

Mortality, morbidity, and long-term survival depend on the selection of patients and on proper management. The reported operative mortality rate ranges from zero to 43% (Belcher and Pulmmer, 1960; Estridge et al, 1972; Karas et al, 1976; Kilman et al, 1969; Saab and Almond, 1974). Daly and colleagues (1986) reported on 53 patients surgically treated for aspergilloma. Operative mortality was 23%. The majority of deaths occurred in patients with complex aspergilloma (34% in patients with complex vs. 5% patients with simple aspergilloma). Postoperative morbidity was also significantly higher in patients with complex aspergillomas (78% in patients with complex vs. 33% in patients with simple aspergilloma). These outcomes could be the results of the widespread pulmonary disease and the secondary bacterial infection. Patients with simple aspergilloma had good results, and their survival rates were comparable to those of the general population (Daly et al, 1986). However, the long-term survival rate of patients with complex aspergilloma is poor because many die as result of the underlying lung disease (Fig. 23–47).

Recurrence of aspergilloma after resection has been reported in 7% of patients (Jewkes et al, 1983). Therefore, careful long-term follow-up is recommended (Daly et al, 1986). If there is evidence on the specimen of parenchymal invasion, the use of antifungal drugs is indicated to prevent subsequent dissemination of the invasive aspergillosis (Suen et al, 1993).

Invasive Pulmonary Aspergillosis. In an immunocompromised patient, invasive pulmonary aspergillosis is a devastating complication. It produces a necrotizing bronchopneumonia with invasion of the pulmonary parenchyma and blood vessels, which leads to thrombosis, hemorrhage and, eventually, dissemination. It occurs in 4.5% of all bone marrow transplant patients and in 20% of allogenic bone marrow transplant patients and has been diagnosed antemortem in 21% of neutropenic acute leukemia patients undergoing standard chemotherapy (Kibbler et al, 1988; Peterson et al, 1983). Among patients with neutropenia for more than 34 days, the risk increases to as much as 70% (Gerson et al, 1984). Other risk factors include age over 30 years, mismatching of bone marrow allograft recipients, cytomegalovirus infection, the presence of high-grade graft-versus-host disease, and corticosteroid therapy (Armstrong, 1993; Gerson et al, 1984; Meyers, 1990; Peterson et al, 1983).

Clinical Features and Diagnosis. Individuals with invasive aspergillosis commonly present with unexplained and unremitting fever that is not responsive to antibacterial agents. This occurs during the period of neutropenia.

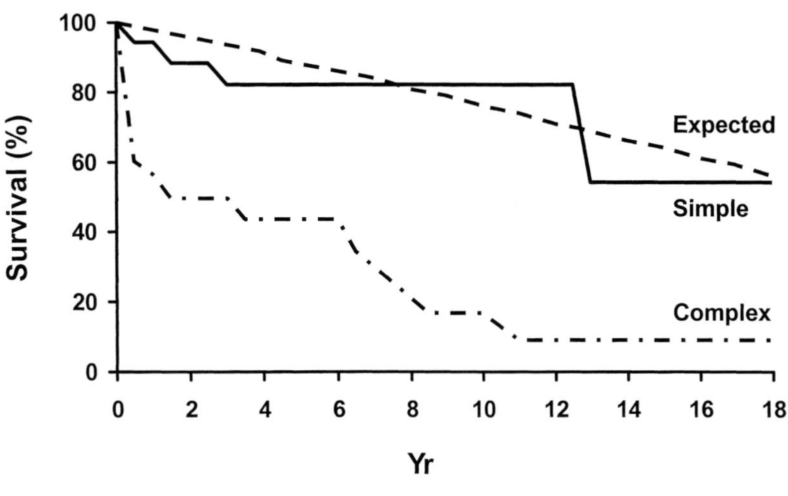

FIGURE 23–47 ■ Long-term survival of simple versus complex aspergilloma. (Courtesy of the Mayo Clinic.)

Other signs and symptoms include pleuritic chest pain, dyspnea, cough, and hemoptysis. *Aspergillus* species have a tropism for the vascular wall. Hemoptysis is seen in about 31% of patients with invasive aspergillosis (Lupinetti et al, 1992) and the risk is higher after the recovery of granulocytes (Albelda et al, 1985).

The characteristic finding on chest radiographs of a rounded infiltrate accompanied by fever in an immunocompromised patient strongly suggests invasive pulmonary aspergillosis (Lupinetti et al, 1992). A CT scan of the chest is helpful for diagnosis as it can show two typical findings: (1) a nodular pattern with or without a surrounding halo, which usually appears during early periods when there is lower absolute neutrophil count; and (2) a cavitary pattern with or without an air-crescent sign, which is generally seen after engraftment (Mori et al, 1991). Sputum cultures and bronchoscopic lavage tend to be nondiagnostic and are usually not helpful because positive results for *Aspergillus* species may indicate only colonization (Wong et al, 1992). Although percutaneous needle biopsy of nodular infiltrates may be helpful, its high risk for bleeding in these commonly thrombocytopenic patients means the procedure is rarely used. The sensitivity of serodiagnosis for invasive aspergillosis has been very poor (Henze et al, 1982; Schaefer et al, 1976; Young and Bennett, 1971). In addition, false-positive results may occasionally occur.

A test kit for the detection of the *Aspergillus* species galactomannan antigen in serum and urine was reported to facilitate early detection and early start of empiric antifungal therapy in high-risk patients (Rogers et al, 1990). However, false-positive results may occur in patients receiving cyclophosphamide.

Diagnosis of invasive aspergillosis therefore depends mainly on clinical suspicion and radiologic finding. Baron and colleagues (1998) described five criteria that are highly suggestive of invasive pulmonary aspergillosis: (1) neutropenia, (2) pneumonia, (3) persistent fever despite broad-spectrum antibiotics, (4) hemoptysis, and (5) and air-crescent sign on a CT scan of the chest.

Treatment. As treatment delay can be uniformly fatal and early definitive diagnosis is often difficult, it is entirely appropriate to institute empiric antifungal therapy with amphotericin B when invasive aspergillosis is clinically suspected (Iwen et al, 1993). Unfortunately, however, even early aggressive medical treatment of invasive aspergillosis results in a high mortality rate. For bone marrow transplant patients, mortality rates as high as 93% to 100% have been reported (Denning and Stevens, 1990; Meyer et al, 1973; Wingard et al, 1987). The mortality rate in liver transplant patients also approaches 100% (Kusne et al, 1992). The other problem is the risk of delaying further treatment for primary disease during the period of medical treatment. Although the mortality rate in renal transplant patients is better (38%), 60% of survivors lose the allograft kidney because of rejection, which occurs during the period when treatment to minimize the likelihood of rejection is not being performed because of ongoing antifungal therapy (Weiland et al, 1983). To improve the results of medical treatment, early diagnosis by means of prompt use of chest CT scan followed by earlier institution of empiric antifungal therapy for febrile neutropenic patients is necessary. Use of lipid formulations of amphotericin B that can provide higher dosages of antifungal drugs and less toxicity, or azole antifungal agents such as intraconazole may be helpful. To reduce the duration of the neutropenic period, hematopoietic growth factors, such as granulocyte colony-stimulating factor (G-CSF), granulocyte-macrophage colony-stimulating factor (GM-CSF), and erythropoietin can also be used (Robinson, 1999).

The poor outcome of medical treatment has introduced surgical removal of the pulmonary focus of infection as a treatment option. Wingard and colleagues (1987) reported that only one patient among their bone marrow transplantation survivors suffered from invasive aspergillosis, and that the patient underwent pulmonary resection of the infection site in addition to amphotericin B therapy. In 1988, Kibbler and colleagues reported a total of eight surgical cures of invasive aspergillosis, with no surgical mortality in neutropenic leukemia patients. Since then, various investigators have reported successful cure of invasive aspergillosis with very low mortalities in patients who had hematologic malignancies that were treated with high-dose chemotherapy or bone marrow transplantation. For solid organ transplant patients, Weiland and colleagues (1983) reported three survivals of invasive aspergillosis after lung resection and antifungal therapy in renal transplant patients. Robinson and colleagues (1995) reported two liver transplant patients who achieved long-term cure of invasive aspergillosis after lung resection. Results of these surgical series suggest that early, complete resection for smaller fungal lesions, along with excision of sufficient normal lung tissue to prevent contamination of uninfected lung, should be performed as soon as the characteristic clinical and radiographic picture appears (Robinson, 1999). There are still controversies about the indications for and timing of the surgical intervention. To achieve a good surgical result, the lesion should be localized so that the resection is feasible. If the lesions are multiple or bilateral, or if there is evidence of extrapulmonary spread to other organs, the surgical resection would not be beneficial. Ventilator dependency is also a relative contraindication for surgery.

Pleural Aspergillosis. Pleural aspergillosis is rare and occurs as a result of advanced pulmonary infection with an *Aspergillus* species and direct spread to the pleural cavity. Denning and Stevens (1990) reported that 88% of 16 cases responded well to treatment, which included antifungal therapy in most, combined with surgical drainage in selected patients who had empyema complicated by bronchopleural fistula. Massard and colleagues (1992), however, reported poor surgical results, including high rates of mortality and morbidity. Among the 13 patients treated surgically, 2 died perioperatively, 9 required prolonged hospitalization, 8 developed pleural-space problems, and 1 developed respiratory failure. With these considerable complications, the author advised that surgery should be limited to symptomatic patients.

Coccidioidomycosis

Coccidioidomycosis is a fungal disease caused by *Coccidioides immitis*. This dimorphic fungus is found in soil and dust and is endemic to the deserts of the southwestern United States. It can occur in several forms and can include persistent or chronic pneumonia, miliary disease, and pulmonary infiltrates, and nodules with or without cavitation. Asymptomatic coccidioidomycosis requires no treatment. However, disseminated disease may be fatal. Amphotericin B is the standard medical therapy for this disorder; pulmonary resection is rarely indicated but may come into play in granulomatous disease to rule out neoplasm or for cavitation, which is much less common but could cause hemoptysis. Whether to use perioperative amphotericin B is controversial; but it currently appears prudent to consider its use, particularly if the lesion is cavitary.

History

Coccidioidomycosis has been recognized as a distinct disease in humans since 1892, when Posadas first described the disease in a patient suffering from multiple cutaneous granulomatous lesions. In the early 1900s, coccidioidomycosis was known as a fatal infectious disease manifested by widely disseminated granulomatous lesions, primarily of the meninges, bone, and skin. After Dickson and Gifford (1938) connected a relatively benign pneumonitis with erythema nodosum, fever, and arthralgias as the usual clinical syndrome caused by *C. immitis*, the disease has been thought of as a pulmonary disease. Thereafter, coccidioidomycosis was appreciated as a relatively benign infection under most circumstances. However, disseminated coccidioidomycosis remained fatal and it was not until the late 1950s, with the development of amphotericin B, that the disease could be treated.

Epidemiology

C. immitis is endemic to California, Arizona, Texas, Mexico, and Central and South America. The fungus lives in soil. During the rainy season, the soil becomes a luxurious environment for growth. Arthroconidia, the form of *C. immitis* infectious to animals and humans, are formed during the following dry season and break off contaminating the air. Outdoor activities such as horseback riding, dirtbike riding, walking, and excavations to install utilities or to build houses may lead to infection. Dust storms also can increase the number of cases. Large numbers of people apparently contact the disease, although many of them are entirely asymptomatic, with skin test conversion being the only manifestation.

Pathophysiology

In nature, *C. immitis* is a saprophyte and grows as a mycelium. As the mycelium grows, it comprises a series of separate hyphae, which ultimately develop into a series of arthroconidia. Mature arthroconidia are quite resistant to drying and are easily detached and easily become airborne. These arthroconidia infect mammals when they are inhaled. Once inhaled into the lung, *C. immitis* develops a distinctly different morphology and becomes a parasite form. Within the lung, arthroconidia swell into a spherule, which is the organism that is histologically identified in infected tissue by its characteristic doubly refractile cell wall (Fig. 23–48). This large (10 to 80 μm) spherule undergoes internal cleavage into many endospores (2 to 5 μm). The spherule matures and then ruptures, releasing endospores into the surrounding tissue. Each endospore then matures into a spherule and the process repeats itself. Unlike the arthroconidia, the spherule is not infective. Because the only form of the fungus to exist in human is the spherule/endospore, *C. immitis* is not usually transmissible from human to human. Patients with coccidioidomycosis do not have to be isolated, but care must be taken in disposing of materials contaminated with secretions (Stevens, 1995).

In response to *C. immitis* infection, host defense mechanisms, including complement activation and chemotactic factors, are generated (Galgiani et al, 1978, 1980). Macrophages and neutrophils accumulate and attempt phagocytosis. However, arthroconida, endospores, and especially spherules are resistant to killing by such cells (Frey and Drutz, 1986; Galgiani, 1986). The infection stimulates T lymphocytes, which are central to immune response against *C. immitis*. With the influx of lympho-

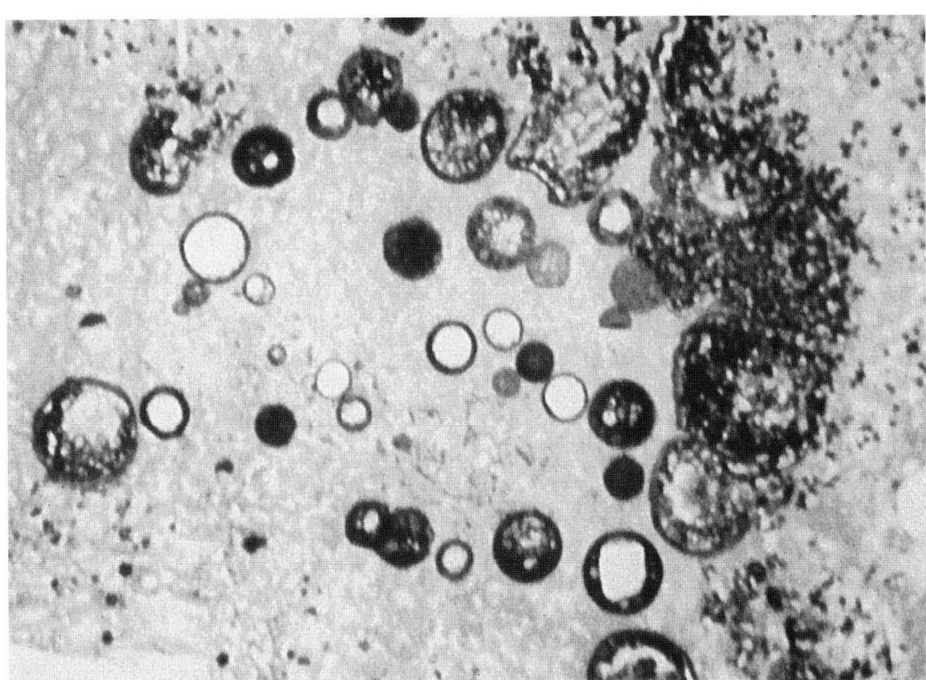

FIGURE 23–48 ■ *Coccidioides immitis* spherule showing a characteristic doubly refractile cell wall.

cytes and macrophages, classic granuloma formation occurs. Intense neutrophil infiltration produces extensive surrounding suppuration and microabscess formation. As the disease progresses, cell-mediated immune responses may become deficient (Catanzaro et al, 1975; Cox et al, 1976). The depression of the cell-mediated immunity is probably due to antigen overload, suppressor cells, immune complexes, or fungal immunosuppressive substances (Brass et al, 1982; Catanzaro, 1981; Cox et al, 1982; Harvey and Stevens, 1981; Ibrahim and Pappagianis, 1973; Opelz and Scheer, 1975).

Clinical Features

Primary Coccidioidomycosis. In the United States, accidental inhalation of airborne arthroconidia causes an estimated 100,000 infections per year. Of the people who inhale them, 60% have no symptoms or have an illness indistinguishable from an upper respiratory infection. In such people, the infection is indicated only by a positive coccidioidal skin test (Smith et al, 1946). In another 40% of people, symptoms develop 1 to 3 weeks after exposure and at least 90% have symptoms that are limited to the pulmonary system. The typical symptoms include fever, sweating, anorexia, weakness, arthralgia, cough, sputum production, and pleuritic chest pain (Werner et al, 1972). When erythema nodosum or erythema multiforme accompanies the other symptoms, the disease has traditionally been called valley fever. When associated with arthralgias, it has been called *desert rheumatism*.

Persistent Coccidioidomycosis. When the symptoms remain present and positive chest radiographic findings exist for more than 6 to 8 weeks, the disease is considered to be persistent coccidioidal pneumonia. The symptoms may last for several months, and chest radiographic findings may take as long as 8 months to clear. These patients experience protracted symptoms of cough, fever, hemoptysis, dyspnea, and weight loss lasting 7 to 162 months (Sarosi et al, 1970). The chest radiograph usually reveals bilateral apical nodular lesions and multiple cavities resembling tuberculosis or chronic histoplasmosis.

Asymptomatic pulmonary residua can be left in 5% of people infected by coccidioidomycosis. These residua are found as nodules or thin-walled cavities on chest radiography. Coccidioidal nodules (coccidioma) have gelatinous centers and often the spherules are identifiable (Fullerton, 1993). It was reported that as many as 30% to 50% of solitary pulmonary nodules are coccidiomas in the southwestern United States (Read, 1972). As the coccidiomas usually do not calcify, surgical resection may be indicated because of suspected carcinoma.

A pulmonary coccidioidal cavity may develop; as primary coccidioidal pneumonitis consolidates, it is followed by central necrosis leading to cavity formation. A patient with diabetes or a compromised immune system may be susceptible to a chronic form of *C. immitis* infection that is characterized by the development of a cavity in the lungs. During the necrosis and cavity formation, mild hemoptysis may occur in 70% of patients. The cavity usually remains asymptomatic and is found on routine chest radiography, on which it appears as a single, thin-walled cavity in the upper lung field, with little surrounding infiltrate. Spontaneous closure occurs in 27% of patients within 4 years (Winn, 1968). Major complications of a coccidioidal cavity include secondary infection by either pyogenic organisms and the development of a lung abscess or the formation of a fungus ball. Fungus balls are most commonly caused by *Aspergillus* species but they may be composed of mycelial elements of *C. immitis*. Other complications are cavity rupture, including bronchopleural fistula and empyema, and hemoptysis, which is common but rarely massive (Drutz and Catanzaro, 1978).

Disseminated Coccidioidomycosis. In about 0.5% of infected people, extrapulmonary disease, may occur in the meninges, bones and joints, skin, or soft tissues. The bones of the skull, hands, feet and spine and the tibia are common sites of infection. Joint lesions are unifocal in 90% of cases, and the ankles and knees are most commonly involved. Wart-like nodules are common skin lesions. When it involves the meninges, basilar meningitis is common (Bouza et al, 1981). Without treatment, 90% of patients with meningitis die within 12 months (Einstein et al, 1961). Cerebrospinal fluid (CSF) shows a mononuclear pleocytosis with a low glucose level and an elevated protein level. The CSF culture is usually negative. The demonstration of IgG antibody in CSF is another way to confirm the diagnosis.

Along with immunocompromised patients, infants, pregnant women, and nonwhite people are especially susceptible to disseminated *C. immitis* infection. Conditions that decrease T cell immunity, such as thymectomy or corticosteroid therapy, also increase susceptibility to infection. Organ transplant recipients, patients with malignancies (especially leukemics), and HIV-infected patients are at great risk. The mortality rate in the immunosuppressed population is usually above 40% (Robinson, 1999). The incidence of coccidioidomycosis among HIV-infected patients is increasing; such patients present with a fulminant course that includes diffuse pulmonary involvement in addition to disseminated infection (Kirkland and Fierer, 1996).

Diagnosis

The diagnosis of coccidioidomycosis can be made by several methods, including histology, culture, and serology. In tissue specimens, a mature spherule of *C. immitis* with endospore is pathognomonic of infection. The surrounding tissue often shows a granulomatous reaction. Early diagnosis of coccidioidomycosis can be made easily on the basis of clinical specimens such as pus, sputum, and aspirates of infected areas. A wet preparation can be examined repeatedly to identify hyphae that develop on the spherules. Sometimes bronchoscopy or needle aspiration is necessary to obtain an adequate specimen. The culture of sputum or BAL fluid is commonly negative in patients with HIV infection, so a lung biopsy may be needed.

C. immitis grows best on Sabouraud's glucose agar, forming colonies in 3 to 4 days. Mature colonies are extremely infectious and should be handled only by experienced personnel using appropriate equipment. *C. immitis* cannot be definitively identified in its mycelial form, so the mycelia should be converted into the parasitic form by inoculation of an animal, special culture conditions, or the detection of extracellular coccidioidal antigens produced by the growing fungus in culture. The last method seems safest because less handling of the cultures is required (Medical Section of the American Lung Association, 1985).

Serologic testing using the mycelial-phase antigen, coccidioidin, is a reliable method of detecting antibody (Pappagianis and Zimmer, 1990). Serum IgM is detected in 75% of patients with primary infection during the initial 1 to 3 weeks, then it disappears after 4 to 6 weeks but may reappear with the spread or relapse of the disease. Serum IgG antibody is detected at 4 to 6 weeks, attains its maximal level at 2 to 3 months, then disappears in several months if infection resolves. The severity of the disease and the prognosis for the patient are reflected by high or rising titers (American College of Chest Physicians, 1973; Medical Section of the American Lung Association, 1985; Penn et al, 1983). An elevated IgG serum antibody titer is a marker of disseminated, extrapulmonary disease. Changes in the serum antibody titer also reflect the course of the disease. False-positive serologic tests are rare.

Skin test responses to coccidioidal antigens become positive soon after the development of symptoms in all people with primary infections. Cross-reactions with other infections are rare. If the patient presents with erythema nodosum, the skin test should be involve a diluted agent so as to avoid severe reactions to the test. In a patient with progressive infection anergy is common and the skin test can be used to follow its course. The skin test does not interfere with serologic tests. Because anergy may develop and because a positive test indicates only in prior infection, the diagnostic role of the skin test is limited in coccidioidomycosis.

Treatment

For asymptomatic immunocompetent patients, no treatment is necessary. However, in an endemic area, patients may be treated with 200 to 400 mg fluconazole daily for variable periods. Occasionally patients in high-risk groups, such as blacks, Filipinos, and immunocompromised patients, are given more aggressive treatment. Some clinicians use fluconazole or ketoconazole for 6 months in all high-risk patients with acute coccidioidomycosis. Sometimes a total dose of 1000 to 2000 mg of amphotericin B is used in an attempt to prevent progression of the infection in members of high-risk groups (American Thoracic Society, 1979).

Chronic pulmonary coccidioidomycosis has been handled surgically with some success but with high complication rates because many of these patients have diminished pulmonary reserve, so it is probably best treated by administering antifungal agents.

The most common surgery performed for coccidioidomycosis is the resection of indeterminate solitary pulmonary nodules to rule out malignancy. In endemic areas, it has been reported that at least 60% of solitary pulmonary nodules are coccidioidomycosis (Cohen et al, 1972; Read, 1972). However, as the incidence of malignancy in the same studies was as high as 26% to 35%, the resection of these nodules appears to be prudent, even in endemic areas, especially with the development of the minimally invasive thoracoscopic technique.

Because the natural history of cavitary lesions in coccidioidomycosis is relatively benign, the indications for surgery remain unclear. In a large percentage of patients with cavitary disease, the lesions, especially if they are smaller than 2 cm, close spontaneously. Both late dissemination and intrapulmonary spread of chronic cavities are rare. When cavities enlarge or when symptoms such as a productive cough or hemoptysis develop, treatment with fluconazole in a dose of 400 mg for at least 6 months or with amphotericin B in a total dose of 1000 to 1500 mg has been recommended (American Thoracic Society, 1979).

Another option in this situation is surgical resection. Hyde and colleagues (1968) proposed that cavitary disease should not be operated on except in the case of repeated and severe hemoptysis, citing a high rate of bronchopleural fistula, empyema, and disability as a result of the operation. They also found a 20% rate of development of new cavities. In the nonoperated cases, one half of the cavities closed spontaneously, with a median closure time of 2 years (Hyde, 1968). As in cases of coccidioidal nodules, the most clear-cut indication for resection of cavitary coccidioidomycosis is the possibility of malignancy. Surgery may also have a role if the infection is complicated by severe hemoptysis, if the cavity has a thick wall, if it is secondarily infected, if it ruptures, or if it enlarges significantly during treatment. Even though the practice is controversial, it seems prudent to administer perioperative amphotericin B in a case of a ruptured cavity, particularly with pyopneumothorax and in immunocompromised patients with high risk for dissemination.

For coccidioidal meningitis, intrathecal amphotericin B is always necessary. Oral fluconazole (400–800 mg) or itraconazole (300–400 mg) may have a role in this situation (Galgiani et al, 1993; Tucker et al, 1990). In patients with extrapulmonary disseminated coccidioidomycosis, if immunocompetent, oral fluconazole 400 mg daily for 6 to 12 months can be tried, reserving amphotericin B for use if that treatment fails. If the disease progresses rapidly or if the patient is in a high-risk group, amphotericin B should be given immediately at minimum dose of 3000 mg. If the patient is immunocompromised, a higher dose is recommended. Life-long suppression therapy may be prudent in patients with permanent immunodepression.

Blastomycosis

Blastomycosis is caused by the fungus *Blastomyces dermatitidis*. It can occur in pulmonary, cutaneous, and disseminated form. The pulmonary form is often occult and has no particular features. Patients are usually asymptomatic; the fungus is usually discovered because of the finding of infiltrate on a chest radiograph. Treatment of blastomycosis has greatly improved with the use of drugs such as amphotericin B and other antifungal agents. If the disease is extremely mild, it may be merely observed. Surgery is performed only to rule out malignancy.

History

The first clinical description of blastomycosis was made by Gilchrist of Johns Hopkins University in 1894. Although he originally attributed a case of cutaneous blastomycosis to infection by a protozoan, he later correctly isolated the fungus in a patient with a long history of blastomycosis of the facial skin. When several additional cases were reported by Hektoen in the Cook County Hospital, the infection became known as Chicago's disease for several decades (Hektoen, 1907).

Epidemiology

Blastomycosis was referred to as North American blastomycosis when it was thought to exist only in North America. However, well-documented cases of blastomycosis have been reported in South America, Africa, and Asia, indicating more widespread existence of the organism (Bhagwandeen, 1974; Emmons et al, 1964; Fragoyannis et al, 1977).

B. dermatitidis has proved difficult to isolate from soil, and early attempts to develop a sensitive and reproducible skin test have failed; thus, the exact area which blastomycosis is endemic has not been defined, and reported cases have been used as markers for defining the endemic area (Furcolow et al, 1970; Klein et al, 1986; Sarosi and Davies, 1979). The central United States and Africa are the most heavily endemic areas. The western border lies in the Canadian province of Manitoba; the line of demarcation then moves south along the North Dakota–Minnesota border and continues to east Texas and Louisiana. The endemic area extends eastward across central Canada, the Midwest, and the southern United States (Allen et al, 1993).

The fungus is thought to grow well in nitrogen-rich soil close to streams, rivers, and lakes. Its growth is facilitated by rapidly increasing soil temperature. Disturbance of contaminated soil, as by rainfall or excavation, facilitates aerosolization of the fungus. Sporadic cases of blastomycosis are most common in middle-aged males with heavy vocational or recreational exposure to woods and streams. In highly endemic areas, cases are also linked to residences in close proximity to recreational water (Baumgardner et al, 1992).

Pathophysiology

In nature, the organism grows as an aerial mycelium in which the microconidia, the infecting particles, are lined up. If the contaminated soil is disturbed, an aerosol of particles is formed; inhaled, they eventually reach the alveoli. There, the organism converts to a parasitic form of yeast. The yeast begins to multiply, and the neutrophilic reaction results in an area of pneumonitis. The regional lymph nodes are commonly involved. Macrophages are also involved in the initial response; they interact with T lymphocytes, developing specific cell-mediated immunity. Histologically, the area of infiltrate shows a mixed neutrophilic and mononuclear cell infiltration. The inflammatory response to blastomycosis includes a mixture of pyogenic and granulomatous components (Sarosi and Davies, 1979). Therefore, the neutrophilic component remains, even after granuloma formation. After all organisms are contained, the infiltrate begins to round off and fibrosis takes place. This healed area of pneumonitis may be found incidentally as a coin lesion on a chest radiograph. Calcification is less common than histoplasmosis or coccidioidomycosis.

If delayed hypersensitivity does not develop, the fungus may disseminate throughout the body and involve the skin, bones, meninges, and prostate or adrenal glands,

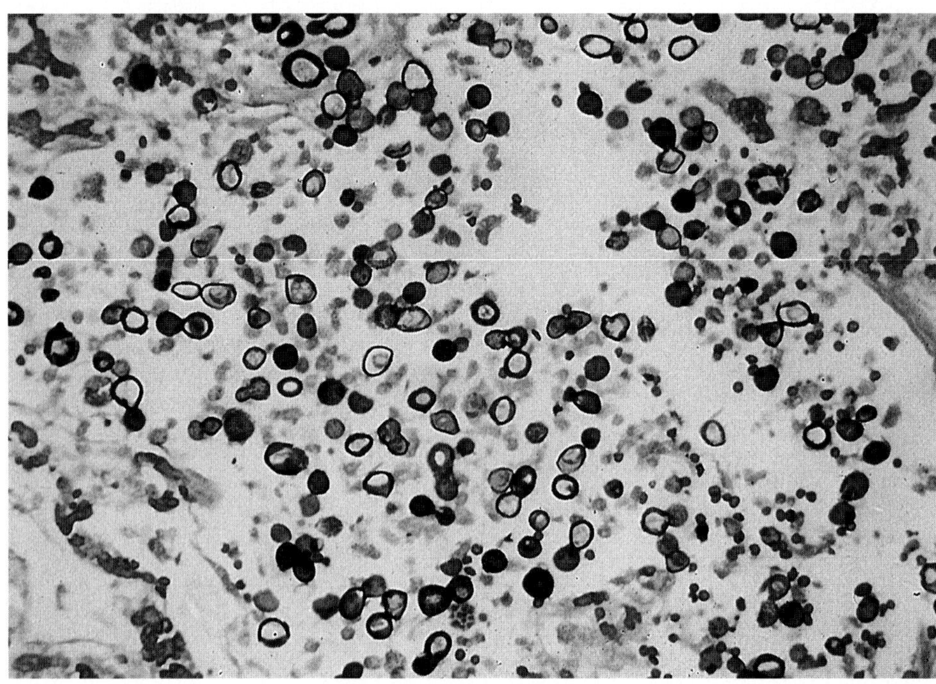

FIGURE 23–49 ■ Transbronchial lung biopsy specimen demonstrating *Blastomyces dermatitidis* in pulmonary tissue. Note the thick walls and broad-based budding.

producing progressive disease. In patients with T cell defects, such as transplant recipients, AIDS patients, and patients receiving high-dose glucocorticoid therapy for malignant or nonmalignant disease, blastomycosis can present as a progressive infection (Pappas et al, 1992). However, blastomycosis is much less common than is histoplasmosis in immunocompromised hosts.

Clinical Features

Several forms of blastomycosis exist: pulmonary, cutaneous, and disseminated. Most cases of pulmonary blastomycosis are sporadic and only a few cases have been recognized. some evidence suggests that asymptomatic infections can occur, although how commonly they occur is unknown (Vaaler et al, 1990). People may have brief flu-like illness that include fever, chills, headache, myalgias, and nonproductive cough and usually resolves rapidly (Sarosi et al, 1974). Usually, this group of patients is detected only during an outbreak. The initial symptoms resemble those of bacterial pneumonia: patients present with acute-onset high fever, productive cough, and pleuritic chest pain, and are usually first treated for bacterial pneumonia. Occasionally, patients may have scanty hemoptysis. With high fever, patients are likely to have shaking chills, tachycardia, and high white blood cell count with neutrophilia. The physical examination is usually negative. However, if patients have segmental or lobar disease, signs of lung consolidation may exist. Patients are usually not diagnosed correctly until more aggressive diagnostic strategies are employed after the failure of antibacterial therapy. Sputum examinations, including sodium-potassium-hydroxide (KOH)–digested smears and fungal cultures normally allow the diagnosis to be made. Other, more invasive diagnostic methods, such as bronchoscopy, needle aspiration, or thoracoscopic or open lung biopsy may be required for the correct diagnosis to be made (Fig. 23–49). Chest radiographs may show multiple nodules, raising early suspicion of a nonbacterial cause, but sometimes blastomyosis presents as a focal, even lobar, alveolar infiltrate. Although not common, a scattering of new skin lesions during unsuccessful antibacterial treatment may provide a clue to the correct diagnosis. Sometimes the disease can improve spontaneously concomitant with antibacterial therapy, when the sputum culture report reveals blastomycosis.

Most cases of sporadic blastomycosis fall into the categories of subacute or chronic illness. These patients may have low-grade fever, productive cough, night sweats, and weight loss as in tuberculosis. Others present with mass-like infiltrates, chronic cough, and weight loss, mimicking lung cancer. In approximately 25% of patients, extrapulmonary lesions such as skin or bone diseases are present. Direct smears, cultures, or histologic examinations of these lesions are helpful for diagnosis. However, the other 75% of patients have isolated pulmonary illness, and a specific diagnosis is necessary to rule out tuberculosis and other fungal diseases. When a patient has few symptoms but a radiograph of the chest reveals a mass, the aim of the diagnostic work-up is to differentiate the disease from possible malignancy. Serodiagnostic tests have a limited role in diagnosis. The immunodiffusion test has low sensitivity, so negative results are never helpful, but it has reasonable specificity, and a positive test result should lead to aggressive diagnostic procedures that will confirm or rule out the diagnosis. A direct smear or culture of material obtained by bronchoscopy or another technique may be diagnostic.

Rarely, a patient with pulmonary blastomycosis may present with a fulminant, infectious acute respiratory distress syndrome and show such symptoms as high fever, chills, productive cough, diffuse infiltrates, and hypoxemic respiratory failure. Pleuritis and pleural effusions may be present. Aspiration of pleural fluid may reveal the organism. The gas exchange is usually impaired and ventilatory support is commonly necessary. Air-space consolidation is present on chest radiographs. Such a patient has more than a 50% chance of dying, and survival may depend on rapid diagnosis and early therapy with a full dose of amphotericin B.

Cutaneous lesions are the next most common manifestation of pulmonary blastomycosis. Although infection can be contracted by direct skin inoculation in extremely rare conditions, the cutaneous manifestation is thought to represent dissemination from an initial pulmonary focus. Most lesions occur in patients with untreated or inadequately treated pulmonary infections. However, as many pulmonary infections are occult, skin lesions may arise without any pulmonary signs or symptoms. With direct inoculation, skin lymphatics are usually involved, and the infection may resolve spontaneously. In contrast, the disseminated form presents as one or more subcutaneous nodules that eventually break through to the skin surface. Most commonly, they appear on exposed skin such as the face, upper lip, cheek, hand, or wrist (Witorsch and Utz, 1968). The initial lesion may take weeks or months to evolve and after time may spread to the trunk. If untreated, the ulcers spread by slow advancement, often taking years to evolve. The pustule can be aspirated for identification of the organism.

Disseminated blastomycosis can involve the bones. The most common sites of bony infection are vertebrae, ribs, and skull (Witorsch and Utz, 1968). The long bones may be involved in one third of cases (Schwarz, 1984). Bone infection presents as a chronically draining sinus or as an abscess. Débridement may be required for cure, but most bone lesions resolve with antifungal therapy alone. The infection may also affect the genitourinary system. Prostatitis and epididymo-orchitis have been the most common infections reported. When the genitourinary tract is involved, other systemic manifestations of the disease are usually present.

Infection occurs in the central nervous system in 5% to 10% and presents either as an abscess or as meningitis. The diagnosis of meningitis is more difficult because the organism is not always recovered in a lumbar puncture. Aspiration of ventricular fluid is often necessary to obtain a positive culture (Kravitz et al, 1981). Blastomycosis can also involve the oropharynx and the larynx, usually as hematogenous spread (Durnich and Neel, 1983).

Diagnosis

Radiographic findings are extremely variable in pulmonary blastomycosis. A review of Mayo Clinic cases revealed that a mass was the most common finding (Fig. 23–50), whereas in other series, an infiltrate was reported to be the most common finding (Brown et al, 1991; Sheflin et al, 1990). In acute pulmonary disease, a chest radiograph shows a pattern of consolidation resembling bacterial pneumonia, either unilateral or bilateral, with or without regional lymph node enlargement. Sometimes there is a diffuse miliary pattern. The infiltration is typically patchy, with poorly defined borders. The density may become mass-like or may cavitate. After the acute process resolves, the patterns change to granuloma formation, fibrosis, and volume loss (Cush et al, 1976). In chronic pulmonary blastomycosis, a chest radiograph can reveal nodular densities with extensive fibrosis and contraction. Although the majority show fibronodular densities with or without cavitation, a pneumonic infiltrate may persist (Cush et al, 1976). The organism has a predilection for the upper lobes but can affect any lobe. Pleural effusions may be seen in the chronic form of blastomyeosis, but it is not a common finding (Kinasewitz et al, 1984). The infiltrate often extends to the hilum and may mimic bronchogenic carcinoma. In the review of 35 Mayo Clinic patients with blastomycosis 55% of patients were found to have undergone thoracotomy because radiographs suggested carcinoma. Findings in CT scans of the chest include air bronchogram, consolidation, intermediate-sized nodules, satellite lesions, lymphadenopathy, and pleural disease. However, radiologic studies alone cannot exclude carcinoma.

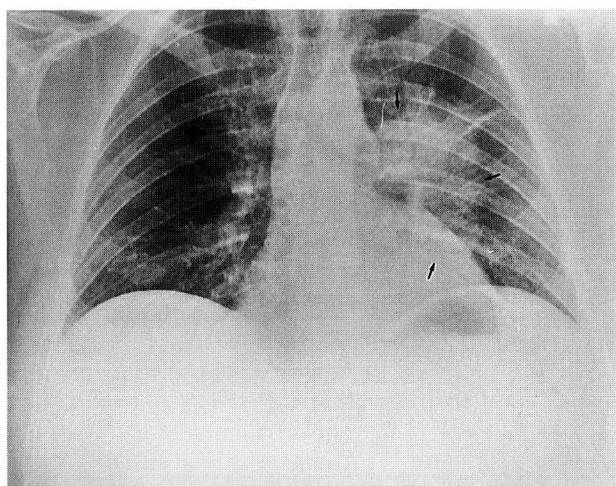

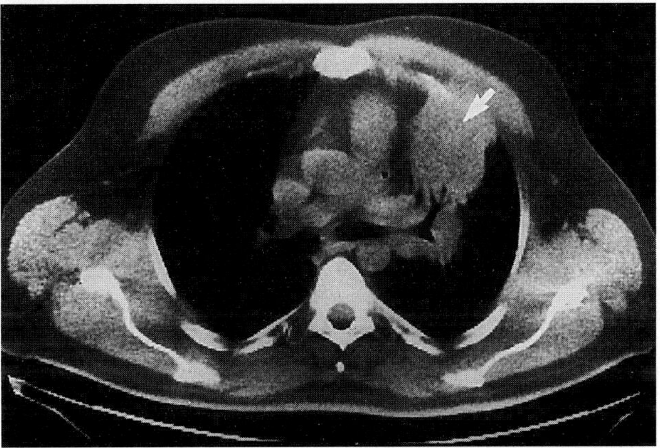

FIGURE 23–50 ■ Chest radiograph and computed tomography scan of a left hilar mass. Transbronchial biopsy was positive for *Blastomyces dermatitidis*.

Although early serologic tests for blastomycosis were disappointing, a recent use of more specific *B. dermatitidis* cell wall antigens and DNA probes have significantly improved their sensitivity and specificity. At present, the most reliable serologic tests are the sandwich enzyme immunoassay and the 120-kd antigen radioimmunoassay, which have a sensitivity of 85% to 88% and specificity of 100% (Klein and Jones, 1990; Lo and Notenboom, 1990).

However, a negative serologic test cannot be used to exclude blastomycosis.

A definitive diagnosis of blastomycosis depends on demonstration of the presence of *B. dermatitidis* in body fluids or tissue specimens by staining or culture. Because the inflammatory response to a blastomycotic infection is predominantly a polymorphonuclear leukocyte reaction, a patient usually produces large amounts of sputum or pus in the infected area. Also, because the organism is relatively large in its tissue phase (5–20 μm in diameter) and shows a characteristic wide-based budding with double refractile walls, direct microscopic diagnosis of blastomycosis is much more common than is that of other fungal infections. Repeated microscopic examination of early-morning sputum samples commonly reveal the organism. Fiberoptic bronchoscopy with brushing, washing, and transbronchial biopsy may be used to obtain an adequate specimen. When bronchoscopy is performed, the concentration of lidocaine used for local anesthesia should not exceed 1 g/dl so as to reduce the its antifungal effect (Taylor et al, 1983). If pleural effusion is present, fluid from thoracentesis should be sent for fungal smears and cultures. Specimens of other body fluids and tissues may also yield the diagnosis. Sputum or prostatic fluid should be prepared with a 10% KOH solution and examined under a microscope using reduced illumination. The multi-nucleated yeast cells vary in diameter from 5 to 20 μm and are so thick-walled that they appear to be double-walled or encapsulated budding from mother cells with broad bases. Various techniques, such as the periodic acid–Schiff methenamine silver, and Papanicolaou stains, are used to demonstrate the organism on histopathologic section.

Even when initial smears do not reveal the organism, cultures are commonly positive. The growth may be detected as early as 5 to 7 days or as late as 30 days, depending on the size of the inoculum. Therefore, specimens should not be considered negative until 4 weeks of incubation have passed. Growth is usually suspected based on the detecting of grayish-white or beige colonies. If the isolate does not produce arthroconidia or tuberculate macroconidia but produces filamentous colonies revealing uniform septate hyphae, conversion to the yeast form at 37°C should demonstrate yeasts forming broad-based buds (Kaufman, 1992). When the number of *B. dermatitidis* organisms is small, the use of specific immunofluorescent reagents is recommended for accurate and specific identification (Areno et al, 1997). If a more rapid identification is needed, 24-hour exoantigen tests or even more rapid 2-hour DNA probes are commercially available (Kaufman, 1992).

Treatment

For the subclinical disease, antifungal agents may not be necessary. Many immunocompetent patients with acute blastomycosis recover without therapy. However, controversies exist on how to treat patients with symptomatic blastomycosis.

The drug of choice for acute, non–life-threatening infection is itraconazole 400 mg orally daily for at least 6 months (Dismukes et al, 1992). Ketoconazole (400–800 mg daily for 6 months) is also effective therapy for acute symptomatic blastomycosis (National Institute of Allergy and Infection Diseases, 1983). However, itraconazole is usually recommended because of its higher efficacy and lower toxicity.

If a patient has diffuse infiltrates and severe hypoxemia, the drug of choice would be amphotericin B. Amphotericin B should be administered until the patient's condition is stable. The usual total cumulative dose is 500 to 1000 mg. Once the patient's condition has stabilized, the antifungal medication can be switched to itraconazole or ketoconazole and then continued for a minimum of 6 additional months. In immunocompromised hosts, acute pulmonary blastomycosis should be treated with 1000 mg of amphotericin B as a primary therapy followed by oral azoles for 6 months (Pappas et al, 1993).

For extrapulmonary disease, if the patient is immunocompetent and the lesion is nonmeningeal, ketoconazole and itraconazole are highly effective, and amphotericin B can be reserved for cases of rapid progression and for refractory cases. If blastomycosis involves the meninges, the treatment of choice is amphotericin B, usually a total dose of 2000 to 3000 mg (Sarosi et al, 1986). For the immunocompromised patient with meningeal disease, ketoconazole is not effective, as it poorly penetrates the CSF. A prolonged course of amphotericin B should be followed by either a weekly administration of 50 mg of amphotericin B or an extended course (6 to 12 months) of itraconazole, with a dose of 400 mg daily (Pappas et al, 1993).

Reactivation has been discovered after initial pulmonary infection both treated and untreated (Landis and Varkey, 1976; Recht et al, 1979). If therapy is not given, a patient should be monitored for a prolonged period. In a patient with life-threatening or central nervous system blastomycosis, amphotericin B should be given. The role of surgery in blastomycosis is only to confirm the disease or to rule out malignancy. The indications for resective pulmonary surgery are few because of the effectiveness of medical therapy.

Pulmonary Cryptococcosis

Cryptococcosis is caused by *Cryptococcus neoformans*, an encapsulated, yeast-like, budding saprophyte that is found in soil and avian excrement especially that of the pigeon. It used to be known as torulosis and European blastomycosis. Although the port of entry seems to be the respiratory tract, it can also involve the central nervous system. A pulmonary disease does not receive as much attention as a disease of the central nervous system, perhaps because it is less dramatic and is rarely life-threatening. The diagnosis of pulmonary cryptococcosis is usually made in retrospect or when the organism has been recovered from some other body site.

History

The first clinical case of pulmonary cryptococcosis without involvement of the central nervous system was reported by Sheppe in 1924. Greening and Menville (1947) described spontaneous healing of pulmonary lesions while disease was progressing in the central nervous system. It was noted that pulmonary disease rarely disseminated in untreated immunocompetent hosts, whereas it almost always disseminated in untreated immunosuppressed individuals (Kerkering et al, 1981). The association of cryptococcosis with AIDS was reported in 1988 (Snider et al, 1983).

Epidemiology

C. neoformans exists as a yeast both in nature and in tissue. With its distinguishing capsule, *C. neoformans* can range from 5 to 20 μm in size. Occasionally, however, noncapsulated strains can be encountered in the clinical setting (Harding et al, 1979). This organism is found worldwide; it grows in soil heavily contaminated with pigeon droppings and in dried bird excreta on windowsills and in church steeples.

The incidence of cryptococcosis has steadily increased over the past decade mainly because of the existence of AIDS, and cryptococcosis is now the fourth most common opportunistic infection in AIDS patients (Currie and Casadevall, 1994).

Pathophysiology

C. neoformans infects the respiratory tract through inhalation. The organism has a thick, sticky capsule, which makes it difficult to be aerosolized or to reach the alveolar space. To reach the alveoli, an organism must have a diameter of less than 2 μm. The naturally aerosolized organisms are not encapsulated, and organisms in desiccated pigeon droppings are commonly smaller than 2 μm (Neilson et al, 1977). There have been no reports of animal-to-human transmission of this disease, and human-to-human transmission is also extremely rare, possibly because of the size of the organism and the presence of the capsule. Similarly, there have never been any reports of infection by means of exposure in the laboratory.

The immunity of the individual host influences the course of the clinical disease. The spectrum of this disease is diverse—signs and symptoms may range from none to overt pneumonia. The histopathologic findings also range from complete absence of inflammatory cells to the presence of exuberant granuloma. This diverse clinical picture seems to be related to varying forms of immunopathogenesis. Cell-mediated immunity is the major defense against the organism (Kerkering et al, 1981; Kovacs et al, 1985; Schimpff and Bennett, 1975). Therefore, patients with AIDS, patients with malignancies of the lymphoreticular system, patients on chronic corticosteroid therapy, solid organ transplant recipients, and sarcoidosis patients are more commonly diagnosed and present more commonly with disseminated disease.

Instead of producing a toxin to destroy the surrounding tissue, these organisms affect tissue by means of mechanical pressure, as the number of yeast cells increases. It has been demonstrated that the cryptococcal antigen can reduce the production of anticryptococcal antibodies (Diamond and Erickson, 1982) and also can induce suppressor lymphocytes (Murphy and Moorhead, 1982). Therefore, if large numbers of organisms are inoculated, the host immune mechanism may be suppressed, allowing the organism to proliferate and cause disease even in an immunocompetent host. This can explain the occasional cases of cryptococcal meningitis in normal hosts. In patients with deficiencies in cell-mediated immunity, the proliferation of the organism can proceed unchecked. An increase in antigens can further suppress the remaining function of the immune system, resulting in overwhelming disseminated disease. Corticosteroid therapy was also noted to increase susceptibility to cryptococcosis, and conditions causing a severely immunocompromised host are significant.

Clinical Features

The clinical features of pulmonary cryptococcosis are nonspecific. Immunocompetent patients may be asymptomatic or may experience low-grade fever, cough, vague chest pain, mild dyspnea, hemoptysis, night sweats, fatigue, and weight loss (Bates, 1970; Campbell, 1966; Kerkering et al, 1981; Warr et al, 1968; Wasser and Talavera, 1987). Patients are commonly found to have extrapulmonary disease. The diagnosis of cryptococcosis is made retrospectively based on abnormalities seen on radiographs of the chest. Patients with deficient cell-mediated immunity, however, may present with marked dyspnea and hypoxia and show diffuse interstitial infiltrates on chest radiographs.

Physical examination reveals no specific finding that suggests pulmonary cryptococcosis. Evidence of extrapulmonary involvement such as lesions of the skin, central nervous system, or prostate should make cryptococcosis the most probable differential diagnosis.

Diagnosis

Radiographic findings vary. Immunocompetent patients are usually seen to have single or multiple pulmonary nodules (Feigin, 1983; Khoury et al, 1984). Symptomatic immunocompetent patients may present with large single masses that have gelatinous collections in them. More than 90% of patients with HIV infection show diffuse interstitial infiltrates (Miller et al, 1990). In the third group of patients, those with partially responsive immune systems (including individuals on chronic corticosteroid therapy, those with hematologic malignancies, organ transplant recipients, and patients with sarcoidosis) radiographic findings may vary widely. Single or multiple nodular lesions are most common. Sometimes a nodule may cavitate and a large cavitary nodule can mimic an abscess. Hilar adenopathy may be concomitant. The next most common lesions are patch alveolar infiltrates which are seen primarily in patients who are more immunosuppressed than patients with nodules. Pleural effusion rarely occurs.

When *C. neoformans* organisms are isolated in the sputum, it must be determined whether their presence represents simple colonization of the airway or true cryptococcal disease. Reiss and colleagues found *C. neoformans* in the sputum of 6 of 92 patients with malignant disease, but no member of the group showed evidence of overt cryptococcal disease (Reiss and Szilazyl, 1965). This suggested that a carrier state does exist in humans. Therefore, specimens from the deeper portion, such as

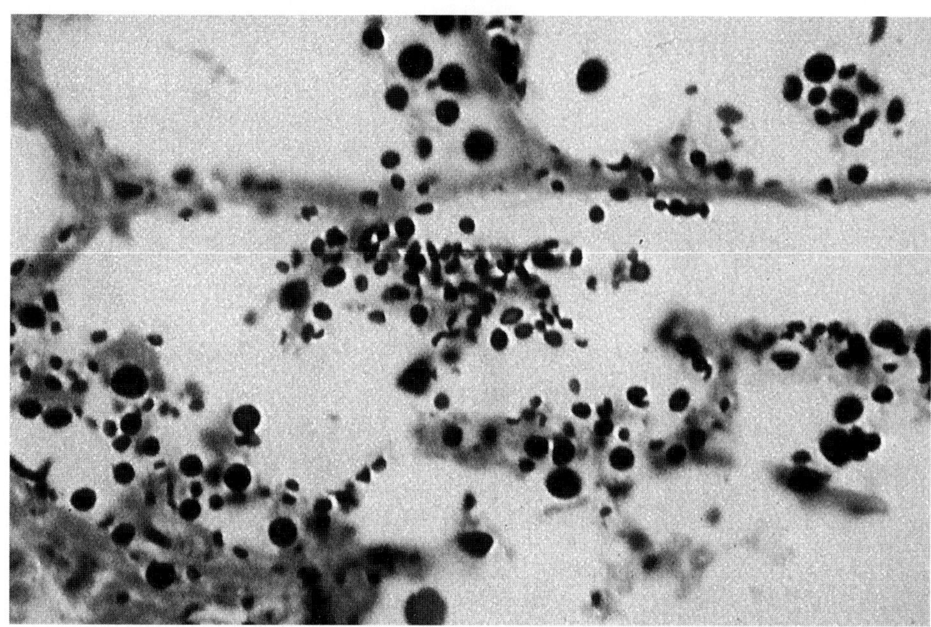

FIGURE 23–51 ■ *Cryptococcus neoformans* showing the characteristic capsule and the narrow budding.

BAL, fine-needle aspiration, and thoracentesis are sometimes necessary (Randhawa and Pal, 1977). BAL provide the highest diagnostic yield in AIDS patients in whom the lesion is usually alveolar or interstitial (Malabonga et al, 1991). For a nodular or mass-like lesion, CT scans should be made to localize the lesion and, if it is feasible, CT-guided fine-needle aspiration should be used to make the diagnosis. If the needle does not reach, transbronchial biopsy, thoracoscopy, or conventional open-lung biopsy can be helpful, depending on the clinical circumstances. If the patient has a skin ulcer, a swab of the lesion stained with India ink reveals yeast under microscopic examination.

Routine hematoxylin and eosin stain does not stain the yeast but is helpful for ascertaining the inflammatory response. Periodic acid–Schiff stain with a pale background may be used to stain the organism. If *C. neoformans* is suspected based on the presence of a capsule and narrow budding (Fig. 23–51), mucicarmine stain will color the capsule yellow to red. Although Gomori-methenamine-silver stains the organism black, it does not stain the capsule. If capsule-deficient cryptococcus is suspected, especially in patients with AIDS a Fontana-Masson stain can be helpful (Ro et al, 1987).

Cryptococcal skin tests have not been standardized, so they are not recommended. The cryptococcal antigen has a higher than 95% sensitivity and specificity (Currie et al, 1993; Tanner et al, 1994). The serum cryptococcal antigen is positive in 99% of patients with cryptococcal meningitis and in those with HIV infection. Although a positive result does not necessarily indicate that invasion into the central nervous system has occurred it indicates the need to perform a lumbar puncture. The serum cryptococcal antigen is usually not detected in patients with pulmonary cryptococcosis unless there is extrapulmonary dissemination. Therefore, a negative result for the serum cryptococcal antigen does not rule out pulmonary cryptococcosis. However, a negative serum antigen test suggests that it is unlikely that there is disease in the central nervous system and the test may be helpful in screening symptomatic patients.

A definitive diagnosis can be made by culturing the specimen. *C. neoformans* is readily cultured in a routine fungal medium that does not contain cycloheximide. Growth is more rapid at temperatures below 37°C and is usually visible by 72 to 96 hours.

Treatment

Although surgical therapy played a prominent role in the early treatment of localized disease, it seldom comes into play today. There still may be selected cases in which resection will be helpful, but usually the role of the thoracic surgeon remains limited to diagnosis or ruling out neoplasm.

The treatment strategy for the pulmonary cryptococcosis is determined by the immune status of the patient and the presence of extrapulmonary dissemination. Once the diagnosis of pulmonary cryptococcosis has been made, an evaluation for extrapulmonary dissemination must be undertaken. If there is extrapulmonary dissemination, the antifungal therapy should be based on the primary site and the immunologic state of the host. In immunocompetent patients, treatment can be accomplished by administering amphotericin B 0.4 mg/kg daily in combination with 100 to 150 mg/kg flucytosine daily for 4 to 6 weeks (Utz et al, 1975). In severely immunocompromised patients, Sarosi and Davies recommend significantly increased doses of amphotericin B for therapy of meningitis or invasive pulmonary disease. Flucytosine is potentially toxic to bone marrow, particularly in patients with AIDS, so its blood level must be monitored to maintain serum levels below 100 μg/ml (Sarosi and Davies, 1994).

When cryptococcal pneumonia has been diagnosed in an immunocompetent patient without extrapulmonary dissemination, a period of observation is indicated. However, because a minor risk of meningitis does exist, treatment with fluconazole may be recommended (Davies, 1994). The optimal duration of oral antifungal therapy is still undetermined for this group of patients. Because immunocompromised patients with pulmonary cryptococcosis usually progress to meningitis, 0.7 mg/kg intravenous amphotericin B daily (usually a total cumulative dose of 1000 to 2000 mg) with or without 100 to 150 mg/kg flucytosine daily should be given to prevent meningitis (Kerkering et al, 1981; Sugar and Saunders, 1988). AIDS patients with positive cultures of sputum or other respiratory specimens usually have positive serum antigens as well as positive cerebrospinal fluid. If the patient shows depressed consciousness, initial therapy is 0.7 mg/kg intravenous amphotericin B combined with 100 mg/kg flucytosine if tolerated, followed by lifetime fluconazole (Sugar and Saunders, 1988). All others may be treated with 200 mg fluconazole daily from the onset, and it should be continued for life (Davies, 1994).

Mucormycosis

Pulmonary mucormycosis is a rare but commonly fatal disease caused by fungi of the subclass Zygomycetes. Other names, such as zygomycosis or phycomycosis, are also used.

History

The first perimortem diagnosis was described by Harris in 1955 and the first surgical cure of pulmonary mucormycosis was reported by Dillon and colleagues in 1958.

Epidemiology and Pathophysiology

Mucor species are ubiquitous and are usually found in soil, manure, or decaying food, with no particular geographic distribution. Infection occurs by inhalation of spores and is commonly found in immunocompromised hosts. The risk factors that predispose for this infection include prolonged neutropenia, acidosis, hyperglycemia, and chelation therapy involving deferoxamine. *Mucor* species grow best in acidic, high-glucose media, which explains the susceptibility of diabetic, ketoacidotic patients. Pathogenic *Mucor* species produce very few siderophores, and it is thought that their infectivity may be greatly enhanced by the iron delivery of deferoxamine.

The clinical manifestations and rate of development are determined by the port of entry and by underlying factors in the host. Once the organism invades the blood vessels, vascular thrombosis, tissue ischemia, and infarction of adjacent tissue occurs. Necrotic debris and infected tissue form a black pus that can be seen in rhinocerebral mucormycosis. The infarcted tissue promotes rapid extension of infection.

Clinical Features

Manifestations have traditionally been divided into six separate syndromes: (1) rhinocerebral, (2) pulmonary, (3) cutaneous, (4) gastrointestinal, (5) disseminated into the central nervous system, and (6) miscellaneous (bones, kidneys, heart, and mediastinum). Patients with poorly controlled diabetes usually have rhinocerebral mucormycosis but may also have pulmonary infection. Patients with prolonged neutropenia usually have the pulmonary form but occasionally have rhinocerebral infection. Although spore inhalation may result in colonization, healthy individuals are not infected because inhaled spores are eliminated by pulmonary macrophages. Pulmonary mucormycosis in neutropenic patients resembles pulmonary aspergilloma, involving persistent fever and pulmonary infiltrates refractory to antibacterial therapy. Pulmonary infection presents initially with bronchopneumonia. The infection progresses to invade pulmonary vasculature, forming thrombosis and subsequent infarction, with late dissemination to extrapulmonary tissues. The organism can directly invade the chest wall, diaphragm, pericardium, myocardium and, rarely, trachea, causing airway obstruction (Schwartz et al, 1982).

Diagnosis

Radiographic findings in the chest are variable; they include bronchopneumonia, segmental or lobar consolidation, cavity formation and, occasionally, pleural effusion and fungus ball formation (Bartrum et al, 1973; Meyer et al, 1972; Silver et al, 1989) (Fig. 23–52). The infection usually progresses rapidly. An important aid to diagnosis is recognition by the attending physician that the disease occurs in patients with predisposing clinical factors and almost never occurs in their absence. Pulmonary infection is heralded by the onset of fever, cough, sputum production, and respiratory distress, which is commonly severe. Hemoptysis is an ominous sign. Other opportunistic fungi (*Aspergillus* and *Candida* species) may colonize the same respiratory tract and confuse the picture. Culture results are commonly negative but if positive, they strongly suggest invasive disease. A diagnosis of pulmonary mucormycosis is usually made by means of histopathology. Because in the clinical setting patients often present with prolonged neutropenia and pulmonary lesions, the initial clinical suspicion is aspergillosis. If the clinical specimen, such as KOH-digested sputum, shows characteristic broad, aseptate hyphae with stubby, right-angled, fingerlike, 45-degree branches, the diagnosis of mucormycosis can be made. However, if the sputum is negative, BAL, bronchial brushing, or transbronchial biopsies may be required to obtain an adequate specimen. It was observed that in the lung, the fungus penetrated bronchial walls and had a propensity to penetrate artery and vein walls, with the fungus invading living, rather than necrotic, tissue. Occasionally, thoracoscopic or open lung biopsy is the only test that will allow the diagnosis to be made. Rhinocerebral mucormycosis is diagnosed by clinical syndrome and confirmed by tissue biopsy. *Mucor* species are difficult to culture in the laboratory, so culture of the organism plays a smaller role in diagnosis. There are currently no routinely available serum immunologic assays for the detection of mucormycosis. An undiagnosed patient can progress to respiratory failure and death.

Treatment

Initial treatment consists of correcting underlying factors, instituting appropriate antifungal therapy, and performing

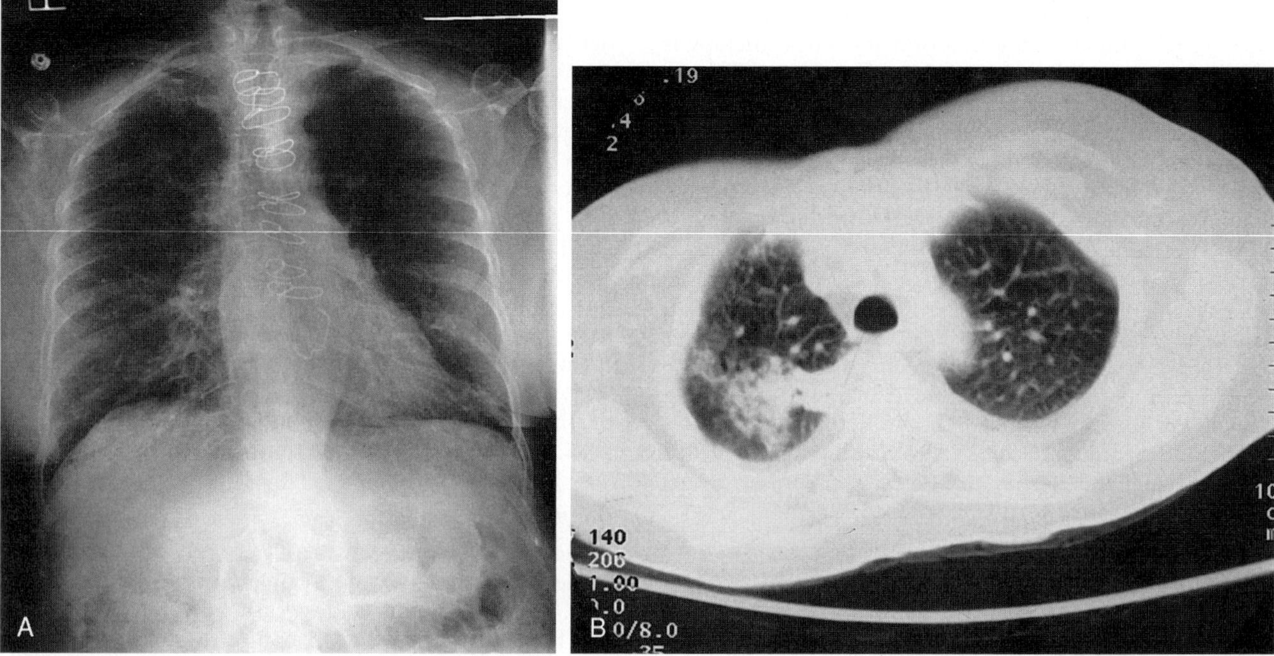

FIGURE 23–52 ■ Chest radiograph *(A)* and computed tomography scan *(B)* of a 70-year-old diabetic female who presented with hemoptysis. Surgical resection revealed pulmonary mucormycosis.

surgical resection when it is indicated. The overall mortality rate of patients with pulmonary mucormycosis is 56%. Patients with renal insufficiency or metabolic acidosis have the worst prognosis. Because diabetes is one of the most common predisposing factors, the correction of ketoacidosis is a vital component of therapy. Reversal of immunosuppression is also imperative for resolution of infection. To recover granulocytopenia, which is essential for survival, various hematopoietic growth factors such as granulocyte colony stimulating factor (G-CSF) and granulocyte-macrophage colony stimulating factor (GM-CSF) can be used (Antman et al, 1988; Brandt et al, 1988; Bronchud et al, 1987). Corticosteroids should be reduced in dosage or discontinued. Amphotericin B is the only effective antifungal agent at this time. Patients should be started on amphotericin B at the time of diagnosis, with a dose of 1.0 to 1.5 mg/kg/day (Walsh and Pizzo, 1988). The optimal duration of administration of amphotericin B is unknown. Therefore, the treatment should be individualized according to the patient's clinical response and the rate of clearing of the infection. The total dose of amphotericin B for the treatment of mucormycosis is not defined either. In most cases, a total dose of 2000 mg has been administered, although some patients have received up to 4000 mg. If there is no response, pulmonary resection of any localized disease should be performed. As much devitalized tissue and necrotic debris as possible should be removed. Although several cases have been cured by surgery alone, even when localized mucormycosis has apparently been completely excised, amphotericin B may still be required. Moreover, lobar or segmental resection of pulmonary mucormycotic lesions restricted to one region of the lung may be as effective in controlling progression of pneumonia as high-dose amphotericin B.

Actinomycosis and Nocardiosis

The Actinomycetales includes the families Actinomycetaceae and Nocardiaceae; they were once considered fungi but are currently classified as bacteria.

The diagnosis of actinomycosis can be difficult. Patients commonly present with progressive pulmonary fibrosis in the periphery of the lung, often in the lower lobes. Associated with this pulmonary fibrosis is a dull, aching pain caused by infection that permeates the pleura and creates periostitis around ribs. This periostitis should indicate the diagnosis. It is common for surgeons to be called upon to treat such patients after a diagnosis of empyema or pulmonary neoplasm has not been confirmed. At thoracotomy, massive, highly vascular fibrosis is usually encountered, and biopsies fail to reveal the diagnosis. Unless actinomycosis is suspected, the appropriate bacteriologic examination will not be made. The classic sulphur granules are rarely encountered in lung involvement. Even with a high index of suspicion, the clinician must order the appropriate testing on biopsy material to make the diagnosis. Because of the extremely intense fibrosis that is encountered, resection of the affected area is usually futile.

Actinomycosis should be considered a possible diagnosis in a patient with poor oral hygiene who has suspected aspiration pneumonia. An aggressive diagnostic approach and a high index of suspicion have resulted in increased survival rates. Medical therapy consists of long-term penicillin.

Nocardiosis should be suspected in any immunocompromised patient who has antibiotic-refractory pneumonia. Concomitant cerebral and pulmonary abscess is also suggestive of this diagnosis. Detailed sputum analysis may be diagnostic, but usually bronchial washings or tissue are needed. Sulfamethoxazole-trimethoprim is the treatment of choice.

Candidiasis

Although *Candida* species are among the most prevalent fungi, candidiasis is not commonly encountered by the thoracic surgeon. These opportunistic fungi usually infect all immunocompromised hosts and patients enduring long-term hospitalization who are receiving prolonged antibiotic therapy, allowing fungal overgrowth, and have indwelling urinary catheters, intravenous tubes, or endotracheal tubes (Penn et al, 1983).

Special clinical situations seen by the thoracic surgeon are the rare *Candida* pneumonia, esophagitis, or endocarditis. *Candida* meningitis also may be seen.

Diagnosis

Diagnosis of invasive candidiasis presents special problems. Species of *Candida* are present in 50% to 60% of respiratory secretions drawn from uninfected patients. Cultures cannot separate colonization from tissue invasion. Positive blood culture findings for *Candida* species require a careful search for the source. Vascular catheters should be removed or moved. Candidemia should be treated to improve survival and abort late metastatic infections by *Candida* species (Terrell and Hughes, 1992). Positive central nervous system cultures are diagnostic because that is a normally sterile site (Sarosi et al, 1985).

Although reports of useful serologic tests have been common, no reliable serologic test is available. Assessment of metabolites of *Candida* species may be useful in the future.

Treatment

Candidemia should be treated with amphotericin B to a total dose of 250 to 1000 mg. *Candida* pneumonia requires a lung biopsy before therapy because the tracheobronchial tree in hospitalized patients is usually colonized with *Candida* species (American Thoracic Society, 1979).

Mild cases of esophagitis may be treated with oral nystatin. Ketoconazole and itraconazole are useful in this situation, but fluconazole may be the best form of therapy for significant esophageal candidiasis. Failure to respond promptly should lead to therapy with amphotericin B alone or in synergy with flucytosine.

Candida endocarditis has been described by Norenberg and colleagues (1975). Fungal endocarditis on a prosthetic valve is usually caused by *Aspergillus* or *Candida* species and requires intensive amphotericin B therapy and prompt valve replacement (Cowgill et al, 1986). Because of the tendency of vegetations of *Candida* species to be bulky, there is always a risk that a large fungal thrombus will be released into the bloodstream as an embolus. Special care must be exercised in such cases to avoid this occurrence when the patient is undergoing cardiopulmonary bypass for replacement of an infected valve.

Sporotrichosis

The causative agent of sporotrichosis is *Sporothrix schenckii*. It is a biphasic fungus and is found worldwide in soil. Because it regularly inhabits plants and thorned bushes, the cutaneous form is usually seen in gardeners and florists. Pulmonary infection is rare, and van Trigt (1990) noted that it mimics tuberculosis in its manifestations in the lung. Hilar adenopathy, a persistent pulmonary infiltrate, and cavitary disease are the most common radiographic findings.

The rarity of pulmonary infection is emphasized by the early article of Ridgeway and colleagues (1962) who reported successful resection of cavitary disease in two patients. They could find only 10 other cases in the literature, none of which had been operated on. Scott and associates (1961) found 20 cases in a literature search, but only 6 had been adequately documented.

Diagnosis

Suspicion of pulmonary sporotrichosis should be aroused in the physician when a patient who works in gardening activities presents with a chronic respiratory illness. The onset is insidious. Low-grade fever and gradual weight loss are common. Chest radiographs show chronic pneumonitis with fibrosis and cavitation and most closely resemble films of histoplasmosis or tuberculosis. Serologic tests are not usually performed, although a tube agglutination test is useful in diagnosing the rare extracutaneous infection (Sarosi et al, 1985).

The organism is commonly found in the sputum and may be easily grown in culture within 3 to 5 days. Culture at 37°C yields the yeast form in 1 or 2 additional days, and this evidence of dimorphism is also diagnostic (Sarosi et al, 1985). Recognition of the characteristic yeast cell in pathologic specimens is accomplished only with difficulty (Baum et al, 1969) even with the use of special stains (Sarosi et al, 1985).

Treatment

Although potassium iodide has been used effectively for antifungal therapy in the cutaneous form for many years, amphotericin B is effective and should be used in the pulmonary variety. Mohr and coworkers (1979) observed cases that were not cured by amphotericin B but responded to iodide therapy. Baum and colleagues (1969), Takaro (1989), and Van Trigt (1990) recommend combined surgical and amphotericin B therapy. Pluss and Opal (1986) also concluded that pulmonary disease should be resected with adjuvant pre- and postoperative amphotericin B and that imidazoles have been ineffective in a few patients. They do not completely dismiss the use of iodide as adjuvant therapy.

Terrell and Hughes (1992) indicate that itraconazole is effective against cutaneous and lymphangitic forms of the disease and suggest, based on isolated case reports, that deep-seated infections might also respond to this agent.

The American Thoracic Society (1988) report suggests that the response to a saturated solution of potassium iodide, amphotericin B, and ketoconazole has been variable and that itraconazole is effective in a small number of cases. Because early authors (Takaro 1967; Michelson, 1977); noted that surgical resection of localized pulmonary infection had produced successful outcomes, the role of adjuvant antifungal agents is difficult to assess in the rare patient with pulmonary infection. No nonsurgical form of therapy is clearly effective; therefore, resectional therapy should be used in localized pulmonary infection.

CONCLUSION

It is important for the general thoracic surgeon to remain aware of the spectrum of presentations of pulmonary mycoses. Surgical intervention, although not commonly performed, can be challenging.

■ *REFERENCES*

Albelda SM, Talbot GH, Gerson SL et al: Pulmonary cavitation and massive hemoptysis in invasive pulmonary aspergillosis: Influence of bone marrow recovery in patients with acute leukemia. Am Rev Respir Dis 131:115, 1985.

Allen M, Trastek V, Descahmps C et al: Blastomycosis. In Faber L (ed): Chest Surgery Clinics of North America. Philadelphia, WB Saunders, 1993, p 627.

Allendoerfer R, Biovin GP, Deepe GS Jr: Modulation of immune responses in murine pulmonary histoplasmosis. J Infect Dis 175:905, 1997.

al-Majed SA, Ashour M, el-Kassimi FA et al: Management of post-tuberculous complex aspergilloma of the lung: Role of surgical resection. Thorax 45:846, 1990.

al-Zeerah M, Jeyasingham K: Limited thoracoplasty in the management of complicated pulmonary aspergillomas. Thorax 44:1027, 1989.

American College of Chest Physicians. The current status of serologic, immunologic and skin tests in the diagnosis of pulmonary mycoses. Report of the Committee on Fungus Diseases and Subcommittee on Criteria for Clinical Diagnosis—American College of Chest Physicians. Chest 63:259, 1973.

American Thoracic Society. Am Rev Respir Dis 120:1393, 1979.

American Thoracic Society. Clinical usefulness of skin testing in histoplasmosis, coccidioidomycosis, and blastomycosis. Am Rev Respir Dis 138:1081, 1988.

Ampel NM, Wieden MA, Gagliani JN: Coccidioidomycosis: Clinical update. Rev Infect Dis 11:897, 1989.

Antman KS, Griffin JD, Elias A et al: Effect of recombinant human granulocyte-macrophage colony-stimulating factor on chemotherapy-induced myelosuppression (Comments). N Engl J Med 319:593, 1988.

Areno JP, Campbell GD Jr, George RB: Diagnosis of blastomycosis. Semin Respir Infect 12:252, 1997.

Armstrong D: Treatment of opportunistic fungal infections. Clin Infect Dis 16:1, 1993.

Baker RD: Pulmonary mucormycosis. Am J Pathol 32:287, 1956.

Baker RD, Severance AO: Mucormycosis with report of acute mycotic pneumonia (abstract). Am J Pathol 24:716, 1948.

Baron O, Guillaume B, Moreau P et al: Aggressive surgical management in localized pulmonary mycotic and nonmycotic infections for neutropenic patients with acute leukemia: Report of eighteen cases. J Thorac Cardiovasc Surg 115:63, 1998.

Bartrum RJ Jr, Watnick M, Herman PG: Roentgenographic findings in pulmonary mucormycosis. Am J Roentgenol Radium Ther Nucl Med 117: 810, 1973.

Bates JH: Pulmonary cryptococcosis: Special problems in diagnosis and treatment. Mod Treat 7:596, 1970.

Baum GL, Donnerberg RL, Stewart D et al: Pulmonary sporotrichosis. N Engl J Med 280:410, 1969.

Baumgardner DJ, Buggy BP, Mattson BJ et al: Epidemiology of blastomycosis in a region of high endemicity in north central Wisconsin (Comments). Clin Infect Dis 15:629, 1992.

Belcher J, Pulmmer N: Surgery in broncho-pulmonary aspergillosis. Br J Dis Chest 54:335, 1960.

Bennett J: On the parasitic vegetable structures found growing in living animals. Trans R Soc Edinburgh, 1842.

Bhagavan BS, Rao DR, Weinberg T: Histoplasmosis producing broncholithiasis. Arch Pathol Lab Med 91:577, 1971.

Bhagwandeen SB: North American blastomycosis in Zambia. Am J Trop Med Hyg 23:231, 1974.

Bonfils-Roberts EA, Nickodem A, Healon TF Jr: Retrospective analysis of the efficacy of open lung biopsy in acquired immunodeficiency syndrome. Ann Thorac Surg 49:115, 1990.

Bouza E, Dreyer JS, Hewitt WL et al: Coccidioidal meningitis: An analysis of thirty-one cases and review of the literature. Medicine 60:139, 1981.

Brandt SJ, Peters WP, Atwater SK et al: Effect of recombinant human granulocyte-macrophage colony-stimulating factor on hematopoietic reconstitution after high-dose chemotherapy and autologous bone marrow transplantation. N Engl J Med 318:869, 1988.

Brass C, Levine HB, Stevens DA: Stimulation and suppression of cell-mediated immunity by endosporulation antigens of *Coccidioides immitis*. Infect Immun 35:431, 1982.

British Tuberculosis Association. Aspergillus in persistent lung cavities after tuberculosis: A report from the Research Committee of the British Tuberculosis Association. Tubercle 49:1, 1968.

Brodsky A, Gregg M, Kaufman L et al: Outbreak of histoplasmosis associated with the 1970 Earth Day activities. Am J Med 54:333, 1973.

Bronchud MH, Scarffe JH, Thatcher N et al: Phase I/II study of recombinant human granulocyte colony-stimulating factor in patients receiving intensive chemotherapy for small cell lung cancer. Br Cancer 56:809, 1987.

Brown LR, Swensen SJ, Van Scoy RE et al: Roentgenologic features of pulmonary blastomycosis. Mayo Clin Proc 66:29, 1991.

Buechner HA, Furcolow ML, Farness OJ et al: Epidemiology of the pulmonary mycoses: Report of the committee on fungus diseases and subcommittee on epidemiology, American College of Chest Physicians. Chest 58:68, 1970.

Buechner HA, Seaburg JH, Campbell CC et al: The current status of serologic, immunologic, and skin tests in the diagnosis of pulmonary mycoses: Report of the Committee on Fungus Diseases and Subcommittee on Criterion for Clinical Diagnosis. Chest 63:259, 1973.

Campbell GD: Primary pulmonary cryptococcosis. Am Rev Respir Dis 94:236, 1966.

Catanzaro A: Suppressor cells in coccidioidomycosis. Cell Immunol 64:235, 1981.

Catanzaro A, Spitler LE, Moser KM: Cellular immune response in coccidioidomycosis. Cell Immunol 15:360, 1975.

Chase HV: Histoplasmosis. Md State Med J 19:65, 1970.

Chechani V, Zaman MK, Finch PJ: Chronic cavitary *Pneumocystis carinii* pneumonia in a patient with AIDS. Chest 95:1347, 1989.

Chuck SL, Sande MA: Infections with *Cryptococcus neoformans* in the acquired immunodeficiency syndrome. N Engl J Med 321:794, 1989.

Clark RA, Greer D, Atkinson W et al: Spectrum of *Cryptococcus neoformans* infection in 68 patients infected with human immunodeficiency virus. Rev Infect Dis 12:768, 1990.

Cohen SL, Gale AM, Liston HE: Report of a pilot study on noncalcified discrete pulmonary coin lesions in a coccicioidomycosis endemic area. Az Med 29:40, 1972.

Conces DJ Jr, Schwenk GR Jr, Doering PR et al: Thoracic needle biopsy: Improved results utilizing a team approach. Chest 91:813, 1987.

Conen P, Walker G, Turner J et al: Invasive primary pulmonary aspergillosis of the lungs with cerebral metastasis and complete recovery. Dis Chest 42:88, 1962.

Connell JV, Muhm JR: Radiographic manifestations of pulmonary histoplasmosis: A 10-year review. Radiology 121:281, 1976.

Coss K, Wheat L, Conces DJ et al: Esophageal fistula complicating mediastinal histoplasmosis: Response to amphotericin B. Am J Med 83:343, 1987.

Cowgill LD, Addonizio UP, Mopeman AR, Harken AM: Prosthetic valve endocarditis. Curr Probl Cardiol 11:617, 1986.

Cox RA, Pope RM, Stevens DA: Immune complexes in coccidioidomycosis: Correlation with disease involvement. Am Rev Respir Dis 126:439, 1982.

Cox RA, Vivas JR, Gross A et al: In vivo and in vitro cell-mediated responses in coccidioidomycosis. I. Immumologic responses of persons with primary, asymptomatic infections. Am Rev Respir Dis 114:937, 1976.

Currie BP, Casadevall A: Estimation of the prevalence of cryptococcal infection among patients infected with the human immunodeficiency virus in New York City. Clin Infect Dis 19:1029, 1994.

Currie BP, Freundlich LF, Soto MA et al: False-negative cerebrospinal fluid cryptococcal latex agglutination tests for patients with culture-positive cryptococcal meningitis. J Clin Microbiol 31:2519, 1993.

Cush R, Light RW, George RB: Clinical and roentgenographic manifestations of acute and chronic blastomycosis. Chest 69:345, 1976.

Daly RC, Pairolero PC, Piehler JM et al: Pulmonary aspergilloma: Results of surgical treatment. J Thorac Cardiovasc Surg 92:981, 1986.

Darling S: Protozoon general infection producing pseudotubercles in lung and focal necrosis in liver, spleen, and lymph nodes. JAMA 46:1283, 1906.

Dartevelle P, Chapelier A, Navajas M et al: Replacement of the superior vena cava with polytetrafluoroethylene grafts combined with resection of mediastinal-pulmonary malignant tumors: Report of thirteen cases. J Thorac Cardiovasc Surg 94:361, 1987.

Davies SF: Fungal pneumonia. Med Clin North Am 78:1049, 1994.

DeMonbreum WA: The cultivation and cultural characteristics of Darling's Histoplasma Capsulatum. Am J Trop Med 14:93, 1934.

Denning DW, Stevens DA: Antifungal and surgical treatment of invasive aspergillosis: Review of 2,121 published cases (Erratum Rev Infect Dis 13:345, 1991) Rev Infect Dis 12:1147, 1990.

Deschamps C, Allen M, Daly R et al: Histoplasmosis. In Faber L (ed): Chest Surg Clin North Am. Philadelphia, WB Saunders, 1993, p 639.

Deve F: Une nouvelle forme anatomoradiologique de mycose pulmonaire primitive: Le megamycetome intra bronchiectatique [French]. Arch Med Chir Appar Respir 13:337, 1938.

Diamond RD, Erickson NF: Chemotaxis of human neutrophils and monocytes induced by *Cryptococcus neoformans*. Infect Immun 38:380, 1982.

Dickson E, Gifford M: *Coccidioides* infection (coccidioidomycosis). II. The primary type of infection. Arch Intern Med 62:853, 1938.

Dillon M, Sealy W, Fetter B: Mucormycosis of the bronchus successfully treated by lobectomy. J Thorac Cardiovasc Surg 35:464, 1958.

Dines D, Payne W, Bernatz P et al: Mediastinal granuloma and fibrosing mediastinitis. Chest 75:320, 1979.

Dismukes WE, Bradsher RW Jr, Cloud GC et al: Itraconazole therapy for blastomycosis and histoplasmosis. NIAID Mycoses Study Group. Am J Med 93:489, 1992.

Dixon G, Donnerberg R, Schonfeld S et al: Advances in the diagnosis and treatment of broncholithiasis. Am Rev Respir Dis 129:1028, 1984.

Dodd K, Tompkins E: Case of histoplasmosis of Darling in infant. Am J Trop Med 14:127, 1934.

Doty DB: Bypass of superior vena cava: Six years' experience with spiral vein graft for obstruction of superior vena cava due to benign and malignant disease. J Thorac Cardiovasc Surg 83:326, 1982.

Doty JR, Flores JH, Doty DB: Superior vena cava obstruction: Bypass using spiral vein graft. Ann Thorac Surg 67:1111, 1999.

Draheim JH, Mitchell JR, Elton NW: Histoplasmosis: Fourth case report from the Canal Zone. Am J Trop Med 31:753, 1951.

Drutz DJ, Catanzaro A: Coccidioidomycosis. II. Am Rev Respir Dis 117:727, 1978.

Dumich PS, Neel HB: Blastomycosis of the larynx. Laryngoscope 93:1266, 1983.

Dye TE, Saab SB, Almond CH et al: Sclerosing mediastinitis with occlusion of pulmonary veins: Manifestations and management. J Thorac Cardiovasc Surg 74:137, 1977.

Eastridge CE, Young JM, Cole F et al: Pulmonary aspergillosis. Ann Thorac Surg 13:397, 1972.

Ein ME, Wallace RJ Jr, Williams TW Jr: Allergic bronchopulmonary aspergillosis-like syndrome consequent to aspergilloma. Am Rev Respir Dis 119:811, 1979.

Einstein H, Holeman CJ, Sandidge L et al: Coccidioidal meningitis: The use of amphotericin B in treatment. Calif Med 94:339, 1961.

Emmons CW, Murray IG, Lurie HI et al: North American blastomycosis: Two autochthonous cases from Africa. Sabouraudia 3:306, 1964.

Faulkner SL, Vernon R, Brown PP et al: Hemoptysis and pulmonary aspergilloma: Operative versus nonoperative treatment. Ann Thorac Surg 25:389, 1978.

Feigin DS: Pulmonary cryptococcosis: Radiologic-pathologic correlates of its three forms. AJR Am J Roentgenol 141:1262, 1983.

Ferguson M, Lee E, DB S et al: Selective operative approach for diagnosis and treatment of anterior mediastinal masses. Ann Thorac Surg 44:583, 1987.

Fojtasek MF, Sherman MR, Garringer T et al: Local immunity in lung-associated lymph nodes in a murine model of pulmonary histoplasmosis. Infec Immun 61:4607, 1993.

Fougner K, Gjonr E: Pulmonary aspergilloma in a case of Boeck's sarcoidosis. Nord Med 59: 303, 1958.

Fragoyannis S, van Wyk G, de Beer M: North American blastomycosis in South Africa: A case report. So Afr Med J 51:169, 1977.

Frey CL, Drutz DJ: Influence of fungal surface components on the interaction of *Coccidioides immitis* with polymorphonuclear neutrophils. J Infect Dis 153:933, 1986.

Fullerton D: Coccidioidomycosis. In Faber L (ed): Chest Surgery Clinics of North America. Philadelphia, WB Saunders, 1993.

Furbringer P: Beobachtungen über Langenmycose beim Menschen. Virchows Arch A Pathol Anat Histopathol 66:330, 1876.

Furcolow ML, Brasher CA: Chronic progressive (cavitary) histoplasmosis as a problem in tuberculosis sanitoriums. Am Rev Respir Dis 73:609, 1956.

Furcolow ML, Chick EW, Busey JF et al: Prevalence and incidence studies of human and canine blastomycosis. 1. Cases in the United States, 1885–1968. Am Rev Respir Dis 102:60, 1970.

Galgiani JN: Inhibition of different phases of *Coccidioides immitis* by human neutrophils or hydrogen peroxide. J Infec Dis 153:217, 1986.

Galgiani JN, Catanzaro A, Cloud GA et al: Fluconazole therapy for coccidioidal meningitis. The NIAID-Mycoses Study Group. Ann Intern Med 119:28, 1993.

Galgiani JN, Isenberg RA, Stevens DA: Chemotaxigenic activity of extracts from the mycelial and spherule phases of *Coccidioides immitis* for human polymorphonuclear leukocytes. Infect Immun 21:862, 1978.

Galgiani JN, Yam P, Petz LD et al: Complement activation by *Coccidioides immitis*: In vitro and clinical studies. Infect Immun 28:944, 1980.

Garrett H Jr, Roper CL: Surgical intervention in histoplasmosis. Ann Thorac Surg 42:711, 1986.

Garvey J, Crastnopol P, Weisz D et al: The surgical treatment of pulmonary aspergillomas. J Thorac Cardiovasc Surg 74:542, 1977.

Garvey J, Crastnopol P, Weisz D et al: Surgical treatment of pulmonary aspergillomas. N Y St J Med 78:1722, 1978.

Genoe GA, Morello JA, Fennessy JJ: The diagnosis of pulmonary aspergillosis by the bronchial brushing technique. Radiology 102:51, 1972.

George RB, Jenkinson SG, Light RW: Fiberoptic bronchoscopy in the diagnosis of pulmonary fungal and nocardial infarctions. Chest 73:33, 1978.

Gerson SL, Talbot GH, Hurwitz S et al: Prolonged granulocytopenia: The major risk factor for invasive pulmonary aspergillosis in patients with acute leukemia. Ann Intern Med 100:345, 1984.

Gilchrist T: Protozoan dermatitis. J Cut Gen Dis 12:496, 1894.

Giron J, Poey C, Fajadet P et al: CT-guided percutaneous treatment of inoperable pulmonary aspergillomas: A study of 40 cases. Eur J Radiol 28:235, 1998.

Gloviczki P, Pairolero PC, Toomey BJ et al: Reconstruction of large veins for nonmalignant venous occlusive disease. J Vasc Surg 16:750, 1992.

Gold W, Stout HA, Pagano JF, Donovich R: Amphotericins A & B, antifungal antibiotics produced by a streptomycete. I. In vitro studies. Antibiot Annu 3:579, 1955–1956.

Goodwin R, Nickell J, Des Prez R: Mediastinal fibrosis complicating healed primary histoplasmosis and tuberculosis. Medicine 51:227, 1972.

Goodwin RA Jr, Des Prez RM: State of the art: Histoplasmosis. Am Rev Respir Dis 117:929, 1978.

Goodwin RA, Loyd JE, Des Prez RM: Histoplasmosis in normal hosts. Medicine 60:231, 1981.

Gottlieb MS, Schroff R, Shanker HM et al: *Pneumocystis carinii* pneumonia and mucosal candidiasis in previously healthy homosexual men: Evidence of a newly acquired cellular immunodeficiency. N Engl J Med 305:1425, 1981.

Greening R, Menville L: Roentgen findings in torulosis. Report of four cases. Radiology 48:381, 1947.

Greenwood MF, Holland P: Tracheal obstruction secondary to histoplasma mediastinal granuloma. Chest 62:642, 1972.

Harding SA, Scheld WM, Feldman PS et al: Pulmonary infection with capsule-deficient cryptococcus neoformans. Virchows Arch A, Pathol Anat Histol 382:113, 1979.

Hargis JL, Bone RC, Stewart J et al: Intracavitary amphotericin B in the treatment of symptomatic pulmonary aspergillosis. Am J Med 68:389, 1980.

Harris J: Mucormycosis: Report of case. Pediatrics 16:857, 1955.

Harvey RP, Stevens DA: In vitro assays of cellular immunity in progressive coccidioidomycosis: Evaluation of suppression with parasiticphase antigen. Am Rev Respir Dis 123:665, 1981.

Hektoen L: Systemic blastomycosis and coccidioidal granuloma. JAMA 49:1070, 1907.

Henderson RD, Deslaurier J, Ritcey EL et al: Surgery in pulmonary aspergillosis. J Thorac Cardiovasc Surg 70:1088, 1975.

Henze G, Aldenhoff P, Stephani U et al: Successful treatment of pulmonary and cerebral aspergillosis in an immunosuppressed child. Eur J Pediatr 138:263, 1982.

Hinson K, Moon A, Plummer N: Bronchopulmonary aspergillosis: Review and report of eight cases. Thorax 7:317, 1952.

Hodgson CH, Weed LA, Clagett OT: Pulmonary histoplasmosis. JAMA 145:807, 1951.

Hyde L: Coccidioidal pulmonary cavitation. Dis Chest 54:273, 1968.

Ibrahim AB, Pappagianis D: Experimental induction of anergy to coccidioidin by antigens of *Coccidioides immitis*. Infect Immun 7:786, 1973.

Israel HL, Ostrow A: Sarcoidosis and aspergilloma. Am J Med 47:243, 1969.

Iwen PC, Reed EC, Armitage JO et al: Nosocomial invasive aspergillosis in lymphoma patients treated with bone marrow or peripheral stem cell transplants (Comments). Infect Control Hosp Epidemiol 14:131, 1993.

Jenkins DW, Fisk DE, Byrd RB: Mediastinal histoplasmosis with esophageal abscess: Two case reports. Gastroenterology 70:109, 1976.

Jewkes J, Kay PH, Paneth M et al: Pulmonary aspergilloma: Analysis of prognosis in relation to haemoptysis and survey of treatment. Thorax 38:572, 1983.

Johnson D: Pulmonary aspergilloma. Br J Clin Pract 31:207, 1977.

Kahanpaa A: Bronchopulmonary occurrence of fungi in adults especially according to cultivation material. Acta Pathol Microbiol Scand B. Microbiol Immunol 227:1, 1972.

Karas A, Hankins JR, Attar S et al: Pulmonary aspergillosis: An analysis of 41 patients. Ann Thorac Surg 22:1, 1976.

Kataria YP, Campbell PB, Burlingham BT: Acute pulmonary histoplasmosis presenting as adult respiratory distress syndrome: Effect of therapy on clinical and laboratory features. South Med J 74:53, 1981.

Kaufman L: Laboratory methods for the diagnosis and confirmation of systemic mycoses. Clin Infect Dis 14:S23, 1992.

Kerkering TM, Duma RJ, Shadomy S: The evolution of pulmonary cryptococcosis: Clinical implications from a study of 41 patients with and without compromising host factors. Ann Intern Med 94:611, 1981.

Khoury MB, Godwin JD, Ravin CE et al: Thoracic cryptococcosis: Immunologic competence and radiologic appearance. AJR Am J Roentgenol 142:893, 1984.

Kibbler CC, Milkins SR, Bhamra A et al: Apparent pulmonary mycetoma following invasive aspergillosis in neutropenic patients. Thorax 43:108, 1988.

Kilman JW, Ahn C, Andrews NC et al: Surgery for pulmonary aspergillosis. J Thorac Cardiovasc Surg 57:642, 1969.

Kinasewitz GT, Penn RL, George RB: The spectrum and significance of pleural disease in blastomycosis. Chest 86:580, 1984.

Kirkland TN, Fierer J: Coccidioidomycosis: A reemerging infectious disease. Emerg Infect Dis 2:192, 1996.

Klein BS, Jones JM: Isolation, purification, and radiolabeling of a novel 120-kD surface protein on *Blastomyces dermatitidis* yeasts to detect antibody in infected patients. Clin Invest 85:152, 1990.

Klein BS, Vergeront JM, Davis JP: Epidemiologic aspects of blastomycosis, the enigmatic systemic mycosis. Sem Respir Infect 1:29, 1986.

Klingman AM, Mescon H: The periodic acid-Schiff stain for the demonstration of fungi in animal tissues. J Bacteriol 60:415, 1950.

Kovacs JA, Kovacs AA, Polis M et al: Cryptococcosis in the acquired immunodeficiency syndrome. Ann Intern Med 103:533, 1985.

Krakowka P, Halweg H, Podsiadlo B: Mycological and serological studies in the diagnosis of various forms of puimonary aspergillosis. Scand J Respir Dis (Suppl) 102:213, 1978.

Kravitz GR, Davies SF, Eckman MR et al: Chronic blastomycotic meningitis. Am J Med 71:501, 1981.

Kusne S, Torre-Cisneros J, Manez R et al: Factors associated with invesive lung aspergillosis and the significance of positive *Aspergillus* culture after liver transplantation. J Infect Dis 166:1379, 1992.

Landis FB, Varkey B: Late relapse of pulmonary blastomycosis after adequate treatment with amphotericin B: Case report. Am Rev Respir Dis 113:77, 1976.

Larsen RA, Bozzette S, McCutchan JA et al: Persistent *Cryptococcus neoformans* infection of the prostate after successful treatment of meningitis. Ann Intern Med 111:125, 1989.

Levin E: Pulmonary intracavitary fungus ball. Radiology 66:9, 1956.

Libshitz HI, Atkinson GW, Israel HL: Pleural thickening as a manifestation of *Aspergillus* superinfection. Am Roentgenol Rad Ther Nucl Med 120:883, 1974.

Lipinski JK, Weisbrod GL, Sanders DE: Unusual manifestations of pulmonary aspergillosis. J Can Assoc Radiol 29:216, 1978.

Lo CY, Notenboom RH: A new enzyme immunoassay specific for blastomycosis. Am Rev Respir Dis 141:84, 1990.

Loyd JE, Tillman BF, Atkinson JB et al: Mediastinal fibrosis complicating histoplasmosis. Medicine 67:295, 1988.

Lupinetti FM, Behrendt DM, Giller RH et al: Pulmonary resection for fungal infection in children undergoing bone marrow transplantation. J Thorac Cardiovasc Surg 104:684, 1992.

Mahajan V, Strimlan V, Ordstrand H et al: Benign superior vena cava syndrome. Chest 68:32, 1975.

Malabonga VM, Basti J, Kamholz SL: Utility of bronchoscopic sampling techniques for cryptococcal disease in AIDS. Chest 99:370, 1991.

Massard G, Roeslin N, Wihlm JM et al: Pleuropulmonary aspergilloma: Clinical spectrum and results of surgical treatment (Comments). Ann Thorac Surg 54:1159, 1992.

Mathisen DJ, Grillo HC: Clinical manifestation of mediastinal fibrosis and histoplasmosis. Ann Thorac Surg 54:1053, 1992.

McCarthy DS, Pepys J: Pulmonary aspergilloma—clinical immunology. Clin Allerg 3:57, 1973.

McKinsey DS, Gupta MR, Riddler SA et al: Long-term amphotericin B therapy for disseminated histoplasmosis in patients with the acquired immunodeficiency syndrome (AIDS). Ann Intern Med 111:655, 1989.

McKinsey DS, Kauffman CA, Pappas PG et al: Fluconazole therapy for histoplasmosis. National Institute of Allergy and Infectious Diseases Mycoses Study Group. Clin Infect Dis 23:996, 1996.

Medical Section of the American Lung Association. Laboratory diagnosis of mycotic and specific fungal infections. Am Rev Respir Dis 132:1373, 1985.

Medoff G, Kobayashi GS: Strategies in the treatment of systemic fungal infections. N Engl J Med 302:145, 1980.

Melick DW: Excisional surgary in palmonary coccidioidomycosis. J Thorac Cardiovasc Surg 20:66, 1950.

Meyer RD, Rosen P, Armstrong D: Phycomycosis complicating leukemia and lymphoma. Ann Intern Med 77:871, 1972.

Meyer RD, Young LS, Armstrong D et al: Aspergillosis complicating neoplastic disease. Am J Med 54:6, 1973.

Meyers JD: Fungal infections in bone marrow transplant patients. Sem Oncol 17:10, 1990.

Micheli P: Nova plantarum genera juxta tournefortii methodum disposita. Florence, Italy, 1729.

Michelson E: Primary pulmonary sporotrichosis. Ann Thorac Surg 24:83, 1977.

Miller R, Sullivan F: Superior vena caval obstruction secondary to fibrosing mediastinitis. Ann Thorac Surg 15:483, 1973.

Miller WT Jr Edelman JM, Miller WT: Cryptococcal pulmonary infection in patients with AIDS: Radiographic appearance. Radiology 175:725, 1990.

Mohr JA, Griffiths W, Long H: Pulmonary sporotrichosis in Oklahoma and susceptibilities in vitro. Am Rev Respir Dis 119:961, 1979.

Mori M, Galvin JR, Barloon TJ et al: Fungal pulmonary infections after bone marrow transplantation: Evaluation with radiography and CT. Radiology 178:721, 1991.

Murphy JW, Moorhead JW: Regulation of cell-mediated immunity in cryptococcosis. I. Induction of specific afferent T suppressor cells by cryptococcal antigen. J Immunol 128:276–283, 1982.

National Institute of Allergy and Infectious Diseases, Mycoses Study Group. Treatment of blastomycosis and histoplasmosis with ketoconazole: Results of a prospective randomized clinical trial. Ann Intern Med 103:861, 1985b.

Neilson JB, Fromtling RA, Bulmer GS: *Cryptococcus neoformans*: Size range of infectious particles from aerosolized soil. Infect Immun 17:634, 1977.

Norenberg R, Sethi GK, Scott SM, Takaro T: Opportunistic endocarditis following open heart surgery. Ann Thorac Surg 19:592, 1975.

Opelz G, Scheer MI: Cutaneous sensitivity and in vitro responsiveness of lymphocytes in patients with disseminated coccidioidomycosis. J Infect Dis 132:250, 1975.

Pappagianis D, Zimmer BL: Serology of coccidioidomycosis. Clin Mierobiol Rev 3:247, 1990.

Pappas PG, Pottage JC, Powderly WG et al: Blastomycosis in patients with the acquired immunodeficiency syndrome. Ann Intern Med 116:847, 1992.

Pappas PG, Threlkeld MG, Bedsole GD et al: Blastomycosis in immunocompromised patients. Medicine 72:311, 1993.

Parish JM, Marschke RF Jr, Dines DE et al: Etiologic considerations in superior vena cava syndrome. Mayo Clin Proc 56:407, 1981.

Paya CV, Roberts GD, Cockerill FR: Transient fungemia in acute pulmonary histoplasmosis: Detection by new blood-culturing techniques. J Infect Dis 156:313, 1987.

Penn RL, Lambert RS, George RB: Invasive fungal infections: The use of serologic tests in diagnosis and management. Arch Intern Med 143:1215, 1983.

Pennington J: *Aspergillus*. In Sarosi G, Davies S (eds): Fungal Diseases of the Lung. New York, Raven Press, 1993, p 133.

Pesle G, Monod O: Bronchiectasis due to aspergilloma. Dis Chest 25:172, 1954.

Peterson EA, Friedman BA, Crowder EO, Rifkind D: Coccidioiduria: Clinical significance. Ann Intern Med 85:34, 1976.

Peterson PK, McGlave P, Ramsay NK et al: A prospective study of infectious diseases following bone marrow transplantation: Emergence of *Aspergillus* and cytomegalovirus as the major causes of mortality. Infect Control 4:81, 1983.

Pimentel JC: Pulmonary calcification in the tumor-like form of pulmonary aspergillosis Pulmonary aspergilloma. Am Rev Respir Dis 94:208, 1966.

Pluss JL, Opal SM: Pulmonary sporotrichosis: Review of treatment and outcome. Medicine (Baltimore) 65:143, 1986.

Posadas A: Ensayo enetomopatologico sobre una neoplasis considerado como micosis funcoides [Spanish]. An Circ Med Argent 15:481, 1892.

Prechter GC, Prakash UB: Bronchoscopy in the diagnosis of pulmonary histoplasmosis. Chest 95:1033, 1989.

Prior J, Saslaw S, Cole C: Experiences with histoplasmosis. Ann Intern Med 40:221, 1959.

Procknow JJ, Page MI, Loosli CG: Early pathogenesis of experimental histoplasmosis. Arch Pathol 69:413, 1960.

Puckett TF: Pulmonary histoplasmosis. Ann Rev Tuberc 67:453, 1953.

Quinones CA, Reuben AG, Hamill RJ et al: Chronic cavitary histoplasmosis: Failure of oral treatment with ketoconazole. Chest 95:914, 1989.

Randhawa HS, Pal M: Occurrence and significance of *Cryptococcus neoformans* in the respiratory tract of patients with bronchopulmonary disorders. J Clin Microbiol 5:5, 1977.

Read CT: Coin lesion, pulmonary: In the Southwest (solitary pulmonary nodules). Ariz Med 29:775, 1972.

Recht LD, Philips JR, Eckman MR et al: Self-limited blastomycosis: A report of thirteen cases. Am Rev Respir Dis 120:1109, 1979.

Reddy P, Gorelick DF, Brasher CA, et al: Progressive disseminated histoplasmosis as seen in adults. Am J Med 48:629, 1970.

Reiss F, Szilazyl G: Ecology of yeast like fungi in a hospital population: Detailed investigation of *Cryptococcus neoformans*. Arch Dermatol 91:611, 1965.

Restrepo A, Gomez I, Cano LE et al: Treatment of paracoccidioidomycosis with ketoconazole: A three year experience. The Second Annual International Symposium on Ketoconazole. Am J Med 74(suppl):48, 1983.

Ribi E, Salvin S: Antigen from the yeast phase of *Histoplasma cansulatum*:: I. Morphology of the cell as revealed by eletron microsope. Exp Cell Res 10:394, 1956.

Ridgeway NA, Whitcomb FC, Erickson EE, Law SW: Primary pulmonary sporotrichosis. Am J Med 32:153, 1962.

Riley W, Watson C: Histoplasmosis of Darling with report of a case originating in Minnesota. Am J Trop Med Hyg 6:271, 1926.

Ro JY, Lee SS, Ayala AG: Advantage of Fontana-Masson stain in capsule-deficient cryptococcal infection. Arch Pathol Lab Med 111:53, 1987.

Robinson LA: *Aspergillus* and other fungi. Chest Surg Clin North Am 9:193, 1999.

Robinson LA, Reed EC, Galbraith TA et al: Pulmonary resection for invasive *Aspergillus* infections in immunocompromised patients. J Thorac Cardiovasc Surg 109:1182, 1995.

Rogers TR, Haynes KA, Barnes RA: Value of antigen detection in predicting invasive pulmonary aspergillosis (Comments). Lancet 336:1210, 1990.

Rosenberg RS, Creviston SA, Schonfeld AJ: Invasive aspergillosis complicating resection of a pulmonary aspergilloma in a nonimmunocompromised host. Am Rev Respir Dis 126:1113, 1982.

Rosenthal J, Brandt K, Wheat L et al: Rheumatologic manifestations of histoplasmosis in the recent Indianapolis epidemic. Arthritis Rheum 26:1065, 1983.

Rubin H, Furcolow M, Yates J et al: The course and prognosis of histoplasmosis. Am J Med 27:278, 1959.

Saab SB, Almond C: Surgical aspects of pulmonary aspergillosis. J Thorac Cardiovasc Surg 68:455, 1974.

Saag MS, Dismukes WE: Treatment of histoplasmosis and blastomycosis. Chest 93:848, 1988.

Sakulsky S, Harrison E, Dines D et al: Mediastinal granuloma. J Thorac Cardiovasc Surg 54:279, 1967.

Sarosi GA, Armstrong D, Davies SF et al: Laboratory diagnosis of mycotic and specific fungal infections: Official statement—American Thoracic Society. Am Rev Respir Dis 132:1373, 1985.

Sarosi GA, Davies SF: Blastomycosis. Am Rev Respir Dis 120:911, 1979.

Sarosi GA, Davies SF: Therapy for fungal infections. Mayo Clin Proc 69:1111, 1994.

Sarosi GA, Davies SF, Phillips JR: Self-limited blastomycosis: A report of 39 cases. Sem Respir Infect 1:40, 1986.

Sarosi GA, Hammerman KJ, Tosh FF et al: Clinical features of acute pulmonary blastomycosis. N Engl J Med 290:540, 1974.

Sarosi GA, Parker JD, Doto IL et al: Chronic pulmonary coccidioidomycosis. N Engl J Med 283:325, 1970.

Sathapatayavongs B, Batteiger BE, Wheat J et al: Clinical and laboratory features of disseminated histoplasmosis during two large urban outbreaks. Medicine 62:263, 1983.

Savides T, Gress F, Wheat L et al: Dysphagia due to mediastinal granulomas: Diagnosis with endoscopic ultrasonography. Gastroenterology 109:366, 1995.

Schaefer JC, Yu B, Armstrong D: An *Aspergillus* immunodiffusion test in the early diagnosis of aspergillosis in adult leukemia patients. Am Rev Respir Dis 113:325, 1976.

Schenck BR: On refractory subcutaneous abscesses caused by a fungus possibly related to the sporotricha. Johns Hopkins Hosp Bull 9:286, 1898.

Schimpff SC, Bennett JE: Abnormalities in cell-mediated immunity in patients with *Cryptococcus neoformans* infection. J Allerg Clin Immunol 55:430, 1975.

Schneider R, Reid J: Mediastinal histoplasmosis with abscean. Chest 67:237, 1975.

Schowengerdt C, Suyemoto R, Main F: Granulomatous and fibrous mediastinitis: A review and analysis of 180 cases. J Thorac Cardiovasc Surg 57:365, 1969.

Schwartz JR, Nagle MG, Elkins RC et al: Mucormycosis of the trachea: An unusual cause of acute upper airway obstruction. Chest 81:653, 1982.

Schwarz J: What's new in mycotic bone and joint diseases? Pathol Res Prac 178:617, 1984.

Scott SM, Peasley ED, Aymes TP: Pulmonary sporotrichosis. N Engl J Med 265:453, 1961.

Seabury JH, Buechner HA, Busey J et al: The diagnosis of pulmonary mycoses: Report of the Committee on Fungus Disease and Subcommittee on Criteria for Clinical Diagnosis, American College of Chest Physicians. Chest 60:82, 1971.

Sheflin JR, Campbell JA, Thompson GP: Pulmonary blastomycosis: Findings on chest radiographs in 63 patients. AJR Am J Roentgenol 154:1177, 1990.

Sheppe W: Torula infections in man. Am J Med Sci 167:91, 1924.

Shin M, Ho K: Computed tomography evaluation of bilateral bronchostenosis caused by sclerosing granulomatous mediastinitis: A complication of histoplasmosis. J Comput Tomog 8:345, 1984.

Silver SF, Grymaloski MR, Bosken CH et al: Pulmonary consolidation with an air crescent sign in an immunocompromised woman (Clinical Conference). Can Assoc Radiol J 40:167, 1989.

Sluyter F: De vegetabilibus orgasmi animalis parasitis ac de novo epiphyto in pityriasi versicolore obvio. Berolini, Italy, G. Schade, 1847.

Smith C, Beard R, Whiting E et al: Varieties of coccidioidal infection in relation to the epidemiology and control of the diseases. Am J Public Health 36:1394, 1946.

Smith JW, Utz JP: Progressive disseminated histoplasmosis: A prospective study of 26 patients. Ann Intern Med 76:557, 1972.

Snider WD, Simpson DM, Nielsen S et al: Neurological complications of acquired immune deficiency syndrome: Analysis of 50 patients. Ann Neurol 14:403, 1983.

Sochocky S: Pulmonary aspergillosis. SD J Med 25:19, 1972.

Stevens DA: Coccidioidomycosis. N Engl J Med 332:1077, 1995.

Stoddard JL, Cutler EC: Torula infection in man: Studies from the Rockefeller Institute for Medical Research 6:1, 1916.

Strimlan C, Dines D, Payne W: Mediastinal granuloma. Mayo Clin Proc 50:702, 1975.

Suen H, Wright C, Mathisen DJ: Surgical management of pulmonary aspergillosis. In Faber L (ed): Chest Surgery Clinics of North America. Philadelphia, WB Saunders, 1993, p 671.

Sugar AM, Saunders C: Oral fluconazole as suppressive therapy of disseminated cryptococcosis in patients with acquired immunodeficiency syndrome. Am J Med 85:481, 1988.

Takaro T: Mycotic infection of interest to thoracic surgeons. Ann Thorac Surg 3:71, 1967.

Takaro T: Lung infections and diffuse interstitial disease of the lungs. In Sabiston DC Jr, Spencer FC (eds): Gibbon's Surgery of the Chest. 4th ed. Philadelphia, WB Saunders, 1983.

Takaro T: Fungal infection. In Grillo HC, Austin WG, Wilkins EW Jr et al (eds): Current Therapy in Cardiothoracic Surgery. Philadelphia, BC Decker, 1989.

Tanner DC, Weinstein MP, Fedorciw B et al: Comparison of commerical kits for detection of cryptococcal antigen. J Clin Microbiol 32:1680, 1994.

Taylor MR, Lawson LA, Boyce JM et al: Inhibition of *Blastomyces dermatitidis* by topical lidocaine. Chest 84:431, 1983.

Terrell CL, Hughes CE: Antifungal agents used for deep-seated mycotic infections. Mayo Clin Proc 67:69, 1992.

Trachiotis GD, Hofner GH, Hix WR et al: Role of open lung biopsy in diagnosing pulmonary complications of AIDS. Ann Thorac Surg 54:898, 1992.

Trastek V: Management of mediastinal tumors. Ann Thorac Surg 44:227, 1987.

Trastek V, Pairolero P, Ceithaml E et al: Surgical management of broncholithiasis. J Thorac Cardiovasc Surg 90:842, 1985.

Trastek V, Pichler J, Pairolero P: Mediastinoscopy. Br Med Bull 42:240, 1986.

Tucker RM, Denning DW, Dupont B et al: Itraconazole therapy for chronic coccidioidal meningitis. Ann Intern Med 112:108, 1990.

Urschel HC Jr, Razzuk MA, Netto GJ et al: Sclerosing mediastinitis: Improved management with histoplasmosis titer and ketoconazole. Ann Thorac Surg 50:215, 1990.

Utz JP, Garriques IL, Sande MA et al: Therapy of cryptococcosis with a combination of flucytosine and amphotericin B. J Infect Dis 132:368, 1975.

Vaaler AK, Bradsher RW, Davies SF: Evidence of subclinical blastomycosis in forestry workers in northern Minnesota and northern Wisconsin. Am J Med 89:470, 1990.

Van Trigt P: Fungal infections of the lung. In Sabiston DC Jr, Spencer FC (eds): Gibbon's Surgery of the Chest. 5th ed. Philadelphia, WB Saunders, 1990.

Varkey B, Rose HD: Pulmonary aspergilloma: A rational approach to treatment Am J Med 61:626, 1976.

Virchow R: Beitrage zur Lehre von den beim Menschen vorkommenden pflanzlichen Parasiten [German]. Virchows Arch 9:557, 1856.

Walker JW, Montgomery FH: Further report of a previously recorded case of blastomycosis of the skin: Systemic infection with blastomyces; death; autopsy. JAMA 58:867, 1902.

Walsh TJ, Pizzo A: Treatment of systemic fungal infections: Recent progress and current problems. Eur J Clin Microbiol Infect Dis 7:460, 1988.

Warr W, Bates JH, Stone A: The spectrum of pulmonary cryptococcosis. Ann Intern Med 69:1109, 1968.

Wasser L, Talavera W: Pulmonary cryptococcosis in AIDS. Chest 92:692, 1987.

Weiland D, Ferguson RM, Peterson PK et al: Aspergillosis in 25 renal transplant patients: Epidemiology, clinical presentation, diagnosis, and management. Ann Surg 198:622, 1983.

Werner SB, Pappagianis D, Heindl I et al: An epidemic of coccidioidomycosis among archeology students in northern California. N Engl J Med 286:507, 1972.

Wernicke R: Über einen protozoenbefund Beimycosis fungoides. Zentralb Mikrobiol 12:859, 1892.

Wheat L: Diagnosis and management of histoplasmosis. Eur J Clin Microbiol Infect Dis 8:480, 1989.

Wheat J: Histoplasmosis: Experience during outbreaks in Indianapolis and review of the literature. Medicine 76:339, 1997.

Wheat L, Connolly-Stringfield P, Baker R et al: Disseminated histoplasmosis in the acquired immune deficiency syndrome: Clinical findings, diagnosis and treatment, and review of the literature. Medicine 69:361, 1990.

Wheat LJ, Connolly-Stringfield P, Williams B et al: Diagnosis of histoplasmosis in patients with the acquired immunodeficiency syndrome by detection of *Histoplasma capsulatum* polysaccharide antigen in bronchoalveolar lavage fluid. Am Rev Respir Dis 145:1421, 1992.

Wheat J, French ML, Kohler RB et al: The diagnostic laboratory tests for histoplasmosis: Analysis of experience in a large urban outbreak. Ann Intern Med 97:680, 1982b.

Wheat J, Hafner R, Wulfsohn M et al: Prevention of relapse of histoplasmosis with itraconazole in patients with the acquired immunodeficiency syndrome. The National Institute of Allergy and Infectious Diseases Clinical Trials and Mycoses Study Group Collaborators. Ann Intern Med 118:610, 1993.

Wheat LJ, Kohler RB, Tewari RP: Diagnosis of disseminated histoplasmosis by detection of *Histoplasma capsulatum* antigen in serum and urine specimens. N Engl Med 314:83, 1986.

Wheat L, Slama T, Eitzen H et al: A large urban outbreak of histoplasmosis: Clinical features. Ann Intern Med 94:331, 1981.

Wheat LJ, Slama TG, Norton J et al: Risk factors for disseminated or fatal histoplasmosis. Ann Intern Med 96:159, 1982a.

Wheat L, Stein L, Corya B et al: Pericarditis as a manifestation of histoplasmosis during two large urban outbreaks. Medicine 62:110, 1983.

Wieder S, White TD, Salazar J et al: Pulmonary artery occlusion due to histoplasmosis. Am J Roentgenol 138:243, 1982.

Wingard JR, Beals SU, Santos GW et al: *Aspergillus* infections in bone marrow transplant recipients. Bone Marrow Transplant 2:175, 1987.

Winn WA: A long-term study of 300 patients with cavitary-abscess lesions of the lung of coccidioidal origin: An analytical study with special reference to treatment. Dis Chest 54:268, 1968.

Witorsch P, Utz JP: North American blastomycosis: A study of 40 patients. Medicine 47:169, 1968.

Wong K, Waters CM, Walesby RK: Surgical management of invasive pulmonary aspergillosis in immunocompromised patients. Eur J Cardio-Thorac Surg 6:138, 1992.

Wynne JW, Olsen GN: Acute histoplasmosis presenting as the adult respiratory distress syndrome. Chest 66:158, 1974.

Young RC, Bennett JE: Invasive aspergillosis: Absence of detectable antibody response. Am Rev Respir Dis 104:710, 1971.

Zimmerman LE: A missing link in the history of histoplasmosis in Panama. US Armed Forces Med J 5:1569, 1954.

PARASITIC DISEASES OF THE LUNG AND PLEURA

Andrés Varela
Raul Burgos
Evaristo Castedo

The term *parasite* is derived from a Greek word meaning *he who eats at the table of another.* Although in a broader sense, all infectious microorganisms could be considered parasites, as consensus would have it, the term *parasitic infections* refers to those caused by protozoa and helminths.

Their main feature is their transmission to humans via biologic vectors or intermediate hosts (insects, molluscs, or mammals). Once lodged in the definitive host, they present complex life cycles and produce long-term chronic infections.

Parasitic diseases of the chest can present as hypersensitivity reactions, as eosinophilic lung diseases, or as direct invasion of the lungs or pleura. The clinical profile to watch for is peripheral blood eosinophilia in immunocompetent individuals who have traveled to endemic regions. The other individuals at great risk are immunocompromised individuals, such as organ transplant recipients and patients with autoimmune deficiency syndrome (AIDS), in whom the prevalence is notably higher.

The presence of eggs or larvae in stool, sputum, bronchoalveolar lavage fluid, pleural fluid, or lung tissue generally indicates pleuropulmonary involvement, although this is an exceptional finding. Thus, diagnosis is usually based on serologic evidence provided by enzyme-linked immunosorbent assay (ELISA) or monoclonal antibodies.

This chapter, which is directed particularly to thoracic surgeons, reviews all the parasitic diseases that affect humans, particularly those found in pleura or lungs. They have been grouped into tables for easy referral (Tables 23–15 through 23–18). Hydatid disease, which is endemic not only in the Mediterranean basin but also in regions as widely dispersed as Australia, South America, and elsewhere, is dealt with in particular depth. It occasionally requires surgical intervention, whereas other parasitic infections can almost always be treated successfully without surgery.

HYDATID DISEASE

Hydatidosis is characterized by the development of cysts as a consequence of the parasitization of humans by the larva of *Taenia echinococcus.* In the adult stage, it is a platyhelminthic worm belonging to the class Cestoda and to the family Taenia. Of the four known species, (*Echinococcus granulosus, E. multilocularis, E. oligarthrus,* and *E. vogeli*), only *E. multilocularis* and *E. granulosus* are human pathogens. The latter is the causative organism in most cases of human infection.

In North America, nearly all cases of this disease are seen in immigrants with the classic syndromes outlined in this section. It is colloquially referred to as the "pastoral" variety of hydatid disease. The "sylvatic" form is most commonly seen in indigenous North Americans, mostly in northern Canada and Alaska. In this type, a different strain of tapeworm is implicated, and the dog, deer, and moose are the usual intermediate hosts. In this form, lung cysts occur more commonly than liver cysts.

Epidemiology

Hydatid disease, known in the times of Galen, was described by Thebesius in the 17th century. It is thought to have originated in Iceland and to have been brought to continental Europe by dogs accompanying whaleboats in the 18th century. Infestation is confined to geographic areas in which there is continuous contact between humans and certain domestic carnivores such as dogs and cats and some ungulates such as sheep.

Echinococcosis is endemic to the Mediterranean region, South America, Australia, New Zealand, the Middle East, Alaska, and Canada, where it is widespread among Native American tribes (Wilson et al, 1995). In Spain, the epidemiologic data on hydatid disease have improved considerably and, at the present time, the number of cases reported is minimal, as illustrated by the fact that in 1966, surgical treatment for this disease was performed in 4.62 patients per 100,000 population per year, whereas in 1988, the incidence had dropped to 1.77 patients per 100,000 population per year, and in 1997 was recorded at 0.78 patients per 100,000 population per year. The number of hospital admissions for hydatid disease each year has decreased over the course of time from 6690 in 1966, to 2343 in 1988, and down to 986 in 1997. These data were obtained from the *Boletin Epidemiológico (Epidemiological Bulletin),* which bases its reports on the Survey of the Obligatory Declaration of Infectious Diseases and the Survey on Hospital Morbidity carried out by the Spanish National Statistical Institute.

Life Cycle

In its adult stage, the parasite lives in the intestinal tract of carnivores. The head is composed of a double crown of hook-like structures, and the body is formed by three

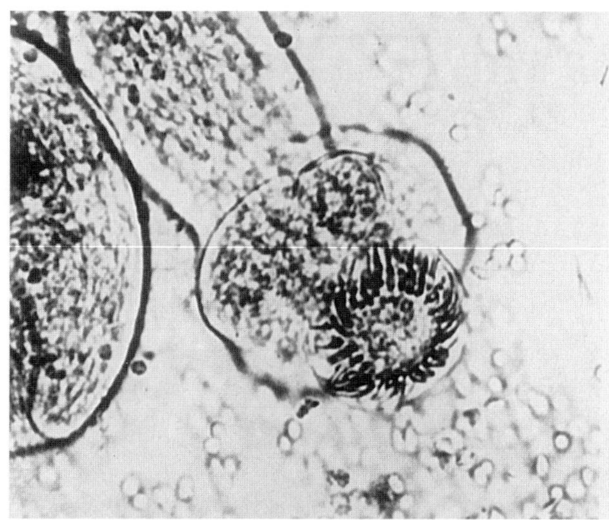

FIGURE 23–53 ■ Microscopic preparation of the scolex of a hydatid cyst showing the ring of hooks.

or four rings, the last of which bears the eggs (Fig. 23–53). After being eliminated with the feces, the eggs contaminate fields, irrigated land, and wells. Herbivores ingest the eggs (see Fig. 23–53), which develop into larvae, or hydatids, within the viscera of these animals. The cycle is completed with the ingestion of the infected viscera by carnivores. Humans contract the disease from water or food or by direct contact with dogs. Once the eggs reach the stomach, the hexacanth embryos are released. They pass through the intestinal wall and reach the tributary veins of the liver where they undergo a vesicular transformation and develop into the hydatid. If they overcome the hepatic obstacle, they may become lodged in the lung, where they would also be transformed into hydatids. If they advance beyond the lung, they may remain in any organ to which they are carried by the bloodstream. It has been shown that the embryos can reach the lung via the lymphatic vessels, bypassing the liver, and there is also evidence that the disease can be contracted through the bronchi (Jerray et al, 1992).

Within the thorax, the lung is the organ most commonly colonized, especially the lower lobes, as was observed in the authors' series (Alvarez Ayuso et al, 1981). If the hexacanth embryo manages to get past the pulmonary filter, it reaches the left heart and, by way of the aorta, the remainder of the organism. According to Devé (1934), the prevalence of the various locations in which hydatid cysts can develop in humans is as follows: liver, 55.6%; lung, 26%; muscles and connective tissue, 6.8%; spleen, 2.1%; kidney, 2.1%; brain, 1.4%; heart, 1.2%; and other organs, such as thyroid glands, bones, breast, pancreas, ovaries, and eyes, 4.2%.

Complications

The natural course of a hydatid cyst is progressive growth over a long period, although at times it may appear to remain static. The growth is usually slow and depends to a large degree on the resistance of the structure of the organ in which it develops. Thus, it is more rapid in organs like lung and peritoneum and slower in others of greater consistency such as heart and liver. Throughout its development, the pulmonary hydatid cyst can compress bronchial structures and produce pulmonary atelectasis accompanied by pneumonia. Various circumstances, such as calcification, infection, or rupture, can affect its course. Spontaneous cure of a pulmonary cyst is rare and should not be considered, from the therapeutic point of view.

Calcification is caused by the deposition of calcium salts in necrotic foci in the adventitial layer. The necrosis may be caused by several circumstances, such as ischemia due to compression, inflammatory or toxic processes, or immune responses. The calcifications are initially microscopic but become macroscopic over the course of time, partially or totally affecting the adventitial layer and appearing in diagnostic imaging studies. This eventuality, which is common in slow-growing cysts located in liver, spleen, or heart, is rare in pulmonary cysts, perhaps because of their more rapid growth. Calcification is not synonymous with the death of the parasite, although these two circumstances can be associated, in that adventitial calcification leads to the malnutrition of the metacestode, which first becomes dehydrated and later establishes hyaline degeneration on the germinal membrane and daughter vesicles.

Infection of the cyst usually produces its suppuration. Its expansion can result in the compression of blood vessels and bronchi, leading to wall necrosis. This makes it possible for pathogens to reach the perivascular lymphatic space, producing infection. Another possible cause is septic puncture, an extremely rare event owing to the fact that diagnostic puncture is contraindicated when pulmonary hydatidosis is suspected. Cyst suppuration leads to the death of the metacestode, although some daughter vesicles may survive. The clinical signs include chills, fever, tachycardia, local pain, and leukocytosis. Suppuration may facilitate the rupture of the cyst, which complicates the situation even more. When rupture occurs, the contents of the cyst may escape into an open space such as the pleural cavity or drain via the bronchi.

Rupture of a pulmonary cyst is one of the most severe complications, and it can occur under many circumstances: accident, progressive growth of the cyst, infection, and surgery. Dissemination of the fluid produces general symptoms that vary widely from one patient to another: in one they may go undetected, whereas in another, they can result in death due to anaphylactic shock. If the cyst is infected at the time of rupture, the general symptoms are accompanied by those of infection.

The intensity of the general symptoms is dependent on the characteristics of the tissue exposed to the hydatid cyst fluid because they determine the amount of fluid and the speed with which it is absorbed. In pulmonary hydatid cysts, the general reaction is severe when the fluid comes into contact with the pleural serosa or reaches the bloodstream. It is less intense when it is eliminated via the airways.

Another problem resulting from the rupture of a pulmonary cyst, especially over the long term, is the possible development of secondary hydatidosis. This occurs primarily in cases in which the rupture is not due to infection because when infection is present, suppuration eliminates the fertile elements that could contaminate another organ.

Secondary echinococcosis is caused by protoscolices, which undergo vesiculation to become hydatid, or daughter, vesicles, which can detach from the mother cyst and nest in a new location, thus growing as autonomous cysts. If a cyst opens toward the pleura, secondary pleural hydatidosis can develop. In contrast, if a ruptured cyst releases its fluid toward the airway, the patient eliminates it in the form of vomica, which can be accompanied by hydatid membranes. The elimination of the cyst in this way may lead to cure, to secondary infection of the residual cavity, or to seeding, which results in the development of multiple pulmonary cysts, all of the same size. If a cyst ruptures toward a blood vessel or the heart, the protoscolices may be carried by the blood simultaneously to a number of sites, forming what is referred to as metastatic hydatidosis.

The rupture of a cyst sometimes occurs gradually, through a fissure, releasing only small amounts of hydatic fluid. In sensitized patients, this can produce urticaria or pruritus. However, some authors consider that the fissure of a cyst may immunize the patient, impeding secondary hydatidosis should the cyst suddenly rupture.

Laboratory Tests

The laboratory tests utilized for the biologic diagnosis of hydatid disease are based primarily on the detection of immune or cellular responses (immunodiagnosis) to the presence of the parasite in the host.

Peripheral Blood Eosinophilia

This factor is neither specific nor constant because not all patients with hydatidosis present eosinophilia and, on the other hand, eosinophilia can exist in patients with other parasites or allergic processes. Relative eosinophilia is considered evaluable when eosinophils represent more than 5% on a differential leukocyte count. Absolute eosinophilia is more constant and is evaluable when there are more than 200 to 300 eosinophils per cubic millimeter. The authors have observed a statistically significant correlation between peripheral blood eosinophilia and ruptured pulmonary hydatid cyst, a finding that they have confirmed intraoperatively. However, there is no such correlation when the hydatid cyst is intact (Alvarez Ayuso et al, 1981).

Weinberg Reaction

This test is also referred to as complement deposition or complement fixation. It is based on the existence, in the plasma of hydatid cyst carriers, of circulating reagins. When a patient's serum is mixed with fluid from a sheep hydatid cyst, which serves as an antigen, the antibody and patient serum complement bond with the hydatid antigen. If rabbit red blood cells and guinea pig serum sensitized against the rabbit red cells are added to this mixture, hemolysis does not occur because the complement necessary for this process is fixed to the antigen and to the antihydatid antibodies.

The Weinberg reaction is positive in 70% to 80% of cases and false-positive reactions are rare. A negative result does not rule out the diagnosis of hydatidosis. Although it is not employed very much anymore, it can be useful in the follow-up of patients under treatment because the test results become negative within 1 year of freedom from the disease.

Casoni Intradermal Test

This test consists of the intradermal injection of 0.1 to 0.3 ml of hydatid fluid from sheep cysts, filtered and undiluted, into the anterior aspect of the patient's forearm. The fixation of circulating reagins produces a local papular rash measuring 1 to 2 cm in diameter. This reaction may appear 5 or 10 minutes after injection (the early reaction) and persist for over 24 hours and may reappear after the early reaction disappears (the late reaction). Occasionally, in addition to this local reaction, focal phenomena can occur (pain in upper quadrant, hemoptysis, and so forth) or even generalized signs that enhance the diagnostic value of the test.

The Casoni reaction is positive in 80% to 95% of cases, but its negativity does not rule out the presence of hydatid disease. On the other hand, false-positive reactions can occur in patients with other parasitic and nonparasitic diseases. This test may remain positive for a long time, even years after the cyst has been treated surgically.

Praunitz-Kustner Reaction or Passive Anaphylaxis

This test consists of the detection of circulating reagins by their transmission to a person who is free of hydatidosis. Serum from the patient (the presumed carrier of hydatidosis) is injected into the forearm of a healthy individual. Hydatid antigen is then injected into the same site. The development of a papular rash, similar to that of the Casoni test, indicates a positive reaction.

Serologic Diagnosis

Serologic diagnosis is usually more reliable than that based on the aforementioned tests. Moreover, it is useful in the follow-up of surgically or medically treated patients. In any case, negative serologic results do not invalidate the diagnosis of hydatidosis because some patients do not have detectable antibodies. On the other hand, the immune response depends on a wide range of factors:

(1) the patient's age, because serologic tests are less effective in children under 15 years of age than in adults; (2) the location of the hydatid cysts, because the reactions are more intense in cases of hepatic and peritoneal cysts than in cases of pulmonary and cerebral cysts; (3) the vitality of the metacestode, because when the parasite dies, the serologic results become negative; (4) the integrity of the cystic sac because when it tears or bursts as a consequence of the massive release of the antigen, there is a spectacular increase in the number of antibodies in a matter of days; and (5) the surgical excision of the cyst or pharmacologic treatment also modifies serologic reactions.

The tests most widely employed are as follows:

Indirect or Passive Hemagglutination. This approach consists of the agglutination of sheep red blood cells coated with hydatid antigen when mixed with serum of patients with antibodies. The test is positive in 70% of patients with pulmonary hydatidosis and in 95% of patients with liver hydatidosis.

Latex Agglutination. Similar to the preceding test, this test consists of the flocculation of latex particles coated with hydatid antigen in the presence of specific antibodies in the patient's serum. Although other, similar tests using ebonite and a colloidal dye as particles have also been carried out, latex agglutination is the one most widely applied. The results are positive in 70% of patients with pulmonary hydatidosis and in 90% of those with liver hydatidosis.

Immunoelectrophoresis. This test determines the serum concentration of each immunoglobulin; patients with hydatid disease have been shown to present IgG, IgM, IgA, and IgE antibodies against *Taenia echinococcus* antigens. Within 6 months of the surgical extirpation of pulmonary hydatid cysts, plasma IgM levels return to normal, whereas IgG remains abnormally high for a longer period of time. These patients often exhibit hypergammaglobulinemia, and when the cyst is infected, the levels of α_1 and α_2 globulins are elevated.

Double-Diffusion Immunoelectrophoresis. Special importance is given to "arc 5," considered specific for antibodies to antigen 5, one of the 10 or more antigens found in *E. granulosus*. It is present in the fluid and structures of the cyst. The presence of antibodies to this antigen in a patient's serum is of great diagnostic value in hydatid disease, although they are also detected in some cases of human cysticercosis and of hydatidosis caused by *E. multilocularis* or *E. vogeli*. The double-diffusion technique, which detects antibodies to antigen 5, is as specific as and more sensitive than immunoelectrophoresis.

Total IgE or Specific IgE. These immunoglobulins, which are usually abnormally high in patients with hydatid disease, are detected by radioimmunoassay. Specific IgE concentrations decrease after pharmacologic or surgical treatment but generally do not return to normal levels.

Indirect Immunofluorescence. This method is based on the fixation of the antibodies in patient serum to protoscolices obtained from hydatid cysts using a fluorescein-labeled human antiglobulin. It is a highly sensitive test but can result in false-positive results in some cases of cysticercosis.

Enzyme-Linked Immunosorbent Assay or Western Blot. This approach consists of the detection of an antigen-antibody complex using an enzyme-bound rabbit antihuman IgG that, acting on a specific substrate, produces a color change that can be measured and is proportional to the amount of antibody present. The complex antigen comes from the cystic fluid of sheep, pig, or rabbit, smeared on a polystyrene surface; the antibody is provided by the patient's serum. This serologic test has a sensitivity of 80% to 100% and a specificity of 88% to 90% in the case of hepatic hydatid cysts, but is less sensitive in detecting hydatid cysts in the lung (50% to 56%) and other organs (25% to 26%). New techniques involving the use of recombinant antigens to *Echinococcus* species may prove more specific.

Imaging studies such as ultrasound, computed tomography (CT), and magnetic resonance imaging (MRI) are more sensitive than serodiagnostic techniques. When these tests suggest hydatidosis, the diagnosis can be confirmed by means of serodiagnosis.

Diagnosis

The authors assessed some of the diagnostic tests for hydatid disease, such as the eosinophil count, the Casoni test, the Weinberg test, and the erythrocyte sedimentation rate, to determine whether any of them showed a statistically significant correlation with the presence of the disease. No correlation was found when the cyst remained intact during the preoperative evaluation or the surgical procedure. However, when rupture of the cyst occurred, an eosinophil level of more than 3%, episodes of vomiting, expectoration of "spring water" and small particles of hydatid cyst membrane with the appearance of grape skin, and the existence of three or more clinical symptoms showed statistically significant correlations according to Student's t test ($P < .05$).

In clinical practice, plain radiographs of the chest have been shown to be most reliable in the diagnosis of pulmonary hydatid disease (Lobinger et al, 1994). Numerous images have been described: those typical of the intact cyst (Fig. 23–54); round or oval shapes, solitary or multiple (Fig. 23–55); homogeneous density and perfectly defined margins as though drawn with a marking pen; ruptured or complicated cysts with membranes floating in fluid resembling a "water-lily" sign (Fig. 23–56); an incarcerated membrane folded back in the form of a barricade which appears as a fluid-filled abscess (Fig. 23–57), with or without air-fluid levels; images of pneumonitis of the lung; and areas of lung atelectasis. In these cases, the differential diagnosis with certain lesions such as bronchial tumors, sarcomas, and tuberculomas is a difficult challenge.

In the authors' series, plain radiographs of the chest and clinical assessment of the symptoms made it possible to establish the correct diagnosis preoperatively in 228 cases (95%). In six (2.5%), imaging studies such as ultrasonography, CT (Fig. 23–58) and MRI (Fig. 23–59) were required, and in the remaining six cases (2.5%), the diagnosis was established intraoperatively or in the subsequent histopathologic study. The preoperative diagnosis of hydatid disease of the lung was incorrect in six cases; the correct diagnoses were lung abscess ($n = 3$), tumor ($n = 2$) and bronchogenic cyst ($n = 1$).

Bronchoscopy was utilized in the diagnosis of pulmonary hydatidosis with considerable success prior to ultrasound and other imaging techniques such as CT and

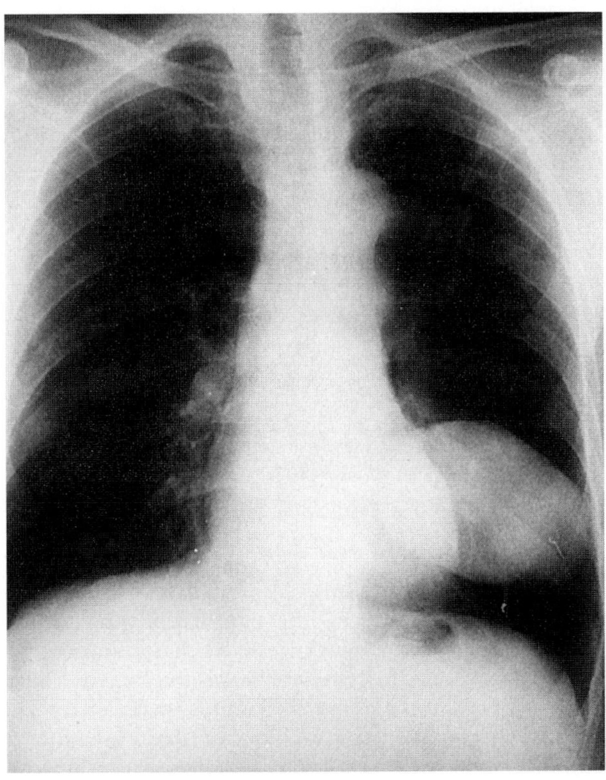

FIGURE 23–54 ■ Plain chest radiograph showing a hydatid cyst located in the lower left lobe of the lung.

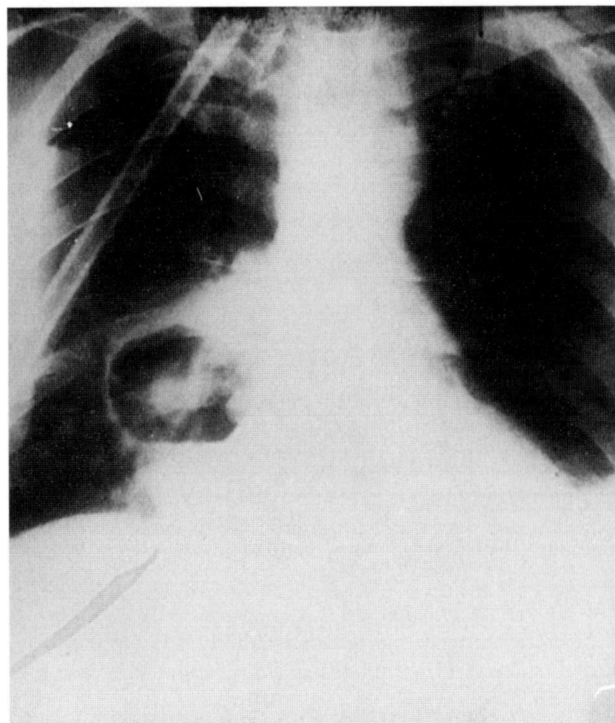

FIGURE 23–56 ■ "Water-lily sign." Radiographic image of a complicated hydatid cyst.

MRI; its use has been limited by the risk of rupture of the cyst and the subsequent development of severe complications. It still may be useful in cases of ruptured hydatid cyst of the lung because it enables the visualization of the hydatid membrane, which resembles the shininess of cooked egg white, and small fragments of the cystic membrane can even be removed during bronchoscopic examination using the technique of Coll and Collomé (Paterson and Blyth, 1996). Bronchography, the approach employed years ago, has followed in the steps

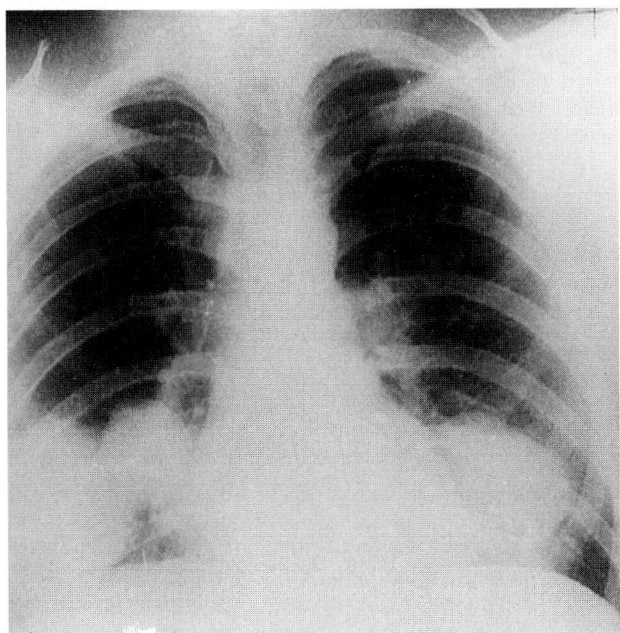

FIGURE 23–55 ■ Plain chest radiograph showing multiple hydatid cysts located in the lower lobes of the lung.

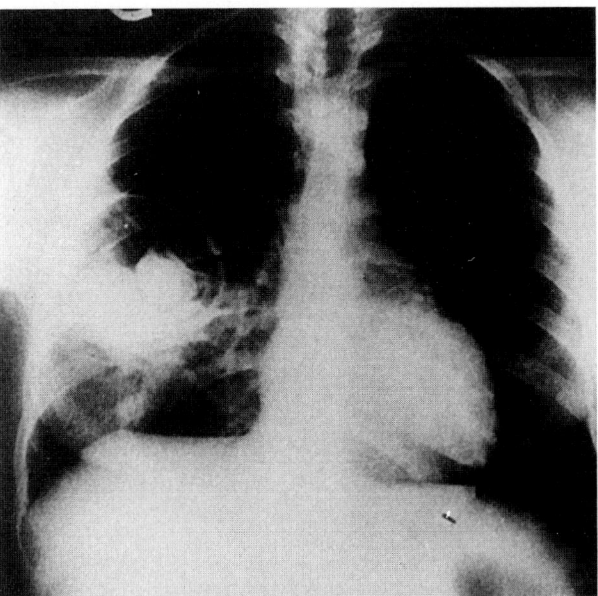

FIGURE 23–57 ■ Radiographic image of an incarcerated hydatid membrane.

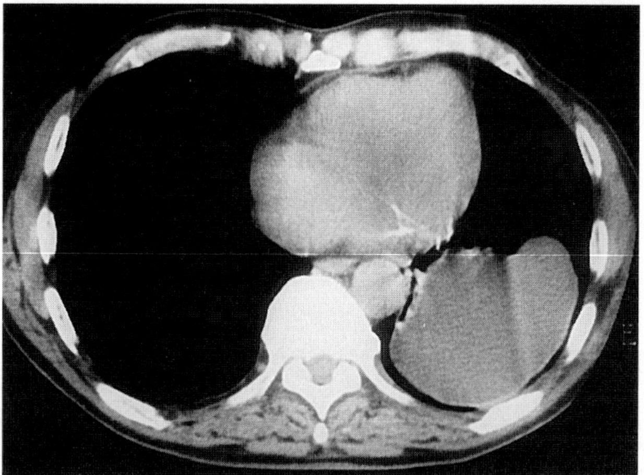

FIGURE 23–58 ■ Chest computed tomography scan showing a hydatid cyst located in the lower left lobe of the lung containing fragments of the hydatid membrane.

of bronchoscopy, being replaced entirely by imaging techniques such as CT and MRI (Prieto et al, 1996; Elburjo and Gani, 1995).

Surgical Treatment

The incision most commonly used in cases of solitary pulmonary cysts is a lateral thoracotomy. In earlier cases, when bilateral cysts were present, the operation was done in two stages, with the first thoracotomy being performed on the side on which the risk of rupture appeared to be greater or on which the cyst was more complicated (Taha et al, 1996). These cases are now treated in a single procedure, using a median sternotomy for cysts located in the anterior position and a trans-sternal bilateral thoracotomy for cysts in the anterior or posterior position or associated with hydatid disease of the heart. In some cases, the authors have performed an anterior bilateral thoracotomy in a single procedure.

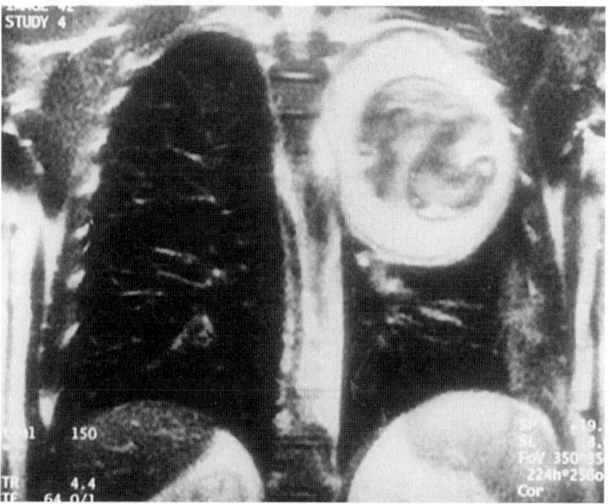

FIGURE 23–59 ■ Chest magnetic resonance image showing a hydatid cyst located in the upper left lobe of the lung, containing fragments of the hydatid membrane.

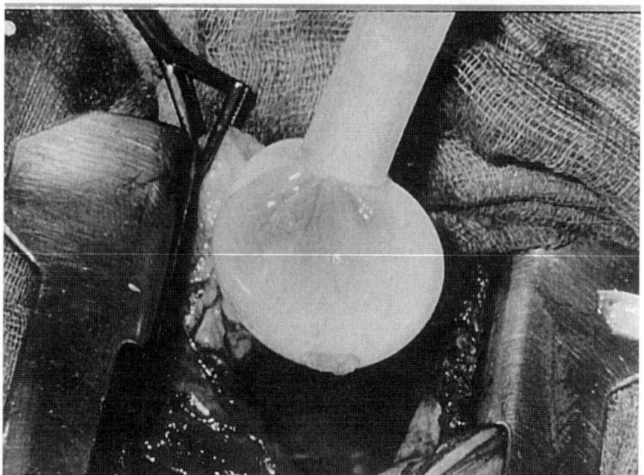

FIGURE 23–60 ■ Cystectomy (method of Posadas).

The objective of the surgical treatment of pulmonary hydatidosis is to eradicate the parasite, to prevent the intraoperative rupture of the cyst with its subsequent dissemination, and to remove the residual cavity. Most authors agree that the attempt should be made to remove as little lung tissue as possible and that resection of pulmonary parenchyma is indicated only when the adjacent tissue is seriously damaged or infected or when the atelectatic areas are presumed to be irrecoverable.

Initially, surgical treatment of pulmonary hydatidosis involved the marsupialization of the cyst after it was attached to the pleura, which was done in two stages: first pleurodesis was produced, followed by marsupialization in a second procedure. These techniques have since been abandoned.

Simple cystectomy with capitonnage (suture approximation of the pericystic tissue, the method of Posadas) (Fig. 23–60), or with cystopericystectomy have also been carried out. When the cyst is small and there is no risk of rupture, its complete removal can be attempted by incising the pleura and delivering the complete cyst, aided by an increase in airway pressure provided by the anesthetist (the Ugón technique).

In 276 cases (92%) treated surgically, after thoracotomy, we performed needle aspiration of the cyst using a trocar-suction device (Fig. 23–61) designed by Prof. D. Figuera (Figuera, 1953). The device is composed of a trocar containing a needle connected to a negative-pressure aspiration system and surrounded by a suction cup that fits over the convex part of the cyst wall. When the device is applied to the cyst, the negative pressure makes the suction cup adhere hermetically to the cyst wall, thus impeding the extravasation of the content as it is sucked out and eliminating the possibility of intraoperative contamination (Fig. 23–62). This surgical technique has been shown to be effective in preventing the rupture and dissemination of the cyst, and it facilitates the excision of the residual cavity. With this approach, we have observed no recurrences of pulmonary hydatidosis in those cases in which the cysts remained intact at the time of the operation.

In patients with hydatid cysts at nonpulmonary sites, the authors treat the other cyst in a second surgical

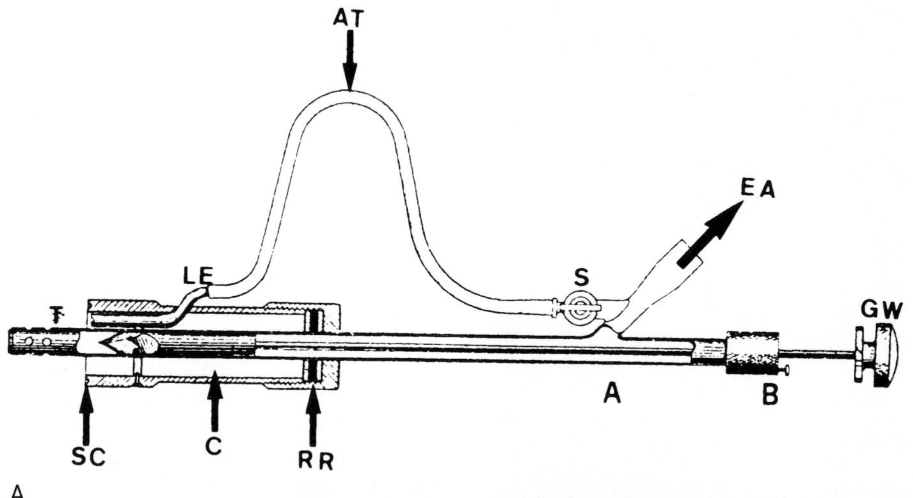

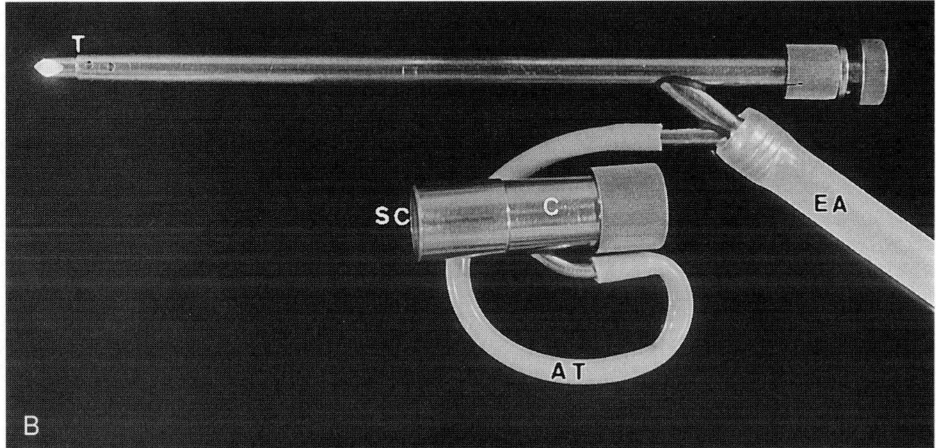

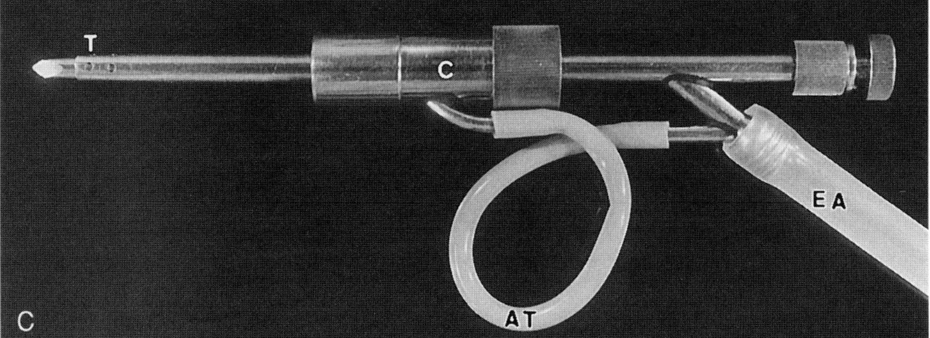

FIGURE 23–61 ■ *A*, Illustration of the trocar-suction device designed by Figuera. This device consists of a chamber (C) that acts like a suction cup (SC) as it generates negative pressure by means of a source of external aspiration (EA), which is transmitted to the chamber via an auxiliary tube (AT). The distal portion of the chamber is open to allow the suction cup to be applied to the convex surface of the hydatid cyst. A trocar (T) with a guidewire (GW) runs through it. The chamber also has a lateral exit (LE) connected by an auxiliary rubber tube. A switch (S) makes it possible to interrupt the emptying of the chamber at any time. The guidewire is cut irregularly, and its thicker distal end fits exactly into the trocar lumen. Its length is calculated so that when it is totally withdrawn, it remains in segment A–B, allowing external aspiration via the trocar and the lateral exit.

The proximal end of the chamber has a rubber ring (RR) that is situated between two metallic rings, all of which have a hole in the center. They allow the trocar to glide smoothly through them, but prevent air from entering the chamber. *B*, Photograph of the device showing the trocar (T) disconnected from the chamber (C), which remains connected to the source of external aspiration (EA) by means of an auxiliary tube (AT). *C*, Photograph of the trocar-suction device assembled for use.

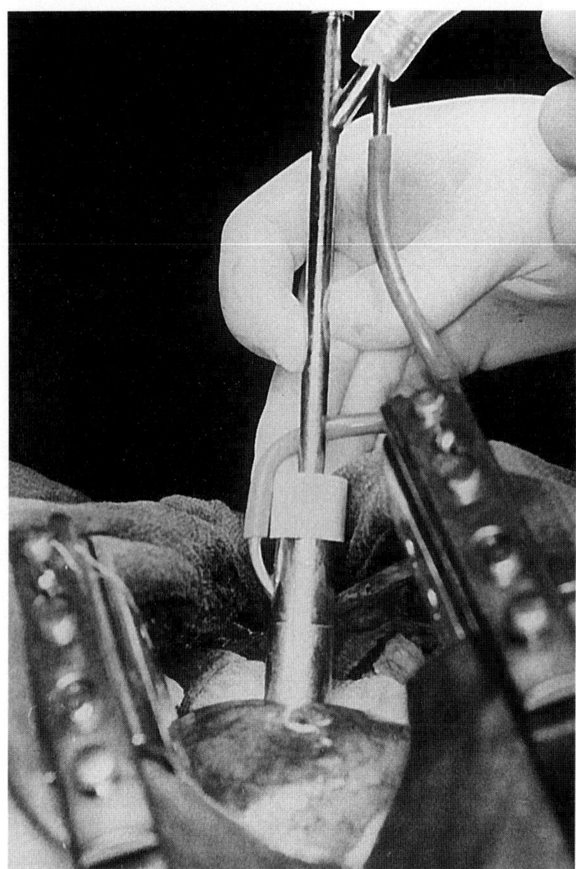

FIGURE 23–62 ■ Surgical technique using the trocar-suction device shown in Figure 23–61.

procedure. The decision as to which cyst should be removed first is based on the susceptibility of each to rupture, on their size, on the risk of dissemination, and on the vital importance of the organ in which each is located (Salih et al, 1998a).

Cysts in the lower right lung lobe may be connected to hepatic cysts that have passed through the diaphragm and resemble an hour glass (Eren and Ozgen, 1990; Gómez et al, 1995; Kir and Baran, 1995). Controversy exists as to the best surgical approach to these lesions. The authors choose thoracotomy or laparotomy, depending on the size of the cyst and the existence of signs of complications. When the cyst appears to affect the lung predominantly, thoracotomy is performed; if the liver is at risk, laparotomy is attempted, although on occasion, the approach must be extended to include thoracotomy because of the need to perform a right lower lobectomy. If thoractomy alone has been used, it is sometimes necessary to extend the incision to include a laparotomy so as to allow for T-tube placement when a hepatic cyst involves the bile ducts.

An atypical resection is usually performed when rupture or peripheral infection is detected. However, pulmonary lobectomy is commonly required when the cyst is associated with abscesses or severe pulmonary changes or with atelectasis that remains unresolved by standard surgical procedures, or when there is evidence that a given lobe contains infected hydatid membranes or several cysts. All authors agree on the need to preserve as much of the lung tissue as possible and to perform resection only when the lung is found to be destroyed (Burgos et al, 1991; Salih et al, 1998b).

Whenever possible, we opt for complete resection of the pericystic tissue and total eversion of the cavity, performing capitonnage in only 13.7% of patients because that approach has been found to result in the persistence of residual cavities. The surgical area should always be protected with hypertonic saline solution or formaldehyde-soaked sponges so as to avoid anaphylaxis and seedings if spillage should occur.

Since the first pilot studies with mebendazole in 1974, we have employed this drug as perioperative therapy according to the protocol proposed by Bekhti and his team (1977)—400 to 600 mg every 8 hours, as follows. Administration commences 7 to 10 days prior to surgery. When the cyst is intact and there appears to be no risk of its rupture during the surgical procedure, the treatment is administered for 1 month. When the cyst has ruptured or the possibility of its intraoperative dissemination is suspected, treatment is continued for 3 to 6 months. When dissemination is confirmed and total or partial resection of the lesions is not feasible, it is necessary to excise as many of the cysts as possible, attempting to conserve a maximum of lung parenchyma, and to administer mebendazole until there is no radiologic evidence of the lesions. Albendazole has been substituted for mebendazole, using the same regimen.

INFECTIONS THAT SOMETIMES REQUIRE SURGERY

Protozoal Infections

Amebiasis

Amebiasis is a parasitic infection produced by *Entamoeba histolytica*. Amebic dysentery is of worldwide distribution. It is estimated that about 500 million people are infected and that 10% will eventually develop the disease. Whereas amebic dysentery shows no age or sex predominance, pleuropulmonary involvement develops most commonly between the ages of 20 and 40 years and is 10 to 15 times more common in men. Pleuropulmonary complications in amebic dysentery have been estimated to occur in 0.1% of patients, but when a liver abscess is present, the incidence may be as high as 20% to 30%.

Amebiasis is acquired by ingesting the cysts in fecally contaminated food or water. In the small bowel, each cyst produces four trophozoites that invade the intestinal epithelium and enter the venous circulation. Although any organ may be affected, the liver is the most common site of secondary amebic abscesses. Pulmonary amebiasis can occur in two ways. The most common way is the direct spread of an amebic liver abscess through the liver capsule, peritoneum, diaphragm, and pleura. In fact, pleuropulmonary contamination is the most common complication of amebic hepatic abscesses. Less commonly, pulmonary involvement can occur by means of hematogenous spread. The right lower lobe of the lung is most commonly involved because of its contiguity with a liver abscess. The majority of amebic hepatic abscesses develop over the superior and posterior surfaces of the right lobe, and as the abscess enlarges, it includes the diaphragm in its wall. If the abscess develops slowly, it may produce a pleural reaction that generates adhesions at the base of the right lung, right pleural effusion, pulmonary consolidation, and sometimes a hepatobronchial fistula. If, on the other hand, the abscess enlarges rapidly, it may rupture in the pleural cavity with consequent empyema and lung abscess. Less commonly, amebic hepatic abscesses may extend into the pericardium and cause amebic pericarditis.

The most common presenting symptom of pleuropulmonary amebiasis is right-sided chest pain with radiation to the shoulder. The dry cough characterizes the early stages of pleuropulmonary disease, but later it may become productive of "chocolate sauce" material, indicating hepatobronchial communication. Expectoration of bile (biloptysis) may occur as a result of a bronchohepatic or bronchobiliary fistula. Fever is more pronounced with pleural involvement, and there often is general malaise, weakness, anorexia, and weight loss.

Diagnostic tests and treatment of this parasitic disease are summarized in Table 23–18. Adequate drug therapy is essential for the management of hepatic and pleuropulmonary amebiasis, but there are some situations in which invasive procedures are required. Massive pleural or pericardial effusions and empyemas must be drained. Postural drainage is useful in cases of hepatobronchial fistulas.

The prognosis of pulmonary amebiasis is poorer than that of uncomplicated liver abscess and becomes even worse if the pleura is involved. Empyema kills one in five patients, and the overall mortality rate associated with thoracic amebiasis ranges from 11% to 14%.

Helminthic Infections

Dirofilariasis

Dirofilaria immitis, the dog heartworm, produces pulmonary dirofilariasis in humans. The typical clinical manifestation of this disease is a solitary pulmonary nodule. Radiographs of the chest show a solitary, well-circumscribed spherical or wedge-shaped nodule, 2 to 3 cm in diameter. It is usually located at the periphery of the lung, attached to the pleura. Most patients are asymptomatic, and only 30% may have cough, chest pain, and hemoptysis. Eosinophilia is uncommon. Excisional lung biopsy with identification of the worm is required for diagnosis and is, at the same time, the treatment of choice. Most of the time, the diagnosis is made after pulmonary resection has been carried out because of suspected pulmonary carcinoma.

INFECTIONS THAT DO NOT REQUIRE SURGICAL INTERVENTION

Protozoal Infections

Toxoplasmosis

Toxoplasmosis is caused by *Toxoplasma gondii*, an obligate intracellular coccidian protozoan. This parasitic disease is of worldwide distribution and is a common human infestation. Most infected immunocompetent individuals are asymptomatic. Disseminated disease is common in immunocompromised patients (those with AIDS or malignancy or in immunosuppressive therapy). This disseminated form commonly involves the lung, producing interstitial pneumonitis with dyspnea, fever, cough, hemoptysis, acidosis, and even respiratory failure, hypotension, and disseminated intravascular coagulation. Pulmonary involvement is rare in the transplacentally transmitted congenital form of this disease, but it may occur in the form of pneumonitis.

Malaria

Malaria caused by *Plasmodium falciparum* can be associated in 3.5% to 7% of cases with acute noncardiogenic pulmonary edema and adult respiratory distress syndrome. The prognosis for patients with pulmonary involvement is very poor, and more than 80% of them die within 1 day of developing pulmonary edema, despite intensive therapy. Less commonly, patients may develop milder forms of pulmonary involvement, including interstitial edema, pleural effusion, and lobar consolidation.

Visceral Leishmaniasis (Kala-azar)

Leishmania donovani, the cause of visceral leishmaniasis, can be found as an amastigote in pulmonary macrophages. Pulmonary disease that causes symptoms is rare, but a few cases of pneumonitis have been reported, especially in untreated patients and AIDS patients.

Helminthic Infections

Trematodes (Flukes)

Lung Flukes: Paragonimiasis (Lung Dwelling Trematodes). Paragonimiasis is an infection caused by a lung fluke, most commonly *Paragonimus westermani*, the Asian lung fluke. Acute disease is rare and is characterized clinically by fever, cough, hepatosplenomegaly, pleural effusion, pneumothorax, and eosinophilia. The chronic form is more common and, classically, patients present a diagnostic triad of cough, hemoptysis, and eggs of *Paragonimus* species in sputa or feces. Radiographs may show transient, diffuse pulmonary infiltrates, pleural effusion, empyema, calcified lesions, pleural thickening, and nodular, cystic, or cavitary patterns. Pulmonary involvement tends to mimic postprimary tuberculosis.

Blood Flukes: Schistosomiasis. Schistosomiasis is caused by blood flukes of the genus *Schistosoma*, three of which (*S. mansoni*, *S. japonicum*, and *S. haematobium*) are traditionally regarded as the most important in human infestation. The acute form of the disease is associated with an eosinophilic Loeffler-like pneumonitis. Chronic schistosomiasis leads to the development of periportal or Symmer's fibrosis with portal hypertension. Schistosomal cor pulmonale with pulmonary hypertension occurs in 15% of patients with periportal fibrosis and is most commonly reported in *S. mansoni* infections from Egypt and Brazil. Patients present with hemoptysis and right ventricular hypertrophy, and the prognosis is poor.

Cestodes

Cysticercosis. Cysticercosis is a parasitic infection caused by the larval stage of *Taenia solium*, a human tapeworm. Humans acquire the disease by ingesting infected undercooked pork. Cysticerci can lodge anywhere in the body, but the usual sites are subcutaneous or intramuscular. Thoracic involvement results from deposition of cysticerci in the respiratory muscles, where their presence may occasion pain. Lung and pleural lesions are uncommon and usually asymptomatic.

Nematodes that Attack the Intestines

Ascariasis (Roundworm). Ascariasis is one of the most common helminthic infections of humans. In the great majority of cases, it is caused by *Ascaris lumbricoides*. Most patients infected by this nematode have no pulmonary symptoms. Only allergic patients with heavy infection are at risk of developing an eosinophilic pneumonitis, an asthma-like reaction, during the lung phase of larval migration. The symptoms usually resolve spontaneously in 2 to 3 weeks, when the larvae migrate out of the lungs.

Ancylostomiasis (Hookworm). Ancylostomiasis is caused by the nematodes *Ancylostoma duodenale* and *Necator americanus*. During the lung phase of larval migration, patients may develop mild, transient eosinophilic pneumonitis. Pulmonary disease appears less commonly than it does with infection by species of *Ascaris* or *Strongyloides*, but severe infestation may give rise to transient cough, hemoptysis, and pulmonary consolidation.

Strongyloidiasis. *Strongyloides stercoralis*, the threadworm, produces strongyloidiasis in humans. Pulmonary disease is caused by the migration of larvae through alveolar capillaries into air spaces. In most cases, pulmonary symptoms are mild or absent. It is only in disseminated strongyloidiasis in an immunocompromised host that the infection can lead to life-threatening pneumonia, with dyspnea, hemoptysis, and bronchospasm. Fatal adult respiratory distress syndrome is uncommon but can occur despite treatment.

Nematodes that Attack Tissue

Visceral Larva Migrans. Visceral larva migrans results from infestation by larvae of dog and cat roundworms *Toxocara canis* and *Toxocara cati*. The disease occurs predominantly in children who swallow soil containing eggs passed in the feces of dogs and cats. The larvae travel throughout the body and can lodge in any organ, particularly the liver, brain, eyes, lungs, cardiac muscle, and lymph nodes. Most children are asymptomatic and only those with severe disease and a significant number of larvae may develop transient pulmonary infiltrates and Loeffler's syndrome. Severe lung disease is rare.

Trichinosis. Trichinosis is caused by the ingestion of larvae of the roundworm *Trichinella spiralis*. Pulmonary manifestations in humans are rare. It is only in heavy and severe infections that patients may develop pneumonitis during the larval migration phase. The phase of larval encystment is characterized by myositis. Any muscle of the body may be parasitized, including the diaphragm and intercostal muscles. When these respiratory muscle are affected, patients may complain of dyspnea and tachypnea. Calcified walls of larval cysts within the respiratory muscles may be visible in radiographs of the chest.

Nematodes of the Filarioidea Superfamily

Tropical Pulmonary Eosinophilia. Tropical pulmonary eosinophilia is a distinct syndrome that develops in some individuals infected by lymphatic filarial species. The organisms most strongly implicated as the causative agents of this parasitic disease are the mosquito-transmitted *Wuchereria bancrofti* and *Brugia malayi*. Patients present with an asthma-like syndrome, malaise, episodes of nocturnal cough and wheezing, low-grade fever, weight loss, and adenopathy. Leukocytosis is usually severe and extreme eosinophilia and high IgE levels persist for weeks. In addition to a geographic history of filarial exposure, a characteristic triad of this disease is nocturnal wheezing, high titers of filarial antibodies, and a rapid response to diethylcarbamazine. Radiographs of the chest usually show a diffuse reticulonodular pattern. Pleural effusions are rare; pulmonary fibrosis may develop in untreated patients.

COMMENTS AND CONTROVERSIES

Since our last edition, we have increased the scope of this chapter to include all parasitic diseases but to specifically deal with those lesions most frequently seen by thoracic surgeons. It is fair to say that, in North America, physicians rarely encounter hydatid disease, but it is still very frequent in southern European countries and South America. The North American variety is mainly the "sylvatic" form, seen mostly in northern Canada and Alaska, and it is caused by a different strain of the tapeworm. Dogs, deer, and moose are the intermediate hosts, and, in this form of disease, lung cysts occur more frequently than do liver cysts.

The treatment of hydatid disease is well outlined by the authors. They prefer the Prez Fontana method of pericystectomy, whereas other surgeons simply enucleate the cyst from the surrounding lung. Certainly, smaller cysts can be wedge excised.

As we continue to increase our worldwide travel, thoracic surgeons everywhere must be aware of hydatid disease and its management approaches. Tables 23–15 through 23–18 are a convenient summary of the most common protozoal infections and their management.

R. J. G.

REFERENCES

Agrawal RL, Jain SK, Gupta SC et al: Hydropneumothorax secondary to hydatid lung disease. Indian J Chest Dis Allied Sci 35:93, 1993.

Alvarez Ayuso L, Téllez de Peralta G, Burgos Lazaro R et al: Surgical treatment of pulmonary hydatidosis. J Thorac Cardiovasc Surg 82:569, 1981.

Bekhti A, Schaaps JP, Capron M et al: Treatment of hepatic hydatid disease with mebedazole: Preliminary results in four cases. BMJ 2:1047, 1977.

Beshear JR, Hendley JO: Severe pulmonary involvement in visceral larva migrans. Am J Dis Child 125:599, 1973.

Botella de Maglia J, Espacio-Casanovas A: Malaria grave y complicada. Estudio de seis casos [Spanish]. Rev Clin Esp 198:509, 1998.

Burgos L, Baquerizo A, Muñoz W et al: Experience in the surgical treatment of 331 patients with pulmonary hydatidosis. J Thorac Cardiovasc Surg 102:427, 1991.

Charoenpan P, Indraprasit S, Kiatboonsri S et al: Pulmonary edema in severe falciparum malaria: Hemodynamic study and cliniphysiologic correlation. Chest 98:10, 1990.

Chitkara Rk, Sarinas PS: Dirofilaria, visceral larva migrans, and tropical pulmonary eosinophilia. Semin Respir Infect 12:138, 1997.

Choi JH, Chung SI, Whang YS et al: A case of pulmonary cysticercosis. Korean J Intern Med 6:38, 1991.

Cordero M, Munoz MR, Muro A et al: Transient solitary pulmonary nodule caused by Dirofilaria immitis. Eur Respir J 3:1070, 1990.

Cosgriff TM: Pulmonary edema in falciparum malaria: Slaying the dragon of volume overload. Chest 97:1190, 1990.

Devé F: Comp Rand Soc Biol 115:1025, 1934.

Elburjo M, Gani EA: Surgical management of pulmonary hydatid cysts in children. Thorax 50:396, 1995.

Eren N, Ozgen G: Simultaneous operation for right pulmonary and liver echinococcosis. Scand J Thorac Cardiovasc Surg 24:131, 1990.

Evans TG, Schwartzman JD: Pulmonary toxoplasmosis. Semin Respir Infect 6:51, 1991.

Figuera D: Trócar-ventosa para el tratamiento quirúrgico de los quistes hidatídicos y para la evacuación de colecciones sépticas [spanish]. Rev Clin Esp 50:373, 1953.

Furst SR, Weinger MB, Simons SM: Pleuropulmonary amebiasis. Chest 100:293, 1991.

Gallant JE, Ko AH: Cavitary pulmonary lesions in patients infected with human immunodeficiency virus. Clin Infect Dis 22:671, 1996.

Garcia LW, Hemphill RB, Marasco WA et al: Acquired immunodeficiency syndrome with disseminated toxoplasmosis presenting as an acute pulmonary and gastrointestinal illness. Arch Pathol Lab Med 115:459, 1991.

Goel MK, Nath J, Mukerji PK et al: A case of bilateral pulmonary hydatid cysts. Indian J Chest Dis Allied Sci 36:163, 1994.

Goldwater LJ, Steinberg I, Most H et al: Hemoptysis in trichiniasis. N Engl J Med 213:849, 1935.

Gómez R, Moreno E, Loinaz C et al: Diaphragmatic or transdiaphragmatic thoracic involvement in hepatic hydatid disease: Surgical trends and classification. World J Surg 19:714, 1995.

Gompels MM, Todd J, Peters BS et al: Disseminated strongyloidiasis in AIDS: Uncommon but important. AIDS 5:329, 1991.

Hashimoto H, Toshima S, Hashimoto H et al: Falciparum malaria in an overseas traveller complicated by disseminated intravascular coagulation and pulmonary edema. Intern Med 32:395, 1993.

Hotez PJ, Pritchard DI: Hookworm infection. Sci Am 272:68, 1995.

Ibarra-Perez C, Seiman-Lama M: Diagnosis and treatment of amebic empyema: Report of 88 cases. Am J Surg 134:283, 1977.

Jerray M, Benzarti M, Garrouche A et al: Hydatid disease of the lungs: Study of 386 cases. Am Rev Respir Dis 146:185, 1992.

Johnson RJ, Johnson JR: Paragonimiasis in Indochinese refugees: Roentgeographic findings with clinical correlation. Am Rev Respir Dis 128:534, 1983.

Jokipii L, Salmela K, Saha H et al: Leishmaniasis diagnosed from bronchoalveolar lavage. Scand J Infect Dis 24:677, 1992.

Kir A, Baran E: Simultaneous operation for hydatid cyst of right lung and liver. Thorac Cardiovasc Surg 43:62, 1995.

Lobinger B, Pfannenberg AC, Brambs HJ: Radiologic diagnosis in echinococcosis. Rontgenpraxis 47:144, 1994.

Magnussen P, Makunde W, Simonsen PE et al: Chronic pulmonary disorders, including tropical pulmonary eosinophilia, in villages with endemic lymphatic filariasis in Tanga region and in Tanga town, Tanzania. Trans R Soc Trop Med Hyg 89:406, 1995.

Marshall BG, Wilkinson RJ, Davidson RN: Pathogenesis of tropical pulmonary eosinophilia: Parasitic alveolitis and parallels with asthma. Respir Med 92:1, 1998.

Matzner Y, Behar A, Beeri E et al: Systemic leishmaniasis mimicking malignant histiocytosis. Cancer 43:398, 1979.

Moore RD, Urschel JD, Fraser RE et al: Cystic hydatid lung disease in northwest Canada. Can J Surg. 37:20, 1994.

Neafie RC, Connor DH: Ascariasis. In Binford CH, Connor DH (eds): Pathology of Tropical and Extraordinary Diseases. Washington, D.C., Armed Forces Institute of Pathology, 1976.

Oksenhendler E, Cadranel J, Sarfati C et al: *Toxoplasma gondii* pneumonia in patients with the acquired immunodeficiency syndrome. Am J Med 88:18N, 1990.

Ong RK, Doyle RL: Tropical pulmonary eosinophilia. Chest 113:1673, 1998.

Paterson HS, Blyth DF: Thoracoscopic evacuation of dead hydatid cyst. J Thorac Cardiovasc Surg 111:1280, 1996.

Prieto A, Díaz A, Calvo J et al: MR imaging of pulmonary hydatid disease. Eur J Radiol 23:85, 1996.

Quah BS, Anuar AK, Rowani MR et al: Cor pulmonale: An unusual presentation of tropical eosinophilia. Ann Trop Paediatr 17:77, 1997.

Ro JY, Tsakalakis PJ, White VA et al: Pulmonary dirofilariasis: The great imitator of primary or metastatic lung tumor. A clinicopathologic analysis of seven cases and a review of the literature. Hum Pathol 20:69, 1989.

Sadigursky M, Andrade ZA: Pulmonary changes in schistosomal cor pulmonale. Am J Trop Med Hyg 31:779, 1982.

Salih OK, Topcuoglu MS, Celik SK et al: Surgical treatment of hydatid cysts of the lung: Analysis of 405 patients. Can J Surg 41:131, 1998a.

Salih OK, Topcuoglu MS, Celik SK et al: Surgical treatment of hydatid cysts of the lung: Analysis of 405 patients with pulmonary hydatidosis. J Thorac Cardiovasc Surg 102:427, 1998b.

Schaberg T, Rahn W, Racz P, Lode H: Pulmonary schistosomiasis resembling acute pulmonary tuberculosis. Eur Respir J 4:1023, 1991.

Schad GA, Warren KS (eds): Hookworm Disease: Current Status and New Directions. London, Taylor & Francis, 1990.

Singh TS, Mutum SS, Razaque MA: Pulmonary paragonimiasis: Clinical features, diagnosis and treatment of 39 cases in Manipur. Trans R Soc Trop Med Hyg 80:967, 1986.

Singh RS, Sridhar MS, Bhaskar CJ: Tropical pulmonary eosinophilia presenting as eosinophilic pleural effusion. Indian J Chest Dis Allied Sci 34:225, 1992.

Stone WJ, Schaffner W: Strongyloides infections in transplant recipients. Semin Respir Infect 5:58, 1990.

Taha AM, Shabb B, Nassar H: Surgical therapy for pulmonary hydatidosis. Int Surg 81:187, 1996.

Tatke M, Malik GB: Pulmonary pathology in severe malaria infection in health and protein deprivation. J Trop Med Hyg 93:377, 1990.

Thompson JR, Berger R: Fatal adult respiratory distress syndrome following successful treatment of pulmonary strongyloidiasis. Chest 99:772, 1991.

Wilson JF, Rausch RL, Wilson FR: Alveolar hydatid disease: Review of the surgical experience in 42 cases of active disease among Alaskan Eskimos. Ann Surg 221:315, 1995.

Wreghitt TG, Hakim M, Gray JJ et al: Toxoplasmosis in heart and lung transplant recipients. J Clin Pathol 42:194, 1989.

TABLE 23–15 ■ **Epidemiology and Clinical Features of Helminthic Infections that May Involve Lung and Pleura**

Parasite	References	Geographic Distribution	Life-Cycle Hosts: Intermediary (transmission)	Life-Cycle Hosts: Definitive	Clinical Manifestations*	Incidence of Pulmonary or Pleural Involvement
TREMATODES (FLUKES)						
Lung flukes						
Paragonimus westermani (lung-dwelling trematodes)	Singh et al, 1986 Johnson et al, 1983	Far East	Snails—crabs, crayfish	Humans, other mammals	Acute (uncommon): **Fever, cough,** hepatosplenomegaly, **pleural effusion, pneumothorax,** eosinophilia Chronic: **Cough, hemoptysis;** chest radiograph: infiltrates, empyema, pleural effusion, calcification, pleural thickening, nodular, cystic, cavitary patterns	Common
Blood flukes						
Schistosoma mansoni	Schaberg et al, 1991 Sadigursky et al, 1982	South America, Caribbean, Middle East, Africa	Snails	Humans	Acute: **Loeffler-like pneumonitis** Chronic: Periportal or Symmers' fibrosis, portal hypertension; **cor pulmonale, pulmonary hypertension;** glomerulonephritis	Acute: Common in visitors to an endemic area. Chronic: 15% of patients with periportal fibrosis
Schistosoma japonicum	Schaberg et al, 1991 Sadigursky et al, 1982	Far East	Snails	Humans	Acute: **Loeffler-like pneumonitis** Chronic: Periportal or Symmers' fibrosis, portal hypertension; **cor pulmonale, pulmonary hypertension;** glomerulonephritis	Acute: Common in visitors to an endemic area. Chronic: 15% of patients with periportal fibrosis
Schistosoma haematobium	Schaberg et al, 1991 Sadigursky et al, 1982 Magnussen et al, 1995	Africa, Middle East	Snails	Humans	Acute: **Loeffler-like pneumonitis** Chronic: Bladder and ureteral fibrosis; **cor pulmonale**	Acute: Common in visitors to an endemic area. Chronic: Uncommon

Cestodes						
Echinococcus granulosus (hydatid disease)	Salih et al, 1998a Moore et al, 1994 Goel et al, 1994 Agrawal et al, 1993	Sheep-raising and hunting areas	Sheep, cattle, humans, goats, camels, horses	Dogs	Liver cyst: Abdominal pain, palpable mass, jaundice **Pulmonary cyst: Cough, chest pain, hemoptysis, pneumothorax, empyema**	25% of adults infected by *E. granulosus*
Taenia solium (cysticercosis)	Choi et al, 1991	Worldwide	Swine, dogs, cats, sheep, humans	Humans	Neurologic symptoms: Seizures, focal deficits, hydrocephalus, meningitis. Skeletal muscle cysticerci: **Thoracic pain if respiratory muscles involved.** Intraocular cyst. Calcified subcutaneous nodules. **Lung lesions** (uncommon and asymptomatic)	Uncommon
Nematodes						
Intestinal						
Ascaris lumbricoides (roundworm)	Neafie et al, 1976	Tropical and subtropical zones, rural southeastern U.S.	Soil, fecal–oral	Humans	Lung phase of larval migration: **Eosinophilic pneumonitis (fever, irritating cough, burning substernal discomfort, dyspnea, blood-tinged sputum, eosinophilia, infiltrates in chest radiograph)** Intestinal phase: Rarely gastrointestinal or biliary obstruction	Only in heavy infections in patients with pulmonary hypersensitivity
Necator americanus, Ancylostoma duodenale (hookworm)	Schad et al, 1990 Hotez et al, 1995	U.S., equatorial Africa *(Necator)* southern Europe, northern Africa, northern Asia *(Ancylostoma)*	Soil–skin	Humans	Lung phase of larval migration: **Mild transient pneumonitis** Intestinal phase: Abdominal pain, diarrhea; eosinophilia, iron-deficiency anemia, hypoproteinemia, dermatitis	Only in heavy infections (less common than with *Ascaris*)

Table continued on following page

TABLE 23–15 ■ **Epidemiology and Clinical Features of Helminthic Infections that May Involve Lung and Pleura** *Continued*

Parasite	*References*	*Geographic Distribution*	*Life-Cycle Hosts*		*Clinical Manifestations**	*Incidence of Pulmonary or Pleural Involvement*
			Intermediary (transmission)	*Definitive*		
Strongyloides stercoralis (strongyloidiasis)	Stone et al, 1990 Gompels et al, 1991 Thompson et al, 1991	Moist tropics and subtopics, southern U.S.	Soil–skin	Humans	Uncomplicated: Urticaria, abdominal symptoms, eosinophilia Complicated or disseminated strongyloidiasis in immunocompromised host: **Pneumonia**, meningitis, sepsis	Only in disseminated form in immunocompromised host
Tissue						
Toxocara canis and *cati* (visceral larva migrans)	Beshear et al, 1973 Chitkara et al, 1997	Tropical and temperate zones	Soil, fecal–oral	Dogs, cats, humans (zoonotic)	Fever, malaise, anorexia, weight loss, cough, wheezing, rash, hepatosplenomegaly, **transient pulmonary infiltrates–pneumonitis**, myocarditis, encephalitis	Only in severe disease
Trichinella spiralis (trichinosis)	Goldwater et al, 1935	Worldwide	Swine–humans	Swine, humans (zoonotic)	Enteric invasion: Abdominal symptoms Larval migration: Fever, hypereosinophilia, periorbital edema, hemorrhages, myocarditis, **pneumonitis**, encephalitis. Larval encystment: Myositis (**if diaphragm involved: dyspnea)**	Only in heavy and severe infections
Filariasis						
Wuchereria bancrofti, Brugia malayi (tropical pulmonary eosinophilia)	Singh et al, 1992 Quah et al, 1997 Chitkara et al, 1997 Marshall et al, 1998 Ong et al, 1998	Coastal in tropics and subtropics *(W. bancrofti)*; Asia, Indian subcontinent *(B. malayi)*	Mosquito	Humans	**Nocturnal cough and wheezing,** low-grade fever, weight loss, adenopathy, eosinophilia, elevated IgE, leukocytosis. **Pulmonary fibrosis** (nontreated), **pleural effusion** (rare)	Common
Dirofilaria immitis (dirofilariasis)	Ro et al, 1989 Cordero et al, 1990 Chitkara et al, 1997	Worldwide	Mosquito	Dogs, cats, humans (zoonotic)	**Solitary pulmonary nodule; cough, chest pain, hemoptysis** (less common)	In 30–40% of infected patients

*Pleuropulmonary involvement is indicated by boldface.

TABLE 23–16 ■ **Epidemiology and Clinical Features of Protozoal Infections that May Involve Lung and Pleura**

Parasite	*References*	*Geographic Distribution*	*Life-Cycle Hosts*		*Clinical Manifestations**	*Incidence of Pulmonary or Pleural Involvement*
			Intermediary (transmission)	*Definitive*		
Entamoeba histolytica (amebiasis)	Ibarra-Perez et al, 1997 Furst et al, 1991	Worldwide, esp. tropics	Fecal–oral	Humans	Intestinal: Colitis, toxic megacolon, ameboma; liver abscess; **right pleural effusion, empyema, hepatobronchial fistula, pulmonary consolidation (right lower or middle lobe), lung abscess;** genital ulcers	0–1%, but 20%–30% of patients with liver abscess
Toxoplasma gondii (toxoplasmosis)	Wreghitt et al, 1989 Oksenhendler et al, 1990 Garcia et al, 1991 Evans et al, 1991 Gallant et al, 1996	Worldwide	Humans, other mammals (orally, transplacentally, in organ transplantation)	Cats	Immunocompetent: Lymphadenopathy Immunocompromised: Encephalitis, chorioretinitis, **interstitial pneumonitis (dyspnea,fever, cough, hemoptysis, acidosis, respiratory failure, hypotension, DIC)** Congenital: Mental sequelae, chorioretinitis, **pneumonitis**	Common in immunocompromised patients (AIDS, malignancy, immunosuppressive therapy)

Table continued on following page

TABLE 23–16 ■ **Epidemiology and Clinical Features of Protozoal Infections that May Involve Lung and Pleura** Continued

Parasite	*References*	*Geographic Distribution*	*Life-Cycle Hosts*		*Clinical Manifestations**	*Incidence of Pulmonary or Pleural Involvement*
			Intermediary (transmission)	*Definitive*		
Plasmodium spp. (malaria)	Charoenpan et al, 1990 Cosgriff et al, 1990 Tatke et al, 1990 Hashimoto et al, 1993 Botella et al, 1998	Subtropics and tropics	Mosquito	Humans	Nonsevere: Nonspecific *Severe:* coma, anemia, renal failure, **acute noncardiogenic pulmonary edema, ARDS**, lactic acidosis, hypoglycemia, DIC	3.5%–7% of patients with *P. falciparum* malaria
Leishmania donovani (visceral leishmaniasis, kala-azar)	Matzner et al, 1979 Jokipii et al, 1992	Widespread in tropics and subtropics	Sand flies (phlebotomus), percutaneous, congenital	Humans, dogs, wild carnivores	Hepatosplenomegaly, fever, diarrhea, cough, lymphadenopathy, cachexia, pancytopenia, hypoalbuminemia, hypergammaglobulinemia, cutaneous lesion, **pneumonitis**	Uncommon (nontreated patients, AIDS patients)

*Pleuropulmonary involvement is indicated by boldface.
ARDS, adult respiratory distress syndrome; DIC, disseminated intravascular coagulation.

TABLE 23–17 ■ **Diagnosis and Treatment of Helminthic Infections that May Involve Lung and Pleura**

	Diagnosis				Treatment	
Parasite	*Main Features*	*Serologic Test*	*Other*	*Differential Diagnosis*	*Choice*	*Alternative*
TREMATODES (FLUKES)						
Lung flukes *Paragonimus westermani* (Lung-dwelling trematodes)	Identification of eggs in stool or sputum*	WB	Chest radiograph, CT, MRI	TB	PZQ 75 mg/kg/day in 3 doses for 2 days	BTH
Blood flukes *Schistosoma mansoni*	Identification of eggs in feces, liver or rectal biopsies*	EIA, WB	Ultrasound	Loeffler's syndrome; other causes of cor pulmonale; TB	PZQ 40 mg/kg in 2 doses for 1 day	OXM
Schistosoma japonicum	Identification of eggs in feces or liver biopsy*	EIA, WB	Ultrasound, CT	Loeffler's syndrome; other causes of cor pulmonale; TB	PZQ 60 mg/kg in 3 doses for 1 day	—
Schistosoma haematobium	Identification of eggs in urine or bladder biopsy*	EIA, WB	Ultrasound	Loeffler's syndrome; other causes of cor pulmonale; TB	PZQ 40 mg/kg in 2 doses for 1 day	MTF
CESTODES						
Echinococcus granulosus (hydatid disease)	Microscopic examination of cyst content*	WB	Chest radiograph, CT, MRI, ultrasound	Pulmonary carcinoma	Surgical excision plus ABZ 400 mg bid for 20 days, repeated as necessary	ABZ 400 mg bid for 28 days, repeated from 1 to 8 times
Taenia solium (cysticercosis)	Identification of the cysticercus within an involved tissue (muscle, CNS)*	WB	CT, MRI radiograph	—	Asymptomatic: no treatment Neurocysticercosis: PZQ 50 mg/kg/day in 3 doses for 15 days or ABZ 15 mg/kg/day in 3 doses for 8–30 days plus glucocorticoids	Surgery (ocular, ventricular, or spinal involvement)

Table continued on following page

TABLE 23–17 ■ **Diagnosis and Treatment of Helminthic Infections that May Involve Lung and Pleura** *Continued*

	Diagnosis				*Treatment*	
Parasite	*Main Features*	*Serologic Test*	*Other*	*Differential Diagnosis*	*Choice*	*Alternative*
NEMATODES						
Intestinal						
Ascaris lumbricoides (roundworm)	Detection of eggs in fecal samples*	—	Chest radiograph, ultrasound, ERCP	Other causes of eosinophilic pneumonitis, Loeffler's syndrome	MBZ 100 mg bid for 3 days or PPZ 75 mg/kg (max 3.5 g) for 2 days	ABZ, PP
Necator americanus, Ancylostoma duodenale (hookworm)	Identification of eggs in fresh stool or larvae in old stool*	—	Chest radiograph	Other causes of eosinophilic pneumonitis, Loeffler's syndrome	MBZ 100 mg bid for 3 days	PP, ABZ
Strongyloides stercoralis (strongyloidiasis)	Detection of larvae in stool, duodenal aspirate, or sputum*	EIA	Chest radiograph	Other causes of pneumonia in immunocompromised host	TBZ 25 mg/kg bid for 2 days; for disseminated disease continue for 7 days of longer	IVR, ABZ
Tissue						
Toxocara canis and *cati* (visceral larva migrans)	Eosinophilia, leukocytosis, hypergammaglobulinemia	EIA*	Chest radiograph	Other eosinophilic pneumonitis	Glucocorticoids (in severe myocardial, CNS, or pulmonary involvement)	—
Trichinella spiralis (trichinosis)	Eosinophilia, elevated IgE, CPK, LDH	BF*	Surgical muscle biopsy*, chest radiograph (infiltrates, calcified cysts within respiratory muscles)	Other eosinophilic pneumonitis	Glucocorticoids (in severe myositis or myocarditis); MBZ or TBZ (enteric stages)	—
Filariasis						
Wuchereria bancrofti, Brugia malayi (tropical pulmonary eosinophilia)	Nocturnal wheezing, high levels of antifilarial antibodies, rapid response to treatment	—	Chest radiograph (reticulonodular pattern); pulmonary function test (restrictive pattern)	Asthma, Loeffler's syndrome, allergic bronchopulmonary aspergillosis, Churg-Strauss and Wegener's vasculitis, chronic eosinophilic pneumonia	DEC 6 mg/kg/day in 3 doses for 21 days	—
Dirofilaria immitis (dirofilariasis)	Excisional lung biopsy*	—	Chest radiograph	Pulmonary carcinoma	Excisional lung biopsy	—

*Definitive diagnostic test

ABZ, albendazole; BF, bentonite flocculation: BTH, bithionol; CNS, central nervous system; CPK, creatine phosphokinase; CT, computed tomography; DEC, diethylcarbamazine; EIA, enzyme immunoassay; ERCP, endoscopic retrograde cholangiopancreatogram; IVR, ivermectin; LDH, lactate dehydrogenase; MBZ, mebendazole; MRI, magnetic resonance imaging; MTF, metrifonate; OXM, oxamniquine; PP, pyrantel pamoate; PPZ, piperazine; PZQ, praziquantel; TB, tuberculosis; TBZ, thiabendazole; WB, Western blot.

TABLE 23–18 ■ **Diagnosis and Treatment of Protozoal Infections that May Involve Lung and Pleura**

	Diagnosis				*Treatment*	
Parasite	*Main Features*	*Serologic Test*	*Other*	*Differential Diagnosis*	*Choice*	*Alternative*
Entamoeba histolytica (amebiasis)	Demonstration of trophozites or cysts in stool, liver aspirate, or pleural exudate*	ID, IHA	Intestinal biopsy; liver CT; ultrasound, MRI; chest radiograph	Other causes of basal pleuropulmonary disease	Asymptomatic: Diloxanide furoate 500 mg tid for 10 days Colitis-liver abscess: Metronidazole 750 mg tid for 5–10 days plus iodoquinol 650 mg tid for 20 days	Aspiration of liver abscess, drainage of pleural effusion (if massive)
Toxoplasma gondii (toxoplasmosis)	Isolation of the parasite after subinoculation of body fluids into mice or in tissue biopsy*	Sabin-Feldman EIA, IIF	Cerebral CT, MRI; chest radiograph	*Pneumocystis carinii* pneumonia	Pyrimethamine 75 mg/day plus sulfadiazine 4–6 g/day plus calcium folinate 10–15 mg/day for 4–6 weeks	Clindamycin plus pyrimethamine plus calcium folinate; spiramycin
Plasmodium spp. (malaria)	Demonstration of asexual form in peripheral blood smears stained with Giemsa*	Little use	PCR, chest radiograph	Other causes of ARDS	Severe malaria: Chloroquine-resistant: Quinidine gluconate 10 mg of base/kg IV over 1 hr followed by 0.02 mg/kg per min for 3 days maximum Chloroquine-sensitive: Chloroquine 10 mg of base/kg IV over 8 hr followed by 15 mg of base/kg over 24 hr	Exchange transfusion (high parasitemia and altered mental status); treatment of complications
Leishmania donovani (visceral leishmaniasis, kala-azar)	Demonstration of amastigotes in aspirates or biopsy (bone marrow, spleen, liver, lymph node)*	EIA	Chest radiograph	Malaria, brucellosis, TB, typhoid, leukemia, lymphoma	Stibogluconate sodium 20 mg/kg/day IV or IM for 28 days	Meglumine antimoniate, amphotericin B, pentamidine

*Definitive diagnostic test.

ARDS, adult respiratory distress syndrome; CT, computed tomography; EIA, enzyme immunoassay; ID, immunodiffusion; IHA, indirect hemagglutination; IIF, indirect immunofluorescence; IV, intravenous; IM, intramuscular; MRI, magnetic resonance imaging; PCR, polymerase chain reaction; TB, tuberculosis

PULMONARY INFECTIONS AND THE IMMUNOCOMPROMISED HOST

Diane E. Stover
M. Patricia Rivera

Immunosuppression can be defined as a relative or absolute defect in the function of antigen-processing cells or effector cells (B lymphocyte, T lymphocyte, macrophage, or neutrophil). Clinically, it is defined by the susceptibility to infection of certain populations rather than by specific laboratory tests of white blood cell or antibody function. These populations include patients with cancer, those who are receiving chemotherapeutic or immunosuppressive agents, those with autoimmune deficiency syndrome (AIDS), and those who have undergone organ transplantation.

HISTORICAL NOTE

Over the past several decades the number of immunosuppressed patients and the spectrum of disorders that they develop have markedly expanded. The reasons for these increases include more effective yet more intensive therapy for patients with cancer, the great success and widespread use of organ transplantation, and the AIDS epidemic. Radiotherapy and chemotherapy almost certainly have an impact on the natural defense mechanisms of the lung, thereby increasing susceptibility to pulmonary infections. The multiple quantitative and functional abnormalities of the cellular and humoral immune systems that occur in patients with the human immunodeficiency virus (HIV) account for the marked increase in incidence of routine and opportunistic infections in the lungs of patients with AIDS.

With the expanding immunosuppressed population and often with the need to make a specific diagnosis urgently, physicians must choose the test or procedure that is most likely to yield a diagnosis quickly and at the lowest cost in morbidity. Probably the single most important technique that has revolutionized the diagnosis of pulmonary infections in the immunocompromised host is fiberoptic bronchoscopy. In 1967 Shigeto Ikeda of the National Cancer Institute in Tokyo designed and standardized the instrument that is now known as the flexible fiberoptic bronchoscope. This instrument has vastly expanded clinicians' ability to diagnose pulmonary infections in all patient populations, and it is well tolerated and engenders few complications. It is particularly important in the immunocompromised host because it can be performed safely in the setting of mechanical ventilation, thrombocytopenia, and platelet dysfunction.

■ *HISTORICAL READINGS*

Fanta CH, Pennington JE: Pulmonary infections in the transplant patient. In Morris PJ, Tilney NL (eds): Progress in Transplantation, Vol 2. New York, Churchill Livingstone, 1985.

Martin WJ, Smith TF, Sanderson DR et al: Role of bronchoalveolar lavage in the assessment of opportunistic pulmonary infections: Utility and complications. Mayo Clin Proc 62:549, 1987.

Pizzo PA, Robichaud KJ, Gill FA et al: Empiric antibiotic and antifungal therapy for cancer patients with prolonged fever and granulocytopenia. Am J Med 72:101, 1982.

Stover DE: Diagnosis of pulmonary disease in the immunocompromised host. Semin Respir Med 10:89, 1989.

Stover DE, Zaman MB, Hajdu SL et al: Bronchoalveolar lavage in the diagnosis of diffuse pulmonary infiltrates in the immunocompromised host. Ann Intern Med 101:1, 1984b.

White DA, Stover DE: Pulmonary complications of HIV infection. Clin Chest Med 17:621, 1996.

EPIDEMIOLOGY

Classically, textbooks divide infectious diseases that immunosuppressed patients acquire according to their underlying disease and in vitro immunologic abnormalities. However, not only intrinsic B cell or T cell immunologic defects but also other factors, such as environmental exposure, travel history, iatrogenic procedures, recent antibiotic therapy, and specific organ transplantation, must be considered when a clinician tries to identify the likely causative agent of pulmonary infection in an immunocompromised host (Shelhamer et al, 1991).

Adults with HIV infection in the United States are primarily homosexual or bisexual men. Intravenous drug abuse is the second largest risk factor for the development of AIDS, and it is the leading source of heterosexual and perinatal transmission in the United States and Europe. A smaller percentage of total AIDS cases is caused by the transfusion of infected blood or blood products, especially in hemophiliac patients. New cases from the latter group have practically disappeared with HIV testing of all blood products.

Although some epidemiologic features of HIV disease are common to all patients with AIDS, geographic variability in the disease patterns does occur. For example, in the United States, bacterial and *Pneumocystis carinii* pneumonia (PCP) are the most common HIV-related pulmonary diseases, whereas in Africa tuberculosis is seen with much greater frequency (Wallace et al, 1993). Tuberculosis is also considerably more common in intravenous drug abusers, blacks, Hispanics, and patients from nonindustrialized countries than in white homosexual men. Some of these differences in infection patterns may be explained by environmental and geographic exposure and the prevalence of infection among various patient populations, but other poorly defined and unknown risk factors also appear to influence the pulmonary manifestations of HIV infection throughout the world.

CAUSES OF PULMONARY INFILTRATES IN THE NON-HIV IMMUNOCOMPROMISED HOST

- Infectious causes
  - Bacterial
    - *Streptococcus pneumoniae*
    - *Haemophilus influenzae*
    - *Staphylococcus aureus*
    - Gram-negative bacilli
    - *Legionella* species
    - *Nocardia* species
  - Mycobacterial
    - *Mycobacterium tuberculosis*
    - Atypical mycobacteria
  - Fungal (opportunistic)
    - *Pneumocystis carinii*
    - *Aspergillus* species
    - *Mucor* species
    - *Candida* species
  - Fungal (pathogenic)
    - *Cryptococcus neoformans*
    - *Histoplasma capsulatum*
    - *Coccidioides immitis*
  - Viral
    - Cytomegalovirus
    - Herpes simplex
    - Varicella-zoster
  - Parasitic
    - *Strongyloides stercoralis*
    - *Toxoplasma gondii*
- Noninfectious causes
  - Pulmonary edema (cardiogenic and noncardiogenic)
  - Neoplastic disorders
  - Toxic lung injury (drug- and radiation-induced)
  - Leukostasis
  - Leukoagglutinin reaction
  - Pulmonary hemorrhage
- Unknown causes
  - Bronchiolitis obliterans with organizing pneumonia (BOOP)
  - Nonspecific interstitial pneumonia
  - Chronic organizing pneumonia

CLINICAL FEATURES

General Considerations

The magnitude of pulmonary problems in the non-HIV immunocompromised host is broad (Murray and Mills, 1990; Williams et al, 1976; Matthay et al, 1980). A listing of common pulmonary disorders found in this patient population is shown in the box.

The purpose of this section is not only to discuss the most common infections that occur in the immunocompromised host but also to provide a framework for approaching the diagnosis of pulmonary infections, especially with regard to the selection of available diagnostic procedures.

When the diagnosis of specific pulmonary diseases is considered in this population, several factors should be evaluated. The underlying immunocompromising condition and the immunologic defect that it imparts are important features (Singer et al, 1979; Matthay and Greene, 1980) (Table 23–19). For example, patients with cell-mediated immune deficiencies, such as those that occur in lymphomas, organ transplantation, and high-dose corticosteroid therapy, are prone to infection by PCP, cytomegalovirus (CMV), *Mycoplasma tuberculosis*, and *Cryptococcus neoformans* and to pathogenic (endemic) fungal infections, such as *Histoplasma capsulatum* and *Coccidioides immitis*. On the other hand, patients immunocompromised by virtue of granulocytopenia are susceptible to infection by gram-negative bacilli, *Staphylococcus aureus*, and opportunistic fungi such as species of *Aspergillus*. A patient with breast carcinoma who is receiving high-dose corticosteroid therapy because of central nervous system metastases and then develops diffuse bilateral pulmonary infiltrates is suspected of having PCP. A neutropenic patient with leukemia who is receiving a course of empiric broad-spectrum antibiotics for a fever and then has a new pulmonary infiltrate is more likely to have a fungal pneumonia, especially one caused by an *Aspergillus* species (Pizzo et al, 1982).

The radiographic patterns, denoted in the box, are helpful for focusing the differential diagnosis on a certain

RADIOGRAPHIC APPEARANCE ASSOCIATED WITH PULMONARY INFECTIONS IN THE IMMUNOCOMPROMISED HOST*

- Localized infiltrates (segmental or lobar)
  - Bacteria
  - *Mycobacterium* species (especially *tuberculosis*)
  - Fungi
- Diffuse infiltrates
  - *Pneumocystis carinii*
  - Viral pneumonia
  - Adult respiratory distress syndrome (sepsis with bacteria or fungus)
- Hilar or mediastinal adenopathy
  - Tuberculosis and atypical mycobacteria
  - Pathogenic fungi
  - *Cryptococcus* species (occasionally)
- Cavitation
  - Bacteria (gram-negative bacilli, anaerobes, and *Nocardia*, *Actinomyces*, and *Legionella* species)
  - Tuberculosis and atypical mycobacteria
  - Septic emboli (bacterial and fungal)
- Pleural effusion
  - Bacteria
  - Tuberculosis
  - Fungi (occasionally)
- Nodules
  - *Nocardia* and *Actinomyces* species
  - Atypical mycobacteria
  - Opportunistic fungi (especially *Aspergillus* species)

*This applies to patients with and without HIV.

TABLE 23–19 ■ **Relationship of Immune Defects to Pulmonary Infections**

*Immune Defect**	*Examples of Disease with Immune Defect*	*Organisms Commonly Seen with Immune Defect*
B cell defect (decreased quantity or impaired function)	Some lymphoproliferative disorders (especially acute and chronic lymphatic leukemia) Multiple myeloma Some drugs (especially corticosteroids, antimetabolites, and alkylating agents)	Common *S. pneumoniae* *H. influenzae* Other gram-negative bacilli Less common *P. carinii*
T cell defect (impaired cell-mediated immunity)	Some lymphoproliferative disorders (especially Hodgkin's disease) Renal insufficiency Some drugs (especially corticosteroids)	Common *P. carinii* Mycobacteria *Cryptococcus* species and other pathogenic fungi Herpesviruses (especially cytomegalovirus) Less common *Legionella* species *Nocardia* species
Granulocyte defect (decrease in number or impaired function)	Myeloproliferative disorders (especially acute myelogenic leukemia) Most chemotherapeutic agents	Common *S. aureus* Gram-negative bacilli Enteric bacilli Opportunistic fungi (especially *Aspergillus* species)

*During organ transplantation the immune defect that develops depends on the organ transplanted, the underlying disease, and the drugs used pre- or post-transplant. Pulmonary infections often occur at a predictable amount of time after certain transplants.

subset of likely agents and for estimating the urgency of making a specific diagnosis. A distinction is often made between processes localized to a lobe or segment and those that involve multiple lobes bilaterally, commonly described as diffuse. The presence of segmental or lobar infiltrates combined with a clinical history that suggests an acute illness would favor the diagnosis of bacterial pathogens, whereas diffuse infiltrates suggest opportunistic infections (such as PCP) or noninfectious processes (such as drug toxicity or lymphangitic spread of tumor) (Tenholder and Hooper, 1980). The presence of pleura-based, wedged-shaped infiltrates, cavitation, nodules, hilar adenopathy, or pleural effusions can also be helpful in focusing the physician's attention on certain disorders.

The seriousness of the illness and the rate of the patient's deterioration can influence such decisions as whether there is time to wait for a response to empiric therapy or whether an invasive procedure should be performed. Consideration of the disease's tempo can also narrow the differential diagnosis. Bacterial infections, particularly in the neutropenic host, can be acute in onset and may be heralded by fever with shaking chills. The acute, often fulminant onset of PCP is notorious in the non–HIV-infected patient. CMV pneumonia more commonly evolves over a period of weeks, a tempo similar to that of infection by *Aspergillus* or *Mucor* species. Nocardiosis, tuberculosis, and some fungal infections such as cryptococcosis usually follow an insidious course; their development over weeks to months may mimic noninfectious processes, such as metastatic disease, drug-induced lung injury, or radiation-induced fibrosis.

Other important considerations in the differential diagnosis of pulmonary disorders include the temporal relationship of the pulmonary disease to the underlying disease. For example, an HIV-infected patient in whom a pulmonary disorder develops early in the course of illness (when the CD4 lymphocyte count is greater than 500 cells/mm^3) is unlikely to have PCP and more likely to have either bacterial pneumonia or tuberculosis (Masur et al, 1989). A patient who has undergone a bone marrow transplant and has pulmonary disease within the first month after the transplant is more likely to have bacterial or fungal pneumonia than CMV pneumonia, which usually develops several months after a bone marrow transplant (Fanta and Pennington, 1985) and almost always after engraftment occurs.

Prophylactic measures are being taken to prevent pulmonary infections among many types of immunocompromised patients, including those who receive solid organ and bone marrow transplants or who have HIV. Low, intermittent doses of trimethoprim-sulfamethoxazole (TMP/SMZ), dapsone, or aerosolized pentamidine are commonly administered to these patients producing a consequently marked reduction in the incidence of PCP. As a result, the differential diagnosis of new pulmonary infiltrates must be strongly influenced by the history of previous antibiotic prophylaxis.

Patient History

Besides these considerations, other points in a clinical history that are worthy of emphasis include the travel history of the patient, an evaluation of the activity of the underlying disease, and a careful evaluation of the patient's fluid balance. If an HIV-infected patient with a CD4 lymphocyte count lower than 100 cells/mm^3 recently traveled to the San Joaquin Valley, an area highly endemic for *Coccidioides immitis*, and did not receive antifungal prophylaxis, invasive disease by this organism should be strongly considered in the differential diagnosis of a pulmonary disorder. A female patient with breast cancer whose bibasilar interstitial infiltrates appear in combination with new hepatic and bony lesions should be suspected of having lymphangitic spread of her cancer, whereas in a woman whose breast cancer is responding to therapy, the appearance of the same infiltrates should prompt a search for a different cause. Pulmonary edema occurs in any patient, regardless of age. Large fluid volumes are often given with certain chemotherapeutic agents or for resuscitation of the hypotensive septic patient. Abnormal renal function and other poorly defined factors impair the body's ability to compensate for large fluid loads. Pulmonary edema can develop, and it may be difficult to differentiate radiographically from PCP or viral pneumonia.

Fever is a nonspecific sign of infection. Many noninfectious processes, including malignancy, radiation pneumonitis, cytotoxic drug-induced lung disease, bronchiolitis obliterans with organizing pneumonia (BOOP), and nonspecific interstitial pneumonitis, cause fever as part of the response to inflammation. However, because fever is the most common sign of pulmonary infection, its absence strongly argues against infectious pneumonia. Cough and dyspnea are common nonspecific symptoms and occur in both infectious and noninfectious processes.

Physical Examination

Although the physical examination of an immunocompromised host with pneumonia may be unrevealing, in the face of life-threatening dyspnea, hypoxemia, and diffuse infiltrates, to conclude that it is inconsequential would be an error. Rales can be heard before infiltrates appear. In addition, when the chest radiograph shows a unilateral infiltrate, the physical examination may reveal the presence of bilateral disease, which would alter diagnostic considerations. A pleural friction rub with a pulmonary infiltrate suggests a virulent bacterial or fungal infection, (usually by a species of *Aspergillus*). Localized wheezing suggests a partially obstructed bronchus, which may be due to a neoplasm or to mucus, to fungal bronchitis (especially if caused by an *Aspergillus* species), or to a blood clot. The presence of wheezing or a pleural friction rub is also strong evidence against certain diagnoses such as PCP and CMV. Finally, the physical examination is often superior to the findings on the chest radiograph in suggesting the overall severity of the illness. Quantitation of the respiratory rate alone may provide critical information about the seriousness of the illness and can help direct the timing and course of the diagnostic evaluation.

Occasionally, extrapulmonic manifestations may be the best clue to the cause of a pulmonary disease. Of particular importance is a detailed examination of the skin, eyes, and neurologic system. Finally, and most important, in the patient with diffuse bilateral pulmonary infiltrates, fluid balance should be evaluated. A physical examination that shows peripheral edema, jugular venous distention, and an early diastolic gallop could lead to the diagnosis of congestive heart failure and spare a patient an unnecessary lung biopsy. In the authors' experience, this is a commonly missed diagnosis.

Noninvasive Procedures

Laboratory Diagnoses

In the immunologically competent patient with pneumonia, sputum smear and culture, blood culture and, at times, acute and convalescent antibody titers are the standard tools for diagnosis. Making an etiologic diagnosis in the immunocompromised host is more complex. The spectrum of potential infectious pathogens is broader, sputum is often not available, and antibody titers are insensitive. Furthermore, the utility of sputum analysis to diagnose bacterial pneumonia in this patient population is controversial. Although many experts believe that sputum cultures are inaccurate, others believe a Gram stain is helpful (Sickles et al, 1973).

Besides the routine Gram and acid-fast stains, special preparations can be applied to sputum that can occasionally provide immediate diagnostic information. India ink staining of a wet preparation of sputum can show the encapsulated budding yeast forms of *Cryptococcus* species; a wet mount of sputum, the parasitic larvae of *Strongyloides* species; and methenamine silver nitrate, Gram-Weigert, and toluidine blue, O, stains of air-dried smears, the cyst walls of *Pneumocystis* species (Fig. 23–63). Direct fluorescent antibody (DFA) staining provides a specific means of identifying *Legionella* species, but the organisms are not often expectorated in the sputum, and antibodies to all serotypes are not widely available.

If spontaneously expectorated sputum cannot be obtained, sputum induction using nebulized hypertonic saline may be useful to diagnose *P. carinii* and *M. tuberculosis*. The diagnostic yield from sputum induction for *P. carinii* in HIV-infected patients ranges from 55% to 92%. The highest yields are obtained with the use of immunofluorescent monoclonal antibodies. In non–HIV-infested patients, the yield for pneumocystis on induced sputum is exceedingly low. If tuberculosis is suspected, sputum induction should be reserved for patients who do not have expectorated sputum or who have negative smears on expectorated sputum.

Polymerase chain reactions (PCR) and DNA probes are techniques being developed for the rapid diagnosis of many infections. Studies using PCR for the diagnosis of *M. tuberculosis* report sensitivities equal to or greater than cultures—ranging from 89% to 100%—and specificities greater than 90%. Preliminary studies suggest that an oral wash is a potential noninvasive method of obtaining a diagnostic specimen during PCP infection both in HIV and in non-HIV patients. In the HIV patient, a sensitivity of 89% and a specificity of 94% have been reported using this method (Helweg-Larsen et al, 1998).

Sputum cultures that grow *Cryptococcus* and *Nocardia* species are almost always pathogenic in an immunocompromised host; other organisms, such as *Staphylococcus* species, gram-negative bacilli, and *Candida* species, may represent contamination or colonization of the upper respiratory tract rather than true pulmonary infections. If metastatic cancer is suspected, it is always worthwhile to submit sputum for cytologic examination.

In summary, although sputum collection for direct examination and culture has limited value and its results must be interpreted with caution, in any patient with pulmonary disease, sputum should be examined because the procedure is simple and safe and may provide valuable information.

Skin Tests and Serology

In general, skin testing is of little value in the diagnosis of acute infections in an immunocompromised host.

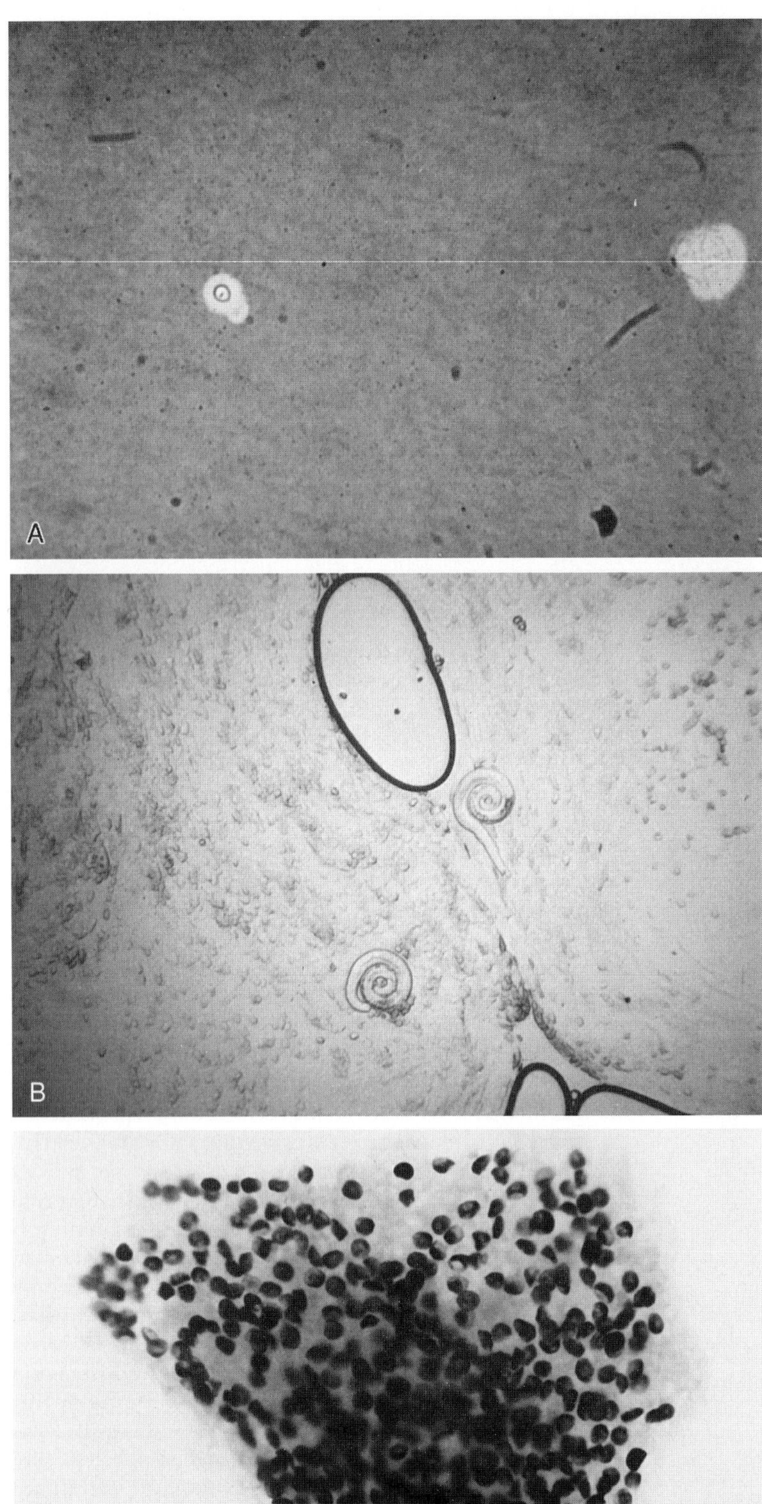

FIGURE 23–63 ■ *A*, India ink staining of a wet preparation of sputum showing the budding yeast form of *Cryptococcus neoformans*. *B*, A wet mount of sputum containing the larvae of *Strongyloides stercoralis*. *C*, A Gram-Weigert stain of an air-dried smear of induced sputum demonstrating the typical crescent-shaped cysts of *Pneumocystis carinii*.

However, when tuberculosis is suspected, a tuberculin skin test with controls should always be placed. Similarly, serologic tests have not been useful in the diagnosis of pulmonary infections in these patients. Exceptions to this include the presence of serum cryptococcal antigen, which is considered highly useful in the diagnosis of disseminated and meningeal cryptococcosis (Goodman et al, 1971). Skin testing may also be helpful in the diagnosis of isolated cryptococcal pneumonia (Baugham et al, 1992; Jensen et al, 1985). The detection of *Aspergillus* species antigenemia by radioimmunoassay is highly specific and moderately sensitive in the diagnosis of invasive aspergillosis; however, a reliable test kit is not commercially available (Weiner et al, 1983).

Imaging Techniques

Although chest radiographs and other radiologic techniques used to evaluate pulmonary disease in an immunocompromised host are nonspecific, they may be helpful in narrowing the diagnosis to a certain subset of likely agents. Occasionally, the radiographic pattern of pulmonary infiltrates is so characteristic that the cause is apparent. Examples of this phenomenon include radiation pneumonitis or fibrosis, which causes infiltrates with linear margins that defy anatomic boundaries and are confined to the radiation portals. Another example is the air-crescent sign, a radiographic finding that is highly suggestive of pulmonary aspergillosis. Computed tomography (CT) scans of the chest can show a similar finding, called the halo sign, weeks before a chest radiograph shows abnormality (Kulhman et al, 1985).

Common causes of pleural effusions in an immunocompromised patient include congestive heart failure, malignancy, pulmonary embolism, and bacterial pneumonia. It is worth emphasizing that pulmonary edema is commonly mistaken for an opportunistic infection.

Gallium scanning of the lungs is a sensitive technique for detection of active inflammatory lung disease, but it is nonspecific. It is especially helpful when a patient has pulmonary symptoms with a normal chest radiograph (Siemsen et al, 1978). This situation can be seen in infection, especially by *Pneumocystis* species; in drug toxicity; and in lymphangitic spread of a tumor (Turbiner et al, 1978). High-resolution CT scans are also helpful in detecting early diffuse lung disease when the chest radiograph is still normal. Spiral CT scanning of the chest is helpful as a diagnostic tool in cases of inconclusive diagnosis of pulmonary emboli.

Pulmonary Function Testing

Pulmonary function testing, especially measurement of the diffusing capacity and of exercise arterial blood gases, provides a sensitive indicator of diffuse pulmonary disease and is useful for evaluating an immunocompromised patient with pulmonary symptoms and a normal chest radiograph (Stover and Meduri, 1988). The findings of a positive gallium lung scan, abnormal diffusing capacity, or exercise desaturation in an immunocompromised patient with pulmonary symptoms and a normal chest radiograph necessitate further investigation.

Invasive Procedures

Invasive investigation becomes necessary when the establishing of a specific diagnosis is mandated so as to optimize management of the patient. The available invasive techniques for obtaining respiratory secretions or lung tissue include transtracheal needle aspiration (TTA), transthoracic needle aspiration (TTNA) or biopsy, bronchoscopy with transbronchial biopsy, and bronchoalveolar lavage (BAL), and thoracoscopic or open lung biopsy (Table 23–20) (Stover, 1989). Of these, bronchoscopy is the most commonly used procedure, followed by TTNA and open lung biopsy (Castellino and Blank, 1979; Cunningham et al, 1977; Davidson et al, 1976; Levine and Stover, 1991; Stover et al, 1984a; Toledo-Pereya et al, 1990). TTA and transthoracic needle biopsy have become obsolete because of nonspecific results or high complication rates.

Bronchoscopy

The most common indication for fiberoptic bronchoscopy in the immunocompromised host is the need to determine the cause of diffuse pulmonary infiltrates, which often occur in association with fever and new respiratory symptoms. Fiberoptic bronchoscopy with transbronchial biopsy, bronchial washings, brushings, and BAL has a relatively high yield in the diagnosis of diffuse pulmonary

TABLE 23–20 ■ **Results of Various Invasive Procedures for the Diagnosis of Pulmonary Infiltrates in the Immunocompromised Host**

				Complications			
		Specific Diagnosis		*Pneumothorax*		*Hemorrhage*	
Procedure	*No. Patients**	*No.*	*%*	*No.*	*%*	*No.*	*%*
Bronchoscopy							
Transbronchial biopsy	584	265	45	29	4.9	20	3.4
Bronchial brushings/washings	328	98	30	NA		NA	
Bronchoalveolar lavage	327	173	55	0		0	
Needle aspirate	178	116	65	35	20	10	6
Needle biopsy	147	85	58	42	29	16	11
Open lung biopsy†	334	238	71	32	10	6	2

NA, not available; AIDS, acquired immunodeficiency syndrome.

*Excludes patients with AIDS.

†Other complications of open lung biopsy include hemothorax, pleural effusion or empyema, subcutaneous emphysema, wound infection or hematoma, and bronchopleural fistula. These are seen in 2%–9% of the patients.

(Data from Davidson M, Tempest B, Palmen DL: Bacteriologic diagnosis of acute pneumonia. JAMA 235:158, 1976; and DeSouza R, MacKinnon S, Spagnola SV et al: Treatment of localized pulmonary phycomycosis. South Med J 72:609, 1979.)

infiltrates in immunosuppressed patients without HIV (Levine and Stover, 1991; Stover, 1989) (see Table 23–20). In fact, when an infection other than bacterial pneumonia is suspected, investigators have reported the sensitivity and specificity of this procedure to range from 80% to 90% (Martin et al, 1987; Meduri et al, 1991; Stover et al, 1984a). The infections most commonly diagnosed by bronchoscopy include PCP (Martin et al, 1987; Meduri et al, 1991; Stover et al, 1984a,b); viral pneumonia, especially when caused by CMV (Emanuel et al, 1986); and mycobacterial disease (Sarkar et al, 1982; Willcox et al, 1987). The bronchoscopic yield for the diagnosis of infection in HIV-infected patients is greater than 90% because of the strong prevalence of PCP in this group (Broaddus et al, 1985; Ognibene et al, 1984; Stover et al, 1984a). Bronchoscopy may also be diagnostic for *Legionella pneumophila*, so appropriate DFA staining should be done on BAL fluid when legionnaires' disease is suspected (Kohorst et al, 1983).

The use of a protected specimen brush and protected BAL has been reported to improve the yield from bacterial infections by allowing accurate aerobic and anaerobic cultures of bronchial secretions to be made (Fagon et al, 1988; Wimberly et al, 1982). For these techniques to have adequate specificity and sensitivity, quantitative bacterial culture counts have to be performed, and patients cannot be on concurrent antibiotic therapy. Because of these limitations, the procedure has not gained widespread use in immunocompromised patients. The problem of reaching a distal localized lesion or a mediastinal lesion may be alleviated as a result of the development of needles that can be placed transbronchially or transtracheally (Wang et al, 1984), but use of this technique is often limited because of thrombocytopenia.

Despite the variability of the yield of fiberoptic bronchoscopy with transbronchial biopsy, especially for noninfectious processes, its extremely low morbidity supports its use as the initial invasive procedure in immunocompromised patients with pulmonary infiltrates.

Bronchoalveolar Lavage

BAL is an effective technique that is used to diagnose diffuse pulmonary disease by means of fiberoptic bronchoscopy. It is estimated that as many as 1 million alveoli are sampled by this method, as opposed to the 20 to 50 alveoli that are included in a successful transbronchial forceps biopsy. Another advantage of BAL over fiberoptic bronchoscopy with transbronchial biopsy is that it is safe in the thrombocytopenic patient and in those who require mechanical ventilation (Levine and Stover, 1991; Stover, 1989; Stover et al, 1984b). It is most helpful in the diagnosis of opportunistic infections, especially *P. carinii* (Broaddus et al, 1985; Meduri et al, 1991; Martin et al, 1987; Ognibene et al, 1984; Stover et al, 1984a,b); CMV pneumonia (Emanuel et al, 1986); and intraparenchymal pulmonary hemorrhage (Drew et al, 1977). Stover and colleagues (1984b) reported making a specific diagnosis by analysis of BAL fluid alone in 66% of 97 non–HIV-immunosuppressed patients with diffuse pulmonary infiltrates. Of the 46 opportunistic infections, 38 (83%) were correctly diagnosed by examination and culture of the BAL fluid. Complications of the procedure are few; the most common is arterial oxygen desaturation, which can be effectively monitored by means of oximetry (Meduri et al, 1991). The incidence of respiratory failure after bronchoscopy is about 1.6%; whether this is a matter of cause and effect is difficult to ascertain from the data available (Levine and Stover, 1991).

Transthoracic (Percutaneous) Needle Aspiration

Fluoroscopically guided TTNA is particularly valuable for the diagnosis of peripheral nodular or cavitary infiltrates. The main advantages of TTNA are that it directly samples the pathologic area, and a small core of lung tissue or lung fluid is obtained, which can be examined microbiologically and cytologically (Castellino and Blank, 1979; Zavala and Schoell, 1981).

Open Lung Biopsy and Video-Assisted Thoracoscopic Surgery

When lung biopsies are performed on immunosuppressed patients by means of open or video-assisted thorascopic surgery (VATS), tissue is obtained in 100% of cases, and a definite diagnosis is made in 65% to 75% of patients, with a 5% to 8% morbidity rate and a 0.5% to 2% mortality rate (Cockerill et al, 1985; Rossiter et al, 1979; Satterfield and McLaughlin, 1979). This technique has been used with a low complication rate in critically ill and thrombocytopenic patients (see Table 23–20) (Levine and Stover, 1991; Stover, 1989). The greatest advantage of an open lung biopsy in an immunocompromised patient is the rapidity with which a diagnosis can be achieved.

In our experience, VATS has a diagnostic yield and complication rate similar to those of conventional thoracotomy. It also appears to be safe in thrombocytopenic patients but can be done only in those who can tolerate single-lung ventilation. Large studies are necessary to further evaluate its limitations and complication rate in this patient population.

PULMONARY INFECTIONS IN THE IMMUNOCOMPROMISED HOST

Many of the infections are presented in greater detail by other authors in earlier sections of this chapter. The purpose of this discussion is to review the presentation, diagnosis, and therapy of the most common infectious disorders as they apply to the immunosuppressed patient.

Bacteria

Common Bacterial Pneumonias

Streptococcus pneumoniae and *Haemophilus influenzae* are common, not only in the immunocompetent patient but also in those who are immunocompromised by B cell defects such as those found in multiple myeloma. Other patients who are immunocompromised by virtue of granulocyte defects commonly get bacterial pneumonias caused by gram-negative organisms, including *Pseudomonas aeruginosa*, *Escherichia coli*, and *Klebsiella* species, and by certain gram-positive organisms. In fact, gram-positive organisms have been recovered at a notably increased rate during the past decade in neutropenic patients with cancer and pneumonia. In a recent study of 40 episodes of bacteremic pneumonia in these patients, 42% of the causative agents were gram-positive organisms (12 cases of *S. pneumoniae* and 3 cases of *Streptococcus mitis*). Of these, 47% were penicillin-resistant and 2 of the 3 stains of *S. mitis* were resistant to ceftazidime (Carratala et al, 1998).

The clinical signs and symptoms of pneumonia in the immunocompromised host may be typical, with acute onset of shaking chills, fever, and productive cough. This type of presentation often accompanies bacterial pneumonia in the HIV-infected patient (Polsky et al, 1986). In the setting of granulocytopenia, clinical signs and symptoms of pneumonia may be atypical or absent (Sickles et al, 1975). Cough is usually present, but 30% of cases report no cough. Sputum production is seen in less than 60% of cases, and in patients with absolute neutrophil counts lower than 100 cells/mm^3, purulent sputum has been reported in only 8% (Sickles et al, 1973). The most sensitive sign of bacterial pneumonia, although nonspecific, is the presence of fever, which is seen in almost 100% of cases; rales and signs of consolidation are inconsistently present (Sickles et al, 1973). The chest radiograph, however, is abnormal in 93% to 97% of cases and commonly shows localized infiltrates (Singer et al, 1979; Tenholder and Hooper, 1980). The incidence of bacteremia is higher, as is the mortality rate in HIV-infected patients and patients with absolute neutrophil counts lower than 100 cells/mm^3, as compared to other immunocompromised hosts with pneumonia (Sickles et al, 1973; Singer et al, 1977).

Because bacterial pneumonias in immunocompromised patients may progress rapidly, empiric broad-spectrum antibiotic coverage should be initiated as soon as the diagnosis is suspected. In non-neutropenic immunosuppressed hosts (e.g., HIV-infected patients), a second-generation cephalosporin or amoxicillin/clavulanate is usually adequate. In seriously ill HIV patients, a third- or fourth-generation cephalosporin (e.g., ceftriaxone and cefepime, respectively) or a fluoroquinolone (e.g., levofloxacin, trovafloxacin) should be considered. In individuals who are neutropenic and have community-acquired pneumonia or nosocomial bacterial pneumonia, an aminoglycoside together with a third- or fourth-generation cephalosporin, an extended-spectrum penicillin β-lactam, or imipenem are choice combinations because both gram-negative and gram-positive organisms are common. In patients with renal insufficiency, aztreonam may be substituted for an aminoglycoside; however, the known synergistic killing of many bacteria by an aminoglycoside together with either a third-generation cephalosporin or β-lactam penicillin has not been demonstrated with aztreonam.

The duration of antibiotic therapy in an immunocompromised host for the therapy of bacterial pneumonias is controversial. A 2-week course of broad-spectrum antibiotics may be sufficient in many patients, especially if there is rapid clinical improvement and recovery of the white blood cell count. When prolonged neutropenia is present, longer courses may be required. The administration of growth factors such as granulocyte colony-stimulating factor or granulocyte-macrophage colony-stimulating factor have helped in preventing and overcoming serious infectious complications associated with neutropenia by accelerating neutropenic recovery.

Aspiration Pneumonia

The term *aspiration pneumonia* describes anaerobic bacterial infections of the lung and pulmonary disease resulting from aspiration of gastric juice or solid particles. Dysphagia related to surgery and radiotherapy for head and neck tumors or mucositis caused by infection, chemotherapy, or radiotherapy places immunocompromised patients at risk for aspiration (Logemann, 1985).

The acute complications of aspiration include bronchospasm and clinical pneumonitis, which presents with fever, tachypnea, cough, hypoxemia, and leukocytosis. Pulmonary infections after aspiration usually occur days after the acute event. Anaerobes are the most common isolates found in out-of-hospital aspiration; nosocomial aspirations include anaerobes, gram-negative bacilli, and *Staphylococcus aureus* (Rotstein et al, 1988).

The diagnosis of infection shortly after the aspiration of gastrointestinal contents is often difficult because fever, leukocytosis, and pulmonary infiltrates can be due to the chemical injury. Persistent fever, radiographic abnormalities, or any other signs of infection after aspiration warrant prompt use of empiric antibiotic therapy in an immunocompromised host. At least two antibiotics directed toward coverage of anaerobes, *S. aureus*, and gram-negative bacilli should be used. Recommended regimens include ticarcillin/clavulanate for gram-positive organisms and anaerobic coverage and an aminoglycoside for gram-negative bacilli. Other regimens include combinations of clindamycin or metronidazole for anaerobic coverage and vancomycin or a semisynthetic penicillin for gram-positive coverage in combination with an aminoglycoside. Between 10 and 14 days of therapy are indicated in immunosuppressed patients, and it should be continued until myelosuppression has resolved.

Less Common Bacterial Pneumonias

Legionnaires' disease and *Mycoplasma pneumoniae* are atypical bacterial pneumonias that can occur in immunocompromised patients. Sporadic cases and community-acquired outbreaks of legionnaires' disease have been reported in these patients, but infection is more commonly acquired from a nosocomial source. Few studies have evaluated this disease in the immunosuppressed patient population. A study by Saravoltz and Colleagues (1979) reported fever and malaise in all their immunocompromised patients, a productive cough in 66%, and hemoptysis in 38%. It is interesting to note that gastrointestinal complaints were uncommon. Radiographically, a unilateral patchy alveolar infiltrate was seen, and it progressed to consolidation and involved contiguous and noncontiguous areas of the lung. The presence of bilateral infiltrates and cavitation is relatively common. The diagnosis of infection by a species of *Legionella* is difficult to make in immunocompromised patients. Although culture of the organism from the respiratory tract, blood, tissue, or pleural fluid is diagnostic, DFA tests are quicker and clinically more applicable in this patient population (Kohorst et al, 1983; Winn et al, 1980). The use of DFA tests has certain drawbacks, including serogroup dependence, limited sensitivity, and the need to have an expert interpret the slides (Winn et al, 1980).

The therapy for disorders resulting from *Legionella* species requires the use of antibiotics than can kill intracellularly by entering alveolar macrophages, and macrolides are the mainstay (Edelstein and Meyer, 1988; Kirby et al, 1980).

Although infections by *Mycoplasma pneumoniae* in normal adults are common and relatively mild, severe pulmonary disease has been described in patients with antibody deficiencies and in those with malignancy (Perez and Leigh, 1991). The clinical manifestations include headache, fever, myalgias, malaise, and anorexia followed by sore throat and a dry, protracted cough that at times may yield nonpurulent sputum (Murray et al, 1975). Radiographic findings are variable but often show patchy or reticular interstitial infiltrates in the lower lobe. Because few laboratories culture for *Mycoplasma* species, the diagnosis is usually not made, and patients are treated empirically. The antibiotics that have proven to be efficacious are tetracycline and erythromycin (Murray et al, 1975).

Although *Nocardia* species can be present in immunocompetent patients, an immunocompromised host, particularly one with impairment of cell-mediated immunity, is most susceptible to this type of infection (Palmer et al, 1974). The lung is the primary site of infection; other organs commonly involved include the brain, skin, spleen, liver, kidney, bones, and lymph nodes. The symptoms and chest radiographs are nonspecific; however, chest pain may be present because of an extension of infection to the pleura or chest wall (Simpson et al, 1981). Although simple colonization and subclinical infection can occur, isolation of *Nocardia* species from the sputum of an immunocompromised host should always be considered diagnostically significant. Sulfonamides are the therapy of choice. Because relapse is common, prolonged therapy lasting at least 6 to 12 months is indicated, and parenteral therapy should be continued for at least 4 to 8 weeks.

Moraxella catarrhalis (formerly called *Neisseria catarrhalis* and *Branhamella catarrhalis*) occasionally causes pulmonary infections in patients with HIV infection and gamma-globulin dyscrasias (Diamond and Lorber, 1984; Polsky et al, 1986). The infection can vary from an acute febrile tracheobronchitis to a rapidly fatal pneumonia. Cephalosporins, macrolides, tetracycline, and TMP/SMX are the antibiotics of choice because 75% of isolates are penicillin-resistant (Doern et al, 1980). Infections caused by *Chlamydia* species, *Rhodococcus equi* (formerly known as *Corynebacterium equi*), and group B streptococci are uncommon causes of pulmonary infections in the immunocompromised host.

Mycobacteria

The genus *Mycobacterium* includes the tubercle bacilli (*M. tuberculosis* and *M. bovis*), Hanson's bacillus (*M. leprae*), and the nontuberculous (or atypical) mycobacteria.

Tuberculosis

The prevalence of tuberculosis is reported to be higher in immunocompromised patients, particularly those with lung cancer, head and neck cancer, lymphoproliferative disorders, and HIV infection (Ortbals and Marr, 1978; Selwyn et al, 1989). Because tuberculosis in the HIV-infected patient is unique, it is discussed later. In most immunocompromised patients, tuberculosis develops from reactivation of a latent pulmonary infection. The symptoms and signs are nonspecific, and the fever and constitutional symptoms that usually accompany tuberculosis are often attributed to the underlying neoplasm, which delays the diagnosis.

Immunocompromised patients are at increased risk for rapidly progressive pulmonary tuberculosis. In a series of 201 patients with cancer and tuberculosis, 9 had tuberculous pneumonia, which was uniformly fatal (Kaplan et al, 1974). In the same series, 34 patients had disseminated tuberculosis, which had a mortality rate of 91%. Patients at greatest risk for severe tuberculosis were those who were receiving antineoplastic therapy.

Chest radiographs can show the typical upper lobe cavitation; however, masses or nodules that mimic cancer and complicate both the diagnosis and the staging of the existing neoplastic disease can occur (Kaplan et al, 1974). In addition, opportunistic infections, such as histoplasmosis, nocardiosis, and cryptococcosis, are diagnostic possibilities in patients with tuberculosis and nodular infiltrates or a solitary cavitary lesion. Pulmonary tuberculosis can be confirmed in most cases by sputum examination; in miliary tuberculosis, however, sputum cultures are positive in only two-thirds of cases and smears are positive in less than one-third (Munt, 1971). In some patients bronchoscopy may be necessary, and this technique has been reported to have a diagnostic yield of more than 90% for the diagnosis of tuberculosis in immunocompromised hosts (Sarkar et al, 1982; Willcox et al, 1987).

Because of the increasing incidence of isoniazid (INH)-resistant tuberculosis, initial therapy for most patients consists of a four-drug regimen that includes INH, rifampin (RIF), ethambutol (EMB), and pyrazinamide (PZA). The official recommendation of the American Thoracic Society/Centers for Disease Control and Prevention is to treat for a total of 6 months. PZA is generally given for the first 2 months and if the organisms are sensitive to INH and RIF, EMB can be discontinued. Because there are no controlled studies in the immunocompromised host (ICH), many practitioners prefer to continue therapy for a longer-time in these patients. If the organism is sensitive; INH and RIF can be continued for a total of 9 to 12 months or at least 6 months after sputum conversion (Kuritzkes and Simon, 1991).

Although the anergy caused by the underlying disease may interfere with the purified protein derivative tuberculin test, it is reported to be positive in 60% to 75% of non—HIV-infected ICH. To increase sensitivity, tuberculin skin tests should be performed before immunosuppressive therapy is instituted, and a reaction size of 5 mm of induration should be used to define a positive reaction. Non-HIV immunocompromised patients with positive tuberculin reactions should probably receive 9 to 12 months of prophylaxis with INH (300 mg/day). Bacillus Calmette-Guérin, an attenuated vaccine strain of *Mycobacterium bovis*, is not recommended for tuberculosis prophylaxis because disseminated disease and death have been reported in immunocompromised patients.

Tuberculosis in HIV-Infected Patients. Tuberculosis in HIV-infected persons results primarily from reactivation of latent infection. The highest incidence of active tuberculosis occurs in those with positive tuberculin skin tests or known tuberculosis exposure and in groups with a high background prevalence of tuberculosis, such as immigrants from countries with endemic tuberculosis, blacks, Hispanics, and intravenous drug users (Pitchenik et al, 1987; Sunderam et al, 1986).

Because *M. tuberculosis* is a more virulent organism than opportunistic pathogens, it tends to occur earlier in the course of HIV disease, often preceding or coinciding with the diagnosis of AIDS. If it occurs at a time when cell-mediated immunity is relatively intact, the disease presents clinically in a manner similar to that of tuberculosis in the immunocompetent patient (Hopewell, 1989). Tuberculosis that develops later in the course of HIV disease tends to present atypically, which may cause a delay in diagnosis and initiation of appropriate therapy (Chaisson et al, 1987; Pitchenik et al, 1984).

The signs, symptoms, and physical examinations in HIV-infected patients with tuberculosis are nonspecific. A chronic wasting syndrome may be the sole presenting sign of the disease. Fever is the most common symptom; it occurs in approximately 90% of cases. Night sweats, cough, sputum production, and dyspnea are also common; hemoptysis and pleuritic chest pain occur less commonly. Extrapulmonary disease (involving the lymph nodes, bone marrow, and central nervous system, with or without pulmonary involvement) has been found in up to 70% of patients, particularly in those with more advanced immunosuppression (Pitchenik and Fertel, 1992).

In patients with higher T helper cell counts and intact tuberculin skin reactivity, the classic findings of upper lobe infiltrates, with or without cavitation, are common. In more severely HIV-infected immunosuppressed patients, radiographs reveal diffuse infiltrates, intrathoracic adenopathy, with or without infiltrates, and pleural effusions. Cavitary lesions in patients with advanced HIV disease are rare, and these patients may even present with normal chest radiographs (Barnes et al, 1991).

The finding of acid-fast bacilli in body secretions or tissue is sufficient evidence to begin empiric therapy in an HIV-infected person suspected of having tuberculosis. However, confirmation by culture is necessary because many cases have nontuberculous mycobacterial disease. Furthermore, the results of drug susceptibility studies are useful in planning definitive therapy. Sputum smears have been reported to be positive for acid-fast bacilli in 30% to 100% of HIV-infected patients, and the yield is higher in less severely immunocompromised patients. Positive sputum cultures for tuberculosis occur in 60% to 100% of cases. The overall positive yield by acid-fast staining and culture of bronchoscopic washings and lavage appears to be approximately 90% (Baugham et al, 1991). Because granulomas may not be present in a severely immunocompromised patient, transbronchial biopsy is helpful in only a small percentage of HIV-infected patients. The use of rapid diagnostic tests known as nucleic acid amplification (NAA) tests has increased sensitivity and specificity, and results are available within 4 to 5 hours. The NAA tests are 20% more sensitive than acid fast bacilli smears; in smear-positive cases, the specificity is 100% and in smear-negative cases it is 97% (Bradley et al, 1996).

Generally, therapy for tuberculosis caused by susceptible or single-drug–resistant organisms is similar and equally effective in the HIV-infected host and in the normal population. An important exception is that rifabutin should be used instead of RIF in all patients taking either reverse transcriptase inhibitors or protease inhibitors because RIF can seriously impair the effectiveness of these therapies. In contrast, no specific drug combination is effective in the therapy of multiple-drug–resistant strains of tuberculosis (Fischl et al, 1992a). In this setting, persistently positive acid-fast stains, disease dissemination, and high mortality rates have been observed. In cases of multiple-drug resistance, drug regimens are individualized and are based on patterns of drug sensitivity within particular areas. Although antituberculous medications are well tolerated in the general population, adverse reactions, mostly to RIF are common in HIV-infected patients. The drugs should not be discontinued for mild symptoms or laboratory abnormalities alone.

The initial evaluation of all HIV-infected patients should include tuberculin skin testing with 5 tuberculin units of purified protein derivative and at least two recall antigens (*Candida species*, mumps, or tetanus toxoid). Any HIV-positive individual with a positive tuberculin test (i.e., 5 mm or more of induration) should be given prophylaxis, regardless of age (Centers for Disease Control, 1989). Recent studies have found that a 2-month regimen of RIF (or rifabutin) and PZA is as effective as a 1-year long course of INH for tuberculosis chemoprophylaxis in people coinfected with HIV and tuberculosis (Centers for Disease Control, 1998).

Atypical Mycobacteria

The nontuberculous or atypical mycobacteria, mycobacteria other than tubercle bacilli (MOTT), are widely distributed in nature and are easily isolated from various environmental sources. Infection is not acquired by person-to-person spread as it is with *M. tuberculosis*. Pulmonary infection by MOTT can occur in those with lung cancer, head and neck cancer, hairy cell leukemia and, less commonly, AIDS (MacDonnell and Glassroth, 1989; Ortbals and Marr, 1978; Rolston et al, 1985).

A chronic pulmonary disease that resembles tuberculosis is the most important clinical problem associated with MOTT in the non–HIV-infected immunosuppressed host. *Mycobacterium avium-intracellulare* (also called *Mycobacterium avium* complex), *Mycobacterium kansasii*, and *Mycobacterium fortuitum* are the most commonly isolated organisms in patients with cancer (Ortbals and Marr, 1978; Rolston et al, 1985). The clinical signs and symptoms are often nonspecific and include cough, dyspnea, and weight loss; fever and hemoptysis are less common.

The chest radiograph may show nodules, thin-walled cavities in the upper lobes, infiltrates, and intrathoracic adenopathy. The therapy given in the presence of these organisms is the same in the non–HIV-infected immunocompromised patient as it is in the immunocompetent patient.

In contrast to the localized pulmonary disease seen in non–HIV-infected patients, MOTT species cause disseminated infection and only rarely cause clinically significant pulmonary disease, even when isolated from lung secretions in patients with AIDS (MacDonnell and Glassroth, 1989). HIV-infected patients with disseminated *M. avium-intracellulare* have a syndrome characterized by fever, weakness, diarrhea, abdominal pain, and general debilitation. It is commonly seen late in the course of HIV infection when the CD4 lymphocyte counts are less than 200 cells/mm^3. The organism usually grows in blood cultures. A three-drug regimen including clarithromycin, EMB, and rifabutin is about 60% effective in clearing bacteremia. If clinical and bacteriologic improvement occur, therapy should be continued for the lifetime of the patient. It appears that clarithromycin is an effective prophylactic agent against disseminated *M. avium-intracellulare* and should be considered in patients with CD counts equal to or less than 200 cells/μL.

Fungi

Patients with neutropenia as their primary immunologic defect (e.g., those with acute myelogenous leukemia) more commonly develop infections by *Aspergillus* species and, less commonly, by *Candida* and *Mucorales* species. These organisms are called opportunistic fungi because they generally infect only patients with abnormalities in host defenses. Patients who have primarily T cell defects (e.g., patients with Hodgkin's disease and those who are receiving corticosteroid therapy) are more often infected by *Cryptococcus* species and the endemic fungi, such as species of *Histoplasma*, *Coccidioides*, and *Blastomyces*. These organisms are called pathogenic fungi because they also commonly infect immunologically normal individuals.

For many years *P. carinii* was classified as a protozoon based on its morphologic features and its response to antiprotozoal drugs. However, ultrastructural studies suggest a phylogenetic relationship between *P. carinii* and higher fungi, so it is now classified as a fungus.

Opportunistic Fungi

Pneumocystosis. *P. carinii* has been recognized since the 1940s as a cause of severe pneumonia in immunocompromised hosts (Vanek, 1951). It occurs in patients with both B cell and, more commonly, T cell deficiencies—especially those with Hodgkin's disease, acute or chronic lymphatic leukemia, organ transplantation, HIV infection, and solid tumors—who are receiving high doses of corticosteroids. The organism exists globally; it occurs in all climates and in all mammalian species. Extensive study of these organisms has been hampered by the inability to grow them in vitro. Based entirely on morphology, three forms have been identified: the cyst (which is the most commonly identified form in human tissue); the sporozoite (which is an intracystic structure); and the free-floating trophozoite. Although asymptomatic infection is thought to occur in normal hosts early in life, active disease with pneumonia occurs only when an infected individual becomes immunosuppressed months or years after the primary infection (Pifer et al, 1978). Reports of person-to-person spread and cluster outbreaks in hospitals suggest that horizontal transmission may also occur (Singer et al, 1975). The natural history of PCP in immunocompromised hosts is characterized by progressive involvement of the lungs, culminating in death if it is untreated.

Nonproductive cough, dyspnea, and fever are the typical symptoms of PCP. It can be subclinical or chronic in HIV-infected patients or rapidly progressive in patients with cancer or transplants (Kovacs et al, 1984; Levine and White, 1988). Lungs may appear to be normal, but dry rales can be present. Wheezing and signs of consolidation are unusual. If they are present, other causes of pulmonary disease should be considered. Routine laboratory and radiographic studies do not provide specific information about the diagnosis of PCP. Measurement of lactate dehydrogenase, arterial blood gases, oxygen saturation with rest and exercise, and diffusing capacity provide sensitive but nonspecific markers for the disease (Jules-Elysee et al, 1992; Masur, 1991).

The typical radiographic appearance of PCP is that of diffuse bilateral, symmetric, interstitial infiltrates, which characteristically progress to fluffy alveolar infiltrates as the disease worsens (Forrest, 1972; Naidich and McGuinness, 1991). In 10% to 15% of patients, chest radiographs are normal. In HIV-infected patients who are receiving aerosolized pentamidine, there have been reports of atypical radiographic manifestations, most commonly the predominance of upper-lobe infiltrates, cavitary lesions, and pneumothoraces (Jules-Elysee et al, 1990). These atypical findings have been attributed to the deposition patterns of aerosolized pentamidine (Jules-Elysee et al, 1990). Pneumothoraces associated with PCP are difficult to manage, usually require surgical intervention, and are associated with a high mortality rate (Sepkowitz et al, 1991; Tietjen et al, 1989).

The diagnosis of PCP can be established only by demonstrating the organism in respiratory secretions or body tissues (see Fig. 23–63). Although induced sputum has been shown to produce a high yield for the diagnosis of PCP in HIV-infected patients, its usefulness in other immunosuppressed populations has been limited to a few medical centers (Kovacs et al, 1988; Masur et al, 1988; Zaman et al, 1988). The application of the polymerase chain reaction to sputum samples or oral washes for the diagnosis of PCP may eventually enhance the yield in non-HIV immunocompromised individuals. (Helweg-Larsen et al, 1998). At present, bronchoscopic diagnosis is more sensitive than induced sputum and it remains the procedure of choice for the diagnosis of PCP in non–HIV-infected patients when suspicion for PCP is high (Martin et al, 1987). The introduction of BAL has increased the sensitivity to detection of *P. carinii* to more than 80% in immunocompromised hosts, and the use of bilateral lavage has been shown to produce an even higher yield (Meduri et al, 1991; Stover et al, 1984b). In HIV-infected patients, an induced sputum should be done first.

There are two conventional drugs for the therapy of PCP—TMP-SMZ and parenteral pentamidine (Hughes et al, 1978). Some clinicians are reluctant to use TMP-SMZ in neutropenic patients because of the possibility of worsening or prolonging neutropenia. Intravenous pentamidine is a reasonable therapeutic choice in this setting, although it is not clear whether TMP-SMZ really causes neutropenia. Therapy in non–HIV-infected patients is usually given for a total of 2 weeks; the success rate varies from 50% to 70% (Sepkowitz et al, 1992). In patients with AIDS, TMP-SMZ (15 to 20 mg/kg/day of trimethoprim) or pentamidine (3 to 4 mg/kg/day) for a total of 3 weeks is recommended. The success rate with both of these agents in AIDS patients is 75% to 90% higher than it is in other immunocompromised hosts. Unfortunately, the rate of adverse reactions in AIDS patients can be as high as 80% with either drug (Sattler et al, 1988). Less-toxic alternatives for mild to moderate PCP include the combination of dapsone and trimethoprim (Medina et al, 1990); the combination of clindamycin and primaquine; and atovaquone, which appears to kill pathogens rather than suppress them. Aerosolized pentamidine has not been shown to be highly effective in the therapy of PCP (Conte et al, 1990; Falloon et al, 1991; Soo Hoo et al, 1990).

In HIV-infected patients with PCP and a Po_2 of less than 70 mm Hg during room-air breathing, the addition of corticosteroids to antimicrobial agents has been shown to decrease the likelihood of respiratory failure, need for mechanical ventilation, and death (Bozzette et al, 1990). Although controlled randomized trials that add corticosteroids to conventional agents are not available for the non–HIV-infected population, it has been our experience that adding or increasing the dose of corticosteroids has a beneficial effect. Effective prophylaxis against PCP can be achieved by the administration of TMP-SMZ orally in two daily doses, on 3 consecutive days per week (Hughes et al, 1987). In patients with AIDS, aerosolized pentamidine has been shown to offer protection against PCP but appears to be less effective than TMP-SMZ (Hardy et al, 1992; Leong et al, 1992). Other disadvantages of the use of aerosolized pentamidine include breakthrough infection by *Pneumocystis* species with atypical presentations and an increase in the incidence of extrapulmonary infection by *Pneumocystis* species because the aerosol affords no protection outside the lung; because of the vigorous coughing associated with its administration, the spread of tuberculosis has occurred in patients in whom active tuberculosis was unsuspected (Fischl et al, 1992b; Pearson et al, 1992).

Aspergillosis. These infections are difficult to diagnose antemortem and to treat effectively. Early diagnosis and therapy may improve the outcome, although the overall prognosis remains poor. *Aspergillus* species, ubiquitous fungi are commonly found in soil, water, and decaying vegetable matter. Common species that cause disease in humans are *Aspergillus fumigatus* and *Aspergillus flavus*. Immunosuppressed patients at risk for invasive pulmonary aspergillosis include those with prolonged neutropenia; those who are receiving chronic corticosteroids, antibiotic therapy, or chemotherapy; and those with a prior history of pneumonia caused by a species of *Aspergillus*.

Infection by one of these species commonly presents as an invasive necrotizing pneumonitis or a pulmonary infarct in an immunocompromised patient because of its propensity to erode blood vessels. The clinical features of pulmonary aspergillosis include fever, dyspnea, nonproductive cough, and acute pleuritic chest pain with or without a friction rub. Although the chest pain may be severe enough to require therapy with narcotics, the simultaneous chest radiograph may appear normal. Massive hemoptysis is a rare complication and tends to occur during the stage of bone marrow recovery and cavity formation (Albelda et al, 1985). Often, the only evidence of the presence of an *Aspergillus* species is prolonged fever with pulmonary infiltrates that do not respond to antibiotics.

Generally, chest radiographs become abnormal as the symptoms escalate. The earliest radiographic manifestation of invasive aspergillosis may be the presence of a single or of multiple nodules. Chest radiographs may then progress to show cavitation of these nodules, progression and enlargement of the nodules to produce a single or multiple areas of homogeneous consolidation, or the rapid development of large, wedge-shaped, pleural-based lesions that mimic pulmonary infarction. Cavitation may occur with or without a mycetoma, and chest CT scans can show the halo sign weeks before the chest radiograph becomes abnormal.

Because noninvasive tests lack specificity and sensitivity, invasive techniques are the mainstay for establishing a diagnosis of pulmonary aspergillosis. The success rate of fiberoptic bronchoscopy is about 50%, and transbronchial biopsy adds little to the yield of bronchial washings, brushings, and lavage (Freeberg et al, 1990). However, if the results are positive, transbronchial biopsy can establish the diagnosis of tissue invasion rather than simple colonization. Although open lung biopsy is the reference standard for the diagnosis of pulmonary aspergillosis, correlation with autopsy findings indicates that up to 25% of leukemic patients with pulmonary aspergillosis have negative findings on lung biopsy (Crawford et al, 1988). Because of the difficulty in the diagnosis of aspergillosis and because it is common in neutropenic patients, empiric therapy for aspergillosis in the proper setting has become commonplace (Pizzo et al, 1982).

Amphotericin B is the drug of choice for invasive aspergillosis, with dosages in the range of 0.6 to 1.25 mg/kg/day, depending on the severity of the infection. Surgical resection should be considered in patients with acute aspergillosis in whom hemoptysis develops and in leukemic patients and bone marrow transplant recipients who, after therapy, have residual disease, especially with mycetomas. Flucytosine appears to have additive or synergistic effects when combined with amphotericin B against aspergillosis. Because its main adverse effect is bone marrow suppression, it is usually avoided. Most of these patients are granulocytopenic.

Itraconazole has been approved for treatment of aspergillosis, and successful treatment with this azole has been reported (Longman and Martin, 1987). It can also be used for prophylaxis in a patient with a history of aspergillosis who is neutropenic. Another drug innovation is liposomal amphotericin B. This is produced by attaching amphotericin B to a liposomal vehicle, which allows higher drug doses to be given, with reduced toxicity. Whether it is more effective than conventional amphotericin B remains in question but current data suggest that it is not (Lopez-Berenstein et al, 1989). The clearest correlation with survival in invasive aspergillosis seems to be remission of the underlying malignancy with recovery of functioning neutrophils. The role of granulocyte colony-stimulating factors in the therapy and prophylaxis of pulmonary aspergillosis in neutropenic patients is unclear (Roilides and Pizzo, 1992).

Mucormycoses. Although fungi of the order Mucorales (which includes the genera *Mucor, Absidia*, and *Rhizopus*) share several common clinical and histologic features with *Aspergillus* species, especially their predilection for infecting the lung and vasculature, these fungi are uncommon in immunocompromised patients (Meyer et al, 1972). Antemortem diagnosis of mucormycosis is difficult to confirm. Sputum cultures are rarely positive; however, if these fungi are found in sputum, invasive disease is likely. As with aspergillosis, the only reliable antifungal therapy for mucormycosis is amphotericin B. The patient's response to therapy depends largely on early diagnosis, aggressive surgical débridement, remission of the underlying disease, and high cumulative doses of amphotericin B (DeSouza et al, 1979).

Candidiasis. It is interesting that despite the high incidence of oral and pharyngeal infection by *Candida species*, pneumonia is rare, even in severely neutropenic patients. The reason is probably that the alveolar macrophage rather than the neutrophil is the lung's major defense against *Candida* species (Baccari et al, 1985). Because the isolation of this fungus from respiratory secretions is so common, a conclusive diagnosis of invasive disease requires confirmation by lung biopsy. The drug of choice for pulmonary candidiasis is amphotericin B.

Cryptococcosis. *Cryptococcus neoformans* is ubiquitous worldwide and is commonly recoverable from the environment. The fungi appear to grow best in desiccated pigeon feces. Because most patients with cryptococcosis give no history of contact with pigeons, it is most likely acquired as an airborne pollutant. Fewer than 25 years ago, 50% of the cases of disseminated cryptococcosis occurred in patients who were immunologically intact. Now the disease is more commonly associated with patients who have defects in cell-mediated immunity, such as those who are receiving chronic corticosteroid therapy and those with chronic lymphocytic leukemia, chronic myelogenous leukemia, Hodgkin's disease, or AIDS (Kaplan et al, 1974; Chuck and Sande, 1989).

Disseminated cryptococcosis, clinically dominated by the occurrence of meningitis, is the most common presentation in immunocompromised patients. Although pulmonary involvement occurs in up to 50% of patients with disseminated infection, isolated pulmonary cryptococcosis is less common (Drutz, 1991).

The clinical manifestations of pulmonary cryptococcosis are usually minimal or absent; when symptoms do occur they include fever, cough, dyspnea, and pleuritic pain. Hemoptysis occurs uncommonly; occasionally, acute cryptococcosis can mimic adult respiratory distress syndrome.

Radiographically, cryptococcal pneumonia usually presents as a single well-defined mass that ranges from 2 to 10 cm in diameter and resembles primary lung cancer. Multiple nodules or miliary densities may also be found on chest radiographs. Cavitation, intrathoracic adenopathy, and pleural effusions are rare in patients without AIDS; however, in HIV-infected patients, hilar or mediastinal adenopathy and pleural effusions, with or without parenchymal involvement, are common features (Kovacs et al, 1985).

Because the disease is usually disseminated, cerebral spinal fluid, blood, and urine cultures provide excellent sources for diagnosis. Although only 20% of immunosuppressed patients with pulmonary cryptococcosis have sputum cultures that are positive, invasive disease should be considered present if the organism is retrieved from the sputum. In this setting, the patient should be fully evaluated for disseminated infection, including a lumbar puncture.

The latex agglutination test for cryptococcal polysaccharide antigen is one of the most useful of all fungal serologic tests. It is highly sensitive and specific for invasive *C. neoformans* in patients with and without AIDS (Chuck and Sande, 1989; Goodman et al, 1971). Besides its diagnostic usefulness, cryptococcal antigen levels in both serum and cerebrospinal fluid should be followed to measure the efficacy of therapy.

Amphotericin B is the mainstay of therapy for cryptococcal infection, and flucytosine is synergistic with this drug. This combination is recommended for most patients with cryptococcal meningitis. In non-HIV immunocompromised patients with pulmonary cryptococcosis, a course of drug therapy is indicated, but there is no agreement as to its nature or duration. In seriously ill patients with HIV, amphotericin B alone or with flucytosine is the best validated initial treatment. Fluconazole administered from the onset can be considered for stable patients. Fluconazole is the treatment of choice for long-term suppression, in a dosage of 200 to 400 mg daily and is given for life to prevent relapse in the HIV-infected patient.

Pathogenic Fungi

Histoplasmosis. *Histoplasma capsulatum*, a fungus endemic in the river valleys of the central and southeastern United States, causes pulmonary and disseminated infections in patients whose cell-mediated immunity is impaired, such as those with Hodgkin's disease, acute and chronic lymphocytic leukemia, and AIDS. In such patients, histoplasmosis is characterized by progressive illness with evidence of extrapulmonary spread of infection. The clinical manifestations include fever, weight loss, malaise, hepatosplenomegaly, and cough. In disseminated disease, bone marrow cultures have the highest yield. They are reported to be positive in 75% of cases, and blood cultures may be positive in more than 50% of cases (Wheat, 1989). BAL and transbronchial biopsy have disclosed the presence of *H. capsulatum* in 25% to 75% of cases; most of them are patients with AIDS (Prechter and Prakash, 1989). A diagnosis of fungemia can be quickly established in up to 30% of patients with AIDS, and disseminated histoplasmosis can be diagnosed by visualization of the characteristic organisms on the buffy coat of peripheral blood smears after Wright or Giemsa staining. Radioimmunoassay of the *H. capsulatum* antigen also offers a rapid method of diagnosing disseminated histoplasmosis. Antigen can be detected in the blood in 50% and in the urine in 90% of patients with disseminated histoplasmosis (Wheat et al, 1986). In an immunosuppressed patient with cancer who is undergoing histoplasmosis therapy with amphotericin B, a total dose of at least 35 mg/kg is indicated. Because relapse is so common, particularly in patients with AIDS, maintenance of suppressive therapy with itraconazole 200 mg twice daily is currently recommended (Wheat et al, 1993). It appears that stable HIV patients with histoplasmosis can be treated safely with itraconazole as the primary treatment (Como and Dismukes, 1994).

Coccidioidomycosis. *Coccidioides immitis* is a fungus that is endemic in the southwestern United States, northern Mexico, and portions of Central and South America. Most infections occur in endemic areas by means of inhalation. Because the fungus does not colonize tissues, isolation of the organism signifies active infection. In an immunocompromised host with or without HIV, disseminated coccidioidomycosis is the most common manifestation of the disease; it may occur as a complication of the primary illness or as a result of reactivation of latent disease. The presenting symptoms are often nonspecific, but pulmonary symptoms, including cough and dyspnea, and chest radiographic abnormalities occur in up to 40% of patients. Sputum smears or cultures are positive in only 20% to 30% of patients, and fiberoptic bronchoscopy has a diagnostic yield of about 50% (Wallace et al, 1981). Serologic tests are generally positive during an active infection and, in the immunocompromised host, may be valuable not only in the diagnosis but also in the management of coccidioidomycosis because the titers usually fall with successful therapy. Amphotericin B is recommended for all forms of coccidioidomycosis. In HIV disease, relapses are common, and maintenance therapy is recommended (Galgiani and Ampel, 1990).

Uncommon Endemic Fungi. Blastomycosis (caused by *Blastomyces dermatitidis*) and paracoccidioidomycosis (caused by *Paracoccidioides brasiliensis*) have occurred sporadically in immunocompromised patients with impaired cell-mediated immunity. The former organism is commonly found in the Mississippi and Ohio River valleys, and the latter is found principally in Central and South America and Mexico. Diagnosis of the presence of these organisms depends on visualization of the fungi on smear and tissue culture. Severely immunocompromised patients should be treated with amphotericin B (Drutz, 1991); milder illness can be treated with itraconazole.

Viruses

Herpesviruses

In patients who are immunocompromised, especially, those with deficiencies of cellular immunity, severe morbidity and death can occur during primary infection or reactivation of herpesviruses.

Cytomegalovirus Pneumonia. CMV pneumonia is the major cause of viral morbidity and death in bone marrow transplant recipients (Neiman et al, 1977). CMV may be reactivated in the host, or it may be transmitted in donor marrow or by transfusion of CMV-infected blood products. It is clinically manifested by interstitial pneumonitis that begins 8 to 12 weeks after bone marrow transplantation and after engraftment has taken place.

The clinical signs, symptoms, and radiographic findings of CMV pneumonia are nonspecific and indistinguishable from those of other common pneumonias seen in this patient population, such as idiopathic interstitial pneumonitis and PCP. Because of the ubiquity of the organism, CMV pneumonia is often difficult to document. The diagnosis can be made reasonably if the following criteria are met: clinical and radiographic evidence of interstitial pneumonia; demonstration of CMV antigen or nucleic acids in alveolar macrophages or epithelial cells obtained by BAL or open lung biopsy; isolation of CMV by culture from BAL fluid or lung tissue; and absence of any other pathogens that might cause interstitial pneumonia (Emanuel et al, 1986). BAL fluid provides an excellent source of cells that are representative of the lower respiratory tract and allow detection of CMV antigens (Emanuel et al, 1986). For most bone marrow transplant patients with CMV pneumonia, this technique has replaced the need to obtain tissue samples through closed or open lung biopsies.

Until recently therapy for CMV pneumonia in allogeneic bone marrow transplant recipients was unsuccessful. However, two uncontrolled studies have suggested that the combined use of ganciclovir and intravenous Ig is associated with a significant decrease in the mortality rate of those with CMV pneumonia (Emanuel et al, 1988; Reed et al, 1988). Using this regimen, the mortality rate of patients with CMV pneumonia at our institution has decreased from 90% to 30%.

Unlike the situation in bone marrow transplantation, the degree to which solid organ recipients experience CMV-associated illness is related to whether the infection is primary or is a reactivation of a previous infection. In those with reactivation of CMV, the incidence of symptomatic disease is much lower than in those with primary CMV infection. The approach to diagnosis is similar to that recommended diagnosis in those with bone marrow transplants. The overall prevalence of CMV infection or disease in lung transplant patients is 50%. Ganciclovir is the drug of choice for treatment of CMV disease in the solid organ transplant recipient (Ettinger et al, 1993). Most episodes of CMV pneumonia respond to a 2 to 3 weeks course of therapy. There are several important considerations concerning patients who fail therapy. First, resistance to ganciclovir should be entertained and susceptibility studies should be done. Second, the intensity of immunosuppression can be decreased, but this poses a risk of rejection. Third, treatment can be augmented by adding intravenous IgG. Foscarnet is effective against CMV and is the best alternative for ganciclovir-resistant infection or treatment failures (Trulock, 1997).

Although CMV has been well-documented pathogen in the eyes and gastrointestinal tracts of patients with HIV infection, it is an uncommon pulmonary pathogen in these patients (Jacobson et al, 1991).

Varicella. In immunocompromised hosts, both primary and reactivated varicella can be a devastating illness; it is associated with hematogenous visceral dissemination in up to 20% of cases. Although the histologic and cytologic features of varicella pneumonia are identical to those of herpes simplex virus, the diagnosis of varicella pneumonia is generally straightforward because the symptoms of pneumonia usually occur 3 to 7 days after the onset of the cutaneous lesions. Therapy of varicella pneumonia is recommended in both immunocompetent and immunocompromised patients because of the high mortality rate involved. Acyclovir is effective in both groups and is preferred over lymphoblastoid interferon or vidarabine because it has the lowest toxicity (Shepp et al, 1986). Because untreated primary varicella and shingles may rapidly disseminate and cause death in immunocompromised patients, prompt therapy for this entity even in the absence of any evidence of pneumonia is also highly recommended. In addition, a reduction in the level of immunosuppressive therapy may hasten the resolution of lesions and limit dissemination. Several studies show that postexposure prophylaxis (before signs of disease occur) with varicella-zoster Ig is highly effective in decreasing the morbidity rate in such patients (Centers for Disease Control, 1984).

Herpes Simplex Virus. Herpes simplex virus is a common cause of mucocutaneous disease in immunocompromised patients, but lung involvement is uncommon. Pulmonary disease caused by herpesvirus type I and II has been noted to include tracheobronchitis and bronchopneumonia. The presence of facial, oral, or esophageal herpetic lesions may be clues to the diagnosis because in one study, mucocutaneous lesions occurred in 85% of patients with pulmonary disease (Ramsey et al, 1982). Cough, dyspnea, and fever are common symptoms. Chest radiographs can show focal lesions, which often denote oropharyngeal aspiration of organisms into the lung. Diffuse infiltrates correlate with hematogenous spread to the lung (Ramsey et al, 1982). The diagnosis of pulmonary infection by the herpes simplex virus depends on isolation of the organism from respiratory specimens in the absence of contamination by oral or upper airway lesions. Bronchoscopy may suggest the diagnosis when a necrotizing tracheitis is noted. Acyclovir is the drug of choice.

Other Viruses

Influenza. Influenza has not been well studied in immunocompromised hosts. Some centers have reported a higher incidence of influenza A among children with cancer; others have reported more prolonged illness, especially in HIV-infected patients, and a particularly high mortality rate among patients with a variety of neoplasms. In immunocompromised patients, the differential diagnosis may be wide, and laboratory studies are usually necessary to arrive at a specific diagnosis (Dowdle et al, 1979). Influenza can be isolated from respiratory secretions, pulmonary tissue, or throat cultures within 1 to 2 days after they are obtained. To detect viruses sooner, immunofluorescent techniques can be used in tissue culture or directly in exfoliated nasopharyngeal cells. Antiviral therapy with amantadine or rimantadine has a beneficial effect on the symptoms of influenza A infections. However, their effectiveness in influenza pneumonia has not been studied. Prevention of influenza A and B involves the use of inactivated influenza vaccines, and although the immune response in these patients is variable, it is recommended that such patients receive vaccination, preferably before chemotherapy (Centers for Disease Control, 1988).

Respiratory Syncytial Virus. Respiratory syncytial virus (RSV) pneumonia can occur in immunocompromised children as well as adolescents and adults, particularly transplant recipients. Epidemics occur in late fall and spring. Cough is invariably present and chest radiographs usually show bilateral infiltrates. RSV can be isolated from respiratory secretions, throat swabs, or naso-oropharyngeal washes. Ribavirin, which is the treatment of choice, has given varying results.

Protozoans

Parasites

Strongyloides Stercoralis. *Strongyloides stercoralis* and *Toxoplasma gondii* are parasites that can affect the lung in immunocompromised patients. Disseminated strongyloidiasis usually occurs in patients with cellular immune defects who come from endemic areas and develop the so-called hyperinfection syndrome (Ingra-Siegman et al, 1981). Although the pulmonary signs and symptoms of disseminated strongyloidiasis are nonspecific, the diagnosis should be entertained in an immunosuppressed patient who comes from an endemic area and has vague abdominal symptoms of pain, diffuse tenderness, or distention and then pneumonia. The diagnosis is made by demonstrating the larvae in sputum or in other respiratory secretions, especially after BAL (Fig. 23–64). The therapy for hyperinfection syndrome is thiabendazole. In our experience, toxoplasmosis is an uncommon cause of pulmonary infiltrates in these patients. When it does occur, it is usually in the setting of HIV infection or organ transplantation.

CONCLUSION

Although the spectrum of infectious pathogens that occurs in the lungs of immunocompromised patients is broad, a general strategy for management of these patients is possible. An algorithm that illustrates these diagnostic and therapeutic options appears in Figure 23–65.

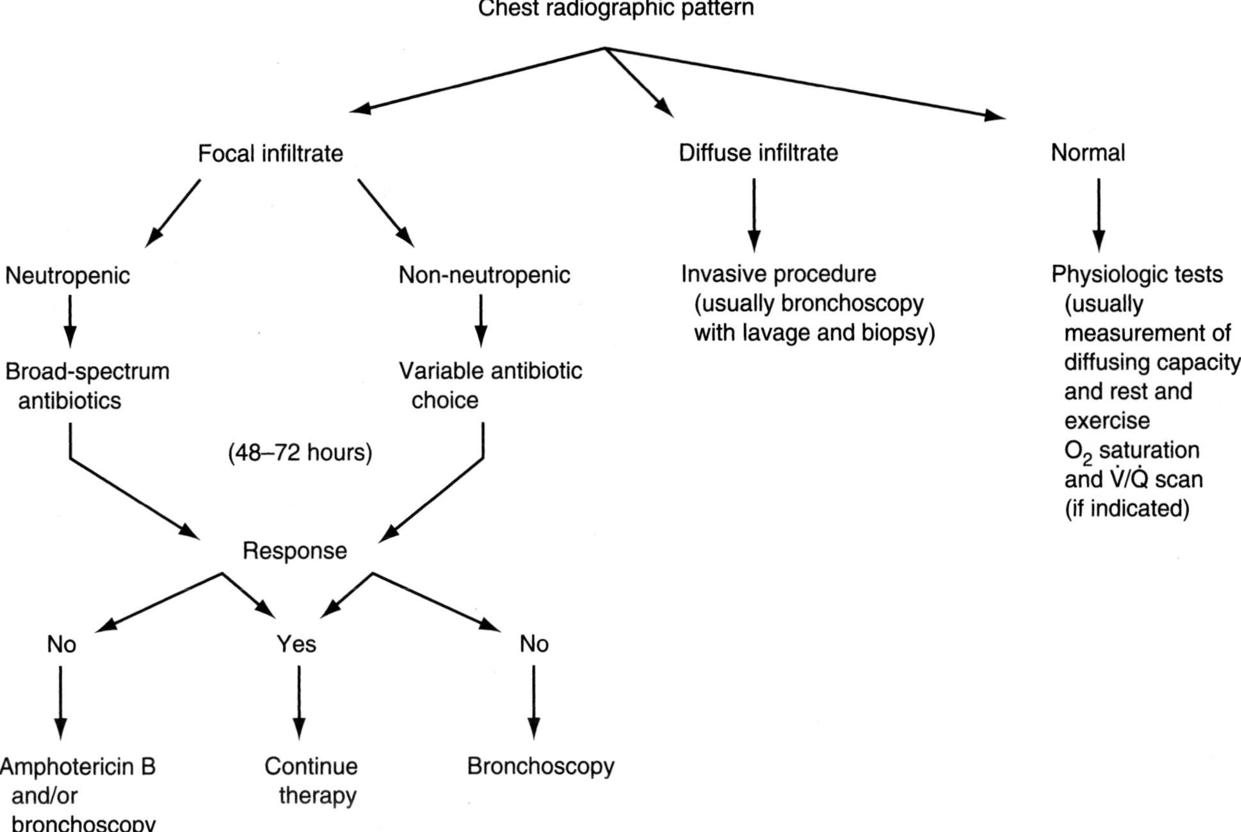

FIGURE 23–64 ■ Algorithm for approach to immunocompromised patients with pulmonary infections based on presenting chest radiograph.

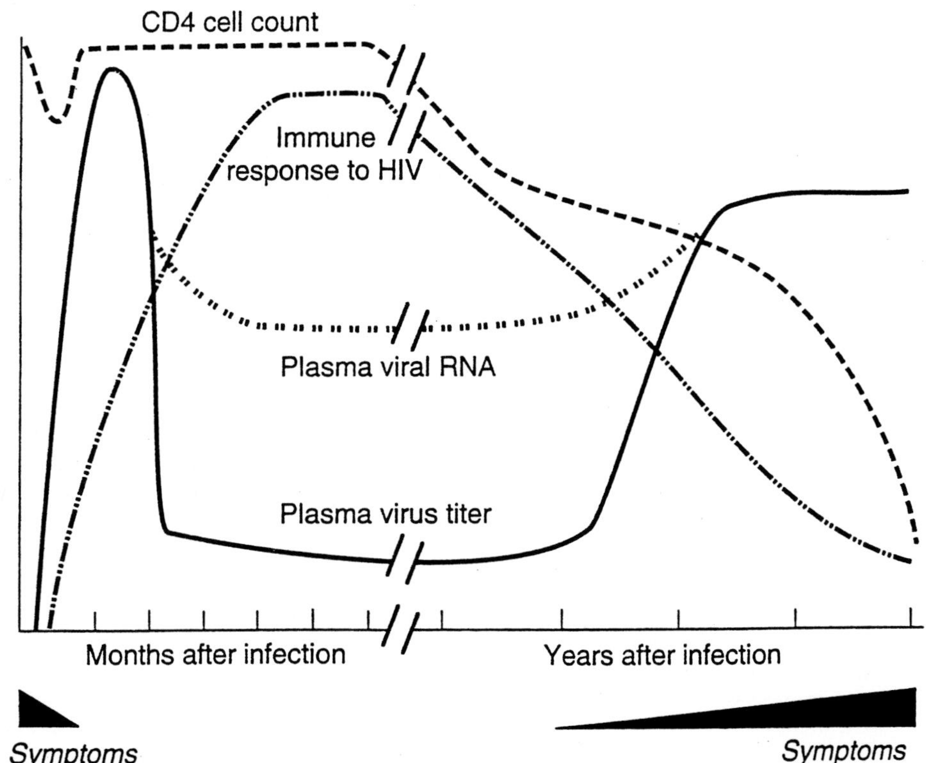

FIGURE 23–65 ■ Course of HIV infections. (From Lyerly HK, Bartlett JA, DiMaio JM: Thoracic disorders in the immunocompromised host. In Sabiston DC Jr, Spencer FC (eds): Surgery of the Chest, 6th ed. Philadelphia, WB Saunders, 1995.)

COMMENTS AND CONTROVERSIES

Surgeons are often called on to aid in the diagnosis of these dreaded pulmonary complications in immunocompromised hosts. In many patients, severe hypoxemia has already occurred. In such instances, when transbronchoscopic techniques do not yield a diagnosis, open lung biopsy is the only rational option. Video-assisted techniques or conventional open lung biopsy (see Chapter 32) is a safe and effective means of obtaining a diagnosis.

Less frequently, the surgeon is called on to participate in therapy, including the resection of localized lesions, in some instances before the induction of immunosuppression (e.g., high-dose chemotherapy with bone marrow rescue), lest these lesions proliferate as a result of immunosuppression. On occasion, even in progressive infections, lesions isolated to one lobe (e.g., progressive aspergillosis) can be treated successfully only by pulmonary resection, albeit with greater risk to the patient.

With the increasing prevalence of AIDS and immunosuppression caused by transplantation and high-dose chemotherapy, there is no doubt that surgeons will continue to be involved in the management of such patients. For further information, the reader should consult the following subchapter.

R. J. G.

KEY REFERENCES

Levine SJ, White DA: Pneumocystis carinii. Clin Chest Med 9:395, 1988.

The biology of the organism and the epidemiology, pathology, clinical presentation, course and outcome, diagnosis, and therapy of pneumonia caused by *Pneumocystis* species in HIV-infected patients are presented in detail.

Murray JF, Mills J: Pulmonary infectious complications of human immunodeficiency virus infection. 1, 2: Am Rev Respir Dis 5:1356, 1990.

A comprehensive review of the infectious complications found in HIV-infected patients is presented.

Shelhamer J, Pizzo PA, Parrillo JE, Masur H: Respiratory Disease in the Immunosuppressed Host. Philadelphia, JB Lippincott, 1991.

To date, this book is the most comprehensive on the subject of pulmonary disease in the immunocompromised host. A general prospective on pulmonary host defenses, the utility of various diagnostic procedures, disease processes that occur in specific patient populations (e.g., recipients of transplants and patients with HIV and cancer), and presentations of respiratory disease in these patients are discussed in detail.

Williams DM, Krick JA, Remington JS: Pulmonary infection in the immunocompromised host. 1, 2. Am Rev Respir Dis 114:359, 1976.

A comprehensive review of infectious complications in the non–AIDS-infected immunocompromised host is presented.

REFERENCES

Albelda SM, Talbot GH, Gerson SL et al: Pulmonary consolidation and massive hemoptysis in invasive pulmonary aspergillosis: Influence of bone marrow recovery in patients with acute leukemia. Am Rev Respir Dis 131:115, 1985.

Baccari MA, Bistoni F, Lohmann-Mathes ML: In vitro natural and cell-mediated cytotoxicity against *Candida albicans*: Macrophage precursors as effector cells. J Immunol 134:2658, 1985.

Barnes PF, Bloch AB, Davidson PT et al: Tuberculosis in patients with human immunodeficiency virus infection. N Engl J Med 324:1644, 1991.

Baugham RP, Dohn MN, Loudon RG et al: Bronchoscopy with bronchoalveolar lavage in tuberculosis and fungal infections. Chest 99:92, 1991.

Baugham RR, Rhodes JC, Dohn MN et al: Detection of cryptococcal antigen in bronchoalveolar lavage fluid: A prospective study of diagnostic utility. Am Rev Respir Dis 145:1226, 1992.

Bozzette SA, Sattler FA, Chiu J et al: A controlled trial of early adjunctive treatment with corticosteroids for *Pneumocystis carinii* pneumonia in the acquired immunodeficiency syndrome. N Engl J Med 323:1451, 1990.

Bradley SP, Reed SL, Catanzaro A: Clinical efficacy of the amplified *M. tuberculosis* direct test for the diagnosis of pulmonary tuberculosis. Am J Respir Crit Care Med 153:1606, 1996.

Broaddus C, Dake MD, Stulberg MS et al: Bronchoalveolar lavage and transbronchial biopsy for the diagnosis of pulmonary infections in the acquired immune deficiency syndrome. Ann Intern Med 102:747, 1985.

Carratala J, Roson B, Fernandez-Sevilla A et al: Bacteremic pneumonia in neutropenic patients with cancer. Arch Intern Med 158:868, 1998.

Castellino RA, Blank N: Etiologic diagnosis of focal pulmonary infection in immunocompromised patients by fluoroscopically guided percutaneous needle aspiration. Radiology 132:563, 1979.

Centers for Disease Control: Varicella-zoster immune globulin for the prevention of chicken pox: Recommendations of the Immunization Practices Advisory Committee. Ann Intern Med 100:859, 1984.

Centers for Disease Control: Prevention and control of influenza. MMWR Morb Mortal Wkly Rep 37:361, 1988.

Centers for Disease Control: Tuberculosis and human immunodeficiency virus infection: Recommendation of the advisory committee for the elimination of tuberculosis (ACET). MMWR Morb Mortal Wkly Rep 38:235, 1989.

Centers for Disease Control: Prevention and treatment of tuberculosis among patients infected with human immunodeficiency virus: Principles of therapy and revised recommendations. MMWR Morb Mortal Wkly Rep 47:40, 1998.

Chaisson RE, Schecter GR, Theuer CP et al: Tuberculosis in patients with the acquired immunodeficiency syndrome: Clinical features, response to therapy and survival. Am Rev Respir Dis 136:570, 1987.

Chuck SL, Sande M: Infections with *Cryptococcus neoformans* in the acquired immunodeficiency syndrome. N Engl J Med 321:794, 1989.

Cockerill FR, Wilson WR, Carpenter HA et al: Open lung biopsy in immunosuppressed patients. Arch Intern Med 145:1398, 1985.

Como J, Dismukes WE: Oral azole drugs as systemic antifungal therapy. N Engl J Med 330:263, 1994.

Conte JE Jr, Chernoff D, Feigal DW Jr et al: Intravenous or inhaled pentamidine for treating *Pneumocystis carinii* pneumonia in AIDS. Ann Intern Med 113:203, 1990.

Crawford SW, Hackman RC, Clark JG: Open lung biopsy diagnosis of diffuse pulmonary infiltrates after bone marrow transplantation. Chest 94:949, 1988.

Cunningham JH, Zavala DC, Corry RJ, Keim LW: Trephine air drill, bronchial brush and fiberoptic transbronchial lung biopsies in immunosuppressed patients. Am Rev Respir Dis 115:213, 1977.

Davidson M, Tempest B, Palmen DL: Bacteriologic diagnosis of acute pneumonia. JAMA 235:158, 1976.

DeSouza R, MacKinnon S, Spagnola SV et al: Treatment of localized pulmonary phycomycosis. South Med J 72:609, 1979.

Diamond LA, Lorber B: *Branhamella catarrhalis* pneumonia and immunoglobulin abnormalities: A new association. Am Rev Respir Dis 129:876, 1984.

Doern CV, Siebers KG, Hallick LM et al: Antibiotic susceptibility of beta-lactamase-producing strains of *Branhamella (Neisseria) catarrhalis*. Antimicrob Agents Chemother 17:24, 1980.

Dowdle W, Kendal AP, Noble GR: Influenza viruses. In Lennette EH, Schmidt NJ (eds): Diagnostic Procedures for Viral, Rickettsial and Chlamydial Infections. Washington, D.C., APHA, 1979, p 585.

Drew WL, Finely TN, Golde DW: Diagnostic lavage and occult pulmonary hemorrhage in the thrombocytopenic immunocompromised patients. Am Rev Respir Dis 116:215, 1977.

Drutz DJ: Pneumonia due to endemic fungi. In Shelhamer J, Pizzo PA, Parrillo JE, Masur H (eds): Respiratory Disease in the Immunosuppressed Host. Philadelphia, JB Lippincott, 1991, p 335.

Dummer JS, White LT, Ho M et al: Morbidity of cytomegalovirus infection in recipients of heart or heart-lung transplants who received cyclosporine. J Infect Dis 152:1182, 1984.

Edelstein PH, Meyer RD: Legionella pneumonias. In Pennington JE (ed): Respiratory Infections: Diagnosis and Management. New York, Raven Press, 1988, p 381.

Edman JC, Kovacs JA, Masur H et al: Ribosomal RNA sequences show *Pneumocystis carinii* to be a member of the fungi. Nature 334:519, 1988.

Emanuel D, Cunningham I, Jules-Elysee K et al: Cytomegalovirus pneumonia after bone marrow transplantation successfully treated with the combination of ganciclovir and high-dose intravenous immune globulin. Ann Intern Med 109:777, 1988.

Emanuel D, Peppard J, Stover DE et al: Rapid immunodiagnosis of cytomegalovirus (CMV) pneumonia by bronchoalveolar lavage using human and murine monoclonal antibodies. Ann Intern Med 104:476, 1986.

Ettinger NA, Bailey TC, Trulock EP et al: Cytomegalovirus infection and pneumonitis: Impact after isolated lung transplantation. Am Rev Respir Dis 147:1017, 1993.

Fagon J, Chastre J, Hance AJ et al: Detection of nosocomial lung infection in ventilated patients. Am Rev Respir Dis 138:110, 1988.

Falloon J, Kovacs J, Hughes W et al: A preliminary evaluation of 566C80 for the treatment of *Pneumocystis* pneumonia in patients with the acquired immunodeficiency syndrome. N Engl J Med 325:1534, 1991.

Fanta CH, Pennington JE: Pulmonary infections in the transplant patient. In Morris PJ, Tilney NL (eds): Progress in Transplantation, Vol 2. New York, Churchill Livingstone, 1985, p 207.

Fischl MA, Daikos GL, Uttamchandandi RB et al: Clinical presentation and outcome of patients with HIV infection and tuberculosis caused by multiple drug resistant bacilli. Ann Intern Med 117:184, 1992a.

Fischl MA, Uttamchandani RB, Daikos GL et al: An outbreak of tuberculosis caused by multiple drug resistant tubercle bacilli among patients with HIV infection. Ann Intern Med 117:177, 1992b.

Forrest JV: Radiological findings in *Pneumocystis carinii* pneumonia. Radiology 103:539, 1972.

Freeberg G, Stover DE, Levine S et al: Spectrum of pulmonary aspergillosis in immunocompromised hosts. Chest 98:31S, 1990.

Galgiani JN, Ampel NM: Coccidioidomycosis in human immunodeficiency virus infected patients. J Infect Dis 162:1165, 1990.

Goodman JS, Kaufman L, Koenig MG: Diagnosis of cryptococcal meningitis: Value of immunologic detection of cryptococcal antigen. N Engl J Med 285:434, 1971.

Hardy WD, Feinberg J, Finkelstein DM et al: A controlled trial of trimethoprim-sulfamethoxazole or aerosolized pentamidine for secondary prophylaxis of *Pneumocystis carinii* pneumonia in patients with the acquired immunodeficiency syndrome—AIDS Clinical Trials Group protocol 021. N Engl J Med 327:1842, 1992.

Helweg-Larsen J, Jensen JS, Berfield T et al: Diagnostic use of PCR for detection of *Pneumocystis carinii* in oral wash samples. J Clin Microbiol 36:2068, 1998.

Hopewell PC: Tuberculosis and the human immunodeficiency virus infection. Semin Respir Infect 4:11, 1989.

Hughes WT, Feldman S, Chaudhary SC et al: Comparison of pentamidine isethionate and trimethoprim-sulfamethoxazole in the treatment of *Pneumocystis carinii* pneumonia. J Pediatr 92:285, 1978.

Hughes WT, Rivera GK, Schell MJ et al: Successful intermittent chemoprophylaxis for *Pneumocystis carinii* pneumonitis. N Engl J Med 316:1627, 1987.

Ingra-Siegman Y, Kapila R, Sen P et al: Syndrome of hyperinfection with *Strongyloides stercoralis*. Rev Infect Dis 3:397, 1981.

Jacobson MA, Mills J, Rush J et al: Morbidity and mortality of patients with AIDS and first-episode *Pneumocystis carinii* pneumonia unaffected by concomitant pulmonary cytomegalovirus infection. Am Rev Respir Dis 144:6, 1991.

Jensen WA, Rose RM, Harmmer SM, Karchmen AW: Serologic diagnosis of focal pneumonia caused by *Cryptococcus neoformans*. Am Rev Respir Dis 132:189, 1985.

Joint Statement of American Thoracic Society and Centers for Disease Control. Treatment of tuberculosis infection in adults and children. Am J Respir Crit Care Med 149:1359, 1994.

Jules-Elysee K, Santamauro J, Vander Els N et al: Use of noninvasive tests in the diagnosis of PCP in non-AIDS patients. Am Rev Respir Dis 145:A543, 1992.

Jules-Elysee K, Stover DE, Zaman MB et al: Effect of aerosolized pentamidine: Effect on diagnosis and presentation of *Pneumocystis carinii*. Ann Intern Med 112:750, 1990.

Kaplan MH, Armstrong D, Rosen P: Tuberculosis complicating neoplastic disease. Cancer 33:850, 1974.

Kirby BD, Snyder KM, Meyer RD et al: Legionnaires' disease: Report of sixty-five nosocomial acquired cases and review of the literature. Medicine (Baltimore) 59:188, 1980.

Kohorst WR, Schonfeld SA, Macklin JE, Whitcomb ME: Rapid diagnosis of legionnaires' disease by bronchoalveolar lavage. Chest 84:186, 1983.

Kovacs JA, Hiemenz JW, Macher AM et al: *Pneumocystis carinii* pneumonia: A comparison between patients with the acquired immunodeficiency syndrome and patients with other immunodeficiencies. Ann Intern Med 100:663, 1984.

Kovacs JA, Kovacs AA, Polis M et al: Cryptococcosis in the acquired immunodeficiency syndrome. Ann Intern Med 103:533, 1985.

Kovacs JA, Ng VL, Masur H et al: Diagnosis of *Pneumocystis carinii* pneumonia: Improved detection in sputum with use of monoclonal antibodies. N Engl J Med 318:589, 1988.

Kulhman JE, Fishman EK, Siegelman SS: Invasive pulmonary aspergillosis in acute leukemia: Characteristic findings on CT: The CT halo sign, and the role of CT in early diagnosis. Radiology 157:611, 1985.

Kuritzkes DR, Simon HB: Pneumonia due to *M. tuberculosis* and to atypical mycobacteria. In Shelhammer J, Pizzo PA, Parrillo JE, Masur H (eds): Respiratory Diseases in the Immunosuppressed Host. Philadelphia, JB Lippincott, 1991, p 312.

Leong GS, Feigal DW, Montgomery AB et al: Aerosolized pentamidine for prophylaxis against *Pneumocystis carinii* pneumonia. The San Francisco Community Prophylaxis Trial. N Engl J Med 323:769, 1990.

Levine SJ, Stover DE: Bronchoscopy and related techniques. In Shelhamer J, Pizzo A, Parrillo JE, Masur H (eds): Respiratory Disease in the Immunocompromised Host. Philadelphia, JB Lippincott, 1991, p. 73.

Levine SJ, White DA: *Pneumocystis carinii*, Clin Chest Med 9:395, 1988.

Logemann J: Aspiration in head and neck surgical patients. Ann Otol Rhinol Laryngol 94:373, 1985.

Longman LP, Martin MV: A comparison of the efficacy of itraconazole, amphotericin B and 5-fluorocytosine in the treatment of *Aspergillus fumigatus* endocarditis in the rabbit. J Antimicrob Chemother 20:719, 1987.

Lopez-Berenstein G, Bodey GP, Fainstein V et al: Treatment of systemic fungal infections with liposomal amphotericin B. Arch Intern Med 149:2533, 1989.

MacDonnell KB, Glassroth J: *Mycobacterium avium* complex and other nontuberculous mycobacteria in patients with HIV infection. Semin Respir Infect 4:123, 1989.

Martin WJ, Smith TF, Sanderson DR et al: Role of bronchoalveolar lavage in the assessment of opportunistic pulmonary infections: Utility and complications. Mayo Clin Proc 62:549, 1987.

Masur H, Gill VJ, Ognibene FP et al: Diagnosis of *Pneumocystis* pneumonia by induced sputum technique in patients with immunologic disorders other than acquired immunodeficiency syndrome. Ann Intern Med 109:755, 1988.

Masur H, Ognibene FP, Yarchoan R et al: CD4 cells are predictors of opportunistic pneumonias in human immunodeficiency virus (HIV) infection. Ann Intern Med 111:223, 1989.

Masur H: *Pneumocystis carinii* pneumonia. In Shelhamer J, Pizzo PA, Parrillo JC, Masur H (eds): Respiratory Disease in the Immunocompromised Host. Philadelphia, JB Lippincott, 1991, p. 409.

Matthay RA, Greene WH: Pulmonary infections in the immunocompromised patient. Med Clin North Am 64:529, 1980.

Medina I, Mills J, Leoung G et al: Oral therapy for *Pneumocystis carinii* pneumonia in the acquired immunodeficiency syndrome. N Engl J Med 323:776, 1990.

Meduri GU, Stover DE, Greeno RA et al: Bilateral bronchoalveolar lavage in the diagnosis of opportunistic pulmonary infection. Chest 100:1272, 1991.

Meyer RD, Rosen P, Armstrong D: Phycomycosis complicating leukemia and lymphoma. Ann Intern Med 77:871, 1972.

Munt PW: Miliary tuberculosis in the chemotherapy era: With a clinical review of 69 American adults. Medicine (Baltimore) 51:139, 1971.

Murray JF, Mills J: Pulmonary infectious complications of human immunodeficiency virus infection. 1, 2. Am Rev Respir Dis 5:1356, 1990.

Murray HW, Masur H, Senterfit LB et al: The protean manifestations of *Mycoplasma pneumoniae* infection in adults. Am J Med 58:229, 1975.

Naidich DP, McGuinness G: Pulmonary manifestations of AIDS: CT and radiographic correlations. Radiol Clin North Am 29:999, 1991.

Neiman PE, Reeves W, Ray G et al: A prospective analysis of interstitial pneumonia and opportunistic viral infection among recipients of allogeneic bone marrow grafts. J Infect Dis 136:754, 1977.

Ognibene FP, Shelhamer J, Gill V et al: The diagnosis of *Pneumocystis carinii* in patients with the acquired immune deficiency syndrome using subsegmental bronchoalveolar lavage. Am Rev Respir Dis 129:933, 1984.

Ortbals DW, Marr JJ: A comparative study of tuberculosis and other mycobacterial infections and their associations with malignancy. Am Rev Respir Dis 117:39, 1978.

Palmer DL, Harvey RL, Wheeler JK: Diagnostic and therapeutic considerations in *Nocardia asteroides* infection. Medicine 53:391, 1974.

Pearson ML, Jereb JA, Frieden TR et al: Nosocomial transmission of multidrug-resistant *Mycobacterium* tuberculosis. Ann Intern Med 117:191, 1992.

Perez CR, Leigh MW: *Mycoplasma pneumoniae* as the causative agent for pneumonia in the immunocompromised host. Chest 100:860, 1991.

Pifer LL, Hughes WT, Stagno S, Woods D: *Pneumocystis carinii* infection: Evidence for high prevalence in normal and immunosuppressed children. Pediatrics 61:35, 1978.

Pitchenik AK, Burr J, Suarez M et al: Human T-cell lymphotropic virus-III (HTLV-III) seropositivity and related disease among 71 consecutive patients in whom tuberculosis was diagnosed. Am Rev Respir Dis 135:875, 1987.

Pitchenik AK, Cole C, Russell BW et al: Tuberculosis, atypical mycobacteriosis and the acquired immunodeficiency syndrome among Haitian and non-Haitian patients in South Florida. Ann Intern Med 101:641, 1984.

Pitchenik AK, Fertel D: Tuberculosis and nontuberculosis mycobacterial disease (medical management of AIDS patients). Med Clin North Am 76:121, 1992.

Pizzo PA, Robichaud KJ, Gill FA et al: Empiric antibiotic and antifungal therapy for cancer patients with prolonged fever and granulocytopenia. Am J Med 72:101, 1982.

Polsky B, Gold JW, Whimbey E et al: Bacterial pneumonia in patients with the acquired immunodeficiency syndrome. Ann Intern Med 140:38, 1986.

Prechter GC, Prakash VBS: Bronchoscopy in the diagnosis of pulmonary histoplasmosis. Chest 95:1033, 1989.

Ramsey PG, Fife KH, Hackman RC et al: Herpes simplex virus pneumonia: Clinical, virologic and pathologic features in 20 patients. Ann Intern Med 97:813, 1982.

Reed EC, Bowden RA, Dandliker PS et al: Treatment of cytomegalovirus pneumonia with ganciclovir and intravenous cytomegalovirus immunoglobulin in patients with bone marrow transplants. Ann Intern Med 15:783, 1988.

Roilides E, Pizzo PA: Modulation of host defenses by cytokines: Evolving adjuncts in prevention and treatment of serious infections in the immunocompromised host. Clin Infect Dis 15:508, 1992.

Rolston KVI, Jones PG, Fainstein V et al: Pulmonary disease caused by rapidly growing mycobacteria in patients with cancer. Chest 87:503, 1985.

Rossiter SJ, Miller DC, Churg AM et al: Open lung biopsy in the immunosuppressed patient: Is it really beneficial? J Thorac Cardiovasc Surg 77:338, 1979.

Rotstein C, Cummings K, Nicolaou A et al: Nosocomial infection rates at an oncology center. Infect Control Hosp Epidemiol 9:13, 1988.

Saravoltz LD, Burch KH, Fisher E et al: The compromised host and legionnaires' disease. Ann Intern Med 90:533, 1979.

Sarkar SK, Sharma TN, Puroket SD et al: The diagnostic value of routine culture of bronchial washings in tuberculosis. Br J Dis Chest 76:358, 1982.

Satterfield JR, McLaughlin JS: Open lung biopsy in diagnosing pulmonary infiltrates in immunosuppressed patients. Ann Thorac Surg 28:359, 1979.

Sattler FR, Cowan R, Nielsen DM et al: Trimethoprim-sulfamethoxazole compared with pentamidine for treatment of *Pneumocystis carinii* pneumonia in the acquired immunodeficiency syndrome. Ann Intern Med 109:200, 1988.

Selwyn PA, Hartel D, Lewis VA et al: A prospective study of the risk of tuberculosis among intravenous drug users with human immunodeficiency virus infection. N Engl J Med 320:545, 1989.

Sepkowitz KA, Brown AK, Telzak EE et al: *Pneumocystis carinii* pneumonia among patients without AIDS at a cancer hospital. JAMA 267:832, 1992.

Sepkowitz KA, Telzak EE, Gold JW et al: Pneumothorax in AIDS. Ann Intern Med 114:455, 1991.

Shelhamer J, Pizzo PA, Parrillo JE, Masur H: Respiratory Disease in the Immunosuppressed Host. Philadelphia, JB Lippincott, 1991.

Shepp DH, Dandliker PS, Meyers JD: Treatment of varicella zoster virus infection in severely immunocompromised patients: A randomized comparison of acyclovir and vidarabine. N Engl J Med 314:208, 1986.

Sickles EA, Greene WH, Wiernik PH: Clinical presentation of infection in granulocytopenic patients. Arch Intern Med 135:715, 1975.

Sickles EA, Young VM, Greene WH et al: Pneumonia in acute leukemia. Ann Intern Med 79:528, 1973.

Siemsen JK, Grebe SF, Waxman AD: The use of gallium-67 in pulmonary disorders. Semin Nucl Med 8:235, 1978.

Simpson GL, Stinson EB, Egger MJ et al: Nocardial infections in the immunocompromised host: A detailed study in a defined population. Rev Infect Dis 3:492, 1981.

Singer C, Armstrong D, Rosen PP et al: Diffuse pulmonary infiltrates in immunocompromised patients: Prospective study of 80 cases. Am J Med 66:110, 1979.

Singer C, Armstrong D, Rosen PP et al: *Pneumocystis carinii* pneumonia: A cluster of eleven cases. Ann Intern Med 82:772, 1975.

Singer C, Kaplan MH, Armstrong D: Bacteremia and fungemia complicating neoplastic disease: A study of 364 cases. Am J Med 62:731, 1977.

Soo Hoo GW, Mohenifar Z, Meyer RD: Inhaled or intravenous pentamidine therapy for *Pneumocystis carinii* pneumonia in AIDS. Ann Intern Med 113:195, 1990.

Stover DE: Diagnosis of pulmonary disease in the immunocompromised host. Semin Respir Med 10:89, 1989.

Stover DE, Meduri GU: Pulmonary function tests. Clin Chest Med 9:473, 1988.

Stover DE, White DA, Romano PA et al: Diagnosis of pulmonary disease in acquired immune deficiency syndrome (AIDS): Role of bronchoscopy and bronchoalveolar lavage. Am Rev Respir Dis 130:659, 1984a.

Stover DE, Zaman MB, Hajdu SI et al: Bronchoalveolar lavage in the diagnosis of diffuse pulmonary infiltrates in the immunosuppressed host. Ann Intern Med 101:1, 1984b.

Sunderam G, McDonald RJ, Maniatis T et al: Tuberculosis as a manifestation of the acquired immunodeficiency syndrome (AIDS). JAMA 256:362, 1986.

Tenholder MF, Hooper RG: Pulmonary infiltrates in leukemia. Chest 78:468, 1980.

Tietjen PA, Jules-Elysee K, Stover DE: Increased incidence of pneumothoraces with aerosolized pentamidine. Chest 96:1875, 1989.

Toledo-Pereya LH, De Miester TR, Kinealy A et al: The benefits of open lung biopsy in patients with previous nondiagnostic transbronchial lung biopsy. Chest 77:647, 1990.

Trulock EP: Lung transplantation: State-of-the art. Am J Respir Crit Care Med 155:789, 1997.

Turbiner KG, Yeh SD, Rosen PP et al: Abnormal gallium scintigraphy in *Pneumocystis carinii* pneumonia with a normal chest radiograph. Radiology 127:437, 1978.

Vanek J: Atypical interstitial pneumonia of infants produced by *Pneumocystis carinii*. Cas Lek Cesk 90:1121, 1951.

Wallace JM, Cantanzaro A, Moser KM et al: Flexible fiberoptic bronchoscopy for diagnosing pulmonary coccidioidomycosis. Am Rev Respir Dis 123:286, 1981.

Wallace JM, Rao AV, Glassroth J et al: Respiratory illness in persons with acquired immunodeficiency virus infection. Am Rev Respir Dis 148:1523, 1993.

Wang KP, Haponik EF, Britt EJ et al: Transbronchial needle aspiration of peripheral pulmonary nodules. Chest 86:819, 1984.

Weiner MH, Talbot GH, Gerson SL et al: Antigen detection in the

diagnosis of invasive aspergillosis: Utility in controlled blinded trials. Ann Intern Med 99:777, 1983.
Wheat LJ: Histoplasmosis. Infect Dis Clin North Am 3:843, 1989.
Wheat LJ, Hafner R, Wulfsohn M et al: Prevention of relapse of histoplasmosis with itraconazole in patients with the acquired immunodeficiency syndrome. Ann Intern Med 118:610, 1993.
Wheat LJ, Kohler RB, Tewari RP: Diagnosis of disseminated histoplasmosis by detection of *Histoplasma capsulatum* antigen in serum and urine specimens. N Engl J Med 314:83, 1986.
White DA, Stover DE: Pulmonary complications of HIV infection. Clin Chest Med 17:621, 1996.
Willcox PA, Benatar SR, Potgieter PD: Use of the flexible fiberoptic bronchoscope in diagnosis of sputum-negative pulmonary tuberculosis. Thorax 37:598, 1987.
Williams DM, Krick JA, Remington JS: Pulmonary infection in the immunocompromised host. 1, 2. Am Rev Respir Dis 114:359, 1976.
Wimberly NW, Bass JB, Boyd BW et al: Use of bronchoscopic protected catheter brush for the diagnosis of pulmonary infections. Chest 81:556, 1982.
Winn WC, Cherry WB, Frank RO et al: Direct immunofluorescent detection of *Legionella pneumophila* in respiratory specimens. J Clin Microbiol 11:59, 1980.
Zaman MK, Wooten OJ, Suprahmanya B et al: Rapid noninvasive diagnosis of *Pneumocystis carinii* pneumonia from induced liquefied sputum. Ann Intern Med 109:7, 1988.
Zavala DC, Schoell JE: Ultrathin needle aspiration of the lung in infectious and malignant disease. Am Rev Respir Dis 123:123, 1981.

THORACIC SURGERY IN THE AIDS PATIENT

Arthur D. Boyd
Lawrence R. Glassman

Acquired immunodeficiency syndrome (AIDS) was recognized in 1981 as a new and unique clinical condition affecting young, otherwise healthy, homosexual men. Clusters of homosexual men were found to have Kaposi's sarcoma and *Pneumocystis carinii* pneumonia (Gottlieb et al, 1981; Hymes et al, 1981; Masur et al, 1981). Similar clusters were soon recognized in other groups, including intravenous drug users and hemophiliacs (Centers for Disease Control, 1982; Davis et al, 1983; Elliot et al, 1983; Poon et al, 1983). The cause of the immunodeficiency in these patients was unknown. Soon extensive clinical and laboratory studies commenced, bringing an initial understanding of the condition. In 1997, Essex, Gallo and colleagues (Gallo et al, 1983; Gelman et al, 1983), and Montagnier (Barre-Sinovasi et al, 1983) postulated that the etiology was infectious and might be caused by a variant of the T lymphotropic retrovirus, the human T cell leukemia lymphoma virus (HTLV). At that time, Montagnier and colleagues (Barre-Sinovasi et al, 1983) isolated a T lymphotropic retrovirus, now called the human immunodeficiency virus, type 1 (HIV-1), and Gallo and associates (Gallo et al, 1984; Popovic et al, 1984; Schupbach et al, 1984) conclusively demonstrated that this virus was the cause of these infections in humans. The hallmark of AIDS, the end stage of infection by the human immunodeficiency virus (HIV), is a marked deficiency in the cellular immune system, which leads to the development of opportunistic infectious diseases and neoplasms. The most common site of localized opportunistic infections in patients with AIDS is the chest; consequently, thoracic surgeons are frequently consulted concerning the diagnosis and treatment of these infections (Essex, 1997; Lyerly et al, 1995; Saag, 1997).

THE HUMAN IMMUNODEFICIENCY VIRUS

HIV—a single-stranded plus sense RNA virus approximately 100 nm in diameter with a nucleoid core that contains proteins, genomic RNA, and reverse transcriptase and that is surrounded by a lipid capsule (Folks and Hart, 1997; Gourla et al, 1986; Ratner et al, 1985)—is a retrovirus with the ability to transport genetic information from RNA to DNA. The unique enzyme reverse transcriptase (RT), which is common to all retroviruses and which is encoded within the retroviral genome, makes this transfer possible (Folks and Hart, 1997; Lyerly et al, 1995).

Pathogenesis

An HIV infection begins with the binding of an infectious virion to a susceptible cell, usually a CD4 lymphocyte (T helper cell), a macrophage, or a monocyte (Lyerly et al, 1995). The surface gp 120 ENV protein of the virus attaches to a cellular CD4 molecule, resulting in fusion of the viral lipid capsule and the cell membrane of the host cell. Genomic RNA of the retrovirus then penetrates into the cytoplasm of the host cell. RT converts RNA into double-stranded DNA, which is carried to the cell nucleus where it is integrated into the host's chromosomal DNA. Proviral DNA can then replicate along with the host's chromosomal genes. Virus-specific proteins are produced and are assimilated into infectious virions that leave the host cells, completing the life cycle of the virus (Folks and Hart, 1997).

Epidemiology

It is estimated that between 1981 and 1997, 1,125,000 people in the United States were infected with HIV and that 612,078 of those infected developed AIDS. A full 70% of the infections resulted from sexual contact; 27% resulted from intravenous drug abuse; 2% from transfusions of contaminated blood or blood products; and 1% from perinatal transmissions. Of the infections resulting from sexual contacts, 87% occurred in gay men (Bartlett, 1999). It is encouraging to note that the number of gay men becoming infected with HIV has dropped, suggesting that education in the gay community concerning infection by HIV has been effective (Lyerly et al, 1995), and that the number of persons infected with HIV in the United States has stabilized (68,473 new cases in 1996; 64,357 in 1997) (Bartlett, 1999).

Natural History

Between 2 and 4 weeks after exposure to HIV, the acute, or first, phase of the infection develops and lasts 1 to 3 weeks. This acute retroviral syndrome is infectious and mononucleosis-like and consists of fever, sore throat, fatigue, malaise, weight loss, and a fleeting morbilliform rash. At this stage, diffuse lymphatic hyperplasia develops (Lyerly et al, 1995; Saag, 1997).

The acute phase is followed by a prolonged, asymptomatic second phase that lasts approximately 10 years, during which diffuse lymphatic hyperplasia persists (Lefson et al, 1988). In this second phase, there is a gradual decrease in the CD4 lymphocyte count and an increase in the plasma concentration of HIV RNA. When the CD4 count drops to approximately 200/mm^3, opportunistic infections and tumors soon follow, along with the onset of fullblown AIDS (Lyerly et al, 1995). The median survival time after the CD4 count falls to 200/mm^3 is 3.1 years (Bartlett, 1999; Centers for Disease Control, 1993a) (Fig. 23–66).

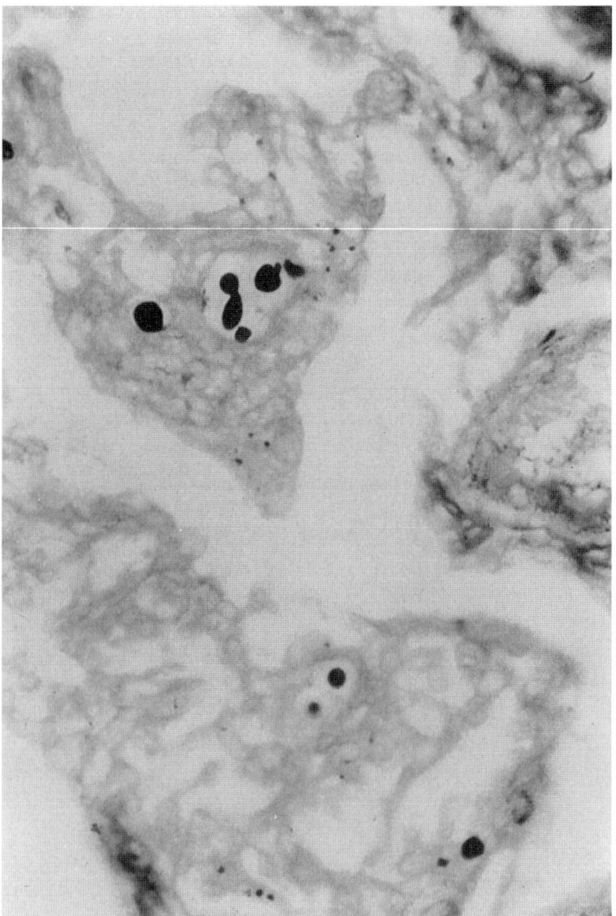

FIGURE 23–66 ■ *Pneumocystis carinii* organisms stained with methenamine silver in fluid obtained at bronchoscopy.

This natural history of HIV infection has been dramatically altered by the introduction of effective antiretroviral therapy. With treatment, CD4 counts may remain in the normal range and plasma HIV RNA may be undetectable for a prolonged period. Infectious complications, hospitalizations, and deaths have all decreased since the introduction of these new drugs (Bartlett, 1999).

Diagnosis of HIV Infections

The Centers for Disease Control in Atlanta recommends that serologic testing for HIV be offered as a routine admission test to patients 15 to 54 years of age in hospitals with seroprevalence rates exceeding 1% and with rates of HIV exceeding 1 in 1000 discharges (Centers for Disease Control, 1993b; Gürtler, 1996). Serologic testing for AIDS should also be highly recommended to patients in high-risk categories and to patients with unusual infections and tumors (Bartlett, 1999). The standard serologic tests for HIV include the enzyme-linked immunosorbent assay (ELISA) as a screening test and the Western blot as the confirmatory test (Bartlett, 1999). Extensive experience with these serologic tests have shown them to be among the most accurate tests in medicine, with sensitivity and specificity higher than 99% (Centers for Disease Control, 1990).

False-negative test results usually occur when the tests are carried out during the period between transmission and seroconversion, an interval rarely lasting more than 3 months (Imazawa and Detels, 1991). If an HIV infection is suspected but the serologic test results are negative or indeterminate, the tests should be repeated after a 3-month period.

In some instances a non–antibody-dependent assay is needed to confirm or clarify serologic results. Qualitative plasma, HIV DNA polymerase chain reaction (Owens et al, 1996), is usually used in these circumstances (sensitivity, 97%–98%; specificity, 98%). Quantitative plasma, HIV RNA, is a more readily available but somewhat less sensitive alternative (Bartlett, 1999)

Serologic screening of blood donated for transfusions has also been shown to be effective. It is estimated that the risk of developing HIV is 1 in 450,000 to 660,000 per unit of screened blood (Lackritz et al, 1995).

Treatment of HIV Infections

Between 1995 and 1997, non-nucleoside reverse transcriptase inhibitors and protease inhibitors became available for the treatment of HIV infections. This was approximately a decade after the introduction of nucleoside analogues, the first effective agent against HIV (Bartlett, 1999). These newer drugs are the most active agents available against HIV, and their availability introduced the era of highly active antiretroviral therapy (HAART). Although these drugs are effective, they have made the treatment of HIV more complex, largely because of their high cost and their toxicity, which makes patient compliance with taking them more difficult. The possibility that strains resistant to these drugs might develop has become a real concern (Bartlett, 1999). HAART, however, has been effective. AIDS-defining complications have decreased by 60% to 80%; hospitalizations by 60% to 80%; and mortality rates by 44% (Bartlett, 1999).

There is hope for the future in the United States and other industrialized countries, but in the Third World the future is bleak, especially in Africa where HIV has reached epidemic proportions and drug therapy remains prohibitively expensive.

Prophylaxis for Health Care Workers Exposed to HIV

A total of 52 health care workers in the United States had acquired HIV infection as a result of occupational exposure as of June 1997. No surgeons had seroconverted as of that date (Bartlett, 1999). The risk factors for seroconversion include: (1) a deep injury; (2) visible blood on an instrument or device; (3) penetration of an artery or vein; and (4) exposure to a source who is in the late stage of the disease (Centers for Disease Control, 1996). Prophylaxis in the form of zidovudine (Retrovir) has been shown to decrease the transmission rate of HIV by 79%. On the basis of this evidence, it is now recommended that prophylaxis be initiated as soon as possible after exposure and that Retrovir plus lamivudine be used (Centers for Disease Control, 1998). Serologic testing should be performed immediately, at 6 and 12 weeks, and again at 6 months after exposure (Bartlett, 1999).

Protection of a Surgical Team Against HIV Infection

When operating on a patient with HIV infection or another highly contagious infection such as hepatitis, the surgical team (surgeons, anesthesiologists, nurses, medical students, and technicians) must be made aware of the potential for transmission of these diseases, and appropriate changes must be made in the method of performing the procedure. The passage of all "sharps" must be announced loudly and clearly so that all members of the operative team are aware that such instruments are being passed. The scrub nurse alone should remove and replace instruments from and to the Mayo stand and back table. The use of a magnetic tray for passing instruments to and from the operative field decreases the likelihood of injury by sharp instruments or needles (Gerberding, 1993). Only one person at a time should be working, so that accidental penetration of the skin by a sharp instrument is minimized.

Instruments such as the electrocautery unit, ultrasonic dissector, lasers, and staplers, which are unlikely to cause skin penetration, may be used when appropriate (Lewis et al, 1995). Blunt-tipped needles also have been shown to decrease the risk of skin penetration, and their use should be considered (Miller and Subharwal, 1994; Montz et al, 1991).

Personal protective clothing is also essential for the operative team. Double or triple gloving and the use of Kevlar gloves, waterproof gowns, face visors, and waterproof shoe covers or boots are effective protective paraphernalia (Short et al 1997).

Most important, the entire surgical team must remain alert and cautious. This will minimize the possibility of exposing any member of the team to the HIV or hepatitis virus.

Acquired Immunodeficiency Syndrome

AIDS, the final stage of HIV infection, is defined by the development of opportunistic infections and tumors, such as Kaposi's sarcoma (KS) and B cell lymphomas, as well as other conditions listed in Table 23–21. Clinically, AIDS patients have a CD4 lymphocyte count of 200/mm^3 or less (Centers for Disease Control, 1992) and they commonly develop pneumonia, esophagitis, diarrhea, central nervous system infections, and wasting (Saag, 1997). Because the chest is the most common site for opportunistic infections and is a common location for these tumors, thoracic surgeons are frequently involved in the diagnosis and treatment of patients with AIDS (Lyerly, 1995).

Until recently, patients with AIDS had short life expectancies (median survival: 1.3 years) (Bartlett, 1999) and were considered, essentially, to be terminally ill, which precluded aggressive therapy for many of the complications that occurred in these patients. With the introduction of HAART, it has become possible for the CD4 count in an HIV-infected patient to increase by 150 to 200/mm^3; for HIV RNA to become undetectable in the peripheral blood; for progression of HIV infection to AIDS to be delayed; and for AIDS-defining complications to decrease by 60% to 80% (Bartlett, 1999).

TABLE 23–21 ■ **AIDS-Defining Conditions According to the Centers for Disease Control, 1993**

CD4 count below 200/mm^3
Candidiasis, pulmonary or esophageal
Cervical cancer
Coccidioidomycosis
Crypotosporidiosis
Cytomegalovirus infection
Herpes esophagitis
HIV encephalopathy
Histoplasmosis
Isosporiasis
Kaposi's sarcoma
Lymphoma
Mycobacterial disease
Pneumocystis carinii infection
Pneumonia, bacterial
Progressive multifocal leukoencephalopenia
Salmonellosis

Any HIV-infected patient who develops infectious or neoplastic complications should be receiving HAART. The patient should be carefully evaluated, taking care to see that the HAART is optimal. Judgment as to the nature and aggressiveness of treatment of a complication should be made on a case-by-case basis. If the patient's general condition is satisfactory and surgical therapy for the complication is indicated, an aggressive surgical approach should be carried out just as it would be in a patient not infected with HIV.

AIDS-DEFINING CONDITIONS

Infections

Pneumocystis Carinii

Pneumocystis carinii pneumonia (PCP) is the most common pulmonary infection to affect patients with HIV. First identified by Chagas in 1905, *P. carinii* was initially classified as a protozoan but now is thought to be more closely related to fungi (Masur et al, 1989). The primary cystic form of *P. carinii* is 4 to 6 μm in diameter and contains as many as 8 pleomorphic intracyst cells called saporozoetes. *P. carinii* is ubiquitous in the environment. Serologic data in the United States suggest that most humans are subclinically infected with *P. carinii* during childhood. When the host becomes immunosuppressed as a result of drugs or illness, the latent infection may then reactivate and develop into clinically apparent PCP (Lyerly et al, 1995).

Fever, dyspnea, cough, and thoracic tightness are the usual presenting symptoms of PCP. Many patients may initially have normal chest radiographs. Diffuse infiltrates varying from interstitial to alveolar develop in adults with AIDS (DeLorenzo et al, 1987).

Because *P. carinii* cannot be cultured, its diagnosis requires the demonstration of the presence of cysts or trophozoites in tissue or body fluids. With Giemsa or methenamine silver staining, organisms can be demonstrated in induced sputum in 50% to 60% of patients with PCP (Pitchenick et al, 1986). Immunofluorescent monoclonal antibodies make the diagnostic capabilities even more accurate—about 90% (Kovacs, 1988). Bronchoalveolar lavage (BAL) and transbronchial biopsy (TBB) increase the diagnostic yield still further (Fig. 23–67), to close to 100% in patients with PCP (Broadelus et al, 1995).

Trimethoprim-sulfamethoxazole (TMP-SMZ), the treatment of choice in cases of PCP, can be given orally or intravenously. Dapsone and trimethoprim, atovaquone or clindamycin and primaquine are other oral regimens that are effective against PCP. Pentamidine can be given intravenously to patients who do not tolerate oral medicine. Steroids are recommended for patients who are hypoxic and have arterial oxygen tensions of less than 70 mm Hg (Lyerly et al, 1995).

PCP is usually seen in patients whose CD4 lymphocyte count is less than 200/mm^3. Because the PCP recurrence rate approaches 60% during the first year following initial treatment and recovery (Fischl et al, 1990), PCP prophylaxis is strongly recommended (Lyerly et al, 1995). Although aerosolized pentamidine is a widely used prophylaxis, TMP-SMZ is judged to be superior in preventing PCP recurrence (Hardy et al, 1992). The diagnosis of PCP in patients receiving prophylactic drugs is clearly more difficult because fewer organisms are present in these patients (Jules-Elysee et al, 1990).

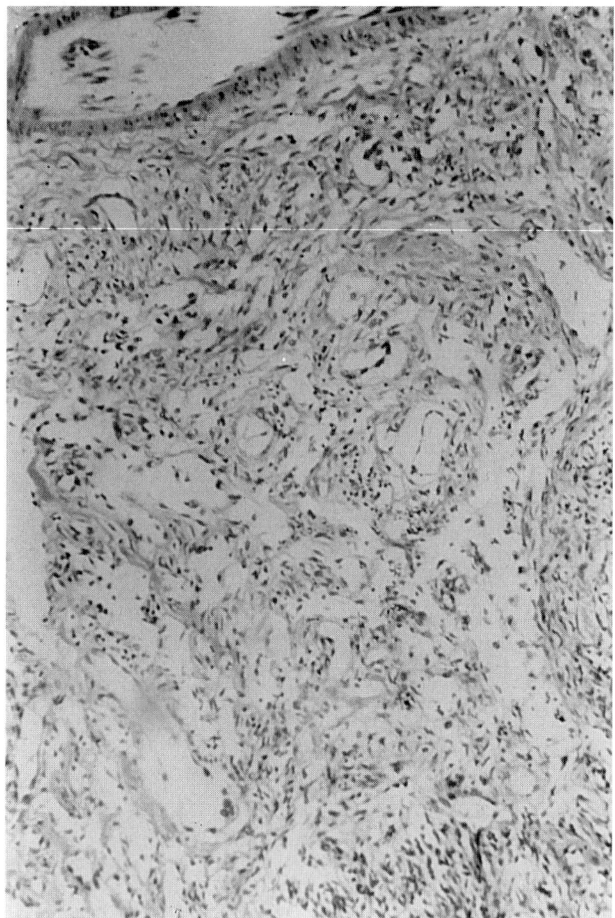

FIGURE 23–67 ■ Microscopic view of AIDS-related Kaposi's sarcoma showing irregularly shaped vascular channels and spindle cells.

Thoracic surgeons are often asked to help in the diagnosis of PCP by performing bronchoscopy with BAL and TBB and, rarely, with open lung biopsy. Spontaneous pneumothorax, which is caused by the rupture of necrotic subpleural lung tissue (Beers et al, 1990), is a complication seen in 3% of cases (Pastores et al, 1996) and is treated by closed-tube thoracotomy. It is common for a prolonged air leak to result, requiring long and expensive care. In a patient with PCP and a bronchopleural fistula, treatment of the PCP must be instituted promptly and a chest tube inserted. If the lung does not re-expand or if the air leak continues for more than 10 days, surgical closure of the leak and partial pleurectomy should be carried out, assuming the patient can withstand surgery (Crawford et al, 1992). Chemical pleurodesis using doxycycline (Read et al, 1994) and early videoscopic talc poudrage (Wait and Dal Nogaic, 1994) have also been recommended.

Bacterial Infections

The lungs are among the most common sites of bacterial infection in HIV-infected patients. These pneumonias usually occur in patients with CD4 lymphocyte counts of less than $200/mm^3$ and can be community-acquired or nosocomial in nature. *Streptococcus pneumoniae* and *Haemophilus influenzae* are the most common causative organisms, but *Strephylococcus aureus, Pseudomonas aeruginosa*, and other *Haemophilus* and *Streptococcus* organisms can be the cause of pneumonia (Burack et al, 1994; Zurlo and Lane, 1997). Fever, dyspnea, productive cough, and chest pain are the usual presenting signs and symptoms. The patients with pneumococcal infections commonly develop bacteremia. Radiographs of the chest can show lobar consolidation and unilateral or bilateral lobar infiltrates. Pleural effusions and empyemas can occur but are uncommon. The diagnosis is usually obtained by examining and culturing sputum and from blood cultures if bacteremia is present. TMP-SMZ is an appropriate initial treatment in patients with bacterial pneumonias. When sensitivity results become available, therapy should be adjusted as necessary. In most cases of community-acquired pneumonias the prognosis is good, but in càses of nosocomial and *Pseudomonas* species infections, the morbidity and mortality rates are higher (Zurlo and Lane, 1997).

Tuberculosis

Mycobacterium Tuberculosis. With the onset of the HIV epidemic in the early 1980s, the steady downward trend in the number of cases of tuberculosis in the United States was reversed (Bloom and Murray, 1992). Many of the patients developing tuberculosis were also infected with HIV. Among the estimated 1 million patients infected with HIV, it is thought that 100,000, or approximately 10%, were also infected with tuberculosis (Centers for Disease Control, 1993a). At least 40% of the coinfected patients were infected with multiple-drug–resistent tuberculous organisms (Frieden et al, 1993). It is estimated that 8% of coinfected patients will develop active tuberculosis each year (Selwyn et al, 1989).

Active tuberculosis is usually an early complication of AIDS that occurs when the CD4 lymphocyte count is $300/mm^3$ or less. These coinfected patients commonly develop extrapulmonary disease involving multiorgan systems. The pulmonary presentation may vary from typical upper lobe disease to miliary patterns to pulmonary nodules to patchy infiltrates involving any portion of the lungs. Pleural and nodal involvement are also encountered. The presence of tuberculosis must be considered in every HIV-infected patient who develops pneumonia (Lyerly et al, 1995).

Acid-fast smears and cultures on multiple 24-hour sputum specimens should be performed in an effort to confirm the diagnosis of tuberculosis. If necessary, sputum can be induced so that adequate specimens are available for examination. Bronchoscopy with BAL and TBB provide the best material for making an immediate diagnosis of pulmonary tuberculosis.

Tuberculous pleural infections are diagnosed by smear and culture of aspirated pleural fluid or histologic examination and cuture of pleural tissue. Mediastinal node involvement can be confirmed by examination of lymph nodes obtained at mediastinoscopy.

An HIV-infected patient who is without evidence of active tuberculosis but who has a positive purified protein derivative (PPD) reaction of 5 mm or larger should be considered to be infected with tuberculosis and treated with isoniazid. Active tuberculosis in HIV-infected patients must be treated with a four-drug regime—isoniazid, rifampin, ethambutol, and pyrazinamide. When drug sensitivity studies become available, alterations in therapy are made if indicated. Regimens for the treatment of multiple-drug–resistent organisms are based on the results of drug sensitivity tests and commonly require the use of second-line drugs (Lyerly et al, 1995). Prolonged drug treatment and occasional surgical resection of localized disease are necessary to cure tuberculosis in patients infected with drug-resistent organisms (Lyerly et al, 1995; Rigsby and Friedland, 1997).

Massive or severe recurrent hemoptysis, persistent positive sputum, a mass lesion that is possibly a carcinoma, and a bronchopleural fistula with a mixed tuberculous and pyogenic empyema are other tuberculous conditions for which surgical therapy should be considered (Boyd et al, 1996). If the HIV-infected patient's condition is satisfactory and there is adequate cardiopulmonary reserve, treatment should be the same as it would be for patients not infected with HIV.

Atypical Tuberculosis. At least 50% of AIDS patients eventually become infected by atypical tuberculous organisms (Masur, 1993). *Mycobacterium avium* complex is the most common causative organism, but *Mycobacterium kansasii* and *Mycobacterium xenopi* can also be causes. These atypical mycobacterial infections usually occur during the late stages of AIDS when the CD4 count is below $100/mm^3$. These infections tend to be widely disseminated and involve multiple organ systems; they are usually diagnosed by means of blood culture (Lyerly et al 1995).

The pulmonary involvement can be typically upper lobe in nature and can be unilateral or bilateral. It can also be nodular, miliary, or diffuse and can affect any of the lobes of the lung.

A macrolide (clarithromycin, azithromycin) combined with at least one other drug has demonstrated some success in the treatment of these patients (Dautzenberg et al, 1991). Rifabutin prophylaxis against short-term dissemination in high-risk patients can now be offered (Nightengale et al, 1993).

Fungal Infections

Histoplasma capsulatum, Coccidioides immitis, Cryptococcus neoformans, and, rarely, *Aspergillus* species cause pneumonia in patients infected with HIV. These infections usually occur as the HIV infection progresses and the CD4 count falls below $250/mm^3$. These pneumonias can be unilateral or bilateral; they are commonly focal in nature but can also be diffuse and, rarely, nodular. The heart and the mediastinal and hilar nodes can be involved (Lyerly et al, 1995; Palis and Kovacs, 1997).

A diagnosis is important so that specific therapy can be started as soon as possible. Sputum examination and culture, bronchoscopy with BAL and TBB, or an open lung biopsy should provide diagnostic material. Amphotericin B is the drug typically used to treat these fungal infections; some authors suggest flucytosine be added for the treatment of cryptococcal infections (Palis and Kovacs, 1997).

Viral Pneumonias

Cytomegalovirus. Between 45% and 80% of the U.S. population harbors the cytomegalovirus (CMV). It is common for the virus to become activated in patients infected with HIV as they become immunocompromised. The CD4 count in these patients is usually below 100/mm^3. The lungs are commonly affected, but clinically significant pneumonitis is unusual. The diagnosis is usually made by finding the characteristic perivascular exudative retinitis on a funduscopic examination, but is often made only at autopsy. Ganciclovir or foscarnet are used to treat these viral infections (Elliot et al, 1983; Schacker and Corey, 1997).

Noninfectious Pulmonary Conditions

Kaposi's Sarcoma

In 1982, Moritz Kaposi first recognized the condition now known as KS. It was found in older people of European and Jewish backgrounds, and it behaved in an indolent manner. Reddish-brown, blue, or purple plaques or nodules involved mainly the lower extremities of these patients, especially the ankles and soles of the feet. These lesions tended to coalesce over a long period and eventually ulcerate (Kaposi, 1982; Safai, 1997).

AIDS-related KS was first recognized in 1981 (Barre-Sinovasi, 1983). This form of the sarcoma is more aggressive, is multifocal, and can involve the skin, mucous membranes, lymph nodes, and visceral organs, most commonly the respiratory and gastrointestinal tract. AIDS-related KS is usually found in homosexual or bisexual men or women who become infected through sexual contact with bisexual men, suggesting that there is a sexually transmitted causative agent involved with this sarcoma (Digiovanna and Safai, 1981; Levine and Shelhamer, 1997; Lyerly et al, 1995).

Histologically, KS is a vascular tumor consisting of nodular collections of plump or elongated spindle cells in a network of reticular fibers. The tumor cells form multiple vascular clefts that are filled with erythrocytes (Fig. 23–68). An inflammatory infiltrate consisting of lymphocytes and plasma cells is often seen in these KS lesions (Levine and Shelhamer, 1997; Lyerly et al, 1995).

Within the chest, KS can involve the lung parenchyma, the airways, the visceral pleura (Fig. 23–69), or mediastinal or hilar nodes. The pulmonary involvement is usually multifocal and courses along the lymphatic pathways of the bronchovascular bundles, the interlobar septa, and the pleura. Nodular lesions may develop around bronchi and vessels (Levine and Shelhamer, 1997).

KS lesions can develop anywhere within the tracheobronchial tree, but usually are located at segmental bifurcations (Garay et al, 1987). Pleural involvement is limited to the visceral pleura and is commonly associated with pleural effusions (Levine and Shelhamer, 1997).

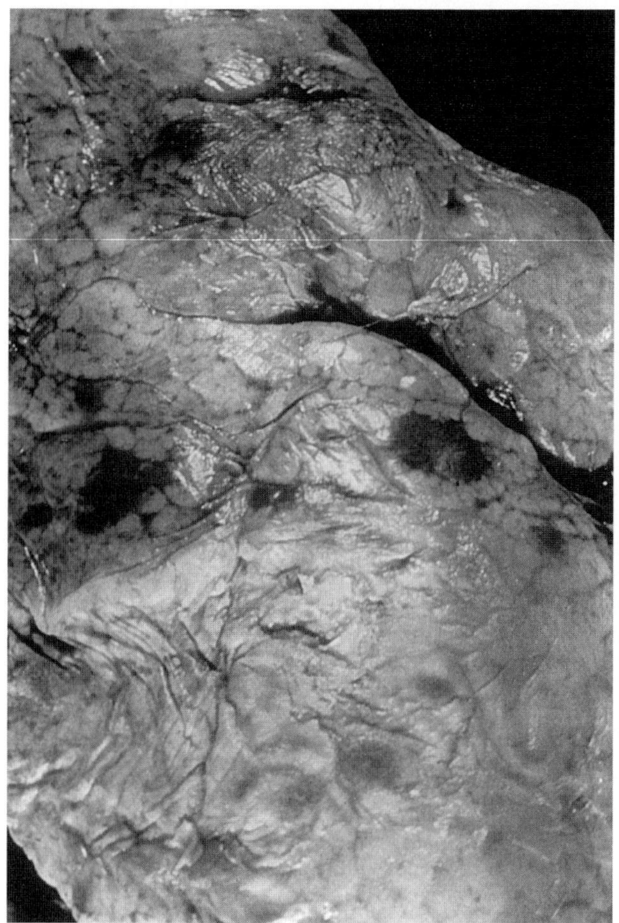

FIGURE 23–68 ■ Multiple subpleural Kaposi's sarcoma nodules of the lung.

The clinical presenting symptoms are usually nonspecific and may mimic those of an opportunistic infection. Kaposi's lesions involving the skin or mucous membranes suggest that intrathoracic involvement is related to KS. Therefore, the lack of such involvement makes it unlikely that intrathoracic lesions are associated with KS (Levine and Shelhamer, 1997).

Radiographically, pulmonary involvement is usually patchy, multifocal, bilateral, and perihilar in location. The infiltrates are interstitial, alveolar, or a mixture, and tend to radiate from the hilum (Figs. 23–70 and 23–71). Often hilar masses are present (Garay et al, 1987; Naidich et al, 1989).

The diagnosis of KS usually requires an invasive procedure such as bronchoscopy or open lung biopsy. Thoracentesis and parietal pleural biopsy are generally not diagnostic. Endobronchial and transbronchial lung biopsies have been associated with severe hemorrhage, making biopsies dangerous. BAL is unlikely to be diagnostic. Bronchoscopy, therefore, provides only a presumptive diagnosis when endobronchial and tracheal lesions are observed (Levine and Shelhamer, 1997). Usually, an open lung biopsy is performed to obtain diagnostic tissue. This can be done either videoscopically or through a small muscle-sparing thoracotomy.

Pulmonary KS has been treated with cytotoxic chemo-

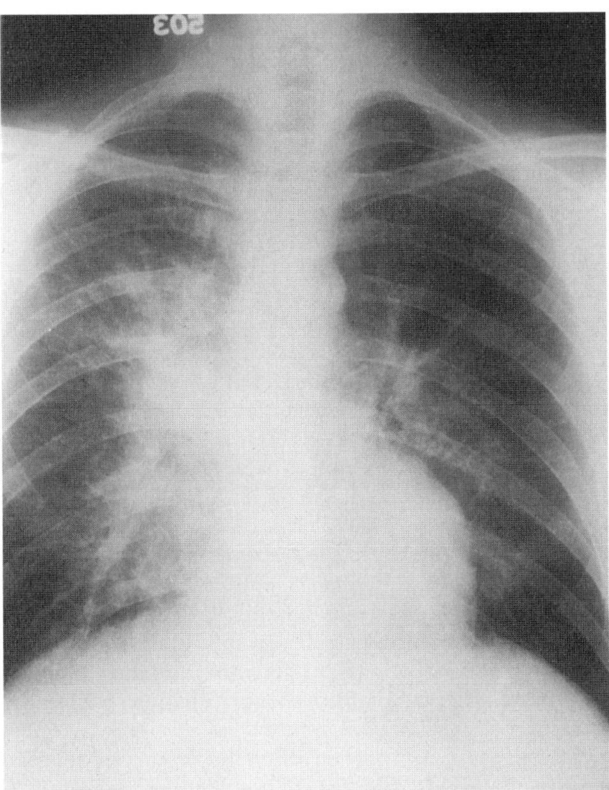

FIGURE 23–69 ■ Chest radiograph showing patchy infiltrates radiating peripherally from a right hilar mass, which is typical of Kaposi's sarcoma.

therapeutic regimes, radiation therapy, and immunomodulatory therapy (interferon alfa-2a) (Naidich et al, 1989). The YAG laser has been used effectively to open obstructing lesions of the tracheobronchial tree (Nathan et al, 1990). It is difficult to evaluate the effectiveness of these treatments because the course of KS is so variable. Palliation and prolonged survival may be achieved, but long-term cure has not been demonstrated. In the past, patients with demonstrated KS had a median survival time of 15 months, but current therapy has increased that time (Levine and Shelhamer, 1997).

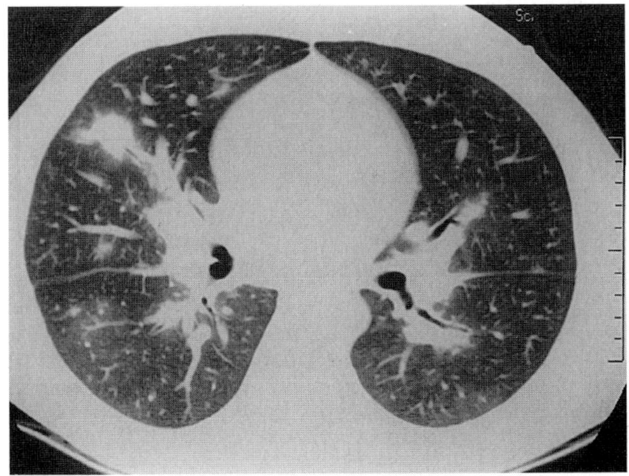

FIGURE 23–70 ■ A computed tomography scan corresponding to the radiograph in Figure 23–69 showing multiple pulmonary nodules with extension along tracheobronchial bundles extending toward the hilum.

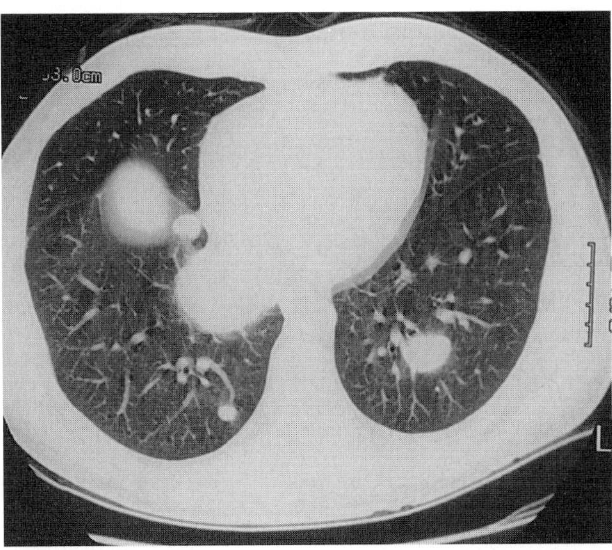

FIGURE 23–71 ■ Bilateral non-Hodgkin's lymphomatous nodules of the lung.

Lymphoma

Non-Hodgkin's Lymphoma. Non-Hodgkin's lymphoma is the second most common malignancy encountered in AIDS patients. These lymphomas are intermediate and high-grade B cell lymphomas and are not limited to any particular risk group of HIV-infected patients (Fraire and Awe, 1992). They are considered to be an AIDS-defining condition (Centers for Disease Control, 1992). These lymphomas are usually aggressive, have high-grade histologic features, and are widely disseminated, with extranodal involvement at the time of presentation. Patients with intrathoracic involvement, which occurs in only 9% of patients (Levine and Shelhamer, 1997), usually present with cough, dypsnea, and chest pain, along with systemic-B symptoms—fever, night sweats, and weight loss (Levine et al, 1984). The pulmonary parenchyma is the most common site of involvement (Fig. 23–72), but the pleura and the mediastinum, including the heart, can be involved too (Levine et al, 1984).

Rarely, a patient presents with AIDS-related primary pulmonary lymphoma. These unusual patients present with single or multiple pulmonary nodules or a mass, but have no mediastinal or hilar adenopathy on radiography, nor any evidence of extrathoracic lymphoma (Cadranel et al, 1999; Ray et al, 1998).

A specific diagnosis of intrathoracic non-Hodgkin's lymphoma is imperative. Bronchoscopy is unlikely to be helpful; cytologic examination of pleural fluid occasionally is diagnostic, and transthoracic needle biopsy of pulmonary nodules and masses is diagnostic in approximately 50% of cases. If these procedures are not diagnostic, an open lung biopsy is required. Surgical intervention has not been shown to be curative (Cadranel et al, 1999; Fraire and Awe, 1992; Ray et al, 1998).

Multiple-drug chemotherapeutic regimens are the

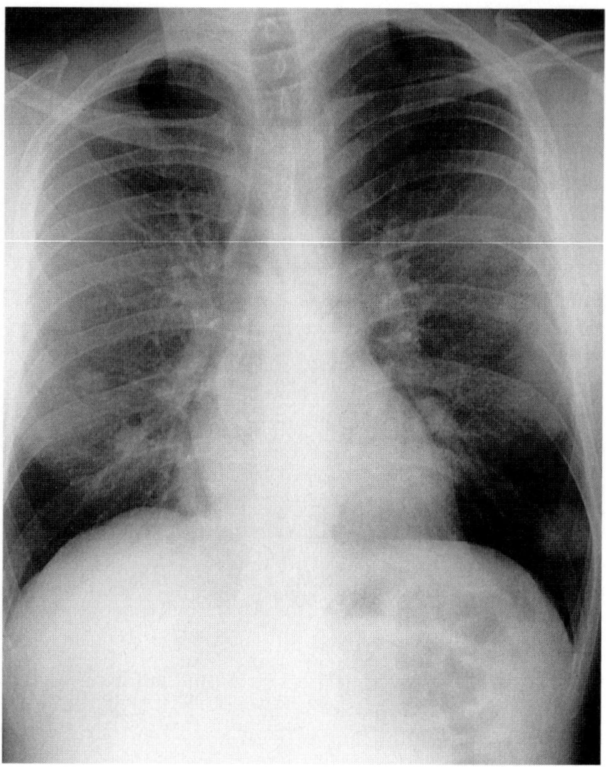

FIGURE 23–72 ■ Chest computed tomography scan corresponding to the radiograph in Figure 23–71 showing multiple bilateral non-Hodgkin's lymphomatous pulmonary nodules.

standard treatment in patients with non-Hodgkin's lymphomas. There is some evidence that reduced-dose chemotherapy is superior to conventional-dose therapy. The prognosis is poor for these patients; usual survival time is less than a year. Longer survival is possible, but cures have not been reported (Cadranel et al, 1999; Ray et al, 1998).

Hodgkin's Lymphoma. It is unclear whether the incidence of Hodgkin's disease is higher in HIV-infected patients than in the normal population, but when it does occur, it is usually aggressive and widely disseminated at presentation. Pulmonary involvement often occurs as a lobar infiltrate. Hilar and mediastinal lymph node involvement is encountered infrequently. The clinical course of Hodgkin's disease in these patients tends to be rapidly progressive, with frequent opportunistic infectious complications and short survival times (Kaplan et al, 1991; Levine and Shelhamer, 1997; Serraino et al, 1990).

Bronchogenic Carcinoma

The relationship between bronchogenic carcinoma and HIV infections has been the subject of numerous articles in the literature. Initially, it was thought that there was no increased incidence (Chan et al, 1993), but later reports suggested that the incidence of bronchogenic carcinoma in HIV-infected patients is higher than in the general population. Parker and associates (1998) found the incidence of carcinoma of the lung in a group of 26,181 HIV-infected patients to be 6.5 times higher than would have been expected. These authors postulate that the increased incidence of lung cancer is related to the recent availability of HAART, which prolongs the symptom-free interval of HIV infections, allowing time for lung cancers to develop.

These cancers are usually non–small cell carcinomas and most commonly are adenocarcinomas (Fraire and Awe, 1992). They develop primarily in young men (average age 49 years) with a history of heavy cigarette smoking, and they commonly occur early in the course of HIV infection. Bronchogenic carcinomas are aggressive and are usually far advanced when initially diagnosed; 80% are stage III or stage IV tumors. Hilar, mediastinal, and pleural involvement is common, and survival time is usually short in these patients (Alshafie et al, 1997; Cadranel et al, 1999; Parker et al, 1998; Rostislav and Remick, 1996).

Resection of localized lung cancers in HIV-infected patients has been reported to allow survival times of up to 77 weeks (Rostislav and Remick, 1996). Because of the small numbers available, meaningful survival data for HIV-infected patients undergoing surgical resection, chemotherapy, or radiation therapy are not available at present.

Opportunistic infections often mask the presence of these tumors, and because of the young ages of these HIV-compromised patients, carcinoma of the lung is not considered as a possible diagnosis. When bronchogenic carcinoma is suspected, an aggressive approach to its diagnosis should be pursued and the carcinoma treated in the same manner as it would be in a patient without HIV infection.

Interstitial Pneumonitis

Lymphocytic Interstitial Pneumonitis. Lymphocytic interstitial pneumonitis (LIP) and pulmonary lymphoid hyperplasia (PLH) are a spectrum of benign pulmonary lymphocytic infiltrative diseases that occur commonly in children with AIDS and only rarely in adult AIDS patients (Levine and Shelhamer, 1997). LIP and PLH develop insidiously but can occasionally progress to cause respiratory failure. Small pulmonary nodules (1–5 mm) in a background of interstitial pulmonary infiltrates are seen on radiographs of the chest (Levine et al, 1984). A definite diagnosis of LIP/PLH requires histologic examination of involved pulmonary parenchymal tissue. Diagnostic tissue can be obtained by means of transbronchial biopsy but, especially in children, an open biopsy is usually required. The clinical course in children varies from spontaneous resolution to slow progression to respiratory failure. If progression of disease occurs, corticosteroids should be administered, but their usefulness is not entirely clear. The outlook for children with AIDS and LIP/PLH seems to be better than that of other children with AIDS who do not have LIP/PLH (Levine and Shelhamer, 1997).

Nonspecific Interstitial Pneumonitis. Adult patients with AIDS often develop nonspecific interstitial pneumonitis, a self-limited pulmonary condition (Levine and Shelhamer,

1997). The pneumonitis consists of infiltrates of lymphoid and plasma cells with edema, fibrin deposits, alveolar lining cell hyperplasia, and alveolar septal thickening. Radiographs of the chest may be normal or may show diffuse interstitial infiltrates. It is usually a chronic, indolent condition that tends to stabilize and then to resolve without therapy (Saffredini et al, 1987). Invasive diagnostic procedures are usually carried out to exclude opportunistic infection when symptoms worsen or radiographic findings progress (Levine and Shelhamer, 1997).

Esophageal Diseases in HIV-Infected Patients

The presence of diseases that affect the esophagus in HIV-infected patients indicate that the infection has reached an advanced stage. In the past, it was estimated that one third of HIV-infected patients would develop esophageal disease at some point during the illness (Connolly et al, 1989). Currently, HAART is effective in delaying and diminishing HIV-defining complications, so esophageal involvement is probably encountered less often than in the past (Bartlett, 1999).

Odynophagia (painful swallowing), dysphagia (difficulty in swallowing), and singultus (hiccups) are the most common symptoms of esophageal disease (Dieterich, 1994). *Candida albicans*, herpes simplex, and cytomegalovirus are the most common infectious agents to involve the esophagus in HIV-infected patients. Bacterial and mycobacterial infections, KS, lymphomas, and aphthous, or idiopathic, ulcers are encountered much less commonly (Dieterich, 1994; Lyerly et al, 1995).

If a patient with symptoms of esophagitis is found on examination to have thrush of the mouth and pharynx, *Candida* esophagitis is the presumptive diagnosis and treatment with fluconazole or ketoconazole is begun. If, after a week of therapy, there has been improvement, treatment is continued for 2 more weeks. If no improvement is recognized, esophagoscopy should be performed in an effort to obtain a definitive diagnosis (Lyerly et al, 1995).

The most common viral infections of the esophagus in HIV-infected patients are caused by CMV. Without strong evidence of a CMV infection, such as characteristic retinal lesions, however, empiric treatment is not justified. Esophagoscopy should be performed (Lyerly et al, 1995).

Shallow ulcers found on examination of the mouth suggest a herpes infection. Empiric treatment with acyclovir is begun. If improvement results, treatment is continued. If not, again, esophagoscopy is indicated (Lyerly et al, 1995).

Radiographic contrast examination of the esophagus is unlikely to provide a specific diagnosis in AIDS patients with esophagitis. If, however, an esophageal ulcer is found on an esophagram, esophagoscopy is clearly indicated. Esophagoscopy is also indicated when empiric therapy is unsuccessful and when the cause of the symptoms is unclear.

At esophagoscopy, infections caused by *Candida* species usually present as small white plaques or as a diffuse, severe inflammatory process. CMV usually presents as a single ulcer, whereas herpes infections present as vesicles or "small discrete volcanic ulcers" (Lyerly et al, 1995). Lesions seen at esophagoscopy should be biopsied. Biopsies are best taken from the periphery of a lesion where viable tissue is most likely to be present. The pathologist should be alerted as to the possible diagnosis so that appropriate immunofluorescent stains can be performed. With a definitive diagnosis, appropriate therapy can be started.

Esophageal perforations and tracheoesophageal fistulas have been encountered in patients with AIDS. Tuberculous lymphadenitis in subcarinal nodes and severe infections of the esophagus and trachea are the usual causes (Adkins et al, 1990; Rusconi et al, 1994; Temes et al, 1995). Perforations are usually treated by esophagectomy or defunctionalization of the esophagus. In severely ill patients who are poor candidates for surgery, endoesophageal stenting with a covered, expandable stent might be tried. Esophageal stenting has also been used in cases of tracheoesophageal fistulas (Temes et al, 1995). Esophageal strictures resulting from esophageal ulcerations have been encountered, and they have been treated with steroids with some success (Wilcox, 1999).

Cardiac Disease in HIV-Infected Patients

Cardiac involvement is now being recognized in greater numbers of AIDS patients. Pericardial effusions and myocarditis are the most commonly encountered conditions, but cardiomyopathies and myocardial vasculopathies have also been recognized (Estok and Wallach, 1998). The causes of these conditions may be infectious or neoplastic, but frequently no cause can be demonstrated. Most patients with cardiac involvement have few or no symptoms and require no treatment, but some have severe cardiac involvement that can result in a fatal outcome. When cardiac tamponade is encountered, pericardial drainage by means of catheter or window formation is indicated in spite of the very poor outlook for these patients (Estok and Wallach, 1998; Gouny et al, 1998; Yunis and Stone, 1998).

CONCLUSION

The AIDS epidemic has been and continues to be devastating for large numbers of patients worldwide. Much has been learned about the human immunodeficiency virus, and effective drugs for its treatment are now available. With the availability of HAART in developed countries, HIV-infected patients now have longer asymptomatic periods before developing AIDS-defining complications, so they have prolonged life expectancies. The need to perform thoracic surgery in these patients has decreased dramatically. In the Third World, however, where these expensive drugs are not available, the number of HIV-infected patients who progress to AIDS continues to escalate, and thoracic surgical care will continue to be needed in those areas.

COMMENTS AND CONTROVERSIES

The complications that a thoracic surgeon may encounter in AIDS patients are summarized in this chapter. The message is quite clear—with modern therapies, AIDS patients have a significant long-term survival, and complications of AIDS, whenever appropriate, should be treated aggressively. Thoracic surgeons will be called upon to diagnose and treat these complications. The standard methods of prophylaxis and precautions recommended for the operating room should be adhered to. AIDS patients should not be relegated to palliative care only!

R.J.G.

REFERENCES

Adkins MS, Raccua JS, Acinapura GJ: Esophageal perforation in a patient with acquired immunodeficiency syndrome. Ann Thorac Surg 50:299, 1990.

Alshafie MT, Donaldson B, Oluwole SF: Human immunodeficiency virus and lung cancer. Br J Surg 88:1068, 1997.

Barre-Sinovasi F, Chermann JC, Rey F et al: Isolation of T-lymphotropic retrovirus from a patient at risk for acquired immune deficiency syndrome (AIDS). Science 220:868, 1983.

Bartlett JG: The Johns Hopkins Hospital 1998–1999 Guide to Medical Care of Patients with HIV Infection, 8th ed. Baltimore, Williams & Wilkins, 1999, p 1.

Beers MF, John M, Swartz M: Recurrent pneumothorax in AIDS patients with pneumocystis pneumonia: A clinopathologic study of these cases and review of the literature. Chest 98:266, 1990.

Bigby TD, Margolskii D, Curtis JL et al: The usefulness of induced sputum in the diagnosis of *Pneumocystis carinii* pneumonia in patients with the acquired immundeficiency syndrome. Am Rev Respir Dis 133:315, 1986.

Bloom BR, Murray CJ: Tuberculosis: Commentary on a reemergent killer. Science 257:1055, 1992.

Boyd AD, Crawford BK, and Glassman L: Surgical therapy of tuberculosis. In Rom WN, Garay SM (eds): Tuberculosis. Boston, Little Brown, 1996, p 513.

Broadelus VC, Dake MD, Stulbargms MS et al: Bronchoalveolar lavage and transbronchial biopsy for the diagnosis of pulmonary infections in patients with the acquired immunodeficiency syndrome. Ann Intern Med 102:747, 1995.

Burack JH, Hahn JA, Saint-Maurice D et al: Microbiology of community-acquired bacterial pneumonia in persons with and at risk for human immunodificiency virus type 1 infection. Ann Intern Med 154:2589, 1994.

Cadranel J, Naccache J, Wislez M et al: Pulmonary malignancies in the immunocompromised patient. Respiration 66:289, 1999.

Centers for Disease Control. Centers for Disease Control task force on Kaposi's sarcoma and opportunistic infections. N Engl J Med, 306:248, 1982.

Centers for Disease Control. Update: Serologic testing for HIV-1 antibody, United States, 1988 and 1989. MMWR Morb Mortal Wkly Rep 391:380, 1990.

Centers for Disease Control. 1993 Revised classification system for HIV infections and expanded surveillance of definition of AIDS among adolescents and adults. MMWR Morb Mortal Wkly Rep 41:17, 1992.

Centers for Disease Control. HIV, AIDS surveillance report. Atlanta, Centers for Disease Control, 1993a.

Centers for Disease Control. Recommendations for HIV testing services for inpatients and outpatients in acute-care hospital settings. MMWR Morb Mortal Wkly Rep 42:2, 1993b.

Centers For Disease Control. Update: Provisional public health service recommendations for chemoprophylaxis after occupations exposure to HIV. MMWR Morb Mortal Wkly Rep 45:468, 1996.

Centers for Disease Control. Public Health guidelines for the management of Health care workers exposed to HIV and Recommendations for postexposure prophylaxis. MMWR Morb Mortal Wkly Rep 47:7, 1998.

Chan TK, Aranda CP, Rom WN: Bronchogenic carcinoma in young patients at risk for acquired immunodeficiency syndrome. Chest 103:862, 1993.

Connolly GM, Hawkeiser D, Harcourt-Webster J et al: Esophageal symptoms: Their cause, treatment and prognosis in patients with the acquired immunodeficiency syndrome. Gut 30:1033, 1989.

Crawford BK, Galloway AC, Boyd AD et al: Treatment of AIDS-related bronchopleural fistula by pleurectomy. Ann Thorac Surg 54:212, 1992.

Dautzenberg B, Truffat C, Ligris S et al: Activity of clarithromycin against *Mycobacterium avium* infection in patients with the acquired immunodeficiency syndrome: A controlled clinical trial. Am Rev Respir Dis 144:564, 1991.

Davis KC, Horsburch CK Jr, Hasiba U et al: Acquired immunodeficiency syndrome in a patient with hemophilia. Ann Intern Med:98:284, 1983.

Dietrich DT, Poles MA, Lew FA: Gastrointestinal manifestation of HIV disease. In Broder S, Mergin TC Jr, Bolognesi D (eds): Textbook of Aids Medicine. Baltimore, 1994, p 542.

Digiovanna JJ, Safai B: Kaposi's sarcoma: Retrospective study of 90 cases, with particular emphasis on the familial occurrence, ethnic background and prevalence of other disease. Am J Med 71:770, 1981.

DeLorenzo IJ, Huang CT, Maguire GP et al: Carinii roentgenography patterns of *Pneumocyctis carinii* pneumonia in 104 patients with AIDS. Chest 91:323, 1987.

Elliot JL, Hoppes WL, Platt NS et al: The acquired immunodeficiency syndrome and *Mycobacterium avium–intracellulare* bacteria in a patient with hemophilia. Ann Intern Med: 98:290, 1983.

Essex M, McLane MF, Lee TH et al: Antibodies to cell membrane antigens associated with human T cell leukemia virus in patients with AIDS. Science 220:859, 1983a.

Essex M, McLane MF, Lee TH et al: Antibodies to human T cell leukemia virus membrane antigens (HTLV-MA) in hemophiliacs. Science 221:1061, 1983b.

Essex ME: Origin of acquired immunodeficiency syndrome. In De Vita VT Jr, Hellman S, Rosenberg SA (eds): AIDS: Biology, Diagnosis, Treatment and Prevention, 4th ed. Philadelphia, Lippincott-Raven, 1997, p 3.

Estok I, Wallach F: Cardiac tamponade in a patient with AIDS: A review of pericardial disease in patients with HIV infection. Mt Sinai J Med, 65:33, 1998.

Fischl MA, Parker CB, Pettinelli C et al: A randomized controlled trial of a reduced dose of zidovudine in patients with the acquired immunodeficiency syndrome. N Engl J Med 323:1009, 1990.

Fraire AE, Awe RJ: Lung cancer in association with human immunodeficiency virus infections. Cancer 70:432, 1992.

Frieden TR, Sterling J, Pablos-Menog et al: The emergence of drug-resistant tuberculosis in New York City. N Engl J Med 328:921, 1993.

Folks TM, Hart CF: The life cycle of human immunodeficiency virus type 1. In De Vita VT Jr, Hellman S, Rosenberg SA (eds): AIDS: Biology, Diagnosis, Treatment and Prevention. 4th ed. Philadelphia, Lippincott-Raven, 1997, p 29.

Gallo RC, Sarion PS, Gelmann EP et al: Isolation of human T cell leukemia virus in acquired immune deficiency syndrome (AIDS). Science 220:865, 1983.

Gallo RC, Salahuddin SZ, Popovic M et al: Frequent detection and isolation of cytopathic retroviruses (HTLV-111) from patients with AIDS and at risk for AIDS. Science 224:500, 1984.

Garay SM, Belenko M, Faggini E et al: Pulmonary manifestation of Kaposi's sarcoma. Chest 91:39, 1987.

Gelmann EP, Popovic M, Blayney D et al: Proviral DNA of a retrovirus, human T cell leukemia virus, in two patients with AIDS. Science 220:862, 1983.

Gerberding JL, Procedure-specific infection control for preventing intraoperative blood exposure. Am J Infect Control 21:364, 1993.

Gottlieb MS, Schroff R, Schanker HM et al: *Pneumocystis carinii* pneumonia and mucosal candidiasis in previously healthy homosexual men: Evidence of a new acquired immunodeficiency. N Engl J Med 305:1425, 1981.

Gouny P, Lancelin C, Girard PM et al: Pericardial effusion and AIDS: Benefits of surgical drainage. Euro J Card Thor Surg 13:165, 1998.

Gourla MA, Braun MJ, Clements JE et al: Human T-cell lymphotropic virus type III shares sequence homology with a family of pathogenic lentivirus. Proc Natl Acad Sci U S A. 83:4007, 1986.

Gürtler L. Difficulties and strategies of HIV diagnosis. Lancet 348:176, 1996.

Hardy WD, Feinberg J, Finkelstein DM et al: A controlled trial of trimethoprim-sulfamethoxazole or aerosolized pentamidine for secondary prophylaxis of *Pneumocystis carinii* pneumonia in patients with the aquired immunodeficiency syndrome. N Engl J Med 327:1842, 1992.

Hymes KB, Cheung T, Greene JB et al: Karposi's sarcoma in homosexual men: A report of eight cases. Lancet 2:598, 1991.

Imazawa D, Detels R: HIV-1 in sero-negative homosexual men. N Eng J Med 325:1250, 1991.

Jules-Elysee KM, Steven DE, Zaman MB et al: Aerosolized pentamidine: Effect on diagnosis and presentation of *Pneumocystis carinii* pneumonia. Ann Intern Med 172:750, 1990.

Kaplan L, Kahn J, Northfelt D et al: Novel combination chemotherapy for Hodgkins disease in HIV-infected individuals. Proc Am Soc Clin Oncol 10:33, 1991.

Kaposi M: Classes in oncology: Idiopathic multiple-pigmented sarcoma of the skin. Cancer 31:3, 1982.

Kovacs JA, Ng VI, Masure et al: Diagnosis of *Pneumocystis carinii* pneumonia: Improved detection in sputum with the use of monoclonal antibodies. N Engl J Med 318:589, 1988.

Lackritz EM, Satten GA, Aberle–Grasse MPH et al: Estimated risk of transmission of the human immunodeficiency virus by screened blood in the United States. N Eng J Med 333:1721, 1995.

Lefson AR, Rutherford GW, Jaffe HW et al: The natural history of human immunodeficiency virus infection. J Infect Dis 158:1360, 1988.

Levine AM. Lymphoma in acquired immunodeficiency syndrome. Semin Oncol 104:12, 1990.

Levine AM, Meyer PR, Begndy et al: Development of B cell lymphoma in homosexual men: Clinical and immunology findings. Ann Intern Med 100:7, 1984.

Levine SJ, Shelhamer JH: Noninfectious pulmonary complications of human immunodeficiency virus infections. In De Vita VT Jr, Hellman S, Rosenberg SA (eds): AIDS: Biology, Diagnosis, Treatment and Prevention, 4th ed. Philadelphia, Lippincott-Raven, 1997, p 409.

Lewis F, Short L, Howard J et al: Epidemiology of injuries by needles and other sharp instruments: Minimizing sharp injuries in gynecological and obstetric operations. Surg Clin North Am 75:1105, 1995.

Lyerly HK, Bartlett JA, DiMaio JM: Thoracic disorders in the immunocompromised host. In Sabiston DC Jr, Spencer FC (eds): Surgery of the Chest, 6th ed. Philadelphia, WB Saunders, 1995, p 731.

Masur H, Lane HC, Kovacs JA et al: Advances in *Pneumocystis* pneumonia: From bench to clinic. Ann Intern Med 111:813, 1989.

Masur H, Michelis MA, Greene JB et al: An outbreak of community-acquired *Pneumocystis carinii* pneumonia: Initial manifestations of cellular immune dysfunction. N Engl J Med 305:1431, 1981.

Masur H and the Public Health Service Task Force on Prophylaxis and Therapy for *Mycobacterium Avium* Complex: Special report—recommendations on prophylaxis and therapy for disseminated *Mycobacterium avium* complex disease in patients infected with the human immunodeficiency virus. N Engl J Med 329:898, 1993.

Miller SS, Subharwal A. Subcuticular skin closure using a blunt needle. Ann R Coll Surg Engl 76:281, 1994.

Montz FJ, Fowler JM, Farias-Eisner R et al.: Blunt needles in fascial closure. Surg Gynecol Obstet 173:147, 1991.

Naidich DP, Tarias M, Garay SM et al: Kaposi's sarcoma: CT—radiographic correlation. Chest 96:723, 1989.

Nathan S, Vaghaiwalla R, Mohsenifar Z: Use of Nd: YAG laser in endobronchial Kaposi's sarcoma. Chest 98:1299, 1990.

Nightengale SD, Cameron DW, Gordin FM et al: Two controlled trials of rifabutin prophylaxis against *Mycobacterium avium* complex in AIDS. N Engl J Med 329:828, 1993.

Owens DK, Holodniy M, Garber AM et al: Polymerase chain reaction for the diagnosis of HIV infection in adults. Ann Intern Med 124:803, 1996.

Palis MA, Kovacs JA: Fungal infections in patients with the acquired immodeficiency syndrome. In De Vita VT Jr, Hellman S, Rosenberg SA (eds): AIDS: Biology, Diagnosis, Treatment and Prevention, 4th ed. Philadelphia, Lippincott-Raven, 1997, p 231.

Parker MS, Levino DM, Tamsia JC et al: AIDS-related bronchogenic carcinoma: Fact or fiction? Chest 113:154, 1998.

Pastores S, Garay SM, Naidich DP et al: Spontaneous pneumothorax in patients with AIDS-related PC pneumonia. Am J Med Sci 312:229, 1996.

Pitchenick AE, Ganjei P, Torris A et al: Sputum examinations for the diagnosis of *Pneumocystis carinii* pneumonia in the acquired immune deficiency syndrome. Ann Rev Resp Dis 133:226, 1986.

Poon MC, Landay A, Prasthofer EF et al: Acquired immunodeficiency syndrome with *Pneumocystis carinii* pneumonia and *Mycobacterium avium*: Intracellular infection in a previously healthy patient with classic hemophilia: clinical, immunologic and virologic findings. Ann Intern Med 98:287, 1983.

Popovic M, Sarngadharan MG, Read E et al: Detection, isolation, and continuous production of cytopathic retroviruses (HTLV-III) from patients with AIDS and pre-AIDS. Science 224:497, 1984.

Ratner L, Haseltine W, Patarca R et al: Complete nucleotide sequence of the AIDS virus HTLV-111. Nature 313:217, 1985.

Ray P, Antoine M, Mary-Krause M et al: Aids-related primary pulmonary lymphoma. Am J Respir Crit Care Med 158:1221, 1998.

Read CA, Reddy UD, O'Mara TE et al: Doxycycline pleurodesis for pneumothorax in patients with AIDS. Chest 105:823, 1994.

Rigsby MO, Friedland G: Tuberculosis and human immunodeficiency virus infections. In DeVito VT Jr, Hellman S, Rosenberg SA (eds): AIDS: Biology, Diagnosis, Treatment and Prevention, 4th ed. Philadelphia, Lippincott-Raven, 1997, p 245.

Rubinstein A, Moreski R, Silverman B et al: Pulmonary disease in children with acquired immune deficiency syndrome and AIDS-related complex. J Pediatr 108:498, 1986.

Rusconi S, Merone L, Galli M: Tracheoesophageal fistula in an HIV-I—positive man due to dual infection of *Candida albicans* and cytomegalovirus. Chest 106:284, 1994.

Saag MS: Clinical spectrum of human immunodeficiency viral disease. In De Vita VT Jr, Hellman S, Rosenberg SA (eds): AIDS: Biology, Diagnosis, Treatment and Prevention, 4th ed. Philadelphia, Lippincott-Raven, 1997, p 203.

Safai B: Kaposi's sarcoma and acquired immunodeficiency syndrome. In De Vita VT Jr, Hellman S, Rosenberg SA (eds): AIDS: Biology, Diagnosis, Treatment and Prevention. 4th ed. Philadelphia, Lippincott-Raven, 1997, p 295.

Saffredini AF, Ognebene FP, Lack EF et al: Nonspecific interstistal pneumonitis: A common cause of pulmonary disease in the acquired immunodeficiency syndrome. Ann Intern Med 107:7, 1987.

Schacker T, Corey L. Herpesvirus infections in human immunodeficiency virus—infected persons. In De Vita VT Jr, Hellman S, Rosenberg SA (eds): AIDS: Biology, Diagnosis, Treatment and Prevention. 4th ed. Philadelphia, Lippincott-Raven, 1997 p 272.

Schupbach J, Popovic M, Gilden RV et al: Serological analysis of a subgroup of human T-lymphotropic retroviruses (HTLC-111) associated with AIDS. Science 224:503, 1984.

Selwyn PA, Harrtel D, Lewis JA et al: A prospective study of the risk of tubuculosis among intravenous drug users with human immunodefiency viral infections. N Engl J Med 320:545, 1989.

Serraino M, Bellas C, Compo E et al: Hodgkin's disease in patients with antibodies to human immunodeficiency virus: A study of 22 patients. Cancer 65:2248, 1990.

Short LJ, Benson DR: Safety precautions: Special considerations for surgeons. In De Vita VT Jr, Hellman S, Rosenberg SA (eds): AIDS: Biology, Diagnosis, Treatment and prevention. 4th ed. Philadelphia, Lippincott-Raven, 1997, p 665.

Temes RT, Wong RS, Davis M et al: Esophago-airway fistula in AIDS. Ann Thorac Surg 60:440, 1995.

Vyzula R, Remick SC: Lung cancer in patients with HIV infection. Lung Cancer 15:325, 1996.

Wait MA, Dal Nogaic AR: Treatment of AIDS-related spontanous pneumothorax: A decade of experience. Chest 106:693, 1994.

Wilcox CM: Esophageal strictures complicating ulcerative esophagitis in AIDS. Am J Gastroenterol 94:339, 1999.

Yunis NA, Stone VE: Cardiac manifestations of HIV/AIDS: A review of disease spectrum and clinical management. J Acquir Immune Defic Syndr Hum Retrovirol 18:145, 1998.

Zibrak JD, Silvestri RC, Costello P et al: Bronchoscopic and radiologic features of Kaposi's sarcoma involving the respiratory system. Chest 90:476, 1986.

Zurlo JJ, Lane HC: Other bacterial infections. In De Vita VT Jr, Hellman S, and Rosenberg SA (eds): AIDS: Biology, Diagnosis, Treatment and Prevention, 4th ed. Philadelphia, Lippincott-Raven, 1997, p259.

CHAPTER **24**

Interstitial Lung Disease

Ronald F. Grossman
Mitra Niroumand

Interstitial lung disease (ILD) is a generic term for almost 200 heterogeneous lung diseases that have several features in common. These disorders are called ILDs because on histologic examination, the interstitium is usually thickened secondary to infiltration with inflammatory cells and fibrosis.

This term, however, is misleading because patients can demonstrate both interstitial, alveolar wall, vascular, or air space involvement secondary to their disease process; therefore, an alternative name is "diffuse infiltrative lung disease" (Crystal et al, 1981).

BASIC SCIENCE

Epidemiology

The prevalence of ILD has been estimated to be 5 to 10 cases per 100,000 people in the United States (Crystal et al, 1984). The most common conditions are sarcoidosis, idiopathic pulmonary fibrosis (IPF), drug-induced disease, pneumoconiosis secondary to inhalation of inorganic dust, ILD associated with collagen-vascular disease, and extrinsic allergic alveolitis. There are several methods of classification of the ILDs. The most common of these are (1) by known and unknown causes, (2) by acute and chronic causes, and (3) by pathologic reaction.

In this chapter, we classify ILD by known and unknown causes.

Anatomy and Pathogenesis

The walls of the alveoli are lined by a layer of epithelial cells lying on a thin basement membrane. Type 1 epithelial cells constitute 95% of these cells, and the rest are type 2 pneumocytes, the surfactant-producing epithelial cell (Murray, 1976). In the gas-exchanging areas of the alveolus, the capillaries are in close proximity to the basement membrane of the type 1 cell and are lined by a single layer of endothelium that rests on its own basement membrane. The area between the endothelial and epithelial basement membranes is the interstitium and contains structures such as fibroblasts, collagen, elastic fibers, and glycoproteins. The normal alveolar wall is only 5 to 10 μm wide but increases with disorders characterized by cellular infiltration (Fulmer, 1982a).

The exact process initiating the development of interstitial pneumonitis is not well understood. The inflammation may be initiated by an agent or agents that injure the epithelial wall and activate inflammatory cells. With the release of mediators by inflammatory cells, an inflammatory reaction (an alveolitis) is initiated and perpetuated (Keogh and Crystal, 1982).

Normally, approximately 80 cells can be identified per alveolus, and, of these, about 90% are macrophages, 10% are lymphocytes, and less than 1% are neutrophils and eosinophils (Reynolds, 1987). In ILD there is a general increase in the number of the inflammatory cells and an alteration in their proportions (Daniele et al, 1985). For example, in sarcoidosis, there is T helper cell alveolitis (Hunninghake and Crystal, 1981). Regardless of the type of initial triggering factor, alveolar macrophages release chemoattractants for neutrophils such as leukotriene B_4 and interleukin-8, as well as oxidants, which induce parenchymal injury. They also release various growth factors for mesenchymal cells that are important in fibrogenesis (Hunninghake and Kalica, 1995). Connective tissue growth factor, induced by transforming growth factor-β, is present in very high concentration in the lungs of these patients (Chan-Yeung and Muller, 1997). T lymphocytes are also involved in the pathogenesis of ILD, through production of cytokines such as tumor necrosis factor and interleukin-1, which seems to play a part in initiating the inflammatory process (Chan-Yeung and Muller, 1997). With influx of inflammatory and immune effector cells (i.e., "alveolitis"), alveolar and interstitial architecture becomes deranged, resulting in loss of alveolar gas exchange units. Reduction of surfactant may also contribute to alveolar collapse in these disorders, leading to distortion of lung architecture and impairment of healing (Burkhardt, 1989).

DIAGNOSIS

Clinical Features

The patient with ILD presents a problem of diagnosis and management because there are numerous conditions associated with ILD, and the majority are rare. Few therapeutic modalities are available, and controlled clinical trials are infrequent because of the rarity and the slowly progressive nature of these disorders. A practical approach is to obtain a careful history and physical examination, study the chest radiograph, and then determine the best approach for additional diagnostic testing (Raghu, 1987). Acute disorders that can mimic ILD should be ruled out, such as viral or bacterial infections, *Pneumocystis carinii* infection, aspiration, or pulmonary edema. The tests with the best diagnostic yield can be selected for the suspected disease.

History

Most patients with ILD seek medical advice because of pulmonary symptoms or abnormal routine chest radiographs. The most common symptoms are progressive shortness of breath on exertion and fatigue (Dill et al, 1975). Other common presenting symptoms include cough and, less commonly, fever and weight loss. Chest pain and ankle edema may occur late in the disease with the development of right heart failure.

A careful occupational and medication history including nonprescription drugs is then obtained to ascertain clues to the cause. Patients' hobbies should be reviewed to determine whether the patients have been exposed to environmental agents, such as toxins or animal danders. The duration and severity of exposure should be documented. A full functional inquiry with particular attention to extrapulmonary symptoms must be taken to reveal the presence of a systemic disorder. The family history may expose hereditary disorders, such as tuberous sclerosis or familial pulmonary fibrosis.

Physical Examination

The vital signs are frequently normal, but patients may demonstrate tachypnea and tachycardia. Clubbing of the fingers and toes is common, especially in IPF and asbestosis; cyanosis, if present, typically occurs late (Scadding and Hinson, 1974). Chest expansion is classically reduced, reflecting the reduction in the total lung capacity. The lung volumes may be normal or paradoxically increased in sarcoidosis, lymphangioleiomyomatosis (LAM), or tuberous sclerosis. Fine, end-inspiratory crackles are audible at the posterior lung bases. Wheezes may be heard if there is a coincident obstructive component, which is often seen in sarcoidosis. Coarse crackles and bronchial breathing are less commonly heard. In the presence of diffuse pulmonary infiltrates seen radiographically, perfectly normal chest examination results suggest sarcoidosis (Baughman et al, 1991).

The general physical examination may reveal evidence of uveitis or cutaneous lesions in sarcoidosis, malar rash in systemic lupus erythematosus (SLE), or the cutaneous findings of dermatomyositis. The cardiac examination is typically normal early in the course of the disease, but pulmonary hypertension may develop later. Signs of pulmonary hypertension include an audible and palpable second component of the second heart sound (increased P2), right ventricular heave, hepatic enlargement, and peripheral edema.

Laboratory Studies

The blood count and differential are not usually contributory to diagnosis, except in the presence of eosinophilic lung disease. The sedimentation rate may be elevated in many of these disorders and is not specific. Rheumatoid factor, antinuclear antibody (ANA), and complement levels may be strikingly abnormal in connective tissue disease, but low titers of ANA and rheumatoid factor are common in patients with IPF (Holgate et al, 1983). The serum angiotensin-converting enzyme (ACE) level is elevated in most patients with sarcoidosis, but this finding is not pathognomonic of this disease (Studdy et al, 1978). Antibodies against specific organic antigens may be elevated in cases of clinically suspected extrinsic allergic alveolitis, but these antigens are not specific and may simply indicate past exposure to the antigen (Reynolds, 1982). Antinuclear cytoplasmic antibodies (ANCAs) are elevated in most patients with Wegener's granulomatosis, and antibasement membrane antibody levels may be present in patients with Goodpasture's syndrome (Briggs et al, 1979; Nolle et al, 1989).

Radiologic Findings

Chest Radiograph

The routine chest radiograph is limited in the etiologic diagnosis of ILD. As many as 10% of patients with biopsy-proven ILD have a normal chest radiograph (Epler et al, 1978). The normal pulmonary interstitium is usually not visible by chest radiography. However, in the presence of fibrosis or edema of the interstitium, the attenuation of the interstitium increases, and it becomes detectable on the radiograph. Early involvement may manifest as perivascular or peribronchial thickening. A typical radiograph of a patient with ILD shows a linear, reticular, or nodular interstitial pattern that is characteristically more prominent at the bases (Fig. 24–1). The infiltrate becomes coarser as the disease progresses, and, finally, cysts and honeycombing develop. Thickening of the interstitium and the interlobular septa can produce a linear pattern on chest radiography.

A specific diagnosis is difficult to make on the basis of the chest radiograph alone. The appearance and distribution of the lung infiltrate may be helpful. For example,

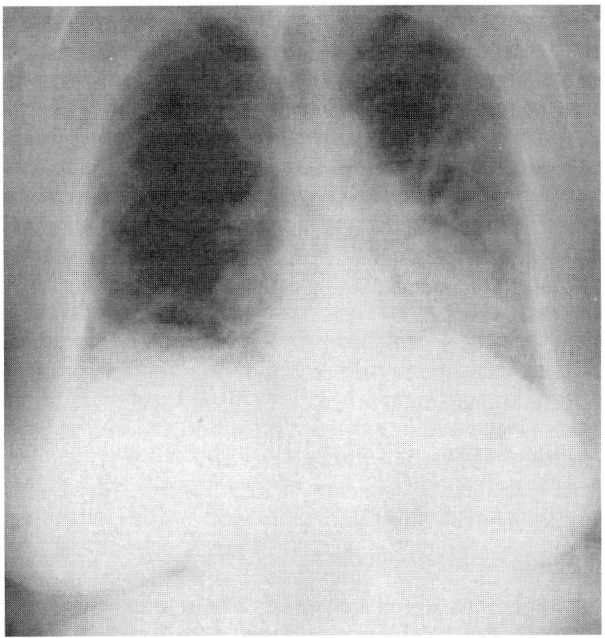

FIGURE 24–1 ■ Posteroanterior chest radiograph from a patient with idiopathic pulmonary fibrosis. Reticular nodular infiltrates are present diffusely with a predominance at the lung bases.

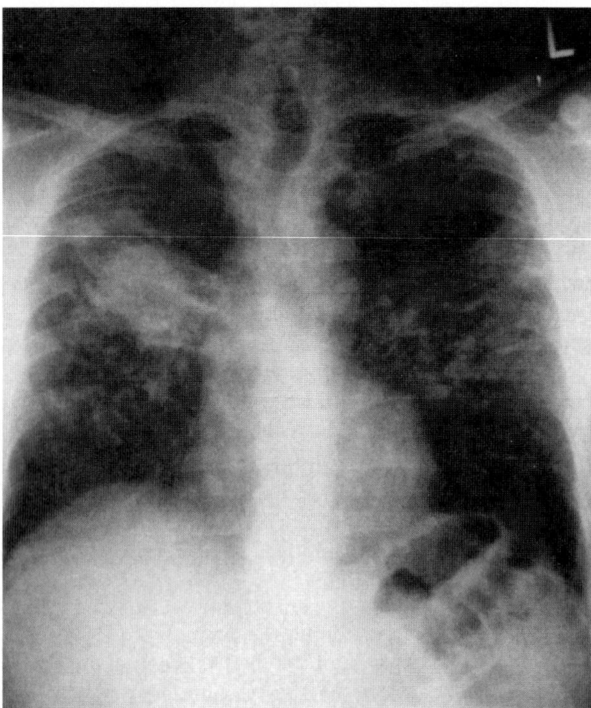

FIGURE 24–2 ■ Posteroanterior chest radiograph from a patient with sarcoidosis. Reticular nodular infiltrates are present with an upper zone predominance.

nodular disease is seen in Wegener's granulomatosis. A predominantly upper lobe distribution is seen with eosinophilic granuloma, sarcoidosis, and fibrosis associated with ankylosing spondylitis (Fig. 24–2). The presence of lymphadenopathy or pleural involvement may help characterize a specific ILD. For example, pleural effusions are often seen in association with pulmonary edema, malignancy, or rheumatoid arthritis. Chylous effusions may be present in patients with LAM. Patients with eosinophilic granuloma or LAM may present with a spontaneous pneumothorax. Bilateral hilar lymphadenopathy favors a diagnosis of sarcoidosis or lymphoma. It is important that previous radiographs be examined to document the progression of disease. In many cases, the appearance on plain radiography is nonspecific and may mislead the clinician. The introduction of high-resolution computed tomography (HRCT) has highlighted the limitations of the routine chest radiograph.

Despite these problems, the chest radiograph is valuable in the detection of ILD. It is the radiographic procedure of choice for the initial assessment of the patient with suspected ILD and is a simple and practical way of following the course of the disease.

Computed Tomography

Computed tomography (CT) and HRCT scans are useful adjuncts. The conventional CT scan is performed by imaging 8- to 10-mm thick slices at 10-mm intervals. The combination of 1- to 2-mm collimation and a high-frequency resolution algorithm is referred to as an HRCT scan. This technique improves spatial resolution by 40%. HRCT scanning can identify abnormalities of lung parenchyma better than the chest radiograph can (Muller and Ostrow, 1991). This is possible because CT eliminates superimposition of pulmonary structures. HRCT can show the details of normal pulmonary anatomy, such as pulmonary vessels, bronchi, and secondary lobules. Additionally, because these diseases are often patchy in distribution, the CT scan can be a useful guide to the best biopsy site. Certain abnormalities on CT scan support the diagnosis of ILD, including irregular linear opacities; thickened interlobular septa; nodules; abnormal interfaces between vessels, bronchi, and the visceral pleura; and air space opacification (Muller et al, 1986). The specific diagnosis is helped by noting the distribution and the pattern of the specific abnormalities. CT scan interpretations are most accurate in silicosis, IPF, lymphangitic carcinomatosis, and sarcoidosis (Mathieson et al, 1989; Muller et al, 1986). Although it is clear that HRCT detects and clarifies the pattern and extent of abnormalities in the chest, the issue of whether it can substitute or decrease the need for open lung biopsy (OLB) or thoracoscopy-guided lung biopsy (TGLB) is currently unsettled. Although certain characteristic image features such as bibasilar subpleural fibrotic changes of IPF supplement other conventional findings, the ground-glass attenuation that has been increasingly recognized in HRCT images has not been satisfactorily correlated with pathology (Raghu, 1995). Moreover, although CT is clearly more sensitive than conventional chest radiography in detecting pulmonary fibrosis, it is nonspecific, as similar patterns may be seen in patients with collagen-vascular disease–associated ILD, IPF, or drug toxicity (Johkoh et al, 1994; Padley et al, 1992). However, certain characteristic HRCT findings, such as pulmonary parenchymal cystic changes, can narrow the differential diagnoses of ILD to the rare disorders of LAM, tuberous sclerosis, or pulmonary histiocytosis X, which can then be distinguished based on supportive clinical history (Raghu, 1995). A CT scan also shows occult parenchymal, pleural, and mediastinal abnormalities. This information is helpful in selecting biopsy sites or suggesting other procedures, which may eliminate the need for lung biopsy such as biopsy of a pleural lesion or sampling of an enlarged mediastinal lymph node by mediastinoscopy. Therefore, it is prudent to obtain a preoperative HRCT scan of the chest in any patient who is to be subjected to surgical lung biopsy (Raghu, 1995).

Radionuclide Imaging

The use of radionuclide to evaluate interstitial lung disease has a long history. In the middle and late 1970s, it was appreciated that gallium uptake was enhanced in the lungs of patients with sarcoidosis (Fig. 24–3) or IPF, and the amount of uptake correlated with other measures of inflammation in the lung. Therefore, it was suggested to use gallium scanning for diagnosis and evaluation of response to therapy. However, several limitations to gallium scanning (including the high cost, the nonspecific nature of a positive gallium scan, the fact that it requires 48 to 72 hours for proper interpretation, and the fact that the uptake reverses quickly during corticosteroid therapy) were soon identified. Therefore, the gallium scan

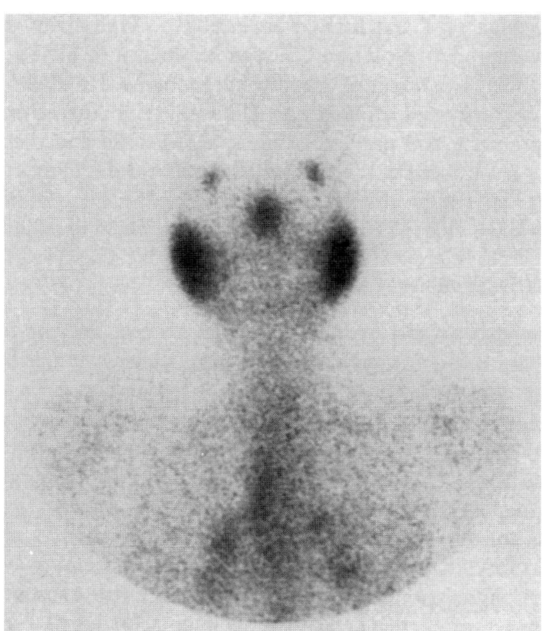

FIGURE 24–3 ■ Gallium scan from a patient with sarcoidosis. Note the increased uptake of gallium in the conjunctival tissue, parotid glands, and hilar and mediastinal lymph nodes.

is no longer used routinely in patients with ILD (Baughman and Fernandez, 1996). The clearance of aerosol ^{99m}Tc diethylenetriamine pentaacetic acid (^{99m}Tc DTPA) is greatly increased in sarcoidosis and other inflammatory lung diseases. However, the major limitation of this method is that cigarette smoking will also cause increased clearance. Therefore, it is not used currently in diagnosis or follow-up of patients with ILDs (Baughman and Fernandez, 1996).

Magnetic Resonance Imaging

Magnetic resonance imaging (MRI) is not routinely used in the assessment of ILD, mainly because of its high cost and limited accessibility. Preliminary data show that MRI has potential use in the assessment of disease activity in the lung parenchyma. It is, however, still largely an experimental tool and is not routinely used (Greaves and Batra, 1995).

Invasive Investigations

Bronchoscopy and Bronchoalveolar Lavage

Patients with ILD are usually investigated with bronchoscopy and bronchoalveolar lavage (BAL) (Strumpf et al, 1981). The flexible fiberoptic bronchoscope is wedged in a peripheral segment where alveolitis is expected. Typically 100 ml of sterile saline is injected through the bronchoscope in 20-ml aliquots, and then samples of the alveolar fluid are recovered. Specimens are sent for cell count, cytologic examination, lymphocyte subtyping, and microbiologic studies. In cases in which eosinophilic granuloma is suspected, electron microscopy can be done to detect typical intracellular X bodies (Basset et al, 1977). The finding of lipoproteinaceous material is consistent with the diagnosis of alveolar proteinosis in appropriate clinical context, and iron-laden macrophages can be highly suggestive of pulmonary hemorrhage (Drew et al, 1977; Martin et al, 1980). The finding of oil-laden macrophages in large numbers suggests a diagnosis of mineral oil aspiration (Corwin and Irwin, 1985). Alternatively, in cases of suspected occupational lung disease, the lavage sample can be analyzed for particles of inorganic material or by electron probe for dust particles (Davison et al, 1983).

BAL can be used as a single diagnostic tool only in some selected lung diseases, such as opportunistic lung infections, malignant conditions, alveolar proteinosis, histiocytosis X, and lung hemorrhagic syndrome (American Thoracic Society, 1990). In other clinical settings, cellular lavage findings can only contribute to the diagnosis of specific lung diseases, provided sufficient diagnostic criteria such as chest radiography, lung function, or serologic parameters are available. There are no consistent quotations in the literature regarding normal values for the relative distribution of BAL cells. Certain ILDs are associated with a specific increase in cell type. For example, an increased percentage of lymphocytes is seen in granulomatous diseases of the lung, such as hypersensitivity pneumonitis, sarcoidosis, tuberculosis, and berylliosis. Predominance of neutrophils is usually observed in adult respiratory distress syndrome and IPF. Eosinophilic predominance of BAL cells is usually seen in patients with eosinophilic lung diseases such as allergic bronchopulmonary aspergillosis, eosinophilic pneumonia, or Churg-Strauss syndrome (American Thoracic Society, 1990). However, there is considerable variation among the absolute cell numbers and their relative percentages within the classic types of alveolitis. This makes it very clear that differential cytology of BAL cells can give only some clinical orientation toward the differential diagnosis of the underlying ILD. There is little evidence to suggest that the cell count and differential obtained from BAL are useful in predicting clinical response to therapy or the natural history of the disease in most patients (Helmers and Hunninghake, 1989). BAL is generally not used to guide therapy and should be regarded as a research tool.

Biopsy

Despite thorough clinical evaluation, the specific diagnosis of ILD may remain unclear. Examination of samples of lung tissue will provide the following: (1) confirmation of a specific diagnosis or exclusion of a particular occupational lung disease; (2) prediction of survival and response to therapy; (3) justification for long-term therapy with drugs that have significant adverse effects or the decision to enroll the patient in a new therapeutic trial; and (4) facilitation of earlier planning for lung transplantation in the appropriate patient (Raghu, 1995). The diagnosis of IPF requires exclusion of other specific entities. Therefore, in a symptomatic or functionally impaired patient with unexplained physiologic and radiographic features of ILD, the presence of the following clinical features, which are suggestive of specific diagnoses other than IPF, should be considered an indication for surgical lung biopsy (Raghu, 1995): relatively young age at the time of presentation; history of systemic symptoms (e.g., fever, weight loss, night sweats) and hemoptysis; family history of apparent ILD; clinical features suggestive of peripheral vasculitis; history of pneumothorax; atypical radiographic features of IPF or a normal chest radiograph; unexplained extrapulmonary manifestations, pulmonary hypertension, or cardiomegaly at the time of presentation; and rapidly progressive disease or rapid deterioration in a patient with long-standing stable ILD. The cost-effectiveness and risk with OLB/TGLB have to be weighed against the benefits in the elderly patient with long-standing, typical clinical features of IPF. Transbronchial biopsy through the bronchoscope may provide sufficient tissue for the diagnosis of sarcoidosis, carcinoma, infections, or alveolar proteinosis. The diagnostic yield in sarcoidosis approaches 80%, but this procedure is less helpful in the other disorders (Thrasher and Briggs, 1982). The samples are generally too small to allow a definitive diagnosis in other disorders, but they can give clues to the disease's cause. Mediastinoscopy with biopsy of enlarged mediastinal lymph nodes may be worthwhile in patients with diffuse infiltrates, especially in sarcoidosis, tuberculosis, lymphoma, and histoplasmosis. Thoracoscopic or open lung biopsies (Fig. 24–4) are usually required to obtain sufficient tissue in the ILDs (Flint, 1982). TGLB is increasingly being substituted for the conventional OLB in many centers. This is due mainly to equivalent diagnostic accuracy and significantly reduced perioperative morbidity associated with TGLB (Bensard et al, 1993). Samples should be sent from the operating room to the microbiology laboratory for assessment for bacteria, fungi, viruses, and parasites. Other specimens should be fixed for light and electron microscopy and immunofluorescence testing. Tissue should also be frozen pending further investigations, such as viral studies or flow cytometry. It is important to discuss the tests required with the referring physician prior to the operative procedure. It is best to take at least two biopsies from areas with early and intermediate disease. In most cases, it is recommended that the lingula be avoided because tissue from this area tends to exhibit end-stage changes.

Patient Assessment

A functional assessment of each patient with ILD is mandatory. It is often performed after the diagnosis of ILD is confirmed and an assessment of the disease's activity has been made. This is best done by complete pulmonary function studies (lung volumes, flow rates, and diffusing capacity), measurement of arterial blood gases, and, in selected cases, exercise studies. In most instances, a restrictive ventilatory pattern is identified that is associated with a decrease in diffusing capacity (Fulmer, 1982b). In a subset of patients, the physiologic abnormalities suggest an obstructive ventilatory defect, despite the presence of a diffuse pulmonary infiltrate (Sharma and Johnson, 1988). This narrows the differential diagnosis to such disorders as sarcoidosis, eosinophilic granuloma, LAM, tuberous sclerosis, and ILD secondary to intravenous drug abuse. Arterial blood gases typically demonstrate hypoxemia with a mild respiratory alkalosis. Exercise studies reveal a pattern of rapid shallow breathing associated with oxygen desaturation, which may be profound (Crystal et al, 1976).

After careful review of clinical information, laboratory data, and pathologic findings, the physician determines whether therapy is indicated. The age and general health of the patient should be considered prior to sending the patient for a lung biopsy or embarking on a long course of therapy. If possible, it is advantageous to make a definitive tissue diagnosis before commencing toxic therapy.

INTERSTITIAL LUNG DISEASES OF UNKNOWN CAUSE

Idiopathic Pulmonary Fibrosis

IPF (also called cryptogenic fibrosing alveolitis) occurs most commonly in patients between the ages of 50 and 60 years. A rapidly progressive fatal illness was originally described by Hamman and Rich (1944), but the syndrome was renamed IPF when the heterogeneous nature of the disorder was identified. Liebow and colleagues

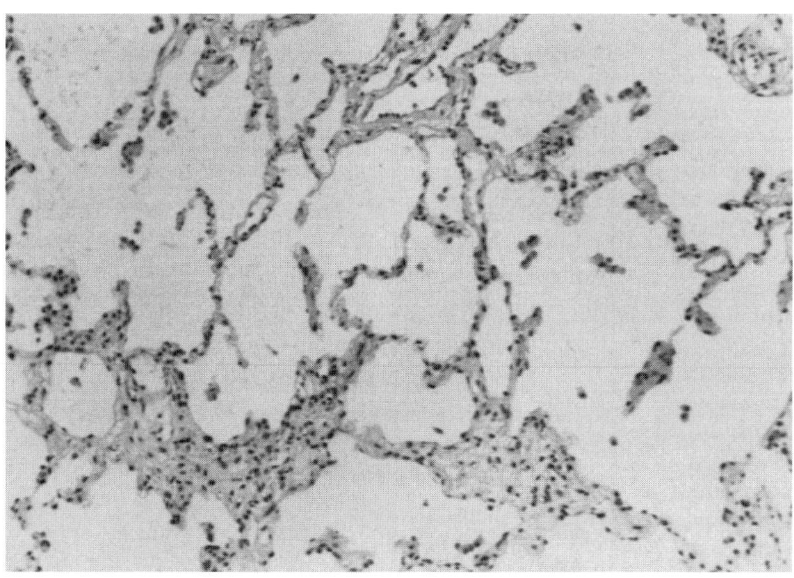

FIGURE 24–4 ■ Open lung biopsy from a patient with idiopathic pulmonary fibrosis. Note the interstitial fibrosis with architectural restructuring (H & E, ×100).

(1965) later subdivided these disorders into usual interstitial pneumonitis (UIP), desquamative interstitial pneumonitis (DIP), lymphocytic interstitial pneumonitis (LIP), giant cell interstitial pneumonitis (GIP), and bronchiolitis obliterans with interstitial pneumonia (BIP). More recently, a new classification scheme was suggested that identifies four histologically distinct forms of idiopathic interstitial pneumonia (Katzenstein and Myers, 1998). This classification scheme maintains UIP and DIP from Liebow's original classification and includes two additional entities: acute interstitial pneumonia (AIP or Hamman-Rich disease) and nonspecific interstitial pneumonia (NSIP). The new classification scheme excludes LIP and GIP from the category of IPF, because they are not idiopathic; LIP is a lymphoproliferative disorder often associated with immunodeficiencies, and GIP is usually a manifestation of hard-metal pneumoconiosis. This classification also excludes BIP from the category of IPF, because BIP pathologically is an intraluminal rather than an interstitial abnormality, and, radiographically, it is mainly an air space rather than a diffuse interstitial process (Katzenstein and Myers, 1998). The proposed advantage of this classification scheme is its clinical implication and its ability to explain the perplexing variation in presentation, response to steroid therapy, and clinical course that has been noted in patients with IPF. In this classification, the term IPF is reserved for cases of UIP, which constitute the most common histologic form. UIP has an insidious onset, is chronically progressive, does not usually respond to therapy, and is fatal in most cases (Katzenstein and Myers, 1998). DIP, on the other hand, is a rare form of idiopathic interstitial pneumonia, which also has an insidious onset but usually has a good prognosis. DIP may be related to cigarette smoking. It is suggested that the term DIP be replaced with respiratory bronchiolitis interstitial lung disease (RBILD), which is a more accurate anatomic and pathologic description (Katzenstein and Myers, 1998). AIP is an acute, fulminant form of IPF that corresponds to the cases described by Hamman and Rich in 1944. It has a rapidly evolving course with high mortality. The pathologic changes are those seen in severe extensive acute lung injury (Katzenstein and Myers, 1998). NSIP is a temporally uniform interstitial pneumonia with predominantly interstitial inflammation, beneficial response to steroids, and generally a good prognosis in most patients (Katzenstein and Myers, 1998).

Patients with IPF present with progressive dyspnea and a nonproductive cough. Physical examination may reveal fine crackles at the lung bases and finger clubbing (Scadding, 1974). The chest radiograph typically shows decreased lung volumes, bilateral interstitial infiltrates, and honeycombing in advanced disease. A reduced diffusion capacity and a restrictive ventilatory defect are found on pulmonary function testing. There are no specific blood tests that are diagnostic of IPF. The sedimentation rate may be elevated, and mild increases in rheumatoid factor and ANA titers are common. There may also be elevated levels of immune complexes (Dreisen et al, 1978). The median survival of all patients is less than 5 years (Stack et al, 1972).

IPF is a difficult condition to manage because the prognosis is unpredictable and therapeutic responses are unusual (Scadding and Hinson, 1967). Assessment and therapeutic protocols therefore differ in content between centers. A large sample of tissue, such as that obtained in an open lung biopsy, is essential both for a confident diagnosis and for staging. It is important to document a definitive diagnosis and rule out other possible causes for fibrosis before committing the patient to a course of corticosteroids or immunosuppressants. Prior to commencing therapy, the patient should be staged for the level of the disease's activity. Symptoms, progression of radiographic abnormalities, gallium scan positivity, and reduction in pulmonary function over a follow-up period have all been used to determine activity. Those whose diseases are classified as inactive are generally followed at regular intervals. Patients whose diseases are deemed to be active are started on a course of corticosteroids. Those who do not respond to a 3-month trial may benefit

INTERSTITIAL LUNG DISEASES OF UNKNOWN CAUSE

- Idiopathic pulmonary fibrosis
- Bronchiolitis obliterans organizing pneumonia
- Sarcoidosis
- Lymphangioleiomyomatosis
- Eosinophilic granuloma
- Pulmonary vasculitis
- Wegener's granulomatosis
- Churg-Strauss vasculitis
- Lymphomatoid granulomatosis
- Interstitial lung disease associated with connective tissue disease
- Rheumatoid arthritis
- Systemic sclerosis
- Sjögren's syndrome
- Systemic lupus erythematosus
- Polymyositis/dermatomyositis
- Ankylosing spondylitis
- Pulmonary renal syndromes
- Goodpasture's syndrome
- Idiopathic pulmonary hemosiderosis
- Eosinophilic pneumonia
- Alveolar proteinosis
- Inherited disorders
- Tuberous sclerosis
- Neurofibromatosis
- Familial idiopathic pulmonary fibrosis
- Gaucher's disease
- Niemann-Pick disease
- Hermansky-Pudlak syndrome
- Amyloidosis
- Lymphocytic disorders
- Pseudolymphoma
- Lymphocytic interstitial pneumonitis
- Immunoblastic lymphoma
- Bronchocentric granulomatosis
- Pulmonary veno-occlusive disease
- Graft-versus-host disease
- Sequelae of adult respiratory distress syndrome

by the addition of azathioprine or cyclophosphamide. Two randomized trials showed that the long-term survival rate may be improved by the early addition of immunosuppressants, such as azathioprine or cyclophosphamide, and early treatment for affected patients has been advocated by some investigators (Johnson et al, 1989; Raghu et al, 1991). Success was also reported with cyclosporine therapy in a limited number of patients, but there are no clinical trials to support its usage (Moolma et al, 1991). Characteristics that support a better prognosis include female gender, younger age, cellular biopsy (DIP), fewer symptoms on first consultation, and an increased amount of type 3 collagen in the biopsy specimen (Raghu, 1987). The prognosis of those who respond to therapy is better than that of nonresponders. This variation in the response to therapy has been explained by the fact that responders may be in an earlier phase of their disease or that responders are a unique subset of patients (Hunninghake and Kalica, 1995). Despite some success with therapy, the lung disease in most patients eventually worsens. This observation supports the recommendation by those who advocate treating all patients early in the course of disease when they are most likely to respond to therapy (Hunninghake and Kalica, 1995). There is ongoing research studying newer modes of therapy including pharmocologic agents such as cytokine inhibitors, growth factor inhibitors, antifibrotic agents, antiproteases, newer anti-inflammatory agents, and antioxidants. Other potential future therapeutic modalities using the increasing knowledge about regulation of white cell traffic and gene therapy are currently being investigated (Hunninghake and Kalica, 1995). Single-lung transplantation is the best option for patients with severe IPF refractory to medical therapy. Unfortunately, many patients with severe IPF die while waiting for organs; therefore, early listing for transplantation is essential in patients with progressive IPF in whom medical therapy has failed. The 3-year survival rate following single-lung transplantation is approximately 51% (Trulock, 1997).

Bronchiolitis Obliterans Organizing Pneumonia

Bronchiolitis obliterans organizing pneumonia (BOOP) is associated with a short period (less than 2 months) of progressive dyspnea, cough, fever, and weight loss (Epler et al, 1985). Physical examination typically reveals bibasilar crackles but may show clubbing, bronchial breathing, and fever. Arterial blood gases reveal a widened alveolar-arterial gradient, and chest radiographs show interstitial or alveolar opacities. The main feature of BOOP is patchy air space consolidation with small nodular opacities. The histologic hallmark of BOOP is an intense inflammatory process involving the terminal and respiratory bronchioles. Aggregates of granulation tissue, neutrophils, edema, debris, fibrin, connective tissue, myofibroblasts, and fibroblasts plug the terminal bronchioles and extend into the peribronchiolar region, alveolar ducts, and alveolar spaces. The disease process is patchy and has a peribronchiolar distribution. The alveolar structure is preserved, and fibrosis is notably absent (Colby and Myers, 1992) (Fig. 24–5). The distribution of air space disease is subpleural in 50% of patients. The sedimentation rate is elevated, and pulmonary function tests show a restrictive ventilatory defect. Open lung biopsy is usually required to establish the diagnosis. It is important to distinguish this illness from IPF because most patients with BOOP recover from their illness. Prednisone is given in a dosage of 1 mg/kg/day for about 3 months until a clinical response is obtained. Then the drug is slowly tapered to a maintenance dose of 20 mg on alternate days. However, no comparative dosing trials have been performed. Prednisone should be tapered slowly because recurrences have been observed. Progressive disease that may ultimately be fatal, despite therapy with high-dose corticosteroids, immunosuppressive therapy, and mechanical ventilation, develops in a subset of patients (Cohen et al, 1994; Cordier et al, 1989).

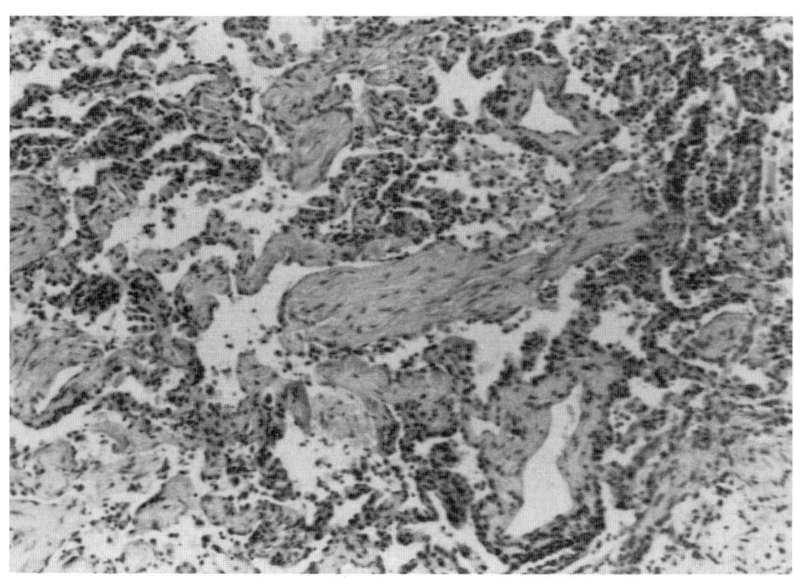

FIGURE 24–5 ■ Open lung biopsy demonstrating bronchiolitis obliterans with organizing pneumonia. Note the presence of loose connective tissue obliterating the small airways with microscopic lipoid pneumonia (H & E, ×100).

Sarcoidosis

Sarcoidosis, a multisystem granulomatous disease, can develop in most organ systems and lead to varied clinical presentations (Fig. 24–6). It was first recognized as a dermatologic disorder in 1877 by Sir Jonathan Hutchinson (1877), a British dermatologist. The pathologic condition was described in 1899 by Caesar Boeck (1899), a Norwegian dermatologist. Almost 40 years after the first description of the disease, the true systemic nature and the associated pulmonary involvement were clearly described (Kuznitsky and Bittorf, 1915).

The cause of the disease is unknown. Many putative agents have been identified, but none so far has withstood rigorous scrutiny. The most recent candidate is once again mycobacteria because some investigators detected minute quantities of mycobacterial DNA in clinical samples from patients with sarcoidosis (Saboor et al, 1992). However, even these provocative findings cannot be confirmed by other investigators (Bocart et al, 1992).

There is an increased prevalence and severity of the disease in the black population (Johns, 1989). The organs that are most commonly involved include the lungs, skin, eyes, nervous system, heart, kidneys, and musculoskeletal system.

Specific syndromes of sarcoidosis include Löfgren's syndrome (Löfgren, 1953), which is characterized by the abrupt onset of hilar lymphadenopathy, fever, and erythema nodosum, and Heerfordt's syndrome (Heerfordt, 1909) or uveoparotid fever, which is distinguished by fever, parotid gland swelling, uveitis, and cranial nerve palsies. The lungs are the most commonly involved organ in sarcoidosis, but up to one third of patients with pulmonary sarcoidosis are asymptomatic. Their disease is discovered by routine chest radiography (Maycock et al, 1963). The symptoms, if present, include dyspnea on exertion, wheezing, and a nonproductive cough.

Traditionally, patients are staged radiographically. Stage 0 reveals no chest radiographic abnormalities. Stage 1 radiographs show hilar adenopathy alone. Stage 2 shows hilar adenopathy and diffuse interstitial infiltrates. Stage 3 is denoted by interstitial infiltrates without adenopathy. Stage 4 disease demonstrates advanced chronic changes with coarse interstitial markings, honeycombing, and hilar retraction (Geraint James, 1984). Radiographic changes, when present, commonly appear as diffuse reticular nodular infiltrates with a predilection for the lung apices but occasionally as a fluffy alveolar pattern. Infrequent findings include large nodules, which rarely cavitate, bullous disease, pleural effusions, eggshell calcification of lymph nodes, pneumothorax, and mycetomas in areas of advanced disease (Rockoff and Rohatgi, 1985). The value of radiographic staging is that the rate of radiographic resolution is inversely related to the radiographic stage at presentation; the mortality rate is directly correlated with the radiographic stage (DeRemee, 1983).

A CT scan can clearly demonstrate anterior mediastinal and subcarinal lymph node enlargement. The usual abnormality on the CT scan is nodules along the bronchovascular bundles, interlobar septa, major fissures, and subpleural region (Muller et al, 1989). The nodules can be focal or diffuse and smooth or irregular. They are less than 5 mm in diameter. The granulomas can cause thickening of the interlobar septa, pulmonary vessels, and bronchial vessels. If fibrosis develops, linear opacities appear that are usually peribronchovascular. Hazy increases in pulmonary densities correlate with active alveolitis, as assessed by gallium scanning (Line et al, 1978).

Pulmonary function test results may be normal or demonstrate a restrictive or obstructive ventilatory defect and a reduction in the diffusing capacity (Boushy et al, 1965). The pulmonary function tests, although defining the level of functional impairment, correlate poorly with the presence and intensity of the alveolitis (Lin et al, 1985). There may be evidence of hypoxemia at rest or with exercise.

The diagnosis of sarcoidosis is often made clinically, especially in an asymptomatic patient with negative physical examination findings and bilateral hilar adenopathy (Winterbauer et al, 1973). Many clinicians prefer to obtain tissue confirmation in all cases of possible sarcoidosis to avoid the possibility of missing a potentially treatable

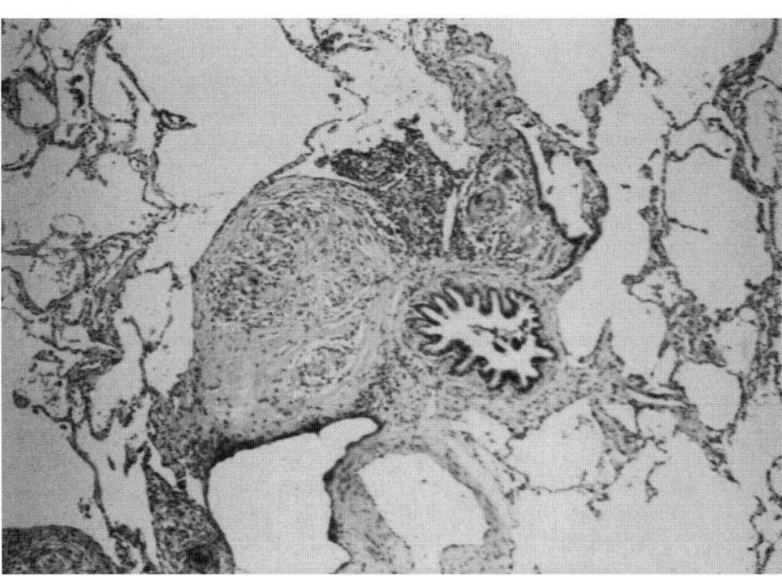

FIGURE 24–6 ■ Open lung biopsy showing sarcoidosis. Note the granuloma present in the microvascular bundle (H & E, ×100).

condition other than sarcoidosis, such as tuberculosis. Bronchoscopy with transbronchial lung biopsy is the preferred diagnostic test, with a yield of noncaseating granulomata in 70% to 90% of cases (Gilman and Wang, 1980; Rothe et al, 1980). Cutaneous lesions and enlarged lymph nodes or lacrimal glands may be biopsied preferentially, if easily accessible (Sharma, 1985). Mediastinoscopy and open lung biopsy are reserved for the most difficult cases when other measures have not yielded the diagnosis.

The serum ACE levels are often elevated in sarcoidosis and can be used to follow disease activity in those patients in whom the test result is abnormal (Lieberman, 1975). Serum ACE concentrations may also be elevated in tuberculosis, leprosy, and Gaucher's disease (Studdy and Bird, 1989). Changes in serum ACE levels correlate poorly with changes in routine clinical parameters, such as chest radiographs or pulmonary function (Hollinger et al, 1985). The pretreatment serum ACE level does not predict improvement in pulmonary function with therapy (Baughman et al, 1984). In most patients, serum ACE levels cannot be used to make therapeutic decisions.

BAL was advocated as a tool to predict the clinical response to therapy (Keogh et al, 1983). Unfortunately, other studies have not confirmed the initial observations, and the clinical utility of this investigation is limited (Foley et al, 1989; Turner-Warwick et al, 1986).

Over a 3-year period, many patients with sarcoidosis have a spontaneous remission (Smellie and Hoyle, 1960). Patients with Löfgren's syndrome or hilar lymphadenopathy alone have the highest rates of spontaneous remission. It is rare for the disease to recur if it has regressed spontaneously. Untreated, the disease can stop at moderate fibrosis or progress to end-stage lung disease. Therapy is usually reserved for patients with symptomatic pulmonary disease; systemic symptoms; hypercalcemia; or involvement of the eyes, kidneys, heart, or central nervous system (Muthiah and Macfarlane, 1990). In patients with stage I disease, therapy is withheld unless evidence of clinical, radiographic, or physiologic deterioration is documented. In patients with stage II or III disease and normal pulmonary function, therapy is usually withheld and introduced when deterioration is documented. In patients with stage II or III disease with abnormal lung function, therapy is usually started immediately. Prednisone in a dose of 0.5 to 1 mg/kg of body weight is initiated until an appropriate clinical response is reached, and then it is tapered gradually. A multicenter, randomized trial of stage II or III sarcoidosis sponsored by the British Thoracic Society found after an initial 6-month observation period that patients with persistent radiographic infiltrates who were treated with corticosteroids showed improved lung function, chest radiographs, and symptoms, as compared with untreated controls (Gibson et al, 1996). We have found that the best monitors to follow include serum ACE levels, chest radiographs, and pulmonary function tests. The role of inhaled steroids in the therapy of sarcoidosis is not clear at this writing. There are some data supporting use of inhaled steroids in pulmonary sarcoidosis, as they may reduce deterioration and postpone the need for systemic steroids (Alberts et al, 1995). Other therapeutic modalities that have been tried include chloroquine, chlorambucil, methotrexate, and cyclosporine (Kataria, 1980; Lower and Baughman, 1990; Martinet et al, 1988; O'Leary et al, 1986). Few controlled clinical trials have been performed, and the role of these medications is uncertain. Transplantation is an option for the patient with end-stage disease. Survival rates following single- and double-lung transplantation are similar, approximately 70% at 2 years. Recurrence of sarcoid granuloma within the lung allografts has been noted in most cases but rarely causes clinical symptoms (Johnson et al, 1993).

Lymphangioleiomyomatosis

In 1937, von Stossel described diffuse cystic changes in the lung and lymphadenopathy in a woman who died of respiratory failure. He commented on the proliferation of smooth muscle cells throughout the lung and called the process "muscular cirrhosis of the lungs." LAM occurs typically in women of reproductive age. The presenting symptoms include cough, slowly progressive dyspnea, and hemoptysis; affected women may develop spontaneous pneumothorax with chylous pleural effusion. Chest radiographs show normal or increased lung volumes with reticulonodular shadows and small cyst-like areas.

The lung's surface is covered with tiny cysts, which are found throughout the lung substance. Smooth muscle cells proliferate in the lung tissue throughout lymphatic, vascular, and bronchial structures. These lesions can cause (1) local airway obstruction, leading to airflow obstruction and cyst formation; (2) blood vessel obstruction, leading to venular congestion and bleeding; and (3) lymphatic obstruction, leading to chylothorax. With HRCT, there is a combination of normal lung tissue and areas filled with numerous thin-walled cystic air spaces of multiple sizes (Merchant et al, 1985) (Fig. 24–7). The cysts are made by muscle cell proliferation in the

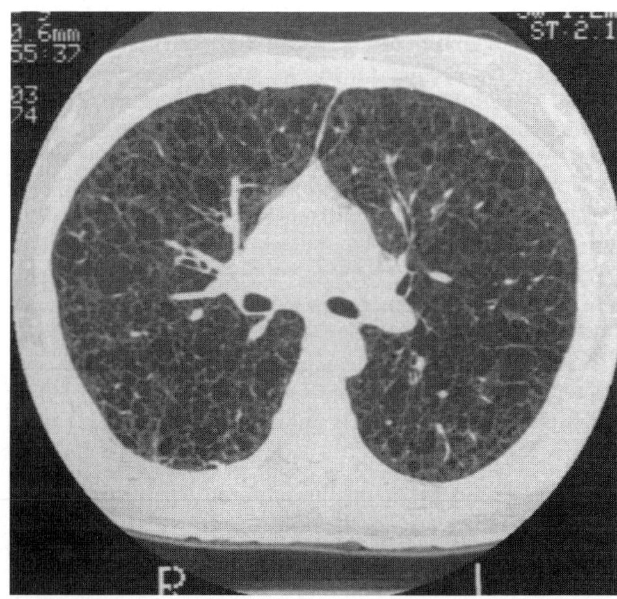

FIGURE 24–7 ■ Lung window of a high-resolution computed tomography scan of the thorax from a patient with lymphangioleiomyomatosis. Note the presence of cystic spaces throughout the lung parenchyma.

bronchioles and subsequent air trapping. LAM can be distinguished from IPF on CT scans because in IPF there are abnormalities in the subpleural areas and the bases, unlike in LAM, in which there are diffuse abnormalities. Additionally, most cysts in LAM are surrounded by areas of normal lung, whereas the honeycombing in IPF is surrounded by abnormalities in the parenchyma.

Although the natural history of this disorder is not known, the general view is that most patients die within 10 years of the onset of disease (Corrin et al, 1975). This view has been challenged, and hormonal manipulation may lead to prolonged survival in some patients (Taylor et al, 1990). Progesterone or oophorectomy appears to produce remissions in about 50% of patients; however, it is difficult to assess the response because the disease's course is variable (Eliasson et al, 1989). Other therapy with androgens and tamoxifen is less successful. Interferon alfa-2b, an antiproliferative agent, has been used with anecdotal success. Successful lung transplants have been done in a select group of patients. Recurrence of LAM in the lung allograft has been noted.

Eosinophilic Granuloma

Eosinophilic granuloma, Letterer-Siwe disease, and Hand-Schüller-Christian disease all traditionally have been called histiocytosis X; the latter two are diseases of children and are not discussed further here. Eosinophilic granuloma is a rare condition of unknown cause that is characterized by histiocytic infiltration of the lung. In a few patients, there are also lesions of the bone, posterior pituitary, and skin.

The disease is usually diagnosed in the third decade, and most series report a male predominance (Friedman et al, 1981). More than 90% of patients report a smoking history. Patients present with cough, dyspnea on exertion, fever, and weight loss. Spontaneous pneumothorax is common. The physical examination may be normal or reveal wheezing. Despite the name, there is no peripheral eosinophilia in this condition. Patients with systemic involvement can develop diabetes insipidus, diffuse lymphadenopathy, rashes, or bone lesions. Chest radiographs show preserved or enlarged pulmonary volumes with reticular nodular and nodular interstitial infiltrates involving the upper and middle lobes and sparing the costophrenic angles (Lacronique et al, 1982). The nodules typically have a stellate shape and a tendency to cavitate when enlarged. The cavitated nodules can progress to honeycombing and bullae. A frequent finding is fine honeycombing of the central portions of the upper lobes. HRCT scanning can identify small and large cysts and micronodules that are not apparent by chest radiography (Brauner et al, 1989). CT findings correlate better with physiologic abnormalities than do radiographic findings (Moore et al, 1989).

Histiocytes containing X bodies (i.e., pentalaminate rods 40 to 45 nm in width with central striations that resemble impressions from a tennis racket) can be seen with electron microscopic examination of bronchoalveolar lavage fluid (Basset et al, 1977). The identification of X bodies is not pathognomonic for eosinophilic granuloma, because they are found in Langerhans cells in the skin, lung cancer, and pulmonary fibrosis. In the appropriate clinical setting, they may be diagnostic. The disease is of variable course and can spontaneously regress or progress rapidly to death (Basset et al, 1978). Factors that suggest a progressive downhill course include extremes of age, multiple pneumothoraces, multisystem generalized disease, prolonged constitutional disturbance, extensive initial pulmonary radiologic involvement with formation of cysts, and a low carbon monoxide–diffusing capacity. Patients must be urged to discontinue smoking. In most patients, the disease will stabilize or even improve following cessation of smoking (Van Essen et al, 1990). Corticosteroids and immunosuppressants have been used, but there is no evidence that they alter the course of the disease (Prophet, 1982). Large compressive masses were reduced with radiation therapy. Pleurodesis can prevent recurrent pneumothoraces. Lung transplantation is an option for selected patients with end-stage disease.

Pulmonary Vasculitis

Wegener's Granulomatosis

Wegener's granulomatosis was first described in the 1930s by Klinger (1931) and then described by Wegener (1936) as a form of periarteritis in which granulomatous inflammation of the nose and paranasal sinuses was prominent. It is characterized by granulomatous vasculitic inflammation of the nose, paranasal sinuses, and lungs and necrotizing glomerulitis. A limited form of the disease, in which there is no evidence of renal disease, was described by Carrington and Liebow (1966). Presenting symptoms include sinusitis, arthralgias, fever, otitis, cough, nasal symptoms, hemoptysis, and weight loss. Other, less common presentations include ocular inflammation, rash, epistaxis, chest discomfort, malaise, dyspnea, hearing loss, and headache (Fauci et al, 1978). Initially, affected individuals may show pulmonary infiltrates, sinus tenderness, renal failure, proptosis, oral ulcers, or pleural effusions. At presentation, pulmonary disease is evident in 94% of patients; renal disease is apparent in 85% (Fauci et al, 1983).

ANCA has been found to be a highly specific marker for active Wegener's granulomatosis. ANCA in Wegener's granulomatosis is associated with a characteristic cytoplasmic staining pattern of neutrophils (c-ANCA) by indirect immunofluorescence. Positive c-ANCA titers occur in more than 90% of patients with generalized Wegener's granulomatosis, 75% of patients with Wegener's granulomatosis without renal involvement, and 50% of patients with vasculitic overlap syndrome including microscopic polyarteritis (Kallenburg et al, 1992). ANCA positivity drops to approximately 40% during remission, and c-ANCA titers have been found to have a direct correlation to the activity of the disease (Kallenberg et al, 1992). The chest radiograph most commonly demonstrates bilateral multiple nodules with cavitation. Up to 40% of patients present with a solitary nodule. Other radiographic patterns include atelectasis secondary to endobronchial lesions, pleural effusions, and diffuse interstitial or alveolar patterns (Cordier et al, 1990). The diagnosis is made from tissue obtained at open lung biopsy. The classic pathologic findings are a necrotizing granulomatous vasculitis involving the small and medium-sized veins and arteries. The histologic finding of capillary inflammation distinguishes Wegener's granulomatosis from Goodpasture's syndrome in the case of acute pulmonary hemorrhage. Biopsy of the nose or sinuses tends not to be useful because specimens often demonstrate nonspecific granulomatous inflammation without frank vasculitis. Furthermore, biopsy of the kidneys does not reveal specific pathologic findings; glomerulitis rather than graulomatous vasculitis is usually seen.

Prior to the introduction of cytotoxic drug therapy, more than 90% of patients with Wegener's granulomatosis died within 2 years. Currently, standard therapy for Wegener's granulomatosis includes high-dose corticosteroids and cyclophosphamide. Therapy is continued until 1 year after recovery and then tapered over the following year. A rise in ANCA titers often precedes the clinical relapse, and it has been proposed that therapeutic decisions should be based on the results of this test (Cohen Tervaert et al, 1990). Treatment with trimethoprim-sulfamethoxazole reduces the incidence of relapses in patients with Wegener's granulomatosis in remission (Stegeman et al, 1996). High-dose pooled intravenous immunoglobulin is used to treat systemic vasculitis, but its exact role has yet to be defined (Jayne and Lockwood, 1996).

Churg-Strauss Vasculitis

Allergic angiitis and granulomatosis is a systemic vasculitis first described by Churg and Strauss (1951), involving the lung, skin, heart, and gastrointestinal tract. The pulmonary syndrome that affects most patients consists of atopy, asthma, and diffuse pulmonary infiltrates. The peripheral eosinophil count and sedimentation rate are often markedly elevated. The diagnosis is made on tissue from an open lung biopsy, and the histologic findings characteristically show granulomas, eosinophilic infiltrates, and necrotizing vasculitis. Most patients respond with steroids; a subgroup requires immunosuppressant drugs.

Lymphomatoid Granulomatosis

Lymphomatoid granulomatosis, originally described by Liebow and colleagues (1972), is a disease characterized by infiltration of various organs with a polymorphic infiltrate consisting of atypical lymphocytoid and plasmacytoid cells with granulomatous inflammation in an angiocentric pattern. Although the lung is most frequently involved, cutaneous, renal, and central nervous system involvement is common (Fauci et al, 1982). The clinical manifestations are nonspecific and include cough, dyspnea, chest pain, fever, and weight loss. Spontaneously clearing multiple bilateral nodules that may cavitate characterize the radiographic findings (Israel et al, 1977). Open lung biopsy shows invasion of small and medium-sized vessels by atypical lymphocytes, monocytes, and granulomas. Many classify lymphomatoid granulomatosis as a lymphoproliferative disorder rather than an inflammatory disease because of the tendency to transform into lymphoma. The lung disease usually responds to steroids and cyclophosphamide; however, some patients require therapy with chemotherapeutic agents. Patients must be closely followed to detect the development of lymphoma.

Interstitial Lung Disease Associated with Connective Tissue Disease

Rheumatoid Arthritis

Until the early 1980s, rheumatoid arthritis was associated with five pulmonary complications: (1) pleurisy with or without effusion, (2) necrobiotic nodules (rheumatoid nodules), (3) Caplan's syndrome (rheumatoid pneumoconiosis), (4) interstitial pneumonitis and fibrosis, and (5) pulmonary arteritis (Hunninghake and Fauci, 1979). In the early 1980s, bronchiolitis obliterans, whether occurring de novo or secondary to drugs used in the treatment of rheumatoid disease, such as penicillamine or gold, was described (Holness et al, 1983; Penny et al, 1982). Ellman and Ball (1948) first noticed the association of rheumatoid disease and ILD. Patients with rheumatoid arthritis develop an ILD similar to IPF. Between 1.6% and 4.5% of patients have radiographic evidence of diffuse pulmonary fibrosis, but up to 40% of patients show pulmonary function abnormalities compatible with this syndrome (Jurik et al, 1982; Roschmann and Rothenberg, 1987). Patients present with dyspnea and cough, and examination reveals basal crackles without clubbing. Pulmonary findings may precede the development of rheumatologic manifestations of the disease by several years. Pulmonary involvement is associated usually with seropositive, erosive, nodular rheumatoid disease (Walker and Wright, 1969). Bibasilar interstitial infiltrates are found on the radiograph, which may eventually progress to honeycombing. Patients with upper lobe bullous disease without basilar infiltrates have been reported, but this presentation is rare. Pulmonary function studies reveal a restrictive ventilatory pattern with an abnormality of gas transfer. Exercise studies indicate a pattern of rapid shallow breathing and exercise-induced oxygen desaturation. The disease may be progressive, but few patients with rheumatoid arthritis die of progressive respiratory failure. In those patients hospitalized for rheumatoid ILD, the prognosis is poor, with a median survival of 3.5 years and a 5-year survival rate of 39% (Hakala, 1988). There is no established therapy for this disease. There are occasional reports of treatment success with corticosteroids, penicillamine, methotrexate, and azathioprine. However, ILD can infrequently develop as a result of methotrexate therapy.

Systemic Sclerosis

Systemic sclerosis (scleroderma) is a generalized disease of connective tissue that is characterized by inflammation and degeneration leading to fibrosis. Shortly after the description of the original disease, pulmonary involvement was noted (Day, 1870). The organs that are most commonly affected include the skin, blood vessels, synovium, skeletal muscles, lungs, gastrointestinal tract, and kidneys. Women are affected three to four times more frequently than are men. Patients present with Raynaud's phenomenon, swelling of the fingers, or arthritis of the small joints of the hand. Many patients have esophageal involvement, and recurrent aspiration may play a role in the pathogenesis of the lung disease. Up to 70% of patients with scleroderma develop pathologic evidence of lung disease, although a minority are clinically symptomatic (Owens and Follansbee, 1987). The pathologic findings are similar to those in IPF. ILD is the most common manifestation and is seen as bibasilar linear or nodular infiltrates. BAL shows an intense alveolitis with macrophages and granulocytes (neutrophils and eosinophils) in about one half of patients (Silver et al, 1990). Pulmonary function testing reveals first a reduction in the diffusing capacity and then a reduction in vital capacity. The relative risk for the development of pulmonary fibrosis in patients with systemic sclerosis is increased more than 16-fold if the major histocompatibility antigen class DR3/DRw52a or the autoantibody to topoisomerase I (Scl-70 autoantibody) is present (Briggs et al, 1991). A few patients develop pulmonary arterial hypertension, and most of these patients have little or no evidence of fibrosis on chest radiography. These patients complain of marked dyspnea and fatigue, and a striking reduction in the diffusing capacity is usually found (Owens et al, 1983). Most patients have a gradually progressive course, but occasionally a patient may have a rapid onset and progression (Schneider et al, 1982). There is no single agent that has been shown to be effective in clinical trials. Penicillamine interferes with the cross-linking of mature collagen. Two studies using this agent have indicated a trend toward improvement, but their design flaws render a definitive statement regarding the efficacy of this agent impossible (de Clerck et al, 1987; Steen et al, 1985). Patients with pulmonary arterial hypertension may respond to vasodilator therapy. There may be an increased frequency of lung cancer, especially bronchoalveolar and small cell carcinoma, in patients with scleroderma, but this remains controversial (Wiedemann and Matthay, 1989).

Sjögren's Syndrome

Sjögren's syndrome is an autoimmune chronic inflammatory disease of which the main features are xerostomia and keratoconjunctivitis sicca; a secondary form includes other connective tissue disease. Diffuse ILD occurs in up to 25% of patients (Constantopoulos et al, 1985). There may be diffuse bilateral reticular or nodular infiltrates on the chest radiograph. Occasionally the pathologic findings reveal LIP (Strimlan et al, 1976). The course of ILD in patients with Sjögren's syndrome is unpredictable, and the condition can stabilize or progress to severe disease. Corticosteroids appear to be efficacious in about one half of the patients treated. LIP can transform to "pseudolymphoma" or malignant lymphoma, which appear as mass lesions on the chest radiograph.

Systemic Lupus Erythematosus

SLE is a disease of unknown cause characterized by multiorgan inflammation. It is associated with the production of autoantibodies against nuclear, cytoplasmic, and cell membrane antigens. The clinical manifestations of SLE include fatigue, anemia, rashes, fever, pericarditis, pleurisy, nephritis, vasculitis, and central nervous system disease. The pulmonary manifestations of SLE were recognized by Osler (1904), who reported a persistent lung infiltrate that varied with the clinical activity of the underlying disease. The respiratory system is involved more commonly in SLE than in the other collagen-vascular diseases. SLE can affect the pleura, interstitium, vasculature, larynx, airways, and respiratory musculature (Hunninghake and Fauci, 1979). Unlike rheumatoid arthritis and scleroderma, ILD is uncommon, occurring in fewer than 3% of patients (Eisenberg et al, 1973). The pathologic findings in SLE include interstitial fibrosis, vasculitis, hematoxylin bodies, and interstitial pneumonitis. Other findings (including pulmonary hemorrhage, edema, and hyaline membranes), although reported, are often related to coincident illnesses (Haupt et al, 1981). Electron microscopic evaluation of lung biopsy specimens from patients with SLE and ILD reveal intracellular tubuloreticular structures within pulmonary vascular endothelial cells that may represent evidence of previous viral infection (Fraire et al, 1971). It is highly probable that the pulmonary fibrosis in patients with SLE represents the sequelae of episodes of acute pneumonitis, because most patients who survive the acute phase have functional abnormalities (Matthay et al, 1974). Corticosteroids are the recommended therapy for ILD in SLE, and the response is variable.

Polymyositis/Dermatomyositis

Polymyositis is an inflammatory myopathy of unknown cause that is called *dermatomyositis* in the presence of a characteristic rash. Pulmonary involvement was first noted 1956 by Mills and Matthews. Traditionally three types of pulmonary involvement have been described: (1) aspiration pneumonia, (2) ventilatory insufficiency, and (3) ILD (Hepper et al, 1964). Involvement of the posterior pharyngeal muscles can lead to dysphonia and dysphagia. Interstitial pneumonitis occurs in 5% of patients and precedes the muscular disease in one third of patients (Schwarz et al, 1976). The ILD in polymyositis/dermatomyositis can be asymptomatic; insidious, with the gradual development of dyspnea and other symptoms; or acute in onset, with dyspnea and lung infiltrates (Frazier and Miller, 1974). Patients with extensive fibrosis on lung biopsy fare poorly; those with evidence of active inflammation respond well to corticosteroids (Duncan et al, 1974). Overall, corticosteroids are helpful in 50% of affected patients (Schwarz et al, 1976).

Ankylosing Spondylitis

Ankylosing spondylitis is a chronic disease that can result in progressive stiffening of the sacroiliac joints and spine. Significant pulmonary disease is uncommon, with a reported incidence of 1.3% (Rosenow et al, 1977). Common pulmonary manifestations include chest wall restriction and fibrobullous disease. Upper lobe fibrobullous disease develops in 1% of the population. Cavities may form and become superinfected with *Aspergillus* or atypical mycobacterial species. In the late stages, patients may develop hemoptysis and recurrent pneumothorax. There are no effective medications for this disease.

Pulmonary-Renal Syndromes

Goodpasture's Syndrome

In 1919, Goodpasture described the occurrence of pulmonary hemorrhage and glomerulonephritis 6 weeks after influenza. The term "Goodpasture's syndrome" was not introduced until 1958 (Stanton and Tange, 1958). Goodpasture's syndrome is an autoimmune disorder in which antiglomerular basement membrane autoantibody is implicated. The patients typically present with pulmonary hemorrhage and glomerulonephritis and show linear deposits of immunoglobulin along the renal basement membrane (Wilson and Dixon, 1979). Antiglomerular basement membrane antibodies recognize an epitope in the $\alpha3$(IV) chain of type IV collagen (Saus et al, 1988). Upper respiratory tract infections and exposure to volatile hydrocarbons precede the illness in some patients (Bierne and Brennan, 1972). Male patients predominate, and most cases occur in patients between 20 and 50 years of age. Sixty percent to 80% of patients have clinically observed pulmonary and renal disease; in 10% the disease is limited to the lung (Rees, 1984). In most patients, hemoptysis is the presenting complaint. Less commonly, the patients present with nonspecific symptoms of renal failure. Laboratory examination reveals iron-deficiency anemia, mildly elevated sedimentation rate, and evidence of renal impairment. Urinalysis shows proteinuria, hematuria, and red blood cell casts. The single-breath diffusing capacity may be elevated because intra-alveolar blood binds inhaled carbon monoxide; an elevation of this test finding may precede the onset of clinical pulmonary hemorrhage (Addleman et al, 1985). Chest radiographs typically demonstrate a bilateral acinar filling pattern, but they can show a mixed interstitial-alveolar pattern or a reticulonodular pattern in persistent disease. In the appropriate clinical setting, a positive test result for circulating antiglomerular basement membrane antibodies establishes the diagnosis (Young, 1989). If the diagnosis is in question, a renal biopsy should be performed and the biopsy specimen should be stained for light microscopy, immunofluorescent studies, and electron microscopy. Focal nephritis or crescentic glomerulonephritis is usually seen on light microscopy. Direct immunofluorescence testing stains linear deposits of immunoglobulin (usually IgG) along the glomerular basement membrane. The recommended therapy for Goodpasture's syndrome includes plasma exchange, high-dose parenteral corticosteroids, and cyclophosphamide. Plasma exchange reduces the level of antibody to the glomerular basement membrane, and immunosuppression inhibits its further synthesis, although it is not established that plasma exchange affects survival (Shumak and Rock, 1984). The use of pulse corticosteroid therapy has also been proposed, but its efficacy compared with standard doses of corticosteroids has not been examined (Leatherman, 1987).

Idiopathic Pulmonary Hemosiderosis

Idiopathic pulmonary hemosiderosis refers to alveolar hemorrhage that occurs in the absence of hemodynamic abnormality, infection, coagulopathy, or systemic disorders, such as SLE, antiglomerular basement membrane antibody disease, or vasculitis. This rare disease occurs mainly in children younger than 10 years of age and adults in their 20s and 30s. Adult male patients are affected more than are female patients. The most common presentations include hemoptysis and iron-deficiency anemia (Leatherman et al, 1984). Other symptoms include dyspnea, cough, malaise, pallor, and fever. Transient alveolar opacities develop during the acute phase of the illness, and, with repetitive episodes, an interstitial pattern develops with progressive dyspnea, crackles, clubbing, and pulmonary hypertension. Antiglomerular basement membrane antibodies are not usually present. BAL fluid supports the diagnosis if hemosiderin-laden macrophages are demonstrated. On open lung biopsy, the alveoli are seen to be filled with blood and hemosiderin-filled macrophages, with nonspecific septal thickening and alveolar lining cell hyperplasia. Immunoglobulin deposition along the alveolar capillary basement membrane has not been demonstrated. Corticosteroids and immunosuppressants have been anecdotally reported to be successful in some patients (Leatherman, 1987).

Chronic Eosinophilic Pneumonia

Historically, chronic eosinophilic pneumonia was described in the group of diseases characterized by pulmonary infiltrates and eosinophilia (Crofton et al, 1952). Women are twice as likely as men to be affected with the disorder. They present with asthmatic symptoms and systemic features, such as fever, night sweats, and weight loss (Jederlinic et al, 1988). Laboratory investigations show marked eosinophilia, an elevated sedimentation rate, and high levels of IgE. The chest radiograph shows a characteristic pattern of peripheral infiltrates, the photographic negative of pulmonary edema (Gaensler and Carrington, 1977). Open lung biopsy is not usually required, but, if performed, it reveals alveolitis with eosinophils and macrophages, multinucleated giant cells, and angiitis with diffuse pulmonary fibrosis. The diagnosis is often made on clinical information, and steroid therapy is usually successful, although relapses are common (Pearson and Rosenow, 1978).

Pulmonary Alveolar Proteinosis

Pulmonary alveolar proteinosis (PAP), first described by Rosen and colleagues (1958), is characterized by the accumulation of PAS (periodic acid–Schiff)–positive, phospholipid-rich material in the alveolar spaces, with minimal fibrosis and inflammation of the interstitium. Pulmonary macrophages exhibit morphologic abnormalities, including excessive lipid accumulation and giant secondary lysosome formation, and function abnormally (Golde et al, 1976; Gonzalez-Rothi and Harris, 1986). PAP has been associated with silica and aluminum dust, malignancy, fungal infection, and parasitic disease. Several cases of PAP have been reported with *P. carinii* infection (Israel and Magnussen, 1989). The patient typically presents with dyspnea on exertion. The chest radiograph reveals interstitial and fine alveolar densities. The serum lactate dehydrogenase level is frequently elevated in this disorder (Martin et al, 1978). BAL and transbronchial biopsy are usually diagnostic, but open lung biopsy may be required (Martin et al, 1980). The recommended treatment for PAP is whole lung lavage under general anesthesia. The disease is of unpredictable course; it may resolve spontaneously or alternatively progress, ultimately leading to death (Claypool et al, 1984).

Inherited Lung Disorders

Neurofibromatosis (von Recklinghausen's Disease)

Neurofibromatosis is an autosomal dominant disorder characterized by café au lait spots and neurofibroma of the nervous system and skin. Interstitial fibrosis occurs in up to 20% of patients.

Tuberous Sclerosis

Tuberous sclerosis is an autosomal dominant disorder associated with the development of multiple tumors of ectodermal and mesodermal origin. They have been described in the retina, skin, kidneys, brain, gingiva, heart, thyroid, pancreas, ovaries, uterus, and spleen. In 0.1% to 1% of patients, there is pulmonary involvement, which pathologically is identical to that seen in patients with LAM (Dwyer et al, 1971). Chest radiographs show normal or large lung volumes, with a diffuse microreticulonodular pattern or honeycombing, and occasionally pneumothorax. Pulmonary function testing typically reveals airway obstruction with gas trapping and a decreased single-breath, carbon monoxide–diffusing capacity (Slingerland et al, 1989). The course is usually progressive, and death from respiratory failure is quite common.

Familial Idiopathic Pulmonary Fibrosis

Familial IPF is an autosomal dominant disorder that is identical to IPF.

Amyloidosis

Three distinct forms of pulmonary amyloidosis have been described: (1) focal deposits of amyloid within the mucosa and adventitia of the major airways; (2) single or multiple parenchymal nodules; and (3) diffuse parenchymal infiltrates involving the alveolar septa and the walls of small blood vessels. Patients present with dyspnea, wheezing, chronic cough, or hemoptysis, and a restrictive ventilatory defect is found on pulmonary function testing. The chest radiograph typically shows diffuse reticulonodular infiltrates, but various other radiographic appearances may be present (Himmelfarb et al, 1977). There is no treatment for systemic amyloidosis, and the disease is usually fatal.

Human Immunodeficiency Virus Disease and Interstitial Lung Disease

ILD was described in patients with human immunodeficiency virus (HIV) disease. *P. carinii* pneumonia and viral pneumonitis are the most common reasons for ILD. Kaposi's sarcoma and LIP, two causes of ILD seen occasionally in the HIV population, are discussed next.

Kaposi's Sarcoma

Kaposi's sarcoma occurs in 10% to 30% of patients with the acquired immunodeficiency syndrome (AIDS), and pulmonary involvement occurs in 21% to 40% of those with cutaneous involvement (White and Matthay, 1989). Common presenting symptoms are cough, dyspnea, stridor, fever, hoarseness, and hemoptysis. Arterial blood gas measurements reveal a reduction in the partial pressure of oxygen and a widened alveolar-arterial gradient. The chest radiograph is usually abnormal and shows four major patterns: (1) interstitial, (2) alveolar, (3) mixed alveolar-interstitial, and (4) nodular disease. Mediastinal, hilar, and paratracheal adenopathy may also be present in Kaposi's sarcoma, and up to 30% of patients have unilateral or bilateral effusions. Nodular lung infiltrates accompanied by pleural effusions and intrathoracic lymphadenopathy in the right clinical setting are highly predictive of pulmonary Kaposi's sarcoma (Davis et al, 1987). Thoracentesis and pleural biopsy do not contribute to the diagnosis of Kaposi's sarcoma. The CT scan may define the distribution of the tumor and demonstrate nodules, lymphadenopathy, and pleural disease, but these findings are not specific. Bronchoscopy may reveal the characteristic lesions of Kaposi's sarcoma in the tracheobronchial tree. The lesion appears as a flat or raised plaque with a violaceous color, but the absence of endobronchial lesions does not exclude the disease (Gill et al, 1989). Bronchial washings do not contribute information to the diagnosis. Transbronchial biopsy is not recommended because the diagnostic yield is low. Crush artifact, hemorrhage, granulation tissue, and fibrosis may mimic the histologic findings of Kaposi's sarcoma. Open lung biopsy has the highest diagnostic yield, but it is not 100% sensitive because lesions have been found at autopsy that were not seen by open lung biopsy (Ognibene et al, 1985). The histologic findings of Kaposi's sarcoma consist of swollen endothelial cells in vascular lumina, loose aggregations of spindle cells, hemorrhage, and stromal hemosiderin deposits with interstitial inflammation. There is no known effective treatment for Kaposi's sarcoma; however, short-term palliation can be produced with interferon alfa, radiotherapy, or combined chemotherapy (White and Matthay, 1989). A high incidence of infections occurs in patients with Kaposi's sarcoma; therefore, new symptoms should be investigated. New antiretroviral strategies incorporating nucleoside analogues with a protease inhibitor, also referred to as highly active antiretroviral therapy (HAART), are noted to result in regression of pulmonary lesions of Kaposi's sarcoma (Aboulafia, 1998).

Lymphocytic Interstitial Pneumonia

LIP is so common as a complication of HIV infection in children that its presence is used as an AIDS-defining illness, but it is less prevalent in adults (Centers for Disease Control and Prevention [CDC], 1985). In HIV-infected adults, LIP is more common in blacks who have an excess of HLA-DR5 (Itescu et al, 1990). LIP occurs in association with HIV-type 2 (HIV-2) as well as HIV-1. In adults, LIP is not a criterion for the CDC definition of AIDS. Clinical features include cough, dyspnea, fever,

INTERSTITIAL LUNG DISEASE ASSOCIATED WITH HUMAN IMMUNODEFICIENCY VIRUS INFECTIONS

Viral
- Cytomegalovirus
- Herpes

Fungal
- *Pneumocystis carinii*
- *Mycobacterium tuberculosis*
- *Mycobacterium avium-intracellulare*

Lymphocytic interstitial pneumonitis
Nonspecific interstitial pneumonitis
Kaposi's sarcoma
Lymphoma
Bronchogenic carcinoma
Alveolar proteinosis

and bilateral reticulonodular or micronodular infiltrates that are diffuse or predominant in the lower lobes on the chest radiograph (Fig. 24–8) (Oldham et al, 1989). BAL demonstrates increased lymphocytes in patients with LIP, but this finding is not specific for this condition (Turner-Warwick and Haslam, 1987). Open lung biopsy is usually necessary for establishing the diagnosis. Typical histologic findings include a diffuse infiltration of the interstitium with lymphocytes and plasma cells. Immunologic stains show a predominance of T lymphocytes, without necrosis or evidence of vasculitis. The course of LIP is variable, and some patients recover without therapy. The results of therapy with steroids have been disappointing, and responders ultimately die with other conditions. LIP is not limited to HIV-positive patients and may be seen in other patients, such as those with Sjögren's syndrome. However, the lymphocytic infiltration is due to $CD8^+$ cells in patients with AIDS, rather than to $CD4^+$ infiltration classically seen in Sjögren's syndrome (Itescu et al, 1990).

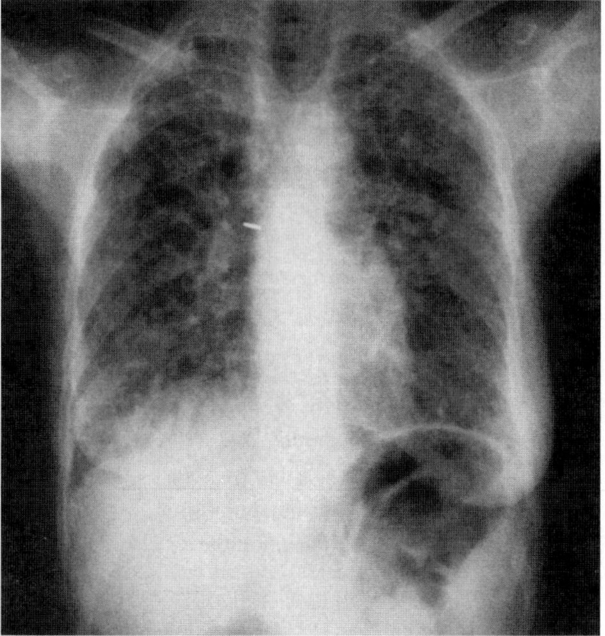

FIGURE 24–8 ■ Posteroanterior chest radiograph from a patient with lymphocytic interstitial pneumonitis.

DISEASES OF KNOWN ORIGIN

Extrinsic Allergic Alveolitis

The term *extrinsic allergic alveolitis* (EAA, or hypersensitivity pneumonitis) refers to a group of disorders characterized by a response of the lung to fine dusts of organic origin that penetrate into the distal lung parenchyma (Reynolds, 1982). EAA has acute, subacute, and chronic forms, which are determined by the frequency and intensity of exposure. In the acute disease, chills, fever, dyspnea, and malaise occur 4 to 6 hours after exposure. A careful history should be taken to determine whether the patient has been exposed to an offending antigen at work (e.g., hay, sugar cane, or malt) or at home (e.g., air conditioning or sauna) or has special hobbies (e.g., parakeet or pigeon breeding). Examination classically reveals crackles in the bases and, in severe cases, fever and cyanosis. In the subacute form of this disease, there is an insidious onset of malaise, cough, sputum production, dyspnea, fatigue, and anorexia, with weight loss. The patient with the chronic form of this disease may develop respiratory failure. Patients with EAA typically exhibit precipitating antibodies against the organic dust or antigen. BAL may reveal a lymphocytic alveolitis with a predominance of T suppressor cells with impaired function (Hughes et al, 1984). Biopsy show both alveolar and interstitial inflammation with lymphocytes, plasma cells, and macrophages with a foamy cytoplasm. Common histologic findings include granulomas, foreign body material, and bronchiolitis obliterans (Reyes et al, 1982). An HRCT scan may define subacute disease by demonstrating areas of hazy increased density (Silver et al, 1989). In 50% of patients, small ill-defined nodules are seen in the areas of air space disease. Treatment of EAA consists of recognizing the offending antigen and eliminating patient contact. This may involve wearing protective masks, alteration in handling the antigen, or changes in occupation. Moderate and severely ill patients should be treated with high-dose corticosteroids.

Radiation-Induced Lung Disease

The first cases of radiation-induced lung injury were published in the 1920s (Hines, 1922). Radiation-induced

INTERSTITIAL LUNG DISEASES OF KNOWN CAUSE

Extrinsic allergic alveolitis (hypersensitivity pneumonitis)
Radiation-induced lung disease
Drug-induced lung disease
Pneumoconiosis
Lymphangitic carcinomatosis

EXAMPLES OF DISEASES CAUSED BY INHALED ORGANIC DUSTS

Bird breeder's lung
Air conditioner lung
Farmer's lung
Cheese handler's lung
Malt worker's lung
Bagassosis
Sequoiosis
Maple bark stripper's disease
Sauna taker's disease
Pituitary snuff lung
Paprika splitter's lung
Wood pulp worker's disease
Detergent worker's lung
Dry rot disease
Mummy unwrapper's disease
Mushroom worker's disease

lung injury presents as ILD in patients with cancer and is difficult to differentiate from malignancy. Radiation-induced lung injury is classified into two clinical syndromes: radiation-induced pneumonitis and radiation-induced fibrosis, which follows pneumonitis. Radiation-induced pneumonitis, which is reported as early as 2 weeks following the completion of therapy, occurs typically 2 to 6 months after the last dose. Radiographic changes can be expected 8 weeks after 4000 cGy and 1 week earlier for each 1000-cGy increment above 4000 (Libshitz and Southard, 1974). Radiographic changes consistent with radiation-induced pneumonitis can be seen in 50% to 70% of patients who receive radiotherapy for carcinoma of the breast, but symptoms develop in less than 10% (Fleming et al, 1961). The symptoms include a nonproductive cough, progressive dyspnea on exertion, low-grade fever, and pleuritic pain. An intractable cough may develop, with thick sputum production. Examination of the lungs is usually normal. The first abnormality noted on chest radiography is often a diffuse haze that quickly progresses to patchy alveolar opacities (Gross, 1977). Later, the opacities form sharp boundaries to redefine the treated areas. In some cases, the changes may extend outside the radiation field, and abnormalities in the contralateral lung have been reported. BAL demonstrates an increase in total cells and a marked lymphocytosis in both relative and absolute terms (Gibson et al, 1988). The acute pneumonitis can resolve or alternatively progress to respiratory failure.

EXAMPLES OF INORGANIC DUSTS THAT CAUSE INTERSTITIAL LUNG DISEASE

Silicates	Cadmium
Talc	Tungsten
Asbestos	Titanium
Aluminum silicates	Hafnium
Mica	Cobalt
Kaolin	Niobium
Diatomaceous earth	Titanium oxide
Silicas	Tin
Metals	Rare earths
Aluminum	Scandium
Beryllium	Cerium
Iron	Yttrium
Barium	Lanthanum

Radiation-induced fibrosis develops in most patients with the radiation-induced pneumonitis syndrome within 1 year of therapy. Although most patients are asymptomatic, the condition in a minority of patients progresses to chronic respiratory failure. Chemotherapeutic agents, such as bleomycin, vincristine, cyclophosphamide, and dactinomycin, increase the toxicity of radiation-induced injury. Pulmonary function tests show a decline in all lung volumes and a reduction in the diffusing capacity for carbon monoxide (Cudkowitz et al, 1969). Lymphangitic spread can mimic radiation damage but can be distinguished by certain characteristics; lymphangitic disease involves the lung bases and shows prominent septal lines with symptoms more severe than the radiographic abnormality would indicate. Corticosteroids are used in severe cases of pneumonitis, although there are no clinical trials to validate their use in humans. During episodes of severe pneumonitis, prednisone (1 mg/kg/day) should be started (Gross, 1977). After a complete response has been documented, a slow taper is advised to prevent recurrent pneumonitis.

Drug-Induced Lung Disease

More than 50 drugs have been reported to cause pulmonary fibrosis (Rosenow et al, 1992). Some drugs injure the lung in an idiosyncratic and sporadic fashion; others cause dose-dependent injury to the lung. Drugs may injure the lung through both direct and indirect mechanisms. The direct effects on the pulmonary parenchyma include oxidant injury, cytotoxic effects on the capillary endothelial cells, deposition of phospholipids, and immune injury. Drugs may indirectly damage the pulmonary parenchyma by altering antioxidant defenses or by amplification of endogenous inflammatory responses. No laboratory tests exist that are diagnostic for drug-induced pulmonary disease. If a drug is suspected of causing disease, it should be discontinued. Most drug reactions are reversible; however, fatalities are not uncommon. Therapy with corticosteroids may be necessary in severe disease. Amiodarone, paraquat, and bleomycin are drugs that induce damage by different mechanisms. They are discussed in detail next.

Amiodarone-Induced Disease

Amiodarone is an antiarrhythmic agent useful in the treatment of serious ventricular arrhythmias.

Approximately 6% of patients who receive more than 400 mg/day of amiodarone for 2 or more months develop pulmonary toxicity (Martin and Rosenow, 1988). Symptoms of toxicity include exertional dyspnea, cough, fever, and chest pain. Malaise and weight loss have been re-

EXAMPLES OF DRUGS AND OTHER AGENTS THAT CAUSE INTERSTITIAL LUNG DISEASE

Antibiotics	Allopurinol
Penicillin	Endocrine drugs
Sulfonamides	Tolbutamide
Nitrofurantoin	Chlorpropamide
Tetracycline	Oncologic drugs
Erythromycin	Bleomycin
Isoniazid	Cyclophosphamide
Para-amino-salicylic acid	Azathioprine
Cardiac drugs	Busulfan
Amiodarone	Chlorambucil
Hydralazine	Methotrexate
Procainamide	Nitrosoureas
Tocainamide	Melphalan
β-Blockers	Procarbazine
Hydrochlorothiazide	Mitomycin C
Neurologic drugs	Mercaptopurine
Phenytoin	Thioguanine
Carbamazepine	Other drugs/agents
Chlorpromazine	Mineral oil
Imipramine	Talc (intravenous drug abuse)
Dantrolene	Silicon
Amitriptyline	Nose drops
Methylphenidate	Paraquat
Pentolinium	Radiation
Mecamylamine	Oxygen
Hexamethonium	Sulfur dioxide
Rheumatologic drugs	Chlorine gas
Phenylbutazone	Fats/oils
Corticosteroids	Vinyl chloride
Gold	Metal fumes
Naproxen	Hydrocarbon or mercury vapors
Penicillamine	
Cromolyn sodium	

corded. Patients may present in two ways. There is a subacute illness characterized by cough, dyspnea, weight loss, and diffuse pulmonary infiltrates. There is also an acute syndrome with diffuse alveolar opacities that mimics pulmonary edema and pneumonia. Pleural effusions and localized infiltrates may be present. Physical findings of amiodarone-induced toxicity include fever, tachypnea, and inspiratory crackles. The presence of abnormalities on chest radiography may predict a higher risk for pulmonary toxicity. Routine pulmonary function testing reveals an impairment of the DLCO. Gallium scans may also be positive in amiodarone-induced pulmonary toxicity; however, they lack sensitivity and specificity (Zhu et al, 1988). BAL may reveal foamy alveolar macrophages containing intracytoplasmic lamellar inclusions. These cells are markers of amiodarone exposure and not diagnostic of toxicity. In most cases, discontinuation of therapy results in the complete reversal of the pulmonary abnormalities (Cooper et al, 1986). Treatment with systemic steroids is indicated in some cases. In patients for whom amiodarone is the only available option for the treatment of serious cardiac dysrhythmia, corticosteroid is added to the lowest effective dose of amiodarone, and patients are maintained on the combination regimen (Rosenow, 1994).

Bleomycin-Induced Disease

Bleomycin is a chemotherapeutic agent derived from a strain of *Streptomyces verticillus*, with a potential to produce pulmonary toxicity. Pulmonary fibrosis, the most common manifestation, can lead to respiratory failure and death. The true incidence of bleomycin toxicity is between 2% and 5%. There is a dose-toxicity relationship such that with doses exceeding 400 to 450 U of bleomycin, there are significant numbers of cases of toxicity (Ginsberg and Comis, 1982). There is evidence that suggests that the combination of radiation or oxygen with bleomycin increases the risk of pulmonary toxicity (Goldiner et al, 1978). Symptoms of toxicity occur at 4 to 10 weeks following therapy but have been reported up to 6 months later. The most prevalent symptoms are nonproductive cough, dyspnea, and fever. Fine crackles are commonly heard at the lung bases. As the disease advances, the crackles coarsen and occupy the lower two thirds of the lung. Monitoring of total lung capacity seems to be a more specific indicator of toxicity than is the DLCO (Wolkowicz et al, 1992). The chest radiograph demonstrates bibasilar reticular or nodular infiltrates. An early change is a triangular infiltrate in the costophrenic angles. With advanced disease, the infiltrates may progress to the middle and upper areas of the lungs. Some patients show a peripheral distribution of infiltrates in a subpleural allocation. Bilateral, focal, and asymmetric patterns and normal radiographs may be seen. A common finding is elevation of the diaphragm secondary to the loss of lung volume. Occasionally, large nodules may be visualized. This can present difficulties in the differentiation from metastatic disease. CT scans commonly show changes that were not seen on plain radiographs, especially subpleural, ill-defined, nodular densities at the posterior lung bases (Bellamy et al, 1985). The evaluation of these nodules discovered on CT presents a diagnostic dilemma, and each patient must be evaluated on an individual basis. In patients with mild toxicity, discontinuation of the bleomycin may reverse the pulmonary disease, but corticosteroid therapy may be necessary. A smaller group will have progressive disease, and a fulminant course leading to death has been reported.

Talc Granulomatosis

Talc granulomatosis occurs in intravenous drug abusers who inject crushed tablets. Talc (magnesium silicate) deposits in the pulmonary arterioles, arteries, and interstitium. Patients present with cough, dyspnea, cor pulmonale, or sudden death. The chest radiograph may be normal in one half of the affected patients, or it may show 1-mm micronodules. The nodules eventually coalesce, and extensive midlung zone fibrotic changes, as in progressive massive fibrosis, can develop. The lower lobes become relatively translucent, often with bullous formation (Pare et al, 1989). Many of these patients demonstrate an obstructive ventilatory defect (Pare et al, 1979). At a late stage, pathologic examination of the lung reveals emphysema, granulomatous inflammation, and fibrosis surrounding the talc particles.

Oxygen Toxicity

Oxygen in high concentrations is toxic to the human lung. The mechanism of damage is postulated to be the inability of antioxidant enzymes to rid the lung of toxic free radicals from the oxygen therapy (Deneke and Fanburg, 1980). Damage occurs acutely (exudative phase), with an increase in alveolar-capillary permeability that may be reversible, and chronically (proliferative phase) (Davis et al, 1983). An ILD may develop with hyperplasia of type 2 cells and deposition of collagen in the interstitium.

Paraquat Toxicity

Ingestion of only 1 teaspoonful of liquid concentrate of the herbicide paraquat can be fatal. One to 5 days after paraquat poisoning, there is an acute syndrome of fever, dyspnea, fatigue, and gastrointestinal problems. Paraquat can induce an ILD because toxic oxygen radicals are generated, which causes secondary alveolitis and subsequent fibrosis (Schoenberger et al, 1984). Ultimately, there is respiratory failure. In acute cases, the paraquat should be removed by gastric lavage, charcoal, and hemoperfusion. Vitamin E is often given as antioxidant therapy; however, there are no clinical trials to support its use. Oxygen should be kept at low concentrations because hyperoxia may accelerate injury.

Pneumoconiosis

Pneumoconiosis is defined by the International Labor Organization as the accumulation of inorganic dust in the lungs and the reactions of tissue to its presence. The type of injury depends on the type of inorganic dust and the length and intensity of exposure. The most common syndromes include silicosis, coalworker's pneumoconiosis, asbestosis, and beryllium-induced disease.

Silicosis is caused by inhalation of silicon dioxide or crystalline silica. Patients characteristically present with dyspnea on exertion and an abnormal chest radiograph (Graham, 1992). Miners, foundry workers, tunnelers, casters, and ceramic molders are at risk. In simple silicosis, chest radiographs typically show rounded opacities with an upper lobe predominance. These nodules can progress and form large lung masses (progressive massive fibrosis) and destroy lung tissue. Eggshell calcification of the intrapulmonary, hilar, or mediastinal lymph nodes is common. Patients with silicosis are at increased risk for the development of tuberculosis, which often causes an increase in the opacities or cavitation.

Another common occupational ILD is asbestosis, which is characterized by interstitial pulmonary fibrosis manifested by dyspnea, cough, basal crepitations, clubbing, and, ultimately, right heart failure (Mossman and Gee, 1989). Patients at risk include shipbuilders, boiler makers, miners, and brake-lining installers. BAL or biopsy may reveal evidence of dust deposition, which can support the diagnosis (Sebastian et al, 1988). In the patient with an appropriate occupational history, an abnormal chest radiograph has been accepted as evidence of asbestosis. The findings of asbestosis on high-resolution CT scans resemble those of UIP, including subpleural lines, parenchymal bands, thickening of the interlobular septal lines, thickening of structures in the secondary pulmonary lobule, and honeycombing.

Pulmonary Lymphangitic Carcinomatosis

Pulmonary lymphangitic carcinomatosis can mimic ILD. In pulmonary lymphangitic carcinomatosis, there is tumor growth along the pulmonary lymphatic channels. The major lymph vessels are found in the bronchovascular bundles, interlobular septa, and subpleural regions of the lung. There is a pathognomonic appearance of uneven thickening of bronchovascular bundles and the interlobular septa, giving these structures a beaded appearance. The thickening may be seen extending to the pleural surfaces or it may form a polygonal arcade. The chest radiograph is normal in 50% of patients with biopsy-proven disease (Trapnell, 1964). The high-resolution CT scan shows characteristic polygonal lines that are not seen on conventional 10-mm cuts (Stein et al, 1987). The diagnosis can usually be made by BAL or transbronchial biopsy (Levy et al, 1988). Open lung biopsy should be done if these tests are not diagnostic. Because the disease is focal in about 50% of patients, the CT scan can be used to guide the biopsy by the surgeon. Occasionally, the diagnosis may be made by determining the cytologic characteristics of blood drawn through a wedged pulmonary artery catheter (Masson et al, 1989).

COMMENTS AND CONTROVERSIES

Thoracic surgeons continually encounter ILD in their practices, and frequently patients with ILD require definitive diagnosis. In most cases, transbronchial lung biopsy is sufficient. However, when this fails or is contraindicated, a thoracoscopic or open lung biopsy is required. As the authors indicate, in assessing chronic ILD, the lingula should be avoided, and biopsy specimens from severely affected and less severely affected areas should be obtained.

These patients can present with massive hemoptysis, pneumothorax, or focal lesions requiring differentiation from malignancy. Because of the underlying restrictive disease, and often severely impaired DLCO*, management can be difficult when patients present with complications such as pneumothorax or require a resection. In such patients, if a pneumothorax requires treatment, pleurodesis should be considered even in the first instance. In the terminal phase of many of these diseases, patients can now be considered for lung transplantation.*

R.J.G.

■ KEY REFERENCES

Chan-Yeung M, Muller NL: Cryptogenic fibrosing alveolitis. Lancet 350:651, 1997.

A review of various aspects of IPF, including epidemiology, pathology, clinical presentation, diagnosis, and treatment of IPF.

Cooper JAD Jr, White DA, Matthay RA: Drug induced pulmonary disease. Am Rev Respir Dis 133:321, 1986.

This is a comprehensive review of the complications in the lung induced by a wide variety of therapeutic agents.

Crystal RG, Gadek JE, Ferrans VJ et al: Interstitial lung disease: Current concepts of pathogenesis, staging and therapy. Am J Med 70:542, 1981.

This is a review of the proposed pathogenesis of ILD, including the role of BAL and gallium scanning.

DeRemee RA: The roentgenographic staging of sarcoidosis: Historical and contemporary perspectives. Chest 83:128, 1983.

The author offers a defense of the traditional approach to the classification of patients with sarcoidosis.

Epler G, Colby T, McLoud T et al: Bronchiolitis obliterans organizing pneumonia. N Engl J Med 312:152, 1985.

A description of the clinical, radiographic, physiologic, and pathologic features of BOOP in a large series of patients. The authors emphasize the importance of the pathologic diagnosis, because the prognosis of this disorder is different from that of IPF, with which it is commonly confused.

Fauci AS, Haynes BF, Costa J et al: Lymphomatoid granulomatosis—prospective clinical and therapeutic experience over 10 years. N Engl J Med 306:68, 1982.

In this landmark article, the response to chemotherapy and the development of lymphoma in patients who do not respond to therapy are described.

Hunninghake GW, Kalica AR: Approaches to the treatment of pulmonary fibrosis: Work summary. Am J Respir Crit Care Med 151:915, 1995.

A brief but comprehensive review of various pharmacotherapeutic approaches to treatment of IPF, with proposed modes of action. A workshop summary emphasizing the basic science as it applies to treatment of IPF and other inflammatory disorders.

Johnson MA, Kwan SK, Snell NJC et al: Randomised controlled trial comparing prednisolone alone with cyclophosphamide and low dose prednisolone in combination in cryptogenic fibrosing alveolitis. Thorax 44:280, 1989.

Prednisolone given in a dose of 60 mg/day for 1 month followed by a tapering regimen to 20 mg on alternate days was compared with cyclophosphamide 100 to 120 mg/day plus prednisolone 20 mg on alternate days. Many patients did not respond to either regimen, but there were responders in each group. It does not appear from this study that the cyclophosphamide regimen was significantly better than was the prednisolone alone.

Katzenstein AA, Myers JL: Idiopathic pulmonary fibrosis: Clinical relevance of pathologic classification: State of the art. Am J Respir Crit Care Med 157:1301, 1998.

A landmark paper that outlines the new pathologic classification of idiopathic pulmonary fibrosis, the rationale for the proposed changes to the old classification scheme, clinical presentation of various pathologic types of IPF, their natural history, and response to therapy.

Raghu G: Idiopathic pulmonary fibrosis: A rational clinical approach. Chest 92:148, 1987.

A reasonable approach to the management of a difficult group of patients is offered. The author is conservative with respect to the use of immunosuppressive agents.

Raghu G: Interstitial lung disease: A diagnostic approach: Are CT scan and lung biopsy indicated in every patient? Am J Respir Crit Care Med 151:909, 1995.

A proposed approach to diagnosis of ILDs with review of indications for surgical lung biopsy and the position of CT scan in the diagnostic algorithm.

Raghu G, Depaso WJ, Cain K et al: Azathioprine combined with prednisone in the treatment of IPF: A prospective double-blind, randomized, placebo-controlled trial. Am Rev Respir Dis 144:291, 1991.

In this study prednisone combined with azathioprine was compared with prednisone alone in a prospective, double-blind, randomized, placebo-controlled trial. The number of patients enrolled was small, but there appeared to be a slight advantage for the azathioprine-prednisone group.

Reynolds HY: Diagnostic and management strategies for diffuse interstitial lung disease. Chest 113:192, 1998.

A review paper in which the approach and use of adjunctive modalities for diagnosis of IPF and options for treatment and monitoring response to treatment are described.

Taylor JR, Ryu J, Colby TV, Raffin TA: Lymphagioleiomyomatosis: Clinical course in 32 patients. N Engl J Med 323:1254, 1990.

This Stanford University group followed a large number of patients with a rare disease. The survival of these patients was better than had been previously understood.

Trulock EP: Lung transplantation: State of the art. Am J Respir Crit Care Med 155:789, 1997.

A comprehensive review of indications and timing of lung transplantation, posttransplant management, outcomes, complications, technical aspects (including organ retrieval), and surgical approach to lung transplantation.

Wiedenmann HP, Matthay RA: Pulmonary manifestations of collagen vascular diseases. Clin Chest Med 10:677, 1989.

The spectrum of disease caused by SLE, rheumatoid arthritis, scleroderma, polymyositis-dermatomyositis, mixed connective tissue disease, ankylosing spondylitis, relapsing polychondritis, and Sjögren's syndrome is reviewed.

Young KR Jr: Pulmonary-renal syndromes. Clin Chest Med 10:655, 1989.

This is an extensive review article on a heterogeneous group of disorders.

■ REFERENCES

Aboulafia DM: Regression of acquired immunodeficiency syndrome–related pulmonary Kaposi's sarcoma after highly active antiretroviral therapy. Mayo Clin Proc 73:439, 1998.

Addleman M, Logan AS, Grossman RF: Monitoring intrapulmonary hemorrhage in Goodpasture's syndrome. Chest 87:119, 1985.

Alberts C, van der Mark TW, Jansen HM, the Dutch Study Group on Pulmonary Sarcoidosis: Inhaled budesonide in pulmonary sarcoidosis: A double-blind, placebo-controlled study. Eur Respir J 8:682, 1995.

American Thoracic Society: Clinical role of bronchoalveolar lavage in adults with pulmonary disease. Am Rev Respir Dis 142:481, 1990.

Basset F, Corin B, Spencer H et al: Pulmonary histiocytosis X. Am Rev Respir Dis 118:811, 1978.

Basset F, Soler P, Jaurand MC et al: Ultrastructural examination of bronchoalveolar lavage for diagnosis of pulmonary histiocytosis X: Preliminary report on 4 cases. Thorax 32:303, 1977.

Baughman RP, Fernandez M: Radionuclide imaging in interstitial lung disease (Review). Curr Opin Pulm Med 2:376, 1996.

Baughman RP, Fernandez M, Bosken CH et al: Comparison of gallium-67 scanning, bronchoalveoloar lavage, and serum angiotensin-converting enzyme levels in pulmonary sarcoidosis. Am Rev Respir Dis 129:676, 1984.

Baughman RP, Shipley RT, Loudon RG, Lower EE: Crackles in interstitial lung disease: Comparison of sarcoidosis and fibrosing alveolitis. Chest 100:96, 1991.

Bellamy EA, Husband JE, Blaquiere RM, Law MR: Bleomycin-related lung damage: CT evidence. Radiology 156:155, 1985.

Bensard DD, McIntyre RC, Simon JS et al: Comparison of video thoracoscopic lung biopsy to open lung biopsy in the diagnosis of interstitial lung disease. Chest 103:765, 1993.

Bierne GJ, Brennan JT: Glomerulonephritis associated with hydrocarbon solvents: Mediated by antiglomerular basement membrane antibody. Arch Environ Health 25:365, 1972.

Bitterman PB, Rennard SI, Hunninghake GW, Crystal RG: Human alveolar macrophage growth factor for fibroblasts: Regulation and partial characterization. J Clin Invest 70:806, 1982.

Bocart D, Lecossier D, De Lassence A et al: A search for mycobacterial DNA in granulomatous tissues from patients with sarcoidosis using the polymerase chain reaction. Am Rev Respir Dis 145:1142, 1992.

Boeck C: Multiple benign sarcoid of the skin. J Cutan Genitourin Dis 17:543, 1899.

Boushy SF, Kurtzman RS, Martin ND et al: The course of pulmonary function in sarcoidosis. Ann Intern Med 62:939, 1965.

Brauner MW, Grenier P, Mouelhi MM et al: Pulmonary histiocytosis X: Evaluation with high-resolution CT. Radiology 172:255, 1989.

Briggs DC, Vaughan RW, Welsh KI et al: Immunogenetic prediction of pulmonary fibrosis in systemic sclerosis. Lancet 338:661, 1991.

Briggs WA, Johnson JP, Teichman S et al: Antiglomerular basement membrane antibody-mediated glomerulonephritis and Goodpasture's syndrome. Medicine 58:348, 1979.

Burkhardt A: Alveolitis and collapse in the pathogenesis of pulmonary fibrosis. Am Rev Respir Dis 140:513, 1989.

Carrington CB, Liebow AA: Limited forms of angiitis and granulomatosis of Wegener's type. Am J Med 41:497, 1966.

Centers for Disease Control: Revision of case definitions of acquired immunodeficiency syndrome for national reporting—United States. MMWR Morb Mortal Wkly Rep 34:373, 1985.

Churg J, Strauss L: Allergic granulomatosis, allergic angiitis and periarteritis nodosa. Am J Pathol 27:277, 1951.

Claypool WD, Rogers RM, Matuschak GM: Update on the clinical diagnosis, management, and pathogenesis of pulmonary alveolar proteinosis (phospholipidosis). Chest 85:550, 1984.

Cohen A, King TE, Downey GP: Rapidly progressive bronchiolitis obliterans with organizing pneumonia. Am J Respir Crit Care Med 149:1670, 1994.

Cohen Tervaert JW, Huitema MG, Hene RJ et al: Prevention of relapses in Wegener's granulomatosis by treatment based on antineutrophil cytoplasmic antibody titer. Lancet 336:709, 1990.

Colby TV, Myers JL: The clinical and histologic spectrum of bronchiolitis obliterans including bronchiolitis obliterans organizing pneumonia. Semin Respir Med 13:119, 1992.

Constantopoulos SH, Papadimitriou CS, Moutsopoulos HM: Respiratory manifestations in primary Sjögren's syndrome: A clinical, functional and histologic study. Chest 88:226, 1985.

Cooper JAD Jr, White DA, Matthay RA: Drug-induced pulmonary disease. Am Rev Respir Dis 133:321, 1986.

Cordier JF, Loire R, Brune J: Idiopathic bronchiolitis obliterans organizing pneumonia: Definition of characteristic clinical profiles in a series of 16 patients. Chest 96:999, 1989.

Cordier JF, Valeyre D, Guillevin L et al: Pulmonary Wegener's granulomatosis: A clinical and imaging study of 77 cases. Chest 9:906, 1990.

Corrin B, Liebow AA, Friedman PJ: Pulmonary lymphangiomyomatosis: A review. Am J Pathol 79:348, 1975.

Corwin RW, Irwin RS: The lipid-laden alveolar macrophage as a marker of aspiration in parenchymal lung disease. Am Rev Respir Dis 132:576, 1985.

Crofton JW, Livingstone JL, Oswald NC, Roberts ATM: Pulmonary eosinophilia. Thorax 7:1, 1952.

Crystal RG, Bitterman PB, Rennard ST et al: Interstitial lung diseases of unknown cause: Disorders characterized by chronic inflammation of the lower respiratory tract. N Engl J Med 310:154, 1984.

Crystal RG, Fulmer JD, Roberts WC et al: Idiopathic pulmonary fibrosis: Clinical, histologic, radiographic, physiologic, scintigraphic, cytologic, and biochemical aspects. Ann Intern Med 85:769, 1976.

Crystal RG, Gadek JE, Ferrans VJ et al: Interstitial lung disease: Current concepts of pathogenesis, staging and therapy. Am J Med 70:542, 1981.

Cudkowitz L, Cunningham M, Haldane EV: Effects of mediastinal irradiation on respiratory function following mastectomy for carcinoma of breast: A five-year follow-up study. Thorax 24:359, 1969.

Daniele RP, Elias JA, Epstein PE, Rossman MD: Bronchoalveolar lavage: Role in the pathogenesis, diagnosis, and management of interstitial lung disease. Ann Intern Med 102:93, 1985.

Davis SD, Henschke CI, Chamides BK, Wescott JL: Intrathoracic Kaposi sarcoma in AIDS patients: Radiographic-pathologic correlation. Radiology 163:495, 1987.

Davis WB, Rennard SI, Bitterman PB, Crystal RG: Pulmonary oxygen toxicity: Early reversible changes in human alveolar structures induced by hyperoxia. N Engl J Med 309:878, 1983.

Davison AG, Haslam PL, Corrin B et al: Interstitial lung disease and asthma in hard-metal workers: Bronchoalveolar lavage, ultrastructural, and analytic findings and results of bronchial provocation tests. Thorax 38:119, 1983.

Day W: Case of scleroderma or sclerema with the autopsy and results. Am J Med Sci 59:350, 1870.

de Clerck LS, Dequeker J, Francx L et al: D-Penicillamine therapy and interstitial lung disease in scleroderma: Long-term follow-up study. Arthritis Rheum 3:643, 1987.

Deneke SM, Fanburg BL: Normobaric oxygen toxicity of the lung. N Engl J Med 303:76, 1980.

DeRemee RA: The roentgenographic staging of sarcoidosis: Historical and contemporary perspectives. Chest 83:128, 1983.

DeRemee RA, McDonald TJ, Weiland LH: Wegener's granulomatosis: Observations on treatment with antimicrobial agents. Mayo Clin Proc 60:27, 1985.

Dill J, Ghose T, Landrigan P et al: Crytogenic fibrosing alveolitis. Chest 67:411, 1975.

Dreisen RB, Schwarz MI, Theofilopoulos AN, Stanford RE: Circulating immune complexes in the idiopathic interstitial pneumonias. N Engl J Med 298:353, 1978.

Drew WL, Finley TN, Golde DW: Diagnostic lavage and occult pulmonary hemorrhage in thrombocytopenic immunocompromised patients. Am Rev Respir Dis 116:215, 1977.

Duncan PE, Griffin JP, Garcia A, Kaplan SB: Fibrosing alveolitis in polymyositis: A review of histologically confirmed cases. Am J Med 57:621, 1974.

Dwyer JM, Hickie JB, Garvan J: Pulmonary tuberous sclerosis: Report of three patients and a review of the literature. Q J Med 40:115, 1971.

Eisenberg H, Dubois EL, Sherwin RP, Balchum OJ: Diffuse interstitial lung disease in systemic lupus erythematosus. Ann Intern Med 79:37, 1973.

Eliasson AH, Phillips YY, Tenholder MF: Treatment of lymphangioleiomyomatosis: A meta-analysis. Chest 196:1352, 1989.

Ellman P, Ball RE: "Rheumatoid disease" with joint and pulmonary manifestations. BMJ 2:816, 1948.

Epler GR, McLoud TC, Gaensler EA et al: Normal chest roentgenogram in chronic diffuse infiltrative lung disease. N Engl J Med 298:934, 1978.

Fauci AS, Haynes BF, Katz P: The spectrum of vasculitis: Clinical, pathologic, immunologic, and therapeutic considerations. Ann Intern Med 89:660, 1978.

Fauci AS, Haynes BF, Katz P, Wolff SM: Wegener's granulomatosis: Prospective clinical and therapeutic experience with 85 patients for 21 years. Ann Intern Med 98:76, 1983.

Fleming JA, Filbee JF, Wiernik G: Sequelae to radical irradiation in carcinoma of the breast. Br J Radiol 34:713, 1961.

Flint A: The interstitial lung diseases: A pathologist's view. Clin Chest Med 3:491, 1982.

Foley NM, Coral AP, Tung K et al: Bronchoalveolar lavage cell counts as a predictor of short term outcome in pulmonary sarcoidosis. Thorax 44:732, 1989.

Fraire AK, Smith MN, Greenberg SD et al: Tubular structures in pulmonary endothelial cells in systemic lupus erythematosus. Am J Clin Pathol 56:244, 1971.

Frazier RA, Miller RD: Interstitial pneumonitis in association with polymyositis and dermatomyositis. Chest 65:403, 1974.

Friedman PJ, Liebow AA, Sokoloff L: Eosinophilic granuloma of lung: Clinical aspects of pulmonary histiocytosis in the adult. Medicine 60:385, 1981.

Fulmer JD: An introduction to the interstitial lung diseases. Clin Chest Med 3:457, 1982a.

Fulmer JD: The interstitial lung diseases. Chest 82:172, 1982b.

Gaensler EA, Carrington CB: Peripheral opacities in chronic eosinophilic pneumonia: The photographic negative of pulmonary edema. AJR 128:1, 1977.

Geraint James D: Sarcoidosis. Postgrad Med J 60:234, 1984.

Gibson GJ, Prescott RJ, Muers MF et al: British Thoracic Society Sarcoidosis study: Effect of long term corticosteroid treatment. Thorax 51:238, 1996.

Gibson PG, Bryant DH, Morgan GW et al: Radiation-induced lung injury: A hypersensitivity pneumonitis? Ann Intern Med 109:288, 1988.

Gill PS, Akil B, Colletti P et al: Pulmonary Kaposi's sarcoma: Clinical findings and results of therapy. Am J Med 87:57, 1989.

Gilman MJ, Wang KP: Transbronchial lung biopsy in sarcoidosis: An approach to determine the optimal number of biopsies. Am Rev Respir Dis 122:721, 1980.

Ginsberg SJ, Comis RL: The pulmonary toxicity of antineoplastic agents. Semin Oncol 9:34, 1982.

Golde DW, Territo M, Finley TN, Cline MJ: Defective lung macrophages in pulmonary alveolar proteinosis. Ann Intern Med 85:304, 1976.

Goldiner PL, Carlon GC, Cvitkovic E et al: Factors influencing postoperative morbidity and mortality in patients treated with bleomycin. BMJ 1:1664, 1978.

Gonzalez-Rothi RJ, Harris JO: Pulmonary alveolar proteinosis: Further evaluation of abnormal alveolar macrophages. Chest 90:656, 1986.

Goodpasture EW: The significance of certain pulmonary lesions in relation to the etiology of influenza. Am J Med Sci 158:863, 1919.

Graham WCB: Silicosis. Clin Chest Med 13:253, 1992.

Greaves SM, Barta P: High-resolution computed tomography, magnetic resonance imaging, and positron emission tomography in interstitial lung disease. Curr Opin Pulm Med 1:351, 1995.

Gross NJ: Pulmonary effects of radiation therapy. Ann Intern Med 86:81, 1977.

Grossman RF, Frost A, Zamel N et al: Improvement in pulmonary function, graft perfusion, and exercise tolerance following single lung transplantation for pulmonary fibrosis. N Engl J Med 322:727, 1990.

Hakala M: Poor prognosis in patients with rheumatoid arthritis hospitalized for interstitial lung disease. Chest 93:114, 1988.

Hamman L, Rich AR: Acute diffuse interstitial fibrosis of the lungs. Bull Johns Hopkins Hosp 74:177, 1944.

Haupt HM, Moore GW, Hutchins GM: The lung in systemic lupus erythematosus: Analysis of the pathologic changes in 120 patients. Am J Med 71:791, 1981.

Heerfordt CF: Über eine "Febris uveoparotidea subchronica." Graefe's Arch Clin Exp Ophthalmol 70:254, 1909.

Helmers RA, Hunninghake GW: Bronchoalveolar lavage in the nonimmunocompromised patient. Chest 96:1184, 1989.

Hepper NG, Ferguson RH, Howard FM: Three types of pulmonary involvement in polymyositis. Med Clin North Am 48:1031, 1964.

Himmelfarb E, Wells S, Rabinowitz JG: The radiologic spectrum of cardiopulmonary amyloidosis. Chest 72:327, 1977.

Hines LE: Fibrosis of the lung following roentgen-ray treatments for tumor. JAMA 79:720, 1922.

Holgate ST, Haslam P, Turner-Warwick M: The significance of antinuclear and DNA antibodies in cryptogenic fibrosing alveolitis. Thorax 38:67, 1983.

Hollinger WM, Staton GW Jr, Fajman WA et al: Prediction of therapeutic response in steroid-treated pulmonary sarcoidosis: Evaluation of clinical parameters, bronchoalveolar lavage, gallium-67 scanning and serum angiotensin-converting enzyme levels. Am Rev Respir Dis 132:65, 1985.

Holness L, Tenenbaum J, Cooter NBE, Grossman RF: Fatal bronchiolitis obliterans associated with chrysotherapy. Ann Rheum Dis 42:593, 1983.

Hughes DA, Haslam PL, Townsend PJ, Turner-Warwick M: Blood and bronchoalveolar lavage T-subsets in sarcoidosis and extrinsic allergic alveolitis. Thorax 39:708, 1984.

Hunninghake GW, Crystal RG: Pulmonary sarcoidosis: A disorder mediated by excess helper T-lymphocyte activity at sites of disease activity. N Engl J Med 305:429, 1981.

Hunninghake GW, Fauci AS: Pulmonary involvement in the collagen vascular diseases. Am Rev Respir Dis 119:471, 1979.

Hunninghake GW, Gadek JE, Kawanami O et al: Inflammatory and immune processes in the human lung in health and disease: Evaluation by bronchoalveolar lavage. Am J Pathol 97:149, 1979.

Hutchinson J: Anomalous disease of the skin of the fingers: Papillary psoriasis. In Illustrations of Clinical Surgery. London, J and A Churchill, 1877.

Israel HL, Patchefsky AS, Saldana MJ: Wegener's granulomatosis, lymphomatoid granulomatosis, and benign lymphocytic angiitis and granulomatosis of lung: Recognition and treatment. Ann Intern Med 87:691, 1977.

Israel RH, Magnussen CR: Are AIDS patients at risk for pulmonary alveolar proteinosis? Chest 96:641, 1989.

Itescu S, Brancato LJ, Buxbaums S, et al: A diffuse infiltrative CD8 lymphocytosis syndrome in human immunodeficiency virus infection: A host immune response associated with HLA-DR5. Ann Intern Med 112:3, 1990.

Jayne DR, Lockwood CM: Intravenous immunoglobulin as sole therapy for systemic vasculitis. Br J Rheumatol 35:1150, 1996.

Jayne DRW, Davies MJ, Fox CJV et al: Treatment of systemic vasculitis with pooled intravenous immunoglobulin. Lancet 337:1137, 1991.

Jederlinic PJ, Sicilian L, Gaensler EA: Chronic eosinophilic pneumonia: A report of 19 cases and a review of the literature. Medicine 67:154, 1988.

Johkoh T, Ikezoe J, Kohno N et al: High resolution CT and pulmonary function tests in collagen vascular disease: Comparison with idiopathic pulmonary fibrosis. Eur J Radiol 18:113, 1994.

Johns CJ: Sarcoidosis. Annu Rev Med 40:353, 1989.

Johnson BA, Duncan SR, Ohori NP, et al: Recurrence of sarcoidosis in pulmonary allograft recipient. Am Rev Respir Dis 148:1373, 1993.

Jurik AG, Davidsen D, Graudal H: Prevalence of pulmonary involvement in rheumatoid arthritis and its relationship to some characteristics of the patients: A radiological and clinical study. Scand J Rheumatol 11:217, 1982.

Kallenberg C, Mulder A, Tervaert J: Antineutrophil cytoplasmic antibodies: A still-growing class of autoantibodies in inflamatory disorders. Am J Med 93:675, 1992.

Kataria YP: Chlorambucil in sarcoidosis. Chest 78:36, 1980.

Keogh BA, Crystal RG: Alveolitis: The key to the interstitial lung disorders. Thorax 37:1, 1982.

Keogh BA, Hunninghake GW, Line BR, Crystal RG: The alveolitis of pulmonary sarcoidosis: Evaluation of natural history and alveolitis-dependent changes in lung function. Am Rev Respir Dis 128:256, 1983.

Klinger H: Grenzformen der Periarteritis nodosa. Frankfurt Z Path 42:455, 1931.

Kuznitsky E, Bittorf A: Boecksches sarkoid mit beteiligung innerer organe. Munch Med Wochenschr 62:1349, 1915.

Lacronique J, Roth C, Battesti JP et al: Chest radiological features of pulmonary histiocytosis X: A report based on 50 adult cases. Thorax 37:104, 1982.

Leatherman JW: Immune pulmonary hemorrhage. Chest 91:891, 1987.

Leatherman JW, Davies SF, Hoidal JR: Alveolar hemorrhage syndromes: Diffuse microvascular lung hemorrhage in immune and idiopathic disorders. Medicine 63:343, 1984.

Levy H, Horak DA, Lewis MI: The value of bronchial washings and bronchoalveolar lavage in the diagnosis of lymphangitic carcinomatosis. Chest 94:1028, 1988.

Libshitz HI, Southard ME: Complications of radiation therapy: The thorax. Semin Roentgenol 9:41, 1974.

Lieberman J: Elevation of serum angiotensin-converting-enzyme (ACE) level in sarcoidosis. Am J Med 59:365, 1975.

Liebow AA, Carrington CRB, Friedman PJ: Lymphomatoid granulomatosis. Hum Pathol 3:457, 1972.

Liebow AA, Steer A, Billingsley JG: Desquamative interstitial pneumonia. Am J Med 39:369, 1965.

Lin YH, Haslam PL, Turner-Warwick M: Chronic pulmonary sarcoidosis: Relationship between lung lavage cell counts, chest radiograph and results of standard lung function tests. Thorax 40:501, 1985.

Löfgren S: Primary pulmonary sarcoidosis. Acta Med Scand 145:424, 1953.

Lower EE, Baughman RP: The use of low dose methotrexate in refractory sarcoidosis. Am J Med Sci 299:153, 1990.

Martin RJ, Coulson JJ, Rogers RM et al: Pulmonary alveolar proteinosis: The diagnosis by segmental lavage. Am Rev Respir Dis 121:819, 1980.

Martin RJ, Rogers RM, Myers NM: Pulmonary alveolar proteinosis. Shunt fraction and lactic acid dehydrogenase concentration as aids to diagnosis. Am Rev Respir Dis 117:1059, 1978.

Martin WJ II, Rosenow EC III: Amiodarone pulmonary toxicity: Recognition and pathogenesis. Chest 93:1067, 1988.

Martinet Y, Pinkston PA, Saltini C et al: Evaluation of the in-vitro and in-vivo effects of cyclosporine on the lung T-lymphocyte alveolitis of active pulmonary sarcoidosis. Am Rev Respir Dis 138:1242, 1988.

Masson RG, Krikorian J, Lukl P et al: Pulmonary microvascular cytology in the diagnosis of lymphangitic carcinomatosis. N Engl J Med 321:71, 1989.

Mathieson JR, Mayo JR, Staples CA et al: Chronic diffuse infiltrative lung disease: Comparison of diagnostic accuracy of CT and chest radiography. Radiology 171:111, 1989.

Matthay RA, Schwarz MI, Petty TL et al: Pulmonary manifestations of systemic lupus erythematosus: Review of twelve cases of acute lupus pneumonitis. Medicine 54:397, 1974.

Maycock RL, Bertrand P, Morrison CE et al: Manifestations of sarcoidosis. Am J Med 35:67, 1963.

Merchant RN, Pearson MG, Rankin RN, Morgan WKC: Computerized tomography in the diagnosis of lymphangioleiomyomatosis. Am Rev Respir Dis 131:295, 1985.

Mills ES, Matthews WH: Interstitial pneumonitis in dermatomyositis. JAMA 160:1467, 1956.

Moolma JA, Bardin PG, Rossouw DJ, Joubert JR: Cyclosporin as a treatment for interstitial lung disease of unknown aetiology. Thorax 46:592, 1991.

Moore ADA, Godwin JD, Muller NL et al: Pulmonary histiocytosis X: Comparison of radiographic and CT findings. Radiology 172:249, 1989.

Mossman BT, Gee JBL: Asbestos-related diseases. N Engl J Med 320:1721, 1989.

Muller NL, Mawson JB, Mathieson JR et al: Sarcoidosis: Correlation of extent of disease at CT with clinical, functional and radiographic findings. Radiology 171:613, 1989.

Muller NL, Miller RR, Webb WR et al: Fibrosing alveolitis: CT-pathologic correlation. Radiology 160:585, 1986.

Muller NL, Ostrow DN: High resolution computed tomography of chronic interstitial lung disease. Clin Chest Med 12:97, 1991.

Murray JF: The Normal Lung. Philadelphia, WB Saunders, 1976.

Muthiah MM, Macfarlane JT: Current concepts in the management of sarcoidosis. Drugs 40:231, 1990.

Nolle B, Specks U, Ludemann J et al: Anticytoplasmic autoantibodies: The immunodiagnostic value in Wegener granulomatosis. Ann Intern Med 111:28, 1989.

Ognibene FP, Steis RG, Macher AM et al: Kaposi's sarcoma causing pulmonary infiltrates and respiratory failure in the acquired immunodeficiency syndrome. Ann Intern Med 102:471, 1985.

Oldham SAA, Castillo M, Jacobson FL et al: HIV-associated lymphocytic interstitial pneumonia: Radiologic manifestations and pathologic correlation. Radiology 170:83, 1989.

O'Leary TJ, Jones G, Yip A et al: The effects of chloroquine on serum 1,25-dihydroxyvitamin D and calcium metabolism in sarcoidosis. N Engl J Med 315:727, 1986.

Osler W: On the visceral manifestations of the erythema group of skin diseases. Am J Med Sci 27:1, 1904.

Owens GR, Fino GJ, Herbert DL et al: Pulmonary function in progressive systemic sclerosis: Comparison of CREST syndrome variant with diffuse scleroderma. Chest 84:546, 1983.

Owens GR, Follansbee WP: Cardiopulmonary manifestations of systemic sclerosis. Chest 91:118, 1987.

Padley SPG, Adler B, Hansell DM et al: High-resolution computed tomography of drug-induced lung disease. Clin Radiol 46:232, 1992.

Pare JAP, Fraser RG, Hogg JC et al: Pulmonary mainline granulomatosis: Talcosis of intravenous methadone abuse. Medicine 58:229, 1979.

Pare JP, Cote G, Fraser RS: Long-term follow-up of drug abusers with intravenous talcosis. Am Rev Respir Dis 139:233, 1989.

Pearson DJ, Rosenow EC: Chronic eosinophilic pneumonia (Carrington's): A follow-up study. Mayo Clin Proc 53:73, 1978.

Penny WJ, Knight RK, Rees AM et al: Obliterative bronchiolitis in rheumatoid arthritis. Ann Rheum Dis 41:469, 1982.

Prophet D: Primary pulmonary histiocytosis X. Clin Chest Med 3:643, 1982.

Rees AJ: Pulmonary injury caused by antibasement membrane antibodies. Semin Respir Med 5:264, 1984.

Reyes CN, Wenzel FJ, Lawton BR, Emanuel DA: The pulmonary pathology of farmer's lung disease. Chest 81:142, 1982.

Reynolds HY: Bronchoalveolar lavage. Am Rev Respir Dis 135:250, 1987.

Reynolds HY: Hypersensitivity pneumonitis. Clin Chest Med 3:503, 1982.

Rockoff SD, Rohatgi PK: Unusual manifestations of thoracic sarcoidosis. AJR 144:513, 1985.

Roschmann RA, Rothenberg RJ: Pulmonary fibrosis in rheumatoid arthritis: A review of clinical features and therapy. Semin Arthritis Rheum 52:174, 1987.

Rosen SH, Castleman B, Liebow AA: Pulmonary alveolar proteinosis. N Engl J Med 258:1123, 1958.

Rosen Y, Athanassiades TJ, Moon S et al: Nongranulomatous interstitial pneumonitis in sarcoidosis: Relationship to development of epitheloid granulomas. Chest 74:122, 1978.

Rosenow E, Strimlan CV, Muhm JR et al: Pleuropulmonary manifestations of ankylosing spondylitis. Mayo Clin Proc 52:641, 1977.

Rosenow EC III: Drug-induced pulmonary disease. Dis Mon 40:253, 1994.

Rosenow EC III, Myers JL, Swensen SJ, Pisani RJ: Drug-induced pulmonary disease: An update. Chest 102:239, 1992.

Rothe RA, Fuller PB, Byrd RB et al: Transbronchoscopic lung biopsy in sarcoidosis: Optimal number and sites for diagnosis. Chest 77:400, 1980.

Saboor SA, Johnson NM, McFadden J: Detection of mycobacterial DNA in sarcoidosis and tuberculosis with polymerase chain reaction. Lancet 339:1012, 1992.

Saus J, Wieslander J, Langeveld JPM et al: Identification of the Goodpasture antigen as the a3(IV) chain of collagen IV. J Biol Chem 263:13374, 1988.

Scadding JG: Diffuse pulmonary alveolar fibrosis. Thorax 29:271, 1974.

Scadding JG, Hinson KFW: Diffuse fibrosing alveolitis (diffuse interstitial fibrosis of the lungs): Correlation of histology at biopsy with prognosis. Thorax 22:291, 1967.

Schneider PD, Wise RA, Hochberg MC, Wigley FM: Serial pulmonary function in systemic sclerosis. Am J Med 73:385, 1982.

Schoenberger CI, Rennard SI, Bitterman PB et al: Paraquat-induced pulmonary fibrosis: Role of the alveolitis in modulating the development of fibrosis. Am Rev Respir Dis 129:168, 1984.

Schwarz MI, Matthay RA, Sahn SA et al: Interstitial lung disease in polymyositis and dermatomyositis: Analysis of six cases and review of the literature. Medicine 55:89, 1976.

Sebastien P, Armstrong B, Monchaux G, Bignon J: Asbestos bodies in bronchoalveolar lavage fluid and in lung parenchyma. Am Rev Respir Dis 137:75, 1988.

Sharma OP: Sarcoidosis: Clinical, laboratory and immunologic aspects. Semin Roentgenol 20:340, 1985.

Sharma OP, Johnson R: Airway obstruction in sarcoidosis: A study of 123 nonsmoking black American patients with sarcoidosis. Chest 94:343, 1988.

Shumak KH, Rock GA: Therapeutic plasma exchange. N Engl J Med 310:762, 1984.

Silver RM, Scott Miller K, Kinsella MB et al: Evaluation and management of scleroderma lung disease using bronchoalveolar lavage. Am J Med 88:470, 1990.

Silver SF, Muller NL, Miller RR et al: Computed tomography in hypersensitivity pneumonitis. Radiology 173:441, 1989.

Slingerland JM, Grossman RF, Chamberlain D, Tremblay CE: Pulmonary manifestations of tuberous sclerosis in first degree relatives. Thorax 44:212, 1989.

Smellie H, Hoyle C: The natural history of pulmonary sarcoidosis. Q J Med 29:539, 1960.

Stack BHR, Choo-Kang FJ, Heard BE: The prognosis of cryptogenic fibrosing alveolitis. Thorax 27:535, 1972.

Stanton MC, Tange JD: Goodpasture's syndrome (pulmonary hemorrhage associated with glomerulonephritis). Aust N Z J Med 7:132, 1958.

Steen VD, Owens GR, Redmond C et al: The effect of D-penicillamine on pulmonary findings in systemic sclerosis. Arthritis Rheum 28:882, 1985.

Stegeman CA, Cohen Tervaert JW, de Jong PE et al: Trimethoprim-sulfamethoxazole(co-trimoxazole) for the prevention of relapses of Wegener's granulomatosis. Dutch Co-trimoxazole Wegener's Study Group. N Engl J Med 335:16, 1996.

Stein MG, Mayo J, Muller N et al: Pulmonary lymphangitic spread of carcinoma; Appearance on CT scans. Radiology 162:371, 1987.

Strimlan CV, Rosenow EC III, Divertie MB, Harrison EG Jr: Pulmonary manifestations of Sjögren's syndrome. Chest 70:354, 1976.

Strumpf IJ, Feld MK, Cornelius MJ et al: Safety of fiberoptic bronchoalveolar lavage in evaluation of interstitial lung disease. Chest 80:268, 1981.

Studdy PR, Bird R: Serum angiotensin converting enzyme in sarcoidosis—its value in present clinical practice. Ann Clin Biochem 26:13, 1989.

Studdy P, Bird R, Geraint James D: Serum angiotensin-converting enzyme (SACK) in sarcoidosis and other granulomatous disorders. Lancet 2:1331, 1978.

Thrasher DR, Briggs DD Jr: Pulmonary sarcoidosis. Clin Chest Med 3:537, 1982.

Trapnell DH: The radiological appearance of lymphangitic carcinomatosa of the lung. Thorax 19:251, 1964.

Turner-Warwick M, Haslam PL: Clinical applications of bronchoalveolar lavage. Clin Chest Med 8:15, 1987.

Turner-Warwick M, McAllister LR, Britten A, Haslam PL: Corticosteroid treatment in pulmonary sarcoidosis: Do serial lavage lymphocyte counts, serum angiotensin converting enzyme measurements and gallium-67 scans help management? Thorax 41:903, 1986.

van der Woude FJ, Rasmussen N, Lobatto S et al: Autoantibodies against neutrophils and monocytes: Tool for diagnosis and marker of disease activity in Wegener's granulomatosis. Lancet 1:425, 1985.

van Essen S, West W, Sitorius M et al: Complete resolution of roentgenographic changes in a patient with pulmonary histiocytosis X. Chest 98:765, 1990.

von Stossel E: Uber muskulare cirrhose der lunge. Beitr Klin Tuberk 90:432, 1937.

Walker WC, Wright V: Diffuse interstitial pulmonary fibrosis and rheumatoid arthritis. Ann Rheum Dis 28:252, 1969.

Wegener F: Uber generalisierte, septische Gefasserkrankungen. Verh Dtsch Ges Pathol 29:202, 1936.

White DA, Matthay RA: Noninfectious pulmonary complications of infection with the human immunodeficiency virus. Am Rev Respir Dis 140:1763, 1989.

Wilson CB, Dixon FJ: Renal injury from immune reactions involving antigens in or of the kidney. In Brenner BM, Stein J (eds): Contemporary Issues in Nephrology, Vol 3. New York, Churchill Livingstone, 1979.

Winterbauer RH, Belic N, Moores KD: A clinical interpretation of bilateral hilar lymphadenopathy. Ann Intern Med 78:65, 1973.

Wolkowicz J, Sturgeon J, Rawji M, Chan CK: Bleomycin-induced pulmonary function abnormalities. Chest 101:97, 1992.

Zerhouni EA, Naidich DP, Stitik FP et al: Computed tomography of the pulmonary parenchyma II: Interstitial disease. J Thorac Imaging 1:54, 1985.

CHAPTER **25**

Lung Volume Reduction Surgery

Stephen Lefrak
Joel D. Cooper

Estimates suggest that more than 12 million Americans have chronic obstructive pulmonary disease (COPD) (Feinleib et al, 1989). As many as 2 million of these have emphysema and many go on to develop severe dyspnea with a subsequent decrement in quality of life (Feinleib et al, 1989; Guyatt, 1988; Higgins and Keller, 1989; McSweeny et al, 1982). Medical therapy is the mainstay of treatment; the major therapeutic modalities consist of smoking cessation (Anthonisen et al, 1994), comprehensive pulmonary rehabilitation, bronchodilator therapy, and if indicated, supplemental oxygen.

HISTORICAL NOTE

Although surgical therapy for emphysema has been offered throughout the 20th century, surgical efforts aimed at diffuse emphysema have almost always been dismissed after circumspect analysis (Deslauriers, 1995; Gaensler et al, 1983; Laforet, 1972). Prior to 1993, surgical therapy for emphysema had been accepted in three situations: (1) localized bullous disease with relatively normal surrounding lung parenchyma, (2) bullous disease associated with a background of generalized emphysema, and (3) lung transplantation for severe end-stage disease. There has been little disagreement about the merits of surgery for localized large bullae, especially if associated with compressed lung, recurrent pneumothoraces, or recurrent infection (Delarue et al, 1977; Gaensler et al, 1983; Knudson and Gaensler, 1965; American Thoracic Society, 1968). However, the indications for surgery for generalized emphysema, with or without a component of bullous disease, have not been well defined or widely accepted.

In 1957, Dr. Otto C. Brantigan proposed a surgical treatment for patients disabled by diffuse pulmonary emphysema (Brantigan and Mueller, 1957). Brantigan resected peripheral lung tissue, anticipating restoration of the elastic recoil of the lung and improved mechanics of the thorax and diaphragm. He performed the procedure with a unilateral thoracotomy and added a radical hilar denervation procedure. He planned to return a few months later to operate on the contralateral side. Overall improvement was reported in 75% of the patients. However, Brantigan provided few quantitative corroborating data, and the in-hospital mortality rate was 19% (Brantigan and Mueller, 1957). As a result, Brantigan's procedure did not gain wide acceptance.

Over the following decades, different groups (Benfield et al, 1966; Brantigan et al, 1959; Brantigan et al, 1961; Delarue et al, 1977; FitzGerald et al, 1974; Gaensler et al, 1986; Nickoladze, 1992; Rogers et al, 1968; Roué et al, 1996), attempted variations on Brantigan's procedure, including laser therapy (Brenner et al, 1994; Lewis et al, 1993; Wakabayashi, 1993; Wakabayashi et al, 1991), with limited success. However, in 1993, Dr. Joel Cooper successfully revitalized Brantigan's procedure and described it as "pneumectomy" or lung "volume reduction" surgery (LVRS). Similar to Brantigan's procedure, Cooper removed approximately 30% of the patient's lung volume by performing peripheral resection of the most emphysematous portions. Distinct from Brantigan's approach, Cooper used linear cutting/stapling devices, buttressed the suture line, and performed a simultaneous bilateral procedure through a median sternotomy. The procedure was considered palliative and was designed to (1) reduce dyspnea, (2) increase exercise tolerance and performance in activities of daily living, and (3) improve quality of life. In most patients, these goals were achieved with concomitant physiologic improvement in airflow limitation, hyperinflation, and alveolar gas exchange (Cooper et al, 1995).

Patients were able to undergo LVRS more safely in 1993 than was previously reported because of significant advances in the evaluation and care of patients with markedly impaired pulmonary function. In addition, the outlook for an improved outcome increased as a result of (1) a more sophisticated understanding of the pathology and physiology of chronic obstructive lung disease; (2) progress in computer-assisted and radionuclide imaging, permitting evaluation of the anatomy and function of the emphysematous lung (Slone, 1996); (3) enhanced techniques in critical care and anesthesia (Triantafillou, 1996); (4) substitution of a median sternotomy incision (Cooper et al, 1978) or video-assisted thoracoscopy (Keenan et al, 1996) for the standard thoracotomy incision; (5) improved methodologies of lung resection (Cooper, 1994); and importantly, (6) bilateral resection of emphysematous lung during the same procedure, generating a greater increment of improvement than can be obtained by unilateral surgery (Brenner et al, 1996; Cooper et al, 1996; Keenan et al, 1996).

LVRS has undergone rapid growth since 1993 for many reasons, not the least of which was the dearth of therapeutic options for patients with severe emphysema. In 1993, the only alternatives for the treatment of disabling emphysema were comprehensive pulmonary rehabilitation and lung transplantation. Unfortunately, pulmonary rehabilitation, although successful in some patients, left many others still disabled by dyspnea. And lung transplantation, although established as an effective treatment for assiduously selected patients with disabling emphysema, is extremely restricted because of (1) the scarcity of donor organs, (2) the complications associated with rejection, and (3) the lifelong requirements for immunosuppression. Consequently, many groups successfully employed similar stapling resection procedures over the ensuing years (Argenziano et al, 1996; Brenner et al, 1996; Eugene et al, 1995; Hazelrigg et al, 1996; Keenan et al, 1996a; McKenna et al, 1996; Miller et al, 1996; Naunheim et al, 1996; O'Donnell et al, 1996; Sciurba et al, 1996), while laser therapy showed little benefit and accordingly has been abandoned (Eugene et al, 1995; Hazelrigg et al, 1996; Little et al, 1995; McKenna et al, 1996b). Selection criteria for surgery were relatively similar at the different centers except for slight variation based on each program's experience and emphasis (Miller et al, 1996). The eligibility criteria and the assessment process have continued to evolve based on analyses of patient outcomes after surgery (Argenziano et al, 1996; Keenan et al, 1996a; McKenna et al, 1996b; Yusen et al, 1996). This chapter reviews (1) the rationale for surgery and current eligibility criteria, (2) patient evaluation procedures and eligibility criteria for surgery, (3) preoperative patient management, and (4) the relationship of outcome after surgery to preoperative characteristics.

BASIC SCIENCE

Dyspnea

The discomfort associated with the act of breathing experienced by patients with emphysema occurs initially with exertion. This progresses to dyspnea at rest only when the disease is far advanced. The fundamental mechanisms for the origin of dyspnea remain poorly understood. Although dyspnea is associated with severe airflow limitation, it is also linked to hyperinflation, respiratory muscle dysfunction, increases in respiratory drive, and abnormalities in alveolar gas exchange. Unfortunately, there is no precise correlation between the symptom of breathlessness and routinely measured physiologic parameters of pulmonary function (Killian, 1993; Killian and Campbell, 1983). The mechanisms by which dyspnea is produced and sensed in patients with far-advanced COPD are likely to be both multifactorial and diverse between patients (Bradley et al, 1979; Campbell, 1975–77; Campbell et al, 1961; Gandevia et al, 1981; Jones et al, 1971; Killian and Campbell, 1983; Levison and Cherniak, 1968; O'Donnell and Webb, 1993). Successful management of dyspnea, either medically or surgically, remains challenging without a more precise understanding of the contribution of each causal component. Nevertheless, the aim of LVRS is primarily to reduce dyspnea; its success is assessed by evaluating the improvements made in pulmonary and thoracic mechanics and respiratory muscle function, changes in ventilatory drive, and improvements in alveolar gas exchange.

EMPHYSEMA

Pulmonary Structure and Function

Emphysema is defined as the dilatation of the terminal lung units beyond the terminal bronchiole associated with alveolar wall destruction with limited, if any, fibrosis present. This remodeling of the peripheral lung units that occurs in emphysema produces a decrease in lung elastic recoil pressure (Christie and McIntosh, 1934; Ebert, 1968). This decrease occurs as a result of both the loss of surface area as alveoli coalesce into larger units and the deterioration of the intrinsic structure of the lung as remodeling takes place. As a result, under static conditions, the emphysematous lung requires less pressure to inflate (increased distensibility), and once inflated, it exerts less pressure toward emptying than does a normal lung. The consequences of this are significant in the production of the physiologic abnormalities of emphysema, which LVRS may address.

First, the increased distensibility of emphysematous lung results in a lung that, although easily inflated, tends to remain inflated. An important consequence of this is that areas of severely emphysematous lung act as essentially nonfunctional, but volume-occupying, areas. Furthermore, these pathologic areas adversely affect the mechanics of the more normal surrounding lung. As a result, this more normal surrounding lung becomes less capable of exerting its better-preserved elastic recoil on its adjoining airways, and the result is an increase in airway resistance (Rogers et al, 1968).

A second effect of the loss of elastic recoil is the decrease in maximum expiratory flow experienced by patients with emphysema. This decreased recoil pressure results in expiratory airflow limitation because of decreases in both the driving pressure for expiratory flow and the transmural pressure, which maintain the patency of intraparenchymal airways (Mead et al, 1966).

Third, emphysema is unevenly distributed throughout the lungs, resulting in regional variation in both structure and function. As a consequence, the lungs, whose regions usually function synchronously and in phase, begin to function dyssynchronously (Mead et al, 1966; Otis et al, 1956). As a result of this, during inspiration and exhalation, the emphysematous lung has regions that are emptying and filling out of phase with one another (Otis et al, 1956). Consequently, more transpulmonary pressure is required for the same tidal volume than with a normal lung; or, for the same transpulmonary pressure, less tidal volume is exchanged. The result is that lung distensibility, or dynamic compliance, decreases as respiratory frequency increases (Woolcock et al, 1969), causing increased work of breathing and increasing dyspnea. Additionally, because lung units are interdependent, the function of the better-conserved lung units adjoining more pathologically affected lung is adversely affected (Mead et al, 1967).

Finally, the heterogeneous distribution of emphysema throughout the lungs also adversely affects alveolar gas exchange (Riley and Cournand, 1951). Portions of the lung that are more affected by the disease process than others ventilate more slowly than do the more normal regions (Briscoe and Cournand, 1959). The relative distribution of blood flow to these poorly ventilating regions determines both the amount of dead space and the venous admixture that are present, thus affecting the overall ventilatory requirement and levels of arterial oxygen and carbon dioxide tension.

Thoracic Hyperinflation and Respiratory Muscle Function

An increase in thoracic volume accompanies the pulmonary abnormalities of emphysema. The hyperinflation (increased total lung capacity) and associated air trapping (increased residual volume) are consequences of the reduction in lung recoil pressure (Christie and McIntosh, 1934) and dynamic airway collapse. This is compounded by an increase in ventilatory drive, producing premature initiation of inspiration. In addition to producing hyperinflation, the premature onset of inspiration results in positive alveolar pressure at end-exhalation. This so-called auto–positive end-expiratory pressure (auto-PEEP) then serves as a threshold inspiratory load to the inspiratory muscles. Initiation of inspiratory flow becomes more difficult because more negative intrathoracic pressures must be generated to overcome this positive pressure. All of these changes increase the work of breathing, which compounds the already increased work secondary to the changes in lung architecture and function.

As thoracic hyperinflation advances, the diaphragm assumes its characteristic flattened position observed on chest radiographs. This has profound effects on inspiratory muscle function (Sharp et al, 1974). First, the zone of apposition between the diaphragm and the abdominal wall is lost as the diaphragm flattens. As a result, any positive abdominal pressure generated during inspiration is not as effectively applied to the chest wall, hindering rib cage movement and impairing inspiration. Second, the flattened diaphragm becomes a less effective lever for moving the rib cage upward and outward. In fact, with severe hyperinflation, the lower rib cage may be observed to move inward during inspiration (Hoover's sign). Third, the muscle fibers of a flattened diaphragm are shorter than those of a more normally curved diaphragm. Because a shorter muscle produces less tension than a longer one, the diaphragm becomes less capable of generating inspiratory pressure as the thorax hyperinflates. Fourth, in accordance with Laplace's law, $P = 2T/r$, as the radius of diaphragm curvature (r) increases with diaphragm flattening, the tension (T) required to develop transpulmonary pressure (P) to generate tidal breathing must increase. This may be perceived as a decrease in efficiency because less transpulmonary pressure is produced by the same tension.

As hyperinflation progresses, the thoracic cage operates at a mechanical disadvantage. Normally, at functional residual capacity, the rib cage is at a lower volume than at its resting position (Rahn et al, 1946). During normal inspiration, the thoracic cage tends to passively expand or recoil outward toward its resting position. This therefore "aids" the inspiratory muscles during tidal inspiration. As thoracic hyperinflation occurs, the rib cage assumes a higher volume, well above its resting volume. As a result, the inspiratory muscles, instead of gaining assistance from the rib cage during tidal inspiration, now must work to overcome the resistance of the rib cage. Thus, hyperinflation, in spite of increasing elastic recoil and decreasing airways resistance, has the following effects: (1) it adversely affects chest wall mechanics and increases the work of breathing (Rochester et al, 1979); (2) it produces a diaphragm that is less capable of generating inspiratory force (Rochester et al, 1979; Sharp et al, 1974); and (3) it results in a diaphragm that works in a less efficient manner than normal with decreased endurance (Rochester et al, 1979). This may result in chronic diaphragmatic fatigue and respiratory failure as well as worsened dyspnea in these patients.

Exercise exaggerates many of these abnormalities. During exercise, patients may maximize expiratory flow by breathing at even higher lung volumes (Henke et al, 1988). Respiratory muscles are then situated in an even more disadvantageous position. Also, inspiratory muscles may experience additional loads (Younes, 1990) produced by the increased ventilatory demand. As respiratory rate increases with exercise, expiratory time shortens, which may lead to increasing dynamic hyperinflation and compression of the airways. The shortened time for exhalation exaggerates the incomplete exhalation, which leads to increasingly positive alveolar pressures at end-exhalation (Pepe and Marini, 1982). All these tend to both increase the work of breathing (McIlroy and Christie, 1954) and impair the muscles required to perform the work.

RATIONALE FOR LUNG VOLUME REDUCTION SURGERY

Removing severely diseased, slowly ventilating, but expanded lung could be expected to decrease hyperinflation and improve thoracic and diaphragmatic function. However, if the most severely diseased lung could be identified and removed, then not only would thoracic function improve by reduced hyperinflation, but lung function would also improve through restored elastic recoil pressure, resulting in increased expiratory flow rates. Importantly, this would also help restore the lung toward more synchronous behavior and would decrease adverse interdependence effects, possibly improving the distribution of ventilation in relation to perfusion. This would cause improved alveolar gas exchange and decreased frequency dependence and improved thoracic mechanics. Additionally, the more normal lung tissue remaining would no longer be adversely affected by the severely diseased tissue, which has been removed. Thus, the work of breathing would be decreased, and the ability of respiratory muscles to meet the demand would be improved. All of these events could be expected to decrease the sensation of dyspnea in these patients and improve their ability to function.

EVALUATION OF PATIENTS FOR LUNG VOLUME REDUCTION SURGERY

The goals of the preoperative assessment are (1) to identify patients who in spite of maximal medical therapy remain disabled by emphysema, (2) to classify which patients will benefit from surgery with an acceptable surgical risk, and (3) to exclude with confidence those patients likely to have a poor outcome. The initial evaluation schema developed at Washington University has been refined by analysis of surgical results and adopted by many centers. As can be expected from our understanding of the pathophysiology of emphysema, this schema (Yusen, 1996) suggests that the patients who will have the best outcome from volume reduction surgery are those patients with marked hyperinflation, whose lungs approach as closely as possible a two-compartment system, with one compartment consisting of emphysematous lung that is volume occupying, relatively nonfunctioning, and surgically accessible. The second compartment is lung that, although emphysematous, is not totally destroyed. The more closely a patient approaches this ideal two-compartment model, the better the outcome appears to be. The patient profile used at Washington University Medical Center for evaluation of patients with COPD is shown in Table 25–1. Some of the most salient points in the evaluation include the following: (1) the classification of patients with airway obstruction produced predominantly by emphysema rather than by intrinsic airways disease, (2) the identification of those patients whose emphysematous lungs have sufficient regional variation in the distribution of emphysema (heterogeneity) to provide target areas of virtually nonfunctioning lung accessible to surgical resection, and (3) the presence of marked hyperinflation of the thorax.

In addition to the very important history and physical examination, the evaluation relies heavily on physiologic and imaging studies. The specific methods for assessing patients for surgery are listed in Table 25–1. Inspiratory chest radiographs are used to evaluate the degree of thoracic hyperinflation as evidenced by downward displacement and flattening of the diaphragm, as well as distention of the thorax with enlarged retrocardiac and retrosternal air spaces. Expiratory films provide additional information and may demonstrate asymmetry of air trapping in one lung, as well as the degree of impairment in movement of the chest wall and diaphragm. The chest radiographs also provide an initial indication of the overall severity and relative distribution of emphysema. Other findings on these films, such as marked pulmonary scarring, pleural disease, infiltrates, adenopathy, effusions, and cardiovascular abnormalities, may be useful for determining ineligibility for surgery.

The standard chest computed tomography (CT) examination without intravenous contrast provides critical information for the selection process. Most important, it provides a detailed depiction of the severity and distribution of emphysema. This is most helpful in characterizing whether the patient's limitations are secondary to emphysema or airways disease. It is also important in establishing whether there are target areas present and in identifying their location. Although high-resolution CT is sensitive for detecting emphysema, detection is most often not problematic in this population with such severe airflow obstruction. Also, high-resolution CT provides increased sensitivity for revealing occult bronchiectasis or underlying interstitial lung disease. In addition, CT may demonstrate evidence of underlying pathology, such as pleural disease, bronchiectasis, infection, cancer, or cardiovascular disease, which might preclude LVRS.

Nuclear medicine ventilation-perfusion lung scans depicting regional blood flow patterns (Fig. 25–1) provide a valuable roadmap for surgery. The absolute severity of emphysema cannot be assessed because the distribution of the perfusion agent is relative, but the presence of diffuse or upper or lower lobe predominant disease can be assessed. Also, a right- or left-sided predominance of lung function may sway a decision toward unilateral surgery if CT corroborates this evidence.

With imaging studies, the degree of emphysema, thoracic hyperinflation, regional heterogeneity (target areas), amount of adequate pulmonary reserve tissue, degree of compressed lung, and other parameters can be quantified using simple grading systems or digital analyses (Bae et al, 1996; Slone, 1996). Further sophistication of computer-based imaging may allow greater objectification of the evaluation process.

In summary, (1) patients with predominant emphysema may be effectively distinguished from those limited by intrinsic airway disease by history, physical examination, and, most useful, pulmonary CT; (2) the degree of regional parenchymal destruction is analyzed by CT of the chest, and the regional distribution of function is assessed by radionuclide ventilation-perfusion lung scanning; and (3) thoracic distention is evaluated by chest radiograph and plethysmographic determination of lung volumes. Eligibility criteria are summarized in Table 25–1.

Review of the surgical results of LVRS reveals several predictors of surgical mortality. These include elevations in $Pa{CO_2}$, marked decreases in diffusing capacity, older patient age, and high supplemental oxygen requirements, at rest or with exercise. These predictors are shown in Table 25–2 and appear to reflect the function of different portions of the respiratory system. The diffusing capacity reflects the distribution of surface areas to perfusion of the lung; a marked decrease in this parameter may well indicate that the lung is so markedly impaired as to be unable to support the patient adequately following LVRS. This should correlate with a marked need for supplemen-

TABLE 25–1 ■ Eligibility Patient Profile

Criteria	*Method*
Disabling COPD despite intensive medical management	History, family interview QOL survey, MRC dyspnea index Intensive pulmonary rehabilitation
Severe airflow obstruction	FEV_1 and lung volumes
Emphysema	CT scan
Hyperinflation	Chest radiograph TLC and RV by plethysmography
Surgically accessible "target areas"	V/Q scan CT scan
Prediction of adequate remaining lung tissue after LVRS	$Pa{O_2}$ at rest Supplemental oxygen with exercise DLCO CT scan
Preserved respiratory muscle function	Normal or minimally elevated $Pa{CO_2}$

COPD, chronic obstructive pulmonary disease; CT, computed tomography; DLCO, carbon monoxide–diffusing capacity of the lung; FEV_1, forced expiratory volume in 1 second; LVRS, lung volume reduction surgery; MRC, maximal respiratory capacity; QOL, quality of life; RV, respiratory volume; TLC, total lung capacity; V/Q, ventilation perfusion.

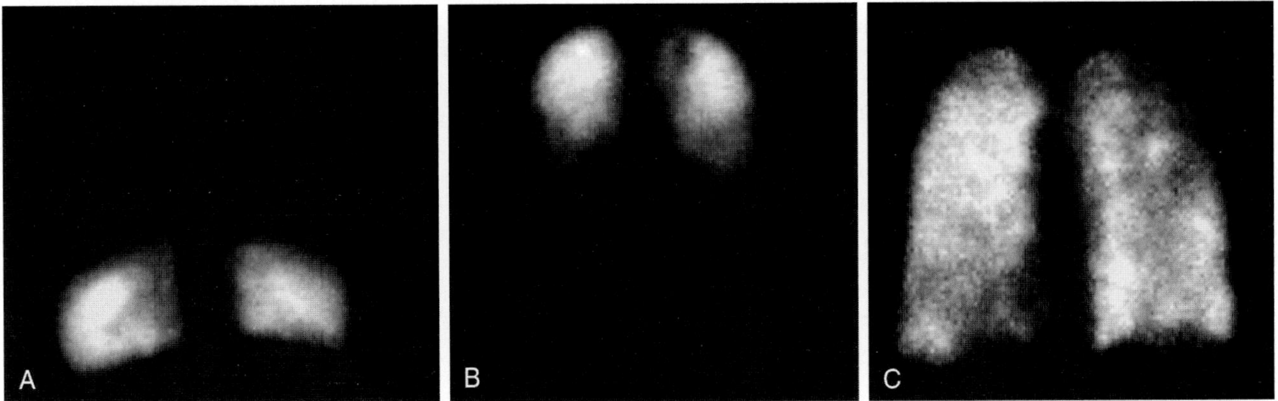

FIGURE 25–1 ■ Perfusion lung scans, posterior view, of three patients evaluated for lung volume reduction surgery. *A*, Virtually absent perfusion of both upper lung zones, providing "target areas" for surgical resection. *B*, Virtually absent perfusion of both lower lung zones providing "target areas" for surgical resection. *C*, Patchy perfusion throughout both lungs, no "target area" accessible (see text).

tal oxygen. Elevated Pa_{CO_2} reflects chronic fatigue of the respiratory muscles caused by the excessive work of breathing. A considerable elevation in Pa_{CO_2} may indicate that the respiratory muscles are too impaired to tolerate the superimposed burden of surgery. It is unclear why resection of the lower lobes for emphysema results in a less impressive improvement than does resection of the upper lobes. Because this is independent of whether patients have alpha$_1$-antitrypsin (AAT) deficiency or not, it may simply reflect the fact that the lower lobes include a relatively greater volume of lung tissue than do the upper lobes; therefore, more lung tissue is lost during lower lobe resection.

Assessment of cardiac function is a critical portion of the evaluation for lung volume reduction surgery. This includes an appraisal for underlying pulmonary hypertension, coronary artery disease, and other significant cardiac dysfunction. Rest and exercise dobutamine echocardiography, radionuclide ventriculograms, thallium imaging, and other similar studies may provide useful information for risk stratification. However, these noninvasive tests of cardiac function are often limited. Exercise testing is often not useful owing to the patient's inability to exercise to heart rate limits. Echocardiography may not provide adequate information because of chest hyperinflation, resulting in poor visualization of the heart. Concern for inducing bronchoconstriction may limit the use of dipyridamole or adenosine. To obtain a definitive answer, many LVRS candidates eventually undergo right and left heart catheterization.

LVRS is a palliative procedure, and criteria should be applied stringently in accepting candidates for surgery. At Washington University Medical Center, approximately 80% of patients referred for this procedure have been excluded from surgery, most commonly because of lack of target areas for surgical resection (30%), insufficient thoracic distention (16%), and the presence of significant co-morbidity (16%). Of note is that 8% of referrals were denied surgery because it was felt that their forced expiratory volume in 1 second (FEV_1) was too well preserved (Richardson et al, 1996). Although limited published data are available (Brenner et al, 1996; Miller et al, 1996) pertaining to selection criteria in other centers, most claim to adhere to similar criteria.

TABLE 25–2 ■ **"Predictors" of Outcome**

Parameter	*Better Result*	*Poorer Result*
Age (years)	<70	<80>70
Pa_{CO_2} mm Hg	<45	>60
FEV_1 (% predicted)	<40%>20%	<15%
DL_{CO} (% predicted)	<50%>20%	<15%
Pa_{O_2} mm Hg	>50	<40
"Target area" location	Upper lobe	Lower lobe >diffuse
Supplemental oxygen with exercise Sp_{O_2} > 88%	<4 L/min	>5 L/min
Ideal body weight	<120%>70%	>130%<60%
Hyperinflation		
RV % predicted	RV>300%	RV<200%
TLC % predicted	TLC>130%	TLC<110%

DL_{CO}, carbon monoxide–diffusing capacity of the lung; FEV_1, forced expiratory volume in 1 second; RV, respiratory volume; TLC, total lung capacity.

PREOPERATIVE MEDICAL MANAGEMENT

Pulmonary Rehabilitation

Comprehensive medical care for the patient with severe obstructive lung disease consists of pulmonary rehabilitation. It is important to assess whether patients who present for LVRS have had an adequate trial of intensive pulmonary rehabilitation, as well as to ensure that those patients who are selected for surgery have undergone an optimal program to prepare them for the rigors of surgery. Pulmonary rehabilitation attempts to return the patient to the highest possible functional capacity. A comprehensive pulmonary rehabilitation program uses pharmacotherapy and provides smoking cessation, education, nutritional counseling, psychosocial support, graded exercise training, and respiratory, physical, and occasional occupational therapy (American Thoracic Society, 1981).

During the initial presurgical evaluation, patients'

medical regimens can be evaluated and individualized, whether or not they are accepted for surgery. For those patients preliminarily accepted for surgery, medical therapy must be optimized after the initial evaluation to ensure that surgery is indicated and to decrease perioperative risk (Gracey et al, 1979). Ideally, medical therapy slows the progression of airflow limitation, corrects secondary physiologic alterations such as pulmonary hypertension and right heart failure, and decreases morbidity and mortality. However, the major achievable goal is palliation with decreased dyspnea, increased exercise tolerance, improved functional status and, an improved quality of life.

Smoking Cessation

Before patients undergo LVRS, they must have ceased smoking tobacco at least 6 months prior to surgery. Because smoking cessation is the only current long-term intervention that has been shown to slow the rate of decline in lung function (Anthonisen et al, 1994; Dockery et al, 1988; Fletcher and Peto, 1977; Hughes et al, 1982; Kanner et al, 1979), cessation is critical to help maintain the postoperative improvement in pulmonary function. In addition, cessation of tobacco use prior to surgery is a representation of the patient's commitment to treatment, a reflection of the severity of the patient's symptoms, and possibly a factor in improving surgical outcomes during the immediate postoperative period, including wound healing (Silverstein, 1992) and postoperative recovery time (Handlin and Baker, 1992; Warner et al, 1989).

Because cigarette smoking remains the most preventable cause of premature death in the United States (American Thoracic Society, 1996), it should be self-evident that smoking cessation should be the first intervention made by the physician (Anthonisen et al, 1994; Burrows et al, 1977). Simple advice to quit smoking from a physician may cause 5% to 10% of smokers to quit each year (Russell et al, 1979), though some studies would suggest otherwise (Wilson et al, 1988).

For those patients who have not ceased smoking, various forms of therapy are available, including group encounters, behavioral modification, hypnosis, and pharmacotherapy. Nicotine replacement therapy has been shown to produce higher cessation rates than those of placebo in clinical trials (Hall et al, 1987; Silagy et al, 1996). Generally, multiple interventions with continued reinforcement are required to achieve long-term success in smoking cessation programs (Kottke et al, 1988), and relapse rates are relatively high (Anthonisen et al, 1994). It is probably counterproductive to monitor cotinine levels as the physician-patient relationship should be established and maintained with mutual trust. However, carboxyhemoglobin data obtained with arterial blood gas analysis are easily available, and abnormal findings should be discussed with the patient.

Vaccinations

During the initial evaluation, a vaccination history is obtained, and appropriate interventions are made. Evidence for benefit from the influenza (Nichol et al, 1995) and pneumococcal (Shapiro et al, 1991) vaccines in this specific population is indirect, but these therapies are generally recommended (Ferguson and Cherniack, 1993) because of the low risk-to-benefit ratio.

PHARMACOTHERAPY

Bronchodilators

Bronchodilator therapy is useful in symptomatic airflow limitation because it optimizes lung function while decreasing dyspnea and increasing exercise tolerance (Guyatt et al, 1987). Although a large proportion of patients with COPD may have partially reversible airways disease (Anthonisen et al, 1994; Eliasson and DeGraff, 1985), aerosolized bronchodilators have not been demonstrated to slow the rate of deterioration of lung function (Anthonisen et al, 1994). A stepwise approach to employing adrenergic receptor agonists, anticholinergics, and possibly methylxanthines is routinely recommended in COPD (Ferguson and Cherniack, 1993); however, the patients evaluated for surgery have markedly compromised pulmonary function, have often already progressed along the stepwise approach, and now require intensified "maximal" therapy. Virtually all patients have previously been prescribed metered-dose inhalers, yet many patients use them incorrectly. Thus, it is imperative to observe inhaler use and then instruct patients on how to correctly use the inhaler, possibly with the addition of a spacer (Newman et al, 1981). In addition, many patients have been prescribed minimal and inadequate doses of ipratropium or β-sympathomimetics. In some cases, longer-acting inhaled bronchodilators such as salmeterol may be useful, especially if the patient is one who is aroused from sleep by dyspnea.

Antibiotics

Antibiotics are not routinely prescribed for our patients awaiting surgery. Antibiotic therapy in COPD should be reserved for those patients with evidence of infection or an acute exacerbation, as there is some evidence that antibiotics may be useful during acute exacerbations that occur without clear evidence of infection (Anthonisen et al, 1987).

Corticosteroids

As many as half of the patients evaluated for LVRS at our medical center use long-term systemic corticosteroid therapy. Unfortunately, most patients with stable COPD do not show a positive response in airflow limitation with oral steroid therapy (Mendella et al, 1982). COPD patients with a large component of reactive airways disease may benefit most from steroid therapy (Weiner et al, 1995), but studies have not definitively supported this suggestion. Therefore, reduction or elimination of dependence on systemic corticosteroids should be the goal of a comprehensive rehabilitation program. Although it seems plausible, there is no definitive evidence suggesting that high-dose inhaled steroids may be used to help wean from, or avoid, the use of oral steroid therapy.

For those patients who are dependent on oral steroids preoperatively, tapering to the lowest possible dose during the rehabilitation phase is mandatory to avoid the associated increased postoperative risks, including poor wound healing (Pessa et al, 1987) and perioperative infection (Glenn and Grafe, 1967). For those patients who remain on long-term systemic corticosteroid therapy within weeks of surgery, supplementation with "stress dose" hydrocortisone is required.

Supplemental Oxygen

Oxygen therapy for the hypoxemic patient is the only therapeutic intervention that increases survival for COPD, as has been demonstrated in randomized controlled trials (Group NOTT, 1980; Medical Research Council Working Party, 1981). In addition, exercise-induced hypoxemia is common in patients with severe COPD, and studies have shown that oxygen supplementation may improve exercise performance (Bye et al, 1985).

Oxygen therapy is indicated for any patient with a $PaO_2 < 55$ mm Hg, or an $SaO_2 < 88\%$. If a patient has evidence of cor pulmonale or a hematocrit of >55%, oxygen therapy is indicated with a PaO_2 of 56 to 59 mm Hg, or an $SaO_2 < 89\%$. Patients should be evaluated during exercise as well as at rest. Oxygen requirements during exercise can be determined by pulse oximetry, using supplemental oxygen to keep arterial oxygen saturation greater than 88% to 90%. If nocturnal oximetry testing is not performed, oxygen should be prescribed at a flow rate of 1 liter per minute above that recommended at rest for patients with a resting daytime PaO_2 of <60 mm Hg, or for those who desaturate with exercise. Patients with evidence of inadequately treated hypoxemia or underlying sleep disorders may be further evaluated with nocturnal oximetry or polysomnography.

Graded Exercise Training

Despite smoking cessation, pharmacotherapy, and oxygen supplementation, many patients with COPD remain breathless and fear overexertion. As a result, these patients become increasingly sedentary, leading to progressive deconditioning. Patients then experience worsened exercise tolerance, and a self-replicating cycle continues. Therefore, a graded exercise program should be initiated for all patients who have severe COPD as a cornerstone of their return to a more active lifestyle.

Exercise training is designed to decrease exertional dyspnea and to increase endurance and maximal exercise capacity (Cockroft et al, 1981; Goldstein et al, 1994; Ries et al, 1995). The mechanisms for improvement have not been fully elucidated, though Casaburi and colleagues have demonstrated reduction in exercise lactic acidosis and ventilation in proportion to the work rate as evidence of a training effect (Casaburi et al, 1991). Improved exercise tolerance may result from (1) improved technique and motivation, (2) improved muscle function and biomechanics, (3) desensitization to dyspnea, and (4) increased aerobic capacity and lactate/ventilatory threshold (Belman, 1986). This improvement in exercise tolerance is not routinely accompanied by improvement in pulmonary mechanics and gas exchange (Casaburi, 1993; Niederman et al, 1991). Given the uncertainties concerning the mechanisms responsible for improved exercise tolerance, controversy exists regarding the ideal training strategy (Patessio et al, 1993). However, aerobic exercise and training of large muscle groups with bicycling or walking may be most useful for mimicking muscle use for daily activities. Other exercise modalities and routines may have some benefit as well. Upper extremity exercise training may improve performance for task-specific arm activities (Lake et al, 1990; Ries et al, 1988), and patients should be encouraged to use arm ergometry equipment and free weights.

Exercise prescription varies based on characteristics of the individual patient, including motivation, lung function, age, and exercise evaluation. Exercise prescription may be defined based on the results of cardiopulmonary exercise testing (Punzal et al, 1991) and scoring of dyspnea during exercise (Borg, 1982; Horowitz et al, 1996). Exercise prescription recommendations vary, and some general guidelines support that individuals should exercise on most days of the week, with the intensity set by tolerance and heart rate limits (Health, 1996). Dyspnea should be assessed before, during, and after participation in a pulmonary rehabilitation program (Borg, 1982; Mahler et al, 1984). Exercise should not be limited by a modest drop in oxygen saturation if oxygen flow rates have not been adjusted upward from resting levels. Supplemental oxygen should be used to keep oxygen saturation above 88% to 90%.

Prior to surgery, patients in the Washington University Medical Center program are required to complete an exercise program that has a minimum goal of 30 minutes of daily continuous exercise (at least 5 days per week) on a treadmill or stationary bicycle. Heart rate limits are set at 80% of the maximum predicted heart rate (220 minus age in years). Supplemental oxygen is provided to maintain the arterial oxygen saturation above 88% to 90%. Patients are periodically re-evaluated throughout the graded exercise program with 6-minute walk tests (Butland et al, 1982). After successful completion of the preoperative program, the average increase in the distance walked in 6 minutes has been 20% (Yusen, 1996). Although a portion of these gains probably occurs initially owing to the "learning effect" (Knox et al, 1988), there is a real training effect. During the preoperative program, patients also experience decreases in dyspnea, as graded by the Medical Research Council of Great Britain Dyspnea Scale and the Mahler Transitional Dyspnea Indices (Yusen, 1996).

An "optimized" preoperative medical status is necessary for multiple reasons. Patients may decide that surgery is not warranted after they experience decreases in dyspnea and improvements in exercise tolerance and functional status related to rehabilitation (Cooper, 1996; Yusen, 1996). Also, preoperative exercise tolerance may predict the risk of perioperative complications (Bechard and Wetstein, 1987; Bolliger et al, 1995), and patients with difficulty meeting rehabilitation goals may warrant further evaluation such as cardiac testing prior to surgery. Finally, it is difficult to claim that postoperative improvements in exercise tolerance have occurred secondary to surgery if patients have not maximized their status prior to surgery. Whether patients who are unable to successfully complete graded exercise programs should be offered the option of lung volume reduction surgery is an area of ongoing debate.

EDUCATION, NUTRITIONAL COUNSELING, AND PSYCHOLOGICAL SUPPORT

Education, which is an important component of pulmonary rehabilitation, may include teaching patients about the basic physiology of COPD, medical management options, and the importance of compliance. This teaching may result in improved understanding and coping, decreased anxiety, and behavioral changes (Make, 1994). Potentially, subsequent improvements in health care utilization may occur (Hudson et al, 1976; Jensen, 1983; Petty et al, 1969; Tougaard et al, 1992). Malnutrition, especially undernutrition, commonly occurs in patients with marked COPD and is associated with increased mortality (Wilson et al, 1989). Patients may benefit from nutritional counseling and the use of nutritional supplements when indicated. Excess production of carbon dioxide due to an increased carbohydrate intake is usually not problematic unless the carbohydrate intake is excessively high (Angelillo et al, 1985).

As part of the initial comprehensive rehabilitation evaluation, counseling may be offered to address coping with anger, depression, and fear related to the chronic illness (Lewis et al, 1993; McSweeny et al, 1982). In addition, counseling provides encouragement and support. Patients may also benefit from enrollment in a support group.

OPERATIVE APPROACH

A bilateral procedure for volume reduction surgery is generally the preferred approach. This is predicated on the goal of achieving maximum benefit at one operation with a minimum of overall morbidity. A comparison of the benefits of bilateral versus unilateral volume reduction was reported by McKenna and associates (1996). Notwithstanding the superior functional results obtained with a bilateral procedure, a unilateral approach may be of significant benefit for certain older, high-risk patients, or for patients with a contraindication to a bilateral procedure (previous thoracotomy or asymmetric involvement of the two lungs). It has also been suggested that a staged sequential approach, with a 1- to 2-year interval between procedures, might produce a longer period of benefit albeit at the expense of a lesser degree of maximum improvement at any one time. For bilateral lung volume reduction procedures, we have employed a standard median sternotomy based on the reduced morbidity associated with sternotomy compared with thoracotomy and long-standing experience with this approach for pulmonary procedures (Cooper et al, 1978). Furthermore, this approach has been successfully employed for many years for patients with severe bullous emphysema undergoing bilateral bullectomy (Gaensler et al, 1983; Lima et al, 1981). Among the advantages of the sternotomy approach are simultaneous bilateral access to both pleural spaces; good exposure for division of adhesions if present; avoidance of injury to chest wall muscles and intercostal nerves from incisions or chest tube sites; reduced postoperative discomfort; and absence of long-term postoperative pain, as may occur with open or video-assisted thoracotomy.

Alternatively, a video-assisted thoracoscopic approach has been adopted by some centers with similar results in terms of short-term improvement, overall morbidity and mortality, and length of hospital stay (Bingisser et al, 1996). The choice of technique will undoubtedly vary from center to center based on experience and the surgeon's preference.

Preoperatively, a thoracic epidural catheter is placed under fluoroscopic guidance to ensure optimum postoperative relief of pain with minimal need for systemic narcotics or respiratory depressants. A left-sided double-lumen tube is used to provide isolated ventilation to either lung. The operative approach we have employed was described by Cooper and Patterson (1996).

Before sternal division, a long, curved sponge forceps holding a rolled gauze is inserted upward behind the sternum from the subxiphoid position and is used to sweep the mediastinal pleura on either side away from the midline. This avoids entry to either pleural space at the time of sternal division. The intact pleura can be deliberately incised following sternotomy, which keeps the opposite lung from protruding into the operative field when reduction of the first lung is taking place.

The initial lung is deflated, and adhesions, if present, are carefully dissected free to avoid laceration of the surface of the lung. Most emphysema patients have few or minimal adhesions, although occasionally, widespread dense adhesions are encountered, usually as a result of a previous pneumonia. Once the lung has become atelectatic, direct visualization of most areas is quite satisfactory. After 5 to 10 minutes of deflation, the less-diseased portions of the lung become atelectatic by the process of absorption atelectasis. However, the more destroyed portions of the lung, those generally targeted for resection, may remain distended owing to the loss of elasticity and the absence of blood flow. Simple cautery puncture of the surface of the region to be excised usually leads to immediate deflation because of the enormous collateral ventilation from one portion of the lung to another in patients with severe emphysema.

Most candidates for bilateral lung volume reduction have a pattern of upper lobe predominant disease. About 80% of the right upper lobe is excised by multiple applications of a linear stapler device buttressed with strips of reinforcing material such as bovine pericardium (Peri-Strips, Bio-Vascular Inc., St. Paul, Minnesota) attached to the surfaces of the stapler before its application. The right pulmonary ligament is usually divided to improve the ability of the remaining lung to fill the apical pleural space.

On the left side, the lingula is generally spared, as it is usually less diseased than the superior subdivision. Thus, about 60% of the left upper lobe is excised with multiple applications of the linear stapler. The pulmonary ligament on the left side is divided when possible, but in older patients, the temporary displacement of the heart needed to visualize this area may be poorly tolerated, in which case the ligament is left intact.

If there is concern that the remaining lung will not easily reoccupy most of the upper portion of the pleural space, then the apical pleura can be released from the chest wall to form a so-called pleural tent, which loosely drapes over the upper surface of the remaining lung. The space above the tent fills with fluid, resulting in a temporary "soft thoracoplasty." It is important to remember that the purpose of LVRS is not to excise all of the grossly diseased lung, but to achieve sufficient volume reduction to improve respiratory mechanics and the function of the remaining lung. An overly aggressive approach may increase postoperative morbidity and mortality, whereas insufficient reduction will diminish the magnitude and duration of benefit achieved.

Virtually all patients are extubated in the operating room. If excessive secretions are present, as indicated by history or by the routine preoperative bronchoscopy, then a minitracheostomy is inserted in the operating room at the time of extubation, to facilitate clearance of secretions.

POSTOPERATIVE CARE

Patients are extubated in the operating room and rarely require reintubation in the initial 48 hours. However, significant hypercarbia and acidosis may be present for several hours owing to the residual effects of the anesthesia or incomplete analgesia. Contrary to the management of other patients undergoing pulmonary resection, the chest tubes in these patients are attached to water-seal drainage without the use of suction. The loss of elastic recoil and the obstructive physiology of the remaining lung make it rather resistant to the usual loss of volume ordinarily associated with a postoperative pneumothorax. The fragile nature of the lungs renders them more susceptible to the adverse effects of increased transpulmonary pressure and overdistention caused by chest tube suction. This has a tendency to increase the magnitude and prolong the duration of air leaks in these patients. Postoperative management is directed at adequate pain relief, early ambulation, vigorous chest physiotherapy and management of secretions, use of inhaled bronchodilators, and use of systemic steroids in the perioperative period to reduce airway reactivity.

Persistent air leakages have been the most frequent source of morbidity, whereas respiratory failure associated with pneumonia has been the most serious source of morbidity and mortality. In our own experience, median length of hospital stay has been 9 days, with a 90-day postoperative mortality rate of 4.5%. This mortality rate is similar to that reported from many other experienced centers.

RESULTS

Several recent reviews have evaluated worldwide results with volume reduction surgery (Stirling et al, 2001; Young et al, 1999). At least five reported randomized clinical trials comparing volume reduction surgery with maximum medical management (including exercise rehabilitation) have demonstrated the improved benefit achieved with volume reduction surgery (Criner et al, 1999; Davies et al, 2000; Geddes et al, 2000; Goodnight-White et al, 2000; Lofdahl et al, 2000; Pompeo et al, 2000). These trials have permitted crossover from medical management to volume reduction surgery after 6 to 12 months. Currently, a long-term trial without crossover is being conducted by the National Institutes of Health in conjunction with the Healthcare Financing Administration in the United States. This trial, known as the National Emphysema Treatment Trial (NETT), is designed to evaluate the effect of volume reduction surgery on long-term mortality, as well as the magnitude and duration of benefit of LVRS compared with outcomes in patients in the control arm who receive standard medical therapy.

The objective benefits achieved with volume reduction surgery have been consistently demonstrated by numerous case-controlled studies (Berger et al, 2001; Young et al, 1999). Maximum improvement is seen within the first year following operation, usually at 3 to 6 months. These improvements include an improvement in first second vital capacity of 50%, a decline in residual volume of 30%, and an improvement in exercise tolerance as reflected in the 6-minute walk test. In addition, many patients showed improved oxygenation with a corresponding decrease, or elimination, of the need for supplemental oxygen. However, this reduction in oxygen requirement may persist for only a year or so. In our own experience, at 6 months, 93% of patients show an improvement in FEV_1, 96% show reduction of residual volume, 83% show improved oxygenation, and 71% demonstrate improvement in the 6-minute walk distance, in comparison with the preoperative, postrehabilitation data.

As these patients inevitably have varying degrees of emphysema throughout their lungs, the early improvement seen following operation gradually diminishes over time, in keeping with the known natural history of emphysema. The duration of improvement is unpredictable; hence the magnitude of the value associated with the procedure remains undefined. There has been sufficient experience to demonstrate that, on average, improvement is provided for at least 2 to 3 years (Stirling et al, 2001; Young et al, 1999). We recently reviewed outcomes through 5 years of follow-up for our initial 200 patients who underwent bilateral LVRS. The improvement in FEV_1 at 6 months averaged 51%, at 3 years 23%, and at 5 years 9%. This analysis, in the context of the known natural history of progressive deterioration in patients with emphysema, confirms significant long-term benefit for the highly selected patients undergoing LVRS. The improvement in FEV_1 observed following volume reduction surgery far exceeds that achievable with any alternative therapy, other than lung transplantation, and contrasts with the observed progressive decline seen in similar emphysema patients denied access to the procedure (Meyers et al, 1998). It appears quite likely that this procedure increases life expectancy as well (Meyers et al, 2001).

In addition to the demonstrable objective benefits, subjective benefits, in terms of reduced dyspnea and overall improved quality of life, have similarly been encouraging. With the use of standard questionnaires to assess quality of life, a significant benefit has been demonstrated for as long as 5 years following operation (Yusen et al, 2001)

The physiologic changes responsible for the subjective and functional improvement experienced by patients remain unclear. Not all objective parameters improve to the same degree. For example, in any individual patient, a minor improvement in FEV_1 may be associated with a marked reduction in residual volume or with a very significant increase in PaO_2. However, the significant improvement observed in virtually all objective parameters for LVRS patients as a whole confirms that the subjective benefits perceived by patients are related to physiologic alterations produced by the procedure. This is in contrast with the "sham effect" produced by numerous procedures performed in the last century, for which no demonstrable objective improvement could be documented. It is likely that the objective measurements employed do not fully reflect the physiologic alterations brought about by the volume reduction procedure. Most likely, the subjective benefit results from reduced dynamic hyperinflation and reduced work of breathing. Whatever the mechanism, the thoracic surgeon will seldom encounter a more grateful group of patients than those who have successfully undergone volume reduction surgery.

COMMENTS AND CONTROVERSIES

The overall concept of lung volume reduction surgery—that "less is more"—seems, at the outset, rather counterintuitive. It is based primarily on the premise that the crippling effects of end-stage emphysema relate in large part to altered mechanics caused by dynamic hyperinflation. This in turn produces both dyspnea and an overall increase in the work of breathing. In this context, reducing overall lung volume to improve chest wall and diaphragmatic mechanics, lessen dyspnea, and secondarily improve function of the remaining lung makes sense. The theoretical objective benefits have in fact been demonstrated to occur, namely, a reduction in residual volume and total lung capacity, improved forced vital capacity, and improved first second vital capacity. Improvements in lung elastic recoil and diaphragmatic function have also been demonstrated. What remains controversial is the appropriate selection of patients, the choice of operative technique, the optimal timing for intervention, and the true value of the procedure. Although comparison with historical controls lacks rigor, long-term denial of surgery to establish a prospective randomized control group for comparison raises serious ethical issues. It is unlikely that a definitive answer will be produced, leaving the appropriate application of this procedure best determined between the surgeon and the individual patient, and the ultimate value of the procedure to be assessed by prospective, comprehensive analysis of results and accurate reporting thereof.

R. J. G.

REFERENCES

American Thoracic Society: Current status of the surgical treatment of pulmonary emphysema and asthma. Am Rev Respir Dis 97:486–489, 1968.

American Thoracic Society: Pulmonary rehabilitation. Am Rev Respir Dis 124:663–666, 1981.

American Thoracic Society: Cigarette smoking and health. Am J Respir Crit Care Med 153:861–865, 1996.

Angelillo V, Bedi S, Durfee D et al: Effects of low and high carbohydrate feedings in ambulatory patients with chronic obstructive pulmonary disease and chronic hypercapnia. Ann Intern Med 103:883–885, 1985.

Anthonisen N, Manfreda J, Warren C et al: Antibiotic therapy in exacerbations of chronic obstructive pulmonary disease. Ann Intern Med 106:196–203, 1987.

Anthonisen N, Connett J, Kiley J et al: Effects of smoking intervention and use of an inhaled anticholinergic bronchodilator on the rate of decline of FEV1. JAMA 272:1497–1505, 1994.

Argenziano M, Moazami N, Thomashaw B et al: Extended indications for lung volume reduction surgery in advanced emphysema. Ann Thorac Surg 62:1588–1597, 1996.

Bae K, Slone R, Gierada D et al: Quantitative CT analysis in emphysema patients before and after lung volume reduction surgery. Radiology (accepted for publication pending revisions), 1996.

Bechard D, Wetstein L: Assessment of exercise oxygen consumption as preoperative criterion for lung resection. Ann Thorac Surg 44:344–349, 1987.

Belman M: Exercise in chronic obstructive pulmonary disease. Clin Chest Med 585–597, 1986.

Benfield J, Cree E, Pellett J et al: Current approach to the surgical management of emphysema. Arch Surg 93:59–70, 1966.

Berger RL, Bartolome RC, Meneghetti AL et al: Limitations of randomized clinical trials for evaluating emerging operations. Ann Thorac Surg 2001 (in press).

Bingisser R, Zollinger A, Hauser M et al: Bilateral volume reduction surgery for diffuse pulmonary emphysema by video-assisted thoracoscopy. J Thorac Cardiovasc Surg 112:875–882, 1996.

Bolliger C, Jordan P, Soler M et al: Exercise capacity as a predictor of postoperative complications in lung resection candidates. Am J Respir Crit Care Med 151:1472–1480, 1995.

Borg G: Psychophysical bases of perceived exertion. Med Sci Sports Exerc 14:377–381, 1982.

Bradley C, Fleetham J, Anthonisen N: Ventilatory control in patients with hypoxemia due to obstructive lung disease. Am Rev Respir Dis 120:21–30, 1979.

Brantigan O, Mueller E: Surgical treatment of pulmonary emphysema. Am Surg 23:789–804, 1957.

Brantigan O, Mueller E, Kress M: A surgical approach to pulmonary emphysema. Am Rev Respir Dis 80:194–202, 1959.

Brantigan O, Kress M, Mueller E: The surgical approach to pulmonary emphysema. Dis Chest 39:485–501, 1961.

Brenner M, Kayaleh R, Milne E et al: Thoracoscopic laser ablation of pulmonary bullae. J Thorac Cardiovasc Surg 107:883–890, 1994.

Brenner M, Yusen R, McKenna R et al: Lung volume reduction surgery for emphysema. Chest 110:205–218, 1996.

Briscoe W, Cournand A: Uneven ventilation of normal and diseased lungs studied by an open-circuit method. J Appl Physiol 14:284–290, 1959.

Burrows B, Knudson R, Cline M et al: Quantitative relationships between cigarette smoking and ventilatory function. Am Rev Respir Dis 115:195–205, 1977.

Butland R, Pang J, Gross E et al: Two-, six-, and 12-minute walking tests in respiratory disease. Br Med J 284:1607–1608, 1982.

Bye P, Esau S, Levy R et al: Ventilatory muscle function during exercise in air and oxygen in patients with chronic air-flow limitation. Am Rev Respir Dis 132:236–240, 1985.

Campbell E. An understanding of breathlessness. Trans Med Soc Lond 92–93:13–17, 1975–1977.

Campbell E, Freedman S, Smith P et al: The ability of man to detect added elastic loads to breathing. Clin Sci 20:223–231, 1961.

Casaburi R: Exercise training in chronic obstructive lung disease. In Casaburi R: Principles and Practice of Pulmonary Rehabilitation. Philadelphia, WB Saunders, 1993.

Casaburi R, Patessio A, Loli F et al: Reductions in exercise lactic acidosis and ventilation as a result of exercise training in patients with obstructive lung disease. Am Rev Respir Dis 143:9–15, 1991.

Christie R, McIntosh C: The measurement of the intrapleural pressure in man. J Clin Invest 13:279–294, 1934.

Cockroft A, Saunders M, Berry G: Randomised controlled trial of rehabilitation in chronic respiratory disability. Thorax 36:200–203, 1981.

Cooper JD: Technique to reduce air leaks after resection of emphysematous lung [see comments]. Ann Thorac Surg 57:1038–1039, 1994.

Cooper JD, Nelems JM, Pearson FG: Extended indication for median sternotomy requiring pulmonary resection. Ann Thorac Surg 26:413, 1978.

Cooper J, Trulock E, Triantafillou A et al: Bilateral pneumectomy (volume reduction) for chronic obstructive pulmonary disease. J Thorac Cardiovasc Surg 109:106–119, 1995.

Cooper JD, Patterson GA: Lung volume reduction surgery for severe emphysema. Semin Thorac Cardiovasc Surg 8:52–60, 1996.

Cooper JD, Patterson GA, Sundaresan RS et al: Results of 150 consecutive bilateral lung volume reduction procedures in patients with severe emphysema. J Thorac Cardiovasc Surg 112:1319–1329, 1996.

Criner GJ, Cordova SC, Furukawa S et al: Prospective randomized trial comparing bilateral lung volume reduction surgery to pulmonary rehabilitation in severe chronic obstructive pulmonary disease. Am J Respir Crit Care Med 160:2021–2027, 1999.

Davies MG, Koyama H, Hansell DM et al: Lung volume reduction surgery in pulmonary emphysema: Results of a randomized controlled trial. International Conference. American Thoracic Society Abstracts. Am J Respir Crit Care Med 161(3):A585, 2000.

Delarue N, Woolf C, Sanders D et al: Surgical treatment for pulmonary emphysema. Can J Surg 20:222–231, 1977.

Deslauriers J: A perspective on the role of surgery in chronic obstructive lung disease. Chest Surg Clin North Am 5:575–602, 1995.

Dockery D, Speizer F, Ferris BJ et al: Cumulative and reversible effects of lifetime smoking on simple tests of lung function in adults. Am Rev Respir Dis 137:286–292, 1988.

Ebert R: Elasticity of the lung in pulmonary emphysema. Ann Intern Med 69:903–908, 1968.

Eliasson O, DeGraff AJ: The use of criteria for reversibility and obstruction to define patient groups for bronchodilator trials. Am Rev Respir Dis 132:858–864, 1985.

Eugene J, Ott R, Gogia H et al: Video-thoracic surgery for treatment of end-stage bullous emphysema and chronic obstructive pulmonary disease. Am Surg 10:934–936, 1995.

Feinleib M, Rosenberg H, Collins J et al: Trends in COPD morbidity and mortality in the United States. Am Rev Respir Dis 140(Suppl):S9–S18,1989.

Ferguson G, Cherniack R: Management of chronic obstructive pulmonary disease. N Engl J Med 328:1017–1022, 1993.

FitzGerald M, Keelan P, Cugell D et al: Long-term results of surgery for bullous emphysema. J Thorac Cardiovasc Surg 68:566–587, 1974.

Fletcher C, Peto R: The natural history of chronic airflow obstruction. Br Med J 1:1645–1648, 1977.

Gaensler EA, Cugell DW, Knudson RJ et al: Surgical management of emphysema. Clin Chest Med 4:443–463, 1983.

Gaensler E, Jederlink P, Fitzgerald M: Patient work-up for bullectomy. J Thorac Imag 1:75–93, 1986.

Gandevia S, Killian K, Campbell E: The effect of respiratory muscle fatigue on respiratory sensation. Clin Sci 60:463–466, 1981.

Geddes D, Davies M, Koyama H et al: Effects of lung volume reduction surgery in patients with severe emphysema. N Engl J Med 343:239–245, 2000.

Glenn F, Grafe W Jr: Surgical complications of adrenal steroid therapy. Ann Surg 165:1023–1034, 1967.

Goldstein R, Gort E, Stubbing D: Randomised controlled trial of respiratory rehabilitation. Lancet 344:1394, 1994.

Goodnight-White S, Jones WJ, Baaklini J et al: Prospective randomized controlled trial comparing bilateral lung volume reduction surgery (LVRS) to medical therapy alone in patients with severe emphysema. Chest 118(suppl 4):102S, 2000.

Gracey D, Divertie M, Didier E: Preoperative pulmonary preparation of patients with chronic obstructive pulmonary disease. Chest 76:123–129, 1979.

Group NOTT: Continuous or nocturnal oxygen therapy in hypoxemic chronic obstructive lung disease: A clinical trial. Ann Intern Med 93:391–398, 1980.

Guyatt G: Measuring health status in chronic airflow limitation. Eur Respir J 1:560–564, 1988.

Guyatt G, Townsend M, Pugsley S et al: Bronchodilators in chronic airflow limitation. Am Rev Respir Dis 135:1069–1074, 1987.

Hall S, Tunstall C, Ginsberg D et al: Nicotine gum and behavioral treatment: A placebo controlled trial. J Consult Clin Psychol 55:603–605, 1987.

Handlin D, Baker T: The effects of smoking on postoperative recovery. Am J Med 93(suppl):32S–37S, 1992.

Hazelrigg S, Boley T, Henkle J et al: Thoracoscopic laser bullectomy: A prospective study with three-month results. J Thorac Cardiovasc Surg 112:319–327, 1996.

Henke K, Sharratt M, Pegelow D et al: Regulation of end-expiratory lung volume during exercise. J Appl Physiol 64:135-146, 1988.

Higgins M, Keller J: Trends in COPD morbidity and mortality in Tecumseh, Michigan. Am Rev Respir Dis 140(suppl):S42–S48, 1989.

Horowitz M, Littenberg B, Mahler D: Dyspnea ratings for prescribing exercise intensity in patients with COPD. Chest 109:1169–1175, 1996.

Hudson L, Tyler M, Petty T: Hospitalization needs during an outpatient rehabilitation program for severe chronic airway obstruction. Chest 70:606–610, 1976.

Hughes J, Hutchison D, Bellamy D et al: The influence of cigarette smoking and its withdrawal on the annual change of lung function in pulmonary emphysema. Q J Med 202:115–124, 1982.

Jensen P: Risk protective factors, and supportive interventions in chronic airways obstruction. Arch Geriatr Psychiatry 40:1203–1209, 1983.

Jones N, Jones G, Edwards R: Exercise tolerance in chronic airway obstruction. Am Rev Respir Dis 103:477–491, 1971.

Kanner R, Renzetti A, Klauber M et al: Variables associated with changes in spirometry in patients with obstructive lung diseases. Am J Med 67:44–50, 1979.

Keenan R, Landreneau R, Sciurba F et al: Unilateral thoracoscopic surgical approach for diffuse emphysema. J Thorac Cardiovasc Surg 111:308–316, 1996a.

Keenan R, Sciurba F, Landreneau R et al: Superiority of bilateral versus unilateral thoracoscopic approaches to lung reduction surgery. Am J Respir Crit Care Med 153:A268, 1996b.

Killian K: Dyspnea: Implications for rehabilitation. Principles and practice of pulmonary rehabilitation. 103–114, 1993.

Killian K, Campbell E: Dyspnea and exercise. Annu Rev Physiol 45:465–479, 1983.

Knox A, Morrison J, Muers M: Reproducibility of walking test results in chronic obstructive airways disease. Thorax 43:388–392, 1988.

Knudson R, Gaensler E: Surgery for emphysema. Ann Thorac Surg 1:332–362, 1965.

Kottke T, Battista R, DeFriese G et al: Attributes of successful smoking cessation interventions in medical practice. JAMA 259:2883–2889, 1988.

Laforet E: Surgical management of chronic obstructive lung disease. N Engl J Med 287:175–177, 1972.

Lake F, Henderson K, Briffa T et al: Upper-limb and lower-limb exercise training in patients with chronic airflow obstruction. Chest 97:1077–1082, 1990.

Levison H, Cherniak R: Ventilatory cost of exercise in chronic obstructive pulmonary disease. J Appl Physiol 25:21–27, 1968.

Lewis R, Caccavale R, Sisler G: VATS—argon beam coagulator treatment of diffuse end-stage bilateral bullous disease of the lung. Ann Thorac Surg 55:1394–1399, 1993.

Lima O, Ramos L, DiBiasi P et al: Median sternotomy for bilateral resection of emphysematous bullae. J Thorac Cardiovasc Surg 82:892–897, 1981.

Little A, Swain J, Nino J et al: Reduction pneumoplasty for emphysema: Early results. Ann Surg 222:365–374, 1995.

Lofdahl CG, Hillerdal G, Strom K: Randomized controlled trial of volume reduction surgery—preliminary results up to 12 months. International Conference. American Thoracic Society Abstracts. Am J Respir Crit Care Med 161(3):A585, 2000.

Mahler D, Weinberg D, Wells C et al: The measurement of dyspnea: Contents, interobserver agreement, and physiologic correlations of two new clinical indexes. Chest 85:751–758, 1984.

Make B: Collaborative self-management strategies for patients with respiratory disease. Respir Care 39:566–569, 1994.

McIlroy M, Christie R: The work of breathing in emphysema. Clin Sci 13:147–154, 1954.

McKenna RJ, Brenner M, Fischel RJ et al: Should volume reduction for emphysema be unilateral or bilateral? J Thorac Cardiovasc Surg 112:1331–1339, 1996a.

McKenna RJ, Brenner M, Gelb AF et al: A randomized, prospective trial of stapled lung reduction versus laser bullectomy for diffuse emphysema [see comments]. J Thorac Cardiovasc Surg 111:317–321, 1996b.

McSweeny A, Grant I, Heaton R et al: Life quality of patients with chronic obstructive pulmonary disease. Arch Intern Med 142:473–478, 1982.

Mead J, Turner J, Macklem P et al: Significance of the relationship between lung recoil and maximum expiratory flow. J Appl Physiol 22:95–108, 1966.

Mead J, Takishima T, Leith D: Mechanical interdependence of distensible units in the lung. Federation Proc 26:551, 1967.

Medical Research Council Working Party (Stuart-Harris CFD, Bishop JM et al): Long-term domiciliary oxygen therapy in chronic hypoxic cor pulmonale complicating chronic bronchitis and emphysema. Lancet 1:681–686, 1981.

Mendella L, Manfreda J, Warren C et al: Steroid response in stable chronic obstructive pulmonary disease. Ann Intern Med 96:17–21, 1982.

Meyers BF, Yusen RD, Lefrak SS et al: Outcome of Medicare patients with chronic emphysema selected for but denied lung volume reduction operation. Ann Thorac Surg 66:331–336, 1998.

Meyers BF, Yusen RD, Lefrak SS, Cooper JD: Letter to the Editor. Ann Thorac Surg 2001 (in press).

Miller J, Lee R, Mansour K: Lung volume reduction surgery: Lessons learned. Ann Thorac Surg 61:1464–1469, 1996.

Naunheim K, Keller C, Krucylak P et al: Unilateral video-assisted thoracic surgical lung reduction. Ann Thorac Surg 61:1092–1098, 1996.

Newman S, Morén F, Pavia D et al: Deposition of pressurized suspension aerosols inhaled through extension devices. Am Rev Respir Dis 124:317–320, 1981.

Nichol K, Lind A, Margolis K et al: The effectiveness of vaccination against influenza in healthy, working adults. N Engl J Med 333:889–893, 1995.

Nickoladze G: Functional results of surgery for bullous emphysema. Chest 101:119–122, 1992.

Niederman M, Clemente P, Fein A et al: Benefits of a multidisciplinary pulmonary rehabilitation program: Improvements are independent of lung function. Chest 99:798–804, 1991.

O'Donnell D, Webb K: Exertional breathlessness in patients with chronic airflow limitation: The role of lung hyperinflation. Am Rev Respir Dis 148:1351–1357, 1993.

O'Donnell D, Webb K, Bertley J et al: Mechanisms of relief of exertional breathlessness following unilateral bullectomy and lung volume reduction surgery in emphysema. Chest 110:18–27, 1996.

Otis A, McKerrow C, Bartlett R et al: Mechanical factors in distribution of pulmonary ventilation. J Appl Physiol 8:427–443, 1956.

Patessio A, Loli F, Donner C: Exercise prescription. Principles and practice of pulmonary rehabilitation. 24:322–335, 1993.

Pepe P, Marini J: Occult positive end expiratory pressure in mechanically ventilated patients with airflow obstruction. Am Rev Respir Dis 126:166–170, 1982.

Pessa M, Bland K, Copeland E III: Growth factors and determinants of wound repair. J Surg Res 42:207–217, 1987.

Petty T, Finigan M, Brink G et al: A comprehensive care program for chronic airway obstruction: Methods and preliminary evaluation of symptomatic and functional improvement. Ann Intern Med 70:1109–1120, 1969.

Physical activity and cardiovascular health. NIH Consensus Development Panel on Physical Activity and Cardiovascular Health. JAMA 276:241–246, 1996.

Pompeo E, Marino M, Nofroni I et al: Reduction pneumoplasty versus respiratory rehabilitation in severe emphysema: A randomized study. Ann Thorac Surg 70:948-954, 2000.

Punzal P, Ries A, Kaplan R et al: Maximum intensity exercise training in patients with chronic obstructive pulmonary disease. Chest 100:618–623, 1991.

Rahn H, Otis A, Chadwick L et al: The pressure-volume diagram of the thorax and lung. Am J Physiol 146:161–178, 1946.

Richardson V, Yusen R, Pohl M et al: Results of initial screening of patients for lung volume reduction surgery (LVRS). Am Rev Respir Crit Care Med 153:A266(suppl), 1996.

Ries A, Ellis B, Hawkins R: Upper extremity exercise training in chronic obstructive pulmonary disease. Chest 93:688–692, 1988.

Ries A, Kaplan R, Limberg T et al: Effects of pulmonary rehabilitation on physiologic and psychosocial outcomes in patients with chronic obstructive pulmonary disease. Ann Intern Med 122:823–832, 1995.

Riley R, Cournand A: Analysis of factors affecting partial pressures of oxygen and carbon dioxide in gas and blood of lungs: Theory. J Appl Physiol 4:77–101, 1951.

Rochester D, Braun N, Arora N: Respiratory muscle strength in chronic obstructive pulmonary disease. Am Rev Respir Dis 119:151–154, 1979.

Rogers R, DuBois A, Blakemore W: Effect of removal of bullae on airway conductance and conductance volume ratios. J Clin Invest 47:2569–2579, 1968.

Roué C, Mal H, Sleiman C et al: Lung volume reduction in patients with severe diffuse emphysema: A retrospective study. Chest 110:28–34, 1996.

Russell M, Wilson C, Taylor C et al: Effect of general practitioner's advice against smoking. Br Med J 2:231–235, 1979.

Sciurba F, Rogers R, Keenan R et al: Improvement in pulmonary function and elastic recoil after lung-reduction surgery for diffuse emphysema. N Engl J Med 334:1095–1099, 1996.

Shapiro E, Berg A, Austrian R et al: The protective efficacy of polyvalent pneumococcal polysaccharide vaccine. N Engl J Med 325:1453–1460, 1991.

Sharp J, Danon J, Druz W et al: Respiratory muscle function in patients with chronic obstructive pulmonary disease: Its relationship to disability and to respiratory therapy. Am Rev Respir Dis 110:154–167, 1974.

Silagy C, Mant D, Fowler G et al: The effect of nicotine replacement therapy on smoking cessation. In Lancaster T, Silagy C, Fullerton D (eds): Tobacco Addiction Module of The Cochrane Database of Systematic Reviews. Oxford: Update Software, 1997.

Silverstein P: Smoking and wound healing. Am J Med 93(suppl):22S–24S, 1992.

Stirling GR, Babidge WJ, Peacock MJ et al: Lung volume reduction surgery in emphysema: A systemic review. Ann Thorac Surg 2001 (in press).

Tougaard L, Krone T, Sorknaes A et al: Economic benefits of teaching patients with chronic obstructive pulmonary disease about their illness. Lancet 339:1517–1520, 1992.

Vigneswaran WT, Podbielski FJ, Halldorsson A et al: Single-stage, bilateral, video-assisted thoracoscopic lung volume reduction surgery for end-stage emphysema. World J Surg 22:799–802, 1998.

Wakabayashi A: Thoracoscopic technique for management of giant bullous lung disease. Ann Thorac Surg 56:708–712, 1993.

Wakabayashi A, Brenner M, Kayaleh R et al: Thoracoscopic carbon dioxide laser treatment of bullous emphysema. Lancet 337:881–883, 1991.

Warner M, Offord K, Warner M et al: Role of preoperative cessation of smoking and other factors in postoperative pulmonary complications: A blinded prospective study of coronary artery bypass patients. Mayo Clin Proc 64:609–616, 1989.

Weiner P, Weiner M, Azgad Y: Inhaled budesonide therapy for patients with stable chronic obstructive pulmonary disease. Chest 108(suppl):107S, 1995.

Wilson D, Taylor W, Gilbert J et al: A randomized trial of a family physician interview for smoking cessation. JAMA 260:1570–1574, 1988.

Wilson D, Rogers R, Wright E et al: Body weight in chronic obstructive pulmonary disease. Am Rev Respir Dis 139:1435–1438, 1989.

Woolcock A, Vincent N, Macklem P: Frequency dependence of compliance as a test for obstruction in the small airways. J Clin Invest 48:1097–1106, 1969.

Younes M: Load responses, dyspnea, and respiratory failure. Chest 97:59S–68S, 1990.

Young J, Fry-Smith A, Hyde C: Lung volume reduction surgery (LVRS) for chronic obstructive pulmonary disease (COPD) with underlying severe emphysema. Thorax 54:179–189, 1999.

Yusen RD, Lefrak SS: Evaluation of patients with emphysema for lung volume reduction surgery. Washington University Emphysema Surgery Group. Semin Thorac Cardiovasc Surg 8:83–93, 1996.

Yusen RD, Trulock EP, Pohl MS et al: Results of lung volume reduction surgery in patients with emphysema. The Washington University Emphysema Surgery Group. Semin Thorac Cardiovasc Surg 8:99–109, 1996.

Yusen RD, Lefrak SS, Gierada DS et al: A prospective evaluation of lung volume reduction surgery in 200 consecutive patients. N Engl J Med 2001 (in press).

CHAPTER **26**

Bullous Disease

Melvyn Goldberg

The surgical treatment for bullous disease has been redefined over the past five decades. The indications for surgical intervention, the types of surgical procedures, and the objectivity of the results have been questioned. This chapter is a discussion of the current practical pathophysiologic findings of bullous disease formation, the specific indicators for surgical intervention, the current operative procedures, and those studies that show definite functional improvement postoperatively. This has been an area of intense clinical activity.

HISTORICAL NOTE

Benfield (1969) summarized the operative procedures that, in the past, were devised to treat bullous emphysema. These included procedures to increase or decrease the size of the thoracic cavity, to increase the flow of pulmonary arterial blood, to denervate the lung, and to stabilize the tracheobronchial tree.

Early in the 20th century, believing that chest wall restriction was an important limiting factor, Freund (1906) and Seidel (1908) devised chest wall operations to reverse rib cage restriction. The intent was to resect several costal cartilages and perform a transverse sternotomy to allow greater pulmonary expansion.

There are reports of operations that were conducted to remove bullae before World War II (Holmes-Sellors, 1933), but it was only when manifestations were gross that surgery was an option. Belcher and colleagues (1974) described 90 patients with large bullae on whom they had operated since the early 1950s. There was a 12% operative mortality rate, and at follow-up, in some cases 10 years after surgery, 35% had died but more than 50% had demonstrably improved. Hugh-Jones and associates (1966) reported a 10% operative mortality rate. Since then, various surgical options for obliteration of bullae have been described. Segmental resection (Head et al, 1960), lobectomy (Woo-Ming et al, 1963), plication (Benfield et al, 1966), and local excision (Wesley et al, 1972) were suggested as suitable techniques for selected cases. Tracheotomy, autonomic denervation, pneumoperitoneum, costochondrectomy, thoracoplasty, tracheal stenting, and intracavitary suction and drainage (MacArthur et al, 1977) have had their advocates (Deslauriers, 1996; Naunheim et al, 1996). Video-assisted thoracoscopic surgery (VATS) and laser technology have been used to ablate both small and large bullae (Wakabayaski, 1993).

■ *HISTORICAL READINGS*

Benfield JR, Cree FM, Pellett JR, et al: Current approach to the surgical management of emphysema. Arch Surg 93:59, 1966.

Brantigan OC, Mueller E, Kress MB: Surgical approach to pulmonary emphysema. Am Rev Respir Dis 80:195, 1959.

Fiore D, Biondetti PR, Sartori F, Calabrio F: The role of computed tomography in the evaluation of bullous lung disease. J Comput Assist Tomogr 6:105, 1982.

Fitzgerald MX, Keelan PJ, Cugall DW, Gaensler EA: Long-term results of surgery for bullous emphysema. J Thorac Cardiovasc Surg 68:566, 1974.

Goldstraw P, Petrou M: The surgical treatment of emphysema: The Brompton approach. Chest Surg Clin North Am 5:777, 1995.

Jensen KM, Miscall L, Steinberg I: Angiocardiography in bullous emphysema: Its role in selection of the case suitable for surgery. AJR Am J Roentgenol 85:229, 1961.

Knudson RJ, Gaensler EA: Surgery for emphysema: Collective review. Ann Thorac Surg 1:332, 1965.

Lefrak SS, Yusen RD, Trulock EP, et al: Recent advances in surgery for emphysema. Annu Rev Med 48:387, 1997.

Monaldi V: Endocavitary aspiration: Its practical applications. Tubercle 28:223, 1947.

BASIC SCIENCE

Pathology

Air Space Disorders

Air space abnormalities may or may not be associated with diffuse underlying lung disease. Such air space abnormalities were precisely defined by Klingman and coworkers (1991).

The anatomic classification of emphysema that is based on acinar involvement was defined by Fitzgerald and associates (1974) and Hugh-Jones and Whimster (1978) (Fig. 26–1). As agreed by the World Health Organization and the American Thoracic Society, pulmonary emphysema is characterized by an abnormal increase in the size of air spaces distal to the terminal nonrespiratory bronchiole that arises from the destruction of their walls (see Fig. 26–1*B*).

Pathologic Classification

Proximal Acinar Emphysema. Proximal acinar emphysema (centrilobular) (see Fig. 26–1*C*) involves the respiratory bronchioles, which are enlarged and destroyed. It is commonly associated with smoking and distal airway inflammation.

Panacinar Emphysema. Panacinar emphysema (panlobular) (see Fig. 26–1*D*) involves the entire acinus uniformly. This form is commonly associated with α_1-antitrypsin deficiency. This association was first described by Laurell and Eriksson (1963).

This type of emphysema is less benign than is distal acinar emphysema and may progress irregularly throughout the lungs. Routine chest radiographic studies identify the stigmata of diffuse emphysema, and the dyspnea that

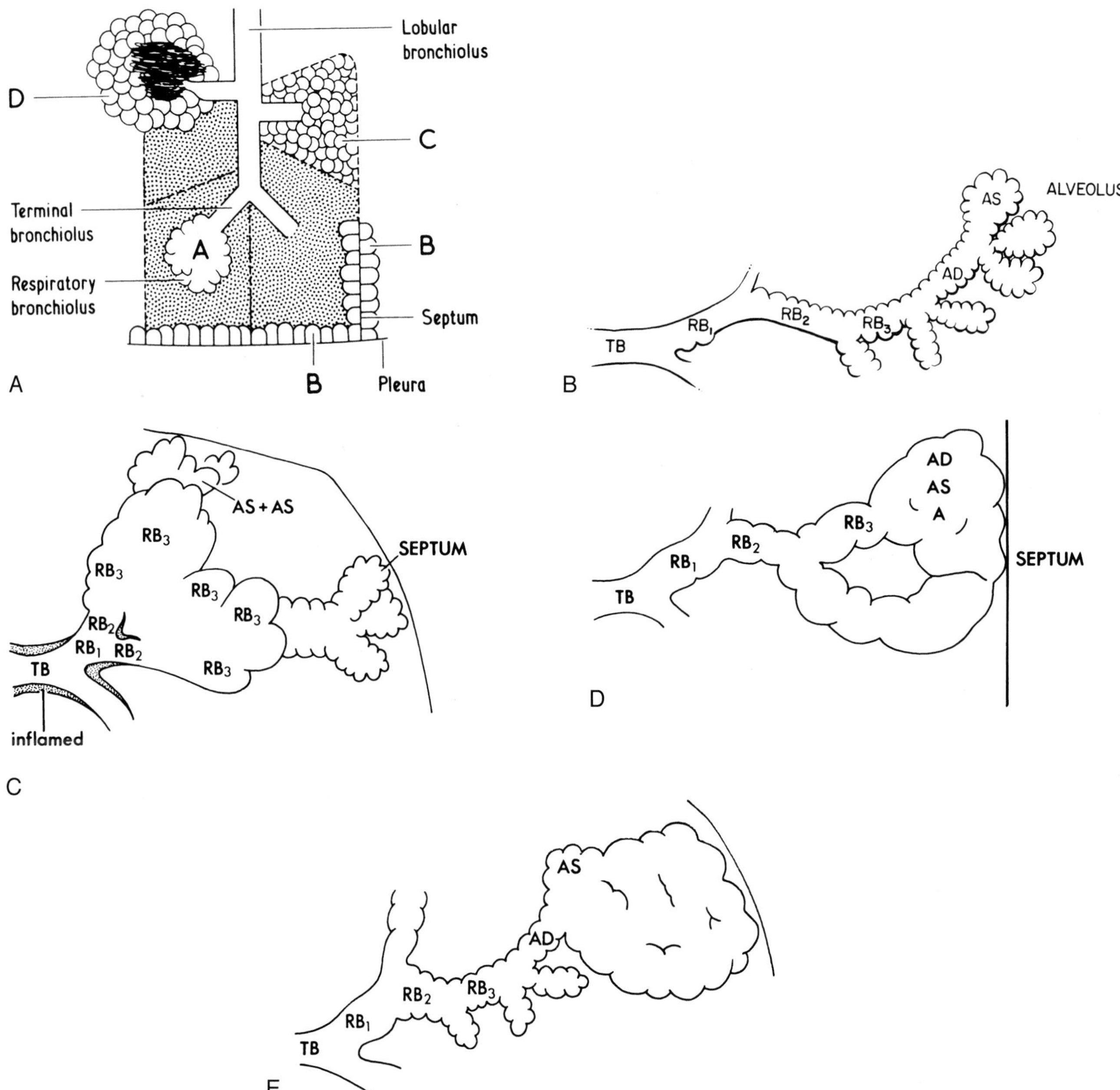

FIGURE 26–1 ■ *A*, Schematic showing various forms of emphysema: A, centriacinar (centrilobular emphysema); B, periacinar or paraseptal emphysema; C, panacinar emphysema; and D, irregular (scar) emphysema. *B*, Component parts of acinus. *C to E*, Specific forms of emphysema: C, proximal acinar (centrilobular) emphysema; *D*, panacinar (panlobular) emphysema; and *E*, distal acinar (paraseptal) emphysema. Periacinar or paraseptal emphysema is probably the most common type among patients referred for surgery for bullous emphysema. The peripheral disruption of the acinus (*B*) is of little consequence deep within the lung, but in acini bordering the pleura, there is coalescence of the tiny spaces, and eventually the lung tissue separates from the visceral pleura to form bullae. (*A*, From Gaensler EA, Cugell DW, Knudson RJ, FitzGerald MX: Surgical management of emphysema. Clin Chest Med 4:443, 1983; *B* through *E*, From Thurlbeck WM: Morphology of Emphysema and Emphysema-Like Conditions in Chronic Airflow Obstructions in Lung Disease. Philadelphia, WB Saunders, 1976.)

the patient experiences is usually much worse than the radiograph might suggest. Pride and colleagues (1970) identified its association with a low diffusion capacity, and Jensen and associates (1961) demonstrated the typical attenuation and pruning of the peripheral vasculature angiographically.

Distal Acinar Emphysema. Distal acinar emphysema (paraseptal) (see Fig. 26–1*E*) involves the distal part of the acinus, ducts, and alveoli. It is usually associated with fibrosis and is subpleural. It is frequently associated with the formation of bullae and pneumothorax. This is the form of bullous disease that surgeons most commonly deal with and fortunately that has the best results after surgical intervention.

This particular type of emphysema is usually benign and confined to the cortex of the lung. It seldom recurs after surgery, and only rarely will this disease progress, allowing the medulla of the lung to retract everywhere with partial obstruction of the communicating airways, air trapping, and resultant giant bulla and adjacent lung compression.

Clinical Classification

A clinical classification of pulmonary emphysema was suggested by Dikjman (1986), identifying three distinct entities: compensatory emphysema, diffuse obstructive emphysema, and bullous emphysema. Compensatory emphysema is not true emphysema, because destruction of the acinus does not occur. It may represent hyperinflation of a portion of the lung to fill a large hemithorax secondary to atelectasis or resective surgery. Diffuse obstructive emphysema is more commonly known as chronic obstructive pulmonary disease and has been discussed in Chapter 25.

Bullous disease is often found with relatively normal underlying tissue and characterized either by bulla or bleb formation. A practical classification of bullous disease was defined by DeVries and Wolfe (1980) (Table 26–1). Group I includes a large single bulla in a normal underlying healthy lung; group II includes multiple bullae of the lung, also with an underlying normal lung; group III comprises bullous disease in the lung in diffuse emphysema; and bullae in patients with other diffuse lung diseases, such as scleroderma, histoplasmosis, pulmonary fibrosis, eosinophilic granuloma, tuberous sclerosis, pneumoconiosis, and talcosis, are included in group IV. Groups I and II are amenable to surgical extirpation with predictably good functional results, whereas the value of surgery is questionable in groups III and IV.

TABLE 26–1 ■ **Classification of Bullous Emphysema**

Group	*Bullae*	*Underlying Lung*
I	Large, single	Normal
II	Multiple	Normal
III	Multiple	Diffuse emphysema
IV	Multiple	Other lung diseases

From DeVries WC, Wolfe WG: The management of spontaneous pneumothorax and bullous emphysema. Surg Clin North Am 60:851, 1980.

Blebs and Bullae

A *bleb* is a subpleural collection of air within the layers of the visceral pleura caused by a ruptured alveolus. The air dissects through the interstitial tissue into the thin fibrous layer of the visceral pleura, where it enlarges to form a bleb. It may produce a pneumothorax. Blebs characteristically occur at the lung apices. Small blebs may coalesce to form larger ones, or they may be multiple, discrete, and scattered diffusely over the upper surfaces of the lungs.

A *bulla* is an air-filled space within the lung parenchyma, resulting from a deterioration of alveolar tissue. Bullae have fibrous walls and are trabeculated by the remnants of alveolar septa. Cooke and Blades (1952) described the following sequence: As the process continues, the cyst-like space is limited at the lung periphery by the visceral pleura. If the visceral pleura is opened over a bulla, the air space beneath it will not be lined by squamous cells but by a disintegrating lung parenchyma, making up the walls and base of the bulla. Fine blood vessels completely stripped of supporting parenchyma cross the air space. Strands of connective tissue and fine denuded bronchioles crisscross the bulla. Multiple small communications with the adjacent bronchi are apparent. Bullae are almost always multiple, but they may be confined to a segment or lobe. The upper lobes are most frequently involved.

Cysts and Cavities

Congenital bronchogenic *cysts* are lined with cuboidal respiratory epithelium. *Acquired cysts* of the lung are thin-walled spaces that remain as an area of lung destruction. They may result from a check valve obstruction of the small bronchioles that distends the distal lung to form a coalescent space or from inflammatory necrosis of the bronchial wall, resulting in the compression of adjacent pulmonary parenchyma to form a large pneumatocele. If a cyst, bleb, or bulla is thicker than 3 mm, it can be called a *cavity.* This almost always occurs after the space has become infected. A thickening of the wall represents a specific or nonspecific inflammatory reaction.

Pathophysiology

Many mechanisms for the pathophysiology of bulla formation have been described. Cooke and Blades (1952) suggested the mechanism that occurs in their development. First, a ball-valve mechanism between the cyst and the bronchus is responsible for progressive enlargement of the bulla. Second, the cyst enlarges because the intracystic pressure increases progressively and thereby collapses the unsupported adjacent pulmonary tissue. Third, inflammation and partial occlusion of the smaller airways produce further breakdown of the bullae with progressive enlargement and further occlusion of the smaller airways. Therefore, the effects of the bulla are to produce an enlarging space-occupying lesion (which is poorly ventilated with no perfusion), which decreases the diaphragmatic and chest wall movements, displaces the mediastinum, and compresses the underlying functional lung and contralateral lung (Table 26–2).

TABLE 26–2 ■ **Classification of Bullous Emphysema**

	Parameter	Type A	Type B
Synonyms		Emphysematous	Bronchitic
		Pink puffer	Blue bloater
		Diffuse	Centrilobular
Subjective	Dyspnea	Severe	Usually severe
	Cough	Occasional	Severe
	Sputum	Scant	Copious
Physical	Breath sounds	Distant	Rales, wheezes
	Cyanosis	None	Frequent
Radiographic findings		Emphysema	Often normal
		Bullae	Fibrosis
Airway resistance		Severely increased	Severely increased
MBC and FEV_1		Severely reduced	Severely reduced
Lung volumes	VC	Normal, reduced	Severely reduced
	RV	Severely increased	Moderate, increased
	TLC	Usual increase	Normal, reduced
Blood gases	Po_2	Normal, reduced	Severely reducced
	Pco_2	Normal, reduced	Increased
Diffusing capacity		Severely decreased	Slightly decreased
Polycythemia		Rare	Frequent
Cor pulmonale		Rare	Frequent
Prognosis		Good	Poor

FEV_1, forced expiratory volume in 1 second; MBC, maximum breathing capacity; Pco_2, partial pressure of carbon dioxide; Po_2, partial pressure of oxygen; RV, residual volume; TLC, total lung capacity; VC, vital capacity.
From Knudson RJ, Gaensler EA: Surgery for emphysema: Collective review. Ann Thorac Surg 1:332, 1965.

Baldwin and associates (1950) demonstrated that large bullae can act as space-occupying lesions that relax or even compress contiguous lung tissue. With the thorax open, either at operation or autopsy, such bullae expand and collapse instantaneously with positive-pressure ventilation. Reid (1967) classified such lesions as "nonobstructive emphysema." The functional residual capacity (FRC) is large, nitrogen washout from the bullae (measured during Monaldi drainage) is slow, physiologic dead space is reduced rather than increased, and ventilation scans show slow turnover within the bullae, as demonstrated by Hugh-Jones and associates (1966). Fitzgerald and colleagues (1974) and Pride and co-workers (1970) elegantly confirmed the following pathophysiologic schema.

1. When the thorax is open, positive pressure allows the lung behind the bulla to expand and radial tension on the airways to be restored. Therefore, bronchial connections leading to bullae become widely patent.
2. When the thorax is closed, surrounding lung tissue is relaxed on positive ventilation; radial tension on the airways is reduced; and all airways (including those connecting with the bullae) have high resistance to flow.
3. After the excision of peripheral bullae, lung tension is restored and the lesion (diffuse obstruction) disappears.
4. The situation in the pulmonary vasculature is similar. Therefore, decreased elastic recoil causes increased vascular resistance in relatively normal regions of the lungs, and pulmonary hypertension is common in patients with giant bullae. There may be as much restoration of the pulmonary vasculature when the lung tension is re-established by surgical excision as there is in the pulmonary parenchyma.

Morgan and colleagues (1989) examined in detail four patients with bullae who underwent resection. They studied intracystic Po_2 and Pco_2, intracystic pressures, and postresection pathologic findings for bronchial communications. They concluded that bullae are not under pressure, there is no obstructive ball-valve effect, and, as a result of parenchymal weakness, bullae are preferentially ventilated (Laplace's law). The elastic recoil of the adjacent lung retracts the lung away from the bulla, thus enlarging it. Their conclusion was that the effect of surgery was not so much to ablate the space as to reconstruct the parenchyma of the surrounding lung, restoring its architecture and mechanical linkage with the chest wall while allowing the lung to regain its elastic properties.

Morgan and colleagues (1989) also suggested that during the operation or in resected specimens there are widely patent bronchi in the floor of the bullae with no valvular mechanisms. The probability of bullae containing gas under positive pressure with resultant compression of adjacent lung is unlikely. The cause of bulla progression is continued intrinsic destruction of lung tissue locally and preferential inflation.

These researchers (1984, 1989) also noted that bullae, as observed by computed tomography (CT), do not change to any appreciable degree in size during inspiration and expiration and the change that does occur is always in phase with the rest of the lung during respiration. The overall gas flow in and out of bullae is small but unimpeded. When bullae and the lung are exposed to the same negative intrapleural pressure, the bullae fill preferentially and always completely before the remainder of the lung is filled. This had been confirmed in vitro by Ting and co-workers (1963). The force of elastic recoil of the surrounding lung produces retraction away from the bulla and enlarges it. Even though the bulla remains in free communication with the airway, it does not participate to any important extent in ventilation (because of its large volume) or in gas exchange (because of its relatively small and avascular internal surface area).

The degree to which bullae contribute to dyspnea depends on the amount of lung that they displace and the extent of the underlying lung disease. Compression appears to have little consequence.

The specific cause of bullous emphysema remains ill defined, although the contributions of smoking and α_1-antitrypsin deficiency have been recognized by Anenback and associates (1972), Hutchison (1978), and Laurell and Eriksson (1963). The most recent theories of the pathophysiology of the formation of bullae were reviewed by Klingman and colleagues (1991).

Patient Selection for Surgical Treatment

Pathology

Although Baldwin and associates (1950) and Siebens and co-workers (1957) thought it important, the differentiation of bullae into those that do and do not communicate with underlying airways has little value in selecting patients for surgery with bullous disease. The only pathologic finding that is important is the size of the cysts and the status of the underlying lung. It has been disproved that cysts in situ in a closed chest are under any tension whatsoever, even when the mediastinum is displaced contralaterally. Siebens and co-workers (1957) identified the importance of the underlying lung in the classification of bullae, with normal underlying lung producing much better functional results than those produced with an underlying emphysematous lung. Wesley and colleagues (1972) pointed out that the type of emphysema is not as important as whether it significantly embarrasses the function of the adjacent lung tissue.

Clinical Presentation

Since the introduction of elective bullectomy in the early 1950s to reduce dyspnea in patients with bullous emphysema, several reports have stressed the importance of careful preoperative selection of patients (Billig et al, 1968; Fitzgerald et al, 1974; Gunstensen and McCormack, 1973; Knudson and Gaensler, 1965; Laros et al, 1986; Pride et al, 1970; Wesley et al, 1972). All patients should be symptomatic with dyspnea. Prophylactic bullectomy in patients with asymptomatic giant bulla cannot be justified. A somewhat quantitative assessment for dyspnea should be used on a consistent basis in preoperative patient analysis. A modified Hugh-Jones and Lambert (1952) grading system for dyspnea is one of several such assessments (Table 26–3). Throughout the literature, there has been uniform agreement that a bulla must occupy more than 30% of a hemithorax before surgery is advised. There are excellent subjective and objective data to suggest that anything less than this produces little, if any, functional improvement after surgery. Clinical improvement and rehabilitation occur in almost all moderately to severely symptomatic patients with bullae that occupy more than 30% of a hemithorax (Billig et al, 1968; Boushy et al, 1969; Foreman et al, 1968; Iwa et al, 1981; Sung et al, 1973; Wesley et al, 1972).

TABLE 26–3 ■ **Hugh-Jones Criteria for Dyspnea (Modified)**

Grade	Definition
0	No dyspnea on exertion
I	Dyspnea on running or climbing two flights of stairs
II	Dyspnea while walking or cycling against the wind
III	Unable to walk or cycle more than 1000 m
IV	Unable to walk more than 100 m
V	Dyspnea on walking in the house, dressing, and washing

From Hugh-Jones P, Lambert AV: A simple exercise test and its use for measuring exertion dyspnea. BMJ 12:65, 1952.

Extreme breathlessness in the presence of a giant bulla is still the best indication for an operation with resultant success (Baldwin et al, 1950; Eschapasse et al, 1980; Fitzgerald et al, 1974; Pride et al, 1970; Weitzenbaum, 1980; Wesley et al, 1972; Witz and Roeslin, 1980). Pulmonary hypertension is not a contraindication to surgery, as outlined by Fitzgerald and co-workers (1974) and Pierce and Growdon (1962). Indeed, the pathophysiologic effect of the bulla on the vasculature of the underlying restricted lung tissue is the same as the effect on the lung tissue itself. With the relief of the space-occupying lesion, the underlying lung expands, the vasculature reopens, and the resistance in both the airway and the vessels may be sizably reduced.

Other clinical and investigational criteria for patient selection are important:

1. Nonfunctioning bullae progressively enlarge (Iwa et al, 1981; Spear et al, 1961; Sung et al, 1973).
2. Bullae should be compressing (and rendering nonfunctional) a significant volume of potentially functional lung parenchyma (Connolly and Wilson, 1989; Fitzgerald et al, 1974; Sung et al, 1973; Wesley et al, 1972).
3. Best results are found in patients with a minimal inflammatory component to the disease process (cough and sputum) (Connolly and Wilson, 1989; Fitzgerald et al, 1974; Wesley et al, 1972).
4. Patients with diffuse emphysema do not tolerate surgical procedures well, and best results occur in patients with localized bullous disease.
5. Removal of a bulla should eliminate the functionless unit and result in re-expansion and return to function of a significant volume of lung.
6. Pneumothorax recurs.
7. Pneumothorax is persistent with bronchopleural fistula (Gaensler et al, 1983).
8. The type of bulla is not as important as whether it significantly embarrasses the function of the adjacent lung tissue.

Functional Status

Much has been written about the differentiation between closed (noncommunicating) and open (communicating) bullae. A differentiation between these two types of bullae can be made based on radiologic and functional studies, which has been described by Billig and co-workers (1968, 1976), Boushy and colleagues (1969), Gunstensen and McCormick (1973), Laros and associates (1986), and

Weisel and Slotnick (1950). Both open and closed bullae are operable, and little or no differentiation between the two needs to be made preoperatively. The assessments have academic value only.

In closed bullae, a small vital capacity (VC) is present because bullae do not contribute to the change in volume. The loss is located on the affected side, which also has only a moderately elevated residual volume (RV) by bronchospirometric assessment. No helium peaks appear on this side with deep expiration at the end of unilateral helium washout. The chest radiograph demonstrates no change in the size of the bulla at maximum expiration.

Open bullae demonstrate a normal VC with spirometry and a normal VC with bronchospirometric assessment of the affected side. The RV is high, and a typical helium peak appears at maximal expiration.

Pride and associates (1973) and Dollery and Hugh-Jones (1963) demonstrated that ventilated cysts are extremely uncommon, and they may function as respiratory dead space. Nonventilated cysts behave as space-occupying lesions, but they seldom produce active positive compression of the adjacent lung.

Jordanogiou and Pride (1968) showed that there is a loss of the elastic recoil pressure, leading to airway collapse during expiration and hyperinflation, as measured by the total lung capacity (TLC) and functional residual capacity (FRC). Ogilvie and Catterall (1959) suggested that overall this increases the work of breathing. Brantigan and colleagues (1959) and Boushy and associates (1968) concluded that elastic recoil can be increased if emphysematous bullae are removed.

Gaensler and co-workers (1986) demonstrated that, with localized bullae, there is good correlation between their size and the forced expiratory volume in 1 second (FEV_1). Therefore, a reduction in FEV_1 that is disproportionate to the size of the bulla suggests significant diffuse disease. There are two indications that the impairment is caused by bullae compressing good lung tissue: (1) a reduction in the forced vital capacity (FVC) almost equal to the reduction in FEV_1, and (2) FRC and TLC that are increased but not to the degree suggested by the lung volume on the chest radiograph.

The difference between the FRC determined by body plethysmographic assessment and that assessed by helium rebreathing indicates accurately the trapped gas volume. Gaensler's group (Fitzgerald et al, 1974; Gaensler et al, 1983) suggested that a large discrepancy is a good indication for surgical improvement. O'Brien and associates (1986) emphasized that it is the nonbullous lung that determines the patient's postoperative function. Vishnevsky and Nickoladze (1990) have shown that a decrease in expiratory flow rates and high respiratory resistance suggests compression of the bronchial tree by bullous areas, the removal of which can cause an increase in FEV_1 and a decrease in bronchial resistance.

The capacity of bullae is assessed from the difference of the RV measured by body box testing and by lung helium dilution (Ichitani, 1985; Laros et al, 1986). After removal of the bullae, the decrease of RV by body box testing indicates a decrease of dead space (Fitzgerald et al, 1974; Gaensler et al, 1983; Ichitani, 1985; Laros et al, 1986). Normal values of diffusing capacity before and after the operation indicate the absence of generalized diffuse emphysema. If the diffusing capacity is reduced preoperatively, it appears to be a reliable test for minimal improvement postoperatively according to Gaensler's group (Fitzgerald et al, 1974; Gaensler et al, 1983, 1986).

Sung and associates (1973) and Parker (1974) showed that, in most instances, patients with resting hypoxemia or resting hypercapnia are not good candidates for surgery. Patients with pulmonary hypertension may also be poor candidates for surgery with resultant poor functional improvement (Fitzpatrick, 1958; Gunstensen and McCormack, 1973; Laforet, 1972). However, the criteria of hypoxemia, hypercapnia, and pulmonary hypertension are not absolute. Harris (1976) has shown that in selected cases, patients can benefit from bullectomy, with the underlying lung function providing the basis for this improvement.

More recently, Tenholder and associates (1980) described progressive incremental exercise testing as a preoperative prognosticator for postoperative improvement. Foreman and co-workers (1968), Fain and colleagues (1967), and others have shown little correlation postoperatively between the clinical improvements and the results of pulmonary function studies. Progressive incremental exercise testing may provide an accurate method for correlating subjective improvement in dyspnea, objective improvement in gas exchange, and increased functional work capacity postoperatively. This exercise testing can also identify the physiologic mechanisms of maximum exercise limitation and abnormal physiologic responses at submaximal exercise levels, as shown by Jones and associates (1975) and Wasserman and Whipp (1975).

The following pulmonary function studies should be performed preoperatively and postoperatively, but there are no magic rules to be derived from the literature to identify the patient who will benefit or who should be refused an operation (Fitzgerald et al, 1974; Pride, 1973; Sung et al, 1973). The tests include spirometric volumes, lung volumes, single-breath diffusing capacity of carbon monoxide, constant volume body plethysmography for airway resistance, specific conductance and FRC, helium alveolar volume, static elastic recoil pressure of the lung, arterial blood gases, and exercise testing.

Clinical assessment in the selection of patients remains problematic. No single lung function test can adequately assess the mechanical and physiologic effects of this disease. Hugh-Jones and Whimster (1978) stated that an overall assessment of the patient preoperatively using many parameters is necessary to determine the candidacy of the patient for surgical intervention.

Imaging

Imaging techniques are used to identify (with as much accuracy as possible) the size, location, and extent of space-occupying lesions. In addition, the technique used identifies the character of the adjacent lung parenchyma that will or should provide improvement in lung function postoperatively.

When an elective operation for bullous emphysema is considered, differentiation between a single giant bulla and vanishing lobes or cysts is important (Billig, 1976;

Billig et al, 1968; Boushy et al, 1969; Fitzgerald et al, 1974; Potgieter et al, 1981).

When simple bullae appear to be present, surgery should not be considered if the bullae occupy one third or less of a hemithorax because, in such cases, an operation seldom improves pulmonary function and validity (Boushy et al, 1969; Fitzgerald et al, 1974; Foreman et al, 1968; Laros et al, 1986; Pearson and Ogilvie, 1983).

Chest Radiography. Burke (1937), a radiologist, coined the term *vanishing lung syndrome*. This expression defines a condition in which bullous disease completely replaces the lung ipsilaterally on the chest radiograph. Fitzgerald and associates (1974) graded lung areas for signs of diffuse emphysema. Each hemithorax was divided into three horizontal zones; and the character, size, and demarcation of the bullae were graded and coded. Vascular crowding, mediastinal shift, and herniation were measured and recorded. Stone and co-workers (1960) showed that such radiographic findings, including severe herniation of the diaphragm on the affected side, mediastinal herniation, and herniation of a bulla to the contralateral side, did not correlate with a patient's symptoms. There was also no identifiable uniformity as to the rate of progression of the bullae over time. No correlation, in addition, was found between the size of the bulla and the symptoms (Fig. 26–2).

Old radiographs might be helpful in so far as they define with some accuracy the natural history and progression of the bullous disease. If the bullous lesion is progressing rapidly, surgical intervention may be more rational than a wait-and-see policy (Gaensler et al, 1986).

Inspiratory and expiratory views are often obtained to differentiate between diffuse emphysema and localized bullous disease. With diffuse emphysema, expiration does not decrease the volume of the hemithorax substantially, whereas with localized bullous disease, expiration dramatically decreases the volume as a result of deflation of the crowded underlying normal lung. For the most part, large well-demarcated bullae are an absolute indication for surgery, with predictable results postoperatively (Capel and Belcher, 1957; Fitzgerald et al, 1974; Sung et al, 1973).

Bullous lesions occupying more than 50% of a hemi-

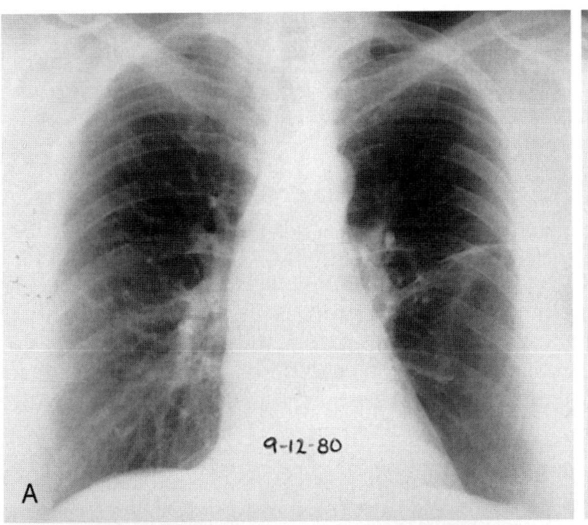

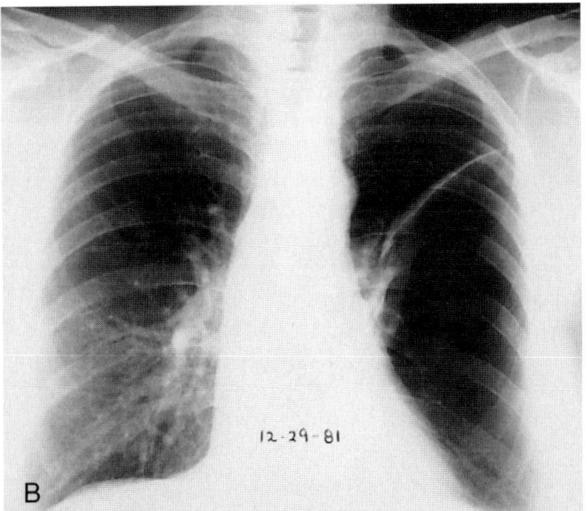

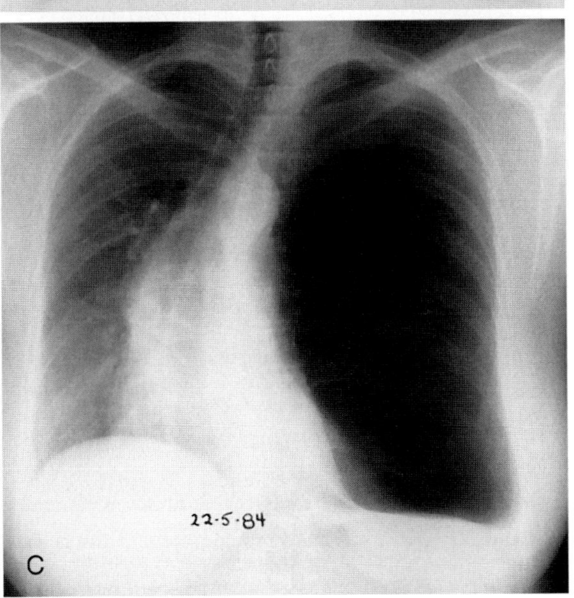

FIGURE 26–2 ■ *A–C*, Chest radiographs showing enlargement serially of a solitary bulla in the left lower lobe over 3.5 years. Ultimately, this produced severe dyspnea and displacement of the diaphragm and mediastinum with additional compromise of the contralateral lung.

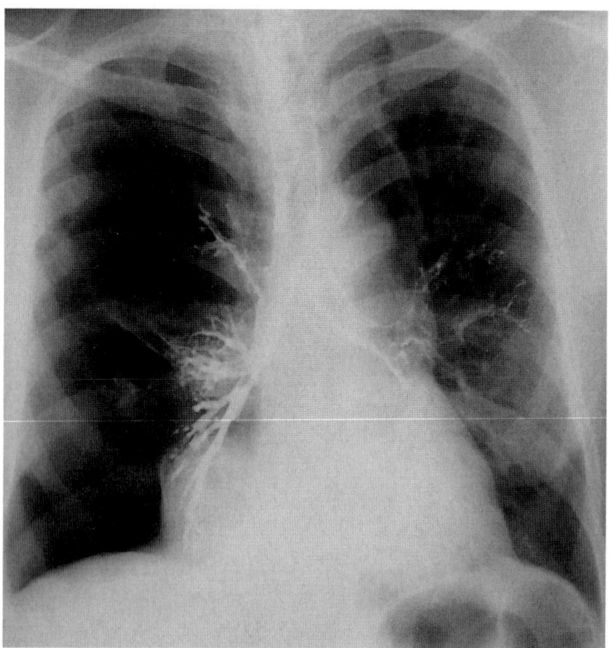

FIGURE 26–3 ■ A bilateral pulmonary bronchogram in a patient with multiple bullae and underlying diffuse disease. The major bullae are on the right, with severe crowding of the bronchi (and presumably vessels) paramediastinally. Excellent symptomatic relief was obtained by multiple right bullectomies.

thorax with normal compressed underlying parenchyma have the best results (Gaensler et al, 1983, 1986; Laros et al, 1986; Morgan and Strickland, 1984; Morgan et al, 1986; Pearson and Ogilvie, 1983). Small bullae occupying one third or less of the radiographic volume with normal lungs have no measurable effect on either lung volume or flow. Ogilvie and Catterall (1959) demonstrated that excision does not improve function or symptoms postoperatively, even in patients with underlying diffuse emphysema.

Bronchography. Before the advent of CT, bronchography was used by several investigators, including Potgieter and co-workers (1981) (Fig. 26–3). This assessment was used preoperatively to identify bronchiectasis and compression of the bronchi by adjacent bullous disease. It is no longer necessary.

Angiography. Before CT, the most accurate definition of areas of functioning lung tissue could only be made by pulmonary angiography. The alveolar "blush" in peripheral lung tissue was the most reliable indicator of persisting capillary circulation. Preservation of vascularity was invariably associated with unimpaired local airflow. Delarue and colleagues (1977) suggested that pulmonary angiography was the most important investigation in determining the feasibility of surgical treatment.

Miscall and Duffy (1953), Steinberg and associates (1950), and Jensen and colleagues (1961) described the effects of bullae on the underlying vasculature. The vasculature may demonstrate the effects of generalized emphysema, which produce a "winter tree" pattern in which arteriolar branches taper abruptly in the midzone and continue in a wiry constricted pattern, causing delayed blood flow to the periphery. Bullae are avascular, and they distort and compress the pulmonary arterial tree. The degree of functional impairment of the surrounding parenchyma can thereby be assessed.

CT contrast studies are now used for this assessment.

Ventilation-Perfusion Scanning. Regional function studies are important in patients with bilateral disease. Asymmetry of function indicates that surgery on the more impaired side entails less risk and is more likely to improve function. Gaensler and associates (1983) demonstrated that perfusion scans are useful to estimate split function but they do not aid in localization because the defects they show generally are already known from ordinary chest radiographs. They concluded that the routinely observed slow entry and poor washout of bullae is predictable without this particular procedure.

However, combined ventilation-perfusion scans, as described by Poe and associates (1973), Polga and colleagues (1984), and Wesley and co-workers (1972), provide a method to evaluate regional pulmonary parameters and may distinguish primary vascular from parenchymal disease. The regional pulmonary function can be identified in both the abnormal and the normal lung, preoperatively, and as a basis for assessing improvement postoperatively.

Computed Tomography. The first description of the use of CT in assessing surgical bullous disease was by Fiore and colleagues (1982). In three cases, this group showed that CT can: (1) differentiate a pneumothorax from a large bulla, (2) identify the extensive nature of the bullous disease in other locations not seen by chest radiography or tomography, and, most important, (3) assess the characteristics of the underlying lung relative to the compression and status of the vasculature (Fig. 26–4).

With its refinements, CT has become the ultimate

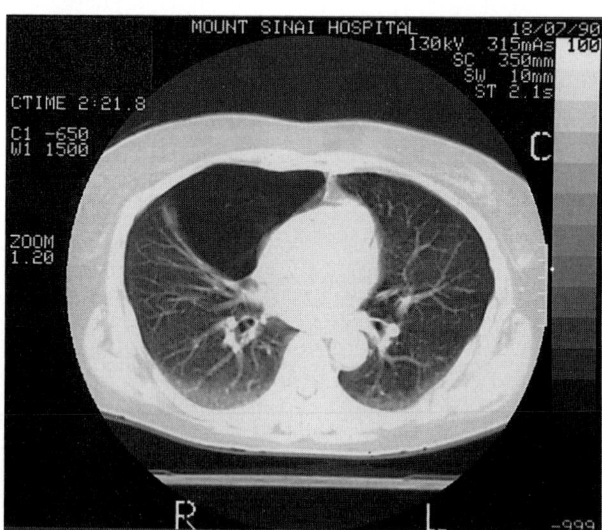

FIGURE 26–4 ■ A computed tomography of the chest with a large solitary bulla in the anterior right hemithorax and crowding of the vasculature in the adjacent normal lung.

imaging technique for assessing patients who have bullous emphysema before surgery. The technique demonstrates the size, location, and extensiveness of bullous disease with increased sensitivity compared with older techniques, such as routine chest radiography, tomography, and angiography. It also provides increased sensitivity and resolution of the pulmonary vasculature and its crowding and the status of the tracheobronchial tree. CT gives useful anatomic information, which should be supplemented by physiologic and functional studies of regional and overall lung function (Carr and Pride, 1984).

In 43 patients, CT was used to assess the distribution, characteristics, size, location, and extent of the bullae; the vasculature of the remaining lung; and the function of the bullae with respect to volume and ventilation. Most bullae were found not to contribute to ventilation, and only patients with true bullae on CT were offered operations (Morgan et al, 1986). Twenty of these patients had generalized emphysema, and 23 had bullous disease only. Operations were performed in 12 patients only with true bullae, with 5 undergoing thoracotomies and 7 undergoing Monaldi procedures.

A reduction in dead space ventilation or a release of lung compression may be unimportant in symptom relief after bullectomy. Practically, demonstrated presence of compressed or dead space ventilation may not be important in justifying surgery. Morgan and associates (1986) and Gaensler and colleagues (1983, 1986) have stated that the mere demonstration by CT that an appreciable space exists may be the only grounds necessary for expecting improvement postoperatively.

Brenner and co-workers (1994) identified a positive correlation between initial radiographic presentation (quantitative assessment of chest radiographs and CT scans) and physiologic function both before and after operation in 24 patients entered into a prospective clinical protocol for evaluation of carbon dioxide laser treatment of emphysematous pulmonary bullae. Patients with large bullae accompanied by crowding of adjacent lung structures, upper lobe predominance, and minimal underlying emphysema showed the greatest improvement in pulmonary function with laser bullae ablation ($P < .05$).

MANAGEMENT

Current Surgical Options

Patients who benefit from the surgical excision of bullae have space-occupying nonfunctioning air spaces or localized nonfunctioning parenchymal areas encroaching on normal or near-normal adjacent lung. Excision removes the space-occupying lesions, allows the compressed lung to expand, permits better ventilation and perfusion similar to the remaining lung, and decreases both dead space and residual volume (Benfield, 1969; Gaensler et al, 1983, 1986).

The surgeon must maximize the preservation of functioning lung tissue or potentially functioning lung tissue by avoiding major resections, such as lobectomies. This is important in patients with diffuse lung disease who have limited overall lung function after bullectomy (DeVries and Wolfe, 1980).

The general indications for surgical intervention are as follows:

1. Moderate to severe dyspnea
2. A bulla occupying more than one third of the lung field
3. A pulmonary angiogram or CT scan demonstrating reduced blood flow to the involved lung field, as defined by Jensen and associates (1961) and Miscall and Duffy (1953)
4. Complications of bullous disease, for example, pneumothorax, infection in a bulla, or massive hemoptysis (Berry and Ochsner, 1972)

Monaldi Procedures

Monaldi (Monaldi, 1947; Monaldi and Tentativi, 1938) introduced a technique using intracavitary drainage for six cases of refractory tuberculous cavitary disease with success. Hennell (1936) and Field and Rosenberg (1937) reported the cure of solitary cysts of the lung by chemical cauterization using the injection of iodized oil or silver nitrate into cysts.

Head and Avery (1949), Head and associates (1960), and Cooke and Schaff (1953) treated several cases of bullous disease successfully with the Monaldi technique in poor-risk patients. The first large series was reported from the Brompton Hospital by MacArthur and Fountain (1977) with 31 patients undergoing such a procedure and an operative mortality of 6.5% in poor-risk patients. Radiographic improvement occurred in 97%, pulmonary function improvement occurred in 83% (FEV_1 and VC), and symptomatic improvement occurred in 90% of patients.

The technique for bullous disease has been attributed to John Alexander in the mid-1940s. A two-stage procedure was initially designed to avoid the risk of pneumothorax and entailed the creation of pleural adhesions over the cyst wall by the insertion of an iodine pack extrapleurally at the first stage and drainage of the cyst 3 weeks later.

Brompton Technique

One-stage procedures (the Brompton technique), as proposed initially by MacArthur (1977) and reviewed by Goldstraw and Petrou (1995), have been successful. A small portion of rib is excised subperiostally over the underlying bulla. A purse-string suture is inserted into the parietal pleura, picking up the visceral pleura and underlying cyst wall. Pleurae and cysts are then opened within the purse-string suture, and a large Foley catheter is inserted. The balloon is inflated with air, the purse-string suture is tightened, and the catheter end is placed underwater to seal and suction. A chest tube is inserted into the free pleural space. Pleurodesis (talc) of both the contents of the bulla and the pleural cavity may aid in the treatment (Uyama et al, 1988; Venn et al, 1988). Rice and colleagues (1987) showed that this technique was excellent in compromised patients and safe with patients whose breathing was supported by ventilators for intracavitary drainage of lung abscesses or expanding cysts.

Venn and associates (1988) accumulated a series of 20 patients in whom this technique was used for 22 bullae.

It was demonstrated that sizable increases in pulmonary function study results occurred postoperatively, with subjective improvement in almost all cases and follow-up of more than 2 years. Shah and Goldstraw (1994) have updated their Brompton experience with this technique in 58 patients with a median age of 56 years. Fifty-two patients (89.6%) noted symptomatic improvement and an objective improvement in lung function. The data have held up for a median follow-up period of 1.9 years. An FEV_1 of less than 500 ml ($P < .05$) and carbon dioxide tension of greater than 6.5 KPa ($P < .05$) were significant predictors of poor prognosis. These authors also recommend the use of talc in the interior of the bulla and the pleural cavity. The rationale for this is based on the reports of Stone and associates (1960), Rubin and Buchberg (1968), and Harada and colleagues (1984), who identified the resolution of bullae after they accumulated fluid spontaneously, whether infected or not.

In an editorial, Ginsberg (1988) described five patients with symptomatic bullae who were all treated successfully. Ginsberg suggested that this technique could replace all other types of procedures performed by open thoracotomy in suitable patients.

Goldstraw and Petrou (1995) defined treatment options for various patient subsets. The surgeon must have a flexible approach and select the optimal procedure for each patient. No single operation is ideal in all circumstances. A major exploratory thoracotomy remains the approach of choice in specific situations:

1. When dealing with the rare patient who has a congenital air cyst in the context of otherwise normal lungs. Local excision normally is possible, but lobectomy may be necessary.
2. When dealing with an infected bulla in which the situation can only be ascertained at operation when adhesions may cause difficulty and drainage may prove inappropriate and when lung resection is necessitated.
3. When operating for a pneumothorax in which the situation can only be assessed at operation and control of an air leak is mandatory by ligation, bullectomy, or intracavitary drainage. The future role of video-assisted operations in this context appears promising and awaits longer follow-up of larger series.

The Brompton technique (intracavitary drainage) offers a simple, safe, and effective therapeutic option in carefully selected patients. The advantages are three-fold:

1. The use of CT scanning allows planning the incision so that a mini-thoracotomy can be performed, reducing the mortality and morbidity formerly associated with thoracotomy in patients with poor respiratory reserve.
2. This approach obviates the need to resect adjacent lung tissue, which in a generalized and progressive disease may be physiologically of disproportionate importance.
3. Pleurodesis allows any future recurrent bullae to be intubated and drained percutaneously under local anesthesia with minimal risk of pneumothorax.

Bullectomy

Most bullectomies were performed through a standard posterolateral approach through the fifth or sixth intercostal space. VATS has developed as an alternative to open thoracotomy. Pedunculated bullae are easily treated through suture ligation of the pedicle and excision of the bulla. For patients with diffuse disease, the basic technique of plication is simple (Fig. 26–5). The development of surgical staplers has made this procedure even easier, and a modification of the method of Naclerio and Langer (1947), as reported by Nelems (1980), is now used routinely.

When an open thoracotomy is used, the largest bulla is opened longitudinally, and the cavity is explored from within. Strands of fibrous septa are excised (Fig. 26–6), and long forceps are applied from inside so that they grasp the pleura at the reflection of relatively normal parenchyma with the cyst cavity. The visceral pleura (cyst wall) is then folded back over the remaining raw surface of the lung, and the stapler is applied along the base of the bulla. The stapler is applied as many times as necessary until the raw surfaces of the entire base of the cyst are closed. This double layer of pleura acts as a buttress for the staples and reduces and prevents air leakage from the stapled margin. Parmar and co-workers (1987) suggested that a Teflon pledget incorporated into the

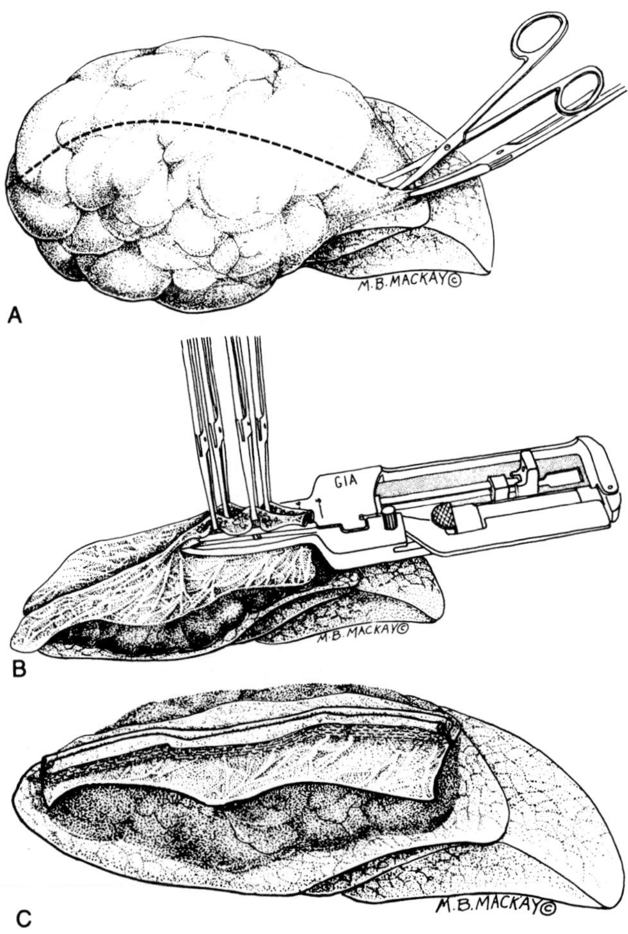

FIGURE 26–5 ■ Operative technique. *A*, Longitudinal opening of the bulla. *B*, Folding of the visceral pleura over the raw surface of the lung and stapling of the entire base of the cyst. *C*, Complete bullectomy. (From Deslauriers J, Leblanc P, McClish A: General Thoracic Surgery, 3rd ed. Philadelphia, Lea & Febiger, 1989.)

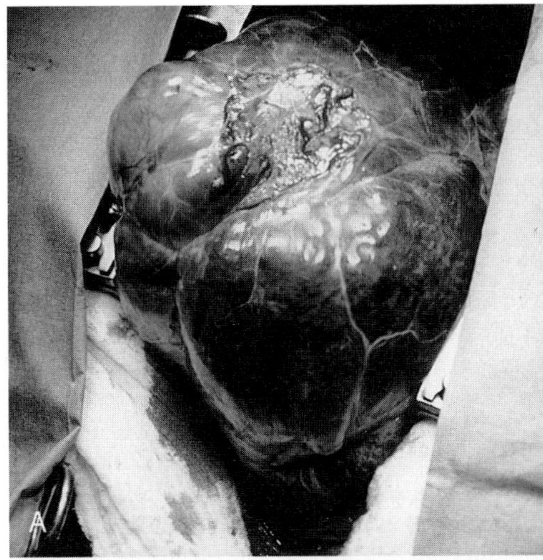

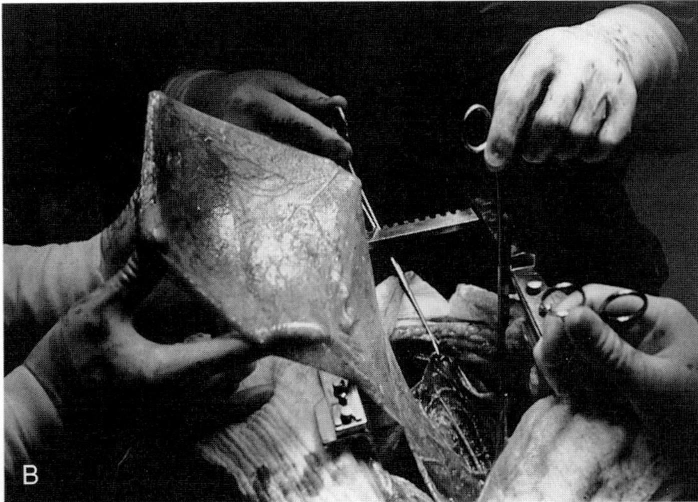

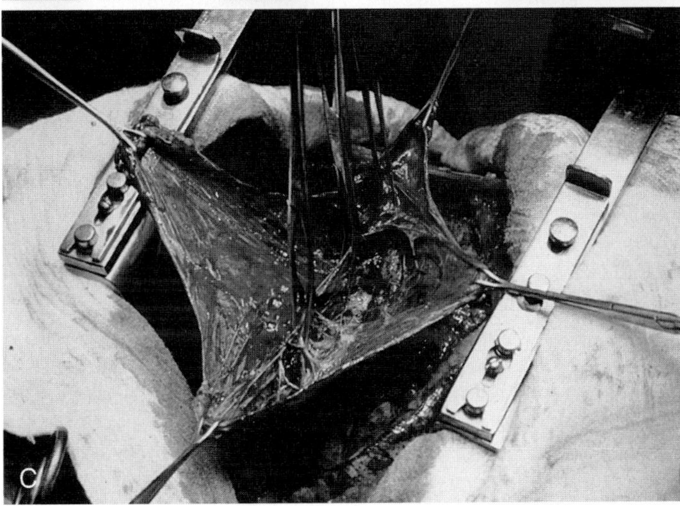

FIGURE 26–6 ■ *A*, A large bulla exposed at thoracotomy, occupying 50% of the hemithorax. *B*, The largest bulla is opened longitudinally, and the cavity is explored from within. The bulla is deroofed, and denuded fibrous strands and vessels are present in its base. *C*, Long Duval forceps are applied from within the bulla so that they grasp the base, which is withdrawn and incorporated into the stapled margin with the folded reflection of the remaining visceral pleura.

bullectomy staple line ensures pneumostasis postoperatively. Cooper (1994) has developed bovine pericardial strips that apply to both sides of the stapling device that help buttress the staple line, preventing air leakage, which otherwise can occur at the staple holes when the lung is reinflated.

After bullectomy, pleural symphysis by poudrage (Cooke and Schaff, 1953), abrasion of the pleural surfaces, introduction of irritating chemicals (Brock, 1948), or parietal pleurectomy (Cabiran and Ziskind, 1964; Gaensler, 1956) has been advocated. It is important to realize that chemical or mechanical pleurodesis is contraindicated, unless there is certainty that, immediately after the procedure, parietal-visceral contact is ensured. This suggests that bronchopleural fistulas must be closed before pleurodesis is attempted, a condition that is rarely satisfied after excision of a bulla in emphysema.

Unilateral bullectomy can be easily performed by a conventional posterolateral thoracotomy with the possible enhancement of postoperative pain reduction and pulmonary function by the addition of a muscle-sparing incision (serratus anterior, latissimus dorsi). If bilateral bullectomies are necessary, the surgeon has two options for open resections—a concurrent bilateral approach by midline sternotomy or bilateral anterior thoracotomies or "clam shell" incision.

Cooper and colleagues (1978), Peters and associates (1969), and Ikeda and co-workers (1988) demonstrated that midline sternotomy (compared with staged thoracotomies) produces slightly better pulmonary function study results postoperatively, with a more rapid restoration over the course of the first week postoperatively. Previous studies were performed by Haughton (1968) and Mattila and associates (1967) that showed little, if any, difference in postoperative lung function when these two types of thoracotomies were compared.

Connolly and Wilson (1989), in a review of 19 patients, preferred staged posterolateral thoracotomies at 4- to 6-week intervals. They suggested that the prolonged air leaks after simultaneous bilateral procedures (sternotomy) are morbid problems that are compounded when the bilateral procedure is performed. Deslauriers and co-workers (1989) and I also prefer bilateral staged operations in which the functional results of the first procedure can be evaluated before proceeding with a contralateral thoracotomy.

Thoracoscopic Approaches

Wakabayashi and colleagues (1991) described the use of thoracoscopy and carbon dioxide laser therapy for bullous emphysema in 22 poor-risk patients. The patients had either diffuse emphysema or multiple bullae. Defocused carbon dioxide laser beams were applied to the external surface of the bullae. Thick intraparenchymal bullae were opened, and the laser beams were applied to the internal surface of the bullae. After complete retraction of all visible bullae, the lung was re-expanded. In contrast to most reports, patients who had less than 50% of the hemithorax replaced by bullae improved after laser ablation. Wakabayashi (1993) has also reported the management of giant bullous lung disease (greater than 50% of the hemithorax) by thoracoscopy and laser therapy. Only 17 of more than 500 cases of thoracoscopic treatment of bullous lung disease over 3 years involved giant bullae. Under general anesthesia with one-lung ventilation, the giant bullae were excised, plicated, or contracted by the laser (carbon dioxide or neodymium:yttrium-aluminum-garnet [Nd:YAG]) thoracoscopically. No procedure was converted to a thoracotomy, and there was no recurrence for up to 3 years of follow-up. This technique has also been used in Russia by Smoljar and Vertianov (1985). Lewis and co-workers (1993) have treated diffuse end-stage bilateral bullous disease of the lung with thoracoscopic argon beam coagulator treatment in 8 patients who were unresponsive to medical therapy and not considered to be candidates for thoracotomy. Complications were uncommonly frequent, but all patients eventually benefited functionally from the unilateral procedure.

Various lasers have been used for bullae ablation including carbon dioxide, Nd:YAG, argon beam coagulation, and holmium:YAG. Both Brenner and co-workers (1997) in the rabbit model and Kaseda and associates (1998) clinically identified the advantages of the holmium:YAG laser as being more effective and resulting in less acute lung injury than the standard Nd:YAG laser. Video-assisted thoracoscopy photoablation may be appropriate therapy for single or multiple superficial bullae because the penetration of the energy source is seldom greater than 2 to 3 mm. Solitary cysts on narrow bases or pedicles can be excised after thoracoscopic ligation or endostapling, but bullae that are more extensive with broad bases and deep parenchymal involvement should be formally excised or plicated by thoracotomy. With this rapidly expanding field, more information on this particular mode of therapy will be available subsequently.

Pulmonary Resection: Lobectomy/Segmental Resection

Lobectomy or segmentectomy is rarely performed for bullous disease, but it may be the procedure of choice when a whole lobe or segment has been replaced by bullae. This may be the initial impression at the thoracotomy when in fact there is merely separation of the lung from the visceral pleura, resulting in a large air space with a relatively normal but atelectatic lobe beneath. Fitzgerald and co-workers (1974), Gaensler and colleagues (1983), and Shaw (1952) showed that, in such cases, lobectomy has had disappointing results because the normal lung tissue that could have been expanded after bullectomy had in fact been removed. Potgieter and co-workers (1981) performed lobectomies in 3 patients of 21 who underwent thoracotomy for bullous disease. All patients had major complications postoperatively, and none of the three had functional or symptomatic improvement postoperatively.

Surgery for Complications

Carcinoma in a Bulla

Tsutsui and associates (1988) have thoroughly reviewed the subject of carcinoma in a bulla. Three patterns of development occur radiographically in the bulla containing the tumor: (1) nodular opacity within or adjacent to the bulla, (2) partial or diffuse thickening of the bulla wall, and (3) secondary signs of the bulla (diameter change, fluid retention, or pneumothorax).

The incidence of bullae in association with bronchogenic carcinoma is 2.5% and is highest in the sixth decade of life (51.6%). Stoloff and colleagues (1971), Korol (1953), Goldstein and co-workers (1968), and Aronberg and associates (1980) have reported this association.

Peabody and co-workers (1957) reinforced the necessity for accurate early radiographic assessment because, in most instances, the diagnosis is made late and is difficult to diagnose. The tumor is seen when it is in an advanced stage in 58.3% of cases.

Infected Bulla

Bullae commonly become infected because they do communicate in most instances with the tracheobronchial tree. Fortunately most can be managed medically, and surgery is limited only to refractory cases that might require surgical drainage or excision. This was the experience of Fain and associates (1967), Ellison and Ellison (1964), and Stone and colleagues (1960). The natural history of a bulla that contains fluid (infected or not) has been described by Lloyd (1949) and Rothstein (1954). Infection in the bulla results in a reduction in its size as a result of fibrotic contraction. The production of fluid produces closure of the connections with the airway and results in the absorption of air and the disappearance of the air spaces. After such infection, bullae often disappear completely.

Hemoptysis

Patients with hemoptysis should undergo mandatory bronchoscopy to rule out endobronchial lesions. *Aspergillus* superinfection should be ruled out. The majority can be treated medically and are commonly associated with infected bullae. With resolution of the infection, the hemoptysis usually resolves. Fitzgerald and co-workers (1974) and Berry and Ochsner (1972) recommended that surgery should be contemplated in those patients who have prolonged, recurrent, or extensive hemoptysis, and the therapy should be bullectomy.

Pneumothorax

Pneumothorax in bullous disease is seldom controlled by tube thoracostomy drainage alone. It commonly produces a persistent bronchopleural fistula and an underlying lung that has not been fully inflated. Therefore, resection of the bulla and closure of the air leaks frequently is the only satisfactory solution. Joress (1956) and others agree that, after a short trial of 5 days of closed-chest tube drainage and suction, thoracotomy should be performed and the bulla and leak should be treated directly.

Tanaka and co-workers (1995) have reviewed the complications of bullous emphysema that require surgical management, including a discussion of the indications, practical aspects, and problems and risks of such surgical treatment.

Preoperative Management

Patients with bullous emphysema usually undergo elective surgery, which allows time for the optimization of pulmonary function. All patients should be required to stop smoking. An active chest physical therapy program is initiated, including deep breathing exercises, coughing exercises, and incentive spirometry. In many centers, a rehabilitation program is available, and a 4-week involvement would be worthwhile in patients who have severely compromised pulmonary function. It has been well established that the objective parameters of the pulmonary function are not improved after rehabilitation, but certainly, both mentally and subjectively, patients are much improved.

These patients commonly have associated reactive airway disease and excessive mucous secretions, which can be treated preoperatively. High airway resistance and bronchospasm should be reduced maximally with appropriate bronchodilators, and antibiotics should be prescribed for intercurrent infections. On occasion, my associates and I pretreat patients with corticosteroids, 5 days preoperatively, to optimize their pulmonary function and bronchodilation. With rehabilitation, the patient's nutrition should be supplemented to provide a positive anabolic effect and an increase in muscle mass.

Anesthesia

Ting and colleagues (1963) showed that, in bullous emphysema, Laplace's law, which relates the expanding force in a hollow structure to the cross-sectional area, applies. The pressure within a bulla equals the mural tension of the bulla divided by its radius multiplied by 2. If positive pressure is applied to the airway, a large bleb can increase in size even more, resulting in a life-threatening situation!

Induction

Hasenbos and Gielen (1985) recommended a spontaneous breathing induction technique and a double-lumen tracheal intubation under sedation and local anesthesia for cases of giant bullae. Myles and Moloney (1994) used this technique to induce anesthesia in a patient with a large leak from a bulla.

Conditions for safe intubation and positioning of a double-lumen tube can be achieved by induction of anesthesia with short-acting opioids and nondepolarizing neuromuscular blocking agents, but it is essential that manual ventilation is commenced cautiously with small tidal volumes, low inspiratory pressures, and deliberate prolonged expiratory phases to atmosphere (Boscoe, 1966; Conacher, 1995, 1997). With such maneuvers, hypoxemia and hypotension are avoided during induction of anesthesia, although carbon dioxide retention occurs, but only in permissive quantities (Quinlan et al, 1993). Deliberate decompression of bullae with intercostal drains preoperatively remains an option, to preempt the development of tension pneumothorax or "breath stacking" and "pulmonary tamponade" effects of positive-pressure ventilation during induction of anesthesia (Eagle and Tang, 1995).

Isenhower and Cucchiara (1976) suggested that premedication should be omitted to prevent preoperative pulmonary depression. To avoid overexpansion of the bulla, intubation can be performed on a conscious patient to omit positive-pressure ventilation during induction. A double-lumen tube is used on a routine basis to achieve split airway control and to ventilate the contralateral isolated lung intraoperatively because most of the ventilation occurs in the bullous lung if both lungs are ventilated simultaneously. Eger and Saidman (1965) suggested that increased concentrations of oxygen are added only after intubation because preoperative increases in oxygen may remove the drive for spontaneous ventilation. These authors showed that the use of nitrous oxide in the presence of an air-filled cavity must be judicious to prevent a further increase in the size of the air space intraoperatively.

Maintenance

The principle is to avoid application of excessive pressure at any point during a respiratory cycle. The safest starting point is to use manual inflation applied cautiously and proceed to a mechanical method with a low-frequency, low-inspiratory pressure (< 20 cm H_2O) and expiratory patterns that are without resistance (no positive end-expiratory pressure) (Bussieres, 1995; Krucylak et al, 1995; Triantafillou, 1996) and prolonged (Conacher, 1995). Various stratagems can be used to maintain the ventilation pattern within the confines that reduce the potential to gas trapping and dynamic hyperinflation. Jet techniques, if not used cautiously, can produce or exacerbate barotrauma (Conacher, 1995), and high-frequency ventilation techniques are potentially dangerous because of the likelihood that high occult positive end-expiratory pressure is generated (Froese et al, 1987). Munson (1974) emphasized the need to avoid nitrous oxide and believed that patients should be breathing spontaneously during the procedure with manual assistance when required. He suggested no positive ventilation and no jet ventilation and avoided inhalant anesthetics. Patients were managed only with intravenous anesthetics to minimize circulatory and ventilatory depressions.

Postoperative Management

Pain control is important postoperatively to allow patients with chronic pulmonary disease and retained secretions to expectorate efficiently with adequate chest physical therapy and minimal pain.

Hasenbos and Gielen (1985) emphasized the value of

intraoperative epidural lidocaine at the T3–T4 level and epidural morphine at least 3 days postoperatively. Most of the afferent nervous input from lungs and airways enters the central nervous system along the sympathetic nerves to the upper four thoracic segments. Brombage (1978), Widdicombe (1963), and Dohi and colleagues (1982) have also shown that afferent blockade with epidural lidocaine at the T3–T4 level can prevent bronchospasm intraoperatively. This also allows intraoperative bronchial toilet to be accomplished with little circulatory depression. Postoperative epidural morphine at the T3–T4 level has been shown by Pinckaers and associates (1981) and Dirksen and colleagues (1984) to produce a rapid onset of analgesia without affecting muscle power or producing ventilatory depression, despite the high position of the thoracic epidural catheter.

Postoperatively, patients may have large-volume air leaks and some difficulty fully aerating the underlying lung and obliterating the pleural space. On returning to the recovery room, an immediate postoperative chest radiograph is obtained to determine the completeness of lung expansion and obliteration of the pleural space. If this problem exists, endotracheal intubation and positive ventilation should be continued at least overnight. If the surgeon can predetermine large air leaks postoperatively, then more than two chest tubes should be used when closing the chest to gain better control of the pleural space. Chest tubes must be drained to underwater sealing, and negative suction can be applied to 20 to 30 cm H_2O, although the exact amount of negative pressure must be optimized in the individual patient. Pain is controlled with epidural morphine for 2 to 3 days postoperatively, which directly promotes effective physical therapy and the removal of retained bronchial secretions. We prophylactically prescribe antibiotics perioperatively to minimize the occurrence of postoperative infection.

Results

Function

Earlier authors (Baldwin et al, 1950; Capel and Belcher, 1957; Fain et al, 1967; Fitzpatrick, 1958; Tabakin et al, 1959) demonstrated that in most cases it is difficult to correlate postoperative subjective findings with postoperative quantitative objective data. Benfield (1969) suggested that one evaluation, which is not done frequently, seems to correlate better than do other parameters, that is, the measurement of the work of breathing. This represents the closest assessment to a patient's subjective dyspnea, which is relied on for subjective assessment of success.

Billig (1976) and Boushy and associates (1969) showed that the values of postoperative pulmonary function depend on the following:

1. The extent to which the bullae contribute to the tests used; therefore, the appropriate test must be performed, and few have value
2. The extent to which ventilated bullae contribute to ventilated space and VC (little change in the VC with resection and replacement by more normal tissue)
3. The extent to which unventilated bullae are resected, producing an increase in VC by filling of the previously compressed lung
4. The extent to which the intrathoracic space occupied by the bullae is replaced by lung tissue
5. The presence of generalized disease

Boushy and associates (1969) and Ogilvie and Catterall (1959) demonstrated that in general after bullectomy, pulmonary function changes toward normal and such alterations are only marked in patients with bullae that occupy most of a hemithorax.

Fitzgerald and co-workers (1974) related early and late pulmonary function to various preoperative assessments (Fig. 26–7). Early functional improvement was related to (1) resection of large bullae (FEV_1 and maximum voluntary ventilation); (2) marked asymmetry of function, with the involved side contributing little, which showed greater improvement (bronchospirometry); and (3) trapped air. The difference between FRC by body box testing and helium rebreathing postoperatively reveals trapped air upon resection. Pride and colleagues (1973) suggested that the large difference preoperatively between FRC by these two measurements favors surgery. In addition, bullectomy for involvement of less than one third of the hemithorax has little benefit as does bullectomy for diffuse disease. Hughes and associates (1984) followed 11 patients who had undergone bullectomy for more than 4

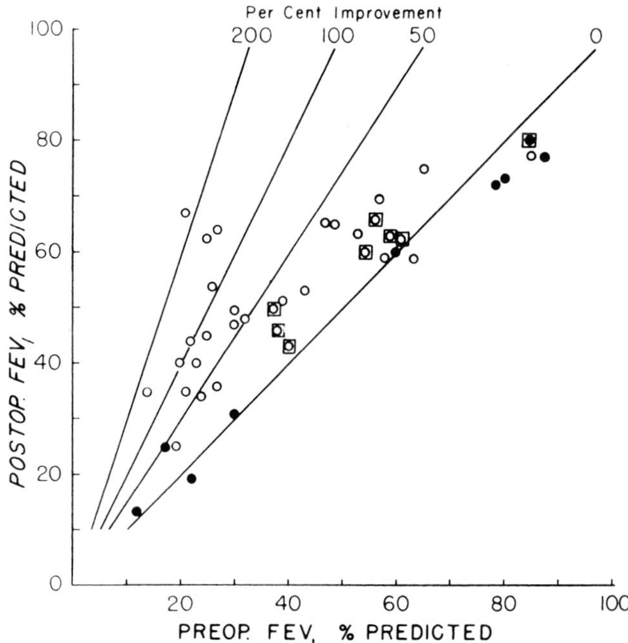

FIGURE 26–7 ■ A comparison of preoperative with postoperative FEV_1 percentages in 42 patients with largely unilateral disease. Resection of small bullae, indicated by black dots, caused little improvement whether overall function initially was severely impaired or nearly normal. Resection of larger bullae, indicated by open circles, generally caused 50% to 200% improvement. Patients who had lobectomies, indicated by squares, showed little increase in FEV_1 after surgery. (From Gaensler EA, Cugell DW, Knudson RJ, FitzGerald MX: Surgical management of emphysema. Clin Chest Med 4:443, 1983.)

years postoperatively with annual pulmonary function tests. Postoperative smokers had a pulmonary function decline, whereas nonsmokers postoperatively had slow, if any, decline in pulmonary function. Pride and colleagues (1970) and Reid (1967) showed that the beneficial effects on symptoms poorly correlated with the objective change.

Iwa and co-workers (1981) performed sternotomy and bilateral resections in 12 patients with bullous disease and showed a good correlation between postoperative subjective and objective results. Nine of 12 patients improved by two functional grades of dyspnea, and 7 of 12 patients had a marked increase in FEV_1 and VC. Improvement was also identified in patients who had preoperative hypoxia and hypercapnia.

Benfield and co-workers (1966) followed 11 of 19 patients who had undergone bullectomy for more than 1 year postoperatively. Initial improvement was seen in all 11, but after 1 year, only 5 had subjective improvement. Eleven of the 19 had increased exercise tolerance several months postoperatively, but this was subjective improvement only.

Wesley and associates (1972) performed bullectomies in 14 patients with 11 long-term follow-ups 2 to 8 years postoperatively. Based on FEV_1, VC, and the transfer factor for carbon monoxide, there was a good correlation between subjective and objective data at the annual follow-up. Long-term follow-up identified good improvement in 6 of 11, fair improvement in 3 of 11, and no improvement in 2.

Fitzgerald and co-workers (1974) reported on 95 operations in 84 patients with bullous disease and found that the best results occurred in localized disease with little generalized obstructive airways disease.

Potgieter and colleagues (1981) concluded that lobectomy should be avoided at all costs and operations should not be offered to bronchitic patients. All patients who had undergone bullectomy with bronchiectasis had major postoperative complications, including empyema, chronic fistula, and chronic collapse. Four of 6 patients with hypercapnia survived.

Pearson and Ogilvie (1983) reaffirmed that successful surgery does not increase the rate of decline of background lung disease or encourage the growth of new bullae. This study also showed that, if patients are selected who have greater than 30% of the hemithorax involved with bullae, both objective and subjective benefits occur for greater than 5 years in most cases. Six of 12 patients had an FEV_1 of less than 1 L preoperatively.

Laros and co-workers (1986) performed bullectomies for single giant bullae in 27 patients in whom more than 50% of the hemithorax was involved. Open, communicating bullae were associated with increases in FEV_1 postoperatively, and the therapy for closed communicating bullae caused increases in VC postoperatively. No difference was identified in those with open or closed bullae, and patients who have chronic purulent bronchitis uniformly do poorly.

Based on the observations made in volume reduction surgery for nonbullous emphysema, Travaline and colleagues (1995) have proposed several mechanisms for improved lung function after bullectomy. By reducing end-expiratory lung volumes, thus diminishing the adverse effects of chronic hyperinflation on chest wall elastic recoil and inspiratory muscle force generation, function is improved. By relocation of the diaphragm after bullectomy to a normalized position, transdiaphragmatic pressure generation, gas exchange, and exercise capacity were sizably improved after unilateral bullectomy.

Fitzpatrick (1958) and Tabakin and associates (1959) understood that specific criteria for surgical intervention are still lacking. The postoperative results are unpredictable, and the most careful studies have shown unpredictable favorable changes and little correlation between subjective and objective improvement.

Laros and associates (1986), Billig and colleagues (1968, 1976), Fitzgerald and associates (1974), Wesley and co-workers (1972), and Pearson and Ogilvie (1983) demonstrated that any improvement shown by spirometric data postoperatively can persist for several years and then gradually decline.

Nickoladze (1992) assessed 46 patients operated on for bullous lung disease. Respiratory function was investigated before and immediately after surgery and during the follow-up to 5 years. The larger the volume of the bullae, the less were the disturbances of lung function caused by their removal immediately after operation. Respiratory function improved significantly during the long-term follow-up after removal of bullae that were more than one third of the hemithorax but did not change when the bullae were less than one third of the hemithorax. No new bullae were revealed roentgenologically at 5 years postoperatively.

Mortality

Data from carefully selected patient studies show that the operative mortality rate for bullous emphysema should be no greater than 5%. In earlier reports of high mortality rates of up to 21% (Delarue et al, 1977; Head et al, 1960), most of the deaths occurred in patients who had generalized diffuse underlying obstructive airways disease, multifocal bullous disease, advanced age, or the presence or absence of pulmonary hypertension. The overall mortality rate in a series of 95 patients was 2.1%; a 1.5% mortality rate occurred with localized disease and a 9% mortality rate occurred with generalized diffuse disease (Witz and Roeslin, 1980). In a study of 50 patients by Head and associates (1960), no deaths occurred in 31 patients with focal disease and a 21% mortality rate was found in 19 patients with either multifocal disease or diffuse emphysema. When the Brompton approach is used, intracavitary drainage has a negligible mortality of less than 1% and a significantly decreased mortality compared with resection in patients who have severely compromised respiratory reserve (Goldstraw et al, 1995).

Morbidity

Fifty percent of complications are related to either poor remaining lung expansion or pleural space problems, as defined by Delarue and colleagues (1977). Fitzgerald and co-workers (1974) subclassified complications into those that were serious or minor. Serious complications occurred in 10.5% of this series, and these included acute respiratory failure, empyema, and chronic bronchopleural fistulae secondary to prolonged air leaks. The incidence of minor complications was 13.6%. Laros and associates (1980) described severe subcutaneous emphysema postoperatively in 12 of 27 cases and also a prolonged air leak greater than 14 days in 12. Potgieter and colleagues (1981) demonstrated that 100% of patients with bronchiectasis who had undergone bullectomy had major postoperative complications in the form of empyema, chronic pneumothorax, or chronic collapse of the remaining lung. This was associated with a mortality rate of 9.5%. A patient's postoperative care should be optimal, with aids in expectoration of retained secretions and cardiovascular maintenance. This procedure should be reserved only for those patients who develop prolonged respiratory failure.

The Brompton approach affords few local or distant morbidities postoperatively, and persistent air leak can easily be managed by outpatient Heimlich valve control (Goldstraw et al, 1995).

SUMMARY

The clear indications for surgery in bullous disease are mainly large or increasing bullae that result in compression of apparently good lung tissue and the complications of bullous disease, such as pneumothorax and infection.

The results of resection of localized giant bullae are dramatic. Lobectomy should not be done until bullae have been removed locally and the remaining lung has been tested by positive ventilation. The resection of small bullae generally has little effect on lung function.

The indications for the resection of large bullae in the presence of severe diffuse emphysema require careful individual study. In such cases, small increments of function may be of great benefit.

Finally, Monaldi-type intracavitary drainage may be indicated in those instances in which open thoracotomy cannot be tolerated. There is some evidence to date that perhaps this particular form of therapy is the procedure of choice in all instances of bullous disease requiring surgical resolution. In the future it is possible that more bullae will be treated electively in this particular fashion.

In general, asymptomatic patients, those whose disease is not localized, and those without radiographic evidence of compression should not undergo an operation.

Pulmonary function tests are mandatory, but CT is the single most useful method of assessing the extent of the bullous disease and the underlying lung disease. If the underlying lung architecture is diffusely cystic, then any surgical option is of a palliative nature only. Nevertheless, these patients should not be precluded from surgical consideration.

Potentially functional lung tissue must not be sacrificed during the operation. Limited resections that preserve all functioning lung tissue ensure maximal improvement. Postoperative complications can be minimized with postoperative intensive care, including tracheobronchial toilet, adequate pain control, and excellent chest physical therapy.

COMMENTS AND CONTROVERSIES

The exact indications and long-term results of surgery for bullous disease are still not completely clear. A patient with an expanding solitary bulla that compresses the lung and produces pulmonary symptoms is certainly helped by bullectomy. The value of surgery in diffuse noncompressive bullous disease is less clear. Lung transplantation has provided another method of treating such terminally ill patients. Since the 1990s there has been a growing interest in "lung volume reduction" procedures to decrease the volume of the hemithorax, thus improving the respiratory mechanics of the chest wall and diaphragm. Whether this "physiologic" approach will alter the management of bullous disease in the future is totally unknown.

I have been especially impressed with the Bimpton technique as a method of treating expanding bullae in exceptionally ill individuals, using local anesthetics and sedation with the patient breathing spontaneously. The reader is referred to Chapter 42 for further information on the management of blebs and bullae complicated by a spontaneous or traumatic pneumothorax and to Chapter 25 for further information on the management of emphysema by lung volume reduction surgery and transplantation.

R. J. G.

■ KEY REFERENCES

Klingman RR, Angelillo A, DeMeester TR: Cystic and bullous lung disease. Ann Thorac Surg 52:576, 1991.

The authors successfully resolve many of the controversies related to the pathophysiologic findings and surgery of bullous lung disease. The review is current and represents a summation and the basis for four decades of interest and ambiguity. It is an excellent source for state-of-the-art information.

Morgan MDL, Denison DM, Strickland B: Value of computed tomography for selecting patients with bullous lung disease for surgery. Thorax 41:855, 1986.

This is the first large series of 43 patients assessed preoperatively with computed tomography for bullous lung disease. The volume and ventilation of the true bullae were measured by computed tomography, and it was confirmed that most did not contribute to ventilation. Computed tomography can be used to accurately predict the functional improvement in patients postbullectomy and is a desired preoperative assessment in selecting appropriate candidates for surgery.

Morgan MDL, Edwards CW, Morris J et al: Origin and behaviour of emphysematous bullae. Thorax 44:533, 1989.

A long-believed hypothesis was that giant bullae produce symptoms of pulmonary compression and collapse by containing gas under pressure that has been generated through valvular feeding airways. This article disproves this postulate and suggests that bullae develop after retraction and collapse of surrounding lung away from a region of weakness that is produced by the pathologic process associated with emphysema.

Shah SS, Goldstraw P: Surgical treatment of bullous emphysema: Experience with the Brompton technique. Ann Thorac Surg 58:1452, 1994.

This article updates a previous report on a series of 58 patients undergoing a modern Monaldi procedure for bullous disease in high-risk patients with low mortality rates and excellent long-term results. The technique is described in detail, and a recommendation is made that all bullae might electively be treated by this minimally invasive procedure.

REFERENCES

Anenback O, Hammond EC, Garfinkel L, Benante C: Relation of smoking and age to emphysema. N Engl J Med 286:853, 1972.

Aronberg DJ, Sagel SS, LeFrak S: Lung cancer associated with bullous lung disease in young men. AJR Am J Roentgenol 134:249, 1980.

Baldwin E, Harden KA, Greene DG et al: Pulmonary insufficiency. IV: A study of 16 cases of large pulmonary air cysts or bullae. Medicine 29:169, 1950.

Belcher JR: Bullous cysts of the lung. In Smith RE, Williams WG (eds): Surgery of the Lung. London, Butterworth, 1974, pp 219–236.

Benfield JR: Clinical Cardiopulmonary Physiology, 3rd ed. New York, Grune & Stratton, 1969.

Benfield JR, Cree FM, Pellett JR et al: Current approach to the surgical management of emphysema. Arch Surg 93:59, 1966.

Berry BE, Ochsner A: Massive hemoptysis associated with localized pulmonary bullae requiring emergency surgery. J Thorac Cardiovasc Surg 63:94, 1972.

Billig DM: Surgery for bullous emphysema. Chest 70:572, 1976.

Billig DM, Boushy SF, Kohen R: Surgical treatment of bullous emphysema. Arch Surg 97:744, 1968.

Boscoe MJ: Anesthesia for heart-lung and lung transplantation. In Prys-Roberts C, Brown BR (eds): International Practice of Anesthesia. Oxford, Butterworth Heinemann, 1966, pp 1–67.

Boushy SF, Billig DM, Kohen R: Changes in pulmonary function after bullectomy. Am J Med 47:916, 1969.

Boushy SF, Kohen R, Billig DM, Heiman MJ: Bullous emphysema: Clinical, roentgenologic and physiologic study of 49 patients. Chest 54:327, 1968.

Brantigan OC, Mueller E, Kress MB: Surgical approach to pulmonary emphysema. Am Rev Respir Dis 80:195, 1959.

Brenner M, Kayaleh RA, Milne EN et al: Thoracoscopic laser ablation of pulmonary bullae: Radiographic selection and treatment response. J Thorac Cardiovasc Surg 107:883, 1994.

Brenner M, Wong H, Yoong B et al: Comparison of Ho:YAG versus Nd:YAG thoracoscopic laser treatment of pulmonary bullae in the rabbit model. J Clin Laser Med Surg 15:103, 1997.

Brock RC: Recurrent and chronic spontaneous pneumothorax. Thorax 3:88, 1948.

Brombage PR: Epidural Analgesia. Philadelphia, WB Saunders, 1978.

Burke RM: Vanishing lungs: A case report of bullous emphysema. Radiology 28:367, 1937.

Bussieres JS: Anesthesia for patients undergoing surgery for emphysema. Chest Surg Clin North Am 5:869, 1995.

Cabiran LR, Ziskind MM: Spontaneous pneumothorax in pulmonary emphysema. Dis Chest 46:571, 1964.

Capel LH, Belcher JR: Surgical treatment of large air cysts of the lung. Lancet 272:759, 1957.

Carr DH, Pride NB: Computed tomography in preoperative assessment of bullous emphysema. Clin Radiol 35:43, 1984.

Conacher ID: Anesthesia for the surgery of emphysema. Br J Anesth 79:530, 1997.

Conacher ID: Prolonged interval jet ventilation. Anesthesia 50:518, 1995.

Connolly JE, Wilson A: The current status of surgery for bullous emphysema. J Thorac Cardiovasc Surg 97:351, 1989.

Cooke FN, Blades BB: Cystic disease of lungs. J Thorac Surg 23:546, 1952.

Cooke FN, Schaff B: Surgical management of emphysematous blebs and bullae. South Med J 46:474, 1953.

Cooper JD: Technique to reduce air leaks after resection of emphysematous lung. Ann Thorac Surg 57:1038, 1994.

Cooper JD, Nelems JM, Pearson FG: Extended indications for median sternotomy in patients requiring pulmonary resection. Ann Thorac Surg 26:413, 1978.

Delarue NC, Woolf CR, Sanders DE et al: Surgical treatment for pulmonary emphysema. Can J Surg 20:222, 1977.

Deslauriers J: History of surgery for emphysema. Semin Thorac Cardiovasc Surg 8:43, 1996.

Deslauriers J, Leblanc P, McClish A: General Thoracic Surgery, 3rd ed. Philadelphia, Lea & Febiger, 1989.

DeVries WC, Wolfe WG: The management of spontaneous pneumothorax and bullous emphysema. Surg Clin North Am 60:851, 1980.

Dikjman JH: Morphological aspects, classification and epidemiology of emphysema. Bull Eur Physiopathol Respir 22:241, 1986.

Dirksen R, Pinckaers JWM, VanEgmond J: Indicators for perispinal opiates. In Gomez DJ, Egay LM, de la Cruz-Odi MF (eds): Anesthesia—Safety for All. New York, Elsevier Science Publishing, 1984, p 397.

Dohi S, Nishikowa T, Ujike Y, Mayumi T: Circulatory responses to airway stimulation and cervical epidural blockade. Anesthesiology 57:359, 1982.

Dollery G, Hugh-Jones P: Gas and blood distribution in lung disease. Br Med Bull 19:59, 1963.

Eagle C, Tang T: Anesthetic management of a patient with a descending thoracic aortic aneurysm and severe bilateral bullous pulmonary disease. Can J Anesth 42:168, 1995.

Eger EL, Saidman LJ: Hazards of nitrous oxide anesthesia with bowel obstruction and pneumothorax. Anesthesiology 26:61, 1965.

Ellison LT, Ellison RG: Surgery of bullae, blebs and cysts of the lung: A six year review. Am Surg 30:774, 1964.

Eschapasse H, Fabre J, Joffa R: Intérét de la pleurectomie comme complement des resections de bulles d'emphysème. Rev Mal Respir 8:155, 1980.

Fain WR, Conn JH, Campbell GD et al: Excision of giant pulmonary emphysematous cysts: Report of 20 cases without deaths. Surgery 62:552, 1967.

Field W, Rosenberg L: Cystic disease of the lung: Cure of a solitary cyst by chemical cauterization. J Thorac Surg 7:218, 1937.

Fiore D, Biondetti PR, Sartori F, Calabrio F: The role of computed tomography in the evaluation of bullous lung disease. J Comput Assist Tomogr 6:105, 1982.

Fitzgerald MX, Keelan PJ, Cugell DW, Gaensler EA: Long-term results of surgery for bullous emphysema. J Thorac Cardiovasc Surg 68:566, 1974.

Fitzpatrick MJ: Prolonged observation of patients with cor pulmonale and bullous emphysema after surgical resection. Am Rev Respir Dis 77:387, 1958.

Foreman S, Weil H, Duke R: Bullous disease of the lung: Physiologic improvement after surgery. Ann Intern Med 69:757, 1968.

Freund WA: Zur operativen Behandlung gewissen Lungenkrankheiten insbesondere des auf starrer Thoraxdilatation bernhenden alveolaren Emphysems. Z Exp Pathol Ther 3:479, 1906.

Froese AB, Bryan AC: High frequency ventilation. Am Rev Respir Dis 135:1363, 1987.

Gaensler EA: Parietal pleurectomy for recurrent spontaneous pneumothorax. Surg Gynecol Obstet 102:293, 1956.

Gaensler EA, Cugell DW, Knudson RJ et al: Surgical management of emphysema. Clin Chest Med 4:443, 1983.

Gaensler EA, Jederlinic PJ, Fitzgerald MX: Patient workup for bullectomy. J Thorac Imaging 1:75, 1986.

Ginsberg RJ: Tube thoracostomy drainage. Chest 94:1125, 1988.

Goldstein MJ, Snider GL, Liberson M et al: Bronchogenic carcinoma and giant bullous disease. Am Rev Respir Dis 97:1062, 1968.

Goldstraw P, Petrou M: The surgical treatment of emphysema: The Brompton approach. Chest Surg Clin North Am 5:777, 1995.

Gunstensen J, McCormack RJM: The surgical management of bullous emphysema. J Thorac Cardiovasc Surg 65:920, 1973.

Harada K, Shimada Y, Saoyama N et al: Postinflammatory reduction of giant bullae and changes of the opposite lung bullae after unilateral bullectomy. Rinsho Geka 39:377, 1984.

Harris J: Severe bullous emphysema: Successful surgical management despite poor preoperation blood gas levels and marked pulmonary hypertension. Chest 70:658, 1976.

Hasenbos MAWM, Gielen MJM: Anaesthesia for bullectomy. Anaesthesia 40:977, 1985.

Haughton V: Changes in pulmonary compliance in patients undergoing cardiac surgery. Dis Chest 53:617, 1968.

Head JR, Avery EF: Intracavitary suction (Monaldi) in the treatment of emphysematous bullae and blebs. J Thorac Surg 18:761, 1949.

Head JM, Head LR, Hudson TR, Head JR: The surgical treatment of emphysematous blebs and localized vesicular and bullous emphysema. J Thorac Cardiovasc Surg 40:443, 1960.

Hennell H: Acquired giant air cysts of the lung. Mt Sinai J Med 3:155, 1936.

Holmes-Sellors T: Surgery of the Thorax. London, Constable, 1933, pp 393–395.

Hugh-Jones P, Lambert AV: A simple exercise test and its use for measuring exertion dyspnea. BMJ 12:65, 1952.

Hugh-Jones P, Ritchie BC, Dollery CT: Surgical treatment of emphysema. BMJ 1:1133, 1966.

Hugh-Jones P, Whimster W: The etiology and management of disabling emphysema. Am Rev Respir Dis 117:343, 1978.

Hughes JA, MacArthur AM, Hutchinson DCS, et al: Long-term changes in lung function after surgical treatment of bullous emphysema in smokers and ex-smokers. Thorax 39:140, 1984.

Hutchison DCS: Alpha-1-antitrypsin deficiency and pulmonary emphysema: The role of proteolytic enzymes and their inhibitors. Br J Dis Chest 67:171, 1978.

Ichitani Y: The pathophysiology and surgical indications of gigantic bullae. Nippon Kyobu Shikkan Gakkai Zasshi 132:1055, 1985.

Ikeda M, Uno A, Yamane Y et al: Median sternotomy with bilateral bullous resection for unilateral spontaneous pneumothorax, with special reference to operative indications. J Thorac Cardiovasc Surg 96:615, 1988.

Isenhower N, Cucchiara RF: Anesthesia for vanishing lung syndrome. Anesth Analg 55:750, 1976.

Iwa T, Watanabe Y, Fukatani G: Simultaneous bilateral operations for bullous emphysema by median sternotomy. J Thorac Cardiovasc Surg 81:732, 1981.

Jensen KM, Miscall L, Steinberg I: Angiocardiography in bullous emphysema: Its role in selection of the case suitable for surgery. AJR Am J Roentgenol 85:229, 1961.

Jones NL, Campbell ESM, Edwards RHT: Clinical Exercise Testing. Philadelphia, WB Saunders, 1975.

Jordanogiou J, Pride NB: A comparison of maximum inspiratory and expiratory flow in health and in lung disease. Thorax 23:38, 1968.

Joress MH: Pulmonary cystic disease: Observations in cases treated by exploratory thoracotomy. Dis Chest 35:256, 1956.

Kaseda S, Aoki T, Hangai N et al: Treating bullous lung disease with Holmium:YAG laser in conjunction with fibrin glue and Dexon mesh. Lasers Surg Med 22:219, 1998.

Klingman RR, Angelillo A, DeMeester TR: Cystic and bullous lung disease. Ann Thorac Surg 52:576, 1991.

Knudson RJ, Gaensler EA: Surgery for emphysema: Collective review. Ann Thorac Surg 1:332, 1965.

Korol E: Correlation of carcinoma and congenital cystic emphysema, 10 cases. Dis Chest 23:403, 1953.

Krucylak PE, Naunheim KS, Keller CA, et al: Anesthetic management of patients undergoing thoracoscopic lung reduction for treatment of end stage emphysema. Anesth Analg 80:SCA80, 1995.

Laforet KG: Current concepts in surgical management of chronic obstructive lung disease. N Engl J Med 287:175, 1972.

Laros CD, Gelissen JH, Bergstein PG: Bullectomy for giant bullae in emphysema. J Thorac Cardiovasc Surg 91:63, 1986.

Laurell CB, Eriksson S: The electrophoretic alpha-1-globulin pattern of serum in alpha-1-antitrypsin deficiency. Scand J Clin Lab Invest 15:132, 1963.

Lewis RJ, Caccavale RJ, Sisler GE: VATS-Argon Beam Coagulator treatment of diffuse end-stage bilateral bullous disease of the lung. Ann Thorac Surg 55:1394, 1993.

Lloyd MS: Bullous emphysema: Case report. J Thorac Surg 18:532, 1949.

MacArthur AM, Fountain SW: Intracavity suction and drainage in the treatment of emphysematous bullae. Thorax 32:668, 1977.

Mattila T, Laustela E, Tala P: On the effect of sternotomy and thoracotomy incision on pulmonary function after open-heart operations. Ann Chir Gynaecol 56:58, 1967.

Miscall L, Duffy RW: Surgical treatment of bullous emphysema: Contributions of angiocardiography. Dis Chest 24:489, 1953.

Monaldi V: Endocavitary aspiration: Its practical applications. Tubercle 28:223, 1947.

Monaldi V, Tentativi D: Aspirazione endocavitaria nelle caverne tuberculari del pulmone. Lotta Contra la Tuberculosi 9:910, 1938.

Morgan MDL, Denison DM, Strickland B: Value of computed tomography for selecting patients with bullous lung disease for surgery. Thorax 41:855, 1986.

Morgan MDL, Edwards CW, Morris J et al: Origin and behaviour of emphysematous bullae. Thorax 44:553, 1989.

Morgan MDL, Strickland BS: Computed tomography in the assessment of bullous lung disease. Br J Dis Chest 78:10, 1984.

Munson ES: Transfer of nitrous oxide into body air cavities. Br J Anaesth 46:202, 1974.

Myles PS, Moloney J: Anesthetic management of a patient with severe bullous lung disease complicated by air leak. Anesth Intens Care 22:201, 1994.

Naclerio E, Langer L: Pulmonary cysts: Special reference to surgical treatment of emphysematous blebs and bullae. Surgery 22:516, 1947.

Naunheim KS, Keller CA, Krucylak PE et al: Unilateral video assisted thoracic surgical lung reduction. Ann Thorac Surg 61:1092, 1996.

Nelems JMB: A technique for controlling bullous cysts of lungs (Abstract). In Postgraduate Course in General Thoracic Surgery. University of Toronto, May 1980.

Nickoladze GD: Functional results of surgery for bullous emphysema. Chest 101:119, 1992.

O'Brien CJ, Hughes CF, Gianoutsos P: Surgical treatment of bullous emphysema. Aust N Z J Surg 56:241, 1986.

Ogilvie C, Catterall M: Patterns of disturbed lung function in patients with emphysematous bullae. Thorax 14:216, 1959.

Parker JP: Surgery in chronic lung disease. Surg Clin North Am 54:1193, 1974.

Parmar JM, Hubbard WG, Matthews HR: Teflon strip pneumostasis for excision of giant emphysematous bullae. Thorax 42:144, 1987.

Peabody JW Jr, Katz S, Davis EW: Bronchial carcinoma arising in a lung cyst. AJR Am J Roentgenol 77:1048, 1957.

Pearson MG, Ogilvie C: Surgical treatment of emphysematous bullae: Late outcome. Thorax 38:134, 1983.

Peters RM, Wellons HA, Htwe TM: Total compliance and work of breathing after thoracotomy. J Thorac Cardiovasc Surg 57:348, 1969.

Pierce JA, Growdon JH: Physical properties of the lungs in giant cysts: Report of a case treated surgically. N Engl J Med 267:169, 1962.

Pinckaers JWN, Nijhuis GMM, Dirksen R: Postoperative nicomorphine analgesia by spinal or epidural application. In Bruckner JB (ed): Anesthesiology and Intensive Medicine, Vol 153. Heidelberg, Springer-Verlag, 1981, p 16.

Poe PH, Wellman HN, Berke RA et al: Perfusion-ventilation scintiphotography in bullous disease of the lung. Am Rev Respir Dis 107:946, 1973.

Polga JP, Spencer RP, Raman TK et al: Radionuclide demonstration of improvement of spatial distribution of pulmonary function after removal of bullous lesion. Clin Nucl Med 9:725, 1984.

Potgieter PD, Benatar SR, Hewitson R et al: Surgical treatment of bullous lung disease. Thorax 36:885, 1981.

Pride NB, Barter CE, Hugh-Jones P: Ventilation of bullae and the effect of their removal on thoracic gas volumes and tests of overall pulmonary function. Am Rev Respir Dis 107:83, 1973.

Pride NB, Hugh-Jones P, O'Brien E, Smith LA: Changes in lung function following surgical treatment of bullous emphysema. Q J Med 153:49, 1970.

Quinlan JJ, Buffington CW: Deliberate hypoventilation in a patient with air trapping during lung transplantation. Anesthesiology 78:1177, 1993.

Reid L: The Pathology of Emphysema. Chicago, Year Book Medical, 1967.

Rice TW, Ginsberg RJ, Todd TRJ: Tube drainage of lung abscesses. Ann Thorac Surg 44:356, 1987.

Rothstein E: Infected emphysematous bullae: 5 cases. Am Rev Respir Dis 69:287, 1954.

Rubin EH, Buchberg AJ: Capricious behaviour of pulmonary bullae developing fluid. Dis Chest 54:546, 1968.

Seidel H: Bemerkungen zur Chondrektomie bei Emphysem infolge starrer Thoraxdilatation. Beitr Klin Chir 58:808, 1908.

Shah SS, Goldstraw P: Surgical treatment of bullous emphysema: Experience with the Brompton technique. Ann Thorac Surg 58:1452, 1994.

Shaw RR: Localized hypertrophic emphysema. Pediatrics 9:220, 1952.

Siebens AA, Grant AR, Kent DC et al: Pulmonary cystic disease: Physiologic studies and results of resection. J Thorac Surg 33:185, 1957.

Smoljar VA, Vertianov VA: Laser photocoagulation in the treatment of bullous lung disease. Grud Serdechnososudistaia Khir 5:44, 1985.

Spear HG, Daughty DC, Chesney JG et al: The surgical management of large pulmonary blebs and bullae. Am Rev Respir Dis 84:186, 1961.

Steinberg I, Dotter CT, Andrus DeW: Angiocardiography in thoracic surgery. Surg Gynecol Obstet 90:45, 1950.

Stoloff IL, Kanofsky P, Magilner L: The risk of lung cancer in males with bullous disease of the lungs. Arch Environ Health 22:163, 1971.

Stone DJ, Schwartz A, Feltman JA: Bullous emphysema: A long-term study of the natural history and effects of therapy. Am Rev Respir Dis 82:493, 1960.

Sung DT, Payne S, Black LF: Surgical management of giant bullae associated with obstructive airway disease. Surg Clin North Am 53:913, 1973.

Tabakin BS, Adhikari PK, Miller DB: Objective long term evaluation of the surgical treatment of diffuse obstructive emphysema. Am Rev Respir Dis 80:825, 1959.

Tanaka F, Wada H, Hitomi S et al: Surgery for complications of chronic obstructive lung disease. Chest Surg Clin North Am 5:797, 1995.

Tenholder F, Jones PA, Matthews JI et al: Bullous emphysema: Progressive incremental exercise testing to evaluate candidates for bullectomy. Chest 77:802, 1980.

Ting KY, Klopstock R, Lyons HA: Mechanical properties of pulmonary cysts and bullae. Am Rev Respir Dis 87:538, 1963.

Travaline JM, Addonizio VP, Criner GJ: Effect of bullectomy on diaphragmatic strength. Am J Respir Crit Care Med 152:1697, 1995.

Triantafillou AN: Anesthetic management for bilateral volume reduction surgery. Semin Thorac Cardiovasc Surg 8:94, 1996.

Tsutsui M, Araki Y, Shirakusa T, Inutsuka S: Characteristic radiographic features of pulmonary carcinoma associated with large bullae. Ann Thorac Surg 46:679, 1988.

Uyama T, Monden Y, Harada K et al: Drainage of giant bulla with balloon catheter using chemical irritant and fibrin glue. Chest 94:1289, 1988.

Venn GE, Williams PR, Goldstraw P: Intracavity drainage for bullous, emphysematous lung disease: Experience with the Brompton technique. Thorax 43:998, 1988.

Vishnevsky AA, Nickoladze GD: One-stage operation for bilateral bullous lung disease. J Thorac Cardiovasc Surg 99:30, 1990.

Wakabayaski A: Thoracoscopic technique for management of giant bullous lung disease. Ann Thorac Surg 56:708, 1993.

Wakabayashi A, Brenner M, Kayalek RA et al: Thoracoscopic carbon dioxide laser treatment of bullous emphysema. Lancet 337:881, 1991.

Wasserman K, Whipp BJ: Exercise physiology in health and disease. Am Rev Respir Dis 112:219, 1975.

Weisel W, Slotnick L: Emphysematous bullae complicated by hemorrhage and infection. Am Rev Respir Dis 61:742, 1950.

Weitzenbaum E: Physiopathologie de l'emphysème diffus et de l'emphysème bulleux. Rev Mal Respir 8:109, 1980.

Wesley JR, MacLeod WM, Mullard KS: Evaluation and surgery of bullous emphysema. J Thorac Cardiovasc Surg 63:945, 1972.

Widdicombe JG: Regulation of tracheobronchial smooth muscle. Physiol Rev 43:1, 1963.

Witz JP, Roeslin N: La chirurgie de l'emphysème bulleux chéz l'adulte: Ses résultats éloignés. Rev Mal Respir 8:121, 1980.

Woo-Ming M, Capel LH, Belcher JR: The results of surgical treatment of large air cysts of the lung. Br J Dis Chest 57:79, 1963.

CHAPTER **27**

Massive Hemoptysis

Carlos Alberto Guimarães

Hemoptysis is defined as the expectoration of blood that originates from the tracheobronchial tree or the pulmonary parenchyma (Thompson et al, 1992). Massive bleeding into the airways is an imminent threat to life because asphyxiation occurs as the tracheobronchial tree fills with blood. Exsanguination itself is rarely the cause of death (Cahill and Ingbar, 1994; Conlan, 1985).

Although many reviews on the subject of hemoptysis have focused on massive bleeds, there is no generally accepted definition of the term "massive hemoptysis" (Cahill and Ingbar, 1994). It has been variably defined as 100 to more than 1000 ml of blood expectorated from the lung over 24 to 48 hours. Many patients cough up only small amounts of the blood but aspirate massively. Expectorated blood is often swallowed and cannot be measured. In evaluating these patients, our experience has led us to emphasize the presence or risk of aspiration rather than the volume of blood expectorated. Many patients with hemoptysis have compromised lung function, and even a small quantity of blood in the bronchial tree can lead to acute airway obstruction and asphyxiation.

A pivotal study by Crocco and colleagues (1968) showed that the greater the rate of bleeding, especially when greater than 600 ml in 16 hours, the higher the mortality rate. This has been accepted as the definition of "massive hemoptysis."

I divide massive hemoptysis into two groups: quantitative massive hemoptysis—expectoration of a volume of 400 ml or more of blood over 24 hours; and qualitative massive hemoptysis—expectoration of any volume of blood that puts a patient with poor lung function at significant risk, whether caused by a previous disease or by the hemoptysis itself.

The coughing up of blood prompts most people to seek medical attention. Although fewer than 5% of patients with hemoptysis expectorate large volumes, the incidence of acutely fatal bleeds in this group ranges from 7% to 32%. Rapid bleeding leaves no opportunity for meaningful intervention (Cahill and Ingbar, 1994).

The incidence of massive hemoptysis is difficult to ascertain from the medical literature. Amirana and colleagues (1968) reported 17 patients with significant hemoptysis among 150 cases of hemoptysis in a group of 722 patients with tuberculosis. Crocco and colleagues (1968) studied 67 patients with massive hemoptysis, which represented 1.5% of the 4331 patients admitted to a pulmonary division.

I have had experience with 514 patients, seen at the Instituto de Doenças do Tórax da Universidade Federal do Rio de Janeiro from 1978 through 1998, who had expectorated blood in a volume of 400 ml or more over 24 hours, excluding 13 patients who had undergone palliative or diagnostic surgical procedures (Tables 27–1 and 27–2).

The etiologies of massive hemoptysis are shown in Table 27–3. Pulmonary tuberculosis was the cause in 420 (85.5%) patients; in 216 of these (44%), acid-fast bacilli were recovered from the sputum. There were 29 cases of multidrug-resistant tuberculosis. In 37 patients (7.5%), bronchiectasis was the source of bleeding. Eleven patients had pulmonary carcinomas and 23 patients had miscellaneous conditions: lung abscess (9); pneumonia (6); atypical mycobacteriosis (4); chronic bronchitis(2); aortic aneurysm (1); and benign tumor (1).

HISTORICAL NOTE

At the time of Hippocrates (circa 460 to 375 BC), hemoptysis was pathognomonic of advanced phthisis. The Hippocratic aphorism, "The spitting of pus follows the spitting of blood, consumption follows the spitting of this, and death follows consumption," provides ancient documentation of the significance of hemoptysis in intrathoracic disease. Although Aretaeus and the Greek physicians recognized many causes as early as 1800 years ago, for centuries the expectoration of blood was regarded as etiologic in tuberculosis (Pursel and Lindskog, 1961).

At the 20th annual meeting of the American Association for Thoracic Surgery, Eloesser (1938) read observations on sources of pulmonary hemorrhage and attempts at its control. He performed mass ligation at the hilum of seven patients. Only two recovered. He suggested that it might be less dangerous to remove the lobe from which the hemorrhage comes.

Pitkin (1941) reported the first pneumonectomy for

TABLE 27–1 ■ **Patients with Massive Hemoptysis by Gender**

	*Group 1**	*Group 2†*	*Total*
	No. (%)	*No. (%)*	*No. (%)*
Male	247	137	384 (76.6)
Female	75	42	117 (23.4)
Total	322 (64.3)	179 (35.7)	501 (100)

*Patients underwent no surgery at all.
†Patients underwent curative surgeries.

TABLE 27–2 ■ **Patients with Massive Hemoptysis by Age***

	Group 1†	Group 2‡	Total
Age (years)	No. (%)	No. (%)	No. (%)
10 to 29	81	32	113 (22.6)
30 to 49	137	91	228 (45.5)
50 to 69	86	54	140 (27.9)
70 to 89	18	2	20 (4.0)
Total	322 (64.3%)	179 (35.7%)	501 (100)

*Mean = 42 years
†Patients underwent no surgery at all.
‡Patients underwent curative surgeries.

massive hemoptysis in a bronchiectatic patient; Ryan and Lineberry (1950) related the first pneumonectomy for tuberculosis associated with massive hemoptysis; and Feldman and Gusmão (1954) described a successful right upper lobectomy in a case of pulmonary tuberculosis. Bracco (1956) studied a series of five patients operated on for massive hemoptysis. They underwent three lobectomies (one for bronchiectasis, one for hydatidosis, and one for tuberculosis) and two pneumonectomies (both for tuberculosis). One patient died postoperatively after a pneumonectomy.

Remy and colleagues (1973) reported the first bronchial artery embolization in four patients with massive or repeated hemoptysis. In all patients, the bleeding stopped. Hiebert (1974) described the successful use of a Fogarty balloon catheter through a rigid bronchoscope to tamponade bleeding in a patient with massive bronchial hemorrhage. Sahebjami (1976) mentioned the first iced-saline lavage during bronchoscopy to treat active (but not massive) bleeding during fiberoptic bronchoscopic examination, and Yang and Berger (1978) documented the first important series of conservative management of life-threatening hemoptysis. They treated 17 patients and found a mortality rate of 17.6%. Shneerson and colleagues (1980) reported the first case of massive hemoptysis and aspergilloma treated successfully with radiotherapy.

■ *HISTORICAL READINGS*

Eloesser L: Observations on sources of pulmonary hemorrhage and attempts at its control. J Thorac Surg 7:671, 1938.

TABLE 27–3 ■ **Causes of Massive Hemoptysis**

	Group 1*	Group 2†	Total‡
Diagnosis	No. (%)	No. (%)	No. (%)
Tuberculosis			
Active	174	42	216 (44)
Inactive	96	108	204 (41.5)
Bronchiectasis	17	20	37 (7.5)
Carcinoma	9	2	11 (2.3)
Others	16	7	23 (4.7)
Total‡	312 (64.3)	179 (35.7)	491 (100)

*Patients underwent no surgery at all.
†Patients underwent curative surgeries.
‡Ten patients had no diagnosis.

Hiebert CA: Balloon catheter control of life-threatening hemoptysis. Chest 66:308, 1974.
Pitkin CE: Repeated severe hemoptysis necessitating pneumectomy. Ann Otol Rhinol Laryngol 50:914, 1941.
Remy J, Voisin C, Ribet M et al: Traitement, par embolisation, des hémoptysies graves ou répétées liées à un hypervascularisation systemique. Presse Med 2:2060, 1973.
Sahebjami H: Iced saline lavage during bronchoscopy. Chest 69:131, 1976.

BASIC SCIENCE

Anatomy

The lungs are supplied by two relatively independent circulations. The pulmonary circulation performs the specialized function of oxygenation and the excretion of carbon dioxide from the body. The pulmonary arteries carry blood from the right ventricle across the highly vascular pulmonary capillary bed and return it via the pulmonary veins to the left atrium (Cahill and Ingbar, 1994).

The bronchial artery circulation is quite variable and complex. Arterial origins arise mainly from the thoracic aorta or its branches. As many as 20% arise from various other vessels, and the remaining 10% originate from the anterior surface of the aortic arch. The same vessels that supply the bronchial arteries may also supply the esophagus, the mediastinal lymph nodes, and the spinal arteries through a complex anastomotic network (Fraser et al, 1997).

Cauldwell and colleagues (1948) studied the bronchial arteries in 150 human cadavers. They originate, with few exceptions, from the proximal part of the thoracic aorta. The right bronchial arteries arise from the lateral or dorsolateral aspect of the aorta, frequently in common with an intercostal artery (intercostobronchial trunk). The left bronchial arteries usually originate from the anterior surface of the thoracic aorta or from the concavity of the aortic arch. They pursue a tortuous course along the surface of the bronchi. Peripherally, it is common to see two bronchial arteries for each bronchus (Pump, 1972). Uflacker and colleagues (1985) studied bronchial angiograms and encountered 10 different anatomic patterns.

Furuse and colleagues (1987) conducted a study to determine the visibility of the bronchial arteries with dynamic computed tomography (CT). They believe that a bronchial artery larger than 2 mm is suggestive of an abnormality.

Remy-Jardin and Remy (1990) reviewed the nonbronchial systemic circulation of the lung in relation to lung diseases and hemoptysis. In most situations that led to nonbronchial systemic arterial hypervascularization, there was pleural symphysis, allowing pulmonary penetration of thoracic parietal vessels. They examined the contribution of the transpleural nonbronchial systemic vessels and the role of the arteries of the pulmonary ligament. This latter circulation can be the source of hemoptysis in a proportion similar to that of the pulmonary circulation (7% of all cases of massive hemoptysis).

Normally, the bronchial and pulmonary circulations anastomose at three anatomic levels. Larger anastomoses, called "bronchopulmonary arteries," arise from medium-sized bronchial arteries and anastomose with the alveolar microvasculature. Bronchial capillaries merge with pulmonary capillaries. These anastomoses multiply as the airways become increasingly smaller. Anastomoses between bronchial arteries and pulmonary veins also occur at the precapillary level, primarily between small bronchial arteries in the bronchial walls and pleural and pulmonary veins (Thompson et al, 1992).

For most etiologies, massive hemoptysis involves disruption of the high-pressure bronchial circulation or pulmonary circulation pathologically exposed to the high pressures of bronchial circulation (Thompson et al, 1992).

Control of bronchial blood flow is poorly understood, but it varies directly with systemic arterial pressure. In addition, there is regulatory input from the autonomic nervous system (Cahill and Ingbar, 1994).

The bronchial circulation plays an important role in hemoptysis because of its intimate association with the tracheobronchial tree. In many cases of hemoptysis, the bronchial arterial tree becomes hyperplastic and tortuous. Because the arterioles associated with the airways are under systemic pressure, they have a propensity to bleed profusely when airways are diseased (Cahill and Ingbar, 1994).

Etiology

Inflammatory Disease

Tuberculosis. Descriptions of abnormalities of the lung vasculature in pulmonary tuberculosis derive from the original observations by Rasmussen in 1868 of aneurysmal dilatations of pulmonary arteries (Rasmussen aneurysms) (Yeoh et al, 1967). Rasmussen analyzed 11 deaths from hemoptysis; eight patients had suffered a rupture of a vessel in the wall of a tuberculous cavity. Rasmussen aneurysms may be single or multiple. They are false aneurysms, corresponding to dilatations of branches of the pulmonary artery or, most frequently, of the bronchial artery, which crosses the wall of a tuberculous cavity.

Cudkowicz (1968) studied the vasculature of tuberculous lungs in five postmortem examinations. The most uniform feature observed was the tortuosity and proliferation of the bronchial arteries to diseased areas. Tuberculous cavities have a rich bronchial blood supply. The pulmonary artery branches do not contribute to the blood supply of caseating tuberculous areas because they undergo thrombosis in the early stages of the disease; this can be demonstrated by angiography. Extensive arterial capillaries in the adhesions between the pleural surfaces and the tendency of these capillaries to recanalize the obliterated pleural arteries indicate that a profuse quantity of arterial blood is present near the tuberculous foci in the periphery of such lungs.

In tuberculosis the mechanism of bleeding varies with the stage, type, and location of the disease. First to be considered is hemoptysis, which occurs in the acute exudative lesion. Owing to the softening of the lung tissue, bleeding results from necrosis of a small branch of the pulmonary artery or vein. A second type of hemorrhage in tuberculosis is that which occurs in a chronic fibroulcerative type of the disease. This type of bleeding is often caused by the rupture of a pseudoaneurysm of an artery traversing the wall of a thick-walled cavity. A third type occurs when a healed and calcified lymph node impinges on the wall of a bronchus. The pressure of the calcific mass causes erosion of the bronchus with ulceration into the lumen (broncholith). An acute ulceration of the bronchial mucosa may also cause hemoptysis. Tracheobronchial tuberculosis may be part of widespread parenchymal involvement or, rarely, it may occur as a primary bronchial infection. Finally, repeated small episodes of hemoptysis occur in patients whose radiographs show small fibrotic or calcific areas.

Normal lung architecture is destroyed by tuberculosis, predisposing to the development of bronchiectasis with its attendant hypervascularized, dilated, tortuous bronchial circulation and anastomoses between the bronchial and pulmonary circulations (Cahill and Ingbar, 1994).

Broncholithiasis. Tuberculosis and histoplasmosis are the most common causes of broncholith formation. The lymph nodes involved may become calcified when healing. The normal movements of the airways during respiration and cough and the pulsation of bronchial arteries can lead to erosion of these structures if they impinge on a calcified lymph node. If a large bronchial artery is eroded by the broncholith, expectoration of the broncholith may be accompanied by massive hemoptysis (Thompson et al, 1992).

Aspergillosis. An intracavitary fungal ball is one of the most important causes of systemic hypervascularization. Many have tried to explain the mechanism of hemorrhage; for example, friction of the fungus ball against the hypervascularized walls of the cavity, toxins or fibrinolytic enzymes elaborated by the fungus, and antigen-antibody reactions in the cavity wall. The blood vessels that line the cavity are branches of the bronchial artery network. The fungal ball complicates the chronic pulmonary, pleural, or bronchial cavities, or it may appear during the evolution of aspergillosis—that is, invasive allergic bronchopulmonary or chronic necrotizing pulmonary aspergillosis. Because most cavities are in the posterior portions of the upper lobes, there is a great contribution of blood from the branches of axillary or subclavian arteries in the area of fused pleura.

Bronchiectasis. Pathologically, bronchiectasis is the destruction of the cartilaginous support of the bronchial wall by infection or bronchial dilatation owing to parenchymal retraction from alveolar fibrosis (Cahill and Ingbar, 1994).

In bronchiectasis, there is evidence of proliferation and enlargement of the bronchial arteries, and precapillary bronchopulmonary anastomoses have been demonstrated. These communications are most widespread near the diseased third- or fourth-order bronchi and the bronchiectatic sacs. At these levels of the bronchial tree, the bronchial arteries are normally small and can be recognized in the adventitial coat of the pulmonary arteries as vasa vasorum, which do not communicate with the lumen of the pulmonary artery. There are also large bronchopulmonary anastomoses (Cudkowicz, 1968; Thompson et al, 1992).

Necrotizing Pneumonitis. Patients with chronic necrotizing pneumonitis can bleed massively; alcoholism is often a predisposing factor. Conlan and colleagues (1983) reported 11 cases of chronic necrotizing pneumonitis in a group of 123 patients with massive hemoptysis.

Cystic Fibrosis. Approximately 5% to 7% of patients with cystic fibrosis have massive bleeds. Bleeding from the lung in this disease is multifactorial but usually originates in the bronchial arteries (Cahill and Ingbar, 1994).

Patients with cystic fibrosis are susceptible to hemoptysis for several reasons. The lungs are focally and diffusely involved with retained secretions, bronchiolar obstruction, pulmonary abscesses, pneumonias, and bronchiectasis. The increased bronchial circulation is tortuous and dilated. There are also bronchiopulmonary artery shunts in areas of bronchiectasis.

Lung Abscess. Bleeding occurs in 11% to 15% of patients with lung abscesses, and 20% to 50% develop massive hemoptysis. The bacterial infection that causes the abscess heals only if the cavity is adequately drained. The bacterial infection destroys lung tissue by the processes of suppuration and necrosis. In the healing of the abscess, granulation tissue forms, and leukocytes infiltrate. When necrosis involves vascular granulation tissue, the capillaries bleed into the cavity of the abscess and a clot forms, blocking the communicating bronchus. This poor drainage allows the infection to go unchecked, and further necrosis of the wall of the abscess and epithelial lining results. When this necrosis involves the larger tertiary branches of the pulmonary arteries, severe hemorrhage occurs, either filling the cavity rapidly or causing an episode of massive hemoptysis. These pathologic descriptions of the necrosis of capillaries in the wall of the abscess and focal necrosis of tertiary pulmonary arteries explain the gradual refilling of abscessed cavities with blood clots during periods of lesser hemoptysis and episodes of massive hemoptysis (Philpott et al, 1993; Thompson et al, 1992; Thoms et al, 1972).

Neoplasm

Although as many as 20% of all patients with lung cancer expectorate blood some time in the course of their disease, massive hemoptysis is rare (Cahill and Ingbar, 1994).

Lung cancer usually causes massive bleeding by direct invasion of central pulmonary arteries (Thompson et al, 1992). There is also proliferation of the bronchial arteries in primary pulmonary neoplasms. This systemic vascularization is thought to be responsible for the frequency of hemoptysis associated with bronchial carcinomas. Some authors think that metastatic lung tumors show no such pattern; others believe that the blood supply of metastases in the lungs is similar.

Miller and McGregor (1980) published a retrospective analysis of 877 cases of lung cancer. Massive terminal hemoptysis (29 cases) was found to be significantly associated with cavitated squamous cell carcinoma, arising in either the right or left main bronchi. Radiotherapy, although used more frequently in the population with massive hemoptysis, did not appear to be causally related to bleeding of any degree.

Bronchial carcinoids frequently cause hemoptysis because of their marked vascularity and endobronchial locations.

Tumors of the mediastinum, particularly esophageal carcinoma, may extend directly into the tracheobronchial tree, resulting in massive hemoptysis.

Trauma

Trauma to the airways is not uncommon following deceleration injuries and penetrating chest trauma. The adjacent main bronchus and the main trunk of the pulmonary artery may be injured. There is little time for management when there is a hemorrhage into the tracheobronchial tree (Conlan, 1983; Thompson et al, 1992).

A case of false left ventricular aneurysm with ventriculobronchial fistula and massive hemoptysis 10 years after a penetrating cardiac injury was reported (Camero and Cushing, 1997). The clinical course suggested that the aneurysm became infected and that the inflammatory process weakened the aneurysmal sac and led to the development of fistula.

Iatrogenic

Pulmonary Artery Catheterization

The introduction of the Swan-Ganz catheter has allowed rapid catheterization of the pulmonary artery at the bedside in the critically ill patient. Perforation of the pulmonary artery with associated hemorrhage has been reported by several groups. Barash and colleagues (1981) evaluated the mechanisms by which perforation of the pulmonary artery occurs. Anticoagulation, hypothermia, and pulmonary hypertension place the patient at higher risk. One or more of three separate mechanisms can be responsible for vascular perforation. First, the balloon can disrupt the pulmonary artery. Second, balloon inflation (eccentric or distorted) can cause the tip to be propelled through the vessel wall. Third, the catheter tip (with the balloon deflated) can be advanced too far distally and perforate the vessel.

Boyd and colleagues (1983) reported a prospective study of complications of pulmonary artery balloon catheterizations in 500 patients. To decrease pulmonary artery injury, after the tip of the catheter was positioned in the superior or inferior vena cava, its balloon was inflated with 1.5 ml of air and advanced while the distal pressure and the electrocardiograph were being monitored. Fluoroscopic guidance was used in only 24 cases. The catheter was advanced with the balloon inflated until a wedge pressure was obtained. Then the balloon was deflated, the pulmonary artery pressure was identified, and the catheter was fixed in this position. Whenever the balloon was reinflated, the pressure tracing was carefully observed. If a wedge pressure appeared with a volume of less than 1 ml, distal migration was assumed to have occurred. The balloon was immediately deflated; the catheter was withdrawn centrally; and the balloon was reinflated and rewedged. This technique minimized the occurrence of pulmonary artery injury by ensuring that the catheter tip was located as centrally as possible. Only one patient had hemoptysis following inflation of the balloon. After it was promptly deflated and the catheter was withdrawn, hemoptysis stopped.

Catheter-induced pulmonary artery rupture is a well-recognized complication of invasive monitoring, commonly associated with cardiopulmonary bypass, but also occurring in the intensive care unit (ICU) (Mullerworth et al, 1998).

Bronchoscopy

Bleeding may occur in the course of bronchoscopy when brush, endobronchial, or transbronchial biopsies are performed. Massive hemorrhage occurring as a complication of bronchoscopy is uncommon. However, there are few experienced endoscopists who have not faced this problem. Because the patient's cough reflex has been abolished by anesthesia, the tracheobronchial tree fills quickly with blood, and ventilation is no longer possible. The massive hemoptysis usually causes death in a few minutes (Cahill and Ingbar, 1994).

Pulmonary Embolism

Ligation of the main pulmonary artery does not cause pulmonary necrosis because of anastomosis between the bronchial and the pulmonary artery systems. Infarction following distal pulmonary embolism, however, is common. After impaction of the embolus, hemorrhage and alveolar edema occur, followed by necrosis and true infarction. A rapid influx of bronchial arterial blood, through anastomoses, into a small segment of peripheral lung can cause extravasation of blood. The resultant hemoptysis may assume massive proportions because of systemic heparinization. Reversal of the heparinization usually stops the bleeding (Conlan, 1985; Thompson et al, 1992).

Sarcoidosis

Massive hemoptysis rarely occurs in sarcoidosis. Most cases occur in patients with advanced disease and major fibrosis. *Aspergillus* colonization of a cavity is the most frequent aggravating factor. Other causes of bleeding are rare. Systemic hypervascularization of sarcoidosis lesions has been proposed as one mechanism other than infection. The cause may also be a simple granuloma. Finally, massive hemoptysis can occur by erosion of the pulmonary artery owing to a necrotic sarcoidosis lesion (Lemay et al, 1995).

Arteriovenous Fistulas

Pulmonary arteriovenous malformations are rare, direct, low-pressure, arterial-to-venous communications in the lung, which may be single or multiple. Usually congenital, acquired lesions are rare and have been reported following surgery, trauma, pulmonary infection, metastatic carcinoma, and hepatic cirrhosis (Najarian and Morris, 1998).

Arteriovenous fistulas constitute a rare cause of massive hemoptysis, accounting for approximately 2% of cases in a large series (Conlan, 1985). Pulmonary arteriovenous fistulas were recently recognized as a manifestation of hereditary hemorrhagic telangiectasis (Rendu-Osler-Weber disease). In cases of pulmonary arteriovenous fistulas, 60% had associated telangiectasis of the skin or superficial mucous membranes. The precapillary pulmonary arteriovenous fistula communicates with the pulmonary arteries and veins, giving rise to a right-to-left shunt. The walls of these vascular structures are thin and may rupture. An angiodysplastic disorder that may involve any vessel appears to be the pathologic basis for the clinical findings.

Pouwels and colleagues (1992) reported a case of life-threatening hemoptysis in which a right bronchial angiogram revealed a hypertrophic and tortuous right bronchial artery, with hypertrophic branches running toward a large malformation in the right lower and middle lobes. The venous drainage of this occurred through the pulmonary veins from the middle and lower lobes toward the left atrium (left-to-left shunt was established, forming a communication between the right bronchial artery and the pulmonary vein, through a vascular mass).

Cardiovascular Disorders

Hemoptysis is a well-known complication of mitral stenosis and may be related to the rupture of smaller vessels from extreme congestion and hypertension in the pulmonary vessels. With increased pulmonary pressure, the gradient of blood flow is reversed through the bronchopulmonary venous connections; therefore, the submucosal bronchial veins dilate and are liable to rupture. Bland or septic embolization of the lungs from tricuspid valve vegetations, which are common in drug abusers, may produce pulmonary infarction and hemoptysis or a more chronic form, which may itself develop into a massive hemoptysis.

Other cardiovascular disorders that may complicate with massive hemoptysis include congenital heart disease and septic pulmonary emboli (Thompson et al, 1992).

Among patients with congenital heart disease, hemoptysis occurs with primary or secondary pulmonary hypertension and with severe pulmonic stenosis (Cahill and Ingbar, 1994).

Hemoptysis is one of the hallmarks of primary pulmonary hypertension, Eisenmenger's complex, and secondary pulmonary hypertension from Blalock-Taussig shunting for cyanotic heart disease. The longstanding state of high flow or pressure (or both) in the pulmonary artery circuit leads to rupture of pulmonary artery atherosclerotic plaques, rupture of smaller pulmonary arteriolar vessels, and subsequent hemoptysis (Cahill and Ingbar, 1994).

In extreme cases of tetralogy of Fallot, in which pulmonic stenosis is severe or the pulmonary outflow tract is atretic, the bronchial artery system and the bronchopulmonary anastomotic network are augmented. Massive hemoptysis may occur from aneurysmal dilatation of hypertrophied bronchial vessels, erosion of varicose bronchial vessels into the airway, or rupture of bronchopulmonary anastomoses (Cahill and Ingbar, 1994).

Bronchovascular Fistulas

Bronchovascular communications may be preceded by minor warning hemorrhages before the final engulfing fatal bleeding. They may be caused by trauma, neoplasm, or intrinsic disease of large vascular structures adjacent to the tracheobronchial tree (Conlan, 1985).

Aortobronchial fistula is a rare but highly lethal condition related in most cases to an expanding aortic aneurysm and, rarely, to tuberculous aortitis. If not diagnosed, it is uniformly fatal, with death caused by massive hemoptysis (Girard et al, 1997; Julià-Serdà et al, 1996). Demeter and Cordasco (1980) reviewed 30 cases in world literature. Seventy-nine percent of the patients had massive hemoptysis.

González Noguera and colleagues (1993) discussed a right bronchial artery aneurysm in its intrapulmonary trajectory, which manifested itself by repeated mild hemoptysis. At that time, they reviewed the literature and found 17 cases of bronchial artery aneurysms with intrapulmonary or mediastinal localization.

A case of left subclavian artery aneurysm was reported that ruptured and penetrated through the left upper lung parenchyma, causing massive hemoptysis and a left hemothorax (Wu et al, 1993).

An aortobronchial fistula, which resulted in fatal massive hemoptysis, developed in a man 13 months after unilateral lung transplantation. His post-transplantation recovery was complicated by bronchial dehiscence requiring revision and subsequent stricture formation treated by granulation tissue excision, placement of endobronchial stents, dilatation, and laser photoablation (Hoff et al, 1993).

Tracheoinnominate artery fistula is a relatively rare but highly lethal complication that can occur in patients with recent tracheostomies. When massive hemorrhage begins, immediate arterial compression, control of the airway, and subsequent treatment of the injured artery may be lifesaving (Keçeligil et al, 1995).

Diffuse Parenchymal Diseases

Massive hemoptysis can also be caused by abnormalities that diffusely affect the pulmonary vasculature. They can be mediated by immunologic mechanisms as in pulmonary hemorrhage owing to systemic lupus erythematosus, Goodpasture's syndrome, idiopathic pulmonary hemosiderosis, polyarteritis nodosa, Wegener's granulomatosis, Takayasu's arteritis, or Behçet's disease (Patel et al, 1994; Rocha et al, 1994; Thompson et al, 1992).

Regardless of the underlying cause, the cardinal manifestations of alveolar hemorrhage include hemoptysis, anemia, and alveolar infiltrates on chest radiographs (Cahill and Ingbar, 1994).

Herb and colleagues (1998) described a case of severe hemoptysis related to aneurysms of the bronchial arteries in Hughes-Stovin syndrome (multiple pulmonary aneurysms and peripheral venous thrombosis).

Cryptogenic Massive Hemoptysis

Cryptogenic or idiopathic hemoptysis refers to hemoptysis in which the cause remains undiagnosed despite a thorough evaluation, including bronchoscopy. Of patients with massive bleeding, 8% to 15% ultimately are given the diagnosis of cryptogenic hemoptysis (Cahill and Ingbar, 1994).

DIAGNOSIS

Clinical Features

A thorough history is imperative. Hematemesis from a peptic ulcer or esophageal varices is rarely confused with hemoptysis, but epistaxis and bleeding from the gums or nasopharynx may be. The history should include: (1) the amount and appearance of blood and clots; (2) the duration of bleeding; (3) chest pain; (4) the relationship of bleeding to rest, exertion, position, or cough; (5) localized wheezing or bubbling; (6) previous lung and heart diseases; and (7) cigarette smoking.

The diagnostic approach to patients with massive hemoptysis should be directed toward determining the site of bleeding to provide rational management (Thompson et al, 1992). Surprisingly, patients can often accurately localize the source of hemoptysis to one lung or the other, experiencing an ipsilateral "heaviness."

In our series of massive hemoptysis, 307 (61%) patients gave a history of pulmonary tuberculosis. Fifty-eight percent of the patients with massive hemoptysis had an episode of hemoptysis before the onset of massive hemoptysis (Table 27–4). The chief clinical manifestations of the 501 patients with massive hemoptysis at admission were hemoptysis (66.2%), cough (34.8%), expectoration (27.1%), and weight loss (10.8%).

Radiography

A clear chest radiograph, even with portable equipment, should be obtained. Localized pulmonary infiltration, atelectasis, cavitation, cyst formation, or a mass may indicate the source of bleeding, especially if it is unique. The mitral configuration of the heart shadow and Kerley B lines may also be helpful (Boren et al, 1966). Massive pulmonary hemorrhage may occur from an area that appears normal on a routine chest radiograph (McCollum et al, 1975).

Special radiographic studies must not be neglected. CT can demonstrate both cavities and solid lesions that are not clearly outlined on posteroanterior and lateral films. The pattern of an "air bronchogram" can be most helpful. Bronchograms or CT scans (after bleeding has ceased for several days) can help identify an obstruction, stenosis, and signs of chronic bronchitis or bronchiectasis. Using CT, Millar and colleagues (1992) investigated 40 patients with a history of hemoptysis, normal chest radiographs apart from evidence of chronic airflow limita-

TABLE 27–4 ■ **Previous Hemoptysis in Patients with Massive Hemoptysis**

Previous Hemoptysis	*Nonsurgical* No. (%)	*Surgical* No. (%)	*Total* No. (%)
Yes	177	115	292 (58.3)
No	145	64	209 (41.7)
Total	322 (64.3)	179 (35.7)	501 (100)

tion, and normal fiberoptic bronchoscopy (or blood alone in the bronchial tree). Abnormalities were seen in 20 (50%) of the CT scans. In some cases, angiography or perfusion scanning studies may confirm the location of a pulmonary embolus.

In our experience with 501 cases of massive hemoptysis, the patients had the following more common chest radiographic abnormalities at admission: destroyed lung or lobe (31.4%), cavities (26.9%), infiltrates (26.7%), fibroatelectasis (16.7%), and condensation (10.7%). Of these radiologic alterations, 54.2% were unilateral. In group 1, 49% of patients had bilateral lesions, and in group 2, 42.6% had the same changes.

Even before bleeding has subsided, the clinician can proceed with appropriate skin testing (tuberculin); sputum cultures for fungi, mycobacteria, and pyogens; and Papanicolaou smears. Chest radiographs are useful, not only because they help in locating the site of hemoptysis but also because they may demonstrate the presence of aspiration. The physical findings may be misleading and must be interpreted with caution when there is aspiration. Frequently, localized wheezes, rales, or rhonchi reflect the presence of aspirated blood, whereas the primary lesion may remain clinically silent (Amirana et al, 1968). The radiologic abnormality of aspiration is usually seen first in the lobe or area that is causing the hemorrhage. Therefore, it occurs ipsilateral to the site of origin but may become bilateral (Bobrowitz et al, 1983).

Thoms and colleagues (1972) discussed the radiologic findings in massive hemoptysis in primary lung abscesses. They looked for clues in the radiographs that would predict recurrent bleeding. If such clues could be found, they would then have a sound basis for resecting the involved lobe before the second episode of bleeding. In some cases, the chest radiographs showed abscessed cavities that were emptying and refilling. The cavities emptied during an episode of massive hemoptysis and partially or completely refilled prior to the next and more severe episode of hemoptysis. The radiographs showed that bleeding was continuing into the abscessed cavity even when there was no indication of it in the sputum, visualizing an emptying and refilling pattern (Fig. 27–1). There was another feature when a patient showed a cavity with an air-fluid level. As the hemoptysis progressed, the air-fluid level became a rounded density that moved around with changes in the patient's position. This change of the air-fluid level to movable mass constituted another radiologic pattern. Another radiographic characteristic was one of persistent radiodensity. Thoms and colleagues called it a persistent radiodensity pattern. All these signs were recognized as "possessing all the dangers of a time bomb."

Bronchoscopy

Bronchoscopy is almost always the appropriate first invasive step in the evaluation of massive hemoptysis (Cahill and Ingbar, 1994; Thompson et al, 1992).

Beyond plain chest radiography, bronchoscopy is the key to localizing the lesion. Our experience shows no ill effects from bronchoscopy in patients with hemoptysis, and it was helpful in the radiographic localization of the site of bleeding, especially in bilateral disease.

Questions have been raised regarding two concerns with this procedure: (1) what type of bronchoscope to use, and (2) the optimum time for endoscopy. Some clinicians claim that in massive hemoptysis only the rigid bronchoscope can provide adequate clearing of the blood from the tracheobronchial tree and maintain a satisfactory airway. Others noted the safety of evaluation of hemoptysis with fiberoptic bronchoscopy. I agree with Garzon and colleagues (1982) that if it is possible to see the site of the bleeding with the flexible bronchoscope, the patient probably is not bleeding massively. The flexible bronchoscope can be used in concert with the rigid scope by passing it through the lumen to examine more selected parts of the bronchial tree (Cahill and Ingbar, 1994).

The most valuable procedure to localize the site of hemorrhage is the rigid bronchoscopy during active bleeding because of its wide conduit that allows ventilation, suctioning of blood, and an excellent view. It also allows the passage of suction cannulas, balloon-bearing catheters, cold-infusion solutions, and snug cannulation of the bronchus of the nonbleeding lung for ventilation. Bronchoscopy enables clinicians to decide whether or not a patient should receive medical therapy, an endoscopic control measure, or surgical treatment. It is the procedure of choice in the management of massive hemoptysis and should be carried out by an endoscopist skilled in the use of both types of bronchoscopes (Conlan, 1985). I performed rigid bronchoscopy during massive hemoptysis in 323 patients, localizing the site of bleeding in 299 (92.6%).

It may be difficult at times to differentiate blood that has spilled over into a bronchus from blood originating distally, but repeated suctioning and careful observation often identifies the segment from which the bleeding originated (Borer et al, 1966; Cahill and Ingbar, 1994). Garzon and Gourin (1978) advise the use of two sets of suction machines during the bronchoscopy of a patient with massive hemoptysis to prevent suffocation.

When bronchoscopy is performed, the hemorrhage is occasionally so rapid that the site of origin cannot be identified immediately. Under these circumstances, the bronchoscope should not be removed but should be used to clear blood from the tracheobronchial tree and to intubate the nonbleeding side for ventilation. Light sedation without depressing the cough reflex and topical oropharyngeal anesthesia are used, and the Trendelenburg position may be helpful for adequate evacuation of blood (McCollum et al, 1975).

Bronchial Arteriography

Massive hemoptysis involves bleeding from the bronchial artery system in most patients. On occasion, the major source of bleeding is the nonbronchial systemic collateral vessels, particularly the subclavian, axillary, intercostal, and phrenic arteries (Cahill and Ingbar, 1994).

With selective catheterization of the bronchial arteries, arteriograms of high quality may be obtained, and a precise anatomic diagnosis is possible (Fig. 27–2). In tuberculosis, there is hyperplasia of the bronchial artery, with numerous branches reaching the tuberculous lesions, especially the walls of the cavities and the adjacent

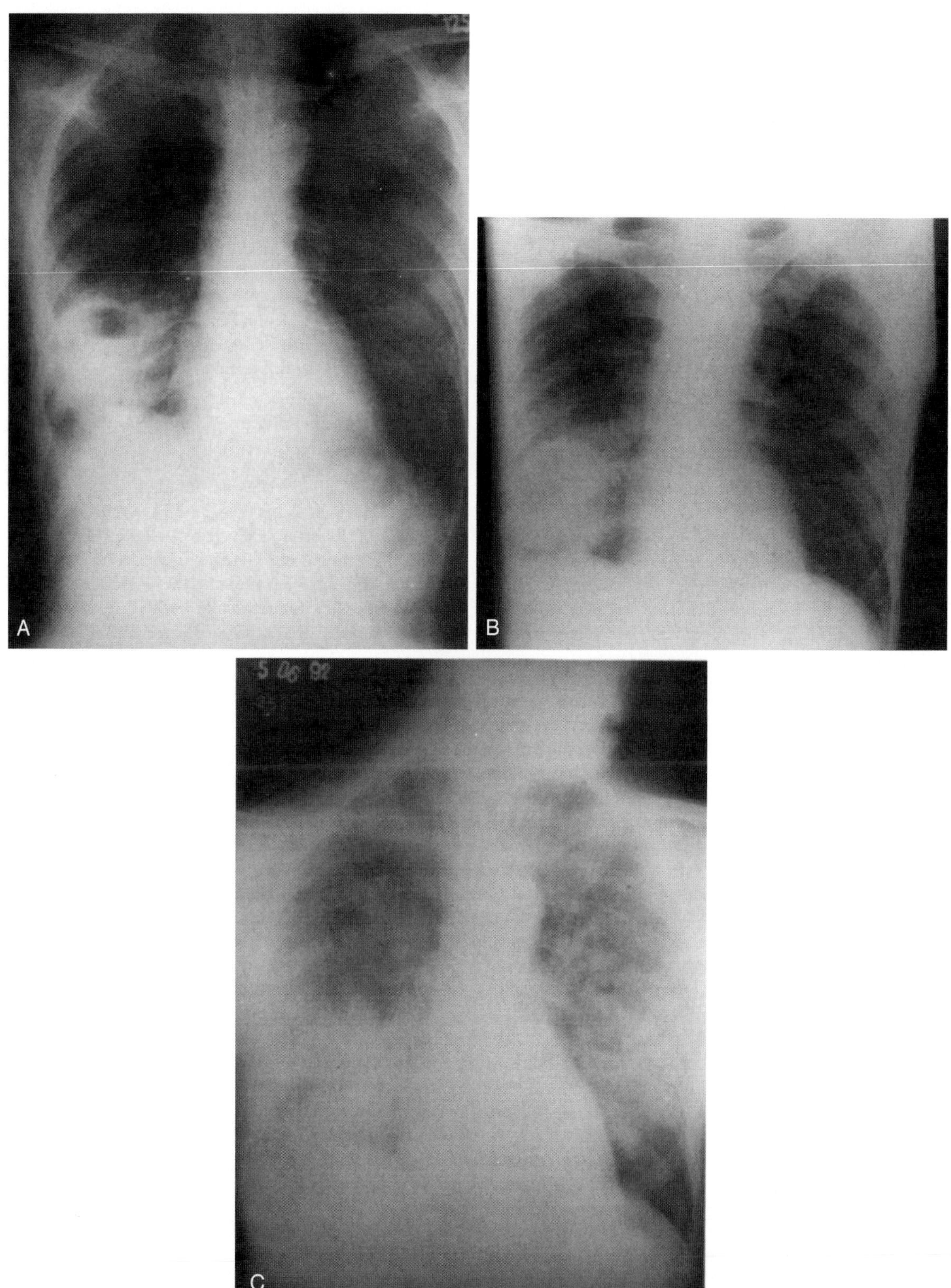

FIGURE 27–1 ■ A lung abscess *(A)*, filling *(B)*, and then emptying *(C)*, producing bilateral massive aspiration of blood.

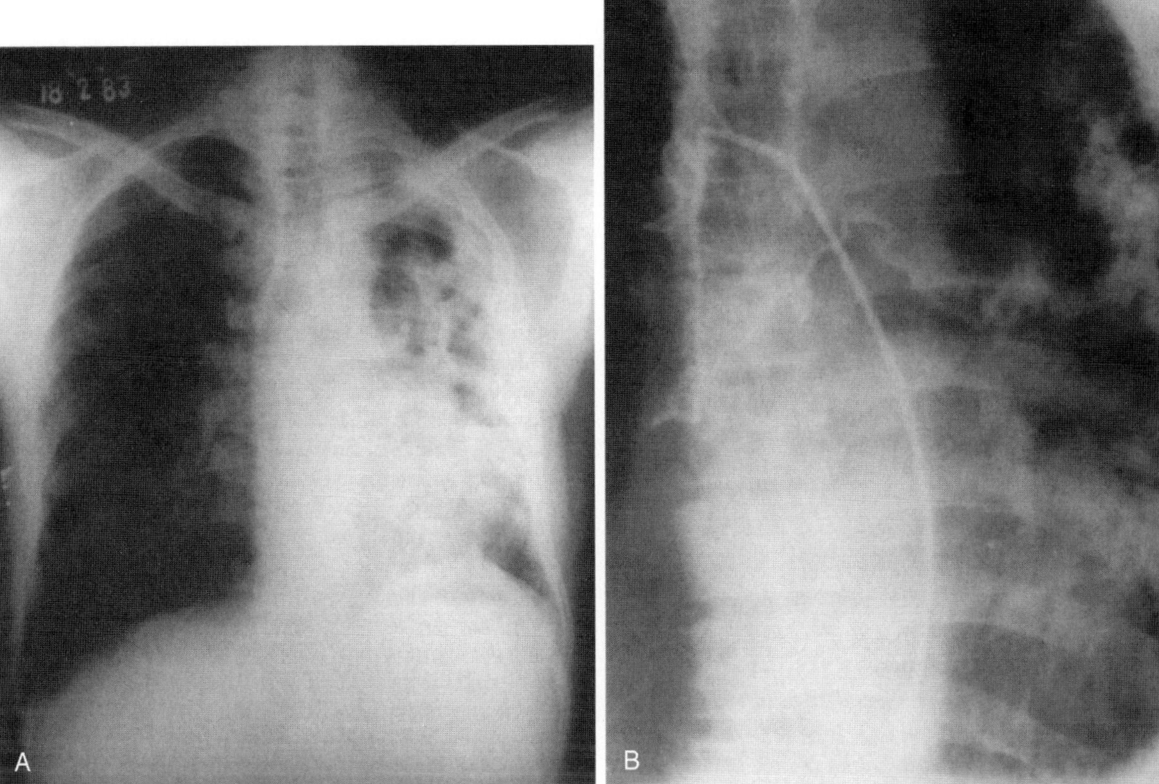

FIGURE 27–2 ■ *A,* A left lung destroyed by tuberculosis. *B,* A bronchial arteriogram demonstrating the bleeding site.

regions; the angiogram may depict bronchopulmonary communications. In bronchiectasis, there is an enlargement of the proximal portion of the bronchial artery, which winds around the ectatic bronchi, running in a twisting course and splitting off into numerous branches. On arteriography, a pulmonary carcinoma has a characteristic pattern. Enlargement of the main bronchial artery is minimal, but many irregular branches develop within and surrounding the tumor.

Bronchoscopy should be performed in all patients prior to bronchial arteriography to identify the side and site of bleeding to allow successful angiographic evaluation (Cremaschi et al, 1993). When bronchoscopy fails to localize bleeding, however, systematic bilateral arteriographic examination of the bronchial and nonbronchial collateral arteries or the pulmonary artery bed can be used to look for evidence of bleeder vessels.

Arteriographic findings suggestive of a bleeding vessel include parenchymal hypervascularity, vascular hypertrophy, tortuosity, capillary stasis, bronchopulmonary shunting, aneurysm formation, and thrombosis of vessels. Rarely is extravasation of contrast from the vasculature to the bronchi seen, and it occurs only when there is active bleeding during the procedure (Cahill and Ingbar, 1994).

Pulmonary Angiography

Bleeding originates from the pulmonary artery bed in fewer than 10% of patients with massive hemoptysis (Cahill and Ingbar, 1994).

In some cases, especially those associated with acute or chronic lung abscess, tuberculosis with Rasmussen's aneurysm formation, pulmonary arteriovenous malformation, or pulmonary artery tears, pulmonary angiography may be indicated (Cahill and Ingbar, 1994; Thompson et al, 1992).

Computed Tomography

CT of the chest is another second-order diagnostic procedure. Routine use of chest CT in the evaluation of patients with massive hemoptysis, however, is not usually necessary. CT scanning during active bleeding may be misleading because aspirated blood may obscure underlying disease or incorrectly appear as a parenchymal mass. Chest radiographs and bronchoscopy provide all the information essential for diagnosis and therapeutic decision making in 94% of my patients. The overall impact of the additional information provided by chest CT is small.

MANAGEMENT

The management of a patient with massive hemoptysis has five main objectives: (1) to prevent asphyxiation, (2) to localize the site of bleeding, (3) to arrest the hemorrhage, (4) to determine the cause of the hemoptysis, and (5) to treat the patient definitively (Cahill and Ingbar, 1994; Jones and Davies, 1990). A patient with massive hemoptysis requires treatment in an ICU. The modalities used to treat massive hemoptysis are listed in the box entitled Treatment of Massive Hemoptysis.

TREATMENT OF MASSIVE HEMOPTYSIS

Medical treatment
Bed rest
  Trendelenburg position
  Affected side down
Wide intravenous line
Arterial blood-gas monitoring
Sedatives
Cough suppressants (antitussives)
Oxygen
Broad-spectrum antibiotics
Blood transfusion
Reversal of anticoagulation (embolism)
Specific disease therapy
Corticosteroids (immunologic diseases)
Antituberculous medication
Endobronchial control measures
Ice-cold saline lavage
Balloon tamponade
Pulmonary separation
Tamponade with vasoconstrictive substances
Miscellaneous control measures
Selective coagulative treatment
  Laser
  Topical thrombin
Arterial embolization
External tubular drainage
Positive end-expiratory pressure
Pneumoperitoneum
Pneumothorax
Intravenous angiotensin
Radiotherapy
Intracavitary treatment
Surgical therapy

Medical Therapy

A complete history and physical examination are essential, but frequently the bleeding has stopped before the patient is examined. The workup in an emergency situation should include a chest radiograph, hematocrit, blood count, blood urea nitrogen and creatinine, coagulation profile, and an arterial blood gas study. A bleeding time should be performed when the patient is suspected of having a bleeding diathesis or a history of aspirin or nonsteroidal anti-inflammatory drug use. Type- and cross-matched blood should be available in the blood bank.

Before the bleeding is considered to be uncontrolled, medical therapy should be promptly initiated. If therapy is successful, even massive hemoptysis will decrease steadily. After 4 days, 87% of patients have decreased hemorrhages (Bobrowitz et al, 1983).

Position the patient in bed with the head lower than the chest and the side of the bleeding dependent to prevent aspiration and asphyxiation. A wide-bore intravenous cannula is inserted (I use the internal jugular vein), and whole blood is kept on standby. Arterial blood gases are monitored.

Sedatives, such as diazepam 5 to 10 mg every 6 hours, and antitussive agents (e.g., small doses of codeine) may be used to depress the excessive or violent coughing that keeps aggravating or stimulating the hemoptysis. However, if the cough reflex is completely suppressed, blood will be retained, and aspiration can occur, promoting pneumonitis and atelectasis (Bobrowitz et al, 1983). If the partial arterial pressure of oxygen is less than 60 mm Hg, supplemental oxygen should be used.

Some clinicians recommend that all patients with massive hemoptysis are given broad-spectrum antimicrobial agents empirically to limit complications or infections caused by aspiration. Others advise antibiotics if the patient has a history of bronchitis or chronic obstructive pulmonary disease, evidence of leukocytosis, or any suggestion of a bacterial complication (Bobrowitz et al, 1983). Pursel and Lindskog (1961) stated that all patients with continuing hemoptysis of significant proportions should receive antimicrobial agents empirically to limit the possible infectious complications of aspiration into the uninvolved lung. I use penicillin with gentamicin for all patients in an attempt to reduce the incidence of pneumonia and sepsis from the aspiration of blood.

In patients with tuberculosis, it is imperative to initiate antituberculous therapy with drugs to which the bacilli are sensitive. This is an effective measure in controlling the hemoptysis of active tuberculosis because such lesions are reversible. For each day that the patient receives new effective drugs, the prognosis improves. If surgery becomes necessary, the morbidity and mortality rates are minimized. I advocate the use of streptomycin with the standard drugs, especially when there is a cavitary lesion. In my experience, most patients with active pulmonary tuberculosis and massive hemoptysis stop bleeding within 1 week after treatment with antituberculous drugs; none bled after the 10th day.

Blood transfusions may be required to keep the hematocrit above 30%, but excessive transfusion to raise the blood pressure to "normal" levels may actually promote bleeding.

Bronchodilators should not be administered, because these may have vasodilator actions and precipitate renewed bleeding (Wedzicha and Pearson, 1990). An assessment of pulmonary function should be carried out promptly, even at the bedside.

Teklu and Felleke (1982) reported a series of cases of massive hemoptysis in tuberculosis. They studied 74 patients at a sanatorium in Addis Ababa that had no surgical facilities. There were 17 deaths. All patients who died, except one who was operated on at another hospital, were managed conservatively (mortality rate of 16 of 73 or 21.9%).

Methods of Control

Endobronchial Control Measures

The introduction and spread of endobronchial control measures revolutionized the management of massive hemoptysis. The measures may be combined with either surgical or medical management, and they gain time for the restoration of clinical stability and the performance of essential diagnostic and management procedures (Conlan, 1985).

Ice-Cold Saline Lavage. The mural musculature of the bronchial vessels is identical to that of peripheral vessels, and it responds to cold by vasoconstriction. The systematic lavage of the bleeding lung with large volumes of ice-cold saline solution can induce slowing and ultimate cessation of the bleeding by hypothermic vasospasm of the bronchial arterial branches that supply it (Conlan, 1985). I use a technique similar to the one reported by Conlan and colleagues (1983). The requirements are as follows: (1) a rigid bronchoscope, (2) a large-bore suction catheter (which allows rapid suctioning of blood, clots, and irrigation fluid; it is better to use two separate sets of suction catheters), (3) ice-cold saline solution with ice blocks floating in it, and (4) an effective light source. I use topical anesthesia or no anesthesia at all in cases of respiratory arrest. Sedation when necessary can be achieved with 10 to 15 mg lorazepam IV. The rigid bronchoscope is rapidly inserted with 100% oxygen pumped through it. All blood and clots are suctioned from the trachea and major bronchi. The bleeding side is identified, and the nonbleeding main bronchus is snugly cannulated with the rigid bronchoscope; ventilation is begun. The Trendelenburg position is used to facilitate the evacuation of blood from the trachea. After the patient is clinically stable, the bleeding bronchus is cannulated; blood and clots are suctioned out; and 50-ml aliquots of iced-saline solution are injected into the endobronchial tree on that side. The iced solution is allowed to remain in contact for approximately 15 seconds and is then rapidly suctioned back. The nonbleeding lung is recanalized, and gas exchange is begun. Using this method, the process of ice-cold irrigation, alternating with periods of ventilation, can proceed quickly. After bleeding has slowed, it is possible to withdraw the bronchoscope into the trachea between periods of irrigation and use both lungs for ventilation. More than 1L of ice-cold saline solution may be used for irrigation. I have used ice-cold saline lavage in 303 patients with massive hemoptysis, and the bleeding stopped in 291 (96%). At this point, I may use the flexible bronchoscope to increase the accuracy of the diagnosis. After the bleeding lobe or segment has been identified, appropriate pathologic and bacteriologic specimens or biopsies can be taken.

After termination of the irrigation procedure, the patient is placed with the bleeding lung dependent and returned to the ICU where medical therapy is continued. It is important to repeat flexible or rigid bronchoscopy in the next 2 days, even if the bleeding has stopped, to aspirate old clots in the tracheobronchial tree. Ice-cold saline lavage allows time to evaluate the disease, to localize the bleeding, to perform the necessary pulmonary function tests, and to facilitate the planning of a safe and precise resection, if necessary. It remains, however, a transitory holding procedure, and definitive therapy should not be delayed. Ice-cold saline lavage should be included as part of the rigid bronchoscopic technique initially used in all patients with massive hemoptysis. Nevertheless, it is not appropriate therapy for a bronchovascular fistula, for which other methods of endobronchial control should be used. At the end of the endoscopy, we decide whether to perform a tracheostomy. This procedure is valuable in cases of bilateral aspiration or for patients with minimal pulmonary reserve.

Balloon Tamponade

Massive hemoptysis can be controlled by the placement of Fogarty-type embolectomy catheters and subsequent balloon inflation in the bleeding segmental bronchus, using the flexible fiberoptic bronchoscope. Since 1974 this technique has been applied to patients with bleeding from nonsurgical causes (e.g., bilateral extensive pulmonary disease; terminal malignant disease; severe associated cardiac, renal, hepatic, or metabolic diseases; and severe cystic fibrosis). It can be used preoperatively in surgical candidates. It allows an accurate localization of disease and subsequent appropriate and concise pulmonary resections. The limitations of the flexible fiberoptic bronchoscope in massive hemoptysis have already been emphasized, and most actively hemorrhaging patients require rigid bronchoscopy. If flexible endoscopy is carried out during a fortuitous pause in the bleeding or when bleeding has slowed spontaneously, it is indeed valuable. It can localize bleeding to the subsegmental bronchus level, especially in upper lobe disease.

Saw and colleagues (1976) described their experience in 10 patients with massive hemoptysis, using selective endobronchial tamponade with the Fogarty balloon through the flexible bronchoscope. Tamponade was achieved in all cases.

A double-lumen, bronchus-blocking catheter has been developed that can be introduced through the working channel of a standard bronchofiberscope, for the management of moderate hemoptysis (Freitag, 1993; Freitag et al, 1994).

Marsico (1991) created an endobronchial blocker that can be made in a few minutes for an adult. He uses a 6 French (F) Foley catheter and an 8F nasogastric tube. The nasogastric tube is cut distally above the side holes and about 3 cm apart from the proximal end. From the Foley catheter, he uses the proximal end and the distal end (approximately 5 cm above the balloon). The proximal end of the Foley catheter is connected to the proximal end of the nasogastric tube. The distal end of the Foley catheter is inserted into the distal end of the nasogastric tube. The exterior surface of the proximal end of the Foley catheter can be smoothed with sandpaper and thus easily passed through the rigid bronchoscope. All connections are reinforced with glue, which is also used to close the distal hole of the Foley catheter. In this way, the balloon can be filled with contrast medium (Fig. 27–3). The Marsico blocker has the following advantages: (1) it is cheap, (2) it is resistant, (3) there is a good adaptation to various diameters of the tracheobronchial tree, and (4) it is available in all hospitals.

When I use an endobronchial balloon, I perform a fiberoptic bronchoscopy 24 hours later. If bleeding does not recur immediately on deflation, secretions are aspirated to avoid postobstructive pneumonia, and if no further blood is observed after several more hours of observation, the balloon can be removed.

Infrequently, the Marsico blocker is used as an endobronchial balloon tamponade because almost all patients

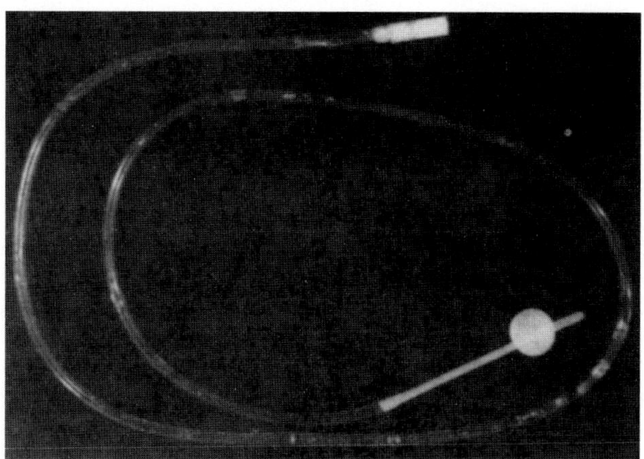

FIGURE 27–3 ■ An example of a homemade endobronchial blocker, as described by Marsico.

stop bleeding with the ice-cold saline lavage. It is sometimes used as a bronchial blocker during operations (see Surgical Therapy).

This technique may be particularly helpful in preserving gas exchange in the nonbleeding lung when patients have persistent massive hemoptysis (Cahill and Ingbar, 1994).

Kato and colleagues (1996) reported a massive hemoptysis successfully treated by modified bronchoscopic balloon tamponade technique. A wire for angiography was inserted into a lobar bronchus to guide a 7F balloon catheter.

Pulmonary Isolation

Isolation of the bleeding lung from the healthy one can be achieved by the use of either a double-lumen tracheal tube of the Carlens type or an ordinary balloon-bearing endotracheal tube to selectively intubate the nonbleeding lung. Both procedures should be preceded by rigid bronchoscopy to allow correct localization or lateralization of the source of bleeding and the suctioning of blood and all its products.

The double-lumen endotracheal tubes carry significant risks and are difficult to place properly, even under controlled circumstances. Their inner diameter is small and not suitable for the removal of large volumes of blood and clots from the airways. In addition, it may be impossible to pass a fiberoptic scope through the small lumen to verify tube position or explore the airway. Other complications include loss of lung separation owing to dislodgment of the tube; traumatic laryngitis from improper insertion of the carinal hook (present in some models); and tracheobronchial rupture from a tube that is too large or from overinflation of the balloon (Cahill and Ingbar, 1994).

Selective intubation of the main bronchus of either lung with a long endotracheal tube (8 mm in diameter) is an attractive and useful option. It can be used for either right- or left-sided bleeding. The techniques for each lung are different because of the variation in anatomy of the main bronchi (Cahill and Ingbar, 1994; Conlan, 1985) (see Surgical Therapy).

If significant quantities of blood have been aspirated and hypoxemia is severe, it may not be feasible to oxygenate and ventilate a bleeding patient using a single lung. Intrapulmonary shunting through the nonventilated lung and ventilation-perfusion mismatching from aspirated blood in the ventilated lung may leave an inadequate surface area for gas exchange, especially in the patient with limited pulmonary reserve (Cahill and Ingbar, 1994).

Packing of the bronchus with swabs or tampons soaked in vasoconstrictive drugs can be used in emergency circumstances when other effective therapy is not available. However, the dangers of an uncontrolled, mobile, endobronchial foreign-body mass must be weighed against the possible benefits (Conlan, 1985). I did not use pulmonary separation or vasoconstrictive drugs as methods of endobronchial control in my series of patients with massive hemoptysis.

Selective Coagulative Treatment

Topical thrombin and fibrinogen-thrombin solutions have been used with reported success in the treatment of patients with massive bleeds (Cahill and Ingbar, 1994; De Gracia et al, 1995).

Tsukamoto and colleagues (1989) studied 19 patients with massive hemoptysis in whom hemostasis was achieved in 6 of 10 (60%) patients using topical thrombin alone and 9 of 9 (100%) patients using a topical fibrinogen-thrombin solution.

Bense (1990) reported three patients with hemoptysis in whom fibrin precursors were sprayed into the bronchus selectively to the site of bleeding. The immediate formation of a fibrin clot, which plugged the bronchus, was observed; hemoptysis ceased promptly. The pressure of the propellant (20 to 30 millibars) is higher than the intracapillary pressure, a fact that might also have a favorable effect on hemoptysis by compressing these small vessels if they are the source of bleeding. Other indirect modes of this treatment should be considered. Total occlusion of a bronchus by plugging causes regional hypoxic vasoconstriction. This decreases the regional blood flow at the site of the vascular damage and thus promotes the arrest of bleeding.

A bleeding endobronchial tumor can be successfully coagulated using neodymium:yttrium-aluminum-garnet laser ablation after the massive bleeding has been controlled.

Arterial Embolization

Bronchial artery embolization has been popularized as both a temporizing and a definitive treatment of patients with massive hemoptysis. Embolotherapy is commonly performed when a bleeding site is identified by arteriography, because it can be done as part of the same procedure. Embolization is an attractive alternative to surgery in patients with bilateral disease, multiple bleeding sites, or borderline pulmonary reserve (Cahill and Ingbar, 1994).

Remy and colleagues (1977) published a study of 104 patients presenting with either massive or repeated hemoptysis who were treated by embolization of the bronchial arteries with a resorbable material (Spongel).

The procedure was performed by selective catheterization of the abnormal arteries. Forty-nine patients were treated during (and 55 after) hemoptysis. Of the 49 patients treated during hemoptysis, an immediate arrest of bleeding was achieved in 41, but 6 of these patients had relapses 2 to 7 months after the procedure. There was no recurrence of bleeding in the remaining 35 patients.

Transverse myelitis is a known complication of bronchial artery embolization because of the anatomic variation of a shared origin of bronchial arteries with intercostal vessels, which supply radiculomedullary branches to the anterior spinal circulation. The anterior spinal cord is supplied by the anterior spinal artery, which originates from branches of the vertebral arteries and from anterior medullary branches of intercostal and lumbar arteries. In the thoracic area, the supply to the anterior spinal artery is usually from a single anterior medullary branch (Fraser et al, 1997).

Remy and colleagues (1984) believed that hemoptysis treatable only by embolization must be approached from the standpoint that most bronchial bleeding has a systemic origin, and, consequently, both the bronchial arteries and the nonbronchial transpleural systemic arteries of the lung must be investigated and occluded. Persistent bleeding after a technically good embolization suggests an origin from vessels other than those previously obstructed, and the pulmonary circulation should be studied. A destructive process of the lung, whatever its pathogenesis, can erode any vessel in its vicinity, whether pulmonary or systemic.

Jardin and Remy (1988) studied a group of seven patients in whom bronchial bleeding persisted despite previous bronchial embolization. In five cases, arrest of bleeding was only obtained when the internal mammary arteries and other systemic nonbronchial arteries were occluded. In two cases, the internal mammary artery was the only systemic nonbronchial vessel that was embolized percutaneously, followed by the immediate and complete cessation of bleeding. They stated that recognition of the numerous collateral vessels and anastomoses of the internal mammary arteries are essential for successful percutaneous embolization for hemoptysis.

Uflacker and colleagues (1985) reported 35 patients with massive bleeding treated by bronchial artery embolization with absorbable gelatin sponge (Gelfoam) particles. Immediate control of hemoptysis was achieved in 31 patients (87%). Bronchial artery embolization alone caused long-term control of bleeding in 13 of 17 patients (76.5%) with massive bleeding. These authors do not consider the presence of anterior and posterior radicular arteries and posterior spinal arteries on the angiogram to be an absolute contraindication for bronchial artery embolization. However, when the anterior spinal artery is demonstrated, embolization should be avoided, or special care should be undertaken to avoid obstruction of this vessel by using larger particles for embolization.

Recurrent hemoptysis results from incomplete embolization, revascularization (progression of the basic disease), or recannulation of embolized vessels. Incomplete embolization is often caused by inadequate evaluation of nonbronchial systemic collaterals (Cahill and Ingbar, 1994).

Bronchial artery embolization is ineffective in treating bleeding from diffuse pulmonary involvement. Occasionally, persistent, recurrent bleeding arises from the pulmonary artery, and examination of this arterial system is mandatory when other possibilities are excluded. A fungal ball in a pulmonary cavity is a frequent cause of rebleeding, which is a major drawback to the interventional therapy for this cause of massive hemoptysis. In most patients, acute bleeding stops after bronchial artery embolization, but most rebleed after some time if they are not treated surgically. Bronchial artery embolization must, therefore, be considered a temporary treatment for massive hemoptysis in patients with aspergilloma.

Rabkin and colleagues (1987), by means of bronchial arteriography, studied a group of 306 patients with acute pulmonary hemorrhage who were treated with transcatheter embolization. In 120 patients, the hemoptysis was massive, with volumes exceeding 500 ml/day. The majority ($n = 225$) were treated during peak hemorrhages. Effective hemostasis was obtained initially in 278 (90.8%) patients, including 87.5% of those treated during peak hemorrhages. In 26 of 28 cases without an initial response, the pulmonary artery was the source of bleeding. Recurrent bleeding within 1 to 4 days, which required surgery, was observed in 39 patients who had initially successful hemostasis. Of 158 patients who were treated without surgery, subsequent episodes of hemoptysis occurred in 36.

Remy and colleagues (1988) reviewed the technique for management of hemoptysis caused by arteriovenous aneurysms of the lung. They called it "vaso-occlusion" of the pulmonary artery and defined it as ". . . an angiographic technique that involves the voluntary and precise obstruction, temporary or permanent, of one or several branches of the pulmonary artery, utilizing coil springs or detachable balloons." They thought that this could not be called "embolization" because with embolization the migration of emboli is uncontrolled and depends on the blood flow.

Tamura and colleagues (1993) pointed out that embolotherapy was consistently more effective in patients who had no pleural abnormalities compared with those with pleural thickening.

Concerning embolic agents, the large Gianturco coils lodge too proximally to be effective in occluding arteries at the peripheral level. The minicoils are more suitable but are very expensive. To handle the numerous pathologic vessels stemming from one origin, particles or liquid material are more suitable for peripheral embolization. Gelfoam, due to its nonpermanence, is not a good embolic agent for embolization in hemoptysis. Polyvinyl alcohol particles (Ivalon), dura particles, ethibloc, and tissue adhesives such as isobutyl-2-cyanoacrylate (IBC) and *N*-butyl-2-cyanoacrylate (NBC) can be used safely and effectively to treat the bleeding site (Lampmann and Tjan, 1994).

Ramakantan and colleagues (1996) studied 140 patients who presented with significant hemoptysis (>300 ml of blood in 24 hours) owing to pulmonary tuberculosis. They underwent bronchial artery embolization, using gelatin sponges, on the side with the greater abnormality on the chest radiograph. Almost complete control of hemoptysis was achieved in 102 (73%) patients.

Carlsen and colleagues (1997) reported the first successful treatment with microcoil embolization of massive hemoptysis following lung transplantation related to proliferated and enlarged tortuous bronchial arteries (possibly owing to pre-existing bronchiectasis in the donor lungs). It occurred 26 months after an en bloc, double-lung transplantation with direct bronchial artery revascularization.

In our series, bronchial artery embolization was attempted in 36 patients as a control method for massive hemoptysis. In only one patient was the catheterization technically impossible. Among the 35 patients who underwent bronchial artery embolization, bleeding stopped immediately in 32 (91.4%); however, 22 patients (62.8%) had recurrences.

Percutaneous Abscess Drainage

There are relatively few indications for urgent percutaneous tube drainage of a cavitary pulmonary lesion in a patient with massive hemoptysis. I use this type of drainage when any cavity shows the radiologic patterns described by Thoms and colleagues (1972) (see Imaging Studies) and the patient has a contraindication to thoracotomy (see Fig. 27–1).

Mechanical Ventilation with Positive End-Expiratory Pressure

Some authors believe that all patients with massive hemoptysis should have an endotracheal tube in place to clean the tracheobronchial tree and, if necessary, to use mechanical ventilation with positive end-expiratory pressure (PEEP). This not only enhances oxygenation but also increases the intrathoracic pressure, which serves as a tamponade for the site of bleeding.

Pneumoperitoneum and Pneumothorax

Collapse therapy with pneumoperitoneum or pneumothorax may be used in selected cases. In the collapsed lung, there is a great decrease in blood flow. Pneumothorax is contraindicated when there are pleural adhesions, which happens in many cases of massive hemoptysis. The most efficient collapses with pneumoperitoneum are obtained with elastic cavities located in pulmonary bases.

Vasoactive Drugs

Bilton and colleagues (1990) reported a conservative measure to control profuse hemoptysis in a critically ill patient with poor lung function who had cystic fibrosis. He was given an intravenous infusion of vasopressin 20 U over 15 minutes, with immediate cessation of the bleeding. In view of this success, an infusion of vasopressin 0.2 U/min was started and continued for 36 hours. The site of action is probably arteriolar smooth muscle, through an increase in the intracellular concentration of inositol phosphates, which mobilize intracellular calcium, causing contraction. I do not have experience with this method of control, but it seems simple and reliable enough to be recommended for further study.

Radiotherapy

Several case reports document the successful use of radiation therapy to treat massive hemoptysis in special circumstances.

Shneerson and colleagues (1980) reported on a patient with massive hemoptysis and a fungal ball. He was irradiated with a ^{60}Co unit with a single anterior field to a total dose of 2000 cGy in five fractions over 7 days. His bleeding ceased completely 3 days after radiotherapy was started. However, 8 weeks later, he had three episodes of hemoptysis, totaling about 150 ml, for which he received an additional 1000-cGy midline dose with opposing fields to the left upper zone in five fractions over 7 days. He had no additional bleeding during 8 months of follow-up. The fungal ball did not change in size after therapy. Presumably, the radiation had no net effect on the growth of the fungus but was acting on the vascular lining of the cavity. The early effects of radiation on small blood vessels include swelling, necrosis, and possibly hyperplasia of the endothelial cells, resulting in thrombosis and compression of the vessels by perivascular edema. Eventually, perivascular and medial fibroses occlude the vessels and impair the capacity of microcirculation to regenerate and remodel in the presence of injury or infection. These effects are dose dependent. The radiation may have acted similarly in this patient.

Intracavitary Treatment

Rumbak and colleagues (1996) reported the efficacy of topical treatment for 12 episodes of severe, life-threatening hemoptysis from a pulmonary aspergilloma (underlying diseases were bronchiectasis, sarcoidosis, tuberculosis, or histoplasmosis) in 11 poor surgical risk patients. A local intracavitary instillation of sodium or potassium iodide was performed. The transcricothyroid approach was used in six patients and the percutaneous approach in five. Hemoptysis ceased within 72 hours in all patients, and all of them were alive at least 1 year later.

Surgical Therapy

The surgical management of massive hemoptysis has been described extensively in the medical literature over the past few decades. Pulmonary resection has been shown to be the most effective method for the control and prevention of recurrent bleeding in most patients, and it has been shown that surgical rather than medical methods reduce mortality rates from massive hemoptysis. In most such reports concerning massive hemoptysis, the recommendation is made that an aggressive surgical approach with immediate or early pulmonary resection is the definitive therapy. Other papers emphasize the role of conservative treatment in massive or life-threatening hemoptysis (Amirana et al, 1968; Bobrowitz et al, 1983; Bracco, 1956; Conlan et al, 1983; Espinosa et al, 1983; Garzon et al, 1982; McCollum et al, 1975; Thoms et al, 1972; Yang and Berger, 1978; and Yeoh et al, 1967).

Comparison of series of medically and surgically treated patients is difficult for several reasons. First, the definition of massive hemoptysis varies between series. Second, the number of operable patients in each series is variable, probably reflecting differences in the population of patients studied. Third, the number of patients undergoing surgery varies considerably between series and is probably the result of institutional or personal bias. Fourth, some of the series place all patients who are not surgical candidates among those in the medical therapy group. Therefore, patients judged inoperable because of limited ventilatory reserve, advanced bilateral pulmonary disease, inoperable carcinoma, a nonlocalized bleeding site, and bleeding so brisk that no intervention is possible are included in the medical therapy group. Because all of these conditions are risk factors for a poor prognosis, the mortality rates for medical treatment are unfairly biased. A more appropriate comparison of the medical versus surgical mortality rates in these series requires a determination of those patients deemed operable but treated medically.

Emergency surgical therapy still carries substantial mortality and morbidity rates compared with elective pulmonary resection. The mortality rate is related to ongoing bleeding at the time of the operation. The spillage of blood, pus, or infected material into the dependent lung during an operation is the prime cause of death and postoperative respiratory morbidity. Likewise, the performance of a pulmonary resection in patients with poor lung function is a major contributory factor to postoperative mortality rates. Elective operations performed on nonbleeding patients whose disease and lung function are known is the ideal situation. Delaying surgical treatment until a spontaneous resolution of the hemorrhage occurs is not a reliable or ethical choice of management. However, the preoperative control of bleeding in every patient undergoing surgical treatment for massive hemoptysis is possible today. The use of endobronchial control techniques and the accurate identification of disease and its extent allow the precise planning of pulmonary resection to conserve functioning lung tissue (Conlan, 1985).

Patient Selection and Choice of Surgical Technique

The criteria for selecting surgical therapy include: (1) localized site of bleeding, (2) adequate pulmonary function, (3) no medical contraindications, (4) resectable carcinoma without distant metastases, and (5) no mitral disease (required of cardiac surgery). In elective cases, we select patients for pulmonary resection based on the forced expiratory volume in 1 second (FEV_1). Patients who have a minimum FEV_1 of 2 or 1.7 L are considered fit for pneumonectomy or lobectomy, respectively. I do not perform any resection when the FEV_1 is less than 850 ml. When the FEV_1 is between 850 ml and 2L, I use perfusion pulmonary scanning to calculate the predicted postoperative FEV_1. With a predicted FEV_1 of less than 850 ml, no resection is done. With a predicted FEV_1 of more than 1.2 L, even pneumonectomy may be performed. Finally, when the predicted FEV_1 is between 850 ml and 1.2 L, I verify the mean pulmonary artery pressure; if the pressure is more than 25 mm Hg, resection is not advisable.

Surgery is also contraindicated when, at the patient's baseline, there is carbon dioxide retention, dyspnea at rest, or severe dyspnea on exertion. Lung resection in patients with inadequate pulmonary reserve has no beneficial effect on outcome; the cause of death is merely changed from asphyxiation or exsanguination to respiratory insufficiency. Bilateral parenchymal disease, unresectable carcinoma, or the inability to lateralize the bleeding site also prohibit surgical resection (Cahill and Ingbar, 1994).

With the introduction of ice-cold saline lavage and arterial embolization, we can control almost all cases of massive hemoptysis. Urgent surgery (i.e., within 24 to 48 hours after initial control) is required only in the following circumstances.

1. Fungus ball (almost all cases will rebleed after any control method)
2. Lung abscess (generally an erosion of a large vessel)
3. Failure of the control method (rare)
4. Presence of a cavity with the following radiologic patterns: emptying and refilling, a movable mass, or a persistent radiodensity (rare)
5. Obstruction of the main or lobar bronchus with a clot that cannot be suctioned during rigid bronchoscopy (rare)

In cases of urgent surgery for continuing bleeding, major resections should be avoided. I prefer a method of collapse (plombage and thoracoplasty), cavernostomy, parietopleuropulmonary devascularization, or even simple bronchial artery ligature. In our series, 21 (11.8%) patients were bleeding at the time of the pulmonary surgery, 40 (22.3%) patients were operated on up to 30 days after the episode of massive hemoptysis, and 118 patients (65.9%) were operated on after 30 days.

The surgical procedures required may be classified into four groups as follows: (1) pulmonary resections (pneumonectomy, lobectomy, or segmentectomy); (2) collapse therapy (thoracoplasty or plombage); (3) cavernostomies; and (4) intrathoracic vascular ligatures. In our series, four patients underwent wedge resection in association with lobectomies. One patient underwent a two-stage left thoracoplasty and a right upper lobectomy at different times. Three patients underwent bronchial artery ligature, two of them as the sole procedure and another concomitantly with a contralateral pneumonectomy. Finally, seven patients had recurrent hemoptysis after bronchial artery embolization; they underwent a thoracotomy, and the lung was mobilized in the same way as for a resection with ligature of all the vessels between the lung and the chest wall and the vessels of the pulmonary ligament. I called this procedure "parietopleuropulmonary devascularization."

Technique

Various techniques have been advocated to facilitate anesthesia for emergency thoracotomy in the patient with endobronchial bleeding. Gauze tamponade of the bleeding bronchus through the bronchoscope, the use of endobronchial blocking devices, and the use of occlusive double-lumen tubes, such as the Robert Shaw type, have been advised (Borer et al, 1966).

I prefer to operate under unilateral lung ventilation. If the right lung is bleeding, an endotracheal tube or double

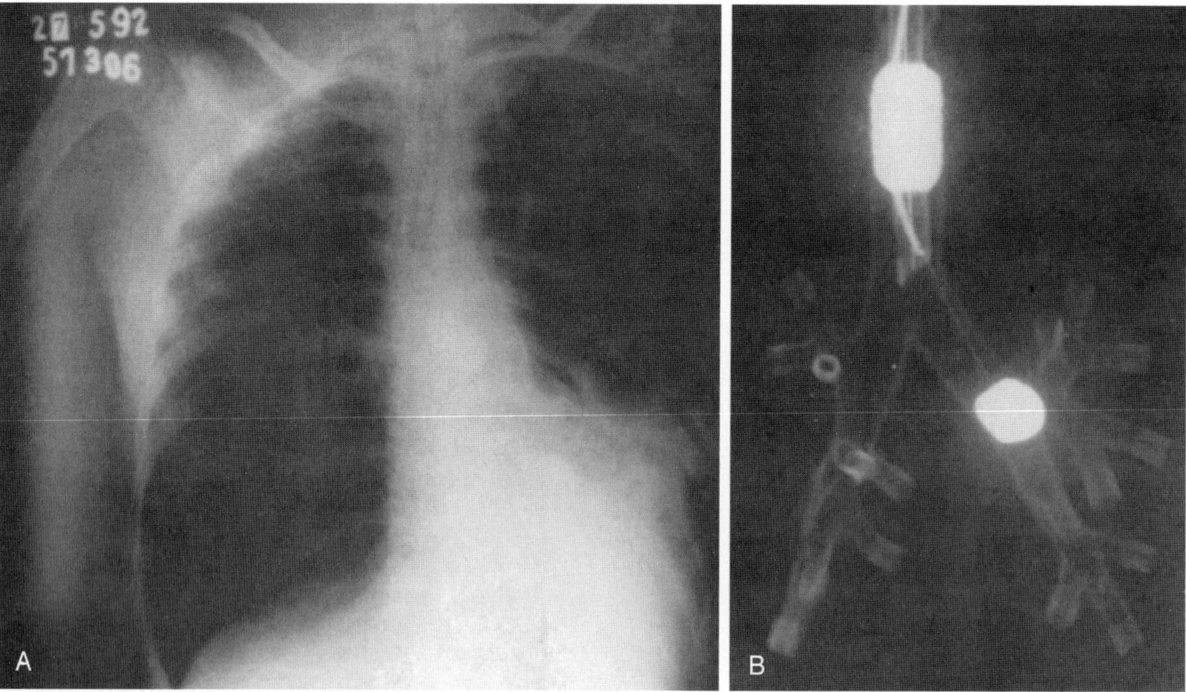

FIGURE 27–4 ■ *A,* Marsico endobronchial blocker in the left main bronchus. *B,* Diagrammatic representation of a Marsico endobronchial blocker in the left mainstem bronchus.

lumen is advanced into the left main bronchus, preventing spillage of blood from the right to the left side. For left-sided bleeding there are three options: (1) a double-lumen tube is used; (2) an endotracheal tube with a ventilation slot for the right upper lobe is advanced into the right main bronchus; or (3) an endobronchial blocker can be performed at the time of rigid bronchoscopy through the lumen. After the blocker is positioned properly, the balloon is inflated (Fig. 27–4). Most blockers do not cause any problem during removal of the bronchoscope. After the bronchoscope is removed, an endotracheal tube is placed, and its cuff is inflated. This helps to hold the blocker against the wall of the trachea and avoid displacement of the balloon. The patient is then given general anesthesia and positioned for a thoracotomy. The anesthesiologist should be aware of the possibility of displacement of the blocker. Displacement of the inflated balloon blocker can produce obstruction of the trachea; if this occurrence is suspected, the balloon should be deflated immediately.

Complications related to one-lung ventilation may be technical or physiologic. Because of the shape and large size of double-lumen tubes, the incidence of difficult tracheal intubation is higher than that with the use of single-lumen tubes. Unsuccessful or difficult intubation has been the only technical complication that I have encountered; I have had no cases of trauma, improper positioning, or tube dislodgment. The physiologic complication of hypoxemia may be the result of increased venous admixture, alteration of hypoxic pulmonary vasoconstriction, increased intra-alveolar pressure, decreased cardiac output, or atelectasis of the dependent lung.

Technique

The basic principle of excisional surgery, maximal elimination of disease with minimal sacrifice of functional lung tissue, must be observed. I currently prefer a muscle-sparing vertical axillary thoracotomy incision. In most of my patients, there is extensive pleural disease coexisting with parenchymal disease, frequently necessitating a pleuropneumonectomy. A plane of cleavage is developed between the endothoracic fascia and the parietal pleura, thus freeing the pleura and the lung as one from the chest wall, diaphragm, and mediastinal structures down to the hilus. From this stage on, the vessels and bronchus are managed as in a standard pneumonectomy. In some cases, when the adhesions between the lung and the chest wall are firm, we perform the "bird-cage" procedure described by Ribeiro-Netto (1988), which consists of liberating the pleura and lung from the chest wall by the extrafascial route, creating a space between the ribs and thoracic fascia or the freed periosteal and intercostal

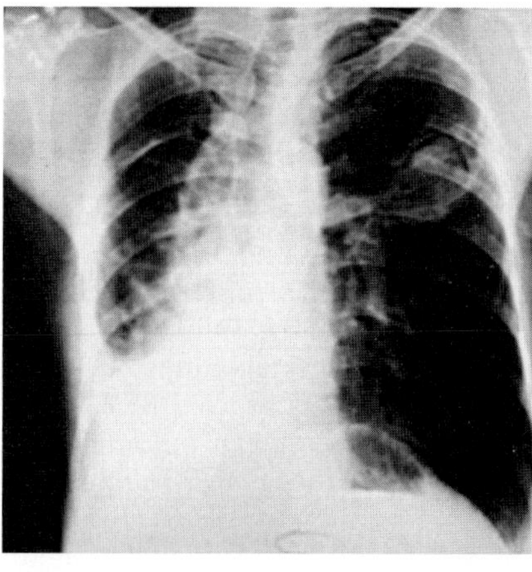

FIGURE 27–5 ■ Left upper lobe cavity with a fungus ball.

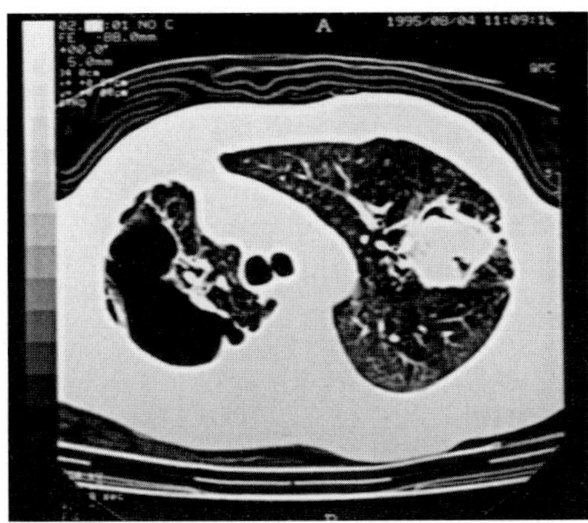

FIGURE 27–6 ■ CT scan; same case shown in Figure 27–5.

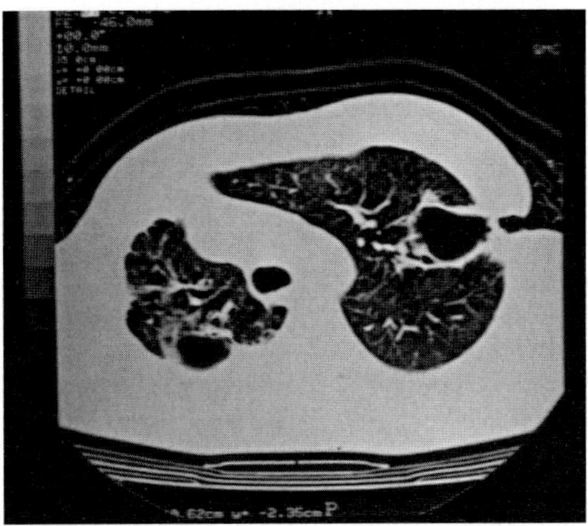

FIGURE 27–8 ■ CT scan; closed cavernostomy; same patient shown in Figure 27–5.

musculature, similar to a plombage thoracoplasty. I always cover the bronchial stump with intercostal muscle.

Flexible bronchoscopy should be performed at the end of the surgical procedure. The postoperative course is smoother if the aspirated blood clots and secretions are removed completely from the tracheobronchial tree immediately after surgery.

Cavernostomy is a method of marsupialization by a direct opening of the chest wall over the cavity. The operation is conducted under general anaesthesia after exact radiologic localization of the cavity. One or two short rib segments over the suspected area are removed through a vertical axillary thoracotomy. (The location of the cavity is demonstrated by inserting a large-bore needle mounted on a syringe: when the plunger is withdrawn, portions of the fungus ball or air from the cavity will come into the syringe.) The posterior periosteum is removed and, through the adherent overlying pleura (if the lung moves beneath the parietal pleura and formal resection is impossible, gauze packing can be inserted to induce pleural symphysis for 10 days), a wide opening is made with removal of the fungal mass. Then, stitches are placed between the skin and the edges of the cavity wall. The walls of the wound leading down to the cavity must be widely exposed. Otherwise great difficulty will be experienced in applying the dressings. In most cases, spontaneous closure of cavernostomy occurs after weeks or months. When necessary, a pedicled muscle flap can be used to close the space (Figs. 27–5, 27–6, 27–7, 27–8).

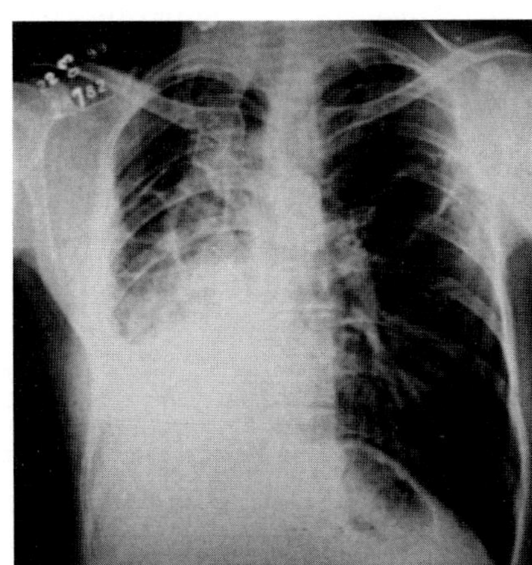

FIGURE 27–7 ■ Cavity three years after cavernostomy; same patient shown in Figure 27–5; no symptoms at all.

I performed 18 cavernostomies in patients with large cavities and blood aspiration. Six patients had active tuberculosis, and 12 had inactive tuberculosis (fungal ball). Six patients underwent cavernostomies during massive bleeding. Four patients died postoperatively. One patient had a prolonged bronchocutaneous fistula, and another had respiratory insufficiency.

Early Results

In my own series of 501 patients with massive hemoptysis, 31 of 179 (17.3%) patients treated surgically died during the hospitalization period; of the 322 patients treated medically, 60 died (18.6%) (Table 27–5).

The 179 surgically treated patients underwent 189 procedures (Table 27–6). Postoperative complications occurred in 72 patients (40.2%). The major complication was pleural empyema (occurring in 27 patients), followed by respiratory failure (occurring in 20 patients) (Table 27–7). No complications occurred in 107 patients (59.8%) who were operated on.

Among the 63 patients who underwent pneumonectomy, 18 (28.6%) had no postoperative complications; 20 (31.7%) had pleural empyema, 16 (25.4%) had respiratory insufficiency, and 25 (39.7%) had miscellaneous complications. In the lobectomy group, 25 patients (47.2%) had no postoperative complications. Ten (18.9%) patients had pleural empyema; eight (15.1%) had respira-

TABLE 27–5 ■ **Mortality Rate in 501 Patients with Massive Hemoptysis**

Type of Treatment	*No. of Patients*	*Mortality Rate*
		No. (%)
Medical	322	60 (18.6)
Surgical	179	31 (17.3)
Total	501	91 (18.2)

TABLE 27–6 ■ **Surgical Procedures in 179 Patients with Massive Hemoptysis**

Type of Prodedure	*Patients* No. (%)
Pneumonectomy	63 (33.3)
Lobectomy	53 (28)
Plombage	20 (10.6)
Cavernostomy	18 (9.5)
Thoracoplasty	12 (6.4)
Segmentectomy	9 (4.8)
Devascularization	7 (3.7)
Wedge resection	4 (2.1)
Bronchial artery ligature	3 (1.6)
Total	189 (100)

tory failure; and 27 (50.9%) had other complications (Table 27–8; see also Table 27-7).

When the surgical mortality rates were analyzed in relation to the timing of the operation, it was found that when pneumonectomy is performed, there is a statistically significant difference ($P < .05$) in mortality rates between the patients operated on emergently during or electively after the massive hemoptysis. Among nine patients who underwent pneumonectomies during bleeding, the mortality rate was 66.7%. Whenever possible, total resection during massive hemoptysis should be avoided.

Late Results

An attempt was made to follow all patients after discharge, but clinic records were available for only 328 patients (80%). A follow-up period of 1 to 48 months was obtained in 183 (55.8%) cases; 145 (44.2%) had a follow-up of more than 48 months.

There was a statistically significant difference ($P <$ .05) between the surgical and nonsurgical groups in relation to the proportions of patients who rebled. In the nonsurgical group, 36.9% of the patients had another episode of hemoptysis, and in the surgical group, only 9.2% did.

TABLE 27–7 ■ **Postoperative Complications in 72 Patients with Massive Hemoptysis**

Type of Complication	*Patients* No. (%)
Pleural empyema	27 (23.1)
Respiratory failure	20 (17.1)
Bronchopleural fistula	20 (17.1)
Pneumonia	12 (10.3)
Hypovolemia	10 (8.5)
Intracavitary clot syndrome	6 (5.1)
Pulmonary edema	3 (2.6)
Miscellaneous	19 (16.2)
Total	117 (100)

TABLE 27–8 ■ **Mortality Rates and Types of Operation in Massive Hemoptysis**

Type of Operation	*Patients (No.)*	*Mortality Rates* No. (%)
Pneumonectomy	63	14 (22.2)
Lobectomy	53	6 (11.3)
Segmentectomy	9	1 (11.1)
Plombage	20	7 (35)
Thoracoplasty	12	1 (8.3)
Cavernostomy	18	4 (22.2)
Devascularization	7	1 (14.3)
Wedge resection	4	— —
Bronchial artery ligature	3	— —

SUMMARY

I believe that endobronchial control measures and artery embolization have radically changed the management of patients with massive hemoptysis. With the control of the hemorrhage, the clinician is able to identify nonsurgical patients and assess surgical candidates accurately, thus allowing an elective, less morbid operation. I await improved techniques for embolization of the nonbronchial system to avoid failures in the follow-up period.

COMMENTS AND CONTROVERSIES

In the reported series by Dr. Guimarães most patients had tuberculosis with pleural fusion, necessitating either pleuropneumonectomy or, when indicated, cavernostomy. In North America, we most frequently encounter massive hemoptysis in patients with totally free pleural spaces. I have never used cavernostomy as a method of treatment in patients suffering massive hemoptysis, but in selected patients in whom pleural fusion has occurred, this might well be something to remember.

The author's message is well worth reiterating: whenever possible, attempt to control the massive hemoptysis before embarking on surgery. Urgent or elective surgery yields far fewer complications and mortality. An experienced angiographer as part of your team is obviously very valuable!

The author defines massive hemoptysis to be 400 ml over 24 hours. The classic definition is 600 ml, although I cannot argue with the author's lowering this figure, especially since the total airway dead space is only 150 ml—three times that volume certainly would asphyxiate anybody!

The Marsico catheter is an ingenious homemade device. Much easier than this is the use of an IVC Foley catheter, angled at the tip to allow placement into virtually any lobar or even segmental bronchus. These catheters are commercially available in most countries (Ginsberg, 1975).

REFERENCE

Ginsberg R.J.: A New Technique for one-lung anesthesia using an endoblocker blocker. J Thorac and Cardiovasc Surg 82:542, 1981.

R.J.G.

■ *KEY REFERENCES*

Cauldwell EW, Siekert RG, Lininger RE, Anson BJ: The bronchial arteries: An anatomic study of 150 human cadavers. Surg Gynecol Obstet 48:395, 1948.

This is the most complete anatomic study about bronchial arteries. It is a superb reference for physicians interested in massive hemoptysis.

Conlan AA: Massive hemoptysis: Diagnostic and therapeutic implications. Surg Annu 17:337, 1985.

This is the most in-depth article available about the causes, diagnostic procedures, and management methods in massive hemoptysis.

Crocco JA, Rooney JJ, Fankushen DS et al: Massive hemoptysis. Arch Intern Med 121:495, 1968.

These are the first authors to correlate the rate of bleeding to the mortality rate.

Remy J, Arnaud A, Fardou H et al: Treatment of hemoptysis by embolization of bronchial arteries. Radiology 122:33, 1977.

The first reported large series of patients undergoing embolization of the bronchial arteries in massive hemoptysis.

Remy-Jardin M, Remy J: La vascularisation systémique non bronchique du poumon. Rev Mal Respir 7:95, 1990.

This is a general review of the nonbronchial systemic arterial circulation of the lung and its pathologic significance as an important source of hemoptysis.

■ REFERENCES

Amirana M, Frater R, Tirschwell P et al: An aggressive surgical approach to significant hemoptysis in patients with pulmonary tuberculosis. Am Rev Respir Dis 97:187, 1968.

Barash PG, Nardi D, Hammond G et al: Catheter-induced pulmonary artery perforation: Mechanisms, management, and modifications. J Thorac Cardiovasc Surg 82:5, 1981.

Bense L: Intrabronchial selective coagulative treatment of hemoptysis. Report of three cases. Chest 97:990, 1990.

Bilton D, Webb AK, Foster H et al: Life threatening haemoptysis in cystic fibrosis: An alternative therapeutic approach. Thorax 45:975, 1990.

Bobrowitz I, Ramakrishna S, Shim Y: Comparison of medical v. surgical treatment of major hemoptysis. Arch Intern Med 143:1343, 1983.

Boren J, Busey J, Corpe RF et al: The management of hemoptysis. Am Rev Respir Dis 93:471, 1966.

Boyd KD, Thomas SJ, Gold J et al: A prospective study of complications of pulmonary artery catheterizations in 500 consecutive patients. Chest 84:245, 1983.

Bracco AN: Resecciones pulmonares urgentes por hemoptisis incoercibles. Bol Soc Cir Bs As 40:107, 1956.

Cahill BC, Ingbar DH: Massive hemoptysis: Assessment and management. Clin Chest Med 15;147, 1994.

Camero LG, Cushing FR: False left ventricular aneurysm with ventriculo-bronchial fistula and massive hemoptysis. Scand Cardiovasc J 31:117, 1997.

Carlens J, Svendsen UG, Efsen F et al: Treatment of massive haemoptysis with microcoil embolization after en bloc double-lung transplantation with bronchial artery revascularization. Eur Respir J 10:492, 1997.

Cauldwell EW, Siekert RG, Lininger RE, Anson BJ: The bronchial arteries: An anatomic study of 150 human cadavers. Surg Gynecol Obstet 48:395, 1948.

Conlan AA: Massive hemoptysis: Diagnostic and therapeutic implications. Surg Annu 17:337, 1985.

Conlan AA, Hurwitz SS, Krige L et al: Massive hemoptysis: Review of 123 cases. J Thorac Cardiovasc Surg 85:120, 1983.

Cremaschi P, Nascimbene C, Vitulo P et al: Therapeutic embolization of bronchial artery: A successful treatment in 209 cases of relapse hemoptysis. Angiology 44:295, 1993.

Crocco JA, Rooney JJ, Fankushen DS et al: Massive hemoptysis. Arch Intern Med 121:495, 1968.

Cudkowicz L: The Human Bronchial Circulation in Health and Disease. Baltimore, Williams & Wilkins, 1968.

De Gracia J, Mayordomo C, Catalán E et al: Utilización de fibrinógeno-trombina por vía endoscópica en el tratamiento de la hemoptisis masiva. Arch Bronconeumol 31:227, 1995.

Demeter SL, Cordasco EM: Aortobronchial fistula: Keys to successful management. Angiology 31:431, 1980.

Eloesser L: Observations on sources of pulmonary hemorrhage and attempts at its control. J Thorac Surg 7:671, 1938.

Espinosa JIC, Fernandez JAC, Perez CN et al: Cirugia en tuberculosis pulmonar por hemoptisis incoercible (analisis de 200 caves). Cir Ciruj 51:269, 1983.

Feldman J, Gusmao RH: Lobectomia de urgência no tratamento de hemoptise causada por tuberculose pulomonar (urgent lobectomy in treatment of hemoptysis caused by pulmonary tuberculosis). Rev Bras Tuber 22:119, 1954.

Fraser KL, Grosman H, Hyland RH et al: Transverse myelitis: A reversible complication of bronchial artery embolisation in cystic fibrosis. Thorax 52:99, 1997.

Freitag L: Development of a new balloon catheter for management of hemoptysis with bronchofiberscopes. Chest 103:593, 1993.

Freitag L, Tekolf E, Stamatis G et al: Three years experience with a new balloon catheter for the management of haemoptysis. Eur Respir J 7:2033, 1994.

Furuse M, Saito K, Kunieda E et al: Bronchial arteries: CT demonstration with arteriographic correlation. Radiology 162:393, 1987.

Garzon AA, Cerruti MM, Golding ME: Exsanguinating hemoptysis. J Thorac Cardiovasc Surg 84:829, 1982.

Garzon AA, Gourin A: Surgical management of massive hemoptysis: A ten-year experience. Ann Surg 187:267, 1978.

Girard Ph, Boquel V, Fournel P et al: Une cause rare de fistule aorto-bronchique: l'aortite tuberculeuse. Rev Mal Resp 14:221, 1997.

González Noguera PJ, Mayol Martínez JÁ, Hernández Villaverde A et al: Hemoptisis por aneurisma de la arteria bronquial. Rer Clin Esp 192:329, 1993.

Herb S, Hetzel M, Hetzel J et al: An unusual case of Hughes-Stovin syndrome. Eur Respir J 11:1191, 1998.

Hiebert CA: Balloon catheter control of life-threatening hemoptysis. Chest 66:308, 1974.

Hoff SJ, Johnson JE, Frist WH: Aortobronchial fistula after unilateral lung transplantation. Ann Thorac Surg 56:1402, 1993.

Jardin M, Remy J: Control of hemoptysis: Systemic angiography and anastomoses of the internal mammary artery. Radiology 168:377, 1988.

Jones DK, Davies RJ: Massive haemoptysis. Medical management will usually arrest the bleeding. BMJ 300:889, 1990.

Julià-Serdà G, Freixinet J, Abad C et al: Massive hemoptysis as a manifestation of fistulized thoracic aortic aneurysms into the bronchial tree. J Cardiovasc Surg 37:417, 1996.

Kato R, Sawafuji M, Kawamura M et al: Massive hemoptysis successfully treated by modified bronchoscopic balloon tamponade technique. Chest 109:842, 1996.

Keçeligil HT, Erk MK, Kolbakir F et al: Tracheoinnominate artery fistula following tracheostomy. Cardiovasc Surg 3:509, 1995.

Lampmann LEH, Tjan TG: Embolization therapy in haemoptysis. Eur J Radiol 18:15, 1994.

Lemay V, Carette MF, Parrot A et al: Les hémoptysies des sarcoïdoses. Rev Pneumol Clin 51:61, 1995.

Marsico GA: Controle da hemoptise maciça com broncoscopia e soro gelado (control of massive hemoptysis with bronchoscopy and ice-cold saline lavage) (thesis). Rio de Janeiro, Universidade Federal Fluminense, 1991.

McCollum WB, Mattox KL, Guinn GA et al: Immediate operative treatment for massive hemoptysis. Chest 67:152, 1975.

Millar AB, Boothroyd AE, Edwards D et al: The role of computed tomography (CT) in the investigation of unexplained haemoptysis. Respir Med 86:39, 1992.

Miller RR, McGregor DH: Hemorrhage from carcinoma of the lung. Cancer 46:200, 1980.

Mullerworth MH, Angelopoulos P, Couyant MA et al: Recognition and management of catheter-induced pulmonary artery rupture. Ann Thorac Surg 66:1242, 1998.

Najarian KE, Morris CS: Arterial embolization in the chest. J Thorac Imaging 13:93, 1998.

Patel U, Pattison CW, Raphael M: Management of massive hemoptysis. Br J Hosp Med 52:74, 1994.

Philpott NJ, Woodhead MA, Wilson AG et al: Lung abscess: A neglected cause of life threatening haemoptysis. Thorax 48:674, 1993.

Pitkin CE: Repeated severe hemoptysis necessitating pneumonectomy. Ann Otol Rhinol Laryngol 50:914, 1941.

Pouwels HM, Janevski BK, Penn OC et al: Systemic to pulmonary vascular malformation. Eur Respir J 5:1288, 1992.

Pump KK: Distribution of bronchial arteries in the human lung. Chest 62:447, 1972.

Pursel SE, Lindskog GE: Hemoptysis: A clinical evaluation of 105 patients examined consecutively on a thoracic surgical service. Am Rev Respir Dis 84:329, 1961.

Rabkin JE, Astafjev VI, Gothman LN et al: Transcatheter embolization in the management of pulmonary hemorrhage. Radiology 163:361, 1987.

Ramakantan R, Bandekar VG, Gandhi MS et al: Massive hemoptysis due to pulmonary tuberculosis: Control with bronchial artery embolization. Radiology 200:691, 1996.

Remy J, Arnaud A, Fardou H et al: Treatment of hemoptysis by embolization of bronchial arteries. Radiology 122:33, 1977.

Remy J, Lemaitre L, Lafitte JJ et al: Massive hemoptysis of pulmonary arterial origin: Diagnosis and treatment. Radiology 143:963, 1984.

Remy J, Remy-Jardin M, Wallaert B et al: La vaso-occlusion de l'artère pulmonaire. Rev Mal Respir 5:429, 1988.

Remy J, Voisin C, Dupuis C et al: Traitement, par embolisation, des hémoptysies graves ou répétées liées à une hypervascularisation systémique. Presse Med 2:2060, 1973.

Remy-Jardin M, Remy J: La vascularisation systémique non bronchique du poumon. Rev Mal Respir 7:95, 1990.

Ribeiro-Netto A: A ressecção extramusculoperiostal "em gaiola de passarinho" (procedimento de Ribeiro-Netto) dos tumores pulmonares malignos invasores da face costal da parede toracica, dos tumores primários ou secundários da parede torácica, do pulmão patológico e dos empiemas pleurais cronicos (extramusculo periosteal resection "en cage d'oiseau" or "bird-cage"-Ribeiro-Netto procedure) (thesis). Universidade Estadual do Rio de Janeiro, Rio de Janeiro, 1988.

Rocha MP, Guntupalli KK, Moise KJ Jr et al: Massive hemoptysis in Takayasu's arteritis during pregnancy. Chest 106:1619, 1994.

Ryan TC, Lineberry WT Jr: Pneumonectomy for pulmonary hemorrhage in tuberculosis. Am Rev Respir Dis 61:426, 1950.

Rumbak M, Kohler G, Eastrige C et al: Topical treatment of life threatening haemoptysis from aspergillomas. Thorax 51:253, 1996.

Sahebjami H: Iced saline lavage during bronchoscopy. Chest 69:131, 1976

Saw EC, Gottlieb LS, Yokoyama T et al: Flexible fiberoptic bronchoscopy and endobronchial tamponade in the management of massive hemoptysis. Chest 70:589, 1976.

Shneerson JM, Emerson PA, Phillips RH: Radiotherapy for massive haemoptysis from an aspergilloma. Thorax 35:953, 1980.

Tamura S, Kodama T, Otsuka N et al: Embolotherapy for persistent hemoptysis: The significance of pleural thickening. Cardiovasc Intervent Radiol 16:85, 1993.

Teklu B, Felleke G: Massive haemoptysis in tuberculosis. Tubercle 63:213, 1982.

Thompson AB, Teschler H, Rennard SI: Pathogenesis, evaluation, and therapy for massive hemoptysis. Clin Chest Med 13:69, 1992.

Thoms NW, Wilson RF, Puro HE et al: Life-threatening hemoptysis in primary lung abscess. Ann Thorac Surg 14:347, 1972.

Tsukamoto T, Sasaki H, Nakamura H: Treatment of hemoptysis patients by thrombin and fibrinogen-thrombin infusion therapy using a fiberoptic bronchoscope. Chest 96:473, 1989.

Uflacker R, Kaemmerer A, Picon PD: Bronchial artery embolization in the management of hemoptysis: Technical aspects and long-term results. Radiology 157:637, 1985.

Wedzicha JA, Pearson MC: Management of massive haemoptysis. Respir Med 84:9, 1990.

Wu MH, Lai WW, Lin MY et al: Massive hemoptysis caused by a ruptured subclavian artery aneurysm. Chest 104:612, 1993.

Yang CT, Berger HW: Conservative management of life-threatening hemoptysis. Mt Sinai J Med 45:329, 1978.

Yeoh CB, Hubaytar RT, Ford JM et al: Treatment of massive hemorrhage in pulmonary tuberculosis. J Thorac Cardiovasc Surg 54:503, 1967.

CHAPTER **28**

Chronic Pulmonary Embolism

Pat O. Daily

DEFINITION

Chronic pulmonary embolism is characterized by persistent elevation of pulmonary vascular resistance secondary to pulmonary arterial obstruction from unresolved chronic pulmonary emboli. The cause of chronic pulmonary embolism remains insufficiently defined. Possible contributors are a hypercoagulable state, compromise of the fibrinolytic system, embolization of organized thrombi, and multiple episodes of pulmonary embolism. Similarly, the incidence of chronic pulmonary embolism among patients has not been determined. It is estimated that 0.1% to 4% of patients with acute pulmonary embolism develop chronic pulmonary embolism. Symptoms and survival vary according to the degree of pulmonary vascular obstruction. Although some patients may be asymptomatic, typically dyspnea is present with minimal exertion. With lesser degrees of pulmonary vascular obstruction, survival may be compromised only slightly. Greater levels of obstruction result in significantly shortened longevity.

HISTORICAL NOTE

As related by Chitwood and colleagues (1984), the first description of some of the clinical characteristics associated with chronic pulmonary emboli was reported by Ljungdahl in 1928. However, after that, some time elapsed before the first successful attempt at surgical relief of chronically occluded pulmonary arteries was reported by Snyder and coworkers (1963). The presumptive diagnosis was pulmonary neoplasm. The authors encountered thrombotic occlusion of the right pulmonary artery and removed the obstructions, at least in part, using endarterectomy spoons. Furthermore, the authors emphasized that the pulmonary alveolar membrane was not irreversibly damaged; therefore, future surgical attempts were feasible because there was functional return of the affected pulmonary parenchyma.

In 1980, our group reported the results of four patients who underwent bilateral pulmonary thromboendarterectomy with median sternotomy (Daily et al, 1980). Endarterectomy in the first patient was performed without deep hypothermia and circulatory arrest. Severe bronchial backbleeding during endarterectomy was encountered in the three subsequent patients, necessitating periods of circulatory arrest so that visualization could be maintained during the process of thromboendarterectomy.

Reidel and associates (1982) reported the only natural history study of chronic pulmonary embolism that correlated the degree of pulmonary vascular obstruction, as evidenced by mean pulmonary artery pressure, with the duration of survival. Obtaining this information is essential before recommendation of pulmonary thromboendarterectomy can be considered. By 1984, Chitwood and colleagues (1984) were able to find only 85 reported cases of surgical procedures for chronic pulmonary embolism in an extensive review of the world literature. Most of these patients had undergone lateral thoracotomy with only one lung approached. The overall operative mortality rate was 22%.

In 1987, we described modifications of the procedure reported in 1980 (Daily et al, 1987). These modifications included the use of a cooling jacket to maintain myocardial temperatures at or below 10°C throughout the aortic cross-clamp period and especially to provide protection of the right ventricle. In addition, dissection was carried out completely within the pericardial and pulmonary hilar tissues. Thus, the possible accumulation of pleural effusions and the dissection of potential vascular adhesions were eliminated by preventing entrance into the pleural spaces. We reported an operative mortality rate of 9% (3 of 33) in the 33 patients who underwent pulmonary thromboendarterectomy with this method. Saline slush, contained in a laparotomy pad, was used in seven patients (group B) for myocardial hypothermia and was identified as a major risk factor for phrenic nerve paresis.

An important consideration with the technique of pulmonary thromboendarterectomy, wherein deep hypothermia with circulatory arrest is used, is the development of delirium as characterized by disruption of attention and cognition and occasionally by disturbances of psychomotor behavior. Wragg and colleagues (1988) reported a cohort of 22 patients in which 77% of the patients manifested delirium as described earlier. In this group of patients, total pulmonary bypass time was not a predictor; however, deep hypothermia time and circulatory arrest time were significantly correlated with the development of delirium. Specifically, as was described previously, circulatory arrest exceeding 55 minutes in duration is strongly associated with the development of delirium. It is important to note, however, that essentially all patients ultimately recover from delirium and return to their previous psychiatric and neurologic status.

Additional experience with pulmonary thromboendarterectomy was reported by Jault and Cabrol (1989), which extended the previous experience of 16 patients of Cabral to 33 patients undergoing pulmonary thromboendarterectomy. Furthermore, Jault and Cabral found that common complications associated with pulmonary thromboendarterectomy were congestive heart failure and hemorrhagic pulmonary edema. The overall mortality for pulmonary thromboendarterectomy in this group of 33 patients was 30%.

A comparison of pulmonary thromboendarterectomy and lung or heart-lung transplantation for chronic pulmonary embolism was reported by Dembitsky and co-workers in 1989. The 5-year survival data with pulmonary thromboendarterectomy were markedly improved compared with heart-lung transplantation.

The technique of pulmonary thromboendarterectomy was essentially standardized in a report by Daily and associates in 1989. From 1984 to 1988, 103 consecutive patients underwent pulmonary thromboendarterectomy using median sternotomy and myocardial protection, which consisted of a single dose of cold blood cardioplegic solution and then maintenance of myocardial hypothermia with the cooling jacket. All myocardial temperatures were maintained at 10°C throughout the period of aortic cross-clamping. Additionally, intermittent periods of 20 minutes of circulatory arrest at 20°C were used to obtain an ischemic field so that pulmonary thromboendarterectomy could be performed.

Subsequently, Daily and colleagues (1990) reported risk factors for pulmonary thromboendarterectomy in a group of 127 patients. Two end points were evaluated with respect to results. The first of these was ventilator dependency requiring 5 or more days of mechanical ventilation, and the second was hospital mortality. Multivariate analysis was performed, which revealed that ascites and the need for 4 or more units of blood predicted ventilator dependency. Predictors of hospital death included increased cardiopulmonary bypass time and failure to achieve at least a 50% reduction in pulmonary vascular resistance. Other factors such as related surgical procedures, other associated diseases, patient age, and degree of pulmonary vascular resistance did not predict an adverse outcome. Also in 1990, Daily and co-workers (1990) reported that from October 1, 1984 to September 18, 1989, 149 consecutive patients underwent pulmonary thromboendarterectomy with an overall hospital mortality rate of 11.4%. In this group, the most common causes of death were respiratory failure and multi-organ failure.

A significant improvement for the performance of pulmonary thromboendarterectomy was the development of surgical instruments specifically designed for this procedure (Daily et al, 1991). In addition, with simultaneous continual aspiration, blood is easily removed from the operative field during pulmonary thromboendarterectomy. These devices have substantially decreased the period of circulatory arrest required for complete pulmonary thromboendarterectomy.

Jamieson and associates (1993) reported a series of 150 patients who underwent pulmonary thromboendarterectomy using the methodology described previously with an operative mortality of 8.7%.

The long-term follow-up evaluation of a group of patients undergoing pulmonary thromboendarterectomy was reported by Fedullo and colleagues (1999). In this group, cardiac output increased from a preoperative level of 3.7 ± 1.2 L to 4.8 ± 1.0 L. Also, the patients were improved significantly with respect to New York Heart Association Functional Classification. With follow-up of 117 patients, 63 patients who were previously in class IV all improved so that no patients remained in class IV. In class III, there had been 49 patients; postoperatively, only 6 patients remained in class III. In class II, there were 5 patients preoperatively and 26 postoperatively. Also, although there were no patients in class I preoperatively, there were 85 in class I postoperatively. Therefore, functional improvement after pulmonary thromboendarterectomy was shown to be significant.

In 1996, Hartz and co-workers reported results in a cohort of 34 patients undergoing pulmonary thromboendarterectomy. The operative mortality for this group of patients was 23%. Hartz and associates suggested that patients with severe pulmonary hypertension as defined by 1100 dynes/s/cm^{-5} or greater and mean pulmonary artery pressure greater than 50 mm of mercury should not undergo pulmonary thromboendarterectomy because of associated excessively high operative mortality.

Simonneau and colleagues (1995) described their experience with a group of 72 patients with chronic pulmonary embolism. Eight of these patients underwent lung transplantation, 55 were treated medically, and 9 of 11 patients had successful pulmonary thromboendarterectomy with excellent functional improvement.

Mayer and co-workers (1996) described 119 patients undergoing pulmonary thromboendarterectomy. The operative mortality for this group of patients was 24%. After follow-up of 13 to 48 months, 65 patients were assessed and the decrease in pulmonary vascular resistance ranged from 1015 ± 454 dynes/s/cm^{-5} to 198 ± 72 dynes/s/cm^{-5}. Echocardiography revealed substantial reduction in right ventricular dimensions.

Archibald and associates (1999) reported a group of 1049 patients managed by pulmonary thromboendarterectomy at the University of California, San Diego. For this group, the overall mortality was 9.2%.

■ HISTORICAL READINGS

Archibald CJ, Auger WR, Fedullo PF et al: Long-term outcome after pulmonary thromboendarterectomy. Am J Respir Crit Care Med 160:523, 1999.

Chitwood WR, Sabiston DC, Wechsler AS: Surgical treatment of chronic unresolved pulmonary embolism. Clin Chest Med 5:507, 1984.

Daily PO, Dembitsky WP, Daily RP: Dissectors for pulmonary thromboendarterectomy. Ann Thorac Surg 51:842–843, 1991.

Daily PO, Dembitsky WP, Iversen S: Technique of pulmonary thromboendarterectomy for chronic pulmonary embolism. J Card Surg 4:10–24, 1989.

Daily PO, Dembitsky PO, Iversen S et al: Current early results of pulmonary thromboendarterectomy for chronic pulmonary embolism. Eur J Cardiothorac Surg 4:117–123, 1990.

Daily PO, Dembitsky WP, Iversen S et al: Risk factors for pulmonary thromboendarterectomy. J Thorac Cardiovasc Surg 99:670–678, 1990.

Daily PO, Dembitsky WP, Peterson KL, Moser KM: Modifications of techniques and early results of pulmonary thromboendarterectomy for chronic pulmonary embolism. J Thorac Cardiovasc Surg 93:221, 1987.

Daily PO, Johnston GG, Simmons CJ, Moser KM: Surgical management of chronic pulmonary embolism. J Thorac Cardiovasc Surg 79:523, 1980.

Dembitsky WP, Daily PO, Moser KM, et al: Pulmonary thromboendarterectomy as the preferred alternative to heart-lung transplantation for chronic pulmonary embolism. In Belfus (ed): Cardiac Surgery: State of the Art Reviews. Philadelphia, Hanley & Belfus, 1989, pp 577–582.

Fedullo PF, Moser KM: Advances in acute pulmonary embolism and chronic pulmonary hypertension. Adv Intern Med 42:67–104, 1997.

Hartz RS, Byrne JG, Levitsky S, et al: Predictors of mortality in pulmonary thromboendarterectomy. Ann Thorac Surg 62:1255–1260, 1996.

Jamieson SW, Auger WR, Fedullo PF et al: Experience and results with 150 pulmonary thromboendarterectomy operations over a 29-month period. J Thorac Cardiovasc Surg 106(1):116–127, 1983.

Jault F, Cabrol C: Surgical treatment for chronic pulmonary thromboembolism. Herz 14:192–196, 1989.

Mayer E, Dahm M, Hake U: Mid-term results of pulmonary thromboendarterectomy for chronic thromboembolic pulmonary hypertension. Ann Thorac Surg 61:1788–1792, 1996.

Reidel M, Stanek V, Widimsky J, Preroesky I: Long-term follow-up of patients with pulmonary thromboembolism. Late prognosis and evolution of hemodynamic and respiratory data. Chest 81:151, 1982.

Simonneau G, Azarian R, Brenot F: Surgical management of unresolved pulmonary embolism. Chest 107(Suppl 1):52S–55S, 1995.

Snyder WA, Kent DC, Baisch BF: Successful endarterectomy of chronically occluded pulmonary artery. J Thorac Cardiovasc Surg 45:482, 1963.

Wragg RE, Dimsdale JE, Moser KM, et al: Operative predictors of delirium after pulmonary thromboendarterectomy. A model for postcardiotomy delirium? J Thorac Cardiovasc Surg 96:524–529, 1988.

BASIC SCIENCE

Surgical Anatomy

Visualization of the origin of each bronchopulmonary segmental artery is essential in the performance of relatively complete thromboendarterectomy. Thus, placing incisions distally in the pulmonary arteries by extending the incisions beyond the pericardial reflections of both the right and left sides is necessary in most cases. The superior vena cava anterior to the right pulmonary artery must be mobilized extensively to allow exposure of the right pulmonary artery.

Another consideration is the division of the pericardial reflection over the right pulmonary artery as it passes posterior to the right phrenic nerve. The line of incision through the pericardium should be placed immediately anterior to the right pulmonary artery to avoid the course of the right phrenic nerve. The incision is extended inferiorly 2 to 3 cm over the pulmonary veins and superiorly 2 to 3 cm to allow the frequently necessary distal extension of the right pulmonary artery incision. In some patients, the right middle lobe arterial branches may arise from the upper lobe branch rather than from the main trunk of the pulmonary artery. In this case, a separate incision is usually required in the right pulmonary artery 1 to 2 cm proximal to the origin of the right upper lobe branch, with extension of the incision into the upper lobe artery to its trifurcation.

The primary incision is initiated in the right pulmonary artery somewhat more inferiorly and 3 to 4 cm proximal to the pericardial reflection. This incision is extended laterally until it reaches the right superior pulmonary vein, which crosses anterior to the pulmonary artery. The superior pulmonary vein can be retracted inferiorly and to the right to allow further extension of the incision. Through these two incisions, it is possible to visualize each of the origins of the bronchopulmonary segmental arteries. At all times, the path of the right phrenic nerve must be kept in mind because it courses a few millimeters anterior to the area of dissection. Furthermore, retraction in the area of the right phrenic nerve must be minimized to avoid injury and possible paresis. On the left side, the dissection is simpler because of the need to divide only the pericardial reflection over the left pulmonary artery as it exits the pericardium. Again, the incision is extended inferiorly from over the pulmonary veins, passing immediately over the pulmonary artery, and reaching superiorly for a distance of 1 to 2 cm. As on the right side, the phrenic nerve passes anteriorly approximately 1 cm to the pulmonary artery. Again, its course must be kept in mind so that injury may be avoided.

The incision on the left side is initiated 4 to 5 cm within the pericardium in the pulmonary artery and is extended distally to the pericardial reflection. The left upper lobe bronchus on the left side crosses anterior to the left pulmonary artery and essentially limits the distal extent of the incision. Through this single incision, it is possible to visualize all bronchopulmonary segmental arteries, except perhaps the anteromedial segment, which is variably visualized.

Physiology

Chronic obstruction of the pulmonary arteries, resulting in elevated pulmonary vascular resistance, is the primary consideration with respect to physiologic findings. It has been demonstrated by Gibbon and colleagues (1932) that more than 60% of the pulmonary vasculature must be occluded before measurable increases in pulmonary vascular resistance occur. Initially, pulmonary physiologic disturbances may be minimal. Relatively normal gas exchange is maintained as is pulmonary function. With worsening obstruction of the pulmonary vasculature, variable degrees of hypoxemia occur. A decrease in diffusion capacity may result, and progressive imbalance of perfusion and ventilation may occur.

The initial cardiac change is right ventricular hypertrophy secondary to the progression of pulmonary hypertension. As pulmonary hypertension worsens, right heart failure may ensue. In addition, hepatic congestion occurs along with associated ascites, peripheral edema, and end-stage development of anasarca. In some patients, the persistence of deep venous thrombosis may contribute to lower extremity edema.

Pathology

The great majority of patients experience substantial resolution of emboli without significant residual pulmonary vascular obstruction after an acute embolic episode (Dalen et al, 1969). However, major pulmonary vascular obstruction persists when resolution is deficient. In the absence of resolution, there is a rapid ingrowth of fibrous and elastic tissue into the embolus, which results in attachment of the embolus to the pulmonary arterial wall. This may occur within 1 week of the acute embolic episode. Significant ingrowth of elastic and fibrous tissue at 2 weeks is seen in Figure 28–1. It is this attachment of embolic material to the pulmonary arterial wall that necessitates endarterectomy rather than simple embolec-

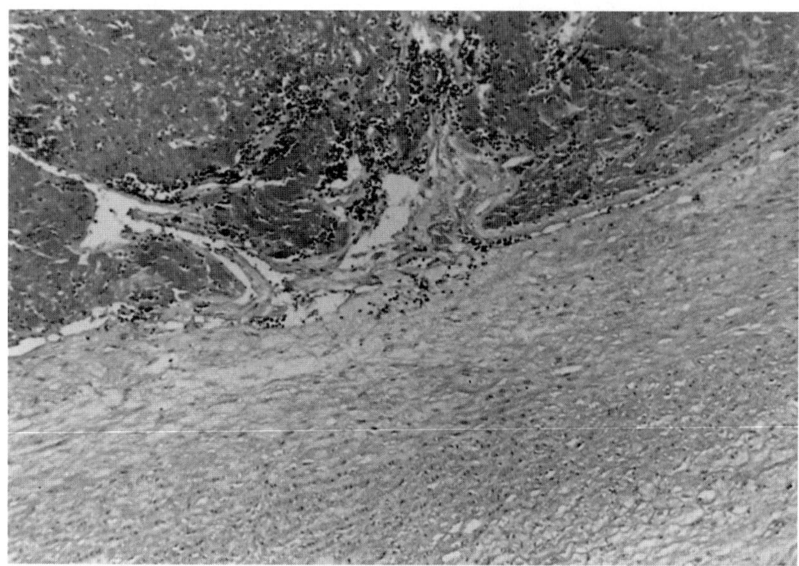

FIGURE 28–1 ■ Cross section of a pulmonary artery approximately 2 weeks after embolization. Significant ingrowth of fibrous tissues from the arterial wall into the embolus can be seen. Consequently, embolectomy by simple removal is no longer possible and thromboendarterectomy techniques are necessary (H&E). (From Daily PO: Chronic pulmonary embolism. In Karp RB [ed]: Advances in Cardiac Surgery. Chicago, Mosby–Year Book, 1993.)

tomy. Establishing the correct plane of dissection is essential to facilitate removal of the pulmonary arterial obstruction and to avoid perforation of the relatively thin residual pulmonary arterial wall. The embolus and intima with some media are removed together. This plane of dissection is seen in Figure 28–2. The inner media of the pulmonary arterial wall shows the embolic material along with the intima and the inner media of the pulmonary arterial wall. After endarterectomy, the remaining pulmonary arterial wall consists of most of the media, as is seen in Figure 28–3. Additional pathologic changes include medial hypertrophy, plexiform lesions, formation of webs, arteriosclerotic plaques, and superimposed thrombus.

Infrequently, there may be considerable distention, possibly to aneurysmal proportions, of the more proximal pulmonary arteries, especially the main pulmonary artery and the proximal right and left pulmonary arteries, before the obstructing material is found. It is important to recognize that total occlusion from pulmonary embolism of either the left or the right pulmonary artery may be mistaken for agenesis of the pulmonary artery. Also, the syndrome of atrial septal defect with pulmonary hypertension and subsequent thrombosis—rather than embolization—of the pulmonary artery must be distinguished and surgical treatment avoided because the underlying pathologic condition may be Eisenmenger's syndrome.

DIAGNOSIS

Clinical Features

Approximately 80% of patients present with an established diagnosis of one or more episodes of pulmonary embolism. Associated evidence of deep vein thrombosis occurs in about 50% of patients. However, 20% have absolutely no history of either pulmonary embolism or deep vein thrombosis. The most prevalent symptom in both groups of patients is dyspnea with relatively minimal degrees of exertion. In most cases, the severity of

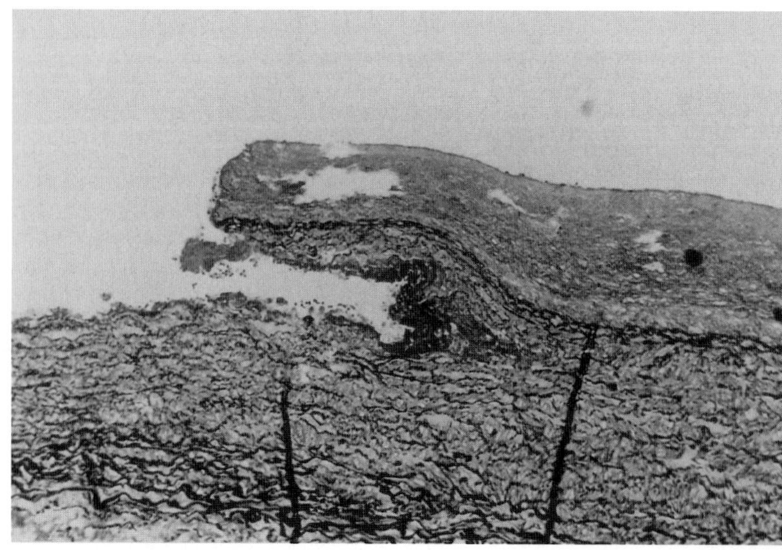

FIGURE 28–2 ■ When the correct plane of dissection is established, the embolus is intimately attached to the media. The plane of dissection occurs in the superficial layer of the media. Consequently, a small amount of media and intima are removed with the embolus.

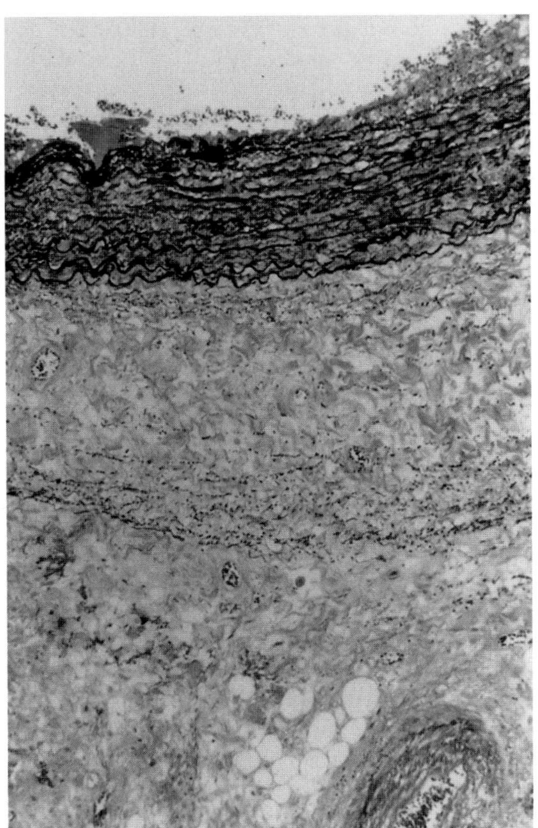

FIGURE 28–3 ■ Endarterectomized pulmonary artery. The pulmonary artery after endarterectomy consists of most of the media. The embolus and the intima and inner media have been removed.

the dyspnea has been progressive. Another associated complaint is that of easy fatigability. Lesser numbers of patients experience near-syncope with exertion, and about 25% have angina with exertion. Other less frequent symptoms include hemoptysis and chest pain. About 50% of patients have received anticoagulation at some point in the past.

Physical examination usually reveals normal chest findings. Occasionally, decreased breath sounds are noted in the lower chest, which are consistent with pleural effusions. Infrequently, rales may be heard. Another less frequent but distinctive finding is that of murmurs over the lung fields, best heard posteriorly. These murmurs are most obvious during periods of breath-holding and are analogous to those associated with pulmonary branch stenosis. It is important to note that these murmurs are *not* present in primary pulmonary hypertension.

Cardiac examination frequently reveals right ventricular hypertrophy. Right ventricular failure, characterized by elevated jugular venous pressure, left parasternal heave, a third heart sound, and a loud P_2, is present in more severe cases. In addition, a murmur of tricuspid regurgitation may be present. Patients with more severe pulmonary vascular obstruction may have hepatojugular reflux, liver enlargement with tenderness, and ascites. The lower extremities may be normal but often reveal evidence of chronic venous thrombosis with bilateral lower extremity edema. In other patients, evidence of chronic venous stasis, including brownish discoloration of the skin with bilateral ankle edema, is present.

Natural History

The overall incidence of acute pulmonary embolism has been estimated by Dalen and Alpert (1975) to exceed 500,000 patients per year. Both the incidence and the cause of chronic pulmonary embolism, however, are unknown. The percentage of patients with acute pulmonary embolism whose conditions progress to chronic pulmonary embolism has been reported to range from 0.1% to 4% (Chitwood et al, 1984; Moser, 1990), with the lower figure probably being more accurate; in the United States, it is estimated that 500 patients per year develop chronic pulmonary embolism. However, this number is discrepant with the 85 cases of pulmonary thromboendarterectomy reported by Chitwood and co-workers (1984) in their review of the world literature because more surgical cases would be expected. Possible reasons for this discrepancy are (1) failure to establish the correct diagnosis of chronic pulmonary embolism, rather than primary pulmonary hypertension; and (2) lack of awareness that pulmonary thromboendarterectomy is an effective procedure (Tilkian et al, 1967). The cause of chronic pulmonary embolism likewise is ill defined. This subset of patients may develop a hypercoagulable state, which may be associated with decreased levels of proteins C and S and antithrombin III. Incomplete resolution may be caused by some defect in the fibrinolytic system or, possibly, the nature of the emboli may play a role. Some emboli are of relatively recent formation and are therefore more prone to fibrinolysis. Other emboli may be fibrotic and more resistant to resolution. Controversy continues as to whether single massive pulmonary embolism can lead to chronic pulmonary embolism, or whether multiple episodes are required.

The survival rate of individuals with severe pulmonary hypertension is shortened significantly. There has been one natural history study to date relating survival to the level of pulmonary vascular obstruction, as evidenced by the mean pulmonary artery pressure (Reidel et al, 1982). Patients with mean pulmonary artery pressures less than or equal to 30 mm Hg remained relatively stable with respect to progression and had a 5-year survival rate of greater than 90%. However, patients with mean pulmonary artery pressures greater than 30 mm Hg had a 5-year survival rate of only 50%. When the mean pulmonary artery pressure was 50 mm Hg or greater, the survival rate was only 10%. Furthermore, patients who had levels of pulmonary artery pressure above 30 mm Hg tended to demonstrate progressive pulmonary hypertension (Table 28–1). The significance of these data is that patients who have mean pulmonary artery pressures lower than 30 mm Hg, which correlates with pulmonary vascular resistance of 300 dynes/s/cm^{-5} or less, are usually not considered surgical candidates because of the high mortality rates associated with the procedure of pulmonary thromboendarterectomy.

Differential Diagnosis

The differential diagnosis of chronic pulmonary embolism is essentially a distinction of this entity from other

TABLE 28–1 ■ **Pulmonary Arterial Pressure in Relation to Survival**

Mean Pulmonary Arterial Pressure (mm Hg)	*5-Year Survival (%)*
≤30	>90
31–40	45
41–50	35
≥50	10

Data from Reidel M, Stanek V, Widimsky J, Preroesky I: Long-term follow-up of patients with pulmonary thromboembolism. Late prognosis and evolution of hemodynamic and respiratory data. Chest 81:151, 1982.

causes of pulmonary hypertension. It is convenient to divide causes of pulmonary hypertension into several categories. These include hypoxic vasoconstriction, pulmonary vascular occlusion, pulmonary parenchymal disease, and primary pulmonary hypertension. Hypoxic vasoconstriction of the pulmonary arteries may be secondary to chronic bronchitis, emphysema, cystic fibrosis, chronic hypoventilation, or high-altitude exposure. The most common causes of pulmonary vasoconstriction—emphysema and chronic bronchitis—account for more than 50% of all pulmonary hypertension cases.

Pulmonary vascular obstruction may be the result of pulmonary thromboemboli or embolic occlusion secondary to parasitic ova or tumors. Additional causes are secondary to pulmonary angiitis associated with collagen-vascular disorders or certain drugs. Parenchymal pulmonary disease may result in pulmonary hypertension by virtue of the destruction of the pulmonary vascular surface. These diseases include chronic bronchitis, emphysema, bronchiectasis, and cystic fibrosis. Also, diffuse interstitial disease may be caused by pneumoconiosis, sarcoidosis, tuberculosis, chronic fungal disease, and adult respiratory distress syndrome. The diagnosis of primary pulmonary hypertension, therefore, remains one of exclusion; that is, it is decided by elimination of the foregoing potential causes of pulmonary hypertension.

CAUSES OF PULMONARY HYPERTENSION

- Hypoxic vasoconstriction
  - Chronic bronchitis
  - Emphysema
  - Cystic fibrosis
  - Chronic hypoventilation
  - High altitude exposure
  - Pulmonary vascular occlusion
  - Pulmonary thromboemboli
  - Embolic occlusion
    - Parasitic ova
    - Tumor
  - Pulmonary angiitis
    - Collagen-vascular disorders
    - Certain drugs
- Pulmonary parenchymal disease
  - Destruction of pulmonary vascular surface
    - Chronic bronchitis
    - Emphysema
    - Bronchiectasis
    - Cystic fibrosis
  - Diffuse interstitial disease
    - Pneumoconiosis
    - Sarcoidosis
    - Tuberculosis
    - Chronic fungal disease
    - Adult respiratory distress
    - Primary pulmonary hypertension
  - Exclusion of the foregoing

Investigative Techniques

The chest radiograph usually reveals clear lung fields. However, there may be areas of hypoperfusion and other small areas of increased perfusion of the pulmonary vasculature. Significant right ventricular enlargement is often present (Fig. 28–4) and can be associated with bilateral dilatation of the proximal pulmonary arteries in the hilar areas. The electrocardiogram is occasionally normal but can reveal changes characteristic of right ventricular enlargement and hypertrophy with right axis deviation. In advanced stages of chronic pulmonary embolism, diffuse ST segment and T wave changes may be representative of myocardial ischemia. Routine blood chemical study findings are typically normal. However, the presence of proteins C and S and deficiencies of antithrombin III should be evaluated; at times, "lupus anticoagulant" is found. Other potential causes of thrombogenicity include factor V Leiden, anticardiolipin antibodies, prothrombin gene mutation 20210/6A, and excessive blood levels of homocysteine.

Study results of pulmonary function at rest are within

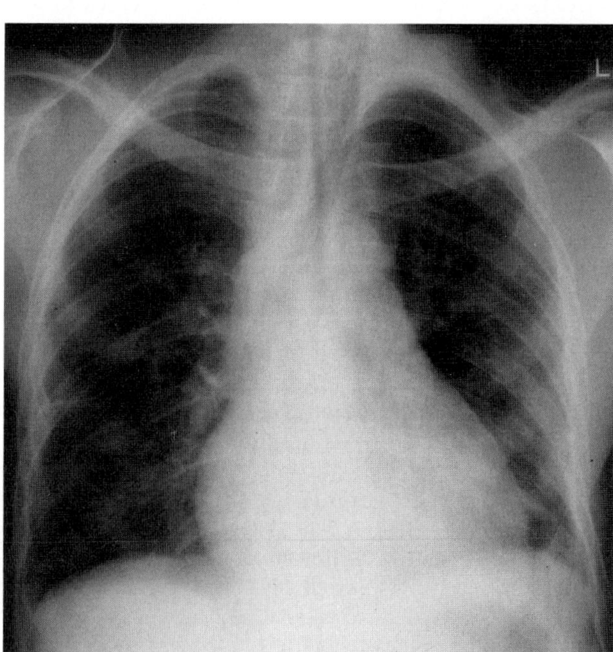

FIGURE 28–4 ■ Chest radiograph taken 4 weeks preoperatively. There is significant enlargement of the right ventricle and the pulmonary hilar regions.

normal limits in approximately 80% of patients. When abnormal, the usual changes are characteristic of restrictive defects, that is, there is a reduction in vital capacity, total lung capacity, and the forced expiratory volume in 1 second (FEV_1). Also, carbon monoxide diffusion may be reduced. Frequently, arterial gas levels are normal at rest. With only moderately increased levels of exercise, arterial desaturation typically occurs.

Echocardiography has been used recently as a routine diagnostic study. The findings of echocardiography that suggest pulmonary hypertension include right ventricular enlargement and abnormal motion of the interventricular septum. It is possible to estimate the level of pulmonary artery systolic pressure using Doppler techniques.

Pulmonary perfusion scanning is an important screening study. In virtually all patients with significant chronic pulmonary embolism, there are multiple segmental or even lobar defects in perfusion, which are present bilaterally. Ventilation scanning reveals a "mismatch" with the perfusion defects. However, in primary pulmonary hypertension, the perfusion defects are much smaller and do not occur at the lobar or even the segmental level. It should be emphasized that the perfusion scan may underestimate the degree of pulmonary vascular obstruction. Consequently, in patients with significant perfusion defects, pulmonary arteriography should be performed to further define the degree and cause of obstruction.

The technique of the pulmonary arteriogram is important for obtaining essential diagnostic information and, at the same time, minimizing risk. Nicod and coworkers (1987) and more recently Auger and associates (1999) described the technique of positioning the catheter in the right pulmonary artery beyond the upper lobe branch. Large "cut-films" are taken in the anteroposterior projection. On the left side, the catheter is positioned similarly, but the preferred plane is the left anterior oblique. With this method, complications have been minimal, and no deaths have occurred in more than 1200 patients to date. The pulmonary arteriogram is critical for diagnosing the presence or absence of intra-arterial obstructions and for determining whether these obstructions are proximal enough to allow pulmonary thromboendarterectomy. If the obstructions begin in the pulmonary arteries proximally in the lobar branches, pulmonary thromboendarterectomy is feasible. Patients with obstructions that begin only at the orifices of the bronchopulmonary artery possibly are operative candidates, but it is highly likely that endarterectomy in these patients will be less complete than in those with more proximally located obstructions.

Other potential diagnostic entities that can simulate obstructions to the pulmonary arteries (as seen by pulmonary arteriography) include fibrosing mediastinitis, tumor invasion of the major pulmonary arteries, and primary tumors of the pulmonary arteries, such as leiomyosarcomas. Also, Takayasu's disease may cause pulmonary artery obstructions. Fibrosing mediastinitis is ordinarily evaluated by computed tomography (CT). Frequently, surgery must be undertaken to distinguish neoplastic from thrombotic obstructions. Systemic arterial obstructions may suggest Takayasu's disease. CT with contrast is capable of demonstrating intraluminal lesions, which are not typical of thromboembolic disease. Furthermore, helical CT may be useful in differentiating pulmonary hypertension secondary to chronic pulmonary embolism because helical CT has been demonstrated to be more accurate for such clarification than magnetic resonance imaging (Auger et al, 1999). Pulmonary intravascular ultrasound is being evaluated as a means to determine the location of chronic thromboemboli. Preliminary data suggest that there is good correlation between ultrasound findings and thromboemboli removed at surgery (Auger et al, 1999).

Right heart catheterization is performed with pulmonary angiography to assess the elevation of pulmonary vascular resistance based on the pulmonary artery pressures and cardiac output. If the foregoing studies suggest operative candidacy, left heart catheterization with coronary arteriography is performed in all patients older than 35 years of age to delineate associated coronary artery disease or other cardiac defects (e.g., congenital and valvular lesions). Correction of associated defects is performed during cooling or rewarming.

Angioscopy is of diagnostic value when thrombotic material can be visualized in the pulmonary arteries. However, chronic pulmonary obstructions frequently are not associated with visible thrombus. In these instances, angioscopy does not distinguish whether or not the patient is a suitable candidate for pulmonary thromboendarterectomy. Lung biopsies, in spite of previous comments to the contrary, unfortunately do not sufficiently differentiate primary pulmonary hypertension from chronic pulmonary embolism. Specifically, plexiform lesions, thought to rule out chronic pulmonary embolisms (Kay, 1990), have been identified in patients with chronic pulmonary embolisms (Moser et al, 1990b). Bronchial arteriography has been recommended for evaluating patients with chronic pulmonary embolism, especially to determine operability. However, complications such as paraplegia have been reported with this procedure. Furthermore, a negative finding would not rule out pulmonary thromboendarterectomy. Therefore, in our clinical experience, this procedure has not been performed.

MANAGEMENT

Principles

After the diagnosis of chronic pulmonary embolism is established as the cause of pulmonary hypertension, it is necessary to select which patients might benefit from pulmonary thromboendarterectomy. Three criteria have been defined to determine operability. The first is significant symptoms, primarily dyspnea with minimal levels of exertion or dyspnea at rest, requiring oxygen and typically associated with a New York Heart Association function classification III or IV. The second criterion incorporates the results of Reidel and associates (1982) regarding the natural history of this disorder based on the level of pulmonary vascular obstruction. Specifically, patients with a mean pulmonary artery pressure less than 30 mm Hg, which approximates a pulmonary vascular resistance less than 300 dynes/s/cm^{-5}, generally are not surgical candidates. However, in rare instances, patients with lower levels of elevation of pulmonary vascular resistance may be candidates for pulmonary thromboendarterectomy if their pulmonary vascular resistance rises substantially above 300 dynes/s/cm^{-5} with relatively minimal exercise. The third essential criterion is pulmonary angiographic demonstration of the degree and location of pulmonary arterial obstructions. These obstructions must be located at least as proximal as the origin of the bronchopulmonary segmental artery and preferably at the lobar or even the main pulmonary arterial level.

The presence of irreversible entities, including various malignant neoplasms or other end-stage diseases, such as diabetes, severe myocardial dysfunction of an irreversible nature, and chronic renal failure requiring dialysis, represents a contraindication to pulmonary thromboendarterectomy. Renal failure in some patients may be secondary to right heart failure and thereby reversible with pulmonary thromboendarterectomy. It is also important to evaluate lower extremity venous status by impedance plethysmography or, in some instances, venography. Patients with evidence of peripheral venous disease should undergo insertion of an inferior vena caval device to minimize the probability of recurrent pulmonary embolism. This can be done either before or during pulmonary thromboendarterectomy.

Operative Technique

Pulmonary Artery Dissection Plane

In a substantial percentage of patients, direct visualization of the pulmonary arterial lumen does not reveal apparent thrombotic material. Often, it appears that the pulmonary arterial wall is essentially normal although perhaps thickened slightly. It must be recognized that obstruction exists even though at first glance there may be no apparent obstruction. This material cannot be removed by embolectomy techniques, including simple extraction or balloon methods. It is necessary to begin dissection in the wall of the pulmonary artery to establish the correct plane of dissection.

Circulatory Arrest

After the correct plane for endarterectomy has been determined, backbleeding associated with bronchial artery hyperplasia is seen in virtually all patients with significant obstruction of their pulmonary vasculature secondary to chronic pulmonary embolism. Because endarterectomy can be performed more completely and accurately with direct visualization, it is necessary to use deep hypothermia and periods of circulatory arrest. In anticipation of circulatory arrest, thiamylal sodium, methylprednisolone, and phenytoin are given.

Controversy exists regarding tolerable circulatory arrest times, but it is usually agreed that in adults, periods in excess of 50 minutes at 20°C or less are associated with significant irreversible neurologic damage (Kirklin and Barrett-Boyes, 1993). We use intermittent periods of 20 minutes of circulatory arrest followed by periods of 10 minutes of reperfusion with blood at less than 20°C (Daily et al, 1989). An alternative is to reperfuse until the mixed venous oxygen saturation has been restored to the pre-arrest level, which usually takes 8 to 10 minutes. With this method, total circulatory arrest times of 120 minutes were reached without permanent neurologic damage (Daily et al, 1990b).

Myocardial Protection

Although the relief of elevated pulmonary vascular resistance is often significant, it usually is not complete. Therefore, it is necessary to optimize protection of the right ventricle during aortic cross-clamping. Our current approach for myocardial protection consists of administering 1 L of cold blood cardioplegic solution initially and then maintaining myocardial hypothermia at 10°C or less with a myocardial cooling jacket (Daily and Kinney, 1991a). A typical temperature curve is seen in Figure 28–5. With this approach, early postoperative myocardial dysfunction has been minimal, evidenced by an adequate cardiac index with minimal need for inotropic agents.

Associated Diseases

Concomitant coronary artery bypass grafting or correction of aortic and mitral valvular lesions may be performed during the process of cooling or rewarming. Management of tricuspid regurgitation is problematic. We evaluate tricuspid regurgitation intraoperatively after discontinuation of cardiopulmonary bypass. Even with se-

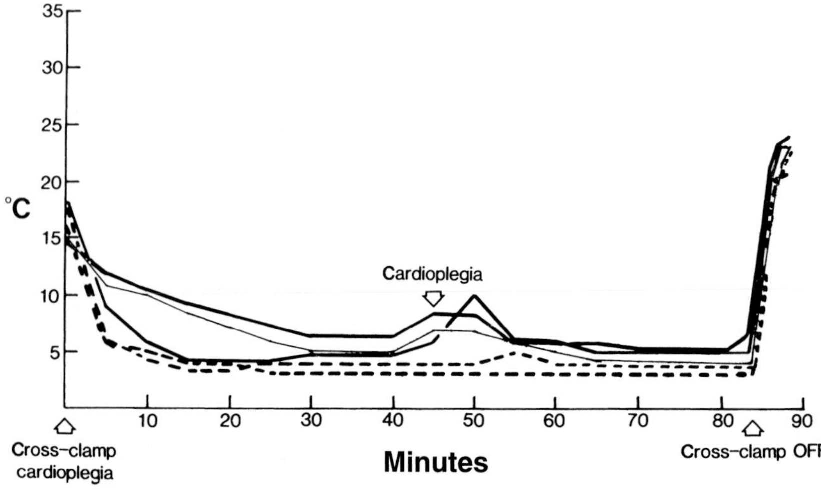

FIGURE 28–5 ■ Myocardial temperature *curves* during cardiac ischemia, with cardioplegia and cooling jacket in use during pulmonary thromboendarterectomy. All myocardial temperatures are consistently maintained at 10°C or less; note the relative lack of temperature difference between *curves*. *Curves* shown are right ventricular epicardium, left ventricular epicardium, right ventricular myocardium, left ventricular myocardium, and septal.

vere tricuspid regurgitation, a specific tricuspid procedure, such as valvuloplasty, is not performed if the cardiac index is adequate. Dittrich and colleagues (1989) reported significant resolution of tricuspid regurgitation relatively early in the postoperative period. If compromise of the cardiac index is associated with severe tricuspid regurgitation, valvuloplasty is performed. Inspection of the atrium and atrial septum is essential because thrombi that could embolize may be found within the atrium. Any atrial septal defect requires closure to preclude significant arterial desaturation secondary to right-to-left shunting and to eliminate the possibility of paradoxical embolization.

Surgical Procedure

Patients undergoing pulmonary thromboendarterectomy are positioned supine on the operating table on a mattress that allows both cooling and rewarming. The entire chest and upper abdomen are prepared and draped in typical fashion for a median sternotomy. The lower extremities are prepared and draped free to allow access to the groin for the potential removal of a saphenous vein for coronary bypass grafting. After median sternotomy and pericardiotomy, caval cannulas are placed through the right atrial wall and directly into the superior and inferior venae cavae. Caval tapes are always used (Daily and Kinney, 1991a). An arterial cannula is placed in the ascending aorta. Just prior to initiation of cardiopulmonary bypass, the left atrial pressure is measured directly, and the cardiac output is determined to calculate the pulmonary vascular resistance. During the process of cooling, the superior vena cava is mobilized superiorly and anteriorly as far as the innominate vein, and posteriorly as far cephalad as the azygous vein. The superior vena cava is dissected free posteriorly and inferiorly to the level of the right atrium. This allows sufficient mobilization of the vena cava and exposure of the right pulmonary artery. Additional dissection is carried out over the right pulmonary artery, starting intrapericardially. The dissection is extended distally to the pericardial reflection; at this point, the pericardium is incised both inferiorly and superiorly, immediately anterior to the pulmonary artery. This allows further extension of the incision and, at the same time, minimizes the risk of damage to the right phrenic nerve. At this phase, it is feasible to open the right atrium, correct any septal defects, and remove any atrial thrombi. After ventricular fibrillation occurs secondary to hypothermic perfusion, a 14-mm sump tube is placed in the pulmonary artery, and a second similar sump tube is inserted through the left superior pulmonary vein and directed into the left ventricle to minimize left ventricular distention and to remove excessive bronchial artery flow. Before reaching a temperature of 20°C, as was mentioned previously, phenytoin, methylprednisolone, and thiamylal sodium are given intravenously. A cooling jacket is placed around the right and left ventricles, and the aorta is cross-clamped. One liter of cold blood cardioplegic solution is delivered through the ascending aorta.

An incision is started in the right pulmonary artery proximal to the pericardial reflection and extended beyond the pericardial reflection. Pathologic findings are noted. It is possible to perform limited dissection during the final stages of cooling if adequate visualization can be maintained. A separate incision may be necessary in the right pulmonary artery with extension into the upper lobe branch to facilitate endarterectomy of more distally located obstructions in the right upper lobe. When a 20°C core temperature (as manifested by bladder and nasopharyngeal temperature) is reached, circulatory arrest occurs with exsanguination of the patient into the cardiopulmonary bypass reservoir. Several hyperinflations of the lungs during exsanguination facilitate the removal of blood from the pulmonary parenchyma, thus minimizing pulmonary backbleeding. Even so, substantial backbleeding does occur in the early stages of endarterectomy because of residual blood.

Using a Penfield elevator or a scalpel, dissection is started away from the incision site in the pulmonary artery to avoid compromising arteriorrhaphy. The correct plane is that which allows relatively easy distal dissection and leaves most of the media intact. Direct visualization of the adventitia indicates that the plane of dissection is too deep. After the correct plane is established, the dissection is performed circumferentially with aspirating dissectors at 360 degrees before distal extension is obtained. It is necessary to always dissect 360 degrees circumferentially simultaneously with distal extension. Otherwise, the obstructing material may not be completely removed. When subsegmental branches are reached, endarterectomy is directed out through each of these until the specimen can be removed. The same procedure is carried out for the middle and upper lobe branches. If necessary, an incision can be made separately in the upper lobe, as was indicated previously. After the specimen has been removed or after 20 minutes of circulatory arrest, reperfusion is initiated with blood temperatures of 16°C to 18°C, and the pulmonary arteriotomy is closed with two rows of continuous 6–0 polypropylene. After reperfusion, an incision is made in the left pulmonary artery intrapericardially with extension beyond the pericardial reflection down to the left upper lobe bronchus. The same procedure is carried out to identify the correct plane and the distal extension of the dissection.

On the left side, the anteromedial segment is particularly difficult to visualize directly. Otherwise, the orifices of the bronchopulmonary segmental arteries can be seen. Figure 28–6 demonstrates performance of the endarterectomy procedure. Figure 28–7 illustrates an endarterectomized pair of bronchopulmonary segmental arteries. A typical specimen is seen in Figure 28–8. To facilitate simultaneous dissection and removal of bronchial backbleeding, dissectors have been elaborated that contain small suction ports at the tips (Fig. 28–9). These tips are spherical in shape and allow simultaneous dissection and suction, as can be seen in Figures 28–10 and 28–11.

When endarterectomy of the left pulmonary artery is complete, rewarming is initiated, and closure of the left pulmonary arteriotomy, as has been previously described, is performed. Associated defects that were not addressed during cooling are corrected during rewarming. After discontinuation of cardiopulmonary bypass and correction of any surgical bleeding, sternotomy closure is routine. Just prior to sternotomy closure, a left atrial pressure

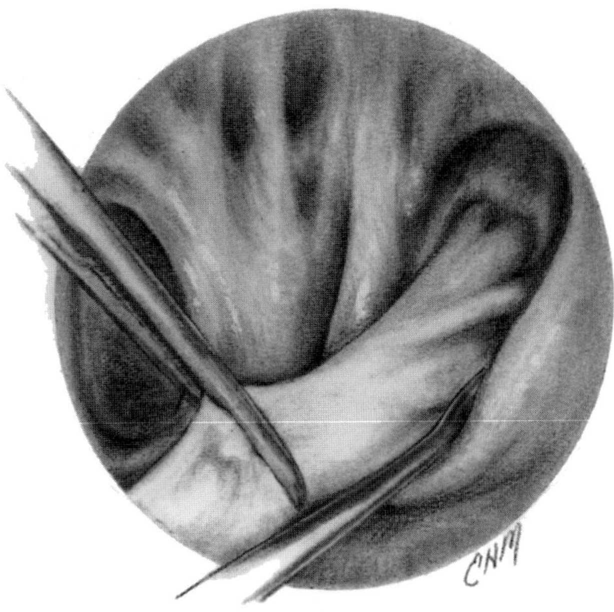

FIGURE 28–6 ■ An endoscope has been passed through the pulmonary arteriotomy to demonstrate the appearance of the endarterectomy process. A vascular forceps is used to grasp material obstructing the bronchopulmonary segmental artery, and an aspirating dissector is passed distally 360 degrees circumferentially. The specimen is grasped more distally, and the process is repeated. It is necessary to use a hand-over-hand technique with the forceps alternating with dissection to remove the material completely. (From Daily PO, Dembitsky WP, Iversen S: Technique of pulmonary thromboendarterectomy for chronic pulmonary embolism. J Cardiovasc Surg 4:10, 1989.)

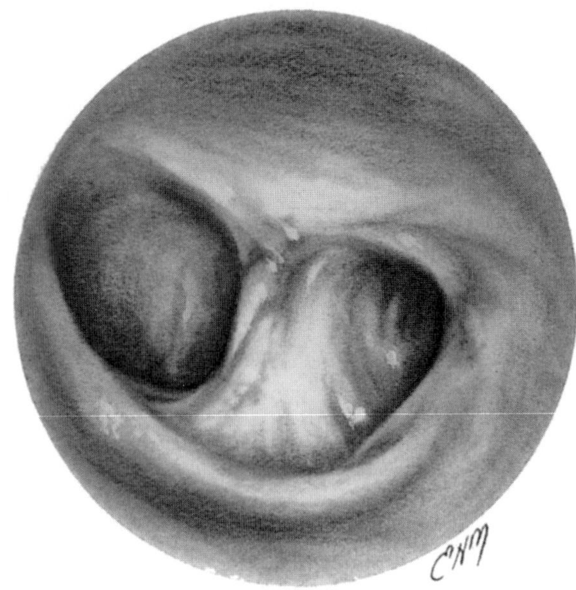

FIGURE 28–7 ■ An endoscopic view of the previous location in Figure 28–6 after endarterectomy reveals the relatively glistening smooth wall of the bronchopulmonary segmental arterial branch and a previously endarterectomized branch to the viewer's *left*. (From Daily PO, Dembitsky WP, Iversen S: Technique of pulmonary thromboendarterectomy for chronic pulmonary embolism. J Cardiovasc Surg 4:10, 1989.)

line is placed, and the intraoperative pulmonary vascular resistance is determined.

Perioperative Care

Perioperative care centers around the maintenance of adequate cardiac function and sufficient oxygenation. The adequacy of cardiac function is evaluated using the cardiac index and the level of left atrial pressure. Because significant residual pulmonary vascular obstruction frequently is present after pulmonary thromboendarterectomy, pulmonary artery wedge pressure is not always indicative of left heart filling pressure. Therefore, direct measurement of left atrial pressure allows a more precise determination of the need for volume expansion. An inadequate cardiac index is first managed by expansion of the volume to optimal levels, as is evidenced by the mean left atrial pressure. After it is optimized, additional incremental improvement in myocardial function can be attained through the use of inotropic agents, including dopamine, dobutamine, and amrinone.

The most significant pulmonary problem during the perioperative period is reperfusion pulmonary edema, which occurs in essentially all patients. The severity of reperfusion pulmonary edema may vary from minimal evidence on a chest radiograph with no measurable hypoxemia to severe pulmonary edema with marked hypoxemia (Daily et al, 1990a). In the most severe form, actual hemorrhagic pulmonary edema may result in exsanguination of the patient (Daily et al, 1990a and 1990b). Pathologic examination after this event reveals no gross defects in the pulmonary vasculature. Instead, an apparent breakdown in the alveolar capillary membrane allows hemorrhagic pulmonary edema to occur. The cause of this problem has not been elucidated but may be related to the reperfusion-caused release of anaphylatoxins and the damage associated with oxygen free

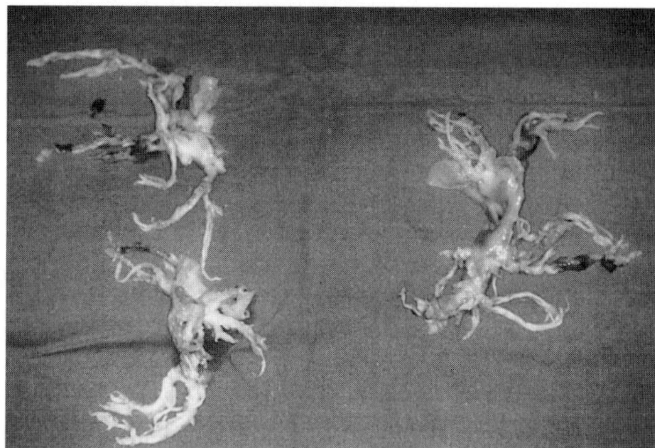

FIGURE 28–8 ■ Surgical specimen from pulmonary thromboendarterectomy of both pulmonary arteries. This specimen is oriented with the patient's right side to the viewer's left. Essentially all of the bronchopulmonary segmental arteries have been endarterectomized, resulting in a cast of the pulmonary arterial tree. (From Daily PO: Surgical treatment of acute and chronic pulmonary embolism. In Ernst CB, Stanley JC [eds]: Current Therapy in Vascular Surgery. II. Philadelphia, BC Decker, 1991.)

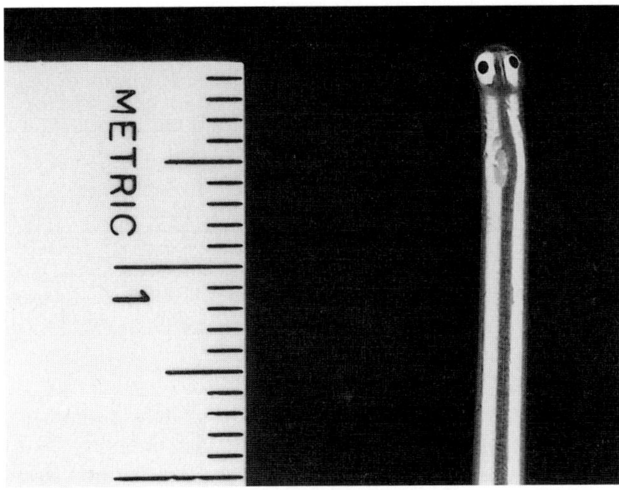

FIGURE 28–9 ■ Detail of dissector tips. The tip of the dissector is spherical and 2 mm in outside diameter. Four holes, 0.5 mm in diameter, are drilled at 90 degrees to each other to permit simultaneous aspiration of blood during dissection. (From Daily PO, Dembitsky WP, Daily RP: Dissection for pulmonary thromboendarterectomy. Ann Thorac Surg 51:842, 1991b.)

radicals. Currently, there is no direct therapeutic approach for minimizing the effect of oxygen free radicals or preventing the release of anaphylatoxins. Frequent determination of arterial oxygen tension levels allows assessment of the adequacy of pulmonary function. When necessary, ventilator settings are optimized to minimize reperfusion edema and facilitate oxygenation. In particular, prostaglandin E_1 (PGE_1) is routinely given to further decrease pulmonary vascular resistance. It is also important that pulmonary hemodynamics be evaluated frequently. An unexplained rise in pulmonary vascular resistance may be associated with pulmonary artery thrombosis. On two occasions, postoperative patients were successfully treated by surgical exploration and removal of in situ pulmonary artery thromboses. Inflatable pneumatic boots are used in all patients to minimize lower extremity venous stasis. Attempts at early extubation are resisted until the patient meets all criteria for extubation, to minimize the severity of reperfusion pulmonary edema.

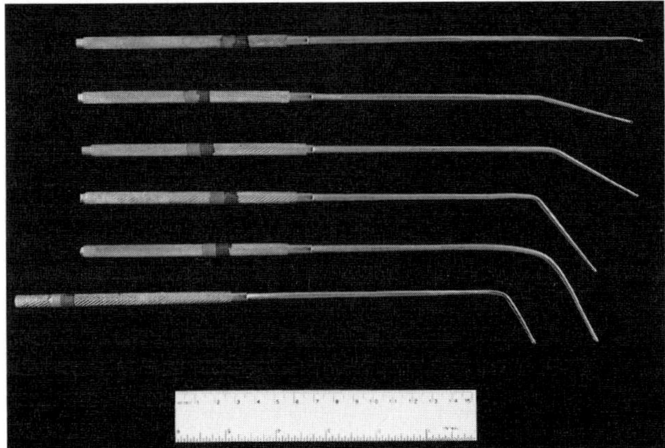

FIGURE 28–10 ■ Array of dissectors. The various angles of the dissectors and tip lengths facilitate dissection of all bronchopulmonary segmental arteries. (From Daily PO, Dembitsky WP, Daily RP: Dissection for pulmonary thromboendarterectomy. Ann Thorac Surg 51:842, 1991b.)

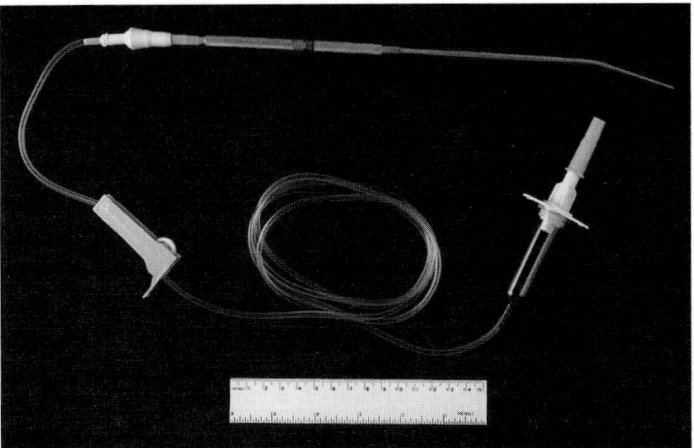

FIGURE 28–11 ■ Connection to intravenous tubing. Standard intravenous tubing is inserted into the end of the handle. The opposite end can be connected to wall suction, a cell saver device, or cardiotomy suction to conserve blood. (From Daily PO, Dembitsky WP, Daily RP: Dissection for pulmonary thromboendarterectomy. Ann Thorac Surg 51:842, 1991b.)

Early Results

Prior to 1984, the results associated with pulmonary thromboendarterectomy were essentially anecdotal, as was manifested by several series of 12 or fewer patients. However, Chitwood and co-workers (1984), in an extensive review of the world literature, described results in 85 patients. The overall operative mortality rate was 22%, and in most patients, unilateral thoracotomy with endarterectomy of a single lung was performed. Dor and associates (1981) reported a 25% mortality rate in a series of 12 patients undergoing unilateral pulmonary thromboendarterectomy. Jault and Cabrol (1989) added 17 cases to the original 16 reported by Cabrol and colleagues (1978). The overall mortality rate was 20%. In the first series, Cabrol and co-workers (1978) recommended unilateral thoracotomy and endarterectomy; currently, this group prefers median sternotomy with normothermic cardiopulmonary bypass and a beating heart (Jault and Cabrol, 1989). All other previous reports had included 12 or fewer patients.

In 1987, we reported (Daily et al, 1987) results and modifications of the procedure described in 1980. A review of our patient series, extending from February 1, 1975 until September 9, 1989, revealed three distinct groups of patients with respect to methods of myocardial protection and pulmonary artery dissection (Daily et al, 1990b). In the first group of 16 patients, myocardial protection consisted of the initiation of cardiac arrest and myocardial hypothermia with crystalloid cardioplegia and maintenance of myocardial hypothermia with saline irrigated into the pericardial cavity, as was described by Shumway and associates (1959). In the next group of 7 patients, the methods of dissection and exposure of the pulmonary arteries were the same as in the first group.

TABLE 28–2 ■ **Hospital Mortality and Morbidity Rates**

	No. of Patients	*Hospital Mortality Rate**	*Phrenic Nerve Paresis*	*Mean No. of Days on Respirator*
Group A (02/01/75–10/20/83)	16	3 (18.7%)	0 (0%)	8.4
Group B (03/12/84–09/11/84)	7	1 (14.3%)	5 (71%)	32.2
Group C (10/01/84–09/18/89)	149	17 (11.4%)	2 (1.34%)	4.5

*All deaths within 30 days or during hospitalization.
Data from Daily PO, Dembitsky WP, Peterson KL, Moser KM: Modifications of techniques and early results of pulmonary thromboendarterectomy for chronic pulmonary embolism. J Thorac Cardiovasc Surg 93:221, 1987, and Daily PO, Dembitsky WP, Iversen S et al: Current early results of pulmonary thromboendarterectomy for chronic pulmonary embolism. Eur J Cardiothorac Surg 4:117, 1990.

Myocardial protection was obtained by initiating cardiac arrest with cold blood cardioplegia, but myocardial hypothermia was maintained by the use of saline slush in a laparotomy pad placed around the heart. It was assumed that the laparotomy pad would minimize the risk of phrenic nerve paresis. However, 5 of these 7 patients sustained paresis of one or both phrenic nerves. In a third cohort of patients, group C, myocardial protection consisted of the use of cold blood cardioplegic solution and maintenance of myocardial hypothermia with a cooling jacket. This resulted in the maintenance of myocardial temperatures at 10°C to 11°C, or less, throughout the duration of aortic cross-clamping. Table 28–2 summarizes these cohorts. We emphasize that the use of saline slush, even if contained in a laparotomy pad, should be rigorously avoided to minimize or eliminate the risk of phrenic nerve paresis. As is seen in Table 28–2, phrenic nerve paresis was associated with a mean number of 32.2 days on a respirator, which represents an unacceptable and preventable complication.

Intraoperative hemodynamic changes in a consecutive series of 13 patients are seen in Figure 28–12. Postoperative complications are listed in Table 28–3 and causes of death in Table 28–4. Hospital mortality rates for the three cohorts of patients are seen in Table 28–2.

In a separate study, various preoperative and operative factors were considered to be potential determinants of hospital mortality rates and ventilator dependency (Daily et al, 1990a). Ventilator dependency was defined arbitrarily as the need to ventilate a patient for 5 or more days postoperatively. Ventilator dependency occurred in 31.5% (39 of 124 patients), and the hospital mortality rate was 12.6% (16 of 127). Multivariate analysis revealed independent predictors of ventilator dependency to be the preoperative presence of ascites, the need for 4 or more units of blood or blood products, and increased cardiopulmonary bypass time. Predictors of death in the hospital included increased cardiopulmonary bypass time and a failure to decrease pulmonary vascular resistance by 50% or more. Potential predictors of ventilator dependency, which did not reach statistical significance but suggested trends, were the duration of symptoms, the New York Heart Association functional classification, and the presence of associated diseases. Potential preoperative predictors associated with death in the hospital also included the New York Heart Association functional classification IV, the presence of associated diseases, and advanced age.

A complication of circulatory arrest is the occurrence of postoperative delirium. A study reported by Wragg and colleagues (1988) suggested that 77% of patients

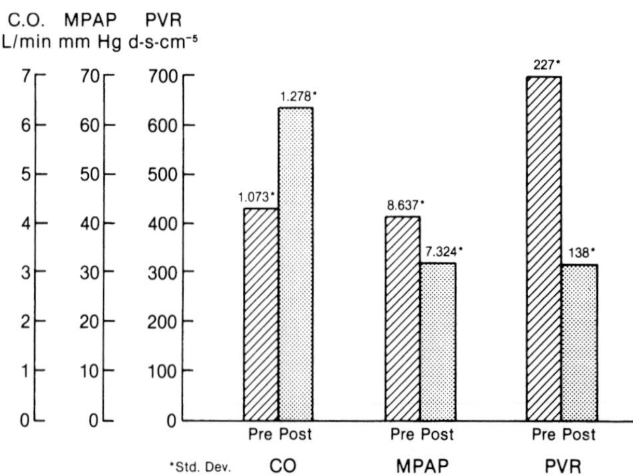

FIGURE 28–12 ■ Intraoperative hemodynamic changes in group C (n = 13). A concomitant increase in cardiac output and decrease in mean pulmonary artery pressure account for a greater net decrease in pulmonary vascular resistance (mean decrease, 59%).

TABLE 28–3 ■ **Postoperative Complications (n = 124*)**

	No. of Patients	%	
New myocardial infarction	2	1.6	
Reintubation	12	9.7	
Tracheostomy	6	4.8	
Phrenic nerve paresis (transient)	1	0.8	
Pneumonia (positive culture)	19	15.3	
Sternal wound infection	6	4.8	
Sepsis (positive blood culture)	9	7.3	
Bleeding requiring reoperation	7	5.6	
Postoperative low cardiac output (cardiac index <2.0 >6 h)	6	4.8	
Focal cerebral deficit	5	4.0	
Requiring dialysis	5	4.0	
No. of days in hospital (hospital survivors)	19.8 ± 12.5	(2–71)	
Total number of blood components (units)	14.5 ± 37.0	(0–300)	n = 118
Average number of days on ventilator	4.7 ± 5.7	(1–35)	

*Intraoperative deaths excluded.

TABLE 28–4 ■ **Causes of Death**

	No. of Patients	%	Postoperative Day(s) Before Death
Respiratory and multi-organ failure	10	58.8	19.9 (range, 4–47)
Pulmonary hemorrhage*	3	17.6	1 (range, 0–3)
Acute myocardial infarction	1	5.9	3
Right heart failure*	1	5.9	0
Pulmonary artery thrombosis	1	5.9	6
Late cardic tamponade	1	5.9	17

*Intraoperative deaths.
Data from Daily PO, Dembitsky WP, Iversen S et al: Current early results of pulmonary thromboendarterectomy for chronic pulmonary embolism. Eur J Cardiothorac Surg 4:117, 1990.

(18 of 22) developed delirium, defined as confusion, disorientation, agitation, and somnolence. An analysis of independent risk factors suggested that the most significant predictor of postoperative delirium was a circulatory arrest time of 55 minutes or longer. However, in essentially all patients, delirium had disappeared by the time of discharge, and no permanent neurologic defects were observed in this group. As of April 1998, 1049 patients at the University of California had undergone pulmonary thromboendarterectomy with an operative mortality of 9.2%, as was reported by Archibald and co-workers (1999). The surgical approach described in 1987 has remained essentially unchanged (Daily et al, 1987).

Late Results

Most patients are able to return to a level of activity appropriate for their ages. Some younger patients have engaged in competitive sports. Moser and associates (1990a) updated the late results of pulmonary thromboendarterectomy. A group of 117 patients were evaluated for a change in the New York Heart Association functional classification, as can be seen in Table 28–5. Hemodynamic data for 47 patients are illustrated in Table 28–6. Pulmonary vascular resistance decreased from a mean level of 971 dynes/s/cm^{-5} preoperatively to 282 dynes/s/cm^{-5} in the follow-up period. The decrease in pulmonary vascular resistance is usually associated with a substantial increase in pulmonary arterial flow, as is seen by comparing preoperative (Fig. 28–13) and late postoperative (Fig. 28–14) pulmonary arteriograms. This reduction in pulmonary vascular resistance suggests that late survival should be significantly enhanced if pulmonary vascular resistance has the same implications after pulmonary thromboendarterectomy as in the natural history of chronic pulmonary embolism, as was reported by Reidel and colleagues (1982).

TABLE 28–5 ■ **New York Heart Association Functional Classification (n = 79)**

Class	Before Surgery	After Surgery
IV	48	0
III	30	3
II	1	16
I	0	60

Data from Moser KM, Auger WR, Fedullo PF: Chronic major-vessel thromboembolic pulmonary hypertension. Circulation 81:1735, 1990.

COMMENTS AND CONTROVERSIES

Pulmonary thromboendarterectomy continues to be a relatively infrequently performed procedure. Undoubtedly, the lack of a high index of suspicion of the diagnosis is at least in part responsible. Until it has been specifically eliminated, the diagnosis of chronic pulmonary embolism should be considered in all patients with pulmonary hypertension. An additional factor related to the relative rarity of pulmonary thromboendarterectomy is a lack of awareness of this procedure, its effectiveness, and the current level of risk.

One of the most significant continuing problems is the inability to predict accurately which patients will have enough obstructive thromboembolic material removed to cause a significant reduction in pulmonary vascular resistance. In our experience to date, 3% to 5% of patients have inadequate relief, as evidenced by a less than 50% reduction in pulmonary vascular resistance or failure to reduce pulmonary vascular resistance to less than 300 dynes/s/cm^{-5}.

Operative mortality rates substantially increase in these patients and approach 100% when pulmonary vascular resistance remains at 800 dynes/s/cm^{-5} *or greater. It was anticipated that endoscopy could be of assistance in this small group of patients in whom operability could not be accurately determined. To date, that has not been the case. Perhaps with the development of other techniques, such as intravascular echocardiography and Doppler sonography, more precise diagnoses can be obtained. It should be emphasized that, although long-term functional capability and survival results are excellent when a significant reduction in pulmonary vascular resistance is obtained, there is a smaller cohort of patients in whom lesser degrees of reduction of pulmonary vascular resistance are associated with persistent significant symptoms. We hope a detailed analysis of a larger database will allow the preoperative identification of patients, usually with more*

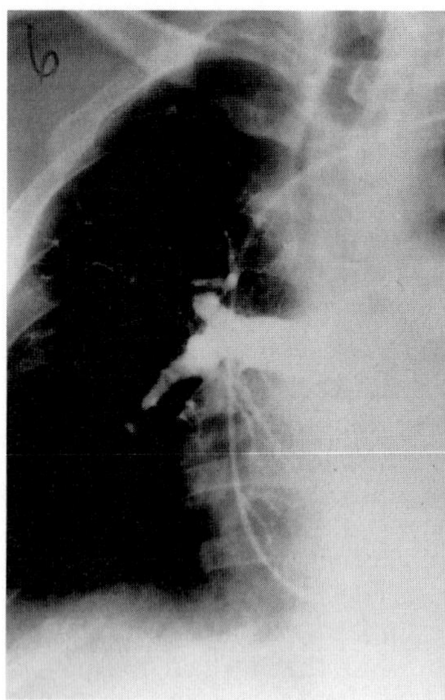
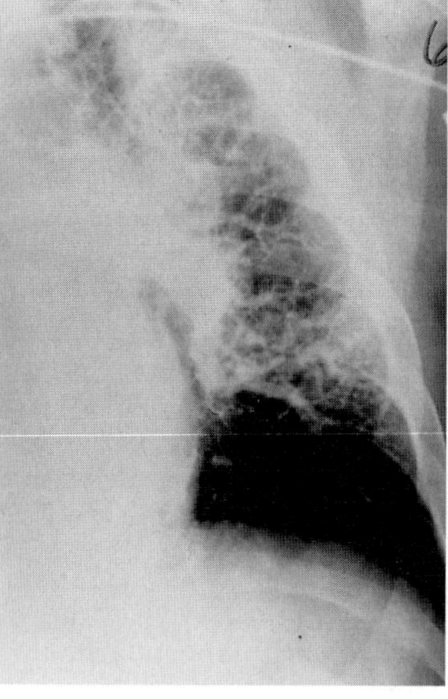

FIGURE 28–13 ■ Preoperative pulmonary arteriogram. The pulmonary arteriogram of the right lung is to the viewer's *left*. There is diffuse obstruction of all the bronchopulmonary segmental arteries, except the left upper lobe and lingula, representing more than 60% total obstruction of the pulmonary vasculature. (From Daily PO, Dembitsky WP, Peterson KL, Moser KM: Modifications of techniques and early results of pulmonary thromboendarterectomy for chronic pulmonary embolism. J Thorac Cardiovasc Surg 93:221, 1987.)

TABLE 28–6 ■ **Hemodynamics (n = 34)**

	Preoperative	*Immediate Postoperative*	*Follow-Up*
Mean pulmonary arterial pressure (mm Hg)	48.5 ± 12.4	26.6 ± 7.5	24.3 ± 10.0
Cardiac output (L/min)	3.82 ± 1.29	5.92 ± 1.15	4.85 ± 1.01
Pulmonary vascular resistance, (dynes/s/cm^{-5})	997 ± 624	230 ± 110	272 ± 256

Data from Moser KM, Auger WR, Fedullo PF: Chronic major-vessel thromboembolic pulmonary hypertension. Circulation 81:1735, 1990.

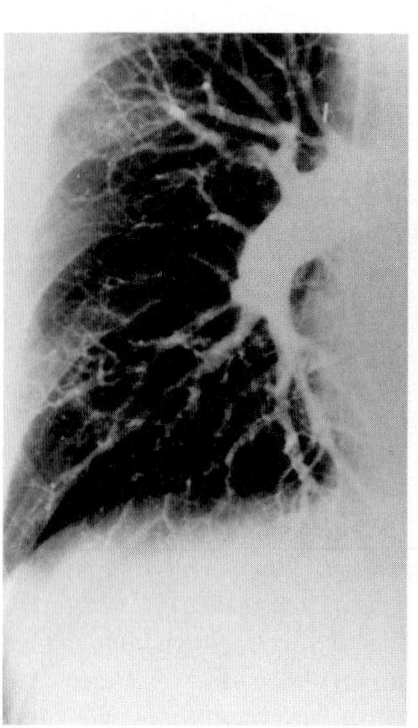
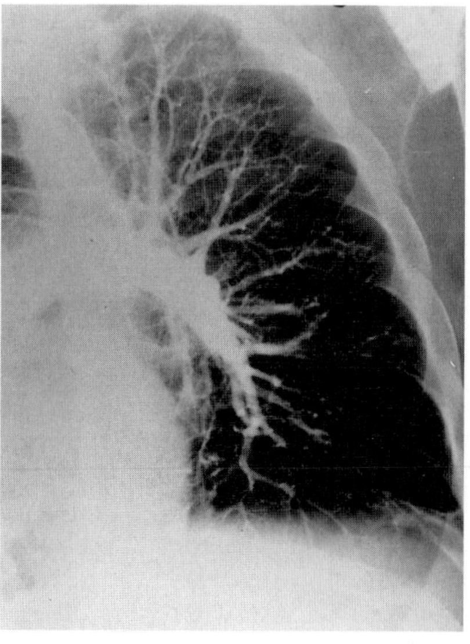

FIGURE 28–14 ■ Postoperative pulmonary arteriogram at 8 months. There is significantly increased perfusion, but some bronchopulmonary subsegmental arterial defects persist. (From Daily PO, Dembitsky WP, Peterson KL, Moser KM: Modifications of techniques and early results of pulmonary thromboendarterectomy for chronic pulmonary embolism. J Thorac Cardiovasc Surg 93:221, 1987.)

distally located obstructions, who are likely to have an inadequate reduction in pulmonary vascular resistance.

Severe reperfusion pulmonary edema in some patients during the early postoperative period is another major problem. In three patients, severe hemorrhagic pulmonary edema occurred intraoperatively, resulting in their deaths on the operating table. To date, neither predictors nor therapeutic options for this disastrous complication have been defined. Perhaps therapeutic attempts to decrease the formation of oxygen free radicals and chemical blockage of anaphylatoxins will be beneficial.

The choice of pulmonary thromboendarterectomy rather than pulmonary transplantation as the primary therapeutic approach is worthy of some discussion. In the majority of patients in whom sufficient relief of pulmonary vascular resistance can be attained, pulmonary thromboendarterectomy is the treatment of choice. The operative mortality rate is lower and the long-term survival is significantly improved compared with both lung and heart-lung transplantation (Registry of the International Society for Heart and Lung Transplantation, 1992). However, those patients deemed inoperable or at especially high risk by virtue of the distal location of their pulmonary obstructions with high pulmonary vascular resistance findings (800 dynes/s/cm^{-5} *or more) should be considered for transplantation as the primary therapeutic approach.*

Potential future trends in managing pulmonary thromboendarterectomy include the development of endoscopic techniques to remove more distally located pulmonary vascular obstructive material. To date, the use of an endoscope for visualization of the distal pulmonary arteries suggests that this might be an effective avenue of approach. However, this method has not been developed. It is also conceivable that the future development of transvenous methods of pulmonary thromboendarterectomy is within the realm of possibility.

P.O.D.

Dr. Daily is one of the world experts in the surgical management of chronic pulmonary embolism. Few surgeons have significant experience in the surgical management of this entity. This is a frequently undiagnosed or misdiagnosed condition, and as the author rightly points out, a high index of suspicion is often required. A patient with signs of pulmonary hypertension or right ventricular failure should be investigated appropriately so that this potentially reversible problem will not be missed.

In the future, prospective studies will be necessary to define the respective roles of pulmonary thromboendarterectomy and lung transplantation in the quest for the most effective therapeutic approach. Future developments in angioscopy and fluoroscopically guided ablation techniques may allow a less invasive, effective therapy for this disease.

Throughout this textbook, in most instances, explanations of surgical techniques have been separated from discussions of disease entities. However, in this instance, we thought that this unique disease and its surgical approach were best presented by combining the disease entity and its surgical therapy into one chapter.

The entity of acute pulmonary embolism is discussed in the introductory chapter on perioperative management (see Chapter 6), and readers are referred to this chapter for its discussion.

R.J.G.

■ KEY REFERENCES

Archibald CJ, Auger WR, Fedullo PF: Outcome after pulmonary thromboendarterectomy. Semin Thorac Cardiovasc Surg 4:164, 1999.

Auger WR, Channick RN, Kim M et al: Evaluation of patients with suspected chronic thromboembolic pulmonary hypertension. Semin Thorac Cardiovasc Surg 4:179, 1999.

Chitwood WR, Sabiston DC, Wechsler AS: Surgical treatment of chronic unresolved pulmonary embolism. Clin Chest Med 5:507, 1984.

In this publication, the authors extensively reviewed the literature concerning chronic pulmonary embolism and its surgical management prior to 1984. They identified 85 patients who underwent pulmonary thromboendarterectomy, with an overall mortality rate of 22%.

Daily PO, Dembitsky WP, Iversen S: Technique of pulmonary thromboendarterectomy for chronic pulmonary embolism. J Cardiovasc Surg 4:10, 1989.

This article presents a complete and detailed description of the technique of pulmonary thromboendarterectomy. In addition, several important perioperative considerations are described. Sufficient illustrations are included to facilitate comprehension of the steps for exposure of the distal pulmonary arteries. Also, the technique of endarterectomy itself is described in detail.

Daily PO, Dembitsky WP, Iversen S et al: Risk factors for pulmonary thromboendarterectomy. J Thorac Cardiovasc Surg 99:670, 1990a.

Daily PO, Dembitsky WP, Jamieson SW: The evolution and the current state of the art of pulmonary thromboendarterectomy. Semin Thorac Cardiovasc Surg 11:152, 1999.

In this symposium, all aspects of the management of chronic pulmonary embolism are updated.

Fedullo PF, Auger WR, Dembitsky WP: Postoperative management of the patient undergoing pulmonary thromboendarterectomy. Semin Thorac Cardiovasc Surg 4:172, 1999.

In this article, various factors are defined that are related to the operative mortality rate or the development of respiratory failure, as characterized by the need for mechanical ventilator use for 5 or more days.

Moser KM, Auger WR, Fedullo PF: Chronic major-vessel thromboembolic pulmonary hypertension. Circulation 81:1735, 1990a.

In this publication, the natural history, diagnosis, and patient selection are discussed in detail. In addition, late follow-up is presented in which the functional classification change is described in 79 patients; late cardiac catheterization data are presented for 34 patients.

Reidel M, Stanek V, Widimsky J, Preroesky I: Long term followup of patients with pulmonary thromboembolism. Late prognosis and evolution of hemodynamic and respiratory data. Chest 81:151, 1982.

This is a critical article with regard to recommending whether or not pulmonary thromboendarterectomy should be performed because it correlates long-term survival with the level of pulmonary vascular obstruction, as manifested by the mean pulmonary artery pressure.

■ REFERENCES

Archibald CJ, Auger WR, Fedullo PF: Outcome after pulmonary thromboendarterectomy. Semin Thorac Cardiovasc Surg 4:164, 1999.

Archibald CJ, Auger WR, Fedullo PF et al: Long-term outcome after pulmonary thromboendarterectomy. Am J Respir Crit Care Med 160:523, 1999.

Auger WR, Channick RN, Kim M et al: Evaluation of patients with suspected chronic thromboembolic pulmonary hypertension. Semin Thorac Cardiovasc Surg 4:179, 1999.

Cabrol C, Cabrol A, Acar J et al: Surgical correction of chronic postembolic obstructions of the pulmonary arteries. J Thorac Cardiovasc Surg 76:620, 1978.

Chitwood WR, Sabiston DC, Wechsler AS: Surgical treatment of chronic unresolved pulmonary embolism. Clin Chest Med 5:507, 1984.

Daily PO, Dembitsky WP, Daily RP: Dissection for pulmonary thromboendarterectomy. Ann Thorac Surg 51:842, 1991a.

Daily PO, Dembitsky WP, Iversen S: Technique of pulmonary thromboendarterectomy for chronic pulmonary embolism. J Card Surg 4:10–24, 1989.

Daily PO, Dembitsky WP, Iversen S et al: Current early results of pulmonary thromboendarterectomy for chronic pulmonary embolism. Eur J Cardiothorac Surg 4:117, 1990a.

Daily PO, Dembitsky WP, Iversen S et al: Risk factors for pulmonary thromboendarterectomy. J Thorac Cardiovasc Surg 99:670–678, 1990b.

Daily PO, Dembitsky WP, Jamieson SW: The evolution and the current state of the art of pulmonary thromboendarterectomy. Semin Thorac Cardiovasc Surg 11:152-163, 1999.

Daily PO, Dembitsky WP, Peterson KL, Moser KM: Modifications of techniques and early results of pulmonary thromboendarterectomy for chronic pulmonary embolism. J Thorac Cardiovasc Surg 93:221, 1987.

Daily PO, Johnston GG, Simmons CJ, Moser KM: Surgical management of chronic pulmonary embolism. J Thorac Cardiovasc Surg 79:523, 1980.

Daily PO, Kinney TB: Optimizing myocardial hypothermia: II. Cooling jacket modifications and clinical results. Ann Thorac Surg 51:284, 1991b.

Dalen JE, Alpert JS: Natural history of pulmonary embolism. Prog Cardiovasc Dis 17:259, 1975.

Dalen JE, Banas JS, Brooks HL et al: Resolution rate of acute pulmonary embolism in man. N Engl J Med 280:194, 1969.

Dembitsky WP, Daily PO, Moser KM, et al: Pulmonary thromboendarterectomy as the preferred alternative to heart-lung transplantation for chronic pulmonary embolism. In Belfus (ed): Cardiac Surgery: State of the Art Reviews. Philadelphia, Hanley & Belfus, 1989, pp 577–582.

Dittrich HC, Chow LC, Nicod PH: Early improvement in left ventricular diastolic function after relief of chronic right ventricular pressure overload. Circulation 80:823, 1989.

Dor V, Jourdan J, Schmitt R et al: Delayed pulmonary thrombectomy via a peripheral approach in the treatment of pulmonary embolism and sequelae. Thorac Cardiovasc Surg 29:227, 1981.

Fedullo PF, Auger WR, Dembitsky WP: Postoperative management of the patient undergoing pulmonary thromboendarterectomy. Semin Thorac Cardiovasc Surg 4:172, 1999.

Fedullo PF, Moser KM: Advances in acute pulmonary embolism and chronic pulmonary hypertension. Adv Intern Med 42:67–104, 1997.

Gibbon JH Jr, Hopkinson M, Churchill ED: Changes in the circulation produced by gradual occlusion of the pulmonary artery. J Clin Invest 11:543, 1932.

Hartz RS, Byrne JG, Levitsky S et al: Predictors of mortality in pulmonary thromboendarterectomy. Ann Thorac Surg 62:1255, 1996.

Jamieson SW, Auger WR, Fedullo PF et al: Experience and results with 150 pulmonary thromboendarterectomy operations over a 29-month period. J Thorac Cardiovasc Surg 106:116, 1983.

Jault F, Cabrol C: Surgical treatment for chronic pulmonary thromboembolism. Herz 14:192, 1989.

Kay JM: Risk and benefit of lung biopsy in primary pulmonary hypertension [Letter]. Circulation 81:2029, 1990.

Kirklin JW, Barrett-Boyes BG: Cardiac Surgery, 2nd ed. New York, Churchill Livingstone, 1993.

Mayer E, Dahm M, Hake U: Mid-term results of pulmonary thromboendarterectomy for chronic thromboembolic pulmonary hypertension. Ann Thorac Surg 61:1788, 1996.

Moser KM: Venous thromboembolism. Am Rev Respir Dis 141:235, 1990.

Moser KM, Auger WR, Fedullo PF: Chronic major-vessel thromboembolic pulmonary hypertension. Circulation 81:1735, 1990a.

Moser KM, Nicod PH, Bloor CM: Risk and benefit of lung biopsy in primary pulmonary hypertension [Letter]. Circulation 81:2030, 1990b.

Nicod P, Peterson KM, Levine MS et al: Pulmonary angiography in severe chronic pulmonary hypertension. Ann Intern Med 107:565, 1987.

Registry of the International Society for Heart and Lung Transplantation: Ninth official report—1992. J Heart Lung Transplant 11:599, 1992.

Reidel M, Stanek V, Widimsky J, Preroesky I: Long-term follow-up of patients with pulmonary thromboembolism. Late prognosis and evolution of hemodynamic and respiratory data. Chest 81:151, 1982.

Shumway NE, Lower RR, Stofer RC: Selective hypothermia of the heart in anoxic cardiac arrest. Surg Gynecol Obstet 109:750, 1959.

Simonneau G, Azarian R, Brenot F: Surgical management of unresolved pulmonary embolism. Chest 107(Suppl 1):52S–55S, 1995.

Snyder WA, Kent DC, Baisch BF: Successful endarterectomy of chronically occluded pulmonary artery. J Thorac Cardiovasc Surg 45:482, 1963.

Tilkian AG, Schroeder JS, Robin ED: Chronic thromboembolic occlusion of main pulmonary artery or primary branches. Am J Med 60:563, 1967.

Wragg RE, Dimsdale JE, Moser KM et al: Operative predictors of delirium after pulmonary thromboendarterectomy. A model for postcardiotomy delirium? J Thorac Cardiovasc Surg 96:524, 1988.

CHAPTER **29**

Benign Lung Tumors

Joseph B. Shrager
Larry R. Kaiser

Most benign tumors of the lung are rare neoplasms. Although many of these lesions present as solitary pulmonary nodules, and occasionally as multiple nodules, slightly less than 15% of such nodules are benign neoplasms (Oldham, 1980). The classification of benign tumors remains somewhat controversial because of disagreement regarding the origin and prognosis of some of the more common lesions. A modification of the classification proposed originally by Liebow (1952) seems to be the simplest and most elegant scheme and serves our purposes well.

The Liebow classification organizes lesions according to their presumed origin, whether epithelial or mesodermal. A number of the benign lesions must be classified as unknown in origin and some as inflammatory. Electron microscopy provides more accurate detail than does light microscopy with regard to ultrastructure. The availability of this technique led to a revision in the classification of several lesions that were previously thought to be benign. Intravascular bronchoalveolar tumor, also known as "sclerosing hemangioendothelioma," and pulmonary blastoma were both considered to be benign but now are known to behave in a malignant fashion. Hemangiopericytoma is a tumor that probably straddles the line between benign and malignant and should perhaps be labeled "benignant." The names themselves imply the benign nature originally attributed to these tumors. The situation with the lesion formerly known as pseudolymphoma is slightly more complex, as discussed later.

In this chapter, we discuss the diagnosis and management of the benign neoplasms encountered in the lung and focus in particular on the influence that thoracoscopic excision plays now that it is firmly established in the armamentarium of the general thoracic surgeon.

CLASSIFICATION OF BENIGN LUNG TUMORS

- Origin unknown
  - Hamartoma
  - Clear cell ("sugar") tumor
  - Teratoma
- Epithelial tumors
  - Papilloma
  - Polyps
- Mesodermal tumors
  - Fibroma
  - Lipoma
  - Leiomyoma
  - Chondroma
  - Granular cell tumor
  - Sclerosing hemangioma (alveolar pneumocytoma)
- Other
  - Inflammatory myofibroblastic tumor (histiocytoma, plasma cell granuloma, inflammatory pseudotumor, fibroxanthoma)
  - Xanthoma
  - Amyloid
  - Mucosa-associated lymphoid tumor—formerly pseudolymphoma (probably not a benign neoplasm)

HISTORICAL NOTE

The history of the surgical treatment of pulmonary neoplasms encompasses less than 60 years. The greatest attention has been paid to malignant neoplasms, which account for the overwhelming majority of lesions. In a landmark report published in 1963, Steele, writing on behalf of the Veterans Administration Armed Forces Cooperative Study of Resected Asymptomatic Solitary Pulmonary Nodules, presented the data obtained from 887 resected lesions collected beginning in 1959. There were 316 malignant tumors, 65 hamartomas, 474 granulomas, and 32 miscellaneous lesions, which included one hemangiopericytoma and five benign pleural mesotheliomas. This sums to a 12.5% incidence of benign lung tumors if the mesotheliomas are included. Most patients in this study (61%) were older than 50 years of age, and all patients were male. Certainly, these numbers will vary depending on the histories of those in the study group—in particular, whether or not they are smokers. The author concluded that the data confirmed the then generally accepted fact that most solitary pulmonary nodules must be resected if cancer is to be ruled out. Radiographic evidence of dense or concentric calcification was thought to be the only finding that eliminated the possibility of malignancy.

Little has changed in the intervening years despite the advent of computed tomography (CT) scans and the refinement of needle biopsy (both percutaneous and transbronchial). The principle remains intact that unless a new nodule can be proved to be benign, it should be removed. We are unable in most cases to prove a nodule benign. The development of videothoracoscopic techniques of pulmonary resection may result in the resection of a few more benign lesions, but it virtually eliminates physicians' reluctance to refer a patient with a possible malignancy for surgical treatment owing to the morbidity of a thoracotomy.

In a review of a 10-year experience of 1822 cases at

TABLE 29–1 ■ Spectrum of Benign Lung Tumors and Their Relative Frequency of Occurrence

Tumor	*No. (%)*
Hamartoma	101 (76.9)
Benign mesothelioma	16 (12.3)
Xanthomatous and inflammatory pseudotumors	7 (5.4)
Lipoma	2 (1.5)
Leiomyoma	2 (1.5)
Hemangioma	1 (0.8)
Adenoma of mucous glands	1 (0.8)
Mixed tumor	1 (0.8)

the Mayo Clinic, Clagett and colleagues (1964) found only 86 (4.7%) benign pulmonary tumors, most of which (66) were hamartomas. Included in this series were 11 benign mesotheliomas. A subsequent 10-year period at the same institution yielded 130 patients who underwent surgical resection of benign lung tumors (Arrigoni et al, 1970). The spectrum of benign lung tumors seen and their relative frequency of occurrence is listed in Table 29–1. Hamartomas account for most of these benign lesions, a finding that is true in all series.

In any series of resected lesions, there is and should be an incidence of resection of benign neoplasms. These lesions grow over time, often do not have characteristic calcification, and were not present on a previous radiograph; either the patient or the referring physician (or both) also were sufficiently anxious to seek a surgical opinion. When there is any doubt, the safest course to follow has been and remains complete removal of the lesion.

■ *HISTORICAL READINGS*

Arrigoni MG, Woolner LB, Bernatz PE et al: Benign tumors of the lung: A ten-year surgical experience. J Thorac Cardiovasc Surg 60:589, 1970.

Clagett OT, Allen TH, Payne WS, Woolner LB: The surgical treatment of pulmonary neoplasms: A 10-year experience. J Thorac Cardiovasc Surg 48:391, 1964.

Steele JD: The solitary pulmonary nodule: Report of a cooperative study of resected asymptomatic solitary pulmonary nodules in males. J Thorac Cardiovasc Surg 46:21, 1963.

SPECIFIC BENIGN TUMORS OF THE LUNG

Hamartoma

The most common benign tumor of the lung is the hamartoma, found in about 0.25% of patients at autopsy. It accounts for about 8% of pulmonary neoplasms (McDonald et al, 1954). These lesions represent an abnormal proliferation and mixing of the normal components of the lung. On histologic section, they are composed mainly of cartilage and gland-like formations and may include a significant amount of fat (Fig. 29–1). Most hamartomas are asymptomatic and come to clinical attention because they must be differentiated from carcinomas following their identification on a routine chest radiograph. They occur most commonly in male patients (2:1 or 3:1 predominance) and are distributed across a spectrum of age ranges, but most are seen in patients between 30 and 60 years of age (Hansen et al, 1992). Hamartomas occur in all parts of the lung, but most commonly they are found in the periphery. They occasionally occur as endobronchial lesions with manifestations of obstruction, such as volume loss.

Radiographically, the majority present as solitary pulmonary nodules and rarely as multiple nodules. They tend to be well-circumscribed lesions, ranging usually between 1 and 2 cm in diameter, although larger ones, in the 5- to 6-cm range, are occasionally seen. Calcification may be present but may not be obvious on the plain chest radiograph. The CT scan may be more useful for demonstrating calcification, and in up to 50% of cases it may also show fat (Siegelman et al, 1986). The presence of fat density in a well-demarcated lesion is certainly suggestive of a benign neoplasm. In an older patient, this finding might conclude the diagnostic evaluation and

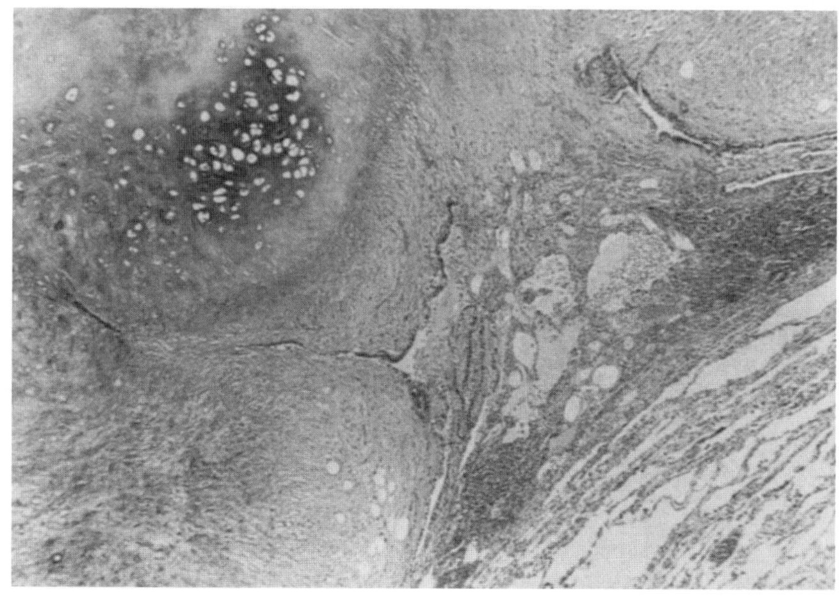

FIGURE 29–1 ■ Microscopic section of a hamartoma demonstrating a mixture of cartilage, fat cells, and undifferentiated mesenchymal cells. There are clefts lined by a single layer of cuboidal epithelial cells.

prompt the clinician to follow the patient with serial chest radiographs. In the past, needle aspiration biopsies were done with great frequency. It has been our experience, however, that rarely are positive findings obtained from an aspiration biopsy of a hamartoma. The use of a larger needle designed to obtain a core biopsy increases the likelihood of success because the clinician must obtain cartilage or fat to make a definitive diagnosis and spare the patient an operation (Ramzy, 1976).

Slow growth is the norm for these tumors. In a series reported by Hansen and colleagues (1992), tumor growth was observed in 48% of patients during a mean observation period of 4.1 years with an average increase in diameter of 3.2 ± 2.6 mm/year. Based on this finding, it is not unreasonable to watch these lesions if the clinician is fairly certain that a lesion is a hamartoma. Malignancy is rare, if it occurs at all, and only a few cases have been reported (Poulsen et al, 1979).

Endobronchial hamartomas occur in 3% to 20% of cases (Bergh et al, 1967; Mateson, 1965). In the series reported by Hansen and colleagues (1992), only 1 patient in a series of 89 had an endobronchial hamartoma, but lesions in this location would be expected to be symptomatic. Figure 29–2*A* is the chest radiograph of a young woman presenting with dyspnea and cough who was found to have a hamartoma in the left main bronchus at bronchoscopy. Note the volume loss on the left with mediastinal shift and hyperinflation of the right lung. Figure 29–2*B*, a perfusion lung scan, demonstrates a paucity of perfusion to the left lung, probably secondary

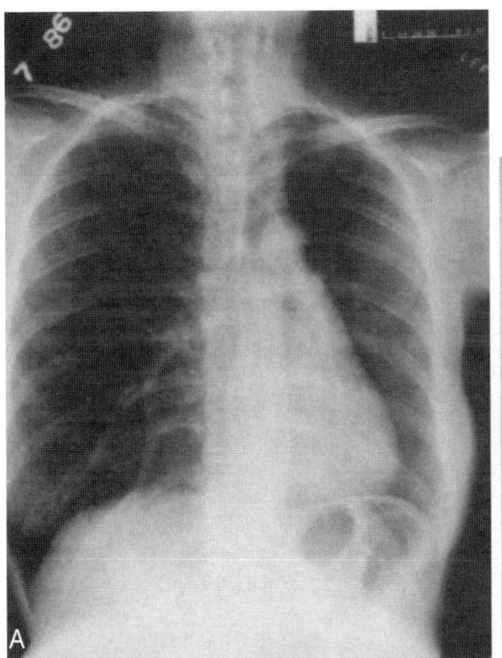

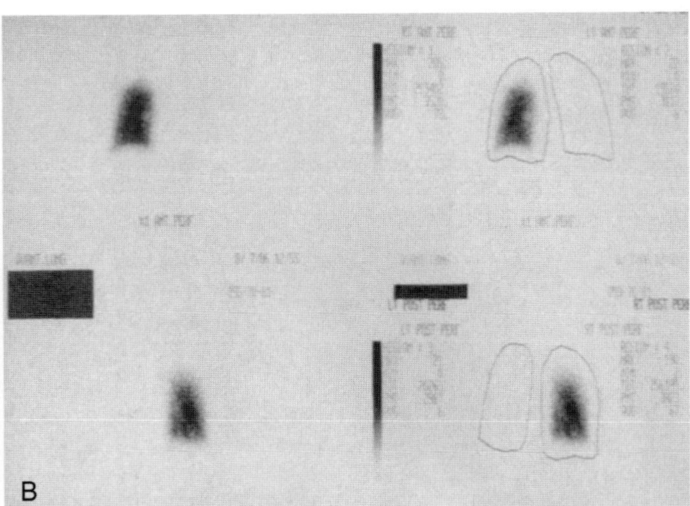

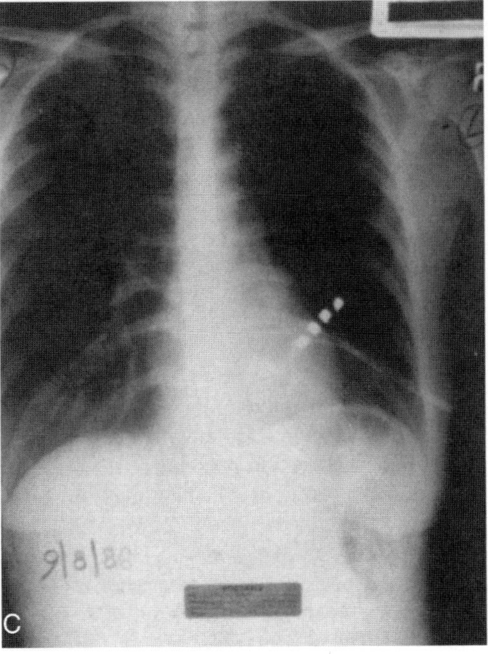

FIGURE 29–2 ■ *A*, Preoperative chest radiograph of a young woman with a hamartoma in the left mainstem bronchus. Note the loss of volume evident on the left as manifested by the mediastinal shift and the hyperinflation of the right lung. *B*, Perfusion lung scan of the same patient demonstrating significantly diminished blood flow to the left lung. *C*, Following bronchoscopic removal of the hamartoma, the chest radiograph returns to a completely normal appearance.

to hypoxic vasoconstriction. Following bronchoscopic removal of the lesion, the chest radiograph returns to normal (see Fig. 29–2C).

Hemangiopericytoma

Hemangiopericytoma is a difficult diagnosis in any site because the histologic pattern is often consistent with that of other sarcomas. Pulmonary hemangiopericytoma can occur at almost any age. These tumors are similar in appearance to lesions that are found in several other sites. The name was originally suggested because these are vascular tumors composed of capillary pericytes. They can be of any size, and in Meade and colleagues' (1974) report, they ranged from 2 to 15 cm in diameter. Approximately one half were asymptomatic at the time of presentation. The signs and symptoms included hemoptysis, dyspnea, and chest pain. Pathologically, the tumor is characterized by its vascularity and the peritheliomatous arrangement of the tumor cells. There are well-preserved vascular channels, although in larger tumors there may be significant central necrosis. These vascular channels are surrounded by sheets of rounded or spindle-shaped cells that have pale cytoplasms and large vesicular nuclei. Mitoses are infrequently seen. This tumor may behave in a benign or malignant fashion, and complete excision is the treatment of choice. The prognosis seems to be best in female patients with small tumors. Meade and colleagues (1974) found 25 cases in the world literature with 4 deaths in 16 female patients and 6 deaths in 9 male patients. Whether this tumor should even be considered in a discussion of benign lung lesions is questionable.

Sclerosing Hemangioma

Sclerosing hemangioma was first described by Liebow and Hubbell (1974). This is an uncommon benign lung tumor that occurs most frequently in middle-aged women, who are usually asymptomatic. The lesion presents as a solitary, peripheral, well-circumscribed nodule that may be partially calcified (Fig. 29–3). Grossly, the

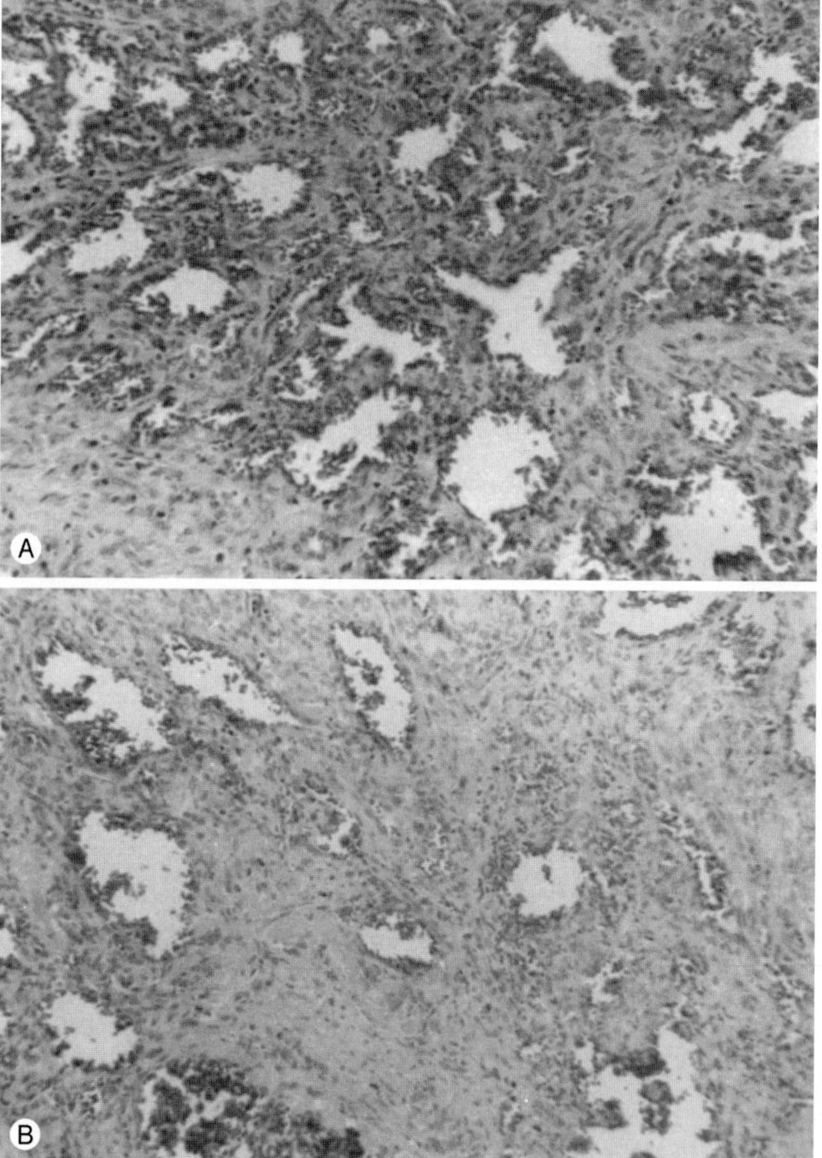

FIGURE 29–3 ■ *A*, Histologic section of sclerosing hemangioma demonstrating the vascular pattern marked by the finding of multiple dilated vascular spaces often filled with blood cells and surrounded by tumor cells of fibrous tissue. *B*, Sclerosing hemangioma showing a pattern more consistent with the fibrous type.

lesion may appear hemorrhagic. In a study by Sugio and colleagues (1992), this tumor was the second most common neoplasm seen among the benign lesions (n = 45) resected from a cohort of 919 patients over a 17-year period. Ten patients (22.2%) had sclerosing hemangiomas compared with 22 with hamartomas. The tumors ranged in size from 1.3 to 8 cm in diameter. Radiographically these lesions appeared to be well-defined, homogeneous, round or oval masses in all patients.

The histologic features of sclerosing hemangioma vary, and four major patterns may be found in the same tumor: solid, papillary, vascular (see Fig. 29–3*A*), and sclerotic (see Fig. 29–3*B*).

As Yousem (1992) points out in his invited commentary following Sugio and colleagues' (1992) article, there has been a significant evolution in our understanding of this tumor. There may be malignant variants of this tumor that present as multiple nodules, in contradistinction to the benign form, which presents as a solitary nodule. The cell of origin, as suggested by immunohistochemical studies, is most likely a primitive respiratory epithelial cell, not a mesenchymal cell. The tumor should perhaps be more appropriately labeled an alveolar pneumocytoma, based on this recent information. Surgical resection would be expected to result in a cure in the overwhelming majority of cases.

Granular Cell Tumor

Granular cell tumors, formerly called *myoblastomas* and now perhaps more appropriately called *schwannomas*, may occur as solitary pulmonary nodules or they may occur in the trachea or mainstem bronchi, occasionally as multiple lesions (Schuster et al, 1975; Thomas et al, 1984). Despite the name, skeletal muscle cells are not identified in most myoblastomas. Pearse (1950) proposed that the cells represent granular degeneration of perineural fibroblasts. They occur with equal frequency in both sexes, and the median age of patients with these tumors is 38 years, younger than that typically seen in patients with endobronchial malignancies. Patients typically present with cough or other symptoms suggestive of bronchial obstruction; hemoptysis occurs occasionally. Valenstein and Thurer (1978) reported only one recurrence of myoblastoma (6 years after bronchoscopic excision) in 46 cases of granular cell tumor. Treatment ranged from bronchoscopic removal to open, anatomic resection.

Pseudolymphoma

Pseudolymphomas, bronchial-associated lymphoid tumors, are fascinating lesions that for many years were thought to be entirely benign. Most manifest as asymptomatic pulmonary nodules noted on a routine chest radiograph. Grossly, they appear to be well-demarcated masses with smooth, soft, pale cut surfaces (Fig. 29–4*A*). A few patients may complain of chest pain or fever. In their original report of pseudolymphoma of the lung, Hutchinson and colleagues (1964) commented on the radiographic finding of air bronchograms within the lesion that resulted from this presumed inflammatory mass surrounding a small bronchus without constricting it. This is not a consistent finding, however, and there are no distinct radiologic criteria to distinguish these lesions from any other neoplasm.

There is a growing body of evidence based on immunohistochemical, molecular, and cytogenetic study that these lesions are actually low-grade, primary B-cell lymphomas of mucosa-associated lymphoid tissue (MALT). Microscopically, the lesion consists of small lymphoid cells interspersed among clusters of plasma cells (see Fig. 29–4*B*). Tumor cells infiltrate along the alveolar septa, resulting in the characteristic lymphoepithelial lesion. The tumor usually has a nodular appearance because of its tendency to localize around lymphoid follicles. Wotherspoon and colleagues (1990) described a case of a lung lesion with the definitive histologic features of a pseudolymphoma in which cytogenetic studies revealed an abnormal karyotype with a t(1;14) translocation characteristic of B cell lymphomas.

Following excision of these lesions, we carry out a complete lymphoma staging workup to rule out the presence of systemic disease. If no other evidence of lymphoma exists, we recommend follow-up only, fully recognizing that a percentage of these patients may develop disseminated lymphoma over a period of years. Despite Saltzstein's (1963) contention that these were reactive lesions, most are probably bona fide lymphomas, albeit low grade, and the term *pseudolymphoma* has probably outlived its usefulness.

Fibroma

Bronchopulmonary fibromas may occur in either the tracheobronchial tree or within the pulmonary parenchyma. Pure fibromas are infrequently diagnosed in the lung or in the soft tissues. There may be myxomatous elements intermixed in these lesions. An endobronchial fibroma would be expected to produce atelectasis or other signs and symptoms of obstruction (Corona and Okeson, 1974). Lesions of this type in this location lend themselves to easy removal through the rigid bronchoscope, or they may be excised with the laser. Similar to other benign tumors, fibromas occurring in the pulmonary parenchyma usually are asymptomatic and appear as well-circumscribed nodules without specific characteristics to differentiate them from other lesions. Wedge excision is both diagnostic and curative and can usually be undertaken thoracoscopically. Histologically, these lesions show an abundance of collagen and bland spindle cells, which are also typical of fibromas seen elsewhere in the body.

Lipoma

Most lipomas are bronchial in origin, arising from the submucosal fat present between cartilaginous rings. Parenchymal lipomas are rare. In the classic study of 130 benign lung tumors from the Mayo Clinic, only 2 were bronchopulmonary lipomas (Arrigoni et al, 1970). The symptoms and signs associated with this lesion depend on its size and location. Because most are endobronchial in origin, manifestations of obstruction predominate with the larger lesions. Cough is especially common. Endobronchial lipomas are usually pedunculated tumors with

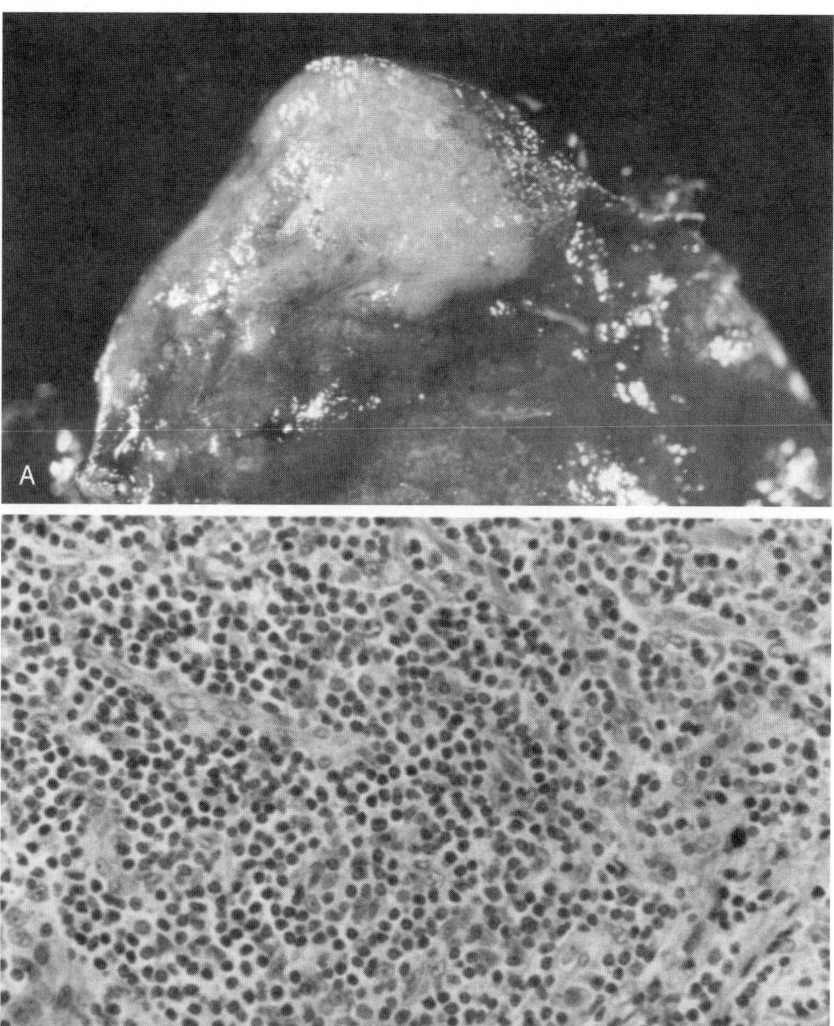

FIGURE 29–4 ■ *A*, Gross appearance of the cut surface of a bronchial-associated lymphoid tumor (BALT) demonstrating a clear demarcation from the surrounding lung tissue. *B*, Microscopic appearance of BALT showing the small lymphoid cells interspersed among clusters of plasma cells. These cells tend to localize around lymphoid follicles, often replacing the mantle zone and invading the follicle's center.

a narrow stalk that are covered by normal respiratory mucosa (Jensen and Petersen, 1970). If there is significant destruction of lung tissue distal to one of these lesions, lobectomy or segmentectomy may be required, despite the ability to remove the lipoma bronchoscopically. Lipomas of both the visceral and parietal pleura may also be seen but are much less common than are the endobronchial variety (Politic et al, 1979).

Leiomyoma of the Lung

Although rare, leiomyoma is the most common soft tissue tumor of the lung. It is composed essentially of smooth muscle fibers (Gal et al, 1989). Women account for two thirds of the affected patients, and the mean age of all reported cases is 35 years (Orlowski et al, 1978). Approximately one third of patients are younger than 20 years of age. As with other benign tumors, the location of the lesion dictates the symptoms. Most of these lesions are solitary, peripheral, pulmonary nodules and, therefore, asymptomatic. They are found incidentally on plain chest radiographs or CT scans of the chest. There are no specific characteristics that distinguish this lesion from other pulmonary nodules. A few patients present with symptoms secondary to endobronchial involvement.

There is substantial controversy regarding the origin of these tumors of the lung. Hypotheses include origination from the bronchial wall smooth muscle or the wall of bronchial arteries. On histologic section, they resemble the smooth muscle tumors seen in several other sites. There is some support for the hypothesis that these tumors are metastatic myomas of uterine origin, despite their bland cytologic appearance (Mackay et al, 1991). These so-called benign metastasizing leiomyomas have a bland histologic pattern with minimal mitosis or necrosis and seem identical to myomas found in the uterus. Because these tumors would by this theory have disseminated by a hematogenous route, many would argue against the designation of benign, no matter what the histologic appearance.

Clear Cell (Sugar) Tumor of the Lung

Clear cell tumors of the lung are rare neoplasms originally described by Liebow and Castleman (1963). In a detailed review of this tumor, Gaffey and colleagues (1990) added 8 additional cases to the 21 cases of this tumor that had previously been reported. The patients were usually asymptomatic and presented with a peripheral solitary pulmonary nodule found incidentally on a plain chest radiograph. There was no predilection according to sex, and most patients were in their 40s or 50s. Until recently these tumors were universally considered benign, but a report by Sale and Kulander (1988) describes one patient who died of metastatic clear cell tumor of the lung.

These tumors bear a striking microscopic resemblance to metastatic renal cell carcinoma, and Gaffey and colleagues (1990) attempt to clarify the pathologic distinctions between clear cell tumors of the lung and renal cell carcinomas by clinical, histologic, immunohistochemical, and ultrastructural features. They are characterized by sheets and cords of polygonal cells separated by a prominent fibrovascular stroma. The "clear cells" may indeed have a clear cytoplasm, but they often have a granular eosinophilic cytoplasm. Based on their intense periodic acid–Schiff positivity, the granules are most likely glycogen, and the eosinophilic appearance of the cytoplasm is imparted when granules are present in large numbers. The nuclei are characteristically bland and vary in size; mitoses are usually absent. The chromatin is finely granular, and intranuclear cytoplasmic invaginations are seen occasionally. Although not distinctly encapsulated, the lesions easily "shell out" of the surrounding lung tissue, are usually peripherally located, and generally are 2 cm or less in size. Immunohistochemical analysis allows for the definitive diagnosis of clear cell tumors of the lung and their distinction from renal cell carcinomas.

Inflammatory Myofibroblastic Tumor

This term is applied to a group of tumors that have been described by a variety of terms including plasma cell granuloma, histiocytoma, fibroxanthoma, and inflammatory pseudotumor (Pettinato et al, 1990). These lesions are thought to be reactive in nature because many of the patients who develop them have a history of previous infection, inflammation, or neoplasm of the lung. The tumors are nonencapsulated and contain varying proportions of plasma cells and histiocytes constituting an abundant inflammatory infiltrate with a large spindle cell component of, primarily, myofibroblasts (Fig. 29–5). In one of the largest series of these lesions, consisting of 20 patients (Pettinato et al, 1990), 40% were asymptomatic whereas 60% had symptoms consisting of cough, fever, chest wall pain, or dyspnea. The average age was 30 years, but the lesion represents 57% of benign lung tumors in children. There were nine peripheral coin lesions, three more irregular lesions, and one endobronchial lesion. Two patients had more than one nodule. Three patients had extrapulmonary extension into the mediastinum, and one was felt to be a primary mediastinal tumor, but even these patients were cured by resection or had only local recurrence (one patient).

Germ Cell Tumors

Benign teratomas presenting in the lung are distinctly uncommon, but they have been reported (Holt et al, 1976). Some of the reported cases may be mediastinal lesions that involve contiguous lung.

Rarer Tumors

Other benign tumors that have been reported in the lung in a few patients include pulmonary meningioma, ganglionoma, and lymphangioma.

DIAGNOSIS

Most benign tumors present as asymptomatic nodules found on a routine chest radiograph. This is almost universally the case with lesions located in the peripheral lung parenchyma. The presence of multiple nodules most commonly represents metastatic disease, which was the case in 73% of 114 patients reported by Gross and colleagues (1985). A small percentage of benign lesions,

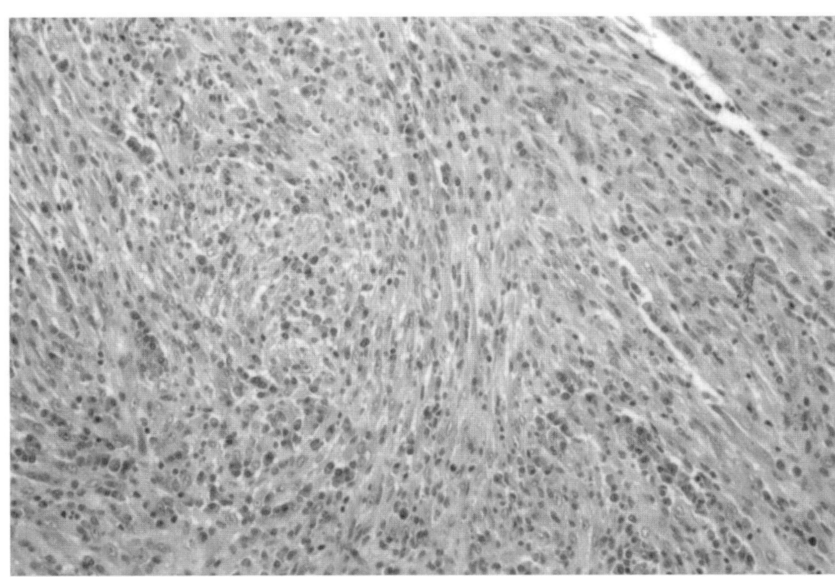

FIGURE 29–5 ■ Inflammatory myofibroblastic tumor (H & E, ×100). The tumor consists of a mix of fibroblasts and chronic inflammatory cells, including conspicuous numbers of plasma cells. (Photomicrograph courtesy of Leslie A. Litzky, MD, Department of Pathology and Laboratory Medicine, University of Pennsylvania Medical Center, Philadelphia, PA.)

however, are located in an endobronchial location and may be manifested by lobar or whole lung collapse, hyperinflation secondary to a ball-valve mechanism, cough, pneumonia, and, occasionally, hemoptysis. Infrequently, a wheeze may be audible. In a series of 130 benign lung tumors, Arrigoni and colleagues (1970) noted eight endobronchial lesions. It should be noted that carcinoid tumors, which frequently present in this fashion, are in fact malignant lesions and are discussed elsewhere in this text.

A definitive diagnosis may be made only by obtaining tissue. This is easily accomplished by bronchoscopy when there is an endobronchial lesion, but the much more common peripheral lesions present more of a challenge. Although no criteria are absolute, a number of factors point to a benign diagnosis (Webb, 1990). Lesions in nonsmokers younger than 30 years of age are extremely unlikely to be malignant, and if the lesion has not changed in size over 2 years or more it is also generally safe to consider the lesion benign. The importance of review of a prior chest radiograph cannot be overemphasized. Dense or central calcification on the chest radiograph is considered to be a reliable indicator that a lesion is benign. The recent application of quantitative CT densitometry (Siegelman et al, 1986) has taken this concept a step further, but this technique will identify benignity in only 22% to 28% of those nodules that show no diagnostic calcification on a plain radiogram (Khouri et al, 1987; Zerhouni et al, 1986). Positron emission tomography (PET) has been advanced as a means of separating benign from malignant pulmonary nodules by virtue of the differing intensity with which they process glucose, but there is clearly some overlap between the two groups. Therefore, despite these noninvasive methods of attempting to determine the nature of a solitary pulmonary nodule, a large number of such lesions remain indeterminate and, therefore, require tissue obtained by one means or another to establish a diagnosis.

Only 10% to 20% of patients with malignant solitary pulmonary nodules will have sputum that is positive for cancer (Khouri et al, 1987). Furthermore, the preponderance of benign tissue fragments obtained from a nodule by one of the two other available nonoperative diagnostic studies—bronchoscopy and transthoracic needle biopsy (TTNB)—do not guarantee that the lesion is, in fact, benign. A specific benign diagnosis is made only 10% of the time at bronchoscopy (Fletcher et al, 1986) and between 12% and 67% of the time by TTNB (Calhoun et al, 1986; Fletcher et al, 1986). Because as many as 29% of patients without a diagnosis of malignancy on TTNB are found ultimately to have carcinoma (Calhoun et al, 1986), only a definitive benign diagnosis by cytology can, in our view, avert a further procedure. Specific benign findings would include cartilage or fat suggestive of a hamartoma or fungal elements diagnostic of an infectious process. Most "negative" results from TTNBs have no benefit to the patient and simply mandate a further diagnostic procedure, whereas a diagnosis of malignancy merely confirms that complete excision should be carried out. Furthermore, the risk of morbidity from TTNB is considerable, with the rate of chest tube placement for significant pneumothorax at approximately 5%.

For these reasons, many groups currently do not perform TTNB for the indeterminate pulmonary nodule except in the patient with multiple nodules who needs a tissue diagnosis and in whom the diagnosis is highly likely to be malignant, or in the patient with an absolute contraindication to operation. The practice used by these groups is complete removal of the lesion by video-assisted thoracic surgery (VATS) wedge resection.

MANAGEMENT

In general, simple excision of a benign lesion is curative. Often, excision may be done without the need for an anatomic resection, although the type of resection is obviously dependent on the location of the lesion. The guiding principle, however, when dealing with a benign lesion is conservation of lung tissue. This may include the use of segmental resections and bronchoplastic procedures. Bronchoscopic excision may suffice for some lesions.

Advances in minimally invasive techniques make it less important to look for ways to avoid removing a lesion that may be benign. The advent of VATS has significantly changed our thinking regarding solitary pulmonary nodules (Kaiser et al, 1995). No longer must a patient be subjected to a formal posterolateral thoracotomy to make a diagnosis or definitively treat a large proportion of benign lesions. Wedge excision through a thoracoscopic approach provides adequate therapy for many benign pathologic conditions with less morbidity than a thoracotomy. Patients leave the hospital sooner and return to normal activities in a shorter period than that following thoracotomy (Landreneau et al, 1993; Santambragio et al, 1995).

The therapy for parenchymal hamartomas is guided more by the fact that the diagnosis usually cannot be definitively established until the lesion is removed. It is easy to visualize these lesions at the time of thoracoscopy and either perform a wedge excision or enucleate them, as has been classically done during an open procedure. These lesions do not invade the surrounding parenchyma, and they shell out with ease following an incision into the visceral pleura. Benign pulmonary lesions presenting in an endobronchial location often may be treated with bronchoscopic excision. This usually requires performing rigid bronchoscopy to ensure complete removal of the lesion. With complete excision, a recurrence is unusual; a repeat bronchoscopic removal is indicated for a recurrence. Pulmonary resection is occasionally indicated for benign endobronchial lesions when there is significant destruction of pulmonary parenchyma distal to an obstructing lesion or when the lesion occurs in a more peripheral endobronchial location.

COMMENTS AND CONTROVERSIES

I disagree with the authors concerning the accuracy of TTNB for benign diagnoses. Most hamartomas and infec-

tious granulomas can be diagnosed in this fashion using cytopathology and bacteriology, thus avoiding an unnecessary thoracotomy or thoracoscopy. My own practice is to perform TTNB when a hamartoma is suspected and simply follow the patient if the TTNB confirms this diagnosis (unless the patient requests that it be removed).

For further information on the use of PET imaging in confirming a benign diagnosis, please see Chapter 21. In the future, a negative nonspecific needle biopsy together with a definite benign result with PET scan (no uptake) may avoid further invasive procedures.

R.J.G.

■ KEY REFERENCES

Hansen CP, Holtveg H, Francis D et al: Pulmonary hamartoma. J Thorac Cardiovasc Surg 104:674, 1992.

The authors report a series of 89 cases of pulmonary hamartoma; 75 patients underwent operations. This is an excellent review on the topic of hamartoma—by far the most common benign lung tumor encountered. The authors obtained a diagnostic result in 34 of 40 patients (85%) who underwent needle biopsy, a higher percentage than would be expected.

Liebow AA: Tumors of the lower respiratory tract. In Atlas of Tumor Pathology, Section V. Fascicle 17. Washington DC, Armed Forces Institute of Pathology, 1952.

This article includes the classic description of the pathologic findings of benign and malignant tumors of the lung and bronchi. A classification scheme, essentially still in use today, is proposed in this monumental work.

Mackay B, Lukeman JM, Ordóñez NG: Tumors of the lung. In Major Problems in Pathology, Vol 24. Philadelphia, WB Saunders, 1991.

This is an outstanding monograph on both benign and malignant tumors of the lung based on the authors' experience at M.D. Anderson Cancer Center in Houston, Texas. An excellent discussion on the pathologic findings of the benign lung tumor is included in the chapter on uncommon lung tumors, which also has an excellent up-to-date bibliography.

Oldham HN: Benign tumors of the lung and bronchus. Surg Clin North Am 60:825, 1980.

This is an excellent overview of the topic that deals with the entire spectrum of benign lung tumors.

Zerhouni EA, Stitik FP, Siegelman SS et al: CT of the pulmonary nodule: A cooperative study. Radiology 160:319, 1986.

This is the definitive study detailing the CT findings of the solitary pulmonary nodule, which includes criteria for establishing or at least suspecting benignity.

■ REFERENCES

Arrigoni MG, Woolner LB, Bernatz PE et al: Benign tumors of the lung: A ten-year surgical experience. J Thorac Cardiovasc Surg 60:589, 1970.

Bergh NP, Hafstrom LO, Schersten T: Hamartoma of the lung: With special reference to the endobronchial localization. Scand J Respir Dis 48:201, 1967.

Calhoun P, Feldman PS, Armstrong P et al: The clinical outcome of needle aspirations of the lung when cancer is not diagnosed. Ann Thorac Surg 41:592, 1986.

Clagett OT, Allen TH, Payne WS, Woolner LB: The surgical treatment of pulmonary neoplasms: A 10-year experience. J Thorac Cardiovasc Surg 48:391, 1964.

Corona FE, Okeson GC: Endobronchial fibroma: An unusual cause of segmental atelectasis. Am Rev Respir Dis 110:350, 1974.

Fletcher EC, Levin DC: Flexible fiber-optic bronchoscopy and fluoroscopically guided transbronchial biopsy in the management of solitary pulmonary nodules. West J Med 136:477, 1982.

Gaffey MJ, Mills SE, Askin FB et al: Clear cell tumor of the lung: A clinicopathologic, immunohistochemical, and ultrastructural study of eight cases. Am J Surg Pathol 14:248, 1990.

Gal AA, Brooks JS, Pietra GG: Leiomyomatous neoplasms of the lung: A clinical, histologic, and immunohistochemical study. Mod Pathol 2:209, 1989.

Gross BH, Glazer GM, Bookstein FL: Multiple pulmonary nodules detected by computed tomography: Diagnostic implications. J Comput Assist Tomogr 9:880, 1985.

Holt S, Deverall PB, Boddy JE: A teratoma of the lung containing thymic tissue. J Pathol 126:85, 1976.

Hutchinson WB, Friedenberg MJ, Saltzstein S: Primary pulmonary pseudolymphoma. Radiology 82:42, 1964.

Jensen MS, Petersen AH: Bronchial lipoma. Three cases and review of the literature. Scand J Thorac Cardiovasc Surg 4:131, 1970.

Kaiser LR, Shrager JB: Video-assisted thoracic surgery: The current state of the art. Am J Roentgen 165:1111, 1995.

Khouri NF, Meziane MA, Zerhouni EA et al: The solitary pulmonary nodule: Assessment, diagnosis and management. Chest 91:128, 1987.

Landreneau RJ, Hazelrigg RS, Mack MJ et al: Postoperative pain-related morbidity: Video-assisted thoracic surgery versus thoracotomy. Ann Thorac Surg 56:1285, 1993.

Landreneau RJ, Mack MJ, Hazelrigg SR et al: Video-assisted thoracic surgery: Basic technical concepts and intercostal approach strategies. Ann Thorac Surg 54:800, 1992.

Liebow AA, Castleman B: Benign clear cell tumors of the lung. Am J Pathol 43:13a, 1963.

Liebow AA, Hubbell DS: Sclerosing hemangioma (histiocytoma, xanthoma) of the lung. Thorax 29:1, 1974.

Mateson EM: Relationship between intrapulmonary and endobronchial cartilage-containing tumors (so-called hamartoma). Thorax 20:447, 1965.

McDonald JR, Harrington SW, Clagett OT et al: Solitary circumscribed lesions of the lung. Arch Intern Med 93:842, 1954.

Meade JB, Whitwell F, Bickford BJ et al: Primary hemangiopericytoma of lung. Thorax 29:1, 1974.

Orlowski TM, Stasiak K, Kolodziej J: Leiomyoma of the lung. J Thorac Cardiovasc Surg 76:257, 1978.

Pettinato G, Manivel JC, DeRosa N, Dehner LP: Inflammatory myofibroblastic tumor (plasma cell granuloma), clinicopathologic study of 20 cases with immunohistochemical and ultrastructural observations. Am J Clin Pathol 94:538, 1990.

Politis J, Funahashi A, Gehisen JA et al: Intrathoracic lipomas: Report of three cases and a review of the literature with emphasis on endobronchial lipoma. J Thorac Cardiovasc Surg 77:550, 1979.

Poulsen JT, Jacobsen M, Francis D: Probable malignant transformation of a pulmonary hamartoma. Thorax 34:557, 1979.

Ramzy I: Pulmonary hamartomas: Cytologic appearance of fine needle aspiration biopsy. Acta Cytol 20:15, 1976.

Sale GE, Kulander BG: "Benign" clear-cell tumor (sugar tumor) of the lung with hepatic metastases ten years after resection of pulmonary primary tumor. Arch Pathol Lab Med 112:1177, 1988.

Saltzstein SL: Pulmonary malignant lymphomas and pseudolymphomas: Classification, therapy, and prognosis. Cancer 16:928, 1963.

Santambrogio L, Nosotti M, Bellaviti N, Mezzetti M: Videothoracoscopy versus thoracotomy for the diagnosis of the indeterminate solitary pulmonary nodule. Ann Thorac Surg 59:868, 1995.

Schuster PL, Khan FA, Azueta V: Asymptomatic pulmonary granular cell tumor presenting as a coin lesion. Chest 68:256, 1975.

Siegelman SS, Khouri NF, Leo FP et al: Solitary pulmonary nodules: CT assessment. Radiology 160:307, 1986.

Siegelman SS, Khouri NF, Scott WW et al: Pulmonary hamartoma: CT findings. Radiology 160:313, 1986.

Steele JD: The solitary pulmonary nodule: Report of a cooperative study of resected asymptomatic solitary pulmonary nodules in males. J Thorac Cardiovasc Surg 46:21, 1963.

Steen-Hansen E: The diagnostic value of chest x-ray combined with fine-needle aspiration biopsy in patients suspected for pulmonary hamartomas. Roentgenblatter 40:321, 1987.

Sugio K, Yokoyama H, Kaneko S et al: Sclerosing hemangioma of the lung: Radiographic and pathological study. Ann Thorac Surg 53:295, 1992.
Thomas L, Risbud M, Gabriel JB et al: Cytomorphology of granular cell tumor of the bronchus: A case report. Acta Cytol 28:129, 1984.
Valenstein SL, Thurer RJ: Granular cell myoblastoma of the bronchus: Case report and literature review. J Thorac Cardiovasc Surg 76:465, 1978.
Webb WR: Radiologic evaluation of the solitary pulmonary nodule. Am J Roentgen 165:111, 1995.
Wotherspoon AC, Soosay GN, Diss TC et al: Low-grade primary B-cell lymphoma of the lung: An immunohistochemical, molecular, and cytogenetic study of a single case. Am J Clin Pathol 94:655, 1990.
Yousem SA: Invited commentary of Sugio et al. Ann Thorac Surg 53:300, 1992.
Zerhouni EA, Boulkadourn M, Siddiky et al: Quantitative CT analysis of pulmonary nodules. Radiology 149:667, 1983.
Zerhouni EA, Stitik FP, Siegelman SS et al: Computed tomography of the pulmonary nodule. A national cooperative study. Radiology 160:319, 1986.

CHAPTER **30**

Bronchial Gland Tumors

Paul M. Kirshbom

David H. Harpole, Jr.

The term "bronchial adenoma" refers to a group of tumors arising beneath the bronchial epithelium or in bronchial glands. They are characterized by a clinical course that is relatively more benign than that for bronchogenic carcinomas. However, this suggestion of benignity is accurate only in a relative sense because these tumors represent a spectrum of biologic activity that is quite broad. Therefore, these tumors are called "bronchial gland tumors." Three distinct entities make up the majority of bronchial gland tumors: bronchial carcinoids, adenoid cystic carcinomas (cylindromas), and mucoepidermoid carcinomas. These lesions account for 1% to 2% of all lung tumors in retrospective reports (Attar, 1985; Donahoe, 1968; Rozenman, 1987).

HISTORICAL NOTE

The first clear description of a bronchial carcinoid was made by Laennec in 1831. Oberndorfer (1907) subsequently introduced the term "Karcinoide," meaning "resembles carcinoma." In 1930, Kramer grouped bronchial carcinoids with cylindromas as bronchial adenomas because of the marked difference in prognosis between these tumors and bronchogenic carcinoma. In the last 25 to 30 years, the underlying biochemical and genetic differences between these tumors have been discerned.

■ *HISTORICAL REFERENCES*

Engelbreth-Holm J: Benign bronchial adenomas. Acta Chir Scand 90:383, 1944.

Heschl R: Über ein Zylindrom der Lunge. Wien Med Wochenschr 17:385, 1877.

Kramer R: Adenoma of bronchus. Ann Otol Rhinol Laryngol 39:689, 1930.

Laennec RTH: Traité de L'Auscultation Médiate et des Maladies des Poumons et du Couer, 3rd ed. Paris, Chaud, 1831.

Muller H: Zur Entstehungsgeschichte der Bronchialerweiterungen, Vol 15. 1nausg. Diss. Univ. Halle. A. Busch, Ermsleben am Halle, Germany, 1882.

Oberndorfer S: Karzinoide: Ergebnisse der allgemeinen Pathologie und pathologischen Anatomie des Menschen und der Tiere. 13:527, 1909.

BASIC SCIENCE

Bronchial gland tumors are similar in that they arise or occur in the trachea and bronchi, and they are typically less aggressive than are bronchogenic carcinomas; however, the similarities end there. Adenoid cystic carcinoma, typical and atypical carcinoids, mucoepidermoid carcinoma, and mucous gland adenoma can be distinguished from one another on the basis of histology, immunostaining, histochemistry, genetics, and clinical activity. Each of these tumors is discussed in greater detail later in the chapter.

Of the bronchial gland tumors, the neuroendocrine tumors can be the most difficult to distinguish on the basis of light microscopy alone. Typical and atypical carcinoids, large cell neuroendocrine carcinoma (LCNC), and small cell lung carcinoma all display features of neuroendocrine differentiation, and they represent a wide spectrum of clinical activity. Because of the significant differences in prognosis and therapy for these tumors, it is important that physicians are able to accurately diagnose these tumors. Several reports have provided new tools that may be useful.

Rusch and colleagues (1996) have reported that the higher-grade neuroendocrine tumors, including LCNC, mixed small-LCNC, and small cell lung carcinoma can be distinguished from the lower-grade typical and atypical carcinoids on the basis of immunohistochemical staining against the molecular genetic markers *Ki67*, *p53*, and *Rb*. These differences in immunohistochemical staining are supported and complemented by reports of chromosomal abnormalities that also can be used to differentiate these tumors. Walch and colleagues (1998) reported that both typical and atypical carcinoids frequently lack a portion of the 11q chromosome including the *MEN I* gene locus, whereas LCNC and small cell lung carcinomas demonstrated a different pattern of genomic loss. Interestingly, there was also a difference between typical and atypical carcinoids in chromosomes 10 and 13.

BRONCHIAL CARCINOID TUMORS

Bronchial carcinoids account for 85% of bronchial gland tumors and 1% to 2% of all lung malignancies. They are seen in patients of all ages (median age of 55 years) with no gender predominance (Harpole, 1992; McCaughan, 1985; Rea, 1989).

In 1972, Arrigoni and colleagues identified a subset of bronchial carcinoids that exhibited more aggressive biology than expected. These atypical carcinoids were found to have a variety of histologically distinct features and were associated with metastatic disease in 70% of cases as opposed to 5.6% of typical carcinoids.

Pathology

The embryonic origin of bronchial carcinoid tumors has been a subject of debate in the literature. The belief that these tumors arise from amine precursor uptake and

TABLE 30–1 ■ **Peptide Hormones Produced by Carcinoid Tumors**

Bombesin	Leu-enkephalin
Bradykinin	Melanocyte-stimulating hormone
Calcitonin	Neuron-specific enolase
Corticotropin	Norepinephrine
Epinephrine	Serotonin
Gastrin	Somatostatin
Glucagon	Substance P
Growth hormone	Vasoactive intestinal polypeptide
Histamine	Vasopressin
Insulin	

From Blobel GA, Gould VE, Moll R et al: Coexpression of neuroendocrine markers and epithelial cytoskeletal proteins in bronchopulmonary neuroendocrine neoplasms. Lab Invest 52:39, 1985; and from Warren WH, Memoli VA, Gould VE: Immunohistochemical and ultrastructural analysis of bronchopulmonary neuroendocrine neoplasms. I: Carcinoids. Ultrastruct Pathol 6:15, 1984.

decarboxylation (APUD) cells originating in the neural crest has been challenged by experimental evidence that suggests a bronchial epithelial stem cell origin (Blobel et al, 1985; Churg, 1988; Gould, 1983). Regardless of the cell of origin, cytoplasmic neurosecretory granules can be identified in these tumors using either argyrophilic staining or electron microscopy (Blobel et al, 1985; Feldman, 1988; Warren, 1984). Carcinoid tumors have been shown to produce peptide hormones (Blobel et al, 1985; Warren, 1984). Several of these hormones are listed in Table 30–1.

Eighty percent to 85% of carcinoids display "typical" histology, which consists of clusters of homogeneous, polyhedral cells in a fibrovascular stroma. Atypical carcinoids are histologically distinguishable by their increased cellularity, "moderate" mitotic activity (1 mitosis every 1 to 2 high-powered field), nuclear hyperchromasia, heterogeneity of cell size and shape, disorganized architecture, and necrosis (Figs. 30–1 to 30–3) (Arrigoni, 1972). Atypical carcinoids require a more aggressive clinical course than do typical carcinoids.

Because of the ultrastructural and histochemical similarities between carcinoids and small cell lung carcinomas, Paladugu and associates (1985) have proposed a classification system that groups these tumors under the rubric of Kulchitsky cell carcinomas (KCC) including KCC-I (typical carcinoids), KCC-II (atypical carcinoids), and KCC-III (small cell cancers). The authors propose that these tumors represent a spectrum of apudomas that arise from Kulchitsky cells and exhibit the full range of clinical aggressiveness from the relatively benign typical carcinoids to the aggressive small cell lung cancers. It is important to note that the literature is not entirely consistent with regard to the terminology used to refer to these tumors. At times, pathologists have referred to carcinoid tumors as low-grade neuroendocrine carcinomas. Although this expression may be correct in that carcinoid tumors represent one end of the spectrum of neuroendocrine tumors, it adds unnecessary confusion to the issue. Typical and atypical carcinoids can be clearly differentiated from neuroendocrine carcinomas on the basis of histology, immunohistochemistry, genetics, and clinical activity. These are distinct entities that should be considered alternatives on the differential diagnosis rather than interchangeable expressions.

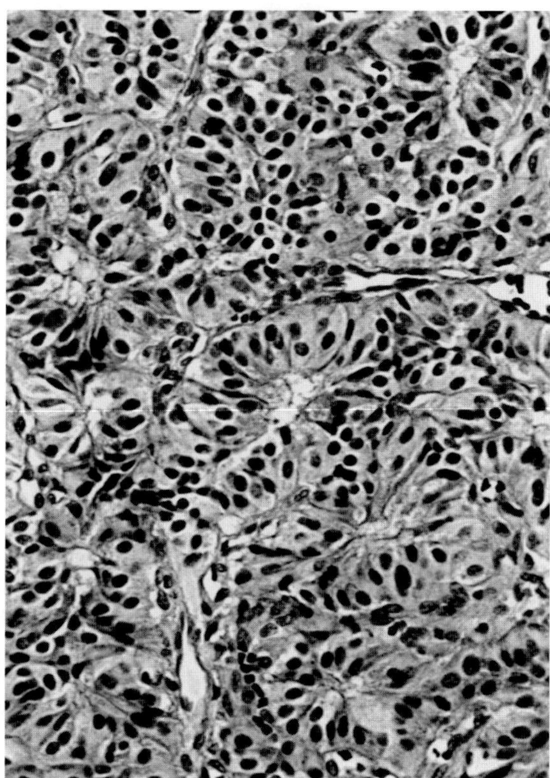

FIGURE 30–1 ■ Histopathologic examination of a typical carcinoid (H & E, × 325).

There are two rare subtypes of carcinoid tumors seen pathologically: a melanotic carcinoid (pigmented) and an oncocytic carcinoid with large eosinophilic cells (Gal, 1993; Ghadially, 1985).

Clinical Presentation

Carcinoids can be found throughout the tracheobronchial tree, with 37% to 60% occurring in the central airways (Harpole, 1992; McCaughan, 1985; Todd, 1980). In many patients, a long history of recurrent pneumonia or "asthma" may precede the diagnosis. The most common presenting symptoms of bronchial carcinoids are shown in Table 30–2. These symptoms are generally caused by

TABLE 30–2 ■ **Symptoms of Bronchial Carcinoids**

Symptom	*% Population (n = 126)*
No symptoms	39
Nonproductive cough	25
Productive cough	27
Hemoptysis	30
Dyspnea or wheezing	25
Chest pain	18
Sweating/flushing	12
Diarrhea	10

From Harpole DH, Feldman JM, Buchanan S et al: Bronchial carcinoid tumors: A retrospective analysis of 126 patients. Ann Thorac Surg 54:50, 1992.

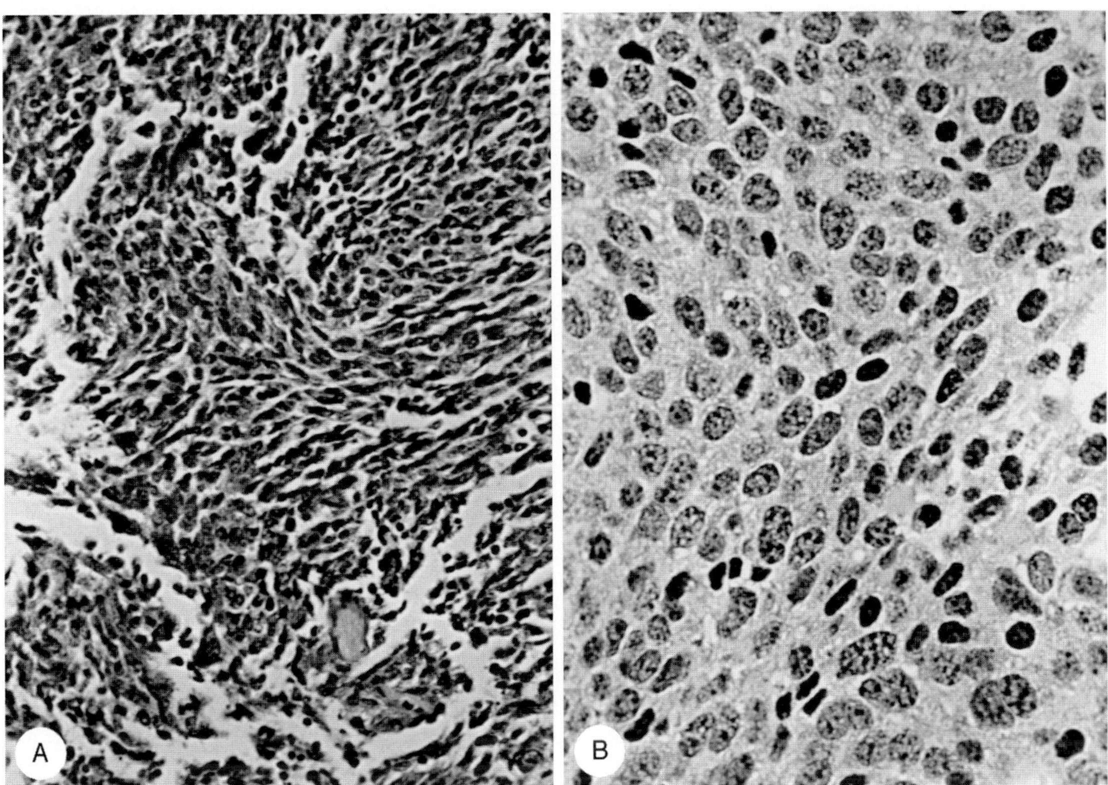

FIGURE 30–2 ■ *A*, Histopathologic examination of an atypical carcinoid (H & E, × 325); *B*, Higher magnification of an atypical carcinoid showing mitotic figures, nuclear pleomorphism, and granular chromatin (H & E, × 680).

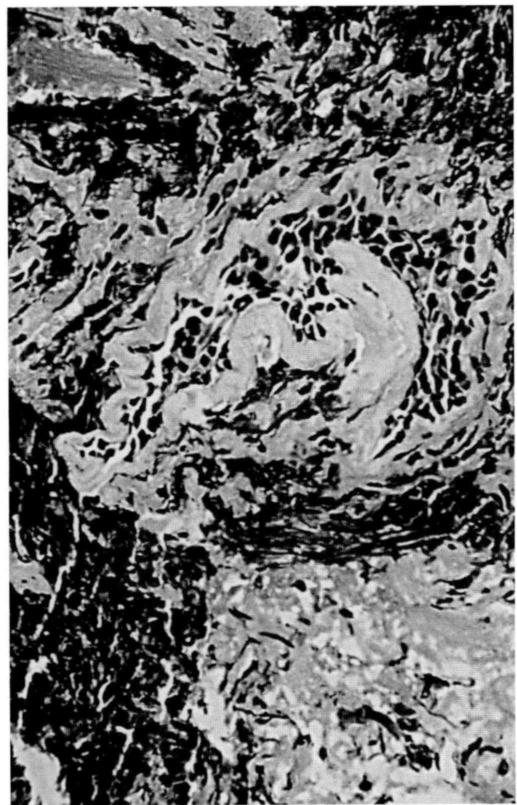

FIGURE 30–3 ■ Histopathologic examination of small cell carcinoma of the lung (H & E, × 325).

central tumors. Peripheral tumors, on the other hand, are often asymptomatic unless they overproduce an active peptide hormone. Approximately 5% to 10% of all patients with bronchial carcinoids will exhibit symptoms that are consistent with the carcinoid syndrome (flushing, change in facial pigmentation, and diarrhea) (Harpole, 1992; Rea, 1989). Carcinoid syndrome is typically seen in patients with very large tumors or liver metastases. The etiology of carcinoid syndrome is a matter of debate, but the most commonly implicated peptides are serotonin (or one of the serotonergic metabolites) and bradykinin (Toole, 1972). Serum levels of either serotonin or its metabolite 5-HIAA (5-hydroxyindoleacetic acid) were elevated in 35 of 106 patients (34%) with pulmonary carcinoids in one series (Harpole, 1992). Unlike other neuroendocrine tumors of the lung, smoking is an infrequent association with these carcinoids.

An interesting but infrequent phenomenon that occurs with pulmonary carcinoids is left-sided cardiac valvular disease. Unlike gastrointestinal carcinoids, which can cause right-sided cardiac valvular thickening and fibrosis, the pulmonary carcinoids can affect the left heart valves. This valve disease is also presumed to be caused by a tumor product.

Other endocrine disorders are occasionally associated with this tumor including Cushing's syndrome (elevated adrenocorticotropic hormone), excessive pigmentation (elevated melanocyte-stimulating hormone), inappropriate antidiuretic hormone secretion, and hypoglycemia.

Diagnosis

In patients with central lesions, more than 90% of chest radiographs will demonstrate a mass with or without atelectasis or postobstructive pneumonia (Attar, 1985; Ducrocq, 1998; Harpole, 1992). Following the initial history, physical examination, and routine chest radiograph, computed tomography (CT) of the chest is the most commonly used study for evaluating the local extent and extrapulmonary metastases.

Bronchoscopy can provide useful anatomic information as well as the opportunity to biopsy many of these lesions; however, due to the vascularity of carcinoid tumors, biopsy can result in considerable hemorrhage. Because of this risk, bronchoscopy with biopsy is best performed in the operating room where rigid bronchoscopy can be used for control of hemorrhage, if necessary. In peripheral tumors, fine needle aspiration may be diagnostic but could lead to a misdiagnosis of small cell carcinoma.

Several nuclear imaging techniques have been applied to endocrine tumors to identify primary and metastatic lesions. One scan that can be useful in the diagnosis and treatment of carcinoid tumors is the octreotide scan. This study employs a radiolabeled somatostatin analogue that binds to and identifies the location of the tumor (Musi, 1998).

Treatment

The treatment of choice for most carcinoids is complete surgical resection. The goal of resection should be complete excision of the tumor while sparing as much lung tissue as possible. Although endoscopic resection or ablation can be useful to open obstructed airways and clear postobstructive pneumonias prior to resection, the extensive extrabronchial component of most carcinoid tumors does not allow complete endoscopic extirpation in most cases (Dusmet, 1996). However, carcinoid tumors occasionally present on a stalk, and in such cases they can be amenable to endoscopic treatment alone (e.g., mechanical removal or laser ablation). If this course of therapy is employed, careful endoscopic follow-up is required.

Typical carcinoids located in the periphery of the lung are often amenable to limited resections such as large wedge resections or segmentectomies, but care must be taken with atypical carcinoids because of their increased frequency of lymphatic invasion. Atypical carcinoids in the periphery should, therefore, undergo lobectomy with removal of first-order lymph nodes (Wilkins, 1984). More extensive resections may be required for central tumors because of either postobstructive parenchymal damage or involvement of the mainstem bronchi. The increasing use of bronchial sleeve resections has decreased the frequency of pneumonectomy for resection of tumors involving the mainstem bronchi (see Fig. 30–1). Sleeve resection should be used only if histologically negative margins can be obtained and the distal lung has not been irreversibly damaged (Ducrocq, 1998; Harpole, 1992; Jensik, 1974; Lowe, 1982; Wilkins, 1984).

Approximately 10% to 15% of patients with pulmonary carcinoids have lymph node metastases at presentation. Martini and associates (1994) reported that although there was a trend of poor survival for patients with N2 nodal disease as opposed to N1 disease, the difference was not statistically significant. Even with nodal metastases, the 5-year survival was approximately 65% to 90%. The factor that most significantly affected prognosis was histologic subtype, with atypical carcinoids faring considerably worse than typical carcinoids. Because the role of chemotherapy has not been established and the presence of nodal metastases would not preclude surgical resection, mediastinoscopy does not add clinically useful information for these tumors as it does for bronchogenic carcinoma. Resection of the tumor with mediastinal lymph node dissection provides excellent local control regardless of lymph node status. However, even in cases of typical carcinoids with no clinical evidence of metastases, lymph node sampling from all potential drainage beds should be undertaken at the time of resection to allow for proper staging of the tumor. There have been no studies demonstrating a clear benefit from postoperative radiation therapy.

Results

Patients with typical bronchial carcinoids have an excellent long-term prognosis with 5- and 10-year survival in the 90% to 97% and 82% to 95% range, respectively (Table 30–3). Factors associated with a worse prognosis include the presence of symptoms at presentation, atypical histology (see Fig. 30–2), size greater than 2 cm in diameter, expression of serotonin, central location, and the presence of lymph node metastases (Harpole, 1992).

TABLE 30–3 ■ **Survival for Typical Carcinoid Tumors**

Institution	*Date*	*Patients* (n)	*Survival (%)*	
			5-year	*10-year*
NCI (Godwin, 1975)	1974	151	96	
Mayo Clinic (Okike, 1976)	1976	190	94	87
Massachusetts General (Wilkins, 1984)	1984	111	90	82
Memorial Sloan-Kettering (McCaughan, 1985)	1985	95	92	87
Los Angeles County Registry (Paladugu, 1985)	1985	115	95	
Emory/State of Iowa (Greenberg, 1987)	1990	210	97	95
Duke University (Harpole, 1992)	1992	106	93	90
Strasbourg/Marseille (Ducrocq, 1998)	1998	139	92	88

The strongest, independent predictors of poor outcome from a multivariate analysis include atypical histology, nodal metastases, and symptomatic presentation (Harpole, 1992).

On the other hand, atypical carcinoids have a much poorer prognosis with a 5-year disease-free survival rate no greater than 60%. Ultimate prognosis depends on the stage of the disease, with nodal involvement affecting it adversely. The role of adjuvant chemotherapy or postoperative irradiation is unknown. The best treatment is surgical excision with complete ipsilateral mediastinal lymph node dissection when nodes are involved.

Although the role of surgical resection in the treatment of bronchial carcinoid tumors is clear, the success of chemotherapy for the treatment of metastatic carcinoids is questionable. It is clear that the long-acting somatostatin analogues such as octreotide can provide symptomatic relief for patients with symptoms of carcinoid syndrome. Although several chemotherapeutic regimens have been shown to have efficacy in the treatment of neuroendocrine carcinomas, they have been shown to have relatively little effect in the treatment of well-differentiated carcinoids (Arnold, 1996). Given the similarities between carcinoids and small cell lung cancers, many oncologists choose to treat metastatic carcinoids with combined radiation and chemotherapy regimens, which have proved to be effective in the latter tumor (Todd, 1980; Harpole, 1992; McCaughan, 1985).

It is important to differentiate between the true carcinoids, discussed earlier and an entity known as "carcinoid tumorlets." The latter are benign pulmonary tumors located in the pulmonary periphery and seem to have no malignant potential. As such, these tumorlets can be followed expectantly with resection reserved for tumors showing signs of rapid growth.

ADENOID CYSTIC CARCINOMA (CYLINDROMA)

Adenoid cystic carcinoma (ACC), also called adenocystic basal cell carcinoma, adenomyoepithelioma, cylindroma, and pseudoadenomatous basal cell carcinoma, is a slow-growing, malignant tumor that most commonly arises in the salivary glands. ACCs arising in the bronchi are less common than carcinoids, constituting only 10% of bronchial gland tumors. Although these are very slow-growing tumors, they have a propensity for submucosal and perineural invasion as well as distant metastases at presentation (Le-Tian, 1983; Moran, 1994; Toole, 1972). ACCs typically present with both tracheal and bronchial involvement. Additional information is included in Chapter 18. These tumors demonstrate no gender predominance and have been observed in all age ranges, although the fifth decade is most common.

Pathology

ACCs have three distinct histologic patterns of growth, which occur with approximately equal frequency: cribriform, tubular, and solid (Figs. 30–4 and 30–5) (Azumi, 1987; Moran, 1994; Nomori, 1988). Cribriform and tubular forms commonly display perineural and lymphatic

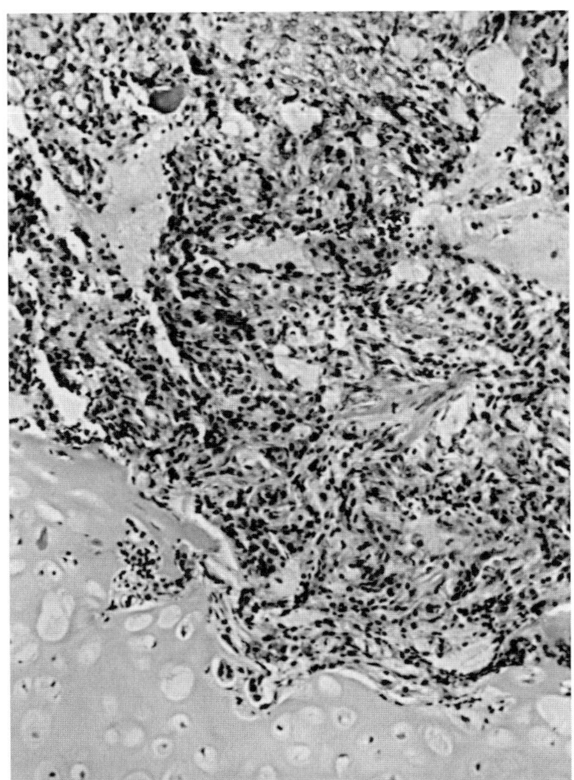

FIGURE 30–4 ■ Adenoid cystic carcinoma of the bronchus featuring classic infiltrating cribriform "cylindromatous" architecture (H & E, × 130).

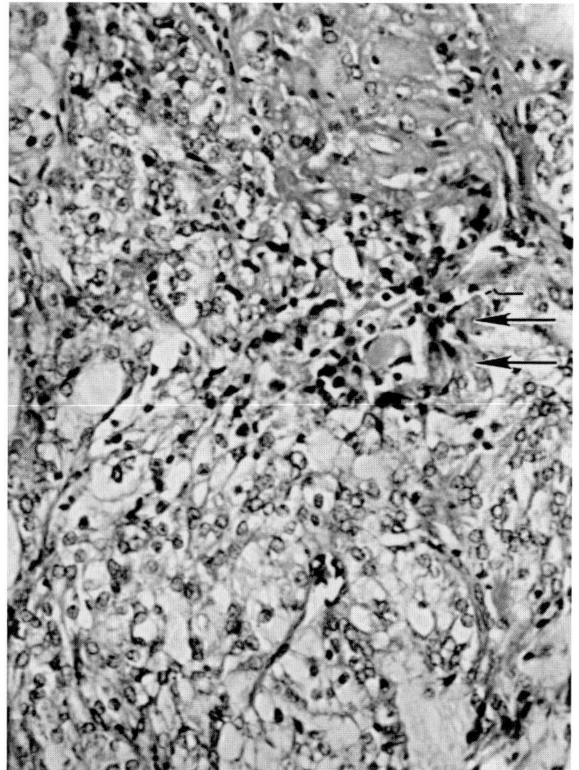

FIGURE 30–5 ■ Adenoid cystic carcinoma of the bronchus demonstrating the propensity to invade perineurium and nerve proper. Characteristic spread along neural routes makes this tumor extremely difficult to eradicate (H & E, × 250).

invasion, whereas the less differentiated solid type is associated with extensive extraluminal growth and distant metastases (Nomori, 1988). Other reports have found no correlation between histologic subtype and clinical activity (Conlan, 1978; Moran, 1994).

Presentation

Because the majority of ACCs are centrally located, the most common symptoms are the result of airway stenosis. Cough, hemoptysis, and stridor progressing to respiratory distress are the typical presenting symptoms. Some patients can present with dysphagia because extraluminal tumors can compress or directly invade the esophagus.

Diagnosis

Radiologic examination of an ACC can demonstrate a centrally located mass that is indistinguishable from bronchogenic carcinoma; however, the most frequent radiologic findings are subtle airway abnormalities or pulmonary changes owing to obstruction. CT and magnetic resonance imaging can be useful in delineating the extent of local invasion and locations of metastases (Shaney, 1991; Spizarny, 1986). Bronchoscopy with biopsy of the mass is usually required to make the diagnosis.

Treatment

Surgery is the primary treatment for ACC, although preoperative radiation therapy has been reported to increase resectability and decrease the rate of positive margins (Pearson, 1974). Because of the propensity of ACCs to extend into the submucosal plane and perineural lymphatics, frozen section evaluation of the bronchial margins is important.

As with most malignancies, complete resection of the tumor should be the primary goal of therapy. However, reports have suggested that only about 60% of ACCs are amenable to complete resection. When complete resection is not possible, palliation can be pursued through tumor debulking using limited resections or endoscopic débridement, with or without laser ablation. The role of newer modalities such as photodynamic therapy has not been defined in this group of rare tumors. Chemotherapy has been relatively ineffective in the treatment of head and neck ACC, suggesting that current chemotherapeutic agents will prove to be similarly ineffective for bronchial ACC.

Results

Because of the relative rarity of this tumor, even the largest series in the literature include no more than 20 patients, and most arise on the trachea. As a result, there have been no randomized trials studying the effects of neoadjuvant or adjuvant radiation or chemotherapy. The resectability rate is in the range of 60%, although there has been a trend toward earlier presentation with concomitant increases in resectability rates in the most recent series. Those patients who undergo resection and subsequently recur most commonly do so as either pulmonary metastases or local recurrence. Some patients can survive for prolonged periods even with metastatic or recurrent disease (Table 30–4) (Conlan, 1978; Moran, 1994; Nomori, 1988; Pearson, 1974). It is important to remember that the patients described in the studies included in Table 30–4 underwent a variety of treatment protocols over a span of 65 years. The merged survival data represent a rough estimate of prognosis at best.

MUCOEPIDERMOID CARCINOMA

Mucoepidermoid carcinoma is a rare tumor constituting 0.1% to 0.2% of all lung tumors and only 1% to 5% of bronchial gland tumors (Archer, 1987; Heitmiller, 1989). As with the other bronchial gland tumors, this tumor is seen across a wide age range, most commonly in the fifth decade. There is no gender predominance.

Pathology

Unlike ACCs, most mucoepidermoid carcinomas arise in the proximal bronchi rather than in the trachea. Histologically, these tumors are composed of squamous, mucous, and intermediate cell types with varying proportions depending on the grade of the tumor. Tumors are classified as low or high grade depending on the number of mitoses present, level of necrosis, and nuclear pleomorphism (see Figs. 30–6 and 30–7) (Heitmiller, 1989; Klacsmann, 1979). Low-grade tumors tend to contain a higher proportion of mucous cells as opposed to the high-grade

TABLE 30–4 ■ **Adenoid Cystic Carcinoma Series**

Institution	*Date*	*Patients* (n)	*Overall Survival (%)*	
			5-Year	*10-year*
Toronto, Canada (Pearson, 1974)	1952–1972	16	5/13 (39)	2/10 (20)
Mayo Clinic (Conlan, 1978)	1927–1977	20	11/18 (61)	6/17 (35)
Tokyo, Japan (Nomori, 1988)	1964–1988	12	5/6 (83)	0/3 (0)
Armed Forces Institute of Pathology (Moran, 1994)	1970–1992	16	7/10 (70)	3/8 (38)
Merged data	1927–1992	64	28/47 (60%)	11/38 (29%)

tumors, which contain more squamous cells (Heitmiller, 1989; Yousem, 1987).

Diagnosis, Treatment, and Results

As with the other bronchial gland tumors, mucoepidermoid carcinomas usually present with signs of bronchial irritation or obstruction (cough, hemoptysis, wheezing, and postobstructive pneumonia) (Heitmiller, 1989). Radiologic studies demonstrate either the tumor itself or signs of airway obstruction.

Surgical resection with negative margins is curative for most low-grade tumors. High-grade tumors tend to be more aggressive with larger tumor size and higher incidence of lymphatic and distant metastases at presentation. These should be investigated and treated in a fashion similar to that for non–small cell tumors with hilar and mediastinal lymph node sampling or dissection. The prognosis is worse for high-grade tumors than for low-grade tumors (Table 30–5).

As with carcinoid tumors, mucoepidermoid carcinomas can arise peripherally and extend centrally. In such cases, lung preservation through the use of lobectomies or sleeve resections should be considered. Adjuvant radiation therapy may play a role in the management of high-grade mucoepidermoid carcinomas; however, the best treatment regimens for radiation and chemotherapy have not been clearly delineated for this rare tumor (Turnbull, 1971; Yousem, 1987).

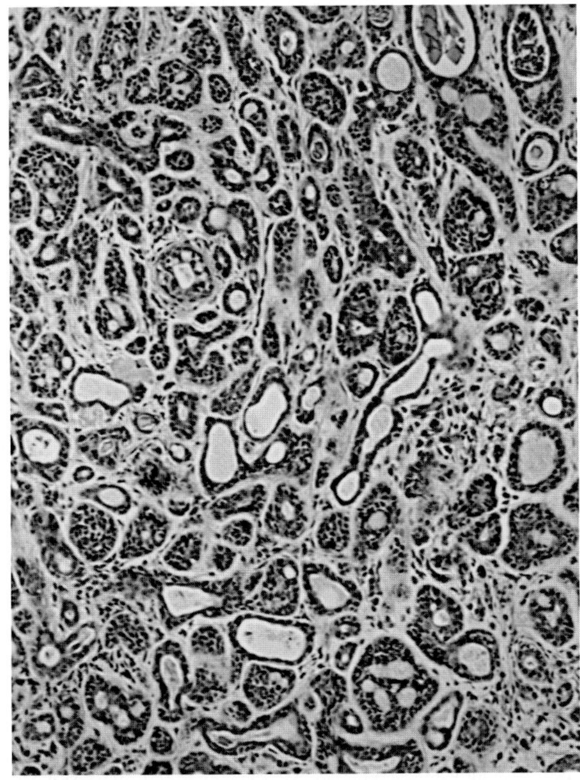

FIGURE 30–6 ■ Mucoepidermoid carcinoma of the bronchus, low grade, composed of squamous, glandular, and intermediate elements. Note invasion of bronchial cartilage (H & E, × 130).

MUCOUS GLAND ADENOMA

The least common of the bronchial gland adenomas is the mucous gland adenoma. There have been several reports of this entirely benign tumor in the literature. It arises most commonly from the submucosal mucous glands of the bronchi, but it can also occur in the trachea (Ferguson, 1988). Histologically, mucous gland adenomas are composed of regular, columnar, mucus-secreting cells in a papillary formation. The tumor commonly extends into the lumen of the airway. Patients present with

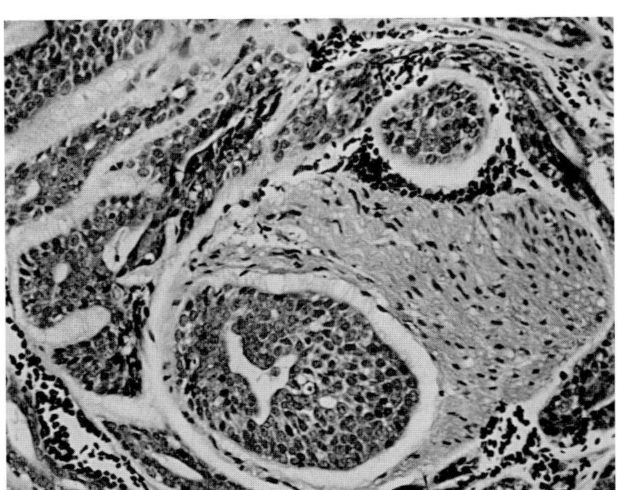

FIGURE 30–7 ■ Mucoepidermoid carcinoma of bronchus, low grade, with predominance of intermediate cells—large size with clear cytoplasm and bland nuclei. These stand in contrast to cells with more eosinophilic and hyperchromatic nuclei *(arrows)* (H & E, × 250).

TABLE 30–5 ■ **Mucoepidermoid Carcinoma Series**

Institution	*Date*	*Patients* (n)	*Overall Survival (%)*	
			5-year	*10-Year*
Memorial Sloan-Kettering (Turnbull, 1971)	1948–68	12	0/12 (0)	0/12 (0)
Results: All were reported as high-grade tumors. Some question whether these were adenosquamous carcinomas rather than mucoepidermoid.				
Mayo Clinic (Conlan, 1978)	1927–77	12	5/9 (56)	3/7 (43)
Armed Forces Institute of Pathology (Yousem, 1987)	1960–86	58	?	?
Results: Low-grade: 39/41 alive at follow-up (mean, 88 months) with 2/41 dead from other causes. High-grade: 9/13 alive (median, 31 months), 3/13 died of cancer (at 1, 12, and 72 months).				
Massachusetts General (Heitmiller, 1989)	1948–88	18	?	?
Results: Low-grade: 15/15 alive at follow-up (mean, 4.5 years). High-grade: 0/3 alive (mean, 12 months).				

symptoms of progressive airway obstruction. These tumors should be completely excised with a negative margin, because there have been reports of recurrences after local excisions (Kroe, 1967). If diagnosed preoperatively, endoscopic resection should be considered. If successful, close follow-up with repeat bronchoscopy is advised.

COMMENTS AND CONTROVERSIES

Bronchial gland tumors are diverse. Bronchial carcinoids usually present as typical N0 tumors with an exceptionally good prognosis following surgical resection. Very superficial carcinoids, usually on a stalk, have been treated endoscopically with neodymium:yttrium-aluminum-garnet laser ablation. Close follow-up for signs of local recurrence is important. One of the most disturbing aspects to these tumors is the prevalence of pathologists now referring to them as "well-differentiated neuroendocrine tumors," which can confuse the clinician. The management of these tumors is totally different from that for neuroendocrine carcinomas. Adenocystic carcinomas are seen mainly in the trachea, but occasionally these are located in the proximal bronchi or peripheral lung. Except for the very low-grade, mucoepidermoid adenomas, these tumors should be considered to be lung cancers and treated accordingly.

R.J.G.

■ REFERENCES

Archer RL et al: Mucoepidermoid bronchial adenoma in a 6-year-old girl: A case report and review of the literature. J Thorac Cardiovasc Surg 94:452, 1987.

Arnold R: Medical treatment of metastasizing carcinoid tumors. World J Surg 20:203, 1996.

Arrigoni MG et al: Atypical carcinoid tumors of the lung. J Thorac Cardiovasc Surg 64:413, 1972.

Attar S et al: Bronchial adenoma: A review of 51 patients. Ann Thorac Surg 40:126, 1985.

Azumi N, Battifora H: The cellular composition of adenoid cystic carcinoma: An immunohistochemical study. Cancer 60:589, 1987.

Blobel GA, Gould VE, Moll R et al: Coexpression of neuroendocrine markers and epithelial cytoskeletal proteins in bronchopulmonary neuroendocrine neoplasms. Lab Invest 52:39, 1985.

Churg A: Tumors of the lungs. Pathology of the Lung. Stuttgart, Thieme Medical Publishers, 1988.

Conlan AA et al: Adenoid cystic carcinoma (cylindroma) and mucoepidermoid carcinoma of the bronchus: Factors affecting survival. J Thorac Cardiovasc Surg 76:369, 1978.

Donahoe JK et al: Bronchial adenoma. Ann Surg 167:873, 1968.

Ducrocq X et al: Operative risk and prognostic factors of typical bronchial carcinoid tumors. Ann Thorac Surg 65:1410, 1998.

Dusmet ME, McKneally MF: Pulmonary and thymic carcinoid tumors. World J Surg 20:189, 1996.

Engelbreth-Holm J: Benign bronchial adenomas. Acta Chir Scand 90:383, 1944.

Feldman JM et al: Biochemical and ultrastructural differences between muco-epidermoid and carcinoid tumors of the bronchus. J Surg Oncol 37:227, 1988.

Ferguson CJ, Cleeland JA: Mucous gland adenoma of the trachea: Case report and literature review. J Thorac Cardiovasc Surg 95:347, 1988.

Gal AA, Koss MN, Hochholzer L et al: Pigmented pulmonary carcinoid: an immunohistochemical and ultrastructural study. Arch Pathol Lab Med 117:832–836, 1993.

Ghadially FN, Block HJ: Oncocytic carcinoid of the lung. J Submicrosc Cytol Pathol 17:435–442, 1985.

Godwin JD: Carcinoid tumors: An analysis of 2837 cases. Cancer 36:560, 1975.

Gould VE et al: Neuroendocrine components of the bronchopulmonary tract: Hyperplasias, dysplasias, and neoplasms. Lab Invest 48:519, 1983.

Greenberg RS et al: Prognostic factors for gastrointestinal and bronchopulmonary carcinoid tumors. Cancer 60:2476, 1987.

Harpole DH et al: Bronchial carcinoid tumors: A retrospective analysis of 126 patients. Ann Thorac Surg 54:50, 1992.

Heitmiller RF et al: Mucoepidermoid lung tumors. Ann Thorac Surg 47:394, 1989.

Heschl R: Über ein Zylindrom der Lunge. Wien Med Wochenschr 17:385, 1877.

Jensik RJ et al: Bronchoplastic and conservative resectional procedures for bronchial adenoma. J Thorac Cardiovasc Surg 668:556, 1974.

Klacsmann PG et al: Mucoepidermoid carcinoma of the bronchus: An electron microscopic study of the low grade and the high grade variants. Cancer 43:1720, 1979.

Kroe DJ, Pitcock JA: Benign mucous gland adenoma of the bronchus. Arch Pathol 84:539, 1967.

Laennec RTH: Traité de L'Auscultation Médiate et des Maladies des Poumons et du Coeur, 3rd ed. Paris, Chaud, 1831.

Le-Tian X et al: Tracheobronchial tumors: An eighteen-year series from Capital Hospital, Peking, China. Ann Thorac Surg 35:590, 1983.

Lowe JE et al: The role of bronchoplastic procedures in the surgical management of benign and malignant pulmonary lesions. J Thorac Cardiovasc Surg 83:227, 1982.

McCaughan BC et al: Bronchial carcinoids: Review of 124 cases. J Thorac Cardiovasc Surg 89:8, 1985.

Moran C A et al: Primary adenoid cystic carcinoma of the lung. Cancer 73:1390, 1994.

Muller H: Zur Entstehungsgeschichte der Bronchialerweiterungen. Vol 15. 1nausg. Diss. Univ. Halle. A. Busch, Ermsleben am Halle, Germany, 1882.

Musi M, Carbone RG, Bertocchi C et al: Bronchial carcinoid tumors: A study on clinicopathological features and role of octreotide scintigraphy. Lung Cancer 22:97–102, 1998.

Nomori H et al: Adenoid cystic carcinoma of the trachea and mainstem bronchus: A clinical, histopathologic, and immunohistochemical study. J Thorac Cardiovasc Surg 96:271, 1988.

Okike N et al: Carcinoid tumors of the lung. Ann Thorac Surg 22:270, 1976.

Paladugu RR et al: Bronchopulmonary Kulchitsky cell carcinomas: A new classification scheme for typical and atypical carcinoids. Cancer 55:1303, 1985.

Pearson FG et al: Adenoid cystic carcinoma of the trachea. Ann Thorac Surg 18:16, 1974.

Rea F et al: Bronchial carcinoids: A review of 60 patients. Ann Thorac Surg 47:412, 1989.

Rozenman J et al: Bronchial adenoma. Chest 92:145, 1987.

Shaney DJ et al: Adenoid cystic carcinoma of the airway. Am J Radiol 156:1322, 1991.

Spizarny DL et al: CT of adenoid cystic carcinoma of the trachea. Am J Radiol 146:1129, 1986.

Todd TR et al: Bronchial carcinoid tumors: Twenty years experience. J Thorac Cardiovasc Surg 79:532, 1980.

Toole AL, Stern H: Carcinoid and adenoid cystic carcinoma of the bronchus. Ann Thorac Surg 13:63, 1972.

Turnbull AD et al: Mucoepidermoid tumors of bronchial glands. Cancer 28:539, 1971.

Warren WH, Memoli VA, Gould VE et al: Immunohistochemical and ultrastructural analysis of bronchopulmonary neuroendocrine neoplasms. I: Carcinoids. Ultrastruct Pathol 6:15, 1984.

Wilkins EW et al: Changing times in surgical management of bronchopulmonary carcinoid tumor. Ann Thorac Surg 38:339, 1984.

Yousem S, Hochholzer L: Mucoepidermoid tumors of the lung. Cancer 60:1346, 1987.

CHAPTER **31**

Lung Cancer

BIOLOGY OF LUNG CANCER

Jack A. Roth

DEFINITION

Lung cancer is generally classified into two major types: non–small cell lung cancer (NSCLC) and small cell lung cancer (SCLC). NSCLC is further subdivided into three major histologic types: squamous carcinoma, adenocarcinoma, and large cell carcinoma. This classification has been useful because the therapeutic approach to these two types is different. SCLC is usually disseminated at the time of presentation and, therefore, needs systemic therapy. It is highly responsive to chemotherapy, although most patients relapse within 1 year following treatment. Conventional therapy for localized NSCLC consists of treatment of the local tumor with either surgery or radiation therapy. It responds poorly to chemotherapy, and surgical resection is the preferred treatment. The biologic basis for these differences in natural history and responsiveness to therapy is one of the topics discussed in this chapter.

HISTORICAL NOTE

Primary carcinoma of the lung was an uncommon cancer until the 1930s. At that time, a dramatic increase in the incidence of lung cancer began that has not yet abated. Lung cancer is now the most common cause of cancer death in both men and women. As described by Hoover (1978), the positive association between cigarette smoking and lung cancer was first suspected more than 60 years ago by Muller, Ochsner, and DeBakey. Modern epidemiologic studies confirm these observations. Lung cancer is one of the few human cancers in which the carcinogen is known. However, only since the 1980s have the molecular events in lung carcinogenesis been identified. The length of time between the initial exposure to tobacco carcinogens and the development of clinical lung cancer suggests that several steps are required for the expression of the malignant phenotype.

It is generally thought that the carcinogenic effects of tobacco are the result of the polycyclic aromatic hydrocarbons from tars, which are produced during combustion. Tobacco also contains specific carcinogens that are related to nicotine. Nicotine can form nitrosamines such as 4-(methylnitrosamino)-1-(3-pyridyl)-1-butanone (NNK), which was identified in tobacco smoke by Hoffmann and Hecht (1974). This substance is a strong carcinogen in rodents.

The observation that the genes that are responsible for carcinogenesis were altered forms of genes normally present in eukaryotic cells, reported by Stehelin and colleagues (1976), initiated many of the advances in molecular biology that have increased our understanding of lung carcinogenesis at the molecular level (Bishop, 1991; Cross and Dexter, 1991; Vinocour and Minna, 1989). Shih and colleagues (1981) and Murray and associates (1981) were among the first to identify and sequence human cancer genes (oncogenes). Subsequently, as discussed in this chapter, many of these genes have been implicated in the development of human cancer. Direct links between tobacco carcinogens and gene mutations have emerged (Denissenko et al, 1996).

HISTORICAL READINGS

Hoffmann D, Hecht SS: N'nitrosonornicotine in tobacco. Science 186:265, 1974.

Hoover R: Epidemiology: Tobacco and geographic pathology. In Harris CC (ed): Pathogenesis and Therapy of Lung Cancer. New York, Marcel Dekker, 1978.

Murray MJ, Shilo BZ, Shih C et al: Three different human tumor cell lines contain different oncogenes. Cell 25:355, 1981.

Shih C, Padhy LC, Murray MJ, Weinberg RA: Transferring genes of carcinomas and neuroblastomas introduced into mouse fibroblasts. Nature 290:261, 1981.

Stehelin D, Varnus HE, Bishop JM, Vogt PK: DNA related to the transforming gene(s) of avian sarcoma viruses is present in normal avian DNA. Nature 260:170, 1976.

LUNG CARCINOGENESIS

Models of multi-step carcinogenesis were most extensively studied in the mouse skin and rat liver models by Stehelin and associates (1976) and Goldsworthy and colleagues (1986). A series of well-defined events occurs in these models. Cells exposed to a carcinogen undergo an initiation event. Following exposure to a carcinogen, the cells are irreversibly altered in their heritable structure. Exposure to a second agent or promoter causes a reversible expansion of the initiated cells. Additional changes may cause the cells to enter the progression stage with expression of features of the malignant phenotype, including metastatic potential.

The formation of metastases is a complex phenomenon that occurs in several steps, including growth and invasion of the primary malignant cells, penetration of the cells into the blood and lymphatic circulation, implantation into distant tissues, and proliferation in the new environment, as described by Nicolson (1988). A metastasis suppressor gene has been identified. The absence of this gene correlates with increased metastasis formation in murine tumors. The locus of this gene was deleted in 42% of lung cancers in a study by Leone and colleagues (1991).

Studies in mice with carcinogen-induced lung cancers implicate genes of the *ras* family in the carcinogenic process, as reviewed by Malkinson (1989). Mouse lung tumors induced by tetranitromethane contained mutated *K-ras* genes. Mice harboring the mutated H-*ras* transgene developed tumors exclusively in the lungs within weeks following birth. Belinsky and colleagues (1989) induced lung tumors in mice with the tobacco-specific NNK or N-nitrosodimethylamine. Ninety percent of these tumors had transforming genes in the National Institutes of Health (NIH) 3T3 mouse assay, and in all lung tumors, this was K-*ras*. The mutations were generally guanine-cytosine to adenine-thymine transitions, indicating that DNA methylation is the most likely pathway to the induction of neoplasia by these carcinogens. This model is of interest because *ras* mutations are commonly found in human lung cancers.

CELL BIOLOGY

The cell of origin for lung cancers is controversial. The NSCLC histologic types all have the phenotypic features of the differentiated cell types in normal or injured bronchial epithelium. SCLC cells have neuroendocrine markers, including high levels of the polypeptide hormones (e.g., gastrin-releasing peptide and calcitonin), creatine kinase isoenzyme BB, L-dopa decarboxylase, and neuron-specific enolase. Endocrine cells can be found in normal bronchial mucosa. Thus, one possibility is that each of the four major histologic types arises from alterations in its pre-existing normal counterpart.

As described by Mabry and associates (1991), an alternative hypothesis is that the four types of lung cancer arise from a common stem cell and are related through a common differentiation pathway of the normal bronchial epithelium. This is supported by the clinical observation that SCLC tumors can contain mixtures of SCLC and NSCLC histologic types. These transitions have been observed in vitro following insertion of the appropriate oncogene. For example, insertion of a mutated H-*ras* oncogene in SCLC cells with overexpression of c-*myc* causes transition to the large cell undifferentiated phenotype.

GENETIC FACTORS

Only 15% of cigarette smokers, including heavy smokers, develop lung cancer, as described by Hoover (1978). This suggests that an inherited predisposition or cofactors, such as additional carcinogens, may predispose some individuals to the development of lung cancer. Lynch and colleagues (1986) evaluated 254 individuals with lung cancer and 231 individuals with other smoking-related cancers. There was a lack of increased risk of developing lung cancer when only lung cancer in relatives was considered. However, there was a significant excess of cancers at all sites for relatives of the patients with lung cancer. This suggests a heritable variation in response to carcinogens. A familial risk for lung cancer was found in studies by Ooi and colleagues (1986) and Samet and associates (1986). Respiratory diseases also predispose to the development of lung cancer, as described by Samet and associates (1986) and Skillrud and colleagues (1986). Sellers and coworkers (1990) analyzed 337 families, each of which was ascertained through a proband with lung cancer. The development of lung cancer in young individuals (50 years of age or younger) was compatible with mendelian codominant inheritance or a rare autosomal gene. This gene was not involved in older persons, reflecting the noncarriers who had long-term exposure to tobacco. The arylhydrocarbon hydroxylase gene product can metabolize promutagenic and procarcinogenic compounds in cigarette smoke. McLemore and colleagues (1990) showed that the aromatic hydrocarbon-inducible cytochrome *P4501A1* gene is highly expressed at the RNA level in the normal lungs from active cigarette smokers but not in the normal lungs from nonsmokers. The ability to metabolize debrisoquin is genetically determined and is associated with susceptibility to lung cancer, as described by Caporaso and colleagues (1990). This group showed that the ability to metabolize debrisoquin is independently associated with a susceptibility to lung cancer in a case-control study.

ONCOGENE ACTIVATION

Numerous genetic alterations have been identified in human lung cancer (Table 31–1). The relative importance of individual genetic lesions, the preferred order (if any) for genetic events, and the pathways by which altered genes mediate their action are not completely known for lung cancer. SCLC is the most extensively studied of all lung cancer histologic types. This is the result in part of the availability of many established SCLC cell lines, which can be grown in serum-free chemically defined media, as described by Gazdar and associates (1985); Gazdar and Oie (1986); and Carney and colleagues (1981, 1985). The biologic behavior of SCLC is distinct from that of NSCLC. SCLC disseminates early in its course and exhibits a marked sensitivity to chemotherapy, followed by early recurrence. It is possible that genetic events may differ between SCLC and NSCLC. Recent studies, which are discussed later, indicate that differences exist at the molecular level. Thus, it may not be possible to generalize molecular mechanisms among the different forms of lung cancer.

TABLE 31–1 ■ **Lung-Cancer Oncogenes and Tumor Suppressor Genes**

Dominant	***Tumor Suppressor***
K-*ras*	*p53*
Myc family	3p
c-*jun*	*rb*
Growth factor	Protein tyrosine phosphatase-γ
Transforming growth factor-α	nm23
Epidermal growth factor receptor	c-*erb*B2

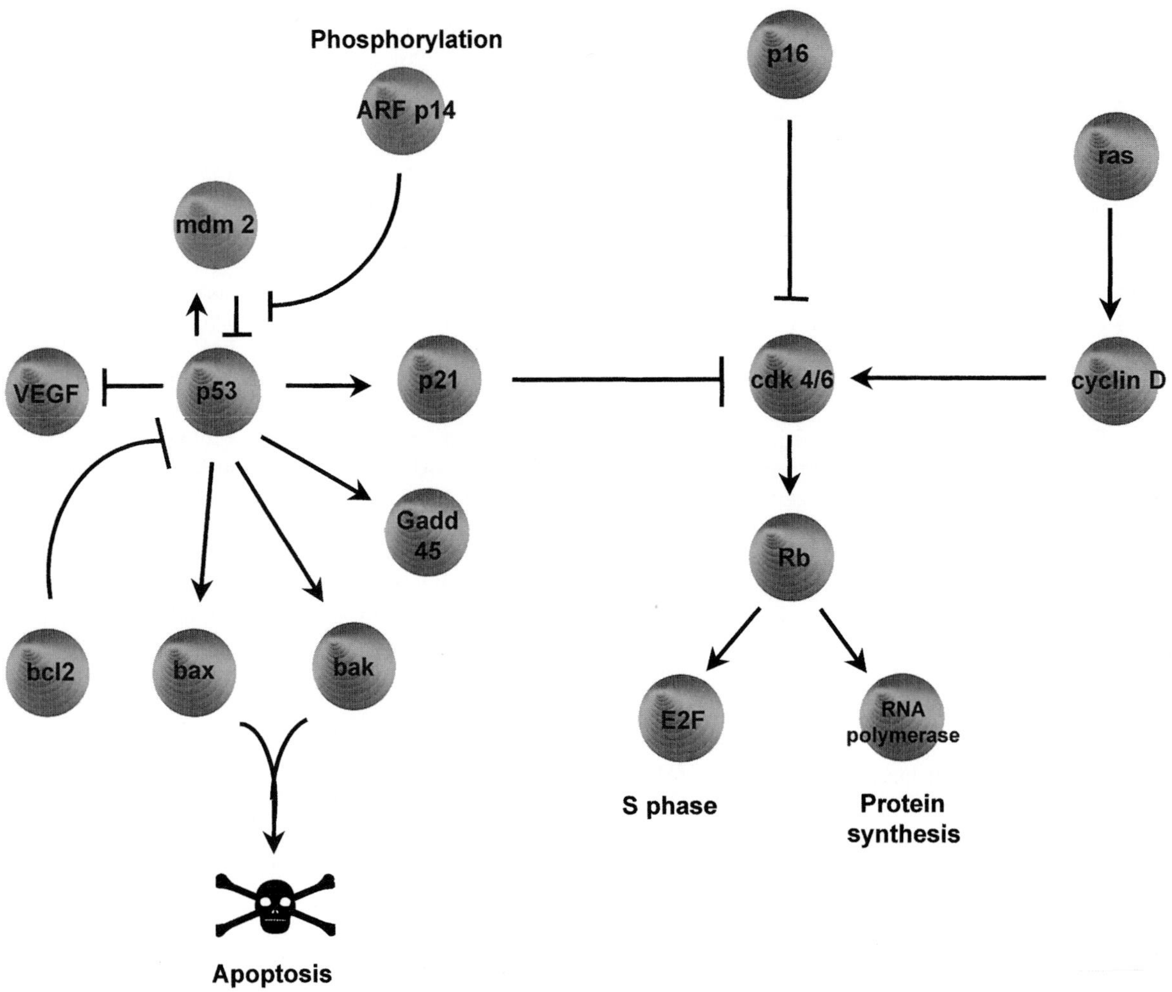

FIGURE 31–1 ■ Molecular pathways in oncogenesis. Shown are the interrelationships between tumor suppressor genes, oncogenes, and other genes that regulate cell cycle progression and apoptosis. These genes and their pathways represent potentially important targets for gene replacement strategies.

The genes that are altered in cancer cells can be classified as having a positive or negative influence on cell growth (Fig. 31–1). Mutations or defects in gene expression have been detected in families of genes that regulate cell cycle progression (*p16, cdk4/6*), DNA repair (*p53*), and apoptosis (*p53, bax*). Genes with a positive influence on cell growth are designated as proto-oncogenes in their unaltered form. Once activated, a single altered allele is sufficient to transform cells, and thus these genes are considered dominant in their action. Potential mechanisms of activation include mutation, amplification, and translocation (Fig. 31–2). Genes of this family may also encode for growth factors and their receptors. Genes that negatively influence cell growth and proliferation are called tumor-suppressor genes. The retinoblastoma gene is the most extensively characterized of this group. The loss or inactivation of both alleles is required for tumor formation, and therefore, these are called recessive genes.

ONCOGENES MEDIATING STIMULATION OF GROWTH

Growth Factors and Their Receptors

Growth factors mediate their action by specific binding to cell receptors (Fig. 31–3). A signal is transduced from the extracellular domain of cell surface receptors to the cytoplasmic domain, usually resulting in the phosphorylation of this region of the receptor. This triggers a cascade of events that may include binding of other cytoplasmic molecules to the receptor and activation of protein kinase C. This in turn may activate "early" genes,

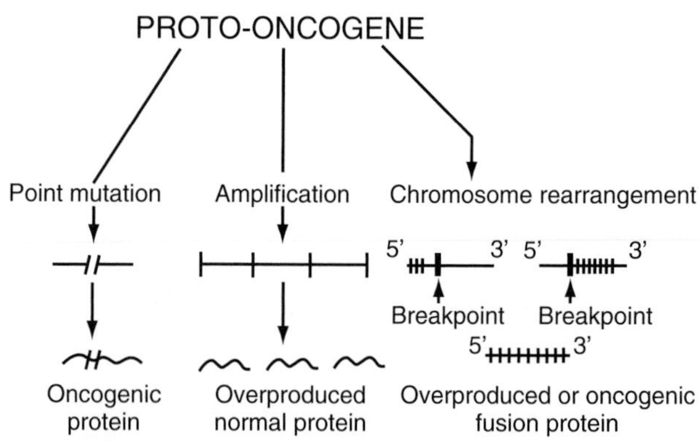

FIGURE 31–2 ■ Mechanisms of gene activation for dominant oncogenes.

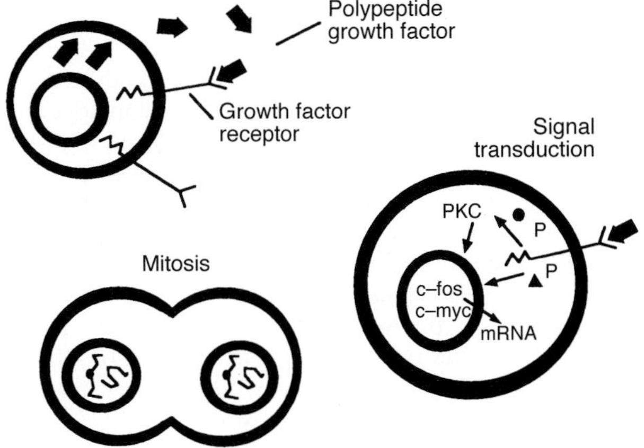

FIGURE 31–3 ■ Schematic representation of growth factor ligand and receptor interaction and the possible effects of this interaction on the cell. mRNA, messenger RNA; PKC, protein kinase C.

such as c-*fos* and c-*jun*. The cell is then stimulated to proceed through the cell cycle.

Tumor cells that make a growth factor and express the receptor for that growth factor may stimulate their own growth (autocrine growth). Cells that have an autocrine loop have several features. They secrete a biologically active growth factor and demonstrate increased proliferation of that factor. Antibodies that bind specifically to the growth factor inhibit cell growth. Growth factors may act to stimulate growth in adjacent cells in a paracrine manner. The interaction of ligand and receptor in the cytoplasm of the cell may form an internal autocrine loop, as described by Browder and associates (1989).

Autocrine growth factors have been implicated in the stimulation of SCLC cell growth. Most SCLC cell lines produce bombesin (BB), as described by Carney and associates (1987). This 14–amino acid peptide is identical to a carboxy-terminal heptapeptide sequence of a mammalian analog, gastrin-releasing peptide. SCLC cell lines express a single class of high-affinity, saturable binding receptors for bombesin. BB is also a potent stimulator of clonal growth for human SCLC. BB receptors are not present on NSCLC.

Epidermal Growth Factor Receptor

Oncogene products that phosphorylate tyrosine residues (tyrosine kinases) are implicated in retrovirally induced neoplasia. For example, v-*erb*B, the transforming gene of avian erythroblastosis virus, codes for a truncated version of the epidermal growth factor receptor (EGFR). Activation of the overexpressed normal receptor gene is sufficient for transformation of NIH 3T3 cells, as described by Riedel and colleagues (1988). NSCLC, but not SCLC, cells express high levels of functional EGFR and have amplification of the *EGFR* gene, as described by Haeder and colleagues (1988) and Sakiyama and associates (1986). This suggests that growth factors and their receptors may play an important role in the development and maintenance of the malignant phenotype.

Schneider and coworkers (1988, 1990a) investigated the EGFR (*erb*B1) structure in fresh NSCLC cells. Southern analysis showed amplification (more than 2-fold) of the *EGFR* gene in 6 of 60 tumors. However, 24 of 60 tumors showed an absence of a 4.2-kilobase EcoRI restriction enzyme fragment that was present in all normal lung specimens. This was detected specifically by a probe that recognizes the intracellular tyrosine kinase domain of *erb*B1. The absence of the fragment in tumor specimens did not correspond to the appearance of new lower molecular weight fragments detected by a complementary DNA probe, suggesting that the fragment corresponds to a genomic region, possibly at an intron-exon junction. Schneider and colleagues (1988, 1990a) showed that an alteration is present that leads to an increased cleavage efficiency of the restriction endonuclease EcoRI for a specific EcoRI site in this 4.2-kilobase fragment. Samples of lymphocyte DNA from 13 normal donors did not show the 4.2-kilobase fragment. The fragment was present in normal muscle DNA samples and could be cleaved with 40 U of enzyme/μg DNA with spermidine, in contrast to corresponding normal lung, which was not completely digested. Thus, this phenomenon is tissue specific. A possible explanation for this is the existence of tissue-specific methylation differences at the restriction enzyme cleavage site. The methylation of one base in a recognition sequence may inhibit cleavage.

The expression of EGFR by lung cancer cells suggests that the production of a ligand by these cells could mediate an autocrine or paracrine growth stimulation loop. The lung cancer cell lines studied did not produce EGF. However, they did produce transforming growth factor-α (TGF-α), which binds to the EGFR. TGF-α is a single polypeptide of 50 amino acids that is derived from a 160–amino acid transmembrane precursor by proteolytic cleavage. It is structurally and functionally related to EGF and binds to the EGFR. TGF-α alone does not transform normal rat kidney (NRK) cells.

Anchorage-independent growth is seen when pro-TGF-α and TGF-α are added together. TGF-α is a candidate autocrine growth factor for NSCLC. Previous studies indicated that a medium conditioned from A549-1 lung carcinoma cells can promote the growth of human NSCLC cells in culture. This conditioned medium is known to contain TGF-α; exogenous TGF-α added to cultures increased colony formation, as described by Siegfried and Owens (1988).

TGF-α does not need to be cleaved from its conserved integral membrane glycoprotein to have biologic activity. Wong and associates (1989) transfected BHK cells with an expression vector containing altered sequences such that the cells did not secrete TGF-α but expressed the pro-TGF-α on the cell surface, as described by Bringman and associates (1987). The membrane-bound pro-TGF-α bound to EGFR on A431 cells and induced receptor autophosphorylation. Brachmann and colleagues (1989) solubilized pro-TGF-α and found that it induced tyrosine autophosphorylation of EGFR in intact receptor-expressing cells and stimulated anchorage-independent growth of NRK fibroblasts. Thus, both pro-TGF-α and TGF-α could function as autocrine growth factors. The possibilities include interactions of pro-TGF-α with a cytoplasmic form of the EGFR and EGFR expressed on adjacent cells.

The presence of EGFR on lung cancer cells suggests an autocrine-paracrine growth mechanism may be operative. This was investigated in vitro with cloned NSCLC cell lines by Putnam and colleagues (1992). Four NSCLC cell lines expressed the EGFR. None of the cell lines expressed EGF by Northern analysis. However, all cell lines expressed TGF-α messenger RNA, which can bind to the EGFR. Therefore, the investigators studied the biologic response to and production of TGF-α by these cell lines. Each cell line expressed EGFR by phosphorylation and by ^{125}I-labeled EGF competitive binding and Scatchard analysis. The receptors were functionally active, as determined in immune complex kinase assays. The cells showed stimulated ^{3}H-labeled thymidine uptake in response to both TGF-α and EGF. Exogenously added TGF-α increased colony formation in soft agar for three of the four cell lines in media containing serum. All cell lines expressed some TGF-α messenger RNA, although to differing degrees. Possible differences were observed in the mechanism of autocrine growth stimulation among the four cell lines. Two cell lines were specifically growth inhibited by the anti-TGF-α monoclonal antibody AB-3 at a low cell density, suggesting that the antibody blocks an autocrine growth loop. However, the AB-3 antibody did not alter the growth of two of the cell lines, even though these cells express EGFR and secrete TGF-α. Suramin, which blocks the binding of ligands to receptors in other autocrine systems, inhibited the growth of both cell lines, as described by Keating and Williams (1988) and Browder and colleagues (1989). The addition of TGF-α, but not platelet-derived growth factor, specifically reversed the inhibition by suramin. This suggests that autocrine activation for this cell line occurred exclusively in the intracellular compartment between unprocessed receptor and unsecreted ligand. TGF-α appears to be an autocrine growth factor for NSCLC cells of both squamous and adenocarcinoma histologic types. Another strategy, now in clinical trials, is to use an antibody to the EGFR, which can inhibit cancer cell proliferation (Peng et al, 1996).

*erb*B2

The gene *erb*B2 is a member of the *EGFR* family. This family includes three genes with a receptor-like structure, including an external ligand-binding domain, a transmembrane domain, and a cytoplasmic tyrosine kinase domain. Drebin and colleagues (1984) and Schechter and associates (1984) first identified the *neu/erb*B2 oncogene in an ethylnitrosourea-induced rat neuroblastoma. The rat oncogene is activated by a point mutation, but the mechanism in human cells appears to be overexpression, as described by Di Fiore and colleagues (1987) and Slamon and associates (1987). The gene has homology with the *EGFR* gene, and the gene product (molecular weight, 185 kDa) is a tyrosine kinase. Although the structure of this protein is receptor-like, a functional ligand was not conclusively identified by Lupu and associates (1990). Schneider and colleagues (1989, 1990b) in our laboratory were the first to identify activation of *erb*B2 in NSCLC. Amplification of *erb*B2 occurred in 10% of 60 paired samples of NSCLC and normal lung. However, adenocarcinomas showed high messenger RNA levels of *erb*B2. In contrast, SCLC cells did not express *erb*B2. A study of freshly excised surgical specimens confirmed and extended these findings, as described by Schneider and colleagues (1990b). NSCLC specimens showed high levels of *erb*B2 RNA expression in 6 of 16 samples compared with those in paired normal lung samples. Increased expression occurred in both early and advanced stages. Fresh SCLC showed minimal or no expression. Kern and colleagues (1990) found that the expression of the *erb*B2 gene product, p185, occurred at higher levels in the tumor than in the bronchiolar epithelium. They found that *erb*B2 expression in adenocarcinomas was independently correlated with diminished survival.

Insulin-Like Growth Factor

Studies by Minuto and colleagues (1988) and Natale and associates (1988) suggest that insulin-like growth factor-I (IGF-I) may participate in autocrine growth stimulation. Shigematsu and colleagues (1990) observed IGF-I immunostaining in primary NSCLC tumors removed at surgery. ^{125}I-labeled IGF-I competitive binding studies showed the presence of IGF-I receptors. The secretion of IGF-I by SCLC cell lines was shown by Macaulay and colleagues (1990). Two classes of IGF-I receptors were identified by Scatchard analysis. Cell lines and fresh SCLC cells showed increased ^{3}H-labeled thymidine uptake in response to IGF-I, and this was specifically inhibited by an anti-IGF-I monoclonal antibody.

Dominant Oncogenes

ras *Family*

Oncogenes of the *ras* family (homologous to the rat sarcoma virus) have three primary members (H-*ras*, K-*ras*, and N-*ras*), and they are among the most common activated oncogenes found in human cancer, as described by Bos (1989). The *ras* genes code for a protein that is located on the inner surface of the plasma membrane, has guanosine triphosphatase activity, and may participate in signal transduction. The *ras* oncogenes are activated by point nucleotide mutations that alter the amino acid sequence of the protein p21. The presence of a single mutated allele is sufficient to transform some immortalized cell lines, such as NIH 3T3 cells, or other cells, such as rat primary embryo fibroblasts, in the presence of a cooperating oncogene.

Amplification of *ras* oncogenes is uncommon in lung cancer. Heighway and Hasleton (1986) found no amplification of K-*ras* in 25 primary specimens. A lymph-node metastasis showed 30-fold amplification of K-*ras*. Expression of p21, as measured by binding of the monoclonal antibody rp-35 increased with the increasing size of the primary tumor, as described by Dosaka and colleagues (1988).

Activation of the K-*ras* oncogene by point mutation occurs in lung cancer cell lines, as described by Yamamoto and associates (1985) and Shimizu and colleagues (1983). A mutation in codon 12 (glycine to cysteine) occurs in Calu-1 cells and in codon 61 in PR310 cells (glutamine to histidine). Restriction fragment length polymorphism analysis for a codon 12 mutation (glycine to arginine) did not show any mutations in 24 primary NSCLC lung cancers, as described by Milici and colleagues (1986). Rodenhuis and associates (1987, 1988) detected other mutations in the 12th K-*ras* codon by using a highly sensitive technique based on amplification with the polymerase chain reaction and detection with a panel of oligonucleotide probes. The K-*ras* mutations were confined to adenocarcinomas of the lung and occurred in 9 of 35 tumors. Mutations were not observed in adenocarcinomas from nonsmokers. Another study by the same group showed that K-*ras* mutations were an independent prognostic factor, indicating a poor prognosis (Rodenhuis et al, 1990). In all patients, mutations occurred in a single allele. Reynolds and colleagues (1991), using an NIH 3T3 cotransfection-nude mouse tumorigenicity assay, found activated proto-oncogenes of the *ras* family in 86% of lung cancers from smokers. Activated *ras* genes were present in 8 of 10 metastatic adenocarcinomas. No *ras* mutations have been identified in any SCLC tumors or cell lines, as described by Gazdar and associates (1991). Infection of SCLC cell lines with the Harvey murine sarcoma virus altered the phenotype of the variant but not the classic cells, as described by Mabry and associates (1988). Following infection, the variant SCLC cell line developed features of a large cell undifferentiated lung carcinoma, including increased carcinoembryonic antigen and keratin expression.

Studies done to date favor the interpretation of *ras* activation as a progression factor in lung cancer. It apparently is activated in approximately one third of adenocarcinomas arising in patients with a heavy smoking history. However, studies of premalignant lung lesions have not been done to determine whether such mutations exist at the precancerous stage, as is the case for adenocarcinoma of the colon, as described by Vogelstein and colleagues (1988).

Any therapy aimed at the reversal of oncogene function must be highly specific. However, many oncogenes are members of multigene families, the function of which is critical for cell viability. Techniques that globally inhibit the expression of all family members are lethal to the cell. Both tumor and normal cells are affected, as described by Debus and associates (1990). In our laboratory, Mukhopadhyay and associates (1990, 1991b) used antisense technology to find the effects of eliminating expression of a mutant K-*ras* oncogene in NSCLC cells. A homozygous mutation at codon 61 was identified in the NCIH460a large cell undifferentiated NSCLC cell line clone with a normal glutamine residue (cytosine-adenine-adenine) substituted by histidine (cytosine-adenine-thymine), using hybridization with specific oligonucleotide probes and direct polymerase chain reaction DNA sequencing. An antisense K-*ras* RNA construct selectively blocked the production of mutant p21 so that the contribution of the mutated p21 protein to the malignant phenotype could be studied. A recombinant plasmid clone was constructed by using a wild-type 2-kilobase K-*ras* genomic DNA segment carrying second and third exons with flanking intron sequences subcloned into an Apr-1-neo expression vector in the antisense orientation. The intron sequence used has a low degree of homology, with other *ras* genomic sequences, so that specific inhibition of K-*ras* with preservation of H-*ras* and N-*ras* expression would occur. Previous studies with the uptake of ras antisense oligonucleotide by cancer cells resulted in cell death instead of regulated growth. This is probably because functioning p21 is necessary for cell viability, and the oligonucleotide blocked all p21 expression. Blockade of oncogene expression, which is not selective, can therefore be toxic to both normal and cancer cells. An additional novel feature of this construct was the use of a β-actin promoter that can constitutively direct synthesis of RNA in a human tumor cell.

The 2-kilobase DNA insert was stably integrated into H406a cells by Southern hybridization, and Northern blot analysis detected the expression of antisense RNA. Western blot analysis showed a 95% reduction in specific K-*ras* p21 protein synthesis in the clones expressing the antisense RNA; H460a cells and sense K-*ras* clones showed unchanged levels of the K-*ras* p21 protein. The total p21 detected with a pan-*ras* monoclonal antibody showed only a slight decrease in the antisense clones, suggesting other *ras* genes were not affected. Antisense transfectants showed a three-fold reduction in growth compared with sense transfectants and parental H460a cells but continued to grow in culture. The expression of antisense K-*ras* RNA significantly reduced the growth rate of H460a tumors in nu/nu mice. These experiments showed that, in H460a cells engineered to synthesize antisense K-*ras* RNA, the level of K-*ras* messenger RNA and K-*ras* p21 protein were dramatically reduced. Therefore constructs can be made that distinguish among members of the *ras* family. Inhibition of K-*ras* reduced the growth rate of H460a cells but did not alter cell viability or continued growth in culture. This suggests that redundancy in p21 expression may compensate for an absence of expression by one member of this family so that functions essential for maintenance of cell viability are preserved. These observations raise the intriguing possibility of specific molecular therapy for cancer. Sequences could be delivered to tumor cells through viral vectors that would specifically inhibit expression of the oncogenes activated in the cancer cell. Such constructs would be relatively nontoxic because, as in the example cited earlier, they could target a single gene whose function might be subsumed by other redundant genes of the same family. Thus, repeated infusions of immunologically distinct vectors could be performed. Retroviral vectors have the added advantage of being incorporated in the genome only of cells that replicate, thus favoring integration in cancer cell DNA. Similar results have been shown with a single chain antibody against ras p21 protein expressed intracellularly by an adenovirus vector (Cochet et al, 1998).

Sporadic alterations in a variety of other oncogenes are described by Shiraishi and colleagues (1989). Cline and Battifora (1987) found amplification of c-*erb*B-1, c-*myc*, and c-*myb* and deletions in c-H-*ras* and c-*myb*. The expression of proto-oncogenes in SCLC was determined by Kiefer and associates (1987) using Northern analysis. An increased expression of *myc* family genes was confirmed. The *ras* family and c-*raf*1 were expressed in all cell lines. Other oncogenes, including c-*fes*, c-*fos*, c-*erb*B-1, c-*mos*, c-*sis*, c-*erb*A, c-*src*, and c-*abl*, were expressed weakly or not at all.

myc Family

A subgroup of SCLC cell lines have an amplified c-*myc* gene, as described by Little and associates (1983). The SCLC cell lines with an amplified c-*myc* gene are morphologic and biochemical variants of SCLC (SCLC-V). SCLC-V have a rapid doubling time, higher cloning efficiency, increased tumorigenicity, and increased resistance to radiation compared with SCLC, as described by Carney and colleagues (1985). In addition, SCLC-V do not express L-dopa decarboxylase or peptide hormones. They do have elevated levels of the bombesin (BB) isoenzyme or creatine kinase and neuron-specific enolase, which distinguishes them from NSCLC, as described by Gazdar and colleagues (1980). Little and associates (1983) reported that five SCLC-V cell lines showed high levels of c-*myc* amplification and c-*myc* messenger RNA levels. Only one NSCLC cell line of five showed c-*myc* amplification. The c-*myc* gene was transfected into the H209 classic SCLC cell line, as described by Johnson and associates (1986). One of the transfectants expressing high levels of c-*myc* had an increase in doubling time and increased cloning efficiency, but L-dopa decarboxylase levels and BB-like immunoreactivity were unchanged. Kiefer and colleagues (1987) observed amplification of c-*myc* in both classic and variant SCLC cell lines. However, c-*myc* messenger RNA levels were more elevated in the variant cell lines. Three classic lines had amplification of N-*myc* messenger RNA and one variant line had amplification of N-*myc* and *myb*. Three SCLC-V cell lines showed high levels of a v-*fms*–related transcript, which is related but not identical to the colony stimulating factor (CSF)-1 receptor. Bepler and colleagues (1989) identified a subpopulation of SCLC with intermediate neuroendocrine differentiation. The cell lines expressed some neuroendocrine markers, such as L-dopa decarboxylase, but not others, such as BB and neurotensin. These cell lines also had high levels of c-myc protein. Expression of c-myb protein was seen for two cell lines in which c-myc expression was low or not detectable. Expression of c-raf1 protein was low in 11 of the 12 cell lines. Four of five NSCLC cell lines expressed c-myc protein at high levels, and these were all of the large cell undifferentiated morphology. Cline and coworkers (1984) and Cline and Battifora (1987) found that 3 of 27 NSCLC cell DNA from primary tumors had amplification of the c-*myc* gene. Yoshimoto and associates (1986) identified high levels of c-*myc* messenger RNA in an NSCLC cell line in the absence of DNA amplification. Runyon transcription studies showed the transcriptional rate for c-*myc* was high.

Analysis of SCLC cell lines for c-*myc* amplification revealed additional EcoRI restriction fragments, suggesting *myc*-related genes. A third gene in the *myc* family, L-*myc*, was cloned and showed homology to c-*myc* and N-*myc*, as described by Nau and associates (1985). Four SCLC cell lines had amplified L-*myc* genes. The L-*myc* gene was cloned and sequenced and consists of three exons and two introns that span 6.6 kilobases of human DNA, as described by Kaye and associates (1988). There is homology with discrete regions of N-*myc* and c-*myc*. The L-*myc* gene encodes a series of nuclear phosphoprotein that arise by alternative messenger RNA processing, as described by Kaye and associates (1988). L-*myc* can cooperate with an activated c-Ha-*ras* to transform primary rat embryo fibroblasts. However, Birrer and associates (1988) revealed that the transforming efficiency was 1% to 10% of that seen with c-*myc*. One study by Kawashima and colleagues (1988) found a correlation between restriction fragment length polymorphisms of the L-*myc* gene and lymph node metastases in NSCLC. The presence of either the S band (6-kilobase) or the S and L (10-kilobase) bands was associated with lymph node metastases.

Amplification and increased expression of the N-*myc* gene occurs in SCLC and NSCLC. Funa and colleagues (1987) measured the expression of N-*myc* in SCLC biopsies by in situ hybridization. Increased expression was associated with a poor response to chemotherapy and short survival. Amplification of N-*myc* gene sequences, ranging from 5- to 170-fold, was observed in SCLC cell lines by Nau and associates (1986). Both c-*myc* and N-*myc* were amplified, but only one member of the *myc* family was amplified in any one cell line. Saksela and colleagues (1986) reported amplification of N-*myc* in an adenocarcinoma. Ibson and associates (1987) found amplification of one of the *myc* family in 2 of 12 SCLC cell lines. Again only one member of the family was amplified in each cell line. All cell lines had deletions of chromosome 3. When fresh tumor specimens were analyzed by Yokota and colleagues (1987), amplification and rearrangement of *myc* genes was heterogeneous. N-*myc* or L-*myc* amplification was noted in 4 of 17 small cell cancers. Amplification of c-*myc* was seen in 3 of 12 NSCLC specimens. In some cases, amplification was seen in the primary tumor but not in the metastases. In two cases amplification was seen only in cell lines but not in the original tumors. Gu and colleagues (1988) demonstrated expression of *myc* family genes in SCLC cell lines and nude mouse xenografts by using in situ hybridization techniques.

The molecular mechanisms regulating the expression of each of the *myc* family genes are complex, as described by Krystal and colleagues (1988). Both c-*myc* and L-*myc* messenger RNA showed a loss of transcriptional attenuation, which correlated with the overexpression seen in cell lines without gene amplification. Regulation of N-*myc* expression correlated with promoter activity and gene amplification. Sausville and coworkers (1988) found an interesting association between responsiveness to BB and *myc* family expression. SCLC cell lines that were responsive to BB showed constitutive expression of L-*myc*. Nonresponsive cell lines expressed N-*myc* or c-*myc*.

The significance of increased expression in *myc* family genes remains uncertain. Initially c-*myc* amplification was described in SCLC cell lines with variant morphology. This variant morphology is also called small cell/large cell carcinoma and is thought to indicate an unfavorable prognosis. Cell lines with the variant morphology have relatively more resistance to chemotherapy and radiation therapy, as described by Carney and colleagues (1983). However, a study by Aisner and associates (1990), reviewing pathologic specimens of patients with extensive-disease SCLC, showed that the variant cell type was rare, occurring in only 4.4% of 550 specimens. There were no significant differences in response rates to chemotherapy or prognosis for patients with classic compared with variant morphology. Amplification of the c-*myc* gene was more frequent in cell lines from patients with SCLC who had tumor relapses compared with that in untreated patients, as described by Johnson and associates (1987). Amplification of c-*myc* was associated with shorter survival in patients who had relapses. Brennan and colleagues (1991) found that c-*myc* amplification was more frequent in tumors from treated (28%) compared with untreated (8%) patients with SCLC.

It is likely that increased *myc* expression leads to the progression of SCLC. It appears unlikely to be a primary event because it is detected in a minority of tumors. Its association with the variant cell type and the significance of this cell type requires additional study. Increased expression may occur by several mechanisms and is not always associated with gene amplification. Alterations in *myc* expression in NSCLC have not been extensively studied, but in one case several NSCLC showed increased expression of c-*myc* (Bepler et al, 1989).

TUMOR-SUPPRESSOR GENES

The presence of certain gene products appears necessary for the maintenance of controlled cell growth. The inactivation or loss of certain genes may thus contribute to tumor growth. Both copies of the gene must be eliminated or inactivated to eradicate the growth suppressive function of the gene in the classic model. Because both copies must be eliminated, the tumor-suppressor gene is called "recessive." The retinoblastoma (*rb*) gene was one of the first tumor-suppressor genes to be identified. Patients with the familial predisposition have a germ line inactivation of one copy of the *rb* gene. The tumor develops when the wild-type allele is either inactivated or deleted. Sporadic retinoblastoma cases have somatic mutations or deletions, which eliminate the expression of the gene product. This model has stimulated studies searching for consistent chromosomal deletions in human tumors.

Deletions in the short arm of chromosome 3 (p14-p23) are frequently present in SCLC. Cytogenetic studies of fresh tumors confirmed the observations on cell lines, as described by DeFusco and associates (1989). Allelic loss in this region was documented with polymorphic DNA probes, as described by Naylor and colleagues (1987). Specific suppressor genes at the 3p locus have not yet been identified. A loss of heterozygosity for alleles on chromosomes 3, 11, 13, and 17 occurs in NSCLC, as was described by Kok and colleagues (1987); Yokota and associates (1987); Weston and coworkers (1989); and Skinner and colleagues (1990). The frequency of 3p deletions in NSCLC is controversial. Kok and colleagues (1987) and Brauch and associates (1987) found this deletion in all SCLC and NSCLC specimens; others found it in a minority of NSCLC specimens. The high frequency of deletions for both SCLC and NSCLC suggests that loss of specific gene function may be a critical step in the development of lung cancer. Two candidate suppressor genes are the nuclear oncogenes *p53* and *rb*.

Loss of heterozygosity on chromosome 13q suggests that the *rb* locus, located at 13q14, may be deleted. Harbour and associates (1988) found that 60% of SCLC and 75% of carcinoid cell lines did not express *rb* messenger RNA. However, 90% of NSCLC cell lines expressed *rb*. Horowitz and colleagues (1990) and Hensel and associates (1990) confirmed the absence of rb protein expression by SCLC cell lines. Hensel and associates (1990) confirmed that the inactivation of the *rb* gene is frequent in SCLC. Six of six patients who were informative had lost one *rb* allele. Of 13 SCLC cell lines, only 3 expressed more than a trace amount of *rb* messenger RNA. Xu and colleagues (1991) found that the rb protein was absent by immunostaining in 10 of 36 primary NSCLC tumors.

p53

The *p53* gene encodes a 375–amino acid phosphoprotein that can form complexes with viral proteins, such as large T antigen and E1B as described by Lane and Benchimol (1990). Missense mutations are the most common gene mutation yet identified for lung cancer. The mechanism of *p53* transformation is controversial. The wild-type *p53* gene may directly suppress or indirectly activate genes that suppress uncontrolled cell growth. The wild-type *p53* is dominant over the mutant form and thus suppresses the transformed phenotype, as described by Baker and colleagues (1990) and Chen and associates (1990). Thus, the absence of the wild-type *p53* or inactivation of wild-type *p53* may therefore contribute to transformation. However, some studies indicate the presence of the mutant *p53* may be necessary for full expression of the transforming potential of the gene. The presence of the mutant *p53* gene can confer a growth advantage to some cells, as described by Chen and associates (1990) and Finlay and colleagues (1989). Studies by Mukhopadhyay and coworkers (1991a) and Roth and colleagues (1991) in our laboratory show that the absence of *p53* is not sufficient for transformation of NSCLC cells. A lung cancer cell line expressing only the mutant *p53* was transfected with an antisense *p53* construct. A marked reduction in colony formation occurred compared with that in control transfections with vector alone or sense *p53*. The only colonies isolated continued to express *p53*. This suggests that the presence of the mutant *p53* contributed to the maintenance of the transformed phenotype. The wild-type *p53* also suppressed colony formation in cell lines expressing mutant *p53*.

Mutations of *p53* are common in a wide spectrum of tumors. These mutations occur in both NSCLC and SCLC cell lines and fresh tumors, as described by Nigro and colleagues (1989); Takahashi and colleagues (1989); and Chiba and coworkers (1990). Hollstein and associates (1991) and Jones and colleagues (1991) showed that two types of mutations occur as follows: transitions, in which a purine is substituted for a purine or a pyrimidine for a pyrimidine, and transversions, in which a purine is substituted for a pyrimidine or vice versa. Transversions have been identified in association with carcinogens such as benzo[*a*]pyrene. Transitions that have a predilection for cytosine paired with guanine (CpG) dinucleotides (frequently having 5-methylcytosine residues) are indicative of the spontaneous mutation rate. Most mutations in lung cancer are guanine-cytosine to thymine-adenine transversions distributed over 10 codons. This suggests a strong influence of tobacco carcinogens as the cause of these mutations. It has been shown that the potent cigarette smoke carcinogen benzo[*a*]pyrene diol epoxide forms adducts along the exons of the *p53* gene. These adducts occurred at codons that are known to be "hot-spot" mutations in human lung cancers. This establishes the "smoking gun" that links tobacco carcinogens with *p53* mutation formation in human lung cancer (Denissenko et al, 1996).

Other genes are candidates for tumor-suppressor genes in lung cancer. The *p16* gene is a G_1-specific regulatory gene for the cell cycle that blocks progression through the cell cycle by binding cell-cycle–dependent kinases 4 and 6 and inhibiting the action of cyclin D (Liggett and Sidransky, 1998). Although mutations of *p16* are infrequent in lung cancer, protein expression is frequently absent because of methylation of the promoter (Kinoshita et al, 1996). Expression of the *nm23* gene is reduced in rodent tumor cells with the highly metastatic phenotype. The *nm23* gene is located near the centromere of chromosome 17. Allelic deletion was shown in 5 of 12 informative cases, all of which were adenocarcinomas, as described by Leone and colleagues (1991). The protein, tyrosine phosphatase-α, maps to 3p21, a region frequently deleted in lung cancers (LaForgia et al, 1991). Five of 10 lung cancers studied had evidence of allelic deletion of this gene. These studies suggest a possible role for both genes as tumor suppressors. A definitive demonstration of this will require reversal of the malignant phenotype following insertion of these genes into human lung cancer cells.

Clinical Trials Targeting Tumor-Suppressor Genes

Based on these studies, clinical protocols to replace a defective *p53* gene with intratumor injection of recombinant retrovirus or adenovirus expressing normal *p53* were developed (Roth, 1996a; Roth, 1996b). Patients with unresectable NSCLCs that are obstructing a bronchus, are extensive local-regional tumors, or are isolated metastases that have a *p53* mutation and have failed conventional therapy underwent direct intratumor injections with the retroviral supernatant. Successful treatment of local-regional lung cancer has important implications, because as many as one third of patients die with only local disease, and radiation therapy is successful in eradicating the tumor only 20% of the time. Nine patients were entered on this protocol (Roth et al, 1996). Vector-derived *p53* DNA is present in post-treatment biopsies by polymerase chain reaction (PCR) techniques. In situ hybridization studies show nuclear localization of the vector. Post-treatment biopsies show increased apoptosis by TUNEL staining. Three patients have shown tumor regression. No grade II or higher vector-related toxicity was observed.

We evaluated the safety and gene transfer efficacy of monthly intratumoral injections of a recombinant adenovirus containing wild-type *p53* (Adp53) in patients with advanced NSCLC who failed conventional treatments. Adp53 doses were escalated from 10^6 plaque-forming units (pfu) in log increments to 10^{10} pfu with the final level being 10^{11}. Patients were treated with (n = 28) or without (n = 24) cisplatin (CDDP) 80 mg/m^2 IV given three days prior to Adp53 injection because of previous animal studies showing synergistic cancer cell kill with the combination of *p53* gene replacement and DNA damaging agents (Fujiwara et al, 1994; Nguyen et al, 1996). Adp53 vector was injected monthly into the same primary or metastatic tumor under computed tomography (CT) guidance. No significant vector-related toxicity has been seen in up to 6 monthly injections. Clinical responses were evaluated with monthly abdominal and chest CT scans. Prolonged (up to 18+ months) disease stabilization (63%) and regression of tumors more than 50% (8%) has been observed in some patients including those previously treated with CDDP (see Fig. 31–2). Of 12 patients with a major airway obstruction, six showed opening of the airway. Evaluable post-treatment tumor biopsies in patients receiving *Adp53* alone showed adenoviral vector sequences by DNA polymerase chain reaction in 18 out of 21 (86%) patients and vector-specific *p53* messenger RNA sequences by reverse transcription PCR (RT-PCR) in 12 out of 26 (46%) patients. Apoptosis was demonstrated by increased TUNEL staining in post-treatment biopsies from 11 patients. Vector-related toxicity was minimal. Transgene expression occurred in post-treatment tumor biopsies in patents with circulating antibodies to adenovirus. There was little in the inflammatory cells infiltrating the tumor suggesting that non-specific inflammation was not responsible for the therapeutic effects. Actuarial survival at 1 year was 40% for those patients treated with Adp53 alone, which compares favorably with chemotherapy-naive patients who were treated with chemotherapy alone. These results suggest that retroviral- and adenoviral-mediated *p53* gene transfer can be successfully accomplished with minimal toxicity in cancer patients. Preclinical studies in *nu/nu* mouse models with lung colonies from human tumors suggest that systemic administration of *Adp53* combined with 2-methoxyestradiol, which increases the *p53* transgene expression, can successfully eradicate metastases (Kataoka et al, 1998). Thus, gene replacement may have a role in the treatment of both local and systemic cancer.

COMMENTS AND CONTROVERSIES

An understanding of the molecular mechanisms underlying the development and progression of lung cancer may allow the development of rational approaches to prevention, early diagnosis, and therapy. Molecular markers of bronchial epithelial cells may allow the identification of individuals at highest risk for lung cancer. These markers could improve the accuracy of diagnosis by sputum cytologic examination and provide intermediate end-point markers for chemoprevention trials. Molecular markers of prognosis may allow a better selection of patients for aggressive multimodality therapy.

Although much has been learned about molecular events in lung cancer, our knowledge about the mechanism of carcinogenesis is still fragmentary. Many more genetic abnormalities are probably present in lung cancer cells. The nature of these changes and their biologic significance is unknown. A major area of controversy is whether there is a necessary or preferred order for these genetic changes. One theory by Fearon and Vogelstein (1990) proposes that it is an accumulation of genetic alterations rather than a specific order that is critical. The identification of the pathways by which these genes mediate their effects is critical. This may allow the identification of accessible target molecules for prevention and therapy. It is important to know if it is necessary to reverse all or many of these genetic changes to alter the malignant phenotype of the cell. The evidence presented in this chapter suggests that it may be necessary to reverse only one or two abnormalities to have a profound effect on tumor cell growth and tumorigenicity. This is promising from the perspective of applying these findings to therapy. For example, the tracheobronchial tree is readily accessible to direct therapeutic manipulation. Thus, a high-priority research area is the identification of genetic alterations in premalignancy and early malignancy. The development of viral vectors with a high efficiency of gene transduction given regionally in the tracheobronchial tree is one possible approach to altering oncogene expression in high-risk individuals. The potential low toxicity and specificity of this type of therapy makes this an exciting field for future study.

J. A. R.

An understanding of the biology of lung cancer is becoming increasingly important for the surgeon. Not only does it appear to impact on prognosis but soon may impact on therapy strategies. The field is growing rapidly, and the understanding of the biology of lung cancer increases logarithmically every year.

It is hoped that all these advances in our understanding will convert to improved methods of prevention, early identification, estimation of prognosis, and, ultimately, therapeutic intervention. For all these reasons, thoracic surgeons who manage patients with lung cancer must have a basic understanding of the biology of the disease.

R. J. G.

■ *KEY REFERENCES*

Bishop JM: Molecular themes in oncogenesis. Cell 64:235, 1991.

In this comprehensive review, the major molecular mechanisms implicated to date in the development of cancer are discussed. The topics include dominant oncogenes and tumor-suppressor genes.

Cross M, Dexter TM: Growth factors in development, transformation, and tumorigenesis. Cell 64:271, 1991.

The authors review the molecular aspects of growth factors. They discuss the biologic responses of cells to growth factors and their role in the development of malignancy.

Vinocour M, Minna JD: Cellular and molecular biology of lung cancer. In Roth JA, Ruckdeschel JC, Weisenburger TH (eds): Thoracic Oncology. Philadelphia, WB Saunders, 1989.

This chapter presents a comprehensive review of molecular biology as it applies to lung cancer.

■ *REFERENCES*

Aisner SC, Finkelstein DM, Ettinger DS et al: The clinical significance of variant-morphology small-cell carcinoma of the lung. J Clin Oncol 8:402, 1990.

Baker SJ, Markowitz S, Fearon ER et al: Suppression of human colorectal carcinoma cell growth by wild-type p53. Science 249:912, 1990.

Belinsky SA, Devereux TR, Maronpot RR et al: Relationship between the formation of promutagenic adducts and the activation of the K-ras protooncogene in lung tumors from A/J mice treated with nitrosamines. Cancer Res 49:5305, 1989.

Bepler G, Bading H, Heimann B et al: Expression of p64c-myc and neuroendocrine properties define three subclasses of small cell lung cancer. Oncogene 4:45, 1989.

Birrer MJ, Segal S, DeGreve JS et al: L-myc cooperates with *ras* to transform primary rat embryo fibroblasts. Mol Cell Biol 8:2668, 1988.

Bos JL: Ras oncogenes in human cancer: A review. Cancer Res 49:4682, 1989.

Brachmann R, Lindquist PB, Nagashima M et al: Transmembrane TGR-alpha precursors activate EGF/TGF-alpha receptors. Cell 56:691, 1989.

Brauch H, Johnson B, Hovis J et al: Molecular analysis of the short arm of chromosome 3 in small cell and non-small cell carcinoma of the lung. N Engl J Med 317:1109, 1987.

Brennan J, O'Connor T, Makuch RW et al: Myc family DNA amplification in 107 tumors and tumor cell lines from patients with small cell lung cancer treated with different combination chemotherapy regimens. Cancer Res 51:1708, 1991.

Bringman TS, Lindquist PB, Derynck R: Different transforming growth factor-alpha species are derived from a glycosylated and palmitoylated transmembrane precursor. Cell 48:429, 1987.

Browder TM, Dunbar CE, Nienhuis AW: Private and public autocrine loops in neoplastic cells. Cancer Cells 1:9, 1989.

Caporaso NE, Tucker MA, Hoover RN et al: Lung cancer and the debrisoquine metabolic phenotype. J Natl Cancer Inst 82:1264, 1990.

Carney DN, Bunn PA Jr, Gazdar AF et al: Selective growth in serum-free hormone-supplemented medium of tumor cells obtained by biopsy from patients with small cell carcinoma of the lung. Proc Natl Acad Sci U S A 78:3185, 1981.

Carney DN, Cuttitta F, Moody TW, Minna JD: Selective stimulation of small cell lung cancer clonal growth by bombesin and gastrin-releasing peptide. Cancer Res 47:821, 1987.

Carney DN, Gazdar AF, Bepler G et al: Establishment and identification of small cell lung cancer cell lines having classic and variant features. Cancer Res 45:2913, 1985.

Carney DN, Mitchell JB, Kinsella TJ: In vitro radiation and chemotherapy sensitivity of established cell lines of human small cell lung cancer and its large cell morphological variants. Cancer Res 43:2806, 1983.

Chen P-L, Chen Y, Bookstein R, Lee W-H: Genetic mechanisms of tumor suppression by the human p53 gene. Science 250:1576, 1990.

Chiba I, Takahashi T, Nau MM et al: Mutations in the p53 gene are frequent in primary, resected non-small cell lung cancer. Oncogene 5:1603, 1990.

Cline MJ, Battifora H: Abnormalities of proto-oncogenes in non-small cell lung cancer. Cancer 60:2669, 1987.

Cline MJ, Slamon DJ, Lipsick JS: Oncogenes: Implications for the diagnosis and treatment of cancer. Ann Intern Med 101:223, 1984.

Cochet OK, Kenigsberg M, Delumeau I et al: Intracellular expression of an antibody fragment-neutralizing p21 ras promotes tumor regression. Cancer Res 58:1170–1176, 1998.

Debus N, Berdichevsky FB, Gryasnov SM: Effects of antisense oligodeoxyribonucleotides complementary mRNA of the human c-Harvey-ras oncogene on cell proliferation (Abstract). J Cancer Res Clin Oncol 116(Suppl, part 1):S-162, 1990.

DeFusco PA, Frytak S, Dahl RJ et al: Cytogenetic studies in 11 patients with small cell carcinoma of the lung. Mayo Clin Proc 64:168, 1989.

Denissenko MF, Pao A, Tang M et al: Preferential formation of benzo[a]-pyrene adducts at lung cancer mutational hotspots in p53. Science 274:430–432, 1996.

Di Fiore PP, Pierce JH, Kraus MH et al: ErbB-2 is a potent oncogene when overexpressed in NIH/3T3 cells. Science 237:178, 1987.

Dosaka H, Harada M, Kizumaki N et al: The relationship of clinical classification to ras p21 expression in human non-small cell lung cancer. Oncology 45:396, 1988.

Drebin J, Stern DF, Link VC et al: Monoclonal antibodies identify a cell surface antigen associated with an activated cellular oncogene. Nature 312:545, 1984.

Fearon ER, Vogelstein B: A genetic model for colorectal tumorigenesis. Cell 61:759, 1990.

Finlay CA, Hinds PW, Levine AJ: The p53 proto-oncogene can act as a suppressor of transformation. Cell 57:1083, 1989.

Fujiwara T, Grimm EA, Mukhopadhyay T et al: Induction of chemosensitivity in human lung cancer cells *in vivo* by adenoviral-mediated transfer of the wild-type p53 gene. Cancer Res 54:2287–2291, 1994.

Funa K, Steinholtz L, Nou E, Bergh J: Increased expression of N-myc in human small cell lung cancer biopsies predicts lack of response to chemotherapy and poor prognosis. Am J Clin Pathol 88:216, 1987.

Gazdar AF, Carney DN, Nau MN, Minna JD: Characterization of variant subclasses of cell lines derived from small cell lung cancer having distinctive biochemical, morphological, and growth properties. Cancer Res 45:2924, 1985.

Gazdar AF, Carney DN, Russell EK et al: Establishment of continuous clonable cultures of small-cell carcinoma of the lung which have amine precursor uptake and decarboxylation cell properties. Cancer Res 40:3502, 1980.

Gazdar AF, Giaccone G, Mitsudomi T: The association between drug resistance of lung cancer cell lines and neuroendocrine differentiation and oncogene activation. J Cell Biochem 15F(Suppl):16, 1991.

Gazdar AF, Oie HK: Cell culture methods for human lung cancer. Cancer Genet Cytogenet 19:5, 1986.

Goldsworthy TL, Hanigan MH, Pitot HC: Models of hepatocarcinogenesis in the rat: Contrasts and comparisons. Crit Rev Toxicol 17:61, 1986.

Gu J, Linnoila RI, Seibel NL et al: A study of myc-related gene expression in small cell lung cancer by in situ hybridization. Am J Pathol 132:13, 1988.

Haeder M, Rotsch M, Bepler G et al: Epidermal growth factor receptor expression in human lung cancer cell lines. Cancer Res 48:1132, 1988.

Harbour JW, Lai S-L, Whang-Peng J et al: Abnormalities in structure and expression of the human retinoblastoma gene in SCLC. Science 241:353, 1988.

Heighway J, Hasleton PS: c-Ki-ras amplification in human lung cancer. Br J Cancer 53:285, 1986.

Hensel CH, Hsieh CL, Gazdar AF et al: Altered structure and expression of the human retinoblastoma susceptibility gene in small cell lung cancer. Cancer Res 50:3067, 1990.

Hoffmann D, Hecht SS: N'nitrosonornicotine in tobacco. Science 186:265, 1974.

Hollstein M, Sidransky D, Vogelstein B, Harris CC: p53 mutations in human cancers. Science 253:49, 1991.

Hoover R: Epidemiology: Tobacco and geographic pathology. In Harris CC (ed): Pathogenesis and Therapy of Lung Cancer. New York, Marcel Dekker, 1978.

Horowitz JM, Park SH, Bogenmann E et al: Frequent inactivation of the retinoblastoma anti-oncogene is restricted to a subset of human tumor cells. Proc Natl Acad Sci U S A 87:2775, 1990.

Ibson JM, Waters JJ, Twentyman PR et al: Oncogene amplification and chromosomal abnormalities in small cell lung cancer. J Cell Biochem 33:267, 1987.

Johnson BE, Battey J, Linnoila I et al: Changes in the phenotype of human small cell lung cancer cell lines after transfection and expression of the c-myc proto-oncogene. J Clin Invest 78:525, 1986.

Johnson BE, Ihde DC, Makuch RW et al: Myc family oncogene amplification in tumor cell lines established from small cell lung cancer patients and its relationship to clinical status and course. J Clin Invest 79:1629, 1987.

Jones PA, Buckley JD, Henderson BE et al: From gene to carcinogen: A rapidly evolving field in molecular epidemiology. Cancer Res 51:3617, 1991.

Kataoka M, Schumacher G, Cristiano RJ et al: An agent that increases tumor suppressor transgene product coupled with systemic transgene delivery inhibits growth of metastatic lung cancer in vivo. Cancer Res 58:4761–4765, 1998.

Kawashima K, Shikama H, Imoto K et al: Close correlation between restriction fragment length polymorphism of the L-myc gene and metastasis of human lung cancer to the lymph nodes and other organs. Proc Natl Acad Sci U S A 85:2353, 1988.

Kaye F, Battey J, Nau M et al: Structure and expression of the human L-myc gene reveal a complex pattern of alternative mRNA processing. Mol Cell Biol 8:186, 1988.

Keating MT, Williams LT: Autocrine stimulation of intracellular PDGF receptors in v-sis-transformed cells. Science 239:914, 1988.

Kern JA, Schwartz DA, Nordberg JE et al: P185-neu expression in human lung adenocarcinomas predicts shortened survival. Cancer Res 50:5184, 1990.

Kiefer PE, Bepler G, Kubasch M, Havemann K: Amplification and expression of proto-oncogenes in human small cell lung cancer cell lines. Cancer Res 47:6236, 1987.

Kinoshita I, Dosaka-Akita H, Mishina T et al: Altered p16(INK4) and retinoblastoma protein status in non-small cell lung cancer: Potential synergistic effect with altered p53 protein on proliferative activity. Cancer Res 56:5557–5562, 1996.

Kok K, Osinga J, Carritt B et al: Deletion of a DNA sequence at the chromosomal region 3p21 in all major types of lung cancer. Nature 330:578, 1987.

Krystal G, Birrer M, Way J et al: Multiple mechanisms for transcriptional regulation of the myc gene family in small-cell lung cancer. Mol Cell Biol 8:3373, 1988.

LaForgia S, Morse B, Levy J et al: Receptor protein-tyrosine phosphatase gamma is a candidate tumor suppressor gene at human chromosome region 3p21. Proc Natl Acad Sci U S A 88:5036, 1991.

Lane DP, Benchimol S: P53: Oncogene or anti-oncogene? Genes Dev 4:1, 1990.

Leone A, McBride OW, Weston A et al: Somatic allelic deletion of nm23 in human cancer. Cancer Res 51:2490, 1991.

Liggett WH Jr, Sidransky D: Role of the p16 tumor suppressor gene in cancer. J Clin Oncol 16:1197–1206, 1998.

Little CD, Nau MM, Carney DN et al: Amplification and expression of the c-myc oncogene in human lung cancer cell lines. Nature 306:194, 1983.

Lupu R, Colomer R, Zugmaier G et al: Direct interaction of a ligand for the erbB2 oncogene product with the EGF receptor and p185erbB2. Science 249:1552, 1990.

Lynch HT, Kimberling WJ, Markvicka SE et al: Genetics and smoking-associated cancers. Cancer 57:1640, 1986.

Mabry M, Nakagawa T, Nelkin BD et al: V-Ha-ras oncogene insertion: A model for tumor progression of human small cell lung cancer. Proc Natl Acad Sci U S A 85:6523, 1988.

Mabry M, Nelkin BD, Falco JP et al: Transitions between lung cancer phenotypes: Implications for tumor progression. Cancer Cells 3:53, 1991.

Macaulay VM, Everard MJ, Teale JD et al: Autocrine function for insulin-like growth factor I in human small cell lung cancer cell lines and fresh tumor cells. Cancer Res 50:2511, 1990.

Malkinson AM: The genetic basis of susceptibility to lung tumors in mice. Toxicology 54:241, 1989.

McLemore TL, Adelberg S, Liu MC et al: Expression of CYP1A1 gene in patients with lung cancer: Evidence for cigarette smoke-induced gene expression in normal lung tissue and for altered gene regulation in primary pulmonary carcinoma. J Natl Cancer Inst 82:1333, 1990.

Milici A, Blick M, Murphy E, Gutterman JU: c-K-ras codon 12 GGT-CGT point mutation: An infrequent event in human lung cancer. Biochem Biophys Res Commun 140:699, 1986.

Minuto F, DelMonte P, Barreca A et al: Evidence for autocrine mitogenic stimulation by somatomedin-C/insulin-like growth factor I on an established human lung cancer cell line. Cancer Res 48:3716, 1988.

Mukhopadhyay T, Cavender A, Tainsky M, Roth JA: Expression of antisense K-ras message in a human lung cancer cell line with a spontaneous activated K-ras oncogene alters the transformed phenotype. Proc Am Assoc Cancer Res 31:304, 1990.

Mukhopadhyay T, Cavender AC, Branch CD, Roth JA: Expression and regulation of wild type p53 gene (wtp53) in human non-small cell lung cancer (NSCLC) cell lines carrying normal or mutated p53 gene. J Cell Biochem 15F(Suppl):22, 1991a.

Mukhopadhyay T, Tainsky M, Cavender AC, Roth JA: Specific inhibition of K-ras expression and tumorigenicity of lung cancer cells by antisense RNA. Cancer Res 51:1744, 1991b.

Murray MJ, Shilo BZ, Shih C et al: Three different human tumor cell lines contain different oncogenes. Cell 25:355, 1981.

Natale RB, Cuttitta F, Nakanishi Y et al: IGF-I can stimulate proliferation of non-small cell lung cancer cell lines in vitro (Abstract). Proc Am Soc Clin Oncol 7:197, 1988.

Nau MM, Brooks BJ, Battey J et al: L-myc, a new myc-related gene amplified and expressed in human small cell lung cancer. Nature 318:69, 1985.

Nau MM, Brooks BJ, Carney DN et al: Human small-cell lung cancers show amplification and expression of the N-myc gene. Proc Natl Acad Sci U S A 83:1092, 1986.

Naylor SL, Johnson BE, Minna JD, Sakaguchi AY: Loss of heterozygosity of chromosome 3p markers in small-cell lung cancer. Nature 329:451, 1987.

Nguyen DM, Spitz FR, Yen N et al: Gene therapy for lung cancer: Enhancement of tumor suppression by a combination of sequential systemic cisplatin and adenovirus-mediated p53 gene transfer. J Thorac Cardiovasc Surg 112:1372–1377, 1996.

Nicolson GL: Cancer metastasis: Tumor cell and host organ properties important in metastasis to specific secondary sites. Biochim Biophys Acta 948:175, 1988.

Nigro JM, Baker SJ, Preisinger AC et al: Mutations in the p53 gene occur in diverse human tumor types. Nature 342:705, 1989.

Ooi WL, Elston RC, Chen VW et al: Increased familial risk for lung cancer. J Natl Cancer Inst 76:217, 1986.

Peng D, Fan Z, Lu Y et al: Anti-epidermal growth factor receptor monoclonal antibody 225 up-regulates p27KIP1 and induces G1 arrest in prostatic cancer cell line DU1451. Cancer Res 56:3666–3669, 1996.

Putnam EA, Yen N, Gallick GE et al: Autocrine growth stimulation by transforming growth factor alpha in human non-small cell lung cancer. Surg Oncol 1:49, 1992.

Reynolds SH, Anna CK, Brown KC et al: Activated protooncogenes in human lung tumors from smokers. Proc Natl Acad Sci U S A 88:1085, 1991.

Riedel H, Massoglia S, Schlessinger J, Ullrich A: Ligand activation of overexpressed epidermal growth factor receptors transforms NIH 3T3 mouse fibroblasts. Proc Natl Acad Sci U S A 85:1477, 1988.

Rodenhuis S, Slebos FJC, Kibbelaar RE et al: Mutational activation of the Kirsten-ras oncogene is associated with early relapse and poor survival in adenocarcinoma of the lung. Proc Am Soc Clin Oncol 9:228, 1990.

Rodenhuis S, Slebos RJC, Boot AJM et al: Incidence and possible clinical significance of K-ras oncogene activation in adenocarcinoma of the human lung. Cancer Res 48:5738, 1988.

Rodenhuis S, Van De Wetering ML, Mooi WJ et al: Mutational activation of the K-ras oncogene. N Engl J Med 317:929, 1987.

Roth JA, Mukhopadhyay T, Yen N et al: Molecular approach to lung cancer therapy. J Cell Biochem Suppl 15F:4, 1991.

Roth JA: Clinical protocol: Modification of tumor suppressor gene expression and induction of apoptosis in non-small cell lung cancer (NSCLC) with an adenovirus vector expressing wildtype p53 and cisplatin. Hum Gene Ther 7:1013–1030, 1996a.

Roth JA: Clinical protocol: Modification of tumor suppressor gene expression in non-small cell lung cancer (NSCLC) with a retroviral vector expressing wildtype (normal) p53. Hum Gene Ther 7:861–874, 1996b.

Roth JA, Nguyen D, Lawrence DD et al: Retrovirus-mediated wild-type p53 gene transfer to tumors of patients with lung cancer. Nat Med 2:985–991, 1996.

Sakiyama S, Nakamura Y, Yasuda S: Expression of epidermal growth factor receptor gene in cultured human lung cancer cells. Jpn J Cancer Res 77:965, 1986.

Saksela K, Bergh J, Nilsson K: Amplification of the N-myc oncogene in an adenocarcinoma of the lung. J Cell Biochem 31:297, 1986.

Samet JM, Humble CG, Pathak DR: Personal and family history of respiratory disease and lung cancer risk. Am Rev Respir Dis 134:466, 1986.

Sausville EA, Moyer JD, Heikkila R et al: A correlation of bombesin responsiveness with myc-family gene expression in small cell lung carcinoma cell lines. Ann N Y Acad Sci 547:310, 1988.

Schechter AL, Stern DF, Vaidyanathan L et al: The neu oncogene: An erb-B-related gene encoding a 185,000-Mr tumour antigen. Nature 312:513, 1984.

Schneider PM, Hung M-C, Ames RS et al: Novel alteration in the epidermal growth factor receptor gene is frequently detected in human non-small cell lung cancer. Lung Cancer 6:65, 1990a.

Schneider PM, Hung M-C, Chiocca SM et al: Differential expression of the c-erbB-2 gene in human small cell and non-small cell lung cancer. Cancer Res 49:4968, 1989.

Schneider PM, Hung M-C, Tainsky MA et al: Epidermal growth factor receptor gene abnormalities in human non-small cell lung cancer. J Cell Biochem Suppl 12A:113, 1988.

Schneider PM, Praeuer HW, Fink U et al: Comparison of neu (c-erbB2) gene expression in small cell lung cancer (SCLC), non-small cell lung cancer (NSCLC), and normal lung. Proc Am Assoc Cancer Res 31:312, 1990b.

Sellers TA, Bailey-Wilson JE, Elston RC et al: Evidence for mendelian inheritance on the pathogenesis of lung cancer. J Natl Cancer Inst 82: 1272, 1990.

Shigematsu K, Kataoka Y, Kurihara M et al: Partial characterization of insulin-like growth factor-I in primary human lung cancers using immunohistochemical and receptor autoradiographic techniques. Cancer Res 50:2481, 1990.

Shih C, Padhy LC, Murray MJ, Weinberg RA: Transferring genes of carcinomas and neuroblastomas introduced into mouse fibroblasts. Nature 290:261, 1981.

Shimizu K, Birnbaum D, Ruly MA et al: Structure of the Ki-ras gene of the human lung carcinoma cell line Calu-l. Nature 304:497, 1983.

Shiraishi M, Noguchi M, Shimosato Y, Sekiya T: Amplification of protooncogenes in surgical specimens of human lung carcinomas. Cancer Res 49:6474, 1989.

Siegfried JM, Owens SE: Response of primary human lung carcinomas to autocrine growth factors produced by a lung carcinoma cell line. Cancer Res 48:4976, 1988.

Skillrud DM, Offord KP, Miller RD: Higher risk of lung cancer in chronic obstructive pulmonary disease. Ann Intern Med 105:503, 1986.

Skinner MA, Vollmer R, Huper G et al: Loss of heterozygosity for genes on 11p and the clinical course of patients with lung carcinoma. Cancer Res 50:2303, 1990.

Slamon DJ, Clark GM, Wong SG et al: Human breast cancer correlation of relapse and survival with amplification of the HER-2/neu oncogene. Science 235:177, 1987.

Stehelin D, Varnus HE, Bishop JM, Vogt PK: DNA related to the transforming gene(s) of avian sarcoma viruses is present in normal avian DNA. Nature 260:170, 1976.

Takahashi T, Nau MM, Chiba I et al: P53: A frequent target for genetic abnormalities in lung cancer. Science 246:491, 1989.

Vogelstein B, Fearon ER, Hamilton SR et al: Genetic alterations during colorectal-tumor development. N Engl J Med 319:525, 1988.

Weston A, Willey JC, Modali R et al: Differential DNA sequence deletions from chromosomes 3, 11, 13, and 17 in squamous-cell carcinoma, large-cell carcinoma, and adenocarcinoma of the lung. Proc Natl Acad Sci U S A 86:5099, 1989.

Wong ST, Winchell LF, McCune BK et al: The TGF-alpha precursor expressed on the cell surface binds to the EGF receptor on adjacent cells leading to signal transduction. Cell 56:495, 1989.

Xu H-J, Hu S-X, Cagle PT et al: Absence of retinoblastoma protein expression in primary non-small cell lung carcinomas. Cancer Res 51:2735, 1991.

Yamamoto F, Nakano H, Neville C, Perucho M: Structure and mechanisms of activation of c-K-ras oncogenes in human lung cancer. Prog Med Virol 32:101, 1985.

Yokota J, Wada M, Shimosato Y et al: Loss of heterozygosity on chromosomes 3, 13, and 17 in small-cell carcinoma and on chromosome 3 in adenocarcinoma of the lung. Proc Natl Acad Sci U S A 84:9252, 1987.

Yoshimoto K, Hirohashi S, Sekiya T: Increased expression of the c-myc gene without gene amplification in human lung cancer and colon cancer cell lines. Jpn J Cancer Res 77:540, 1986.

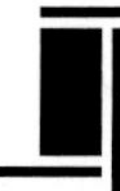

EPIDEMIOLOGY OF LUNG CANCER

Anthony B. Miller

DEFINITION

Epidemiology is the science that identifies the distribution and determinants (causes) of disease. Descriptive epidemiology documents the changes in the incidence of and mortality rate from disease with time and the differences in the rates of disease in different populations. Analytic epidemiology evaluates disease determinants, mainly using two types of studies: case-control and cohort. In case-control studies, the histories of cases (patients with the disease) and controls (those without the disease), who are drawn from the same population as the cases, are compared. In cohort studies, the status of large numbers of individuals is ascertained, and participants are followed to determine the subsequent incidence or mortality rate from the disease. Case-control studies usually consider one cancer site, but they can simultaneously evaluate the effect of multiple exposures to different hazards. Cohort studies usually consider limited numbers of exposures (e.g., occupation or tobacco use), but they can evaluate the effect of these exposures on many different diseases.

In this subchapter, I refer to two different measures of the risk of disease in humans, derived from analytic epidemiology: the relative risk and the attributable risk. The relative risk is the multiple of disease risk in one group (e.g., smokers of cigarettes) relative to that in a referent group (e.g., nonsmokers of cigarettes). When the risk is increased, the relative risk is greater than 1; when the risk is less than that in the referent group, the relative risk is less than 1. A relative risk of 1.0 means no increased risk; one of 1.5 is a 50% increase in risk; one of 2.0 is a doubling of risk; and one of 10.0 is a 10-fold increase in risk. In a well-conducted study, a finding of a relative risk of more than 2.0 is very suggestive of a causal association; one greater than 5.0 is almost certainly causal. The attributable risk is the amount of disease attributable to (or caused by) a factor. In a cohort study, the amount of disease attributable to a factor can be directly determined. In a population-based case-control study, the amount of disease in that population that was attributable to the exposure can be estimated.

HISTORICAL NOTE

In the 19th century, lung cancer was a rare disease. Throughout most of the 20th century, the incidence of and mortality rate from lung cancer in men in North America and Europe rose, and is now rising in the rest of the world. The rates started rising in women approximately 30 years later than in men. Initially there was confusion as to the cause of this epidemic. Although some suspected tobacco, the potential causes also under consideration in the late 1940s were increased automobile exhaust fumes and general air pollution. However, the early case-control studies published in the 1950s (Doll and Hill, 1952; Wynder and Graham, 1950), followed by several cohort studies in Britain and North America (Doll and Peto, 1976; Hammond and Horn, 1958; Kahn, 1966), confirmed that the cause is tobacco, largely cigarette smoking. In the British doctors study (Doll and Peto, 1976), after a 20-year follow-up, the mean annual death rate from lung cancer in nonsmokers was 10 per 100,000; that in smokers of 15 to 24 cigarettes/day was 127 per 100,000. The risk in these smokers relative to the nonsmokers was therefore 12.7. The number of deaths from lung cancer attributable to smoking 15 to 24 cigarettes/day among those with this intensity of smoking is derived by subtracting the rate of death from lung cancer in the nonsmokers from that in the smokers, under the assumption that the smokers would have had the same death rate as the nonsmokers if they had not smoked. In this instance, the attributable risk is 127 minus 10 per 100,000 = 117 (i.e., 117/127 x 100%, or 92%). Numerous studies confirmed that 80% to 90% of the lung cancer in developed countries is attributable to tobacco use. The risk of lung cancer is dependent on the age at which smoking starts, the intensity of smoking, and the duration of the habit. Of these factors, duration is the most important.

■ *HISTORICAL READINGS*

Doll R, Hill AB: A study of the aetiology of carcinoma of the lung. BMJ 2:1271, 1952.

Doll R, Peto R: Mortality in relation to smoking: 20 years observations on male British doctors. BMJ 2:1525, 1976.

Hammond EC, Horn D: Smoking and death rates: Report on forty-four months of follow-up of 187,783 men. II. Death rates by cause. JAMA 166:1294, 1958.

Kahn HA: The Dorn study of smoking and mortality among US veterans: Report on eight and one-half years of observation. Monogr Natl Cancer Inst 19:1, 1966.

Wynder EL, Graham EA: Tobacco smoking as a possible etiologic factor in bronchiogenic carcinoma: A study of six hundred and eighty-four proved cases. JAMA 143:329, 1950.

DESCRIPTIVE EPIDEMIOLOGY

It is well recognized that lung cancer is now the most important cancer in men in terms of both incidence and mortality (Parkin et al, 1999) and although it is not the most important cancer in women in terms of incidence (breast cancer still holds this position), it is now the number one cancer in terms of mortality in North America. With the decline in the cardiovascular disease mortality rate, lung cancer is the number one cause of death attributable to tobacco in the United States (Shopland et al, 1991), having supplanted coronary heart dis-

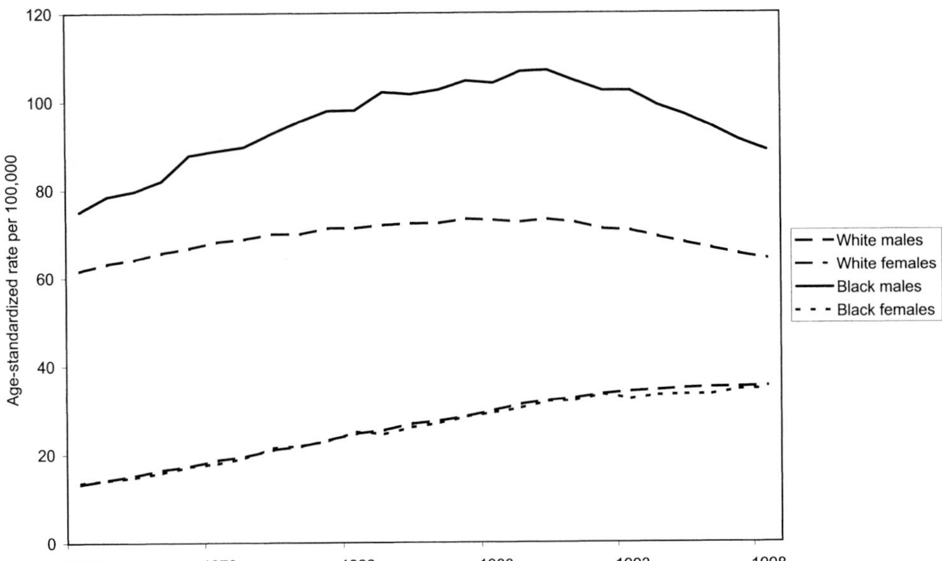

FIGURE 31–4 ■ Trends in mortality from lung cancer—United States. (Data from SEER Cancer Statistics, Review 1973–1978.) (www.seer.ims.nci.nih.gov)

ease as the leading cause of death among smokers in 1987.

For most of the 20th century, lung cancer rates were rising in men, with the rise in women occurring largely in the latter half of the century. Brown and Kessler (1988) analyzed trends in smoking and projections of resulting long-term (to 2025) lung cancer mortality rates in men and women for the United States. Although the age-adjusted rates in women are expected to almost reach those in men during this time period, they are not expected to exceed them. However, in women the age-standardized rate will not begin to decline until about 2020. Within age groups, the decline in the lung cancer mortality rate for men is occurring for all ages up to about 60 years, but for women, the rate declines only up to age 45 years. The decline in the age-specific mortality rate for women is expected to remain about 20 years behind that for men. With declining smoking rates (Marcus et al, 1989), there was anticipation that a downturn of the rates in men might be about to occur (Devesa et al, 1989). This has now been confirmed. Figure 31–4 shows that the age-standardized mortality rate from lung cancer in men peaked in 1988 in white males and in 1992 in black males in the United States, and has been falling since. As yet there is no decline for women, although there is a suggestion that rates may be beginning to plateau.

In men in North America, lung cancer rates rise throughout life, most steeply at ages older than 50 years, except at extreme old age (Fig. 31–5). In women in North America, the age-specific incidence of lung cancer does not yet express the full effect of smoking, hence the downturn in rates at younger ages than men. It is of interest that at nearly every age, the incidence of lung cancer in black men is higher than that in whites, whereas for black and white women, the rates are similar. This probably represents higher smoking rates in black men than in white men, but also higher exposure to other causes of lung cancer, such as carcinogens in the occupational environment.

Internationally, as for other cancers, there are substantial differences in the incidence of lung cancer. Figure 31–6 depicts this for selected cancer registries. The highest rates in the world in 1990 were recorded in blacks in the United States' central Louisiana. The lowest were recorded from a rural cancer registry in India, although the rates in Native Americans in New Mexico were also low. Within countries there are substantial differences by race and ethnicity. Nearly all of these differences reflect differences in the prevalence of cigarette smoking about 40 years ago. As the smoking prevalence changes, international differences will change, with a similar delay. It seems probable that in the 21st century the country with the highest rates will be China, with possibly Japan not far behind. The numbers of lung cancers diagnosed each year in many other countries of Asia, Africa, and South America will also increase substantially, with falls continuing in Europe and North America. Thus lung cancer

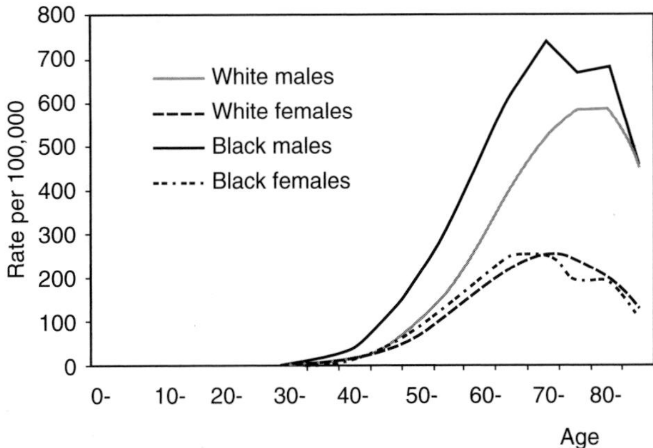

FIGURE 31–5 ■ Age-specific rates of lung cancer—United States. (From Parkin DM, Whelan SL, Ferlay J et al: Cancer incidence in five continents, Vol VII. IARC Scientific Publications no. 143. Lyon, International Agency for Research on Cancer, 1997, pp 314–321, 842, 843.)

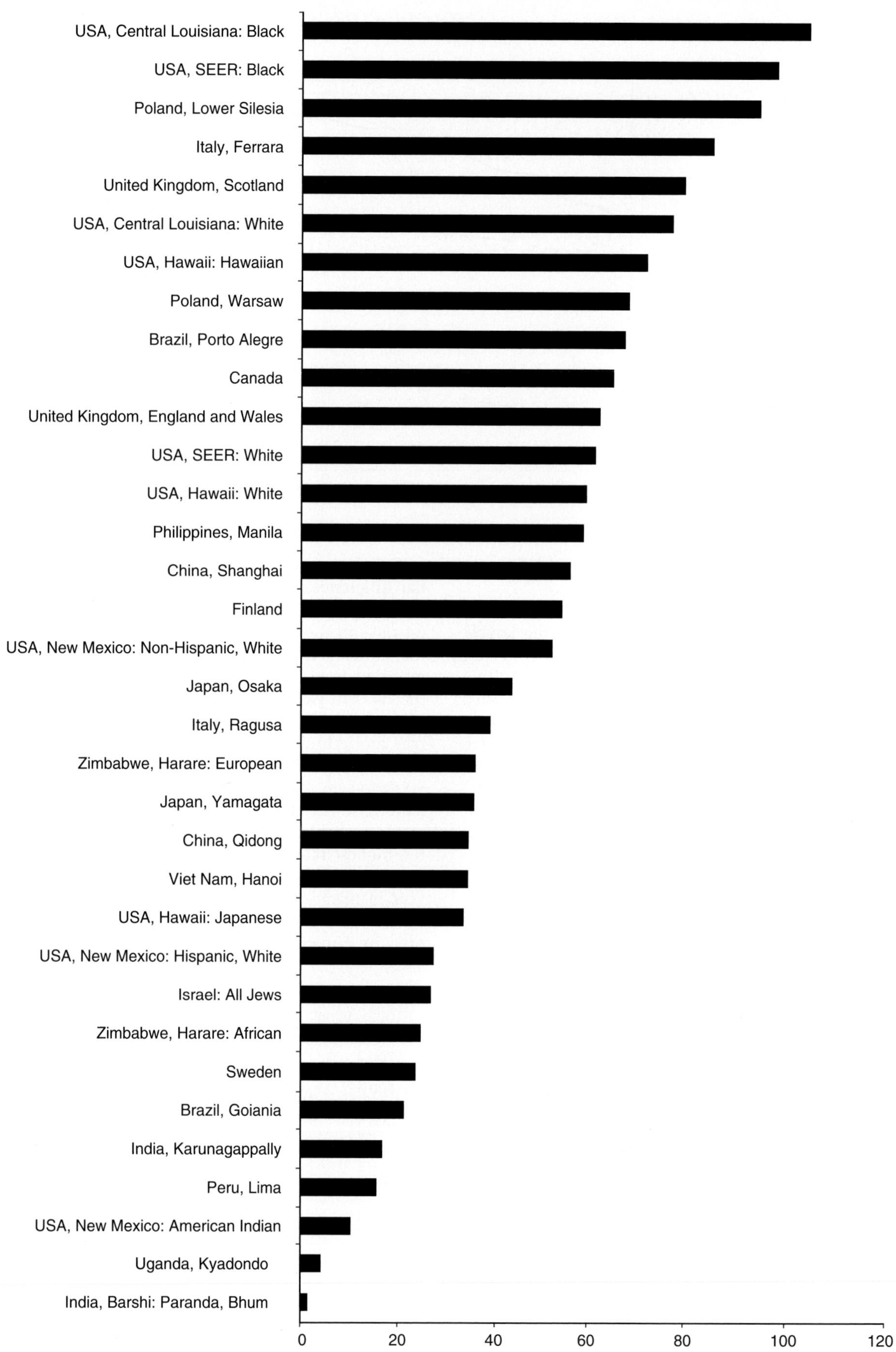

FIGURE 31–6 ■ Age-standardized incidence of lung cancer in men—selected cancer registries. SEER, Surveillance, Epidemiology, and End Results [Program]. (From Parkin DM, Whelan SL, Ferlay J et al: Cancer incidence in five continents, Vol VII. IARC Scientific Publications no. 143. Lyon, International Agency for Research on Cancer, 1997, pp 314–321, 842, 843.)

will have been the predominant cancer in the developed world in the 20th century, but it will become the predominant cancer in the developing world in the 21st century.

LUNG CANCER AND ACTIVE SMOKING

More evidence is available on tobacco smoking as a cause of lung cancer than for any other complex mixture of carcinogens, such as is present in mainstream tobacco smoke (International Association for Research on Cancer [IARC], 1986). The evidence relating to exposure to passive or environmental tobacco smoke is reviewed in a later section of this chapter. The risk varies according to the type of tobacco smoked, amount of tobacco smoked, duration of smoking, and tar content of the tobacco smoked. The risk remains relatively constant, however, when individuals stop smoking. The evidence increasingly shows that women have at least as great a risk as men per amount smoked.

Type of Tobacco Smoked

The risk is greater for cigarette smoking than for smoking any other type of tobacco. For example, in the British doctors cohort study, the risk for pipe or cigar smokers relative to the risk for nonsmokers who had never previously smoked cigarettes was 5.8, that for pipe or cigar smokers who also smoked cigarettes, 8.2; and that for cigarette smokers only, 14.0 (Doll and Peto, 1976). Similar differences in the risk with the type of tobacco were found in other major cohort studies, with the risk consistently higher for smokers of cigarettes only (IARC, 1986). In the 40-year follow-up of the British doctors study, the risk for current smokers of cigarettes was approximately double that of smokers of other types of tobacco, although the risk in former smokers was similar (Doll et al, 1994).

Amount of Tobacco Smoked

All studies consistently show a dose-response relationship; that is, the risk of lung cancer increases with the amount smoked, usually expressed as the number of cigarettes smoked per day. In the Canadian Veterans study, for example, the risk for those who smoked 1 to 9 cigarettes per day was 10.0 relative to nonsmokers, 16.4 for those who smoked 10 to 20 cigarettes per day, and 17.3 for those who smoked 21 or more cigarettes per day (Lossing et al, 1966). Even higher risks for heavy smokers relative to nonsmokers have been found in some studies. For example, a 25-fold risk for smokers of 25 or more cigarettes per day was found in the British doctors study (Doll and Peto, 1976; Doll et al, 1994), and a risk of 23.7 for smokers of 40 or more cigarettes per day was found in the U.S. Veterans study (Rogot and Murray, 1980).

Duration of Smoking

One of the key features of the relationship between cigarette smoking and lung cancer is the relevance of the duration of regular cigarette smoking to lung cancer risk. Using a statistical model fitted to data from the British doctors study, Peto and Doll (1984) estimated that the excess annual lung cancer incidence rates after about 45, 30, and 15 years of cigarette smoking were in the ratio of approximately 100:20:1. The long delay that is seen between an increase in cigarette smoking and its full effect on national lung cancer rates is caused by this critical dependence on the duration of smoking (Doll and Peto, 1981). One effect of this dependence on duration is that the lifetime risk of lung cancer varies substantially according to whether cigarette smoking starts at the age of 15 years (or earlier) or is delayed until 20 or 25 years of age (IARC, 1986).

Effect of Different Levels of Tar

There are two major difficulties in assessing the risk of cigarettes of different tar contents (and the risk of filter versus nonfilter cigarettes). The first relates to the reduction in the tar content in the last 30 years in North America and Europe. Most people who developed lung cancer in the late 20th century started smoking with much higher tar–level cigarettes than are generally available now. The second relates to the fact that the main driving force for individuals in the amount they smoke is the level of nicotine to which they are addicted (Surgeon General, 1988). Nicotine reduction usually accompanies a reduction in the tar levels in cigarettes. Thus, on switching to lower tar–level brands, smokers compensate by adopting smoking practices that have the effect of increasing the amount of nicotine absorbed, and hence the amount of tar inhaled, and by increasing the numbers of cigarettes smoked per day (Gritz, 1988). Nevertheless, both the Surgeon General (1982) and the IARC Working Group (1986) concluded that reduced tar levels were followed by a reduced lung cancer risk, although the risk for smoking low-tar cigarettes was still substantially greater than the risk for not smoking at all. One large, case-control study of 7804 cases of lung cancer and 15,207 hospital-based controls that demonstrated this reduction in risk was conducted in seven centers in western Europe (Lubin et al, 1984). In this study, lifetime smokers of nonfiltered cigarettes had nearly twice the risk of lung cancer compared with lifelong filtered cigarette smokers, after controlling for the duration of cigarette use and the number of cigarettes smoked per day. The same study indicated that male smokers of high-tar cigarettes had about 1.7 times the risk of smokers of low-tar brands. For women, the corresponding estimate was 7.7. Changes in tobacco content of cigarettes that began in approximately the mid-1950s have contributed to declines in tar levels and may have contributed to the decline in the lung cancer mortality rate (Walker and Brin, 1988). Nevertheless, in one study in the United States, careful control for differences in age and total amount smoked resulted in an insignificant risk reduction for smokers of low-tar cigarettes (Wilcox et al, 1988). Those who smoked low-tar cigarettes had compensated by increasing the number of cigarettes they smoked by almost one-half pack per day; a similar effect was not noted in the controls or in those who smoked high-tar cigarettes.

Effect of Cessation of Smoking

The risk among ex-smokers is usually compared with that of continuing smokers or nonsmokers. On the basis of the former comparison, it is usually concluded that the risk among ex-smokers decreases the longer the time since smoking was given up. However, this comparison has to include the fact that continuing smokers incur a substantial increase in risk the longer they continue to smoke. Once this is appreciated, it is clear that the risk among ex-smokers does not fall but stays at approximately the same level it had reached at the time smoking ceased. The level of risk is determined by the duration of smoking up to the time of cessation and the intensity of smoking (IARC, 1986; Miller, 1984). This relationship was most clearly seen from the analyses of the British doctors study. There was a longer follow-up period in this study than in other cohort studies, because the investigators sought information on smoking habits at 5-year intervals during the course of the study and were thus able to classify the changes of cigarette smoking that occurred with time. The study also demonstrated that the risk among ex-smokers exceeded the risk among nonsmokers throughout the 40-year follow-up period (Doll et al, 1994). There were similar findings in the U.S. Veterans study (Rogot and Murray, 1980). In the American Cancer Society study, the risk among ex-smokers appeared to fall to the same level as that for nonsmokers 10 or more years after the cessation of smoking (Freedman and Navidi, 1990); however, this was based on only five deaths from lung cancer in ex–heavy smokers and one in former light smokers (Hammond, 1966). Furthermore, the data on cessation of smoking were based only on those obtained on enrollment in the study.

In most clinical series, a high proportion of the lung cancers are found in male ex-smokers.

LUNG CANCER AND OTHER RISK FACTORS

Female Gender

Although most of the earlier studies of lung cancer involving women suggested lower risks from cigarette smoking in women than in men, the study of female British doctors suggested that, for equivalent amounts smoked, women had as great a risk of lung cancer as did men (Doll et al, 1980). The earlier studies showing lower risks in women than in men were conducted in populations in which women had not been smoking long enough to show the full effect of smoking, a problem largely avoided in the female British doctors study, which had a 22-year follow-up.

In a case-control study in Los Angeles County, risks were assessed in relation to the main histologic types of lung cancer in women (Wu et al, 1985). Approximately two thirds of the patients had adenocarcinomas, and the risks for cigarette smokers relative to nonsmokers were increased 6.5-fold for those who smoked more than 20 cigarettes/day and 8-fold for those who began smoking at 18 years of age or earlier. For the patients with squamous cell carcinoma (well recognized as largely caused by smoking in men; IARC, 1986), the corresponding relative risks were 94.4 and 115.7, respectively. A similar differential effect was found in a French case-control study (Benhamou et al, 1987). However, the estimated risks were substantially lower, perhaps because only recently have a great number of French women begun to smoke, and, at that time, lung cancer in women in France was rare.

In the Surgeon General's (1989) report, preliminary findings from the new large American Cancer Society Cancer Prevention Study II (CPS-II), based on more than 1.2 million American men and women followed from 1982 to 1986, were presented. This study, conducted in all 50 states, had the same design and methods as did the earlier large American Cancer Society cohort study of more than 1 million men and women conducted in 25 states, beginning in 1959 (Hammond, 1966). This earlier study is now called the Cancer Prevention Study I (CPS-I) and is directly comparable to CPS-II. It is clear that there has been a substantial increase in the risk of lung cancer in women as a result of the increased proportion of women in the population who have smoked for long periods. For example, the risk for women smokers in CPS-II relative to nonsmokers (11.94) was similar to that for men in CPS-I (11.35) (Surgeon General, 1989).

In a study done in New Jersey, particularly high risks were found for small cell carcinoma of the lung (Schoenberg et al, 1989). Compared with that in nonsmokers, the risk was increased 62-fold for small cell carcinoma, 11-fold for squamous cell carcinoma, and 4-fold for adenocarcinoma. Similar risk levels were found in a study of lung cancer in women in Sweden (Svensson et al, 1989). This reminds us that although the risks are lower for adenocarcinoma with smoking than for other histologic types, in both sexes, most such cancers are caused by cigarette smoking (Brownson et al, 1987).

In our case-control study in southern Ontario, 469 women with lung cancer were interviewed (315 in person and 154 by proxy) as were 472 men matched to the women by age and selected at random from the larger pool of men (335 in person and 137 by proxy). A matched population control was interviewed for each case. The risk of lung cancer per 10 pack-years relative to that in nonsmokers was 9.77 for the women and 7.18 for the men. The risk was higher for the women within each smoking intensity category and for each histologic type of carcinoma, except large or giant cell and unspecified carcinomas (Risch et al, 1993).

Passive Smoking

The first studies to indicate a possible increased risk of lung cancer from passive smoking came from Japan and Greece, countries with a larger proportion of female nonsmokers than in North America. From a large cohort study, Hirayama (1981) reported a relative risk of 1.8 for female nonsmokers married to husbands who smoked relative to those whose husbands did not smoke, which included a total of 108,906 women, 346 of whom died from lung cancer during a 14-year follow-up period, with 17,366 cigarette smokers, 69,645 nonsmokers married to smoking husbands, and 21,895 nonsmokers married to nonsmoking husbands. Although the relative risk for female smokers was 3.8, the amount of lung cancer attributable to passive smoking in women was potentially greater than that from active smoking because four times as many women in the study were exposed to passive smoke than were active smoking women. Analysis of the amount of smoking by the husbands suggested a dose-response relationship. Trichopoulos and colleagues (1981), in a hospital-based, case-control study, had almost identical findings. Thus, the risk for nonsmoking women married to smoking husbands was 3.4 for husbands who smoked 20 or more cigarettes a day, 2.4 for those who smoked 1 to 19, and 1.8 for those married to ex-smokers, relative to nonsmoking women married to nonsmoking husbands.

These early studies were greeted with some skepticism because of the potential for misclassification of smoking status. It would only be necessary for a few active female smokers to be misclassified as nonsmokers for the effects observed to be produced. The potential for this was particularly great in Hirayama's (1981) study because it was not as socially acceptable for women to smoke in Japan in 1966, when the data were collected, as it became later. However, a case-control study based on the atomic bomb survivors in Japan and performed later showed similar findings (Akiba et al, 1986). Thus, the risk for nonsmoking women married to husbands who smoked 30 or more cigarettes a day relative to women married to nonsmoking husbands was 2.1 (95% confidence interval [CI], 0.7, 2.5). There was also a suggestion of a dose-response relationship (*P* for trend, 0.06).

The publication of the early results led to a succession of studies. Some were largely negative (Garfinkel, 1981; Kabat and Wynder, 1984; Koo et al, 1985). Part of the difficulty is related to the overwhelming importance of active smoking as a cause of lung cancer, even in women, and the rarity of lung cancer in nonsmokers. Thus, to obtain sufficient subjects in a case-control study, Garfinkel and colleagues (1985) had to identify cases from four hospitals over an 11-year period. Patients with colorectal cancer served as controls. A significantly increased doubling in risk was found for nonsmoking women with husbands who smoked 40 or more cigarettes a day or 20 or more at home, relative to nonsmoking women with nonsmoking husbands. This excess risk was largely restricted to cases with squamous cell carcinoma.

Excess risk for cases with histologic types recognized as being smoking related, such as squamous or small cell carcinomas, was found in a number of other studies, adding to the biologic plausibility of the association. Thus, Dalager and associates (1986), in a joint analysis of the results of two case-control studies in the United States, found that the relative risk for the occurrence of squamous and small cell carcinomas in nonsmoking women married to smoking husbands was 2.88 (95% CI, 0.91, 9.10), with women married to nonsmoking husbands as the reference group. A similar effect was found in a nested case-control study set within a cohort of 27,409 nonsmoking Swedish women (Pershagen et al, 1987). In this study, it was possible to examine the effect of both the intensity of husbands' smoking and the histologic type simultaneously. The relative risk for the occurrence of squamous or small cell carcinoma among nonsmoking women married to husbands' who smoked 15 or more cigarettes a day was 6.4 (95% CI, 1.1, 34.7). The risk for the occurrence of other histologic types with similar intensity of the husbands' smoking was 2.4 (0.6, 8.7), relative to nonsmoking women married to nonsmoking husbands.

Wald and colleagues (1986) published the results of a meta-analysis of the 13 studies along with results that were then available that had been contributed to a report of the National Research Council on passive smoking (1986). There was a consistent tendency for an excess risk to be seen from passive exposure to environmental tobacco smoke. The conjoint risk from 10 case-control studies was 1.27 (95% CI, 1.05, 1.53) and from 3 cohort studies, 1.44 (1.20, 1.72), the latter heavily influenced by Hirayama's (1981) results. For all 13 studies, the combined estimate of relative risk was 1.35 (1.19, 1.54). An adjustment for misclassification reduced this risk to 1.30, but adjustment for the fact that the referents (largely nonsmoking women married to nonsmoking husbands) were in fact exposed to some environmental tobacco smoke from others raised the relative risk to 1.53.

Since this analysis, the results of additional studies have been reported. Lam and colleagues (1987) in Hong Kong included in their study a larger number of subjects than had been included in the earlier negative studies in Hong Kong (Koo et al, 1985, 1987). They found a significant positive association among never-smoking women for passive smoking caused by a smoking husband (relative risk, 1.65; 95% CI, 1.16, 2.35). Svensson and associates (1989) attempted to evaluate the role of passive smoking in Sweden with risk estimates of a similar order to those found in studies elsewhere. Passive smoking was further evaluated in a case-control study of nonsmoking women in Greece (Kalandidi et al, 1990). The marriage of a nonsmoking woman to a smoker was associated with a doubling of the risk of lung cancer. In New York State, in a study of 191 patients with lung cancer who had never smoked (Janerich et al, 1990), no effect of exposure to a spouse's smoking was found, but household exposure to 25 or more smoker-years during childhood and adolescence doubled the risk of lung cancer. Although other positive and negative studies have been reported (Gao et al, 1987; Holowaty et al, 1991; Humble et al, 1987; Lee et al, 1986), it seems probable that the earlier combined estimate of risk still stands. Indeed, a review conducted for the Environmental Protection Agency (1992) produced a pooled estimate of risk from 22 studies of 1.41 (95% CI, 1.26, 1.57).

Nevertheless, in a report of a meta-analysis of nine studies conducted in America, apparently financed by the tobacco industry, a nonsignificant combined estimate of risk of 1.12 (95% CI, 0.95, 1.30) was derived (Fleiss and Gross, 1991). This analysis included four U.S. studies not available in 1986 (but included in the EPA 1992 estimate). One of these, however, was a 1987 doctoral dissertation, which, at that time, reported negative findings but which, on further analysis, was found to show significant risks for household exposure to passive smoke (Janerich et al, 1990). This was the only unpublished study cited as justification for the claim in a commentary supported by the RJR Nabisco Company (Butler, 1991), that the Working Group on Passive Smoking (1990) (itself supported by the tobacco industry) failed to cite unpublished relevant studies. The Working Group on Passive Smoking (1990) had concluded that passive smoke was hazardous to health and significantly increased the risk of lung cancer in nonsmokers.

The largest case control study yet conducted in nonsmoking women in the United States on the relationship of environmental tobacco smoke to lung cancer confirmed the previous estimates of risk (Fontham et al, 1994). The odds ratio (OR) for exposure to all types of environmental tobacco smoke was 1.29, the OR for 80 or more pack-years of exposure from the spouse was 1.79.

In a recent case-control study with 650 cases and 1542 controls conducted in several centers in Europe, subjects were included who had smoked up to 400 cigarettes in their lifetime. The OR for spousal exposure to environmental tobacco smoke was 1.16 (95% CI, 0.93–1.44), and for workplace exposure 1.17 (0.93–1.45) (Boffetta et al, 1998). Although interpreted by some as a negative study, these slight elevations of risk are in fact compatible with those of other studies and may reflect some misclassification because the subjects were not pure nonsmokers.

Passive smoking may also increase the risk of lung cancer in active smokers. A possible particularly critical time may be exposure in childhood. Correa and colleagues (1983) attempted to evaluate the effect of parental smoking, adjusting for active smoking. There was no increased risk if the father was a smoker (relative risk, 0.83), but the relative risk was 1.36 if the mother was a smoker ($P < 0.05$). Sandler and associates (1985) also found evidence of a greater cancer risk for individuals with household exposure to cigarette smoke during both childhood and adulthood than for individuals with exposures during only one period. Fontham and associates (1994) found that in women with childhood exposure in addition to spousal exposure, the OR was 3.25 (95% CI, 2.42–7.46), and in women without such exposure the OR was 1.77 (0.98–3.19). However, no increased risk for exposure to passive smoke in childhood was found in a study by Boffetta and colleagues (1998).

Lung Cancer in Asia

One of the largest cohort studies ever performed was initiated in 1966 in Japan by Hirayama (1982). This largely confirmed the findings from the studies in the West that implicated cigarette smoking as the major cause of lung cancer. A report from Japan of a large case-control study of the lung cancer risk in ex-smokers also confirms previous reports from cohort and case-control studies (Sobue et al, 1991). The risks of lung cancer in exsmokers compared with those in continuing smokers diminished progressively with an increasing duration after the cessation of smoking.

China is also one of the countries in Asia where smoking rates are now high and where lung cancer is becoming more and more frequent as a consequence. Until recently, however, there was a widespread disbelief in China that smoking was hazardous. In a study among Chinese women, cigarette smoking was a strong risk factor, but it accounted for only approximately one quarter of the cases (Gao et al, 1987). The remainder were adenocarcinomas, with various associated factors, including previous chest diseases and cooking with rapeseed oil at high temperatures. Cigarette smoking was found to be the principal cause of lung cancer in Shenyang, an industrial city in northeastern China, accounting for 55% of the lung cancers in men and 37% in women (Xu et al, 1989). Increased risks were also found among those who reported exposure to outdoor environments smoky from air pollution and those with many years of sleeping on beds heated by coal-burning stoves. In another case-control study involving 965 female patients with lung cancer and 959 population controls conducted in two industrial cities of northeast China, cigarette smoking was found to be the main causal factor, accounting for about 35% of the cases (Wu-Williams et al, 1990). Other factors found to be relevant in this population included air pollution from coal-burning stoves, exposure to indigenous smoky heating stoves, and prior chronic bronchitis. In a more recent study in China, an effect of passive smoke was demonstrated (Sun et al, 1996) that was similar to the effect found earlier by Lam and colleagues (1987) in Hong Kong. In both these studies, a higher risk was found for adenocarcinomas than was found in other studies.

Substantially increased risk for tobacco-associated disease, and especially for lung cancer in male patients, has been found in a recent study in China (Liu et al, 1998). In this study, the family members of a million people who died between 1986 and 1988 in eight areas of China were interviewed to determine whether the deceased person had been a smoker before 1980. There was a threefold greater risk of death from lung cancer among male smokers aged 35 to 69 years than there was among nonsmokers. This excess risk is expected to increase substantially in the 21st century as the full effect of smoking in China is manifested.

Radon Exposure

A series of studies in uranium miners in the United States, Canada, and Czechoslovakia confirmed that radon daughters released in poorly ventilated uranium mines increase the risk of lung cancer, with an approximate doubling of risk after a 5- to 10-year latent period (Committee on the Biological Effects of Ionizing Radiations, 1988). The risk levels were considerably raised for those with substantial cumulative exposure (Howe et al, 1986; Woodward et al, 1991), although there is some evidence that the effect is greatest at low-dose rates (Howe et al, 1987). Because the joint effect of smoking and radon exposure has been difficult to quantify (L'Abbé et al, 1991), there has been residual suspicion that part of the radon effect may actually be the result of smoking. This suspicion was put to rest with a study of lung cancer deaths in nonsmoking uranium miners from Colorado (Roscoe et al, 1989). Fourteen deaths from lung cancer were observed during a 34-year observation period of 516 never-smoking uranium miners; only 1.1 such deaths were expected, giving a standardized mortality ratio of 12.7. This confirms that, in the absence of cigarette smoking, radon daughter exposure increases the risk of lung cancer.

There is interest in indoor radon exposure as a possible risk factor for lung cancer (Edling et al, 1986; Samet, 1989). Elevated lung cancer rates have been noted in U.S. counties with Precambrian granite deposits, which are known to result in raised radon daughter concentrations in homes (Archer, 1987). In a study in China, the effect of indoor radon was evaluated (Blot et al, 1990). No relationship to lung cancer was found. However, in tin miners in a different area of China, lung cancer was found to be related to both water-pipe smoking and radon exposure in the mines (Qiao et al, 1989). A quantitative analysis of the effect of radon showed that a long duration of exposure at a low rate may be more deleterious than a short duration of exposure at a high rate; the joint effects of water-pipe smoking and radon exposure were intermediate between additive and multiplicative (Lubin et al, 1990).

In a case-control study of lung cancer among New Jersey women, a significant trend of increasing lung cancer risk with increasing radon exposure was found (Schoenberg et al, 1990). The risk gradient was similar to that estimated for uranium miners. Even so, the risk was largely related to the highest exposure levels, which were measured in the homes of only 6 of the 433 cases and in 2 of the 402 controls with measurements. Consequently, in this population, it seems that high levels of radon exposure account for less than 2% of the cases of lung cancer.

Several studies of lung cancer in relation to radon exposure in homes have now been completed, but not all have found excess risk, including a study conducted in Winnipeg, Manitoba, the city in Canada with the highest radon exposure in homes (Letourneau et al, 1994). However, a meta-analysis of eight of these studies including 4263 cases and 6612 controls found a relative risk of 1.14 (95% CI, 1.0–1.3) for exposure to radon at 150 becquerels per meter squared (Lubin and Boice, 1997). This is similar to the estimates of risk from domestic radon exposure that were derived from extrapolation of the studies in uranium miners.

Diet

Interest in diet and lung cancer began with a cohort study in Norway, which showed that an index of vitamin A intake was negatively associated with the incidence of lung cancer (Bjelke, 1975; Kvale et al, 1983). Others had similar findings (Gregor et al, 1980; Mettlin et al, 1979).

With the finding of a negative association of beta carotene, but not preformed vitamin A, with the incidence of lung cancer (Shekelle et al, 1981) and some understanding on how beta carotene might be protective (Peto et al, 1981), attention shifted to beta carotene. Several authors found evidence of the protective effects of beta carotene (Byers et al, 1987; Hinds et al, 1984; Samet et al, 1985; Wu et al, 1985; Ziegler et al, 1986). Furthermore, some of the strongest associations in earlier work were with "vitamin A" indices derived from plant foods. Others also found evidence of a protective effect of vegetables against lung cancer (Hirayama, 1986; MacLennan et al, 1979; Ziegler et al, 1986). Our study in Toronto did not show a protective effect for beta carotene, retinol, or total vitamin A consumption, but it did show a protective effect for estimated nitrate ingestion in foods, considered as an index of the consumption of a number of nitrate-containing vegetables (Jain et al, 1990). Additional evidence came from a study in Athens in which a protective effect of a high consumption of fruits but not carotenoids was found (Kalandidi et al, 1990). In Hawaii, although a protective effect of beta carotene intake was found, the protective effect of all vegetables, including dark green vegetables, cruciferous vegetables, and tomatoes, was stronger (Le Marchand et al, 1989). The studies in Hawaii and Toronto used quantitative dietary questionnaires and, therefore, may have more accurately computed the relative importance of various dietary factors than simpler frequency-based instruments. In a small study in Australia, a protective effect of fish consumption was noted but not one for foods containing retinol or beta carotene (Pierce et al, 1989). However, in a small case control study in England, there was some confirmation that dietary carotene was protective for lung cancer, with a nonsignificant protective effect for carotene-rich fruits and vegetables (Harris et al, 1991). The serum beta carotene level was also lower in lung cancer cases than in controls. Additional evidence of lower lung cancer risk in people who consume higher frequencies of vegetables and sometimes of fruit has come from case-control studies in China (Swanson et al, 1992), Japan (Gao et al, 1993), and the United States (Candelora et al, 1992; Dorgan et al, 1993; Mayne et al, 1994).

An analysis of data from a cohort study of California Seventh-Day Adventists (who have low rates of smoking and alcohol consumption) with a 6-year follow-up period showed associations with both smoking and dietary factors, which are independent of each other (Fraser et al, 1991). There was a strong statistically significant protective association with fruit consumption. Foods included in the data set that have a substantial content of beta carotene showed no consistent association. In another cohort study in the United States, which was conducted among postmenopausal women, an inverse association for high levels of fruits and vegetables and of vegetables alone was found, but a weaker effect was found for fruit consumption considered alone (Steinmetz et al, 1993).

All investigators have been careful to adjust their analyses for smoking. Several also attempted to evaluate the interaction with smoking. In one study, the reduced relative risk of lung cancer associated with vitamin A was most evident among men who smoked heavily (Kvale et al, 1983). Hirayama (1986) suggested that green-yellow vegetable consumption might hasten the effect of the cessation of cigarette smoking and might also affect the risk caused by passive smoking. Samet and associates (1985) found effects only in whites rather than in Hispanics and only in former rather than current cigarette smokers. Ziegler and associates (1986) found the protective effect of vegetables was limited to current and recent cigarette smokers. Pisani and colleagues (1986) found an increased risk of lung cancer for smokers who did not consume carrots, but no corresponding effect for ex-smokers or nonsmokers. Byers and associates (1987) found the risk reduction that was associated with vitamin A from fruits and vegetables was most evident for light or ex-smokers. Bond and associates (1987) found the strongest inverse association of a vitamin A index with the lung cancer risk among cigarette smokers.

Some investigators also attempted to evaluate the differential risks for dietary factors, according to histologic type. Several found associations that were strongest for squamous cell cancer (Byers et al, 1984, 1987; Gregor et al, 1980; Ziegler et al, 1986). Byers and associates (1984) also found associations with small cell cancer and Ziegler and colleagues (1986), with adenocarcinoma for current and recent smokers.

Interest in beta carotene as a possible agent for chemoprevention of lung cancer abruptly ended with the publication of the findings from two randomized trials of beta carotene supplementation (Alpha-Tocopherol, Beta Carotene Lung Cancer Prevention Study Group, 1994; Omenn et al, 1996). Both found excess incidence of lung cancer in heavy smokers taking beta carotene supplements and one found such in asbestos-exposed workers. In retrospect, it appears that there was insufficient evidence from experimental models to support a major chemopreventive effect of beta carotene on lung cancer in humans (IARC, 1998a). Evaluation of the chemopreventive efficacy of vitamin A in lung cancer has also resulted in a conclusion of the absence of a cancer-preventive effect (IARC, 1998b). However, these conclusions do not negate the efficacy of fruits and vegetables in lowering the risk of lung cancer.

Three correlation studies demonstrated an association between lung cancer mortality rates and per capita consumption of dietary fat (Carroll and Khor, 1975; Wynder et al, 1987; Xie et al, 1991). Two of these attempted to adjust for the consumption of tobacco (Wynder et al, 1987; Xie et al, 1991). Both found independent contributions from smoking and dietary fat consumption. Xie and colleagues (1991) found that animal but not vegetable fat contributed significantly to the risk. Some studies found increased risks for dietary cholesterol (Goodman et al, 1988; Hinds et al, 1983; Jain et al, 1990), but not others (Alvanja et al, 1993; Byers et al, 1987). Two case-control studies in men and women found increased risks for total fat (Byers et al, 1987; Goodman et al, 1988) and a case-control study of lung cancer in nonsmoking women found increased risks for fat consumption, specifically saturated fat (Alvanja et al, 1993). This effect was not seen in Toronto (Jain et al, 1990) or Iowa (Wu et al, 1994).

In summary, although it is clear that cigarette smoking is far and away the most important risk factor for lung cancer, there appear to be modulating factors in plant foods and perhaps risk factors in animal foods. It is now clear that no protective effect is derived from supplemental beta carotene. However, there are other inhibitors of carcinogenesis in fruits and vegetables, although those important for reducing lung cancer risk have not yet been identified.

Occupational Factors

Occupational factors have long been recognized as increasing the risk of lung cancer (Tomatis et al, 1990).

TABLE 31–2 ■ Factors Encountered in the Occupational Environment with Sufficient Evidence for Carcinogenicity in Humans that Increase the Risk of Lung Cancer

Occupational Circumstance or Chemical	*Reference*
Aluminum production	IARC, 1987
Arsenic	IARC, 1987
Asbestos	IARC, 1987
Beryllium (refining, machining, and producing beryllium)	IARC, 1994
Bis(chloromethyl) ether	IARC, 1987
Chromium compounds as encountered in the chromate production, chromate pigment production, and chromium plating industries	IARC, 1990
Coal gasification	IARC, 1987
Coal tar, coal-tar pitches	IARC, 1987
Coke production	IARC, 1987
Crystalline silica (inhaled in the form of quartz or cristobalite)	IARC, 1997
Iron and steel founding	IARC, 1987
Nickel sulphate and the combinations of nickel sulphides and oxides encountered in the nickel refining industry	IARC, 1990
Occupational exposure as a painter	IARC, 1989
Radon	IARC, 1988

IARC, International Agency for Research on Cancer.

The classic factors (other than uranium mining) that are unequivocally related to an occupational risk of lung cancer include exposure to asbestos (in mining, manufacturing, and insulating); occupations involving the inhalation of polycyclic aromatic hydrocarbons; iron and steel founding; and exposure to arsenic, chromates, and bis(chlormethyl)ether. Table 31–2 lists the factors encountered in the occupational environment for which there is *sufficient* evidence for carcinogenicity in inducing lung cancer in humans according to the IARC. Although compounding by smoking has often been suspected as explaining some of the occupational associations, the difference in smoking prevalence between the occupational group and the comparison group must be large to explain the associations observed (Blair et al, 1985).

In the last two decades, attention has shifted to try to identify new and possibly unexpected causes for lung cancer risk in occupational groups. A large international study evaluated the risk of exposure to human-made mineral fibers (Simonato et al, 1987). The lung cancer mortality rate increased with the time since the first exposure, both in rock wool, slag wool, and glass wool production, but only the rock wool and slag wool excess was seen when local reference populations were substituted for national reference populations. These findings were confirmed in a subsequent update of the study (Boffetta et al, 1997). In northern Sweden, a case-control study found excess risks in occupations with exposures to known carcinogens (radon daughters, arsenic, and asbestos) (Damber and Larsson, 1987). In Sweden as a whole, trends of occupationally induced lung cancer were assessed by means of a special register (Carstensen et al, 1989). Decreasing trends for blacksmiths and members of the armed forces and increasing trends for foundry workers and construction machine operators were noted. In a case control study within a cohort of Swedish smelter workers, strong associations were found for both estimated arsenic exposure and cigarette smoking (Järup and Pershagen, 1991). Both exposures appeared to increase the risk with an interaction between additive and multiplicative. The relationship with arsenic was strongest for the estimated average exposure, less strong for cumulative exposure, and absent for the duration of exposure. There was some suggestion of a weaker effect of arsenic among heavy smokers than among light and medium smokers. The possibility that occupational lung cancer might be identified through specific histologic types was evaluated in a large census-derived data base in Finland (Sankila et al, 1990). In general, this was not confirmed, although miners and quarriers had a high risk of small cell carcinoma compared with other economically active men. In a combined analysis of three U.S. case control studies, 10 years or more exposure to motor exhaust–related occupations was found to increase the lung cancer risk by 50% (Hayes et al, 1989). Among specific occupations, the risk was elevated for truck drivers. Diesel exhaust exposure was further evaluated in another large U.S. study (Boffetta et al, 1990). Although a 30% increase in the risk for probable exposure was found, this was accounted for by an adjustment for smoking and other compounders. Another potential risk exposure for lung cancer is formaldehyde, assessed in a cohort study of 26,561 workers employed in 10 facilities (Blair et al, 1990). Although a 30% excess had been noted, this did not appear to be consistent within plants, nor could a dose-response relationship to formaldehyde be found. It appeared that other substances to which the workers were also exposed (including phenol, melamine, urea, and wood dust) might have been responsible for the excess number of lung cancer cases in the cohort. In contrast, occupational exposure to silica is being recognized more and more frequently as increasing the risk of lung cancer. In Quebec, Canada, men who had received compensation for silicosis had more than three times the risk of death from lung cancer than that expected from population rates in Quebec (Infante-Rivard et al, 1989). A doubling of the lung cancer risk was also found in a cohort of men in a silicosis register in Hong Kong (Ng et al, 1990). Although there is some selection bias in relation to the inclusion of workers in such registers (Abraham, 1990; Spivack, 1990), the degree of elevation of risk found, especially in the Quebec study, seems unlikely to be the result of such factors (Infante-Rivard et al, 1990a, 1990b). Excess risk of lung cancer in those with silicosis has also been found in studies in California (Goldsmith et al, 1995), Italy (Merlo et al, 1995) and China (Wang et al, 1996). IARC (1997) has concluded that there is *sufficient* evidence in humans for the carcinogenicity of inhaled crystalline silica in the form of quartz or cristobalite from occupational sources.

Excess deaths from lung cancer were found in the melting department of two Ontario steel manufacturers (Finkelstein and Wilk, 1990; Finkelstein et al, 1991). In the second plant (Finkelstein et al, 1991), the excess risk was confined to men who had worked in the pouring pit department. No polycyclic aromatic hydrocarbons were detected in the environment of the work process. Indeed, no definitive cause of the excess lung cancer risk in these two plants has yet been identified. In an investigation of lung cancer risk in three midwestern U.S. plants that manufactured heavy equipment, no significant excess risk was found for either welders or nonwelders of mild steel compared with that in the general population; neither was there an increased risk in welders compared with nonwelders (Steenland et al, 1991). Although it is reassuring, this finding contrasts with a finding of an increased risk of lung cancer of 2.43 (95% CI, 1.56, 3.79) among workers in the ferrous primary metal manufacturing industry in an Occupational Cancer Incidence Surveillance study in metropolitan Detroit (Burns and Swanson, 1991). This large, case control study, which was based on data collected by the Detroit cancer registry, was designed to evaluate lung cancer risk, and it also found an excess risk among furnace and steel workers (and in several other occupational groups). As was reported first many years ago for coke plant workers (Lloyd, 1971), it is clear that iron and steel refining and manufacturing have several component groups in which an excess lung cancer risk can be identified. The causal factors are likely to be diverse and probably do not include iron itself, but rather additives, contaminants, and other substances in the work environment (including arsenic, silica, and polycyclic aromatic hydrocarbons) that will have to be specifically identified in the relevant plants for appropriate preventive actions to be taken.

Attempts have been made to quantify the amount of lung cancer that can be attributable to occupation. In two industrialized areas of northern Italy (Ronco et al, 1988), when only occupations known to be causally associated with lung cancer were included in the estimate of the attributable risk, the percentage was 12% in one area and 5% in the other. When suspect occupations were also included, the attributable risks rose to 36% and 12%, respectively. In the United States, occupational data from five case-control studies were considered by Vineis and colleagues (1988). The percentage of lung cancer that was attributable to occupations with potential exposure to well-recognized carcinogens ranged from 3% to 17% by study area. The authors believed that errors in exposure classification made these estimates conservative.

Air Pollution

In the early stages of the investigations in the 1950s concerning the reasons for the increase in lung cancer, air pollution was strongly suspected as a possible cause. Over the years, however, it has become clear that general air pollution adds only a small component to the effect of individual air pollution through tobacco use. One of the earliest studies to demonstrate this was conducted in heavily polluted areas in the north of England. The risk of lung cancer, adjusted for smoking, was at most increased two-fold in the heavily polluted areas compared with the less polluted areas (Dean et al, 1978). A similar differential was found in an analysis of lung cancer mortality rates in a Scottish town that was related to degrees of pollution from two iron foundries (Smith et al, 1987). However, in most studies, it has been difficult to exclude the effects of occupation, social class, and differential smoking, which seemed to be more likely to explain area differences in Contra Costa County, California, in spite of exposure to emissions from petroleum and chemical plants (Kaldor et al, 1984). Indeed, such factors may have explained the findings in the other studies. A similar effect was noted in a study in Texas in which air pollution accounted for less than 5% of the total variation in the interurban lung cancer mortality rate (Buffler et al, 1988). Furthermore, a study in the heavily polluted town of Hamilton, Ontario, showed little effect of air pollution in increasing the risk after smoking was taken into account (Shannon et al, 1988).

Nevertheless, when local air pollution is extreme, an increased risk of lung cancer appears to be related to it. This is the case for an area of China with severe exposure indoors to the emissions of smoky coal (Mumford et al, 1987), as has also been noted for external air pollution in other areas of China (Wu-Williams et al, 1990; Xu et al, 1989). These findings are compatible with the conclusion of Tomatis and colleagues (1990) that "it seems probable that, in heavily polluted areas, air pollution may contribute to mortality from lung cancer."

Recently, this conclusion has been confirmed for occupational cohorts exposed to air pollution. Peluso and associates (2001), as a result of a meta-analysis of 13 studies, found that there was a significant association between levels of DNA adducts and air pollution exposure in heavily exposed industrial workers and less heavily exposed urban workers.

Familial Aspects of Lung Cancer and the Role of Genetics

An association of lung cancer with a positive family history was noted several years ago (Tokuhata and Lilienfeld, 1963). In a report on a study in the Texas Gulf Coast region, a risk of 2.8 for lung cancer in two or more relatives was reported (Shaw et al, 1991). However, the association was stronger for the histologic types associated with smoking. A similar finding arose from a study in Canada in which a family history of any neoplastic disease was evaluated (McDuffie, 1991). Most of the sites with the highest elevations of risk were smoking associated, supporting an ecogenetic cause of cancer within the affected families (i.e., a strong influence of smoking, possibly superimposed on some genetic base, but requiring the environmental factor [smoking] to induce the disease).

For some time there has been a suspicion that a genetic susceptibility to certain carcinogens may play a role in the cause of lung cancer (Minna et al, 1988). Markers for susceptibility to lung cancer related to drug metabolism have been described (Ayesh et al, 1984). Law (1990) reviewed the evidence and concluded that genetic factors must contribute to the lung cancer risk because it is the metabolites of environmental carcinogens that usually initiate a cancer and the metabolic pathways are genetically controlled. One of the metabolic pathways identified is associated with the drug debrisoquin, with fewer participants with lung cancer than controls being poor metabolizers of debrisoquin, although the proportions of poor metabolizers in both groups was low in one study (1.9 versus 8.7%) (Law et al, 1989). The association seems stronger in those who are occupationally exposed to asbestos and polycyclic aromatic hydrocarbons. In such individuals, extensive metabolizers of debrisoquin had a four-fold increase in the risk of lung cancer in comparison with poor metabolizers (Caporaso et al, 1989). Another possible genetic marker that has been identified is the class mu phenotype of glutathione transferase, which appears to be more frequent in non–cancer-affected smokers than in patients with lung cancer (Seidegard et al, 1990). Perhaps more convincing, however, is the fact that evidence for mendelian inheritance of lung cancer was obtained through a segregation analysis of 337 families, who were ascertained through lung cancer probands (Sellers et al, 1990). The data were compatible with codominant inheritance of a rare autosomal gene that produces an earlier age of onset of lung cancer in individuals who are exposed to the appropriate carcinogenic stimulus, particularly smoking.

d'Errico et al (1996) reviewed the evidence on genetic polymorphisms associated with lung cancer. They found a high level of heterogeneity in the studies, such that conclusions were not possible, and that more carefully designed studies including sound methodologic validation are necessary.

CONCLUSION

Surprisingly, we continue to learn of etiologically relevant factors for what is the most important potentially preventable cancer in the world. Smoking remains the preeminent cause of lung cancer, but factors that interact with smoking, such as occupation, diet, genetics, and possibly radon, are relevant. Much of the emerging knowledge can be incorporated into cancer control programs, especially the protective effect of smoking cessation. It is important that increased understanding of the possible effect of other factors (e.g., as for other cancers, the protective effect of plant foods) not result in diverting attention from smoking control policies. In this respect, the almost unanimous agreement that passive smoking increases the risk of lung cancer in nonsmokers has moved smoking control out of the realm of individual action into general public health. Occupational factors that increase the risk of lung cancer should continue to be sought and controlled. For radon daughter exposure in homes, however, the public health significance seems slight.

Internationally, the most important action that could be taken to halt the epidemic of lung cancer would be to agree on appropriate smoking control policies, even though they sometimes seem to be in conflict with international trade. It is reprehensible that short-term financial gain should take precedence over long-term health.

■ *KEY REFERENCES*

Committee on the Biological Effects of Ionizing Radiations of the National Research Council: BEIR IV. Health Risks of Radon and Other Internally Deposited Alpha-Emitters. Washington, DC, National Academy Press, 1988.

This is an important review of the health risks from radon daughters. Although it is most clearly relevant to the risks from uranium mining, it has substantial implications for the possible adverse effect of radon daughter exposure in homes.

Doll R, Peto R, Wheatley K et al: Mortality in relation to smoking: 40 years observations on male British doctors. BMJ 309:901, 1994.

This is the report on the 40-year follow-up of the male British doctors cohort study. Probably one of the best known cohort studies ever conducted, it has the considerable advantage that information on current smoking was collected every 5 years after the cohort was established.

IARC: Tobacco Smoking. In IARC (eds): IARC Monographs on the Evaluation of the Carcinogenic Risk of Chemicals to Humans, Vol 38. Lyon, International Agency for Research on Cancer, 1986.

This is the most detailed and authoritative compilation of the carcinogenicity of tobacco available. It contains an extensive literature review of the data available on the epidemiology of tobacco and lung (and other) cancers up to 1985.

Surgeon General: Reducing the health consequences of smoking: 25 years of progress. Rockville, MD, US Department of Health and Human Services, 1989.

This is the 25-year anniversary issue of the annual Surgeon General's reports on the health consequences of tobacco since the series commenced in 1964. It contains an extensive review of changes in smoking rates in the United States and an update on lung cancer and tobacco epidemiology, including the preliminary results of the large American Cancer Society CPS-II.

Tomatis L, Aitio A, Day NE et al (eds): Cancer: Causes, Occurrence and Control. IARC Scientific Publications, No. 100. Lyon, International Agency for Research on Cancer, 1990.

This is an extensive review of the causes of cancer and the approaches available for its control. It contains summaries of the effects of many different factors on the risk of lung and other cancers. It provides for the world what Doll and Peto (1981) attempted to do for the United States—that is, a summary of the principal causes of cancer and the amount of disease attributable to these causes.

■ *REFERENCES*

Abraham JL: Silicosis and lung cancer. Lancet 335:1163, 1990.

Akiba S, Kato H, Blot WJ: Passive smoking and lung cancer among Japanese women. Cancer Res 46:4804, 1986.

Alpha-Tocopherol, Beta Carotene Lung Cancer Prevention Study Group: The effect of vitamin E and beta carotene on the incidence of lung cancer and other cancers in male smokers. N Engl J Med 330: 1029, 1994.

Alvanja MC, Brown CC, Swanson C, Brownson RC: Saturated fat intake and lung cancer risk among nonsmoking women in Missouri. J Natl Cancer Inst 85:1906, 1993.

Archer VE: Association of lung cancer mortality with Precambrian granite. Arch Environ Health 42:87, 1987.

Ayesh R, Idle JR, Ritchie JC et al: Metabolic oxidation phenotypes as marker for susceptibility to lung cancer. Nature 312:169, 1984.

Benhamou E, Benhamou S, Flamant R: Lung cancer and women: Results of a French case-control study. Br J Cancer 55:91, 1987.

Bjelke E: Dietary vitamin A and human lung cancer. Int J Cancer 15:561, 1975.

Blair A, Hoar S, Walrath J: Comparison of crude and smoking adjusted standardized mortality ratios. J Occup Med 27:881, 1985.

Blair A, Stewart PA, Hoover RN: Mortality from lung cancer among workers employed in formaldehyde industries. Am J Ind Med 17:683, 1990.

Blot WJ, Xu ZY, Boice JD et al: Indoor radon and lung cancer in China. J Natl Cancer Inst 82:1025, 1990.

Boffetta P, Agudo A, Ahrens W et al: Multicenter case-control study of exposure to environmental tobacco smoke and lung cancer in Europe. J Natl Cancer Inst 90:1440, 1998.

Boffetta P, Harris RE, Wynder EL: Case-control study on occupational exposure to diesel exhaust and lung cancer risk. Am J Ind Med 17:577, 1990.

Boffetta P, Sarraci R, Andersen A et al: Cancer mortality among man-made vitreous fiber production workers. Epidemiology 8:259, 1997.

Bond GG, Thompson FE, Cook RR: Dietary vitamin A and lung cancer: Results of a case-control study among chemical workers. Nutr Cancer 9:109, 1987.

Brown CC, Kessler LG: Projections of lung cancer mortality in the United States: 1985–2025. J Natl Cancer Inst 80:43, 1988.

Brownson RC, Reif JS, Keefe TJ et al: Risk factors for adenocarcinoma of the lung. Am J Epidemiol 125:25, 1987.

Buffler PA, Cooper SP, Stinnett S et al: Air pollution and lung cancer mortality in Harris county, Texas, 1979–1981. Am J Epidemiol 128:683, 1988.

Burns PB, Swanson GM: The Occupational Cancer Incidence Surveillance Study (OCISS): Risk of lung cancer by usual occupation and industry in the Detroit metropolitan area. Am J Ind Med 19:655, 1991.

Butler WJ: Commentary on "Links between passive smoking and disease: A best evidence synthesis. A report of the Working Group on Passive Smoking." [CIM 13:17–42, 1990]. Clin Invest Med 14:484, 1991.

Byers TE, Graham S, Haughey BP et al: Diet and lung cancer risk: Findings from the Western New York diet study. Am J Epidemiol 125:351, 1987.

Byers T, Vena J, Mettlin C et al: Dietary vitamin A and lung cancer risk: An analysis by histologic subtypes. Am J Epidemiol 120:769, 1984.

Candelora EC, Stockwell HG, Armstrong AW, Pinkham PA: Dietary intake and risk of lung cancer in women who never smoked. Nutr Cancer 17:263, 1992.

Caporaso N, Hayes RB, Dosemeci M et al: Lung cancer risk, occupational exposure, and the debrisoquin metabolic phenotype. Cancer Res 49:3675, 1989.

Carroll KK, Khor HT: Dietary fat in relation to tumorigenesis. Prog Biochem Pharmacol 10:308, 1975.

Carstensen JM, Pershagen G, Eklund G: Time trends in occupational risks of lung cancer among Swedish men from 1961–1979. Am J Ind Med 15:441, 1989.

Committee on the Biological Effects of Ionizing Radiations of the National Research Council: BEIR IV: Health Risks of Radon and Other Internally Deposited Alpha-Emitters. Washington, DC, National Academy Press, 1988.

Correa P, Pickle LW, Fontham E et al: Passive smoking and lung cancer. Lancet 2:595, 1983.

Dalager NA, Pickle LW, Mason TJ et al: The relation of passive smoking to lung cancer. Cancer Res 46:4808, 1986.

Damber LA, Larsson LG: Occupation and male lung cancer: A case-control study in Northern Sweden. Br J Ind Med 44:446, 1987.

Dean G, Lee PN, Todd GF, Wicken AJ: Report on a second retrospective mortality study in north-east England. Part II. Changes in lung cancer and bronchitis mortality and in other relevant factors occurring in areas of north-east England 1963–72. Research Paper 14, Part II. London, Tobacco Research Council, 1978.

d'Errico A, Taioli E, Chen X, Vineis P: Genetic metabolic polymorphisms and the risk of cancer: A review of the literature. Biomarkers 1:149, 1996.

Devesa SS, Blot WJ, Fraumeni JF: Declining lung cancer rates among young men and women in the United States: A cohort analysis. J Natl Cancer Inst 81:1568, 1989.

Doll R, Peto R, Wheatley K et al: Mortality in relation to smoking: 40 years observations on male British doctors. BMJ 309:901, 1994.

Doll R, Gray R, Hofner B, Peto R: Mortality in relation to smoking: 22 years observations on female British doctors. BMJ 1:967, 1980.

Doll R, Hill AB: A study of the aetiology of carcinoma of the lung. BMJ 2:1271, 1952.

Doll R, Peto R: Mortality in relation to smoking: 20 years observations on male British doctors. BMJ 2:1525, 1976.

Doll R, Peto R: The causes of cancer: Quantitative estimates of avoidable risks of cancer in the United States today. J Natl Cancer Inst 66:1191, 1981.

Dorgan JF, Zeigler RG, Schoenberg JB et al: Race and sex differences in associations of vegetables, fruits, and carotenoids with lung cancer risk in New Jersey (USA). Cancer Causes Control 4:273, 1993.

Edling C, Wingren G, Axelson O: Quantification of the lung cancer risk from radon daughter exposure in dwellings: An epidemiological approach. Environ Int 12:55, 1986.

Environmental Protection Agency: Respiratory health effects of passive smoking: Lung cancer and other disorders. Washington, DC, U.S. Environmental Protection Agency, 1992.

Finkelstein MM, Boulard M, Wilk N: Increased risk of lung cancer in the melting department of a second Ontario steel manufacturer. Am J Ind Med 19:183, 1991.

Finkelstein MM, Wilk N: Investigation of a lung cancer cluster in the melt shop of an Ontario steel producer. Am J Ind Med 17:483, 1990.

Fleiss JL, Gross AJ: Meta-analysis in epidemiology, with special reference to studies of the association between exposure to environmental tobacco smoke and lung cancer: A critique. J Clin Epidemiol 44:127, 1991.

Fontham ETH, Correa P, Reynolds P et al: Environmental tobacco smoke and lung cancer in nonsmoking women. JAMA 271:1752, 1994.

Fraser GE, Beeson WL, Phillips RL: Diet and lung cancer in Seventh-Day Adventists. Am J Epidemiol 133:683, 1991.

Freedman DA, Navidi WC: Ex-smokers and the multistage model for lung cancer. Epidemiology 1:21, 1990.

Gao C, Tajima K, Kuroishi T et al: Protective effects of raw vegetables and fruit against lung cancer among smokers and ex-smokers: A case-control study in the Tokai area of Japan. Jpn J Cancer Res 84:594, 1993.

Gao YT, Blot WJ, Zheng W et al: Lung cancer among Chinese women. Int J Cancer 40:604, 1987.

Garfinkel L: Time trends in lung cancer mortality among nonsmokers and a note on passive smoking. J Natl Cancer Inst 66:1061, 1981.

Garfinkel L, Auerbach O, Joubert L: Involuntary smoking and lung cancer: A case-control study. J Natl Cancer Inst 75:463, 1985.

Goldsmith DF, Beaumont JJ, Morin LA, Schenker MB: Respiratory cancer and other chronic disease mortality among silicotics in California. Am J Ind Med 28:459, 1995.

Goodman MT, Kolonel LN, Yoshizawa CN, Hankin JH: The effect of dietary cholesterol and fat on the risk of lung cancer in Hawaii. Am J Epidemiol 128:1241, 1988.

Gregor A, Lee PM, Roe FJC et al: Comparison of dietary histories in lung cancer cases and controls with special reference to vitamin A. Nutr Cancer 2:93, 1980.

Gritz ER: Cigarette smoking: The need for action by health professionals. CA Cancer J Clin 38:194, 1988.

Hammond EC: Smoking in relation to the death rates of one million men and women. Monogr Natl Cancer Inst 19:127, 1966.

Hammond EC, Horn D: Smoking and death rates: Report on forty-four months of follow-up of 187,783 men. II. Death rates by cause. JAMA 166:1294, 1958.

Harris RWC, Key TJA, Silcocks PB et al: A case-control study of dietary carotene in men with lung cancer and in men with other epithelial cancers. Nutr Cancer 15:63, 1991.

Hayes RB, Thomas T, Silverman DT et al: Lung cancer in motor exhaust-related occupations. Am J Ind Med 16:685, 1989.

Hinds MW, Kolonel LN, Hankin JH et al: Dietary vitamin A, carotene, vitamin C and risk of lung cancer in Hawaii. Am J Epidemiol 119:227, 1984.

Hinds MW, Kolonel LN, Lee J, Hankin JH: Dietary cholesterol and lung cancer risk among men in Hawaii. Am J Clin Nutr 37:192, 1983.

Hirayama T: Nutrition and cancer: A large scale cohort study. In Knudsen I (ed): Genetic Toxicology of the Diet. New York, Alan R Liss, 1986.

Hirayama T: Smoking and cancer in Japan: A prospective study on cancer epidemiology based on census in Japan: Results of 13 years follow up. In Tominaga S, Aoki K (eds): The UICC Smoking Control Workshop, Nagoya, Japan. Nagoya, The University of Nagoya Press, 1982.

Hirayama T: Non-smoking wives of heavy smokers have a higher risk of lung cancer: A study from Japan. BMJ 282:183, 1981.

Holowaty EJ, Risch HA, Miller AB, Burch JD: Lung cancer in women in the Niagara region, Ontario: A case-control study. Can J Public Health 82:304, 1991.

Howe GR, Nair RC, Newcombe HB et al: Lung cancer mortality (1950–80) in relation to radon daughter exposure in a cohort of workers at the Eldorado Port Radium uranium mine: Possible modification of risk by exposure rate. J Natl Cancer Inst 79:1255, 1987.

Howe GR, Nair RC, Newcombe HB et al: Lung cancer mortality (1950–80) in relation to radon daughter exposure in a cohort of workers at the Eldorado Beaverlodge uranium mine. J Natl Cancer Inst 77:357, 1986.

Humble CG, Samet JM, Pathak DR: Marriage to a smoker and lung cancer risk. Am J Public Health 77:598, 1987.

IARC Handbooks of Cancer Prevention, Volume 2: Carotenoids. Lyon, International Agency for Research on Cancer, 1998a.

IARC Handbooks of Cancer Prevention, Volume 3: Vitamin A. Lyon, International Agency for Research on Cancer, 1998b.

IARC Monographs on the evaluation of carcinogenic risk to humans, Supplement 7: Overall evaluations of carcinogenicity: An updating of monographs, Vol 1 to 42. Lyon, International Agency for Research on Cancer, 1987.

IARC Monographs on the evaluation of carcinogenic risk to humans, Volume 43: Man-made mineral fibres and radon. Lyon, International Agency for Research on Cancer, 1988.

IARC Monographs on the evaluation of carcinogenic risk to humans, Volume 47: Some organic solvents, resin monomers and related compounds, pigments and occupational exposures in paint manufacture and painting. Lyon, International Agency for Research on Cancer, 1989.

IARC Monographs on the evaluation of carcinogenic risk to humans, Volume 49: Chromium, nickel and welding. Lyon, International Agency for Research on Cancer, 1990.

IARC Monographs on the evaluation of carcinogenic risk to humans, Volume 58: Beryllium, cadmium, mercury and exposures in the glass manufacturing industry. Lyon, International Agency for Research on Cancer, 1994.

IARC Monographs on the evaluation of carcinogenic risk to humans, Volume 68: Silica, some silicates, coal dust and *para*-Aramid fibrils. Lyon, International Agency for Research on Cancer, 1997.

IARC Monographs on the evaluation of the carcinogenic risk of chemicals to humans, Volume 38. Lyon, International Agency for Research on Cancer, 1986.

Infante-Rivard C, Armstrong B, Petitclerc M et al: Response to Dr. Spivack. Lancet 335:1163, 1990a.

Infante-Rivard C, Armstrong B, Petitclerc M et al: Response to Dr. Abraham. Lancet 335:854, 1990b.

Infante-Rivard C, Armstrong B, Petitclerc M et al: Lung cancer mortality and silicosis in Québec, 1938–1985. Lancet 2:1504, 1989.

Jain M, Burch JD, Howe GR et al: Dietary factors and risk of lung cancer: Results from a case-control study, Toronto, 1981–1985. Int J Cancer 45:287, 1990.

Janerich DT, Thompson WD, Varela LR et al: Lung cancer and exposure to tobacco smoke in the household. N Engl J Med 323:632, 1990.

Jârup L, Pershagen G: Arsenic exposure, smoking, and lung cancer in smelter workers: A case-control study. Am J Epidemiol 134:545, 1991.

Kabat GC, Wynder EL: Lung cancer in nonsmokers. Cancer 53:1214, 1984.

Kahn HA: The Dorn study of smoking and mortality among US veterans: Report on eight and one-half years of observation. Monogr Natl Cancer Inst 19:1, 1966.

Kalandidi A, Katsouyanni K, Voropoulou N et al: Passive smoking and diet in the etiology of lung cancer in non-smokers. Cancer Causes Control 1:15, 1990.

Kaldor J, Harris JA, Glazer E et al: Statistical association between cancer incidence and major-cause mortality, and estimated residential exposure to air emissions from petroleum and chemical plants. Environ Health Perspect 54:319, 1984.

Koo LC, Ho JHC, Lee N: An analysis of some risk factors for lung cancer in Hong Kong. Int J Cancer 35:149, 1985.

Koo LC, Ho JHC, Saw D, Ho CY: Measurements of passive smoking and estimates of lung cancer risk among non-smoking Chinese females. Int J Cancer 39:162, 1987.

Kvale G, Bjelke E, Gart JJ: Dietary habits and lung cancer risk. Int J Cancer 31:397, 1983.

L'Abbé KA, Howe GR, Burch JD et al: Radon exposure, cigarette smoking, and other mining experience in the Beaverlodge uranium miners cohort. Health Phys 60:489, 1991.

Lam TH, Kung ITM, Wong CM et al: Smoking, passive smoking and histological types in lung cancer in Hong Kong Chinese women. Br J Cancer 56:673, 1987.

Law MR: Genetic predisposition to lung cancer. Br J Cancer 61:195, 1990.

Law MR, Hetzel MR, Idle JR: Debrisoquin metabolism and genetic predisposition to lung cancer. Br J Cancer 59:686, 1989.

Lee PN, Chamberlain J, Alderson MR: Relationship of passive smoking to risk of lung cancer and other smoking-associated diseases. Br J Cancer 54:97, 1986.

Le Marchand L, Yoshizawa CN, Kolonel LN et al: Vegetable consumption and lung cancer risk: A population-based case-control study in Hawaii. J Natl Cancer Inst 81:1158, 1989.

Letourneau EG, Krewski D, Choi NW et al: Case-control study of residential radon and lung cancer in Winnipeg, Manitoba, Canada. Am J Epidemiol 140:310, 1994.

Liu B-Q, Peto R, Chen Z-M et al: Emerging tobacco hazards in China: 1. Retrospective proportional mortality study of one million deaths. BMJ 317:1411, 1998.

Lloyd JW: Long-term mortality study of steelworkers. V. Respiratory cancer in coke plant workers. J Occup Med 13:53, 1971.

Lossing EH, Best EWR, McGregor JT et al: A Canadian Study of Smoking and Health. Ottawa, Department of National Health and Welfare, 1966.

Lubin JH, Blot WJ, Berrino F et al: Patterns of lung cancer risk according to type of cigarette smoked. Int J Cancer 33:569, 1984.

Lubin JH, Boice JD: Lung cancer risk from residential radon: Meta-analysis of eight epidemiological studies. J Natl Cancer Inst 89:49, 1997.

Lubin JH, Qiao YL, Taylor PR et al: Quantitative evaluation of the radon and lung cancer association in a case-control study of Chinese tin miners. Cancer Res 50:174, 1990.

MacLennan R, Da Costa J, Day NE et al: Risk factors for lung cancer in Singapore Chinese, a population with high female incidence rates. Int J Cancer 20:854, 1979.

Marcus AC, Shopland DR, Crane LA, Lynn WR: Prevalence of cigarette smoking in the United States: Estimates from the 1985 current population survey. J Natl Cancer Inst 81:409, 1989.

Mayne ST, Janerich DT, Greenwald P et al: Dietary beta carotene and lung cancer risk in U.S. nonsmokers. J Natl Cancer Inst 86:33. 1994.

McDuffie HH: Clustering of cancer in families of patients with lung cancer. J Clin Epidemiol 44:69, 1991.

Merlo F, Fontana L, Reggiardo G et al: Mortality among silicotics in Genoa, Italy, from 1961 to 1987. Scand J Work Environ Health 21(Suppl 2):77, 1995.

Mettlin C, Graham S, Swanson MJ: Vitamin A and lung cancer. J Natl Cancer Inst 62:1435, 1979.

Miller AB: The information explosion: The role of the epidemiologist. Cancer Forum 8:67, 1984.

Minna JD, Battey JF, Birrer MJ et al: Genetic changes involved in the pathogenesis of human lung cancer including oncogene activation, chromosomal deletions, and autocrine growth factor production. In Fortner JG, Rhoads JE (eds): Accomplishments in Cancer Research, 1987. Philadelphia, JB Lippincott, 1988.

Mumford JL, He XZ, Chapman RS et al: Lung cancer and indoor air pollution in Xuan Wei, China. Science 235:217, 1987.

National Research Council: Environmental Tobacco Smoke: Measuring Exposures and Assessing Health Effects. Washington, DC, National Academy Press, 1986.

Ng TP, Chan SL, Lee J: Mortality of a cohort of men in a silicosis register: Further evidence of an association with lung cancer. Am J Ind Med 17:163, 1990.

Omenn GS, Goodman GE, Thornquist MD et al: Effects of a combination of beta carotene and vitamin A on lung cancer and cardiovascular disease. N Engl J Med 334:1150, 1996.

Parkin DM, Pisani P, Ferlay J: Estimates of the worldwide incidence of 25 major cancers in 1990. Int J Cancer 80:827, 1999.

Parkin DM, Whelan SL, Ferlay J et al (eds): Cancer incidence in five continents, Vol VII. IARC Scientific Publications No. 143. Lyon, International Agency for Research on Cancer, 1997, pp 314–321 and 842–843.

Peluso M, Ceppi M, Munnia A et al: Analysis of 13 ^{32}P-DNA postlabelling studies on occupational cohorts exposed to air pollution. Am J Epidemiol 153:546, 2001.

Pershagen G, Hrubec Z, Svensson S: Passive smoking and lung cancer in Swedish women. Am J Epidemiol 125:17, 1987.

Peto R, Doll R: The control of lung cancer. In Mizell M, Correa P (eds): Lung Cancer, Causes and Prevention. New York, Verlag Chemie International, 1984.

Peto R, Doll R, Buckley JD et al: Can dietary beta-carotene materially reduce human cancer rates? Nature 290:201, 1981.

Pierce RJ, Kune GA, Kune S et al: Dietary and alcohol intake, smoking pattern, occupational risk, and family history in lung cancer patients: Results of a case-control study in males. Nutr Cancer 12:237, 1989.

Pisani P, Berrino F, Macaluso M et al: Carrots, green vegetables and lung cancer: A case-control study. Int J Epidemiol 15:463, 1986.

Qiao YL, Taylor PR, Yao SX et al: Relation of radon exposure and tobacco use to lung cancer among tin miners in Yunnan Province, China. Am J Ind Med 16:511, 1989.

Risch HA, Howe GR, Jain M et al: Are female smokers at higher risk for lung cancer than male smokers? A case-control analysis by histologic type. Am J Epidemol 138:281, 1993.

Rogot E, Murray JL: Smoking and causes of death among U.S. veterans: 16 years of observation. Public Health Rep 95:213, 1980.

Ronco G, Ciccone G, Mirabelli D et al: Occupation and lung cancer in two industrialized areas of northern Italy. Int J Cancer 41:354, 1988.

Roscoe RJ, Stennland K, Halperin WE et al: Lung cancer mortality among nonsmoking uranium miners exposed to radon daughters. JAMA 262:629, 1989.

Samet JM: Radon and lung cancer. J Natl Cancer Inst 81:745, 1989.

Samet JM, Skipper BJ, Humble CG et al: Lung cancer risk and vitamin A consumption in New Mexico. Am Rev Respir Dis 131:198, 1985.

Sandler DP, Wilcox AJ, Everson RB: Cumulative effects of lifetime passive smoking on cancer risk. Lancet 1:312, 1985.

Sankila RJ, Karjalainen ES, Oksanen HM et al: Relationship between occupation and lung cancer as analyzed by age and histologic type. Cancer 65:1651, 1990.

Schoenberg JB, Klotz JB, Wilcox HB et al: Case-control study of residential radon and lung cancer among New Jersey women. Cancer Res 50:6520, 1990.

Schoenberg JB, Wilcox HB, Mason TJ et al: Variation in smoking-related lung cancer risk among New Jersey women. Am J Epidemiol 130:688, 1989.

Seidegard J, Pero RW, Markowitz MM et al: Isoenzyme(s) of glutathione transferase (class mu) as a marker for the susceptibility to lung cancer: A follow-up study. Carcinogenesis 11:33, 1990.

Sellers TA, Bailey-Wilson JE, Elston RC et al: Evidence for mendelian inheritance in the pathogenesis of lung cancer. J Natl Cancer Inst 82:1272, 1990.

Shannon HS, Hertzman C, Julian JA et al: Lung cancer and air pollution in an industrial city: A geographical analysis. Can J Public Health 79:255, 1988.

Shaw GL, Falk RT, Pickle LW et al: Lung cancer risk associated with cancer in relatives. J Clin Epidemiol 44:429, 1991.

Shekelle RB, Lepper M, Lui S et al: Dietary vitamin A and risk of cancer in the Western Electric study. Lancet 2:1185, 1981.

Shopland DR, Eyre HJ, Pechacek TF: Smoking-attributable cancer mortality in 1991: Is lung cancer now the leading cause of death among smokers in the United States? J Natl Cancer Inst 83:1142, 1991.

Simonato L, Fletcher AC, Cherrie JW et al: The International Agency for Research on Cancer historical cohort study of MMMF production workers in seven European countries: Extension of the follow-up. Ann Occup Hyg 31:603, 1987.

Smith GH, Williams FLR, Lloyd OL: Respiratory cancer and air pollution from iron foundries in a Scottish town: An epidemiological and environmental study. Br J Ind Med 44:795, 1987.

Sobue T, Suzuki T, Fujimoto I et al: Lung cancer risk among exsmokers. Jpn J Cancer Res 82:273, 1991.

Spivack SD: Silica and lung cancer. Lancet 335:854, 1990.

Steenland K, Beaumont J, Elliot L: Lung cancer in mild steel welders. Am J Epidemiol 133:220, 1991.

Steinmetz KA, Potter JD, Folsom AR: Vegetables, fruit, and lung cancer in the Iowa women's health study. Cancer Res 53:536, 1993.

Sun XW, Dai XD, Lin CY et al: Passive smoking and lung cancer among nonsmoking women in Harbin, China. Lung Cancer 14(Suppl 1):S237, 1996.

Surgeon General: Reducing the health consequences of smoking: 25 years of progress. Rockville, MD, U.S. Department of Health and Human Services, 1989.

Surgeon General: The health consequences of smoking: Nicotine addiction. Rockville, MD, U.S. Department of Health and Human Services, 1988.

Surgeon General: The health consequences of smoking: Cancer. Rockville, MD, U.S. Department of Health and Human Services, 1982.

Svensson C, Pershagen G, Klominek J: Smoking and passive smoking in relation to lung cancer in women. Acta Oncol 28:623, 1989.

Swanson CA, Mao BL, Li JY et al: Dietary determinants of lung cancer risk: Results from a case-control study in Yunnan Province, China. Int J Cancer 50:876, 1992.

Tokuhata GK, Lilienfeld AM: Familial aggregation of lung cancer in humans. J Natl Cancer Inst 30:289, 1963.

Tomatis L, Aitio A, Day NE et al (eds): Cancer: Causes, Occurrence and Control. IARC Scientific Publications No. 100. Lyon, International Agency for Research on Cancer, 1990.

Trichopoulos D, Kalandidi A, Sparros L, MacMahon B: Lung cancer and passive smoking. Int J Cancer 27:1, 1981.

Vineis P, Thomas T, Hayes RB et al: Proportion of lung cancers in males, due to occupation, in different areas of the USA. Int J Cancer 42:851, 1988.

Wald NJ, Nanchahal K, Thompson SG, Cuckle HS: Does breathing other people's tobacco smoke cause lung cancer? BMJ 293:1217, 1986.

Walker WJ, Brin BN: U.S. lung cancer mortality and declining cigarette tobacco consumption. J Clin Epidemiol 41:179, 1988.

Wang Z, Dong D, Liang X et al: Cancer mortality among silicotics in China's metallurgical industry. Int J Epidemiol 25:913, 1996.

Wilcox HB, Schoenberg JB, Mason TJ et al: Smoking and lung cancer: Risk as a function of cigarette tar content. Prev Med 17:263, 1988.

Woodward A, Roder D, McMichael AJ et al: Radon daughter exposures at the Radium Hill uranium mine and lung cancer rates among former workers, 1952–87. Cancer Causes Control 2:213, 1991.

Working Group on Passive Smoking: Links between passive smoking and disease: A best-evidence synthesis. Clin Invest Med 13:17, 1990.

Wu AH, Henderson BE, Pike MC et al: Smoking and other risk factors for lung cancer in women. J Natl Cancer Inst 74:747, 1985.

Wu Y, Zheng W, Seller T et al: Dietary cholesterol, fat, and lung cancer incidence among older women: The Iowa women's health study (United States). Cancer Causes Control 5:395, 1994.

Wu-Williams AH, Dai XD, Blot W et al: Lung cancer among women in northeast China. Br J Cancer 62:982, 1990.

Wynder EL, Graham EA: Tobacco smoking as a possible etiologic factor in bronchiogenic carcinoma: A study of six hundred and eighty-four proved cases. JAMA 143:329, 1950.

Wynder EL, Hebert JR, Kabat GC: Association of dietary fat and lung cancer. J Natl Cancer Inst 79:631, 1987.

Xie J, Lesaffre E, Kesteloot H: The relationship between animal fat intake, cigarette smoking, and lung cancer. Cancer Causes Control 2:79, 1991.

Xu ZY, Blot WJ, Xiao HP et al: Smoking, air pollution, and the high rates of lung cancer in Shenyang, China. J Natl Cancer Inst 81:1800, 1989.

Ziegler RG, Mason TJ, Stemhagan A et al: Carotenoid intake, vegetables, and the risk of lung cancer among white men in New Jersey. Am J Epidemiol 123:1080, 1986.

PATHOLOGY OF LUNG CANCER

Mark R. Wick
Jon H. Ritter

In the early 1900s, the first attempt at morphologic classification of lung cancer was undertaken by Marchesani. This scheme, outlining the now-classic categories of carcinoma—squamous cell carcinoma, adenocarcinoma, small cell "undifferentiated" carcinoma, and large cell "undifferentiated" carcinoma—is still widely recognized and has gone through several iterations over the ensuing decades. In recent times, a pragmatic, clinically attuned movement has been enjoined wherein a more simplified system is embraced, dividing malignant epithelial tumors of the lung into "small cell" and "non–small cell" carcinomas. At the same time, research by pathologists has resulted in ever-greater refinement of morphologic categorization, and the interface between the practical needs of the operating suite and data generated in the clinical laboratory has therefore become problematic. In light of this situation, a prognostically oriented nosologic scheme for lung cancer was devised by the Veterans Administration Lung Group in 1991 (Yesner et al, 1991), and it has since been modified by other organizations.

The pathologist should choose to use these systems, or not, only after consultation with clinical colleagues. In any event, nonstandard designations for pulmonary carcinomas (i.e., those that are not sanctioned by the World Health Organization [Travis et al, 1999]) (Table 31–3) should be well-defined in surgical pathology reports, with pertinent references being provided in cases that are particularly uncommon or conceptually contentious.

A particular problem that must be recognized forthrightly by everyone involved in treating lung cancer is the common heterogeneity that it may demonstrate at a light microscopic level. The literature is now well-supplied with reports of admixtures of virtually all of the lung carcinoma histotypes with one another in the same tumor mass (Fraire et al, 1992; Olcott, 1955). An analysis by Roggli and colleagues (1985) demonstrated such heterogeneity in 66% of a consecutive series of lung cancers, and others have reported similar findings. This biologic diversity may attain prognostic importance in the future, particularly in light of recent work that appears to affirm the impact of histologic features on tumor evolution (Fraire et al, 1987). In any event, neoplastic heterogeneity is a practical diagnostic problem for surgeons and other oncologists, because small biopsies will often fail to represent "divergent" tumor elements as a consequence of sampling bias. At a time when ever more limited methods of tissue procurement are being advanced, it is clear that substantial discrepancies will be observed be ween biopsy results and examination of resection specimens in the surgical pathology laboratory. That is not to imply that such techniques as fine-needle aspiration bi-

TABLE 31–3 ■ 1999 WHO/IASLC Histologic Classification of Lung and Pleural Tumors

1. Epithelial Tumors

1.1 Benign

1.1.1 Papillomas
1.1.1.1 Squamous cell papilloma
1.1.1.1.1 Exophytic
1.1.1.1.2 Inverted
1.1.1.2 Glandular papilloma
1.1.1.3 Mixed squamous cell and glandular papilloma

1.1.2 Adenomas
1.1.2.1 Alveolar adenoma
1.1.2.2 Papillary adenoma
1.1.2.3 Adenomas of salivary gland type
1.1.2.3.1 Mucous gland adenoma
1.1.2.3.2 Pleomorphic adenoma
1.1.2.3.3 Other
1.1.2.4 Mucinous cystadenoma
1.1.2.5 Others

1.2 Preinvasive Lesions

1.2.1 Squamous dysplasia/carcinoma in situ
1.2.2 Atypical adenomatous hyperplasia
1.2.3 Diffuse idiopathic pulmonary neuroendocrine cell hyperplasia

1.3 Invasive Malignant

1.3.1 Squamous cell carcinoma
Variants:
1.3.1.1 Papillary
1.3.1.2 Clear cell
1.3.1.3 Small cell
1.3.1.4 Basaloid

1.3.2 Small cell carcinoma
Variant:
1.3.2.1 Combined small cell carcinoma

1.3.3 Adenocarcinoma
1.3.3.1 Acinar
1.3.3.2 Papillary
1.3.3.3 Bronchioloalveolar carcinoma
1.3.3.3.1 Nonmucinous
1.3.3.3.2 Mucinous
1.3.3.3.3 Mixed mucinous and nonmucinous or indeterminate
1.3.3.4 Solid adenocarcinoma with mucin formation
1.3.3.5 Mixed
1.3.3.6 Variants:
1.3.3.6.1 Well-differentiated fetal adenocarcinoma
1.3.3.6.2 Mucinous ("colloid")
1.3.3.6.3 Mucinous cystadenocarcinoma
1.3.3.6.4 Signet ring
1.3.3.6.5 Clear cell

1.3.4 Large cell carcinoma
Variants:
1.3.4.1 Large cell neuroendocrine carcinoma
1.3.4.1.1 Combined large cell neuroendocrine carcinoma
1.3.4.2 Basaloid carcinoma
1.3.4.3 Lymphoepithelioma-like carcinoma
1.3.4.4 Clear cell carcinoma
1.3.4.5 Large cell carcinoma with rhabdoid phenotype

1.3.5 Adenosquamous carcinoma

1.3.6 Carcinomas with pleomorphic, sarcomatoid, or sarcomatous elements
1.3.6.1 Carcinomas with spindle and/or giant cells
1.3.6.1.1 Pleomorphic carcinoma
1.3.6.1.2 Spindle cell carcinoma
1.3.6.1.3 Giant cell carcinoma
1.3.6.2 Carcinosarcoma
1.3.6.3 Blastoma (pulmonary blastoma)
1.3.6.4 Others

1.3.7 Carcinoid tumor
1.3.7.1 Typical carcinoid
1.3.7.2 Atypical carcinoid

1.3.8 Carcinomas of salivary gland type
1.3.8.1 Mucoepidermoid carcinoma
1.3.8.2 Adenoid cystic carcinoma
1.3.8.3 Others

1.3.9 Unclassified carcinoma

2. Soft Tissue Tumors

2.1 Localized fibrous tumor
2.2 Epithelioid hemangioendothelioma
2.3 Pleuropulmonary blastoma
2.4 Chondroma
2.5 Calcifying fibrous pseudotumor of the pleura
2.6 Congenital peribronchial myofibroblastic tumor
2.7 Diffuse pulmonary lymphangiomatosis
2.8 Desmoplastic small round cell tumor
2.9 Other

3. Mesothelial tumors

3.1 Benign

3.1.1 Adenomatoid tumor

3.2 Malignant

3.2.1 Epithelioid mesothelioma
3.2.2 Sarcomatoid mesothelioma
3.2.2.1 Desmoplastic mesothelioma
3.2.3 Biphasic mesothelioma
3.2.4 Other

4. Miscellaneous Tumors

4.1 Hamartoma
4.2 Sclerosing hemangioma
4.3 Clear cell tumor
4.4 Germ cell neoplasms
4.4.1 Teratoma, mature or immature
4.4.2 Malignant germ cell tumor
4.5 Thymoma
4.6 Melanoma
4.7 Others

5. Lymphoproliferative Diseases

5.1 Lymphoid interstitial pneumonia
5.2 Nodular lymphoid hyperplasia
5.3 Low-grade marginal-zone B-cell lymphoma of the mucosa-associated lymphoid tissue (MALT)
5.4 Lymphomatoid granulomatosis

6. Secondary Tumors

7. Unclassified Tumors

8. Tumor-Like Lesions

8.1 Tumorlet
8.2 Multiple meningothelioid nodules
8.3 Langerhans cell histiocytosis
8.4 Inflammatory pseudotumor (inflammatory myofibroblastic tumor)
8.5 Organizing pneumonia
8.6 Amyloid tumor
8.7 Hyalinizing granuloma
8.8 Lymphangioleiomyomatosis
8.9 Multifocal micronodular pneumocyte hyperplasia
8.10 Endometriosis
8.11 Bronchial inflammatory polyps
8.12 Others

IASLC, International Association for the Study of Lung Cancer; WHO, World Health Organization.

opsy should not be used, because they are extremely helpful in planning therapy in many cases. Nonetheless, the potential limitations of all sampling procedures must be weighed carefully against their benefits.

CLINICOPATHOLOGIC FEATURES OF NONENDOCRINE PULMONARY CARCINOMAS

Squamous Cell Carcinoma

Morphogenesis

Squamous cell carcinoma (SCC) is no longer the most common type of lung cancer and has been eclipsed by adenocarcinoma in recent years (Fraire et al, 1992; Vincent et al, 1977). However, SCC has retained its classic clinicopathologic attributes in most instances. SCC shows a tendency for multifocal but clonal in situ disease in the bronchial mucosa, often preceding the appearance of a discrete mass by several years, and it has a propensity to arise in large central airways that are proximal to the subsegmental bronchi. Because of the common presence of an endobronchial tumor mass, obstructive pneumonia is a relatively common accompaniment of this neoplasm, albeit by no means pathognomonic of it. "Pure" SCC may certainly take origin in the peripheral pulmonary parenchyma as well, and rare examples are subpleural (Fraire, 1992).

Morphologic Findings

Squamous cancer of the lung has an irregular, often-friable, grey-white cut surface, commonly showing a large area of central necrosis, with or without cavitation (Fig. 31–7). The surrounding pulmonary parenchyma is frequently tethered to the mass, giving it a "spiculated" appearance that may be well-seen on radiographic images. Microscopically, SCC is defined by its resemblance to stratified squamous epithelium of the upper airway but with disordered architectural and cytologic maturation. Anucleate keratin and squamous pearls are observed in only the better differentiated of these lesions, which account for a minority of pulmonary carcinomas (Fig. 31–8). Poorly differentiated SCC may be extremely difficult for the pathologist to distinguish from high-grade adenocarcinomas or large cell undifferentiated carcinomas, inasmuch as all of them commonly take the form of nondescript proliferations of primitive epithelioid cells, arranged in nests and sheets with no other distinguishing features. In the absence of special studies, one may have to use the default terminology of "non–small cell carcinoma, not further specified," in the frozen section laboratory and in reference to small biopsies of such lesions. Other recognized and distinct subtypes of poorly differentiated SCC include spindle-cell and pleomorphic forms (Fishback et al, 1994) (see "Sarcomatoid Carcinoma"); adenoid (pseudoglandular) variants (Nappi et al, 1994); a pseudovascular (angiosarcoma-like) subtype (Nappi et al, 1994; Ritter et al, 1995); "lymphoepithelioma-like" carcinoma (Frank et al, 1997); and a basaloid form ("small cell squamous carcinoma" or "basaloid carcinoma") (Brambilla et al, 1992) that is analogous to primary poorly differentiated squamous carcinoma of the anorectum, hypopharynx, thymus, and other anatomic sites. Other than confronting the pathologist with special problems in microscopic differential diagnosis, these tumor variants have no singular clinical significance.

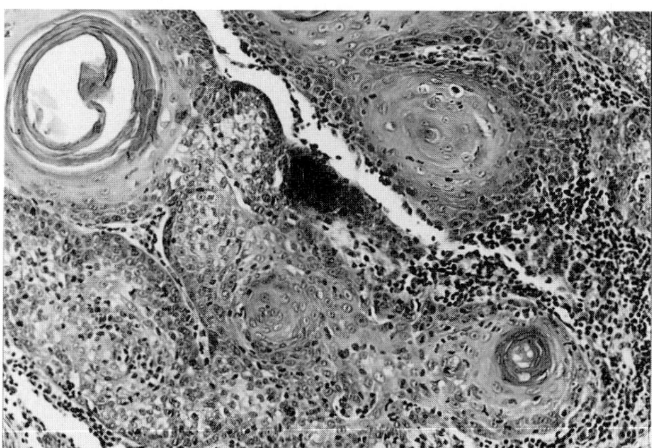

FIGURE 31–8 ■ Keratinization, with formation of squamous "pearls," is seen in a small number of pulmonary squamous cell carcinomas, as shown in this photomicrograph.

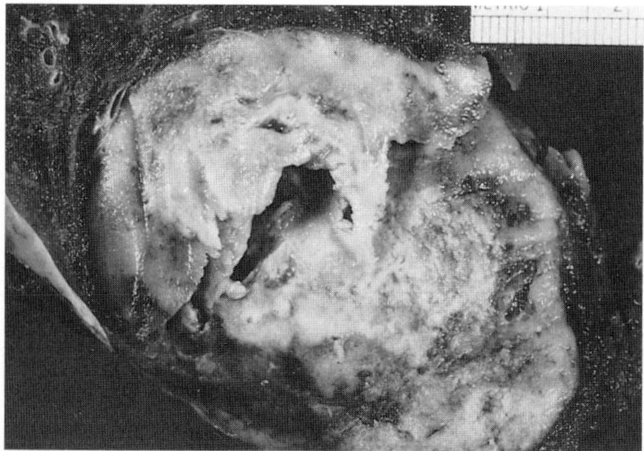

FIGURE 31–7 ■ Central cavitary necrosis in a squamous cell carcinoma of the lung.

Adenocarcinoma

Morphogenesis

Adenocarcinoma (ACA) has now successfully rivaled SCC as the most common form of monodifferentiated lung cancer. In North America and Europe, most ACAs are predominantly peripheral parenchymal masses; however, interestingly, histologically identical lesions in India and Asia are as likely to be central as peripheral in location.

Morphologic Findings

Grossly, ACA typically has an irregularly lobulated configuration, with a grey-white cut surface (Fig. 31–9). Anthracotic pigment is commonly entrapped in the tumor mass as well, but foci of necrosis and hemorrhage are seen only in large (>5 cm) lesions. A relationship to tubular airways is only rarely obvious. Close inspection

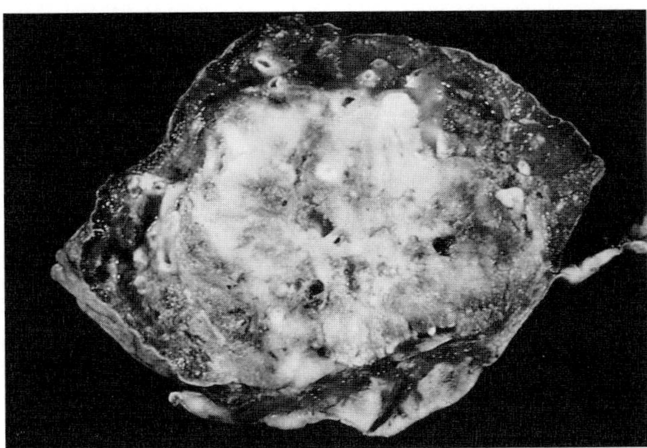

FIGURE 31–9 ■ Peripheral adenocarcinomas of the lung are usually solid, lobulated masses that often closely approach the pleural surfaces.

also may demonstrate the presence of "satellitotic" nodules around the main tumor mass; in fact, however, this phenomenon may be a reflection of the tendency for pulmonary ACA to be synchronously or metachronously multifocal, either in one lobe of the lung or in both lungs. The latter statement particularly applies to a special subtype of ACA: namely, bronchioloalveolar carcinoma (BAC) (see later). One peculiar and uncommon macroscopic presentation of pulmonary ACA merits special mention: that is, its "pseudomesotheliomatous" form, wherein the pleurotropic growth of extremely peripheral intrapulmonary tumors creates a "rind" of tumor tissue surrounding the lung. This virtually perfectly simulates the appearance of mesothelioma, both intraoperatively and on radiographic imaging studies (Dessy and Pietra 1991; Koss et al, 1992; Lin et al, 1980).

Microscopically, there are four major subtypes of pulmonary ACA: acinar (the most common) (Fig. 31–10), papillary, bronchioloalveolar, and solid (DaCosta et al, 1993). However, additional variants exist, such as sarcomatoid, well-differentiated mucinous ("colloid"); signet-ring cell; clear cell; and enteric (intestinal-like) (Gaffey et al, 1997; Hayashi et al, 1999; Moran et al, 1992; Nakatani et al, 1998; Weidner, 1992). In some cases, because of the overlap between these histologic groups and the appearances of metastatic adenocarcinomas in the lung, it may be extremely difficult for the pathologist to separate primary from secondary lesions. This is particularly true of enteric and signet-ring cell tumors, which can closely imitate the attributes of gastric or colorectal carcinomas. Psammoma bodies also can be seen in primary papillary adenocarcinomas of the lung (Colby et al, 1995), and these structures therefore raise the question of whether one is instead viewing a solitary metastasis from an occult tumor of the thyroid, ovary, or other locations wherein psammomatous carcinomas are potentially found. Special studies, including electron microscopy and immunohistology, are not particularly helpful in resolving this differential diagnosis. Needless to say, in cases featuring multifocality of adenocarcinoma in more than one lobe, this problem is even more striking.

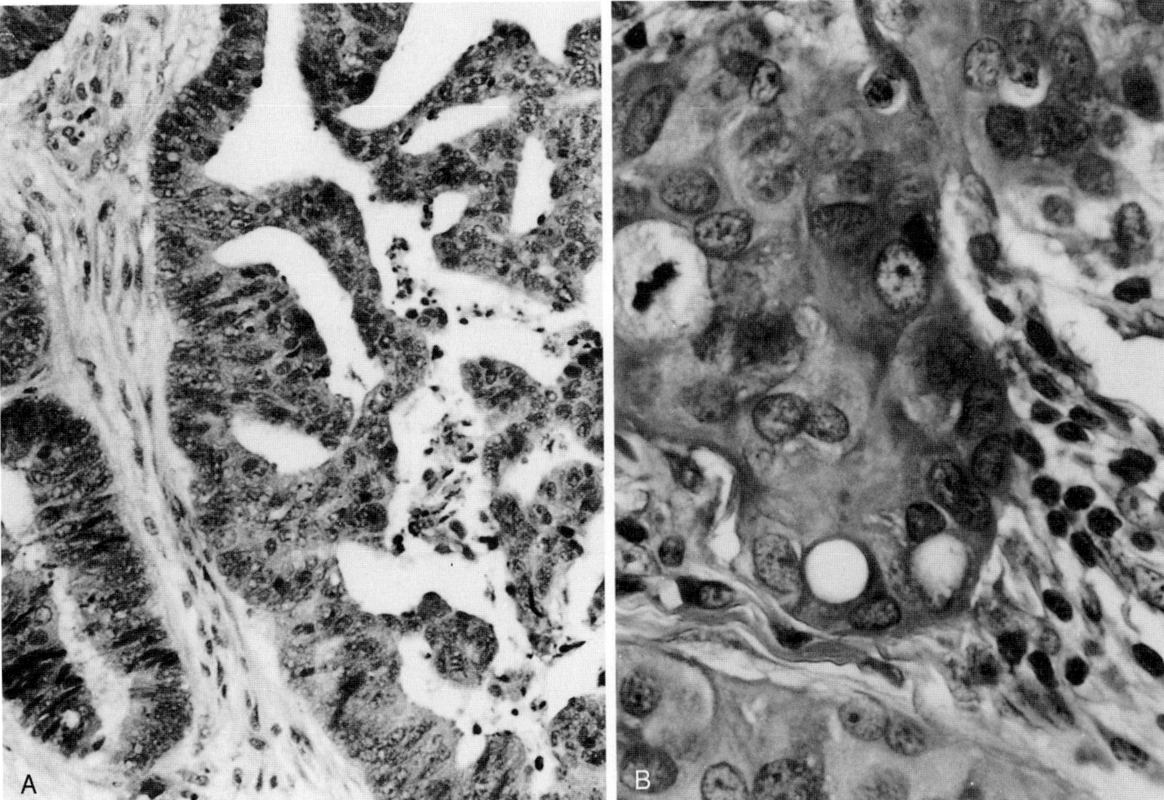

FIGURE 31–10 ■ Adenocarcinoma of the lung demonstrating obvious gland-like formations (*A*) and nucleoli and mitotic figures (*B*).

Ultimately, reliance is usually placed on such banal characteristics as peritumoral fibrosis and inflammation, which are generally more common in primary pulmonary lesions than in metastases.

Pulmonary ACA may rarely involve the bronchial epithelium diffusely in a pagetoid fashion (Higashiyama et al, 1991). Whether this represents intraepithelial spread of the tumor or multifocal synchronous growth is an open question, but pagetoid lesions are excruciating management problems because of the difficulty in obtaining tumor-free bronchial margins.

"Pseudomesotheliomatous" (pleurotropic) adenocarcinomas are indeed separable from true mesotheliomas using adjuvant pathologic techniques, particularly immunophenotyping (Wick, 1997). Nonetheless, whether this exercise has any more than academic significance is an open question. At present, available therapies for both of these tumor types are suboptimal to say the least, and the only real significance of the differential diagnosis in question may be a medicolegal one.

Bronchioloalveolar Carcinoma

Morphogenesis

BAC of the lung was initially described in the 1800s but was most fully characterized as a distinct entity by Liebow in 1960. Since that time, BAC has been the subject of intense interest and controversy. In particular, the pathologic criteria that apply to the diagnosis of this tumor entity, and how its histologic attributes relate to prognosis, represent perhaps the two most contentious issues (Clayton, 1986, 1988; Feldman et al, 1992; Grover and Piantadosi, 1989; Lozowski and Hajdu, 1987; Manning et al, 1984; Marcq and Galy, 1973; Rosenblatt et al, 1967; Schulze et al, 1994).

There are no particular distinguishing demographic features that are associated with BAC, vis-à-vis other adenocarcinomas of the lung. They tend to occur in elderly individuals, with an essentially equal distribution by gender (Clayton, 1988; Schulze et al, 1994). Contrary to reports made in the 1970s (Marcq and Galy, 1973), before such phenomena as "passive" tobacco exposure were recognized, there is a definite relationship between cigarette smoking and the genesis of this tumor, as is true of virtually all pulmonary carcinomas. Nonetheless, BAC is indeed over-represented (with regard to other histotypes of lung cancer) in patients who have never smoked and who have never lived with smokers. Radiologically and clinically, three discrete subsets of patients with BAC are recognized (Schulze et al, 1994; Sutton et al, 1989). These include individuals who have chest radiograph findings and clinical complaints that suggest the presence of pneumonia (fever, productive cough, and lobar or segmental consolidation) (Fig. 31–11), as well as some with a solitary peripheral mass lesion and others with multiple, rounded densities throughout one or both lung fields. On computed tomograms, the latter lesions may assume a "Cheerio" shape, in that they commonly demonstrate small central areas of cavitation. Hence, BAC may simulate an infectious disease, represent a nondescript "coin" lesion of the lung, or imitate the pattern of metastases to the lung from an occult visceral neoplasm.

Morphologic Findings

Histologically, two distinct cytologic subtypes of BAC are recognized: mucinous and nonmucinous (Clayton, 1986, 1988; Manning et al, 1984). These are important because of their clinical associations. Mucinous tumors are those that tend to assume a pseudopneumonic or multifocal/multinodular clinical appearance, whereas nonmucinous BAC (Fig. 31–12) is more usually a solitary lesion. Furthermore, stage for stage, nonmucinous variants may show a more favorable clinical evolution (Manning et al, 1984). The criteria for distinction of BAC from type ordinaire pulmonary adenocarcinoma have been debated. The authors restrict the use of this diagnosis to neoplasms that demonstrate a mantling of pre-existing airspaces ("lepidic growth") by single layers or by limited

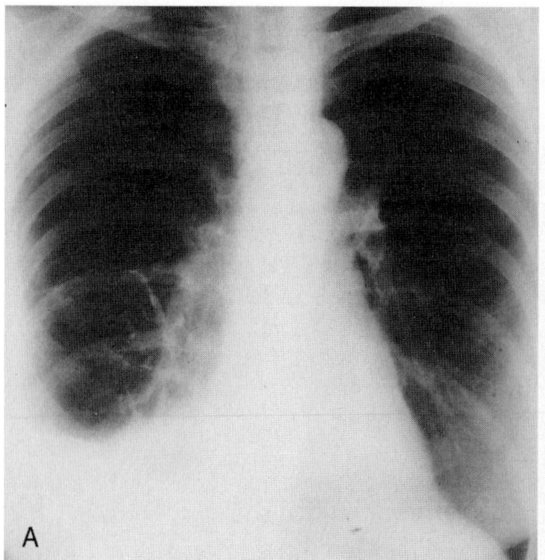

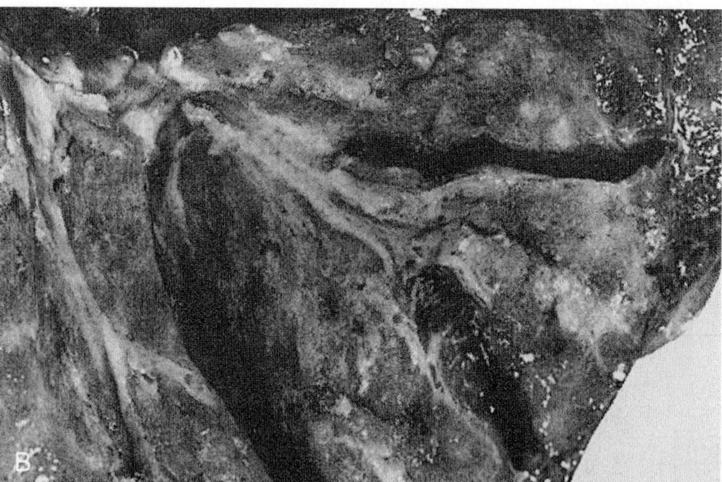

FIGURE 31–11 ■ Diffuse consolidation of the pulmonary parenchyma is apparent in radiographic (*A*) and morphologic (*B*) images of this pseudopneumonic bronchioloalveolar carcinoma of the lung.

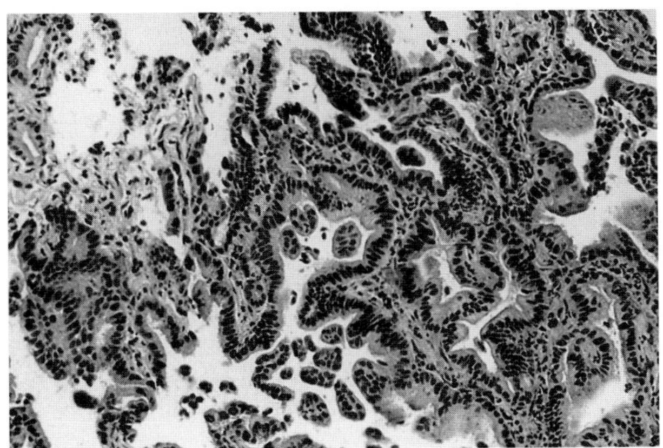

FIGURE 31–12 ■ A "lepidic" growth pattern, conforming to the pre-existing pulmonary architecture, is evident in this nonmucinous bronchioloalveolar carcinoma of the lung.

strata and micropapillae of only modestly atypical cuboidal or columnar epithelial cells, with or without intracellular or extracellular mucin production. Intranuclear inclusions of cytoplasm containing surfactant proteins are also common (Mizutani et al, 1988). Save for mucin production, such characteristics are shared by both of the forms of BAC: namely, mucinous and nonmucinous (serous). Moreover, there must be no sclerosis or inflammation within or around the lesion if it is to be considered a bona fide BAC. This demanding definition differs from that of other observers, who have accepted the existence of a "sclerosing" BAC subtype (Sorensen et al, 1993). Justification for more narrow requirements is gained from biologic data, which show that "sclerosing" BAC behaves worse than do nonfibrotic tumors (Clayton, 1986). Indeed Clayton, who has devoted much attention to BAC, has stated that "bronchioloalveolar carcinomas with sclerosis should be classified with other peripheral adenocarcinomas" (Clayton, 1988).

Another traditional point of discussion pertaining to the microscopic features of BAC (particularly its mucinous form) is that this neoplasm is said to disseminate within the lung by "aerogenous" means. That is to say, it appears that tumor cells are detached from a "mother lesion" and spread to other foci in the pulmonary parenchyma by the process of inhalation and exhalation. Molecular analyses, however, have cast doubt on that premise and instead suggest that the lesions are multiclonal (Barsky et al, 1994).

Other lesions that may be confused pathologically with BAC include foci of florid type II pneumocytic hyperplasia surrounding areas of diffuse alveolar damage (Grotte et al, 1990) and interstitial fibrosing pneumonitides or organizing pulmonary infarcts (Ritter et al, 1995); the proliferation known as "atypical adenomatous alveolar hyperplasia" (see later) (Mori et al, 1993); and the unicentric neoplasm known as "papillary alveolar adenoma" (Hegg et al, 1992). The latter entity is extremely bland cytologically and shows a sharp interface with the surrounding pulmonary parenchyma, unlike BAC. Another point that was often raised in the older literature on BAC concerned the great difficulty with which metastases to the lung could be distinguished from the former neoplasm. It is still true that there are currently no immunohistologic or ultrastructural markers that can be used with absolute certainty to distinguish BAC from all extrapulmonary adenocarcinomas. This separation must ultimately rest on careful analysis of conventional clinicopathologic data.

Prognostically, patients with multifocal BACs have a much worse outlook than that of others with unicentric tumors of this type, quite simply because the former lesions are inoperable. Furthermore, mucinous tumors tend to behave more aggressively—with a higher incidence of extrapulmonary metastasis—than nonmucinous BAC when they are matched by size and stage (Clayton, 1986, 1988). Overall, nonmucinous tumors measuring under 3 cm in maximum dimension have a good prognosis, approximating 90% survival at 5 yrs. Note that the natural history of BAC is more protracted than that of more conventional pulmonary adenocarcinomas, and tumor-related fatalities will continue to accrue even at 10 years after diagnosis (Clayton, 1986; Marcq and Galy, 1973). Nevertheless, in an often-cited study by Manning and colleagues, the 5-year survival of nonmucinous BAC was 72%, whereas only 26% of patients with mucinous tumors survived to that point (Manning et al, 1984).

Atypical Adenomatous Alveolar Hyperplasia and Its Relationship to BAC

Kitamura and colleagues (1999) have addressed the conceptual mechanistic relationship between topographically small, atypical glandular proliferations of the lung—"atypical adenomatous alveolar hyperplasia" (AAAH)—and BAC. Their model appears to demonstrate a stepwise progression from atypical adenomatous hyperplasia (AAH) to BAC, with further evolution to invasive growth. This concept has been advanced before, especially by Miller and colleagues (1988), who postulated that such a stepwise process existed in the lung in analogy to the adenoma-carcinoma sequence in the colon.

Atypical adenomatous hyperplasia must be differentiated from reactive or regenerative pneumocytic lesions, at one end of the spectrum, and from small bona fide adenocarcinomas, at the other. With regard to separation of AAAH from various reactive lesions, Kitamura and coworkers have emphasized the tendency of reactive lesions to include multiple cell types, including type II pneumocytes, ciliated cells, and mucinous cells, and they have described the relatively more conspicuous interstitial inflammation and edema in localized interstitial pneumonitis (Kitamura et al, 1999). Additional criteria that are helpful in this context involve assessment of the lesional borders and patterns of fibrosis. There is a tendency for lesions of AAAH to be more sharply circumscribed and for the mild interstitial fibrosis and inflammation to stop at the same boundary as the atypical alveolar cells. Conversely, reactive lesions tend to be less well defined, and the interstitial scarring extends beyond the areas of alveolar cell atypia. The individual cells in AAAH, although they are less homogeneous than those in BAC, tend to be more uniformly atypical than those of reactive hyperplasias (Fig. 31–13). Notably, a variety of chemotherapeutic agents can induce striking degrees

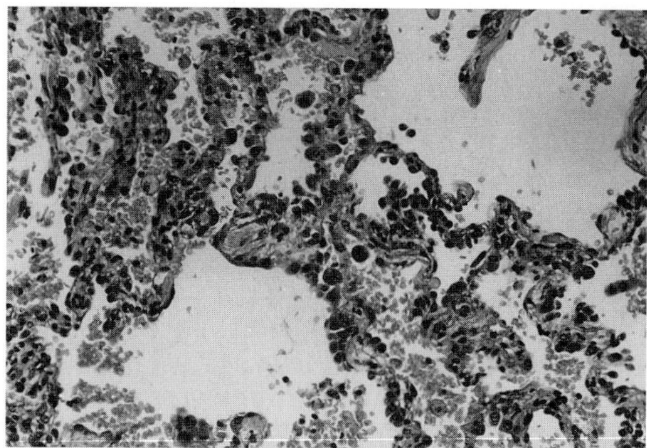

FIGURE 31–13 ■ Atypical adenomatous alveolar hyperplasia (AAAH) is conceptually related to bronchioloalveolar carcinoma and probably represents its precursor. Note the striking similarity between this photomicrograph of AAAH and the features shown in Figure 31–12.

of cytologic atypia; this phenomenon is a well-documented pitfall in exfoliative cytology (Huang et al, 1989; Ritter et al, 1995). The authors have also seen several examples of pneumocytes with intranuclear cytoplasmic inclusions in clear-cut cases of organizing phase diffuse alveolar damage; hence, their presence should not be viewed as pathognomonic of neoplasia.

It is the authors' view that the distinction of AAAH from small BAC is a conceptually arbitrary one. Standard criteria that are useful in this task include uniformly atypical nuclei, large lesional size, and complex growth with budding or tufting of tumor cells in the alveolar spaces in BAC but not AAAH (Mori et al, 1993; Rao and Fraire, 1995). Kitamura and colleagues (1999) suggested that a nuclear area of less than 40 μm^2 and a lesional diameter of less than 5 mm could effectively distinguish AAAH from small BAC. Miller (1990) also proposed a cut-off of 5 mm to separate "bronchioloalveolar cell adenoma" from BAC.

Nevertheless, morphometric and immunohistologic analyses have shown a synonymity rather than a disparity between AAAH and BAC (Nakanishi, 1990; Travis et al, 1988). Similarly, molecular studies, although showing some differences in statistical groups, have demonstrated many more shared features than differences (Niho et al, 1999).

The most important consideration of this discussion concerns the clinical significance of AAAH. In practice, this lesion is not appreciated until microscopic sections arrive on the pathologist's desk, and they are seen in four main contexts: in sections of a wedge biopsy specimen of a non-neoplastic disease; in wedge resection margins of a peripheral carcinoma; in "random" sections of a lobe with another, discrete carcinoma; and as suspected nodules of multifocal tumor along with at least one other documented peripheral adenocarcinoma. To develop some understanding of the importance of atypical lesions, several points must be kept in mind. First, inasmuch as most AAAH lesions are found in patients undergoing resection of an obvious cancer, it is nearly an insurmountable challenge to arrive at any conclusions concerning their biology. This is so because the outcome of those cases will be determined by the characteristics of the macroscopically obvious tumors. AAAH lesions tend to be multifocal throughout both lungs but may be inapparent on gross examination and can easily be missed even with modern radiologic imaging techniques. Therefore, short of bilateral lung transplantation, it is impossible to say what would constitute adequate surgical resection of such lesions. Given these realities, it is best for pathologists to be pragmatically conservative in the diagnosis of clinically inapparent AAAH as small BACs, despite the previously cited conceptual considerations. It is important to emphasize, however, that such lesions can be multifocal and have a relationship with subsequent multicentric BAC, underscoring the need for close follow-up to identify the possible appearance of metachronous tumors. On the other hand, proliferations that represent grossly observed lesions with compellingly atypical cytology should be designated as outright carcinomas.

Adenocarcinomas Associated with Scars

In the past, it was taught that fibrous scarring in the lung—seen as a consequence of pneumonia, interstitial fibroproliferative diseases, or pneumoconioses—predisposed to adenocarcinoma and had a directly causative role in the genesis of that tumor type (Meyer and Liebow, 1965). Nevertheless, several investigators have concluded that the central fibrosis seen in "scar adenocarcinomas" is formed *following* initiation of the carcinoma and is the product of the tumor cells themselves (Barsky et al, 1996; Cagle et al, 1985; Shimosato et al, 1993). At a practical level, there is no reason to suspect that fibrosing conditions in the lung are, in and of themselves, preneoplastic. With particular reference to asbestosis and silicosis, special forms of pulmonary interstitial fibrosis, the authors' redaction of the aggregated literature leads to the conclusion that carcinomas of the lung arise *only* in patients with those conditions who also are, or have been, cigarette smokers. In that scenario, it is further believed that smoking is the principal carcinogenic factor.

ADENOSQUAMOUS CARCINOMA

Morphogenesis and Morphologic Findings

Adenosquamous carcinoma (ASC) is a "composite" tumor exhibiting simultaneous squamous and glandular differentiation in the same mass. It accounts for no more than 5% of all lung cancers in most surgical series (Ishida et al, 1992; Sridhar et al, 1990; Takamori et al, 1991). The clinical, radiographic, and gross pathologic attributes of ASC are most similar to those of "pure" adenocarcinomas of the lung. A point of contention in regard to this lesion is whether it is synonymous with high-grade mucoepidermoid carcinoma of the salivary glandular type. The authors' opinion is that those two neoplasms are typically separable from one another. Salivary gland analog tumors in the lung tend to arise in the large central airways, in contrast to the propensity of ASC to be peripheral. In addition, foci of lower-grade mucoepidermoid carcinoma are often present in the former, but not the latter, of these tumor types. The prognosis of pulmonary ASC is said to be rather adverse. In series reported by Ishida and colleagues (1992) and Takamori and associates (1991), the survival of patients with adenosquamous tumors was statistically worse than that of individuals with "pure" adenocarcinomas or squamous cell carcinomas.

LARGE CELL UNDIFFERENTIATED CARCINOMA

Morphogenesis

Large cell undifferentiated carcinomas (LCUCs) account for approximately 15% of all lung cancers (Carter and Patchefsky, 1998). As discussed, diagnostic use of the term "non–small cell carcinoma" has produced some confusion between poorly differentiated SCC, poorly differentiated ACA, poorly differentiated ASC, and true LCUC. Accordingly, it has been suggested that the designation of "large cell carcinoma" should be employed restrictively as a synonym for LCUC.

Morphologic Findings

LCUCs are typically larger than 5 cm in maximum dimension, have a white-grey cut surface (which may be lobulated and may resemble "fish flesh," thus potentially simulating the appearance of a sarcoma or a hematolymphoid lesion), and are rarely multicentric. Internal necrosis is a relatively common feature. Approximately 50% demonstrate a connection to a large tubular airway.

Histologically, LCUCs comprise large polygonal cells with vesicular chromatin, prominent nucleoli, discernible cytoplasmic borders, and a lack of glandular differentiation or keratinization (Fig. 31–14). They are typically arranged in sheets or large clusters, potentially exhibiting foci of central necrosis. Two distinctive subtypes of large cell carcinoma also exist—giant cell carcinoma and clear cell carcinoma.

Giant cell carcinoma was initially thought to be a separate clinicopathologic entity unto itself (Ginsberg et al, 1992; Nash and Stout, 1958), but that philosophy is no longer thought to be valid (Attanoos et al, 1988). Microscopically, this variant group of LCUC includes extremely pleomorphic large tumor cells, which are often multinucleated. There is a regular admixture of polymorphonuclear leucocytes with the neoplastic elements, even in the absence of necrosis, suggesting tumoral synthesis of leucocyte cytokines such as granulocyte colony stimulating factor (Sawyers et al, 1992). Parenthetically, this phenomenon can also be associated with systemic neutrophilia in association with giant cell LCUC. Neoplastic "cannibalism" may also be observed, wherein the giant tumor cells appear to engulf one another microscopically.

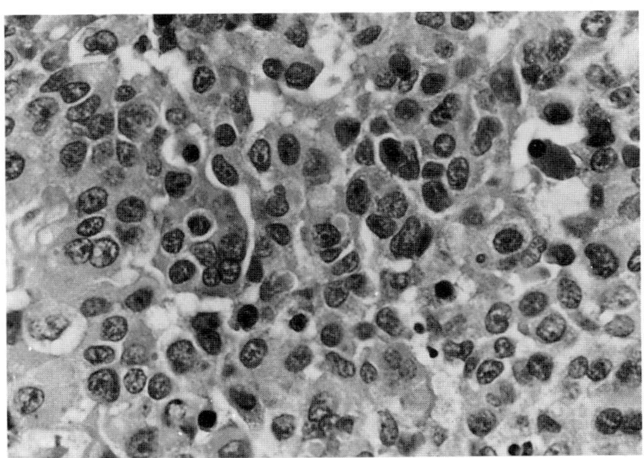

FIGURE 31–14 ■ Large cell, undifferentiated carcinoma of the lung that comprises polygonal cells with prominent nucleoli and no evidence of lineage-related differentiation.

Primary clear cell carcinoma of the lung (CCCL) is a diagnosis of exclusion. That is so because a number of other clear cell neoplasms of the lung, including some "carcinoids," the so-called benign sugar tumor, metastatic renal cell carcinoma, and metastatic "balloon cell" melanoma, must be considered before making an interpretation of CCCL (Bonetti et al, 1994; Gaffey et al, 1997, 1998; Nowak et al, 1998; Shimosato, 1995; Yoshida et al, 1995). This can be accomplished by a combination of radiographic, electron microscopic, and immunohistologic evaluations, which should be done invariably in each instance. The overall clinicopathologic attributes of CCCL are comparable to those of LCUC that are not otherwise specified.

In recent years, it has been suggested that a subset of pulmonary large cell carcinomas that show neuroendocrine differentiation (as detected by electron microscopy or immunohistology) should be nosologically separated from truly undifferentiated large-cell tumors (Hammond and Sause, 1985; MacDowell et al, 1981; Piehl et al, 1988; Wick et al, 1992). Hence, the terms "exocrine large cell carcinoma" (another synonym for LCUC) and "endocrine large cell carcinoma" have entered use (Piehl et al, 1988). In the authors' opinion, "endocrine large cell carcinomas" are best specified as either large cell neuroendocrine carcinomas or large cell carcinomas with occult neuroendocrine differentiation.

SARCOMATOID CARCINOMAS (INCLUDING "CARCINOSARCOMAS" AND "BLASTOMAS")

Morphogenesis

Neoplasms of the lung with histologic appearances featuring the presence of fusiform and pleomorphic cells, like those of sarcomas, are uncommon. A review of malignant pulmonary tumors seen during a 12-year study period at the authors' institution showed that roughly 2400 such neoplasms were treated overall; sarcomatoid carcinomas (SCs) (a term that the authors use to encompass lesions called "carcinosarcomas" [CSs] and pulmonary "blastomas" [PBs] by others) accounted for 1% of these cancers (Nappi et al, 1994). During the same interval, however, only one example of well-documented primary pulmonary sarcoma was observed, excluding examples of Kaposi's sarcoma in patients with the acquired immunodeficiency syndrome (AIDS). Therefore, a diagnosis of carcinoma is far more likely than one of true mesenchymal neoplasia when confronted with a primary spindle-cell and pleomorphic tumor of the lung (Huang et al, 1996; Keel et al, 1999; Suster, 1995; Zeren et al, 1995).

SCs, PBs, and CSs show a similar male-to-female ratio of 2:1. The age range at discovery of the tumors is 44 to 78 years, with a mean of 65. Virtually all patients with such lesions are cigarette smokers, and they usually complain of cough, dyspnea, or hemoptysis. The anatomic distribution of these lesions potentially includes all of the pulmonary lobes; they may be either central or peripheral, although PB is typically a centrifugal tumor and may even be subpleural.

Radiographically, the neoplasms are represented by irregularly marginated (often spiculated) masses that range in maximum dimension between 1.5 and 12 cm. A few show variable internal radiographic attenuation that is consistent with the presence of intratumoral hemorrhage or necrosis.

Morphologic Findings

Grossly, most CSs, PBs, and SCs are large lesions that often exhibit internal necrosis and hemorrhage, as well as an irregular permeative interface with the surrounding lung parenchyma. Occasional tumors of this type, however, are small (<3 cm) and peripherally located, suggesting the appearance of "usual" pulmonary adenocarcinomas. Some examples of CS and SC have a discernibly polypoid endobronchial component, whereas PB is usually a peripheral lesion.

Microscopically, a range of histologic appearances can be observed in such neoplasms, including monodifferentiated spindle cell and pleomorphic lesions that closely resemble sarcomas; biphasic tumors composed of recognizable carcinoma morphotypes admixed with nondescript spindle-cell elements; other biphasic lesions in which the sarcoma-like components demonstrate heterologous (e.g., osteosarcoma-like, chondrosarcoma-like, angiosarcoma-like, or rhabdomyosarcoma-like) differentiation (these are the lesions that are still called carcinosarcomas by other observers (Fig. 31–15); biphasic neoplasms showing admixtures of fetal-like glands and nondescript blastema-like small cells (traditionally called blastomas) (Francis and Jacobsen, 1983; Koss, 1995; Souza et al, 1965), and still other proliferations that are deceptively bland and simulate the appearance of inflammatory pseudotumors of the lung (Wick et al, 1995). Cavazza and associates (1996) also have described examples of "composite" rhabdoid tumors of the lung, in which elements resembling malignant rhabdoid tumor of other sites were admixed with ordinary adenocarcinoma of the lung. These neoplasms probably represent additional examples of sarcoma-like change in pulmonary cancers.

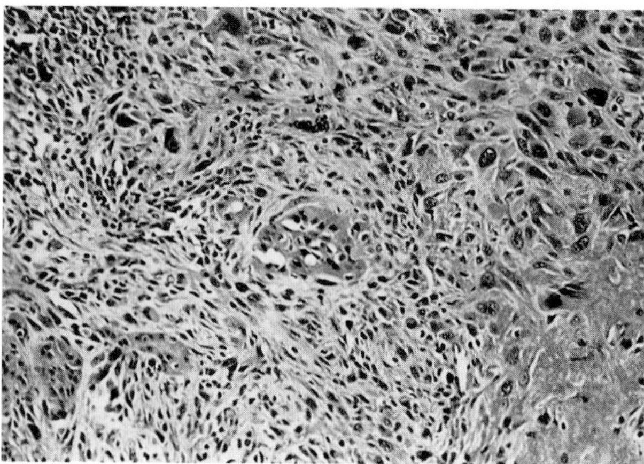

FIGURE 31–15 ■ Carcinosarcoma (sarcomatoid carcinoma) of the lung in which the foci of recognizable, poorly differentiated, squamous carcinoma (*center* and *bottom left*) are admixed with sarcoma-like spindle cells.

Despite its relative rarity, sarcomatoid pulmonary cancer has been the object of intense interest for many decades. Several papers have been written on the clinicopathologic features of carcinosarcoma, pulmonary blastoma, and spindle-cell carcinoma of the lung, with histologic descriptions of such entities paralleling those discussed earlier. Although it was suggested in early communications that carcinosarcomas were merely carcinomas showing pseudomesenchymal metaplasia, other authors appear to have adopted the premise that such lesions were "collision" tumors with truly sarcomatous components (Wick and Swanson, 1993). Some definitions of CS have not mandated the presence of heterologous mesenchymal elements, so that neoplasms simply showing admixtures of overt carcinoma and spindle-cell foci were included in this nosologic category.

Recent reports on CS, PB, and SC have revealed four reproducible observations that link these proliferations together conceptually. First, one relatively commonly finds areas in all three tumor types where obviously epithelioid foci merge imperceptibly with others having sarcomatoid patterns, provided that the lesions are sampled thoroughly. Second, conjoint immunoreactivity for several potential markers of carcinomatous differentiation has been seen in both of the components just mentioned. Third, microscopically obvious carcinomas have been identified that appear to lack keratin production—at least as detected in routinely processed tissues—providing a link to those examples of SC with a similar immunophenotype. Fourth, there is little if any difference in the biologic behaviors of pulmonary SC, PB, and CS, regardless of the histologic nuances of such tumors (Wick et al, 1997).

There is growing evidence that carcinomas undergoing divergent sarcomatoid evolution may demonstrate immunohistologic co-labelling for epithelial and mesenchymal markers in the same cell populations, some of which may have acquired a mesenchymal-like phenotype (e.g., of myogenous or chondro-osseous tissue) microscopically (Wick and Swanson, 1993). In view of these findings, other authors also have suggested that CS and SC are merely points in the same neoplastic spectrum of lung tumors, the basic nature of which is epithelial (Humphrey et al, 1988; Ro et al, 1992). We strongly endorse this construct. Moreover, in our desire to eliminate confusing diagnostic terminology whenever possible, we suggest that the terms "biphasic sarcomatoid carcinoma" and "monophasic sarcomatoid carcinoma" should be adopted to replace "carcinosarcoma"/"pulmonary blastoma" and "spindle cell carcinoma," respectively. Using this paradigm, biphasic neoplasms may or may not display evidence of a divergent cell line, either on conventional microscopy, ultrastructural studies, or immunohistology.

Such proliferations may be regarded as examples of clonal evolution, as acknowledged in "de-differentiated" malignancies of various types (Brooks, 1986). Parenthetically, this general concept can also be implemented to explain the existence of pulmonary tumors with mixed-carcinomatous (e.g., adenosquamous or mixed small cell/non–small cell) phenotypes, as mentioned above.

CLINICOPATHOLOGIC FEATURES OF NEUROENDOCRINE NEOPLASMS OF THE LUNG

The concept of a "diffuse neuroendocrine system" is not a new one. Feyrter developed this paradigm in 1938, in a philosophical attempt to unify tumors in several anatomic locations that had potential secretory functions and similar morphologic characteristics (Feyrter, 1938). Pearse (1974) refined and renamed the cellular network in question 35 years later, coining the designation of "APUD system" (for Amine Precursor Uptake and Decarboxylation) to describe its shared biochemical attributes. Inherent in the latter scheme was the presumption that all "APUD" cells—and tumors deriving from them (i.e., "APUDomas")—emanated from the remnants of the neural crest.

There is, perhaps, no other single aspect of neuroendocrine pulmonary neoplasia that is as exasperating as the pathologic terminology that has been used to describe it. Such terms as "bronchial adenoma," "carcinoid," "atypical carcinoid," "Kulchitsky cell carcinoma," "argentaffinoma," "APUDoma," "atypical endocrine carcinoma," "oat cell carcinoma," "small cell carcinoma," "large cell neuroendocrine carcinoma," and "large cell carcinoma with neuroendocrine features" have all been employed in the past in this context.

A crucial concept in understanding the categorization and clinical behavior of neuroendocrine neoplasms is that all of them are at least potentially malignant tumors. Therefore, it follows logically that the modifier "benign" should not ever be applied in conjunction with any of the diagnostic terms discussed earlier. For example, in reference to classic bronchial "carcinoids"—generally regarded as defining the "low" end of the spectrum of biologic behavior in this context—there are many well-documented examples of metastasizing lesions that can be found in the literature on these tumors. The following sections consider discrete members of the family of neuroendocrine lung tumors, as defined by the World Health Organization.

Classic Carcinoid

Morphogenesis

Pulmonary carcinoids were initially labeled as "adenomas" of the bronchus (Dramer, 1930), a term that most unfortunately persists in clinical usage. Their similarity to gastrointestinal carcinoids, so named as "carcinoma-like tumors," was noted many decades ago. Although most classic carcinoids are centrally located, a few are found in the periphery of the lung (Abdi et al, 1988; Skinner and Ewen, 1976). The criterion commonly used to distinguish these two locations is the relationship of the lesion to a cartilaginous airway; tumors that are so associated are considered central, whereas those without such a relationship to a tubular airway are considered peripheral.

Morphologic Findings

Carcinoids with classic histology are rarely a diagnostic dilemma. They typically grow as polypoid intraluminal masses, with an intact overlying epithelium, or one demonstrating squamous metaplasia. This pattern explains the usual clinical presentation, which is largely that of localized obstruction, manifested by wheezing, cough, or pneumonia. These patients almost never exhibit the carcinoid syndrome; rarely, patients have had associated Cushing's syndrome or other endocrinopathies. Localized obstruction also dominates the radiographic picture, with evidence of localized pneumonia, or atelectasis. Rarely, a central mass growing with a dumbbell-like configuration will be seen on plain films, and computed tomography scans will usually demonstrate a lesion within and adjacent to a large airway. Men and women are approximately equally affected, and young to middle-aged adults account for most cases. The lesions are thus usually seen in patients who are substantially younger than those with ordinary bronchogenic carcinomas.

Gross features include a lesion size of 2 to 4 cm. Carcinoids are usually tan to dark red and should lack obvious necrosis or hemorrhage. Both central and peripheral tumors display a variety of growth patterns, including trabecular, ribbon-like, nested, and solid sheet (Fig. 31–16). The cytoplasm is relatively abundant and may be strikingly oncocytic. Spindle cell change is rarely noted in central lesions and is more usual in peripheral carcinoids (Ranchod and Levine, 1980); it should be emphasized that fusiform cells are not, in and of themselves, evidence of more aggressive biologic potential. Mitotic activity is very limited, and necrosis is absent (Travis et al, 1998).

The behavior of central and peripheral carcinoids of the lung is generally good. Complete excision is the treatment of choice, which may necessitate lobectomy or a more complicated sleeve resection. Endobronchial

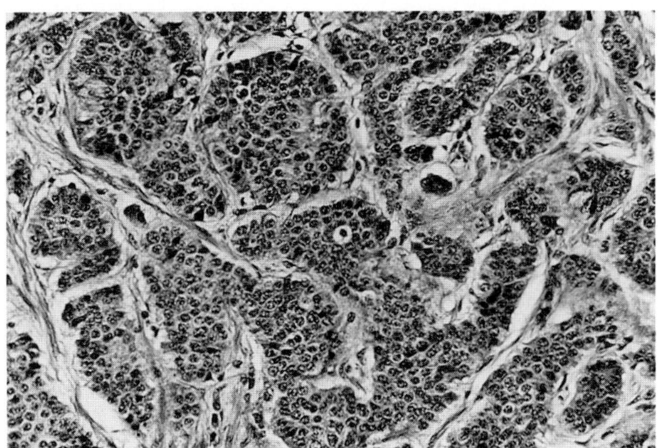

FIGURE 31–16 ■ Classic carcinoid of the lung that manifests organoid growth of uniform tumor cells with minimal mitotic activity and no necrosis.

excisions are associated with an unacceptable rate of local recurrence. Metastatic rates vary from 1% to 20%; true incidence is approximately 5% to 10%, and, when present, secondary deposits are usually seen in adjacent peribronchial or hilar lymph nodes (McCaughan et al, 1985). It is this observation that leads the authors to consider these lesions as undeniable carcinomas. Moreover, distant metastases of prototypical grade I pulmonary neuroendocrine carcinomas (NECs) have been well documented, although they are rare (McBurney et al, 1953). These show a tendency for involvement of the skin, bones, liver, or brain. Overall, survival is in excess of 90% to 95% at 5 years.

Atypical Carcinoid

Morphogenesis

Few areas of pathology arouse the combination of angst, confusion, and controversy as the discussion surrounding the proper labelling of atypical carcinoid. That term was first used by Arrigoni and colleagues in 1972. They reviewed 216 pulmonary "carcinoids" and found 23 with unusual features, including pleomorphism, increased mitotic activity, hyperchromatic nuclei, high nucleocytoplasmic ratios, and evidence of spontaneous necrosis or hemorrhage. In this original series, 70% of the lesions metastasized, and 7 individuals (30%) died of their tumors.

Morphologic Findings

The following criteria are used to define atypical carcinoma: a mitotic rate of 5 or more per 10 high-power fields; at least moderate nuclear pleomorphism; spontaneous necrosis; and at least a focal loss of the organoid growth pattern associated with low-grade NECs of the lung (Fig. 31–17). As indicated by Yousem (1991), to avoid overgrading, a requirement for two or more of these criteria is a reasonable one before the designation of "atypical" is used.

Atypical carcinoids are slightly larger than their "typical" relatives, often greater than 3 cm in diameter. Lymph-node metastases are present at diagnosis in 30% to 50% of cases, and roughly 25% will have remote metastatic disease.

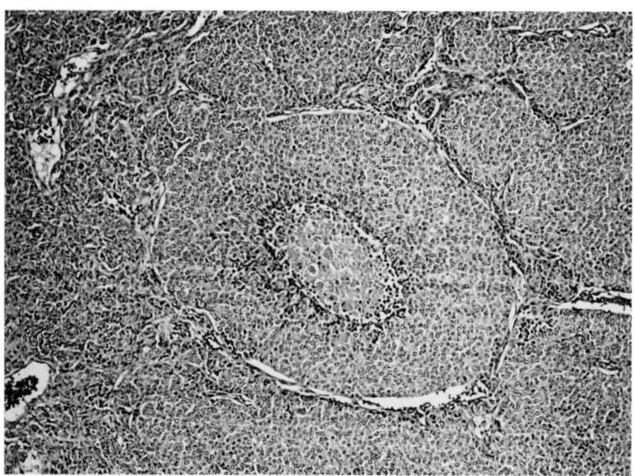

FIGURE 31–17 ■ Atypical carcinoid of the lung that shows central en masse necrosis and brisk mitotic activity.

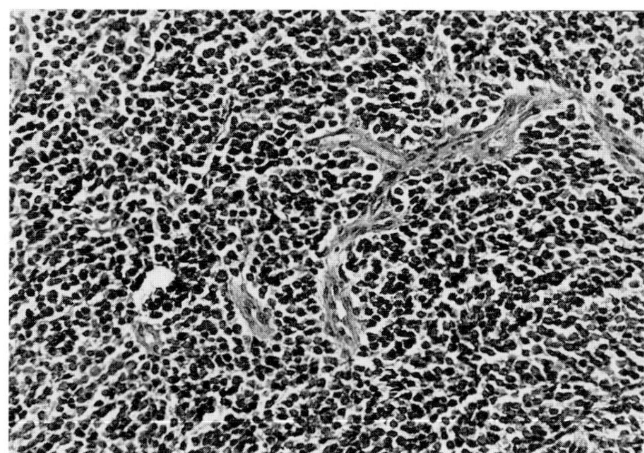

FIGURE 31–18 ■ Small cell neuroendocrine ("oat-cell") carcinoma comprising sheets and nests of tumor cells with little cytoplasm and abundant mitoses.

Small Cell Carcinoma

Morphogenesis

Small cell carcinoma (SmCC) is probably the best-recognized neoplasm in the family of neuroendocrine lung tumors, accounting for about 20% of all pulmonary carcinomas (Azzopardi, 1959; Carter, 1983; Cook et al, 1993; Yesner, 1983). Most SmCCs arise in the large central airways, but peripheral examples are also well documented.

Morphologic Findings

The classic morphologic appearance of this lesion features small, hyperchromatic, molded cells; almost no visible cytoplasm; inconspicuous or absent nucleoli; single cell necrosis; and a relative absence of stromal desmoplasia (Azzopardi, 1959) (Fig. 31–18). En-masse (coagulative) necrosis is not uncommon, and the tumor cells of SmCC may be focally pleomorphic as well.

A difficulty that may be encountered is the identification of cells that have the appearance of small cell carcinoma in a fine-needle aspirate of an apparently solitary peripheral lung nodule. As mentioned earlier, peripheral lesions of this type account for 10% of cases (Gephardt et al, 1988). Another problem relating to SmCC is that although they are definable as high-grade tumors, their small cell nature may not be obvious in limited biopsy material (Thomas et al, 1993; Vollmer, 1982)

Large Cell Neuroendocrine Carcinoma

Morphogenesis and Morphologic Findings

The diagnosis of "large cell NEC" is a relatively new entry to the nomenclature of pulmonary carcinomas. Travis and associates (1991, 1998) proposed that this term should be used for tumors that have obvious features of neuroendocrine differentiation by light microscopy, but that do not

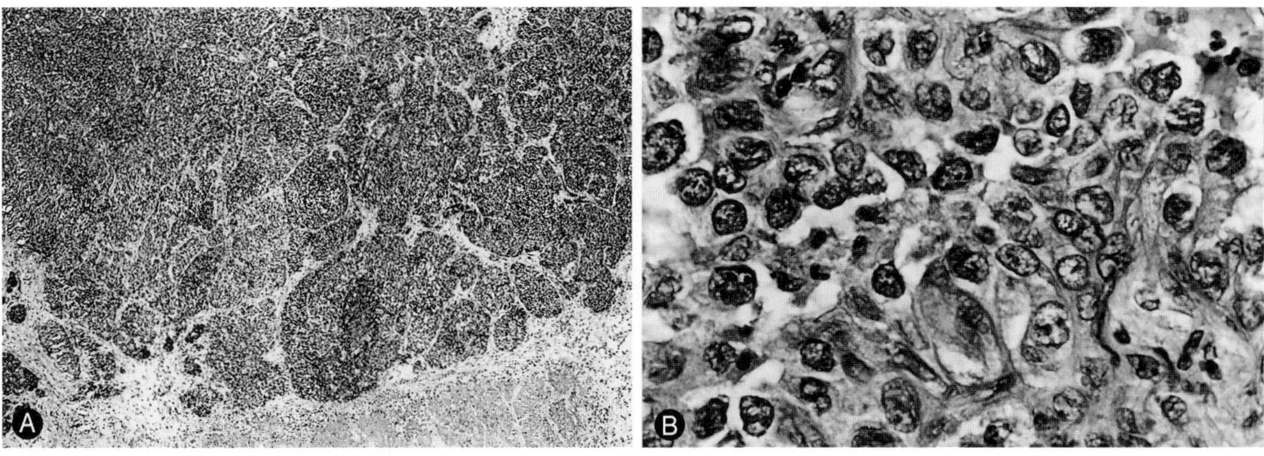

FIGURE 31–19 ■ Large cell neuroendocrine carcinoma demonstrating an organoid growth pattern and geographic necrosis (*A, bottom*). The tumor cells have dispersed chromatin and inconspicuous nucleoli (*B*), and they are much larger than those of small cell carcinoma (note contrasts with Figure 33–18).

fit into the diagnostic categories of "carcinoid," "atypical carcinoid," or "small cell carcinoma." The histologic attributes in question include a cell size that is at least three times that of small cell NEC; the presence of an organoid growth pattern; cellular palisading or rosette-like areas; geographic necrosis; a high mitotic rate (approximating that of small cell NEC); and a variably granular chromatin pattern (Travis et al, 1998) (Fig. 31–19).

The clinical features of large cell NECs (LCNECs) are distinctive. In reports by Travis and associates (1991, 1998) and others (Dresler et al, 1997; Jiang et al, 1998), these lesions almost always occur in heavy smokers, as does small cell NEC. Although a few cases are central masses, most tend to be located in the more peripheral lung parenchyma. Many examples of LCNEC are T1 or T2 tumors pathologically, but the aggressive potential of these lesions cannot be overstated. Only 10% of patients are alive at 2 years, despite the fact that many of them have stage I tumors. All patients in series published by Travis and co-workers (1991, 1998) were dead of disease or had distant metastases at 2 years' follow-up. We have studied a series of 23 institutional LCNECs. The survival for stage I cases in that experience was 18% at 40 months (Dresler et al, 1997). Thus, the behavior of LCNEC is significantly worse than that of poorly differentiated adenocarcinoma or squamous carcinoma, or LCUC. Surprisingly, the survival of patients with resected, low-stage small cell NECs is *better* than that of individuals with LCNEC (Smit et al, 1994).

STYLIZED SURGICAL PATHOLOGY REPORTS ON CARCINOMA OF THE LUNG

Not all pulmonary carcinomas are resectable. Colby and Deschamps (1996) have summarized the clinicopathologic features of these tumors, including that subset that is surgically approachable (Table 31–4). For those lesions that can be completely excised, pathology organizations such as the College of American Pathologists and the Association of Directors of Anatomic and Surgical Pathology (ADASP) have published guidelines for reporting morphologic findings (Association of Directors of Anatomic and Surgical Pathology, 1995; Nash et al, 1995). In the authors' opinion, the most tenable is that provided by the latter of those two organizations, which is reproduced in slightly modified form below.

COMMENTS AND CONTROVERSIES

A knowledge of basic pathologic findings as they relate to lung cancer is of supreme importance to the clinician. Since the first edition of this book, a new 1999 World Health Organization (WHO) classification has emerged and in some respects has made things a bit more confusing, especially with regards to the "neuroendocrine" group of tumors including small cell lung cancer, large undifferentiated lung cancer with neuroendocrine features, and neuroendocrine large cell carcinoma. These, according to the WHO, are three different tumors—I am not sure the

TABLE 31–4 ■ **Comparison of Clinicopathologic Features by Histologic Types of Carcinoma of the Lung**

Tumor Type	*Cases (%)*	*Smokers (%)*	*Central Lesions (%)*	*Localized (%)*	*5-Yr Survival (%)*
Squamous cell	30	98	64	21.5	15.4
Adenocarcinoma	31	82	5	22.2	16.6*
Small cell carcinoma	19	99	74	8.2	4.6
Other**	15	95	42	15	11.5

*Bronchioloalveolar carcinomas are associated with a 42% 5-year survival.
**Statistics in this group encompass large cell "undifferentiated" carcinoma, large cell neuroendocrine carcinoma, and sarcomatoid carcinoma.
From Colby TV, Deschamps C: The lung and pleura. In Banks PM, Kraybill WG (eds): Pathology for the Surgeon. Philadelphia, WB Saunders, 1996.

SUGGESTED ADASP REPORTING FORMAT FOR RESECTED LUNG CARCINOMAS

A. Gross Description

1. How the specimen was received—fresh, in formalin, opened, unopened, and so on.
2. How the specimen was identified—labeled with (name, number) and designated as (e.g., right upper lobe).
3. Part(s) of lung included—including measurements in three dimensions and weights and description of other attached structures (i.e., parietal pleura, hilar lymph nodes, etc.).
4. Tumor description
   —Tumor location, including relationship to lobe(s), segment(s), and, if pertinent, major airway(s) and pleura. Involvement of lobar or mainstream bronchus should be specified.
   —Proximity to bronchial resection margin and to other surgical margins (i.e., chest wall, soft tissue, hilar vessels) as appropriate.
   —Tumor size (three dimensions, if possible).
   —Presence or absence of satellite tumor modules.
5. Description of non-tumorous lung—that is, presence or absence of postobstructive changes or other abnormalities (e.g., bronchiectasis, mucus plugs, obstructive pneumonia, atelectasis).

B. Diagnostic Information

1. Site of tumor (i.e., side, lobe, specific segment, if appropriate) and surgical procedure (i.e, segmentectomy, lobectomy, pneumonectomy), including portion of lung resected.
2. Histologic type—that is, a modified World Health Organization (WHO) classification (Travis et al, 1999) is recommended. Although the WHO classification is based on light microscopic criteria, the results of ancillary studies (i.e., histochemistry, immunohistochemistry, electron microscopy) should be reported when appropriate (e.g., large cell neuroendocrine carcinoma).
   —Squamous cell carcinoma (keratinization or intercellular bridges). Variant: spindle cell (squamous carcinoma).
   —Adenocarcinoma (tubular, acinar, or papillary growth pattern, or mucus production; acinar adenocarcinoma (i.e., adenocarcinoma, not otherwise specified); papillary adenocarcinoma; solid carcinoma with mucus formation; and variants including bronchioloalveolar adenocarcinoma and spindle cell adenocarcinoma.
   —Large cell carcinoma (large nuclei, prominent nucleoli, abundant cytoplasm, without characteristic features of squamous cell, small cell, or adenocarcinoma) including variants of giant cell carcinoma and clear cell carcinoma (large cell carcinomas composed extensively [>90%] of large cells with clear or foamy cytoplasm without mucin; clear cell features also can be prominent in squamous cell carcinomas and adenocarcinomas and in metastatic renal cell carcinoma).
   —Adenosquamous carcinoma.
   —Neuroendocrine tumors including "carcinoid tumor"; "atypical carcinoid"; "large cell neuroendocrine carcinoma"; and "small cell carcinoma." Variants can be mixed small cell/large cell carcinoma or composite small cell carcinoma (typical small cell carcinoma intimately admixed with areas of squamous cell carcinoma or adenocarcinoma).
   —Bronchial gland (salivary gland analogue) carcinomas (adenoid cystic carcinoma, mucoepidermoid carcinoma, acinic cell carcinoma).
   —Other specific carcinoma types
3. Histologic grade—WHO classification (i.e., well, moderately, and poorly differentiated) recommended for squamous cell carcinoma and adenocarcinomas of acinar (i.e., adenocarcinoma, not further specified) or papillary type.
4. Histologic assessment of surgical margins—Include comment regarding involvement of lobar or mainstem bronchi by invasive or in situ carcinoma, and microscopic relationship of tumor to bronchial or vascular margin(s).
5. Pleural involvement—Specify whether tumor invades into but not through visceral pleura without involving parietal pleura (T2) or into parietal pleura (T3) (elastic tissue stains can be helpful in defining the limiting elastic layer of visceral pleura).
6. Lymph node metastases—Indicate the number of involved nodes and the total number of nodes received. (Precise node counts may be difficult for fragmented specimens such as those received from mediastinoscopy.) The nodal groups (N) should be specifically identified using the American Joint Committee on Cancer intraoperative staging system for regional lymph nodes (Fleming et al, 1997). N2 lymph nodes (with the exception of level 11 interlobar nodes) are generally received separately and must be appropriately identified by the submitting surgeon; these are to be reported separately. Pneumonectomies are usually accompanied by attached N2 lymph nodes, which should be specifically identified by location. If the nodal involvement is only by direct extension, this feature should be noted.
7. Non-neoplastic lung—Any significant abnormalities (e.g., granulomas, pneumonia) should be recorded.

SUGGESTED ADASP REPORTING FORMAT FOR RESECTED LUNG CARCINOMAS *Continued*

C. Optional Features

The following features are considered optional in the final report because they represent specific institutional preferences or they are considered inconclusive vis-à-vis prognostic significance.

1. Stage—Surgical pathology reports containing the previously listed information will contain all of the necessary data to establish the International TNM (tumor, node, metastasis) Staging System for lung carcinoma. It should be emphasized that pathologic tumor stage may be based on incomplete information and therefore may differ from clinical tumor stage.
2. Angiolymphatic invasion—Whenever possible, it should be specified whether the structures involved are blood vessels or lymphatic vessels and whether the involved blood vessels are muscular arteries, elastic arteries, or veins.
3. Perineural invasion.
4. Presence or absence of extranodal (extracapsular) tumor invasion.
5. Results of ancillary investigations (e.g., molecular pathology evaluations).

first and last are that much different, although their response to chemotherapy seems to be somewhat different. I note, with dismay, that the WHO Panel contained not one clinician; only pathologists were consulted for the new classification, which impacts so significantly on management issues.

Although it is less important clinically to distinguish the various types of non–small cell lung cancer, immunohistochemical testing, and, to a lesser extent, electron microscopy can differentiate midline tumors in which the site of origin (e.g., mediastinum versus lung) is in doubt.

The tumor, necrosis, metastasis (TNM) classification and cell type (non–small cell versus small cell) remain the most important prognostic factors, but large cell neuroendocrine tumors (considered to be a non–small cell tumor) also display poorer prognoses, much like their small cell counterpart. In the future, biologic prognostic factors will become more significant and, hopefully, will augment the TNM system and cell typing in the determination of treatment.

The authors discuss the reporting format for resected lung carcinomas. I certainly support this and every hospital should adopt this as a minimum. Surgeons should understand that pathologists need information to complete the pathologic reporting. Most of that information must come from the surgeon!

R. J. G.

■ REFERENCES

Abdi EA, Goel R, Bishop S, Bain GO: Peripheral carcinoid tumors of the lung: A clinicopathologic study. J Surg Oncol 39:190–196, 1988.

Arrigoni MG, Woolner LB, Bernatz PE: Atypical carcinoid tumors of the lung. J Thorac Cardiovasc Surg 64:413–421, 1972.

Association of Directors of Anatomic & Surgical Pathology: Recommendations for the reporting of resected primary lung carcinomas. Am J Clin Pathol 104:371–374, 1995.

Attanoos RL, Papagiannis A, Suttinont P et al: Pulmonary giant cell carcinoma: Pathological entity or morphological phenotype? Histopathology 32:225–231, 1998.

Azzopardi JG: Oat cell carcinoma of the bronchus. J Pathol Bacteriol 78:513–519, 1959.

Barsky SH, Grossman DA, Ho J, Holmes EC: The multifocality of bronchioloalveolar lung carcinoma: Evidence and implications of a multiclonal origin. Mod Pathol 7:633–640, 1994.

Barsky SH, Huang SJ, Bhuta S: The extracellular matrix of pulmonary scar carcinomas is suggestive of a desmoplastic origin. Am J Pathol 124:412–419, 1996.

Bonetti F, Pea M, Martignoni G et al: Clear cell ("sugar") tumor of the lung is a lesion strictly related to angiomyolipoma—the concept of a familiy of lesions characterized by the presence of the perivascular epithelioid cell (PEC). Pathology 26:230–236, 1994.

Brambilla E, Moro D, Veale D et al: Basal cell (basaloid) carcinoma of the lung: A new morphologic and phenotypic entity with separate prognostic significance. Hum Pathol 23:993–1003, 1992.

Brooks JJ: The significance of double phenotypic patterns and markers in human sarcomas. Am J Pathol 125:113–123, 1986.

Cagle PT, Cohle SD, Greenberg SD: Natural history of pulmonary scar cancers: Clinical and prognostic implications. Cancer 56:2031–2035, 1985.

Carter D: Small-cell carcinoma of the lung. Am J Surg Pathol 7:787–795, 1983.

Carter D, Patchefsky AS: Tumors and Tumor-like Conditions of the Lung, Philadelphia, WB Saunders, 1998, pp. 266–285.

Cavazza A, Colby TV, Tsokos M et al: Lung tumors with a rhabdoid phenotype. Am J Clin Pathol 105:182–188, 1996.

Clayton F: Bronchioloalveolar carcinomas: Cell types, patterns of growth, and prognostic correlates. Cancer 57:1555–1564, 1986.

Clayton F: The spectrum of significance of bronchioloalveolar carcinomas. Pathol Annu 23:361–394, 1988.

Colby TV, Deschamps C: The lung and pleura. In Banks PM, Kraybill WG (eds): Pathology for the Surgeon. Philadelphia, WB Saunders, 1996, pp. 155–168.

Colby TV, Koss MN, Travis WD: Tumors of the lower respiratory tract. In Armed Forces Institute of Pathology: Atlas of Tumor Pathology (Series 3, Fascicle 13), Washington, DC, 1995, pp. 203–234.

Cook RM, Miller YE, Bunn PA Jr: Small cell lung cancer: Etiology, biology, clinical features, staging, and treatment. Curr Probl Cancer 17:69–141, 1993.

DaCosta N, Sivararnan A, Kinare SG: Carcinoma of lung with special reference to adenocarcinoma: An autopsy study of 122 cases. Ind J Cancer 30:42–47, 1993.

Dessy E, Pietra GG: Pseudomesotheliomatous adenocarcinoma of the lung: An immunohistochemical and ultrastructural study of three cases. Cancer 68:1747–1753, 1991.

Dramer R: Adenomas of the bronchus. Ann Otol Rhinol Laryngol 39:689–695, 1930.

Dresler CM, Ritter JH, Patterson GA et al: Clinical-pathologic analysis of 40 patients with large cell neuroendocrine carcinoma of the lung. Ann Thorac Surg 63:180–185, 1997.

Feldman ER, Eagan RT, Schaid J: Metastatic bronchioloalveolar carcinoma and metastatic adenocarcinoma of the lung: Comparison of clinical manifestations, chemotherapeutic responses, and prognosis. Mayo Clin Proc 67:27–32, 1992.

Feyrter F: Über Diffuse Endokrine Epitheliale Organe. Leipzig, Germany, JA Barth, 1938.

Fishback NF, Travis WD, Moran CA et al: Pleomorphic (spindle/giant-cell) carcinoma of the lung: A clinicopathologic correlation of 78 cases. Cancer 73:2936–2945, 1994.

Fleming ID, Cooper JS, Henson DE et al (eds): American Joint Committee on Cancer: Cancer Staging Manual, 5th ed. Philadelphia, Lippincott-Raven, 1997, pp. 127–137.

Fraire AE, Cooper SP, Greenberg SD, Buffler PA: Carcinoma of the lung: Changing cell distribution and histopathologic cell types. Prog Surg Pathol 12:129–149, 1992.

Fraire AE, Roggli VL, Vollmer RT et al: Lung cancer heterogeneity: Prognostic implications. Cancer 60:370–379, 1987.

Francis D, Jacobsen M: Pulmonary blastoma. Curr Top Pathol 73:265–294, 1983.

Frank MW, Shields TW, Joob AW et al: Lymphoepithelioma-like carcinoma of the lung. Ann Thorac Surg 64:1162–1164, 1997.

Gaffey MJ, Mills SE, Frierson HF Jr et al: Pulmonary clear cell carcinoid tumor: Another entity in the differential diagnosis of pulmonary clear cell neoplasia. Am J Surg Pathol 22:1020–1025, 1998.

Gaffey MJ, Mills SE, Ritter JH: Clear cell tumors of the lower respiratory tract. Semin Diagn Pathol 14:222–232, 1997.

Gephardt GN, Grady KJ, Ahmad M et al: Peripheral small cell undifferentiated carcinoma of the lung: Clinicopathologic features of 17 cases. Cancer 61:1002–1008, 1988.

Ginsberg SS, Buzaid AC, Stern H, Carter D: Giant cell carcinoma of the lung. Cancer 70:606–610, 1992.

Grotte D, Stanley MW, Swanson PE et al: Reactive type II pneumocytes in bronchoalveolar lavage fluid from acute respiratory syndrome can be mistaken for cells of adenocarcinoma. Diagn Cytopathol 6:317–322, 1990.

Grover FL, Piantadosi S: Recurrence and survival following resection of bronchioloalveolar carcinoma of the lung: The Lung Cancer Study Group experience. Ann Surg 209:779–790, 1989.

Hammond ME, Sause WT: Large cell neuroendocrine tumors of the lung. Cancer 56:1624–1629, 1985.

Hayashi H, Kitamura H, Nakatani Y et al: Primary signet-ring-cell carcinoma of the lung: Histochemical and immunohistochemical characterization. Hum Pathol 30:378–383, 1999.

Hegg CA, Flint A, Singh G: Papillary adenoma of the lung. Am J Clin Pathol 97:393–397, 1992.

Higashiyama M, Doi O, Kodama K et al: Extramammary Paget's disease of the bronchial epithelium. Arch Pathol Lab Med 115:185–188, 1991.

Huang JC, Ritter JH, Wick MR: Malignant nonepithelial neoplasms of the lungs and pleural surfaces. In Aisner J, Arriagada R, Green MR et al (eds): Comprehensive Textbook of Thoracic Oncology. Baltimore, Williams & Wilkins, 1996, pp. 815–849.

Huang MS, Colby TV, Goellner JR et al: Utility of bronchoalveolar lavage in the diagnosis of drug-induced pulmonary toxicity. Acta Cytol 33:533–538, 1989.

Humphrey PA, Scroggs MW, Roggli VL, Shelbourne JD: Pulmonary carcinoma with a sarcomatoid element. Hum Pathol 19:155–165, 1988.

Ishida T, Kaneko S, Yokohama H et al: Adenosquamous carcinoma of the lung: Clinicopathologic and immunohistochemical features. Am J Clin Pathol 97:678–695, 1992.

Jiang SX, Kameya T, Shoji M et al: Large cell neuroendocrine carcinoma of the lung: A histologic and immunohistochemical study of 22 cases. Am J Surg Pathol 22:526–537, 1998.

Keel SB, Bacha E, Mark EJ et al: Primary pulmonary sarcoma: A clinicopathologic study of 26 cases. Mod Pathol 12:1124–1131, 1999.

Kitamura H, Kameda Y, Ito T et al: Atypical adenomatous hyperplasia of the lung: Implications for the pathogenesis of peripheral lung adenocarcinoma. Am J Clin Pathol 111:610–622, 1999.

Koss MN: Pulmonary blastomas. Cancer Treat Res 72:349–362, 1995.

Koss MN, Hochholzer L, Frommelt RA: Carcinosarcomas of the lung: A clinicopathologic study of 66 patients. Am J Surg Pathol 23:1514–1526, 1999.

Koss MN, Travis WD, Moran CA, Hochholzer L: Pseudomesotheliomatous adenocarcinoma: A reappraisal. Semin Diagn Pathol 9:117–123, 1992.

Liebow AA: Bronchioloalveolar carcinoma. Adv Intern Med 10:329–358, 1960.

Lin JI, Tseng CH, Tsung SH: Pseudomesotheliomatous carcinoma of the lung. South Med J 73:655–657, 1980.

Lozowski W, Hajdu SI: Cytology and immunocytochemistry of bronchioloalveolar carcinoma. Acta Cytol 31:717–725, 1987.

MacDowell EM, Wilson TS, Trump BF: Atypical endocrine tumors of the lung. Arch Pathol Lab Med 105:20–28, 1981.

Manning JT Jr, Spjut HJ, Tschen JA: Bronchioloalveolar carcinoma: The significance of two histopathologic types. Cancer 54:525–534, 1984.

Marcq M, Galy P: Bronchioloalveolar carcinoma: Clinicopathological relationships, natural history, and prognosis in 29 cases. Am Rev Respir Dis 107:621–629, 1973.

McBurney RP, Kirklin JW, Woolner LB: Metastasizing bronchial adenomas. Surg Gynecol Obstet 96:482–492, 1953.

McCaughan BC, Martini N, Bains MS: Bronchial carcinoids: Review of 124 cases. J Thorac Cardiovasc Surg 89:8–17, 1985.

Meyer EC, Liebow AA: Relationship of interstitial pneumonia honeycombing and atypical epithelial proliferation to cancer of the lung. Cancer 18:322–351, 1965.

Miller RR: Bronchioloalveolar cell adenomas. Am J Surg Pathol 14:904–912, 1990.

Miller RR, Nelerris B, Evans KG et al: Glandular neoplasia of the lung: A proposed analogy to colonic tumors. Cancer 61:1009–1014, 1988.

Mizutani Y, Nakajima T, Morinaga S et al: Immunohistochemical localization of pulmonary surfactant apoproteins in various lung tumors, with special reference to lung adenocarcinoma subtypes. Cancer 61:532–537, 1988.

Moran CA, Hochholzer L, Fishback N et al: Mucinous (so-called colloid) carcinomas of lung. Mod Pathol 5:634–638, 1992.

Mori M, Chiba R, Takahashi T: Atypical adenomatous hyperplasia of the lung and its differentiation from adenocarcinoma: Characterization of atypical cells by morphometry and multivariate cluster analysis. Cancer 72:2331–2340, 1993.

Nakanishi K: Alveolar epithelial hyperplasia and adenocarcinoma of the lung. Arch Pathol Lab Med 114:363–368, 1990.

Nakatani Y, Kitamura H, Inayama Y et al: Pulmonary adenocarcinomas of the fetal lung type: A clinicopathologic study indicating differences in histology, epidemiology, and natural history of low-grade and high-grade forms. Am J Surg Pathol 22:399–411, 1998.

Nappi O, Glasner SD, Swanson PE, Wick MR: Biphasic and monophasic sarcomatoid carcinomas of the lung: A reappraisal of "carcinosarcomas" and "spindle cell carcinomas." Am J Clin Pathol 102:331–340, 1994.

Nappi O, Swanson PE, Wick MR: Pseudovascular adenoid squamous cell carcinoma of the lung: Clinicopathologic features of three cases and comparison with true pleuropulmonary angiosarcoma. Hum Pathol 25:373–378, 1994.

Nash G, Hutter RVP, Henson DE: Practice protocol for the examination of specimens from patients with lung cancer. Cancer Committee Task Force on the Examination of Specimens from Patients with Lung Cancer. Arch Pathol Lab Med 119:695–700, 1995.

Nash G, Stout AP: Giant cell carcinoma of the lung: Report of 5 cases. Cancer 11:369–376, 1958.

Niho S, Yokose T, Suzuki K et al: Monoclonality of atypical adenomatous hyperplasia of the lung. Am J Pathol 154:249–254, 1999.

Nowak MA, Fatteh SM, Campbell TE: Glycogen-rich malignant melanomas and glycogen-rich balloon cell malignant melanomas: Frequency and pattern of PAS positivity in primary and metastatic melanomas. Arch Pathol Lab Med 122:353–360, 1998.

Olcott CT: Cell types and histologic patterns in carcinoma of the lung: Observations on the significance of tumors containing more than one type of cell. Am J Pathol 31:975–995, 1955.

Pearse AGE: The APUD cell concept and its implications in pathology. Pathol Annu 9:27–41, 1974.

Piehl MR, Gould VE, Warren WH et al: Immunohistochemical identification of exocrine and neuroendocrine subsets of large cell lung carcinomas. Pathol Res Pract 183:675–682, 1988.

Ranchod M, Levine GD: Spindle cell carcinoid tumors of the lung: A clinicopathologic study of 35 cases. Am J Surg Pathol 4:315–331, 1980.

Rao SK, Fraire AE: Alveolar cell hyperplasia in association with adenocarcinoma of the lung. Mod Pathol 8:165–169, 1995.

Ritter JH, Mills SE, Nappi O, Wick MR: Angiosarcoma-like neoplasms of epithelial organs: True endothelial tumors or variants of carcinoma? Semin Diagn Pathol 12:270–282, 1995.

Ritter JH, Wick MR, Reyes AR et al: False-positive interpretations of carcinoma in exfoliative respiratory cytology: Report of two cases and a review of underlying disorders. Am J Clin Pathol 104:133–140, 1995.

Ro JY, Chen JL, Lee JS et al: Sarcomatoid carcinoma of the lung: Immunohistochemical and ultrastructural studies of 14 cases. Cancer 69:376–386, 1992.

Roggli VL, Vollmer RT, Greenberg SD et al: Lung cancer heterogeneity: A blinded and randomized study of 100 consecutive cases. Hum Pathol 16:569–579, 1985.

Rosenblatt MB, Lisa JR, Collier F: Primary and metastatic bronchioloalveolar carcinoma. Chest 52:147–152, 1967.

Sawyers CL, Golde DW, Quan S, Nimer SD: Production of granulocyte-macrophage colony stimulating factor in two patients with lung cancer, leukocytosis, and eosinophilia. Cancer 69:1342–1346, 1992.

Schulze ES, Mattia AR, Chew FS: Bronchioloalveolar carcinoma. Am J Roentgenol 162:1294, 1994.

Shimosato Y: Lung tumors of uncertain histogenesis. Semin Diagn Pathol 12:185–192, 1995.

Shimosato Y, Noguchi M, Matsuno Y: Adenocarcinoma of the lung: Its development and malignant progression. Lung Cancer 9:99–108, 1993.

Skinner C, Ewen SWB: Carcinoid lung: Diffuse pulmonary infiltration by a multifocal bronchial carcinoid. Thorax 31:212–219, 1976.

Smit EF, Croen HJ, Timens W et al: Surgical resection for small cell carcinoma of the lung: A retrospective study. Thorax 49:20–22, 1994.

Sorensen JB, Hirsch FR, Gazdar A, Olsen JE: Interobserver variability in histopathologic subtyping and grading of pulmonary adenocarcinoma. Cancer 71:2971–2976, 1993.

Souza RC, Peasley ED, Takaro T: Pulmonary blastomas: A distinctive group of carcinosarcomas of the lung. Ann Thorac Surg 1:259–268, 1965.

Sridhar KS, Bounassi MJ, Raub W, Richman SP: Clinical features of adenosquamous lung carcinoma in 127 patients. Am Rev Respir Dis 142:19–23, 1990.

Suster S: Primary sarcomas of the lung. Semin Diagn Pathol 12:140–157, 1995.

Sutton LN, Morrison JF, Rees MR: Radiographic features and prognosis in bronchioloalveolar carcinoma: A local experience. Resp Med 83:471–477, 1989.

Takamori S, Noguchi M, Morinaga S et al: Clinical pathologic characteristics of adenosquamous carcinoma of the lung. Cancer 67:649–654, 1991.

Thomas JS, Lamb D, Ashcroft T et al: How reliable is the diagnosis of lung cancer using small biopsy specimens? Report of a UKCCCR Lung Cancer Working Party. Thorax 48:1135–1139, 1993.

Travis WD, Colby TV, Corrin B et al: Histological Typing of Lung and Pleural Tumours (International Histological Classification of Tumours). Geneva, World Health Organization, 1999, pp. 1–55.

Travis WD, Linnoila RI, Horowitz M et al: Pulmonary nodules resembling bronchioloalveolar carcinoma in adolescent cancer patients. Mod Pathol 1:372–377, 1988.

Travis WD, Linnoila RI, Tsokos MG et al: Neuroendocrine tumors of the lung with proposed criteria for large-cell neuroendocrine carcinoma: An ultrastructural, immunohistochemical, and flow cytometric study of 35 cases. Am J Surg Pathol 15:529–553, 1991.

Travis WD, Rush W, Flieder DB et al: Survival analysis of 200 pulmonary neuroendocrine tumors with clarification of criteria for atypical carcinoid and its separation from typical carcinoid. Am J Surg Pathol 22:934–944, 1998.

Vincent RG, Pickren JW, Lane NVW et al: The changing histopathology of lung cancer: A review of 1682 cases. Cancer 39:1617–1655, 1977.

Vollmer RT: The effect of cell size on the pathologic diagnosis of small and large cell carcinomas of the lung. Cancer 50:1380–1383, 1982.

Weidner N: Pulmonary adenocarcinoma with intestinal-type differentiation. Ultrastruct Pathol 16:7–10, 1992.

Wick MR: Immunophenotyping of malignant mesothelioma. Am J Surg Pathol 21:1395–1398, 1997.

Wick MR, Berg LC, Hertz M: Large cell carcinoma of the lung with neuroendocrine differentiation: A comparison with large cell "undifferentiated" pulmonary tumors. Am J Clin Pathol 97:796–805, 1992.

Wick MR, Ritter JH, Humphrey PA: Sarcomatoid carcinoma of the lung: A clinicopathologic review. Am J Clin Pathol 108:40–53, 1997.

Wick MR, Ritter JH, Nappi O: Inflammatory sarcomatoid carcinoma of the lung: Report of three cases and clinicopathologic comparison with inflammatory pseudotumors in adult patients. Hum Pathol 26:1014–1021, 1995.

Wick MR, Swanson PE: "Carcinosarcomas:" Current perspectives and a historical review of nosological concepts. Semin Diagn Pathol 10:118–127, 1993.

Yesner R: Small cell tumors of the lung. Am J Surg Pathol 7:775–785, 1983.

Yesner R, Seydel G, Asbell SO et al: Biopsies of non-small cell lung cancer: Central review in cooperative studies of the Radiation Therapy Oncology Group. Mod Pathol 4:432–440, 1991.

Yoshida J, Nagai K, Hasebe T et al: Pulmonary metastasis of renal cell carcinoma resected sixteen years after nephrectomy. Jpn J Clin Oncol 25:20–24, 1995.

Yousem SA: Pulmonary carcinoid tumors and well-differentiated neuroendocrine carcinomas: Is there room for an atypical carcinoid? Am J Clin Pathol 95:763–764, 1991.

Zeren H, Moran CA, Suster S et al: Primary pulmonary sarcomas with features of monophasic synovial sarcoma: A clinicopathological, immunohistochemical, and ultrastructural study of 25 cases. Hum Pathol 26:474–480, 1995.

CLINICAL FEATURES, DIAGNOSIS, AND STAGING OF LUNG CANCER

Michael A. Maddaus
Robert J. Ginsberg

HISTORICAL NOTE

The staging of cancer began with the development of the TNM (tumor, node, metastasis) classification system by Denoix in 1946 and acceptance by the Union Internationale Contre Cancer (UICC). Although modified, it remains the basis of staging systems for many tumors, including lung cancer. In 1959, the American Joint Committee on Cancer (AJCC) Staging and End Results Reporting was formed by several organizations, including the American College of Surgeons, the National Cancer Institute, and the American Cancer Society. The goal of these organizations was to develop staging systems for different cancers by assigning a task force to each particular cancer. The AJCC lung cancer staging system that the lung cancer task force developed was based on the original TNM descriptors (Mountain et al, 1974) but initially differed from the UICC.

Although the AJCC lung cancer staging system functioned well, several problems became apparent when significant survival differences were noted between subsets of patients at the same clinical stage. For example, stage I included one subset with N1 disease, subsequently shown to have a poorer prognosis than subsets with N0 disease. Stage III included an array of patients with disease that was more advanced than N1 nodal involvement, such as those with isolated mediastinal nodal disease and chest wall involvement and no nodal disease. It did not separate operative from nonoperative candidates.

The original AJCC lung cancer staging system was used in North America through 1985. A significantly different UICC system was used elsewhere. In 1986, a new international staging system, developed jointly by the AJCC lung cancer task force and the UICC, was introduced (Mountain, 1986). It corrected problems with the AJCC system and has been in use worldwide since. In 1997, additional modifications were made to more accurately reflect survival patterns.

Surgical exploration of the mediastinum as a staging procedure was first developed by Harken and colleagues (1954). Through a supraclavicular incision, a Jackson laryngoscope was inserted into the mediastinum, and lymph node biopsies were performed. Cervical mediastinoscopy, through a pretracheal suprasternal notch incision, was developed by Carlens (1959) in Sweden and was subsequently popularized by Pearson in North America (Pearson, 1965).

■ *HISTORICAL READINGS*

Carlens E: Mediastinoscopy: A method for inspection and tissue biopsy in the superior mediastinum. Dis Chest 36:343, 1959.

Denoix PF: Enquete permanent dans les centres anticancereux. Bull Inst Nat Hyg (Paris) I:70, 1946.

Harken DE, Black H, Clauss R, Ferrand RE: Simple cervicomediastinal exploration for tissue diagnosis of intrathoracic disease. N Engl J Med 251:1041, 1954.

Mountain CF, Carr DT, Anderson WA: A system for the clinical staging of lung cancer. AJR Am J Roentgenol 120:130, 1974.

Pearson FG: Mediastinoscopy: A method of biopsy in the superior mediastinum. J Thorac Cardiovasc Surg 49:11–21, 1965.

CLINICAL FEATURES

Over 160,000 new cases of lung cancer are diagnosed in the United States every year. Ninety-five percent of patients with lung cancer are symptomatic at the time of diagnosis. Of these, 27% have symptoms secondary to the primary tumor, 32% secondary to metastatic spread, and 34% have nonspecific symptoms (malaise, weight loss, and anorexia) (Carbone et al, 1970). A high percentage of patients already have clinical evidence of systemic spread. At most, only 5% are asymptomatic with an abnormal chest radiograph, and still fewer have occult carcinomas with a normal chest radiograph.

The clinical presentation of lung cancer is one of the most varied and unpredictable in all of medicine. Such a wide range of symptoms and signs is related to several factors: (1) the stage at presentation, ranging from asymptomatic to widely disseminated metastatic disease; (2) the tumor's anatomic location, which determines its mechanical effects; (3) tumor histology, which often influences anatomic location; and (4) intrinsic tumor biology, leading to differing growth rates and the production of a variety of paraneoplastic syndromes (Fig. 31–20).

The impact of tumor location and histologic subtype on the clinical presentation of lung cancer must be emphasized. In general, squamous cell and small cell carcinomas frequently arise in the proximal bronchi and often produce symptoms of airway irritation or obstruction. Common symptoms include cough, hemoptysis, wheezing (because of high-grade airway stenosis), dyspnea secondary to bronchial occlusion (with or without postobstructive atelectasis), and postobstructive pneumonia (caused by secretion retention and atelectasis). In contrast, adenocarcinomas and their variant, large cell carcinomas are often peripherally located. They less frequently cause the airway symptoms seen with squamous and small cell carcinomas. Instead, they are often found to be asymptomatic peripheral nodules on the chest radiograph or, when symptomatic, with parietal pleural or chest wall invasion (resulting in pleuritic or chest wall pain). Pleural seeding and development of a malignant effusion (with progressive dyspnea) can also occur. Because of their peripheral location, these tumors are often not visible on flexible bronchoscopic examination.

Bronchoalveolar carcinomas are highly variable and arise peripherally from alveolar-lining cells. They may be solitary nodules, multifocal nodules, or diffuse infiltrating processes that can be easily confused with a consolidating pneumonia (Donaldson et al, 1978). In the diffuse infiltrating or pneumonic form, marked shortness of breath and hypoxia may develop; occasionally, extreme bronchorrhea with expectoration of massive volumes (more than 1 L/day) of light-tan fluid can lead to dehydration and electrolyte imbalance. Unlike peripheral squamous or adenocarcinomas, chest wall invasion is unusual. A unique radiologic feature of bronchoalveolar carcinomas is the presence of air bronchograms, resulting from the tendency of the tumor to fill alveolar air spaces instead of destroying and compressing the surrounding normal lung.

Pulmonary Manifestations

Pulmonary symptoms of lung cancer result from bronchus or lung involvement by the primary tumor or extrinsic compression by enlarged metastatic lymph nodes.

Cough

Cough may result from either bronchial irritation or compression and is the most common pulmonary symptom, occurring in 75% of patients (Cromartie et al, 1980). Initially attributed (in smokers) to a chronic cigarette cough, with persistence or worsening, it eventually defines itself as significant.

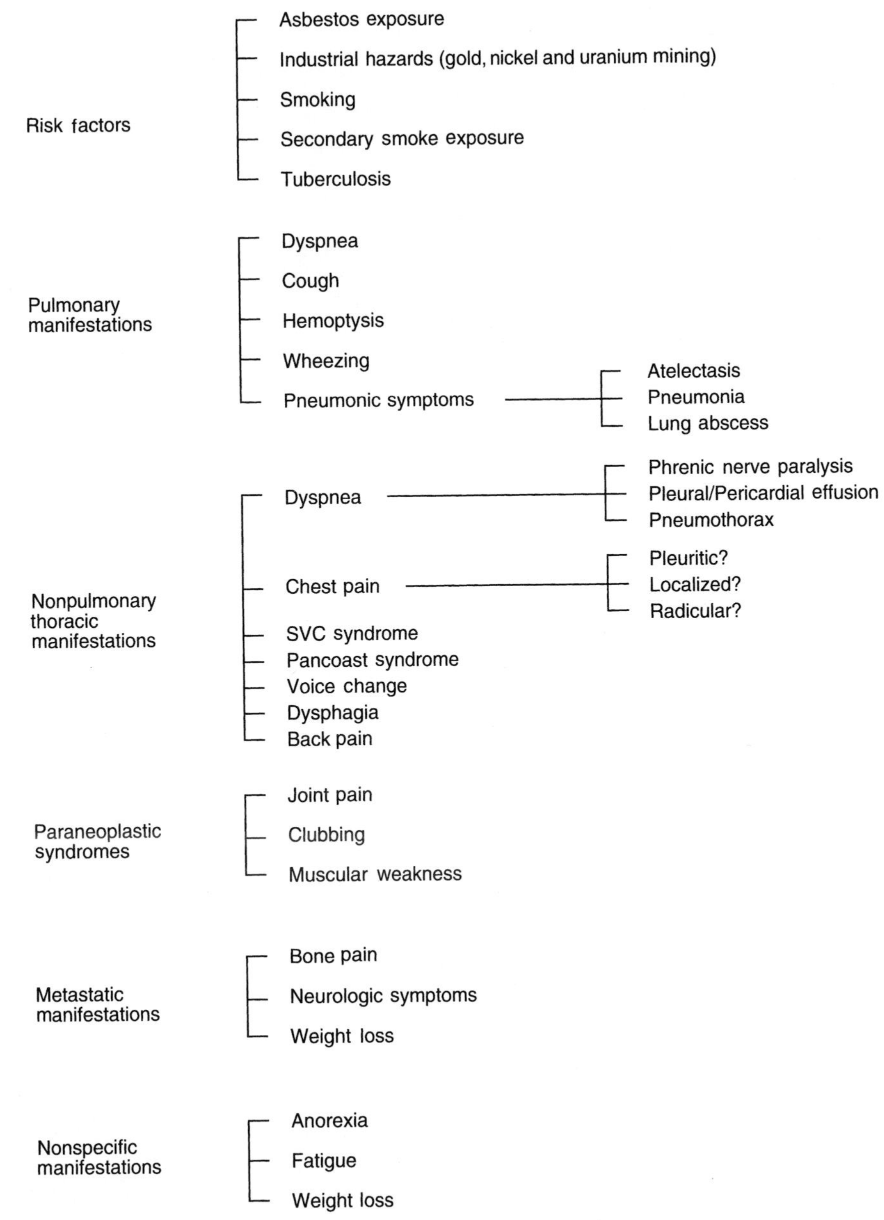

FIGURE 31–20 ■ Risk factors and symptoms to be evaluated in patients with suspected or proved lung cancer. SVC, superior vena cava.

Dyspnea

Dyspnea, the second most frequent pulmonary symptom, occurs in 50% to 60% of patients (Cromartie et al, 1980). With central tumors, or hilar lymph node spread, dyspnea results from partial or complete bronchial occlusion, with or without postobstructive atelectasis. With peripheral tumors, dyspnea, if present, may be the result of lymph-node spread (a malignant pleural effusion caused by pleural seeding) or lymphatic obstruction but can also be due to diffuse lymphangetic spread or, in the case of bronchoalveolar disease, diffuse alveolar spread of tumor. Rarely, a pneumothorax can occur from this visceral pleural invasion.

Wheezing and Stridor

Wheezing, seen with partial occlusion of a proximal bronchus, occurs when the airway is narrowed to less than 50% of its normal diameter. In proximal mainstem bronchi, an inspirating stridor, rather than a wheeze, may be present.

Hemoptysis

Hemoptysis occurs in 25% to 40% of patients. It usually involves simple blood streaking of sputum. It occurs most frequently with centrally located tumors that are degenerating or that invade and ulcerate surrounding bronchial tissue. Massive hemoptysis is rare.

Pneumonic Symptoms

These occur as a result of bronchitis, atelectasis, or post-obstructive pneumonia. With postobstructive atelectasis or pneumonia, a combination of symptoms may occur: cough, sputum production, fever, and pleuritic chest pain (caused by contact of inflamed lung with parietal pleura).

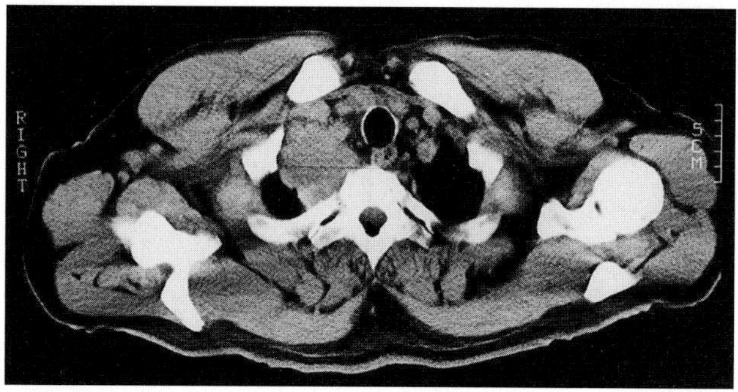

FIGURE 31–21 ■ A computed tomography scan demonstrating a right apical Pancoast tumor.

Lung Abscess

Lung abscess results from postobstructive pneumonia or from secondary infection of a necrotic tumor cavity, which occurs most frequently with squamous or large cell anaplastic cancer.

Nonpulmonary Thoracic Manifestations

When the primary tumor directly invades contiguous structures (e.g., chest wall, diaphragm, pericardium, phrenic nerve, recurrent laryngeal nerve, superior vena cava, esophagus) or when enlarged tumor-bearing lymph nodes mechanically compress a structure (e.g., superior vena cava), specific signs and symptoms evolve.

Chest Wall Involvement

Chest wall involvement of the primary tumor by extension into the parietal pleura or into deeper structures (intercostal muscles, ribs, and neurovascular bundle) occurs most often with peripherally located adenocarcinomas. Chest pain may be due either to parietal pleural contact (without invasion) with a tumor that has invaded the visceral pleura (often pleuritic) or to true parietal invasion into rib or muscle, which produces a gnawing localized pain; invasion of a neurovascular bundle may produce radicular chest wall pain. The Pancoast syndrome occurs with extension of apical lung tumors superiorly into the thoracic outlet (Fig. 31–21). These superior sulcus tumors cause variable combinations of shoulder pain (from direct invasion of the ribs and muscles), radicular arm pain (from invasion of the C8 and T1 nerve roots of the brachial plexus), and Horner's syndrome (unilateral enophthalmos, ptosis, myosis, and anhidrosis of the face resulting from invasion of the stellate sympathetic ganglion). This triad of symptoms is indicative of the Pancoast syndrome.

Diaphragm Invasion

Invasion of the diaphragm is often asymptomatic but may lead to diaphragmatic dysfunction with an enhanced sense of dyspnea on exertion or pleural effusion. The diaphragm's extensive lymphatic plexus (which normally drains fluid from the peritoneal cavity), with invasion, can lead to early lymphatic spread.

Involvement of Mediastinal Structures

Tumors on the medial lung surface may invade mediastinal structures. *Phrenic nerve invasion* leads to diaphragmatic paralysis or hiccups with dyspnea on exertion. The diagnosis is usually confirmed by plain chest x-ray (showing elevation of one diaphragm radiograph [Fig. 31–22]), or by fluoroscopic examination of the diaphragm with breathing and sniffing maneuvers. Phrenic

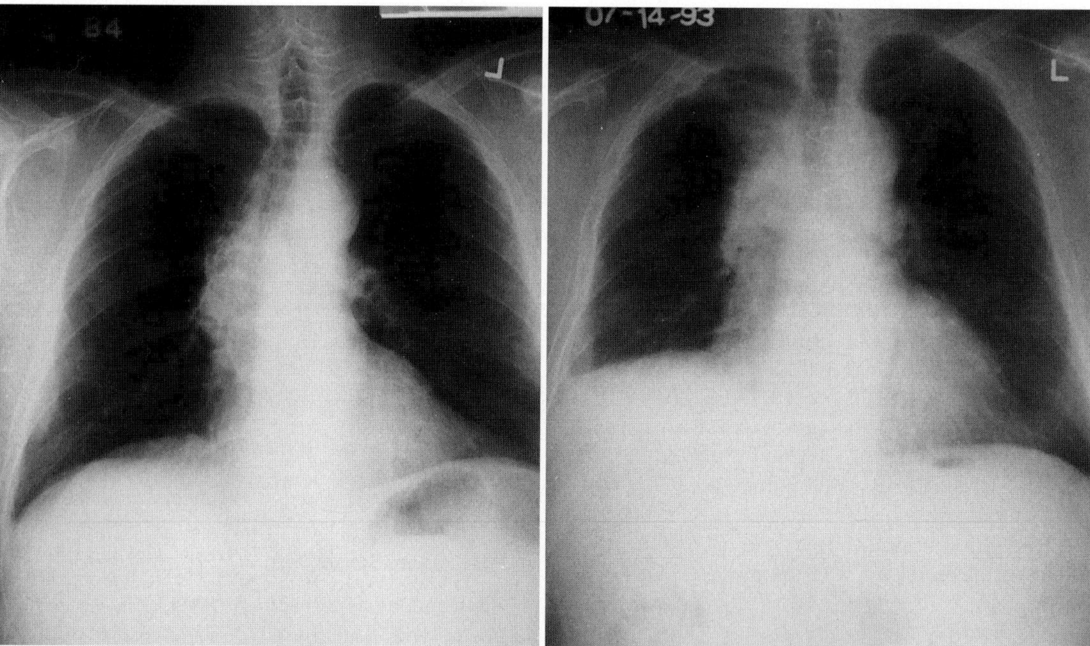

FIGURE 31–22 ■ Phrenic nerve paralysis. The *left* chest radiograph shows a previously normal right hemidiaphragm. The *right* chest radiograph shows an elevated right hemidiaphragm that is secondary to invasion of the right phrenic nerve by a hilar tumor.

nerve or diaphragmatic involvement may also cause referred shoulder pain due to its origin from the C3, C4, and C5 nerve roots. *Recurrent laryngeal nerve* dysfunction occurs predominantly on the left side (because of the proximity of the left recurrent laryngeal nerve to the pulmonary hilum and to the left upper lobe as it passes under the aortic arch). Paralysis can occur with extension of a medially based primary left upper lobe tumor into the vagus nerve as it descends toward the pulmonary hilum, with invasion or compression of the vagus nerve by aortopulmonary and anterior mediastinal lymphatic metastases or with invasion or compression of the recurrent nerve by a hilar mass. Recurrent laryngeal nerve involvement resulting in vocal cord palsy alters the voice, ranging from subtle tone changes to distinct hoarseness and results in pulmonary dysfunction owing to an inadequate cough and loss of intrinsic positive end-expiratory pressure (PEEP).

Superior vena cava syndrome can occur with invasion of the superior vena cava by a medially based right upper lobe tumor, or more commonly, with extrinsic compression of the superior vena cava by enlarged tumor-bearing mediastinal lymph nodes. Small cell carcinomas, with their propensity to early and widespread lymphatic dissemination, are the predominant cause. Overall, this syndrome occurs in 4% of lung cancer patients. Up to one third of patients with this syndrome can have acute symptoms secondary to acute thrombosis of the vena cava, but with time most patients develop sufficient venous collaterals, allowing at least partial decompression and symptom relief.

Pericardial involvement can result in pericardial effusions occasionally associated with pericardial tamponade. Tamponade often presents subtly with increasing dyspnea or with a new arrhythmia (sinus tachycardia or atrial fibrillation). Diagnosis requires a high index of suspicion based on the primary tumor's location, evidence of increased cardiac size on the chest radiograph, and ultimately, echocardiography. Because a pleural effusion is often simultaneously present, recognition of a pericardial effusion is often delayed. Such an effusion should be suspected when the patient has persistent dyspnea or cough, particularly after successful management of a pleural effusion.

Esophageal invasion by a primary tumor is rare. Dysphagia more commonly results from extrinsic esophageal compression by enlarged tumor-bearing subcarinal or posterior mediastinal lymph nodes. Such compression usually occurs with lower lobe tumors and indicates advanced disease. With time, tumor-bearing subcarinal lymph nodes may erode through the esophagus and trachea, creating a tracheoesophageal fistula with subsequent recurrent aspiration pneumonitis.

A posterior-based tumor can directly extend into a *vertebral body*, resulting in persistent, gnawing, and often severe localized back pain. Growth into the epidural space though the intervertebral foramen can produce symptoms of spinal cord compression.

Paraneoplastic Syndromes

Paraneoplastic syndromes related to lung cancer are unusual (occurring in about 2% of patients); most are caused by small cell lung cancer (SCLC) and squamous cell carcinomas. These syndromes frequently predate thoracic symptoms, and the clinician must recognize them to diagnose early, surgically treatable lung cancer. Unfortunately, paraneoplastic symptoms are often inaccurately attributed to metastatic or advanced disease (particularly neurologic symptoms), thus delaying recognition and treatment of the primary tumor. The many paraneoplastic syndromes seen with lung cancer are listed in Table 31–5. The most common ones are reviewed.

TABLE 31–5 ■ Paraneoplastic Syndromes in Patients with Lung Cancer

Endocrine
Ectopic parathyroid hormone–induced hypercalcemia
Ectopic adrenocorticotropic syndrome
Syndrome of inappropriate antidiuretic hormone secretion
Carcinoid syndrome
Gynecomastia
Hypercalcitoninemia
Elevated growth hormone
Elevated prolactin, follicle-stimulating hormone, luteinizing hormone
Hypoglycemia
Hyperthyroidism
Neurologic
Lambert-Eaton myasthenic syndrome
Subacute cerebellar degeneration
Progressive multifocal leukoencephalopathy
Peripheral neuropathy
Polymyositis autonomic neuropathy
Encephalopathy
Optic neuritis
Skeletal
Clubbing
Hypertrophic pulmonary osteoarthropathy
Hematologic
Anemia
Leukemoid reactions
Thrombocytosis
Thrombocytopenia
Eosinophilia
Pure red cell aplasia
Leukoerythroblastosis
Disseminated intravascular coagulation
Cutaneous
Hyperkeratosis
Dermatomyositis
Acanthosis nigricans
Hyperpigmentation
Erythema gyratum repens
Hypertrichosis lanuginosa acquisita
Other
Nephrotic syndrome
Hypouricemia
Secretion of vasoactive intestinal peptide with diarrhea
Hyperamylasemia
Anorexia or cachexia

Hypertrophic Pulmonary Osteoarthropathy and Clubbing

Hypertrophic pulmonary osteoarthropathy (HPO) is characterized by a proliferating periostitis of the distal ends of the long bones, particularly the tibia, the fibula, and the radius. The periostitis leads to tenderness and swelling; with progression, it may involve the metacarpals and metatarsals and may also be associated with acute polyarthritis. Occasionally the symptoms are debilitating. HPO is always associated with clubbing of the digits. However, clubbing often occurs independent of HPO in patients with non–small cell lung cancer (NSCLC): Sridhar and colleagues (1998) found clubbing in 32 (29%) of 111 patients with lung cancer. Of 88 cases of NSCLC, 31 (35%) had clubbing whereas only one case occurred in 23 patients with SCLC.

As in other paraneoplastic syndromes, HPO may precede the diagnosis of the primary lung tumor by many months. Unlike the endocrinopathies, it is rare in SCLC. Owing to the periostitis, alkaline phosphatase levels are often elevated, but serum hepatic enzyme levels are normal. Plain radiographs of the affected bones demonstrate periostitis; radionuclide bone scans reveal an intense and symmetrical generalized uptake, particularly in the distal long bones. The symptoms can respond dramatically to aspirin and other nonsteroidal anti-inflammatory agents. Complete symptom relief usually occurs immediately on resection of the primary tumor. In unresectable cases, ipsilateral vagotomy proximal to the pulmonary hilum has been reported to be of some benefit.

Syndrome of Inappropriate Antidiuretic Hormone Secretion

Elevated levels of antidiuretic hormone are commonly found in lung cancer patients, but symptoms are infrequent. The full syndrome of inappropriate antidiuretic hormone secretion syndrome is seen primarily with small cell cancer (Odell and Wolfsen, 1978), occurring in 11% to 46% of patients (List et al, 1986). Secretion of large quantities of antidiuretic hormone leads to hyponatremia; symptoms of anorexia, nausea, and vomiting; and increased neurologic dysfunction (confusion, lethargy, and seizures). Diagnosis is made by demonstrating hyponatremia, which is associated with low serum osmolality (<275 mOsm/kg), high urinary excretion of sodium (>25 mEq/L), and an inappropriately high urine osmolality (urine osmolality > serum osmolality).

The primary treatment in most instances is chemoradiotherapy of the small cell tumor. In most cases, as the tumor shrinks, the syndrome resolves. Before induction of chemoradiotherapy, fluid restriction is appropriate—unless neurologic symptoms are present, in which case hypertonic saline infusion combined with diuretic administration may be necessary. Patients with relapsed tumors and recurrent SIADH may require treatment with demeclocycline, an antibiotic that blocks the action of ADH on the renal tubule.

Another more recently recognized cause of hyponatremia in patients with SCLC is the secretion of atrial natriuretic peptide (ANP), a peptide hormone that is normally secreted by the cardiac atria (Campling et al, 1995). Like SIADH patients, patients with ANP secretion have hyponatremia, high urine sodium levels, and inappropriate antidiuresis; however, they have normal serum levels of ADH. Elevated plasma levels of ANP have been documented in these patients. Chemoradiation treatment is indicated in such patients as well.

Hypercalcemia

Approximately 10% of lung cancer patients will develop hypercalcemia during the course of their disease. However, only 15% of cases of hypercalcemia are secondary to production of parathyroid hormone (PTH) or other humoral substances, including prostaglandin E_2 (Cryer and Kissaine, 1979). Secretion of ectopic PTH occurs most often with squamous cell carcinomas. A diagnosis of ectopic PTH secretion is supported by hypophosphatemia (secondary to the action of PTH on renal tubules) and confirmed by elevated serum levels of PTH. However, the clinician must also rule out concurrent metastatic bone disease by bone or positron emission tomography (PET) scan. Because of its more chronic nature, the hypercalcemia of ectopic PTH secretion causes primarily neurologic symptoms (lethargy and a depressed level of consciousness) and dehydration. Most important, patients with ectopic PTH secretion often have resectable tumors, and after complete resection, the calcium level normalizes. However, an elevated serum calcium is an independent poor prognostic sign. Tumor recurrence following resection is extremely frequent and may manifest as recurrent hypercalcemia.

Ectopic Adrenocorticotropic Syndrome

Cushing's syndrome secondary to ectopic production of an adrenocorticotropic (ACTH)-like substance occurs primarily with SCLC. ACTH production is autonomous and not suppressible by dexamethasone. Immunoreactive ACTH is present in nearly all extracts of SCLC and a high percentage of patients with small cell carcinomas have elevated ACTH levels by radioimmunoassay, yet fewer than 5% have symptoms of Cushing's syndrome (Richardson et al, 1978; Shepard et al, 1992). Due to the rapidity of ACTH elevation, the physical stigmata of Cushing's syndrome (e.g., truncal obesity, buffalo hump, striae) are rare. Rather, symptoms are primarily due to the metabolic consequences of severe hypokalemia, metabolic alkalosis, and hyperglycemia. The diagnosis is made by demonstrating hypokalemia (<3.0 mMol/L); nonsuppressible elevated plasma cortisol levels that lack the normal diurnal variation; elevated blood ACTH levels; or elevated urinary 17-hydroxycorticosteroids, all of which are not suppressible by administration of exogenous dexamethasone.

Neurologic Paraneoplastic Syndromes

Many peripheral neuropathies (sensory, sensorimotor, and autonomic) and central neuropathies (cerebellar degeneration, dementia, brainstem encephalitis, and encephalomyelitis) occur in lung cancer patients. SCLC and (to a lesser extent) squamous carcinomas are the leading causes of these syndromes. Unlike other paraneoplastic syndromes involving secretion of an ectopic hormone or hormone-like substance, neurologic paraneoplastic syndromes are thought to be immune-mediated. It is hypothesized that the cancer cells aberrantly express antigens normally expressed only by the nervous system. A subsequent immune response to the tumor-associated antigen develops. Antibodies (e.g., anti-Yo, anti-Hu, anti-Ri antibodies) are produced, which leads either to interference with neurologic function or to immunologically mediated neurologic destruction (Posner, 1997).

Peripheral neuromyopathies are the most common paraneoplastic syndromes related to lung cancer. When carefully sought, evidence of neuromuscular disability can be found in up to 16% of lung cancer patients; of these, 56% have small cell carcinomas, 22% have squamous cell carcinomas, 16% have large cell carcinomas, and 5% have adenocarcinomas (Morton et al, 1966). Unlike the endocrinopathies, neuromyopathies occur later in the course of the disease and tend to occur in patients who already have significant weight loss making it difficult to differentiate between neuromuscular weakness secondary to neuromyopathy and the generalized disability secondary to metastatic disease. As well, in patients with neurologic or muscular symptoms, central nervous system (CNS) metastases must be ruled out with computed tomography (CT) or magnetic resonance imaging (MRI) of the head.

Lambert-Eaton myasthenic syndrome (most frequent in SCLC) is a myasthenia-like syndrome related to a defect in neuromuscular conduction. Symptoms include proximal muscle weakness and fatigability (particularly of the thighs), with waddling gait and dry oral mucosa; they can occur before the onset of any symptoms of the primary tumor and may precede the radiographic evidence of the tumor by up to 4 years (McEvoy, 1994). The syndrome is produced by immunoglobulin (IgG) antibodies that target voltage-gated calcium channels, which function in the release of acetylcholine from presynaptic sites at the motor endplate. The antibodies appear to be generated through an immune response to similar voltage-gated calcium channels that are present in the tumor cells (Lennon and Lambert, 1989).

Therapy is directed at the primary tumor with resection, radiation, or chemotherapy. Many patients have dramatic improvement after resection or successful medical therapy. For patients with refractory symptoms, treatment consists of guanidine hydrochloride, immunosuppressive agents such as prednisone and azathioprine, and, occasionally, plasma exchange. Unlike with myasthenia gravis patients, neostigmine is usually ineffective.

Metastatic Symptoms

Metastases occur most commonly in the CNS, spinal cord, bones, liver, adrenal glands, lungs, and skin and soft tissues.

Central Nervous System Metastases

At diagnosis, 10% of lung cancer patients have CNS metastases; another 10% to 15% of patients develop CNS metastases over the course of their disease and are often asymptomatic. The symptoms when present are primarily caused by increased intracranial pressure, leading to headache, nausea, vomiting, and changes in the level of consciousness. Focal neurologic signs, such as weakness and seizures, are less common.

Bone Metastases

Bone metastases occur in up to 25% of all lung cancer patients. Most skeletal metastases (55%) occur in the axial skeleton (spine, pelvis, sternum, and ribs); 12% occur in the extremities or appendicular skeleton (Krishnamurthy et al, 1977). The metastases are primarily osteolytic, producing localized pain when symptomatic; thus, any localized skeletal complaints warrant radiologic evaluation.

Hepatic and Adrenal Metastases

Hepatic metastases usually are an incidental finding on routine CT scans or, when symptomatic, are part of a premorbid state. Adrenal metastases are also primarily asymptomatic, typically discovered by routine CT scans, and rarely lead to adrenal hypofunction even with bilateral metastases.

Skin and Soft Tissue Metastases

Skin and soft tissue metastases, which occur in up to 8% of patients dying of lung cancer, generally occur late in the course of the disease as painless subcutaneous or intramuscular masses. Occasionally, the tumor erodes through the overlying skin, with necrosis and creation of a chronic wound; excision may then be necessary for both mental and physical palliation.

Nonspecific Symptoms

Lung cancer often produces a variety of nonspecific symptoms, such as anorexia, weight loss, fatigue, and malaise. The cause of these symptoms is often unclear, but as outlined later, they should raise concern about possible metastatic disease.

STAGING SYSTEM

Staging measures the extent of lung cancer in any given patient. Assigning patients to a particular clinical TNM subset and stage facilitates the most appropriate individual therapeutic decisions, tailored to different stages of the disease. Staging also provides prognostic information and allows more reliable comparison of data between studies. In addition, the impact of new therapeutic interventions can be evaluated, and the expected survival curves can be compared.

Staging is a continuous process: First, a clinical estimate of disease stage (cTNM) is determined by the history, physical examination, and radiologic and invasive studies. If surgery takes place, the stage is either confirmed or revised, based on the operative findings. After surgery, a final pathologic stage is determined, based on the pathologic results (pTNM).

As previously mentioned, the current international staging system evolved from the 1946 TNM classification and has been adopted worldwide. To understand the nodal descriptors N1, N2, and N3, it is necessary to be fully conversant with the lymph node mapping schema devised by Naruke and colleagues (1978), subsequently modified for North Americans by the American Thoracic Society (1983), by the Lung Cancer Study Group (LCSG)

(1985), and by Mountain (1997). In this schema, lymph nodes are placed into well-defined stations based on clearly defined anatomic boundaries (Figs. 31–23 and 31–24).

The international staging system was originally applied (based on clinical estimates of the extent of disease) to a database of more than 3000 patients from the M. D. Anderson Hospital in Texas and the LCSG (Mountain, 1986). This database study produced a series of 5-year survival curves for each stage, which verified the significant survival differences between each stage. This study has been confirmed by other investigators (Martini et al, 1983; Naruke et al, 1978, 1988; Watanabe et al, 1991).

The 1987 international staging system significantly improved the staging of NSCLC. It became clear that, within each stage, marked differences existed in postoperative 5-year survival rates. For example, within stage I, patients with T2N0M0 tumors were shown to have 5-year survival rates that were 10% to 30% or more below those for patients with T1N0M0 tumors (Mountain, 1986; Naruke et al, 1988; Watanabe et al, 1991). Similarly, within stage IIIa, extreme differences were seen in post-resection 5-year survival rates: 40% to 50% for T3N0 tumors versus 5% to 25% for T1 to T3 tumors with N2 nodal involvement.

In 1997, Mountain reviewed survival data from an additional 1524 patients beyond the original LCSG/M. D. Anderson database. After reviewing data on this combined total of 5319 patients, multiple revisions in the staging system were subsequently adopted by the AJCC and UICC (see later). Important changes included dividing stage I into IA and IB, dividing stage II into IIA and IIB, and incorporating T3N0 tumors into stage IIB. These changes have brought staging into much closer alignment with survival rates, rather than with the tumor's anatomic location, the site of intrathoracic spread, or potential surgical resectability (Figs. 31–25 and 31–26).

Despite these improvements, significant variability still exists within stage groups. For example, tumors that are 1 cm or less in diameter have a significantly better prognosis than tumors that are 2 to 3 cm in diameter. Also, the wide range of postoperative 5-year survival rates (5% to 25%) for tumors with N2 nodal involvement is affected by the number and location of nodal stations involved and perhaps by whether the metastatic tumor within the node has grossly replaced the node, is growing into surrounding tissues, or both (Luke et al, 1986). Such variations within stage groups should play a role in how the surgeon tailors preoperative decision making to individual patients.

OTHER PROGNOSTIC FACTORS

A whole host of prognostic factors affecting survival have not been incorporated in any staging system (Table 31–6). These have been discussed in detail in previous chapters. In the future, a TNM staging system may well have to be augmented by a "P" system of prognostic factors, thus developing a TNMP staging system. Staging decisions may then be based on such a TNMP model rather than on TNM alone. Verification of these prognostic factors is required before incorporation into such a system.

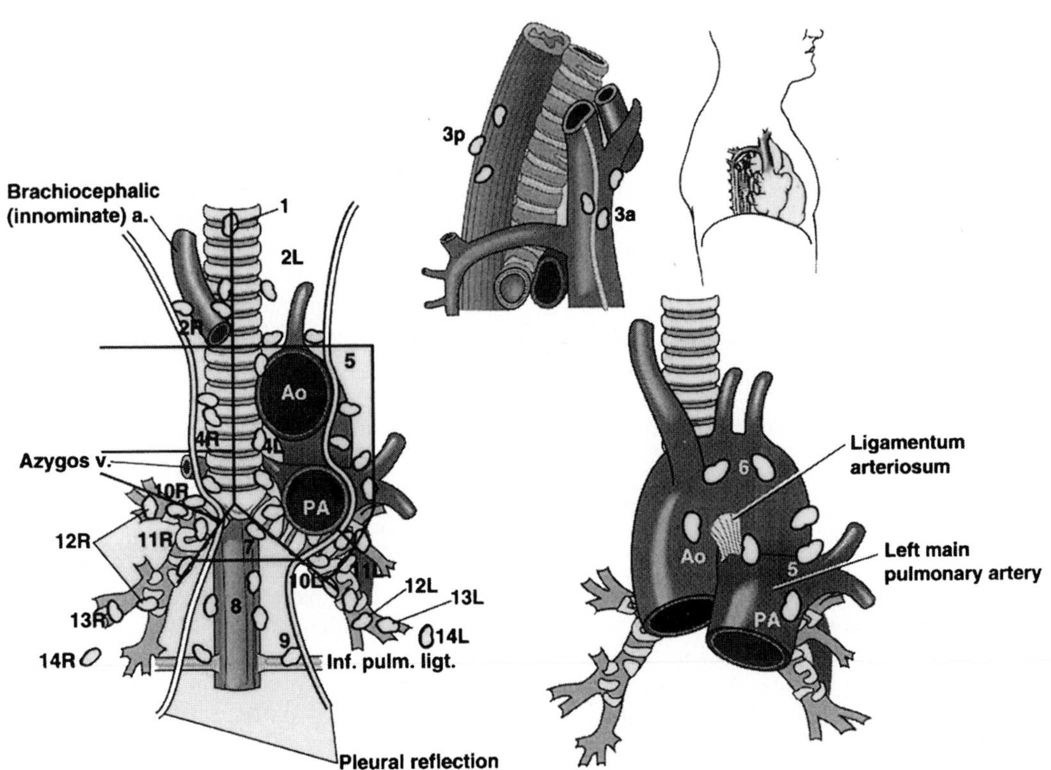

FIGURE 31–23 ■ American College of Surgeons Oncology Group lymph node mapping schema showing anatomic boundaries of each lymph node station. (Reprinted with permission from the American College of Surgeons.)

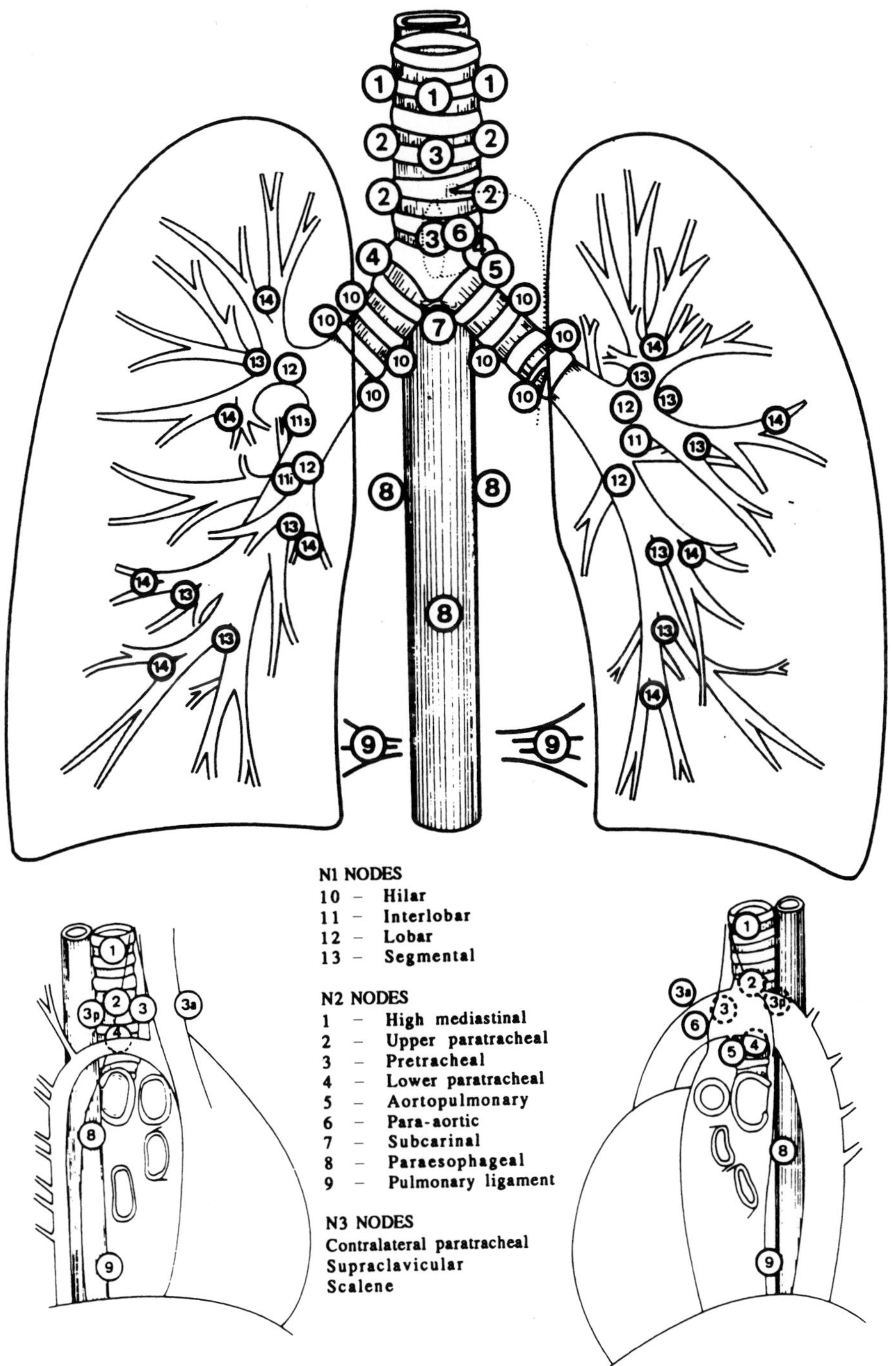

N1 NODES
10 – Hilar
11 – Interlobar
12 – Lobar
13 – Segmental
N2 NODES
1 – High mediastinal
2 – Upper paratracheal
3 – Pretracheal
4 – Lower paratracheal
5 – Aortopulmonary
6 – Para-aortic
7 – Subcarinal
8 – Paraesophageal
9 – Pulmonary ligament
N3 NODES
Contralateral paratracheal
Supraclavicular
Scalene

FIGURE 31–24 ■ Union Internationale Contre Cancer map. Sites of pulmonary lymph node drainage with numeric designations for each site. (From Naruke T, Suemasu K, Ishikawa S: Lymph node mapping and curability at various levels of metastasis in resected lung cancer. J Thorac Cardiovasc Surg 76:832, 1978.)

TABLE 31–6 ■ International System for Staging Lung Cancer: TNM Classification

Primary Tumor (T)

TX: Primary tumor cannot be assessed, or the tumor has been proved by the presence of malignant cells in sputum or bronchial washings but not visualized by imaging or bronchoscopy.
T0: No evidence of primary tumor.
TIS: Carcinoma in situ.
T1: Tumor <3 cm in greatest dimension, surrounded by lung or visceral pleura, without bronchoscopic evidence of invasion more proximal than the lobar bronchus* (i.e., not in the main bronchus).
T2: Tumor with any of the following features of size of extent.
>3 cm in greatest dimension.
Involves main bronchus, >2 cm distal to the carina
Invades the visceral pleura.
Associated with atelectasis or obstructive pneumonitis that extends to the hilar region but does not involve the entire lung.
T3: Tumor of any size that directly invades any of the following:
Chest wall (including superior sulcus tumors), diaphragm, mediastinal pleura, parietal pericardium; or
Tumor in the main bronchus <2 cm distal to the carina but without involvement of the carina; or
Associated atelectasis or obstructive pneumonitis of the entire lung.
T4: Tumor of any size that invades any of the following:
Mediastinum, heart, great vessels, trachea, esophagus, vertebral body, carina; or
Tumor with a malignant pleural or pericardial effusion,† or
Tumor with satellite tumor nodules(s) within the ipsilateral primary-tumor lobe of the lung.

Regional Lymph Nodes (N)

NX: Regional lymph nodes cannot be assessed.
N0: No regional lymph node metastasis.
N1: Metastasis to ipsilateral peribronchial or ipsilateral hilar lymph nodes and intrapulmonary nodes involved by direct extension of the primary tumor.
N2: Metastasis to ipsilateral mediastinal or subcarinal lymph node(s).
N3: Metastasis to contralateral mediastinal, contralateral hilar, ipsilateral, or contralateral scalene or supraclavicular lymph node(s).

Distant Metastasis (M)

M0: No distant metastases detected.
M1: Distant metastasis present.‡

*The uncommon superficial tumor of any size with its invasive component limited to the bronchial wall, which may extend proximal to the main bronchus, is also classified T1.

†Most pleural effusions associated with lung cancer are due to tumor. However, there are a few patients in whom multiple cytopathologic examinations of pleural fluid show no tumor. In these cases, the fluid is nonbloody and is not an exudate. When these elements and clinical judgment indicate that the effusion is not related to the tumor, the effusion should be excluded as a staging element and the patient's disease should be staged T1, T2, or T3. Pericardial effusion is classified according to the same rules.

‡Separate metastatic tumor nodule(s) in the ipsilateral nonprimary-tumor lobe(s) of the lung are also classified M1.

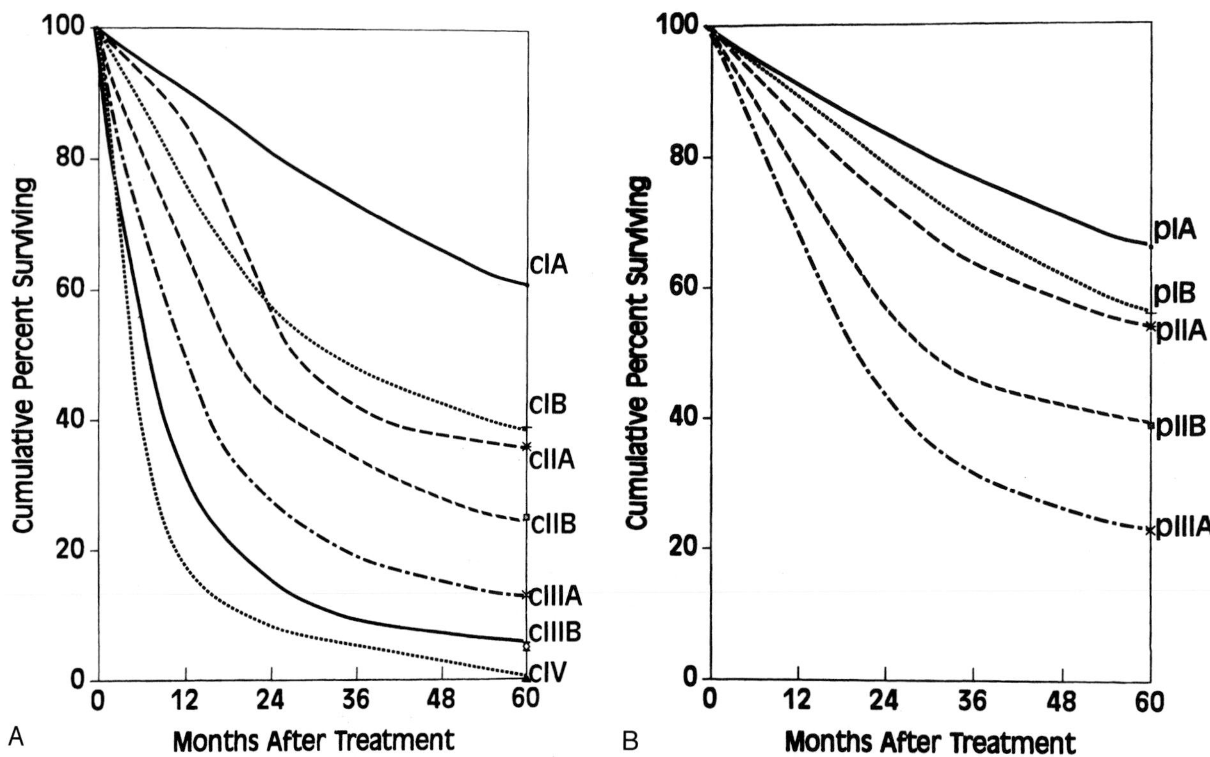

FIGURE 31–25 ■ Cumulative proportion of patients surviving 5 years based on clinical stage (*A*) and surgical pathologic stage of disease (*B*). Pairwise comparisons are significant. (From Mountain CF: Lung Cancer—A Handbook for Staging, Imaging, and Lymph Node Classification. Austin, University of Texas Press, 1999.)

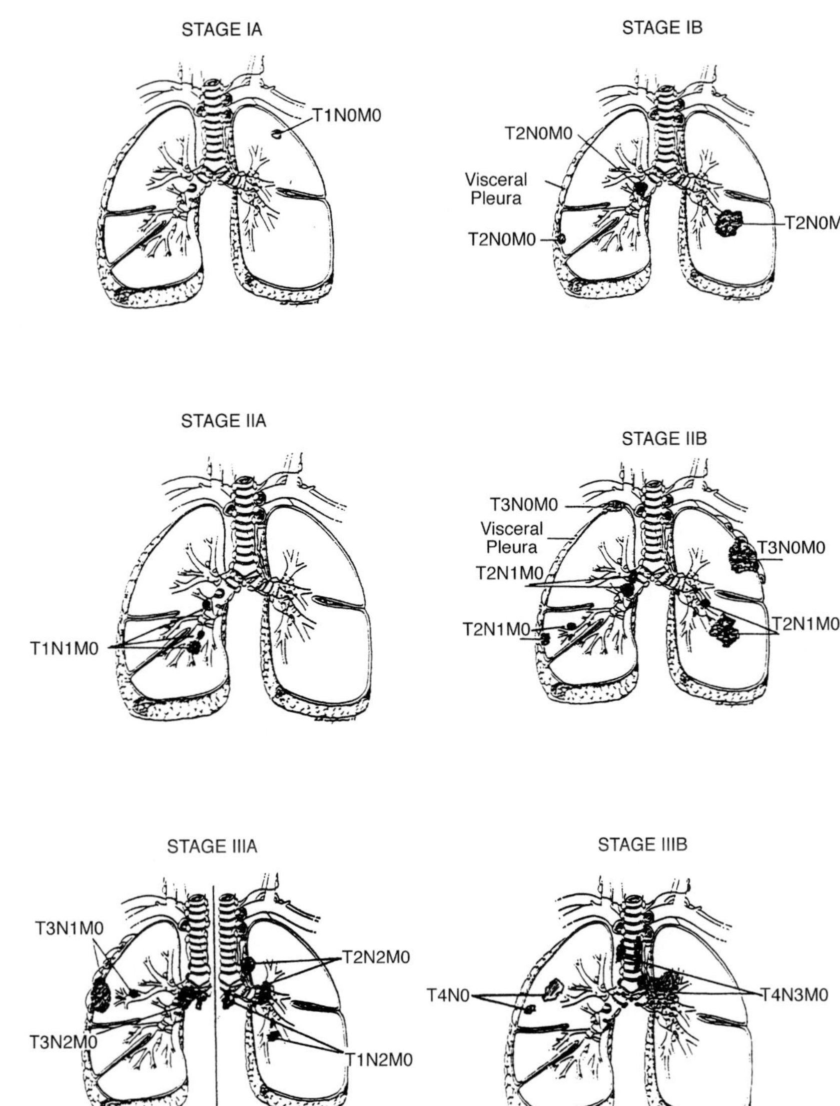

FIGURE 31–26 ■ The categories of stage I, II, and III disease and their subdivisions are illustrated. Note the changes in stage IIB disease (T3–N0) and IIIB disease (satellite nodules).

STAGING MAPS

Two somewhat different staging maps are utilized, one by the AJCC and one by the UICC. The former is based on an American Thoracic Society's map with multiple modifications and the latter is based on Naruke's original proposal in 1976. There are subtle differences between the two staging systems. In the AJCC's system, level 1 nodes are supraclavicular whereas in the Naruke system they also include any node within the thorax above the level of the left innominate vein. As well, in the AJCC system, level 3 lymph nodes are limited to those anterior lymph nodes found in front of the superior vena cava (3a) and periesophageal lymph nodes (3p) from the carina to the thoracic inlet. In the UICC system, midline superior mediastinal lymph nodes are also considered to be level 3, whereas, in the AJCC system, there are no midline superior mediastinal lymph nodes but only left and right (2 and 4). As well, the definitions of "hilar" (level 10) lymph nodes differ in the two systems. Lymph nodes along the left and right mainstem bronchi down to the reflection of the mediastinal pleura, arbitrarily identified as the take-off of the upper lobe bronchi, are all considered to be level 4 in the new AJCC map. In the UICC map, only a portion of the left and right mainstem bronchi lymph nodes are considered to be level 10.

DIAGNOSIS AND STAGING

The diagnosis and clinical staging of lung cancer are two processes that occur simultaneously, beginning with the history and physical examination. An accurate initial clinical estimate of the extent of disease can often be based solely on the history and physical examination. To obtain a tissue diagnosis and to further determine the clinical stage of the disease, directed radiologic and invasive studies can be performed. Many of these studies (e.g., chest radiography, CT scan, bronchoscopy, and mediastinoscopy) serve both purposes.

History and Physical Examination

The history and physical examination are the most important initial steps in evaluating a lung cancer patient.

DEFINITIONS OF REGIONAL NODAL STATIONS FOR PRETHORACOTOMY STAGING

1: Supraclavicular nodes (AJCC), nodes above innominate vein (UICC)
2R: Right upper peritracheal (suprainnominate) nodes: nodes to the right of the midline of the trachea, between the intersection of the caudal margin of the innominate artery with the trachea and the apex of the lung (includes highest right mediastinal node). (Radiologists may use the same caudal margin as in 2L.)
2L: Left upper peritracheal (supra-aortic) nodes: nodes to the left of the midline of the trachea between the top of the aortic arch and the apex of the lung (includes highest left mediastinal node).
3: Midline superior mediastinal nodes (UICC)
3a: Anterior mediastinal lymph nodes along the superior vena cava (AJCC)
3p: Posterior, retrotracheal, and upper periesophageal nodes (AJCC)
4R: Right lower paratracheal nodes: nodes to the right of the midline of the trachea between the cephalic border of the azygos vein and the intersection of the caudal margin of the brachiocephalic artery with the right side of the trachea (includes some pretracheal and pericaval nodes). (Radiologists may use the same cephalic margin as that in 4L.)
4L: Left lower paratracheal nodes: nodes to the left of the midline of the trachea between the top of the aortic arch and the level of the carina, medial to the ligamentum arteriosum (includes some pretracheal nodes).
5: Left aortopulmonary nodes: subaortic and para-aortic nodes, lateral to the ligamentum arteriosum or the aorta or left pulmonary artery, proximal to the first branch of the left pulmonary artery.
6: Left anterior mediastinal nodes: nodes anterior to the ascending aorta or the innominate artery (includes some pretracheal and preaortic nodes).
7: Subcarinal nodes: nodes rising caudal to the carina of the trachea, but not associated with the lower lobe bronchi or arteries within the lung.
8: Paraesophageal nodes: nodes dorsal to the posterior wall of the trachea and to the right or left of the midline of the esophagus (includes retrotracheal but not subcarinal nodes).
9: Right or left pulmonary ligament nodes: nodes within the right or left pulmonary ligament.
10R: Right tracheobronchial nodes: nodes to the right of the midline of the trachea from the level of the cephalic border of the azygos vein to the origin of the right upper lobe bronchus.
10L: Left hilar nodes: nodes to the left of the midline of the trachea between the carina and the left upper lobe bronchus, medial to the ligamentum arteriosum.
11: Interlobar nodes: nodes lying between the lobar bronchi (sump nodes).
12: Lobar nodes: nodes adjacent to the distal lobar bronchi.

Post-thoracotomy staging: nodes could be divided into stations 11, 12, or 13, according to the AJCC classification.

AJCC, American Joint Committee on Cancer; UICC, Union Internationale Contre Cancer.

From American Thoracic Society: Clinical staging of primary lung cancer. Am Rev Respir Dis 127:659, 1983.

Several features of the history deserve special emphasis. A history of tobacco smoking increases the risk of developing lung cancer, based on the number of years of smoking. Recent evidence also implicates secondary exposure to tobacco smoke, particularly in children raised with tobacco-smoking relatives. Asbestos exposure is also a risk factor; the risk increases with the length and intensity of the exposure. A history of both asbestos exposure and tobacco smoking actually has a multiplicative rather than an additive effect on the risk of developing lung cancer. Other industrial exposures (e.g., gold, nickel, and uranium mining) have a similar co-carcinogenic effect. Weight loss of more than 5% of body weight is significant and should alert the clinician to the possible presence of locally advanced disease or metastatic spread.

The complete physical examination first assesses the overall status of the patient. Is the patient vigorous or debilitated? Is there evidence of weight loss with muscle wasting? Are these neurologic signs of tumor involvement or paraneoplastic syndromes? Further examination focuses on the oropharynx for evidence of other tumors associated with tobacco use; on the neck and supraclavicular areas for evidence of lymph node metastases; on the lungs to detect localized rhonchi, areas of consolidation, pleural effusion, or localized chest wall discomfort; and on the digits for evidence of clubbing.

NONINVASIVE LABORATORY TESTING

Sputum Cytology

Microscopic examination of the sputum for tumor cells is a simple diagnostic technique. However, with the availability of bronchoscopy and percutaneous needle biopsy, sputum cytologic examination is now infrequent, and often forgotten. The diagnostic yield depends on several factors: sputum production, tumor location, tumor size, tumor histologic type, and the cytopathologist's ability and experience. Central tumors have the highest yield. Sputum samples may be obtained either spontaneously or by induction with a saline nebulization. Ideally, samples should be immediately fixed and stained. Spontaneous sputum samples can also be obtained by pooling early morning sputum samples for 3 consecutive days and preserving them in Saccamanno's solution (50% ethanol and 2% polyethylene glycol) or 70% ethanol. Saccamanno's solution is preferred over 70% ethanol because of the better admixture and preservation of the cells.

In a consecutive series of 449 cases of lung cancer, Ng and Horak (1983) demonstrated the diagnostic sensitivity of the sputum examination to be 82.8% overall. The number of specimens collected and the diagnostic yield were correlated (83% for three and 90% for five or more specimens). Both Pilotti and colleagues (1982) and Liang (1989) confirmed that the number of specimens necessary for optimal diagnostic sensitivity is three; increasing the number to five or more does not significantly improve the diagnostic yield.

Other factors influencing diagnostic sensitivity are tumor location, size, and histologic type. Because of their proximal bronchial location and endobronchial site, central tumors have a higher probability of shedding tumor cells into the sputa that will be expectorated. Kato and colleagues (1983) demonstrated a diagnostic yield of 77% for central tumors versus 47% for peripheral tumors. They also found that large tumors, and those associated with collapse or consolidation and a lower lobe location, had higher diagnostic yields. The poorest diagnostic yield occurred with small peripheral tumors: as low as 20% for those less than 3.0 cm. Histologic findings have less influence over the diagnostic yield. In general, squamous cell tumors, most likely because of their central location, are more frequently diagnosed than are adenocarcinomas or large cell carcinomas. Potentially premalignant dysplastic cells can also be detected in the sputum. Risse and coworkers (1988), on follow-up of 46 patients with dysplastic sputum cytologic findings but no other evidence of lung cancer, found that 21 (46%) developed lung cancer. Patients with dysplastic changes should undergo bronchoscopy, with brushing and biopsy of any abnormalities in addition to segmental bronchial washings. Tockman and associates (1988) appear to have improved the sensitivity of cancer detection techniques in dysplastic cells by staining with a monoclonal antibody (not yet commercially available) to neoplastic antigens. They detected tumor antigens up to 2 years before lung cancer developed. If proved to be accurate, such techniques may allow early resection if the site of such changes can be localized.

Finally, false-positive sputum cytologic findings occur in 1% to 3% of examinations. The primary causes (Truong et al, 1985) are viral infections (which can produce cellular changes that are difficult to distinguish from malignancy, particularly adenocarcinoma) and any acute inflammatory process (e.g., asthma, tuberculosis, or bronchitis). Clinical correlation is, therefore, always necessary.

Chest Radiograph

A high-quality posteroanterior and lateral chest radiograph is the most important study in diagnosing lung cancer. It localizes the site of peripheral or central pulmonary lesions and detects evidence of hilar and mediastinal enlargement (suggestive of lymphatic spread), pleural effusion, and areas of atelectasis or consolidation. A completely normal chest radiograph essentially rules out lung cancer, except in the rare instance of a tiny endobronchial lesion or a subcentimeter peripheral lesion that is usually hidden by other structures.

The presence of pleural effusion on chest radiography (or CT scan) does not necessarily denote a T4 tumor. A malignant pleural effusion can only be diagnosed by finding malignant cells in a sample of pleural fluid examined microscopically. A pleural effusion associated with a peripherally based tumor, particularly one that abuts the visceral or parietal pleural surface, has a higher probability of being malignant. However, pleural effusions are often exudate secondary to the atelectasis or consolidation seen with central tumors. No pleural effusion should be considered to be malignant until proved so by cytologic examination despite the suggestion that a "bloody" effusion is proof-positive of malignancy.

Excluding massive mediastinal involvement, plain chest radiographs are unreliable in detecting tumor spread to hilar or mediastinal lymph nodes. Even with mediastinal lymph node enlargement, mediastinoscopy or another method of lymph biopsy is necessary to confirm metastases.

Elevation of a hemidiaphragm can be the result of volume loss (from atelectasis) or paralysis of the hemidiaphragm secondary to involvement of the phrenic nerve by the primary tumor, particularly if it abuts the mediastinum. Evidence of rib destruction (caused either by metastasis or by direct invasion by a peripheral tumor contiguous with the chest wall) or vertebral body involvement by metastasis may also be identified.

Computed Tomography

In developed countries, CT scanning of the chest and upper abdomen is now a standard part of evaluating any patient with suspected or documented lung cancer. CT provides information about the primary lesion, including its size, any signs of benignity (e.g., calcification, density), its relationship to surrounding structures, and any invasion of contiguous structures. However, it must be strongly emphasized that, without unequivocal evidence of invasion of contiguous structures (e.g., rib or vertebral body destruction), no conclusion can be made. In general, thoracotomy should not be denied based on presumptive evidence of unresectable invasion of chest wall, vertebral body, or mediastinal structures; proof of invasion may require thoracotomy.

CT also provides detailed information about the remaining lung parenchyma and pleural space. Other pulmonary nodules (not seen by chest radiography), bullae, emphysematous changes, pleural thickening or masses, and unsuspected pleural effusion may be identified. When chest CT includes the upper abdomen, unsuspected metastases may be found in the liver or adrenal gland; as shown by Pagani (1984), such metastases occur in the liver in 3% to 6% of lung cancer patients (with normal hepatic function) and in the adrenal glands in 3% to 7%. Therefore, upper abdominal CT should be a routine part of every chest CT performed for suspected malignancy.

Finally, of greatest value in evaluating lung cancer, CT assesses the mediastinal lymph nodes for the possible presence of metastatic tumor. CT is the most effective radiologic method available to assess the nodes for enlargement (McCloud et al, 1992). However, a "positive" CT result (nodal diameter more than 1 cm) predicts actual metastatic involvement in only about 70% of lung cancer patients. Accordingly, no patient should be denied an attempt at curative resection based on this finding. Any CT finding of metastatic nodal involvement must be confirmed histologically.

A "negative" CT result (lymph nodes less than 1.0 cm) is, in general, much more accurate. With a "negative" CT and a T1 or T2 lesion, the false-negative rate is less than 10%, and histologic confirmation by mediastinoscopy is omitted by many surgeons. However, as demonstrated by Daly and coworkers (1987), the false-negative rate increases to 28% with central T3 tumors; in this situation, mediastinoscopy is recommended. In addition, Vallieres and Waters (1987) and others have demonstrated that T1 adenocarcinomas or large cell carcinomas have a higher rate of early micrometastasis; therefore, we believe that all such patients should undergo mediastinoscopy.

Magnetic Resonance Imaging

MRI of pulmonary lesions and mediastinal nodes has been disappointing, offering no real improvement over CT in diagnosis or staging except in specific situations. Lung cancers that are adjacent to either the vertebral body or the spinal canal are best assessed with MRI—it provides superior detail of the spinal canal and detects changes in the bone marrow that may be suggestive of involvement by carcinoma with greater accuracy than does CT. Heelan and colleagues (1985) found MRI to be more accurate than CT in assessing possible invasion of mediastinal structures. However, as demonstrated by Stiglbauer and associates (1991), this enhanced ability may also overdiagnose mediastinal invasion, with a high incidence of false-positive results. Because of its superb imaging of vascular structures, MRI can be useful in defining a tumor's relationship to a major vessel. It is particularly useful when contrast material is contraindicated.

Radionuclide Scanning

Bone Scans

The ability of radionuclide scans to diagnose and stage lung cancer has been limited by their lack of specificity. Routine nuclide scanning with gallium citrate or cobalt-bleomycin was used mainly for detecting unsuspected mediastinal spread after an initial diagnosis. However, the rate of incorporation of the radioisotope by the primary tumor and its metastatic foci was variable, limiting its clinical use in either diagnosis or staging (Kies et al, 1978; Little et al, 1986). Isotope-labelled monoclonal antibodies have also been investigated as a tool for staging and diagnosing lung cancer. Specific monoclonal antibodies that are directed at lung cancer cells may be valuable in the future for diagnosis and staging in conjunction with the newer modality, PET scanning.

Positron Emission Tomography Scanning

PET scanning is based on the detection of positrons emitted by isotopes of atoms with low atomic weight such as carbon, fluorine, oxygen, and nitrogen. The agent used most for imaging is fluorodeoxyglucose (FDG), which is a D-glucose analogue that is labeled with positron-emitting ^{18}F. After cellular uptake and phosphorylation, FDG is not metabolized further, leading to intracellular accumulation. This accumulation, coupled with a malignancy's intrinsically higher rate of glucose metabolism, leads to preferential accumulation and subsequent visualization. Thus, PET is a physiologic imaging modality. A significant potential advantage is that it enables whole-body imaging after a single injection of FDG, allowing simultaneous evaluation of the primary lung lesion, mediastinal lymph nodes, and distant organs.

A full review of PET scanning in the diagnosis and staging of lung cancer can be found in the Imaging section of this book (Chapter 21). PET scanning is being actively investigated for use as a diagnostic and staging tool. Like all other imaging (and most invasive) diagnostic and staging techniques, false-negative and false-positive examinations can occur. PET scanning appears to be exceptionally valuable in detecting occult distant metastases.

The exact role of PET scanning in the routine diagnosis and staging of lung cancer is yet to be determined. PET scanning is limited by the size of the lesion, and lesions less than 5 mm in diameter often go undetected. Similarly, granulomatous inflammation of the mediastinum can be "hot" on a PET scan. For these reasons, mediastinoscopy remains a valuable tool when confirmation or denial of mediastinal metastases is required for treatment planning.

In summary, PET scanning shows significant promise in both the diagnosis and the staging of patients with NSCLC. It complements conventional imaging. A more extensive discussion of PET scanning can be found in Chapter 21.

INVASIVE EXAMINATIONS

Transthoracic Needle Aspiration

Fine-needle aspiration biopsy of pulmonary nodules is an excellent method for obtaining cytologic or histologic material for a positive identification of malignancy. Fluoroscopic or CT-guided techniques are used. Its value is operator-dependent, however. The positive yield in experienced hands can be as high as 95%. The accuracy of cytologic examination in identifying histologic subtypes, however, is only 75%. An indeterminate biopsy result cannot be accepted as negative. False-negative examinations are frequent and must be considered indeterminate, unless a positive benign diagnosis (e.g., hamartoma or granuloma) can be made (Wescott, 1980). An algorithm for investigating a solitary pulmonary nodule is presented in Figure 31–27.

Bronchoscopy

Visualization of the tracheobronchial tree with the rigid or flexible bronchoscope is, in addition to chest radiogra-

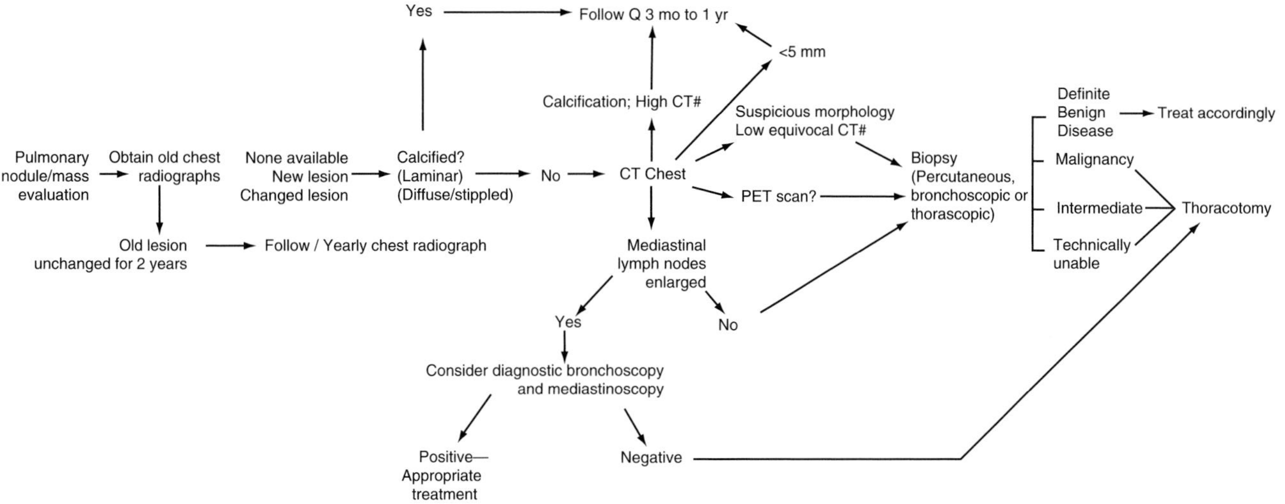

FIGURE 31–27 ■ Algorithm for evaluation of a pulmonary nodule or mass.

phy and CT, a standard part of evaluating patients with suspected or known lung cancer. Flexible bronchoscopy with video-imaging capabilities has replaced rigid bronchoscopy, except in select circumstances, and allows visualization of the proximal tracheobronchial tree up to the second, and occasionally the third, subsegmental bronchus. In general, bronchoscopy serves three invaluable purposes: (1) diagnosis, (2) staging, and (3) assessment of the remaining bronchial tree.

Diagnosing lung cancer by bronchoscopy can be pursued by one of five techniques: direct biopsy; transbronchial needle aspiration; brushing; saline lavage (for cytologic testing); and fluoroscopically guided biopsy, brushing, or needle aspiration. Using more than one technique often improves the diagnostic yield; in particular, after performing any biopsies, routine brushing and washing of the area should be done to retrieve cells "liberated" by the biopsy. In addition, after any diagnostic bronchoscopic procedure, the yield of sputum cytologic testing appears to increase, making this technique of value as an added diagnostic tool.

Three findings may be encountered at bronchoscopy: visible endobronchial tumor or suspicious lesion; bronchial distortion; and a normal examination. Endobronchial tumor is seen in 25% to 50% of patients, usually with small cell and squamous tumors because of their central location. If three or four biopsy specimens are obtained followed by brushings and washings, the diagnostic yield for endobronchial tumors should be greater than 90%.

Bronchial distortion (usually thickening or blunting of either the tracheal carina or minor carina, or evidence of extrinsic compression), secondary to the tumor or enlarged lymph nodes extrinsic to the airway, may be all that is evident. Transbronchial needle aspiration (TBNA) can be useful in this circumstance. First introduced by Schiepatti (1958) and subsequently refined and popularized by Wang and Terri (1983), TBNA is performed by passing a rigid needle, usually 20 to 22 gauge, through the channel of the fiberoptic bronchoscope and then puncturing through the airway wall into the area of interest; thus, aspirates of either lymph nodes or tumor extrinsic to the bronchus are obtained. The aspirate is placed on slides, stained, and examined microscopically.

Although useful, TBNA has significant limitations. As a diagnostic technique, it may be of value in obtaining a histologic diagnosis. As a staging procedure, however, TBNA must be approached with caution. Although TBNA of subcarinal or paratracheal lymph nodes can verify the presence of N2 disease, such results need to be interpreted carefully (Shure and Fedullo, 1984). As noted by Cropp and colleagues (1984), false-positive results can occur if tumor cells are incorporated into the needle from the epithelial surface. Also, because of the need to assess multiple nodal stations, the presence of contralateral (N3) disease, and the degree of nodal involvement (microscopic, node replaced by tumor, extranodal tumor extension) in most circumstances, it will still be necessary to perform formal mediastinal staging by mediastinoscopy. For these reasons, we feel TBNA has limited application in staging mediastinal nodes in all but the massively involved cases.

A normal bronchoscopic examination is seen most often with peripheral lesions, typically solitary pulmonary nodules. With the aid of fluoroscopy, the lesion can be identified and a transbronchial biopsy can be performed. Guided by the image intensifier, the lesion is biopsied under direct fluoroscopic vision, and samples are obtained. Similarly, brushings and needle aspiration can be carried out to increase the yield. Successful diagnosis depends on lesion size: those less than 2 cm have diagnostic yields of 35% or less (Stringfield et al, 1977) compared with rates of 50% to 60% for lesions greater than 2 cm. Improved diagnostic yields of up to 80% can be obtained through the use of fluoroscopically guided TBNA and bronchoalveolar lavage (Schenk et al, 1987). Many studies affirm that a combination of techniques ensures the best chance of making a diagnosis.

Bronchoscopy is also an important staging tool, often providing invaluable information for preoperative planning, such as the tumor location, the length of the normal bronchus proximal to the tumor, the tumor's relationship to the tracheal carina (T3 versus T2 or T1), any evidence of extrinsic compression of proximal airways (by extrinsic tumor or enlarged lymph nodes), and, as noted by Shure and Fedullo (1985), any evidence of submucosal or peribronchial spread. Suggestive of such spread, they found, were concentric bronchial narrowing, bronchial indentation, and either the absence of mucosal markings or the presence of a hypervascular-appearing mucosa.

Autofluorescence Bronchoscopy

There has been significant interest in the detection of premalignant and malignant lesions by taking advantage of the different degrees of autofluorescence seen when different tissues are exposed to specific wavelengths of light. It appears that dysplastic and malignant bronchial epithelial cells show a significant decrease in autofluorescence, particularly in the green region of the visible spectrum, compared with normal bronchial epithelium (Lam and Becker, 1996). A fluorescence endoscope (Lung Imaging Fluorescence Endoscope [LIFE]) uses a helium-cadmium laser as a light source with wavelengths of 442 nm. It allows one to visually distinguish between normal mucosa and dysplasia or carcinoma. Normal tissue fluoresces green while dysplastic tissue or carcinoma fluoresces brown or reddish brown, allowing directed biopsies or brushings. The examination can be done under local anesthesia on an outpatient basis. LIFE bronchoscopy may play a role in preoperative screening for synchronous carcinomas and in the follow-up of postoperative patients with squamous cell tumors for either recurrence or the development of second primary tumors.

Esophageal Ultrasonography and Fine-Needle Aspiration

Endoscopic ultrasonography in the area of subcarinal and peritracheal lymph nodes has been used to guide needles into enlarged lymph nodes. Like TBNA with bronchoscopy, this will prove the diagnosis of tumor involvement but does not have the sensitivity to identify resectable versus unresectable lymph node disease and, therefore, should be used with caution in determining resectability.

Cervical Mediastinoscopy

Cervical mediastinoscopy is the most accurate way (short of thoracotomy) to stage superior mediastinal lymph nodes. A thorough cervical mediastinal exploration has several advantages over CT: (1) it enables a histologic diagnosis; (2) it accurately determines the presence or absence of N2 disease with a precise anatomic mapping by nodal station; (3) it identifies extranodal extension of the tumor and any involvement of contiguous structures (trachea or aorta); and (4) it can identify N3 disease. Because mediastinal lymphadenopathy may affect treatment decisions, accurate assessment is important.

The indications for mediastinoscopy are debated. In general, lymph nodes larger than 1 cm on CT should undergo biopsy by mediastinoscopy, because the CT's accuracy in predicting metastasis in enlarged nodes is only 70%. Conversely, a negative CT result (lymph nodes smaller than 1 cm) is, in many centers, sufficient to prove operability. In this circumstance, mediastinoscopy is omitted, and pulmonary resection and mediastinal lymph node dissection or sampling are performed, yielding a high rate of complete resection. Because of the poor prognosis (even with complete resection) conferred by high paratracheal (station 2) node involvement, by multiple sites of N2 disease, or by N3 disease, others believe that mediastinoscopy is routinely indicated to preoperatively identify such patients.

The results of routine mediastinoscopy as a staging procedure were examined by Luke and associates (1986) in a retrospective analysis of 1000 consecutive mediastinoscopies. Positive lymph nodes were found in 296 examinations (29.6%) and negative lymph nodes in 704 (70.4%)—rates consistent with other large series of mediastinoscopy. Of 590 patients with a negative mediastinoscopy result who underwent thoracotomy, 93% also underwent complete tumor resection (85% curative, 7% palliative). Unsuspected N2 disease was found in 52 patients, for a false-negative rate of 8.9%. However, most of these false-negative results were at sites that are inaccessible by mediastinoscopy, such as posterior subcarinal, periesophageal, and anterior mediastinal regions, all of which allow complete resectability.

What, then, are the current indications for mediastinoscopy in the staging of lung cancer? The answer depends on the training, experience, and philosophy of the thoracic surgeon. Most clinicians agree that the absolute indications for mediastinoscopy are: (1) lymph node enlargement more than 1 cm on CT prior to thoracotomy and (2) potential entry into neoadjuvant therapy protocols. Relative indications are a negative CT result and either a T2 or T3 primary tumor or a T1 adenocarcinoma or large cell carcinoma (Vallieres and Waters, 1987).

The issue of routine mediastinoscopy for patients with negative CT scans is highly controversial. Proponents of routine mediastinoscopy cite its low complication rate; the ability to select patients with N2 disease who are most likely to benefit from resection without neoadjuvant therapy (single station, ipsilateral, lower paratracheal, and no extracapsular extension); the higher rate of thoracotomies that lead to curative resection; and CTs with 10% to 15% false-negative rates. Proponents of selectively applying mediastinoscopy cite the high rate of negative mediastinoscopy examinations (70%) and the ability to completely resect patients with unsuspected N2 disease (assuming routine performance of a mediastinal lymph node dissection). Both approaches have merit and are supported by available data. Our practice, for the reasons outlined earlier, is routine mediastinoscopy with rare exceptions.

The emerging utility of PET scanning must be entered into the argument for and against invasive versus noninvasive mediastinal staging. However, as yet, its exact role in replacing invasive staging is undefined.

Left Anterior Mediastinotomy or Extended Cervical Mediastinoscopy

These techniques, when applied to lung cancer staging, are used to evaluate lymph node stations 5 and 6 in patients with left hilar or left upper lobe tumors. If enlargement of station 5 or 6 lymph nodes is detected on CT, cervical mediastinoscopy should precede mediastinotomy (or extended cervical mediastinoscopy), even in the absence of paratracheal lymph node enlargement. If results are negative, left anterior mediastinotomy or extended cervical mediastinoscopy (Ginsberg, 1987) should be done. Indications for prethoracotomy assessment of station 5 and 6 are: (1) potential entry into an adjuvant therapy protocol for N2 disease preoperatively; (2) a CT suggestion of bulky nodal metastases or extracapsular spread, which may preclude complete resection; and (3) the need for tissue diagnosis in a patient with recurrent laryngeal nerve paralysis caused by extracapsular nodal extension, with contiguous involvement of the nerve. Alternatively, if cervical mediastinoscopy gives negative results, the surgeon may proceed directly to thoracotomy with the intent of resecting the primary tumor and all enlarged lymph nodes in stations 5 and 6; even if nodal metastases are present, a reasonable 5-year survival rate is possible (Patterson et al, 1987).

Scalene Node Biopsy

Routine scalene node biopsy of nonpalpable lymph nodes, previously the only available nodal staging procedure, is no longer used. However, palpable cervical lymph nodes should be assessed, preferably by needle aspiration biopsy. Scalene node biopsy is valuable to rule out N3 disease in patients with proven N2 disease. Lee and Ginsberg (1996) demonstrated the ability to perform scalene node biopsy at the time of mediastinoscopy with minimal additional dissection. They found that 6 (15.4%) of 39 patients with N2 disease at mediastinoscopy had positive scalene node biopsies; all "positive" cases had centrally located tumors (visible on bronchoscopy) and nonsquamous histology. Thus, scalene node biopsy during mediastinoscopy in patients with N2 disease may identify inoperable N3 disease.

Thoracoscopy

Video-assisted thoracoscopy (VATS) has been used to diagnose and stage lung cancer. VATS is often used in excising and diagnosing indeterminate pulmonary nodules. Lesions most suitable for such an approach are those that are located in the outer one third of the lung and those that are less than 3 cm in diameter (Landreneau et al, 1992). Certain principles must be followed when excising potentially malignant lesions via VATS. The nodule should not be directly manipulated with instruments, care must be taken not to violate the visceral pleura overlying the nodule, and the excised nodule must be extracted from the chest within a bag to prevent seeding of the chest wall. As an aid to staging tumors, VATS may be useful to sample anterior mediastinal lymph nodes (most notably, stations 5 and 6) for histologic examination (Lewis et al, 1992; Mack et al, 1992; Miller et al, 1992b), to look for unsuspected pleural disease, to assess the status of pleural effusion, and to biopsy ipsilateral or contralateral pulmonary nodules that may represent metastases. As a tool to assess T4 invasion of the mediastinum, VATS has proved less useful.

Thoracotomy

Diagnostic thoracotomies are still occasionally necessary to diagnose and stage lung cancer. However, given the availability of less invasive procedures, more than 95% of tumors can now be accurately diagnosed and staged without thoracotomy. Nonetheless, a few patients with a high probability of having cancer cannot be diagnosed with certainty without thoracotomy. At the time of thoracotomy, fine-needle aspiration, a Tru-Cut biopsy, or (preferably) an excisional biopsy can make a diagnosis with frozen-section analysis. All these techniques provide tissue that can be rapidly assessed by pathologists. As noted earlier, a determination that a tumor is either T3 or T4 often cannot be made until thoracotomy. If lung cancer is diagnosed at the time of thoracotomy, further staging by mediastinal lymph node sampling or complete lymph node dissection is mandatory.

EVALUATION FOR METASTATIC DISEASE

Because distant metastases are found in about 40% of patients with newly diagnosed lung cancer, and because the presence of metastases usually confers inoperability, a patient's risk of harboring metastatic disease must be carefully considered by the surgeon.

The most important initial evaluations are the history, physical examination, and laboratory studies. Constitutional symptoms of anorexia, malaise, and unintentional weight loss of more than 5% of body weight suggest either a large tumor burden or the presence of metastases. Focal skeletal discomfort, particularly if new and unassociated with trauma, suggests skeletal metastases. Neurologic symptoms of metastases are typically nonfocal and consist of headaches (new or changed pattern), mental status changes (e.g., poor attentiveness, drifting thought processes, excessive sleepiness), personality change, nausea, and seizures. Less frequent are focal neurologic signs. Signs of metastases on physical examination include supraclavicular or cervical adenopathy, localized bone pain on palpation, and soft tissue or skin mass (up to 8% of patients with NSCLC develop skin metastases). Routine laboratory studies should include hepatic enzymes (serum glutamic oxaloacetic transaminase and alkaline phosphatase levels) and calcium levels (to detect bone metastases or the ectopic parathyroid syndrome); elevation of either typically occurs with extensive metastases.

Patients with a positive clinical evaluation, with either non–organ-specific or organ-specific symptoms or signs, should undergo multi-organ scanning consisting of radionuclide bone scan, intravenous contrast–enhanced abdominal CT, and either intravenous contrast–enhanced CT or MRI of the brain (Hooper et al, 1978; Quinn et al, 1986).

Routine Multi-Organ Scanning of Asymptomatic Patients

Although controversial, several studies have demonstrated that preoperative routine organ scanning (bone, brain, and abdomen) in asymptomatic patients appears to yield a low percentage (3% to 10%) of positive scans. Sider and Horejs (1988) reviewed the records of 95 patients with NSCLC who had no evidence of hilar or mediastinal adenopathy on CT scan (clinical stage I); 24 (25%) proved to have extrathoracic metastases. However, only 4 (4%) had clinically silent disease. Quinn and associates (1986) found that 3 of 20 (15%) patients with a negative clinical evaluation had silent metastases. Salvatierra and coworkers (1990) performed a prospective study of routine multi-organ scanning in 146 patients with potentially resectable NSCLC; the incidence of detecting asymptomatic (or silent) metastases was 2.7% each for head CT and bone scan.

To more accurately determine the value of the clinical evaluation (history, physical examination, and laboratory studies) in predicting the presence of metastatic disease, Silvestri and colleagues (1995) performed a meta-analysis. They reviewed studies with data on both the clinical evaluation and the documented presence or absence of metastatic disease discovered on CT or bone scan. They calculated the mean negative predictive value of the clinical evaluation (i.e., the probability a scan will be negative given a negative clinical evaluation). For CT of the brain and abdomen and bone scan, it was 95%, 94%, and 89%, respectively. For example, in a patient whose neurologic symptoms and physical examination were deemed normal, the probability of having a negative head CT is 95%.

Although a negative clinical evaluation is reliable, a small percentage of patients will harbor metastatic disease, which will be undetected without scanning. We feel the risk of not detecting these metastases is balanced by the risk of a false-positive scan. Patchell and associates (1990) found that 6 (11%) of 54 lesions thought to be brain metastases on CT were either inflammatory lesions or synchronous primary brain tumors. Adrenal adenomas, which are found in 2% of the general population and in up to 8% of patients with hypertension, may be mistakenly assumed to represent metastasis (Gajraj and Young, 1993). Bone scans are notorious for their high sensitivity but low specificity, with a known overall false-rate of 40% (Quinn et al, 1986) and with only 50% of solitary foci of uptake representing a metastasis (Rosenthal, 1997). False-positive scans of any organ often lead to further noninvasive and invasive evaluation and may even lead to denial of surgical resection. For these reasons, we do not recommend routine preoperative multi-organ scanning of patients with a negative clinical evaluation and clinical stage I or II disease.

Under certain circumstances, we believe multi-organ scanning of patients with a negative clinical evaluation should be considered. Patients with stage IIIA disease proved by mediastinoscopy are at higher risk of harboring metastatic disease. Unfortunately, given the small number of patients, few data (including the meta-analysis by Silvestri et al, 1995) can be used to determine the predictive value of a negative clinical evaluation in patients with stage IIIA disease. However, because patients with stage IIIA disease are often subjected to intense multimodal therapy, it seems reasonable to routinely perform multi-organ scanning in this group. Finally, given the well-documented higher incidence of brain metastasis with adenocarcinoma, as opposed to squamous carcinoma (Silvestri et al, 1995), some clinicians advocate routine brain CT or MRI for patients with this cell type. The value of this is unproven. However, brain CT or MRI scans in squamous cell carcinoma patients with normal neurologic clinical evaluations are very rarely positive (Salvatierra et al, 1990); therefore, in this subgroup, they are probably unnecessary.

In summary, we feel the two primary indications for multi-organ scanning in patients with negative clinical evaluations are: (1) clinical stage I or II disease in marginally acceptable operative candidates with poor pulmonary function or other medical illness and (2) stage IIIA disease in patients being considered for surgical resection, curative radiotherapy, or multimodal therapy. Finally, any patient—regardless of clinical stage—who has a positive clinical evaluation, whether organ-specific or not, should also undergo multi-organ scanning.

In the future, with the imminent arrival of fusion CT-PET scans, one-stop shopping may be available to help diagnose and stage patients with lung cancer.

The Positive Scan: Is It Truly Positive?

A common problem clinicians face with a positive scan is whether it is true- or false-positive. Because a false-positive scan can have a dramatic impact on a patient's therapy, the physician must ensure the accuracy of every scan. If any doubt about the accuracy of a scan exists, the patient must be afforded the benefit of the doubt, and the scan must be proved to be true-positive.

Bone scans, as noted earlier, are highly sensitive but nonspecific. Increased radionuclide uptake occurs with increased osteoblastic activity and depends on the concomitant increase in blood flow. Most skeletal metastases (55%) occur in the axial skeleton (spine, pelvis, sternum, and ribs); 12% occur in the extremities (Krishnamurthy et al, 1977). Bone scan findings that are consistent with metastases include the presence of a new lesion, irregular or asymmetrical appearance in a bone, randomly scattered lesions, and extension of the lesion into the bone's medullary cavity (Krasnow et al, 1997). Thus, a classic pattern of metastatic spread on a bone scan is multiple areas of increased activity in the axial skeleton (Fig. 31–28). The final determination as to whether a bone scan is true-positive depends on the appearance of the bone scan findings combined with the patient's history (e.g., trauma) and current symptoms. Frequently, confidence in the bone scan findings is shaky, and further evaluation of a "positive" or "cannot rule out mets" reading of a bone scan will be required.

Figure 31–29 is an algorithm for the evaluation of bone scans. With an equivocal bone scan result, plain radiographs of the area of increased isotope uptake may determine if other pathology (most commonly degenerative arthritis) is present and whether its distribution correlates with the bone scan abnormalities. If no explanation for the increased uptake is found, MRI is performed next. The sensitivity and specificity of MRI for metastatic disease is higher than that for a bone scan, because MRI directly visualizes and characterizes focal abnormalities

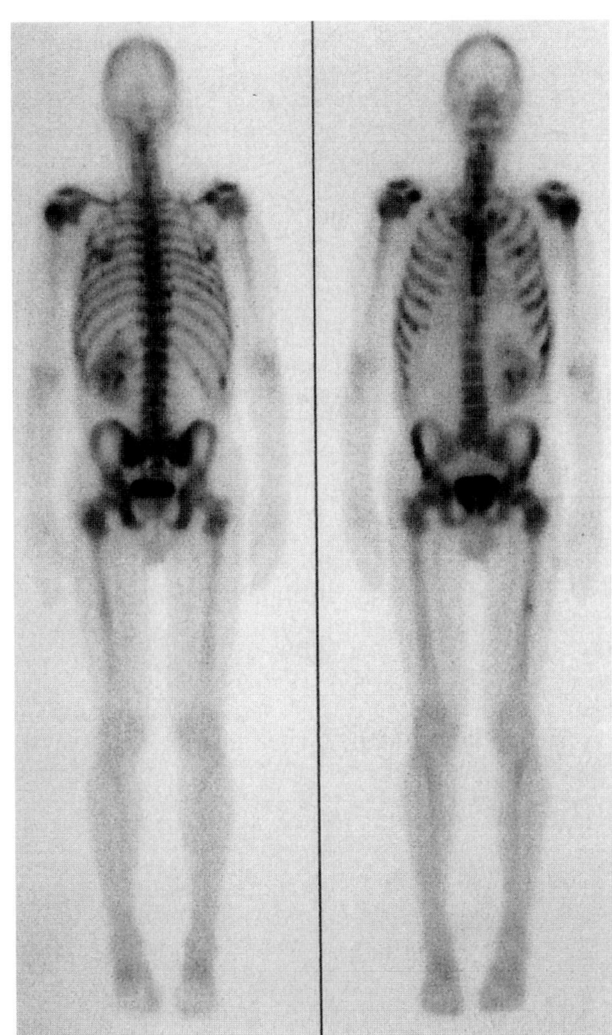

FIGURE 31–28 ■ Bone scan showing multiple foci of increased uptake in the axial skeleton (spine and ribs) that is consistent with diffuse osseous metastases.

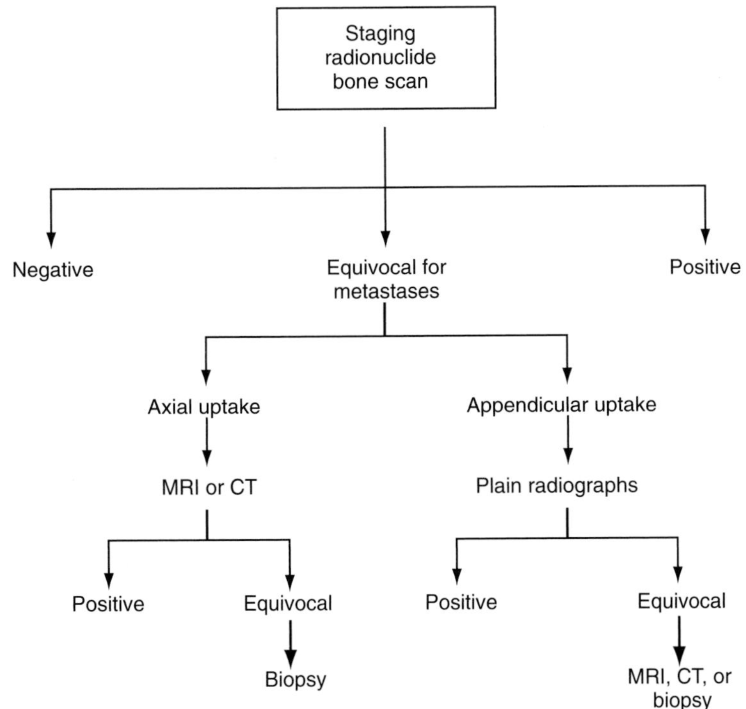

FIGURE 31–29 ■ An algorithm for the evaluation of bone scan results. MRI is preferred over CT unless contraindicated. CT, computed tomography; MRI, magnetic resonance imaging.

including the bone marrow, which is frequently the site where bone metastases begin.

Occasionally, percutaneous or open bone biopsy may still be required. Open biopsies may be difficult to localize intraoperatively. To aid intraoperative localization, the skin overlying the area of increased isotope uptake can be injected with ink preoperatively. Alternatively, the patient can be reinjected with 25 mCi of a ^{99m}Tc-labeled bone scanning agent 2 hours before the planned biopsy, and an intraoperative gamma probe can be used to localize the area of increased uptake (Robinson et al, 1998).

Adrenal masses or enlargement also pose a frequent dilemma, as they are often discovered on an intravenous contrast–enhanced chest CT that includes the liver and adrenal glands. As noted, adrenal adenomas occur in 2% of the general population and in up to 8% of patients with hypertension (Gajraj and Young, 1993), whereas in patients with NSCLC, the incidence of adrenal metastases is as high as 40% at autopsy. Thus, there is a high probability that the adrenal lesion may be malignant.

The size of the adrenal lesion is first evaluated. In a prospective study of 27 unilateral adrenal masses in patients with operable NSCLC, all of which were histologically verified by percutaneous biopsy or adrenalectomy, Burt and colleagues (1994) found that adrenal lesion size correlated significantly ($P < .001$) with risk of malignancy. Benign lesions (n = 22, 81%) had a mean size of 0.4 to 2.0 cm (median 2.0, range 1.2 to 2.8); malignant lesions (n = 5, 19%), a mean size of 1.9 to 3.8 cm (median 3.1, range 2.5 to 7.1). Therefore, size plays an important role in assessing the risk of malignancy, and lesions greater than 3 cm have a significant risk of being malignant.

Most incidentally discovered adrenal masses are 1 to 4 cm in diameter and cannot be determined to be malignant or benign on the original chest CT. In the subsequent radiologic evaluation of an adrenal mass, the chemical makeup of an adenoma versus a malignant lesion should be exploited as a clue. Adrenal adenomas originate from the adrenal cortex and have a high lipid content (secondary to steroid production), whereas metastases and most primary adrenal malignancies contain little if any lipid. This difference is the basis for the ability to distinguish adenomas from malignancies on CT and MRI (Choyke, 1998).

Noncontrast CT has been used to distinguish between benign and malignant adenomas based on density as measured by the lesion's Hounsfield units (HU). Numerous studies have shown that lesions that are less than 10 HU are nearly always benign, with specificities of 95% to 100%. Conversely, lesions greater than 10 HU do not imply malignancy; in fact, such a result is nondiagnostic. Because of the lower density and lower vascularity of benign adenomas compared with malignant tumors, delayed-contrast CT has been used to distinguish between them based on densities of less than 25 HU. Sensitivities of 96% to 100% and specificities of 92% to 100% have been reported (Boland et al, 1997; Brodeur et al, 1995; Szolar and Kammerhuber, 1997). However, the technique appears to depend on the type of contrast (ionic vs. nonionic), the amount of contrast injected, and the timing of scanning after contrast injection. Because this technique is less standardized and usually requires the patient to return for a repeat CT, it is less common than MRI.

Adrenal adenomas contain approximately equal mixtures of lipid and water, so chemical shift MRI can be used to reliably determine whether a lesion is an adenoma. Adenomas demonstrate a strong signal on in-phase images, but show a dramatic loss of signal on out-of-phase images (Fig. 31–30). Metastases have little lipid, so no such chemical shift is observed. Comparisons then need to be made with another tissue (typically spleen) and a ratio computed. Using this technique, sensitivities and specificities as high as 80% and 100% have been reported (Schwartz et al, 1995). Thus, as with noncontrast CT, an adenoma can be reliably diagnosed with certain measured values, but values found outside this range require histologic verification.

CT-guided biopsy is safe and, in experienced centers, has a low rate of complications (primarily pneumothorax). Tissue diagnosis is accurate in approximately 85% of cases, but depends on specimen adequacy and pathologic

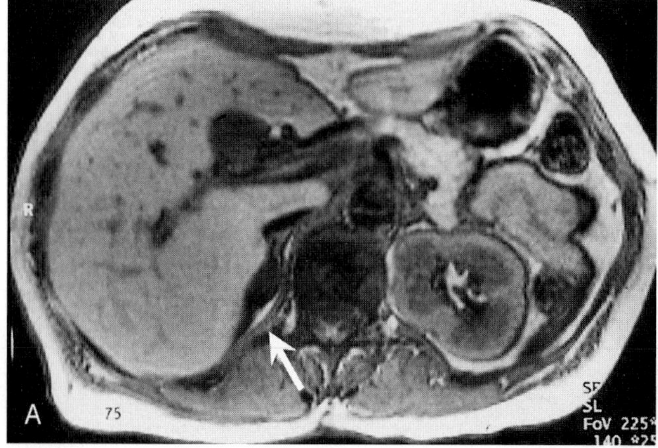

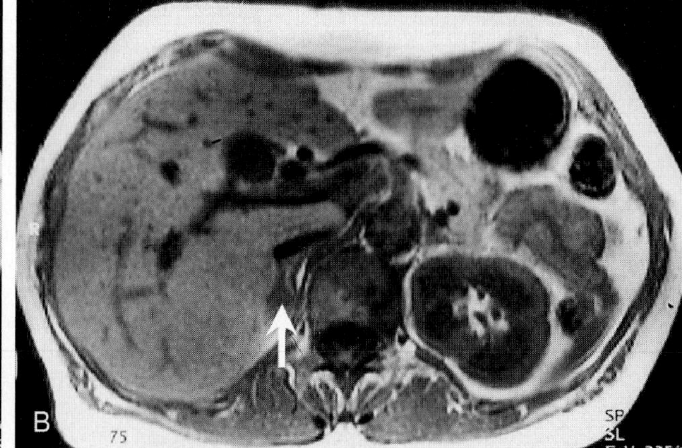

FIGURE 31–30 ■ Nonhyperfunctioning adrenal adenoma. *A*, Signal intensity of right adrenal mass on an in-phase T_1-weighted image is comparable with adjacent liver. *B*, Opposed-phased T_1-weighted image shows relative signal loss of the adrenal mass compared with the liver as a result of lipid content and suppression of fat signal. PET scans can also be used to differentiate benign from malignant masses in the adrenals. PET, positron emission tomography.

interpretation. If needle biopsy is technically impossible or yields an indeterminate result (neither malignant cells nor adrenal cells), then adrenalectomy through a posterior approach may be required. In some centers, PET scanning has replaced invasive procedures to identify adrenal malignancy in the face of a "positive" CT scan.

Abnormalities of the liver that are suspicious for metastases may require repeat abdominal CT scanning with intravenous contrast. Ultrasound is often useful to distinguish between cystic and solid lesions. Ultimately, if uncertainty exists, needle biopsy or laparoscopy may be necessary. Contrast-enhanced brain CT or MRI also have, as noted, a false-positive rate as high as 11% (Patchell et al, 1990). Typical features of a metastatic lesion are contrast enhancement (diffuse or in the periphery of the lesion), edema, and mass-effect. As with other organs, should the history or scan raise doubt about the nature of a lesion, biopsy or excision may be required.

Where PET scans are available, confirmation of these indeterminate abnormalities of bone scans and CT scans may be confirmed by this new imaging modality. However, in many cases histologic confirmation will still be required.

Immunohistochemical and Molecular Staging

Given the limitations of standard histochemistry for detecting submicroscopic or occult micrometastases (OM), the use of monoclonal or polyclonal antibodies has been introduced for detecting tumor cells in bone marrow and lymph nodes. With the use of primarily monoclonal antibodies to cytokeratin, single-cell occult bone marrow and lymph node metastases have been detected in several epithelial tumors, including melanomas, renal cell carcinomas, and colon, breast, gastric, and bladder cancers. In general, a correlation has been found between detection of occult bone marrow or lymph node metastases and prediction of poorer clinical outcome—for example, higher relapse rates and decreased survival.

In patients with NSCLC, several studies suggest a role for immunohistochemistry in detecting OM. Passlick and colleagues (1994) used monoclonal antibody Ber-EP4 (a monoclonal antibody directed against a cell-surface glycoprotein of epithelial cells) to detect OM in 391 lymph nodes in 72 patients with T1 to T3, N0, and M0 tumors who had complete tumor resection. Staining of 99% of the primary tumors with Ber-EP4 was seen. Ber-EP4–positive cells were detected in 15 (3.8%) of the 391 lymph nodes in 11 (15.2%) of 72 patients. Tumors recurred in 5 (50%) of the 10 patients with positive lymph nodes (3 local, 2 distant), compared with 8 (14%) of the 56 lymph nodes (4 local, 4 distant). Survival in the "positive" group was significantly worse ($P < 0.05$)—3 (30%) of 10 patients in this group died versus 4 (7%) the 56 patients in the negative group.

Pantel and colleagues (1996) used monoclonal antibody CK2 (reactive with cytokeratin component CK18) to detect bone marrow OM in patients with NSCLC. CK18 was detected in 95% of the primary tumors, with equal staining of both adenocarcinomas and squamous cell carcinomas. The incidence of detecting cells that were positive for CK18 was the same for adenocarcinomas and squamous cell carcinomas. The incidence of bone marrow aspirates that were positive for CK18 was 60%. The presence of positive cells in bone marrow predicted systemic relapse significantly earlier.

Recently, interest has developed in the use of reverse transcriptase-polymerase chain reaction (RT-PCR) to detect tumor-specific mRNA as a means to detect OM. Experimentally, RT-PCR can detect a single cancer cell in as few as 100 million background cells in vitro, demonstrating its enormous sensitivity.

RT-PCR has been used to detect tumor cells from prostate carcinomas (blood), melanomas (blood), and breast carcinomas (lymph nodes). *MUC1* is one of 10 genes that encode for mucinous glycoproteins in the lung and other organs. Nguyen and colleagues (1996) found that expression of the MUC1 gene product, MUC1 mRNA and its protein, are highly conserved in patients with NSCLC. Using the RT-PCR assay for MUC1 mRNA, Salerno and colleagues (1998) demonstrated a high rate of detecting OM in histologically negative lymph nodes in 18 patients with surgically resected stage I NSCLC. Of 72 lymph nodes examined, 29 (40%) were positive for MUC1 mRNA; these 29 positive lymph nodes were in 13 (72%) of the 18 patients.

The prognostic value of detecting OM by immunohistochemistry and RT-PCR awaits statistical verification by larger trials. Because PCR is so sensitive, detecting OM by this method may only represent the functional effectiveness of the immune system in filtering and clearing tumor cells. However, if detection of OM by either immunohistochemistry or RT-PCR proves to be of prognostic value, detecting OM may allow better selection of patients for both preoperative and postoperative adjuvant therapies.

CONCLUSIONS

Both noninvasive and invasive techniques are used to diagnose and stage lung cancer. Effective treatment planning requires accurate diagnosis and a valid clinical estimate of tumor stage.

COMMENTS AND CONTROVERSIES

As one reads this chapter, there is no doubt of the importance of an accurate history and physical examination in making the diagnosis and staging patients with lung cancer. Although accurate clinical staging does require having noninvasive and invasive testing, surgeons should not pass their responsibility to perform and complete a thorough history and physical examination to their pulmonary or oncologic medical colleagues. If the latter is done, I am concerned that important diagnostic and staging elements affecting the individual patient's management outcome may be lost. The very exciting modality of PET scanning still requires further study before accepting the results of such a study without histologic confirmation.

The symptoms of patients with lung cancer are extremely variable but I would estimate that at least 10% to 15% of cases are asymptomatic at presentation. This high incidence relates not only to the liberal use of routine chest radiographs but also to the rising number of periph-

eral adenocarcinomas. As pointed out by the authors, worsening of pre-existing cough or changes in the pattern of coughing habits are some of the most common early symptoms of lung cancer, as is hemoptysis. Worsening of dyspnea is usually a late symptom.

In general, the incidence of paraneoplastic syndromes is higher than 2% if one takes into account all patients with lung cancer. Hypertrophic pulmonary osteoarthropathy and clubbing, for instance, can be seen in up to 25% of cases. As a rule, the presence of paraneoplastic syndromes indicates a more advanced disease which often cannot be cured by surgical intervention. As mentioned by the authors, hypertrophic pulmonary osteoarthropathy often disappears within hours of surgical excision if the carcinoma has been completely resected. Vagotomy, which in the past has been reported to be of some use to reduce symptoms related to paraneoplastic syndrome, is no longer done. It is interesting to note that recurrent cancer will often initiate recurrence of the paraneoplastic syndrome.

Pretreatment staging of lung cancer is very important because it will determine the best therapy for a given patient. Unfortunately, not everybody agrees on which methods should be used to achieve that goal, and there is a great deal of controversy over the extent to which staging should be done, especially in asymptomatic patients. Even the TNM staging system is imperfect despite all of its recent modifications. The presence of a cytologically negative pleural effusion, for instance, is a sign of poor prognosis but yet the terminology of the TNM staging system is vague on this issue. This is even worse when one tries to determine the nodal status because three different nodal maps are currently available. Despite these difficulties, I believe that it is inconceivable to operate without having made an effort to adequately clinically stage the patient. It would also be inconceivable to deny surgery to a patient with lung cancer without proper documentation of the stage of disease.

How important it is to document lung cancer preoperatively remains a major controversy because many surgeons have the attitude that abnormal densities have to be resected whether you have or do not have a positive diagnosis beforehand. In my view, every effort should be made to establish a diagnosis prior to resection not only because it will determine which staging tests should be done but also because it facilitates an open discussion with the patient. In addition, it avoids having to rely on frozen sections which at times can be misleading. With the help of sputum cytology, transthoracic needle biopsy, and bronchoscopy, one can achieve that goal in over 95% of patients who are to undergo resectional surgery.

What should be done with a patient who has dysplastic cells in the sputum is also unclear because as of now, no specific marker has been proved to be accurate in determining which patient with dysplasia will eventually develop an invasive carcinoma. I do not think, however, that segmental bronchial washings and biopsies should routinely be done in all patients with dysplasia, especially if it is mild or moderate. It is possible that in the future, inhalation chemotherapy might be useful to stop the process of malignant degeneration in such individuals.

J. D.

■ KEY REFERENCES

Cooper JD, Ginsberg RJ: The use of mediastinoscopy in lung cancer: Preoperative evaluation. In Kittle FC: Current Controversies in Thoracic Surgery. Philadelphia, WB Saunders, 1986.

An in-depth review of the debate about the role of mediastinoscopy and CT scanning in staging lung cancer. The accompanying chapter by Shields should also be read. Fifteen years later, the arguments are still valid!

Deslauriers J, Gregoire J: Clinical and surgical staging of non-small cell lung cancer. Chest 117(Suppl):96S–103S, 2000.

An excellent review of staging lung cancer.

Feins RH: Thoracic endoscopy. Chest Surg Clin N Am 6:2, 1996.

An excellent mini-text covering all aspects of the endoscopic diagnosis and management of lung cancer.

Marchioli CC, Graziano SL: Paraneoplastic syndromes associated with small cell lung cancer. Chest Surg Clin N Am 7:65, 1997.

An in-depth review of the neurologic and endocrine paraneoplastic syndromes seen in small cell lung cancer.

McCloud TC, Bourgouin PM, Greenberg RW et al: Bronchogenic carcinoma: Analysis of staging in the mediastinum with CT by correlative lymph node mapping and sampling. Radiology 182:319, 1992.

An excellent prospective study comparing CT scanning and mediastinoscopy. Particularly interesting is the comparison of CT and mediastinoscopy by nodal stations.

Miller JD, Gorenstein LA, Patterson GA: Staging: The key to rational management of lung cancer. Ann Thorac Surg 53:170, 1992a.

A review of the new international staging system and the radiologic and invasive techniques used in staging.

Mountain CF: A new international staging system for lung cancer. Chest 89(Suppl):225S, 1986.

Mountain CF: Revisions in the international system for staging lung cancer. Chest 111:1710–1717, 1997.

The original and updated description of the new international staging system.

■ REFERENCES

American Thoracic Society: Clinical staging of primary lung cancer. Am Rev Respir Dis 127:659, 1983.

Boiselle PM, Patz EF, Vining DJ et al: Imaging of mediastinal lymph nodes: CT, MR, and FDG PET. Radiographics 18:1061, 1998.

Boland GW, Hahn PF, Pena C et al: Adrenal masses: Characterization with delayed contrast enhanced CT. Radiology 202:693, 1997.

Brodeur FJ, Korobkin MT, Francis IR et al: Delayed enhanced CT: A method of differentiating adrenal adenomas from non-adenomas. Radiology 166:197:185, 1995.

Burt M, Heelan RT, Coit D: Prospective evaluation of unilateral adrenal masses in patients with operable non-small cell lung cancer. J Thorac Cardiovasc Surg 107:584, 1994.

Campling BG, Sarda IR, Baer KA et al: Secretion of atrial natriuretic peptide and vasopressin by small cell lung cancer. Cancer 75:2442, 1995.

Carbone PP, Frost JK, Feinstein AR et al: Lung cancer: Perspective and prospects. Ann Intern Med 73:1024, 1970.

Carlens E: Mediastinoscopy: A method for inspection and tissue biopsy in the superior mediastinum. Dis Chest 36:343, 1959.

Choyke PL: From needles to numbers: Can noninvasive imaging distinguish benign and malignant adrenal lesions? World J Urol 16:29, 1998.

Cromartie RS, Parker EF, May JE et al: Carcinoma of the lung: A clinical review. Ann Thorac Surg 30:30, 1980.

Cropp AJ, DiMarco AF, Lankerani M: False-positive transbronchial needle aspiration in bronchogenic carcinoma. Chest 85:696, 1984.

Cryer PE, Kissaine JM: Clinicopathologic conference: Malignant hypercalcemia. Am J Med 65:486, 1979.

Daly BDT, Faling LJ, Bite G et al: Mediastinal lymph node evaluation

by computed tomography in lung cancer. J Thorac Cardiovasc Surg 94:664, 1987.
Denoix PF: Enquete permanent dans les centres anticancereux. Bull Inst Nat Hyg (Paris) 1:70, 1946.
Donaldson JC, Kaminsky DB, Elliot RC: Bronchiolar carcinoma: Report of 11 cases and review of the literature. Cancer 41:250, 1978.
Gajraj H, Young AE: Adrenal incidentaloma. Br J Surg 80:422, 1993.
Ginsberg RJ: Extended cervical mediastinoscopy: A single staging procedure for bronchogenic carcinoma of the left upper lobe. Thorac Cardiovasc Surg 94:673, 1987.
Harken DE, Black H, Clauss R, Ferrand RE: Simple cervicomediastinal exploration for tissue diagnosis of intrathoracic disease. N Engl J Med 251:1041, 1954.
Heelan R, Martini N, Westcot JW et al: Carcinomas involving the hilum and mediastinum: Computed tomographic and magnetic resonance evaluation. Radiology 156:111, 1985.
Hooper RG, Beechler CR, Johnson MC: Radioisotope scanning in the initial staging of bronchogenic carcinoma. Am Rev Respir Dis 118:279, 1978.
Kato H, Konako C, Ono J et al: Cytology of the Lung: Techniques and Interpretation. Tokyo, Igaku-Shoin, 1983.
Kies MS, Baker AW, Kennedy PS: Radionuclide scans in staging of carcinoma of lung. Surg Gynecol Obstet 147:175, 1978.
Krasnow AZ, Hellman RS, Timins ME et al: Diagnostic bone scanning in oncology. Semin Nucl Med 27:2, 1997.
Krishnamurthy GT, Tubis M, Miss J et al: Distribution pattern of metastatic bone disease: A need for total body skeletal imaging. JAMA 237:2504, 1977.
Lam S, Becker HD: Future diagnostic procedures. Chest Surg Clin N Am 6:363, 1996.
Landreneau RJ, Mack MJ, Hazelrigg SR et al: Video-assisted thoracic surgery: Basic technical concepts and intercostal approach strategies. Ann Thorac Surg 54:800, 1992.
Lee JD, Ginsberg RJ: Lung cancer staging: The value of ipsilateral scalene lymph node biopsy performed at mediastinoscopy. Ann Thorac Surg 62:338, 1996.
Lennon VA, Lambert EH: Autoantibodies bind solubilized calcium channel-omega-conotoxin complexes from small cell lung carcinoma: A diagnostic aid for Lambert-Eaton myasthenic syndrome. Mayo Clin Proc 64:1498, 1989.
Lewis P, Griffin S, Marsden P et al: Whole-body 18F-fluorodeoxyglucose positron emission tomography in preoperative evaluation of lung cancer. Lancet 344:1265, 1994.
Lewis RJ, Caccavale RJ, Sisler GE, Mackenzie JW: One hundred consecutive patients undergoing video-assisted thoracic operations. Ann Thorac Surg 54:421, 1992.
Liang XM: Accuracy of cytologic diagnosis and cytotyping of sputum in primary lung cancer: Analysis of 161 cases. J Surg Oncol 40:107, 1989.
List AF, Hainsworth JD, Davis BW et al: The syndrome of inappropriate secretion of antidiuretic hormone (SIADH) in small-cell lung cancer. J Clin Oncol 4:1191, 1986.
Little AG, DeMeester TR, Ryan JW: The use of radionuclide scans in lung cancer: Gallium-67 scanning for preoperative staging. In Kittle FC: Current Controversies in Thoracic Surgery. Philadelphia, WB Saunders, 1986.
Lowe VJ, Naunheim KS: Current role of positron emission tomography in thoracic oncology. Thorax 53:703, 1998.
Luke WP, Pearson FG, Todd TRJ et al: Prospective evaluation of mediastinoscopy for assessment of carcinoma of the lung. J Thorac Cardiovasc Surg 91:53, 1986.
Mack MJ, Aronoff RJ, Acuff TE et al: Present role of thoracoscopy in the diagnosis and treatment of diseases of the chest. Ann Thorac Surg 54:403, 1992.
Martini N, Flehinger BJ, Nagasaki F, Hart B: Prognostic significance of N1 disease in carcinoma of the lung. J Thorac Cardiovasc Surg 86:646, 1983.
McCloud TC, Bourgouin PM, Greenberg RW et al: Bronchogenic carcinoma: Analysis of staging in the mediastinum with CT by correlative lymph node mapping and sampling. Radiology 182:319, 1992.
McEvoy KM: Diagnosis and treatment of Lambert-Eaton myasthenic syndrome. Neurol Clin 12:387, 1994.
Miller DL, Allen MS, Trastek VF et al: Videothoracoscopic wedge excision of the lung. Ann Thorac Surg 54:410, 1992b.
Morton DL, Itabashi HH, Gromes OF: Nonmetastatic neurologic complications of bronchogenic carcinoma: The carcinomatous myopathies. J Thorac Cardiovasc Surg 51:14, 1966.
Mountain CF, Carr DT, Anderson WA: A system for the clinical staging of lung cancer. AJR Am J Roentgenol 120:130, 1974.
Mountain CF: A new international staging system for lung cancer. Chest 89(4 Suppl):225S, 1986.
Mountain CF: Revisions in the international system for staging lung cancer. Chest 111:6, 1997.
Naruke T, Goya T, Tsuchya R et al: Prognosis and survival in resected lung cancer based on the new international staging system. J Thorac Cardiovasc Surg 96:440, 1988.
Naruke T, Suemasu K, Ishikawa S: Lymph node mapping and curability at various levels of metastasis in resected lung cancer. J Thorac Cardiovasc Surg 76:832, 1978.
Ng A, Horak GC: Factors significant to the diagnostic accuracy of lung cytology in bronchial washing and sputum samples. II. Sputum samples. Acta Cytol 27:397, 1983.
Nguyen PL, Niehans GA, Cherwitz DL et al: Membrane-bound (MUC1) and secretory (MUC2, MUC3, and MUC4) mucin gene expression in human lung cancer. Tumour Biol 17:176, 1996.
Odell WD, Wolfsen AR: Humoral syndromes associated with cancer. Annu Rev Med 29:379, 1978.
Pagani JJ: Non-small cell lung carcinoma adrenal metastases: Computed tomography and percutaneous needle biopsy in their diagnosis. Cancer 53:1058, 1984.
Pantel K, Izbicki J, Passlick B et al: Frequency and prognostic significance of isolated tumor cells in the bone marrow of patients with NSCLC without overt metastases. Lancet 347:649, 1996.
Passlick B, Izbicki RJ, Kubuschok B et al: Immunohistochemical assessment of individual tumor cells in lymph nodes of patients with non-small cell lung cancer. J Clin Oncol 12:1827, 1994.
Patchell RA, Tibbs PA, Walsh JW et al: A randomized trial of surgery in the treatment of single metastases to the brain. N Engl J Med 322:494, 1990.
Patterson GA, Piazza D, Pearson FG et al: Significance of metastatic disease in subaortic lymph node. Ann Thorac Surg 43:155, 1987.
Pearson FG: Mediastinoscopy: A method of biopsy in the superior mediastinum. J Thorac Cardiovasc Surg 49:11–21, 1965.
Pilotti S, Rilke F, Gribaudi D et al: Sputum cytology for the diagnosis of carcinoma of the lung. Acta Cytol 26:649, 1982.
Posner JB: Paraneoplastic syndromes. Curr Opin Neurol 10:471, 1997.
Prauer HW, Weber WA, Romer W et al: Controlled prospective study of positron emission tomography using the glucose analogue ^{18}F-fluorodeoxyglucose in the evaluation of pulmonary nodules. Br J Surg 85:1506, 1998.
Quinn DL, Ostrow LB, Porter DK et al: Staging of non-small cell bronchogenic carcinoma: Relationship of the clinical evaluation to organ scans. Chest 89:270, 1986.
Richardson RI, Greco FA, Oldham RK et al: Tumor products and potential markers in small cell lung cancer. Semin Oncol 5:253, 1978.
Risse EKJ, Vooijs GP, van't Hof MA: Diagnostic significance of "severe dysplasia" in sputum cytology. Acta Cytol 32:629, 1988.
Robinson LA, Preksto D, Muro-Cacho C et al: Intraoperative gamma probe-directed biopsy of asymptomatic suspected bone metastases. Ann Thorac Surg 65:1426, 1998.
Rosenthal DI: Radiologic diagnosis of bone metastases. Cancer 80(Suppl):1595, 1997.
Salerno CT, Neihans GA, Kratske RA, Maddaus MA: Detection of occult micrometastases in non-small cell lung carcinoma by reverse transcriptase polymerase chain reaction. Chest 113:1526, 1998.
Salvatierra A, Baamonde C, Llamas JM et al: Extrathoracic staging of bronchogenic carcinoma. Chest 97:5, 1990.
Schenk DA, Bryan CL, Bower JH et al: Transbronchial needle aspiration in the diagnosis of bronchogenic carcinoma. Chest 92:83, 1987.
Schiepatti E: Mediastinal lymph node puncture through the tracheal carina. Surg Gynecol Obstet 110:243, 1958.
Schwartz LH, Panicek DM, Koutcher JA et al: Adrenal masses in patients with malignancy: Prospective comparison of echo-planar, fast spin-echo, and chemical shift MR imaging. Radiology 197:421, 1995.
Shepard FA, Laskey J, Evans WK et al: Cushing's syndrome associated with ectopic corticotropin production and small cell lung cancer. J Clin Oncol 10:21, 1992.
Shure D, Fedullo F: The role of transcarinal needle aspiration in the staging of bronchogenic carcinoma. Chest 86:5819, 1984.

Shure D, Fedullo F: Transbronchial needle aspiration in the diagnosis of submucosal and peribronchial bronchogenic carcinoma. Chest 88:49, 1985.

Sider L, Horejs D: Frequency of extrathoracic metastases from bronchogenic carcinoma in patients with normal-sized hilar and mediastinal lymph nodes on CT. AJR Am J Roentgenol 151:893, 1988.

Silvestri GA, Littenberg B, Colice GL: The clinical evaluation for detecting metastatic lung cancer. Am J Respir Crit Care Med 152:225, 1995.

Sridhar KS, Lobo CF, Altman RD: Digital clubbing and lung cancer. Chest 114:1535, 1998.

Stiglbauer R, Schurawitzki H, Klepetko W et al: Contrast-enhanced MRI for the staging of bronchogenic carcinoma: Comparison with CT and histopathologic staging: Preliminary results. Clin Radiol 44:293, 1991.

Stringfield JT, Markowitz DJ, Bentz RR et al: The effect of tumor size and location on diagnosis by fiberoptic bronchoscopy. Chest 72:474, 1977.

Szolar DH, Kammerhuber F: Quantitative CT evaluation of adrenal gland masses: A step forward in the differentiation between adenomas and non-adenomas. Radiology 202:517, 1997.

Tockman MS, Gupta PK, Myers JD et al: Sensitive and specific monoclonal antibody recognition of human lung cancer antigen on preserved sputum cells. J Clin Oncol 6:1685, 1988.

Truong L, Underwood R, Greenberg S et al: Diagnosis and typing of lung carcinomas by cytopathologic methods. Acta Cytol 29:379, 1985.

Valk PE, Pounds TR, Hopkins DM et al: Staging non-small cell lung cancer by whole-body positron emission tomographic imaging. Ann Thorac Surg 60:1573, 1995.

Vallieres E, Waters PF: Incidence of mediastinal node involvement in clinical T1 bronchogenic carcinomas. Can J Surg 30:341, 1987.

Vansteenkiste JF, Stroobants SG, De Leyn PR et al: Lymph node staging in non-small-cell lung cancer with FDG-PET scan: A prospective study on 690 lymph node stations from 68 patients. J Clin Oncol 16:2142, 1998.

Wang JP, Terri TB: Transbronchial needle aspiration in the diagnosis or staging of bronchogenic carcinoma. Am Rev Respir Dis 127:344, 1983.

Watanabe Y, Shimizu J, Oda M et al: Proposals regarding some deficiencies in the new international staging system for non-small cell lung cancer. Jpn J Clin Oncol 21:160, 1991.

Weder W, Schmid RA, Bruchhaus H et al: Detection of extrathoracic metastases by positron emission tomography in lung cancer. Ann Thorac Surg 66:886, 1998.

Westcott JL: Direct percutaneous needle aspiration of localized pulmonary lesions: Results in 422 patients. Radiology 137:31, 1980.

CHAPTER **32**

Non–Small Cell Lung Cancer

SURGICAL MANAGEMENT

Robert J. Ginsberg
Nael Martini

Surgical resection for lung cancer is still regarded as the most effective method of controlling the primary tumor, provided it is resectable for cure and the risks of the procedure are low. Radiation therapy, when used alone or with chemotherapy, has been effective in palliation and has resulted in occasional cure but has not achieved the success rate of surgery. At present, except for treatment of small cell lung cancer, chemotherapy as a single modality is reserved for palliation of advanced tumors because almost no cures have been reported unless it is combined with surgery or irradiation.

The incidence of lung cancer is still at epidemic proportions. The American Cancer Society (2001) projected a lung cancer incidence of 169,500 new cases for the year 2000, with a male-to-female ratio of 1.2:1 (1). Unfortunately, 86% of these cases were expected to die ultimately of their disease, despite the fact that approximately 35% of such patients are surgical "candidates."

HISTORICAL NOTE

Surgery for lung cancer was first discussed in the literature before the turn of the last century. Sauerbruch (1926) reported that Heidenhan had performed a partial resection for lung cancer using cautery, with the patient surviving 2 months. Pean (1895) reported success in the removal of lung cancer by partial excision, including the chest wall; the actual operation was performed 30 years previously. In 1912, Hugh Morriston Davies (1913–1914) completed the first dissection lobectomy for lung cancer, with the patient unfortunately dying 8 days later from empyema.

The modern era of surgical resection for lung cancer required the development of underwater drainage. The first one-stage lobectomy was reported by Brunn (1929), followed by Allan and Smith (1932) who used a two-stage resection in 1930. The production of adhesions by pleural abrasion was followed by lobectomy and mass ligature. Following Graham's (Graham and Singer, 1933) historic pneumonectomy in 1932, surgical resection quickly became prevalent, with pneumonectomy being the procedure of choice (Churchill, 1933). The technique of segmentectomy was described by Churchill and Belsey (1939). Radical pneumonectomy with en bloc removal of mediastinal lymph nodes was first proposed by Alison in 1946. Subsequent to this, more refined techniques were developed, including sleeve resection by Price-Thomas (1956) in 1947, carinal resection by Mathey and associates (1966) and Thompson (1966), and en bloc resection of the chest wall by Coleman (1947) and for a superior sulcus tumor in 1956 (Chardak and MacCallun, 1956); this latter procedure was popularized in 1961 by Shaw and colleagues (Shaw et al, 1961). Although lesser resections had been performed by a variety of authors as compromise procedures in patients with poor pulmonary function, Jensik and colleagues (1973) reported the first series of segmental resections as intentional curative procedures.

HISTORICAL READINGS

Alison PR: Intrapericardial approach to the lung root in the treatment of bronchial carcinoma by dissection pneumonectomy. J Thorac Surg 15:991, 1946.
Allan CI, Smith FJ: Primary carcinoma of the lung with report of case treated by operation. Surg Gynecol Obstet 55:151, 1932.
Brunn HB: Surgical principles underlying one-stage lobectomy. Arch Surg 18:490, 1929.
Chardak WM, MacCallun JD: Pancoast tumor (5 yr survival without recurrence or metastases following radical resection and postoperative irradiation). J Thorac Surg 31:535, 1956.
Churchill E, Belsey HR: Segmental pneumonectomy in bronchiectasis. Ann Surg 109:481, 1939.
Churchill ED: The surgical treatment of carcinoma of the lung. J Thorac Surg 2:254, 1933.
Coleman FP: Primary carcinoma of the lung with invasion of ribs: Pneumonectomy and simultaneous block resection of chest wall. Ann Surg 126:156, 1947.
Davies HM: Recent advances in the surgery of the lung and pleura. Br J Surg 1:228, 1913.
Graham EA, Singer JJ: Successful removal of the entire lung for carcinoma of the bronchus. JAMA 101:1371, 1933.
Jensik RJ, Faber LP, Milloy FJ, Monson DO: Segmental resection for lung cancer. A fifteen year experience. J Thorac Cardiovasc Surg 66:563, 1973.
Mathey J, Binet JP, Galey JJ et al: Tracheal and tracheobronchial resections: Technique and results in 20 cases. J Thorac Cardiovasc Surg 51:1, 1966.
Pean J: Chirurgie des poumons. Discussion Ranc Chir Proc Verh Paris 9:72, 1895.
Price-Thomas C: Conservative resection of the bronchial tree. J R Coll Surg Edinb 1:169, 1956.
Sauerbruch F: Die Operation Entfernung von Lungengesch-wulste. Zentralbl Chir 53:852, 1926.
Shaw RR, Paulson DL, Kee JL Jr: Treatment of the superior sulcus tumor by irradiation followed by resection. Ann Surg 154:29, 1961.
Thompson DT: Tracheal resection with left lung anastomosis following right pneumonectomy. Thorax 21:560, 1966.

PREOPERATIVE ASSESSMENT

It is now standard practice to carefully stage all cancers of the lung at the time of their initial diagnosis (see preceding section). Since 1986, the international tumor-node-metastasis (TNM) staging system has been used by most oncologists (AJCC, 1997; UICC, 1997). Briefly stated, tumors confined to the lung without any metastases, regional or distant, are classified as stage I, and tumors associated with only hilar or peribronchial lymph node involvement (N1), or extension to chest wall, mediastinum, or diaphragm, as stage II. Locally advanced tumors with mediastinal or cervical lymph node metastases or invasion of adjacent "unresectable" structures are classified as stage III tumors, and tumors presenting with distant metastases are classified as stage IV tumors. For a complete discussion of staging, see previous chapter.

The 5-year survival rate following complete resection (R0) of a lung cancer is stage dependent (Table 32–1). Incomplete resection (R1,R2) rarely, if ever, cures the patient. Most recent series show that 60% to 70% of patients with T1N0 resected lung cancer survive for 5 years, and 80% never have recurrences (almost 20% of patients dying within 5 years of resection die of unrelated causes without recurring tumor) (Martini et al, 1995; Mountain, 1987; Rami Porta, 2000; Williams et al, 1981). At the other extreme, unless they are highly selected, only a handful (less than 10%) of patients resected with stage IIIB disease are ever cured.

SURGICAL PRINCIPLES AND MANAGEMENT

It is no longer acceptable for surgically curable lung cancer to be treated by a slapdash resection without regard to oncologic principles. The following principles of oncologic surgery must be employed:

1. Whenever possible, the tumor and all intrapulmonary lymphatic drainage should be removed completely, most frequently by lobectomy or pneumonectomy.
2. Care must be taken not to transgress the tumor during the resection to avoid tumor spillage.
3. En bloc resection of closely adjacent or invaded structures is preferable to discontinuous resection.
4. Resection margins should be assessed by frozen-section analysis (where available), including bronchial, vascular, and any other margins with close proximity to the tumor. Re-excision is preferred whenever possible if positive resection margins are encountered.
5. All accessible mediastinal lymph node stations should be removed or sampled for pathologic evaluation (we prefer mediastinal lymph node dissection); these should be identified and properly labeled by the surgeon.

TABLE 32–1 ■ **5-Year Survival Rates by Stage Following Complete Resection for Lung Cancer at Memorial Sloan-Kettering Cancer Center**

Stage	*Survival (%)*
Stage I (n = 539)	76
T1N0	84
T2N0	68
Stage II (n = 214)	47
Stage IIIA	
T3N0 (chest wall)	56
T3N0 (carina)	36
T3N0 (mediastinum)	29
N2 (surgery) (n = 151)	30
N2 (chemotherapy + surgery) (n = 89)	26

Martini N, Bains MS, Burt ME et al: Incidence of local recurrence and second primary tumors in resected stage I lung cancer. J Thorac Cardiovasc Surg 109:120, 1995.

Surgical resection is the therapy of choice for early-stage non–small cell lung cancer and is generally offered to all patients with stage I and II disease, specific groups of patients with stage III disease, and those with solitary metastases and completely resectable primary disease.

Occult Lung Cancer

An occult lung cancer is defined as that tumor not evident on radiologic imaging but discovered by sputum cytology or incidentally at bronchoscopy.

Localization

Few patients (less than 1% of the lung cancer population) have their lung cancer diagnosed by sputum cytology before it becomes apparent radiographically. These include individuals who participate in early lung cancer detection programs and patients who present to institutions with hemoptysis in the absence of any abnormal findings on routine chest radiographs. Prior to consideration of therapy, occult carcinomas presenting in this fashion require a careful investigation for localization of the site of the cancer. The fact that the patient has a normal chest radiograph and a positive sputum on cytologic examination does not necessarily mean that the patient has lung carcinoma, let alone an early lung carcinoma. In most instances, the cytologic examination indicates a squamous cell cancer. A complete aerodigestive examination is essential for ruling out carcinoma in other sites. It has been our experience that one of three patients who have positive sputum cytologic results and negative chest radiographs has a carcinoma in the head and neck region (Martini and Melamed, 1980). Following a detailed examination of the head and neck, a careful diagnostic bronchoscopy is performed initially under local anesthesia to examine the pharynx, larynx, and proximal airway. With the advent of the flexible bronchoscope, it has become possible to extend the inspection of the tracheobronchial tree from the mainstem and lobar bronchi to segmental and subsegmental bronchi. By this method alone, the clinician can usually identify the specific site of a radiographically occult lung cancer. If the lesion is located centrally in a main or lobar bronchus, it is readily visualized, and a biopsy can be easily obtained. However, in instances in which the tracheobronchial tree appears normal at bronchoscopy, a meticulous sampling of each segmental bronchus by endoscopic brushings and cytologic analysis becomes necessary, unless a tumor has been identified in the head and neck region. Careful attention to detail to avoid cross-contamination has resulted in localization of even these peripheral tumors in nearly all instances. Only repeated positive brushings from an isolated segment are acceptable for such localization.

Recently, more sophisticated techniques of in vivo fluorescent staining of mucosal malignancy with hematoporphyrin derivatives or, more recently, laser-induced fluorescence excitation (LIFE) have enhanced the sensitivity and specificity of the bronchoscopic localization (Edell and Cortese, 1989; Hayata et al, 1984; Lam et al, 1993; Weigel et al, 1999). These techniques are helpful in identifying and localizing occult malignancy that is not apparent to the naked eye during bronchoscopy. The clinician must always be wary of "field cancerization" with multiple in situ aerodigestive tumors.

Therapy

Following localization, the therapy of choice for a radiographically occult carcinoma of the lung remains surgical extirpation of the primary tumor by segmentectomy, lobectomy, or pneumonectomy, with or without a sleeve resection as necessary. Because most occult lung cancers are relatively central in position, lesser resections usually are not possible. Photodynamic therapy, using transbronchoscopic laser–induced photoexcitation of hematoporphyrin derivative, has been shown by Hayata and coworkers (1984) and Cortese and associates (1997) to be effective in eradicating occult in situ endobronchial lung cancer, and the short-term follow-up has been encouraging with only about 20% of highly selected patients recurring (Kato et al, 1996). However, once invasive carcinoma has been identified, resection is usually necessary. Endobronchial brachytherapy or three-dimensional (3D) conformal radiotherapy may also offer curative treatment, although long-term results with these modalities have not been reported.

The 5-year survival of patients treated surgically for a radiographically occult carcinoma approaches 100%. Recurrences are rare, but new lung primaries are frequently observed in this group of patients. As many as 45% of these patients develop new carcinomas, the majority of which are new endobronchial squamous cell cancers (Martini and Melamed, 1980). It becomes essential, therefore, that continued surveillance of these patients be carried out at frequent intervals. The LIFE bronchoscope technique is particularly suited for this type of surveillance (Weigel et al, 1999). For further information, see subchapters: Brachytherapy and Intraoperative Radiotherapy, and Photodynamic Therapy for Endobronchial Lesions.

A new form of "chest radiograph–occult" lung cancer is being identified. These are lesions picked up on routine computed tomography (CT) scanning or "low-dose" scanning used for screening (Henschke et al, 1999). Many of these tumors are only a few millimeters in diameter and are difficult to diagnose as carcinoma. CT-guided needle aspiration biopsy, growth over a period of months, positron emission tomography (PET) scanning, or wedge resection may be required for diagnosis. Whether or not these lesions, often 5 to 10 mm in diameter, can be excised by less than a lobectomy or treated primarily by radiotherapy is a moot point. Often at surgery, these lesions are difficult to localize within a lobe and lobectomy is required to ensure their removal. Others, found in a very peripheral site, may be suitable for lesser resection for cure, although the question has not been completely addressed scientifically as yet.

Since the adverse reports on lesser resection for stage I lung cancer appeared in the literature (Ginsberg, 1995; Warren and Faber, 1994), many authors, especially those from Japan, have addressed the role of limited resection in very early peripheral disease. It has been found that even in tumors less than 1 cm in diameter, lymphatic permeation and lymph node metastases within the lung can occur. A lesser resection, especially wedge resection, necessarily ignores this lymphatic permeation. If a wedge resection is required because of compromised pulmonary function, it appears that postoperative radiotherapy decreases the local-regional recurrence rate (Errett, 1985; Miller, 1987). The role of postoperative radiotherapy using video-assisted thoracoscopic surgery (VATS) limited resection has been studied by the CALGB Cooperative Group in North America. A recent report suggests that this VATS approach is less than satisfactory (Shennib et al, in press). In Japan, where spiral CT screening has been prevalent for almost 20 years, many centers have employed wedge resection and segmentectomy for these very early subcentimeter lesions. Many of these lesions that are detected early are pure bronchoalveolar carcinomas and are identified by their ground-glass appearance on CT scanning. In these highly selected individuals, especially those with ground-glass appearance indicating noninvasive pure bronchoalveolar carcinoma, limited resections, both wedge and segmentectomy, have yielded up to a 90% 5-year tumor-free survival (Kodama et al, 1997; Konaka et al, 1998; Takizawa et al, 1999; Tsubota et al, 1998).

STAGE I DISEASE (T1N0, T2N0)

This is the most common form of early lung cancer seen by most physicians. Many patients in this stage are detected on routine chest radiographs or CT scans of the chest and upper abdomen performed for unrelated medical conditions. Most are discrete peripheral tumors, presenting as a coin lesion. CT scans are routinely done on these patients to assess the mediastinum, the liver, and the adrenal glands. Full-organ scanning beyond the CT scan has not been shown to be cost effective. PET scanning as a method of staging is still under investigation. Routine mediastinoscopy remains controversial if the CT scan is "negative." (See Chapter 31 subchapter on diagnosis and staging of lung cancer.) If no mediastinal involvement is suspected and the patient is fit, surgical therapy is the recommended treatment of choice. At the time of thoracotomy, systematic lymph node dissection or sampling is carried out to ensure that no hilar or mediastinal nodal metastasis is present.

Lesser resections such as wedge excision or segmentectomy have been advocated by some for small peripheral tumors. Jensik (1987) and Kulka and Forai (1985) reported on a large series of patients with stage I carcinoma treated in this conservative fashion. More recently, the Lung Cancer Study Group (LCSG) completed a randomized clinical trial of lobectomy versus a lesser resection by wedge or segmentectomy in stage I carcinomas presenting as small peripheral tumors (Ginsberg, 1995). This study suggests a 3-fold increased incidence of local recurrence in patients treated by lesser resections than lobectomy. This was confirmed by an updated analysis of the Rush-Presbyterian segmental resection data by Warren and Faber (1994). In the LCSG analysis, overall survival was decreased in the limited resection group. Although the apparent advantage of a lesser resection is the conservation of lung tissue, this was not evident in the long-term pulmonary function assessment. An important disadvantage is the 10% to 15% risk of local recurrence in the local-regional area. We use this form of therapy only for patients with a limited lung reserve (McCormack and Martini, 1980). In more central nodules, therapy necessarily requires lobectomy or pneumonectomy. A recent Japanese study has demonstrated virtually no loss of pulmonary function 1 year following lobectomy and no significant differences in function following segmentectomy (Takizawa et al, 1999). The role of ipsilateral mediastinal lymph node dissection (vs lymph node sampling) in this early stage of disease remains to be decided. However, there is no doubt that the formal type of complete dissection provides the most accurate postsurgical staging, unless preoperative mediastinoscopy is combined with complete intraoperative lymph node sampling. A randomized comparative trial of these two modalities (Izibicki et al, 1994) demonstrated no survival nor local recurrence advantage to either therapeutic arm in stages I and II disease if mediastinoscopy was used in conjunction with intraoperative sampling.

This question is now being addressed in a very large North American trial, which may provide the answer as to whether or not mediastinal lymph node dissection in stage I and nonhilar stage II lung cancer is of added value (vs sampling). Based on experiences with lymph node mapping for breast cancer and melanoma, investigators are now assessing the value of intraoperative radioisotope and blue dye identification of sentinel lymph nodes. Whether this type of approach will have value in deciding whether or not a lymph node dissection is required awaits significant further study (Liptay, 2000; Sugi et al, 2000; Tiffet et al, 2000).

For tumors protruding from a lobar orifice into the main bronchus, a sleeve lobectomy should be considered whenever possible. This procedure conserves the pulmonary parenchyma and offers lower morbidity and mortality rates than are associated with a pneumonectomy, with comparable curability when a complete resection is done (Gaissert et al, 1984).

Survival

Patients with small tumors that are 3 cm or less in diameter and are confined to the lung parenchyma without evidence of regional lymphatic metastases or extension to chest wall, diaphragm, or pleura have a 5-year disease-free survival rate of 60% to 80% when treated by primary surgical resection (Martini et al, 1995). Tumors greater than 3 cm in diameter that are still confined to lung without metastasis to nodes or distant sites (stage IB) also have a favorable prognosis with a 5-year disease-free survival rate of 68%. The overall 5-year survival rate in stage I carcinoma of the lung, whether T1 or T2 in size, that is surgically treated in our institution is currently 75% (Fig. 32–1; see Table 32–1). This has been confirmed by other investigators as well (Rami-Porta, 2000; Mountain, 1988; Naruke et al, 1988a) (Table 32–2). No adjuvant treatment is recommended for patients with stage I disease following resection, although this continues to be investigated in clinical trials. Patterns of recurrence at this stage of disease suggest that, of the 20% to 30% of patients who ultimately do have recurrences, the majority have relapses at distant sites, with more than 20% of all recurrences being solitary brain metastases. Close follow-up for the detection of solitary recurrences or second primaries is advised.

Stage II Disease

T1–2N1

Tumors confined to the lung or bronchus with involvement of hilar or bronchopulmonary lymph nodes as the sole site of tumor spread (T1–2N1 disease) account for less than 5% of the lung cancer population and less than 10% of all resected lung cancers. We recently reviewed our experience at Memorial Sloan-Kettering Cancer Center on the surgical treatment of stage II lung cancer (Martini et al, 1992). From 1973 to 1989, 214 patients had undergone complete resection of their stage II lung cancer with a mediastinal lymph node dissection. Of these, 35 patients had T1N1 lesions and 179, T2N1 tumors. Eighty-three percent of those patients with T1 lesions had adenocarcinomas; however, this difference in histologic findings was not apparent in T2 lesions in which adenocarcinomas and squamous cancers were of equal frequency.

Lobectomy is the procedure of choice in most patients. In our series, 68% of patients underwent lobectomy; 31%, pneumonectomy; and only 1%, wedge resection or segmentectomy. A lobectomy was sufficient to encompass all disease in 34 of the 35 T1N1 lesions. Of interest was the fact that one half of the patients had a single N1 node involved, and 85% of the patients had nodal involvement at a single N1 level. At this stage of disease, we believe it is imperative that a complete lymph node dissection be performed because occult mediastinal metastases occur with increasing frequency. This is espe-

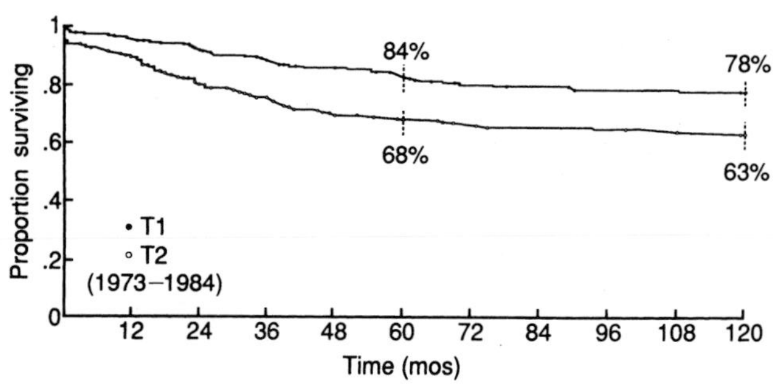

FIGURE 32–1 ■ Survival at MSKCC following complete resection in stage I non-small cell lung cancer (T1N0M0–T2N0M0).

TABLE 32–2 ■ **The 5-Year Survival Rates in the Three Largest Series Reporting Stage-by-Stage Survival According to the 1997 Stage Classification***

	Naruke		*Mountain*		*Rami-Porta*	
	# Pts	*% 5-Yr Survival*	*# Pts*	*% 5-Yr Survival*	*# Pts*	*% 5-Yr Survival*
STAGE I						
T1N0 (IA)	245	75	511	67	235	58
T2N0 (IB)	291	57	549	57	817	50
STAGE II						
T1N1 (IIA)	66	52	76	55	31	66
T2N1 (IIB)	153	38	288	39	290	42
T3N0 (IIB)	106	33	87	38		
STAGE IIIA						
T3N1 (IIIA)	85	139	55	38	389	25
T1–3N2 (IIIA)	368	15	344	23		
T1–3N3 (IIIB)	55	0	572	3	138	28
T4 any N (IIIB)	104	8	458	6		
STAGE IV						
TN any M1	293	7	1427	1	27	25

*In the Naruke and Mountain series, the stage IV survival includes unresected patients as well, whereas the Rami-Porta series includes only resected patients. Similarly, in the stage IIIB patients, the Mountain series includes all patients whether resected or not.

Mountain CF: Revisions in the International System for Staging Lung Cancer 111:1710, 1997.

Rami-Porta, for the Bronchogenic Carcinoma Cooperative Group of the Spanish Society of Pneumonology and Thoracic Surgery. Lung Cancer 29 (suppl 1):133, 2000.

Naruke T, Goya T, Tsuchiya R, Suemasu K: Prognosis and survival in resected lung cancer based on the new international staging system. J Thorac Cardiovasc Surg 96:440, 1988a.

cially true if the nodal involvement is hilar. A recent report by Keller and associates (2000b) appears to indicate a survival advantage to this approach (vs sampling).

The role of sleeve lobectomy and vascular sleeve resection for N1 disease has been addressed recently. It appears that if a complete resection can be performed by sleeve lobectomy with or without a vascular sleeve resection, the results of surgical treatment appear identical to those seen following pneumonectomy (Icard et al, 1999; Lausberg et al, 2000). Therefore, in patients for whom a sleeve resection with ipsilateral mediastinal lymphadenectomy will encompass all involved disease, it should be considered so that lung function may be preserved.

The overall survival rate following resection, calculated by the Kaplan-Meier method and considering all deaths, was 39% at 5 years at our institution. There was no difference in survival between T1 and T2 lesions. However, there was a distinct difference in survival between tumors that were 3 cm or smaller in size and those that were 5 cm or greater. There was a trend in the survival rate by histologic type that favored epidermoid carcinoma over adenocarcinoma with a *P* value of .07. The location of the primary tumor, the location of the N1 nodes, the extent of the surgical resection, and the presence or absence of visceral pleural involvement had no appreciable impact on survival rate. However, in our series, the number of lymph nodes involved was significant. The survival rate following resection in patients with involvement of a single lymph node was 45% compared with 31% in patients with multiple lymph node involvement (Fig. 32–2).

The patterns of recurrence differed by histologic type. As is seen in many other series, local or regional recurrences were more numerous in patients with squamous cancer, and distant metastases occurred more frequently in patients with adenocarcinoma. The incidence of local or regional recurrence was reduced by the administration of postoperative radiation therapy. However, the addition of postoperative radiation therapy in this group of patients had no impact on survival; this confirms the Lung

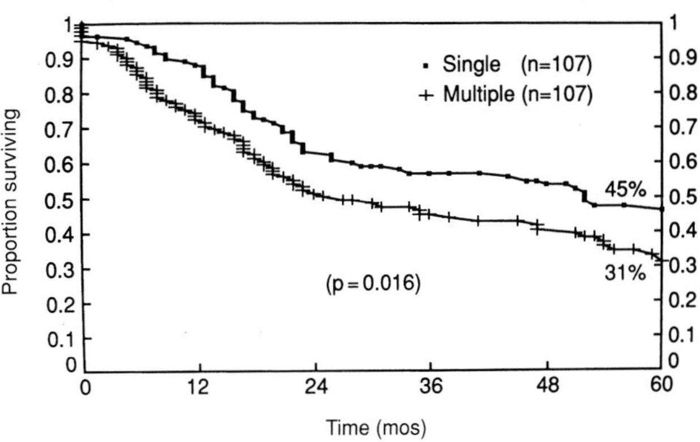

FIGURE 32–2 ■ Survival by number of N1 nodes involved following complete resection in stage II non-small cell lung cancer (Martini et al, 1995).

Cancer Study Group (1986) report and more recent analyses of postoperative radiotherapy (PORT analysis, 1998). Recurrence rates were high despite R0 resections. Prognostic factors were limited to the number of involved nodes and the size of the lesion.

At this stage of disease, most patients developed distant metastases, suggesting the need for an effective systemic treatment, but few studies have demonstrated any benefit of systemic treatment for this group of patients. The Lung Cancer Study Group, in a trial comparing postoperative irradiation with chemoradiation, reported some advantages in the time to recurrence using combined adjuvant radiation and chemotherapy in adenocarcinoma (Holmes et al, 1986). However, this latter study did not compare or assess adjuvant treatment with chemotherapy alone nor the outcome with no adjuvant treatment. A recent Eastern Cooperative Oncology Group (ECOG) study, replicating the LCSG trial, has also failed to show an advantage of postoperative chemoradiation over radiation alone (Keller et al, 2000a). Postoperative adjuvant trials of chemotherapy, immunotherapy, or combinations of the two have had little effect on the survival rate in randomized studies (Holmes et al, 1986; Lung Cancer Study Group, 1986). Induction (neoadjuvant and preoperative) chemotherapy has recently been tested in this subset of patients (Pisters et al, 2000). Although confirmation and larger follow-up are needed, a French phase III trial (Depierre et al, 1999) suggests a survival advantage in clinical stage II patients treated with induction therapy.

The role of adjuvant or neoadjuvant therapies in the treatment of patients with N1 disease has yet to be defined, despite 30 years of intensive study. Currently, there are ongoing trials in North America and Europe that are addressing this question. At present, except for inclusion in clinical trials, at this stage of disease adjuvant therapies cannot be recommended following complete resection, even though in practice, many patients are offered such therapy. Neoadjuvant approaches remain investigational.

T3N0 Disease

Tumors invading adjacent structures that can be completely resected by simple en bloc resection techniques are classified as T3. Because of their favorable survival following surgical resection, they have been recategorized as stage IIB disease, as long as no lymph node involvement is present. Once this occurs, the overall survival following resection of T3 tumors is lessened such that T3N1–2 tumors remain in the stage IIIA category.

Tumors Invading Chest Wall. Cancers of the lung that invade the chest wall are usually peripheral in position. Hilar or mediastinal lymph node metastases are less likely to occur in this group of patients. These tumors extend to invade the parietal pleura, and some involve the muscles and ribs of the chest wall. Even with chest wall invasion, significant numbers of these patients are amenable to treatment by resection. Factors that appear to influence survival in this group of patients include (1) completeness of resection of the tumor, (2) the extent of invasion of the chest wall, and (3) the presence or absence of regional lymph node metastases. We recently reviewed 334 patients with carcinoma of the lung invading the chest wall who were treated surgically (Downey et al, 1999) (Table 32–3). Of these, 175 had a complete resection with an overall 5-year survival rate of 50% in those T3N0 patients completely resected. A recent Mayo Clinic report suggests a 35% 4-year survival in this stage of disease (Gould et al, 1999). In those in whom resection was incomplete (macroscopic or microscopic disease) or not possible, the 5-year survival in both series was virtually zero. Postoperative radiation therapy in this group of patients does not have an impact on their ultimate survival. This was confirmed by the Mayo experience (Gould et al, 1999; Piehler et al, 1982) and that of others.

Unlike the findings in other series, in our experience the extent of chest wall involvement by the tumor did not appear to affect survival. In patients in whom the tumor extended to the parietal pleura but did not penetrate beyond the parietal pleura into the soft tissues of the chest wall and the ribs, the 5-year survival rate following complete resection was not statistically better than in patients with deeper involvement of the chest wall.

Our series suggested that a significant number of patients whose tumors are confined to involvement of the parietal pleura can be treated by extrapleural mobilization of the tumor without necessarily resecting en bloc the adjoining segments of ribs, as long as the resection margins are negative. On the other hand, Pairolero and Arnold (1985) stressed the need for a routine chest wall resection whenever adherence of a peripheral tumor to the chest was identified at thoracotomy. However, many of their patients did not demonstrate any involvement beyond the parietal pleura. Whether or not en bloc resection of chest wall (versus parietal pleura only) is required in every instance remains a contentious issue.

We favor chest wall reconstruction with a Marlex mesh/methyl methacrylate sandwich technique whenever there is anticipated chest wall instability, but we rarely find this necessary with the resection of fewer than three contiguous rib segments. For these smaller defects, a taut Marlex mesh patch closure ensures acceptable cosmetic results and chest wall stability (McCormack et al, 1981, 1987). Others prefer a Gore-Tex patch for larger defects (Pairolero and Arnold, 1985). Very small defects of one to two rib segments may require no reconstruction, especially if they are located posteriorly beneath large muscles or scapula.

Superior Sulcus Tumors. Superior sulcus tumors (Pancoast tumors) represent a subset of carcinomas of the lung invading the chest wall. By reason of their location in the pleural apex, they invade adjoining structures early. Patients are generally symptomatic. Early invasion of the lower brachial plexus, especially the T1 nerve root, is common. Shoulder and arm pain radiating to the inner aspect of the upper arm (T1) and the ulnar distribution in the fourth and fifth fingers of the hand (C8) is a common presenting symptom. Extension to the stellate ganglion with consequent Horner's syndrome is seen in at least one third of patients. Extension to the ribs or vertebrae is common.

TABLE 32–3 ■ **The Recent Series Reporting Survivals for Tumors Involving the Chest Wall Following Surgical Resection**

Author	No. Patients	5-Yr Survival	R0	R1–2	Mortality
Piehler (1982)	55	33%	NS	NS	NS
Allen (1991)	52	26%	NS	NS	NS
Gould (1999)		35%	NS	NS	NS
Downey (1999)	334	NS	32%	4%	6% (R0)

NS, not stated.

Most superior sulcus tumors are initially diagnosed histologically or cytologically by transcutaneous needle biopsy performed under fluoroscopic or CT guidance. Diagnostic bronchoscopy is less helpful in establishing a tissue diagnosis in this group of patients because of the peripheral position of the lesion, although transbronchoscopic biopsy using image intensification has been successful. The majority of tumors are squamous carcinomas or adenocarcinomas, but 3% to 5% are small cell carcinomas with vastly different therapeutic implications, hence the importance of a tissue diagnosis before treatment.

Shaw and associates (1961) and Paulson (1982, 1985) first advocated the combined use of preoperative radiation and resection and demonstrated a 31% 5-year survival rate. They also noted that, in a small percentage of these patients, mediastinal lymph node metastases (N2) may coexist, and few patients in this group survive longer than 1 year. Mediastinoscopy is thus recommended in the preoperative evaluation of these patients to rule out the presence of N2 disease.

The current standard therapy for this group of patients continues to be preoperative radiation followed by resection. Therapy begins with a preoperative course of external radiation therapy to a dose of 3000 to 4000 cGy to the tumor (Hilaris et al, 1987; Paulson, 1985). This is usually given in 200-cGy fractions per day for a period of 3 to 4 weeks. The radiation portal traditionally included the primary tumor, the adjacent mediastinum, and the ipsilateral supraclavicular area. Following a rest period of 1 month, these patients are assessed for surgical treatment. If no distant disease is evident, these patients are then offered surgical exploration for removal of the residual tumor. The presence of Horner's syndrome is not an absolute contraindication for this combined therapy, but the results are less satisfactory. The standard resection described by Paulson encompasses en bloc removal of the affected lobe and chest wall, including the entire first rib and the posterior segments of ribs two, three, and often four; the transverse processes of the contiguous thoracic vertebrae; the nerve roots C8 and T1 to T3; the lower trunk of the brachial plexus; and the dorsal sympathetic chain with mediastinal node dissection. Paulson's (1982, 1985) latest series suggest that nearly 90% of the patients explored have undergone complete resection. The 5-year survival rate results obtained by us following complete resection were confirmed by those of other series (Paulson, 1985 and others) (Table 32–4). The determinants of unresectability have generally included involvement of the subclavian artery or the vertebral body with or without cord compression and widespread invasion of the major divisions of the brachial plexus (T4). As is discussed later in the subchapter (see later section, Stage IIIB Disease [T4 or N3]), aggressive surgeons have successfully resected subclavian vessels, vertebral bodies, and so forth with some suggestion of long-term benefit following such extended operations. Magnetic resonance imaging is extremely valuable for assessing this involvement. In many of our patients in whom the tumor is incompletely resected or is found unresectable, interstitial implantation of radioisotopes (brachytherapy) was used to complete the radiation therapy of the tumor. However, in analyzing our results of intraoperative brachytherapy, we found no distinct advantage over postoperative irradiation in dealing with R1 or R2 resections (Ginsberg et al, 1994); less than 10% survived for 5 years, no matter which adjuvant therapy was used.

We initially reviewed our results in 1994 (Ginsberg et al) and added a further 100 patients in a report recently published (Rusch et al, 2000). In both series, our 5-year survival following complete surgical resection was 41%, and 5-year survival following an R1 or R2 resection was only 9%. In the latter series, the adverse effects of stage and nodal status were quite evident (Figs. 32–3, 32–4, and 32–5).

Whether preoperative treatment enhances surgical therapy has been questioned by some. Many surgeons are now offering primary surgery for superior sulcus tumors preoperatively identified as T3N0. A recent North American Intergroup trial has assessed the role of preoperative chemoradiation prior to resection for superior sulcus

TABLE 32–4 ■ **Survival Following Resection for Superior Sulcus Tumors According to the Largest Series Reported**

Author	No. Patients	% 5-yr Survival Overall	R0	R1–2	% Mortality
Paulson (1985)	78	35%	NS	NS	3
Satori (1992)	42	25%	NS	NS	2.3
Dartevelle (1999)	70	34%	NS	NS	0
Ginsberg (1994)	124	26%	41%	9%	4
Maggi (1994)	60	17%	24%	0%	5
Rusch (2000)	225	NS	41%	9%	NS
Hogan (1999)	34	33%	NS	NS	0

NS, not stated.

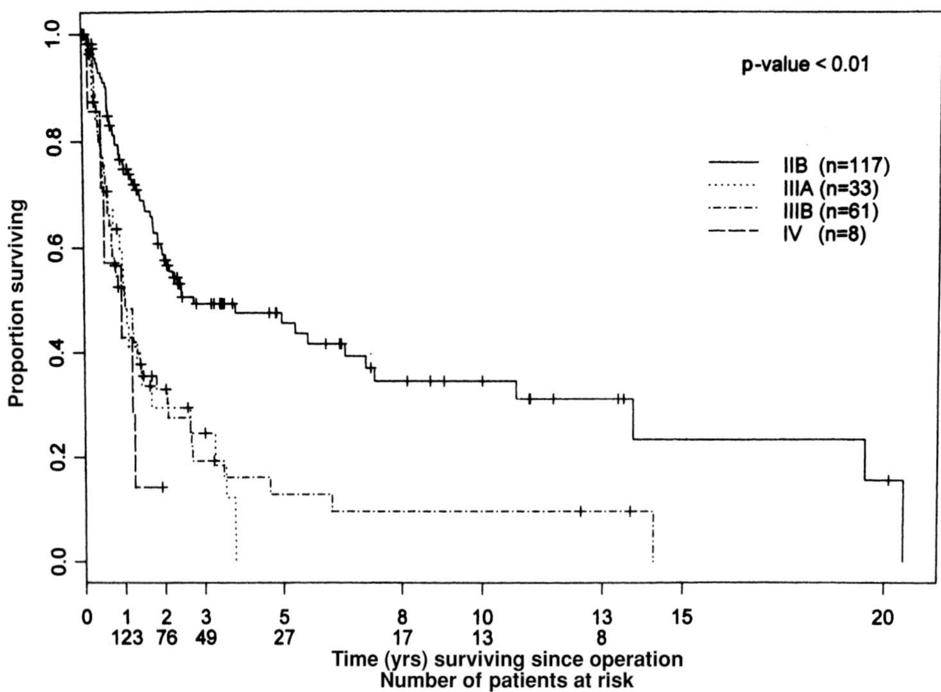

FIGURE 32–3 ■ Survival curve of superior sulcus tumors stratified by stage (IIB, IIIA, IIIB, IV).

tumors. The results of this trial have just been analyzed (Rusch, 2001). This report suggests that both T3 and T4 tumors appear to benefit from preoperative chemoradiation with very high complete resection rates and apparently improved 3-year survival compared with historical controls. Shahian and colleagues (1987) reported improved results with "sandwich irradiation," that is, addition of postoperative therapy to full therapeutic doses. The adverse prognostic factors we identified included N1 or N2 disease, incomplete resection, and wedge (vs lobectomy) resection of the pulmonary component.

Tumors in Proximity to Carina. Another subset of stage IIB carcinomas that benefits from surgical management includes patients with central tumors that extend within 2 cm of the carina without carinal involvement. In most instances, surgical extirpation of the tumor is possible. Nodal involvement severely affects prognosis, which em-

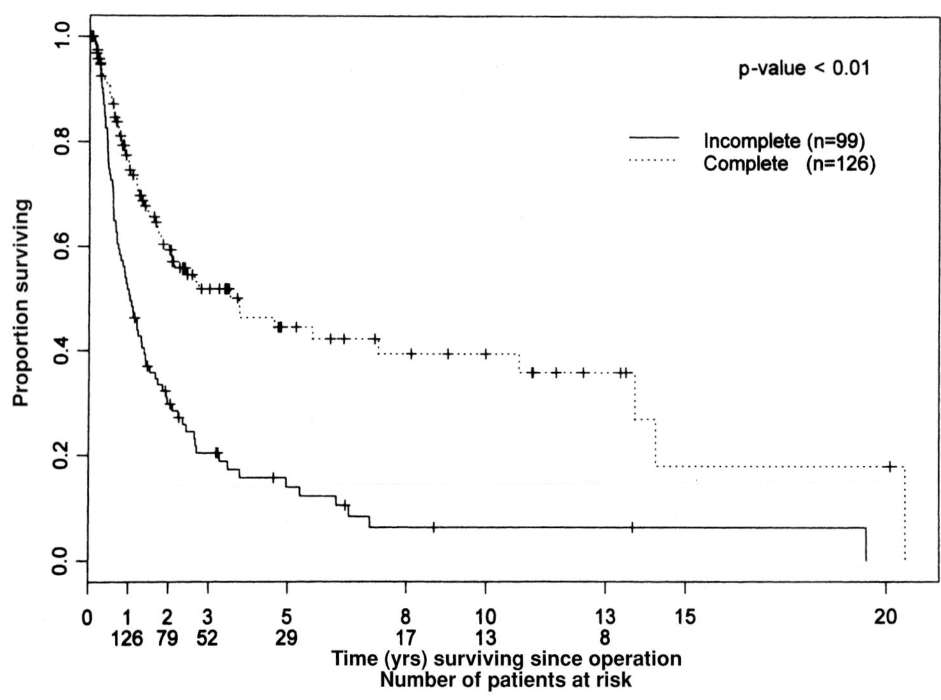

FIGURE 32–4 ■ Survival curve of superior sulcus tumors stratified by complete resection.

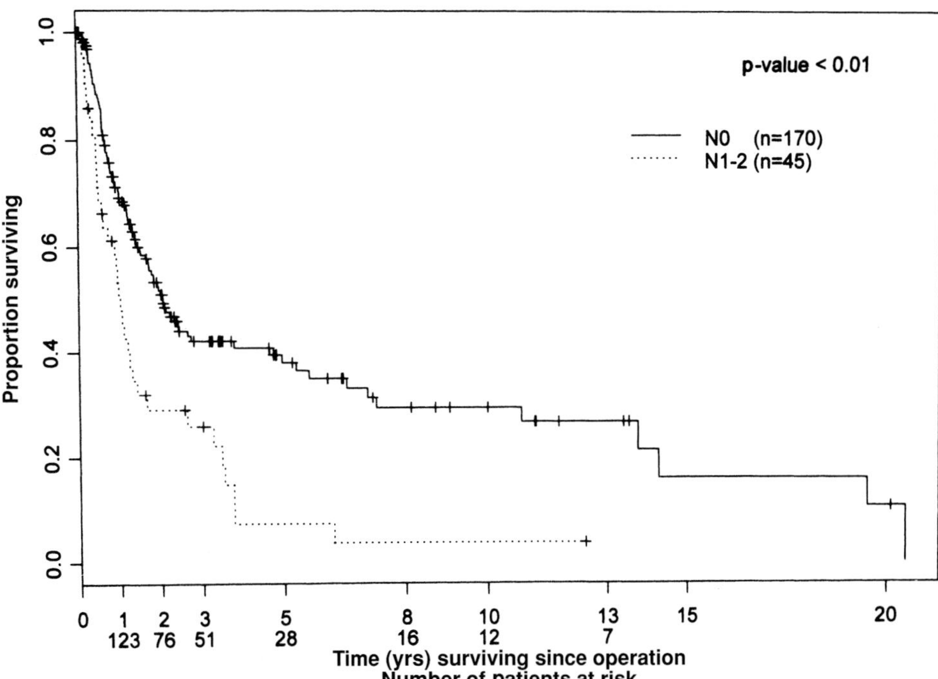

FIGURE 32–5 ■ Survival curve of superior sulcus tumors stratified by nodal status (N0, N1–2).

phasizes the need for preoperative mediastinoscopy. In patients in whom resection can be undertaken despite the proximity of the lesion to the carina but without its involvement, the 5-year anticipated survival rate following resection is 30% to 40% (Martini et al, 1988a and others).

Because most series report the results of either sleeve lobectomies or sleeve pneumonectomies, there are no definitive series reporting the results of surgical resection of T3 tumors because of their proximity to the carina. Pitz and co-workers (1996) reported on 75 such patients with a 40% 5-year survival for proximal bronchial tumors.

Although pneumonectomy is the common resection in these situations, a sleeve lobectomy is a very worthwhile alternative when possible; it provides lower mortality and morbidity and preserves pulmonary function. When complete excision is possible, the curability rate by sleeve lobectomy appears comparable to that obtained by pneumonectomy. Faber and associates (1984) performed 101 sleeve lobectomies over a 21-year period, with only two postoperative deaths in the entire series. The survival rate in this group of patients was 30% at 5 years and 22% at 10 years. When tumor involves not only the mainstem bronchus but also the proximal pulmonary artery, vascular sleeve resection combined with bronchial sleeve resection can be performed. Early authors reported a much higher mortality rate with very poor survival. However, more recent reports, with improved techniques, suggest results equivalent to sleeve lobectomy alone and pneumonectomy (Rendina et al, 1999). Mehran and associates (1994) reported on the adverse effects of nodal disease managed by sleeve lobectomy. In this latter group, pneumonectomy should be considered, when complete resection cannot be performed using a sleeve technique. A recent analysis, however, comparing N1–2 disease treated by pneumonectomy with that treated by sleeve lobectomy suggests that the overall outcome is identical, and that sleeve lobectomy does not compromise curative treatment (Icard et al, 1999; Lausberg et al, 2000). On occasion, sleeve pneumonectomy is required in T3 tumors approaching but not involving the carina.

Tumors Invading Mediastinum. Patients presenting with invasion of the primary tumor into the mediastinum generally have poor outcomes if treated by surgery alone. Two thirds of these patients also have mediastinal lymph node metastases. Few centers have reported their results in this subset of patients. From 1974 to 1984, 225 patients underwent thoracotomy at Memorial Sloan-Kettering Cancer Center for non–small cell carcinoma invading only the mediastinum (T3) (Burt et al, 1987). Of these, only 49 patients (22%) underwent complete resection of all intrathoracic disease. The 5-year survival rate in this group of patients was only 9%. Partial resection and implantation of isotopes to the residual disease, along with external radiation therapy, was carried out in 33 patients (15%) with surprising 3- and 5-year survival rates of 22%. Partial resection without implantation was performed in 42 patients (19%), and implantation without resection in 101 patients (45%). There were no 5-year survivors in the latter two groups. In a more recent update of this experience, we analyzed only N0 patients. Of 102 patients resected, a 19% 5-year survival was achieved. However, when complete resection was possible, 36% of T3 patients and only 12% of T4 patients survived for 5 years. The only other large series in the literature (Pitz et al, 1996) reported a 25% 5-year survival in 40 patients with disease invading the mediastinum. Once again, as in our original series, the adverse effect of N2 disease was apparent in that no survivors were reported in the 9 patients with mediastinal invasion and concomitant N2 disease.

Pulmonary resection combined with postoperative radiation therapy may offer some survival advantage in this specific subset of patients. However, only a few benefit from this combined approach. This group of patients may benefit from the newer approaches using combined modality therapy, including induction chemotherapy + radiotherapy.

Stage III Disease

The majority of lung cancers presenting for therapy are advanced tumors. When distant metastases are absent, but lymphatic metastases to the mediastinum are present, they are classified as stage III disease (N2 or N3 disease). Tumors invading "unresectable" adjacent organs (T4) are also included in this stage. Many of these locally advanced tumors, particularly T4 or N2 disease, are amenable to surgical resection or combined modality therapy that includes surgery. At this stage of disease, it is important that distant metastases be ruled out with preoperative organ scanning. It should be noted, however, that, once disease is clinically staged as T4 or N2, the current accepted therapy, in most instances, is nonsurgical. The importance of preoperative mediastinoscopy in this subset is obvious.

T3N1–2

The presence of hilar or mediastinal nodes adversely affects survival in this group of patients with T3 tumors despite complete resection. The survival rate following complete resection in the presence of nodal disease is less than 20% at 5 years (N1, 20%; N2, 40%). When identified preoperatively, many of these patients are currently being offered neoadjuvant approaches with re-evaluation following a response. There is no evidence that preoperative radiation therapy alone for clinical N1 or N2 disease benefits patients with tumors invading the chest wall. Postoperative radiation therapy in patients who have evidence of mediastinal lymph node metastases or residual disease is usually advised in an attempt to decrease the incidence of local recurrence (Patterson et al, 1982), although the efficacy of this treatment is unknown. A randomized trial by the Lung Cancer Study Group to assess the value of postoperative radiotherapy in this group of patients was abandoned because of low accrual. Preoperative mediastinoscopy identifies those patients unlikely to benefit from primary surgical resection when their tumors have been clinically staged as T3. PET scans may reveal hilar nodal involvement.

N2 Disease

Metastasis to mediastinal lymph nodes (N2 disease) is probably the most frequent deterrent to cancer cure despite a "localized" presentation. Mediastinal metastasis is present in nearly one half of all limited disease patients at presentation with non–small cell lung carcinoma. Many view this large group of patients as having a "nonsurgical" disease despite the best efforts of surgery and radiation therapy (Paulson and Urschel, 1971; Pearson, 1985) because the majority probably have occult micrometastatic disease already present elsewhere.

Not Clinically Evident—"Resectable"

Selected patients with ipsilateral N2 disease identified at thoracotomy can benefit from effective management by primary surgery. From 1974 to 1981, 1598 patients with non–small cell lung cancer were seen at Memorial Sloan-Kettering; 706 of them had mediastinal lymph node metastases. Of these, only 151 (21%) were completely resectable (Martini et al, 1983). Mediastinoscopy at that time was not routinely performed as part of staging before thoracotomy. Clinical evidence of N2 disease was based largely on radiographic and bronchoscopic findings. Patients with a normal-appearing mediastinum on routine chest radiographs and CT scan and a normal carina at bronchoscopy without compression or distortion of the trachea or main bronchi were classified as having N0 or N1 disease. Patients who had an abnormal mediastinum on chest radiographs, which was suggestive of N2 disease, and those with findings at bronchoscopy suggestive of carinal involvement were considered to have clinically manifested N2 disease.

Of 151 patients with N2 disease that was not clinically evident who were treated by complete resection (10% of the entire group), the overall 5-year survival rate was 30% (Martini and Flehinger, 1987). There was no difference in survival at 5 years between patients with adenocarcinoma (30%) and those with squamous cell carcinoma (32%). However, the survival rate was affected by tumor size. Better survival rates at 5 years were noted in patients with small tumors (T1, 46%) compared with those with large tumors (T2, 27%) or those with extension outside the lung or in proximity to the carina (T3, 14%; $P = .003$).

The survival rate was also calculated by nodal size and the number of involved nodes. When nodal involvement was present, the size per se did not affect the survival rate because patients with normal-sized nodes, nodes of 2 cm or less in size, and nodes greater than 2 cm had essentially similar survival rates ($P = .17$). This suggests that patients with encapsulated lymph nodes, regardless of their size, can have prolonged survival if the nodes are completely removed. However, the number of nodes affected was significant. Patients with a single involved N2 node did better than those with multiple nodal involvement at one or more levels ($P = .005$). Many other studies have identified improved survival in patients with single-station nodal disease (versus multistation).

On the other hand, patients presenting with radiologic or endoscopic evidence of clinical N2 disease had a very poor survival rate. In our series, only 18% of such patients had resectable disease, and only 9% of those treated by resection survived 5 years. None ultimately survived their cancer. The survival of patients following completely resected N2 disease is dependent on the number of mediastinal nodal stations involved with the tumor. This has been confirmed by many authors (Suzuki, 1999; Thomas, 1988; Watanabe 1991). In all retrospective analyses, single-station mediastinal lymph node involvement yielded a better prognosis than multi-station involvement and showed the adverse effects of multiple levels of involved lymph nodes assessed at the time of surgery and assessed clinically. Only those patients with clinical N1 disease had a survival greater than 10% following complete surgical resection (Fig. 32–6). This result has been repeated over and over in the literature. The importance of preoperative mediastinoscopy in any patient suspected to have clinical hilar or N2 disease cannot be overestimated. The identification of N2 disease preoperatively suggests the need to consider a combined modality therapeutic approach because primary surgery yields such a poor survival outcome when clinically evident N2 disease is noted by imaging or invasive staging.

The role of primary surgery in the management of N2 disease can be summarized as follows: Patients found at thoracotomy to have unsuspected N2 disease (clinical N1 disease) that can be completely resected should be offered that opportunity. If, at mediastinoscopy, one microscopic focus of N2 disease is identified in one station only, primary surgery can be considered, although presently, most surgeons offer patients combined modality therapy. Patients who do best are those in whom, following a negative mediastinoscopy, N2 disease is discovered serendipitously at surgery. In these instances, usually only one station of mediastinal nodal disease is present. In all of these cases, ipsilateral mediastinal lymph node dissection (vs sampling) is strongly advised, and has been found in a recent analysis to improve survival (Keller et al, 2000). In this interesting subset analysis of an intergroup study assessing postoperative radiation therapy, the authors identify the fact that an ipsilateral mediastinal lymph node dissection on the right side improved survival in patients with N2 disease, but no such improvement was noted when left-sided mediastinal nodal dissection (levels V, VI, and VII) was carried out. This suggests the very important role of mediastinoscopy, especially in suspected left hilar nodal involvement. It does appear that these patients may well have had unsuspected and mediastinoscopy-accessible superior mediastinal nodal involvement that was not identified at the time of surgery. Whether or not an extended lymph node dissection that includes superior mediastinal nodal stations when left-sided tumors are present is worthwhile awaits further study.

Unfortunately, adjuvant therapies in patients with resected N2 disease that has been completely or incompletely resected have not shown much benefit. Postoperative radiotherapy appears to decrease the incidence of local-regional recurrence but does not affect survival. Adjuvant chemotherapy and chemoradiotherapy have not been impressive in improving long-term and disease-free survival. Studies are continuing that use more "modern" chemotherapy, but it is highly unlikely that major improvements will be demonstrated. (See next chapter.)

Clinically Evident—"Unresectable"

CT scanning has now become an integral part of the staging and presurgical evaluation of the mediastinum

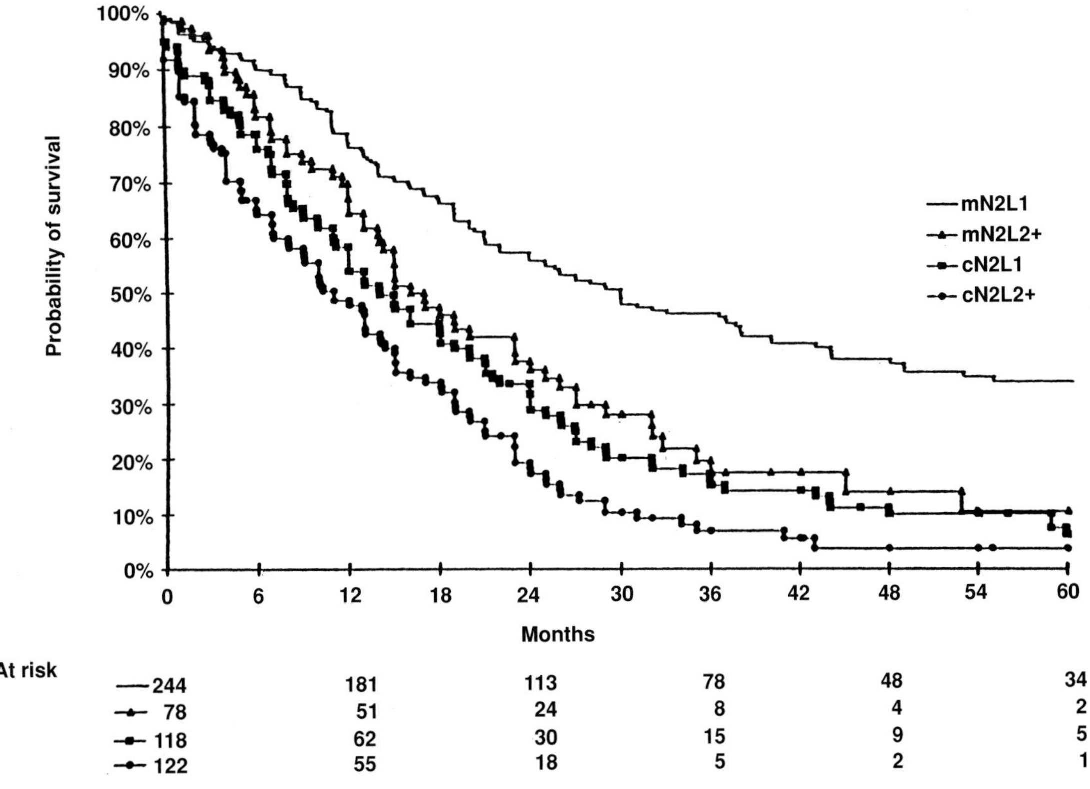

FIGURE 32–6 ■ Lymph node involvement and survival based on pathologic and clinical staging. In this analysis, N2 disease identified clinically (CN) had an extremely poor prognosis as did more than one level of mediastinal lymph nodes (L24) found at pathologic analysis. This confirms multiple other studies reported in the past 30 years.

(Ferguson et al, 1986; Graves et al, 1985; Martini et al, 1985). CT scanning correlates well (80% to 90% accuracy) with negative nodes less than 1 cm in transverse diameter. Many centers accept this as evidence of mediastinal "negativity" and proceed with surgical resection based on this negative result. Enlarged mediastinal lymph nodes (greater than 1 cm in shortest diameter) detected on CT scans should be confirmed to be positive by mediastinoscopy or other invasive staging before therapy is begun because 30% of such cases do not contain tumors in the mediastinal nodes, and patients can be offered primarily surgical therapy.

The role of PET scanning in providing confirmatory evidence of N2 disease without the need for invasive mediastinal staging has yet to be defined. Unfortunately, "positive" PET scans in the mediastinum may reflect inflammatory changes, and "negative" PET scans may be falsely negative. (See Chapter 31.)

When hilar N1 disease or microscopic N2 disease is discovered at the time of surgery or is identified prior to induction therapy, complete ipsilateral mediastinal lymph node dissection is warranted and, we believe, necessary, although its exact role in curing such patients has never been tested scientifically.

In summary, the patients with N2 disease who benefit best from surgery as their primary therapy are those who present with peripheral tumors, an apparently normal mediastinum on plain chest radiographs and at bronchoscopy, and a normal mediastinum on CT scan and mediastinoscopy with a single, but encapsulated, discrete ipsilateral lymph node involvement that is discovered at surgery. The importance of CT scanning and mediastinoscopy, we believe, is to identify significant mediastinal disease (i.e., involvement at multiple stations of N2 nodes, invasion of mediastinal structures by nodal disease, or contralateral [N3] nodal disease), thus avoiding primary surgery and poor outcomes. Unfortunately, neither CT scan nor plain radiography correlates well with N2 disease when the tumor in the lung is central or hilar in location or extends to the mediastinum, making it difficult to separate T3 from N2 disease. In these groups of patients, invasive mediastinal evaluation by mediastinoscopy is helpful.

The role of preoperative radiation therapy alone for clinically evident N2 disease has been extensively evaluated in the past, and there is general agreement that this does not improve survival (Shields et al, 1970; Warram, collaborative study, 1975). This is so despite a reported increase in resectability, local-regional control, and apparent sterilization of some of the tumors, as evidenced in the resected specimens following preoperative radiation therapy, because most patients die of distant metastases.

Several centers have assessed the benefit of preoperative chemotherapy or combined chemotherapy and radiation therapy in these locally advanced tumors that are usually considered incurable by primary surgery (Burkes et al, 1992; Taylor et al, 1987). Phase II studies have suggested an improved survival compared with that in historical controls, and two randomized trials confirmed the benefit of induction therapy compared with primary surgery (Burkes et al, 1992; Kris et al, 1987; Rosell et al, 1994; Roth et al, 1994).

When N2 disease is discovered preoperatively, the current standard of care is nonsurgical (chemoradiation). However, when the disease is potentially completely resectable, but is considered "unresectable" because of the poor results of primary surgery, the role of induction therapies (preoperative radiotherapy, chemotherapy, or chemoradiation) continues to be investigated, along with their combination with ultimate surgery.

Over the past 20 years, innumerable phase II trials have investigated a variety of induction chemotherapy regimens, most containing cisplatinum and mitomycin, and a huge variety of chemoradiation regimens. Most recently, attempts have been made to shorten the chemoradiation approaches with hyperfractionation techniques. The results of these phase II trials suggest that, when used as induction therapy, chemotherapy and chemoradiation produce similar outcomes, similar morbidity, and similar long-term survival (see subsequent subchapter of Chapter 33, Chemotherapy, for further information).

The role of surgeons in managing such patients must begin prior to any induction therapy and must include preoperative assessment of the T (bronchoscopy) and N (mediastinoscopy) stages and a predetermination of the expected resection that might follow the induction therapy. After completion of such preoperative treatment, a careful reassessment is required to determine whether the patient's disease is potentially resectable and whether the patient has the cardiopulmonary capability to tolerate such a resection, keeping in mind the adverse cardiopulmonary toxicities of specific agents and radiotherapy. Following induction therapy, resection is possible in most responders, and complete mediastinal lymph node dissection is essential. Survival following these regimens is contingent on attainment of a complete resection (Fig. 32–7). Despite the preoperative regimens, surgical morbidity and mortality rates have not exceeded those expected following resection of locally advanced stage III lung cancer. One caveat should be noted: In a recent analysis at Memorial Sloan-Kettering Cancer Center of almost 500 resections following induction therapy, the only significant factor predicting morbidity and mortality was the use of right pneumonectomy. Whereas left pneumonectomy resulted in no postoperative mortality in more than 50 patients, a similar number of patients undergoing right pneumonectomy suffered a 20% postoperative mortality rate (Abolhoda et al, 2000)!

The two early phase III trials of induction chemotherapy (Rosell et al, 1994; Roth et al, 1994) suggested that there is significant improvement in survival with this modality. However, a recent trial (Ichinose, 2000) has failed to confirm these results. When one takes into account all of these trials, it is evident that persisting N2 disease following induction therapy is an adverse prognostic factor, whereas a complete response or downstaging is a positive prognostic factor.

All reports on preoperative treatment to date can be viewed only as feasibility studies because of the small number of patients studied in each report, but all demonstrate high responses to induction treatment with increased resectability in responders. The early survival data of these trials were sufficiently encouraging to support the initiation of large-scale randomized studies,

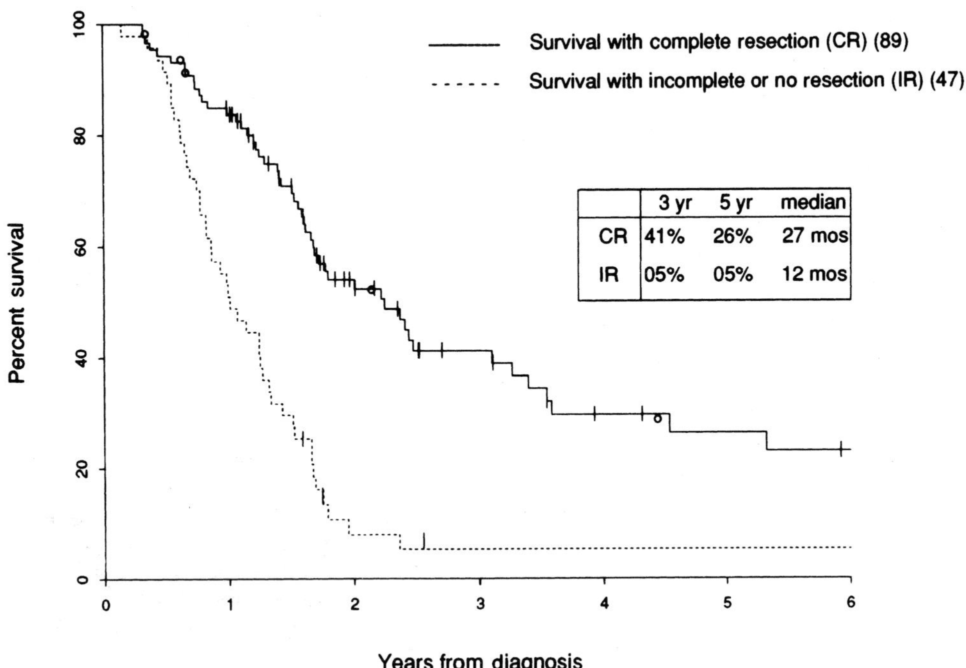

	3 yr	5 yr	median
CR	41%	26%	27 mos
IR	05%	05%	12 mos

FIGURE 32-7 ■ Survival by the extent of resection following induction chemotherapy in stage IIIA (N2) non–small cell lung cancer (P = 0.00002).

which are currently in progress to assess fully the role of induction therapy and surgery versus the current standard therapy, radiotherapy (with or without chemotherapy), in these "unresectable" N2 patients. Recent reports suggest up to a 15% 5-year survival rate with chemoradiotherapy as the primary treatment (Dillman et al, 1996; Schaake-Koning et al, 1992). These primary chemoradiation results are equivalent to those seen following induction therapy and surgery. Currently, a North American trial is being completed that compares these two approaches. As well, in North America and Europe, induction chemotherapy is now being tested in phase III trials that compare primary surgery with this combined modality approach in earlier stage (IB, II, and II–III,N1) disease.

A complete discussion of the role and use of induction therapies can be found in subsequent chapters on radiotherapy and chemotherapy.

Stage IIIB Disease (T4 or N3). Patients presenting with (1) supraclavicular or contralateral mediastinal lymph node metastases (N3); (2) invasion of the spine, trachea, carina, esophagus, aorta, or heart (T4), or satellite lesions within the same lobe; or (3) malignant pleural effusion (T4) are currently grouped under stage IIIB disease and are considered inoperable. Most of these patients are treated by radiotherapy or chemoradiation. Few at present are considered for surgical therapy, although a small group of T4N0 tumors can be completely resected. Currently, phase II clinical trials are assessing the potential role of combined modality therapy, including surgery, for this subset of patients. Occasionally, patients are found at thoracotomy to have completely resectable T4 disease because they have been clinically understaged. These comprise most of the reported long-term survivors. In a telling report by Stamatis and associates (1999) in which the authors used induction chemoradiation followed by surgery for stage IIIB tumors, 9 of the 13 R0 resections for T4 disease had complete pathologic responses, and 8 of the 14 R0 resections with N3 disease had complete pathologic responses at the time of the surgery. The 5-year survival rate of the various subgroups is identical to the number of patients who have complete responses and one wonders about the impact of surgery (vs induction chemoradiation) in this report.

One real concern is clinical overstaging of these patients. Before a patient is assigned to a T4 or N3 category on clinical grounds, there should be incontrovertible evidence of this involvement. All too often, such patients, clinically staged as T4 or N3, are of lower stage at the time of invasive staging or thoracotomy. If these invasive approaches are not used for staging, inappropriate (nonsurgical) therapy is frequently prescribed for totally resectable tumors.

T4 Disease. *Carinal Involvement.* Lesions that extend to and invade the carina have a much poorer prognosis than those in the mainstem bronchi. Pneumonectomy with tracheal sleeve resection and direct reanastomosis of the trachea to the contralateral mainstem bronchus has been offered to young patients who are good surgical risks with up to a 20% 5-year survival rate, often in the face of 13% to 30% operative mortality rates (Deslauriers, 1985; Jensik et al, 1982). In a recent update of the Massachusetts General experience, Mitchell and colleagues (1999) performed carinal resections or sleeve pneumonectomies on 58 primary bronchogenic carcinomas. The operative mortality for right carinal pneumonectomy was 15.9% (7 of 44) and for left carinal pneumonectomy was 30.8% (4 of 13). The therapy (sleeve pneumonectomy) should be reserved for young healthy patients with clinical N0 disease, as determined by mediastinoscopy, who have completely resectable disease. All other patients should be treated primarily with chemoradiation without resection. On occasion, tiny tumors around the carina but originating in the mainstem bronchus, usually squamous cell cancers, can be treated with carinal resection alone or carinal resection combined with lobectomy. If tiny tumors are involving the carina, nonsurgical approaches may be valuable (Cortese et al, 1997; Kato et al, 1996). Transbronchoscopic brachytherapy or photodynamic therapy may play an important adjuvant role in the future management of such localized tracheal invasion (Oho et al, 1983).

In the report by Stamatis and co-workers (1999) of 33 patients resected, only 5 patients had an en bloc resection of a T4 structure. Similarly, in another report by Rendina and associates (1999), despite the fact that the authors documented tumor invasion preoperatively, at the time of surgery only four patients underwent an en bloc resection of an adjacent organ. Either the induction therapy is sterilizing the T4 involvement or the patients were overstaged initially. The mortality rates for this aggressive surgery approach 10%, although in the Stamatis series, only 6% of patients succumbed postoperatively.

Satellite Nodules. Although ipsilobar satellite nodules are now considered T4, the 5-year survival following resection of a tumor with an ipsilobar satellite lesion still warrants surgical resection. In many instances, the satellite lesion is discovered only at the time of pathologic examination. One cannot conclude that a satellite nodule seen on CT scan represents cancer (vs an inflammatory lesion). For this reason, we believe that, although satellite lesions may be discovered preoperatively (e.g., PET scanning), unless there is evidence of disease elsewhere, the approach for these patients should be surgical because the 5-year survival of this subset of T4 disease is significant (>20%). Reports of survival in patients with ipsilobar satellite nodules vary. In most reports, although the presence of satellite nodules is a poor prognostic factor, it does not have the same prognosis as other T4 lesions.

Organ Involvement. Other T4 lesions can be completely resected in selected instances, offering an occasional cure. This includes direct invasion of the vertebra, superior vena cava, esophagus, and atrium. It is this group of patients for whom induction therapy, either chemotherapy or chemoradiotherapy, is currently being investigated. Early reports have suggested down-staging of such patients, allowing less than radical resections (Rendina et al, 1999). One has to wonder whether or not these patients were clinically overstaged. Other authors (Dartevelle and Macchiarini, 1999) approach such lesions without preoperative treatment, using imaging and invasive staging to assess operability and resectability of the involved adjacent structure.

With improved surgical techniques and the use of cardiopulmonary bypass where indicated, reports are emerging of patients having had main pulmonary arteries reconstructed, superior venae cavae reconstructed, and total vertebrectomies being performed for this stage of disease. The rare, fortunate patient who has had an R0 resection can be cured of his or her tumor with this very aggressive approach (Spaggiari, 2000; Putnam, 1999). If one highly selects such patients, up to a 25% 5-year survival can be expected in the presence of an R0 resection.

N3 Disease. Contralateral mediastinal lymph node metastases are considered by most surgeons to be an absolute contraindication to surgery because long-term survival with surgery is rare and anecdotal. However, the Southwest Oncology Group has completed a phase II induction chemotherapy and radiotherapy program followed by surgery for this group of patients. The early results of this trial suggested a complete resection rate similar to that seen with induction therapy for N2 disease (Rusch et al, 1993). Long-term results, including survival rates, in patients treated for N3 disease by this aggressive fashion have been reported. None of the patients with N3 disease due to contralateral mediastinal involvement survived 5 years. The only survivors were two patients with preoperatively proven scalene node involvement. At the time of surgery, no attempt was made to remove the cervical lymph nodes. One has to conclude that, in this form of combined modality therapy, it was the radiotherapy that cured the extrathoracic disease. Many centers in Japan use a median sternotomy to accomplish an extended lymph node dissection that includes contralateral mediastinal and ipsilateral or bilateral neck node dissection for patients with N3 involvement. There have been occasional long-term survivors using this aggressive approach (Hata et al, 1988; Naruke et al, 1988b; Watanabe et al, 1988). Although unlikely to provide substantial long-term benefit, these approaches are worthy of well-constructed clinical trials. At the present time, however, the standard of care for patients with proven N3 involvement is a chemoradiation approach without surgery.

In a recent update by Hata of 232 patients undergoing bilateral mediastinal lymph node dissection over a 20-year period, the overall survival of patients ultimately staged as having N3 disease was 41% (47 patients). This was identical to that seen with those patients ultimately found to have N2 disease. The postoperative mortality was somewhat higher than one would expect for a similar resection without bilateral mediastinal lymphadenectomy (7.1%) (Hata, personal communication, 2000). Of the 16 patients preoperatively identified as having N3 disease, there was a similar (46%) 5-year survival following bilateral lymphadenectomy. In patients identified as having supraclavicular nodal disease, Hata extended his resection to include not only bilateral mediastinal lymph nodes but also a bilateral neck dissection. In these patients (40 patients), a very satisfactory 20% 5-year survival was achieved. Spurred by this information, other surgeons in Japan are now exploring this very extended lymph node dissection. It is unknown what adjuvant therapies were used in the Hata series. As yet, surgeons in Europe and North America have not adopted this very aggressive approach, offering primary chemoradiation for those patients with preoperatively identified N3 disease. As one can see from Figure 32–8, when bilateral mediastinal lymphadenectomy is used with or without cervical

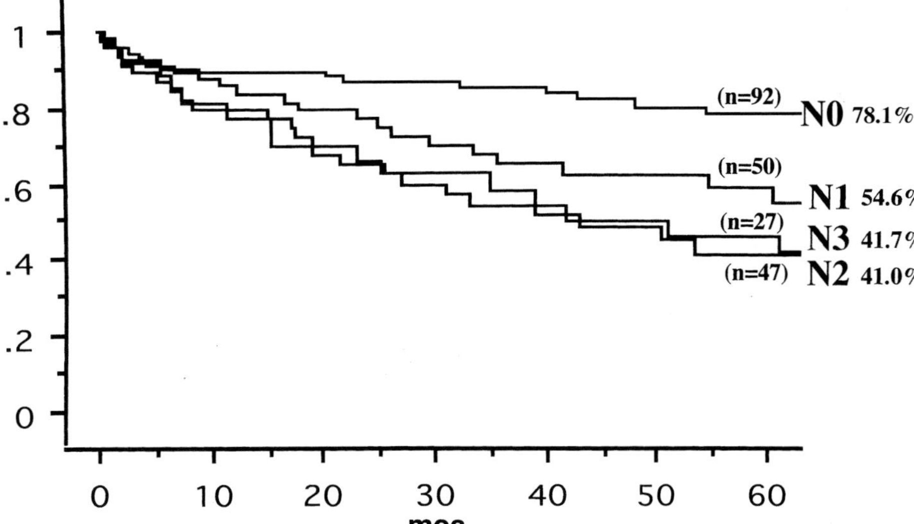

FIGURE 32-8 ■ Survival according to nodal involvement following extended (2-field) lymphadenectomy. (Courtesy of Dr. Hata—unpublished data).

lymphadenectomy, the overall survival according to pathologic stage far exceeds that achieved by other surgical approaches, with or without combined modality treatment.

Although the value of postoperative treatment in this group of aggressively treated patients is unknown, most surgeons advocate postoperative radiotherapy if an induction approach has not been used.

Solitary Metastases (M1)

Brain

Occasionally, patients present with resectable lung cancer and evidence of a solitary metastasis on complete organ scanning. These patients can and should be considered for a combined approach, removing the primary tumor and the solitary metastasis. In these patients, PET scanning should prove to be extremely useful for ruling out other sites of disease.

Brain metastases constitute nearly one third of all observed distant recurrences in patients with resected non–small cell lung cancer; twice that incidence is found at autopsy of all patients dying with lung cancer. Most brain metastases occur in those patients with a histologic diagnosis of adenocarcinoma as opposed to squamous or large cell carcinoma.

Therapy

When local and regional control is achieved or achievable but brain metastases develop as the sole site of metastasis, the therapy employed for the brain metastasis determines the ultimate survival. Untreated patients with brain metastases have a median survival of less than 3 months. When brain metastases are multiple or advanced, or other metastatic disease is present, the therapy of choice is whole-brain irradiation. However, one third of patients presenting with brain metastases have solitary lesions. Therapy with surgery or radiation can be effective (Burt et al, 1992). Those most likely to receive long-term benefit from surgical resection, or stereotactic or gamma knife radiosurgery, are patients with a single surgically accessible brain metastasis and no other evident systemic disease. However, a recent randomized trial suggests that surgery offers the best form of palliation despite other noncerebral metastases (Patchell et al, 1990).

High-dose corticosteroid therapy reduces edema, causing regression of neurologic symptoms that is sometimes complete. It is the initial treatment prescribed for all patients. Surgery or radiation therapy is usually initiated after 3 to 4 days of such therapy.

Magilligan and associates (1986) reported on 41 patients treated surgically for their brain metastases. All had solitary metastases, and in 14 of 41, or one third of the patients, the neurologic symptoms preceded the diagnosis of lung cancer, which is in keeping with our experience. Improvement in neurologic symptoms was noted in most patients, the operative mortality rate was low, and there was a clear survival advantage over patients treated by nonsurgical means, all of which is also in accord with the findings of most recent reports.

Two studies now have demonstrated conclusively that surgical extirpation followed by whole-brain irradiation is superior to whole-brain irradiation alone in managing solitary cerebral metastases with regard to survival and quality of life. As yet, no such study has compared the newer forms of stereotactic radiosurgery directed solely at the solitary metastatic focus, although the results of such nonsurgical therapies are encouraging.

When the brain lesion is detected first and the search for the primary tumor is negative, resection of the cranial metastasis is the therapy of choice (Burt et al, 1992; Martini, 1986). Even when the brain metastasis presents subsequent to the resection of the lung carcinoma (metachronous) and no other site of recurrence is present, or the patient has minimal disease elsewhere, resection of the intracranial lesion is again the therapy of choice. When both brain and lung lesions are detected simultaneously (synchronous), if both lesions are resectable, craniotomy is done first and thoracotomy shortly thereafter, unless dominating symptoms from the primary tumor dictate otherwise. If either the lung or brain lesion is suspected to be unresectable, surgical therapy is directed first to the site where resectability is questioned most; otherwise, therapy by nonsurgical means is recommended.

Postoperative brain irradiation has usually been prescribed for all patients who have had resected brain metastases because of its potential ability to sterilize the tumor bed, even in patients who have had an apparent complete surgical excision.

Survival

The 1-year survival of 55% and the mean survival of 2.3 years reported by Magilligan and colleagues (1986) were similar to our results (Burt et al, 1992). The overall 5-year survival rate for such patients approaches 20%. Surgical therapy should be offered to patients with single surgically accessible brain metastases, no evident systemic disease elsewhere, and a primary cancer confined to the lung.

Lung

Despite the possibility that a second lung lesion may be a metastatic deposit, many second lesions represent synchronous primary tumors and should be considered as such; resection of both tumors should be evaluated whenever possible. The long-term results of those patients even with solitary lung metastases suggest that many patients are salvaged. Deslauriers and co-workers (1989a) reviewed the solitary metastatic lesions identified in resected specimens and reported a 22% 5-year survival rate. Similarly, in those patients with synchronous primary pulmonary metastases, about 25% have similar long-term survival when treated surgically.

Adrenal Gland

Solitary adrenal metastases are being detected with increasing frequency because of routine upper abdominal CT scanning in the preoperative workup (Allard et al, 1990; Burt et al, 1994; Nielsen et al, 1982; Sandler et al, 1982). Resection of the primary tumor and the solitary metastatic focus should be considered if both are completely resectable (Raviv et al, 1990; Reyes et al, 1990; Twomey et al, 1982). The long-term results of such aggressive therapy are unknown, although 5-year survivors have been reported, whereas no survivors have been reported with nonsurgical therapy.

Bone and Other Sites

It is rare for truly solitary metastases to occur in the bone, liver, and other common metastatic sites, such as the skin. However, if thorough preoperative staging procedures do not reveal any other sites of metastasis, and if both lesions (primary and solitary metastatic focus) are completely resectable, surgical therapy can be offered if the risks are low.

PALLIATIVE RESECTION

For surgery to be effective in controlling lung cancer, it must be complete and potentially curative. The role of surgery for the palliation of patients with unresectable tumors is debatable. There are specific situations, such as an unremitting lung abscess distal to an obstructing tumor, massive hemoptysis, or painful invasion of the chest wall (ribs or vertebrae), that have led surgeons to consider and perform palliative or incomplete resection in the hope of improving the patient's symptoms; on occasion, long-term palliation has been achieved.

Lung Abscess

An unresolving lung abscess, caused by either a necrotizing tumor (usually a squamous cell carcinoma) or a lung abscess distal to an obstructing tumor, rarely requires surgical resection. Other options, such as endobronchial laser therapy to relieve the proximal obstruction followed by external radiotherapy or percutaneous drainage of the abscess, usually suffice to alleviate the symptoms. However, if complete resection is probable, a surgical approach should be considered. Otherwise, the lesser measures described may relieve all symptoms and result in satisfactory palliation without noncurative surgery.

Massive Hemoptysis

Massive uncontrolled hemoptysis is a rare feature of untreated lung cancer. Most frequently, it is the result of the development of a vascular-bronchial fistula following radiotherapy. The pulmonary artery, aorta, or eroded bronchial vessels can be the source of the bleeding. In most of these instances, exsanguination or suffocation leads to the instantaneous death of the patient. On occasion, persisting but significant hemoptysis (usually from bronchial vessels) allows time for the situation to be controlled. Bronchoscopic treatment by laser coagulation or the placement of an endobronchial blocker or selective bronchial artery embolization by percutaneous angiography may relieve the problem. Rarely is thoracotomy required, despite the tumor's resectability. In completely unresectable cases, at the time of thoracotomy, hilar division of all bronchial vessels may relieve the problem. Occasionally, palliative resection is possible and can control the bleeding.

Chest Wall Invasion

When a patient with an otherwise unresectable tumor as a result of extensive nodal involvement or distant metastases presents with excruciating chest wall pain caused by invasion of the ribs or vertebrae, in exceptional instances, consideration can be given to resection of the primary tumor for palliative purposes by combining incomplete resections with radiotherapy, although this modality has usually already failed. In almost all cases, it is preferable for other nonsurgical measures to be used, such as external beam irradiation (if possible) or pain-relieving techniques, either local or systemic. When thoracic vertebrae are invaded and destroyed, causing extradural compression, resection of the primary tumor invading the vertebra together with vertebral body resection has been used, with or without the addition of brachytherapy, to avoid impending paralysis, thus protecting the spine from high-dose external irradiation. Short-term pain relief can also be obtained in this fashion. Unfortunately, in most instances, the tumor recurs within 3 to 6 months. The palliative benefit obtained through these surgical approaches has never been prospectively compared with that of less aggressive alternatives for pain control.

In summary, palliative resection should be avoided when less aggressive nonsurgical approaches are available that provide similar palliative results.

POSTOPERATIVE MORBIDITY AND MORTALITY RATES

Because most reported cures in carcinoma of the lung have occurred in patients treated surgically, it is natural for clinicians to want to expand the role of surgery, either alone or combined with radiation, chemotherapy, or both. Many nonsurgical physicians are justifiably concerned with the reported postoperative mortality rates, which can range from 5% to 20%, as well as morbidity rates of up to 40%.

Proper case selection and careful preoperative and perioperative management can minimize postoperative complications. Major complications occur in nearly 10% of patients with stage I or II disease and in 20% of those requiring extended resection for the treatment of locally advanced tumors (stage III) (Deslauriers et al, 1989b).

In most series, the total morbidity following surgical resection for lung cancer approaches 40%, 20% being major. Mortality rates, however, vary and are affected by a variety of factors. In a recent analysis by Reed and colleagues (1998), it was apparent that surgeons properly trained in cardiothoracic surgery perform these resections with less morbidity and less mortality. From other reports (Begg et al, 1998), it does not appear that the total volume of surgery performed has any bearing on these postoperative outcomes. Multimodality treatments have been implicated to increase these adverse outcomes. A recent analysis in our own hospital suggests that, although morbidity may be increased slightly with multimodality treatment, overall mortality is not. One specific adverse factor is right pneumonectomy combined with preoperative chemotherapy. In this specific subset, a 20% postoperative mortality rate has been reported at Memorial Sloan-Kettering Cancer Center (MSKCC) (Abolhoda et al, 2000).

The Lung Cancer Study Group analyzed 2000 consecutive resections for lung cancer and reported an overall postoperative mortality rate of 3.3% (Ginsberg et al, 1983). More recent retrospective analyses confirm that pneumonectomy carries an overall 6% to 7% mortality rate, whereas lobectomy and lesser resections should not exceed a 2% postoperative mortality figure. A recent Japanese survey suggests a much improved 30-day mortality rate (pneumonectomy 3.2%, lobectomy 1.2%, and lesser resection 0.8%) (Wada et al, 1998). To minimize complications, a lesser resection may be considered in elderly patients and in all physiologically compromised persons who present an increased risk for surgery.

SPECIFIC CONSIDERATIONS

Intraoperative Tumor Spillage

Transgression of the tumor with intraoperative spillage of cells theoretically could lead to pleural implants and local recurrence. If such tumor spillage occurs, the hemithorax should be copiously irrigated with large quantities of saline. Whether cell-lysing agents (e.g., hypertonic saline, water, absolute alcohol, or chemotherapeutic agents) have any role to play in such irrigations is unknown.

Positive Resection Margins

Bronchial, vascular, and close-proximity margins should be always monitored by frozen-section analysis at the time of surgery. Resection to negative margins is advised whenever a positive margin is identified. Although a 2-cm bronchial resection margin is ideal, we accept a negative margin, no matter the distance from the tumor. In situ disease at the resection margin carries a much better prognosis than that caused by invasive disease, or submucosal or adventitial lymphatic involvement (Kaiser et al, 1989). In these instances, because of the potential value of minimizing local-regional occurrence, most surgeons advocate postoperative irradiation when close margins are encountered. Residual in situ disease can be treated with endoluminal brachytherapy or photocoagulation using hematoporphyrins.

Perioperative Blood Transfusion

Retrospective data have not confirmed the adverse prognostic effect of perioperative blood transfusions in the long-term survival of patients with resected lung cancers. Tartter and associates (1984) reported that perioperative blood transfusion adversely affects the prognosis after resection of stage I non–small cell lung cancer. In 165 patients with stage I disease, using disease-free survival rates as the end point, they found a significantly decreased disease-free survival rate in transfused patients. Hyman and co-workers (1985) also reported a significantly increased relative risk of dying in transfused patients among their 105 patients with stage I or II resected lung cancer.

To determine the impact of perioperative transfusion on the recurrence-free interval, the status of 352 patients treated by resection for stages I and II non–small cell lung cancer at MSKCC was investigated (Keller et al, 1988). The recurrence rate was not significantly different in transfused patients compared with those who received no blood, even when stratified for stage. Furthermore, the number of units transfused was not associated with the time to tumor recurrence. Our results did not support the contention that perioperative blood transfusion is associated with a decreased recurrence-free interval. Despite this, we avoid unnecessary blood transfusions and encourage autologous blood donations whenever possible.

Lobectomy Versus Pneumonectomy

Intraoperatively, especially with central lesions by virtue of the primary tumor or involved lymph nodes, a decision has to be made whether a lobectomy or pneumonectomy should be performed. Incomplete resections never cure. Before a lobectomy is considered to be complete, all resection margins should be confirmed by frozen-section analysis. The "sump" lymph nodes lying on the pulmonary artery between the upper and lower lobes should be examined. If there is any question that these contain tumor, indicating that a larger resection (e.g., pneumonectomy) is required, frozen-section analysis of such lymph nodes should be performed. When an upper lobectomy is performed, involvement of the sump lymph nodes between the upper and lower lobes may necessitate a completion pneumonectomy. Following right lower lobectomy, involvement of the sump nodes around the middle lobe requires the addition of a middle lobectomy, necessitating a bilobectomy for complete resection. In upper lobectomy, any lymph involvement proximal to the upper lobe takeoff along the mainstem bronchi requires consideration of sleeve resection or pneumonectomy, as does involvement of the lymph nodes around the main pulmonary artery. In all instances, the surgeon must remember that there is only one chance to cure the patient, and a complete resection is required for this.

Local Recurrence Following Initial Pulmonary Resection

Following surgical resection for lung cancer, the majority of patients do recur, especially those proven to have greater than stage I disease. No matter the stage of disease, approximately two thirds of recurrences are in distant sites, but one third are initially local. In most patients, unfortunately, local recurrence is a very poor prognostic sign and the patient ultimately succumbs to his or her disease. When these patients are symptomatic, surgical interventions can afford palliation. In highly selected patients, the local recurrence can be resected with a hope of ultimate cure if there is no evidence of significant regional or widespread metastases. Unfortunately, in most instances, locally recurrent disease cannot be completely excised, and, in the majority of patients, surgery is not an option. Before a curative surgical approach is considered for the rare patient who warrants it, an extensive search for occult regional and distant metastases is mandatory.

Tumors can recur locally within the remaining lung parenchyma following limited resection; endobronchially (in the residual stump); in the node, pleura, and chest wall; pericardially; and, as a solitary metastasis in the remaining lobe.

Local Recurrence Following Limited Resection

A limited resection (less than lobectomy) is usually reserved for patients who cannot tolerate a larger procedure. Unfortunately, following such a limited resection, there is an increased rate of local recurrence. Except for those with severe restrictive disease, most patients can tolerate a lobectomy despite even poor pulmonary function. When a local resectable recurrence does occur, serious consideration should be given to reoperation and completion lobectomy. At thoracotomy, if this is not possible, the surgeon has the option of working with the radiotherapy team to apply brachytherapy to the local area. This can be augmented postoperatively with external beam radiotherapy.

Endobronchial Recurrence

On occasion, endobronchial recurrences at the stump of the previous resection are limited to the mucosa and submucosa rather than occurring in peribronchial lymphatics, which augurs a much poorer prognosis and is usually accompanied by more proximal lymphatic involvement. Endobronchial recurrences can be treated locally using photodynamic therapy or brachytherapy; alternatively, in selected postlobectomy patients, a sleeve resection or completion pneumonectomy may be indicated. Although the morbidity and mortality of completion pneumonectomy are somewhat higher than with primary pneumonectomy, it certainly is worthwhile in selected patients and can be curative. In recent series, the postoperative mortality for completion pneumonectomy ranges from 0% to 15%, and 5-year survival averages 25%. There appears to be no difference whether the operation was performed for locally recurrent disease or for a second primary tumor (Table 32–5). On rare occasions, following pneumonectomy, re-resection of the bronchial stump may be worthwhile—this usually requires a concomitant carinal resection. The procedure does carry a high postoperative mortality (up to 20%) and should be carried out only by experienced surgeons.

Nodal Recurrence

Following surgical resection, the remaining lymph nodes within the hilum or within the mediastinum can harbor occult metastases, and recurrences can be isolated to these areas. On very rare occasions, the recurrence is limited to intraparenchymal or hilar lymph nodes. If this can be proved with noninvasive or invasive staging (PET scan and mediastinoscopy) and disease has not recurred in mediastinal lymph nodes, a completion pneumonectomy can be considered with the hope of ultimate cure. In such patients, induction therapies prior to resection or postoperative adjuvant therapies may be beneficial, although this is not known. On very rare occasions, mediastinal nodal recurrence can be treated surgically with some expectation of complete disease control. In these cases, combined modality therapy is usually employed.

When nodal recurrence presents as a symptomatic recurrent nerve palsy, consideration should be given to augment the affected vocal cord (see Chapter 16). This will have an exceptionally salutary effect on the patient's

TABLE 32–5 ■ **Mortality and Actuarial 5-Yr Survival Following Completion Pneumonectomy for Recurrent or Second Primary Lung Cancer**

Author	*No. Patients*	*Mortality*	*5-Yr Survival*
McGovern (1988)	84	9.4%	26.4%
Gregoire (1993)	41	11.6%	33%
Terzi (1995)	32	3.6%	28.7%
Al-Kattan (1995)	26	0%	23%
Verhagen (1996)	33	15.2%	18.3%
Muysoms (1998)	76	13.2%	32.3%
Regnard (1999)	62	5%	35%

general well-being by improving speech, the ability to cough, and the ability to ventilate properly.

Most instances of nodal recurrence present in the mediastinum or supraclavicular regions with massive involvement. Such patients may have symptoms related to tracheal, esophageal, or superior vena caval compression. With all of these complications, endoluminal stenting may offer relief and is usually combined with, or follows, radiotherapy treatment.

Pleural and Chest Wall Recurrence

Apparent solitary pleural and chest wall recurrences usually augur a more diffuse process within the pleural space. The most common indication for surgical management of a pleural recurrence is the development of a malignant pleural effusion significant enough to cause symptoms. In such instances, pleural drainage and pleurodesis are often worthwhile if the residual lung is expandable. More recently, ambulatory pleural drainage has been advocated as the simplest approach. In many cases, because of the previous surgery, the patient will require a general anesthetic and proper placement of chest tubes to achieve permanent pleurodesis, rather than a bedside approach. If the lung cannot be expanded following drainage, ambulatory pleural catheters can be used to relieve symptoms. On rare occasions, a truly solitary pleural or chest wall recurrence may warrant resection in the hope of cure, but in most instances, local radiotherapy is the treatment of choice.

Solitary Ipsilateral Pulmonary Metastases

Following resection that is less extensive than pneumonectomy, a solitary nodule may appear in the residual lung. This may represent a second primary tumor or a metastasis. No matter the etiology, it is our belief that these patients should be considered for curative re-resection, which often necessitates completion pneumonectomy.

SUMMARY

Most patients presenting with local recurrent disease will be found to have concurrent metastatic disease as well. However, on occasion, the local recurrence may be isolated, can be treated with curative intent, and may require a re-resection. For those patients with locally recurrent disease that causes symptoms, surgical approaches may be necessary for palliation.

COMMENTS AND CONTROVERSIES

Role of Thoracoscopic Surgery

The role of video-assisted thoracoscopic surgery in the management of lung cancer is still being investigated in many centers; in other centers, it has been accepted for the management of T1–2N0 tumors. In those centers where standard oncologic techniques are being used, the early and midterm results appear favorable. However, the value of this technique in decreasing postoperative pain and promoting early discharge from hospital has, as yet, been unproven. It is still a concern of ours that there is a temptation to do less when a minimal access operation is performed. When mediastinal lymph node dissection is required (e.g., hilar N1 disease), thoracoscopic approaches have proved to be very difficult and time consuming. There continue to be reports of local recurrences in port sites and access incisions, despite steps taken to avoid this problem. When a lesser resection is required, we certainly prefer segmentectomy, which can be a daunting procedure when performed thoracoscopically. If this approach is to be used, surgeons should always respect the oncologic principles that have been developed over the past 50 years (see Surgical Principles in this chapter).

Induction Chemotherapy in Patients With Earlier Stage Disease and Poor Prognosis

The result of surgical resection for stage II disease and stage I disease with poor prognosis (e.g., T2N0) have led investigators to evaluate the role of adjuvant chemotherapy and radiotherapy for these patients. Neither approach appears to be beneficial, although postoperative radiotherapy decreases local recurrence rates. The long-term survival of such patients is not affected by adjuvant treatment. With the encouraging results of induction therapy in more advanced disease, investigation of the role of such treatment in these earlier stage tumors with poor prognosis is currently under way in North America and Europe, following encouraging reports of a North American phase II trial (Pisters et al, 2000) and a European phase III trial (Depierre et al, 1999).

Mediastinal Lymph Node Dissection

There is no doubt that routine mediastinal lymph node dissections provide the best surgical staging at the time of operation and may on occasion contribute to long-term survival in patients with occult N2 disease. A current North American trial may ultimately resolve the role of routine mediastinal lymph node dissection (vs sampling) in early-stage, including N0 and nonhilar N1, tumors. In hilar N1 and N2 disease, mediastinal lymphadenectomy is advised and is supported by a recent report of a North American intergroup trial (Keller et al, 2000). The result of extending this lymph node dissection in patients with N2 disease to include two-field lymphadenectomies (mediastinal and cervical) is being explored by our Japanese colleagues (Hata, 1988; Naruke, 1988b; Watanabe, 1988; Hata, personal communication, 2000). On occasion, it does appear that, with occult N3 disease, long-term survival using this approach is possible. Most patients, however, are also treated with adjuvant chemoradiotherapy. Whether or not surgical treatment of N3 disease by induction chemotherapy, chemoradiotherapy, or extended lymphadenectomy will ever be proved to be beneficial for patients is unknown (see previous discussion of N3 disease in this chapter).

R. J. G.

KEY REFERENCES

AJCC Cancer Staging Manual, Chap 19, 5th ed. Philadelphia, Lippincott-Raven, 1997.

Cortese DA, Edell ES, Kinsey JH: Photodynamic therapy for early stage squamous cell carcinoma of the lung. Mayo Clin Proc 72:595, 1997.

Errett LE, Wilson J, Chiu RC, Monroe DD: Wedge resection as an alternative procedure for peripheral bronchogenic carcinoma in poor-risk patients. J Thorac Cardiovasc Surg 90:656, 1985.

Lung Cancer Study Group (Prepared by Robert J. Ginsberg and Lawrence V. Rubinstein, PhD): Randomized trial of lobectomy versus limited resection for T1 N0 non-small cell lung cancer. Ann Thorac Surg 60:615, 1995.

Martini N, Bains MS, Burt ME et al: Incidence of local recurrence and second primary tumors in resected stage I lung cancer. J Thorac Cardiovasc Surg 109:120, 1995.

Martini N, Burt ME, Bains MS et al: Survival after resection in stage II non-small cell lung cancer. Ann Thorac Surg 54:460, 1992.

Miller JI, Hatcher CR: Limited resection of bronchogenic carcinoma in the patient with marked impairment of pulmonary function. Ann Thorac Surg 44:340, 1987.

Non–Small Cell Collaborative Group: Chemotherapy in non-small cell lung cancer: A meta analysis using updated data on individual patients from 52 randomized clinical trials. BMJ 311:899, 1995.

Postoperative radiotherapy in non-small-cell lung cancer: Systematic review and meta-analysis of individual patient data from nine randomized controlled trials. PORT meta-analysis Trialists Group. Lancet 352:257, 1998.

Van Raemdonck DE, Schneider A, Ginsberg RJ: Surgical Treatment for Higher Stage Non-small Cell Lung Cancer—"A Collective Review." Ann Thorac Surg 54:999, 1992.

These key references summarize the current concepts in the surgical treatment of lung cancer. They include the best treatment by stage and focus on multimodality therapy in the more advanced stages of disease. They should be valuable references for the practicing clinician.

■ REFERENCES

Abolhoda A, Martin J, Ginsberg R et al: Morbidity and mortality for pulmonary resections in lung cancer after induction treatment. Presented at the 9th World Conference on Lung Cancer, Tokyo, Japan, September 12, 2000.

AJCC Cancer Staging Manual, Chapter 19, 5th ed. Philadelphia, Lippincott-Raven, 1997.

Alison PR: Intrapericardial approach to the lung root in the treatment of bronchial carcinoma by dissection pneumonectomy. J Thorac Surg 15:991, 1946.

Al-Kattan K, Goldstraw P: Completion pneumonectomy: Indications and outcome. J Thorac Cardiovasc Surg 110:1125, 1995.

Allan CI, Smith FJ: Primary carcinoma of the lung with report of case treated by operation. Surg Gynecol Obstet 55:151, 1932.

Allard P, Yankaskas BC, Fletcher RH et al: Sensitivity and specificity of computed tomography for the detection of adrenal metastatic lesions among 91 autopsied lung cancer patients. Cancer 66:457, 1990.

American Cancer Society: Cancer Facts and Figures—2001. Atlanta, American Cancer Society.

Begg CB, Cramer LD, Hoskins WJ, Brennan MF: Impact of hospital volume on operative mortality for major cancer surgery. JAMA 280:1747, 1998.

Brunn HB: Surgical principles underlying one-stage lobectomy. Arch Surg 18:490, 1929.

Burkes RL, Ginsberg RJ, Shepard FA et al: Induction chemotherapy with mitomycin, vindesine, and cisplatin for stage III unresectable non-small-cell lung cancer: Results of the Toronto phase II trial. J Clin Oncol 10:580, 1992.

Burt M, Wronski M, Arbit E et al: Resection of brain metastases from non-small cell lung carcinoma: Results of therapy. J Thorac Cardiovasc Surg 103:399, 1992.

Burt ME, Heelan R, Coit D et al: Prospective evaluation of unilateral adrenal metastases in patients with operable non-small cell lung cancer: Impact of magnetic resonance imaging. J Thorac Cardiovasc Surg 107:584, 1994.

Burt ME, Pomerantz AH, Bains MS et al: Results of surgical treatment of stage III lung cancer invading the mediastinum. Surg Clin North Am 67:987, 1987.

Chardak WM, MacCallun JD: Pancoast tumor (5 yr survival without recurrence or metastases following radical resection and postoperative irradiation). J Thorac Surg 31:535, 1956.

Churchill E, Belsey HR: Segmental pneumonectomy in bronchiectasis. Ann Surg 109:481, 1939.

Churchill ED: The surgical treatment of carcinoma of the lung. J Thorac Surg 2:254, 1933.

Coleman FP: Primary carcinoma of the lung with invasion of ribs: Pneumonectomy and simultaneous block resection of chest wall. Ann Surg 126:156, 1947.

Cortese DA, Edell ES, Kinsey JH: Photodynamic therapy for early stage squamous cell carcinoma of the lung. Mayo Clin Proc 72:595, 1997.

Dartevelle P, Macchiarini P: Surgical management of superior sulcus tumors. The Oncologist 4:398, 1999.

Dartevelle PG, Chapelier AR, Macchiarini P et al: Anterior transcervical-thoracic approach for radical resection of lung tumors invading the thoracic inlet. J Thorac Cardiovasc Surg 105:1025, 1993.

Davies HM: Recent advances in the surgery of the lung and pleura. Br J Surg 1:228, 1913.

Depierre A, Milleron B, Moro D et al: Phase III trial of neoadjuvant chemotherapy (NCT) in resectable stage I (except T1N0), II, IIIa non-small cell lung cancer (NSCLC): The French experience (Abstract No. 1792). Proc ASCO 18:465a, 1999.

Deslauriers J: Involvement of the main carina. In Delarue NC, Eschapasse H (eds): International Trends in General Thoracic Surgery. Philadelphia, WB Saunders, 1985.

Deslauriers J, Brisson J, Cartier R et al: Carcinoma of the lung: Evaluation of satellite nodules as a factor influencing prognosis after resection. J Thorac Cardiovasc Surg 97:504, 1989a.

Deslauriers J, Ginsberg RJ, Dubois P et al: Current operative morbidity associated with elective surgical resection for lung cancer. Can J Surg 32:335, 1989b.

Dillman RO, Herndon J, Seagran SL et al: Improved survival in stage III non-small cell lung cancer: Seven-year follow-up of cancer and leukemia group B (CALGB) 8433 trial. J Natl Cancer Inst 88:1210, 1996.

Downey RJ, Martini N, Rusch VW et al: Extent of chest wall invasion and survival in patients with lung cancer. Ann Thorac Surg 68:188. 1999.

Edell ES, Cortese DA: Bronchoscopic localization and treatment of occult lung cancer. Chest 96:919, 1989.

Errett LE, Wilson J, Chiu RC, Monroe DD: Wedge resection as an alternative procedure for peripheral bronchogenic carcinoma in poor-risk patients. J Thorac Cardiovasc Surg 90:656, 1985.

Faber LP, Bonomi PD: Neoadjuvant treatment in locally advanced non-small cell lung cancer. Semin Surg Oncol 6:255, 1990.

Faber LP, Jensik RJ, Kittle CF: Results of sleeve lobectomy for bronchogenic carcinoma in 101 patients. Ann Thorac Surg 37:279, 1984.

Faber LP, Kittle CF, Warren WH et al: Preoperative chemotherapy and irradiation for stage III non-small cell lung cancer. Ann Thorac Surg 47:669, 1989.

Ferguson MK, MacMahon H, Little AG et al: Regional accuracy of computed tomography of the mediastinum in staging of lung cancer. J Thorac Cardiovasc Surg 91:498, 1986.

Gaissert HA, Mathisen DJ, Grillo HC et al: Comparison of survival and lung function following sleeve lobectomy and pneumonectomy for lung cancer. Presented at the 73rd Annual Meeting of the American Association for Thoracic Surgery, Chicago, April 25–28, 1993.

Ginsberg R, Rubinstein L, Lung Cancer Study Group: A randomized trial of lobectomy versus limited resection in patients with TIN0 non-small cell lung cancer. Ann Thorac Surg 60:615–622, 1995.

Ginsberg RJ: Surgery and small cell lung cancer: An overview. Lung Cancer 5:232, 1989.

Ginsberg RJ, Hill LD, Eagan RT et al: Modern thirty-day operative mortality for surgical resections in lung cancer. J Thorac Cardiovasc Surg 86:498, 1983.

Ginsberg RJ, Martini N, Zaman M et al: The influence of surgical resection and intraoperative brachytherapy in the management of superior sulcus tumor. Ann Thorac Surg 57:1440, 1994.

Gould PM, Bonner JA, Sawyer TE et al: Patterns of failure and overall survival in patients with completely resected T3 N0 M0 non-small cell lung cancer. Int J Radia Oncol Biol Phys. 45:91–5, 1999.

Graham EA, Singer JJ: Successful removal of the entire lung for carcinoma of the bronchus. JAMA 101:1371, 1933.

Gralla RJ, Kris MG, Martini N et al: Adjuvant chemotherapy approaches in non-small cell lung cancer. In Salmon SE (ed): Adjuvant Therapy of Cancer. Orlando, Grune & Stratton, 1987.

Graves WG, Martinez MJ, Carter PL et al: The value of computed tomography in staging bronchogenic carcinoma: A changing role for mediastinoscopy. Ann Thorac Surg 40:57, 1985.

Gregoire J, Deslauriers J, Guodin L, Rouleau J: Indications, risks, and results of completion pneumonectomy. J Thorac Cardiovasc Surg 105:918, 1993.

Hagan MP, Choi NC, Mathisen DJ et al: Superior sulcus tumors: Impact of basal control on survival. J Thorac Cardiovasc Surg 117:1086, 1999.

Hata E, Hayakawa K, Miyamoto H et al: The incidence and prognosis of the contralateral mediastinal node involvement of the left lung cancer patients who underwent bilateral mediastinal dissection and pulmonary resection through a median sternotomy [Abstract]. Lung Cancer 4:A87, 1988.

Hayata Y, Kato H, Konaka C et al: Photoradiation therapy with hematoporphyrin derivative in early and stage I lung cancer. Chest 86:169, 1984.

Henschke CI, McCauley DI, Yankelovitz DF et al: Early lung cancer action project: Overall design and findings from baseline screening. Lancet 354:99, 1999.

Higgins GA: Use of chemotherapy as an adjuvant to surgery for bronchogenic carcinoma. Cancer 30:1383, 1972.

Hilaris BS, Martini N: Interstitial brachytherapy in cancer of the lung: A 20-year experience. Int J Radiat Oncol Biol Phys 5:1951, 1979.

Hilaris BS, Martini N: Multimodality therapy of superior sulcus tumors. In Bonica J (ed): Advances in Pain Research and Therapy. New York, Raven Press, 1982.

Hilaris BS, Martini N, Wong GY, Nori D: Treatment of superior sulcus tumors (pancoast tumor). Surg Clin North Am 67:965, 1987.

Holmes EC, Gail M for the Lung Cancer Study Group: Surgical adjuvant therapy for stage II and III adenocarcinoma and large cell undifferentiated carcinoma. J Clin Oncol 4:710, 1986.

Hyman NH, Foster RS Jr, DeMeules JE, Costanza MC: Blood transfusions and survival after lung cancer resection. Am J Surg 149:502, 1985.

Icard P, Regnard JF, Guibert L et al: Survival and prognostic factors in patients undergoing parenchymal saving bronchoplastic operation for primary lung cancer: A series of 110 consecutive patients. Eur J Cardiothorac Surg 15:426, 1999.

Ichinose Y, Tsuchiya R, Kato H: Randomized trial of chemotherapy versus surgery for stage IIIA non-small cell lung cancer. Lung Cancer 29(Suppl. 2):173, 2000.

Izibicki JR, Thetter O, Habekost M et al: Radical systematic mediastinal lymphadenectomy in non-small cell lung cancer: A randomized trial. Br J Surg 81:229, 1994.

Jensik RJ: Miniresection of small peripheral carcinomas of the lung. Surg Clin North Am 67:951, 1987.

Jensik RJ, Faber LP, Kittle CF et al: Survival in patients undergoing tracheal sleeve pneumonectomy for bronchogenic carcinoma. J Thorac Cardiovasc Surg 84:489, 1982.

Jensik RJ, Faber LP, Milloy FJ, Monson DO: Segmental resection for lung cancer: A fifteen year experience. J Thorac Cardiovasc Surg 66:563, 1973.

Kaiser LR, Fleshner P, Keller S, Martini N: The significance of extramucosal residual tumor at the bronchial resection margin. Ann Thorac Surg 47:265, 1989.

Kato H, Okunaka T, Shimatani H: Photodynamic therapy for early stage bronchogenic carcinoma. J Clin Laser Med Surg 14:235, 1996.

Keller SM, Adak S, Wagner H et al: A randomized trial of postoperative adjuvant therapy in patients with completely resected stages II and IIIa non-small cell lung cancer: An Intergroup Trial (E3590) [Abstract No. 1793]. N Engl J Med 343:1217, 2000.

Keller SM, Adak S, Wagner H et al: The J. Maxwell Chamberlain Memorial Paper: Complete mediastinal lymph node dissection improves survival in patients with resected stages II and IIIa non-small cell lung cancer. Ann Thorac Surg 70:358, 2000.

Keller SM, Groshen S, Martini N, Kaiser LR: Blood transfusion and lung cancer recurrence. Cancer 62:606, 1988.

Kodama K, Doi O, Higashiyama M, Yokouchi H: Intentional limited resection for selected patients with T1N0M0 non-small cell lung cancer: A single-institution study. J Thorac Cardiovasc Surg 114:347, 1997.

Konaka C, Ikeda N, Hiyoshi T et al: Peripheral non-small cell lung cancers 2.0 cm or less in diameter: Proposed criteria for limited pulmonary resection based upon clinicopathological presentation. Lung Cancer 27:185, 1998.

Kris M, Cohen E, Gralla R: An analysis of 134 phase II trials in non-small cell lung cancer [Abstract]. In Proceedings of the IV World Conference on Lung Cancer, Toronto, Canada, 1985a, p 39.

Kris MG, Gralla RJ, Clark RA et al: Consecutive dose finding trials adding lorazepam to the combination of metoclopramide plus dexamethasone: Improved subjective effectiveness over the combination of diphenhydramine plus metoclopramide plus dexamethasone. Cancer Treat Rep 69:1257, 1985b.

Kris MG, Gralla RJ, Martini N et al: Preoperative and adjuvant chemotherapy in patients with locally advanced non-small cell lung cancer. Surg Clin North Am 67:1051, 1987.

Kulka F, Forai I: The segmental and apical resection of primary lung cancer. In Proceedings of the IV World Conference on Lung Cancer, Toronto, Canada, 1985, p 81.

Lam S, MacAulay C, Hung J et al: Detection of dysplasia and carcinoma in situ with a lung imaging fluorescence endoscopic device. J Thorac Cardiovasc Surg 105:1035, 1993.

Lausberg HF, Graeter TP, Wendler O et al: Bronchial and bronchovascular sleeve resection for treatment of central lung tumors. Ann Thorac Surg 70:367, 2000.

Liptay MJ, Masters BA, Freed BH, Bakshay AG: Intraoperative radioisotope sentinal lymph node mapping in non-small cell lung cancer. Lung Cancer 29(Suppl. 1):138, 2000.

Lung Cancer Study Group: Effects of postoperative mediastinal radiation on completely resected stage II and stage III epidermoid cancer of the lung. N Engl J Med 315:1377, 1986.

Lung Cancer Study Group: Postoperative T1N0 non-small cell lung cancer. Squamous versus non-squamous recurrences. J Thorac Cardiovasc Surg 94:349, 1987.

Lung Cancer Study Group (prepared by Robert J. Ginsberg and Lawrence V. Rubinstein): Randomized trial of lobectomy versus limited resection for T1 N0 Non-Small Cell Lung Cancer. Ann Thorac Surg 60:615, 1995.

Lynch TJ Jr, Clark JR, Kalish LA et al: Continuous-infusion cisplatin, 5-fluorouracil, and bolus methotrexate in the treatment of advanced non-small cell lung cancer. Cancer 70:1880, 1992.

Maggi G, Casadio C, Pischedda F et al: Combined radiosurgical treatment of Pancoast tumor. Ann Thorac Surg 57:198, 1994.

Magilligan DJ Jr, Duvernoy C, Malik G et al: Surgical approach to lung cancer with solitary cerebral metastasis: Twenty-five years' experience. Ann Thorac Surg 42:360, 1986.

Martini N: Rationale for surgical treatment of brain metastasis in non-small cell lung cancer. Ann Thorac Surg 42:357, 1986.

Martini N, Bains MS, Burt ME et al: Incidence of local recurrence and second primary tumors in resected stage I lung cancer. J Thorac Cardiovasc Surg 109:120, 1995.

Martini N, Bains MS, McCormack PM et al: Surgical treatment in non-small cell carcinoma of the lung: The Memorial Sloan-Kettering experience. In Hoogstraten B, Addis BJ, Hansen HH et al (eds): (UICC) Current Treatment of Cancer, Lung Tumors. Heidelberg, Springer-Verlag, 1988a.

Martini N, Burt ME, Bains MS et al: Survival after resection in stage II non-small cell lung cancer. Ann Thorac Surg 54:460, 1992.

Martini N, Flehinger BJ: The role of surgery in N2 lung cancer. Surg Clin North Am 67:1037, 1987.

Martini N, Flehinger BJ, Zaman MB, Beattie EJ Jr: Results of resection in non-oat cell carcinoma of the lung with mediastinal lymph node metastases. Ann Surg 198:386, 1983.

Martini N, Heelan R, Westcott J: Comparative merits of conventional, computed tomographic and magnetic resonance imaging in assessing mediastinal involvement in surgically confirmed lung carcinoma. J Thorac Cardiovasc Surg 90:639, 1985.

Martini N, Kris MG, Gralla RJ et al: The effects of preoperative chemotherapy on the resectability of non-small cell lung carcinoma with mediastinal lymph node metastases (N2M0). Ann Thorac Surg 45:370, 1988b.

Martini N, McCaughan BC, McCormack P, Bains MS: Lobectomy for stage I lung cancer. In Kittle CF (ed): Current Controversies in Thoracic Surgery. Philadelphia, WB Saunders, 1986.

Martini N, Melamed MR: Occult carcinomas of the lung. Ann Thorac Surg 30:215, 1980.

Mathey J, Binet JP, Galey JJ et al: Tracheal and tracheobronchial resections: Technique and results in 20 cases. J Thorac Cardiovasc Surg 51:1, 1966.

McCormack P, Martini N: Primary lung cancer. N Y State J Med 80:618, 1980.

McCormack PM, Bains MS, Beattie EJ Jr, Martini N: New trends in skeletal reconstruction after resection of chest wall tumors. Ann Thorac Surg 31:45, 1981.

McCormack PM, Bains MS, Martini N et al: Methods of skeletal reconstruction following resection of lung carcinomas invading the chest wall. Surg Clin North Am 67:979, 1987.

McGovern EM, Trastek VF, Pairolero PC, Payne WS: Completion pneumonectomy: Indications, complications and results. Ann Thorac Surg 46:141, 1988.

Mehran R, Deslauriers J, Guojin L et al: Survival related to nodal status after sleeve resection for primary lung cancer. J Thorac Cardiovasc Surg 107:1087, 1994.

Meyer JA: Indications for surgical treatment in small cell carcinoma of the lung. Surg Clin North Am 67:1103, 1987.

Miller JI, Hatcher CR: Limited resection of bronchogenic carcinoma in the patient with marked impairment of pulmonary function. Ann Thorac Surg 44:340, 1987.

Mitchell JD, Mathisen DJ, Wright CD et al: Clinical experience with carinal resection. J Thorac Cardiovasc Surg 117:39, 1999.

Mountain CF: The new international staging system for lung cancer. Surg Clin North Am 67:925, 1987.

Mountain CF: Prognostic implication of the international staging system for lung cancer. Semin Oncol 15:236, 1988.

Muysoms FE, de la Riviere AB, Defauw JJ et al: Completion pneumonectomy: Analysis of operative mortality and survival. Ann Thorac Surg 66:1165, 1998.

Nagasaki F, Flehinger BJ, Martini N: Complications of surgery in the treatment of carcinoma of the lung. Chest 82:25, 1982.

Naruke T, Goya T, Tsuchiya R, Suemasu K: Prognosis and survival in resected lung carcinoma based on the new international staging system. J Thorac Cardiovasc Surg 96:440, 1988a.

Naruke T, Goya T, Tsuchiya R, Suemasu K: Extended radical operation for N2 left lung cancer through median sternotomy [Abstract]. Lung Cancer 4(suppl):A87, 1988b.

Nielsen ME Jr, Heaston DK, Dunnick NR, Korobkin M: Preoperative CT evaluation of adrenal glands in non-small cell bronchogenic carcinoma. AJR Am J Roentgenol 139:317, 1982.

Non–Small Cell Collaborative Group: Chemotherapy in non-small cell lung cancer: A meta-analysis using updated data on individual patients from 52 randomized clinical trials. BMJ 311:899, 1995.

Oho K, Ogawa I, Amemiya R et al: Indications for endoscopic Nd-YAG laser surgery in the trachea and bronchus. Endoscopy 15:302, 1983.

Osterlind K, Hansen M, Hansen HH, Dombemowsky P: Influence of surgical resection prior to chemotherapy on long-term results in small cell lung cancer: A study of 150 operable patients. Eur J Cancer 5:589, 1989.

Pairolero PC, Arnold PG: Chest wall tumors. Experience with 100 consecutive patients. J Thorac Cardiovasc Surg 90:367, 1985.

Pass HI, Pogrebniak HW, Steinberg SM et al: Randomized trial of neoadjuvant therapy for lung cancer: Interim analysis. Ann Thorac Surg 53:992, 1992.

Patchell RA, Cirrincione C, Thaler HT et al: Single brain metastases: Surgery plus radiation or radiation alone. Neurology 36:447, 1986.

Patchell RA, Tibbs PA, Walsh JW et al: A randomized trial of surgery in the treatment of single metastases to brain. N Engl J Med 322:494, 1990.

Patterson GA, Ilves R, Ginsberg RJ et al: The value of adjuvant radiotherapy in pulmonary and chest wall resection for bronchogenic carcinoma. Ann Thorac Surg 34:692, 1982.

Paulson DL: Combined preoperative irradiation and extended resection for carcinoma in the superior pulmonary sulcus. In Bonica JJ et al (eds): Advances in Pain Research and Therapy. New York, Raven Press, 1982.

Paulson DL: The "superior sulcus" lesion. In Delarue NC, Eschapasse H (eds): International Trends in General Thoracic Surgery. Philadelphia, WB Saunders, 1985.

Paulson DL, Urschel HC Jr: Selectivity in the surgical treatment of bronchogenic carcinoma. J Thorac Cardiovasc Surg 62:554, 1971.

Pean J: Chirurgie des poumons. Discussion Ranc Chir Proc Verh Paris 9:72, 1895.

Pearson FG: Mediastinal adenopathy—the N2 lesion. In Delarue NC, Eschapasse H (eds): International Trends in General Thoracic Surgery. Philadelphia, WB Saunders, 1985.

Piehler JM, Pairolero PC, Weeland LH et al: Bronchogenic carcinoma with chest wall invasion: Factors affecting survival following en-bloc resection. Ann Thorac Surg 34:684, 1982.

Pisters KMW, Ginsberg RJ, Bunn PA et al (For the Bimodality Lung Oncology Team BLOT): Induction chemotherapy prior to surgery for early-stage lung cancer: A novel approach. J Thorac Cardiovasc Surg 119:429, 2000.

Pitz CC, Brutel de la Riviere A, Elbers HR et al: Results of resection of T3 non-small cell lung cancer invading the mediastinum or main bronchus. Ann Thorac Surg 62:1016, l996.

Postoperative therapy in non-small cell lung cancer: Systematic review and meta-analysis of individual patient data from nine randomized controlled trials. PORT Meta-analysis Trials Group. Lancet 352:257, 1998.

Price-Thomas C: Conservative resection of the bronchial tree. J R Coll Surg Edinb 1:169, 1956.

Raviv G, Klein E, Yellin A et al: Surgical treatment of solitary adrenal metastases from lung cancer. J Surg Oncol 43:124, 1990.

Regnard JF, Icard P, Magdeleinat P et al: Completion pneumonectomy: Experience in eighty patients. J Thorac Cardiovasc Surg 117:1095, 1999.

Rendina EA, Venuta F, DeGiacomo T et al: Induction chemotherapy for T4 centrally located non-small cell lung cancer. J Thorac Cardiovasc Surg 117:225, 1999.

Reyes L, Parvez Z, Nemoto T et al: Adrenalectomy for adrenal metastasis from lung carcinoma. J Surg Oncol 44:32, 1990.

Rosell R, Gomez-Codina J, Camps C et al: A randomized trial comparing preoperative chemotherapy plus surgery with surgery alone in patients with non-small cell lung cancer. N Engl J Med 330:153, 1994.

Roth JA, Fosella F, Komaki R et al: A randomized trial comparing perioperative chemotherapy and surgery with surgery alone in resectable stage IIIA non-small-cell lung cancer. J Natl Cancer Inst 86:673, 1994.

Rowland K, Bonomi P, Taylor SG IV et al: Phase II trial of etoposide, cisplatin, 5-FU and concurrent split course radiation in stages 3A and 3B non-small cell lung cancer (NSCLC) [Abstract]. Proc Am Soc Clin Oncol 7:203, 1988.

Rusch VW, Albain KS, Crowley JJ et al: Surgical resection of stage IIIA and stage IIIB non-small cell lung cancer after concurrent induction chemoradiotherapy: A Southwest Oncology Group trial. J Thorac Cardiovasc Surg 105:97, 1993.

Rusch VW, Giroux DJ, Kranton J et al: Induction chemoradiation and surgical resection for non-small cell carcinomas of the superior sulcus: Initial results of Southwest Oncology Group Trial 9916 (Intergroup Trial 0160). J Thorac Cardiovasc Surg 121:472, 2001.

Rusch VW, Parekh KR, Leon L et al: Factors determining outcome after surgical resection of T3 and T4 lung cancers of the superior sulcus. J Thorac Cardiovasc Surg 119:1147, 2000.

Salazar OM, Creech RH: "The state of the art" toward defining radiation therapy in the management of small cell bronchogenic carcinoma. Int J Radiat Oncol Biol Phys 6:1103, 1980.

Sandler MA, Paerlberg JL, Madrazo BL et al: Computed tomographic evaluation of the adrenal gland in the preoperative assessment of bronchogenic carcinoma. Radiology 145:733, 1982.

Sartori F, Rea F, Calabro F et al: Carcinoma of the superior pulmonary sulcus: Results of irradiation and radical resection. J Thorac Cardiovasc Surg 104:679, 1992.

Sauerbruch F: Die Operation Entfernung von Lungengesch-wulste. Zentralbl Chir 53:852, 1926.

Schaake-Konig C, Van Den Bogaert W, Dalesio O et al: Effects of concomitant cisplatin and radiotherapy on inoperable non-small-cell lung cancer. N Engl J Med 326:524, 1992.

Shah SS, Thompson J, Goldstraw P: Results of operations without adjuvant therapy in the treatment of small cell lung cancer. Ann Thorac Surg 54:498, 1992.

Shahian DM, Neptune WB, Ellis FH: Pancoast tumors: Improved survival with preoperative and postoperative radiotherapy. Ann Thorac Surg 43:32, 1987.

Shaw RR, Paulson DL, Kee JL Jr: Treatment of the superior sulcus tumor by irradiation followed by resection. Ann Surg 154:29, 1961.

Shennib H, Bogart J, Kohman L et al: Video-assisted wedge resection and local radiotherapy for peripheral lung cancer in high risk patients. CALGB 9335: A Phase II multi-institutional cooperative group study. J Thorac Cardiovasc Surg (in press).

Shepherd FA, Ginsberg RJ, Feld R et al: Surgical treatment for limited small-cell lung cancer. J Thorac Cardiovasc Surg 101:385, 1991.

Shepherd FA, Ginsberg RJ, Patterson GA et al: A prospective for adjuvant surgical resection after chemotherapy for limited small cell lung cancer. J Thorac Cardiovasc Surg 97:177, 1989.

Shields TW, Higgins GA, Lawton R et al: Preoperative x-ray therapy as an adjuvant in the treatment of bronchogenic carcinoma. J Thorac Cardiovasc Surg 59:49, 1970.

Spaggiari L, Solli P, Leo F: Tracheal sleeve and superior vena cava resection for bronchogenic carcinoma. Lung Cancer 29(Suppl. 1):135, 2000 (Abstract).

Stamatis G, Eberhardt W, Stuben G et al: Preoperative chemoradiotherapy and surgery for selected non-small cell lung cancer IIIB subgroups: Long-term results. Ann Thorac Surg 68:1144, 1999.

Strauss GM, Herndon JE, Sherman DD et al: Neoadjuvant chemotherapy and radiotherapy followed by surgery in stage IIIA nonsmall cell carcinoma of the lung: Report of a Cancer and Leukemia Group B phase II study. J Clin Oncol 10:1237, 1992.

Sugi K, Kaneda Y, Esato K: The identification of sentinel lymph node by staining in lung cancer patients. Lung Cancer 29(suppl 1):139, 2000.

Suzuki K, Nagai K, Yoshida Y et al: The prognosis of surgically resected N2 non-small cell lung cancer: The importance of clinical N status. J Thorac Cardiovasc Surg 118:145, 1999.

Takizawa T, Haga M, Yagi N et al: Pulmonary function after segmentectomy for small peripheral carcinoma of the lung. J Thorac Cardiovasc Surg 118:536, 1999.

Takizawa T, Terashima M, Koike T et al: Lymph node metastasis in small peripheral adenocarcinoma of the lung. J Thorac Cardiovasc Surg 116:276, 1998.

Tartter PE, Burrows L, Kirschner P: Perioperative blood transfusion adversely affects prognosis after resection of stage I (subset N0) non-oat cell lung cancer. J Thorac Cardiovasc Surg 88:659, 1984.

Taylor SG IV, Trybula M, Bonomi PD et al: Simultaneous cisplatin fluorouracil infusion and radiation followed by surgical resection in regionally localized stage III, non-small cell lung cancer. Ann Thorac Surg 43:87, 1987.

Terzi A, Furlan G, Terrini A, Magnanelli G: Completion pneumonectomy: Experience with 47 cases. Thorac Cardiovasc Surg 43:52, 1995.

Thomas PA, Piantadosi S, Mountain CF: Should subcarinal lymph nodes be routinely examined in patients with non-small cell lung cancer? J Thorac Cardiovasc Surg 95:883, 1988.

Thompson DT: Tracheal resection with left lung anastomosis following right pneumonectomy. Thorax 21:560, 1966.

Tiffet O, Davies T, Jenc O: Preoperative detection of the sentinel lymph node in non-small cell lung cancer with radioisotope and blue dye technique. Lung Cancer 29(suppl 1):138, 2000.

Tsubota J, Ayabe K, Doi O et al: Ongoing prospective study of segmentectomy for small lung tumors. Study Group of Extended Segmentectomy for Small Lung Tumor. Ann Thorac Surg 66:1787, 1998.

Twomey P, Montgomery C, Clark O: Successful treatment of adrenal metastases from large-cell carcinoma of the lung. JAMA 248:581, 1982.

Van Raemdonck DE, Schneider A, Ginsberg RJ: Surgical treatment for higher stage non-small cell lung cancer: A collective review. Ann Thorac Surg 54:999, 1992.

Verhagen AFTM, Lacquet LKMH: Completion pneumonectomy: A retrospective analysis of indications and results. Eur J Cardiothorac Surg 10:238, 1996.

Vogt-Moykopf I, Fritz TH, Meyer G et al: Bronchoplastic and angioplastic operation in bronchial carcinoma: Long-term results of a retrospective analysis from 1973 to 1983. Int Surg 71:211, 1986.

Wada H, Nakamura T, Nakamoto K: Thirty-day operative mortality for thoracotomy in lung cancer. J Thorac Cardiovasc Surg 115:70, 1998.

Warram J (collaborative study): Preoperative irradiation of cancer of the lung: Final report of a therapeutic trial. Cancer 36:914, 1975.

Warren WH, Faber LP: Segmentectomy vs. lobectomy in patients with stage I pulmonary carcinoma: Five year survival and patterns of intrathoracic recurrence. J Thorac Cardiovasc Surg 107:1087, 1994.

Watanabe Y, Ichihashi T, Iwa T: Median sternotomy as an approach for pulmonary surgery. Thorac Cardiovasc Surg 36:227, 1988.

Watanabe Y, Shimizu J, Oda M et al: Proposals regarding some deficiencies in the new international staging system for non-small cell lung cancer. Jpn J Clin Oncol 21:160, 1991.

Weigel TL, Kosco PJ, Dacic S et al: Fluorescence bronchoscopic surveillance in patients with a history of non-small cell lung cancer. Diagn Ther Endosc 6:1, 1999.

Williams DE, Pairolero PC, Davis CS et al: Survival of patients surgically treated for stage I lung cancer. J Thorac Cardiovasc Surg 82:70, 1981.

Yashar J, Weitberg AB, Glicksman AS et al: Preoperative chemotherapy and radiation therapy for stage IIIa carcinoma of the lung. Ann Thorac Surg 53:445, 1992.

CHEMOTHERAPY FOR NON–SMALL CELL LUNG CANCER

Frances A. Shepherd

Lung cancer is now the leading cause of cancer-related death for both men and women in North America (Boring et al, 1992). Adenocarcinoma, squamous cell carcinoma, and large cell anaplastic carcinoma, referred to collectively as non–small cell lung cancer (NSCLC), together represent more than three quarters of all pulmonary neoplasms. The relative proportions of these three histologic cell types have changed during the last two decades, and currently, adenocarcinoma is seen most frequently (in approximately 35% of patients), followed by squamous (30%), and large cell (10% to 15%). At the time of initial diagnosis, almost 50% of patients with tumors of these cell types have clinically detectable spread beyond the thorax, and a further 10% to 15% have locally advanced unresectable tumors. Furthermore, more than 50% of patients who undergo surgical resection have recurrences with either localized unresectable disease or hematogenous metastases. This means that more than 80% of patients with NSCLC are potential candidates for systemic chemotherapy at some time during the course of their disease. This represents more than 100,000 patients per year in North America.

HISTORICAL NOTE

Despite the large patient base for clinical trials, the role of systemic chemotherapy in the management of NSCLC remains one of the most controversial issues in medical oncology today (Vokes et al, 1991). The therapeutic philosophy varies from one extreme of chemotherapy for all patients (Buccheri, 1991) to outright therapeutic nihilism and the view that chemotherapy is unjustified outside a clinical trial (Haskell, 1991). Although this controversy was applied initially only to patients with advanced unresectable tumors, the incorporation of chemotherapy into combined modality therapeutic programs in early-stage resectable disease has broadened the debate to include virtually all stages of NSCLC.

The application of chemotherapy to NSCLC was reviewed more than a decade ago by Bakowski and Crouch (1983) and Joss and associates (1984). These authors identified ifosfamide, vindesine, cisplatin, and mitomycin C as the most active agents against NSCLC; until the 1990s, these agents formed the nucleus for most combination chemotherapeutic regimens. The first reports of single-agent activity against NSCLC appeared in the 1960s (Green et al, 1969). These observations quickly led to trials of combination chemotherapy, and in the mid-1970s, encouraging response rates of more than 40% were reported with a variety of regimens (Bitran et al, 1976; Chahinian et al, 1979; Eagan et al, 1977). Sadly, little has changed since that time despite the introduction of several new agents and classes of agents, and the overall contribution of chemotherapy to the prolongation of a patient's survival is modest in those with NSCLC.

■ *HISTORICAL READINGS*

Bailor JC, Smith EM: Progress against cancer! N Engl J Med 314:1226, 1986.

Vokes EE, Bitran JD, Vogelzang NJ: Chemotherapy for non-small cell lung cancer. The continuing challenge. Chest 99:1326, 1991.

PROGNOSTIC FACTORS

Tumor stage is one of the most important determinants of both prognosis and survival in NSCLC, and tumor staging has recently been revised to enable better stage-by-stage depiction of prognosis.

Although it is clear that stage is an important determinant of survival in NSCLC, several other prognostic factors have been identified that may have a significant influence on the natural history of the disease, the response to therapy, treatment-related morbidity and mortality, and survival. In all studies of chemotherapy for NSCLC, it is crucial, therefore, that the patient population in the trial be clearly defined and the prognostic variables identified that may have a significant impact on the results obtained (Takigawa et al, 1996). This is particularly important in the reporting of phase II trials, which represent the most common type of clinical trials for NSCLC published in the literature.

Prognostic factors in operable patients will be more important for future trials because chemotherapy is now being applied to earlier stages of NSCLC, as either adjuvant therapy following surgical resection or as preoperative induction therapy in locally advanced disease. An analysis of patients with stage I (including T1N1) disease from Lung Cancer Study Group (LCSG) trials showed that pathologic subtype and tumor-node-metastasis (TNM) stage were the strongest predictors for recurrence, whereas preoperative performance status and postoperative infection added importantly to the histologic type and TNM status with respect to the prediction of overall survival (Gail et al, 1984). Some, but not all, retrospective reviewers have suggested that the need for postoperative blood transfusions may have a negative effect on recurrence and survival (Keller et al, 1983).

A meta-analysis of 6247 patients entered in chemotherapeutic trials in NSCLC identified several variables that were important for the response to therapy (Donnadieu et al, 1991). The overall and complete response rates correlated strongly with stage or disease extent (limited disease, 39%; extensive disease, 25%). The response rates were significantly lower for single-agent chemotherapy than for combination chemotherapy, and the best results were obtained when combination chemotherapy included cisplatin, a vinca alkaloid, mitomycin C, or ifosfamide. A review of chemotherapeutic trials in 699 patients with stage IV disease treated by Eastern Cooperative Oncology Group (ECOG) protocols demonstrated lower response rates in patients with liver, bone, and bone marrow involvement and a poor initial performance status (Bonomi et al, 1989).

With respect to survival, almost all studies have confirmed that the extent of disease (stage) and performance status have a statistically significant impact on survival rate. Weight loss and an elevated lactic dehydrogenase (LDH) level have also been found to be significant, whereas age and histologic subtype do not seem to alter the survival rate significantly (Maki and Feld, 1991). Female sex has been associated with a longer survival in several studies (Ferguson et al, 1990; Maki and Feld, 1991). In a retrospective study of 478 men and 294 women with primary lung cancer, the survival time of women was found to be longer than that of men for all histologic subtypes and all stages of disease at presentation (Ferguson et al, 1990).

Most large series evaluating prognostic factors have focused on the clinical characteristics of the patients at presentation and the histologic subtypes of their tumors. For patients undergoing surgical resection, adequate tissue is frequently available for more sophisticated in vitro testing, and several laboratory parameters have now been identified that may provide prognostic information in certain subsets of patients. In a retrospective analysis of DNA content and ploidy in 146 cases of resected NSCLC, patients with diploid squamous cell carcinomas survived significantly longer than did those with aneuploid tumors ($P = .002$), irrespective of stage (Sahin et al, 1990). The tumor's proliferative activity, as measured by the thymidine-labeling index, was found to be prognostic in univariate analysis, although in multivariate analysis, stage was found to be significantly more important

(Alama et al, 1990). In some, but not all, studies, the presence of neuroendocrine markers (Berendsen et al, 1989) and the ability of tumor cell lines to be established in vitro have both been associated with an adverse prognosis (Carney, 1991, 1992; Stevenson et al, 1990). The identification of K-*ras* mutations in tumor cell lines has also been associated with shortened survival times, irrespective of the extent of disease (Mitsudomi et al, 1991). Enhanced *ras* expression, which was identified in surgical resection specimens analyzed immunohistochemically, was also found to correlate with shortened survival times (Harada et al, 1992). It has been observed recently that the survival time of patients with blood type A or AB who had primary tumors that were negative for the blood group antigen A was significantly shorter than that of patients with antigen A–positive tumors (Lee et al, 1991).

The degree of angiogenesis as measured by blood vessel density or number has recently been shown to correlate with survival, and poorer outcome has been seen in patients whose tumors are highly vascularized (Giatromanolaki et al, 1996). This is likely to be a more important pathologic marker of outcome as new antiangiogenesis agents are being developed for clinical use.

It is clear, therefore, that many variables other than the therapy selected may influence both the response and survival rates in patients with NSCLC.

AVAILABLE AGENTS

Although several dozen single agents have been evaluated during the last three decades, far fewer have demonstrated adequate activity to justify their continued use in combination regimens (Table 32–6).

Cisplatin and Other Platinum Analogs

Although other chemotherapeutic drugs have demonstrated higher single-agent activity than cisplatin, it remains an important drug in combination chemotherapeutic protocols (Bunn, 1989b). In phase II trials, response rates from 6% to 32% (average, 20%) were achieved when cisplatin was used alone in varying dosing schedules (Bakowski and Crouch, 1983). It may be administered in divided doses over 3 to 5 days, or as a single large dose of up to 120 mg/m^2 on a single day. The optimal dose and schedule remain controversial. At least two studies suggest that the high dose (100 to 120 mg/m^2) is superior with respect to both response rate (Donnadieu et al, 1991; Sculier et al, 1994) and duration of response (Gralla et al, 1981), but this was not confirmed in a recent study undertaken by the Southwest Oncology Group (SWOG) (Gandara et al, 1993). Cisplatin is important in the therapy of NSCLC, not only because of its significant single-agent activity, but also because it is associated with only modest myelosuppression and has demonstrated both in vivo and in vitro synergy with several other chemotherapeutic agents that are active against NSCLC. For these reasons, it forms the backbone of most combination regimens. Cisplatin can also be administered concurrently with thoracic radiotherapy without undue toxicity (Schaake-Konig et al, 1992; Soresi et al, 1988).

Other platinum analogs have been evaluated, including carboplatin, iproplatin, and zeniplatin (Bonomi et al, 1989; Bunn, 1989a; Green et al, 1992; Jones and Smith, 1991). These agents have low single-agent response rates. However, despite a response rate of only 9%, a prospective randomized ECOG study demonstrated significantly prolonged survival for a cohort of patients with stage IV disease who were treated with carboplatin alone compared with other combination regimens (Bonomi et al, 1989). Carboplatin is associated with less gastrointestinal toxicity, neurotoxicity, and nephrotoxicity, although it is more myelosuppressive than is cisplatin, and this may limit its usefulness in combination regimens.

TABLE 32–6 ■ **Single Agents with Activity in Non–Small Cell Lung Cancer**

- Agents with response rates >15%
  - Cisplatin
  - Epirubicin (high dose)
  - Ifosfamide
  - Mitomycin C
  - Vinca alkaloids
    - Vinblastine
    - Vindesine
    - Vinorelbine
  - Taxanes
    - Paclitaxel
    - Docetaxel
  - Gemcitabine
- Agents with response rates <15%
  - Carboplatin
  - Cyclophosphamide
  - Doxorubicin
  - Etoposide
  - 5-Fluorouracil
  - Methotrexate
- New or investigational agents
  - Camptothecins
    - CPT-11
    - Topotecan
  - Tirapazamine

Ifosfamide

Ifosfamide is an alkylating agent that can be used in significantly higher doses than its parent compound cyclophosphamide. Although it has been available for clinical use since the early 1970s, hemorrhagic cystitis, which was identified as the dose-limiting toxicity in phase I trials, limited the usefulness of ifosfamide until the introduction of the uroprotective agent, mesna. The role of ifosfamide in the therapy of lung cancer was reviewed recently (Eberhardt and Niederle, 1992; Johnson, 1990). It has been evaluated in varying doses and schedules, and as a single agent, it produces responses in more than 20% of patients.

Vinca Alkaloids

Vinblastine and vinorelbine are the vinca alkaloids most frequently used in combination chemotherapeutic regimens for NSCLC.

Vinorelbine is a semisynthetic vinca alkaloid (Depierre et al, 1991). Like other vinca alkaloids, it acts by inhibiting microtubule assembly. Its dose-limiting toxicity is leukopenia and neutropenia, but it appears to be less neurotoxic than the other vinca alkaloids. In phase II and III trials of untreated patients with NSCLC, response rates of 20% to 33% have been reported when the drug is given on a weekly schedule, starting at 30 mg/m^2. At this dose, granulocytopenia is the dose-limiting toxicity, and dose delays or reductions are required for approximately one third of patients.

Mitomycin C

Mitomycin C has demonstrated reproducible single-agent activity of 15% to 20% when given at maximal single-agent doses. Unfortunately, however, at these high doses, this drug has been associated with pulmonary fibrosis, cumulative marrow suppression, prolonged thrombocytopenia, and the hemolytic-uremic syndrome in a small number of patients. Pulmonary toxicity may be reduced by the administration of a steroid with mitomycin (Spain, 1988), and bone marrow toxicity may be avoided by reducing the dose and prolonging the interval between therapeutic courses.

Etoposide and Analogs

The epipodophyllotoxin etoposide has only modest activity when used as a single agent (Bakowski and Crouch, 1983; Donnadieu et al, 1991), but because of in vivo and in vitro synergy, it has been used extensively in combination with cisplatin and often in combination with radiotherapy (Albain et al, 1995; Friess et al, 1987). A prospective randomized trial demonstrated convincingly that a 5-day schedule was superior to a 1-day schedule of equal doses of etoposide given to patients with SCLC (Slevin et al, 1989), and so multiple-day dosing is also employed for patients with NSCLC.

Teniposide, another epipodophyllotoxin that is active against NSCLC, is not available in North America. In combination with cisplatin, teniposide produces response rates that are similar to those of etoposide-cisplatin combinations, but it is considerably more myelosuppressive (Splinter et al, 1996).

Taxanes

Paclitaxel is a novel cytotoxic agent that exerts its antitumor activity by inducing excessive polymerization of tubulin, thereby interfering with normal mitotic activity. In phase II trials of advanced NSCLC, paclitaxel showed consistent single-agent response rates of 20% or greater (Ettinger, 1993). It has been administered as a continuous infusion over 24 hours in doses up to 250 mg/m^2 every 3 weeks. Dose-limiting toxicities included neutropenia and peripheral neuropathy. Paclitaxel may also be administered over a shorter infusion time of 3 hours, or even 1 hour. Response rates appear to be similar with shorter infusion times, but the toxicity profile changes considerably. Myelosuppression is less severe, but neurotoxicity and myalgia increase substantially. In combination chemotherapy regimens, doses of 175 to 225 mg/m^2 are usually used.

Docetaxel is a semisynthetic taxane that has the same mechanism of action and a similar spectrum of activity as paclitaxel (Cortes and Pazdur, 1995). In phase II trials in which doses of 60, 75, and 100 mg/m^2 were evaluated, response rates of approximately 25% were seen in previously untreated patients, but no clear evidence of a dose–response effect was seen in this dosing range. The dose-limiting toxicity of docetaxel is myelosuppression. Nonhematologic side effects are usually mild. As with paclitaxel, premedication with corticosteroids is required to prevent allergic reactions. With prolonged use, docetaxel may cause edema and pleural effusions, but this toxicity may be lessened by corticosteroid administration.

Gemcitabine

Gemcitabine, 2′2′-difluorodeoxycytidine, a pyrimidine antimetabolite, is a new deoxycytidine analog that has shown considerable activity against NSCLC. In several phase II trials comprising over 600 patients, overall response rates consistently were 20% or higher (Shepherd, 1995). Gemcitabine produces only mild to moderate nausea and vomiting; grade IV myelosuppression is rare, and it does not cause alopecia. It is usually administered weekly for 3 weeks at a dose of 1000 to 1250 mg/m^2 followed by a 1-week rest period. A recent review of the phase II trials of gemcitabine showed that it was well tolerated and very effective in elderly patients (Shepherd et al, 1997); because of its favorable toxicity profile, it has been suggested as a possible alternative for the treatment of this population of patients with NSCLC.

Camptothecins

The camptothecins are a new family of natural products that exert their anticancer activity through inhibition of the enzyme topoisomerase I. In phase II trials of camptothecin-11 (CPT-11), response rates of 30% or greater were seen in previously untreated patients with NSCLC (Asakawa et al, 1991; Fukuoka et al, 1992). The dose-limiting toxicities of CPT-11 are leukopenia and diarrhea. The diarrhea may be quite severe, which may limit its usefulness in this patient population.

Topotecan has also been evaluated in patients with NSCLC, but the single-agent response rate of approximately 15% appears to be lower than that seen in patients with NSCLC treated with CPT-11 (Lynch et al, 1994; Perez-Solar et al, 1996).

Tirapazamine

Tirapazamine is a benzotriazine compound that exhibits differential toxicity for hypoxic cells. Under hypoxic conditions, tirapazamine undergoes one-electron reduction by cytochrome P-450 and P-450 reductase to a cytotoxic free radical. The free radical is believed to abstract hydrogen ions from DNA, thereby causing DNA strand cleavage and selective hypoxic cell cytotoxicity. Tirapazamine causes acute nausea and vomiting and diarrhea. Muscle cramping has been seen in some patients, as well as acute, and usually rapidly reversible, hearing loss. Despite the unusual ototoxicity seen with this agent, phase I and II trials have shown that it may be combined safely with cisplatin (Rodriguez et al, 1996).

Other Agents

Other agents with less than 10% single-agent activity include cyclophosphamide, lomustine, 5-fluorouracil (5-FU), methotrexate, doxorubicin, and epirubicin. Response rates up to 19% may be achieved with epirubicin in a high dose (135 to 150 mg/m^2), but this is at the expense of greater myelosuppression and potentially greater cardiotoxicity. These doses would not be suitable for incorporation into most combination chemotherapeutic regimens (Feld et al, 1992).

COMBINATION CHEMOTHERAPY

As is the case in other tumor types, response rates in NSCLC are higher when combination chemotherapy is used compared with single-agent therapy. It should also be noted that the response in most patients is a partial response. A complete clinical response is seen in only 10% to 15% of patients with localized disease and in less than 5% of patients with hematogenous metastases.

Although many chemotherapeutic regimens result in significant responses, the contribution of such therapy to the prolongation of survival remains controversial. In general, survival gains have been small in both locally advanced and disseminated disease trials. Even in the trials that have demonstrated a statistically significant prolongation of survival, it is questionable whether the short weeks or months gained are clinically relevant in view of the potential toxicity and cost of the therapy involved. In advanced disease, chemotherapy is never curative, and the survival curves remain exponential, with no sign of a "plateau" or "tail" on the curve. As chemotherapy is administered in earlier stages of NSCLC, combined modality therapeutic programs should not be considered successful if they result merely in a shift of the survival curve to the left, with prolongation only of the median survival but without an accompanying increase in the level of the plateau and cure rate.

At this time, it is fair to say that cisplatin still forms the cornerstone of most combination chemotherapeutic regimens that are active against NSCLC. However, cisplatin is associated with considerable toxicity, and is responsible for much of the cumulative debility that is seen in patients undergoing chemotherapy for NSCLC. The activity and toxicity profiles of the new chemotherapy agents introduced in the 1990s suggest that it may be possible now to develop new regimens that do not contain cisplatin. Such combinations are under phase I and II study, but have not yet been subjected to randomized phase III trials. Specific combination chemotherapy regimens are presented in more detail in the following sections, which discuss the application of chemotherapy to various stages of NSCLC.

ADJUVANT CHEMOTHERAPY FOLLOWING SURGICAL RESECTION FOR STAGES I, II, AND IIIA

The poor survival rates following surgical resection for patients with stage II and III disease have led several groups to investigate the usefulness of adjuvant chemotherapy after complete or partial resection of NSCLC. In general, to be effective in the adjuvant setting, combination chemotherapeutic regimens should result in response rates of greater than 50% in patients with advanced disease, and a significant proportion of patients should achieve complete clinical responses. The most active regimens result in responses in only 30% to 40% of patients with advanced disease, and complete clinical responses are rare. It is not surprising, therefore, that a major survival advantage has not been seen in most of the prospective randomized trials of adjuvant therapy to date.

The results from several prospective trials of adjuvant chemotherapy are summarized in Table 32–7. The LCSG was formed in 1977 to evaluate the role of adjuvant therapy after surgery for NSCLC. The trials undertaken by this group are particularly important because all patients underwent meticulous mediastinal node sampling at the time of surgery to allow for precise staging. The first chemotherapy trial of the LCSG evaluated postoperative cyclophosphamide, doxorubicin, and cisplatin (CAP) or immunotherapy with bacillus Calmette-Guérin (BCG) in patients with completely resected stage II or III adenocarcinoma or large cell undifferentiated carcinoma (Holmes et al, 1986). The recurrence rate was significantly lower in the chemotherapeutic arm. The median survival was approximately 7 months longer, and the 2-year survival rate was also greater, although this did not reach statistical significance by the two-sided log-rank test. This trial has been criticized because it did not have a no-therapy control arm.

In another trial, the LCSG also observed a benefit in patients with incompletely resected tumors who received postoperative CAP and radiotherapy compared with those treated with radiotherapy alone (Lad et al, 1988). Once again, the median survival time was prolonged by approximately 7 months, but the 3-year survival rate was equal in both therapeutic arms. The last LCSG study evaluated the usefulness of CAP chemotherapy following complete resection of early-stage tumors (T1N1 and T2N0) compared with no additional therapy. This study was disappointing because no improvement was seen for patients treated with CAP with respect to either the median survival or long-term survival time (Feld et al, 1993). The Finnish lung cancer group undertook a similar trial of adjuvant CAP chemotherapy in patients with early-stage (T1–3N0) NSCLC (Niiranen et al, 1992). In contrast to the last LCSG study reported by Feld and associates, this study did demonstrate a survival advantage for patients in the chemotherapy arm at 5 and 10 years (P = .05). The greatest benefit was seen in patients with T2N0 tumors, but because of the small number of patients in this subgroup, the difference did not reach statistical significance (72.5% vs 50.3%; P = .15).

The CAP regimen was expanded to include vincristine and lomustine (COPAC) in a multicenter French trial (Dautzenberg et al, 1995). At a minimum follow-up time of 6 years, no difference in either disease-free or overall survival was seen between the group who received thoracic radiotherapy alone and those who received three courses of COPAC followed by radiation.

When these trials were designed up to 20 years ago,

TABLE 32–7 ■ **Randomized Trials of Adjuvant Chemotherapy After Surgical Resection**

Author	*Stage*	*Treatment*	*No. Patients*	*Median Survival*	*Survival*		
					1 yr	*2 yr*	*3 yr*
Holmes et al, 1986	Completely resected Stage II–III	CAP BCG	62 68	23 mo 16 mo	75% 64%	41% 30%	— —
Lad et al, 1988	Incompletely resected Stage I–III	CAP-RT RT	78 86	20 mo 13 mo	60% 54%	41% 32%	24% 20%
Niiranen et al, 1992	Completely resected T1–3N0	CAP No Rx	54 56	5+ yr 7+ yr	— —	— —	67% (5 yrs) 56% (5 yrs)
Feld et al, 1993	Completely resected T2N0, T1N1	CAP No Rx	136 133	76 mo 83 mo	89% 88%	80% 73%	60% (5 yrs) 52% (5 yrs)
Ohta et al, 1993	Completely resected Stage III	VdsP No Rx	90 91	31 mo 37 mo	— —	— —	35% (5 yrs) 41% (5 yrs)
Dautzenberg et al, 1995	Completely resected Stage I–III	COPAC and RT RT	138 129	1.3/1.2 yr* 2.1/0.8 yr*	— —	38/36%* 54/22%*	17/19%* 34/6%*
Wada et al, 1996	Completely resected Stage I–III	CVUft Uft No Rx	115 108 100	— — —	— — —	— — —	61% (5 yrs) 64% (5 yrs) 49% (5 yrs)

*Stage I–II/stage III.
BCG, bacillus Calmette Guerin; CAP, cyclophosphamide, doxorubicin, cisplatin; COPAC, cyclophosphamide, doxorubicin, cisplatin, vincristine, lomustine; CVUft, cisplatin, vindesine, tegafur, uracil; No Rx, no treatment control arm; RT, radiotherapy; Uft, tegafur, uracil; VdsP, vindesine, cisplatin.

CAP chemotherapy was the most active regimen available for the treatment of non–small cell lung cancer. However, a National Cancer Institute of Canada (NCI-C) study demonstrated a higher response rate and longer survival for patients with advanced disease who received vindesine and high-dose cisplatin compared with CAP (Rapp et al, 1988). In a Japanese study (Wada et al, 1996), three cycles of vindesine and low-dose cisplatin, 50 mg/m^2, were administered, followed by 1 year of tegafur and uracil. The control arms received either 1 year of uracil alone or no therapy. The 5-year survival rates for the chemotherapy and uracil groups were 60.6% and 64.1%, respectively, compared with 49% for the no-treatment group (P = .053, log-rank, and P = .044, Wilcoxon). A comparison of the overall survival of the two treatment arms combined with that of the surgery-alone group showed a significant advantage for treatment (P = .022). In another Japanese trial limited to patients with completely resected stage III tumors, postoperative vindesine and cisplatin was compared with no further treatment (Ohta et al, 1993). These results were similar to those of the LCSG trials in that the median survival was prolonged by approximately 6 months, but long-term survival was not significantly improved (5-year rates of 41% and 35%). Other platinum-based regimens have been evaluated by the National Kyushu Cancer Center in Japan, but no improvement in median survival or overall survival was seen in the trial (Ichinose et al, 1991).

ECOG, SWOG, and Radiation Therapy Oncology Group (RTOG) have just completed a trial of postoperative etoposide and cisplatin plus radiotherapy versus radiotherapy alone in patients with completely resected stages II and IIIA non–small cell lung cancer. This trial did not show any evidence of advantage to either arm (Keller et al, 2000).

Although these studies demonstrated a definite biologic effect for adjuvant chemotherapy, the survival gains have been modest at best, and frequently, the benefit was reflected only in median survival, without a long-term benefit. In addition, the CAP generation of studies encountered significant problems with both patient and physician compliance, with the result that only half of the intended chemotherapy was actually administered in most of the trials. Because most of the trials were relatively small, they lacked the statistical power to show significant differences. To determine whether small but meaningful survival gains could actually be attributed to the administration of chemotherapy after surgery, a large meta-analysis was performed by the Non–Small Cell Lung Cancer Collaborative Group (1995). To evaluate the addition of chemotherapy to surgery, 14 trials, which included 4357 patients, were studied. The results for the use of long-term alkylating agents were negative with a combined hazard ratio of 1.15 (P = .005). However, for regimens that contained cisplatin, the overall hazard ratio was 0.87 (P = .08), with an absolute benefit from chemotherapy of 3% at 2 years and 5% at 5 years. When chemotherapy was added to surgery plus thoracic irradiation, the benefits were less, with an overall hazard ratio of 0.94 (P = .46) and a 2% survival benefit at both 2 and 5 years.

Several groups currently are evaluating the usefulness of adjuvant chemotherapy for completely resected non–small cell lung cancer, and despite the results presented earlier, this is justified for several reasons. First, since the CAP or vindesine and cisplatin studies of the 1970s and 1980s, the introduction of the serotonin ($5HT_3$) antagonist class of drugs has changed the delivery of cisplatin-based chemotherapy dramatically. These new agents are much more effective at controlling chemotherapy-induced emesis, and therefore, may improve patient compliance in the current adjuvant chemotherapy trials. The second reason to continue to evaluate adjuvant chemotherapy is the availability of more active agents and chemotherapy combinations within the last decade. Some of these regimens have already been shown to be superior to previous combinations of cisplatin with either an epipodophyllotoxin (Bonomi et al, 1996; Giaccone et al, 1996) or a vinca alkaloid (Le Chevalier et al, 1996). At least three large randomized trials of adjuvant chemotherapy have now completed accrual in Europe and North America and await survival analysis in the next 2 to 3 years.

Induction Chemotherapy and Surgery

Although radiation with or without chemotherapy is standard therapy for patients with "unresectable" locally advanced tumors, there has been recent interest in combined modality treatment programs of chemotherapy followed by surgery. Neoadjuvant or induction chemotherapy before surgery has theoretical appeal for several reasons. Response to chemotherapy may allow an otherwise unresectable tumor to be surgically resected. However, this should not be viewed as the primary goal of treatment because other treatment modalities can achieve local control and most patients die of distant failure. If this form of combined modality treatment is to result in a significant prolongation of long-term survival, it will likely be as a result of eradication of micrometastatic tumor deposits. Surgical resection following chemotherapy provides a true pathologic assessment of response to induction therapy, which may be used to guide subsequent treatment. In a sense, the preoperative treatment may be viewed as an "in vivo chemosensitivity test," with postoperative chemotherapy recommended only for those patients who demonstrate a response to their initial treatment.

There have been several phase II feasibility trials of induction chemotherapy followed by surgical resection, and the results of these studies have been reviewed by several authors (Albain, 1993; Friedland and Comis, 1995; Johnson and Piantidosi, 1994; Shepherd, 1993). It is impossible for firm conclusions to be drawn from these trials because they included mixed populations of stage IIIA and IIIB disease, and even some patients with earlier stage tumors. Chemotherapeutic regimens were not standardized, and some patients had both combination chemotherapy and radiation before surgical resection. However, important observations may be made from these studies. The response rates achieved by these early-stage, good-performance-status patients were significantly higher than those seen with the same combinations administered to patients with advanced stage IV tumors. Responses ranged from 39% to as high as 76%, and complete pathologic response was documented in up to 15% of patients (predominantly with squamous pathology). Median survival ranged from 9 months to 30+ months with an average of approximately 18 months. This, on the surface, might appear to be better than the median survival of approximately 1 year, which is achieved with radiotherapy alone, but it should be emphasized that all of these studies represent a select subgroup of stage III patients, and that most patients with poor prognostic findings such as superior vena caval obstruction, involvement of mediastinal structures, and so forth, were excluded from these trials. Long-term survival and cure rates are much more difficult to interpret from the literature. The most optimistic interpretation would be approximately 25% to 35% survival at 3 to 5 years.

It is not possible to draw firm conclusions with respect to the optimal chemotherapeutic regimen to be employed as induction treatment before surgery. No single combination chemotherapy regimen nor any of the trials that administered both chemotherapy and radiotherapy have demonstrated apparent superiority with respect to response rate, complete resection rate, and median or long-term survival.

These studies all showed that induction chemotherapy before surgical resection is feasible, but the absence of standards with respect to patient selection, induction regimens, and reporting of results makes it impossible to compare these studies with historical data. The results of five prospectively randomized trials of induction chemotherapy and surgery have been published to date, and these have been summarized in Table 32–8. All of the studies were small with 60 patients each in two (Rosell et al, 1994; Roth et al, 1998), 57 in one (Elias et al, 1997), and only 31 (Shepherd et al, 1998) and 27 (Pass et al, 1992) in the others.

Although different chemotherapy regimens were used in the trials reported by Roth (1998), Rosell (1994), and Pass (1992), they all had similar results. Both median and 3-year survival rates were superior in the treatment arms, which included chemotherapy, and the differences were statistically significant in the trials reported by Rosell (1994) and Roth (1998). In fact, the differences were so great that a decision was made to close these two studies prematurely. Despite the similarity of results, these studies are not felt to be definitive for several reasons. In part because of the small sample sizes, both studies suffered from major imbalances in critical prognostic variables between the two arms. In the surgery-alone arm of the Roth study (1998), ten patients (31%) had stage IIIB tumors, and an additional three (9%) had stage IV tumors. This means that 40% of patients in that arm were not truly eligible for the trial compared with 11% in the combined modality chemotherapy arm, which included only three patients with stage IIIB tumors and none with stage IV. In view of the small sample size, this serious stage imbalance alone could have accounted for much of the difference in outcome. In the Rosell trial (1994), all patients had stage IIIA tumors, and both arms were well balanced for clinical prognostic factors. However, in the surgery-alone group, 42% of patients were found to have mutations of the *K-ras* gene, which is known to be a significant adverse prognostic factor, compared with only 15% of the patients in the combined modality arm. In addition, the survival in the surgery-alone arm was particularly poor with no patient surviving to 2 years. Based on many historical surgical series, this survival is very much less than would be expected in a population of potentially resectable patients with stage IIIA tumors, especially because several patients had T3N0 tumors without mediastinal node involvement.

TABLE 32–8 ■ **Randomized Trials of Induction Chemotherapy and Surgery**

Author	*Treatment*	*Number*	*Survival*		*P*
			Median	*Long Term*	
Pass et al, 1992	EP and surgery	13	28.7 mo	42% (3 yr)	.095
	versus				
	Surgery and Thoracic radiotherapy	14	15.6 mo	18% (3 yr)	
Rosell et al, 1994	MIC, Surgery, and Thoracic radiotherapy	30	26 mo	30% (3 yr)	<.001
	versus				
	Surgery and Thoracic radiotherapy	30	8 mo	0	
Elias et al, 1997	EP, Surgery, and Thoracic radiotherapy	23	19 mo	?	.64
	versus				
	Surgery and Thoracic radiotherapy	24	23 mo	?	
Roth et al, 1998	CEP and Surgery	28	22 mo	36% (5 yr)	.048
	versus				
	Surgery	32	14 mo	15% (5 yr)	
Shepherd et al, 1998	PV and Surgery	16	—	40% (2 yr)	n.s.
	versus				
	Thoracic radiotherapy	15	—	40% (2 yr)	

CEP, cyclophosphamide, etoposide, and cisplatin; EP, etoposide and cisplatin; MIC, mitomycin C, ifosfamide, and cisplatin; PV, cisplatin, vinblastine; n.s., not significant.

The results of a small aborted study from the Cancer and Acute Leukemia Group B (CALGB) have been reported recently (Elias et al, 1997). In this trial, patients received thoracic irradiation and surgical resection with or without chemotherapy with cisplatin and high-dose etoposide with growth factor support. Median survival for the chemotherapy arm was actually lower than that for the control arm (19 vs 23 months, respectively), although the differences were not significant ($P = .64$).

A small Canadian trial, which was also closed early, had a slightly different design. In this study, patients in the control arm received thoracic irradiation alone, and the study arm consisted of induction chemotherapy with high-dose cisplatin and vinblastine followed by surgery and postoperative chemotherapy. Although the median and progression-free survival rates showed a slight trend in favor of chemotherapy and surgery, 2-year survival was identical at 40% in each arm (Shepherd et al, 1998).

Results of a large French trial have been presented only in preliminary form (Depierre et al, 1994). In this trial, patients were randomized to proceed to immediate surgery, or to receive two courses of chemotherapy consisting of mitomycin, ifosfamide, and cisplatin followed by surgical resection and postoperative chemotherapy for responding patients only. It should be noted that patients with stage I (T2N0) and stage II disease were eligible for this study; they constituted more than 50% of the patients in the surgery-alone arm and, in this early report, this group appears to have a more favorable prognosis than those treated with surgery alone.

These trials certainly suggest that surgery alone may be inferior treatment for patients with potentially resectable lung tumors. They do not, however, tell us that induction chemotherapy followed by surgery is the best treatment for stage III patients. Several investigators have questioned whether surgery is necessary at all, and whether thoracic irradiation, either alone or combined with chemotherapy, might be equivalent to induction chemotherapy and surgery. Three large trials designed to answer this question are currently ongoing in Europe and North America. It will be several years before the results of these trials are available.

CHEMOTHERAPY FOR LOCALLY ADVANCED (STAGE IIIA AND IIIB) DISEASE

Up to one third of patients with non–small cell lung cancer present with disease that remains localized to the thorax but is thought to be too extensive for surgery with curative intent. Standard management for these patients with locally advanced stages IIIA and IIIB tumors is thoracic irradiation, which produces objective tumor regression in a significant proportion of patients. This almost always results in palliation of symptoms, but 5-year survival is usually 10% or less.

The observation that death for most patients with stage III tumors is caused by distant metastases has led to the development of combined modality treatment programs that incorporate chemotherapy. The intent of such treatment is to eradicate the micrometastatic deposits, which obviously are present at the time of initial diagnosis even though they are undetectable clinically. Chemotherapy has the potential to be most effective against these subclinical deposits because their growth kinetics should theoretically be faster than those of the primary tumor, which should increase their sensitivity to the effects of the drugs. In addition, chemotherapy has been shown to be more active against the primary tumor when it is administered at this early stage of the disease before drug-resistant clones have had a chance to emerge and metastasize. This is confirmed by the observation that response rates are almost 2-fold higher in patients with locally advanced disease compared with patients with clinically detectable hematogenous metastases.

In addition to causing the previously described systemic effects, chemotherapy may improve local control. Chemotherapeutic agents may act as radiation sensitizers when given concurrently with radiotherapy, and radiation has the potential to be more effective when administered sequentially to smaller bulk tumors that have responded to induction chemotherapy.

Chemotherapy and Radiotherapy

Several trials were performed in the early 1980s and 1990s to determine whether the sequential administration of combination chemotherapy followed by thoracic radiotherapy could prolong survival for patients with locally advanced non–small cell lung cancer. The results of some of the larger and more recent trials are summarized in Table 32–9. In one trial (Morton et al, 1991), a cisplatin-based regimen was not employed, and in another (Mattson et al, 1988), the CAP regimen included only low-dose cisplatin. In four studies (Dillman et al, 1990, 1996; Le Chevalier et al, 1992; Planting et al, 1996; Sause et al, 1998), high-dose cisplatin (100 to 120 mg/m^2) was used. In the European Organization for Research and Treatment of Cancer (EORTC) trial (Planting et al, 1996), the radiotherapy was delivered as a split course with 30 Gy in 10 fractions followed by 25 Gy in 10 fractions. In most of the other trials, the radiotherapy was uninterrupted at a dose of 60 Gy delivered over 6 weeks, and in the RTOG trial (Sause et al, 1998), there was also a hyperfractionated radiotherapy arm.

Even in the studies that employed high-dose cisplatin, the median survival in the chemotherapy arms was only in the range of 1 year. Furthermore, even though the prolongation of median survival achieved statistical significance in some of the trials, the actual survival gain was less than 1 month for two studies, approximately 2 months for three, and 4 months for the other. Two-year survival was similar in all studies and ranged from 12% to 15% for the radiation-alone arms, and 20% to 26% for the radiation and chemotherapy arms. No or minimal survival benefit was seen at 3 years and 5 years in most of the studies, and only two studies continued to show a small survival advantage beyond the 2-year mark (Dillman et al, 1996; Le Chevalier et al, 1992).

Concurrent Chemotherapy and Radiotherapy

The optimal sequence for the administration of chemotherapy and radiation for locally advanced non–small cell lung cancer has not yet been determined. The concurrent administration of chemotherapy and radiotherapy offers all the benefits of early administration of systemic treatment, with the added potential benefit of improved local control as a result of synergy between the chemotherapeutic agents and radiation.

There have been only two randomized trials that compared radiation therapy alone with radiation therapy with concurrent chemotherapy. In a study at the National Tumor Institute of Milan, patients were randomized to receive radiotherapy, 50 Gy in 28 fractions, or the same radiation with cisplatin, 15 mg/m^2 weekly (Soresi et al, 1988). Patients in the combination arm had a higher response rate (64% vs 50%), but no statistical differences were observed in disease-free or overall survival. In an EORTC trial (Schaake-Konig et al, 1992), patients were randomized to split-course radiotherapy, 55 Gy in 20 fractions, or to the same treatment with cisplatin, either 30 mg/m^2 per week or 6 mg/m^2 daily. Response rates in the three arms were similar, but the daily cisplatin group had significantly longer survival than the no-chemotherapy group (P = .009). The weekly cisplatin group was

TABLE 32–9 ■ **Randomized Trials of Radiation Therapy With or Without Chemotherapy for Stages IIIA and IIIB**

Author	Radiotherapy (Gy)	Chemotherapy	No. Patients	Median (mo)	Survival 1 yr	Survival 2 yr	Survival 3 yr
Mattson et al, 1988	55	—	119	10.3	41%	15%	11%
	55	CAP	119	11.0	41%	20%	7%
Morton et al, 1991	60	—	58	9.6	43%	12%	7% (5 yr)
	60	MACC	56	10.4	47%	23%	5% (5 yr)
Dillman et al, 1990, 1996	60	—	77	9.7	40%	13%	11%
	60	PV	79	13.8	55%	26%	23%
Le Chevalier et al, 1992	65	—	177	10.0	41%	14%	4%
	65	VCPC	176	12.0	51%	21%	12%
Sause et al, 1998	60	—	153	11.4	46%	—	5%
	60	PV	152	3.8	60%	—	8%
	60.9 HF	—	156	12.2	51%	—	6%
Planting et al, 1996	55	—	33	12.0	—	20%	0
	55	PVds	37	12.0	—	20%	8%
Soresi et al, 1988	50*	—	50	11.0	48%	40%	—
	50*	Weekly-P	45	16.0	73%	25%	—
Schaake–Konig et al, 1992	55*	—	108	—	46%	13%	2%
	55*	Weekly-P	98	—	44%	19%	13%
	55*	Daily-P	102	—	54%	26%	16%

*Thoracic irradiation administered concurrently with chemotherapy.
CAP, cyclophosphamide, doxorubicin, cisplatin; HF, hyperfractionated; MACC, methotrexate, doxorubicin, cyclophosphamide, lomustine; P, cisplatin; PV, cisplatin, vinblastine; PVds, cisplatin, vindesine; VCPC, vindesine, cyclophosphamide, cisplatin, lomustine.

intermediate between the other two groups and was not significantly different from either.

Studies of sequential and concurrent chemotherapy and radiotherapy are ongoing using some of the new chemotherapy agents now available. Phase I trials have shown that radiation may be combined safely with paclitaxel, docetaxel, gemcitabine, and vinorelbine tartrate (Navelbine). The CALGB is performing a very interesting randomized phase II trial of both sequential and concurrent administration of chemotherapy. All patients receive cisplatin and they are randomized to receive one of paclitaxel, vinorelbine tartrate, docetaxel, or gemcitabine. The cisplatin is given on days 1 and 22, and the other drugs on days 1 and 8, then 22 and 29. At the beginning of the seventh week, thoracic radiotherapy starts, and the same chemotherapy drugs are continued using the same schedule of administration, but with attenuated doses. Based on the results of this phase II trial, future phase III studies will be designed (Vokes et al, 1997).

Whether the concurrent administration of chemotherapy and radiotherapy is superior to sequential administration has been studied in only one randomized trial to date (Furuse et al, 1997). All patients received chemotherapy with mitomycin C, vindesine, and cisplatin either before or concurrently with thoracic radiotherapy. Thoracic radiation was administered as 28 Gy in 14 fractions followed by a 10-day rest period and another 28 Gy in 14 fractions. Three hundred fourteen patients entered the study, and the overall response rate was higher in the concurrent arm (84% vs 66%). Median (16.5 months vs 13.3 months), 2-year (37% vs 25.6%), and 3-year (27% vs 12.5%) survival times were all higher for concurrent therapy (P = .473). Marrow toxicity was higher with concurrent therapy, but this was not associated with an increased toxic death rate.

All of the studies discussed here showed improvement in both median and 2-year survival, but this was not always accompanied by prolongation of long-term survival or increased cure rates. Because most trials were relatively small, they may have lacked the power to show small but meaningful differences in survival, and so several groups have undertaken meta-analyses, which have been published recently.

The Non–Small Cell Lung Cancer Collaborative Group (1995) included trials of chemotherapy and radiotherapy for locally advanced disease in their extensive review of chemotherapy for NSCLC. According to data from only seven trials (807 patients), of which six used a cisplatin-based regimen, the overall hazard ratio of 0.98 was only marginally in favor of chemotherapy. For the six cisplatin trials, the hazard ratio was 0.94, with an absolute benefit of only 2% at both 2 and 5 years. Two other analyses, which included the results from 14 trials, had similar results. An Italian study (Marino et al, 1995) reported reduction in mortality at 1 and 2 years of 5% and 18%, but no differences were detectable at the 3- and 5-year points. Pritchard and Anthony (1996) also reported a slightly reduced risk of death with chemotherapy with a relative risk of death of 0.87 at 2 years. This corresponded to a mean gain in life expectancy for the entire group of 2 months.

CHEMOTHERAPY FOR ADVANCED DISEASE

The role of chemotherapy in advanced (stage IV) disease remains controversial to this day. Because patients are not curable at this stage, the primary goals of therapy must be palliation of symptoms and prolongation of survival. Response rate alone is an inadequate measure of the usefulness of combination chemotherapy. Response must be accompanied by meaningful prolongation of survival without unacceptable toxicity. Recently, it has been suggested that prolongation of median survival for only a few weeks is also not adequate justification for treatment, and that the success of chemotherapy for advanced disease should be based on the proportion of patients who achieve long-term survival of 1 year or longer. With the new agents and combinations that are now available, at least 35% to 40% of patients should achieve 1-year survival. However, it is recognized that a major proportion of patients may experience improvement in symptoms even in the absence of a 50% reduction in tumor mass (Ellis et al, 1995). Despite response rates as low as 25% to 30%, improvement in major lung cancer–related symptoms such as cough, chest pain and shortness of breath may be seen in as many as two thirds of patients.

There seems to be little doubt that response to chemotherapy is associated with prolongation of survival. Despite this, the overall contribution that chemotherapy makes to survival remains modest. There have been eight prospectively randomized trials of chemotherapy versus best supportive care for patients with advanced non–small cell lung cancer, and their results are summarized in Table 32–10 (Cellerino et al, 1991; Cormier et al, 1982; Ganz et al, 1989; Kassa et al, 1991; Perrone et al, 1998; Quoix et al, 1991; Rapp et al, 1988; Woods et al, 1990). In only the studies of Quoix and associates (1991), Rapp and colleagues (1988), and Cormier and co-workers (1982) were statistically significant prolongations of survival achieved with chemotherapy. However, it should be noted that in the Cormier trial, the patients in the best supportive care arm had a very short median survival of only 8.5 weeks. Furthermore, in the Rapp study, survival for patients in the high-dose cisplatin and vindesine arm was less than 4 months longer than that for patients in the control arm.

The most recent trial of chemotherapy versus best supportive care was limited to elderly patients over age 70 (Perrone et al, 1998). The treatment arm consisted of single-agent vinorelbine, 30 mg/m^2 days 1 and 8 every 3 weeks. Patients on chemotherapy had significantly longer median survival (27 vs 21 weeks) and 1-year survival rates (27% vs 5%, P = .04), and this was achieved without significant toxicity.

The Non–Small Cell Lung Cancer Collaborative Group (1995) also assessed the benefit of chemotherapy for advanced disease in their meta-analysis. Data were available from 11 trials and a total of 1190 patients. Eight of the studies used cisplatin in doses that ranged from 40 to 120 mg/m^2 and either a vinca alkaloid or etoposide. The analysis showed a benefit from chemotherapy with a hazard ratio of 0.73 (P = .095). Although the overall increase in median survival was only 1½ months, there

TABLE 32–10 ■ Randomized Trials of Chemotherapy versus Supportive Care for Patients with Advanced Non–Small Cell Lung Cancer

Author	Chemotherapy	No. Patients	Median Survival (wk)	P
Cormier et al, 1982	MACC	20	30.5	.0005
	BSC	19	8.5	
Rapp et al, 1988	VP	44	32.6	.01 (VP vs BSC)
	CAP	43	24.7	.05 (CAP vs BSC)
	BSC	50	17.0	
Ganz et al, 1989	VblP	22	18.6	.26
	BSC	26	14.4	
Woods et al, 1989	VdsP	97	27.0	.33
	BSC	91	17.0	
Cellerino et al, 1991	CEP/MEC	58	34.3	.135
	BSC	57	21.1	
Kassa et al, 1991	VdsP	44	22.0	.29
	BSC	43	16.5	
Quoix et al, 1991	VdsP	24	28	<.0013
	BSC	22	10	
Perrone et al, 1998	Vinorelbine	161 Total	27 (27% 1-yr)	.04
	BSC	All ≥ age 70	21 (5% 1-yr)	

BSC, best supportive care; CAP, cyclophosphamide, doxorubicin, and cisplatin; CEP, cyclophosphamide, epirubicin, and cisplatin; MACC, methotrexate, doxorubicin, cyclophosphamide, and CCNU; MEC, methotrexate, etoposide, and CCNU; VP, vindesine and cisplatin; VblP, vinblastine and cisplatin; VdsP, vindesine and cisplatin.

was an absolute increase in 1-year survival of 10%. This long-term survival benefit has not been confirmed by all authors. In a slightly smaller meta-analysis of seven studies and 700 patients (Souquet et al, 1993), chemotherapy was reported to result in a significant reduction in mortality at 6 months, but no benefit at 12 and 18 months.

Because of concerns that the small survival benefit seen in the combination chemotherapy arms of the Canadian trial might be associated with unacceptable financial cost, a formal economic evaluation of this study was undertaken (Jaakkimainen et al, 1990). It is interesting, and perhaps surprising, that this evaluation demonstrated that the use of combination chemotherapy *was* cost effective. This was due to the high costs of supporting patients in the supportive care arm, who actually spent *more* time in hospital than patients on either of the chemotherapy arms. Economic analyses of other clinical trials have also been reported (Smith et al, 1995). The European trial, which compared vinorelbine alone with cisplatin in combination with either vinorelbine or vindesine, showed a significant survival advantage for the cisplatin-vinorelbine arm over the other two arms at a cost of only U.S. $17,700 per year of life gained. The cost for vindesine-cisplatin was U.S. $22,100 per year of life gained. These two studies suggest, therefore, that chemotherapy should not be withheld for financial reasons from patients with non–small cell lung cancer.

Combinations incorporating some of the new chemotherapeutic agents have now been evaluated in randomized trials, some of which have been summarized in Tables 32–11, 32–12, and 32–13.

Although it is clear that chemotherapy exerts a biologic effect in patients with advanced non–small cell lung cancer, broad generalizations cannot be made for the treatment of this group of patients as a whole. Whenever possible, patients with stage IV disease should be treated on clinical trials of either new agents or new combinations of drugs. Continued research in patients with advanced disease is essential for identifying regimens that may have sufficient activity to justify their future use in patients with earlier stages of disease. At this time, chemotherapy is sufficiently active to justify its use in patients who want treatment and who understand its limitations. Treatment must be individualized and should be offered to patients who have the greatest chance to benefit from therapy and the least potential to develop toxicity. It seems that combinations incorporating the new agents are modestly superior to the standard regimens used until the early 1990s. Improvements have been seen in response rates, although on the whole, survival gains have been small. Some agents such as gemcitabine have resulted in response and survival rates equivalent to combination chemotherapy, but with significantly less toxicity. In a patient population in which the aim of treatment is mainly palliation, this could be viewed as an important improvement over current standard therapy.

COMMENTS AND CONTROVERSIES

New Drugs

The enthusiasm engendered by the spectacular phase II study results of the new agent combinations reported in the 1980s and early 1990s has now been tempered by the results of several multicenter randomized trials. It appears that the new agents provide response and survival rates that are modestly better than the combinations of the last two decades. Unfortunately, this improvement has been accompanied by significant increases in cost, with most of the new combinations falling in the range of $1000 to $2000 per cycle. Some of the new agents have demonstrated very favorable toxicity profiles, which may further enhance the therapeutic index of the new regimens and

TABLE 32–11 ■ **Randomized Trials of New Chemotherapy Combinations Versus Single-Agent Cisplatin**

Author	*Cisplatin Dose*	*Dose of Study Drugs*	*No. Patients*	*Response Rate (%)*	*Survival*	
					Median	*1-Yr*
Wozniak et al, 1998	100 mg/m²	None	218	10	6 mo	16%
	100 mg/m²	Vinorelbine 25 mg/m² weekly	214	25	7 mo	35%
Sandler et al, 1998	100 mg/m²	None	154	10	32 wk	28%
	100 mg/m²	Gemcitabine 1000 mg/m²/wk × 3	155	32	39 wk	39%
von Pawel et al, 1998	75 mg/m²	None	219	14	28 wk	22%
	75 mg/m²	Tirapazamine 390 mg/m²	218	28	35 wk	33%
Gatzemeier et al, 1998	100 mg/m²	None	205	17	37 wk	32%
	80 mg/m²	Taxol 175 mg/m² (3 hr)	202	26	35 wk	35%

TABLE 32–12 ■ **Randomized Trials of New Single Agents Versus Standard or New Chemotherapy Combinations**

Author	*Cisplatin Dose*	*Doses of Study Drugs*	*No. Patients*	*Response Rate (%)*	*Survival*	
					Median	*1-Yr*
Depierre et al, 1994	None	Vinorelbine 30 mg/m² weekly	119	16	32 wk	10%
	80 mg/m²	Vinorelbine 30 mg/m² weekly	121	43	33 wk	15%
Gil Deza et al, 1996	None	Vinorelbine 30 mg/m² weekly	73	42	32 wk	—
	100 mg/m²	Vinorelbine 30 mg/m² weekly	89	42	41 wk	—
Le Chevalier et al, 1996	None	Vinorelbine 30 mg/m² weekly	188	14	31 wk	30%
	120 mg/m²	Vinorelbine 30 mg/m² weekly	182	30	40 wk	35%
	120 mg/m²	Vindesine 3 mg/m² weekly	179	19	32 wk	30%
Manegold et al, 1997	None	Gemcitabine 1000 mg/m²/wk × 3	72	18	6.6 mo	26%
Phase II study	100 mg/m²	Etoposide 100 mg/m² × 3	75	15	7.6 mo	24%
Perng et al, 1997	None	Gemcitabine 1250 mg/m²/wk × 3	27	19	37 wk	40%
Phase II study	80 mg/m²	Etoposide 80 mg/m²/wk × 3	25	21	48 wk	33%

TABLE 32–13 ■ **Randomized Trials of Standard Chemotherapy Combinations Versus New Chemotherapy Combinations**

Author	*Cisplatin Dose*	*Doses of Study Drugs*	*No. Patients*	*Response Rate (%)*	*Survival*	
					Median	*1-Yr*
Bonomi et al, 1996	75 mg/m²	Paclitaxel 135 mg/m² (24 hr)	189	27	9.6 mo	37%
	75 mg/m²	Paclitaxel 250 mg/m² (24 hr)	191	32	10 mo	39%
	75 mg/m²	Etoposide 100 mg/m² × 3	194	12	7.7 mo	32%
Giaccone et al, 1996	80 mg/m²	Paclitaxel 175 mg/m² (3 hr)	155	44	9.4 mo	41%
	80 mg/m²	Teniposide 100 mg/m² × 3	157	30	9.7 mo	43%
Belani et al, 1998	75 mg/m²	Etoposide 100 mg/m² × 3	179	15	39 wk	37%
	None	Carboplatin AUC 6	190	23	33 wk	32%
		Paclitaxel 223 mg/m² (3 hr)				
Le Chevalier et al, 1996	None	Vinorelbine 30 mg/m² weekly	188	14	31 wk	30%
	120 mg/m²	Vinorelbine 30 mg/m² weekly	182	30	40 wk	35%
	120 mg/m²	Vindesine 3 mg/m² weekly	179	19	32 wk	30%
Cardenal et al, 1997	100 mg/m²	Gemcitabine 1250 mg/m²/wk × 3	69	41	8.7 mo	32%
(Phase II trial)	100 mg/m²	Etoposide 100 mg/m² × 3	62	22	7.2 mo	26%
Crino et al, 1998	100 mg/m²	Gemcitabine 1000 mg/m²/wk × 3	155	38	37 wk	33%
	100 mg/m²	Mitomycin C 6 mg/m²	152	26	39 wk	34%
		Ifosfamide 3 g/m²				
Comella et al, 1997	50 mg/m²	Gemcitabine 1000 mg/m²/wk × 2	55	62	—	—
(Phase II trial)	weekly × 2	Vinorelbine 25 mg/m²/wk × 2				
		Epirubicin 60 mg/m² × 1	50	35	—	—
	60 mg/m² × 1	Vindesine 3 mg/m² × 1				
		Lonidamine 75 mg PO daily				

AUC, area under the curve.

may allow treatment of elderly or poor-performance patients who would previously not have been offered cisplatin-based therapy.

Adjuvant Chemotherapy

The large meta-analysis of the Non–Small Cell Lung Cancer Collaborative Group showed that adjuvant chemotherapy after complete surgical resection improves 5-year survival by approximately 5% in early-stage NSCLC. Despite this clear demonstration of benefit, adjuvant chemotherapy is not considered standard practice at this time. It is to be hoped that with more efficacious and better tolerated combination chemotherapy, the adjuvant trials that have closed recently now will confirm that adjuvant chemotherapy is justified and appropriate for NSCLC patients.

Combined Modality Therapy

It is clear that no single therapeutic modality, be it surgery, radiotherapy, or chemotherapy, is able to achieve cure for most patients with NSCLC. Whether combined modality therapy will be able to improve long-term survival and cure rates still remains undetermined. The addition of systemic chemotherapy to radiotherapy for patients with locally advanced disease has resulted in modest, but statistically significant, prolongation of survival times in some, but not all, trials. The magnitude of the survival benefit is small, but combined modality therapy has been adopted as standard practice for good-performance-status patients in most centers. The issue of the sequential versus the concurrent administration of chemotherapy and radiotherapy remains unresolved and awaits the results of some of the cooperative group studies currently under way.

Although phase II pilot studies confirmed the feasibility of induction chemotherapy followed by surgical resection for patients with locally advanced NSCLC, the role of surgery in stage III disease remains unclear. The phase III studies published to date have produced conflicting results. These studies all suffered from small numbers with some having major imbalances in critical prognostic factors between the treatment arms. Hopefully, the three large North American, British, and European trials that are currently active will provide the definitive answer to this important therapeutic question in locally advanced NSCLC.

F. A. S.

Since our last edition, many new drugs have demonstrated effectiveness in phase II trials in treating non–small cell lung cancer. In fact, it seems that the newer two- and three-drug combinations tested so far (usually platinum-based) are relatively equivalent. The only difference seems to be cost, patient tolerance, and, perhaps, morbidity. Occasionally, complete responses occur, and, in induction therapy trials, it is expected that 7% to 10% of patients will have a complete response at the time of surgery. Very few reports record chemotherapy as the only treatment used for a non–small cell lung cancer with a resultant total cure. Unlike radiotherapy and surgery, at this writing, chemotherapy alone cannot be considered curative treatment.

Despite the availability of new drugs, the overall management of non–small cell lung cancer following surgical resection has not changed significantly. The indications for adjuvant chemotherapy are still unclear. Large trials in North America and Europe, hopefully, in the near future, will finalize whether or not adjuvant therapy should be advised and at what resected stage of disease it should be advised. An interesting phenomenon in the adjuvant treatment of stage I disease is the positive result using oral 5-fluorouracil as described by Japanese investigators. This trial is being repeated in Japan and, hopefully, in North America in early stage disease. Perhaps low-dose chemotherapy for a prolonged period of time has a salutary effect. It does appear to decrease the incidence of second primaries in the only reported trial.

With newer biologic agents, a whole new adjuvant treatment strategy is being investigated—that is, adjuvant chemotherapy combined with biologic agents such as anti-angiogenesis factors and tyrosine kinase inhibitors. Hopefully, these biologic targeting agents will improve the adjuvant treatment of this disease, because, except for stage I tumors, fewer than 50% of patients survive 5 years following surgical resection.

In unresectable, locoregional disease, there is no doubt that chemotherapy plus radiation is better than radiation alone and is now the standard of care. In stage IV disease, median survivals are improving as we better understand supportive care that can minimize the toxicity of drugs, making chemotherapy extremely tolerable.

Now that the genome project has been completed, we are looking forward to using this information to help target therapy and improve the survival of resectable, locally advanced, and stage IV lung cancer.

R. J. G.

■ KEY REFERENCES

Donnadieu N, Paesmans M, Sculier J-P: Chemotherapy of non-small cell lung cancer according to disease extent: A meta-analysis of the literature. Lung Cancer 7:243, 1991.

These articles provide good overviews of prognostic factors.

Maki E, Feld R: Prognostic factors in patients with non-small cell lung cancer. A critique of the world literature. Lung Cancer 7:27, 1991.

Mountain C: A new international staging system for lung cancer. Chest 89:225S, 1986.

This article is important because it provides all the survival data that led to the new staging system.

Non–Small Cell Lung Cancer Collaborative Group: Chemotherapy in non-small cell lung cancer: A meta-analysis using updated data on individual patients from 52 randomized clinical trials. Br Med J 311:899, 1995.

This is the most important meta-analysis of chemotherapy for NSCLC.

■ REFERENCES

Alama A, Costantini M, Repetto L et al: Thymidine labelling index as prognostic factor in resected non-small cell lung cancer. Eur J Cancer 25:622, 1990.

Albain KS: Induction chemotherapy followed by definitive local control for stage III non-small cell lung cancer. A review with focus on recent trimodality trials. Chest 103:43s, 1993.

Albain KS, Rusch VW, Crowley JJ et al: Concurrent cisplatin etoposide plus chest radiotherapy followed by surgery for stages IIIA (N2) and IIIB non-small cell lung cancer: Mature results of Southwest Oncology Group phase II study 8805. J Clin Oncol 13:1880, 1995.

Asakawa M, Fujita A, Fukuoka M et al: Phase II study of CPT-11, a new camptothecin derivative in previously untreated non-small cell lung cancer [Abstract]. Lung Cancer 7:125, 1991.

Bailor JC, Smith EM: Progress against cancer! N Engl J Med 314:1226, 1986.

Bakowski MT, Crouch JD: Chemotherapy of non-small cell lung cancer: A reappraisal and a look to the future. Cancer Treat Rep 10:159, 1983.

Belani CP, Natale RB, Lee JS et al: Randomized Phase 3 Trial comparing cisplatin/etoposide versus carboplatin/paclitaxel in advanced and metastatic non-small cell lung cancer (NSCLC) [Abstract No. 1751]. Proc ASCO 17:455a, 1998.

Berendsen HH, de-Leij L, Poppemma S et al: Clinical characterization of non-small cell lung cancer tumors showing neuroendocrine differentiation features. J Clin Oncol 11:1614, 1989.

Bitran JD, Desser RK, DeMeester TR et al: Cyclophosphamide, Adriamycin, methotrexate and procarbazine (CAMP): Effective four-drug combination chemotherapy for metastatic non-oat cell bronchogenic carcinoma. Cancer Treat Rep 60:1225, 1976.

Bonomi P, Kim K, Chang A et al: Phase III trial comparing etoposide (E) cisplatin (C) versus taxol (T) with cisplatin-G-CSF (G) versus taxol-cisplatin in advanced non-small cell lung cancer. An Eastern Cooperative Oncology Group (ECOG) trial [Abstract No. 1145]. Proc Am Soc Clin Oncol 15:382, 1996.

Bonomi PD, Finkelstein DM, Ruckdeschel JD et al: Combination chemotherapy versus single agents followed by combination chemotherapy in stage IV non-small cell lung cancer: A study of the Eastern Cooperative Oncology Group. J Clin Oncol 17:1602, 1989.

Borges M, Sculier JP, Paesmans M et al: Prognostic factors for response to chemotherapy containing platinum derivatives in patients with unresectable non-small cell lung cancer. Lung Cancer 16:21, 1996.

Boring CC, Squires TS, Tong T: Cancer statistics 1992. CA Cancer J Clin 42:19, 1992.

Buccheri G: Chemotherapy and survival in non-small cell lung cancer: The old vexata questio. Chest 99:1328, 1991.

Bunn PA: Review of therapeutic trials of carboplatin in lung cancer. Semin Oncol 16(suppl 5):27, 1989a.

Bunn PA: The expanding role of cisplatin in the treatment of non-small cell lung cancer. Semin Oncol 16(suppl 6):10, 1989b.

Cahill A, White INH: Reductive metabolism of 3-amino-1,2,4-benzotriazine-1,4-dioxide (SR4233) and the induction of unscheduled DNA synthesis in rat and human derived cell lines. Carcinogenesis 11:1407, 1990.

Cardenal F, Rosell, R, Anton A et al: Gemcitabine + cisplatin versus etoposide + cisplatin in advanced non-small cell lung cancer patients: Preliminary randomized phase III results [Abstract 1648]. Proc Am Soc Clin Oncol 16:458a, 1997.

Carney D: Lung cancer biology. Curr Opin Oncol 3:288, 1991.

Carney DN: The biology of lung cancer. Curr Opin Oncol 4:292, 1992.

Cellerino R, Tummarello D, Guidi F: A randomized trial of alternating chemotherapy versus best supportive care in advanced non-small cell lung cancer. J Clin Oncol 9:1453, 1991.

Chahinian AP, Mandel EM, Holland JK et al: MACC (methotrexate, Adriamycin, cyclophosphamide and CCNU) in advanced lung cancer. Cancer 43:1590, 1979.

Comella P, Panza N, Frasci G et al: Gemcitabine (GEM)-cisplatin (CDDP)-vinorelbine (VNR) combination in advanced non-small cell lung cancer (NSCLC): A phase II randomized study [Abstract No. 1616]. Proc Am Soc Clin Oncol 16:449a, 1997.

Cormier Y, Bergeron D, La Forge J et al: Benefits of polychemotherapy in advanced non-small cell bronchogenic carcinoma. Cancer 50:845, 1982.

Cortes JE, Pazdur R: Docetaxel. J Clin Oncol 13:2643, 1995.

Crino L, Conte P, De Marinis F et al: A randomized trial of gemcitabine cisplatin (GP) versus mitomycin, ifosfamide and cisplatin (MIC) in advanced non-small cell lung cancer (NSCLC) A multi-centre phase III study [Abstract No. 1751]. Proc ASCO 17:455a, 1998.

Cullen MH, Joshi R, Chetiyawardna A: Mitomycin, ifosfamide and cisplatin in non-small cell lung cancer: Treatment good enough to compare. Br J Cancer 9:359, 1988.

Dautzenberg B, Chastang C, Arriagada R et al: Adjuvant radiotherapy versus combined sequential chemotherapy followed by radiotherapy in the treatment of resected non-small cell lung carcinoma. Cancer 75:779, 1995.

Depierre A, Chastang C, Quoix E et al: Vinorelbine versus vinorelbine plus cisplatin in advanced non-small cell lung cancer: A randomized trial. Ann Oncol 5:37, 1994.

Depierre A, Milleron B, Lebeau B et al: An ongoing randomized study of neoadjuvant chemotherapy in resectable non-small cell lung cancer. Semin Oncol 21(suppl l4):16, 1994.

Depierre R, Lemarie E, Dabouis G et al: A phase II study of navelbine (vinorelbine) in the treatment of non-small cell lung cancer. Am J Clin Oncol 14:115, 1991.

Dillman RO, Herndon J, Seagren SL et al: Improved survival in stage III non-small cell lung cancer: Seven-year follow-up of Cancer and Acute Leukemia Group B (CALGB) 8433 trial. J Natl Cancer Inst 88:1210, 1996.

Dillman RO, Seagren SL, Propert KJ et al: A randomized trial of induction chemotherapy plus high-dose radiation vs. radiation alone in stage III non-small cell lung cancer. N Engl J Med 323: 940, 1990.

Donnadieu N, Paesmans M, Sculier J-P: Chemotherapy of non-small cell lung cancer according to disease extent: A meta-analysis of the literature. Lung Cancer 7:243, 1991.

Drings P: European experience with ifosfamide in non-small cell lung cancer. Semin Oncol 26:294, 1989.

Eagan RT, Ingle JN, Frytak S et al: Platinum-based polychemotherapy versus dianhydrogalacitol in advanced non-small cell lung cancer. Cancer Treat Rep 61:1339, 1977.

Eberhardt W, Niederle N: Ifosfamide in non-small cell lung cancer: A review. Semin Oncol 19(suppl 1):40, 1992.

Elias A, Herndorn J, Kumar P et al, for the Cancer and Acute Leukemia Group B: A phase III comparison of "best local-regional therapy" with or without chemotherapy (CT) for stage IIIA Tl–3N2 non-small cell lung cancer (NSCLC): Preliminary results (Abstract No. 1611). Proc Am Soc Clin Oncol 16:448a, 1997.

Ellis PA, Smith IE, Hardy JR et al: Symptom relief with MVP (mitomycin C, vinblastine and cisplatin) chemotherapy in advanced non-small cell lung cancer. Br J Cancer 71:366, 1995.

Ettinger D: Overview of paclitaxel (Taxol) in advanced lung cancer. Semin Oncol 4(suppl 3):46, 1993.

Feld R, Rubenstein L, Thomas P (Lung Cancer Study Group): Adjuvant chemotherapy with cyclophosphamide, doxorubicin, and cisplatin in patients with completely resected Stage I non-small cell lung cancer. J Natl Cancer Inst 85:299, 1993.

Feld R, Wierzbicki R, Walde D et al: Phase I–II study of high dose epirubucin in advanced non-small cell lung cancer. J Clin Oncol 20:297, 1992.

Ferguson MK, Skosey C, Hoffman PC et al: Sex-associated differences in presentation and survival in patients with lung cancer. J Clin Oncol 8:1402, 1990.

Frasci G, Panza N, Comella P et al: Cisplatin, gemcitabine and vinorelbine in locally advanced or metastatic non-small cell lung cancer: A phase I study. Ann Oncol 8:1045, 1997.

Friedland DM, Comis RL: Perioperative therapy of non-small cell lung cancer: A review of adjuvant and neoadjuvant approaches. Semin Oncol 22:571, l995.

Friess GG, Balkadi M, Harvey WH: Concurrent cisplatin and etoposide with radiotherapy in locally advanced non-small cell lung cancer. Cancer Treat Rep 71:681, 1987.

Fukuoka M, Niitani H, Sizuki A et al: A phase II study of CPT-II, a new derivative of camptothecin, for previously untreated non-small cell lung cancer. J Clin Oncol 10:16, 1992.

Furuse K, Fukuoka Y, Takada Y et al, for the West Japan Lung Cancer Group: A randomized phase III study of concurrent versus sequential thoracic radiotherapy (TRT) in combination with mitomycin (M), vindesine (V), cisplatin (P) in unresectable stage III non-small cell lung cancer (NSCLC) (Abstract No. 1649). Proc Am Soc Clin Oncol 16:459a, 1997.

Gail MH, Eagan RT, Feld R et al: Prognostic factors in patients with resected stage I non-small cell lung cancer: A report from the Lung Cancer Study Group. Cancer 54:1802, 1984.

Gandara D, Crowley J, Livingston R et al: Evaluation of cisplatin intensity in metastatic non-small cell lung cancer: A phase III study of the Southwest Oncology Group. J Clin Oncol 11:873, 1993.

Ganz PA, Figlin RA, Haskell CM: Supportive care versus supportive care and combination chemotherapy in metastatic non-small cell lung cancer. Cancer 63:1271, 1989.

Gatzemeier U, von Pawel J, Gottfried M et al: Phase III comparative study of high-dose cisplatin (HD-Cis) versus a combination of paclitaxel (TAX) and cisplatin (Cis) in patients with advanced non-small cell lung cancer (NSCLC) [Abstract No. 1748]. Proc ASCO 17:454a, 1998.

Giaccone G, Splinter T, Postmus P et al: Paclitaxel-cisplatin versus teniposide-cisplatin in advanced non-small cell lung cancer [Abstract No. 1109]. Proc ASCO 15:373, 1996.

Giatromanolaki A, Koukourakis M, O'Byrne K et al: Prognostic value of angiogenesis in operable non-small cell lung cancer. J Pathol 179:80, 1996.

Gil Deza E, Balbiani L, Coppola F et al: Phase II study of navelbine (NVB) vs NVB plus cisplatin in non-small cell lung cancer stage III or IV [Abstract No. 1193]. Proc ASCO 15:394, 1996.

Gralla RJ, Casper ES, Kelsen DP et al: Cisplatin and vindesine combination chemotherapy for advanced carcinoma of the lung: A randomized trial investigating two dosage schedules. Ann Intern Med 95:414, 1981.

Green M, Kreisman H, Soll D et al: Carboplatin in non-small cell lung cancer: An update on the Cancer and Leukemia Group B experience. Semin Oncol 19(suppl 2):44, 1992.

Green R, Humphrey E, Close H et al: Alkylating agents in bronchogenic carcinoma. Am J Med 46:516, 1969.

Harada M, Dosaka-Akita H, Miyamoto H et al: Prognostic significance of the expression of ras oncogene product in non-small cell lung cancer. Cancer 69:72, 1992.

Haskell CM: Chemotherapy and survival of patients with non-small cell lung cancer. A contrary view. Chest 99:1325, 1991.

Holmes EC, Gail M, for the Lung Cancer Study Group: Surgical adjuvant therapy for stage II and stage III adenocarcinoma and large-cell undifferentiated carcinoma of the lung. J Clin Oncol 4:710, 1986.

Ichinose Y, Hara N, Ohta M et al: Postoperative adjuvant chemotherapy in non-small cell lung cancer: Prognostic value of DNA ploidy and post-recurrent survival. J Surg Oncol 46:15, 1991.

Jaakkimainen L, Goodwin PJ, Pater J et al: Counting the costs of chemotherapy in a National Cancer Institute of Canada randomized trial in non-small cell lung cancer. J Clin Oncol 8:1301, 1990.

Johnson DH: Overview of ifosphamide in small cell and non-small cell lung cancer. Semin Oncol 17(suppl 4):24, 1990.

Johnson DH, Piantidosi S: Chemotherapy for resectable stage III non-small cell lung cancer: Can *that* dog hunt? J Natl Cancer Inst 86:650, 1994.

Jones AL, Smith IE: Zeniplatin (CL286,558), an active new platinum analog in advanced non-small cell lung cancer (NSCLC): A phase II study [Abstract]. Proc ASCO 10:268, 1991.

Joss RA, Cavalli F, Goldhirsch A et al: New agents in non-small cell lung cancer. Cancer Treat Rev 11:205, 1984.

Kassa S, Lund E, Thorud E et al: Symptomatic treatment versus combination chemotherapy for patients with extensive non-small cell lung cancer. Cancer 67:2443, 1991.

Keller S, Adak S, Wagner H et al: A randomized trial of postoperative adjuvant therapy in patients with completely resected stage II or IIIA non-small cell lung cancer. N Engl J Med 343:1217, 2000.

Keller S, Groshen S, Martini N et al: Blood transfusion and lung cancer recurrence. Cancer 62:606, 1983.

Lad T, Rubinstein L, Fadeghi A: The benefit of adjuvant treatment for resected locally advanced non-small cell lung cancer. J Clin Oncol 6:9, 1988.

Le Chevalier T, Arriagada R, Tarayre M et al: Significant effect of adjuvant chemotherapy on survival in locally advanced non-small cell lung cancer. J Natl Cancer Inst 84:58, 1992.

Le Chevalier T, Brisgand D, Douillard JY et al: Randomized trial of vinorelbine and cisplatin versus vindesine and cisplatin versus vinorelbine alone in advanced non-small cell lung cancer. J Clin Oncol 14:687, 1996.

Lee JS, Ro JY, Sahin AA et al: Expression of blood-group antigen A: A favorable prognostic factor in non-small cell lung cancer. N Engl J Med. 324:1084, 1991.

Lynch T, Kalish L, Strauss G et al: Phase II study of topotecan in non-small cell lung cancer. J Clin Oncol 12:347, 1994.

Maki E, Feld R: Prognostic factors in patients with non-small cell lung cancer. A critique of the world literature. Lung Cancer 7:27, 1991.

Manegold C, Bergman B, Chemaissani A et al: Single-agent gemcitabine versus cisplatin-etoposide: Early results of a randomized phase II study in locally advanced metastatic non-small cell lung cancer. Ann Oncol 8:513, 1997.

Marino P, Preatone A, Cantone A: Randomized trials of radiotherapy alone versus combined chemotherapy and radiotherapy in stages IIIa and IIIb non-small cell lung cancer: A meta-analysis. Cancer 76:593, 1995.

Mattson K, Holsti LR, Holsti P et al: Inoperable non-small cell lung cancer: Radiation with or without chemotherapy. Eur J Clin Oncol 24:477, 1988.

Mitsudomi T, Steinberg SM, Oielt K et al: Rat gene mutations in non-small cell lung cancer are associated with shortened survival irrespective of treatment intent. Cancer Res 51:4999, 1991.

Morton RF, Jett JR, McGinnis WL et al: Thoracic radiation therapy alone compared with combined chemoradiotherapy for locally unresectable non-small cell lung cancer. Ann Intern Med 115:681, 1991.

Mountain C: A new international staging system for lung cancer. Chest 89:225S, 1986.

Mountain CF: Revisions in the International System for Staging Lung Cancer. Chest 113:1728, 1997.

Niiranen A, Niitamo-Korhonen S, Kouri A et al: Adjuvant chemotherapy after radical surgery for non-small-cell lung cancer: A randomized study. J Clin Oncol 10:1927, 1992.

Non–Small Cell Lung Cancer Collaborative Group: Chemotherapy in non-small cell lung cancer: A meta-analysis using updated data on individual patients from 52 randomized clinical trials. Br Med J 311:899, 1995.

Ohta M, Tsuchiya R, Shimoyama M et al: Adjuvant chemotherapy for completely resected stage III non-small-cell lung cancer. Results of a randomized prospective study. The Japan Clinical Oncology Group. J Thorac Cardiovasc Surg 106:307, 1993.

Pass H, Pobgrebniak H, Steinberg S et al: Randomized trial of neoadjuvant therapy for lung cancer: Interim analysis. Ann Thorac Surg 53:992, 1992.

Perez-Solar R, Fossella F, Glisson BS et al: Phase II study of topotecan in patients with advanced non-small cell lung cancer not treated previously with chemotherapy. J Clin Oncol 14:503, 1996.

Perng RP, Chen Y, Ming-Liu J et al: Gemcitabine versus the combination of cisplatin and etoposide in patients with inoperable non-small cell lung cancer in a phase II randomized study. J Clin Oncol 15:2097, 1997.

Perrone F, Rossi A, Ianniello GP et al: Vinorelbine plus best supportive care (BSC) versus BSC in the treatment of advanced non-small cell lung cancer patients: Results of a phase III randomized trial [Abstract 1752]. Proc ASCO 17, 1998.

Planting A, Helle P, Drings P et al: A randomized study of high-dose split course radiotherapy preceded by high-dose chemotherapy versus high-dose radiotherapy only in locally advanced non-small cell lung cancer. An EORTC Lung Cancer Cooperative Group trial. Ann Oncol 7:139, 1996.

Pritchard R, Anthony S: Chemotherapy plus radiotherapy in the treatment of locally advanced, unresectable non-small cell lung cancer: A meta-analysis. Ann Intern Med 125:723, 1996.

Quoix E, Dietemann A, Charbonneau J et al: La chimiotherapie comportant du cisplative est-elle utile dans le cancer bronchique non microcelluleve au stad IV? Resultats d'une etude randomisee. Bull Cancer 78:341, 1991.

Rapp E, Pater J, Willan A et al: Chemotherapy can prolong survival in patients with advanced non-small cell lung cancer. A report of the Canadian multicenter trial. J Clin Oncol 6:633, 1988.

Rodriguez G, Valdivvieso M, Von Hoff D et al: A phase I/II trial of the combination of tirapazamine and cisplatin in patients with non-small cell lung cancer [Abstract 1144]. Proc ASCO 15:382, 1996.

Rosell R, Gomez-Codina J, Camp C et al: A randomized trial comparing preoperative chemotherapy plus surgery with surgery alone in patients with non-small cell lung cancer. N Engl J Med 330:153, 1994.

Roth JA, Atkinson EN, Fossella F et al: Long-term follow-up of patients enrolled in a randomized trial comparing perioperative chemotherapy and surgery with surgery alone in resectable stage IIIA non-small cell lung cancer. Lung Cancer 21:1, 1998.

Rowland KM Jr, Bonomi P, Taylor SG IV et al: Phase II trial of etoposide, cisplatin, 5-FU and concurrent split course radiation in stage IIIA and IIIB non-small cell lung cancer. Proc ASCO 7:203, 1988.

Rusch V, Klimstra D, Venkatraman E et al: Aberrant p53 expression predicts clinical resistance to cisplatin-based chemotherapy in locally advanced non-small cell lung cancer. Cancer Res 55:5038, 1995.

Sahin AA, Ro JY, el-Naggar AK et al: Flow cytometric analysis of the DNA content of non-small cell lung cancer. Ploidy as a significant prognostic indicator in squamous cell carcinoma of the lung. Cancer 65:530, 1990.

Sandler A, Nemunaitis J, Denham C et al: Phase III study of cisplatin (C) with or without gemcitabine (G) in patients with advanced non-small cell lung cancer (NSCLC) (Abstract No. 1747). Proc ASCO 17:454a, 1998.

Sause W, Kolesar P, Taylor S et al: Five-year results; phase III trial of regionally advanced, unresectable non-small cell lung cancer, RTOG 8808, ECOG 4588, SWOG 8992 [Abstract No. 1743]. Proc ASCO 17:435a, 1998.

Schaake-Konig C, van den Bogaert W, Dalesio O et al: Effects of concomitant cisplatin and radiotherapy on inoperable non-small cell lung cancer. N Engl J Med 326:524, 1992.

Sculier JP, Klastersky J, Giner V et al: A phase II randomized trial comparing high-dose cisplatin with moderate-dose cisplatin and carboplatin in patients with advanced non-small cell lung cancer. J Clin Oncol 12:353, 1994.

Shepherd F, Johnston M, Payne D et al: A randomized trial of chemotherapy and surgery versus radiotherapy: A National Cancer Institute of Canada Clinical Trials Group study. Br J Cancer 78:683, 1998.

Shepherd FA: Induction chemotherapy for locally advanced non-small cell lung cancer. Ann Thorac Surg 55:1585, 1993.

Shepherd FA: Phase II trials of single-agent activity of gemcitabine in patients with advanced non-small cell lung cancer: An overview. Anticancer Drugs 6:19, 1995.

Shepherd FA, Abratt RP, Anderson H et al: Gemcitabine in the treatment of elderly patients with non-small cell lung cancer. Semin Oncol 24:S70, 1997.

Shepherd FA, Evans WK, Goss PE et al: Ifosfamide, cisplatin and etoposide (ICE) in the treatment of advanced non-small cell lung cancer. Semin Oncol 19(suppl 1):54, 1992.

Slevin ML, Clark PI, Joel SP et al: A randomized trial to evaluate the effect of schedule on the activity of etoposide in small cell lung cancer. J Clin Oncol 7:1333, 1989.

Smith TJ, Hillner BE, Neighbors DM et al: Economic evaluation of a randomized clinical trial comparing vinorelbine, vinorelbine plus cisplatin and vindesine plus cisplatin for non-small cell lung cancer. J Clin Oncol 13:2166, 1995.

Soresi E, Clerici M, Grilli R et al: A randomized clinical trial comparing radiation therapy versus radiation therapy plus cis-dichlorodiammine-platin (II) in the treatment of locally advanced non-small cell lung cancer. Semin Oncol 15(suppl 7):20, 1988.

Souquet P, Chauvin F, Boissel JP et al: Polychemotherapy in advanced non-small cell lung cancer: A meta-analysis. Lancet 342:19, 1993.

Spain RC: Neo-adjuvant mitomycin C, cisplatin and infusion vinblastine in locally and regionally advanced non-small cell lung cancer: Problems and progress from the perspective of long-term follow-up. Semin Oncol 15(suppl 4):6, 1988.

Splinter TAW, Sahmoud T, Festen J et al: Two schedules of teniposide with or without cisplatin in advanced non-small-cell lung cancer: A randomized study of the European Organization for Research and Treatment of Cancer Lung Cancer Cooperative Group. J Clin Oncol 14:127, 1996.

Stevenson H, Gazdar A, Phelp S et al: Tumor cell lines established in vitro, an independent prognostic factor for survival in non-small cell lung cancer. Ann Intern Med 113:764, 1990.

Takigawa N, Segawa Y, Okahara M et al: Prognostic factors for patients with advanced non-small cell lung cancer: Univariate and multivariate analyses including recursive partitioning and amalgamation. Lung Cancer 15:66, 1996.

Vokes EE, Bitran JD, Vogelzang NJ: Chemotherapy for non-small cell lung cancer. The continuing challenge. Chest 99:1326, 1991.

Vokes EE, Leopold KA, Herndon JE et al: A CALGB randomized phase II study of gemcitabine or paclitaxel or vinorelbine with cisplatin as induction chemotherapy (Ind CT) and concomitant chemoradiotherapy (XRT) in stage IIIB non-small cell lung cancer (NSCLC): Feasibility data [Abstract No. 1636]. Proc ASCO 16:455a, 1997.

von Pawel J, von Romeleling R: Survival benefit from Tirazone (tirapazamine and cisplatin) in advanced non-small cell lung cancer (NSCLC) patients: Final results from the international phase III CATAPULT 1 trial [Abstract 1747]. Proc ASCO 17:454a, 1998.

Wada H, Hitomi S, Teramatsu T: Adjuvant chemotherapy after complete resection in non-small cell lung cancer. J Clin Oncol 14:1048, 1996.

Woods RL, Williams CJ, Levi J et al: A randomized trial of cisplatin and vindesine versus supportive care only in advanced non-small cell lung cancer. Br J Cancer 61:608, 1990.

Wozniak AJ, Crowley JJ, Balcerzak GR et al: Randomized trial comparing cisplatin with cisplatin plus vinorelbine in the treatment of advanced non-small cell lung cancer: A Southwest Oncology Group study. J Clin Oncol 16:2459, 1998.

RADIOTHERAPY FOR NON–SMALL CELL LUNG CANCER

Thomas H. Weisenburger

Cancer of the lung, which was a rare disease in the early part of the 20th century, has become the leading cause of cancer-related death in men and women in the United States. Approximately 171,500 cases were diagnosed in 1998 (Landis et al, 1999), of which 80% had non-small cell lung cancer (NSCLC). Approximately 55% of these patients were expected to have distant metastases, 30% regional lymphatic involvement, and 15% had a tumor that was confined to the lung (LaRoux, 1968; Paulson, 1968). Only 15% of patients could be offered resection for cure (Shields and Robinette, 1973).

Patients who present without clinically apparent distant metastatic disease (approximately 40,000 to 45,000 patients per year) present a challenging problem to the oncologist. Unfortunately, the overall cure rate in this population remains low, however, and there has been a debate about whether radiotherapy should be offered to *all* patients in this category (Berry et al, 1977; Brashear, 1978; Cohen, 1983; Cox et al, 1983; Krant, 1966; Payne, 1988; Pett et al, 1986; Phillips and Miller, 1978; Rubin et al, 1970).

Radical radiotherapy (RT) for lung cancer has some associated morbidity, and it should not be considered a "soft alternative to surgery" (Ash, 1984). The same is true for combinations of chemotherapy and radiotherapy. Physicians caring for these patients must base their decisions regarding therapeutic recommendations on their clinical assessment of the many prognostic factors pertaining to each patient and on their understanding of the benefits and morbidities of the various therapeutic modalities.

To cure sometimes,
To relieve often,
To comfort always.
—Anonymous
(quoted in Lee, 1974)

HISTORICAL NOTE

In 1940, Leddy and Moersch (1940) reported one of the first series documenting long-term survival with radiotherapy. Of 250 patients with primary lung cancer, 125 were followed without therapy, and 125 received orthovoltage radiotherapy. None of the untreated patients survived 1 year. Twenty-five of the treated group survived 1 year, and 5 (4%) survived 5 years. Smart and Hilton (1956) treated 40 patients with orthovoltage radiotherapy alone following biopsy. These were selected patients who had localized lesions with no radiographic or clinical evidence of lymph node metastases. They were in good general condition and were considered operable. Nine patients (22.5%) were alive at 5 years and 3 (7.5%) at 10 years. This clearly established radiotherapy as a potentially curative modality in selected patients. Morrison and associates (1963) compared surgery versus radiotherapy in 37 patients who had epidermoid carcinomas. Patients undergoing radiotherapy received 45 Gy in 4 weeks delivered with 8-MeV photons. The 4-year survival rate was 30% versus 6% for surgery and radiotherapy, respectively, establishing early that surgery is the therapy of choice for operable patients and also demonstrating again, despite the low dose, that radiotherapy can provide a small but real opportunity for cure. Since these pioneering articles were written, much work has been, and continues to be, done to define the optimum dose and fractionation scheme and to integrate radiotherapy with surgery or chemotherapy. The difficulties have been the high rate of pre-existing occult metastatic disease in locally advanced NSCLC (which often obscures any effect of local therapy, either surgical or radiotherapeutic) and the lack of comparability of the treated population in many reported combined modality series (Cox et al, 1990; Holmes, 1990).

■ *HISTORICAL READINGS*

Cox JD, Azarnia N, Byhart RW et al: A randomized phase I/II trial of hyperfractionated radiation therapy with total doses of 60.0 Gy to 79.2 Gy: Possible survival benefit with 69.6 Gy in favorable patients with Radiation Therapy Oncology Group stage III nonsmall-cell lung carcinoma: Report of Radiation Therapy Oncology Group 83-11. J Clin Oncol 8:1543, 1990.

Holmes EC: Adjuvant therapy of non small cell lung cancer. In Salmon SE (ed): Adjuvant Therapy of Cancer, Vol IV. Philadelphia, WB Saunders, 1990, p 119.

Leddy E, Moersch HJ: Roentgen therapy for bronchogenic carcinoma. JAMA 15:2239, 1940.

Morrison R, Deeley TJ, Cleland WP: The treatment of carcinoma of the bronchus. A clinical trial to compare surgery and supervoltage radiotherapy. Lancet 1:683, 1963.

Smart J, Hilton G: Radiotherapy of cancer of the lung: Results in a selective group of cases. Lancet 1:880, 1956.

BASIC SCIENCE

An understanding of the lymphatic pathways of the lung is necessary when patients with lung cancer are evaluated for radiation therapy. The lymphatic channels of the left upper lobe drain to the nodes between the aortic arch and the pulmonary artery (Lee, 1977). Metastatic nodes in this area may cause paralysis of the left vocal cord by involving the recurrent nerve. The right upper lobe drains to the mediastinal node at the junction of the superior vena cava and the azygous vein. The inferior portions of the lungs drain to nodes in the inferior pulmonary ligaments, communicating with the subcarinal nodes superiorly and the nodes near the cisterna chyli inferiorly (Weinberg, 1972), perhaps explaining the worse prognosis for lower lobe carcinoma described by Deeley (1974). The remaining portions of the lung drain to the hilar lymph nodes. Involvement of the parietal pleura allows the direct spread to regional lymph nodes outside the thorax (axillary, supraclavicular, or subdiaphragmatic lymph nodes, depending on location). The location of the primary tumor and lymphatic metastases, if present, must be determined in relation to the sensitive structures of the thorax. The arrangement of treatment portals is usually designed to include the primary tumor and the lymph node regions while limiting the dose delivered to normal tissues (normal lung, heart, esophagus, and spinal cord) to tolerable levels.

Each fraction of radiotherapy eliminates a percentage of the tumor cells treated, leaving a surviving fraction of cells. The goal of therapy is to reduce the probability of survival of the last clonogenic cell to as low a level as possible. The effect of radiotherapy on tumor cells depends on the basic radiosensitivity of the cells and the biologic factors that influence the response to fractionated radiotherapy. These include repair from radiation damage, reoxygenation of the tumor during the course of treatment, redistribution of the cells in the cell cycle, and repopulation of the cells between fractions (the four R's of radiobiology). Withers and colleagues (1988) noted that there is accelerated repopulation of clonogenic cells in response to therapy that occurs during therapy. Delays in completing a course of therapy once started (as in split-course therapy) are to be avoided. They also noted that chemotherapy prior to radiotherapy may induce the same effect, which could decrease the likelihood of local control with radiotherapy.

Radiotherapy for patients with NSCLC can be used as an adjunct to surgery, as primary therapy in the medically inoperable or unresectable patient (either alone or combined with chemotherapy), as "prophylactic" therapy of subclinical disease to prevent the development of clinical disease, or as palliative therapy.

PRIMARY RADIOTHERAPY

Although surgery is the preferred treatment for localized, resectable disease, radiotherapy (primary or "radical" radiotherapy) is used with curative intent for those patients unable or unwilling to undergo surgery, or in treating local-regional stage IV mass disease that is deemed "unresectable."

DIAGNOSIS AND STAGING

Following histologic confirmation of the diagnosis of NSCLC, the patient must be carefully evaluated for the anatomic extent of both local and distant disease and for the prognostic indicators important in selection of candidates for radiotherapy. A computed tomographic (CT) scan of the chest and upper abdomen, including the adrenal glands and liver, should be performed. If adrenal enlargement is noted, a biopsy is recommended because of the high false-positive rate of CT. Nielson and co-workers (1982) reported that only 4 of 15 adrenal masses seen on a CT scan in 84 patients were confirmed by biopsy. Oliver and associates (1984) noted 32 adrenal masses on CT scan in 330 patients with NSCLC, and only 8 of the 25 that underwent biopsy were positive (32%). Positron emission tomography (PET) may be useful for identifying metastatic disease to the adrenals (Nabi and Steinbrenner, 1996). CT scans of the brain have a low yield in asymptomatic patients. Hillers and colleagues (1994) reviewed 16 selected citations of staging methods for NSCLC and reported that only 4% (14/353) of asymptomatic patients had positive brain scans. They also reported only a 3% (9/301) incidence of positive bone scans in asymptomatic patients. Hooper and coworkers (1984) observed that none of 28 asymptomatic patients with NSCLC had a positive brain scan. They noted that, as the number of clinical and laboratory indicators of disease increased, the likelihood of a positive scan increased. Salvatierra and associates (1990) reported the results of whole-body bone scanning and CT scan of the brain and upper abdomen in 146 patients with NSCLC who had potentially resectable disease. Metastatic disease was found in 44 patients (30%). Brain metastases were found in 19 patients (13%), only 4 of whom (2.7%) were asymptomatic. Bone scans were positive in only 3.4% of asymptomatic patients. They found that, if head CT scans had been performed on symptomatic patients with squamous cell carcinomas and all patients with adenocarcinomas and large cell carcinomas; bone scans had been obtained on symptomatic patients; and abdominal CT had been performed on all patients, only one patient would have been understaged, and 80% of bone scans and 53% of brain scans would have been avoided.

PET scanning may significantly improve our ability to correctly stage patients with NSCLC prior to radiotherapy. Whole-body PET detected extrathoracic metastases in 13 of 94 (14%) patients with non–small cell lung cancer of stage IIIA or lower who were otherwise eligible for operation (Weder et al, 1998). As well, PET may be useful for delineation of lung cancer volumes that are poorly defined by chest radiograph or CT scan (Hebert et al, 1996). In a series of 15 patients analyzed retrospectively, 26.7% (four patients) would have had their RT volume influenced by PET findings (Kiffer et al, 1998)

Selection criteria for radical primary radiotherapy have included evidence of adequate pulmonary function based on a forced expiratory volume at 1 second of 700 ml, ability to climb one flight of stairs without severe dyspnea, no evidence of hypercapnia at rest, and a maximum breathing capacity of at least 50% of predicted (Lee, 1974). These criteria are guidelines only because pulmonary function may improve significantly with response of the tumor. The hemoglobin level should be above 10 g/dl (Lee, 1977). The presence of a malignant pleural effusion is a contraindication to radical therapy (Ash, 1984).

Evaluation of patients for the presence of various prognostic factors identified with survival may help in deciding whether primary radiotherapy is indicated, although none of the negative indicators alone should preclude the decision to proceed. Patients with good performance status, inoperability because of medical reasons, unresectability determined at thoracotomy, no significant weight loss, and more limited disease stage had a better prognosis (Komaki et al, 1985; Scott et al, 1997; Stanley, 1980). In a Stanford series evaluating prognostic factors in 269 patients treated with radiotherapy, the presence of pain or hemoptysis or the requirement of fields larger than 200 cm^2 was associated with lower survival rates (Caldwell and Bagshaw, 1968). None of the 34 patients with vocal cord paralysis survived 2 years. Recursive partitioning analysis (RPA) (Ciampi and Triffault, 1988) can assist in stratifying patients based on known prognostic variables, and may allow for a more appropriate therapeutic intervention. Using RPA, Scott and colleagues (1997) evaluated 1592 patients with inoperable non–small cell lung cancer who were treated with radiotherapy in a number of RTOG trials (Scott et al, 1997). They reported four classes of patients whose median survival varied from 12.6 months for those in class I to as little as 3.3 months for those in class IV. The inclusion of class IV patients in clinical trials may obscure the outcome (Komaki et al, 1998).

MANAGEMENT

Radiotherapy for patients with NSCLC can be used as an adjunct to surgery, as primary therapy in the medically inoperable or unresectable patient (either alone or combined with chemotherapy), as "prophylactic" therapy of subclinical disease to prevent the development of clinical disease, or as palliative therapy.

Primary radical radiotherapy alone for NSCLC provides long-term survival in approximately 6% of patients with unresectable disease (Caldwell and Bagshaw, 1968), 11% of patients with more favorable prognostic indicators (Cox et al, 1980), and as many as 17% to 33% (Haffty et al, 1988; Sibley et al, 1998; Smart and Hilton, 1956; Talton et al, 1990; Zhang et al, 1989) when early-stage resectable patients are treated.

Despite the numerous studies that have been reported using many varied dose and time combinations, the optimal fractionation schedule remains to be defined (Perez, 1985). Several conclusions can be drawn, however, concerning radiotherapy as primary therapy. The RTOG protocol 73-01 compared 40-Gy continuous and split-course therapy with 50- and 60-Gy continuous course. Higher doses and the use of a continuous as opposed to a split course were associated with greater local control at 3 years (Perez et al, 1987). The survival time was longer in those patients who achieved local control, but there was no significant difference in the overall survival rate or local failure rate between the groups at 5 years. The dose of 60 Gy in 6 weeks, limiting the spinal cord dose to approximately 45 Gy, became the RTOG standard therapeutic arm in studies of altered fractionation schemes. This schedule results in clinical local control of approximately 60% at 3 years. However, a report by Arriagada and co-workers (1991), which incorporated aggressive re-staging with bronchoscopy, yielded a much lower incidence of local control of 17% in patients with stage III disease who were treated with radiotherapy alone. Because of the disappointing local control and survival results of standard radiotherapy, attempts have been made to improve local control by adding chemotherapy and by altering the delivery of radiotherapy.

The combination of chemotherapy and primary radiotherapy continues to be actively investigated and is considered to be the standard of care for good-performance patients with locally advanced disease (Turrissi, 1991). The CALGB (8433) (Dillman et al, 1996) studied 180 patients, comparing radiotherapy alone with radiotherapy preceded by a course of cisplatin on days 1 and 29 and five weekly cycles of vinblastine (neoadjuvant chemotherapy). There was a significant increase in median survival time (13.7 vs 9.6 months, $P = .012$) and 5-year survival rate (17% vs 7%) for the neoadjuvant group compared with those in the conventional radiotherapy-alone group. This study has established induction chemotherapy as the standard of care for good-performance patients. Arriagada and associates (1991) reported a randomized trial of 353 patients who received either radiotherapy alone, consisting of 65 Gy in 26 fractions of 2.5 Gy each over 45 days, or induction chemotherapy with vindesine, cyclophosphamide, cisplatin, and lomustine for three cycles, followed by the same radiotherapy followed by the same chemotherapy for three more cycles if there was no progression. The 2-year survival rates of 14% and 21% for the control and experimental groups, respectively, were not statistically significantly different ($P = .08$). Schaake-Konig and colleagues (1992) compared a split course of radiotherapy alone (giving 30 Gy in 10 fractions of 3 Gy, followed by a 3-week rest, and then 25 Gy in 10 2.5-Gy fractions over 2 weeks) with the same regimen combined with cisplatin either weekly or daily with the irradiation. The 2-year survival rates in the daily cisplatin plus radiotherapy group were increased compared with those in the radiotherapy-alone group (26% vs 13%, $P = .009$); the survival rate in the weekly cisplatin group of 19% was not different from either group. They reported a significant decrease in local failure in the daily cisplatin group. The authors note that the split course may have been suboptimal because of the possibility of accelerated repopulation during the rest period, but they point out that the daily cisplatin did increase local control in spite of the split-course regimen.

Several groups have evaluated altered fractionation schemes. The RTOG (Cox et al, 1990) reported increased survival rates using a hyperfractionated course of radiotherapy that delivered doses of 69.2 Gy with a 1.2-Gy twice-a-day schedule compared with the results from previous RTOG studies using 60 Gy in 30 daily fractions over 6 weeks. The 3-year survival rate was 20% compared with 7% in the standard fractionation arm ($P = .002$). A phase III randomized study (RTOG 8808 and ECOG 4588) compared standard radiation therapy (STD RT) with 60 Gy at 2.0 Gy per day, hyperfractionated radiation therapy (HFX RT) with 69.6 Gy at 1.2 Gy twice a day, and induction chemotherapy with cisplatin 100 mg/m^2 days 1 and 29 with vinblastine 5 mg/m^2 weekly for 5 weeks followed by 60 Gy at 2.0 Gy per day (CT + RT) (Sause et al, 1995). One-year survival and median survival (months) were as follows: STD RT—46% and 11.4; CT + RT—60% and 13.8; and HFX RT—51% and 12.3. The chemotherapy plus radiotherapy arm was statistically superior to the other two treatment arms (log-rank $P = .03$). Saunders and co-workers (1997) randomized 563 patients to continuous hyperfractionated accelerated radiotherapy (CHART) consisting of 1.5-Gy fractions given every 6 hours over 12 consecutive days or 60 Gy in 2-Gy fractions over 6 weeks. Overall, there was a 24% decrease in the relative risk of death (RRD) using CHART, with a 2-year survival increase from 20% to 29%. The greatest reduction in RRD was 34% in the squamous cell group with an improvement in 2-year survival from 19% to 33%. Other than increased severe dysphagia in the CHART group, there were no significant differences in short- or long-term morbidity.

The RTOG recently completed accrual for a three-arm phase III study of induction chemotherapy and thoracic radiotherapy consisting of 63 Gy in 7 weeks in 34 daily fractions (1.8 Gy × 25 fx, then 2.0 Gy × 9 fx) beginning on day 50, versus concomitant chemotherapy with the same radiotherapy, versus concomitant chemotherapy with hyperfractionated radiotherapy (69.6 Gy in 6 weeks in 58 × 1.2-Gy twice-daily fractions at least 6 hours apart) beginning day 1 for patients with locally advanced, inoperable non–small cell lung cancer (RTOG 9410).

Dose escalation studies using a three-dimensional (3D) conformal technique have been reported by several groups (Armstrong et al, 1997; Graham et al, 1996; Robertson et al, 1997; Sibley et al, 1995). This technique appears to be feasible from a tolerance standpoint and promising with respect to local control. The RTOG is currently conducting a phase I–II dose escalation study (9301).

Intraoperative radiotherapy (IORT) using an electron beam has been evaluated clinically by several investigators (Abe et al, 1980; Calvo et al, 1990; Juettner et al, 1990; Pass et al, 1987) and has been assessed in the laboratory setting (Tochner et al, 1992). The experience with IORT is too limited at this time for conclusions to be drawn about its usefulness in combination with, or instead of, more conventional therapy.

Surgical Adjuvant Radiotherapy

Radiotherapy, as part of combined modality therapy that includes surgery, has been investigated as preoperative or postoperative treatment with or without chemotherapy.

Preoperative Radiotherapy

Prospective studies of preoperative radiotherapy in clinically resectable patients have not shown an increase in survival compared with surgery alone (Komaki et al, 1985). Bromley and Szur (1955) found 47% of 66 patients had no tumors after preoperative radiotherapy, but the mortality rate was high (15%). There were significant complications. Bloedorn and associates (1961) studied 37 patients who received doses up to 60 Gy, with a finding of 46% sterilization at the time of surgery. The operative mortality rate of 22% exceeded the 5-year survival rate of 20%. Shields (1972) reported on 300 clinically resectable patients who were randomized to surgery alone or preoperative radiotherapy. The 4-year survival rate of the surgery-alone group was 21% compared with the combined modality group rate of only 13%. In addition, postoperative complications were more frequent in the combined therapy group. A Collaborative Study (Warram, 1975) of the National Cancer Institute (NCI) reported on 550 patients who were randomly assigned to surgery alone or preoperative radiotherapy plus surgery with survival rates of 14% and 16%, respectively, at 5 years. It should be remembered that these studies included some patients with small cell lung cancer and and that staging of patients was inadequate by modern standards. Though not considered routine for resectable patients, preoperative irradiation is routinely considered in the therapy of patients with superior sulcus tumors (Ginsberg, 1995).

Preoperative Chemotherapy and Radiotherapy

The optimal application of surgery, chemotherapy, and radiotherapy for locally advanced disease remains controversial (Ginsberg, 1995). Several phase III trials have shown an increase in survival when neoadjuvant chemotherapy was used in patients with potentially resectable stage IIIA disease (Pass et al, 1992; Rosell et al, 1994; Roth et al, 1994). Chemotherapy appears to reduce the incidence of distant metastases (Arriagada et al, 1991; Cox et al, 1999) and to improve survival in patients with NSCLC treated in combination with radiotherapy. Preoperative radiotherapy was compared with preoperative chemotherapy in a randomized trial of 57 patients (CALGB 9134). With a minimum follow-up of 34.2 months, the median survival was 23.5 and 18 months, respectively (not statistically significant) (Kumar et al, 1997). Fowler and colleagues (Fowler et al, 1993) reported on 13 patients who received concurrent preoperative chemotherapy and radiotherapy to 60 Gy. Although the six patients who underwent lobectomy tolerated the regimen, there were three postoperative deaths (two with adult respiratory distress syndrome) among the seven pneumonectomy patients. Preoperative chemoradiotherapy using doses of 45 Gy or less has been evaluated in a number of phase II trials (Faber et al, 1989; Rusch et al, 1993; Skarin et al, 1989; Strauss et al, 1992; Weiden and Piantadosi 1994) (Table 32–14).

A randomized phase III comparison between concurrent chemotherapy plus radiotherapy and concurrent chemotherapy plus radiotherapy followed by surgical resection for stage IIIA (N2) non–small cell lung cancer is ongoing (INT 0139). The effectiveness of the routine use of preoperative therapy for advanced stage III disease remains unproven (Ruckdeschel, 1997).

Postoperative Radiotherapy

The role of postoperative radiotherapy has been controversial for many years. Analysis of the various nonrandomized and randomized studies of postoperative radiotherapy demonstrates the significant heterogeneity of the patient populations and therapeutic parameters studied, including stage, mediastinal evaluation, radiation fields, and doses delivered, which makes it difficult for definitive conclusions to be drawn (Weisenburger, 1991). Postoperative radiotherapy in patients without evidence of lymphatic metastasis provides no significant survival benefit (Bangma, 1972; Green et al, 1975; Paterson and Russell, 1962; Van Houtte et al, 1980) and may be detrimental to survival (Anonymous, 1998).

Retrospective studies by Green and co-workers (1975) and Kirsh and Sloan (1982) reported that postoperative radiotherapy significantly increased the survival rate for patients with lymph node metastases from epidermoid carcinoma. Choi and associates (1980) did not show an increased survival rate with postoperative radiotherapy for epidermoid carcinoma patients, but the groups were not comparable because the postoperative radiotherapy group included 52% of patients with T3 or N2 involvement versus 24% in the surgery-only group. In addition, systematic mediastinal lymph node evaluation had not been performed, leading to a potential bias in the distribution of patients with an uneven distribution of subclinical N2 involvement. The randomized prospective trial by the LCSG (LCSG 773) (Weisenburger and Gail, 1986) showed a substantial decrease in local recurrences, indicating that the desired effect of control of intrathoracic disease had been achieved but without a significant increase in survival time. The study, however, included only 44 patients with mediastinal metastatic disease, and as stated by the authors, this is a subgroup in which irradiation may be beneficial. They reported a higher number of deaths caused by cardiac or respiratory causes in the treated group (11 of 108 vs 5 of 108 in the control group), but the difference was not statistically significant. It should also be noted that these patients had complete resections, as defined by negative margins and thorough mediastinal sampling, and that the most proximal lymph node was not involved. The conclusions from this study apply to similarly staged patients.

Several retrospective studies have also shown increased survival rates in patients with adenocarcinoma with node-positive (Choi et al, 1980; Green et al, 1975) or N2 disease (Kirsh and Sloan, 1982) who have received postoperative radiotherapy. There has not been a prospective randomized trial in patients with adenocarcinomas who have had adequate presurgical evaluation and extensive mediastinal staging. A more recent study by Sawyer and colleagues (1997) evaluated in a retrospective fashion the 4-year actuarial survival and local recurrence rate of 224 unrandomized N2 patients, 88 of whom received postoperative radiotherapy and 136 of whom did not. The median dose was 50.4 Gy. The local recurrence rate was 17% for the treated group and 60% for the surgery-alone group, and the 4-year survival was 43% versus 22%, respectively.

Postoperative radiotherapy appears to contribute sig-

TABLE 32–14 ■ **Selected Studies of Neoadjuvant Chemotherapy and Radiotherapy* for Stage III, Mostly N2, Non–Small Cell Lung Cancer**

Reference	*No. Patients*	*Chemotherapy*	*Response Rate (%)*	*Median Survival (months)*	*OP Mortality*
Rush-Presbyterian (Faber, 1989)	83	FP+/−E	72	20	7%
Lung Cancer Study Group (Weiden, 1994)	76	FP	42	11	8%
CALGB (Strauss, 1992)	32	FVP	62	15	15%
SWOG (Rusch, 1993)	75	EP	76	17	9%
Dana-Farber** (Skarin, 1989)	41	CAP	88	32	

*Radiotherapy doses ranged from 30 to 45 Gy.
**CT administered before RT.
A, adriamycin; C, cyclophosphamide; E, etoposide; F, 5-fluorouracil; M, mitomycin; OP, operative; P, cis-platinum; V, vindesine or vinblastine.
From Ginsberg RJ: Neoadjuvant (induction) treatment for non–small cell lung cancer [Review]. Lung Cancer 12(Suppl 2):S33, 1995.

nificantly to local-regional control in patients who have lymph node metastases to either hilar or mediastinal lymph nodes. There will be no significant increase in survival time in patients with negative lymph nodes, and any increased survival in those patients with positive nodes is likely to be small because of the tendency of these patients to develop disseminated disease (Tubiana, 1989). As more effective systemic therapy becomes available, local control will have a greater impact on survival. It seems reasonable in view of the definite decrease in local recurrence and the possible survival benefit that postoperative radiotherapy be considered in patients with positive mediastinal nodes. Care must be exercised, however, in the selection and therapy of these patients because the additional loss of pulmonary volume after the lung resection may make a critical difference in clinical pulmonary performance (see later section, Complications of Radiotherapy).

RADIOTHERAPY COMBINED WITH CHEMOTHERAPY

Prophylactic Cranial Irradiation

Brain metastases from NSCLC are frequent, developing in 16% of patients with squamous cell carcinomas and 30% of those with adenocarcinomas and large cell carcinomas, according to RTOG data (Perez et al, 1987). Russell and co-workers (1991) reported a delay in the appearance of metastatic disease but no significant difference in the incidence of brain metastases or survival in a randomized study of elective brain irradiation for patients with adenocarcinomas or large cell carcinomas. Prophylactic cranial irradiation is not considered routine practice in NSCLC that has been treated with curative intent by surgery, radiotherapy, or combined modality treatments. In stage III patients treated for cure, brain as a solitary site of first metastasis is a frequent occurrence (up to 30%), and prophylactic cranial irradiation in this group of patients is worthy of investigation.

Palliative Radiotherapy

Radiotherapy can provide effective palliation of the symptoms produced by lung cancer in the majority of patients. Slawson and Scott (1979) reported a 61% response rate overall in 330 patients who had symptoms. Hemoptysis was relieved in 84% (95 of 113), chest pain in 61% (66 of 108), dyspnea in 60% (51 of 85), superior vena cava syndrome in 86% (36 of 42), and vocal cord paralysis in only 6% (3 of 54). Reddy and Marks (1991) reported complete or partial re-expansion of the lung in 74% of 48 patients with malignant obstruction. Patients treated within 2 weeks of onset had a complete response rate of 71% as opposed to 23% if treated after that time.

The doses and fields of radiotherapy that are prescribed depend on the individual circumstances surrounding the need for palliation. The expected survival, the extent of disease, the severity of symptoms, the expected side effects of therapy, and the desire to deliver the therapy as efficiently as possible all factor into the decision regarding dose, time, and field management. A dose of 30 Gy in 10 fractions of 3 Gy each over 2 weeks is frequently initially prescribed, with re-evaluation for additional therapy according to the patient's condition and response. Rapidly progressive symptoms in a patient with a limited life expectancy may be treated with larger fractions over a shorter time (20 Gy in five daily fractions of 4 Gy), with consideration of additional therapy as noted previously. Patients with a longer life expectancy may benefit from higher doses. The RTOG reported on the response of patients treated for painful bone metastases and noted that, although short, intense courses of radiotherapy (15 to 25 Gy in 1 week) can give meaningful palliation, more highly fractionated schemes using higher total doses (30 to 40 Gy in 2 to 3 weeks) produced greater pain relief (Blitzer, 1985; Tong et al, 1982). The American College of Radiology published guidelines for palliative radiotherapy for various presentations of bone metastases as part of their Appropriateness Criteria Program (Leibel, 1999). Patients with superior vena cava syndrome without evidence of metastatic disease may benefit from a course of radical radiotherapy even when the intent is palliative (Lokich and Goodman, 1975).

Technical Aspects of Radiotherapy

CT scans of the chest have become established in the management of patients with NSCLC when they are treated with radiotherapy. Mira and associates (1982) compared chest CT with conventional radiographs for therapeutic planning in 45 patients. Eleven of 14 patients whose radiographs were considered to demonstrate the tumor volume satisfactorily had greater tumor extension on CT scan. Of the 31 patients whose radiographs did not show the tumor volume, 21 (68%) could be defined by CT scan. There are limitations to CT scans because atelectasis cannot always be distinguished from a tumor and the resolution of the best scanners is 0.5 mm, allowing for undetected subclinical involvement outside the irradiation portals. As note above, PET scans may be useful in treatment planning for lung cancer (Kiffer et al, 1998).

CT scans can provide the attenuation characteristics of the tissues being irradiated. Correcting for the decreased attenuation as the beam passes through aerated lung can result in doses 5% to 28% higher than those calculated without correction (van't Reit et al, 1985). The clinical usefulness of this correction has not yet been demonstrated, and it is not currently being used in clinical practice.

The therapeutic volume for patients with locally advanced disease should have a minimum 2-cm and a maximum 2.5-cm margin around the appreciable tumor and should include the ipsilateral hilar nodes and mediastinum (Bleehen and Cox, 1985). The inferior border should be at least 5 cm below the carina. If the lower lobes or inferior mediastinal lymph nodes are involved, the field should extend to the bottom of T-10. Both hilar regions should be included, with a 1-cm margin around the contralateral hilar region (Perez et al, 1987). The ipsilateral supraclavicular region is generally included if the tumor is in the upper lobe, or if there is significant mediastinal adenopathy. This reduces the incidence of supraclavicular metastasis but has not been shown to influence survival (Cox, 1985). In patients with marginal pulmonary function, it is reasonable to exclude the supraclavicular fossae. The superior portion of the anteroposterior/posteroanterior field is usually thinner because of the slope of the chest wall (Lambert, 1978), and a wedge or compensating filter may be necessary to provide a uniform distribution of dose. The fields are reduced to exclude the spinal cord at approximately 45 Gy with the aid of a simulator and CT-guided therapeutic planning. The fields of radiotherapy are usually delineated by individual, focused blocks that are fashioned for each portal used. Spinal cord blocks placed in the posterior field to limit the dose to the cord also limit the dose to the mediastinum and are to be avoided (Cox, 1985).

The issue of elective nodal irradiation was addressed by Krol and colleagues (1996) in a study of 108 patients with clinical stage I disease treated at the primary tumor only. They reported a cancer-specific survival of 42% and 31% at 3 and 5 years, and concluded that the low regional relapse rate did not support the need for the use of large fields encompassing regional lymph nodes. Sawyer and co-workers (1999) studied 346 patients undergoing complete resection for non–small cell lung cancer and compared the preoperative assessment with the operative findings in order to estimate the risk of mediastinal node involvement. They concluded that mediastinal radiation therapy is most likely indicated in those with a positive preoperative bronchoscopy and grade III and IV tumors larger than 3 cm.

COMPLICATIONS OF RADIOTHERAPY

The most frequent symptomatic side effect is esophagitis, which occurs in 50% of patients (Lee, 1977). This usually begins 2 weeks after the initiation of therapy and subsides 1 to 2 weeks after its completion. Radiographic evidence of radiation-induced pneumonitis occurs in almost all patients treated for lung cancer with radiation therapy. Hellman and associates (1964) reported a 100% incidence of radiographic evidence of radiation-induced pneumonitis but only a 5% incidence clinically. Data from the RTOG indicate a risk of 2.7% of life-threatening pneumonitis with doses of 60 Gy (Cox et al, 1990). Monson and colleagues (1998) reported a 20% incidence and noted an increased risk with low performance status, comorbid lung disease, smoking history, and low pulmonary performance tests. Kwa and co-workers (1998) have developed a formula that takes into account the fractional and the total dose and the total and treated lung volume to calculate a mean lung dose as a predictor of radiation pneumonitis risk. Plasma transforming growth factor-β_1 tends to be elevated in patients with radiation pneumonitis; therefore, it may be useful as a predictor of radiation pneumonitis and may identify candidates for dose escalation (Anscher et al, 1998). The severity of the symptoms of dry cough, dyspnea, and chest tightness, and occasionally a mild fever vary with the dose and volume of the lung treated. If a small volume was treated, the symptoms usually subside. However, as the volume irradiated increases, the cough can be productive of thick, whitish to uniformly pink sputum, and the dyspnea can become severe and life-threatening. The differential diagnosis includes bacterial or viral infection, recurrent cancer, lymphangitic spread, or metastatic disease (Roswit and White, 1977). A review of the chest radiographs with the radiation therapy portal films is necessary to determine if the involved lung was in the treated volume, although the changes may extend outside the field (Monson et al, 1998). The risks of radiation-induced myocarditis and pericarditis relate directly to the volume of the heart treated (Ruckdeschel et al, 1975). Lawson and co-workers (1972) reported a 4% incidence if one half of the heart received 45 to 50 Gy in 4 to 5 weeks. With respect to acute effects, Lagrange and associates (1992) demonstrated a temporary decrease of approximately 10% in the left ventricle ejection fraction 2 weeks after mediastinal radiation, with recovery of pre-therapy function within 2 months. Radiation-induced myelitis is the most devastating complication from thoracic radiotherapy and can be avoided by careful administration of the radiotherapy. Doses to the cord of 45 Gy in 4.5 to 5 weeks in a continuous course of 1.8 to 2 Gy per day are generally considered safe (Phillips and Buschke, 1969; Wara et al, 1975).

COMMENTS AND CONTROVERSIES

Radiotherapy is the best single agent, aside from surgery, for the management of NSCLC. It is a curative modality in patients with local-regional disease, but only in a small minority, and it is an effective palliative therapy in a majority of patients with symptomatic disease. Despite advances in the delivery of therapy using CT scans, computer-generated dosimetry, and simulators, local control remains an elusive goal in the majority of patients. Radiotherapy combined with chemotherapy is now the standard in good-performance patients with unresectable disease.

The optimal chemotherapy, radiotherapy, and combination will continue to evolve as newer drugs become available and technical advances allow more sophisticated targeting of the beams of radiation.

The controversies that remain include the selection criteria for radical treatment in unresectable patients and for postoperative radiotherapy in patients with nodal metastases. After local control is achievable in the majority of patients, it may be reasonable to reconsider the question of prophylactic cranial irradiation.

Areas of active investigation include the aforementioned hyperfractionation studies and dose escalation conformal studies, which may lead to increased local control. Because the majority of patients develop metastatic disease, however, improved systemic chemotherapeutic agents are needed before there can be substantial improvement in overall survival rates in NSCLC.

T.H.W.

Like surgery, radiotherapy is effective only as a local treatment. In patients with potentially curable localized disease, when surgery cannot be offered, primary radiotherapy remains the therapy of choice. The addition of concomitant or induction chemotherapy appears to improve the ultimate results of this nonsurgical therapy. In North America, concomitant chemotherapy with a minimum radiotherapy dose of 60 Gy is the standard treatment if radiotherapy is the primary treatment of choice. In very small T1N0 tumors, it does appear that radiotherapy has a significant curative role to play. Indeed, when clinically staged disease treated this way is compared with surgical results, primary radiotherapy has a significant curative benefit. With the newer techniques of 3D conformal radiotherapy, this may be a real option (vs surgery) in the future for treating these very early stage patients.

The role of adjuvant radiotherapy is still debated. Other than decreasing the incidence of local recurrence, adjuvant radiotherapy, even in locally advanced disease or incompletely resected disease, does not appear to improve the ultimate survival rate. This is not unexpected considering the fact that the preponderant type of recurrence following resection for lung cancer is systemic. The very disappointing results of a recent North American trial comparing postoperative radiotherapy with postoperative chemoradiation (no apparent difference) further substantiate the whole question of whether postoperative radiotherapy is indicated in any patient. In this trial (Keller, 2000), the incidence of local-regional recurrence was not insignificant, unlike in other trials of postoperative radiotherapy. The destructive complications related to postoperative radiotherapy and the long-term effects on pulmonary function have not been well delineated. The cost benefit, therefore, of adjuvant radiotherapy following surgical resection is extremely questionable.

The use of external beam irradiation for palliation is unquestioned. Focal areas that cause symptoms can certainly be managed effectively by radiotherapeutic means. Whether or not full-dose radiotherapy is required for this palliative therapy is still unknown.

R.J.G.

■ KEY REFERENCES

Dillman RO, Herndon J, Seagren SL et al: Improved survival in stage III non-small-cell lung cancer: Seven-year follow-up of cancer and leukemia group B (CALGB) 8433 trial. (Comment in J Natl Cancer Inst Sep 4;88(17):1175, 1996.) J Natl Cancer Inst 88(17):1210, 1996.

Report of CALGB 8433, which established combined modality therapy as the standard for good-performance patients with unresectable stage III disease.

Ginsberg RJ: Neoadjuvant (induction) treatment for non-small cell lung cancer [Review[. Lung Cancer 12(suppl 2):S33, 1995.

Good review of neoadjuvant therapy for non–small cell lung cancer.

Perez CA, Stanley K, Grundy G et al: Impact of irradiation technique and tumor extent in tumor control and survival of patients with unresectable non-oat cell carcinoma of the lung: Report of the Radiation Therapy Oncology Group. Cancer 50:1091, 1982.

RTOG report 73-01 compares various fractionation schemes.

Sause WT, Scott C, Taylor S et al, for the Radiation Therapy Oncology Group (RTOG) 88–08 and Eastern Cooperative Oncology Group (ECOG) 4588: Preliminary results of a phase III trial in regionally advanced, unresectable non-small-cell lung cancer. J Natl Cancer Inst 87(3):198, 1995.

This report details the results of the three-arm trial of 60 Gy in 6 weeks versus induction chemotherapy, then 60 Gy in 6 weeks versus hyperfractionated radiotherapy of 69.6 Gy in 6 weeks.

■ REFERENCES

Abe M, Takehishi M, Yabumoto E et al: Clinical experiences with intraoperative radiotherapy of locally advanced cancers. Cancer 45:40, 1980.

Anonymous: Postoperative radiotherapy in non-small-cell lung cancer: Systematic review and meta-analysis of individual patient data from nine randomised controlled trials. PORT Meta-analysis Trialists Group [see comments]. Lancet 352:257, 1998.

Anscher MS, Kong FM, Andrews K et al: Plasma transforming growth factor beta1 as a predictor of radiation pneumonitis. Int J Radiat Oncol Biol Phys 41:1029, 1998.

Armstrong J, Raben A, Zelefsky M et al: Promising survival with three-dimensional conformal radiation therapy for non-small cell lung cancer. Radiother Oncol 44:17, 1997.

Arriagada R, le Chevalier T, Quoix E et al: ASTRO Plenary: Effective chemotherapy on locally advanced non-small cell lung cancer: A randomized study of 353 patients. Int J Radiat Oncol Biol Phys 20:1183, 1991.

Ash D: Role of radiotherapy. Recent results. Cancer Res 92:99, 1984.

Bangma PJ: Postoperative radiotherapy. In Deeley TJ (ed): Modern Radiotherapy: Carcinoma of the Bronchus. New York, Appleton-Century-Crofts, 1972, p 163.

Berry RJ, Laing AH, Newman CR et al: The role of radiotherapy in treatment of inoperable lung cancer. Int J Radiat Oncol Biol Phys 2:443, 1977.

Bleehen NM, Cox JD: Radiotherapy for lung cancer. Int J Radiat Oncol Biol Phys 11:1001, 1985.

Blitzer P: Reanalysis of the RTOG study of palliation of symptomatic osseous metastases. Cancer 55:1468, 1985.

Bloedorn FG, Cowley RA, Cuccia CA et al: Combined therapy: Irradiation and surgery in the treatment of bronchogenic carcinoma. AJR Am J Roentgenol 85:175, 1961.

Brashear RE: Should asymptomatic patients with inoperable bronchogenic carcinoma receive immediate radiotherapy? No. Am Rev Respir Dis 117:411, 1978.

Bromley LI, Szur L: Combined radiotherapy and resection of carcinoma of the bronchus: Experiences with 66 patients. Lancet 2:937, 1955.

Caldwell WL, Bagshaw MA: Indications for end results of irradiation for carcinoma of the lung. Cancer 22:99, 1968.

Calvo FA, Ortiz de Urbina D, Abuchaibe O et al: Intraoperative radiotherapy during lung cancer surgery: Technical description and early clinical results. Int J Radiat Oncol Biol Phys 19:103, 1990.

Choi NCH, Grillo HC, Gardiello M et al: Basis for new strategies in postoperative radiotherapy of bronchogenic carcinoma. Int J Radiat Oncol Biol Phys 6:31, 1980.

Ciampi A, Triffault J: Recurative partition and amalgamation (RECPAM) for censored survival data: Criteria for tree selection. Stat Soft News 14:78, 1988.

Cohen MH: Is immediate radiation therapy indicated for patients with unresectable non-small cell cancer? No. Cancer Treat Rep 67:333, 1983.

Cox JD: Current role of radiation therapy for inoperable carcinoma of the lung. In Cox JD (ed): A Categorical Course in Radiation Therapy of Lung Cancer. New York, Radiologic Society of North America, 1985.

Cox JD: Induction chemotherapy for non-small cell carcinoma of the lung: Limitations and lessons. Int J Radiat Oncol Biol Phys 20:1375, 1991.

Cox JD, Azarnia N, Byhardt RW et al: A randomized phase I/II trial of hyperfractionated radiation therapy with total doses of 60.0 Gy to 79.2 Gy: Possible survival benefit with 69.6 Gy in favorable patients with Radiation Therapy Oncology Group stage III nonsmall-cell lung carcinoma: Report of Radiation Therapy Oncology Group 83-11. J Clin Oncol 8:1543, 1990.

Cox JD, Komaki R, Byhardt RW: Is immediate chest radiotherapy obligatory for any or all patients with limited-stage non-small cell carcinoma of the lung? Yes. Cancer Treat Rep 67:327, 1983.

Cox JD, Komaki R, Eisert D et al: Irradiation for inoperable carcinoma of the lung and high performance status. JAMA 244:1931, 1980.

Cox JD, Scott CB, Byhardt RW et al: Addition of chemotherapy to radiation therapy alters failure patterns by cell type within non-small cell carcinoma of lung (NSCCL): Analysis of Radiation Therapy Oncology Group (RTOG) trials. Int J Radiat Oncol Biol Phys 43:505, 1999.

Deeley TJ: Radiotherapy for carcinoma of the bronchus. Cancer Treat Rev I:39, 1974.

Dillman RO, Herndon J, Seagren SL et al: Improved survival in stage III non-small-cell lung cancer: Seven-year follow-up of cancer and leukemia group B (CALGB) 8433 trial (see comments). (Comment in J Natl Cancer Inst September 4;88:1175, 1996.) J Natl Cancer Inst 88:1210, 1996.

Faber LP, Kittle CF, Warren WH et al: Preoperative chemotherapy and irradiation for stage III non-small cell lung cancer. Ann Thorac Surg 47:669, discussion 676, 1989.

Fletcher GH: Subclinical disease. Cancer 53:1274, 1984.

Fowler WC, Langer CJ, Curran WJ et al: Postoperative complications after combined neoadjuvant treatment of lung cancer. Ann Thorac Surg 55:986, 1993.

Ginsberg RJ: Neoadjuvant (induction) treatment for non-small cell lung cancer [Review]. Lung Cancer 12(suppl 2):S33, 1995.

Graham MV, Purdy JA, Emami B et al: 3-D conformal radiotherapy for lung cancer. The Washington University experience. Front Radiat Ther Oncol 29:188, 1996.

Green N, Kurohara SS, George FW III, Crews QE Jr: Post resection irradiation for primary lung cancer. Radiology 116:405, 1975.

Haffty BG, Goldberg MB, Gerstley J et al: Results of radical radiation therapy in clinical stage I technically operable non-small cell lung cancer. Int J Radiat Oncol Biol Phys 15:69, 1988.

Hebert ME, Lowe VJ, Hoffman JM et al: Positron emission tomography in the pretreatment evaluation and follow-up of non-small cell lung cancer patients treated with radiotherapy: Preliminary findings. Am J Clin Oncol 19:416, 1996.

Hellman S, Kligerman MM, von Essen CF et al: Sequelae of radical radiotherapy of carcinoma of the lung. Radiology 82:1055, 1964.

Hillers TK, Sauve MD, Guyatt GH: Analysis of published studies on the detection of extrathoracic metastases in patients presumed to have operable non-small cell lung cancer (see comments). Thorax 49:14, 1994.

Holmes EC: Adjuvant therapy of non small cell lung cancer. In Salmon SE (ed): Adjuvant Therapy of Cancer, Vol IV. Philadelphia, WB Saunders, 1990.

Holmes EC, Gail MH, for the Lung Cancer Study Group: Surgical adjuvant therapy for stage II and III adenocarcinoma and large cell undifferentiated carcinoma. J Clin Oncol 4:710, 1986.

Hooper RG, Tenholder MF, Underwood GH et al: Computed tomographic scanning of the brain in the initial staging of bronchogenic carcinoma. Chest 85:774, 1984.

Juettner FM, Arian-Schad K, Porsch G et al: Intraoperative radiation therapy combined with external irradiation in non-resectable non-small cell lung cancer: Preliminary report. Int J Radiat Oncol Biol Phys 18:1143, 1990.

Keller S, Adak S, Wagner H et al: A randomized trial of postoperative adjuvant therapy in patients with completely resectable Stage II or IIIA non–small cell lung cancer. N Engl J Med 343:1217, 2000.

Kiffer JD, Berlangieri SU, Scott AM et al: The contribution of 18F-fluoro-2-deoxy-glucose positron emission tomographic imaging to radiotherapy planning in lung cancer. Lung Cancer 19:167, 1998.

Kirsh MM, Sloan H: Mediastinal metastases in bronchogenic carcinoma: Influence of postoperative irradiation, cell type and location. Ann Thorac Surg 33:459, 1982.

Komaki R: Preoperative and postoperative irradiation for cancer of the lung. J Belge Radiol 68:195, 1985.

Komaki R, Cox J, Hartz AJ et al: Characteristics of long-term survivors after treatment for inoperable carcinoma of the lung. Am J Clin Oncol 8:362, 1985.

Komaki R, Scott CB, Byhardt R et al: Failure patterns by prognostic group determined by recursive partitioning analysis (RPA) of 1547 patients on four radiation therapy oncology group (RTOG) studies in inoperable nonsmall-cell lung cancer (NSCLC). Int J Radiat Oncol Biol Phys 42:263, 1998.

Krant MJ: The question of irradiation therapy in lung cancer. JAMA 195:177, 1966.

Krol AD, Aussems P, Noordijk EM et al: Local irradiation alone for peripheral stage I lung cancer: Could we omit the elective regional nodal irradiation? (Review). Int J Radiat Oncol Biol Phys 34:297, 1996.

Kumar PJ, Herndon J, Elias AD, et al: Comparison of pre-operative thoracic radiation therapy (TRT) to pre-operative chemotherapy (CT) in surgical staged IIIA (N2) non-small cell lung cancer (NSCLC): Initial results of Cancer and Leukemia Group B (CALGB) phase III Protocol 9134. Int J Radiat Oncol Biol Phys 36(suppl 2):195, 1997.

Kwa SL, Lebesque JV, Theuws JC et al: Radiation pneumonitis as a function of mean lung dose: An analysis of pooled data of 540 patients. Int J Radiat Oncol Biol Phys 42:1, 1998.

Lagrange JL, Darcourt J, Benoliel J et al: Acute cardiac effects of mediastinal irradiation: Assessment by radionuclide angiography. Int J Radiat Oncol Biol Phys 22:897, 1992.

Lambert PM: Radiation myelopathy of the thoracic spinal cord in long-term survivors treated with radical radiotherapy using conventional fractionation. Cancer 41:1751, 1978.

Landis SH, Murray T, Bolden S, Wingo PA: Cancer statistics, 1998. CA Cancer J Clin 46:6, 1999.

LaRoux BT: Bronchial carcinoma. Thorax 23:136, 1968.

Lawson RAM, Ross WM, Gold RJ et al: Post radiation pericarditis: Report on four more cases with special reference to bronchogenic carcinoma. J Thorac Cardiovasc Surg 63:841, 1972.

Leddy E, Moersch HJ: Roentgen therapy for bronchogenic carcinoma. JAMA 15:2239, 1940.

Lee RE: Radiotherapy of bronchogenic carcinoma. Semin Oncol 1:245, 1974.

Lee RE: Radiotherapy for lung cancer. In Strauss MJ (ed): Lung Cancer Clinical Diagnosis and Treatment. New York, Grune and Stratton, 1977.

Leibel SA: ACR appropriateness criteria. Expert Panel on Radiation Oncology. American College of Radiology. Int J Radiat Oncol Biol Phys 43:125, 1999.

Lokich J, Goodman R: Superior vena cava syndrome. JAMA 231:58, 1975.

Marks LB: A standard dose of radiation for "microscopic disease" is not appropriate. Cancer 66:2498, 1990.

Mira JG, Potter JL, Thorton GD et al: Advantages and limitations of computed tomography scans for treatment planning of cancer. Int J Radiat Oncol Biol Phys 8:1617, 1982.

Monson JM, Stark P, Reilly JJ et al: Clinical radiation pneumonitis and radiographic changes after thoracic radiation therapy for lung carcinoma. Cancer 82:842, 1998.

Morrison R, Deeley TJ, Cleland WP: The treatment of carcinoma of the bronchus. A clinical trial to compare surgery and supervoltage radiotherapy. Lancet 1:683, 1963.

Nabi HA, Steinbrenner L, Lamonica D et al: The use of positron emission tomography in the pre-operative work-up of patients with resectable non-small cell lung cancer [Meeting abstract]. Proc Annu Meet Am Soc Clin Oncol, 1996.

Nielson ME, Heiston DK, Dunnick NR: Preoperative CT evaluation of adrenal glands in non-small cell bronchogenic carcinoma. AJR Am J Roentgenol 139:317, 1982.

Oliver TW Jr, Bernardino ME, Miller JI et al: Isolated adrenal masses in non-small cell bronchogenic carcinoma. Radiology 153:217, 1984.

Pass HI, Pogrebniak HW, Steinberg SM et al: Randomized trial of neoadjuvant therapy for lung cancer: Interim analysis. Ann Thorac Surg 53:992, 1992.

Pass HI, Sindelar WF, Kinsella TJ et al: Delivery of intraoperative radiation therapy after pneumonectomy: Experimental observations and early clinical results. Ann Thorac Surg 44:14, 1987.

Paterson R, Russell MH: Clinical trials in malignant disease IV. Lung cancer: Value of postoperative radiotherapy. Clin Radiol 13:141, 1962.

Paulson DL: A philosophy of treatment for bronchogenic carcinoma. Ann Thorac Surg 5:289, 1968.

Payne DG: Non-small cell lung cancer: Should unresectable stage III patients routinely receive high-dose radiation therapy? J Clin Oncol 6:552, 1988.

Perez CA: Non-small cell carcinoma of the lung: Dose-time parameters. Cancer Treat Symp 2:131, 1985.

Perez CA, Pajak TF, Rubin P et al: Long-term observations of the patterns of failure in patients with unresectable non-oat cell carcinoma of the lung treated with definitive radiotherapy. Cancer 59:1874, 1987.

Perez CA, Stanley K, Grundy G et al: Impact of irradiation technique and tumor extent in tumor control and survival of patients with unresectable non-oat cell carcinoma of the lung: Report of the Radiation Therapy Oncology Group. Cancer 50:1091, 1982.

Pett SB Jr, Wernly JA, Akl BF: Lung cancer: Current concepts and controversies. West J Med 145:52, 1986.

Phillips TL, Buschke F: Radiation tolerance of the spinal cord. AJR Am J Roentgenol 105:659, 1969.

Phillips TL, Miller RJ: Should asymptomatic patients with inoperable bronchogenic carcinoma receive immediate radiotherapy? Yes. Am Rev Respir Dis 117:404, 1978.

Reddy SP, Marks JE: Total atelectasis of the lung secondary to malignant airway expansion. Am J Clin Oncol 13:394, 1991.

Robertson JM, Ten Haken RK, Hazuka MB et al: Dose escalation for non-small cell lung cancer using conformal radiation therapy. Int J Radiat Oncol Biol Phys 37:1079, 1997.

Rosell RJ, Gomez-Codina J, Camps C et al: A randomized trial comparing preoperative chemotherapy plus surgery with surgery alone in patients with non-small-cell lung cancer (see comments). (Comment in N Engl J Med Jan 20;330:206, 1994; Comment in N Engl J Med Jun 16;330:1756, 1994, discussion 1757; Comment in N Engl J Med Jun 16;330:1757, 1994.) N Engl J Med 330:153, 1994.

Roswit B, White DC: Severe radiation injuries of the lung. AJR Am J Roentgenol 129:127, 1977.

Roth JA, Fossella F, Komaki R et al: A randomized trial comparing perioperative chemotherapy and surgery with surgery alone in resectable stage IIIA non-small-cell lung cancer (see comments). (Comment in J Natl Cancer Inst May 4;86:650, 1994.) J Natl Cancer Inst 86:650, 1994.

Rubin P, Ciccio S, Setisarn B: Controversial status of radiation therapy in lung cancer. In Proceedings of The Sixth National Cancer Conference, Philadelphia, JB Lippincott, 1970.

Ruckdeschel JC: Combined modality therapy of non-small cell lung cancer (Review). Semin Oncol 24:429, 1997.

Ruckdeschel JC, Chang P, Morton RG et al: Radiation related pericardial effusions in patients with Hodgkin's disease. Medicine 54:245, 1975

Rusch VW, Albain KS, Crowley JJ et al: Surgical resection of stage IIIA and stage IIIB non-small-cell lung cancer after concurrent induction chemoradiotherapy. A Southwest Oncology Group trial. J Thorac Cardiovasc Surg 105:97, discussion 104, 1993.

Russell AH, Pajak TE, Selim HM et al: Prophylactic cranial irradiation for lung cancer patients at high risk for development of cerebral metastasis: Results of a prospective randomized trial conducted by the Radiation Therapy Oncology Group. Int J Radiat Oncol Biol Phys 21:637, 1991.

Salvatierra A, Baamonde C, Llamas JM et al: Extrathoracic staging of bronchogenic carcinoma. Chest 97:1052, 1990.

Saunders M, Dische S, Barrett A et al: Continuous hyperfractionated accelerated radiotherapy (CHART) versus conventional radiotherapy in non-small-cell lung cancer: A randomised multicentre trial. CHART Steering Committee (see comments). (Comment in Lancet Jul 19;350:156, 1997.) Lancet 350:161, 1997.

Sause WT, Scott C, Taylor S et al: Radiation Therapy Oncology Group (RTOG) 88–08 and Eastern Cooperative Oncology Group (ECOG) 4588: Preliminary results of a phase III trial in regionally advanced, unresectable non-small-cell lung cancer. J Natl Cancer Inst 87:198, 1995.

Sawyer TE, Bonner JA, Gould PM et al: The impact of surgical adjuvant thoracic radiation therapy for patients with nonsmall cell lung carcinoma with ipsilateral mediastinal lymph node involvement. Cancer 80:1399, 1997.

Sawyer TE, Bonner JA, Gould PM et al: Predictors of subclinical nodal involvement in clinical stages I and II non-small cell lung cancer: Implications in the inoperable and three-dimensional dose-escalation settings. Int J Radiat Oncol Biol Phys 43:965, 1999.

Schaake-Konig C, Van den Bogaert W, Dalesio O et al: Effects of concomitant cisplatin and radiotherapy on inoperable non-small cell lung cancer. N Engl J Med 326:524, 1992.

Scott CW, Sause WT, Byhardt R et al: Recursive partitioning analysis of 1592 patients on four Radiation Therapy Oncology Group studies in inoperable non-small cell lung cancer. Lung Cancer 17(suppl 1):S59, 1997.

Shields TW: Preoperative radiation therapy in the treatment of bronchial carcinoma. Cancer 30:1388, 1972.

Shields TW, Robinette CD: Long term survivors after resection of bronchial carcinoma. Surg Gynecol Obstet 136:759, 1973.

Sibley GS, Jamieson TA, Marks LB et al: Radiotherapy alone for medically inoperable stage I non-small-cell lung cancer: The Duke experience. Int J Radiat Oncol Biol Phys 40:149, 1998.

Sibley GS, Mundt AJ, Shapiro C et al: The treatment of stage III nonsmall cell lung cancer using high dose conformal radiotherapy. Int J Radiat Oncol Biol Phys 33:1001, 1995.

Skarin AM, Jochelson M, Sheldon T et al: Neoadjuvant chemotherapy in marginally resectable stage III M0 non-small cell lung cancer: Long-term follow-up in 41 patients. J Surg Oncol 40:266, 1989.

Slawson RG, Scott RM: Radiation therapy in bronchogenic carcinoma. Radiology 132:175, 1979.

Smart J, Hilton G: Radiotherapy of cancer of the lung: Results in a selective group of cases. Lancet 1:880, 1956.

Stanley KE: Prognostic factors for survival in patients with inoperable lung cancer. J Natl Cancer Inst 65:25, 1980.

Strauss GM, Herndon JE, Sherman DD et al: Neoadjuvant chemotherapy and radiotherapy followed by surgery in stage IIIA non-small-cell carcinoma of the lung: Report of a Cancer and Leukemia Group B phase II study. J Clin Oncol 10(8):1237, 1992.

Talton BM, Constable WC, Kersh CR: Curative radiotherapy in non-small cell carcinoma of the lung. Int J Radiat Oncol Biol Phys 19:1521, 1990.

Tochner ZA, Pass HI, Sindelar WF et al: Long term tolerance of thoracic organs to intraoperative radiotherapy. Int J Radiat Oncol Biol Phys 22:65, 1992.

Tong C, Gillick L, Hendrickson FR: The palliation of symptomatic osseous metastases: Final results of the study by the Radiation Therapy Oncology Group. Cancer 50:893, 1982.

Tubiana M: Radiotherapy in non-small cell lung cancer. Chest 96(suppl):85s, 1989.

Turrissi AT: The integration of platinum and radiotherapy in the treatment of lung cancer. Semin Oncol 18(suppl 3):81, 1991.

Van Houtte P, Rockmans P, Smets P et al: Postoperative radiation therapy in lung cancer: A controlled trial after resection of curative design. Int J Radiat Oncol Biol Phys 6:983, 1980.

van't Reit A, Stam HC, Mak ACA et al: Implications of lung corrections for dose specification in radiotherapy. Int J Radiat Oncol Biol Phys 11:621, 1985.

Wara WM, Phillips TL, Sheline GE et al: Radiation tolerance of the spinal cord. Cancer 35:1558, 1975.

Warram J: Preoperative irradiation of cancer of the lung: Final report of a therapeutic trial collaborative study. Cancer 36:914, 1975.

Weder W, Schmid RA, Bruchhaus H et al: Detection of extrathoracic metastases by positron emission tomography in lung cancer. Ann Thorac Surg 66:886, discussion 892, 1998.

Weiden PL, Piantadosi S: Preoperative chemotherapy (cisplatin and fluorouracil) and radiation therapy in stage III non-small cell lung cancer. A phase 2 study of the LCSG. Chest 106(suppl 6):344S, 1993.

Weinberg JA: The intrathoracic lymphatics. In Haagensen CD, Feind CR, Herter FP et al (eds): The Lymphatics in Cancer. Philadelphia, WB Saunders, 1972.

Weisenburger T: Postoperative radiotherapy for non-small-cell lung cancer. Chest Surg Clin North Am 1:71, 1991.

Weisenburger T, Gail M: Postoperative mediastinal radiation for cancer of the lung (Letter). N Engl J Med 316:1476, 1987.

Weisenburger T, Gail M, for the Lung Cancer Study Group: Effects of postoperative mediastinal radiation on completely resected stage II and III epidermoid carcinoma of the lung. N Engl J Med 315:1377, 1986.

Withers HR, Taylor JMG, Maciejewski B: The hazard of accelerated tumor clonogen repopulation during radiotherapy. Acta Oncol 27:131, 1988.

Zhang HX, Yin WB, Zhang LJ et al: Curative radiotherapy of early operable non-small cell lung cancer. Radiother Oncol 14:89, 1989.

BRACHYTHERAPY AND INTRAOPERATIVE RADIOTHERAPY FOR NON–SMALL CELL LUNG CANCER

Carol McGibney
John G. Armstrong

The principal types of radiation used for the therapy of tumors are external beam and brachytherapy. With external beam radiotherapy (EBRT), the source of radiation is outside the patient and the radiation must pass through superficial tissues to arrive at its destination. Examples of external beam machines include linear accelerators that can produce photons or electrons and isotopic cobalt-based machines that produce photons. External beam radiation may also be delivered intraoperatively (IORT). While still anesthetized and draped, the patient is transported to the linear accelerator (as described earlier), and the machine is pointed directly into the operative field and is oriented toward the tumor bed. Retractors can be used to remove normal tissues from the pathway of the radiation. Brachytherapy is the therapy of tumors provided by the direct application of radioactive sources, either into a tumor (interstitial) or into a naturally occurring cavity (intracavitary) such as the airways. In contrast to external beam radiotherapy, the source of radiation is an isotope that emits radiation in a localized manner and delivers a high dose to the tissues from within (*brachy* means short).

HISTORICAL NOTE

The interstitial implantation of radioactive isotopes—preoperatively—for lung cancer began in 1941 at Memorial Sloan-Kettering Cancer Center in New York (Henschke, 1958). Initially, encapsulated radon (^{222}Rn) was used. Radioactive isotopes encapsulated in metal seeds were placed through hollow needles into tumors, one seed at a time. There was no mechanism for calculating the optimal distribution of seeds or for ensuring that the seeds could be evenly distributed throughout the tumor. In addition, the dose to the tumor could not be calculated, and therapy was prescribed solely in terms of the total amount of "activity" of the radioisotope. Subsequently, encapsulated radioactive iodine (^{125}I) seeds were used. The development of the Mick applicator permitted accurate spacing of the ^{125}I seeds, which were evenly distributed throughout the tumor. An intraoperative nomogram was devised to permit the delivery of uniform doses to tumors of varying sizes and shapes. By measuring the tumor intraoperatively, a nomogram could be used to calculate the total activity required, the optimal placement of the Mick applicator needles, and the spacing of the individual seeds along the needles. Dose calculations are now computerized and reflect the actual dose delivered to the tumor, which can be displayed in a three-dimensional format.

Intracavitary brachytherapy for lung cancer consists of intraluminal therapy for cancers in the major airways. The first intraluminal (endoscopic) brachytherapy treatment was reported by Yankauer in 1922. Two patients were treated with radon seeds, which were inserted through a rigid bronchoscope at the tumor location. Later, the use of radon was replaced by the use of cobalt-60 beads and ultimately, by the isotope iridium-192, initially in the form of iridium wire (Aygun and Blum, 1995; Mehta et al, 1998). Catheters were positioned in the lumen of the bronchus beyond the site of the tumor in the airway. The iridium wire, which was of sufficient length to span the tumor with several additional centimeters on either side, was inserted into the catheter under bronchoscopic guidance and was positioned at the site of the tumor. After the removal of the bronchoscope, the catheter containing the wire was left in place for 1 day or longer. The typical dose 1 cm from the center of the source was 30 to 40 Gy over 1 to 2 days. The disadvantages of this technique were its duration, the discomfort for the patient, and the need to protect the staff from the radiation exposure associated with this prolonged therapy (Raben and Mychalczak, 1996). The development of high-activity remote afterloading machines, initially driven manually (Henschke, 1964) and later by computer (Macha et al, 1987), removed these practical disadvantages and led to great interest in the use of this technology for the palliation of obstructing airway malignancies. The development of fiberoptic bronchoscopy, which enhances access to the more distal bronchi, and the yttrium-aluminum-garnet (YAG) laser, which can create a channel through an obstructing tumor, and the advent of more effective local anesthetic agents, antitussive agents, and reversible sedation have increased the use of pulmonary brachytherapy to treat many more patients (Aygun and Blum, 1995; Mehta et al, 1998). Several studies have confirmed that high-dose radiotherapy (HDR) can achieve the same results as low-dose radiotherapy (LDR) in palliation, in terms of European Cooperative Oncology Group (ECOG) performance status, decreased symptoms, radiographic response, and percentage of lifetime rendered symptom free (Lo et al, 1995; Mehta, 1992). A hyperfractionated treatment regimen that is administered over 2 to 3 days may be even more appropriate in the palliative setting because only one bronchoscopy is necessary for insertion of the afterloading brachytherapy catheter (Mehta, 1992).

■ *HISTORICAL READINGS*

Henschke UK: Interstitial implantation in the treatment of primary bronchogenic carcinoma. AJR Am J Roentgenol 79:981, 1958.

Henschke UK, Hilaris BS, Mahan GD: Remote afterloading for intracavitary applicators. Radiology 83:344, 1964.

Hilaris BS, Martini N: The current state of intraoperative interstitial brachytherapy in lung cancer. Int J Radiat Oncol Biol Phys 15:1347, 1988.

Macha HN, Koch K, Stadler M et al: New technique for treating occlusive and stenosing tumours of the trachea and main bronchi: Endobronchial irradiation by high dose iridium-192 combined with lasar canalization. Thorax 42:511, 1987.

Nori D, Hilaris B, Martini N: Intraluminal irradiation in bronchogenic carcinoma. Surg Clin North Am 67:1093, 1987.

Yankauer S: Two cases of lung tumour treated bronchoscopically. N Y Med J 21:741, 1922.

BASIC SCIENCE

Radiobiology

Radiobiology is the study of the action of ionizing radiation on living cells. The effect is mediated indirectly by the formation of chemically reactive free radicals that attack the base pairs of DNA, leading to chemical changes and biologic damage. The interval between the chemical damage and the expression of biologic effects may be hours, days, months, or even years. A number of factors contribute to the timing and magnitude of the biologic effect and are described as the "4 R's" of radiobiology.

The impact of a given dose of radiation on the target cell is related to the cell's ability to repair radiation damage. Although the biologic mechanisms of repair have not been elucidated, they have been quantified mathematically. It appears that a minimum of 4 to 6 hours is required for the optimal repair of damage to normal tissues. Tumor cells may repair radiation damage less well than normal cells, hence, the preferential killing of malignant cells. If the repair is complete before cell division occurs, then there is no untoward effect on the cell or its progeny. However, if the repair is incomplete or severe, the damage is lethal and the cell dies on attempting division. Because radiation-induced death occurs when mitosis is attempted, the response to radiation may occur a long time after the therapy is completed. In the interval between two fractions of radiation exposure, both tumor and normal cells repopulate. This has an adverse effect on the potential for tumor control (particularly if it is rapidly growing). In contrast, this allows compensatory proliferation of actively dividing normal tissues (e.g., mucosal membrane) but has no beneficial effect on slowly dividing normal tissues (such as spinal cord).

Because molecular oxygen is required to stabilize radiation damage, large tumors with central hypoxic zones are relatively radioresistant. It has been shown that these hypoxic areas disappear throughout a course of fractionated radiotherapy, and this phenomenon (described as reoxygenation) explains why large tumors can be cured despite the presence of hypoxic areas. The most radiosensitive phases of the cell cycle are G_2 and M. As a fractionated course of radiotherapy proceeds, the tumor's cells tend to accumulate in these phases (perhaps because sublethal radiation-induced damage has not been repaired and control mechanisms prevent mitosis), and therefore, they become radiosensitive. This is referred to as *redistribution*.

Physics

The physical characteristics of isotopes determine their biologic effects. The typical energy of radiation emitted from isotopes ranges from a high of 1.25 MeV for ^{60}Co to a low of 0.028 MeV for ^{125}I. At the high end of the energy spectrum, the emitted radiation penetrates tissue well, to such an extent that ^{60}Co can be used as the radiation source for external beam radiotherapy machines. In contrast, the low-energy emissions penetrate tissue poorly. In addition, the dose decreases in proportion to the square root of the distance from the source. Therefore, the majority of the dose is released into the immediately adjacent tissues. Because of this physical advantage of brachytherapy, high activities of isotopes can be placed directly into the tumor with a powerful localized antitumor effect.

Radioactive Iodine

The rate of radioactive decay of an isotope is indicated by its half-life, which is the time required for it to decay to one half of its original activity. Radioactive iodine (^{125}I) has a half-life of 60 days. It can be calculated that it will decay to 1.5% of its original activity within 1 year after a permanent implant has been placed. Thus, the majority of the biologic effect is delivered in the first 2 months, and ^{125}I is safe to use as a permanent interstitial implant. The disadvantage of this low dose rate (8 cGy/hr) is that it facilitates complete repair of radiation-induced damage, in theory negating the antitumor effect. In addition, if the tumor contains rapidly cycling cells (such as a histologically high-grade neoplasm), they may repopulate during this protracted therapy. In defense of ^{125}I, the low dose rate may facilitate redistribution and increase tumor cell death. The reality is that tumors respond in a heterogeneous manner, and ^{125}I can permanently eradicate some tumors. Another disadvantage of ^{125}I is that the poor penetrance of the beam requires that the seeds be placed within (or in close proximity to) the tumor.

Iridium-192

Iridium-192 (^{192}Ir) is the other important isotope used for lung cancer brachytherapy. Unlike ^{125}I, the emitted radiation from this isotope has a higher energy (0.38 MeV). Consequently, this radiation penetrates more deeply and can effectively treat to a distance of 1 cm from the location of the source. In addition, the dose rate from this isotope is higher, and it can be used for temporary brachytherapy. The most common use of this isotope is in high-dose-rate machines that use a source of 10 Ci, which can deliver a dose of 500 cGy at 1 cm from the source in a matter of minutes. Thus ^{192}Ir is used for repeated intraluminal therapy of tumors accessible by bronchoscopy. This approach appears to have a greater antitumor effect than do numerically similar total doses of fractionated external beam radiotherapy. This is probably because the large fraction size (500 cGy vs 180 to 200 cGy with external beam) exceeds the repair potential of tumor cells. In addition, there are components of the tumor (closer than 1 cm to the source) that receive much higher doses than the prescription dose of 500 cGy.

MANAGEMENT

The use of brachytherapy by means of interstitial implants or endoluminal treatment can be intended as a curative or adjuvant treatment depending on the situation. Frequently, this type of therapy is an adjunct to other treatments, including surgical excision or thermal destruction of endobronchial tumors. Similarly, intraoperative radiotherapy is very occasionally used, in conjunction with surgery, to ablate potential micrometastatic disease at resection margins, or as primary therapy when resection is impossible.

In all of these instances, the potential advantage of these local therapies (vs external beam radiotherapy) is the preciseness with which the treatment can be delivered, thereby theoretically increasing the radiation dose without injuring adjacent vital structures (e.g., esophagus, spinal cord).

Interstitial Implants

Indications

Interstitial implants may be inserted intraoperatively if the patient has an early-stage, technically resectable tumor but cannot tolerate the required resection because of limited pulmonary reserve. In addition, they are used as adjuncts in incompletely resectable tumors or as primary therapy for unresectable tumors caused by advanced disease or at the site of the tumor (near large pulmonary vessels).

Interstitial implantation may be undertaken endoscopically in the palliative setting for recurrent disease (Tomberlin et al, 1992), or percutaneously, under CT control, for the treatment of primary lesions, recurrent disease, or secondary lesions from other sites, for example, thyroid, breast, melanoma, or sarcoma (Brach et al, 1994).

Technique

Intraoperative, Permanent Interstitial Implants. An intraoperative, permanent implant is performed at thoracotomy under general anesthesia. The unresected tumor is measured, and the area or volume to be covered is identified. This includes a margin around the clinically evident tumor. If the tumor is a palpable mass, the appropriate nomogram for volume implants is consulted to determine the total activity required and the separation of the needles. The lesion is then firmly grasped, and the Mick needle is inserted into the tumor. The hand grasping the tumor is used to palpate the deepest extent of the tumor and to determine the depth of insertion. The required number of needles is inserted into the tumor; these are usually placed 1 cm apart. The Mick applicator is then used to deposit the seeds—usually ^{125}I—in the tissue at predetermined intervals along the track of the needle as it is withdrawn.

Plaques of residual disease or areas of possible microscopic disease are covered with a planar implant, attached either by directly suturing ^{125}I seeds encapsulated in Vicryl or by evenly spacing suture seeds in a premeasured Dexon mesh and suturing the mesh directly onto the area at risk (Hilaris et al, 1988). The latter technique is well suited to areas such as the major vessels or the paraspinal region (Armstrong et al, 1991). Postoperatively, when the chest tubes are removed, plain radiographs are taken to determine the location of the seeds and to produce computerized dose distribution calculations. The typical dose delivered with ^{125}I is 16,000 cGy minimal peripheral dose. When used by experienced practitioners, this approach is remarkably safe. It has not increased postoperative morbidity or mortality rates to any appreciable extent. In one instance at Memorial Hospital, a seed migrated into the pulmonary vein and eventually lodged in the circle of Willis, with ensuing neurologic sequelae.

The majority of patients treated with permanent ^{125}I implants have also received supplemental postoperative external beam radiotherapy. The usual dose is 5040 cGy in conventional fractions (180 to 200 cGy). An example of a patient with a T4N0 unresectable squamous cancer is presented in Figure 32–9.

Palladium-103 (^{103}Pd) has also been used in both volume and planar implants. A technique whereby a Gelfoam plaque has been impregnated with ^{125}I or ^{103}Pd seeds was introduced in 1981 (Marchese et al, 1981). Again, based on nomograph calculation, a matrix is drawn on the Gelfoam with mesh points corresponding to where each seed should be placed. The radioactive sources are placed using the Mick applicator or a long forceps. The entry sites are closed with Surgilube, and another layer of Gelfoam, equal in dimension, is sandwiched to the radioactive layer. The plaque is either clipped or sutured into place or is placed within a Dexon or Vicryl mesh onto the tumor bed. The preparation of the Gelfoam plaque with Vicryl mesh is undertaken outside of the patient; thus measurements and seed placement can be carried out with a high degree of accuracy (Nori, 1993).

Percutaneous, Permanent Interstitial Implants. The percutaneous, permanent implantation of ^{125}I seeds has been reported by Heelan and associates from the Memorial Sloan-Kettering Cancer Center (MSKCC) (Heelan et al, 1987). The procedure was carried out as an outpatient procedure in 5 of 7 patients. Two of the seven had been admitted initially for radical surgery. This technique was restricted to peripherally sited tumors, which included two primary lung tumors in two patients with poor respiratory reserve, two recurrent localized lung tumors, one contralateral localized tumor, one subpleural adenocarcinoma of unknown origin, and one subpleural metastasis from a thymoma. All were discrete lesions and were measurable in three dimensions on diagnostic computed tomography (CT) scan. Tracks were initially developed under biplane fluoroscopic control, the trajectories having been calculated on a computerized planning model. Smaller needles were then placed in the tracks and were

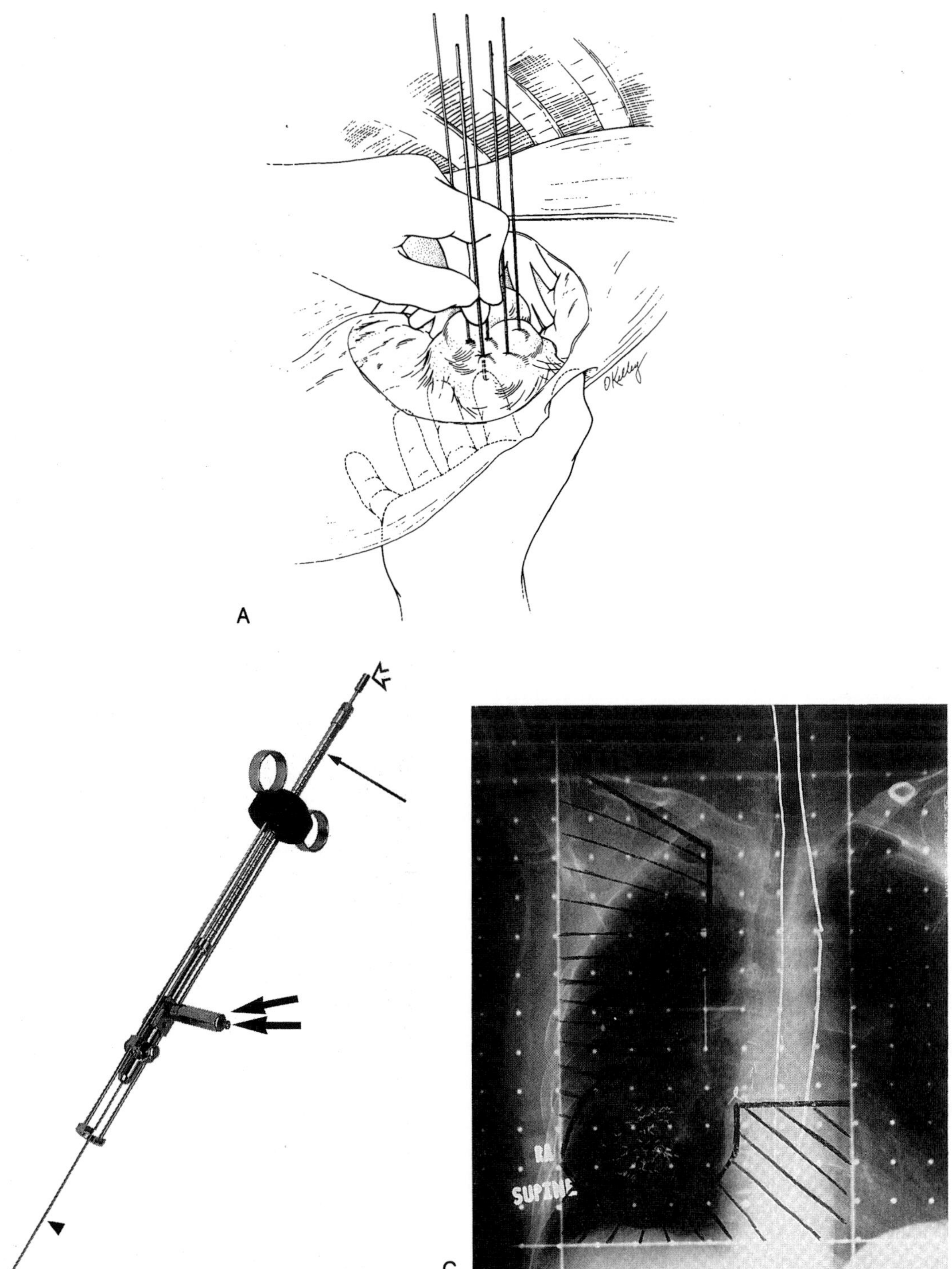

FIGURE 32–9 ■ A non-small cell lung carcinoma invading the right pulmonary artery was unresectable because the results of the patient's pulmonary function tests were too poor to permit pneumonectomy. The implant was performed with ^{125}I. *A*, At thoracotomy, the afterloading trocars are placed in the tumor one at a time, spaced approximately 1 cm apart (see text). When all the trocars are inserted, the Mick afterloader is used, and the radioactive seeds are deposited along the length of each trocar as it is withdrawn by the applicator. *B*, The Mick applicator. The cartridge of radioactive ^{125}I seeds (*double arrows*) is inserted into the applicator. The plunger is used to advance the seeds (one by one) into the tumor, withdrawing the central applicator (*long slender arrow*) to space the seeds. *C*, After recovery from surgery, the patient received external beam radiotherapy, consisting of 5040 cGy to the primary tumor, ipsilateral hilum, mediastinum, and ipsilateral supraclavicular area. The radioactive seeds are seen within the tumor on the simulation radiograph.

loaded with radioactive sources through use of the Mick applicator.

Temporary Interstitial Implants. The afterloading catheters for temporary, interstitial implantation may also be inserted intraoperatively. With this technique, either ^{192}Ir (low dose rate or remote afterloading high dose rate) or high-activity ^{125}I has been used to deliver additional radiation dose to the mediastinum or paravertebral or chest wall resection sites for areas of unresected tumor or with positive margins. The skin of the anterior chest wall between the nipple and the anterior axillary line is marked to indicate the points through which the catheters will be passed into the chest. A hollow, straight, stainless steel needle is passed through the chest wall at the marked site (17 gauge, 15 cm long), and the closed end of a plastic catheter is threaded through the needle until it emerges from the end of the needle. The latter is then removed while the catheter is held in place. This process is repeated until all afterloading catheters are in place and are sutured or clipped in the desired position. A system of metallic clips is placed at the closed ends of the catheters for later identification. The catheters are then sutured to the skin in situ via a system of plastic hemispheres and stainless steel buttons. The number of catheters is determined using the planar implant guide. The radioactive sources are afterloaded into the catheters 3 to 5 days post surgery in order to facilitate immediate postoperative care and to promote healing (Aye et al, 1993; Hilaris, 1994; Nori, 1993).

In low-dose-rate ^{192}Ir temporary implants, a minimal dose of 3000 cGy is prescribed and is supplemented with 4000 to 5000 cGy of external beam radiation. If high-dose-rate afterloading implantation is undertaken, a minimal peripheral dose of 1000 cGy is delivered in 3 to 4 minutes, and the afterloaded catheters are removed following treatment. Temporary interstitial implants using high dose-rate remote afterloading (HDR-RAL) brachytherapy are prescribed in fractions of 400 to 500 cGy × 3 or 4, over 2 days (Aye et al, 1993).

The HDR-RAL technique is a flexible technique, the source of which is readily available (unlike ^{125}I seeds). There is no limitation to the size that may be treated, dosimetry optimization is good, and there is no exposure to personnel. The extra time required to suture catheters post resection is decreased by using the Multi-Fire Endoscopic stapler (Aye et al, 1993). With this technique, one has the benefit of reviewing the pathology report before the actual radiation is administered.

Temporary interstitial implantation of ^{192}Ir active sources may also be inserted percutaneously. Brach and associates (1994) reported their results of high-dose-rate remote afterloading percutaneous brachytherapy technique, undertaken in a small group with either primary lung tumors or metastatic deposits in the lung and chest wall. Multiple fine-gauge afterloading needles were first inserted percutaneously, under CT guidance, and the positions were checked with CT with or without orthogonal views on radiograph; the resulting volume was then planned. A dose of 2000 cGy in four fractions was administered over 2 days, but in some instances the dose ranged from 1000 to 2000 cGy in 1 to 3 fractions (Brach, 1994).

Results

Medically Inoperable Tumors. Some patients with T1–2N0–1 resectable disease have medical contraindications or refuse surgery. For such patients, external beam radiotherapy alone is a potentially curative therapy (Armstrong and Minsky, 1989). An alternative approach has been reported by the Memorial Sloan-Kettering group. Between 1958 and 1984, they used brachytherapy for 55 patients with borderline pulmonary function test results (Hilaris, 1994; Hilaris et al, 1987b). Preoperatively, the tumors were considered resectable by lobectomy or a lesser procedure. At the time of surgery, however, a more radical procedure that the patient could not tolerate was considered necessary. Consequently, the gross tumor was implanted with ^{125}I seeds intraoperatively. Following brachytherapy, 24 patients received external beam radiotherapy. Local-regional control was 100% in T1N0 tumors and 70% in large T2N0 or T2N1 lesions. The actuarial 5-year survival rate was 32% (cause-specific survival was not calculated), suggesting that this approach is reasonable for patients whose conditions are found to be medically inoperable at the time of surgery. Multivariate analysis indicated that patient age (i.e., younger than 58 years) and tumor site (i.e., those with right-sided tumors) were important; these criteria were associated with an improved prognosis (4.5 yr vs 1.2 yr for worst prognosis group). Postoperative radiotherapy did not influence the prognosis overall but did appear to improve local control in those with N1 disease who received postoperative radiotherapy, 86% vs 57%, respectively (Hilaris et al, 1986). Fleischman and colleagues (1992) also treated a group of stage I to stage II tumors with permanent ^{125}I implants. The patients were selected for this therapy if they had node-negative, technically resectable tumors that were medically inoperable, as was described earlier. With a minimum follow-up of 12 months, the mean and median survival times were 16.7 months and 15.1 months, respectively, in this group. The survival rate of the 14 patients was approximately 32% at 2 years. Local control was obtained in 10 of 12 patients with tumors 5 cm or less in maximum dimension. Local failures occurred in stage III tumors and in those with tumors greater than 5 cm. Both patients with larger tumors had local recurrences. No radiation pneumonitis occurred; there was one operative mortality and two postoperative complications (Fleischman et al, 1992).

Locally Advanced Lung Cancer. ***Patients with N0 Disease.*** Hilaris and Martini (1988) reported on 101 patients with unresectable primary tumors invading the major vessels, pericardium, or esophagus, who were treated with biopsy, brachytherapy, or external beam radiotherapy. These patients had no evidence of mediastinal metastasis at thoracotomy. The median survival time was 11 months, and the 2-year survival rate was 21%. A contemporary group of 44 patients with locally advanced primary tumors and a clinically negative mediastinum were treated with external beam radiotherapy (with or without chemotherapy); they had a median survival time of 8 months and a 2-year survival rate of 10%.

Patients with N0–N2 Disease. In 100 patients with stage III NSCLC (T1–T3, N0–N2, 86% with N2 disease), ^{125}I implants were used in 45 patients for unresected or incompletely resected primary tumors, and temporary ^{192}Ir implants were placed in 55 patients with subclinical disease in the superior mediastinum or chest wall. All patients had received postoperative mediastinal radiation therapy to a median dose of 40 Gy 4 to 6 weeks after surgery. The local control rate was greater than 70% at 5 years, but the extent of surgical resection, the presence or absence of positive margins, and the dose of postoperative external beam radiation therapy significantly influenced local control rates. Overall survival was 22%, but this was reduced to 13% in those who had incomplete surgical resection and rose to 30% in those with complete resection (Hilaris et al, 1985).

Burt and co-workers (1987) at the MSKCC reported on a study of 225 patients who had T3 (52%) or T4 (48%) disease with N1–N2 nodal metastases and who underwent exploration, resection, or brachytherapy. Forty-nine patients underwent complete resection, and the rest fell into three categories: those with incomplete resection and brachytherapy (33), those with biopsy and brachytherapy (101), and those who had incomplete or no resection and no brachytherapy (33). When those who had complete resection were compared with those who had resection plus brachytherapy for residual disease, the 2-year survival figures were 30% and 29%, respectively—the 3-year survival figures were 22% and 21%, respectively. Those who had brachytherapy only with biopsy had 2-year and 3-year survival figures of 21% and 9%, respectively. Local control, which may be due in part to the external beam radiation therapy also used, was 70%, and most failures occurred as distant +/− local failures (Burt et al, 1987).

Lewis and associates (1990) treated 82 patients with intraoperative brachytherapy as an adjunct to surgical resection. In general, temporary implants with ^{192}Ir were used for microscopic residual disease, and permanent ^{125}I implants were used for gross disease. Supplemental external beam radiotherapy was used (approximately 50 Gy). The techniques of the Memorial group were used. The tumor stage was IIIA or IIIB in 89% of cases, and the implanted volume was 6 cm or less in maximum dimension. The overall survival rate was 40% at 2 years. The survival rate at 2 years was 50% if microscopic residual disease was implanted and 30% if gross residual disease was implanted.

The selected use of intraoperative brachytherapy for residual disease appears advantageous in those with N2 non–small cell lung cancer who have undergone aggressive induction chemotherapy, surgical resection, and postoperative external beam radiotherapy. Median survival figures are not significantly different when those requiring intraoperative brachytherapy for residual disease are compared with those who do not require it—19 months versus 22 months, respectively (Armstrong et al, 1992).

The results of CT-guided, percutaneous implantation brachytherapy (high-dose-rate remote afterloading procedure) with radical intent have been reported (Brach et al, 1994). This subgroup consisted of 10 patients with small, localized N0 disease who had refused surgery or with residual disease post external beam radiation therapy or surgery. Seven of the ten patients had N0 disease, two had N1 disease, and one had N2 disease. The median tumor size was 4 cm with a range of 1.3 to 11 cm. At follow-up (6–30 months), 50% of patients had complete resolution of tumor, and a further 50% had a significant response. Complications included a 30% incidence of pneumothorax; minor, untreated hemoptysis in 30%; asymptomatic central tumor necrosis in one instance; and one case of pericarditis, the pericardium having received 1000 cGy in 2 fractions. Long-term survival has not been reported.

Metastatic Cancer in Lung or Chest Wall. Heelan and colleagues (1987) reported the results of a pilot study of percutaneous, permanent interstitial therapy (^{125}I seed sources). Seven patients with a variety of tumors, all of which were at the periphery of the lung, were treated with a dose of 160 Gy to the periphery of each tumor. There were no complications. Complete response occurred in four of seven patients, partial response resulted in two of seven patients, and one patient was lost to follow-up.

Pancoast Tumors. The management of Pancoast tumors is controversial. Radiotherapy is considered to be an essential component of therapy—as sole therapy, as preoperative therapy, postoperatively, or as intraoperative brachytherapy (Anderson et al, 1986; Attar et al, 1979; Komaki et al, 1981; Miller et al, 1979; Neal et al, 1991; Paulson, 1985). Preoperative radiotherapy, pioneered by Shaw and co-workers (1961), is used to reduce the volume of the tumor, thus facilitating complete resection. Subsequent reports of preoperative radiotherapy demonstrated 5-year survival rates in the range of 20% to 30%.

Hilaris and associates (1987a) treated 82 patients with 2000 to 4000 cGy of preoperative radiotherapy followed by resection and permanent interstitial implantation of ^{125}I in the majority. The fatal complication rate was 1%, and the 5-year survival rate was 29%. In addition to this experience with preoperative radiotherapy, this group (Hilaris et al, 1987b) employed initial surgery with intraoperative brachytherapy for 36 patients, followed by postoperative radiotherapy, and reported 20% 5-year survival rates. Univariate analysis suggested that completeness of resection and histologic type, as well as nodal status and preoperative radiation, were significant for outcome; however, multivariate analysis indicated that mediastinal nodal status and preoperative radiation were independent prognostic variables. Although the results achieved with combined brachytherapy, surgery, and external beam radiotherapy are impressive, they are not strikingly different from the survival rates reported in series without brachytherapy.

The results of surgical treatment of 124 patients with Pancoast tumors at the Memorial Sloan-Kettering Cancer Center have been reported (Ginsberg et al, 1994). Ninety-four patients had stage IIIA disease, and 30 had stage IIIB. Of the 124 patients, 117 received EBRT. Intraoperative brachytherapy was used in 102 patients with either (1) permanent implantation of ^{125}I or ^{103}Pd seeds at a median dose of 160 cGy, or (2) temporary implantation of afterloading catheters containing ^{192}Ir at a dose of 30 to 40 Gy over 3 to 5 days.

Local control and 5-year survival (41%) were comparable for patients who had completely resected tumors, with (n = 49) and without (n = 20) the addition of brachytherapy. The true impact of brachytherapy was unclear as the local failure rate was comparable in those completely resected with no additional brachytherapy (69%) when compared with those with incompletely resected (n = 31) or nonresectable (n = 24) tumors in whom brachytherapy was used (77%).

Intraluminal Brachytherapy

Direct permanent implantation of ^{125}I seeds into endobronchial tumors was also pioneered at Memorial Sloan-Kettering Cancer Center in the 1960s. Relief of symptoms was achieved in about 60% of patients, but there was significant morbidity as a result of perforation of the airway, hemorrhage, and ventilatory arrest (Nori et al, 1987). Subsequent workers avoided direct implantation into tissues (interstitial) and used temporary intraluminal placement of 60 Co or ^{192}Ir to deliver one or more large fractions over a few days (Mehta et al, 1989; Schray et al, 1985). High-dose-rate fractionated intraluminal brachytherapy (HDR-ILBRT) was later developed to avoid such prolonged therapeutic times, which were uncomfortable for the patient and required hospitalization with its attendant expense and radiation risk to personnel (Macha et al, 1987).

Indications

The use of HDR-ILBRT has increased over the past decade. The generally accepted criteria for HDR-ILBRT are previous external beam radiotherapy, intraluminal recurrence in the bronchus or trachea, and significant symptoms caused by the local disease. Other indications include those with life-threatening symptoms prior to definitive treatment of locally advanced disease and those with small (<1 cm) endobronchial tumors who are not candidates for other forms of therapy (Nomoto et al, 1997; Perol et al, 1997; Taulelle et al, 1998). The role of HDR-ILBRT in the definitive management of stage I to stage III NSCLC is evolving (Gaspar, 1998; Raben and Mychalczak, 1996).

Technique

If endobronchial laser resection is planned at the time of the first HDR-ILBRT, then general anesthesia and rigid bronchoscopy are required (Fig. 32–10). When endobronchial laser resection is not used, the bronchoscopy is performed as an outpatient procedure with sedation, local anesthesia, cardiac monitoring, and pulse oximetry. The bronchoscope is inserted transnasally, and a routine examination of the airway is performed. The brachytherapy catheter is placed through the working channel of the bronchoscope and is lodged at least 3 cm distal to the obstruction. With the catheter left in place, the bronchoscope is withdrawn, and the catheter is taped to the nose, thus securing it in position. Another useful technique is to pass a guidewire through a cannula through the midline of the neck into the upper trachea and a Seldinger-type dilator over this wire. The brachytherapy catheter can be passed through the dilator into the airway. When the position of the catheter in the trachea is verified by the bronchoscope, the dilator can be withdrawn and peeled off the catheter, but left in the airway. With the use of fiberoptic bronchoscopy, the catheter is then manipulated into position and is secured to the overlying skin.

A "dummy" source is placed in the catheter and pushed to its distal end. The dummy is a wire that has radiopaque beads located at 0.25- to 1-cm intervals, which can be occupied by the radiation source. Radiographs are taken to assist in verifying the location of the catheter and in deciding which potential source locations are to be treated. It is important to treat the entire tumor and a margin of 3 cm proximally and distally. Computerized planning is used to calculate the dwell time of the source at the various locations along the treated length of airway. (The newer machines can use a number of catheters and can be programmed to modify dwell times to create an envelope of dosing volume around the tumor.) The therapeutic time is calculated to determine the prescribed dose at a distance of 1 cm from the source. When the planning is complete, the catheter is connected to the afterloading machine, which contains a high-activity ^{192}Ir source (10 Ci) that travels along the catheter and is programmed to remain at specific locations for delivery of a precisely controlled dose over several minutes.

The optimal radiotherapeutic parameters for HDR-ILBRT are being sought. These variables include the use of initial laser debulking, external radiotherapy, the number of brachytherapy procedures, dose per fraction, the interval between procedures, and the total dose. The most commonly used approach is to deliver a total of three courses, spaced 1 week apart. The dose per fraction is prescribed at 1 cm from the source and varies between 5 and 10 Gy. Doses in the low range of this scale may be more appropriate for patients previously treated with high doses of external radiotherapy (60 Gy or more).

Assessment of Response to HDR-ILBRT

Response to ILBRT can be assessed with the use of clinical or endoscopic parameters, depending on the context in which ILBRT is used (Mehta et al, 1998). The clinical response in patients treated palliatively may be assessed using symptom control, percentage of remaining time rendered symptom free, or improvement in Karnofsky performance status (KPS) and ECOG performance status (Cotter et al, 1993; Mehta, 1998).

The degree of reduction in bronchial obstruction post HDR-ILBRT may be scored in different ways and may be used as an objective parameter of response, as may the radiographic response to therapy. The latter is important as re-aeration of the lung volume not only may decrease symptoms in those requiring palliation but also may reduce the thoracic volume, which needs to be irradiated in those being treated with radical intent (Bastin et al, 1993; Cotter et al, 1993). The percentage of those patients with atelectasis and postobstructive pneumonia demonstrating re-aeration of the lung post HDR-ILBRT

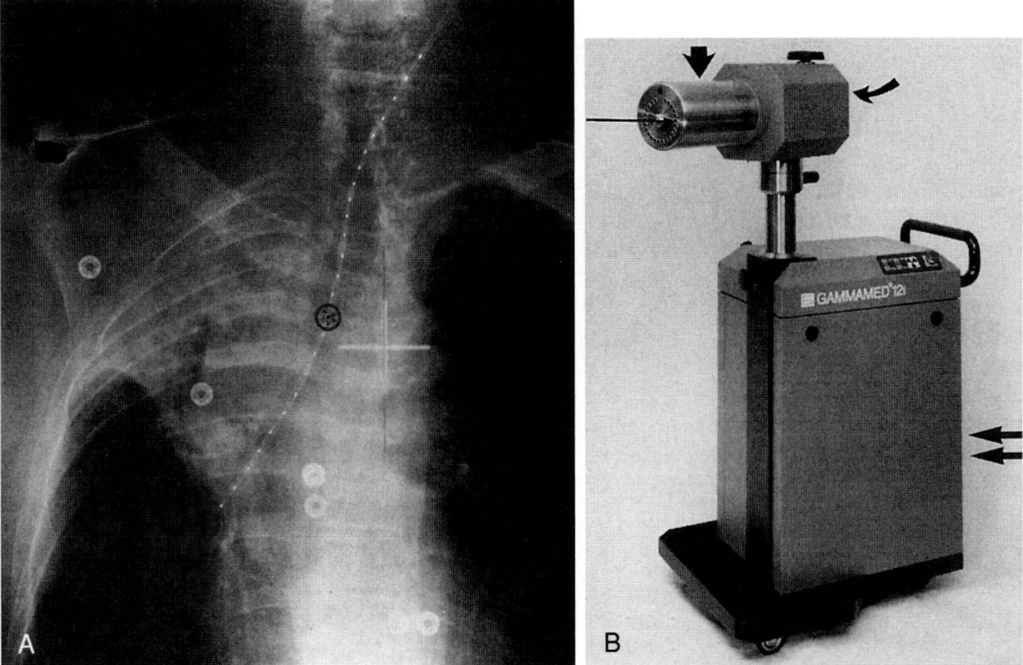

FIGURE 32–10 ■ *A*, A 68-year-old man with medically inoperable (poor pulmonary function) T2N0 squamous cancer of the right mainstem bronchus who was treated with primary external beam radiotherapy to a total dose of 5960 cGy. Seven months later, the tumor had progressed. The localization radiograph shows the afterloading catheter. *B*, A remote afterloading device. The main portion of the device (*double arrows*) contains a power supply, electronics, and most of the cables. The radioactive source is kept in the safe (*single thick arrow*) when not in active use. Cable-driving devices (*curved arrow*) are used to propel both a dummy cable and source and the real cable and source. The cable controls the location of the real source, which exits the machine through any one of 24 channels (*long slender arrow*) and enters the catheter (applicator), which is situated in the airway.

averages 45%, range 11% to 88% (Chang et al, 1994; Goldman et al, 1993; Nori, 1993; Ofiara et al, 1997).

The timing of such objective assessments has a bearing on response reports and can vary from the last brachytherapy session to 6 weeks (Goldman et al, 1993; Stout et al, 1995), to 2 or 3 months (Huber et al, 1995, 1997), to 1 year later (Zajac et al, 1993).

The duration of such responses as clinical symptoms in the palliative context or of endoscopic responses in the curative setting is clearly relevant and may be reported as the number of months during which the disease did not progress (e.g., 7.5 months or 4.5 months [Bedwinek et al, 1991; Delclos et al, 1986]), as the percentage having 6 months disease progression–free interval (Nori, 1993), or as the percentage of patients remaining symptom free until death (e.g., 67%, 76%, 78%) (Gollins et al, 1994; Ornadel et al, 1997; Zajac et al, 1993).

Assessment of Toxicity of HDR-ILBRT

The serious complications include hemorrhage, fistula formation, pneumonitis, soft tissue necrosis, tracheal perforation, and radiation-induced bronchitis.

Speiser and Spratling (1993b) described the bronchial tree changes—radiation bronchitis and stenosis (RBS)—that occurred in 342 patients treated with different schedules of medium dose-rate–ILBRT (MDR-ILBRT) and HDR-ILBRT between 1986 and 1991. They described RBS as a series of endobronchial changes, graded I to IV, seen at follow-up bronchoscopy, usually 6 weeks post treatment. The grades progressed according to the severity of the inflammatory response, the associated degree and completeness of a circumferential membranous exudate and fibrotic reaction in the lumen, the presence of symptoms, and the extent of medical intervention required.

During the long-term follow-up of those treated definitively with intent to cure, the same group found that duration of survival was the single most important predictor of radiation pneumonitis.

Results

Intraluminal Disease Only. Intraluminal brachytherapy may be used alone or in conjunction with external beam radiotherapy in the definitive treatment of early-stage disease when surgery is refused or contraindicated. The doses prescribed and the results of such studies using HDR-ILBRT and low dose-rate–ILBRT (LDR-ILBRT) are detailed in Tables 32–15 and 32–16.

Pathologic complete response rates have varied from 72% to 96% in those treated with ILBRT only (Taulelle et al, 1998; Tredanial et al, 1994), and from 67% to 100% in those treated with ILBRT and concurrent external beam (photon) therapy (EBRT) (Ardiet et al, 1992; Saito et al, 1996).

Median survival in those treated with ILBRT only varied from 17 months to 28 months, with 2-year survival

TABLE 32–15 ■ **Brachytherapy for Endoluminal, Node-Negative Disease: Methods***

Study	*T & N Stage*	*n*	*EBRT*	*BTD Gy*	*Gy‡*	*Fraction Number*	*Interval*	*PP*
Taulelle, 1998	†T1–2, med inop	22/189	Nil	30–35	10–7	3–5	1–2 wk	1 cm
Hennequin, 1998	†T<2 cm	73/149	40–60 Gy in 60% P	35–42	7	5–6	1 wk	0.5–1.5 cm
Perol, 1997	†T_1≤1 cm med inop in 5/18	18	7 had EBRT P	21–35	7	3–5	1 wk	1 cm
Nomoto, 1997	Tis-T4, N0–N2: All curative intent	9/39	40–60 Gy in 3/9 P	18	6	3	1 wk	0.3–1 cm
Saito, 1996	†T1, med inop	40	40–60 No ENI CT	25–35	5	5	2 wk	3–9 mm
Stout, 1995	†T1<2 cm med inop	37	Nil	15 Gy in 40% 20 Gy in 60%	1	1	1 dy	1 cm
Tredanial, 1994	†Endoluminal	25/63	Most had RT or surg, P	28–42	7	4–6	2 wk	1 cm
Sutedja, 1994	†T1, med inop	2	Nil	30	10	3	2 wk	1 cm
Aygun, 1992	Stage I, med inop	19/62	50–60 Gy with or after ILBRT, CT	15–25	5	3–5	1 wk	1 cm
Ardiet, 1992	†T_1≤1 cm	28	Nil	21–35	7	3–5	1 wk	1 cm

*All HDR-ILBRT except Saito, 1996 and 2000, who used LDR.
† = node-negative disease (N0).
‡Gy = fraction size.
BTD, brachytherapy dose; CT, external beam radiation part of current treatment plan; EBRT, external beam radiation; ENI, elective neck irradiation; P, previous radiation therapy; PP, prescription point.

varying from 18% to 78%. The low survival rates at approximately 2 years are disappointing when compared with the initial size of the tumors and the pathologic complete response rates but may be due to the increased number of non-neoplastic deaths occurring in a population for whom surgery is already contraindicated because of poor performance status or respiratory insufficiency (Gaspar, 1998; Perol, 1997; Aygun, 1992). The discrepancy between response rate and survival may also be due to the fact that some patients had intraluminal recurrence after surgery or EBRT, but no other evidence of disease beyond the lumen at the time of treatment. Metastases may have developed soon afterward, thus undermining the survival figures (Hennequin, 1998; Perol et al, 1997; Tredanial et al, 1994).

Toxicity rates are reported as overall rates, usually of severe complications requiring treatment or leading to death. Severe (grade III–IV) complication rates can vary from 14% to 22% and include rates for radiation bronchitis, fatal hemoptysis, and fistula formation (see Table 32–16). However, it is worth noting that the rates reported pertain to the whole study in some cases and not just the group with early-stage disease (Aygun et al, 1992; Taulelle et al, 1998).

Definitive Treatment of Locally Advanced Disease. The role of HDR-ILBRT in the management of locally advanced lung cancer is evolving. Only those studies with uniform radiation treatment or reporting specific results of toxicity and survival have been included in Tables 32–17 and 32–18.

The average (median) brachytherapy fraction dose was 5 Gy, and the mean number of fractions was three. The average external beam dose varied between 50 and 60 Gy.

Overall, the range of biopsy-proven complete response (pCR) is less than in those with endoluminal disease only and varies from 48% to 76%. Nori (1993) reported a local control rate of 88% at 6 months, but only 5 of 17 had endoscopic assessment at an average follow-up of 9.3 months, range 6 to 24 months. Median survival was also less than that of the endoluminal disease–only group and varied from 8 to 24.6 months, averaging 11.8 months. A prospective, randomized study, which assessed the addition of HDR-ILBRT to EBRT in those with advanced lung cancer, confirmed that the addition of ILBRT to external beam therapy can improve local control rates in those with stage III and some stage IV disease who were not previously treated with any modality, when compared with those treated with external beam therapy

TABLE 32–16 ■ **Brachytherapy for Endoluminal, Node-Negative Disease: Methods**

Study	*n*	*pCR*	*Med Surviv month*	*Overall survival (years)*	*Overall, Delayed Toxicity Rate (grade III–IV)*	*RB‡*	*Hemoptysis‡*
Taulelle, 1998	22/189	96%	17	71% (1) 46% (2)	*17%	33%	6.8%
Hennequin, 1998	73/149	48% pCR, 31% PR	14.4	45% (2)	17.7%	15%	2.7%
Perol, 1997	18	83%	28	78% (1) 58% (2)	16%	66%	11%
Nomoto, 1997	9/39	67	12	64% (3)	22%	22%	0%
Saito, 1996	40	100%	†24.5	100% (1), 100% (2), 95% (3)	5%	5%	0%
Stout, 1995	37	92%	23.3	49% (2), 14% (5)	NA	NA	NA
Tredanial, 1994	25/63	72%	†23	55% (2)	11.4%	20%	4%
Aygun, 1992	19/62	NA	20	40% (1), 18% (2), 8% (3)	*16.5%	1.5%	15%
Ardiet, 1992	28	84%	†7	N/A	14%	14%	3.8%

*The % toxicities refer to the whole study.
†Median survival had not been reached in these studies at these median follow-up times. In the studies by Taulelle, Hennequin, Nomoto, Tredanial and Aygun, n, the number in the subgroup, is given, as well as the total number in the study.
‡The % in RB (radiation bronchitis) and hemoptysis refer to all grades.
pCR, biopsy-proven complete response; PR, partial response; NA, not available.

TABLE 32–17 ■ **Brachytherapy for Radical Treatment of Locally Advanced Lung Cancer: Methods**

Study	*T & N Stage*	*n*	*EB Gy*	*BTD Gy*	**Gy*	*Fraction Number*	*Interval*	*PP*
Hennequin, 1998	I–IIIB	29/149	≤60 Gy (17) >60 Gy (12)	10–14 Gy	5–7	2	1 wk post RT	0.5–1.5
Huber, 1997	III 70%	56	50 ± 12.5 vs	7.4±2.6	4.8	2	1 wk before EBRT and 2 weeks after EBRT	1 cm
	IV 30%	42	50 ± 14					
Cotter, 1993	T1N1 T4N2	65	55–66	6–35	2.7–10	2–4	1 wk	1 cm
Nori, 1993	Stage IIIB	17/32	50–60 Med-50	15	5	3	1 wk	1 cm
Aygun, 1992	I–IIIA	62	59	90%≥20 Gy	5	3–5	1 wk	1 cm

*Fraction.
All HDR apart from Cotter, 1993: HDR 74%, IDR 26%; and Speiser and Spratling, 1993: HDR 86%, MDR 14%.
BTD, brachytherapy total dose; EBRT, external beam radiation therapy; HDR, high dose rate; IDR, intermediate dose rate; MDR, medium dose rate; PP, prescription point.

TABLE 32–18 ■ **Brachytherapy for Radical Treatment of Locally Advanced Lung Cancer: Results**

Study	*n*	*pCR*	*PR*	*Median Survival (months)*	*Overall Survival (years)*	*RB% Grade 3–4 (%)*	*FH (%)*
Hennequin, 1998	29/149	48%	31%	24.6	52% (2)	3.5	3.5
*Huber, 1997	56/98	58%	NA	10.6	28% (1)	NA	19.6
	42/98	48%	NA	7.5	17% (1)	NA	15
Cotter, 1993	65	63%	23%	8	38% (1) 23% (2)	12.3	1.5
Nori, 1993	17/32	88% LC at 14 months	NA	—	NA	0	0
Aygun, 1992	62	76%	NA	13 (10–20)	16% at 1.5 yr	≥1.6	15

*98 patients in 2 groups: Group 1 (ILBRT+EBRT) 58%, Group 2 (EBRT only) 48%. The results in the study by Hennequin refer to the whole study group.
EBRT, external beam radiotherapy; FH, fatal hemoptysis; ILBRT, intraluminal brachytherapy; LC, local control; NA, not available; pCR, biopsy-proven complete response; PR, partial response; RB, radiation bronchitis and stenosis.

alone (Huber et al, 1997). Median survival time was also longer in those receiving both modalities, but this did not reach statistical significance. The previous survival figures and those in Huber's study are not significantly different from the survival rates post external beam therapy alone. Furthermore, in the study by Cotter and associates (1993), 65 patients, presenting with stage T1N1, T4N3 disease, were treated with external beam radiation therapy averaging 55 to 66 Gy (including elective nodal irradiation) with ILBRT. The response rates, the median survival, and the 2-year survival were not significantly different from those reported by Huber and colleagues (1997). The disappointing survival results may have been due to the selection and inclusion within the studies of patients with stage I to stage IV disease.

The rate of significant radiation bronchitis (grade III–IV) varied from 0% to 12.3%, and the rate of fatal hemoptysis varied from 0% to 19.6% between the studies, but again in the one prospective trial by Huber and coworkers (1997), there was no significant difference in the incidence of fatal hemoptyses between those receiving ILBRT in addition to EBRT and those receiving EBRT alone. The total treatment dose, the selection of patients, and the precise sequencing of the treatment varied between and within the studies, all of which may account for the difference in rates of fatal hemoptysis and grade III to IV radiation bronchitis (Cotter et al, 1993; Huber et al, 1997; Nori, 1993).

Conformal, three-dimensional (3D) therapy for lung cancer may be improved with HDR-ILBRT when the latter is used to reduce postobstructive atelectasis and pneumonia. The amount of ipsilateral thoracic volume irradiation may be reduced by re-aeration of the lung and the more accurate definition of tumor and lung parenchyma. Escalation of the total dose may then be possible if the limits of lung tolerance are restored by re-aeration of the lung (Bastin et al, 1993). The percentage of those affected with atelectasis showing an improvement varied from 44% to 88% (Chang et al, 1994; Cotter et al, 1993; Nori, 1993).

Palliation. HDR-ILBRT is an effective method by which to palliate lung cancer that is causing airway obstruction or other problems related to intraluminal disease. Clinical response varies according to the parameter being assessed, and overall varies between 28% and 100%. The lower figures for clinical response in Table 32–19 refer to the percentage of those with cough gaining relief with HDR-ILBRT. Relief of hemoptysis is achieved in 60% to 100% of patients, cough is relieved in 24% to 93% of patients, and dyspnea is relieved in 54% to 100% of patients. The median duration of symptomatic response is often not well documented but would appear to be in the 4- to 5-month range, which is a significant proportion of the expected survival time in this group of patients with such a bad prognosis.

An objective assessment of response using bronchoscopy after HDR-ILBRT is difficult because of the inability of conventional bronchoscopic video equipment to measure visible disease or to assess the response of extrinsic disease. With the use of subjective visual criteria, the typical range of responses observed is 41% to 99%. Biopsy-proven complete response rates reported vary from 33% to 54%. The percentage of those with atelectasis and postobstructive pneumonia responding with visibly improved aeration of lung or improved respiratory function ranges from 18% to 99% and averages 40%.

Predicting Response to HDR-ILBRT

Several factors may influence the rate and degree of response to HDR-ILBRT:

External Beam Radiation Therapy. The comparative roles of HDR-ILBRT and EBRT for relief of endobronchial obstruction have yet to be established, particularly in comparison with other "local" treatment modalities. A trial set up to address this issue was recently closed owing to poor recruitment (Moghissi, 1998).

However, when used in a complementary way, in patients with stage III and IV disease, external beam therapy plus intraluminal brachytherapy have improved local control when compared with outcomes in those receiving radical EBRT alone (Huber et al, 1997). In the latter study, the radical combination of modalities was associated with comparable rates of fatal hemoptysis. There was also an advantage in median survival for those treated with both—43 weeks versus 30 weeks in those with squamous cell cancers. Taulelle and associates (1998) did, however, show that the incidence of fatal hemoptysis (FH) was 20% with previous EBRT, but 12% in those without EBRT provided previously.

Total Treatment Dose. A dose–response relationship has been demonstrated in those patients receiving definitive therapy, part of which is achieved with HDR-ILBRT. Cotter and colleagues (1993) showed that a higher dose predicted an improvement in performance status. Performance status improved in 39% of patients if the total dose was less than 70 Gy, but it improved in 70% if the total dose was 85 Gy or more.

Dose Fractionation. It is clear that when used with external beam therapy, 15-Gy fractions exceed lung tolerance (Van Zandwijk, 1995). Even when used alone in the palliative setting, the raising of the total dose to greater than 14 Gy does not significantly increase the total number of responders but does introduce 19.5% grade III to IV toxicity when compared with those receiving between 5 and 14 Gy (Laing, 1994). Taulelle and co-workers (1998) reported that FH occurred at a rate of 18% in those receiving fractions of 8 to 10 Gy versus 13% in those with lower fractions, but response rates were similar.

Those receiving an even lower weekly fraction dose of 5 Gy × 3 have the same response rate and local failure rate when compared with those receiving 10 Gy × 3 fractions or 7 Gy × 3 fractions (Zajac et al, 1993). However, in this study, there was no toxicity encountered in those treated with the 5 Gy-per-fraction regimen when compared with the 10% toxicity encountered by those receiving the higher regimens. In another study of HDR-ILBRT, when the fraction size of 10 Gy was compared with a slightly lower fraction size of 7.5 Gy, the response rate and the toxicity rate were similar, but the percentage of grade III or IV RBS was 15% in those receiving 7.5-Gy fractions; this was increased to 76% in those receiving the 10 Gy-per-fraction regimen (Speiser and Spratling,

TABLE 32–19 ■ **Role of ILBRT in Palliation of Advanced Lung Cancer**

Study	*Year*	*n*	*% with Additional Laser Rx*	*% Endo Response (% CR)*	*% X-ray Response*	*% Clinical Response*	*% Fatal Hemoptysis*	*% RBS (grade III–IV)*
Taulelle	1998	87/189	*25	78 (54)	—	*54–74	*6.9	*12
Hennequin	1998	47/149	12.8	*79 (48)	—	*60.3	17	2
Nomoto	1997	30/39	0	—	—	77	10	0
Ofiara	1997	24	0	62	45	30–60	—	20
Ornadel	1997	102	50	—	—	43–75	9.4	11
Kochbati	1997	16	0	83 (50)	—	—	19	38 (all grades)
Burt	1997	100	—	—	—	†Decrease in survival	—	—
Hernandez	1996	29	10	42	28	24–69	27	0
Delclos	1986	81	0	84	—	84	1.2	6.2
Huber	1995	44	33	41	—	KPS unchanged	10	—
		49	46	48	—		10	—
Macha	1995	346	?%	—	—	—	21	2
Gollins	1994	406	*1.7	—	46	62–88	*7.9	*0.3
Chang	1994	20/76	*2.6	*87 (35)	88	79–95	*4	*4
Laing	1994	40	57.5	75	—	66	12	7.5
Kohek	1994	40/79	33	*89 (6)	70	*65	4	4
Speiser	1993b	259	*24	—	99	*88–99	*7.3	*11
Nori	1993	15/32	0	70	44	85.7–100	0	0
Zajac	1993	58/82	0	24	—	30–94	*1.2	*12.4
Goldman	1993	20	0	85 (40)	—	85	—	—
Seagren	1986	18	20	99 (33)	—	93–100	0	0
Sutedja	1992	31	45	71	—	81	3.2	35.5
Grawitz	1992	24	33	100	83	88	4	32
Bedwinek	1991	38	0	76 (42)	64	71–80	32	0

*Percentages for total study group.
†A randomized trial of 30 Gy in 8 fractions EBRT vs 15 Gy HDR-ILBRT. A 6-week survival advantage with EBRT associated with more morbidity.
—, not available, n, number of patients treated palliatively (numerator) and the total study group (denominator).
CR, complete response; EBRT, external beam radiotherapy; HDR, high dose rate; ILBRT, intraluminal brachytherapy; KPS, Karnofsky performance score; RBS, radiation bronchitis and stenosis; Rx, therapy.

1993a). Perol and associates (1997) used an escalating protocol of 7 Gy × 3, 4, or 5 fractions. The numbers were small but toxicity occurred in 75% of those with the higher regimens.

Clearly, the optimal fraction size for both response rate and toxicity lies between 5 and 7 Gy. Huber and colleagues (1995) have shown that a scheme of 2 × 7.2-Gy fractions with a 3-week interval is equivalent to a 4 × 3.8-Gy regimen for palliation, given on a weekly basis. It is clearly more convenient for patients, has the same local control and survival rates, and does not produce a greater number of side effects (Huber et al, 1995).

Site, Macroscopic Appearance, and Degree of Obstruction of the Tumor. HDR-ILBRT increases local control in locally advanced central tumors (Huber et al, 1997). However, it would appear that those tumors located in the periphery show a greater response in both microscopic control and symptomatic control than those situated centrally, in both the palliative and radical settings (Ofiara et al, 1997).

The appearance of the tumor (i.e., whether it is endoluminal disease or extrinsic disease with submucosal infiltration) is not predictive of who will or will not respond to therapy (Ofiara et al, 1997). However, if the tumor is mainly extrabronchial, then the extent of extrabronchial disease is important. If the amount of extrinsic disease is less than 50% of the tumor burden, then the pCR is 62%, but if it is greater than 50%, the pCR is 44%, $P = .02$ (Taulelle et al, 1998). Bedwinek and coworkers (1991) have also shown that if extrabronchial disease is less than 5 cm, 67% will have a complete response and 33% a partial response. However, if extrabronchial disease is greater than or equal to 5 cm, then only 60% will respond and only partially (Bedwinek et al, 1991). The degree of obstruction also influences the response rates (Cotter et al, 1993; Taulelle et al, 1998). Cotter and colleagues demonstrated that if the bronchial obstruction is greater than 50% in one mainstem bronchus or in two segmental bronchi of the same lung, the complete response rate is 65%. If the obstruction is less than 50% in any of the larger airways, then a complete response rate of 100% is possible.

Performance Status. In patients with good performance status (0–1), the frequency of pCR is greater than that occurring in those with a performance status of greater than or equal to 2, $P = .0001$; 76% vs 35%, respectively (Taulelle et al, 1998).

Predicting Toxicity of HDR-ILBRT

Fatal hemoptysis and radiation bronchitis are the major toxicities that can occur post HDR-ILBRT.

In those studies reporting group-specific complication rates, the percentage of those suffering fatal hemoptysis—whether due to disease or toxicity—ranges from 0% to 21% (median, 10%). From Tables 32–19, 32–18, and 32–17, it can be seen that fatal hemoptysis occurred at a rate of 11% (0%–21%) in those treated palliatively;

at a rate of 9% (0%–19.6%) in those treated with curative, definitive therapy; and at a rate of 3.7% (0%–11%) in those with disease limited to the lumen. The rate appears greater in those with more extensive disease when compared with that for disease limited to the endobronchial lumen. These are much less than the earlier reported figures of 32% and 50% for this complication in the palliative setting (Bedwinek et al, 1991; Khanavkar et al, 1991). However, the discrepancy may be due to inaccurate reporting, variable follow-up, patient selection, or additional treatment before, during, or after HDR-ILBRT (Mehta et al, 1998).

Similarly, the rate of grade III to IV radiation bronchitis varies from 0% to 20% in reports from 1993 onward, the median being 3%. Prior to that, the range reported varied from 0% to 35.5%

Analysis of toxicity frequency and therefore the factors that influence or predict for it is complicated by lack of agreement on terminology and differences in patient selection, with inclusion of different stages of disease and associated therapies (Perol et al, 1997; Taulelle et al, 1998). Long-term follow-up is important as duration of survival appears to be the single most important predictor of radiation pneumonitis (Speiser and Spratling, 1993b).

Several factors associated with increased risk of FH have been reported. Either prior laser treatment or a prior ILBRT treatment at the same site increases the risk of FH (Gollins, 1994). A risk of 20% for FH was found in those with previous EBRT to the lung, but the rate was only 12% in those who had no previous EBRT (Gollins et al, 1994). If the fraction size is greater than 8 Gy, or if the length of the treatment area is more than 3 cm, there is an increased risk of FH (Gollins et al, 1994; Hennequin et al, 1998; Taulelle et al, 1998).

The influence of treatment length was also demonstrated in the study by Khanavkar and associates (1991), in which the area of treatment length of those with FH averaged 5.3 cm, but the length of treatment area in those with no complications was significantly less, that is, 3.5 cm. Tumor location in the upper lobes has also been cited as predicting for toxicity. This is thought to occur because the left pulmonary artery is close to the anterior and superior surface of the left upper lobe bronchus and is therefore at increased risk of invasion by left upper lobe tumor (Bedwinek et al, 1991; Khanavkar et al, 1991; Taulelle et al, 1998). Miller and McGregor (1975) have further demonstrated that, because of its anatomy, the wall of the pulmonary artery could fall within a hot spot of 20 to 30 Gy when a single fraction of 6 Gy is prescribed with ILBRT alone. If this is added to the dose received at this site from previous conventional EBRT, the patient could be at increased risk of FH. However, 80% to 100% of cases of FH may still be due to disease recurrence (Gollins et al, 1994; Speiser and Spratling, 1993b).

Radiation Bronchitis. Speiser and Spratling have demonstrated that survival was the main predictor of RBS. Tumor location in the trachea and mainstem bronchus increases the relative risk to 5.35, $P = .0001$, when compared with other sites: The rate was 18% for the trachea and mainstem bronchus versus 2% to 3.5% for all other sites (Hennequin et al, 1998). The performance status also influences the rate of RBS. Those with better KPS survive longer and are therefore more at risk to develop RBS; the rate for the curative therapeutic subgroup was 15% vs 2% to 3.5% for all other groups (Hennequin et al, 1998).

Dose Rate and Toxicity

Dose rate does not appear to influence or predict for toxicity. The evolution from LDR-ILBRT to HDR-ILBRT was based on patient convenience, resource economy, and radiation protection. Studies on the efficacy of LDR-ILBRT indicate that satisfactory palliation can be achieved with this technique, that is, 67% to 100% response rates can be achieved using LDR-ILBRT, and response rates of 70% to 94% using HDR-ILBRT (Mehta et al, 1998). Both systems are similar in terms of symptom relief, radiographic re-aeration, and percentage of lifetime rendered symptom free. Response rates and complication rates were also reported to be similar in those treated with LDR-ILBRT to those treated with a hyperfractionated HDR-ILBRT regimen. In this last study, the results of treatment of 31 patients with 4 Gy × 4 fractions prescribed at 2 cm and administered over 48 hours, using an HDR-ILBRT afterloading system, were compared with those of 66 patients treated with 20 Gy at 2 cm using LDR-ILBRT (Mehta, 1998). More recently, Lo and associates (1995) compared the results of 110 patients treated with LDR-ILBRT with those of 59 patients treated with HDR-ILBRT and showed that clinical or bronchoscopic response rates were significantly greater in those with HDR-ILBRT: 72% and 85%, respectively, $P = .05$. Survival and complication rates were similar.

Huber and associates (1995) also assessed the influence of dose rate applied and the potential for possible toxicity produced by varying dose rates of the actual source in HDR-ILBRT, by assessing the impact on complication rates of the time lapse between the source replacement of the afterloading unit and actual treatment. After 2.5 months, the source has half the dose rate of a freshly replaced one. However, no relationship was found between the higher interval, the diminished dose rate, and the cause of death or survival time.

Laser and ILBRT

Studies on the use of HDR-ILBRT for palliation include a percentage—0% to 57.5%—of patients in whom laser therapy has been used, but the precise contribution of laser treatment to the overall effect remains unclear in most (see Table 32–19). Endobronchial laser resection provides immediate relief of symptoms, facilitates catheter placement beyond the obstruction, which may increase response rates and duration of response.

Seagren and Harrell (1990) reported significantly improved response rates among a population of 36 patients who underwent laser resection versus 14 who did not. In another series in which laser resection was used for some patients, bronchoscopic responses occurred in 90% (19 of 21) of the patients receiving laser resection and HDR-ILBRT compared with 75% (50 of 67) of those treated with HDR-ILBRT alone, P = .08 (Miller and Phillips, 1990). Similarly, Schray and colleagues (1985) have demonstrated that HDR-ILBRT adds to the quality and duration of palliation when compared with laser therapy alone. Shea and co-workers (1993) have demonstrated increased survival (i.e., 10 months vs 4 months, P = .001) when those treated with a combination of EBRT, laser therapy, and LDR-ILBRT (n = 13) were compared with those treated with EBRT and laser therapy alone (n = 33). However, this was a retrospective study, and although both groups were similar in age, they were not similar in the number of laser treatments they received, the number being greater in the EB + ILBRT subgroup. Neither were the site and size of tumors, the presence or absence or degree of extrinsic disease, nor the actual symptom response addressed. There is also conflicting evidence that suggests that laser therapy may or may not be associated with an increased risk of FH (Bedwinek et al, 1991; Gollins et al, 1994; Ornadel et al, 1997).

Intraoperative Radiotherapy

Intraoperative radiation therapy (IORT) using linear accelerators with modified cones has been described by a number of investigators (Abe et al, 1980). The cone is applied to the area of unresected residual tumor, and normal structures that are not involved by the cancer are retracted or covered with custom-made blocks. Electron energies are selected to cover the required depth appropriately. Doses in the range of 10 to 25 Gy are given in a single fraction in the operating room.

The NCI ran a phase I trial and reported that two of four patients died as a result of esophageal complications, and the other two had life-threatening fistulas (Pass et al, 1987).

In Austria, 21 patients with negative nodes after mediastinal dissection received 10 to 20 Gy IORT with electrons to unresected primary tumors. Postoperatively, this was supplemented by 45 to 46 Gy external beam radiotherapy. The authors report CT scan–documented responses as early as 4 weeks, which improved with time, eventually leading to a 33% complete response rate and a disease-free survival rate of 90% (19 of 21) at a median follow-up of 1 year. The good results in this group of patients may be due to the N0 nodal status and the fact that many of the tumors were resectable early-stage tumors in medically unfit patients. Only one patient died as a result of therapy (Juettner et al, 1990). This experience was updated in 1994. A pilot study on IORT combined with EBRT in nonresectable NSCLC was performed in 31 patients—21 functionally unresectable and 10 were also anatomically unresectable. On staging of mediastinal lymph node dissection, 11 had positive nodes. Seven were staged as T1, 16 were staged as T2, and 8 were staged as T3. Ten to twenty Gy was given as IORT, using 7- to 20-MeV electrons. EBRT (average, 46 Gy) was also prescribed postoperatively using 8- to 20-MeV photons to the mediastinum and primary tumor, but if the mediastinum was positive, then 56 Gy was given to this area. There were 13 complete responses and 8 partial (50%–90% regression) and 2 minor responses among the 23 evaluable patients. The 5-year survival rate was 34%. The recurrence-free survival was 41% (Smolle-Juettner et al, 1994).

At the Graduate Hospital in Philadelphia, a further pilot study was undertaken in 10 patients with locally advanced disease. The study group comprised three patients with T3N0 disease, three with T3N1 disease, and four with T2–T3N2 disease (Fallah-Nejad et al, 1994). Six of the 10 patients had chemotherapy as well as preoperative radiation. All tumors were resected (7 pneumonectomies and 3 lobectomies) with tumor staging. IORT was undertaken in all in whom 10 Gy was administered using 6- to 9-MeV electrons. Six patients were alive at a median of 11 months post therapy. Four died with distant metastases but no local recurrence. This study therefore demonstrated that the technique is feasible, safe, and without obvious associated mortality or morbidity. It may prevent local recurrence as part of combined therapy.

Less favorable results were obtained in Spain where 34 patients with unresected or incompletely resected primary or nodal tumors received an intraoperative dose of 10 to 15 Gy with electrons followed by 46 to 50 Gy of external beam radiotherapy postoperatively (Calvo et al, 1990). Acute pneumonitis occurred in 35% (12 of 34), the median survival time was only 12 months, and the freedom from thoracic progression rate was only 30%.

Dubois and associates (1992) used kilovoltage x-rays (100-Kv photons) in 170 patients following complete surgical excision of cancers at different primary sites. Those with NSCLC included 18 patients, 15 of whom were evaluable. They were treated with 10- to 20-Gy single doses of IORT following excision of their tumors, using 100-kV photons at 15 cm source to skin distance. Six had stage III disease. EBRT (45 Gy) was also given to the mediastinum post surgery. At follow-up, local control was achieved in 86% of patients. (The length of follow-up was not stated.) Median survival was 30 months, and the 3-year actuarial survival was 66%. Six patients had died, two with persistent disease, two with recurrences locally but outside the IORT field, and two with distant metastases but with local control.

In conclusion, the relatively limited experience with IORT added to external beam radiotherapy for NSCLC did not demonstrate that it is superior to radical external beam radiotherapy alone (Table 32–20). In view of its frequent toxicity, its use must be regarded as experimental.

COMMENTS AND CONTROVERSIES

Despite the large experience at Memorial Sloan-Kettering, intraoperative interstitial brachytherapy has not been widely adopted. The series reported have good local control and survival for the various disease categories. Although it is a theoretically attractive technique, its superiority to external beam radiotherapy alone has not been clearly demonstrated. An attempt to conduct a randomized trial of external beam radiotherapy with and without brachytherapy for incompletely resected NSCLC was closed because of accrual failure (Armstrong, unpublished data). There is now sufficient evidence demonstrating the feasibility of intraluminal brachytherapy for lung cancer.

TABLE 32–20 ■ **Results of Intraoperative Radiotherapy**

Author, yr	*n*	*Surgery*	*IORT*	*EBRT*	*LC*	*Survival*	*Comment*
Pass, 1987 (Electrons)	4 (stage not defined)	Yes	25 Gy to superior and inferior mediastinum	No	25%	25%	2 died from complications; I died with brain metastases; I alive and well
Juettner, 1990 (Electrons)	21 All N0 disease	No	10–20 Gy	45–46 Gy	90% @ 1 yr	N/A	All N0 disease 1/21 died of complications
Smolle-Juettner, 1994 (Electrons)	31 11 N pos 20 N neg	No	10–20 Gy, with 7–20 MeV electrons	46 Gy with 8–20 MeV photons	42% CR 26% PR	5-yr survival 34.1%	N0 to N1–2 disease patients not compared
Fallah-Nejad, 1994 (Electrons)	10 3 stage II (T3N0) and 7 stage III	Yes 6/10 had preop chemo + RT also	10 Gy using 6–9 MeV electrons	Preop RT in 6/10 ? dose	N/A	60% alive and disease free at 11 (1–21) months	4/10 died with distant metastases but no local rec
Calvo, 1990 (Electrons)	34 All stage III disease	Incomplete or unresectable	10–15 Gy	46–50 Gy	30% free from disease progression	Median survival 1 yr	12/34 acute pneumonitis
Martinez-Monge, 1994	18 Pancoast tumors	Yes plus pre- and postop chemo	10–15 Gy	46–50 Gy	70% pCR	Overall survival 56% at 4 yr	Toxic 16.6% mortality from treatment
Dubois, 1992 (kilo-voltage)	18 (15/18 evaluable—6/15 had stage III disease)	Yes—assume complete	10–20 Gy, 100 Kv photons, @ 15 cm SSD	No	86.6%	Median survival 30 months; 3 yr survival 66%	

EBRT, external beam radiation therapy; IORT, intraoperative radiotherapy; LC, local control; N/A, not available; pCR, biopsy-proven complete response; PR, partial response.

Predictors of response and toxicity have been identified. Standardization of technical details is necessary to allow prospective, multi-institutional trials to further define the role of this approach.

J.G.A.

The use of intraoperative brachytherapy remains controversial and has never been tested in a prospective randomized trial that would compare it with routine postoperative irradiation. Its main indications are for residual gross tumor, residual microscopic tumor, or "close" resection margins. Its theoretical advantages include less pulmonary toxicity and the application of higher doses to areas close to vital structures (e.g., spinal cord). An analysis performed at Memorial Sloan-Kettering suggests no distinct advantage for the use of intraoperative brachytherapy in the management of superior sulcus tumors for the above reasons. (Ginsberg 1994.)

The role of intraoperative external beam radiotherapy to either supplement or treat unresectable tumors has also not been tested in a controlled fashion. The initial reports have been somewhat encouraging when combined with EBRT to the mediastinum.

Brachytherapy used intraluminally for the palliation of obstructing tumors of the airway and for augmentation of primary radiotherapy for the management of lung cancer, appears to be the best use of this type of therapy. It has certainly been proved to have a distinct advantage in palliating previously irradiated obstructing tumors and, when combined with EBRT in radiation-naive patients, does produce greater local control. Its use, in combination with photodynamic therapy as palliation for endobronchial obstruction is being investigated.

R.J.G.

■ KEY REFERENCES

Henschke UK: Interstitial implantation in the treatment of primary bronchogenic carcinoma. AJR Am J Roentgenol 79:981, 1958.

This is a report of the initial experience with interstitial implantation at Memorial Sloan-Kettering.

Hilaris BS, Martini N: The current state of intraoperative interstitial brachytherapy in lung cancer. Int J Radiat Oncol Biol Phys 15:1347, 1988.

This is a review of the long-term experience with interstitial implantation at Memorial Sloan-Kettering.

Mehta MP, Lamond JP, Nori D, Speiser BL: Brachytherapy for lung cancer. In Nag S (ed): Principles and Practice of Brachytherapy. New York, Futura Publishing, 1998.

This is an update on current practice of brachytherapy in lung cancer.

■ REFERENCES

Abe M, Takahishi M, Yabumoto E et al: Clinical experiences with intraoperative radiotherapy of locally advanced cancers. Cancer 45:40, 1980.

Aird EG, Williams JR: Brachytherapy. In Williams JR, Thwaites DIR (eds): Radiotherapy Physics in Practice. Oxford, Oxford Medical Publications, 1993.
Anderson T, Moy P, Holmes E: Factors affecting survival in superior sulcus tumors. J Clin Oncol 4:1589, 1986.
Ardiet JM, Perol M, Mornex F et al: Curative irradiation of limited endobronchial epidermoid carcinomas with HDR endoluminal brachytherapy. A pilot study. Ann Oncol 3(suppl 5):1992.
Armstrong JG, Fass DE, Bains M et al: Paraspinal tumors: Techniques and results of brachytherapy. Int J Radiat Oncol Biol Phys 20:787, 1991.
Armstrong JG, Martini N, Kris MG et al: Induction chemotherapy for non-small cell lung cancer with clinically evident mediastinal node metastases: The role of post-operative radiotherapy. Int J Radiat Oncol Biol Phys 23:605, 1992.
Armstrong JG, Minsky BD: Primary radiation therapy for stage I and II medically inoperable non-small cell lung cancer. Cancer Treat Rev 16:247, 1989.
Attar S, Miller J, Satterfield J et al: Pancoast's tumor: Irradiation or surgery? Ann Thorac Surg 28:578, 1979.
Aye RW, Mate TP, Anderson HN et al: Extending the limits of lung cancer resection. Am J Surg 165:572, 1993.
Aygun C, Blum JE: Treatment of unresectable lung cancer with brachytherapy. World J Surg 19:823, 1995.
Aygun C, Weiner S, Scariato A et al: Treatment of non-small cell lung cancer with external beam radiotherapy and high dose rate brachytherapy. Int J Radiat Oncol Biol Phys 23:127, 1992.
Bastin KT, Mehta MP, Kinsella TJ: Thoracic volume radiation sparing following endobronchial brachytherapy: A quantitative analysis. Int J Radiat Oncol 25:703, 1993.
Bedwinek J, Petty A, Bruton C et al: The use of high dose rate endobronchial brachytherapy to palliate symptomatic endobronchial recurrence of previously irradiated bronchogenic carcinoma. Int J Radiat Oncol 22:23, 1991.
Brach B, Buhler C, Hayman MH et al: Percutaneous computed tomography-guided fine needle brachytherapy of pulmonary malignancies. Chest 106:268, 1994.
Burt M, Pomerantz AH, Bains MS et al: Results of surgical treatment of stage II lung cancer invading the mediastinum. Surg Clin North Am 67:997, 1987.
Burt P, O'Driscoll R, Notley M et al: Intraluminal irradiation for the palliation of lung cancer with the high dose rate Micro-Selectron. Thorax 45:765, 1990.
Burt PA: High dose rate brachytherapy in endobronchial tumours. Lung Cancer 18(suppl 2):35, 1997.
Calvo F, Ortiz de Urbina D, Abuchaibe O et al: Intraoperative radiotherapy during lung cancer surgery: Technical description and early clinical results. Int J Radiat Oncol Biol Phys 19:103, 1990.
Chang LL, Horvath J, Peyton W, Ling SS: High dose rate afterloading intraluminal brachytherapy in malignant airway obstruction of lung cancer. Int J Radiat Oncol Biol Phys 28:589, 1994.
Cotter GW, Lariscy C, Ellingwood K, Herbert D: Inoperable endobronchial obstructing lung cancer treated with combined endobronchial and external beam irradiation: A dosimetric analysis. Int J Radiat Oncol 27:531, 1993.
Delclos ME, Komaki R, Morice RC et al: Endobronchial brachytherapy with high dose rate remote afterloading for recurrent endobronchial lesions. Radiology 201:279, 1986.
Dubois JB, Gu SD, Hay MH et al: Intraoperative radiation therapy (IORT) with 100 KV X photons on 170 patients. Pathol Biol Paris 39(9):884, 1992.
Fallah-Nejad M, Fisher S, Mason B et al: Intraoperative radiation therapy in the treatment of lung cancer. Chest 106(suppl 2):70S, 1994.
Fass DE, Armstrong JG, Harrison LB, Nori D: Fractionated high dose endobronchial treatment for recurrent lung cancer. Endocuriether Hyperthermia Oncol 6:211, 1990.
Fleischman EH, Kagan AR, Streeter OE et al: Iodine (125) interstitial brachytherapy in the treatment of carcinoma of the lung. J Surg Oncol 49:25, 1992.
Gasper LE: Brachytherapy in lung cancer. J Surg Oncol 67:60, 1998.
Ginsberg RJ, Martine N, Zaman M et al: Influence of surgical resection and brachytherapy in the management of superior sulcus tumor. Ann Thorac Surg 57:1440, 1994.
Goldman JM, Bulman AS, Rathmell AJ et al: Physiological or endobronchial radiotherapy in patients with major airway occlusion by carcinoma. Thorax 48:110, 1993.
Gollins SW, Burt PA, Barber PV, Stout R: High dose rate intraluminal radiotherapy for carcinoma of the bronchus: Outcome of treatment of 406 patients. Radiother Oncol 33:31, 1994.
Gollins SW, Ryder WDJ, Burt PA et al: Massive haemoptysis and other morbidity associated with high dose rate intraluminal radiotherapy for carcinoma of the bronchus. Radiother Oncol 39:105, 1996.
Grafton C, Lam S, Voss N et al: High dose rate endobronchial brachytherapy using the Microselection. Lung Cancer 7(suppl 1):97, 1991.
Grawitz M, Ellerbroek N, Komaki R et al: High dose endobronchial irradiation in recurrent bronchogenic carcinoma. Int J Radiat Oncol Biol Phys 23:397, 1992.
Hatlevoll R, Karlsen K, Aamdal S, Bohman T: Endobronchial radiotherapy for malignant bronchial obstruction or recurrence. Lung Cancer 7(suppl 1):95, 1991.
Heelan RT, Hilaris BS, Anderson LL et al: Lung tumours: Percutaneous implantation of I-125 sources with CT treatment planning. Radiology 164:735, 1987.
Hennequin C, Tredanial J, Chevret S et al: Predictive factors for late toxicity after endobronchial brachytherapy: A multivariate analysis. Int J Radiat Oncol Biol Phys 42:21, 1998.
Henschke UK: Interstitial implantation in the treatment of primary bronchogenic carcinoma. AJR Am J Roentgenol 79:981, 1958.
Henschke UK, Hilaris BS, Mahan GD: Remote afterloading for intracavitary applicators. Radiology 83:344, 1964.
Hernandez P, Gursahaney A, Roman T et al: High dose rate brachytherapy for the local control of endobronchial carcinoma following external irradiation. Thorax 51(4):354, 1996.
Hilaris B, Gomez J, Nori D et al: Combined surgery, intraoperative brachytherapy, and postoperative external radiation in stage III non-small cell lung cancer. Cancer 55:1226, 1985.
Hilaris B, Martini N, Wong G, Nori D: Treatment of superior sulcus tumor (Pancoast tumor). Surg Clin North Am 67:965, 1987a.
Hilaris BS: Lung brachytherapy. An overview and current indications. Chest Surg Clin North Am 4:45, 1994.
Hilaris BS, Martini N: The current state of intraoperative interstitial brachytherapy in lung cancer. Int J Radiat Oncol Biol Phys 15:1347, 1988.
Hilaris BS, Nori D, Anderson LL: Brachytherapy techniques. In Hilaris BS, Nori D, Anderson LL (eds): Atlas of Brachytherapy. New York, Macmillan, 1988.
Hilaris BS, Nori D, Martini N: Results of radiation therapy in stage I and II unresectable non-small cell lung cancer. Endocuriether Hypertherm Oncol 2:15, 1986.
Hilaris BS, Nori D, Martini N: Intraoperative radiotherapy in stage I and II lung cancer. Semin Surg Oncol 3:22, 1987b.
Huber RM, Fischer R, Hautmann H et al: Palliative endobronchial brachytherapy for central lung tumors: A prospective, randomized comparison of two fractionation schedules. Chest 107:463, 1995.
Huber RM, Fischer R, Hautmann H et al: Does additional brachytherapy improve the effect of external irradiation? A prospective randomized study in central lung tumors. Int J Radiat Oncol Biol Phys 38:533, 1997.
Juettner FM, Arian-Schad K, Porsch G et al: Intraoperative radiation therapy combined with external irradiation in nonresectable non-small-cell lung cancer: Preliminary report. Int J Radiat Oncol Biol Phys 18:1143, 1990.
Khanavkar B, Stern P, Alberti W et al: Complications associated with brachytherapy alone or with laser in lung cancer. Chest 99:1062, 1991.
Kochbati L, Baldeyrou P, Coupkova H et al: Endobronchial high dose rate brachytherapy (HDRBT) in prior irradiated non small cell lung carcinoma: Is there a real benefit? Lung Cancer 18(suppl 1):128, 1997.
Kohek PH, Pakisch B, Glanzer H: Intraluminal irradiation in the treatment of malignant airway obstruction. Eur J Surg Oncol 20:674, 1994.
Komaki R, Mountain C, Holbert J et al: Superior sulcus tumors: Treatment selection and results for 85 patients without metastases (M0) at presentation. Int J Radiat Oncol Biol Phys 19:31, 1990.
Komaki R, Roh J, Cox J, Lopes da Conceicao A: Superior sulcus tumors: Results of irradiation of 36 patients. Cancer 48:1563, 1981.
Laing S, Ajlouni M, Kvale P: Clinical efficacy of endobronchial irradiation for airway obstruction utilizing a high dose rate afterloading system (meeting abstract). Proc Ann Mtg ASCO 13:A1188, 1994.

Lewis J, Ajlouni M, Kvale P et al: Role of brachytherapy in the management of pulmonary and mediastinal malignancies. Ann Thorac Surg 49:728, 1990.

Lo TCM, Beamis JF, Weinstein RS et al: Intraluminal low-dose rate brachytherapy for malignant endobronchial obstruction. Radiother Oncol 23:16, 1992.

Lo TCM, Girshovich L, Healey GA et al: Low dose rate versus high dose rate intraluminal brachytherapy for malignant endobronchial tumors. Radiother Oncol 35:193, 1995.

Macha H, Koch K, Stadler M et al: New technique for treating occlusive and stenosing tumours of the trachea and main bronchi: Endobronchial irradiation by high dose iridium-192 combined with laser canalization. Thorax 42:511, 1987.

Macha HN, Wahlers B, Reichle C, von Zwehl D: Endobronchial radiation therapy for obstructing malignancies: Ten years' experience with Iridium-192 high dose radiation brachytherapy afterloading technique in 365 patients. Lung 173:271, 1995.

Marchese M, Nori D, Anderson LL, Hilaris BS: A versatile permanent planar implant technique utilising I-125 seeds embedded in Gelfoam. Int J Radiat Oncol Biol Phys 194:747, 1981.

Martinez-Monge R, Herreros J, Aristu JJ et al: Combined treatment in superior sulcus tumors. Am J Clin Oncol 17:317, 1994.

Mehta M, Shahabi S, Jarjour N, Kinsella T: Endobronchial irradiation for malignant airway obstruction. Int J Radiat Oncol Biol Phys 17:847, 1989.

Mehta MP, Lamond JP, Nori D, Speiser BL: Brachytherapy for lung cancer. In Nag S (ed): Principles and Practice of Brachytherapy. New York, Futura Publishing, 1998, p 323.

Mehta M, Petereit D, Chosy L et al: Sequential comparison at low dose rate and hyperfractionated high dose rate endobronchial radiation for malignant airway occlusion. Int J Radiol Oncol Biol Phys 23:133, 1992.

Miller J, Mansour K, Hatcher C: Carcinoma of the superior pulmonary sulcus. Ann Thorac Surg 28:44, 1979.

Miller J, Phillips T: Neodymium-YAG laser and brachytherapy in the management of inoperable bronchogenic carcinoma. Ann Thorac Surg 50:190, 1990.

Miller R, McGregor D: Hemorrhage from carcinoma of the lung. Cancer 36:904, 1975.

Moghissi K, Bond MG, Sawbrook RJ et al: Treatment of endobronchial or endotracheal obstruction by non-small cell lung cancer. Clin Oncol R Coll Radiol 11:79, 1999.

Neal C, Amdur R, Mendenhall W et al: Pancoast tumor: Radiation therapy alone versus preoperative radiation plus surgery. Int J Radiat Oncol Biol Phys 21:651, 1991.

Nomoto Y, Shouji K, Toyota S et al: High dose rate endobronchial brachytherapy using a new applicator. Radiother Oncol 45:33, 1997.

Nori D: Role of intraoperative brachytherapy in non-small cell lung cancer. In Nori D (ed): Proceedings of the International Conference on Thoracic Oncology. New York, Booth Memorial Medical Center, 1991.

Nori D: Intraoperative brachytherapy in non-small cell lung cancer. Semin Surg Oncol 9:99, 1993.

Nori D, Hilaris B, Martini N: Intraluminal irradiation in bronchogenic carcinoma. Surg Clin North Am 67:1093, 1987.

Nori D, Li X, Pugkhem T: Intraoperative brachytherapy using Gelfoam radioactive plaque implants for resected stage III non small cell lung cancer with positive margin: A pilot study. J Surg Oncol 60:257, 1995.

Ofiara L, Roman T, Schwartzman K, Levy RD: Local determinants of response to endobronchial high dose rate brachytherapy in bronchogenic carcinoma. Chest 112:946, 1997.

Ornadel D, Duchesne G, Wall P et al: Defining the roles of high dose rate endobronchial brachytherapy and laser resection for recurrent bronchial malignancy. Lung Cancer 16:203, 1997.

Pass HI: Delivery of intraoperative radiation therapy after pneumonectomy: Experimental observations and early clinical results. Ann Thorac Surg 58:269, 1994.

Pass HI, Sindelar W, Kinsella T et al: Delivery of intraoperative radiation therapy after pneumonectomy: Experimental observations and early clinical results. Ann Thorac Surg 44:14, 1987.

Paulson D: The "superior sulcus" lesion. In Delarue N, Eschapasse H (eds): International Trends in General Thoracic Surgery, Vol 1. Philadelphia, WB Saunders, 1985.

Perol M, Caliandro R, Pommier P et al: Curative irradiation of limited endrobronchial carcinomas with high-dose rate brachytherapy. Chest 111:1417, 1997.

Raben A, Mychalczak B: Brachytherapy for non-small cell lung cancer and selected neoplasms of the chest. Chest 112(suppl 4):276S, 1996.

Saito M, Yokoyama A, Kurita Y et al: Treatment of roentgenographically occult endobronchial carcinoma with external beam radiotherapy and intraluminal low dose rate brachytherapy. Int J Radiat Oncol Biol Phys 34:1029, 1996.

Schray M, McDougall J, Martinez A et al: Management of malignant airway obstruction: Clinical and dosimetric considerations using an iridium-192 afterloading technique in conjunction with the neodymium-YAG laser. Int J Radiat Oncol Biol Phys 11:403, 1985.

Seagren S, Harrell J: Prospective trial of palliative high dose rate endobronchial irradiation with or without laser for recurrent nonsmall cell lung cancer. Proc Am Soc Clin Oncol 9:224, 1990.

Seagren SL: Endobronchial irradiation: A review. Endocuriether Hypertherm Oncol 2:87, 1986.

Shaw R, Paulson D, Kee J: Treatment of the superior sulcus tumor by irradiation followed by resection. Ann Surg 154:29, 1961.

Shea JM, Allen RP, Tharratt RS et al: Survival of patients undergoing Nd:YAG laser therapy compared with Nd:YAG laser therapy and brachytherapy for malignant airway disease. Chest 103:1028, 1993.

Smolle-Juettner FM, Geyer E, Kapp KS et al: Evaluating intraoperative radiation therapy (IORT) and external beam radiation therapy (EBRT) in non-small cell lung cancer. Eur J Cardiothorac Surg 8:511, 1994.

Speiser B, Spratling L: Remote afterloading brachytherapy for the local control of endobronchial carcinoma. Int J Radiat Oncol Biol Phys 25:579, 1993a.

Speiser B, Spratling L: Radiation bronchitis and stenosis secondary to high dose rate endobronchial irradiation. Int J Radiat Oncol Biol Phys 25:589, 1993b.

Stout R, Barber PV, Burt PA, Gollins SW: Intraluminal brachytherapy and cure of small bronchial carcinomas. In International Brachytherapy, 8th International Brachytherapy Conference, Nice, France, 1995, p 216.

Sutedja G, Baris G, Schaake-Konig C, Van Zandwijk N: High dose rate brachytherapy in patients with local recurrences after radiotherapy of non small cell lung cancer. Int J Radiat Oncol Biol Phys 24:551, 1992.

Sutedja G, Baris G, Van Zandwijk N, Postmus PE: High dose rate brachytherapy has a curative potential in patients with intraluminal squamous cell lung cancer. Respiration 61:167, 1994.

Taulelle M, Chauvet B, Vincent P et al: High dose rate endobronchial brachytherapy: Results and complications in 189 patients. Eur Respir J 11:162, 1998.

Tomberlin JK, Halperin EC, Kusin P et al: Endobronchial interstitial Au-198 implantation in the treatment of recurrent bronchogenic carcinoma. J Surg Oncol 49:21, 1992.

Tredanial J, Hennequin C, Zalcman G et al: Prolonged survival after high dose rate endobronchial radiation for malignant airway obstruction. Chest 105:767, 1994.

Van Zandwijk N, Baas P, Schaake-Konig C et al: Pulmonary hemorrhage after intensive combined treatment with endobronchial irradiation and external radiotherapy in advanced non-small cell lung cancer (NSCLC) (meeting abstract). Proc Ann Mtg ASCO 14:A1061, 1995.

Yankauer S: Two cases of lung tumour treated bronchoscopically. N Y Med J 21:741, 1922.

Zajac AJ, Kohn ML, Heiser D, Peters JW: High dose rate intraluminal brachytherapy in the treatment of endobronchial malignancy. Radiology 187:571, 1993.

PHOTODYNAMIC THERAPY FOR ENDOBRONCHIAL LESIONS

Tracey L. Weigel
Pamela J. Kosco
James D. Luketich

HISTORICAL NOTE

The concept of harnessing the energy of light to treat disease was reported by Kime more than 100 years ago in *JAMA* when he described the use of phototherapy to treat tuberculosis of the lungs (Kime, 2000). Kime felt that "the actinic rays of the sun were desired rather than the heat rays," thus a blue glass was placed in front of the phototherapy reflector, which was positioned 8 feet in front of the patient. Kime believed that, "the action of the light was not limited to its local effects alone on the parts diseased. The blood, every drop of which passes a number of times through the area bathed in the powerful light during each treatment, is without doubt beneficially influenced by the chemical action of the light upon it" (Kime, 2000).

Photodynamic therapy (PDT) as referred to today involves administration of a photosensitizing agent, which, when exposed to a certain wavelength of light, results in the formation of toxic oxygen radicals and subsequently in cell death. Photodynamic therapy, as defined previously, was first described in 1900 when paramecia were killed by sequential exposure to acridine and then light (Edell and Cortese, 1995). Case reports of treatment of skin cancer with PDT date back to 1903, and the porphyrin-based photosensitizers most commonly used today were first employed in 1911 (Edell and Cortese, 1995). In the 1950s, Lipson and colleagues (1960) at the Mayo clinic observed that hematoporphyrin derivative (HpD, Photofrin I) had better tumor localization than did hematoporphyrin, and it preferentially accumulated in most squamous carcinomas and adenocarcinomas (Lipson, 1960). HpD contains several porphyrins, monomers, dimers, and oligomers. Photofrin II (dihematoporphyrin ether, DHE), a refinement of HpD derived from the removal of less-active porphyrin monomers, is more efficacious and is currently the most common clinically used photosensitizer.

BASIC SCIENCE

Two types of photo-oxidative reactions are associated with PDT: Type I involves the generation of a free radical reaction by an excited photosensitizer, and type II results from the transfer of a photon to ground-state triplet oxygen to generate singlet oxygen. The resultant cell death from photodynamic therapy is attributed predominantly to singlet oxygen generation. In vitro experiments have demonstrated that cells are relatively resistant to PDT in low-oxygen-tension environments (Lee See et al, 1984; Mitchell et al, 1985). In addition, in vivo murine data have demonstrated singlet oxygen production secondary to PDT (Sery et al, 1987). The initial cellular damage from PDT appears to occur at the plasma membrane level and can be observed within minutes after light exposure. Membrane blebs consistent with apoptosis can be seen protruding from the cell membrane after PDT. Intracellular membrane damage secondary to PDT is evidenced by injury to mitochondria, inhibition of electron transport enzymes and oxidation phosphorylation, and reduction in adenosine triphosphate levels (Hilf et al, 1984, 1986). In summary, PDT appears to directly initiate an apoptotic response, without obligate intermediate signal transduction pathways that can be absent in drug-resistant populations of neoplastic cells (Dougherty et al, 1998). Tumor neovasculature endothelium appears to be a key target for PDT damage, resulting in alterations in capillary integrity, in neutrophil and platelet aggregation, and eventually in intravascular coagulation (Reed et al, 1989; Stern et al, 1991; Weiman et al, 1988).

FDA-APPROVED ENDOBRONCHIAL INDICATIONS FOR PHOTODYNAMIC THERAPY WITH PHOTOFRIN

Photofrin II first received FDA approval for the palliation of obstructing esophageal carcinomas in 1995; however, it was not until January 1998 that Photofrin II was approved for the treatment of microinvasive non–small cell lung carcinomas (NSCLCs). Microinvasive lesions are defined as those that do not appear to extend transmurally through the bronchial wall and that appear to be node negative, as defined by computed tomography of the chest. In December 1998, Photofrin II received approval by the FDA for use in endobronchial palliation of NSCLC in patients who were not candidates for chemotherapy or radiation, although the possible reasons for patient ineligibility for the latter two conventional therapies were not further specified.

METHODOLOGY

The requisite wavelength of light employed in PDT is determined both by the absorption spectrum of the photosensitizer administered and by the absorption of the tissue being treated. Both HpD (Photofrin) and DHE

(Photofrin II) have absorption peaks at 405 nm, and light of this wavelength would be absorbed within 1 mm of tissue penetration. A wavelength of 630 nm is used for PDT treatment, however, in order to afford deeper tissue (tumor) penetration. Laser light allows a uniform spectral wavelength and coherence that can be focused into a fiberoptic bundle for use with a flexible bronchoscope (Edell and Cortese, 1995). The lasers most commonly employed for endobronchial PDT are the argon dye pump laser using rhodamine-B (Laserscope, San Jose, CA) and the excimer laser (Cogent, Santa Clarita, CA). A potassium titanyl phosphate/yttrium-aluminum-garnet (KTP/YAG) laser can be used with a dye module to derive the requisite 630 nm red light for PDT with Photofrin II. Commercially available cylindrical diffusing fibers are used to deliver endobronchial PDT. These fibers come in 1-cm and 2.5-cm lengths and diffuse light 360 degrees over the length of the fiber.

DOSE SCHEDULE AND TREATMENT

Endobronchial PDT is readily performed with a combination of topical anesthesia and conscious sedation with a flexible bronchoscope. A power density of 200 to 400 milliwatts/cm^2 is used to deliver a tumor dose of 200 to 400 joules/cm-fiber length. The location and volume of the lesion influence the dose and manner of delivery of PDT. For superficial, sessile lesions, the fiber is frequently laid on the surface of the lesion and the lesion is treated sequentially over its full extent. Alternatively, bulky or polypoid lesions are commonly impaled with the fiber, which allows for deeper tumor-parenchyma light delivery and relative sparing of the surrounding normal bronchial mucosa. For a tracheal lesion, a dose as high as 300 J/cm-fiber with the longer, 2.5-cm fiber might be used. For mainstem bronchial lesions, doses of 200 to 300 J/cm-fiber are common, and for lobar lesions, a dose of 100 to 200 J/cm-fiber is used. Additionally, overlapping dose(s) of 50 to 100 J/cm-fiber may be used for lesions that appear to extend into subsegmental bronchi.

The PDT treatment schedule employed is dependent on both the performance status of the patient and the anatomic location of the lesion. Some investigators prefer general anesthesia for both the PDT laser application and débridement (McCaughan and Williams, 1997); however, both are readily performed using conscious sedation and topical anesthesia. The latter avoids multiple intubations and general anesthesia in patients who frequently have significant pulmonary compromise (Weigel et al, 1999). Many investigators advocate an outpatient treatment regimen for healthy patients with injection of Photofrin II on Monday, followed by PDT treatment on Wednesday, and débridement on Friday. Others prefer a condensed schedule with injection on Monday or Tuesday followed by a same-day admission on the subsequent day after PDT treatment. Débridement is performed on postoperative day #1 (POD #1) with discharge later the same day. With either regimen, an additional PDT treatment can be performed following débridement, that is, on the same day, if viable tumor is still present, but another débridement is required 24 hours later. McCaughan and Williams (1997), in one of the largest U.S. experiences with endobronchial PDT, reported that PDT is efficacious as early as 10 minutes and as late as 1 week after injection of Photofrin II.

The inpatient schedule described earlier is safe for patients with marginal pulmonary status and proximal lesions who may experience further deterioration in their performance status after the PDT treatment, prior to the planned débridement session. The PDT-treated lesion routinely completely occludes the bronchus within which it resides between 8 and 24 hours post treatment because of the resultant tumor necrosis and edema. A significant amount of the tumor debris or cast can be elevated off the bronchial wall with simple, forceful irrigation using a 10-ml slip-top syringe. The flexible laser bronchoscope with its larger, 3-mm, working channel (Olympus, Melville, NY) facilitates and hastens débridement by affording rapid removal of large pieces of tumor debris.

INTERVAL BETWEEN PHOTODYNAMIC THERAPY TREATMENTS

The minimum time interval between PDT treatments is dictated by the half-life of Photofrin II and its attendant side effects such as skin photosensitivity. The FDA and manufacturer recommendations are that PDT treatments should be separated by at least 1 month.

BASIC ADVANTAGES OF PHOTODYNAMIC THERAPY OVER YTTRIUM-ALUMINUM-GARNET LASER THERAPY

PDT is associated with a significantly lower perforation rate than is yttrium-aluminum-garnet (YAG) laser therapy, and PDT can be performed in severely compromised patients with high oxygen requirements. The nonthermal mechanism of action can be used with high FIO_2 and is associated with a low risk of endobronchial fire. Using a cylindrical diffusing fiber, up to 2.5 cm of tumor length can be treated simultaneously. Owing to the limited depth of penetration (0.5–1.0 cm) of PDT and the cylindrical diffusing fiber used to deliver the laser light, lobar and subsegmental bronchial lesions can be safely treated with PDT in contrast to YAG laser therapy. In addition, because of its nonthermal, photochemical mechanism of tumor destruction, pinpoint precision is not necessary nor is a completely immobile patient. PDT can thus be performed with the patient under conscious sedation with topical anesthesia, rather than with general anesthesia as is commonly used with YAG laser therapy.

BASIC DISADVANTAGES OF PHOTODYNAMIC THERAPY OVER YTTRIUM-ALUMINUM-GARNET LASER THERAPY

PDT, in contrast to YAG laser therapy, requires the administration of a costly photosensitizer. Photofrin II (Axcan Pharma Inc, Mont Saint-Hilaire, Quebec) costs approximately $2000 per 75-mg vial; based on the recommended dose of 2 mg/kg, most patients require 2 vials ($4000) per course of PDT. Costly débridements, in either the pulmonary suite or the operating room, are required following the PDT treatment owing to its delayed, photochemical-dependent mechanism of tumor destruction. Patients who present with severely compromised respiratory status frequently can experience further deterioration after completion of PDT, prior to subsequent débridement sessions. Lastly, PDT with Photofrin II is associated with approximately 6 weeks of photosensitivity; however, this was not considered a major morbidity by patients who presented for endobronchial palliation with PDT at the University of Pittsburgh. Patient indifference to photosensitivity reflects the severity of their illness at the time of presentation, as evidenced by their median life expectancy of 2.3 months (Weigel et al, 1999).

RESULTS OF CURATIVE PHOTODYNAMIC THERAPY FOR MICROINVASIVE CARCINOMA

The strategy of treating early NSCLCs with curative endoluminal ablative therapy is attractive because of the magnitude of the resections required to eradicate these proximal lesions and their attendant morbidity. In addition, data that correlate the metastatic potential of these lesions to their diameter enable investigators to predict with reasonable success which lesions may be amenable to nonresectional approaches. Specifically, in 127 surgical specimens examined, there were 55 specimens with lesions smaller than 10 mm in diameter in whom no lymph node metastases were identified; only a 9% (4/46) rate of nodal metastases was documented in lesions whose diameters ranged from 10 to 20 mm (Usuda et al, 1993).

In 1993, Hayata published phase I and phase II clinical data documenting that 90% of superficial tumors smaller than 1 cm had a complete response (CR) to PDT, with a similar response rate in patients with nodular lesions smaller than 0.5 cm in diameter. Of 81 complete responders in this study with long-term follow-up, 15 patients had no evidence of disease (NED) at 5 years, 3 patients were NED after 10 years, and 2 patients were dead of disease. The overall complete response rate in Hayata's series was 71% (Hayata, 1993; Kato et al, 1993). In the same year, Furuse and associates (1993) published the results of The Japan Lung Cancer Photodynamic Therapy Study Group, a prospective phase II trial of PDT with Photofrin II for centrally located early stage NSCLCs. In this study, 50 of 59 (85%) cancers had a CR; best results were seen in tumors smaller than 1 cm whose distal margin was visible on bronchoscopy. Median durability of CR in this study was 14 months, and 5 of 59 cancers recurred locally at 6, 10, 12, 16, and 18 months after PDT (Furuse et al, 1993).

The third, perhaps most definitive, series on curative PDT for early NSCLC was reported initially by Edell and Cortese at the Mayo Clinic in 1992 (Edell and Cortese, 1992) and was updated in 1997 (Cortese et al, 1997). These investigators treated 23 lesions in 21 patients and recommended surgical resection if a cancer persisted after no more than 2 sessions of PDT. A CR was identified in 15 patients with 16 lesions, and it lasted longer than 12 months in 52% (11 patients). A new lung primary was diagnosed in 5 of the 21 patients during follow-up. Surgical resection was recommended to 12 patients: Two patients refused, 10 ultimately underwent surgical resection, and N1 disease was identified in 3 (30%). At a mean of 68 months follow-up, 9 patients (43%) remained NED and were thus spared surgical resection.

In an attempt to improve local control, one group of Japanese investigators treated 39 roentgenologically occult lung cancers with PDT in 29 patients and added external beam radiation therapy to lesions that demonstrated less than a complete response (Imamura et al, 1994). Sixty-four percent of lesions achieved a CR after initial PDT; 10 of 14 of the noncomplete responders were subsequently treated with external beam radiation, and all achieved a CR. The remaining four patients underwent surgical resection. Only one patient died of primary lung cancer at a median of 47 months follow-up, and 2- and 3-year survivals were 93% and 72%, respectively (Imamura et al, 1994).

In 1999, Patelli reported on 26 early-stage central-type squamous cancers with maximum diameters between 5 and 20 mm treated with PDT in 23 patients: Twenty were not operative candidates and three refused surgery. Patients in this study received a dose of 5 mg/kg of hematoporphyrin (HP) and were treated with an average of 360 J/cm^2; a CR was seen in 62% (16/26) with a partial response (PR) in 10 of 26 patients. A CR was subsequently achieved in two of three patients in this study who received endobronchial brachytherapy after a documented PR from PDT (Patelli et al, 1999). Although Perol reported an 83% response with high-dose-rate brachytherapy alone for endobronchial lesions with diameters greater than 10 mm, this was complicated by a hemorrhage rate of 13%. In one additional small series of seven nonsurgical patients with 11 microinvasive NSCLCs treated with curative intent, an average of 1.1 PDT sessions were required to achieve a durable CR in 70% of lesions, with a median follow-up of 34 months (Weigel et al, 2000).

RESULTS OF PHOTODYNAMIC THERAPY FOR PALLIATION OF ENDOBRONCHIAL OBSTRUCTION

Multiple phase I and II studies on PDT for endobronchial obstruction in the United States, Japan, and Canada documented re-establishment of lumen patency with symptomatic, radiographic, and lung function improvement in 70% of patients (Lam, 1994). PDT is fairly expensive because of the need for a photosensitizer ($2000/75-mg vial; with a standard dose of 2 mg/kg, most patients require two vials) and multiple débridements, which are required after PDT in either a bronchoscopy suite or the operating room. Therefore, PDT must be proven superior with respect to its efficacy or applicability if the less costly, conventional endobronchial palliation with yttrium-aluminum-garnet (YAG) laser is to be replaced.

A prospective trial of PDT versus YAG laser therapy demonstrated that, although both had equal efficacy with respect to relieving endobronchial obstruction, the risk of local recurrence was three times higher with YAG laser therapy (McCaughan, 1992).

McCaughan, in one of the largest experiences with

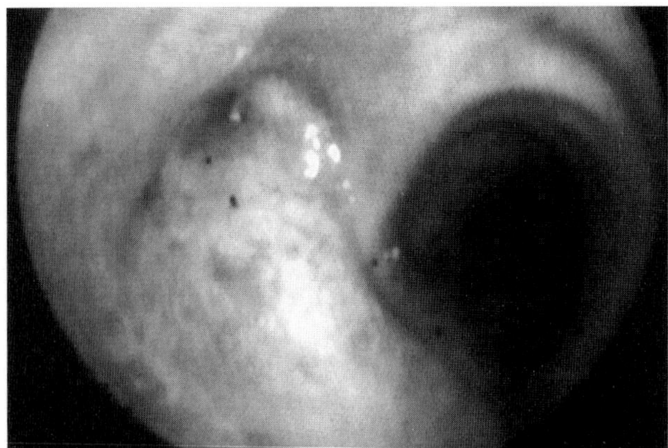

FIGURE 32–11 ■ Obstructed right mainstem bronchus (prior to photodynamic therapy).

endobronchial PDT, noted that the median survival for patients with endobronchial obstruction secondary to stage IIIA, IIIB, or IV NSCLC was only between 2.0 and 4.0 months for patients with Karnofsky performance scores greater than 50% (McCaughan and Williams, 1997). Recognizing the limited life span of these patients, investigators at the University of Pittsburgh focused on symptom relief and noted that 59% (20/34) of patients treated for shortness of breath subjectively experienced good palliation at 1 month post PDT (Figs. 32–11 through 32–14). Although ten patients required a second PDT treatment, in this series at a mean of 2.3 months after their initial PDT, the majority (24/34 patients) succumbed to their disease prior to the need for additional PDT (Weigel et al, 2000).

Although both PDT and YAG are successful in relieving endobronchial obstruction due to intraluminal tumor, neither is effective against bronchial obstruction secondary to submucosal tumor extension or extraluminal compression. Recognizing that obstruction is frequently multifactorial, Lam and colleagues performed a randomized phase III study comparing PDT followed by external beam radiation therapy (EBRT) with EBRT alone (Lam et al, 1991). In patients who received PDT plus EBRT, 70% of bronchial obstructions were relieved versus only 10% of those treated with EBRT alone, with a doubling of the time to local recurrence seen in the combined therapy group (Lam, 1994).

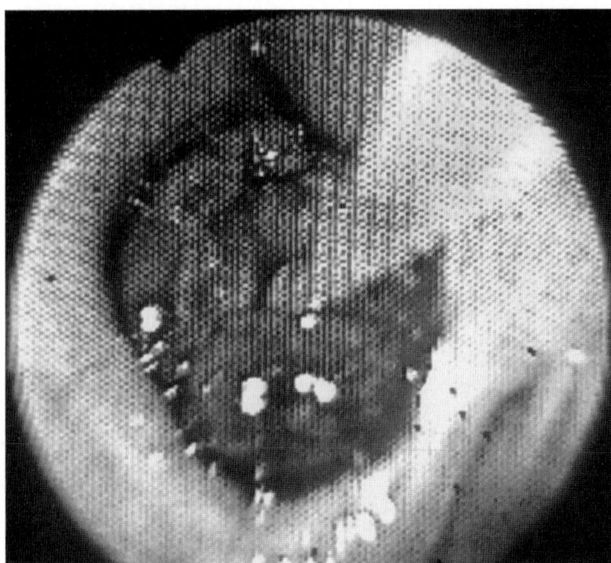

FIGURE 32–12 ■ Obstructing melanoma metastasis impaled with a 1-cm cylindrical-diffusing fiber for photodynamic therapy.

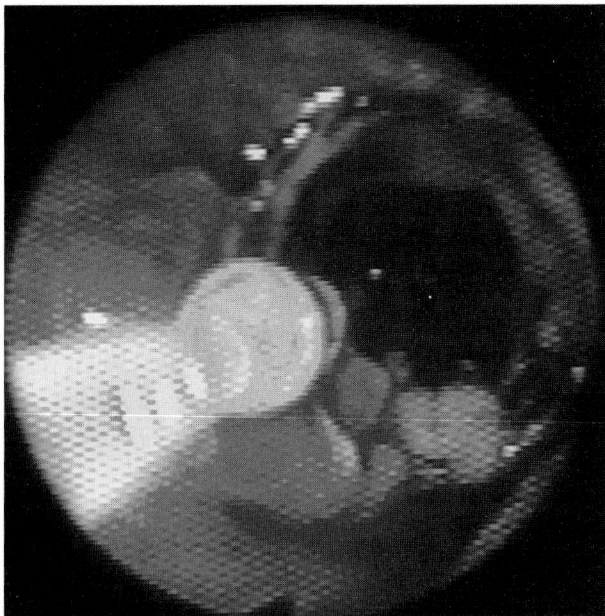

FIGURE 32–13 ■ Palliative photodynamic therapy to open obstructed microvasive stent in bronchus intermedius.

DISCUSSION

Photodynamic therapy with Photofrin II is now approved by the FDA for the treatment of early NSCLC and for palliation of advanced endobronchial lesions. PDT is safer, more versatile, and more user-friendly than YAG

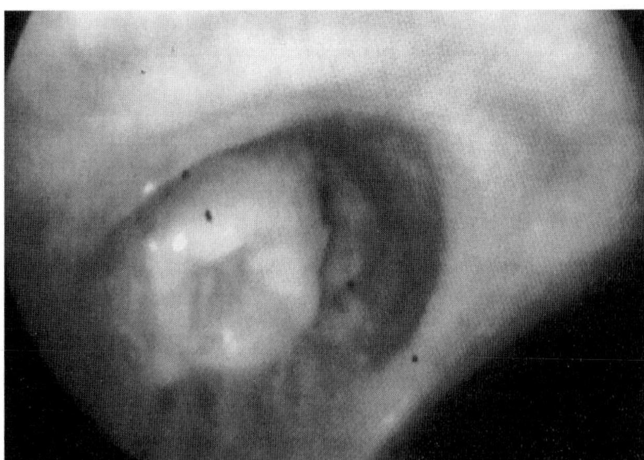

FIGURE 32–14 ■ Tumor cast in left mainstem bronchus after rigorous irrigation, 24 hours after photodynamic therapy treatment.

laser therapy. PDT can be performed under conscious sedation with high FIO_2, making it particularly useful for endobronchial palliation of high-risk patients. PDT, however, is significantly more expensive than YAG because of the requisite photosensitizer and the multiple post-treatment débridements required. In addition, PDT has an attendant morbidity of 6 weeks of photosensitivity. Photodynamic therapy, like YAG laser therapy, should be a part of the armamentarium of all general thoracic surgeons.

COMMENTS AND CONTROVERSIES

Although photodynamic therapy for the curative management of lung cancer has a small but specific role to play, its role in the palliative treatment of endobronchial disease has yet to be defined.

As a method of curative therapy for in situ or very minimally invasive mucosal squamous cell tumors, its efficacy has been substantiated by multiple reports. Patients receiving such treatment must be followed very closely with repeated bronchoscopies, and all patients with persisting or recurrent disease in the local site require other treatments. There certainly are other options for treating in situ and minimally invasive disease, which include continued observation (in situ disease only) and endobronchial brachytherapy, Nd-Yag laser destruction, or surgical resection. It does appear that PDT therapy and endobronchial brachytherapy are becoming the favored approaches, reserving surgical resection for more invasive lesions or those that don't respond to the local approach. The risk of nodal involvement in this early-stage tumor is minimal if the disease is noninvasive.

With regard to palliative therapy, there certainly are multiple options. These include other methods of tumor destruction such as mechanical débridement and a variety of methods of thermal destruction, including neodymium-yttrium-aluminum-garnet (Nd-YAG) treatment and cryotherapy. It is quite likely that no single approach will satisfy all surgeons and all patients. Possibly the combination of hematoporphyrin therapy with radiotherapy will prolong the patient's symptom-free period. One must always remember that these local ablation techniques are valuable only in endobronchial obstructions. Those caused by external compression due to extrinsic tumor require endobronchial stenting if symptomatic—few of these local ablative techniques will have any impact.

R.J.G.

REFERENCES

Cortese DA, Edell ES, Kinsey JH: Photodynamic therapy for early stage squamous cell carcinoma of the lung. Mayo Clin Proc 72:595, 1997.

Dougherty TJ, Gomer CJ, Henderson BW et al: Photodynamic therapy. J Natl Cancer Inst 90:891, 1998.

Edell ES, Cortese DA: Photodynamic therapy in the management of early superficial squamous cell carcinoma as an alternative to surgical resection. Chest 102:1319, 1992.

Edell ES, Cortese DA: Photodynamic therapy is used in the management of bronchogenic carcinoma. Clin Chest Med 16:455, 1995.

Furuse K, Fukuoka M, Kato H et al: A prospective phase II study of photodynamic therapy with Photofrin II for centrally located early-stage lung cancer. J Clin Oncol 11:1852, 1993.

Hayata Y: The indications of photodynamic therapy in early stage lung cancer. Chest 103:262S, 1993.

Hilf R, Murant RS, Narayanan U et al: Hematoporphyrin derivative-induced photosensitivity of mitochondrial succinate dehydrogenase and selected cytosolic enzymes of R3230AC mammary adenocarcinomas of rats. Cancer Res 44:1483, 1984.

Hilf R, Murant RS, Narayanan U et al: Relationship of mitochondrial function and cellular adenosine triphosphate levels of hematoporphyrin derivative-induced photosensitization in R3230AC mammary tumors. Cancer Res 46:211, 1986.

Imamura S, Kusunoki Y, Takifuji N, et al: Photodynamic therapy and/or external beam radiation therapy for roentgenologically occult lung cancer. Cancer 73:1608, 1994.

Kato H, Konaka C et al: Photodynamic therapy (PDT) in early stage lung cancer [Abstract]. Lung Cancer 9:287,1993.

Kime JW: Instrument for use in phototherapy. JAMA 283(18):2365, 2000.

Lam S: Photodynamic therapy of lung cancer. Semin Oncol 21(6 suppl 15):18, 1994.

Lam S, Grafton C, Coy P et al: Combined photodynamic therapy (PDT) using Photofrin and radiotherapy (XRT) versus radiotherapy alone in patients with inoperable obstructive non-small cell bronchogenic carcinoma. SPIE Proc 1616:L20, 1991.

Lee See K, Forbes IJ, Betts WH: Oxygen dependency of photocytotoxicity with haematoporphyrin derivative. Photochem Photobiol 39:631, 1984.

Lipson RL, Baldes EJ: The photodynamic properties of a particular hematoporphyrin derivative. Arch Dermatol 82:508, 1960.

McCaughan JS Jr: Photodynamic therapy versus Nd:YAG laser treatment of endobronchial or esophageal malignancies. In Spinelli P (ed): Photodynamic Therapy and Biomedical Lasers. Proceedings of the International Conference on Photodynamic Therapy and Medical Laser Applications, Milan, Italy, June 25–27, 1992, p 23.

McCaughan JS, Williams TE: Photodynamic therapy for endobronchial malignant disease: A prospective fourteen-year study. J Thorac Cardiovasc Surg 114:940, 1997.

Mitchell JB, McPherson S, DeGraff W et al: Oxygen dependence of hematoporphyrin derivative-induced photoinactivation of Chinese hamster cells. Cancer Res 45:2008, 1985.

Patelli M, Lazzariagli L, Poletti V et al: Photodynamic laser therapy for the treatment of early stage bronchogenic carcinoma. Monaldi Arch Chest Dis 54:315, 1999.

Reed MW, Schuschke DA, Ackermann DM et al: The response of rat urinary bladder microcirculation to photodynamic therapy. J Urol 142:865, 1989.

Sery TV, Shields JA, Augsburger JJ et al: Photodynamic therapy of human ocular cancer. Ophthalmic Surg 18:413, 1987.

Stern SJ, Flock S, Small S et al: Chloraluminum sulphonated phthalocyanine versus dihematoporphyrin ether: Early vascular events in the rat window chamber. Laryngoscope 101:1219, 1991.

Usuda K, Saito Y, Kanma K et al: Resected roentgenographically occult bronchogenic squamous cell carcinoma tumor size, survival and recurrence. Nippon Geka Gakkai Zasshi 94:631, 1993.

Weigel TL, Fernando HC, Ferson PF et al: Palliation of tracheobronchial lesions with photodynamic therapy. Chest 116:2595, 1999.

Weigel TL, Kosco PJ, Christie NA et al: Photodynamic therapy for early non-small cell lung carcinoma in high-risk patients. Chest 118:905, 2000.

Weiman TJ, Mang TS, Fingar VS et al: Effect of photodynamic therapy on blood flow in normal and tumor vessels. Surgery 104:512, 1988.

BIOLOGIC THERAPY OF LUNG CANCER

Robert K. Bright
Helen A. Pass
Harvey I. Pass

Biologic therapy, or immunotherapy, refers to a treatment that elicits an immune response that augments the host's antitumor defenses. Biologic therapy can be specific or nonspecific and active or passive. Specific immunotherapy is treatment with specific reactivity to tumor-associated antigens such as monoclonal antibody therapy, the use of tumor cell vaccines, or treatment with tumor-infiltrating lymphocytes (TILs). Nonspecific immunotherapy is treatment that augments or restores the host's immune system but lacks tumor specificity, such as immune adjuvants and cytokines. Active immunotherapy refers to treatment that actively elicits an immune response such as tumor cell vaccines, adjuvants, and cytokines, whereas passive immunotherapy is the transfer to the host of immunologic reagents that mediate tumor regression.

The basis for an immunologic approach to cancer is grounded in the increasing genetic evidence that cancers arise from molecular changes that lead to transformation and unrestrained cellular growth, often resulting in death. These changes can be manifested as "aberrant" expressions of proteins (e.g., mutated, upregulated, or expressed by those normally silent) by the tumor cells targeting them as potentially foreign, dangerous, or at least "altered" in contrast to the "normal" tissue cells from which the tumor(s) arose. The immune system may be able to sort out these changes and distinguish between healthy and diseased, hence "normal" and malignant, cells. Thus, the proteins encoded by the aberrantly expressed genes of a tumor cell represent targets for the cells of the immune system, serving as tumor rejection or regression antigens. In this light, much effort has turned to the study of the manipulation of the immune response to tumors in the clinical setting. Transfer of immune cells and therapeutic vaccination represent two areas of active research that use methods of eliciting lymphocytes with specificity for antigens aberrantly expressed by tumor cells.

It is evident after a review of the literature that hundreds if not thousands of studies have been published on some aspect of tumor immunology or immunotherapy, from animal tumor models to human malignancies. Any attempt to compile all that has been investigated in the field would be an impossible task and beyond the scope of this chapter. Therefore, the following text represents at best an overview of specific endeavors in immunotherapy.

HISTORICAL NOTE

A prevailing question that puzzled investigators (Rous, 1910) in the early days of tumor immunology (prior to the 1950s) was whether or not the tumor rejection observed in experimental animals was due to rejection of the tissue transplant or of the tumor itself (with awareness of the fact that a tumor arose from once-healthy tissue). During the late 19th century, while tumor transplantation rejection was being studied in animals, a surgeon, William Coley, was testing a vaccine preparation known as "Coley's toxin" on lymphoma and sarcoma patients at New York's Memorial Hospital (known today as the Memorial Sloan-Kettering Cancer Center). Coley had observed tumor regression and remission in patients who suffered a nosocomial bacterial infection following resection of their tumors. He subsequently isolated the bacterium (later the active component) and demonstrated that this "toxin," when administered to sarcoma and lymphoma patients, could mediate tumor regression in nearly 50% of his cases (Coley, 1893). The mechanism of action of this toxin-based vaccine is now believed to be mediated by cytokines that are induced following its administration, an observation that likely influenced the current tumor cell vaccine strategies involving the engineering of tumor cells to express cytokine transgenes. Regardless, Coley recorded perhaps the earliest example of cancer therapy based on the deliberate manipulation of the immune system. However, with the advent of radiation therapy and chemotherapy, and because of the difficulties inherent in reproducing Coley's results, immunotherapy was sidelined for nearly 50 years.

In 1953, the paradigm was challenged when E.J. Foley (1953) published his landmark work on the antigenic properties of methylcholanthrene (MCA)-induced tumors in mice. Foley demonstrated that when MCA tumors were ligated to induce necrosis, protection from a subsequent challenge with the same tumor was observed, but tumors grew quite well in unmanipulated animals. Certainly this phenomenon could not be attributed to differences in major histocompatibility complex (MHC) molecules (i.e., graft rejection) because the experiments were conducted using syngeneic mice. Excitement grew over the observation that tumors could be rejected by (presumed) immune recognition of antigens uniquely expressed on tumor cells. Four years later, Prehn and Main confirmed and extended Foley's results by demonstrating that skin grafts were tolerated when mice of the same inbred strain were used. Moreover, ligated and necrosing syngeneic tumors induced protection from subsequent tumor challenge (Prehn and Main, 1957).

The conclusive proof of tumor antigenicity came in 1960 when George Klein and co-workers published a series of experiments in which surgical removal of tumors (as opposed to ligation) followed by tumor challenge resulted in protection (Klein et al, 1960). More striking was their demonstration that tumor protection was obtained by injection of irradiated (inactivated) tumor cells prior to challenge (this experiment remains today as the standard for assessing tumor cell immunogenicity in vivo). Collectively, these experiments established that immune-mediated tumor rejection in inbred strains of mice was not a consequence of histocompatibility differences, but rather a result of tumor antigen recognition.

Numerous studies expounding the complexities of the immunologic rejection of solid tumors were published during the decades of the 1960s and 1970s. The majority of these studies focused on experimental tumor models in mice. As progress was made toward the feasibility of employing the immune system against human cancer, theories concerning the biology and progression of cancer as these relate to incidence and natural control of occurrence were also being developed. At the forefront was the immune surveillance theory (Burnet, 1971). This theory holds that all tumor cells express antigenic markers capable of eliciting immune responses that result in tumor destruction, and that this process occurs continuously, thus preventing the outgrowth of malignant cells in most healthy individuals. As a person ages, the immune system declines, allowing the growth of tumors, hence one explanation for the increased incidence of cancer in people over the age of 50. Conceptually, this theory would be difficult to prove in vivo, and certainly other mechanisms may participate in controlling cellular transformation and tumor formation in the healthy individual (e.g., events at the molecular and genetic levels within the nascent tumor cell).

Nevertheless, the power of the immune system lies within its ability to discriminate between self and nonself, or more appropriately, to differentiate a normal cell from a tumor cell, thereby selectively and specifically eliminating tumor cells while leaving normal cells intact. The arm of the immune system that is primarily responsible for tumor-specific immunity is classically referred to as the *adaptive immune response*. Adaptive immunity employs a subset of cells of the lymphocyte lineage as the primary effectors responsible for the mechanisms of tumor-specific killing. Interest in the response of lung cancer to immunotherapies was initiated when Takita (1970), and then Ruckdeschel (1972), reported an improved survival in lung cancer patients who survived postoperative empyemas versus uninfected patients. The improvement in survival was thought to be due to the adjuvant, immunostimulatory effect of the bacterial products.

BASIC SCIENCE

T Cell–Mediated Immune Responses

Immunologic rejection of tumors is believed to be executed primarily by lymphocytes, and the most widespread idea is that T lymphocyte (cell)–mediated immunity is essential for the destruction of most solid tumors. T cells are subdivided into two main groups: (1) "helper" function ($CD4^+$ T cells) for immune responses following recognition of peptide antigens processed and presented in the context of class II major histocompatibility antigens (MHC-II) on professional antigen-presenting cells, or APCs (e.g., dendritic cells, macrophages, and B lymphocytes); and (2) $CD8^+$ cytotoxic T cells that directly mediate tumor destruction resulting from recognition of peptide antigens (usually derived from endogenously expressed proteins) in the context of MHC-I molecules expressed on the surface of the tumor cells. MHC-I molecules are normally expressed on all somatic cells in the body, including fibroblasts and epithelial cells, which give rise to sarcomas and carcinomas, respectively.

Typically, $CD4^+$ T cells are noncytolytic, yet have been shown to play a role in tumor rejection by providing the necessary help for $CD8^+$ cytotoxic T-lymphocyte (CTL) activation and lytic activity. For example, tumor immunity was attributed to the induction of $CD4^+$ T cells in a murine melanoma model wherein tumors were engineered to express the human p97 gene (Kahn et al, 1991), as well as a model for disseminated MHC-II negative lymphoma (Greenberg, 1990). Topalian and colleagues (1996) identified $CD4^+$ T cells with specificity for tyrosinase, a shared tumor antigen associated with human malignant melanoma. Although there is evidence for the role of $CD4^+$ MHC-II restricted T cells in tumor immunity, the vast majority of tumor-reactive T cells defined for human systems and in animal models are $CD8^+$ MHC-I–restricted CTLs (Boon et al, 1994; Rosenberg, 1995).

CTLs recognize peptide fragments (8–10 amino acids in length) of intracellular protein antigens in the context of MHC-I molecule heavy chains in association with β_2-microglobulin. These tri-molecular complexes are expressed on the tumor (target) cell surface, giving an extracellular presentation of endogenously expressed and enzymatically processed protein fragments for a CTL to engage using its antigen-specific receptor(s) (T cell receptors, TCRs) (Davis et al, 1998). The role of CTLs in tumor destruction has been demonstrated in numerous murine tumor models by the induction of tumor antigen–specific immune responses following immunization with antigen-coated beads (Kovacsovics-Bankowski et al, 1993), recombinant viruses (Roa et al, 1996), synthetic peptides (Feltkamp et al, 1993), or naked plasmid DNA (Bright et al, 1996). The presence of tumor antigen–specific $CD8^+$ CTLs within a developing tumor was first demonstrated for humans by the process of growing the tumor-infiltrating lymphocytes (TILs) from resected melanomas (Rosenberg et al, 1994). The in vitro growth and adoptive transfer of TILs have become a viable and available therapy for patients with malignant melanoma. These studies (and numerous others) have clearly demonstrated that CTLs can be recruited (via immunization or in vitro manipulation) and deployed against tumors, resulting in complete protection or treatment of tumors in murine models or in objective clinical responses for cancer patients. Unfortunately, much of the skepticism regarding tumor immunology is based on the contention that the immune system has been taught to fight infection (foreign), not cancer (self), and that it cannot be educated otherwise. Mounting data, however, indicate that the cellular arm of the immune system can be taught to kill cancer and that tumors themselves are often actively involved in the tactics of immunologic escape and evasion.

Escape of Tumors from Immunologic Rejection

Tumors express *unique* antigenic targets capable of inducing tumor-destructive immune responses, and it is possible that the clinical occurrence of cancer represents those "not-so-usual" circumstances in which the immune system is ineffective at recognizing these targets. The process of tumor progression in the absence of an apparent immune response is classically referred to as *tumor escape*. Much speculation is given to the mechanism(s) by which tumors escape and evade immune destruction. Although there exist a number of studies describing many possible mechanisms of tumor escape (few, however, without accompanying contradictory reports), we focus here on mechanisms most likely to impact the development of immunotherapies, such as vaccines and adoptive cell transfer.

Downregulation of MHC-I Expression

As alluded to previously, $CD8^+$ CTLs constitute the primary and perhaps the most important arm of immune-mediated defense against solid tumors. The removal or downregulation of MHC-I molecules from the surface of a tumor cell renders that tumor incapable of presenting MHC-I molecules complexed with antigenic peptides, and as such, removes the means by which a CTL could recognize the tumor cell and subsequently destroy it. Some clinical studies have demonstrated that primary tumors can exhibit detectable decreases in MHC-I expression compared with adjacent normal tissue. Metastatic tumors, however, do not seem to differ from their parent (primary) tumor with respect to the level of MHC-I expression, although they have escaped immune destruction, as evidenced by the metastatic event. Examination of multiple human and experimental tumors has demonstrated that MHC-I expression is often retained on tumors from patient to patient or between tumor histologies, thus it has proven difficult to correlate tumorigenicity, or lack thereof, with MHC-I expression or downregulation. Nonetheless, animal studies have demonstrated that tumorigenic cell lines (capable of forming tumors in vivo) become less tumorigenic in immunocompetent hosts when MHC-I expression is increased (typically accomplished by cytokine induction or MHC-I gene transfection [Wallich et al, 1985]). The corollary assumption (again supported by data) is that MHC-I expression leaves a tumor cell nontumorigenic (owing to increased immunogenicity) in syngeneic, immunocompetent animals. Often tumor models in murine systems include a tumorigenic cell line that expresses MHC-I, as well as an immunogenic tumor antigen capable of eliciting tumor-destructive immunity (Bright et al, 1998; Kast et al, 1989). Although there exist some conflicting conclusions concerning MHC-I downregulation and its role as a mechanism of tumor escape, caution directs that it be given careful consideration when immunologic therapies are developed for cancer that rely on induction of MHC-I–restricted CTLs.

Absence of Co-stimulation

T cells require secondary signals in addition to those obtained through TCR-MHC-peptide engagement (the primary signal, or signal 1) in order to become active effector cells. The B7 family of gene products (including B7.1 and B7.2) have been identified as key elements that provide the second signal known as co-stimulation. The B7 ligand is found primarily on professional APCs such as dendritic cells and B cells, and has not been demonstrated on somatic cells, such as those giving rise to most solid tumors. The receptor for B7 is the CD28 molecule, which is found on T cells. When CD28 on a T cell is engaged by B7, following TCR engagement of an MHC–peptide complex, the necessary 1 and 2 signals are delivered to the T cell, resulting in its activation and proliferation (Fig. 32–15). Experiments have demonstrated that the first (MHC–peptide) and second (B7–CD28) signals are most efficiently delivered when expressed on the same APC (Schwartz, 1992). When resting or naive T cells are engaged with a specific MHC–peptide complex through their TCR in the absence of B7 and CD28 engagement, the result is peripheral tolerance or anergy (Schwartz, 1990). Because tumors do not express B7 molecules (B cell malignancies are an exception), tumor cell antigen presentation to T cells results in anergy (or functional unresponsiveness), hence the premise for absence of co-stimulation as a mechanism for tumor escape. Tumor cells that lack B7 expression and fail to stimulate T cells can be engineered to express B7 and successfully stimulate tumor-specific T cells (Townsend and Allison, 1993). Indeed, tumor cells expressing a B7 transgene are being explored as a "new generation" of whole tumor cell vaccines.

Tolerance

The absence of co-stimulation represents a mechanism of immunologic tolerance to tumor cells. The primary mechanism of establishing peripheral tolerance is neonatal exposure to antigens during ontogeny. This process (involving thymic mechanisms of positive and negative selection) (Kappler et al, 1987) provides the necessary environment for immunologic tolerance of self antigens and the prevention of autoimmune disease. Studies have demonstrated that tumor antigens encountered early enough in fetal development are tolerated by the adult animal and thus are no longer immunogenic. Virally induced breast tumors in virus-bearing versus virus-free animals represent one example (Le Bon et al, 1995). Another example is Simian virus 40 (SV40) Tag transgenic mice that develop spontaneous tumors that remain Tag positive and grow unchecked, even though Tag is highly immunogenic in mice (Husler et al, 1998). Tumor formation in the SV40 Tag transgenic system is difficult to define as *tolerance* to Tag because Tag-positive tumors transplanted to syngeneic adult immunocompetent mice grow progressively, resulting in death, unless

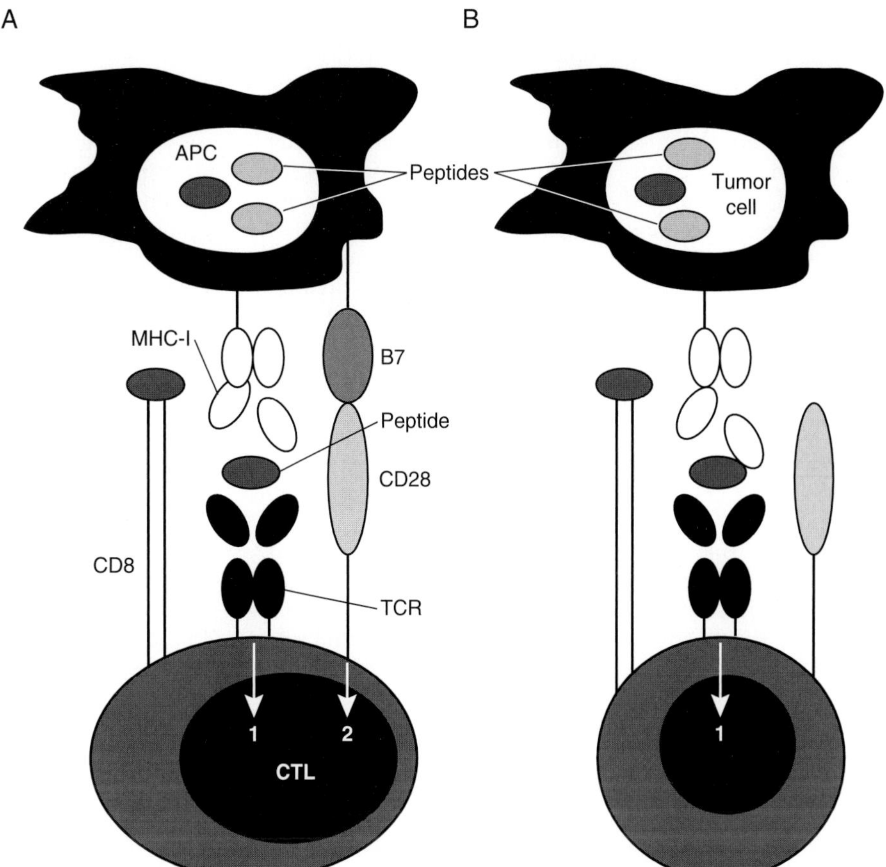

FIGURE 32–15 ■ Schematic representation of T-cell recognition of an antigenic peptide in the context of an MHC-I molecule. *A*, An illustration of the events leading up to successful T-cell activation following effective delivery of signal 1 and signal 2, *co-stimulation* (see text for details). *B*, An illustration of the induction of T-cell anergy following delivery of signal 1 in the absence of signal 2 (see text for details). APC, antigen presenting cell (e.g., dendritic cells); CTL, CD8$^+$ cytotoxic T cell; MHC-I, class I major histocompatibility antigen; TCR; T-cell antigen receptor. From Pass HI et al (eds): Lung Cancer: Principles and Practice, 2nd ed, Philadelphia, Lippincott, Williams & Wilkins, 1995.

an immune response to Tag is induced prior to transplantation (Bright et al, 1998). In addition, when hemagglutinin (HA) of influenza virus was expressed in the pancreas (driven by a tissue-specific promoter) of transgenic mice, the viral antigen was well tolerated and no autoimmune disease was evident, even when the animals were immunized against HA. Interestingly, when these HA-transgenic mice were immunized with HA followed by a lethal challenge with HA expression of tumor cells, the tumors were rejected and HA-specific immunity was demonstrated, yet the pancreas was left healthy and functional (Morgan et al, 1998). Conversely, when a viral glycoprotein (GP) was expressed in the pancreas of transgenic mice for study of the induction of autoimmunity against a defined antigen, tolerance was broken, resulting in autoimmune diabetes following immunization with dendritic cells that express GP (Ludewig et al, 1998). The implication here for cancer treatment is that therapeutic immunization against antigens that are not tumor specific (most of the candidate tumor antigens for human cancer defined thus far are not tumor specific) could result in autoimmune disease. Though tolerance is clearly an obstacle in the path of many tumor immunotherapy approaches, complete understanding surrounding the involvement of tolerance in tumor immunity and methods to overcome or manipulate it require further investigation.

Tumor-Secreted Factors

Cultured tumor cells secrete numerous cytokines and various growth factors that are suppressive to the cells of the immune system, including transforming growth factor-β (TGF-β). TGF-β is a family of molecules first identified as supporting transformation, defined by cell growth in soft agar. Many tumor cells secrete TGF-β, which sets up an immunosuppressive microenvironment by inhibiting T cell proliferation and CTL maturation. Tumors make other cytokines as well, which influence or drive T-helper cell function to support either cellular (CTL) or humoral (antibody) immunity (Mossman and Coffman, 1989). Because CTLs are important for tumor cell killing, a cytokine profile (influenced by cytokines secreted by the tumor) that favors humoral versus cellular immunity could be detrimental to the successful immunologic rejection of the tumor. Therapies employed in such an environment may be aided by administration of anticytokine antibodies, recombinant cytokines (or tumor cells engineered to secrete cytokines), or cytokine analogs that block cytokine receptors on immune cells (e.g., T cells), which drive a cellular immune response.

Active Manipulation of the Immune Response for Eliminating Tumors

A realistic goal for the immunologic treatment of cancer is to administer immunotherapy as an adjuvant therapy to surgical resection of the primary tumor. Immunotherapy can be divided into two categories—active and passive strategies. Active approaches comprise both specific and nonspecific strategies, and passive methods involve the transfer of antigen-specific antibodies. Antibodies have been useful clinically as diagnostic tools in the context of enzyme-linked immunosorbent assay (ELISA) or immunocytochemistry performed on tissue sections. The power of antibodies in this capacity comes by exploitation of their ability to recognize surface proteins either unique on tumor tissues or overexpressed on tumor cells compared with normal cells. Antibodies have demonstrated potential as immunotherapeutic agents as well (by complexing the antibody with toxins [immunotoxins] [Krolick et al, 1982] or radioactive molecules [Goldenberg, 1994]) or as free antibody, presumably inducing mechanisms of antibody dependent cell-mediated cytotoxicity (ADCC) (Bright et al, 1994). ADCC, for example, is a possible mechanism that is employed during therapy with trastuzumab (Herceptin), a new passive immunotherapy that targets the HER-2/neu tumor antigen on breast cancer cells with an antigen-specific monoclonal antibody.

Active nonspecific immunotherapy of cancer involves the induction of immune cells that do not rely on tumor antigen recognition and MHC-I restriction. Generally, the therapy involves administration of cytokines or immune stimulatory adjuvants such as bacillus Calmette-Guerin (BCG) or *Corynebacterium parvum*, resulting in the subsequent activation of nonspecific effectors such as natural killer (NK) cells or lymphokine-activated killer (LAK) cells. LAK cells have demonstrated limited efficacy as immunotherapeutic agents when activated in vitro and adoptively transferred back to the patient. Countless studies have demonstrated that protective immune responses can be elicited by vaccination with candidate synthetic tumor antigens or peptide fragment(s) (epitopes) from the tumor antigen (Melief et al, 1996). In this light, strategies for the development of new therapies for the treatment of human cancer based on the identification and characterization of a target tumor antigen(s) and the MHC-I–binding peptides from the tumor antigen(s) include (1) in vitro generated antitumor -$CD8^+$ CTLs that may be useful for adoptive cellular transfer immunotherapy, and (2) active immunization with synthetic peptide epitope(s) as subunit therapeutic cancer vaccines.

Adoptive Transfer of Tumor-Specific T Cell

Adoptive immunotherapy has been defined as the acquisition of immunity in a naive subject as the result of the administration of immunologically activated lymphoid cells (Shu et al, 1997). The process of adoptive transfer of tumor-specific lymphocytes involves obtaining T cells from the patient to be treated, culturing the T cells in vitro to activate and expand them, and finally infusing them back into the patient. As alluded to previously, T cells that infiltrate solid tumor masses (e.g., melanomas and renal cell carcinomas) have proven to be a powerful source of tumor-reactive T cells for adoptive cellular transfer. These T cells, designated tumor-infiltrating lymphocytes (TILs), have been used successfully to treat patients with malignant melanoma. However, there are reasons why TIL transfer therapy has not seen wider application: (1) Not all solid tumors are a source of TILs; (2) Administration of cytokines such as the T cell growth factor interleukin-2 (IL-2) with the TILs is often necessary to maintain the T cells in vivo; and (3) It is often difficult to acquire enough autologous tumor cells for use as a source of tumor antigen for in vitro activation and expansion. One alternative is to collect lymph node–draining T cells, following immunization with autologous tumor and adjuvant, and stimulate them in vitro with anti-CD3 (the signalling portion of the TCR) antibody (Chang et al, 1997; Yoshizawa et al, 1991). This provides an effective method for generating sufficient numbers of tumor-reactive CTLs for adoptive transfer.

Active Specific Induction of Tumor Immunity

The identification of human tumor antigens and the availability of synthetic peptides have made possible the generation of human tumor-specific CTLs. For example, repeated exposure of peripheral blood lymphocytes (PBLs) from melanoma patients to an immunodominant peptide from the shared melanoma antigen MART-1 (methods for antigen identification are discussed later) resulted in the generation of CTLs that were from 50 to 100 times more potent in specific tumor killing than activated infiltrating lymphocytes harvested from the patient's tumor (Parkhurst et al, 1996). A separate study demonstrated the generation of CTL with specificity for the shared human melanoma antigen gp100 by in vitro stimulation of the patient's PBL with synthetic peptides representing CTL epitopes on gp100 (Salgaller et al, 1995). In addition, a number of studies demonstrated the feasibility of inducing tumor-reactive CTLs in vitro by co-culturing PBLs from cancer patients with tumor cell lines expressing matched or autologous MHC-I antigens (Crowley et al, 1990; Herin et al, 1987; Slingluff et al, 1989; Stevens et al, 1995). Most striking were the results from a recent clinical trial involving melanoma CTL-MHC-I peptides as a therapeutic vaccine administered to patients with advanced metastatic disease. Therapeutic peptide vaccination resulted in a higher percentage of clinical responses (to include complete responses) in patients than has previously been seen for any other therapy for melanoma (Rosenberg et al, 1998). Indeed, this and other studies under way are clearly demonstrating the power and potential of therapeutic peptide–based vaccines for the treatment of advanced cancer. In spite of the evidence for the existence of tumor-reactive CTLs in patients with cancer and in murine tumor models, as well as the potential of peptide-based therapeutic vaccines, most efforts to demonstrate an ongoing CTL response against tumor antigens in humans have failed. However, it is of the utmost importance to remember that in most murine tumor models (e.g., the Balb/c SV40 tumor model), the tumor of interest, though it expresses a highly immunogenic tumor-specific antigen (e.g., SV40 Tag) and MHC-I molecules, grows rapidly and aggressively in vivo, ultimately killing the immunocompetent host if an antigen-specific immune response is not present prior to or concurrent with tumor transplantation (Bright et al, 1998).

IMMUNOTHERAPY RELATED TO LUNG CANCER

Despite newfound optimism for high-dose chemotherapy for certain types of lung cancer (namely, small cell lung cancer) (Thatcher et al, 1997), overall treatment options are limited. This seemingly desperate situation demands investigation into new treatments and re-evaluation of treatments such as immunotherapy with the application of new advances in technology. Typically, immunotherapies for lung cancer can be divided into nonspecific and specific approaches. Nonspecific therapies primarily involve the administration of bacterium or components of bacterium with the expectation that an ensuing inflammatory immune response will result in accompanying immunity against the tumor. Specific immunotherapy involves either the passive transfer of tumor-reactive immune cells or antibodies that target and destroy the tumor, or active induction of tumor-destroying immunity following injection (vaccination) with inactivated tumor cells or molecular components of tumor cells (antigens).

Nonspecific Immunotherapy

The nonspecific immunotherapy of lung cancer dates back to the 1970s and 1980s, with trials showing little to no benefit (Al-Moundhri et al, 1998). Most efforts focused on the administration of BCG or *C. parvum* with limited clinical success. Adjuvant therapies attempt to overcome the immunosuppressive effects of malignancies in a generalized nonspecific manner. BCG stimulates both the cellular and humorally mediated immune responses, whereas *C. parvum* primarily augments cell-mediated immunity. Unlike BCG and *C. parvum*, the anthelmintic drug levamisole only restores the immune response to normal, and does not stimulate it above the normal level. Levamisole augments T cell function and number, as well as enhances the phagocytosis and chemotaxis of macrophages and neutrophils. O'Brien and associates (1997) began trials to evaluate the efficacy of treating lung cancer patients with a different species of *Mycobacterium, M. vaccae*, which is devoid of toxicity, in combination with chemotherapy.

The discovery that immune cells produce cytokines, secretory products that regulate the immune response, greatly expanded the potential number of anticancer agents. Administration of cytokines represents another arm of nonspecific immunotherapy for cancer. The effects of the interferons (IFNs), tumor necrosis factor-α (TNF-α), and IL-2 against lung cancer have been studied.

The interferons were the first cytokines discovered as new polypeptides secreted by virally infected cells. Clinically, IFN-α has been the most extensively studied cytokine and the first to be successfully cloned and mass-produced by recombinant technology. There are three types of interferons. IFN-α (produced by leukocytes) and IFN-β (produced by fibroblasts) together are called type I interferons. They have considerable similarities in amino acid sequence and are both elicited in response to viral infections. IFN-γ, or type II interferon, has little homology to the type I interferons and is produced by T lymphocytes in response to antigenic or mitogenic stimuli.

Interferon may have anticancer activity through direct or host-mediated mechanisms. Interferon has direct antitumor activity through inhibition of tumor cell growth, transformation suppression, angiogenesis inhibition, and induction of differentiation. Equally important are interferon's immunomodulatory activities. Interferon enhances host-mediated anticancer activity through upregulation of tumor-associated antigens, natural killer cell function, and macrophage activity.

Since its discovery in 1976, interleukin-2 (IL-2) has been identified as a critically important molecule in immune regulation. IL-2 has a variety of functions, including selective expansion of T lymphocytes, enhancement of natural killer activity, generation of LAK cells (see Adoptive Immunotherapy in earlier section, Adoptive Transfer of Tumor-Specific T Cell), and induction of the release of a variety of other cytokines. Because T lymphocytes, natural killer cells, and LAK cells are all involved in the immune responses mediating tumor regression, the anticancer effects of IL-2 have been extensively studied in a number of cancer histologies.

Tumor necrosis factor (TNF) was originally described as an endotoxin-derived serum factor that caused the regression of meth-A sarcomas in experimental animals. The mechanisms of TNF's antitumor action are unknown. TNF is both an activator and a cytotoxic product of macrophages. Additionally, it activates lymphocytes and NK cells, promotes leukocyte adherence, disrupts vascular integrity, and induces the secretion of other cytokines, specifically interleukin-1 and interleukin-6.

Clinically, TNF has failed to meet expectations when administered as a single agent. In human phase I trials, systemic side effects, including hypotension, fever, rigors, thrombocytopenia, and neutropenia, have been dose limiting. The maximum tolerated dose of TNF is 40-fold less on a per-kilogram basis than the dose that is required to generate a significant antitumor response in mice. Thus, current trials are exploring the use of TNF in combination with other cytokines.

IFN, TNF, and IL-2 have been evaluated alone and in combination in a limited number of lung cancer patients. Since 1981, these phase I trials have demonstrated that cytokine therapy can be administered safely and occasionally may mediate regression of lung cancer. Many of the studies have combined the cytokine with chemotherapy or radiation therapy. These studies have provided the impetus for further ongoing trials; however, the contribution of the cytokine to these dramatic results is unclear, and unfortunately, a phase III trial has not been designed. In recent years, recombinant IFN-α has been re-evaluated clinically as a maintenance therapy following chemotherapy. Overall, the use of nonspecific approaches to immunotherapy has been disappointing and the hope in such treatments has waned. As the use of nonspecific immunotherapy declines, efforts to actively and specifically target tumors with cytolytic immune responses are on the rise.

Passive Specific Immunotherapy

As was alluded to earlier, passive immunotherapy has traditionally involved either the infusion of tumor-specific antibodies or the transfer of tumor-reactive immune cells. For passive antibody therapy, monoclonal antibodies (mAbs) have seen the greatest utility. Antibodies have been administered alone (e.g., L6 mAb, which recognizes a surface carbohydrate antigen on NSCLC) (Goodman et al, 1993) or complexed to toxic molecules like *Pseudomonas* exotoxin-A (Pai et al, 1991) or ricin for SCLC (Lynch, 1993). Antibodies, for the most part, have not demonstrated much usefulness as therapies for lung cancer, but they remain valuable as diagnostic and prognostic tools.

The adoptive transfer of tumor-reactive immune cells into patients with advanced cancer was pioneered by Rosenberg and colleagues (1985). The earliest efforts involved the ex vivo expansion of lymphocytes in the presence of high-dose IL-2; the resulting effectors were designated lymphokine-activated killer cells, or LAK cells. LAK cells behave somewhat like natural killer (NK) cells in that they are not MHC-restricted T cells but they do exhibit an increased propensity to kill tumor cells. In time, LAK cells were replaced by more potent tumor-specific, MHC-I–restricted cytotoxic T lymphocytes (CTLs) isolated from resected tumor following culture of the tumor in the presence of IL-2. Again pioneered by Rosenberg and colleagues, these CTLs, known as tumor-infiltrating lymphocytes (TILs), have demonstrated objective clinical responses when transferred into patients with malignant melanoma or renal cell carcinoma (Topalian et al, 1987).

In the past, adoptive transfer trials for lung cancer involved LAK cells alone or with IL-2, or in combination with different chemotherapies. The generation of patient-specific LAKs or TILs is labor and resource intensive; hence, only a few patients with lung cancer have received adoptive immunotherapy in a phase II setting. Although most of these efforts were disappointing, it was reported by Kimura and Yamaguchi (1995) that LAK cells and IL-2 showed a significant survival benefit over radiotherapy, chemotherapy, or radiochemotherapy when administered to 105 randomized patients undergoing noncurative resection for lung cancer. Adoptive transfer trials for melanoma have demonstrated that TILs are more potent than LAK cells; however, TILs have been difficult to isolate from malignancies other than melanoma (examples include breast, prostate, and lung cancer). A recent strategy for generating tumor-specific CTLs is to immunize the patient with his or her own tumor cells in the presence of an immunostimulant like the cytokine granulocyte-macrophage colony-stimulating factor (GM-CSF); then CTLs from the patient's draining lymph nodes or peripheral blood should be isolated and cultured for expansion in vitro and subsequent transfer back to the patient (Wakimoto et al, 1996). Small-scale studies to evaluate this strategy for the therapy of lung cancer are just beginning, thus time will reveal their usefulness. Because most of the more common and deadly tumors do not easily (if at all) give rise to TILs, and because the generation of CTLs in vivo (as alluded to earlier) is labor intensive, taking weeks to accomplish, much effort has turned to active specific immunotherapy involving tumor vaccines.

Active Specific Immunotherapy

The early work of Klein and co-workers (1960), as well as others, demonstrating that immunization of mice with inactivated tumor cells resulted in protection from a subsequent lethal tumor challenge, prompted trials to evaluate whole tumor cell vaccines in lung cancer patients. This early approach to tumor vaccination usually involved injection of irradiated autologous or allogeneic tumor cells alone or with an adjuvant such as BCG (more recently, cytokines such as GM-CSF have been used). Unfortunately, like the nonspecific immunotherapy approaches to treating lung cancer, whole tumor vaccines have not produced very promising results (Hollinshead et al, 1987). One explanation is that there are components of whole tumor cells that are at the very least detrimental if not suppressive to concomitant immunity. In this light, much effort has turned to the development of molecularly defined tumor vaccines. For example, Carbone and colleagues (1994) have recently begun evaluation of lung cancer vaccines comprising either mutated *ras* oncogene products or mutated *p53* tumor suppressor gene products in an attempt to take advantage of the aberrant expression of these proteins in human lung cancers (Gabrilovich et al, 1997). These and other studies are beginning to reveal the importance of identifying tumor-associated antigens (TAAs) toward their development as defined therapeutic tumor vaccines.

Tumor-Associated Antigens

A hallmark of active immunity that has formed the foundation of the field of vaccinology (pioneered for infectious diseases such as polio and smallpox) is the ability of the immune system to specifically target and destroy invaders or diseased cells while leaving adjacent healthy cells intact. Specificity arises from immune cell recognition of defined targets or antigens on diseased cells (as described earlier, T cell antigens comprise a peptide in the groove of an MHC molecule). As was mentioned previously, the first evidence for antigens on tumor cells came from the pioneering work of Foley, Prehn, and Main. For decades since, researchers have hunted for evidence of tumor-associated antigens (TAAs) on human tumors with the hope of employing the power and specificity of the immune system to specifically destroy tumor cells. The premise was that if TAAs could be identified that were exclusively expressed on tumor cells, then the immune response could be manipulated against these TAAs much as had been demonstrated for infectious agents, namely viruses. In this light, the hunt for tumor viruses began.

Viral Proteins

Certain cancers are thought to be caused by viral infection, although a direct causal relationship is difficult to define. Some viruses considered to be associated with human malignancies include the following: hepatitis B virus (HBV) with hepatocellular carcinoma, human T cell leukemia/lymphoma virus (HTLV-I) with T cell lymphoma, Epstein-Barr virus (EBV) with Burkitt's lymphoma, and the human papovavirus (HPV) with cervical carcinoma (Rudden, 1995). Viruses by nature possess the ability to alter host cell function and directly influence the multistep process that leads to transformation. Virally induced transformation may occur through the induction of genetic aberrations resulting from physical interaction of viral DNA with the host genome, or through viral gene products expressed following infection. Because viral infection (in permissive as well as nonpermissive hosts) often results in the expression of virally encoded protein antigens, cancers with true viral etiologies or associations represent prime candidates for the development of targeted, specific immunologic therapies.

The foremost example of targeting viral antigens for the immunotherapy of human cancer is that of HPV and cervical carcinoma. Clinical studies of malignant lesions indicate that more than 90% of cervical carcinomas contain HPV genetic sequences (Resnick et al, 1990). The induction of tumor-killing CTLs by vaccination with MHC-I peptides from E6 or E7 has been demonstrated, most notably in murine models for HPV-16–induced cervical carcinoma (Melief and Kast, 1995). Taken together, such information has led to clinical trials involving the vaccination of cervical carcinoma patients with peptides from the E6 or E7 oncoproteins of HPV. A second virus from the papovavirus family, simian virus 40, has recently been implicated with several different human malignancies.

Simian virus 40–like DNA sequences (in particular the SV40 large tumor antigen, *Tag*, gene) have been amplified from human tumors of the bone (osteosarcomas), brain (ependymomas and glioblastomas), and mesothelium, with more than 60% of ependymomas exhibiting expression of the SV40 Tag protein (Bersagel et al, 1992). Further, reports have demonstrated that 60% of malignant pleural mesotheliomas (MPMs) contain SV40 Tag genetic sequences and proteins (Carbone et al, 1994; Pass et al, 1996). The viral genes and gene products, though present in MPM tumors, could not be found in the normal mesothelium of the same patient. Studies involving other papovaviruses like HPV as targets for immunotherapy of cervical carcinoma, along with data from murine models demonstrating the immunotherapeutic potential of SV40 Tag against Tag-positive tumors (Bright et al, 1998), suggest that SV40 Tag represents a shared tumor-specific antigen that may be a target for the immunotherapy of MPM in humans. In spite of the enthusiasm surrounding the immunologic targeting of HPV and SV40 for the therapy of certain human cancers, it has become clear that viruses do not represent candidates for immunotherapy in the majority of human malignancies.

Oncogene and Tumor Suppressor Gene Products

The products of oncogenes may impart the desired tumor-specific expression, and they have the potential for being a target that is shared among tumors of multiple histologies. The following are a few of the more common examples of TAAs from expressed oncogenes or tumor suppressor genes (Table 32–21).

The transmembrane tyrosine kinase HER2/neu has been demonstrated to be overexpressed in several clinically important human malignancies, including cancers of the breast, ovary, colon, and lung. Although HER2/neu is expressed on some "normal" tissues and cells, it exhibits a significant increase in expression in some tumors compared with the corresponding normal tissue. This overexpression or upregulation has been demonstrated to be sufficient to elicit an immune response against HER2/neu. CTLs with specificity for HER2/neu epitopes have been identified in the peripheral blood of breast cancer patients (Linehan et al, 1995), and antibodies against an extracellular domain of HER2/neu have formed the basis for a recently FDA-approved antibody-based therapy (Herceptin) for certain breast cancers.

TABLE 32–21 ■ **Tumor Antigens Associated with Human Lung Cancer**

Tumor Antigen	*Tumor Association*
K-ras	NSCLC
p53	NSCLC, SCLC
HER2/neu	NSCLC
CEA	NSCLC, SCLC
MUC-1	NSCLC, SCLC

CEA, carcinoembryonic antigen; NSCLC, non–small cell lung cancer (may include histologies such as squamous cell and adenocarcinoma); SCLC, small cell lung cancer.

Oncogenes of the *ras* family are the most frequently expressed oncogenes in human cancers, including lung cancer. Ras proteins that are involved in malignant transformation often differ from the normally expressed gene products by a single amino acid substitution. Studies have demonstrated that CTLs can be generated that recognize an epitope (containing a single amino acid substitution) on tumor cells that express mutated-activated *ras*, resulting in tumor protection in vivo (Fenton and Longo, 1997). Yet another tumor-specific antigen derived from a mutation in the normal protein and resulting in a single amino acid substitution is that of β-catenin (Robbins et al, 1996). This candidate TAA, a cell adhesion protein, was cloned from melanoma cells using TILs generated in vitro from a surgically resected melanoma. Similarly, mutations in the tumor suppressor p53 have been identified in an increasing number of human cancers, making it the leading shared TAA discovered for human malignancies to date (Levine et al, 1991). The single amino acid substitutions that account for the increased immunogenicity of "mutated" p53 come with the same caution as that discussed earlier for mutated Ras proteins, that is, a limited number of potential targets for immunotherapy. However, a more recent study demonstrated that CTL immunity can be directed against nonmutated or "normal" epitopes in the p53 protein, suggesting that tolerance can be broken against p53, making it a more viable shared candidate TAA (Vierboom et al, 1997). Moreover, immunologic reactivity to normal p53, as well as other normal self TAAs to be discussed later, in the absence of apparent autoimmune-related pathology, expands the list of potential TAAs beyond that of foreign or tumor specific/unique to include normal tissue differentiation antigens.

Antigens Cloned from Melanoma

The majority of TAAs discovered thus far for human cancers have been cloned from malignant melanoma.

The melanoma antigens can be divided into two main categories. One group includes the MAGE, BAGE, and GAGE gene family of TAAs expressed on melanomas and a variety of other tumors, including lung cancers, but not on normal cells (the exceptions are the testes) (Boon and van der Bruggen, 1996); the other group comprises normal melanocyte differentiation or lineage antigens (involved in skin pigmentation), which include tyrosinase, MART-1, gp100, and tyrosinase-related protein-1 (TRP-1) (Rosenberg, 1997). Several tumor antigens from each of the groups are currently being evaluated in clinical trials as therapeutic vaccines for melanoma (expanded on later).

Other Antigens

The mucin family of genes and carcinoembryonic antigens (CEAs) are examples of such TAAs. MUC-1 is a mucin found on malignant as well as normal ductal epithelial cells of the breast, ovary, pancreas, lung, and prostate (Wei et al, 1998; Zhang et al, 1998). These tumors express an MUC-1 that is aberrantly glycosylated compared with MUC-1 on normal tissues. The altered glycosylation renders MUC-1 immunogenic, as has been demonstrated in animal tumor models (Henderson et al, 1998). CEA is normally silent in healthy adults but is expressed on many of the same tumors as MUC-1. This dual association (Coveney et al, 1995) could lead to vaccine trials targeting CEA and MUC-1 in breast cancer patients.

CANCER VACCINES

The two-fold premise for the development of therapeutic cancer vaccines (Table 32–22) is that (1) there are differences between tumor and normal cells, differences that are manifested as abnormally expressed genes (TAAs); and that (2) there exist in patients the immune cells (CTLs) capable of discriminating between the normal and tumor cells because of TAA recognition, resulting in CTL-mediated tumor killing. It is reasonable to speculate that these conditions exist for all human tumors and for the patients who harbor the disease. With candidate TAAs in hand (for a limited number of cancers) and empirical evidence that antigen-specific tumor-killing CTLs exist in cancer patients, the challenge for investigators is to use the TAAs to elicit therapeutic immune responses in patients. However, in order to expand the study of cancer vaccines beyond tumors such as melanoma, investigators are faced with an additional challenge—to develop methods for identifying TAAs in the more common cancers, including cancers of the lung.

TABLE 32–22 ■ Tumor Vaccine Strategies

Vaccine Source	*Vaccine Design*
Cell-based	Whole tumor cells (modified with cytokine genes) DC-pulsed with peptide, protein, mRNA, or transduced with recombinant retrovirus
Protein-based	HSPs Recombinant protein in adjuvant
Peptide-based	T cell epitopes in adjuvant B cell epitopes in adjuvant
Plasmid DNA	Naked plasmid DNA DNA-coated particles (ballistic*)
Viral vectors	Recombinant vaccinia, other pox viruses Recombinant adenovirus Recombinant AAV

**Gene Gun.*
AAV, adeno-associated virus (AAV is a less immunogenic vector); DC, dendritic cell; HSP, heat-shock protein.

Whole Tumor Cells

As was alluded to earlier for the immunotherapy of lung cancer, trials with inactivated whole tumor cells administered as vaccines have been at best disappointing. It has been surmised that the reason for the ineffectiveness of whole tumor cell vaccines in humans is the lack of co-stimulatory molecules on tumor cells, or the lack of secretion of the cytokines necessary for activating professional APCs (e.g., dendritic cells). To this end, tumor cells have been modified to express co-stimulatory molecules like B7.1 or cytokines such as GM-CSF, TNF, IFN, or one of several interleukins (Jaffee et al, 1995). Animal studies have demonstrated that immunization with GM-CSF–secreting inactivated tumor cells resulted in increased antitumor immunity in vivo (Dranoff et al, 1993). Data such as these have led to the recent evaluation of GM-CSF–modified tumor cells as vaccines for several human cancers, including renal cell carcinoma.

Proteins or Peptides

Purified protein vaccines against cancer have primarily consisted of artificially engineered tumors with model antigens in murine tumor systems, for example, solid tumors expressing ovalbumin (OVA) (Young and Inaba, 1996) or the bacterial enzyme beta-galactosidase (β-gal) (Wang et al, 1995). Although these TAAs are completely artificial and the tumor models are irrelevant to real-life cancers, the information gained through these studies has been and will continue to prove invaluable to the field of cancer vaccine development. Recombinant viral proteins (e.g., SV40 Tag and HPV) have also been tested as protein vaccines in animal tumor models (Ji et al, 1998; Shearer et al, 1993). Information gathered from these studies may be directly applied to human cancers with the corresponding viral association (see earlier section, Viral Proteins).

Synthetic peptide epitopes from cloned tumor antigens would be valuable for clinical trials for the following reasons: (1) Peptides that are stable and free of contaminating substances can be easily produced in large quantities with minimal cost; (2) Such peptide(s) could be used to stimulate and expand CTLs from patients ex vivo for therapeutic transfer back to the same patient; and (3) These anticancer CTL-inducing peptides could be developed as vaccines to be delivered parenterally for therapeutic treatment of cancer. A striking example is a recent clinical trial involving melanoma-derived TAA peptides as a therapeutic vaccine administered to patients with advanced metastatic disease. Peptide immunization resulted in a higher percentage of clinical responses (including complete responses) in patients than has previously been seen for any other therapy for melanoma (Rosenberg et al, 1998). Investigators are hopeful that peptide vaccine studies currently under way will demonstrate the power and potential of therapeutic peptide–based vaccines for the treatment of cancer.

Nucleic Acids and Recombinant Viruses

Advances in recombinant DNA technology have ushered in some novel and exciting approaches for anticancer vaccine development, namely nucleic acid vaccination (Xiang et al, 1997). Injection of plasmid DNA–encoding TAAs has been successful in inducing tumor immunity in animal models when administered either ballistically as DNA-coated gold particles (Irvine et al, 1996) or as "naked" DNA in saline (Bright et al, 1996).

Viruses have long been known to be potent inducers of CTL-mediated immunity (Irvine and Restifo, 1995). Efforts to deliver TAAs as vaccines with the greatest potential for CTL induction have employed recombinant viruses. Some examples include recombinant adenoviruses that express murine homologs to human melanoma antigens (Zhai et al, 1996) and recombinant pox viruses, including vaccinia, canary pox, or modified vaccinia viruses (MVAs). Recombinant vaccinia viruses expressing model tumor antigens not only have been successful at inducing protective immunity to tumor challenge, but also have been successful in treating established tumors in mice (Bronte et al, 1995; Xie et al, 1999).

Heat-Shock Proteins

Srivastava and Udono (1994) have demonstrated that heat-shock proteins (HSPs) chaperone peptides from the cytosol of tumor cells to the endoplasmic reticulum, thereby playing an active role in the process of antigen presentation. Moreover, purified heat-shock proteins (bearing peptides from intracellularly digested TAAs) effectively serve as vaccines against the tumor from which they were purified. These studies have led to trials involving the extraction of HSPs from tumors resected from patients followed by therapeutic immunization with the purified HSPs.

Dendritic Cells

Dendritic cells (DCs) are the most potent of antigen-presenting cells, expressing both MHC-I and MHC-II molecules, as well as a full complement of co-stimulatory molecules (Steinman, 1991); DCs have been a recent focus of experimental cell-based cancer vaccines. Briefly, DC-based tumor vaccines include DCs pulsed with recombinant protein TAAs, synthetic peptides (Porgador and Gilboa, 1995) or mRNA-encoding TAAs (Boczkowski et al, 1996), DCs transduced with retroviruses expressing TAAs (Specht et al, 1997), and DCs fused to tumor cells, thus forming a DC–tumor hybrid cell vaccine (Wang et al, 1998).

CONCLUDING COMMENTS

The overall rise in cancer incidence (Fig. 32–16), coupled with a high mortality rate for many forms of cancer, necessitates the need for alternative therapies for treatment and prevention. Immunotherapeutic strategies for cancer treatment represent attractive alternatives to standard protocols for the following reasons: (1) The immune system has the ability to recognize changes as small as a single amino acid in a complex protein, as well as to distinguish "normal self" from "nonself" or "diseased self," thereby eliminating the overwhelming and sometimes fatally toxic side effects associated with most of the available conventional therapies; (2) The immune system is by nature systemic, that is, the cells and products of an immune response possess the ability to reach tissue sites harboring microscopic metastatic deposits of tumor cells not detectable or resectable using standard procedures. In this capacity immunotherapy holds great promise in the near future as a follow-up therapy for surgical resection of primary tumors; and (3) Possibly the most powerful hallmark of the immune system is its unique ability to mount an amnestic response. This attribute has made possible, through vaccination, the eradication of deadly viral diseases such as polio and smallpox.

It is evident that a single, shared TAA that could be applied against cancer in general does not exist. It is also becoming clear that there may be multiple candidate TAAs for any one type of cancer (e.g., melanoma). Taken together, this information supports the possibility of multiple TAAs that may be clinically useful for specific tumor immunotherapy. However, it is likely that the number of candidate TAAs is finite and definable for a given type of cancer. Future clinical application may consist of early detection screening at which time a tissue specimen could be examined for expression (molecular biology techniques, perhaps microchip arrays) of any one or more of the defined TAAs for that type of cancer. The patient could then be treated with a vaccine (made up of TAAs

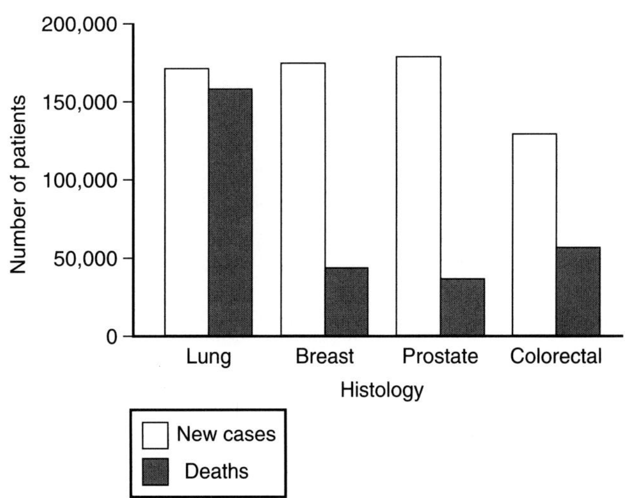

FIGURE 32–16 ■ Cancer Statistics, United States, 1999. Overall cancer incidence and mortality for the four most prevalent primary cancer histologies. (Adapted from http://www.cancer.org/statistics/cff99.)

expressed by the tumor) at a time point at which tumor burden (minimal, perhaps following resection of primary lesion) and immune status of the patient would not undermine the efficacy of the therapy and the subsequent response.

COMMENTS AND CONTROVERSIES

For the past 30 years, scientists and clinicians have attempted to deploy biologic therapies in conjunction with surgery in the management of non–small cell lung cancer. As well, in small cell lung cancer, adjuvant biologic therapies together with chemotherapy have been investigated. As yet, in lung cancer, no biologic therapy has proven efficacious other than one recent report of an adjuvant treatment following complete response in the management of small cell lung cancer. However, much has been learned. For the first time, in the past decade, there is a scientific basis for using biologic therapies, altering the host immunocompetence, and directing therapies toward the cancer cell by applying information gathered about the genetic alterations within the various malignant cells. It is highly unlikely that this type of therapy will provide a "magic bullet." However, it is hoped that in the future, biologic treatment as a coadjuvant will lead to the breakthrough required for an effective result.

R.J.G.

REFERENCES

Al-Moundhri M, O'Brien M, Souberbielle BE: Immunotherapy of lung cancer. Br J Cancer 78:282, 1998.

Bersagel DJ, Finegold MJ, Butel JS et al: DNA sequences similar to those of simian virus 40 in ependymomas and choroid plexus tumors of childhood. N Engl J Med 326:988, 1992.

Boczkowski D, Nair SK, Snyder D et al: Dendritic cells pulsed with RNA are potent antigen-presenting cells in vitro and in vivo. J Exp Med 184:465, 1996.

Boon T, Cerottini J-C, Van den Eynde B et al: Tumor antigens recognized by T lymphocytes. Annu Rev Immunol 12:337, 1994.

Boon T, van der Bruggen P: Human tumor antigens recognized by T lymphocytes. J Exp Med 183:725, 1996.

Bright RK, Beames B, Shearer MH et al: Protection against a lethal tumor challenge with SV40-transformed cells by the direct injection of DNA-encoding SV40 large tumor antigen. Cancer Res 56:1126, 1996.

Bright RK, Shearer MH, Kennedy RC: Immunization of BALB/c mice with recombinant SV40 large tumor antigen induces antibody-dependent cell-mediated cytotoxicity (ADCC) against SV40 transformed cells: An antibody based mechanism for tumor immunity. J Immunol 153:2064, 1994.

Bright RK, Shearer MH, Pass HI et al: Immunotherapy of SV40-induced tumors in mice: A model for vaccine development. Dev Biol Stand 94:341, 1998.

Bronte V, Tsung K, Rao JB et al: IL-2 enhances the function of recombinant poxvirus-based vaccines in the treatment of established pulmonary metastases. J Immunol 154:5282, 1995.

Burnet FM: Immunologic surveillance in neoplasia. Transplant Rev 7:3, 1971.

Carbone M, Pass HI, Rizzo P et al: Simian virus 40-like DNA sequences in human pleural mesothelioma. Oncogene 9:1781, 1994.

Chang AE, Aruga A, Cameron MJ et al: Adoptive immunotherapy with vaccine-primed lymph node cells secondarily activated with anti-CD3 and IL-2. J Clin Oncol 15:796, 1997.

Coley WB: The treatment of malignant tumors by repeated inoculums of erysipelas. Am J Med Sci 105:487, 1893.

Coveney EC, Geraghty JG, Sherry F et al: The clinical value of CEA and CA15-3 in breast cancer management. Int J Biol Markers 10:35, 1995.

Crowley NJ, Slingluff CL, Darrow TL, Seigler HF: Generation of human autologous melanoma-specific cytotoxic T-cells using HLA matched allogeneic melanomas. Cancer Res 50:492, 1990.

Davis MM, Boniface JJ, Reich Z et al: Ligand recognition by $\alpha\beta$ T cell receptors. Annu Rev Immunol 16:523, 1998.

Dranoff G, Jaffee E, Lazenby A et al: Vaccination with irradiated tumor cells engineered to secrete murine granulocyte-macrophage colony-stimulating factor stimulates potent, specific, and long-lasting anti-tumor immunity. Proc Natl Acad Sci 90:3539, 1993.

Feltkamp MCW, Smits HL, Vierboom MPM et al: Vaccination with a cytotoxic T lymphocyte-containing peptide protects against a tumor induced by human papillomavirus type 16-transformed cells. Eur J Immunol 23:2242, 1993.

Fenton RG, Longo DL: Danger versus tolerance: Paradigms for future studies of tumor-specific cytotoxic T lymphocytes. J Natl Cancer Inst 89:272, 1997.

Foley EJ: Antigenic properties of methylcholanthrene-induced tumors in mice of the strain of origin. Cancer Res 13:835, 1953.

Gabrilovich D, Kavanaugh D, Ishida T et al: Induction of p53/ras specific cellular immunity in patients with common solid tumors. Lung 18:90, 1997.

Goldenberg DM: New developments in monoclonal antibodies for cancer detection and therapy. CA Cancer J Clin 44:43, 1994.

Goodman GE, Hellstrom I, Yelton D et al: Phase I trial of chimeric monoclonal antibody L6 in patients with non small cell lung, colon, and breast cancer. Cancer Immunol Immunother 36:267, 1993.

Greenberg PD: Adoptive T cell therapy of tumors: Mechanisms operative in the recognition and elimination of tumor cells. Adv Immunol 49:281, 1990.

Henderson RA, Konitsky WM, Barratt-Boyes SM et al: Retroviral expression of MUC-1 human tumor antigen with intact repeat structure and capacity to elicit immunity in vivo. J Immunother 21:247, 1998.

Herin M, Lemoine C, Weynants P et al: Production of stable cytolytic T-cell clones directed against autologous human melanoma. Int J Cancer 39:390, 1987.

Hollinshead A, Stewart TH, Takita H et al: Adjuvant specific active lung cancer immunotherapy trials. Tumor-associated antigens. Cancer 60:1249, 1987.

Husler MR, Kotopoulis KA, Sundberg JP et al: Lactation-induced WAP-SV40 Tag transgene expression in C57BL/6J mice leads to mammary carcinoma. Transgenic Res 7:253, 1998.

Irvine KR, Rao JB, Rosenberg SA et al: Cytokine enhancement of DNA immunization leads to effective treatment of established pulmonary metastases. J Immunol 156:238, 1996.

Irvine KR, Restifo NP: The next wave of recombinant and synthetic anticancer vaccines. Semin Cancer Biol 6:337, 1995.

Jaffee EM, Hurwitz, Pardoll DM: Gene modification of tumors. In DeVita VT, Hellman S, Rosenberg SA (eds): Biological Therapy of Cancer. 2nd ed. Philadelphia, JB Lippincott, 1995, p 774.

Ji H, Chang EY, Lin KY et al: Antigen-specific immunotherapy for murine lung metastatic tumors expressing human papillomavirus type 16 E7 oncoprotein. Int J Cancer 78:41, 1998.

Kahn M, Sugawara H, Mcgowan P et al: CD4+ T cell clones specific for the human p97 melanoma-associated antigen can eradicate pulmonary metastases from a murine tumor expressing the p97 antigen. J Immunol 146:3235, 1991.

Kappler JW, Roehm N, Marrack P: T cell tolerance by clonal elimination in the thymus. Cell 49:273, 1987.

Kast WM, Offringa R, Peters PJ et al: Eradication of adenovirus E1-induced tumors by E1a-specific cytotoxic T lymphocytes. Cell 59:603, 1989.

Kimura H, Yamaguchi Y: Adjuvant immunotherapy with interleukin-2 and lymphokine-activated killer cells after noncurative resection of primary lung cancer. Lung Cancer 13:31, 1995.

Klein G, Sjogren HO, Klein E, Hellstrom KE: Demonstration of resistance against methylcholanthrene-induced sarcomas in the primary autochthonous host. Cancer Res 20:1561, 1960.

Kovacsovics-Bankowski M, Clark K, Benacerraf B, Rock KL: Efficient major histocompatibility class I presentation of exogenous antigen upon phagocytosis by macrophages. Proc Natl Acad Sci 90:4942, 1993.

Krolick KA, Uhr JW, Slavin S, Vitetta ES: In vivo therapy of a murine B cell tumor BCL1 using antibody-ricin A chain immunotoxins. J Exp Med 155:1797, 1982.

Le Bon A, Desaymard C, Papiernik M: Neonatal impaired response to viral superantigen encoded by MMTV(SW) and Mtv-7. Int Immunol 12:1897, 1995.

Levine AJ, Momand J, Finlay CA: The p53 tumour suppressor gene. Nature 351:453, 1991.

Linehan DC, Goedegebuure PS, Peoples GE et al: Tumor-specific and HLA-A2-restricted cytolysis by tumor-associated lymphocytes in human metastatic breast cancer. J Immunol 155:4486, 1995.

Ludewig B, Odermatt B, Landmann S et al: Dendritic cells induce autoimmune diabetes and maintain disease via de novo formation of local lymphoid tissue. J Exp Med 188:1493, 1998.

Lynch TJ: Immunotoxin therapy of small cell lung cancer: N901 blocked ricin for relapsed small cell lung cancer. Chest 103:436s, 1993.

Melief CJ, Offringa R, Toes RE, Kast WM: Peptide-based cancer vaccines. Curr Opin Immunol 8:651, 1996.

Melief CJM, Kast WM: T-cell immunotherapy of tumors by adoptive transfer of cytotoxic T lymphocytes and by vaccination with minimal essential epitopes. Immunol Rev 146:167, 1995.

Morgan DJ, Kreuwel HTC, Fleck S et al: Activation of low avidity CTL specific for a self epitope results in tumor rejection but not autoimmunity. J Immunol 160:643, 1998.

Mossman TR, Coffman RL: Th1 and Th2 cells: Different patterns of lymphokine secretion lead to different functional properties. Annu Rev Immunol 7:145, 1989.

O'Brien MER, Bromelow K, Prendiville J et al: A study of SRL 172 (*Mycobacterium vaccae*) as the first component of a tumour vaccine with immunological changes and clinical activity in patients with lung cancer. Lung 18:163, 1997.

Pai L, Batra J, Fitzgerald D: Antitumor activities of immunotoxin made of mab B3 and various forms of pseudomonas exotoxin. Proc Natl Acad Sci 88:3358, 1991.

Parkhurst MR, Salgaller ML, Southwood S et al: Improved induction of melanoma-reactive CTL with peptides from the melanoma antigen gp100 modified at HLA-A*0201-binding residues. J Immunol 157:2539, 1996.

Pass HI, Kennedy RC, Carbone M: Evidence for and implications of SV40-like sequences in human mesotheliomas. In DeVita V, Hellman S, Rosenberg SA (eds): Important Advances in Oncology. Philadelphia, Lippincott-Raven, 1996.

Porgador A, Gilboa E: Bone marrow-generated dendritic cells pulsed with a class I-restricted peptide are potent inducers of cytotoxic T lymphocytes. J Exp Med 182:255, 1995.

Prehn RT, Main JM: Immunity to methylcholanthrene-induced sarcomas. J Natl Cancer Inst 18:769, 1957.

Resnick RM, Cornelissen MT, Wright DK et al: Detection and typing of human papillomavirus in archival cervical cancer specimens by DNA amplification with consensus primers. J Natl Cancer Inst 82:1477, 1990.

Roa JB, Chamberlain RS, Bronte V et al: IL-12 is an effective adjuvant to recombinant vaccinia virus-based tumor vaccines. J Immunol 156:3357, 1996.

Robbins PF, El-Gamil M, Li YF et al: A mutated beta-catenin gene encodes a melanoma-specific antigen recognized by tumor infiltrating lymphocytes. J Exp Med 183:1185, 1996.

Rosenberg SA: The development of new cancer therapies based on the molecular identification of cancer regression antigens. Cancer J Sci Am 2:90, 1995.

Rosenberg SA: Cancer vaccines based on the identification of genes encoding cancer regression antigens. Immunol Today 18:175, 1997.

Rosenberg SA, Lotze MT, Muul LM et al: Observations on the systemic administration of autologous lymphokine-activated killer cells and recombinant interleukin-2 to patients with metastatic cancer. N Engl J Med 313:1485, 1985.

Rosenberg SA, Yang JC, Schwartzentruber DJ et al: Immunologic and therapeutic evaluation of a synthetic peptide vaccine for the treatment of patients with metastatic melanoma. Nat Med 4:269, 1998.

Rosenberg SA, Yannelli JR, Yang JC et al: Treatment of patients with metastatic melanoma using autologous tumor-infiltrating lymphocytes and interleukin-2. J Natl Cancer Inst 86:1159, 1994.

Rous P: An experimental comparison of transplanted tumor and a transplanted normal tissue capable of growth. J Exp Med 12:344, 1910.

Rudden RW: Tumor immunology: Immunologic approaches to the diagnosis and treatment of cancer. In Rudden RW (ed): Cancer Biology, 3rd ed. New York, Oxford University Press, 1995, p 442.

Salgaller ML, Afshar A, Marincola FM et al: Recognition of multiple epitopes in the human melanoma antigen gp 100 by peripheral blood lymphocytes stimulated in vitro with synthetic peptides. Cancer Res 55:4972, 1995.

Schwartz RH: A cell culture model for T lymphocyte clonal anergy. Science 248:1349, 1990.

Schwartz RH: Costimulation of T lymphocytes: The role of CD28, CTLA-4, and B7/BB1 in interleukin-2 production and immunotherapy. Cell 71:1065, 1992.

Shearer MH, Bright RK, Lanford RE, Kennedy RC: Immunization of mice with baculovirus-derived recombinant SV40 large tumor antigen induces protective tumor immunity to a lethal challenge with SV40-transformed cells. Clin Exp Immunol 91:266, 1993.

Shu SS, Plautz GE, Krauss JC, Chang AE: Tumor immunology. JAMA 278:1972, 1997.

Slingluff CL, Darrow TL, Seigler HF: Melanoma-specific cytotoxic T cells generated from peripheral blood lymphocytes. Ann Surg 210:194, 1989.

Specht JM, Wang G, Do MT et al: Dendritic cells retrovirally transduced with a model antigen gene are therapeutically effective against established pulmonary metastases. J Exp Med 186:1213, 1997.

Srivastava PK, Udono H: Heat shock protein-peptide complexes in cancer immunotherapy. Curr Opin Immunol 6:728, 1994.

Steinman RM: The dendritic cell system and its role in immunogenicity. Annu Rev Immunol 9:271, 1991.

Stevens EJ, Jacknin L, Robbins PF et al: Generation of tumor-specific CTLs from melanoma patients by using peripheral blood stimulated with allogeneic melanoma tumor cell lines. J Immunol 154:762, 1995.

Thatcher N, Sambrook RJ, Stephens RJ: First results of a randomized trial of dose intensification with G-CSF in small cell lung cancer. Lung 18:7, 1997.

Topalian SL, Gonzales MI, Parkhurst M et al: Melanoma-specific CD4+ T cells recognize nonmutated HLA-DR-restricted tyrosinase epitopes. J Exp Med 183:1965, 1996.

Topalian SL, Muul LM, Solomon D et al: Expansion of human tumor infiltrating lymphocytes for use in immunotherapy trials. J Immunol Methods 102:127, 1987.

Townsend SE, Allison JP: Tumor rejection after direct costimulation of CD8+ T cells by B7-transfected melanoma cells. Science 259:368, 1993.

Vierboom MPM, Nijman HW, Offringa R et al: Tumor eradication by wild-type p53-specific cytotoxic T lymphocytes. J Exp Med 186:695, 1997.

Wakimoto H, Abe J, Tsunoda R et al: Intensified antitumor immunity by a cancer vaccine that produces granulocyte-macrophage colony-stimulating factor plus interleukin-4. Cancer Res 56:1828, 1996.

Wallich R, Bulbuc N, Hammerling GJ et al: Abrogation of metastatic properties of tumor cells by de novo expression H-2^k antigens following *H-2* gene transfection. Nature 315:301, 1985.

Wang J, Saffold S, Cao X et al: Eliciting T cell immunity against poorly immunogenic tumors by immunization with dendritic cell-tumor fusion vaccines. J Immunol 161:5516, 1998.

Wang M, Bronte V, Chen PW et al: Active immunotherapy of cancer with a non-replicating recombinant fowlpox virus encoding a model tumor-associated antigen. J Immunol 154:4685, 1995.

Wei WZ, Pauley R, Lichlyter D et al: Neoplastic progression of breast epithelial cells: A molecular analysis. Br J Cancer 78:198, 1998.

Xiang ZQ, Pasquini S, He Z et al: Genetic vaccines: A revolution in vaccinology? Springer Semin Immunopathol 19:257, 1997.

Xie YC, Hwang C, Overwijk W et al: Induction of tumor antigen-specific immunity in vivo by a novel vaccinia vector encoding safety-modified simian virus 40 T antigen. J Natl Cancer Inst 91:169, 1999.

Yoshizawa H, Chang AE, Shu S: Specific adoptive immunotherapy mediated by tumor-draining lymph node cells sequentially activated with anti-CD3 and IL-2. J Immunol 147:729, 1991.

Young JW, Inaba K: Dendritic cells as adjuvants for class I major histocompatibility complex-restricted antitumor immunity. J Exp Med 183:7, 1996.

Zhai Y, Zang JC, Kawakami Y et al: Development and characterization of recombinant adenoviruses encoding MART1 or gp100 for cancer therapy. J Immunol 156:700, 1996.

Zhang S, Zhang HS, Cordon-Cardo C et al: Selection of tumor antigens as targets for immune attack using immunohistochemistry: Protein antigens. Clin Cancer Res 4:2669, 1998.

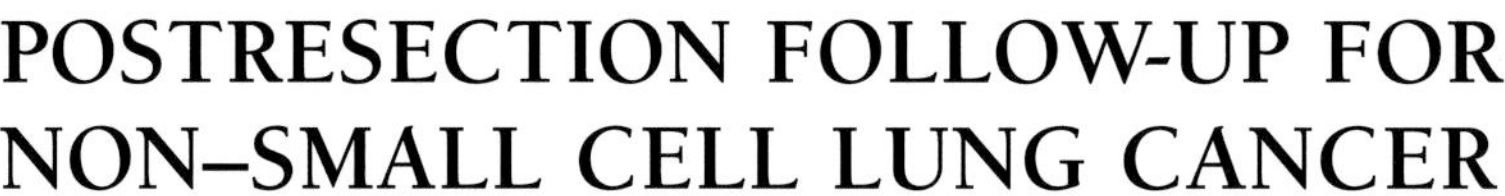

POSTRESECTION FOLLOW-UP FOR NON–SMALL CELL LUNG CANCER

Joe B. Putnam, Jr.

The need for postresection follow-up and improved postresection screening for recurrence is evident in the limited survival found after primary treatment of primary non–small cell lung carcinoma (NSCLC). Lung cancer is a significant public health problem in the United States and the world.

Despite optimal resection, 5-year survival for stage I NSCLC is approximately 57% to 80%, and for stage II disease, 45% (Martini et al, 1993; Mountain, 1997; Naruke et al, 1988; Nesbitt et al, 1995). In patients with mediastinal (N2) lymph node metastasis (stage IIIA), the 5-year survival may be only 20% even with aggressive treatment (Table 32–23).

Although local and systemic interventions may improve survival after primary therapy in these patients, additional survival advantage from treatment of recurrent disease or from treatment of a second primary is less clear (Pisters et al, 2000). Molecular changes that predispose to the development of lung cancer may provide strategies for chemoprevention or other treatments directed at genetic alterations in the cancer itself. Currently, numerous prospective protocols are ongoing in an attempt to better understand and evaluate various combinations of multidisciplinary treatments.

Postresection follow-up of a thoracic malignancy requires a careful balance of clinical examination, diagnostic imaging examination, and cost effectiveness. After resection for early-stage lung cancer, second lung cancers develop at a rate of about 2% to 5% per year (Johnson, 1998; Johnson et al, 1997). The clinician must evaluate those factors that will provide for the patient and the health care system an advantage, in health and cost, for those services provided. For that reason, multiple scans to identify early recurrence or metastasis may not be consistently effective and may yield false-positive examinations requiring further costly evaluation or surgical intervention. The optimal postresection follow-up protocol has not been defined, and this is complicated by other medical and social needs of the patient and the patient's family. A balance of specialty care from the thoracic surgeon and general medical care by the patient's regular physician appears to optimize the specific needs of the patient following resection of lung cancer.

Postresection follow-up of the patient begins in the immediate postoperative period with the patient's normal convalescence from surgery. The in-hospital recovery phase, including the first 30 days after surgery, is usually considered the early follow-up period from which surgical morbidity and mortality (defined as ≦30 days after resection, or >30 days if the patient has been continuously in hospital) are calculated. Routine follow-up usually begins about 1 month after discharge (approximately 5 to 6 weeks after the date of surgery). New symptoms or sequelae of early events related to the operation, or those noted during the in-hospital convalescence, are evaluated and treated. Typically, the first postresection follow-up visit includes an interim history, a physical examination, and a baseline chest roentgenogram (posteroanterior and lateral). This chapter discusses the various options available to the physician and the patient for postresection follow-up after resection of thoracic malignancy, and the value of such follow-up.

TABLE 32–23 ■ Postresection Survival in Patients with Primary Non–Small Cell Lung Cancer

TNM	*Mountain, 1997*		*Naruke, 1988*	
Subset	*N*	*% 5-Year Survival*	*N*	*% 5-Year Survival*
T1N0M0	511	67	245	75.5
T2N0M0	549	57	241	57.0
T1N1M0	76	55	66	52.5
T2N1M0	288	39	153	40.0
T2N0M0	87	38	106	33.3
T3N1M0	55	25	85	39.0
Any N2M0	344	23	368	15.1

TNM, tumor necrosis metastasis.

THE NEED FOR POSTRESECTION FOLLOW-UP

Postresection follow-up not only benefits the patient but assists the thoracic surgeon in evaluating the benefits as well as the disadvantages of a particular operation. With follow-up, the surgeon can determine the value of a specific operation and evaluate the need for changes or modifications in the operation. This process of continuous self-education and improvement (by the thoracic surgeon's personal evaluation of his or her patients) is critical to the specialty of thoracic surgery and thoracic surgical oncology. Although larger multi-institutional studies may be required to prove the advantage of one operation over another, for the individual surgeon, close follow-up provides immediate feedback on the relative value of specific operations. For example, resection for lung cancer should consist of anatomic resections such as lobectomy and mediastinal lymph node dissection. The value of lobectomy over a more limited resection (wedge resection or segmentectomy) was shown by a prospective study performed by the Lung Cancer Study Group, which evaluated lobectomy or limited resection with mediastinal lymph node dissection in patients with stage T1N0 lung cancer. Patients with lesser resections tended to have a greater number of local recurrences (which were not second primary cancers), more second primary cancers (P = .079), more frequent local-regional metastases, and a trend (P = .094) toward increased likelihood of death from cancer. The study validated the concept of lobectomy as the procedure of choice in patients with lung cancer (Ginsberg and Rubinstein, 1995).

Frequently, tumors occur in the lung after resection of primary lung cancer. This recurrence may be a second primary lung cancer, a local recurrence, or metastatic disease to the lung. In the presence of limited disease, a physiologically fit patient, and a clinical stage I or II tumor, resection may be considered. If it is detected early, these patients may be subsequently cured of their recurrent lung cancer.

The location of recurrent disease may be modified by radiation therapy or surgery techniques. Recurrence patterns may vary depending on the treatment provided. In the North American Intergroup Trial 3590, postoperative adjuvant therapy was given to patients with completely resected stages II and IIIA NSCLC. The patients had concomitant adjuvant therapy with four cycles of cisplatin plus radiotherapy over radiotherapy alone. Sites of intrathoracic recurrences were similar in both groups: 42% in the combination arm and 49% in the radiotherapy arm.

Second Primary Lung Cancer

After curative (R0) resection with pathologically negative margins and no involved lymph nodes, a new lesion in the lung may well represent a second primary, which may occur at any time in the patient's postresection course. Generally, when the same histology occurs within a 2-year period, this is classified as a metastasis. Still, resection is frequently offered to these patients, as a second primary tumor cannot be absolutely excluded. When doubt exists, the benefit is given to the patient, and the patient is treated for the most favorable stage of the disease, that is, early-stage second primary lung cancer. Histologic diagnosis and appropriate clinical staging are critical in the planning of subsequent treatment.

Second primary tumors have been defined as (1) a different histologic cell type, (2) a tumor-free interval of 24 months, and (3) location in the contralateral lung, or a new tumor in a separate and distinct ipsilateral lobe for tumors within the same thorax. In a study from Memorial Sloan-Kettering, 118 patients who had survived 10 or more years were reviewed. Second primary lung cancers developed in 16% (19/118) of patients between 6 and 22 years after resection. Thirteen of these had a different histology (Temeck et al, 1984). The results of treatment of these tumors were recently reviewed. This study evaluated second thoracotomy in 114 patients with second primary tumors of the lung. Eighteen patients underwent thoracotomy for a third primary lung cancer. Of 132 thoracotomies, a conservative resection was emphasized to minimize postoperative complications reflected in the 73 sequential resections performed. Operative mortality was 8.8% (10/114) for second primary tumors and 5.5% for those undergoing a third resection. Cumulative survival rates for 114 patients with metachronous tumors were 33% at 5 years and 20% at 10 years. The authors recommend early detection and resection as a means of enhancing survival (Faber, 1993).

ROUTINE FOLLOW-UP: AN EVOLVING PROCESS

The thoracic surgeon requires a simple, consistent, and cost-effective method of evaluating the patient. Various outcomes must be identified and catalogued. Although the patient's regular physician can conduct routine health care, the thoracic surgeon's knowledge of various oncologic and physiologic variables after resection and the myriad presentation of normal and abnormal events are critical to the patient's health and well-being.

Each follow-up visit should include discussion with the patient as to his or her general health, and whether problems exist. Follow-up to these questions by the discerning physician may elicit symptoms of early local or regional recurrence, or potentially, the presence of metastatic disease. The patient may also describe other problems related to the surgery, or other new medical problems. These problems should be evaluated further by the surgeon and communicated appropriately to the patient's primary or referring physician. The signs and symptoms of local recurrence are shown in Table 32–24.

Evaluation of the patient's physical condition includes a physical examination, with note taken of changes in weight and changes in performance status. The history should include the onset or persistence of specific symptoms, and the presence or occurrence of late events.

TABLE 32–24 ■ **Signs and Symptoms of Local Recurrence**

Chest pain—localized or pleuritic	Pleural effusion
Thoracic rib or vertebral/back pain	Phrenic nerve paralysis
Cough	Superior vena caval obstruction
Hoarseness	Weight loss
Horner's syndrome	Anorexia
Dysphagia	Fatigue
	Decreased performance status

Other evaluation for a new primary tumor, or for recurrent disease, typically includes a screening chest roentgenogram that should be reviewed by the surgeon. Often the surgeon has clinical information, personally obtained, that may not be available to the radiologist interpreting the films.

Most commonly, patients have stopped smoking over the months following the re-resection of a thoracic neoplasm. If not, aids to this smoking cessation, including smoking cessation clinics and counseling, biofeedback, nicotine patches, nicotine gum, pharmaceuticals, and physician counseling, should be offered.

Symptoms of local recurrence are shown in Table 32–24. Nonspecific symptoms such as anorexia, malaise, fatigue, and weight loss may occur in up to 70% of patients. Paraneoplastic syndromes are distant manifestations of lung cancer (not metastases) as revealed in extrathoracic nonmetastatic symptoms (Table 32–25). Lung cancer affects these extrathoracic sites by producing one or more biologic or biochemical substances. These various effects are grouped into paraneoplastic syndromes.

PHYSICAL EXAMINATION AND ROUTINE RADIOGRAPHIC STUDIES

Physical Examination

A limited physical examination with specific attention to the cervical and supraclavicular nodal beds may demonstrate the presence of metastatic disease in these lymph nodes. Additional examination of the surgical wound for healing or local recurrence, as well as those areas influenced or changed by the operation, should also be performed.

Chest Radiography

The standard chest radiograph and computed tomography of the chest and upper abdomen (including the adrenals) are the most frequent diagnostic imaging studies performed in patients with lung cancer. Routinely, a plain chest radiograph is obtained at the first postoperative visit and at every visit thereafter. The purpose of this chest radiograph is to serve as a baseline for future changes within the chest. With the plain posteroanterior and lateral chest roentgenogram ("chest x-ray"), the surgeon can evaluate the postoperative appearance and can assess for local, regional, or metastatic disease. After the first visit, chest radiographs are reviewed as serial films in time order (e.g., 1999, 2000, 2001, etc.). This serial comparison may enable detection of subtle changes that may be evident only after review of two or three sequential chest radiographs; however, the abnormality may not be identified within the most recent films. If abnormalities are identified, the patient may require further evaluation directed by the patient's history, physical examination, signs and symptoms, or other findings.

TABLE 32–25 ■ **Manifestations of Extrathoracic Paraneoplastic Syndromes**

General
Fatigue
Malaise
Other constitutional symptoms
Endocrine
Cushing's syndrome
Inappropriate antidiuretic hormone secretion (hyponatremia)
Carcinoid syndrome
Hypercalcemia
Hypoglycemia
Skeletal
Clubbing
Hypertrophic pulmonary osteoarthropathy
Neuromuscular (more common with small cell lung carcinoma)
Polymyositis
Eaton-Lambert syndrome (myasthenia-like syndrome)
Peripheral neuropathy
Subacute cerebellar degeneration
Encephalopathy
Vascular
Vascular thrombophlebitis
Thrombosis

SCREENING STUDIES

Serial Computed Tomography of the Chest

The value of routine screening studies beyond chest radiography is not known, but they do not appear to be helpful, nor do they contribute to the patient's overall care. False-positives are occasionally found and may be a source of significant anxiety to the patient and to the family. Still, various screening studies are being developed in an attempt to identify recurrent disease that may be more effectively treated, with improved survival.

Investigations of other screening modalities for patients at high risk for lung cancer may be of even greater benefit for patients after resection of lung cancer. Initial favorable reports on computed tomographic (CT) screening for patients at high risk for lung cancer have suggested a significant cost benefit associated with CT screening in patients at high risk for lung cancer. Patients with previous lung cancer are at the most increased risk for developing a second lung cancer. Use of screening CT in patients following pulmonary resection of lung cancer may be effective in identifying recurrences at an earlier (and potentially curable) stage of disease, but this requires further study.

Spiral CT scanning is a technique that allows a low-resolution image of the entire thorax to be obtained during a single breath-holding with low radiation exposure. Various centers throughout the world are now involved in evaluating large numbers of patients with screening CT scans. The purpose of screening CT scans is to increase the frequency of curable lung cancer. A criticism of screening CT scans is that small benign nodules are identified with increasing frequency. These observations may result in increased numbers of surgical procedures for benign disease, increased cost of care, and as well, complications as a result of this care. Patients involved in such a screening program following curative therapy should continue to be evaluated by traditional methods for comparison purposes to assess the value of these studies for improved survival, reduced recurrence rate, and improved health.

An evaluation of 1500 patients with no prior diagnosis of lung cancer but at high risk (>50 years of age, smoking history of 20 or more pack-years, and no prior cancer within the last 5 years [except skin, localized prostate cancer, or cervical carcinoma in situ]) is being conducted by physicians at the Mayo Clinic. They are evaluating the possibility of detecting 75% or more of lung cancers while they are at stage I (Henschke et al, 1999; Henschke and Yankelevitz, 2000).

Sputum Cytology

In the absence of smoking, most patients do not produce sputum. In the postresection follow-up period with the absence of spontaneous sputum production or hemoptysis, induced sputum cytologies are frequently negative and are not cost efficient.

Sputum cytology may yield a diagnosis if the patient is a poor operative risk or has symptoms suggestive of cancer, or if a transthoracic needle biopsy may cause increased risk. A fine-needle aspiration via a transthoracic route (FNA) may be approximately 95% accurate in patients with a poor operative risk, or it may be used to obtain a biopsy prior to definitive therapy. Screening of patients at high risk of lung cancer by sputum cytology does not consistently provide a sensitive examination for the presence of small resectable lung cancer.

METASTATIC DISEASE FROM PRIMARY LUNG CANCER

Metastatic disease is common after curative resection of lung cancer and may occur in up to two thirds of patients (Martini et al, 1993). Most patients with recurrent or metastatic disease have symptoms; only a minority are identified with asymptomatic recurrence. Even fewer patients with asymptomatic recurrence have isolated localized recurrence amenable to resection. Criteria for nonresectability are presented in Table 32–26.

If neurologic problems, jaundice, or other suspected signs or symptoms of metastatic disease are present, the patient should be screened for the presence of metastatic disease in all areas. Typically, this screening consists of bone scan, computed tomography of the abdomen and the chest, and a computed tomographic evaluation or a magnetic resonance image of the brain. More recently, these scans have been suggested as a means of postresection follow-up for individuals having prior radiation therapy, or those in whom an infectious process or other process cannot be completely excluded.

Surgical resection of metastasis from lung cancer generally is a curiosity, although many patients with resectable brain metastases do quite well. After excision, patients with a solitary brain metastasis may have up to 15% 5-year survival (Burt et al, 1992).

TABLE 32–26 ■ General Criteria for Nonresectability

Recurrent laryngeal nerve paralysis
Superior vena cava syndrome
Involvement of main pulmonary artery
Contralateral or supraclavicular node involvement
Ipsilateral mediastinal nodes if high (2R)
Malignant (or bloody) pleural effusion
Malignant pericardial effusion
Phrenic nerve paralysis (relative contraindication)
Extrathoracic metastatic disease typically involving the brain, bone, adrenals, or liver
Involvement of trachea, heart, great vessel
Insufficient pulmonary reserve
Tracheoesophageal fistula
Other signs may suggest a more advanced tumor:
- Chest wall pain
- Horner's syndrome
  - Compression of the splanchnic nerve with unilateral ptosis, miosis, anhidrosis, and enophthalmos
- Phrenic nerve paralysis
- Esophageal compression with dysphagia from extrinsic compression from enlarged subcarinal lymph nodes

TABLE 32–27 ■ Surveillance for Non–Small Cell Lung Cancer After Resection

Stage I and II
- Postoperative visits every 6 months for 2 years, then annually. CXR annually

Stage III
- History and physical examination, CXR, and laboratory tests every 3 months for 2 years, then every 6 months for 3 years, and then annually. CXR with each visit

Stage IV (not on treatment or in-home hospice)
- History and physical examinations, CXR, CBC, and other tests as clinically indicated every 2–3 months

*The postresection follow-up guidelines as suggested by The University of Texas M.D. Anderson Cancer Center (Houston) for non–small cell lung cancer

CBC, complete blood count; CXR, chest radiograph.

POSTRESECTION FOLLOW-UP GUIDELINES

In general, the routine visits to the thoracic surgeon should be straightforward, simple, and consistent. The postresection follow-up guidelines suggested by the University of Texas M.D. Anderson Cancer Center are shown in Table 32–27.

The frequency of the postoperative follow-up depends on the extent of the resection, and whether the resection was complete or incomplete. An incomplete resection may be defined as R1 (microscopic) or R2 (gross tumor). If all identifiable disease, including lymph nodes, is completely resected, then the extent of resection may be defined as complete (R0). An incomplete resection leaves a positive margin, which predisposes to earlier local, or local-regional, recurrence. These patients may have received adjuvant therapy to decrease local or local-regional recurrence, to prevent worsening systemic metastasis, or to improve quality of life.

Follow-up for early-stage lung cancer (stages I and II) includes a history, a limited regional physical examination, and screening chest radiography (after baseline) every 6 months for 2 years, then yearly thereafter. For later stage lung cancer that has been resected, these patients are often on a clinical protocol that prescribes the required follow-up period—usually every 3 or 4 months with a chest radiograph and blood work for the first 2 years, every 6 months for the next 3 years, and every year thereafter. These recommendations have been incorporated into the guidelines of care for patients with lung cancer as published by the University of Texas M.D. Anderson Cancer Center (see Table 32–27).

A recent comparison was made between postresection follow-up guidelines developed by the National Comprehensive Cancer Network (NCCN) and those developed by the American Society of Clinical Oncology (ASCO) (Winn et al, 1999). The premise of the author's paper was that guidelines would be reproducible if "two groups of experts, presented with the same evidence and methods, derive a similar set of recommendations." The authors point out that current medical knowledge is incomplete and cannot provide the hard data on which to base recommendations. The role of expert opinion may be to fill the gap where hard evidence is not available. Combinations of medical care, clinical need, patient demands, medical-legal responsibilities, general health care issues, family concerns, and cost effectiveness must all be weighed during the physician's care of the patient. A mathematical model complex enough to solve this multivariable equation would require data from a large number of patients, objectively defined, prospectively collected, and analyzed in a valid manner. Unfortunately, these data do not exist. Therefore, comparison of guidelines may be considered an appropriate alternative.

The National Comprehensive Cancer Network recommended monitoring, including a history and physical examination every 4 months for the first 2 years, and then every 6 months for the next 3 years. A chest radiograph would be obtained at each visit during this period generally, and annual chest radiographs would be obtained thereafter. This panel did not recommend any additional scans. The American Society of Clinical Oncology panel recommended a history and physical examination every 3 months for the first 2 years, and then every 6 months for the next 3 years. A chest radiograph was recommended on an annual basis. The guidelines proposed by ASCO recommended fewer chest radiographs. Neither group recommended screening computed tomography of chest or abdomen, nor MRI brain imaging, as part of the surveillance program.

EVALUATION OF EFFECTIVENESS OF POSTOPERATIVE FOLLOW-UP

Guidelines for the appropriate follow-up of lung cancer patients after surgery have been proposed; however, few studies exist in which the value of this follow-up has been evaluated.

In a retrospective study of 358 patients undergoing complete resection of lung cancer, recurrence, secondary primary, and survival were studied (Walsh et al, 1995). Median follow-up was 76 months. The authors found that recurrences developed in 135 patients—local only in 32, distant only in 90, and local and distant in 13. Most patients (n = 102) were symptomatic, and only 33 were asymptomatic. New primary tumors developed in 35 patients. Asymptomatic diagnosis was most commonly made by chest radiography. Ninety-five patients were treated palliatively, and only 40 were treated with curative intent with radiation or surgery. Surprisingly, median survival from time of recurrence was 8 months for symptomatic patients and 16 months for asymptomatic patients. Multivariate analysis revealed that longer disease-free interval (greater than 12 months) was the most favorable predictor of survival. The authors concluded that although a lead-time bias was noted, survival was not significantly affected by early detection of lung cancer. In addition, the authors concluded that frequent follow-up and radiologic evaluations may be unnecessary.

Problems with this study include the retrospective nature of the analysis and the exclusion of patients with incomplete resection, superior sulcus tumors, mixed tumor histology, or follow-up outside of the home institution. A role for screening for second primary tumors (either aerodigestive tract or other) in patients with completely resected early-stage disease was suggested. Thirty-five patients developed 36 new malignancies. About half of these patients had aerodigestive tract cancers. Of all patients in the study, 80 of 358 patients had additional primary malignancies either before or after the index pulmonary resection for cancer. Physical examination detected a recurrence in only 2 of 33 asymptomatic patients. The charge associated with curative treatment was $1256/month, compared with $859/month for palliative care. Median survival was 27.7 months for patients treated with curative intent and 18.3 months for patients treated with palliative intent (P = .03). This study suggests that follow-up of patients with pulmonary resection may not be a cost-effective clinical practice given the end points of survival and identification of recurrent disease; still, other outcomes of care were not measured. In addition, the financial impact of identification and management of new or concurrent medical problems, the improvement in our understanding of the biology of lung cancer or the effectiveness of certain treatments, and the evaluation of the effectiveness of specific operations cannot be quantified.

A nonrandomized comparison of intensive versus symptom-related follow-up in patients with NSCLC did not identify a significant difference in median survival after diagnosis of recurrent disease (7.9 months vs 6.6 months, respectively) (Younes et al, 1999).

MOLECULAR PREDICTORS OF RECURRENCE AND SURVIVAL

No generally accepted blood study or molecular characteristic is being routinely used to diagnose a patient's recurrent tumor or metastasis, although various serum and molecular characteristics exist that are negatively associated with survival. Postresection survival may be modified by specific molecular characteristics of the patient's individual tumor. Although clinical stage and lymph node status are strong predictors of survival, other clinical and cancer-related factors are associated with poorer stage-for-stage outcome; these include male gender, weight loss, decreased performance status, and increased age. Adenocarcinoma tends to have a poorer survival than squamous cell carcinoma.

Molecular alterations in lung cancer include increased expression of specific oncogenes (upregulation of *myc, ras, c-erb,* and *BCL-2*) and decreased expression of specific tumor suppressor genes (downregulation of *p53,* RB, etc.). Kwiatkowski evaluated 244 resected stage I tumors and noted that predictors of diminished (poor) cancer-free survival included age older than 60, male gender, limited resection of lung (wedge resection), large tumor size (>4 cm), adenocarcinoma with mucin subtype, lymphatic invasion, *k-ras* mutation, *p53* expression, and lack of h-ras expression (Kwiatkowski et al, 1998). D'Amico and associates (1999) evaluated 408 early (stage I) lung cancers with immunohistochemical staining of 10 common molecular markers. Markers associated with increased risk of recurrence and death include *p53* (associated with apoptosis), factor VIII (angiogenesis), erb-b2 (growth regulation), CD-44 (adhesion), and radiation bronchitis (cell cycle regulation). In other studies evaluating stage I lung cancer tumors from patients with histologically negative lymph nodes, early relapse and decreased survival could be predicted by immunostaining techniques for p53 protein (Dobashi et al, 1997) and for cytokeratin (Maruyama et al, 1997). Molecular assays may be more advantageous and more sensitive than immunostaining techniques in predicting postresection survival or recurrence. Molecular techniques to evaluate p53 mutations, k-ras mutations, p16 methylation, and microsatellite markers in tumor cells were found in 53% of patients who underwent bronchoalveolar lavage at the time of surgical resection. Sputum cytology is not a sensitive test for occult lung cancer; however, DNA biomarkers may indicate premalignant changes (Ahrendt et al, 1999; Belinsky et al, 1998; Sozzi et al, 1998; Wistuba et al, 1997).

SUMMARY

Follow-up after resection for lung cancer should be directed toward identifying those patients with recurrent disease in the earliest stage possible, in the most cost-efficient manner possible. The techniques of low-dose spiral computed tomography of the chest and molecular markers either in primary lung cancer or in sputum cytology specimens may prove to be more efficient and sensitive means of identifying recurrent lung cancer than the more traditional methods of history (symptoms), physical examination, and chest radiography. Although some studies have failed to demonstrate an objective improvement in survival with clinical follow-up by retrospective analysis, prospective confirmation of this finding has not been confirmed nor attempted, and may be medically inappropriate. Techniques identified by population screening in patients without prior history of lung cancer may provide clues that enable us to more efficiently identify patients at high risk of recurrence after resection of lung cancer.

Follow-up of patients after resection of lung cancer requires a simple, consistent clinical protocol to optimize the health of the patient. Improvements in survival as a result of improved primary therapy are required to lessen the need for postoperative follow-up. Improved survival will result from better understanding of the molecular events leading to lung cancer and modulation of those events. Until then, routine clinical follow-up of the lung cancer patient and evaluation of new screening techniques for those patients at increased risk of recurrence will be required to optimize survival and decrease recurrence.

COMMENTS AND CONTROVERSIES

Dr. Putnam reviews in detail the reasons for postresection follow-up, its limitations and the arguments suggesting it has no practical value either for the care of the patient or economically. One of the most important aspects of postresection follow-up is that it enables the surgeon to evaluate his treatment strategies over the long term. Any surgeon who simply performs the pulmonary resection and never follows the patient cannot learn from his successes or errors.

Whether or not postresection follow-up benefits the patient is very questionable, at least in retrospective studies that have addressed this question. A recent analysis suggests that follow-up by family physicians is less expensive than that performed by thoracic surgeons and, for economic reasons, patients should be offered this type of follow-up. Despite all the uncertainties, on occasion, second primary tumors are discovered early and solitary sites of metastases are aggressively treated with beneficial results for the patient because of the follow-up performed by the thoracic surgeon. How to quantitate this is unclear.

With regard to spiral CT screening for follow-up of surgically resected lung cancer patients, an ACOSOG trial is planned to evaluate this. At the moment, the standard recommendation remains chest radiography only.

R.J.G.

REFERENCES

Ahrendt SA, Chow JT, Xu LH et al: Molecular detection of tumor cells in bronchoalveolar lavage fluid from patients with early stage lung cancer (see comments). J Natl Cancer Inst 91:332, 1999.

Belinsky SA, Nikula KJ, Palmisano WA et al: Aberrant methylation of p16(INK4a) is an early event in lung cancer and a potential biomarker for early diagnosis. Proc Natl Acad Sci USA 95:11891, 1998.

Burt M, Wronski M, Arbit E, Galicich JH: Resection of brain metastases from non-small-cell lung carcinoma. Results of therapy. J Thorac Cardiovasc Surg 103:399, 1992.

D'Amico TA, Masse M, Herndon JE et al: A biological risk model for stage I lung cancer: Immunohistochemical analysis of 408 patients with the use of ten molecular markers. J Thorac Cardiovasc Surg 117:736, 1999.

Dobashi K, Sugio K, Osaki T et al: Micrometastatic p53-positive cells in the lymph nodes of non-small cell lung cancer: Prognostic significance. J Thorac Cardiovasc Surg 114:339, 1997.

Faber LP: Resection for second and third primary lung cancer. Semin Surg Oncol 9:135, 1993.

Ginsberg RJ, Rubinstein LV: Randomized trial of lobectomy versus limited resection for T1 N0 non-small cell lung cancer. Lung Cancer Study Group. Ann Thorac Surg 60:615, discussion 622, 1995.

Henschke CI, McCauley DI, Yankelevitz DF et al: Early Lung Cancer Action Project: Overall design and findings from baseline screening. Lancet 354:99, 1999.

Henschke CI, Yankelevitz DF: Screening for lung cancer. J Thorac Imaging 15:21, 2000.

Johnson BE: Second lung cancers in patients after treatment for an initial lung cancer. J Natl Cancer Inst 90:1335, 1998.

Johnson BE, Cortazar P, Chuste JP: Second lung cancers in patients successfully treated for lung cancer. Semin Oncol 24:492, 1997.

Kwiatkowski DJ, Harpole DH, Godleski J, et al: Molecular pathological substaging in 244 stage I non-small cell lung cancer patients: Clinical implications. J Clin Oncol 16:2468, 1998.

Landis SH, Murray T, Bolden S, Wingo PA: Cancer statistics, 1999 CA Cancer J Clin 49:8, 1999.

Martini N, Bains MS, Burt ME et al: Incidence of local recurrence and second primary tumors in resected stage I lung cancer. J Thorac Cardiovasc Surg 109:120, 1995.

Martini N, Kris MG, Flehinger BJ et al: Preoperative chemotherapy for stage IIIa (N2) lung cancer: The Sloan-Kettering experience with 136 patients. Ann Thorac Surg 55:1365, 1993.

Maruyama R, Sugio K, Mitsudomi T et al: Relationship between early recurrence and micrometastases in lymph nodes of patients with stage I non-small cell lung cancer. J Thorac Cardiovasc Surg 114:535, 1997.

Mountain CF: Revisions in the International System for Staging Lung Cancer. Chest 111:1710, 1997.

Naruke T, Tomoyuki G, Tsuchiya R, Suemasu K: Prognosis and survival in resected lung carcinoma based on the new international staging system. J Thorac Cardiovasc Surg 96:440, 1988.

Nesbitt JC, Putnam JBJ, Walsh GL: Survival in early-stage non-small cell lung cancer. Ann Thorac Surg 60:466, 1995.

Patz EFJ, Lowe VJ, Hoffman JM et al: Persistent or recurrent bronchogenic carcinoma: Detection with PET and 2-F-[18]-2-deoxy-D-glucose. Radiology 191:379, 1994.

Pisters KM, Ginsberg RJ, Giroux DJ et al, on behalf of the Bimodality Lung Oncology Team (BLOT): Induction chemotherapy before surgery for early-stage lung cancer: A novel approach. J Thorac Cardiovasc Surg 119:429, 2000.

Sozzi G, Pastorino U, Moiraghi L et al: Loss of FHIT function in lung cancer and preinvasive bronchial lesions. Cancer Res 58:5032, 1998.

Temeck BK, Flehinger BJ, Martini N: A retrospective analysis of 10 year survivors from carcinoma of the lung. Cancer 53:1405, 1984.

Walsh GL, O'Connor M, Willis KM et al: Is follow-up of lung cancer patients after resection medically indicated and cost-effective? Ann Thorac Surg 60:1563, 1995.

Winn RJ, Brown NH, Botnick WZ: A comparison of the NCCN and ASCO lung cancer guidelines. Oncology (Huntingt) 13:35, 1999.

Wistuba II, Lam S, Behrens C et al: Molecular damage in the bronchial epithelium of current and former smokers. J Natl Cancer Inst 89:1366, 1997.

Younes RN, Gross JL, Deheinzelin D:. Follow-up in lung cancer: How often and for what purpose. Chest 115:1494, 1999.

CHAPTER **33**

Small Cell Lung Cancer

Ronald Feld

Robert J. Ginsberg

Small cell lung cancer once included oat cell and intermediate cell types. The term *intermediate cell*, however, has been abandoned. With the advent of immunohistochemical staining, many pathologists now include this latter group with large cell neuroendocrine carcinomas. Not all pathologists agree that these two lesions are identical. When the true clinical behavior of large cell neuroendocrine tumors is identified, all of these tumors may be called neuroendocrine carcinomas, small and large cell variants. The clinical courses of these variants (small and large cell neuroendocrine tumors) may not be identical, and their responses to chemotherapy may not be similar. However, perhaps these two tumors should be considered identical with regard to treatment. In the past, most reports dealing with small cell lung cancer (SCLC) included the intermediate cell variant that is now often included in the large cell neuroendocrine category. The most confusing issue is that many pathologists identify another subgroup of large cell carcinomas that have neuroendocrine features. These tumors, unlike neuroendocrine large cell carcinomas, have features that are suggestive of neuroendocrine carcinoma but they do not stain appropriately with neuroendocrine markers and are not considered in this discussion.

HISTORICAL NOTE

Although chemotherapy is the major form of therapy in SCLC and is discussed in detail, it is often useful to review how therapy evolved to its present approach. Initially, surgery was the therapy of choice for patients with all types of lung cancer, but it was abandoned in patients with SCLC after the results of a randomized trial done in the United Kingdom by the Medical Research Council, which compared radiotherapy alone with surgery alone in patients with limited disease (Fox et al, 1973; Miller et al, 1969). Even though the mean survival time for all these patients was short (10 months), with only 5% of patients alive at 5 years, the fact that all surviving patients were being treated in the radiation therapy arm made this the standard form of therapy thenceforth.

Green and colleagues (1969) demonstrated the activity of cyclophosphamide against SCLC compared with placebo. In this study, the median survival time for patients with extensive disease who were receiving placebo was about 6 weeks, and for patients with limited disease, it was only 12 weeks. These data must be remembered perspectively when observing the modest improvements in the treatment of this disease during the 1970s, 1980s, and early 1990s.

Many single agents have been tested in patients with SCLC and have given response rates of 20% or more (Feld et al, 1988). A review of all studies from 1970 to 1990 identified 11 active drugs (Grant et al, 1992). Newer agents were found to be active, adding more drugs to earlier lists. When active drugs were combined, an improved response rate was observed, with complete response rates ranging from 20% to 50% and rising even higher in patients with limited disease (Minna et al, 1989). Retrospective reviews of the median survival times of patients who were treated with either single agents or combination chemotherapy showed that those receiving combinations survived longer. Randomized trials comparing single agents with combination chemotherapy with or without chest irradiation have demonstrated a benefit for the combinations.

Bergsagel and associates (1972) showed that the addition of cyclophosphamide to standard thoracic irradiation in patients with limited disease resulted in a survival benefit. This was confirmed by others and led to the use of combined modality therapy in the early 1970s (Smyth, 1984). Thoracic irradiation is added to combination chemotherapy in patients with limited disease, but it is not usually given to patients with extensive disease. Some groups add thoracic irradiation in patients with extensive disease who achieve a complete response.

When a large number of patients had relapses in the central nervous system (CNS), prophylactic cranial irradiation (PCI) was tested in randomized trials and showed a reduced failure rate in the brain without a survival advantage (Feld et al, 1988). Subsequently, it became routine to add PCI for all patients with SCLC, regardless of the stage. In the 1980s, signs of neurologic toxicity that was associated with either the radiation therapy or the combined treatment (radiotherapy and chemotherapy) were noted, and more stringent criteria for the use of PCI have been advocated since that time. In particular, PCI should be limited to patients who have shown a complete response because they are the most likely to benefit. In this subpopulation, the potential disadvantage of PCI, that is, CNS toxicity (not observed in all studies) (Lishner et al, 1990), is probably worth risking.

The controversial theory, based on the results of a meta-analysis of randomized trials (Arriagada et al, 1991), that thoracic irradiation adds to combination chemotherapy in patients with limited SCLC, is discussed later. Most centers treat patients who achieve a complete response, and many treat patients who achieve at least a partial response with this therapeutic modality. There are also arguments about how best to give thoracic irradiation. The issues include dose, fractionization, portal size, and the point at which the radiation therapy should be given in reference to the beginning of combination chemotherapy. These questions are discussed in more detail later.

Significant interest has also been shown in the use of surgery in this disease. Most groups recommend operating on peripheral lesions in early-stage disease (clinical stage I). These patients often receive thoracic irradiation and possibly PCI with or without chemotherapy along with their surgery. In patients with more advanced disease, the only well-designed randomized trial, which was carried out by the Lung Cancer Study Group, did not show a benefit from the addition of surgery to radiation and chemotherapy (Lad et al, 1991a). Consequently, this is not a standard approach, although some centers around the world still use it as part of their therapy in selected patients.

In general, immunotherapy (biologic response modifiers) has not shown a major benefit in this disease. One study using thymosin fraction V (Cohen et al, 1979) showed a survival benefit, but this was not confirmed (Shank et al, 1983). A later study by Mattson and colleagues (1991) from Finland suggested a benefit to maintenance therapy with interferon-α in patients who responded to standard therapeutic modalities. Cooperative groups in the United States have attempted to confirm this information, but the final analysis of these data is not yet available. This form of therapy should not be considered standard. Tumor vaccines are under investigation.

■ *HISTORICAL READINGS*

Albain KS, Crowley JJ, LeBlanc M et al: Determinants of improved outcome in small-cell lung cancer: An analysis of the 2,580-patient Southwest Oncology Group data base. J Clin Oncol 8:1563, 1990.

Arriagada R, Pignon JP, LeChevalier TL: Thoracic radiotherapy in small cell lung cancer: Rationale for timing and fractionation. Lung Cancer 5:237, 1989.

Campling B, Quirt IC, DeBoer G et al: Is bone marrow examination in small-cell lung cancer really necessary? Ann Intern Med 105:508, 1986.

Carney DN: The biology of lung cancer. Curr Opin Oncol 4:292, 1992.

Crawford J, Ozer H, Stoller R et al: Reduction by granulocyte colony stimulating factor of fever and neutropenia induced by chemotherapy in patients with small-cell lung cancer. N Engl J Med 325:164, 1991.

Ettinger DS: Evaluation of new drugs in untreated patients with small-cell lung cancer: Its time has come. J Clin Oncol 8:390, 1990.

Feld K: Late complications associated with the treatment of small cell lung cancer. Cancer Treat Res 45:301, 1989.

Fukuoka M, Furuse K, Saijo N et al: Randomized trial of cyclophosphamide, doxorubicin and vincristine versus cisplatin and etoposide versus alternation of these regimens in small cell lung cancer. J Natl Cancer Inst 83:855, 1991.

STAGING

Staging plays a key role in the choice of therapeutic modalities for the treatment of SCLC. Although chemotherapy is the main therapeutic modality used in SCLC, thoracic irradiation or surgery may also be valuable, depending on the stage of the tumor before therapy. The most important reason for staging, however, is its potential effect on prognosis.

Less advanced cases of SCLC have better long-term survival rates than have more advanced cases. In non–small cell lung cancer (non-SCLC), tumor–node–metastasis (TNM) staging with the older International Union Against Cancer–American Joint Committee on Cancer classification (Mountain, 1986) has been routinely used and has been replaced by the new 1997 version of the staging system (Mountain, 1997), but TNM staging has not been found to be the most useful approach for staging in patients with SCLC. Most patients with this disease have stage III or IV disease at the time of diagnosis, making the TNM staging system less likely to be predictive of long-term survival.

Most therapeutic trials in the treatment of SCLC have involved a very simple two-stage system, as originally suggested by the Veterans Administration Lung Cancer Study Group. This divides patients into those with limited and those with extensive disease. Limited disease is defined as a tumor that is confined to one hemithorax and its regional lymph nodes, including the ipsilateral mediastinal, ipsilateral supraclavicular, and contralateral hilar nodes, and it should all be easily encompassed within a tolerable radiotherapy portal (Zelen, 1973). Ipsilateral pleural effusions, left laryngeal nerve involvement, and superior vena caval obstruction are considered limited; pericardial involvement and bilateral pulmonary involvement are considered to be extensive because they would require too large a radiotherapy portal.

Some confusion occurs when considering how to stage patients with contralateral mediastinal or supraclavicular lymph node metastases and patients with ipsilateral pleural effusions. Investigators often handle these differently. A consensus report prepared at the International Association for the Study of Lung Cancer Workshop on SCLC in 1989 suggested that limited disease should include patients with disease that is restricted to one hemithorax with regional lymph node metastases (including hilar, ipsilateral, and contralateral mediastinal, ipsilateral, and contralateral supraclavicular nodes) and with ipsilateral pleural effusions whether cytologic findings are positive or negative (Stahel et al, 1989). The inclusion of contralateral mediastinal and supraclavicular metastases and ipsilateral pleural metastases in limited disease is recommended because the prognosis of patients with these sites of disease (which includes ipsilateral pleural effusions) is superior to that of patients with distant sites of metastases.

One other variation in staging among investigators results because of the number and type of staging procedures used. If one investigator carries out more exhaustive staging than does another, a higher yield of patients with extensive disease results, but, surprisingly, the outcome in both groups of patients (limited and extensive disease) improves, not affecting the overall survival. This has usually been *stage migration,* or the *Will Rogers phenomenon* (Pfister et al, 1990). Although it is virtually impossible to correct for this effect, the clinician must be aware of its possibility when unusually good results are reported.

The two-stage system generally separates patients with different outcomes well. Those with limited disease have a higher objective regression rate, a higher complete response rate, and significantly longer disease-free and long-term survival rates compared with patients who have extensive disease. Patients who achieve complete response in either stage do relatively well. Table 33–1 lists staging procedures for patients not involved in clinical trials.

The Toronto group has identified a subgroup called *very limited disease*. This arose during a retrospective study of 180 patients with limited disease in which the 33 patients without mediastinal involvement, supraclavicular node involvement, or pleural effusions had a projected 25% 5-year survival rate (Shepherd et al, 1984).

Subgroups may also be important for patients with extensive disease. Patients with single sites of extensive disease have longer survival times than do patients with multiple sites of metastases and are not dissimilar from those with limited disease (Ihde et al, 1981). Patients with specific sites of involvement, including the liver and brain, do particularly poorly (Ihde, 1985). In most series, the outcome for 50% to 65% of patients who turn out to have extensive disease is to some degree dependent on how exhaustive the staging is at a particular center. The staging procedures that are most appropriate and necessary for patients who are not being treated in clinical trials are shown in Table 33–1. Excessive staging procedures in this setting can be a burden for individual patients and can also unnecessarily increase the cost of medical care. More exhaustive staging is probably indicated only in clinical trials, as shown later. These stages are similar to those that were noted in a review on the staging of patients with SCLC (Stahel, 1991). Another study suggests that a simpler approach to staging may be as good and cheaper (Richardson et al, 1991). This requires confirmation.

TABLE 33–1 ■ **Staging Procedures for Patients with Small Cell Lung Cancer**

Patients Not in a Clinical Trial
Complete physical examination
Chest radiograph, thorax and upper abdominal computed tomography scan
Routine hematologic tests (complete blood count, differential, and platelet count)
Liver function tests
Lactate dehydrogenase level
Alkaline phosphatase level (for bony metastases)
Serum electrolyte concentration (looking for low sodium)
Ultrasonography or abdominal computed tomography scan (for liver and adrenals)
Radionuclide bone scan
Skeletal radiographic examinations if bone scan not definite
Brain computed tomography scan or magnetic resonance imaging study (if symptoms)
Patients Being Treated in Clinical Trials
Computed tomography scan of thorax (for mediastinum and measurement of primary lesion)
Ultrasonography or computed tomography scan of abdomen (for liver and adrenals)
Liver biopsy (by peritoneoscopy or possibly with ultrasound guidance)
Routine computed tomography scans of brain (possibly magnetic resonance imaging)
Fiberoptic bronchoscopy
Mediastinoscopy (rarely necessary)
Neuron-specific enolase (serum and possibly cerebrospinal fluid)
Serum arginine vasopressin level
Lumbar puncture for cytologic examination

Areas of Controversy

Intrathoracic Tumors

Although chest radiographs are useful for the evaluation of disease in the lungs, chest wall, and mediastinum, they may still underestimate the extent of disease in these sites. Computed tomography (CT) scanning of the thorax may be more accurate in detecting tumors within the lung itself, and it is useful for radiation therapy planning, although it probably adds little to the evaluation of the mediastinum, unless the chest radiograph findings are negative (Hirsch, 1989; Lewis et al, 1990). Enlarged nodes in the mediastinum may not be indicative of tumor and may mislead the investigator into raising the stage of the patient being evaluated. CT scans of the thorax are often extended to include the abdomen, which, of course, may help in defining metastases in the liver or the adrenal glands.

Abnormalities in the adrenal glands are not uncommon, but available data have not clearly established that patients with abnormalities (metastases or adenoma) at this site have a worse outcome than do patients with limited disease. Magnetic resonance imaging (MRI) has not shown a benefit over CT scanning in patients with SCLC or non-SCLC (Hirsch, 1989). Fiberoptic bronchoscopy is not necessarily beneficial unless surgery is being contemplated. A baseline may be useful if re-evaluation is to be considered after a possible response to therapy (Stahel, 1991). Positron emission tomography (PET) scanning, although already used in some centers in patients with non-SCLC, has not yet been shown to be beneficial in patients with SCLC. This may change with the greater availability of this technology worldwide.

Hepatic Metastases

Hepatic metastases are common in patients with SCLC. Liver function tests alone are not useful unless the results are completely normal, in which case there is rarely evidence for a tumor at this site (Hirsch, 1989). Ultrasound or CT scanning of the liver usually is the preferred approach because both these techniques may also detect adrenal metastases. Some investigators also recommend an ultrasound-guided needle biopsy. With its potential morbidity, the use of peritoneoscopy to prove involvement of the liver is probably unnecessary in most patients (Table 33–2).

Bone Marrow

During clinical trials, it was customary to do bone marrow aspirates and biopsies in patients with SCLC. Usually, single iliac crest aspirations and biopsies are carried out, but in some series, this has been done bilaterally. Even more sophisticated techniques increase the likelihood of

TABLE 33–2 ■ Established Active Single Agents in the Treatment of Small Cell Lung Cancer

Agents	*Approximate Single-Agent Activity (%)*
Carmustine	20
Carboplatin*	40
Lomustine	15
Cisplatin*	15
Cyclophosphamide*	40
Doxorubicin*	30
Epirubicin (high dose)	50
Etoposide intravenous*	40–50
Etoposide oral*	50
Hexamethylmelamine	30
Ifosfamide	40–50
Methotrexate	35
Nitrogen mustard	35
Teniposide	40–50
Vincristine*	35
Vindesine	30

*Agents most commonly used today.

finding bone marrow involvement by the tumor, for example, using specific monoclonal antibodies (Berendsen et al, 1988; Stahel et al, 1985). The latter approach may be important for the screening of patients who are being considered for potential autologous bone marrow transplantation along with intensive chemotherapy, but it is probably less important for patients who are not undergoing this type of aggressive therapy. Even MRI has been used, with early data suggesting it may be more sensitive (Carney et al, 1989).

A more controversial issue is whether bone marrow involvement should be sought. Some studies have found few patients with metastases at this site (less than 10%); even less commonly, it is the only site that classifies the patient as having extensive disease and therefore potentially changes the prognosis (Campling et al, 1986; Hirsch, 1989). Some investigators found that lactate dehydrogenase (LDH) might also give similar information without a relatively uncomfortable invasive procedure (Hirsch, 1989; Sagman et al, 1991a). This is still controversial, but most centers have abandoned doing bone marrow aspirate and biopsies.

Central Nervous System Metastases

CNS metastases may be detected clinically in approximately 10% of patients with SCLC but are found at autopsy in up to 65% (Hirsch, 1989; Klastersky, 1990). The standard investigation for this site has been CT scanning, although MRI is probably superior to CT, as it is for most brain abnormalities. The role of PET scans is as yet unknown (Klastersky, 1990). Carcinomatous meningitis is a rare presenting feature of this disease. When symptoms occur, a sample of cerebrospinal fluid is used to demonstrate malignant cells, usually by cytocentrifugation (Feld et al, 1988). Nodular filling defects along the root sleeves may be seen by myelography or with MRI of the cord when the spinal cord is compressed.

Biomarkers

Many biomarkers have been studied in SCLC, and they are usually measured before, during, and after treatment. Corticotropin-releasing hormone, calcitonin, neuron-specific enolase, plasma neurophysins, and antidiuretic hormone have not been clearly useful prognosticators in these patients (Feld et al, 1988; Hansen, 1990). Pretreatment carcinoembryonic antigen levels correlate with the stage of the disease and may actually constitute an independent prognostic factor (Sculier et al, 1985). The disadvantage of depending on these levels is that the antigen concentration is only elevated in about one third of patients, thereby making it a less valuable indicator. Pretreatment LDH levels may provide a useful prognostic factor, based on a number of older publications (Albain et al, 1990; Rawson and Peto, 1990; Sagman et al, 1991a; Stahel, 1992), but these levels continue to be important in this disease (Sagman et al, 1997).

Several groups have reported that rising levels of biomarkers sometimes precede clinical evidence of tumor relapse by weeks or months (Biran et al, 1991; Feld et al, 1988). Good therapy is usually unavailable for relapses of this disease; therefore, the value of an early knowledge about the relapse of these tumors is questionable. The consensus at the moment is that biomarkers are probably of little value in the pretreatment prognosis or as early evidence of relapse; however, additional research is ongoing on this subject. A relatively new biomarker is the C-terminal flanking peptide of human gastrin-releasing peptide (Holst et al, 1989), which may indicate a worse prognosis, but again, more data are necessary.

Restaging

Restaging is a definite area of controversy. A retrospective study that was carried out by the National Cancer Institute of Canada found that routine restaging in patients with limited disease who had responded to treatment was probably of little value (Feld, 1994). Although a small survival benefit was demonstrated in a subgroup of patients who had negative, repeat bronchoscopic results compared with those patients with positive results, the investigators found that this approach should be considered only in a clinical trial. Economic analysis also supported the concept of not proceeding with restaging. Others still recommend restaging, especially with repeat bronchoscopy (Stahel et al, 1989; Stahel, 1991).

Prognostic Factors

Prognostic factors may be useful for assessing individual patients and for proper stratification in clinical trials. The factors that have been deemed important by most groups include the stage of disease (limited versus extensive), the performance status, and whether patients have received previous chemotherapy previously (Albain et al, 1990; Ihde, 1971; Rawson et al, 1990; Stahel et al, 1989; Stahel, 1991). Many other prognostic factors have been noted. Female gender has become an accepted good prognostic factor by a number of investigators (Stahel, 1992). Consensus is yet to be reached on which factors are the most important; however, the information derived from staging and prognostic factors must be carefully considered when comparing the results of therapy in published articles on clinical trials in this disease. Newer methods, such as recursive partitioning and amalgamation, may be useful, as evidenced by two recent articles (Albain et al, 1990; Sagman et al, 1991b). A simplified approach using a large database suggests that the extent of the disease, the performance status, and LDH levels may be all that are required to determine the initial prognosis in patients with SCLC (Sagman et al, 1997).

CHEMOTHERAPY

Single Agents

Chemotherapy is the mainstay of therapy for all stages of SCLC. Green and colleagues (1969) demonstrated improved survival rates in patients with extensive SCLC after three courses of cyclophosphamide compared with placebo. Since that time, many active drugs have been identified. A partial list of the most active single agents in SCLC is shown in Table 33–2. The most frequently used include etoposide, cisplatin, cyclophosphamide, doxorubicin, and vincristine. New agents that look promising include gemcitabine (Carmichael, 1998; Postmus, 1998) and paclitaxel (Ettinger et al, 1995; Zochbauer-Muller, 1999) and derivatives such as docetaxel (Taxotere) (Laetrille et al, 1996).

Single-agent chemotherapy produces objective responses but rarely complete regression, even in previously untreated patients with SCLC. Based on studies that were carried out by the National Cancer Institute of Canada and the Eastern Cooperative Oncology Group, it is ethical and appropriate to treat previously untreated patients with extensive SCLC by using an experimental agent (Ettinger, 1990; Evans et al, 1990). The evaluation should occur early if this is done, and if no response is observed, patients should be switched to an active regimen before their condition is irretrievable. This may be less of a problem when the clinician uses derivatives of known active agents, such as anthracyclines (Blackstein et al, 1990) and platinum compounds. Both previously mentioned cooperative groups have had experiences with both active and inactive agents and reasonable response and survival rates were observed, irrespective of the activity of the new drug. Treating previously treated patients may result in prematurely negative data with potentially useful drugs. One recent review suggested the use of a lower response rate (10%) as evidence of activity in previously treated patients may still be a useful approach (Grant et al, 1992).

In addition to the active agents mentioned, a large number of phase II trials have found that many agents show little or no activity (Table 33–3) in patients with SCLC (Grant et al, 1992). A recent review describes some newer data on chemotherapy in patients with SCLC (Sorensen et al, 1998).

TABLE 33–3 ■ Activity of Recently Tested Single Agents in Small Cell Lung Cancer

*Active Agents**	*Possibly Active Agents†*	*Inactive Agents‡*
Epirubicin (high dose)	Iproplatin	Mitoguazone
Carboplatin	Gemcitabine	Mitomycin C
Hexamethylmelamine	Lonidamine	Aclarubicin
Ifosfamide	Paclitaxel	Diaziquone
Vindesine		Bisantrene
Teniposide		Cytarabine
		Idarubicin
		Mitoxantrone
		Vinblastine
		PCNU
		Esorubicin

*At least 20% single-agent activity.
†10% to 20% single-agent activity.
‡<10% single-agent activity.

Combination Chemotherapy

Despite partial responses and occasional complete responses, the relatively poor results with single-agent chemotherapy led to attempts at combining these agents in patients with SCLC, as has been done with other malignancies. Just less than 20% of 753 patients given single-agent chemotherapy had an objective response, and less than 3% obtained a complete response in a study carried out by Bunn and Ihde (1981). In contrast, among 1236 patients who received combination chemotherapy, a 70% objective response rate was seen, with 31% of those responses being complete. In addition, those who received combination chemotherapy survived longer than did those who received single agents. A number of randomized trials compared single agents and combination chemotherapy, with or without chest radiotherapy, and demonstrated a slight benefit of combination chemotherapy in both objective tumor response and median survival (Minna et al, 1989). Bunn and Ihde (1981) also reviewed the literature regarding the appropriate number of drugs to be included in combinations for this disease. They found that there was no significant difference in the complete response rate nor the long-term disease-free survival rate when more than three drugs were used in patients with limited disease.

The most commonly used and highly active combinations for the treatment of SCLC worldwide are shown in Table 33–4. Of these, the most prevalent are etoposide and cisplatin, but alternating cyclophosphamide, doxorubicin (Adriamycin), plus vincristine (CAV) with etoposide plus cisplatin is still used in many centers. Although these are among the most common regimens, virtually any combination of the most active agents has been used with reasonable results. Any of these regimens should result in response rates in excess of 80% (50% to 60% complete response) in patients with limited disease and of 65% to 70% in patients with extensive disease (10% to 20% complete response) (Feld et al, 1988).

If adequate staging procedures are done, the median survival for patients with limited disease should be 15 to 18 months or more. In recent trials of combined-modality therapy, median survival times in excess of 18 to 20 months occurred (Johnson, 1990; Johnson et al, 1991; Murray et al, 1991a; Tourani et al, 1991). The median survival time for patients with extensive disease is 10

TABLE 33–4 ■ **Frequently Used Chemotherapeutic Combinations for Small Cell Lung Cancer†**

Chemotherapeutic Combination	*Possible Abbreviation*
Cyclophosphamide, Adriamycin (doxorubicin)	CA
Adriamycin (doxorubicin), etoposide (VP-16)	AE
Etoposide (VP-16), cisplatin	V_pP
Cyclophosphamide, Adriamycin (doxorubicin), vincristine, etoposide (VP-16)	CAVE
Cyclophosphamide, Adriamycin (doxorubicin), vincristine	CAV
Etoposide (VP-16), carboplatin	V_pCP
Ifosfamide, cisplatin, etoposide (VP-16)	ICE (VIP)
Cisplatin, vincristine (Oncovin), doxorubicin, etoposide	CODE

†All regimens give response rates of 70% to 90% in patients with limited disease and 55% to 75% in patients with extensive disease.

months or less, with a range of 8 to 12 months (Ihde et al, 1991; Kristjansen, 1991). Approximately 15% to 20% of patients with limited disease and less than 5% of those with extensive disease remain disease free for more than 2 years. Patients who achieve a complete response usually live longer than do those who show only a partial response, the former being the only group with the potential for long-term disease-free survival. Patients with limited disease usually live significantly longer than do those with extensive disease. Patients who have a better performance status at the time of diagnosis also have greater survival rates.

Intensity of Chemotherapy

Cohen and associates (1977), comparing low-dose intensive induction therapies consisting of cyclophosphamide, CCNU (lomustine), and methotrexate (CCM), showed that a more intensive regimen resulted in a higher response rate and a longer median survival time. In a review of nonrandomized trials by Morstyn and coworkers (1984), there was a suggestion of benefit with more intense regimens but it was a relatively minor increment. Although it was retrospective, the review did not show a major improvement in survival. In fact, the more intensive regimens often increased toxicity. An Eastern Cooperative Oncology Group study, using cyclophosphamide, methotrexate, and etoposide without dosage reductions for myelosuppression, showed results that were similar to those of other series but with increased hematologic and pulmonary toxicity (Bonomi et al, 1985).

Ihde and coworkers (1991) reported an attempt at testing both intensity and "dose intensity," as it is frequently called by the Canadian investigator Hryniuk (1987) from the Hamilton Cancer Centre. They compared the outcome in patients with either low-dose or high-dose etoposide and cisplatin and found no benefits of the high-dose regimen. They found an increase in toxicity. Attempts at using autologous bone marrow transplantation with high doses of agents such as cyclophosphamide or combinations gave results that were similar to those achieved with standard-dose combination chemotherapy (Souhami et al, 1982; Souhami, 1985b). This might be the result of the emergence of early drug-resistant clones of SCLC.

In summary, moderate-dose therapy using the available drugs is necessary to achieve a response and reasonable survival in patients with SCLC. Although there appears to be a dose-response curve for some drugs (e.g., cyclophosphamide) with this disease, the administration of high doses of the most active drugs does not appear to be beneficial. The issue of dose intensity has been addressed in a number of tumors, and to date, no prospective trials have shown a clear benefit of a more dose-intensive approach, although retrospective studies have shown a benefit with this approach (Hryniuk et al, 1987).

The merit of pharmacologic approaches with known active drugs is exemplified by the interest in the use of relatively low-dose oral etoposide on a continuous 14- or 21-day schedule with about 1 week off and then restarting this therapy. This was pioneered by Johnson and Greco (Johnson, 1990; Johnson et al, 1991), Einhorn and colleagues (1990), and Clark and associates (1990, 1991). The toxicity in previously untreated patients appears tolerable and makes this a reasonable approach in elderly patients in whom an aggressive approach with a more standard regimen is contraindicated or refused by the patient (Carney et al, 1990). In addition, there are instances of responses in patients who received previous injectable etoposide and who have either responded in the past or not responded at all. Two studies from the United Kingdom suggest that survival is worse in patients taking oral etoposide than it is in those taking the standard parenterally administered combination therapy (Girling et al, 1996; Souhami et al, 1997); therefore, it is infrequently used even in frail or elderly patients. This information suggests that we have much work to do to learn how to use the available drugs properly. In addition to looking at new agents, oral etoposide has been combined with cisplatin and carboplatin, but data do not suggest a major benefit over the oral etoposide alone by continuous daily treatment (Evans et al, 1991; Murphy et al, 1991).

One reason that intensive therapy has not been extensively studied is the severe myelosuppression that is associated with aggressive approaches to this disease. With the availability of colony-stimulating factors (granulocyte [G-CSF] and granulocyte-macrophage [GM-CSF]), studies have been done to determine whether this approach may also be useful in patients with SCLC. These studies allow greater dose escalation with possibly improved results. A landmark study in patients with extensive SCLC, which allowed Food and Drug Administration approval of G-CSF (Amgen) in the United States, compared the regimen CAE (cyclophosphamide, doxorubicin [Adriamycin], and etoposide), a seldom-used combination in the 1990s, with or without G-CSF. The biologic effects of the growth factor were documented, with a marked reduction in febrile episodes, patient days in the hospital, and granulocytopenia, and no negative effect on survival (Crawford et al, 1991). An almost identical study was carried out by a European group and reported in abstract form, showing virtually identical results (Green et al, 1991). Studies are ongoing with GM-CSF but are not yet as optimistic as the data observed with G-CSF (Anderson et al, 1991a; Bishop et al, 1991).

It is questionable whether this is an advance in the treatment of SCLC. Survival in the various studies that showed a clear biologic effect of the growth factor was not better than that achieved by far less toxic regimens that are available to all practitioners in the community. These regimens include alternating CAV with etoposide and cisplatin or just etoposide and cisplatin, among others. To establish real value for the new growth factors in this disease, studies must either (1) demonstrate a major reduction in toxicity by using a standard regimen with or without growth factors or (2) demonstrate a reduction of the likelihood of serious toxicity and an improvement in survival by comparing a dose-intensive regimen using growth factors with a non–dose-intensive regimen.

A randomized trial using G-CSF showed improved survival with increased dose intensity (Thatcher et al, 2000). Because most other studies are negative, it is difficult to decide how to interpret this apparently positive result. Confirmation of this observation is required before this approach becomes part of standard treatment. As previously mentioned, without growth factors, etoposide plus cisplatin used in a more dose-intensive way was not superior (Ihde et al, 1991). It is possible that most of the benefits of febrile episode reduction and decreased days in the hospital can be achieved by using only oral prophylactic antibiotics, such as co-trimoxazole or a fluoroquinolone antibiotic. Additional studies need to be done to address these issues; however, standard-dose regimens without growth factor still seem reasonable for community-based physicians.

Late Intensification Therapy

Based on data acquired from patients with acute leukemia, more aggressive therapy may be better tolerated when patients are in remission than when a large tumor burden is present (Thomas et al, 1979). Therapy after an initial response might include the same agents that are used for induction, or it might include totally different chemotherapy. Although a number of studies have looked at this approach in SCLC, the results are not strikingly different from those obtained in trials using conventional doses of chemotherapy along with thoracic irradiation when appropriate in patients with SCLC. A Belgian study was more optimistic (Prignot et al, 1985). Patients were randomized in this study at week 18 to receive late intensification therapy or not. The 2-year survival rate with intensification was 17% and without it, only 4%, although the overall survival from the time of randomization was not significantly improved. A review of other studies on this subject was less optimistic (Feld et al, 1988).

In many of these studies, most patients are not eligible for randomization (if patients with extensive disease are included in sufficient numbers) because they must achieve complete response to be considered for this approach. For most studies, in limited disease less than half of the patients achieved a complete response. The major difficulty with this approach may be the large tumor burden that is present in patients with SCLC, even after initial induction therapy, or it may be the relative ineffectiveness of the agents currently used, the relative unimportance of high doses of moderately active agents, and the possible infusion of tumor cells when autologous marrow is used, even when the best purging approaches are employed.

Alternating Non–Cross-Resistant Chemotherapy

Tumor resistance to chemotherapy is probably a significant cause of therapeutic failure in SCLC (Goldie and Coldman, 1984). This resistance may be present at the start of therapy or it may be acquired during it.

During the 1980s, the Goldie-Coldman hypothesis, which is an approach to early resistance, became popular. The authors proposed a mathematical model based on the hypothesis that tumor-cell kill displays a logarithmic pattern and tumors continuously develop resistant mutations during therapy. Their assumption was that alternating two combinations of non–cross-resistant drugs early in the course of therapy might decrease the development of drug-resistant clones and increase the chance of cure (Goldie and Coldman, 1984; Goldie et al, 1982). In their model, it was necessary that the combinations tested be truly clinically non–cross resistant and that both non–cross-resistant combinations be as active as initial treatment of the disease being evaluated. Most frequently, the benefit of this approach was noted in the treatment of Hodgkin's disease, in which it appeared that treatment with mechlorethamine (nitrogen mustard), vincristine (Oncovin), procarbazine, and prednisone (MOPP) alternating with doxorubicin (Adriamycin), bleomycin, vinblastine (ABVD), and dactinomycin (DTIC) was superior to MOPP alone (Bonadonna, 1982). Some studies show, however, that ABVD may be superior to MOPP, which may mean that another explanation for the observation is still necessary (Santoro et al, 1987). In addition, preliminary data may actually suggest that ABVD is equivalent to alternating MOPP and ABVD (Canellos, 1990), again emphasizing the difference in the two regimens rather than the superiority of the alternating approach.

Because of the encouraging data in Hodgkin's disease and the availability of many active agents, resulting in possible non–cross-resistant combinations to test, the alternating therapy approach has been used frequently in the treatment of patients with SCLC. A review by Elliott and coauthors (1984) showed some of the shortfalls in trial designs but also showed that in general there were not many clearly positive studies. A Canadian study compared CAV alone with alternating CAV and etoposide plus cisplatin for a total of six courses in previously untreated patients with extensive SCLC. In this large trial, a 6-week difference in median survival was observed (Evans et al, 1987) and was believed to be cost-effective (Goodwin et al, 1988).

A Canadian study in patients with limited disease compared three courses of CAV followed by three courses of etoposide and cisplatin with six courses of the alternating regimen. No difference in outcome was found (Feld et al, 1987). It may be difficult, however, to detect the small potential benefit of different approaches to alternating therapy. On the other hand, etoposide and cisplatin may be the superior combination, so that no differences could be observed between the two therapeutic arms.

Other studies, such as those done by the Southeast Cooperative Oncology Group (Roth et al, 1992) and a Japanese cooperative group (Fukuoka et al, 1991), do not totally support the concept that alternating combination chemotherapy is superior to standard regimens, although the Japanese study shows a significant survival advantage to alternation in patients with limited disease. A review on this subject (Havemann, 1990) supports the view that there are conflicting results in the literature, but no clear superiority to alternating chemotherapy can be demonstrated.

Some (Evans et al, 1987) believe that the results from the Canadian study mean that alternating chemotherapy should be standard treatment. Most investigators think that the alternating approach is reasonable but not necessarily superior to other approaches.

Another approach came from the pioneering efforts of the Vancouver group. Murray and colleagues (1991b) showed that the use of a four-drug intensive regimen, such as cisplatin, vincristine (Oncovin), doxorubicin, and etoposide (CODE)—most of the major active agents, for a short time (9 to 12 weeks) gave apparent superior results in patients with extensive SCLC and also possibly in those with non-SCLC (Murray et al, 1989). This includes additional prophylactic supportive agents, such as corticosteroids, oral antifungals, and oral antibiotics. The results to date are promising in SCLC but may in part be caused by selection bias. To address this issue, in an intergroup study, the Southwest Oncology Group and the National Cancer Institute of Canada tested the CODE regimen against a more standard approach in patients with extensive SCLC. The study had to be stopped early because of toxicity, with no survival advantage documented for CODE (Murray et al, 1999).

Duration

Until the middle or late 1980s, it was not uncommon to treat patients with chemotherapy for a minimum of 12 to 24 months. More recently, there has been more concern about the quality of life of patients receiving such treatments.

A number of retrospective studies, including a large one from Toronto (Feld et al, 1984), suggested no benefit to prolonged therapy. A large randomized trial carried out by the European Organization for Research on the Treatment of Cancer (EORTC) Lung Group showed no benefit in survival, at least in patients with limited disease, although there may have been the suggestion of a benefit in patients with extensive disease (Splinter et al, 1986; Splinter, 1988, 1989). The update of a French trial that was testing this hypothesis showed a small survival benefit in patients with SCLC who were maintained on therapy (LeBeau et al, 1991). Few studies support the use of prolonged therapy in this disease. In addition, an update on a trial by the United Kingdom's Medical Research Council showed no superiority in six courses of therapy over three courses (Girling, 1991).

Other studies confirm the lack of benefit of maintenance therapy after four to six courses of standard combination therapy (Beith et al, 1996; Sculier et al, 1996; Velemes et al, 1998). Maintenance therapy exploring a new concept is being tested in an international multicenter randomized trial. In this trial, marimastat, which inhibits angiogenesis by acting as a matrix metalloproteinase inhibitor, is being compared to placebo in patients with both limited and extensive SCLC who have achieved at least a partial response on standard chemotherapy. Hopefully, this will reduce the metastatic potential of this tumor and hence prolong survival. Its main toxicities are musculoskeletal (arthralgia, myalgia, tendinitis, and tenosynovitis). Because these problems are usually reversible if the dose is lowered or the drug is withdrawn, this agent is generally well tolerated. We await the results of this study and hope a major advance in the therapy of this disease is forthcoming.

Four to six courses of chemotherapy for patients who show a complete response should be adequate; available maintenance chemotherapy does not appear to provide any additional benefit. It is still unclear whether maintenance with long-term interferon-α therapy will be beneficial in this disease, as suggested by the Finnish trial (Mattson et al, 1991). Therefore, until this is confirmed, this should not be part of standard care.

New Drug Development

One of the most important approaches in the treatment of SCLC is the procurement of new active agents for managing the disease and defining better ways of using presently available therapy, as already described with the recent interest in using daily oral etoposide. We re-emphasize the concept of using new agents in previously untreated patients. As previously mentioned, this appears to be safe as long as a crossover design is used with early crossover to an established regimen to avoid patients' becoming too ill to receive potentially valuable treatment after waiting too long. Lower response rates are expected in previously treated patients (Grant et al, 1992).

Although many new agents have become available for testing in SCLC, few have appeared promising. High-dose epirubicin was found by several groups to be active in both SCLC and non-SCLC (Banham et al, 1990; Blackstein et al, 1990; Eckhardt et al, 1990; Feld, 1992; Johnson, 1989; Meyer et al, 1982; Wils et al, 1990). It probably should replace doxorubicin in SCLC. Although not used routinely, carboplatin has been established as an active agent in this disease (Grant et al, 1992; Johnson, 1989; Thatcher and Lind, 1990). It is not clear whether it is as active as cisplatin, but it is a reasonable alternative to prevent or reduce neurotoxicity and nephrotoxicity in selected patients at high risk (e.g., patients with preexisting kidney or hearing problems). Ifosfamide is also active in SCLC (Johnson, 1989, 1990), but its superiority to cyclophosphamide has not yet been proved. Expense, the required use of mesna, and its usual requirement for administration in a hospital all make it a more difficult agent to use in SCLC than are most of the other available active agents.

The only other agents that look promising at this stage of development are gemcitabine and paclitaxel (Taxol) and perhaps its derivatives, along with topotecan. Gemcitabine appears to be active in non-SCLC (Anderson et al, 1991b; Lund et al, 1991). In preliminary data, both agents appear active in SCLC, but larger phase II trials are required to determine their relative activity compared with other available agents. Topotecan appears to be equivalent to CAV as second-line treatment in this disease (Ormrod and Spencer, 1999). Derivatives of paclitaxel are also likely to be tested in the near future and are likely to be active. No other obvious chemotherapeutic agents are on the horizon for this disease. Agents that were designed to bypass established drug resistance, such as verapamil, have not proved helpful in patients with SCLC (Figueredo et al, 1990; Milroy et al, 1991). A correlation of in vitro drug sensitivity with potentially active agents may be useful. Preliminary data from the National Cancer Institute are not encouraging but show that this approach is feasible (Gazdar et al, 1990).

RADIATION THERAPY

Although it was hoped that chemotherapy would be adequate to control this disease, patients with SCLC frequently relapse first in the thorax. In initial trials, it was hoped that thoracic irradiation in patients with limited disease would reduce local failure and result in improved median and long-term disease-free overall survival.

As previously mentioned, the Medical Research Council Trial carried out in the United Kingdom (Fox et al, 1973; Miller et al, 1969) showed that thoracic irradiation was superior to surgery, and as a result, it became the standard therapy. When chemotherapeutic regimens were developed that resulted in significant prolongation of survival, it became unclear whether radiation therapy added to the beneficial effects of combination chemotherapy. There was also the potential for additional toxicity as a result of radiotherapy to the thorax, bone marrow, esophagus, and cardiovascular system. A number of randomized trials were carried out in patients with limited disease, comparing combination chemotherapy alone with combination chemotherapy plus radiotherapy. Details of the major trials are shown in Table 33–5 with references. Recent meta-analyses done by Warde and Payne (1992) and by Arriagada and colleagues (1991) both showed a significant but small survival benefit of combined modality therapy. A detailed discussion of these data is beyond the scope of this chapter.

From these meta-analyses, it may be concluded that combining chemotherapy and radiation therapy, using current approaches, has only a modest effect on long-term survival. More aggressive approaches, as exemplified by a National Cancer Institute trial (Bunn et al, 1987), resulted in a number of therapy-related deaths, which were sufficient to offset some of the survival advantage of the combined modality regimen that otherwise might not have been seen (Brooks et al, 1986). In addition to decreased failure in the lung, resulting in a slight prolongation of survival, there is also likely to be an improvement in the quality of life in patients who receive this modality of therapy. Newer fractionation schemes, particularly multiple daily fractions, as initially piloted by Turrisi (1991), actually show even greater benefit from the addition of radiation therapy to combination chemotherapy. A randomized trial comparing more standard fractionation with multiple daily fractions demonstrated a major improvement in survival in this serious disease using daily fractionation twice (Turrisi et al, 1999).

Timing, Dose, and Volume of Thoracic Irradiation

Although the Cancer and Leukemia Group B study did not show a clear benefit of early thoracic irradiation (Perry et al, 1987), a large multicenter Canadian trial carried out by the National Cancer Institute of Canada found an advantage to early thoracic irradiation (Murray et al, 1991a). This trial used standard alternating chemotherapy—CAV alternating with etoposide plus cisplatin. The thoracic irradiation was given either early (concurrently with the second course of etoposide and cisplatin) or late with the sixth (final) course of chemotherapy and again with etoposide and cisplatin. Thoracic irradiation was given with the cisplatin-containing regimen because it was believed there would not be any enhancement of pulmonary toxicity. The survival results were impressive, with 25% 4-year survival rates in the early treatment group versus 15% in the late treatment group (Murray et al, 1991a). Even more encouraging was the fact that these differences appeared to be getting larger with the passage of time. Obviously, this study may need to be confirmed before this approach is adopted as standard therapy, but this appears to be an observation that reflects benefits for early thoracic irradiation in this disease. If multiple daily fractions are superior, such a regimen should probably be tested early in therapy to maximize its possible beneficial effect.

Although a dose-response effect probably exists, a Canadian randomized study comparing 25 versus 37.5 Gy in responding patients showed only a modest delay in intrathoracic progression and no overall survival benefit from the higher dose (Coy et al, 1988). Despite this study, most practitioners tend to use higher doses of at least 40 Gy within 3 weeks or even higher doses if the fractionation scheme is prolonged over 5 to 6 weeks.

Prophylactic Cranial Irradiation

Many randomized trials comparing PCI with no additional treatment have been carried out, and although most of them showed a significant reduction in CNS relapse for patients receiving PCI, none showed a survival advantage. A summary of the older radiation studies is shown in Table 33–6. Kristjansen (1989) from Copenhagen reviewed this subject extensively.

A number of recently completed studies have also addressed this problem. These studies consistently showed fewer brain metastases with no increase in neuropsychological complications, with inconclusive data on whether PCI provides a benefit in terms of survival. A meta-analysis involving 987 patients entered in seven trials provides further support for this approach (Auperin et al, 1999). This study showed that in cases in which PCI was given to patients in complete remission, there

TABLE 33–5 ■ **Randomized Trials of Thoracic Radiotherapy in Limited Small Cell Lung Carcinoma* Treated by Chemotherapy: Design and Results**

Author (yr)	Radio-CT Sequence	Chemotherapeutic Regimen	Beginning of RT†	Chest (Gy Fraction)	Radiotherapy	No. Randomized	No. Analyzed	Median Survival Time (wk)	2-Year Survival Rate (%)	No. of Lethal Toxicities
Bunn et al, 1987	C	CYC, MTX, CCNU	D1–3	40/15	No	49	49	50	12	4
		alt VCR, ADR, PCB			Yes					
Greco et al, 1986	C	CYC, ADR, VCR‡	D1	45/15	No	373	210	54	—	—
				split	Yes			64	—	—
Osterlind et al, 1986	C	CYC, VCR, MTX, CCNU	D43	40/10		148	76	52	12	0
							69	44	4	6
Perry et al, 1987	C	CYC, VCR, VP-16	D1 or D64	50/24	No	426	129	102	15	2
		alt CYC, ADR, VCR			Yes (D1)		125	98	24	3
					Yes (D64)		145	110	30	1
Stevens et al, 1979	C	CYC, ADR, VCR	D22	35/10	No	18	18	50	—	—
		alt CYC, MTX		split	Yes	14	14	56	—	—
Perez et al, 1984	A	CYC, ADR, VCR	D29¶	40/14	No	148	142	49	19	—
				split	Yes	156	146	60	28	—
Fox et al, 1980, 1981	S	CYC, ADR, VCR	D63	40/20	No	44	44	64	—	—
					Yes	40	40	63	—	—
Kies et al, 1987	S	VCR, MTX, VP16	D85+	48/22	No	56	53	68	28	0
		alt CYC, ADR, VCR		split	Yes	47	40	68	33	2
Nou et al, 1988	S	CYC, ADR, VCR, MTX	D77	40/20	No	31	31	64	15	2
		alt CYC, VCR, MTX, CCNU			Yes	25	25	67	26	2
Ohnoshi et al, 1986	S	CYC, VCR, MTX, PCB	D30	40/20	No	26	26	65	16	0
		alt VP-16, ADR, CCNU			Yes	24	24	52	25	2
Souhami et al, 1984	S	VCR, ADR	D85**	40/20	No	139	73	41	—	2
		alt CYC, MTX			Yes		57	46	—	2
Creech et al, 1988	S	CYC, CCNU, MTX§	D43	50/?	No	243	243	62††	—	3
					Yes			75	—	

A, alternating; alt, alternating chemotherapy; ADR, doxorubicin (Adriamycin); C, concurrent chest RT and CT; CCNU, lomustine; CT, chemotherapy; CYC, cyclophosphamide; D, day; MTX, methotrexate; PCB, procarbazine; PCI, prophylactic cranial irradiation; RT, chest radiotherapy; S, sequential; VCR, vincristine; VP-16, etoposide.

*Only results obtained in patients with limited disease (even if extensive disease patients included in the trial).

†D1, beginning of chemotherapy (day 1).

‡Second randomization of patients in CR or PR: intensification CT (etoposide + cisplatin) versus no CT—significant result on survival preliminary report.

§In the radiotherapy group, only patient with complete, partial response or with stable disease after chemotherapy were treated by radiotherapy.

¶In responders to induction chemotherapy: CYC, MTX, CCNU alternating with ADR, VP-16.

**In the chemotherapy group, some nonresponders received thoracic RT.

††Median survival in responders.

Adapted from Arriagada R, Pignon JP, LeChevalier TL: Thoracic radiotherapy in small cell lung cancer: Rationale for timing and fractionation. Lung Cancer 5:237, 1989.

TABLE 33–6 ■ **Randomized Prophylactic Cranial Irradiation (PCI) Trials**

Author (yr)	*No. Patients*		*Stage of Disease*	*PCI Time/ Dose Fraction*	*CNS Relapse (No./%)*		*Sole Brain Relapse (No./%)*		*Systemic Treatment*	*Observation Time*	*Survival*
	−PCI	*+PCI*			*−PCI*	*+PCI*	*−PCI*	*+PCI*			
Jackson et al, 1977	15	14	All	Day 1: 30 Gy/10	4 (27)*	0 (0)*	NR		VAC or LM	NR	NS
Cox et al, 1978	21	24	LD	Day 1: 20 Gy/10	5 (24)†	4 (17)†	NR		None	NR	NR
Beiler et al, 1979	31	24	LD	Week 3: 24 Gy/8	5 (16)*	0 (0)*	NR		LMCV	NR	NR
Maurer et al, 1980	84	79	All	Week 9: 30 Gy/10	15 (18)*	3 (4)*	NR		C, CVM, CVM, or CM	NR	NR
Hansen et al, 1980	55	54	LD	Week 12: 40 Gy/20	6/20 (30)†	4/26 (15)†	2 (4)	2 (4)	LMC	>18 mo.	NS
Eagan et al, 1981	15	15	LD	Week 20: 36 Gy/10	11 (73)*	2 (13)*	NR		CAVED	16 mo.	NS
Katsenis et al, 1982	18	17	All	Day 1: 40 Gy/25	8 (44)*	2 (12)*	NR		CVM, CAM, or LMC	>10 mo.	NS
Seydel et al, 1983	112	107	LD	Day 1: 30 Gy/10	22 (20)*	5 (5)*	NR		LC (50%)	>24 mo.	NS
Aroney et al, 1983	15	18	All	At CR: 30 Gy/10	4 (27)†	0 (0)†	NR		ACE/CLVP	NR	NS
Total	366	350			80 (22)	20 (6)					

A, doxorubicin; C, cyclophosphamide; D, cisplatin, E, etoposide; L, lomustine; LD, limited disease; M, methotrexate; NR, not reported; NS, not significant; P, procarbazine; V, vincristine.

*$P < .05$.

†Not significant.

Adapted from Kristjansen PEG: The role of cranial irradiation in the management of patients with SCLC. Lung Cancer 5:148, 1989.

was a 5.4% increase in overall survival at 3 years (15.3% in the control group versus 20.7% in the treatment group). There was a trend in favor of higher doses of PCI, but the effect on survival was not significant. There was also a trend in favor of earlier administration of PCI after the initiation of chemotherapy. An accompanying editorial (Carney, 1999) suggested that these data should change practice. All patients with limited or extensive disease (with only one site of metastasis) should be offered PCI as part of standard treatment. The issues of dose, fractionation, and when to administer PCI in the course of treatment can be decided only on the basis of the results of ongoing and future multicenter randomized clinical trials.

The clinician must also take into consideration the morbidity of the therapy because acute effects are probably more severe with regimens that include larger fractions and those given with concurrent chemotherapy, particularly when they contain an anthracycline. Some studies of PCI show significant toxicities, including a virtual incapacity to carry out the activities of daily living; in other studies, it did not produce this effect (Fleck et al, 1990; Lishner et al, 1990). Better measures of toxicity, quality of life, and so forth were recorded in many of the current studies, and PCI was well tolerated. Most authorities would at this time recommend PCI for patients with limited disease who achieve a complete response; other patients with SCLC would not normally receive this modality of therapy.

Palliation

A major role for radiation therapy in patients with SCLC is palliation of symptoms (Klastersky, 1990). A situation in which radiation therapy is used palliatively is superior vena caval obstruction. This may be given as the first and only form of therapy or it may be given after chemotherapy; the latter is more common. In addition, radiation therapy may be used to treat recurrent laryngeal or phrenic nerve palsy, hemoptysis, esophageal compression, pleural effusions, and painful bony lesions. Standard therapy for spinal cord compression is usually radiation therapy, although surgery may be used in selected cases. The use of concomitant steroid therapy has largely supplanted escalating fraction sizes during therapy. Cerebral metastases are often treated with radiation therapy. Patients with meningeal disease may benefit occasionally from craniospinal irradiation. Other localized masses in unusual sites may benefit from local radiation therapy, either to unblock a hollow organ, such as the ureter or bronchus, or to relieve pain. Appropriate palliative radiotherapy may make a marked difference to the quality of life of these patients when the tumor progresses and cure is not a reasonable possibility.

SURGERY

As previously suggested in the historical perspective, surgery, once the main form of therapy for SCLC until the United Kingdom's Medical Research Council trial changed its place in this disease, remains a controversial and as yet undecided issue despite re-examination of its role over the past 15 years (Fox et al, 1973; Miller et al, 1969). Chemotherapy is the standard therapy for limited-stage SCLC (Livingston, 1986). The Veterans Administration Lung Group recommended that SCLC presenting as a solitary pulmonary nodule is treated with pulmonary resection (Higgins et al, 1975). This is standard therapy around the world and is often combined with a number of courses of combination chemotherapy with or without thoracic irradiation and PCI (Ginsberg, 1989; Ginsberg and Karrer 1989). It is mainly carried out in patients with peripheral stage T1, N0 lesions that are determined to be SCLC at pathologic review. Reports in the late 1970s and early 1980s demonstrated that surgery alone could provide curative therapy in up to 25% of such patients (Mountain, 1978; Shields et al, 1982).

With the addition of postoperative chemotherapy, even better long-term survival in this early stage of disease has been reported. In a retrospective analysis of patients with stage I disease who receive postoperative chemotherapy, especially those with T1, N0 disease, there was an up to 80% survival rate for more than 5 years (Myer et al, 1982). Postoperative thoracic irradiation is usually given only in situations in which the lesion is classified as N1. Five-year survival rates in the range of 20% to 30% have also been reported in patients with more advanced stage I, II, and IIIa SCLC when the lesions were totally excised and the patient treated with postoperative chemotherapy. Some of these patients did extremely well with only chemotherapy and radiotherapy in this setting (Shepherd et al, 1984).

In fact, this led to a randomized study in patients with limited SCLC by the Lung Cancer Study Group in conjunction with the Eastern Cooperative Oncology Group and EORTC, which compared induction chemotherapy plus radiation to the chest and brain with and without surgery. As previously mentioned, however, the results of this study suggested no benefit from the addition of surgery in that setting (Lad et al, 1991b, 1991c). Although most of the 144 patients randomized were preoperatively staged as having limited (versus very limited) disease, the results of this trial show no difference in either therapeutic arm and no difference when a subset analysis attempted to isolate the very limited group.

Other authors confirmed these equivalent results in nonrandomized retrospective analyses. It would probably be impossible for another large-scale trial to be carried out to evaluate this issue critically. There may in fact be a benefit for patients with less disease in the chest. This is especially important because the Lung Cancer Study Group trial included patients with bulky mediastinal disease, which may have skewed the results and may partially account for the negative outcome. It cannot be recommended, however, that surgery be used routinely in this group of patients with SCLC, except as part of clinical trials. We believe that it is still appropriate to investigate adjuvant surgery in a prospective randomized trial confined to this limited SCLC group.

Another important point is that although a histologic biopsy or cytologic analysis may demonstrate SCLC in certain cases, these may be inaccurate or there may be mixed cell types. Some patients who have limited disease and do not respond to chemotherapy may still have a non-SCLC tumor that may benefit from surgical resection, even possibly resulting in cure. This is also a major issue to be addressed when there are isolated recurrences more than 18 months to 2 years after the original diagnosis of limited SCLC. Again, these may be second primary tumors and should be totally evaluated for the possibility of curative resection (salvage surgery).

The final role that has been suggested for surgery in the treatment of SCLC is that of salvage therapy when primary chemoradiation does not control the local disease or when there are recurrences and only the primary site is affected. In these cases, surgical therapy after reinduction chemotherapy has been used as a salvage procedure.

Primary Surgery

SCLC that has been resected, usually without prior knowledge of the cell type, results in significant 5-year survival rates in completely resected patients. One series reported that postoperative chemotherapy is a necessary part of treatment (Table 33–7). In most centers, after surgical resection, a minimum of five to six courses of an adequate two- or three-drug regimen of chemotherapy is advised. If hilar and mediastinal lymph node disease is found at the time of surgery, postoperative mediastinal irradiation is also advised. The role of PCI is yet to be decided.

It is difficult to compare this multimodality surgical approach with chemoradiation alone because medical oncologists usually do not classify these very limited tumors as a separate entity (Shepherd et al, 1984); however, some retrospective analyses have been performed despite this. Osterlind and associates (1986), in their retrospective analysis, did not demonstrate a beneficial effect for surgical resection. On the other hand, Shepherd and colleagues suggested a two-fold improvement in survival when surgery was used as part of therapy and control of the primary site was improved (Salzer et al, 1990a).

Not all authors support the use of adjuvant chemotherapy after surgical resection for SCLC. The Brompton group (Shaw et al, 1992) reported 57% and 55% 5-year survival rates after surgical resection alone in stage I and stage II SCLC. However, most other authors support its use. Karrer and Ulsperger (1995) reported on 183 patients: the overall 5-year survival rate for N0 was 63% and for N2 disease, 37% with the use of adjuvant treatment.

The results of primary surgery for SCLC are listed in Table 33–8.

Induction Chemotherapy Plus Adjuvant Surgery

As previously discussed, the role of surgery in more proximal tumors with clinical N1 or minimal N2 disease (but still resectable by non-SCLC criteria) is less apparent. Few induction chemotherapeutic trials in very limited disease have been reported. The experiences of the Toronto group (Shepherd et al, 1989) and the Innsbruck group (Salzer et al, 1990) suggest that with this combined modality therapy using surgery as an adjuvant 5-year survival rates in the range of 40% can be obtained (Table 33–9). Tumors with good responses to chemotherapy that are down-staged by the time of surgery to the N0 level have as high as a 60% to 70% 5-year survival rate. Persisting nodal disease yields a less satisfactory 20% to 30% 5-year survival rate. An interesting sidelight of such

TABLE 33–7 ■ **Review of Studies of Primary Surgery for Small Cell Lung Cancer**

Study	*Number of Patients*	*Median Survival Time (mo)*	*Five-Year Survival Rate (%)*
SURGERY ALONE			
Coolen et al, 1995	15		13
Shaw et al, 1992	28		43.3
Sorensen et al, 1988	76		12
Shore and Paneth, 1980	40		27
SURGERY WITH OR WITHOUT CHEMOTHERAPY			
Lucchi et al, 1997	127	18	22.6
Merkle et al, 1986	170		18
Maassen and Greschuchna, 1986	124		20
SURGERY AND CHEMOTHERAPY			
Asamura and Ginsberg, 2000	183		37*
Coolen et al, 1995	15		27
Davis et al, 1993	37	17	36
Muller et al, 1992	45	18	36
Shepherd et al, 1991	79	21	40
Salzer et al, 1990	79		25 (N2 disease)
Osterlind et al, 1986	25		23*
Ohta et al, 1986	52		31
Friess et al, 1985	15	25	44

*Three-year survival rate.
Adapted from Asamura H, Ginsberg RJ: Treatment of small cell lung cancer: Surgery. In Hansen HH (ed): The International Association for the Study of Lung Cancer Textbook of Lung Cancer. London, Martin Dunitz, 2000, pp 243–249.

therapy is the fact that many of the resected tumors contain no remaining SCLC, but they do contain persisting elements of non-SCLC.

Salvage Surgery

The Toronto group promulgated the concept of salvage surgery for SCLC that persists in the primary site after induction treatment or that recurs only in the primary site after a complete response. In both instances, mediastinoscopy is used to identify patients with unresectable disease (Shepherd et al, 1991). Although this salvage type of operation has led to only a handful of long-term survivors, it is rare for reinduction chemotherapy and radiotherapy in locally recurrent or persistent disease to result in long-term disease-free survival.

TABLE 33–8 ■ **Results of Primary Surgery for Small Cell Lung Cancer**

Authors (yr)	*No. Patients*	*Mean Survival Time (mo)*	*5-Year Survival Rate (%)*
Surgery + chemotherapy			
Karrer and Shields 1991	183	26	45
Shepherd et ai, 1991	79	21	40
Ohta et al, 1986	25		31
Osterlind et al, 1989	52		23*
Surgery ± chemotherapy			
Merkle et al, 1986	170		18
Maassen and Greschuchna, 1986	124		20*
Surgery			
Sorensen et al, 1986	76		12
Miyazawa et al, 1986	25		8

*3-year survival rate.

BIOLOGIC RESPONSE MODIFIERS

As Induction Therapy

Many agents, including bacillus Calmette-Guérin (BCG) or the methanol extraction residue of BCG and *Corynebacterium parvum*, have been tested in all types of lung cancer, with no clear evidence that they are beneficial (Shank and Sher, 1985). The only encouraging study, as previously mentioned, is from the U.S. National Cancer Institute, where a randomized trial using thymosin fraction V was carried out (Cohen et al, 1979). A significant increase in survival was noted with the highest dose, but has not been confirmed (Shank et al, 1983). Woll and Rozengurt (1989) reviewed the literature on this subject.

Antibodies directed against bombesin (a gastrin-like peptide hormone) were evaluated in phase I studies. Additional work is being done with this approach, as reviewed by Carney (1991, 1992), but so far, these anti-

TABLE 33–9 ■ **Induction Chemotherapy Followed by Surgery for Small Cell Lung Cancer: The Toronto Results**

Stage	*No. Patients*	*Mean Survival Time (yr)*	*Estimated 5-Year Survival Rate (%)*
Overall	38	1.8	38
N0	11	Not reached	45
N1	13	1.3	30
N2	14	1	40

bodies are not clinically useful, although they continue to be investigated (Kelley et al, 1997). Interferons, interleukins, and other similar agents have not been found to be useful as therapy in lung cancer; therefore, we can say that biologic response modifiers alone have no place in standard induction therapy for patients with SCLC.

As Maintenance Therapy

As previously mentioned, the only significantly positive study using maintenance therapy is the one by Mattson and associates (1991) from Finland, who seemed to show a survival advantage with long-term interferon-α maintenance. This study was repeated by the Southwest Oncology Group, but the data are not yet available. The use of interferon-γ was tested by the North Central Oncology Group, but the data from this study are still unpublished.

In Combination with Other Therapies

The best example of using biologic response modifiers in combination with other therapy is using growth factors, such as G-CSF and GM-CSF. These were mentioned in detail earlier. In summary, G-CSF appears to reduce myelosuppression, febrile episodes, and number of days of hospitalization. GM-CSF may also do this, but it has many other inherent toxicities, including the possibility of enhanced thrombocytopenia. In fact, thrombocytopenia that is not dealt with by either G-CSF or GM-CSF may present serious difficulties. If the clinician wants to use myelosuppressive therapy, the dose-limiting hematologic toxicity will in fact be thrombocytopenia, rather than granulocytopenia, as is the case when other CSF preparations are used. New growth factors, alone or in combination, may help avoid this problem in the future; however, as of 1999, CSFs are not a required part of therapy in patients with SCLC that is treated with moderate-dose chemotherapy.

A concept that has been tested only in non-SCLC is chemotherapy plus biologic response modifiers, such as cisplatin and interferon-α. A combination of cisplatin and interferon-α was shown to be active in a pilot study by Smyth and coworkers (1990) in patients with non-SCLC and extensive disease. Similar results were observed in about 100 patients who were treated by an international cooperative group funded by Hoffman-LaRoche (Holdener E, personal communication, 1992). Randomized trials have yet to be presented or published regarding the clear value of interferon-α in this setting. Whether this approach will be useful in SCLC has yet to be determined.

Another potential use for one type of biologic response modifier (monoclonal antibodies to SCLC antigens) may be in the detection of these tumors. Imaging techniques are already available and look promising. The same monoclonal antibodies may be useful as possible therapeutic interventions in the future, as discussed in a review by Stahel (1992), but clinical studies are just beginning.

COMPLICATIONS OF TREATMENT

Early Complications

All modalities of therapy can result in significant individual toxicities. Those associated with individual modalities of therapy are shown in Table 33–10, and these are divided into those that occur early after treatment and those that occur late. Possible toxicity must always be considered when offering such treatment to patients who have SCLC and should be discussed with the patient in detail. A detailed description of these problems is beyond the scope of this chapter but can be found elsewhere (Feld, 1981, 1989, 1990, 1992a). Although these data come from studies in patients with SCLC, similar complications would be expected with non-SCLC.

New approaches and supportive care may offset many of these toxicities. For example, nausea and vomiting are a frequent and serious problem in patients with SCLC because cisplatin is a commonly used agent, along with other agents that cause moderate emesis. The use of dexamethasone in combination with serotonin antagonists, such as ondansetron and granisetron, has alleviated nausea substantially (Aaproms, 1991). Early nausea is virtually eliminated, although delayed-onset nausea is still a potential problem in some patients. The use of more potent antiemetics (substance P inhibitors) is an exciting development in supportive care. These agents may augment the effects of 5-HT3 inhibitors or replace them, and the chemotherapy-induced nausea and vomiting experienced by these patients may be reduced or eliminated. This should improve the compliance with chemotherapy, the quality of life, and the survival of patients with SCLC.

Myelosuppression, with its potential for infection, has been a serious problem in the treatment of SCLC. As previously discussed, a common regimen that was used in the 1980s was CAE. This resulted in severe and prolonged myelosuppression, leading to as high as a 40% to 50% admission rate for febrile neutropenia in these patients. Therapeutic results were reasonable, but the complication rate was probably unacceptable. This regimen was supplanted by regimens, such as etoposide and cisplatin, that have less than 5% admission rates for this complication. Another approach to this problem was the use of growth factors, particularly G-CSF, to reduce the degree and length of neutropenia, hence reducing the infection and hospitalization rates. In addition, patients in the hospital are discharged sooner. In the landmark study discussed previously (Crawford et al, 1991), the CAE regimen was compared with the CAE regimen plus G-CSF. The costly addition of CSF substantially reduced the myelosuppressive and subsequent infectious complications; this result was confirmed in a similarly designed European study (Green et al, 1991). The other options include using less myelosuppressive but equally effective chemotherapy, as previously suggested, or possibly oral prophylactic antibiotics, such as co-trimoxazole or various marketed fluoroquinolones.

Cardiotoxicity can usually be avoided by the use of less cardiotoxic anthracyclines such as epirubicin, which is active in both SCLC (Blackstein et al, 1990; Eckhardt et al, 1990) and non-SCLC (Feld et al, 1992). In addition,

TABLE 33–10 ■ **Early and Possible Late Toxicities in Patients with Small Cell Lung Cancer**

Therapy	*Early Toxicities*	*Possible Late Toxicities*
Chemotherapy	Nausea and vomiting Alopecia Peripheral neuropathy Myelosuppression with possible resulting bleeding (cisplatin) Anemia Constipation Electrolyte disturbances Cardiotoxicity Nephrotoxicity and ototoxicity Hemorrhagic cystitis Mucositis Hypotension or hypertension (etoposide) Bronchoesophageal fistulas	Unusual infections (e.g., herpes zoster) Anthracycline-induced cardiomyopathy Pulmonary fibrosis Central nervous system toxicity (especially in conjunction with prophylactic cranial irradiation) Second malignancies Second lung primaries Other solid tumors Acute leukemia
Radiotherapy		
Thoracic	Esophagitis ± stricture Pneumonitis Cardiac toxicity	Pulmonary fibrosis Late cardiac effects Myelitis ?Predisposition to second primary
Cranial	Erythema of the scalp Otitis externa Prolongation of chemotherapy-induced myelosuppression	Somnolence, confusion, problems with concentration, and memory deficits Tremor, dysarthria, slurred speech, and ataxia Frank dementia
Surgery	Immediate postoperative problems (can be fatal) Pain at thoracotomy incision site Bronchopleural fistulas	Continued long-term pain at incision site Bronchopleural fistulas Respiratory failure secondary to removal of functioning lung

the use of only four to six courses of therapy, which is now standard throughout the world, reduces the frequency of this problem and many of the other side effects, thereby improving the quality of life of patients with SCLC. The use of mesna, especially when combined with ifosfamide, has virtually eliminated the problem of hemorrhagic cystitis associated with this agent (Johnson, 1990). It can also be used with high-dose cyclophosphamide to avoid this complication. If nephrotoxicity, ototoxicity, or emesis is a problem, the cisplatin-containing regimen can be switched to one with carboplatin. This usually either prevents or stabilizes these side effects, but it causes more myelosuppression. Carboplatin is also far more expensive and possibly less active than cisplatin in this disease (Green et al, 1992). The use of the Calvert formula (area under the curve) in patients with SCLC when determining the dosage of carboplatin, if it is part of their treatment, can reduce myelosuppression and possibly infections and bleeding.

Peripheral neuropathy remains a common problem. Of particular concern is the late-onset neuropathy that is associated with cisplatin. This can come on even a few months after the final course of cisplatin and can be disabling. New approaches to this problem are needed. Possible new approaches include the prophylactic use of amifostine and the use of new growth factors.

Modern radiotherapy planning despite higher doses can help avoid many of the complications of this treatment. Radiation myelitis can occur in 1% to 5% of patients within 5 years after a spinal cord dose of 50 Gy given in 25 fractions over 5 weeks (Rubin and Casarett, 1972). Because large fractions may increase this risk, an increased number of smaller fractions is frequently used.

PCI is commonly used in patients with SCLC, although it is not usually used in patients with non-SCLC. The frequency and seriousness of long-term toxicities constitute a controversial subject. The Toronto experience of PCI in SCLC was relatively positive, with a low incidence of significant abnormalities, which were similar to those in patients who did not receive PCI (Lishner et al, 1990). A study from Indiana University published at the same time, however, showed serious long-term complications (Fleck et al, 1990). In an editorial, Turrisi (1990) tried to rationalize why this might be and indicated that it may be related to the fractionation schemes used.

A number of large trials, along with a recent meta-analysis and an accompanying editorial (Auperin et al, 1999), as already discussed, suggested that PCI is both safe and efficacious (survival advantage) in patients who achieve a complete remission. Toxicity is difficult to demonstrate without sophisticated psychometric testing, and the individual studies in which these tests were performed as part of the trial (before and after treatment) found no long-term statistically significant differences between the treated and untreated patients, suggesting that safety is not likely a serious issue. In fact, the authors of the meta-analysis wondered whether patients with good partial responses could also benefit from PCI, but the data are not yet available for this conclusion.

Late Complications

Although numerous late complications of therapy are shown in Table 33–10, the one that is of most concern is the development of second malignancies in potentially cured patients. Second primary lung tumors are relatively common in patients with SCLC who survive long enough (Sagman et al, 1992). These may go unnoticed or be assumed to be a relapse of the initial tumor, which may prevent possible surgical removal with the potential for cure. A second primary tumor must always be considered when new lesions are seen in patients, particularly if it is 2 years or less since diagnosis. Other solid tumors also occur with reasonable frequency as second primaries, probably partly related to therapy but more likely associated with patient age (median, 60 years of age or older). Smoking cessation may reduce the likelihood of these patients' developing second solid tumors. Acute leukemia is a rare event and will become less common with the discontinued use of nitrosoureas and procarbazine for SCLC in recent years and the far shorter duration of treatment. Second primary lung tumors and acute leukemia are occasionally seen in patients with non-SCLC but are less of a problem.

FUTURE DIRECTIONS IN THERAPY

A paucity of new agents appear to be potentially active in SCLC. The promising new drugs that already appear active include gemcitabine, paclitaxel, and topotecan. Docetaxel is also likely to be active. Hopefully, these new agents can be successfully added to our already useful armamentarium. The recent addition of ifosfamide to the list of active agents may be helpful, but its neurotoxicity and its usual requirement for inpatient administration to prevent hemorrhagic cystitis may make it a less desirable agent than are some of the others already in common use (Eberhardt and Niederle, 1992). Because of these inherent problems, evidence that it is superior to other agents, particularly cyclophosphamide, is needed before it becomes part of standard therapy.

The use of early radiotherapy with concurrent chemotherapy was superior to late radiotherapy in the limited SCLC study by the National Cancer Institute of Canada (Murray et al, 1991a). Some of the new chemotherapeutic agents and combinations discussed previously should also be tested in conjunction with concurrent early radiotherapy in future trials, which should evaluate both single and multiple daily fractionation techniques. In both SCLC and non-SCLC, studies should be designed to confirm the European trial, which demonstrated superiority of daily low-dose cisplatin with concurrent radiation (Schaake-Koenig et al, 1992). Consideration could also be given to the addition of chronic oral etoposide to the regimen to improve the antitumor effects of cisplatin.

The ability of growth factors to permit dose intensification without the need for autologous bone marrow transplantation will certainly be further explored in this disease. Future studies should be designed to identify significant survival benefits associated with dose-intense regimens and should not focus primarily on second end points, such as nadir granulocyte counts or the incidence of fever, as has been the case in most studies to date.

Toxicity is a common problem in patients with lung cancer; however, if all the side effects are considered and appropriate management is initiated to either prevent or treat them, they are usually manageable, taking into account the seriousness of the disease being treated. Short-duration chemotherapy (four to eight courses), proper use of antiemetics, good radiation therapy planning, and rapid hospitalization and therapy for patients with febrile neutropenia or bleeding episodes will all help to alleviate this problem in the future.

Acknowledgment

We gratefully acknowledge the assistance provided by Anne Burrows Faulkner in the careful preparation of the manuscript for this chapter.

COMMENTS AND CONTROVERSIES

Since the first edition of this title (1995), there is very little new in the management of small cell lung cancer. It has been established that early local control (early radiotherapy) in the overall management of limited disease has some beneficial effect. As well, it has been established that more intensive chemotherapy has not proved as beneficial as one might have hoped.

The newer drugs that are available for the management of non–small cell lung cancer have shown no great benefit in the treatment of small cell lung cancer other than perhaps the comptothecans. Biologic response modifiers, as in every other cancer, are being intensely investigated.

With regard to the role of surgery in small cell lung cancer, little new has been added to the information obtained prior to the first edition. Surgeons continue to operate on small cell lung cancer, especially in previously undiagnosed malignancies, and the results of surgery followed by chemotherapy are as good as those seen with nonsurgical treatment and may, in fact, be somewhat better, although this is not known. Except in very early stage I peripheral tumors, the recommended treatment for most limited small cell lung cancer remains a nonsurgical approach, reserving surgery for the indications outlined in this chapter.

R.J.G.

■ KEY REFERENCES

Asamura H, Ginsberg RJ: Treatment of small cell lung cancer: Surgery. In Hansen HH (ed): The International Association for the Study of Lung Cancer Textbook of Lung Cancer. London, Martin Dunitz, 2000, pp 243–249.

In this chapter, the current role of surgery in the management of SCLC and the experience from collected series are summarized.

Evans WK, Feld R, Murray N et al: Superiority of alternating noncross-resistant chemotherapy in extensive small cell lung cancer: A multicenter randomized clinical trial by the National Cancer Institute of Canada. Ann Intern Med 107:451, 1987.

The results of a National Cancer Institute of Canada trial in patients with extensive non–SCLC are reported. There were two arms of therapy: standard cyclophosphamide, doxorubicin (Adriamycin), and vincristine (CAV) or six courses of CAV alternating with etoposide and cisplatin for a total of six cycles. The best response was seen in the patients receiving alternating chemotherapy, and the progression-free survival time for patients receiving the alternating chemotherapy was significantly longer (median, 6 weeks). In addition, the overall survival time was significantly longer in this therapeutic arm, despite the fact that major toxicities were about equal. These results showed a modest superiority of alternating chemotherapy over standard therapy. This article is the basis for making alternating chemotherapy one of the standard approaches in the treatment of extensive small cell lung cancer.

Feld R: Complications in the treatment of small cell carcinoma of the lung. Cancer Treat Rev 8:5, 1981.

The complications of treatment of SCLC, primarily early, are reviewed in this article, but some mention is made of late complications in all studies reported to that time. This is one of the classic articles on this subject. From this study it was concluded that combining radiation with chemotherapy containing doxorubicin may increase the incidence of esophagitis, radiation-induced pneumonitis, and skin toxicity. In general, combined modality therapy is relatively safe, although it causes a slight increase in the frequency of infectious complications compared with chemotherapy alone. Chemotherapy adds significant toxicity to radiation but is a necessary part of therapy. Reporting of toxicity should be a key part of reporting data on studies involving this patient population.

Feld R, Evans WK, Coy P et al: Canadian multicentre randomized trial comparing sequential and alternating administration of two non-cross resistant chemotherapy combinations in patients with limited small cell carcinoma of the lung. J Clin Oncol 5:1401, 1987.

The results of a randomized trial carried out by the National Cancer Institute of Canada comparing the use of alternating cyclophosphamide, doxorubicin (Adriamycin) and vincristine (CAV) with etoposide and cisplatin for six courses, with three courses of initial CAV followed by three courses of etoposide and cisplatin in patients with limited disease are described. In addition, patients were randomized to two doses of thoracic irradiation. The data showed no difference in outcome between the two regimens.

Fox W, Scadding JG: Medical Research Council comparative trial of surgery and radiotherapy for primary treatment of small celled or oat celled carcinoma of the bronchus: Ten year follow-up. Lancet 2:63, 1973.

The 10-year results of a controlled trial of surgery versus a policy of radical radiotherapy in the treatment of small cell lung cancer are reported. The analysis includes 144 patients: 71 patients were allocated at random to surgery and 73 were allocated to radiotherapy. There were no 10-year survivors in the surgical series, but on the radiotherapeutic series, 11 remained well. The mean survival for the surgical series was 199 days and that for the radical radiotherapeutic series was 100 days, which was statistically significant. This reinforced the 5-year report on the same study and became the basis for making radiotherapy standard treatment for SCLC at the time of this trial.

Fukuoka M, Furuse K, Saijo N et al: Randomized trial of cyclophosphamide, doxorubicin and vincristine versus cisplatin and etoposide versus alternation of these regimens in small cell lung cancer. J Natl Cancer Inst 82:855, 1991.

In this article the multicenter randomized comparison of cyclophosphamide, doxorubicin (Adriamycin), and vincristine (CAV) alone versus etoposide and cisplatin alone versus an alternating regimen, starting with the CAV regimen, is described. The alternating and the etoposide and cisplatin regimens gave a higher response rate, but the complete response rates were similar. The response duration on the alternating version was significantly longer than that noted with CAV alone. The survival time was also of borderline significance, but it seemed to be longer with the alternating regimen than with the CAV alone in patients with limited disease. Survival in the alternating therapeutic arm was significantly superior to that in the only CAV arm in patients with limited disease, although it was not superior in those with extensive disease. The authors concluded that alternating chemotherapy was superior to standard chemotherapy.

Gazdar AF, Steinberg SM, Russell EK et al: Correlation of in vitro drug-sensitivity testing results with response to chemotherapy in survival in extensive-stage small cell lung cancer: A prospective clinical trial. J Natl Cancer Inst 82:117, 1990.

The results of a clinical protocol in which specimens were obtained from metastatic sites during routine staging procedures in a group of patients undergoing treatment for proven extensive small cell lung cancer are described. After initial staging procedures including biopsy, patients were treated with etoposide and cisplatin. During the initial 12 weeks of therapy, tumor cells from tumor-containing specimens were examined and in vitro drug sensitivity testing was carried out. When possible, after 12 weeks, the patients were restaged, and where appropriate tissue was available, post-therapy samples were taken for in vitro sensitivity testing. When the in vitro drug sensitivity testing data were available, the patients with partial or no response and those who had relapses after complete response to primary therapy were switched to the best in vitro regimen. If these data were not available, an empiric combination of cyclophosphamide, doxorubicin, and vincristine was administered. The authors concluded that the selection of individual chemotherapy is labor intensive but feasible.

Ginsberg RJ: Surgery and small cell lung cancer: An overview. Lung Cancer 5:232, 1989.

This article is an overview of the role of surgery in the management of patients with SCLC. Surgery in very early disease and its role after neoadjuvant chemotherapy in patients who do not respond to induction chemotherapy are examined.

Karrer K, Ulsperger E: Surgery for cure followed by chemotherapy in small cell carcinoma of the lung. For the ISC Lung Cancer Study Group. Acta Oncol 34:899–906, 1995.

This manuscript summarizes the experience of a multi-institutional prospective data collection group in the management of SCLC in patients who received surgery followed by chemotherapy. The authors indicate that complete surgical resection followed by chemotherapy has relatively satisfactory 5-year survival rates when compared with similarly staged groups of patients with resected non–small cell lung cancer.

Miller AB: Epidemiology, prevention and prognostic factors, and natural history of lung cancer. Curr Opin Oncol 4:286, 1992.

Data on active and passive smoking, occupational hazards, and diet as causes of lung cancer are described. Information on prognostic factors is also presented. The author concludes that additional and larger studies are needed to prove that passive smoking causes lung cancer in this disease but that a reasonable conclusion remains that passive smoking is a health risk. The author added that lactate dehydrogenase has been proved to be a significant prognostic factor and that additional markers should be sought.

Perry MC, Eaton WL, Propert KJ et al: Chemotherapy with or without radiation therapy in limited small-cell carcinoma of the lung. N Engl J Med 316:916, 1987.

This randomized controlled trial was designed to clarify the role of thoracic radiotherapy in patients with limited SCLC. The chemotherapy used consisted of cyclophosphamide, etoposide, and vincristine, with doxorubicin subsequently replacing etoposide in alternating cycles 7 through 18. Chemotherapy was given every 3 weeks for 18 months. Radiotherapy was given either initially (starting on day 1 of cycle 1), after three initial cycles of chemotherapy, or not at all. There was a significant survival benefit for those receiving radiotherapy but not according to the order in which they received it. This is one of the classic articles describing a positive outcome of thoracic irradiation therapy, which proved to be the correct observation based on a meta-analysis of many such studies.

Stahel RA: Morphology, surface antigens, staging and prognostic factors of small cell lung cancer. Curr Opin Oncol 4:308, 1992.

Advances in the field of SCLC are described. The author concludes that the morphologic and biologic properties of SCLC change with chemotherapy toward a non–SCLC and well-differentiated neural endocrine phenotype. This may in part be responsible for drug resistance. The author emphasizes that these data suggest a benefit to irradiating patients with limited disease, and therefore, it becomes important to focus on cost-effective ways of anatomic staging. He recommends that efforts to analyze pretreatment prognostic factors be continued.

Tsai CM, Ihde DC, Kadoyami C et al: Correlation of in vitro sensitivity testing of long-term small cell lung cancer cell lines with response and survival. Eur J Cancer 26:1148, 1990.

The authors gave patients four 3-week cycles of etoposide and cisplatin and performed in vitro sensitivity testing using the Weisenthal dye exclusion assay on material collected during pretherapy diagnostic staging procedures. They found that the in vitro sensitivity of long-term SCLC cell lines predicted the clinical response and survival. They concluded that the use of human tumor cell lines to screen for the in vitro sensitivity of new drugs might be done in a similar manner.

Turrisi AT: Brain irradiation and systemic chemotherapy for small cell lung cancer: Dangerous liaisons? J Clin Oncol 8:196, 1990.

This is an editorial comment on two articles in the specified issue of this journal. One shows significant long-term toxicity from prophylactic cranial irradiation (PCI) in patients with SCLC, and the other shows little compared with similar-aged patients who did not receive such treatment. Turrisi attempts to identify reasons for the differences in the two articles. He suggests that the timing of the PCI may be the important variable. He also implicates the difference in the systemic agents that were used as possible causes of this problem. He concludes that PCI should probably be reserved for selected patients because it does not affect survival, and he recommends additional randomized trials to address this subject.

■ REFERENCES

Aapro MS: 5-HT3 receptor antagonists: An overview of their present status and future potential in cancer therapy–induced emesis. Drugs 42:551, 1991.

Albain KS, Crowley JJ, LeBlanc M et al: Determinants of improved outcome in small-cell lung cancer: An analysis of the 2,580-patient Southwest Oncology Group data base. J Clin Oncol 8:1563, 1990.

Anderson H, Gurney H, Thatcher N et al: Recombinant human GMCSF in small cell lung cancer: A phase I/II study. Recent Results Cancer Res 121:155, 1991a.

Anderson H, Lund B, Hansen HH et al: Phase II study of gemcitabine in non small cell lung cancer (NSCLC) (Abstract). Proc Am Soc Clin Oncol 10:247, 1991b.

Aroney RS, Aisner J, Wesley MN et al: Value of prophylactic cranial irradiation in prevention of central nervous system metastases in small cell lung cancer: Potential benefit restricted to patients with complete response. Cancer Treat Rev 67:675, 1983.

Arriagada R, Ihde DC, Johnson DH et al: Meta-analysis of randomized trials evaluating the role of thoracic radiotherapy in limited small cell lung carcinoma (SCLC) (Abstract). Presented at the 6th World Conference on Lung Cancer, Melbourne, November 10–14, 1991. Lung Cancer 7(Suppl):98, 1991.

Arriagada R, Pignon JP, Le Chevalier TL: Thoracic radiotherapy in small cell lung cancer: Rationale for timing and fractionation. Lung Cancer 5:237, 1989.

Asamura H, Ginsberg RJ: Treatment of small cell lung cancer: Surgery. In Hansen HH (ed): The International Association for the Study of Lung Cancer Textbook of Lung Cancer. London, Martin Dunitz, 2000, pp 243–249.

Auperin A, Arriagada R, Pignon JP, Le Pechoux C et al. Prophylactic cranial irradiation for patients with small-cell lung cancer in complete remission. N Engl J Med 341:476, 1999.

Banham SW, Henderson AF, Bicknell S et al: High dose epirubicin chemotherapy in untreated poorer prognosis small cell lung cancer. Respir Med 84:241, 1990.

Beiler DD, Kane RC, Bernath AM et al: Low dose elective brain irradiation in small cell carcinoma of the lung. Int J Radiat Oncol Biol Phys 5:941, 1979.

Beith J, Clark SJ, Woods RL et al: Long term followup of a randomized trial of combined chemoradiotherapy induction therapy with and without maintenance chemotherapy in patients with small cell carcinoma of the lung. Eur J Cancer 32A:438, 1996.

Berendsen HH, de-Leij L, Postmus PE et al: Detection of small cell lung cancer metastases in bone marrow aspirates using monoclonal antibody directed against neuroendocrine differentiation antigen. J Clin Pathol 41:273, 1988.

Bergsagel DE, Jenkin RDT, Pringle JF et al: Lung cancer: Clinical trial of radiotherapy alone vs. radiotherapy plus cyclophosphamide. Cancer 30:621, 1972.

Biran H, Feld R, Malkin A: Circulating arginine-vasopressin, calcitonin, carcinoembryonic antigen, neuron-specific enolase, and beta-2 microglobulin fluctuations during combined modality induction therapy for small-cell bronchogenic carcinoma: Association of postchemotherapy AVP surge with high tumor response rate and durable remission. Tumour Biol 12:131, 1991.

Bishop JF, Morstyn G, Stuart-Harris R et al: Dose and schedule of granulocyte macrophage colony stimulating factor (GM-CSF) carboplatin and etoposide in small cell lung cancer (SCLC) (Abstract). Proc Am Soc Clin Oncol 10:240, 1991.

Blackstein M, Eisenhauer EA, Wierzbicki R et al: Epirubicin in extensive small-cell lung cancer: A phase II study in previously untreated patients. A National Cancer Institute of Canada Clinical Trials Group Study. J Clin Oncol 8:385, 1990.

Bonadonna G: Chemotherapy strategies to improve the control of Hodgkin's disease: The Richard and Hinda Rosenthal Foundation Award Lecture. Cancer Res 42:4309, 1982.

Bonomi P, O'Reilly WO, Vogl SE et al: Intensive induction treatment of small cell bronchogenic carcinoma with cyclophosphamide, methotrexate and etoposide. Cancer Treat Rev 69:1007, 1985.

Brooks BJ Jr, Seifler EJ, Walsh TE et al: Pulmonary toxicity with combined modality therapy for limited stage small-cell lung cancer. J Clin Oncol 4:200, 1986.

Bunn PA, Lichter AS, Makuch RW et al: Chemotherapy alone or chemotherapy with chest radiation therapy in limited stage small cell lung cancer. Ann Intern Med 106:655, 1987.

Bunn PA Jr, Ihde DC: Small cell bronchogenic carcinoma: A review of therapeutic results. In Livingston BB (ed): Lung Cancer. 1. Boston, Martinus Nijhoff, 1981, p 169.

Campling B, Quirt IC, DeBoer G et al: Is bone marrow examination in small-cell lung cancer really necessary? Ann Intern Med 105:508, 1986.

Canellos GP: Can MOPP be replaced in the treatment of advanced Hodgkin's disease? Semin Oncol 17:2, 1990.

Carmichael J: The role of gemcitabine in the treatment of other tumours. Br J Cancer 3:21, 1998.

Carney D: Lung cancer biology. Curr Opin Oncol 3:288, 1991.

Carney D: The biology of lung cancer. Curr Opin Oncol 4:292, 1992.

Carney DN: Prophylactic cranial irradiation and small-cell lung cancer (Editorial). N Engl J Med 341:524–526, 1999.

Carney DN, Grogan L, Smit EF et al: Single-agent oral etoposide for elderly small cell lung cancer patients. Semin Oncol 17(Suppl 2):49, 1990.

Carney DN, Redmond 0, Harford P et al: Bone marrow involvement (BMI) by small cell lung cancer (SCLC) using magnetic resonance imaging (MRI) (Abstract). Proc Am Soc Clin Oncol 9:228, 1989.

Clark PI, Cottier B, Joel S et al: Prolonged administration of single agent oral etoposide in patients with untreated small cell lung cancer (SCLC) (Abstract). Proc Am Soc Clin Oncol 9:226, 1990.

Clark P, Cottier B, Joel S et al: Two prolonged schedules of single agent oral etoposide of differing duration and dose in patients with untreated small cell lung cancer (SCLC) (Abstract). Proc Am Soc Clin Oncol 10:268, 1991.

Cohen MH, Chretien PB, Ihde DC et al: Thymosin fraction V and intensive combination chemotherapy: Prolonging the survival of patients with small cell lung cancer. JAMA 241:1813, 1979.

Cohen MH, Creaven PJ, Fossieck BE Jr et al: Intensive chemotherapy of small cell bronchogenic carcinoma. Cancer Treat Rev 61:349, 1977.

Coolen L, van den Eeckhout A, Deneffe G et al: Surgical treatment of small cell lung cancer. Eur J Cardiothorac Surg 9:59–64, 1995.

Cox JD, Petrovich A, Paig C et al: Prophylactic cranial irradiation in patients with inoperable carcinoma of the lung: Preliminary report of a cooperative trial. Cancer 42:1135, 1978.

Coy P, Hodson I, Payne DG et al: The effect of dose of thoracic irradiation on recurrence in patients with limited stage small cell lung cancer: Initial results of a Canadian multicenter randomized trial. Int J Radiat Oncol Biol Phys 14:219, 1988.

Crawford J, Ozer H, Stoller R et al: Reduction by granulocyte colony stimulating factor of fever and neutropenia induced by chemotherapy in patients with small-cell lung cancer. N Engl J Med 325:164, 1991.

Creech R, Richter M, Finkelstein D: Combination chemotherapy with or without consolidation radiation therapy (RT) for regional small cell carcinoma of the lung (Abstract). Proc Am Soc Clin Oncol 7:196, 1988.

Davis S, Crino L, Tonato M et al: A prospective analysis of chemotherapy following surgical resection of clinical stage I–II small-cell lung cancer. Am J Clin Oncol 16:93, 1993.

Eagen RT, Frytak S, Lee RE et al: A case for preplanned thoracic and prophylactic whole brain irradiation therapy in limited small cell lung cancer. Cancer Clin Trials 4:261, 1981.

Eberhardt W, Niederle N: Ifosfamide in non-small cell lung cancer: A review. Semin Oncol 19(Suppl 1):40, 1992.

Eckhardt S, Kolaric K, Vukas D et al: Phase II study of 4′-epidoxorubicin in patients with untreated, extensive small cell lung cancer. Med Oncol Tumor Pharmacother 7:19, 1990.

Einhorn LH, Pennington K, McClean J: Phase II trial of daily oral VP-16 in refractory small cell lung cancer: A Hoosier Oncology Group study. Semin Oncol 17(Suppl 2):32, 1990.

Elliott JA, Osterlind K, Hansen HH: Cyclic alternating "non-cross resistant" chemotherapy in the management of small cell anaplastic carcinoma of the lung. Cancer Treat Rev 11:103, 1984.

Ettinger DS: Evaluation of new drugs in untreated patients with small-cell lung cancer: its time has come. J Clin Oncol 8:374, 1990.

Ettinger DS, Finkelstein DM, Sarma RP et al: Phase II study of paclitaxel in patients with extensive disease small cell lung cancer: An Eastern Cooperative Oncology Group study. J Clin Oncol 13:1430–1435, 1995.

Evans WK, Eisenhauer EA, Cormier Y et al: Phase II study of amonafide: Results of treatment and lessons learned from the study of an investigational agent in previously untreated patients with extensive small-cell lung cancer. J Clin Oncol 8:390, 1990.

Evans WK, Feld R, Murray N et al: Superiority of alternating noncross-resistant chemotherapy in extensive small cell lung cancer: A multicenter randomized clinical trial by the National Cancer Institute of Canada. Ann Lat Med 107:450, 1987.

Evans WK, Stewart DJ, Maroun J et al: Oral VP-16 and carboplatin for small cell lung cancer (Abstract). Proc Am Soc Clin Oncol 10:247, 1991.

Feld R: Complications associated with the treatment of small cell lung cancer. Lung Cancer 10(Suppl):S307, 1994.

Feld R: Complications in the treatment of small cell carcinoma of the lung. Cancer Treat Rev 8:5, 1981.

Feld R: Late complications associated with the treatment of small cell lung cancer. Cancer Treat Res 45:301, 1989.

Feld R: Lung and mediastinum: Editorial overview. Curr Opin Oncol 2:309, 1990.

Feld R: Lung and mediastinum: Editorial overview. Curr Opin Oncol 4:283, 1992.

Feld R, Evans WL, Coy P et al: Canadian multicentre randomized trial comparing sequential and alternating administration of two non-cross resistant chemotherapy combinations in patients with limited small cell carcinoma of the lung. J Clin Oncol 5:1401, 1987.

Feld R, Evans WK, DeBoer G et al: Combined modality induction therapy without maintenance chemotherapy for small cell carcinoma of the lung. J Clin Oncol 2:294, 1984.

Feld R, Ginsberg R, Payne DG: Treatment of small cell lung cancer. In Roth JA, Ruckdeschel JC, Weisenburger TH (eds): Thoracic Oncology. Philadelphia, WB Saunders, 1988, p 229.

Feld R, Wierzbicki R, Walde D et al: Phase I–II study of high dose epirubucin in advanced non-small cell lung cancer. J Clin Oncol 20:297, 1992.

Figueredo A, Arnold A, Goodyear M et al: Addition of verapamil and tamoxifen to the initial chemotherapy of small cell lung cancer: A phase I/II study. Cancer 65:1895, 1990.

Fleck JF, Einhorn LH, Lauer RC et al: Is prophylactic cranial irradiation indicated in small-cell lung cancer? J Clin Oncol 8:209, 1990.

Fox RM, Tattersall MHN, Woods RL: Radiation therapy as an adjuvant in small cell lung cancer treated by combination chemotherapy: A randomized study (Abstract). Proc Am Soc Clin Oncol 22:502, 1981.

Fox RM, Woods RL, Brodie GN et al: A randomized study: Small cell anaplastic lung cancer treated by combination chemotherapy and adjuvant radiotherapy. Int J Radiat Oncol Biol Phys 6:1083, 1980.

Fox W, Scadding JG: Medical Research Council comparative trial of surgery and radiotherapy for primary treatment of small celled or oat celled carcinoma of the bronchus: Ten year follow-up. Lancet 2:63, 1973.

Friess GG, McCracken JD, Troxell ML et al: Effect of initial resection of small-cell carcinoma of the lung: A review of Southwest Oncology Group Study 7628. J Clin Oncol 3:964, 1985.

Fukuoka M, Furuse K, Saijo N et al: Randomized trial of cyclophosphamide, doxorubicin, and vincristine versus cisplatin and etoposide versus alternation of these regimens in small cell lung cancer. J Natl Cancer Inst 83:855, 1991.

Gazdar AF, Steinberg SM, Russell EK et al: Correlation of in vitro drug-sensitivity testing results with response to chemotherapy in survival in extensive-stage small cell lung cancer: A prospective clinical trial. J Natl Cancer Inst 82:117, 1990.

Ginsberg RJ: Surgery and small cell lung cancer: An overview. Lung Cancer 5:232, 1989.

Ginsberg RJ, Karrer K: Surgery in small cell lung cancer. Lung Cancer 5:139, 1989.

Girling DJ: Prospective randomised trial of 3 or 6 courses of etoposide, cyclophosphamide, methotrexate and vincristine and of 6 courses of etoposide and ifosfamide in small cell lung cancer (SCLC) (Abstract). For the British Medical Research Council Lung Cancer Working Party. Presented at the 6th World Conference on Lung Cancer, Melbourne, November 10–14, 1991. Lung Cancer 7(Suppl):103, 1991.

Girling DJ, Thatcher N, Clark PI et al: Comparison of oral etoposide and standard intravenous multidrug chemotherapy for small cell lung cancer: A stopped multicentre randomized trial. Lancet 348:563, 1996.

Goldie JH, Coldman AJ: The genetic origin of drug resistance in neoplasms: Implications for systemic therapy. Cancer Res 44:3643, 1984.

Goldie JH, Coldman AJ, Gudavskas GA: Rationale for the use of alternating non-cross resistant chemotherapy. Cancer Treat Rev 66:439, 1982.

Goodwin PJ, Feld R, Evans WK: Cost-effectiveness of cancer chemotherapy: An economic evaluation of a randomized trial in small cell lung cancer. J Clin Oncol 6:1537, 1988.

Grant SC, Gralla RJ, Kris MG et al: Single-agent chemotherapy trials in small-cell lung cancer, 1970 to 1990: The case for studies in previously treated patients. J Clin Oncol 10:484, 1992.

Greco FA, Perez C, Einhorn LH et al: Combination chemotherapy with or without concurrent thoracic radiotherapy (RT) in limited stage (LD) small cell lung cancer (SCLC): A phase III trial of the Southeastern Cancer Study Group (SEG) (Abstract). Proc Am Soc Clin Oncol 5:178, 1986.

Green JA, Trillet VN, Manegold C: 4-MetHuG-CSf (G-CSF) with CDE chemotherapy (CT) in small cell lung cancer (SCLC): Interim results from a randomized, placebo controlled trial (Abstract). For the European G-CSF Lung Cancer Study Group. Proc Am Soc Clin Oncol 10:243, 1991.

Green RA, Humphrey E, Close H et al: Alkylating agents and bronchogenic carcinoma. Am J Med 46:516, 1969.

Hansen HH, Dombornowsky P, Hirsch FR et al: Prophylactic irradiation in bronchogenic small cell anaplastic carcinoma. Cancer 46:279, 1980.

Hansen M: Paraneoplastic syndrome and tumor markers for small cell and non–small cell lung cancer. Curr Opin Oncol 2:345, 1990.

Havemann MWK: Alternating chemotherapy in small cell lung cancer. Onkologie 13:157, 1990.

Higgins GA, Shields TW, Keehn RJ: The solitary pulmonary nodule: Ten-year follow-up of Veterans Administration–Armed Forces Cooperative study. Arch Surg 110:570, 1975.

Hirsch F: Staging and prognostic factors. 1. Staging procedures. Lung Cancer 5:152, 1989.

Holst JJ, Hansen M, Bork E et al: Elevated plasma concentration of C-flanking gastrin-releasing peptide in small cell lung cancer. J Clin Oncol 7:1831, 1989.

Hryniuk WM, Figueredo A, Goodyear M: Applications of dose intensity to problems of chemotherapy of breast and colorectal cancer. Semin Oncol 14:3, 1987.

Ihde DC: Staging evaluation and prognostic factors in small cell lung cancer. p. 241. In Aisner J (ed): Lung Cancer. Contemporary Issues in Clinical Oncology, Vol. 3. New York, Churchill Livingstone, 1985, p 241.

Ihde DC, Makuch RW, Carney DN et al: Prognostic implications of stage of disease and sites of metastases in patients with small cell carcinoma of the lung treated with intensive combination chemotherapy. Am Rev Respir Dis 123:500, 1981.

Ihde DC, Mulshine J, Kramer B et al: Randomized trial of high vs. standard dose etoposide (VP16) and cisplatin in extensive small cell lung cancer (SCLC) (Abstract). Presented at the 6th World Conference on Lung Cancer, Melbourne, November 10–14, 1991. Proc Am Soc Clin Oncol 10:240, 1991.

Jaakkimainen L, Goodwin PJ, Pater J et al: Counting the costs of chemotherapy in a National Cancer Institute of Canada randomized trial in non-small cell lung cancer. J Clin Oncol 8:1301, 1990.

Jackson DV, Richards F, Cooper R et al: Prophylactic cranial irradiation in small cell carcinoma of the lung: A randomized study. JAMA 237:2730, 1977.

Johnson BE, Salem C, Nesbitt J et al: Limited (Ltd) stage small cell lung cancer (SCLC) treated with concurrent BID chest radiotherapy (RT) and etoposide cisplating (VP/PT) followed by chemotherapy (CT) selected by in vitro drug sensitivity testing (DST) (Abstract). Presented at the 6th World Conference on Lung Cancer, Melbourne, November 10–14. Lung Cancer 7(Suppl):152, 1991a.

Johnson DH: New drugs in the management of SCLC. Lung Cancer 5:221, 1989.

Johnson DH: Overview of ifosphamide in small cell and non-small cell lung cancer. Semin Oncol 17(Suppl 4):24, 1990.

Johnson DH, Turrisi AT, Chang AY et al: Alternating chemotherapy (CT) and thoracic radiotherapy (TRT) in limited small cell lung cancer (LSCLC): A test of the Looney hypothesis (Abstract). For the Eastern Cooperative Oncology Group. Proc Am Soc Clin Oncol 10:243, 1991b.

Karrer K, Denck H, Karnicka-Mlofkowska H et al: Multi-modality treatment after surgery for cure of small cell lung cancer (SCLC) (Abstract). Lung Cancer 4:A153, 1988.

Karrer K, Shields T: The importance of complete resection in the multimodality treatment of SCLC (Abstract). For ISC-Lung Cancer Study Group. Presented at the 6th World Conference on Lung Cancer, Melbourne, November 10–14, 1991. Lung Cancer 7(Suppl):71, 1991.

Karrer K, Ulsperger E: Surgery for cure followed by chemotherapy in small cell carcinoma of the lung. For the ISC-Lung Cancer Study Group. Acta Oncol 34:899, 1995.

Katsenis AT, Karpasitis N, Giannakakis J et al: Elective brain irradiation in patients with small-cell carcinoma of the lung: Preliminary report. In Lung Cancer International Congress Series. Excerpta Medica, 1982, p 277.

Kelley MJ, Linnoila RI, Avis IL et al: Antitumor activity of a monoclonal antibody directed against gastrin-releasing peptide in patients with small cell lung cancer. Chest 112:256–261, 1997.

Kies MS, Mira JC, Livingston RB et al: Multimodal therapy for limited small cell lung cancer: A randomized study of induction chemotherapy with or without thoracic radiation in complete responders and with wide field versus reduced volume radiation in partial responders. J Clin Oncol 5:592, 1987.

Klastersky J: Diagnosis and staging in small cell lung cancer. Curr Opin Oncol 2:331, 1990.

Kristjansen PEG: The role of cranial irradiation in the management of patients with SCLC. Lung Cancer 5:264, 1989.

Kristjansen PEG, Osterland K, Dombernowsky P et al: A three armed randomized trial in small cell lung cancer (SCLC) of two induction regimens with tenoposide and cisplatin or carboplatin followed by alternating chemotherapy versus alternating chemotherapy (Abstract). Lung Cancer 7(Suppl):121, 1991.

Lad T, Thomas P, Piantadosi S: Surgical resection of small cell lung cancer: A prospective randomized evaluation (Abstract). Presented at the 6th World Conference on Lung Cancer, Melbourne, November 10–14, 1991. Lung Cancer 7(Suppl):162, 1991b.

Lad T, Thomas P, Piantadosi S et al: Thoracotomy staging of small cell lung cancer (Abstract). Presented at the 6th World Conference on Lung Cancer, Melbourne, November 10–14, 1991. Lung Cancer 7(Suppl):53 1991a.

Lad T, Wagner H, Piantadosi S: Randomized phase II evaluation of preoperative chemotherapy alone and radiotherapy alone in stage IIIA non-small cell lung cancer (Abstract). Proc Am Soc Clin Oncol 10:258, 1991c.

Laetrille J, Cormier Y, Martins H et al: Phase II study of docetaxel (Taxotere) in patients with previously treated extensive small cell lung cancer. Invest New Drugs 13:342–345, 1996.

LeBeau B, Chastang CL, Brechot JM: Small cell lung cancer (SCLC): Long term results of a randomized trial assessing chemotherapy continuation in patients reaching complete remission after six courses (Abstract). For the "Petites Cellules" Group (02PC 83 protocol). Presented at the 6th World Conference on Lung Cancer, Melbourne, November 10–14, 1991. Lung Cancer 7(Suppl):130, 1991.

Lewis JW Jr, Pearlberg JL, Beute GH et al: Can computed tomography of the chest stage lung cancer? Yes and no. Ann Thorac Surg 49:591, 1990.

Lishner M, Feld R, Payne DG et al: Late neurological complications after prophylactic cranial irradiation in patients with small-cell lung cancer: The Toronto experience. J Clin Oncol 8:215, 1990.

Livingston RG: Current chemotherapy of small cell lung cancer. Chest 89:258S, 1986.

Lucchi M, Mussi A, Chella A et al: Surgery in the management of small cell lung cancer. Eur J Cariothorac Surg 12:689–693, 1997.

Lund B, Anderson H, Walling J et al: Phase II study of gemcitabine in non-small cell lung cancer (NSCLC) (Abstract). Presented at the 6th World Conference on Lung Cancer Melbourne, November 10–14, 1991. Lung Cancer 7:121, 1991.

Maassen W, Greschuchna D: Small cell carcinoma of the lung: To operate or not? Surgical experience and results. Thorac Cardiovasc Surg 34:71, 1986.

Mattson K, Nilranen A, Holsti LR et al: Natural alpha interferon as maintenance therapy for small cell lung cancer (Abstract). Presented at the 6th World Conference on Lung Cancer, Melbourne, November 10–14, 1991. Lung Cancer 7(Suppl):127, 1991.

Maurer LH, Tulloh M, Weiss RB et al: A randomized combined modality trial in small cell carcinoma of the lung: Comparison of combination chemotherapy-radiation therapy versus cyclophosphamide-radiation therapy. Effects of maintenance chemotherapy and whole brain irradiation. Cancer 45:30, 1980.

Merkle NM, Mickisch GH, Kayser K et al: Surgical resection and adjuvant chemotherapy for small cell carcinoma. Thorac Cardiovasc Surg 34:71–76, 1986.

Meyer JA, Comis RL, Ginsberg SJ: Selective surgical resection in small cell carcinoma of the lung. J Thorac Cardiovasc Surg 84:641, 1982.

Meyer JA, Gullo JJ, Ikins PM et al: Adverse prognostic effect of N2 disease in treatment of small cell carcinoma of the lung. J Thorac Cardiovasc Surg 88:495, 1984.

Miller AB: Epidemiology, prevention and prognostic factors, and natural history of lung cancer. Curr Opin Oncol 4:286, 1992.

Miller AB, Fox W, Tall R: Five-year follow-up of the Medical Research Council's comparative trial of surgery and radiotherapy for the primary treatment of small celled carcinoma or oat celled carcinoma of the bronchus. Lancet 12:501, 1969.

Milroy R, Paul J, Cram L et al: Randomised clinical study of verapamil in addition to chemotherapy in small cell lung cancer (SCLC) (Abstract). Presented at the 6th World Conference on Lung Cancer, Melbourne, November 10–14, 1991. Lung Cancer 7(Suppl):114, 1991.

Minna JD, Pass H, Glatstein H et al: Cancer of the lung. In De Vita VT Sr, Hellman S, Rosenberg S (eds): Cancer: Principles and Practice of Oncology, 3rd ed. Philadelphia, JB Lippincott, 1989, p 591.

Miyazawa N, Tsuchiya R, Naruke T et al: A clinicopathological study of surgical treatment of small cell carcinoma of the lung. Jpn J Clin Oncol 16:297–307, 1986.

Morstyn G, Ihde DC, Lichter AS et al: Small cell lung cancer 1973–1983: Early progress and recent obstacles. Int J Radiat Oncol Biol Phys 10:515, 1984.

Mountain C: Clinical biology of small cell lung cancer: Relationship to surgical therapy. Semin Oncol 5:272, 1978.

Mountain C: A new international staging system for lung cancer. Chest 89:225S, 1986.

Mountain C: Revisions in the international system for staging lung cancer. Chest 111:1710, 1997.

Muller LC, Salzer G, Huber H, et al: Multimodal therapy of small cell lung cancer in TNM stage I through IIIa. Ann Thorac Surg 54:493–497, 1992.

Murphy PB, Hainsworth JD, Greco FA et al: Cisplatin (P) and prolonged administration of oral etoposide (E) in extensive small cell lung cancer (ESCLC) patients (PT): A phase II trial (Abstract). Proc Am Soc Clin Oncol 10:257, 1991.

Murray N, Coy P, Pater J et al: The importance of timing for thoracic irradiation (TI) in the combined modality treatment of limited stage small cell lung cancer (LSCLC) (Abstract). Proc Am Soc Clin Oncol 10:243, 1991a.

Murray N, Livingston RB, Shepherd FA et al: Randomized study of

CODE versus alternative CAV/EP for extensive-stage small cell lung cancer: An intergroup study of the National Cancer Institute of Canada Clinical Trials Group and the Southwest Oncology Group. J Clin Oncol 17:8, 1999.

Murray N, Shah A, Osoba D et al: Dose-intensive chemotherapy (CODE) for non-small cell lung cancer (NSCLC) (Abstract). Proc Am Soc Clin Oncol 8:219, 1989.

Murray N, Shah A, Osoba D et al: Intensive weekly chemotherapy for the treatment of extensive-stage small-cell lung cancer. J Clin Oncol 9:1632, 1991b.

Myer JA, Comis RL, Ginsberg RJ et al: Phase II trial of extended indications for resection in small cell carcinoma of the lung. J Thorac Cardiovasc Surg 83:12, 1982.

Nou E, Brodin O, Bergh J: A randomized study of radiation treatment in small cell bronchial carcinoma treated with two types of four drug chemotherapy regimens. Cancer 62:1079, 1988.

Ohnoshi T, Hiraki S, Kawahara S et al: Randomized trial comparing chemotherapy alone and chemotherapy plus chest irradaition in limited stage small cell lung cancer: A preliminary report. Jpn J Clin Oncol 16:271, 1986.

Ohta M, Hara N, Ichinose Y: The role of surgical resection in the management of small cell carcinoma of the lung. Jpn J Clin Oncol 16:289–296, 1986.

Ormrod D, Spencer CM: Topotecan: A review of its efficacy in small cell lung cancer. Drugs 58:3, 1999.

Osterlind K, Hansen HH, Hansen H et al: Chemotherapy versus chemotherapy plus irradiation in limited small cell lung cancer: Results of a controlled trial with 5 years follow-up. Br J Cancer 54:7, 1986.

Osterlind K, Hansen M, Hansen H et al: Influence of surgical resection prior to chemotherapy on long-term results in small cell lung cancer: A study of 150 operable patients. Eur J Cancer Clin Oncol 5:589–593, 1989.

Osterlind K, Hansen M, Hansen H et al: Treatment policy of surgery in small cell carcinoma of the lung: Retrospective analysis of a series of 874 consecutive patients. Thorax 40:272, 1985.

Perez CA, Einhorn L, Oldham RK et al: Randomized trial of radiotherapy to the thorax in limited chemotherapy and elective brain irradiation: a preliminary report. J Clin Oncol 2:1200, 1984.

Perry MC, Eaton WL, Propert KJ et al: Chemotherapy with or without radiation therapy in limited small-cell carcinoma of the lung. N Engl J Med 316:916, 1987.

Pfister DG, Wells CK, Chan CK et al: Classifying clinical severity to help solve problems of stage migration in nonconcurrent comparisons of lung cancer therapy. Cancer Res 50:4664, 1990.

Postmus PE, Schramel FM, Smit EF et al: Evaluation of new drugs in small cell lung cancer: The activity of gemcitabine. Semin Oncol 9:79–82, 1998.

Prignot J, Humblet Y, Francis C et al: A randomized trial for small cell lung cancer: Late intensification chemotherapy or not (Abstract). Proceedings of the IV World Conference on Lung Cancer, Toronto, August 25–30, 1985.

Rapp E, Pater J, Willan A et al: Chemotherapy can prolong survival in patients with advanced non-small cell lung cancer. A report of the Canadian Multicentre Trial. J Clin Oncol 6:633, 1988.

Rawson NSB, Peto J: An overview of prognostic factors in small cell lung cancer: A report of prognostic factors in small cell lung cancer. A report of the Subcommittee for the Management of Lung Cancer in the United Kingdom, Co-ordinating Committee on Cancer Research. Br J Cancer 61:597, 1990.

Richardson GE, Venzon DJ, Steinberg SM et al: An algorithm for staging patients (PTS) with small cell lung cancer (SCLC) can save 40% of the initial evaluation costs (Abstract). Proc Am Soc Clin Oncol 10:242, 1991.

Roth BJ, Johnson DH, Einhorn LH et al: Randomized study of cyclophosphamide, doxorubicin, and vincristine versus etoposide and cisplatin versus alternation of these two regimens in extensive small cell lung cancer: A phase III trial of the Southeastern Cancer Study Group. J Clin Oncol 10:282, 1992.

Rubin P, Casarett GI: A direction for clinical radiation pathology. Front Radiat Ther Oncol 6:1, 1972.

Sagman U, Feld R, Evans WK et al: The prognostic significance of pretreatment serum lactate dehydrogenase in patients with small cell lung cancer. J Clin Oncol 9:954, 1991a.

Sagman U, Feld R, Evans WK et al: The prognostic significance of pretreatment serum lactate dehydrogenase in patients with small cell lung cancer. J Clin Oncol 2:1, 1997.

Sagman U, Lishner M, Maki E et al: Second primary malignancies following the diagnosis of small cell lung cancer. J Clin Oncol 10:1525, 1992.

Sagman U, Maki E, Evans WK et al: Small cell carcinoma of the lung: Derivation of a prognostic staging system. J Clin Oncol 9:1639, 1991b.

Salzer GM, Muller LC, Huber H et al: Operation for N2 small-cell lung carcinoma. Ann Thorac Surg 49:759, 1990.

Santoro A, Bonadonna G, Valagussa P et al: Long-term results of combination chemotherapy-radiotherapy approach in Hodgkin's disease: Superiority of ABVD plus radiotherapy versus MOPP plus radiotherapy. J Clin Oncol 5:27, 1987.

Schaake-Konig C, van den Bogaert W, Dalesio O et al: Effects of concomitant cisplatin and radiotherapy on inoperable non-small cell lung cancer. N Engl J Med 326:524, 1992.

Sculier JP, Feld R, Evans WK et al: Carcinoembryonic antigen: A useful prognostic marker in small cell lung cancer. J Clin Oncol 3:1349, 1985.

Sculier JP, Paesmans M, Bureau G, et al: Randomized trial comparing induction chemotherapy versus induction chemotherapy followed by maintenance chemotherapy in small cell lung cancer. J Clin Oncol 14:2337, 1996.

Seydel JG, Creech R, Pagano M et al: Combined modality treatment of regional small cell undifferentiated carcinoma of the lung: A cooperative study of the RTOG and ECOG. Int J Radiat Oncol Biol Phys 9:1135, 1983.

Shank B, Sher H: Controversies in treatment of small cell carcinoma of the lung. Cancer Invest 3:367, 1985.

Shank B, Sher H, Hilaris B et al: Increased survival with high dose multifield radiotherapy and intensive chemotherapy in limited small cell carcinoma of the lung. Int J Radiat Oncol Biol Phys 10(Suppl 1):122, 1983.

Shaw SS, Thompson J, Goldstraw P: Results of an operation without adjuvant therapy in treatment of small cell lung cancer. Ann Thorac Surg 54:498–501, 1992.

Shepherd FA, Ginsberg RJ, Evans WK et al: Reduction in local recurrence and improved survival in surgically treated patients with small cell carcinoma of the lung. J Thorac Cardiovasc Surg 86:498, 1983.

Shepherd FA, Ginsberg R, Evans WK et al: "Very limited" small cell lung cancer (SCLC): Results of non-surgical treatment (Abstract). Proc Ann Meet Am Soc Clin Oncol 3:223, 1984.

Shepherd FA, Ginsberg RJ, Feld R et al: Surgical treatment for limited small-cell lung cancer: The University of Toronto Lung Oncology Group experience. J Thorac Cardiovasc Surg 101:385–393, 1991.

Shepherd FA, Ginsberg RJ, Patterson GA et al: A prospective study of adjuvant surgical ressection after chemotherapy for limited small cell lung cancer: A University of Toronto Lung Oncology Group study. J Thorac Cardiovasc Surg 97:177, 1989.

Shields TW, Higgins GA, Matthews NJ et al: Surgical resection in the management of small-cell carcinoma of the lung. J Thorac Cardiovasc Surg 84:481, 1982.

Shore DF, Paneth M: Survival after resection of small cell carcinoma of the bronchus. Thorax 35:819–822, 1980.

Slevin ML, Clark PI, Joel SP et al: A randomized trial to evaluate the effect of schedule on the activity of etoposide in small cell lung cancer. J Clin Oncol 7:1333, 1989.

Smyth JF: The management of small cell anaplastic lung cancer. In Smyth JF (ed): The Management of Lung Cancer. London, Edward Arnold, 1984, p 115.

Smyth JF, Bowman A, Fergusson RJ et al: Potentiation of cisplatin by alpha-interferon in advanced non-small cell lung cancer (NSCLC): A phase II study. Ann Oncol 1:351, 1990.

Sorensen HR, Lund C, Alstrup P: Survival in small cell lung carcinoma after surgery. Thorax 41:478–482, 1986.

Sorensen M, Lassen U, Hansen HH: Current therapy of small cell lung cancer. Curr Opin Oncol 10:133–138, 1998.

Souhami RL, Geddes DM, Spiro SG et al: Radiotherapy in small cell cancer of the lung treated with combination chemotherapy: A controlled trial. Br Med J 288:1643, 1984.

Souhami RL, Harper PG, Linch D et al: High-dose cyclophosphamide with autologous marrow transplantation as initial treatment of small cell carcinoma of the bronchus. Cancer Chemother Pharmacol 8:31, 1982.

Souhami RL, Bradbury I, Geddes DM et al: Prognostic significance of laboratory parameters measured at diagnosis in small cell carcinoma of the lung. Cancer Res 45:2878, 1985a.

Souhami RL, Finn G, Gregory WM et al: High-dose cyclophosphamide in small cell carcinoma of the lung. J Clin Oncol 3:958, 1985b.

Souhami RL, Spiro SG, Rudd RM et al: Five day oral etoposide treatment for advanced small-cell lung cancer: Randomized comparison with intravenous chemotherapy. J Natl Cancer Inst 89:577–580, 1997.

Splinter TAW: Chemotherapy of SCLC: Duration of treatment. Lung Cancer 5:186, 1989.

Splinter TAW: EORTC 08825 induction versus induction plus maintenance chemotherapy in small cell lung cancer: Definitive evaluation (Abstract). For the EORTC Lung Co-operative Group. Proc Am Soc Clin Oncol 7:202, 1988.

Splinter TAW, McVie J, Dalesio O et al: EORTC 08825 induction versus induction plus maintenance chemotherapy (CT) in small cell lung cancer (Abstract). Proc Am Soc Clin Oncol 5:188, 1986.

Stahel RA: Diagnosis, staging and prognostic factors of small cell lung cancer. Curr Opin Oncol 3:306, 1991.

Stahel RA: Morphology, surface antigens, staging and prognostic factors of small cell lung cancer. Curr Opin Oncol 4:308, 1992.

Stahel RA, Aisner J, Ginsberg R et al: Staging and prognostic factors in small cell lung cancer. Lung Cancer 5:119, 1989.

Stahel RA, Mabry M, Skarin AT et al: Detection of bone marrow metastasis in small cell lung cancer by monoclonal antibody. J Clin Oncol 3:455, 1985.

Stevens E, Einhorn L, Sohn R: Treatment of limited small cell cancer (Abstract). Proc Am Assoc Cancer Res 20:435, 1979.

Thatcher N, Lind M: Carboplatin in small cell lung cancer. Semin Oncol 17(Suppl 2):40, 1990.

Thatcher N, Girling DJ, Hopwood P et al: Improving survival without reducing quality of life in small-cell lung cancer patients by increasing the dose-intensity of chemotherapy with granulocyte colony-stimulating factor support: Results of a British Medical Research Council multicenter randomized trial. J Clin Oncol 18:2, 2000.

Thomas ED, Buckner CD, Clift RA et al: Bone marrow transplantation for acute non-lymphoblastic leukemia in first remission. N Engl J Med 301:597, 1979.

Tourani JM, Levy R, Even P et al: Short intensive five drug chemotherapy (CT) followed by intensive irradiation for limited small cell lung cancer (LSCLC): Improved response rate and survival. A pilot study (Abstract). Proc Am Soc Clin Oncol 10:245, 1991.

Tsai CM, Ihde DC, Kadoyami C et al: Correlation of in vitro sensitivity testing of long-term small cell lung cancer cell lines with response and survival. Eur J Cancer 26:1148, 1990.

Turrisi AT: Brain irradiation and systemic chemotherapy for small cell lung cancer: Dangerous liaisons? J Clin Oncol 8:196, 1990.

Turrisi AT: The integration of cisplatin and radiotherapy in the treatment of lung cancer. Semin Oncol 18(Suppl 3):81, 1991.

Turrisi AT, Kim K, Blum R et al: Twice-daily compared with once-daily thoracic radiotherapy in limited small-cell lung cancer treated concurrently with cisplatin and etoposide. N Engl J Med 340:4, 1999.

Velemes M, Polyzos A, Latsi P et al: Optimal duration of chemotherapy in small cell lung cancer: A randomized study of 4 versus 6 cycles of cisplatin-etoposide. J Chemother 10:136–140, 1998.

Wadler S, Lembersky B, Atkins M et al: Phase II trial of fluorouracil and recombinant interferon alfa-2a in patients with advanced colorectal carcinoma: An Eastern Cooperative Oncology Group study. J Clin Oncol 9:1806, 1991.

Wadler S, Schwartz EL, Goldman M et al: Fluorouracil and recombinant alpha-2A-interferon: An active regimen against advanced colorectal carcinoma. J Clin Oncol 7:1769, 1989.

Warde P, Payne D: Does thoracic irradiation improve survival or local control in limited stage small cell carcinoma of the lung? A meta-analysis. J Clin Oncol 10:890, 1992.

Wils J, Utama I, Sala L et al: Phase II study of high dose epirubucin in non-small cell lung cancer. Eur J Cancer 26:1140, 1990.

Woll PJ, Rozengurt E: Therapeutic implications of growth factors in small cell lung cancer. Lung Cancer 5:287, 1989.

Zelen M: Keynote address on biostatistics and data retrieval. Cancer Chemother Rep 4:31, 1973.

Zochbauer-Muller S, Pirker R, Huber H: Treatment of small cell lung cancer patients. Ann Oncol 6:83, 1999.

CHAPTER **34**

Rare Primary Malignant Neoplasms

Robert J. Downey
Maureen Zakowski
Michael Burt

Most primary pulmonary neoplasms are malignant, and of these, most are bronchogenic carcinomas. The uncommon primary malignant neoplasms that arise in the lung are of disparate histogenesis and include pulmonary blastoma, thymoma, carcinosarcoma, intravascular bronchioalveolar tumors, melanomas, teratomas, sarcomas, and lymphoreticular disorders. There is no single accepted classification for these neoplasms. In this chapter, we review the available literature concerning each of these rare malignant neoplasms individually.

OVERVIEW OF CLINICAL PRESENTATIONS

Most rare primary pulmonary malignant tumors have clinical features that mimic those of non–small cell lung cancer (NSCLC). Most patients (50% to 85%) are symptomatic, most commonly with cough, dyspnea, chest pain, or hemoptysis and less commonly with wheezing, fever, fatigue, and weight loss. Investigation of these symptoms leads to radiographs that, with the exception of patients with intravascular bronchioalveolar tumors, typically demonstrate a solitary pulmonary nodule. Although the diagnosis may be suspected or, rarely, made prior to surgical exploration, the histologic diagnosis of a rare malignant primary lung tumor is most commonly made during surgery with the intent of resecting locoregional disease. On the whole, management after diagnosis of most rare primary pulmonary malignancies should follow the guidelines for those of patients with non–small cell cancer.

PULMONARY BLASTOMA

Pulmonary blastomas are malignancies that are composed of a mixture of malignant mesenchymal and epithelial cells that morphologically resemble embryonal lung. As such, these tumors are held to be dysembryonic or dysontogenetic neoplasms, other examples of which are hepatoblastoma, neuroblastoma, and Wilms tumors. Pulmonary blastoma is unique within this group as the only tumor to occur consistently in adulthood rather than childhood.

The first description of pulmonary blastoma was made in 1945 by Barrett and Barnard. They described a 40-year-old woman with influenza, fatigue, weight loss, anemia, and a chest radiograph demonstrating "a circumscribed opacity of even density in the middle of the right lung about as large as a small grapefruit," which was removed by pneumonectomy. In 1952, a follow-up report by Barnard revealed that "the patient has had no further trouble attributable to the tumor since its removal in 1943." The microscopic appearance was described, and the tumor labeled an "embryoma of lung." In 1961, Spencer described three additional cases and coined the term *pulmonary blastoma* because of the similarity of this lesion to nephroblastoma (Wilms tumor), suggesting that analogously the tumor arose from primitive blastematous cells. Recent immunologic evidence to support this view has been provided by Yousem and colleagues (1990) who found a remarkable resemblance between the antigenic profile of blastoma and embryonic lung, as others have found between nephroblastoma and fetal kidney (Albeda et al, 1989). Microscopically, this tumor contains a mixture of epithelial and mesenchymal components, either of which may be dominant. Hemorrhage and necrosis are common features. The epithelial component may be arranged on branched tubules and surrounded by spindle or polygonal stromal cells. The stroma may show cartilaginous, osseous, or skeletal muscle (rhabdoid) differentiation, and metastases may be epithelial, stromal, or both (Fraser et al, 1989; Mackay et al, 1990). Fine-needle aspiration biopsy may characterize the lesion in sufficient detail to allow diagnosis (Francis and Jacobsen, 1979).

Attempts to draw histologic distinctions on the basis of the predominant elements have been made and have led to the recognition of two distinct entities in pulmonary blastoma (PB): first, well-differentiated fetal adenocarcinoma (WDFA), which is composed only of epithelial cells and was first described by Kradin and colleagues (1982); and second, pleuropulmonary blastoma (PPB), which is composed primarily of malignant mesenchyme without epithelial cells (Manivel et al, 1988; Priest et al, 1997).

A second source of confusion in the literature has to do with the similarities between pulmonary blastoma and carcinosarcoma, as both demonstrate features of epithelial and mesenchymal differentiation. For a complete discussion of this controversial area, the reader is referred to the recent review by Berho and colleagues (1995).

Pulmonary blastomas are uncommon. Jacobson and

Francis (1980) reviewed their experience at one hospital in Sweden over the 8-year period from 1971 to 1978 and found 11 cases, representing 0.5% of all lung neoplasms seen during that period. In a review of the English language literature published since the first reported case in 1945, 156 cases of pulmonary blastoma have been sufficiently described to allow analysis, and they have been reviewed in two comprehensive reports by Larsen and Sorensen (1996) and Berho and colleagues (1995). The largest report from a single institution was by Koss and colleagues (1991) from the Armed Forces Institute of Pathology (AFIP) who described 52 patients with pulmonary blastoma. The following discussion summarizes the available information concerning presentation, therapy, and survival contained in these reports.

Of the 156 patients described in the literature, 102 (6%) were male and 54 (34%) were female, for a ratio of 1.9:1. The age at diagnosis ranged from neonatal to 80 years (median, 40 years). The distribution of left (45%) versus right lung (54%) was as expected. At presentation, many patients (40%) were asymptomatic, but approximately 60% had symptoms; in the report from the AFIP, 33% presented with cough, 31% with chest pain, 20% with hemoptysis, 14% with dyspnea, 12% with weight loss, 8% with fever, and 4% with recurrent pneumonia. Most pulmonary blastomas were peripheral and ranged in size from 1 to 28 cm in diameter (median, 7 to 8 cm).

Details regarding treatment are difficult to extract coherently from the literature. The review by Larsen notes that series often combine patients with PB, PPB, and WDFA when discussing therapy and, furthermore, do not separate the effects of surgery, chemotherapy, and radiation, which are often coadministered. However, it appears that most patients who present with evidence of locoregional disease underwent only pulmonary resection. Of the patients not undergoing resection, approximately one half had advanced unresectable locoregional disease (i.e., pleural effusion) and the other half, distant disease. Because of the heterogeneous nature of the reports in the literature, pathologic staging cannot be summarized other than to note that there were reports describing hilar and mediastinal nodal metastases.

Larsen and Sorensen's review of the literature (1996) suggests that the overall prognosis for patients with PB, PPB, or WDFA is poor, with 66%, 84%, and 92% of patients dead within 2, 5, and 10 years, respectively. Prognosis varies according to subgroup. Priest and colleagues (1997) record that patients with PPB have a 5-year survival rate of 48%, similar to the overall 5-year survival rate of approximately 50% of the 52 patients with PB reported by Koss and colleagues (1991) from the AFIP. WDFA appears to be associated with a better prognosis; it was reported by Koss and colleagues (1991) to be approximately an 80% survival rate at 10 years. Most patients who experience recurrences after resection do so with distant metastases, many of them occurring in the brain.

In summary, pulmonary blastoma behaves much like a NSCLC. Given the incomplete information available, the evaluation, indications for surgery, and pulmonary resection probably best follow those of a patient with suspected or proved NSCLC; there is insufficient information available to support recommendation of regimens of chemoradiation therapy.

PRIMARY PULMONARY THYMOMA

A total of 19 cases of thymoma arising from the lung have been reported in the English literature since the first report in 1951 (Fukayama et al, 1988; Green et al, 1987; James et al, 1992; Kalish, 1963; Kung et al, 1985; McBurney et al, 1951; Moran et al, 1995; Veynovich et al, 1997; Yeoh et al, 1966); they are well summarized in the recent case report by Veynovich (1997). The mean age at presentation of these 19 cases was 55 years (range, 19–79) with discovery being based on an asymptomatic radiographic finding in most and, less commonly, with symptoms including chest pain, cough, hemoptysis and, in two patients, myasthenia gravis. The gross appearance is that of well-demarcated and encapsulated lesions within the lung, with sizes ranging up to 12 cm in diameter. As with mediastinal thymomas, the histologic appearance of lymphocyte-predominant, epithelioid-predominant, or mixed cellularity may be seen. Distinguishing lymphocyte-predominant thymomas from primary pulmonary lymphomas and epithelioid-predominant from disease metastatic to the lung can be problematic.

The origin of these lesions is unknown. It has been suggested that intrapulmonary thymoma may arise from ectopic descent of thymic tissue during embryogenesis (Moran, 1995) or from the postulated pluripotential cells within the lung parenchyma that could also give rise to other unusual lung neoplasms such as intrapulmonary meningioma and so forth.

Treatment is by surgical resection, with postoperative radiation to be considered if the lesion is found to be unresectable or, as with mediastinal thymomas, if gross or microscopic extension of thymic tissue beyond the capsule is noted.

PRIMARY PULMONARY CARCINOSARCOMA

The first case report of carcinosarcoma is attributed to Kika in 1908, as cited by Herxheimer and Reinke (1912), but there is no information available concerning the patient. Bergmann and colleagues (1951) reviewed eight cases of carcinosarcoma of lung and described the first two cases that were successfully resected, both by pneumonectomy by Dr. Evarts Graham. These two patients represented 0.8% of the 258 resected bronchopulmonary tumors at Barnes Hospital in St. Louis at that time.

The term *carcinosarcoma* is taken to mean a malignancy containing both epithelial and mesenchymal components differentiated into specific tissues. Initially, Virchow considered carcinosarcoma a "manifestation of the multipotentiality of the mother tissue," such that the "sarcoma and carcinoma grow side by side like two branches of the same tree" (Bergmann et al, 1951). The simultaneous development of epithelial and stromal malignancy is another possibility, but it is less likely than differentiation of a malignant tumor into two or more divergent pathways from a single primitive neoplastic cell. Its definition as a malignancy containing both epithelial and mesenchymal components differentiated into specific tissues allows a distinction to be drawn between carcinosarcoma and spindle cell carcinoma, with the latter being a squamous cell carcinoma demonstrating spindling of the squamous components without the presence of sarcomatous elements. The recent review by Nappi and colleagues (1994) presented data on 21 patients and suggested that the two entities should be considered "part of a single clinicopathologic continuum". Wick and coauthors (1997) support this view and propose the designations *biphasic* and *monophasic sarcomatoid carcinomas* as replacements for the terms *carcinosarcoma* and *spindle cell carcinoma*, respectively. Of the patients with carcinosarcomas of the lung, approximately 75% were men, with an average age of 60. The majority of patients are heavy smokers. If the tumor lies in the periphery of the lung, the patients tend to be asymptomatic unless the tumor has invaded adjacent structures; as may be expected, patients with tumors involving the major airways presented with cough, hemoptysis, wheezing, dyspnea, chest pain, or pulmonary infections. Endobronchial disease is common and present in 62% of patients, by bronchoscopy. Chest radiographs generally demonstrate well-circumscribed lesions, with approximately two thirds being in the upper lobes and one third in the lower lobes. Of the patients reported in the literature, approximately 90% presented with evidence for local disease only and underwent pulmonary resection. The one- and 5-year actuarial survival rates are reported as being 46% and 19%, respectively, with a median of 11 months, comparable to the median survival time of 12 months reported by the Mayo group (Davis, 1984).

Patients who have recurrences after resection do so in a pattern similar to that of patients with NSCLC, with distant metastases predominating. Metastases to the lung, liver, adrenal gland, brain, bone, and heart have been described. Histologically, carcinosarcomas can show significant necrosis, especially when peripheral in location. The epithelial component of carcinosarcoma is usually squamous cell carcinoma and less often adenocarcinoma, with large cell undifferentiated carcinoma found with the lowest frequency. Small cell carcinoma has not been reported in these tumors (Fraser et al, 1989). The mesenchymal component may be made up of undifferentiated spindle cells, but areas of cartilaginous, osteoid, or rhabdoid differentiation (Ishizuka et al, 1988) and pleomorphic areas resembling malignant fibrous histiocytoma (Fraser et al, 1989) have been reported. Metastases, which may be present at the time of diagnosis, may be sarcomatous, epithelial, or both.

As it appears that its pattern of locoregional spread and distant metastasis mimics that of NSCLC, the evaluation and treatment of carcinosarcoma of the lung should be similar to that of NSCLC.

INTRAVASCULAR BRONCHIOALVEOLAR TUMOR

Intravascular bronchioalveolar tumor (IVBAT) is a rare malignant tumor of the lung first described by Dail and Liebow in 1975 in an abstract and later in a full report (Dail et al, 1983). In early reports, IVBAT was thought to be a peculiar form of bronchioloalveolar carcinoma with a high rate of vascular involvement. Although recent electron microscopic and immunologic studies (Azumi and Churg, 1981; Corrin et al, 1979; Dail et al, 1983; Sherman et al, 1981; Weldon-Linne et al, 1981) have demonstrated that this tumor is of endothelial, not alveolar cell, origin, the name has been retained to indicate tumor growth in alveoli, bronchioles, and vessels. This tumor is typically multifocal, and there is some evidence to suggest that the multiple foci arise synchronously (Eggleston, 1985). Grossly, the well-demarcated pulmonary nodules of IVBAT have a firm cartilaginous cut surface, and microscopically, the almost acellular central portion of the tumor is surrounded by a cellular periphery that consists of an intra-alveolar collection of plump spindle cells and looser myxomatous tissue. The interstitial tissue can become hyalinized and sclerotic, and calcification and ossification can occur. The tumor can extend to adjacent alveoli and into peribronchial lymphatic channels. This tumor is probably best categorized as a low-grade sarcoma (Fraser et al, 1989).

A review of the English literature yielded 36 patients with sufficient data to analyze the demographics and survival rates (Azumi and Churg, 1981; Borlee-Hermans et al, 1985; Corrin et al, 1979; Dail et al, 1983; Eggleston, 1985; Emery et al, 1982; Gledhill and Kay, 1984; Marsh et al, 1982; Mata et al, 1991; Miettinen et al, 1987; Sherman et al, 1981; Sicilian et al, 1983; Sweeney et al, 1986; Weldon-Linne et al, 1981; Yanagawa et al, 1994; Yi et al, 1995).

Of the patients, 85% were female, with ages of patients ranging from 12 to 69 years (median 35). One half of the patients were asymptomatic at presentation, with the diagnosis suggested by radiographs. Of those with symptoms, two thirds had relatively minor complaints, such as mild cough or mild chest discomfort, and one third had major symptoms, such as dyspnea or weight loss. All but three patients presented with multiple, bilateral pulmonary nodules; of the three, one presented with unilateral multiple nodules, and two with unilateral lung nodules. All patients underwent open lung biopsy (by lobectomy in two) to make the diagnosis. Of the 36 patients, 9 (24%) presented with or subsequently developed metastases: liver (6), retroperitoneum (1), small bowel (1).

Recommendations about therapy are difficult to make based on the literature. Varying chemotherapeutic regimens have been attempted but usually only in symptomatic patients near death (Dail et al, 1983). Radiation therapy was unsuccessful in two patients (Azumi and Churg, 1981; Yanagawa, 1994). The disease tends to be indolent, with death usually resulting from slowly progressive pulmonary compromise secondary to replacement of the lung parenchyma by the tumor, although death due to diffuse metastases can occur (Yanagawa, 1994). Overall survival rates of 5 and 10 years are 61% and 55%, respectively, with the median survival not reached at 10 years. IVBAT should be considered in the differential diagnosis of any patient with multiple bilateral pulmonary nodules, especially if the patient is a young woman.

PRIMARY PULMONARY MELANOMA

Primary melanoma at any site except the skin and juxtacutaneous mucous membranes, eye, and leptomeninges is extremely uncommon, and primary malignant melanoma of the lung is extremely rare. Generally accepted criteria for a primary pulmonary melanoma include (1) the absence of a current or previous primary melanoma elsewhere or the absence of a previously resected or cauterized cutaneous lesion of unknown type; (2) no ocular tumor resection; (3) a solitary tumor in the surgical specimen from the lung; (4) tumor morphology consistent with a primary melanoma; (5) no demonstrable melanoma in other organs at time of operation; and (6) autopsy findings without primary malignant melanomas being demonstrated elsewhere (Jensen and Egedorf, 1967). The first reported case of primary malignant melanoma of the lung has been attributed to Todd in 1888. Subsequent cases were reported by Kunkel and Torrey (1916), Carlucci and Schleussner (1942), and Allen and Spitz (1953). Although some believe these cases were actually primary pulmonary melanomas, others contend that there was not enough evidence to support such a conclusion and consider the first adequately documented case of primary melanoma of lung to be that reported by Salm in 1963.

The histologic appearance of malignant melanoma of the lung is identical to that of a melanoma at any site. Large pleomorphic cells, sometimes with prominent nucleoli, are seen; intranuclear inclusions may be present, and a search for pigment should be made. Immunohistochemical stains and electron microscopy may be helpful. Because cutaneous or mucosal malignant melanoma can spontaneously regress (Mackay et al, 1990), some authors believe that the diagnosis of primary (as opposed to secondary) pulmonary melanoma of the lung cannot be made unless the lesion is located in the bronchial epithelium only (Bagwell et al, 1989; Cagle et al, 1984; Carstens et al, 1984; Gepharat, 1981; Robertson et al, 1980; Taboada et al, 1972). Other investigators suggest that melanoma can be primary within the lung parenchyma, suggesting derivation from cells of the primitive foregut that migrate to the tracheobronchial tree in fetal life (Cagle et al, 1984; Jensen and Egedorf, 1967; Robertson et al, 1980; Salm, 1963).

Once the diagnosis has been established, an exhaustive examination of the skin, eyes, and mucosa, including the pharynx, vagina, esophagus, and anal canal, has been conducted in an attempt to locate an alternative primary site, with careful radiographic evaluation (which today should probably include a PET scan) for other possible sites of disease. If no other site can be found, then it is reasonable to proceed with surgical resection if possible.

Since Salm's report in 1963, 14 additional cases of primary malignant melanoma of the lung have been reported in the English language literature (Alghanem et al, 1987; Allen and Drash, 1968; Bagwell et al, 1989; Cagle et al, 1984; Farrell et al, 1996; Jensen and Egedorf, 1967; Pasquini et al, 1994; Reed and Kent, 1964; Reid and Mehta, 1966; Robertson et al, 1980; Salm, 1963; Santos et al, 1987; Taboada et al, 1972). There were eight men and seven women (male-to-female ratio, 1), whose ages ranged from 40 to 80 years (median, 60 years). Approximately 25% were asymptomatic; the rest had cough, hemoptysis, chest pain, dyspnea, or pneumonia. No predilection for side or upper or lower lobes was present. The tumors ranged in size from 1 to 10 cm in diameter (median, 4 cm). Four (28%) were endobronchial. Twelve patients (86%) underwent complete resection (seven by lobectomy, three by pneumonectomy, one by segmentectomy, and one by wedge resection). The 5-year survival rate was approximately 50%. Those who died did so primarily of distant metastases (brain, liver, bone, adrenal, heart, or lung).

PRIMARY MALIGNANT GERM CELL TUMORS

Primary malignant germ cell tumors of the lung are exceedingly rare. Two types have been described: malignant teratoma and choriocarcinoma.

Malignant Teratoma

Benign intrapulmonary teratomas (Jamieson and McGowan, 1982) are exceedingly uncommon, with only 20 cases documented by 1978 (Day and Taylor, 1975; Holt et al, 1978; Kakkar et al, 1996), and primary malignant teratomas of the lung are very rare. Intraparenchymal tumors are more common than endobronchial tumors (Jamieson and McGowan, 1982). Histologically endoderma-, ectoderma-, and mesoderma-derived tissue is present, usually in a cystic mass, and pancreatic tissue may be identified.

A review of the literature yielded only five cases with enough information to confirm the diagnosis of a malignant intrapulmonary teratoma Gautam, 1969; Kakkar 1996; Pound and Willis, 1969; Ruland, 1956; Schiodt and Jensen, 1960). The case of Barrett and Barnard (1945) has been recorded in multiple reviews as a malignant teratoma, but it has been classified by Spencer (1961) as a pulmonary blastoma. In the report of Ruland (1956), little clinical information is presented. The case of Schiodt and Jensen (1960) was a 66-year-old man who underwent an apicoposterior segmentectomy of the left upper lobe for a "walnut-sized" malignant teratoma. The patient had a recurrence locally and died approximately 1 year after the operation. The case of Gautam (1969) was a 68-year-old man who underwent a pneumonectomy for a 5-cm malignant teratoma with an endobronchial component completely obstructing the left upper lobe bronchus. No follow-up after discharge was presented. The case of Pound and Willis (1969) was a 10-month-old boy who presented with supraclavicular lymphadenopathy that on biopsy revealed an undifferentiated large cell carcinoma. There was complete opacification of the right chest. He died 6 days after admission, and the autopsy revealed a 9-cm malignant teratoma within the right lower lobe, with associated hilar and mediastinal lymph node metastases. The patient reported by Kakkar and colleagues (1996) was a 20-year-old male who presented with recent onset of hemoptysis and a longer history of fever and cough. Radiographs revealed consolidation of a portion of the right lung; the patient died shortly thereafter, with final pathologic diagnosis being consistent with elements from all the germ cell layers as well as yolk sac components.

Like other germ cell tumors, primary intrapulmonary malignant teratoma is exceptionally rare, and little information is available to guide management. Most malignant teratomas are treated as one would treat other germ cell tumor sites.

Choriocarcinoma

Elevations of human chorionic gonadotropin in patients with lung tumors is not uncommon, but primary pulmonary choriocarcinoma is rare. Approximately 175,000 patients are diagnosed with primary bronchogenic carcinoma of the lung in the United States each year, and secretion of human chorionic gonadotropin occurs in approximately 6% of these lung cancers (Braunstein et al, 1973; Fukuda et al, 1990; Hattori et al, 1979; Miyake et al, 1987; Muggia et al, 1975). Primary extragonadal choriocarcinoma of the lung, by comparison, is extremely uncommon; in a review of the literature in 1962, Fine and colleagues did not record a single case of primary pulmonary choriocarcinoma in 109 reported cases of primary extragonadal choriocarcinoma in male patients.

The first reported case of primary choriocarcinoma of the lung was by Gerber in 1935. Since then, at least eight other cases have been reported in the English language literature (Berman, 1940; Gerin-Lajoie, 1954; Kay and Reed, 1953; Pushchak and Farhi, 1987; Sridhar et al, 1989; Sullivan, 1989; Tanimura et al, 1985; Uwatoko et al, 1997; Zapatero et al, 1982). Of these 10 cases, 6 were female patients and 4 were male (male-to-female ratio, 0.4), with ages ranging from 7 months to 67 years (median, 37 years). Six patients (67%) presented with hemoptysis, and one patient died after a bronchoscopic biopsy as a result of endobronchial bleeding. Six patients underwent pulmonary resection (four by pneumonectomy and two by lobectomy). Two of the patients died postoperatively following pneumonectomy. Of the remaining six patients, four died of disease at 1, 4, 4, and 15 months after the diagnosis, with metastases to the brain, liver, lung, or spleen. The remaining two patients were alive and well at 6 and 36 months after lobectomy. One patient, who later died of disease, had a partial response to chemotherapy (5-fluorouracil, etoposide, and cisplatin) (Sridhar et al, 1989). Choriocarcinoma may be misdiagnosed as adenocarcinoma; however, staining for human chorionic gonadotropin or α-fetoprotein (or the presence of serum elevation of these proteins) may assist in making the diagnosis. Intensive chemotherapy is probably the treatment of choice either preoperatively (if diagnosed) or postoperatively.

PRIMARY SARCOMA OF THE LUNG

Primary malignant mesenchymal tumors (sarcomas), although rare, can arise in the lung, just as they do in all other anatomic sites. Most reports of primary sarcomas of the lung describe soft tissue sarcomas, but primary chondrosarcomas and osteosarcomas, although even more rare, do occur. The area has been extensively reviewed by Suster (1995).

Chondrosarcoma

Primary extraskeletal chondrosarcoma of the lung is an extremely uncommon entity. Using the strict criteria of Morgan and Salama (1972), only 10 well-documented cases were available for review (Bini, 1942; Daniels et al, 1967; Filho and Pasqualucci, 1963; Greenspan, 1933; Lowell and Tuhy, 1949; Rees, 1970; Sedlezky, 1955; Sun et al, 1982; Yellin et al, 1983). There were four men and six women (male-to-female ratio, 0.7), whose ages ranged from 23 to 74 years (median, 44 years). Most presented with cough. Two had hemoptysis, and two had chest pain. All presented with a solitary, usually large pulmonary mass. Of those 10 patients, 3 received no therapy and died of locoregional disease at 6, 6, and 20 months following the onset of symptoms. Seven patients underwent resection (two by pneumonectomy, three by lobectomy, one by wedge resection, and one by endobronchial resection). Of those resected, one died of metastatic disease to the lung 24 months after the lobectomy. The remaining six patients were alive and well 1 to 48 months following resection. Two patients (20%) had metastases to their mediastinal lymph nodes.

As noted by Morgan and Salama (1972), primary extraskeletal chondrosarcoma of the lung occurs as a solitary, well-circumscribed, slow-growing tumor that, if left untreated, may spread within the thorax and cause death. Distant metastases are uncommon (10%). If diagnosed preoperatively, these tumors should be resected because resection appears to translate into long-term survival. Because 20% of these tumors have metastasized to mediastinal lymph nodes, a mediastinal lymph node dissection at the time of resection appears to be advisable.

Primary pulmonary chondrosarcoma may be derived from tracheobronchial cartilage, but an origin from bronchial chondroma or hamartoma is possible (Fraser et al, 1989). Grossly, the tumor may appear to be a round, lobulated mass within the lung (Morgan and Salama, 1972). The histologic appearance is of plump, somewhat pleomorphic chondrocytes, some showing binucleation. Calcification or ossification may be present (Morgan and Salama, 1972). Surgical resection is the treatment of choice.

Osteosarcoma

Primary osteosarcoma of the lung is also extremely rare; in two of the largest series of extraosseous osteosarcomas, not a single case of primary osteosarcoma of the lung was reported (Fine and Stout, 1956; Sordillo et al, 1983). In a review of the literature, only eight reports containing 10 cases that were considered primary osteosarcoma of the lung (Bhalla et al, 1992; Colby et al, 1989; Connolly et al, 1991; Nascimento et al, 1982; Nosanchuk and Weatherbee, 1969; Petersen, 1990; Reingold and Amromin, 1971; Yamashita et al, 1964). Of these 10 patients, there were 7 men and 3 women whose ages ranged from 51 to 93 years (median, 62 years). Most patients presented with cough; one had hemoptysis. All lesions were solitary by chest radiography, and most were greater than 4 cm in diameter. Of the 10 reported patients, 4 received no therapy, 3 of them dying of the disease; the fourth, with a follow-up of only 1 month, was alive with disease. One patient was treated with cyclophosphamide and died 6 months after the start of therapy secondary to neutropenia and sepsis. Of the five patients who underwent resection (one by pneumonectomy and four by lobectomy), one patient was alive and well at 6 months, one was alive with disease at 14 months, and two died of unrelated causes at 4 and 6 months. Three of the seven developed distant metastases (two in the lung and one in the liver). In addition, two patients developed hilar lymph node metastases, and both also had distant metastases.

Histologically, spindle cells with myxoid, chondroid, or osteoid tissue are present. The osteoid tissue must be cytologically malignant and must be present to make the diagnosis of osteosarcoma.

Primary osteogenic sarcoma of the lung occurs as a large solitary lesion on chest radiography. If no distant disease is documented, resection appears to be the treatment of choice. Because 29% of these patients had hilar lymph node metastases, a mediastinal lymph node dissection appears advisable. The role of adjuvant or neoadjuvant chemotherapy is unknown.

Soft Tissue Sarcoma

Primary soft tissue sarcomas of the lung are not quite as rare as other pulmonary sarcomas. In a review of the experience at Memorial Sloan-Kettering Cancer Center, Martini and colleagues (1971) reported on 22 patients with primary soft tissue sarcomas who were evaluated over a 42-year period (1926 to 1968). During that time, 5714 patients with primary lung cancer were seen, a relative incidence of primary pulmonary sarcoma to lung cancer of 0.4%. In the literature, the descriptions of patients with "primary sarcoma of the lung" prior to 1975 are confusing; for example, reports such as those of Hochberg and Crastnopol (1955) include the lymphoproliferative disorders under the term *lymphosarcoma*. In this 1955 review of 77 "primary sarcomas of the bronchus and lung," 44 (57%) were soft tissue sarcomas, 26% were lymphoproliferative disorders (including Hodgkin's disease, lymphosarcoma, malignant lymphoma, and reticulum cell sarcoma), 5 (6%) were carcinosarcomas, and 2 (3%) were chondrosarcomas.

However, since 1931, 288 primary soft tissue sarcomas of the lung have been reported (Allan et al, 1987; Avagnina et al, 1984; Bacha et al, 1999; Ball, 1931; Bartley and Arean, 1965; Bedrossian et al, 1979; Beluffi et al, 1986; Cameron, 1975; Capewell et al, 1986; Carswel and Kraeft, 1949; Caves and Jacques, 1971; Chowdhury et al, 1980; Conquest et al, 1965; Crane and Sutton, 1972; Eriksson et al, 1982; Gebauer, 1982; Goldthorn et al, 1986; Guccion and Rosen, 1972; Hochberg and Crestnopol, 1955; Janssen et al, 1994; Kalus et al, 1973; Kern et al, 1979; Lee et al, 1984; Martini et al, 1971; McDonnell et al, 1988; Meade et al, 1974; Nascimento et al, 1982; Neilson, 1958; Ott et al, 1987; Pedersen et al, 1984; Pettinato et al, 1989; Regnard et al, 1999; Rusch et al, 1989; Shariff et al, 1988; Shuman, 1984; Silverman and Coalson, 1984; Spragg et al, 1983; Thomas et al, 1981; Ueda et al, 1977; Van Assendelft et al, 1984; Venn et al, 1986; Wick et al, 1982; Yousem, 1986; Yousem and Hochholzer, 1987a, 1987b). The number of patients per report is small, ranging from 1 to 42 patients per report, with a median of 1. The largest single report was by McCormack and Martini (1989). The raw data from the 42 patients in this report from Memorial Sloan-Kettering Cancer Center were re-analyzed and, because they are representative of other reports in the literature, they are presented in the following paragraph.

Of the 42 patients with primary soft tissue sarcomas of the lung, 19 were male and 23 were female (male-to-female ratio, 0.8); their ages ranged from 1.5 to 78 years (median, 52 years). Approximately 25% of the patients were asymptomatic, and the lesions were detected by routine chest radiograph. Seven patients (17%) presented with hemoptysis. The remaining patients presented with cough, dyspnea, chest pain, or systemic symptoms, such as fatigue, malaise, fever, or weight loss. All lesions were solitary masses, the diameter of which ranged in size from 1 to 17 cm (median, 5.5 cm). The histologic subtypes of soft tissue sarcomas in these 42 patients were leiomyosarcoma (16), rhabdomyosarcoma (6), spindle cell carcinoma (13), angiosarcoma (2), malignant fibrous histiocytoma (3), fibrosarcoma (2), hemangiopericytoma (1), and blastoma (1). Although not specified, the spindle cell sarcomas probably contained a number of malignant peripheral nerve tumors.

Twenty-nine (69%) of these patients underwent resection of their primary pulmonary soft tissue sarcomas (lobectomy 15, pneumonectomy 7, wedge resection 6, and segmentectomy 1). Of those not resected, five received no therapy, six received radiation therapy, and two received radiation and chemotherapy.

These 42 patients with primary soft tissue sarcomas of the lung experienced overall 1-, 3-, and 5-year survival rates of 55%, 31%, and 25%, respectively, with a median survival of 13 months. In a report from the Mayo Clinic (Nascimento et al, 1982), size was thought to affect survival; in the Memorial Sloan-Kettering Cancer Center experience, there was a trend, although not significant, toward improved rate of survival in patients with tumors 5 cm or smaller.

Leiomyosarcoma is the most common histologic subtype, with approximately 41 having been reported in the series above. It is probably likely that a certain proportion of these arise from unrecognized leiomyosarcoma of the uterus in women, particularly if the patient has undergone a hysterectomy for "fibroids" in the past. Having said this, the male-to-female ratio in the series was 2.5:1. The reported cases presented primarily as a solitary mass, with even distribution among the regions of the lung. Treatment has consisted mainly of surgical removal.

Malignant fibrous histiocytoma is the most common soft tissue sarcoma, but it is only a subgroup of tumors arising in the lung, and has been well reviewed by Yousem and Hochholzer (1987a). The histologic classification of this sarcoma dates back only about 20 years, and it is possible that pulmonary sarcomas previously diagnosed as fibrosarcomas, leiomyosarcomas, myxosarcomas, or unclassified sarcomas would be called malignant fibrous histiocytomas today (Fraser et al, 1989). Four histologic subtypes are described: (1) storiform pleomorphic, (2) myxoid, (3) giant cell, and (4) inflammatory (Weiss, 1982). Storiform pleomorphic is the type most commonly found in the lung (Yousem and Hochholzer, 1987a). It consists of bundles of spindle cells arranged in a cartwheel, or storiform, pattern. Present in this background are pleomorphic, often giant, cells with many mitotic figures. The most important predictor of survival is complete resection of the primary tumor. The patients undergoing resection survived significantly longer (36% alive at 5 years) than those receiving radiation therapy or no therapy (no one survived longer than 2 years).

MISCELLANEOUS MALIGNANT TUMORS

There have been case reports of primary ependymoma (Crotty et al, 1992), Ewing's sarcoma (Palmer et al, 1981), lymphoepithelioma-like carcinoma (Miller et al, 1991), and pseudomesotheliomatous carcinoma (Dessy and Pietra, 1991) of the lung. Because of the scarcity of data concerning these extraordinarily rare primary malignant tumors of the lung, the reader is referred to the reference section for more information.

PRIMARY MALIGNANT LYMPHORETICULAR DISORDERS OF THE LUNG

All the components of the lymphoreticular system are found in the normal lung and can give rise to primary tumors of the lymphoreticular system. Although extremely uncommon, primary Hodgkin's disease, non-Hodgkin's lymphoma, and plasmacytoma of the lung are seen and are estimated to be approximately 0.5% of all primary lung tumors. Involvement of the lung as one site of disease in a patient with extrapulmonary Hodgkin's or non-Hodgkin's lymphoma is, of course, much more common and has been reported to be found in 40% (Kern et al, 1961) and 49% (Mentzer et al, 1993; Risdall et al, 1979), respectively. In this section, we focus on primary Hodgkin's disease, non-Hodgkin's lymphoma, and plasmacytoma of the lung.

Solitary Plasmacytoma

Plasma cell malignancies are a group of related disorders characterized by the proliferation of plasma cells, which are immunoglobulin-secreting B cells. The most common is multiple myeloma. Of patients with plasma cell malignancies, 4% present with a solitary malignant plasma cell neoplasm of the soft tissues (called an *extramedullary plasmacytoma*) (Woodruff et al, 1979). Most extramedullary plasmacytomas occur in the nasopharynx, the upper respiratory tract, or the oropharynx; a primary plasmacytoma of the lung is extremely uncommon. In a review of six collected series, only 4% of extramedullary plasmacytomas were found to occur in the lung (Corwin and Lindberg, 1979; Holland et al, 1992; Knowling et al, 1983; Meis et al, 1987; Wiltshaw, 1976; Woodruff et al, 1979).

The first reported case of an extramedullary plasmacytoma of the lung was noted by Gordon and Walker (1944). A review of the English literature since then revealed 15 cases for which sufficient data were available for analysis (Amin, 1985; Baroni et al, 1977; Childress and Adie, 1950; Cotton and Penido, 1952; Hill and White, 1953; Joseph et al, 1993; Kazzaz, 1992; Kennedy and Kneafsey, 1959; Kerren and Meyer, 1966; Mazumdar et al, 1969; Rozsa and Frieman, 1953; Wang, 1999; Wlle et al, 1976). Primary plasmacytoma of the lung occurs more frequently in men, with a male to female ratio of 2:1. Patient age ranges from 3 to 72 years (median, 43). Of these patients, 13 were treated with pulmonary resections (10 lobectomies and 3 pneumonectomies); in 3 of them, radiation therapy was added, and in 1, chemotherapy. Two patients underwent biopsy followed by medical therapy alone. The overall 5-year survival rate was approximately 40% (although it should be noted that only limited follow-up was reported). It is notable that two patients (17%) developed multiple myeloma at intervals of 7 and 26 months after resection.

Primary pulmonary plasmacytoma can present as a parenchymal lesion or within the airway as an endotracheal or endobronchial lesion with airway obstruction (Mazumdar et al, 1969). Microscopically, specimens demonstrate sheets of atypical plasma cells, similar to multiple myeloma. Ossification can be seen (Kinare et al, 1965), and amorphous eosinophilic material representing immunoglobulin or amyloid may be present (Morinaga et al, 1987). This type of tumor must be distinguished from a plasmacytoid B cell lymphoma, and immunohistochemical stains for immunoglobulins may be helpful in doing so. Most pulmonary plasmacytomas are not associated with abnormal serum or urine immunoglobulin levels (Fraser et al, 1989).

If diagnosed at thoracotomy, a complete resection of all apparent disease should be performed. If no other sites of disease are found, if serum electrophoresis is normal, and if Bence Jones proteinuria is absent, such a patient may be followed expectantly (Corwin and Lindberg, 1979; Holland et al, 1992; Knowling et al, 1983; Meis et al, 1987; Wiltshaw, 1976).

Hodgkin's Disease

The occurrence of Hodgkin's disease as extranodal disease is extremely uncommon (Wood and Coltman, 1973), and primary extranodal Hodgkin's disease was found to represent only 0.6% of all patients with Hodgkin's disease seen at Yale-New Haven Hospital from 1980 to 1987 (Radin, 1990) and 0.0756% of 1470 patients seen at Stanford Medical Center from 1960 to 1980 (Johnson et al, 1983).

To be defined as primary pulmonary Hodgkin's disease, the following criteria are to be met: (1) histologic features of Hodgkin's disease; (2) restriction of the disease to the lung, with no nodal involvement (although some authors accept "minimal" local nodal involvement) (Radin, 1990); and (3) clinical or pathologic exclusion of disease at distant sites (Johnson et al, 1983; Yousem et al, 1986;

Zulian et al, 1986). According to the Ann Arbor staging system (Carbone et al, 1971), a patient with primary pulmonary Hodgkin's disease would be either stage IE (involvement of a single extranodal site) or IIE (localized involvement of an extranodal site and its contiguous lymph node chain).

To summarize the presentation, therapy, and outcome, a literature search was performed; it revealed reports detailing 64 patients with sufficient data to be analyzed (Boshnakova et al, 2000; Dhingra and Flance, 1970; Guttman and Saavedra, 1968; Kern et al, 1961; Monahan 1965; Nelson et al, 1983; Pinson et al, 1992; van der Schee et al, 1990; Yousem et al, 1986; Zulian et al, 1986). The excellent reviews of Radin (1990) and Habermann (1999) are the sources of much of the data presented subsequently.

Of 64 patients with primary Hodgkin's disease of the lung, 40% were male and 60% female, with ages ranging from 12 to 82 years (median, 37 years). Of those, 15% were asymptomatic; 85% had symptoms, in decreasing frequency, of cough, weight loss, chest pain, dyspnea, hemoptysis, fatigue, rash, night sweats, and wheezing. Of those with symptoms, approximately 50% had the B-type symptoms of Hodgkin's disease (weight loss, fever, and night sweats).

The location of the finding on chest radiograph was unilateral in 49 patients (72%) and bilateral in 15 (25%). Two patients with normal chest radiographs had endobronchial Hodgkin's disease diagnosed by bronchoscopy. All bilateral disease demonstrated multiple nodules; unilateral disease presented as a single nodule in 85% and as multiple nodules in 15%. Of the solitary nodules, 31% demonstrated cavitation.

Intrathoracic Hodgkin's disease, either primary or with contiguous mediastinal spread, is most often of the nodular sclerosing type. The histologic appearance of primary pulmonary Hodgkin's disease is identical to that seen in extrapulmonary sites (Fraser et al, 1989) and is characterized by the presence of Reed-Sternberg cells (or their variants) in the appropriate background of inflammatory cells, such as lymphocytes, plasma cells, histiocytes, and eosinophils. Granulomas may also be present.

In all but one patient reviewed, tissue was obtained by thoracotomy, with either open biopsy (59%) or resection (41%) by pneumonectomy ($n = 9$); lobectomy ($n = 11$); segmentectomy ($n = 2$); or wedge resection ($n = 3$). The remaining patient was diagnosed at autopsy. A diagnosis of Hodgkin's disease can be made by percutaneous transthoracic needle biopsy or bronchoscopy, but the accuracy of these methods is debated by pathologists (Flint et al, 1988; Moralles and Matthews, 1987; Wisecarver et al, 1989). There are reports of the diagnosis being made by sputum cytology (Reale et al, 1983).

The therapy of patients with primary Hodgkin's disease of the lung has varied considerably by decade and institution. Of the 64 patients reviewed, approximately 40% underwent complete resection of their intrathoracic disease, 40% radiotherapy, and 50% chemotherapy.

Many patients with primary Hodgkin's disease of the lung may have their disease diagnosed during thoracotomy for a "coin" lesion. It is reasonable to subject these patients to formal pulmonary resections with mediastinal lymph node dissection if it appears that all evident disease can be removed. Other patients present with multiple bilateral or unilateral nodules, and although an attempt at diagnosis by less invasive methods may be made, most undergo open biopsy because of concerns that the transthoracic needle biopsy or bronchoscopy may not be sufficiently accurate. Once a diagnosis of pulmonary Hodgkin's disease has been made by biopsy or resection, a search for other sites of disease should be performed. If no other disease is found (patient's disease stage is IE or IIE), radiotherapy is added to the treatment. It is debatable whether chemotherapy should also be given for patients with unilateral disease; patients with bilateral disease could be considered as having stage IV disease and they should be offered chemotherapy in the hope of long-term survival.

Non-Hodgkin's Lymphoma

Although primary extranodal non-Hodgkin's lymphoma is not uncommon (10% of 380 untreated patients with non-Hodgkin's lymphoma at Tufts University School of Medicine between 1966 and 1976) (Rudders et al, 1978), primary non-Hodgkin's lymphoma of the lung is rare. In the Tufts series, there were no cases of primary extranodal pulmonary non-Hodgkin's lymphoma. However, another large series found that 3.6% of extranodal non-Hodgkin's lymphoma occurred in the lung (Freeman et al, 1972). The series from Memorial Sloan-Kettering Cancer Center (1949 to 1982) reported 36 cases of primary non-Hodgkin's lymphoma of the lung (L'Hoste et al, 1984). During this period, 5030 patients with non-Hodgkin's lymphoma were seen; thus, the estimated frequency of this lymphoma's arising in the lung was 0.34% of all cases (L'Hoste et al, 1984).

A review of the published literature from 1940 to the present revealed that approximately 550 patients with primary non-Hodgkin's lymphoma of the lung were reported (Asherson et al, 1987; Baas and van Herwaarden, 1986; Ben-Ezra et al, 1987; Bosanko et al, 1991; Chow, 1996; Dahlgren and Ovenfors, 1979; Davis and Gadek, 1987; Ehrenstein, 1966; Eliasson et al, 1990; Ellison et al, 1964; Farquhar et al, 1988; Ferraro, 2000; Greenberg et al, 1972; Hansen et al, 1989; Hardy, 1995; Herbert et al, 1984; Hilbun and Chavez, 1967; Kennedy et al, 1985; Koss et al, 1983; Le Tourneau et al, 1983; L'Hoste et al, 1984; Marchevsky et al, 1983; Mark, 1977; McCormack and Martini, 1989; Papaiannou and Watson, 1965; Peterson et al, 1985; Poelzleitner et al, 1989; Polish et al, 1989; Rabiah, 1968; Reverter et al, 1987; Roggeri, 1993; Rubin, 1968; Rush, 2000; Sakula, 1979; Saltzstein, 1963; Schwaiger et al, 1991; Sinclair et al, 1978; Sprague and deBlois, 1989; Sugarbaker and Craver, 1940; Tan et al, 1988; Turner et al, 1984; Wotherspoon et al, 1990). This total includes the 90 cases from the prior literature reviewed by Saltzstein (1963) and by Papaiannou and Watson (1965) in addition to their cases. If these summary cases are excluded, there have been approximately 460 patients with primary pulmonary non-Hodgkin's lymphoma reported in 41 articles from 1963 to 2000; the median number of patients per report was two.

In the Memorial Sloan-Kettering Cancer Center series

published in 1984 (n = 36) (L'Hoste et al, 1984), 44% were asymptomatic, with the abnormality first being detected by incidental chest radiograph. Of the symptomatic patients, 30% had cough, 11% chest pain, 11% malaise, and 7% diagnoses of pneumonia. There were 18 men and 18 women, with ages ranging from 12 to 75 years (mean, 53 years). The AFIP report (Koss et al, 1983) enumerated the radiographic findings in 124 patients with primary non-Hodgkin's lymphoma of the lung: a solitary nodule in 58%, a solitary infiltrate in 27%, multiple nodules in 9%, and multiple infiltrates in 6%.

Primary non-Hodgkin's lymphoma has been associated with acquired immunodeficiency syndrome (Gibson et al, 1987). Similar to most non-Hodgkin's lymphomas, most primary pulmonary non-Hodgkin's lymphoma is of the B cell type. The diagnosis may be made by fine-needle aspiration or transbronchoscopic biopsy.

Primary pulmonary non-Hodgkin's lymphomas probably arise from bronchus-associated lymphoid tissue. Grossly, the parenchymal lesions of lymphoma are white to tan in color and may be well-defined or diffuse. The malignant cells are found predominantly in interstitial tissues (Fraser et al, 1989), and extension into the pleura can occur. Tumor necrosis is uncommon.

After a histologic diagnosis of non-Hodgkin's lymphoma is made, the patient should be thoroughly evaluated for any evidence of extrathoracic disease. Once this is completed, the patient's disease is then staged according to a modification of the Ann Arbor Staging Classification (Carbone et al, 1971; L'Hoste et al, 1984) as follows: (1) stage IE, lung only involved; (2) stage II1E, lung and hilar nodes involved; (3) stage II2E, lung and mediastinal nodes involved; and (4) stage II2EW, lung and adjacent chest wall or diaphragm involved.

Although the disease in patients with primary non-Hodgkin's lymphoma of the lung can be histologically classified by one of the four classification systems—Nathwani (1979); Lukes-Collins (1974); Kiel (Lennert, 1978); or the International Working Formulation (Non-Hodgkin's Lymphoma Pathologic Classification Project, 1982)—a simpler approach is to group the disease in patients with primary non-Hodgkin's lymphoma of the lung into small cell (lymphocytic) and large cell (histiocytic) lymphomas. In the Memorial Sloan-Kettering Cancer Center experience (L'Hoste et al, 1984), 58% of the patients could be classified as having small cell lymphoma and 42% large cell lymphoma. Of those with small cell lymphomas, 90% underwent complete resection, and 10% had a biopsy only; 35% received chemotherapy, and 40% experienced recurrence. In the large cell non-Hodgkin's lymphoma group, 33% underwent resection, and 67% underwent biopsies alone; 89% received chemotherapy. The overall recurrence rate was 50%. Overall, 5-year survival rates can be anticipated to be approximately 85% and 45% for patients with primary small cell and large cell non-Hodgkin's lymphoma, respectively, with treatment (Freeman et al, 1972; Koss et al, 1983; Saltzstein, 1963; Turner et al, 1984).

Primary non-Hodgkin's lymphoma of the lung usually presents as an asymptomatic pulmonary nodule in a 40- to 60-year-old patient. If an extent-of-disease evaluation fails to disclose other sites of disease, it is reasonable to suggest resection. General recommendations for medical therapy are as follows: patients with large cell non-Hodgkin's lymphoma should receive chemotherapy; patients with stage IE small cell non-Hodgkin's lymphoma of the lung may be watched expectantly; but those with stage IIE should probably be offered chemotherapy.

COMMENTS AND CONTROVERSIES

This chapter, originally written by Drs. Burt and Zakowski, has been updated by Drs. Downey and Zakowski. It remains the ultimate compendium of these types of tumors because of the extensive literature search. In the course of practice, a surgeon undoubtedly will encounter a few of these rare primary malignancies, diagnosed preoperatively or intraoperatively. If diagnosed preoperatively, some of these tumors may be best treated by primary chemoradiotherapy (e.g., myeloma, B cell lymphoma), although surgery may be the treatment of choice when the lesion is solitary. In most cases, the diagnosis is made at the time of surgery, and because of inadequacies of frozen section, the true diagnosis may not be available in the operating room. For this reason, these lesions, if believed to be solitary or within one lung, should be resected and a lymph node dissection should be accomplished. This approach may seem radical, but the ultimate diagnosis may not confirm the frozen section diagnosis.

An example of this dilemma is seen in pulmonary lymphomas. Although surgeons continue to offer resection to these patients when they have been diagnosed preoperatively, it is unknown whether surgical resection is required to effect the best therapy. Like lymphomas elsewhere, these tumors are chemoresponsive and radioresponsive. However, because of lack of firm evidence to the contrary, it appears that, where possible, total surgical excision remains the mainstay of treatment.

Unfortunately, the reports in the literature are so few that once resection has been performed, the prognosis of an individual patient is difficult to estimate. Adjuvant therapies must be considered on a per patient basis because there is very little to guide the practitioner. In most instances, one must look to other sites where these primary lesions occur and follow the examples of treatment of these sites. Most important, however, is that at the time of surgery, a complete resection should be accomplished whenever possible.

R.J.G.

KEY REFERENCES

Bagwell SP, Flynn SD, Cox PM, Davison JA: Primary malignant melanoma of the lung. Am Rev Respir Dis 139:1543, 1989.

This is a case report of one patient with primary malignant melanoma of the lung. It is also the best review of the literature available.

Colby TB, Bilbao JE, Battifora H, Unni K: Primary osteosarcoma of lung: A reappraisal following immunohistologic study. Arch Pathol Lab Med 113:1147, 1989.

This report from the Mayo Clinic describes three patients with primary osteosarcomas of the lung and reviews the limited literature in detail.

Dail DH, Liebow AA, Gmelich IT et al: Intravascular, bronchiolar, and alveolar tumor of the lung (IVBAT): An analysis of twenty cases of a peculiar sclerosing endothelial tumor. Cancer 51:452, 1983.

This report summarizes the collected series of 20 patients with IVBAT from the AFIP. It is the largest report in the literature.

Davis MP, Eagan RT, Weiland LH, Pairolero PC: Carcinosarcoma of the lung: Mayo Clinic experience and response to chemotherapy. Mayo Clin Proc 59:598, 1984.

This is the largest report about carcinosarcomas of the lung from a single institution. It describes the clinical findings in 17 patients from the Mayo Clinic and details the clinical presentation, therapy, and outcome.

Ferraro P, Trasteck VF, Adlakha H, et al: Primary non-Hodgkin's lymphoma of the lung. Ann Thorac Surg 69:993, 2000.

This report details one institution's extensive experience with the surgical management of 48 patients with primary non-Hodgkin's lymphoma of the lung, emphasizing the diffuse nature of presenting symptoms and the lack of prognostic factors.

Joseph G, Pandit M, Korfhage L: Primary pulmonary plasmacytoma. Cancer 71:721, 1993.

This case report and review of the literature succinctly summarizes the literature.

Koss MN, Hochholzer L, O'Leary T: Pulmonary blastomas. Cancer 67:2368, 1991.

This is the largest report about pulmonary blastomas from a single institution. It describes the clinical and pathologic findings in a collected series of 52 patients from the AFIP.

L'Hoste RJ, Filippa DA, Lieberman PH, Bretsky S: Primary pulmonary lymphomas: A clinicopathologic analysis of 36 cases. Cancer 54:1397, 1984.

This report, which is the largest reported series from a single institution, describes the presentations, therapies, and clinical outcomes of 79 patients seen at Memorial Sloan-Kettering Cancer Center.

McCormack PM, Martini N: Primary sarcomas and lymphomas of lung. In Martini N, Vogt-Moykopf I (eds): Thoracic Surgery: Frontiers and Uncommon Neoplasms, Vol 5. St. Louis, CV Mosby, 1989.

This report from Memorial Sloan-Kettering Cancer Center reviews the clinical presentation, therapy, and outcome of 42 patients with primary soft tissue sarcomas of the lung.

Mentzer SJ, Reilly JJ, Skarin AT, Sugarbaker DJ: Patterns of lung involvement by malignant lymphoma. Surgery 113:507, 1993.

This retrospective review details one institution's experience with both primary pulmonary lymphomas and secondary lung involvement; correlation between the anatomic pattern of lung involvement and patient outcome is described.

Pound AW, Willis RA: A malignant teratoma of the lung in an infant. J Pathol 98:111, 1969.

In this report, the literature concerning primary malignant teratoma of the lung, of which there are few reports, is reviewed.

Sridhar KS, Saldana MJ, Thurer RJ, Beattie EJ: Primary choriocarcinoma of the lung: Report of a case treated with intensive multimodality therapy and review of the literature. J Surg Oncol 41:94, 1989.

This report describes one patient with primary choriocarcinoma of the lung. It also is an excellent review of the sparse data available in the literature.

Veynovich B, Masetti P, Kaplan PD, et al: Primary pulmonary thymoma. Ann Thorac Surg 64:1471, 1997.

This report summarizes very well the available literature, describing 18 patients, to which they add one of their own. In particular, the authors provide detailed suggestions for distinguishing primary pulmonary thymoma from either primary pulmonary lymphoma or malignancies metastatic to the lung.

Yellin A, Schwartz L, Hersho E, Lieberman Y: Chondrosarcoma of the bronchus: Report of a case with resection and review of the literature. Chest 84:224, 1983.

This report describes a patient with a primary chondrosarcoma of the lung and reviews the limited literature available concerning this rare neoplasm.

Yousem SA, Weiss LM, Colby TV: Primary pulmonary Hodgkin's disease: A clinicopathologic study of 15 cases. Cancer 57:1217, 1986.

This report from Stanford University is the largest single institutional series of primary Hodgkin's disease of the lung. The clinical data from 15 patients are reviewed, as is the literature.

■ *REFERENCES*

Addis BJ, Corrin B: Pulmonary blastoma, carcinosarcoma and spindle-cell carcinoma: An immunohistochemical study of keratin intermediate filaments. J Pathol 147:291, 1985.

Albeda RW, Monenaar WH, deLey L, Ipema AH: Heterogeneity of Wilms' tumor blastoma: An immunohistological study. Virchows Arch A Pathol Anat Histopathol 414:263, 1989.

Alghanem AA, Mehan J, Hassan AA: Primary malignant melanoma of the lung. J Surg Oncol 34:109, 1987.

Allan BT, Day DL, Dehner LP: Primary pulmonary rhabdomyosarcoma of the lung in children: Report of two cases presenting with spontaneous pneumothorax. Cancer 59:1005, 1987.

Allen AC, Spitz S: Malignant melanoma: A clinicopathological analysis of the criteria for diagnosis and prognosis. Cancer 6:1, 1953.

Allen MS, Drash EC: Primary melanoma of the lung. Cancer 21:154, 1968.

Amin R: Extramedullary plasmacytoma of the lung. Cancer 56:152, 1985.

Asherson RA, Muncey F, Pambakian H et al: Sjögren's syndrome and fibrosing alveolitis complicated by pulmonary lymphoma. Ann Rheum Dis 46:701, 1987.

Ashworth TG: Pulmonary blastoma, a true congenital neoplasm. Histopathology 7:585, 1983.

Avagnina A, Elsner B, DeMarco L et al: Pulmonary rhabdomyosarcoma with isolated small bowel metastasis: A report of a case with immunohistochemical and ultrastructural studies. Cancer 53:1948, 1984.

Azumi N, Churg A: Intravascular and sclerosing bronchioalveolar tumor: A pulmonary sarcoma of probable vascular origin. Am J Surg Pathol 5:587, 1981.

Baas AAF, van Herwaarden CLA: Primary non-Hodgkin's lymphoma of the lung. Eur J Respir Dis 68:218, 1986.

Bacha EA, Wright CD, Grillo HC et al: Surgical treatment of primary pulmonary sarcomas. Eur J Cardiothoracic Surg 15:456, 1999.

Bagwell SP, Flynn SD, Cox PM, Davison JA: Primary malignant melanoma of the lung. Am Rev Respir Dis 139:1543, 1989.

Ball HA: Primary pulmonary sarcoma: A review, with report of an additional case. Am J Cancer 15:2319, 1931.

Barnard WG: Embryoma of lung. Thorax 7:299, 1952.

Barrett NR, Barnard WG: Some unusual thoracic tumors. Br J Surg 32:447, 1945.

Baroni CD, Mineo TC, Ricci et al: Solitary secretory plasmacytoma of the lung in a 14-year-old boy. Cancer 40:2329, 1977.

Barson AJ, Jones AW, Lodge KV: Pulmonary blastoma. J Clin Pathol 21:480, 1968.

Bartley TD, Arean VM: Intrapulmonary neurogenic tumors. J Thorac Cardiovasc Surg 50:114, 1965.

Bauermeister DE, Jennings ER, Beland AH, Judson HA: Pulmonary blastoma, a form of carcinosarcoma: Report of a case of 24 years' duration without treatment. Am J Clin Pathol 46:322, 1966.

Bedrossian CWM, Verani R, Unger KM, Salman J: Pulmonary malignant fibrous histiocytoma. Chest 75:186, 1979.

Beluffi G, Bertolotti P, Mietta A et al: Primary leiomyosarcoma of the lung in a girl. Pediatr Radiol 16:240, 1986.

Ben-Ezra J, Winberg CD, Wu A et al: Concurrent presence of two clonal populations in small lymphocytic lymphoma of the lung. Hum Pathol 18:399, 1987.

Bergmann M, Ackerman LV, Kemler RL: Carcinosarcoma of the lung: Review of the literature and report of two cases treated by pneumonectomy. Cancer 4:919, 1951.

Berman L: Extragenital chorioepithelioma with report of a case. Am J Cancer 38:23, 1940.

Berho M, Moran CA, Suster S: Malignant mixed epithelial/mesenchymal neoplasms of the lung. Semin Diagn Pathol 12:123, 1995.

Bhalla M, Thompson BG, Marley RA, McLoud TC: Primary extraosseous pulmonary osteogenic sarcoma: CT findings. J Comput Assist Tomogr 16:974, 1992.

Bini G: Osservailioni anatomiche ed istopatologiche sopra particolari forme di tumori (polmonari maligni) di nature mesenchimale. Pathologica 34:77, 1942.

Borlee-Hermans G, Bury TH, Grand JL et al: Intravascular bronchioloalveolar tumour. Eur J Respir Dis 66:341, 1985.

Bosanko CMM, Korobkin M, Fantone JC et al: Lobar primary pulmonary lymphoma: CT findings. J Comput Assist Tomogr 15:679, 1991.

Boshnakova T, Michailova V, Koss M, et al: Primary pulmonary Hodgkin's disease: report of two cases. Resp Med 94:830, 2000.

Braunstein GD, Vaitukaitis JL, Carbone PP, Ross GT: Ectopic production of human chorionic gonadotropin by neoplasms. Ann Intern Med 78:39, 1973.

Bull JC, Grimes OR: Pulmonary carcinosarcoma. Chest 65:9, 1974.

Cagle P, Mace ML, Judge DM et al: Pulmonary melanoma: Primary vs. metastatic. Chest 85:125, 1984.

Cameron EWJ: Primary sarcoma of the lung. Thorax 30:516, 1975.

Capewell S, Webb JN, Crompton GK: Primary leiomyosarcoma of the lung presenting with a persistent pneumothorax. Thorax 41:649, 1986.

Carbone PP, Kaplan HS, Mussholf K et al: Report of the committee on Hodgkin's disease staging classification. Cancer Res 31:1860, 1971.

Carlucci GA, Schleussner RC: Primary (?) melanoma of lung: A case report. J Thorac Surg 11:643, 1942.

Carstens PHB, Kuhns JG, Ghazi C: Primary malignant melanomas of the lung and adrenals. Hum Pathol 15:910, 1984.

Carswell J, Kraeft NH: Fibrosarcoma of the bronchus: Report of a case diagnosed by bronchoscopy and treated by pneumonectomy. J Thorac Surg 19:117, 1949.

Caves PK, Jacques J: Primary intrapulmonary neurogenic sarcoma with hypertrophic pulmonary osteoarthropathy and asbestosis. Thorax 26:212, 1971.

Chaudhuri MR: Bronchial carcinosarcoma. J Thorac Cardiovasc Surg 61:319, 1971.

Childress WG, Adie GC: Plasma cell tumors of the mediastinum and lung: Report of two cases. J Thorac Cardiovasc Surg 19:794, 1950.

Chow WH, Ducheine Y, Milfer J, Brandstetter RD: Chronic pneumonia: Primary malignant non-Hodgkin's lymphoma of the lung arising in mucosa-associated lymphoid tissue. Chest 110:838, 1996.

Chowdhury LN, Swerdlow MA, Jao W et al: Postirradiation malignant fibrous histiocytoma of the lung: Demonstration of alpha-antitrypsin-like material in neoplastic cells. Am J Clin Pathol 74:820, 1980.

Colby TB, Bilbao JE, Battifora H, Unni K: Primary osteosarcoma of lung: A reappraisal following immunohistologic study. Arch Pathol Lab Med 113:1147, 1989.

Connolly JP et al: Intrathoracic osteosarcoma diagnosed by CT scan and pleural biopsy. Chest 100:265, 1991.

Conquest HF, Thornton JL, Massie JR, Coxe JW III: Primary pulmonary rhabdomyosarcoma: Report of three cases and literature review. Ann Surg 161:688, 1965.

Corrin B, Manners B, Millard M, Weaver L: Histogenesis of the so-called "intravascular bronchioalveolar tumour." J Pathol 128:163, 1979.

Corwin J, Lindberg RD: Solitary plasmacytoma of bone vs. extramedullary plasmacytoma and their relationship to multiple myeloma. Cancer 43:1007, 1979.

Cotton BH, Penido JRF: Plasma cell tumors of the lung: Report of a case. Dis Chest 21:218, 1952.

Cox JL, Fuson RL, Daly JT: Pulmonary blastoma: A case report and review of the literature. Ann Thorac Surg 9:364, 1970.

Crane M, Sutton JP: Primary sarcoma of the lung. South Med J 65:850, 1972.

Crotty TB, Hooker RP, Swenson SJ et al: Primary malignant ependymoma of the lung. Mayo Clin Proc 67:373, 1992.

Dahlgren SE, Ovenfors CO: Primary malignant lymphoma of the lung. Acta Radiol 8:401, 1969.

Dail DH, Liebow AA: Intravascular bronchioalveolar tumor (Abstract). Am J Pathol 78:6a, 1975.

Dail DH, Liebow AA, Gmelich JT et al: Intravascular, bronchiolar, and alveolar tumor of the lung (IVBAT): An analysis of twenty cases of a peculiar sclerosing endothelial tumor. Cancer 51:452, 1983.

Daniels AC, Conner GH, Straus FH: Primary chondrosarcoma of the tracheobronchial tree: Report of a unique case and brief review. Arch Pathol Lab Med 84:615, 1967.

Davis MP, Eagan RT, Weiland LH, Pairolero PC: Carcinosarcoma of the lung: Mayo Clinic experience and response to chemotherapy. Mayo Clin Proc 59:598, 1984.

Davis WB, Gadek JE: Detection of pulmonary lymphoma by bronchoalveolar lavage. Chest 91:787, 1987.

Day DW, Taylor SA: An intrapulmonary teratoma associated with thymic tissue. Thorax 30:582, 1975.

Dessy E, Pietra GG: Pseudomesotheliomatous carcinoma of the lung: An immunohistochemical and ultrastructural study of three cases. Cancer 68:1747, 1991.

Dhingra HK, Flance IJ: Cavitary primary pulmonary Hodgkin's disease presenting as pruritus. Chest 58:71, 1970.

Dixon DS, Breslow A: Pulmonary blastoma. Am Rev Respir Dis 108:968, 1973.

Eggleston IC: The intravascular bronchioalveolar tumor and the sclerosing hemangioma of the lung: Misnomers of pulmonary neoplasia. Semin Diagn Pathol 2:270, 1985.

Ehrenstein F: Primary pulmonary lymphoma: Review of the literature and two case reports. J Thorac Cardiovasc Surg 52:31, 1966.

Eliasson AH, Ragopal KR, Dow NS: Respiratory failure in rapidly progressing pulmonary lymphoma: Role of immunophenotyping in diagnosis. Am Rev Respir Dis 141:231, 1990.

Ellison RG, Bailey AW, Yeh TJ et al: Primary lymphosarcoma of the lung. Am Surg 30:737, 1964.

Emery RW, Fox AL, Raab DE: Short reports: Intravascular bronchioloalveolar tumour. Thorax 37:472, 1982.

Engel AF, Groot G, Bellot S: Carcinosarcoma of the lung. A case history of disseminated disease and review of the literature. Eur J Surg Oncol 17:94, 1991.

Eriksson A, Thuneil M, Lundqvist G: Pendulating endobronchial rhabdomyosarcoma with fatal asphyxia. Thorax 37:390, 1982.

Farquhar DL, Crompton GK, McIntyre MA, Leonard RCF: Non-Hodgkin's lymphoma of the lung. Scott Med J 33:243, 1988.

Farrell DJ, Kashyap AP, Ashcroft T, Morritt GN. Primary malignant melanoma of the bronchus. Thorax 51:223, 1996.

Ferraro P, Trasteck VF, Adlakha H, et al: Primary non-Hodgkin's lymphoma of the lung. Ann Thorac Surg 69:993, 2000.

Filho BG, Pasqualucci MEA: Sarcoma condroblastico primitivo do pulmao. Rev Bras Cir 45:293, 1963.

Fine G, Smith RW, Pachter MR: Primary extragenital choriocarcinoma in the male subject. Am J Med 32:776, 1962.

Fine G, Stout AP: Osteogenic sarcoma of the extraskeletal soft tissues. Cancer 9:1027, 1956.

Flint A, Kumar NB, Naylor B: Pulmonary Hodgkin's disease: Diagnosis by fine-needle aspiration. Acta Cytol 32:221, 1988.

Francis D, Jacobsen M: Pulmonary blastoma: Preoperative cytologic and histologic findings. Acta Cytol 23:437, 1979.

Fraser RG, Paré JA, Fraser RS, Genereux GP: Diagnosis of Diseases of the Chest, 3rd ed. Philadelphia, WB Saunders, 1989.

Freeman C, Berg JW, Cutler SJ: Occurrence and prognosis of extranodal lymphomas. Cancer 29:252, 1972.

Fukayama M, Maeda Y, Funata N et al: Pulmonary and pleural thymoma: Diagnostic application of lymphocyte markers to the thymoma of unusual site. Am J Clin Pathol 89:617, 1988.

Fukuda M, Sasaki Y, Morita M et al: Large cell carcinoma of the lung secreting human chorionic gonadotropin which responded to combination chemotherapy: Case report. Jpn J Clin Oncol 20:299, 1990.

Fung CH, Lo JW, Yonan TN et al: Pulmonary blastoma: An ultrastructural study with a brief review of literature and a discussion of pathogenesis. Cancer 39:153, 1977.

Gautam HP: Intrapulmonary malignant teratoma. Am Rev Respir Dis 100:863, 1969.

Gebauer C: The postoperative prognosis of primary pulmonary sarcomas: A review with a comparison of the histological forms and the other primary endothoracal sarcomas based on 474 cases. Scand J Thorac Cardiovasc Surg 16:91, 1982.

Gepharat GN: Malignant melanoma of the bronchus. Hum Pathol 12:671, 1981.

Gerber IE: Ectopic chorioepithelioma. Mt Sinai J Med 7:135, 1935.

Gerin-Lajoie L: A case of chorioepithelioma of the lung. Am J Obstet Gynecol 68:391, 1954.

Ghaffar A, Vaidynathan SV, Elguezabal A, Levowitz BS: Pulmonary blastoma: Report of two cases. Chest 67:600, 1975.

Gibbons JRP, McKeown F, Field TW: Pulmonary blastoma with hilar lymph node metastases: Survival for 24 years. Cancer 47:152, 1981.

Gibson PG, Bryant DH, Harkness J et al: Pulmonary manifestations of the acquired immunodeficiency syndrome. Aust N Z J Med 17:551, 1987.

Gledhill A, Kay JM: Hepatic metastases in a case of intravascular bronchioalveolar tumour. J Clin Pathol 37:279, 1984.

Goldthorn JF, Duncan MH, Kosloske AM, Ball WS: Cavitating primary pulmonary fibrosarcoma in a child. J Thorac Cardiovasc Surg 91:932, 1986.

Gordon J, Walker G: Plasmacytoma of the lung. Arch Pathol Lab Med 37:222, 1944.

Green WR, Pressoir R, Gumbs RV, et al: Intrapulmonary thymoma. Arch Pathol Lab Med 111:1074, 1987.

Greenberg SD, Heisler 1G, Gyorkey F, Jenkins DE: Pulmonary lymphoma versus pseudolymphoma: A perplexing problem. South Med J 65:775, 1972.

Greenspan EB: Primary osteoid chondrosarcoma of the lung: Report of a case. Am J Cancer 18:603, 1933.

Guccion JG, Rosen SH: Bronchopulmonary leiomyosarcoma and fibrosarcoma: A study of 32 cases and review of the literature. Cancer 30:836, 1972.

Guttman RF, Saavedra A: Primary Hodgkin's disease of the lung: Report of a case. Dis Chest 53:660, 1968.

Habermann TM, Ryo JH, Inwards DJ, Kurtin PJ: Primary pulmonary lymphoma. Semin Oncol 26:307, 1999.

Hansen LA, Prakash UBS, Colby TV: Pulmonary lymphoma in Sjögren's syndrome. Mayo Clin Proc 64:920, 1989.

Hardy K, Nicholson DP, Schaefer RF, Hsu SM: Bilateral endobronchial non-Hodgkin's lymphoma. South Med J 88:367, 1995.

Hattori M, Imura H, Matsukura S et al: Multiple-hormone producing lung carcinoma. Cancer 43:2429, 1979.

Henry K, Keal EE: Pulmonary blastoma with a striated muscle component. Br J Dis Chest 60:87, 1966.

Herbert A, Wright DH, Isaacson PG, Smith JL: Primary malignant lymphoma of lung: Histopathologic and immunologic evaluation of nine cases. Hum Pathol 15:415, 1984.

Herxheimer G, Reinke F: Pathologie des krebses. Ergebn D Allg Path U Path Anat 16:280, 1912.

Hilbun BM, Chavez CM: Lymphoma of the lung. J Thorac Cardiovasc Surg. 53:721, 1967.

Hill LD, White ML Jr: Plasmacytoma of the lung. J Thorac Cardiovasc Surg 25:187, 1953.

Hochberg LA, Crastnopol P: Primary sarcoma of the bronchus and lung. Arch Surg 73:74, 1955.

Holland J, Trenkner DA, Wasserman TH, Fineberg B: Plasmacytoma: Treatment results and conversion to myeloma. Cancer 69:1513, 1992.

Holt S, Deverall PB, Boddy JE: A teratoma of the lung containing thymic tissue. J Pathol 126:85, 1978.

Ishida T, Tateishi M, Kaneko S et al: Carcinosarcoma and spindle cell carcinoma of the lung: Clinicopathologic and immunohistochemical studies. J Thorac Cardiovasc Surg 100:844, 1990.

Ishizuka T, Yoshitake J, Yamada T et al: Diagnosis of a case of pulmonary carcinosarcoma by detection of rhabdomyosarcoma cells in sputum. Acta Cytol 32:658, 1988.

Iverson RE, Straehley CJ: Pulmonary blastoma: Long-term survival of juvenile patient. Chest 63:436, 1973.

Jacobson M, Francis D: Pulmonary blastoma: A clinicopathologic study of 11 cases. Acta Pathol Microbiol Scand 88:151, 1980.

James CL, Iyer PV, Leong ASY: Intrapulmonary thymoma. Histopathology 21:175, 1992.

Jamieson MPG, McGowan AR: Endobronchial teratoma. Thorax 37:157, 1982.

Janssen JP, Mulder JJ, Wagenaar SS, et al: Primary sarcoma of the lung: A clinical study with long-term follow-up. Ann Thorac Surg 58:1151, 1994.

Jenkins BJ: Carcinosarcoma of the lung: Report of a case and review of the literature. J Thorac Cardiovasc Surg 55:657, 1968.

Jensen OA, Egedorf J: Primary malignant melanoma of the lung. Scand J Respir Dis 48:127, 1967.

Jetley NK, Bhatnagar V, Krishna A et al: Pulmonary blastoma in a neonate. J Pediatr Surg 23:1009, 1988.

Jimenez JF: Pulmonary blastoma in childhood. J Surg Oncol 34:87, 1987.

Johnson DW, Hoppe RT, Cox RS et al: Hodgkin's disease limited to intrathoracic sites. Cancer 52:8, 1983.

Joseph G, Pandit M, Korfhage L: Primary pulmonary plasmacytoma. Cancer 71:721, 1993.

Kakkar N, Vasishta RK, Banerjee AK et al: Primary pulmonary malignant teratoma with yolk sac element associated with hematologic neoplasia. Respiration 63:52, 1996.

Kakos GS, Williams TE, Assor D, Vasko JS: Pulmonary carcinosarcoma: Etiologic, therapeutic, and prognostic considerations. J Thorac Cardiovasc Surg 61:777, 1971.

Kalish PE: Primary intrapulmonary thymoma. NY State J Med 63:1705, 1963.

Kalus M, Rahman F, Jenkins DE, Beall AC Jr: Malignant mesenchymoma of the lung. Arch Pathol Lab Med 95:199, 1973.

Karcioglu ZA, Someren AO: Pulmonary blastoma: A case report and review of the literature. Am J Clin Pathol 61:287, 1974.

Kay S, Reed WG: Chorioepithelioma of the lung in a female infant seven months old. Am J Pathol 21:555, 1953.

Kazzaz B, Dewar A, Corrin B: An unusual pulmonary plasmacytoma. Histopathology 21:285, 1992.

Kennedy A, Prior AL: Pulmonary blastoma: A report of two cases and a review of the literature. Thorax 31:776, 1976.

Kennedy JD, Kneafsey DV: Two cases of plasmacytoma of the lower respiratory tract. Thorax 14:353, 1959.

Kennedy JL, Nathwani BN, Burke JS et al: Pulmonary lymphomas and other pulmonary lymphoid lesions: A clinicopathologic and immunologic study of 64 patients. Cancer 56:539, 1985.

Kern WH, Crepeau AG, Jones JC: Primary Hodgkin's disease of the lung: Report of 4 cases and review of the literature. Cancer 14:1151, 1961.

Kern WH, Hughes RK, Meyer BW, Harley DP: Malignant fibrous histiocytoma of the lung. Cancer 44:1793, 1979.

Kern WH, Stiles QR: Pulmonary blastoma. J Thorac Cardiovasc Surg 72:801, 1976.

Kernen JA, Meyer BW: Malignant plasmacytoma of the lung with metastases. J Thorac Cardiovasc Surg 51:739, 1966.

Kinare SG, Parulkar GB, Panday SR et al: Extensive ossification in a pulmonary plasmacytoma. Thorax 20:206, 1965.

Knowling MA, Harwood AR, Bergsagel DE: Comparison of extramedullary plasmacytomas with solitary and multiple plasma cell tumors of bone. J Clin Oncol 1:255, 1983.

Kodama T, Shimosato Y, Watanabe S et al: Six cases of well-differentiated adenocarcinoma simulating fetal lung tubules in pseudoglandular stage: Comparison with pulmonary blastoma. Am J Surg Pathol 8:735, 1984.

Koss MN, Hochholzer L, Nichols PW et al: Primary non-Hodgkin's lymphoma and pseudolymphoma of lung: A study of 161 patients. Hum Pathol 14:1024, 1983.

Koss MN, Hochholzer L, O'Leary T: Pulmonary blastomas. Cancer 67:2368, 1991.

Kradin RI, Young RH, Dickersin GIC et al: Pulmonary blastoma with argyrophylic cells lacking sarcomatous features (pulmonary endodermal tumor resembling fetal lung). Am J Surg Pathol 6:165, 1982.

Kummet TD, Doll DC: Chemotherapy of pulmonary blastoma: A case report and review of the literature. Med Pedatr Oncol 10:27, 1982.

Kung ITM, Loke SL, So SY et al: Intrapulmonary thymoma: Report of two cases. Thorax 40:471, 1985.

Kunkel OF, Torrey E: Report of a case of primary melanotic sarcoma of lung presenting difficulties in differentiating from tuberculosis. N Y State J Med 16:198, 1916.

Larsen H, Sorensen JB. Pulmonary blastoma: A review with special emphasis on prognosis and treatment. Cancer Treat Rev 22:145, 1996.

Lee JT, Shelburne JD, Linder J: Primary malignant fibrous histiocytoma of the lung: A clinicopathologic and ultrastructural study of five cases. Cancer 53:1124, 1984.

Lennert K: Malignant Lymphomas Other than Hodgkin's Disease. Springer-Verlag, New York, 1978

Le Tourneau A, Audouin J, Garbe L et al: Primary pulmonary malignant lymphoma, clinical and pathological findings, immunocytochemical and ultrastructural studies in 15 cases. Hematol Oncol 1:49, 1983

L'Hoste RJ, Filippa DA, Lieberman PH, Bretsky S: Primary pulmonary lymphomas: A clinicopathologic analysis of 36 cases. Cancer 54:1397, 1984.

Lowell LM, Tuhy JE: Primary chondrosarcoma of the lung. J Thorac Cardiovasc Surg 18:476, 1949.

Lukes RJ, Collins RD: Immunologic characterization of human malignant lymphomas. Cancer 34:1488, 1974.

Mackay B, Lukeman JM, Ordonez NG: Tumors of the Lung. Philadelphia, WB Saunders, 1990.

Manivel JC, Priest JR, Watterson J et al: Pleuropulmonary blastoma: The so-called pulmonary blastoma of childhood. Cancer 62:1516, 1988.

Manning JT, Ordonez NG, Rosenberg HS et al: Pulmonary endodermal tumor resembling fetal lung: Report of a case with immunohistochemical studies. Arch Pathol Lab Med 109:48, 1985.

Marchevsky A, Padilla M, Kaneko M, Kleinerman J: Localized lymphoid nodules of lung: A reappraisal of the lymphoma versus pseudolymphoma dilemma. Cancer 51:2070, 1983.

Marcus PB, Dieb TM, Martin JH: Pulmonary blastoma: An ultrastructural study emphasizing intestinal differentiation in lung tumors. Cancer 49:1829, 1982.

Mark LK: Primary lymphoma of the lung. JAMA 237:895, 1977.

Marsh K, Kenyon WE, Earis JE, Pearson MG: Intravascular bronchioloalveolar tumour. Thorax 37:474, 1982.

Martini N, Haddu SI, Beattie EJ Jr: Primary sarcoma of the lung. J Thorac Cardiovasc Surg 61:33, 1971.

Mata JM, Caceres J, Prat J, et al: Intravascular bronchio-alveolar tumor: Radiographic findings. Eur J Radiol 12:95, 1991.

Mazumdar P, Abraham S, Damodaran VN, Saha NC: Pulmonary plasmacytoma: A case report. Am Rev Respir Dis 100:866, 1969.

McBurney RP, Claggett OT, McDonald JR: Primary intrapulmonary neoplasm (?thymoma) associated with myasthenia gravis: Report of a case. Proc Mayo Clin 26:345, 1951.

McCann MP, Fu YS, Kay S: Pulmonary blastoma: A light and electron microscopic study. Cancer 38:789, 1976.

McCormack PM, Martini N: Primary sarcomas and lymphomas of lung. In Martini N, Vogt-Moykopf I (eds): Thoracic Surgery: Frontiers and Uncommon Neoplasms, Vol 5. St. Louis, CV Mosby, 1989, p 269.

McDonnell T, Kyriakos M, Roper C, Mazonjian G: Malignant fibrous histiocytoma of the lung. Cancer 61:137, 1988.

Meade JB, Whitwell F, Bickford BJ, Waddington JKB: Primary haemangiopericytoma of lung. Thorax 29:1, 1974.

Meade P, Moad J, Fellows D, Adams CW: Carcinosarcoma of the lung with hypertrophic pulmonary osteoarthropathy. Ann Thorac Surg 51:488, 1991.

Medbery CA III, Bibro MC, Phares JC et al: Pulmonary blastoma: Case report and literature review of chemotherapy experience. Cancer 53:2413, 1984.

Meis JM, Butler JJ, Osborne BM, Ordonez NG: Solitary plasmacytomas of bone and extramedullary plasmacytomas: A clinicopathologic and immunohistochemical study. Cancer 59:1475, 1987.

Mentzer SJ, Reilly JJ, Skarin AT, Sugarbaker DJ: Patterns of lung involvement by malignant lymphoma. Surgery 113:507, 1993.

Miettinen M, Collan Y, Halttunen P et al: Intravascular bronchioloalveolar tumor. Cancer 60:2471, 1987.

Miller B, Montgomery C, Watne AL et al: Lymphoepithelioma-like carcinoma of the lung. J Surg Oncol 48:62, 1991.

Miyake M, Ito M, Mitsuoka A et al: Alpha-fetoprotein and human chorionic gonadotropin-producing lung cancer. Cancer 59:227, 1987.

Monahan DT: Hodgkin's disease of the lung. J Thorac Cardiovasc Surg 49:173, 1965.

Moore T: Carcinosarcoma of the lung. Surgery 50:886, 1961.

Moralles FM, Matthews JI: Diagnosis of parenchymal Hodgkin's disease using bronchoalveolar lavage. Chest 91:785, 1987.

Moran CA, Suster S, Fishback NF, Koss MN: Primary intrapulmonary thymoma: A clinicopathologic and immunohistochemical study of eight cases. Am J Surg Pathol 1995;19:304–12.

Morgan AD, Salama FD: Primary chondrosarcoma of the lung: Case report and review of the literature. J Thorac Cardiovasc Surg 64:460, 1972.

Morinaga S, Watanabe H, Gemma A et al: Plasmacytoma of the lung associated with nodular deposits of immunoglobulin. Am J Pathol 11:989, 1987.

Muggia FM, Rosen SW, Weintraub BD, Hansen HH: Ectopic placental proteins in nontrophoblastic tumors. Cancer 36:1327, 1975.

Muller-Hermelink MK, Kaiserling E: Pulmonary adenocarcinoma of fetal type: Alternating differentiation argues in favor of a common endodermal stem cell. Virchows Arch A Pathol Anat Histopathol 409:195, 1986.

Nappi O, Glasner SD, Swanson PE, Wick MR: Biphasic and monophasic sarcomatoid carcinomas of the lung: A reappraisal of "carcinosarcomas" and "spindle-cell carcinomas". Am J Clin Pathol 102:331, 1994.

Nascimento NG, Unni UK, Bernatz PE: Sarcomas of the lung. Mayo Clin Proc 57:355, 1982.

Nathwani BN, Kim H, Rappaport H, Solomon J et al: Non-Hodgkin's lymphomas: A clinicopathologic study comparing two classifications. Cancer 41:303, 1978.

Neilson DB: Primary intrapulmonary neurogenic sarcoma. J Pathol 76:419, 1958.

Nelson S, Prince D, Terry P: Primary Hodgkin's disease of the lung: Case report. Thorax 38:310, 1983.

Non-Hodgkin's Lymphoma Pathologic Classification Project. National Cancer Institute sponsored study of classifications of non-Hodgkin's lymphoma. Cancer 49:2112, 1982.

Nosanchuk JS, Weatherbee L: Primary osteogenic sarcoma in lung: Report of a case. J Thorac Cardiovasc Surg 58:242, 1969.

Ott RA, Eugene J, Kollin J et al: Primary pulmonary angiosarcoma associated with multiple synchronous neoplasms. J Surg Oncol 35:269, 1987.

Ozkaynak MF, Ortega JA, Laug W et al: Role of chemotherapy in pediatric pulmonary blastoma. Med Pediatr Oncol 18:53, 1990.

Palmer RN, Saini N, Guccion J: Ewing's-like sarcoma appearing as a primary pulmonary neoplasm. Arch Pathol Lab Med 105:277, 1981.

Papaiannou AN, Watson WL: Primary lymphoma of the lung: An appraisal of its natural history and a comparison with other localized lymphomas. J Thorac Cardiovasc Surg 49:373, 1965.

Parker JC, Payne WS, Woolner LB: Pulmonary blastoma (embryoma): Report of two cases. J Thorac Cardiovasc Surg 51:694, 1966.

Pasquini E, Rastelli E, Muretto P, et al: Primary bronchial malignant melanoma: A case report. Pathologica 86:546, 1994.

Pedersen VM, Schulre S, Madsen KH, Krogdahl AS: Primary pulmonary leiomyosarcoma: Review of the literature and report of a case. Scand J Thorac Cardiovasc Surg 18:251, 1984.

Petersen M: Radionuclide detection of primary pulmonary osteogenic sarcoma: A case report and review of the literature. J Nucl Med 31:1110, 1990.

Peterson H, Snider HL, Yam LT et al: Primary pulmonary lymphoma: A clinical and immunohistochemical study of six cases. Cancer 56:805, 1985.

Pettinato G, Manivel JC, Saldana MJ et al: Primary bronchopulmonary fibrosarcoma of childhood and adolescence: Reassessment of a low-grade malignancy. Pathol 20:463, 1989.

Pinson P, Joos G, Praet M, Pauwels R: Primary pulmonary Hodgkin's disease. Respiration 59:314, 1992.

Poelzleitner D, Huebsch P, Mayerhofer S et al: Primary pulmonary lymphoma in a patient with the acquired immune deficiency syndrome. Thorax 44:438, 1989.

Polish LB, Cohn DL, Ryder JW et al: Pulmonary non-Hodkin's lymphoma in AIDS. Chest 96:1321, 1989.

Pound AW, Willis RA: A malignant teratoma of the lung in an infant. J Pathol 98:111, 1969.

Priest JR, McDermott MB, Bhatia S, et al: Pleuropulmonary blastoma: A clinicopathologic study of 50 cases. Cancer 80:147, 1997.

Prive L, Tellem M, Meranze DR, Chodoff RD: Carcinosarcoma of the lung. Arch Pathol Lab Med 72:119, 1961.

Pushchak MJ, Farhi DC: Primary choriocarcinoma of the lung. Arch Pathol Lab Med 111:477, 1987.

Rabiah FA: Primary lymphocytic lymphoma (lymphosarcoma) of the lung. Am Surg 34:275, 1968.

Radin AJ: Primary pulmonary Hodgkin's disease. Cancer 65:550, 1990.

Razzuk MA, Urschel HC, Race GJ et al: Carcinosarcoma of the lung: Report of two cases and review of the literature. J Thorac Cardiovasc Surg 61:541, 1971.

Reale FR, Variakojis D, Compton J et al: Cytodiagnosis of Hodgkin's disease in sputum specimens. Acta Cytol 27:258, 1983.

Reed RJ, Kent EM: Solitary pulmonary melanomas: Two case reports. J Thorac Cardiovasc Surg 48:226, 1964.

Rees GM: Primary chondrosarcoma of lung. Thorax 25:366, 1970.

Regnard J-F, Icard P, Guibert L, et al: Prognostic factors and results after surgical treatment of primary sarcomas of the lung. Ann Thorac Surg 68:227, 1999.

Reid JD, Mehta VT: Melanoma of the lower respiratory tract. Cancer 19:627, 1966.

Reingold IM, Amromin GD: Extraosseous osteosarcoma of the lung. Cancer 28:491, 1971.

Reverter JC, Coca A, Font J, Ingelmo M: Erythema nodosum and pulmonary solitary nodule as the first manifestations of a non-Hodgkin's lymphoma. Br J Dis Chest 81:397, 1987.

Risdall R, Hoppe RT, Warnke R: Non-Hodgkin's lymphoma: A study of the evolution of the disease based upon 92 autopsied cases. Cancer 44:529, 1979.

Robertson AJ, Sinclair DJM, Sutton PP, Guthrie W: Primary melanocarcinoma of the lower respiratory tract. Thorax 35:158, 1980.

Roggeri A, Agostini L, Vezzani G, Sabattini E et al: Primary malignant non-Hodgkin's lymphoma of the lung arising in mucosa-associated lymphoid tissue (MALT). Eur Respir J 6:138, 1993.

Roth JA, Elquezabal A: Pulmonary blastoma evolving into carcinosarcoma. Am J Surg Pathol 2:407, 1978.

Rozsa S, Frieman H: Extramedullary plasmacytoma of the lung. AJR Am J Roentgenol 70:982, 1953.

Rubin M: Primary lymphoma of lung. J Thorac Cardiovasc Surg 56:293, 1968.

Rudders RA, Ross ME, DeLellis RA: Primary extranodal lymphoma: Response to treatment and factors influencing prognosis. Cancer 42:406, 1978.

Ruland L: Malignant teratoblastoma of the lung. Thorac Cardiovasc Surg 4:119, 1956.

Rusch VW, Shuman WP, Schmidt R, Laramore GE: Massive pulmonary hemangiopericytoma: An innovative approach to evaluation and treatment. Cancer 64:1928, 1989.

Rush WL, Andriko JA, Taubenberger JK et al: Primary anaplastic large cell lymphoma of the lung: A clinicopathologic study of five patients. Mod Pathol 13:1285, 2000.

Sakula A: Primary malignant lymphoma of lung. Postgrad Med J 55:46, 1979.

Salm R: A primary malignant melanoma of the bronchus. J Pathol 85:121, 1963.

Saltzstein SL: Pulmonary malignant lymphomas and pseudolymphomas: Classification, therapy, and prognosis. Cancer 16:928, 1963.

Santos F, Entrenas LM, Sebastian F et al: Primary bronchopulmonary malignant melanoma: Case report. Scand J Thor Cardiovasc Surg 21:187, 1987.

Schiodt T, Jensen KG: Malignant teratoid tumour of the lung: ? malignant hamartoma. Thorax 15:120, 1960.

Schwaiger A, Prior C, Weyrer K et al: Non-Hodgkin's lymphoma of the lung diagnosed by gene rearrangement from bronchoalveolar lavage fluid: A fast and noninvasive method. Blood 77:2538, 1991.

Sedlezky 1: Malignant pulmonary lesion with calcification. Can Assoc Radiol J 6:65, 1955.

Shariff S, Thomas JA, Shetty N, D'Cunha S: Primary pulmonary rhabdomyosarcoma in a child, with a review of literature. J Surg Oncol 38:261, 1988.

Sherman JL, Rykwalder PJ, Tashkin DP: Intravascular bronchioalveolar tumor. Am Rev Respir Dis 123:468, 1981.

Shuman RL: Primary pulmonary sarcoma and left atrial extension via left superior pulmonary vein: En bloc resection and radical pneumonectomy on cardiopulmonary bypass. J Thorac Cardiovasc Surg 88:189, 1984.

Sicilian L, Warson F, Carrington CB et al: Intravascular bronchioalveolar tumor (IV-BAT). Respiration 44:387, 1983.

Silverman JF, Coalson JJ: Primary malignant myxoid fibrous histiocytoma of the lung: Light and ultrastructural examination with review of the literature. Arch Pathol Lab Med 108:49, 1984.

Sinclair RA, Sullivan JR, McConchie J: Primary lymphoma of lung. Med J Aust 1:356, 1978.

Sordillo PP, Hajdu SI, Magill GB, Golbey RB: Extraosseous osteogenic sarcoma: A review of 48 patients. Cancer 51:727, 1983.

Spencer H: Pulmonaty blastoma. J Pathol 82:161, 1961.

Spragg RG, Wolf PL, Haghighi P et al: Angiosarcoma of the lung with fatal pulmonary hemorrhage. Am J Med 74:1072, 1983.

Sprague RI, deBlois GG: Small lymphocytic pulmonary lymphoma: Diagnosis by transthoracic fine-needle aspiration. Chest 96:929, 1989.

Sridhar KS, Saldana MJ, Thurer RJ, Beattie EJ: Primary choriocarcinoma of the lung: Report of a case treated with intensive multimodality therapy and review of the literature. J Surg Oncol 41:94, 1989.

Stackhouse EM, Harrison KG, Ellis FH: Primary mixed malignancies of lung: Carcinosarcoma and blastoma. J Thorac Cardiovas Surg 57:385, 1969.

Sugarbaker ED, Craver LF. Lymphosarcoma: Study of 196 cases with biopsy. JAMA 115:17, 1940.

Sullivan LG: Primary choriocarcinoma of the lung in a man. Arch Pathol Lab Med 113:82, 1989.

Sun CCJ, Kroll M, Miller JE: Primary chondrosarcoma of the lung. Cancer 50:1864, 1982.

Suster S: Primary sarcomas of the lung. Sem Diagn Pathol 12:140, 1995.

Sweeney WB, Vesoulis Z, Blaum LC Jr: Intravascular bronchioloalveolar tumor: A distinctive surgical and pathological entity. Ann Thorac Surg 42:702, 1986.

Taboada CF, McMurray JD, Jordan RA, Seybold WD: Primary melanoma of the lung. Chest 62:629, 1972.

Tamai S, Kameya T, Shimosato Y et al: Pulmonary blastoma: An ultrastructural study of a case and its transplanted tumor in athymic nude mice. Cancer 46:1389, 1980.

Tan TB, Spaander PJ, Blaisse M, Gerritzen FM: Angiotropic large cell lymphoma presenting as interstitial lung disease. Thorax 43:578, 1988.

Tanimura A, Natsuyama H, Kawano M et al: Primary choriocarcinoma of the lung. Hum Pathol 16:1281, 1985.

Thomas WJ, Koenig HM, Ellwanger FR, Lightsey AL: Primary pulmonary rhabdomyosarcoma in childhood. Am J Dis Child 135:469, 1981.

Todd FW: Two cases of melanotic tumors in lungs. JAMA 11:53, 1888.

Turner RR, Colby TV, Doggett RS: Well-differentiated lymphocytic lymphoma: A study of 47 patients with primary manifestation in the lung. Cancer 54:2088, 1984.

Ueda K, Gruppo R, Unger F et al: Rhabdomyosarcoma of lung arising in congenital cystic adenomatoid malformation. Cancer; 40:383, 1977.

Uwatoko K, Kajita M: Primary choriocarcinoma of the lung: A case report involving a male. J Jpn Assoc Chest Surg 11:662, 1997.

Van Assendelft AHW, Strengell-Usanov L, Kastarinen S: Pulmonary haemangiopericytoma with multiple metastases. Eur J Respir Dis 65:380, 1984.

van der Schee AC, Dinkla BA, van Knapen A: Primary pulmonary manifestation of Hodgkin's disease. Respiration 57:127, 1990.

Venn GE, Gellister J, DaCosta PE, Goldstraw P: Malignant fibrous histiocytoma in thoracic surgical practice. J Thorac Cardiovasc Surg 91:234, 1986.

Veynovich B, Masetti P, Kaplan PD, et al: Primary pulmonary thymoma. Ann Thorac Surg 64:1471, 1997.

Wang J, Pandha HS, Trelearen J, Powles R: Metastatic extramedullary plasmacytoma of the lung. Leuk Lymphoma 35:423, 1999.

Weinblatt ME, Siegel SE, Isaacs H: Pulmonary blastoma associated with cystic lung disease. Cancer 49:669, 1982.

Weiss SW: Malignant fibrous histiocytoma: A reaffirmation. Am J Surg Pathol 6:773, 1982.

Weldon-Linne CM, Victor TA, Christ ML, Fry WA: Angiogenic nature of the "intravascular bronchioalveolar tumor" of the lung: An electron microscopic study. Arch Pathol Lab Med 105:174, 1981.

Wick MR, Ritter JH, Humphrey PA: Sarcomatoid carcinomas of the lung: A clinicopathologic review. Am J Clin Pathol 108:40, 1997.

Wick MR, Scheithauer BW, Piehler JM, Pairolero PC: Primary pulmonary leiomyosarcomas. Arch Pathol Lab Med 106:510, 1982.

Wile A, Olinger G, Peter JB, Dornfeld L: Solitary intraparenchymal pulmonary plasmacytoma associated with production of an Mprotein: Report of a case. Cancer 37:2338, 1976.

Wiltshaw E: The natural history of extramedullary plasmacytoma and its relation to solitary myeloma of bone and myelomatosis. Medicine 55:217, 1976.

Wisecarver J, Ness MJ, Rennard SJ et al: Bronchoalveolar lavage in the assessment of pulmonary Hodgkin's disease. Acta Cytol 33:527, 1989.

Wood N, Coltman CA: Localized primary extranodal Hodgkin's disease. Ann Intern Med 78:113, 1973.

Woodruff RK, Whittle JM, Malpas JS: Solitary plasmacytoma. I: Extramedullary soft tissue plasmacytoma. Cancer 43:2340, 1979.

Wotherspoon AC, Soosay GN, Diss TC, Isaacson PG: Low-grade primary B-cell lymphoma of the lung: An immunohistochemical, molecular, and cytogenic study of a single case. Am J Clin Pathol 94:655, 1990.

Yamashita T, Kiyota T, Ukishima G et al: Autopsy case of chondro-osteoid sarcoma originating in the lung. J Shonai Med Assoc 23:472, 1964.

Yanagawa H, Hashimoto Y, Bando H, et al: Intravascular bronchioloalveolar tumor with skin metastases. Chest 105:1882, 1994.

Yellin A, Schwartz L, Hersho E, Lieberman Y: Chondrosarcoma of the bronchus: Report of a case with resection and review of the literature. Chest 84:224, 1983.

Yeoh CB, Ford JM, Lattes R, Wylie RH: Intrapulmonary thymoma. J Thorac Cardiovasc Surg 51:131, 1966.

Yi ES, Auger WR, Friedman PJ, et al: Intravascular bronchioloalveolar tumor of the lung presenting as pulmonary thromboembolic disease and pulmonary hypertension. Arch Pathol Lab Med 119:255, 1995.

Yousem SA: Angiosarcoma presenting in the lung. Arch Pathol Lab Med 110:112, 1986.

Yousem SA, Weiss LM, Colby TV: Primary pulmonary Hodgkin's disease: A clinicopathologic study of 15 cases. Cancer 57:1217, 1986.

Yousem SA, Hochholzer L: Malignant fibrous histiocytoma of the lung. Cancer 60:2532, 1987a.

Yousem SA, Hochholzer L: Primary pulmonary hemangiopericytoma. Cancer 59:549, 1987b.

Yousem SA, Wick MR, Randhawa P, Manivel JC: Pulmonary blastoma: An immunohistochemical analysis with comparison with fetal lung in its pseudoglandular stage. Am J Clin Pathol 93:167, 1990.

Zapatero J, Bellon J, Baamonde C et al: Primary choriocarcinoma of the lung: Presentation of a case and review of the literature. Scand J Thorac Cardiovasc Surg 16:279, 1982.

Zulian GB, Jacot-des-Combes E, Aapro MS: Primary pulmonary Hodgkin's disease and the dilemma of E stage. Eur J Surg Oncol 12:307; 1986.

CHAPTER 35

Pulmonary Metastases

Ugo Pastorino

Dominique Grunenwald

Near the end of the 20th century, pulmonary metastasectomy gradually became a standard treatment in properly selected patients. However, the curative potential of surgical resection of pulmonary metastases is still dismissed by many oncologists on the grounds that systemic disseminated disease is already present at the time of diagnosis.

The first resection of a single lung metastasis was reported by Weinlechner in 1882, as a consequence of intraoperative assessment for a chest wall sarcoma (Weinlechner, 1882). During the following 50 years and more, elective surgery was offered to a limited number of patients (Barney and Churchill, 1939) who presented with single pulmonary metastases or a long disease-free interval (Alexander and Haight, 1947).

Initial criticism of surgical treatment, based on the judgment that pulmonary metastasis was an indication of widespread end-stage disease, restricted the indication to those patients with solitary lesions occurring many years after the initial tumor. With the improvement of surgical techniques and the proven safety and efficacy of limited pulmonary resections, metastasectomy gained greater popularity. Nonetheless, it was only in the last 2 decades of the 20th century, and in selected oncologic departments, that metastasectomy was offered systematically to patients with multiple or bilateral lesions on the basis of favorable results achieved in metastatic sarcomas (Martini et al, 1979; Vogt-Moykopf et al, 1994).

Major proof of the curative potential of metastasectomy was achieved in the management of childhood osteosarcoma, in which fatal lung metastases occurred in 80% of patients after amputation of the primary tumor. (Marcove and Huvos, 1971). In a consecutive series of 27 patients presenting at Memorial Sloan-Kettering cancer center with lung metastases from osteosarcoma, systematic lung resection resulted in complete eradication of the disease in more than 80% of cases and a 45% survival at 5 years (Martini et al, 1971).

New chemotherapy regimens, which are potentially effective on micrometastatic foci but are usually unable to totally eradicate the component of the disease that is clinically detectable, have further expanded the role of adjuvant or salvage surgery aimed at excising the residual tumor after induction chemotherapy or confirming a complete pathologic remission.

HISTORICAL READINGS

Alexander J, Haight C: Pulmonary resection for solitary metastatic sarcomas and carcinomas. Surg Gynec Obstet 85:129, 1947.

Barney JD, Churchill EJ: Adenocarcinoma of the kidney with metastasis to the lung. J Urol 42:269, 1939.

Martini N, Huvos AG, Mike V et al: Multiple pulmonary resections in the treatment of osteogenic sarcoma. Ann Thorac Surg 12:271, 1971.

Weinlechner: Tumoren an der Brustwand und deren Behandlung (Resection der Rippen) Eroffnung der Brusthohle und partielle Entfernung der Lunge. Wien Med Wschr 32:590, 1892.

BASIC MECHANISMS

The basic mechanisms controlling the process of metastatic spread remain largely unknown. Recent research on angiogenesis and growth factors has provided new insight into some aspects of tumor progression, but a proper biologic explanation of the selectivity and specificity of distant metastases is still lacking.

Studies performed on large series of autopsies demonstrated that in 29% of patients who died of malignancies, the lung was the second most common metastatic locus (Wills, 1967). Weiss and Gilbert (1978) showed that in 20% of autopsied patients, the lungs were the sole site of detectable cancer.

The clinical incidence of isolated pulmonary metastasis varies with the primary tumor site. Lung metastases represent the main reason for treatment failure in 50% to 80% of osteosarcomas (Friedman and Carter, 1972; Marcove et al, 1970) and in 30% to 50% of soft tissue sarcomas (Lawrence et al, 1987; Potter, Glenn et al, 1985; Potter, Kinsella et al, 1985; Rosenberg et al, 1986). In the experience of the National Cancer Institute (Potter, Glenn et al, 1985), median survival time of patients with unresected lung metastases from soft tissue sarcomas was 7.4 months.

For the majority of patients with pulmonary metastases, resection may represent the sole chance of permanent cure, but the number of surgical candidates is relatively small. The cases that are amenable to surgical resection for cure are determined by the primary tumor and a number of clinical factors, such as the risk of metastases to other organs, the sensitivity to chemotherapy or hormone treatment, and the probability of new primary tumors (Table 35–1). In sarcomas and germ cell or pediatric malignancies, many patients presenting with lung metastases may be candidates for metastasectomy, but in most epithelial cancers only a small fraction (1% to 2%) of patients may be so treated because most present with concurrent distant metastases in other organs (Mayo and Schlicke, 1978; McCormack and Attiyeh, 1979).

The efficacy of chemotherapy in treating pulmonary metastases varies with the primary tumor site. In germ

TABLE 35–1 ■ **Rationale of Metastasectomy in Various Primary Tumors**

Primary Site	*Aim of Metastasectomy*	*Usual Application*
Sarcoma	Permanent cure	Whenever possible
Teratoma	Confirm complete remission, residual teratoma	Systematic
Colon-rectum	Permanent cure, ± liver resection	Selective
Kidney	Occasional cure	Highly selective
Melanoma	Occasional cure, new primary	Only single lesion
Breast	Hormone receptors, new primary	Only single lesion

cell tumors and osteogenic sarcomas, systemic therapy alone may sometimes achieve complete eradication of the disease. Radiotherapy has a limited role in the management of pulmonary metastases and is usually reserved for palliation of local symptoms.

SURGICAL RESECTION FOR PULMONARY METASTASES

Diagnosis and Staging

The probability of detecting pulmonary metastases depends on the modality used and intensity of clinical follow-up after primary tumor management. If the risk of pulmonary metastasis is high and the chances of successful salvage therapy are good (germ cell tumors and sarcomas), more frequent surveillance of a patient is justified, including serial computer tomography (CT) scans.

Lung metastases may occur with symptoms that mimic primary lung cancer, such as pain due to pleural or chest wall extension, cough and hemoptysis secondary to bronchial or vessel erosion, and mediastinal syndrome resulting from nodal metastases. Extensive pulmonary dissemination, pleural effusion, or central airway obstruction can cause dyspnea, whereas severe shortness of breath and a limited radiologic picture is suggestive of lymphangitic spread.

Nonetheless, most pulmonary metastatic lesions are detected on routine chest radiography in otherwise asymptomatic patients (Fig. 35–1). CT is the appropriate procedure to use for clarifying the nature of any suspicious nodular density found on chest radiograph (Chang et al, 1979; Mintzer et al, 1979). It provides accurate information on the number, dimension, and site of each individual lesion (Table 35–2). For patients with germ cell tumors or sarcomas, CT scans have been adopted as routine follow-up in many centers.

Conventional CT can identify up to 80% of all pulmonary nodules greater than 3 mm detected at surgical exploration (25% more than linear tomography) (Chang et al, 1979; Mintzer et al, 1979; Roth et al, 1986). Spiral CT scanning has further improved the diagnostic yield of radiologic staging, in terms of minimum size of parenchymal nodules detectable (less than 3 mm) and of significant hilar or mediastinal adenopathies. With such a high sensitivity, however, the rate of false-positive lesions has also increased.

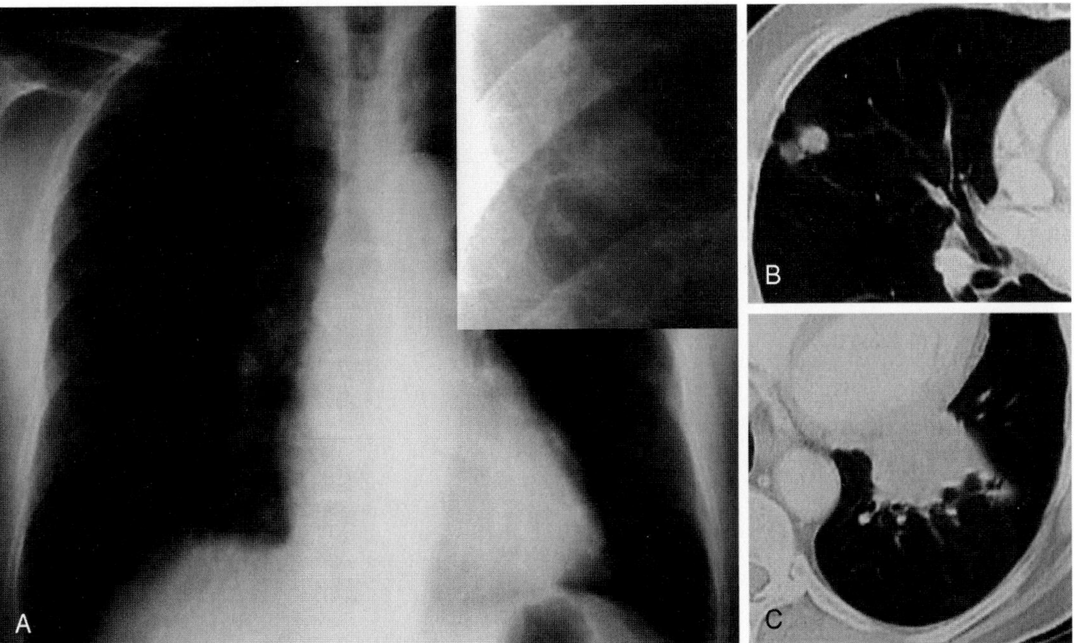

FIGURE 35–1 ■ Follow-up chest radiograph of a patient who was radically resected for colon cancer shows a solitary lesion on the right lung (enlarged) *(A)*; however, the chest computed tomography scan demonstrates, in addition to the lesion in the right upper lobe *(B)*, a metastasis in the left lower lobe *(C)*.

TABLE 35–2 ■ **Relevant Questions in Clinical Staging**

Probability of a false-positive result
Single versus multiple lesions
Unilateral versus bilateral disease
Lung primary or single metastasis
Involvement of hilar or mediastinal lymph nodes
Total required volume of resection

A survey covering 4 decades of surgical metastasectomy and various radiologic techniques showed an overall accuracy in the radiologic assessment of lung metastases of 61% with 25% of cases showing more metastases at the time of surgery and 14% showing fewer lesions than detected preoperatively (Pastorino et al, 1997). However, in the subset of patients who underwent bilateral surgical exploration, the number of radiologic metastases was accurate in only 37% of cases and underestimated the number in 39% of cases. Particularly in patients with multiple pulmonary lesions, a liver ultrasound, a bone scan, and a CT or magnetic resonance imaging (MRI) scan of the brain should be part of the preoperative staging. In sarcomas and gastrointestinal tumors in which the probability of local relapse is high, full examination of the primary tumor site, including CT, MRI, or endoscopy, may be necessary to exclude local recurrence or to assess its resectability before undertaking lung metastasectomy. Where tumor markers are available, they, too, should be assessed (e.g., germ cell or gastrointestinal).

The role of positron emission tomography (PET) is under evaluation. The data concerning the specificity of PET are promising, particularly in epithelial tumors, which have a higher risk for extrapulmonary metastasis and locoregional relapse (Fig. 35–2), but the minimum size of detectable pulmonary lesions (approximately 5 mm) remains a problem. High cost and limited resources are a further restraint on the use of PET.

A solitary lesion seen on a chest radiograph should not be considered a metastasis unless it is histologically confirmed as such (Cahan et al, 1978). A primary lung cancer or a benign lesion is not an uncommon finding in middle-aged patients. As illustrated in Table 35–3, the probability that a new solitary lesion is a new primary tumor is related to the type, and also to the stage, of the previous primary cancer. In germ cell tumors, specific tumor markers can help to confirm the diagnosis.

Preoperative tissue diagnosis through bronchoscopy, percutaneous needle-aspiration biopsy, or thoracoscopy may be useful for planning the best surgical approach and the appropriate resection volume in the case of a solitary lesion that may be a primary cancer, and also in the presence of multiple pulmonary lesions, when systemic chemotherapy may be considered before resection.

Selection of Patients

The selection criteria for pulmonary metastasectomy are listed in Table 35–4. Adequate control of the primary tumor is an essential requirement. In the case of synchronous metastases, lung surgery may be done first if complete metastasectomy is a prerequisite to justify a radical approach to the primary tumor such as limb amputation. When lung metastases are associated with local recurrence of the primary tumor, the resectability of local

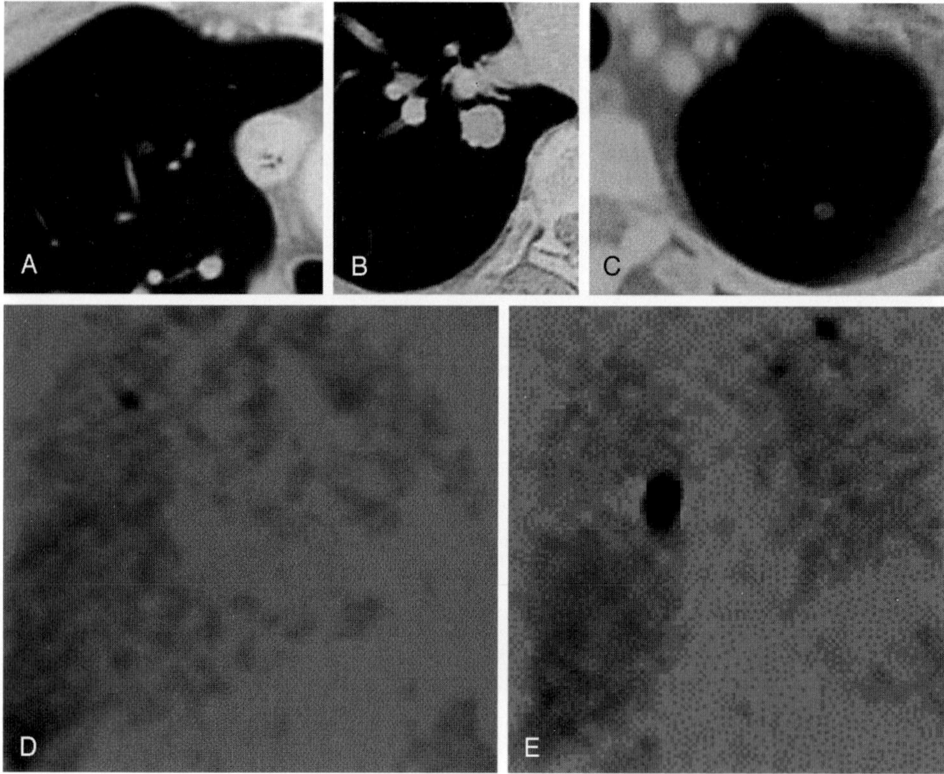

FIGURE 35–2 ■ The routine computed tomography scan of the chest performed in a patient treated for endometrial cancer revealed a 2 cm lesion in the right lower lobe *(B)* as well as two small lesions of less than 1 cm in the right *(A)* and left *(C)* upper lobes. All these metastases were detected by positron emission tomography scan *(D, E)* and pathologically confirmed at thoracotomy.

TABLE 35–3 ■ **Probability of New Primary Cancer Versus Metastasis in Patients Presenting with a Solitary Lung Opacity after Prior Treatment for Malignant Tumor**

Prior Tumor	*New Primary (%)*	*Metastasis*	*Total*
Wilms	0	8	8
Sarcoma	5 (8)	55	60
Melanoma	7 (19)	29	36
Testis	6 (33)	12	18
Kidney	11 (55)	9	20
Colon-rectum	30 (58)	22	52
Breast	40 (63)	23	63
Ovary	6 (66)	3	9
Uterus	32 (74)	11	73
Bladder	25 (89)	3	28
Lung	47 (92)	4	51
Head and neck	158 (94)	10	168
Other*	140 (100)	0	140
Total	507 (73)	189	696

*Esophagus, prostate, stomach, pancreas, skin, lymphoma, leukemia.
Modified from Cahan WG, Shah JP, Castro EB: Benign solitary lung lesions in patients with cancer. Ann Surg 187:241, 1978.

relapse must be assessed before lung resection is undertaken.

A full clinical restaging based on the nature of the primary site must be completed before pulmonary resection to exclude the presence of extrapulmonary metastases. However, in primary colon carcinoma occuring with liver and lung metastases, resection of both sites has been successful, achieving long-term survival in a significant proportion of cases (McAfee et al, 1992; Sauter et al, 1990; Spaggiari et al, 1998).

In chemosensitive tumors such as germ cell tumors, first- or second-line chemotherapy should be considered prior to pulmonary resection. The evaluation of a patient for metastasectomy should always include an assessment of the risk benefit ratio of surgery alone versus chemotherapy or combined modalities. For less chemosensitive tumors such as soft tissue sarcomas the clinical decision is more difficult because complete disappearance of pulmonary metastases is uncommon and relapse at multiple lung sites is common when chemotherapy stops.

In patients presenting with multiple bilateral lesions detected on CT scan, when resectability is questionable and prognosis poorer, the absence of new pulmonary metastasis during the previous 2 months may be a further selection criterion.

The medical condition of the patient has to be assessed in terms of ability to tolerate general anesthesia, adequate cardiac and renal function, and sufficient lung reserve with respect to the anticipated resection volume. The final requirement is that all visible lesions on the CT scan must be resectable with adequate margins. Incomplete resections yield little benefit for the patient.

TABLE 35–4 ■ **Selection of Patients for Pulmonary Resection**

The primary tumor is controlled or is controllable
No extrapulmonary tumor exists
No better method of proven treatment value is available
Adequate medical status for the planned resection exists
Complete resection is possible based on CT scan evaluation

INDICATIONS FOR SYSTEMIC THERAPY

In some tumor types, induction chemotherapy has proved moderately effective. In osteogenic sarcoma, primary tumor regression after chemotherapy contributes to limb-sparing surgery in a large number of cases. Similarly, chemotherapy may eradicate many, if not all, lung metastases, and residual disease can be resected, resulting in long-term survival in about 30% of cases (Al-Jilaiharui et al, 1988; Bar et al, 1992).

The outcome of metastatic testicular carcinoma has changed in the past 3 decades as a consequence of highly effective chemotherapy (Vugrin et al, 1982). Complete clinical remission of lung metastases can be achieved in the majority of patients, and resection of residual pulmonary lesions reveals the presence of viable tumor in only 20% to 25% of cases.

For these reasons, in cases of losteosarcoma and testicular carcinoma presenting with pulmonary metastates, chemotherapy should be given initially. If a complete remission is achieved, as observed on a CT scan, surgical metastasectomy can be avoided in germ cell tumors, whereas in osteosarcoma, a thoracotomy may still be considered to confirm pathologic remission and prevent later relapses. On the other hand, in most epithelial tumors and soft tissue sarcomas, induction chemotherapy has proven ineffective, with the possible exception of metastases from colon cancer.

The value of adjuvant systemic therapies after lung metastasectomy is not well established. In tumors in which chemotherapy shows definite activity for disseminated disease (e.g., breast cancer), adjuvant systemic treatment is a logical option after metastasectomy unless the same therapy has been fully explored before lung surgery. In non-pretreated patients, when the risk of relapse is high because of multiple resected lesions, adjuvant therapy may be considered as part of the treatment plan. Adjuvant radiotherapy may be indicated when incomplete resection occurs at a single site, such as chest wall or mediastinal adenopathy, particularly if the primary tumor has proven sensitive to radiation.

SURGICAL APPROACHES

The surgical approach to metastasectomy remains controversial. Two main questions still have to be answered: What is the relative value of open versus thoracoscopic surgery? and What is the relative value of bilateral versus unilateral exploration? Long-term survival has been obtained using radical metastasectomy techniques, but no randomized trial has proven the advantage of early resection of occult disease. On the other hand, it is possible that spiral CT and other diagnostic tools will improve the accuracy of clinical staging and patient selection to the extent that intraoperative assessment will lose most of its relevance. At this time, it is appropriate to test innovative treatment policies with prospective clinical trials.

Unilateral Thoracotomy

Posterolateral thoracotomy has for a long time been the standard approach to pulmonary metastasectomy. Two sequential operations were utilized for bilateral lesions, during one or two hospitalizations (Roth et al, 1986). Since the 1990s, more conservative approaches combining a limited skin incision and a muscle-sparing thoracotomy have become popular. Compared with posterolateral thoracotomies, these approaches produce less functional damage of thoracic muscles and nerves, lessen postoperative pain, facilitate early mobilization of the patient, and reduce pleural adhesions, thus facilitating future reoperation, if needed (Pastorino et al, 1994).

Median Sternotomy

The median sternotomy incision as an alternative approach for the resection of bilateral metastases has some distinct advantages: both lungs can be examined at the same time, and the midsternal split prevents surgical damage of thoracic muscles and nerves and disruption of the chest wall parietal pleura, and it causes fewer pleural adhesions—all features that prove useful if reoperation must be performed (Johnston, 1983; Roth et al, 1986).

In sarcomas, sternotomy allows the exploration of both lungs, even in cases of single or unilateral metastases. In fact, it has been demonstrated that in 30% to 50% of cases presenting with unilateral lesions, median sternotomy revealed bilateral lung metastases (Johnston, 1983; Pastorino et al, 1990; Vogt-Moykopf et al, 1994; Winkler, 1986).

Most cases of metastasic sarcomas can be operated on through the median approach, although this incision is best for superficial nodules located anteriorly in the lungs. A left lower lobe segmentectomy or lobectomy, if required, is technically demanding with this approach, as the necessary mobilization of the lung may trigger transient arrhythmias.

Bilateral Anterior Thoracotomy

In patients presenting with numerous or centrally located lesions involving both lungs or with mediastinal adenopathies, a sequential lateral approach may facilitate resection and prevent acute lung injury. Bilateral anterior thoracotomy with or without transverse sternotomy, also called the clamshell incision, may be preferred in selected cases to combine the advantages of the sternotomy, which allows access to both lungs, with those of the lateral thoracotomy, which provides adequate exposure to all lobes of both lungs (Bains et al, 1994).

TECHNIQUES OF RESECTION

The objectives of lung metastasectomy with curative intent are the excision of all detectable lesions, allowing clear surgical margins and preserving as much functional tissue as possible. To achieve a macroscopically complete resection, the surgeon must be able to palpate the lung, in both the inflated and the deflated state, to identify and remove any radiologically occult lesions. The hilar lymph nodes should be examined and sampled if involvement is suspected.

The appropriate resection volume depends on the number, sites, and dimensions of the lung lesions. A sublobar resection (an atypical tangential or wedge resection) is generally adequate, as most metastatic lesions are small and peripherally located. It is usually sufficient to resect 1 cm of normal lung around the palpable tumor. A variety of mechanical staplers are available to achieve a quick and easy resection. However, the so-called precision resection may be more volume-effective in the case of multiple or deeper metastases. This technique consists of cutting out a uniform layer (5 to 10 mm) of normal lung tissue around the nodule, usually making a cone-shaped excision with the larger base on the pleural surface, using a diathermy needle or a laser (yttrium-aluminum-garnet [YAG]) or argon beam. Small intrapulmonary vessels and bronchi that are encountered during such a precision resection may easily be controlled by electrocautery or metal clips.

For multiple metastases that are centrally located and for larger solitary lesions suggestive of primary lung tumors, segmentectomy or lobectomy may be necessary to obtain a complete resection (Fig. 35–3). A frozen section may occasionally help in the choice of the proper resection volume. The presence of nodal metastases may require a lobectomy or even a larger volume of resection, but this is uncommon. Pneumonectomy is an exceptional indication for metastasectomy and should be considered only if preoperative pulmonary function tests guarantee a good quality of life after surgery. Nonetheless, in properly selected cases, long-term survival can be achieved after pneumonectomy for metastasis (Koong, 1999; Martini et al 1971; Wilkins et al, 1961).

En Bloc Resections

If a pulmonary metastatic lesion invades adjacent structures and these structures are completely resectable, the surgeon should not be deterred from offering a surgical excision when the other criteria for metastasectomy can be satisfied. En bloc resections of chest wall, pericardium, or diaphragm during lung metastasectomy are still associated with satisfactory long-term survival.

Video-Assisted Thoracic Surgery

Video-assisted thoracic surgery (VATS) gained popularity during the last decade of the 20th century as a safe alternative to open thoracotomy when performing small resections, as it allows for small incisions and thus less subsequent pain (Dowling et al, 1992; Landreneau et al, 1992; Lewis et al, 1992). However, the majority of thoracic surgeons, believing that a thorough palpation of the entire lung is necessary to perform a complete metastasectomy, have maintained substantial skepticism about the advantages and safety of the thoracoscopic approach (Mack et al, 1992). There is little question that creating adequate surgical margins requires palpation of the lesion

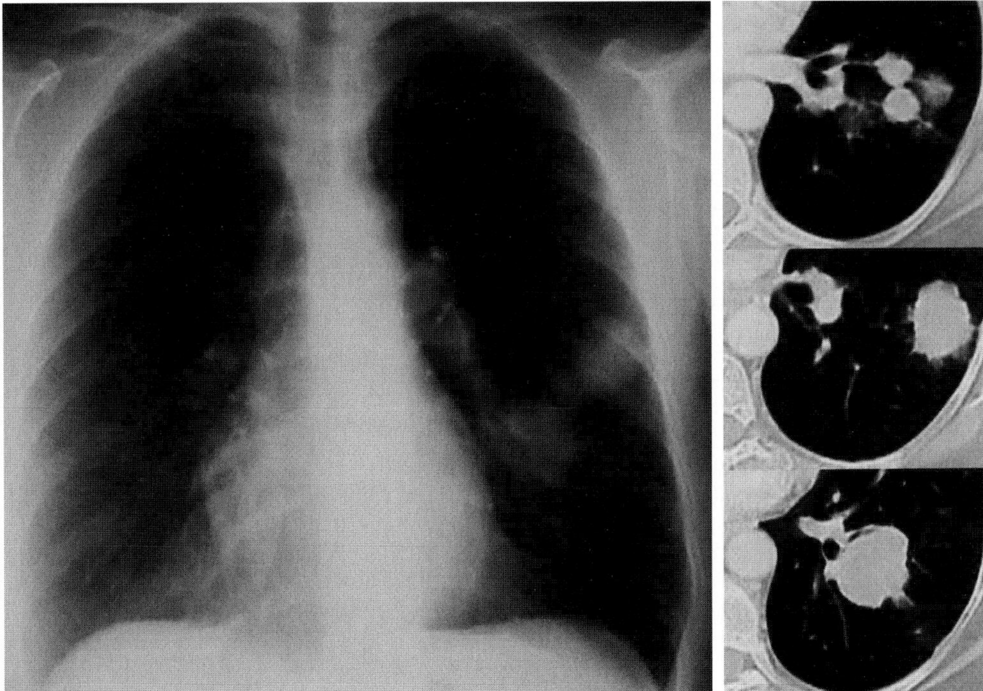

FIGURE 35–3 ■ These large and centrally located metastases from breast carcinoma required a left lower lobectomy for radical excision.

so the stapler may be placed properly, and open manual suture or precision dissection may better fit the size and location of the nodule. Moreover, small nodules located deeper in the lung parenchyma are frequently missed. As demonstrated by McCormack and colleagues (1996), in patients who underwent thoracoscopy followed by immediate thoracotomy, open surgical exploration allowed resection of additional metastases in 56% of the cases.

The aim of lung metastasectomy is not cytoreduction or debulking but complete removal of detectable disease. This fundamental principle applies to any type of salvage surgery with curative intent and is critical in pulmonary metastases, in which preoperative staging is grossly inaccurate. Complete resection of all metastatic nodules is the only operation that will help the patient. However, current prospective trials employing VATS may resolve the issue and indicate its value in pulmonary metastasectomy.

RESULTS OF SURGERY

In experienced hands, morbidity rates are low, and overall perioperative mortality ranges between zero and 2% (Pastorino et al, 1997). The history of pulmonary metastasectomy indicates that permanent cure can be achieved in less than one third of cases. Five-year survival results vary with the primary site and depend on the site and the pattern of metastases.

The International Registry of Lung Metastases (IRLM) analyzed 5206 patients who had undergone lung metastasectomy in 18 departments of thoracic surgery in Europe, the United States, and Canada; 4572 (88%) achieved complete surgical resection (Pastorino et al, 1997). Despite the large number, this is clearly a highly selective series of patients, and the denominator population is not known. In the experience of the IRLM, the actuarial survival rate after complete metastasectomy was 36% at 5 years, 26% at 10 years, and 22% at 15 years (median 35 months) (Table 35–5). The corresponding values for incomplete resection were 13% at 5 years and 7% at 10 years (median 15 months). The overall 30-day mortality rate after complete resection was only 0.8%.

Prognostic Factors

Selecting appropriate patients for metastasectomy based on the prediction of a successful outcome in an individual patient can be difficult. A number of adverse prognostic factors have been suggested, but the number of patients analyzed in each individual series has been relatively small, giving rise to conflicting results (Putnam et al, 1984).

Tumor doubling time (TDT), based on serial chest radiographs, has been suggested as a factor by a number of investigators. This calculation, unfortunately, may prove impractical when assessable radiographs are not available and tumor growth rates are not constant (Joseph et al, 1971).

The disease-free interval (DFI), defined as the time from the treatment of the primary tumor to the appearance of metastases, correlates differently with survival in various series. Depending on the series, DFIs from as little as 8 months to as long as 5 years have been significant positive prognostic factors, but on the whole, results are inconclusive.

The number of metastases had been initially considered an important variable in predicting outcome. However, in the past 20 years a number of authors have

TABLE 35–5 ■ **International Registry of Lung Metastases Analysis of Long-Term Survival after Complete Resection**

		No.	5-Year (%)	10-Year (%)	Median (months)
Overall		4572	36	26	35
Disease-free interval	0–11 months	1384	33	27	29
	12–35 months	1662	31	22	30
	36+ months	1416	45	29	49
Number	1	2169	43	31	43
	2–3	1226	34	24	31
	4+	1123	27	19	27
	10+	342	26	17	26

reported long-term survival after resection of multiple lesions in both lungs (McCormack et al, 1989; Pastorino et al, 1994; Roth et al, 1986). The probability of survival tends to decrease proportionally with the number of resected lesions; however, a firm cut-off point beyond which resection is useless has not been defined. The data of the Institut Montsouris in Paris showed that the survival time of 44 patients who underwent resection of eight or more pulmonary metastases was not significantly different from that of the other 412 patients operated on during the same period (Girard et al, 1994). The prognostic value of the number of pulmonary metastases seemed to be more dependent on associated resectablity than on the number per se. Similarly, the results of the Memorial Sloan-Kettering Cancer Center study of metastatic colorectal cancer suggested that complete resection provided the only significant variable (McCormack et al, 1993). Occasionally, at thoracotomy, patients show widespread dissemination of multiple small nodules in the lung. This is an obvious contraindication to metastasectomy and, whenever detectable by CT, should exclude the patient from thoracotomy.

The occurrence of hilar or mediastinal lymph node metastasis varies with the primary tumor and has only rarely been identified in the metastasectomy reports. The prognostic influence of this type of lymphatic spread is unknown. The role of concurrent lymph node dissection and pulmonary metastasectomy is under investigation.

The IRLM was established with the specific purpose of defining by multivariate analysis the prognostic factors for the various primary tumors. In the analysis by the IRLM, the DFI, the number of metastases, and the tumor type were highly significant independent prognostic variables at univariate as well as multivariate analysis. However, the achievement of a macroscopically complete resection was the most important independent prognostic factor. Such a large series of patients presented a unique opportunity to build up a system of prognostic groupings that could take into account all the relevant prognostic factors simultaneously.

As a result of this analysis, a novel classification was proposed, combining three prognostic indicators—DFI, number of metastases, and radicality (Table 35–6). Figure 35–4 shows the actuarial survival rate of the four prognostic groups. Median survival was 61 months for group I, 34 months for group II, 24 months for group III, and 14 months for group IV ($P < 0.00001$). The discriminatory power of this prognostic grouping was tested in terms of the various primary tumors and proved to be highly significant in each specific tumor type.

Other potential tumor-specific prognostic factors have been proposed and now must be investigated by prospective studies: grading and local recurrence in soft tissue sarcomas; persistent malignant disease and elevated β-human chorionic gonadotropin (β-HCG) following induction therapy in teratoma; carcinoembryonic antigen (CEA) and liver resection in colorectal cancer; and hormone receptors in breast cancer (Girard et al, 1996; Van Geel et al, 1996).

Relapse after Metastasectomy and Surgical Rescue

The pattern of relapse after lung metastasectomy depends on the primary tumor's histology as well as on the extent of pulmonary disease. A significant proportion of these patients may be suitable for surgical rescue. As an example, in the historical series of 22 carefully selected children with metastatic osteosarcoma treated at Memorial Sloan-Kettering Cancer Center, four of the six 10-year survivors lived more than 19 years after as many as nine thoracotomies, and three of six (50%) developed second primary cancers during the second decade of follow-up (Beattie et al, 1991).

In the experience of the IRLM, a recurrence was documented in 53% of patients after complete lung metastasectomy, with a median time to recurrence of 10 months. The probability of relapse at all sites was higher for sarcomas and melanomas (64%) than for epithelial (46%)

TABLE 35–6 ■ **International Registry of Lung Metastases System of Prognostic Grouping**

Group	Characteristics
I	Resectable, no risk factors: DFI 36 months and single metastasis
II	Resectable, 1 risk factor: DFI < 36 months or multiple metastases
III	Resectable, 2 risk factors: DFI < 36 months and multiple metastases
IV	Unresectable

DFI, disease-free interval.

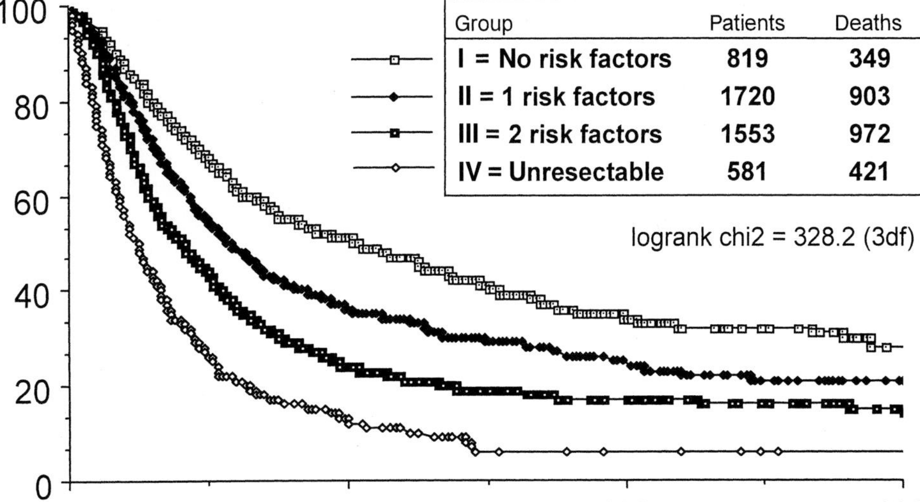

FIGURE 35–4 ■ Survival according to the four prognostic groups defined by the IRLM classification system. A disease-free interval shorter than 36 months or multiple metastases represent the risk factors.

or germ cell (26%) tumors. Limited intrathoracic relapse accounted for 66% of recurrences in sarcomas, 44% in epithelial tumors, and only 27% in melanomas. The proportion of relapsed patients who underwent a second metastasectomy was higher in those with sarcomas than in those with epithelial tumors (53% versus 28%), and the median interval was shorter (10 versus 17 months). The long-term survival rate of patients treated by a second metastasectomy was 44% at 5 years and 29% at 10 years, little different from that seen following initial metastasectomy.

Clinical follow-up after pulmonary resection should be tailored according to the expected time and site of relapse, including chest radiographs every month and a chest CT scan every 3 months during the first year, followed by chest radiographs every 3 to 4 months up to the third year. In sarcomas, for which salvage surgery is more commonly needed and the size of the pulmonary lesions is a critical factor for resectability, a more intense follow-up may be appropriate after primary tumor treatment if the risk of relapse is high. This may include, in selected cases, routine chest radiographs every 2 to 3 months and a chest CT scan every 6 months for a prolonged period.

MANAGEMENT OF SPECIFIC CANCERS

The purpose and applicability of lung metastasectomy varies with the primary tumor according to a number of clinical factors, such as the risk of metastases in other organs, the sensitivity to chemotherapy or hormone treatment, and the probability of new primary tumors. Carcinomas as a group have a different pattern of metastatic spread from sarcomas, and within this group each major primary site has a distinctive behavior. The results found by the IRLM for the main primary tumor sites are summarized in Table 35–7.

Sarcoma

Osteosarcoma metastasizes mainly to the lungs, and in the days before effective chemotherapy 80% of patients treated by radical resection of their primary tumors developed lung metastases (Friedman and Carter, 1972; Marcove et al, 1970). A surgical approach was therefore advocated by Marcove, and a strategy of resection was introduced at Memorial Sloan-Kettering Cancer Center with encouraging results—a 30% 5-year survival rate (Martini et al, 1971). More recently, the pattern of metas-

TABLE 35–7 ■ **International Registry of Lung Metastases Analysis of Long-Term Survival Based on Primary Tumor**

		No.	*5-Year (%)*	*10-Year (%)*	*Median (months)*
Epithelial	Overall	1894	37	21	40
	Colorectal	653	37	22	41
	Breast	411	37	21	37
	Kidney	402	41	24	41
Sarcoma	Overall	1917	31	26	29
	Osteosarcoma	734	33	27	40
	Soft tissue	938	30	22	27
Melanoma		282	21	14	19
Germ cell		318	68	63	

tasis appears to be changing, with metastases of bone and other sites occurring more commonly.

Despite the efficacy of intensive chemotherapy, lung metastases have remained the main reason for failure in 40% to 50% of osteosarcomas (Edmonson et al, 1977; Rosenberg et al, 1959). More recent studies have provided further evidence that employing systematic surgical resection of pulmonary metastases might contribute more to sustained improvement in survival rates than the use of chemotherapy (Rosenberg et al, 1959).

In a consecutive series of 174 primary childhood osteosarcomas, the authors reported that in the years 1982 to 1988, after the introduction of systematic bilateral metastasectomy, the total proportion of patients who underwent complete resections of their pulmonary metastases rose to 55%, compared with 17% in the years 1970 to 1981 (Pastorino et al, 1991). This change of strategy lead to an improvement in 5-year survival rates of all metastatic patients from zero to 28%, with a 47% survival rate occurring after complete metastasectomy in the latter period (Fig. 35–5).

Patients presenting with metastases at the time of initial diagnosis may still be eligible for metastasectomy. The best timing for metastasectomy is unclear. In most centers, control of the primary tumor takes precedence while the response of the metastases to chemotherapy is assessed. Other centers have advocated immediate operation, if possible. Lung exploration may rule out false-positive lesions, avoid unnecessary amputation in cases of disseminated disease, and possibly improve the chances of permanent eradication of disease. In the IRLM analysis, 108 osteosarcoma patients with synchronous lung metastases showed a 38% 5-year survival rate after complete resection.

Primary soft tissue sarcomas also produce both synchronous and metachronous metastases to the lungs, although their incidence is lower. Chemotherapy has a less important role in the management of these tumors than in cases of osteogenic tumor. Therefore, metastasectomy may be particularly important for eligible patients. A meta-analysis by the European Organization for Research and Treatment of Cancer (EORTC)-Soft Tissue and Bone Sarcoma Group based on 255 patients showed a 5-year survival rate of 30% (Van Geel et al, 1996). These figures were confirmed by the IRLM data (see Table 35–7). No controlled trials exist that compare metastasectomy with no treatment or with chemotherapy or radiation therapy alone. However, the data concerning the results of untreated lung metastases suggest that they are usually fatal in 2 years (McCormack et al, 1989; McKenna et al, 1978; Potter et al, 1985). Poor median survival may, to some extent, be biased by the number of patients with more advanced disease ("unresectable"), but observed survival beyond 3 years is unlikely to be influenced by such a selection bias.

Germ Cell Tumors

Germ cell tumors are very sensitive to chemotherapy, and the use of cisplatin-based regimens has greatly improved the cure rate from around 10% in the 1960s to the current 85% to 90% (Horwich, 1996), even in the presence of metastatic disease.

Resection of any residual disease after chemotherapy is considerably important because there is no reliable way to predict histology (necrosis, mature teratoma, persisting tumor), and survival depends on the elimination of active disease (Williams et al, 1987).

In an analysis of 141 patients who underwent resection of thoracic metastases at the Royal Brompton Hospital of London, complete resection was achieved in 123 cases (87%), and pathology showed viable malignant elements in 46 patients (32%), necrosis or fibrosis in 32 patients, and differentiated teratoma in the remaining 63

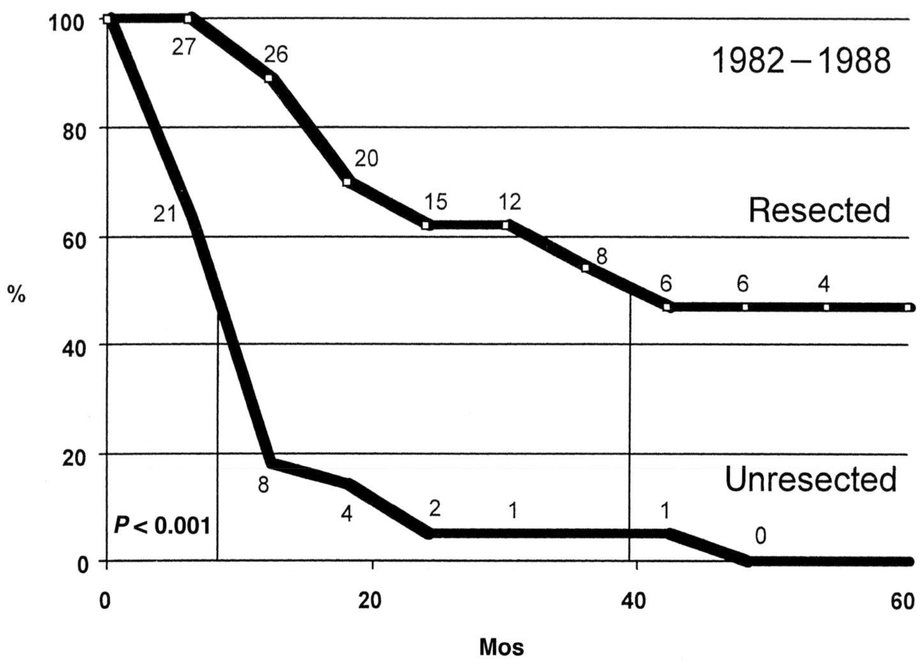

FIGURE 35–5 ■ Lung metastasectomy in a consecutive series of childhood osteosarcomas; overall survival from detection of pulmonary metastases according to salvage surgery, in the years 1982 to 1988.

(Cagini et al, 1998). The overall survival rate was 77% at 5 years and 65% at 15 years, and was significantly shorter in patients with malignant teratomatous elements. However, in the last group, metastasectomy still achieved a 51% survival rate at 5 years.

Colorectal Tumors

Metastatic spread of colorectal cancer typically involves regional lymph nodes, liver, and lung. However, lung metastases may occur in the absence of disease below the diaphragm. Primary rectal tumors show the distinct capability of bypassing the liver through an alternative venous drainage and giving direct metastases to the lungs. For patients with isolated pulmonary metastases, chemotherapy can provide palliation and a small survival benefit. However, it is unable to provide permanent cure. In the study at Memorial Sloan-Kettering Cancer Center, in which 144 carefully selected patients were treated by lung metastasectomy, the 5-year survival rate was 44% and the 10-year survival rate 25% (McCormack et al, 1992). Chemotherapy alone for colorectal metastases to lung without metastasectomy had no survivors beyond 24 months (McAfee et al, 1992; McCormack et al, 1992). In the report of the Institut Montsouris in Paris, the survival rate was significantly better in patients with normal CEA at the time of metastasectomy (Girard et al, 1996), whereas the series at Memorial did not show that CEA levels have any prognostic value. Given the reported good results from an aggressive approach to simultaneous liver and lung metastases, such an approach is worth considering in selected individuals (Okumura et al, 1996; Spaggiari et al, 1998).

Breast Tumors

Breast cancer metastases to the lungs are rarely amenable to resection with curative intent. In this disease, pulmonary spread is likely to occur through the internal mammary or mediastinal lymph nodes, rather than through limited hematogenous deposits. Bone, pleura, or liver metastases are often associated. Solitary or few nodules have been resected with good results (Morrow et al, 1980), but they represent less than 1% of all mammary carcinomas. For the majority of patients with lung metastases, it is not certain to what extent surgical approach may be better than medical management only. However, almost 50% of solitary pulmonary nodules in patients with prior breast cancer do not represent metastasis but secondary primary lung malignancy or benign disease. Often, a clear distinction between primary and secondary tumors is impossible even after surgery, as pathologic features are ambiguous. Therefore, resection is warranted in the case of solitary lesions, and long-term survival rates approach 40%. In the IRLM series, based on 411 patients, the overall survival rates of those with solitary and multiple metastases were 37% at 5 years and 21% at 10 years (median 37 months).

Hypernephroma

Metastatic renal cancer shows very limited sensitivity to systemic chemotherapy or immunotherapy. In the few selected cases, in which no other distant or nodal metastases can be detected, pulmonary metastasectomy may contribute to long-term survival. However, lung metastases are often multiple and not suitable for complete resection at the time of initial diagnosis. Spontaneous regression of these metastatic foci may rarely occur, but the probability is so low that the event has no clinical relevance. Only 67 cases are reported in the world literature, by Freed and colleagues (1977) and Fairlamb (1981). Of these cases, only 12 have documented 5-year follow-up.

The survival rates (24% to 44%) reported in the literature after metastasectomy for hypernephroma have been confirmed by the IRLM data (see Table 35–7) (Dernevik et al, 1985). Solitary lesions appear to have better results, but re-do surgery yields similar results in selected candidates (Pogrebniak et al, 1991; Tolin and Whitmore, 1975).

Head and Neck Tumors

The occurrence of a pulmonary opacity in a patient previously treated for head and neck tumors is a common event. If the pulmonary nodule is solitary, it is virtually impossible to distinguish a metastasis from a primary lung tumor. Such a patient has a high risk of multiple aerodigestive tract malignancies because of the long history of smoking and is prone to developing second primary lung tumors. In all such cases, if the lesion is resectable, it should be treated as a primary lung tumor, with curative intent. If, on the contrary, multiple pulmonary nodules are detectable on CT scans, a needle aspiration or thoracoscopic biopsy usually demonstrates a metastatic squamous cell carcinoma. The real efficacy of pulmonary metastasectomy for metastatic head and neck carcinoma is unclear. A recent analysis of data from Memorial Sloan-Kettering Cancer Center suggests that a 20% 5-year survival rate is obtained when complete resection of all nodules can be achieved (Liu and Ginsberg; unpublished data).

Salivary gland and thyroid tumors may present with solitary lesions in the lung. As with other head and neck tumors, the clinician must differentiate between a primary lung cancer and a solitary metastasis. Radioisotope studies or needle-aspiration biopsy can be helpful. Although many of these solitary metastases are resected, it is difficult to estimate whether metastasectomy is really able to improve the life expectancy of these patients, as long-term survival can be observed even with conservative management.

Melanoma

The clinical behavior of metastatic melanoma is often unpredictable. Metastatic foci can be stable for many years and then give rise to disseminated spread through both the hematogenous and the lymphatic routes. Systemic chemotherapy and immunotherapy are still being used with mixed results (Harpole et al, 1992). Approximately one quarter of patients affected by malignant melanoma develop pulmonary metastases, but the role of metastasectomy is controversial. Resection of pulmonary metastases was advocated by some for solitary metastases, but the overall results did not appear to be significantly better than with other treatment modalities (McCormack, 1978; Vogt-Moykopf et al, 1994; Wilkins, 1978). The data from the IRLM revealed favorable outcomes in patients with fewer than two risk factors according to the proposed classification system: the 5-year survival rate was 29% for group I (a solitary lesion and a long DFI) and 20% for group II (multiple lesions or a short DFI).

THE FUTURE

Prospects for better management of pulmonary metastases rely on effective systemic therapy to prevent their occurrence. At present, induction and adjuvant systemic therapies play a small role in managing resectable and unresectable metastases, but innovative and possibly more effective systemic treatments will become available in the near future. New antimetastatic agents, such as metallo-proteinase inhibitors and antibodies against vascular endothelial growth factors, are very promising drugs that can be used in adjuvant or neoadjuvant therapy in this set of patients. Intra-arterial infusion of high-dose chemotherapy agents directly into the pulmonary artery after isolating the lung in order to increase the dose without toxicity have shown some encouraging results in animal models (Abolhoda et al, 1997; Weksler, Blumberg et al, 1994; Weksler, Lenert et al, 1994).

Currently, the best therapeutic results can be obtained by surgical resection of pulmonary metastases in properly selected candidates. Treatment should be offered to patients who appear likely to benefit from this aggressive approach. The authors have attempted to present selection criteria in this chapter but acknowledge the limitations of current predictors.

The classification proposed by the IRLM combines essential indicators of tumor biology (DFI), anatomic extent (number) and radicality of treatment into a simplified system that reliably predicts long-term survival rates of patients with various tumor types. This classification may be useful in the future to stratify patients into randomized trials to test new systemic treatments and to further define the role of surgery in the treatment of pulmonary metastases.

COMMENTS AND CONTROVERSIES

The authors have outlined in exquisite detail the role of surgery in the management of pulmonary metastases. During my own career, this role has expanded from the very occasional resection of a solitary metastasis to an aggressive approach in patients with resectable metastases in which the primary tumor is controlled or controllable. Yet with experience resecting both hepatic and pulmonary metastases in the treatment of colorectal disease, we now have to consider treatment of "oligo" metastases, that is, a finite number of metastases in more than one organ. Whether the experience with colorectal disease will be transferable to other metastatic tumors in two sites awaits further investigation. Newer imaging techniques such as PET scans may allow us to identify those patients who may benefit from an aggressive treatment of oligo metastatic disease.

In my own practice, with increasing frequency we are using bilateral anterior thoracotomies with or without transverse sternotomy in the management of bilateral lesions. In most instances, we have found that the transverse sternotomy is not required unless there are bulky lesions in the left lower lobe. These bilateral anterior thoracotomies are relatively painless, provide good exposure, and allow an even earlier discharge from the hospital than does the bilateral clamshell approach.

R.J.G.

REFERENCES

Abolhoda A, Brooks A, Nawada S et al: Isolated lung perfusion with doxorubicin prolongs survival in a rodent model of pulmonary metastases. Ann Thorac Surg 64:181, 1997.

Al-Jilaiharui AN, Bullemore J, Mott M, Wisheart JD: Combined chemotherapy and surgery for pulmonary metastases from osteogenic sarcoma: Results of 10 years' experience. Eur J Cardiothorac Surg 2:37, 1988.

Alexander J, Haight C: Pulmonary resection for solitary metastatic sarcomas and carcinomas. Surg Gynec Obstet 85:129, 1947.

Bains MS, Ginsberg RJ, Jones WGH et al: The clamshell incision: An improved approach to bilateral pulmonary and mediastinal tumor. Ann Thorac Surg 58:30, 1994.

Bar LC, Skene AI, Thomas JM: Metastasectomy. Rev Br J Surg 79:1268, 1992.

Barney JD, Churchill EJ: Adenocarcinoma of the kidney with metastasis to the lung. J Urol 42:269, 1939.

Beattie EJ, Harvey JC, Marcove R, Martini N: Results of multiple pulmonary resections for metastatic osteogenic sarcoma after two decades. J Surg Oncol 46:154, 1991.

Cagini L, Nicholson AG, Horwich A et al: Metastasectomy for germ cell tumors: Long-term survival and prognostic factors. Ann Oncol 9:1185, 1998.

Cahan WG, Shah JP, Castro EB: Benign solitary lung lesions in patients with cancer. Ann Surg 187:241, 1978.

Chang AE, Schaner EG, Conkle DM et al: Evaluation of computed tomography in the detection of pulmonary metastases. Cancer 43:913, 1979.

Dernevik L, Berggren H, Larsson S, Roberto D: Surgical removal of pulmonary metastases from renal cell carcinoma. Scand J Urol Nephrol 19:133, 1985.

Dowling RD, Ferson PF, Landreneau RJ: Thoracoscopic resection of pulmonary metastases. Chest 102:1450, 1992.

Edmonson JM, Green SJ, Inins JC et al: Methotrexate as adjunct treatment for primary osteosarcoma. N Engl J Med 303:642, 1977.

Fairlamb DJ: Spontaneous regression of metastases from renal cancer. Cancer 47:2102, 1981.

Freed SZ, Halperin JP, Gordon M: Idiopathic regression of metastases from renal cell carcinoma. Scand J Urol Nephrol 118:538, 1977.

Friedman MA, Carter SK: The therapy of osteogenic sarcoma: Current status and thoughts for the future. J Surg Oncol 4:482, 1972.

Girard P, Baldeyrou P, Le Chevalier T et al: Surgical resection of pulmonary metastases. Up to what number? Am J Respir Crit Care Med 149:469, 1994.

Girard P, Ducreux M, Baldeyrou P et al: Surgery for lung metastases from colorectal cancer: Analysis of prognostic factors. J Clin Oncol 14:2047, 1996.

Harpole DH, Johnson CM, Wolfe WG et al: Analysis of 945 cases of pulmonary metastatic melanoma. J Thorac Cardiovasc Surg 103:743, 1992.

Horwich A. Testicular germ cell tumours: An introductory overview. In Horwich A (ed): Testicular Cancer: Investigation and Management, 2nd ed. London, Chapman & Hall Medical, 1996, p 1.

Johnston MR: Median sternotomy for resection of pulmonary metastasis. J Thorac Cardiovasc Surg 85:516, 1983.

Joseph WL, Morton DL, Adkins PC: Prognostic significance of tumor doubling time in evaluating operability in pulmonary metastatic disease. J Thorac Cardiovasc Surg 61:23, 1971.

Koong HN, Pastorino U, Ginsberg RJ: Is there a role for pneumonectomy in pulmonary metastases? International Registry of Lung Metastases. Ann Thorac Surg 68:2039, 1999.

Landreneau RJ, Hazelrigg SR, Ferson PF et al: Thoracoscopic resection of 85 pulmonary lesions. Ann Thorac Surg 54:415, 1992.

Lawrence W Jr, Donegan WL, Natarajan N et al: Adult soft tissue sarcomas. A pattern of care survey of the American College of Surgeons. Ann Surg 205:349, 1987.

Lewis RJ, Caccavale RJ, Sisler GE, Mackenzie JW: Video-assisted thoracic surgical resection of malignant lung tumors. J Thorac Cardiovasc Surg 104:1679, 1992.

Liu D, Ginsberg R: unpublished data.

Mack MJ, Aronoff RJ, Acuff TE et al: Present role of thoracoscopy in the diagnosis and treatment of lesions of the chest. Ann Thorac Surg 54:403, 1992.

Marcove RC, Huvos AG: Osteogenic sarcoma in childhood. NY State J Med 71:857, 1971.

Marcove R, Mike V, Hajek JV et al: Osteogenic sarcoma under the age of 21: A review of 145 operative cases. J Bone Joint Surg 52A:411, 1970.

Martini N, Huvos AG, Mike V et al: Multiple pulmonary resections in the treatment of osteogenic sarcoma. Ann Thorac Surg 12:271, 1971.

Martini N, McCormak PM, Bains MS: Indications for surgery for intrathoracic metastases in testicular carcinoma. Semin Oncol 6:99, 1979.

Mayo CW, Schlicke CP: Carcinomas of the colon and rectum: A decade of experience at the Lahey Clinic. Dis Colon Rectum 22:717, 1978.

McAfee MK, Allen MS, Trastek VF et al: Colorectal lung metastases: Results of surgical excision. Ann Thorac Surg 53:780, 1992.

McCormack P, Ginsberg KB, Bains MS et al: Accuracy of lung imaging in metastases with implications for the role of thoracoscopy. Ann Thorac Surg 56:863, 1993.

McCormack PM, Attiyeh FF: Resected pulmonary metastases from colorectal cancer. Dis Colon Rectum 22:583, 1979.

McCormack PM: Surgical treatment of pulmonary metastases: Memorial Hospital experience. In Weiss L, Gilbert HA (eds): Pulmonary Metastases. Boston, GK Hall, 1978, p 260.

McCormack PM, Burt ME, Bains MS et al: Lung resection for colorectal metastases: 10-year results. Arch Surg 127:1403, 1992.

McCormack PM, Bains MS, Martini N: Surgical management of pulmonary metastases. In Shiu M, Brennan M (eds): Surgical Management of Soft Tissue Sarcoma. Philadelphia, Lea & Febiger, 1989, p. 263.

McCormack PM, Bains MS, Begg CB et al: Role of video-assisted thoracic surgery in the treatment of pulmonary metastases: Results of a prospective trial. Ann Thorac Surg 62:213, 1996.

McKenna RJ, McKenna RJ Jr: Patterns of pulmonary metastases: An orthopedic hospital experience. In Weiss L and Gilbert HA [eds]: Pulmonary Metastasis. Boston, GK Hall, 1978.

Mintzer RA, Malave SR, Neiman HL et al: Computed vs. conventional tomography in evaluation of primary and secondary pulmonary neoplasms. Radiology 132:653, 1979.

Morrow CE, Vassilopoulos PP, Grage TB: Surgical resection for metastatic neoplasms of the lung: Experience at the University of Minnesota Hospitals. Cancer 45:2981, 1980.

Okumura S, Kondo H, Tsuboi M et al: Pulmonary resection for metastatic colorectal cancer: Experience with 159 patients. J Thorac Cardiovasc Surg 112:867, 1996.

Pastorino U, Valente M, Gasparini M et al: Median sternotomy and multiple lung resections for metastatic sarcomas. Eur J Cardiothorac Surg 4:477, 1990.

Pastorino U, Valente M, Muscolino G et al: Muscle-sparing anterolateral thoracotomy for pulmonary or mediastinal resections. In Motta G (ed): Lung Cancer. Frontiers in Science and Treatment. Genos, Grafica LP, 1994, p 337.

Pastorino U, Buyse M, Friedal et al for The International Registry of Lung Metastases: Long-term results of lung metastasectomy: Prognostic analyses based on 5,206 cases. J Thorac Cardiovasc Surg 113:37, 1997.

Pastorino U, Gasparini M, Tavecchio L et al: The contribution of salvage surgery to the management of childhood osteosarcoma. J Clin Oncol 9:1357, 1991.

Pogrebniak HW, Roth JA, Steinberg SM et al: Re-operation for pulmonary metastases. Ann Thorac Surg 52:197, 1991.

Potter DA, Glenn J, Kinsella T et al: Patterns of recurrence in patients with high-grade soft-tissue sarcomas. J Clin Oncol 3:353, 1985.

Potter DA, Kinsella T, Glatstein E High-grade soft tissue sarcomas of the extremities. Proceedings of the ASCO 4:144, 1985.

Putnam JB, Roth JA, Wesley MN et al: Analysis of prognostic factors in patients undergoing resection of pulmonary metastases from soft tissue sarcomas. J Thorac Cardiovasc Surg 87:260, 1984.

Rosenberg SA, Suit HD, Baker LH: Sarcomas of the soft tissue and bone. In DeVita VT Jr, Hellman S, Rosenberg SA (eds): Cancer: Principles & Practice of Oncology. Philadelphia, JB Lippincott, 1985.

Rosenberg SA, Chabner BA, Young RC et al: Treatment of osteogenic sarcoma. 1: Effect of adjuvant high-dose methotrexate after amputation. Cancer Treat Rep 63:739, 1959.

Roth JA, Pass HI, Wesley MN et al: Comparison of median sternotomy and thoracotomy for resection of pulmonary metastases in patients with adult soft tissue sarcomas. Ann Thorac Surg 42:134, 1986.

Sauter ER, Bolton JS, Gladden WW et al: Improved survival after pulmonary resection of metastatic colorectal carcinoma. J Surg Oncol 43:135, 1990.

Spaggiari L, Grunenwald D, Regnard JF: Resection of hepatic and pulmonary metastases in patients with colorectal carcinoma. Cancer 83:1049, 1998.

Tolin BM, Whitmore WF: Solitary metastasis from renal cell carcinoma. J Urol 114:836, 1975.

van Geel AN, Pastorino U, Jauch KW et al: Surgical treatment of lung metastases: The European Organization for Research and Treatment of Cancer-Soft Tissue and Bone Sarcoma Group study of 255 patients. Cancer 77:675, 1996.

Vogt-Moykopf I, Krysa S, Bulzebruck H, Schirren J: Surgery for pulmonary metastases: The Heidelberg experience. Chest Surg Clin N Am 4:85, 1994.

Vugrin D, Whitmore WF, Bains MS, Golbey RB: Role of chemotherapy and surgery in the treatment of thoracic metastases from nonseminomatous germ cell testis tumor. Cancer 50:1057, 1982.

Weinlechner: Tumoren an der Brustwand und deren Behandlung (Resection der Rippen) Eroffnung der Brusthohle und partielle Entfernung der Lunge. Wien Med Wschr 32:590, 1892.

Wiener Med Wrsch 20, 21, 1882.

Weiss L, Gilbert HA: In Weiss L, Gilbert HA (eds): Pulmonary Metastasis. Boston, GK Hall, 1978, p 142.

Weksler B, Blumberg D, Lenert JT et al: Isolated single-lung perfusion with tumor necrosis factor: Effects of pulmonary metastases from sarcoma. Ann Thorac Surg 58:328, 1994.

Weksler B, Lenert J, Ng B, Burt M: Isolated single lung perfusion with doxorubicin is effective in eradicating soft tissue sarcoma lung metastases in a rat model. J Thorac Cardiovasc Surg 107:50, 1994.

Wilkins EW: The status of pulmonary resection of metastases: Experience at Massachusetts General Hospital. In Weiss L, Gilbert HA (eds): Pulmonary Metastasis. Boston, GK Hall, 1978, p 271.

Wilkins EW, Burke JF, Head JM: The surgical management of metastatic neoplasms in the lung. J Thorac Cardiovasc Surg 42:298, 1961.

Williams S, Birch R, Einhorn LH et al: Treatment of disseminated germ cell tumors with cisplatin, bleomycin, and either vinblastine or etoposide. N Engl J Med 316:1435, 1987.

Wills RA: Pathology of Tumors. 4th ed. London, Butterworth, 1967.

Winkler K: Surgical treatment of pulmonary metastases in childhood. Thorac Cardiovasc Surg 34:133, 1986.

CHAPTER **36**

Surgical Techniques

PNEUMONECTOMY

Paul F. Waters

HISTORICAL NOTE

The first successful one-stage pneumonectomy was performed by Graham and Singer in 1933 for a patient with bronchogenic carcinoma. This followed the first pneumonectomy in multiple stages in a patient with tuberculosis and empyema, achieved by Macewen in 1895. Earlier attempts had not met with success. In 1910, Kummel performed a pneumonectomy for lung cancer by clamping the pedicle and leaving the clamps in situ; that patient survived 6 days. The first individual hilar ligation was accomplished by Hinz in 1922, and that patient succumbed to heart failure on the third postoperative day. Churchill in 1930, Archibald in 1931, and Ivanissevich in 1933 had also attempted removal of a whole lung with no survival beyond a few days. Churchill left a tube in the residual bronchus, bringing it out through the chest wall. Reinhoff first described the modern-day technique of individual ligation of the pulmonary vessels and suturing of the bronchus. By the 1940s, the standard operation for resectable lung cancer became pneumonectomy.

■ *HISTORICAL READINGS*

Abbey Smith R, Nigam BK: Resection of proximal left main bronchus carcinoma. Thorax 43:616, 1979.

Graham EA, Singer JJ: Successful removal of an entire lung for carcinoma of the bronchus. JAMA 101:1371, 1933.

Meade RH: A History of Thoracic Surgery. Springfield, IL, Charles C Thomas, 1961.

INDICATIONS

Historically, removal of an entire lung was the suggested therapy for all bronchogenic carcinomas, although in many cases lesser resections such as lobectomy or segmentectomy could be considered appropriate. It is generally accepted that with careful patient selection and staging, pneumonectomy is the correct treatment for lung cancer that cannot be treated by lobectomy. Pneumonectomy for inflammatory lung disease, bronchiectasis, tuberculosis, and other nonmalignant conditions is uncommon in modern-day pulmonary medicine following the advances in antibiotics (Sarot and Gilbert, 1949).

Incision

The most common incision used for the removal of the lung is the posterolateral thoracotomy with access to the pleural cavity via the fifth intercostal space. This approach allows access to all areas of the lung, both posterior and anterior and therefore is the most popular. Although many surgeons routinely remove a rib, this is not necessary. If the rib is excised, then in the rare instance when empyema and infection cause dehiscence of the thoracotomy incision, it may be difficult to eventually close the incision because of the loss of tissue the rib represents. Also removal of a rib may hamper the use of the intercostal muscle, if needed, to protect the bronchial stump.

Posterior thoracotomy with the patient in the prone position was popular in the early days of thoracic surgery, when control of airway secretions was a major problem in the removal of lungs for septic inflammatory diseases such as tuberculosis. The techniques of airway control with reliable endobronchial intubation and one-lung anesthesia are such that the prone position is not necessary. Moreover, access to the vascular structures of the hilum is less convenient, such that the approach is very rarely employed. Anterolateral thoracotomy with the patient in a supine position results in an incision that is poorly tolerated cosmetically, and access to the necessary hilar structures is suboptimal. This approach also is rarely employed for pneumonectomy.

Median sternotomy carries with it the advantage of less postoperative compromise of pulmonary function, and some practitioners favor it for that reason. It allows good access to the hilar structures for right pneumonectomy. It can be very difficult and sometimes impossible to perform left pneumonectomy through this approach because the heart prevents access to the inferior veins. Although it is preferred by some surgeons, there is also the theoretic risk of sternal infection, which might be increased when this approach is used for clean contaminated cases such as those involving pulmonary resection (Cooper et al, 1978; Takita et al, 1977).

Video-assisted or thoracoscopic (VATS) approaches have been employed in a limited manner to perform pneumonectomy. There are only a few scattered reports in the literature (Craig et al, 1996; Podbielski et al, 1997; Roviaro et al, 1999). Thoracoscopy can provide better visualization of the necessary structures in some cases. An additional thoracotomy incision is by definition required to remove the specimen once the resection is complete. This has been accomplished using a limited standard thoracotomy incision—the so-called "utility" thoracotomy. The VATS approach has been more widely applied for lesser resections and has been met with mixed enthusiasm. The expected decrease in pain, length of hospital stay, and subsequent costs have not lived up to expectations. Therefore, VATS pneumonectomy cannot be recommended for widespread use, given the current state of the technology.

ANESTHESIA

It is very important for the surgeon performing thoracic surgery and pulmonary resections to maintain very clear communication with the attending anesthesiologist. It is also important that the anesthesiologist be experienced in thoracic anesthesia and be comfortable with the various techniques of one-lung anesthesia. Careful monitoring of blood pressure (using an arterial line), of blood gases, of end-tidal carbon dioxide, and of pulmonary arterial pressures with a Swan-Ganz line, as well as urine output measurement and pulse oximetry, will all be required depending on the preoperative condition of the patient.

Single-lung anesthesia is best provided with the use of a standard disposable Robert-Shaw double-lumen endotracheal tube. Some surgeons prefer to use either a bronchial blocker in combination with a standard endotracheal tube or one of the newer commercially available tubes that have a built-in blocker, especially for left pneumonectomy.

OPERATIVE TECHNIQUE

Often, the decision to perform pneumonectomy has been made preoperatively on the basis of the type or location of the pathology. On other occasions, the need for pneumonectomy is determined intraoperatively. In either situation, the possibility of performing a lesser resection without compromising the intended purpose of the procedure should always be kept in mind. It is not uncommon, for example, to find a situation in which a bronchoplastic sleeve resection with or without a concomitant vascular sleeve resection can be performed instead of pneumonectomy. This determination may sometimes not be possible until the intraoperative assessment is made. Once thoracotomy has been performed, a determination of the extent of the disease, its resectability, and the appropriate resection is made (Brock and Whitehead, 1955; Cahan et al, 1951). If the need for pneumonectomy is confirmed, the approach to the resection should be flexible, depending on the circumstances of each particular case. In any event, the hilum is first dissected to identify the pulmonary artery and the two (inferior and superior) pulmonary veins to assess resectability (Fig. 36–1).

Pulmonary Veins

Although theoretically (for oncologic reasons) the division of the veins should occur early in the procedure and before the division of the artery, this may not always be possible, depending on the intraoperative situation (Miller et al, 1968). In my opinion, much of the dissection is best performed bluntly with an "educated" finger to complete the vessel identification. The inferior pulmonary veins are best-exposed by retracting the lung anteriorly and superiorly. When not involved with tumor, they are easily dissected and isolated. I prefer to staple or oversew the main trunk. Other surgeons doubly ligate or suture-ligate branches separately. The superior pulmonary vein is in close proximity to the pulmonary artery anteriorly on both sides and is handled similarly to the inferior vein. Although the vessels may be closed in various ways, the most popular method seems to be the use of vascular staples, which are especially designed for this purpose. They are safe and extremely convenient.

Before the veins are manipulated in central tumors, the veins should be gently palpated to be sure they do not contain extension of the tumor. If tumor is present, a determination should be rapidly made as to its extent and resectability. Tumor released from such veins can result in a potentially disastrous tumor embolus. When suspected, it is best to examine the intrapericardial portion of the veins to make this determination. If necessary, several millimeters of atrium may be encompassed in the resection (see Fig. 36–4). Under these circumstances, I prefer to use an atrial clamp rather than mechanical staples, oversewing the atrium following its division. As a clamp is applied to the atrium in such circumstances, venous return from the contralateral lung may be compromised, rapidly resulting in hemodynamic instability requiring a less central application. Under these circumstances, the clamp should be applied for 1 or 2 minutes before any incision in the vessels is made, so that if instability is noted, the clamp can be reapplied. Although there is sufficient atrium on the left side, on the right side, mobilization of the interatrial groove may be required to provide sufficient atrium to apply a clamp.

Pulmonary Artery

Where the tumor is close to the origin of the pulmonary artery, it may not be possible to obtain enough room to safely apply staplers. In this situation, use of a proximal atraumatic vascular clamp, with oversewing of the vessel in a more traditional way, is perfectly acceptable.

When possible, division of the first branch of the pulmonary artery on either the left side or the right side allows greater length for ultimate division of the main trunk. When the tumor is not very central, dissection of the pulmonary artery is not difficult and can be carried out intrapericardially. With the more frequent use of Swan-Ganz catheters, it is important to be sure the device is not included in the artery when it is divided. The pulmonary artery is weakened by application of staples in continuity. It is, therefore important to avoid traction on the vessel once it has been stapled but before it is divided.

Difficulty can occur when the tumor is "tight" on the pulmonary artery and obtaining sufficient length for safe control presents a problem. There are a few techniques available to deal with this. On either side, the pericardium should be opened anterior to the pulmonary artery, and the intrapericardial portion of the pulmonary artery should be identified (Allison, 1946). This maneuver will produce 1 or 2 cm of additional length. It is important to avoid injury to the phrenic nerve when doing this and

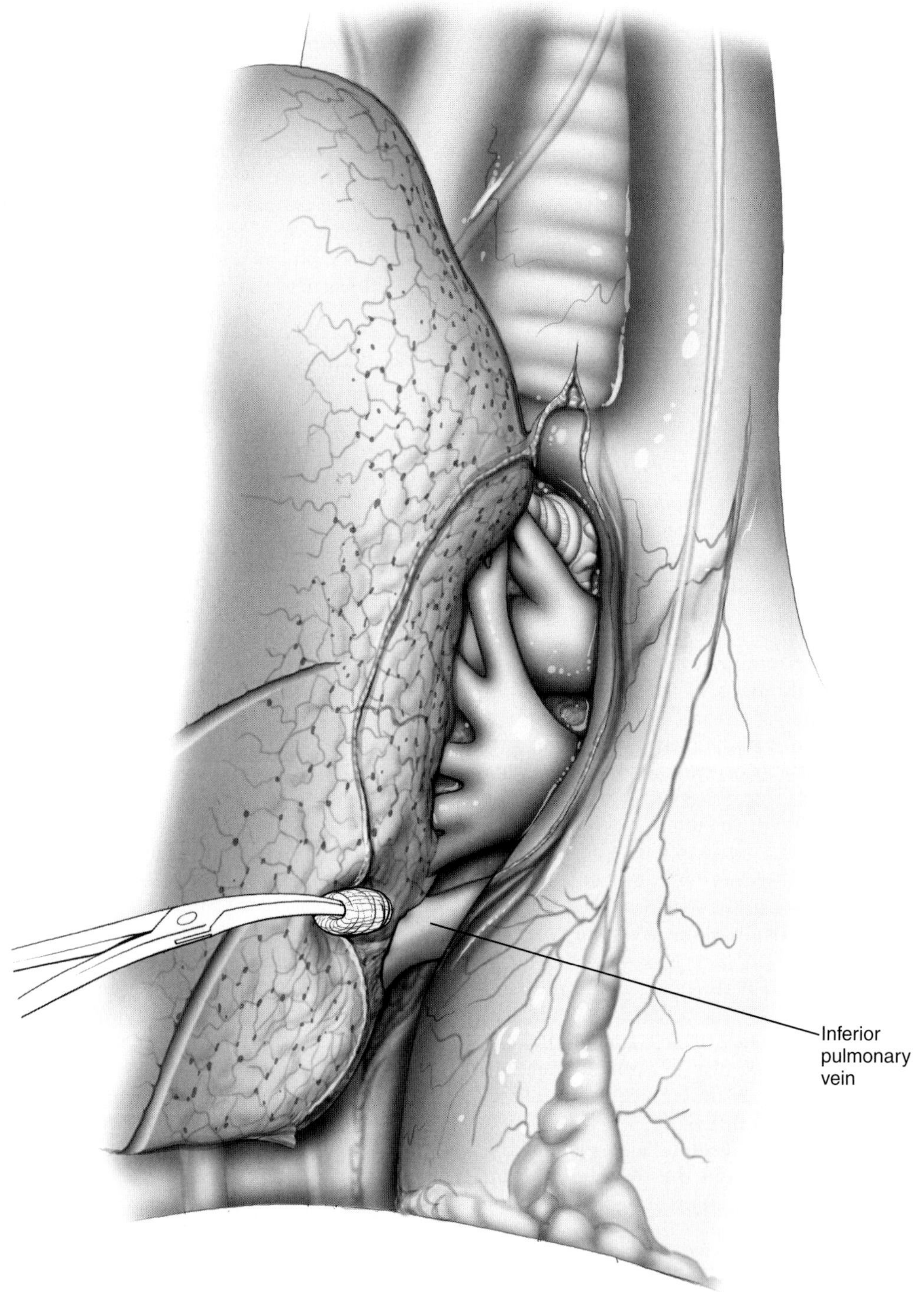

FIGURE 36–1 ■ The hilum of the right lung has been dissected completely, showing an anterior view of the right mainstem bronchus, the right pulmonary artery, and the pulmonary veins.

also to ensure that adequate hemostasis on the pericardiotomy is secured. Postoperative bleeding from this area can be troublesome and can result in unacceptable blood loss requiring re-exploration and may cause pericardial tamponade. The size of the pericardial defect should be considered at the end of the procedure and the necessary steps taken to prevent cardiac herniation and compromise to venous return.

On the left side, dissection may be continued proximally, and the remnant of the ductus (ligamentum arteriosus) may be divided to obtain additional length on the left main pulmonary artery (Fig. 36–2). The left recurrent laryngeal nerve is vulnerable here, and care should be taken to avoid injury to it, cautery to nearby structures, or traction on the nerve. As one proceeds centrally, it is possible to divide the left pulmonary artery at its origin (Fig. 36–3). Care must be taken to avoid compromise to the contralateral right pulmonary artery when the vessel is divided. It is also wise to loop a vessel around the main right or left pulmonary artery during the dissection. This will allow control of a potentially lethal problem and salvage the situation if the artery is entered or torn. Where extensive intrapericardial dissection is contemplated, the possibility of requiring cardiopulmonary bypass should be considered. This is exceedingly rare, but the surgeon should be prepared to institute it, if necessary.

On the right side, control of the intrapericardial artery may require mobilization of the superior vena cava and dissection of the artery that is medial to it, allowing a greater length of artery for control. The pulmonary artery is unforgiving and does not tolerate undue traction or rough handling. The veins are much tougher, and inadvertent injury is less frequent.

On occasion, when the bulk of tumor is anterior and large, the vessels may be divided after isolation and division of the main bronchus (Fig. 36–4). Resectability should be determined with certainty before this approach is used, although considerable experience is sometimes required to make such a judgment. Once the great pulmonary vessels have been divided, the suture or staple lines are carefully examined for satisfactory hemostasis.

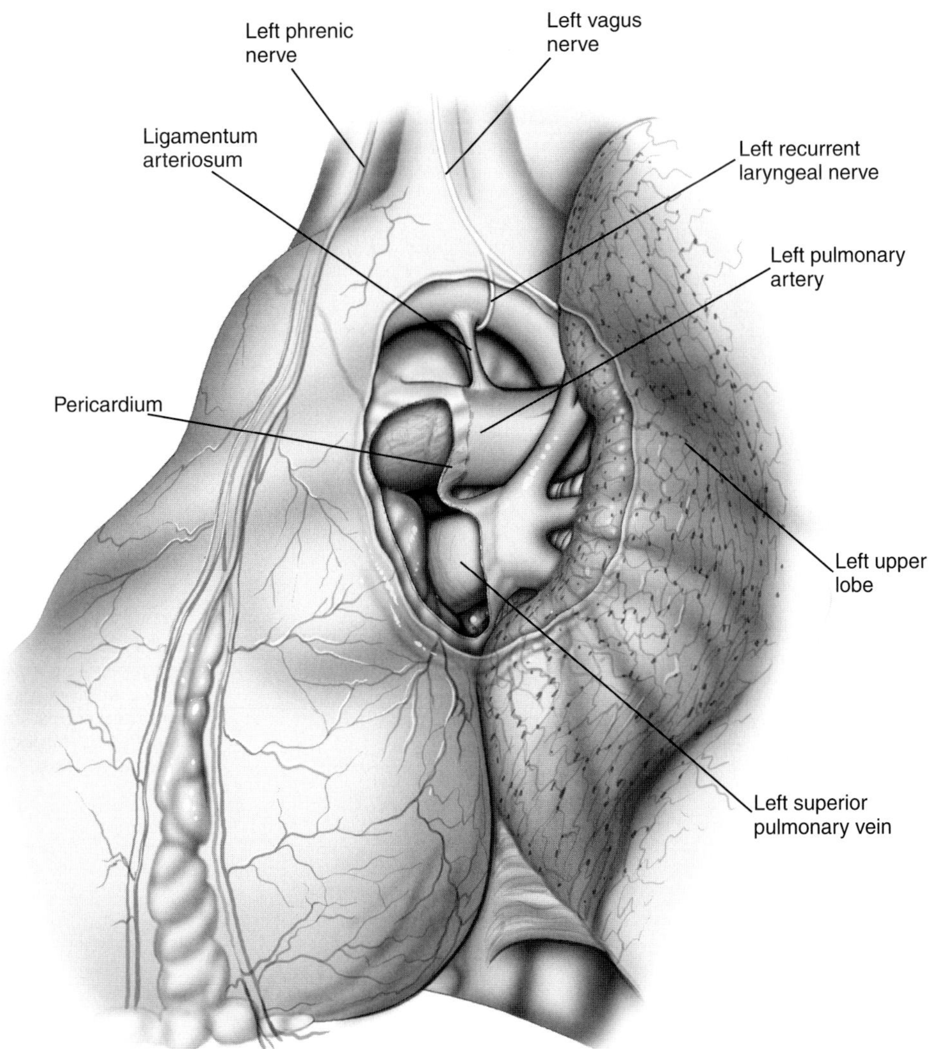

FIGURE 36–2 ■ The left pulmonary hilum has been totally exposed intrapericardially. The ligamentum arteriosum can be divided to provide further length on the left main artery. The recurrent nerve must always be protected.

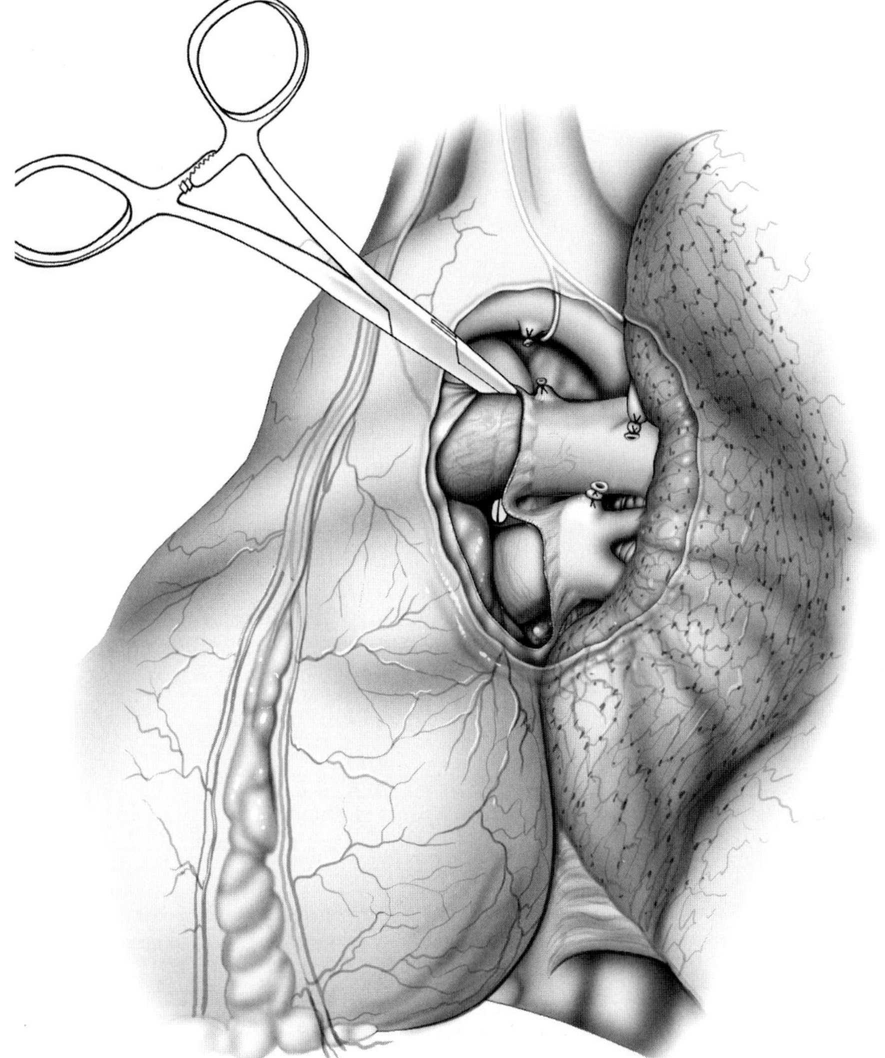

FIGURE 36–3 ■ Following division of the ligamentum arteriosum, a Satinsky clamp is applied just distal to the pulmonary conus. Care must always be taken not to impinge on the right pulmonary artery.

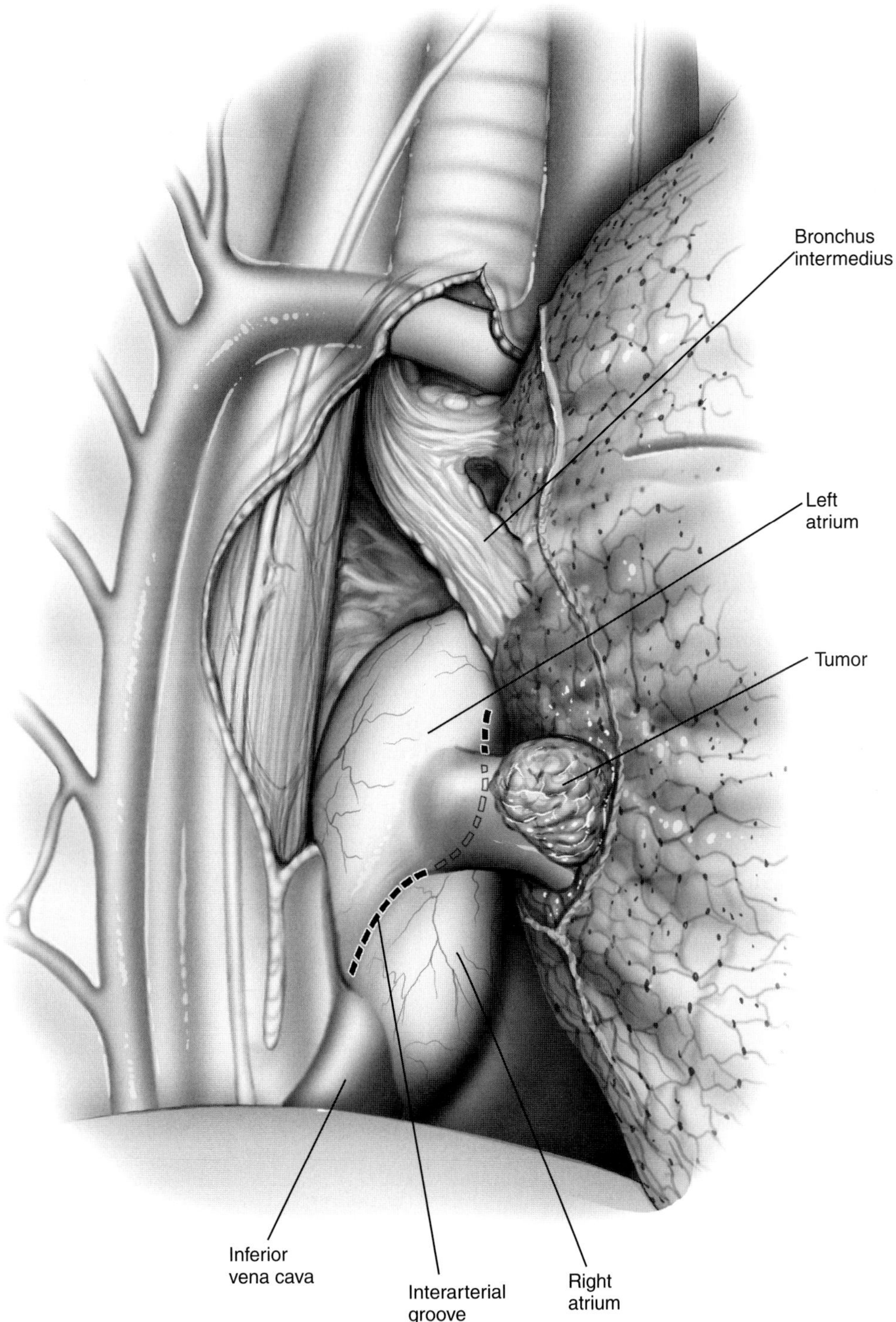

FIGURE 36–4 ■ The right lung is retracted anteriorly, exposing the right mainstem bronchus. With difficult hilar dissection, often the bronchus can be dissected first and divided, exposing the pulmonary artery from behind. With a tumor approximating the pulmonary veins, greater length can be obtained by opening up the interarterial groove *(dotted lines)* with careful sharp dissection.

Where the dissection has been very central, the site of division may retract, and small amounts of bleeding may not be readily apparent.

Bronchus

The handling of the main left or right bronchus is also a function of experience and personal preference. Dissection of the bronchus proximal to the resection margin should be kept to a minimum to preserve as much as possible of its blood supply. The goal of the process is to divide the mainstem bronchus as proximally as possible to avoid the problem of a long bronchial stump. On the right side, it is very easy to judge the point of bronchial division in relation to the trachea and avoid a long stump. It is a little more difficult on the left side, and particular care should be taken to follow the left main bronchus centrally to the carina. Sometimes this requires an initial distal division of the bronchus, removal of the specimen, and a subsequent revision, taking the bronchus a little more proximally. If staplers are not available, possible, or desired, the bronchus may be closed by standard suturing techniques. Nonabsorbable suture material is to be avoided because of the incidence of suture granuloma and troublesome hemoptysis later. I prefer to use Vicryl or a similar suture. Sutures are interrupted, in an anterior-posterior orientation. They are placed approximately 1 mm apart, encompassing the first cartilaginous ring. At the completion of the bronchial closure, the suture line is tested under water for air leaks, with the anesthesiologist's help. A Valsalva maneuver with about 30 to 35 cm H_2O static airway pressure is sufficient. If there are any air leaks, they should be dealt with and obliterated. This may require additional suture or additional tissue depending on the circumstances. Additional tissue implies the mobilization of neighboring vascularized tissues such as the pleura, the pericardium, the pericardial fat, the omentum, and the intercostal bundle, to suggest a few possibilities. The routine use of additional tissue to patch the bronchial suture line is controversial. Some believe it is necessary in every case; others think that it provides an enclosed area to encourage local infection. I do not routinely cover the bronchus.

Postpneumonectomy Space

Before closure, the usual checklist should be covered: satisfactory hemostasis, the absence of air leak, the condition and size of any pericardial defect, and, if applicable, an examination for possible esophageal or thoracic duct injuries. The phrenic nerve should not be crushed or otherwise intentionally damaged unless it is involved with the tumor.

The thoracotomy is closed in standard fashion, with consideration to the location of the mediastinum. If the incision has been a posterolateral thoracotomy, the mediastinum will fall away during the procedure with resulting compromise of contralateral lung function and even possible impairment of venous return. Once the chest is closed and the patient is supine, steps should be taken to evacuate air from the operated hemithorax to return the mediastinum to the midline (Suarez et al, 1969). Once the patient is placed supine, a sterile needle can be introduced into the chest in the operating room, and air can be evacuated until the sensation of resistance to evacuation is obtained. I have left a 16-gauge soft catheter in the hemithorax during the closure, bringing it out through the front of the incision. The catheter is positioned and the closure conducted in such a way to allow immediate removal of the catheter without a defect in the chest wall. With the catheter in place, a member of the surgical team and the necessary equipment (a "Christmas tree," 50-ml syringe, and three-way stopcock) remain sterile while the patient is returned to the supine position. Sufficient air is then evacuated in a sterile fashion to accomplish the goal; this is usually about 1 L of air in the average adult patient. The changes in position may be accompanied by arrhythmia and hypotension, and, therefore, it is necessary for a member of the surgical team to remain in the operating room for this. Some surgeons leave a chest tube in the hemithorax following pneumonectomy to achieve balancing of the mediastinum and to announce promptly any significant blood loss. This tube, if used, should receive no more than 5 cm H_2O suction, and personnel caring for the patient should be warned that additional suction may have disastrous consequences. Alternatively, commercially available "pneumonectomy" drainage systems allow for balanced drainage, maintaining the pneumonectomy space at -1 cm H_2O. Other surgeons leave the tube clamped after the mediastinum has been repositioned. The tube should be removed within 12 to 24 hours of the surgery. I have not used a tube because of the risk of introducing microorganisms via this route, with subsequent infection.

COMMENTS AND CONTROVERSIES

In this chapter, the author reviews the surgical steps involved in the performance of a pneumonectomy. Of all these steps, the most important is the actual decision to perform a pneumonectomy rather than a more limited procedure such as a sleeve resection. This decision is most important because pneumonectomy carries a significantly higher operative morbidity and mortality but often does not facilitate a better oncologic operation. It is, therefore, important to evaluate the possibilities of bronchial or pulmonary artery reconstruction before deciding on doing a pneumonectomy.

The actual sequence of division of hilar structures can be flexible, but unless the tumor invades the pulmonary veins, we prefer to start with the pulmonary artery and then move on to the veins and bronchus. We do not hesitate to open the pericardium to gain a few extra centimeters of artery and, indeed, more than 50% of pneumonectomies are done with intrapericardial division of pulmonary artery and veins. As mentioned by the author, the phrenic nerve should be preserved, although its division may not have a major impact because the lung will be removed. The pericardium should always be closed even if the opening does not appear to be large enough for cardiac herniation, which is usually a fatal complication. We currently staple all blood vessels, and I find that the "roticulator vascular stapler" is very useful

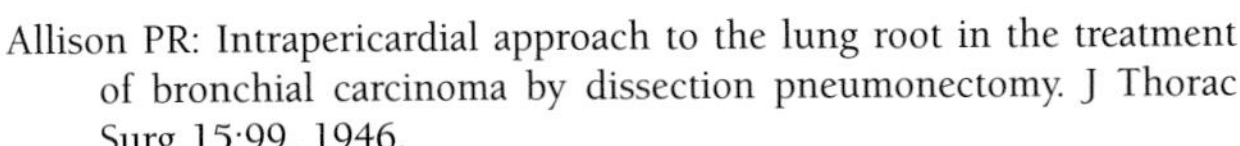

to deal with short stumps. The stapler line should always be inspected before dividing the vessel.

The bronchus is also stapled because we find this method to be expedient and very safe. On the right side, we recommend covering the stump with local tissues because after right pneumonectomy, the stump is left bare within the pleural space. On the left side, the bronchus retracts underneath the aorta and therefore coverage is not as important. Overall, the incidence of bronchopleural fistula should be less than 2% to 3% after pneumonectomy.

There is a great deal of controversy regarding drainage of the pneumonectomy space. We currently do not drain the space, but we remove approximately 1 L of air once the chest wall cavity is closed. If necessary, more air can be removed after a portable chest radiograph has been seen. The important thing is to keep the mediastinum as central as possible to avoid hemodynamic instability as well as acute overexpansion of the remaining lung.

In my opinion, pneumonectomy is a physiologically bad operation that should be reserved for patients with carcinomas that cannot be resected by lesser operations.

J.D.

■ REFERENCES

Abbey Smith R, Nigam BK: Resection of proximal left main bronchus carcinoma. Thorax 43:616, 1979.

Allison PR: Intrapericardial approach to the lung root in the treatment of bronchial carcinoma by dissection pneumonectomy. J Thorac Surg 15:99, 1946.

Brock R, Whitehead LL: Radical pneumonectomy for bronchial carcinoma. Br J Surg 43:8, 1955.

Cahan GC, Watson WL, Pool JL: Radical pneumonectomy. J Thorac Surg 22:449, 1951.

Cooper JD, Nelems JM, Pearson FG: Extended indications for median sternotomy in patients requiring pulmonary resection. Ann Thorac Surg 26:413, 1978.

Craig SR, Hamzah M, Walker WS: Video-asisted thoracoscopic pneumonectomy for bronchial carcinoid tumor in a 14-year-old girl. J Pediatr Surg 31:1724, 1996.

Graham EA, Singer JJ: Successful removal of an entire lung for carcinoma of the bronchus. JAMA 101:1371, 1933.

Meade RH: A History of Thoracic Surgery. Springfield, Charles C Thomas, 1961.

Miller GE, Aberg THJ, Gerbode F: Effect of pulmonary vein ligation on pulmonary artery flow in dogs. J Thorac Cardiovasc Surg 55:668, 1968.

Podbielski FJ, Marquez GD, Nelson DG et al: Thoracoscopic assisted pneumonectomy. J Soc Laparoendosc Surg 1:75, 1997.

Roviaro G, Varolli F, Vergani C, Maciocco M: Techniques of pneumonectomy: Video-assisted thoracic surgery pneumonectomy. Chest Surg Clin North Am 9:419, 1999.

Sarot IA, Gilbert L: Extrapleural pneumonectomy and pleurectomy in pulmonary tuberculosis. Thorax 4:173, 1949.

Suarez J, Clagett OT, Brown AL Jr: The post-pneumonectomy space. J Thorac Cardiovasc Surg 57:539, 1969.

Takita H, Merrin C, Didolkar MS et al: The surgical management of multiple lung metastases. Ann Thorac Surg 24:359, 1977.

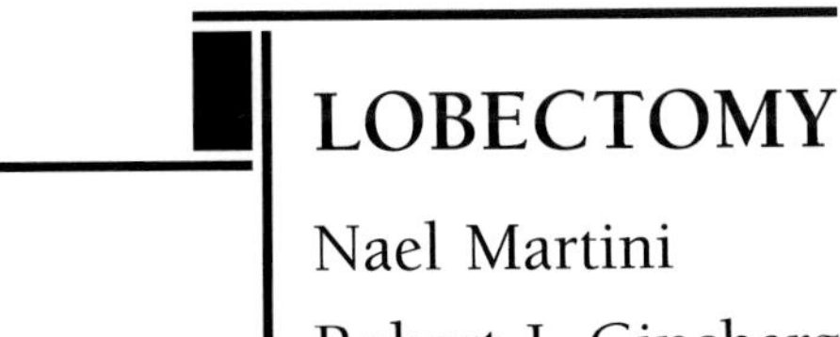

LOBECTOMY

Nael Martini
Robert J. Ginsberg

HISTORICAL NOTE

The first proper dissection lobectomy was performed by Davies in 1912. Before that, most pulmonary resections were performed by hilar ligation and cautery dissection of the surrounding lung. Although the operation was technically successful, Davies' patient died 8 days later of an empyema. For the next 15 years, surgeons continued to remove lung by nonanatomic means. In 1929, Brunn reported a one-stage lobectomy and demonstrated the value of underwater drainage in anticipation of a bronchopleural fistula. Despite these early successes with dissection lobectomy, pneumonectomy remained the treatment of choice following Graham's successful report in 1933. It was not until Churchill's report of long-term survival following lobectomy for peripheral lung cancer in the early 1950s that this procedure became acceptable in the management of lung cancer. Before this, lobectomy had been reserved for inflammatory diseases such as tuberculosis and bronchiectasis.

■ HISTORICAL READINGS

Brunn HB: Surgical principle underlying one stage lobectomy. Arch Surg 18:490, 1929.

Churchill ED: Lobectomy and pneumonectomy in bronchiectasis of cystic disease. J Thorac Surg 6:286, 1937.

Churchill ED, Sweet RH, Sutter L, Scannel JG: The surgical management of carcinoma of the lung: A study of cases treated at the Massachusetts General Hospital from 1930–50. J Thorac Cardiovasc Surg 20:349, 1950.

Davies HM: Recent advances in the surgery of lung and pleura. Br J Surg 1:228, 1913–1914.

Lobectomy remains the preferred excision for the surgical therapy of lung cancer. Pneumonectomy is reserved for the more centrally placed tumors, and resections that are less extensive than lobectomy are carried out in patients with compromised pulmonary function or, less frequently, electively in those with small peripheral tumors. There is a 10% to 15% risk of local recurrence within the remaining portion of the resected lobe when lesser resections are performed, particularly in patients with adenocarcinomas. Indications for lobectomy in benign disease include pulmonary tuberculosis, chronic lung abscess, and bronchiectasis, benign tumors, fungal infections, and congenital anomalies.

GENERAL CONSIDERATIONS

Although the techniques of lobectomy have been amply described, the main emphasis in lung cancer surgery has been focused on complete resection with regional lymph node excision for better staging and local control. We prefer complete mediastinal lymph node dissection (vis-à-vis lymph node sampling) to accomplish this.

The reader is referred to the chapters on anatomy (see Chapter 57) and the technique of mediastinal lymph node dissection (see Chapter 63). Prior to any lobectomy or other pulmonary resection, we believe that the surgeon shall perform his/her own bronchoscopy to ensure that endobronchial disease, which would negate the possibility of a lobectomy, and that congenital anomalies of the bronchial tree are not present.

Operative Positions

For lobectomy, the lateral approach through a posterolateral incision is the gold standard. Entry into the pleural space is usually gained through the fifth intercostal space or through the periosteal bed of the fifth rib when an upper or middle lobectomy is contemplated and through the sixth intercostal space or the bed of the sixth rib when a lower lobectomy is planned. This is particularly true for tumors in the periphery of the lobes. In more centrally placed lower lobe tumors, it may be advantageous to expose the pleural space through the fifth intercostal space to provide better access to the hilum for a safe dissection. More recently, anterolateral muscle-sparing incisions have been increasingly used and usually require an approach that is one interspace higher because the anterior aspect of the ribs is positioned more inferiorly.

An anterior approach, via a median sternotomy or anterior thoracotomy, provides excellent access to the superior pulmonary veins and the main pulmonary arteries but somewhat poorer access to the major bronchi and the inferior pulmonary veins. Access for safe pulmonary resections has been facilitated by the use of double-lumen endobronchial intubation and one-lung anesthesia.

Initial Mobilization

After the pleural space is entered, adhesions, if present, are divided by either blunt or sharp dissection. Any free pleural fluid is aspirated for cytologic study and culture. The entire lung is then inspected and palpated to assess the extent of involvement, to identify occult tumors, and to determine if lobectomy is possible. The mediastinum is inspected also to rule out the presence of any disease outside the lung that needs to be attended to or biopsied before any pulmonary resection is carried out. The mediastinal pleura at the hilum is then completely incised to facilitate hilar and lymph node dissection. The inferior pulmonary ligament is incised to the inferior pulmonary vein, thus totally mobilizing the lung.

Adhesions and Fissures

Two problems, adhesions and incomplete fissures, are common to many lobectomies, especially when performed for inflammatory lesions, in which adhesions between the visceral and parietal pleurae are common. When the adhesions are thin and avascular, division with scissors or blunt dissection with the fingers or a sponge stick is a simple matter. For dense adhesions, sharp dissection by scalpel or electrocautery is required to develop the pleural planes. Despite best efforts, it may be difficult to avoid injuring lung parenchyma, in which case dissecting extrapleurally is advisable. An incision is made in the parietal pleura adjacent to the adherent area, and an extrapleural fascial plane is developed by blunt dissection with the index finger or a sponge. The parietal pleura overlying the densely adherent area is then excised.

The lobar fissures are often not completely open from the periphery to the hilum. Incomplete fissures may be caused by inflammatory adhesions, congenital failure of complete development, or extension of a tumor from one lobe to another. If the problem is solely that of inflammatory adhesions, blunt dissection should be tried first. If the adhesions are filmy, a gentle sweeping motion with a sponge stick will suffice. Dense adhesions and completely fused fissures are more problematic. Classic anatomic stripping of the fissure, as with segmental resection, may be useful but can result in significant oozing and air leakage. Division with a linear stapler, which staples and divides, is generally more secure and more efficient. Refer to the section on anatomy (Chapter 57) in which a detailed description of division of fissures is available.

Hilar Dissection

Dissection of the secondary hilar structures for a lobectomy is often more tedious and time consuming than is dissection of the hilar structures for a pneumonectomy. Anomalies are much more frequent, and in many cases, the fissures between the lobes are incomplete. When the lobectomy is performed in the presence of significant inflammatory disease, the fibrosis, lymph node scarring, and calcification can make the dissection difficult. In performing a lobectomy, classically one first divides the artery, then the veins, and then the bronchus. For lung cancer surgery, some surgeons have favored division of the veins first to prevent the escape of circulating tumor cells lest they implant elsewhere. This rarely, if ever, occurs. More importantly, when the veins are ligated first, the lobe may become more congested and retain blood that is unnecessarily sacrificed with the resected specimen, although peribronchial venous channels usually prevent this.

Division of the bronchus before ligating the vessels was classically described for patients with associated lung abscesses to prevent spillage into the main bronchus and to the opposite lung. This approach may be used to advantage where vessel dissection is difficult. Except for the case of a left upper lobectomy, once the bronchus has been divided, the interlobar vessels are immediately in view, anterior to the bronchus. In patients with central tumors, it is occasionally advantageous not to adhere to the recommended ligation sequence of artery, vein, then bronchus but rather to remove that structure whose absence provides better exposure to the remaining structures.

When encountering an extremely difficult dissection, in which injury to pulmonary arteries is possible, dissecting and encircling the main pulmonary artery and lobar veins prior to the segmental arterial dissection is advised. Using this technique, if problems arise, the main pulmonary artery and lobar pulmonary vein can be cross-clamped to prevent unnecessary blood loss.

Management of Vessels

The segmental pulmonary arteries have a significant media and intima. These are usually divided between ligatures. Some surgeons prefer transfixion ligatures whereas others use a simple, non-absorbable ligature. Other surgeons prefer double ligation or ligation and transfixion of arteries, although this does not appear necessary. When the tumor approaches the main trunk of the pulmonary artery, frequently a small portion of it requires removal with the affected segmental vessel. When this appears to be the case, it is best to isolate and tape the main pulmonary artery for control before dissecting so close to the take-off of an individual segmental artery. In cases of short, thick arteries, the use of stapling devices can be valuable, rather than ligation and division or clamping and sewing.

Unlike segmental arteries, the pulmonary veins, whether lobar or segmental, have a tendency to slip from a single ligature. Therefore, double ligation or ligation and transfixion is the rule. Many surgeons prefer suturing or stapling the main lobar pulmonary vein, dividing it at its origin, rather than individually dissecting segmental vessel.

Bronchial Closure

For most surgeons, resection includes the liberal use of staplers instead of hand sewing, particularly for the bronchus and frequently also for the main pulmonary artery and veins. Adequate closure can be achieved by the manual suturing techniques, but closure by stapling is equally safe, clearly more expedient, and currently the most widely used form of bronchial closure. A few precautions can lead to safe closure without consequent complications:

1. Avoid excessive devascularization of the bronchial stump.
2. When using staples, make sure the right "leg length" of stapler is used. Although the 3.5-mm stapler is adequate for most bronchial stumps, in individuals in whom the bronchial wall is thick, larger staplers such as the 4.8-mm may be more appropriate.
3. Make sure that there is an adequate stump to staple to avoid impingement on the main bronchus or other lobar bronchi and also that the margins are clear of tumor and inflammatory tissues.
4. In cancer surgery, obtain frozen section margins of any questionable area.
5. We continue to oversew the staple line with a running absorbable suture to avoid the occasional catastrophe of individual staples misfiring and springing loose at a later time.
6. Vascularized material (e.g., pericardium, pleura, pleurocardial fat pad, intercostal muscle) should be used to cover the bronchus in special circumstances in which a risk of fistula formation is significant.
7. Before the bronchus is divided, it should be clamped at the anticipated site of division, and a test of patency of the remaining bronchus should be carried out by gently inflating the remaining lobe and observing it deflate.

Lobectomy versus Pneumonectomy

In more centrally placed endobronchial lesions, lobectomy still may be the procedure of choice. In cancer surgery, it is extremely important for the surgeon to perform preoperative bronchoscopy to identify the proximal extent of the tumor and to determine whether the bronchus proximal to the lobar bronchus is involved. In these cases, consideration must be given to either a sleeve lobectomy or a pneumonectomy. Frequently, one encounters involved lymph nodes at the most proximal lobar level. In such cases, extensive lymph node sampling and frozen section analysis is required to ensure that lymph nodes more proximal or distal are not involved, a situation which could result in converting the lobectomy to a pneumonectomy ("sump nodes"). Although the surgeon frequently encounters patients for whom a lobectomy is preferred, if the proximity of the tumor or involved lymph nodes necessitates a pneumonectomy, one should not hesitate to perform one, assuming the patient has adequate pulmonary function. If the lobe remaining is destroyed or severely shrunken by long-standing infection or obstruction, completion pneumonectomy should be considered.

Prevention and Control of Air Leaks

Significant air leaks following lobectomy can be disastrous resulting in postlobectomy air spaces, chronic bronchopleural fistulae and chronic empyemas. This occurs most frequently following bilobectomies and left upper lobectomies when the residual remaining lung is small and air leaks are present.

A variety of techniques have been used to minimize the leaking lung. Although this is not a dissertation on the prevention of air leaks, several maneuvers have been advocated and are valuable. They include: careful dissection of adhesions, to avoid lung injury, using an extrapleural dissection where necessary; careful dissection of fissures, employing staples or clamps and oversewing where necessary; buttressing of "thick" areas of divided lung using bovine pericardium or other reinforcing materials; suturing with nonabsorbable monofilament material of any large exposed terminal bronchi; covering large raw areas with adjacent lung (e.g., middle lobe applied to upper lobe) or pleural flaps; cauterizing exposed surfaces (the Argon beam laser is valuable for this); application of fibrin glue or other newer aerostatic materials to raw surfaces; decreasing the hemithorax by maneuvers described below; and consideration of "no suction" or very low suction following the lobectomy. The use of such maneuvers varies with the individual patients. In many instances more than one of these maneuvers will be used in attempts to decrease air leakage postoperatively.

Placement of Chest Tubes and Their Management

There are no hard and fast rules for the management of chest tubes following lobectomy. With increasing frequency, much smaller chest tubes are being placed. We (RJG) currently use number 20 siliconized. The smaller size causes less postoperative pain. Whether one or two chest tubes are necessary is debatable and varies from surgeon to surgeon. For upper lobectomies, apical chest tube placement is the rule, and for lower lobectomies, an angled chest tube placed above the diaphragm is preferred. With increasing frequency, we use a single chest tube when there is absolutely no air leakage following the lobectomy, two chest tubes when raw surfaces or air leakage from the remaining lung is present, and three or more chest tubes when dense adhesions have required marked dissection of the chest wall and lung surface resulting in extensive open surfaces and oozing.

Prevention of Postlobectomy Spaces

Frequently, the remaining lobe or lobes are considered insufficient to fill the ipsilateral hemithorax. This can be especially true in pulmonary fibrotic diseases or following left upper lobectomy or right bilobectomy. In such cases, several maneuvers can be used to attempt to decrease the size of the hemithorax. These include: temporary paralysis of the phrenic nerve by crushing or injection of local anesthetic; a "soft thoracoplasty" or "pleural tent" of the upper chest and mediastinum by mobilizing the apical pleura, allowing it to fall down over the remaining lobe (this produces an extrapleural space, which ultimately can fill with fluid); insertion of more than two chest tubes with high postoperative suction; repositioning of the diaphragm to a higher level; and intraoperative or postoperative creation of a pneumoperitoneum, which is increased gradually over a few days to elevate the ipsilateral diaphragm. In most cases, attention to detail, with closure of large leaking areas in the residual lobe, accurate placement of chest tubes, and fastidious attention in the postoperative period will result in fewer problematic postoperative spaces. Rarely, a "tailoring thoracoplasty" may be required.

SPECIAL FEATURES OF THE VARIOUS LOBES

There are many atlases of thoracic surgery that discuss in detail the various approaches to lobectomy. In the following discussion, we are not trying to replace these atlases but to add "tricks" that we have found useful in performing the various lobectomies.

Right Upper Lobectomy

The pleura over the anterior aspect of the right hilum is incised to provide exposure to the pulmonary artery and its branches to the upper lobes. The mediastinal pleura is incised posterior to the phrenic nerve which is protected, and the incision is extended down to the superior pulmonary vein which is exposed and mobilized by sharp and blunt dissection, [and encircled with a heavy ligature] protecting the middle lobe vein which is preserved (Fig. 36–5). The anterior and apical segmental arteries are then dissected and also encircled with a heavy ligature. It is preferable not to ligate the vessels to be sacrificed until all have been identified and the surgeon is satisfied that a lobectomy will completely encompass all the diseased tissue to be removed.

The dissection is then directed toward the major or oblique fissure; the interlobar portion of the pulmonary artery is identified, and the posterior ascending branch to the right upper lobe is exposed (Fig. 36–6). It is often necessary to separate the upper and lower lobes by completing the dissection of the posterior aspect of the oblique fissure to identify the vessels. This can be done by dividing the fused fissure between clamps or by stapling. The minor or transverse fissure between the upper and middle lobes is frequently incomplete but rarely requires division to identify upper lobe vessels and must ultimately must be divided. Care must be taken to avoid injury to the middle lobe and the superior segmental arteries.

The right upper lobe bronchus is then exposed posteriorly to ascertain that no disease is at its margin that will preclude a lobectomy. Once that is done, the segmental arteries to the right upper lobe are individually ligated and divided. The superior pulmonary vein is either doubly ligated and divided or secured by stapling or suturing. The right upper lobe bronchus is then completely dissected, stapled at its takeoff, and divided distal to the staples or divided and sutured, which completes the lobectomy. At the completion of the right upper lobectomy, care must be taken to reposition the middle lobe correctly. With a complete minor fissure, the middle lobe should be secured to the adjoining lobe by staple or suture to avoid volvulus. Hemostasis is secured, and if two chest tubes are used, they are placed through separate incisions, one directed to the pleural apex and another over the diaphragm. The tubes are connected to water seal drainage and the thoracic incision is closed in layers in the usual fashion.

If access to the arteries is difficult, the anterior and apical arteries can be exposed more readily if the apical division of the superior pulmonary vein is divided—this often crosses these first branches of the pulmonary artery. The posterior ascending artery may come off the superior segmental artery, and injury to this latter vessel should be avoided. When the fissure is difficult to dissect, careful dissection and division of the upper lobe bronchus using a posterior approach will reveal the posterior ascending artery, which is often surrounded by lymph nodes just deep (anterior) to the bronchus. Another approach to the posterior ascending artery is, following division of the vein and anterior and apical arteries, to dissect on the

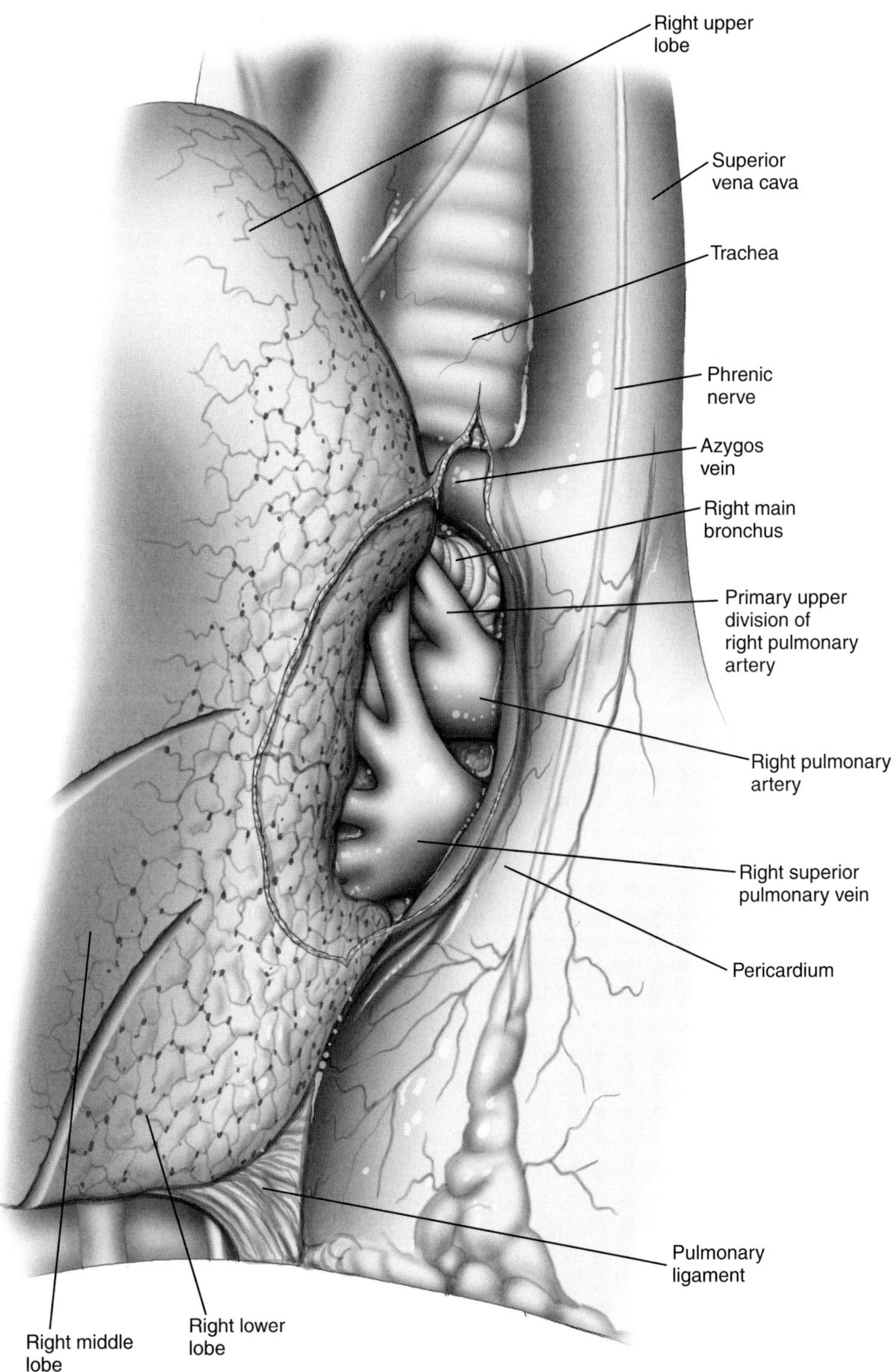

FIGURE 36–5 ■ Anterior view of the right hilum. The lung is retracted posteriorly. The mediastinal pleura is open widely posterior to the phrenic nerve, exposing the pulmonary artery with its branches to the right upper lobe, the superior pulmonary vein, and the azygos tributary of the superior vena cava. Dividing the apical segmental vein first will improve exposure to pulmonary artery branches. Note the middle lobe vein, which is to be protected during the upper lobectomy.

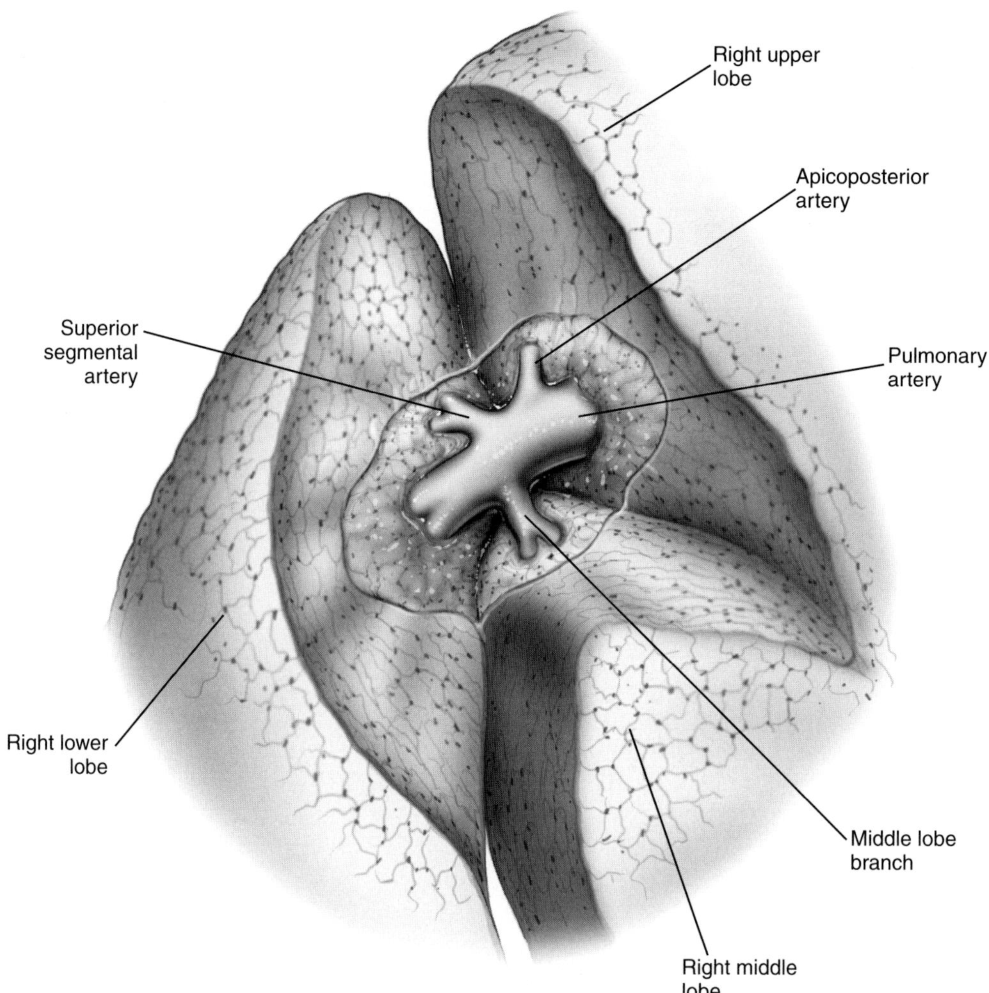

FIGURE 36–6 ■ View into the right major fissure from the front. The fissure has been opened widely to expose and identify the segmental arteries to the upper, middle, and lower lobes. Anomalies of these vessels are common. The location of the posterior segmental artery to the right upper lobe is most variable; this artery may be a branch of the superior segmental artery. Occasionally, this segmental arterial branch is absent.

surface of the remaining main pulmonary trunk anteriorly, lifting the pulmonary parenchyma until the posterior ascending artery is revealed within the depths of the upper lobe. When all else fails in attempting to isolate the arteries to the upper lobe, the best approach is early division of the upper lobe bronchus after dissecting the right main bronchus and bronchus intermedius completely. When the superior vein is engulfed in tumor or inflammation, an intrapericardial approach is valuable, always protecting the middle lobe vein.

Right Middle Lobectomy

Dissection usually begins at the minor or transverse fissure, which is often fused and necessitates division by electrocautery or by stapling. The arterial supply to the middle lobe is found at the junction of the transverse and oblique fissures. There are usually two middle lobe vessels supplying the medial and the lateral segments (see Fig. 36–6). Exposure, mobilization followed by ligation, and division of each of these vessels will lead to exposure of the middle lobe bronchus. As a rule, it is preferable to expose the venous branches to the middle lobe before dissecting the middle lobe bronchus. The middle lobe veins are easily accessed from the superior pulmonary vein; each is mobilized, doubly ligated, and divided. The middle lobe bronchus is then readily mobilized by blunt or digital dissection, stapled at its takeoff, and divided distal to the stapled line. Completion of the lobectomy may necessitate completing the fissures to the upper and lower lobes by blunt dissection or by stapling the lung at the fissures. Occasionally, with difficult fissures, division of all structures from the anterior approach is easier (i.e., divide vein, then bronchus, then arteries before dividing the fissures) and many surgeons use this anterior approach (vein, then bronchus, then artery) as the preferred one.

Right Lower Lobectomy

Following division of the inferior pulmonary ligament, the inferior pulmonary vein is exposed, dissected, and encircled (Fig. 36–7). Dissection then begins in the central portion of the major fissure at its junction with the minor fissure to identify the arteries to the lower lobe and ensure that both middle and upper lobes can be separated and are free of disease. Dissection is carried out along the pulmonary artery, identifying its major basilar division and the superior segmental division (see Fig. 36–6). Once that is done, the two main arteries to the right lower lobe (superior segmental and common basal) are ligated and divided. The inferior pulmonary vein is also doubly ligated, transfixed, and divided or secured by stapling or oversewing. The lower lobe bronchus is thus exposed and mobilized to ensure an adequate cuff for stapling distal to the right middle lobe bronchial takeoff. It then is stapled and divided distal to the stapled line or divided and sutured, which completes the lobectomy. Occasionally, a high takeoff of the superior segmental bronchus requires separate closure of the basilar and

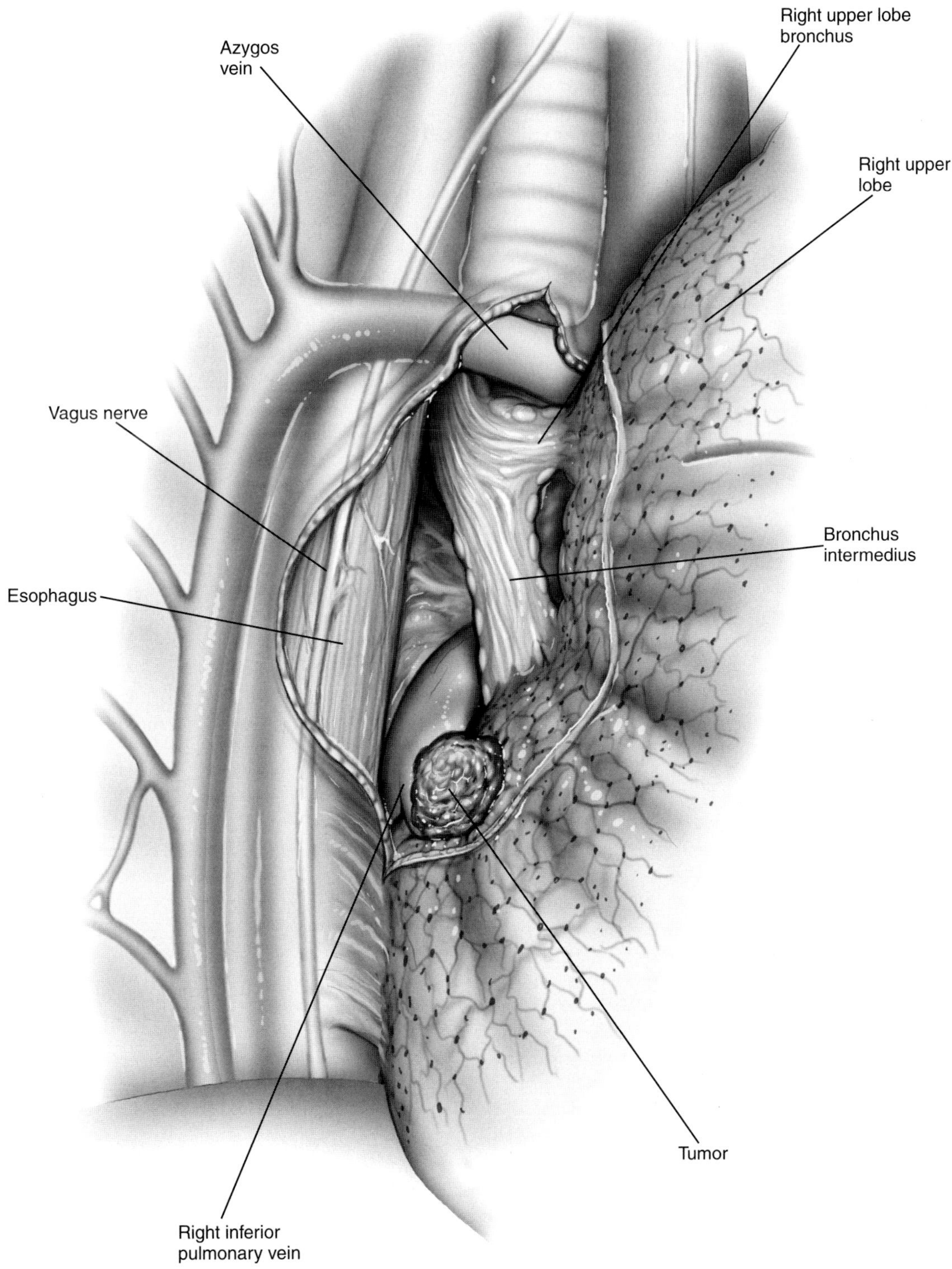

FIGURE 36–7 ■ View of the pulmonary hilum from behind.

superior segmental stumps to avoid impingement on the middle lobe. The placement of the chest tubes has already been discussed.

Bilobectomy

In diseases affecting the right lung, bilobectomy becomes necessary when a tumor is peripheral but crosses fissures: Involvement of the minor fissure will necessitate an upper and middle lobectomy to encompass all disease invasion of the posterior portion of the major fissure. This will necessitate a lobectomy and wedge resection or segmentectomy of the involved lung of the adjoining lobe. Involvement of the anterior portion of the major fissure will dictate the need for a middle and lower lobectomy. Bilobectomy is also necessary when a tumor is endobronchial at or near the takeoff of the middle or lower lobes, extending into the intermediate bronchus, or when lymph node involvement in lower lobe tumors dictates removal of the middle lobe as well. Some of these patients will benefit from a sleeve lobectomy if pulmonary compromise is at issue, thus preserving the lower lobe (for proximal middle lobe tumors) or the middle lobe (for proximal lower lobe tumors). In middle lobectomies or bilobectomies, division of the bronchus is distal to the upper lobe take-off, ensuring that it is not compromised. In difficult cases, division of the bronchus intermedius first will facilitate arterial dissection. A bilobectomy involving the middle and lower lobes has the highest risk for bronchopleural fistula and empyema. We (RJG) cover the bronchus with vascularized tissue (e.g., pleura, pericardial fat pad) and perform maneuvers to decrease the likelihood of space problems, hoping to lessen the risk of this morbid complication.

Left Upper Lobectomy

Two distinctive anatomic features are involved in performing a left upper lobectomy—the recurrent laryngeal

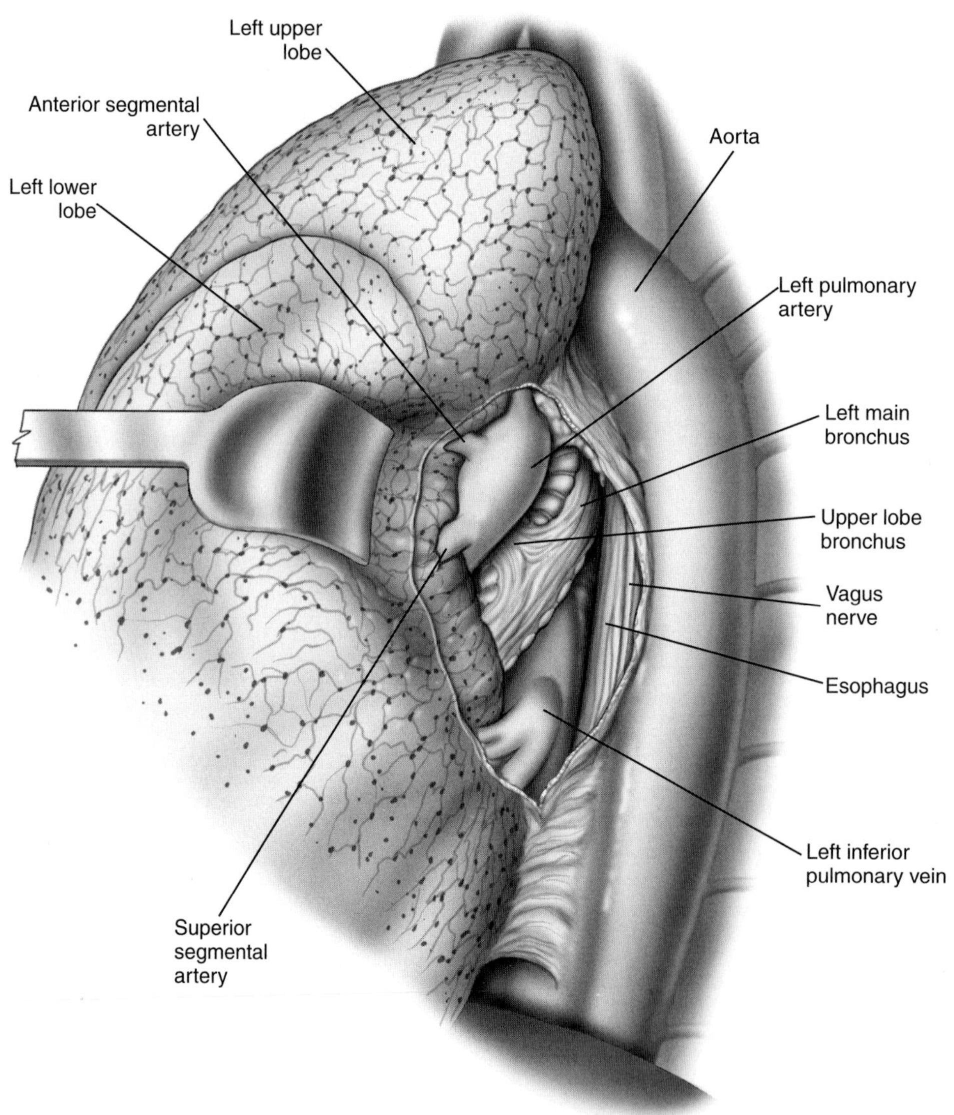

FIGURE 36–8 ■ Posterior view of the left hilum. The pulmonary arteries that are accessible posteriorly have been dissected as has the inferior pulmonary vein.

nerve at the aortopulmonary window and the variable arterial supply to the left upper lobe. Following hilar mobilization, dissection is first directed to the aortopulmonary window, where the mediastinal pleura is divided beginning anterior to the descending aorta just past the arch. The pleural incision is then continued inferiorly to the pulmonary vein and then proximally to the arch, exposing and protecting the vagus nerve and identifying the recurrent laryngeal nerve (Fig. 36–8). This exposes the main pulmonary artery. Following division of the anterior hilar pleura, the dissection is then focused on the major fissure, and all arterial branches to the left upper lobe are sequentially exposed and mobilized. It is preferable to first identify the lingular vessels and then move cephalad to isolate the apical posterior segmental and anterior segmental vessels (Fig. 36–9). These vessels may number from three to seven. By retracting the upper lobe inferiorly, access to the dangerous (usually short) anterior segmental artery can be improved. Unless one is careful to avoid undue traction, injury by traction alone to that vessel at its takeoff from the main pulmonary artery may occur. In difficult dissections, initial control of the main pulmonary artery is advised. The apicoposterior segmental vein often limits adequate exposure of this artery and can be divided first. For these two reasons, it is generally preferred to begin dissection of the lingular vessels and move proximally.

Mobilization, ligation, and division of the lingular ar-

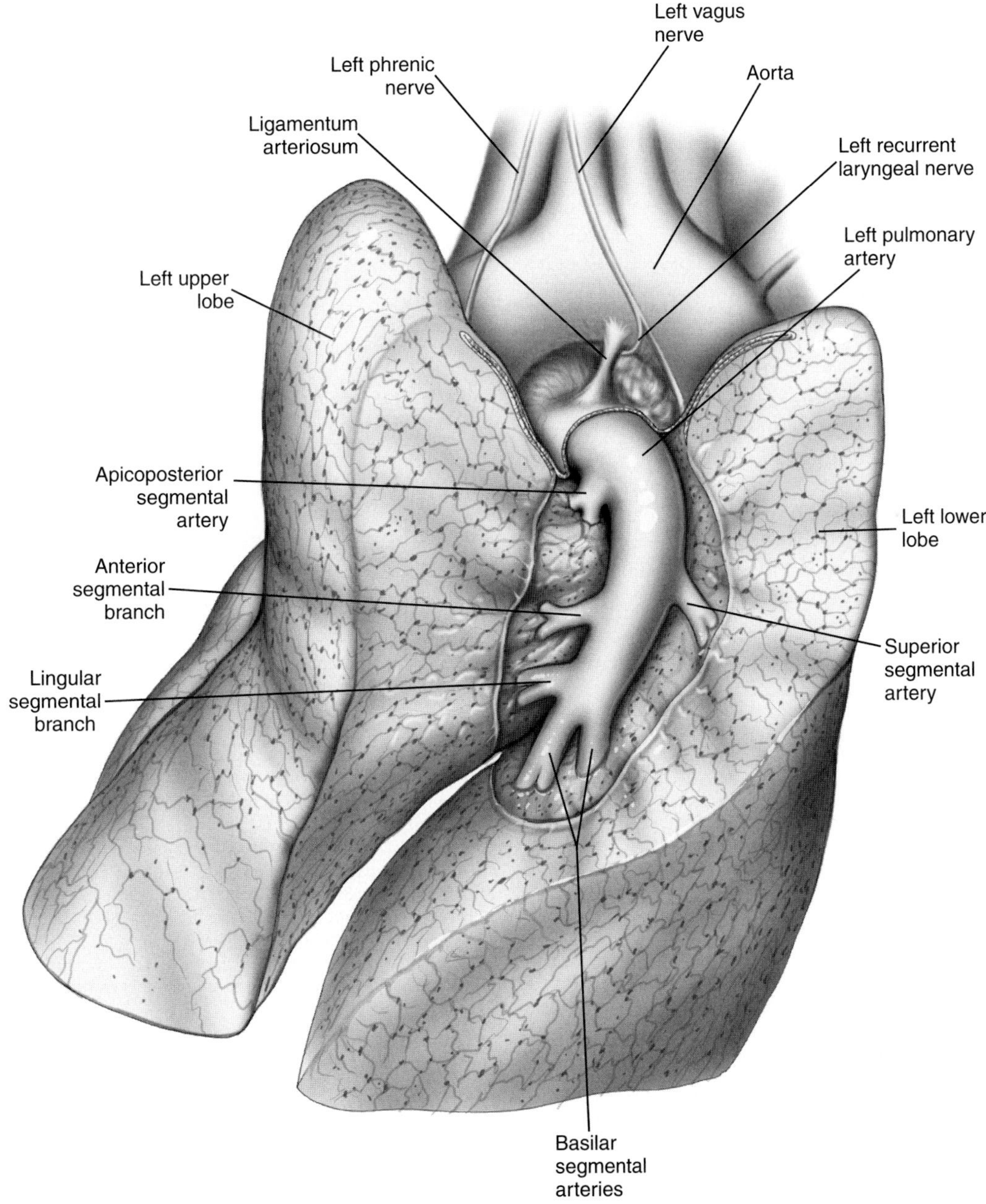

FIGURE 36–9 ■ Exposure or the left hilum, interlobar view. The patient's head is to the top, and the back is to the right. The segmental arterial supply to both the upper and the lower lobes is detailed. Note the ligamentum arteriosum, which can be divided to facilitate difficult dissections.

teries and more proximal segmental arteries are usually carried out once the major fissure has been opened before dissecting the "artery of sorrow" (anterior segmental). The upper lobe is retracted posteriorly to expose the pericardium and phrenic nerve and to provide access to the superior pulmonary vein. The latter is readily dissected out, its segmental veins are individually ligated and divided, or the whole superior pulmonary vein is stapled proximally or divided after a vascular clamp is placed and oversewn. This usually provides excellent exposure to the remaining anterior segmental artery and facilitates its dissection and safe division. Because a large common pulmonary vein can be encountered, care must be taken to ensure that injury to the inferior pulmonary vein does not occur when dividing the superior pulmonary vein.

The upper lobe bronchus is then easily visualized in the major fissure. It is skeletonized and stapled at its takeoff and divided distal to the staple line or divided and sutured, which completes the lobectomy.

Left Lower Lobectomy

In contrast to the left upper lobe, considered to be technically the most difficult and dangerous lobe to resect, the left lower lobe is viewed as the easiest. Dissection begins in the major fissure. The arterial supply to the superior and basilar segments is visualized and dissected out. Each of the branches are individually ligated and divided. The mediastinal pleura anterior to the descending aorta is incised to the level of the inferior pulmonary ligament. Division of the ligament provides exposure to the inferior pulmonary veins. The left lower lobe bronchus lies immediately posterior to the arterial branches and is easily exposed. Both vein and lobar bronchus are managed in a manner that is similar to that used in a right lower lobectomy, with avoidance of any impingement on the upper lobe bronchus.

COMMENTS AND CONTROVERSIES

Perhaps one of the most important aspects of lobectomy for lung cancer is its indication (as opposed to pneumonectomy) when sump nodes are positive for metastatic disease. Although there is no clear answer to this question, we generally do not hesitate to carry out a pneumonectomy for left-sided tumors, whereas we prefer a sleeve resection of the upper or lower lobe on the right side where the bronchus intermedius allows for greater maneuverability.

As discussed by the authors, most postoperative spaces can be prevented by careful technique, which includes stapling of fissures and closure of significant parenchymal leaks. We have found that the use of sealant products is not very helpful. I would also caution against crushing the phrenic nerve, because more than likely it will result in permanent damage. We prefer the instillation of bupivacaine hydrochloride (Marcaine) in the fatty tissues around the nerve just above the diaphragm. It is worth noting that elevation of the diaphragm and thoracoplasty are no longer done, largely because they add much to the procedure and are unnecessary. If a space is anticipated, we use a pleural tent after upper lobectomy and a pneumoperitoneum after lower lobectomy. This latter maneuver is done by inserting a catheter through the diaphragm and bringing it out through the chest wall. Air can then be injected as needed to decrease the "boundaries" of the pleural space. Perhaps the most important technique in preventing postlobectomy spaces is the use of adequate analgesia, usually through an epidural catheter. This allows the patient to have a more productive cough, therefore encouraging lung re-expansion.

For space management, I feel that one chest tube is adequate in most cases. Because I still believe that lung re-expansion is most important in sealing air leaks, this tube is always connected to an active drainage system with a negative pressure of −20 cm of water.

J.D.

■ KEY REFERENCES

Beattie EJ, Economou SG: An Atlas of Advanced Surgical Techniques. Philadelphia, WB Saunders, 1968.

Hood RM: Techniques in general thoracic surgery. Philadelphia, WB Saunders, 1985.

Ravitch MM, Steichen FM: Atlas of General Thoracic Surgery. Philadelphia, WB Saunders, 1988.

Urschel H, Cooper JD (eds): Atlas of Thoracic Surgery. New York, Churchill Livingstone, 1995.

Waldhausen JA, Pierce WS: Johnson's Surgery of the Chest, 5th ed. Chicago, Year Book Medical Publishers, 1985.

These key references encompass detailed descriptions and step-by-step illustrations of the techniques of the more common thoracic surgical procedures.

■ REFERENCES

Brunn HB: Surgical principals underlying one stage lobectomy. Arch Surg 18:490, 1929.

Churchill ED: Lobectomy and pneumonectomy in bronchiectasis of cystic disease. J Thorac Surg 6:286, 1937.

Churchill ED, Sweet RH, Sutter L, Scannell JG: The surgical management of carcinoma of the lung: A study of cases treated at the Massachusetts General Hospital from 1930–50. J Thorac Cardiovasc Surg 20:349, 1950.

Davies HM: Recent advances in the surgery of lung and pleura. Br J Surg 1:228, 1913–1914.

SEGMENTAL RESECTION

Stanley C. Fell
Thomas J. Kirby

Anatomic segmental resection is the excision of one or more bronchopulmonary segments of a lobe, with individual ligation and division of the corresponding bronchovascular structures. Although portions of lobes may be excised by use of clamps, stapling devices, cautery, or lasers, these nonanatomical methods are properly classified as wedge resections.

HISTORICAL NOTE

Clinical application of the known detailed knowledge of human bronchovascular anatomy did not occur until Kramer and Glass originated the term *bronchopulmonary segment* in their study of lung abscess in 1932.

Segmental resection was first proposed and performed by Churchill and Belsey in 1939. These authors stated that "the bronchopulmonary segment may replace the lobe as the surgical unit of the lung." The surgical and anatomic study of Kent and Blades in 1942 popularized the technique of individual ligation of hilar structures. Subsequently, Overholt and Langer (1949) systematized the operative methods for resection of all bronchopulmonary segments.

Segmental resection was developed for the surgical management of tuberculosis and bronchiectasis. Both are often multisegmental and bilateral diseases. Segmental resection made it possible to extirpate irreversible disease with minimal loss of functioning lung parenchyma. An additional advantage claimed for segmental resection in resections for tuberculosis was that it minimized compensatory hyperinflation of the residual lung, a phenomenon believed (erroneously) in the preantibiotic era to accelerate the reactivation of quiescent residual disease. Segmental resection has more recently been applied to the surgical therapy of primary or metastatic lung cancer.

■ *HISTORICAL READINGS*

Churchill ED, Belsey R: Segmental pneumonectomy in bronchiectasis. Ann Surg 109:481, 1939.

Kent EM, Blades B: The anatomic approach to pulmonary resection. Ann Surg 116:782, 1942.

Kramer R, Glass A: Bronchoscopic localization of lung abscess. Ann Otol Rhinol Laryngol 41:1210, 1932.

Overholt RH, Langer L: The Technique of Pulmonary Resection. Springfield, Charles C Thomas, 1951.

The authors gratefully acknowledge the support of the Feldesman Fund for Thoracic Surgery at the Montefiore Medical Center, Bronx, New York, in the preparation of this chapter.

PRINCIPLES OF SEGMENTAL RESECTION

General Considerations

Segmental resection is technically more difficult than lobectomy, requiring intimate three-dimensional knowledge of the relevant bronchoarterial relationships and possible arterial anomalies. Preoperative bronchoscopy is required to ensure that segmental bronchi are free of disease. Following thoracotomy, lysis of adhesions, and hemostasis, complete mobilization of the lung is required to facilitate the exposure required for resection and subsequent pulmonary re-expansion.

In cases of lung cancer, sampling of hilar and mediastinal lymph nodes with frozen section analysis is mandatory to determine the applicability of segmentectomy. Ideally, the tumor is 2 cm or less in diameter and deeply seated in the segment with surrounding normal lung tissue. Subpleural tumors near the edge of a lobe are generally amenable to generous wedge resection with a stapling device. Visual examination and palpation determine whether the residual segments are of sufficient volume to warrant their preservation. In surgery for inflammatory disease, a shrunken fibrotic basilar segment, for example, is usually associated with compensatory hypertrophy of the superior segment, which makes salvage of this segment worthwhile. In carcinoma, this phenomenon is not noted.

The most reliable landmark of a segment is its bronchus, which is rarely anomalous. Identification of the segmental bronchus may be facilitated by repeated traction on the tumor and finger palpation in the hilar area for the resultant tautening of the segmental bronchus. The segmental bronchi of the right upper and lower lobes and left lower lobe are usually identifiable prior to the division of any segmental arteries This situation does not occur in the left upper lobe, in which the segmental bronchi are obscured by the segmental arteries.

The order of division of the segmental hilar structures may vary; generally the arterial branches are divided first, which allows identification of the segmental bronchus. The segmental veins may then be identified. Because the venous drainage may not be readily apparent, venous ligation is best performed last, after the intersegmental plane has been delineated and developed. The *intersegmental* veins define the perimeter of a bronchopulmonary segment and drain contiguous segments. Dissection in the intersegmental plane, sparing the intersegmental vein and thus preserving the venous drainage of adjacent segments, is a stringent requirement of segmental resection if complications are to be avoided.

Identification and separation of the intersegmental

plane is performed by differential inflation, in which occlusion of the segmental bronchus in a deflated lung is followed by expansion of the lung. The excluded segment remains airless and can be readily delineated. Occasionally, collateral ventilation will fill the diseased segment. The reverse procedure may then be employed; the lung is expanded and, following occlusion of the segmental bronchus, the lung is deflated. The expanded, diseased segment is thus demarcated. The bronchus is transected, leaving a stump of sufficient length so that closure will not occlude other segmental orifices. Manual closure of the segmental bronchus, using a few fine polyglactin or silk sutures, is preferred. Stapling devices are often difficult to apply at the tertiary hilum, and their application may compromise adjacent segmental orifices or leave a long stump.

A right-angled clamp is applied to the specimen end of the bronchus, elevated, and retracted under the left thumb (by a right-handed surgeon). Traction is applied to the clamp with the lung partially inflated. Dissection of the segmental plane by scissors is commenced inferior to the bronchus. Fine fibrous strands, possibly representing tiny bronchi or veins, that impede the development of the intersegmental plane are clipped and divided. Finger dissection along the path of least resistance completes the intersegmental plane to the pleura, using the intersegmental vein as a guide.

Alternatively, the bronchus clamp is held by the left thumb and pressure is applied to the pleural surface of the segment using the fingers of the left hand, thus everting the deep surface of the segment along the intersegmental plane. Again, the fibrous strands that impede the progress of the dissection are individually clipped and divided. The segmental vein, if not conveniently demonstrated and divided earlier in the procedure, is now readily identified and ligated.

Pressure applied with a gauze pad to the raw lung surface for several minutes will usually control bleeding; if not, cautery is used. Small air leaks are controlled with fine sutures. Air leaks may also be controlled by suturing the raw surface down to a contiguous segment, but this method may induce distortion and kinking of bronchi and thus limit re-expansion of the residual segments, a major goal of segmental resection. A pedicled pleural flap applied to the raw surface also may be useful, particularly following resection of apical or superior segments.

The previous description is that of segmental resection as classically performed; however, the development of stapling devices has added a new dimension to the technique. The prevalence of obstructive emphysema in cancer patients mandates stringent control of air leak, for which staples have no equal at this time. Biologic adhesives are not readily available and require further evaluation.

If stapling devices are to be used, they are best applied along the intersegmental plane in the partially inflated lung after division of the segmental artery and bronchus to avoid excessive distortion of the residual lobe. Stapling facilitates extending the resection into an adjacent subsegment if this is required to obtain an adequate margin about the tumor.

Two large-bore intercostal catheters are inserted prior to closure, one placed apical and anterior and the other placed postero-laterally lying on the diaphragm. The anterior tube should be sutured to the apical pleura to ensure continued evacuation of air leak. Suction of 20 cm H_2O is applied to the drainage apparatus. If necessary, nasotracheal suction and bronchoscopy are performed to achieve complete expansion of the residual lung, thus preventing late pleural space problems.

Prolonged air leak is the most common complication of segmental resection, occurring in approximately 10% of cases; its management depends on the severity of the leak, the extent of lung expansion and the condition of the patient. Small alveolopleural fistulas may seal, leaving a "neutral air space," which usually reabsorbs with gradual lung expansion. If empyema supervenes, drainage and later obliteration of the space by muscle flap transposition or limited thoracoplasty will be required. A large air leak associated with radiographic evidence of opacification of the residual lobe suggests that complete lobectomy may be indicated.

Technical Considerations

Right Upper Lobe

Apical Segment. The mediastinal pleura is incised about the hilus of the right upper lobe, the incision extending from the superior pulmonary vein anteriorly and continuing about the branches of the right upper lobe to its lower border. Anteriorly, the superior pulmonary arterial trunk is demonstrated; the apical segmental artery is its uppermost branch (Fig. 36–10). The lower branch is the anterior segmental artery, which is crossed by the apical segmental vein. The apical segmental vein and artery are ligated and divided. If the artery is short, additional length may be obtained by dissecting with a right-angle clamp into the pulmonary parenchyma and dividing the parenchyma with cautery.

Scissors dissection exposes the posterior surface of the lobar bronchus. Several branches of the bronchial artery require division. Pledget dissection will demonstrate the posterior aspects of the segmental bronchi (Fig. 36–11). The apical segmental bronchus arises from the upper portion of the right upper lobe bronchus. Traction on the segment and palpation of the bronchus, as well as bronchial occlusion and differential inflation, confirm that the appropriate bronchus has been isolated. Closure of the bronchus and excision of the segment are performed as previously described (Figs. 36–12 and 36–13).

Posterior Segment. The posterior segment is often removed with the apical segment of the right upper lobe in resections for inflammatory disease. The posterior segmental bronchus arises from the midportion of the right upper lobe bronchus. The posterior portion of the major fissure is opened to demonstrate the origin of the posterior segmental artery from the anterior aspect of the interlobar artery, just above the origin of the superior segmental artery. Rarely, the superior segmental artery of the lower lobe gives rise to the posterior segmental artery of the upper lobe. If it is not possible to complete the major fissure readily, the posterior segmental artery may be demonstrated after division of the posterior segmental

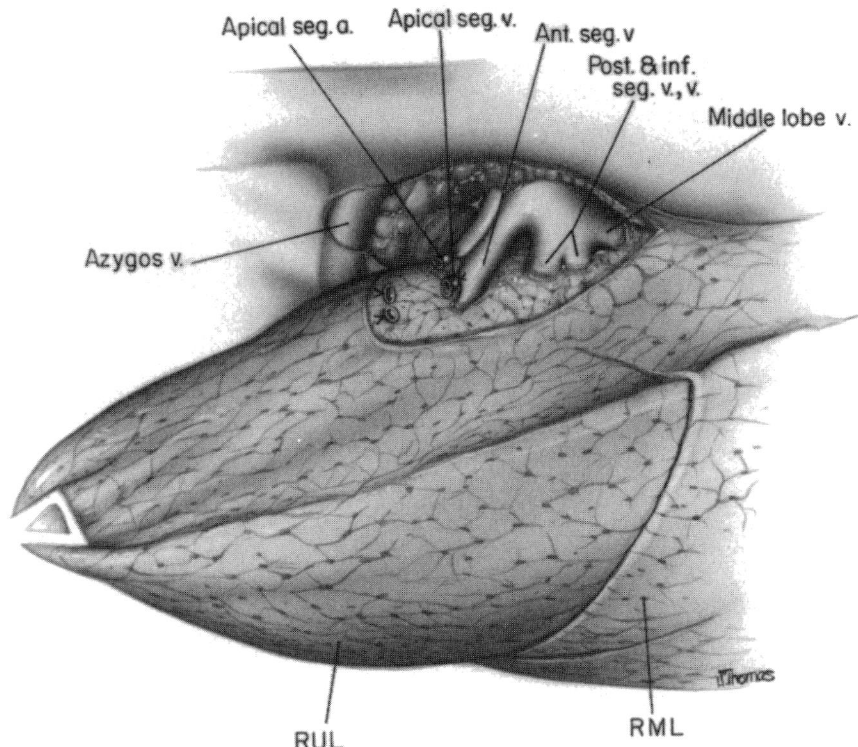

FIGURE 36–10 ■ The apical segmental artery and vein have been ligated and divided. RML, right middle lobe; RUL, right upper lobe (head of patient at left).

bronchus. Dissection of the bronchus must be performed with great care because the artery lies directly anterior to it and is vulnerable to injury. Elevation of the stump of the divided bronchus will demonstrate the posterior segmental artery. Traction on the distal stump of the bronchus and differential inflation will demonstrate the line of demarcation between the posterior and the anterior segments.

The posterior segmental vein is best identified and divided following completion of the retrograde dissection, so that injury to the anterior and inferior segmental veins is avoided.

Anterior Segment. Dissection of the anterior segment is the most technically difficult of all segmental resections. Its bronchus is not easily accessible from the posterior

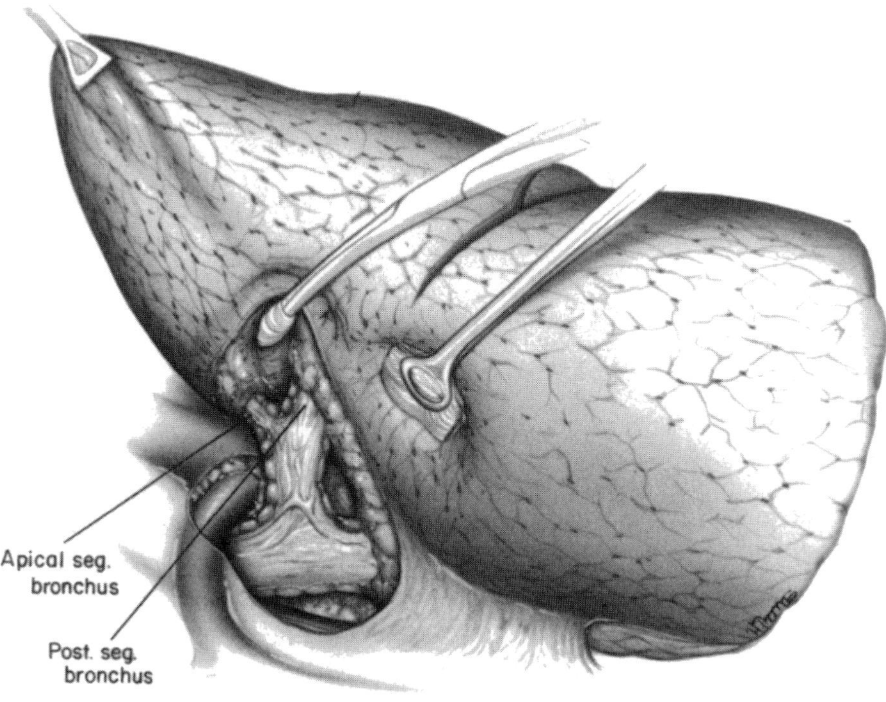

FIGURE 36–11 ■ Following medial retraction of the right upper lobe, the apical segmental bronchus is dissected.

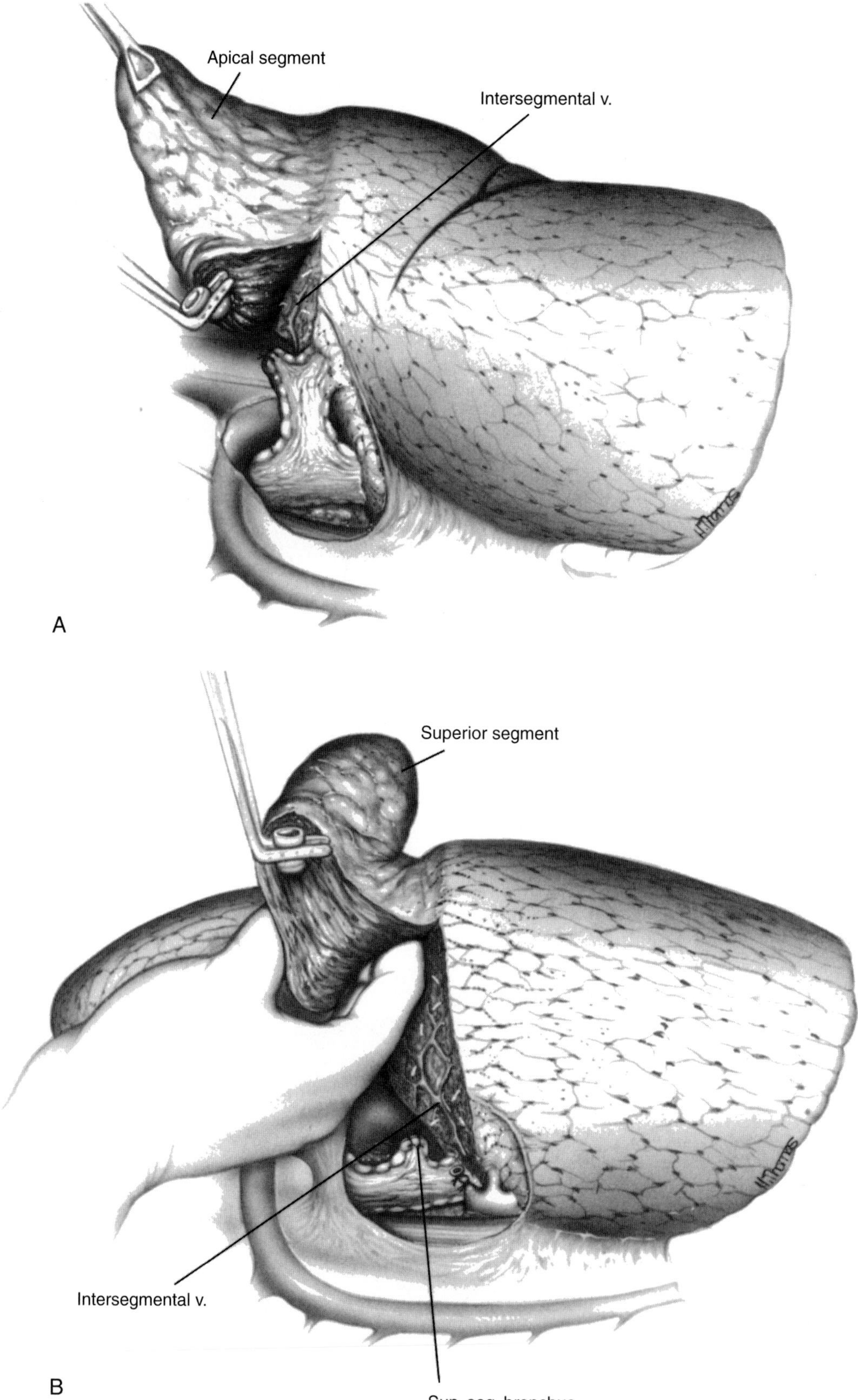

FIGURE 36–12 ■ *A*, Dissection of the intersegmental plane between apical and posterior segments is commenced. *B*, Finger dissection of intersegmental plane, preserving the intersegmental vein.

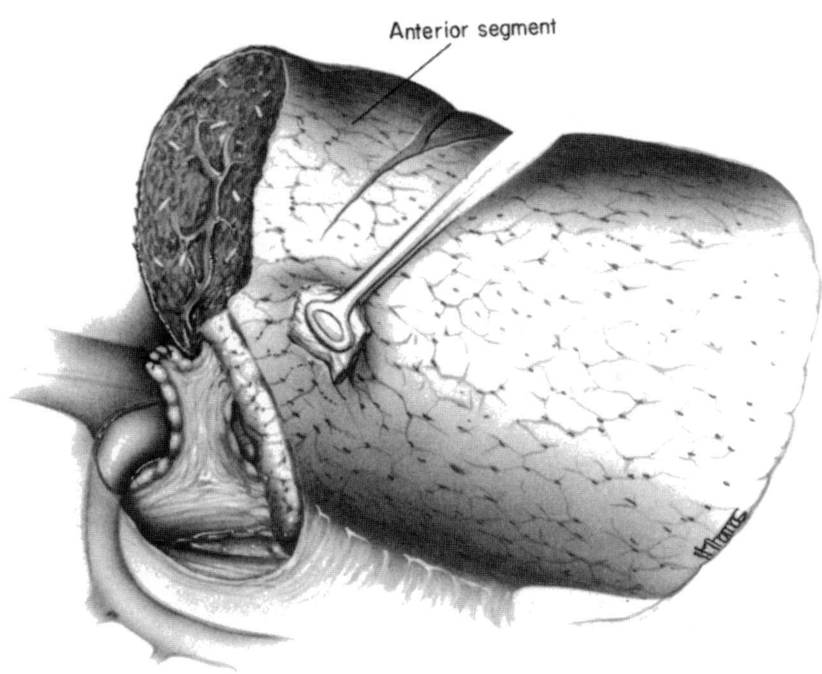

FIGURE 36–13 ■ Completed apical segmentectomy.

aspect, as it is obscured by the posterior segmental vein. Dissection of the arterial supply and preservation of the venous drainage of contiguous segments is tedious.

The mediastinal pleura is incised about the anterior aspect of the hilus of the right upper lobe to below the level of the middle lobe vein. The superior trunk of the pulmonary artery is identified; its lower branch, crossed by the apical vein, is the anterior segmental artery. The apical segmental vein joins the anterior segmental vein to form the upper trunk of the superior pulmonary vein and must be preserved. It is generally convenient to ligate and divide the anterior segmental vein prior to ligation and division of the segmental artery. The interlobar pulmonary artery is closely applied to the undersurface of the vein, and careless dissection may be disastrous. The middle lobe vein originating at the lower border of the superior pulmonary vein is identified and preserved. The inferior segmental vein is ligated and divided, with care taken to avoid injury to the posterior segmental vein lying deep to it.

The horizontal fissure is then completed by using a stapling device. The interlobar pulmonary artery is visualized. Occasionally accessory arteries to the anterior segment are noted and require division. The anterior segmental bronchus, originating near the lower border of the lobar bronchus, is then divided and closed, and the segment is excised.

Given the setting of a voluminous anterior segment and small apical and posterior segments, lobectomy may be preferable to segmental resection. Lobectomy is technically easier, and the patient's postoperative course is likely to be smoother.

Right Lower Lobe

Superior Segment. The oblique fissure is opened to expose the interlobar pulmonary artery, which is deeply situated in the region where the oblique and horizontal fissures meet (Fig. 36–14). The middle lobe artery originates from the anteromedial surface of the interlobar artery, while the superior segmental artery originates posterolaterally at a slightly lower level. Rarely, the posterior ascending artery to the upper lobe originates from the superior segmental artery, and occasionally there are two superior segmental branches. The basal segmental arteries may have a short common trunk from which two branches originate, or all four basal segmental arteries may originate separately distal to the middle lobe artery. Following division of the superior segmental artery, the superior segmental vein, which is the uppermost tributary of the inferior pulmonary vein, is divided (Fig. 36–15). It lies at a slightly lower level than and posterior to the superior segmental bronchus. The superior segmental bronchus is divided, leaving a stump that is long enough that ventilation of the middle lobe bronchus is not compromised. The segment is then excised as previously described (Figs. 36–16 and 36–17).

Basal Segments. Exposure and anatomy are as described earlier. The basal segmental bronchi follow the arterial distribution closely, being situated posterior and medial to their respective segmental arteries.

Following division of the basal segmental arteries, the inferior pulmonary ligament is divided. Three or four basal segmental veins join the inferior pulmonary vein, either individually or via two trunks. Following division of the basal segmental veins, the basal bronchi are divided and sutured distal to the superior segmental bronchus, and the segment is excised.

Left Upper Lobe

Commonly performed segmental resections involving the left upper lobe are excision of the apicoposterior segment, upper division (apicoposterior and anterior segment) resections, and lingulectomy.

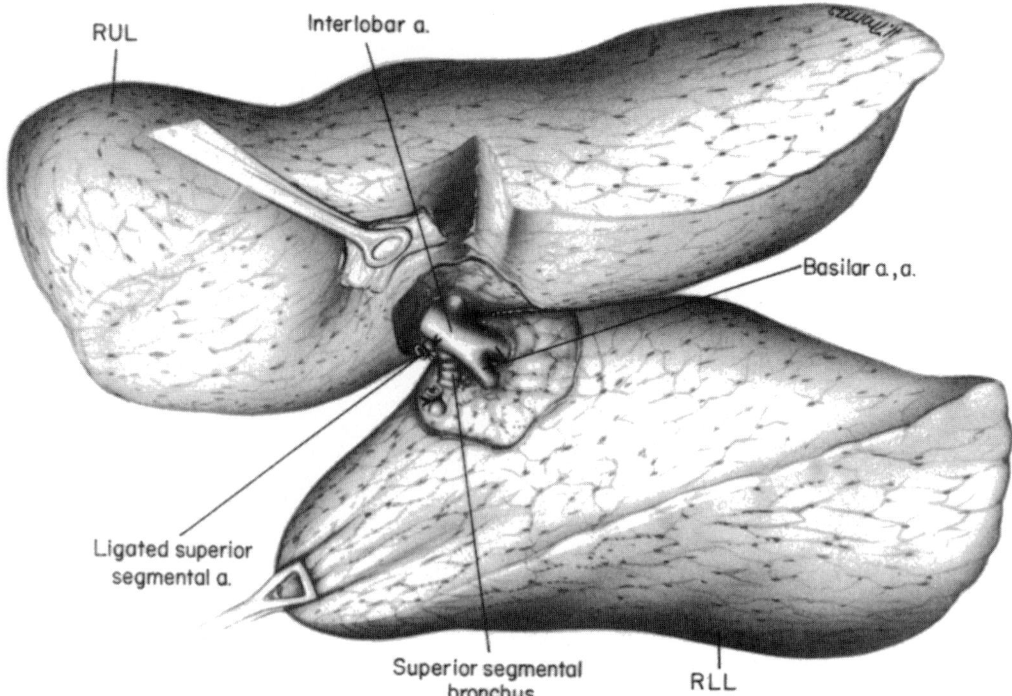

FIGURE 36–14 ■ The oblique fissure has been opened, and the interlobar pulmonary artery has been exposed. The superior segmental artery has been ligated and divided. RLL, right lower lobe; RUL, right upper lobe.

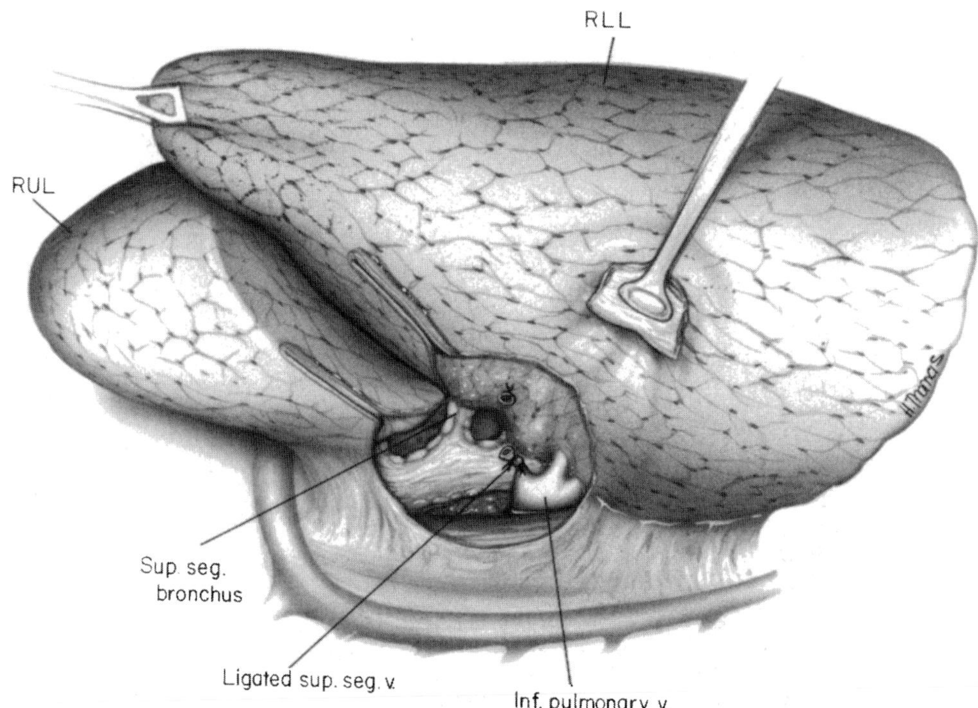

FIGURE 36–15 ■ Posterior aspect of right lower lobe hilum. The superior segmental vein has been divided, and the superior segmental bronchus, has been identified. RLL, right lower lobe; RUL, right upper lobe.

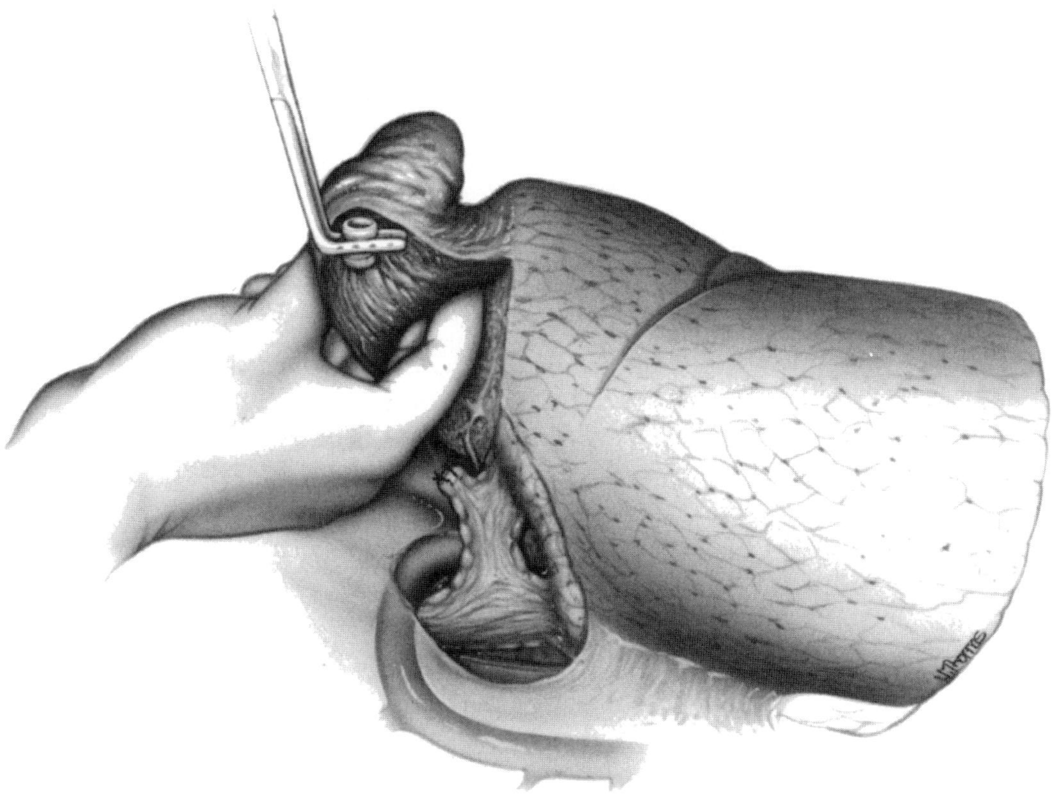

FIGURE 36–16 ■ Traction on the specimen bronchus and finger dissection of the intersegmental plane, sparing the intersegmental vein.

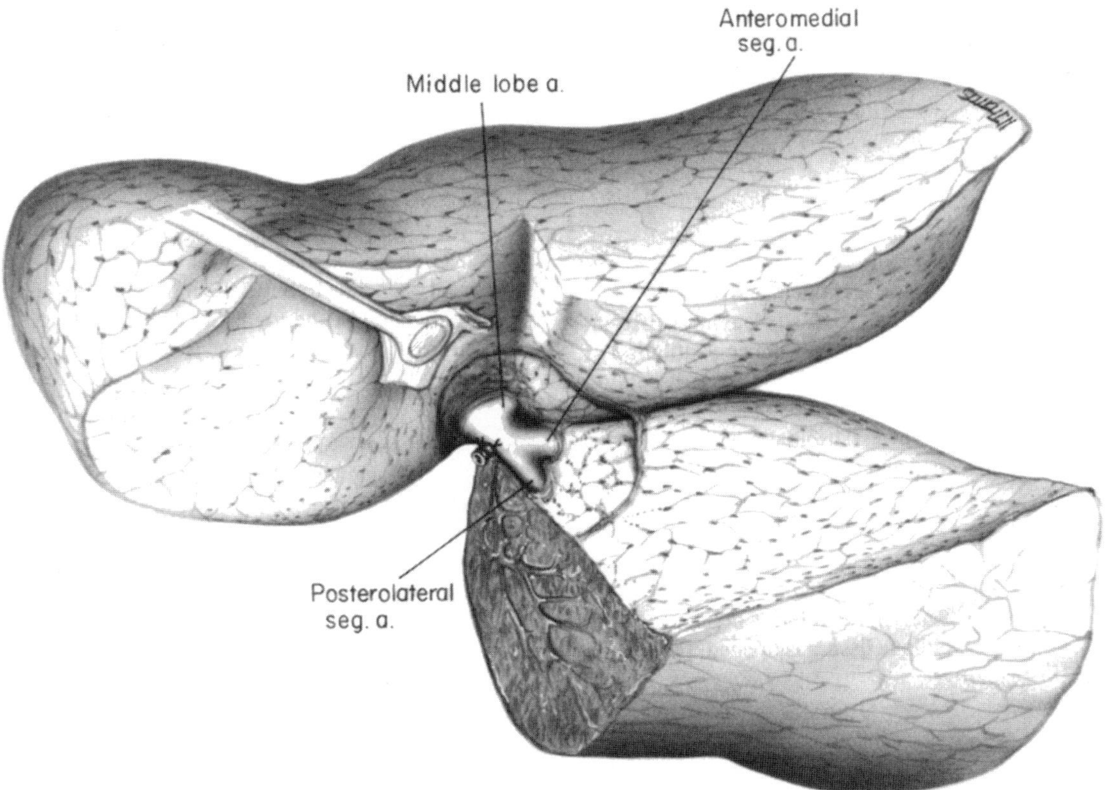

FIGURE 36–17 ■ Completed superior segmentectomy.

The key to segmental resection of the left upper lobe is control of the left pulmonary artery. It is best dissected in its subadventitial plane and encircled with a Silastic loop for proximal control. Isolation of the left pulmonary artery allows easier dissection of its apical and anterior segmental branches, which are often short and broad and, therefore, susceptible to injury. Anterior and inferior to the pulmonary artery, the superior pulmonary vein and its tributaries are demonstrated: the superior venous trunk drains the apicoposterior segment, the middle trunk drains the anterior segment, and the lowermost trunk drains the lingula.

The oblique fissure is completed by sharp dissection or with a stapling device with the pulmonary artery visualized. Dissecting the pulmonary artery from its perivascular sheath over the midpoint of its presenting surface as it enters the fissure facilitates this dissection. Additional posterior segmental arteries may be demonstrated, as well as the lingular arteries arising as terminal branches from the upper border of the interlobar pulmonary artery. The segmental bronchi of the left upper lobe are concealed by arteries. Because of possible anatomic variations, no arteries to the apicoposterior segment should be divided until all arteries to the left upper lobe have been demonstrated. Traction on the tumor and the distal bronchus will demonstrate which arteries require division. Division of the appropriate segmental arteries exposes the segmental bronchus, which is then divided and sutured. Traction is applied to the specimen end of the bronchus, and the intersegmental plane is delineated as previously described. The venous drainage is generally best divided when it is most easily identified—that is, after the segmental dissection has been completed.

Lingula

The oblique fissure is open for its entire length, and the interlobar pulmonary artery is exposed (Fig. 36–18). As noted above, in the presence of a fused or incomplete fissure, the pulmonary artery is at risk of injury, and proximal isolation of the main pulmonary artery is indicated. The lingular arteries, generally two in number, are identified and divided. The bronchus is readily isolated and divided, leaving sufficient length so that its closure does not compromise ventilation of the upper division bronchi (Fig. 36–19). Retrograde dissection is then performed as previously described (Fig. 36–20). The lingula vein, which is the lowest tributary of the superior pulmonary vein, is identified and transected as the final step (Fig. 36–21).

Left Lower Lobe

Superior Segment. The posterior mediastinal pleura is incised medial to the vagus nerve, the inferior pulmonary ligament is divided, and the oblique fissure is opened. Dissection of the pulmonary artery commences as it enters the oblique fissure. The superior segmental artery arises from the posterolateral surface of the interlobar artery at a slightly lower level than the posterior segmental artery to the upper lobe. There may be two superior segmental arteries. They are divided after demonstrating the lingula arteries originating anteriorly and the basal arterial trunks. The uppermost tributary of the inferior pulmonary vein is the superior segmental vein, which lies slightly inferior to the bronchus. It crosses the basal bronchus to enter the inferior pulmonary vein. Following division of the vein, the bronchus is readily divided and sutured, and the segment is removed as previously described.

Basal Segments. The dissection proceeds as described for the superior segment. After the superior segmental and lingula arteries have been demonstrated, the basal arterial trunk with its three branches is dissected and divided. Posteriorly, basal segmental veins are divided, with care taken to preserve the superior segmental vein. Following division of the vein, the basal bronchi are divided and sutured, and the segment is excised.

COMMENTS AND CONTROVERSIES

Segmental resection was designed for and is admirably suited to the surgical management of bronchiectasis and tuberculosis, which are benign diseases with multisegmental and bilateral distribution. Salvage of functional parenchyma is of paramount importance in such cases.

These diseases have largely disappeared from thoracic surgery services in developed nations by virtue of improvements in social hygiene and the availability of antibiotics. Considering also the dismal reality that thoracic surgery training is an atrophied appendage to many cardiothoracic programs and the attrition in the ranks of thoracic surgeons who have mastered segmental resection, McElvein's (1991) comment that "few of these resections are now being performed and many thoracic surgeons are not familiar with this method" is understandable. Fortunately, a few major teaching institutions have kept the technique of segmental resection alive and have used it not only in patients with compromised respiratory reserve but also in patients who could tolerate lobectomy.

The development of single-lung anesthesia and improved stapling devices has made wedge resection an almost irresistible alternative to anatomic segmental resection. Huge wedges of parenchyma may be excised without regard to anatomic planes. Despite warnings that distortion of residual parenchyma might lead to pleural complications, such as empyema and bronchopleural fistula, documentation of these events is lacking in the surgical literature. Commonly, the stapled residual lobe has a grotesque appearance in the open chest, but the postoperative radiograph is quite satisfactory (Kittle, 1989).

Ravitch and Steichen (1988) state that "with the advent of mechanical sutures, the classic anatomical segmental resection has become a technique of the past." They acknowledge, however, that preliminary ligation of the segmental artery and the bronchus may still be useful. It is our opinion that stapling devices are a useful adjunct to the classic technique of segmental resection, especially in patients with marginal pulmonary function. It is in this group that avoidance of prolonged air leak is critical. Careful sequential application of a stapler along the demonstrated intersegmental plane of a partially expanded

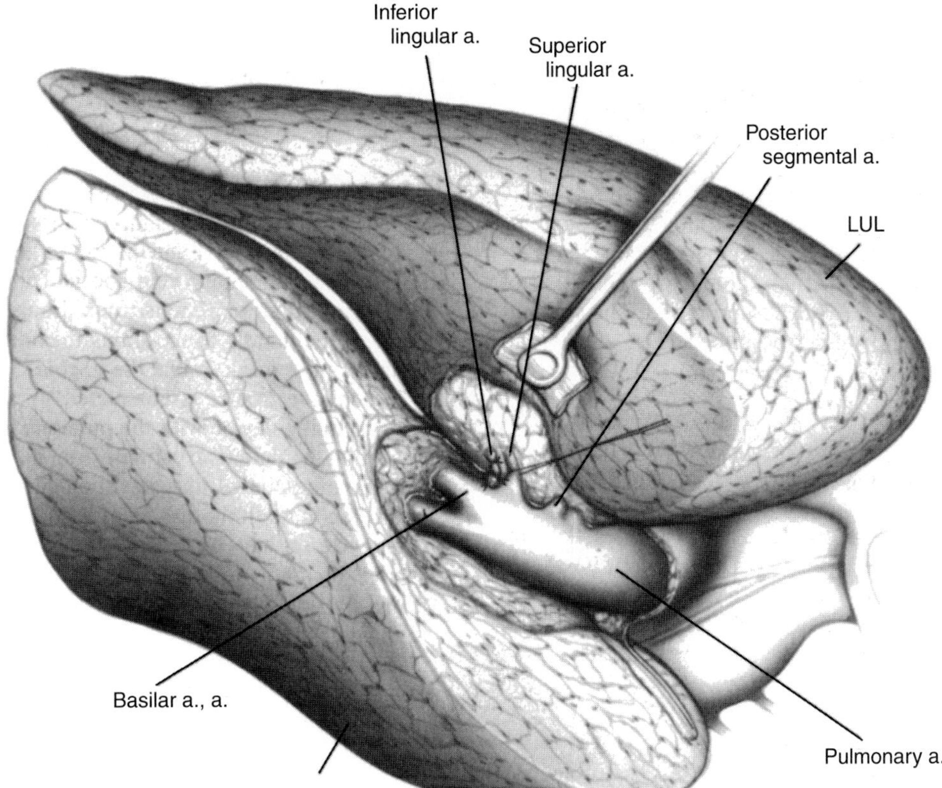

FIGURE 36–18 ■ The oblique fissure has been opened, and the branches of the interlobar pulmonary artery have been demonstrated. One lingular artery has been ligated. LLL, left lower lobe; LUL, left upper lobe (head of patient to right).

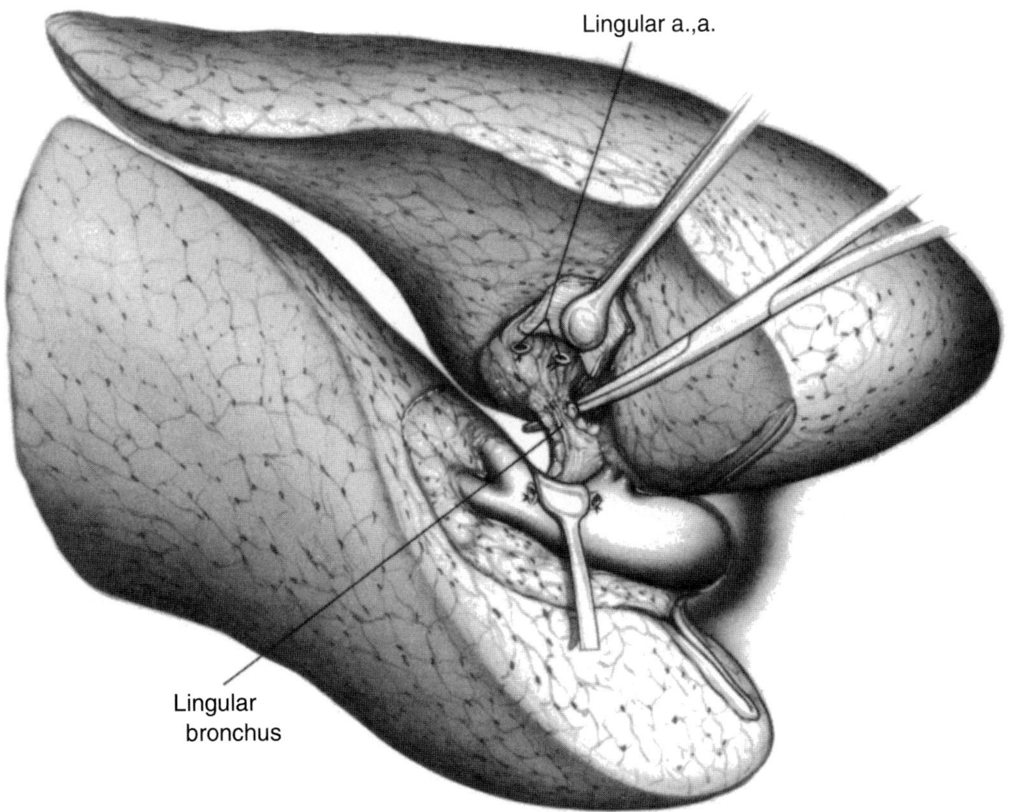

FIGURE 36–19 ■ Following the division of the lingular arteries, the lingular bronchus is dissected.

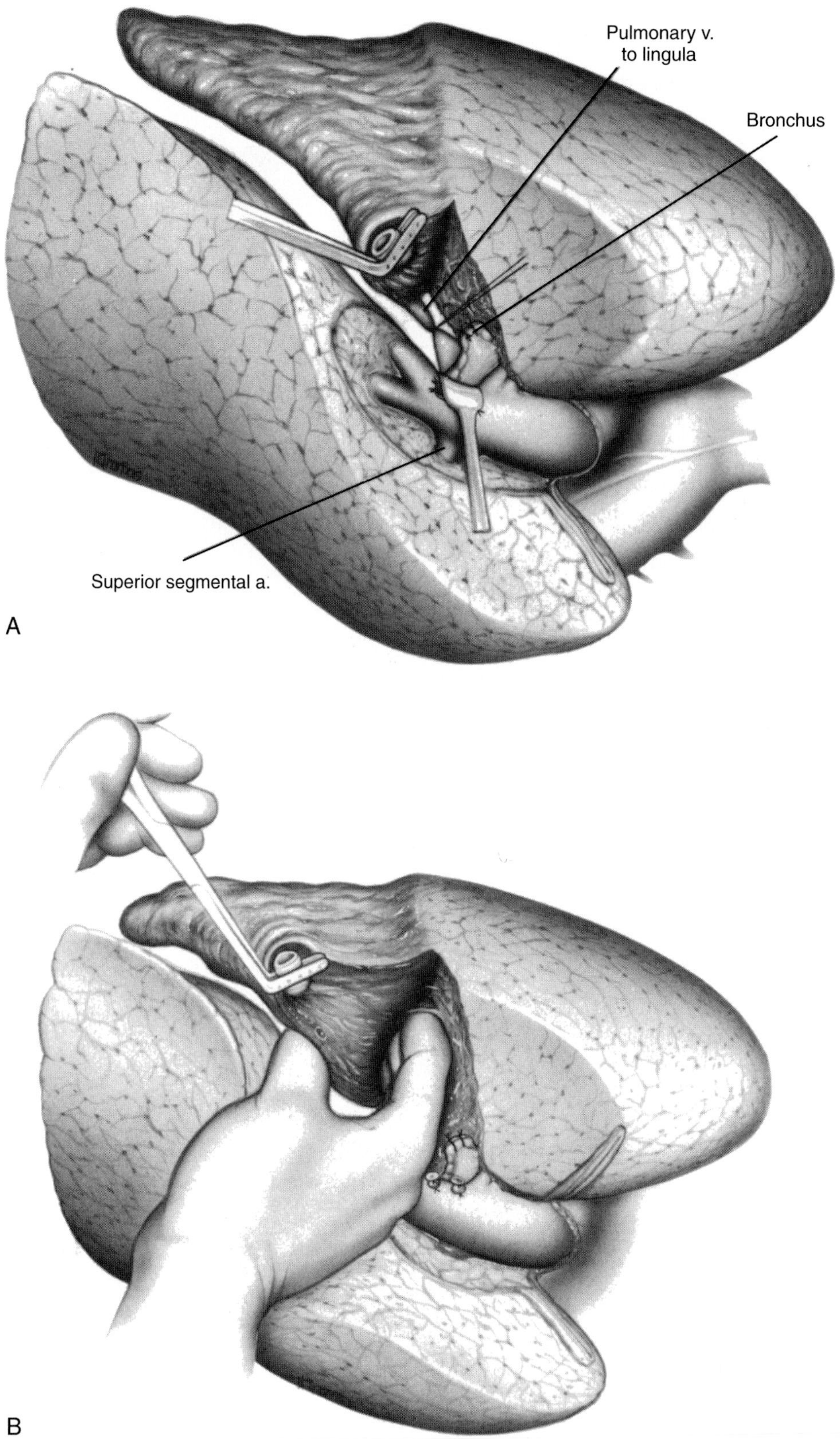

FIGURE 36–20 ■ *A* and *B*, Traction on specimen bronchus and dissection of the intersegmental plane.

lobe minimizes distortion and loss of volume of the remaining lobar segments. If air leak is controlled and the bronchi are patent, pleural space problems are unlikely to occur. There is general agreement that patients with compromised pulmonary function caused by intrinsic lung disease or prior resection should be offered limited resection, if this is feasible. Miller and Hatcher (1987) have defined the criteria: maximum breathing capacity greater than 35% of predicted, forced expiratory volume in 1 second (FEV_1) greater than 0.6 L, and forced expiratory

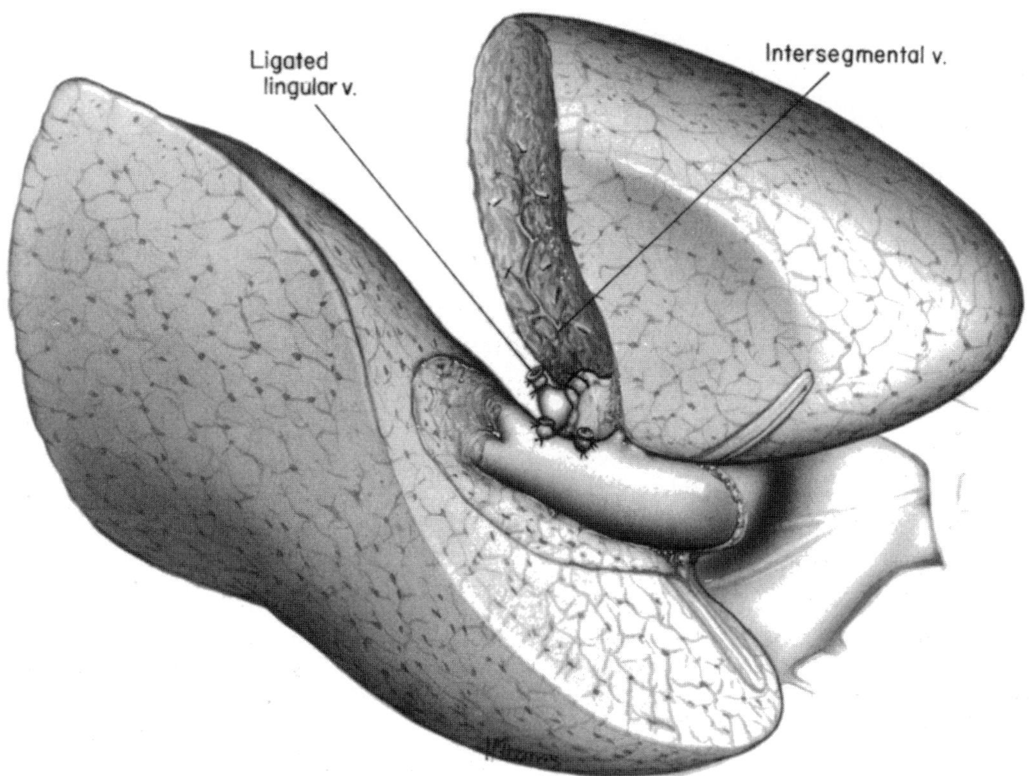

FIGURE 36–21 ■ Completed lingulectomy. The divided lingular vein is demonstrated.

volume between 25% and 75% of expiration (FEV_{25-75}) greater than or equal to 0.6 L. If pulmonary function values are less, the patient is not considered a candidate for limited resection.

Local recurrence following segmental resection has been reported to be from 12% to 35% and commonly occurs in patients in whom the tumor has crossed an intersegmental plane (Miller and Hatcher, 1987). Jensik (1986) reported a 55% 5-year survival with a 12% local recurrence rate. In some of these cases, completion lobectomy was possible, which suggests that lobectomy could have been tolerated at the initial operation. Wain and colleagues (1991) reported a 5% local recurrence rate in 128 cases in which limited resections were performed by choice—that is, in patients who could tolerate lobectomy.

The incidence of local recurrence following segmental resection has led to controversy regarding its applicability if lobectomy could be tolerated. Proponents of segmental resection reason that incomplete fissures between lobes do not afford lobectomy a wider margin about the tumor than does segmental resection (Jensik, 1986). Nevertheless, their 12% local recurrence rate for T1N0 lung cancer (with tumor size <3 cm) is disturbing. Martini and others (1986) reported a local recurrence rate of 19% following segmental resection or wedge excision and no local recurrences after lobectomy. We agree with those who state that segmental resection should be restricted to T1N0 tumors in patients with compromised pulmonary function who would not otherwise be surgical candidates. Segmental resection is, however, a useful method for excision of benign tumors, metastases, and inflammatory lesions.

S.C.F.
T.J.K.

■ REFERENCES

Jensik RJ: The extent of resection for localized lung cancer: Segmental resection. In Kittle CF (ed): Current Controversies in Thoracic Surgery. Philadelphia, WB Saunders, 1986.

Kittle CF: Atypical resections of the lung: Bronchoplasties, sleeve sections, and segmentectomies—their evolution and present status. Curr Probl Surg 26:109, 1989.

Martini N, McCaughan BC, McCormack PM et al: The extent of resection for localized lung cancer: Lobectomy. In Kittle CF (ed): Current Controversies in Thoracic Surgery. Philadelphia, WB Saunders, 1986.

McElvein RB: Commentary on Landreneau SR, Johnson JA, Hazelrigg SR: Neodymium:yttrium-aluminum garnet laser-assisted pulmonary resections. Ann Thorac Surg 51:973, 1991.

Miller JI, Hatcher CR: Limited resection of bronchogenic carcinoma in the patient with marked impairment of pulmonary function. Ann Thorac Surg 44:340, 1987.

Ravitch MM, Steichen FM: Atlas of General Thoracic Surgery. Philadelphia, WB Saunders, 1988, p 200.

Wain JC, Mathisen DJ, Hilgenberg AD et al: Wedge and segmental resection for primary lung carcinomas: Presented at Am Assoc Thorac Surg Meeting, May 1991.

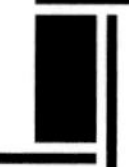

LIMITED PULMONARY RESECTION

Stanley C. Fell

Thomas J. Kirby

A limited pulmonary resection is one performed in a nonanatomic fashion, without regard to intersegmental or interlobar planes and without individual ligation of segmental bronchovascular structures. The actual volume of lung parenchyma resected in this fashion may exceed that of a single segment, because the "limited" resection often crosses segmental planes. This approach is indicated for excisional biopsy of indeterminate lesions that, if benign, require no further treatment. If the lesion is a primary malignancy, anatomic resection (lobectomy) is preferred in patients with adequate pulmonary function. Limited resection of primary lung cancer should be done for patients deemed so compromised in pulmonary function that lobectomy or segmentectomy are contraindicated. Resection of pulmonary metastasis, single or multiple, is usually accomplished by limited pulmonary resection.

HISTORICAL NOTE

In 1861, Pean removed a portion of a lung after first suturing the parietal pleura to the adjacent lung to avoid a pneumothorax. He employed "galvanocautery" for excision of the lesion whose pathology was not reported. In 1891, Tuffier performed the first pulmonary resection for tuberculosis. Using chloroform anesthesia and a second intercostal space incision, he initially performed an extrapleural dissection, however, an extrapleural pneumothorax developed. He then applied a clamp across the lung and dissected pleura beneath the lesion. A continuous suture was employed 2 cm beneath the clamp, and a 5 cm mass was excised. It reportedly contained a caseous nodule "the size of a nut."

■ *HISTORICAL READINGS*

Pean J: Chirurgie des poumon. Discussion Assoc, Ranc. Chir Proc Verb (Paris) 9:72, 1895.

Tuffier T: De la resection du sommet du poumon. Semin Med 2:202, 1891.

APPROACHES

Limited pulmonary resection may be performed via conventional posterolateral thoracotomy or via muscle sparing lateral thoracotomy. Median sternotomy and bilateral thoracosternotomy ("clam shell") incisions are usually reserved for cases in which bilateral metastatic lesions are to be resected simultaneously. Video-assisted thoracic surgery (VATS) has also been employed for excisions (Landreneau, 1991); VATS techniques are discussed later in this text.

Unilateral thoractomy provides the best exposure of the lung but necessitates a second stage if bilateral metastatic disease is present. Median sternotomy provides poor access to posterior and central lesions, especially those involving the left lower lobe, which may be distorted and compromised in function.

The VATS approach, although useful for peripheral superficial lesions that are less than 3 cm in diameter, has intrinsic disadvantages during resection for metastatic disease. Deep lesions and those larger than 3 cm tax the ability of the stapling devices that are used to achieve bronchovascular control in the residual lobe. The major disadvantage of the VATS approach is the inability to manually palpate the lung. In a retrospective study, McCormack and colleagues (1993) demonstrated that more lesions are found by palpation during thoracotomy than are demonstrated by computed tomography (CT) scan, an incidence of 12.5% in 144 cases. In 18 prospective cases, McCormack and colleagues (1996) followed VATS resection by thoracotomy and resected additional metastatic lesions in 10 of 18 cases, an incidence of 56%. Additionally, there have been reports of intrathoracic seeding of malignancy following VATS excision (Fry et al, 1995; Walsh et al, 1995), but this can be minimized by using appropriate safeguards.

WEDGE RESECTION

Until the advent of mechanical stapling devices (Fig. 36–22), wedge resection was performed in a manner that is remarkably similar to that of Tuffier in 1891. The lesion, with a margin of normal parenchyma of at least 1 cm in the deflated lung, is isolated using long, crushing clamps, or vascular clamps, and then excised. A continuous horizontal suture of nonabsorbable material is then placed beneath the clamp. Following removal of the clamp, judicious application of the cautery may be required for any bleeding points. A continuous over and over suture of nonabsorbable material completes the closure. The use of absorbable suture material is not recommended because its premature dissolution may cause delayed air leak. Ideally, the lesion to be resected is superficial and is close to the edge of a lobe. Lesions located on the broad surface of a lobe may not be amenable to wedge resection, because application of a clamp or stapling device to the deflated lobe causes excessive distortion and volume loss, and the staples tend to tear out of the lung parenchyma. In these cases, segmentectomy, lobectomy, or cautery excisions, as described later, are required.

Supported by the Feldesman Fund for Thoracic Surgery.

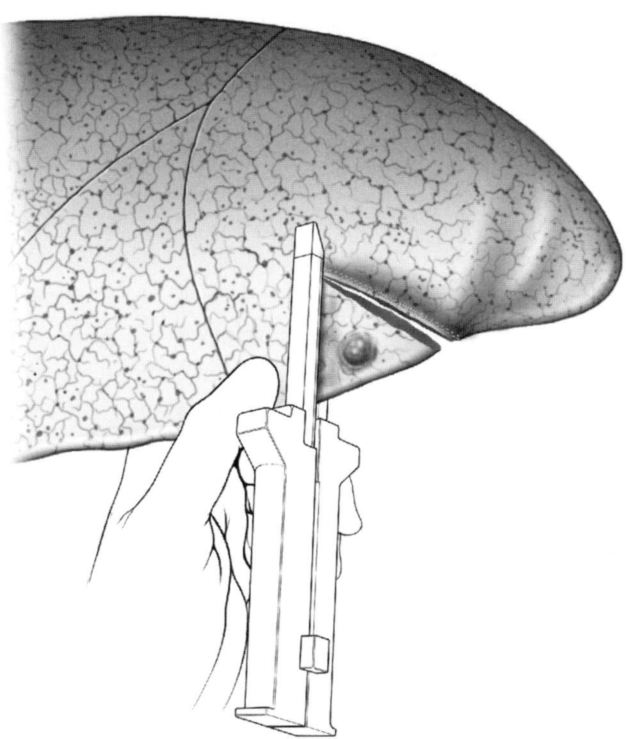

FIGURE 36–22 ■ Stapled wedge resection.

When performing multiple limited resections for metastatic disease, the technique of Ollila and Morton (1998) should be employed. Visual inspection and palpation of the lung in both the inflated and the deflated condition is performed by both the surgeon and the first assistant, correlating the findings with the CT scan on the operating room view box. Each metastatic lesion is marked with a suture prior to performing any resections, because deformity of the lung resulting from staple lines may be mistaken for additional lesions.

PRECISION CAUTERY EXCISION

In patients who are not considered candidates for segmentectomy or lobectomy, deep-seated lesions or those on the broad surface of the lung may be excised by coring them out of the lung parenchyma using cautery (Fig. 36–23). A modification of this method, described by Perelman (1983) in the Russian literature and later by Cooper and others (1986), consists of a painstakingly slow coagulation of all lung parenchyma with individual ligation of small vessels and bronchi in the depth of the resultant cavity. In their experience, using this approach, the resultant coagulated surface did not demonstrate significant air leak and was usually left open. Fibrin glue has been used to line the cavity to prevent delayed air leak (Vincent, 1990); others have closed the resultant cavity using a spiral stitch or by filling the cavity with fibrin glue and closing the parietal pleura over it.

VAPORIZATION

The neodymium:yttrium-aluminum-garnet (Nd:YAG) laser has been demonstrated to seal pulmonary vessels and minor bronchi, (LoCicero et al, 1989; Moghissi, 1989) and has been employed successfully for the resection of multiple pulmonary metastasis (Harvey et al, 1993). Superficial metastasis may be vaporized. Ueda and associates (1993) reported resection or vaporization of 110 metastases in a patient who was still alive 50 months following Nd:YAG laser resection. It has been especially useful as an aid to cautery dissection because the coring out of deep lesions would otherwise require lobectomy (Landreneau et al, 1991). When laser vaporization is used for metastatic nodules that are 1 cm or less in diameter, the tissue that is 2 to 4 mm adjacent to the lesion is destroyed, thus increasing the margin of resection.

The cavitron ultrasonic surgical aspirator (CUSA) is another device that has been applied to the management of multiple metastases, especially those deep within the lung. Following fragmentation and aspiration of tumor, carrying the CUSA applicator into normal lung, the adjacent vessels and minor bronchi are ligated or clipped. Nevertheless, prolonged air leak has been noted postoperatively in some cases (Vergin, 1991). The use of the Nd:YAG laser and CUSA has been limited because of the expense of these devices, the training required for their proper use, and the failure to demonstrate that their use holds only significant advantage over electrocautery dissection.

SUMMARY

Refinements in the invasive diagnostic techniques of transbronchial lung biopsy and CT-guided needle aspiration of the lung, together with increasingly sophisticated pathologic analysis of specimens thus obtained, will surely decrease the incidence of wedge resection of benign lesions. Is there really any need for excisional biopsy of a lesion with the radiologic criteria of hamartoma, when pathologic evidence supporting the diagnosis is obtained by fine-needle aspiration? The dictum "when in doubt take it out" no longer applies indiscriminately. In

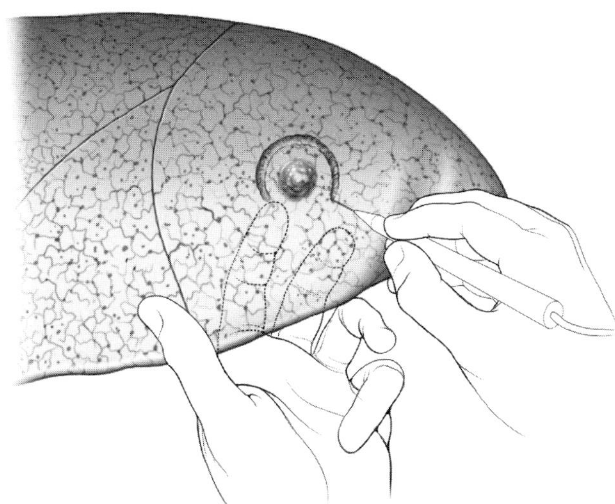

FIGURE 36–23 ■ Cautery excision of a lesion on the broad surface of a lobe.

the appropriate clinical setting (non-smoker, lesion present on previous radiograph), transbronchial needle biopsy and fine needle aspiration will dispense with the need for thoracotomy and wedge resection in many instances.

The local recurrence rate following limited resection for primary carcinoma is discussed in the preceding section of this chapter, Segmental Resection. The Lung Cancer Study Group demonstrated the locoregional recurrence rate to be increased three times with wedge resection and 2.4 times with segmental resection as compared with lobectomy (Ginsberg, 1995). Therefore, wedge resection and segmental resection must be considered salvage procedures in lung cancer patients with compromised pulmonary function who are not otherwise surgical candidates. Similarly, wedge resection and its modifications are, in most instances, adjuncts to chemotherapy and radiotherapy for treatment of pulmonary metastases.

COMMENTS AND CONTROVERSIES

The exact margins that are required for excision of a malignant lesion, using either a wedge resection in the deflated lung or precision cautery dissection in an inflated lung, has never been adequately assessed. In the deflated lung, we generally accept a 1.5-cm margin and a 2-cm margin in the inflated lung. Whenever there is any doubt, biopsies of the remaining resected margin on the lung should be sent for frozen section. Unfortunately, when the pathologist assesses margins on a resected small specimen, it is extremely difficult to identify whether or not the margin is truly "clear."

Except for very small subpleural lesions, I prefer the precision cautery dissection when a limited excision is required. This is performed on the inflated lung. When dealing with malignancies, a 2-cm margin is inscribed on the pleural surface by the cautery surrounding the lesion. Precision cautery dissection is then carried out on the inflated lung, maintaining a 2-cm margin until the dissection has passed beyond the depths of the lesion by 2 cm. Only at that time should the feeding vessels in the depths of the lesion be divided and ligated. In carrying out the dissection, any large structures transgressing the margin of dissection should also be divided and ligated.

R.J.G.

REFERENCES

Cooper JD, Perelman MI, Todd TRJ et al: Precision cautery excision of pulmonary lesions. Ann Thorac Surg 41:51, 1986.

Fry WA, Siddiqui A, Pensler JM et al: Thoracoscopic implantation of cancer with a fatal outcome. Ann Thorac Surg 59:42, 1995.

Ginsberg RJ, Rubinstein LV: Randomized trial of lobectomy versus limited resection of T1 N0 nonsmall cell lung cancer. Lung Cancer Study Group. Ann Thorac Surg. 60:615, 1995.

Harvey JC, Beattie EJ: Aggressive pulmonary metastasectomy facilitated by use of median sternotomy and Nd:Yag laser. Cancer 72:1807, 1993.

Landreneau RJ, Hazelrigg SR, Johnson JA et al: Neodymium: yttrium-aluminum garnet laser assisted pulmonary resections. Ann Thorac Surg 51:973, 1991.

LoCicero J III, Frederiksen JW, Hartz RS, Michaelis LL: Laser assisted parenchyma sparing pulmonary resection. J Thorac Cardiovasc Surg 97:732, 1989.

McCormack PM, Bains MS, Begg CB et al: Role of video assisted thoracic surgery in the treatment of pulmonary metastases: Results of a prospective trial. Ann Thorac Surg 62:213, 1996.

McCormack PM, Ginsberg KB, Bains MS et al: Accuracy of lung imaging in metastases with implications for the role of thoracoscopy. Ann Thorac Surg 56:863, 1993.

Moghissi K: Local excision of pulmonary nodular (coin) lesion with noncontact yttrium-aluminum-garnet laser. J Thorac Cardiovasc Surg 97:147, 1989.

Ollila DW, Morton DL: Surgical resection as the treatment of choice for melanoma metastatic to the lung. Chest Surg Clin North Am 8:183, 1998.

Perelman MI: A precision technic of removing pathological structures from the lungs. (Russian) Khirurgiia 46(11):12, 1983.

Ueda T, Uchida A, Kodorno K et al: Aggressive pulmonary metastectomy for soft tissue sarcomas. Cancer 72:1919, 1993.

Verzin GT, Regal AM, Antowiak JG et al: Ultrasonic surgical aspirator for lung resection. Ann Thorac Surg 52:787, 1991.

Vincent JM, van de Wal HJ, Meijer JM et al: Postponing the limits: Multiple and repeated pulmonary metastectomy by parenchyma sparing electrocautery excision. Helv Chir Acta 57:295, 1990.

Walsh GL, Nesbitt JC: Tumor implants after thoracoscopic resection of a metastatic sarcoma. Ann Thorac Surg 59:216, 1995.

BRONCHOPLASTIC TECHNIQUES

Ryosuke Tsuchiya

Sleeve resection of the bronchus was described by Paulson and Shaw in 1955 as a bronchoplastic procedure. The combined procedure of bronchoplasty, resection, and anastomosis of the pulmonary artery is known as bronchovasculoplasty.

HISTORICAL NOTE

In 1932, Bigger (1935) performed the first bronchotomy to remove a tumor of the left main bronchus in a 14-year-old boy; because the tumor could not be completely resected by the bronchotomy alone, a completion pneumonectomy was also performed. Unfortunately, the patient developed purulent pericarditis and died.

In 1939, Eloesser (1940) successfully removed an adenoma that originated at the orifice of the lower left lobe bronchus. In 1944, Belsey (1946) removed an adenoma with segments of bronchus and successfully repaired the defects of the bronchial wall using fascia. In 1947, Price-Thomas (1955) performed the first sleeve resection of the bronchus to remove an adenoma that originated in the right main bronchus; in 1949, D'Abreu and MacHale (1951) performed a similar operation for removal of an adenoma; and in 1951, Gebauer (1951) performed the first elective excision (sleeve resection) of a whole main bronchus with severe tuberculous stenosis. In 1949, Carlens reported the development of a flexible double-lumen catheter for bronchospirometry, which was later used for one-lung anesthesia in bronchoplastic procedures.

Price-Thomas credited Allison with performing the first sleeve resection for therapy of lung cancer in 1952. In 1955, Paulson and Shaw, who first used the term *bronchoplastic* to describe these operations, reported their results in treating a series of 16 patients, including 4 with traumatic rupture, 3 with tuberculous bronchostenosis, 2 with bronchial adenoma, and 7 with bronchogenic carcinoma. Johnston and Jones (1959) and Paulson and Shaw (1960) reported the long-term results of lobectomy and sleeve resection of the main bronchus in the treatment of patients with bronchial carcinoma. Six years later, Jensik (1966) recommended irradiation prior to bronchopulmonary sleeve resection for lung cancer to improve results. Several other reports on the results of bronchoplastic procedures for bronchogenic carcinomas, as well as for benign tumors and adenomas, of the proximal bronchi followed throughout the 1970s and 1980s (Alp et al, 1987; Bennett and Smith, 1978; Jensik et al, 1972; Lowe et al, 1982; Naruke et al, 1977; Rea et al, 1989; Weisel et al, 1979).

Hsieh and colleagues (1988), reporting an experimental study on the influence of suture material in bronchial anastomosis in growing puppies, concluded that absorbable suture was superior to nonabsorbable suture in pediatric bronchoplasty.

■ *HISTORICAL READINGS*

Alp M, Ucanok D, Dogan R et al: Surgical treatment of bronchial adenomas: Results of 29 cases and review of the literature. Thorac Cardiovasc Surg 35:290, 1987.

Belsey R: Stainless steel wire suture technique in thoracic surgery. Thorax 1:39, 1946.

Bennett WF, Smith RA: A twenty-year analysis of the results of sleeve resection for primary bronchogenic carcinoma. J Thorac Cardiovasc Surg 76:840, 1978.

Bigger IA: The diagnosis and treatment of primary carcinoma of the lung. South Surg 4:401, 1935.

Carlens E: A new flexible double-lumen catheter for bronchospirometry. J Thorac Cardiovasc Surg 18:742, 1949.

D'Abreu AL, MacHale SJ: Bronchial "adenoma" treated by local resection and reconstruction of the left main bronchus. J Surg 39:355, 1951.

Eloesser L: Transthoracic bronchotomy for removal of benign tumors of the bronchi. Ann Surg 112:1067, 1940.

Gebauer PW: Reconstructive surgery of the trachea and bronchi: Late results with dermal grafts. J Thorac Cardiovasc Surg 22:568, 1951.

Hsieh C, Tomita M, Ayabe H et al: Influence of suture on bronchial anastomosis in growing puppies. J Thorac Cardiovasc Surg 95:998, 1988.

Jensik RJ: Preoperative irradiation and bronchopulmonary sleeve resection for lung cancer. Surg Clin North Am 46:145, 1966.

Jensik RJ, Faber LP, Milloy FJ, Amato JJ: Sleeve lobectomy for carcinoma. J Thorac Cardiovasc Surg 64:400, 1972.

Johnston JB, Jones PH: The treatment of bronchial carcinoma by lobectomy and sleeve resection of the main bronchus. Thorax 14:48, 1959.

Lowe JE, Bridgman AH, Sabiston DC Jr: The role of bronchoplastic procedures in the surgical management of benign and malignant pulmonary lesions. J Thorac Cardiovasc Surg 83:227, 1982.

Naruke T, Yoneyama T, Ogata T, Suemasu K: Bronchoplastic procedures for lung cancer. J Thorac Cardiovasc Surg 73:927, 1977.

Paulson DL, Shaw RR: Results of bronchoplastic procedures for bronchogenic carcinoma. Ann Surg 151:729, 1960.

Paulson DL, Shaw RR: Bronchial anastomosis and bronchoplastic procedures in the interest of preservation of lung tissue. J Thorac Cardiovasc Surg 29:238, 1955.

Price-Thomas C: Conservative resection of the bronchial tree. J R Coll Surg Edinburgh 1:169, 1955.

Rea F, Binda R, Spreafico G et al: Bronchial carcinoids: A review of 60 patients. Ann Thorac Surg Surg 47:412, 1989.

Weisel RD, Cooper JD, Delarue NC et al: Sleeve lobectomy for carcinoma of the lung. J Thorac Cardiovasc Surg 78:839, 1979.

BASIC SCIENCE

Surgical Anatomy of the Bronchi and the Pulmonary Artery

Bronchi may be classified into two categories—extrapulmonary and intrapulmonary. Both main bronchi and the right intermediate bronchus are extrapulmonary.

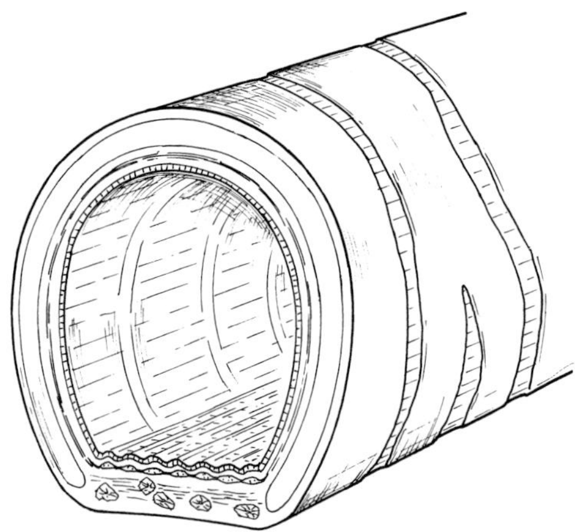

FIGURE 36–24 ■ The extrapulomnary bronchus, like the trachea, comprises a horseshoe-shaped, cartilaginous portion and a membranous portion.

Structurally, the extrapulmonary bronchi are practically identical to the trachea, consisting of cartilaginous, horseshoe-shaped rings and a membranous portion (Fig. 36–24). In the intrapulmonary bronchi, the rings are replaced by irregularly shaped cartilaginous plates, which are distributed around the bronchus in a paving stone configuration (Fig. 36–25). These structural differences are important in the creation of the anastomosis in a sleeve resection, because adjustments must be made for the difference in luminal size of the two bronchial segments. The right pulmonary artery gives rise to branches that supply the upper lobe and cross in front of the intermediate bronchus. The left pulmonary artery runs across the left main bronchus and the carina of the left upper lobe (Fig. 36–26). Therefore, a neoplasm in the upper division of the left lung, which has invaded the upper lobe carina, necessitates a sleeve lobectomy and possibly a sleeve resection of the pulmonary artery.

Blood Supply of the Bronchi

Cauldwell and colleagues (1948), in a review of the bronchial arterial blood supply in 300 specimens, reported nine variations. Salassa and others (1977) examined the gross and microscopic blood supply of 21 tracheal specimens and found rich anastomoses in the paracarinal nodes that interconnected the circulation of the upper thoracic trachea with the superior, the middle, and possibly the inferior bronchial arteries. Inui and coworkers (1990), in evaluating the healing of bronchial anastomosis by laser Doppler velocimetry, reported that the state of healing of the anastomosis site was closely related to bronchial mucosal blood flow. Excessive devascularization of the bronchus should be avoided to maintain a good blood supply at the bronchial anastomosis.

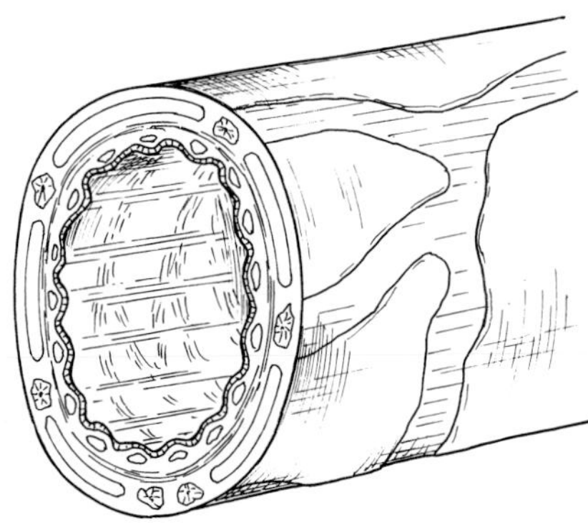

FIGURE 36–25 ■ The intrapulmonary bronchus is made up of cartilaginous plates that are distributed in a paving-stone configuration but it has no membranous portion.

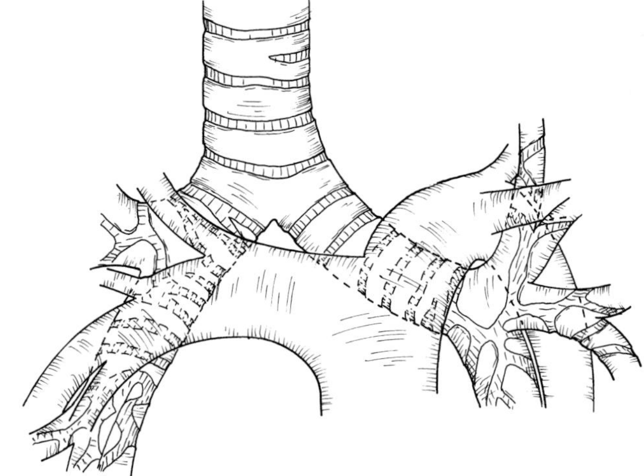

FIGURE 36–26 ■ The relationship between the bronchial tree and the pulmonary arteries. The right pulmonary artery branches to the right upper lobe bronchus and extends across the intermediate bronchus. The left pulmonary artery courses over the left upper lobe bronchus. A lung cancer located in the left upper lobe bronchus, therefore, has already invaded the left pulmonary artery by the time the tumor invades the left second carina. Such a tumor necessitates not only sleeve lobectomy but also sleeve resection of the pulmonary artery.

Bronchial Innervation

Both vagus nerves enter the thoracic cavity through the thoracic outlet along with the internal carotid artery. The right vagal nerve branches to the bronchi and lung and extends along the bronchial artery at its crossing with the azygos vein. The left vagal nerve courses toward the root of the left subclavian artery and branches into the left recurrent nerve and then extends to the bronchi and lungs before exiting along the esophagus as the posterior vagus.

PREOPERATIVE ASSESSMENT

Preoperative assessment is very important, not only to determine the limit of the resection but also to estimate the functional status of the residual lung. The extent of bronchial resection is usually determined by the bronchoscopic findings; computed tomography (CT), magnetic resonance imaging (MRI), and pulmonary arteriography may provide added information about the anatomic and functional status of each lobe of the lung.

Bronchoplastic procedures are most commonly performed for squamous cell carcinomas. The border of the central (hilar) type of squamous cell carcinoma can be easily recognized with the fiberoptic bronchoscope because the epithelial layer of the bronchus is usually involved. When the lesion only involves the epithelium, as in carcinoma in situ or intraepithelial spreading carcinoma, the luster of the epithelium disappears, and the surface becomes cloudy. With further involvement, widening, fusion of longitudinal bundles, and surface irregularities appear. The border between the abnormal findings and the normal tissue is usually very distinct. Preoperative bronchoscopic biopsies ensure accuracy in the endoscopic assessment. In cases of submucosal invasion by lymphatics, it is often difficult to determine the extent of invasion of the carcinoma, and intraoperative frozen section analysis is required.

Patients with carcinoid tumors or adenoid cystic carcinoma may also require bronchoplastic procedures. Central carcinoids and some adenoid cystic carcinomas grow as polypoid lesions with distinct borders. Removal of the polypoid lesion may be required to determine the distal limit of resection. Most adenoid cystic carcinomas, however, have ill-defined borders and spread extratracheally and submucosally along perineural lymphatics. In these cases, the limit of resection of the bronchus cannot be determined grossly prior to surgery, or even during the operation, which mandates intraoperative frozen-section analysis.

Intrabronchial ultrasound examination has given us valuable information concerning submucousal extension of lung cancer and adenoid cystic carcinoma.

PREOPERATIVE MANAGEMENT

Preoperative administration of antibiotics and endoscopic removal of any bronchial obstruction will help treat or prevent the development of pneumonia, which often occurs as a result of retention of purulent sputum. Even if there is no evidence of infection, polypoid lesions should be removed if possible to facilitate assessment of the extent of invasion by the tumor. Although proximal and distal biopsies aid in assessing the extent of tumor invasion and in determining the procedure required, the final determination depends on intraoperative frozen-section assessment of the cut surface of the surgical specimen.

INTRAOPERATIVE MANAGEMENT OF THE AIRWAY

There are several methods for managing the airway during bronchoplastic procedures. Right- and left-sided double-lumen tubes are widely used in bronchoplasty. Fogarty occlusion catheters may be used to produce endobronchial blockade; especially for left-sided surgery, as reported by Ginsberg (1981) and Tsuchiya and colleagues (1981). Inoue developed the "Univent" tube, which incorporates a blocker for unilateral ventilation.

High-frequency jet ventilation can also be used with a conventional single-lumen tracheal tube (El-Baz et al, 1983; Klain and Smith, 1977).

OPERATIVE TECHNIQUE

A standard posterolateral thoracotomy is generally the most suitable incision for bronchoplasty, as it affords the best exposure for safe dissection of the proximal bronchus, the tracheal carina, and the pulmonary arteries and veins. Paulson and colleagues (1970) and Bennett and Smith (1978), however, have emphasized the excellent exposure of the hilum achieved with a posterior approach. We usually resect the fifth rib from the transverse process to the cartilage, as well as 1-cm segments of the fourth and sixth ribs posteriorly to obtain a very wide operating field.

After the thorax has been opened, the surgeon must confirm the preoperative findings, including the location and the extent of primary tumor, the status of the lymph nodes, and the presence of pleural dissemination, intrapulmonary metastasis, or lymphatic spread. Paulson and colleagues (1970) and Weisel and others (1979) have stated that, in general, the finding of extensive nodal involvement of the bronchial wall or extension of tumor across fissure lines should be considered a contraindication to bronchoplasty.

We then perform a complete mediastinal and hilar lymph node dissection and isolate the pulmonary arteries and veins as for a pneumonectomy before resecting of the bronchus.

Right Upper Sleeve Lobectomy

The hilum of the right lung is dissected, and the branches of the superior pulmonary vein draining the right upper lobe of the lung, the superior trunk of the right pulmonary artery, and the ascending pulmonary artery are divided. The anterior surface of the main and intermediate bronchi and the interlobar lymph nodes are then dissected. The pulmonary ligament is divided by electrocautery, the subcarinal lymph nodes are dissected, and the posterior surfaces of both main bronchi, the intermediate bronchus, and the carina are exposed. The upper mediastinal lymph nodes are then dissected, with division of the azygos vein and exposure of the anterior and right lateral surfaces of the trachea and carina. Extensive dissection of the left lateral wall of the trachea and separation of the trachea from the esophagus are avoided to preserve the vascular supply of the trachea. Incomplete fissures are separated by electrocautery or stapler. Interlobar lymph node dissection is performed to completely expose the bronchus and confirm the extent of invasion of the bronchial wall by tumor. Stay sutures are placed in the right main and intermediate bronchi. Proper positioning of the bronchial cuts is confirmed by pulling the sutures toward each other. The site of dissection of the main bronchus is determined according to the spread of the tumor. The intermediate bronchus is usually cut at the orifice of the middle lobe bronchus to obtain bronchial ends of approximately the same caliber and to avoid having to use a long intermediate bronchus with a poor blood supply for the anastomosis, even if the lower border of tumor invasion is more proximal.

The margins of the resected main and intermediate bronchi are examined by frozen section to confirm the border of tumor invasion. If cancerous tissue is found at the margin, further resection is performed whenever possible. We perform the anastomosis (Fig. 36–27) of the main and intermediate bronchi using subepithelial

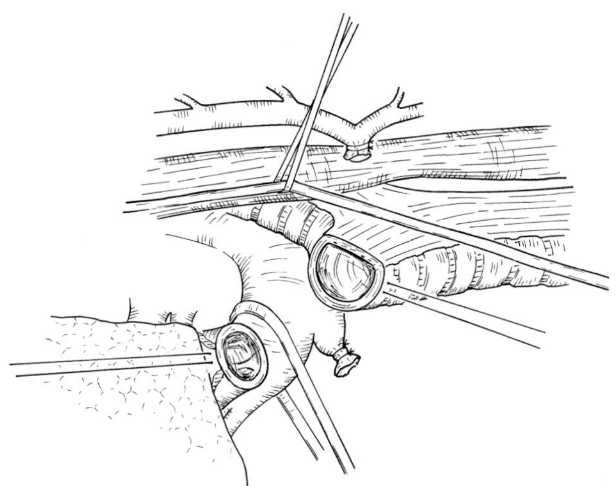

FIGURE 36–27 ■ A right upper sleeve lobectomy is the most commonly performed bronchoplastic procedure. During reanastomosis, the pulmonary artery must be protected.

interrupted sutures for the cartilaginous portion and either full-layer or subepithelial interrupted sutures for the membranous portion (4–0 Prolene [Ethicon Inc., Somerville, NJ] or Maxon [Davis & Geck, Danbury, CT]) (Tsuchiya et al, 1990). We find that a subepithelial interrupted suture affords the best coadaptation of the bronchial epithelium at the anastomosis, preventing granuloma formation, ulcers, and deformity of the bronchial stumps. Double-needle sutures are used and passed exactly through the subepithelial layer from the cut surface to the adventitia of the bronchus (Fig. 36–28). Suturing is begun at the medial edge and stopped at the lateral edge of the cartilaginous portion. Suturing of the membranous portion is begun at the medial edges of the membranous portions of the main and intermediate bronchi. The membranous portion of the main bronchus is slightly gathered and that of the intermediate bronchus is slightly stretched by each suture to adjust for any difference in caliber.

Three methods are used to compensate for the difference in caliber between the larger central bronchus and the smaller peripheral bronchus. First, the interval between sutures of the central bronchus may be made slightly larger than that of the peripheral bronchus. A second technique is to adjust for the difference by gathering or stretching the membranous portions of both bronchi. The third method is used in right upper sleeve lobectomy; because both bronchi are extrapulmonary and, therefore, have a structure that is similar to that of the trachea, suturing is started at the edge of the cartilaginous portion of the intermediate bronchus and 1 to 2 mm from the edge of the right main bronchus and is stopped at the other edge of the cartilaginous portion of the intermediate bronchus and 1 to 2 mm from the edge of the cartilaginous portion of the right main bronchus (Fig. 36–29).

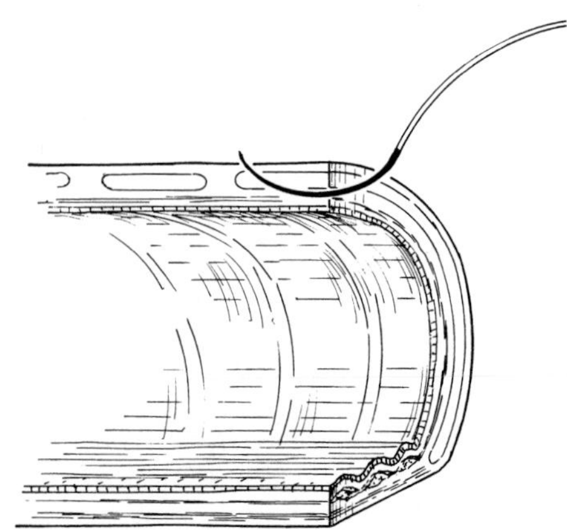

FIGURE 36–28 ■ A double-needle technique is used to pass interrupted sutures through the subepithelial layer from the cut surface to the adventitia of the bronchus.

When the sutures are tied, the stay sutures are pulled toward each other to decrease tension on the anastomosis, and the lobes connected to the central bronchus by the bronchial anastomosis are pushed toward the central bronchus (Fig. 36–30). These procedures prevent cutting of the bronchial wall by decreasing tension (Fig. 36–31). Mobilization of the hilum by intrapericardial release can be helpful.

The anastomosis is examined for air leakage by a water seal test. The anastomosis is protected by a pedicled pericardial fat pad that is nourished by the internal thoracic artery and vein. Two chest tubes are inserted into the thoracic cavity: one is placed in the apicoanterior dead space created by the right upper lobe defect for the escape of air leaking from the interlobar cut surface of the lung, and the other is placed in the lower back thoracic cavity to allow pleural drainage.

Left Upper Sleeve Lobectomy with Resection of the Pulmonary Artery

A tumor located in the left upper lobe may infiltrate the arch of the left pulmonary artery before invading the left main bronchus or left upper lobe carina, depending on the anatomic relationship between the tumor and the pulmonary artery and bronchial tree. Therefore, left upper sleeve lobectomy combined with resection of the pulmonary artery is the most frequent type of bronchovasculoplasty.

After a standard posterolateral thoracotomy has been performed, if the tumor is found to be suitable for bronchoplasty, the anterior hilum of the left lung is dissected, the superior pulmonary vein is ligated, and the anterior surface of the left main bronchus and the interlobar lymph nodes are dissected. A tape passed around the left main pulmonary artery will allow complete control. The anterior mediastinal lymph nodes are dissected to preserve the phrenic, vagal, and recurrent nerves. The ligamentum arteriosum is exposed by the upper mediastinal lymph node dissection and is divided to obtain clear access to the carina and the proximal left main bronchus (Boyd et al, 1970). The aortic arch is retracted, the recurrent nerve is taped and preserved, and the tracheobronchial lymph nodes are dissected. The inferior pulmonary ligament and the subcarinal and posterior hilar lymph nodes are dissected to expose the membranous and medial cartilaginous portions of the left main bronchus. Exposure of the pulmonary artery is continued until

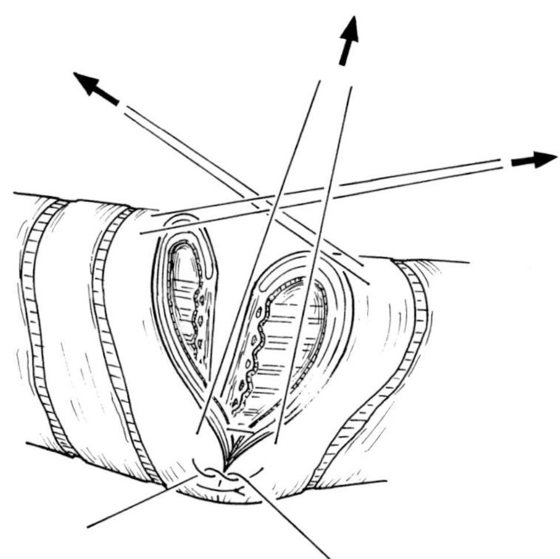

FIGURE 36–29 ■ Adjusting for the difference in caliber of the bronchial segments. Suturing is started at the edge of the cartilaginous portion of the intermediate bronchus and 1 to 2 mm from the edge of the cartilaginous portion of the right main bronchus.

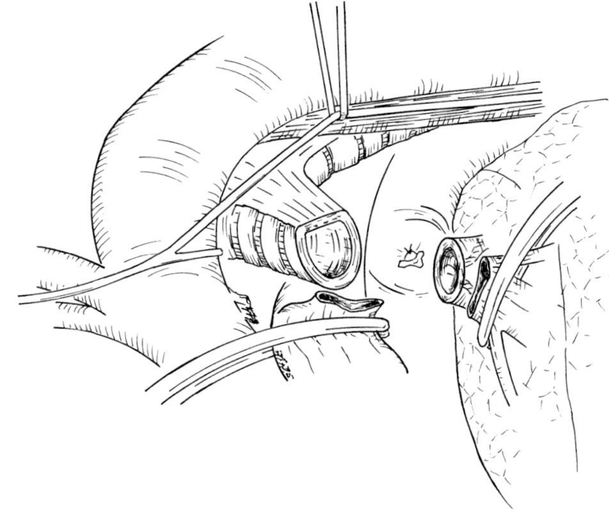

FIGURE 36–31 ■ Cutting of the bronchial wall by sutures is avoided by using stay sutures to draw the segments toward each other and thus decrease tension on the anastomosis. Pulling up the next suture will also serve to decrease tension.

the superior segmental artery of the lower lobe can be identified. The anterior segmental pulmonary artery is exposed from the front or interlobar space. An incomplete fissure between the upper and lower lobes is separated by electrocautery or stapler.

A tape is passed around the interlobar pulmonary artery to facilitate retraction, and the degree of tumor invasion of the pulmonary artery and bronchus is assessed. After invasion of the pulmonary artery and bronchus has been confirmed, the root and interlobar segment of the pulmonary artery are clamped distal to all upper lobe branches, and after the lingular arteries have been divided, the artery is divided with the bronchus. The left main bronchus is divided proximal to the tumor, and the location of the double-lumen catheter or blocker is adjusted through the open left main bronchus to maintain ventilation of the right lung. The lower bronchus of the left lung is then divided, and the tumor is removed along with the affected portions of the left upper lobe, pulmonary artery, main bronchus, and second carina (Fig. 36–32).

The bronchial (first) and arterial anastomoses are performed after the stumps of the bronchi and pulmonary artery have been determined, by frozen section, to be free of tumor invasion. After the medial portion of the bronchi is sutured, the stumps are ligated from the most medial portion of the bronchi laterally, so that the cartilaginous portion of the left main bronchus from the medial edge to the anterolateral angle is approximated. The remaining cartilaginous portion and, finally, the membranous portion are then sutured to adjust for any difference in caliber between the two segments. Because the left lower lobe bronchus is intrapulmonary, it has no

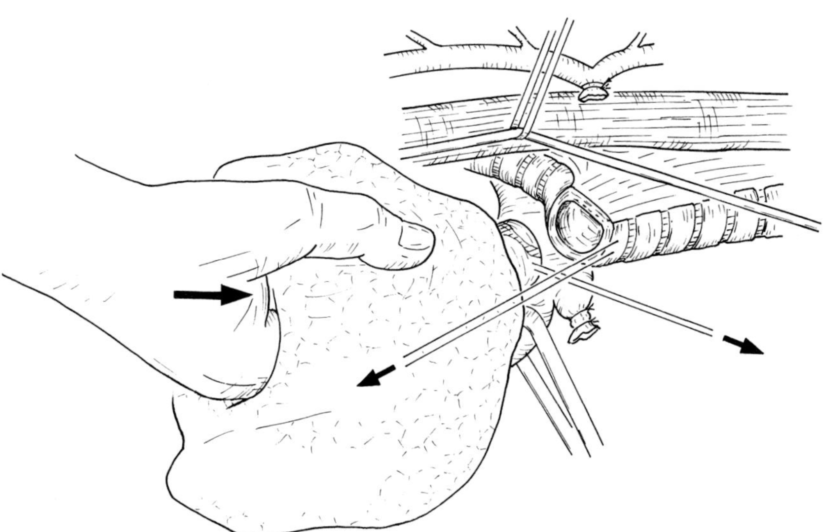

FIGURE 36–30 ■ Mobilization of preserved middle and lower lobes. An assistant standing at the patient's back grasps the preserved right middle and lower lobes and pushes them toward the patient's head to decrease the tension of the anastomosis for right upper sleeve lobectomy.

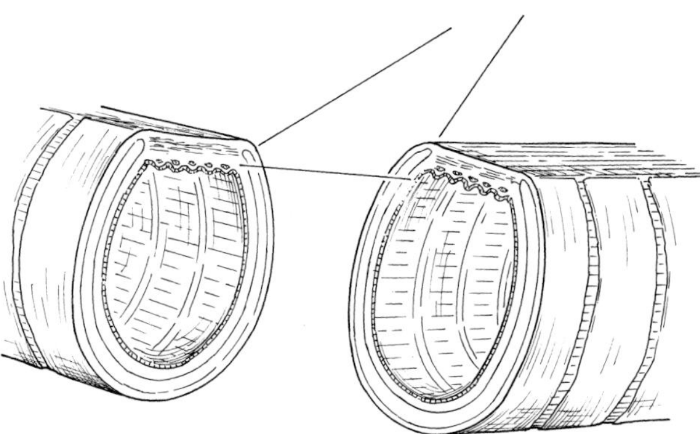

FIGURE 36–32 ■ Left upper sleeve lobectomy. The left main bronchus and pulmonary artery are resected with the cancer, as in bronchovasculoplasty for lung cancer.

membranous portion. After the anastomosis of the bronchi has been completed and tested for patency and leakage, the pulmonary arteries are approximated continuously with use of two or three stay sutures of monofilament nylon. The anastomosis of the bronchi is usually covered by a pedicled fat pad, a pedicled muscle flap, or omentum. Omentum is the best covering material because a large amount is available and it has a good blood supply and good plasticity. However, an extra incision is required for this. We prefer a pedicled pericardial fat pad nourished by the intrathoracic artery and vein (Brewer and Bai, 1955), but when this cannot be used because of poor nutrition or invasion by tumor, a flap of latissimus dorsi muscle may be used. In the case of bronchovasculoplasty, the covering separates the bronchial anastomosis from the anastomosis or plasty of the pulmonary artery and is absolutely necessary to prevent bronchoarterial fistula. (For further details see next chapter.)

POSTOPERATIVE CARE

To ensure success, bronchoplasty must be an uncomplicated, bloodless, and expeditiously performed procedure. Well-organized postoperative care is an important factor, as are a well-trained paramedical staff and a well-informed patient.

The condition of the anastomosis should be checked immediately after completion as well as postoperatively because bleeding from the bronchial stump or inadequate adaptation of the anastomosis is occasionally found. Even when the anastomosis has been performed adequately, sputum retention can be found beyond the anastomosis. Fiberoptic bronchoscopy should be performed in the morning of the first postoperative day to observe the anastomosis and to aspirate sputum even if the patient has no abnormal symptoms. Viscous sputum that adheres to the bronchial wall cannot be detected by auscultation or chest radiography. The need for further fiberoptic bronchoscopic evaluation is determined by the findings of the examination that should be performed on the first postoperative day. In elderly patients, bronchoscope-assisted tracheal toilet is usually needed by the end of the first postoperative week; however, in young patients, it is performed once or twice to confirm the findings in the anastomosis and other bronchial lumina.

COMPLICATIONS AND RESULTS

Operative Mortality

In the first report involving a large number of cases, Johnston and Jones (1959) reported the results of 98 cases of lobectomy and sleeve resection of the main bronchus. Of the 98 patients, 8 died as a direct result of the operation. Two patients died of a combination of sputum retention, bronchopneumonia, and respiratory insufficiency. One patient died of hemoptysis; at necropsy, a communication with the pulmonary artery at the bronchial suture line was found. Another patient died of a cause that was not related to the bronchoplasty. Many other reports have been published, with operative mortality rates ranging from 1.8% to 11.4% (Bennett and Smith, 1978; Jensik et al, 1972; Naef et al, 1974; Paulson et al, 1970; Ree and Paneth, 1970; Tedder et al, 1992; Van Den Bosch et al, 1981; Van Schil et al, 1991; Weisel et al, 1979).

Early Complications

Postoperative bleeding is the most common early complication in lung cancer surgery with or without bronchoplasty. Intrabronchial bleeding from the anastomosis is a complication that is specific to bronchoplasty. Upon completion, the anastomosis should be examined intraoperatively by fiberoptic bronchoscopy to check not only its adaptation but also for any persistent bleeding. Bleeding may cause hemoptysis or aspiration pneumonia. Maladaptation of the anastomosis can cause granulation and stenosis of the bronchus. If bleeding or maladaptation is recognized intraoperatively, it should be corrected immediately by reanastomosis. Rehabilitation, early ambulation, and exercise are useful adjuncts to prevent postoperative pulmonary complications.

Ischemic changes of the peripheral bronchus of the anastomosis can occur when overaggressive lymph node dissection is performed or a long peripheral bronchus is preserved to decrease the tension on the anastomosis. Most of these changes are only temporary, but some may result in stenosis or bronchopleural fistula. Bronchovascular fistula occasionally occurs when an anastomosis exists near a stump or when it involves the pulmonary artery; covering the bronchus is, therefore, helpful.

Bronchoplasty shortens the bronchus and may cause bending and stenosis of the pulmonary artery, especially when the left pulmonary artery is not resected, which occasionally results in pulmonary infarction. Although this is a rare occurrence, it is an important complication of bronchoplasty. When a radical sleeve resection of a long left bronchus is performed, sleeve resection of the pulmonary artery is also required to prevent this complication.

Tedder reviewed 1915 bronchoplastic procedures for carcinoma, reported over 12 years, to determine the incidence of complications and survival. Early complications included pneumonia, 6.7%; atelectasis, 5.4%; empyema, 2.8%; and pulmonary embolism, 1.9%.

Late Complications

The most troublesome late complication is bronchopleural or bronchovascular fistula. Preoperative irradiation, chemotherapy, and ischemic changes caused by dissection of the bronchial artery are the major causes of such fistulas, which usually occur 3 to 4 weeks after operation; fistulas caused by technical failure usually occur within a few days of surgery. When a fistula occurs, surgical repair of the anastomosis is usually futile and completion pneumonectomy is required (Van Schil et al, 1992).

Stenosis of the anastomosis may occur as a late complication of bronchoplasty. Maladaptation of the anastomosis is considered the most common cause of stenosis. The stenosis may be dilated or, if granulations are the cause, managed by laser or cauterized. Stents may be of value. Occasionally, surgical repair or completion pneumonectomy is required in recalcitrant cases.

According to Tedder's review of 1915 bronchoplastic procedures, late complications included local recurrence, 10.3%; benign stricture or stenosis, 5.0%; bronchopleural fistulas, 3.5%; and bronchovascular fistulas, 2.6%.

Long-Term Results

Low and colleagues (1982) summarized reports in the literature on 565 bronchoplastic procedures from 1947 to 1981. Of these, 504 were performed for lung cancer, 51 for adenoma, 6 for bronchial stenosis, and 4 for trauma. They also reported survival data amoung 480 patients undergoing sleeve lobectomy for lung cancer and found that operative mortality was about 7% (32 of 480); 1-year survival was 79% (129 of 162); a 5-year survival was 33% (53 of 159); and 10-year survival was 21% (15 of 71). Tedder and others (1992) reviewed reports on 1915 cases. In this review, the five-year survival of patients undergoing sleeve lobectomy for bronchogenic carcinoma was 40%. Sleeve lobectomy for stage I, II, and III carcinoma yielded 63%, 37%, and 21% five-year survivals, respectively.

Vogt-Moykopf and associates (1986) reported the results of the largest single series of patients undergoing bronchoplasty for lung cancer. Among the 248 patients, the 5-year survival rates were as follows: stage N0 disease, 37%; stage N1 disease, 30%; stage N2 disease, none. Rea and coworkers (1997) reported the second largest single series of 217 patients. Five-year survivals for N0, N1, and N2 were 72.4%, 35.7%, and 22%, respectively. Naruke and others (1989) reported the results of a series of 111 patients and found that the 5-year survival rates of patients with stage N0, N1, and N2 disease were 50%, 46%, and 33%, respectively. Van Schil and others (1991), reporting the results of a series of 112 patients, found 5-year survival rates of patients with stage N0, N1, and N2 disease were 59%, 21%, and 44%, respectively. Watanabe and coworkers (1990) reported the results of a series of 104 patients. Five-year survival rates of patients with stage N0, N1, and N2 disease were 79%, 55%, and 30%, respectively. These results are similar to those of patients treated by lobectomy, as reported by Naruke and colleagues (1988). Therefore, bronchoplastic and bronchovascular procedures are one of the best procedures for the treatment of lung cancer even with hilar or mediastinal lymph node metastases detected by pathologic examination of surgically resected specimen.

COMMENTS AND CONTROVERSIES

Indications for Surgery

Squamous cell carcinoma and low-grade malignant tumors are the most common indications for bronchoplasty. Squamous cell carcinomas with intraepithelial spread do better with bronchoplasty than do carcinomas with submucosal spread, most of which are adenocarcinomas that have lymphatic permeation beyond the limits of resection. The preoperative diagnosis of histologic type and assessment of bronchial extent of cancer are therefore important to determine the usefulness of bronchoplasty in the individual patient.

Covering the Anastomosis

The anastomosis is covered with omentum, a fat pad, or a muscle flap to prevent bronchopleural or bronchovascular fistula formation. It cannot prevent early fistula caused by technical failure, however, nor can it decrease the frequency of anastomotic separation, because these complications occur before the omentum or flap can adhere to and nourish the bronchi. The main purpose of these coverings is to minimize the effect of such complications.

Technique and Materials

The time of onset of the bronchial fistula indicates whether it was caused by technical or predisposing factors. Hsieh and others (1988) concluded that absorbable suture was superior to nonabsorbable suture in pediatric bronchoplasty, and Inui and colleagues (1990) reported that the state of healing of the anastomosis was closely related to the bronchial mucosal blood flow. However, the difference in clinical course of the patients in whom absorbable and nonabsorbable materials were used is minimal. Maladaptation produced granulations, resulting in stenosis of the bronchial lumen. Ischemic changes in the peripheral bronchus affect wound healing and, if prolonged, can result in fistula or stenosis. Therefore, sharp and straight cut edges, accurate adjustment for differences in caliber of the bronchial lumen, proper cutting position of the bronchus, and adequate dissection of lymph nodes around the bronchus are required to prevent bronchial fistula.

R. T.

Bronchial sleeve resection should be in the armamentarium of every thoracic surgeon. Dr. Tsuchiya does not discuss "wedge" bronchoplasty, which occasionally can be of value. However, especially on the right side, kinking of the right main bronchus at the site of wedge bronchoplasty makes this a less desirable approach in dealing with upper lobe tumors.

The extensive posterolateral thoracotomy incision described by Tsuchiya is probably unnecessary—a standard posterolateral thoracotomy is all that is required. On occasion, when the sleeve resection was found to be necessary intraoperatively, I have successfully used a vertical axillary thoracotomy without any problems.

Dr. Tsuchiya does not discuss "hilar release" which is especially valuable in avoiding tension on the anastomosis when there is a long bronchus intermedius resected. Another technique that may avoid tension is the use of "tension-relieving" stay sutures as described by Grillo.

Most surgeons do not use Dr. Tsuchiya's subepithelial suturing technique, believing that the mucosa has strength and aids in avoiding dehiscence. Most surgeons use absorbable polyglycolic acid sutures, either braided or monofilament. There is no doubt that monofilament nylon causes less of a granulomatous reaction, but the disadvantage of this suture is the multiple knots that are required, which, in areas of apposition to the pulmonary artery, potentially aids the production of a bronchovascular fistula.

In my own practice, I rarely bronchoscope patients postoperatively except immediately prior to extubation at the time of surgery. I do not find it necessary to perform daily bronchoscopic toilet except for the usual indications that are required in any patient. However, I do routinely bronchoscope the patient 1 month after surgical procedure to assess healing.

R. J. G.

In this chapter, Dr. Tsuchiya provides a good description of the techniques of bronchoplasty and their usefulness in avoiding pneumonectomy. It is worth remembering that sleeve resection can be done for any segment or lobe in either lung, whereas wedge bronchoplasties are seldom carried out because they have a tendency to kink at the level of the reconstruction.

Our technique of sleeve resection differs somewhat from that of Tsuchiya. For right upper lobe sleeve, the azygos vein is almost never divided, and the anastomosis is done as distally as possible because, at that level, the vascular supply of the bronchus is provided both by the pulmonary artery and the bronchial arteries. The anastomosis is done with absorbable sutures (Vicryl) to prevent granulation tissue. For routine cases, we do not advocate covering the reconstruction, because the incidence of dehiscence or bronchovascular fistula is exceedingly rare. If bronchial covering is advisable, we use pleura, pericardium, or pericardial fat rather than the omentum as suggested by Tsuchiya. (See next chapter.)

In recent years, we have become interested in pulmonary artery reconstructions that can be done with the use of a pericardial patch or through complete circumferential anastomosis. In such cases, clamping the inferior pulmonary vein will stop the backflow while avoiding the presence of a clamp in the immediate vicinity of the operative field.

As noted by Tsuchiya, bronchoplasties are excellent procedures for lung cancer. In all recent publications, 5-year survival figures are similar to those reported after lobectomy.

J. D.

■ KEY REFERENCES

Carlens E: A new flexible double-lumen catheter for bronchospirometry. J Thorac Cardiovasc Surg 18:742, 1949.

A flexible double-lumen catheter was developed for bronchospirometry and later was used in one-lung anesthesia for bronchoplastic procedures. The construction of the catheter is shown.

Cauldwell EW, Siekert RG, Lininger RE, Anson BJ: The bronchial arteries. Surg Gynecol Obstet 86:395, 1948.

The origin, course, and distribution of the bronchial arteries are described for a series of 150 cadavers. The specimens were classified into types (I to IX) in the order of decreasing frequency of occurrence and subclassified on the basis of arterial origin.

Jensik RJ, Faber LP, Milloy FJ, Amato JJ: Sleeve lobectomy for carcinoma. J Thorac Cardiovasc Surg 64:400, 1972.

This is one of the early reports of results of sleeve lobectomy for lung cancer. Preoperative irradiation was used to a greater degree (66% of cases) than previously reported by others in the hope that with reduction in tumor size, more sleeve resections could be carried out.

Tsuchiya R, Goya T, Naruke T, Suemasu K: Resection of tracheal carina for lung cancer. J Thorac Cardiovasc Surg 99:779, 1990.

The suturing technique for anastomosis of bronchi, suture materials, and covering of the anastomosis are discussed. Anastomosis was performed with subepithelial interrupted sutures at the cartilaginous portion and full-layer or subepithelial interrupted sutures at the membranous portion with 3–0 or 4–0 polypropylene or Maxon.

Van Schil PE, de la Riviere AB, Knaepen PJ et al: TNM staging and long-term follow-up after sleeve resection for bronchogenic tumors. Ann Thorac Surg 52:1096, 1991.

The results of sleeve resection for bronchogenic tumors are discussed. Survival is best for carcinoid tumors and squamous cell carcinoma with negative nodes. The presence of N1 or N2 disease significantly worsens prognosis, with no 10-year survivors and no difference between N1 and N2 status.

■ REFERENCES

Alp M, Ucanok K, Dogan R et al: Surgical treatment of bronchial adenomas: Results of 29 cases and review of the literature. Thorac Cardiovasc Surg 35:290, 1987.

Belsey R: Stainless steel wire suture technique in thoracic surgery. Thorax 1:39, 1946.

Bennett WF, Smith RA: A twenty-year analysis of the results of sleeve resection for primary bronchogenic carcinoma. J Thorac Cardiovasc Surg 76:8, 1978.

Bigger IA: The diagnosis and treatment of primary carcinoma of the lung. South Surg 4:401, 1935.

Boyd AD, Spencer FC, Lind A: Why has bronchial resection and anastomosis been reported infrequently for treatment of bronchial adenoma? J Thorac Cardiovasc Surg 59:359, 1970.

Brewer LA, Bai AF: Surgery of the bronchi and trachea. Am J Surg 89:331, 1955.

D'Abreu AL, MacHale SJ: Bronchial "adenoma" treated by local resection and reconstruction of the left main bronchus. Br J Surg 39:355, 1951.

El-Baz N, El-Ganzouri A, Ivankovich AD: One-lung high-frequency ventilation for intrathoracic surgery. In Scheck PA, Sjostrand UH, Smith RB (eds): Perspectives in High-Frequency Ventilation. Dordrecht, The Netherlands, Kluwer Academic, 1983.

Eloesser L: Transthoracic bronchotomy for removal of benign tumors of the bronchi. Ann Surg 112:1067, 1940.

Gebauer PW: Reconstructive surgery of the trachea and bronchi: Late results with dermal grafts. J Thorac Cardiovasc Surg 22:568, 1951.

Gebauer PW: Plastic reconstruction of tuberculous bronchostenosis with dermal grafts. J Thorac Cardiovasc Surg 19:604, 1950.

Ginsberg RJ: New technique for one-lung anesthesia using an endobronchial blocker. J Thorac Cardiovasc Surg 82:542, 1981.

Hsieh C, Tomita M, Ayabe H et al: Influence of suture on bronchial anastomosis in growing puppies. J Thorac Cardiovasc Surg 95:998, 1988.

Inoue H: Univent endotracheal tube: Twelve-year experience. J Thorac Cardiovasc Surg 107:1171, 1994.

Inui K, Wada H, Yokomise H et al: Evaluation of a bronchial anastomosis by laser Doppler velocimetry. J Thorac Cardiovasc Surg 96:614, 1990.

Jensik RJ: Preoperative irradiation and bronchopulmonary sleeve resection for lung cancer. Surg Clin North Am 46:145, 1966.

Johnston JB, Jones PH: The treatment of bronchial carcinoma by lobectomy and sleeve resection of the main bronchus. Thorax 14:48, 1959.

Klain M, Smith RB: High-frequency percutaneus transtracheal jet ventilation. Crit Care Med 5:280, 1977.

Lowe JE, Bridgman AH, Sabiston DC Jr: The role of bronchoplastic procedures in the surgical management of benign and malignant pulmonary lesions. J Thorac Cardiovasc Surg 83:227, 1982.

Naef AP, Schmid de Gruneck J: Right pneumonectomy or sleeve lobectomy in the treatment of bronchogenic carcinoma. Ann Thorac Surg 17:168, 1974.

Naruke T: Bronchoplastic and bronchovascular procedures of the tracheobronchial tree in the management of primary lung cancer. Chest 96(Suppl):535, 1989.

Naruke T, Goya T, Tsuchiya R, Suemasu K: Prognosis and survival in resected lung carcinoma based on the new international staging system. J Thorac Cardiovasc Surg 96:440, 1988.

Naruke T, Yoneyama T, Ogata T, Suemasu K: Bronchoplastic procedures for lung cancer. J Thorac Cardiovasc Surg 73:927, 1977.

Paulson DL, Shaw RR: Results of bronchoplastic procedures for bronchogenic carcinoma. Ann Surg 151:729, 1960.

Paulson DL, Shaw RR: Bronchial anastomosis and bronchoplastic procedures in the interest of preservation of lung tissue. J Thorac Cardiovasc Surg 29:238, 1955.

Paulson DL, Urschel HC Jr, McNamara JJ, Shaw RR: Bronchogenic procedures for bronchogenic carcinoma. J Thorac Cardiovasc Surg 59:38, 1970.

Price-Thomas C: Conservative resection of the bronchial tree. J R Coll Surg Edinburgh 1:169, 1955.

Rea F, Binda R, Spreafico G et al: Bronchial carcinoids: A review of 60 patients. Ann Thorac Surg 47:412, 1989.

Rea F, Loy M, Bortolotti L et al: Morbidity, mortality, and survival after bronchoplastic procedures for lung cancer. European J Cardiothorac Surg 11:201, 1997.

Ree GM, Paneth M: Lobectomy with sleeve resection in the treatment of bronchial tumors. Thorax 25:160, 1970.

Salassa JR, Pearson BW, Payne WS: Gross and microscopical blood supply of the trachea. Ann Thorac Surg 24:100, 1977.

Tedder M, Anstadt MP, Tedder SD, Lowe JE: Current morbidity, mortality, and survival after bronchoplastic procedures for malignancy. Ann Thorac Surg 54:387, 1992.

Tsuchiya R, Hiraga K, Tengan L, Suemasu K: Management of airway by Fogarty occlusion catheter in pulmonary resection. Jpn Ann Thorac Surg 1:642, 1981 (in Japanese, abstract in English).

Van Den Bosch JMM, Laros CD, Schaepkens ALEMS, Wagenaar SJSC: Lobectomy with sleeve resection in the treatment of tumors of the bronchus. Chest 80:154, 1981.

Van Schil PE, de la Riviere AB, Knaepen PJ et al: Completion pneumonectomy after bronchial sleeve resection: Incidence, indications, and results. Ann Thorac Surg 53:1042, 1992.

Vogt-Moykopf I, Fritz TH, Meyer G et al: Bronchoplastic and angioplastic operation in bronchial carcinoma: Long-term results of a retrospective analysis from 1973 to 1983. Int Surg 71:211, 1986.

Watanabe Y, Shimizu J, Oda M et al: Results in 104 patients undergoing bronchoplastic procedures for bronchial lesions. Ann Thorac Surg 50:607, 1990.

Weisel RD, Cooper JD, Delarue NC et al: Sleeve lobectomy for carcinoma of the lung. J Thorac Cardiovasc Surg 78:839, 1979.

RECONSTRUCTION OF THE PULMONARY ARTERY

Erino A. Rendina

Federico Venuta

The pulmonary artery (PA) can be infiltrated by primary lung tumors or by metastatic hilar-mediastinal lymph nodes with extracapsular extension. The right and left PA can be involved to various extents—partial infiltration of the arterial wall may be limited and require simple, tangential resection and direct suture. This technique should be regarded as a variation of standard lobectomy and will not be considered in this chapter.

More extensive defects of the PA (Table 36–1) may require reconstruction by a patch (of various materials), sleeve resection and reconstruction by end-to-end anastomosis, or sleeve resection and reconstruction by a prosthetic conduit. If the main PA is infiltrated by advanced lung cancer, the reconstruction requires the use of cardiopulmonary bypass.

The Authors are greatly indebted to Professor G. Furio Coloni, Chief of Thoracic Surgery, University "La Sapienza" Roma, for his support and advice.

HISTORICAL NOTE

The first report concerning resection and reconstruction of the PA in a patient with lung cancer was made by Allison in 1952. The vessel was partially infiltrated by tumor, and the technique employed was tangential resection and direct suture. Later, scanty descriptions of PA reconstructive procedures came from Thomas in 1956, Petrovsky and Perelman in 1966, and Wurning in 1967. The first study focusing on PA sleeve resection appeared in 1967; Gundersen described two patients with left upper lobe tumors that infiltrated the artery who were treated by PA sleeve resection and end-to-end anastomosis, without complications. In 1971, Pichlmeier and Spelberg reported four successful cases of combined bronchial and vascular sleeve resections, and, in 1974, Vogt-Moykopf published his first series of 39 angioplastic procedures of various types. During the following decade, a limited number of cases were reported in different

TABLE 36–1 ■ **Techniques of Reconstruction of the Pulmonary Artery**

Partial infiltration	Patch reconstruction Autologus pericardium Bovine pericardium Azygos vein Synthetic
Complete circumferential infiltration	Pulmonary artery sleeve End-to-end anastomosis Pericardial conduit Prosthesis
Infiltration of main pulmonary artery	Reconstruction via cardiopulmonary bypass

series (Bennett et al, 1978; Lowe, 1982; Weisel, 1979) however, no real breakthrough was made in PA reconstruction. Thoracic surgeons were concerned about technical difficulties and perioperative complications. Long-term survival did not seem to be advantageous, and pneumonectomy was still considered oncologically more appropriate. The series of 37 PA sleeve resections published by Vogt-Moykopf in 1986 demonstrated that the operation was feasible with acceptable complications and good long-term survival, but it was not until very recently that lobectomy associated with resection and reconstruction of the PA has been demonstrated to be an advantageous alternative to pneumonectomy.

■ *HISTORICAL READINGS*

Allison PR: Course of thoracic surgery in Groningen. Quoted by: Jones PH. Lobectomy and bronchial anastomosis in the surgery of bronchial carcinoma. Ann R Coll Surg Engl 25:20, 1959.

Gundersen AE: Segmental resection of the pulmonary artery during left upper lobectomy. J Thorac Cardiovasc Surg 54:582, 1967.

Kittle FC: Atypical resections of the lung: Bronchoplasties, sleeve resections, and segmentectomies—their evolution and present status. Curr Probl Surg 26:57, 1989.

Petrovsky B, Perelman M, Kuzmichev A: Resection and plastic surgery of bronchi: Translated from the 1966 edition by Askenova L. Moscow, MIR Publishers, 1968.

Thomas CP: Conservative resection of the bronchial tree. J R Coll Surg Edinb 1:169, 1956.

Vogt-Moykopf I: Gefäβplastiken bei bronchusmanschettenresektion. Prax Klin Pneumol 28:1030, 1974.

Wurning P: Technische Vorteile bei der Hauptbronchusresektion rechts und links. Thorax Chir 15:16, 1967.

SURGICAL ANATOMY

The main PA originates in the pericardial sac from the right ventricle, and its axis is oriented in an anteroposterior direction, slightly upward and toward the left. Below the aortic arch, the main PA divides into its right and left branches.

The right PA (Figs. 36–33 and 36–34A) runs horizontally to the right, behind the ascending aorta and the superior vena cava (SVC) and in front of the carina. Lateral to the SVC, the right PA lies in front of the right main bronchus and, almost immediately, it gives rise to its first branch to the right upper lobe (Boyden trunk). Shortly thereafter, the vessel curves inferiorly between the bronchus intermedius posteriorly and the superior pulmonary vein anteriorly. At this level, the artery is closely applied to the undersurface of the vein, and careless dissection may be hazardous. Subsequently, the interlobar PA turns posteriorly behind the origin of the middle lobe bronchus. In this portion, one or two ascending arteries originate posterior to the segment of the upper lobe and the middle lobe artery. The middle lobe artery arises from the anteromedial surface of the interlobar artery, and the ascending arteries originate posteromedially at a slightly lower level. Distal to the latter is the origin of the artery to the apical segment of the lower lobe, and, subsequently, the PA branches into the arteries to the basal pyramid.

The left PA (Figs. 36–33 and 36–34A) is shorter than its right counterpart; at its origin is the ligamentum arteriosum and its relationship with the aortic arch continues posteriorly. At this level (the so-called aortopulmonary window) are the recurrent laryngeal nerve and several mediastinal lymph nodes. The left PA lies above the left main bronchus and surrounds three fourths of the circumference of the left upper lobe bronchus. In fact, the PA abuts the superior, posterior, and inferior aspects of the upper lobe bronchus, leaving its anterior surface in contact with the superior pulmonary vein. The first branches, the apical and the anterior segmental arteries, arise anteriorly and superiorly to the upper lobe bronchus, and posteriorly and superiorly to the superior pulmonary vein. These arteries are often short and broad, and, therefore, susceptible to injury. They are often best exposed after division of the superior pulmonary vein. Throughout its course around the upper lobe bronchus, the interlobar PA delivers branches to the upper lobe that are highly variable in number and location and are usually surrounded by lymph nodes. The most distal of these branches is the lingular artery, which usually arises distally or at approximately the same level as the artery that leads to the superior segment of the lower lobe. The lingular artery arises from the anteromedial surface of the interlobar PA, and the superior segmental artery originates posterolaterally. The PA axis is then oriented anteriorly, and the vessel branches into the arteries to the basal segments.

INDICATIONS

Reconstructive surgery of the PA, often associated with sleeve resection of the bronchus, is intended to obtain complete resection of lung cancer, avoiding pneumonectomy. This is a reasonable approach not only in patients who cannot tolerate pneumonectomy because of impaired cardiopulmonary function but also in any patient in whom the procedure is feasible. Complete resection being the primary goal, extensive use of frozen-section histology should be made on all resection margins, and if tumor infiltration persists, pneumonectomy should be performed without hesitation. It is difficult to establish the indication for a PA reconstruction preoperatively. PA angiography, computed tomography scan with injection of contrast material (Fig. 36–35), and magnetic resonance imaging of the blood vessels (MR-Angio) (Figs. 36–36 and 36–37) can all contribute to clarification of the pattern of infiltration, but the decision is usually made intraoperatively.

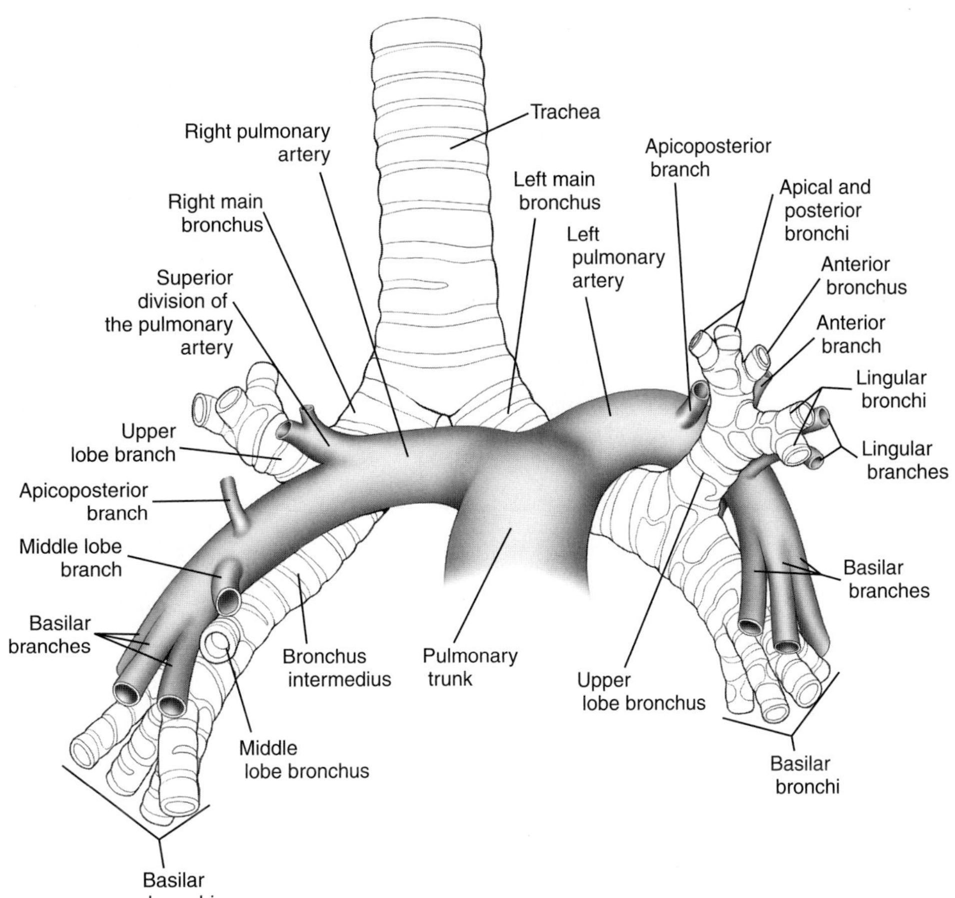

FIGURE 36–33 ■ Anteroposterior view of the pulmonary artery branching and its relationship to the bronchial tree.

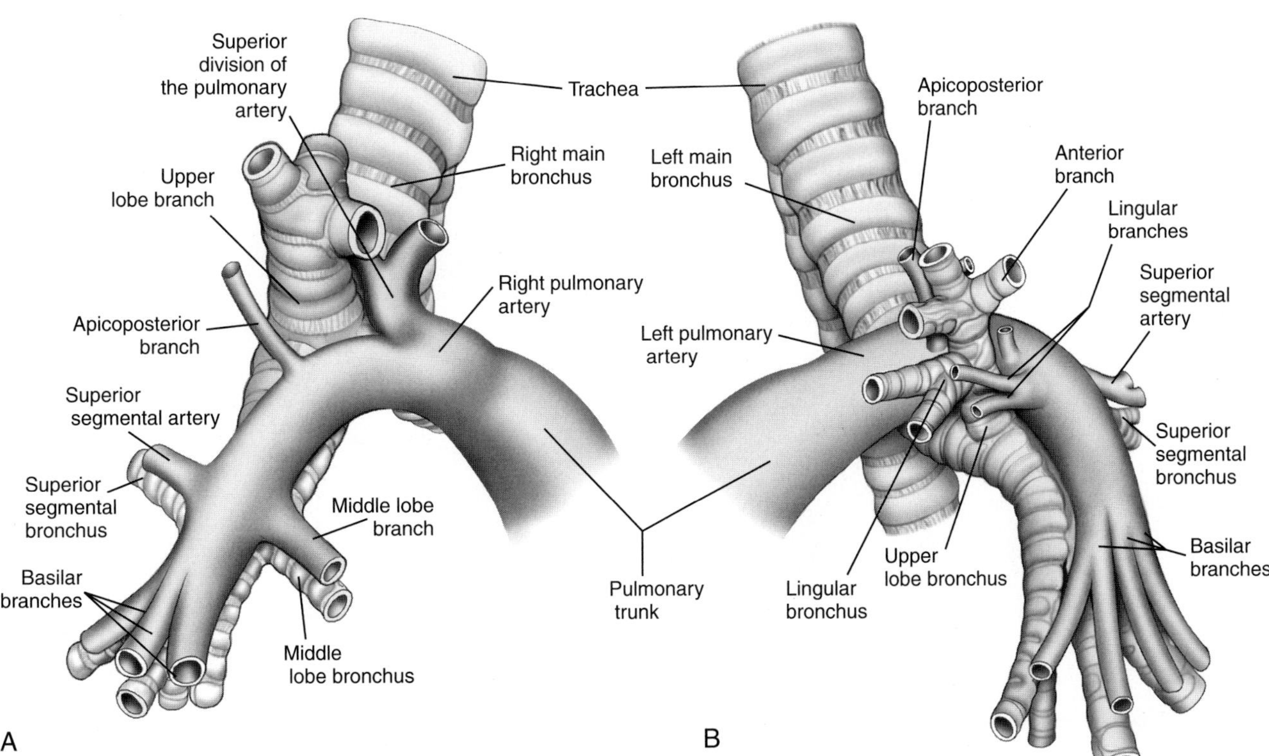

FIGURE 36–34 ■ *A*, Lateral view of the right pulmonary artery. *B*, Lateral view of the left pulmonary artery.

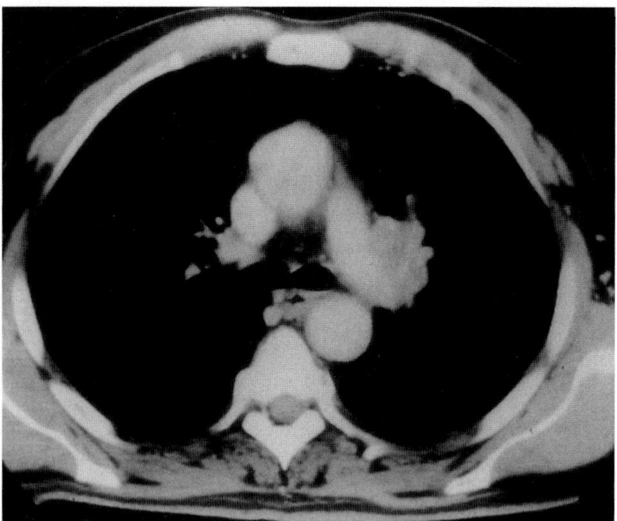

FIGURE 36–35 ■ A computed tomography scan with injection of contrast material of the left pulmonary artery. Extrapericardial tumor infiltration involves the left interlobar pulmonary artery and its branches to the left upper lobe.

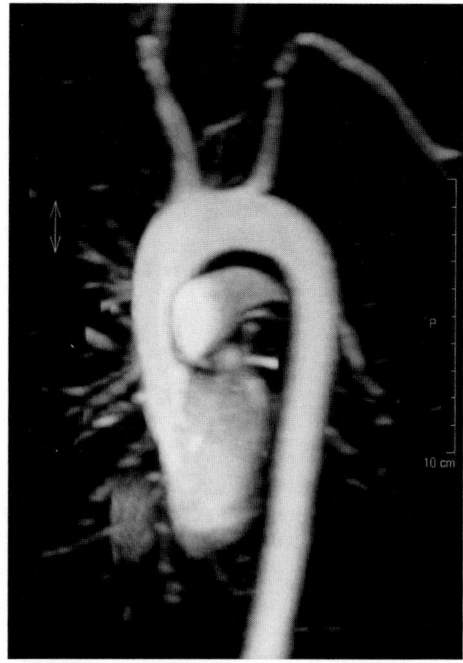

FIGURE 36–37 ■ A three-dimensional reconstruction by angio–magnetic resonance imaging showing caliber reduction of the left pulmonary artery.

The primary indication is direct infiltration of the interlobar PA by the primary tumor (Fig. 36–38); however, extracapsular nodal extension into the vessel can also be treated effectively by this technique. After induction therapy, the PA can be involved to a various extent either by residual tumor or by desmoplastic reaction, scarring tissue, or fibrosis. The concern about an increased complication rate in these patients has been proved to be excessive, and, in our experience, PA reconstructive techniques can be performed in this setting safely and effectively. Approximately 70% of all PA reconstructions are performed for left upper lobe tumors and 20% for right upper lobe lesions. The remaining 10% entails procedures performed on the main PA or on the lower lobes bilaterally.

Reconstruction of the main PA via cardiopulmonary bypass is applicable only in patients with left T4 lung

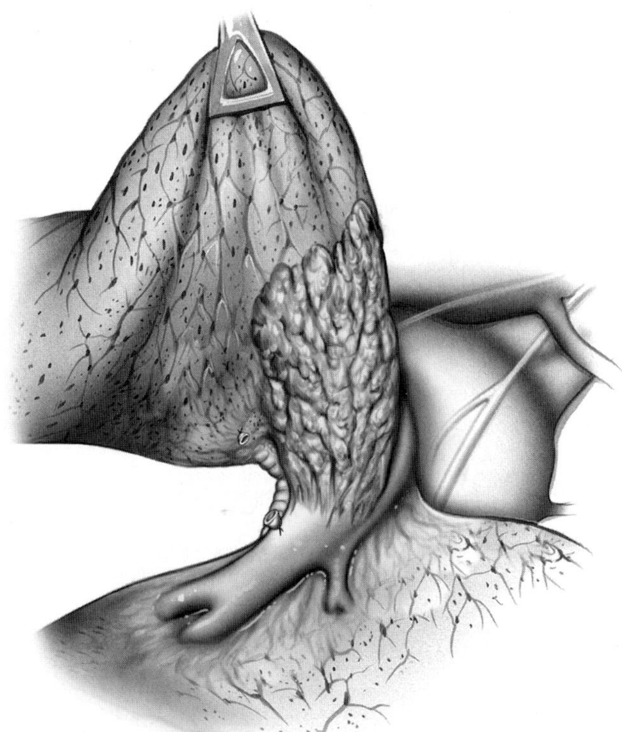

FIGURE 36–38 ■ Typical pattern of a pulmonary artery tumor infiltration requiring pulmonary artery resection and reconstruction. The left upper lobe tumor involves the artery in the interlobar fissure; often, the lingular artery is free of tumor and can be ligated and resected separately as shown in this figure. (Redrawn from Rendina EA, Venuta F, De Giacomo T et al: Safety and efficacy of bronchovascular reconstruction after induction chemotherapy for lung cancer. J Thorac Cardiovasc Surg 114:830, 1997.)

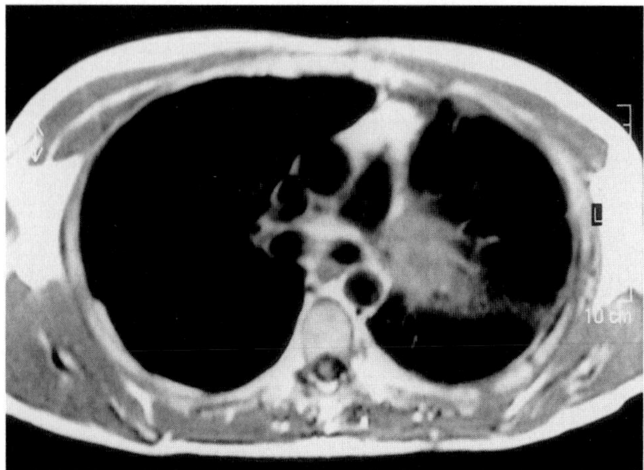

FIGURE 36–36 ■ Magnetic resonance imaging of an intrapericardial tumor infiltration into the left pulmonary artery.

cancer. On the right side, the anatomical relationship of the PA with the SVC, right atrium, and ascending aorta make these tumors invariably unresectable. The long-term results of this approach are uncertain, although the development of effective multimodality protocols for locally advanced lung cancer (i.e., induction therapy) may rejuvenate its use.

OPERATIVE TECHNIQUE

General Principles

The resection phase of the operation and the preparation of the operative field can present pitfalls and difficulties. The first step consists of achieving full control of the PA proximally and will be described in detail later. On both sides, the exposure of the PA and its first branches can be facilitated by the division of the superior pulmonary vein. In general, however, the transection of any vessel or bronchus should be postponed until the feasibility of the procedure is ascertained. The vein should nevertheless be dissected and retracted as much as possible. Once all the elements involved in the resection are duly prepared (main and distal PA; main and distal bronchus; both pulmonary veins), the resection phase begins. The superior pulmonary vein (in the instance of upper lobe tumors) is transected first; subsequently 3000 to 5000 U of heparin sodium are injected intravenously, and the main PA is occluded, inserting a Satinsky clamp from the assistant's side of the table. The artery is not occluded distally, and the backflow is arrested by clamping the inferior pulmonary vein. Moderate backbleeding is easily controlled by suction. As a result, both clamps will be out of the surgeon's way during suturing, and the fragile distal stump of the artery will not be traumatized.

The reconstructive phase of the operation is usually simple, and judicious employment of three basic techniques (patch; end-to-end; conduit) warrants straightforward reconstruction of the arterial lumen. In fact, the only PA defect that would be too extended for reconstruction is one for which pneumonectomy is mandatory for complete tumor resection. The different techniques for reconstruction are described in detail later. After the suture is completed, the venous clamp is removed before the suture is tied, and backflow is restored to allow air drainage. The suture is then tied, and the arterial clamp is removed, but heparin is not reversed by protamine. Before closing the chest, it is very important to check the suture line for oozing sites, which might pass unnoticed owing to low PA pressure. Secondly, lung re-expansion should be carefully tested to ascertain that no kinking or folding of the PA occurs. At the end of the procedure, especially if a bronchial sleeve was also performed, it is advisable to interpose viable tissue between the artery and the bronchus. Our preference is an intercostal muscle flap. In the postoperative period, low dose anticoagulation therapy (10,000 to 15,000 U/day of heparin subcutaneously) is administered for 7 to 10 days.

Arterial Mobilization

Left Upper Lobe. (Figs. 36–38, 36–39, 36–40, and 36–41). If the tumor involves only the interlobar artery (see

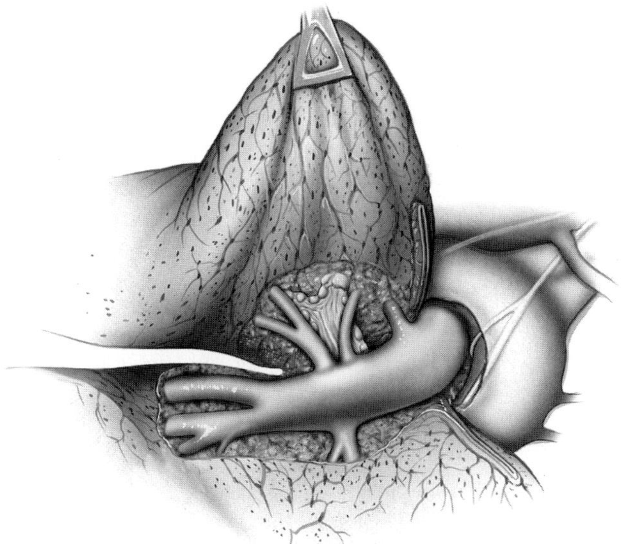

FIGURE 36–39 ■ Surgical anatomy of the interlobar left pulmonary artery from a posterolateral view.

Fig. 36–35), the main PA can be prepared extrapericardially, but in the more common case in which the artery is infiltrated close to its origin (see Figs. 36–36 and 36–37), the pericardium must be opened. The pericardium is incised longitudinally behind the phrenic nerve, and a finger is introduced to palpate the PA. The origin of the left PA may be free of tumor, and it can be encircled by an umbilical tape. Sometimes, tight adhesions below the aortic arch require further dissection before resectability can be ascertained. The aortopulmonary window needs, therefore, to be carefully dissected, dividing the ligamentum arteriosum and the pericardial duplication, and sometimes mobilizing the aortic arch. During this maneuver, the recurrent laryngeal nerve can be injured. If the tumor infiltrates the artery very proximally, the posterior aspect of the vessel is invariably dissected blindly. This maneuver has to be carried out very carefully. In fact, the traction applied on the hilum elevates the main PA bifurcation, and the tip of the clamp passed behind the left PA may injure the right PA with disastrous results. Usually, the anatomical location of the tumor is such that the posterior aspect of the pulmonary hilum, and, in particular, the main bronchus is free of disease. However, when the interlobar PA is infiltrated by tumor behind the upper lobe bronchus, the dissection planes between the posterior mediastinal pleura and the descending aorta might be obliterated. This area must, therefore, be carefully dissected before the hilum can be elevated and the main bronchus exposed and prepared. Once proximal control of the PA is obtained, the interlobar fissure is approached. Clamping the PA proximally may facilitate the dissection in this area. It is important at this stage to expose the artery to the superior segment of the lower lobe arising posterolaterally and the artery to the anterior basal segment of the lower lobe, which continues anteriorly along the curve of the interlobar artery. If these two vessels are tumor free, the vasculature to the lower lobe can be preserved. All along the curve of the PA around the upper lobe bronchus, branches to the upper lobe can

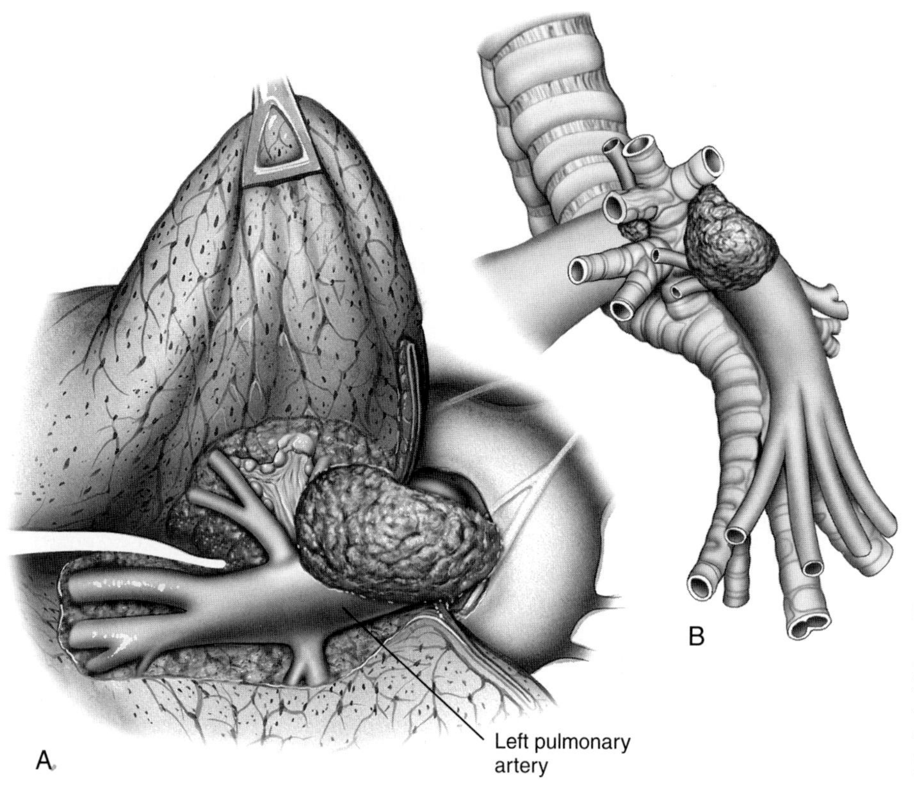

FIGURE 36–40 ■ Full circumference infiltration of the pulmonary artery requiring sleeve resection. *A*, Surgical anatomy of the interlobar artery from a posterolateral view. *B*, A schematic drawing of the infiltrated pulmonary artery from a lateral view.

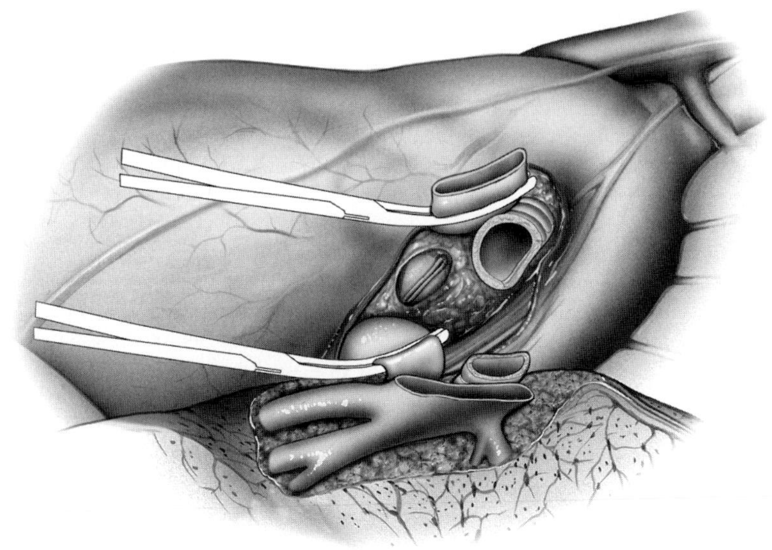

FIGURE 36–41 ■ A posterolateral view of the left hilum after upper lobectomy associated with sleeve resection of the pulmonary artery and the bronchus. Note that the distal stump of the pulmonary artery is not clamped; backflow is avoided by occlusion of the lower pulmonary vein.

arise. These can be separately ligated and transected if tumor free, as is often the case for the lingular artery.

Left Lower Lobe. (Fig. 36–42) tumors in the left lower lobe or infiltrative metastatic lymph nodes located between the lower lobe branches may involve the inferior aspect of the interlobar artery. The procedure is much simpler than that involving the upper lobe, because the proximal PA is free from tumor. After the hilar structures have been prepared and the viability of the lingular artery has been ascertained, the inferior pulmonary vein is transected and the main PA and superior pulmonary vein are clamped. The interlobar artery is then incised obliquely in an anteroposterior and inferosuperior direction, and

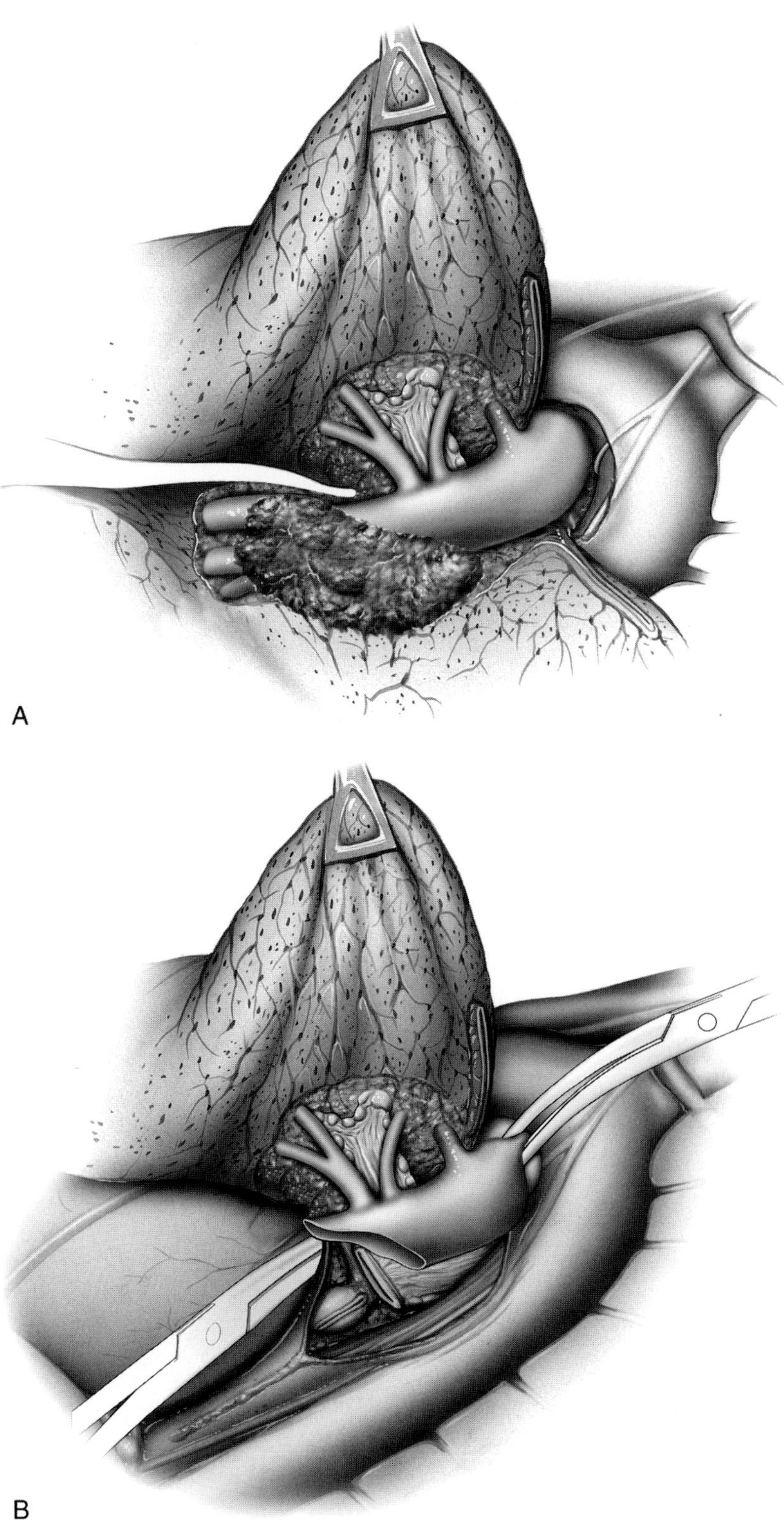

FIGURE 36–42 ■ Infiltration of the pulmonary artery by left lower lobe tumor. *A*, The tumor involves the distal pulmonary artery before its lower lobe branching; the lingular artery is, however, free of disease. *B*, After resection of the lower lobe, the lower pulmonary vein is sutured, and the upper pulmonary vein and main pulmonary artery are clamped. The pulmonary artery defect will be reconstructed by a pericardial patch.

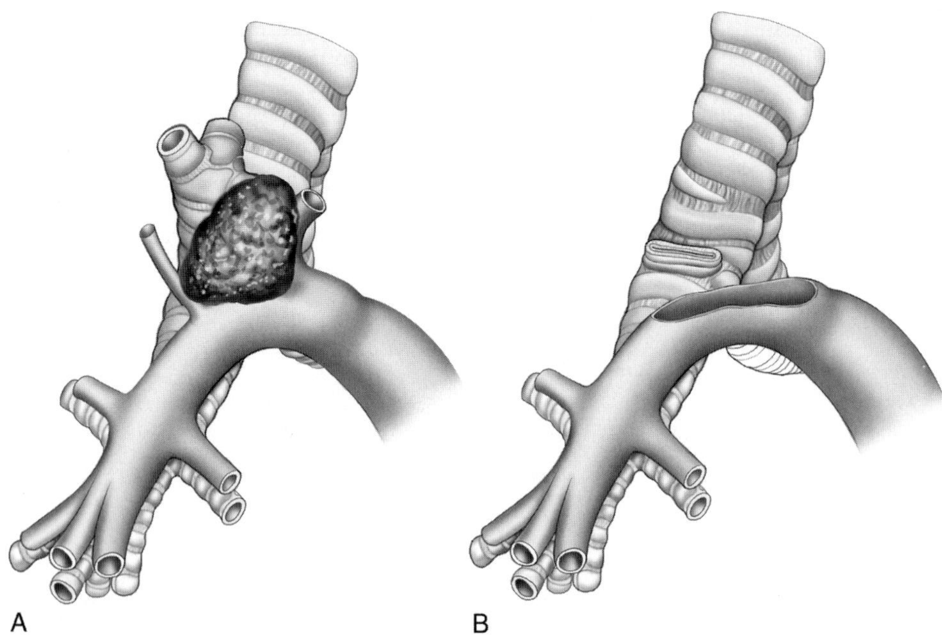

FIGURE 36–43 ■ Partial tumor infiltration of the right pulmonary artery requiring patch reconstruction of the vessel. *A*, The right upper lobe tumor partially infiltrates the artery. *B*, After the resection, the ensuing arterial wall defect can be reconstructed by a patch.

subsequently reconstructed by a tissue patch. The elastic retraction of the arterial wall in this setting is such that the patch must be very carefully trimmed to the appropriate size to preserve the patency of the lingular artery and properly reconstruct the dead-end of the PA. This technique can also be employed during harvesting of the left lower lobe in living donor lobar transplantation.

Right Upper Lobe. (Figs. 36–43 and 36–44) The anatomy of this region makes proximal tumors often unresectable owing to the invasion of the SVC and the right atrium. PA reconstruction is usually feasible for tumors or lymph nodes that are located on the anterior or the inferior aspects of the upper lobe bronchus and involve the PA between the superior trunk and the posterior ascending fissural arteries. The transection of the superior pulmonary vein would greatly facilitate the exposure at this level; this maneuver should, however, be discouraged unless the feasibility of the reconstruction has been ascertained or the patient can withstand right pneumonectomy. Proximal control of the PA can usually be obtained extrapericardially after anterior and medial retraction of the SVC. Alternatively, the PA can be exposed transpericardially between the SVC and the ascending aorta. Distally, it is important to demonstrate the integrity of the arteries to the middle lobe and to the superior segment of the lower lobe. For anatomical reasons, the arterial wall defect resulting after resection is usually extended

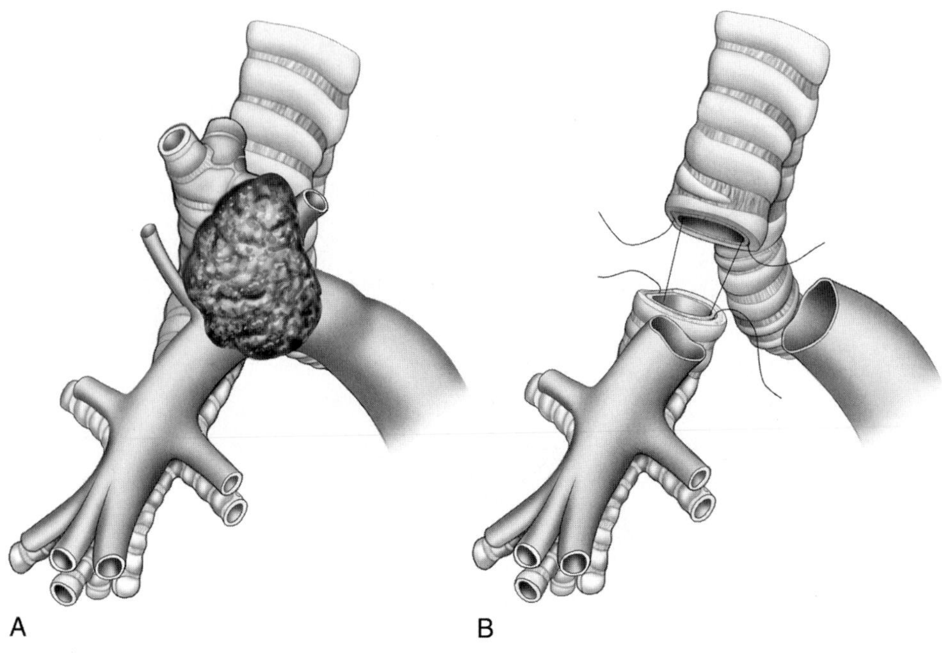

FIGURE 36–44 ■ Full circumference infiltration of the right pulmonary artery requiring sleeve resection. *A*, The right upper lobe tumor involves the pulmonary artery. *B*, After the resection, the ensuing defect can be reconstructed by end-to-end anastomosis.

longitudinally but does not involve the full circumference of the vessel. Sleeve resection is therefore rarely indicated, and a tissue patch is often adequate for reconstruction.

Right Lower Lobe. This is a very unusual situation, similar to its left counterpart. The harvesting of the right lower lobe for living donor lobar transplantation also presents similar features.

RECONSTRUCTION

Partial Resection and Patch Reconstruction

This technique is very versatile and can be used in a variety of circumstances (Fig. 36–45*A* and *B*). These range from limited infiltration involving the origin of segmental arteries to large defects extended longitudinally on one aspect of the PA. The only necessary condition is that the opposite side of the circumference of the PA is free from tumor. If this is not the case, sleeve resection with end-to-end anastomosis or conduit interposition should be performed. After the resection, an oval defect oriented along the PA axis ensues (Fig. 36–46), even if the resected portion is round in shape. Such would be due to the tension applied on the vessel by the lower lobe. The patch should, therefore, be tailored on the resected portion rather than on the PA defect. Different patches can be used; our preference is for biological materials because of better biocompatibility. Azygos vein patches, although adequate, have a number of disadvantages. First, the azygos vein is available only on the right side, where the need for a PA patch is less likely to occur, and harvesting of other venous patches requires a separate procedure. In addition, the amount of tissue is limited. We recommend the use of autologous or bovine pericardium, both of which have none of the aforementioned limits. Autologous pericardium is fresh and unpreserved, cost-free, and biocompatible; it is, however, difficult to use. Conversely, bovine pericardium is less cost effective and less biocompatible, but is very easy to use.

The autologous pericardium is harvested anteriorly to the phrenic nerve, and the pericardial defect is left open. The arterial reconstruction is performed before the bronchial anastomosis to reduce the arterial clamping time. The patch is trimmed appropriately and secured to the artery by two stay sutures (Fig. 36–46*B*). The inferior stay suture is not tied; it is used only to keep the patch in place and will be removed when the suture line reaches its level. Some degree of tension is desirable at this stage; it shows that the patch is not exceedingly long, and tension will disappear after declamping (Fig. 36–46*B*). Suturing (Fig. 36–46*C*) must be done very carefully, because the edge of the pericardium tends to shrink and curl and sutures that are too wide apart may result. The pitfalls of harvesting, trimming, and suturing the autologous pericardium are overcome by the use of bovine pericardium, which displays little if any elasticity, and has even and stiff edges. The patch is sutured using running 5–0 or 6–0 monofilament nonabsorbable material. The right-handed surgeon proceeds from top to bottom "artery first" on the right side while the assistant grasps and stretches the patch, and then continues from bottom to top "patch first."

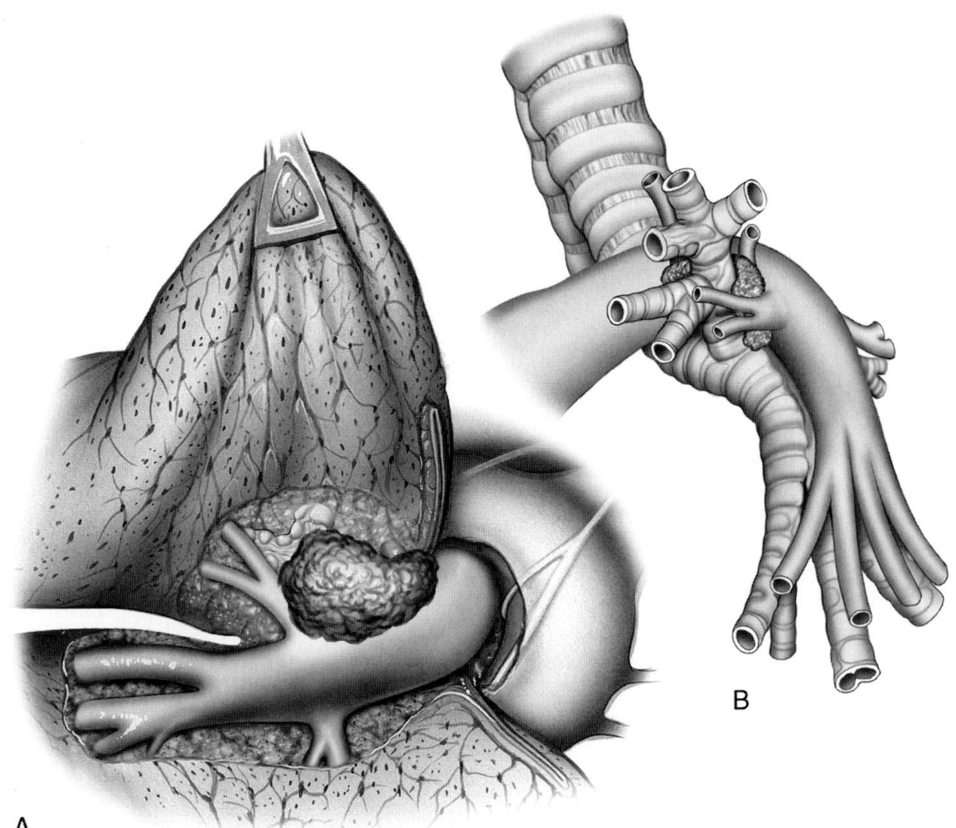

FIGURE 36–45 ■ Posterolateral (*A*) and lateral (*B*) views of the typical indications for patch reconstruction of the pulmonary artery on the left side.

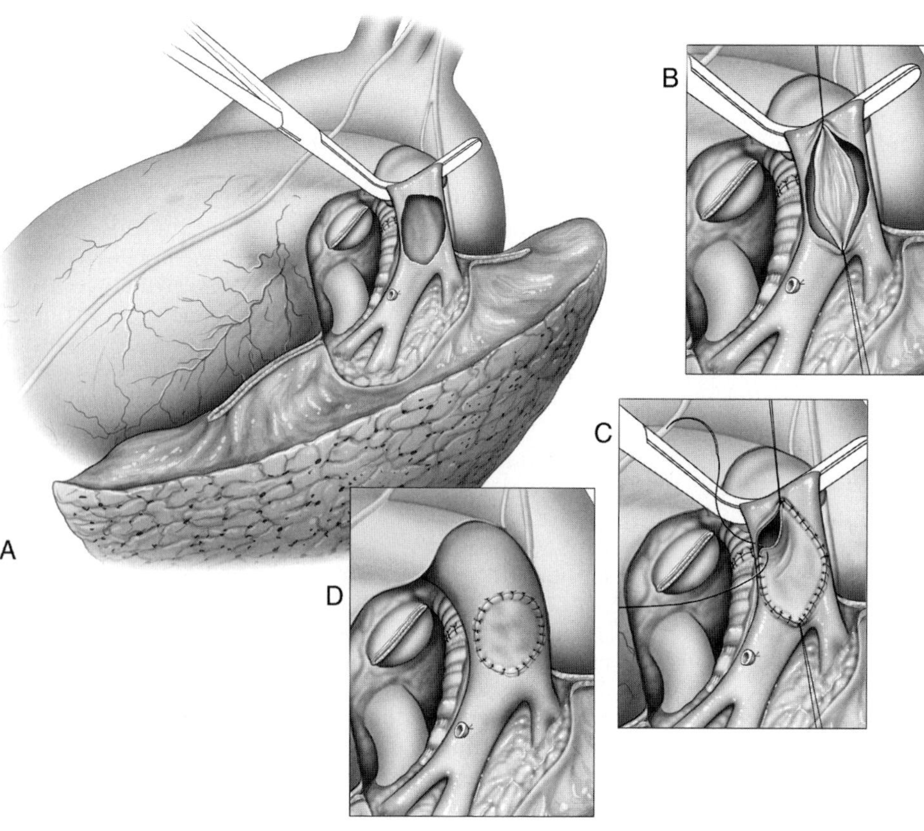

FIGURE 36–46 ■ Patch reconstruction. *A*, After upper lobectomy and partial resection of the pulmonary artery, an oval defect ensues, caused by the tension applied to the vessel by the lower lobe. *B*, The patch is held in place by two stay sutures. Some degree of tension on the patch is desirable at this stage; it shows that the patch is not too long; tension will disappear after declamping. *C*, The lower stay suture is not tied but simply keeps the patch in place. The right-handed surgeon would proceed from top to bottom, "artery first," on the right side and then continue bottom to top, "patch first." *D*, Completed patch reconstruction of the pulmonary artery. The pericardial defect is left open. The ligated stump of the lingular artery can also be seen. (*A* and *D* redrawn from Rendina EA, Venuta F, De Giacomo T et al: Safety and efficacy of bronchovascular reconstruction after induction chemotherapy for lung cancer. J Thorac Cardiovasc Surg 114:830, 1997.)

Sleeve Resection and Reconstruction by End-to-End Anastomosis

When transecting the artery, both proximally and distally, regular and even margins are desirable, even at the cost of some loss of tissue (see Fig. 36–41). This allows proper placement of the stitches and yields an even inside lumen. In addition, regular suture borders facilitate the correction of the large caliber discrepancy that usually occurs. Caliber discrepancy is never a problem owing to the elasticity of the arterial wall. The PA reconstruction is usually performed after completion of the bronchial anastomosis to minimize the manipulation of the vessel (Fig. 36–47*A*). In addition, the exposure of the bronchial stumps is optimal when the artery is divided. When the vascular and bronchial procedures are done simultaneously, the bronchial axis is shortened, and the PA stumps will almost always oppose with acceptable tension (Fig. 36–47*B*). Upon completion of the bronchial anastomosis, the distance between the two arterial ends will be markedly decreased, and can be further reduced by elevating the lower lobe while suturing. Restoration of blood flow and removal of the proximal clamp will almost always relieve any residual tension (Fig. 36–47*C* and *D*). If the distance between the arterial stumps is deemed excessive, the interposition of a prosthetic conduit is indicated. The anastomosis is performed by running 5–0 or 6–0 monofilament nonabsorbable material; especially if some degree of tension exists, it is safer to complete the posterior portion of the suture and subsequently parachute the two stumps together while lifting the lower lobe. Sometimes the distal end of the PA will shrink so that the first branch (apical segmental artery on the left; middle lobe artery on the right) will appear almost separate from the rest of the vessel. The reconstruction is still feasible, but the sutures should be placed very carefully to avoid stenosis.

Sleeve Resection and Reconstruction by a Prosthetic Conduit

In the very unusual case of extended circumferential defects in which end-to-end anastomosis is not feasible, a prosthetic conduit of synthetic or biological material can be used. We prefer the autologous pericardium, because other materials might increase the risk of thrombosis. The conduit interposition may be useful when a left upper lobe tumor infiltrates the PA extensively, but the lobar bronchus is not involved and, therefore, a bronchial sleeve is not indicated. This unusual situation (PA sleeve without bronchial sleeve) may produce a long bronchial segment separating the two widely spaced PA stumps so that an end-to-end anastomosis is not possible (Fig. 36–48*A*). The autologous pericardium is trimmed to rectangular shape, wrapped around a 28 French chest tube with the epicardial surface inside, and sutured longitudinally with 6–0 monofilament nonabsorbable material. A pericardial conduit of approximately 1 to 2 cm is thus created. When sizing the conduit, two points must be considered: the PA stumps can be approximated closer than it seems, and the conduit will stretch more than

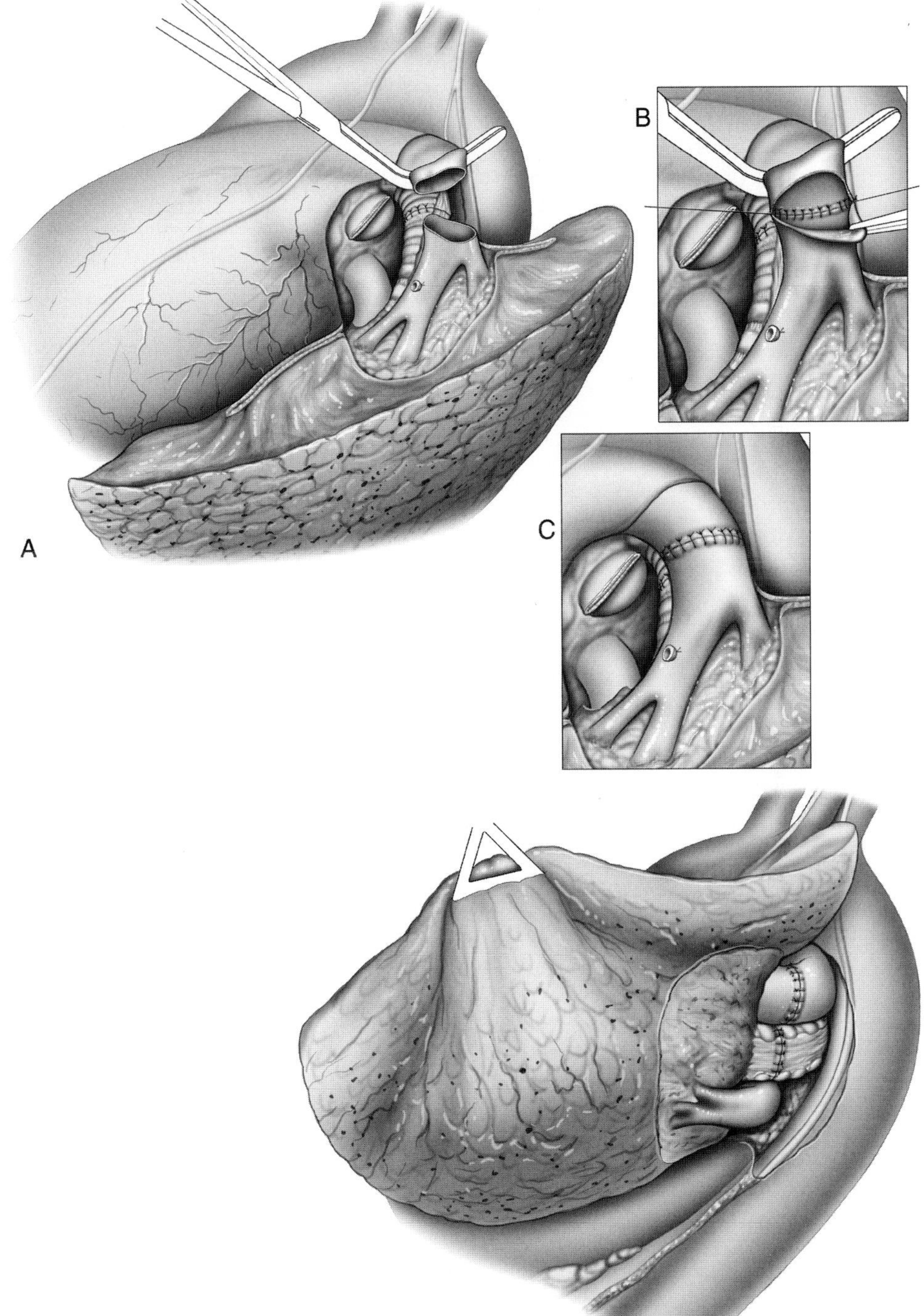

FIGURE 36–47 ■ Sleeve resection with end-to-end anastomosis. *A*, The arterial anastomosis is performed after the bronchial suture to minimize manipulation of the vessel. *B*, Regular and even arterial margins facilitate proper placement of the stitches. When the bronchial and pulmonary artery sleeves are associated, the pulmonary artery stumps will reach with acceptable tension. *C*, After completion of the end-to-end anastomosis, caliber discrepancy is compensated by the elasticity of the pulmonary artery. *D*, A posterior view of the left hilum after bronchial and pulmonary artery sleeve resection. The inferior pulmonary vein is visible on the left side. (*A* and *B* redrawn from Rendina EA, Venuta F, De Giacomo T et al: Safety and efficacy of bronchovascular reconstruction after induction chemotherapy for lung cancer. J Thorac Cardiovasc Surg 114:830, 1997.)

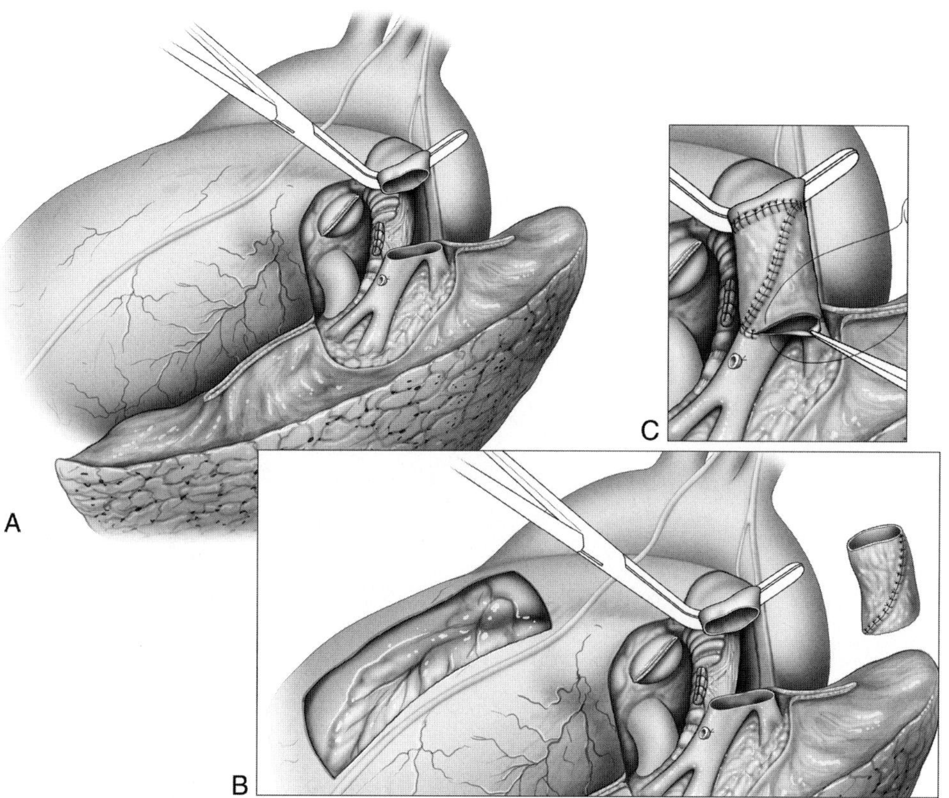

FIGURE 36–48 ■ Sleeve resection and reconstruction by a prosthetic conduit. *A*, The need for a pulmonary artery sleeve without bronchial sleeve produces a long bronchial segment separating the two widely spaced pulmonary artery stumps so that end-to-end anastomosis is not possible. *B*, The proximal anastomosis between the pulmonary artery and the conduit is performed first. *C*, The distal anastomosis is performed last, overlapping the suture margins to create tension, which will be relieved by declamping. (*C* redrawn from Rendina EA, Venuta F, De Giacomo T et al: Safety and efficacy of bronchovascular reconstruction after induction chemotherapy for lung cancer. J Thorac Cardiovasc Surg 114:830, 1997.)

predicted. It is advisable to tailor the length of the conduit on the basis of the resected arterial segment, because the elasticity of the two tissues is comparable. The proximal anastomosis is performed first with running 5–0 monofilament suture (Fig. 36–48*B*). The distal anastomosis is performed last, after the conduit has been trimmed to the appropriate length by overlapping the suture margins. It is advisable to parachute the distal end of the conduit, folding it over itself to obtain some degree of tension, which will disappear after declamping (Fig. 36–48*C*). When the blood flow is restored, the dimension of the conduit will increase by approximately one third. Care must be taken to avoid lengthening of the PA, which may cause kinking of the vessel, impaired blood flow, and ultimately thrombus formation.

Resection and Reconstruction of the Main Pulmonary Artery via Cardiopulmonary Bypass

Cardiopulmonary bypass is instituted via median sternotomy, and the main PA is separated from the ascending aorta and clamped. The right PA is clamped between the aorta and the SVC, as tumor does not allow placement of the clamp on the left side of the aorta (Fig. 36–49*A*). Alternatively, the right heart can be emptied by bicaval cannulation, thus making PA clamping unnecessary. The left PA and part of the main and right PA are resected en bloc with the left lung. The defect is then reconstructed by a tissue patch (Fig. 36–49*B*).

PITFALLS AND COMPLICATIONS

Although the postoperative course of bronchial sleeve resection depends to some extent on patient compliance and judicious clinical management, the short-term results of PA reconstruction depend mostly on operative judgment and technique. If the operation has been correctly performed, specific complications might be expected in no more than 5% of the patients. These essentially consist of leakage from the suture line and thrombosis. Bronchoarterial fistula is much more likely to be associated with bronchial sleeve resection and can be effectively prevented by interposing the intercostal muscle between the two structures.

Because the PA is a low pressure vessel, leakage from the suture line may pass unnoticed intraoperatively. Also, the bleeding may start in the first or second postoperative day after a patch reconstruction. A blood loss of up to 800 to 1000 ml daily may occur after 1 or 2 days of no drainage. This may last for 1 or 2 days and then stop spontaneously independently from anticoagulation. A possible explanation is that the autologous pericardium shrinks and curls markedly after harvesting, and it is difficult to place the suture bites at the appropriate distance. After declamping and distention, bites too wide apart may result. These would not cause bleeding immediately because the PA is stretched downward by the atelectatic lower lobe, and simple apposition of the tissue edges is enough to contrast the low PA pressure. However, in the postoperative period when the re-expansion of the lower lobe elevates the hilum, the rotation and

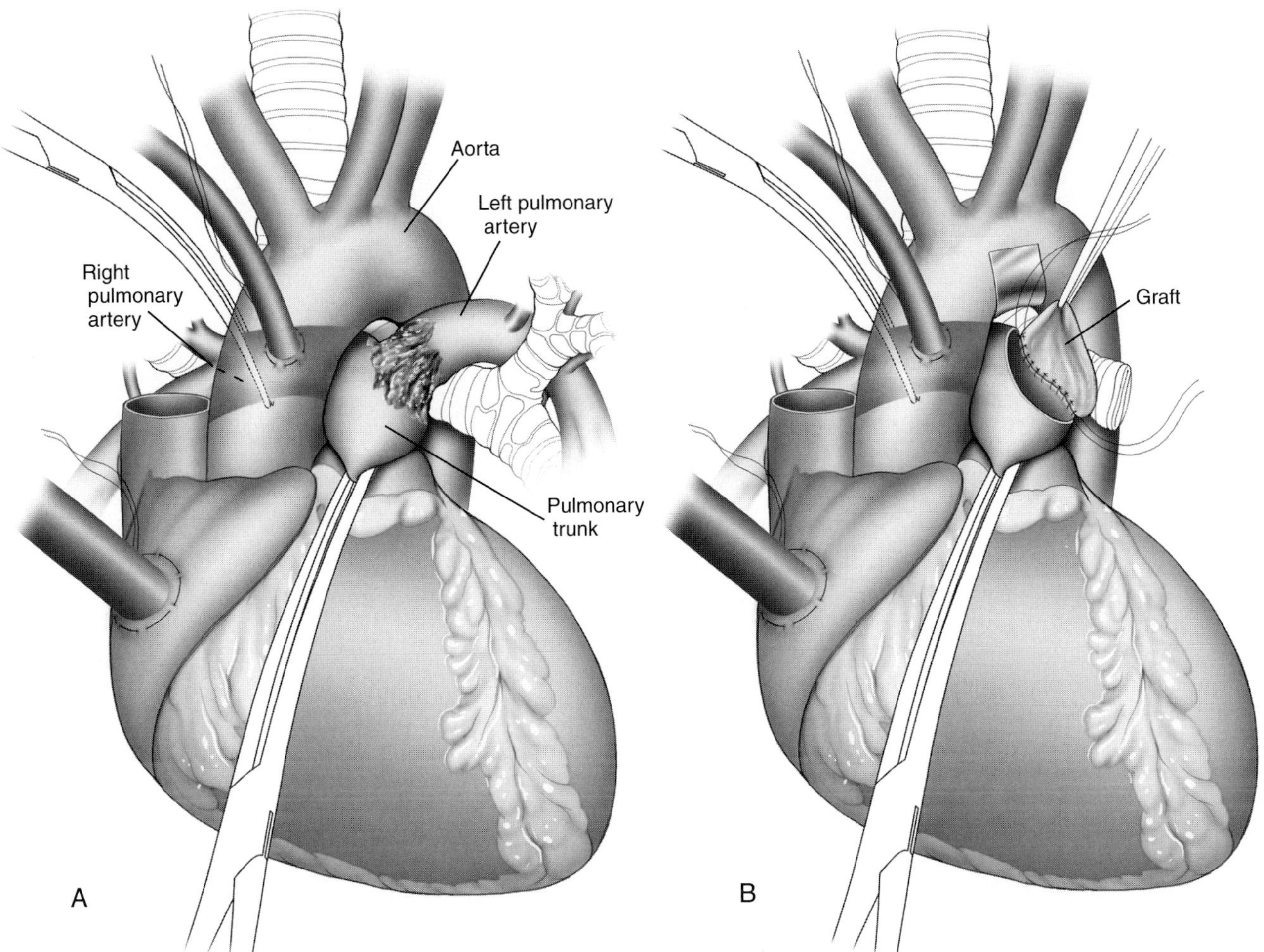

FIGURE 36–49 ■ Resection and reconstruction of the main pulmonary artery via cardiopulmonary bypass (CPB). *A*, The tumor infiltrates the left and main pulmonary artery. CPB is instituted, and the main and right pulmonary artery are clamped. *B*, After left pneumonectomy and en bloc resection of the main pulmonary artery the defect is reconstructed by a pericardial patch. (Redrawn from Ricci C, Rendina EA, Venuta F et al: Reconstruction of the pulmonary artery in patients with lung cancer. Ann Thorac Surg 57:627, 1994.)

kinking of the PA may distort the suture line and reopen the bleeding site. It is, therefore, very important, especially when using autologous pericardial patches, to carefully check the suture line and test the PA position after re-expansion of the residual lobe. The latter maneuver is also important to prevent thrombosis. After a patch reconstruction of the PA associated with a bronchial sleeve, the bronchial axis is shortened, and the length of the artery remains stationary. Some of the discrepancy is compensated by the elasticity of the vessel, but the PA may tend to kink and fold over itself. The aforementioned repositioning of the PA due to the re-expansion of the lower lobe further increases this risk. Impairment of blood flow may ensue, and thrombosis may be facilitated. Under these circumstances, it is better to cut the distorted segment away and proceed to an end-to-end anastomosis.

The pitfalls of sleeve resection and end-to-end anastomosis are of a different nature: sometimes it is anatomically impossible, such as in cases of left upper lobe tumors infiltrating the concave surface of the PA from its origin down to the anterobasal artery. On the right side, the same problem may arise when the posterolateral aspect of the PA is infiltrated from the upper division artery to the artery for the superior segment of the lower lobe. Conversely, sleeve resection is sometimes excessive, if the artery is only partially infiltrated. Additionally, the end-to-end anastomosis can be technically difficult, owing to unexpected traction between the stumps and caliber discrepancy. Tears on the arterial wall while suturing are difficult to repair, and failure to do so may produce disastrous results.

The main pitfall of the use of a conduit is sizing its length. Application of the aforementioned technical insights will prevent this problem.

LONG-TERM RESULTS

Mid-term and long-term evaluation of patients undergoing PA reconstruction are based on three issues:

A. Patency of the PA and perfusion of the residual lobe.
B. Right heart function.
C. Analysis of survival.

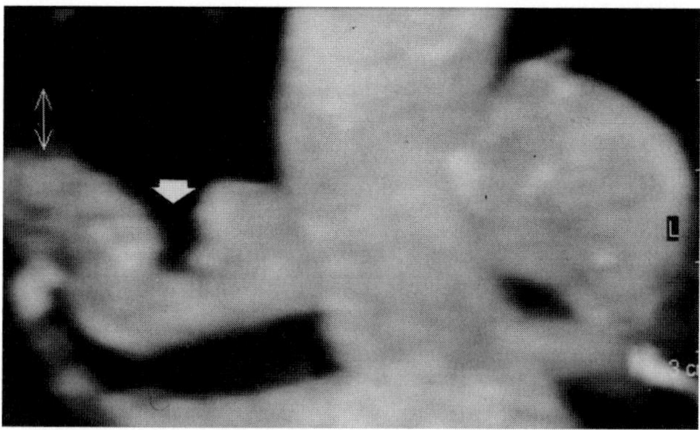

FIGURE 36–50 ■ Pitfalls of tangential resection and direct suture of the pulmonary artery. Postoperative angio–magnetic resonance imaging shows marked caliber reduction and narrowing of the right pulmonary artery (*arrow*).

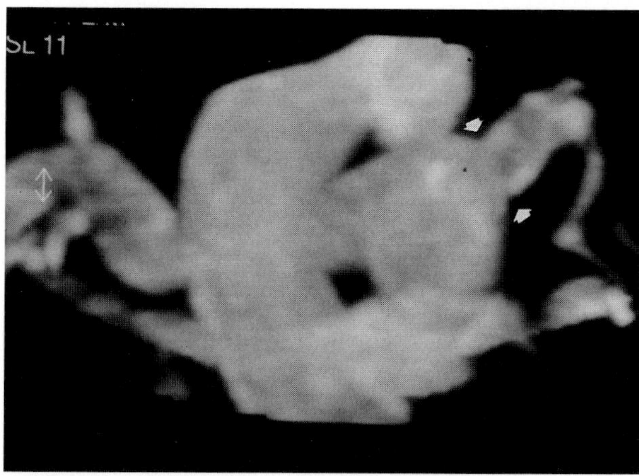

FIGURE 36–52 ■ Postoperative angio–magnetic resonance imaging after sleeve resection with end-to-end anastomosis (*arrows*) of the left pulmonary artery.

1. Immediately after the operation, patency problems occur in less than 5% of cases. Newer noninvasive techniques such as MR-Angio provide outstanding imaging of the PA (Figs. 36–50, 36–51, and 36–52), and may be very useful in demonstrating patency problems even in the immediate postoperative period. However, once the normal blood flow through the PA has been restored, and the new orientation of the PA due to the re-expansion of the residual lobe has taken place without kinking in the early postoperative period, patency impairment is very unlikely to occur. In the absence of clinical symptoms, pulmonary angiograms in addition to perfusion lung scans are, therefore, redundant. In the long term, CT with injection of contrast material has proven a versatile noninvasive diagnostic tool, useful to evaluate both PA patency and distal PA branching, as well as the overall oncologic status of the patient.

2. Standard electrocardiography and echocardiography are useful to confirm the advantages in terms of right heart function and morphology obtained by the preservation of a normally perfused lobe. These tests confirm that, unlike pneumonectomy, the right ventricular size and motility remains normal, and that pulmonary hypertension does not tend to develop. These findings parallel those of spirometry, which indicates that bronchial sleeve lobectomy equals standard lobectomy in terms of pulmonary function.

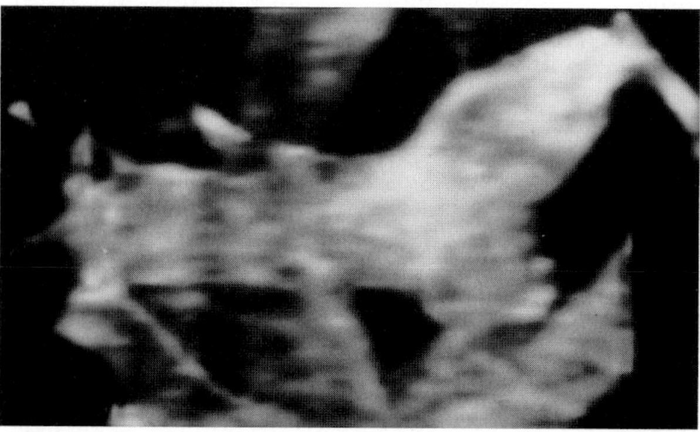

FIGURE 36–51 ■ Postoperative angio–magnetic resonance imaging after patch reconstruction of the left pulmonary artery.

3. Because the reports on PA reconstructions have been rare in the literature so far, the long-term survival of these patients has been uncertain. Recently, it has been indicated that the survival of PA reconstruction is comparable, stage-by-stage, to that reported in the major reviews on lung cancer surgery and sleeve resection in the literature (Fig. 36–53). The impact of the nodal status on survival is also comparable with that reported for bronchial sleeve and standard resection. In the face of N1 or N2 involvement, once the decision to resect the disease with intent to cure is taken, PA reconstruction can, also be proposed as an adequate procedure in this setting. Also, there is no statistically significant difference between PA reconstruction alone or PA reconstruction associated with bronchial sleeve. This suggests that even complex lung-sparing operations can be pursued with intent to cure as long as a complete anatomical resection is achieved.

COMMENTS AND CONTROVERSIES

The techniques outlined by the authors superbly illustrate the various methods of performing vascular sleeve resections on both the right and left lung, thus preserving pulmonary function. I certainly have not extended the indications as much as these authors have. One wonders whether many of these tumors were indeed T4—with regard to the pulmonary artery or vein, a T4 tumor denotes one that involves the main pulmonary artery (not the right or left main pulmonary artery) or invades through the pericardium itself with tumor nodules on the intrapericardial pulmonary artery. In such cases, it is a rare event that an R0 resection can be performed, even utilizing cardiopulmonary bypass. It is highly unlikely that the IIIb patients were staged because of their nodal involvement. Many of Dr. Rendina's patients were clinically staged as T4 only to be found less than T4 at the time of surgery—one must be very wary of clinically overstaging the T4 subset! Be that as it may, I know

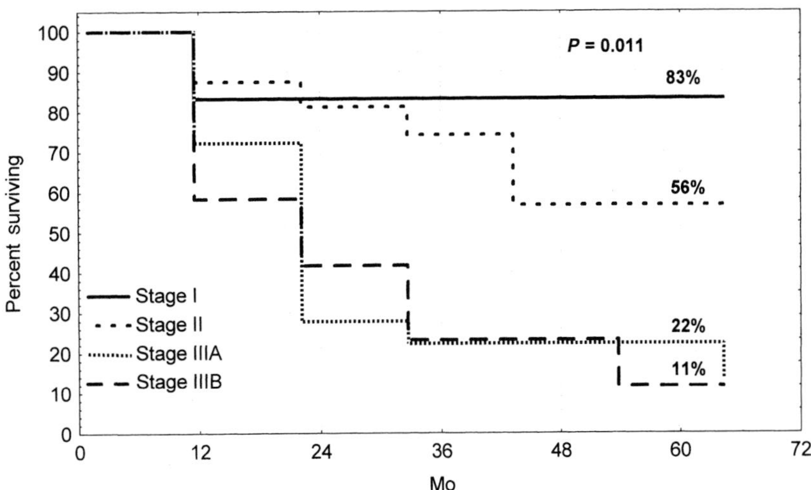

FIGURE 36–53 ■ Five-year survival by stage of 52 patients undergoing pulmonary artery reconstruction. (From Rendina EA, Venuta F, De Giacomo T et al: Sleeve resection and prosthetic reconstruction of the pulmonary artery for lung cancer. Ann Thorac Surg 68:995, 1999.)

of no other technical chapter outlining bronchovascular resections that matches this one!

R.J.G.

■ REFERENCES

Bennett WF, Abbey-Smith R: A twenty-year analysis of the results of sleeve resection for primary bronchogenic carcinoma. J Thorac Cardiovasc Surg 76:840, 1978.

Lowe JE, Bridgman AH, Sabiston DC Jr et al: The role of bronchoplastic procedures in the surgical management of benign and malignant pulmonary lesions. J Thorac Cardiovasc Surg 83:227, 1982.

Rendina EA, Venuta F et al: Safety and efficacy of bronchovascular reconstruction after induction chemotherapy for lung cancer. J Thorac Cardiovasc Surg 114:830, 1997.

Rendina EA, Venuta F, De Giacomo T et al: Sleeve resection and prosthetic reconstruction of the pulmonary artery for lung cancer. Ann Thorac Surg 68:995, 1999.

Ricci C, Rendina EA, Venuta F et al: Reconstruction of the pulmonary artery in patients with lung cancer. Ann Thorac Surg 57:627, 1994.

Vogt-Moykopf I, Frits TH et al: Bronchoplastic and angioplastic operation in bronchial carcinoma: Long-term results of a retrospective analysis from 1973 to 1983. Int Surg 71:211, 1986.

Weisel RD, Cooper JD et al: Sleeve lobectomy for carcinoma of the lung. J Thorac Cardiovasc Surg 78:839, 1979.

SUPERIOR SULCUS TUMOR

Farid Shamji
Robert J. Ginsberg
Harold C. Urschel, Jr.

A true superior sulcus tumor is usually a primary lung cancer, which early on, extends beyond the lung to invade important anatomic structures in the narrow, crowded thoracic inlet. Local tumor invasion may involve the lower trunk of the brachial plexus, including the roots of the first thoracic and first eight cervical nerves, and the sympathetic chain including the stellate ganglion. There may be local extension into adjacent upper ribs and thoracic vertebrae. The subclavian artery may become encased in the tumor mass as it extends into the root of the neck. Spread of the tumor through the adjacent intervertebral foramen may cause epidural spinal cord compression. Although superior pulmonary sulcus tumors were originally considered to be inoperable and incurable because of their relative inaccessibility and extensive local invasion into the thoracic inlet, it has become obvious that in selected patients the therapy that completely eradicates the local growth gives the most appreciable pain relief and survival in terms of both quality and duration.

HISTORICAL NOTE

Pancoast, in his presidential address to the American Medical Association in 1932, described the clinical features of a lung cancer involving the apex of the chest, which is now known as a Pancoast tumor. The syndrome associated with this apical tumor includes pain radiating down the arm, Horner's syndrome, and radiologic destruction of ribs, as well as atrophy of the hand muscles.

Until the reports by Chardack and MacCallum (1956) and Shaw and others (1961), there had been no curative resections of this disease. Subsequently, any apical tumor with associated pain around the shoulder and extending down the arm is termed a *superior sulcus tumor.* Few, if any, patients exhibiting the full-blown Pancoast syndrome are curable because of extensive brachial plexus and subclavian artery involvement.

■ *HISTORICAL READINGS*

Chardack WM, MacCallum JD: Pancoast tumor: Five year survival without recurrence or metastases following radical resection and postoperative irradiation. J Thorac Surg 31:535, 1956.

Pancoast HK: Superior pulmonary sulcus tumors: Tumor characterized by pain, Horner's syndrome, destruction of bone and atrophy of hand muscles. JAMA 99:1391, 1932.

Shaw RR, Paulson DL, Kee JL: Treatment of the superior sulcus tumor by irradiation followed by resection. Ann Surg 154:29, 1961.

THERAPY

When determined to be completely resectable, en bloc surgical excision is the best treatment for superior sulcus tumors. The posterolateral approach as described by Shaw and Paulson is best suited for those tumors situated in the posterior half of the apex without significant involvement of anterior structures such as the subclavian artery. When these anterior structures are involved, other approaches such as the "hook"—extending the incision anteriorly across the axilla to expose the first rib anteriorly or the anterior approach—(described in chapter 36) should be chosen.

Preoperative radiotherapy to a moderate dose, followed by extended en bloc resection in selected patients, is the most common therapeutic protocol for true superior sulcus tumors, although the value of preoperative versus postoperative radiotherapy has never been established. More recently, surgeons are investigating preoperative combined modality approaches (chemoradiation). Resection is carried out 4 to 6 weeks after completion of radiotherapy. For local resection to be complete and curative, it usually includes removal of the following:

1. Chest wall
   a. Entire first rib and posterior parts of other involved ribs, most often the second and third ribs.
   b. Occasionally, portions of upper thoracic vertebrae (up to one quarter of the body can be removed without undue instability), including their transverse processes if necessary.
2. Corresponding thoracic nerve roots up to the intervertebral foramen.
3. A portion of the lower trunk of the brachial plexus, with sacrifice of the first thoracic nerve and usually with preservation of the eighth cervical nerve root.
4. A portion of the stellate ganglion and the thoracic sympathetic chain.
5. A pulmonary resection, usually by lobectomy or occasionally by anatomic segmental or wedge resection, although the latter has recently been shown by us to yield a poorer ultimate survival rate.
6. Mediastinal lymph node dissection or sampling.

It is important to identify those patients who are most likely to benefit from this posterior approach. This requires proper patient selection, careful and thorough staging of the cancer by mediastinal node biopsy and distant organ scanning, and examination of the local findings from noninvasive assessment by computed tomography (CT) scanning and magnetic resonance imaging (MRI).

In most cases, N2 disease discovered at mediastinoscopy, invasion of thoracic vertebral cancellous bone, and involvement of subclavian vessels have been considered to indicate inoperability. This has been questioned with the popularization of the anterior approach (see Dartevelle's discussion of the cervical approach to apical lesions in the next subchapter). When tumors are identified in the anterior compartment of the apex, the anterior approach is more suitable and is described in a separate section.

OPERATIVE TECHNIQUE

Anesthesia and Patient Position

General anesthesia using one-lung anesthesia greatly facilitates exposure within the chest. Full monitoring capacity is established for continuous recording of arterial blood pressure, oxygen saturation, cardiac rhythm, central venous pressure, and urine output. The patient is placed in the full lateral position with the affected side uppermost. The upper arm rests on a support. Conventional draping with sheets provides satisfactory exposure from the nape of the neck to the costal arch and from the nipple to the spinous processes of the thoracic spine.

The Incision

Lateral Thoracotomy Incision for Initial Exploration

The skin incision (Fig. 36–54) is started 3 cm beneath the nipple or just lateral to the breast in women and extends in a gentle arc 2 cm below the inferior angle of the scapula. The incision is carried deeper by use of electrocautery. The latissimus dorsi muscle is divided toward the lower margin of the incision. The fascia posterior to the serratus anterior muscle is incised along its posterior edge, and the muscle is divided along the lower part of the incision. In most cases, the chest is entered through a normal intercostal space between the two highest ribs that have not been invaded by the tumor (usually the fourth or fifth interspace), as determined by the preoperative CT scan or MRI; this allows one intact rib to be removed below the lower extent of the tumor (Fig. 36–55). The chest is explored to determine tumor resectability and the extent of the resection (i.e., the number of ribs and the portions of vertebral bodies and the corresponding transverse processes to be removed [Fig. 36–56]).

Parascapular Incision for Exposure of the Thoracic Inlet and Chest Wall Resection

Once resectability has been determined possible, the skin incision is extended posteriorly in a gentle arc from below

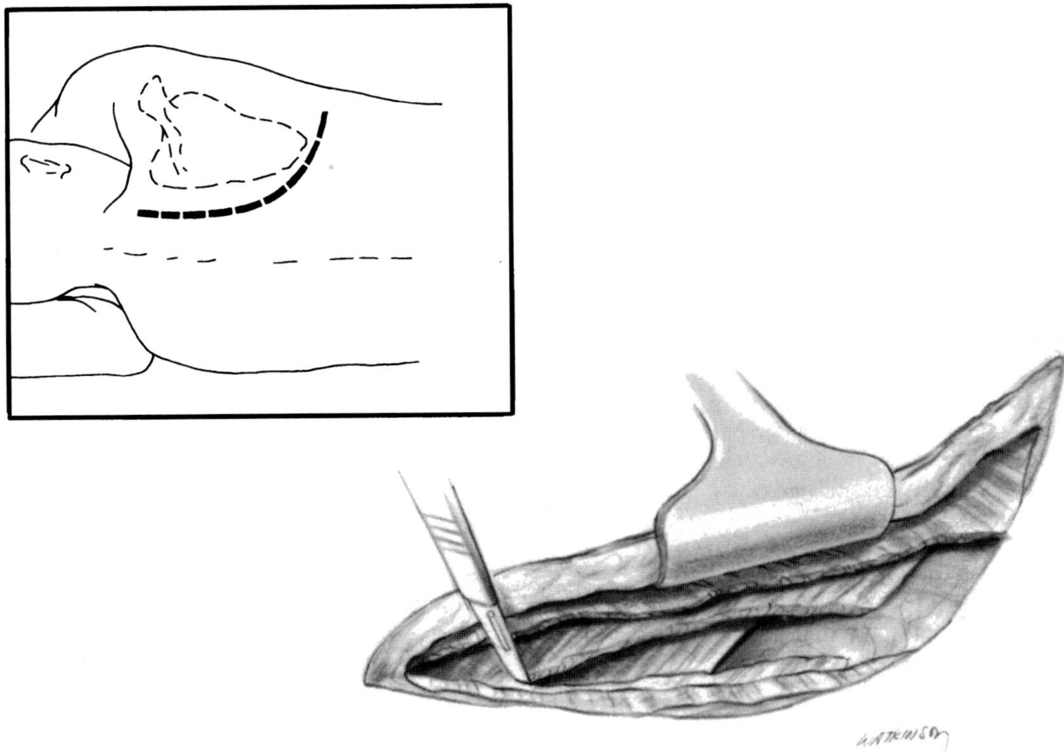

FIGURE 36–54 ■ The posterolateral incision, which should extend proximally to the C7 spinous process. The trapezius has been divided, and the rhomboids are in their final stage of division. (From Cooper JD, Urschel HC Jr: Superior pulmonary sulcus carcinoma resection: Posterior approach. In Urschel HC Jr, Cooper JD [eds]: Atlas of Thoracic Surgery. New York, Churchill Livingstone, 1995, with permission.)

the inferior angle of the scapula to a point midway between the spinous process and the medial border of the scapula. From this point, the incision is carried vertically upward, ending opposite the level of the spinous processes of the seventh cervical vertebra and is then carried deeper with electrocautery, dividing the trapezius muscle for the full length of the incision. Deep to the trapezius are the levator scapulae and rhomboid minor and major muscles (from inferior to superior), which originate on the spinous process and insert into the medial border of the scapula. The rhomboids are divided, with care taken to avoid injury to the underlying dorsal scapular nerve (the nerve to the rhomboids) and the accompanying descending scapular artery; the nerve and artery run down the medial border of the scapula. The division of the rhomboids allows the medial border of the scapula to be elevated from the chest wall, allowing access to the thoracic inlet and en bloc chest wall resection before pulmonary resection.

En Bloc Chest Wall Resection

A rib-spreading retractor is placed in position to allow gentle elevation of the scapula with the lower blade outside the thoracotomy incision on the chest wall and the upper blade under the inferior angle of the scapula. Loose areolar tissue between the dense fascial covering of the subscapularis muscle and the chest wall is divided by a combination of sharp and blunt dissection to allow access to the first rib and the thoracic inlet. The chest wall excision is now outlined. An incision is made along the anterior border of the erector spinae muscle from the fifth to the first thoracic vertebra. The muscle is sharply dissected away from the angles of the ribs and the transverse processes to expose these bony structures for division later on. Hemostasis, deep to the dissected muscle mass, is obtained with temporary packing. The tumor is palpated from inside the chest, and the number of ribs requiring resection and the anterior margin of resection of these ribs with the intervening intercostal muscles are determined and marked on the outer surface of the chest wall by use of electrocautery. This margin should be at least 5 cm anterior to the growth and include one uninvolved rib inferiorly.

Attention is now directed to the thoracic inlet, and its important anatomic relationships are carefully examined to avoid inadvertent injury to the subclavian artery and vein and the brachial plexus during dissection around the first rib. The scalenus anterior and medius muscles are carefully divided with scissors, either at their insertion point on the first rib or higher if indicated by the extent of the tumor. The scalenus posterior muscle, which inserts into the second rib, is divided where it crosses the outer border of the first rib. The superior margin of the first rib is freed where there is no tumor attachment while the subclavian artery and vein and the brachial plexus are protected with the operator's index finger.

The division of the ribs is started anteriorly and inferiorly, along the previously outlined wide margin of resec-

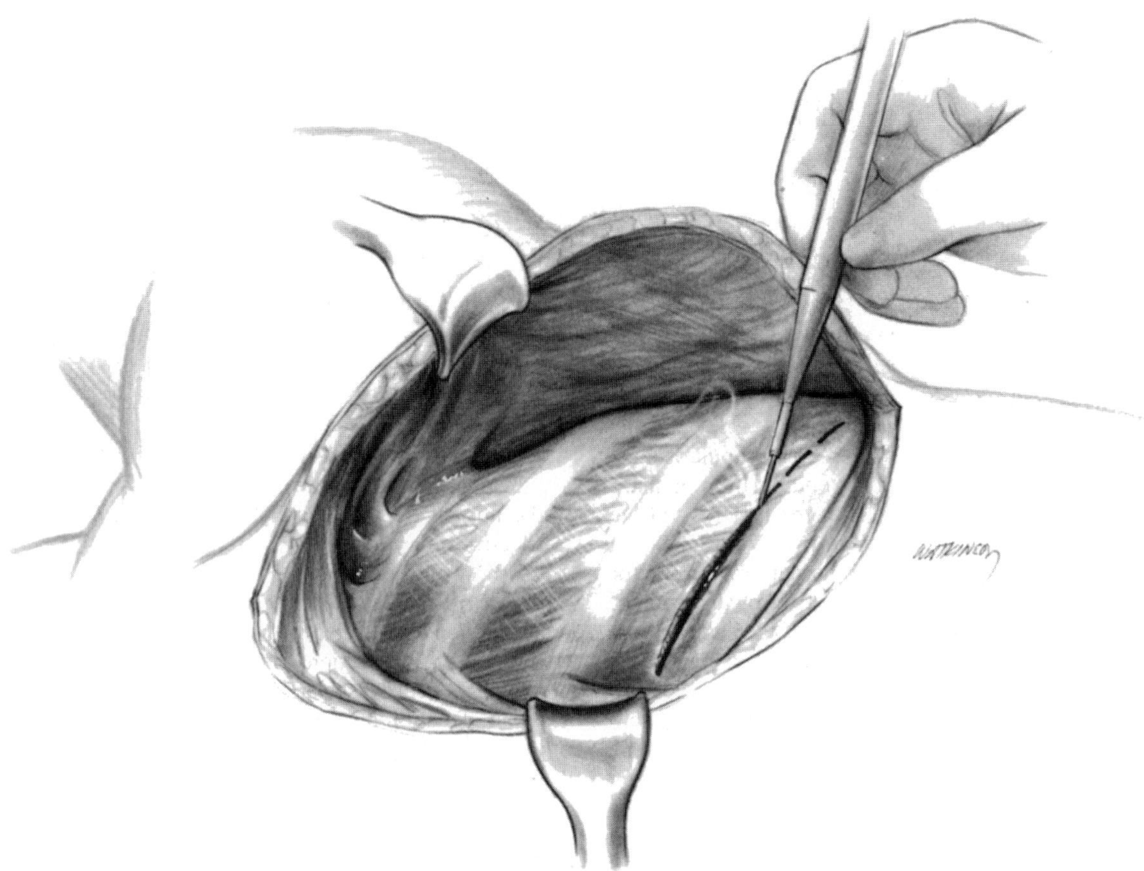

FIGURE 36–55 ■ The interspace selected for initial exploration is opened. (From Cooper JD, Urschel HC Jr: Superior pulmonary sulcus carcinoma resection: Posterior approach. In Urschel HC Jr, Cooper JD [eds]: Atlas of Thoracic Surgery. New York, Churchill Livingstone, 1995.)

tion, beginning with the normal rib immediately below the tumor (Fig. 36–57). Electrocautery is used to score the periosteum over a 1-cm width of all the ribs to be divided, except the first rib. Using rib shears, a short segment of each rib is removed in succession and labeled with adjacent soft tissue as the anterior margin of resection. The intervening intercostal muscles and their neurovascular bundles are suture-ligated and divided. Traction on the specimen side of the chest wall with a sharp towel clip helps to expose the anterior end of the first rib for transection. The lower trunk of the brachial plexus and its nerve roots from the eighth cervical and first thoracic nerves are now more clearly visible, as well as the relationship of the apical lung tumor to these structures.

The intercostal space below the lowest rib to be resected is entered and opened posteriorly to the angle of the rib. The chest wall resection is continued posteriorly, starting with the lowermost rib already divided anteriorly and proceeding upward. The erector spinae muscle is retracted to allow access to the transverse processes and the angles of the corresponding ribs. The transverse process is transected flush with the lamina by use of a curved osteotome, which is held at right angles to the vertebral column to avoid entering the spinal canal (Fig. 36–58). If there is no rib or vertebral invasion, the rib may be disarticulated from the transverse process without transecting the latter structure, preserving spinal stability. When this is possible, the head of the rib is disarticulated at the costovertebral joint with a periosteal elevator. The intervening intercostal nerve is divided after securing it with a hemoclip at the intervertebral foramen, and the intercostal vessels are suture-ligated and divided. The posterior line of resection is continued upwards until, finally, the posterior end of the first rib is reached.

At this point, the roots of the eighth cervical nerve above and the first thoracic nerve below the neck of the first rib, which join to form the lower trunk of the brachial plexus, are clearly seen, as is the extent of their involvement by tumor invasion (Fig. 36–59). The head of the first rib is disarticulated from the costovertebral joint after transecting the transverse process. The first thoracic nerve root is divided at the intervertebral foramen for completeness of tumor resection. If invaded by the tumor, the mass is dissected off the remaining lower trunk of the brachial plexus, keeping intact the eighth cervical nerve component, and resection margins are assessed by frozen section. Division of the T1 nerve root at its entry into the lower trunk completes the resection (Fig. 36–60). Occasionally, the eighth cervical nerve root may also need to be divided because of invasion by the tumor, and, in such a case, the lower trunk of the brachial plexus is also divided distal to the point of invasion

Text continued on page 1035

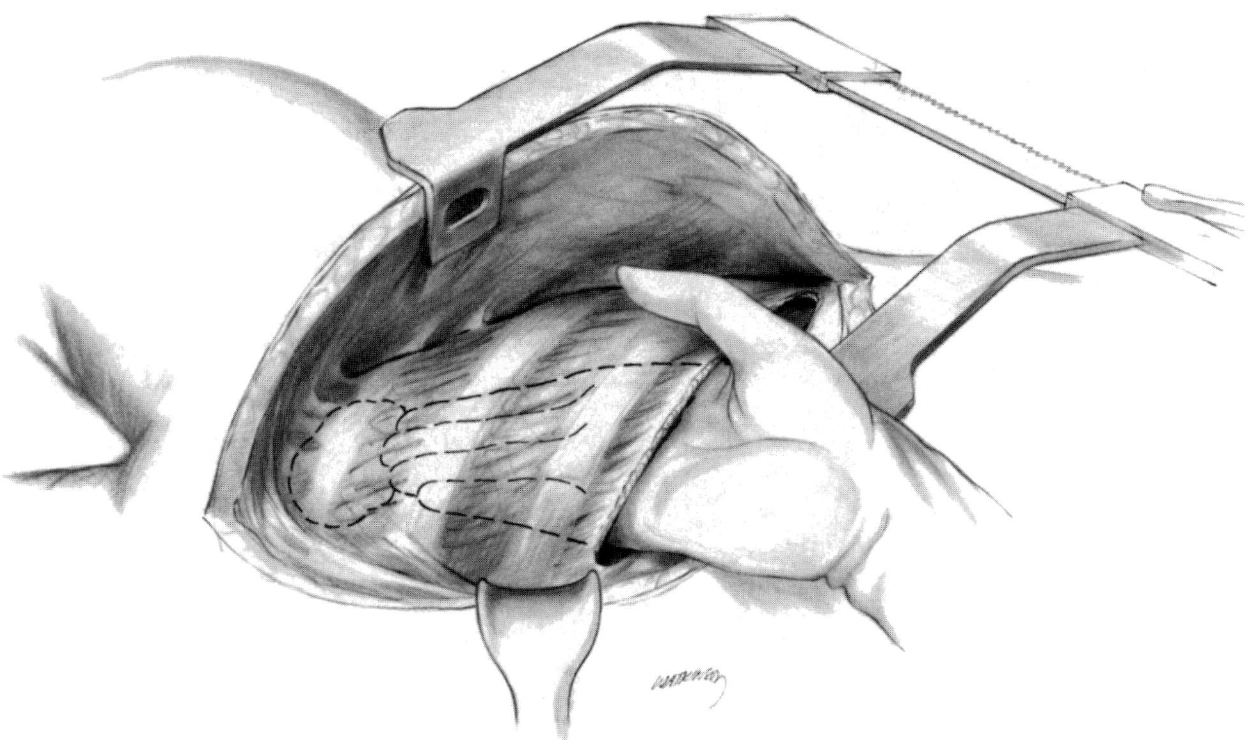

FIGURE 36–56 ■ Palpation of the tumor assesses resectability. (From Cooper JD, Urschel HC Jr: Superior pulmonary sulcus carcinoma resection: Posterior approach. In Urschel HC Jr, Cooper JD [eds]: Atlas of Thoracic Surgery. New York, Churchill Livingstone, 1995.)

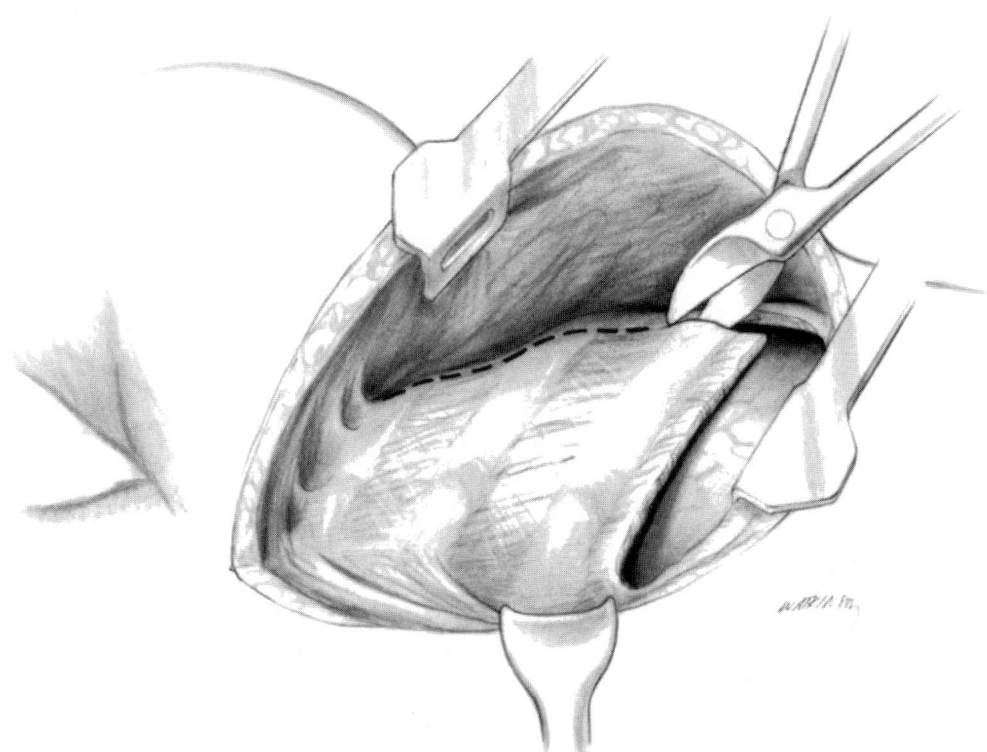

FIGURE 36–57 ■ The resection of the en bloc specimen begins anteriorly by dividing the anterior margin of the wall away from the tumor. (From Cooper JD, Urschel HC Jr: Superior pulmonary sulcus carcinoma resection: Posterior approach. In Urschel HC Jr, Cooper JD [eds]: Atlas of Thoracic Surgery. New York, Churchill Livingstone, 1995.)

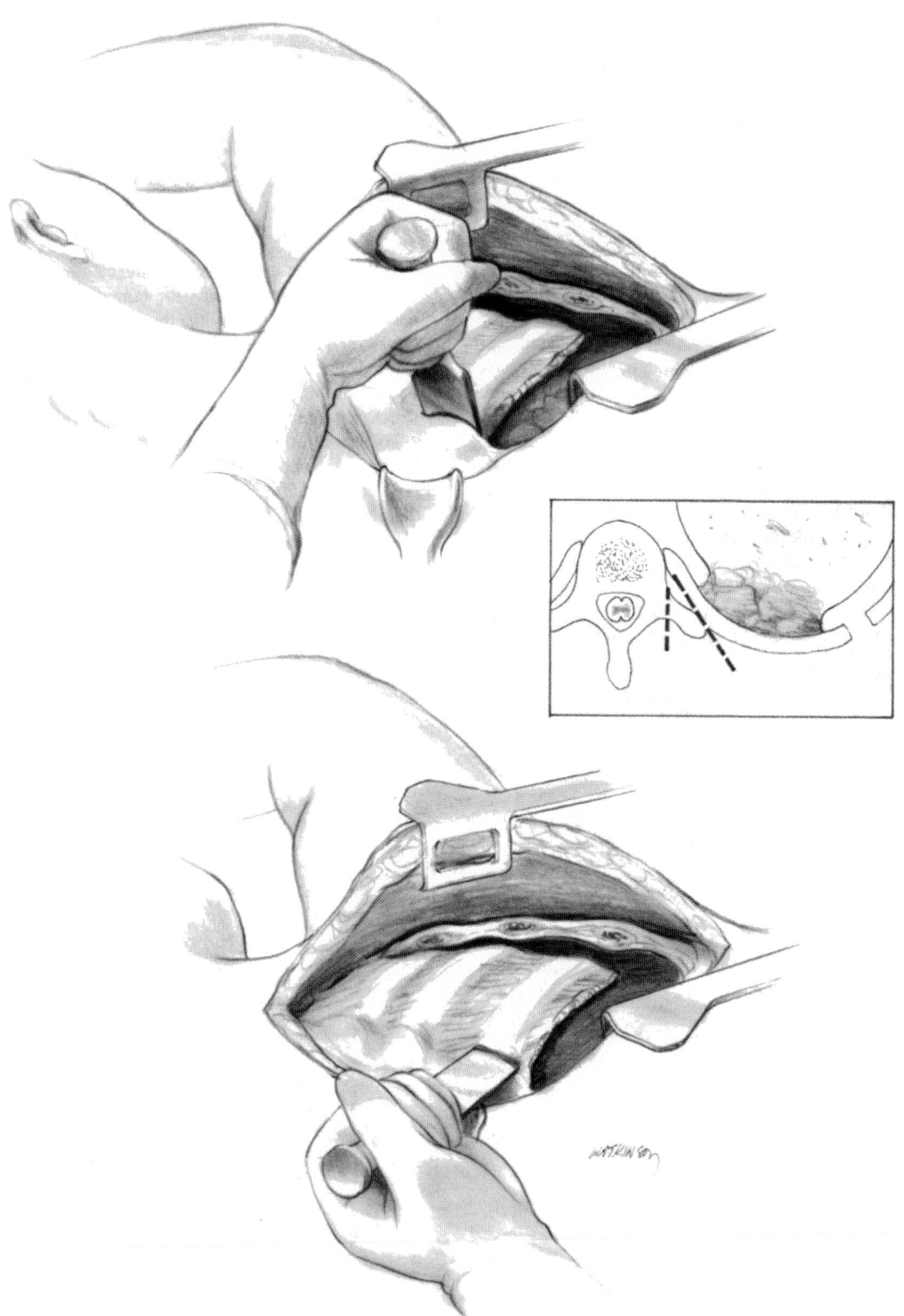

FIGURE 36–58 ■ The rib is resected with or without the transverse process (see text).

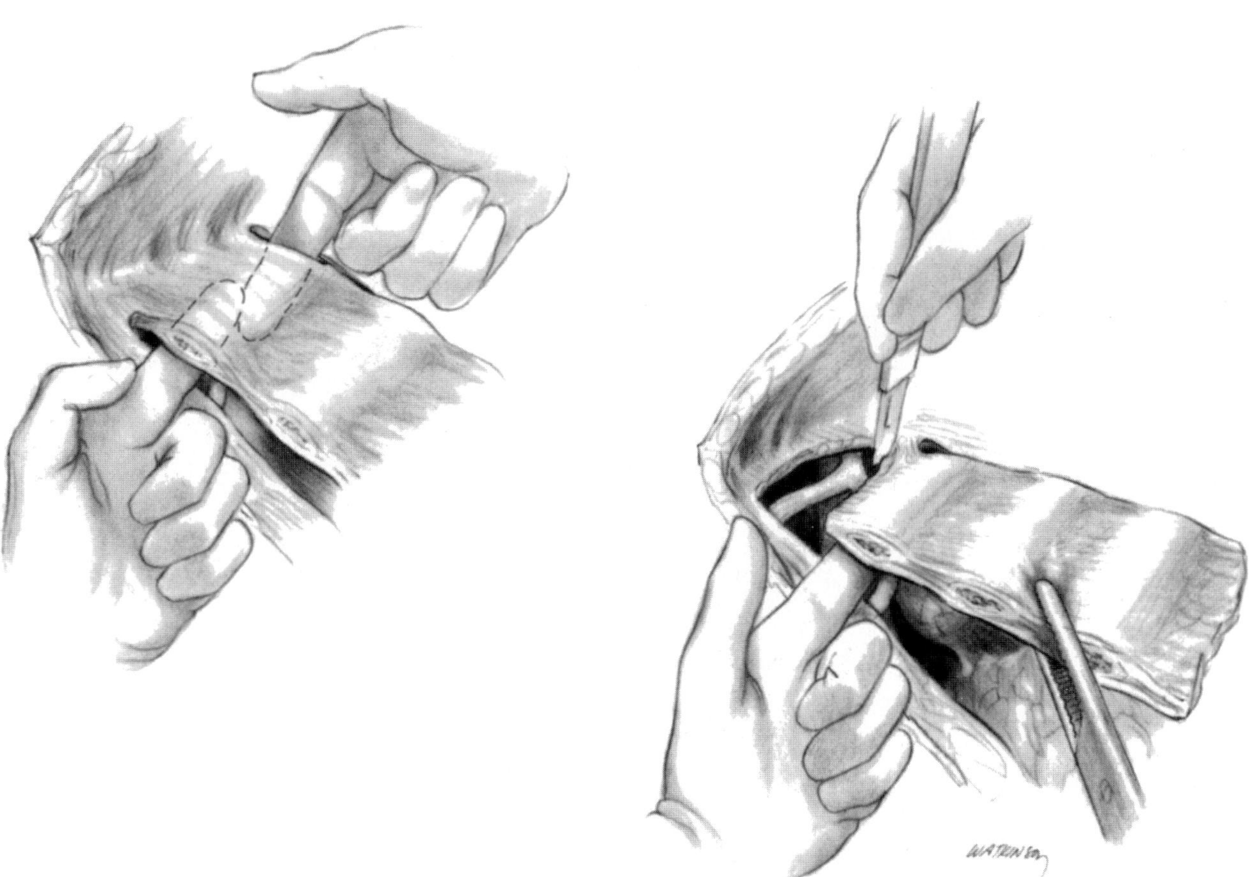

FIGURE 36–59 ■ Removing the superior aspect of the first rib from the subjacent brachial plexus. (From Cooper JD Urschel HC Jr: Superior pulmonary sulcus carcinoma resection: Posterior approach. In Urschel HC Jr, Cooper JD [eds]: Atlas of Thoracic Surgery. New York, Churchill Livingstone, 1995.)

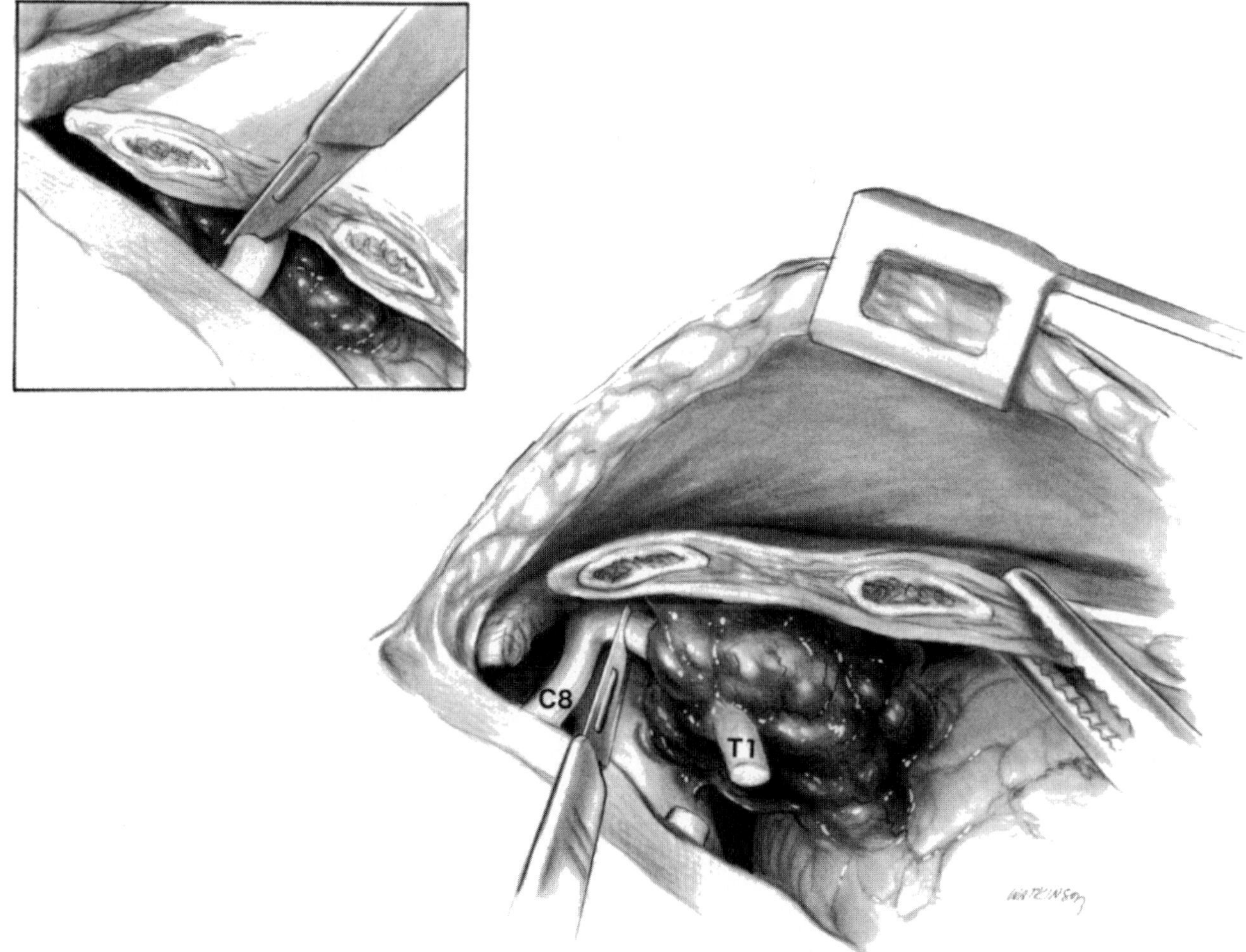

FIGURE 36–60 ■ The T1 nerve root has been divided at the end of the vertebral foramen (*inset*) and is now being divided at a juncture with the C8 nerve root. (From Cooper JD, Urschel HC Jr: Superior pulmonary sulcus carcinoma resection: Posterior approach. In Urschel HC Jr, Cooper JD [eds]: Atlas of Thoracic Surgery. New York, Churchill Livingstone, 1995.)

beyond the T1-C8 fusion. It is important to secure the nerve roots at the neural foramen with hemoclips before dividing to prevent leakage of cerebrospinal fluid (CSF); if this happens, the foramen should be lightly packed with a piece of free muscle, and the erector spinae muscle should be sutured to the lateral aspect of vertebral bodies for tamponade of the leak. Neurosurgical consultation is advised. The dissection is continued into the root of the neck, where the tumor is gradually dissected from the subclavian artery in the adventitial plane; rarely, the arterial wall is invaded, in which case resection and reconstruction will be necessary after obtaining proximal and distal control.

Posteriorly, the relationship of the tumor mass to the upper thoracic vertebral bodies is assessed. Depending on the degree of tumor attachment and the frozen section analysis of the periosteum, the tumor resection may require removal of a portion of the involved vertebral bodies; up to one quarter of the body may be removed without affecting stability. The sympathetic chain is secured with hemoclips and divided both below and above the tumor mass, taking a portion of the stellate ganglion (Fig. 36–61).

Once the chest wall resection is complete, the involved segment of the chest wall, still attached to the apical lung tumor, is allowed to drop into the chest cavity, and pulmonary resection is performed.

Pulmonary Resection

In most cases, a dissection upper lobectomy is carried out with individual ligation of the blood vessels and the bronchus (Fig. 36–62). The superior mediastinal lymph nodes are resected en bloc or sampled through a vertical incision in the superior mediastinum. The posterior subcarinal, lobar, interlobar, and hilar lymph nodes are sampled separately to complete the intraoperative staging.

Chest Reconstruction

The erector spinae muscle mass can be sutured to the lateral aspect of the vertebral bodies with interrupted sutures of 0 Vicryl. This provides good hemostasis and tamponades CSF leak from the intervertebral foramina. When necessary, the chest wall defect is now reconstructed using a Marlex 2-mm Gore Tex patch. The patch is tailored to the size of the defect and is secured and stabilized in place, under tension for a taut cover, with 2–0 Prolene sutures. The sutures are placed through the patch along all the margins of the defect except the superior margin, which is left free to allow free mobility of the plexus, the artery, and the vein. A continuous running suture along the three margins fixes the patch under tension. We only reconstruct larger defects, usually greater than three resected ribs.

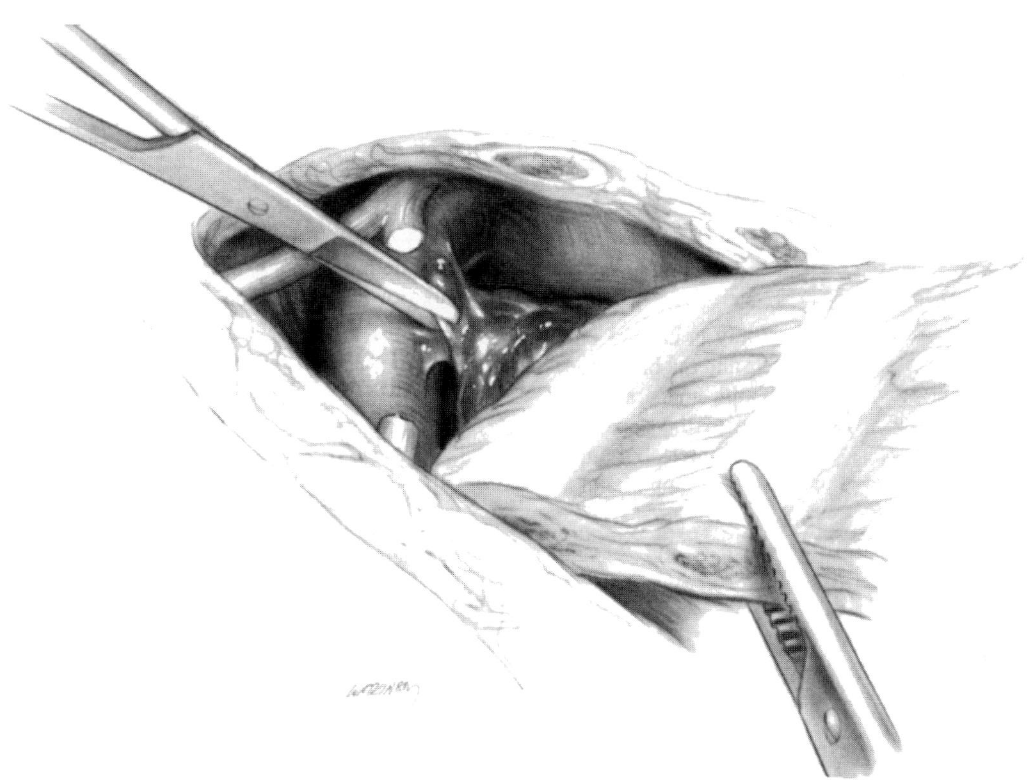

FIGURE 36–61 ■ The inferior half of the stellate ganglion is being dissected from the subclavian artery. (From Cooper JD, Urschel HC Jr: Superior pulmonary sulcus carcinoma resection: Posterior approach. In Urschel HC Jr, Cooper JD [eds]: Atlas of Thoracic Surgery. New York, Churchill Livingstone, 1995.)

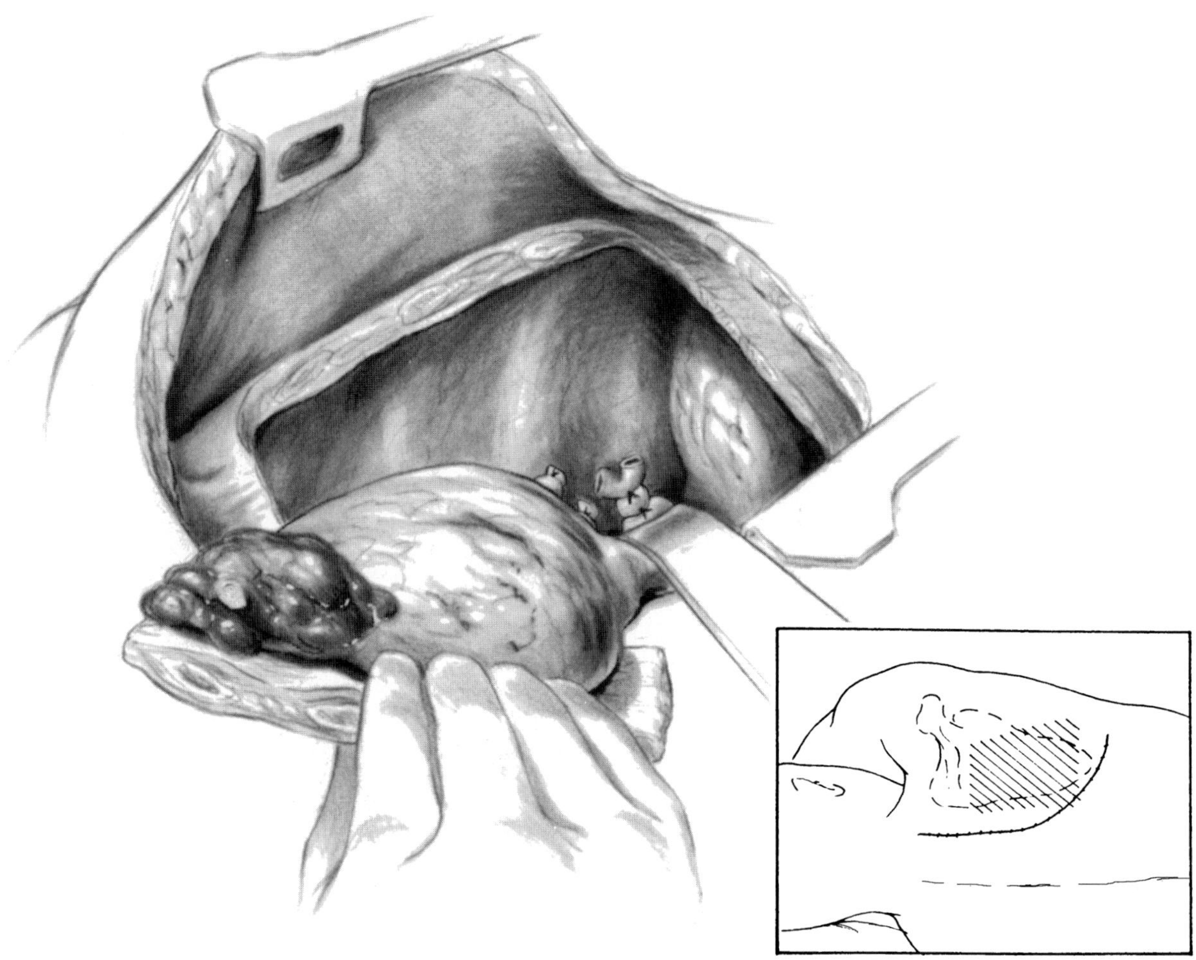

FIGURE 36–62 ■ Following lobectomy, the en bloc specimen is being removed. (From Cooper JD, Urschel HC Jr: Superior pulmonary sulcus carcinoma resection: posterior approach. In Urschel HC Jr, Cooper JD [eds]: Atlas of Thoracic Surgery. New York, Churchill Livingstone, 1995.)

Closure of the Thoracotomy Incision

The chest is drained with two intercostal chest tubes inserted through separate stab incisions. The remaining lung is reinflated, with care taken to avoid torsion. Closure of the chest is then begun using pericostal sutures of 1 Vicryl. The individual muscle layers are reapproximated. The subcutaneous tissue is closed, and the skin is closed with a subcuticular suture.

COMMENTS AND CONTROVERSIES

With the popularization of the anterior approach (see next chapter), fewer superior sulcus tumors are approached in this classic way, unfortunately, because this does provide the best exposure to the posterior side, nerves, and vertebrae. Once this approach is well learned, every structure, except the subclavian vein, can be handled with ease.

ANTERIOR APPROACH TO APICAL LESIONS

Philippe Dartevelle
Paolo Macchiarini

HISTORICAL NOTES

Superior sulcus tumors, or lung neoplasms arising from either upper lobes (Paulson, 1973), may extend through the visceral pleura into the parietal pleura and the surrounding structures of the thoracic inlet and supraclavicular region. They usually are small-sized neoplasms situated at a definite location of the "thoracic inlet" (Pancoast, 1932) that evoke a characteristic clinical picture called Pancoast-Tobias syndrome (Teixeira, 1983; Tobias, 1931). The local nerve and bone involvement produces this syndrome at an early stage of the disease, generally before the mass is well defined radiographically and lymphatic and distant metastasis occurs (Shahian et al, 1987). For many years, these tumors were considered inoperable, and treatment consisted of palliative radiation therapy. However, during the last decades of the 20th century, it became evident that they could be caused by the combination of preoperative radiation therapy (30 Gy) followed by surgical resection (Devine et al, 1986; Miller et al, 1979; Pancoast, 1932; Paulson, 1989; Shaw et al, 1961; Standford et al, 1979). As reported by Shaw, Paulson, and Kee (1961), the operation consisted of an extended en bloc resection of the chest wall (usually including posterior portions of the first three ribs and their transverse processes), the intercostal nerves, and the lower trunk of the brachial plexus, together with the involved lung, resected usually by means of lobectomy or segmental resection and performed through a posterior interscapulovertebral approach. This combined treatment modality usually results in long-term survivals (5-year rates of approximately 30% to 34%) and cure for selected patients (Attar et al, 1998; Devine et al, 1986; Hagan et al, 1999; Miller et al, 1979; Paulson, 1989; Shaw et al, 1961; Standford et al, 1979). Presence of positive mediastinal lymph nodes and extensive vertebral body, brachial plexus, and subclavian vascular invasion represent poor prognostic factors and, thus, relative contraindications for surgical resection (Anderson et al, 1985; Ginsberg et al, 1994; Hagan et al, 1999).

Pancoast (1932) found it necessary to discard the term *apical chest tumors* from the *superior sulcus tumors*, which he had originally used in his paper in 1924 (Pancoast, 1924) "because it has proved to be confusing and has permitted the inclusion of other more common tumors of the upper part of the thorax." Therefore, apical tumors of the upper lobes, which in their natural history invade the thoracic inlet and concur to the Pancoast-Tobias syndrome with signs and symptoms of pulmonary, mediastinal, and inlet involvement, now include lesions of greater extent and stage of involvement than do the classic superior sulcus tumors (Paulson, 1973). Because of their locally advanced stage and impressive tendency to invade the structures lying in the thoracic inlet (Dartevelle et al, 1993), the difficulty and hazards of achieving a complete resection of the tumor-bearing inlet area (Macchiarini et al, 1993), and the surgery-related morbidity and mortality (Paulson, 1973), these larger apical tumors have represented an unresectable and an extremely dismal disease, usually treated by palliation or best supportive care.

Several years ago (Dartevelle et al, 1993), we described a combined cervicothoracic approach for the resection of these extensive apical lesions invading the thoracic inlet. In the course of our 15-year experience, we have learned how to perform the entire resection through the single cervical approach. We describe the procedure as it is done transclavicularly, including the technical modifications we made to resect the upper lobe along with the invaded bony, vascular, and soft tissues by the cervical anterior approach alone, without complementary thoracotomy.

SURGICAL ANATOMY

The insertion of the anterior, middle, and posterior scalenus muscles on the first and second ribs, respectively, divides the thoracic inlet into three compartments: an anterior (prescalenus) compartment containing the platysma and the sternocleidomastoid muscles; the external and anterior jugular veins; the inferior belly of the omohyoid muscle; the subclavian and internal jugular veins, and their major branches and the scalene fat pad; a middle (interscalenus) compartment containing the anterior scalenus muscle with the phrenic nerve lying on its anterior aspect, the subclavian artery with its primary branches except the posterior scapular artery, the trunks of the brachial plexus, and middle scalenus muscle; and a posterior compartment (extrascalenus), lying posteriorly to the middle scalenus muscles and including the long thoracic and external branch of the accessorius spinalis nerves, posterior scapular artery, sympathetic chain and stellate ganglion, vertebral bodies, spinal foramen, and epiduritis.

According to the level of involvement of the first rib, apical tumors might be classified as neoplasms that are anterior (invading the anterior part of the first rib, the subclavian vessels, the anterior scalenus muscle, and the phrenic nerve); middle (invading the middle part of the first rib, the middle scalenus muscle, and the trunks of the brachial plexus); and posterior (invading the vertebral bodies, the posterior part of the first ribs, the lower roots of the brachial plexus, the posterior wall and posterior branches of the subclavian artery).

CLINICAL FEATURES

The clinical features of apical tumors are influenced by their location and type of invasion of the thoracic inlet. Anterior apical tumors generally cause severe pain arising from the anterior chest wall, without radiation to the upper limb, that is related to the invasion of the first intercostal nerve and first ribs. They may cause phrenic nerve palsy and, to a lessen extent, ipsilateral superior vena cava hemisyndrome. These tumors usually do not invade the brachial plexus or other structures of the posterior inlet compartment.

Tumors invading the middle part of the thoracic inlet may cause signs and symptoms that are related to the compression or infiltration of the middle and lower trunks of the brachial plexus and manifest clinically with pain radiating to the shoulder and upper limb. These tumors may spread along the fibers of the middle scalenus muscle.

Posterior tumors usually occur with all the signs and symptoms of the Pancoast-Tobias syndrome and are usually located in the costovertebral groove, invading the nerve roots of T1, the posterior aspect of the subclavian and vertebral artery, the sympathetic chain, the stellate ganglion, and the prevertebral muscles. The severity of this form is linked to their potential spread to the vertebral body or along the neurolemma of the T1 and T2 nerve roots up to the spinal canal through the intervertebral foramina of the first three thoracic vertebrae.

STAGING

Any patient presenting with signs and symptoms evoking the involvement of the thoracic inlet should undergo a careful and detailed preoperative workup to establish a diagnosis of apical carcinoma of the lung and to determine operability, because the Pancoast-Tobias syndrome (Teixeira, 1983) might result from malignancies other than apical lung tumors (Macchiarini et al, 1993), such as metastases.

The diagnosis is established by history and physical examination, biochemical profile, chest radiograph, bronchoscopy and sputum cytology, fine needle transthoracic or transcutaneous biopsy and aspiration, and computed tomography (CT) of the chest. A video-assisted thoracoscopy might be indicated to obtain tissue proof when the other investigations are negative and to eliminate the presence of pleural metastatic diffusion. If there is evidence of mediastinal lymphadenopathy on chest radiograph or CT scanning, mediastinoscopy is mandatory, because patients with clinical N2 disease are not suitable for operation. Neurologic examination, electromyography, and magnetic resonance imaging are often required to delineate the tumor's extension to the brachial plexus, phrenic nerve, and dura, whereas vascular invasion can be studied using venous angiography, subclavian arteriography, doppler ultrasonography (cerebrovascular disorders might contraindicate the sacrifice of the vertebral artery), and magnetic resonance imaging. Fluoroscopy can be performed to search for paralysis of the phrenic nerve. The initial workup also includes all preoperative cardiopulmonary functional tests routinely performed before any major lung parenchymal resection and investigative procedures delineating the extrathoracic extension of the disease.

INDICATIONS

Absolute surgical contraindications are the presence of extrathoracic sites of metastasis and clinically and histologically confirmed mediastinal lymph node involvement. Invasion of the brachial plexus above T1 as supported by sensory or, even worse, motor deficits in the nerve distribution of the median and radial nerves also indicates inoperability. Such extensive invasion of the brachial plexus above T1 should be considered a contraindication. Extensive involvement of the subclavian vessels is not a contraindication provided a complete surgical resection may be anticipated. Patients whose tumors abut the vertebral body should not be deemed inoperable unless invasion of the spinal canal through the intervertebral foramina is confirmed by magnetic resonance imaging. The role of palliative incomplete resection is highly questionable and appears to be without any individual benefit.

OPERATIVE TECHNIQUE

The patient is placed in the supine position with the neck hyperextended and the head turned away from the involved side. A bolster is placed behind the shoulder to elevate the operative field. The skin preparation extends from the mastoid downwards to the xiphoid process and between both middle axillary lines laterally. An adhesive plastic draping is then placed over the skin.

An L-shaped incision cervicotomy is made and includes a vertical presternocleidmastoid incision prolonged horizontally below the clavicle up to the deltopectoral groove. However, to increase the exposure and perform the entire resection through this incision only, the interception between the vertical and horizontal branches of the L-shaped incision is lowered at the level of the second or third intercostal space, as shown in Figure 36–63. The incision is then deepened with cautery. Division of the sternal attachment of the sternocleidomastoid muscle is made, and this muscle, along with the upper muscle fibers of the pectoralis major, is scraped from the clavicle, creating a well-vascularized myocutaneous flap that, once folded back, gives a full exposure of the neck, the thoracic inlet, and the upper part of the anterolateral chest wall. Once the inferior belly of the omohyoid muscle is transected, the scalene fat pad is dissected and pathologically examined to exclude scalene lymph node micrometastasis. Inspection of the ipsilateral superior mediastinum is then made by the operator's finger along the lateral aspect of the tracheoesophageal groove. Extension of tumor to the thoracic inlet is then carefully assessed. We recommend resection of the internal half of the clavicle only if the tumor is deemed resectable.

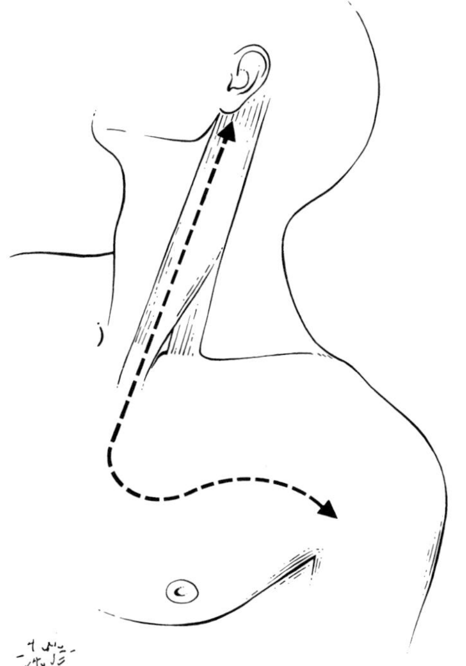

FIGURE 36–63 ■ A left L-shaped cervicotomy incision is made and includes a vertical presternocleidomastoid incision prolonged horizontally below the clavicle up to the deltopectoral groove. However, to increase the exposure and make the entire resection through this incision only, the interception between the vertical and the horizontal branches of the L-shaped incision is lowered at the level of the second or third intercostal space, as indicated by the level of tumoral invasion.

Dissection of the Subclavian Vein

Jugular veins are first dissected, so that branches to the subclavian vein can eventually be divided. On the left side, ligation of the thoracic duct is usually required. Division of the distal part of the internal, external, and anterior jugular veins makes the visualization of the venous confluence at the origin of the innominate vein easier (Fig. 36–64). We do not hesitate to suture-ligate the internal jugular vein to increase the exposure to the subclavian vein. If the subclavian vein is involved, it can be easily resected after proximal and distal control has been achieved. Direct extension to the innominate vein does not preclude resection, because this vessel may be removed.

Next, the scalenus anterior muscle is divided either at its insertion on the scalene tubercle on the first rib or in tumor-free margins with cautery. If the tumor has invaded the upper part of this muscle, it needs to be divided at the insertion on the anterior tubercles of the transverse processes of C3 through C6. Before dealing with the anterior scalenus muscle, the status of the phrenic nerve is carefully assessed, because its unnecessary division has a deleterious influence on the postoperative course. It should be preserved whenever possible (Fig. 36–65).

Dissection of the Subclavian Artery

The subclavian artery is then dissected. To improve its mobilization, its branches are divided (Fig. 36–66); the vertebral artery is resected only if invaded and provided that no significant extracranial occlusive disease was detected on preoperative doppler ultrasound. If the tumor rests against the wall of the subclavian artery, the artery can be freed following a subadventitial plane. If there is an invasion of the arterial wall, resection of the artery, in obtaining at least a 2-cm tumor-free margin is necessary; this will also facilitate further resection. After its proximal and distal cross-clamping, the artery is divided on either side (Fig. 36–67). Revascularization is performed with an end-to-end anastomosis or, less frequently, with a polytetrafluoroethylene ringed graft (6- or 8-mm). During these maneuvers, the pleural space might be opened by dividing the Sibson's fascia (a fascia on the deep surface of the scalenus muscles forming a subpleural membrane arching over the cupola of the pleura).

Dissection of the Brachial Plexus

The middle scalenus muscle is divided above its insertion on the first rib or higher as indicated by the extension of the tumor. It might require, especially for apical tumors invading the middle compartment of the thoracic inlet, division of its insertions on the posterior tubercles of the transverse processes of the second through seventh

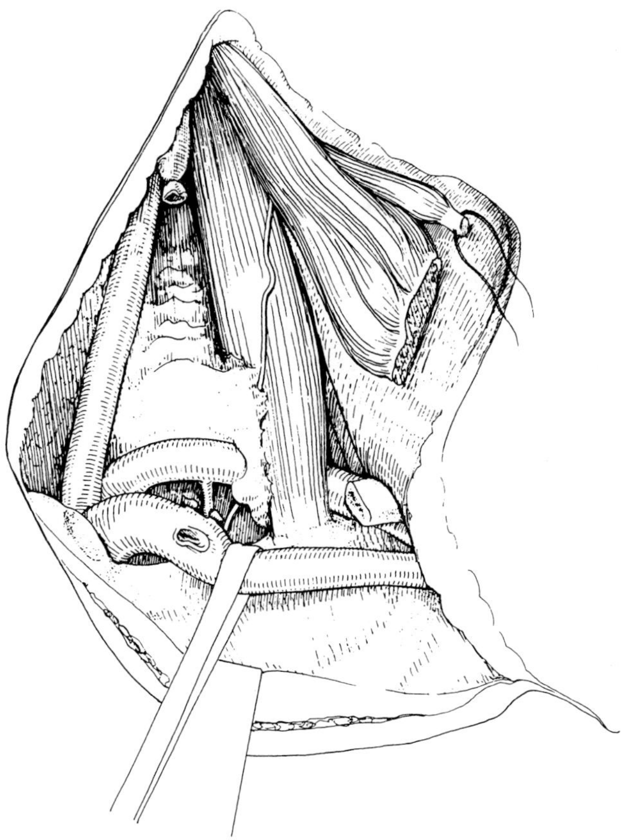

FIGURE 36–64 ■ Illustrative view after division of the sternal head of the sternocleidomastoid and the inferior belly of the omohyoid muscles, with resection of the scalene fat pad and the internal half of the clavicle. Thereafter, the exposure, dissection, and division of the external and internal jugular vein greatly facilitates the exposure of the subclavian vein and permits assessment of tumor resectability.

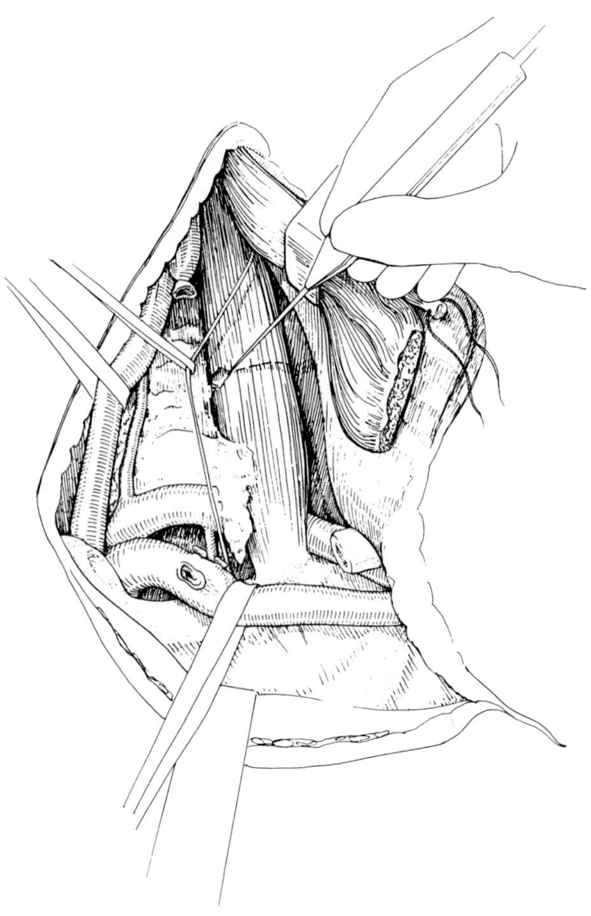

FIGURE 36–65 ■ The subclavian artery is exposed after division of the insertion of the anterior scalenus muscle on the first rib; the phrenic nerve is protected and preserved. (From Dartevelle P, Chapelier A, Macchiarini P et al: Anterior transcervical approach for radical resection of lung tumors invading the thoracic inlet. J Thorac Cardiovasc Surg 105:1025, 1993.)

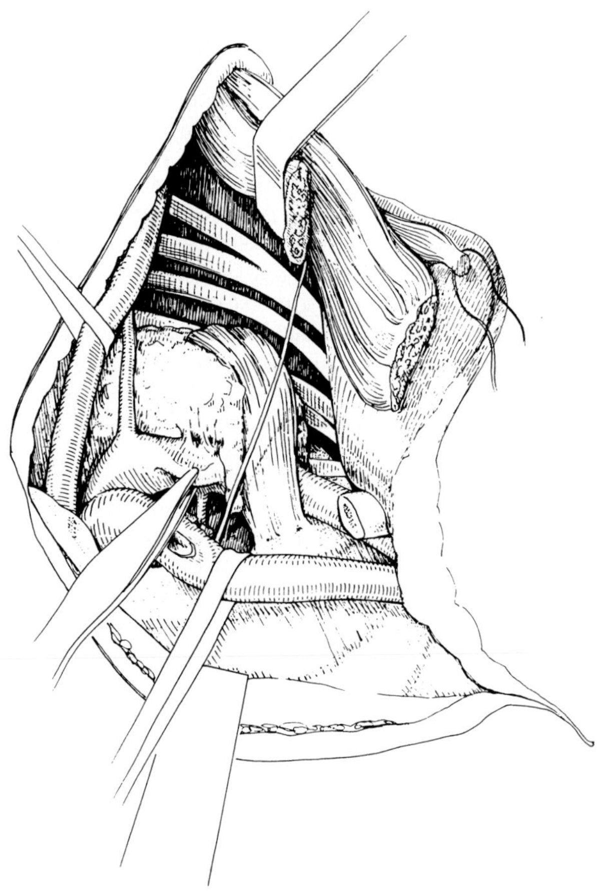

FIGURE 36–66 ■ The retraction of the anterior scalenus muscles allows the identification of the interscalenic trunks of the brachial plexus; the subclavian artery may be gently freed from the tumor by dividing all collateral branches (the vertebral artery is generally preserved, if not invaded). (From Dartevelle P, Chapelier A, Macchiarini P et al: Anterior transcervical approach for radical resection of lung tumors invading the thoracic inlet. J Thorac Cardiovasc Surg 105:1025, 1993.)

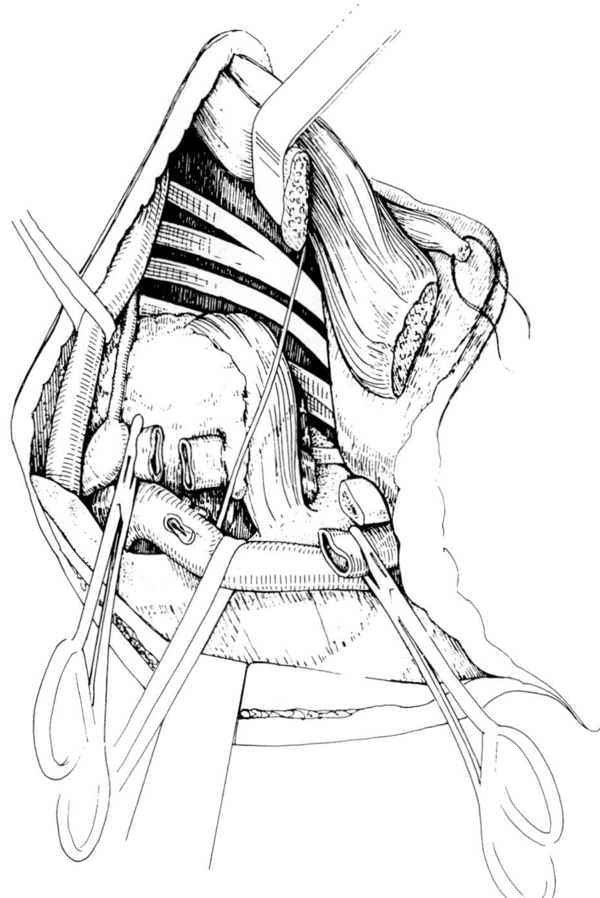

FIGURE 36–67 ■ If involved by the tumor, the subclavian artery might be divided after its proximal and distal control. (From Dartevelle P, Chapelier A, Macchiarini P et al: Anterior transcervical approach for radical resection of lung tumors invading the thoracic inlet. J Thorac Cardiovasc Surg 105:1025, 1993.)

cervical vertebrae. The nerve roots of C8 and T1 are then easily identified and dissected in an "out-to-in-side" fashion from the origin of the lower trunk of the brachial plexus to the emergence of the vertebral foramina.

Thereafter, the prevertebral muscles are systematically detached together with the dorsal sympathetic chain and stellate ganglion from the anterior surface of the vertebral bodies of C7 and T1 (Fig. 36–68). This permits visualization of the intervertebral foramina. The T1 nerve root is usually divided beyond visible tumor, just lateral to the T1 intervertebral foramen. Although tumor spread to the brachial plexus may be extensive, neurolysis can usually be achieved without division of the nerve roots above T1 (Fig. 36–69). Damage of the lateral and long thoracic nerves may result in winged scapula.

Pulmonary Resection

Before performing the pulmonary resection, the chest wall resection is completed. The anterolateral arch of the first rib is divided at the costochondral junction while the second rib, unless involved more anteriorly, is divided at the level of its middle arch and the third is scraped on the superior border toward the costovertebral angle (Fig. 36–70). Then the specimen is progressively freed. The first ribs are then disarticulated from the transverse processes of the first two or three thoracic vertebrae.

It is through this hole created by the bony resection that the operation is completed by an en bloc upper lobectomy (Fig. 36–71). Through experience, we have come to favor upper lobectomies rather than limited resections.

Tumors involving the transverse process (Fig. 36–72*A*) can be resected through the cervical approach; the maneuver used is similar to what is used in the posterior approach, but from the front to the back, with a finger placed behind the transverse process of T1 and T2 to give the correct direction to the chisel. We recommend maintaining meticulous hemostasis throughout the procedure to ensure a clear visual exposure at all times, and careful inspection and verification of all vascular structures previously resected or ligated should be done to prevent postoperative hemorrhage and lymphatic leakage. The cervical incision is closed in two layers after the

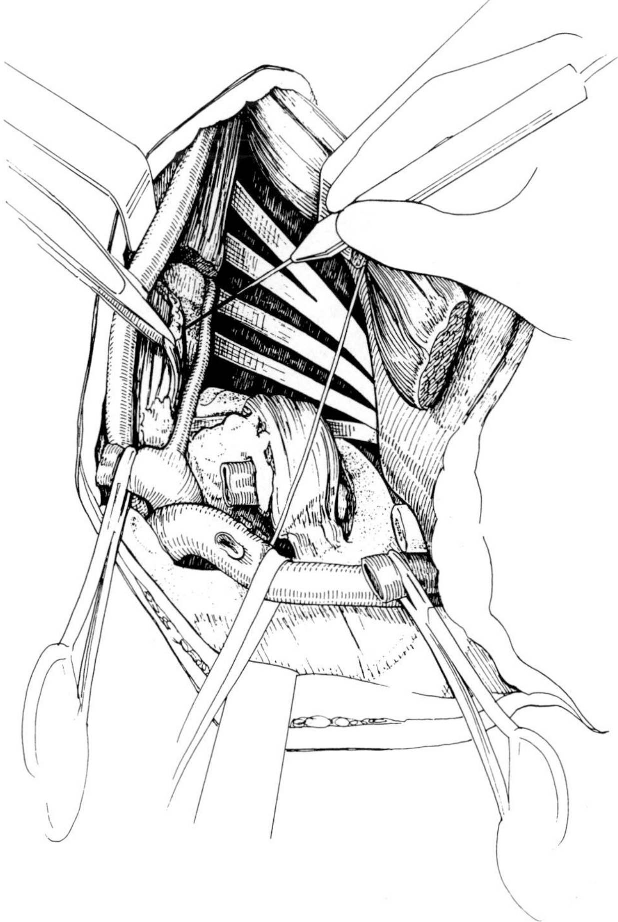

FIGURE 36–68 ■ The prevertebral muscles are extensively detached from the vertebral bodies and both the stellate ganglion and the dorsal sympathetic chain are isolated and finally released, using raspatories, from all surrounding attachments. (From Dartevelle P, Chapelier A, Macchiarini P et al: Anterior transcervical approach for radical resection of lung tumors invading the thoracic inlet. J Thorac Cardiovasc Surg 105:1025, 1993.)

sternal insertion of the sternocleidomastoid muscle is sutured, and a conventional drain for the ipsilateral chest cavity is placed.

Vertebral Resections

One of the limits of the surgery for apical tumors is the spread of the tumor to the vertebral body, as mainly observable in posteriorly located apical lesions. This does not mean, however, that one should resect tumors extending inside the spinal canal but only those abutting the costovertebral angle or extending into the intervertebral foramen without intraspinal extension (Fig. 36–72*B* and *C*). Two (anterior and midline posterior) cervical approaches must be combined to perform a hemivertebrectomy (usually, T1–T3), followed by spinal fixation with metal rods interposed between screws placed into the vertebral pedicles.

The anterior approach is begun first to (1) assess operability; (2) safely dissect the anterolateral aspects of the invaded vertebra(e) in tumor-free margins to be subsequently individualizable from the posterior approach; (3) mark with cautery the anterior aspect of the involved vertebra so that during the posterior operative approach it can be used as a guide of the extent of resection; and (4) perform the lobectomy and the anterior resection of the chest wall as described earlier. Following completion of this anterior approach, the patient is placed in a prone position and a median vertical incision is performed at the level of the cervicothoracic junction. After a unilateral laminectomy on three levels, the nerve roots are divided inside the spinal canal at the emergence of the external sheath covering the spinal cord. After dividing the vertebral bodies in the midline, the specimen is resected en bloc with the lung, ribs, and vessels through this midline posterior incision. On the side of the tumor, the spinal fixation stabilizes the pedicle above and below the resected hemivertebrae; on the contralateral side, all remaining pedicles may be used for fixation.

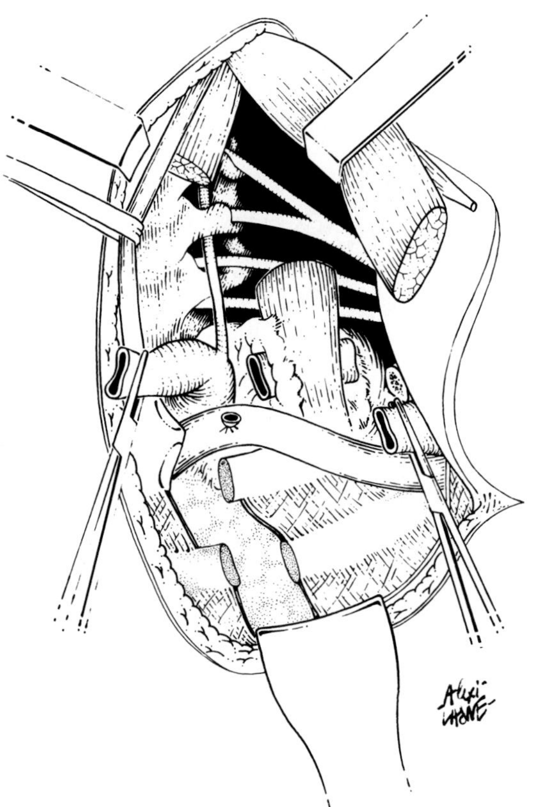

FIGURE 36–70 ■ Once structures above the thoracic inlet are freed from the tumor, the first two ribs can be separated anteriorly at the chondrocostal junction and resected posteriorly in tumor-free margins. The third rib is scraped on its superior border toward the costovertebral angle and retracted inferiorly.

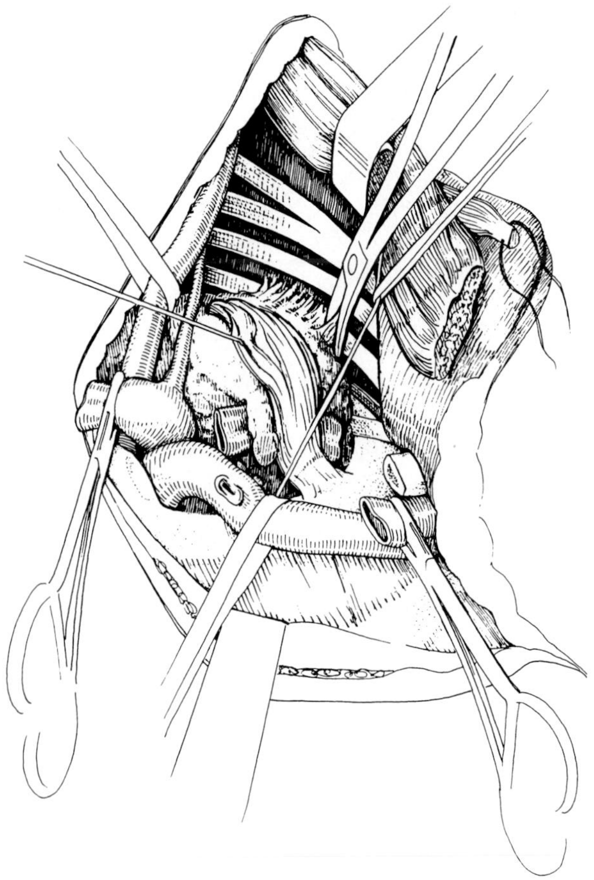

FIGURE 36–69 ■ The tumor's involvement of the brachial plexus requires an inside-out neurolysis, if the upper trunks are involved, or, a resection of T1, if the lower trunk or nerve roots are involved. (From Dartevelle P, Chapelier A, Macchiarini P et al: Anterior transcervical approach for radical resection of lung tumors invading the thoracic inlet. J Thorac Cardiovasc Surg 105:1025, 1993.)

SURGICAL COMPLICATIONS AND POSTOPERATIVE CARE

The surgical complications of patients undergoing resection of apical tumors are similar to any patient undergoing a major pulmonary resection. However, specific complications are:

1. Spinal fluid leakage should be suspected whenever clear fluid drains from the chest tubes. It can have cata-

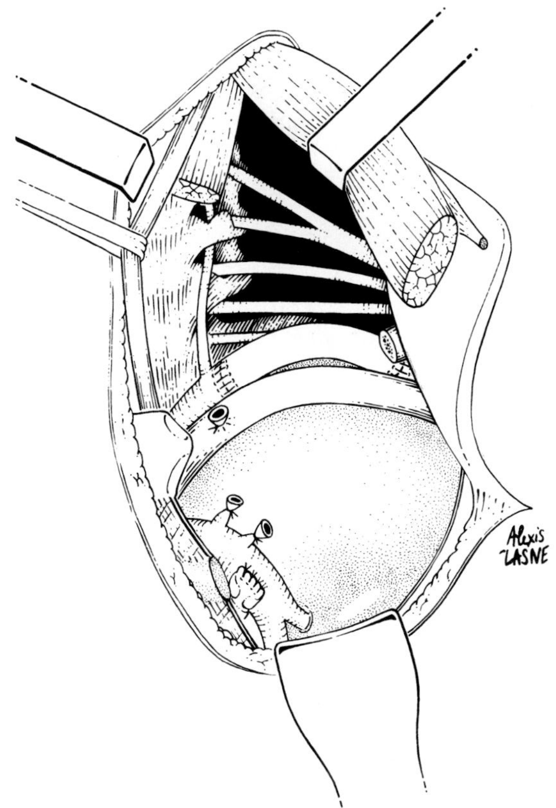

FIGURE 36–71 ■ Completion of the subclavian artery revascularization and upper lobectomy through the cervical incision alone.

strophic consequences, because the direct communication of the intervertebral foramina with the pleural space can facilitate air embolism into the subarachnoid space, ventricles, and central canal of the brain and spinal cord. Reoperation is mandatory and the leakage should be closed with the technical options listed above; exceptionally, a cerebral ventriculovenous derivation may be required.

2. Horner's syndrome and nerve deficits, which should be discussed with the patient preoperatively, may occur. Division of the T1 nerve root is usually well tolerated without significant muscle palsy in the nerve territory. By contrast, the resection of the lower trunk of the brachial plexus (T1 and C8) may result in an atrophic paralysis of the forearm and small muscles of the hand with paralysis of the cervical sympathetic system (Klumpke-Déjérine syndrome). However, relief of the preoperative pain is far more important than the neurologic deficit created by the operation, and adaptation is surprisingly good.

3. Hemothorax may occur as the result of the chest wall resection and difficulty and risks of securing the small veins at the level of the intervertebral foramina.

4. Chylothorax is a possible complication and should be avoided by individual ligation of the thoracic duct and its branches. If it occurs, it usually can be managed by continued chest tube drainage and expansion of the lung.

The postoperative course is usually characterized by atelectasis because patients have an extended chest wall resection associated either with phrenic nerve resection or extensive manipulation. Treatment involves measures to achieve complete lung expansion by ensuring

1. Adequate ventilation using mechanical support if necessary;
2. Satisfactory chest tube function;
3. Clear secretion by mobilizing, coughing, chest physiotherapy, nasotracheal or orotracheal suctioning, or suctioning through a bronchoscope or a temporary tracheostomy;
4. Adequate analgesia (epidural catheter, patient-controlled analgesia);
5. Increased transpulmonary pressure with incentive spirometry or continuous positive airway pressure mask.

Although fluid compensation is necessary, fluid overload should be avoided, and diuretics should be used judiciously to avoid acute respiratory distress. Chest tubes remain in place until all air leaks have stopped, there is complete lung expansion, and drainage is less than 100 ml/24 hr (usually within 24 to 72 h). The presence of an incomplete lung expansion with persistent intrapleural air space will ultimately be filled with serous fluid.

SUMMARY

Over the last 20 years, 70 patients (mean age, 53 ± 12 years) presenting with malignant bronchogenic apical lesions were operated on using this approach. Most of the lesions were of nonsquamous histology (n = 51), right-sided (n = 41), and extending to the anterior (n = 23), middle (n = 5), or posterior (n = 42) compartments of the thoracic inlet. All tumors were completely resected through the anterior approach, either alone (n = 33) or with (n = 37) an additional posterior approach (early on in our experience). Forty-seven lobectomies, 21 wedge resections, and 2 pneumonectomies were employed. Most (n = 55) of the patients were without pathologic diseased lymph nodes, whereas 5, 7, and 3 patients had, respectively, N1, N2, or N3 disease. The 28 invaded subclavian arteries were revascularized 16 times by a synthetic graft and 12 by an end-to-end anastomosis; nine vertebral arteries were also invaded and resected. The T1 nerve root was invaded either alone (n = 25) or along with the phrenic nerve (n = 21). The first rib was invaded and resected in all patients either alone (n = 8) or with the 2nd (n = 29), 3rd (n = 17), 4th (n = 15), and 5th (n = 1) ribs. There were no hospital deaths. The overall 5- and 10-year survivals were 35% and 20%, respectively, and the only predictor of long-term, disease-free survival was the presence of N2 disease. The 2-year survival for 13 patients requiring a hemivertebrectomy was 59%.

CONCLUSIONS

The enhancement of these long-term results reflects the technical improvements and more aggressive surgical attitude that we have had over the last years. The procedure has become a real en bloc exenteration of the lateral cervicothoracic junction including the scalene fat pad,

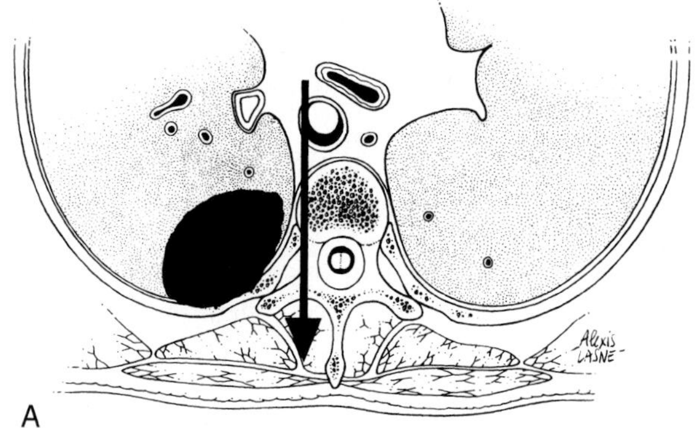

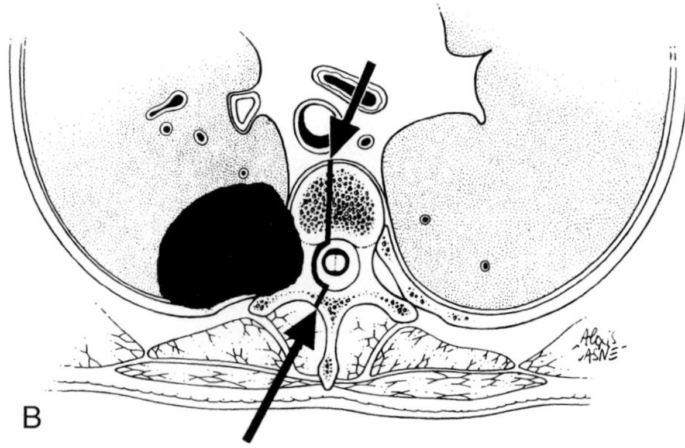

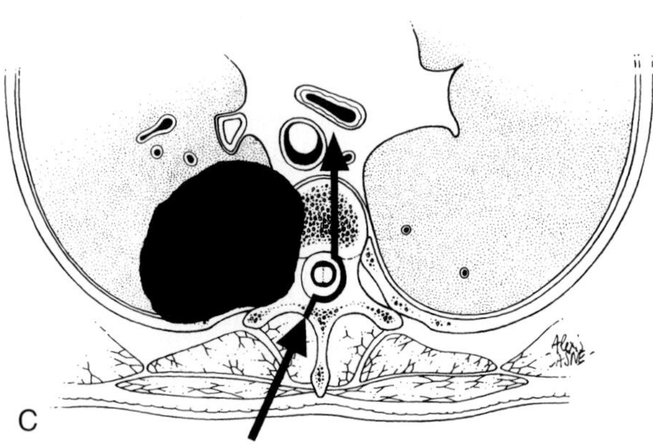

FIGURE 36–72 ■ Different types of vertebral invasion. *A*, A right-sided apical tumor involving the posterior arch of the rib only and resected from the anterior cervical approach by a vertical en bloc resection of part of the lateral vertebral body, the costotransverse space, and the transverse process. This procedure is entirely done through a single anterior approach with a finger placed behind the transverse processes of T1 and T2. *B*, A right-sided apical tumor involving the costotransverse space and the intervertebral foramen and part of the ipsilateral vertebral body; this tumor is first approached anteriorly as described in the text, and the operation is completed through a hemivertebrectomy performed through the posterior midline approach. *C*, A right-sided apical tumor involving the costotransverse space, the intervertebral foramen, and the vertebral body (to a greater extent than that in *B*). Following completion of the anterior step of the procedure, an extended hemivertebrectomy to include part of the contralateral vertebral hemibody is made through a posterior midline approach, as depicted here. The vertebral stability is reaccomplished by spinal fixation with metal rods interposed between screws placed into the vertebral pedicles.

the prevertebral muscles, the dorsal sympathetic chain, and the stellate ganglion from the anterior surface of the vertebral bodies of C7 and T1, the upper mediastinal lymph nodes, and the upper lobectomy. Even the invasion of the extracranial cervical vessels does not contraindicate operation and long-term patency results are now well established (Fadel et al, 1999). Although our preliminary results are encouraging, vertebral invasion limited to less than 2 body levels should not be considered a surgical contraindication. Only when necessary do we remove the internal half of the clavicle, keeping in mind that it may be better to remove it to perform a safe and more radical exenteration and the entire operation through the anterior approach alone.

These technical advances have allowed us to perform the entire procedure through the anterior approach, even for posterior-based lesions, in 15 patients. Because of the evident benefit derived from the avoidance of a complementary posterior thoracotomy, this anterior approach alone has become our standard.

COMMENTS AND CONTROVERSIES

The authors have further refined their anterior approach to superior sulcus tumors and truly have excellent results. With increasing experience, they now perform all of their resections through an anterior approach unless a hemivertebrectomy is required. It is interesting to note that they appear to have significant postoperative pulmonary complications, almost certainly related to the fact that they do not employ a plastic reconstruction when two or more ribs are resected. We certainly prefer this, using either taut Gore-Tex or a Marlex methylmethacrylate sandwich applied to all but the first rib when using the anterior approach.

The anterior approach has been modified by many authors. A hemi-clamshell incision or a modified hemi-clamshell can be used incising the very lateral margins of the sternum. Both of these approaches are more likely to preserve the clavicle. In our own practice, we prefer the hemi-clamshell thoracotomy with a sternomastoid extension. With this anterior approach, the clavicle is always preserved, unless invaded, and only the affected ribs are removed.

Although not stated, the authors do not employ preoperative radiotherapy or chemoradiotherapy and, if the resection is complete, no postoperative treatment. In North America, the most frequent approach is preoperative radiotherapy and, more recently, chemoradiation.

R.J.G.

■ REFERENCES

Anderson TM, Moy PM, Holmes EC: Factors affecting survival in superior sulcus tumors. J Clin Oncol 4:1598, 1985.

Attar S, Krasna MJ, Sonett JR et al: Superior sulcus (Pancoast) tumor: Experience with 105 patients. Ann Thorac Surg 66:193, 1998.

Dartevelle P, Chapelier A, Macchiarini P et al: Anterior transcervical-thoracic approach for radical resection of lung tumors invading the thoracic inlet. J Thorac Cardiovasc Surg 105:1025, 1993.

Devine JW, Mendenhall WM, Million RR, Carmichael MJ: Carcinoma of the superior pulmonary sulcus treated with surgery and/or radiation therapy. Cancer 57:941, 1986.

Fadel E, Chapelier A, Cerrina J et al: Subclavian artery and reconstruction for thoracic inlet cancers. J Vasc Surg 28:581, 1999.

Ginsberg RJ, Martini N, Zaman M et al: Influence of surgical resection and brachytherapy in the management of superior sulcus tumor. Ann Thorac Surg 57:1440, 1994.

Hagan MP, Choi NC, Mathisen DJ et al: Superior sulcus tumors: Impact of local control on survival. J Thorac Cardiovasc Surg 117:1086, 1999.

Macchiarini P, Dartevelle P, Chapelier A et al: Surgical management of non-bronchogenic tumors invading the thoracic outlet. Ann Thorac Surg 55:611, 1993.

Miller JI, Mansour KA, Hatcher CR: Carcinoma of the superior pulmonary sulcus. Ann Thorac Surg 28:44, 1979.

Pancoast HK: Importance of careful roentgen-ray investigations of apical chest tumors. JAMA 83:1407, 1924.

Pancoast HK: Superior sulcus tumors. JAMA 99:1391, 1932.

Paulson DL: The importance of defining location and staging of superior pulmonary sulcus tumors. Ann Thorac Surg 15:549, 1973.

Paulson DL: Carcinomas in the superior pulmonary sulcus. J Thorac Cardiovasc 70:1095, 1975.

Paulson DL: General Thoracic Surgery. Philadelphia, Lea & Febiger, 1989.

Shahian DM, Wildford BN, Ellis FH Jr: Pancoast tumors: Improved survival with preoperative and postoperative radiotherapy. Ann Thorac Surg 43:32, 1987.

Shaw RR, Paulson DL, Kee JL Jr: Treatment of the superior sulcus tumor by irradiation followed by resection. Ann Surg 154:29, 1961.

Standford W, Barnes RP, Tucker AR: Influence of staging in superior sulcus (Pancoast) tumors of the lung. Ann Thorac Surg 29:406, 1979.

Teixeira JP: Concerning the Pancoast tumor: What is the superior pulmonary sulcus? Ann Thorac Surg 35:577, 1983.

Tobias JW: Sindrome apico-costo-vertebral-doloroso por tumor apexiano: Su valor diagnostico en el cancer primitivo del pulmon. Buenos Aires, Tese, Imp. Mercatali., 1931.

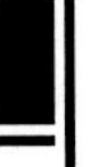

EXTENDED PULMONARY RESECTIONS

G. Alexander Patterson

As neoplasms of the lung grow, they may infiltrate tissues or contiguous organs and structures. The most commonly invaded structures are the chest wall, The vertebral bodies, the diaphragm, the aorta, the left atrium, the pericardium, the esophagus, and the superior vena cava. In those situations in which invasion of lung carcinomas extends beyond the visceral pleura, the ability to resect the contiguous invaded structure or organ varies greatly. The prognosis is directly related to the completeness of the resection and the presence of nodal metastases. Resection techniques for each structure are discussed later.

HISTORICAL NOTE

Carcinoma of the lung is the most frequent cause of cancer deaths in both men and women. Lung cancers invade the chest wall in 5% of cases, which amounted to 8250 cases in 1992. Approximately 1% to 2% invade vertebral bodies, diaphragm, pericardium, esophagus, and superior vena cava.

In 1899, Parham was the first to describe a successful resection of a chest wall tumor in the American literature. He stressed leaving an intact parietal pleura, lest the normal respiratory function be interrupted and death result.

In 1943, Graham and colleagues produced a thoracic surgical manual that standardized the surgical approach for chest wall injuries, on the basis of experience gained during World War I. The gravity of a sucking chest wound was recognized and immediate closure to maintain ventilation was urged. Surrounding soft tissues were used to close the defect. These authors also recommended tube thoracostomy for drainage and ventilation purposes.

Brewer (1983) chronicled his experience during World War II, applying these principles and improving their application. Resection of a portion of the lung in continuity with the chest wall invaded by the tumor is now commonplace. Early chest wall resections were performed when the resulting defect was small. This defect was bridged by a variety of materials, including dura mater, fascia lata, or fascia, and, more recently, Marlex mesh. Rigid materials, including autogenous ribs and metal struts, have also been used. If a large defect occurred, the Marlex mesh and fascia-like materials did not prevent a respiratory flail, and patients remained on respirator support for prolonged periods. This changed in 1974 with the introduction of the Marlex mesh—polymethylmethacrylate prosthesis.

Reconstruction techniques using materials that are readily available, are adaptable to any size and contour needed, and are integrated by the body tissues with little reaction. Low infection rates were reported by McCormack and co-workers (1981) using a mesh with polymethylmethacrylate.

Sundaresan and others (1985) described the technique and results of resections of a vertebral body in continuity with a lung cancer. This requires collaboration among neurosurgeons and orthopedic and thoracic surgeons.

Complete sleeve resections of the vena cava, with reconstruction by varying techniques, uniformly failed until Chu and colleagues in 1974 and Doty in 1982 described the construction of a spiral vein graft. Long-term patency rates improved, but the intrinsic complexity of this technique prevented widespread acceptance. Dartevelle and associates in 1987 detailed the use of a polytetrafluoroethylene (Gore-Tex) graft with proven patency if used as a venous substitute when resecting the superior vena cava because of tumor.

Dartevelle and others (1991) used a Gore-Tex graft for vena cava reconstruction combined with a right pneumonectomy in six patients with lung cancer. Two of the six lived 16 and 51 months, respectively; the median survival of the four others was 13 months. All grafts remained patent in this series.

■ *HISTORICAL READINGS*

Brewer LA III: The contributions of the Second Auxiliary Surgical Group to military surgery during World War II with special reference to thoracic surgery. Ann Surg 197:318, 1983.

Chu CJ, Tazis H, MacRae ML: Replacement of superior vena cava with the spiral composite vein graft. Ann Thorac Surg 17:553, 1974.

Dartevelle P, Chapelier A, Navajas M et al: Replacement of the superior vena cava with polytetrafluoroethylene grafts combined with resection of mediastinal-pulmonary malignancy: Report of 13 cases. J Thorac Cardiovasc Surg 94:361, 1987.

Dartevelle PJ, Chapelier AR, Pastorino U et al: Long-term follow-up after prosthetic replacement of the superior vena cava combined with resection of mediastinal-pulmonary malignant tumors. J Thorac Cardiovasc Surg 102:259, 1991.

Doty DB: Bypass of superior vena cava: Six year's experience with spiral vein graft for obstruction of superior vena cava due to benign and malignant disease. J Thorac Cardiovasc Surg 83:326, 1982.

Graham EV, Bigger IA, Churchill EO, Eloesser L: Thoracic Surgery. Philadelphia, WB Saunders, 1943.

McCormack PM, Bains MS, Beattie EJ et al: New trends in skeletal reconstruction after resection of chest wall tumors. Ann Thorac Surg 31:45, 1981.

Parham DW: Thoracic resections for tumors growing from the bony chest wall. Trans South Surg Assoc 2:223, 1899.

Sundaresan N, Bains MS, McCormack PM: Surgical treatment of spinal cord compression in patients with lung cancer. Neurosurgery 16:350, 1985.

CHEST WALL INVASION

The most reliable predictor of chest wall invasion is chest pain. Radiographic demonstration of chest wall invasion is not reliable unless clear evidence of chest wall soft tissue or bony invasion is demonstrated by computed tomography (CT) or magnetic resonance imaging (MRI) (Fig. 36–73). Occasionally, involved ribs will enhance on nuclear bone scan. If resection is contemplated, accurate staging is essential. N2 disease must be excluded. Several authors have demonstrated that long-term survival will not be achieved in patients undergoing resection of T3 tumors in the presence of N2 disease (Chapelier 2000; Patterson 1982; Trastek 1984). Therefore, mediastinoscopy is mandatory if chest wall invasion is suspected.

The goal of surgery when lung cancer invades the chest wall is complete resection and reconstruction of the chest wall when necessary. Frequently reconstruction is not required because the chest wall defect is often beneath the scapula or chest wall musculature and does not require reconstruction for cosmesis or chest wall stability. However, for anterolateral or anterior defects,

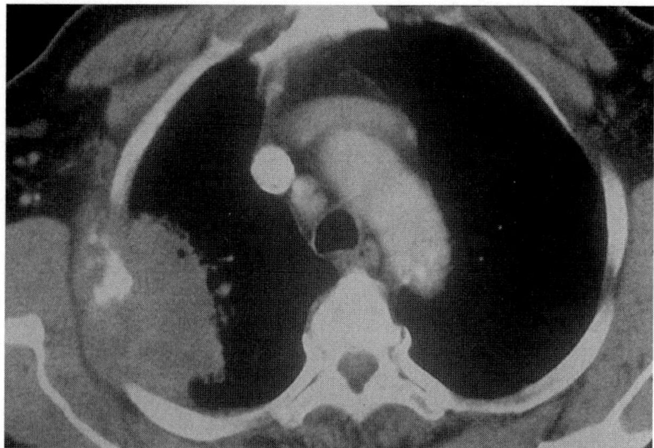

FIGURE 36–73 ■ A computed tomography scan showing obvious extension of a primary bronchogenic carcinoma through full-thickness chest wall. Note the convexity of the tumor mass outside the skeletal chest wall. Also note the large right paratracheal lymph node. In this patient, mediastinoscopy revealed N2 disease, contraindicating any attempt at resection.

standard techniques of reconstruction are employed. These are thoroughly discussed in Chapter 55.

SURGICAL ASSESSMENT

In cases in which chest wall invasion is suspected, the chest should initially be explored through an aspect of the incision that is away from the area of suspected invasion. Careful digital palpation of the pleural surface will confirm the location and extent of the tumor. Chest wall invasion is usually evident by the degree of fixation of the primary tumor to the chest wall. If fixation is not firm, the adhesion is likely due to inflammatory fibrosis. In this situation, an extrapleural plane can easily be developed over the area of adherence. If the parietal pleura dissects away easily, tumor invasion further into the chest wall is usually not present. Frozen section examination of the pleural surface under suspicion is essential to confirm tumor-free margins on the outer pleural surface.

TECHNICAL CONSIDERATIONS

If rigid fixation is present, an extrapleural plane is difficult to accomplish or if there is any doubt, chest wall invasion should be assumed and an en bloc chest wall resection should be performed. It is usually easier from a technical point of view to conduct the chest wall resection first from outside-in with a minimum of 3-cm margins. When the chest wall detachment is complete, the anatomic resection of lung can then be conducted either through the chest wall defect or through the initial exploration thoracotomy. Lesser pulmonary resections by wedge or segmentectomy are associated with an increased likelihood of local recurrence (Ginsberg 1994). The anatomic pulmonary resection should be accompanied by a thorough lymph node sampling or dissection to accurately stage the tumor. For lesions involving the lateral chest wall, resection of one rib above and one rib below plus three to five centimeters anterior and posterior to the tumor should be resected to maximize the opportunity for complete resection. Frozen section confirmation of complete resection should be also obtained. Invasion of rib cancelling bone is not an indication for complete resection of the affected rib because the margins described above are generally sufficient to provide an R0 resection, although this has never been studied.

For posterior and lateral defects beneath the scapula, chest wall reconstruction is not required. However, if the fifth rib is removed, some sort of prosthetic replacement using Marlex, Gore-Tex, or Dacron should be employed to prevent the scapular tip from falling into the chest over the top of the posterior sixth rib. If reconstruction is undertaken for posterior superior defects, curved chest contour is not required. However, for more anterior or lateral defects, a contoured rigid reconstruction is preferable and can be accomplished by a combination of Marlex and methylmethacrylate, which has been described by several authors. Others believe that a taut 2-mm Gore-Tex graft is sufficient. Unless this type of patch is overlayed by a myocutaneous flap, it will cause a deformity. As well, it will cause a temporary flail segment. In the Mayo Clinic experience, using Gore-Tex grafts exclusively, a significant number of patients postoperatively required ventilation and, in fact, the mortality rate of their group's experience was extremely high (Fig. 36–74).

RESULTS

Several reports have demonstrated acceptable long-term survival in patients undergoing resection of bronchogenic carcinoma with chest wall invasion. Patterson and colleagues (1982) reported a 5-year survival rate of 32.9%. Trastek and colleagues (1984) reported a 5-year survival figure of 39.7%. The Memorial Sloan-Kettering Cancer Center reported their experience in 1985. In 125 patients, 5-year survival was directly related to completeness of resection (42% versus 0), the absence of lymph node metastasis (56% versus 20%), and depth of chest wall invasion (50% versus 16% for those with full-thickness chest wall invasion). Chapelier and colleagues (2000) reported their experience in 100 consecutive patients who underwent radical en bloc resection of lung and chest wall. Survival was less satisfactory than it was in other reports with 5-year survival for patients with N0, N1, and N2 disease—22.9% and 0, respectively. In this report, histologic differentiation and depth of chest wall invasion were the major factors affecting long-term survival.

Vertebral Invasion

In the minds of most thoracic surgeons, vertebral involvement by bronchogenic carcinoma has represented a specific contraindication to resection because of the low likelihood of complete margins and the associated morbidity of vertebral resection. However, technical developments have been made that overcome most of the concerns regarding morbidity. However, limited survival suggests that the problem of incomplete resection has not been overcome. Vertebral invasion is usually documented clearly by CT and MRI imaging. Invasion of cortical bone is likely not a specific contraindication to attempt at radical resection. However, cancellous invasion makes resection a contentious issue. DeMeester and his colleagues (1989) reported a series of 12 patients who underwent resection (Fig. 36–75). However, cancellous invasion makes resection a contentious issue.

Technical Considerations

The technical approach to total vertebrectomy is indicated in Figures 36–76*A* and *B* with one method of reconstruction demonstrated in Figures 36–76*C*, *D*, and *E*. There have been many variations of the methods of resection and reconstruction. This is always done in conjunction with orthopedic surgeons and neurosurgeons. The vertebral resection can be performed piecemeal (versus en bloc), although the oncologic result of this is unknown. An en bloc hemivertebrectomy or total vertebrectomy is ideal as described by Grunenwald and colleagues (1996b) (Fig. 36–77).

In a subsequent communication (Grunenwald, 1996b), the same group reported experience with an anterior cervicothoracic and median posterior approach eliminating the need for posterolateral thoracotomy. However, the survival in Grunenwald's original report is less than satisfactory. Among four patients who underwent resection for bronchogenic carcinoma, two were alive without disease and two had died within a short time after resection. In an invited commentary on this report, Dartevelle (1996) cautioned against widespread application of this technique without very careful patient selection. In Dartevelle's experience with partial vertebral resection, five of six patients were alive and disease-free with a median follow up of 10 months. He argued strongly that spinal canal invasion was an absolute contraindication to resection. Most surgeons agree with Dartevelle's opinion and consider invasion of the spinal canal a definite contraindication for attempt at curative resection (Fig. 36–78)

Gandhi and colleagues (1999) from the M.D. Anderson Cancer Center report what is probably the largest experience with resection of superior sulcus tumors with vertebral invasion. Seventeen patients underwent preoperative radiation (3000 cGy) and postoperative radiation to a total dose of 5400 cGy plus postoperative adjuvant cisplatin and etoposide. Seven patients underwent total vertebrectomy, seven patients had partial vertebrectomy, and three patients had resection of the neuroforamen and transverse process. There was no operative mortality and, at the time of the report, all patients were ambulant. Two-year actuarial survival was 54%. Once again, the importance of complete resection is emphasized in this report. Only 1 of 11 patients with negative margins had local recurrence, whereas six of 6 patients with positive margins developed locally recurrent disease.

RECONSTRUCTION METHODS

Many strategies to accomplish spinal fixation have been reported. In Gandhi's report (1999), a novel strategy of spinal fixation consisting of methylmethacrylate to re-

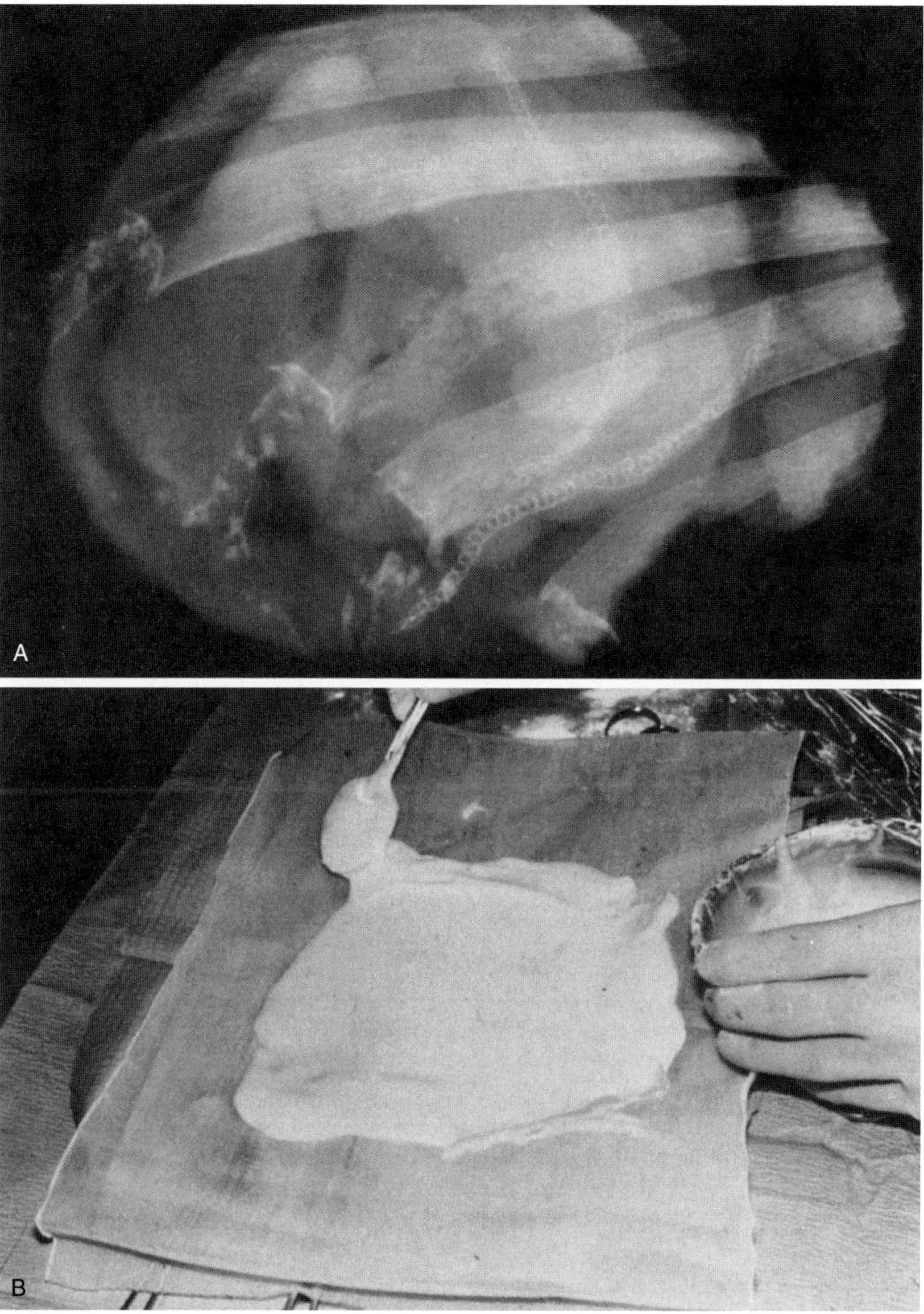

FIGURE 36–74 ■ Chest wall reconstruction. *A*, Radiograph of a resected chest wall tumor. *B*, Spreading methylmethacrylate over mesh.

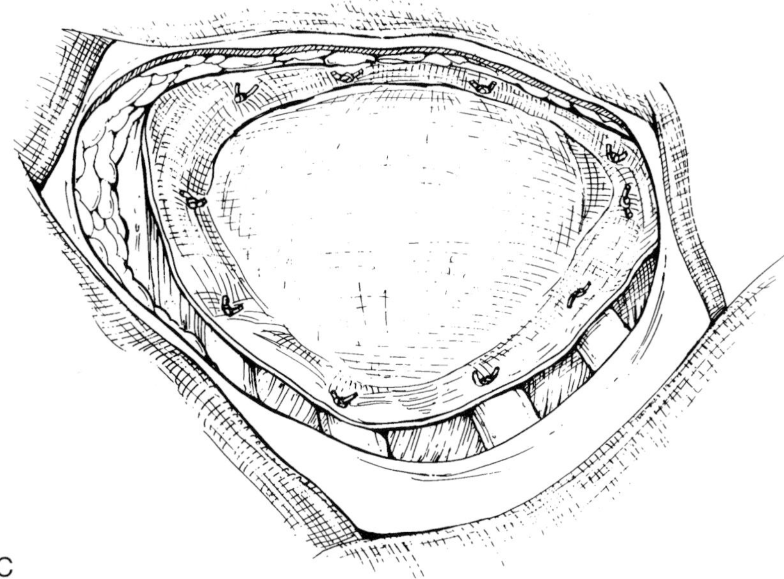

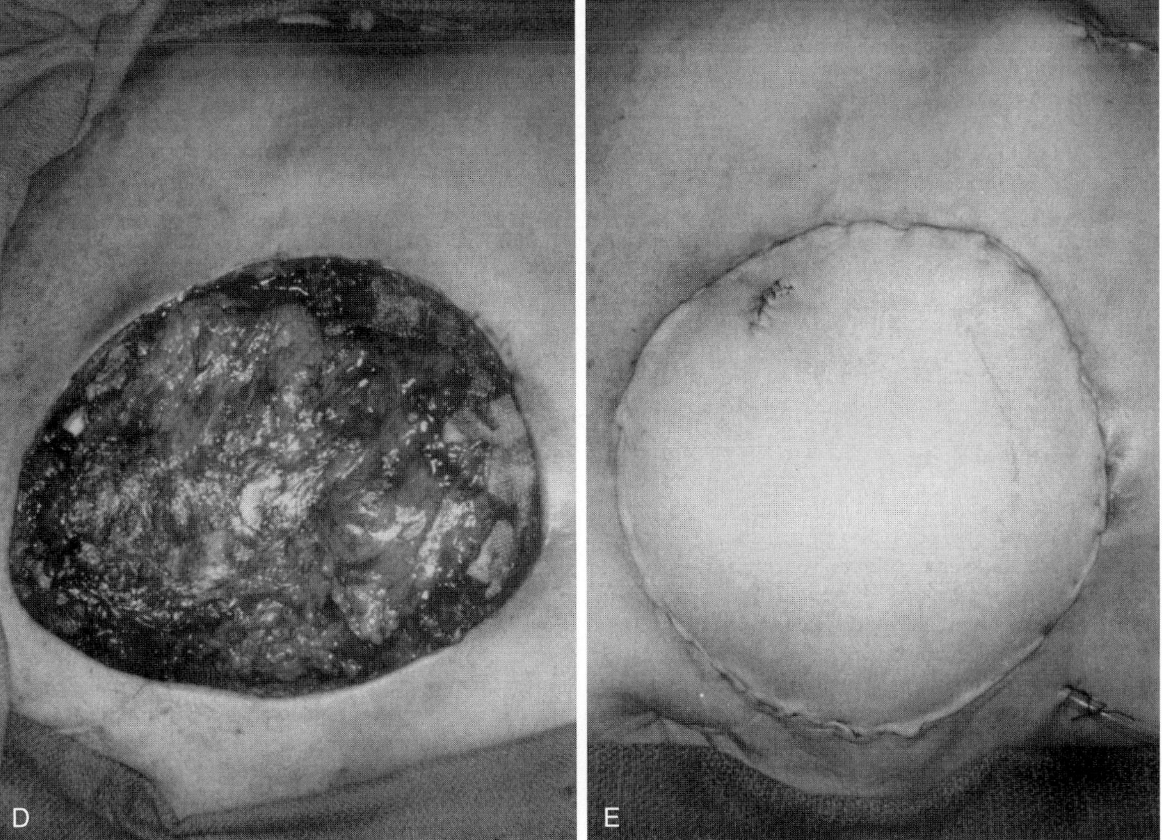

FIGURE 36–74 *Continued* ■ *C*, Prosthesis sutured in place. *D*, Omentum sutured over prosthesis. *E*, Myocutaneous flap sutured to skin.

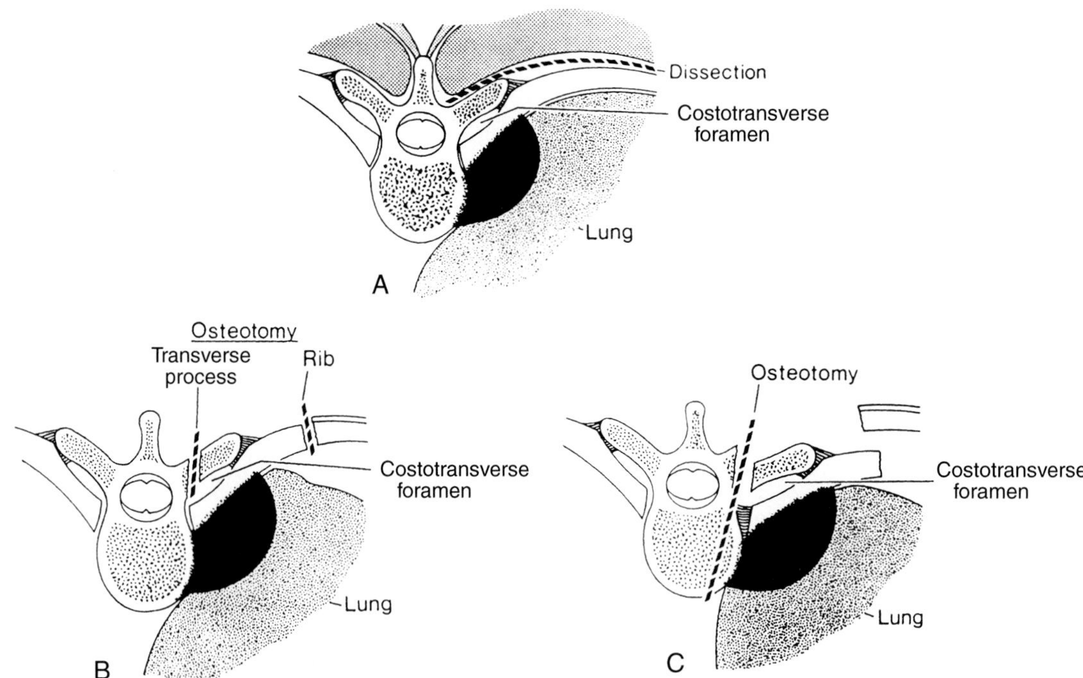

FIGURE 36–75 ■ Transverse section of the thoracic vertebra showing a fixed lung tumor. The costotransverse foramen is free of disease. *A*, The *broken line* shows the plane of dissection posterior to the rib. *B*, The site of osteotomy of the transverse process and rib. *C*, The plane of the tangential osteotomy of the vertebral body. Access to the vertebral body is through the costotransverse foramen. (From DeMeester TR, Albertucci M, Dawson PJ et al: Management of tumor adherent to the vertebral column. J Thorac Cardiovasc Surg 97:373, 1989.)

place vertebral substance was utilized. Spinal fixation was accomplished with a combination of anterior locking plate and screw construct as well as posterior fixation with hooks and rods (Fig. 36–79). Methylmethacrylate was used to reconstruct vertebral bodies (Fig. 36–80). Errico and Cooper (1993) have described a useful technique to control the delivery of methylmethacrylate into the vertebral body above and below the defect while at the same time filling the interval defect with methylmethacrylate (Fig. 36–81).

AORTIC INVASION

Involvement of the aorta is not uncommon for left-sided lung cancers. Aortic invasion can be suspected when the tumor is in apposition to the aorta, more than 25% of aortic circumference, or when the fat plane is lost between the aorta and the tumor (Fig. 36–82). In most patients, resectability cannot be determined until the time of exploration. It may be possible to develop a plane of dissection within the aortic adventitia and to accomplish a complete resection. Full-thickness involvement of the aortic wall is generally considered a contraindication to resection. Unfortunately, determination of such involvement is very difficult prior to resection. For such central lesions, direct aortic invasion and frequent nodal metastasis make complete resection and cure unlikely. In addition, there are a limited number of reports available in the literature from which to draw conclusions.

Surgical Technique

The methods for resecting tumors that invade the aortic area include a subadventitial dissection, a partial resection with patch, or a total tubular resection with reconstruction. The latter approach requires at least partial bypass or other techniques to maintain distal circulation.

Klepetko and colleagues (1999) described a small experience in seven patients undergoing resection of lung tumors involving the aorta. Six of these seven resections were conducted with the assistance of cardiopulmonary bypass and in one patient a temporary interposition graft was employed. Aortic reconstruction was accomplished by tube graft or pericardial patch for small noncircumferential defects. Long-term survival was limited, with only two of seven patients alive without disease. In another report, Tsuchiya and associates (1994) from the National Cancer Center Hospital in Tokyo reported a large experience of resection for tumors involving the aorta in 28 patients. Twenty-one of these patients underwent a subadventitial resection and seven patients underwent full-thickness resection and aortic replacement. Only one of these seven patients with full-thickness resections was a long-term survivor. Interestingly, among the 21 patients with aortic adventitial resection, 11 were incomplete resections, and all of these patients did poorly. Ten patients had a complete subadventitial resection but four of these patients developed recurrent disease.

In another report, Nakahara and colleagues (1989) reported results in three patients who underwent en bloc

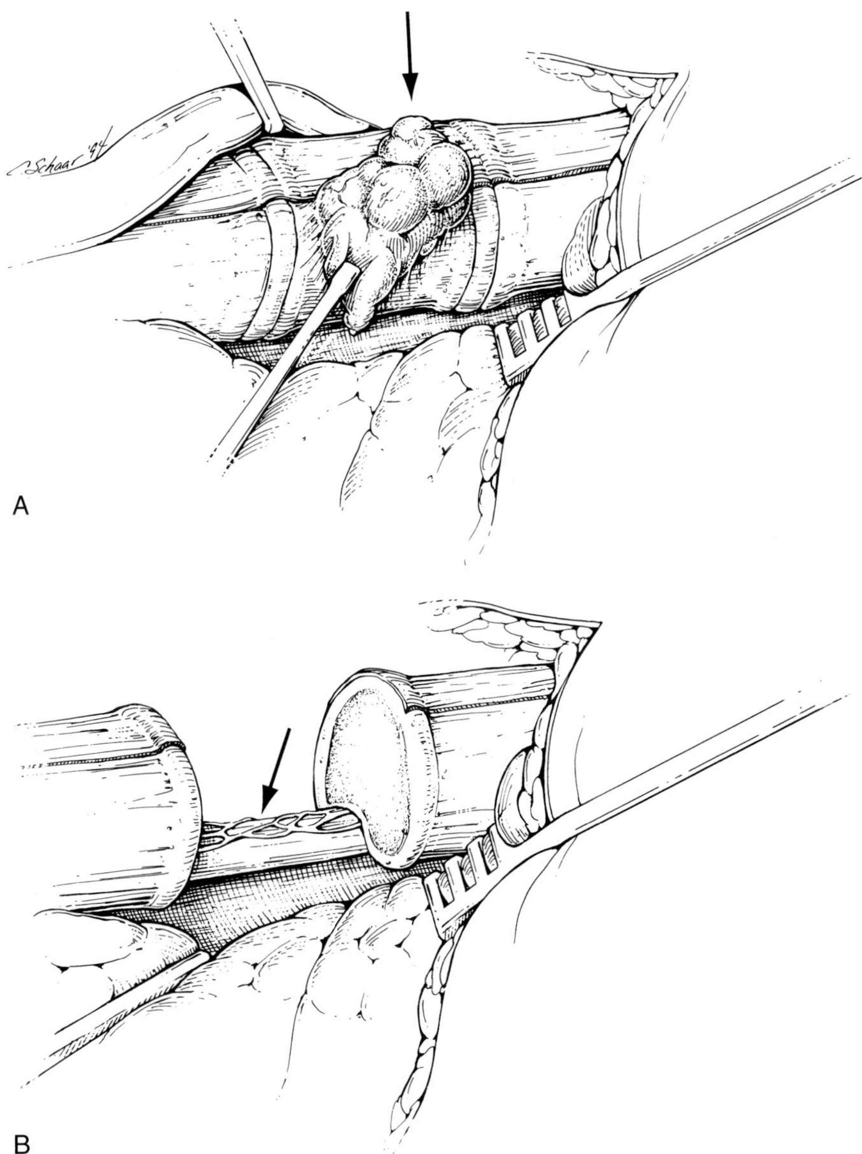

FIGURE 36–76 ■ Vertebral body reconstruction. *A*, Tumor *(arrow)* invading vertebral body. *B*, After resection of tumor and vertebral body (*arrow*, spinal cord).

Illustration continued on following page

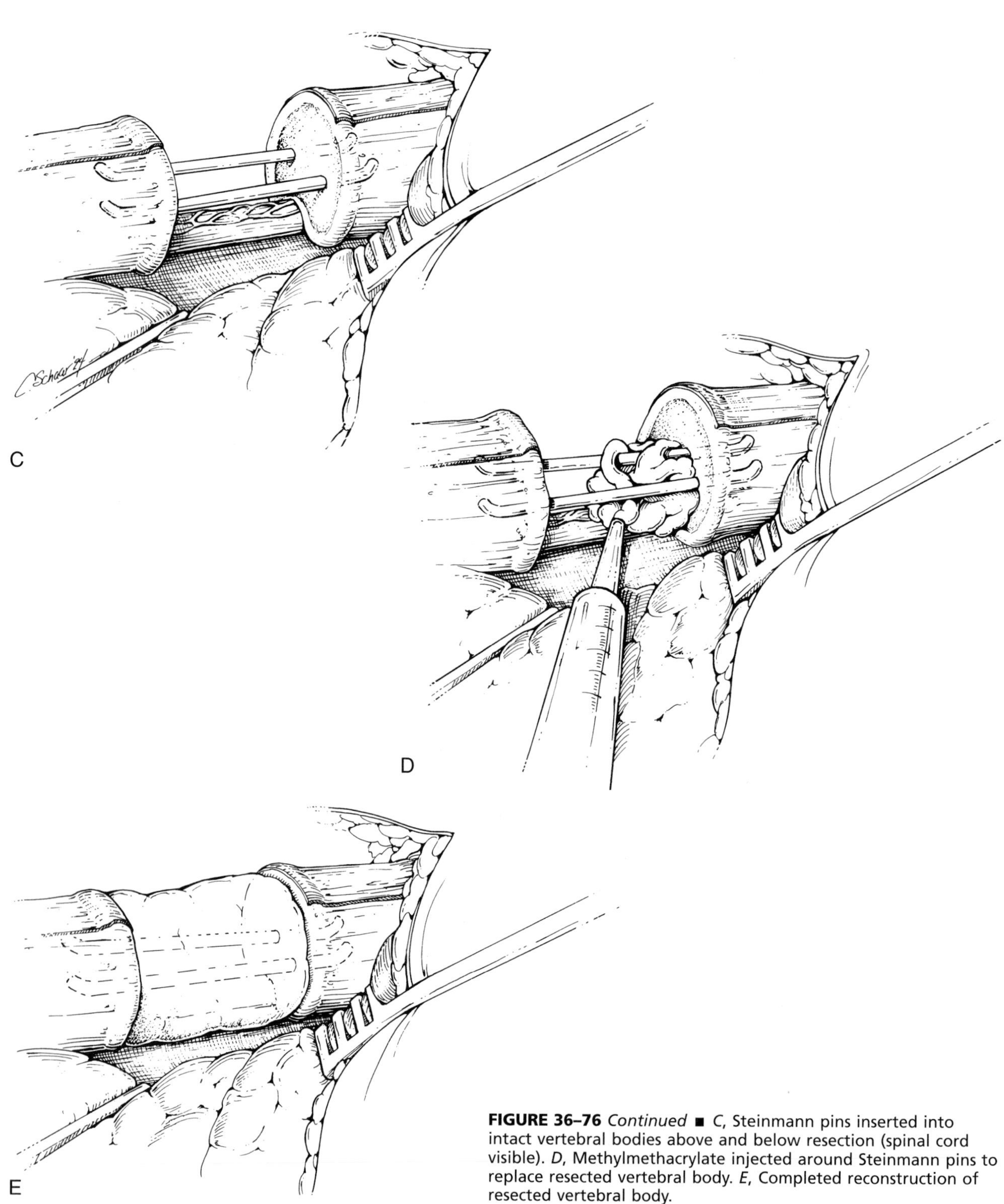

FIGURE 36–76 *Continued* ■ *C*, Steinmann pins inserted into intact vertebral bodies above and below resection (spinal cord visible). *D*, Methylmethacrylate injected around Steinmann pins to replace resected vertebral body. *E*, Completed reconstruction of resected vertebral body.

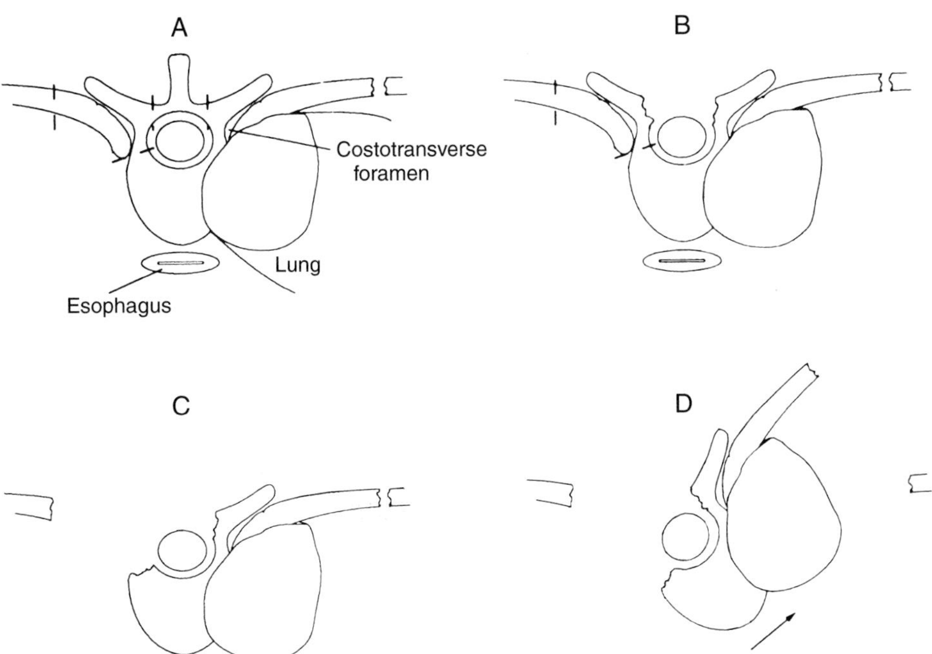

FIGURE 36–77 ■ *A*, The technique of total vertebrectomy with the patient in the ventral position after the chest wall and lung have been sectioned in tumor-free margins. *B*, A laminectomy is performed at the level of the lesion extending one level above and below the involved vertebra. *C*, The lateral dissection is continued to the point of the dissection through the previous thoracotomy and cervicotomy. *D*, Mobilization of the vertebral bodies and transection of the vertebral body end plate using a Gigli saw completes the resection.

resection of left-sided lung cancers and the aorta. Two of these patients died from metastatic disease within 1 year. In their experience, there was only one intermediate-term survivor.

LEFT ATRIAL INVASION

There are limited reports of curative resection for bronchogenic carcinoma involving the left atrium. However, there are techniques described to permit complete and potentially curative resection of selected lesions invading the left atrium. On the right side, the anterior left atrial wall can be lengthened significantly by opening the interatrial groove increasing the margin of resection and the likelihood of an adequate cuff for primary atrial closure. Tsuchiya and colleagues (1994) reported on their experience with 44 patients who underwent resection of left atrium alone or in combination with other major vascular structures. All of these resections were conducted without cardiopulmonary bypass using vascular clamps. The fact that primary repair was conducted in all cases suggested that the extent of atrial wall resection was limited in this series. In one of these patients, a pedunculated tumor growing into the left atrial lumen was grasped from outside with a central clamp (Fig. 36–83).

The atrial wall was opened laterally, and the tumor mass flipped out while the central clamp was secured. A more conventional and safer technique would have been to place the patient on cardiopulmonary bypass, fibrillate the heart, create an atriotomy for resection under direct vision, and primary closure.

Ferguson and Reardon reported a single case in which a "complete" resection was conducted including left atrium, atrial septum, and right atrial wall (Fig. 36–84). Of course, cardiopulmonary bypass was required for this procedure. Primary reconstruction was accomplished. At the time of this report, the patient's survival was 24 months without any evidence of disease.

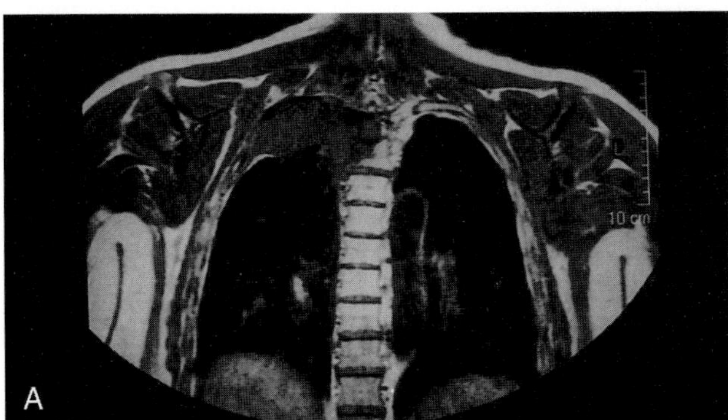

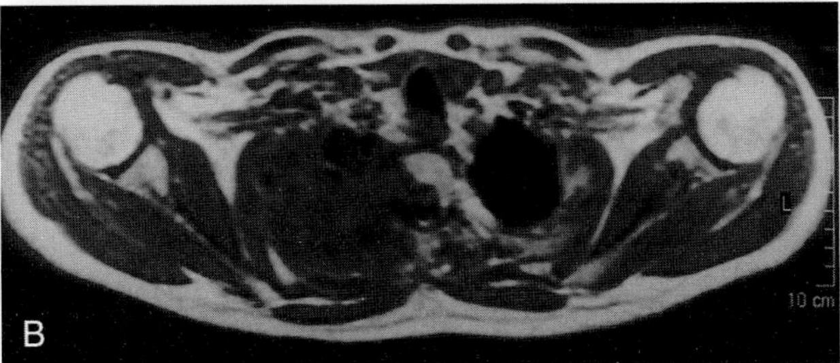

FIGURE 36–78 ■ Coronal (*A*) and axial (*B*) magnetic resonance images demonstrating extensive multilevel vertebral body involvement by a right apical superior sulcus tumor. Obvious invasion of the spinal canal is present.

SUPERIOR AND INFERIOR VENA CAVA

Surgical Technique

Bronchogenic carcinoma can involve the superior vena cava by direct extension of the primary tumor or by

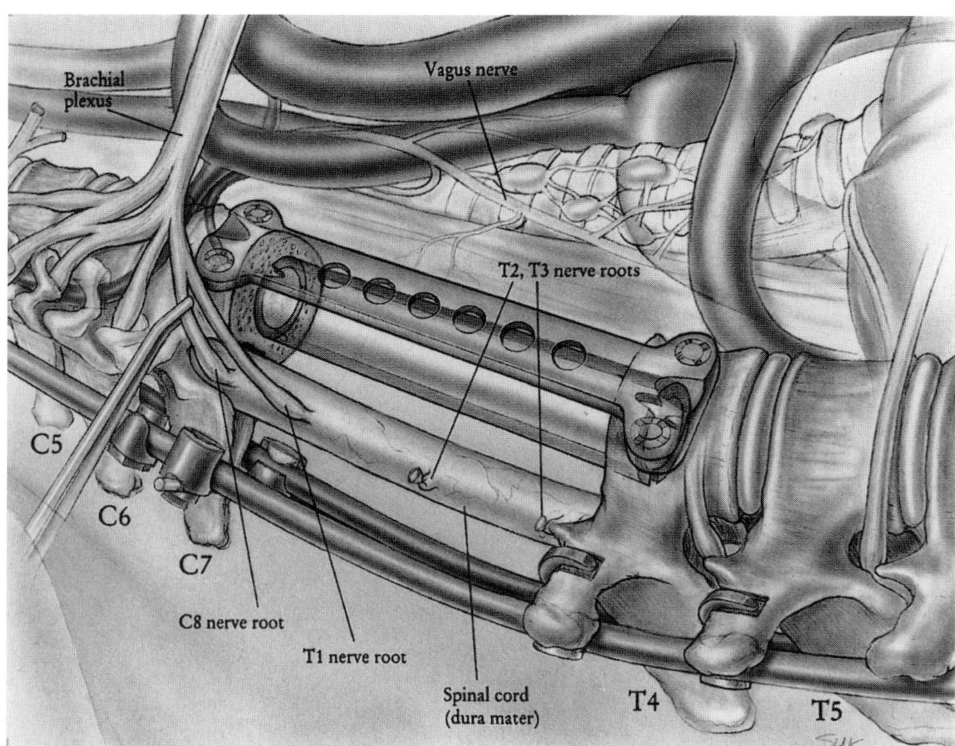

FIGURE 36–79 ■ Multilevel thoracic vertebrectomy and laminectomy, reconstruction with methylmethacrylate, placement of anterior locking plate and screw construct, and posterior fixation with hooks and rods. (From Gandhi S, Walsh GL, Komaki R et al: A multidisciplinary surgical approach to superior sulcus tumors with vertebral invasion. Ann Thorac Surg 68:1778, 1999.)

nodal metastasis. The technical details of superior vena cava resection and reconstruction are covered in detail by Macchiarini and Dartevelle in Chapter 64 and are outlined in Fig. 36–85. There are two possible techniques for resecting a superior vena cava. It may be performed en bloc with the pulmonary resection. For minimal involvement, a side-biting clamp can be applied, and the cava simply oversewn or patched if the lumen is compromised. Patches can include Gore-Tex or pericardium. For full reconstruction, the preferable method is a Gore-Tex sleeve patch as outlined by Dartevelle (see Chapter 64).

Although the ideal approach for superior vena caval reconstruction is a sternotomy or hemi-clamshell, often this is encountered at the time of thoracotomy, and the incision should be appropriately extended to allow appropriate control of vessels.

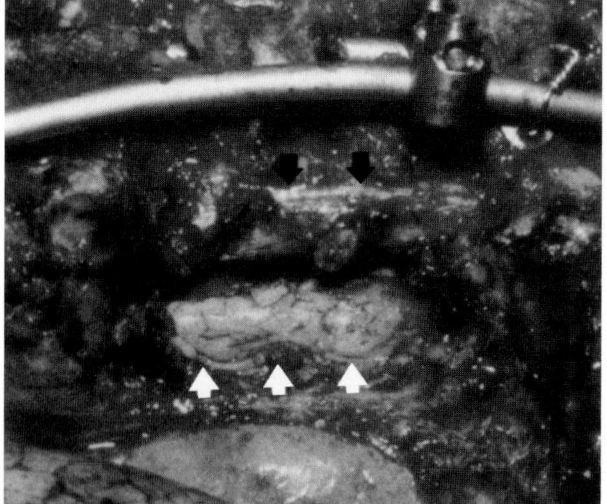

FIGURE 36–80 ■ Operative photograph demonstrating posterior rod fixation. The vertebral body defect is filled with methylmethacrylate (*arrows*). (From Gandhi S, Walsh GL, Komaki R et al: A multidisciplinary surgical approach to superior sulcus tumors with vertebral invasion. Ann Thorac Surg 68:1778, 1999.)

Results

In 1987 Dartevelle first reported a technique of caval reconstruction using Gore-Tex grafts (Fig. 36–86). Subsequently, Dartevelle and colleagues (1991) reported a larger series of patients who had undergone caval resection and replacement, only six of whom had primary bronchogenic carcinoma. Among these patients, two patients with N1 disease were alive at 16 and 51 months and one patient with N1 disease died at 38 months. There were no long-term survivors among patients with N2 disease. In a more recent report of his experience (1997), Dartevelle described a total experience of 14 patients who underwent caval resection for non–small cell carcinoma. Eleven patients had squamous cancer. Most patients required extended pneumonectomy, six of which were sleeve pneumonectomies. Overall survival was 31% with five of 14 patients still alive and disease-free 3 to 65 months post resection.

Spaggiari and colleagues (2000) described their experience in 25 patients who underwent resection of the superior vena caval system for non–small cell lung cancer. Seven patients had complete resection of the superior vena cava with graft interposition. Twelve patients underwent tangential resection of the superior vena cava, and

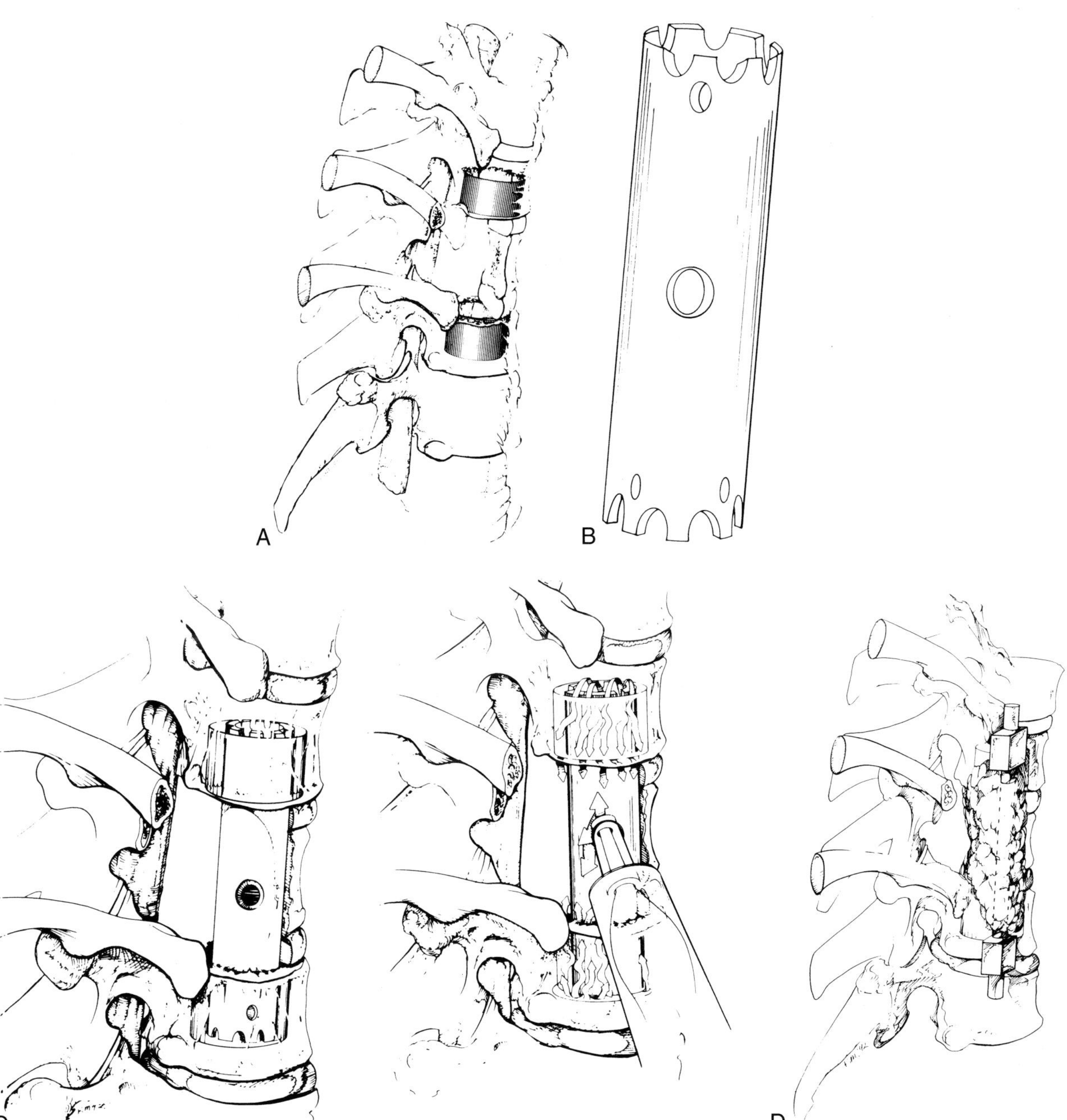

FIGURE 36–81 ■ *A*, The involved vertebral body is resected with decompression of the spinal canal. Carefully leaving the lateral aspect of the vertebral bodies above and below intact, the cancellus bone is excavated with either angled curettes or an angled drill. *B*, A Silastic tube is fashioned to fit into the vertebral body above as well as below. A hole is made with a rongeur and the lateral portion of the tube to accept a syringe filled with methylmethacrylate in a highly liquid phase. Holes are fashioned at the ends of the tube *as shown* to facilitate extrusion of the cement. *C*, The cement is pressurized into the tube until it is seen to exude out of the bodies above and below. Care is taken to avoid migration of the cement into the spinal canal. Cement is then packed all around the tube until it is flush with the lateral aspects of the vertebral bodies. *D*, In the lumbar spine, a threaded rod is placed between the two Kostuik-Harrington screws or Zielke screws that are inserted into the bodies above and below. Cement is packed around the rod thus incorporating the rod and the Silastic tube into a single construct. (From Errico TJ, Cooper PR: A new method of thoracic and lumbar body replacement for spinal tumors: Technical note. Neurosurgery 32:678, 1993.)

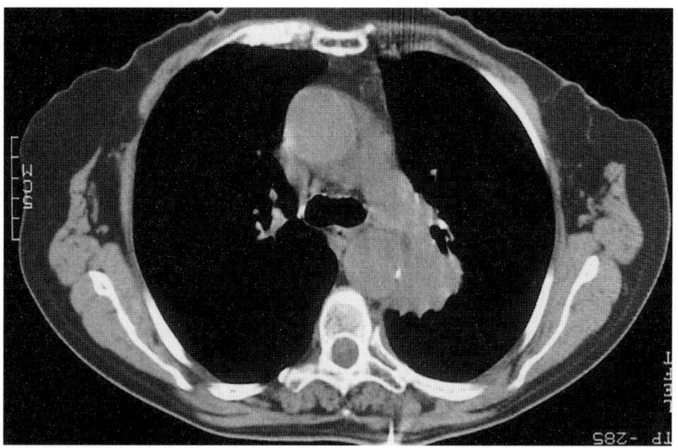

FIGURE 36–82 ■ A computed tomography image depicting a left lower lobe superior segment non–small cell carcinoma with extensive apposition to the descending thoracic aorta. The fat plane between the tumor and the aorta is obliterated. This lesion was resected by subadventitial resection through tumor-free margins.

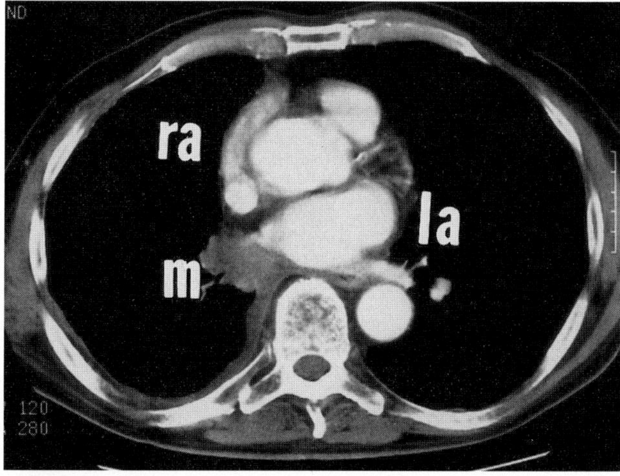

FIGURE 36–84 ■ A computed tomography image of the chest with intravenous contrast demonstrating a central right hilar mass with involvement of the posterior aspect of the left atrium. (From Ferguson ER Jr, Reardon MJ: Atrial resection in advanced lung carcinoma: Under total cardiopulmonary bypass. Tex Heart Inst J 27:110, 2000.)

one patient had a pericardial patch. Five patients underwent resection of the right innominate and subclavian veins without vessel reconstruction. Most patients had N2, and 20% of patients had an incomplete resection. Operative mortality was 12%, median survival was 11.5 months, and 5-year actuarial survival was 29%. There were only four patients alive at 5 years. The central location of non–small cell lung cancers involving vena cava often mandate extended resections of other structures including the airway (Fig. 36–87).

In addition to Dartevelle's description of vena caval and tracheal sleeve resection, Spaggiari and Pastorino (2000) have reported a small experience in six patients who underwent combined superior vena cava resection and tracheal sleeve resection. Muscle-sparing thoracotomy was performed in four patients and a hemi-clamshell approach was used in two patients. There were no postoperative deaths. However, three patients had major postoperative complications. Median survival in this small experience is 14.5 months with a range of 3 to 17 months.

Invasion of the inferior vena cava by resectable bronchogenic carcinoma is exceedingly rare. Roberts and his colleagues (1998) reported their experience with an inter-

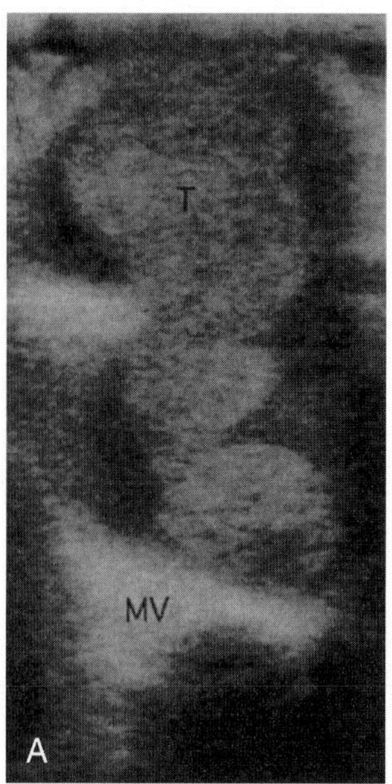

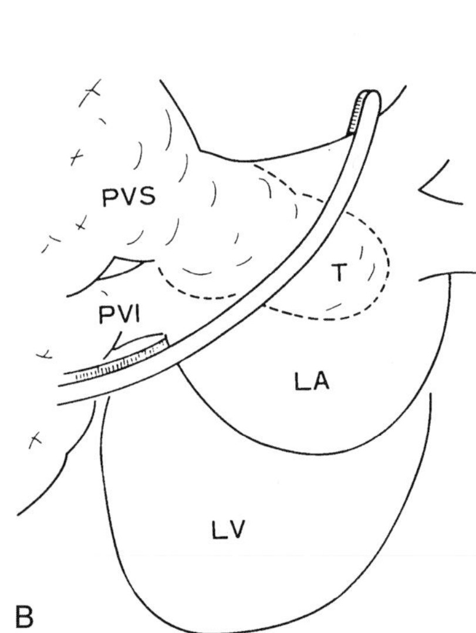

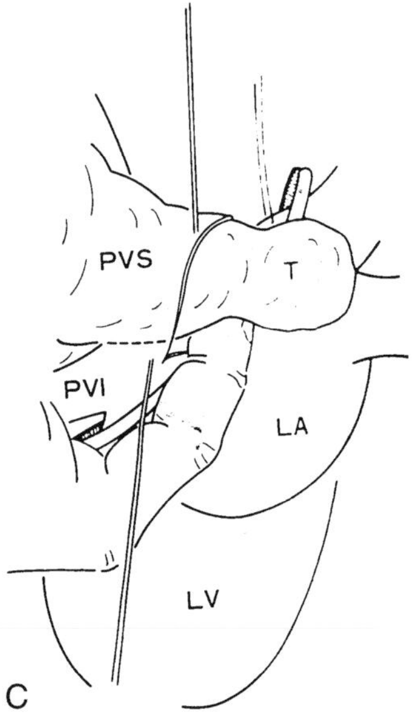

FIGURE 36–83 ■ *A*, An echocardiographic image demonstrating a long tumor polyp (T) with contact to the mitral valve (MV). *B*, The tumor mass was gently grasped within the left atrium by a vascular clamp. *C*, After posterior left atriotomy, the polyp was pulled out with forceps, and the operator's finger, and the atrial clamp were secured. (From Tsuchiya R, Asamura H, Kondo H et al: Extended resection of the left atrium, great vessels, or both, for lung cancer. Ann Thorac Surg 57:960, 1994.)

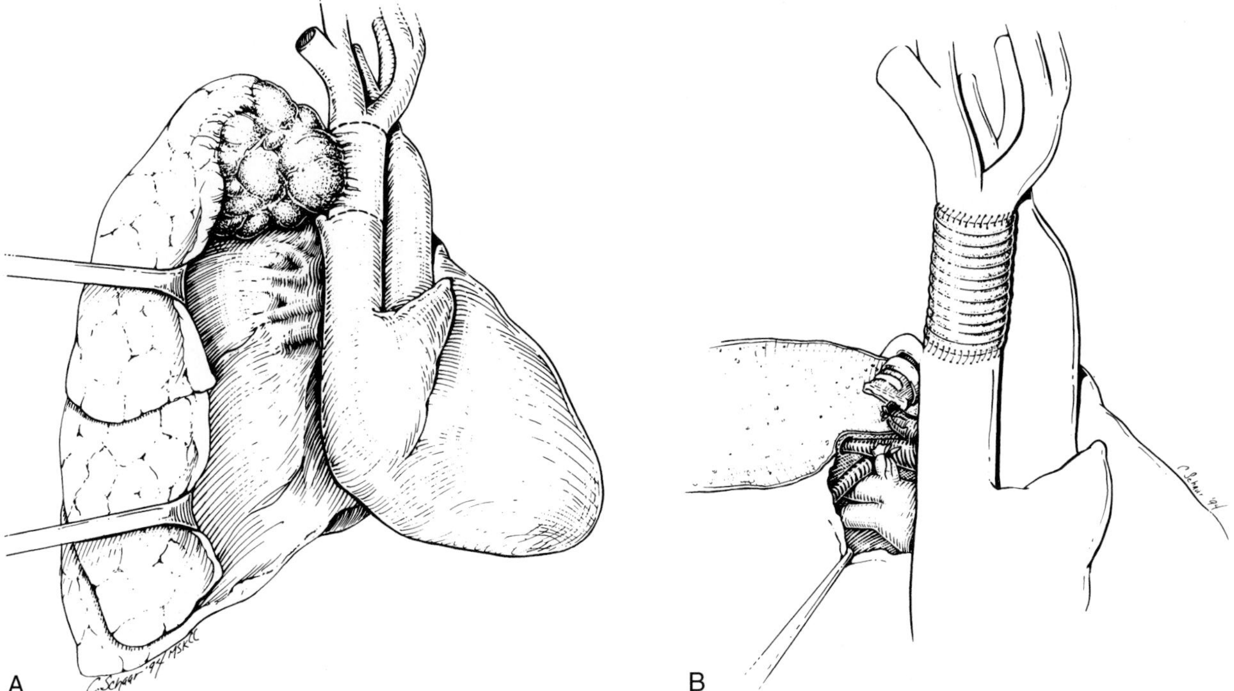

FIGURE 36–85 ■ Caval invasion. *A*, Illustration of a tumor invading the superior vena cava. *B*, Reconstruction with a polytetrafluoroethylene graft.

esting patient who presented with a lesion involving the right lower lobe diaphragm and interpericardial inferior vena cava (IVC). The patient underwent resection and primary replacement of the IVC without cardiopulmonary bypass. The patient was alive and well 8 months following the procedure.

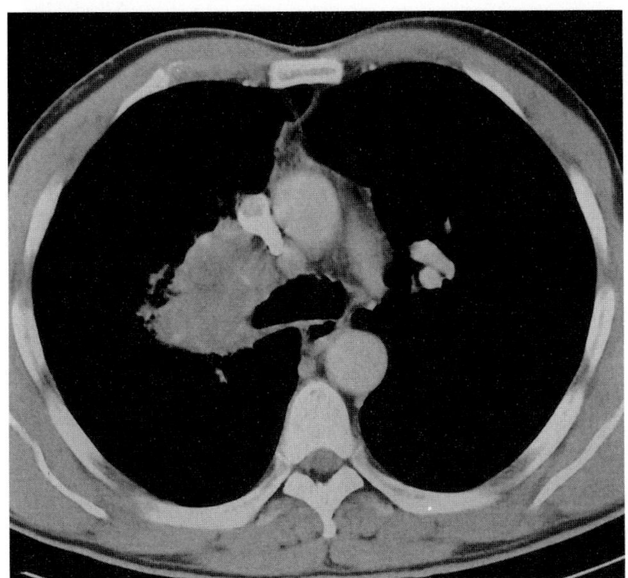

FIGURE 36–86 ■ Central right hilar non–small cell carcinoma with invasion of the proximal right main bronchus and lateral vena cava. This lesion was resected by tracheal sleeve pneumonectomy and vena cava replacement.

TRACHEAL CARINA

The technical details of tracheal carinal resection are covered in detail by Drs. Mathisen and Grillo in Chapter 19.

In the past, sleeve pneumonectomy or carinal resection in treating lung cancer was associated with significant operative mortality that often exceeded any possibility of 5-year survival. However recent advances in anesthetic, operative, and postoperative care have resulted in a dramatic reduction in operative mortality in most published series. Most reported series include all resections, no matter what the underlying disease is. Roviaro and colleagues (1994) reported an experience with 27 right tracheal sleeve resections. There was only one postoperative death in this series. Dartevelle (1997) reported his experience with a larger number of patients. Among 60 patients undergoing carinal resection for non–small cell carcinoma, there were two early and two late postoperative deaths. Overall operative mortality was 6.6%. Mitchell and colleagues (1999) determined that postoperative mechanical ventilation, length of resected airway, and development of anastomotic complication were all significant predictors of postoperative mortality following carinal resection. Several strategies have been developed to maintain viability of the remaining proximal and distal airway and reduce tension on the airway anastomosis. Most authors advocate coverage of the airway anastomosis with vascularized pericardial fat pad, pericardium, or omentum.

Despite these advances, long-term survival remains limited. In Roviaro's (1994) report, among 27 patients

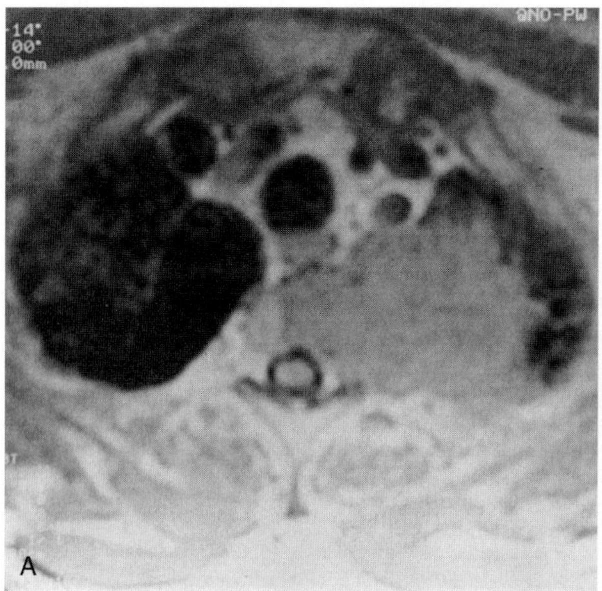

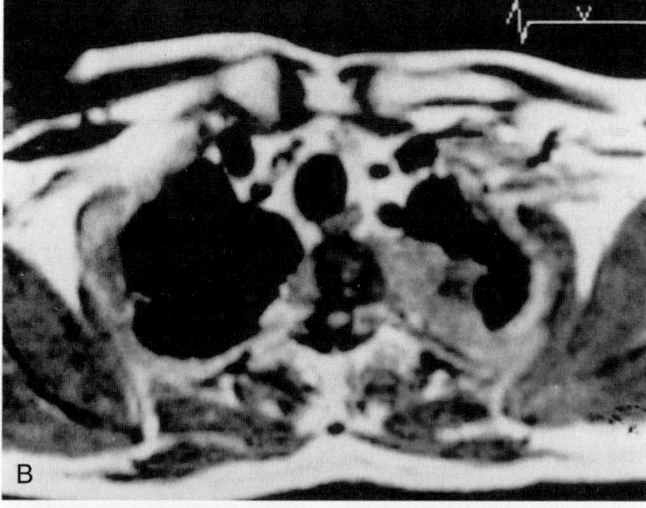

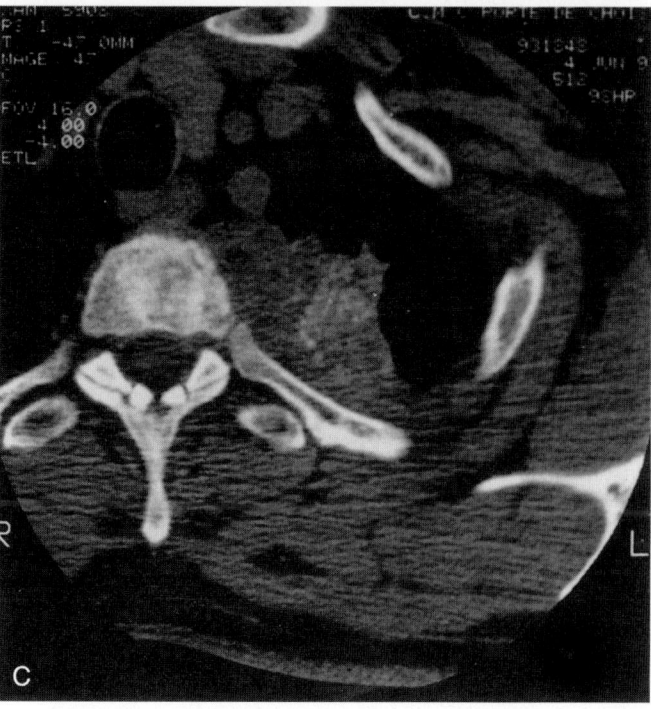

FIGURE 36–87 ■ *A*, A magnetic resonance image of the thoracic apex showing vertebral body involvement of T2 prior to induction chemotherapy. Note that there is no involvement of the spinal canal or spinal cord compression. *B*, A magnetic resonance image and *C*, a computed tomography scan of the thoracic apex after three cycles of chemotherapy showing a slight decrease in tumor size and persistent vertebral body involvement. Note the abnormal bone structure of the body of T2. (From Grunenwald D, Mazal C, Baldeyrou P et al: En bloc resection of lung cancer invading the spine. Ann Thorac Surg 61:1878, 1996.)

undergoing resection, there were only seven patients alive at 4 years and one at 5 years. In Dartevelle's report (1997), the median follow up of 4.3 years median survival was 2.9 years. There were 12 (20%) 5-year and four (6.7%) 10-year survivors. Not surprisingly, long-term survival was significantly influenced by nodal status. Among the 12 N2 patients, there were no survivors beyond 46 months.

DIAPHRAGM INVASION

Diaphragmatic invasion by otherwise resectable non-small cell lung cancer is exceedingly rare. As a result, there are a limited number of reports from which thoracic surgeons can draw conclusions. Diagnosis of isolated diaphragmatic invasion is difficult. Symptoms are usually absent and imaging is of limited value in determining diaphragmatic invasion. Thoracoscopic examination has been suggested as a means to detect diaphragmatic invasion in suspected cases. The available literature suggests a poor prognosis following resection, perhaps because of vascular and lymphatic invasion within the diaphragm.

Weksler and associates (1997) from the Memorial Sloan Kettering Cancer Center reported only eight patients with diaphragmatic invasion from a total experience of 4668 (17%) patients explored for non–small cell carcinoma. Seven of these eight patients had squamous cancers and four had N2 disease. Primary repair was accomplished in seven of eight patients. There was only one long-term survival. All patients with N2 disease developed fatal recurrence.

In a subsequent report, Rocco and colleagues (1999) reported a dual institution experience with 15 patients. Overall, 5-year actuarial survival was 20% and only 27% for patients without nodal metastasis. Interestingly, these authors found a correlation between need for prosthetic diaphragmatic replacement and survival suggesting that wider margins of resection conferred some survival benefit.

Two multi-institutional retrospective reviews have been published. The Japanese group (Yokoi et al, 2000) described an experience with 63 patients who underwent resection of T3 lung cancers invading the diaphragm. Five-year survival following complete resection was only 22.6%. There was no long-term survival in patients undergoing incomplete resection. For patients with T3N0 disease, survival was only 28.3% and 18% if nodal metastases were discovered. In this report, depth of invasion was of prognostic importance. Minimal invasion (parietal pleura or subpleural tissue) had a survival of 33% in comparison with the 14.8% survival noted in patients with deeper invasion (muscle or peritoneum).

In the French multi-institutional report (Riquet et al, 2000), there were 68 patients who underwent exploration for T3 cancers involving the diaphragm. Eight patients had exploration; surprisingly, long-term survival was significantly influenced by nodal status. Among the 12 N2 patients, there were no survivors beyond 46 months.

Localized diaphragmatic invasion by lung cancer is amenable to wide resection in a few selected cases. In light of reports of dismal overall survival, the T3 descriptor assigned to primary tumors with diaphragmatic invasion is inaccurate. These tumors behave much more like T4 tumors. The difficulty of establishing a preoperative diagnosis without thoracoscopic examination makes consideration of induction therapy impractical in most of these patients.

PERICARDIAL INVASION

The pericardium is in contact with the lung over most of its medial surface. Nonetheless, invasion of the pericardium in otherwise resectable lung cancers is somewhat unusual. For medially positioned tumors, if pericardial adherence is noted, the pericardium should be opened away from the phrenic nerve. The phrenic nerve should be spared if at all possible. Digital and visual exploration of the pericardium provides an accurate assessment of the extent of tumor and the magnitude of pericardial resection required. If a pneumonectomy is performed, any pericardial defect should be closed to prevent cardiac torsion or herniation. A variety of patch materials can be used including Marlex, GoreTex, Dacron, bovine pericardium, or Vicryl. Interestingly, a complete defect of the percardium on the left side probably does not need repair, because there is little chance of herniation or torsion.

Occasionally, for central tumors that do not involve the percardium, an intrapericardial dissection will greatly facilitate resection, providing central exposure to the pulmonary vein or pulmonary artery.

ESOPHAGEAL INVASION

Occasionally, the esophagus can be involved by primary bronchogenic carcinoma, although it is far more commonly involved by metastatic spread to periesophageal or subcarinal lymph nodes. Resection of a portion of the musculature wall of the esophagus leaving the mucosa intact is an appropriate strategy for such central tumors. However, long-term prognosis in these patients is poor because most have extensive disease, and complete resection is not probable. Similarly, resection of the esophagus en bloc with a pulmonary resection, although technically feasible, cannot be justified by the experience of any reported series.

Extended Resection Following Induction Therapy

Recent enthusiasm for the use of induction chemotherapy and radiation has led some groups to study the use of this modality in patients with locally advanced tumors. Several reports suggest that there may be a place for induction chemoradiation prior to resection in patients with T4 tumors. Arguments for the use of induction therapy include measurement of tumor response, decrease of tumor size (Fig. 36–88) to facilitate or reduce the magnitude of subsequent resection, increase the likelihood of negative surgical margins, and treatment of micrometastatic disease.

Macchiarini and his colleagues (1994) reported an experience in 23 patients with T4 non–small cell lung cancer. These patients received two courses of cisplatin-based chemotherapy with or without radiation (median dose 4500 cGy). Twenty-one of these 23 patients underwent subsequent complete resection. There were two patients who had incomplete resections. Complete pathologic response was noted in 13 patients. Postoperative complications occurred far more commonly in patients who had combination chemoradiation in comparison with those who received chemotherapy alone. Projected 3-year survival was 54%.

In a subsequent report, Rendina and associates (1999) describe their experience with 57 patients who presented with T4 non-small cell lung cancer. Patients received three cycles of cisplatin, vinblastine, and mitomycin. Forty-two patients (73%) responded to therapy and underwent exploration. Eleven patients did not obtain a

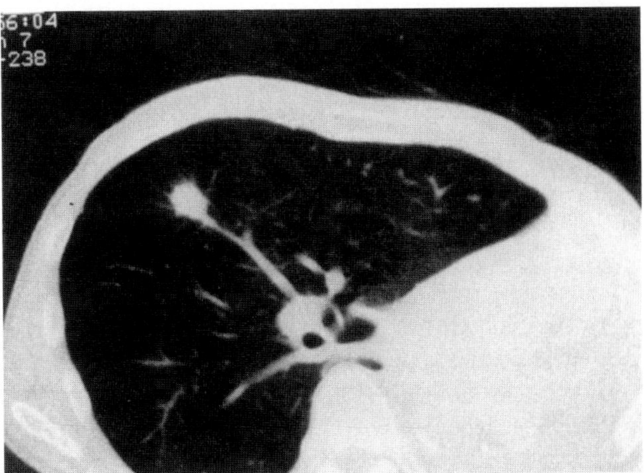

FIGURE 36–88 ■ A computed tomography image demonstrating a metachronous primary non–small cell lung cancer after left pneumonectomy. (From Lewis RJ, Caccavale RJ: Pulmonary resection after pneumonectomy. Ann Thorac Surg 64:583, 1997.)

response, and four patients had major chemotherapy-related toxicity. Thirty-six patients (63% of the entire group) had a complete resection. Only four patients had a complete pathologic response. Overall survival at one and four years was 61.4% and 19.5% respectively. The 36 patients who had complete resection had a 4-year survival of 30.5%. In another recent report, Stamatis and colleagues (1999) reported their experience with an intensive regimen of cisplatin and etoposide chemotherapy and preoperative irradiation (4500 cGy) in patients with stage IIIb lung cancer. Among patients who had T4N0–1 lesions, complete resections were conducted in 80% of patients, and 50% of patients experienced complete pathologic response. Median survival was 26.5 months and 5-year actuarial survival was 37.5%.

Despite the small number of patients in these Phase II studies, a number of speculations can be made. First, treatment toxicity is significant, particularly with concurrent chemoradiation. Postoperative morbidity is increased significantly in patients who receive concurrent chemoradiation in comparison with those receiving chemotherapy alone. T4 lesions can be downstaged, increasing the possibility of complete resection. Unfortunately, there are no Phase III data on which to base any conclusion regarding the merits of this approach with respect to long-term survival.

CONTRALATERAL RESECTION AFTER PNEUMONECTOMY

Metachronous primary lung cancers occur at a rate of 1% to 3% per year in patients who have undergone prior curative resection for lung cancer. If the prior resection was pneumonectomy, resection of a subsequent contralateral lesion is often contraindicated because of the extent of the lesion. Kittle and colleagues (1985) reported an experience among 15 patients who underwent resection of pulmonary malignancies following prior pneumonectomy. At the time of their report, only three patients were alive without disease with a range of follow-up that was 18 months to 70 months. Westerman and colleagues (1993) reported their experience with resection after contralateral pneumonectomy in eight patients. There was one postoperative death due to pulmonary embolism. Resection included one right upper lobectomy, five segmental resections, and two wedge resections. Only four of these patients were alive, one of whom has locally recurrent tumor.

Spaggiari and associates (1996) have reported a series of 13 patients who underwent resection of a new lesion following prior pneumonectomy. Three patients underwent segmentectomy, seven patients had wedge resection, two patients had multiple wedge resection, and one patient was explored without resection. There was no operative mortality. Median survival was 19 months and probability of 3-year survival was 46%. Subsequently, Lewis and Caccavale (1997) reported a single case utilizing video-assisted technology with an excellent early result.

■ REFERENCES

Chapelier A, Fadel E, Macchiarini P et al: Factors affecting long-term survival after en bloc resection of lung cancer invading the chest wall. European J Cardio Thorac Surg 18:513, 2000.

Dartevelle P, Chapelier A, Navajas M et al: Replacement of the superior vena cava with polytetrafluoroethylene grafts combined with resection of mediastinal-pulmonary malignant tumors. J Thorac Cardiovasc Surg 94:361, 1987.

Dartevelle P, Chapelier A, Pastorino U et al: Long-term follow-up after prosthetic replacement of the superior vena cava combined with resection of mediastinal-pulmonary malignant tumors. J Thor Cardiovasc Surg 102:259, 1991.

Dartevelle PG, Missenard G, Macchiarini P et al: Invited commentary. Ann Thorac Surg 61:725, 1996.

Dartevelle PG: Extended operations for the treatment of lung cancer. Ann Thorac Surg 63:12, 1997.

DeMeester TR, Albertucci M, Dawson PJ et al: Management of tumor adherent to the vertebral column. J Thorac Cardiovasc Surg 97:373, 1989.

Errico TJ, Cooper PR: A new method of thoracic and lumbar body replacement for spinal tumors: Technical note. Neurosurgery 32:678, 1993.

Ferguson ER Jr, Reardon MJ: Atrial resection in advanced lung carcinoma: Under total cardiopulmonary bypass. Tex Heart Inst J 27:110, 2000.

Gandhi S, Walsh GL, Komaki R et al: A multidisciplinary surgical approach to superior sulcus tumors with vertebral invasion. Ann Thorac Surg 68:1778, 1999.

Ginsberg RJ, Martini N, Zaman M et al: Influence of surgical resection and brachytherapy in the management of superior sulcus tumor. Ann Thorac Surg 57:1440, 1994.

Grunenwald D, Mazel C, Baldeyrou P et al: En bloc resection of lung cancer invading the spine. Ann Thorac Surg 61:1878, 1996a.

Grunenwald D, Mazel C, Girard P et al: Total vertebrectomy for en bloc resection of lung cancer invading the spine. Ann Thorac Surg 61:723, 1996.

Kittle CF, Faber LP, Jensik RJ et al: Pulmonary resection in patients after pneumonectomy. Ann Thorac Surg 40:294, 1985.

Klepetko W, Wisser W, Birsan T et al: T4 lung tumors with infiltration of the thoracic aorta: Is an operation reasonable? Ann Thorac Surg 67:340, 1999.

Lewis RJ, Caccavale RJ: Pulmonary resection after pneumonectomy. Ann Thorac Surg 64:583, 1997.

Macchiarini P, Chapelier AR, Monnet I et al: Extended operations after induction therapy for stage IIIb (T4) non-small cell lung cancer. Ann Thorac Surg 57:966, 1994.

McCaughan BC, Martini N, Bains MS et al: Chest wall invasion in carcinoma of the lung: Therapeutic and prognostic implication. J Thorac Cardiovasc Surg 89:836, 1985.

Mitchell JD, Mathisen DJ, Wright CD et al: Clinical experience with carinal resection. J Thorac Cardiovasc Surg 117:39, 1999.

Nakahara K, Ohno K, Mastumura A et al: Extended operation for lung cancer invading the aortic arch and superior vena cava. J Thorac Cardiovasc Surg 97:428, 1989.

Patterson GA, Ilves R, Ginsbert RJ et al: The value of adjuvant radiotherapy in pulmonary and chest wall resection for bronchogenic carcinoma. Ann Thorac Surg 24:692, 1982.

Rendina EA, Venuta F, De Giacomo T et al: Induction chemotherapy for T4 centrally located non–small lung cancer. J Thorac Cardiovasc Surg 117:225, 1999.

Riquet M, Porte H, Chapelier A et al: Resection of lung cancer invading the diaphragm. J Thorac Cardiovasc Surg 120:417, 2000.

Roberts JR, Abbot PS, Smythe WR et al: Resection of a pulmonary malignancy invading the intrapericardial inferior vena cava. Ann Thorac Surg 65:263, 1998.

Rocco G, Rendina EA, Meroni A et al: Prognostic factors after surgical treatment of lung cancer invading the diaphragm. Ann Thorac Surg 68:2065, 1999.

Roviaro GC, Varoli F, Rebuffat C et al: Tracheal sleeve pneumonectomy for bronchogenic carcinoma. J Thorac Cardiovasc Surg 107:13, 1994.

Spaggiari L, Grunenwald D, Girard P et al: Cancer resection on the residual lung after pneumonectomy for bronchogenic carcinoma. Ann Thorac Surg 62:1598, 1996.

Spaggiari L, Pastorino U: Combined tracheal sleeve and superior vena cava resections for non–small cell lung cancer. Ann Thorac Surg 70:1172, 2000.

Spaggiari L, Regnard JF, Magdeleinat P et al: Extended resections for bronchogenic carcinoma invading the superior vena cava system. Ann Thorac Surg 69:233, 2000.

Stamatis G, Eberhardt W, Stuben G et al: Preoperative chemoradiotherapy and surgery for selected non–small cell lung cancer IIIB subgroups: Long-term results. Ann Thorac Surg 68:1144, 1999.

Trastek VF, Pairolero PC, Piehler JM et al: En bloc (non-chest wall) resections for bronchogenic carcinoma with parietal fixation. J Thorac Cardiovasc Surg 87:352, 1984.

Tsuchiya R, Asamura H, Kondo H et al: Extended resection of the left atrium, great vessels, or both for lung cancer. Ann Thorac Surg 57:960, 1994.

Weksler B, Bains M, Burt M et al: Resection of lung cancer invading the diaphragm. J Thorac Cardiovasc Surg 114:500, 1997.

Westermann CJJ, van Swieten HA, de la Riviere AB et al: Pulmonary resection after pneumonectomy in patients with bronchogenic carcinoma. J Thorac Cardiovasc Surg 106:868, 1993.

Yokoi K, Tsuchiya R, Mori T et al: Results of surgical treatment of lung cancer involving the diaphragm. J Thorac Cardiovasc Surg 120:799, 2000.

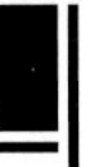

MEDIASTINAL LYMPH NODE DISSECTION

Steven M. Keller

MEDIASTINAL LYMPH NODE DISSECTION

Intraoperative staging is an essential component of the surgical treatment of lung cancer. Though the T category of the primary tumor is readily apparent to both surgeon and pathologist, the presence or absence of tumor within the intrathoracic lymph nodes is frequently not obvious. Indeed, the lymph nodes themselves may not be apparent and must be diligently sought. Microscopic assessment is required to determine accurately the N status. Furthermore, because histologic staging is completely dependent on the material submitted during the operative procedure, the surgeon must *accurately identify* and *properly label* the requisite specimens.

Knowledge of the metastatic patterns of lung cancer provides the rationale for lymph node dissection. Lymph node level definitions and lymph node dissection techniques are best appreciated in their anatomic and historical perspectives. Finally, the utility of mediastinal lymph node dissection can only be fully comprehended through review of the accompanying risks and benefits.

Staging

Appropriate staging of lung cancer can only be accomplished with accurate and thorough lymph node dissection. In the absence of precise staging, comparison of results from different institutions is impossible, as is the conduct of multi-institutional trials. Although most authors believe that the value of mediastinal lymph node dissection results from detailed staging, some investigators (principally from Japan) believe that removal of all intrathoracic and supraclavicular lymph nodes in the likely drainage pathways results in improved survival (Hata et al, 1990; Hata et al, 1994; Nakahara et al, 1993; Watanabe et al, 1991).

Critical assessment of the published literature relating survival to pathologic stage in patients with non–small cell lung cancer (NSCLC) requires knowledge of the investigator's intrathoracic staging technique. In general, *sampling* means that only those lymph nodes that were obviously abnormal were removed. *Systematic sampling* refers to routine biopsy of lymph nodes at levels specified by the author. *Complete mediastinal lymph node dissection* indicates that all lymph node–containing tissue was routinely removed at those levels indicated by the investigators.

Gaer and Goldstraw (1990) reported the results of the only study that directly compares intraoperative visual evaluation of lymph nodes with pathologic examination. Based on inspection and palpation of the lymph nodes after dissection, the surgeon recorded his impression regarding the presence or absence of metastatic tumor in 95 consecutive patients with NSCLC who underwent pulmonary resection and mediastinal lymph node dissection. Two hundred and eighty-seven nodal levels were removed (Table 36–2). Sensitivity was 71%, and the positive predictive value was 64%. If only tactile inspection of the nodal levels through unopened mediastinal pleura would have been performed, these values would presumably have been lower.

The need for routine intraoperative systematic lymph node sampling was further demonstrated by Graham et al (1999), who reported the results of systematic sampling of right levels 2–4 and 7–10 or left levels 4–10 in 240 patients with clinical T1–3N0 NSCLC. Mediastinoscopy was performed prior to thoracotomy if the computed tomography (CT) scan demonstrated mediastinoscope-accessible lymph nodes that were greater than 1.5 cm. No patient with documented N2 disease underwent thoracotomy. Mediastinal lymph node metastases were demonstrated in 20% of patients, most of whom had T1 or T2 tumors.

Haiderer et al (1990) reported the results of routine mediastinal lymph node dissection performed as part of their operation for NSCLC. Enlarged mediastinal lymph nodes were found in 34 out of 83 patients (41%). However, only 19 (56%) contained metastatic disease. Micrometastatic disease was found in two (4.1%) of the 49 patients with normal-appearing mediastinal lymph nodes. Supporting data are contained in a publication by Bollen et al (1993), who found that the discovery ratio (calculated in a fashion similar to the more familiar relative risk ratio) of N2 disease in patients with NSCLC who underwent mediastinal lymph node dissection was 1.9 (confidence interval, 0.9–4) when compared with those patients whose lymph nodes were removed only if they appeared or felt abnormal.

A number of investigators have evaluated the extent of mediastinal biopsy necessary to obtain accurate staging information. Bollen et al (1993) found that systematic

TABLE 36–2 ■ Intraoperative Assessment of Lymph Nodes

Assessment	*No. Node Stations*	*No. Patients*
True negative	238	88
True positive	25	16
False positive	14	11
False negative	10	9
Total number of resections	95	

Accuracy, 91.6%, predictive value: positive, 25/(25 + 14) = 64.1%:negative, 238/(238 + 10) = 96.0%.

From Gaer JAR, Goldstraw P: Intraoperative assessment of nodal staging at thoracotomy for carcinoma of the bronchus. Eur J Cardiothorac Surg 4:207, 1990.

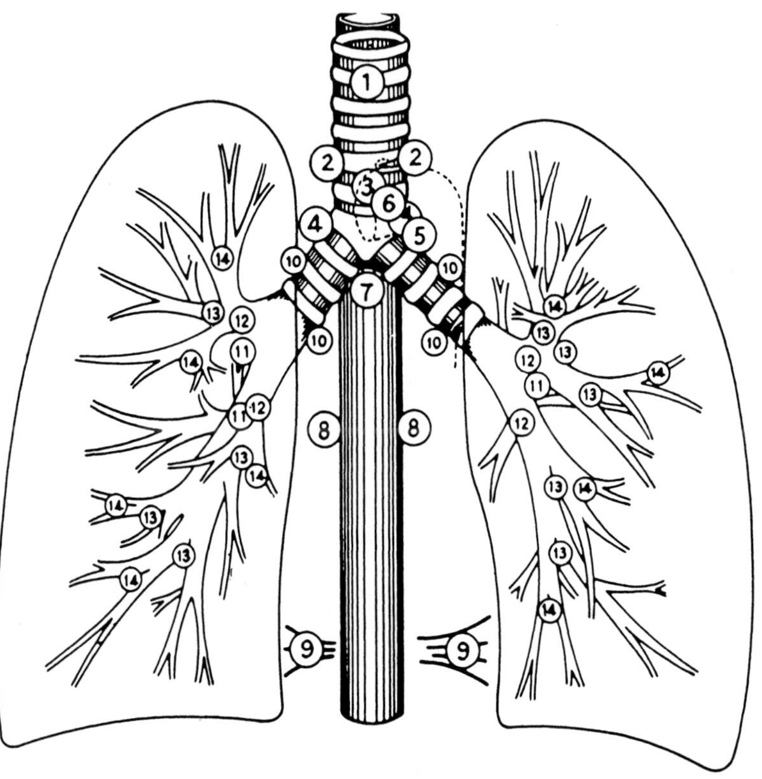

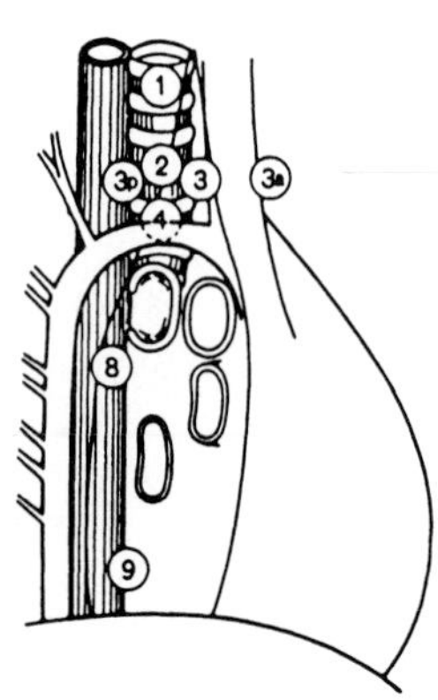

1 Superior mediastinal or highest mediastinal
2 Paratracheal
3 Pretracheal, retrotracheal or posterior mediastinal (3p), and anterior mediastinal (3a).
4 Tracheobronchial
5 Subaortic or Botallo
6 Para-aortic (ascending aorta)
7 Subcarinal
8 Paraesophageal (below carina)
9 Pulmonary ligament
10 Hilar
11 Interlobar
12 Lobar .... Upper lobe, Middle lobe and Lower lobe
13 Segmental
14 Subsegmental

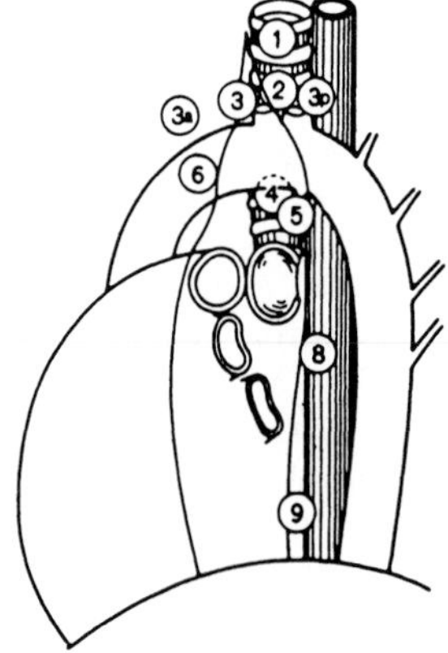

FIGURE 36–89 ■ Lymph node map originally proposed by Naruke. (From Naruke T, Suemasu K, Ishikawa S: Lymph node mapping and curability at various levels of metastasis in resected lung cancer. J Thorac Cardiovasc Surg 76:832, 1978.)

sampling of mediastinal lymph nodes was as successful as mediastinal lymph node dissection in identifying N2 disease (discovery ratio 2.7; confidence interval 1.04–4.2). Izbicki et al (1995) conducted a randomized prospective trial containing 182 patients comparing systematic lymph node sampling with mediastinal lymph node dissection. The number of N2 positive levels was greater in the patients who had full lymph node dissections, although the percentage of patients found to have N1 or N2 disease was not significantly different between the two study arms. A similar study was conducted by Sugi et al (1998) in 115 patients with clinical T1N0 tumors that were less than 2 cm in diameter. Mediastinal metastases were found in 13% of each study group. Thus, it appears that systematic lymph node sampling is as accurate as mediastinal lymph node dissection for staging NSCLC. The survival advantage of mediastinal lymph node dissection, if any, has not been proven.

Biopsy of the sentinel lymph node has been proposed as a selective method for directing mediastinal lymph node staging. Little et al (1999) injected each quadrant of lung tissue surrounding the tumors of 36 clinically N0 patients with Isosulfan blue dye. Following pulmonary resection, a systematic mediastinal lymph node sampling was performed. A sentinel lymph node was identified in 17 patients. Each of the five sentinel lymph nodes found in the mediastinum contained tumor, while only three of 12 within the pleural reflection harbored metastatic cancer. Among the 19 patients in whom no sentinel lymph node could be found, five patients proved to have N1 disease and one patient had N2 disease. The role of this technique in intraoperative lung cancer staging requires additional data.

N Category

The stumbling block of accurate lung cancer staging has been the N of the tumor-node-metastasis (TNM) system. Disagreement about the stage to which lymph node levels should be assigned (e.g., level 10), as well as competing definitions for a number of the N levels (e.g., levels 2–4) has caused much confusion.

The realization that clinical outcome varied with the location of the tumor-containing lymph node influenced the definitions of the N category. The lymph node mapping schema proposed by Naruke et al (1978) (Fig. 36–89) and accepted by the American Joint Committee for Cancer Staging and End Results Reporting (AJCC) achieved universal acceptance after publication in 1978 (see Fig. 36–89). However, interinstitutional as well as intrainstitutional interpretation of lymph node levels varied because of the lack of precise anatomic definitions. For instance, the term *hilar* was utilized for level 10. Were these lymph nodes within the pleural reflection, or were they located in the mediastinum? If they were located outside the pleural reflection, why were they included in the N1 category, and how could they be differentiated from the contiguous level 4 lymph nodes? Similarly, the precise limits of the *superior mediastinal lymph nodes* (levels 1 through 4) and *aortic lymph nodes* (levels 5 and 6) allowed some investigators to report multilevel metastases, whereas others reported only single nodal level involvement.

The American Thoracic Society (ATS) attempted to ameliorate the confusion by issuing an official statement in which the vague terms "hilar" and "mediastinal" were discarded in favor of nodal level definitions based on constant anatomic structures identified in the operating room (Tisi et al, 1983). For instance, right level 4 lymph nodes were defined as those lymph nodes found ". . . to the right of the midline of the trachea between the cephalic border of the azygos vein and the intersection of the caudal margin of the brachiocephalic artery with the right side of the trachea." No decision was made regarding whether level 10 lymph nodes should be considered as N1 or N2. This determination was deferred until survival data of patients who had accurate and thorough intraoperative lymph node dissections could be collected and analyzed. The ATS nodal definitions were not officially accepted by the AJCC, although they were commonly utilized.

The Lung Cancer Study Group initially employed the AJCC lymph node definitions, but later adopted and modified the ATS definitions (Holmes, 1990; Rusch et al, 1993). Level 10 lymph nodes were unequivocally placed in the N2 category. In 1986, a revised international staging system for lung cancer was adopted by the AJCC and the Union Internationale Contre le Cancer (UICC) (Mountain, 1986). Lymph node level definitions remained unchanged, although the components of the N2 nodal group were altered, and an N3 category was created.

The staging system and lymph node level definitions were again significantly modified in 1997 (Mountain, 1997, Mountain and Dresler, 1997). The new mediastinal lymph node level definitions were created to enable accurate and reproducible clinical staging and are based on structures readily identified by CT scans (Figs. 36–90, 36–91; Table 36–3). Unfortunately, the intraoperative identification of some of the lymph node levels has been rendered more difficult (e.g., right levels 2 and 4), because the revised definitions utilize structures that are

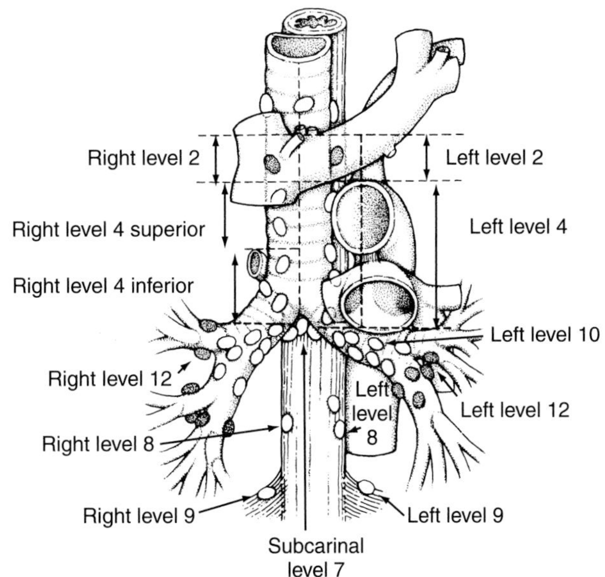

FIGURE 36–90 ■ Graphic representation of lymph node level definitions. (Courtesy of Steven M. Keller, MD.)

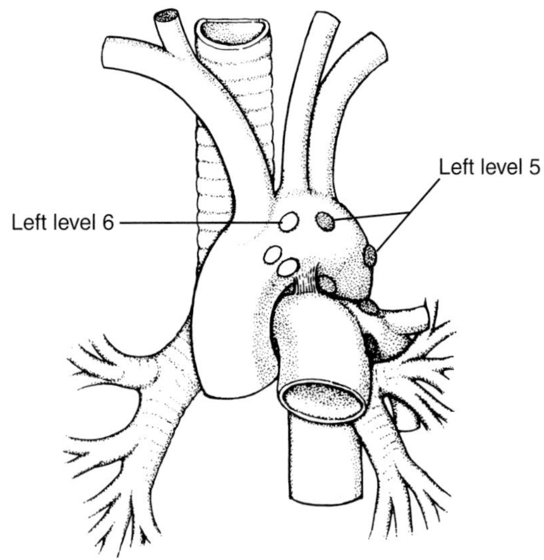

FIGURE 36–91 ■ Details of lymph node definitions in the left hemithorax. (Courtesy of Steven M. Keller, MD.)

not easily identified during surgery. Level 10 lymph nodes were defined as those nodes found along the anterior surface of the mainstem bronchus distal to the pleural reflection and were placed in the N1 category. Mountain (1992) has emphasized the importance of identifying the nodal and stage definitions used by different authors when interpreting and comparing published results. The new revised staging system is utilized in studies conducted under the aegis of the various American national cooperative oncology groups.

BASIC SCIENCE

Patterns of Metastatic Spread

Harvey and Zimmerman (1934–1935) documented the development of the pulmonary lymphatics within the human embryo. The definitive description of the locations of the extrapulmonary intrathoracic adult human lymph nodes was written by Rouviere (1938). Superb summaries of the common intrapulmonary lymphatic anatomy were published by Borrie (1952) and Weinberg (1972).

The patterns of lung cancer dissemination within the intrapulmonary lymphatics of resected specimens were investigated by Borrie (1952). He found that right upper lobe tumors metastasized to the lymph nodes surrounding the right upper lobe bronchus and to those lymph nodes "in the angle between the upper and middle lobe bronchus and also along the medial surface of the right main bronchus." The latter region became known as the *lymphatic sump of Borrie*. Metastases from right upper lobe tumors were not found below the level of the middle lobe bronchus.

Lymph nodes surrounding the middle lobe bronchus and proximal to the previously described bronchial sump were the site of metastases from right middle lobe tumors. Tumors within the right lower lobe metastasized to the peribronchial lymphatics, the lymph nodes contained within the inferior pulmonary ligament, and the sump of Borrie. Metastases to the lymphatic sump have been found to correlate with the presence of endobronchial tumor in the middle or lower lobe orifices (Murray et al, 1982).

Left upper lobe cancers metastasized to lymph nodes surrounding the left upper lobe bronchus and to those surrounding the apical and basilar segmental bronchi of the left lower lobe. Sites of lymphatic metastases of left lower lobe tumors included nodes surrounding the left lower lobe bronchus, the inferior pulmonary ligament, and the left upper lobe bronchus.

These observations were confirmed and extended by Nohl-Oser (1956; 1972) to include the patterns of mediastinal spread. The locations of nodal specimens from 749 patients with stages I–IV NSCLC who underwent mediastinoscopy, scalene node biopsy, or mediastinal lymph node dissection were included in the analysis. Histology was not stated. Right upper lobe tumors spread rarely to the subcarinal region (1%) or to the contralateral scalene nodes or mediastinum (3%), but they commonly spread to the ipsilateral mediastinum (50%). Tumors within the right lower lobe metastasized to the contralateral scalene nodes or mediastinum infrequently (4%), but commonly spread to the subcarinal region (13%) and ipsilateral mediastinum (29%). Insufficient numbers of right middle lobe tumors were present to allow analysis. Left upper lobe tumors metastasized to the subcarinal region (5%) and contralateral mediastinum (7%). Tumors originating within the left lower lobe metastasized to the subcarinal region (3%), as well as the contralateral mediastinum. Greschuchna, cited by Nohl-Oser (1989), documented a much higher prevalence of subcarinal lymph node metastases from upper lobe tumors and a greater occurrence of paratracheal disease from lower lobe neoplasms.

More recently, Asamura et al (1999) documented the patterns of intrathoracic lymph node metastases in 166 patients with proven N2 disease (Table 36–4). All patients had undergone complete mediastinal lymph node dissections at the time of pulmonary resection. He found that upper lobe tumors rarely metastasized to the subcarinal lymph nodes, particularly in the absence of concomitant paratracheal lymph node metastases. He suggested, therefore, that subcarinal node dissection is unnecessary in the absence of documented lymph node level 1–4 metastases.

The intrathoracic metastatic patterns of 124 patients with N2 NSCLC who underwent pulmonary resection and mediastinal lymph node dissection were reported by Watanabe (1990). In contradistinction to Nohl (1956) and Asamura (1999), he found frequent metastases from right upper lobe tumors to the subcarinal lymph nodes (36%). He also demonstrated that tumors originating in the right middle and lower lobes commonly (28%) spread to the ipsilateral paratracheal region (level 4). The subcarinal lymph nodes were a common site of metastases from tumors of the left upper (20%) and left lower (38%) lobes.

Experimental support for these results was provided by Hata (1990). Lymphoscintigraphies were performed in 179 patients who had no evidence of lymph node involvement by transbronchoscopic injection of anti-

TABLE 36–3 ■ American Joint Committee on Cancer and Union Internationale Contre le Cancer 1996 Lymph Node Level Definitions

Nodal Station	*Anatomic Landmarks*
N2 nodes—All N2 nodes lie within the mediastinal pleural envelope.	
1—Highest mediastinal	Nodes lying above a horizontal line at the upper rim of the brachiocephalic (left innominate) vein where it ascends to the left, crossing in front of the trachea at its midline.
2—Upper paratracheal	Nodes lying above a horizontal line drawn tangential to the upper margin of the aortic arch and below the inferior boundary of No. 1 nodes.
3—Prevascular and retrotracheal	Prevascular and retrotracheal nodes may be designated 3A and 3P; midline nodes are considered to be ipsilateral.
4—Lower paratracheal	The lower paratracheal nodes on the right lie to the right of the midline of the trachea between a horizontal line drawn tangential to the upper margin of the aortic arch and a line extending across the right main bronchus at the upper margin of the upper lobe bronchus, and contained within the mediastinal pleural envelope; the lower paratracheal nodes on the left lie to the left of the midline of the trachea between a horizontal line drawn tangential to the upper margin of the aortic arch and a line extending across the left main bronchus at the level of the upper margin of the left upper lobe bronchus, medial to the ligamentum arteriosum and contained within the mediastinal pleural envelope.
	Researchers may wish to designate the lower paratracheal nodes as No. 4S (superior) and No. 4I (inferior) subsets for study purposes; the No. 4S nodes may be defined by a horizontal line extending across the trachea and drawn tangential to the cephalic border of the azygos vein; the No. 4I nodes may be defined by the lower boundary of No. 4S and the lower boundary of No. 4I as described earlier.
5—Subaortic (aorto-pulmonary window)	Subaortic nodes are lateral to the ligamentum arteriosum or the aorta or left pulmonary artery and proximal to the first branch of the left pulmonary artery. They lie with the mediastinal pleural envelope.
6—Para-aortic (ascending aorta or phrenic)	Nodes lying anterior and lateral to the ascending aorta and the aortic arch or the innominate artery, beneath a line that is tangential to the upper margin of the aortic arch.
7—Subcarinal	Nodes lying caudal to the carina of the trachea, but not associated with the lower lobe bronchi or arteries within the lung.
8—Paraesophageal	Nodes lying adjacent to the wall of the esophagus and to the right or left of the midline, excluding subcarinal nodes.
9—Pulmonary ligament	Nodes lying within the pulmonary ligament, including those in the posterior wall and the lower part of the inferior vein.
N1 nodes—All N1 nodes lie distal to the mediastinal pleural reflection and within the visceral pleura.	
10—Hilar	The proximal lobar nodes, distal to the mediastinal pleural reflection, and the nodes, adjacent to the bronchus intermedius to the right; radiographically, the hilar shadow may be created by enlargement of both hilar and interlobar nodes.
11—Interlobar	Nodes lying between the lobar bronchi.
12—Lobar	Nodes adjacent to the distal lobar bronchi.
13—Segmental	Nodes adjacent to the segmental bronchi.
14—Subsegmental	Nodes around the subsegmental bronchi.

From Mountain CF, Dresler CM: Regional lymph node classification for lung cancer staging. Chest 111:1718, 1997.

TABLE 36–4 ■ Pattern of Intrathoracic Metastases in Patients with N2 Disease*

Lymph Node Location	*Right Upper Lobe (n=54)*	*Right Lower Lobe (n=41)*	*Left Upper Lobe (n=44)*	*Left Lower Lobe (n=19)*
Levels 1–4	75	46	27	11
Level 10–14	30	36	37	7
Level 7	7	24	9	11
Level 8	0	0	0	1
Level 9	0	4	0	5
Level 5	—	—	26	3
Level 6	—	—	14	1

*Metastases may be present at more than one lymph node level.

From Asamura H, Nakayama H, Kondo H et al: Lobe-specific extent of systematic lymph node dissection for non-small cell lung carcinomas according to a retrospective study of metastasis and prognosis. J Thorac Cardiovasc Surg 117:1102, 1999.

mony sulfide or rhenium colloid labeled with ^{99m}technetium into the submucosa of each segment. Gamma camera scanning demonstrated patterns of lymphatic drainage that recapitulated the clinical findings of Greschuchna and Watanabe (1990) (Fig. 36–92).

SURGICAL TECHNIQUES

The earliest detailed description of a thorough intrathoracic lymph node dissection as part of an operation for lung cancer was given in 1951 by Cahan et al (1951), although Brock (1948) indicated that it was a routine part of his operative procedure for lung cancer a number of years earlier. En bloc removal of the lymphatics and lung was emphasized. Other authors soon published their techniques describing the lymph node locations in general anatomic terms (Brock and Whytehead, 1955; Cahan 1960; Higginson, 1953; Kirsh et al, 1971; Naruke et al, 1976; Weinberg, 1951). Numbers were first assigned to the lymph node regions by Weinberg (1951).

Martini (1995) has detailed the mediastinal lymph node dissection technique developed at the Memorial Sloan-Kettering Cancer Center. During a right thoracotomy, the right paratracheal and subcarinal regions are routinely cleared of all lymphatic tissue, while during a left thoracotomy, the subcarinal and aortopulmonary window lymph nodes are removed. Lymph nodes were not resected in continuity with the pulmonary specimen. Level numbers were assigned according to Naruke (1978).

Extensive lymphadenectomies have been devised by surgeons who believe that removal of regional lymphatics offers a survival advantage. These have included contralateral mediastinal lymph nodes and, in some cases, supraclavicular lymph nodes. Watanabe (1991) transects the azygos vein to gain access to the upper mediastinal lymph nodes (Naruke levels 1 through 4) during a right thoracotomy. Nodes anterior to the superior vena cava with associated thymic tissue are also removed. In addition, left levels 2–4 are resected by continuing the dissection to the contralateral aspect of the trachea. All lymph node–containing tissue is cleared from the subcarinal region. Both ipsilateral and contralateral levels 8 and 10 lymph nodes are removed.

An equally aggressive lymph node dissection is possible in the left hemithorax. However, such an approach requires mobilization of the arch of the aorta and a portion of the descending aorta. Watanabe's left mediastinal lymph node dissection involves transection of several intercostal arteries. In this fashion, left levels 3 and 4 as well as portions of level 2 can be resected.

Watanabe further modified his operative procedure to

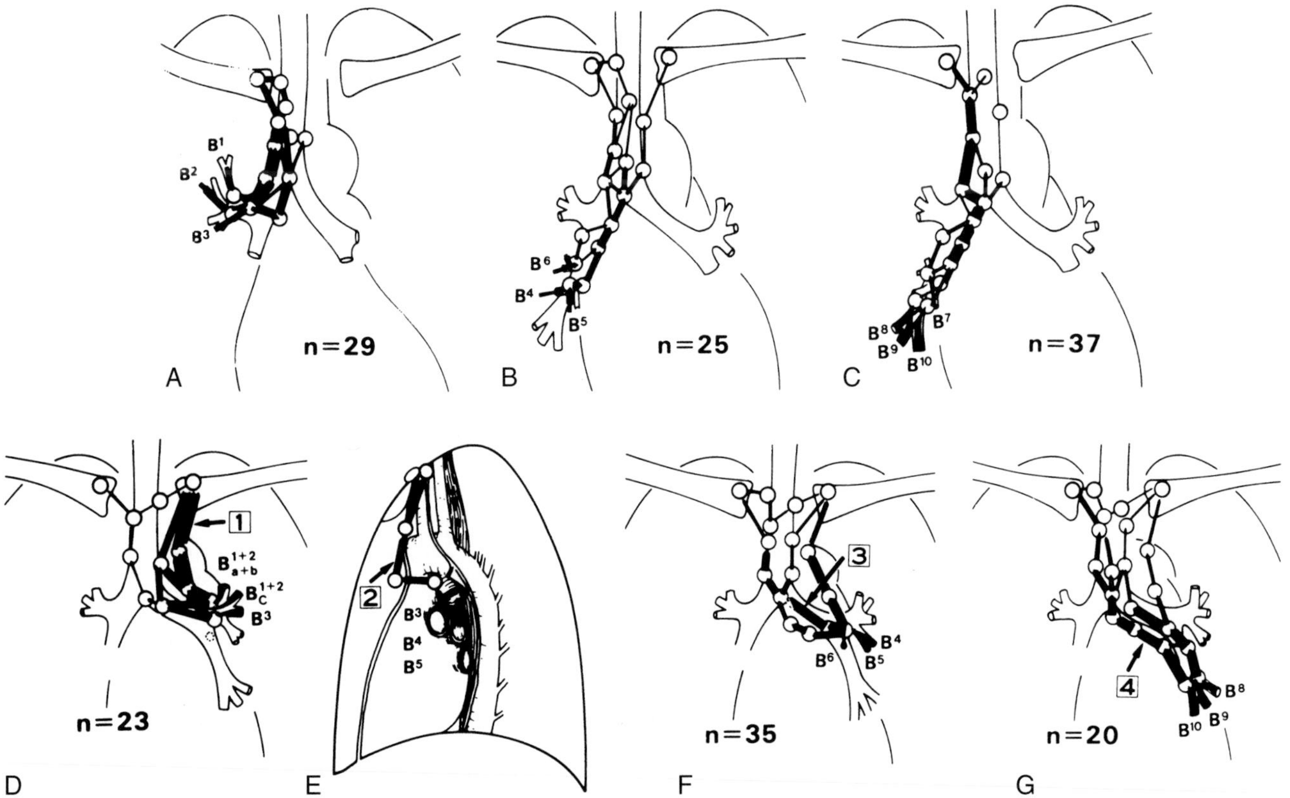

FIGURE 36–92 ■ The width of each arrow corresponds to the relative frequency of lymphatic drainage. *A*, Apical and dorsal segments of the right upper lobe. *B*, Middle lobe and superior segment of the lower lobe. *C*, Basal segments of the lower lobe. *D* through *G*, Four routes of drainage are identified from the left lung: *D*, through the subaortic lymph nodes and then dividing to run proximally along either the vagus nerve to the scalene nodes or along the recurrent laryngeal nerve to the mediastinal nodes; *E*, by way of the phrenic nerve to the scalene nodes; *F*, along the mainstem bronchus to the paratracheal nodes; *G*, under the mainstem bronchus to the subcarinal lymph nodes. (From Hata E, Hayakawa K, Miyamoto H, Hayashida R: Rationale for extended lymphadenectomy for lung cancer. Theor Surg 5:19, 1990.)

permit more thorough dissection of all left mediastinal lymph nodes. Following completion of pulmonary resection by means of a standard posterolateral thoracotomy, a median sternotomy is performed. This permits complete dissection of all left levels 1–4 as well as access to contralateral levels 1–4 and 10. This approach has also been investigated by Mitsuoka (1994).

Nakahara (1993) utilized a similar approach for treatment of right lung cancers. A median sternotomy was not, however, employed for left lung tumors. Rather, the ligamentum arteriosum was transected, the aorta was encircled with a catheter, and traction was applied caudally. The pleura between the left common carotid and subclavian arteries was opened, and the trachea and left mainstem bronchus were exposed, permitting dissection of left levels 2–4.

Hata (1990; 1994) has pursued an even more aggressive approach, extending the right lymphadenectomy performed during posterolateral thoracotomy to include ipsilateral scalene lymph nodes if the most cephalad right paratracheal lymph nodes (Naruke levels 1, 2, and 4) contain metastatic cancer. He advocates broadening the supraclavicular dissection to include the left scalene lymph nodes if anterior mediastinal lymph node (Naruke level 3) involvement is suspected.

The extent of the left lymphadenectomy was determined by both tumor histology and stage. Mediastinal lymph nodes of patients with stage I squamous cell cancers were removed via a left posterolateral thoracotomy. Although the authors did not specifically state the operative details, they appear to include division of the ligamentum arteriosum and mobilization of the aortic arch. Patients with more advanced stages and other histologies undergo median sternotomy followed by anterior and bilateral paratracheal lymphadenectomy (levels 1–4). Exposure is obtained by retracting the ascending aorta to the left and the superior vena cava to the right. The subcarinal nodes are exposed by caudal retraction of the right main pulmonary artery. The left lobe of the thymus is resected to uncover the aortopulmonary window lymph nodes, which are removed to the ligamentum arteriosum. Left upper lobectomy and pneumonectomy are performed via sternotomy, while a left lower lobectomy is accomplished through an additional anteroaxillary thoracotomy.

Hata recommends a cervical dissection if metastatic disease is found in the highest mediastinal, supraclavicular, or scalene lymph nodes. A cervical collar incision is made, the sternocleidomastoid muscles are retracted laterally, and the strap muscles are divided. The fascia over the internal jugular vein is opened, and the vein is skeletonized. The recurrent laryngeal nerve is gently retracted forward, and the cervical paraesophageal lymph nodes are removed.

MEDIASTINAL LYMPH NODE DISSECTION

The author's technique is a variation of the lymph node dissection method originally developed at the Memorial Sloan-Kettering Cancer Center. Modifications reflect current lymph node level definitions as well as changes in surgical technique.

Right Hemithorax

Mediastinal lymphadenectomy can readily be accomplished via either a posterolateral thoracotomy or through a muscle-sparing skin incision. Entry into the chest through the fourth or fifth interspace provides access to the necessary lymph node locations. Although mediastinal lymph node dissection is commonly performed following completion of the pulmonary resection, if the presence of tumor within the lymph nodes will change the operative procedure, the lymph node resection should be performed before lung removal.

The superior mediastinum, encompassed by the trachea, the superior vena cava, and the azygos vein, is exposed by retracting the lung inferiorly (Fig. 36–93).

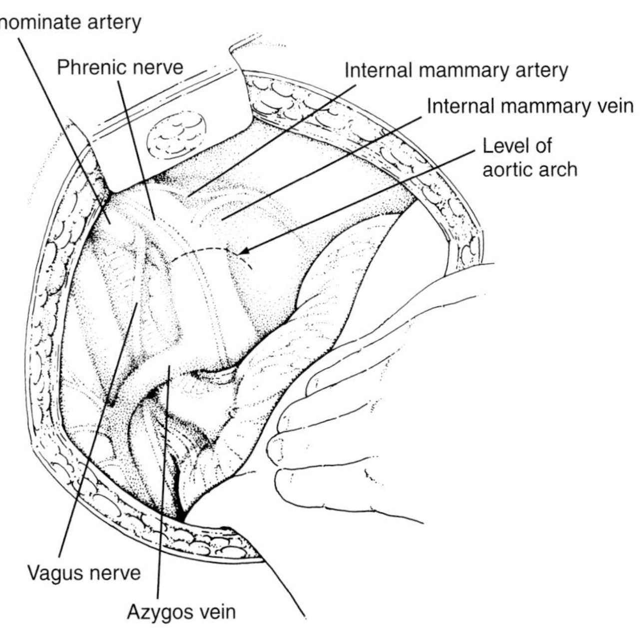

FIGURE 36–93 ■ Exposure of right superior mediastinum with mediastinal pleura intact. (Courtesy of Steven M. Keller, MD.)

The phrenic nerve is identified on the lateral border of the superior vena cava. The vagus nerve traverses the superior mediastinum and is usually visible through the unopened mediastinal pleura. The mediastinal pleura cephalad to the azygos vein (between the trachea and superior vena cava) is grasped with a forceps and incised to the level of the innominate artery. The pleural edge over the trachea is retracted, and using a peanut sponge rolled tightly on a clamp, the mediastinal fat pad is dissected off the anterolateral tracheal surface (Fig. 36–94). Traction is placed on the pleural edge over the superior vena cava, and the mediastinal fat pad is gently dissected from the junction of the superior vena cava and the azygos vein to the level of the innominate artery. A small vein draining from the mediastinal fat pad directly into the superior vena cava is frequently present.

The mediastinal fat pad is removed from the superior vena cava anteriorly to the trachea posteriorly, and from the cephalad border of the azygos vein inferiorly to the caudal border of the innominate artery superiorly. Nonmagnetic clips (to avoid artifacts on future CT scans) are used liberally. *Right level 2* lymph nodes are located between the cephalic border of the aortic arch and the cephalic border of the innominate vein. Lymph nodes distal to the aortic arch and proximal to the azygos vein are labeled *right level 4 superior* (Fig. 36–95).

A vein retractor is used to elevate the azygos vein, and the lymph nodes located between its cephalic border and the origin of the right upper lobe bronchus are removed (Fig. 36–96). During dissection of these *level 4 inferior* lymph nodes, care must be taken not to injure the pulmonary artery. Dissection between the esophagus and membranous portion of the trachea will reveal *level 3 posterior* nodes (Fig. 36–97). *Level 3 anterior* lymph nodes are found anterior and medial to the superior vena cava at the insertion of the azygos vein.

Right level 10 lymph nodes are located along the anterior border of the bronchus intermedius distal to the pleural reflection (Fig. 36–98). *Level 11*, interlobar lymph nodes are found in the sump of Borrie and are exposed

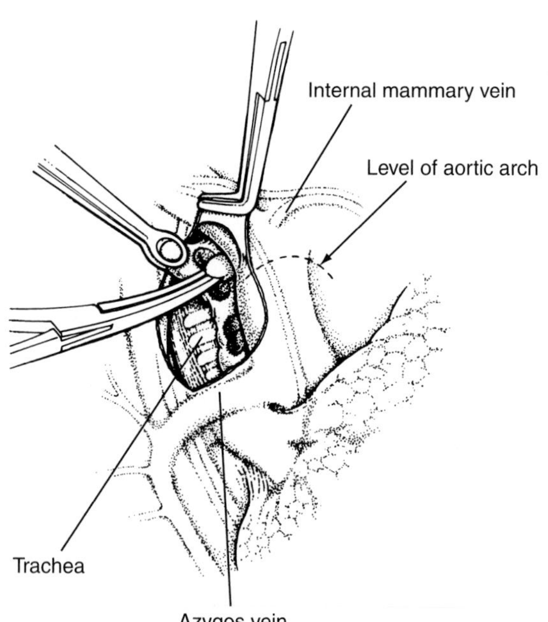

FIGURE 36–94 ■ The internal mammary vein drains into the approximate juncture between the right and the left innominate veins as they combine to form the superior vena cava. It is a reliable structure with which to differentiate the division between level 2 and level 4 lymph nodes. The *dashed line* represents the aortic arch. (Courtesy of Steven M. Keller, MD.)

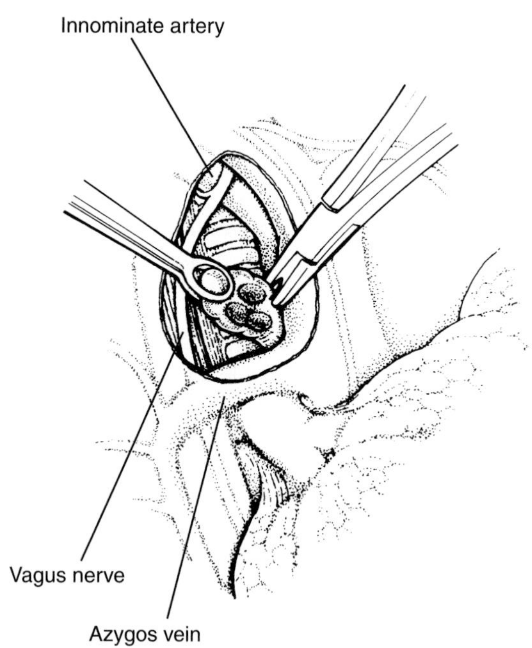

FIGURE 36–95 ■ The lymphadenectomy may be extended to the contralateral lymph node levels (*not shown*). Care must be taken not to injure the left recurrent laryngeal nerve, which is found in the tracheoesophageal groove. (Courtesy of Steven M. Keller, MD.)

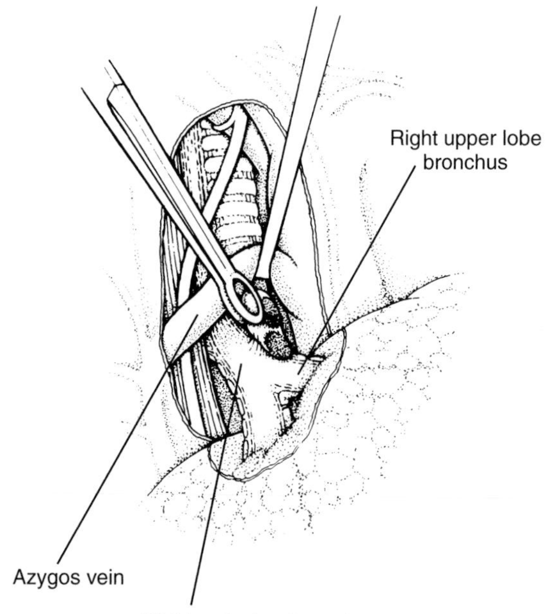

FIGURE 36–96 ■ Division of the azygos vein is rarely necessary. (Courtesy of Steven M. Keller, MD.)

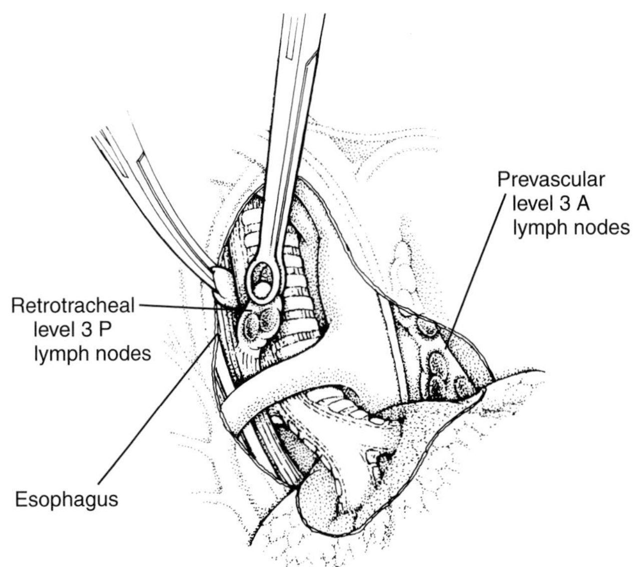

FIGURE 36–97 ■ The location of the membranous portion of the trachea and the phrenic nerve must be determined prior to application of clips. (Courtesy of Steven M. Keller, MD.)

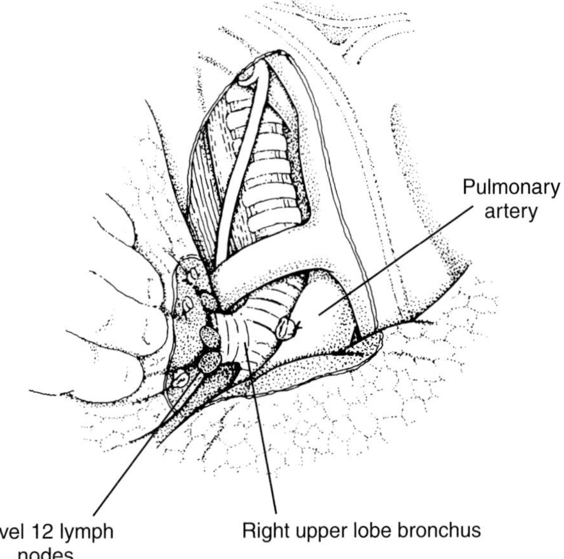

FIGURE 36–99 ■ Peanut forceps are used to dissect the level 12 lymph nodes and include them with the specimen. Cautery is employed to transect soft tissue, because a clip may interfere with the application of a stapling device. (Courtesy of Steven M. Keller, MD.)

by retracting the lung anteriorly. *Level 12* nodes are adjacent to the distal lobar bronchus and are removed with the specimen (Fig. 36–99).

The *level 7* subcarinal region is exposed by retracting the lung anteriorly (Fig. 36–100). The mediastinal pleura is opened, and the edge overlying the esophagus is grasped with a right angle clamp. The esophagus is retracted posteriorly, and the subcarinal lymph node packet is grasped with a ring clamp and elevated from the pericardium. Prior to transection, the attachments to the right and left mainstem bronchi are clipped. Vessels course along the anterior border of the trachea and enter the subcarinal lymph nodes from the region of the carina. These arteries and veins must be identified and controlled prior to transection.

The inferior pulmonary ligament contains the easily visualized *level 9* lymph nodes, which are grasped with a ring forceps and removed with cautery or clips. Paraesophageal, *level 8*, lymph nodes are not always present.

Left Hemithorax

The aortopulmonary (*levels 5 and 6*) and subcarinal (*level 7*) lymph nodes are exposed via a fifth interspace thoracotomy. Beginning at the level of the aortopulmonary window, the pleura is incised in a cephalad direction

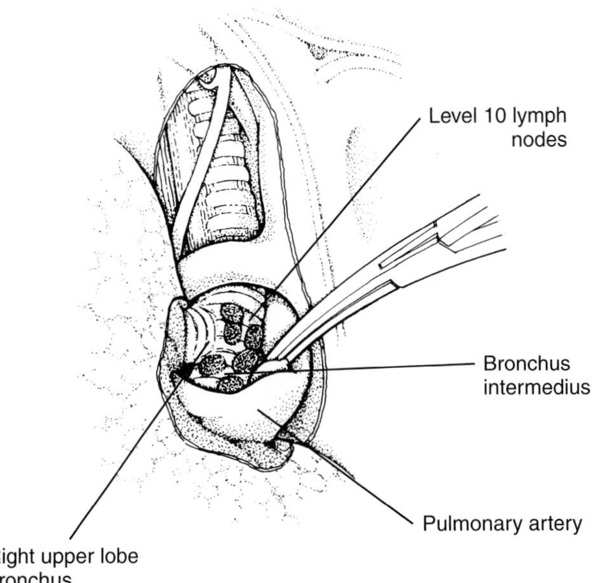

FIGURE 36–98 ■ Exposure of the level 10 lymph nodes is accomplished by retracting the pulmonary artery anteriorly. (Courtesy of Steven M. Keller, MD.)

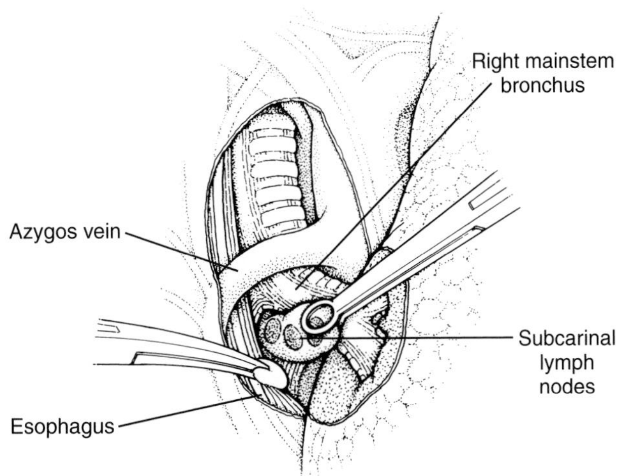

FIGURE 36–100 ■ The esophagus and membranous portion of the bronchus must not be injured when applying clips. (Courtesy of Steven M. Keller, MD.)

midway between and parallel to the vagus and phrenic nerves (Fig. 36–101). The ligamentum arteriosum is not usually seen, but is readily palpated. The pleural edge closest to the phrenic nerve is grasped, and the lymph node–containing fat pad anterior to the ligamentum arteriosum is removed. Dissection of the *level 6* lymph nodes is best accomplished with blunt instruments. To avoid electrical injury to the nearby nerves, vessels should be controlled with clips or ties. The location of the phrenic nerve must be ascertained to avoid iatrogenic diaphragm paralysis. *Level 5* lymph nodes are located posterior to the ligamentum arteriosum and are exposed with blunt dissection. Vocal cord paralysis is a potential but rare complication. Therefore, the recurrent laryngeal nerve and the proximal vagus nerve must be zealously protected.

The *level 7* subcarinal lymph nodes are approached with the lung retracted anteriorly (Fig. 36–102). The left mainstem bronchus is identified, and the pleura is opened anterior and parallel to the aorta. The lymph nodes are grasped with a ring clamp, and clips are liberally applied prior to removal of the nodal packet. The arterial vessel that commonly enters the lymph nodes from the anterior border of the trachea at the level of the carina must be identified and clipped to avoid postoperative hemorrhage.

Level 11 interlobar lymph nodes are best visualized with the lung retracted anteriorly. The pulmonary artery is located immediately anterior and must be avoided when clips or cautery are utilized. *Level 12* lymph nodes are located along the distal lobar bronchus near its junction with the mainstem bronchus and are removed with the specimen (Fig. 36–103). *Level 9* pulmonary ligament lymph nodes are identified within this structure and removed with cautery or clips. The esophagus courses posteriorly, and injury must be avoided.

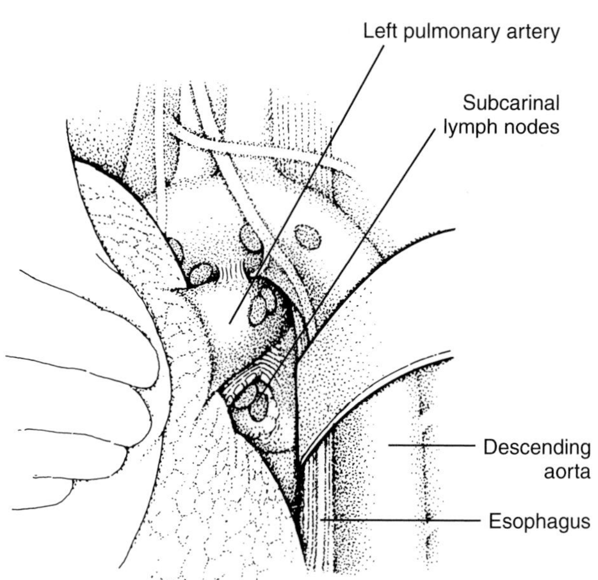

FIGURE 36–102 ■ The subcarinal lymph nodes are more difficult to expose in the left hemithorax than in the right hemithorax. A malleable retractor is used to retract the aorta and the esophagus posteriorly. (Courtesy of Steven M. Keller, MD.)

If the resected specimens are not correctly labeled, even the most detailed lymph node dissection will provide little information. To ensure that each level is reported separately and that levels are not lumped together as "mediastinal lymph nodes," each level must be sent from the operating room as a discrete specimen.

Complications

Some surgeons are hesitant to perform a complete mediastinal lymph node dissection for fear of complications

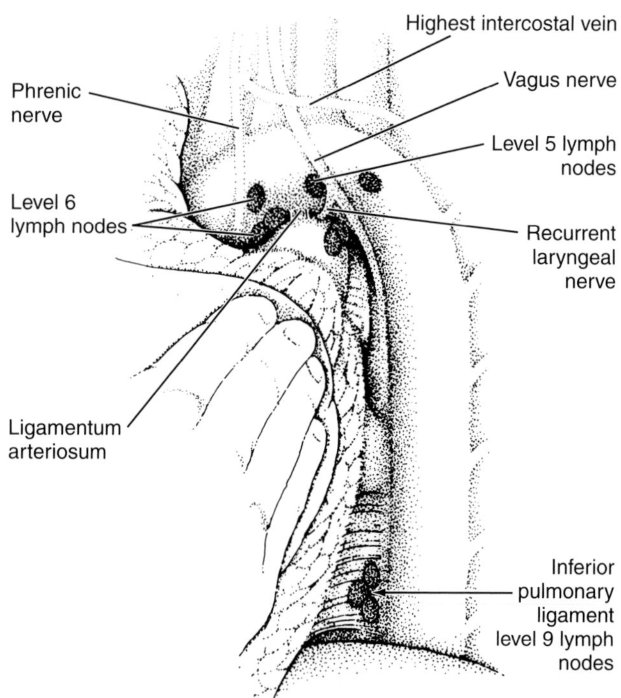

FIGURE 36–101 ■ The left superior mediastinum before opening the mediastinal pleura. Exposure of level 2 or 4 lymph nodes would require mobilization of the aortic arch. (Courtesy of Steven M. Keller, MD.)

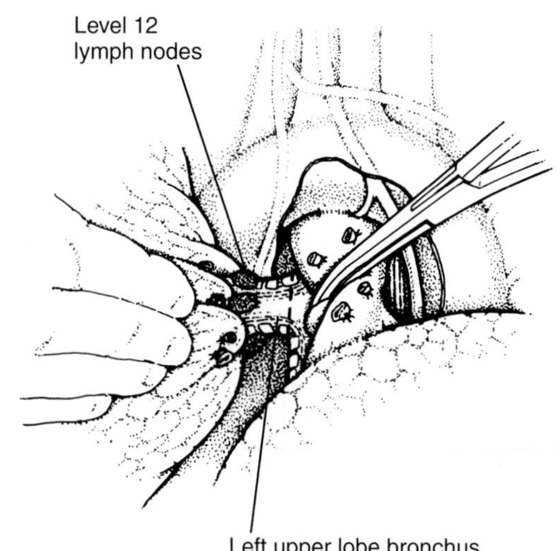

FIGURE 36–103 ■ As the soft tissue is cleared to permit application of the stapling device, the nodes are pushed distally with peanut forceps. (Courtesy of Steven M. Keller, MD.)

that might arise from either interrupting the blood supply to the bronchial stump or removing a large portion of the intrathoracic lymphatics. The postoperative complications of 155 patients with NSCLC who underwent no mediastinal lymph node dissection or sampling (n = 70), complete mediastinal lymph node dissection (n = 65), or systematic mediastinal lymph node sampling (n = 20) were reported by Bollen (1993). Intraoperative blood loss or the need for transfusion was not significantly different among the groups. Three patients (5%) who underwent complete nodal dissection suffered unintentional left recurrent laryngeal nerve injury. Chylothoraces developed in two additional patients. One patient who underwent node dissection required reoperation for bleeding that was not related to the lymphadenectomy. Bronchopleural fistulas developed in two patients who had not undergone node dissection. Hata (1990) reported two left recurrent laryngeal nerve injuries and one phrenic nerve paralysis in 50 patients who underwent extensive mediastinal dissection.

The morbidity and mortality associated with systematic mediastinal sampling and mediastinal lymph node dissection was compared in a randomized prospective study (n = 182) conducted by Izbicki (1994). Although mediastinal lymph node dissection extended the operative procedure by approximately 20 minutes, there was no increase in blood loss, mortality, or need for reoperation. One chylothorax occurred in each group. Six patients who underwent systematic sampling and five patients who underwent mediastinal lymph node dissection had recurrent laryngeal nerve injury. Chest tube drainage and hospitalization were similar in both groups.

Results of Lymph Node Sampling and Dissection

The principle benefit of lymph node dissection is accurate staging. Most investigators make no therapeutic claim for nodal dissection, but rather emphasize the benefits of accurate staging. However, the proponents of the more extensive nodal dissections purport to demonstrate improved survival.

Five-year survival of patients with N2 disease after pulmonary resection and mediastinal lymph node dissection performed as described earlier is reported (Asamura et al, 1999; Maggi et al, 1990; Martini, 1995; Naruke et al, 1988; Regnard et al, 1991; van Klaveren et al, 1993; Watanabe et al, 1991a and b) at 9% to 35%. Following bilateral mediastinal lymph node dissection via sternotomy, a 5-year survival of 66% in 15 patients with N2 disease and 35% in 13 patients with N3 (contralateral mediastinal) disease was reported by Hata (1994). Five-year survival was 33% in 12 patients with scalene or supraclavicular N3 disease who underwent sternotomy and cervical dissection. Nakahara (1993) documented a 3-year median survival for 13 patients with N2 disease who also underwent bilateral mediastinal lymph node dissection. However, no patient with N3 disease survived more than 14 months (n = 4). Watanabe (1991) claimed significantly improved survival in a retrospective study of patients with left upper lobe tumors who underwent bilateral lymph node dissections when compared with those patients who had only suspicious lymph nodes removed.

These reports should be interpreted with some degree of skepticism because they contain small numbers of patients. Indeed, Mitsuoka (1994) found no significant survival advantage for patients with pathologic stage IIIa left lung NSCLCs who underwent sternotomy and nodal dissection when compared with those patients who had resection and node dissection via thoracotomy only. Furthermore, no patients with N3 disease survived 3 years.

FUTURE DIRECTIONS

The American College of Surgeons-Oncology Group has recently activated a randomized prospective trial designed to evaluate the influence of the type of lymph node dissection on patient survival. Following histologic documentation of the absence of N2 disease, patients with T1–2, N0–1 NSCLCs will undergo intraoperative randomization to complete either lymph node dissection or lymph node sampling (ACOS-OG Z0030). Accrual of 1000 patients is underway. A companion study addressing the issue of micrometastatic lymphatic disease has also been opened.

COMMENTS AND CONTROVERSIES

Complete ipsilateral mediastinal node dissection differs in definition among various surgeons. In North America, the lymph node dissection described by Dr. Keller is the one most frequently employed. In Japan, on the left side, the ligamentum arteriosum is always divided and dissection is carried out along the left mainstem bronchus. If lymph nodes are involved in this area, the aorta is mobilized and further dissection is carried out between the subclavian and the carotid arteries along the left peritracheal region. In our own practice, we perform mediastinoscopy for every left-sided tumor, ensuring that left peritracheal and mainstem bronchial lymph nodes (levels 2 and 4) are uninvolved. In such cases, the more limited lymph node dissection as described in this chapter is used. However, if mediastinal lymph nodes are involved, and induction chemotherapy or chemoradiotherapy is employed, we do perform a more extensive mediastinal dissection, dividing the ligamentum described by the Japanese.

It should be noted that the UICC Lymph Node Map defines midline pretracheal nodes as level 3. In the AJCC definition, there are two level 3 lymph node stations—level 3a, which is anterolateral to the superior vena cava (prevascular), and level 3p, which is in the retrotracheal periesophageal region above the carina. There are no pretracheal level 3 lymph nodes in the AJCC interpretation.

R.J.G.

REFERENCES

Asamura H, Nakayama H, Kondo H et al: Lobe-specific extent of systematic lymph node dissection for non-small cell lung carcinomas according to a retrospective study of metastasis and prognosis. J Thorac Cardiovasc Surg 117:1102, 1999.

Bollen ECM, van Duin CJ, Theunissen PHMH et al: Mediastinal lymph node dissection in resected lung cancer: Morbidity and accuracy of staging. Ann Thorac Surg 55:961, 1993.

Borrie J: Primary carcinoma of the bronchus: Prognosis following surgical resection. Ann R Coll Surg Engl 10:165, 1952.

Brock RD: Bronchial carcinoma. Br Med J 2:737, 1948.

Brock R, Whytehead LL: Radical pneumonectomy for bronchial carcinoma. Br J Surg 43:8, 1955.

Cahan WG: Radical lobectomy. J Thorac Cardiovasc Surg 39:555, 1960.

Cahan WG, Watson WL, Pool JL: Radical pneumonectomy. J Thorac Surg 22:449, 1951.

Gaer JAR, Goldstraw P: Intraoperative assessment of nodal staging at thoracotomy for carcinoma of the bronchus. Eur J Cardiothorac Surg 4:207, 1990.

Graham ANJ, Chan KJM, Pastorino U, Goldstraw P: Systematic nodal dissection in the intrathoracic staging of patients with non-small cell lung cancer. J Thorac Cardiovasc Surg 117:246, 1999.

Haiderer O, Wustinger E, Lexer G, Weitensfelder W: Die mediastinale Lymphadenektomie: Anatomische Grundlagen und ihre chirurgische Relevanz beim zentralen Bronchuskarzinom. Wien Med Wochenschr 140:422, 1990.

Harvey DF, Zimmerman, HM: Studies on the development of the human lung. Anat Rec 61:203, 1934–1935.

Hata E, Hayakawa K, Miyamoto H, Hayashida R: Rationale for extended lymphadenectomy for lung cancer. Theor Surg 5:19, 1990.

Hata E, Miyamoto H, Tanaka M et al: Superradical operation for lung cancer: Bilateral mediastinal dissection (BMD) with or without cervical dissection (CD). Lung Cancer 11(Suppl 2):41, 1994.

Higginson JF: Block dissection in pneumonectomy for carcinoma. J Thorac Surg 25:582, 1953.

Holmes EC: Staging non-small cell lung cancer. Evansville, IN, Bristol Meyers Squibb, 1990.

Izbicki JR, Passlick B, Karg O et al: Impact of radical systematic mediastinal lymphadenectomy on tumor staging in lung cancer. Ann Thorac Surg 59:209, 1995.

Izbicki JR, Thetter O, Habekost M et al: Radical systematic mediastinal lymphadenectomy in non-small cell lung cancer: A randomized controlled trial. Br J Surg 81:229, 1994.

Kirsh MM, Kahn DR, Gago O et al: Treatment of bronchogenic carcinoma with mediastinal metastases. Ann Thorac Surg 12:11, 1971.

Little AG, DeHoyos A, Kirgan DM et al: Intraoperative lymphatic mapping for non-small cell lung cancer: The sentinel node technique. J Thorac Cardiovasc Surg 117:220, 1999.

Maggi G, Casadio C, Mancuso M et al: Resection and radical lymphadenectomy for lung cancer: Prognostic significance of lymphatic metastases. Int Surg 75:17, 1990.

Martini N: Mediastinal lymph node dissection for lung cancer. Chest Surg Clin North Am 5:189, 1995.

Mitsuoka M, Hayashi A, Takamori S et al: The significance of lymph nodes (LN) dissection through median sternotomy for left lung cancer. Lung Cancer 11(Suppl 1):149, 1994.

Mountain CF: A new international staging system for lung cancer. Chest 89(Suppl):225S, 1986.

Mountain CF: Revisions in the system for staging lung cancer. Chest 111:1710, 1997.

Mountain CF, Dresler CM: Regional lymph node classification for lung cancer staging. Chest 111:1718, 1997.

Mountain CF, Libshitz HI, Hermes KE: Lung cancer: A handbook for staging and imaging. Houston, TX, Charles P Young, 1992.

Murray GF, Mendes OC, Wilcox BR: Bronchial carcinoma and the lymphatic sump: The importance of bronchoscopic findings. Ann Thorac Surg 34:634, 1982.

Nakahara K, Fujii Y, Matsumura A et al: Role of systematic mediastinal dissection in N2 non-small cell lung cancer patients. Ann Thorac Surg 56:331, 1993.

Naruke T, Goya T, Tsuchiya R, Suemasu K: The importance of surgery to non-small cell carcinoma of lung with mediastinal lymph node metastasis. Ann Thorac Surg 46:603, 1988.

Naruke T, Suemasu K, Ishikawa S: Lymph node mapping and curability at various levels of metastasis in resected lung cancer. J Thorac Cardiovasc Surg 76:832, 1978.

Naruke T, Suemasu K, Ishikawa S: Surgical treatment for lung cancer with metastasis to mediastinal lymph nodes. J Thorac Cardiovasc Surg 71:279, 1976.

Nohl HC: An investigation into the lymphatic and vascular spread of carcinoma of the bronchus. Thorax 11:172, 1956.

Nohl-Oser HC: An investigation of the anatomy of the lymphatic drainage of the lungs. Ann R Coll Surg Engl 51:157, 1972.

Nohl-Oser HC: Lymphatics in the lung. In Shields TW (ed): General Thoracic Surgery, 3rd ed. Philadelphia, Lea & Febiger, 1989.

Regnard JF, Magdeleinat P, Azoulay D et al: Results of resection for bronchogenic carcinoma with mediastinal lymph node metastases in selected patients. Eur J Cardiothorac Surg 5:583, 1991.

Rouviere H: Anatomy of the Human Lymphatic System. (Tobias MJ) (transl): Anatomie des lymphatiques de l'homme.) Ann Harbor, Edward Brothers, 1938.

Rusch VW, Ginsberg RJ, Holmes EC: A thoracic surgery handbook for clinical trials. New York, Memorial Sloan-Kettering Cancer Center, 1993.

Sugi K, Nawata K, Fujita et al: Systematic lymph node dissection for clinically diagnosed peripheral non-small-cell lung cancer less than 2 cm in diameter. World J Surg 22:290, 1998.

Tisi GM, Friedman PJ, Peters RM et al: Clinical staging of primary lung cancer. Am Rev Respir Dis 127:659, 1983.

van Klaveren RJ, Festen J, Ottenn HJAM et al: Prognosis of unsuspected but completely resectable N2 non-small cell lung cancer. Ann Thorac Surg 56:300, 1993.

Watanabe Y, Hayashi Y, Shimizu J et al: Mediastinal nodal involvement and the prognosis of non-small cell lung cancer. Chest 100:422, 1991a.

Watanabe Y, Shimizu J, Oda M et al: Aggressive surgical intervention in N2 non-small cell cancer of the lung. Ann Thorac Surg 51:253, 1991b.

Watanabe Y, Shimizu J, Oda M et al: Improved survival in left non-small-cell N2 lung cancer after more extensive operative procedure. Thorac Cardiovasc Surg 39:89, 1991c.

Watanabe Y, Shimizu J, Tsubota M, Iwa T: Mediastinal spread of metastatic lymph nodes in bronchogenic carcinoma. Chest 97:1059, 1990.

Weinberg JA: Identification of regional lymph nodes in the treatment of bronchogenic carcinoma. J Thorac Surg 22:517, 1951.

Weinberg JA: The intrathoracic lymphatics. In Haagensen CD, Feind CR, Herter FP et al (eds): The Lymphatics in Cancer. Philadelphia, WB Saunders, 1972.

VIDEO-ASSISTED PULMONARY RESECTIONS

Anthony P. C. Yim

HISTORICAL NOTE

Direct thoracoscopy has been in use for almost a century. Jacobaeus from Stockholm first used a cystoscope to examine the pleural cavity under local anesthesia at the turn of the 20th century (Jacobeus, 1910). He primarily used the technique to lyse adhesions to collapse the lungs, as this was the prevailing treatment for tuberculosis at the time. Adhesions were classified by their position, shape, and surgical difficulty. This technique was adopted throughout Europe in the early decades of the 20th century. Specific instruments for thoracoscopy were designed by Davidson (1929) and Cutler (1933). Large clinical experience of adhesiolysis was subsequently reported by pulmonologists from several European centers. The introduction of streptomycin in 1945, however, marked the end of a period of enthusiasm for therapeutic thoracoscopy. Surgical application of this technique was introduced by Lewis to diagnose pleural disease under general anesthesia in the 1970s (Lewis, 1976). This stimulated renewed interest in this approach among some surgeons.

Modern video-assisted thoracic surgery (VATS) was made possible by two technological developments. First, improved endoscopic lens systems coupled with the advent of solid state systems and microcameras in the early 1980s allowed a panoramic view of the hemithorax instead of the previous tunnel-like vision. Second, the availability of new endoscopic instruments such as the linear mechanical staplers opened up new vistas for a spectrum of diagnostic and therapeutic procedures. The tremendous success of laparoscopic cholecystectomy in the mid 1980s gave impetus to surgeons to apply this technique to body cavities beyond the abdomen.

The first major meeting on VATS was held in San Antonio, Texas in conjunction with the Society of Thoracic Surgeons meeting. Over 50 papers were presented, and the proceedings were subsequently published as a 200-page supplement in the *Annals of Thoracic Surgery* under the joint guest editorship of Mack, Hazelrigg, Landreneau, and Naunheim (First International Symposium on Thoracoscopic Surgery, 1993). This represented the baptism of a newborn technique.

In subsequent years, VATS gained popularity, and the technique was further developed and refined independently in several centers in North America, Asia, Europe, Australia and South America (Braimbridge, 2000). Cost-containing strategies for VATS were developed in Hong Kong and Taiwan. Its applications as a diagnostic approach and a therapeutic modality for benign thoracic diseases were gradually accepted into mainstream thoracic surgery. However, VATS major resection, particularly for primary cancer, was met with much initial skepticism. A randomized, prospective study of VATS lobectomy compared with thoracotomy (which retrospectively was premature because the VATS techniques used were neither established nor standardized), presented at the American Association for Thoracic Surgery meeting in 1994, showed no benefits for using VATS. This quelled the interest in this application for most surgeons except for a few who persevered to further develop and refine this approach, which subsequently has been shown to give excellent, reproducible results.

■ *HISTORICAL READINGS*

Braimbridge MV: Thoracoscopy—a historical perspective. In Yim APC, Hazelrigg SR, Izzat MB et al (eds): Minimal Access Cardiothoracic Surgery. Philadelphia, WB Saunders, 2000

Cutler JW: A technique and apparatus for intrapleural pneumonolysis. Am Rev Tuberc 28:528, 1933.

Davidson LR: A simplified operating thoracoscope. Am Rev Tuberc 19:306, 1929.

Jacobaeus HC: Ueber die Möglichkeit die Zystoskopie bei Untersuchung seröser Höhlungen anzuwenden. München Med Wchenschr 57:2090, 1910

Kirby TJ, Mack MJ, Landreneau RJ, Rice TW: Lobectomy—video-assisted thoracic surgery versus muscle-sparing thoracotomy: A randomized trial. J. Thorac Cardiovasc Surg 109:997, 1995

Lewis RJ, Kunderman PJ, Sisler GE, Mackenzie JW: Direct diagnostic thoracoscopy. Ann Thorac Surg 21:536, 1976

Mack MJ, Hazelrigg SR, Landreneau RJ, Naunheim KS (eds): The First International Symposium on Thoracoscopic Surgery. Ann Thorac Surgery 56:605, 1993

Meade RH: A history of thoracic surgery. Springfield, Charles C Thomas, 1961

Since the first lung resection was performed in 1891 by Tuffier, posterolateral thoracotomy and, occasionally, median sternotomy and clam-shell incision for bilateral pulmonary procedures have been the preferred modes of surgical access. Although these incisions generally provide good surgical exposure, they unfortunately are also among the most painful incisions ever to be encountered by patients—not only because of the lengths of the incisions, and division of muscles, but primarily because ribs (or sternum) have to be separated to gain access into the chest.

Although it has been realized for some time that the trauma of access is often worse than that of the procedure itself, the use of smaller incisions alone to access the chest (i.e., without video-assistance), such as the French incision (Heitmiller and Mathisen, 1989) never gained wide popularity in the surgical community. Conventional wisdom relates minimal access to limited surgical exposure, and hence, complicated intrathoracic procedures performed under suboptimal surgical exposure are generally not considered safe. However, any attempt to spread the ribs to compensate for the smaller skin incision would defeat the purpose of minimal access surgery. This situation was changed by the advent of videoendoscopic surgery. Fueled by the success of laparoscopic cholecystectomy in the 1980s, VATS plays a part in a revolution that now affects all surgical disciplines. The thoracoscope–camera unit with its own light source provides a well-illuminated, magnified operative view with very high resolution for details, which surpasses that provided by the conventional headlight and magnifying loops.

However, it is important to be able to be flexible in the application of new technology. Video-assistance has a role to play even in open surgery. Video-assistance or simply making use of the illumination it brings can help with a difficult adhesiolysis in the lung apex or base. Also, when median sternotomy is used for bilateral lung surgery, resection of a posteriorly located nodule could be difficult, and video-assistance could facilitate success in these situations. One can call this thoracotomy/median sternotomy with video-assistance, but irrespective of what names were given, the possibility of combining a new technology with an existing, established surgical technique to improve outcome should not be ignored. This could also serve as an intermediate step for some practicing surgeons who are trying to acquire a new skill (Yim, 1997).

There are few detailed technical descriptions of VATS pulmonary resection. Much of this chapter will be dedicated to anatomical lung resections, with a smaller section to nonanatomical resections. The techniques we have used in our practice will be described.

VATS MAJOR LUNG RESECTIONS

The Concerns and the Controversies

VATS major resection was not well received initially (Mack, 1997). Several concerns have been raised in the thoracic surgical community (including those surgeons who are already practicing VATS). First, anatomical dissection of the hilum in an essentially closed chest immediately raised the issue of safety. Second, oncologic resection with a curative intent raises skepticism regarding adequacy of clearance. Third, although the short-term benefits of VATS to patients were intuitively obvious, its long-term advantages over conventional surgery remained unclear. Fourth, the high cost of the endoscopic equipment, particularly the consumables, cast doubt on the cost-effectiveness of this approach. These issues will be fully addressed in this chapter.

It is important to point out that VATS major resection is not a unified technique, because several variations exist (Yim, 1998a). This is not surprising as this procedure was developed almost simultaneously at different centers, with each unit carrying its own characteristics. There is little consensus over some details of the technique. For example, how long an incision distinguishes "minithoracotomy" from "thoracotomy"? How often should one operate through the minithoracotomy as opposed to the video monitor? How much rib spreading can we afford before the benefits of minimal access surgery are lost? For the sake of description, we define VATS major resection as a video-assisted, minimal access technique in which the surgeon operates primarily by watching the television monitor, and little or no rib spreading is required throughout the entire procedure. For those surgeons who use rib-spreaders and operate primarily by looking through the minithoracotomy wound, we suggest the term *minithoracotomy with video assistance* to describe such a technique (Yim, 1998a). Lewis described a technique of simultaneous stapling of the pulmonary vessels and bronchus with excellent results (Lewis, 1999). This represents not only a new approach, but a new operation altogether. Most surgeons practicing VATS major resections continue with the individual ligation technique as in conventional surgery.

Indications, Patient Selections, and Contraindications

VATS represents a new approach and not a new procedure. Therefore, the indications for VATS major resections remain the same as those for conventional resection. In our institution, close to 80% of the resections are for early, primary lung cancer, with the remaining for benign diseases such as localized bronchiectasis or multi-drug–resistant tuberculosis (Yim, 1996e). For primary lung cancer, preresectional staging (including mediastinoscopy) remains a critically important step in cancer management and should be strictly adhered to.

One major advantage of VATS resection is that it allows recruitment of older and sicker patients with multiple co-morbidity who would otherwise not be suitable candidates for resection through a conventional thoracotomy approach (Demmy and Curtis, 1999; Yim, 1996c). The lowest limits in lung function parameters that would still be considered acceptable for VATS lobectomy have not been scientifically studied (Meyer, 2000), but this would depend on, among other factors, the surgeon's judgment, experience, and techniques, and the exact location of the pathology (for example, upper lobe lesions in patients with emphysema and middle lobe pathology are favorable candidates for resection). We have performed lobectomy on many patients whose forced expiratory volume in 1 second (FEV_1) was less than 1 L or less than 40% predicted with excellent outcome. Patients who are not candidates for an anatomical resection could still be considered for VATS wedge resection as a compromise procedure (see later).

There are few absolute contraindications that are specifically applicable to VATS major resections (Table 36–5). Aside from the inability to tolerate single lung ventilation, all of them are anatomical considerations. We do not recommend VATS for tumors that are larger than 4 cm—not primarily because of technical difficulties, but because ribs have to be excessively spread to retrieve the specimen, and this tends to negate the benefit of minimal access surgery. True pleural symphysis, which would rule out the VATS approach, is uncommon in our experience. Once a space is created when the correct plane in the pleural space is entered, endoscopic adhesiolysis can proceed quickly and safely. As mentioned earlier, VATS has the advantage over conventional thoracotomy in visualiz-

TABLE 36–5 ■ Contraindications for VATS Major Resections

ABSOLUTE CONTRAINDICATIONS
Inability to tolerate single-lung ventilation
Large tumor (above 4 cm maximal diameter)
Pleural symphysis
Established N2 disease
T3 tumor (mainstem bronchial involvement)
Planned sleeve resection
RELATIVE CONTRAINDICATIONS
Hilar lymphadenopathy
Previous surgery (VATS or thoracotomy)
Completely fused fissures
Prior irradiation to the hilum
T3 tumor (chest wall involvement)

VATS, video-assisted thoracic surgery.

ing details in the apex and the base of the hemithorax with high resolution. We have reported our experience on redo-VATS surgery (Yim, 1998b), and, hence, we no longer consider prior surgery an absolute contraindication to VATS resection. The current, available data however does not support that a complete mediastinal lymphadenectomy can be faithfully reproduced through VATS compared with the thoracotomy approach.

Naruke switched several years ago to systematic lymph node sampling instead of lymphadenectomy for stage I cancer (Naruke, 1999). Therefore, patients with pathologically established N2 disease (either through cervical mediastinoscopy or intraoperatively by frozen section) should be treated through an open surgical approach. Fused fissures present a technical challenge to VATS lobectomy. However, with experience and proper intraoperative planning, successful lobectomy can be accomplished—the fused fissure should be divided last following the pulmonary vasculatures and the bronchus. Lobectomy with en bloc chest wall resection through the VATS approach for primary cancer with chest wall invasion has been reported (Widmann et al, 2000). It is anticipated that with increased experience and further refinement of technique, the indication for VATS could be extended to include selected, locally advanced primary lung cancer, beyond the current indication for clinical stage I tumor.

Operative Technique

Compared with conventional surgery, VATS demands a new set of manual skills and eye–hand coordination. However, for someone who is experienced with open surgery, the learning curve is usually very steep. Like any technical procedure, attention to fine details is crucial to success.

Anesthesia

The procedure should be carried out under general anesthesia with selective single lung ventilation. This can usually be accomplished using a double-lumen endobronchial tube (usually left-sided intubation unless a left pneumonectomy is anticipated). We prefer this over the commercially available endotracheal tube with a built-in bronchial blocker, as the latter technique makes it more difficult to collapse the lung, especially in patients who have emphysema. There is currently no endobronchial tube commercially available for young children, and, therefore, for children we use a single-lumen endotracheal tube and position its tip in the appropriate mainstem bronchus (Yim, 1995c). Readers are referred to specific reviews on this topic for details (Low, 2000; Krucylak, 2000).

Patient Positioning

The patient is placed in a full lateral decubitus position. We advocate flexing the operating table at the level of the nipples. This allows the minithoracotomy to naturally "gap," and hence render excessive rib retraction unnecessary (Fig. 36–104). The flexion of the table further opens up the intercostal spaces for insertion of the thoracoscope and instruments (Yim, 1995a). If there is any doubt, the position of the endobronchial tube should be confirmed or reconfirmed at this time using a fine-bore, flexible bronchoscope before the patient is prepared and draped in the same way as for thoractomy.

Instruments

We prefer a 10-mm thoracoscope and a three-chip camera system (Stryker 884TE, Kalamazoo, MI) for major resection. We use two television monitors so that the surgeon and the assistants can view simultaneously without having to turn their heads. Our operating room set up is schematically as shown in Figure 36–105. We use a 0-degree lens for resections of the lower lobes and middle lobe and a 30-degree lens for the upper lobes. The correct

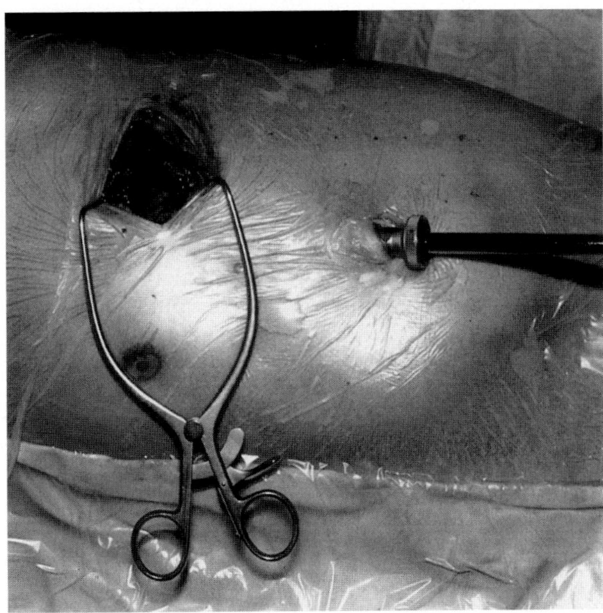

FIGURE 36–104 ■ With the flexion of the operating table to 30 degrees at the level of the nipples, the minithoracotomy naturally opens up rendering rib spreading unnecessary throughout the procedure, and only a soft tissue retractor is used. Note the position of the thoracoscope.

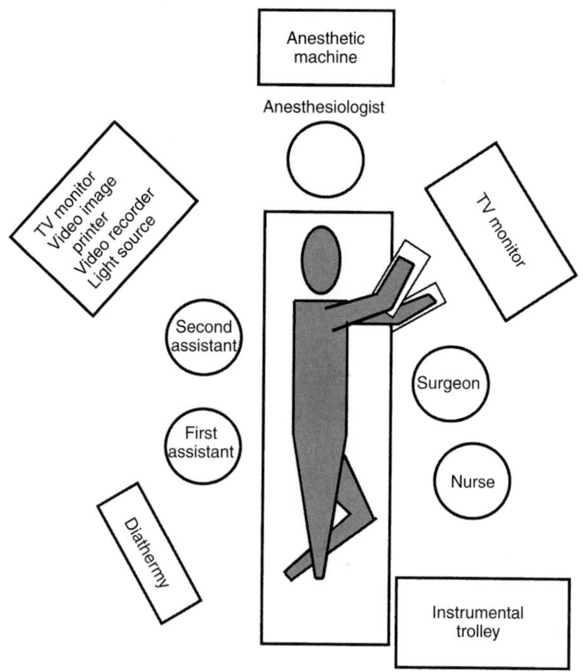

FIGURE 36–105 ■ Schematic view of our operating room set-up. The surgeon stands facing the patient. The first assistant holds the camera.

choice of lens for each operation cannot be overemphasized. It is crucial that the assistant be reminded at all times to avoid torquing the thoracoscope—because of the leverage, even slight torquing could result in significant pressure on the intercostal nerve and, hence, postoperative neuralgia (Yim, 1995a).

We generally do not use ports except for the thoracoscope and for introducing mechanical staplers (Yim APC, 1995b). This is done not just to save money on the ports, but because the presence of a trocar port makes it difficult to use conventional thoracic instruments (Liu, HP et al, 1993). Although complete sets of disposable, endoscopic as well as dedicated, reusable thoracoscopic instruments (such as those designed respectively by Kaiser, Landreneau, and Lewis) are commercially available, our preference is still to use conventional instruments (like sponge-holding forceps and Metzenbaum scissors), which are light, easy to use, familiar to all surgeons, universally available, and inexpensive (Yim, 1996a).

Routine VATS Exploration Prior to Resection

The routine use of VATS exploration to evaluate patients with known primary lung cancer prior to resection has been studied by several authors. The results are summarized in Table 36–6. Among a total of over 650 patients who were clinically staged as resectable, approximately 7% were found to have inoperable disease (pleural metastasis or direct invasion to vital structures) and, hence, were able to avoid an unnecessary thoracotomy (Sonett and Krasna, 2000). VATS exploration adds very little time to the operation and could yield important information that would markedly alter the treatment strategy. We therefore recommend the routine use of VATS exploration in all surgical cases of pulmonary malignancy, including those advanced cases for which thoracotomy is used as the primary mode of access (Yim, 1996b).

Intercostal Strategy and Initial Exploration

The surgeon stands facing the patients (see Fig. 36–105). We generally explore by placing the thoracoscope in the seventh or eighth intercostal space over the midaxillary to anterior axillary line, depending on the build of the patient and the location of the pathology (see Fig. 36–104). From this position, a panoramic view of the hemithorax is obtained. The basic principle is to align the thoracoscope, the pathology, and the television monitor. This allows the surgeon to look straight ahead when he or she operates, thus providing the best ergonomic position for the surgeon (Lin and Landreneau, 2000).

If there is no contraindication to proceed, a minithoracotomy (generally 6 to 8 cm in length) is placed over the fourth intercostal space in the anterolateral chest (Fig. 36–106). In females, the skin incision can be made (if the anatomy allows) over the inframammary fold, for cosmesis. The location of this wound usually means only a small portion, if any, of the latissimus dorsi muscle needs to be divided. The serratus anterior muscle is split along the direction of its fibers. Division of the intercostal muscles permits access into the pleural cavity. There are two main reasons why we choose to place the minithoracotomy in the position described. First, because this provides an easy direct access to the hilum. Second, because the anterior intercostal space is wider than the posterior space, it facilitates later retrieval of the specimen.

A sponge holding forceps is introduced through a separate tiny incision in the seventh or eighth intercostal space in the posterior axillary line (see Fig. 36–107). With two sponge-holding forceps, one through the anterior minithoracotomy and the other through the posterior wound, the collapsed lung can then be moved around, and a thorough assessment can be made to the location and extent of the primary lesion, as well as to search for associated pathology (satellite nodules or mediastinal lymphadenopathy, which could be missed even on high-resolution contrast CT thorax).

Unlike laparoscopic surgery, which generally does not allow digital palpation (because of the need to use valved ports to sustain carbon dioxide insufflation), digital palpation through the minithoracotomy, in addition to in-

TABLE 36–6 ■ **Routine use of VATS Exploration in Lung Cancer Patients who have Potentially Resectable Lesions**

Authors	*No. Patients*	*Inoperable (%)*
Wain (1993)	43	5.0
Yim (1996b)	63	3.3
Loscertales (1996)	151	11.9
Roviaro (1996)	286	5.7
Asamura (1997)	116	4.3

Modified from Sonett JR, Krasna MJ: Thoracoscopic staging for intrathoracic malignancy. In Yim APC et al (eds): Minimal Access Cardiothoracic Surgery. Philadelphia, WB Saunders, 2000.

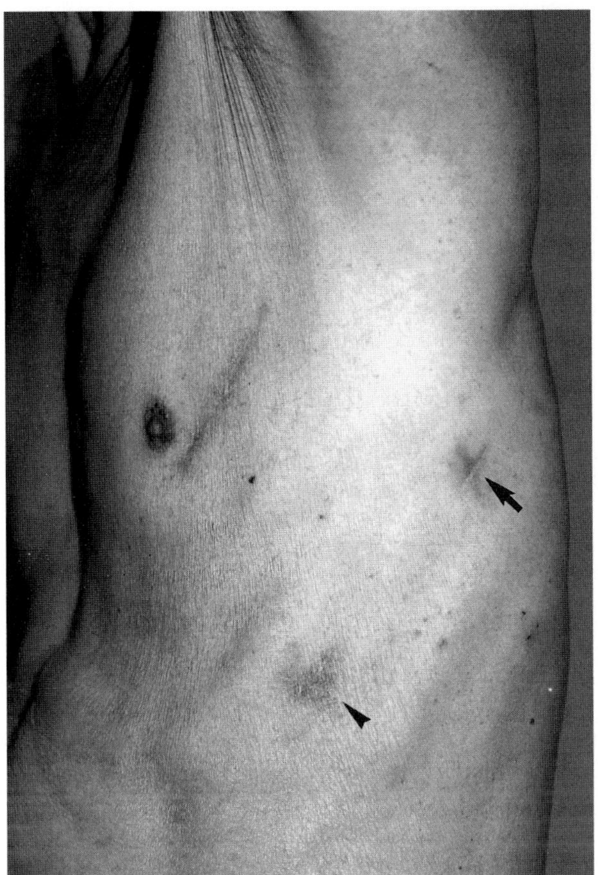

FIGURE 36–106 ■ Postoperative picture of a typical patient who underwent a major resection via video-assisted thoracic surgery (a left pneumonectomy in this case). Note the position of the minithoracotomy scar. The anterior stab wound scar (*arrowhead*) was for the thoracoscope, and the posterior scar (*arrow*) for the sponge holding forceps for lung maneuvering.

strument palpation during VATS exploration, can provide valuable information to the surgeon; this should be encouraged. By bringing the lung towards the palpating finger placed through different sites, a large portion of the lung surface can be palpated. This is important, because small nodules (less than 0.5 cm) that are not subpleurally located would almost certainly go undetected by thoracoscopic examination alone. If a suspicious-looking mediastinal lymph node is detected, it should be biopsied, and a frozen section examination performed (Fig. 36–107*B*). Confirmation of N2 disease mandates conversion to open surgery for complete mediastinal lymphadenectomy (see earlier).

Hilar Dissection

As mentioned earlier, we prefer to use the conventional Metzenbaum scissors and Debakey forceps introduced through the minithoracotomy wound for sharp dissection of the hilum. The sponge-holding forceps from the posterior wound is used to provide appropriate traction and to position the lobes so that the hilum can be easily accessed through the minithoracotomy. If there are adhesions of the lung to the chest wall or mediastinum, these should be separated before starting hilar dissection, as it is essential to be able to freely move the lobes around. Hilar dissection is often a cause of high anxiety for surgeons learning this technique. Although manual (and bimanual) palpation is not possible with VATS, experienced VATS surgeons have learned to feel with the tips of their instruments. One important reason why we advocate using conventional tools is because they are familiar to the surgeons, and they shorten the time needed to acquire this technique. Long (and hence heavier) instruments are generally not necessary for hilar dissection and only decrease the sensitivity of essential tactile feedback. The inherent decrease in tactile information owing to the lack of manual palpation during VATS is compensated by the enhancement of visual information—the monitors provide a magnified view of the operative field with high resolution for details. Subtle displacement of a structure during dissection (which is usually not noticeable in conventional open surgery) provides important clues to an experienced VATS surgeon.

If the interlobar fissure is complete or near complete, sharp incision of the visceral pleura and blunt dissection using a dental pledget mounted on a conventional curved clamp allow easy identification of the pulmonary artery. If the fissure is not complete, a monopolar diathermy forceps (Olsen Electrosurgical, Inc., Concord, CA) at a low setting is useful for hemostasis when a layer of lung parenchyma has to be divided to access the hilar vessel.

Dissecting around a pulmonary vessel is basically the same as in conventional, open surgery. We use a right-angle Mixter clamp (Downs Surgical, Surrey, UK) to go around a vessel, and then loop it with a heavy silk ligature (see Fig. 36–108). With gentle traction on the suture, a dental pledget is used to gently dissect the undersurface of the vessel. A mechanical stapler (Endo-GIA30V, Autosuture, United States Surgical [USSC], Norwalk, CT) is then introduced through one of the other two ports (depending on the alignment), but usually the camera port (with the thoracoscope repositioned to view through the minithoracotomy wound) to staple-transect the vessel. Appropriate traction (using a sponge-holding forceps from the other port) is crucial in aligning the vessel with the stapler for transection.

In recent years, we have been using ligation of pulmonary arterial branches with extracorporeal knots (Yim and Lee, 1995d) instead of mechanical staplers, mainly to reduce cost (Fig. 36–108).

Management of the Bronchus

We divide a lobar bronchus with a linear mechanical stapler with a built-in blade for transection (EndoGIA30, Autosuture, USSC, Norwalk, CT). For a mainstem bronchus, we use a different stapler that requires manual transection (Roticulator 30, Autosuture, USSC, Norwalk, CT). The specifications of these mechanical staplers are summarized in Table 36–7. The integrity of the bronchial stump is then tested to 35 cm of airway pressure in the usual manner under water. Our normal operative sequence for the different major resections is summarized in Table 36–8. As mentioned earlier, fused fissures call for a different operative sequence.

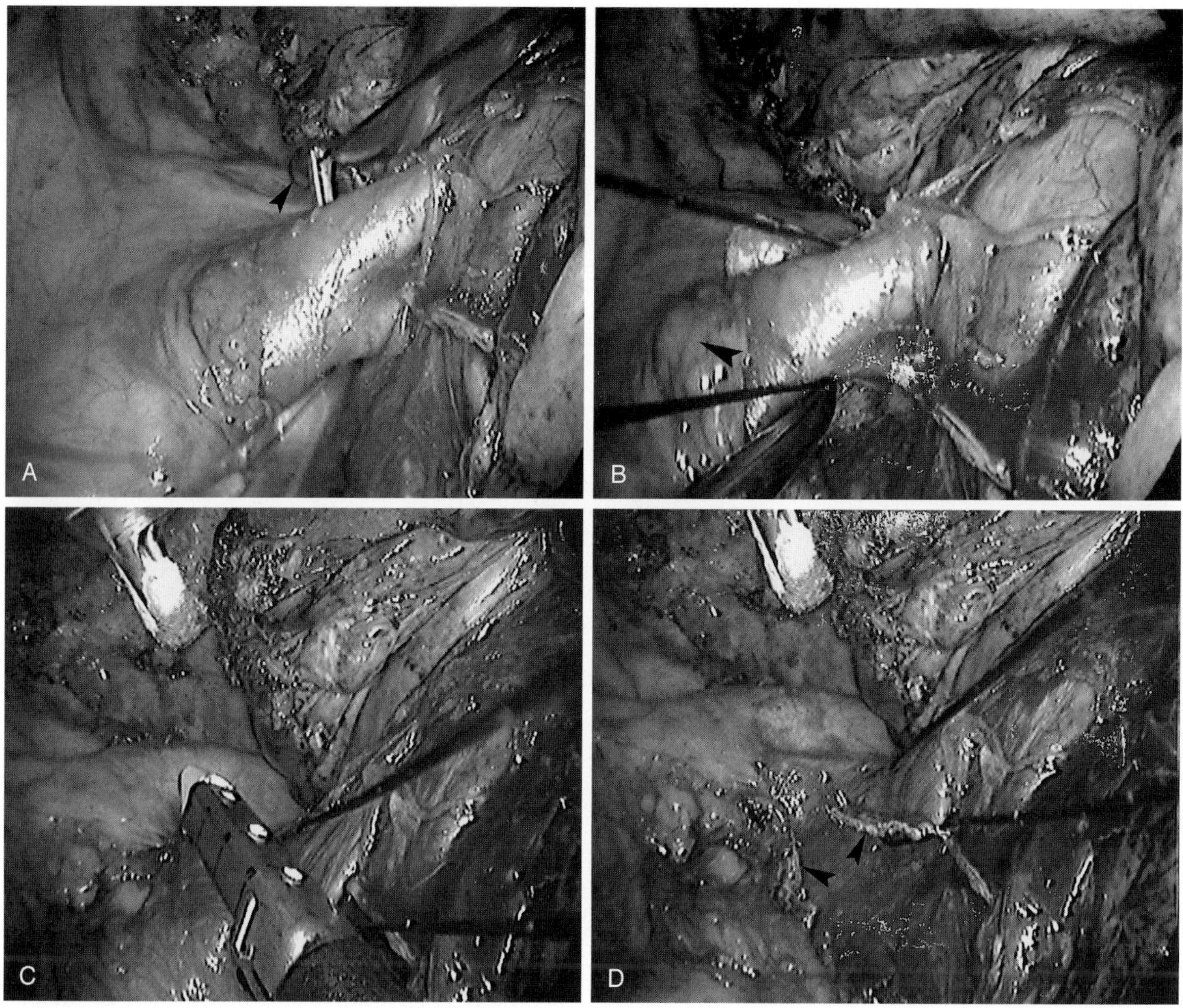

FIGURE 36–107 ■ Management of the left main pulmonary artery (PA) in a pneumonectomy via video-assisted thoracic surgery to illustrate our technique. *A*, Under thoracoscopic vision, the PA was totally dissected with a conventional right angle clamp. A #2 silk tie is about to be pulled around the vessel *(arrow)*. *B*, With traction on the silk tie, a dental pledget mounted on a right angle clamp is used to open up the space behind the PA. Any suspicious mediastinal lymph node, such as level 5 (*arrowhead*), is biopsied, and frozen section is performed before proceeding further. *C*, The frozen section of the level 5 node was benign. A vascular stapler (EndoGIA30V, Autosuture, USSC) was used to staple-transect the PA. *D*, Three rows of staples are left on either side of the transected PA (*arrowheads*).

Release of the Pulmonary Ligament

Release of the inferior pulmonary ligament is required following upper or middle lobectomies. Although this is usually a straightforward maneuver, the positions of the ports and minithoracotomy make paradoxical motion difficult to avoid. Paradoxical motion is generated when the camera and instruments are facing each other. We have found that by turning the camera 180 degrees, a normal spatial relationship is restored for the operator (Yim, et al, 1998d). This simple maneuver allows the surgeon to use the camera and existing ports to the best ergonomic advantage.

Systematic Lymph Node Sampling

Following resection, the mediastinal lymph nodes are systematically sampled. All the accessible nodal stations should be sampled. Because of sentinel lymph nodes, some stations are more likely to be involved for tumor originating from a particular lobe. These stations should be preferentially sampled. Naruke (1999) recently published his recommendations on lymph node sampling: right upper lobe (prevascular and retrotracheal #3 and lower paratracheal #4R); right middle lobe (#3 and subcarinal #7); right lower lobe (#7); left upper lobe (subaortic #5, and para-aortic #6); left lower lobe (#7).

We do not perform VATS mediastinal lymphadenectomy. If a complete lymph node dissection is considered necessary, it should be done through a thoracotomy (see earlier). Nonetheless, there are surgeons who advocate routine VATS lymphadenectomy, but as in open surgery, their results have not been shown to be superior to those who sample (see later).

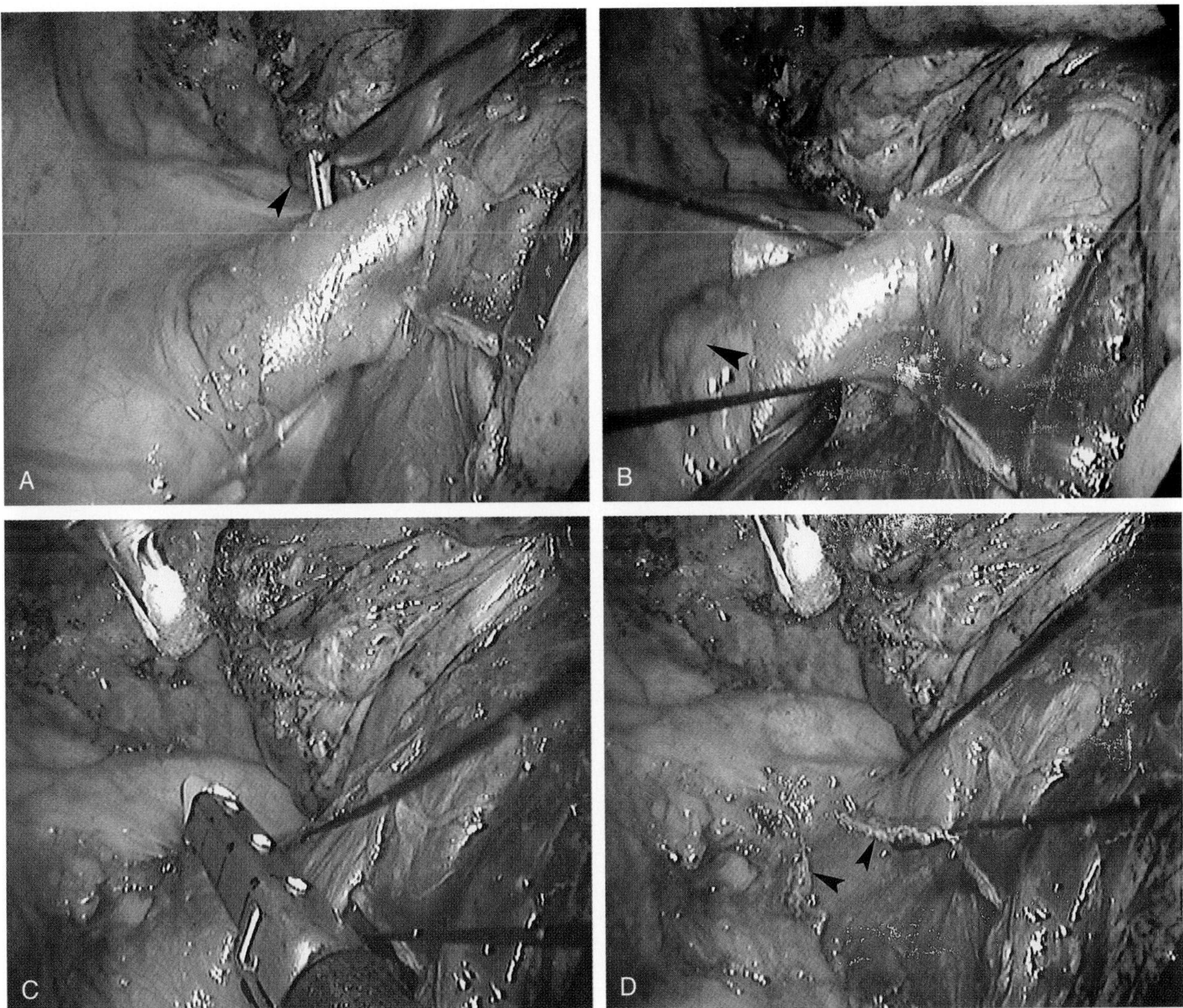

FIGURE 36-107 ■ Management of the left main pulmonary artery (PA) in a pneumonectomy via video-assisted thoracic surgery to illustrate our technique. *A*, Under thoracoscopic vision, the PA was totally dissected with a conventional right angle clamp. A #2 silk tie is about to be pulled around the vessel *(arrow)*. *B*, With traction on the silk tie, a dental pledget mounted on a right angle clamp is used to open up the space behind the PA. Any suspicious mediastinal lymph node, such as level 5 *(arrowhead)*, is biopsied, and frozen section is performed before proceeding further. *C*, The frozen section of the level 5 node was benign. A vascular stapler (EndoGIA30V, Autosuture, USC) was used to staple-transect the PA. *D*, Three rows of staples are left on either side of the transected PA *(arrowheads)*.

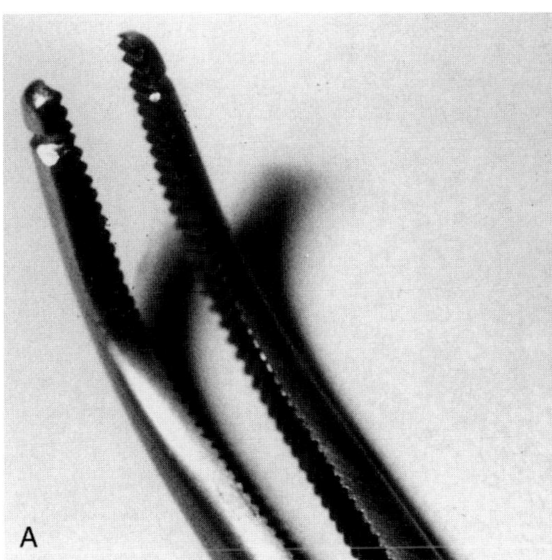

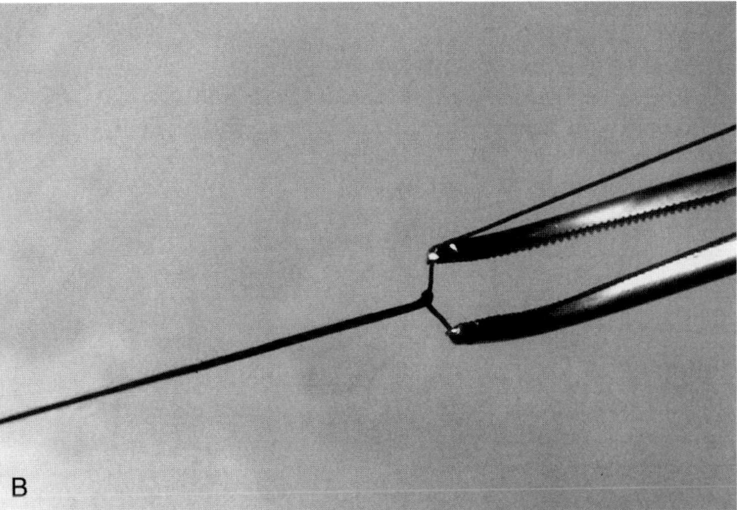

FIGURE 36–108 ■ *A*, A knot pusher was made by engraving a groove on the outside of a right angle Mixter clamp. *B*, The device is used to slide down an extracorporeal knot. This technique was originated by Naruke. (From Yim APC, Lee TWC: 'Homemade' knot pusher for extracorporeal ties. Aus N Z J Surg 65:511, 1995.)

Retrieval of Specimens

We always use a wound protector to avoid any potential implantation of tumor cells on the wound (Fig. 36–109). When the primary tumor is less than 4 cm, we generally have not found that a mechanical rib spreader is necessary for retrieval of the resected lobe, bi-lobe, or even the entire lung (although some manual rib retraction may be needed at the time of retrieval).

The entire hemithorax is copiously irrigated with warm saline. If there is any significant parenchymal leak, we then perform endoscopic suturing using a dedicated needle holder (Fig. 36–110) and conventional 3–0 Prolene on a 25-mm curved needle through the minithoracotomy. Endoscopic suturing using this needle holder (originally designed by Carpentier for mitral valve surgery) is straightforward, and easier than most surgeons think.

We routinely perform intercostal block with about 20 ml of 0.5% bupivacaine with epinephrine (two levels above and below the minithoracotomy) using a spinal needle (Becton Dickinson & Co, Franklin Lakes, NJ) through the minithoracotomy. Placement of two 24 French chest drains (through the previous camera and instrument ports) and closure of the minithoracotomy wound completes the operation (see Fig. 36–106).

Results

Mortality and Morbidity

Some of the larger published series on VATS major resection are summarized in Table 36–9. Despite slight variations in individual techniques, the results universally range from good to excellent. The overall surgical mortality of 0% to 2% for VATS compared favorably with the conventional technique, even though it must be pointed out that the former was for highly selected patients.

Major complications from VATS resections are relatively uncommon (Walker, 2000). Persistent airleak beyond 7 days was the most common morbidity in our earlier experience (Yim et al, 1996d; Yim, 1996f). This was almost certainly related to hilar dissection when the fissures were incomplete. However, like most technical issues, this improved with experience (we have found endoscopic suturing a great asset, as described earlier).

Tumor implantation following VATS has been reported (Downey, et al, 1996). However, this is relatively uncommon and could be further minimized by gentle handling of tissue, routine use of a wound protector, and copious irrigation of the hemithorax prior to closure.

One of the most dreaded complications for surgeons is massive bleeding from pulmonary vessels. Both Walker

TABLE 36–7 ■ **Specifications of Some Mechanical Staplers**

			Staples Specificity						
Device Names	*Color Code*	*Applications*	*Cut Line (mm)*	*Staple Line (mm)*	*Leg Length (mm)*	*Crown Length (mm)*	*Approximate Closed Staple Height (mm)*	*Wire Diameter (mm)*	*No. Staggered Rows**
EndoG1A30	Blue	Lung parenchyma/ Lobar bronchus	27.5	32.5	3.5	3	1.5	0.21	3
EndoGIA30V	White	Pulmonary vessel	27.5	32.5	2.5	3	1.0	0.21	3
Roticulator 30	Green	Mainstem bronchus	Manual	31.5	4.8	4	2.0	0.28	2

*Refers to the number of staggered rows of staples left in patient.

TABLE 36–8 ■ Operative Sequence for VATS Resection of Different Lobes

LEFT UPPER LOBE
Lingular PA
Superior PV
Anterior ascending PA
Bronchus
Posterior PA (variable number)
LEFT LOWER LOBE
Descending PA to LLL (before division into apical and basal branches)
Inferior PV
Fissure
Bronchus
RIGHT UPPER LOBE
Anterior ascending segmental PA
Superior pulmonary vein
Anterior trunk (before division into apical and posterior segmental PA)
Fissure
Bronchus
RIGHT MIDDLE LOBE
Middle lobe PA
Middle lobe tributary to superior PV
Fissure
Bronchus
RIGHT LOWER LOBE
Descending PA to RLL (apical and basal branches usually have to be taken separately)
Inferior PV
Fissure
Bronchus
LEFT PNEUMONECTOMY
Superior PV
PA
Inferior PV
Left main bronchus
RIGHT PNEUMONECTOMY
Superior PV
PA
Inferior PV
Right main bronchus

LLL, left lower lobe; PA, pulmonary artery; PV, pulmonary vein; RLL, right lower lobe; VATS, video-assisted thoracic surgery.

and the author have experienced mechanical failure of the staplers that resulted in massive bleeding (Craig and Walker, 1995; Yim 1995b). This was controlled by pressing on the bleeder with a sponge stick and converting to a thoracotomy. It should be pointed out that these are anecdotal cases, and the mechanical staplers available now are generally very reliable. Having now acquired the skill and experience in endoscopic suturing, we feel comfortable using this technique in the unlikely event of minor to moderate bleeding from the pulmonary vasculature, thus avoiding the need for a conversion.

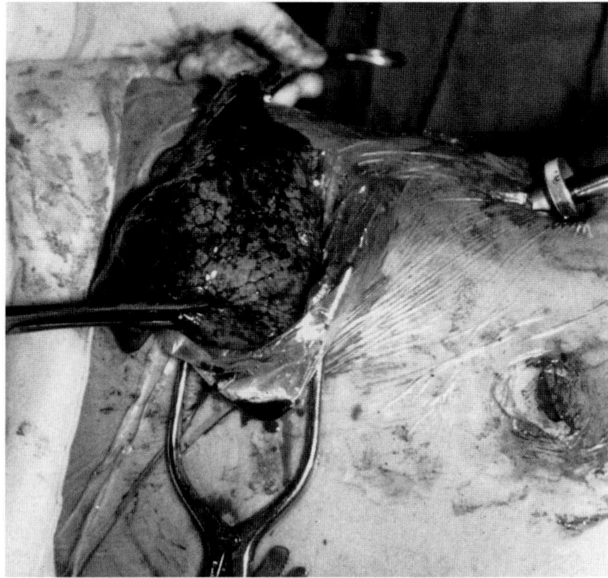

FIGURE 36–109 ■ Retrieval of the resected lung through the minithoracotomy. Note the use of a wound protector. Only a soft tissue retractor was used. Forceful rib spreading was not necessary.

Benefits over Conventional Surgery

The rationale behind using the VATS approach is summarized in the following sections.

Decreased Postoperative Pain

It is now fairly well accepted that patients who undergo VATS resection are expected to experience less immediate postoperative pain compared with those who have undergone the thoracotomy approach. This has been documented in several large case-controlled studies either by objective assessment in terms of analgesic requirements (Walker, 1998; Yim APC 1996d) or subjective assessment in terms of pain score, usually in the form of a visual analogue scale (Demmy and Curtis, 1999; Giudicelli et al, 1994; Yim APC 1996d). A trend in the decrease in

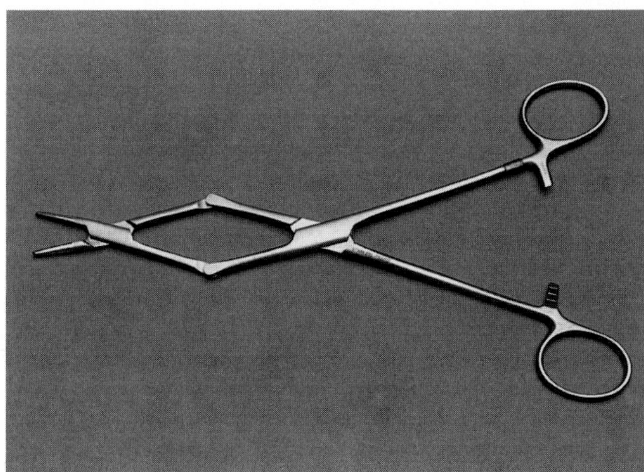

FIGURE 36–110 ■ A specially designed needle holder with the additional double joints for endoscopic suturing (Model 56615–28, Delacroix-Chevalier, Paris, France).

TABLE 36–9 ■ **Large Case Series on VATS Lobectomy**

Authors	*No. of Cases*	*Conversion (%)*	*Postoperation Mortality (%)*	*Follow-up (mos)*	*Survival Stage I (%)*
Walker (1998)	149	13.4	2	36	94
Kaseda (1998)*	145	11.7	0.8	48	94
Roviaro (1998)	211	18.9	0.6	—	—
McKenna (1998)	212	7.0	0.5	28.9	76
Yim (1998d)	266	19.5	0.5	26	95
Lewis (1999)	250	—	0	34	92
Naruke (2000)	79	21.5	0	36	94

*Routine mediastinal lymphadenectomy was included.

analgesic requirement was seen in the early randomized, prospective study comparing VATS with thoracotomy for lobectomy (Kirby et al, 1995). The lack of statistical significance was likely due to the small sample sizes. Landreneau and colleagues (1993) reported earlier that the incidence of chronic postoperative pain beyond 6 months following VATS was not different from thoracotomy. However, this has not been our experience when the above maneuvers (see patient positioning) have been adhered to.

Better Preservation of Pulmonary Function

Kaseda (2000) recently reported that lung function in patients who underwent VATS lobectomy was better preserved than it was in those who underwent a thoracotomy approach when FEV_1 and forced vital capacity (FVC) values were measured both preoperatively and then 3 months postoperatively. The differences were shown to be highly significant ($P < 0.0001$). The same conclusion was reached in a similar, but smaller study (Nakata et al, 2000).

Earlier Return to Normal Activities

Sugiura (1999) recently showed that patients who underwent VATS lobectomy for early cancer could return to activities postoperatively significantly earlier than patients who underwent the thoracotomy approach (2.5 versus 7.8 months). Similarly, Demmy and Curtis (1999), who compared VATS versus conventional major resections in high risk patients, came to the same conclusion (2.2 versus 3.6 months). Our unpublished data of a telephone survey of a large number of patients is in complete agreement with these findings.

Long-Term Survival

The success of a cancer operation is judged by the long-term survival of the patient. The published results to date from several centers on VATS major resection for stage I lung cancer consistently show that the intermediate to long-term survival for some is at least as good, if not superior to that of the conventional thoracotomy approach (see Table 36–9). We prospectively studied our pathologic stage I lung cancer patients who underwent either the VATS or the thoracotomy approach, and we showed that there was a trend of improved disease-free survival in favor of the former (Fig. 36–111). This was very exciting, and our observations were reproduced at several other centers (unpublished results through personal communications). We are cautious in not drawing any premature conclusion that there is a definitive survival advantage until the results from a larger prospective, randomized study with long-term follow-up become available.

We have intensively searched for possible mechanisms behind our observation. There is now a wealth of literature showing that the body's immune function is better preserved following laparoscopic surgery compared with open surgery, although few of these publications exist in the thoracic surgical literature. We prospectively studied two groups of patients with clinical stage I lung cancer who underwent either VATS or conventional resection through a thoracotomy. Significantly reduced postoperative release of both pro-inflammatory (interleukins 6 and 8) and anti-inflammatory (interleukin 10) cytokines in the plasma was found in the VATS group compared with that in the control (Yim et al, 2000). Our findings were consistent with a similar but smaller Japanese study that showed a significantly reduced cytokine release (interleukin 6 and 8) in the pleural fluid in the VATS lobectomy

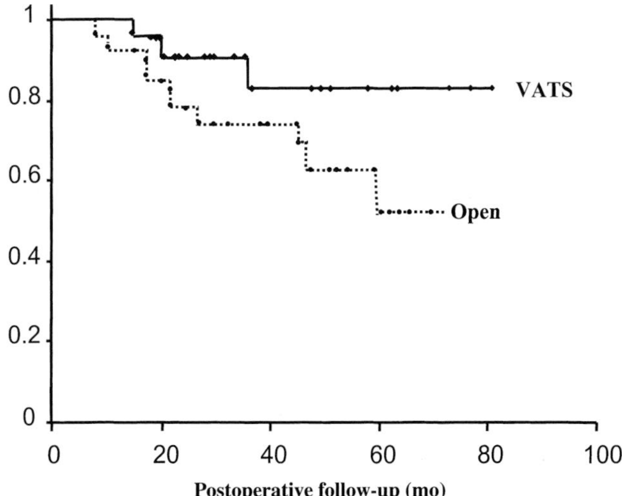

FIGURE 36–111 ■ Disease-free survival of pathologic stage I non–small cell lung cancer patients who underwent either video-assisted thoracic surgery (VATS) or open surgery at the Prince of Wales Hospital, Hong Kong (1994–1999).

group compared with the open thoracotomy group (Sugi et al, 2000). Leaver and colleagues from Edinburgh showed, in a small, randomized, prospective study, that VATS lobectomy was associated with a lesser effect on the postoperative fall in circulating T (CD4) cells and natural killer (NK) cells. Lymphocyte oxidation was also less suppressed by VATS compared with open surgery (Leaver et al, 2000). We have independently studied NK cells in our unit, and our unpublished results were in agreement with the findings described earlier. In essence, there is evidence now to believe that VATS is associated with lesser perturbation in the humoral and cellular immune functions compared with open surgery, at least in the short term (Walker, 2000). As immunosurveillance is still believed by many to be important, surgically induced immunosuppression may predispose to increased tumor growth or recurrence. Whether better preservation of the immune system by minimal access surgery may lead to improved long-term survival is unclear, but it certainly deserves further investigation.

However, a word of caution was raised by Yamashita and colleagues (2000) who studied a tumor marker, carcinoembryonic antigen messenger RNA (CEAmRNA), using reverse transcriptase polymerase chain reaction (RT-PCR) in the peripheral blood in patients with early lung cancer who underwent VATS lobectomy. They found that in a high proportion of patients, CEAmRNA, which was absent before surgery, could be detected in the peripheral blood during the procedure. The proportion was more than that found in a historical group of patients who underwent conventional resection. RT-PCR is an extremely sensitive technique, and the significance of this observation is unclear. However, in several large case series with intermediate to long-term follow-up, VATS has not been shown to be associated with more distant metastasis than conventional surgery for clinical stage I cancer.

Cost Effectiveness

The high cost of the consumables for VATS is a serious concern and represents a major deterrent to adopt VATS in developing countries. However, by choosing the right patients for this technique, as well as relying on ligation and suturing, the consumable costs can be minimized (Yim, 1996e). In experienced hands, VATS major resection is a relatively quick operation, because little time is needed to open and close the chest. Our average time for a VATS lower lobectomy is under 1 hour and only slightly longer for an upper lobectomy. This represents significant cost saving in terms of operating room time. A recent Japanese study comparing VATS versus open resections for cancer showed that the overall hospital charges were lower for the former approach (Nakajima et al, 2000).

NONANATOMICAL PULMONARY RESECTIONS

VATS nonanatomical resections that include wedge resections and nodulectomy are indicated for four main groups of patients. First, patients with diffuse pulmonary infiltrates or indeterminate nodules for diagnosis. Second, patients with early lung cancer but whose pulmonary function or comorbidities would not permit a lobectomy. Limited resections in these situations represent an acceptable but compromised therapy (Ginsberg et al, 1995). Third, selected patients with pulmonary metastasis for therapeutic resections. Fourth, patients with end-stage emphysema for lung-volume reduction surgery.

A detailed discussion on each of these indications is beyond the scope of this chapter, which is primarily intended to focus on surgical technique. Mechanical staplers remain the most frequently used device for VATS wedge resection. They are ideal for small nodules situated in the lung periphery, especially when they are close to a free edge. For bigger nodules (over 3 cm) lying deep to a flat lung surface, wedge resections using endoscopic staplers are often technically difficult or even hazardous. Even if it could be done, it would almost certainly sacrifice more functional lung tissue than would be necessary for the procedure. This could have a major impact on the recovery of patients who are elderly and frail, with multiple comorbidities and borderline lung function.

Although Nd:YAG laser has been advocated for resection of these nodules in conjunction with a mechanical stapler (Landreneau et al, 1993), the former requires specialized equipment and high up-front costs. A monopolar floating ball device (Fig. 36–112) was recently made available (TissueLink Medical, Dover, NH). Used in conjunction with a conventional Bovie generator, it allows an endoscopic Perelman procedure (Cooper et al, 1986) to be carried out with high level of precision. This device differs from the conventional electrocautery in generating less smoke and not charring tissue. The first clinical trial of this device for nodulectomy was carried out in our unit with good to excellent results.

CONCLUSION

VATS pulmonary resections represent an attractive, alternative approach to conventional open surgery for selected patients. VATS major resection has been shown to be a safe operation in experienced hands. Postoperative pain is significantly less following VATS than it is for open surgery. Other documented advantages include better preservation of pulmonary function in the early postoperative period, earlier return to full activities, and possibly better quality of life. Intermediate to long term survival for stage I lung cancer patients who underwent VATS

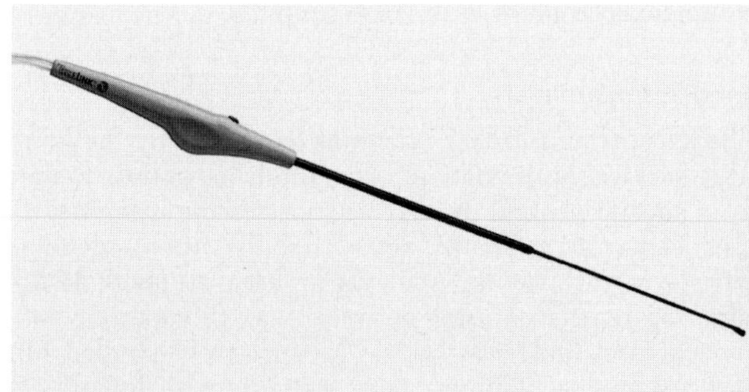

FIGURE 36–112 ■ A TissueLink floating ball device (TissueLink Medical, Dover, NH) designed for endoscopic nodulectomy.

resection appears at least as good, if not superior to open surgery. As the established benefits of VATS resections start to accumulate, it would be increasingly difficult to justify not using VATS as the approach of choice. VATS should be an integral part of thoracic surgery training, and all our thoracic surgical residents are expected to complete their training proficient in VATS major resections.

Acknowledgments

The author wishes to recognize the support and dedication of his colleagues in the development of this technique as we described here: Dr. T. W. Lee, Dr. John Low, Dr. S. K. Ng, Karen Tse, RN and Ying Ying Chiu, RN.

COMMENTS AND CONTROVERSIES

Dr. Yim is a leader in minimally invasive thoracic surgery. In the future, this emerging technology will certainly play an important role in thoracic surgery. When applying this technique to oncologic disease, it is extremely important that short cuts are not taken. For lung cancer, because of the inability of most minimally invasive surgeons to perform adequate superior mediastinal sampling, I would urge that mediastinoscopy always be done. Dr. Yim agrees with this. If one does not use a significant access incision, this approach does have the disadvantage of not being able to palpate tiny nodules (vis-à-vis a larger incision).

I would disagree with Dr. Yim that one can recruit more people with poorer pulmonary function by the use of MIS. Certainly, with the very effective pain-relieving approaches available today, major thoracotomies can be done in patients with very poor pulmonary function—this is evident with the work done in volume reduction surgery etc., by open procedure. Once a chest wall resection has to be performed, it behooves me to accept any advantages for a video-assisted approach. Chest wall resections cause significant pain, and one may as well use an open thoracotomy approach if a chest wall resection has to be performed.

I am quite surprised that once this pain-relieving approach is chosen, Dr. Yim continues to use fairly large chest tubes (No. 24 French). These add to the postoperative pain. In routine thoracotomies, I now use No. 20 French tubes and anticipate further reductions in tube size. I am convinced that this causes less pain and certainly is as effective in removing air and fluid.

R.J.G.

REFERENCES

Asamura H, Nakayma H, Kondo H et al: Thoracoscopic evaluation of histologically/cytologically proven or suspected lung cancer: A VATS exploration. Lung Cancer 16:183, 1997.

Cooper JD, Perelman M, Todd TRJ et al: Precision cautery excision of pulmonary lesions. Ann Thorac Surg 41:51, 1986.

Craig SR, Walker WS: Potential complications of vascular stapling in thoracoscopic pulmonary resection. Ann Thorac Surg 59:736, 1995.

Demmy TL, Curtis JJ: Minimally invasive lobectomy directed toward frail and high-risk patients: A case control study. Ann Thorac Surg 68:194, 1999.

Downey RJ, McCormick P, LoCicero J et al: Dissemination of malignant tumors after video-assisted thoracic surgery: A report of twenty-one cases. J Thorac Cardiovasc Surg 111:954, 1996.

Ginsberg RT, Rubinstein LV: Lung Cancer Study Group Randomized trial of lobectomy versus resection for TN non–small cell lung cancer. Ann Thorac Surg 60:615, 1995.

Giudicelli R, Thomas P, Lonjon T et al: Video-assisted minithoracotomy versus muscle sparing thoracotomy for performing lobectomy. Ann Thorac Surg 58:712, 1994.

Heitmiller RF, Mathisen DJ: French incision. In Grillo HC, Austen WG, Wilkins EW et al (eds): Current Therapy in Cardiothoracic Surgery. Toronto, B.C. Decker, 1989, pp 268–269.

Kaseda S, Aoki T, Hangai N: Video-assisted thoracic surgery (VATS) lobectomy: The Japanese experience. Semin Thorac Cardiovasc Surg 10:300, 1998.

Kaseda S, Aoki T, Hangai N, Shimizu K: Better pulmonary function and prognosis with video-assisted thoracic surgery than with thoracotomy. Ann Thorac Surg 70:1644, 2000.

Kirby TJ, Mack MJ, Landreneau RJ, Rice TW: Lobectomy video-assisted thoracic surgery versus muscle-sparing thoracotomy: A randomized trial. J Thorac Cardiovasc Surg 109:997, 1995.

Krucylak CP: Anesthetic considerations for pediatric thoracoscopic procedures. In Yim APC, Hazelrigg SR, Izzat MB et al (eds): Minimal Access Cardiothoracic Surgery. Philadelphia, WB Saunders, 2000.

Landreneau RJ, Keenan RJ, Hazelrigg SR et al: VATS wedge resection of the lung using the neodymium: yttrium-aluminium garnet laser. Ann Thorac Surg 56:758, 1993.

Landreneau RJ, Mack MJ, Hazelrigg SR et al: Prevalence of chronic pain after pulmonary resection by thoracotomy or video-assisted thoracic surgery. J Thorac Cardiovasc Surg 107:1079, 1994.

Leaver HA, Craig SR, Yap PL, Walker WS: Lymphocyte responses following open and minimally invasive thoracic surgery. Eur J Clin Invest 30:230, 2000.

Lewis RJ, Caccavale RJ, Boncage JP, Widmann MD: Video-assisted thoracic surgical non-rib spreading simultaneously stapled lobectomy: A more patient-friendly oncologic resection. Chest 116:1119, 1999.

Lin JC, Landreneau RJ: Strategic planning for video-assisted thoracic surgery. In Yim APC, Hazelrigg SR, Izzat MB et al (eds): Minimal Access Cardiothoracic Surgery. Philadelphia, WB Saunders 2000.

Liu HP, Lin PJ, Chang JP, Chang CH: Video-assisted thoracic surgery: Manipulation without trocar in 112 consective procedures. Chest 104:1452, 1993.

Loscertales J, Garcia Diaz F, Jimenez Merchan R et al: Valoracion de la resecabilidad del cancer de pulmon mediante videotoracoscopia exploradora. Arch Bronconeumol 32:275, 1996.

Low JM: Anesthesia for video-assisted thoracoscopic surgery. In Yim APC, Hazelrigg SR, Izzat MB et al (eds): Minimal Access Cardiothoracic Surgery. Philadelphia, WB Saunders, 2000.

Mack MJ, Scruggs GR, Kelly KM et al: Video-assisted thoracic surgery: Has technology found its place? Ann Thorac Surg 64:211, 1997.

McKenna RJ Jr, Wolf RK, Brenner M et al: Is VATS lobectomy an adequate cancer operation? Ann Thorac Surg 66:1903, 1998.

Meyer DM: Preoperative assessment for video-assisted thoracic surgery. In Yim APC, Hazelrigg SR, Izzat MB et al (eds): Minimal Access Cardiothoracic Surgery. Philadelphia, WB Saunders, 2000.

Nakajima J, Takamoto S, Kohno T, Ohtsuka T: Costs of video thoracoscopic surgery versus open resection for patients with lung carcinoma. Cancer 89:2497, 2000.

Nakata M, Saeki H, Yokoyama N et al: Pulmonary function after lobectomy: Video-assisted thoracic surgery versus thoracotomy. Ann Thorac Surg 70:938, 2000.

Naruke T, Tsuchiya R, Kando H et al: Lymph node sampling in lung cancer: How should it be done? Eur J Cariothorac Surg 16:S17, 1999.

Roviaro GC, Varoli F, Rebuffat C et al: Videothoracoscopic operative staging for lung cancer. Int Surg 81:252, 1996.

Roviaro G, Varoli F, Vergani C et al: VATS major pulmonary resections: The Italian experience. Semin Thorac Cardiovasc Surg 10:313, 1998.

Sonett JR, Krasna MJ: Thoracoscopic staging for intrathoracic malignancy. In Yim APC, Hazelrigg SR, Izzat MB et al (eds): Minimal Access Cardiothoracic Surgery. Philadelphia, WB Saunders, 2000.

Sugi K, Kaneda Y, Esato K: Video-assisted thoracoscopic lobectomy reduces cytokine production more than conventional open lobectomy. Jpn J Thorac Cardiovasc Surg 48:161, 2000.

Sugiura H, Morikawa T, Kaji M et al: Long-term benefits for the quality of life after video-assisted thoracoscopic lobectomy in patients with lung cancer. Surg Laparosc Endosc 9:403, 1999.

Tuffier T: De la resection du sommet du poumon. Sem Med Paris 2:202, 1891.

Wain JC: Video-assisted thoracoscopy and the staging of lung cancer. Ann Thorac Surg 56:776, 1993.

Walker WS: VATS lobectomy: The Edinburgh experience. Semin Thorac Cardiovasc Surg 10:291, 1998.

Walker WS: Complications and pitfalls in video-assisted thoracic surgery. In Yim APC, Hazelrigg SR, Izzat MB et al (eds): Minimal Access Cardiothoracic Surgery. Philadelphia, WB Saunders, 2000.

Walker WS, Leaver HA, Craig SR, Yap PL: The immune response to surgery: Conventional and VATS lobectomy. In Yim APC, Hazelrigg SR, Izzat MB et al (eds): Minimal Access Cardiothoracic Surgery. Philadelphia, WB Saunders, 2000.

Widmann MD, Caccavale RJ, Bocage JP, Lewis RJ: Video-assisted thoracic surgery resection of chest wall en bloc for lung carcinoma. Ann Thorac Surg 70:2138, 2000.

Yamashita JI, Kurusu Y, Fujino N: Detection of circulating tumor cells in patients with non-small cell lung cancer undergoing lobectomy by video-assisted thoracic surgery: A potential hazard for intraoperative hematogenous tumor cell dissemination. J Thorac Cardiovasc Surg 119:899, 2000.

Yim APC: Minimizing chest wall trauma in video-assisted thoracic surgery. J Thorac Cardiovasc Surg 109:1255, 1995a.

Yim APC, Ho JKS: Malfunctioning of vascular staple cutter during thoracoscopic lobotomy. J Thorac Cardiovasc Surg 109:1252, 1995b.

Yim APC, Low JM, Ng SK et al: Video-assisted thoracoscopic surgery in the pediatric population. J Paed & Child Health 31:192, 1995c.

Yim APC, Lee TWC: 'Home-made' knot pusher for extracorporeal ties. Aust NZJ Surg 65:510, 1995d.

Yim APC: Cost containing strategies in video-assisted thoracoscopic surgery: An Asian perspective. Surg Endosc 10:1198, 1996a.

Yim APC: Routine video-assisted thoracoscopy prior to thoracotomy. Chest 109:1099, 1996b.

Yim APC: Thoracoscopic surgery in the elderly population. Surg Endosc 10:880, 1996c.

Yim APC, Ko KM, Chau WS et al: Video-assisted thoracoscopic anatomic lung resections: The initial Hong Kong experience. Chest 109:13, 1996d.

Yim APC, Ko KM, Ma CC: Thoracoscopic lobectomy for benign disease. Chest 109:554, 1996e.

Yim APC, Landreneau RJ, Izzat MB, Fung ALK: Is video-assisted thoracoscopic lobectomy a unified approach? Ann Thorac Surg 66:1155, 1998a.

Yim APC, Liu HP: Complications and failures from video-assisted thoracic surgery: Experience from two centers in Asia. Ann Thorac Surg 61:538, 1996f.

Yim APC: Training in thoracoscopy in the Asia-Pacific. Int Surg 82:22, 1997.

Yim APC, Liu HP, Hazelrigg SR et al: Thoracoscopic operations on reoperated chests. Ann Thorac Surg 65:328, 1998b.

Yim APC, Liu H, Izzat MB et al: Thoracoscopic major lung resection: An Asian perspective. Semin Thorac Cardiovasc 10:326, 1998c.

Yim APC, Izzat MB, Lee TW: Counteracting paradoxical motion in videoendoscopic operations. Ann Thorac Surg 66:965, 1998d.

Yim APC, Wan S, Lee TW, Arifi AA: VATS lobectomy reduces cytokine responses compared with conventional surgery. Ann Thorac Surg 70:243, 2000.

CHAPTER **37**

Transplantation

LUNG TRANSPLANTATION

Bryan F. Meyers
G. Alexander Patterson

Since the first long-term successful human lung transplant was performed in 1983 (Toronto Lung Transplantation Group, 1986), remarkable progress has been achieved. Lung transplantation is successfully used worldwide. Improved donor and recipient selection, technical advances, superior immunosuppression strategies, and newer antibiotic regimens have improved results dramatically. The operative mortality rate is now in the range of 9%. One- and 2-year survival rates are 80% and 70%, respectively. Problems remain, however. Most notable is chronic rejection, which appears in the pulmonary allograft as the bronchiolitis obliterans syndrome (BOS).

HISTORICAL NOTE

In the early 1950s, Metras (1950) in France and Hardin and Kittle (1954) in the United States demonstrated the technical feasibility of canine lung transplantation. The initial perception that pulmonary vascular resistance increased in the lung allograft was dispelled by reports that meticulous vascular anastomotic technique resulted in normal pulmonary artery pressures. Similar techniques are used today.

Hardy and associates (1963) reported the first human lung transplantation in 1963. Although the patient died after 18 days, this short-lived success demonstrated the technical feasibility of the operation and stimulated worldwide interest in pulmonary transplantation.

During the subsequent 15 years, approximately 40 clinical lung transplants were performed in centers around the world. None of these procedures was successful. Only one recipient was actually discharged from the hospital, a 23-year-old patient (Derom et al, 1971). This patient left the hospital 8 months following transplantation but died a short time thereafter as a result of chronic rejection, sepsis, and bronchial stenosis. Most patients died within the first 2 weeks of transplantation, as a result of primary graft failure, sepsis, or rejection. The most frequent cause of death beyond the second postoperative week was bronchial anastomotic disruption. The initial lung transplant in the Toronto experience was performed for a young ventilator-dependent patient with inhalation burns (Nelems, 1980). The patient died during the third postoperative week after a bronchial anastomotic dehiscence. This problem of bronchial anastomotic dehiscence stimulated the interest of a number of surgical laboratories. Lima and coworkers (1981), working with Cooper and colleagues in Toronto, demonstrated that high-dose corticosteroid therapy (2 mg/kg/day, which at that time was felt to be necessary for adequate immunosuppression) had an adverse effect on bronchial anastomotic healing. That same group also demonstrated that the ischemic donor bronchus could be revascularized within a few days by a pedicled flap of abdominal omentum (Morgan et al, 1982). Not only could the omental pedicle provide new collateral circulation to the ischemic bronchus, but the omentum provided additional benefit by containing anastomotic dehiscence in the event of partial disruption. During this same interval, it became apparent that cyclosporine had impressive immunosuppressive properties and could eliminate the need for high-dose corticosteroid immunosuppression. Furthermore, the Toronto group also demonstrated that cyclosporine had no adverse effect on bronchial anastomotic healing (Goldberg et al, 1983).

In 1981, a Stanford group reported initial clinical experience with combined heart-lung transplantation in patients with pulmonary vascular disease (PVD) (Reitz et al, 1982b). The combined heart-lung transplant was attempted without success by Cooley and associates (1969) and then by Lillehei (1970) and Barnard (1981). The Stanford experience demonstrated conclusively that, with the new immunosuppressive drug cyclosporine, the transplanted lung would provide acceptable long-term function for patients with pulmonary hypertension and right ventricular failure. However, by 1983, successful isolated lung transplantation had not been performed.

Satisfactory patient selection remained the final obstacle to successful clinical lung transplantation. The Toronto group reasoned that end-stage respiratory failure from pulmonary fibrosis provides ideal conditions for single-lung transplantation. The increased resistance to perfusion and ventilation in the native lung preferentially directs both perfusion and ventilation to the transplanted lung. A clinical lung transplant program at the University of Toronto was initiated in 1983 with a policy of careful recipient selection and strict adherence to rigid donor criteria. Bronchial omentopexy was used in every transplant procedure, and early perioperative corticosteroids were avoided. With these strategies, the first successful lung transplant was achieved in 1983 (Toronto Lung

Transplantation Group, 1986) in a 58-year-old man with idiopathic pulmonary fibrosis.

Subsequent development of an experimental (Dark, 1986) and clinical (Patterson et al, 1988) en bloc, double-lung replacement technique enabled bilateral lung replacement in patients for whom a single-lung transplant was not appropriate. Although this procedure allowed the preservation of the recipient heart, it was a technically complex procedure. In addition, it was associated with a high incidence of complications, notably donor airway ischemia (Patterson et al, 1990) and cardiac denervation (Schafers et al, 1990).

Subsequent innovations were achieved in the ensuing years that expanded the application of pulmonary transplantation. In the initial transplant experience, patients with obstructive pulmonary disease had been considered suitable only for bilateral lung replacement. It was subsequently shown that single-lung transplantation offers an attractive option for such patients (Mal et al, 1989). Combined heart-lung transplantation was formerly thought to be the only option for patients with PVD; however, many have shown that single (Pasque et al, 1992) and bilateral (Bando et al, 1994) lung transplantation provide satisfactory functional results in this patient group.

Technical advances have steadily accrued, most notably the development of a simplified method for bilateral sequential lung replacement (Pasque et al, 1990). Anterior thoracotomies and transverse sternal division (the clamshell incision) provide superior exposure for safe division of pleural adhesions. Sequential excision and replacement of both lungs often avoids the need for cardiopulmonary bypass. A logical extension of the clamshell incision is bilateral anterior thoracotomy with the omission of the transverse division of the sternal bone. This approach offers excellent access without the morbidity of sternal complications commonly seen after the clamshell access has been used (Meyers et al, 1998). For single-lung transplants, some groups have adopted muscle sparing thoracotomies to minimize morbidity and improve healing and postoperative function (Pochettino and Bavaria, 1997).

The shortened length of donor bronchus used in single-lung allografts reduces the incidence of bronchial anastomotic complications. Direct bronchial artery revascularization for double-lung (Couraud et al, 1992; Daly et al, 1993) and single-lung (Daly and McGregor, 1994) transplants has been described and is used in a number of programs.

Improved strategies of pulmonary preservation have enabled reliable long-distance procurement and satisfactory early allograft function in most cases. We have also demonstrated that pharmacologic agents such as prostaglandin E_1 (Aoe et al, 1994), pentoxifylline (Okabayashi et al, 1994), and nitric oxide (Date et al, 1996; Fujino et al, 1997) can also lessen reperfusion injury. Retrograde delivery of the perfusate improves the uniformity of the lung perfusion and has been credited with improved results by several investigators (Varela et al, 1997; Venuta et al, 1999).

Advances have also been made in the prevention and therapy of postoperative sepsis. Bacterial infection, which is particularly troublesome in patients with cystic fibrosis, has been lessened by the routine use of broad-spectrum prophylactic antibiotics and inhaled aminoglycosides. Herpes simplex infections have been lessened by routine prophylactic use of acyclovir. Cytomegalovirus (CMV) infection, a potentially fatal complication in recipients of lung transplants, has been markedly reduced by appropriate matching of donor and recipient CMV serologic findings when possible and prophylactic use of ganciclovir.

■ *HISTORICAL READINGS*

Dark JH et al: Experimental en-bloc double-lung transplantation. Ann Thorac Surg 42:394, 1986.

Derom F, Barbier F, Ringoir S: Ten-month survival after lung homotransplantation in man. J Thorac Cardiovasc Surg 61:835, 1971.

Goldberg M et al: A comparison between cyclosporin A and methylprednisolone plus azathioprine on bronchial healing following canine lung allotransplantation. J Thorac Cardiovasc Surg 85:821, 1983.

Hardin CA, Kittle CF: Experience with transplantation of the lung. Science 119:87, 1954.

Hardy JD: Lung homotransplantation in man. JAMA 186:1065, 1963.

Lillehei CW: Discussion of Wildevuur CRH, Benfield JR: A review of 23 human lung transplantations by 20 surgeons. Ann Thorac Surg 9:489, 1970.

Mal H et al: Unilateral lung transplantation in end stage pulmonary emphysema. Am Rev Respir Dis 140:797, 1989.

Metras H: Note préliminaire sur la graffe totale du poumon chéz le chien. Fr Acad Sci 1176[AU1], 1950.

Morgan WE et al: Improved bronchial healing in canine left lung reimplantation using omental pedicle wrap. J Thorac Cardiovasc Surg 85:139, 1983.

Patterson GA et al: Technique of successful clinical double-lung transplantation. Ann Thorac Surg 45:626, 1988.

Reitz BA et al: Heart-lung transplantation: Successful therapy for patients with pulmonary vascular disease. N Engl J Med 306:557, 1982b.

Toronto Lung Transplant Group: Unilateral lung transplantation for pulmonary fibrosis. N Engl J Med 314:1140, 1986.

PATIENT SELECTION

Recipient

General Considerations

General selection criteria are listed in the box titled "Recipient Selection Criteria" and are described in detail in a review by Maurer and associates (1998). For pulmonary transplant, only those patients believed to have a limited life expectancy (12 to 24 months) as a result of their underlying pulmonary disease are listed. As discussed later, the time course of deterioration and subsequent death is highly variable and depends on the specific disease. With the inherent risk of lung transplantation and the acute shortage of suitable donor lungs, we believe that it is inappropriate to offer lung transplantation to patients who are not in imminent danger of death from their underlying pulmonary disease. Patients who have major coexisting dysfunction involving another organ system are not eligible for transplantation. This creates a particular problem in the evaluation of older patients. In general, we do not accept a patient who is older than 60 years of age. Patients with a history of malignant disease within the past 5 years are not eligible for lung transplantation. A patient who is judged to be cured of a more recent malignancy might be considered. An exception to this criterion is the rare patient with bilateral bronchoalveolar carcinoma without metastatic disease, who might be eligible for lung transplantation in some programs (Zorn, 1998). Patients with serious psychological dysfunction are not able to meet the rigorous demands for patient compliance that are necessary for a successful lung transplantation. We do not evaluate patients who continue to smoke.

> **RECIPIENT SELECTION CRITERIA**
>
> Clinically and physiologically severe disease
> Medical therapy ineffective or unavailable
> Substantial limitation in activities of daily living
> Limited life expectancy
> Adequate cardiac function without significant coronary artery disease
> Ambulatory with rehabilitation potential
> Acceptable nutritional status
> Satisfactory psychosocial profile and emotional support system

Previous thoracic surgery or pleurodesis is not a specific contraindication to lung transplantation. With the recent development of lung-volume reduction surgery (Cooper et al, 1996), increasing numbers of patients will be referred for transplantation after unilateral or bilateral reduction pneumoplasty. Adhesions and anatomic distortion from previous surgery complicate the conduct of a transplant procedure, and allowance must be made for this in planning surgery. Patients who are receiving high-dose corticosteroid therapy (e.g., prednisone ≥40 mg/day) are not eligible for lung transplantation. Such high doses of corticosteroids cause a well-documented negative effect on bronchial healing and an increased susceptibility to postoperative infection. Patients who are receiving low- or moderate-dose steroid therapy (e.g., prednisone 10 mg/day or less) are candidates and have undergone pulmonary transplantation without an increased incidence of bronchial anastomotic complications. Ventilator dependency is not a contraindication to transplantation; however, most programs have a highly selective policy concerning such patients to prevent waiting lists from filling with chronic, stable, ventilated patients.

We insist that all patients listed for transplantation (except those with primary pulmonary hypertension [PPH] or Eisenmenger's syndrome) participate in a progressive, monitored exercise rehabilitation program while they await transplantation. Virtually all patients experience a marked improvement in strength and exercise tolerance without any measurable change in pulmonary function. We are convinced that this improved endurance enables patients to better withstand the rigors of a transplant procedure and the subsequent rehabilitation.

Specific Considerations

Obstructive Pulmonary Disease. Obstructive pulmonary disease, notably emphysema and α_1-antitrypsin deficiency, is the most common indication for lung transplantation. More than half of the transplant procedures reported to the International Society for Heart and Lung Transplantation (ISHLT) Registry were performed for obstructive lung disease (Hosenpud et al, 1999). The general criteria for transplantation in these patients have been published (Trulock, 1993). Most patients have deteriorated to a point at which oxygen supplementation is required. In our experience, the mean supplemental oxygen requirement is slightly more than 4 L/min. The obstructive physiology in these patients produces a forced expiratory volume at 1 second (FEV_1) that is well below 1 L, or approximately 15% of predicted normal values. Fortunately, this patient group has a relatively stable course during the inevitable long wait for a suitable donor.

Although obstructive pulmonary disease is the most common indication for single-lung transplantation, the ideal operative procedure for these patients is not yet defined (Bavaria et al, 1997; Sundaresan et al, 1996). The functional outcomes after single- and bilateral-lung transplantation for these patients are discussed later. In general, for young patients, particularly those with α_1-antitrypsin deficiency, we prefer to use bilateral sequential single-lung transplantation. The bilateral option is also more attractive in larger recipients for whom an oversized single donor lung would be difficult to obtain. On the other hand, for smaller recipients, single-lung transplantation offers a more attractive option, particularly when an oversized donor lung can be used. Finally, in the older patient, single-lung transplantation offers an attractive option because it is a technically simple procedure and is associated with a lower operative mortality rate.

Septic Lung Disease. Cystic fibrosis is the most frequently encountered condition in this category (Cooper et al, 1994). Cystic fibrosis is a common inherited disorder resulting in diffuse bronchiectatic destruction of both lungs. Without transplantation, most patients die as a result of progressive respiratory failure in the second or third decade of life. The most reliable predictors of life expectancy in patients with cystic fibrosis have been published (Hayllar et al, 1997; Kerem et al, 1992). A FEV_1 that is less than 30% of predicted, an elevated partial carbon dioxide pressure ($PaCO_2$), a requirement for supplemental oxygen, frequent admissions to the hospital for the control of acute pulmonary infections, and failure to maintain acceptable body weight are reliable predictors of early death. These are the criteria that we use in selecting patients with cystic fibrosis for lung transplantation. After reaching this stage of disease, patients with cystic fibrosis usually have a rapidly progressive downhill course. Indeed, in the Papworth experience, approximately one third of cystic fibrosis patients who were accepted for transplantation died while waiting for a donor (Sharples et al, 1993).

Fibrotic Lung Disease. Pulmonary fibrosis is one of the less common indications for single-lung transplantation. Specific selection criteria for patients with pulmonary fibrosis have not changed significantly since they were originally published by the Toronto Lung Transplant Group (Toronto Lung Transplantation Group, 1986). In our experience, candidates for transplantation have had classic restrictive physiologic findings with a mean forced vital capacity (FVC) and FEV_1 of 1.35 and 1.14, respectively (Meyers, 2000). All were using supplemental oxygen and demonstrated marked impairment of exercise tolerance with oxygen desaturation after minimal exertion. Moderate pulmonary hypertension is common in these patients. In contrast to the stability of patients with obstructive physiology (Trulock, 1993), patients with pulmonary fibrosis who required a transplant have a rapid downhill course. Many prospective recipients will not survive the lengthy wait for a donor lung.

Pulmonary Vascular Disease. Fremes and associates (1990) reported the first successful single-lung transplant in a patient with a patent ductus arteriosus and an associated Eisenmenger syndrome. Since this report, a number of centers have demonstrated that right ventricular function improves immediately following transplantation and that the improvement is maintained in long-term follow-up (Cooper et al, 1994). There are reliable predictors of early death in patients with PPH (D'Alonzo et al, 1991). Mean pulmonary artery pressures above 60 mm Hg, syncopal episodes, clinical evidence of right ventricular failure, significant elevation of central venous pressure, and depression of the cardiac index are predictors of death in patients with PPH. Among our first 22 patients undergoing single-lung transplant for PVD, the mean New York Heart Association functional class pretransplant was 3.4.

In the late 1980s and early 1990s, pulmonary transplantation was the only effective therapy for patients with end-stage pulmonary hypertension. Despite the comparatively short waiting time for donor lungs in that era as compared with the present, death rates were very high for PPH patients waiting for lungs (Gammie et al, 1998). Subsequent work has shown that continuous intravenous infusion of epoprostenol, a vasodilating prostaglandin, produces a symptomatic and hemodynamic benefit as well as improved survival for patients with pulmonary hypertension (Barst et al, 1996). Since that discovery, the absolute number of patients transplanted annually for PPH has decreased dramatically as fewer patients are referred for transplantation. Work in this alternative therapy continues, exploring such modalities as aerosolized prostacylin and inhaled nitric oxide as pulmonary vasodilators. Whether these therapies can eliminate the need for transplant, or simply delay it, remains to be seen.

Despite having degrees of pulmonary hypertension equivalent to those of patients with primary pulmonary hypertension, patients with Eisenmenger's physiology have a less predictable rate of deterioration, and the appropriate timing for transplantation in these patients is less certain. In these patients we rely on the development of intractable and progressive symptoms of right ventricular failure as the predominant selection criterion.

Donor

Rapid progress in transplantation has resulted in a shortage of suitable allografts for all organs. This is a particularly significant problem for lung transplantation because at most only 20% of otherwise suitable organ donors have lungs that meet the standard donor lung criteria. Most of the conditions that result in brain death (trauma or spontaneous intracerebral hemorrhage) are associated with significant pulmonary parenchymal pathologic findings as a result of lung contusion, infection, aspiration, or neurogenic pulmonary edema.

Satisfactory gas exchange is imperative for donor lungs. This can be confirmed by a partial oxygen pressure (PaO_2) that is greater than 300 mm Hg with the ventilator delivering a fraction of inspired oxygen (FIO_2) of 1.0 and 5 cm H_2O positive end-expiratory pressure (PEEP). A PaO_2 to FIO_2 ratio of 300 or greater provides adequate evidence of satisfactory gas exchange. A donor chest radiograph taken shortly prior to harvest must reveal clear lung fields. Bronchoscopic assessment at the donor institution often reveals mucopurulent secretions from which a variety of organisms might be cultured. This finding is commonly observed and is not a contraindication to lung transplantation if the donor is otherwise suitable. However, bronchoscopic evidence of aspiration or frank pus in the airway is a definite contraindication to transplantation.

Donor and recipient ABO compatibility is essential. Donor and recipient histocompatibility antigen (HLA) matching is not currently performed. There is controversy regarding the importance of HLA matching and no data in the literature that support its impact on subsequent graft function. Furthermore, any delay in donor harvest to conduct HLA matching places the donor lungs at risk for deterioration. Unfortunately, we do not have at our disposal satisfactory preservation strategies to permit "postharvest" tissue matching. We prefer to use CMV-negative donors for CMV-negative recipients whenever possible.

STANDARD LUNG DONOR SELECTION CRITERIA

Age less than 55 years
No history of pulmonary disease
Normal serial chest radiographs
Adequate gas exchange (PaO_2 300 mm Hg on FIO_2 1.0 and PEEP 5 cm H_2O)
Normal bronchoscopic examination
Negative serologic screening for hepatitis B and human immunodeficiency virus (HIV)
Recipient matching for ABO blood group
Size matching

PEEP, peak end-expiratory pressure.

A significant consideration is size matching between the donor and recipient. Acceptable size matching depends on the nature of the recipient's pulmonary disease and the type of transplant planned. Size matching can be achieved by a comparison of vertical lung height, transverse chest diameter, and chest circumference. However, we have found these donor measurements are unreliable when made by busy and inexperienced donor coordinators in remote donor hospitals. Much more reliable are predicted donor and recipient pulmonary volumes, which are calculated using standard nomograms that are based on age, sex, and height.

In patients undergoing single-lung transplantation for obstructive pulmonary disease, we attempt to place allografts that are 15% to 20% larger than the predicted recipient lung volume. Implantation of such a large allograft is easily achieved in a patient with obstructive pulmonary disease because of the enormous size of the recipient's pleural space. However, in patients with pulmonary fibrosis or PVD, the pleural spaces are reduced or normal in size. It is, therefore, inadvisable to oversize these patients. In patients who are undergoing bilateral lung replacement, we prefer to match the donor's lung volumes to the estimated volume that the recipient would possess in the absence of disease.

Certain circumstances allow relaxation of the normally strict donor selection criteria. A minor degree of pulmonary infiltrate can be accepted in a donor who is being used for a bilateral transplantation. We analyzed 133 consecutive donor lungs and identified 37 donors with "marginal" quality, as judged by arterial blood gas analysis and radiographic assessment. The marginal donors provided postoperative function that was equivalent to those that were deemed excellent (Sundaresan et al, 1995a) (Fig. 37–1). On occasion, a donor is identified with

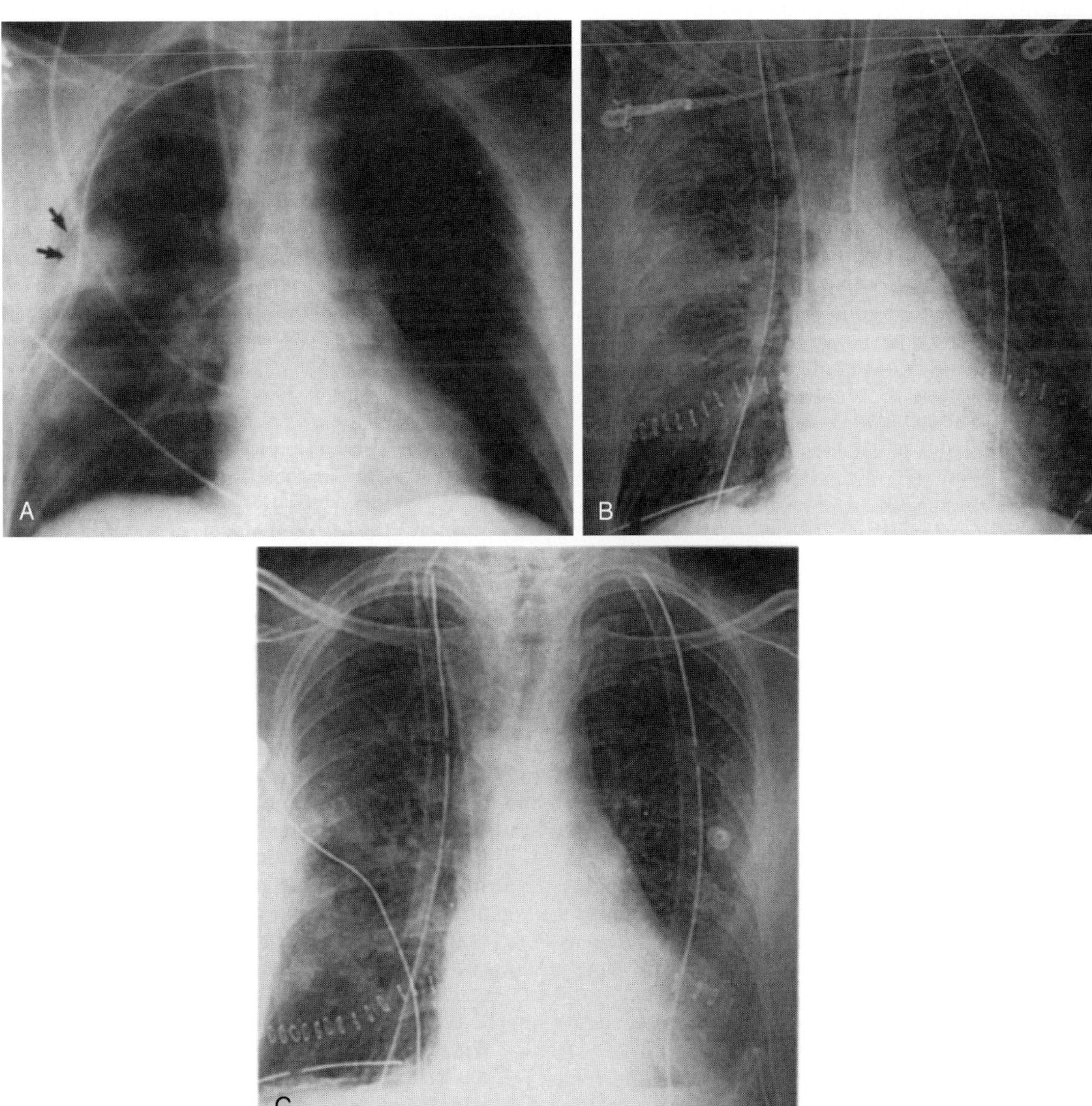

FIGURE 37–1 ■ *A*, An anteroposterior chest radiograph from a patient with brain death as a result of a motor vehicle accident. The right chest tube evacuated a 50% pneumothorax. The *arrows* point to a right upper lobe contusion. Several hours following this radiograph, both lungs were harvested for use as bilateral sequential allografts in a patient with obstructive lung disease. (From Shields TW: General Thoracic Surgery. Philadelphia, Lea & Febiger, 1994.) *B*, Immediate postoperative recipient radiograph demonstrating some progression of the right upper lobe contusion. *C*, Recipient chest radiograph taken 3 days following transplantation. Note the dramatic clearing of the right upper lobe contusion.

marginal gas exchange and radiographic evidence of a unilateral pulmonary infiltrate. In a number of such situations, we have made an intraoperative donor assessment with ventilation and perfusion only to the seemingly normal donor lung, judged that lung to be acceptable, and conducted a successful unilateral transplantation (Puskas et al, 1992c).

Other strategies have been adopted to increase the donor pool. Living, related, bilateral, lobar transplantation has been successfully used in a selected small group of patients with cystic fibrosis (Cohen et al, 1994). The authors reported results for 37 patients including 32 with cystic fibrosis, 2 with pulmonary hypertension, and 2 with pulmonary fibrosis. One-year survival was 68%, and there were no deaths or life-threatening complications to the 76 healthy donors (Starnes et al, 1996). Although innovative and exciting, this procedure is unlikely to have any meaningful impact on the overall shortage of lung allografts. Xenografts offer the only potential hope for a large increase in the supply of suitable donor lungs, although work toward a xenograft lung source remains at the most basic level of investigation (Macchiarini et al, 1997). An innovative method to expand the use of existing donor lungs is pulmonary bipartitioning, described by Couetil (Couetil et al, 1997) as a way to use a single left lung to perform a bilateral transplant in a child or small adult. The seven patients reported demonstrated the feasibility of this approach. Work with non–heart-beating donors has shown acceptable lung function in lungs that were extracted up to 2 hours after cessation of heart function (Van Raemdonck et al, 1997), although this source of donor lungs has not yet become clinically useful.

LUNG PRESERVATION

Lung preservation has been the focus of intense laboratory interest for a number of years. Several detailed reviews of this subject have recently been published (Christie and Waddell, 1993; Novick et al, 1996). Clinical pulmonary preservation has progressed considerably since the Toronto group initially reported unilateral lung transplantation using donor lungs that were harvested in an atelectatic state and stored after topical hypothermic immersion (Todd et al, 1988). There are minor differences in the preservation strategies of most clinical lung transplant programs, but basic principles remain the same.

Following systemic donor heparinization and just prior to circulatory arrest, a pulmonary vasodilator is administered. We use prostaglandin E_1 (PGE_1) 500 mg as a direct bolus injection into the pulmonary artery. Pulmonary arterial flushing is then achieved with the lungs in a state of moderate inflation at an FIO_2 that is greater than room air (usually 100%). Most lung transplant programs use an intracellular flush solution, most commonly modified Euro-Collins solution (4 mEq/mg SO_4 and 3% glucose) or University of Wisconsin solution (Hopkinson et al, 1998). Following extraction, the lung allograft is immersed in iced crystalloid solution and maintained in a semi-inflated state during transport. This technique results in reliable allograft function following ischemic times of up to 6 hours. On occasion, we have extended the ischemic time, particularly for the second lung of a bilateral sequential transplant in which the ischemic time has occasionally reached 8 to 10 hours with satisfactory subsequent function. Work by Snell and associates (1996) has shown an effect on outcome with longer ischemic times, particularly if the time exceeds 5 hours. Novick and coworkers (1999) reported a complex relationship between donor age and ischemic time on outcome, with older donor lungs being more sensitive to prolonged ischemic time than younger lungs.

A detailed review of experimental pulmonary preservation is beyond the scope of this chapter, but there have been several interesting developments.

Inflation

The state of lung inflation during pulmonary artery flush and storage probably has a significant impact on post-transplant pulmonary function. Puskas and colleagues (1992b) demonstrated that canine lungs that are flushed and stored in a hyperinflated state produce more reliable post-transplant lung function after a 30-hour storage period compared with lungs that are stored at low pulmonary volumes. Using the same model, our laboratory demonstrated that hyperinflation during storage and flush is necessary to achieve the maximum benefit. However, when we adopted a policy of donor hyperinflation in our clinical program, we noted a disturbing incidence of allograft dysfunction. Recent evidence from our laboratory obtained by the use of a rabbit model suggests that hyperinflation produces increased pulmonary capillary permeability. We confirmed this finding in a recent series of canine allotransplants. For this reason we recommend that lungs are flushed and stored in a state of moderate inflation that is consistent with normal end-tidal inspiration (Haniuda et al, 1996).

Temperature of Flush and Storage

Clinical lung transplant programs use pulmonary artery flush solutions with temperatures of 1°C to 4°C. Lungs are extracted, immersed in crystalloid, and packed in ice for storage and transport at approximately 1°C. A number of investigators have shown that moderate degrees of hypothermia (10°C) result in superior pulmonary function. This has been demonstrated in our own laboratory in an in vitro rabbit lung perfusion model (Wang et al, 1993), a standard model of canine left-lung allotransplantation (Date et al, 1992), and a bilateral baboon lung transplantation (Sundaresan et al, 1993). However, in a canine allograft study, Mayer and colleagues (1992) were unable to show a difference between storage at 4°C versus 10°C in canine left-lung allografts.

Composition of Flush Solution

There has been considerable controversy as to the optimal composition of the pulmonary flush solution. Various solutions are used clinically at present. Some groups advocate cardiopulmonary bypass to cool the donor, thereby essentially flushing the lungs with cooled autologous donor blood (Yacoub et al, 1989). The Papworth group popularized the use of an extracellular solution that is supplemented with donor blood to achieve a flush hematocrit of approximately 10% (Hakim et al, 1988). During the past several years, a number of experimental studies have demonstrated that an extracellular low-potassium dextran (LPD) solution provided superior function over the standard, intracellular Euro-Collins solution (Keshavjee et al, 1992). It was argued that this LPD solution induced less pulmonary vasoconstriction during flush. However, we have recently shown that, if pulmonary vasodilatation is achieved with PGE_1 prior to flush, Euro-Collins solution provides equivalent preservation to that achieved with LPD (Puskas et al, 1992a).

The Pittsburgh group (Hardesty et al, 1993) conducted a retrospective review of their experience and concluded that the University of Wisconsin solution may actually provide preservation that is superior to that observed with the more commonly used modified Euro-Collins solution. Most programs responding to a recent survey (Hopkinson et al, 1998) reported use of either modified Euro-Collins or University of Wisconsin solution.

Pharmacologic Manipulation

In addition to the apparent benefit gained when prostaglandins are administered prior to pulmonary artery flush (Mayer et al, 1992), recent evidence suggests that infused prostanoids are useful in the early post-transplant period. Matsuzaki and associates (1993) demonstrated that PGE_1 infusion decreased reperfusion injury following 2 hours of warm ischemia in a rabbit lung model. We continued this work, demonstrating that PGE_1 improves canine lung allograft function following an 18-hour ischemic period (Aoe et al, 1994). We use a PGE_1 infusion routinely during the postoperative period in our clinical program. Pentoxifylline and inhaled nitric oxide also ameliorate canine lung allograft reperfusion injury.

Evidence suggests that oxygen-free radicals are important in the genesis of ischemia reperfusion injury in the lung. This subject was concisely reviewed by Christie and Waddell (1993). A number of antioxidant interventions, including enzymatic (superoxide dismutase, catalase, or glutathione peroxidase) and nonenzymatic (allopurinol, glutathione, dimethylthiourea, and lazaroids) have shown impressive results in reducing lung reperfusion injury. Some of these agents have been used with success in clinical lung transplant programs.

The latest in the long series of phamacologic additives is cyclic adenosine monophosphate which, when added to lung preservation solution, provides better results than those seen with traditional preservatives (Kayano et al, 1999).

Metabolism

The lung is unique among the solid organs that are harvested and preserved for transplantation. Oxygen in the inflated alveoli and intracellular glucose that is augmented by glucose in the flushing solution allows the cooled lung to maintain aerobic metabolism and to preserve cellular adenosine triphosphate (ATP) levels during extended periods of preservation (Date et al, 1993). In fact, the lung likely maintains a state of aerobic metabolism within the cadaver for short periods following death. Egan and colleagues (1993) demonstrated satisfactory gas exchange in canine lung allografts that were harvested from canine donors some hours after death. Van Raemdonck showed acceptable lung function in grafts that were procured up to 2 hours after death as long as the lungs were ventilated or kept in a state of static inflation (Van Raemdonck et al, 1997).

Controlled Reperfusion

A recent innovation that was adapted from the experience gained by cardiac surgeons in the reperfusion of ischemic myocardium is the notion of "controlled reperfusion." Many authors have explored the impact of altering pressure (Bhabra et al, 1996; Clark et al, 1998), leukocyte content (Shiraishi et al, 1998), or both (Halldorsson et al, 1998) in the initial 10 minutes of reperfusion of pulmonary grafts after prolonged ischemia. The evidence indicates beneficial effects gained by initial reperfusion with low pressure, leukocyte depleted, substrated enhanced blood to reduce or eliminate reperfusion injury. Clinical studies have yet to verify the exiting potential of this seemingly minor alteration of standard techniques.

TECHNIQUE

Donor Extraction

Our donor extraction technique is the same as that reported by Sundaresan and colleagues (1993). When the harvest team arrives at the donor hospital, the lung extraction team assesses the chest radiographs and performs fiberoptic bronchoscopy. The final assessment is made by gross inspection of the lungs once they are exposed by a median sternotomy in conjunction with the midline laparotomy for the extraction of abdominal organs.

The abdominal organs are prepared for extraction by their respective surgical teams. It is preferable for the liver team to insert a large-caliber cannula in the inferior vena cava for liver flush effluent rather than planning to vent the hepatic flush into the chest through the divided inferior vena cava, thereby obscuring the view of the thoracic organ extraction team.

Both vena cavas are encircled within the pericardium. Care must be taken to avoid injury to the right main pulmonary artery that lies immediately posterior to the superior vena cava and the ascending aorta. The aorta is mobilized and encircled. It is not necessary to dissect the main pulmonary artery.

The donor is heparinized. A cardioplegia cannula is placed in the ascending aorta. A large-bore pulmonary flush cannula is then placed in the main pulmonary artery immediately proximal to its bifurcation. PGE_1 (0.5 mg) is administered directly into the main pulmonary artery and produces an immediate drop in systemic pressure. Double ligation of the superior vena cava with clamping of the inferior vena cava at the diaphragm results in venous inflow occlusion. The aorta is cross-clamped, and cardioplegia is initiated. Cardioplegia is vented through the inferior vena cava, which is divided immediately above the previously placed clamp. After cardioplegic arrest has been achieved, pulmonary flushing is initiated. With the lungs continuously ventilated, pulmonary artery flushing is achieved with 50 ml/kg of modified Euro-Collins solution delivered at a pressure of 30 cm H_2O. This solution is vented through the amputated tip of the left atrial appendage (Fig. 37–2). Cold effluent is allowed to collect in both pleural spaces. Topical hypothermia is supplemented by crushed ice.

It is our preference to extract the donor heart in situ. It should be stated emphatically that satisfactory cardiac and bilateral lung grafts can always be safely extracted with appropriate cooperation between the heart and lung transplant teams. The superior vena cava is divided between the previously placed ligatures, again taking care not to injure the underlying right main pulmonary artery. The aorta is divided distal to the cardioplegia cannula. The main pulmonary artery is then divided through the cannulation site, typically just proximal to the bifurcation. The heart is then elevated and retracted to the right. The left atrium is opened midway between the coronary sinus and the inferior pulmonary vein. The left atrial incision is then continued toward the right. The right side of the left atrial wall is then divided, taking care to preserve a rim of atrial muscle on the pulmonary vein side (Fig. 37–3). This completes the cardiac excision.

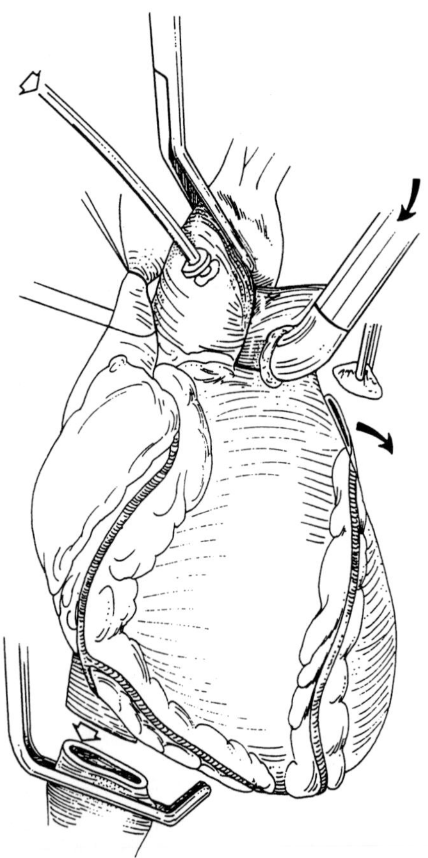

FIGURE 37–2 ■ Cardioplegia is administered proximal to an aortic cross clamp and vented through the transsected inferior vena cava *(open arrow)*. Pulmonary flush solution is administered through the main pulmonary artery and vented through the amputated tip of the left atrial appendage *(solid arrow)*. (From Sundaresen S et al: Donor lung procurement: Assessment and operative technique. Ann Thorac Surg 56:1409, 1993.)

Extraction of the lungs is continued by mobilization and division of the trachea well above the carina. It is our preference to divide the trachea with a stapling instrument and keep the lungs moderately inflated. The great vessels are divided at the apex of the chest, and the esophagus is transsected with a stapling instrument. The remaining thoracic contents are then extracted by lifting and dissecting them off the spine in a cranial-to-caudal direction. The thoracic aorta and esophagus are transsected at the diaphragm. The lung allografts are then immersed in cold crystalloid solution and transported in a semi-inflated state. If the individual lungs are destined for use by different transplant centers, they are separated into separate allografts at the donor hospital. The donor left main bronchus is divided at its origin with a cutting stapling device to leave the airway to both lungs sealed (Fig. 37–4). Otherwise, the grafts should be transported en bloc for separation immediately prior to implantation. On arrival at the recipient hospital, the graft is exposed and kept cold during the remainder of its preparation. The esophagus and aorta are removed, leaving all other soft tissues on the specimen side to maximize bronchial arterial collateral flow to the donor lung. If bronchial revascularization is to be attempted, the anterior wall of the proximal descending aorta is left on the specimen (Couraud et al, 1992).

Viewing the double-lung block from its anterior aspect, the posterior pericardium is divided inferiorly to superiorly. The posterior left atrium is divided, leaving equal atrial cuffs on both sides. The remaining pericardium posterior to the left atrium is then divided. The pulmonary artery is divided at its bifurcation (see Fig. 37–4). It is important to separate the pulmonary artery from its pericardial attachments on each side out to the first pulmonary arterial branch. This prevents postimplantation kinking of the pulmonary artery distal to the pulmonary artery anastomosis.

Subcarinal nodes are divided, and the left main bronchus is transsected. The left main bronchus is then dissected from the nodal tissue and divided two rings proximal to the upper lobe orifice. On the right side, excision of the carina usually provides an adequate length (two rings proximal to the upper lobe origin) for subsequent bronchial anastomosis. It is important during dissection of the bronchus to minimize any nodal dissection at the site of bronchus transsection to maximize retrograde bronchial collateral blood flow to the donor bronchus after transplantation.

Recipient Anesthesia

A successful lung transplant program requires active involvement of expert anesthesiologists who are familiar with complex cardiothoracic anesthesia techniques, bronchoscopy, and cardiopulmonary bypass. Full hemodynamic monitoring is required in every patient. We routinely use a Foley catheter, central venous line, pulmonary artery Swan-Ganz catheter, radial artery cath-

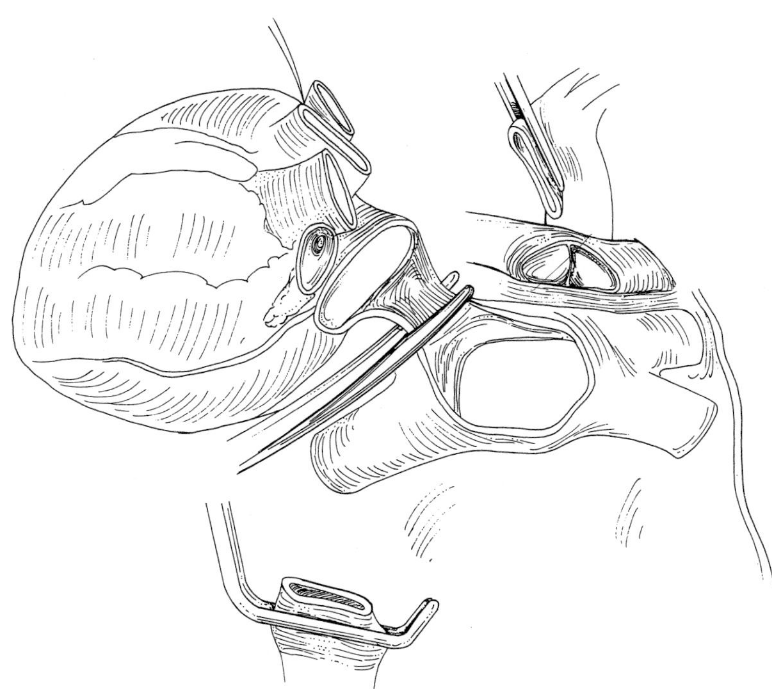

FIGURE 37–3 ■ The ascending aorta is divided. The main pulmonary artery has been transsected at its bifurcation. The heart is retracted upward and to the right to enable safe division of the left atrium leaving suitable cuffs on both cardiac and lung allografts. (From Sundaresen S et al: Donor lung procurement: Assessment and operative technique. Ann Thorac Surg 56:1409, 1993.)

eter, and femoral artery catheter. It is useful to supplement the radial artery catheter with a femoral artery line, especially if cardiopulmonary bypass is anticipated. We routinely use a transesophageal echocardiographic probe and believe it is critical for patients with severe pulmonary hypertension and coexisting right ventricular dysfunction.

The airway is routinely intubated with a left-sided double-lumen endobronchial tube, which enables independent ventilation of either or both lungs. A single-lumen tube with an endobronchial Fogarty catheter provides independent ventilation. However, this technique lacks the reliability of a double-lumen tube. A single-lumen tube can present difficulties, particularly in a bilateral transplant recipient in whom intraoperative maneuvering of the tube can be troublesome. In patients with cystic fibrosis, thick purulent secretions are continuously expressed into the bronchial lumen during manipulation of the lungs for extraction. To aspirate the airway completely prior to placement of the double-lumen tube in these patients, a large-caliber single-lumen tube and a flexible fiberoptic bronchoscopy are necessary.

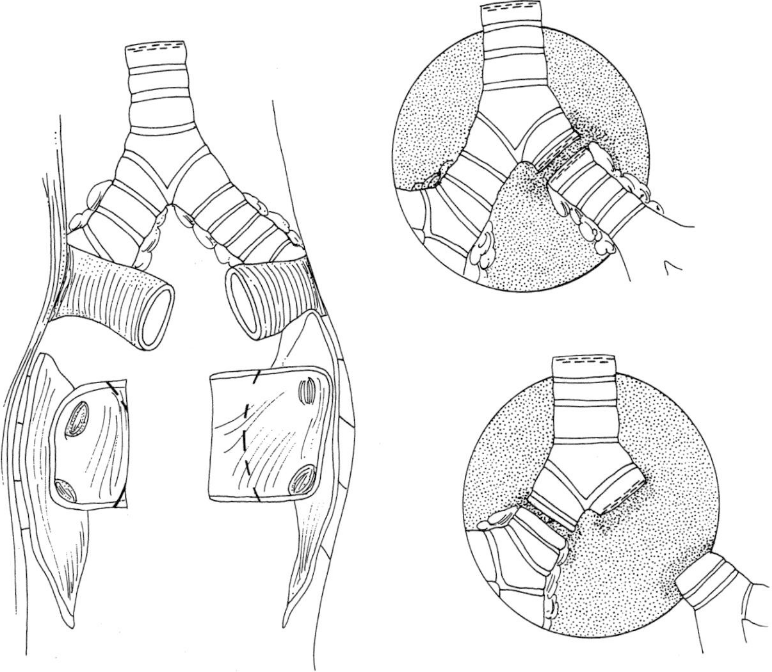

FIGURE 37–4 ■ The pericardium and left atrium are divided with the left atrium further trimmed *(dotted lines)*. The airway is transsected and kept sealed with the use of a gastrointestinal anastomosis stapling device across the proximal left mainstem bronchus. The donor airway is further revised for implantation, as shown in the bottom right. (From Sundaresen S et al: Donor lung procurement: Assessment and operative technique. Ann Thorac Surg 56:1409, 1993.)

In patients of small stature, a single-lumen tube must be used. If a bilateral procedure is planned in such patients, cardiopulmonary bypass should be used routinely during extraction and implantation. This is the standard technique for bilateral transplantation in children (Spray et al, 1994).

It has been our practice to use aprotinin in patients in whom there is an anticipation of dense intrapleural adhesions (e.g., in cases of cystic fibrosis, bronchiectasis, or previous thoracic surgery). This agent effectively reduces perioperative blood loss, especially when cardiopulmonary bypass is required in patients with extensive pleural or mediastinal adhesions (Westaby, 1993).

Single-Lung Transplantation

Choice of Side

In general we prefer to transplant the side with the least pulmonary function, as judged by preoperative quantitative nuclear perfusion scans. It was previously argued that the right side was preferable for patients with obstructive pulmonary disease. However, in our experience and that of others (Levine et al, 1993), there is no difference in functional outcome among single-lung recipients, regardless of the transplanted side. If cardiopulmonary bypass is anticipated, as in patients with PPH or severe pulmonary fibrosis with associated pulmonary hypertension, the right side is the preferred transplant side. For patients with Eisenmenger's syndrome, we prefer the right side to facilitate closure of the coexisting atrial or ventricular septal defects. A patent ductus arteriosus can be repaired in association with a transplant on either side.

Exposure

A generous posterolateral thoracotomy through the fifth interspace is the preferred approach, although a muscle-sparing incision has be advocated by some authors (Pochettino and Bavaria, 1997). For right-sided transplants in which cardiopulmonary bypass is anticipated, cannulation of the ascending aorta is facilitated by the use of a fourth interspace incision. A median sternotomy can be used for right-sided transplants, especially if associated cardiac repair dictates an anterior approach, permitting access to the left side of the heart. The patients are always positioned with the ipsilateral groin in the operative field for subsequent cannulation if necessary. Femoral partial bypass was formerly our technique of choice. However, intrathoracic cannulation avoids a groin incision and the necessary arterial and venous repairs following decannulation. The ascending aorta and right atrium are easily cannulated through the right chest. The cannulas are positioned in the anterior aspect of the incision and remain well out of the operative field throughout the procedure. Through a left posterolateral thoracotomy, the proximal left pulmonary artery and descending aorta are easily cannulated.

Recipient Pneumonectomy

Following adequate exposure of the pleural space, pleural adhesions are divided. These can be extensive in patients with fibrotic or septic lung disease and are ordinarily absent in patients with emphysema and PPH. Extreme care is taken not to injure the phrenic and recurrent laryngeal nerves. The inferior pulmonary ligament is divided. The pulmonary veins and main pulmonary artery are encircled outside the pericardium. During this dissection, the need for cardiopulmonary bypass is determined. The ventilation of the contralateral lung and occlusion of the ipsilateral pulmonary artery determine whether the contralateral native lung provides adequate gas exchange and hemodynamics to tolerate pneumonectomy and implantation without cardiopulmonary bypass. Assessment of right ventricular contractility with the transesophageal echo probe is especially useful at this point (Triantafillou et al, 1995).

Easily accessible upper lobe pulmonary artery branches are ligated and divided. This increases the length of pulmonary artery available for subsequent pulmonary artery anastomosis. It also decreases the caliber of the pulmonary artery to match the donor's size to the recipient's pulmonary artery, particularly when significant pulmonary hypertension is present. Furthermore, having a ligated recipient upper lobe branch helps with proper orientation of the donor and recipient pulmonary arteries. The pulmonary artery just distal to this branch is stapled proximally. A distal pulmonary artery clamp is placed, the vessel is divided, and its distal aspect is ligated to minimize backbleeding, which can be torrential if vigorous bronchial circulation is present.

Pulmonary veins are divided between the stapled lines or between silk ligatures that are placed on each venous branch at the hilum. This latter option increases the size of the subsequent left atrial cuff. Pulmonary artery division is often made easier after division of the superior pulmonary vein.

Peribronchial nodal tissue is divided, and bronchial arterial vessels are secured with ligatures. The bronchus is transsected just proximal to the upper lobe origin, and the lung is excised (Fig. 37–5). The recipient bronchus is then trimmed back up into the mediastinum, taking care to avoid any devascularization of the recipient bronchus at the site of anastomosis. The pericardium around the vein stumps is then widely opened, and hemostasis is achieved in the mediastinum.

Implantation

The donor lung, wrapped in cold, moist gauze, is then placed in the posterior portion of the thorax. In this position, manipulation of the lung can be avoided during the entire implantation. The lung is kept cold with a topical application of crushed ice. This topical hypothermia provides an extended period of cold preservation and gives additional time for meticulous anastomoses.

The bronchial anastomosis is performed first (Fig. 37–6). Various techniques have been described. Our preference is to first close the membranous posterior wall using a continuous suture of 4-0 absorbable monofilament suture. The anterior cartilaginous airway is then closed by using an interrupted suture of absorbable monofilament. Sutures are placed using a figure-eight technique or a simple interrupted technique with no attempt to intussuscept the smaller bronchus. Small-cali-

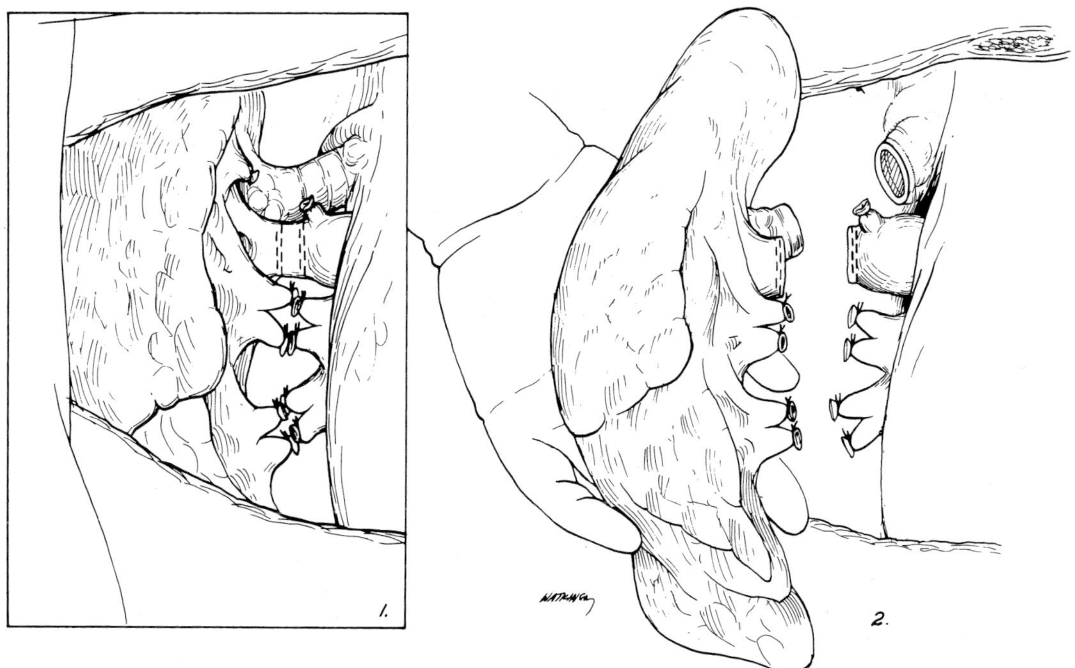

FIGURE 37–5 ■ Excision of the native right lung is depicted. The pulmonary artery is stapled beyond its first upper lobe branch. Pulmonary veins are divided between ligatures, and the bronchus is transsected just proximal to the upper lobe orifice. (From Shields TW: General Thoracic Surgery. Philadelphia, Lea & Febiger, 1994.)

ber bronchi can be narrowed by the figure-eight technique. In this circumstance, an end-to-end closure is obtained by using simple interrupted sutures of monofilament absorbable material. The bronchial anastomosis is covered by using either local peribronchial nodal tissue or, rarely, a pedicle flap of pericardium or thymic fat. We no longer use bronchial omentopexy in routine transplant procedures.

A vascular clamp is then placed as proximal as possible on the ipsilateral main pulmonary artery. The donor and recipient arteries are trimmed to size, and an end-to-end anastomosis is created using 5-0 polypropylene suture (Fig. 37–7). Care must be taken to excise an adequate length of donor and recipient pulmonary artery. Excessive length results in kinking of the pulmonary artery after allograft inflation. Proper orientation of the donor and recipient pulmonary artery is also obviously important.

Lateral traction on the pulmonary vein stumps enables central placement of an angled atrial clamp. For right-sided transplants, it is occasionally necessary to open the interatrial groove to increase the length of recipient left atrium that is available for placement of the clamp. Pulmonary vein stumps are then amputated, and the bridge of tissue between the two is incised to create a suitable cuff for the left atrial anastomosis (Fig. 37–8). Following completion of this anastomosis, but before tightening and tying the final stitch, the lung is gently inflated while the pulmonary artery clamp is temporarily removed, enabling the lung to be "de-aired" through the open left atrial anastomosis. All suture lines are then secured and inspected, and the vascular clamps are removed. It is our practice to initiate reperfusion with the recipient receiving a continuous infusion of PGE_1. This infusion continues for at least a day after the transplant unless pulmonary artery pressures are low and lung function is ideal. Two pleural drains are left in each pleural space, and routine closure is achieved using absorbable suture material. At the termination of the procedure, the double-lumen endotracheal tube is replaced with a large-caliber, single-lumen tube. Flexible bronchoscopy is then performed to inspect the bronchial anastomosis and evacuate the airway of any blood or secretions.

Sequential Bilateral Lung Transplantation

Exposure

Sequential bilateral single-lung transplantations are conducted through bilateral anterolateral fourth or fifth interspace thoracotomies that are connected by a transverse sternotomy (Fig. 37–9). This "clamshell" incision provides adequate exposure for safe division of pleural adhesions. In patients with cystic fibrosis, these can be particularly dense at the apex and posterior aspect of the chest. In addition, this incision provides satisfactory exposure for institution of cardiopulmonary bypass by ascending aortic and right atrial cannulation. Since 1996, we have modified this incision by omitting the transverse sternotomy (Fig. 37–10), thus avoiding frequent major and minor complications that can be encountered with the healing of the sternal closure (Meyers et al, 1998).

Pneumonectomy and Implantation

The techniques of pneumonectomy and implantation are identical to those just described for single-lung transplantation. The side with the worse function (as predicted

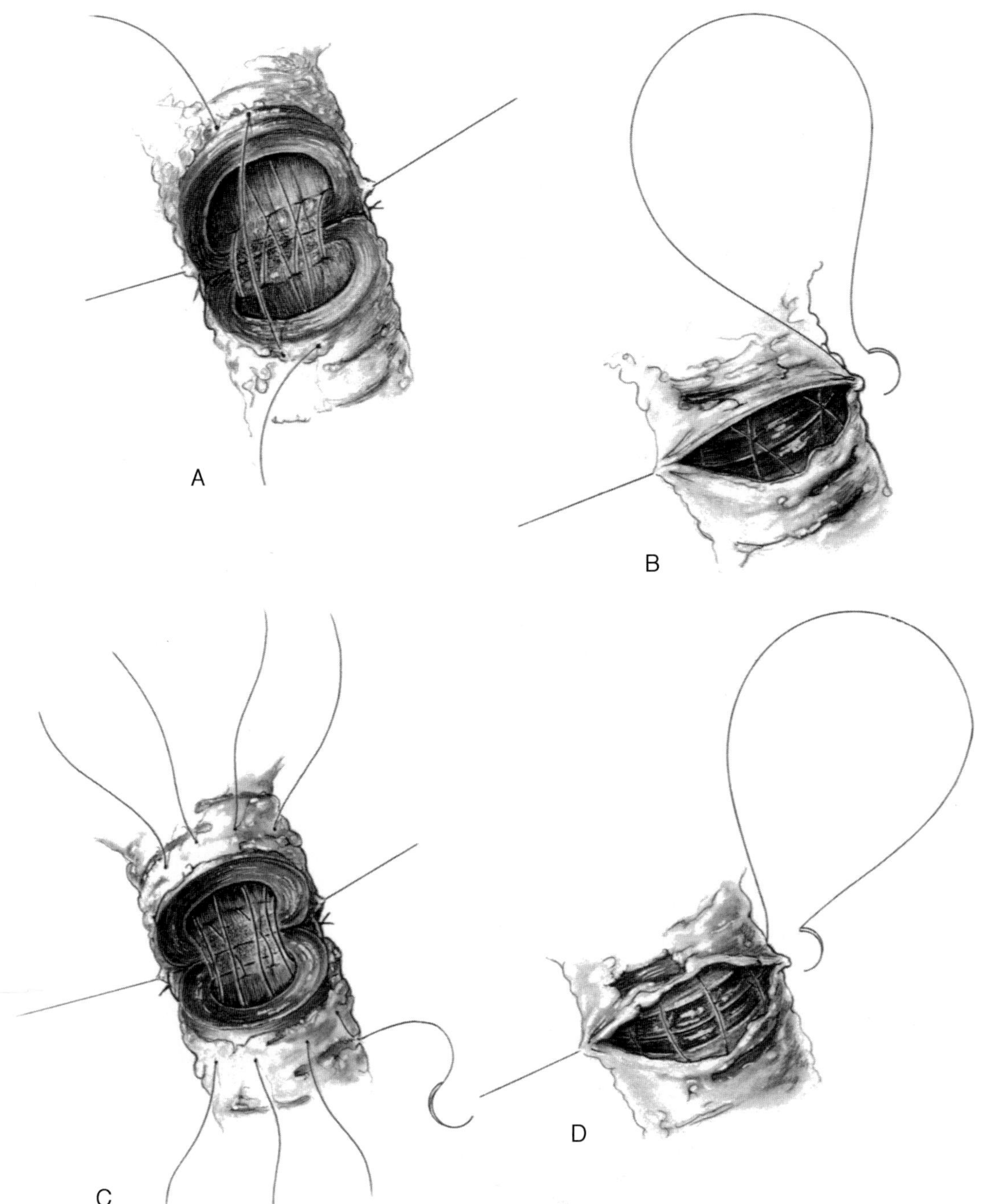

FIGURE 37–6 ■ A bronchial anastomosis is depicted. The membranous wall is approximated *(A* and *C)*. If the airways are large, a figure-eight cartilaginous suture technique can be seen *(A)*. Smaller airways require simple, interrupted sutures *(C)*. Peribronchial mediastinal tissue covers the anastomosis *(B* and *D)*. (From Meyers BF, et al: Op Tech Thorac Surg 4:169, 1999.)

by preoperative ventilation and perfusion nuclear scans) is replaced first. If function is equivalent, the right lung is replaced first. Cardiopulmonary bypass may be necessary at several junctures during bilateral sequential transplant (Triantafillou et al, 1994). First, patients with small airways that are not amenable to double-lumen tube placement require cardiopulmonary bypass to be instituted following mobilization of both lungs and maintained during bilateral extraction and implantation. Some patients with airways that are suitable for double-lumen endotracheal tubes will have inadequate contralateral native lung to allow satisfactory gas exchange or hemodynamics to occur during removal or replacement of the first lung. Cardiopulmonary bypass is instituted at this point. The most common situation that necessitates bypass occurs following implantation of the first lung. An acutely dysfunctional transplanted lung may not support the recipient's circulation and gas exchange. This problem

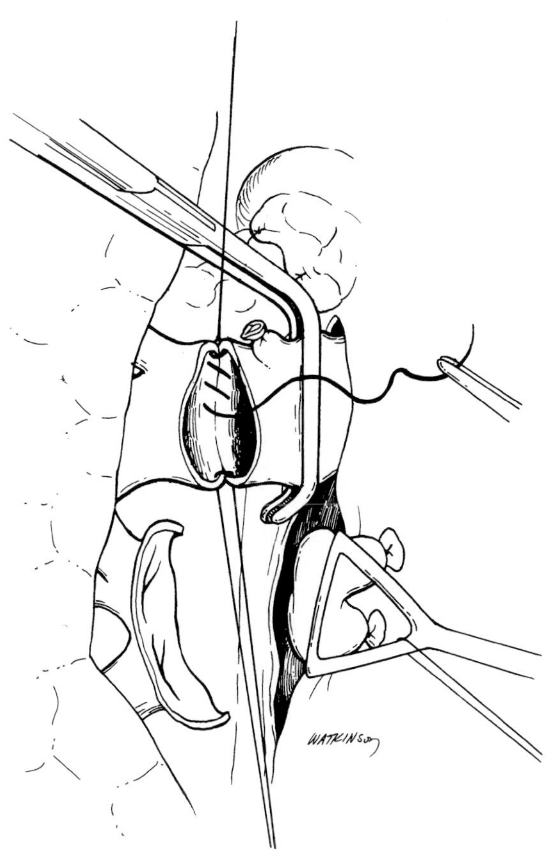

FIGURE 37–7 ■ A central pulmonary artery clamp is placed, the staple line is excised, and an end-to-end anastomosis is constructed with 5–0 polypropylene. (From Meyers BF: Technical aspects of adult lung transplantation. Semin Thorac Cardiovasc Surg 10:213, 1998.)

presents itself as a progressive increase in pulmonary artery pressure. If increased pulmonary artery pressure is genuine and substantial, pulmonary edema will develop and cause hypoxemia. The cause of this typical clinical phenomenon is not well understood, although it is likely to be the result of poor preservation. Alternatively, it may be caused by recipient systemic bacteremia, as it is commonly observed following implantation of the first lung in patients with cystic fibrosis. It is prudent to institute cardiopulmonary bypass for the completion of the procedure as soon as clinical problems arise rather than to wait for an emergent situation in an unstable patient.

POSTOPERATIVE MANAGEMENT

Ventilation

Generally patients are ventilated with standard ventilatory techniques. The FIO_2 is kept at a level to maintain a PaO_2 that is greater than 70 mm Hg. A tidal volume of 12 to 15 mm/kg is usually sufficient, and a PEEP of 5 to 7.5 cm H_2O is used, except in single-lung recipients with obstructive pulmonary disease. Extubation is performed in accordance with standard requirements of satisfactory gas exchange and mechanics. Most patients are extubated between 24 and 48 hours following transplantation. A standard, intermittent, mandatory ventilation or pressure support wean is used in all bilateral lung transplant recipients and in single-lung recipients who are transplanted for pulmonary fibrosis.

Patients who have undergone single-lung transplantation for chronic obstructive pulmonary disease and PVD are managed differently (Davis et al, 1994). In the former condition, we avoid the use of PEEP and select tidal volumes that are lower than would ordinarily be used. These adjustments reduce hyperinflation of the excessively compliant native lung and minimize compression of the less compliant transplanted lung. This trapping of air in the native lung results in major problems including high airway pressures, inadequate removal of carbon dioxide, and hypotension due to reduced venous return to the heart. Some patients have required a volume reduction of the native lung by lobectomy or even pneumonectomy to decompress the contralateral transplanted lung.

In single-lung recipients with PVD, we have elected to use a more prolonged period (48 to 72 hours) of mechanical ventilation. Patients are kept heavily sedated and often paralyzed for that period. We choose to maintain these patients in a position with the native lung dependent to maintain inflation and appropriate drainage of the transplanted lung. Standard tidal volumes are used, but an increased PEEP of 7.5 to 10 cm H_2O is applied. Early graft dysfunction, rejection, or infection necessi-

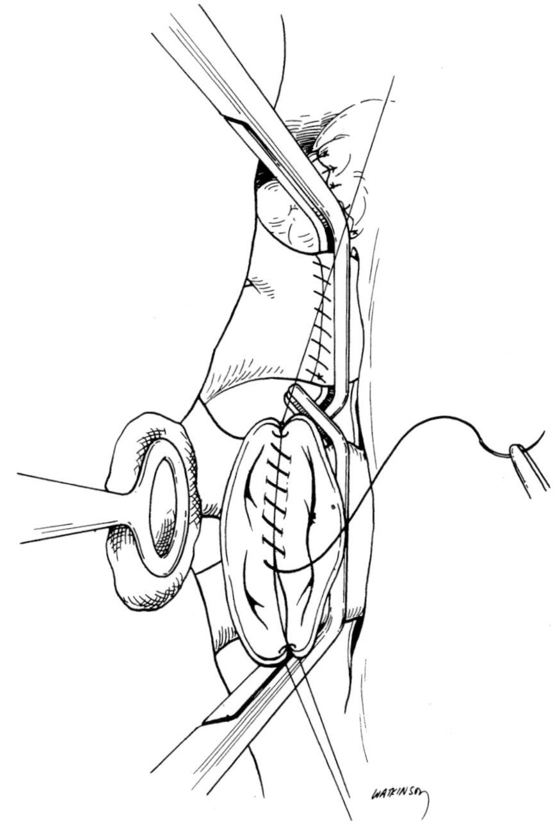

FIGURE 37–8 ■ A central left atrial clamp is in place while the vein stumps are amputated and the bridge of atrial muscle is divided. The 4–0 polypropylene suture is used to complete the anastomosis. (From Meyers BF: Technical aspects of adult lung transplantation. Semin Thorac Cardiovasc Surg 10:213, 1998.)

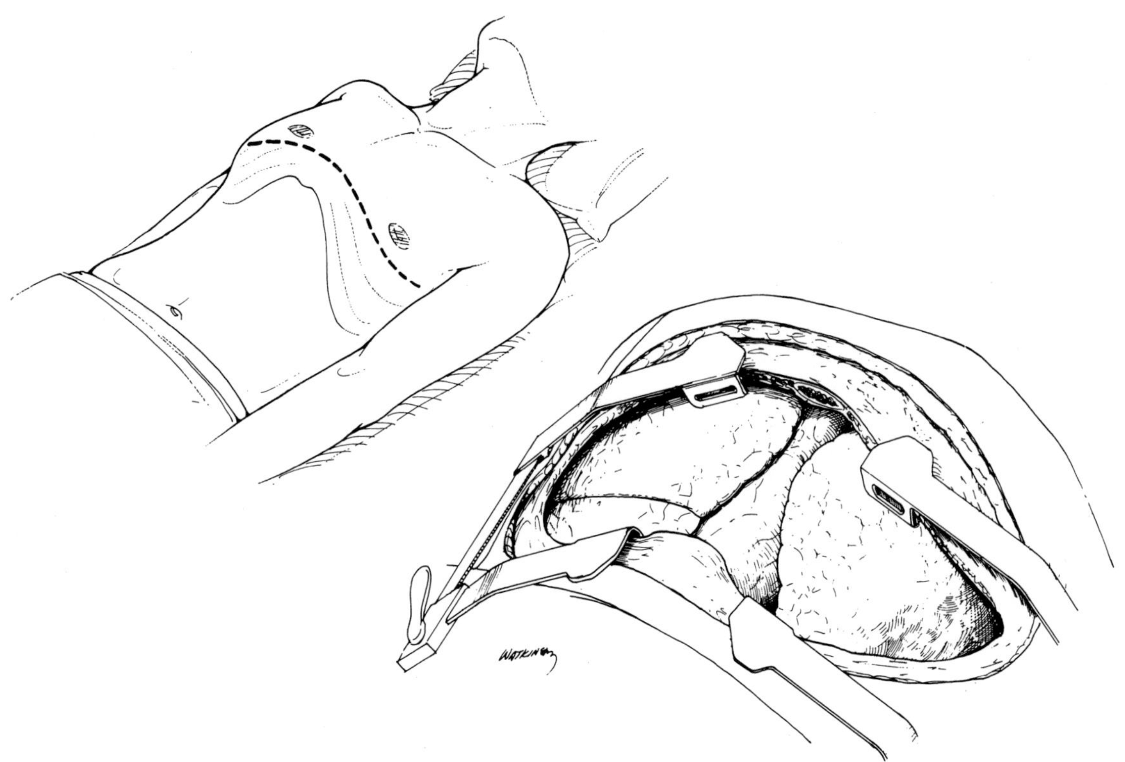

FIGURE 37–9 ■ Bilateral anterolateral thoracotomies are performed through the fourth or fifth interspace with transverse division of the sternum. (From Shields TW: General Thoracic Surgery. Philadelphia, Lea & Febiger, 1994.)

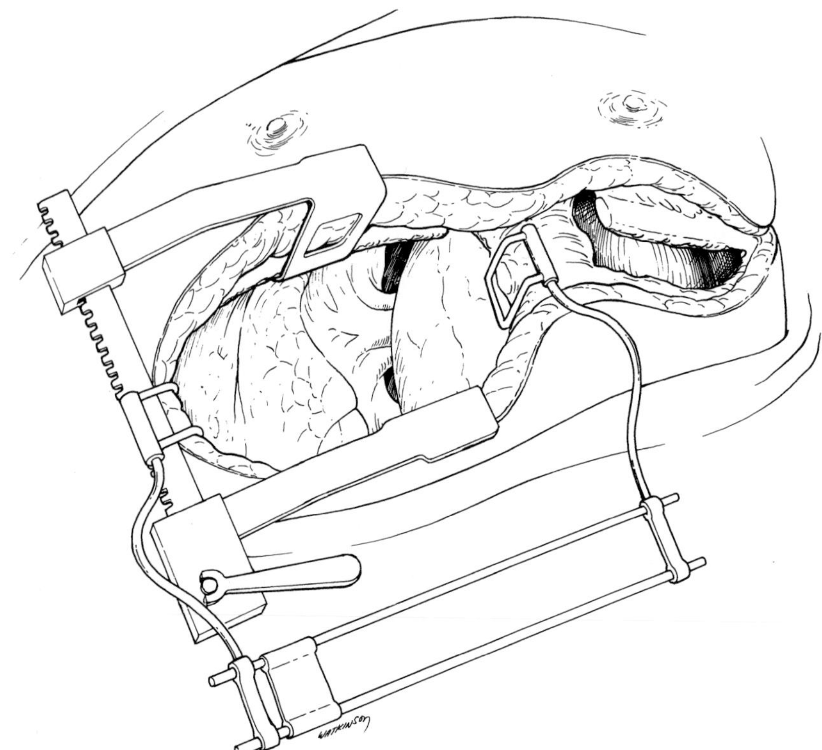

FIGURE 37–10 ■ A chest retractor is used to spread the ribs vertically while a Balfour retractor is used to open the muscle and skin of the lateral chest wall laterally. The combined use of these two retractors results in excellent exposure without sternal division. (From Meyers BF: Technical aspects of adult lung transplantation. Semin Thorac Cardiovasc Surg 10:213, 1998.)

tates a prolonged period of postoperative mechanical ventilation for some patients. We do not hesitate to perform a tracheostomy because a tracheostomy improves patient comfort, facilitates mobilization, permits oral nutrition, and enhances the attitude of the ventilator-dependent patient.

Fluid Management

During the first few postoperative days, fluid management is facilitated by a determination of pulmonary capillary wedge pressure and daily weight. Despite careful management, most patients leave the operating room with a significant positive fluid balance. Diuretics are used aggressively during the early postoperative period. Recipients of single-lung transplants for PPH may develop hemodynamic instability if their right heart filling pressures are excessively reduced.

Sepsis Prophylaxis

Bacterial

All patients are given routine antibacterial prophylaxis with cefepime and vancomycin for several days. If indicated by cultures of bronchial secretions from the donor or recipient, adjustments in these antibiotics are made. In the cystic fibrosis population, aerosolized colistin or tobramycin are also used. These patients also require specific antipseudomonal coverage, as dictated by the sensitivities of their preoperative sputum cultures.

Viral

Herpes simplex was formerly a frequent cause of postoperative morbidity as a result of oral ulcerations and pneumonitis. Routine use of acyclovir prophylaxis has eliminated herpes infection as a frequent postoperative complication. CMV remains a significant problem in pulmonary transplant recipients. Most programs have adopted the strategy of matching seronegative donors with seronegative recipients whenever possible. The highest incidence of severe CMV infection occurs with donor-negative/recipient-positive transplants. In these patients, prophylaxis with intravenous ganciclovir is used routinely according to the following protocol: ganciclovir 5 mg/kg IV twice daily for weeks 2 through 8; once daily for weeks 9 through 12; and three times weekly for weeks 13 through 16.

There is a reasonable argument for using this prophylactic regimen in any circumstance in which either the donor or recipient is seropositive. Although CMV infection or disease is uncommon during prophylaxis, there is a high rate of CMV disease after cessation of prophylactic therapy, especially in the donor-negative recipient-positive combination.

Fungal

It has been our practice not to use routine fungal prophylaxis. However, in the circumstance in which a heavy growth yeast is identified in the donor's bronchial culture post-transplant, prophylactic ketoconazole or low-dose amphotericin B may be justified. There have been anecdotal reports of early systemic candidal septicemia in patients who received lungs from which bronchial cultures grew *Candida*.

Pneumocystis carinii

This parasite was formerly an occasional cause of postoperative pulmonary infection. However, routine use of co-trimoxazole prophylaxis has eliminated this as a significant pathogen. Alternative agents are used when an allergy to sulfa is present.

Immunosuppression

Essentially all clinical lung transplant programs rely on triple-agent immunosuppression, usually consisting of cyclosporine, azathioprine, and corticosteroid therapy. Recent additions to the list of commonly used immunosuppressants are tacrolimus and mycophenolate mofetil, which are now used in more than 20% of lung recipients. In a detailed review by Briffa and Morris (1997), novel approaches to routine immunosuppression and responses to persistent rejection are discussed.

Azathioprine 1.5 mg/kg IV is administered immediately preoperatively. Our clinical program typically withholds early cyclosporine in an attempt to avoid intravenous delivery. This mode of administration often induces a significant increase in serum creatinine, thus necessitating a reduction in the cyclosporine dose. As an alternative, when an oral diet is initiated, oral cyclosporine can be started with twice-daily doses, as determined by the whole blood level. Azathioprine is continued at a dose of 1 to 2 mg/kg IV, and when an oral diet is initiated, the same dose can be administered orally. The dose must be adjusted to maintain a white blood cell count in excess of 3500/dl.

The early use of perioperative corticosteroids is controversial. Some suspect that early steroids contribute to bronchial complications wheras others claim that omission of steroids increases the likelihood of early rejection. We have demonstrated (Miller et al, 1993) that withholding the initial 2 weeks of prednisone has no effect on either bronchial healing or the incidence of acute rejection. As a result, methylprednisolone 10 to 15 mg/kg IV is given intraoperatively just prior to graft perfusion. Most programs have adopted the use of moderate-dose corticosteroid therapy (methylprednisolone 0.5 to 1 mg/kg/day IV) for several days before initiating an oral dose of prednisone of 0.5 mg/kg/day.

A matter of considerable controversy is the use of postoperative cytolytic therapy (antithymocyte globulin or OKT3). These cytolytic agents are in use in a number of programs. The Pittsburgh group reported a reduced incidence of acute rejection in patients who received rabbit antithymocyte globulin (Griffith et al, 1992). We use ATGAM (Upjohn, Kalamazoo, MI). It has been argued that these agents, particularly OKT3, predisposed patients to a higher incidence of CMV infection. However, these observations were made at a time when CMV matching was not widely practiced and CMV prophylaxis was not used. It is probable that the early use of cytolytic therapy does reduce the frequency and severity of early postoperative rejection episodes. These assertions are supported with the experience of Wain and colleagues (1999), who noted decreased acute rejection and an acceptable rate of CMV infections using routine OKT3 induction with gancyclovir prophylaxis.

For most patients, chronic immunosuppression consists of cyclosporine, prednisone, and azathioprine. After the first month post-transplant, the doses of cyclosporine are reduced to maintain blood levels in the range of 250 to 300 ng/ml. Prednisone is also reduced to minimize the well-known complications of long-term steroid use.

Infection and Rejection Surveillance

Acute rejection following lung transplantation is expected. Ninety-seven percent of recipients in our program have been treated for acute rejection on at least one occasion during the first 3 postoperative weeks. Early acute rejection episodes are characterized by dyspnea, low-grade fever, moderate leukocytosis, hypoxemia, and a diffuse perihilar interstitial infiltrate on the chest radiograph. This clinical picture most typically occurs around the fifth to seventh post-transplant day. All these clinical features are also consistent with infection. Clinical examination, radiographic assessment, and fiberoptic bronchoscopy are valuable tools in resolving the frequent dilemma of infection versus rejection in lung transplant recipients (Trulock, 1993). During the early years of our experience, if early acute rejection was suspected, our usual strategy was to administer a trial bolus dose of 500 to 1000 mg of methylprednisolone and to observe the clinical response. If rejection was truly the problem, a dramatic improvement in clinical findings, radiographic appearance (Fig. 37–11), and PaO_2 was observed within 8 to 12 hours. In that case, the patient received two additional daily intravenous bolus doses of methylprednisolone, and the event was recorded as an episode of acute rejection. If improvement did not occur, other causes were sought to explain the clinical findings.

The current approach to the same problem is to perform routine fiberoptic bronchoscopy whenever there is a clinical lung dysfunction in the absence of a recently identified but untreated infection. The advantage of routine flexible bronchoscopy is that it enables the performance of bronchoalveolar lavage and transbronchial biopsy. Although bronchoalveolar lavage has not been useful in the diagnosis of rejection, it is invaluable in the identification of opportunistic infections that are commonly encountered in transplant recipients. Transbronchial biopsy is the procedure of choice in the diagnosis of pulmonary rejection. We have used this modality frequently in patients with unexplained pulmonary infiltrates that are not responsive to corticosteroid therapy. Transbronchial biopsy is a highly sensitive and specific diagnostic tool for the evaluation of acute rejection. Routine bronchoalveolar lavage and transbronchial biopsies are performed at 3 weeks; at 3, 6, 9, and 12 months; and annually thereafter.

COMPLICATIONS

Technical Error

Many technical complications may be encountered during the postoperative period. Formerly, hemorrhage was a frequent complication. In the early experience of some programs that involved heart-lung and en bloc double-lung transplants, approximately 25% of patients required reoperation for postoperative hemorrhage. However, with surgical techniques such as the posterolateral thoracotomy for single-lung transplantation and the clamshell incision for bilateral lung replacement, surgical exposure is superb. In addition, aprotinin has dramatically reduced intraoperative and postoperative bleeding, especially in

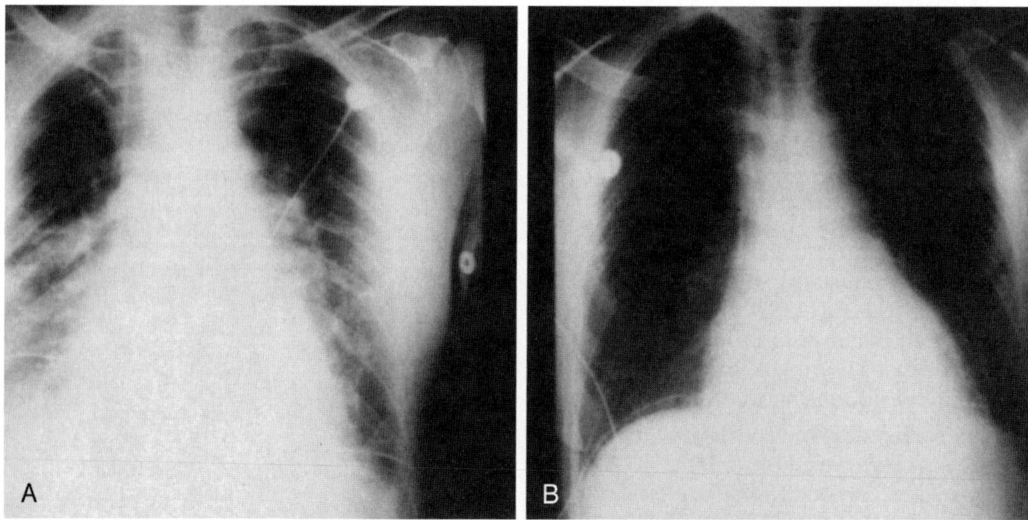

FIGURE 37–11 ■ Posteroanterior chest radiographs from a patient 7 days following bilateral sequential single-lung transplantation. *A*, On the morning of the seventh postoperative days, the radiograph shows a bilateral diffuse infiltrate. A clinical diagnosis of rejection was made, and the patient received methylprednisolone 1 g IV bolus. *B*, A radiograph taken 8 hours later demonstrates a dramatic improvement in the infiltrate, which is consistent with the typical response of acute rejection to steroid bolus therapy. (From Shields TW: General Thoracic Surgery. Philadelphia, Lea & Febiger, 1994.)

patients with extensive pleural adhesions that necessitate cardiopulmonary bypass.

Anastomotic complications can also occur and result in postoperative graft dysfunction. The University of Pittsburgh group (Griffith et al, 1994) reported their experience with anastomotic complications following lung transplantation and made a number of important technical points. An unsatisfactory bronchial anastomosis is routinely identified in the operating room during the postimplantation bronchoscopy. Inadequate anastomotic caliber dictates an immediate surgical revision.

Persistent pulmonary hypertension and unexplained hypoxemia can occur as a result of stenosis at the pulmonary artery anastomosis. This problem may be detected by a nuclear perfusion scan, which will demonstrate the unsatisfactory flow to a single-lung graft or unequal distribution of flow in a bilateral-lung recipient. Occasionally, a stenotic anastomosis can be visualized by transesophageal echocardiography. However, contrast angiography should be performed in any patient in whom there is a concern. At the time of angiography, the pressure gradient across the pulmonary artery anastomosis should be determined. A gradient of 15 to 20 mm Hg is commonly encountered, especially in single-lung recipients in whom most of the cardiac output is directed to the transplanted lung or in bilateral recipients with a high cardiac output. The need for anastomotic revision is dictated by the clinical situation.

Compromise in flow across the atrial anastomosis can also occur as a result of unsatisfactory anastomotic technique. Compression of the anastomosis by a clot or an omental or pericardial flap brought anterior or posterior to the atrial anastomosis for purposes of bronchial anastomotic coverage can also impair ipsilateral pulmonary venous drainage. Impaired venous outflow results in elevated venous pressure and ipsilateral pulmonary edema. Pulmonary artery pressures remain unexpectedly high, and flow through the graft is less than expected. Transesophageal echocardiography can image the atrial anastomosis clearly. Contrast studies may be helpful in demonstrating reduced flow through the anastomosis. Open exploration is occasionally necessary to confirm the diagnosis and conduct an appropriate repair.

Early Graft Dysfunction

Approximately 20% of patients have severe early graft dysfunction (Haydock et al, 1992). This problem may arise as a result of pathologic conditions in the donor lung, such as aspiration, infection, or contusion. Inadequate preservation can occur as a result of technical difficulties at the time of harvest or prolonged warm ischemia during implantation. It is imperative to exclude remedial technical problems. Most commonly, allograft dysfunction occurs unexpectedly in the absence of an obvious cause (Fig. 37–12). The development of immediate postoperative florid pulmonary edema, severe hypoxemia, persistent pulmonary hypertension, and reduced pulmonary compliance can present a formidable management problem.

These patients generally can be managed with aggressive intensive care unit (ICU) ventilatory and pharmacologic intervention. High levels of PEEP and vigorous diuresis are important strategies. However, severe graft dysfunction or coexisting cardiac failure may require extracorporeal membrane oxygenation (ECMO) support. In our experience with 450 lung transplant recipients, only 12 have required ECMO support (arteriovenous) during the immediate postoperative phase. Seven of these 12 patients survived and were discharged from the hospital (Meyers, 2000). In most patients, early allograft dysfunction (and other forms of diffuse alveolar damage) resolves over several days of ICU support, and patients obtain satisfactory long-term allograft function (Haydock et al, 1992).

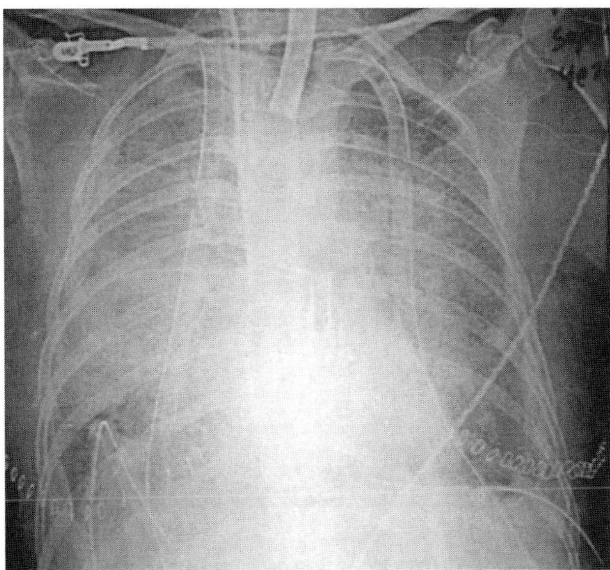

FIGURE 37–12 ■ An anteroposterior chest radiograph taken immediately postoperatively in a patient who underwent bilateral sequential single-lung transplant. Despite satisfactory lung harvest, acceptable ischemic time (*right*, 4.5 hours; *left*, 6 hours), and only 3 hours of cardiopulmonary bypass time, severe allograft dysfunction occurred. All anastomoses were intact. A quantative perfusion scan revealed 40% flow to the right lung and 60% to the left. The patient was euvolemic and recovered from this severe lung injury over a period of 7 days.

Infection

Bacterial

Bacterial pneumonia is the most commonly encountered infection after lung transplantation. An aggressive approach is taken to identify the specific organism. Fiberoptic bronchoscopy with a protected brush should be undertaken if routine sputum cultures do not provide an identifiable organism. Routine intravenous antibiotic therapy is used, and, in most patients, the pneumonia rapidly clears. Patients with cystic fibrosis present a management dilemma during the postoperative period because they are susceptible to recurrent post-transplant pulmonary infections from the same *Pseudomonas* organisms that are harbored in the airway and the paranasal sinuses. This is particularly true of patients with highly resistent *Pseudomonas cepacia* (Snell et al, 1993).

Lung abscess is occasionally encountered in lung transplant recipients. Patients with cystic fibrosis occasionally develop multifocal lung abscesses, presumably as a result of inhaled contamination from an upper airway or sinus infection. In single-lung recipients, the native lung is also susceptible to bacterial infection, which on occasion can cavitate and produce a lung abscess. These patients should be managed as any other patient with a lung abscess. Appropriate broad-spectrum antibiotic therapy is administered, and bronchoscopy is performed to ensure that no airway obstruction is present. Occasionally, external drainage is required (Fig. 37–13).

Viral

Viral pneumonitis can occur during the postoperative period. During the early postoperative phase, herpes simplex infection was encountered frequently. However, with the routine use of acyclovir, it is now an unusual complication. CMV infection is more commonly encountered when the donor, recipient, or both are CMV seropositive. Our experience at Washington University showed that 92% of patients developed CMV infection, with 75% of them having biopsy-proved CMV pneumonitis (Ettinger et al, 1993). A donor-negative recipient-positive combination resulted in more frequent and severe infections. No donor-negative recipient-negative patient developed an infection or disease. Biopsy-proved CMV pneumonitis was associated with radiographic infiltrate in less than 30% of cases. The detection of CMV in bronchoalveolar lavage was not always predictive of CMV pneumonitis. The high incidence of CMV infection and disease in our experience reflects the aggressive viral surveillance that is used in our program.

We do not treat CMV infection without biopsy proof of CMV disease. In this circumstance, ganciclovir 5 mg/kg IV is administered twice daily for 2 to 3 weeks. In severe pneumonitis, CMV hyperimmune globulin is also administered. Most patients respond promptly to this regimen.

Fungal

The most frequent cause of significant fungal infection post-transplant is *Aspergillus*. Unfortunately, once *Asper-*

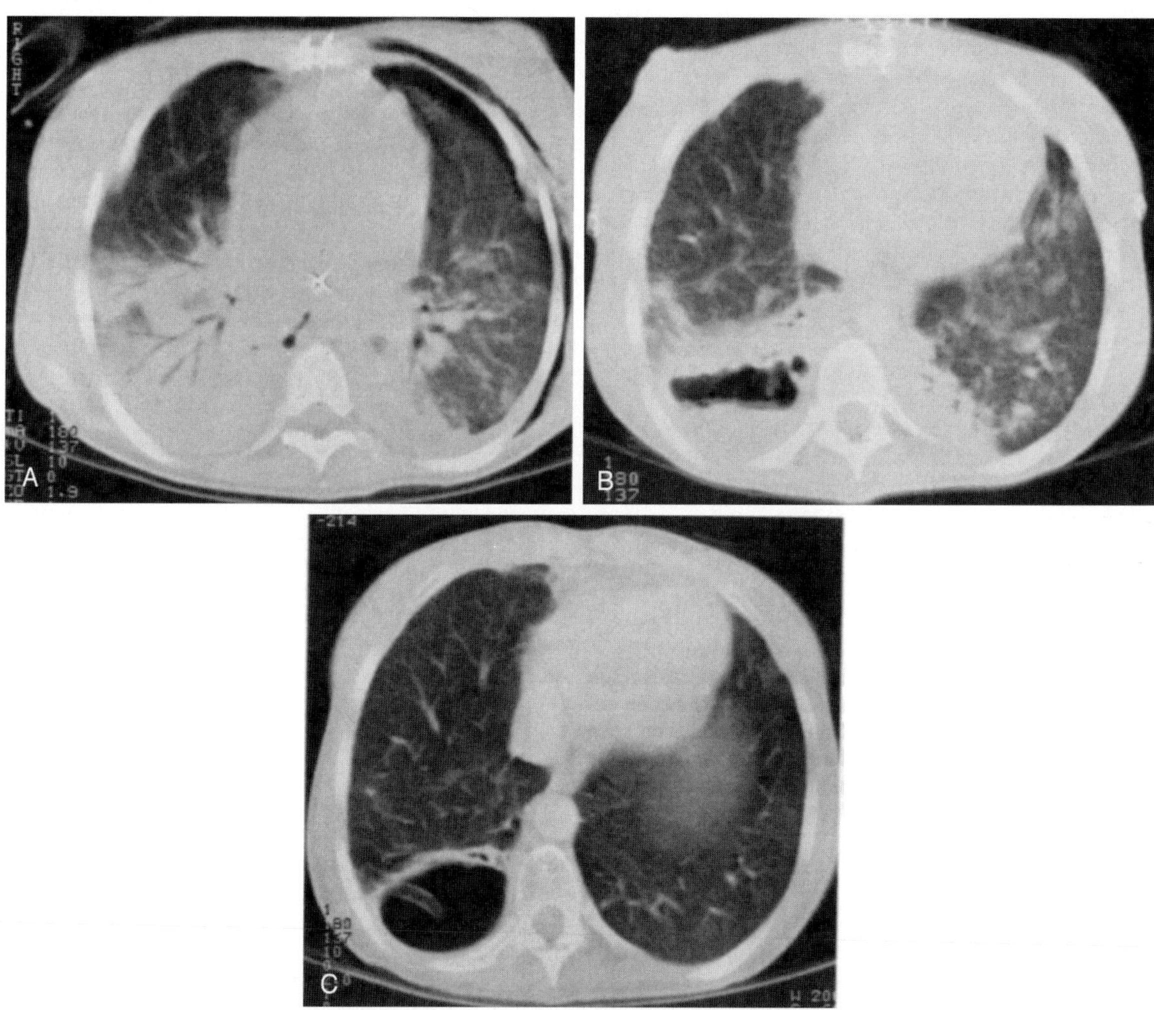

FIGURE 37–13 ■ *A*, Ten days following bilateral sequential single-lung transplantation for cystic fibrosis. The patient was noted to have a right lower lobe pneumonia and an incidental contralateral left pneumothorax with subcutaneous emphysema. *B*, During the ensuing week, the right lower lobe pneumonia cavitated. An obvious air-fluid level was visible. *C*, Satisfactory drainage was achieved with tube thoracostomy while the patient was convalescent. An elective rib resection was performed several months postoperatively.

gillus has become a resident organism, it is difficult to clear. In patients without evidence of active invasive infection, we have administered ketoconazole with reasonable success. However, in patients whose infections do not clear with ketoconazole or who have developed an invasive infection, amphotericin B is required. Invasive *Aspergillus* infection usually is fatal.

A particularly interesting group of patients are those who have had single-lung transplants for pulmonary fibrosis and who develop *Aspergillus* infection in the diseased native lung. These patients should be treated aggressively, with the expectation that the *Aspergillus* will probably not clear from the native lung. In this circumstance, contralateral native lung pneumonectomy is warranted.

Pleural Space Complications

Pleural space complications occur frequently following pulmonary transplantation. Pneumothorax is encountered in two circumstances. It can occur as a result of airway dehiscence with communication into the pleural space (Fig. 37–14). However, this is not a frequent occurrence, and, when present, it is usually readily managed by intercostal tube drainage with appropriate re-expansion of the underlying lung. A more common circumstance is the development of insignificant pneumothoraces in patients with obstructive pulmonary disease, either emphysema or cystic fibrosis, who have undergone bilateral replacement and received lungs that are much smaller than the pleural space into which they were implanted. Often a minimal degree of bilateral pneumothorax occurs subsequent to chest tube replacement. In general, these pneumothoraces can be ignored, the pleural air will eventually resorb, and any remaining space will fill with fluid.

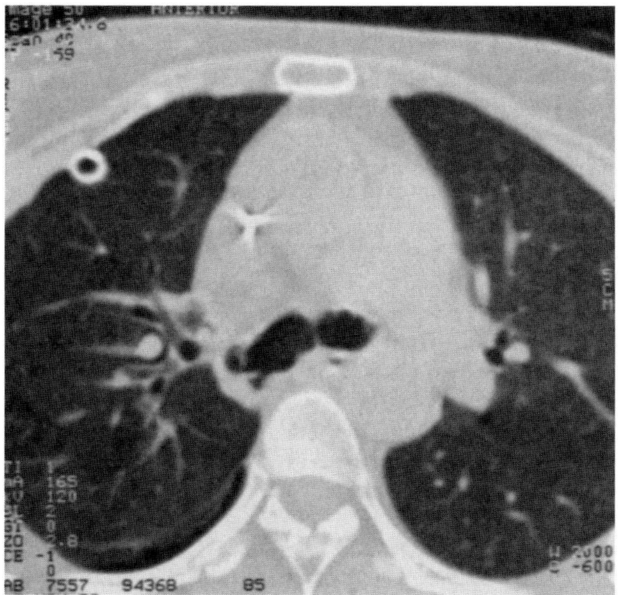

FIGURE 37–14 ■ In a patient receiving bilateral sequential lung allografts for obstructive pulmonary disease, a small right main bronchial dehiscence developed. The dehiscence can be clearly seen in this computed tomography image, and there is a small pneumothorax. The anterior chest tube maintained satisfactory expansion of the lung until the membranous wall healed completely and the air leak ceased.

Pleural effusions are commonly encountered, particularly in the group just noted in whom the pulmonary volume is somewhat smaller than the pleural space. A sympathetic effusion may occur in association with an underlying pulmonary infection or rejection. As with other effusions, these generally clear with appropriate therapy of the underlying parenchymal condition.

Empyema is infrequently encountered in lung transplant recipients. Spontaneous development of an empyema is rare. More commonly, an empyema develops following any prolonged air leak as a result of the open lung biopsy performed on a patient receiving high-dose corticosteroids. Persistent air leak, failure to achieve re-expansion of the lung, and subsequent pleurodesis result in a chronic pleural space that will eventually become infected. A number of these patients have been treated by open drainage, by rib resection, or by a formal creation of a Clagett window or Eloesser flap. An empyema rarely occurs as a result of bronchial dehiscence in communication with the pleural space. In most of these patients, satisfactory intercostal tube drainage with re-expansion of the underlying lung results in satisfactory anastomotic healing and the absence of any significant pleural space infection.

Airway Complications

Airway complications were formerly a major cause of morbidity and mortality following pulmonary transplantation. Using standard methods of implantation, the donor bronchus is rendered ischemic, without reconstitution of its systemic bronchial artery circulation. The donor bronchus thereby relies on collateral pulmonary flow during the first few days following transplantation. It has been demonstrated that pulmonary collateral flow makes a substantial contribution to the viability of the distal main bronchus and lobar bronchi. A shortened donor bronchial length—two rings proximal to the upper lobe takeoff—reduces the length of donor bronchus at risk for ischemia. In addition, improved techniques of preservation have resulted in increased bronchial viability following transplantation. Post-transplant pulmonary parenchymal pathologic change also results in decreased collateral flow that leaves the ischemic donor bronchus at increased risk for necrosis and subsequent dehiscence. The role of perioperative steroids is important in this regard. Davreux and associates (1993) reported our work showing that epithelial regeneration and revascularization of rat heterotopic tracheal allografts are improved by postoperative corticosteroid administration. In addition, Inui and coworkers (1993) of the Hanover group demonstrated that postoperative corticosteroid therapy improves retrograde bronchial blood flow in porcine lung allografts. Superior preservation, improved sepsis prophylaxis, and immunosuppression have reduced the incidence of airway complication. In a review of our experience, Date and colleagues (1995) reported a reduction of the prevalence of anastomotic complications from 14% to 4% of anastomoses at risk. Airway complications resulted in 6 of the 37 postoperative deaths reported in our first 450 lung transplants. The deaths related to anastomotic complications occurred in patients with tracheal anastomoses who underwent the now-abandoned single-airway anastomosis (Meyers et al, 1999).

Airway complications are identified in a number of ways. Routine postoperative bronchoscopic surveillance generally provides early detection of anastomotic complications. On occasion, a CT scan performed for some other indication demonstrates an unexpected airway stenosis or dehiscence. We have learned that the CT scan is a useful diagnostic tool in the evaluation of documented or suspected donor airway complications. Late airway stenoses generally cause symptoms of dyspnea, wheezing, or a decreased FEV_1. Bronchoscopic assessment confirms the diagnosis.

Most airway complications are identified in the first weeks or months following transplantation. A normal bronchial anastomotic suture line demonstrates a narrow rim of epithelial sloughing, which ultimately heals. On occasion, patchy areas of superficial necrosis of the donor bronchial epithelium are observed. These are also of no concern and ultimately heal without incident. Minor degrees of bronchial dehiscence are also of little long-term consequence. Membranous wall defects generally heal without any airway compromise, whereas cartilaginous defects usually result in some degree of late stricture. Significant dehiscence (greater than 50% of the circumference) may result in compromise of the airway. This problem should be managed expectantly by gentle mechanical débridement of the area to maintain satisfactory airway patency. Surgeons who use a laser in an attempt to maintain airway caliber can injure the normal distal donor airway that must be preserved for the subsequent placement of a stent. Occasionally, a significant dehiscence results in direct communication with the pleural space (see Fig. 37–14) or pericardium. However, if the lung remains completely expanded, and the pleural space is evacuated, the leak ultimately seals, and the airway usually heals without stenosis. A dehiscence may communicate directly with the mediastinum and result in mediastinal emphysema. If the lung remains completely expanded and the pleural space is filled, adequate drainage of the mediastinum can be achieved by mediastinoscopy, placing a drain in close proximity to the anastomotic line. This also results in satisfactory healing of the anastomosis, often without stricture.

Surgical revision of the anastomosis is only possible if an adequate length of donor airway is available for resuturing. This type of reconstruction has been successfully performed (Kirk et al, 1990). However, it is rarely possible if the donor bronchus was cut to an appropriate short length at the time of the initial procedure. Massive dehiscence of the airway with uncontrolled leak or mediastinal contamination has been treated by a successful retransplantation in a number of programs.

Chronic airway stenoses can present significant management problems. A right main bronchial anastomotic stricture is generally easily managed by repeated dilatation and ultimate placement of an endobronchial stent. The right main bronchus is easily dilated, and there is generally room for the placement of a right main bronchial orifice stent without impingement of the right upper lobe bronchus.

However, on the left side, strictures can be somewhat more difficult to manage. Dilatation of the distal left main bronchus is technically more difficult because of its angulation. In addition, the lobar bifurcation immediately distal to the usual site of anastomosis does not provide a suitable length of bronchus distal to the stricture for the placement of large-caliber dilating bronchoscopes. Finally, a stent placed across a distal left main bronchial anastomotic stricture may occlude the upper or lower lobe orifice as it bridges the stricture.

We have used Silastic endobronchial stents preferentially. Straight bronchial stents have been used for main bronchial strictures. Y stents have been used for the occasional tracheal stricture that is seen following heart-lung transplantation or more commonly following en bloc double-lung transplantation with tracheal anastomosis. We previously described the technique of insertion (Cooper et al, 1989). Wire-mesh stents can only be used for malacic strictures that are completely lined by epithelium. If a wire stent is placed in a granulating stricture, the wires become embedded by granulation, and a stricture develops within the stent.

Silastic stents are tolerated exceptionally well. However, patients may require daily inhalation of *N*-acetyl cystine to keep the stents patent. Stents have resulted in dramatic improvements in pulmonary function (DeHoyos and Maurer, 1992). Fortunately, most of these stents have been required only temporarily. After several months, most patients are able to maintain satisfactory airway patency without the stent. The advantage of a silastic stent is seen at the time of removal because it is well tolerated without the development of granulation tissue or mucosal overgrowth that is seen with wire mesh stents. Even the coated wire stents have uncoated regions at the ends that offer interstices for the ingrowth of tissue.

Finally, distal bronchial strictures on occasion can be unmanageable by dilatation or stent insertion. In these patients, retransplantation is an option and has been used successfully (Novick et al, 1993).

Rejection

Immunologic matching is crude (ABO blood group only) and immunosuppression strategies are imperfect; therefore, it is not surprising that rejection is a troublesome problem following lung transplantation. Acute rejection is encountered during the early postoperative period in almost all patients (Cooper et al, 1994). This rarely presents a significant clinical problem. However, chronic rejection is the most common underlying cause of late death following lung transplantation. This is a particularly vexing problem because the pathogenesis is poorly understood, and there is no effective means of therapy.

Acute rejection has a typical clinical presentation of dyspnea, low-grade fever, perihilar interstitial infiltrate, hypoxia, and increased white blood cell count. Typically, the first episode occurs within the first 5 to 7 postoperative days. Several episodes during the first 2 months are not unusual. In the early years of lung transplantation, the diagnosis was confirmed by an abrupt favorable re-

WORKING FORMULATION FOR CLASSIFICATION AND GRADING OF PULMONARY REJECTION

A. Acute rejection
   0. Grade 0—no significant abnormality
   1. Grade 1—minimal acute rejection*
   2. Grade 2—mild acute rejection*
   3. Grade 3—moderate acute rejection*
   4. Grade 4—severe acute rejection*
B. Active airway damage without scarring
   1. Lymphocytic bronchitis
   2. Lymphocytic bronchiolitis
C. Chronic airway rejection
   1. Bronchiolitis obliterans, subtotal
      a. Active
      b. Inactive
   2. Bronchiolitis obliterans, total
      a. Active
      b. Inactive
D. Chronic vascular rejection
E. Vasculitis

*Grades 1 to 4 are subdivided according to bronchial inflammation: (a) with evidence of bronchiolar inflammation; (b) without evidence of bronchiolar inflammation; (c) with large airway inflammation; (d) no bronchioles are present.

sponse to a bolus dose of methylprednisolone (500 mg to 1 g). Subsequently, the clinical parameters noted above are the most commonly used indicators of rejection. Intensive laboratory investigation continues in a number of centers to find noninvasive techniques to diagnose rejection. The level of nitric oxide in the exhaled gas from a lung transplant recipient has been studied with some promise for early identification of rejection (Fisher et al, 1998). Nuclear scanning has little value. Various immunologic tests have also been advocated. The Pittsburgh group had initial enthusiasm for a primed lymphocyte test, which we have not found useful. We have demonstrated increased cytotoxicity of bronchoalveolar lavage lymphocytes in patients with biopsy-proved rejection, and there is mounting evidence that cytokines are important mediators in the development of rejection. The manipulation of cytokine expression may be therapeutically important, although it currently has little clinical utility.

The technique of choice in the diagnosis of rejection is transbronchial biopsy that is performed under fluoroscopic control. The Papworth group (Higenbottam et al, 1988) deserves credit for demonstrating the safety and value of this technique in the lung transplantation population. The typical histologic appearance is that of perivascular lymphocytic infiltrate (Fig. 37–15). The internationally accepted classification for pulmonary rejection was reported by Yousem and colleagues (1990; 1996).

The factors that predispose patients to an increased incidence of rejection are unclear. There is experimental evidence that poorly preserved allografts are more likely to suffer subsequent rejection. There is some evidence that expression of major histocompatibility complex class II antigens on bronchial epithelium and pulmonary capillary endothelium is increased following extended periods of preservation. In addition, we demonstrated increased expression of the adhesion molecule ICAM following extended preservation of human lung allografts (Hasegawa et al, 1995). Infection may also predispose to subsequent rejection. A number of groups have reported serious rejection episodes following established bacterial or viral infection.

Acute rejection can be effectively controlled in most patients, irrespective of its cause. Most patients respond promptly to the first course of methylprednisolone. Occasionally, a second course of steroid may be necessary to bring a serious rejection episode under control. Persistent rejection despite this intervention is distinctly unusual. In this circumstance, cytolytic therapy with ATGAM or OKT3 should be considered. Recent evidence suggests that alternative immunosuppressants, such as FK506, may be useful in this situation. There is increasing experimental (Hirai et al, 1993) and clinical evidence that FK506 may offer advantages over cyclosporine as a first-line agent.

It seems intuitive that early rejection increases the likelihood of subsequent chronic rejection and allograft dysfunction. Our experience, however, demonstrates no relationship between the number of early clinical acute rejection episodes and subsequent graft function (Cooper et al, 1994). On the other hand, the Pittsburgh group (Bando et al, 1995a) did show a clear relationship between the frequency and severity of biopsy-proved acute rejection and the subsequent development of chronic rejection.

While acute rejection is commonly manageable, chronic rejection remains a major problem with severe consequences. The clinical presentation of chronic rejection is a progressive fall in FEV_1. This decline actually precedes the clinical symptoms of dyspnea. Chest radiographs and computed tomography scans may be normal despite advanced chronic rejection, but they should be performed to rule out other correctable causes of a decreasing FEV_1. Bronchoscopy is necessary to ensure that there is no bronchial anastomotic compromise. Pulmonary function studies reveal obstructive physiologic find-

BRONCHIOLITIS OBLITERANS SYNDROME SCORING SYSTEM

0 No significant abnormality: FEV_1 80% of baseline value
1 Mild obliterative bronchiolitis syndrome: FEV_1 66% to 80% of baseline value
2 Moderate obliterative bronchiolitis syndrome: FEV_1 51% to 65% of baseline value
3 Severe obliterative bronchiolitis syndrome: FEV_1 50% or less of baseline value

Grades 0 to 3 are subdivided into category A, without pathologic evidence of obliterative bronchiolitis, or category B, with pathologic evidence of obliterative bronchiolitis.

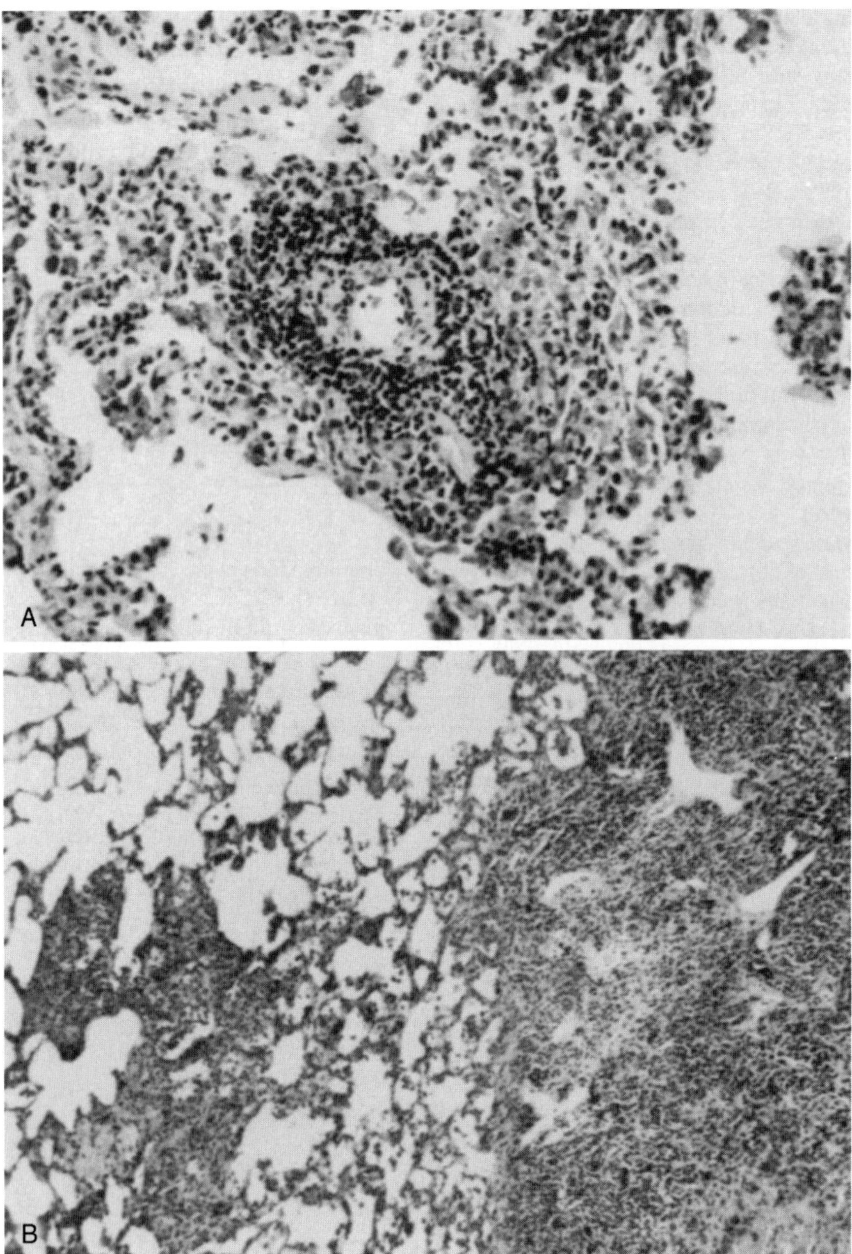

FIGURE 37–15 ■ *A,* A photomicrograph of a transbronchial biopsy specimen showing typical early (A1b) rejection. Isolated perivascular cuffs of lymphocytes are noted. *B,* A more severe degree of rejection is evident in this photomicrograph of a transbronchial biopsy specimen. There are perivascular and interstitial lymphoid infiltrates, which is consistent with grade 3 rejection (A3a). (From Shields TW: General Thoracic Surgery. Philadelphia, Lea & Febiger, 1994.)

ings. The pathologic hallmark of chronic rejection is obliterative bronchiolitis (Fig. 37–16). The term chronic rejection is often used interchangeably with BOS. This practice may cloud the fact that not all post-transplant obliterative bronchiolitis is immunologically mediated. Various other etiologic factors, including aspiration or chronic infection, may result in obliterative bronchiolitis. However, those conducting transplant programs have come to realize that more than 50% of recipients will develop post-transplant allograft dysfunction caused by obstructive physiologic conditions. This problem appears to be unrelated to the underlying disease or the type of transplant (Kroshus et al, 1997; Reichenspurner et al, 1995; Smith et al, 1998; Sundaresan et al, 1995).

A consensus conference sanctioned by the International Heart and Lung Transplant Society termed this chronic allograft dysfunction BOS (Cooper et al, 1993). This clinical terminology was used to reflect the importance of clinical findings (i.e., diminished FEV_1) in its diagnosis. Biopsy is not required to make a diagnosis of BOS. Furthermore, the scoring system noted earlier reflects the fact that patients can move from one score to another. Although most patients' conditions either stabilize or deteriorate, all programs have had patients with BOS who have improved (for whatever reason) with augmentation of immunosuppression (Cooper et al, 1993).

Unfortunately, therapeutic options for established BOS are limited. Standard therapy consists of augmentation of immunosuppression, either by high-dose corticosteroid or cytolytic therapy. On occasion, the obliterative bronchiolitis can be arrested to preserve pulmonary function at a stable, though diminished, level. Unfortunately, most

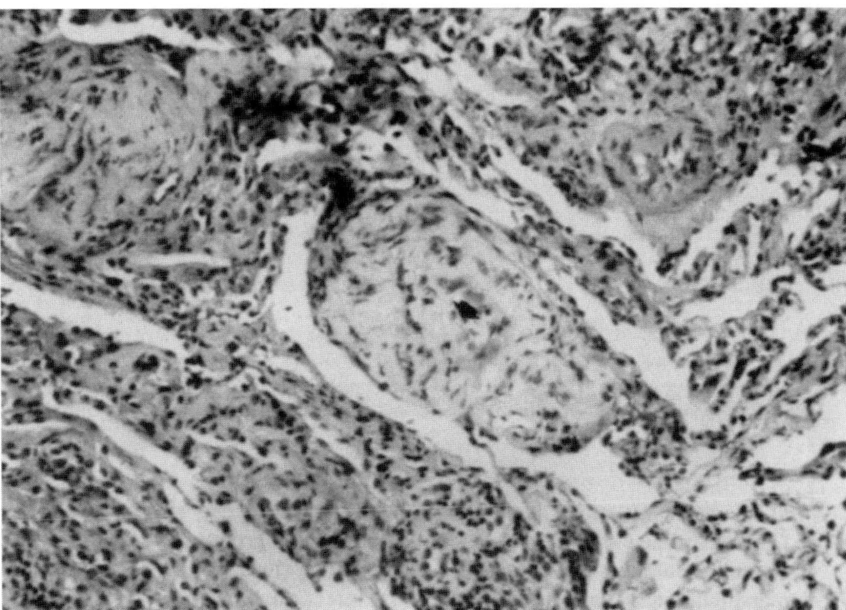

FIGURE 37–16 ■ This photomicrograph of a transbronchial biopsy specimen reveals the typical findings of a bronchiolitis obliterans, which is thought to be the result of chronic rejection. Mature fibrous obliteration of the bronchiolar lumen is evident *(arrow)*. (From Shields TW: General Thoracic Surgery. Philadelphia, Lea & Febiger, 1994.)

patients either develop progressive obliterative bronchiolitis or contract some lethal opportunistic infection as a result of the augmented immunosuppression.

Retransplantation has been offered to a large number of patients with BOS (Novick et al, 1998). However, in most such patients, the process reappears within a short period following retransplantation. Nonetheless, few patients have survived and obtained excellent long-term results following retransplantation for this devastating condition.

RESULTS

Operative Mortality

Improvements in selection, technique, and management have resulted in a dramatic reduction in the operative mortality rate. We recently reported an early mortality rate of only 8.4% in our cumulative experience with 450 single and bilateral transplants (Meyers et al, 1999). Our updated survival data are illustrated in Figure 37–17. The Toronto group experience was reported by De Hoyos and colleagues (1992). Operative mortality for single- and double-lung transplant was 13% and 21%, respectively. Other large programs have reported equally impressive results. Sweet and colleagues (1997) at Washington University have reported exciting results of lung transplantation in children. This group of patients represents a particular challenge, especially those with Eisenmenger's syndrome, in whom technically difficult operative procedures were undertaken with success.

Early mortality rates differ depending on the type of procedure or the underlying disease (Fig. 37–18). The current ISHLT data show that operative deaths comprise 17% of the total fatalities for patients with cystic fibrosis, 12% of the deaths for patients with idiopathic pulmonary

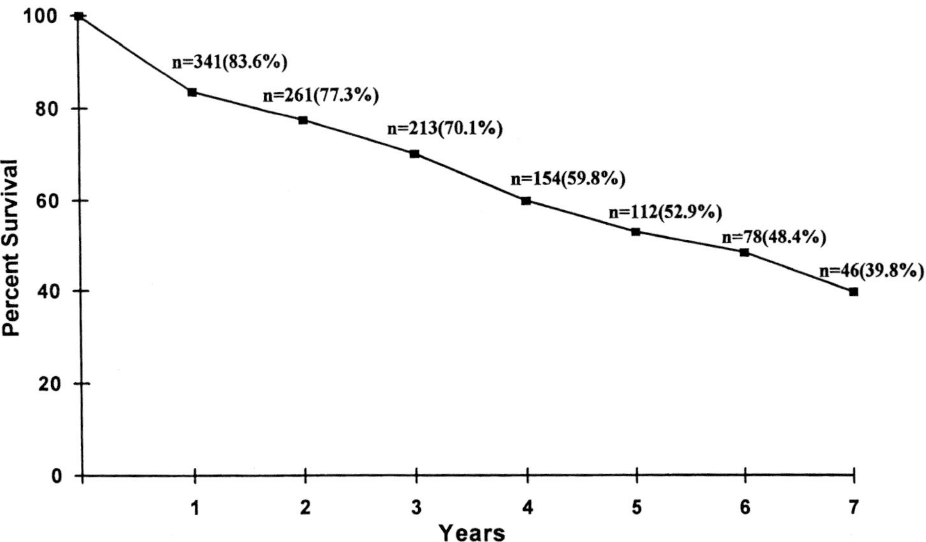

FIGURE 37–17 ■ Graph showing survival after lung transplantation performed on 443 recipients at the Washington University School of Medicine from July 1988 to November 1998. (From Meyers BF: Lung transplantation: A decade of experience. Ann Surg 230:362, 1999.)

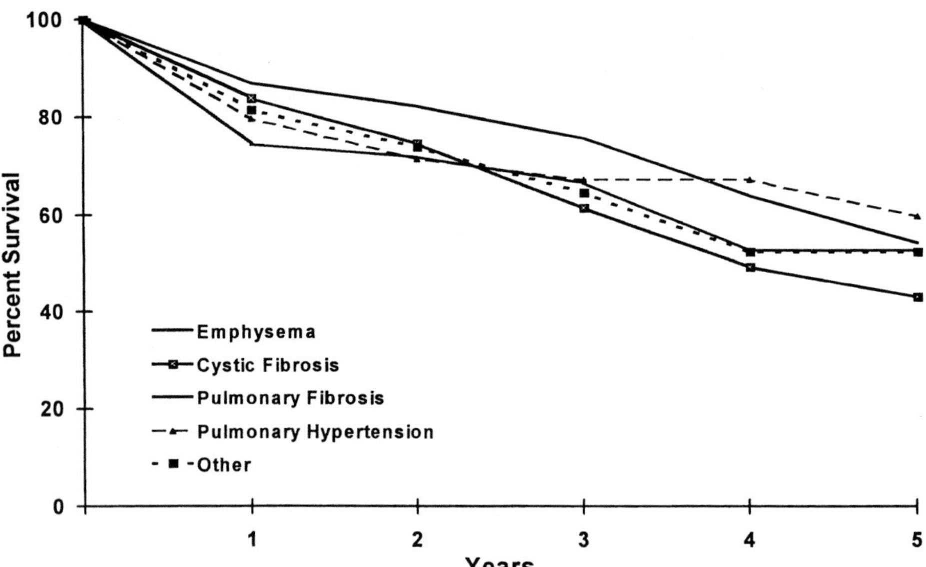

FIGURE 37–18 ■ Graph showing survival of lung transplantation recipients after 443 operations at the Washington University School of Medicine from July 1988 to November 1998. Survival was stratified according to the underlying diagnosis that led to transplant. (From Meyers BF, et al: Ann Surg 230:362, 1999.)

fibrosis, and only 5% of the deaths in patients with emphysema. In contrast, the rate of deaths caused by BOS or infection is comparable for the three groups (Hosenpud et al, 1998a). Bilateral procedures are associated with higher early operative mortality than are single-lung transplantations. This reflects an increase in technical difficulty and the increased risk of septic complications in the cystic fibrosis patients, who make up a large fraction of the bilateral transplant population. The Toronto group (Ramirez et al, 1992) reported a high incidence of postoperative death caused by sepsis. This was particularly frequent in those recipients who harbored highly resistant *P. cepacia* organisms. In our program, we have not found a difference in perioperative mortality rates among the disease categories for which single-lung transplants are undertaken. However, other groups have reported increased mortality rate in patients undergoing single-lung transplantation for PPH in comparison with those suffering from emphysema. This is likely a reflection of the difficulties of the postoperative course of patients with PVD.

Late Mortality

Numerous patients underwent pulmonary transplantation in the last decade of the 20th century. Increasing numbers of these patients have survived 6 to 8 years following lung transplantation (Chaparro et al, 1997; Meyers et al, 1999). Survival data from the ISHLT is shown in Figure 37–19. Considering that many of the programs reporting to the Registry have limited experience, the overall worldwide results are impressive and improving steadily. Causes of late death, as reported to the ISHLT, are shown in Figure 37–20. The ISHLT calculated a multivariate analysis of the risk factors contributing to early and late mortality after lung transplantation. The results are displayed in Table 37–1.

Functional Results

Among operative survivors, the functional results are excellent. Patients usually can return to normal levels of exercise tolerance without oxygen supplementation within 6 to 8 weeks of transplantation (Fig. 37–21).

Obstructive Pulmonary Disease

This is the most frequent indication for lung transplantation. Single- and bilateral-lung transplantations have been used with success. Gas exchange, pulmonary function, and exercise tolerance are dramatically improved, as illustrated in Figures 37–22 to 37–24. Single and bilateral recipients achieve satisfactory postoperative lung volumes. However, there is considerable controversy regarding the long-term functional advantages of bilateral versus single-lung transplants for this disease. Early functional assessment suggests minimal difference between the two procedures. However, bilateral lung replacement offers significant functional advantages long term. This may offset the increased operative risk of bilateral transplantation, especially in younger patients with emphysema (Bavaria et al, 1997; Sundaresan et al, 1996).

Septic Pulmonary Disease

A number of centers have reported satisfactory results with the application of bilateral lung transplantations in these patients. Ramirez and colleagues (1992) from Toronto reported excellent gas exchange, pulmonary function, and exercise capabilities among operative survivors. Our Washington University experience is similar (see Figs. 37–22 to 37–24). Dramatic improvement in chest contour was apparent (Fig. 37–25).

Fibrotic Pulmonary Disease

Whereas this condition was formerly the most frequent indication for pulmonary transplantation, it is now one

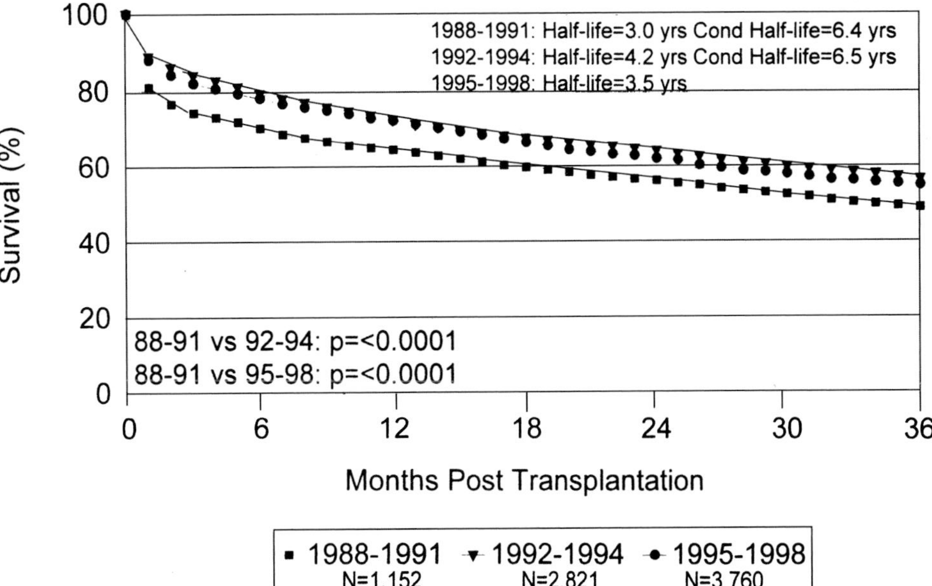

FIGURE 37–19 ■ Graph showing total lung transplant actuarial survival, stratified by era, as reported by the International Society of Heart and Lung Transplantation. (From Hosenpud JD, Bennett LE, Keck BM, et al: The Registry of the International Society for Heart and Lung Transplantation: Sixteenth Official Report, 1999. J Heart Lung Transplant 18:611, 1999.)

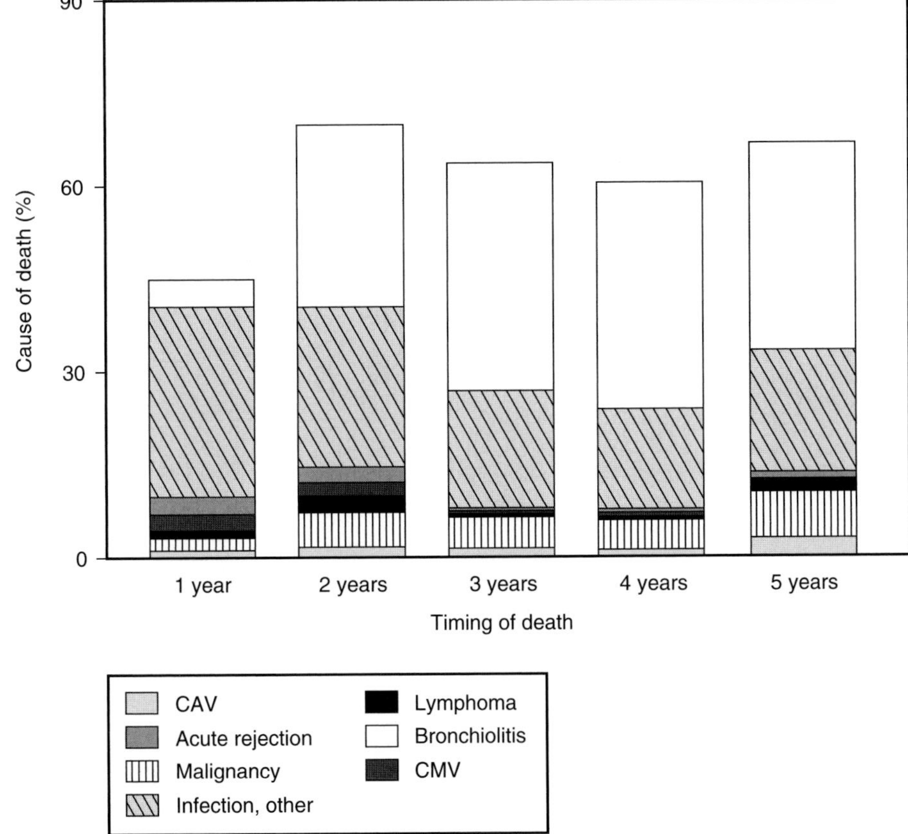

FIGURE 37–20 ■ A bar graph depicting the changes in cause of death over time following lung transplantation. (CAV, cardiac allograft vasculopathy; CMV, cytomegalovirus.) (From Hosenpud JD, Bennett LE, Keck BM, et al: The Registry of the International Society for Heart and Lung Transplantation: Sixteenth Official Report, 1999. J Heart Lung Transplant 18:611, 1999.)

TABLE 37–1 ■ Risk Factors for 1- and 5-Year Mortality After Adult Lung Transplantation According to The International Society of Heart and Lung Transplantation

	1 Year (n = 7086)			*5 Year (n = 2933)*		
Variable	*Odds Ratio*	*95% Confidence Interval*	*P-Value*	*Odds Ratio*	*95% Confidence Interval*	*P-Value*
Repeat TX	2.38	1.81–3.12	<.0001	2.41	1.55–3.75	<.0001
Ventilator	2.3	1.65–3.21	<.0001			
Diagnosis = congenital heart	2.15	1.53–3.02	<.0001			
Diagnosis = PPH	1.45	1.17–1.79	.0006			
Year of TX = 1988–1991	1.42	1.23–1.64	<.0001	1.31	1.11–1.54	.002
Female recipient	0.77	0.69–0.86	<.0001			
Female donor/female recipient				0.81	0.67–0.98	.03
Diagnosis = α_1-antitrypsin	0.72	0.60–0.88	.001	0.68	0.52–0.88	.003
Diagnosis = emphysema	0.52	0.45–0.60	<.0001	0.79	0.64–0.97	.03

PPH, primary pulmonary hypertension; TX, transplant.
From Hosenpud JD, Bennett LE, Keck BM et al: The Registry of the International Society for Heart and Lung Transplantation: Sixteenth official Report — 1999. J Heart Lung Transplant 18:611, 1999.

of the less common indications. Nonetheless, enough data are available to realize that the long-term functional result in this group of patients is excellent. The longest surviving lung transplant recipient lived 13 years following a right single-lung transplant for pulmonary fibrosis. Single-lung transplantation provides satisfactory pulmonary volumes for these patients. Gas exchange and exercise tolerance are maintained during late follow-up (see Figs. 37–22 to 37–24) (Meyers, 2000).

Pulmonary Vascular Disease

Our program has been particularly interested in single-lung transplantation for patients with PPH and Eisenmenger's syndrome (Pasque et al, 1995). It is well documented that the cardiac function of these patients recovers promptly with the reduction in right heart afterload provided by a satisfactory lung allograft. However, the early postoperative course of these patients is complicated because of the impressive ventilation/perfusion mismatch, which can occur because 90% to 95% of right heart output is directed to the transplanted lung, and more than 50% of the ventilation is directed to the native lung. The unique nature of these patients is reflected in the fact that 5 of the 12 patients who require ECMO support post-transplant in our program have been pulmonary hypertension patients, whereas the patients with PPH only make up a small fraction of the overall experience. Our program has evolved a rigorous protocol

FIGURE 37–21 ■ Preoperative and postoperative room air Pa_{O_2} values among adult recipients in the Washington University Barnes Hospital experience, according to disease categories. Note the dramatic and sustained increase in oxygenation in all patient groups. (BLT, bilateral; CF, cystic fibrosis; COPD, chronic obstructive pulmonary disease; IPF, idiopathic pulmonary fibrosis; PH, pulmonary hypertension; SLT, single-lung transplant.) (From Shields TW: General Thoracic Surgery. Philadelphia, Lea & Febiger, 1994.)

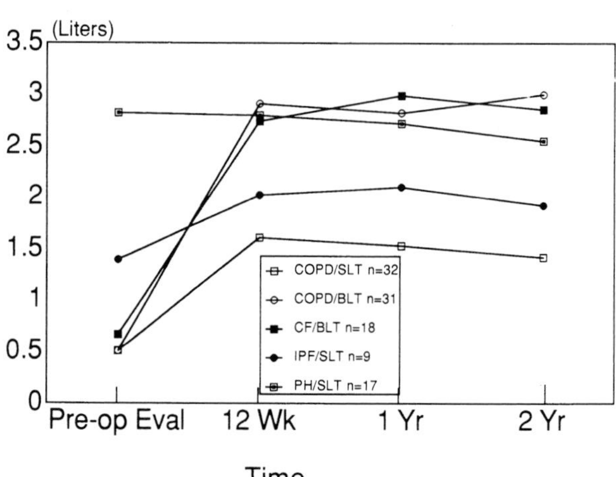

FIGURE 37–22 ■ Preoperative and postoperative forced expiratory volume in one second (FEV_1) among adult recipients in the Washington University Barnes Hospital experience according to disease categories. Dramatic and sustained improvements are noted in bilateral (BLT) recipients with chronic obstructive pulmonary disease (COPD) or cystic fibrosis (CF). Less dramatic improvements in FEV_1 are noted in single-lung recipients (SLT) with COPD or idiopathic pulmonary fibrosis (IPF). Single-lung recipients with pulmonary hypertension (PH) and normal preoperative FEV_1 derived no improvement in that parameter following transplant. (From Shields TW: General Thoracic Surgery. Philadelphia, Lea & Febiger, 1994.)

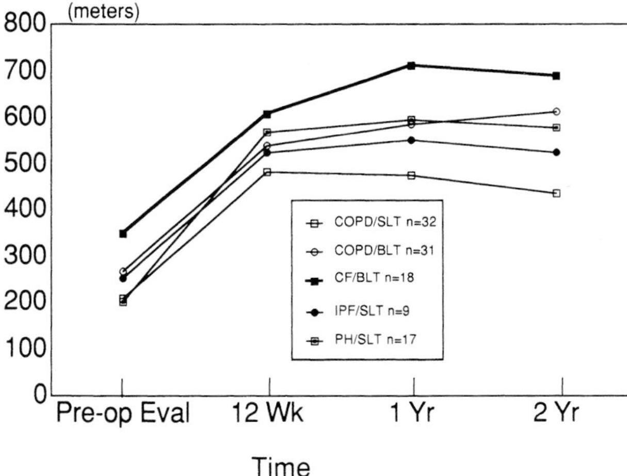

FIGURE 37–23 ■ Preoperative (eval) and postoperative 6-minute walk distances (in meters) for adult recipients in the Washington University Barnes Hospital program according to various disease and transplant categories. Note the dramatic improvement in exercise tolerance in all patient groups. This improvement appears to be sustained, except perhaps in the COPD group who received single-lung transplantation, in which a slight decrease was noted in late follow-up. (BLT, bilateral; CF, cystic fibrosis; COPD, chronic obstructive pulmonary disease; IPF, idiopathic pulmonary fibrosis; PH, pulmonary hypertension; SLT, single-lung recipients.) (From Shields TW: General Thoracic Surgery. Philadelphia, Lea & Febiger, 1994.)

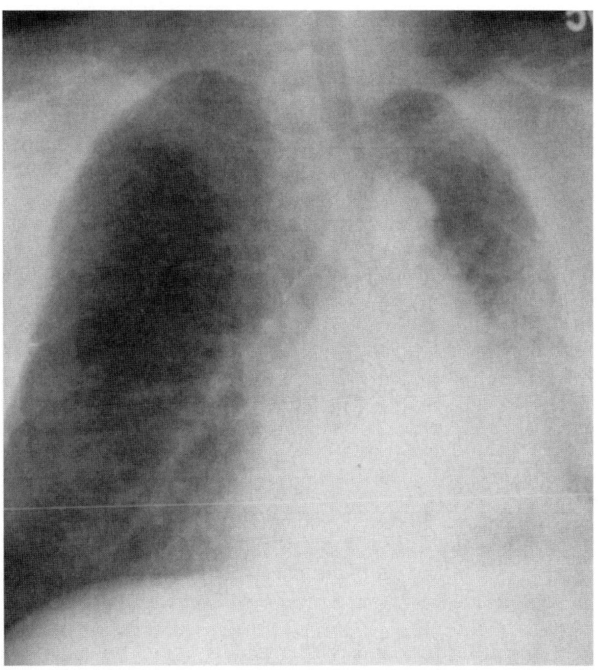

FIGURE 37–25 ■ Chest radiograph from a patient who underwent right single-lung transplantation for idiopathic pulmonary fibrosis in February 1985. At the time of this radiograph in 1993, he continued to enjoy an excellent functional result for 13 years following transplantation.

for the early postoperative management of these patients, with good results. Of 22 patients undergoing transplantation for PVD, there have been only two operative deaths and 3 late deaths, resulting in a 9.1% operative mortality rate and a late survival rate of 77%. The mean New York Heart Functional Class improved from a pretransplant mean value of 3.4 to a post-transplant mean value of 1.3. Gas exchange and exercise tolerance (see Figs. 37–22 to 37–24) demonstrate that these patients have functional results that are equivalent to any other transplant group in our experience.

Other groups have had significant difficulty with the application of single-lung transplantation in these patients. Bilateral lung replacement has been advocated by a

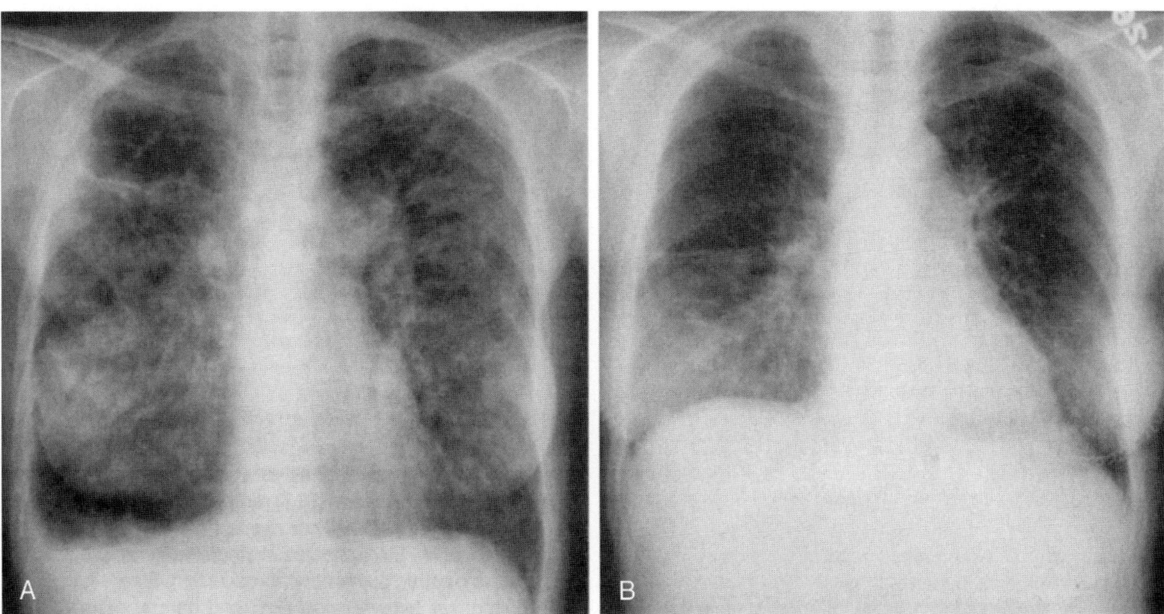

FIGURE 37–24 ■ *A*, Preoperative chest radiograph from a patient with cystic fibrosis. *B*, Postoperative chest radiograph in the same patient following bilateral sequential single-lung transplants. Note the return of a normal chest contour.

number of other programs (Bando et al, 1994), although subsequent reports from the same institution acknowledge equivalent long-term results using single-lung transplantation (Gammie et al, 1998). The standard operation that was offered these patients, combined heart-lung transplant, is still practiced widely, particularly in the United Kingdom. These bilateral lung replacement procedures may have a long-term advantage over single-lung transplantations in this patient group. Patients who have undergone single-lung transplantation for pulmonary hypertension do exceedingly well as long as BOS can be avoided. However, when BOS develops in PPH or Eisenmenger's syndrome patients who have received single-lung transplants, severe functional impairment results.

COMMENTS AND CONTROVERSIES

Lung transplantation has evolved into an effective therapeutic option for many patients with end-stage pulmonary disease. The successful lung transplant programs are those with a dedicated multidisciplinary approach to the investigation and management of patients with pulmonary diseases. A number of major problems await solution; for example, inadequate donor supply, suboptimal strategies of allograft preservation, insufficient selectivity of immunosuppression, and chronic allograft rejection. Prospective trials are required to determine which of the currently used therapeutic strategies is superior. Multi-institution cooperation will be required for their completion.

An acceptable long-term survival rate is still lacking. We have estimated the 5-year survival of our cohort of 450 recipients to be just over 50% (Meyers et al, 1999). There is an urgent need for improved strategies for the management of BOS. The induction of specific tolerance may be possible. Routine xenografting may also evolve as the ultimate solution to the worsening donor shortage. Until that time, the distribution of the limited donor lungs and the management of chronic rejection will remain the most pressing problems of clinical lung transplantation.

B.F.M.
G.A.P.

KEY REFERENCES

Hosenpud JD et al: Effect of diagnosis on survival benefit of lung transplantation for end-stage lung disease. Lancet 351:24, 1998.

This paper uses data from the Joint United Network for Organ Sharing/ International Society for Heart and Lung Transplantation Thoracic Registry to analyze the survival benefit conferred by lung transplantation. The controversial conclusions demonstrate the clearest survival benefit for recipients with cystic fibrosis. Lung transplantation did not confer a survival benefit to patients with emphysema by 2 years post-transplant.

Kroshus TJ et al: Risk factors for the development of bronchiolitis obliterans syndrome after lung transplantation. J Thorac Cardiovasc Surg 114:195, 1997.

This paper is a detailed discusssion of one of the major problems plaguing lung transplantation. The University of Minnesota performed a multivariate proportional hazards model to identify the clinical variables that are associated with the development of BOS. Cumulative episodes of acute rejection, CMV pneumonitis, and HLA mismatch at A loci were implicated as statistically significant risk factors, thus pointing the way for future prevention and intervention.

Meyers BF et al: Lung Transplantation: A Decade of Experience. Ann Surg 239:362, 1999.

This retrospective account of 450 transplants from 1988 to 1998 chronicles the growth years of lung transplantation. The outcomes include a 91.6% hospital survival and 54% five-year survival. This compilation of results from one of the busiest lung transplant centers in the world provides a benchmark for clinical lung transplant at the millennium.

Pasque MK et al: Improved technique for bilateral lung transplantation: Rationale and initial clinical experience. Ann Thorac Surg 49:785, 1990.

This paper by the Washington University Group represents the initial description of the bilateral sequential single-lung transplant technique. The en bloc double-lung procedure that was previously used was a tedious procedure that required cardiopulmonary bypass and cardioplegic arrest. The simpler bilateral sequential single-lung technique has become the procedure of choice and is used worldwide for bilateral lung replacement.

REFERENCES

Aoe M, Trachiotis GD, Okabayashi K et al: Administration of prostaglandin E1 after lung transplantation improves early graft function. Ann Thorac Surg 58:655, 1994.

Bando K, Armitage JM, Paradis IL et al: Indications for and results of single, bilateral and heart-lung transplantation for pulmonary hypertension. J Thorac Cardiovasc Surg 108:1056, 1994.

Bando K, Paradis IL, Similo S et al: Obliterative bronchiolitis after lung and heart-lung transplantation: An analysis of risk factors and management. J Thorac Cardiovasc Surg 110:4, 1995a.

Barnard CN: Clinical transplantation of the heart: A review of 13 years personal experience. J R Soc Med 74:670, 1981.

Barst RJ, Rubin LJ, Long WA et al: A comparison of continuous intravenous epoprostenol (prostacyclin) with conventional therapy for primary pulmonary hypertension. N Engl J Med 334:296, 1996.

Bavaria J, Kotloff R, Palevsky H et al: Bilateral versus single lung transplantation for chronic obstructive pulmonary disease. J Thorac Cardiovasc Surg 113:520, 1997.

Bhabra MS, Hopkinson DN, Shaw TE et al: Critical importance of the first 10 minutes of lung graft reperfusion after hypothermic storage. Ann Thorac Surg 61:1631, 1996.

Briffa N, Morris RE: New immunosuppressive regimens in lung transplantation. Eur Resp J 10:2630, 1997.

Chaparro C, Scavuzzo M, Winton T et al: Status of lung transplant recipients surviving beyond five years. J Heart Lung Transplant 16:511, 1997.

Christie NA, Waddell TK: Lung preservation. Chest Surg Clin North Am 3:29, 1993.

Clark SC, Sudarshan C, Khanna R et al: Controlled reperfusion and pentoxifylline modulates reperfusion injury after single lung transplantation. J Thorac Cardiovasc Surg 115:1335, 1998.

Cohen RG, Barr ML, Schenkel FA et al: Living-related donor lobectomy for bilateral lobar transplantation in patients with cystic fibrosis. Ann Thorac Surg 57:1423, 1994.

Cooley DA, Bloodwell RD, Hallman GL et al: Organ transplantation for advanced cardiopulmonary disease. Ann Thorac Surg 8:30, 1969.

Cooper JD, Billingham M, Egan T: A working formulation for the standardization of nomenclature and for clinical staging of chronic dysfunction in lung allografts. J Heart Lung Transplant 12:713, 1993.

Cooper JD, Patterson GA, Sundaresan RS et al: Results of 150 consecutive bilateral lung volume reduction procedures in patients with severe emphysema. J Thorac Cardiovasc Surg 112:1319, 1996.

Cooper JD, Patterson GA, Trulock EP et al: Results of single and bilateral lung transplantation in 131 consecutive recipients. J Thorac Cardiovasc Surg 107:460, 1994.

Cooper JD, Pearson FG, Patterson GA et al: Use of silicone stents in the management of airway problems. Ann Thorac Surg 47:371, 1989.

Couetil JA, Tolan MJ, Loulmet DF et al: Pulmonary bipartitioning and lobar transplantation: A new approach to donor organ shortage. J Thorac Cardiovasc Surg 113:529, 1997.

Couraud L, Baudet E, Martigne C et al: Bronchial revascularization in double-lung transplantation: A series of 8 patients. Ann Thorac Surg 53:88, 1992.

D'Alonzo GE, Barst RJ, Ayres SM et al: Survival in patients with primary pulmonary hypertension: Results from a National Prospective Registry. Ann Intern Med 115:343, 1991.

Daly R, Tadjkarimi S, Khaghani A et al: Successful double lung transplant with direct bronchial artery revascularization. Ann Thorac Surg 56:885, 1993.

Daly RC, McGregor CGA: Routine immediate direct bronchial artery revascularization for single-lung transplantation. Ann Thorac Surg 57:1446, 1994.

Dark JH: Experimental en-bloc double-lung transplantation. Ann Thorac Surg 42:394, 1986.

Date H, Lima O, Matsumura A et al: In a canine model, lung preservation at 10°C is superior to that at 4°C. J Thorac Cardiovasc Surg, 1992.

Date H, Lynch JP, Sundaresan S. Patterson GA, Trulock EP: The impact of cytolytic threapy on bronchiolitis obliterans syndrome. J Heart Lung Transplant 17:869, 1998.

Date H, Matsumura A, Manchester JK et al: Changes in alveolar oxygen and carbon dioxide concentrations and oxygen consumption during lung preservation: The maintenance of aerobic metabolism during lung preservation. J Thorac Cardiovasc Surg 105:492, 1993.

Date H, Triantafillou A, Trulock E et al: Inhaled nitric oxide reduces human lung allograft dysfunction. J Thorac Cardiovasc Surg 111:913, 1996.

Date H, Trulock EP, Arcidi JM et al: Improved airway healing after lung transplantation: An analysis of 348 bronchial anastomoses. J Thorac Cardiovasc Surg 110:1424, 1995.

Davis RD, Trulock EP, Manley J et al: Differences in early results after single lung transplantation. Ann Thorac Surg 58:1327, 1994.

Davreux C, Chu NH, Waddell TK et al: Improved tracheal allograft viability in immunosuppressed rats. Ann Thorac Surg 55:131, 1993.

DeHoyos A, Maurer JR: Complications following lung transplantation. Semin Thorac Cardiovasc Surg 4:132, 1992.

De Hoyos A, Patterson GA, Maurer J: Pulmonary transplantation: Early and late results. J Thorac Cardiovasc Surg 103:295, 1992.

Derom F, Barbier F, and Ringoir S: Ten month survival after lung homotransplantation in man. J Thorac Cardiovasc Surg 61:835, 1971.

Egan T, Ulicny KS, Lambert CJ et al: Effect of a free radical scavenger on cadaver lung transplantation. Ann Thorac Surg 55:1453, 1993.

Ettinger NA, Bailey TC, Trulock EP et al: Cytomegalovirus infection and pneumonitis: Impact after isolated lung transplanation. Am Rev Respir Dis 147:1017, 1993.

Fisher AJ, Gabbay E, Small T et al: Cross sectional study of exhaled nitic oxide levels following lung transplantation. Thorax 53:454, 1998.

Fremes SE, Patterson GA, Williams WG et al: Single lung transplantation and closure of patent ductus arteriosus for Eisenmenger's syndrome. J Thorac Cardiovasc Surg 100:1, 1990.

Fujino S, Nagahiro I, Triantafillou AN et al: Inhaled nitric oxide at the time of harvest improves early lung allograft function. Ann Thorac Surg 63:1383, 1997.

Gammie JS, Keenan RJ, Pham SM et al: Single- versus double-lung transplantation for pulmonary hypertension. J Thorac Cardiovasc Surg 115:397, 1998.

Goldberg M, Lima O, Morgan E et al: A comparison between cyclosporine A and methylprednisolone plus azathioprine on bronchial healing following canine lung transplantation. J Thorac Cardiovasc Surg 85:821, 1983.

Griffith BP, Hardesty RL, Armitage JM et al: Acute rejection of lung allografts with various immunosuppressive protocols. Ann Thorac Surg 54:846, 1992.

Griffith BP, Magee MJ, Gonzalez IF et al: Anastomotic pitfalls in lung transplantation. J Thorac Cardiovasc Surg 107:743, 1994.

Hakim M, Higgenbottam T, Bethune D et al: Selection and procurement of combined heart and lung grafts for transplantation. J Thorac Cardiovasc Surg 85:474, 1988.

Halldorsson A, Kronon M, Allen BS et al: Controlled reperfusion after lung ischemia: Implications for improved function after lung transplantation. J Thorac Cardiovasc Surg 115:415, 1998.

Haniuda M, Hasegawa S, Shiraishi T et al: Effects of inflation volume during lung preservation on pulmonary capillary permeability. J Thorac Cardiovasc Surg 112:85, 1996.

Hardesty R, Aeba R, Armitage J et al: A clinical trial of University of Wisconsin solution for pulmonary preservation. J Thorac Cardiovasc Surg 105:660, 1993.

Hardin CA, Kittle CF: Experiences with transplantation of the lung. Science 119:97, 1954.

Hardy JD, Webb WR, Dalton ML et al: Lung homotransplantation in man. JAMA 186:1065, 1963.

Hasegawa S, Ritter JH, Patterson GA et al: Expression of intercellular and vascular cell adhesion molecules and class II major histocompatibility antigens in human lungs: Lack of influence by conditions of organ preservation. J Heart Lung Transplant 14:897, 1995.

Haydock DA, Trulock EP, Kaiser LR et al: Management of dysfunction in the transplanted lung: Experience with 7 clinical cases. Ann Thorac Surg 53:635, 1992.

Hayllar KM, Williams SGJ, Wise AE et al: A prognostic model for the prediction of survival in cystic fibrosis. Thorax 52:313, 1997.

Higenbottam T, Stewart S, Penketh A et al: Transbronchial lung biopsy for the diagnosis of rejection in heart-lung transplant patients. Transplantation 46:532, 1988.

Hirai T, Waddell TK, Puskas JD et al: Prolonged lung allograft survival with short course of FK 506. J Thorac Cardiovasc Surg 105:1, 1993.

Hopkinson DN, Bhabra MS and Hooper TL: Pulmonary graft preservation—a worldwide survey of current clinical practice. J Heart Lung Transplant 17:525, 1998.

Hosenpud JD, Bennett LE, Keck BM et al: Effect of diagnosis on survival benefit of lung transplantation for end-stage lung disease. Lancet 351:24, 1998a.

Hosenpud JD, Bennett LE, Keck BM et al: The Registry of the International Society for Heart and Lung Transplantation: Fifteenth Official Report, 1998. J Heart Lung Transplant 17:656, 1998b.

Hosenpud JD, Bennett LE, Keck BM et al: The Registry of the International Society for Heart and Lung Transplantation: Sixteenth Official Report, 1999. J Heart Lung Transplant 18:611, 1999.

Inui K, Schafers HJ, Aoki M et al: Bronchial circulation after experimental lung transplantation: The effect of long term administration of prednisolone. J Thorac Cardiovasc Surg 105:474, 1993.

Kayano K, Toda K, Naka Y et al: Superior protection in orthotopic rat lung transplantation with cyclic adenosine monophosphate and nitroglycerine-containing preservation solution. J Thorac Cardiovasc Surg 118:135, 1999.

Kerem E, Reisman J, Corey M et al: Prediction of mortality in patients with cystic fibrosis. N Engl J Med 326:1187, 1992.

Keshavjee S, Yamazaki F, Yokomise H et al: The role of dextran 40 and potassium in extended hypothermic lung preservation for transplantation. J Thorac Cardiovasc Surg 103:314, 1992.

Kirk JB, Conacher ID, Corris PA et al: Successful surgical management of bronchial dehiscence after single-lung transplantation. Ann Thorac Surg 49:147, 1990.

Kroshus TJ, Kshettry VR, Savik K et al: Risk factors for the development of bronchiolitis obliterans syndrome after lung transplantation. J Thorac Cardiovasc Surg 114:195, 1997.

Levine S, Anzueto A, Gibbons WJ et al: Graft position and pulmonary function after single lung transplantation for obstructive lung disease. Chest 103:444, 1993.

Lillehei CW: Discussion of Wildevuur CRH, Benfield JR: A review of 23 human lung transplantations by 20 surgeons. Ann Thorac Surg 9:489, 1970.

Lima O, Cooper JD, Peters WJ et al: Effects of methylprednisolone and azathioprine on bronchial healing following lung autotransplantation. J Thorac Cardiovasc Surg 82:211, 1981.

Macchiarini P, Mazmanian G, Oriol R et al: Ex vivo lung model of pig to human hyperacute xenograft rejection. J Thorac Cardiovasc Surg 114:315, 1997.

Mal H, Andreasian B and Pamela F: Unilateral lung transplantation in end stage pulmonary emphysema. Am Rev Respir Dis 140:797, 1989.

Matsuzaki Y, Waddell TK, Puskas JD et al: Amelioration of post-ischemic lung reperfusion injury by PGE. Am Rev Respir Dis 148:882, 1993.

Maurer JR, Frost AE, Estenne M et al: International Guidelines for the Selection of Lung Transplant Candidates. J Heart Lung Transplant 17:703, 1998.

Mayer E, Puskas JD, Cardoso PFG et al: Reliable eighteen-hour lung preservation at 4°C and 10°C by pulmonary artery flush after high-dose prostaglandin E1. J Thorac Cardiovasc Surg 103:1136, 1992.

Metras H: Note préliminaire sur la greffe totale du poumon chez le chien. C R Acad Sci (Paris) 231:1176, 1950.

Meyers BF: Lung Transplantation for Pulmonary Fibrosis. J Thorac Cardiovasc Surg 120:99, 2000.

Meyers BF, Lynch J, Trulock EP et al: Lung transplantation: A decade experience. Ann Surg 239:362, 1999.

Meyers BF, Sundaresan RS, Cooper JD et al: Bilateral sequential lung transplant without sternal division eliminates post-transplant sternal complications. J Thorac Cardiovasc Surg 117:358, 1998.

Meyers BF, Sundt TM, Henry S et al: Selective use of extracorporeal membrane oxygenation is warranted after lung transplantation. J Thorac Cardiovasc Surg 120:20, 2000.

Miller JD, DeHoyos A, Group UoTLT et al: An evaluation of the role of omentopexy and of early perioperative corticosteroid administration in clinical lung transplantation. J Thorac Cardiovasc Surg 105:246, 1993.

Morgan E, Lima O, Goldberg M et al: Successful revascularization of totally ischemic bronchial autografts with omental pedicle flaps in dogs. J Thorac Cardiovasc Surg 84:204, 1982.

Nelems W: Human lung transplantation. Chest 78:569, 1980.

Novick RJ, Gehman KE, Ali IS et al: Lung preservation: The importance of endothelial and alveolar type II cell integrity. Ann Thorac Surg 62:302, 1996.

Novick R, Kaye MP, Patterson GA et al: Redo lung transplantation: A North American-European experience. J Heart Lung Transplant 12:5, 1993.

Novick RJ, Bennett LE, Meyer DM et al: Influence of graft ischemic time and donor age on survival after lung transplantation. J Heart Lung Transplant 18:425, 1999.

Novick RJ, Menkis AH and McKenzie FN: New trends in lung preservation: A collective review. J Heart Lung Transplant 11:377, 1992.

Novick RJ, Stitt L: Pulmonary retransplantation. Semin Thorac Cardivasc Surg 10:227, 1998.

Novick RJ, Stitt LW, Alkattan K et al: Pulmonary retransplantation: Predictors of graft function and survival in 230 patients. Ann Thorac Surg 65:227, 1998.

Okabayashi K, Aoe M, DeMeester SR et al: Pentoxifylline reduces lung allograft reperfusion injury. Ann Thorac Surg 58:50, 1994.

Pasque MK, Cooper JD, Kaiser LR et al: An improved technique for bilateral lung transplantation: Rationale and initial clinical experience. Ann Thorac Surg 49:785, 1990.

Pasque MK, Kaiser LR, Dresler CM et al: Single lung transplantation for pulmonary hypertension. J Thorac Cardiovasc Surg 103:475, 1992.

Pasque MK, Trulock EP, Cooper JD et al: Single lung transplantation for pulmonary hypertension: Single institution experience in 34 patients. Circ 92:2252, 1995.

Patterson GA, Cooper JD, Goldman B et al: Technique of successful clinical double-lung transplantation. Ann Thorac Surg 45:626, 1988.

Patterson GA, Todd TR, Cooper JD et al: Airway complications after double lung transplantation. J Thorac Cardiovasc Surg 99:14, 1990.

Pochettino A, Bavaria JE: Anterior axillary muscle-sparing thoracotomy for lung transplantation. Ann Thorac Surg 64:1846, 1997.

Puskas J, Cardoso PFG, Mayer E et al: Equivalent eighteen-hour lung preservation with low-potassium dextran or Euro-Collins solution after prostaglandin E1 infusion. J Thorac Cardiovasc Surg 104:83, 1992a.

Puskas J, Hirai T, Christie N et al: Reliable 30 hour lung preservation by donor hyperinflation. J Thorac Cardiovasc Surg 104:1075, 1992b.

Puskas JD, Winton TL, Miller JD et al: Unilateral donor lung dysfunction does not preclude successful contralateral single lung transplantation. J Thorac Cardiovasc Surg 103:1015, 1992c.

Ramirez JC, Patterson GA and Winton T: Bilateral lung transplantation for cystic fibrosis. J Thorac Cardiovasc Surg 103:287, 1992.

Reichenspurner H, Girgis RE, Robbins RC et al: Obliterative bronchiolitis after lung and heart-lung transplantation. Ann Thorac Surg 60:1845, 1995.

Reitz BA, Wallwork J, Hunt S et al: Heart-lung transplantation: Successful therapy for patients with pulmonary vascular disease. N Engl J Med 306:557, 1982b.

Schafers HJ, Waxman MB, Patterson GA et al: Cardiac innervation after double lung transplant. J Thorac Cardiovasc Surg 99:22, 1990.

Sharples L, Hathaway T, Dennis C et al: Prognosis of patients with cystic fibrosis awaiting heart and lung tranplantation. J Heart Lung Transplant 12:669, 1993.

Shiraishi Y, Lee JR, Laks H et al: Use of leukocyte depletion to decrease injury after lung preservation and rewarming ischemia—an experimental model. J Heart Lung Transplant 17:250, 1998.

Smith MA, Sundaresan S, Mohanakumar T et al: Effect of development of antibodies to HLA and cytomegalovirus mismatch on lung transplantation survival and development of bronchiolitis obliterans syndrome. J Thorac Cardiovasc Surg 116:812, 1998.

Snell G, DeHoyos A, Krajden M et al: Pseudomonas cepacia in lung transplant recipients with cystic fibrosis. Chest 103:466, 1993.

Snell GI, Rabinov M, Griffiths A et al: Pulmonary allograft ischemic time: An important predictor of survival after lung transplantation. J Heart Lung Transplant 15:160, 1996.

Spray T, Mallory GB, Canter CB et al: Pediatric lung transplantation: Indications, techniques and early results. J Thorac Cardiovasc Surg 107:990, 1994.

Starnes VA, Barr ML, Cohen RG et al: Living-donor lobar lung transplantation experience: Intermediate results. J Thorac Cardiovasc Surg 112:1284, 1996.

Sundaresan S, Lima O, Date H et al: Lung preservation with low potassium dextran flush in a primate bilateral transplant model. Ann Thorac Surg 56:1129, 1993.

Sundaresan S, Semenkovich J, Ochoa L et al: Successful outcome of lung transplantation is not compromised by the use of marginal donor lungs. J Thorac Cardiovasc Surg 109:1075, 1995a.

Sundaresan S, Shiraishi Y, Trulock EP et al: Single or bilateral lung transplantation for emphysema? J Thorac Cardiovasc Surg 112:1485, 1996.

Sundaresan S, Trachiotis GD, Aoe M et al: Donor lung procurement: Assessment and operative technique. Ann Thorac Surg 56:1409, 1993.

Sundaresan S, Trulock EP, Mohanakumar T et al: Prevalence and outcome of bronchiolitis obliterans syndrome after lung transplantation. Ann Thorac Surg 60:1341, 1995b.

Sweet S, Spray T, Huddleston C et al: Pediatric lung transplantation at St. Louis Children's Hospital. Am J Respir Crit Care Med 155:1027, 1997.

Todd T, Goldberg M, Koshal A et al: Separate extraction of cardiac and pulmonary grafts from a single organ donor. Ann Thorac Surg 46:356, 1988.

Toronto Lung Transplantation Group: Unilateral lung transplantation for pulmonary fibrosis. N Engl J Med 314:1140, 1986.

Triantafillou A, Pasque MK, Huddleston CB et al: Frequency and indications for cardiopulmonary bypass during lung transplantation in adults. Ann Thorac Surg 57:1248, 1994.

Triantafillou AN: Lung transplantation: Anesthetic considerations. Curr Top Gen Thor Surg 3:171, 1995.

Trulock EP: Lung transplantation. Am J Respir Crit Care Med 155:789, 1997.

Trulock EP: Management of lung transplant rejection. Chest 103:1566, 1993.

Trulock EP: Recipient selection. Chest Surg Clin North Am 3:1, 1993.

Van Raemdonck DEM, Jannis, Rega et al: Extended preservation of ischemic pulmonary graft by postmortem alveolar expansion. Ann Thorac Surg 64:801, 1997.

Varela A, Cordoba M, Serrano-Fiz S et al: Early lung allograft function after retrograde and antegrade preservation. J Thorac Cardiovasc Surg 114:1119, 1997.

Venuta F, Rendina EA, Bufi M et al: Preimplantation retrograde pneumoplegia in clinical lung transplantation. J Thorac Cardiovasc Surg 118:107, 1999.

Wain JC, Wright CD, Ryan DP et al: Induction immunosuppression for lung transplantation with OKT3. Ann Thorac Surg 67:187, 1999.

Wang L, Nakamoto K, Hseih C et al: Influence of temperature of flushing solution on lung preservation. Ann Thorac Surg 55:711, 1993.

Westaby S: Aprotinin in perspective. Ann Thorac Surg 55:1033, 1993.

Yacoub M, Khagani A, Banner N, Tajkarimi S: Distant organ procurement for heart and lung transplantation. Transplant Proc 21:2548, 1989.

Yousem SA, Berry GJ, Brunt EM et al: A working formulation for the standardization of nomenclature in the diagnosis of heart and lung rejection: Lung Rejection Study Group. J Heart Lung Transplant 9:593, 1990.

Yousem SA, Berry GJ, Cagle PT et al: Revision of the 1990 working formulation for the classification of pulmonary allograft rejection: Lung Rejection Study Group. J Heart Lung Transplant 15(1 Pt 1):1, 1996.

Zorn G: Lung transplantation in patients with thoracic malignant disease. In Franco KL, Putnam J (eds): Advanced Therapy in Thoracic Surgery. Hamilton, Ontario, Canada, BC Decker, 1998.

HEART-LUNG TRANSPLANTATION

Axel Haverich
Wolfgang Harringer

Heart-lung transplantation refers to the combined or en bloc allografting of the heart and both lungs for end-stage cardiopulmonary disease.

HISTORICAL NOTE

Alexis Carrel (1907) was the first to attempt transplantation of the heart and both lungs at the beginning of the 20th century, although it was only transplantation into the neck of a cat. In 1946, Demikhov (1962) transplanted the heart and lungs of a dog, and the recipient survived for 2 hours on the allografted organs alone. During the same period, other researchers, notably Marcus and colleagues (1953) were also studying experimental heart-lung transplantation; they developed a technique for transplantating the heart and both lungs into the abdomen and suggested the possibility of using a heterologous heart-lung preparation (xenograft) as an extracorporeal pump in open heart surgery. In 1953, Neptune and colleagues reported the use of hypothermia to protect the recipient during orthotopic cardiopulmonary transplantation. Four years later, the use of a pump oxygenator to perform such operations in dogs was reported by Webb and Howard (1957). These authors found it possible to restore the heart to relatively normal function, and the animals lived from 75 minutes to 22 hours. However, their experimental animals were unable to breathe spontaneously; thus, this group concluded that respiratory dysfunction resulting from simultaneous bilateral pulmonary denervation made cardiopulmonary transplantation impracticable. In 1958, Blanco and co-workers (1958) also reported attempts at orthotopic heart and lung replacement using a pump oxygenator. Spontaneous respiration returned in two dogs after mechanical ventilation was discontinued. Similar findings were made by Lower and colleagues (1961) 3 years later. Still, the respiratory pattern was reported to be altered with increased tidal volumes and slow respiratory rates. In a study of the working heart-lung preparation to examine heart viability after storage, Robicsek and coworkers (1967) repeated Demikhov's experiments, with up to 37 hours of survival. Respiratory difficulties again prevented long-term survival. The experiments of Nakae and colleagues (1967), who performed cardiopulmonary autotransplantation in several species of animals, suggested that denervation of both lungs did not prevent a return of adequate spontaneous respiration in primates, as it did in dogs. These experiments were followed by the studies of Castaneda and co-workers (1972), and later of Reitz and colleagues (1980), in monkeys, which confirmed long-term survival and a normal respiratory pattern in autotransplanted heart-lung grafts. Subsequent experiments using allotransplant in primates definitively confirmed the clinical applicability of combined heart-lung transplantation.

The first clinical attempt was made by Cooley and colleagues (1969) in 1968 in a 2-month-old infant who died 14 hours after the operation. In December 1969, Lillehei (1970) performed the second human heart-lung transplantation in a 43-year-old patient with emphysema. The patient died 8 days later from pneumonia. Barnard (1981) was the third surgeon to try this operation in July 1971. The patient did well initially but died on the twenty-third day from disruption of the bronchial suture line. In this case, bilateral bronchial anastomoses rather than a tracheal suture line had been performed. Ten years later, a fourth transplant was reported by Reitz and colleagues (1982) at Stanford University. The use of cyclosporine and the application of the surgical technique developed in this group's experimental program resulted in the first long-term survivor, a 45-year-old woman with primary pulmonary hypertension (Reitz 1980; 1982b). Since then, more than 2,400 combined heart-lung transplantations have been performed worldwide (Hosenpud et al, 1998).

■ *HISTORICAL READINGS*

Cooley DA, Bloodwell RD, Hallman GL et al: Organ transplantation for advanced cardiopulmonary disease. Ann Thorac Surg 8:30, 1969.

Reitz BA, Burton NA, Jamieson SW et al: Heart and lung transplantation: Autotransplantation and allotransplantation in primates with extended survival. J Thorac Cardiovasc Surg 80:360, 1980.

Reitz BA, Wallwork J, Hunt SA et al: Heart-lung transplantation: Successful therapy for patients with pulmonary vascular disease. N Engl J Med 306:557, 1982b.

Webb WR, Howard HS: Cardio-pulmonary transplantation. Surg Forum 8:313, 1957.

INDICATIONS

Following the first successful clinical application, surgeons reserved heart-lung transplantation for patients with primary and secondary pulmonary hypertension. This selection, based on Reitz and co-workers' (1982b) criteria, was made because of the poor results that were previously obtained in patients with parenchymal lung disease and an infected tracheobronchial tree. With increasing clinical experience, patients who had a number of pulmonary disorders, including restrictive and obstructive pathologic types, were accepted as candidates for the operation (Kaiser et al, 1991; Penketh et al, 1987). In fact, even patients with bronchiectasis and cystic fibrosis were considered for surgery (Leval et al, 1991; Scott et al, 1988).

The established foreseeable results of heart-lung replacement during the first 5 years of its clinical application also resulted in an increase in the number of operations that were performed in patients who actually were not in need of replacement of the heart. In these patients, heart-lung transplantation was performed, and the recipient's heart was given to another patient awaiting isolated heart transplantation (i.e., domino procedure) (Madden et al, 1992; Oaks et al, 1994; Smith et al, 1996). Although this approach is still used by some surgeons, the majority of cardiothoracic transplant centers now perform single- or double-lung transplantation in candidates with adequately preserved cardiac function (Bando et al, 1994; Kramer et al, 1994). The heart of the respective organ donor may be simultaneously transplanted into a cardiac transplant recipient. This change in the indications for heart-lung transplantation has been grossly influenced by the lack of adequate numbers of organ donors for combined heart-lung transplantation. In most countries, the number of potential heart-transplant recipients has grown to such an extent that cardiopulmonary allografts only rarely are offered for transplantation.

This severe restriction in organ supply has recently resulted in two developments in thoracic organ transplantation. First, the number of heart-lung transplantations performed worldwide has reached a plateau since 1988 (Hosenpud et al, 1998). Second, increasing numbers of patients with "classic" indications for heart-lung transplantation (Reitz et al, 1982b), including primary and secondary pulmonary hypertension, are being treated by single- or double-lung transplantation. In patients with Eisenmenger's syndrome, simultaneous repair of the intracardiac or extracardiac shunt followed by single-lung implantation has been reported.

As a result, patients are potential recipients for heart-lung transplantation only if end-stage pulmonary disease coexists with irreversible right or biventricular failure. Because this is rarely the case in parenchymal lung disease, indications for en bloc replacement generally are reserved for end-stage pulmonary hypertension with severely impaired right ventricular function, Eisenmenger's syndrome (especially if combined with complex cardiac anomalies), and thromboembolic pulmonary disease—poor left ventricular function or concomitant coronary artery disease. The threshold of recovery of right ventricular dysfunction is unknown.

DIAGNOSIS

Clinical Features

When the rare cases of parenchymal pulmonary disease that result in end-stage heart failure are excluded, the clinical features of the typical candidate for heart-lung transplantation who has primary or secondary pulmonary hypertension are predominant arterial hypoxemia aggravated by exercise and signs of chronic right heart failure (Maurer et al, 1998). Accepted patients should have reached the New York Heart Association's class III or IV despite maximum medical therapy. In patients with primary pulmonary hypertension, this should include a trial with calcium antagonists, intravenous epoprostenol, or intermittently inhaled iloprost (Rubin, 1997). Because of predominant right heart failure, clinical signs of tricuspid insufficiency, such as extended neck veins and hepatic enlargement, are usually present. Peripheral edema is almost never seen in these patients, even in the late course of the disease. Jaundice caused by hepatic congestion may be an earlier clinical sign.

Natural History

The natural history of pulmonary hypertension may vary significantly according to the pathogenesis in individual patients. Adults with Eisenmenger's syndrome seem to have a more favorable hemodynamic profile and prognosis when compared with patients with primary pulmonary hypertension (Hopkins et al, 1996). We have performed heart-lung transplants in two patients older than 50 years of age who had Eisenmenger's complex (one with an atrioventricular canal and one with a ventricular septal defect) with a history of right heart failure of more than 20 years' duration. Primary pulmonary hypertension, by contrast, especially if occurring postpartum, may lead to a rapid clinical deterioration, sometimes resulting in death within 1 year after the first clinical signs. This large variation in survival after establishing the diagnosis makes it difficult to decide when the patient should be put on the waiting list. Anamnestic features, such as endobronchial bleeding or syncope, both of which suggest a dismal prognosis quoad vitam, may be helpful in regard to this decision. Some candidates, however, may live and remain on a heart-lung waiting list for more than 2 years, which reflects the insecurities of the prognosis in such patients.

Differential Diagnosis

The differential diagnosis of the underlying disease is usually not important if transplantation is clearly indicated owing to arterial hypoxemia combined with end-stage right heart failure. However, thromboembolic pulmonary disease and congenital heart disease should be ruled out in all patients with borderline right ventricular function because either pulmonary thromboendarterectomy or repair of the defect followed by single-lung transplantation may be performed in such cases. If thromboembolic disease is expected, phlebography and pulmonary angiography should be performed to prove or exclude this pathologic condition and to assess the potential risk of recurrent thromboembolic events.

Systemic illness, such as collagen disease, systemic vasculitis, or rheumatoid arthritis, should be ruled out as the underlying disorder associated with pulmonary hypertension. Such entities represent relative contraindications for transplantation because the recurrence of pulmonary hypertension cannot be excluded and vasculitis per se may limit patient survival (Maurer et al, 1998).

Investigative Techniques

Taking into account that the replacement of the heart and both lungs represents a major surgical intervention, comparably little has to be done in terms of preoperative investigations. After the exact diagnosis of pulmonary hypertension and right heart failure has been established by right heart catheterization and echocardiography, little has to be done with respect to cardiopulmonary functional assessment. Only in patients with borderline right ventricular function is a complete assessment of both left and right ventricular function necessary to exclude the option of single-lung transplantation. This assessment should include the right ventricular ejection fraction by echocardiography or multiple-gated blood scan, the degree of pulmonary and tricuspid valve regurgitation, the left ventricular ejection fraction, coronary angiography, and aortic and mitral valve function. If Eisenmenger's syndrome cannot be excluded, an angiocardiographic search for a potential intracardiac shunt should always be complemented by aortography to rule out a patent ductus arteriosus or an aortopulmonary window. In patients with thromboembolic pulmonary hypertension and only moderately impaired right ventricular ejection function (more than 20% as in mild to moderate tricuspid insufficiency or mild pulmonary valve regurgitation on echocardiography), pulmonary angiography is mandatory to exclude the indication for thromboendarterectomy.

Computed tomography (CT) scans or magnetic resonance imaging (MRI) of the chest are helpful to assess the anatomic position of the heart and great vessels and potential pleural and mediastinal thickening, especially in reoperated cases. Cranial CT often shows signs of cortical atrophy of various degree. This investigation is believed to be mandatory in candidates with a history of cerebrovascular accidents. Abdominal sonography is always performed to assess the size and structure of the liver and the biliary system (gallstones), renal anatomy, and the status of the intra-abdominal blood vessels. Peripheral arterial disease is excluded clinically and by noninvasive methods (ultrasound techniques); phlebography is done in patients with histories of deep vein thromboses. Investigations of other organ systems, such as the central nervous system, peripheral nervous system, and gastrointestinal tract, are only indicated if they are substantiated by the medical history.

Blood is drawn to (1) verify the degree of cardiopulmonary failure; (2) assess the renal, hepatic, and hematologic status; and (3) document the immunologic baseline characteristics of the potential recipients.

1. An arterial blood gas analysis is performed with the patient at rest. If it is normal, it is repeated during exercise.

2. Renal and hepatic function are assessed by routine serologic and hematologic examinations (coagulation status). If the status is abnormal, this study is complemented by specific studies (glomerular filtration rate, renal plasma flow, and direct/indirect bilirubin values). Hematologically, a differential white blood count, red blood count, and the hematocrit and platelet counts are performed. A full coagulation status report, including antithrombin III levels, should also be ordered.

3. Blood group, rhesus factor, and preformed reactive antibodies must be known before the patient is placed on the waiting list. If the percentage of preformed antibodies exceeds 10%, a direct cross-match between donor (lymphocytes) and recipient (plasma) will be necessary at the time of transplantation. We do not perform histocompatibility antigen (HLA) typing preoperatively because the supply of organs does not allow for organ allocation according to HLA criteria. The virologic history should be assessed by antibody screening, including Epstein-Barr and herpes simplex viruses. Transplantation-specific infections, most importantly cytomegalovirus (CMV); hepatitis A, B, and C; and human immunodeficiency virus (HIV) serologic testing, should be investigated. Some centers match donor and recipient according to the CMV status. Even if this policy is not followed, knowledge of the preoperative CMV status and potential conversions after the procedure may be helpful in the postoperative management.

MANAGEMENT

Principles of Management

Histocompatibility

Despite ample evidence for the positive influence of HLA-matching on the long-term function of allotransplanted parenchymal organs, this strategy has not become a reality in thoracic organ transplantation. First, there are logistic problems in obtaining donor HLA typing prior to heart and lung retrieval, especially in distant organ procurement. Second, the number of potential recipients, according to blood groups, type of transplantation (heart-lung versus single-lung versus double-lung transplantation), and size of the potential recipients leaves only a few options for HLA-compatible transplantation in most organ-procurement organizations. The practice, therefore, is to perform heart-lung transplantation irrespective of HLA typing. Reports on longstanding hemolysis in blood group A, B, or AB recipients of group O lungs, however, would suggest that ABO identical transplantation is necessary.

CONTRAINDICATIONS TO HEART-LUNG TRANSPLANTATION

Major

Active (nonpulmonary) infection
Severe chest deformity
Malignant disease
Severe renal or hepatic disease
Uncontrolled systemic disease
Severe central nervous system disability
Drug abuse or psychological instability
Positive hepatitis or human immunodeficiency virus serologic findings

Minor

Advanced age: >55 years
Young age: <6 years
Multiple cardiac or thoracic surgical procedures
Insulin-dependent diabetes mellitus
Active peptic ulceration

To minimize hyperacute rejection by preformed cytotoxic antibodies (which is more often seen in postpartum female patients and in those who have undergone previous blood transfusions—e.g., following open heart surgery), the recipient's serum is tested against a random panel of lymphocytes from about 50 blood donors. If more than 10% of the lymphocytes are lysed, presensitization must be suspected, and repeat analysis (after 4 to 12 weeks) is obligatory. If it is still positive, a direct cross-match must be performed prior to transplantation. In any case, a retrospective crossmatch should be initiated postoperatively to estimate the immunologic risk of the respective donor/recipient combination. We also perform HLA typing of both donor and recipient for potential future investigation and management.

Recipient Selection

After the correct diagnosis of the underlying disease and its degree of severity have been confirmed with a pretransplant evaluation, the selection of a patient as a potential recipient only requires the exclusion of contraindications (see earlier).

Specific considerations in regard to patient selection at the time an organ becomes available should include basic immunologic and demographic criteria, such as sex, height, weight, and age. Great care must be taken to avoid any oversizing (more than 10%) of the donor's organs compared with the recipient's chest. In general, transplantation within one gender can be done according to donor/recipient heights only. Routine chest measurements in donor/recipient matching have been abandoned because of the possibility of lung volume reduction by multiple atypical resections. In cases with doubtful intrathoracic volume estimates, such as in pediatric donors, the posteroanterior chest radiograph or measurements should be compared (Fig. 37–26).

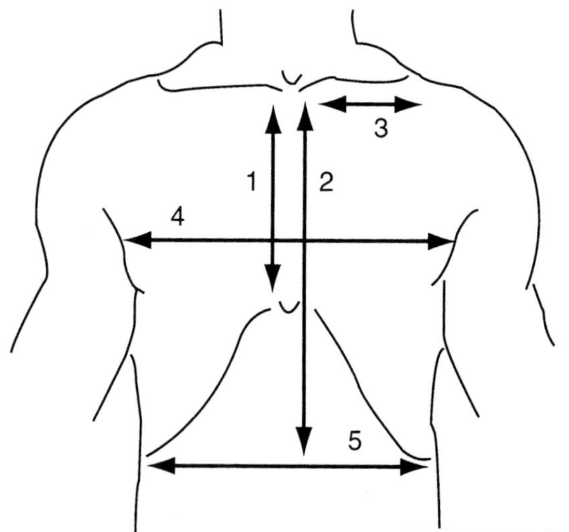

FIGURE 37–26 ■ Thoracic chest measurements that allow for a comparison between donor and recipient prior to explantation: 1, length of the sternum; 2, manubrium to lower thoracic circumference; 3, manubrium to acromion; 4, thoracic circumference at the level of the nipples; 5, at the level of the lower chest circumference. (From Haverich A: Herz und Herz-Lungen Transplantation. In Borst HG, Klinner W, Oelert H [eds]: Herzchirurgie. Berlin, Springer-Verlag, 1978.)

Recipient Preparation

When a potential donor organ becomes available, any febrile illness must be determined during the first contact with the potential recipient, which is usually made by phone. Transportation to the recipient hospital should be by the fastest mode available to ensure sufficient time for a final checkup. This includes preoperative instruction of the patient and obtaining the patient's consent for the procedure, chest radiograph, and immediate blood testing, such as white blood cell count, serum levels of creatinine and hepatic transaminases, coagulation parameters, an arterial blood gas analysis, and an order of blood and blood products for transfusions with the blood bank. If applicable, the recipient may receive the pretransplant dose of immunosuppression therapy, followed by a whole-body shave and scrub. We do not transfer a heart-lung transplant recipient to the operating room before the explanting surgeon has confirmed that the donor organs to be removed are suitable for implantation. Precise timing is crucial in patients with multiple previous cardiac or thoracic procedures, because explantation of organs and control of mediastinal and chest wall bleeding can be time consuming.

Donor Selection

Selection of the appropriate donor organs for heart-lung transplantation remains a critical issue in view of both the limited number of allografts available and their quality, especially of the lungs in the organ donor. Less than 20% of potential heart donors may be suitable for heart-lung donation (Harper and Rosendale, 1996). Pneumonic changes may occur in a brain-dead individual as a result of infection or aspiration, which precludes donation of the lungs. Tracheal intubation, often performed emergently under less than optimal sterile conditions, and neurogenic pulmonary edema both may result in pulmonary dysfunction (Novitzky et al, 1987). To minimize the risk of pulmonary failure or infection after transplantation, the potential donor should meet the following criteria.

Age. Preferably, the donor should be younger than 50 years (male patient) or 55 years of age (female patient) to reduce the risk of coronary artery disease. With the severe shortage of suitable donors, this age limit might be extended if the donor appears to be suitable in other respects. In cases of doubt, coronary angiography should be performed.

Medical History. The donor should ideally be a nonsmoker with no history of significant pulmonary or cardiac disease.

Cardiac and Pulmonary Function. Normal cardiac function is essential, and adequate gas exchange should be present. With a postive end-expiratory pressure (PEEP) of 5 cm H_2O and a fraction of inspired oxygen (F_{IO_2}) of 0.40 (40% O_2 or less), the partial oxygen pressure (P_{aO_2}) should be greater than 100 mm Hg. With an F_{IO_2} of 1 (100% O_2), the P_{aO_2} should be greater than 300 mm Hg. The static pressure should not exceed 20 cm H_2O at an inspiratory volume of 15 ml/kg, which indicates relatively normal lung compliance.

To achieve or maintain such function, fluid restriction may be necessary, especially with respect to crystalloid solutions. Close monitoring of central venous pressure and cautious administration of catecholamines are mandatory, as in cardiac donors. Prolonged artificial ventilation, an FIO_2 that exceeds 0.5 (50%), and PEEP greater than 10 mm Hg should be avoided.

Pulmonary Infection. In view of the risk of nosocomial infections, if mechanical ventilation is used in a brain-dead subject for more than 7 days, the lungs generally cannot be used for transplantation. The chest radiograph should be free of major pulmonary infiltrates, including post-traumatic opacities, which suggest that there are contusion or infection. Minor infiltrates, however, have not precluded donation. Frequent aseptic and thorough endotracheal suction and toilette is mandatory, and a broad-spectrum antibiotic should be administered before the donor undergoes the operation.

The presence of purulent sputum or definite signs of bronchial aspiration at the time of routine pre-explant bronchoscopy are considered to be contraindications to donation; the presence of some pus cells without detectable pathogens on a Gram stain generally will not preclude donation. Postoperative antibiotic treatment must be based on the results of the bacterial culture.

Size Match. In contrast to orthotopic heart transplantation and single-lung transplantation, a close size match between the donor and recipient thoracic cavity is required for heart-lung transplantation because undue compression of the donor lungs within the recipient's thoracic cage will lead to cardiac compression and atelectasis. Although fewer problems result from the use of smaller donor organs, the donor thoracic cavity's dimensions should not be less than 20% of those of the recipient.

To compare the relative sizes of donor and recipient thoracic cavities, simple measurement of weight and height within sex-related transplants will suffice. Some surgeons, however, compare the radiographic dimension of the thorax or measurements of the chests of the donor and the recipient (Hakim et al, 1988). Experience has shown that these techniques are only necessary in pediatric cases and in opposite-gender cardiopulmonary transplantations. In routine adult male-to-male or female-to-female transplantation, the donor should not be more than 5 cm taller or more than 10 cm shorter than the recipient. The limitations of using small-sized organ donors include the necessity to accept a greater size mismatch in the future. In these cases, multiple atypical resections with mechanical staplers or even lobectomy of donor lungs might prevent complications. These techniques have been used successfully in some adult and pediatric lung transplantations (Lillehei et al, 1994; Wisser et al, 1996).

Donor Management. The donor is maintained on a PEEP of 5 cm H_2O with the lowest possible FIO_2 required to maintain a PaO_2 greater than 100 mm Hg. The mean arterial blood pressure is maintained at a minimum of 60 mm Hg. Because most donors have diabetes insipidus, the urinary output is usually excessive. Fluid replacement has to be kept at the minimum necessary to maintain normotension. Following blood volume correction, fluids will be administered to replace those lost by diuresis, but fluid overload must be prevented to avoid overhydration of the donor lungs. Therefore, every effort should be made to maintain a relatively low central venous pressure (approximately 5 cm H_2O). Under these criteria, if an acceptable arterial pressure cannot be maintained, catecholamines (dopamine: maximum dosage 8 μg/kg/min) or vasopressors (norepinephrine and α-adrenergic constrictors) should be administered (Fisher and Alexander, 1992; Okamoto et al, 1992).

Excision of Donor Organs: Surgical Technique. The technique for excising the donor organs is described irrespective of the mode of graft preservation used. In multiorgan donors, the chest is usually opened at the same time as the abdominal surgeons are beginning explantation because this facilitates the dissection of the liver and enables the cardiothoracic surgeon to inspect the heart and lungs.

A median sternotomy is usually preferred. However, a bilateral anterior thoracotomy has also been suggested by Hardesty and Griffith (1985). This practice allows easier dissection of the posterior mediastinum and better control of bleeding in combination with use of extracorporeal circulation and donor cooling for organ procurement. Following a median sternotomy, an anterior longitudinal pericardiotomy is performed, and the heart and aorta are exposed up to the innominate and left carotid arteries (Fig. 37–27). The pericardium, with adjacent pleura, is bilaterally excised. The presence of dense and extensive pleural adhesions usually is a contraindication for using the affected lung for transplantation. The superior vena cava (SVC), inferior vena cava (IVC), ascending aorta, and trachea (between the SVC and aorta) all are mobilized. The ascending aorta is dissected free from the main pulmonary artery. A tape is passed around the ascending aorta; this structure is retracted to the left to expose the trachea. Minimal dissection is carried out around the trachea because it is important to preserve its blood supply through the coronary collaterals.

Two different principles of preservation of the thoracic organs are currently applied for clinical use: simple hypothermic flush perfusion and cooling by extracorporeal circulation, both followed by cold storage. The details are given below. For simple flush perfusion, a 14-French (F) catheter is inserted into the main pulmonary artery, and a cardioplegic infusion line is placed in the ascending aorta. If donor cooling by extracorporeal circulation is preferred, aortic and right atrial cannulation is necessary. Both methods require prior full heparinization (300 IU/kg). For venting of the left heart, the tip of the left atrial appendage may be transsected (flush perfusion) or a vent catheter can be placed into the left atrium through its appendage or the right superior pulmonary vein. The vent catheter can also be placed in the apex of the left ventricle.

Cold (4°C) saline is poured into both pleural cavities

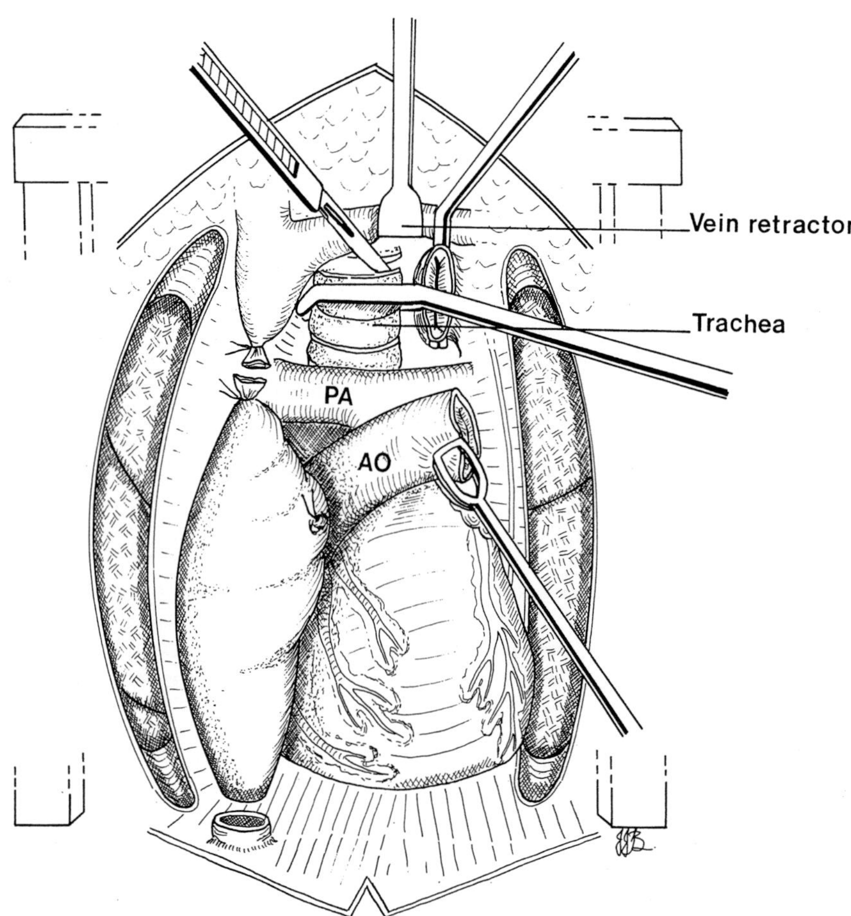

FIGURE 37–27 ■ The ascending aorta has been retracted downward and to the left, exposing the trachea, which has been clamped and divided as high as possible (after withdrawal of the endotracheal tube). (AO, aorta; PA, pulmonary artery.) (From Haverich A: Selection of the donor. In Cooper DKC, Novitzky D [eds]: The Transplantation and Replacement of Thoracic Organs. Dordrecht, The Netherlands, Kluwer Academic Publishers, 1990.)

to cool the lungs, which may or may not be maintained on mechanical ventilation (preferably using unheated room air) during this period. After satisfactory cooling of the organs has been achieved, both caval veins are transsected at the level of the pericardial reflections, the ascending aorta is divided as high as possible, and the trachea is transsected, preserving as much of its length as is available above the carina (see Fig. 37–27) after central closure by a stapled line (remember to pull back the endotracheal tube!). The heart-lung graft is excised en bloc in a craniocaudal direction by dividing the posterior mediastinal tissue anterior to the esophagus and descending aorta (Fig. 37–28). To avoid subsequent post-transplant bleeding in the recipient, electrocautery should be used wherever possible; the inferior pulmonary ligaments should be either stapled or suture ligated. During explantation, the lungs must be handled with maximal care to prevent trauma. Following excision, some surgeons prefer the lungs to remain partially inflated, although others advocate deflation. We prefer partial inflation of the lungs to prevent prolonged post-transplant atelectasis. The heart-lung block is placed in a sterile container or a bag filled with cold (4°C) fluid (blood or Ringer's lactate solution), which in turn is placed in a box of appropriate size that is filled with ice. The organs are then transported to the recipient site.

The alternative to the craniocaudal dissection of the posterior mediastinum is caudocranial explantation. This approach allows for continued intubation of the trachea. In the presence of complete atelectasis, retraction of the heart and lungs is usually much easier. At the end of the procedure, the lungs are reinflated, and the trachea is stapled and dissected above.

Cardiopulmonary Preservation. In the first heart-lung transplants, donor transferral to the transplant center with on-site procurement was felt to be essential. Intensive research resulted in adequate preservation techniques to overcome problems of pulmonary ischemia and reperfusion injury, which allowed for distant organ procurement with several hours of ischemia. Among the many techniques for pulmonary preservation that have been evaluated experimentally and reviewed repeatedly in the literature (Novick et al, 1992; Novick et al, 1996; Unruh, 1995), three methods have emerged and are currently in clinical use. The concept of crystalloid flush perfusion is the method most often used in human lung and heart-lung transplantation (Bando et al, 1989, 1990; Collins et al, 1969; Jurmann et al, 1990; Kennan et al, 1991). The other two modalities include cooling of the lungs with cold blood by either pump oxygenator (Bando et al, 1991; Kontos et al, 1987; Ladowski et al, 1984, 1985; Wahlers et al, 1986) or flush perfusion with cold donor blood (Hakim et al, 1985; Hooper et al, 1990; Jones et al, 1985; Locke et al, 1991). Another alternative, the autoperfusing heart-lung preparation, has been used clinically by only a few groups (Hardesty and Griffith, 1985,

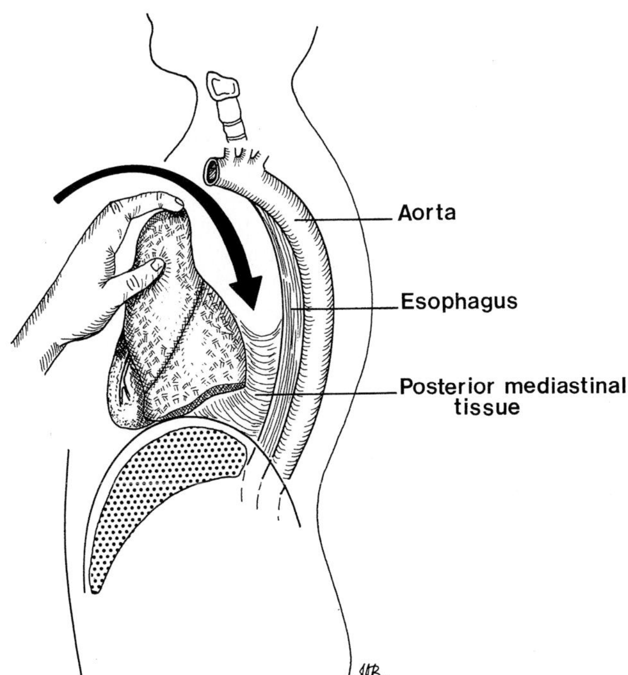

FIGURE 37–28 ■ The plane of the dissection between the heart (and lungs) and posterior mediastinal structures (esophagus and descending aorta) is shown. (From Haverich A: Selection of the donor. In Cooper DKC, Novitzky D [eds]: The Transplantation and Replacement of Thoracic Organs. Dordrecht, The Netherlands, Kluwer Academic Publishers, 1990.)

1987; Miyamoto et al, 1987; Robicsek et al, 1967, 1985) and is now practically abandoned.

Hypothermic Flush Perfusion with Crystalloid Solutions. Hypothermic flush perfusion has been the basis of preservation of solid organs for the purpose of transplantation. Thus, most renal, hepatic, and cardiac allografts are harvested using simple perfusion with a crystalloid solution followed by cold storage. Although numerous biochemical compositions have been suggested for this purpose, buffered solutions with an intracellular ionic composition (high in K^+ and low in Na^+) and slightly increased osmolarity compared with serum, such as the Euro-Collins solution or University of Wisconsin solution, are preferred by many centers. Additionally, an extracellular type solution combined with a nondiffusible colloid (low-potassium dextran solution) has been used clinically after promising results in the laboratory (Hausen et al, 1997; Sakamaki et al, 1997). The ease of application and satisfactory graft function represent the chief advantages of high volume–low pressure crystalloid flush perfusion of the lungs. Euro-Collins solution, modified by the addition of magnesium sulfate and glucose, is most widely used and is administered into the main pulmonary artery following aortic cross-clamping. For this purpose, a 14-F cannula is inserted into the main pulmonary artery. It is advisable to measure the pulmonary artery pressure during perfusion. The pressure should be kept above 15 mm Hg but to facilitate the even distribution of the perfusate within both lungs it should not exceed 25 mm Hg. For the same purpose, pretreatment of the donor using a prostaglandin analog, such as PGE_1 or PGI_2, is used by many centers (Bonser et al, 1990, 1991; Moncada, 1982). In our practice, PGI_2 is given intravenously immediately prior to flush perfusion (500 to 1000 mg until the systolic arterial pressure falls by 30 mm Hg). In addition, PGI_2 may be added to the flush perfusate (50–100 mg/L). Cardiac arrest is performed following standard heart transplantation protocol (University of Wisconsin solution in our center).

Hypothermic Flush Perfusion with Blood. During procurement, the lungs may also be flushed with third-party donor blood, as advocated by the Cambridge group (Hakim et al, 1985; Jones et al, 1985). This approach may be as simple to perform as single crystalloid flush with respect to the technical and instrumental requirement and has also resulted in a predictably adequate lung function after transplantation.

Cooling by Extracorporeal Circulation. This mode of preservation for heart-lung transplantation was first described experimentally in 1984 (Ladowski et al, 1984). It is now used by a number of transplant centers around the world. The major drawback of this technique is the need to transport a relatively large amount of equipment to the donor center. A roller pump, perfusion circuits, heat exchanger, and oxygenator constitute the minimum requirements for this purpose. Also, there is good experimental evidence of a reduced post-transplant gas exchange by lungs preserved with extracorporeal circulation compared with those undergoing flush perfusion with Euro-Collins solution. The pulmonary vasculature, in contrast, however, may be better preserved with the former method (Locke et al, 1991; Wahlers et al, 1986).

Both simple hypothermic flush and extracorporeal circulation offer simple and relatively efficient modes of pulmonary preservation. Heart and lung ischemic intervals of up to 3 to 4 hours have been shown to be safe with either method (Feeley et al, 1986), although the typical reimplantation response (vide infra) may still occur on occasion.

Operative Technique

The induction of anesthesia includes oral tracheal intubation, placement of a peripheral arterial line, one or two central venous lines, a peripheral venous line, and a urinary catheter (Sale et al, 1987). A peripheral oxymetric probe (finger tip) and rectal and nasopharyngeal temperature probes are also applied. The patient is then placed in a supine position, and a median sternotomy is performed. Alternatively, a clamshell approach has been used with good results facilitating exposure to pleural cavities in patients who had several previous operations (Luciani et al, 1997). Following division of the thymus, the left innominate vein is exposed, and the pericardium is opened in the midline. This incision is extended caudally in a Y shape. Four pericardial stay sutures are placed. The ascending aorta is mobilized from the pulmonary arterial trunk and the right pulmonary artery. Purse-string sutures are placed in the aortic arch opposite the origin of the brachiocephalic artery. Following heparinization, the ascending aorta is cannulated. For venous return, two purse-string sutures are placed posteriorly in the right atrium just above the interatrial sulcus. The SVC and IVC cannulas are inserted, and cardiopulmonary bypass is initiated. The rectal temperature is reduced to 28°C. While cooling proceeds and with the heart empty, both the IVC and the SVC are exposed, encircled with tapes, and snared for the total cardiopulmonary bypass. The aorta is cross-clamped proximal to the aortic cannula (Fig. 37–29).

Cardiectomy is first performed on the atrial level. The right and left atrium are divided close to the atrioventricular groove, leaving sufficient remnants of the left and especially the right atrial wall. For this purpose, the right atrium is incised first at its lateral aspect with the appendage included in the tissue that is removed. The interatrial septum is incised at the foramen ovale. The left atrial free wall is transsected along the coronary sinus, and the apex of the heart is lifted anteriorly and to the right. The great vessels are divided at approximately 2 cm above the semilunar valves (leaving the opportunity to harvest them as homografts) (see Fig. 37–29).

Following cardiectomy, the remnant of the pulmonary trunk is divided in the midline, separating the left and right main pulmonary arteries. This incision is extended posteriorly into the pericardium and downward until the posterior remnants of the left atrium are reached. These are also divided in the midline, including the underlying posterior pericardium. The atrial cuffs, including the attached pericardium, are further mobilized on both sides as far as possible toward the pulmonary hilum, taking care not to injure the vagus nerves at this level. Blood vessels arising from the posterior mediastinum are ligated or clipped.

Further dissection of the pulmonary artery includes full mobilization toward the lung hilum on both sides. On the left side, this is done by also excising a "button" that carries the ductus ligament, which is left in place (recurrent nerve!). On the right side, dissection of the right pulmonary artery includes its portion behind the aorta and the SVC.

The operative field now allows for a left-sided pneumonectomy (Fig. 37–30). In preparation for this, the anterior portion of the pericardium on the left is excised, including the anterior pleura. A pedicle of the pericardium carrying the phrenic nerve is left behind by a careful incision that is 3 cm anterior and posterior to the nerve from the pulmonary artery to the diaphragm. The left lung is mobilized; the pulmonary ligament is divided, with all bleeding carefully controlled; and the posterior portion of the hilum is dissected sharply close to the parenchyma of the lung. This dissection is carried out with careful control of collateral vessels until both the pulmonary artery and the remnants of the left atrium (including the adjacent pericardium) can be mobilized toward the pleural space. Then, again with careful control of bleeding, the left main bronchus is dissected free, closed by stapling, and divided distally. The left lung is then removed from the operating field.

On the right, the anterior pleura is opened from the brachiocephalic vein to the diaphragm. With careful visualization of the right-sided phrenic nerve, the pericardium is incised 3 cm anterior to the nerve from the pulmonary artery toward the diaphragm. Here, the anterior portion of the pericardium is divided at the diaphragm but left attached proximally as a pedicle. Again under constant visualization of the phrenic nerve, the pericardium is incised dorsally to the nerve in close proximity to the right hilar structures. This incision is made from the azygos vein to the diaphragm. No electrocautery should be used at this point; instead, bleeding

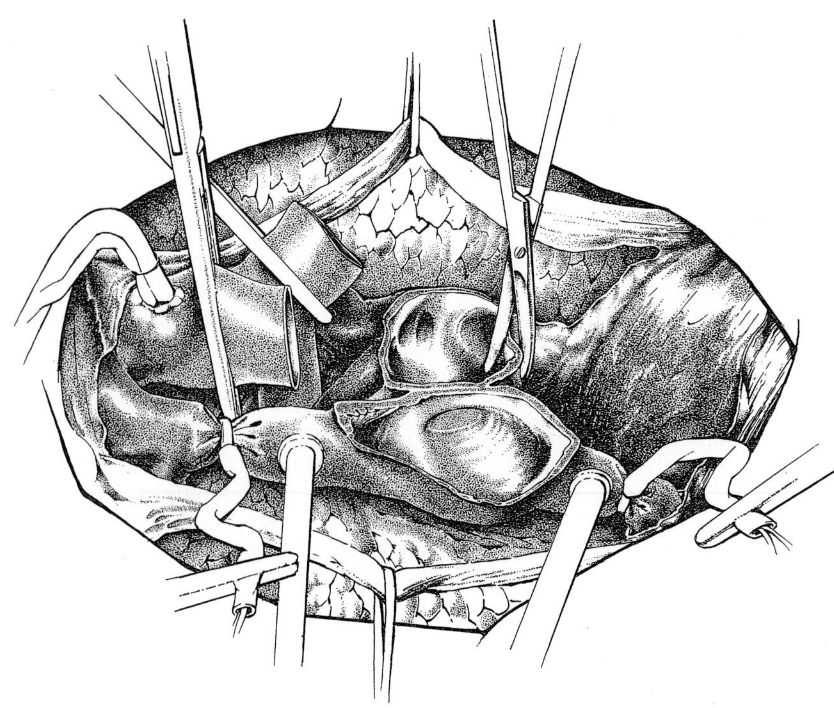

FIGURE 37–29 ■ Operative view following explantation of the recipient's heart during heart-lung transplantation. Both phrenic nerves are isolated, including a pericardial flap. Both the aorta and the pulmonary artery are cross-clamped. To further mobilize both lungs, the dorsal remnant of the left atrium is transsected between left and right pulmonary veins. (From Haverich A: Herz und Herz-Lungen Transplantation. In Borst HG, Klinner W, Oelert H [eds]: Herzchirurgie. Berlin, Springer-Verlag, 1991.)

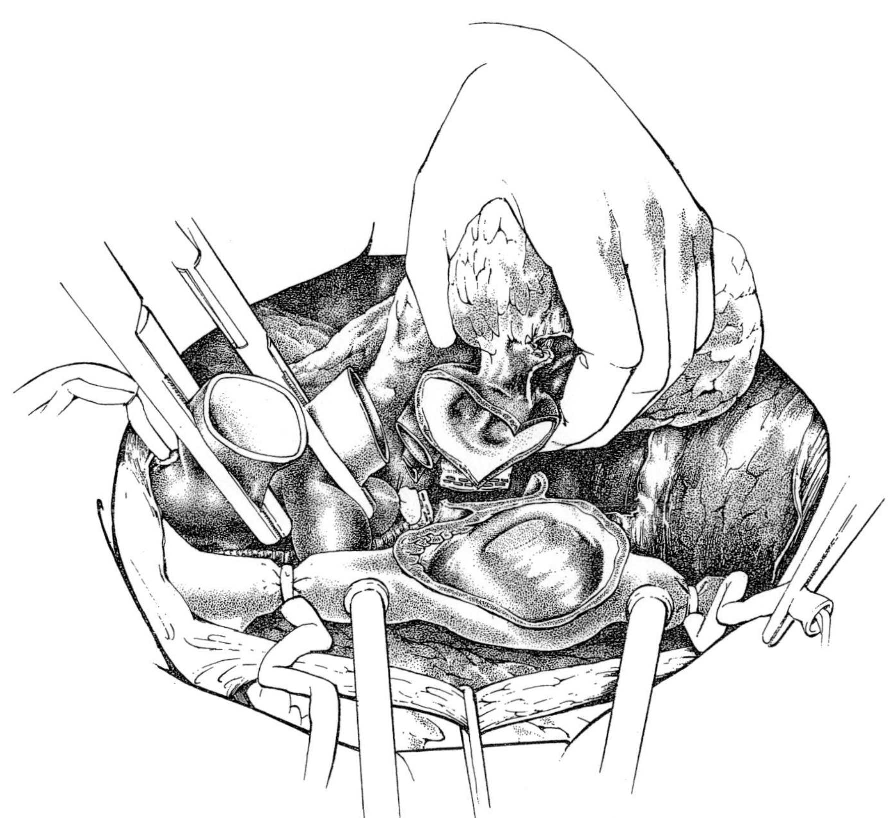

FIGURE 37–30 ■ Following separation of the remnants of the left atrium and transsection of the left pulmonary artery and bronchus, the left recipient lung is removed. (From Haverich A: Herz und Herz-Lungen Transplantation. In Borst HG, Klinner W, Oelert H [eds]: Herzchirurgie. Berlin, Springer-Verlag, 1991.)

vessels are either clipped or ligated. An incision is made posterior to the interatrial groove (as in mitral valve replacement). With careful attention not to injure the SVC or IVC, this incision is directed posteriorly beneath the IVC until the right-sided remnants of the left atrium can be mobilized toward the right pleura. Mobilization of the right lung is carried out according to the technique used on the left, followed by the stapling and the division of the bronchus and removal of the right lung.

At this point, careful bleeding control in the posterior mediastinum should be secured with close attention to the course of both vagus nerves. When the bleeding has been controlled, the remnants of both main bronchi are grasped with Allis clamps and pulled caudally. With the aorta retracted to the left, further dissection of the tracheal carina is performed, carefully preserving the surrounding collateral-rich tissue. The trachea is then divided exactly one cartilage ring cephalad to the carina. Again, bleeding must be controlled because this area will be inaccessible after implantation of the donor organs (Fig. 37–31).

The donor organs are brought to the surgical field with the trachea still closed by a row of staples or by a clamp. The trachea is divided one or two cartilage rings proximal to the carina. In doing so, the trachea should be dissected only in the area where the final division takes place. Mucus secretions are aspirated from both main bronchi. The suction device is then discarded to prevent subsequent contamination of the surgical field. The secretions are collected for bacteriologic culture.

Now the heart-lung block is transferred into the recipient's chest. The left lung is introduced into the left pleura cavity by passing it posteriorly to the phrenic nerve, and the right lung is passed posteriorly to both the right atrial cuff and the phrenic nerve (Fig. 37–32). Proper positioning of the lungs at this stage is ensured by identifying each lung separately and excluding rotation of the organs. Cold laparotomy pads are applied over the heart and lungs to prevent rewarming.

A stay suture (3–0 polydioxanone [PDS]) is placed on each side of the recipient's trachea at the junction of the membranous and the cartilaginous portions. Additional sutures are passed through corresponding points of the recipient's trachea. The tracheal suture line can be accomplished by several different techniques. Our preference is described. A single running suture, 4–0 PDS, is used for the posterior (membranous) part of the trachea (see Fig. 37–32). Both stay sutures also are tied down at this stage. The cartilaginous part is anastomosed with single 3–0 PDS sutures, which are tied outside the trachea. A total of six to eight of these sutures is required. Two- to 3-mm bites of trachea spaced at similar intervals are thought to be adequate. The anastomosis is then tested under saline to rule out the presence of air leaks. We test the anastomosis to a maximum airway pressure of 20 cm H_2O.

It has been our preference to seal this anastomosis with a mixture of antibiotics and fibrin adhesive (Haverich et al, 1989). For this purpose, 2 ml of fibrinogen (component I) and a mixture of neomycin and bacitracin (Nebacetin) and thrombin solution (component II) are applied circumferentially around the tracheal anastomosis. Then the right-sided pericardial patch is passed coun-

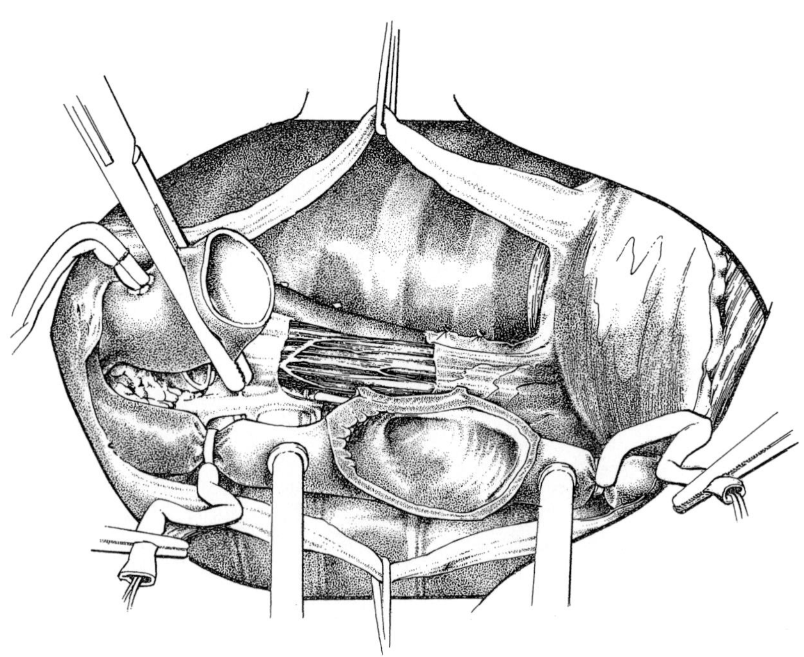

FIGURE 37–31 ■ Operative view following complete resection of the recipient heart-lung, including the main pulmonary artery and the tracheal carina. (From Haverich A: Herz und Herz-Lungen Transplantation. In Borst HG, Klinner W, Oelert H [eds]: Herzchirurgie. Berlin, Springer-Verlag, 1991.)

terclockwise around this anastomosis and again is secured with fibrin sealant and two stay sutures, one on the left and one on the right of the trachea.

The preparation for the right atrial anastomosis includes an oblique incision of the donor atrium from the lateral aspect of the IVC orifice toward the right atrial appendage to preserve the sulcus terminalis and the sinus node (Fig. 37–33). A patent foramen ovale in the recipient can be closed at this stage.

In the presence of a very thin interatrial septum or in cases with an atrial septal defect, the posterior wall of the right-sided left atrium may be pulled through behind the right atrium and serve as a reinforcement for the left lateral aspect of the right atrial suture line.

The right atrial anastomosis is accomplished with a continuous double-armed 3–0 polypropylene suture, starting at the midpoint of the medial wall of both right atria and corresponding to the remnant of the atrial

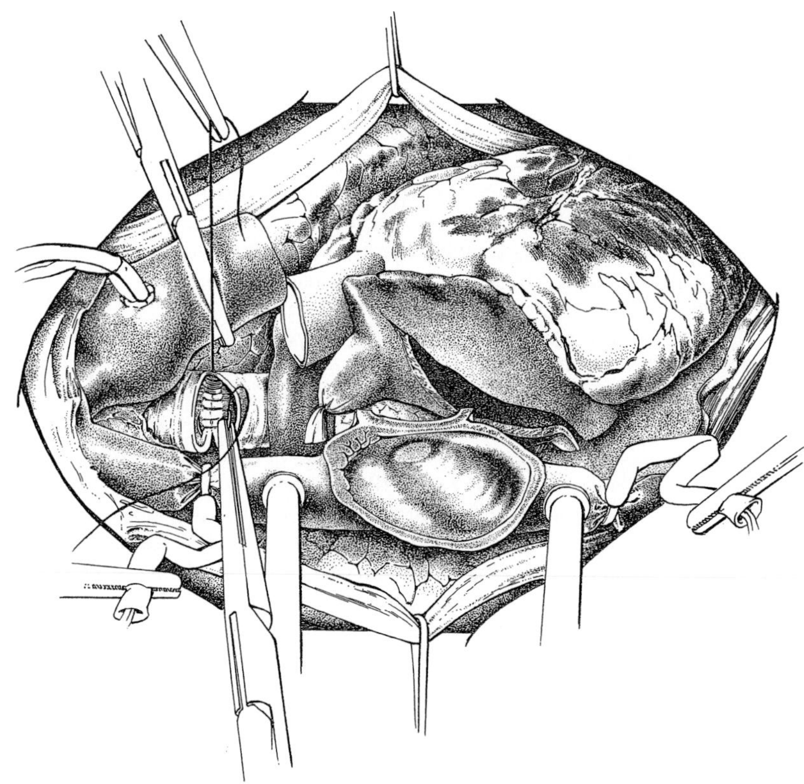

FIGURE 37–32 ■ Implantation of the donor organs is initiated by end-to-end anastomosis of donor and recipient trachea. (From Haverich A: Herz und Herz-Lungen Transplantation. In Borst HG, Klinner W, Oelert H [eds]: Herzchirurgie. Berlin, Springer-Verlag, 1991.)

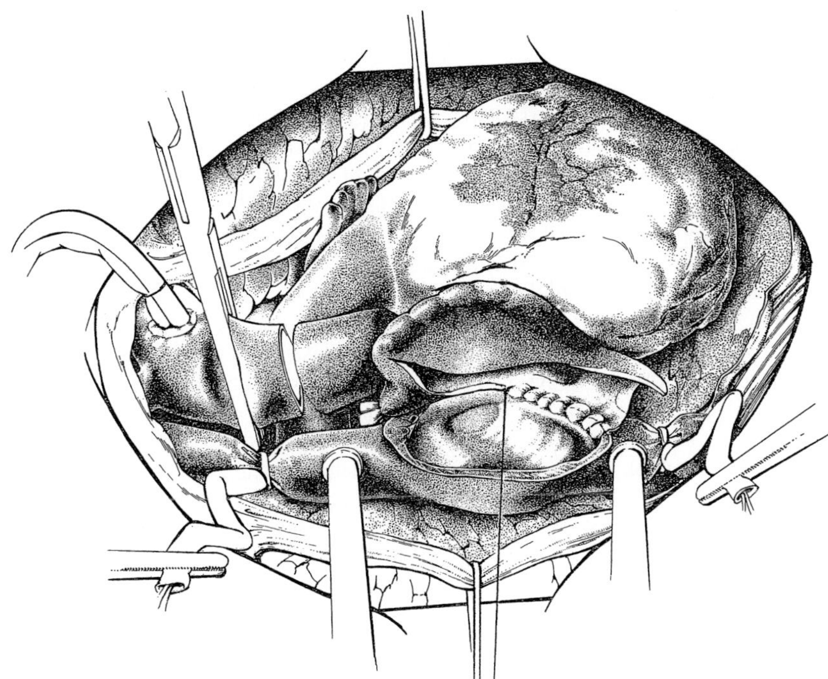

FIGURE 37–33 ■ Side-to-side anastomosis between donor and recipient right atrium using running 3–0 polypropylene suture. The stumps of donor and recipient aorta have not been connected. (From Haverich A: Herz und Herz-Lungen Transplantation. In Borst HG, Klinner W, Oelert H [eds]: Herzchirurgie. Berlin, Springer-Verlag, 1991.)

septum on the recipient side. The right atrial suture line is continued first toward, then around, the IVC, and finally cranially. If necessary, the incision in the donor right atrial wall can be lengthened to match the orifice of the recipient's right atrium. Thereafter, the sutures are carried along the lateral wall of the right atrium. They are tied only after de-airing the right heart (see later). Prior to construction of the aortic suture line, the lengths of the donor and recipient vessels are assessed, and the excess tissue is trimmed from one or both ends. An end-to-end anastomosis is constructed with a continuous double-armed 4–0 polypropylene suture, which is terminated at the most superior aspect of the suture line to allow for de-airing.

Before reperfusion of the heart and lungs, de-airing is performed through the right atrial suture line following the release of SVC and IVC snares. The pulmonary artery is stabbed with a large-bore needle. Ventilation is begun with the venous line of the extracorporeal circulation partially occluded to allow for filling of the pulmonary vasculature. Prior to release of the aortic cross-clamp, the ascending aorta and the apex of the left ventricle are stabbed, and any remaining air is removed by manual compression of the heart.

In many instances, the heart has to be electrically defibrillated. Temporary ventricular pacing may be required at this stage. Also, the "washout phenomenon" of the pulmonoplegic solution results in transient hyperkalemic effects when the coronary arteries are perfused with blood returning through the left atrium. The administration of calcium and catecholamines results in the restoration of normal sinus rhythm, usually within 15 minutes.

During rewarming, ventilation is maintained with 50% oxygen to avoid undue release of oxygen-free radicals from the lung tissue. Following stabilization of cardiac and pulmonary function, the patient can be weaned from extracorporeal circulation, usually after 30 minutes of reperfusion. At this stage, a PEEP of 6 cm H_2O should be maintained, and continuous spontaneous de-airing of the left heart through the ascending aorta should be allowed. Following decannulation of the aorta and the right atrium and bleeding control, two pleural chest tubes are inserted into each side, one to drain the apical portion of each pleura and the second to drain the costophrenic sinus. Normally, no mediastinal tubes are inserted. The sternal incision is closed in a routine fashion. Modifications and simplifications of the standard operative technique have been reported in the literature with limitation of hilar dissection and placement of the heart-lung block anteriorly to the phrenic nerves (Icenogle et al, 1995; Lick et al, 1995).

Perioperative Care

Intensive Care Unit

In general, the postoperative care of heart-lung transplant recipients in the intensive care unit does not differ significantly from that of other patients after major cardiac or thoracic interventions. The cardiac status is usually characterized by a high cardiac output at heart rates between 120 and 140 beats/min because of the denervation of the heart. Right and left ventricular function, unlike the situation after cardiac transplantation, is usually normal, and the requirement for inotropic support is minimal. In cases with doubtful cardiac status, a Swan-Ganz catheter is readily inserted to assess pulmonary artery pressure, cardiac output, and pulmonary capillary wedge pressure. The most common form of circulatory insufficiency in our heart-lung transplant patients has been high-output failure from low peripheral vascular resistance, especially in patients who had preoperative hepatic insufficiency. This situation requires vasoconstrictor therapy.

Pulmonary function usually is adequate; thus, routine postoperative respiratory therapy may be commenced (McGoldrick et al, 1989). This includes ventilatory settings with an FiO_2 greater than 0.5 and a PEEP of 6 to 10 mm Hg. At frequent intervals, arterial gas samples should be taken to ensure an arterial oxygen saturation that is greater than 95%. In rare cases with profound reperfusion injury, a higher FiO_2 may be required for variable time spans. In such cases, vigorous bronchial toilette by frequent endobronchial suction may be required for pulmonary edema. Extubation may be initiated at FiO_2 of 0.3 or less, when the patient is fully awake, cooperative, and able to cough with sufficient strength.

The chest tubes, initially connected to an underwater seal with a negative pressure of −15 to − 20 cm H_2O, should be left in place for at least 5 days because small air leaks may persist or develop, and the transplanted lungs could produce fluid secretions because of the lack of lymphatic channels (as much as 500 to 1000 ml/day).

Reversed isolation used to be the standard care regimen for heart-lung transplant recipients until 1990. Since then, a number of reports have demonstrated no significant differences regarding infectious episodes among those patients with and those without isolation procedures in the intensive care unit. Therefore, at our unit, one-to-one nursing and frequent changes of (nonsterile) gloves represent the only specific measures for organizational infectious prophylaxis after thoracic organ transplantation.

Immunosuppression

Standard immunosuppression has been based on cyclosporine, azathioprine, and prednisolone. Use of cytolytic induction therapy using antithymocyte globulin (ATG; Biotest Diagnostics Corp., Denville, NJ) is limited to the discretion of the surgeon, but is mostly used in patients with significant renal dysfunction. Intravenous cyclosporine is usually administered within 6 hours postoperatively. The initial dose (1 mg/kg) is increased within the following 1 to 2 weeks up to 10 mg/kg depending on renal and hepatic function. Cyclosporine serum levels (monoclonal assay) are aimed at 220 to 300 ng/ml for the first year with reduction to 150 to 200 ng/ml for the following years. Patients also recieve 1 to 2 mg/kg azathioprine with a target white blood cell count of 4000 cells/mm^3 or greater. Prednisolone (1000 mg IV) is administered intraoperatively followed by 3 doses of 250 mg at 12-hour intervals. Prednisolone maintenance therapy is started on the second postoperative day (initially 0.5 mg/kg and tapered to 0.07 mg/kg within 1 year). Recently, tacrolimus and mycophenolate mofetil are assessed in clinical studies for de novo immunosuppression in thoracic organ transplantation either alone or in combination. Additional new immunosuppressants (e.g., rapamycin, leflunomide) await further experimental and clinical evaluation and have the potential to change the immunosuppressive strategy after heart-lung transplantation significantly in the future (Hausen et al, 1997).

Infection Prophylaxis and Therapy

Pulmonary infections represent the most common complication in allograft recipients (Hosenpud et al, 1998). Colonization of the donor lungs as well as the recipient proximal airways, decreased lung defenses (depressed cough reflex, reduced mucociliary clearance, lymphatic disruption), and newly acquired infections together with immunosuppression increase the risk of intrathoracic infection significantly. Bacterial pneumonia accounts for the majority of all infectious episodes with the highest incidence in the first month after transplantation. *Pseudomonas aeruginosa* and other gram-negative bacteria as well as *Staphylococcus* species represent the predominating pathogens (Bando et al, 1995b; Chan et al, 1996; Kramer et al, 1993). Furthermore, CMV infection, toxoplasmosis, and tuberculosis may be transferred by the donor lung, potentially resulting in severe illness if reactivated in the recipient (Hutter et al, 1989). Particularly, transplantation of CMV-positive donor lungs in CMV-negative recipients carries a risk of 71% for CMV infection or disease, typically detected between 3 weeks and 2 months after transplantation (Paradis and Williams, 1993). Manifestation of CMV disease affects the gastrointestinal tract and, more commonly, the lungs. CMV pneumonitis represents a diagnostic dilemma because it mimics acute pulmonary allograft rejection clinically and radiologically, and transbronchial biopsy is often required to demarcate viral infection from acute rejection. The major impact of CMV disease on morbidity and mortality after heart-lung transplantation as well as the possible correlation between obliterative bronchiolitis and CMV infection requires aggressive antiviral treatment with or without immunoglobulin when viremia is present, or in case of CMV mismatch (Duncan et al, 1991; Kroshus et al, 1997; Smith et al, 1996; Soghikian et al, 1996).

Among fungal infections *Aspergillus* and *Candida* represent the most prevalent organisms. High mortality rates with disseminated invasive aspergillosis have led to routine administration of itraconazole as well as aerolized amphotericin after heart-lung transplantation.

Contamination of the operative field in heart-lung transplantation as a result of tracheal transsection can aggravate impaired airway healing with stenosis or disruption of the tracheal anastomosis as well as rupture of the ascending aortic suture line mainly caused by *Pseudomonas, Aspergillus*, and *Candida* infections (Cassart et al, 1994; Colquhuon et al, 1994; Dowling et al, 1990). In general, airway complications are less frequent in heart-lung transplantation than they are in isolated lung transplantation because of the preserved collateral circulation from coronary arteries (Higgins et al, 1994).

With increasing experience, our institution has developed a sophisticated protocol of primary and secondary antimicrobial prophylaxis (Table 37–2). This regimen may not be applicable to all transplant units and may be adapted to local pharmacologic preferences or the endemic microbial environment.

The details of therapy and the huge variety of potential bacterial, viral, protozoal, and fungal infections that may be identified in the postoperative course after heart-lung transplantation, including their management, are beyond

TABLE 37–2 ■ **Antimicrobial Prophylaxis in Heart-Lung Transplantation**

Type of Infection	*Primary Prophylaxis*	*Secondary Prophylaxis (Positive Culture, No Clinical Signs of Infection)*
Viral		
Herpes simplex	Acyclovir	Acyclovir
Cytomegalovirus	Hyperimmune globulin	Ganciclovir
Bacterial	Cefazolin (48 hr) Cefotaxime/ tobramycin (5 days)	According to antibiogram
Tuberculosis	Isoniazid (6 mo)	
Candida albicans	—	Fluconazole or itraconazole
Aspergillus	—	Itraconazole
Pneumocystis	Cotrimoxazole (twice weekly)	Continue therapy

the scope of this chapter. Any suspected infection must result in prompt investigation by radiography, serology, and bronchoscopy with bronchoalveolar lavage. During the first 6 months after transplantation, we recommend immediate administration of a broad-spectrum antibiotic following bronchoalveolar lavage in cases with clinical signs of infection. The therapy is then modified after the infecting organism has been identified. Expedient exclusion of pulmonary infection is especially important because pulmonary rejection represents one differential diagnosis.

Other Prophylactic Measures

When the patient is able to leave the room, he or she should wear a mask and gloves while ambulatory in the hospital. Mobilization outside the room by regular bicycle exercise is allowed, even if supplemental oxygen is required or the chest tubes still are in place. Intensive physical therapy, including regular postural drainage, is maintained, and patients are later taught to manage their own airway clearance.

Diagnosis and Therapy for Rejection

Acute. Acute allograft rejection after heart-lung transplantation focuses primarily on the lungs and is as difficult to diagnose in heart-lung transplantation as it is in isolated lung transplantation. The transplanted heart is protected from acute rejection in this setting, and it usually does not reject at all or only subsequent to rejection of the lungs (Cooper et al, 1986; Novitzky et al, 1986; Prop et al, 1987; Sarris et al, 1994). Routine endomyocardial biopsy, therefore, has been abandoned from the surveillance protocols in most heart-lung transplant centers (Baldwin et al, 1987; Higenbottam et al, 1988; Husain et al, 1996; Madden et al, 1992; Sarris et al, 1994). Instead, all diagnostic measures must concentrate on the pulmonary grafts. As such, fever, a low peripheral oxygen saturation, a reduced vital capacity, and especially a diminished forced expiratory volume in one second (FEV_1) with an obstructive pattern on airflow analysis, are suggestive of pulmonary rejection (Otulana et al, 1990; Trulock, 1993a; van Muylem et al, 1997). Often, a "hilar flare" occurring around day 9 after transplantation represents the first sign of pulmonary rejection. The radiologic signs, however, may be less impressive in acute rejection episodes that occur later in the postoperative course (Millet et al, 1989). Clinical, radiologic, and physiologic criteria do not allow differentiation between rejection and infection. Therefore, many centers perform transbronchial biopsies on a routine basis early after transplantation or during any episode that may herald lung rejection (Guilinger et al, 1995; Kukafka et al, 1997; Scott et al, 1991; Starnes et al, 1989). Rejection monitoring by routine surveillance lung biopsies is currently discussed controversially and has not proved helpful in the management of stable asymptomatic patients more than 2 years after transplantation (Girgis et al, 1995; Kesten et al, 1996; Trulock, 1993). In our institution, routine transbronchial biopsy has achieved a low sensitivity and specificity of the histologic findings in the specimens and very little impact on patient treatment (Sibley et al, 1993). We therefore perform only standard bronchoscopy and alveolar lavage as routine surveillance protocol and to exclude infection in patients with clinical and functional signs of pulmonary deterioration.

During bronchoscopy, the complete airway, including the tracheal anastomosis, is carefully inspected. Unlike purulent bacterial infections, acutely rejecting lungs often exude small amounts of ubiquitous, non-liquid, whitish secretions. The material obtained by bronchoalveolar lavage is analyzed for bacterial and viral organisms and fungi. In patients who are in poor clinical condition and in whom pulmonary infection is unlikely, methylprednisolone is initiated immediately after bronchoscopy. Otherwise, the therapy is withheld until the Gram stain and CMV early antigen test results are available to exclude an infectious episode as the cause of pulmonary deterioration.

In the presence of rejection, 1 g IV of methylprednisolone is given per day for 3 consecutive days. Only recipients with severe rejection refractory to steroids are subsequently treated by anti–T cell antibodies such as rabbit or horse antithymocyte globulin. Concomitant with this therapy, infectious prophylaxis is intensified with antibiotics (e.g., cephalosporins) and anti-CMV hyperimmune globulin.

Chronic. Bronchiolitis obliterans syndrome (BOS) represents the clinical entity of lung allograft dysfunction with the obstructive physiology that is considered to reflect chronic rejection. Histologically, bronchiolitis obliterans—a diffuse, concentric, luminal narrowing of the terminal bronchioli—is the characteristic finding, but it is not mandatory in establishing the diagnosis (Cooper et al, 1993; Reichenspurner et al, 1996). Currently, BOS represents the main obstacle to long-term function of allografts after lung and heart-lung replacement (Hosenpud et al, 1998; Sundaresan et al, 1995; Valentine et al, 1996a). Clinically, BOS is characterized by a progressive loss of vital capacity and FEV_1 with an obstructive airflow pattern that ultimately leads to impaired gas exchange and death from respiratory failure. Frequent acute rejection episodes were identified as the most significant risk factor for development of BOS in several reports (Bando et al, 1995a; Keller et al, 1995; Reichenspurner et al, 1996; Sharples et al, 1996). CMV pneumonitis may be a predisposition for BOS but its significance is still discussed controversially (Kroshus et al, 1997; Smith et al, 1996; Trulock, 1993). A possible mechanism of CMV infection for BOS development is the induced upregulation of major histocompatibility complex (MHC) class II antigens in the transplanted lungs, making them more prone to acute rejection episodes (You et al, 1996). Preventive measures other than aggressive treatment of acute rejection episodes and CMV pneumonitis and, probably, CMV prophylaxis are not evident (Hertz et al, 1998; Soghikian et al, 1996; Trulock, 1997). Once BOS is diagnosed, augmentation and modification of basic immunosuppression is empirically performed by most transplant centers including corticosteroids, polyclonal and monoclonal antibodies, methotrexate, tacrolimus, mycophenolic acid, aerolized cyclosporine and total lymphoid irradiation with modest and often transient improvement of lung function (Dusmet et al, 1996; Iacono et al, 1996; Kesten et al, 1997; Valentine et al, 1996b; Whyte et al, 1997). Retransplantation may ultimately represent the last option for selected patients, although survival results are significantly lower than they are in first-time transplants (Adams et al, 1994; Novick et al, 1992). Unlike single-lung transplantation, en bloc transplantation seems to protect the heart against the development of transplant vasculopathy, which is defined as those changes in coronary arteries that are considered to represent chronic rejection (Lim et al, 1996). In the Stanford series, freedom from transplant vasculopathy was 100%, 90%, and 66% after 1, 5, and 10 years, respectively (Sarris et al, 1994).

EARLY RESULTS

Data on 30-day mortality rates are available, both from the registry of the International Society for Heart and Lung Transplantation (ISHLT) (Hosenpud et al, 1998) and from single-center studies (Conte et al, 1996; Sarris et al, 1994). Prior to 1986, the 30-day mortality rate was reported to be about 30% worldwide (Reitz, 1982a). Since then, significant improvement has been seen with mortality rates of about 10% to 15%. Actuarial 1- and 5-year survival in 2427 patients who were registered in the database of the ISHLT were 60% and 40%, respectively. The main cause of early death was bleeding and pulmonary failure. With improved techniques of donor lung preservation, pulmonary failure appears to be substantially reduced. Bleeding complications can be significantly reduced with improved surgical technique and the use of aprotinin during the operation. Risk factor analysis for 1-year mortality in this patient group revealed retransplantation, a center volume of fewer than five transplants per year, and older donor age as significant predictors for poor patient outcome.

In our experience with 46 heart-lung transplants, no early deaths were related to pulmonary failure or bleeding. In fact, with the routine use of aprotinin from the start of our program, no reoperation for bleeding control has been necessary. Infection, the second most important risk factor for early death, will probably continue to be the major cause of death (Brooks et al, 1985). Improved management of heart-lung transplant recipients in terms of prophylaxis of infection type and the dosing of immunosuppressive therapy will be necessary to allow for improved early survival rates.

LATE RESULTS

At present, 60% of heart-lung transplant recipients live 12 months postoperatively. Much better results than those reported by the ISHLT registry have been obtained in some single-center studies. A 1-year survival rate of 80% has been reported (Scott et al, 1988), which matches our results of a 1-year survival rate of 78% (Harringer et al, 1999). Therefore, 1-year success rates of 80% or more should be obtainable in the future.

Beyond the first 12 months, the death rate after heart-lung transplantation appears to be twice as high as that after heart transplantation alone. Late death occurs at an annual rate of 5%, for a 5-year survival rate of 40% (Hosenpud et al, 1998). This high rate of late lethal complications is also evident by the survival data after single- and double-lung transplantations. Infection and obliterative bronchiolitis are the main causes of mortality beyond 1 year. Compared with the magnitude of these problems, other causes of late death play minor roles and occur at comparable incidence with other organ transplantations.

COMMENTS AND CONTROVERSIES

During the past 10 years, pulmonary allografting has undergone major changes. The limited availability of heart and lungs for en bloc transplantation has resulted in a worldwide stagnate number of operations. The simultaneous increase in surgical activities with respect to isolated lung grafting limits the application of combined cardiopulmonary transplantation to patients with truly irreversible pulmonary and cardiac failure, including those with uncorrectable congenital cardiac anomalies. All other disorders, including pulmonary hypertension of various causes and Eisenmenger's syndrome, will probably continue to be treated by lung transplantation alone. Available single-center results indicate that double-lung transplantation rather than single-lung transplantation represents the more successful approach in such patients. Early and late consequences of the "programmed" ventilation/perfusion mismatch in single-lung transplantation in severe pulmonary hypertension probably will induce a change in favor of double-lung transplantation.

The major impediment to true long-term survival after any type of allogeneic lung replacement and, in fact, any organ transplantation, remains chronic rejection. The high incidence of obliterative bronchiolitis after the first year after transplantation must encourage intensive research to obviate its development or to formulate new regimens of drug therapy. Improved selection of donor/recipient pairs on immunologic grounds by HLA matching appears to be the sole prophylactic measure against chronic rejection. After the diagnosis of obliterative bronchiolitis is made, increased immunosuppression using currently available drugs has repeatedly resulted in a standstill of the course of the disease. True control of this complication in terms of restoration of normal lung function parameters, however, has not been achieved but is the most important aspect of further research in this field.

A. H.
W. H.

■ KEY REFERENCES

Haverich A: Experience with lung transplantation. Ann Thorac Surg 67:305, 1999.

A single-center experience with 283 lung and heart-lung transplantations is provided. Changes and developments in the Hannover lung transplantation program during the last decade are covered.

Lim TT, Botas J, Ross H et al: Are heart-lung transplant recipients protected from developing transplant coronary artery disease? A case-matched intracoronary ultrasound study. Circulation 94:1573, 1996.

The incidence of coronary transplant vasculopathy detected by coronary intravascular ultrasound is determined in 22 heart-lung transplant patients and compared with a case-matched group of heart transplant patients. The incidence and severity of transplant coronary artery disease are fewer and less in patients receiving heart-lung transplants than in those receiving heart transplants alone.

Sarris GE, Smith JA, Shumway NE et al: Long-term results of combined heart-lung transplantation: The Stanford experience. J Heart Lung Transplant 13:940, 1994.

This report summarizes the Stanford experience in 109 patients who underwent heart-lung transplantation. A description of operative techniques and immunosuppressive protocol as well as a detailed analysis of complications and outcome is provided.

Sharples LD, Tamm M, McNeil K et al: Development of bronchiolitis obliterans syndrome in recipients of heart-lung transplantation: Early risk factors. Transplantation 61:560, 1996.

Incidence and risk factors in 126 6-month survivors after heart-lung transplantation at Papworth Hospital are analyzed in this article. The number of acute rejection episodes is the single most important determinant for development and progression of bronchiolitis obliterans syndrome.

■ REFERENCES

Adams DH, Cochrane AD, Khaghani A et al: Retransplantation in heart-lung recipients with obliterative bronchiolitis. J Thorac Cardiovasc Surg 107:450, 1994.

Baldwin JC, Oyer PE, Stinson EB et al: Comparison of cardiac rejection in heart and heart-lung transplantation. J Heart Lung Transplant 6:352, 1987.

Bando K, Armitage JM, Paradis IL et al: Indications for and results of single, bilateral and heart-lung transplantation for pulmonary hypertension. J Thorac Cardiovasc Surg 108: 1056, 1994.

Bando K, Paradis IL, Similo S et al: Obliterative bronchiolitis after lung and heart-lung transplantation: An analysis of risk factors and management. J Thorac Cardiovasc Surg 110: 4, 1995a.

Bando K, Paradis IL, Similo S et al: Analysis of time-dependent risk for infection, rejection and death after pulmonary transplantation. J Thorac Cardiovasc Surg 110:49, 1995b.

Bando K, Schueler S, Cameron De et al: Twelve-hour cardiopulmonary preservation using donor core cooling, leukocyte depletion, and liposomal superoxide dismutase. J Heart Lung Transplant 10:304, 1991.

Bando K, Tago M, Teraoka H et al: Extended cardiopulmonary preservation for heart-lung transplantation: A comparative study of superoxide dismutase. J Heart Lung Transplant 8:59, 1989.

Bonser RS, Fragomeni LS, Jamieson SW et al: Effects of prostaglandin E1 in twelve-hour lung preservation. J Heart Lung Transplant 10:310, 1991.

Bonser RS, Fragomeni LS, Harris K et al: Acute physiologic changes after extended pulmonary preservation. J Heart Lung Transplant 9:220, 1990.

Brooks RG, Hofflin JM, Jamieson SW et al: Infectious complications in heart-lung transplant recipients. Am J Med 79:412, 1985.

Cassart M, Gevenois PA, Knoop C et al: Pseudomonas aeruginosa aortic aneurysm after heart-lung transplantation for cystic fibrosis. Transplantation 58:1051, 1994.

Chan CC, Abi-Saleh WJ, Arrolioa AC, et al: Diagnostic yield and therapeutic impact of flexible bronchoscopy in lung transplant recipients. J Heart Lung Transplant 15:196, 1996.

Collins GM, Bravo-Shugarman M, Terasaki PI: Kidney preservation for transplantation: Initial perfusion and 30 hours ice storage. Lancet 2:1219, 1969.

Colquhoun IW, Gascoigne AD, Au J et al: Airway complications after pulmonary transplantation. Ann Thorac Surg 57:141, 1994.

Conte JV, Robbins RC, Reichenspurner H et al: Pediatric heart-lung transplantation: Intermediate term results. J Heart Lung Transplant 15:692, 1996.

Cooper DKC, Novitzky D, Rose AG, Reichart BA: Acute pulmonary rejection precedes cardiac rejection following heart-lung transplantation in a primate model. J Heart Lung Transplant 5:29, 1986.

Cooper JD, Billingham M, Egan T: A working formulation for the standardization of nomenclature and for clinical staging of chronic dysfunction in lung allografts. J Heart Lung Transplant 12: 713, 1993.

Dowling RD, Baladi N. Zenati M et al: Disruption of the aortic anastomosis after heart-lung transplantation. Ann Thorac Surg 49:118, 1990.

Duncan AJ, Dummer JS, Paradis IL et al: Cytomegalovirus infection and survival in lung transplant recipients. J Heart Lung Transplant 10:638, 1991.

Dusmet M, Maurer J, Winton T, Kesten S: Methotraxate can halt the progression of bronchiolitis obliterans syndrome in lung transplant recipients. J Heart Lung Transplant 15:948, 1996.

Feeley TW, Mihm FG, Downing TP et al: Hypothermic preservation of the heart and lungs with Collins solution: Effect on cardiorespiratory function following heart-lung allotransplantation in dogs. Ann Thorac Surg 41:301, 1986.

Fisher RA, Alexander JW: Management of the multiple organ donor. Clin Transpl 6:328, 1992.

Girgis RE, Reichenspurner H, Robbins RC et al: The utility of annual surveillance bronchoscopy in heart-lung transplant recipeitns. Transplantation 60:1458, 1995.

Guillinger RA, Paradis IL, Dauber JH et al: The importance of bronchoscopy with transbronchial lung biopsy and bronchoalveolar lavage in the management of lung transplant recipients. J Respir Crit Care Med 152:2037, 1995.

Hakim M, Higgenbottam T, Bethune D et al: Selection and procurement of combined heart and lung grafts for transplantation. J Thorac Cardiovasc Surg 85: 474, 1988.

Hakim M, Wreghitt TG, English TAH et al: Significance of donor-transmitted diseasee in cardiac transplantation. J Heart Lung Tranplant 4:302, 1985.

Hardesty RL, Griffith BP: Autoperfusion of the heart and lungs for preservation during distant procurement. J Thorac Cardiovasc Sug 93:11, 1987.

Hardesty RL, Griffith BP: Procurement for combined heart-lung transplantation. J Thorac Cardiovasc Surg 89:795, 1985.

Harper A, Rosendale JD: The UNOS OPTN waiting list and donor registry: 1988–1996. Clin Transpl 69:546, 1996.

Harringer W, Wiebe K, Strüber M et al: Lung transplantation: 10 years experience. Eur J Cardiothorac Surg 16:546, 1999.

Hausen B, Beuke M, Schröder F et al: In vivo measurement of lung preservation solution efficacy: Comparison of LPD, UW, EC and low K+-EC following short and extended ischemia. Eur Cardiothorac Surg 12:771, 1997.

Hausen B, Morris RE: Review of immunosuppression for lung transplantation: Novel drugs, new uses for conventional immunosuppressants and alternative strategies. Clin Con Chest Med 18:353, 1997.

Haverich A, Frimpong-Boateng K, Wahlers T, Schäfers H-J: Pericardial flap-plasty for protection of the tracheal anastomosis in heart-lung transplantation. J Cardiac Surg 4:136, 1989.

Hertz MI, Jordan C, Savik SK et al: Randomized trial of daily versus three-times-weekly prophylactic ganciclovir after lung and heart-lung transplantation. J Heart Lung Transplant 17:913, 1998.

Higenbottam T, Hutter JA, Stewart S, Wallwork J: Transbronchial biopsy has eliminated the need for endomyocardial biopsy in heart-lung recipients. J Heart Lung Transplant 7:435, 1988.

Higgins R, McNeil K, Dennis C et al: Airway stenoses after lung transplantation: Management with expanding metal stents. J. Heart Lung Transplant 13:774, 1994.

Hooper TL, Locke TJ, Fetherston G et al: Comparison of cold flush perfusion with modified blood versus modified Euro-Collins solution for lung preservation. J Heart Lung Transplant 9:429, 1990.

Hopkins WE, Ochoa LL, Richardson GW, Trulock EP: Comparison of the hemodynamics and survival of adults with severe primary pulmonary hypertension or Eisenmenger syndrome. J Heart Lung Transplant 15:100, 1996.

Hosenpud JD, Bennett LE, Keck BM et al: The Registry of the International Society for Heart and Lung Transplantation: Fifteenth Official Report, 1998. J Heart Lung Transplant 17: 656, 1998.

Husain AN, Siddiqui MT, Montoya A et al: Post-lung transplant biopsies: An 8-year Loyola experience. Mod Pathol 9:126, 1996.

Hutter JA, Scott J, Wreghitt T et al: The importance of cytomegalovirus in heart-lung transplantation recipients. Chest 95:627, 1989.

Iacono AT, Keenan RJ, Duncan SR et al: Aerosolized cyclosporine in lung recipients with refractory chronic rejection. Am J Respir Crit Care Med 153:1451, 1996.

Icenogle TB, Copeland JG: A technique to simplify and improve exposure in heart-lung transplantation. J Thorac Cardiovasc Surg 110:1590, 1995.

Jones KD, Cavarocchi N, Hakim M et al: A single flush technique for successful distant organ procurement in heart-lung transplantation. J Heart Lung Transplant 4:614, 1985.

Jurmann MJ, Dammenhayn L, Schäfers H-J, Haverich A: Pulminary reperfusion injury: Evidence for oxygen-derived free radical mediated damage and effects of different free radical scavengers. Eur J Cardiothorac Surg 4:665, 1990.

Kaiser LR, Cooper JD, Trulock EP et al: The evolution of single lung transplantation for emphysema. J Thorac Cardiovasc Surg 102:333, 1991.

Kaye MP: The Registry of the International Society for Heart and Lung Transplantation. Ninth Official Report 1992. J Heart Lung Transplant 11:599, 1992.

Keller CA, Cagle PT, Brown RW et al: Bronchiolitis obliterans in recipients of single, double, and heart-lung transplantation. Chest 107:973, 1995.

Kennan RJ, Griffith BP, Kormos RL et al: Increased perioperative lung preservation injury with lung procurement by Euro-Colins solution flush. J Heart Lung Transplant 10:650, 1991.

Kesten S, Chamberlain D, Maurer J: Yield of surveillance transbronchial biopsies performed beyond two years after lung transplantation. J Heart Lung Transplant 15:384, 1996.

Kesten S, Chaparro C, Scavuzzo M, Gutierrez C: Tacrolimus as rescue therapy for bronchiolitis obliterans syndrome. J Heart Lung Transplant 16:905, 1997.

Kontos GJ, Adachi H, Borkos AM et al: A no-flush, core-cooling technique for successful cardiopulmonary preservation in heart-lung transplantation. J Thorac Cardiovasc Surg 94:836, 1987.

Kramer MR, Marshall Se, Starnes Va et al: Infectious complications in heart-lung transplantation. Arch Intern Med 153:2010, 1993.

Kramer MR, Valentine HA, Marshall S et al: Recovery of the right ventricle after single-lung transplantation in pulmonary hypertension. Am J Cardiol 73:494, 1994.

Kroshus TJ, Kshettry VR, Savik K et al: Risk factors for the development of bronchiolitis obliterans syndrome after lung transplantation. J Thorac Cardiovasc Surg 114: 195, 1997.

Kukafka DS, O'Brien GM, Furukawa S et al: Surveillance bronchoscopy in lung transplant recipients. Chest 111:377, 1997.

Ladowski JS, Hardesty RL, Griffith BP: Protection of the heart-lung allograft during procurement: Cooling of the lungs with extracorporeal circulation or pulmonary artery flush. J Heart Lung Transplant 3:351, 1984.

Ladowski JS, Kapelanski DP, Teodori MF et al: Use of autoperfusion for distant procurement of heart-lung allografts. J Heart Lung Transplant 4:330, 1985.

Leval MR de, Smyth R, Whitehead B et al: Heart and lung transplantation for terminal cystic fibrosis. J Thorac Cardiovasc Surg 101:633, 1991.

Lick SD, Copeland JG, Rosado LJ et al: Simplified technique of heart-lung transplantation. Ann Thorac Surg 59:1592, 1995.

Lillehei CW, Shamberger RC, Mayer JE Jr: Size disparity in pediatric lung transplantation. J Pediatr Surg 29:1152, 1994.

Locke TJ, Hooper TL, Flecknell PA, McGregor CGA: Preservation of the lung: Comparison of flush perfusion with cold modified blood and core cooling by cardiopulmonary bypass. J Heart Lung Transplant 10:1, 1991.

Luciani GB, Starnes VA: The clamshell approach for the surgical treatment of complex cardiopulmonary pathology in infants and children. Eur J Cardiothorac Surg 11:298, 1997.

Madden BP, Hodson ME, Tsand V, Radley-Smith et al: Intermediate-term results of heart-lung transplantation for cystic fibrosis. Lancet 339:1583, 1992.

Maurer JR, Frost AE, Estienne M, et al: International guidelines for the selection of lung transplant candidates. J Heart Lung Transplant 17:703, 1998.

McGoldrick JP, Scott JP, Smyth R et al: The radiographic appearances of infection and acute rejection of the lung following heart-lung transplantation. Am Rev Respir Dis 140:62, 1989.

Millet B, Higenbottam TW, Flower CD et al: The radiographic appearances of infection and acute rejection of the lung following heart-lung transplantation. Am Rev Respir Dis 140:62, 1989.

Miyamoto Y, Lajos TZ, Bhayana JN et al: Physiologic constraints in autoperfused heart-lung preservation. J Heart Lung Transplant 6:261, 1987.

Moncada S: Biology and therapeutic potential of prostacyclin. Stroke 14:157, 1982.

Novick RJ, Menkis AH and McKenzie FN: New trends in lung preservation: a collective review. J Heart Lung Transplant 11: 377, 1992.

Novitzky D, Cooper DKC, Rose AG, Reichart B: Acute isolated pulmonary rejection following transplantation of the heart and both lungs: Experimental and clinical observations. Ann Thorac Surg 42:180, 1986.

Novitzky D, Wicomb WN, Rose AG et al: Pathophysiology of pulmonary edema following experimental brain death in the Chacma baboon. Ann Thorac Surg 43:288, 1987.

Oaks TE, Aravot D, Dennis C et al: Domino heart transplantation: The Papaworth experience. J Heart Lung Transplant 13:433, 1994.

Okamoto K, Kinoshita Y, Yoshioka T et al: Myocardial preservation in brain-dead patients maintained with vasopressin and catecholamine. Clin Transpl 6:294, 1992.

Otulana BA, Higenbottam T, Ferrari L et al: The use of home spirometry in detecting acute lung rejection and infection following heart-lung transplantation. Chest 97:353, 1990.

Paradis IL, Williams P: Infection after lung transplantation. Semin Respir Infect 8:207, 1993.

Penketh A, Higenbottam TW, Hakim M, Wallwork J: Heart and lung transplantation in patients with end-stage lung disease. BMJ 295:311, 1987.

Prop J, Tazelaar HD, Billingham ME: Rejection of combined heart-lung transplants in rats: Function and pathology. Am J Pathol 127:97, 1987.

Reichenspurner H, Girgis RE, Robbins RC et al: Stanford experience with obliterative bronchiolitis after lung and heart-lung transplantation. Ann Thorac Surg 62:1467, 1996.

Reitz BA: Heart-lung transplantation: A review. J Heart Lung Transplant 2:291, 1982a.

Reitz BA, Wallwork J, Hunt S et al: Heart-lung transplantation: Successful therapy for patients with pulmonary vascular disease. N Engl J Med 306: 557, 1982b.

Robicsek F, Lesage A, Sanger PW et al: Transplantation of "live" hearts. Am J Cardiol 20:803, 1967.

Robicsek F, Master TN, Duncan GD et al: An autoperfused heart-lung preparation: Metabolism and function. J Heart Lung Transplant 4:334, 1985.

Rubin LJ: Primary pulmonary hypertension. N Engl J Med 336:111, 1997.

Sakamaki F, Hoffmann H, Müller C et al: Reduced lipid peroxidation and ischemia reperfusion injury after lung transplantation using low-potassium dextran solution for lung preservation. Am J Respir Crit Care Med 156:1073, 1997.

Sale JP, Patel D, Duncan B, Waters JH: Anesthesia for combined heart and lung transplantation. Anesthesia 42:249, 1987.

Scott JP, Fradet G, Smyth RL et al: Prospective study of transbronchial biopsies in the management of heart-lung and single lung transplant patients. J Heart Lung Transplant 10:626, 1991.

Scott JP, Hutter JA, Higenbottam TW, Wallwork J: Combined heart and lung transplantation. Cardiol Pract 6:21, 1988.

Sibley RK, Berry GJ, Tazelaar HD et al: The role of transbronchial biopsies in the management of lung transplant recipients. J Heart Lung Transplant 12:308, 1993.

Smith JA, Roberts M, McNeil K et al: Excellent outcome of cardiac transplantation using domino donor heart. Eur J Cardiothorac Surg 10:628, 1996.

Soghikian MV, Valentine VG, Berry GJ et al: Impact of ganciclovir prophylaxis on heart-lung and lung transplant recipients. J Heart Lung Transplant 15:881, 1996.

Starnes VA, Theodore J, Oyer PE, Billingham ME et al: Evaluation of heart-lung transplant recipients with prospective, serial transbronchial biopsies and pulmonary function studies. J Thorac Cardiovasc Surg 98:683, 1989.

Sundaresan S, Trulock EP, Mohanakumar T et al: Prevalence and outcome of bronchiolitis obliterans syndrome after lung transplantation. Ann Thorac Surg 60: 1341, 1995.

Trulock EP: Management of lung transplant rejection. Chest 103:1566, 1993a.

Trulock EP: Recipient selection. Chest Surg Clin North Am 3:1, 1993b.

Unruh HW: Lung preservation and lung injury. Chest Surg Clin North Am 5:91, 1995.

Valentine VG, Robbins RC, Berry GJ et al: Actuarial survival of heart-lung and bilateral sequential lung transplant recipients with obliterative bronchioliotis. J Heart Lung Transplant 15:371, 1996a.

Valentine VG, Robbins RC, Wehner JH et al: Total lymphoid irradiation for refractory acute rejection in heart-lung and lung allografts. Chest 109:1184, 1996b.

Van Muylem A, Melot C, Antoine M et al: Role of pulmonary function in the detection of allograft dysfunction after heart-lung transplantation. Thorax 52:643, 1997.

Wahlers T, Haverich A, Fieguth HG et al: Flush perfusion using Euro-Collins solution versus cooling by means of extracorporeal circulation in heart-lung preservation. J Heart Lung Transplant 5:89, 1986.

Whyte RI, Rossi SJ, Mulligan MS et al: Mycophenolate mofetil for obliterative bronchiolitis syndrome after lung transplantation. Ann Thorac Surg 64:945, 1997.

Wisser W, Klepetko W, Weckerle T et al: Tailoring of the lung to overcome size disparities in lung transplantation. J Heart Lung Transplant 15:239, 1996.

You XM, Steinmuller C, Wagner TO et al: Enhancement of cytomegalovirus infection and acute rejection after allogeneic lung transplantation in the rat: Virus-induced expression of major histocompatibility complex class II antigens. J Heart Lung Transplant 15:1108, 1996.

Pleura

CHAPTER **38**

Anatomy and Physiology of the Pleural Space

Reza John Mehran
Jean Deslauriers

ANATOMY

The pleura is formed of two serosal membranes, one covering the lung (the visceral pleura) and one covering the inner chest wall (the parietal pleura). One surface glides over the other one, facilitating proper lung movements during the various phases of respiration. The pleural space is the space delimited by the two layers. Under normal conditions, it contains only a small amount of liquid that functions as a lubricator. The total amount of pleural fluid ranges between 0.1 and 0.2 ml/kg, with a thickness of about 10 μm (Staub et al, 1985). The two pleural cavities are independent of each other, but in some conditions the parietal pleura of each side is in contact anteriorly behind the sternum.

The transition between the parietal and visceral pleurae is at the level of the pulmonary hilum. At this level, the reflection covers the constituents of the hilum, except inferiorly where the reflection extends down to the diaphragm. The overall shape of this reflection is a racquet, the handle of which forms the pulmonary ligament, also known as the triangular ligament of the lung. The limits of the triangular ligament are: (1) medially on the right, the esophagus; on the left, the aorta; and the pericardium; (2) superiorly on the inferior pulmonary vein; and (3) inferiorly on the diaphragm. The ligament contains a few small arteries and veins that have little clinical significance and lymph nodes that drain the inferior lobe.

EMBRYOLOGY

During the end of the third week of gestation, the embryonic mesoderm differentiates into the para-axial mesoderm, the intermediate mesoderm, and the lateral plate (Figs. 38–1 to 38–4). The lateral plate forms two different layers: (1) the somatic mesoderm or somatopleure, and (2) the splanchnic mesoderm or splanchnopleure. Gradually, the somatic mesoderm progresses to meet in the midline, in the ventral portion of the embryo, closing the intraembryonic coelom from the extraembryonic coelom. The somatic mesoderm becomes the parietal layer, and

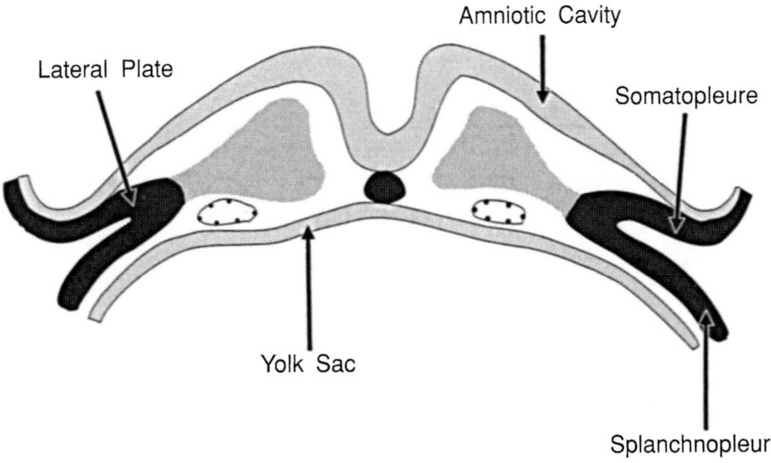

FIGURE 38–1 ■ Differentiation of the lateral plate into the somatopleure and the splanchnopleure, the precursors of the parietal and visceral pleura, respectively (early third week of gestation).

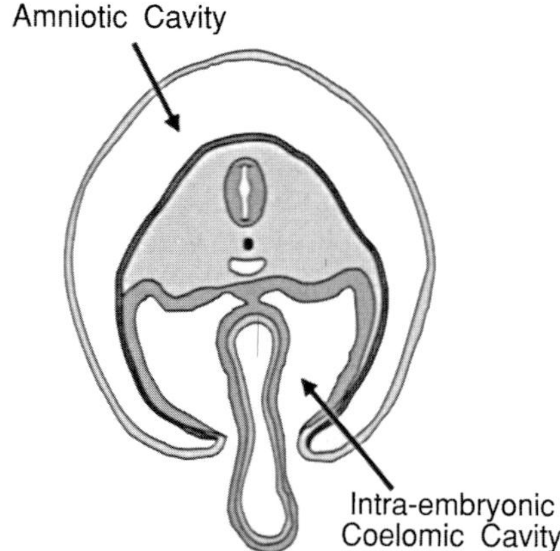

FIGURE 38–2 ■ The creation of the intra-embryonic celomic cavity by ventral migration of the somatopleure toward the midline.

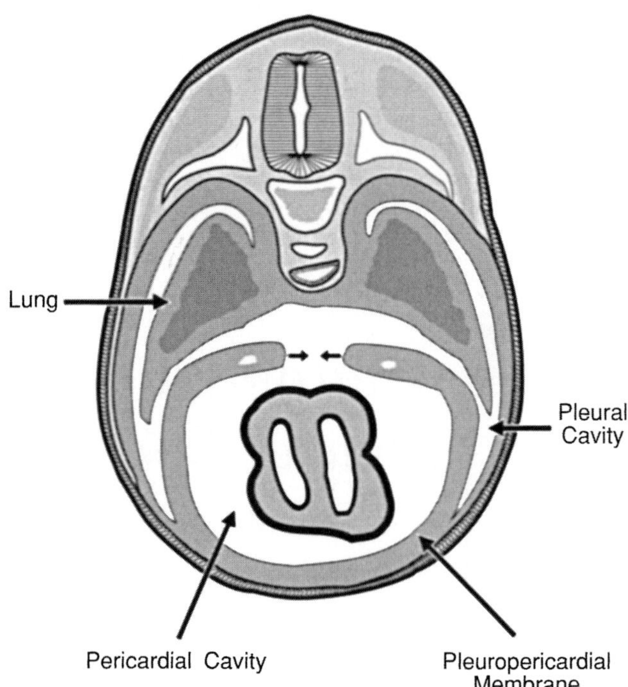

FIGURE 38–4 ■ Midline fusion of the pleuropericardial folds, with separation of the pleural cavity from the pericardial sac. Expansion of the pleural cavity (fifth week to third month).

the splanchnic mesoderm becomes the visceral layer of the intraembryonic coelomic sac.

By the end of the seventh week, the diaphragm separates the pleuropericardial and peritoneal spaces. Meanwhile, the separation of the serosal cavities of the chest starts with the medial growth of the pericardial folds. The folds contain the phrenic nerves and the common cardinal veins (Cuvier's duct), the precursors of the superior vena cava. The folds coalesce in the midline during the fifth week, separating the pericardial from the pleural space. During the same period, the pulmonary buds grow and contribute to the formation of the final shape of the pleural and pericardial cavities (see Figs. 38–3 and 38–4). By the third month, the pleural cavities have expanded cranially, caudally, and ventrolaterally to surround the pericardium.

ADULT PLEURAL SAC

Visceral Pleura

The visceral pleura covers the surface of the lung and extends into the fissures. The visceral pleura is thin, transparent, and tightly adherent, via elastic fibers, to the underlying alveolar wall elastica (Fig. 38–5). Disruption of these elastic fibers results in the formation of pleural blebs (Harley, 1987).

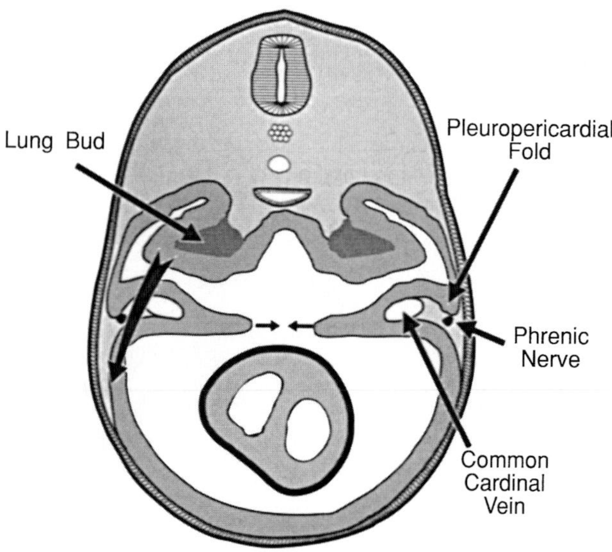

FIGURE 38–3 ■ Creation of the lung bud and the pleuropericardial folds (around fifth week).

Parietal Pleura

The parietal pleura is more complex anatomically. This layer almost completely covers the inner surface of the

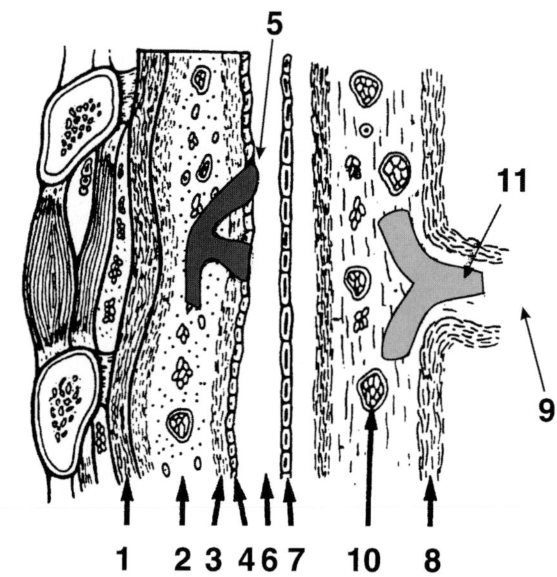

FIGURE 38–5 ■ The different layers of the parietal and visceral pleurae: 1, endothoracic fascia; 2, subpleural connective tissue layer; 3, superficial elastic layer; 4, parietal mesothelial layer; 5, lymphatic stoma; 6, pleural space; 7, visceral mesothelial layer; 8, deep elastic layer; 9, interlobular septa; 10, connective fiber; 11, interlobular lymphatics.

thoracic wall and the medial aspect of the mediastinum. The attachment of the parietal pleura to these structures is via a fibrous layer known as the endothoracic fascia (see Fig. 38–5). The endothoracic fascia is a cleavage layer within which the parietal pleura can be separated from the chest wall. The thickness and strength of the endothoracic fascia vary with location. The fascia is strongest over the inner surface of the ribs. Posterior to the sternum and in the pericardium, the endothoracic fascia is almost nonexistent. This makes the detachment of the pleura in these locations impossible. At the level of the thoracic inlet, the fascia is again strong and forms a diaphragm called the fibrous cervicothoracic septum (Nebut et al, 1982) or the cervicothoracic diaphragm of Bourgery (Bouchet and Cuilleret, 1974). This diaphragm is supported by a number of suspensory ligaments to surrounding structures.

Pleural Sinuses

The parietal pleura can be divided into the costal, mediastinal, and diaphragmatic pleurae. The transition between each segment is done at the level of the pleural sinuses. The pleural sinuses are: (1) the anterior and posterior costomediastinal sinuses, (2) the costophrenic sinus, and (3) the mediastinophrenic sinus. The parietal pleura in the sinuses, especially in the posterior costophrenic sinus, are in contact at rest, but the sinuses fill with lung during inspiration.

In only one order of mammal, the Proboscidea, which includes the elephant, are the fetal pleural cavities replaced by elastic tissue (Lawrence, 1983). In humans, the capacity of the pleura is seen after a pneumonectomy in which the remaining lung expands into the contralateral pleural space.

Pleural Topography

The projection of the pleural sinuses over the chest wall is fairly similar on the right and the left. Anteriorly, the lung extends no lower than the sixth rib in the midclavicular line, whereas the pleural costophrenic sinus extends to the seventh rib. Laterally in the midaxillary line, the lung descends to the eighth rib; the lateral costophrenic sinus descends to the ninth rib. Posteriorly, the lung extends to the eleventh rib and the pleura to the twelfth rib. The pleural space and the lung extend above the bony limits of the thoracic inlet.

Blood Supply

The blood supply of the parietal pleura comes exclusively from the systemic arteries. The costal pleura is supplied by intercostal arteries and branches from the internal mammary arteries; the mediastinal pleura is vascularized by bronchial, upper diaphragmatic, and internal mammary arteries. The blood supply to the cervical pleura (pleural dome) comes from subclavian arteries. For the most part, venous blood drains into peribronchial veins or directly into the venae cavae.

In contrast, the visceral pleura is vascularized by both the systemic (through the bronchial arteries) and the pulmonary circulation. Venous blood is drained into the pulmonary venous system.

Lymphatic Drainage

The pleural space is on the boundary of two lymphatic systems, both of which play a major role in the removal of fluid, cells, and foreign particles from the pleural space.

In the subpleural space of the visceral pleura, large lymphatic capillaries form a meshed network that drains into the pulmonary lymphatic system. These capillaries are more abundant over the lower lobes and are connected to the deep pulmonary plexuses located in the interlobular and peribronchial spaces.

The lymphatic drainage of the parietal pleura is more elaborate, with direct communication between the pleural space and the parietal pleural lymphatic channels. These communications, called stomata (see Fig. 38–5), are 2 to 6 μm in diameter and predominate over the lower portions of the mediastinal, diaphragmatic, and costal pleura. They have endoluminal valves and drain into a network of submesothelial lymphatic lacunae. Over the costal pleura, these collecting vessels run parallel to the ribs to reach the internal mammary nodal chain anteriorly and the intercostal nodal chain posteriorly. At the diaphragm, the drainage is to the retrosternal, mediastinal, and celiac nodes (Wang et al, 1997). The transdiaphragmatic anastomoses allow for the passage of fluid and foreign particles from the peritoneal cavity into the pleural space. The subpleural lymphatics play an important role in the reabsorption of fluid and the removal of proteins, particles, and cells from the pleural space.

Innervation

The visceral pleura is devoid of somatic innervation; in contrast, the parietal pleura is innervated through a rich network of somatic, sympathetic, and parasympathetic fibers. At the costal pleura level, these fibers travel through the intercostal nerves. Pain stimuli at the diaphragm are transmitted through the phrenic nerve.

MICROSCOPIC ANATOMY

Pleural Membrane

The visceral and parietal pleural membrane consists of a single layer of mesothelial cells resting on connective tissue. Mesothelial cells are stretchable, and their size and shape may vary, depending on their location. Abundant microvilli cover their surface. The presence of a rich endoplasmic reticulum points to some secretory capacity. By expanding the cell surface, microvilli favor phagocytosis and fluid absorption (pinocytosis). They are also well adapted for deforming structure and help in sliding. Hills (1992) demonstrated that the pleural surface contains an adsorbed, surface-active, phospholipid coating. Because surfactant molecules are charged, they repulse each other on opposite surfaces. This graphite-like antiwear property is comparable to the best lubricants.

The epithelium lies on a basal membrane with various

amounts of collagen and elastic fibers. It contains blood vessels, nerve endings, and lymphatic channels. In the visceral pleura, this underlayer is directly connected to the fibroelastic network of the lung and thus helps to distribute mechanical stress evenly throughout the structure. Arterial vascularization of the parietal pleura comes from the systemic circulation through the internal mammary and intercostal arteries. The arterial blood supply of the visceral pleura is mixed. It comes in part from the pulmonary circulation, but Gilbert and Hakim (1992) observed that the relative contribution of the systemic circulation through the branches from the bronchial arteries is increased at the subpleural level.

The parietal pleura contains two particular features not present in the visceral pleura. A rich network of lymphatic vessels is concentrated in the posteroinferior portion of the chest. As described earlier, these vessels communicate directly with the pleural space through openings, or "stomata," in the parietal pleura.

Kampmeier's foci, or milky spots, are found in the lower portion of the mediastinal pleura and are covered with slightly different, cuboidal, mesothelial cells. They consist of an aggregate of macrophages, lymphocytes, histiocytes, plasma cells, mast cells, and undifferentiated mesenchymal cells encircling thick blood capillaries and lymphatic channels. Kanazawa (1985) demonstrated that Kampmeier foci participate in the defense of the pleural space in different ways. They exhibit phagocytic activity, trap macrophages and particles, appear to exert some focal suction, and have the capacity to produce leukocytes under the stimulus of inflammation, not unlike the lymphoid tissue in the tonsils.

MECHANICAL PROPERTIES

The lung and the thorax are two elastic structures connected in series and acting in opposite directions. The visceral pleura has a double mechanical action—that is, volume limitation of the lung and the generation of elastic recoil pressure. The pleural contribution to lung elastic recoil pressure originates from the elastic network, which turns back to its resting position when inspiratory pressures are negligible (Lemos et al, 1997).

The mechanisms that hold the lung close to the chest wall are complex and depend mainly on two physiologic processes: (1) those ensuring a constant removal of pleural fluid, and (2) those preventing the accumulation of free gas in the pleural space. These mechanisms involve the interplay of different pressures.

Pleural Pressure

The pressure at the surface of the pleura (P_{PL}) results from the mechanical properties of the respiratory system (Fig. 38–6) and can be described by the following equation:

$$P_{RS} = P_L + P_W$$

where P_{RS} is the pressure of the respiratory system, P_L is the pressure exerted by the lung, and P_W is the pressure developed in the chest wall.

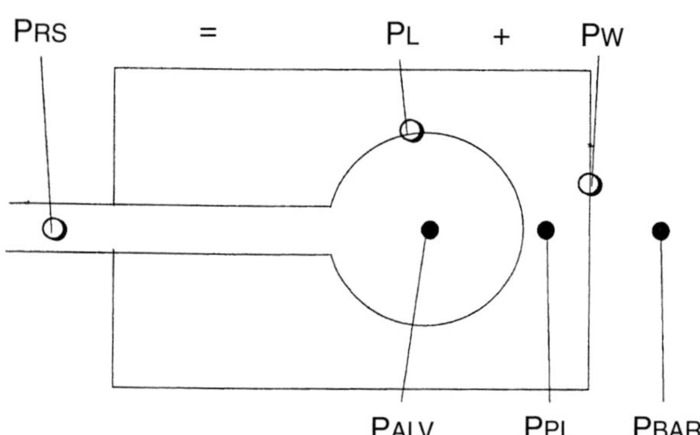

FIGURE 38–6 ■ This model represents the pressures involved in the mechanics of the respiratory system. PRS is the total respiratory system pressure plus the sum of PL, the pressure developed in the lung, and PW, the pressure developed in the chest wall. PALV, alveolar pressure; PBAR, ambient barometric pressure; PPL, pleural pressure.

The pressures measured at the boundaries of these structures are the alveolar pressure (P_{ALV}), the pleural pressure (P_{PL}), and the ambient barometric pressure (P_{BAR}). The P_{PL} is equal to the difference of the alveolar minus the transpulmonary pressure (P_L) as shown in the following equations:

$$P_L = P_{ALV} - P_{PL}$$

$$P_{PL} = P_{ALV} - P_L$$

In static conditions, the alveolar pressure is equal to zero, and the equation becomes:

$$P_{PL} = - P_{PL}$$

The latter equation demonstrates that the pleural pressure is proportional to the pressure developed in the lung. When the pulmonary volume is at its functional residual capacity, the elastic forces of the lung and thorax are in equilibrium, and the pleural pressure equals −2 to −5 cm H_2O. As the pulmonary volume increases during inspiration to the vital capacity, the pleural pressure becomes progressively more negative, −25 to −35 cm H_2O. In any condition in which the elastic recoil of the lung is increased—for example, interstitial fibrosis, edema, atelectasis, or resection of the parenchyma of the lung—the pleural pressure becomes more subatmospheric. In situations in which airway resistance is increased—such as chronic obstructive pulmonary disease, bronchial stenosis, or obstruction by a foreign body or secretions—the negativity of the pleural pressure increases further during inspiration.

Vertical Gradient of Pleural Pressure

The pleural pressure is not uniform around the surface of the lung. Minor local variations of pleural liquid pressure occur in relation to variations in the thickness of the pleural space, but these are of no practical consequence. More important, a vertical pleural pressure gradient exists

TABLE 38–1 ■ **Partial Pressures of Gases in Air and Blood***

Partial Pressure	Atmosphere	Alveolar Gas	Arterial Blood	Pleural Space	Venous Blood
Water	47	47	47		47
Oxygen	150	102	95		40
Carbon dioxide	0	39	40		45
Nitrogen	563	572	575		575
Total	760	760	757		703
				[Gradient + 54 mm Hg]	

*All pressures in millimeters of mercury, assuming temperature at 37°C, saturated in water vapor.

from the top to the bottom of the thoracic cavity. The mechanisms responsible for this gradient have been reviewed by Agostoni (1986). The effect of gravity on the lung is one important determinant. Other factors include the size, volume, shape, and position of the lung. The pleural pressure changes by approximately 0.25 cm H_2O/cm of height and is more negative at the apex (−7 to −9 cm H_2O) than at the base (0 to −2 cm H_2O) of the lung in an upright subject. This is one reason why the upper portion of the lung usually collapses more in partial pneumothorax.

Gas Pressures

Given that the hydrostatic pleural pressure is subatmospheric, there is a theoretic risk that gases dissolved in the blood and interstitial fluid could be freed in the pleural space. The pleural space is influenced by the partial pressures of gas prevailing in the arterial and venous blood that irrigates the pleura. The cascade of partial pressure changes from the atmospheric pressure to the venous blood are summarized in Table 38–1. Oxygen and carbon dioxide are exchanged during respiration. Nitrogen is not consumed or produced during respiration. However, because the respiratory quotient is less than 1, more oxygen is consumed than carbon dioxide is rejected in the alveoli. As a consequence, nitrogen's partial pressure increases slightly from 563 mm Hg in the inspired gas to 572 mm Hg in the alveolar gas. The partial pressure of nitrogen in the blood equals 575 mm Hg and is close to equilibrium with the alveolar gas (Cotes, 1979). The situation is different with oxygen and carbon dioxide. As a result of cellular respiration, the contents of the blood change at the capillary level. The oxygen content decreases, and the carbon dioxide content increases. The repercussions of these gas exchanges are different on the partial pressures for both gases because the dissociation curves of oxygen and carbon dioxide in the blood are not the same. A partial oxygen pressure of 95 mm Hg in arterial blood drops to 40 mm Hg in venous blood, a 55-mm Hg difference. The partial carbon dioxide pressure goes from 40 to 45 mm Hg, a corresponding gain of only 5 mm Hg. The total pressure of dissolved gases equals 757 mm Hg in arterial blood and becomes 703 mm Hg in venous blood, a drop of 54 mm Hg (or 72 cm H_2O) compared with that in arterial blood and the pleural space. This pressure gradient protects the pleural space against the spontaneous formation of gas if the hydrostatic pressure does not exceed −72 cm H_2O. It ensures also that air collected in the pleural space, as in the pneumothorax, will be reabsorbed by the venous side of the circulating blood.

PLEURAL FLUID DYNAMICS

Normal Fluid

Only a small amount of fluid can be recovered from the pleural space under normal conditions (see box for Composition of Normal Pleura Fluid). A volume of 0.1 to 0.3 ml/kg may be extrapolated from experimental data in animals (Miserocchi, 1997). The protein content is low, 10 to 20 g/L, a fact that led Staub and colleagues (1985) to question the mechanisms of fluid reabsorption.

Pleural Fluid Turnover

Pleural fluid is constantly secreted, mostly by filtration from the microvessels in the parietal pleura mainly in the less dependent regions of the cavity. This was confirmed by Broaddus and colleagues (1991). A quantitative assessment is difficult, however. Animal studies reviewed by Pistolesi and colleagues (1990) yield a wide range of values from 0.02 to 2 ml/kg/hr. Comparative studies reveal that pleural fluid turnover decreases with increasing

COMPOSITION OF NORMAL PLEURAL FLUID

Volume: 0.1–0.2 ml/kg
Protein: 10–20 g/L
Albumin: 50%–70%
Glucose: As in plasma
Lactic dehydrogenase: <50% of plasma level
Cells/mm³: 4500
- Mesothelial cells: 3%
- Monocytes: 54%
- Lymphocytes: 10%
- Granulocytes: 4%
- Unclassified: 29%

pH: 7.38 (mixed venous blood + 0.02)
Partial pressure of carbon dioxide: 45 mm Hg (= mixed venous blood)
Bicarbonate: 25 mmol/L (= mixed venous blood)

From Agostini E: Mechanisms of pleural space. In American Physiological Society: Handbook of Physiology, Vol 3, sec. 3, Part 2. Bethesda, MD, American Physiological Society, 1986.

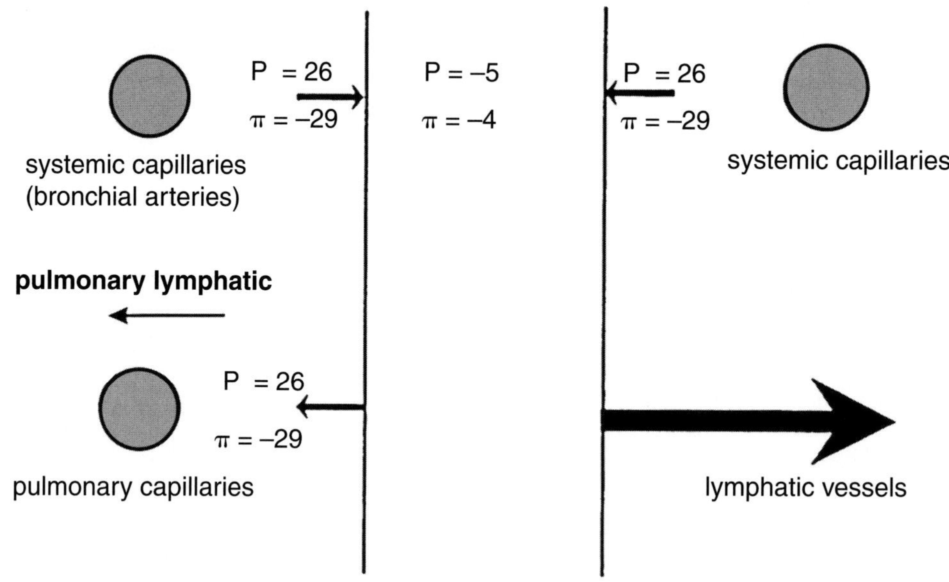

FIGURE 38–7 ■ The mechanisms of pleural fluid exchanges at the level of the parietal and the visceral pleura. P is the hydrostatic pressure, and π is the osmotic pressure (both in centimeters of water). The *arrows* indicate the direction of flow. In areas in which the pleura is vascularized by the systemic circulation, the net balance of pressures, according to Starling's Equation, favors the filtration of fluid toward the pleural space. Capillary hydrostatic pressures are lower in the capillaries of the pulmonary circulation, and the balance of pressures favors pleural fluid resorption through the visceral pleura. However, most of the resorption occurs through the lymphatic channels of the parietal pleura.

size (Miserocchi, 1991). In large mammals such as elephants, there is no production of pleural fluid and the pleural space is actually nonexistent.

Under pathologic conditions, fluid may originate from other sources. In congestive (Broaddus et al, 1990; Wiener-Kronish et al, 1984) and in chemically induced (Miller et al, 1989; Wiener-Kronish et al, 1988) lung edema, liquid may filtrate directly from the pulmonary interstitium into the pleural space. Under such conditions, as much as 25% of pulmonary edema fluid may be cleared through the visceral pleura. Clara cell protein (CC16) is a small protein readily diffusible and secreted by the bronchial Clara cells. Hermans and colleagues (1998) showed an increased concentration of CC16 in the pleural fluid of patients and rat model compared with the serum level. This indicates that the origin of some of the pleural fluid could be leakage from the lung into the pleural space across the semipermeable visceral pleura.

Peritoneal fluid may also leak into the chest through pores in the diaphragm in patients with ascites or in those who are undergoing peritoneal dialysis. Obstruction or narrowing of the lymphatic trunks draining the diaphragm lymph in an experimental rat model cause a hydrothorax, indicating that this is at least one other mechanism causing fluid accumulation during chronic ambulatory dialysis and diseases with ascites (Ohtani and Ohtani, 1997).

Agostoni and colleagues (1957) proposed that pleural fluid exchange could be explained by the balance of hydrostatic and osmotic pressures. The Starling Equation (refer to the box for the equation) states that the flow of fluid through a semipermeable membrane such as the pleura depends on three factors: (1) the permeability coefficient of the pleura, (2) the difference of hydrostatic pressures, and (3) the difference of osmotic pressures across the pleura. Application of this equation shows that, at the level of the parietal pleura, the net difference of pressures favors the passage of fluid into the pleural space. However, recent data show that the system of diffusion of fluids across the parietal pleura is more complicated than the principles of the Starling Equation can explain. Rather, the parietal pleura is a complex membrane that allows selective passage of proteins and solute. This can explain the low protein concentration of the pleural fluid compared with the extrapleural interstitium.

The old theories about the absorption of the pleural fluid by the visceral pleura no longer apply. Particularly in large mammals, the visceral pleura is relatively thick, and the absorption through the visceral pleura is mini-

STARLING'S EQUATION APPLIED TO PLEURAL FLUID DYNAMICS

$$F = K \times [(P_{CAP} - P_{PL}) - (\pi_{CAP} - \pi_{PL})]$$

where: *F* is fluid movement across the pleura; *K* is permeability coefficient; π_{CAP} is hydrostatic capillary pressure; P_{PL} is hydrostatic pleural pressure; π_{CAP} is osmotic capillary pressure; and π_{PL} is osmotic pleural pressure.

mal. In fact, most pleural fluid is reabsorbed by the parietal pleura (Negrini et al, 1994). This absorption is thought to be via the lymphatic stomata. The parietal pleural lymphatics, through the contractile wall, are able to create a negative pressure, sucking in the pleural fluid (Miserocchi et al, 1989). These mechanisms account for most of pleural fluid resorption. The predominance of the lymphatic stomata in the most dependent portion of the chest also creates a flow of pleural fluid from the area of production to the lower portion of the chest cavity.

The mechanisms of pleural fluid turnover are summarized in Figure 38–7.

REFERENCES

Agostoni E: Mechanics of the pleural space. In American Physiological Society: Handbook of Physiology, Vol 3, sec. 3, Part 2. Bethesda, MD, American Physiological Society, 1986.

Agostoni E, Taglietti A, Setnikar I: Absorption forces of the capillaries of the visceral pleura in determination of the intrapleural pressure. Am J Physiol 191:277, 1957.

Bouchet A, Cuilleret J: Anatomie topographique, le thorax. Villwurbanne, France, Simep, 1974.

Broaddus VC, Araya M, Carlton DP, Bland RD: Developmental changes in pleural liquid protein concentration in sheep. Am Rev Respir Dis 143:38, 1991.

Broaddus VC, Wiener-Kronish JP, Staub NC: Clearance of lung edema into the pleural space of volume-loaded anesthetized sheep. J Appl Physiol 68:2623, 1990.

Cotes JE: Lung Function. London, Blackwell, 1979.

Gilbert E, Hakim TS: Relative contribution of bronchial flow to subpleural region in dog lung. J Appl Physiol 73:855, 1992.

Harley R: Anatomy of the pleura. Semin Respir Med 9:1, 1987.

Hermans C, Lesur O, Weynand B et al: Clara cell protein (CC16) in pleural fluids: A marker of leakage through the visceral pleura. Am J Respir Crit Care Med 157:962, 1998.

Hills BA: Graphite-like lubrication of mesothelium by oligolamellar pleural surfactant. J Appl Physiol 73:1034, 1992.

Kanazawa K: Exchanges through the pleura. In Chrétien J, Bignon J, Hirsch A (eds): Pleura in Health and Disease. New York, Marcel Dekker, 1985.

Lawrence GH: Considerations of the anatomy and physiology of the pleural space. In Lawrence GH (ed): Problems of the Pleural Space. Philadelphia, WB Saunders, 1983.

Lemos M, Pozo RM, Montes GS, Saldiva PH: Organization of collagen and elastic fibers studied in stretch preparations of whole mounts of human visceral pleura. Anat Anz 179:447, 1997.

Miller KS, Russell AH, Sahn SA: Pleural effusions associated with ethchlorvynol lung injury result from visceral pleural leak. Am Rev Respir Dis 140:764, 1989.

Miserocchi G: Physiology and pathophysiology of pleural fluid turnover. Eur Respir J 10:219, 1997.

Miserocchi G: Pleural pressures and fluid transport. In Crystal RG, West JB (eds): The Lung: Scientific Foundations. New York, Raven Press, 1991, p 885.

Miserocchi G, Negrini D, Mukenge S et al: Liquid drainage through the peritoneal diaphragmatic surface. J Appl Physiol 66:1579, 1989.

Nebut M, Hirsch A, ChretiÂn J: Embryology and anatomy of the pleura. In ChretiÂn J, Hirsch A (eds): Diseases of the Pleura. Paris, Masson, 1982.

Negrini D, Ballard ST, Benoit JN: Contribution of lymphatic myogenic activity and of respiratory movements to pleural lymph flow. J Appl Physiol 76:2267, 1994.

Ohtani Y, Ohtani O: Obliteration of the lymphatic trunks draining diaphragmatic lymph causes peritoneal fluid to enter the pleural cavity. Arch Histol Cytol 60:503, 1997.

Pistolesi M, Miniati M, Giuntini C: Pleural liquid and solute exchange. Am Rev Respir Dis 140:825, 1990.

Staub NC, Wiener-Kronish JP, Albertine KH: Transport through the pleura. In Chrétien J, Bignon J, Hirsch A (eds): Pleura in Health and Disease. New York, Marcel Dekker, 1985.

Wang QX, Ohtani O, Saitoh M, Ohtani Y: Distribution and ultrastructure of the stomata connecting the pleural cavity with lymphatics in the rat costal pleura. Acta Anat 158:255, 1997.

Wiener-Kronish JP, Albertine KH, Licko V, Staub NC: Protein egress and entry rates in pleural fluid and plasma in sheep. J Appl Physiol 56:459, 1984.

Wiener-Kronish JP, Broaddus VC, Albertine KH et al: Relationship of pleural effusions to increased permeability pulmonary edema in anesthetized sheep. J Clin Invest 82:1422, 1988.

CHAPTER **39**

Diagnostic Procedures for Pleural Diseases

Jean Deslauriers
Guy Carrier
Éric Vallières

Although pleural diseases are relatively common in the practice of thoracic surgery, their diagnosis is often problematic. Pleural effusions, for instance, can be secondary to a number of thoracic, abdominal, or systemic diseases, and their origin can still be unknown after thoracentesis or pleural biopsy.

In such patients, clinical history and physical examination are important because most pleural effusions are manifestations of extrapleural diseases. Imaging of the pleural space also represents first-line investigation, with conventional radiographs, computed tomography (CT), high-resolution CT, ultrasound, isotopic studies, and magnetic resonance imaging (MRI) often providing definitive clues to the cause of the effusion.

More invasive techniques, such as thoracentesis or percutaneous pleural biopsies, have contributed substantially to the investigation of pleural diseases, and with them a diagnosis can be firmly established in 80% to 85% of cases, with minimal morbidity. Patients may also benefit because those procedures will help to rule out specific and treatable diseases such as pleural tumors or tuberculosis. Recent advances in thoracoscopy and video-assisted thoracic surgery (VATS) have further improved the sensitivity and specificity of these diagnostic procedures.

It has been said that the term "idiopathic pleural effusion . . . is idiotic from the standpoint of the physician and pathetic from that of the patient" (Branscomb and Harrison, 1966; Gaensler, 1970). This statement is even more true now because modern diagnostic techniques have simplified access to the pleural space, where fluid and tissue can be sampled and sent for detailed biochemical, bacteriologic, and pathologic analysis.

HISTORICAL NOTE

Thoracentesis is a procedure that involves thrusting a needle into the pleural space for the purpose of removing accumulated air or fluid. It was established as a diagnostic procedure by Bowditch (1852) and since then has been used extensively for the investigation of patients with pleural effusions of unknown origin.

In 1955 De Francis and colleagues reported the use of the Vim-Silverman needle to biopsy the pleura and establish a diagnosis of tuberculosis in two of six patients with pleural effusion. Between 1958 and 1961 Cope (1958), Abrams (1958), and others (Harvey and Harvey, 1958; Skowran, 1960; Carpenter and Lowell, 1961) introduced similar types of needles, which have proved capable of obtaining satisfactory specimens without damage to the lung. In 1958 Mestitz and colleagues reported their experience with the Abrams needle. There were no serious complications related to the procedure, and histologic proof was obtained in 104 (52%) of 200 patients.

Direct visual inspection of the pleural space was first described by Professor H. C. Jacobaeus of Sweden in 1910 in an article titled "Possibility of the Use of the Cystoscope for Investigation of Serous Cavities." A few years later, he reported on the use of the "thorakoscope" and of the two-puncture approach to access and lyse by cautery pleural adhesions so as to facilitate artificial pneumothorax as a treatment for tuberculosis (Jacobaeus, 1921). In 1925, he authored a detailed 30-page document describing his diagnostic and therapeutic experiences with the technique, as applied mainly to tuberculosis (Jacobaeus, 1925). Between 1925 and 1965, references to thoracoscopy as a diagnostic modality were rare and occurred mostly in the European literature (Sergent and Kourilsky, 1939; Delarue and De Pierre, 1956). In 1942 Fabri and Parmeggiani reported the use of thoracoscopy to evaluate pleural exudates, and in 1943 Fourestier and Duret reported three cases of pleural malignancies in which the diagnosis was made by pleuroscopy. During the 1970s and early 1980s diagnostic thoracoscopy was repopularized by Boutin and associates (1981, 1984), who reported on 1000 cases of chronic pleurisy in which the cause remained unknown after the usual investigations. In their series, after thoracoscopy the diagnosis was still unknown in only 4% of patients.

Over the years thoracoscopy has been performed in a number of ways. The instrument could be a simple mediastinoscope, a flexible bronchoscope, a cystoscope, a rigid bronchoscope, or a specially designed thoracoscope with a cold light source. Currently, the thoracoscope is coupled to a microcamera system, which allows for the involvement of the whole surgical team in the procedure by means of video systems. Thoracoscopy has been performed through the neck or through an intercostal space and under local or regional as well as general anesthesia.

■ *HISTORICAL READINGS*

Abrams LD: Pleural-biopsy punch. Lancet 1:30, 1958.
Boutin C, Farisse P, Rey F et al: La thoracoscopie doit-elle être un examen de routine en pratique pneumologique courante? Med Hyg 42:2992, 1984.
Boutin C, Viallat JR, Cargnino P, Farisse P: Thoracoscopy in malignant pleural effusion. Am Rev Respir Dis 124:588, 1981.
Bowditch HI: Paracentesis thoracis. Am J Med Sci 23:103, 1852.
Carpenter RL, Lowell JR: Pleural biopsy and thoracentesis by new instrument. Chest 40:182, 1961.
Cope C: New pleural biopsy needle. JAMA 167:1107, 1958.
De Francis N, Kiosk E, Albano E: Needle biopsy of parietal pleura: Preliminary report. N Engl J Med 252:948, 1955.
Delarue J, De Pierre R: Contribution à l'étude des pleurésies cancéreuses cliniquement primitives: Intérêt de la biopsie sous pleuroscopie. J Fr Med Chir Thorac 6:653, 1956.
Fabri G, Parmeggiani D: Observations on thoracoscopy in pleural exudates. Policlin Sez Prat 5:49, 1942.
Fourestier M, Duret M: Nécessité de la biopsie pleurale pour le diagnostic de l'endothéliome de la plévre. Presse Med 32:467, 1943.
Harvey C, Harvey HPB: Subclavian lymph node, pleural and pulmonary biopsy in diagnosis of intrathoracic disease. Postgrad Med J 34:204, 1958.
Jacobaeus HC: Possibility of the use of the cystoscope for investigation of serous cavities. Munch Med Wochenschr 57:2090, 1910.
Jacobaeus HC: The practical importance of thoracoscopy in surgery of the chest. Surg Gynecol Obstet 32:493, 1921.
Jacobaeus HC: Thoracoscopy and its practical applications. Ergeb Ges Med 7:122, 1925.
Mestitz P, Purves MJ, Pollard AC: Pleural biopsy in diagnosis of pleural effusion: Report of 200 cases. Lancet 2:1349, 1958.
Sergent E, Kourilsky R: Contribution to the study of endothelioma. Presse Med 47:257, 1939.
Skowran CA: Kerrison rongeur: Needle-punch biopsy. Del Med J 32:294, 1960.

INITIAL ASSESSMENT

The initial assessment of a patient with suspected or proven pleural disease is critical not only because history taking and physical examination may provide clues to the diagnosis but also because they may be useful in suggesting the cause of the underlying disease and the likelihood that the disease is related to the pleural effusion (Jay, 1985).

History and Physical Examination

In taking the medical history of a patient with a pleural effusion, the most important questions relate to the possibility of previous asbestos exposure, tuberculous contact, or malignancy. Also important to elucidate is a possible history of recent respiratory symptoms such as may be seen with pulmonary infection or bronchogenic carcinoma.

The typical symptoms associated with pleural diseases are dyspnea and "pleuritic" chest pain radiating to the shoulder and made worse by deep breathing and coughing. It is worth noting that the severity of symptoms does not necessarily reflect the severity of disease or amount of effusion. Patients can be relatively asymptomatic with large effusions or be intensely symptomatic with the smaller effusions associated with intense pleural inflammation. With respect to asymptomatic effusions, Smyrnios and colleagues (1990) have shown that the spectrum of causes is similar to that for symptomatic effusions and that patients should be evaluated in the same fashion.

Chest pain is due to inflammation of the parietal and diaphragmatic pleura, distortion of the mediastinum with phrenic nerve stretching, or frank neoplastic invasion of the parietal pleura or chest wall. Pain stimuli radiating to the shoulder, back, or neck are carried through the sensory part of the phrenic nerve.

As shown by Jay (1985), the physical findings are generally related to the amount of pleural effusion, but they lack sensitivity and specificity (Table 39–1). They include decreased breath sounds, decreased chest expansion, and tracheal shift. Other findings that should be looked for are palpable nodes in the neck, a thoracic mass, red or fluctuant areas in the chest wall, asymmetry of the rib cage, and pain induced by palpation of specific areas of the chest. All these findings will help in the planning of further investigation so that it may proceed in a methodical and controlled fashion.

IMAGING

Conventional Radiographic Examination

Conventional radiographic imaging is the mainstay of the initial evaluation of patients with suspected pleural disease. It is simple, accessible, safe, cheap, and rapid, and in addition it allows bedside examination. It is also easy to reproduce, which makes it a useful tool for follow-up.

Pneumothorax is one of the most common pleural abnormalities, and on an erect chest radiograph, a few milliliters of air in the pleural space can usually be detected (Schabel, 1987). It is seen as a pure air lucency without bronchovascular markings and is limited medially by a thin water density representing the visceral pleura. Small pleural effusions are often associated with pneumothoraces.

Radiographs taken during forced expiration may increase the relative volume and lucency of a pneumothorax and permit its detection when it cannot be seen on a

TABLE 39–1 ■ **Physical Signs of Pleural Effusion**

Amount of Effusion	*Respiratory Rate*	*Chest Expansion*	*Fremitus*	*Breath Sounds*	*Contralateral Tracheal Shift*
Small (<300 ml)	N, ↑	N	N	V	O
Moderate (300–1500 ml)	N, ↑–↑↑	N, ↓	N, ↓	↓, V	O
Large (>1500 ml)	↑↑	↓↓	↓↓	↓↓BV, O	O, +

N, normal; V, vesicular; BV, bronchovesicular; O, absent; +, present.
From Jay SJ: Diagnostic procedures for pleural disease. Clin Chest Med 6:33, 1985.

standard radiograph. This, however, is unusual and does not justify the routine use of both inspiration and expiration films for the documentation of suspected pneumothoraces. On a supine or a portable film, a pneumothorax of small or even of moderate volume may not be visible (Tocico et al, 1985), but it can be suspected on the basis of indirect signs such as an increased lucency of the affected hemithorax, a deep sulcus of increased lucency (Gordon, 1980) (air collected in the anteroinferior costophrenic sulcus), or extremely well-defined diaphragmatic or cardiac contours (Rhea et al, 1979).

The diagnosis of tension pneumothorax usually cannot be made on a plain radiograph taken at total lung capacity (Fraser and Paré, 1977). Rather, it should be documented fluoroscopically by a shift of the mediastinum toward the side of the pneumothorax during inspiration and by restricted inflation of the normal lung with limited movement of the ipsilateral hemidiaphragm during expiration. Standard chest radiographs may also be useful to determine the cause of the pneumothorax, as subpleural blebs, fibrotic lung, or metastatic disease may at times be clearly seen. Misplacement of a chest tube in an interlobar fissure may be definitively documented on lateral chest radiographs.

Normal pleural fluid in the amount of 1 to 5 ml (Black, 1972) is usually not detectable on standard chest radiographs. As shown by Moskowitz and associates (1973), films taken with the patient in the lateral decubitus position are more sensitive and may be able to detect 5 ml of fluid. The earliest sign of pleural effusion on an erect radiograph is the displacement of the normally sharp costophrenic angle away from the lateral chest wall, a feature that may be present with 25 ml of pleural fluid (Rudikoff, 1980). Small amounts (50 ml) of pleural fluid can also be seen on an upright lateral chest radiograph as a meniscus in the posterior costophrenic sulcus (Blackmore et al, 1996). The presence of 200 ml of fluid usually leads to the blunting of the lateral costophrenic angle on posteroanterior (PA) erect films, but on occasion up to 500 ml may not cause any blunting of the costophrenic angle; such is the case with subpulmonic effusions, in which the fluid is located between the lung and the diaphragm. Collins and coworkers (1972) have described four radiologic signs associated with subpulmonic effusions: (1) the apex of the hemidiaphragm migrates laterally from its usual medial location; (2) the medial portion of the diaphragm appears flat, with accentuation on expiration; (3) the upper abdomen appears more dense, owing to the filling of the posterior costophrenic angle with pleural fluid; and (4) on the left side, the apparent distance between the diaphragm and the stomach bubble is increased.

On supine films large quantities of pleural fluid may be missed, especially if the effusion is bilateral. In those cases it may be suspected based on the presence of a veiling density of one hemithorax associated with persistence of vascular markings or the presence of an apical cap, a blunting of the costophrenic angle (Ruskin et al, 1987; Woodring, 1984), a loss of the hemidiaphragm silhouette (Emamian et al, 1997), or a liquid density in a scissural position. Occasionally, pleural fluid collects in atypical locations (Henschke et al, 1989) such as the interlobar fissure, where it presents as a "pseudotumor," which is recognized by its biconvex lenticular shape and scissural position. In cases of pseudotumors, pleural fluid is often present elsewhere in the pleural space.

Standard chest radiographs cannot distinguish between the densities of a transudate, an exudate, an empyema, a hemothorax, and a chylothorax. Transudates associated with congestive heart failure are usually bilateral, but when they are unilateral, they are more common on the right side, a feature that is different from what is seen in constrictive pericarditis, in which the effusion is more often left-sided (Kreel, 1990). Parapneumonic effusions are usually serous exudates that resolve spontaneously once the pneumonia is under control and resolving (Fraser and Paré, 1977). Consequently, a rapid increase in the amount of pleural fluid with an associated pneumonia suggests an impending or established empyema. Exudates and empyemas tend to loculate and accumulate posteroinferiorly, producing the "pregnant lady" or "inverted D" sign (Kreel, 1990) on lateral chest radiographs.

Empyemas may be difficult to distinguish from lung abscesses on standard chest radiographs. Lung abscesses are usually more spherical, with an almost equal length of the air-fluid level in both frontal and lateral views. An empyema forms an obtuse angle as it apposes the chest wall, whereas a lung abscess forms an acute angle. Lung abscesses tend to respect lobar and segmental boundaries, which are frequently crossed by an empyema (Stark et al, 1983a). Empyemas and hemothoraces may ultimately lead to pleural thickening, to distortion of the diaphragm (which may also lose its dome shape), to blunting of the costophrenic angles, and to unilateral pleural calcifications.

Pleural disease is the most common manifestation of asbestos exposure. Pleural plaques, pleural calcifications, benign pleural effusions, and malignant mesotheliomas can all be seen. Pleural plaques are present in 20% to 60% of workers exposed to strong concentrations of asbestos fibers (Schwartz et al, 1990; Schwartz, 1991), and there is a latency period of more than 20 years before radiographically visible calcified plaques appear (Fletcher and Edge, 1970; Schwartz, 1991). These plaques are generally located posterolaterally, where they follow the contours of the 7th to the 10th rib. They are often bilateral but tend to be asymmetric (Fisher, 1985; Gefter and Conant, 1988). In 25% of cases, pleural plaques are unilateral, and in those cases they tend more commonly to be left-sided (Gefter and Conant, 1988; Withers et al, 1984). Pleural plaques are almost always located on the parietal pleura, although at times they can occur on the visceral pleura, usually within the interlobar fissures (Rockoff et al, 1987).

The use of oblique views to detect pleural plaques is controversial (Baker and Greene, 1982; McLoud et al, 1985; Reger et al, 1982) because the increased sensitivity of this view also increases the incidence of false-positive results. Normal muscle and fat shadows may cause false images of pleural thickening, but these are usually more symmetric in distribution than pleural plaques. Hillerdal and Lindgren (1980) have shown that the presence of bilateral pleural plaques at least 5 mm thick or of bilateral calcified diaphragmatic plaques has a 100% positive predictive value for the diagnosis of asbestos-related pleural plaques. Up to 50% of pleural plaques are calcified (Fraser and Paré, 1977), making this the second most common finding in asbestos-related disease.

Benign asbestos pleurisy is a less common manifestation of asbestos-related pleural disease. It is usually recurrent, bilateral, associated with chest pain (Gaensler and Kaplan, 1971), and less than 500 ml in total volume. Because pleural effusion is seldom associated with asbestos exposure alone, its mere presence should raise the possibility of another disease such as a mesothelioma (Fraser and Paré, 1977).

Rounded atelectasis (Mintzer et al, 1981) is a form of atelectasis associated with pleural disease and, more commonly, with asbestos-related pleural disease. It occurs as a well-circumscribed mass abutting a pleura, which is always thickened. In those cases there is also crowding of adjacent bronchi and blood vessels, producing the so-called comet-tail sign (Schneider et al, 1980). The diagnosis of rounded atelectasis may be suspected on the basis of standard radiographs, but characteristic features are often difficult to appreciate.

Diffuse malignant mesotheliomas are uncommon neoplasms, associated in about 60% to 80% of cases with a history of asbestos exposure (Mossman and Gee, 1989). Although calcified pleural plaques may be seen with mesotheliomas, they are not common (Kawashima and Libshitz, 1990). A mesothelioma usually occurs as an irregular or nodular thickening of the pleura with or without a pleural effusion (Fig. 39–1), and typically there is no contralateral shift of the mediastinum because of the constrictive effect of the tumor (Fraser and Paré, 1977) on the underlying lung. Because mesothelioma is a relatively uncommon cause of malignant pleural effusion (5% of cases), pleural metastases or pleural invasion of lung cancer should first be considered, especially if there are associated ribs or pulmonary abnormalities (Godwin, 1984).

Standard chest radiographs may allow detection of local pleural thickening or of localized pleura-based masses. Pleural apical thickening is a common finding, often representing nonspecific fibrous scarring of the lung apex. It is usually bilateral, and calcifications are seldom associated. Old tuberculosis may also be responsible for pleural apical thickening, which, in those cases, is usually unilateral and associated with fibrosis and retraction of the lung parenchyma. Occasionally, Pancoast's tumors can mimic benign pleural thickening, and this should be considered in the differential diagnosis, especially if the finding is unilateral and associated with pain.

Benign pleural tumors are rare, and most are incidental findings on chest radiographs. They present as broad-based masses with rounded margins forming obtuse angles with the pleura. Tangential views may also demonstrate well-defined medial margins and ill-defined lateral margins with the pleura. Accurate diagnosis is generally not possible unless one can appreciate such characteristic features as a change in location of the tumor, which is typical of benign fibrous mesotheliomas (Fig. 39–2) (Weisbrod and Yee, 1983).

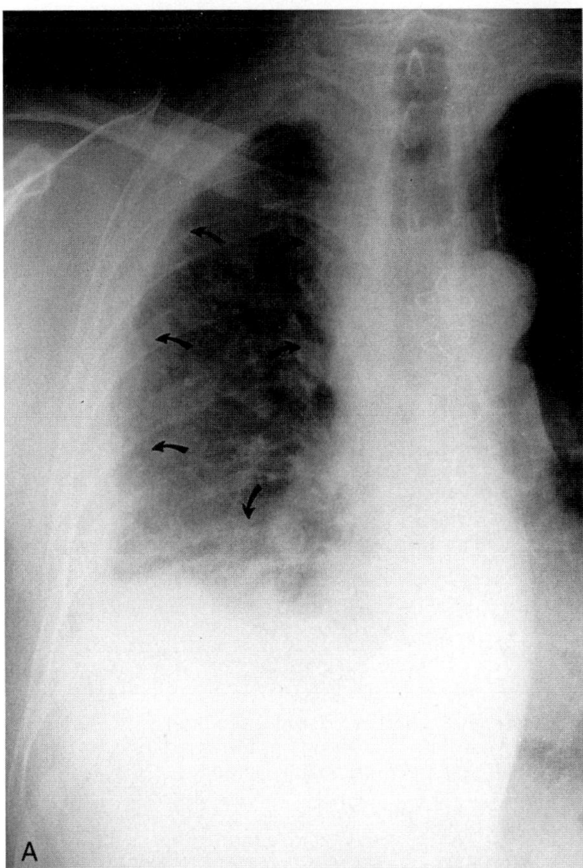

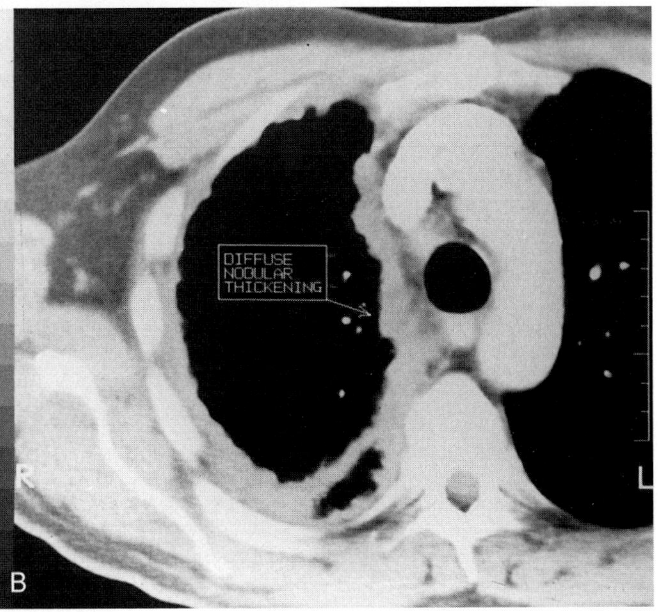

FIGURE 39–1 ■ Malignant mesothelioma. *A*, Standard chest radiograph demonstrating diffuse pleural nodular thickening and loss of volume of the right hemithorax; *B*, same findings on computer tomography scan, where thickening of the tissue can also be seen.

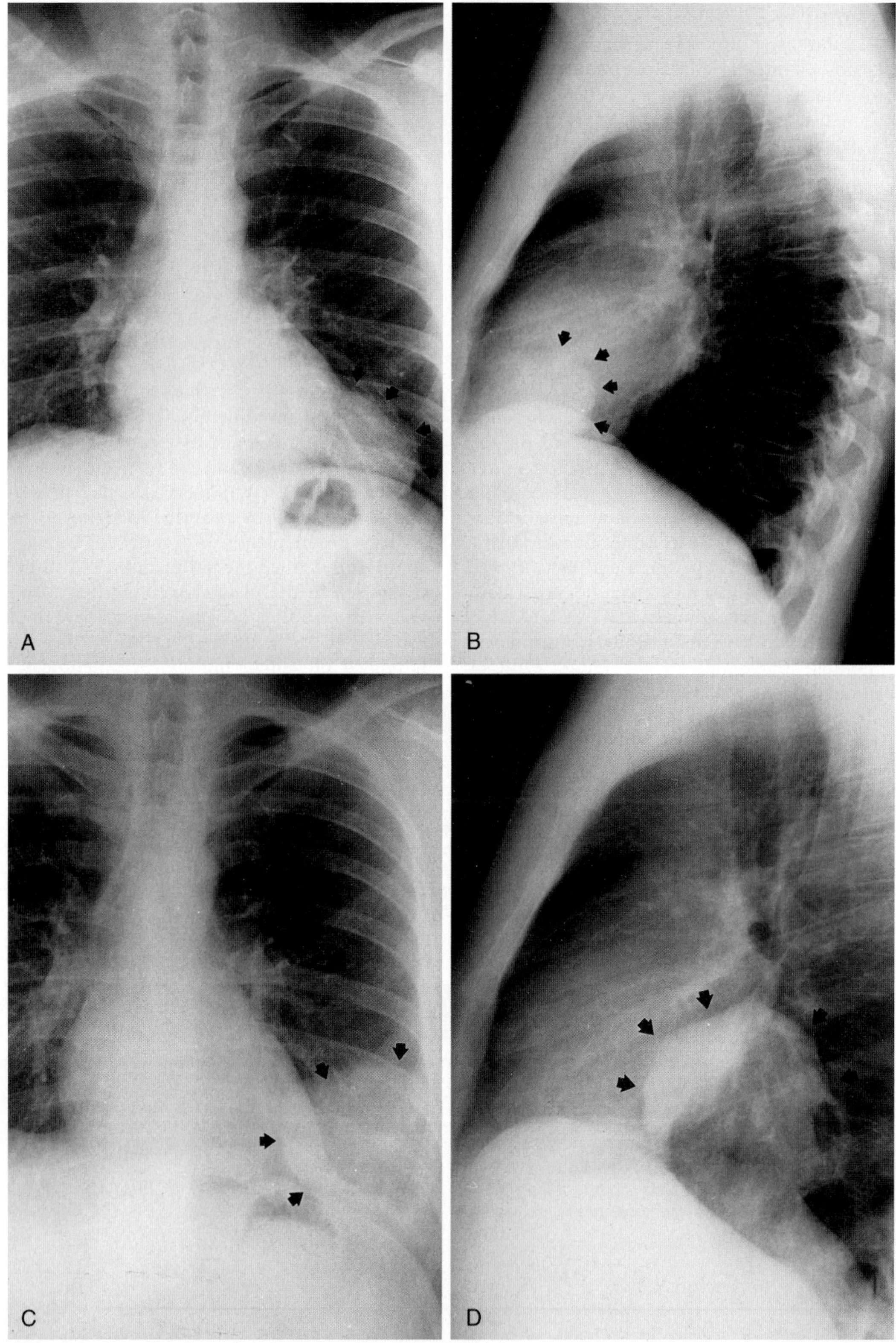

FIGURE 39–2 ■ Benign mesothelioma. Posteroanterior *(A)* and lateral *(B)* chest radiographs showing a well-circumscribed left posterior paracardiac mass. *C* and *D*, Three years later the lesion has increased in size and has moved to the left posterior paracardiac position. At surgery a benign pedunculated mesothelioma originating in the oblique fissure was seen.

Computed Tomography

High-contrast resolution and axial transverse slices, which eliminate confusing superposition of images, have had a major impact on the use of the CT scan to evaluate pleural disease. CT may demonstrate disease at an earlier stage than other imaging techniques can, and characterization of tissue density is possible by the analysis of attenuation coefficient numbers (Hounsfield units). Pleural and parenchymal lesions can easily be separated. Also, CT images can be reproduced, allowing for accurate follow-up of pleural lesions (Rusch et al, 1988).

CT scanning facilitates detection of small pneumothoraces that are sometimes not seen on chest radiographs, and it is also useful for demonstrating underlying parenchymal lesions such as interstitial disease, bullae, lung metastases, and other lesions that are causing the pneumothorax. It can be used to rule out a pneumothorax in a patient with a hyperlucent area on chest radiograph (Bourgouin et al, 1985), and questions about the location of a chest tube can be answered readily.

Pleural fluid is easily seen on CT scans; however, CT is of limited value for differentiating between a transudate and an exudate (Müller, 1993). Hemothoraces can be diagnosed by the presence of a fluid level or by the increased density of the pleural fluid (McLoud and Flower, 1991). Occasionally, loculations develop in hemothoraces. They may appear as "fibrin balls" or pleural pseudotumors with characteristically high attenuation on nonenhanced CT (Armstrong et al, 1995).

Differentiation between a pleural effusion and ascites may be a problem because both are in close proximity on axial images of the lower chest and upper abdomen. In such cases, four radiologic signs may help to establish a correct diagnosis. The interface sign (Teplick et al, 1982) refers to a sharp interface between fluid and spleen or liver in a case of ascites or to an interface that is ill-defined in a case of pleural effusion. The displaced crus sign (Dwyer, 1978) describes diaphragmatic crus displacement away from the spine in a pleural effusion, whereas ascites is seen anterior and lateral to the crus. The diaphragm sign (Müller, 1993) refers to the different positions of pleural fluid and ascites in relation to the diaphragm; pleural fluid usually lies peripheral to the diaphragm; ascites is medial. Finally, the bare-area sign (Halvorsen et al, 1986) refers to the anatomy of the right lobe of the liver. It is attached to the posterior abdominal wall, so ascites cannot extend behind the liver at this level; pleural effusions can be seen posterior to the liver.

Differentiation between an empyema and a sterile effusion may be possible by use of CT with intravenous injection of a contrast agent. Enhancement of the parietal and visceral pleura, thickening of the extrapleural subcostal tissues, and increased attenuation of the extrapleural fat favor the diagnosis of empyema over that of a sterile effusion (Waite et al, 1990).

CT is more accurate than standard radiographs for differentiating an empyema from a lung abscess because a CT scan usually sees the thin and uniform wall of an empyema whereas the wall of a lung abscess is thicker and more irregular (Williford and Godwin, 1983). The split pleural sign (Stark et al, 1983a) is associated with an empyema; it refers to fluid that has collected between the thickened parietal and visceral pleural membranes. The parenchymal compression seen with an empyema and the sharp boundaries between empyema and lung (Stark et al, 1983a) are better demonstrated by CT. Injection of contrast medium, especially by means of the bolus method, also facilitates differentiation between an empyema and a lung abscess (Bressler et al, 1987). A CT scan can demonstrate loculations unsuspected on chest radiographs, and it can also help to explain a failure of tube drainage by showing that the tube is out of the collection, that it is in the lung or in the fissure, or that it has kinked in its entry through the chest wall (Stark et al, 1983b).

In the evaluation of asbestos-related disorders, CT—especially high-resolution CT—has greater sensitivity than chest radiographs (Aberle et al, 1988; Friedman et al, 1988). Because of its high cost, however, CT is not recommended for screening (Müller, 1993) except to rule out a false-positive diagnosis of pleural plaques, intercostal muscles or extrapleural fat. CT allows for differentiation between pleural plaques and pulmonary lesions, and the diagnosis of rounded atelectasis is more easily made on a CT scan than on a radiograph. Contrast enhancement occurs in rounded atelectasis, and this finding alone may facilitate its differentiation from a neoplasm (Blouin et al, 1991) (Fig. 39–3).

CT can be used to diagnose and assess the extent of mesothelioma (see Fig. 39–1) and is also helpful in the postsurgical follow-up of mesothelioma patients, as it may demonstrate tumor recurrence before it is clinically evident or seen on standard radiographs.

CT may also be useful for differentiating between benign and malignant processes (Leung et al, 1990). Circumferential pleural thickening, nodular pleural thickening, parietal pleural thickening greater than 1 cm, and mediastinal pleural involvement all suggest the presence of malignant disease. Mesotheliomas are, however, difficult to differentiate from pleural metastatic disease (Leung et al, 1990). Finally, CT is recommended for the follow-up of patients with previous malignant thymomas treated by radiotherapy or surgery, because pleural seeding is often the first sign of recurrent disease (Zerhouni et al, 1982) and this can be detected easily by CT examination.

In localized pleural tumors, CT can be used but there are no pathognomonic features that allow for differentiation between a benign and a malignant lesion unless the homogeneous fatty density typical of a subpleural lipoma can be seen (McLoud and Flower, 1991) (Fig. 39–4). In bronchogenic carcinoma, standard CT is not accurate for distinguishing between neoplastic contiguity with the pleura and frank invasion, but its accuracy may be increased with the use of artificial CT pneumothorax (Yokoi et al, 1991).

The number of CT-assisted interventional procedures that can be performed to investigate pleural-space pathologies has increased significantly over the past few years and this tendency should continue, especially with the expanded usage of CT-fluoroscopy technology. Biopsies, pleural drainage, spring-hook wire insertion before video-thoracoscopic surgery, and fibrinolytic or sclerosing therapy under CT guidance have, in some cases, improved the investigation and treatment of pleural processes.

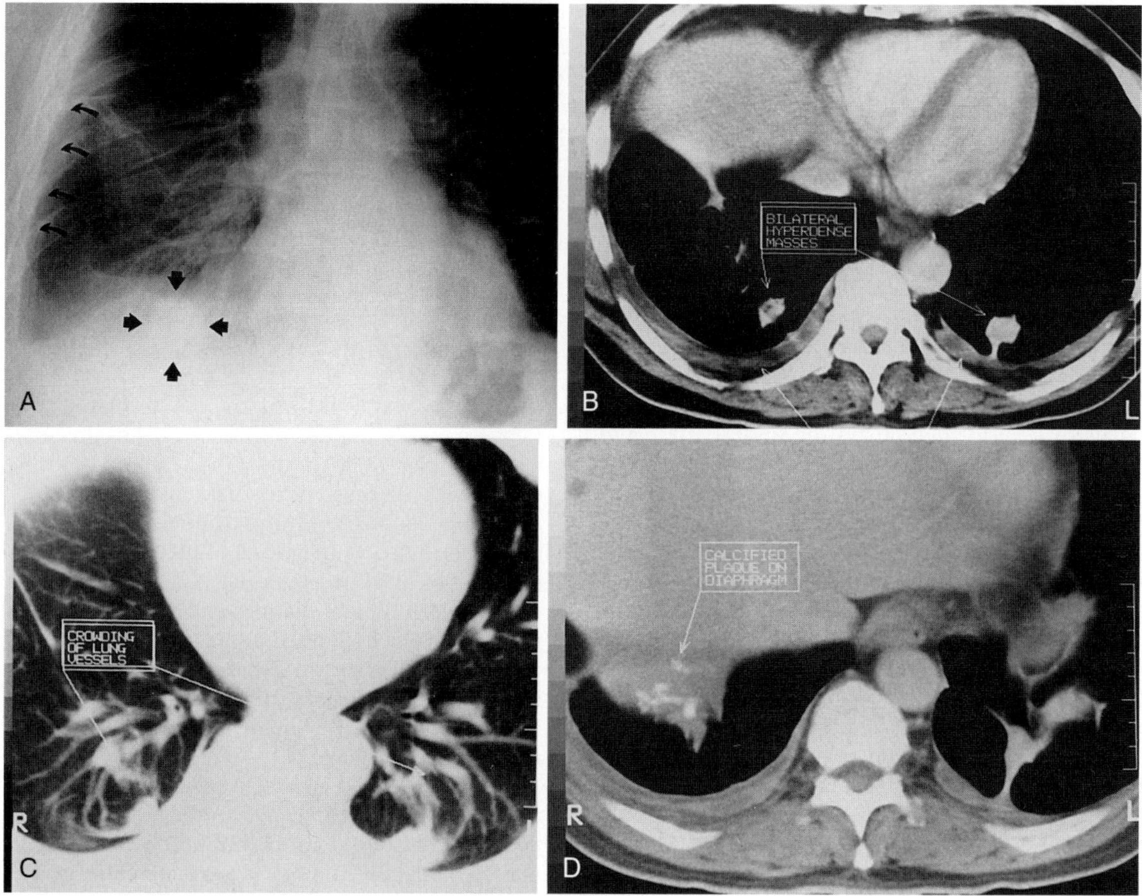

FIGURE 39–3 ■ Asbestos-related disease. *A*, Standard posteroanterior chest radiograph showing bilateral pleural thickening (*small arrows*) and a mass (rounded atelectasis) located behind the right hemidiaphragm (*large arrows*); *B*, computed tomography (CT) scan demonstrating pleural thickening and bilateral rounded atelectasis with typical enhancement after injection of contrast; *C*, CT scan demonstrating crowded lung vessels medially to rounded atelectasis and diaphragmatic pleural calcifications, *D*.

Ultrasound

The superficial location of the pleura makes it easily accessible to ultrasound, a simple, noninvasive imaging technique that, in addition to being much less expensive than CT, does not expose the patient to radiation.

Ultrasound is complementary to standard radiographs for the detection of pleural fluid, especially when the presence of fluid is uncertain, as is often the case when an extensive pulmonary consolidation is present. As little as 3 to 5 ml of pleural fluid can be detected by ultrasound (Mathis, 1997). It may help to characterize the effusion, and the demonstration of septae, sometimes not seen on CT, may suggest possible difficulties with tube drainage. Occasionally, pleural thickening or tumor may be very hypoechogenic and may be mistaken for pleural fluid. For the diagnosis of minimal or loculated effusions, the fluid-color sign may be a useful aid to real-time gray-scale ultrasound (Wu et al, 1994, 1995). Demonstration of highly reflective bronchi in consolidated lungs (McLoud and Flower, 1991) or of a sonographic "fluid bronchogram" (Dorne, 1986) allows differentiation between parenchymal and pleural disease.

Real-time ultrasound imaging usually demonstrates normal movement of the visceral pleura synchronous with that of the underlying lung during the respiratory cycle. Local invasion of the parietal pleura by a peripheral bronchogenic carcinoma can be ruled out, therefore, if one sees the sliding of the visceral pleura over the parietal pleura at the tumor site (Carrier et al, 1987). In the evaluation of chest wall invasion by peripheral lung cancer, Suzuki and colleagues (1993) demonstrated a sensitivity of 100% and a specificity of 98% in the presence of at least two of the three following ultrasound criteria: (1) disruption of the pleura, (2) fixation of the tumor during breathing, and (3) extension through the chest wall.

Multiple-plane imaging with ultrasound allows for easier assessment of the apical and diaphramatic pleura than does CT scanning. Subphrenic abscesses are readily distinguished from pleural effusions. Small Pancoast's tumors can also be seen and biopsied under ultrasound guidance (Carrier et al, 1987).

Ultrasound guidance of interventional pleural procedures is one of the most important contributions of ultrasound to the investigation of pleural diseases. Real-time and multiplane imaging allows for safe and accurate procedures (Fig. 39–5), and the incidence of pneumothorax after ultrasound-guided biopsy is low because the short tract between skin and pleura helps in avoiding the adjacent lung (Carrier et al, 1987). In pleural biopsies,

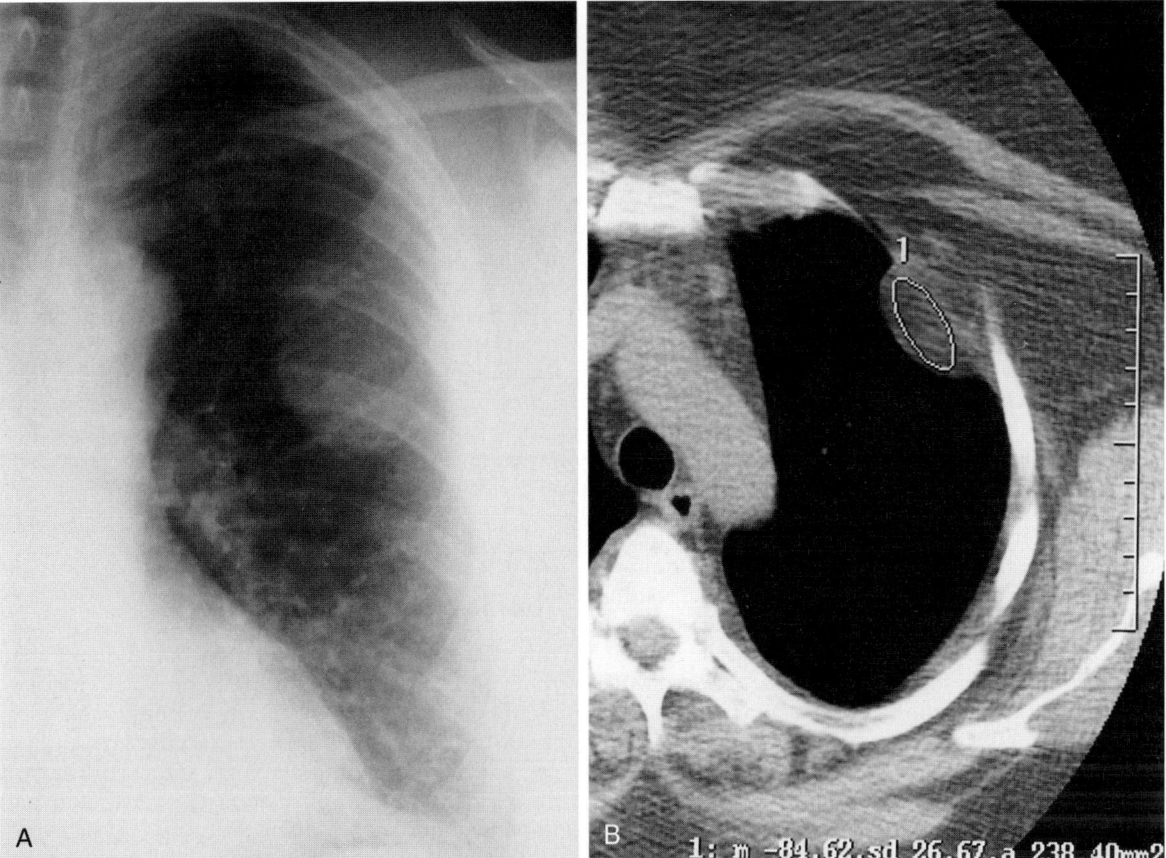

FIGURE 39–4 ■ *A*, Standard chest radiograph showing a well-defined pleural-based mass; and *B*, A computed tomography scan demonstrating the fatty content of this pleural lipoma with negative Hounsfield units (−84 HU).

the development of high-speed, 18- and 20-gauge cutting needles combined with ultrasound guidance provides better histologic samples and helps to differentiate the pathologic processes.

Nuclear Medicine

Radionuclide studies may be useful in the evaluation of pleural diseases. Ventilation-perfusion isotope lung scans

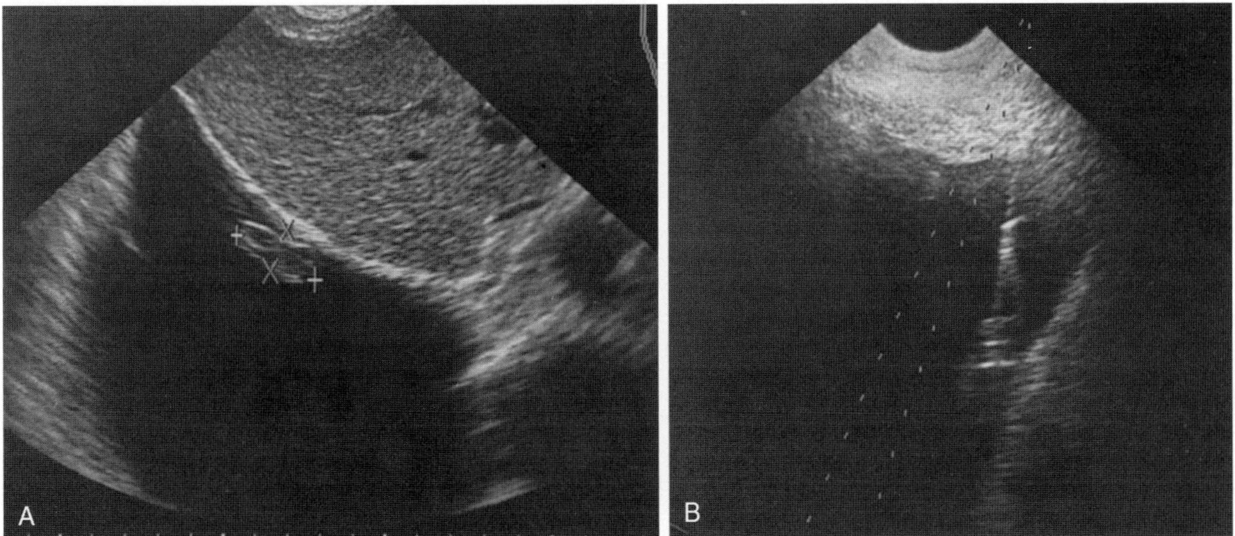

FIGURE 39–5 ■ Diagnosis of malignant pleural effusion documented by ultrasound. *A*, Pleural effusion with a pleural nodule; *B*, biopsy of the pleural nodule under sonographic guidance showed metastatic adenocarcinoma.

can be done when searching for pulmonary embolism as a cause for pleural effusion. Myelography with ^{111}In diethylenetriamine pentaacetic acid (^{111}In DTPA) has been useful in the diagnosis of pleurosubarachnoid fistulas after surgery or trauma (Krasnow et al, 1989). Ventilation scanning may also be useful to demonstrate postpneumonectomy bronchopleural fistulas (Moote et al, 1987), and ^{67}Ga scanning can document whether the pleural fluid is purulent. Suspicion of peritoneopleural communication (Verreault et al, 1986) may be evaluated with either ^{99m}Tc diethylenetriamine pentaacetic acid ^{99m}Tc DTPA sulfur colloid or ^{99m}Tc DTPA macroaggregated albumin (MAA) injected intraperitoneally (Fig. 39–6).

Magnetic Resonance Imaging

MRI, a noninvasive imaging technique, is likely to have an increasingly large role in the evaluation of pleural diseases even though it is expensive and does not allow for bedside examination. Although preliminary results suggest that MRI may help in the characterization of pleural fluid (Davis et al, 1990), it is of little clinical significance at present. Gadolinium-DTPA–enhanced MRI may help in the differentiation between transudative and exudative pleural effusions. The absence of signal enhancement is strongly suggestive of a transudate, although unfortunately it does not completely rule out an exudate (Frola et al, 1997). MRI imaging can also be useful to differentiate a benign from a malignant localized lesion because signal hypointensity on long TR (repetition time) images is an accurate predictor of benign disease (Falaschi et al, 1996).

Because MRI produces images in axial, coronal, and sagittal planes, it may be superior to CT scanning for the evaluation of the apical and diaphragmatic pleura (Fig. 39–7). This is particularly interesting in the assessment of Pancoast's tumors, for which invasion of the spinal canal and of the base of the neck or involvement of the brachial plexus may be demonstrated by MRI (McLoud and Flower, 1991). MRI may be also useful for patients with mesothelioma, especially to document mediastinal invasion or extension into the chest wall or below the diaphragm (McLoud and Flower, 1991). For the work-up of lung cancer abutting the parietal pleura, dynamic-line MRI during breathing is a good technique for documenting whether the tumor invades the chest wall (Sakai et al, 1997).

BIOPSY PROCEDURES

Thoracentesis

Any alteration of the fluid transportation gradients, of the lymphatic drainage, or of the physical integrity of the pleural surfaces can result in accumulation of pleural fluid. In that circumstance, thoracentesis with biochemical, microbiologic, and cytologic studies of the fluid is of great importance in evaluating the cause and nature of the effusion.

Thoracentesis is performed under local anesthesia, and other than a hemorrhagic diathesis, there are virtually

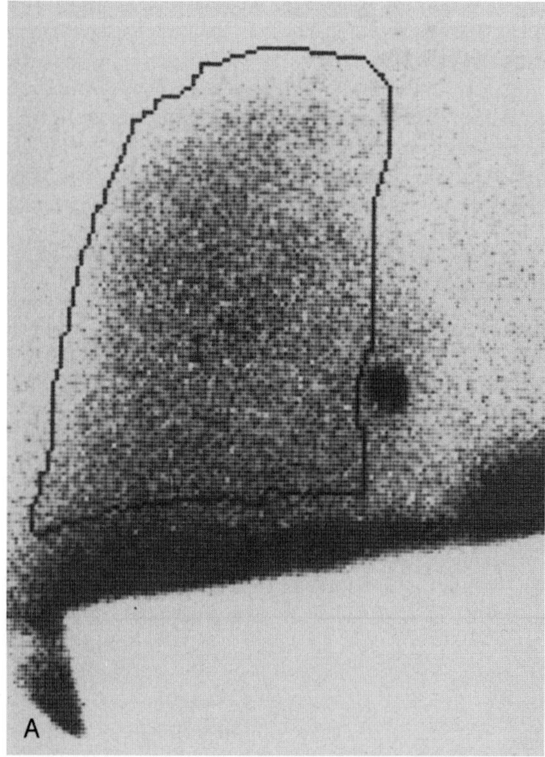

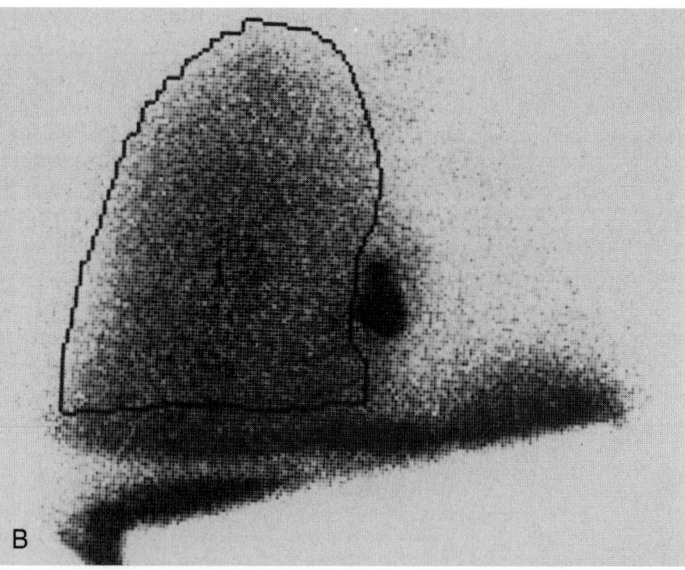

FIGURE 39–6 ■ Peritoneopleural communication documented by nuclear medicine. *A*, ^{99m}Tc macroaggregated albumin injected intraperitoneally flows in the pleural space in this patient with ascites and unilateral pleural effusion. *B*, Same findings with ^{99m}Tc sulfur colloid isotope scan. (Courtesy of Jean Guimond, MD.)

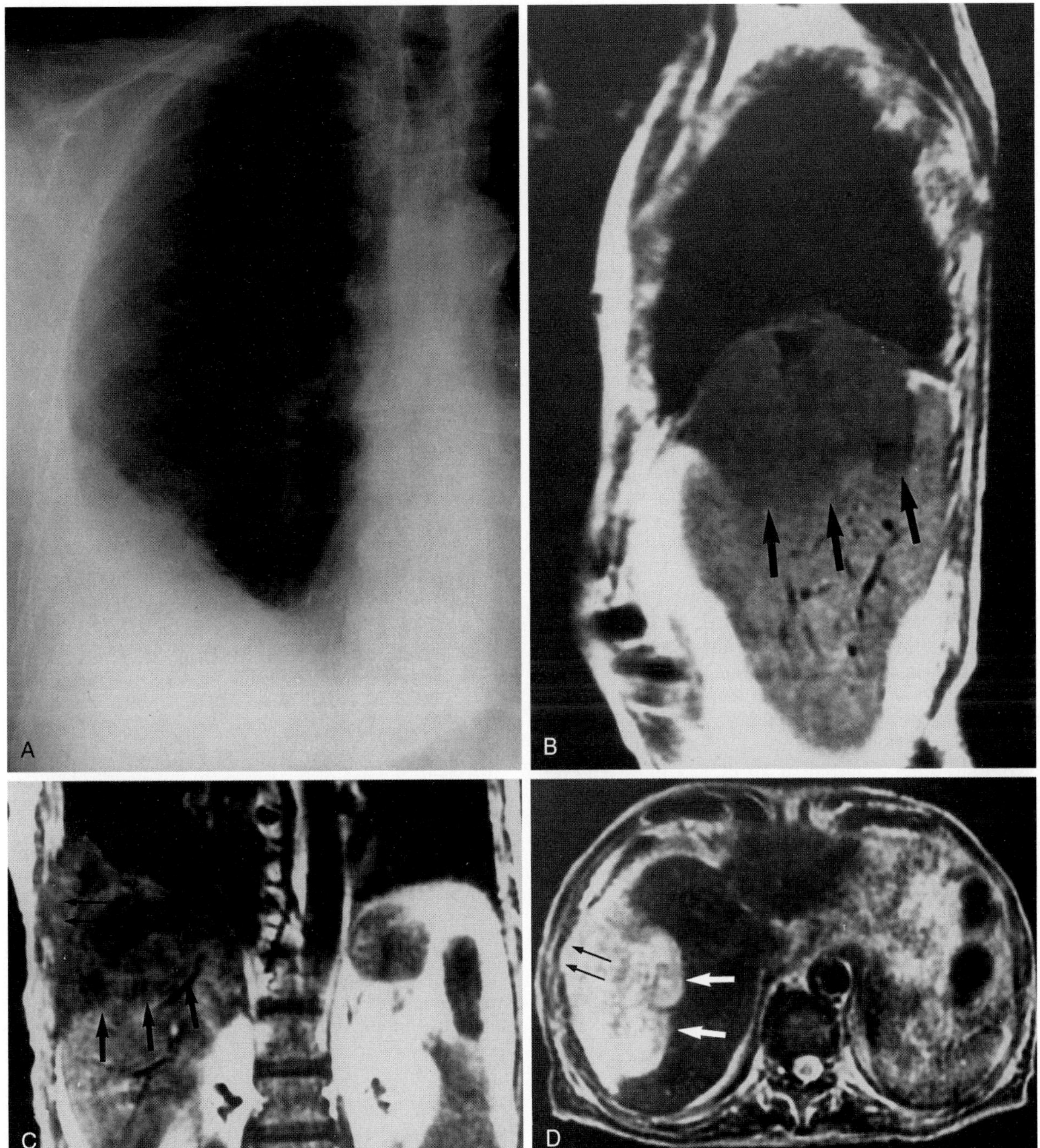

FIGURE 39–7 ■ Magnetic resonance imaging (MRI) imaging of diaphragmatic and chest wall neoplastic invasion by lung carcinoma. *A,* Standard chest radiograph showing a density obscuring the right hemidiaphragm. Chest wall invasion (*small arrows*) and liver invasion (*large arrows*) as demonstrated by MRI: *B,* Sagittal T_1-weighted magnetic resonance image (WMRI). *C,* Coronal T_1-WMRI. *D,* Axial T_2-WMRI. (Courtesy of Gilles Bouchard, MD.)

no absolute contraindications to the procedure. Relative contraindications include an uncooperative patient, a small amount of fluid, and a clinically secure diagnosis (Sahn, 1988). The classic technique of thoracentesis involves good anesthesia of the parietal pleura, entry into the pleural space, aspiration of a small amount of fluid to confirm the proper location of the needle, and fluid removal with a larger needle. Approximately 50 ml of pleural fluid is sufficient to carry out most analyses. Kovarik (1970) and Krausz and Manny (1976) have described modified techniques of thoracentesis, in which they use an Angiocath to provide greater safety for the patient and more flexibility for the physician. In many centers thoracentesis is now performed under ultrasound guidance, a technique that has the advantage of directing the needle into the effusion.

Thoracentesis is diagnostic in 50% to 60% of patients with pleural effusion, and higher yields can be obtained for diseases, such as empyemas, hemothoraces, and chylothoraces, that rely less on cytology and biochemistry for their diagnosis. In 1987 Collins and Sahn reported the results of a prospective study of 129 consecutive thoracenteses in 86 patients. Pleural fluid analysis in conjunction with the clinical presentation placed 78 pleural fluids into diagnostic categories, and 92% of thoracenteses provided clinically useful information.

Cytologic analysis, even with repeated examination of large amounts of pleural fluid, is diagnostic in only 60% to 80% of patients with metastatic disease to the pleura (Light, 1983). It is higher in patients with ovarian or breast cancer and lower in patients with bronchogenic carcinoma or mesothelioma (Miguères et al, 1981). When the cytology is positive for malignant cells, the histologic type of the primary tumor can sometimes be determined (Serre et al, 1990), but up to 5% of patients may have a false-positive cytology reading. In a study of 414 patients with pleural effusion, Prakash and Reiman (1985) were able to show that cytologic analysis has a higher sensitivity ($P < .001$) than needle biopsy for diagnosing malignant pleural effusions. It is also important to note that it is virtually impossible to differentiate between a malignant mesothelioma and a metastatic adenocarcinoma by cytologic examination of the pleural fluid alone.

Although several complications of thoracentesis have been reported, most are minor. They include vasovagal reactions, hemothorax or pneumothorax, contamination of the pleural space, and improper placement of the needle in organs located below the diaphragm. In Collins and Sahn's series (1987), 34 objective complications occurred in 26 of 129 thoracenteses (20%), and 65 subjective complications occurred in 56 of 123 thoracenteses (46%), anxiety and site pain being the most common of these events. In another study of the complications of thoracentesis (Seneff et al, 1986), major complications occurred in 14% of patients and minor complications in 33%. These occurred even when a lecture and printed guidelines on performing thoracentesis had been given, and experienced individuals were in attendance.

Other reported but unusual complications of thoracentesis are hypoxemia, which may worsen temporarily after fluid removal, and re-expansion pulmonary edema, which may follow the development of marked negative pleural pressure during thoracentesis (Light et al, 1980).

Closed Pleural Needle Biopsy

The conventional technique of closed pleural biopsy using an Abrams or a Cope needle provides a diagnosis in 37.5% to 67% of patients with malignancy of the pleura (Rao et al, 1965; Cantó et al, 1977) and in 54% to 75% of patients with tuberculous pleurisy (Tomlinson and Sahn, 1987). Cantó and associates (1977) have further shown that most tumors are located in the lower half of the thorax and that within that portion most are located on the visceral, diaphragmatic, or mediastinal pleura, none of which is readily accessible by conventional techniques of needle biopsy.

Various needles can be used for biopsy of the parietal pleura, but at present the Vim-Silverman, Cope, and Abrams needles are the most extensively used. The Vim-Silverman needle is a puncture type of needle, the Cope a hook type, which cuts inside out, and the Abrams, a guillotine type, which cuts laterally. In general, the results of pleural biopsy depend less on the type of needle than on the experience of the operator and pathologist.

In the series of Poe and colleagues (1984), 211 patients underwent pleural biopsies, and adequate tissue was obtained in 207. Specificity was 100% and sensitivity 90% for tuberculosis and 68% for neoplasia. In another study, Salyer and colleagues (1975) showed that malignant neoplasms involving the pleura could be diagnosed in 90% of cases if both pleural fluid and tissues were examined. Contrary to what is seen with malignant effusions, the diagnosis of pleural tuberculosis is easier to make by pleural biopsy than by cytologic examination (Frist et al, 1979; Scharer and McClement, 1967). In a review of 14 papers from 1958 to 1985, reporting a total of 2893 pleural biopsies, the diagnostic yield was 57% for carcinoma of the pleura and 75% for tuberculous pleurisy (Sahn, 1988; Tomlinson and Sahn, 1987).

Complications of closed pleural biopsy are infrequent if the procedure is performed by or under the direct supervision of a staff pulmonary disease specialist or a thoracic surgeon (Poe et al, 1984). Pneumothorax is the most common complication, having occurred in 8.4% of patients in the series of Poe and colleagues (1984). Fité et al (1989) also described the breakage and detachment of an Abrams needle in the pleural cavity during the performance of a pleural biopsy.

Thoracoscopy

As a consequence of the relatively low yields of thoracentesis and pleural biopsies, in about 20% of patients with pleural effusion, no cause can be found despite exhaustive and expensive testing (Gunnels, 1978; Poe et al, 1984). Of much concern are the 50% of this group who will ultimately show evidence of malignancy. By thoracoscopy 90% to 100% of the surfaces of both visceral and parietal pleura can be explored. This allows direct access for biopsy of suspicious areas, and because the biopsy specimens are bigger and are obtained from different sites, it significantly improves the yield of what is obtained by percutaneous blind biopsy.

Indications and Contraindications

Thoracoscopy is indicated for patients with pleural effusion of causes still unknown after conventional methods such as thoracentesis and needle biopsy have been tried and proven unsuccessful (Table 39–2). It is especially indicated in patients with a known primary tumor at another site, a history of asbestos exposure, a combined pleural and pericardial effusion, or a family history of malignancy (Cantó et al, 1990). It may also be indicated for the diagnosis of pleura-based masses. In all such cases thoracoscopy is not a first-line diagnostic technique, but it should be performed after other methods have failed to provide a positive diagnosis. Occasionally, thoracoscopy can be used to visualize solitary fibrous tumors of the pleura, especially those located in the lower hemichest or over the diaphragm. In such cases, thoracoscopic examination allows visualization of the lesion and optimal placement of the thoracotomy incision. Diagnos-

TABLE 39–2 ■ Indications for Diagnostic Thoracoscopy

Unexplained pleural effusion
Pleural mass biopsy
Thoracic malignancy and associated pleural effusion
Mesothelioma
Diagnosis
Need for additional biopsies to confirm diagnosis
Enlarged mediastinal lymph nodes
Other metastatic effusions or lesions
Need for additional biopsies for pathologic studies
Unexplained pericardial effusion
Pneumothorax
To evaluate at first occurrence
Traumatic hemothorax
Evaluation of intrapleural foreign body
To help placement of unusual thoracotomy incision

tic thoracoscopy can also be used to categorize patients with spontaneous pneumothoraces (Rivas de Andrés and Lanzas, 1993; Vanderschueren, 1990) at the time of the first episode.

Other than the usual contraindications to general anesthesia and surgery, the only true contraindication to diagnostic thoracoscopy is a fused pleural space, a condition seldom seen in patients with significant pleural effusions.

Technique and Instrumentation

The operative technique and instrumentation have evolved enormously since Jacobaeus first performed "thorakoscopy" with the help of a cystoscope in 1910. For the next 80 years, the endoscope used could be a mediastinoscope (Rusch and Mountain, 1987), a flexible bronchoscope (Gwin et al, 1975; Williams and Thomas, 1981); a rigid bronchoscope, a laparoscope, or a working thoracoscope as designed and popularized by Boutin and associates (1981). Nowadays, videoscopic instrumentation has largely replaced these older methods. Videothoracoscopy offers better optics and magnification and allows for the involvement of the whole surgical team through the video system. Certain situations, however, still lend themselves to nonvideo thoracoscopy (Urschel, 1997).

Thoracoscopy is usually performed through the intercostal space under local anesthesia (Boushy et al, 1978; Cantó et al, 1977; Menzies and Charbonneau, 1991; Oldenburg and Newhouse, 1979); regional anesthesia (Rusch and Mountain, 1987); or general anesthesia (Boutin et al, 1981; Weissberg et al, 1980). For simple, uncomplicated examination and biopsy of the pleural surfaces, whether one strategy is preferable to the others remains an unanswered question. However, general endotracheal anesthesia with a double-lumen tube is recommended when a thorough inspection of the whole space, diaphragm, or mediastinum is anticipated; when dense adhesions or loculations may have to be broken down; when multiple visceral pleural biopsies or lung or mediastinal biopsies are required; or when a frozen-section result will be obtained prior to termination of the thoracoscopy (Boutin et al, 1981).

Most thoracoscopic evaluations can be performed through a single trocar, utilizing a zero-degree thoracoscope that incorporates a working channel. Additional trocars may be required to perform more complex procedures. Boutin and colleagues (1981) preferred a 7-mm thoracoscope, arguing that the 9-mm scope was too wide and prevented easy pleural inspection in every direction. The use of 30-degree–, 45-degree–, and 90-degree–angle telescopes may also facilitate the examination of difficult areas. Contrary to laparoscopic surgery in which insufflation of the abdominal cavity requires a closed and hermetic system, during thoracoscopy, it is preferable to keep an open system to minimize reinflation of the deflated lung when applying suction inside the pleural space. At times, a second trocar may have to be inserted to serve as a vent to allow inflow of air into the space while suctioning.

Thoracoscopy is performed with the patient in the full lateral decubitus position. For complete pleural examination, the main trocar is usually placed through the fifth or sixth intercostal space in the midaxillary line. Even when general anesthesia is used, it is recommended that the trocar site or sites be infiltrated and that related intercostal space or spaces be instrumented in an effort to minimize patient discomfort in the early postoperative period. Additional trocar placement, when needed, is directed by the operative findings. Occasionally, the position of the trocar may vary, such as when dealing with a partially fused pleural space or when targeting a particular imaged process.

After complete evacuation of the pleural fluid, which should be sent for cytologic and microbiologic analysis, the cavity is thoroughly inspected. Particular attention is given to visualizing the paravertebral gutter and the costophrenic angles. These areas, being dependent, often harbor pathologic changes (Cantó et al, 1990). Any abnormal area on the parietal or visceral pleural surfaces is sampled and specimens are sent for pathologic and microbiologic analysis, including tuberculosis stain and cultures. Depending on the clinical scenario, additional biopsies may be required to allow electron microscopy, hormonal receptor assays, or immunocytochemistry studies. Frozen-section analyses of the biopsied material is strongly recommended so that, when necessary, additional sampling can be performed. When a process involves both pleural surfaces, the parietal surface should be biopsied first and the results confirmed by frozen section to minimize the need to biopsy the visceral surface, with its risks of postoperative air leak. "Blind" biopsies in the most dependant portion of the chest should be obtained even when the endoscopic appearance of the pleural surface is unremarkable.

Another potential advantage of obtaining a frozen-section diagnosis is to possibly complete the procedure with a talc poudrage when a diagnosis of malignancy is confirmed. In most instances, a single chest drain is left in place. Some have reported a more selective use of chest drains after diagnostic thoracoscopies (Enk and Viskum, 1981).

Operative Findings

One of the most common findings of diagnostic thoracoscopy is a nonspecific inflammation of the pleural membranes. With an acute inflammatory reaction, there is increased vascularization, redness, and edema and disappearance of the pleural transparence, all findings more commonly seen over the diaphragm and in the costovertebral gutters. When inflammation is more chronic, the pleura is thickened, opaque, and whitish-gray in color. Specific benign pleural lesions such as granulomas or pleural plaques can usually be readily recognized. Metastatic lesions are often found over the lower half of the space and are recognized as small nodules, masses, or polypoid lesions. White, patchy lesions of the pleura may also be seen, and these must be differentiated from pleural plaques.

The diagnosis of malignant mesothelioma can be made by gross examination of the pleura. In the epithelial or mixed varieties, multiple small, friable, and vascular lesions, sometimes filled with viscous fluid, can be seen. These can be localized over the diaphragm, scattered over the whole space, or confluent in the more advanced stages of disease. In the sarcomatous and more localized variety, there may be only a thickened pleura, although large nodules and masses can also be found. In a review of 35 cases of mesotheliomas, Boutin and colleagues (1979) showed that pleural biopsy was conclusive in only 40% of cases, whereas a positive diagnosis was obtained in 94% of cases by thoracoscopy. Sgro and colleagues (1991) also obtained a yield of 85.7% after thoracoscopy in 21 cases of proven mesothelioma.

We have seen many cases in which the diagnosis of malignant mesothelioma was obtained by thoracoscopic biopsy of what appeared to be normal pleura or inoffensive pleural plaques often located over the diaphragm or in costophrenic angles. In those cases in which the diagnosis is made at an early stage, it is possible that radical resectional surgery will improve overall survival.

Morbidity

In experienced hands, diagnostic thoracoscopy, particularly when limited to inspection and biopsy, whether it is done under local or general anesthesia, is a safe procedure with very few complications (Table 39–3) (Boutin et al, 1981; Cantó et al, 1977). In the Marseilles series of 150 consecutive thoracoscopies done in the evaluation of pleural effusion, no complication was reported in the subgroup done after 1978 (Boutin et al, 1981). Most reported deaths after thoracoscopy are related to the underlying advanced pathology and not to the procedure itself (Viskum and Enk, 1981). The occurrence of postoperative air leaks usually relates to the need to biopsy the visceral pleura or adjacent lung. In one series, however, it resulted solely from taking down adhesions, without intentional visceral biopsy (Menzies and Charbonneau, 1991). Empyemas will likely result from prolonged pleural drainage in instances complicated by inadequate lung re-expansion after pleural space evacuation. This can be avoided by adopting a policy of early chest tube removal despite ongoing pleural drainage in these situations.

Tumor implant at thoracoscopy sites has been reported by many authors and reflects the ability of mesotheliomas to grow in incisions and needle tracts (Boutin et al, 1981; Cantó et al, 1977; Hucker et al, 1991; Tomlinson and Sahn, 1987). Prophylactic local radiation therapy to the thoracoscopy incision or thoracentesis puncture site has been shown to eliminate this complication completely (Boutin et al, 1995).

TABLE 39–3 ■ **Complications of Diagnostic Thoracoscopy**

Prolonged air leak
Subcutaneous emphysema
Bleeding (entry site, adhesions, biopsy site)
Inadequate lung re-expansion and empyema
Cardiac arrhythmia
Entry-tract implant or metastasis

Results

In 1971, Brandt and Mai reported on 1130 diagnostic thoracoscopies, of which 414 were performed for undiagnosed pleural effusions. When thoracoscopy was combined with cytologic and bacteriologic studies, only 2.5% of effusions were still of unknown cause. In 1991 Wakabayashi reported 315 thoracoscopies performed under general anesthesia, with a mortality of 1% and a diagnostic accuracy of 99%.

In a collective review of 1500 thoracoscopies from different centers, Menzies and Charbonneau (1991) found that the diagnostic accuracy of this technique was around 90% and morbidity, which included arrhythmias, bleeding, and empyema, was under 3%. In their own series of 102 thoracoscopies performed under local anesthesia, the diagnostic accuracy was 96%, the sensitivity was 91%, the specificity was 100%, and the negative predictive value was 93%. Major operative complications occurred in 1.9% of cases. Other recent studies have presented similar data (Buchhotz et al, 1990; Get'man et al, 1989; Hucker et al, 1991; Kimura et al, 1990).

OTHER PROCEDURES

Open Thoracotomy

With the recent development of thoracoscopy techniques, very few circumstances occur in which open thoracotomy is necessary for the diagnosis of pleural diseases (Kirby and Ginsberg, 1990). In our opinion, it is indicated only when the pleural space is obliterated and thoracoscopy is not possible or when the surgeon wishes to proceed immediately with a surgical procedure such as decortication, pleurectomy, or pleuropneumonectomy in the case of a malignant mesothelioma. In all other instances, videothoracoscopy is far better than open thoracotomy for fully exploring the pleural space.

In an interesting paper, Ryan and associates (1981) studied the outcomes of 51 patients in whom the cause of pleural effusion was still unknown after open thoracotomy. In 31 patients (60.8%), there was no recurrence of effusion, and no cause became apparent during a follow-up period of 12 to 15 years. In 18 patients, cause of effusion became apparent between 12 days and 6 years after thoracotomy. In 13 of these 18 patients, malignancy (6 patients with lymphoma, 4 with malignant pleural mesothelioma, and 3 with other malignancy) was ultimately diagnosed.

Bronchoscopy

Although the literature is somewhat controversial concerning the role of bronchoscopy in patients with undiagnosed pleural disease, it is our opinion that most of these patients, especially those who will undergo thoracoscopy or open thoracotomy, should have this examination. In the series of Feinsilver and colleagues (1986), 28 patients with unexplained pleural effusion, no mass on chest radiographs, and no lobar atelectasis underwent fiberoptic bronchoscopy. In this group, the yield was only 4% (1 positive of 28 patients) despite a final diagnosis of tumor in 7. Based on these findings and on their own experience, Tomlinson and Sahn (1987) concluded that the key point for the indication of bronchoscopy appears to be the presence or absence of radiographic abnormalities in addition to the pleural effusion.

By contrast, Williams and Thomas (1981) also reported 28 patients who underwent fiberoptic bronchoscopy as part of the evaluation of an undiagnosed pleural effusion. In four patients the diagnosis was made by this examination, with three patients found to have bronchial carcinoma and one tuberculosis. Williams and Thomas concluded that bronchoscopic examination is of value in the workup of patients with undiagnosed pleural effusions without radiographic evidence of mass lesion or atelectasis.

In our experience most pleural effusions are caused by pulmonary diseases, and in those cases, especially if tuberculosis or malignancy is suspected, the importance of bronchoscopy cannot be overestimated.

CONCLUSION

On the basis of this review it is obvious that the cause of most pleural effusions and of other pleural diseases can be determined by the judicious use of available diagnostic methods. Imaging techniques can readily detect an effusion, but they generally are not very accurate in identifying its cause. Thoracentesis and blind pleural biopsies are diagnostic in 80% of patients, whereas thoracoscopy has a yield of close to 100%.

When investigating a pleural effusion, it is important to have a methodical and structured approach to the use of these techniques. For instance, it is important to begin with simple methods such as careful history taking, standard chest radiographs, and thoracentesis rather than to proceed with thoracoscopy as the first line of investigation. This approach not only reduces the cost of investigation but also minimizes patient morbidity.

■ *KEY REFERENCES*

Collins TR, Sahn SA: Thoracentesis: Clinical value, complications, technical problems and patient experience. Chest 91:817, 1987.

This is an excellent review of the role of thoracentesis in the diagnosis of pleural effusions. It includes a critical evaluation of the complications associated with the procedure.

Jay SJ: Diagnostic procedures for pleural diseases. Clin Chest Med 6:33, 1985.

This article reviews the role and results of all the techniques used for the diagnosis of pleural diseases.

Poe RH, Israel RH, Utell MV et al: Sensibility, specificity and predictive values of closed pleural biopsy. Arch Intern Med 114:325, 1984.

This article shows that closed pleural biopsy with simultaneous fluid analysis is a valuable diagnostic procedure.

Sahn SA: Pleural fluid analysis: Narrowing the differential diagnosis. Semin Respir Med 9:22, 1987.

This article reviews the role and diagnostic yield of thoracentesis. There is an excellent discussion of pleural fluid cells.

Tomlinson JR, Sahn SA: Invasive procedures in the diagnosis of pleural diseases. Semin Respir Med 9:30, 1987.

This excellent article analyzes the role of pleural biopsy, thoracoscopy, and open pleural biopsy.

■ *REFERENCES*

Aberle DR, Gamsu G, Ray CS: High-resolution CT of benign asbestos-related diseases: Clinical and radiographic correlation. AJR Am J Roentgenol 151:883, 1988.

Abrams LD: Pleural-biopsy punch. Lancet 1:30, 1958.

Armstrong P, Wilson AG, Dee P et al: Imaging of the Chest. St. Louis, Mosby–Year Book, 1995, pp 641–703.

Baker EL, Greene R: Incremental value of oblique chest radiographs in the diagnosis of asbestos-induced pleural disease. Am J Ind Med 3:17, 1982.

Black LF: The pleural space and pleural fluid. Mayo Clin Proc 47:493, 1972.

Blackmore CC, Black WC, Dallas RV et al: Pleural fluid volume estimation: A chest radiograph prediction rule. Acad Radiol 3:103, 1996.

Blouin O, Carrier G, Ferland S: Atélectasie ronde: Nouveau critère diagnostique. Proceedings of the French Canadian Association of Radiologists Annual Meeting, Montreal, October 9–11, 1991, p 20.

Bourgouin P, Cousineau G, Lemire P, Hébert G: Computed tomography used to exclude pneumothorax in bullous lung disease. Can Assoc Radiol J 36:341, 1985.

Boushy SF, North LB, Helgason AH: Thoracoscopy: Technique with results in eighteen patients with pleural effusion. Chest 74:386, 1978.

Boutin C, Farisse P, Rey F et al: La thoracoscopie doit-elle être un examen de routine en pratique pneumologique courante? Med Hyg 42:2992, 1984.

Boutin C, Farisse P, Viallat P et al: La thoracoscopie dans le mésothéliome pleural. Intérêt diagnostique, pronostique et thérapeutique. Rev Fr Mal Respir 7:680, 1979.

Boutin C, Rey F, Viallat JR: Prevention of malignant seeding after invasive diagnostic procedures in patients with pleural mesothelioma. A randomized trial of local radiotherapy. Chest 108:754, 1995.

Boutin C, Viallat JR, Cargnino P, Farisse P: Thoracoscopy in malignant pleural effusion. Am Rev Respir Dis 124:588, 1981.

Bowditch HI: Paracentesis thoracis. Am J Med Sci 23:103, 1852.

Brandt HJ, Mai J: Differential diagnosis of pleural effusions using thoracoscopy. Pneumologie 145:192, 1971.

Branscomb BV, Harrison TR: Diseases of the pleura, mediastinum and diaphragm. In Harrison TR, Adams RD, Bennett IL Jr et al (eds): Principles of Internal Medicine, 5th ed. New York, McGraw-Hill, 1966, p 964.

Bressler EL, Francis IR, Glazer GM, Gross BH: Bolus contrast medium enhancement for distinguishing pleural from parenchymal lung disease: CT features. J Comput Assist Tomogr 11:436, 1987.

Buchhotz J, Mayer M, Giesekus D: The diagnosis of pleural effusion using thoracoscopy. Zentralb Chir 115:1565, 1990.

Cantó A, Blasco E, Casillas M et al: Thoracoscopy in the diagnosis of pleural effusion. Thorax 32:550, 1977.

Cantó A, Saumench J, Moya J: Points to consider when choosing a biopsy method in cases of pleuritis of unknown origin with special reference to thoracoscopy. In Deslauriers J, Lacquet LK (eds): International Trends in General Thoracic Surgery. St. Louis, CV Mosby, 1990, p 49.

Carpenter RL, Lowell JR: Pleural biopsy and thoracentesis by new instrument. Chest 40:182, 1961.

Carrier G, Mercier A, Bilodeau S: La place de l'échographie dans la sphère thoracique. Proceedings of the French Canadian Association of Radiologists Annual Meeting, Montreal, November 25–27, 1987, p 64.

Collins JD, Burwell D, Furmanski S et al: Minimal detectable pleural effusions. Radiology 105:51, 1972.

Collins TR, Sahn SA: Thoracentesis: Clinical value, complications, technical problems and patient experience. Chest 91:817, 1987.

Cope C: New pleural biopsy needle. JAMA 167:1107, 1958.

Davis SD, Henschke CI, Yankelevitz DF et al: MR imaging of pleural effusions. J Comput Assist Tomogr 14:192, 1990.

De Francis N, Kiosk E, Albano E: Needle biopsy of parietal pleura: Preliminary report. N Engl J Med 252:948, 1955.

Delarue J, De Pierre R: Contribution à l'ètude des pleurésies cancéreuses cliniquement primitives. Intérêt de la biopsie sous pleuroscopie. J Fr Med Chir Thorac 6:653, 1956.

Dorne HL: Differentiation of pulmonary parenchymal consolidation from pleural disease using the sonographic fluid bronchogram. Radiology 158:41, 1986.

Dwyer A: The displaced crus: A sign for distinguishing between pleural fluid and ascites on computed tomography. J Comput Assist Tomogr 2:598, 1978.

Emamian SA, Kaasbol MA, Olsen JF et al: Accuracy of the diagnosis of pleural effusion on supine chest x-ray. Eur Radiol 7:57, 1997.

Enk B, Viskum K: Diagnostic thoracoscopy. Eur J Respir Dis 62:344, 1981.

Fabri G, Parmeggiani D: Observations on thoracoscopy in pleural exudates. Policlini Sez Prat 5:49, 1942.

Falaschi F, Battola L, Mascalchi M et al: Usefulness of MR signal intensity in distinguishing benign from malignant pleural disease. AJR Am J Roentgenol 166:963, 1996.

Feinsilver SH, Barrows AA, Braman SS: Fiberoptic bronchoscopy and pleural effusion of unknown origin. Chest 90:517, 1986.

Fisher MS: Asymmetrical changes in asbestos-related disease. Can Assoc Radiol J 36:110, 1985.

Fité E, Force L, Casarramowa F, Verdaguer A: Breakage and detachment of an Abrams needle in the pleural cavity during performance of a pleural biopsy. Chest 95:928, 1989.

Fletcher DE, Edge JR: The early radiological changes in pulmonary and pleural asbestosis. Clin Radiol 21:355, 1970.

Fourestier M, Duret M: Nécessité de la biopsie pleurale pour le diagnostic de l'endothéliome de la plèvre. Presse Med 32:467, 1943.

Fraser RG, Paré JAP: Diagnosis of Diseases of the Chest. Philadelphia, WB Saunders, 1977.

Friedman AC, Fiel SB, Fisher MS et al: Asbestos-related pleural disease and asbestosis: A comparison of CT and chest radiography. AJR Am J Roentgenol 150:269, 1988.

Frist B, Kahan AV, Koss LG: Comparison of the diagnostic value of biopsies of the pleura and cytological evaluation of pleural fluids. Am J Clin Pathol 72:48, 1979.

Frola C, Cantoni S, Turtulici I et al: Transudative vs exudative pleural effusions: Differentiation using Gd-DTPA-enhanced MRI. Eur Radiol 7:860, 1997.

Gaensler EA: Idiopathic pleural effusion. N Engl J Med 283:816, 1970.

Gaensler EA, Kaplan AI: Asbestos pleural effusion. Ann Intern Med 74:178, 1971.

Gefter WB, Conant EF: Issues and controversies in the plain-film diagnosis of asbestos-related disorders in the chest. J Thorac Imaging 3:11, 1988.

Get'man VG, Kelemen LL, Kizimenko VM: The importance of thoracoscopy in the differential diagnosis of pleurisy. Vrach Delo 9:49, 1989.

Godwin JD: Computed Tomography of the Chest. Philadelphia, JB Lippincott, 1984, p 130.

Gordon R: The deep sulcus sign. Radiology 136:25, 1980.

Gunnels JS: Perplexing pleural effusion. Chest 74:390, 1978.

Gwin E, Pierce G, Boggan M et al: Pleuroscopy and pleural biopsy with the flexible fiberoptic bronchoscope. Chest 67:527, 1975.

Halvorsen RA, Fedyshin PJ, Korobkin M et al: Ascites or pleural effusion? RadioGraphics 6:135, 1986.

Harvey C, Harvey HPB: Subclavian lymph node, pleural and pulmonary biopsy in diagnosis of intra-thoracic disease. Postgrad Med J 34:204, 1958.

Henschke CI, Davis SD, Romano RM, Yankelevitz DF: Pleural effusions: Pathogenesis, radiologic evaluation, and therapy. J Thorac Imaging 4:49, 1989.

Hillerdal G, Lindgren A: Pleural plaques: Correlation of autopsy findings to radiographic findings and occupational history. Eur J Respir Dis 61:315, 1980.

Hucker J, Bhatnagar NK, Al-Jilaihawi AN, Forrester-Wood CP: Thoracoscopy in the diagnosis and management of recurrent pleural effusions. Ann Thorac Surg 52:1145, 1991.

Jacobaeus HC: Possibility of the use of the cystoscope for investigation of serous cavities. Munch Med Wochenschr 57:2090, 1910.

Jacobaeus HC: The practical importance of thoracoscopy in surgery of the chest. Surg Gynecol Obstet 32:493, 1921.

Jacobaeus HC: Thoracoscopy and its practical applications. Ergeb Ges Med 7:122, 1925.

Jay SJ: Diagnostic procedures for pleural diseases. Clin Chest Med 6:33, 1985.

Kawashima A, Libshitz HI: Malignant pleural mesothelioma: CT manifestations in 50 cases. AJR Am J Roentgenol 155:965, 1990.

Kimura M, Nakamura J, Tomizawa S et al: The role of thoracoscopy in pleural biopsy in cases with pleural effusion. Nippon Kyobo Shikkan Gakkai Zasshi 28:882, 1990.

Kirby TJ, Ginsberg RJ: Role of open thoracostomy in undiagnosed pleural effusions. In Delarue NC, Eschapasse H (eds): Thoracic Surgery: Surgical Management of Pleural Diseases. In Deslauriers J, Lacquet LK (eds): International Trends in General Thoracic Surgery, Vol 6. St. Louis, CV Mosby, 1990, p 62.

Kovarik JL: Thoracentesis: A modified technic. Postgrad Med 48:96, 1970.

Krasnow AZ, Collier BD, Isitman AT et al: The use of radionuclide cisternography in the diagnosis of pleural cerebrospinal fluid fistulae. J Nucl Med 30:120, 1989.

Krausz M, Manny J: A safe method of thoracentesis. J Thorac Cardiovasc Surg 72:323, 1976.

Kreel L: Conventional and new imaging techniques. In Delarue NC, Eschapasse H (eds): Thoracic Surgery: Surgical Management of Pleural Diseases. In Deslauriers J, Lacquet LK (eds): International Trends in General Thoracic Surgery, Vol 6. St. Louis, CV Mosby, 1990, p 19.

Leung AN, Müller NL, Miller RR: CT in differential diagnosis of diffuse pleural disease. AJR Am J Roentgenol 154:487, 1990.

Light RW: Pleural Diseases. Philadelphia, Lea & Febiger, 1983.

Light RW, Jenkinson SG, Minh VD, George RB: Observations on pleural fluid pressures as fluid is withdrawn during thoracentesis. Am Rev Respir Dis 121:799, 1980.

Mathis G: Thoraxsonography. I: Chest wall and pleura. Ultrasound Med Biol 23:1131, 1997.

McLoud TC, Flower CDR: Imaging the pleura: Sonography, CT and MR imaging. AJR Am J Roentgenol 156:1145, 1991.

McLoud TC, Woods BO, Carrington CB et al: Diffuse pleural thickening in an asbestos-exposed population: Prevalence and causes. AJR Am J Roentgenol 144:9, 1985.

Menzies R, Charbonneau B: Thoracoscopy for the diagnosis of pleural disease. Ann Intern Med 114:271, 1991.

Mestitz P, Purves MJ, Pollard AC: Pleural biopsy in diagnosis of pleural effusion: Report of 200 cases. Lancet 2:1349, 1958.

Miguères J, Jover A, Bouissou H et al: Place de la ponction-biopsie à l'aiguille et du cyto-diagnostic dans le diagnostic des pleurésies malignes. Poumon Coeur 37:29, 1981.

Mintzer RA, Gore RM, Vogelzang RL, Holz S: Rounded atelectasis and its association with asbestos-induced pleural disease. Radiology 139:567, 1981.

Moote D, Ehrlich L, Martin RH: Postpneumonectomy bronchopleural fistula imaged by ventilation lung scanning. Clin Nucl Med 12:337, 1987.

Moskowitz H, Platt RT, Schachar R, Mellins H: Roentgen visualization of minute pleural effusion. Radiology 109:33, 1973.

Mossman BT, Gee JBL: Asbestos-related diseases. N Engl J Med 320:1721, 1989.

Müller NL: Imaging of the pleura. Radiology 186:297, 1993.

Oldenburg FA, Newhouse MT: Thoracoscopy: A safe, accurate diagnostic procedure using the rigid thoracoscope and local anesthesia. Chest 75:45, 1979.

Poe RH, Israel RH, Utell MV et al: Sensibility, specificity and predictive values of closed pleural biopsy. Arch Intern Med 114:325, 1984.

Prakash UBS, Reiman HM: Comparison of needle biopsy with cytologic analysis for the evaluation of pleural effusion: Analysis of 414 cases. Mayo Clin Proc 60:158, 1985.

Rao NV, Jones PO, Greenberg SD et al: Needle biopsy of parietal pleura in 124 cases. Arch Intern Med 115:34, 1965.

Reger RB, Ames RG, Merchant JA et al: The detection of thoracic abnormalities using posterior-anterior (PA) vs PA and oblique roentgenograms. Chest 81:290, 1982.

Rhea JT, Van Sonnerberg E, McLoud T: Basilar pneumothorax in the supine adult. Radiology 133:593, 1979.

Rivas de Andrés JJ, Lanzas JT: Thoracoscopy and spontaneous pneumothorax (Letter). Ann Thorac Surg 55:811, 1993.

Rockoff SD, Kagan E, Schwartz A et al: Visceral pleural thickening in asbestos exposure: The occurrence and implications of thickened interlobar fissures. J Thorac Imaging 2:58, 1987.

Rudikoff JC: Early detection of pleural fluid. Chest 77:109, 1980.

Rusch VW, Godwin JD, Shuman WP: The role of computed scanning in the initial assessment and the follow-up of malignant pleural mesothelioma. J Thorac Cardiovasc Surg 96:171, 1988.

Rusch VW, Mountain C: Thorocoscopy under regional anesthesia for the diagnosis and management of pleural disease. Am J Surg 154:274, 1987.

Ruskin JA, Gurney JW, Thorsen MK, Goodman LR: Detection of pleural effusions on supine chest radiographs. AJR Am J Roentgenol 148:681, 1987.

Ryan CJ, Rodgers RF, Unni KK, Hepper NGG: The outcome of patients with pleural effusion of indeterminate cause at thoracotomy. Mayo Clin Proc 56:145, 1981.

Sahn SA: Pleural fluid analysis: Narrowing the differential diagnosis. Semin Respir Med 9:22, 1987.

Sahn SA: The pleura. Am Rev Respir Dis 138:184, 1988.

Sakai S, Murayama S, Murakami J et al: Bronchogenic carcinoma invasion of the chest wall: Evaluation with dynamic cine MRI during breathing. J Comput Assist Tomogr 21:595, 1997.

Salyer WR, Eggleston JC, Erozan YS: Efficacy of pleural needle biopsy and pleural fluid cytopathology in the diagnosis of malignant neoplasm involving the pleura. Chest 67:536, 1975.

Schabel SI: Radiologic techniques in pleural disease. Semin Respir Med 9:13, 1987.

Scharer L, McClement JH: Isolation of tubercule bacilli from needle biopsy specimens of parietal pleura. Am Rev Respir Dis 97:466, 1967.

Schneider HJ, Ferson B, Gonzales LL: Rounded atelectasis. AJR Am J Roentgenol 134:225, 1980.

Schwartz DA: New developments in absestos-related pleural disease. Chest 99:191, 1991.

Schwartz DA, Fuortes LJ, Galvin JR et al: Asbestos-induced pleural fibrosis and impaired lung function. Am Rev Respir Dis 141:321, 1990.

Seneff MG, Corwin RW, Gold LH, Irwin RS: Complications associated with thoracentesis. Chest 90:97, 1986.

Sergent E, Kourilsky R: Contribution to the study of endothelioma. Presse Med 47:257, 1939.

Serre G, Daste G, Vincent C et al: Diagnostic approach to the patient with pleural effusion: Cytologic analysis of pleural fluid. In Delarue NC, Eschapasse H (eds): Thoracic Surgery: Surgical Management of Pleural Diseases. In Deslauriers J, Lacquet LK (eds): International Trends in General Thoracic Surgery, Vol 6. St. Louis, CV Mosby, 1990, p 35.

Sgro B, Gorla A, Tacchi G et al: Thoracoscopy in the diagnosis of pleural mesothelioma. Chir Ital 43:95, 1991.

Skowran CA: Kerrison rongeur: Needle punch biopsy. Del Med J 32:294, 1960.

Smyrnios NA, Jederlinic PJ, Irwin RS: Pleural effusion in an asymptomatic patient: Spectrum and frequency of cases and management considerations. Chest 97:192, 1990.

Stark DD, Federle MP, Goodman PC et al: Differentiating lung abscess and empyema: Radiography and computed tomography. AJR Am J Roentgenol 141:163, 1983a.

Stark DD, Federle MP, Goodman PC: CT and radiographic assessment of tube thoracotomy. AJR Am J Roentgenol 141:253, 1983b.

Suzuki N, Saitoh T, Kitamura S: Tumor invasion of the chest wall in lung cancer: Diagnosis with US. Radiology 187:39, 1993.

Teplick JG, Teplick SK, Goodman L, Haskin ME: The interface sign: A computed tomographic sign for distinguishing pleural and intra-abdominal fluid. Radiology 144:359, 1982.

Tocico IM, Miller MH, Fairfax WR: Distribution of pneumothorax in the supine and semirecumbent critically ill adult. AJR Am J Roentgenol 144:901, 1985.

Tomlinson JR, Sahn SA: Invasive procedures in the diagnosis of pleural disease. Semin Respir Med 9:30, 1987.

Urschel JD: Current applications of nonvideo thoracoscopy. Int Surg 82:131, 1997.

Vanderschueren RGJRA: The role of thoracoscopy in the evaluation and management of pneumothorax. Lung 168 (Suppl):1122, 1990.

Verreault J, Lepage S, Bisson G, Plante A: Ascites and right pleural effusion: Demonstration of a peritoneo-pleural communication. J Nucl Med 27:1706, 1986.

Viskum K, Enk B: Complications of thoracoscopy. Poumon Coeur 37:25, 1981.

Waite RJ, Carbonneau RJ, Balikian JP et al: Parietal pleural changes in empyema: Appearances on CT. Radiology 175:145, 1990.

Wakabayashi A: Expanded applications of diagnostic and therapeutic thoracoscopy. J Thorac Cardiovasc Surg 102:721, 1991.

Weisbrod GL, Yee AC: Computed tomographic diagnosis of a pedunculated fibrous mesothelioma. Can Assoc Radiol J 34:147, 1983.

Weissberg D, Kaufman M, Zurkowski Z: Pleuroscopy in patients with pleural effusion and pleural masses. Ann Thorac Surg 29:205, 1980.

Williams T, Thomas P: The diagnosis of pleural effusions by fiberoptic bronchoscopy and pleuroscopy. Chest 80:566, 1981.

Williford ME, Godwin JD: Computed tomography of lung abscess and empyema. Radiol Clin North Am 21:575, 1983.

Withers BF, Ducatman AM, Yang WN: Roentgenographic evidence for predominant left-sided location of unilateral pleural plaques. Chest 95:1262, 1984.

Woodring JH: Recognition of pleural effusion on supine radiographs: How much fluid is required? AJR Am J Roentgenol 142:59, 1984.

Wu RG, Yang PC, Kuo SH et al: "Fluid color" sign: A useful indicator for discrimination between pleural thickening and pleural effusion. J Ultrasound Med 14:767, 1995.

Wu RG, Yuan A, Liaw YS et al: Image comparison of real-time gray scale ultrasound and color Doppler ultrasound for use in diagnosis of minimal pleural effusion. Am J Respir Crit Care Med 150:510, 1994.

Yokoi K, Mori K, Miyazawa N et al: Tumor invasion of the chest wall and mediastinum in lung cancer: Evaluation with pneumothorax CT. Radiology 181:147, 1991.

Zerhouni EA, Scott WW, Baker RR et al: Invasive thymomas: Diagnosis and evaluation by computed tomography. J Comput Assist Tomogr 6:92, 1982.

CHAPTER **40**

Pleural Effusion: Benign and Malignant

Valerie W. Rusch

Pleural effusions are a common and significant clinical problem. At the end of the 20th century, several advances made possible a more systematic approach to their management, and research, based primarily on animal models, has provided a better understanding of their pathophysiology (Broaddus et al, 1990; Broaddus and Light, 1992; Miserocchi, 1997). Characterization of the biochemical characteristics of pleural fluid has improved our ability to diagnose the cause of an effusion by using the relatively noninvasive approach of thoracentesis (Gázquez et al, 1998; Light, 1983). The advent of computed tomography (CT) in the late 1970s also dramatically improved the noninvasive evaluation of pleural disease. Thoracoscopy, which was always a popular procedure in Europe (Boutin et al, 1991; Deslauriers and Lacquet, 1990), is now widely practiced in North America for the diagnosis and treatment of pleural disease because of the development of video-assisted technology in the early 1990s. Patients who previously were subjected to multiple thoracenteses and percutaneous pleural biopsies are now offered thoracoscopy if the initial noninvasive evaluation is not diagnostic. Finally, pleurodesis for malignant pleural effusions, which was often performed in a highly individualized manner, has been evaluated in well-designed prospective trials.

A better understanding of pathophysiology, better imaging, faster and more accurate methods of diagnosis, and the careful assessment of therapy have improved the diagnosis and therapy of pleural effusions. This chapter covers the current approach to the management of pleural effusions, focusing on malignant pleural effusions, which are the most common problem seen by surgeons.

PATHOPHYSIOLOGY

The anatomy and physiology of the pleural space are described in detail in Chapter 38. Pleural effusions develop because of a disturbance in the mechanisms that normally move 5 to 10 L of fluid across the pleural space every 24 hours and resorb it, leaving only 5 to 20 ml present at any time (Kinasewitz and Fishman, 1981; Miserocchi, 1997). Increased capillary permeability (inflammation or tumor implants), increased hydrostatic pressure (congestive heart failure), decreased oncotic pressure (hypoalbuminemia), increased negative intrapleural pressure (atelectasis), and decreased lymphatic drainage (lymphatic obstruction by a tumor or radiation-induced fibrosis) can all cause a pleural effusion. In patients with cancer, several different mechanisms often contribute to the formation of an effusion (Table 40–1). These mechanisms may relate directly to the presence of the tumor (e.g., obstruction of lymphatic channels), may

TABLE 40–1 ■ **Interaction Among Pathogenetic Mechanisms and Contributing Factors Favoring the Accumulation of Pleural Fluid**

Pathogenetic Mechanisms	*Impaired Lymphatic Drainage*	*Increased Pleural Osmotic Pressure*	*Increased Capillary Permeability*	*Increased Venous Pressure*
Pleural implants	+	+	+	−
Lymphatic metastases				
Mediastinal nodes	+	+	−	−
Lymphangitis	+	+	−	−
Tumor cell suspension	+	+	+	−
Contributing syndromes				
Superior vena cava syndrome	+	+	−	+
Congestive heart failure	+	+	−	+
Pericarditis or effusion	+	+	−	−
Infection	+	+	+	−
Mediastinal irradiation	+	+	−	−
Ascites	+	+	−	+
Hypoalbuminemia	−	+	−	−

+, contributes; −, does not contribute.

Data from Roth JA, Ruckkdeschel JC, Weisenburger TH (eds): Thoracic Oncology. Philadelphia, WB Saunders, 1989, p 596, and Harper GR: Pleural effusions in cancer. Clin Cancer Briefs 1:1, 1979,

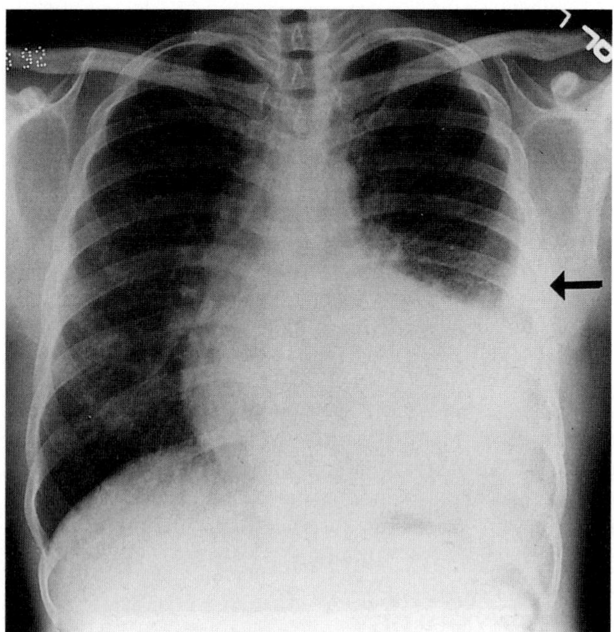

FIGURE 40–1 ■ Posteroanterior chest radiograph of a patient with widely disseminated lung cancer and a left pleural effusion. The retrocardiac region is opacified, and there is a fluid level with a typical meniscus sign (*arrow*).

reflect underlying medical problems (e.g., congestive heart failure or hypoalbuminemia), or may be a combination of both.

CLINICAL PRESENTATION AND DIAGNOSIS

Small pleural effusions are asymptomatic. Larger pleural effusions cause dyspnea, cough, and chest discomfort. Dullness to percussion and diminished breath sounds are present on the physical examination. The clinical diagnosis is confirmed by chest radiography. Small pleural effusions cause blunting of the costophrenic angle. If the pleural space is free, larger effusions produce the classic picture of a fluid level with a meniscus sign (Fig. 40–1). A lateral decubitus radiograph confirms freely flowing fluid (Fig. 40–2). Massive effusions cause a complete opacification of the hemithorax. Rarely, they present as a tension hydrothorax, with a mediastinal shift, respiratory distress, and hemodynamic instability. Loculated pleural effusions are harder to diagnose on a standard chest radiograph. They present as opacities of varying sizes and shapes that can be hard to distinguish from a pulmonary parenchymal process, such as atelectasis or dense consolidation (Fig. 40–3). Lateral decubitus radiographs do not show layering of the fluid. Ultrasound detects a loculated fluid collection and can help determine the proper site for thoracentesis, but the most useful examination under these circumstances is a CT scan. This helps direct therapy by outlining the size and location of fluid collections and by distinguishing underlying parenchymal disease from pleural fluid and thickening (Fig. 40–4). Thin-section CT, with images at 2-mm intervals, is more accurate in identifying pleural metastases than is standard CT because it detects very small pleural nodules (Mori et al, 1998).

The clinical setting in which an effusion occurs influences the approach to diagnosis and therapy. A patient who develops a small effusion in conjunction with pneumonia but is improving while receiving antibiotics is likely to have a parapneumonic effusion and could be treated expectantly. The same would be true of a patient with known cirrhosis and ascites who has a small pleural effusion. These effusions are known to occur in the absence of primary intrathoracic disease and are related to the presence of peritoneopleural communication (Mittal et al, 1996). In contrast, a woman who develops a new pleural effusion several years after treatment for a node-positive breast cancer merits intensive investigation. Before any invasive workup is initiated, the patient with a pleural effusion should have a careful history and physical examination so that all subsequent evaluation is directed toward the clinically likely causes.

Knowledge of the most common causes of pleural effusions is also helpful in defining etiology. The four most common causes of pleural effusions in North America are congestive heart failure, bacterial pneumonia, malignancy, and pulmonary emboli. Viral pneumonia, cirrhosis with ascites, gastrointestinal disease, collagen-vascular disease, and tuberculosis are less common causes (Light, 1983). The most common causes of malignant pleural effusion are lung cancer, breast cancer, and lymphoma. However, the frequency of the type of cancer responsible for a pleural effusion depends on the patient's gender. Lung cancer, lymphoma, and gastrointestinal cancers are the three most common causes in men; breast cancers, gynecologic cancers, and lung cancers are the most common ones in women (Tables 40–2 and 40–3).

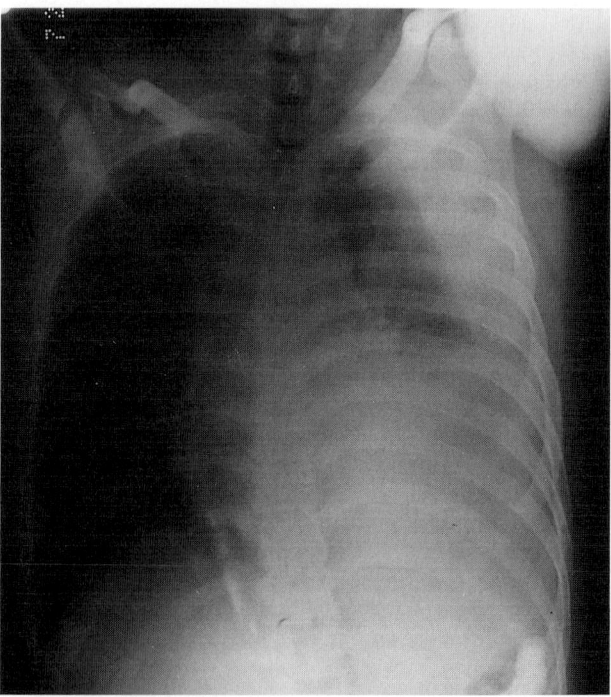

FIGURE 40–2 ■ The lateral decubitus chest radiograph of the patient shown in Fig. 40–1 shows that the pleural effusion layers easily and is, therefore, free flowing.

DIFFERENTIAL DIAGNOSIS OF PLEURAL EFFUSIONS

I. Transudative pleural effusions
  A. Congestive heart failure
  B. Cirrhosis
  C. Nephrotic syndrome
  D. Peritoneal dialysis
  E. Glomerulonephritis
  F. Myxedema
  G. Pulmonary emboli
  H. Sarcoidosis

II. Exudative pleural effusions
  A. Neoplasic diseases
    1. Metastatic disease
    2. Mesothelioma
  B. Infectious diseases
    1. Bacterial infections
    2. Tuberculosis
    3. Fungal infections
    4. Parasitic infections
    5. Viral infections
  C. Pulmonary embolization
  D. Gastrointestinal disease
    1. Pancreatitis
    2. Subphrenic abscess
    3. Intrahepatic abscess
    4. Esophageal perforation
    5. Diaphragmatic hernia
  E. Collagen-vascular diseases
    1. Rheumatoid pleuritis
    2. Systemic lupus erythematosus
    3. Drug-induced lupus
    4. Immunoblastic lymphadenopathy
    5. Sjögren's syndrome
    6. Familial Mediterranean fever
    7. Wegener's granulomatosis
  F. Drug-induced pleural disease
    1. Nitrofurantoin
    2. Dantrolene
    3. Methysergide
    4. Bromocriptine
    5. Procarbazine
    6. Methotrexate
    7. Practolol
  G. Miscellaneous diseases and conditions
    1. Asbestos exposure
    2. Postpericardiectomy or postmyocardial infarction syndrome
    3. Meigs' syndrome
    4. Yellow nail syndrome
    5. Sarcoidosis
    6. Uremia
    7. Trapped lung
    8. Radiation therapy
    9. Electrical burns
    10. Urinary tract obstruction
    11. Iatrogenic injury
  H. Hemothorax
  I. Chylothorax

From Light RW: Pleural Diseases. Philadelphia, Lea & Febiger, 1983, p 62.

If the diagnosis is not clinically obvious, a thoracentesis should be performed, and the character of the fluid should be noted. Bloody fluid occurs with pulmonary emboli, malignancy, or trauma. Clear milky fluid is strongly suggestive of a chylothorax; turbid or purulent fluid is indicative of an empyema.

The pleural fluid should be sent for cytologic examination, culture, and cell count. Simultaneous pleural fluid and serum glucose, protein, and lactic dehydrogenase levels should be obtained. Effusions are classified as exu-

TABLE 40–2 ■ Primary Organ Site or Neoplasm Type in Male Patients with Malignant Pleural Effusions

Primary Site or Tumor Type	*No. of Male Patients*	*% Male Patients*
Lung	140	49.1
Lymphoma/leukemia	60	21.1
Gastrointestinal tract	20	7.0
Genitourinary tract	17	6.0
Melanoma	4	1.4
Miscellaneous less common tumors	10	3.5
Primary site unknown	31	10.9
Total	285	100.0

From Johnson WW: The malignant pleural effusion: A review of cytopathologic diagnoses of 584 specimens from 472 consecutive patients. Cancer 56:905, 1985.

TABLE 40–3 ■ Primary Organ Site or Neoplasm Type in Female Patients with Malignant Pleural Effusions

Primary Site or Tumor Type	*No. of Female Patients*	*% Female Patients*
Breast	70	37.4
Female genital tract	38	20.3
Lung	28	15.0
Lymphoma/leukemia	14	8.0
Gastrointestinal tract	8	4.3
Melanoma	6	3.2
Urinary tract	2	1.1
Miscellaneous less common tumors	3	1.6
Primary site unknown	17	9.1
Total	187	100.0

From Johnson WW: The malignant pleural effusion: A review of cytopathologic diagnoses of 584 specimens from 472 consecutive patients. Cancer 56:905, 1985.

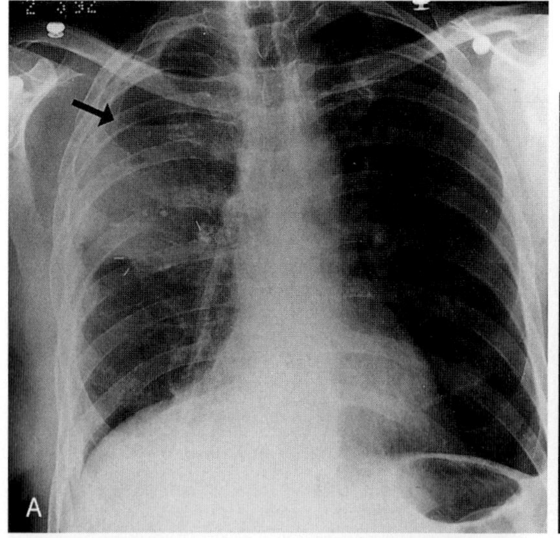

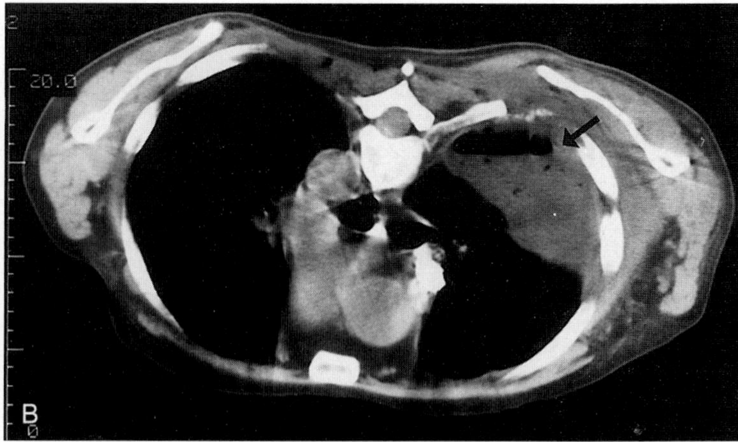

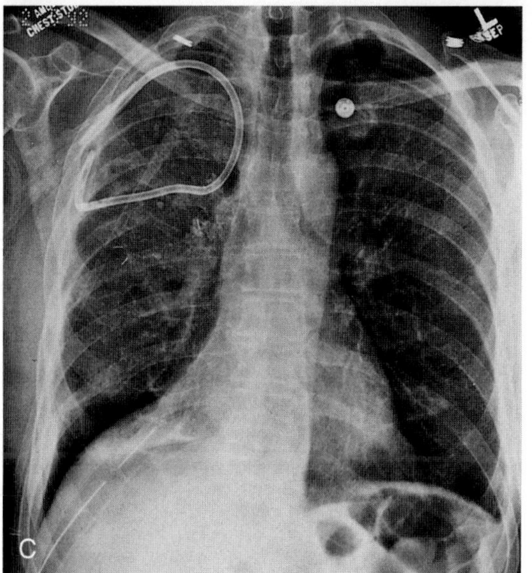

FIGURE 40–3 ■ *A*, Loculated right pleural effusion in patient status postdecortication of the right lung for empyema. There is a hazy density in the right midlung field with a fluid level at its upper margin (*arrow*). *B*, Computed tomography scan of the patient shown in *A*, taken in the prone position, demonstrates a loculated fluid collection with an air-fluid level (*arrow*). *C*, Posteroanterior chest radiograph of the same patient following percutaneous catheter drainage of the fluid collection shows clearing of the hazy density that was seen on the initial chest radiograph.

dative or transudative based on the protein and lactic dehydrogenase (LDH) levels. An effusion is considered an exudate if the pleural fluid to serum ratio of protein is greater than 0.5, and the LDH ratio is greater than 0.6, or the absolute pleural LDH level is greater than two thirds of the normal upper limit for serum (Gázquez et al, 1998). The most common cause of transudative effusions is congestive heart failure. There are many causes of exudative effusions, but the most common ones are malignancy, infection, and pulmonary emboli. The pleural fluid concentration of glucose is also helpful because a level less than 60 mg/dl is seen only in four conditions: malignancy, tuberculous pleuritis, parapneumonic effusions, and rheumatoid pleural effusion (Pettersson and Riska, 1981; Smyrnios et al, 1990; Vladutiu et al, 1981). Thus, a patient who has a bloody exudative effusion with a low glucose level is likely to have a malignancy.

Several other biochemical tests are helpful in specific clinical situations. The amylase level is elevated in three conditions: esophageal perforation, pancreatitis, and malignant effusions. A triglyceride level should be obtained if a chylothorax is suspected. A level above 110 mg/dl is considered diagnostic. Pleural fluid pH and glucose levels have been used in the evaluation of parapneumonic effusions. Light (1983) reported that a pH less than 7.00 in conjunction with a glucose level less than 60 mg/dl indicates that a parapneumonic effusion will progress to a frank empyema. However, other authors have not found the pH and glucose levels to be as reliable in the management of parapneumonic effusions. Complement, rheumatoid factor, and antinuclear antibody levels are often elevated in collagen-vascular disease and should be obtained if this is being considered in the differential diagnosis (Light, 1983).

Other tests have been used to determine the cause of pleural effusions and particularly to distinguish whether an effusion is malignant. The carcinoembryonic antigen level has been the most widely used pleural fluid marker. Levels of this antigen above 5 ng/ml are a specific but relatively insensitive marker of malignancy (Asseo and Tracopoulos, 1982; Rittgers et al, 1978; Sorensen, 1981; Tamura et al, 1988). Creatine kinase isoenzyme BB, adenosine deaminase, and galactosyltransferase have been reported to distinguish benign from malignant effusions in

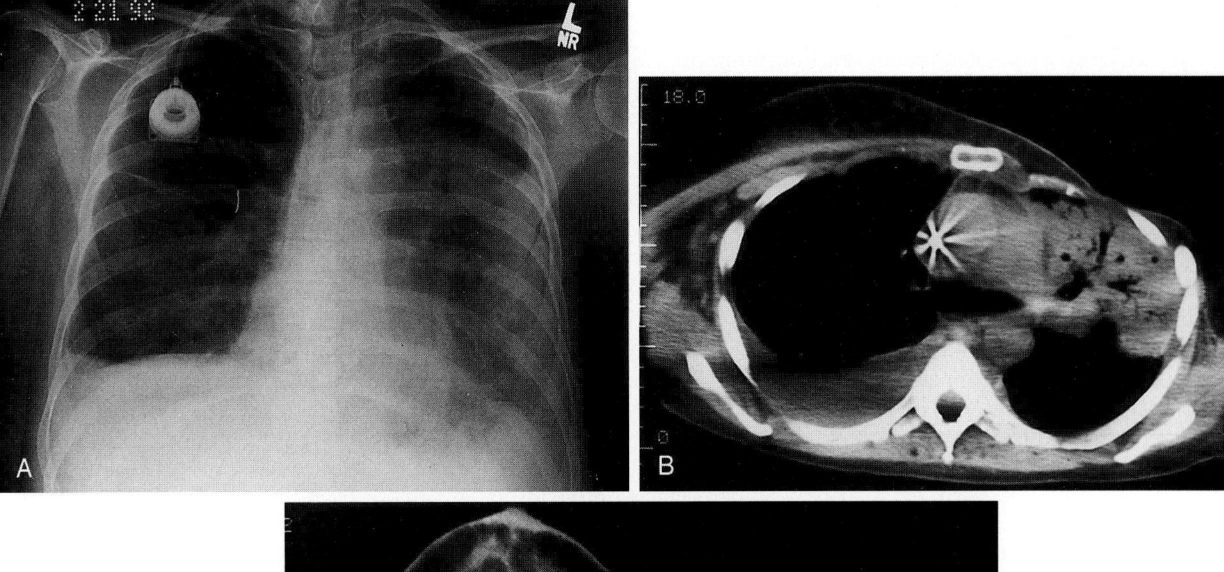

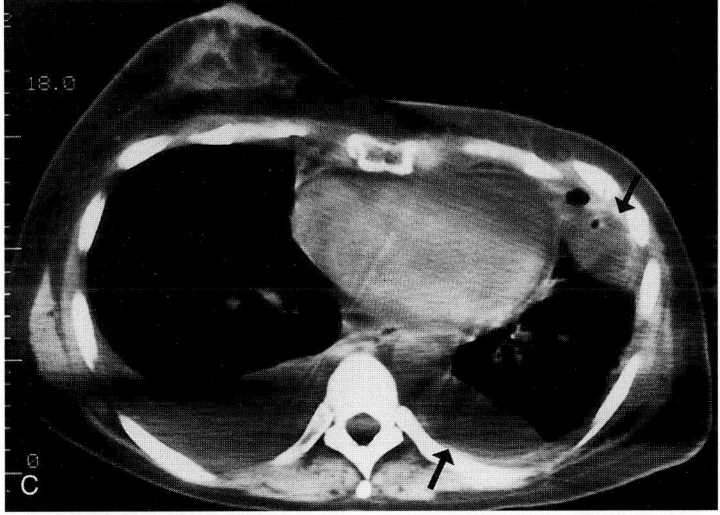

FIGURE 40–4 ■ *A*, Another example of a loculated pleural effusion that is extremely difficult to distinguish from underlying parenchymal disease in a patient who had severe radiation-induced fibrosis. The posteroanterior chest radiograph shows a hazy density in the midlateral aspect of the left lung with an underlying air bronchogram. *B*, Computed tomography (CT) scan of this patient at the level of the carina shows dense consolidation of the left upper lobe with an air bronchogram. There is no pleural fluid at this level. *C*, CT scan of the same patient at the level of the midheart shows a large free-flowing right pleural effusion and a multiloculated left pleural effusion (*arrows*). This combination of parenchymal disease and multiloculated pleural effusion accounts for the abnormalities seen on the plain chest radiograph in *A*. It would be hard to interpret the chest radiograph and make a determination of whether drainage of the pleural effusion were appropriate without the aid of the CT scan.

small series of patients (Kim et al, 1982; Pettersson et al, 1984; Silverman et al, 1979). Various immunohistochemical stains have been used to identify malignant cells and to distinguish them from reactive mesothelial cells (Herbert and Gallagher, 1982). Flow cytometry is relatively inaccurate in diagnosing malignancy because cytologically positive pleural effusions do not always contain aneuploid cells (Schneller et al, 1987). Cytogenetic techniques can diagnose malignant pleural effusions, but they are labor intensive and do not consistently add to the standard cytologic examination (Dewald et al, 1976, 1982; Falor et al, 1982; Monif et al, 1976). Uptake of ^{99m}Tc phosphate in malignant pleural effusions has been anecdotally reported in patients undergoing bone scans to search for osseous metastases (Goldstein and Gefter, 1983; Kida et al, 1984). Although this is not likely to be useful as a routine diagnostic test, its clinical significance as an incidental finding should be remembered.

More recently, molecular biologic techniques have been applied to the diagnosis of pleural effusions. These include the development of a sensitive and specific reverse transcriptase polymerase chain reaction (RT-PCR) assay to detect epithelial tumor cells, which potentially increases the diagnosis of malignancy in cytologically negative effusions (Sakaguchi et al, 1999). The detection of specific molecular alterations, such as K-*ras* mutations, may also enhance the diagnosis of malignancy in pleural effusions (Yamashita et al, 1998). Telomerase activity is frequently observed in malignant effusions but is occasionally seen in some inflammatory conditions, such as tuberculosis (Mu et al, 1999; Yang et al, 1998). The precise benefit of molecular techniques in the diagnosis of pleural effusion requires further investigation.

The long list of tests that can be performed on pleural effusion to pinpoint a cause are of academic rather than practical interest. The character of the fluid (e.g., bloody versus serous), a determination of whether it is an exudate or a transudate, measurement of the glucose level, and culture and cytologic examination are the most important initial tests (Rodriguez-Panadero and Lopez Mejias, 1989; Roth et al, 1990; Xaubet et al, 1985). Additional biochemical or molecular analyses should be used selectively based on the clinical setting. If the examination of the pleural fluid is nondiagnostic, a percutaneous or thoracoscopic pleural biopsy should be considered. A pleural biopsy alone yields a diagnosis of malignancy in 40% to 69% of cases. When pleural fluid cytologic findings and pleural biopsy results are combined, the yield increases to 80% to 90% (Migueres et al, 1981; Poe et al, 1984; Prakash, 1985; Winkelmann and Pfitzer, 1981). Pleural biopsy can also diagnose some benign diseases, such as tuberculous effusion or amyloidosis, in situations in which the pleural fluid analysis is uninformative (Chertow et al, 1991; Kavuru et al, 1990; Seibert et al, 1991).

Patients whose effusions remain undiagnosed after a thoracentesis and percutaneous pleural biopsy should undergo a CT scan of the chest and abdomen, a bronchoscopy, and a thoracoscopy. If the effusion is large, the CT scan should be done after the fluid has been evacuated so that the lung can be imaged when it is fully expanded. CT detects underlying pulmonary parenchymal and abdominal disease that may not be evident otherwise. Bronchoscopy diagnoses endobronchial tumors (primary or metastatic) that may be responsible for an effusion because of postobstructive atelectasis. Thoracoscopy is performed to obtain a tissue diagnosis by directed pleural biopsy and to do a pleurodesis, usually by talc poudrage. Several large series report a diagnostic accuracy of 80% to 100% for thoracoscopy, depending on the reasons for which thoracoscopy was performed. In almost all patients, it is the definitive way of diagnosing a malignancy involving the pleura (Boushy et al, 1978; Faurschou, 1985; Faurschou et al, 1985; Hucker et al, 1991; Page et al, 1989; Rusch and Mountain, 1987; Vanderschueren, 1981; Voellmy, 1995; Weissberg et al, 1980). The exceptions are patients in whom thoracoscopy cannot be performed because of a fused pleural space. The development of video-assisted thoracoscopy (VATS) significantly expanded the diagnostic potential of this technique by making lung biopsies and nodal dissection possible (Lewis et al, 1992; Oakes et al, 1984). In the past, patients often underwent multiple thoracenteses and percutaneous pleural biopsies in an effort to avoid a thoracotomy for diagnosis. Thoracoscopy, widely used in Europe for a long time, was a largely forgotten procedure in North America for the diagnosis of pleural disease (Thermann et al, 1985). With the popularization of VATS, patients with undiagnosed pleural effusions are now referred sooner for this minimally invasive and highly diagnostic procedure.

MANAGEMENT

General Principles

Transudative pleural effusions are managed by therapy for the underlying disease and usually resolve after this has been controlled (Friedman and Slater, 1978; Light, 1983). Occasionally, additive intervention is required, either because the effusion is symptomatic or because the underlying medical problem is refractory to maximal medical treatment. For example, tube thoracostomy might be necessary to drain a large effusion secondary to a pulmonary embolus, or a pleurodesis or pleuroperitoneal shunt might be required to control a symptomatic effusion in a patient with medically refractory ascites.

Some exudative effusions also resolve after therapy for the underlying disease. This is true of effusions caused by gastrointestinal disease, drugs, collagen-vascular disease, and nonbacterial infections (Deslauriers and Lacquet, 1990; Light, 1983; Seibert et al, 1991). Some exudative effusions caused by malignancy are also best managed in this manner if the tumor is highly responsive to chemotherapy or irradiation. The classic example is an effusion or chylothorax caused by a lymphoma, which usually resolves quickly after chemotherapy or irradiation alleviates the lymphatic obstruction (Xaubet et al, 1985). Effusions caused by solid tumors, such as breast cancer and ovarian cancer, for which effective chemotherapy is available, also may resolve spontaneously after chemotherapy is instituted (Deslauriers and Lacquet, 1990; Friedman and Slater, 1978; Reshad et al, 1985).

The most difficult management problem is the malignant pleural effusion caused by a tumor that is refractory to chemotherapy. Traditionally, these have been treated by some form of pleurodesis. Before proceeding with pleurodesis, however, it is important to make certain that the patient does not have a "trapped" lung with a fixed pleural space. The lung is often encased by a peel of visceral pleural tumor that causes chronic collapse of the lung and prevents the parietal and visceral pleural surfaces from coming into apposition with each other. Effective pleurodesis under these circumstances is obviously impossible. Partial entrapment of the lung with smaller loculated effusions is also common in patients with cancer. Sometimes this is not caused by a pleural tumor but is the result of a chronic effusion that contains a lot of protein and fibrinous debris, which create a limited fibrothorax. A trapped lung is readily recognized by a lack of expansion of the lung after therapeutic thoracentesis or chest tube insertion (Fig. 40–5). Complete or near-complete expansion of the lung and evacuation of the pleural space should be documented on a chest radiograph before proceeding with pleurodesis.

Pleurodesis for Malignant Effusions

At one time it was believed that malignant pleural effusions could be controlled by serial thoracentesis or tube thoracostomy alone without pleurodesis. Although Lambert and colleagues (1967) reported a recurrence rate of only 17% for effusions managed by tube thoracostomy alone, subsequent experience with this approach demonstrated that almost all patients experienced a rapid reaccumulation of their effusion (Anderson et al, 1974). Today drainage of the effusion without pleurodesis (usually by serial thoracentesis) is only considered appropriate for terminally ill patients who are unwilling or unable to tolerate other therapies.

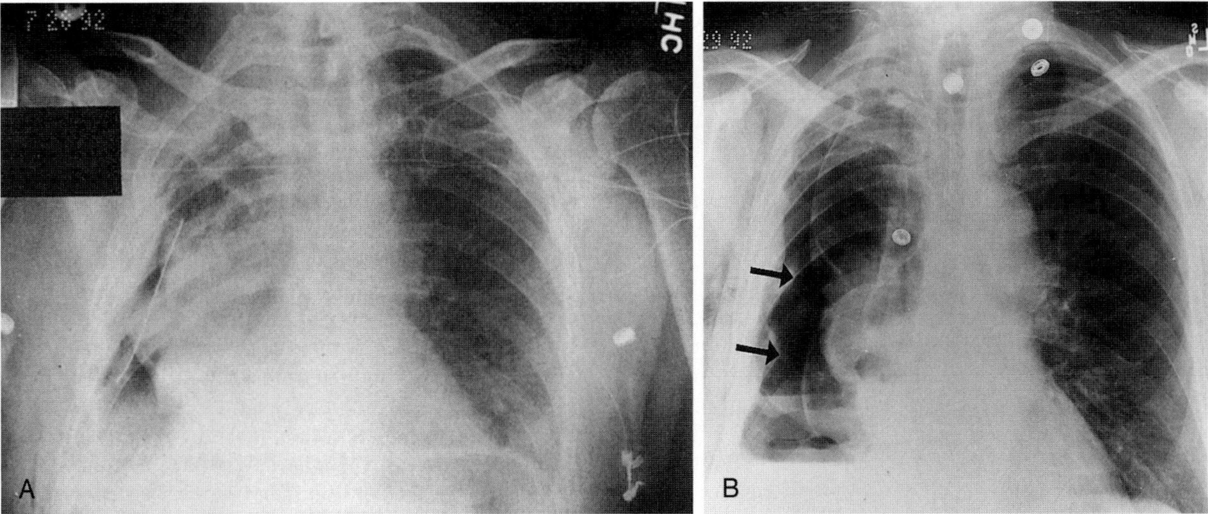

FIGURE 40–5 ■ *A,* Posteroanterior chest radiograph on a patient with malignant mesothelioma who underwent a thoracoscopy for diagnosis. The lung was clearly trapped at thoracoscopy. The initial postoperative portable chest radiograph shows evacuation of the pleural space with an unexpanded lung. *B,* The chest radiograph obtained the following day after removal of chest tube shows this more clearly. There is a fixed pleural space (*arrows*) and lack of re-expansion of the underlying lung. This patient would not be an appropriate candidate for pleurodesis.

A large number of agents have been used intrapleurally to try to control malignant pleural effusions. These agents can be classified in two broad categories according to their modes of action: (1) cytostatic agents, which presumably control the effusion by reducing the tumor volume, and (2) sclerosants, which produce a chemical pleuritis that leads to the formation of adhesions and subsequent obliteration of the pleural space (Frankel et al, 1961). Radioactive colloids and some chemotherapeutic agents (nitrogen mustard, doxorubicin, and bleomycin) may combine both modes of action when administered intrapleurally. However, with the exception of cisplatin and perhaps thiotepa and 5-fluorouracil, most chemotherapeutic drugs act predominantly as sclerosants.

The early experience with pleurodesis for malignant pleural effusions has been comprehensively reviewed (Austin and Flye, 1979; Hausheer and Yarbro, 1985). Nitrogen mustard controlled the effusions in approximately one third of cases but caused significant pleuritic pain and fever and was associated with bone marrow depression (Anderson et al, 1974; Leininger et al, 1969). Thiotepa and 5-fluorouracil have fewer side effects but are no better at controlling effusions (Friedman and Slater, 1978). Response rates as high as 80% have been reported for intrapleural doxorubicin, but the associated problems of pain, fever, and nausea and vomiting preclude its routine use (Ike et al, 1991; Kefford et al, 1980; Masuno et al, 1991). Quinacrine was an effective sclerosant that controlled effusions in up to 80% of patients but caused severe pleuritic pain, fever, nausea, and, occasionally, hypotension, hallucinations, and seizures (Bayly et al, 1978; Taylor et al, 1977). These agents were abandoned, either because of their ineffectiveness or because of significant toxicity. Radioactive colloids including radioactive zinc (^{63}Zn), gold (^{198}Au), and chromium phosphate ($Cr_{32}PO_4$) were associated with little toxicity but were successful in only 50% to 60% of patients (Ariel et al, 1966; Hausheer and Yarbro, 1985). They were also expensive and inconvenient because of the need to shield hospital personnel from radioactivity, and, therefore, they are no longer routinely used. Experience with these agents, however, established that pleurodesis was more likely to be successful if the pleural space was fully evacuated by tube thoracostomy before instillation of the sclerosant, and the chest tube was left in place after the pleurodesis until the drainage was minimal. This remains an important principle in performing a pleurodesis.

Tetracycline pleurodesis was introduced in 1972. It had the advantage of being inexpensive, easily available, and relatively nontoxic. Its major side effect was severe pleuritic pain, which was often difficult to control even with appropriate systemic premedication and the use of intrapleural lidocaine (Landvater et al, 1988; Wallach, 1978; Zaloznik et al, 1983). Success rates ranging from 39% to 83% have been reported with tetracycline in several prospective studies in which it was compared with other agents (Table 40–4). The effectiveness of tetracycline depended on the dose and technique. Tetracycline had so many advantages over other sclerosants that it rapidly became the agent of choice, even though it did not always result in a successful pleurodesis.

TABLE 40–4 ■ **Results of Tetracycline Pleurodesis in Pleural Effusions**

Patient Success (No.)	*Success Rate (%)*
10/12	83
7/7	100
10/12	83
53/60	80
15/25	60
101/108	94

Adapted from Boutin C, Viallat JR, Aelony Y: Practical Thoracoscopy. Berlin, Springer-Verlag, 1991, p 68.

Bleomycin has also become a popular sclerosant (Bitran et al, 1981; Ostrowski, 1986; Paladine et al, 1976). Its success rate is at least as good and perhaps better than that of tetracycline, and it may cause less pain (Ruckdeschel et al, 1991). A prospective randomized trial that compared pleurodesis with 1 g of tetracycline to 60 units of bleomycin found that the median time to recurrence or progression of the effusion was 32 days for tetracycline and 46 days for bleomycin. The recurrence rate within 90 days of instillation was 30% with bleomycin and 53% with tetracycline. Toxicity was similar for the two agents (Ruckdeschel et al, 1991). Although it is usually well tolerated, it can occasionally cause nephrotoxicity in patients with underlying renal insufficiency. Bleomycin is also expensive.

In the early 1990s, the manufacture of tetracycline was discontinued, and in North America this led to a resurgence in the use of talc, a sclerosant first used by Bethune in 1935 that was always popular in Europe (Bethune, 1935). Because it is insoluble, talc is most often administered as a powder by insufflation at thoracoscopy or thoracotomy. Several series, however, report instilling it as a suspension by tube thoracostomy (Adler and Sayek, 1976; Chambers, 1958; Webb et al, 1992). This approach has become increasingly popular, and the success rates with talc slurry approximate those achieved by VATS and talc poudrage (Weissberg and Be-Zeev, 1993; Yim et al, 1996). Experimentally talc was shown to cause an intense chemical pleuritis that exceeds that caused by other agents (Adler and Sayek, 1976; Frankel et al, 1961). Table 40–5 summarizes some of the published experience with talc. Its reported success rate has consistently been 90% or better (Adler and Rappole, 1967; Aelony et al, 1991; Boniface and Guerin, 1989; Camishion et al, 1962; Daniel et al, 1990; Hamed et al, 1989; Harley, 1979; Ladjimi et al, 1985, 1989, 1991; Migueres and Jover, 1981; Ohri et al, 1992; Pearson and MacGregor, 1966; Scarbonchi et al, 1981; Shedbalkar et al, 1971; Srensen et al, 1984; and Todd et al, 1980). Several randomized trials show that talc is superior to tetracycline or bleomycin (Boutin et al, 1991; Fentiman et al, 1986; Hamed et al, 1989; Hartman et al, 1993; Zimmer et al, 1997). Iodine was sometimes added to the talc to keep the talc sterile and to intensify the pleuritis (Jones, 1969; Webb et al, 1992), but this is clearly not necessary in light of the high success rate of noniodized talc.

Fever and pleuritic pain occur after the administration of talc, although pain seems to be much less common and less severe than that with tetracycline. Rare reports have been made of adult respiratory distress syndrome developing after talc pleurodesis (Bouchama et al, 1984; Rinaldo et al, 1983), but given the thousands of patients treated with talc over several decades, the risk of this complication appears to be low (Campos et al, 1997). It has been hypothesized that the development of adult respiratory distress syndrome may be related to the amount of talc used or to contaminants within the talc preparation (Weissberg, 1984). However, published series report using widely varying amounts of talc (usually at least 5 to 10 g), and some do not specify the amount of talc used at all. Moreover, when a talc poudrage is performed, it is hard to estimate the amount of talc remaining in the pleural space because some of it is dissipated into the air during the procedure. There has been some concern in the past that talc pleurodesis might lead to a significant decrease in pulmonary function and

TABLE 40–5 ■ **Results of Studies of Talc Pleurodesis for Malignant Pleural Effusions**

Author (Year)	*Method of Administration*	*No. of Effusions Controlled/No. of Effusions Treated (%)*
Chambers (1958)	Suspension, chest tube	17/20 (85)
Camishion et al (1962)	Poudrage, thoracotomy	30/31 (97)
Roche (1963)	Poudrage, thoracoscopy	6/6 (100)
Pearson and MacGregor (1966)	Poudrage, thoracotomy or trocar	17/19 (89)
Adler and Rappole (1967)	Poudrage, thoracoscopy	4/4 (100)
Jones (1969)	Poudrage, thoracoscopy	22/23 (96)
Shedbalkar et al (1971)	Not stated	22/28 (96)
Adler and Sayek (1976)	Suspension, chest tube	41/44 (93)
Harley (1979)	Poudrage, thoracoscopy	41/44 (93)
Austin and Flye (1979)	Suspension, chest tube	38/41 (91)
Todd et al (1980)	Poudrage, thoracotomy or trocar	158/163 (97)
Scarbonchi et al (1981)	Poudrage, thoracoscopy	70/77 (91)
Migueres et al (1981)	Poudrage, thoracoscopy	15/26 (58)
Srensen et al (1984)	Suspension, chest tube	9/9 (100)
Ladjimi et al (1985)	Poudrage, thoracoscopy	66/78 (85)
Viallat et al (1986)	Poudrage, thoracoscopy	23/25 (92)
Fentiman et al (1986)	Poudrage, thoracoscopy	11/12 (92)
Boniface and Guerin (1989)	Poudrage, thoracoscopy	233/254 (92)
Ladjimi et al (1989)	Poudrage, thoracoscopy	192/218 (88)
Hamed et al (1989)	?Poudrage, thoracoscopy	10/10 (100)
Daniel et al (1990)	Poudrage, thoracoscopy	18/20 (90)
Ladjimi et al (1991)	Poudrage, thoracoscopy	18/21 (84)
Aelony et al (1991)	Poudrage, thoracoscopy	23/28 (82)
Engeler (1992)	Poudrage, thoracoscopy	19/20 (95)
Ohri et al (1992)	Poudrage, thoracoscopy	35/37 (95)
Webb et al (1992)	Suspension, chest tube	37/37 (100)
Hartman et al (1992)	Poudrage, thoracoscopy	22/25 (88)

predispose to the development of malignancy. A mild restrictive defect was seen as a late sequela in patients who underwent talc pleurodesis for spontaneous pneumothorax (Lange et al, 1988). Long-term follow-up (14 to 40 years) by the British Thoracic Association of 210 patients who underwent pleurodesis disclosed no increased incidence of lung cancer or mesothelioma (Chappell et al, 1979). The risk of carcinogenesis from talc may have been related to contamination of the talc preparations with asbestos. Talc prepared for medical use today is asbestos free. Neither one of these issues is important for patients with malignant pleural effusions, who usually have a life expectancy of less than 1 year and who need pleurodesis to palliate their dyspnea.

Several early collective reviewers (Austin and Flye, 1979; Friedman and Slater, 1978; Hausheer and Yarbro, 1985) attempted to assess the relative merits of the various agents used as sclerosants (Table 40–6). This was difficult because many of the published series were retrospective and uncontrolled. Prospective trials have often been poorly designed, because they are based on small numbers of patients and loosely defined eligibility and response criteria. Follow-up is usually short, and a central review of chest radiographs to verify the response data is rare (Rusch, 1991). In addition, patients with malignant pleural effusions represent a difficult patient population in which to carry out clinical trials. They have a limited life expectancy, with about one half of the patients dying within 3 months of therapy. Thus, large numbers of patients must be entered into a study to have statistically adequate numbers of patients available to analyze response rates and toxicity. Many patients require ongoing radiation or chemotherapy, which can make it hard to evaluate the effect and morbidity of pleurodesis. Underlying pleural or pulmonary disease and minor degrees of entrapment of the lung confuse the interpretation of the response on chest radiographs. Assessment of symptoms is rarely meaningful, because patients often have multiple reasons to feel dyspneic (e.g., pleural effusion plus lymphangitic spread of the tumor). Only recently has there been an attempt to develop well-designed clinical trials that include an adequate number of patients.

TABLE 40–6 ■ **Results of the Principal Randomized, Controlled Studies of Pleurodesis in the Treatment of Pleurisy**

Patients (No.)	*Agents Used*	*Success Rates (%)*
25	Quinacrine/Thiot	64/27
22	TCN/quinacrine	83/90
25	TCN/bleomycin	58/54
21	Cory/mustine	56/42
24	TCN/drainage	72/36
37	Mustard/talc	56/90
24	TCN/drainage	77/22
21	Talc/drainage	100/60
40	Talc/TCN	90/50
32	Cory/TCN	88/79
41	Talc/TCN	92/48
32	Cory/bleomycin	65/13
34	TCN/bleomycin	39/31
30	Talc/doxycycline	90/63

Cory, *Corynebacterium parvum*; TCN, tetracycline; Thiot, thiotepa.
Adapted from Boutin C, Viallat JR, Aelony Y: Practical Thoracoscopy. Berlin, Springer-Verlag, 1991.

Intrapleural Cytotoxic Agents

Several different agents have been used to try to control pleural effusions by cytotoxicity rather than sclerosis. Some of these are thought to act indirectly by immunomodulation; others exert direct cytotoxicity. *Corynebacterium parvum* enjoyed a period of popularity as an intrapleural agent after it was found to have antitumoral activity in an animal model (Casali et al, 1988; Felletti and Ravazzoni, 1983; McLeod et al, 1985). Success rates ranging from 56% to 100% were reported, but at least one study found the incidence of pain and fever to be greater than that with tetracycline (Leahy et al, 1985). Tetracycline is not used routinely because the same or better results can be achieved with sclerosants that are more easily available. Intrapleural interleukin-2 was found to control effusions in a small number of patients in whom it induced lymphokine-activated killer cells (Nagashima et al, 1987; Yasumoto et al, 1987). The expense and systemic toxicity of interleukin-2 limit its routine use, and its role outside the research setting remains to be shown.

Cisplatin is the drug that has been the most widely used for intracavitary chemotherapy. Multiple studies of intraperitoneal cisplatin, primarily for the treatment of ovarian cancer, showed that it acts through cytotoxicity rather than sclerosis and that the local pharmacologic advantage achieved by intracavitary administration can lead to tumor regression when systemic treatment has failed (Kirmani et al, 1991; Markman et al, 1991). The depth of penetration of drugs given by the intracavitary route appears to be 5 mm or less; therefore, they are not effective in the setting of bulky tumor (Markman, 1986). Cisplatin-based chemotherapy has also been administered intrapleurally (Markman et al, 1984, 1985), and the pharmacokinetic properties have been found to be analogous to the intraperitoneal route of administration (Rusch et al, 1992). One study of cisplatin-based intrapleural chemotherapy for malignant pleural effusions reported a 49% response rate (Rusch et al, 1991). Intrapleural cisplatin carries the potential of significant toxicity because a significant amount is absorbed systemically (Rusch et al, 1992) and, therefore, is unlikely to be used routinely for the management of malignant pleural effusions. Rather, it may be useful in clinical trials designed to maximize the local intrathoracic effects of chemotherapy (Rusch et al, 1994).

Techniques of Administration

Administration of Sclerosing Agents by Tube Thoracostomy

Good and Sahn (1978) believed strongly that the technique of administration of tetracycline affected the success of pleurodesis. They recommended insertion of a chest tube in the eighth or ninth intercostal space in the posterior axillary line and drainage of the effusion for 24 hours. Complete drainage of the pleural effusion and full expansion of the lung was documented by chest radiography. A dose of 15 to 20 mg/kg of tetracycline mixed in 75 ml of sterile water was then instilled through the chest tube into the pleural space. This was followed by 200 ml of air to facilitate contact of the tetracycline with both visceral and parietal pleural surfaces. The chest tube was clamped, and the patient was rotated to the left and right lateral decubitus, prone, and supine positions every 30 minutes to disperse the tetracycline solution throughout the pleural cavity. At the end of 2 hours, the chest tube was unclamped and placed back on suction. It was removed when the drainage was less than 150 ml per 24 hours.

The methods proposed by Good and Sahn (1978) became widely accepted guidelines for the administration of any sclerosing agent by tube thoracostomy. However, in practice there are some variations in the precise technique used with respect to drug dose and the amount of fluid in which it is mixed. The length of time that the chest tube is left to drainage before instillation of the intrapleural agent also varies. Some physicians believe that drainage should be allowed to decrease 100 to 150 ml/24 hr before instillation of the intrapleural agent; others proceed with instillation as soon as the pleural space is completely evacuated, usually within 48 hours of inserting the chest tube. Some physicians remove the chest tube 24 hours after pleurodesis; others leave it in place until the drainage is less than 150 ml per 24 hours. However, the principles to be considered in performing a pleurodesis by tube thoracostomy remain as follows: First, for a pleurodesis to be effective, the lung must be fully expanded so that the parietal and visceral pleural surfaces are in apposition. Second, there must be good dispersion of the agent throughout the pleural space. This is less likely to occur if the chest tube has been in for several days and loculations have begun to form around the tube. Third, the pleural surfaces must be kept in close apposition after instillation of the agent for the chemical pleuritis to progress to pleural symphysis. This is most likely to happen if the chest tube is left in place and on suction until drainage is minimal.

Talc Poudrage

Talc can be administered as a suspension through a tube thoracostomy, but it is more often insufflated by poudrage. Traditionally, asbestos-free talc was dry heat sterilized by hospital pharmacies and stored in sterile glass containers (test tubes or Petri dishes) in 5- to 10-g aliquots. It was then transferred to a bulb syringe or to a powder blower and insufflated at thoracoscopy or thoracotomy. Attaching the bulb syringe to a red rubber catheter facilitates insufflation at thoracoscopy. Insufflation by a powder blower can also be done by attaching it to a source of pressurized air or oxygen, just as would be done with an atomizer. This produces a finer and more uniform coverage of the pleura than does hand insufflation with a bulb syringe, but either method seems to produce a satisfactory pleurodesis. A spray can containing 4 g of sterile asbestos-free talc is now commercially available. This eliminates many of the logistic problems that were previously faced by hospitals in the preparation of sterile talc. Talc produces a rapid pleural symphysis, and it is helpful to insert two chest tubes (28 French [F] anterior and posterior tubes or 28 F anterior and 32 F right-angle diaphragmatic tubes) to prevent loculated fluid collections. If these develop during the immediate postoperative period, they usually are resorbed over the subsequent 1 to 2 months.

Administration of Cytotoxic Agents

A technique similar to that described by Good and Sahn for tetracycline is used for the administration of cytotoxic agents intrapleurally, but different considerations apply for cytotoxic than for sclerosing agents. Cytotoxic agents are left in the pleural space longer to maximize contact with the pleural tumor. The length of instillation time is dictated by the pharmacokinetic properties of the individual drug. Cisplatin is left in the peritoneal or pleural space for 4 hours, because after that time it has been nearly totally absorbed into the systemic circulation (Markman et al, 1986; Rusch et al, 1992). The chest tube can be removed immediately after instillation of a cytotoxic drug because there is no need to produce pleural symphysis. However, full expansion of the lung before instillation of the drug should be documented because an effusion caused by a trapped lung is no more effectively treated by cytotoxic than it is by sclerosing agents.

Management of an Effusion in Patients with a Trapped Lung

Patients who have a trapped lung are not candidates for therapy with sclerosants and are unlikely to benefit from intrapleural cytotoxic agents because they have bulky tumor. Even though they have a collapsed, unexpandable lung, some of these patients experience relief from dyspnea and chest discomfort when the effusion is evacuated, perhaps because this alleviates mediastinal compression. Some patients have a lung that can re-expand partially and experience a definite improvement in pulmonary function with drainage of the effusion. The insertion of a pleuroperitoneal shunt is one way to palliate such patients (Cimochowski et al, 1986; Little et al, 1988; Petrou et al, 1995; Sade and Wiles, 1990). The device used for this procedure, the Denver pleuroperitoneal shunt (Codman and Shurtleff, Randolph, MA), is a single-unit silicone rubber conduit that consists of a unidirectional valved pumping chamber located between fenestrated pleural and peritoneal catheters. One catheter is introduced into the pleural space by using a Seldinger technique and is directed toward the posterior costophrenic sulcus. The other catheter is placed into the peritoneal cavity by a small upper quadrant muscle splitting incision. The pumping chamber is positioned in a subcutaneous pocket created over the anterolateral costal margin that provides a stable base for shunt compression (Ponn et al, 1991). Pleuroperitoneal shunting is also a therapeutic option for patients with pleural effusions secondary to intractable ascites and has sometimes been combined with peritoneovenous shunting for such patients. However, active participation by the patient or family is required for the shunt to function because the pumping chamber must be actively compressed approximately 25 times every 4 hours. Patients who are unable to cooperate with this routine should not have a shunt implanted. In properly selected patients, pleuroperitoneal shunting provides good palliation with minimal morbidity. The risk of infection is minimal, but shunt occlusion as a result of fibrin deposition over the ends of the catheter occurs occasionally and may require replacement of the shunt.

Another alternative for patients who have a symptomatic pleural effusion and a trapped lung is intermittent drainage via an indwelling catheter (Pleurx; Denver Biomaterials, Golden, CO). The catheter is inserted under local anesthesia and can be used by the patient and family at home as needed to drain pleural fluid whenever the effusion becomes symptomatic. The efficacy and safety of this approach have been shown in both a retrospective study and a prospective multi-institutional trial (Putnam et al, 1999; 2000).

Pleurectomy

Pleurectomy with or without decortication was one of the early approaches used for malignant pleural effusions. Jensik and associates (1963) reported a series of 52 pleurectomies, 15 of which were associated with decortication. The immediate mortality rate was 6%, and the 30-day mortality rate was 18%. Two patients developed recurrent effusions, and the average survival was only 10.4 months. Subsequently, Martini and colleagues (1975) reported on a series of 106 patients whose malignant pleural effusion was treated by pleurectomy. Most patients required 2 to 3 units of blood transfusion intraoperatively, and the overall 30-day mortality rate was 10%. In both of these series, which antedate modern chemotherapeutic regimens, patients with breast cancer had the longest survival. More recently, Fry and Khandekar (1995) reported the results of pleurectomy and decortication in 24 patients who did not respond to standard treatment for malignant pleural effusion. Three patients died postoperatively for an overall mortality of 12.5%, and the other 21 patients all experienced control of their recurrent effusions. The high operative mortality rates undoubtedly reflect the poor performance status and limited reserve of patients who have malignant pleural effusions. With far less morbid therapeutic options now available, pleurectomy for the palliation of malignant pleural effusions has largely been abandoned. Only a highly selected group of patients are candidates for a pleurectomy. This includes patients who have a trapped lung and still have an excellent performance status.

SUMMARY

Patients with pleural effusion should first undergo a thorough clinical evaluation to try to identify the likely cause. The size and location of the effusion and the determination of whether it is free flowing should be made on posteroanterior, lateral, and lateral decubitus chest radiographs. CT is helpful in characterizing effusions that appear loculated and in detecting underlying pulmonary or intra-abdominal disease that may be responsible for the effusion. Thoracentesis with biochemical analysis of the pleural fluid, culture, and cytologic examination should then be performed to determine whether the effusion is a transudate or an exudate, whether it is malignant, and to direct further evaluation. Ultrasound and CT can localize loculated effusions for thoracentesis. If the cytologic findings are negative and malignancy is suggested, percutaneous pleural biopsy and repeat thoracentesis or thoracoscopy is indicated to establish a definitive tissue diagnosis.

Transudative effusions are managed by therapy for the underlying medical condition. Exudative effusions are also treated in this manner if they are not malignant. Patients with malignant effusions must have a determination made as to whether the lung will fully re-expand after evacuation of the effusion. If the lung expands completely, the effusion can be managed by sclerosis. Talc is probably the most effective sclerosant currently available, although tetracycline and bleomycin have also been popular. Intrapleural cytotoxic agents should still be considered investigational. If the lung is trapped and the patient is symptomatic, pleuroperitoneal shunting is an option. The diagnosis and therapy have often been empirical in the past. The increasing use of thoracoscopy and attempts to perform more carefully designed clinical trials are improving the approach to this often debilitating problem.

COMMENTS AND CONTROVERSIES

There really is not much to add to this excellent review on pleural effusion by Valerie Rusch. As discussed, the management of a symptomatic and recurrent malignant pleural effusion remains a difficult problem and at the present time this treatment can only be palliative. Talc pleurodesis is the most efficient method. Although two randomized trials have shown that bedside instillation of talc slurry is as effective as thoracoscopic talc insufflation, we prefer the latter method because it allows for biopsy of the tumor as well as proper positioning of chest tubes at dependent sites. We also think that insufflated talc powder produces a more uniform coverage of pleural surfaces. If the lung does not re-expand, the use of the Pleurx pleural catheter is recommended. This system can also be used if the lung re-expands, because the patient can go home the same day as tube insertion (as opposed to talc instillation). Occasionally, this method alone will produce a pleural symphysis and eventually control the effusion. The main disadvantage of the Pleurx system is the frequent change of drainage bottles, which can lead to increased costs.

■ KEY REFERENCES

Deslauriers J, Lacquet LK: Thoracic Surgery: Surgical Management of Pleural Diseases. St. Louis, CV Mosby, 1990.

This is a multiauthored text that provides an in-depth review of the pathophysiology and management of pleural diseases.

Light RW: Pleural Diseases. Philadelphia, Lea & Febiger, 1983.

This is a comprehensive reference on the diagnosis and treatment of pleural effusions with an emphasis on the biochemical characteristics of pleural fluid.

■ REFERENCES

Adler RH, Rappole BW: Recurrent malignant pleural effusions and talc powder aerosol treatment. Surgery 62:1000, 1967.

Adler RH, Sayek I: Treatment of malignant pleural effusion: A method using tube thoracostomy and talc. Ann Thorac Surg 22:8, 1976.

Aelony Y, King R, Boutin C: Thoracoscopic talc poudrage pleurodesis for chronic recurrent pleural effusions. Ann Intern Med 115:778, 1991.

Anderson CB, Philpott GW, Ferguson TB: The treatment of malignant pleural effusions. Cancer 33:916, 1974.

Ariel IM, Oropeza R, Pack GT: Intracavitary administration of radioactive isotopes in the control of effusions due to cancer: Results in 267 patients. Cancer 19:1096, 1966.

Asseo PP, Tracopoulos GD: Simultaneous enzyme immunoassay of carcinoembryonic antigen in pleural effusion and serum. Am J Clin Pathol 77:66, 1982.

Austin EH, Flye W: The treatment of recurrent malignant pleural effusion. Ann Thorac Surg 28:190, 1979.

Bayly TC, Kisner DL, Sybert A et al: Tetracycline and quinacrine in the control of malignant pleural effusions: A randomized trial. Cancer 41:1188, 1978.

Bethune N: Pleural poudrage: A new technique for the deliberate production of pleural adhesions as a preliminary to lobectomy. J Thorac Surg 4:241, 1935.

Bitran JD, Brown C, Desser RK et al: Intracavitary bleomycin for the control of malignant effusions. J Surg Oncol 16:273, 1981.

Boniface E, Guerin JC: Value of talc administration using thoracoscopy in the symptomatic treatment of recurrent pleurisy: Apropos of 302 cases. Rev Fr Mal Respir 6:133, 1989.

Bouchama A, Chastre J, Gaudichet A et al: Acute pneumonitis with bilateral pleural effusion after talc pleurodesis. Chest 86:795, 1984.

Boushy SF, North LB, Helgason AH: Thoracoscopy: Technique and results in eighteen patients with pleural effusion. Chest 74:386, 1978.

Boutin C, Viallat JR, Aelony Y: Practical Thoracoscopy. Berlin, Springer-Verlag, 1991.

Broaddus VC, Light RW: What is the origin of pleural transudates and exudates? Chest 102:658, 1992.

Broaddus VC, Wiener-Kronish JP, Staub NC: Clearance of lung edema into the pleural space of volume-loaded anesthetized sheep. J Appl Physiol Respir Environ Exerc Physiol 68:2623, 1990.

Camishion RC, Gibbon JH Jr, Nealon TF Jr: Talc poudrage in the treatment of pleural effusion due to cancer. Surg Clin North Am 42:1521, 1962.

Campos JRM, Werebe EC, Vargas FS et al: Respiratory failure due to insufflated talc. Lancet 349:251, 1997.

Casali A, Gionfra T, Rinaldi M et al: Treatment of malignant pleural effusions with intracavitary *Corynebacterium parvum*. Cancer 62:806, 1988.

Chambers JF: Palliative treatment of neoplastic pleural effusion with intercostal intubation and talc instillation. West J Surg Obstet Gynecol 66:26, 1958.

Chappell AG, Johnson A, Charles J et al: A survey of the long-term effects of talc and kaolin pleurodesis. Br J Dis Chest 73:285, 1979.

Chertow BS, Kadzielawa R, Burger AJ: Benign pleural effusions in long-standing diabetes mellitus. Chest 99:1108, 1991.

Cimochowski GE, Joyner LR, Fardin R et al: Pleuroperitoneal shunting for recalcitrant pleural effusions. J Thorac Cardiovasc Surg 92:866, 1986.

Daniel TM, Tribble CG, Rodgers BM: Thoracoscopy and talc poudrage for pneumothoraces and effusions. Ann Thorac Surg 50:186, 1990.

Deslauriers J, Lacquet LK: Thoracic Surgery: Surgical Management of Pleural Diseases. St. Louis, CV Mosby, 1990.

Dewald G, Dines DE, Weiland LH et al: Usefulness of chromosome examination in the diagnosis of malignant pleural effusions. N Engl J Med 295:1494, 1976.

Dewald GW, Hicks GA, Dines DE et al: Cytogenetic diagnosis of malignant pleural effusions: Culture methods to supplement direct preparations in diagnosis. Mayo Clin Proc 57:488, 1982.

Falor WH, Ward RM, Brezler MR: Diagnosis of pleural effusions by chromosome analysis. Chest 81:193, 1982.

Faurschou P: Diagnostic thoracoscopy in pleuro-pulmonary infiltrates without pleural effusion. Endoscopy 17:21, 1985.

Faurschou P, Francis D, Faarup P: Thoracoscopic, histological, and clinical findings in nine cases of rheumatoid pleural effusion. Thorax 40:371, 1985.

Felletti R, Ravazzoni C: Intrapleural *Corynebacterium parvum* for malignant pleural effusions. Thorax 38:22, 1983.

Fentiman IS, Rubens RD, Hayward JL: A comparison of intracavitary talc and tetracycline for the control of pleural effusions secondary to breast cancer. Eur J Cancer Clin Oncol 22:1079, 1986.

Frankel A, Krasna I, Baronofsky ID: An experimental study of pleural symphysis. J Thorac Cardiovasc Surg 42:43, 1961.

Friedman MA, Slater E: Malignant pleural effusions. Cancer Treat Rev 5:49, 1978.

Fry WA, Khandekar JD: Parietal pleurectomy for malignant pleural effusion. Ann Surg Oncol 2:160, 1995.

Gázquez I, Porcel JM, Vives M et al: Comparative analysis of Light's criteria and other biochemical parameters for distinguishing transudates from exudates. Respir Med 92:762, 1998.

Goldstein HA, Gefter WB: Detection of unsuspected malignant pleural effusion by bone scan. AJR Am J Roentgenol 10:556, 1983.

Good JT Jr, Sahn SA: Intrapleural therapy with tetracycline in malignant pleural effusions: The importance of proper technique. Chest 75:602, 1978.

Hamed H, Fentiman IS, Chaudary MA et al: Comparison of intracavitary bleomycin and talc for control of pleural effusions secondary to carcinoma of the breast. Br J Surg 76:1266, 1989.

Harley HRS: Malignant pleural effusions and their treatment by intercostal talc pleurodesis. Br J Dis Chest 73:173, 1979.

Hartman DL, Gaither JM, Kesler KA et al: Comparison of insufflated talc under thoracoscopic guidance with standard tetracycline and bleomycin pleurodesis for control of malignant pleural effusions. J Thorac Cardiovasc Surg 105:743, 1993.

Hausheer FH, Yarbro JW: Diagnosis and treatment of malignant pleural effusion. Semin Oncol 12:54, 1985.

Herbert A, Gallagher PJ: Interpretation of pleural biopsy specimens and aspirates with the immunoperoxidase technique. Thorax 37:822, 1982.

Hucker J, Bhatnagar NK, Al-Jilaihawi AN et al: Thoracoscopy in the diagnosis and management of recurrent pleural effusions. Ann Thorac Surg 52:1145, 1991.

Ike O, Shimizu Y, Hitomi S et al: Treatment of malignant pleural effusion with doxorubicin hydrochloride–containing poly(L-lactic acid) microspheres. Chest 99:911, 1991.

Jensik R, Cagle JE Jr, Milloy F et al: Pleurectomy in the treatment of pleural effusion due to metastatic malignancy. J Thorac Cardiovasc Surg 46:322, 1963.

Jones GR: Treatment of recurrent malignant pleural effusion by iodized talc pleurodesis. Thorax 24:69, 1969.

Kavuru MS, Adamo JP, Ahmad M et al: Amyloidosis and pleural disease. Chest 98:20, 1990.

Kefford RF, Woods RL, Fox RM et al: Intracavitary adriamycin nitrogen mustard and tetracycline in the control of malignant effusions: A randomized study. Med J Aust 2:447, 1980.

Kida T, Hujita Y, Sasaki M et al: Accumulation of ^{99m}Tc methylene diphosphonate in malignant pleural and ascitic effusion. Oncology 41:427, 1984.

Kim D, Weber GF, Tomita JT et al: Galactosyltransferase variant in pleural effusion. Clin Chem 28:1133, 1982.

Kinasewitz GT, Fishman AP: Influence of alterations in Starling forces on visceral pleural fluid movement. J Appl Physiol Respir Environ Exerc Physiol 51:671, 1981.

Kirmani S, Lucas WE, Kim S et al: A phase II trial of intraperitoneal cisplatin and etoposide as salvage treatment for minimal residual ovarian carcinoma. J Clin Oncol 9:649, 1991.

Ladjimi S, Djemel A, Ben Youssef R et al: Thoracoscopie diagnostique et thérapeutique dans 83 cas de pleurésies chroniques. Rev Mal Respir 2:355, 1985.

Ladjimi S, M'Raihi ML, Djemel A, Mathlouthi A: Results of talc administration using thoracoscopy in neoplastic pleurisies: Apropos of 218 cases. Rev Fr Mal Respir 6:147, 1989.

Ladjimi S, M'Raihi ML, Djemel A et al: Pleural talc treatment using thoracoscopy in lymphomatous pleurisy. Rev Fr Mal Respir 8:75, 1991.

Lambert CJ, Shah HH, Urschel HC Jr et al: The treatment of malignant pleural effusion by closed trocar tube drainage. Ann Thorac Surg 3:1, 1967.

Landvater L, Hix WR, Mills M et al: Malignant pleural effusion treated by tetracycline sclerotherapy: A comparison of single vs repeated instillation. Chest 93:1196, 1988.

Lange P, Mortensen J, Groth S: Lung function 22–35 years after treatment of idiopathic spontaneous pneumothorax with talc poudrage or simple drainage. Thorax 43:559, 1988.

Leahy BC, Honeybourne D, Brear SG et al: Treatment of malignant pleural effusions with intrapleural *Corynebacterium parvum* or tetracycline. Eur J Respir Dis 66:50, 1985.

Leininger BJ, Barker WL, Langston HT: A simplified method for management of malignant pleural effusion. J Thorac Cardiovasc Surg 58:758, 1969.

Lewis RJ, Caccavale RJ, Sisler GE et al: Video-assisted thoracic surgical resection of malignant lung tumors. J Thorac Cardiovasc Surg 104:1679, 1992.

Light RW: Pleural Diseases. Philadelphia, Lea & Febiger, 1983.

Little AG, Kadowaki MH, Ferguson MK et al: Pleuro-peritoneal shunting: Alternative therapy for pleural effusions. Ann Surg 208:443, 1988.

Markman M: Intracavitary chemotherapy. Curr Probl Cancer 10:401, 1986.

Markman M, Cleary S, King ME et al: Cisplatin and cytarabine administered intrapleurally as treatment of malignant pleural effusions. Med Pediatr Oncol 13:191, 1985.

Markman M, Cleary S, Pfeifle CE et al: Cisplatin administered by the intracavitary route as treatment for malignant mesothelioma. Cancer 58:18, 1986.

Markman M, Hakes T, Reichman B et al: Intraperitoneal cisplatin and cytarabine in the treatment of refractory or recurrent ovarian carcinoma. J Clin Oncol 9:204, 1991.

Markman M, Howell SB, Green MR: Combination intracavitary chemotherapy for malignant pleural disease. Cancer Drug Delivery 1:333, 1984.

Martini N, Bains MS, Beattie EJ Jr: Indications for pleurectomy in malignant effusion. Cancer 35:734, 1975.

Masuno T, Kishimoto S, Ogura T et al: A comparative trial of LC9018 plus doxorubicin and doxorubicin alone for the treatment of malignant pleural effusion secondary to lung cancer. Cancer 68:1495, 1991.

McLeod DT, Calverley PMA, Millar JW et al: Further experience of *Corynebacterium parvum* in malignant pleural effusion. Thorax 40:515, 1985.

Migueres J, Jover A: Indications for intrapleural talc under pleuroscopic control in malignant recurrent pleural effusions: Based upon 26 cases. Poumon Coeur 37:295, 1981.

Migueres J, Jover A, Bouissou H et al: Place de la ponction-biopsy à l'aiguille et du cyto-diagnostic dans le diagnostic des pleurésies malignes. Poumon Coeur 37:29, 1981.

Miserocchi G: Physiology and pathophysiology of pleural fluid turnover. Eur Respir J 10:219, 1997.

Mittal BR, Maini A, Das BK: Peritoneopleural communication associated with cirrhotic ascites: Scintigraphic demonstration. Abdom Imaging 21:69, 1996.

Monif GRG, Stewart BN, Block AJ: Living cytology: A new diagnostic technique for malignant pleural effusions. Chest 69:626, 1976.

Mori K, Hirose T, Machida S et al: Helical computed tomography diagnosis of pleural dissemination in lung cancer: Comparison of thick-section and thin-section helical computed tomography. J Thorac Imaging 13:211, 1998.

Mu XC, Brien TP, Ross JS et al: Telomerase activity in benign and malignant cytologic fluids. Cancer Cytopathol 87:93, 1999.

Nagashima A, Yasumoto K, Nakahashi H et al: Antitumor activity of pleural cavity macrophages and its regulation by pleural cavity lymphocytes in patients with lung cancer. Cancer Res 47:5497, 1987.

Oakes DD, Sherck JP, Brodsky JB et al: Therapeutic thoracoscopy. J Thorac Cardiovasc Surg 87:269, 1984.

Ohri SK, Oswal SK, Townsend ER et al: Early and late outcome after diagnostic thoracoscopy and talc pleurodesis. Ann Thorac Surg 53:1038, 1992.

Ostrowski MJ: An assessment of the long-term results of controlling the reaccumulation of malignant effusions using intracavity bleomycin. Cancer 57:721, 1986.

Page RD, Jeffrey RR, Donnelly RJ: Thoracoscopy: A review of 121 consecutive surgical procedures. Ann Thorac Surg 48:66, 1989.

Paladine W, Cunningham TJ, Sponzo R et al: Intracavitary bleomycin in the management of malignant effusions. Cancer 38:1903, 1976.

Pearson FG, MacGregor DC: Talc poudrage for malignant pleural effusion. J Thorac Cardiovasc Surg 51:732, 1966.

Petrou M, Kaplan D, Goldstraw P: Management of recurrent malignant pleural effusions: The complementary role of talc pleurodesis and pleuroperitoneal shunting. Cancer 75:801, 1995.

Pettersson T, Ojala K, Weber TH: Adenosine deaminase in the diagnosis of pleural effusions. Acta Med Scand 215:299, 1984.

Pettersson T, Riska H: Diagnostic value of total and differential leukocyte counts in pleural effusions. Acta Med Scand 210:129, 1981.

Poe RH, Israel RH, Utell MJ et al: Sensitivity, specificity, and predictive values of closed pleural biopsy. Arch Intern Med 144:325, 1984.

Ponn RB, Blancaflor J, D'Agostino RS et al: Pleuroperitoneal shunting for intractable pleural effusions. Ann Thorac Surg 51:605, 1991.

Prakash UBS: Comparison of needle biopsy with cytologic analysis for the evaluation of pleural effusion: Analysis of 414 cases. Mayo Clin Proc 60:158, 1985.

Putnam JB Jr, Light RW, Rodriguez RM et al: A randomized comparison of indwelling pleural catheter and doxycycline pleurodesis in the management of malignant pleural effusions. Cancer 86:1992, 1999.

Putnam JB Jr, Walsh GL, Swisher SG et al: Outpatient management of malignant pleural effusion by a chronic indwelling pleural catheter. Ann Thorac Surg 69:369, 2000.

Reshad K, Inui K, Takeuchi Y et al: Treatment of malignant pleural effusion. Chest 88:393, 1985.

Rinaldo JE, Owens GR, Rogers RM: Adult respiratory distress syndrome following intrapleural instillation of talc. J Thorac Cardiovasc Surg 85:523, 1983.

Rittgers RA, Loewenstein MS, Feinerman AE et al: Carcinoembryonic antigen levels in benign and malignant pleural effusions. Ann Intern Med 88:631, 1978.

Rodriguez-Panadero F, Lopez Mejias J: Low glucose and pH levels in malignant pleural effusions: Diagnostic significance and prognostic value in respect to pleurodesis. Am Rev Respir Dis 139:663, 1989.

Roth BJ, O'Meara TF, Cragun WH: The serum-effusion albumin gradient in the evaluation of pleural effusions. Chest 98:546, 1990.

Ruckdeschel JC, Moores D, Lee JY et al: Intrapleural therapy for malignant pleural effusions: A randomized comparison of bleomycin and tetracycline. Chest 100:1528, 1991.

Rusch VW: The optimal treatment of malignant pleural effusions: A continuing dilemma. Chest 100:1483, 1991.

Rusch VW, Figlin R, Godwin D et al: Intrapleural cisplatin and cytarabine in the management of malignant pleural effusions: A Lung Cancer Study Group trial. J Clin Oncol 9:313, 1991.

Rusch VW, Mountain C: Thoracoscopy under regional anesthesia for the diagnosis and management of pleural disease. Am J Surg 154:274, 1987.

Rusch VW, Niedzwiecki D, Tao Y et al: Intrapleural cisplatin and mitomycin for malignant mesothelioma following pleurectomy: Pharmacokinetic studies. J Clin Oncol 10:1001, 1992.

Rusch VW, Saltz L, Venkatraman E et al: A phase II trial of pleurectomy/decortication followed by intrapleural and systemic chemotherapy for malignant pleural mesothelioma. J Clin Oncol 12:1156, 1994.

Sade RM, Wiles HB: Pleuroperitoneal shunt for persistent pleural drainage after Fontan procedure. J Thorac Cardiovasc Surg 100:621, 1990.

Sakaguchi M, Virmani AK, Ashfaq R et al: Development of a sensitive, specific reverse transcriptase polymerase chain reaction-based assay for epithelial tumour cells in effusions. Br J Cancer 79:415, 1999.

Scarbonchi J, Boutin C, Cargino P, Scarbonchi-Efimieff T: Intrapleural talc in malignant pleural effusions. Poumon Coeur 37:283, 1981.

Schneller J, Eppich E, Greenebaum E et al: Flow cytometry and Feulgen cytophotometry in evaluation of effusions. Cancer 59:1307, 1987.

Seibert AF, Haynes J Jr, Middleton R et al: Tuberculous pleural effusion: Twenty-year experience. Chest 99:883, 1991.

Shedbalkar AR, Head JM, Head LR et al: Evaluation of talc pleural symphysis in management of malignant pleural effusion. J Thorac Cardiovasc Surg 61:492, 1971.

Silverman LM, Dermer GB, Zweig MH et al: Creatine kinase BB: A new tumor-associated marker. Clin Chem 25:1432, 1979.

Smyrnios NA, Jederlinic PJ, Irwin RS: Pleural effusion in an asymptomatic patient: Spectrum and frequency of causes and management considerations. Chest 97:192, 1990.

Sorensen PG: Carcinoembryonic antigen in malignant pleural effusions: A negative report. Eur J Respir Dis 62:138, 1981.

Srensen PG, Svendsen TL, Enk B: Treatment of malignant pleural effusion with drainage, with and without instillation of talc. Eur J Respir Dis 65:131, 1984.

Tamura S, Nishigaki T, Moriwaki Y et al: Tumor markers in pleural effusion diagnosis. Cancer 61:298, 1988.

Taylor SA, Hooton NS, Macarthur AM: Quinacrine in the management of malignant pleural effusion. Br J Surg 64:52, 1977.

Thermann M, Loddenkemper R, Schröder D: Thoracoscopy: A forgotten endoscopic procedure? Endoscopy 17:203, 1985.

Todd TRJ, Delarue NC, Ilves R et al: Talc poudrage for malignant pleural effusion. Chest 78:542, 1980.

Vanderschueren RG: Thorascopie sous anesthésie locale. Poumon Coeur 37:21, 1981.

Vladutiu AO, Brason FW, Adler RH: Differential diagnosis of pleural effusions: Clinical usefulness of cell marker quantitation. Chest 79:297, 1981.

Voellmy W: Résultats diagnostiques de la thoracoscopie dans les affections du poumon et de la plèvre. Poumon Coeur 37:67, 1995.

Wallach HW: Intrapleural therapy with tetracycline and lidocaine for malignant pleural effusions. Chest 73:246, 1978.

Webb WR, Ozmen V, Moulder PV et al: Iodized talc pleurodesis for the treatment of pleural effusions. J Thorac Cardiovasc Surg 103:881, 1992.

Weissberg D: Talc and adult respiratory distress syndrome. J Thorac Cardiovasc Surg 87:474, 1984.

Weissberg D, Be-Zeev I: Talc pleurodesis: Experience with 360 patients. J Thorac Cardiovasc Surg 106:689, 1993.

Weissberg D, Kaufman M, Zurkowski Z: Pleuroscopy in patients with pleural effusion and pleural masses. Ann Thorac Surg 29:205, 1980.

Winkelmann M, Pfitzer P: Blind pleural biopsy in combination with cytology of pleural effusions. Acta Cytol 25:373, 1981.

Xaubet A, Diumenjo MC, Marín A et al: Characteristics and prognostic value of pleural effusions in non-Hodgkin's lymphomas. Eur J Respir Dis 66:135, 1985.

Yamashita K, Kuba T, Shinoda H et al: Detection of K-*ras* point mutations in the supernatants of peritoneal and pleural effusions for diagnosis complementary to cytologic examination. Am J Clin Pathol 109:704, 1998.

Yang C-T, Lee M-H, Lan R-S et al: Telomerase activity in pleural effusions: Diagnostic significance. J Clin Oncol 16:567, 1998.

Yasumoto K, Miyazaki K, Nagashima A et al: Induction of lymphokine-activated killer cells by intrapleural instillations of recombinant interleukin-2 in patients with malignant pleurisy due to lung cancer. Cancer Res 47:2184, 1987.

Yim APC, Chan ATC, Lee TW et al: Thoracoscopic talc insufflation versus talc slurry for symptomatic malignant pleural effusion. Ann Thorac Surg 62:1655, 1996.

Zaloznik AJ, Oswald SG, Langin M: Intrapleural tetracycline in malignant pleural effusions: A randomized study. Cancer 51:752, 1983.

Zimmer PW, Hill M, Casey K et al: Prospective randomized trial of talc slurry vs. bleomycin in pleurodesis for symptomatic malignant pleural effusions. Chest 112:430, 1997.

CHAPTER **41**

Empyema and Bronchopleural Fistula

Francisco Paris
Jean Deslauriers
Victor Calvo

Empyema thoracis can be defined as a purulent pleural effusion. Although this infection usually originates from the lung, it may enter through the chest wall or from sources below the diaphragm or in the mediastinum. Complications from elective thoracic surgery or from post-traumatic hemithoraces are other possible causes. Most empyemas are, however, parapneumonic, and infection occurs when the host reaction is overwhelmed by the number and virulence of the innoculum.

Whereas the normal pleural space is resistant to infection, the abnormal space, such as one containing air, blood, or other fluids, is highly susceptible to empyema formation. The therapy for empyema depends on a clear understanding of the pathogenesis of pleural infection.

In this chapter, some of the most controversial issues concerning pathogenesis, diagnosis, and management of postpneumonic empyemas are addressed. The problems associated with posttraumatic or postoperative empyemas are covered extensively in other sections of this textbook.

HISTORICAL NOTES

Empyema of the pleural cavity was recognized approximately 2400 years ago when Hippocrates (Chadwick and Mann, 1950) made the distinction between empyema and hydrothorax. Prior to his description, the terms were used interchangeably, and before the principles of asepsis were defined by Semmelweis and Lister, infection from unsterilized instruments (used to evacuate fluid) occurred often in the treatment of serous pleural effusions.

Hippocrates diagnosed empyema mainly based on its clinical presentation. Fever was constant, but it was slight during the day and increased at night. Patients' coughs were nonproductive. Eyes were hollow, and cheeks showed red spots. When the patient was shaken by the shoulders, splash succussion sounds could be heard from the thorax, depending on the presence of air and fluid. In his book on chest auscultation, Laennec (Lain Entralgo, 1954) translated Hippocrates' description that distinguished hydrothorax from empyema: "When applying the ear on the ribs, during a certain time you hear a noise like boiling wine gar, which suggests that the chest contains water and no pus." Sometimes, the noises were not heard, depending on the quantity and physical characteristics of the intrathoracic liquid.

Hippocrates is also credited with the first drainage operation for empyema by using the cautery or doing the trephination of a rib. As reported by Paget (1897), Hippocrates opened the chest where the pain and swelling were most evident. He packed the wound with a strip of linen cloth, which was changed every day. He observed that this packing allowed fluid to escape around the strip but prevented the incoming of air into the space. Daily irrigations with "warm wine and oil" cleaned the lung surfaces, and when the empyema had healed, metal rods were used to close the wound. He clearly understood the natural history of undrained empyemas when he wrote in a treatise on pleurisy and peripneumonia (Major, 1945): "Patients with pleurisy who, from the beginning, have sputum of different colors or consistencies die on the third or the fifth day, or they become suppurative by the eleventh day." Hippocrates also wrote: "When empyemas are opened by the cautery or by the knife, and the pus flows pale and white, the patient survives, but if it is mixed with blood, muddy, and foul smelling, he will die."

In the 19th century, aspiration of acute pleural effusions was introduced. Wyman (Atwater, 1972) and his colleague, Bowditch (Bowditch, 1852), are credited with establishing this procedure. Wyman described the first therapeutic thoracentesis in a letter addressed to Sir William Osler: "With Dr. Homans' advice and assistance, the chest was punctured with an exploring trocar and cannula between the sixth and seventh ribs about six inches from the spine, and twenty ounces of straw colored serum drawn off slowly with great relief of the symptoms." Needles used for pleural aspiration, cannulas, devices preventing the entry of air, and suctioning systems were developed during the 19th century (Hurt, 1996).

Commenting on infections of the pleural space, Osler (1892) wrote (Moran, 1988): "It is sad to think of the number of lives which are sacrificed annually by the failure to recognize that empyema should be treated as an ordinary abscess by free incision." Historical records indicate that Osler underwent a rib resection at his home for drainage of a postpneumonic empyema (Barondess, 1975; Varkey et al, 1961).

Paget (1896) was distressed because the efforts of Paré, de Chauliac, and Laennec (to explain the principles of drainage in empyema, as reported by Hippocrates) were not understood. He said that because of "whole ages of

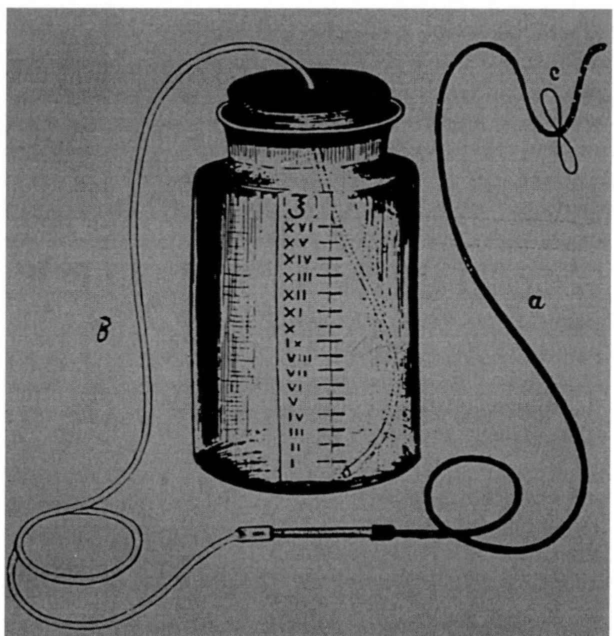

FIGURE 41–1 ■ Water seal drainage of the pleural space as described by Playfair in 1875. "The end of the tube was placed in a vessel of water under the bed" (King's College Hospital). This system was used mostly for children with empyema. (From Hochberg LA: Thoracic Surgery Before the 20th Century. New York, Vantage Press, 1960, p 244.)

neglect and perversion of the truth," Hippocrates' method of treatment for empyema became hopelessly lost. In 1872, Bouchut (Moir and Telander, 1991) described one patient who underwent 122 punctures during an 11-month period. Paget then wrote: ". . . and the worst of it all is that out of 48 patients thus tormented, only 6 were cured."

Thoracentesis was modified by the description of closed-tube thoracostomy by Playfair (1875) (Fig. 41–1) and Hewitt (1876), who performed drainage with a trocar, placing a rubber tube through the cannula in the pleural space. The rubber drain was connected to a glass tube that went through a cork into a bottle with a sealing level of antiseptic solution. It acted like a unidirectional valve, allowing the liquid to leave the thoracic cavity but keeping air from entering the space. The sealing level could be adjusted depending on the type and amount of fluid being drained. This system constituted a true siphon drainage system that also allowed pleural irrigation. In 1891, von Bulaŭ popularized the underwater drainage system throughout Europe. His name is still associated with this "no suction" method of pleural drainage.

The consequences of open pneumothorax and the importance of closed-tube drainage were not truly appreciated until a clear understanding of the pathogenesis of pleural infection was provided by Graham and Bell (1918). They were members of the U.S. Army Medical Corp (USAMC) and of the World War I Empyema Commission, and most of their work was done in Europe during the severe influenza epidemic due to hemolytic *Streptococcus*. Prior to their report, acute empyemas were managed by rib resection, and open drainage, and mortality rates averaged 30%. Death frequently occurred within 30 minutes of the procedure and was attributed to the open pneumothorax and mediastinal instability rather than to the empyema itself. Soon after Graham and Bell recommended closed rather than open drainage to treat early empyemas, the mortality rates decreased from 30% to 5% to 10% (Graham, 1925; Peters, 1989). The principles of empyema management as described by Graham and Bell include: (1) careful avoidance of open pneumothorax during the acute stage; (2) prevention of chronicity by rapid sterilization and obliteration of the space; and (3) careful attention to the patient's nutritional status. Open drainage is indicated only when fibrotic changes have occurred within the space.

In 1935, Eloesser described a tissue flap for the treatment of acute pleural tuberculosis. This flap was constructed as a one-way valve, allowing the exit of pus but preventing the entry of air.

As thoracic surgery evolved rapidly during the end of the 19th century, procedures such as thoracoplasty (Estlander, 1879; Schede, 1890) and decortication (Delorme, 1894; Fowler 1893) were introduced. These procedures described the obliteration of space either by collapsing it over the lung or by attempting to re-expand the lung itself. The results were not always good but, in 1901, Fowler (Yeh et al, 1963) stated that decortication was applicable to all patients with nontuberculous empyemas who could tolerate the procedure. He even said that "decortication could be used instead of Estlander's operation in most cases and should replace the Schede's thoracoplasty in all." In 1923, Eggers reported on 146 patients who submitted to decortication, and he described in full details the procedure as it is still used today.

With the onset of the antibiotics era, the incidence of pneumococcal and streptococcal empyemas fell sharply, and the mortality rate also declined dramatically. Subsequently, the increasing significance of anaerobic infection and the development of new generations of drug-resistant organisms led to a new spectrum of problems. In addition, the increasing frequency of immunosuppression such as seen in patients with acquired immunodeficiency syndrome (AIDS) or in patients undergoing active chemotherapy has somewhat modified the natural history of the disease, because patients are no longer able to produce the inflammatory reaction that is so important to localize the empyema and obliterate the space (Delarue, 1990).

■ *HISTORICAL REFERENCES*

Atwater EC: Morrill Wyman and the aspiration of acute pleural effusions, 1850 (Letter). N Engl Bull Hist Med 36:235, 1972.

Barondess JA: A case of empyema: Notes on the last illness of Sir William Osler. Transactions of the American Clinical and Clinicopathological Association. The 87th Annual Meeting, Vol 86, Baltimore, Waverly Press, 1975.

Bowditch HI: On pleuritic effusions and the necessity of paracentesis for their removal. Am J Med Sci 22:320, 1852.

Chadwick J, Mann WN: The medical works of Hippocrates. Springfield, Charles C Thomas, 1950.

Delarue NC: Empyema: Principles of management—an old problem revisited. In Deslauriers, Lacquet LK (eds): International Trends in General Thoracic Surgery, Vol 6. St. Louis, Mosby–Year Book, 1990.

TABLE 41–1 ■ **Pathologic Findings of Empyema**

Stage	*Phase*	*Characteristics*
Stage 1	Exudative (acute phase)	Swelling of pleura and fluid with low viscosity and cellular content
Stage 2	Fibrinopurulent (transitional phase)	Heavy fibrin deposits with turbid or purulent fluid
Stage 3	Organizing (chronic phase)	Ingrowth of fibroblasts and capillaries with lung trapping by collagen

Delorme E: Nouveau traitement des empyèmes chroniques. Gaz Hôp 67:94, 1894.

Eggers C: Radical operation for chronic empyema. Ann Surg 77:327, 1923.

Eloesser L: An operation for tuberculous empyema. Surg Gynecol Obstet 60:1096, 1935.

Estlander JA: Résection des côtes dans l'empyème chronique. Rev Med Chir (Paris) 3:156, 1879.

Fowler GR: A case of thoracoplasty for the removal of a cicatricial fibrous growth from the interior of the chest, the result of an old empyema. Med Record 44:938, 1893.

Fowler GR: A History of Thoracic Surgery (quoted by R. Meade). Springfield, Illinois, Charles C Thomas, 1961.

Graham EA: Some fundamental considerations in the treatment of empyema thoracis. St. Louis, CV Mosby, 1925.

Graham EA, Bell RD: Open pneumothorax: Its relation to the treatment of acute empyema. Am J Med Sci 156:939, 1918.

Hewitt LF: Thoracentesis: The place of continuous aspiration. BMJ 1:317, 1876.

Hurt R: The diagnosis and treatment of empyemas. In Hurt R (ed): The History of Cardiothoracic Surgery, New York, Parthenon, 1996.

Lain-Entralgo P: Clásicos de le medicina: Laënec. Madrid, CSIC, Instituto Arnaldo de Vilanova, 1954.

Major RH: Classic descriptions of the disease. London, Ballìere, Tindall and Cox, 1945.

Moir C, Telander R: Complications of lower respiratory tract infection, empyema complicating pneumonia, pneumatoceles, and respiratory embarrassment. In Follis, J, Filler M, Lemoine G (eds): Current Topics in General Thoracic Surgery: Pediatric Thoracic Surgery, Vol I. New York, Elsevier, 1991.

Moran JF: Surgical management of pleural infections. Semin Respir Infect 3:383, 1988.

Osler W: The Principles and Practice of Medicine. New York, Appleton, 1892.

Paget S: Empyema. In Paget S (ed): The Surgery of the Chest. New York, EB Treat, 1897, pp 204–229.

Paget S: Surgery of the Chest. Bristol, John Wright and Sons, 1896.

Peters RM: Emyema thoracis: Historical perspective. Ann Thorac Surg 48:306, 1989.

Playfair GE: Case of empyema treated by aspiration and subsequently by drainage: Recovery. BMJ 1:45, 1875.

Ribera y Sans J: Introduccion a le historia de le medicina, Vol 2 (quoted by F.H. Garrison). Madrid, Calpe, 1922.

Schede M: Die Behandlung der Empyema. Verh Dtsch Ges Imm Med 9:41, 1890.

Varkey B, Rose HD, Kulty K, Politis J: Empyema thoracis during a ten-year period: Analysis of 72 cases and comparison to a previous study. Arch Intern Med 141:1771, 1981.

Von Bülau G: Für die Heber Drainage bei Behandlung der Empyema. Z Klin Med 18:31, 1891.

Yeh TJ, Hall DP, Ellison RG: Empyema thoracis: A review of 110 cases. Am Rev Respir Dis 88:785, 1963.

BASIC SCIENCE

An empyema is a collection of pus in a natural body cavity. One of the most common varieties of empyema is the empyema thoracis, which can be localized (i.e., encapsulated) or can involve the entire pleural space (Le Roux et al, 1986).

Stages of Empyema Progression

The American Thoracic Society (1962) divides the formation of an empyema into three distinct stages, indicative of disease progression in the pleural space (Table 41–1). These occur over a 3-to-4-week period. For management purposes, two stages are recognized: an acute process and an organizing phase.

During the exudative phase (stage I), the pleural membranes swell considerably and discharge a thin exudative fluid. Fibrin is deposited over all pleural surfaces, and, despite early angioblastic and fibroblastic proliferation that extends outward from the pleura, the peel is not thickened enough to prevent complete lung re-expansion once the space is emptied. During the fibrinopurulent phase (stage II) (Fig. 41–2), there are heavy fibrin deposits over all pleural surfaces, more over the parietal pleura than over the visceral pleura. The pleural fluid is turbid or frankly purulent and has a large number of polymorphonuclear white cells. At this stage, the pleura is still relatively intact, and the lung, although less mobile, can be re-expanded. Loculations form during this stage (Fig. 41–3).

Within 3 to 4 weeks, organization (stage III) begins with massive ingrowth of fibroblasts and formation of collagen fibers over both parietal and visceral surfaces. The pus is very thick, and the lung, which at this stage is virtually functionless, is imprisoned within a thick fibrous peel (Fig. 41–4). The lung can no longer expand without being decorticated. Within 7 weeks, arterioles infiltrate the peel. In a 10-year retrospective analysis of 101 patients with empyema (Renner et al, 1998), 17 patients had stage I empyema, 8 were in the purulent stage, and 76 (75%) had an organized empyema.

Complications

Complications can occur at any time during the formation of an empyema, but they are more likely to develop during the chronic stage of disease (Table 41–2). One of the most common but often unrecognized complication is increased fibrosis and scar tissue in the lung, which produce pulmonary fibrosis. Scar tissue can also penetrate the parietal pleura and reach the intercostal spaces,

TABLE 41–2 ■ **Complications of Empyema**

Pulmonary fibrosis
Contraction of the chest wall
Spontaneous drainage through the skin: empyema necessitatis
Spontaneous drainage through the bronchus: bronchopleural fistula
Others
- Osteomyelitis (rib, spine)
- Pericarditis
- Mediastinal abscess
- Subphrenic abscess

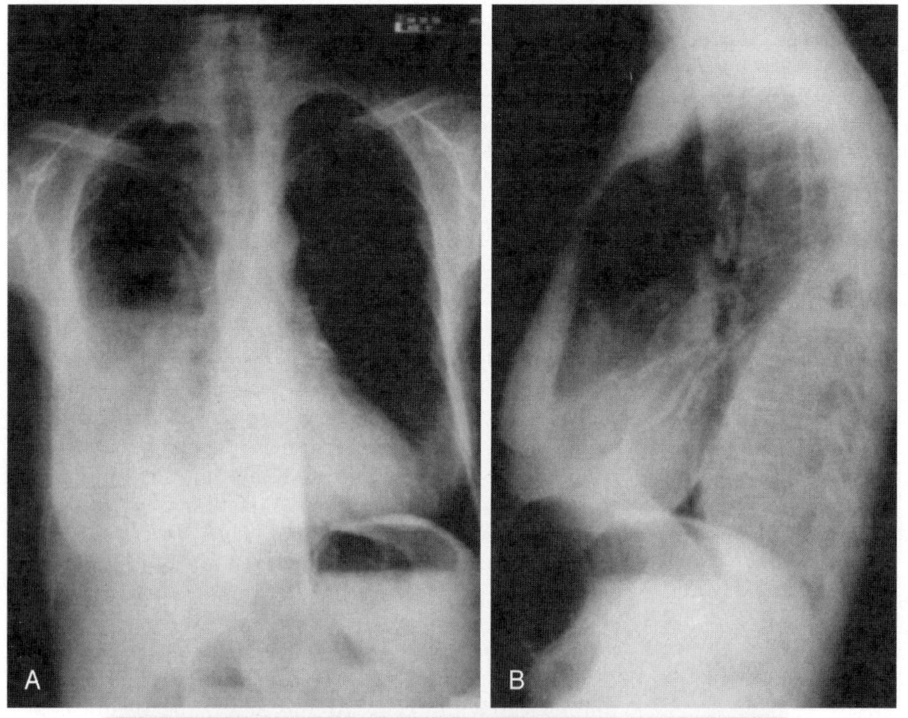

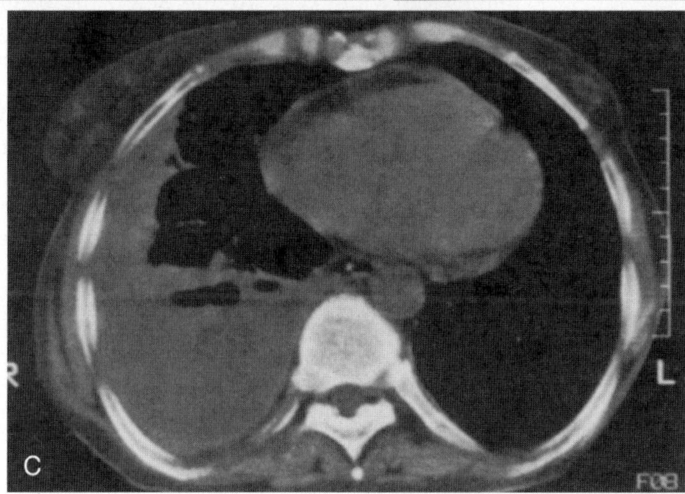

FIGURE 41–2 ■ *(A)*, Posteroanterior, *(B)* lateral chest radiographs, and *(C)* computed tomography scan of a 62-year-old woman with postpneumonic empyema during the fibrinopurulent stage. Note the typical image of a posteriorly located inverted D-shaped density (pregnant lady sign).

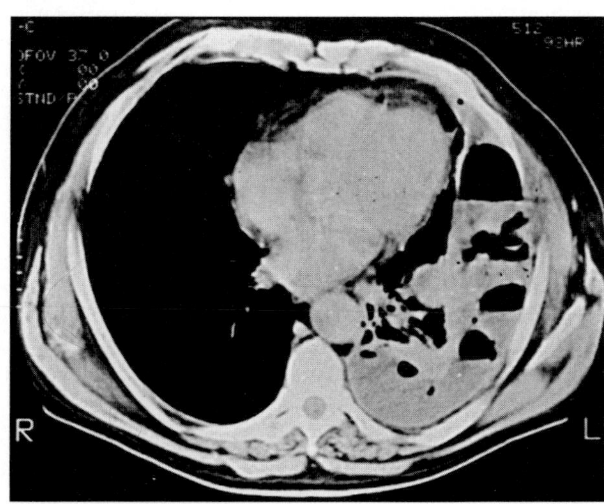

FIGURE 41–3 ■ Computed tomography scan showing a multiloculated empyema.

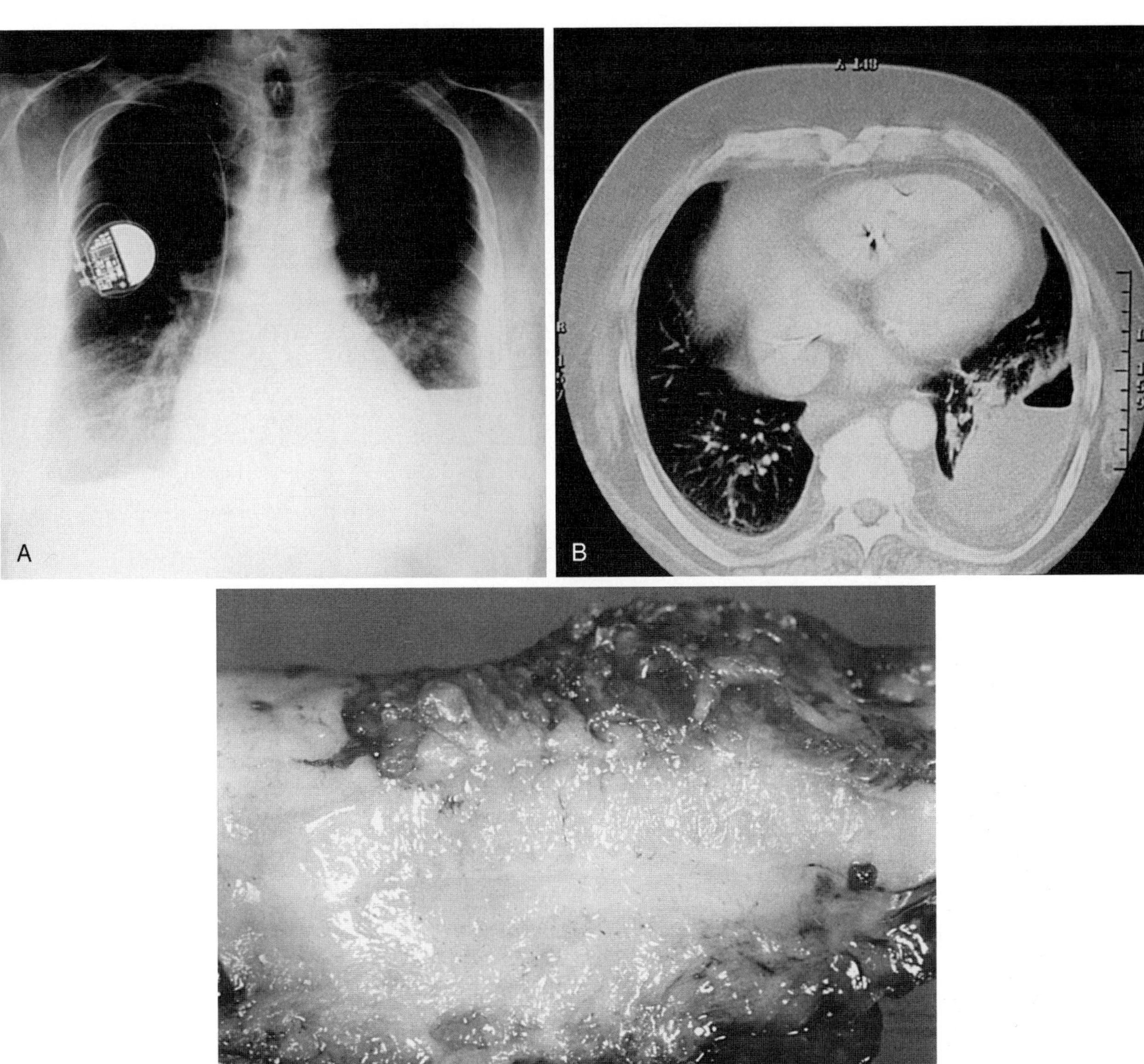

FIGURE 41–4 ■ Standard posteroanterior chest radiograph *(A)* and computed tomography scan *(B)* of a 60-year-old man with chronic empyema. Note the thickening over the visceral pleura. *C*, Thickened fibrotic peel that was resected from the visceral pleura to re-expand the lung.

which become narrowed and contracted, giving the chest wall the appearance of a carapace (LeRoux et al, 1986). In extreme cases, the shape of the ribs is altered, and on cross-section they appear triangular. In other instances, calcifications may develop in the fibrous tissue, and bone may be formed. Empyema necessitatis (Fig. 41–5) is characterized by the dissection of pus through the soft tissues of the chest wall and eventually through the skin. Similarly, the sudden appearance of purulent sputum signals the onset of a bronchopleural fistula with spontaneous drainage of pus into the bronchial tree (Fig. 41–6). In a series of 77 patients with bronchopleural fistula presented by Hankins and colleagues (1978), spontaneous fistulas (n = 28) were secondary to tuberculosis in 23 patients and to bacterial pneumonia or lung abscess in five. Unusual complications include rib or spine osteomyelitis, pericarditis, mediastinal abscesses, or transdiaphragmatic drainage of the empyema into the peritoneal cavity.

Parapneumonic Effusions

Patients with bacterial pneumonia may have an associated pleural effusion, which is called a parapneumonic or a postpneumonic effusion. Uncomplicated effusions are nonpurulent, have a negative Gram stain result and culture, and do not loculate in the pleural space. They resolve spontaneously with antibiotic treatment of the underlying pneumonia (Potts et al, 1978). Complicated effusions are either empyemas or loculated parapneumonic effusions that require surgical drainage for adequate resolution. According to Light and colleagues (1980), the pleural fluid, pH, lactate dehydrogenase (LDH), and glucose levels appear to be useful to differen-

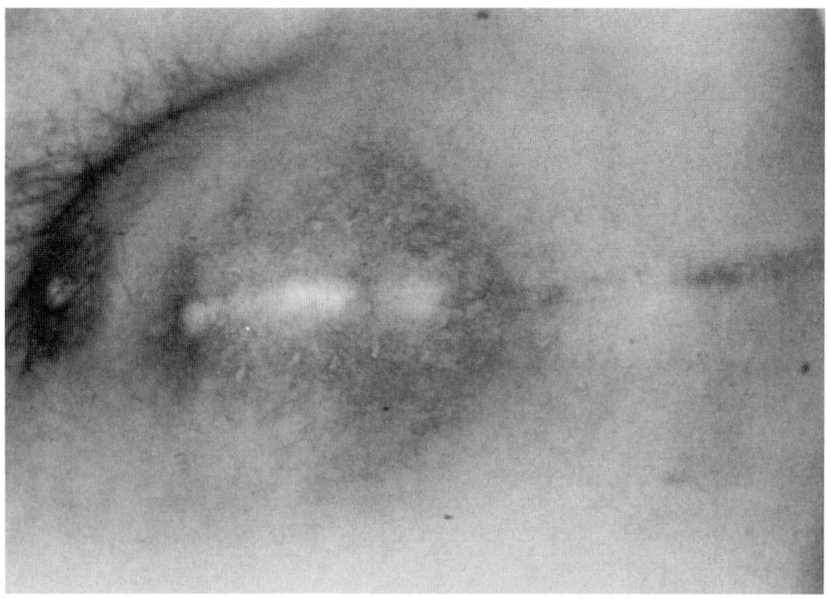

FIGURE 41–5 ■ Patient with an empyema necessitatis that has eroded through the soft tissues of the chest wall.

tiate uncomplicated from complicated parapneumonic effusions.

PATHOGENESIS

Most empyemas are the result of bacterial suppuration in organs that are contiguous to the pleural surface. Among these, the lungs are the most common contaminants. In such cases, empyema occurs by direct bacterial spread across the visceral pleura or by free intrapleural rupture of microscopic and peripherally located lung abscesses. In a classic description of putrid empyemas, Maier and Grace (1942) showed that most were associated with bronchiectasis, pulmonary abscess, and suppurative pneumonia. In most series, empyemas are secondary to bronchopulmonary infections in 50% to 60% of cases (Table 41–3) (Ali and Unruh, 1990; Sherman et al, 1977; Yeh et al, 1963), and nearly all of the so-called primary empyemas are due to subclinical pneumonic processes.

In 1969 and 1970, a severe influenza epidemic occurred in Spain, and several hospitals had the opportunity to treat large numbers of patients with parapneumonic empyemas. In a series reported by Paris and colleagues (1970), the number of empyemas seen during the epidemic (Fig. 41–7) was much larger than what was seen during the following year, indicating the importance of pulmonary infection as a cause of empyema.

Vianna (1971) showed that several patients with post-

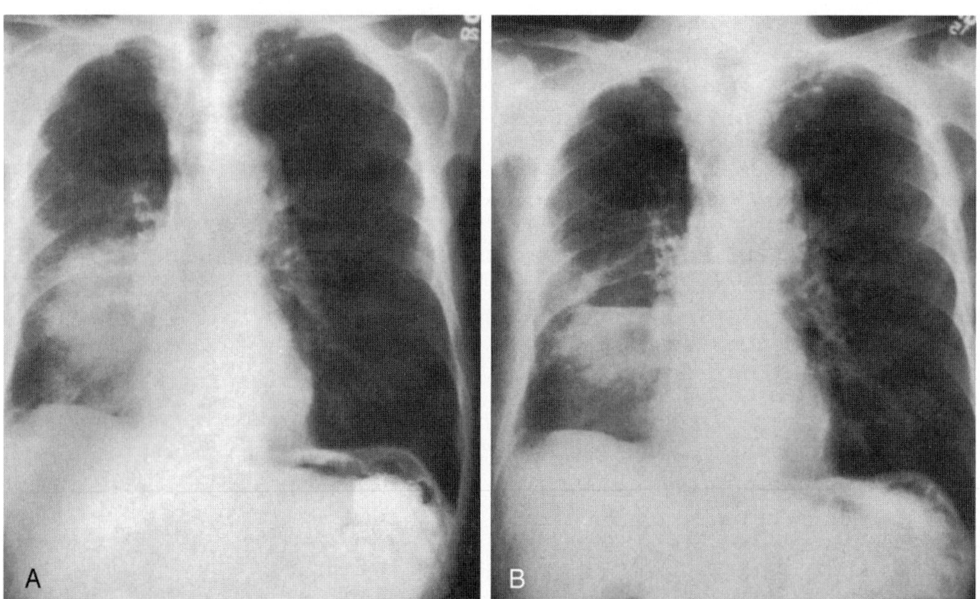

FIGURE 41–6 ■ Bronchopleural fistula. *A*, Chest radiograph of a 75-year-old man showing an empyema over the lower third of the right hemithorax. Three days later, the patient experienced a sudden expectoration of abundant purulent material. *B*, Repeat chest radiograph shows an air-fluid level containing space.

TABLE 41–3 ■ **Pathogenesis of Empyema**

Contamination from a source contiguous to the pleural space (50% to 60%)
- Lung
- Mediastinum
- Deep cervical
- Chest wall and spine
- Subphrenic

Direct inoculation of the pleural space (30% to 40%)
- Minor thoracic interventions
- Postoperative infections
- Penetrating chest injuries

Hematogenous infection of the pleural space from a distant site (<1%)

pneumonic empyemas had various underlying conditions, such as alcoholism or chronic pulmonary disease. Inactive pulmonary tuberculosis, diabetes mellitus, long-term steroid therapy, and various malignancies are other common predisposing conditions. Substance abusers (Hoover et al, 1988) and immunosuppressed individuals, such as patients with AIDS, are also at risk for bacterial and aspiration pneumonia and other pulmonary infections. These may lead to parenchymal destruction with subsequent contamination of the pleural space, which results in either simple empyema or complex infections, including bronchopleural fistula.

Other potential sources of contamination should be sought when the cause of empyema is unclear. Rupture of the esophagus, for instance, nearly always results in empyema formation. Rare causes of contamination include infection in the deep posterior region of the neck and, more infrequently, infections in the chest wall or thoracic spine. Although subphrenic abscesses can occasionally contaminate the pleural space through direct transdiaphragmatic erosion, most effusions associated with these abscesses are sterile exudate. Le Roux (1965) showed that lymph drainage from the subphrenic spaces is cephalad through the diaphragm, and this is the likely route of transferral of subphrenic infections to the pleural space. He also noted that silent paracolic abscesses can occasionally erode through the diaphragm and infect the pleural space. Similarly, hepatic amebic (Whitton, 1990) or hydatid (Nin Vivo et al, 1990) abscesses can erode through the diaphragm and produce secondary empyemas.

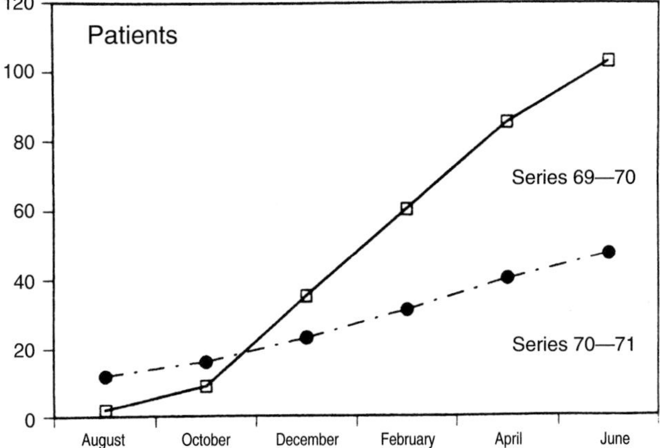

FIGURE 41–7 ■ Graph showing the number of postpneumonic empyemas recorded from 1969 to 1971 at the La Fe University Hospital, Valencia, Spain. The larger number of cases seen from 1969 to 1970 relates to the influenza epidemic that occurred during those years.

Virtually all post-traumatic empyemas are associated with penetration of the chest wall or the presence of a hemothorax. In a large series of trauma patients seen between 1972 and 1996, Mandal and colleagues (1997) reported a 1.6% incidence of empyema. In penetrating thoracic injuries, empyema formation is mostly the result of organic foreign bodies being carried into the pleural space (Thurer and Palatinos, 1987). In an interesting study, Ogilvie (1950) showed that the nature of the missile (e.g., shell splinters, bullets, or bayonets) played little part in determining the rate of infection in empyemas secondary to penetrating injuries. In blunt thoracic injuries, hemothoraces become secondarily infected via contamination through the chest tube or from an infection in the adjacent lung. Risk factors for empyema formation are shown in Table 41–4. In 1977, Arom and colleagues made a distinction between post-traumatic empyemas and infected organizing hemothoraces (clotted hemothoraces) in which masses of blood clot became secondarily infected. Ogilvie (1950) showed that air in the pleural space that is associated with blood is more likely to get infected than is a pneumothorax or a hemothorax alone. In an experimental model for empyema thoracis, Mavroudis and colleagues (1985) showed that concomitant hemothorax increased the incidence of empyema and early death after *Staphylococcus* was inoculated in the pleural space ($P < .05$). In rarer cases, traumatic empyemas follow blunt esophageal rupture, acute diaphragmatic hernia with bowel strangulation and/or necrosis, or aspiration of a foreign body with perforation of the lung (Baethge et al, 1990).

Direct inoculation of the pleural space can occur as a result of minor thoracic interventions, such as thoracentesis, thoracic biopsies, or chest tube drainage. In a series published in the early 1980s (de la Rocha, 1982), empyemas secondary to minor procedures were identified in eight patients.

Postoperative empyemas are seen almost exclusively after operations in which the esophageal or bronchial lumina have been entered. The incidence of this complication is in the range of 2% to 4% after pulmonary

TABLE 41–4 ■ **Risk Factors for Empyema after Blunt Thoracic Injuries**

- Initial large hemothorax (> 500 to 1000 ml)
- Delay in tube drainage
- Drainage in nonsterile conditions
- Incomplete evacuation of the hemithorax
- Loculations in the pleural space
- Prolonged drainage
- Multiple reinsertions of chest tubes
- Excessive manipulations of chest tubes
- Associated bacterial pneumonia
- Presence of pneumohemothorax

resection. In recent years, prophylactic use of antibiotics during the postoperative period and improved surgical technique have played a significant role in lowering the incidence of these events.

There is little evidence that hematogenous infection of the pleural space can occur from a distant infection site (classically, osteomyelitis) without an intermediate lung infection, which then contaminates the pleural space. In Sherman and colleagues' series (1977), only four cases represented true metastatic hematogenous seeding of the pleural space.

BACTERIOLOGY

In the preantibiotic era, the predominant organisms recovered from empyemas were pneumococci and *Streptococcus pneumoniae* (Brown et al, 1956; Keefer et al, 1941). In summarizing a total of 3000 empyemas reported from 1934 to 1939, Ehler (1941) noted that pneumococci had been found in 63.9% of cases, *Streptococcus pyogens* in 9.4%, and *Staphylococcus aureus* in 6.5%. He concluded that other organisms were found rarely and should be considered curiosities (Bartlett et al, 1974). The incidence of empyema was greater (80%) with streptococcal pneumonia than with other types of pneumonia because of greater lung destruction associated with the causative organism. In those cases, myriads of tiny lung abscesses occurred along the lymphatic channels and discharged the infecting organisms into the effusion in great quantities; this converted the effusion into an empyema within a matter of hours (Thomas et al, 1966).

The introduction and increasing use of antibiotics was accompanied not only by a marked reduction in the incidence and mortality rates of empyemas but also by a change in the spectrum of causative organisms. In a study on the changing etiology of acute bacterial empyema, Finland and Barnes (1978) showed that although the incidence of streptococcal pneumonia generally declined from 1950 to 1953, it still continued to occur in community-acquired empyemas. The incidence of *S. aureus*-related empyemas increased, and it became the most frequently found organism in empyemas in 1955. It declined to its original levels after 1965, but gram-negative rods increased in importance.

The predominant isolates in recent years have been *S. aureus* (29% to 69% of culture-positive cases) and enteric gram-negative bacilli (29% to 60% of culture-positive cases) (Bartlett et al, 1974). In a report by Vianna (1971), 41 patients with bacterial pneumonia complicated by empyema were studied, and *S. aureus* was the most common causative organism isolated (14 of 41, 34%). Gram-negative bacteria were isolated in 64% of empyemas that complicated some other underlying disease, probably owing to previous antibiotic therapy. The incidence of *S. aureus*-induced empyema has also increased in children. From 1955 to 1958, it was the causal organism in 92% of cases in children younger than 2 years, as reported by Ravitch and Fein (1961). In countries in which the introduction of new antibiotics and of new techniques of administration were delayed, the changes in the bacteriology of empyemas were seen at a later date. During the epidemic of influenza that occurred in Spain in 1969 and 1970, for instance, 49% of empyemas were still related to streptococcal pneumonias (Paris et al, 1970). During the ensuing years, *S. aureus* empyema became more prevalent (Blasco et al, 1976), especially in children (Paris et al, 1991).

The recovery rates for anaerobes isolated from empyema vary from 19% (Sullivan et al, 1973) to 76% (Bartlett et al, 1974). These micro-organisms are normal inhabitants of the mouth, intestine, and female genital tract. They reach the lung by aspiration from the mouth or bacteremic spread from the intestines or areas of pelvic suppuration. In a series reported by Sullivan and colleagues (1973), 226 culture-proved empyemas were analyzed, and anaerobes were isolated in 44 patients. More than 50 anaerobic bacteria were identified, but the most common was *Streptococcus*.

In a series by Bartlett and colleagues (1974), 76% of patients with empyemas had either anaerobes alone (35%) or in combination with aerobic agents. In most cases, the flora were complex, with an average of three different species of bacteria per case. According to these authors, the paucity of anaerobic isolates in most reports of empyema is due to inadequate methods to preserve oxygen-sensitive forms during transfer to the laboratory and lack of adequate anaerobic culture technique.

Often, a culture of empyema fluid does not establish a microbiologic diagnosis. In the series of Le Roux (1965), a causative organism could not be isolated in 80% of patients. In other series (Bergeron, 1990; Paris et al, 1970), the percentage of negative cultures varied from 25% to 60%. In general, negative cultures are due to inadequate culture techniques or to very effective antibiotics that can penetrate the empyema and prevent bacterial growth.

When empyema necessitatis occurs, the pathogens recovered do not necessarily represent the micro-organism responsible for the disease, because the skin fistula may be contaminated with skin flora or hospital pathogens (Bergeron, 1990).

DIAGNOSIS

The diagnosis of an empyema is made on clinical grounds, the presence of leukocytosis, characteristic findings on chest radiographs, and the recovery of purulent fluid from the pleural space. In several cases, however, the real problem is to distinguish between a noninfected parapneumonic pleural effusion and a true empyema or to correlate radiographic findings and fluid analysis with the stage of empyema.

An empyema should be suspected in patients with acute respiratory illnesses with associated pleural effusion. Typical symptoms, such as pleuritic chest pain, high fever, cough, tachypnea, tachycardia, toxicity, or local tenderness, are often present. Other symptoms include generalized malaise, anorexia, and weight loss. These symptoms can occur very acutely or develop insidiously over a period of a few days or even weeks. Physical examination nearly always shows diminished mobility of the involved hemithorax, decreased breath sounds, and dullness to percussion.

In the series by Varkey and colleagues (1981) of 72

case of empyema, the most common initial manifestations were dyspnea (82%), fever (81%), cough (70%), and chest pain (67%). In addition, a major underlying disease was present in 45 patients. Because the symptoms are related to the cause and stage of empyema, the amount of pus in the pleural space, the status of the host's defense mechanisms, and the virulence of the microorganisms involved, patient experience may vary from a few symptoms to several, with severe toxicity. Symptoms may also vary with the cause of the empyema. Patients with parapneumonic empyemas, for instance, often present with cough and purulent sputum, whereas the symptoms of patients with empyemas secondary to subphrenic abscesses may be exclusively abdominal complaints. On the basis of the clinical history, Maier and Grace (1942) divided cases of putrid anaerobic empyemas into one of two groups. In the first group, expectoration of foul sputum indicated the presence of a pulmonary anaerobic process or of an anaerobic empyema with a bronchopleural fistula. In the second group, the foul sputum was absent, and the symptoms suggested ordinary pneumonia. Most patients with an empyema have leukocytosis with a shift of the cell count to the left.

Chest radiographs show a pleural effusion with or without underlying pneumonia or lung abscess. On lateral radiographs, the empyemas are nearly always posterior and lateral, and most extend to the diaphragm. The classic image is that of a posteriorly located, inverted D-shaped density (pregnant lady sign) as seen in the lateral chest film (see Fig. 41–2C). Decubitus views are useful to determine if the collection is free flowing in the pleural space (stage I) or if it is loculated (stage II). Because it is often difficult to differentiate between lung consolidation and pleural fluid, computed tomographic (CT) scanning is useful to ascertain the underlying pulmonary pathologic condition. It is also useful to stage the empyema as determined by the presence of loculations, thickness of the pleura, and presence or absence of a trapped lung. As reported by Stark and colleagues (1983), visualization of thickened and separated pleural surfaces, compression of the parenchyma, and pleural thickening are specific CT signs of empyema. In 1991, Herna and colleagues described the "split pleural sign," which is indicative of the presence of pleural fluid between the thickened visceral and parietal pleuras (Fig. 41–8).

Ultrasonography may be used to document the presence of fluid or to distinguish between pleural fluid, pleural thickening, or parenchymal consolidation. It is also useful for guided pleural needle aspiration of fluid, especially when the position of the diaphragm cannot be documented with certainty on standard radiographs. As described by Moran (1988) and Orringer (1988), an empyemogram can be done by injecting contrast material at the time of initial thoracentesis and then obtaining posteroanterior (PA) and lateral chest films and decubitus views. Although this technique has seldom been used since the advent of CT scanning, it may provide information about the extent of the empyema cavity and the presence or absence of loculations within the space.

After the presence of pleural fluid has been confirmed, diagnostic thoracentesis should be done, and the aspirate should be sent for cytologic study, biochemical analysis, Gram's stain, and aerobic and anaerobic studies, including bacterial sensitivity tests.

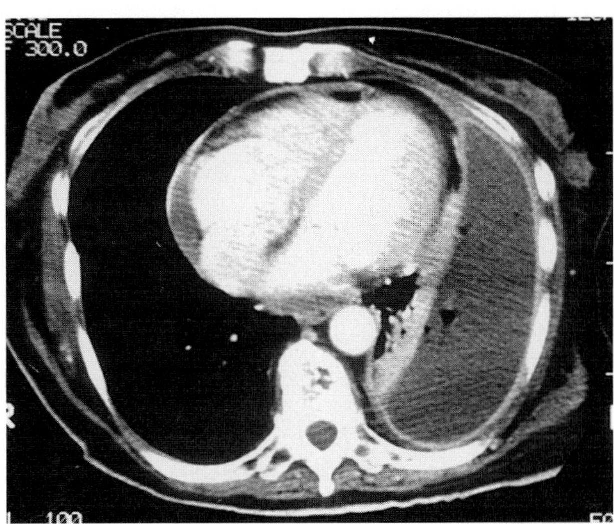

FIGURE 41–8 ■ Computed tomography scan of the chest showing a large empyema compressing the underlying lung.

Orringer (1988) showed that the gross appearance and odor of pleural fluid are among the most significant items of information obtainable by thoracentesis. Thin fluid, even with positive bacteriologic findings, may respond to selective antibiotherapy and thoracentesis; thick pus requires formal surgical drainage. Anaerobic pus is usually foul; aerobic pus has no offensive odor.

Several authors have shown that to recover anaerobes careful attention must be paid to the technique. Varkey and colleagues (1981) noted that the variability in the reported incidence of anaerobic empyemas may be caused by differences in the methods of transportation and processing of the pleural fluid specimens. In addition to standard bacteriologic examinations, pleural fluid should also be sent for viral, tubercular, and fungal cultures.

The relevance of pleural fluid analysis in empyema diagnosis is controversial especially regarding its biochemistry (Table 41–5). Some authors (Houston, 1987; Light, 1985, 1987) believe that pleural effusions with low fluid pH (less than 7.0), low glucose concentration (less than 50 mg/dl), and high LDH contents (more than 1000 IU/L) should be drained because these parameters indicate a complicated effusion or impending empyema. These changes can be detected before organisms are found on Gram's staining or culture, and they usually occur concomitantly. In uncomplicated effusions, the pH is greater than 7.3, the glucose level is higher than 60 mg/dl, and the LDH concentration is less than 1000 IU/L (Sahn and Light, 1989); these do not need to be drained. If the patient has free-flowing, nonpurulent fluid with borderline biochemical parameters, Sahn and Light (1989) recommend appropriate antibiotic therapy and repeated thoracentesis 12 hours later. If the pleural fluid measurements are stable or improving, continued antibiotic therapy is warranted, but if there is worsening of these measurements, chest tube drainage is generally necessary for resolution. In a series by Potts and colleagues (1976), three categories of parapneumonic effusions were

TABLE 41–5 ■ **Analysis of Pleural Effusions and Empyema**

Specimen	*Simple Parapneumonic Effusion*	*Complicated Parapneumonic Effusion*	*Empyema*
Pleura	Thin, leaky	Fibrin deposition/Loculi	Thick granulation tissue
Fluid appearance	Clear	Opalescent	Pus
White blood cell count	PMN +	PMN + +	PMN + +
Bacteria	−/Sterile	±/−	+/+
pH	>7.3	<7.1	<7.1
Lactate dehydrogenase (U/L)	<500	>1000	>1000
Glucose mg/dl	>60	<40	<40
Fluid/serum glucose (U/L)	>0.5	<0.5	<0.5

PMN, Polymorphonuclear cells. +, positive; + +, more positive; −, negative.
From Muers MF: Streptokinase for empyema. Lancet 349:1491, 1997. © by The Lancet Ltd., 1997.

characterized. The pH was greater than 7.3 in all 10 benign effusions, and spontaneous resolution occurred in each case. All 10 empyemas and the four loculated effusions had pH levels that were less than 7.3.

Physiologically, these biochemical changes are explained by an increased leukocytic activity and acid production in the pleural fluid. Based on all these diagnostic parameters, Van Way III and colleagues (1988) proposed a method of regrouping patients with empyemas by diagnostic class. Patients with class I empyemas ($N = 12$) were treated with short-duration chest tubes, and there were no deaths. Patients with class II empyemas ($N = 28$) were treated with chest tubes, and there were 2 deaths (7%). There were 40 patients with class III empyemas, and most required some form of surgical intervention (Table 41–6).

Despite the usefulness of all of these tests, the proper clinical staging of parapneumonic effusions remains difficult. How does one differentiate simple inflammatory reaction likely to respond to antibiotics and drainage from early organization? How does one differentiate between the very acute stage in which pleural fluid is thin and the purulent stage in which fibrin is deposited over pleural surfaces? Values of pleural fluid chemistry, such as a pH less than 7.2, correlate with loculated effusions but not necessarily with the presence of frank empyema (Himelman and Callen, 1986). In experienced hands, CT scan and ultrasonography provide significant information by detecting loculations and thickness of the fibrinous deposits encasing the lung (Cassina et al, 1999).

During the investigation of patients with empyema, it is also important to look for the causative process. Sullivan and colleagues (1973), for instance, showed that decayed teeth, retained roots, or advanced periodontal disease were present in 17 of 24 patients with anaerobic empyemas of pulmonary origin. Bronchoscopy should be performed to rule out foreign bodies or endobronchial tumors, especially if the patient requires surgery.

MANAGEMENT

As emphasized by Cohen and colleagues (1995), empyema management depends on its cause, clinical stage, state of the underlying lung, presence or absence of a bronchopleural fistula, and the patient's clinical and nutritional status.

Acute Empyema

In acute empyemas (Table 41–7), antibiotics are used to control the infection, and intercostal tube drainage is both simple and effective to drain and obliterate the space. Repeated thoracentesis, in conjunction with antibiotic therapy, may be indicated when the fluid is thin and the toxicity is well controlled. According to Moran (1988), antibiotics and thoracentesis can be curative in a large proportion of parapneumonic effusions if the mode of therapy is instituted early enough. Conversely, Personne (1990) suggests that performing thoracentesis alone is usually a mistake, because the chances of complete success are minimal. It often leads to the formation of multiloculated pockets, which eventually become difficult to drain. Ferguson (1990) noted that ". . . although simple drainage and antibiotic therapy remain the norm,

TABLE 41–6 ■ **Regrouping of Patients with Empyema into Diagnostic Classes**

Class	*Type*	*Characteristics*
Class I	Low pH pleural effusion	Postpneumonia effusion, pleural fluid, pH less than 7.2, negative pleural fluid cultures
Class II	Classic empyema	Positive pleural fluid culture, absence of multiple loculations, chest radiograph visualization.
Class III	Complicated empyema	Multiple loculations on chest radiograph, initially or subsequently, or trapped lung.

From Van Way C III, Narrod J, Hopeman A: The role of early limited thoracotomy in the treatment of empyema. J Thorac Cardiovasc Surg 96:434, 1988.

TABLE 41–7 ■ **Principles of Therapy of Acute Empyemas**

Drainage: closed-tube drainage, VATS drainage, open thoracotomy
Antibiotics: appropriate selection
Enzymes: intrapleural fibrinolytic enzymes (streptokinase or urokinase)
Supportive measures: respiratory care, nutrition, therapy of comorbid conditions
Therapy: underlying cause of empyema

VATS, Videoassisted thoracoscopic surgery.

an enlarging group of patients, particularly those with complicated or postoperative empyemas, will require aggressive surgical intervention. Early recognition of these patients and institution of surgical intervention as primary therapy rather than as a last resort will likely result in improved survival and shortened hospital stay." Open drainage plays no role in the therapy of acute empyemas.

Drainage

Surgical removal of pus by proper pleural space drainage remains the gold standard of empyema management. This procedure not only evacuates the pus but also allows for the apposition of pleural surfaces, a feature that eventually leads to obliteration of the space and resolution of the infection. The timing of the surgical drainage and the choice of a drainage procedure must be tailored to the individual patient (Moran, 1988).

Pleural drainage can be accomplished by closed-tube thoracostomy, by videothoracoscopy (VATS), or by open thoracotomy. The technique of intercostal tube drainage is simple and well described in every textbook of thoracic surgery. When inserting a chest tube without proper visualization of the space, the surgeon must be careful not to penetrate the diaphragm, which is often retracted upward. The chest tube, size 18 to 28 French (F), is connected to an active suction system, usually with a negative pressure of −25 cm of water. If the lung expands well, the chest tube is left under suction drainage for a period of 2 to 3 weeks or until the space is permanently obliterated. This is likely to have occurred when the daily amount of drainage is low (less than 10 ml/day), when there are no up-and-down movements of fluid in the tubing, or when no pneumothorax develops if the tube is opened to atmospheric pressure. At this point, the tube can simply be removed or closed drainage can be changed to open drainage by cutting it close to the chest wall. The tube is then shortened at the rate of about 1 in/wk or until granulation tissue and fibrosis lead to its spontaneous expulsion from the pleural space (Fig. 41–9).

When the lung expands well with tube drainage and there is no persistent empyema cavity, intrapleural irrigation of antibiotics (as suggested by Luizy et al, 1966; Dieter et al, 1970; and Rosenfeldt et al, 1981) does not appear to present additional advantages. Intrapleural irrigations were required in 96 of 236 patients (44%) with empyema reported by Blasco and colleagues (1990). In these individuals, initial drainage was inadequate either because fibrin clots occluded the chest tube or because persistent loculations and adhesions prevented adequate lung re-expansion. Several patients (n = 36) required more than one chest tube for these irrigations. In that series, the overall mortality was low (2%), and only 20 patients had permanent radiologic sequelae.

Another option for closed pleural space drainage is to use small-base, pig-tail catheters positioned with ultrasound or CT guidance. This technique is less traumatic but often these patients will need several CT scans and replacement of blocked or misplaced catheters. Lee and colleagues (1991) and Crouch and colleagues (1987) have reported success rates ranging from 70% to 90%. Pig-tail catheters should not be used when thick pus is likely to clog these small bore tubes.

In 1991, Wakabayashi reported on expanded applications of therapeutic VATS. In his series, 20 patients underwent thoracoscopic débridement of chronic empyema; the lungs re-expanded in 18, in whom the duration of empyema had been less than 2 months, and failed to re-expand in two patients who had empyema for 4 and 7 months, respectively. Since then, several authors (Cassina et al, 1999; Landreneau et al, 1995; Lawrence et al, 1997; MacKinlay et al, 1996; Ronson and Miller, 1998; Striffeler et al, 1998) have used this technique as a primary method to drain acute empyemas. Following ultrasound or CT delineation of the location and size of the collection, VATS techniques are used to evacuate the pus, disrupt

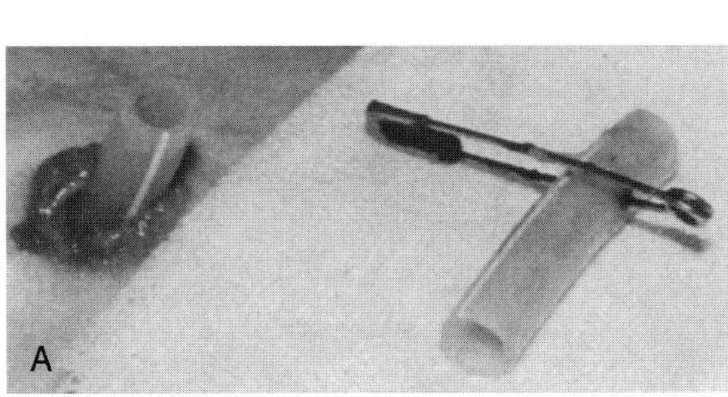

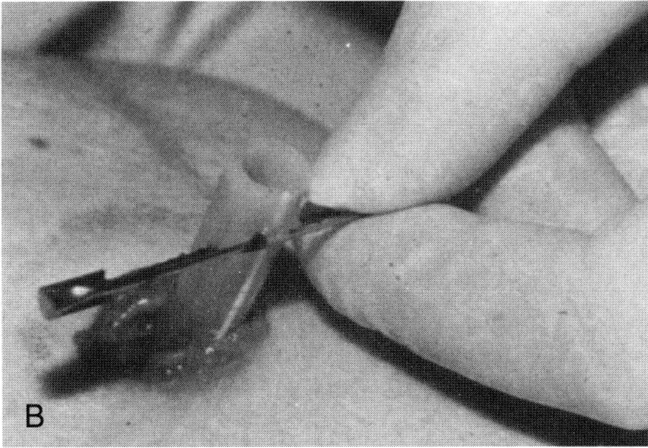

FIGURE 41–9 ■ *A*, A chest tube being shortened by about 1 inch. *B*, A safety pin is used to prevent tube from falling back into the space.

TABLE 41–8 ■ **Thoracoscopic Treatment for Empyema**

Author	No. of Patients	Stage of Empyema	Success Rate (%)	Complications (%)	No. of Deaths
MacKinlay et al	31	2	90	16	3
Landreneau et al	76	2 and 3	83	3	
Striffeler et al	67	2	72	4	4
Cassina et al	45	2 and 3	82	11	0

From Cassina PC, Hauser M, Hillejan L et al: Videoassisted thoracoscopy in the treatment of pleural empyema: Stage-based management and outcome. J Thorac Cardiovasc Surg 117:234, 1999.

the loculations containing fibrin clots and membranes, remove the fibrinous membranes, re-expand the lung, and position the chest tubes in the most dependent portion of the space. Because it is minimally invasive, VATS is also an ideal procedure for most of these critically ill patients, who are at high surgical risk not only because of their illness but also because of a prior debilitating condition or immunosuppressed status. In the authors' view (Deslauriers, 1999), VATS débridement of fibrinopurulent empyemas represents one of the best indications for therapeutic VATS techniques. In 1996, MacKinlay and colleagues reported 64 cases of fibrinopurulent empyemas treated by formal thoracotomy (n = 33) or thoracoscopy (n = 31). The mortality was similar in both groups (3%), but VATS techniques had substantial advantages over thoracotomy in terms of resolution of the disease, hospital stay, and cosmetic outcome. In 1999, Cassina and colleagues presented a prospective, selected single institution series of 45 patients with pleural empyema who underwent operation. In 37 patients (82%), VATS débridement was successful, and there were no complications during the procedure. At follow-up (n = 35), with pulmonary function tests, 86% of the patients treated by VATS showed normal values. A summary of the world's literature on thoracoscopic treatment of empyema is shown in Table 41–8. Overall, these techniques are safe and efficient for stage II empyemas but inefficient for organized disease (Silen and Naunheim, 1996).

Before the advent of VATS techniques, several authors (Hoover et al, 1986; Morin et al, 1972; Personne, 1990; Van Way III, 1988) proposed early open thoracotomy to drain acute empyemas that could not be adequately evacuated by tube thoracostomy because of multiple loculations or inaccessible purulent collections (Mavroudis et al, 1981). This procedure was incorrectly called "early decortication" by many of these authors (Fishman and Ellertson, 1977; Frimodt-Moller and Vejlsted, 1985; Mandal and Tradepalli, 1987). Under general anesthesia, a small incision is made over the cavity, and a short segment of rib is resected. The empyema is then completely evacuated (Fig. 41–10) and, through a separate incision, a large-bore chest tube is secured in the most dependent portion of the space. In Fishman and Ellertson's series (1977), six of eight immunosuppressed patients survived early decortication and were discharged 3 to 6 weeks after the operation. Morin and colleagues (1972) also reported excellent results with early thoracotomy in 23 patients with posteriorly located, D-shaped densities seen on the lateral chest radiograph. Miller (1990) and Pothula and Krellenstein (1994) also advocate early aggressive surgical approach when the standard chest tube does not relieve the loculated fluid, because the surgical risk is low and the expected outcome is good in more than 95% of patients. Of 52 patients reported by Pothula and Krellenstein (1994), there were no operative deaths, and good results were obtained in 50 of 52. In substance abuse patients, exploration thoracotomy is recommended within 24 to 48 hours if the patient has toxic manifestations despite drainage, or if there is evidence of parenchymal destruction, multiple loculations, or trapped lung (Hoover et al, 1988).

Antibiotics

Several factors, such as the pathogen involved, the stage of the empyema, and the immune status of the host,

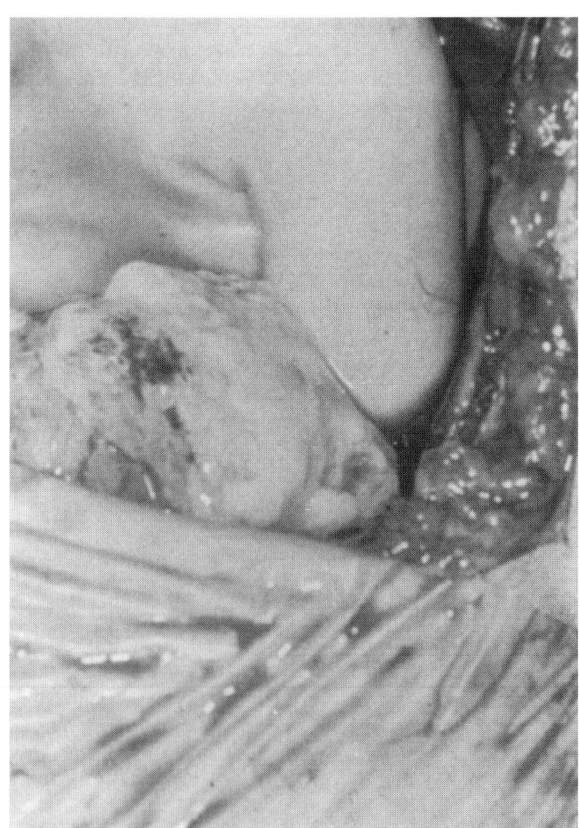

FIGURE 41–10 ■ Operative photograph showing fibrin being removed from an empyema space through a rib resection thoracotomy. (Courtesy of Jean Morin, MD.)

TABLE 41–9 ■ **Choice of Antibiotics for Empyema**

Organism	First Choice	Alternative
GRAM-POSITIVE BACTERIA		
Streptococcus pneumoniae	Penicillin Clindamycin Ceftriaxone	Erythromycin
Staphylococcus aureus (BL−)	Penicillin	Cefazolin Clindamycin
Staphylococcus aureus (BL+)	Oxacillin	Cefazolin Clindamycin
Staphylococcus aureus (methicillin-resistant)	Vancomycin Tricoplanin	Ciprofloxacin Aminoglycosides
Staphylococcus epidermidis (BL−)	Penicillin	Cefazolin Clindamycin
Staphylococcus epidermidis (BL+)	Oxacillin	Cefazolin Clindamycin
Staphylococcus epidermidis (methicillin-resistant)	Vancomycin	Cefazolin Clindamycin
Streptococcus faecalis	Ampicillin Gentamicin	Vancomycin
GRAM-NEGATIVE BACTERIA		
Pseudomonas aeruginosa	Ceftazidime	Imipenem Aminoglycoside Piperacillin Ticarcillin Ciprofloxacin
Escherichia coli	Cefazolin Cefuroxime	Cefamandole Cefoxitin
Proteus mirabilis		Ampicillin (if sensitive)
Haemophilus influenzae	Cefamandole	Cefuroxime Ampicillin (if sensitive) Amoxicillin Clavulanate
Bacteroides fragilis	Amoxicillin Clavulanate Clindamycin Metronidazole	Cefoxitin

BL (+ or −), β-lactamase producer or nonproducer.
Modified from Bergeron MG: The changing bacterial spectrum and antibiotic choice. In Deslauriers J, Lacquet LK (eds): International Trends in General Thoracic Surgery, Vol 6, St. Louis, Mosby–Year Book, 1990.

determine the response to antibiotics. Concentrations of antibiotics in the infected pleural space must be high enough to neutralize the pathogens, a feature possible during the exudative phase of disease but less likely during the fibrinopurulent or organization stages (Bergeron, 1990). Initially, and while awaiting the results of antibiotic susceptibility, a semisynthetic penicillin, such as doxacillin, or clindamycin should be given if the empyema has been acquired in the community or if the Gram staining reveals clusters of gram-positive cocci that are compatible with *S. aureus* (Bergeron, 1990).

A guide to the choice of antibiotics is given in Table 41–9. In patients with anaerobic, gram-negative empyema, penicillin is the antibiotic of choice; clindamycin can also be used. It is generally agreed that antibiotics should be continued for a period of 2 to 4 weeks.

Intrapleural Enzymes and Talc

During the transitional stage of empyema progression, fibrin is deposited in the pleural space, and fibrin strands develop between visceral and parietal pleura, forming loculi and preventing lung re-expansion despite well-placed chest tubes. During that period, the use of intrapleural fibrinolytic enzymes has been described as a method to break up these strands and to improve drainage.

The use of intrapleural streptokinase for the therapy of acute empyemas was first described by Tillett and Sherry (1949). However, allergy and bleeding complications, probably owing to impure preparations and overlong dwelling times, prevented adoption of these techniques (Muers, 1997). In 1977, Bergh and colleagues showed that streptokinase at the dose of 250,000 U diluted in 100 ml of physiologic saline solution stimulates the liquefaction of fibrin clots and, in some cases, facilitates the subsequent drainage of the pleural space. In 1994, Robinson and colleagues presented a series of 13 consecutive patients with fibrinopurulent empyemas who had incomplete drainage. Streptokinase (250,000 U in 100 ml of 0.9% saline solution) or urokinase (100,000 U in 100 ml of 0.9% saline solution) was instilled daily into the chest tube, and the tube was clamped for 6 to 12 hours, followed by suction. This regimen was completely successful in 10 of 13 patients (77%), with resolution of the empyema, eventual withdrawal of the chest tubes, and no recurrence. In 1997, Davies and colleagues reported the benefits of this technique in a randomized, controlled trial. Twenty-four patients with infected, community-acquired, parapneumonia effusions were studied, and all had either frankly purulent or Gram's-stain–positive pleural fluid. These patients were treated by drainage and either intrapleural saline flushes or intrapleural streptokinase given as 250,000 IU in 20 ml of saline with a 2-hour dwelling time daily for 3 days. The streptokinase group drained more fluid and showed greater improvement on chest radiograph at discharge. Surgery was required in three control patients but none in the streptokinase group. Another randomized trial of empyema therapy (Wait et al, 1997) compared pleural drainage and fibrinolytic therapy with VATS with regard to efficacy and duration of hospitalization. In patients with loculated, complex, fibrinopurulent, parapneumonic empyema, this study showed that a primary treatment strategy of VATS was associated with a higher efficacy, shorter hospital duration, and lower cost.

Urokinase, an enzyme isolated from human urine and acting through activation of plasminogen, can also be used for the lysis of loculated pleural effusions (Moulton et al, 1989; Pollack and Passik, 1994). In a prospective, double-blind study, Bouros and colleagues (1997) concluded that urokinase could be the thrombolytic of choice given the potential for dangerous allergic reaction to streptokinase and the relatively small cost of urokinase. In a series by Lopez-Rivero and colleagues (1994), 22 patients with empyema were treated by intrapleural instillation of urokinase (200,000 IU) three times a day. Depending on the clinical and radiologic response, this treatment was continued for 48 hours, sometimes with lower dosage. Ninety-five percent of empyemas were completely drained after an average dose of 900,000 IU, and only one patient had to undergo surgery because of treatment failure.

The use of talc has also been described by Weissberg and Kaufman (1986). They reported on five patients with fibrinopurulent empyema who did not respond to conventional therapy and in whom intrapleurally insufflated talc powder led to pleurodesis. Although no side effects were observed, this technique should clearly be restricted to a few selected patients.

Supportive Measures

Supportive measures, including proper respiratory care with therapy of associated respiratory infection and obstructive pulmonary disease and maintenance of nutrition by enteral feedings, are essential for the successful management of early empyemas. Active chest physiotherapy is particularly important to promote lung re-expansion and prevent chest wall contraction. Because nearly 50% to 60% of patients have a major associated medical illness, it is imperative that this condition is diagnosed and appropriately managed.

Chronic Empyema

Usual causes of chronicity include a delay in diagnosis, inadequate antibiotic therapy, improper drainage during the acute phase, continuing reinfection (such as that which occurs with a bronchopleural fistula or lung abscess), presence of a foreign body, or presence of a specific infection (such as tuberculosis or fungal infection).

In 1986, Paget (Holmes Sellors and Cruickshank, 1951) wrote "One might add a score of cases to show that an unhealed empyema is, as a rule, the direct result of the patient's neglect, or of the surgeon's delay, or of inadequate and useless surgery; but our business now is to inquire how we may most surely and safely cure it." Chronicity is diagnosed by persistent or increasing fever and chest pain, thick pleural fluid, unresolving radiologic findings, and incomplete re-expansion of the lung following closed drainage (Delarue, 1990). When the empyema has reached this stage, simple forms of therapy, such as rib resection, open drainage, or window thoracostomy, may be useful initially, but they are, as a rule, ineffective for definitive space obliteration. Decortication of the lung, space filling by muscle transplants, space collapse,

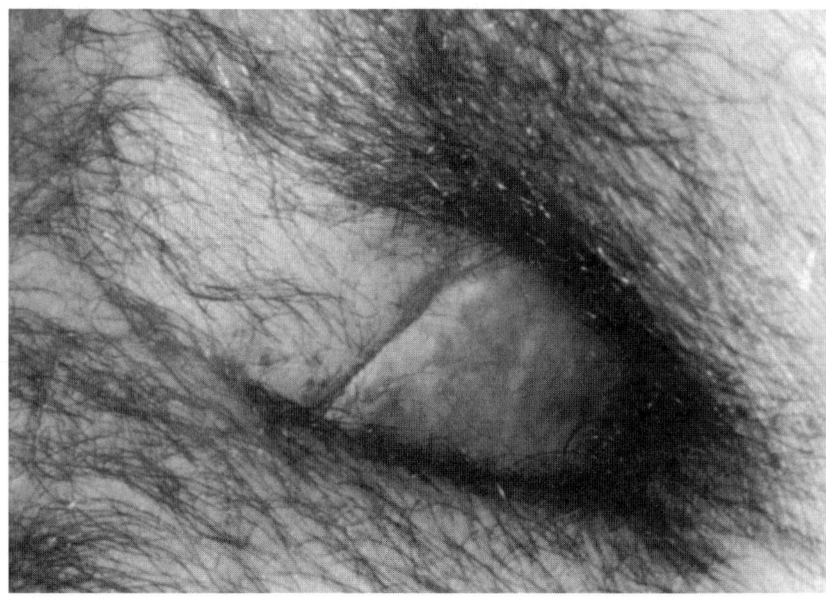

FIGURE 41–11 ■ Open thoracic window that closed spontaneously by re-epithelialization from the skin flaps.

and space sterilization are alternative therapeutic options that should be considered before a final decision is made. It is most important to weigh all options before a decision is reached so that nonreversible procedures are not performed.

Rib Resection Drainage and Open Thoracic Window

The first therapeutic priority is to provide adequate drainage of the empyema. In poor-risk patients, this can be done either by inserting a large drainage tube or by the creation of an open thoracic window. Lemmer and colleagues (1985) noted that early rib resection, especially for postoperative empyemas and for empyemas that have occurred in immunosuppressed patients, was likely to result in fewer therapeutic failures. In their series, control of the empyema was obtained in 10 of 11 patients treated by this method.

Rib resection drainage is a relatively minor procedure, but it should be done only at a time at which sufficient adhesions have formed between the visceral and parietal pleura. When the pleural fluid produces 75% of sediment, the empyema can be considered to be in a chronic stage, and rib resection with open thoracic window can be safely performed. It is primarily indicated for debilitated, poor-risk patients and for patients with small residual spaces that are expected to obliterate early (Samson, 1971). Rib resection is usually performed under general anesthesia. It requires the resection of a short segment of rib over the most dependent part of the cavity, the opening and deloculation of the space, and the insertion of a large multifenestrated tube into the cavity. If the visceral pleura is thin and "stretchable," space obliteration may eventually occur through lung re-expansion, contraction of the space, and filling by granulation tissue. With this technique, the recovery period is long, and frequent dressings and tube changes are usually needed. In Conlan and colleagues' series (1983), 50 patients with chronic empyema without bronchopleural fistula were treated with rib resection, closed-tube drainage, and twice-daily instillation of 2% taurolidine solution into the empyema space through the drainage tube. Forty-one patients underwent further therapy, which consisted of drain removal, decortication, or open-window thoracostomy.

A more permanent form of drainage can be established by the creation of an open-window thoracostomy, a technique originally described by Eloesser (1935) as a drainage procedure for acute, tuberculous empyemas. An open thoracic window is particularly useful for patients in whom long-term drainage may be required (Virkkula and Eerola, 1974). The advantages of the technique are that the cavity can be easily irrigated and cleaned, and the dressings can be changed daily on an outpatient basis. Given time, some of these windows close spontaneously, either by filling of the space with granulomatous tissue or by complete re-epithelialization from the skin flaps (Fig. 41–11). Free skin grafts can also be used to stimulate faster closure. In most cases, however, the space is too large for spontaneous closure to occur (Fig. 41–12). In these cases, the window may have to be left open permanently, or it may be closed at a later stage with muscle transplant on a pedicle.

Space Sterilization

Sterilization of chronic persistent empyema cavities was originally described as a therapeutic option for parapulmonary empyema spaces. According to Virkkula and colleagues (1990), Heuer (1929) first described space sterilization techniques when he discussed the therapy of 24 patients with chronic empyemas, some of which were of tuberculous origin. He used drainage and sterilization of the empyema cavities with antiseptic chemicals. In a number of patients, he tried, in addition to space sterilization, operative maneuvers that involved the parietal pleura.

One of the most important contributions to the therapy of chronic empyema was made by Clagett and Geraci (1963), who reported a technique of sterilization for the treatment of postpneumonectomy empyemas. This technique is effective in 50% to 70% of patients who do not have an associated bronchopleural fistula (Goldstraw, 1979; Stafford and Clagett, 1972).

Space sterilization techniques can also be used in pa-

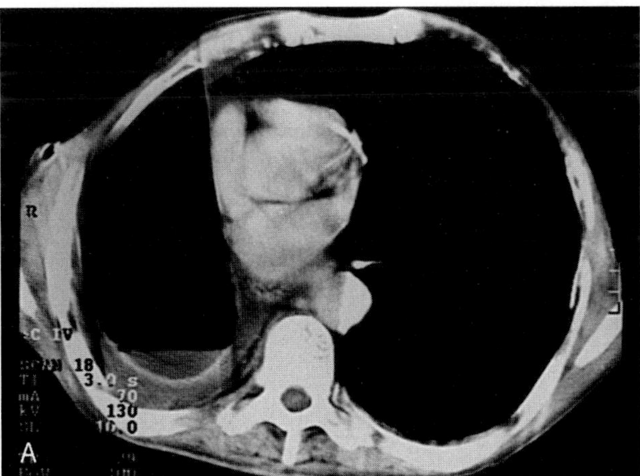

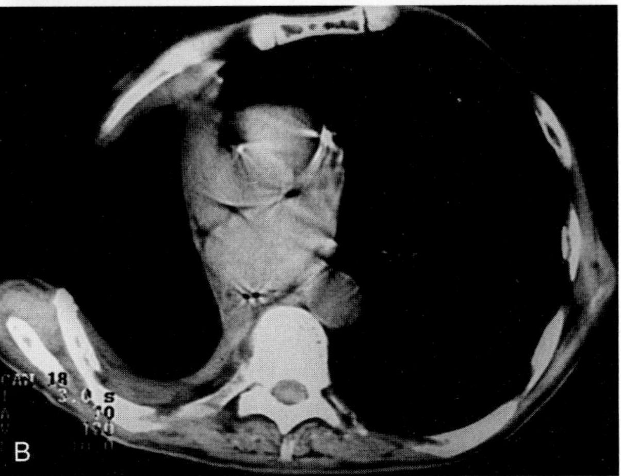

FIGURE 41–12 ■ *A*, A computed tomography scan of a patient with postpneumonectomy empyema before open window thoracostomy. *B*, A computed tomography scan taken 3 months later showing spontaneous reduction of the size of the space.

tients who have empyemas but no previous pneumonectomy (Bayes et al, 1987; Weissberg, 1982). In Weissberg's series, open-window thoracostomy was created in 12 patients with empyema and sepsis after conventional therapy with antibiotics and drainage had failed. Complete obliteration of the empyema cavity by granulation tissue occurred in 11 of 12 patients within 1 to 8 months; the time variation depended on the size of the space. Smolle-Jüttner and colleagues (1992) also showed that open-window thoracostomy is worthwhile because of its potential for rapid and low-risk control of severe, life-threatening, septic conditions in desperate cases of pleural empyema.

Space-Filling Procedures

Decortication and Empyemectomy

Decortication is defined as the removal of a constricting peel over the lung, and empyemectomy is the complete excision of the empyema space and of its contents without entering it. In empyemectomy, both visceral and parietal peels are excised together, avoiding contamination of either the thoracotomy wound or the free pleural space. Although decortication is the procedure most commonly used, both operations are performed to encourage lung re-expansion in the hope of filling the space.

In general, decortication is seldom required because most patients with parapneumonic empyemas are treated before the disease process reaches the chronic organizing stage. In Blasco and colleagues' series (1990), only eight of 236 patients required decortication. Personne (1990) also emphasized that decortication should be reserved for patients with obvious treatment failures.

The timing of decortication in relation to the diagnosis of chronic empyema remains somewhat controversial. Many authors (Personne, 1990; Thurer, 1996) believe that it is best to wait 3 or more months after diagnosis to achieve maximal functional respiratory recovery. Others (Moir and Telander, 1991) recommend decortication at an earlier stage when the peel of the empyema is not excessively adherent to the lung and therefore may be removed without important blood losses or parenchymal tears. In addition, when decortication is performed before significant ingrowth of fibrous tissue into the lung has occurred, the visceral pleura does not need to be removed, thus minimizing the likelihood of lung injuries.

The success rates of decortication depend on an intact visceral pleura, a lung that is expandable, and, most important, a space that can be completely obliterated by pulmonary re-expansion. In a series of 94 patients reported on by Sensening and colleagues (1963), the results of decortication for chronic, nontuberculous empyema were as follows: good, 79; passable, 9; and poor, 2. Four patients died; all were older than 45 years of age. In another report of 25 patients with chronic empyemas, Martella and Santos (1995) showed that decortication should be the preferred treatment for chronic postpneumonic empyemas because it was the only procedure that permitted complete débridement of the space and full re-expansion of the affected lung.

To eradicate any potential source of chronic infection completely, it is occasionally necessary to resect a segment or lobe of the lung adjacent to the empyema. In a few cases when the lung is completely destroyed, total pleuropneumonectomy may be necessary. Several authors (Carroll et al, 1951; Morton et al, 1970; Patton et al, 1952) have also noted that significant functional improvement cannot be achieved after decortication in patients with significant underlying lung disease.

Muscle Transposition

Since first reported by Abrashanoff (1911) and Robinson (1915, 1916), transposing muscle flaps on pedicles has been used extensively (Baena-Montilla and Tarazona, 1987; Borro et al, 1991; Deschamps et al, 1990; Garcia-Yuste et al, 1998; Miller et al, 1984; Pairolero and Arnold, 1980; Pairolero and Arnold, 1990; Pairolero et al, 1983; Miller, 1991; Tarazona et al, 1981; Uri and Nahai, 1990; Virkkula and Eerola, 1973) for the therapy of residual, infected pleural spaces, whether closed or in the form of open-window thoracostomies. The indications for muscle transposition include obliteration of persistent pleural spaces and reinforcement of the bronchial stump following closure of an associated bronchopleural fistula (Deschamps et al, 1990).

Viable tissue in the cavity is essential for successful surgery. The muscle selection should be based not only on its availability but also on the location, size, and shape of the empyema space. The blood supply, innervation, and bulk of the muscle must be preserved, and it must fill the entire space, because empyema is likely to recur if a residual space is left. No attempt to close small bronchopleural fistulas (less than 2 mm) should be made; however, large fistulas must be débrided and closed. The space should always be drained during the first 10 to 12 postoperative days.

Thoracoplasty

The concept of resecting ribs to decrease the size of the thorax and collapse infected spaces was first described by Estlander (1879) and Schede (1890). In 1937, Alexander (1937) redefined some of these principles. He proposed a posterior extramusculoperiosteal approach through which residual spaces could be collapsed in most cases.

During the last 30 years of the 20th century, collapse therapy lost much of its popularity because it is considered by many to be a mutilating and poorly tolerated operation. Two studies have shown, however, that extrapleural thoracoplasty is an excellent therapeutic option for selected patients. In the Hopkins and colleagues (1985) series of 30 patients, the operative mortality was 10%, and permanent space closure was obtained in 82% of the survivors. Grégoire and colleagues (1987) showed that of 17 patients who underwent one-stage thoracoplasties for the therapy of postpneumonectomy empyemas, there were no operative deaths, and immediate control of the empyema was obtained in 15 (88%) patients.

In 1989, Nakaoka and colleagues (1989) presented the cases of 22 patients with chronic empyema thoracis who underwent decortication. In 11 of them, decortication alone did not achieve sufficient lung re-expansion, and the parietal wall was collapsed, without rib resection, to contact the surface of the decorticated lung. All 11 patients had a one-stage cure, and in all, pulmonary function was well preserved. In another series, Laisaar and Ilves (1997) described the use of partial thoracoplasty with omental transplant as a method to treat postpneumonectomy empyemas. In five patients, there were no recurrences of the empyema, and the authors emphasized that the procedure was a one-stage operation without open-window thoracostomy.

SPECIAL PROBLEMS

Empyema in Children

Empyemas that occur in children are usually complications of upper or lower respiratory tract infections. As it is in adults, the pathologic response is divided into three phases, and the principles of therapy are based on appropriate antibiotic therapy, adequate drainage, and maintenance of lung expansion.

Incidence, Pathogenesis, and Bacteriology

Nearly all empyemas that occur in children are of the postpneumonic type, although it is difficult to determine the exact incidence of this complication. Stiles and colleagues (1970) reported on a series of 152 patients (1955 to 1969) with acute pneumonia that was accompanied by a significant amount of pleural fluid. These patients were considered to have acute pneumonia with empyema. Most were secondary to staphylococcal pneumonia, and five deaths occurred—an overall mortality of 3.3%. By contrast, series published in the 1980s nearly always reported on fewer than 40 cases (Gustafson et al, 1990; Kosloke and Cartwright, 1988; Mayo et al, 1982; Raffensperger et al, 1982). Raffensperger and colleagues (1982) noted that "more effective antibiotics have practically eliminated the disease." This apparent decline in the incidence of empyema in children is related not only to better physician education but also to better and more specific medical management of the pneumonia and secondary pleural effusion. It is possible, however, that in the future, the incidence may increase, with the emergence of antibiotic-resistant micro-organisms and of immunosuppression in children with AIDS or other related syndromes. In developing countries, pleural sepsis is still prevalent (Anyanwu and Egbue, 1981; Farpour and Sajedee, 1967). Factors such as malnutrition and poor hygiene complicate the clinical progress and management of children with pneumonia. In Mangele and colleagues' series (1993) of 56 children with empyemas seen in Nigeria, 80% belonged to the lowest social class.

The bacteriologic findings of empyema in children have changed considerably over the years. In the preantibiotic era, pneumococci (Ravitch and Fein, 1961) and streptococci were the most frequent organisms isolated in postpneumonia empyemas (Gustafson et al, 1990). After World War II, *S. aureus* became the most prevalent bacterium, which is well documented in several reports (Henchen and Haggerty, 1958; Koch et al, 1959). In a classic article on empyema, Ravitch and Fein (1961) noted that there had not been any cases of empyema caused by *Haemophilus influenzae* since 1944 nor any as a result of streptococci since 1948. Furthermore, they had seen only five cases caused by pneumococci since 1947. In Cattaneo and Kilman's (1973) report, coagulase-positive staphylococci were the offending organisms in 80% of the positive pleural cultures; only three patients had pneumococci. Stiles and colleagues (1970) also showed that when a definite organism could be identified, staphylococci were recovered in 93% of cases (78 of 84). In recent years, *H. influenzae*, β-hemolytic streptococci, *S. pneumoniae*, and anaerobes have emerged as the leading offending organisms (Foglia and Randolph, 1987; Kosloke, 1986). In Kosloke and Cartwright's (1988) series of 22 patients treated by open drainage, streptococci (n = 5) and *H. influenzae* (n = 3) were the most common single pathogens.

In children, the bacteriologic findings of empyema are important because they affect the speed and severity of loculations that develop in the space. Anaerobic effusions, for instance, loculate quickly and often require aggressive surgical drainage because of a thick pleural peel that is not amenable to conventional therapy (Gustafson et al, 1990). By contrast, staphylococcal effusions are often fibrinoid deposits with little actual fluid. If there is fluid, it is unilocular and amenable to adequate drainage by thoracentesis or conventional tube thoracostomy.

Clinical Presentation and Diagnosis

The most common presenting symptom of an empyema in children is fever. In a series of 42 patients with either parapneumonic effusion (n = 21) or empyema (n = 21), presented by Chonmaitree and Powell (1983), the clinical signs associated with effusion included fever (81%), tactile and vocal fremitus (81%), and respiratory difficulties (52%). For patients with empyema, the clinical signs were also fever (95%), tactile and vocal fremitus (62%), and respiratory difficulties (62%). In a series by McLaughlin and colleagues (1984) of 16 patients aged 1 month to 15 years, fever, cough, and dyspnea were the most common symptoms; all three were present in 12 of 16 patients (75%) on admission. Other signs and symptoms include decreased breath sounds, tachypnea (30 to 40 breaths/min), tachycardia, intercostal retractions, and lethargy (seen in 25% of patients in the series by McLaughlin and colleagues). Middlekamp and colleagues (1969) also noted that symptoms of upper respiratory infection—cough, lethargy, anorexia, malaise, fever, abnormal respiratory rate, and grunting respiration—were commonly associated with empyema. In a series of 131 children with empyema reported by Paris and colleagues (1991), 28 (21%) complained of abdominal pain. In patients aged less than 2 years (n = 44), 11 (25%) had abdominal distention. This percentage increased to 40% when *S. aureus* was cultured from the empyema. In children aged 2 to 15 years (n = 87), 17 (13%) had abdominal distention. Overall, seven patients had symptoms suggestive of appendicitis, and 3 of 7 underwent appendectomy. In that series, 45 patients were admitted in very poor medical condition. This was more notable in younger patients and in those with *S. aureus* empyemas.

The white blood cell count is nearly always elevated (15,000 to 20,000 U) in these children with a shift to the left in the differential count. Radiographic findings include the presence of pleural effusion, encapsulated collections with air fluid levels, pneumonic infiltrates, or pneumatoceles. In Chonmaitree and Powell's series (1983), pneumonic infiltrates associated with empyemas were lobar in distribution in 52% of the patients, segmental in 33%, and bilateral patchy in 14%. Sometimes, it is not possible to distinguish between pulmonary infiltrates and pleural effusion or pleural fibrin deposits (fibrinous pleurisy). Foglia and Randolph (1987) showed the importance of using CT scanning to ascertain more accurately the configuration of the fluid collections and lung compression and to differentiate parenchymal from pleural involvement.

Thoracentesis is a more definitive diagnostic procedure and should be done early in patients with parapneumonic effusion. It may show frank pus, a positive Gram-stain result, or biochemical findings that suggest that an infectious process may be found.

Management

In 1982, Mayo and colleagues (1982) (Table 41–10) described the goals of therapy of acute nontuberculous empyemas in children. These were ". . . to save life with complete elimination of the empyema and avoidance of recurrent empyema pockets; to return respiratory function promptly to normal by re-expansion of the trapped lung and restoration of the mobility of the chest wall and diaphragm; to eliminate complications or chronicity and thereby any need for a crippling or debilitating surgical procedure; to reduce days of hospital stay." Despite these clearly outlined objectives, the management of empyema is controversial in the pediatric literature.

In 1987, Foglia and Randolph showed that the specific therapy for empyema in children should be based on the stage of disease, the type of bacteria that predominate within the pleural fluid, the response to the therapy instituted, and the degree of lung trapping. Most children with empyema recover when treated with parenteral antibiotics, which are selected on the basis of pleural fluid culture and appropriate tube drainage. Drainage may also be required for massive effusions with respiratory distress or when there is a pneumothorax associated with the empyema (pyopneumothorax).

If there is no resolution of the process and radiographs show no persistent fluid loculations or thick pleural shadows for several weeks, persistence of symptoms, leukocytosis, or progression of pulmonary infiltrates despite adequate drainage and antibiotics, open deloculation is recommended by most authors (Gustafson et al, 1990; Kosloke and Cartwright, 1988; Mayo et al, 1982; Raffensperger et al, 1982). Gustafson and colleagues (1990) showed that ". . . early decortication in these highly select patients with symptomatic respiratory empyemas shortened the hospital stay, minimized the risks of long-term use of antibiotics and prolonged chest tube drainage, completely re-expanded the trapped lung, and led to excellent long-term results." In this series, the recoveries of all such treated patients were rapid. The use of thoracentesis alone with antibiotics parenterally or intrapleurally or of streptokinase solutions infused through the chest tube (Rodgers, 1987) is not recommended if a true empyema has been diagnosed.

The second factor of importance for the therapy of empyemas in children is the organism isolated from the pleural fluid (Foglia and Randolph, 1987). *S. aureus* or other gram-positive organisms usually induce unilocular empyemas that are amenable to good drainage by accurate placement of a large, intercostal catheter (Kosloke, 1986). These almost never require early deloculation. By contrast, anaerobic empyemas tend to be loculated, and empyemas produced by β-hemolytic streptococci, *S. pneumoniae*, and *H. influenzae* may rapidly cause a thick, fibrous peel over the lung.

The third factor that may alter therapy is the degree of lung trapping, as documented on the CT scan. Foglia and Randolph (1987) showed that ". . . when the empyema reaches an organized stage and no free fluid remains, there is little excuse for waiting for weeks to see if some resolution of the process will occur. In these instances, formal decortication should be carried out early because lung growth and function may be permanently adversely affected." In another series, Soysal and colleagues (1998) reported 104 children with empyema who required surgical treatment over a period of 20 years (1974 to 1994). In that series, the indications for surgery were severe pleural thickening in 54 cases (51.9%) and trapped lung in 36 cases (34.6%). The authors concluded that re-expansion of the lung is the most important objective of treatment, because residual space will almost certainly lead to accumulation of pleural fluid and reinfection.

There is little role for the conversion of closed-tube thoracotomy to open drainage because the failure rate is notoriously high and the morbidity and mortality rates are unacceptable (Mayo et al, 1982). In a recent series of 131 children with empyemas (Paris et al, 1991), adequate drainage was achieved by thoracentesis in eight and by one or more chest tubes in 123. In that series, there were two deaths and only three children eventually required decortication. Fifteen additional patients had radiologic sequelae, which cleared over a period of months after control of the empyema. To prevent these sequelae, the authors recommend the use of cortisone, which is started as soon as the septic period is over.

The use of fibrinolytic agents is not recommended in children, although it has been shown that they can be used in selected cases of empyemas that are not improving with adequate drainage and antibiotics (Kornecki and Sivan, 1997; Krishnan et al, 1997).

TABLE 41–10 ■ Goals of Therapy in Acute Nontuberculous Empyema in Children

To save lives
To eliminate the empyema
To re-expand the trapped lung
To restore mobility of the chest wall and diaphragm
To return respiratory function to normal
To eliminate complications of chronicity
To reduce the duration of hospital stay

From Mayo P, Saha SP, McElvein RB: Acute empyema in children treated by open thoracotomy and decortication. Ann Thorac Surg 34:401, 1982.

Bronchopleural Fistula

Bronchopleural fistulas aggravate the course of empyemas and present a major therapeutic challenge. The presence of a bronchopleural fistula indicates persistent contamination of the pleural space, difficulties in the re-expansion of the lung, and possible aspiration in the remaining lung. For many patients with empyema, the presence or absence of a fistula makes the difference between recovery, chronicity, or death.

Incidence and Pathogenesis

Bronchopleural fistulas usually follow pulmonary resection. In the series of Malave and colleagues (1971), 1307 resections were done, and in 35 patients (2.7%), bronchopleural fistulas developed. In another study (Vester et al, 1991), the overall incidence of postresection fistulas was 1.6% (35 of 2243 resections), and approximately two thirds of the patients with postoperative fistulas had undergone preoperative radiotherapy, chemotherapy, or both. Postoperative bronchopleural fistulas can either be at the bronchial or at the peripheral level (alveolar peripheral air leak). Pertinent etiologic factors include endobronchial tuberculosis, contamination of the pleural space during the procedure, devascularization of the bronchus, poor surgical technique, or concomitant illnesses.

Patients are considered to have a spontaneous fistula if no previous pulmonary resection has been carried out (Hankins et al, 1978). These usually occur in association with tuberculosis, bacterial pneumonia, or lung abscesses. They also occur with spontaneous pneumothoraces, especially those secondary to chronic obstructive lung disease, or to AIDS. In a series by Crawford and colleagues (1992), 44 patients with AIDS were treated for spontaneous pneumothorax, and in 14 of them a bronchopleural fistula that persisted for more than 10 days developed.

Clinical Presentation and Diagnosis

The most common presenting symptoms of postoperative bronchopleural fistulas are the coughing up of serosanguineous fluid or pus, fever, malaise and general symptoms of toxicity. On chest radiograph, a previously small space may be enlarging or newly formed air fluid may be noted. Other radiologic signs include lowering or sudden disappearance of a pleural effusion or a mediastinal shift toward the contralateral side.

The diagnosis of a bronchopleural fistula is usually made by bronchoscopy or by observing persistent air leak through the chest tube. Occasionally, late occurring fistulas and empyema are overlooked until they drain spontaneously through the skin of the chest wall (empyema necessitatis) or they are misdiagnosed as a cancer recurrence.

Management

The management of patients with postresection fistulas depends on the reason why the bronchial stump or lung tissue has failed to hold the sutures (Perelman and Rymko, 1990). Primary failures result from poor closure technique, persistent pathologic changes in the bronchial wall, or impaired healing, such as that seen in patients who have undergone radiotherapy. In these cases, the therapy may be conservative, with suction drainage of the pleural cavity and possible use of fibrin sealants applied through the rigid bronchoscope (Onotera and Unruh, 1988) or through the flexible fiberoptic bronchoscope (Jensen and Shaira, 1985; Glover et al, 1987; York et al, 1990). In some cases, reclosure of the bronchus, reamputation of the stump, additional sealing of the pulmonary sutures, or additional resection may be advisable (Perelman and Rymko, 1990).

Secondary failures occur in empyemas in which the bronchial stump reopens because of local pressure by the purulent collection (Perelman and Rymko, 1990). In this situation, drainage should be done initially followed by definitive management, which consists of bronchial reclosure, myoplasty, or thoracoplasty. These patients are usually very ill, and definitive therapy should be delayed until the empyema has become chronic and the patient's overall medical condition has improved. Puskas and colleagues (1994) showed that direct surgical repair of chronic bronchopleural fistulas may be achieved in most patients by suture closure and aggressive transposition of vascularized flaps on pedicles.

Immunocompromised Patients and Transplant Recipients

Immunocompromised patients, defined as individuals with impaired immunity from any cause (Robinson, 1999), are at high risk for infectious complications. They include not only patients with AIDS or transplant recipients but also patients on chronic steroid use, patients with malignancies, malnourished patients with congenital or acquired immunoglobulin deficiencies, postoperative patients, and others.

The prevalence of pleural effusion in patients with human immunodeficiency virus (HIV) infections ranges from 1.7% in the series of Joseph and colleagues (1993) to 18.3% in the series of Labadibi and colleagues (1994).

In 1995, Gil Suay and colleagues studied 983 patients with community-acquired pneumonia and compared 99 patients infected with HIV to 884 patients who had not been infected with HIV. Parapneumonic effusions were significantly more common in patients infected with HIV (21 out of 99—21%) than patients who were not infected with HIV (116 out of 884—13%) ($P < .005$). In addition, the clinical course of patients with HIV was more severe with higher rates of bacteremias (58% versus 18%). Pleural fluid from the group infected with HIV showed significantly lower glucose levels, and *S. aureus* was the most common micro-organism isolated. Finally, chest-tube drainage was required more often in patients with HIV (71%) than in patients who were not infected (44%).

There are relatively few actual documented HIV-associated empyemas that have been reported. In 1994, Ambrosi and colleagues presented 16 cases and Mouroux and colleagues (1995) described 18 cases that occurred after chest surgery was done in patients infected with HIV. Fifty percent of patients included in that cohort were treated by tube drainage alone, whereas the other patients required formal decortication.

In 1998, Hernandez and colleagues reviewed 23 empyemas that occurred in 419 patients with HIV infections seen between 1985 and 1993. These were diagnosed by purulent pleural fluid, positive bacteriology, or biochemical abnormalities (pH < 7.10; LDH > 1000 L; glucose < 40 mg/dl). Twenty-one patients developed their empyema secondary to community-acquired pneumonia, and parenteral drug abuse was a predominant risk factor. A single bacteria was isolated from 10 patients (52%), whereas multiple organisms grew in the remaining nine positive cultures. The most common organisms were *S. aureus* (23%) and gram-negative bacilli (36%). It is interesting to note that only 10 patients had been previously diagnosed as HIV patients when the diagnosis of empyema was made.

The treatment of empyema in patients with HIV infection is similar to that described in patients with non-HIV empyemas. Early closed-tube drainage, specific antibiotics, and intrapleural enzymes should be part of the therapy in patients with stage I and stage II empyemas. In the series of Hernandez and colleagues (1998), 18 patients had tube drainage and none required surgery. Eleven complications developed in nine patients and five of these 11 complications were related to chest tubes. The mean duration of hospital stay was 26 days. Patients with empyema and HIV infection require prolonged hospitalization for bacteremias. Prolonged air leaks are more common in patients with HIV than in patients who are not infected with HIV.

Patients who have undergone transplants are more likely to have virulent respiratory infections and empyemas than are individuals who have not undergone transplantation. Pleural empyemas have been reported after renal (Corbett et al, 1996; Spizarny et al, 1993), cardiac (Amber et al, 1990), and lung transplantation (Herridge et al, 1995; Judson et al, 1996; Noyes et al, 1994; Snell et al, 1993; Westney et al, 1996).

Recipients of lung transplants are likely to have pleural complications, mostly because of the prolonged and intense manipulations that occur during surgery. In these cases, the empyema is secondary to bacterial pneumonia or lung abscess. The most common organisms isolated are *S. aureus* and *Pseudomonas aeruginosa*. Empyemas secondary to bacterial pneumonia are often preceded by graft dysfunction and prolonged periods of postoperative mechanical dysfunction. It is also more common in patients for whom lung transplant was performed for septic lung diseases such as cystic fibrosis or chronic bronchiectasis to develop.

In a study by Paris (1999), 8 of 120 lung transplant patients had postoperative empyemas, and all recovered after treatment with closed-tube drainage and specific antibiotherapy. In 1995, Herridge and colleagues reported pleural complications (seven empyemas) in 30 of 138 patients who had lung transplantation. They emphasized that pleural complications are expected in transplant patients because (1) the pleural space is completely exposed; (2) patients receive immunosuppressive agents; (3) patients may have had previous pleural procedures and complications; (4) some patients already have bronchopulmonary infections; and (5) frequent transbronchial biopsies are part of transplant surveillance protocols. In that series, all empyemas occurred after double lung transplant, and the authors found no significant differences in the incidence of postoperative empyemas between patients with previous septic lung disease and patients with noninfected native lungs. Open thoracotomy was necessary in two patients, and three of the seven patients with empyemas eventually died.

CONCLUSION

Empyema thoracis has been a major medical concern throughout recorded medical history. During the 20th century and particularly over the past 2 decades, management has been influenced by the identification of a spectrum of new and more virulent pathogens and by the increasing incidence of immunologically compromised hosts. New antibacteriologic agents have contributed to major advances in the therapy of these infectious problems. In many centers, early decortication by thoracoscopic techniques is also performed to re-expand the lung and prevent the more serious complications associated with chronicity.

The overall mortality rate associated with empyemas ranges between 2% and 30% (Benfield, 1981; Grant and Finley, 1985; Jess et al, 1984; Paris et al, 1991). Most deaths occur in elderly patients or from conditions that predispose patients to the empyema, rather than from the empyema itself. Other important factors include the cause of the empyema, the bacteria involved, the correct use of antibiotics, and the immunologic status of the host.

■ *KEY REFERENCES*

Barrett NR: The treatment of acute empyema. Ann R Coll Surg Engl 15:25, 1954.

This is an excellent discussion of various therapies that have been applied to acute empyema over the years.

Bergeron MG: The changing bacterial spectrum and antibiotic choice. In Deslauriers J, Lacquet LK (eds): International Trends in General Thoracic Surgery, Vol. 6, St. Louis, Mosby–Year Book, 1990.

This is a classic review of the bacteriologic findings in empyema and of the principles to follow when selecting antibiotic therapy.

Foglia RP, Randolph J: Current indications for decortication in the treatment of empyema in children. J Pediatr Surg 22:28, 1987.

The authors present the principles of empyema management in children. This is a good discussion that highlights the controversies.

Light RW: Parapneumonic effusion and empyema. Clin Chest Med 6:55, 1985.

This is a complete review from a medical standpoint of the pathophysiology, investigation, and management of empyemas.

Moran JF: Surgical management of pleural space infections. Semin Respir Infect 3:383, 1988.

This is a good review article on the surgical management of empyemas. The authors analyze all surgical options to manage empyemas in the acute or chronic form.

Robinson LA, Moulton AL, Fleming WA et al: Intrapleural fibrinolytic treatment of multiloculated empyemas. Ann Thorac Surg 57:803, 1994.

This article analyzes the indications, techniques, and results of the intrapleural use of fibrinolytic agents. The authors provide an excellent review of the principles involved in empyema management.

Striffeler H, Gugger M, Imhof V et al: Videoassisted thoracoscopic surgery for fibrino-purulent empyema in 67 patients. Ann Thorac Surg 65:319, 1998.

The authors review the indications for early débridement of fibrinopurulent empyemas by thoracoscopic technique. They conclude that VATS is safe and efficient in stage II empyemas but that open decortication should be performed during the organizing stage.

REFERENCES

Abrashanoff A: Plastishe methode zur Schliessung von Fistel-gangen welche von immeran organen Komman. Zentralbl Chir 38:186, 1911.

Alexander J: The Collapse Therapy of Pulmonary Tuberculosis. Springfield, Illinois, Charles C Thomas, 1937.

Ali L, Unruh H: Management of empyema thoracis. Ann Thorac Surg 50:355, 1990.

Amber IJ, Gilbert EM, Schiffman G, Jacobson JA: Increased risk of pneumococcal infections in cardiac transplant recipients. Transplantation 49:122, 1990.

Ambrosi C, Cianni R, Perona F et al: The percutaneous treatment of purulent intrathoracic fluid collections in HIV-positive patients. Radiol Med (Torino) 87:833, 1994.

American Thoracic Society, Medical Section of the National Tuberculosis Association: Management of nontuberculous empyema. Am Rev Respir Dis 85:935, 1962.

Anyanwu CH, Egbue M: Management of pleural sepsis in Nigerian children. Thorax 36:282, 1981.

Arom KK, Grover FL, Richardson JD, Trinkle JK: Posttraumatic empyema. Ann Thorac Surg 23:254, 1977.

Atwater EC: Morrill Wyman and the aspiration of acute pleural effusions, 1850 (Letter). N Engl Bull Hist Med 36:235, 1972.

Baena-Montilla P, Tarazona V: Bronchopleural fistula: Management with muscle transposition. In Grillo H, Eschapasse H (eds): International Trends in General Thoracic Surgery, Vol 2. Philadelphia, WB Saunders, 1987.

Baethge BA, Eggerstedt JM, Olash FA: Group F streptococcal empyema from aspiration of a grass inflorescence. Ann Thorac Surg 49:319, 1990.

Barondess JA: A case of empyema: Notes on the last illness of Sir William Osler. Transactions of the American Clinical and Clinicopathological Association. The 87th Annual Meeting, Vol 86. Baltimore, Waverly Press, 1975.

Barrett NR: The treatment of acute empyema. Ann R Coll Surg Engl 15:25, 1954.

Bartlett JG, Thadepalli H, Gorbach SL, Finegold SM: Bacteriology of empyema. Lancet 1:338, 1974.

Bayes AJ, Wilson JAS, Chiu RCJ et al: Clagett open-window thoracostomy in patients with empyema who had and had not undergone pneumonectomy. Can J Surg 30:329, 1987.

Benfield GFA: Recent trends in empyema thoracis. Br J Dis Chest 75:358, 1981.

Bergeron MG: The changing bacterial spectrum and antibiotic choice in thoracic surgery: Surgical management of pleural diseases. In Deslauriers J, Lacquet LK (eds): International Trends in General Thoracic Surgery, Vol 6. St. Louis, Mosby–Year Book, 1990, p 197–207.

Bergh NP, Ekroth R, Larsson S, Nagy P: Intrapleural streptokinase in the treatment of haemothorax and empyema. Scand J Thorac Cardiovasc Surg 11:265, 1977.

Blasco E, Paris F, Padilla J: Acute postpneumonic empyema treated by intercostal tube drainage with suction and pleural washing but without rib resection. In Deslauriers J, Lacquet LK (eds): International Trends in General Thoracic Surgery, Vol 6. St. Louis, Mosby–Year Book, 1990.

Blasco E, Tarazona V, Canto A et al: Tratamiento de las pleuresias purulentas no organizadas. Proceedings IX Congreso de la Sociedad Espanola de Patologia Respiratoria. Liade, Sevilla, 1976.

Borro JM, Tarazona V, Paris F: Management of postpneumonectomy empyema of the pleural space. In Peters RM, Toledo J (eds): Current Topics in General Thoracic Surgery: An International Series, Vol 2. New York, Elsevier, 1991.

Bouros D, Schiza S, Patsourakis G et al: Intrapleural streptokinase versus urokinase in the treatment of complicated parapneumonic effusions: A prospective double-blind study. Am J Respir Crit Care Med 155:291, 1997.

Bowditch HL: On pleuretic effusions and the necessity of paracentesis for their removal. Am J Med Sci 22:320, 1852.

Brown B, Ory EM, Meads M et al: Penicillin treatment of empyema: Report of 24 cases and review of the literature. Ann Intern Med 24:343, 1956.

Carroll D, McClement J, Himmelsteen A et al: Pulmonary function following decortication. Am Rev Tuberc 63:231, 1951.

Cassina PC, Hauser M, Hillejan L et al: Video-assisted thoracoscopy in the treatment of pleural empyema: Stage-based management and outcome. J Thorac Cardiovasc Surg 117:234, 1999.

Cattaneo SM, Kilman JW: Surgical therapy of empyema in children. Ann Surg 106:564, 1973.

Chadwick J, Mann WN: The medical works of Hippocrates. Springfield, Charles C Thomas, 1950.

Chonmaitree T, Powell KR: Parapneumonic pleural effusion and empyema in children: Review of a 19-year experience, 1962–1980. Clin Pediatr 22:414, 1983.

Clagett OT, Geraci JE: A procedure for the management of postpneumonectomy empyema. J Thorac Cardiovasc Surg 45:141, 1963.

Cohen RG, DeMeester TR, Lafontaine E: The pleura. In Sabinston DC, Spencer FC (eds): Surgery of the Chest, 6th ed. Philadelphia, WB Saunders, 1995.

Conlan AA, Abramor E, Delikaris O, Hurwitz SS: Taurolidine instillation as therapy for empyema thoracis. S Afr Med J 64:653, 1983.

Corbett CE, Wall BM, Cohen M: Case report: With hydropneumothorax an empyema with hydropneumothorax and bacteremia caused by clostridium sporogenes. Am J Med Sci 312:242, 1996.

Crawford BK, Galloway AC, Boyd AD, Spencer FC: Treatment of AIDS-related bronchopleural fistula by pleurectomy. Ann Thorac Surg 54:212, 1992.

Crouch JD, Keagy BA, Delany DJ: "Pigtail" catheter drainage in thoracic surgery. Am Rev Respir Dis 136:174, 1987.

Davies RJO, Traill ZC, Gleeson FV: Randomized controlled trial of intrapleural streptokinase in community acquired pleural infection. Thorax 52:416, 1997.

de la Rocha AG: Empyema thoracis. Surg Gynecol Obstet 155:839, 1982.

Delarue NC: Empyema: Principles of management—an old problem revisited. In Deslauriers J, Lacquet LK (eds): International Trends in General Thoracic Surgery, Vol 6. St. Louis, Mosby–Year Book, 1990.

Delorme E: Nouveau traitement des empyèmes chroniques. Gaz Hôp 67:94, 1894.

Deschamps C, Trastek VF, Arnold PG, Pairolero PC: Surgical approach to chronic empyema: Decortication and muscle transposition. In Deslauriers J, Lacquet LK (eds): International Trends in General Thoracic Surgery, Vol 6. St. Louis, Mosby–Year Book, 1990.

Deslauriers J: Invited commentary to Cassina PC et al: Video-assisted thoracoscopy in the treatment of pleural empyema: Stage-based management and outcome. J Thorac Cardiovasc Surg 117:238, 1999.

Dieter RA, Pifarré R, Neville WE et al: Empyema treated with neomycin irrigation and closed-chest drainage. J Thorac Cardiovasc Surg 59:496, 1970.

Eggers C: Radical operation for chronic empyema. Ann Surg 77:327, 1923.

Ehler AN: Non-tuberculous thoracic empyema: A collective review of the literature from 1934 to 1939. Int Abstr Surg 72:17, 1941.

Eloesser L: An operation for tuberculous empyema. Surg Gynecol Obstet 60:1096, 1935.

Estlander JA: Résection des côtes dans l'empyème chronique. Rev Med Chir (Paris) 3:156, 1879.

Farpour A, Sajedee M: Empyema in pediatric patients in Iran. Am J Surg 114:856, 1967.

Ferguson MK: The healing hand. Chest 97:4, 1990.

Finland M, Barnes MW: Changing ecology of acute bacterial empyema occurrence and mortality at Boston City Hospital during 12 selected years from 1935 to 1972. J Infect Dis 137:274, 1978.

Fishman NH, Ellertson DG: Early pleural decortication for thoracic empyema in immunosuppressed patients. J Thorac Cardiovasc Surg 74:537, 1977.

Foglia RP, Randolph J: Current indications for decortication in the treatment of empyema in children. J Pediatr Surg 22:28, 1987.

Fowler GR: A case of thoracoplasty for the removal of a large cicatricial fibrous growth from the interior of the chest, the result of an old empyema. Med Record 44:938, 1893.

Fowler GR: A History of Thoracic Surgery (quoted by R. Meade). Springfield, Illinois, Charles C Thomas, 1961.

Frimodt-Moller PC, Vejlsted H: Early surgical intervention in nonspecific pleural empyema. Thorac Cardiovasc Surg 33:41, 1985.

Garcia-Yuste M, Ramos G, Duque JL et al: Open-window thoracostomy and thoracomyoplasty to manage chronic pleural empyema. Am Thorac Surg 65:818, 1998.

Gil Suay V, Cordero PJ, Martinez E et al: Parapneumonic effusions secondary to community-acquired bacterial pneumonia in human immunodeficiency virus-infected patients. Eur Resp J 8:1934, 1995.

Glover W, Chavis TV, Daniel TM et al: Fibrin glue application through the flexible fiberoptique bronchoscope: Closure of bronchopleural fistulas. J Thorac Cardiovasc Surg 93:470, 1987.

Goldstraw P: Treatment of the post-pneumonectomy empyema: The case for fenestration. Thorax 34:740, 1979.

Graham EA: Some fundamental considerations in the treatment of empyema thoracis. St. Louis, CV Mosby, 1925.

Graham EA, Bell RD: Open pneumothorax: Its relation to the treatment of acute empyema. Am J Med Sci 156:839, 1918.

Grant DR, Finley RJ: Empyema: Analysis of treatment techniques. Can J Surg 28:449, 1985.

Grégoire R, Deslauriers J, Beaulieu M, Piraux M: Thoracoplasty: Its forgotten role in the management of non-tuberculous post-pneumonectomy empyema. Can J Surg 30:343, 1987.

Gustafson RA, Murray GF, Warden HE, Hill RC: Role of lung decortication in symptomatic empyemas in children. Ann Thorac Surg 49:940, 1990.

Hankins JR, Miller JE, Altar S et al: Bronchopleural fistula: Thirteen-year experience with 77 cases. J Thorac Cardiovasc Surg 76:755, 1978.

Henchen WH III, Haggerty RJ: Staphylococcic pneumonia in infants and childhood. JAMA 168:6, 1958.

Herna JW, Read JC, Choplin RH: Pleural infections: A clinical radiological review. J Thorac Imaging 6:68, 1991.

Hernandez BJ, Alfageme MI, Muflioz MJ et al: Thoracic empyema in HIV-infected patients: Microbiology, management, and outcome. Chest 113:732, 1998.

Herridge MS, de Hoyos AL, Chaparro A et al: Pleural complications in lung transplant recipients. J Thorac Cardiovasc Surg 110:22, 1995.

Heuer GA: Observations on the treatment of chronic empyema. Ann Surg 72:80, 1929.

Hewitt CF: Thoracentesis: The plan of continuous aspiration. BMJ 1:317, 1876.

Himelman RB, Callen PW: The prognostic value of loculations in parapneumonic pleural effusion. Chest 90:852, 1986.

Hochberg LA: Thoracic surgery before the 20th surgery. New York, Vantage Press, 1960:7, 9–12, 244.

Holmes Sellors T, Cruickshank G: Chronic empyema. Br J Surg 38:411, 1951.

Hoover EL, Hsu HK, Ross MJ et al: Reappraisal of empyema thoracis: Surgical intervention when the duration of illness is unknown. Chest 90:511, 1986.

Hoover EL, Hsu HK, Webb H et al: The surgical management of empyema thoracis in substance abuse patients: A 5-year experience. An Thorac Surg 46:563, 1988.

Hopkins RA, Ungerleider RM, Staub EN, Young WG: The modern use of thoracoplasty. Ann Thorac Surg 40:181, 1985.

Houston MC: Pleural fluid pH: Diagnostic, therapeutic and prognostic value. Am J Surg 154:333, 1987.

Hurt R: The diagnosis and treatment of empyemas. In Hurt R (ed): The History of Cardiothoracic Surgery. New York, Parthenon, 1986.

Jensen C, Sharna P: Use of fibrin glue in thoracic surgery. Ann Thorac Surg 39:521, 985.

Jess P, Brynitz S, Moller AF: Mortality in thoracic empyema. Scand J Thorac Cardiovasc Surg 18:85, 1984.

Joseph J, Strange C, Shan SA: Pleural effusions in hospitalized patients with AIDS. Ann Intern Med 118:856, 1993.

Judson MA, Handy JR, Sahn SA: Pleural effusions following lung transplantation: Time course, characteristics and clinical implications. Chest 109:1190, 1996.

Keefer CS, Rantz LA, Rammelkamp CH: Hemolytic streptococcal pneumonia and empyema: Study of 55 cases with special reference to treatment. Ann Intern Med 14:1533, 1941.

Koch R, Carson M, Donnell G: Staphylococcal pneumonia in children. J Pediatr 55:473, 1959.

Kornecki A, Sivan Y: Treatment of loculated pleural effusion with intrapleural urokinase in children. J Pediatr Surg 32:1473, 1997.

Kosloske AM: Infections of the lungs, pleura and mediastinum. In Welch KJ et al (eds): Pediatric Surgery, 4th ed. Chicago, Year Book Medical Publishers, 1986.

Kosloske AM, Cartwright KC: The controversial role of decortication in the management of pediatric empyema. J Thorac Cardiovasc Surg 96:166, 1988.

Krishnan S, Amin N, Dozor AJ, Stringel G: Urokinase in the management of complicated parapneumonic effusions in children. Chest 112:1579, 1997.

Labadibi HMS, Gupta K, Newman T et al: A retrospective analysis of pleural effusions in human immunodeficiency virus infected patient. Chest 106:86S, 1994.

Lain-Entralgo P: Clàsicas de le medicina: Laënnec. Madrid, CSIC Instituto Arnaldo de Vilanova, 1959.

Laisaar T, Ilves A: Omentoplasty together with partial thoracoplasty: A one-stage operation for post-pneumonectomy pleural empyema. Ann Chir Gynecol 86:319, 1997.

Landreneau RJ, Keenan RJ, Hazelrigg SR et al: Thoracoscopy for empyema and hemothorax. Chest 109:18, 1995.

Lawrence DR, Obri SK, Moxon RE et al: Thoracoscopic débridement of empyema thoracis. Ann Thorac Surg 64:1448, 1997.

Lee IMJG, Kim YH et al: Tretment of thoracic multiloculated empyemas with intra-cavitary urkinase: A prospective study. Radiol 179:771, 1991.

Lemmer JH, Botham MJ, Orringer MB: Modern management of adult thoracic empyema. J Thorac Cardiovasc Surg 90:849, 1985.

Le Roux BT: Empyema thoracis. Br J Surg 52:89, 1965.

Le Roux BT, Mohlala ML, Odell JA, Whitton D: Suppurative diseases of the lung and pleural space. Part 1: Empyema thoracis and lung abscess. Curr Probl Surg 23:6, 1986.

Light RW: Parapneumonic effusions and empyema. Clin Chest Med 6:55, 1985.

Light RW: Parapneumonic effusions and empyema. Semin Respir Med 9:37, 1987.

Light RW, Girard WM, Jenkinson SG, George RB: Parapneumonic effusions. Am J Med 69:507, 1980.

Lopez-Rivero L, Lopez-Pujol J, Quevedo S et al: Urokinase in the management of loculated intrapleural effusion. Abstracts from the 2nd European Conference on General Thoracic Surgery. E.S.T.S. Gotti G, Elias S, Paldini P (eds): Universita degli Studi di Siena, Cattedra de Chirugia Toracica, Siena, Italy, 1994.

Luizy J, Mathey J, Le Brigand H, Galey JJ: Technique d'irrigation pleurale sous dépression continue dans le traitement des pyothorax. Rev Tuberc Pneumol 30:393, 1966.

MacKinlay TAA, Lyons GA, Chimondeguy DJ et al: VATS débridement versus thoracotomy in the treatment of loculated post-pneumonia empyema. Ann Thorac Surg 61:1626, 1996.

Maier AC, Grace EJ: Putrid empyema. Surg Gynecol Obstet 74:69, 1942.

Major RH: Classic descriptions of the disease. London, Ballìere, Tindall and Cox, 1945.

Malave G, Foster ED, Wilson JA, Munro DD: Bronchopleural fistula: Present day study of an old problem. Ann Thorac Surg 11:1, 1971.

Mandal AK, Thadepalli H: Treatment of spontaneous bacterial empyema thoracis. J Thorac Cardiovasc Surg 94:414, 1987.

Mandal AK, Thadepailli H, Mandal AK, Chettipalli U: Post-traumatic empyema thoracis: A 24-year experience at a major trauma center. J Trauma 43:764, 1997.

Mangete EDD, Kombo BB, Leg JTE: Thoracic empyema a study of 56 patients. Arch Dis Child 69:587, 1993.

Martella AT, Santos GH: Decortication for chronic postpneumonic empyema. J Am Coll Surg 180:573, 1995.

Mavroudis C, Ganzel BL, Katzmark S, Polk HC: Effect of hemothorax on experimental empyema thoracis in the guinea pig. J Thorac Cardiovasc Surg 89:42, 1985.

Mavroudis C, Symmonds JB, Minagi H, Thomas AN: Improved survival in management of empyema thoracis. J Thorac Cardiovasc Surg 82:49, 1981.

Mayo P, Saha SP, McElvein RB: Acute empyema in children treated by open thoracotomy and decortication. Ann Thorac Surg 34:401, 1982.

McLaughlin FJ, Goldmann DA, Rosenbaum DM et al: Empyema in children: Clinical course and long-term follow-up. Pediatrics 73:587, 1984.

Middlekamp JN, Purkerson ML, Burford TH: The changing pattern of empyema thoracis in pediatrics. J Thorac Cardiovasc Surg 47:165, 1969.

Miller JI: Empyema thoracis. Ann Thorac Surg 50:343, 1990.

Miller JI, Mansour KA, Nahai F et al: Single-stage complete muscle flap closure of the post-pneumonectomy empyema space: A new method and possible solution to a disturbing complication. Ann Thorac Surg 38:227, 1984.

Miller JI: Management of post-pneumonectomy empyema of the pleural space. In Peters RM, Toledo J (eds): Current Topics in General Thoracic Surgery: An International Series, Vol 2. New York, Elsevier, 1991.

Moir R, Telander RL: Complications of lower respiratory tract infection, empyema complicating pneumonia, pneumatoceles, and respiratory embarrassment. In Fallis JC, Filler RM, Lemoine G (eds): Current Topics in General Thoracic Surgery, Vol 1. New York, Elsevier, 1991.

Moran JF: Surgical management of pleural infections. Semin Respir Infect 3:383, 1988.

Morin JE, Munro DD, MacLean LD: Early thoracotomy for empyema. J Thorac Cardiovasc Surg 64:530, 1972.

Morton JR, Boushy SF, Guin GA: Physiological evaluation of results of pulmonary decortication. Ann Thorac Surg 9:321, 1970.

Moulton JS, Moore PT, Mencini RA: Treatment of loculated pleural effusions with transcatheter intracavitary urokinase. AJR Am J Roentgenol 153:941, 1989.

Mouroux J, Riquet M, Podovani B et al: Surgical management of thoracic manifestations in human immunodeficiency virus positive patients: Indications and results. Br J Surg 82:39, 1995.

Muers MF: Streptokinase for empyema. Lancet 349:1491, 1997.

Nakaoka K, Nakalara K, Iioka S et al: Postoperative preservation of pulmonary function in patients with chronic empyema thoracis: A one-stage operation. Ann Thorac Surg 47:848, 1989.

Nin Vivo J, Brandolino MU, Pomi JA et al: Hydatid pleural disease. In Deslauriers J, Lacquet LK (eds): International Trends in General Thoracic Surgery, Vol 6. St. Louis, Mosby–Year Book, 1990.

Noyes BE, Michaels MG, Kurland G et al: Pseudomonas cepacia empyema necessitatis after lung transplantation in two patients with cystic fibrosis. Chest 105:1888, 1994.

Ogilvie AG: Final results in traumatic haemothorax: A report of 230 cases. Thorax 5:116, 1950.

Onotera RT, Unruh HW: Closure of post-pneumonectomy bronchopleural fistula with fibrin sealant (Tisseel). Thorax 43:1015, 1988.

Orringer MB: Thoracic empyema: Back to basics. Chest 93:901, 1988.

Osler W: The Principles and Practice of medicine. New York, Appleton, 1892.

Paget S: Empyema. In Paget S (ed): The Surgery of the Chest. New York, EB Treat, 1897, pp 204–229.

Paget S: Surgery of the Chest. Bristol, John Wright and Sons, 1896.

Pairolero PC, Arnold PHG: Bronchopleural fistula: Treatment by transposition of pectoralis major. J Thorac Cardiovasc Surg 79:142, 1980.

Pairolero PC, Arnold PHG: Management of empyema: The problems of associated bronchopleural fistula. In Grillo H, Eschapasse H (eds): International trends in general thoracic surgery, Vol 2. Philadelphia, WB Saunders, 1987.

Pairolero PC, Arnold PHG, Piehler JM: Intrathoracic transposition of extrathoracic skeletal muscle. J Thorac Cardiovasc Surg 86:809, 1983.

Paris F: Empyema after lung transplant (Personal Communication), 1999.

Paris F, Blasco E, Tarazona V et al: El empiema pleural como complicacion de la bronchopneumopathia aguda. Proceedings II Symposium International sobre antibioticos. Beecham, Valencia, 1970.

Paris F, Ruiz-Compay S, Asensi F et al: Complications of lower respiratory tract infection: Empyema complicating pneumonia, pneumatoceles, and respiratory embarrassment. In Fallis JC, Miller M, Lemoine G (eds): Current Topics in General Thoracic Surgery: An International Series, Vol 1. New York, Elsevier, 1991.

Patton WE, Warson TR, Gaensler EA: Pulmonary function before and at intervals after surgical decortication of the lung. Surg Gynecol Obstet 95:477, 1952.

Perelman ME, Rymko LP: Management of empyemas: The problems of associated bronchopleural fistulas. In Deslauriers J, Lacquet LK (eds): International Trends in General Thoracic Surgery, Vol 6. St. Louis, Mosby–Year Book, 1990.

Personne C: Role of early thoracotomy in the treatment of empyema. In Deslauriers J, Lacquet LK (eds): International Trends in General Thoracic Surgery, Vol 6. St. Louis, Mosby–Year Book, 1990.

Peters RM: Empyema thoracis: Historical perspective. Ann Thorac Surg 48:306, 1989.

Playfair GE: Case of empyema treated by aspiration and subsequently by drainage: Recovery. BMJ 1:45, 1875.

Pollack JS, Passik CS: Intrapleural urokinase in the treatment of loculated pleural effusions. Chest 105:868, 1994.

Pothula V, Krellenstein DJ: Early aggressive surgical management of parapneumonic empyemas. Chest 105:832, 1994.

Potts DE, Levin DC, Sahn SA: Pleural fluid pH in parapneumonic effusions. Chest 70:328, 1976.

Potts DE, Taryle DA, Sahn SA: The glucose-pH relationship in parapneumonic effusions. Arch Intern Med 138:1378, 1978.

Puskas JD, Mathisen DJ, Grillo HC et al: Treatment strategies for bronchopleural fistula. Presented at the Annual Meeting of the American Association for Thoracic Surgery, New York, April 24–28, 1994.

Raffensperger JG, Luck SR, Shkolnik A, Ricketts RR: Mini-thoracotomy and chest tube insertion for children with empyema. J Thorac Cardiovasc Surg 84:497, 1982.

Ravitch M, Fein R: The changing picture of pneumonia and empyema in infants and children: A review of the experience at the Harriet Lane home from 1934 through 1958. JAMA 175:1039, 1961.

Renner H, Gabor S, Pinter H et al: Is aggressive surgery in pleural empyema justified? Eur J Cardiothorac Surg 14:117, 1998.

Robinson LA: Thoracic disorders in the immunocompromised patient: Preface. Chest Surg Clin North Am 9:1, 1999.

Robinson LA, Moulton AL, Fleming WH et al: Intrapleural fibrinolytic treatment of multiloculated thoracic empyemas. Ann Th Surg 57:803, 1994.

Robinson S: The treatment of chronic non-tuberculous empyema. Surg Gynecol Obstet 22:557, 1916.

Robinson S: The treatment of chronic non-tuberculous empyema (Collected Papers). Mayo Clin 7:618, 1915.

Rodgers BM: Discussion of Foglia RP and Randolph J: Current indications for decortication in the treatment of empyema in children. J Pediatr Surg 22:32, 1987.

Ronson RS, Miller JI: Video-assisted thoracoscopy for pleural disease. Chest Surg Clin North Am 8:919, 1998.

Rosenfeldt FL, McGibney D, Braimbridge MV, Watson DA: Comparison between irrigation and conventional treatment for empyema and pneumonectomy space infections. Thorax 36:272, 1981.

Sahn SA, Light RW: The sun should never set on a parapneumonic effusion. Chest 95:945, 1989.

Samson PE: Empyema thoracis: Essentials of present-day management. Ann Thorac Surg 11:210, 1971.

Schede M: Die Behandlung der Empyema. Verh Dtsch Ges Inn Med 9:41, 141, 1890.

Sensenig DM, Rossi NP, Ehrenhaft JL: Decortication for chronic nontuberculous empyema. Surg Gynecol Obstet 117:443, 1963.

Sherman MM, Subramanian V, Berger RL: Management of thoracic empyema. Am J Surg 133:474, 1977.

Silen ML, Nauheim KS: Thoracoscopic approach to the management of empyema thoracis: Indications and results. Chest Surg Clin North Am 6:491, 1996.

Smolle-Jüttner E, Beuster W, Pinter H et al: Open-window thoracostomy in pleural empyema. Eur J Cardiothorac Surg 6:635, 1992.

Snell GI, de Hoyos A, Karjden M et al: Pseudomona cepacia in lung patients recipients with cystic fibrosis. Chest 103:466, 1993.

Soysal O, Topcu S, Tastepe I et al: Childhood chronic pleural empyema: A continuing surgical challenge in developing countries. Thorac Cardiovasc Surg 46:357, 1998.

Spizarny DL, Gross BH, McLoud T: Enlarging pleural effusion after liver transplantation. J Thorac Imaging 8:85, 1993.

Stafford EG, Clagett OT: Post-pneumonectomy empyema: Neomycin instillations and definitive closure. J Thorac Cardiovasc Surg 63:771, 1972.

Stark DD, Federle MP, Goodman PC et al: Differentiating lung abscess and empyema: Radiography and computed tomography. AJR Am J Roentgenol 141:163, 1983.

Stiles QR, Lindersmith GG, Tucker BL et al: Pleural empyema in children. Ann Thorac Surg 10:37, 1970.

Striffeler H, Gugger M, Im Hof V et al: Video-assisted thoracoscopic surgery for fibrinopurulent pleural empyema in 67 patients. Ann Thorac Surg 65:319, 1998.

Sullivan KM, O'Toole RD, Fisher RH, Sullivan KN: Anaerobic empyema thoracis: The role of anaerobes in 226 cases of culture proven empyemas. Arch Intern Med 131:521, 1973.

Tarazona V, Paris F, Chamorro JJ et al: Comblement des poches résiduelles après pneumonectomie par transposition complète du grand dorsal, du grand dentelé et du grand pectoral: à propos de quatre malades. Ann Chir Thorac Cardiovasc 35:681, 1981.

Thomas DF, Glass JL, Baisch BF: Management of streptococcal pneumonia. Ann Thorac Surg 2:658, 1966.

Thurer RJ: Decortication in thoracic empyema: Indications and surgical technique. Chest Surg Clin North Am 6:461, 1996.

Thurer RJ, Palatinos GM: Surgical aspects of the pleural space. Semin Respir Med 9:98, 1987

Tilett WS, Sherry S: The effect in patients of streptococcal fibrinolysin (streptokinase) and streptococcal desoxyribonuclease on fibrinous, purulent and sanguineous pleural exudations. J Clin Invest 28:173, 1949.

Uri SU, Nahai F: Intrathoracic muscle transposition: Surgical anatomy and techniques of harvest. Chest Surg Clin North Am 6:501, 1996.

Van Way III C, Narrod J, Hopeman A: The role of early limited thoracotomy in the treatment of empyema. J Thorac Cardiovasc Surg 96:436, 1988.

Varkey B, Rose HD, Kesavan-Kutty CP, Politis J: Empyema thoracis during a ten-year period: Analysis of 72 cases and comparison to a previous study (1952 to 1967). Arch Intern Med 141:1771, 1981.

Vester SR, Faber LP, Kittle F et al: Bronchopleural fistula after stapled closure of bronchus. Ann Thorac Surg 52:1253, 1991.

Vianna NJ: Nontuberculous bacterial empyema in patients with and without underlying diseases. JAMA 215:69, 1971.

Virkkula L, Eerola S: The treatment of postpneumonectomy empyema and large fistula. Les Bronches 23:230, 1973.

Virkkula L, Eerola S: Treatment of post-pneumonectomy empyema. Scand J Thorac Cardiovasc Surg 8:133, 1974.

Virkkula L, Eerola S, Varstela E: Surgical approach to the chronic empyema: Space sterilization. In Deslauriers J, Lacquet LK (eds): International Trends in General Thoracic Surgery, Vol 6. St. Louis, Mosby–Year Book, 1990.

Von Bülau G: Für die Heber Drainage bei Behandlung des Empyema. Z Klin Med 18:31, 1891.

Wait MA, Sharma S, Hohn J, Dal Nogare A: A randomized trial of empyema therapy. Chest 111:1548, 1997.

Wakabayashi A: Expanded applications of diagnostic and therapeutic thoracoscopy. J Thorac Cardiovasc Surg 102:721,1991.

Weissberg D: Empyema and bronchopleural fistula: Experience with open window thoracostomy. Chest 82:447, 1982.

Weissberg D, Kaufman M: The use of talc for pleurodesis in the treatment of resistant empyema. Ann Thorac Surg 41:143, 1986.

Westney GE, Kesten S, de Hoyos A et al: Aspergillus infection in single and double lung transplant. Transplantation 61:915, 1996.

Whitton I: Pleural amebiasis. In Deslauriers J, Lacquet LK (eds): International Trends in General Thoracic Surgery, Vol 6. St. Louis, Mosby–Year Book, 1990.

Yeh TJ, Hall DP, Ellison RG: Empyema thoracis: A review of 110 cases. Am Rev Respir Dis 88:785, 1963.

York JEL, Lewall DB, Hidi M et al: Endoscopic diagnosis and treatment of postoperative bronchopleural fistula. Chest 197:1390, 1990.

CHAPTER **42**

Spontaneous Pneumothorax and Pneumomediastinum

Gilles Beauchamp

Denise Ouellette

Pneumothorax is the presence of air in the pleural space with secondary lung collapse. Although the air may originate from different sources, rupture of the visceral pleura with leakage from the lung parenchyma is by far the most common cause.

Most patients with pneumothoraces have significant symptoms such as chest pain and dyspnea but no major physiologic changes. Occasionally, however, a simple and uncomplicated pneumothorax comes under tension, resulting in significant hemodynamic and respiratory instability that requires urgent treatment (Baumann and Sahn, 1993).

Pneumothoraces can be classified as spontaneous, post-traumatic, or iatrogenic (Table 42–1). Whereas primary spontaneous pneumothoraces occur in young people without lung disease, secondary spontaneous pneumothoraces occur in patients with clinical or radiographic evidence of underlying lung disease, most often chronic obstructive pulmonary disease (COPD) (Killen and Gobbel, 1968; Light, 1993). Post-traumatic pneumothoraces are the result of injuries to the bronchi, the lung, or the esophagus. These are said to be open (open pneumothorax) when associated with a disruption of the chest wall.

Iatrogenic pneumothoraces can occur after diagnostic or therapeutic thoracic procedures. They are relatively common in a hospital environment (Despars et al, 1994), but they are not discussed in this chapter. Therapeutic as well as diagnostic pneumothoraces are largely of historical interest.

HISTORICAL NOTE

The presence of abnormal air in the pleural cavity has been known to occur for a long time, but its clinical significance was not recognized until Boerhaave (1724) (Table 42–2) described a relationship between anatomy and clinical presentation (Emerson, 1903). In 1759, Meckel described a tension pneumothorax that was recognized at postmortem examination, and the term "pneumothorax" was suggested by Etard in 1803. Sixteen years later, Laennec (1819) described the clinical signs and symptoms related to a pneumothorax.

Until the early 1930s, tuberculosis was considered to be the principal cause of pneumothoraces. In 1932, however, Kjaergaard speculated that the rupture of isolated blebs located at the apex of the lung may be the cause of pneumothoraces in young, apparently healthy adults. He further described some physical characteristics of these patients such as bimodal age distribution, male predominance, specific body morphology, and association with cigarette smoking.

TABLE 42–1 ■ **Classification of Pneumothorax**

SPONTANEOUS
Primary
Secondary (underlying pulmonary disease):
Chronic obstructive pulmonary disease
Infection
Neoplasm
Catamenial
POST-TRAUMATIC
Blunt
Penetrating
IATROGENIC
Inadvertent
Diagnostic
Therapeutic

TABLE 42–2 ■ **Historical Landmarks**

Authors	*Landmark*
Boerhaave (18th century)	Ruptured esophagus associated with presence of air in the pleural cavity
Meckel (18th century)	Postmortem description of a tension pneumothorax
Etard (19th century)	Autopsy description; introduction of the term pneumothorax
Laennec (19th century)	Description of clinical signs and symptoms
Kjaergaard (1932)	Rupture of lung blebs replacing tuberculosis as the most frequent cause of primary spontaneous pneumothorax
Getz and Beasely (1983)	Chronic obstructive lung disease as a frequent cause of pneumothoraces
Wait and Estrera (1992)	*Pneumocystis carinii* pneumonia, cytomegalovirus pneumonia, and atypical mycobacterial infections associated with AIDS are common causes of pneumothorax

We have now entered a new phase in the pathogenesis of this disease as chronic obstructive and diffuse interstitial lung diseases have become a frequent cause of pneumothoraces in the aging Western population (Getz and Beasely, 1983; Wait and Estrera, 1992). With advances in immunosuppression and the emergence of acquired immunodeficiency syndrome (AIDS), *Pneumocystis carinii* pneumonia, cytomegalovirus pneumonia, and atypical mycobacterial infections have also become more frequently associated with secondary spontaneous pneumothoraces (Suster and Ackerman, 1986).

For a long time, the treatment of spontaneous pneumothoraces consisted solely of several weeks of bed rest. Intercostal tube thoracostomy contributed to accelerating lung re-expansion, and in the early 1960s it became the method of choice for treatment of a first episode (Klassen and Meckstroth, 1962).

In 1937, Bigger advocated thoracotomy for the resection of apical blebs, and soon after, Tyson and Crandall (1941) reported on the results of elective thoracotomy and excision of subpleural blebs (Table 42–3).

According to Killen and Gobbel (1968), Churchill was the first to describe the method of using gauze abrasion of the parietal pleura to generate the formation of pleural adhesions and prevent recurrences. Gaensler (1956) and Thomas and Gebauer (1958) also described parietal pleurectomy as an alternative method to achieve permanent pleurodesis. In his discussion of these two options, Clagett (1968) concluded that pleurectomy was perhaps too aggressive and too radical in the treatment of a benign disease, and he recommended the use of abrasion. In 1970, Youmans and colleagues provided additional clinical and experimental evidence for the efficacy of pleural abrasion in reducing the risks of recurrences, and in 1980 Deslauriers and associates were the first to report the combination of "blebectomy" and limited apical pleurectomy done through a transaxillary incision. In keeping with the tremendous development of minimally invasive surgery that occurred in the 1990s, Levi and coworkers (1990) introduced video-assisted thoracic surgery (VATS) for the surgical treatment of pneumothorax.

■ *HISTORICAL REFERENCES*

Bigger IA: Operative Surgery. St. Louis, CV Mosby, 1937.

Clagett OT: The management of spontaneous pneumothorax (Editorial). J Thorac Cardiovasc Surg 56:761, 1968.

Deslauriers J, Beaulieu M, Després JP et al: Transaxillary thoracotomy for treatment of spontaneous pneumothorax. Ann Thorac Surg 30:35, 1980.

TABLE 42–3 ■ **Evolution of Therapy**

Tyson and Crandall (1951)	Thoracotomy, resection of blebs
Gaensler (1956)	Subtotal parietal pleurectomy
Thomas and Gebauer (1958)	
Deslauriers (1980)	Axillary thoracotomy, bleb resection, and apical pleurectomy
Levi et al (1990)	Video-assisted thoracoscopic surgery for bleb resection, pleural abrasion, or pleurectomy

Emerson CP: Pneumothorax: A historical, clinical, and experimental study. Johns Hopkins Rev 11:1, 1903.

Gaensler EA: Parietal pleurectomy for recurrent spontaneous pneumothorax. Surg Gynecol Obstet 102:293, 1956.

Getz SB, Beasely WE: Spontaneous pneumothorax. Am J Surg 145:823, 1983.

Killen DA, Gobell WG: Spontaneous Pneumothorax. Boston, Little, Brown, 1968.

Kjaergaard H: Spontaneous pneumothorax in the apparently healthy. Acta Med Scand Suppl 43:159, 1932.

Klassen KP, Meckstroth CV: Treatment of spontaneous pneumothorax: Prompt expansion with controlled thoracotomy tube suction. JAMA 182:1, 1962.

Levi JF, Kleinmann P, Riquet M, Debesse B: Percutaneous parietal pleurectomy of recurrent spontaneous pneumothorax. Lancet 336:1577, 1990.

Suster B, Ackerman M: Pulmonary manifestation of AIDS: Review 106 episodes. Radiology 161:87, 1986.

Thomas PA, Gebauer PW: Pleurectomy for recurrent spontaneous pneumothorax. J Thorac Surg 35:117, 1958.

Tyson MD, Crandall WB: The surgical treatment of recurrent idiopathic spontaneous pneumothorax. J Thorac Surg 10:566, 1941.

Wait MA, Estrera A: Changing clinical spectrum of spontaneous pneumothorax. Am J Surg 164:528, 1992.

Youmans CR Jr, Williams RD, Monthy RM: Surgical management of spontaneous pneumothorax by bleb ligation and pleural dry sponge abrasion. Am J Surg 120:644, 1970.

BASIC SCIENCE

Anatomy of the Pleural Space

The visceral pleura covers the entire surface of the lung but has no plane of dissection with the parenchyma; the parietal pleura is a serous membrane that covers the inner surfaces of the mediastinum, the chest wall, the diaphragm, and the apex of the chest cavity. The presence of the endothoracic fascia between pleura and chest wall provides a plane of dissection that makes it easy for surgeons to perform a parietal pleurectomy. The parietal pleura is vascularized through branches originating from intercostal arteries and the apical pleura through branches of the subclavian artery. The parietal pleura, unlike the visceral pleura, has somatic innervation, and pain stimuli are transmitted through the intercostal and phrenic nerves (Desmeules et al, 1990).

Physiology of Pleural Space

When a patient is at rest and relaxed, thus at functional residual capacity, the elastic forces of the chest wall and lung tend to separate the parietal pleura from the visceral pleura, creating a negative pressure with respect to atmospheric and alveolar pressure. This negative intrapleural pressure is, however, not uniform throughout the pleural space; a gradient exists between the apex and the base of the lung. At the apex, the pressure is more negative than at the base; this difference tends to favor greater distention of the apical alveoli. In tall individuals, this gradient may be even greater, thus probably contributing to the development of pneumothoraces through the rupture of apical blebs.

Physiologic Changes Secondary to Pneumothorax

Simple Pneumothorax

When a communication develops between the lung and the pleural space, the positive pressure of intra-alveolar

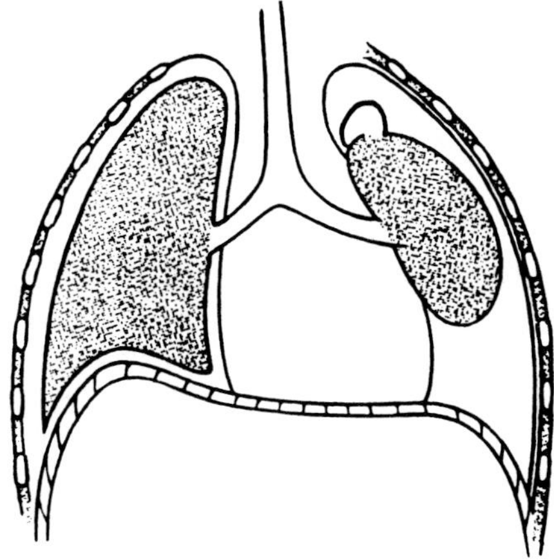

↑ Air flow until no pressure difference.

↓ Apex to base pressure gradient

↓ Lung compliance

↓ FRC

↓ Ventilation

↓ Oxygenation

Slight shunt

FIGURE 42–1 ■ Some of the physiologic characteristics of spontaneous pneumothorax. (FRC, functional residual capacity.)

air makes the air flow from the lung into the pleural space until there is no difference between the negative intrapleural pressure and the atmospheric pressure (Fig. 42–1). The same mechanism of pressure equilibration occurs when there is a communication between the open chest wall and the pleural cavity.

Alveolar hypoventilation and hypoxemia develop in patients with significant (greater than 25%) pneumothoraces (Norris et al, 1968). According to Moran and coauthors (1977), this hypoxemia is related to an alteration of the ventilation-perfusion ratio. Anatomic shunting can also contribute to the low arterial oxygen pressure (Dines et al, 1970). In 1977, Anthonisen suggested that the ventilation mismatch often seen in pneumothoraces was secondary to airway closure at low lung volumes.

A pneumothorax also leads to reductions in lung compliance, vital capacity, total capacity, and functional residual capacity (Gilmartin et al, 1985), and the normal apex-to-base pleural pressure gradient disappears (Agostini, 1986).

Tension Pneumothorax

When a tension pneumothorax develops, a positive intrapleural pressure is created during expiration because the accumulated intrapleural air cannot flow back in the bronchial tree. At each inspiration, more air is brought into the closed chest cavity, increasing the intrapleural pressure (Fig. 42–2).

It was long believed that in cases of tension pneumothoraces, mediastinal compression by accumulated air induced a decrease of the venous return and ultimately of the cardiac output.

According to Gutsman and colleagues (1983), only a fraction of the increased intrapleural pressure is transmitted to the mediastinum, suggesting another explanation for the cardiovascular changes. In an experimental model, Hurewitz and associates (1986) observed a fall in cardiac stroke volume as well as a progressive reduction in systemic oxygen transport and tissue oxygenation during an episode of tension pneumothorax. These alterations were thought to be caused by insufficient tissue oxygenation and inability to increase the cardiac output, which itself was the result of inadequate oxygenation of the heart.

Tension pneumothorax may also create a shunt effect, and in 1968, Rutherford and coworkers showed that hypoxemia was caused by increased pulmonary blood flow in hypoventilated or nonventilated lung zones.

Resorption of Pleural Gas

Although the normal pleural space is free of gas, the pleural membrane is a semipermeable structure through which gases can move by simple diffusion and equilibra-

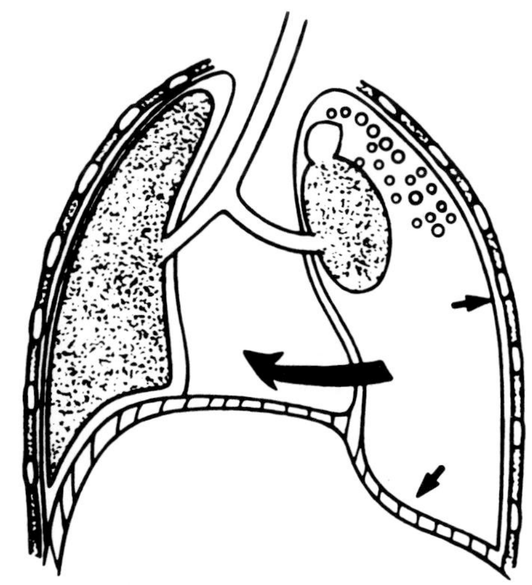

↑ Continuous air flow–one-way valve

↑ Intrapleural pressure

↑ Mediastinal shift: alteration of lung mechanic

↓ Ventilation

↑ Shunt

↓ Oxygenation

↓ Cardiac stroke volume

↑ Heart rate

FIGURE 42–2 ■ Some of the physiologic characteristics of a tension pneumothorax.

tion. In pneumothoraces, the pressure gradient between the gas in the pleural space and the gas in the subpleural venous system is the driving force directing this diffusion process. Each gas is resorbed independent of the others.

Gas resorption from the pleural space takes place gradually and in successive phases. During the first phase, there is equilibration of oxygen and carbon dioxide partial pressures, and during the second phase, there is a progressive resorption of the remaining intrapleural gases. Gradually, the intrapleural pressure recovers its negative pressure favoring lung re-expansion. When the lung does not re-expand, fluid transudates in the pleural space and fills the cavity (Cormier, 1990).

The rate of resorption of a pneumothorax is related to the quality of the pleural membrane. In a fibrotic pleura, for instance, the rate of resorption is slower than it is in a normal pleura. The rate of resorption is also proportionate to the total membrane area of the pleura and to the amount of residual gas in the pleural cavity. The greater the amount of gas, the longer it takes for resorption. Finally, the composition of gases in the pleural space can also vary. For example, oxygen is more diffusible and soluble, and its transfer from pleura to circulation is faster than that of carbon dioxide or nitrogen.

PRIMARY SPONTANEOUS PNEUMOTHORAX

Etiology and Epidemiology

The most common cause of primary spontaneous pneumothorax is the rupture of small subpleural blebs. This rupture may occur when the patient is at rest or during exercise, and it is seen most commonly in young and tall men (Melton et al, 1979) who smoke (Bense et al, 1987). As suggested by Nakamura and coworkers (1986), the increase in smoking that is now seen in women has led to an increased incidence of primary spontaneous pneumothorax in this gender. An increased familial incidence has also been reported by Sugiyama and coauthors (1986).

In North America, the incidence varies from 6 to 7 per 100,000 in men and 1 to 2 per 100,000 women (Melton et al, 1979). Primary spontaneous pneumothorax occurs more commonly on the right side than on the left (Brooks, 1973), and bilateral pneumothoraces occur in less than 10% of patients (Donovan, 1987).

Specific mechanisms by which a pneumothorax develops are still open to discussion, and exertion is probably not a major factor. In 1984, Bense reported interesting observations on the variations of atmospheric pressure in relation to spontaneous pneumothoraces. He noted, for instance, that the hospital admission rate for spontaneous pneumothorax was significantly higher during the first 48 hours after a fall in the atmospheric pressure. Scott and colleagues (1989) also showed a relationship between spontaneous pneumothoraces and changes in atmospheric pressure, although they stated that several other factors were also likely to be contributors. Studies on flight personnel with prior episodes of pneumothoraces showed that small apical bullae increase in size when subjected to decreasing atmospheric pressure in altitude chambers (Dermksian and Lamb, 1959). These studies seem to confirm that rupture of blebs and bullae may occur with variations of intrabronchial and intrathoracic pressures.

Histopathology

The terms blebs and bullae are frequently used in the literature. Blebs are defined as small (less than 2 cm) subpleural collections of air contained within the visceral pleura. They result from ruptured alveoli with air being trapped between the elastica interna and externa of the visceral pleura. Blebs are usually found at the apex of the upper lobes or over the posterior apices of the lower lobes (Edge et al, 1966), and as shown by Lichter (1974), they are often accompanied by apical fibrosis. They are considered to represent the paraseptal variety of emphysema, which can occur independently of widespread centriacinar or panacinar emphysema.

Computed tomographic (CT) findings have contributed to a better understanding of the pathogenesis of pneumothoraces (Muller, 1993). A study of a group of nonsmoking, non–α-antitrypsin–deficient patients showed that 80% of patients suffering from primary spontaneous pneumothorax had so-called emphysema-like changes (ELCs), identified on CT scan as blebs and bullae, whereas no ELCs were found in a control group (Bense et al, 1993). ELCs tend to be located in the upper peripheral zones of the lung and are frequently found bilaterally (Lesur et al, 1990; Mitlehner et al, 1992).

Blebs are well demarcated from the remaining normal lung, although they are still attached to it by a narrow neck. Electron microscopic examination of the outer membrane of a bleb showed absence of mesothelial cells but presence of naked collagen fibers and small pores, which apparently were the cause of air leak (Ohata and Suzuki, 1980). Eosinophilic pleuritis often accompanies the rupture of blebs into the pleural cavity. Histiocytes, eosinophils, fibrin, multinucleated giant cells, and mesothelial cells can also be found on microscopic examination of the pleura.

Bullae are large, air-filled spaces that can be associated with any form of emphysema. Although they usually result from the alveolar wall destruction (Klingman et al, 1990) typically seen in diffuse emphysema, they can also be found in a normal lung.

In 1966, Reid described three types of bullae. Type I bullae have thin walls made of pleura and connective tissue with few blood vessels. These bullae are located at the apices of upper lobes or over the edges of other lobes. They correspond to overinflation of a small volume of parenchyma and communicate with the lung by a narrow neck. In type II bullae, mesothelial cells are relatively well preserved but destroyed alveolar structures are found at their base. The diseased alveoli are in continuity with the bullae through a broad neck (Ohata and Suzuki, 1980). In type III bullae, the base of the bulla is large and extends deep into the lung.

According to Fukuda and associates (1994), the formation of blebs and bullae is probably associated with the degradation of elastic fibers. This process of elastolysis is caused by an imbalance between proteases and antiproteases and between oxidants and antioxidants, in which neutrophils and macrophages play an important role. The bronchiolitis caused by inflammatory cells found in smokers is also associated with bronchiolar wall fibrosis and destruction of the pulmonary parenchyma (Adesina et al, 1991; Kondo et al, 1991; Tetely, 1993).

Smoking produces an increased number of inflammatory cells, especially macrophages, in the small airways (Hunninghake and Crystal, 1983). These macrophages release potent chemotactic factors, resulting in the accumulation of neutrophils. This phenomenon is enhanced by the loss of activity of chemotactic inactivator factors that are associated with cigarette smoke (Robbins et al, 1990).

Endobronchial obstruction by inflammatory cells is probably part of the pathogenesis of blebs and bullae because it generates increased pressure in the alveolar tissue, which may result in the rupture of pulmonary parenchyma. In two studies (Lichter and Gwynne, 1971; Tueller et al, 1977), histopathologic and electron microscopic analysis of tissue from patients with spontaneous pneumothorax showed obstruction and stenosis of distal airways caused by bronchial wall inflammation and peribronchial fibrosis.

According to Swierenga and coauthors (1974), Swierenga (1977), and Vanderschueren (1981), at least four macroscopic presentations of the disease can be found at surgery. The first corresponds to a normal lung without evidence of blebs or bullae, which is seen in mostly 30% to 40% of cases. In 12% to 15% of patients, there is no evidence of blebs or bullae, but there are pleuropulmonary adhesions, suggesting previous pneumothoraces. In 28% to 41% of patients, blebs that are less than 2 cm in diameter are found. Multiple bullae larger than 2 cm are found in the remaining individuals.

Diagnosis

The severity of symptoms such as chest pain and dyspnea usually correlates with the degree of lung collapse. Occasionally, patients also have a nonproductive cough (De Vries and Wolfe, 1981). Physical findings may be totally absent if lung collapse is minimal, but when a substantial pneumothorax is present, there is nearly always a decrease in chest wall movement on the affected side. On percussion, the chest cavity is hyper-resonant, and at auscultation, breath sounds are diminished or absent. A pleural friction rub can sometimes be heard, and tachycardia is almost invariably present.

The diagnosis of pneumothorax is best confirmed by erect posteroanterior (PA) and lateral chest radiographs (see Fig. 42–3). Expiration films are useful in demonstrating a small pneumothorax that may have been missed on a standard film. In a study of induced pneumothoraces in cadavers, Carr and associates (1992) demonstrated that lateral decubitus views may be advantageous in confirming the presence of a pneumothorax.

Pseudopneumothoraces such as skin folds or chest wall alterations must always be ruled out. Occasionally, pulmonary cysts or emphysematous bullae may also be mistaken for a pneumothorax. The diagnosis of a tension pneumothorax is suggested by complete collapse of the

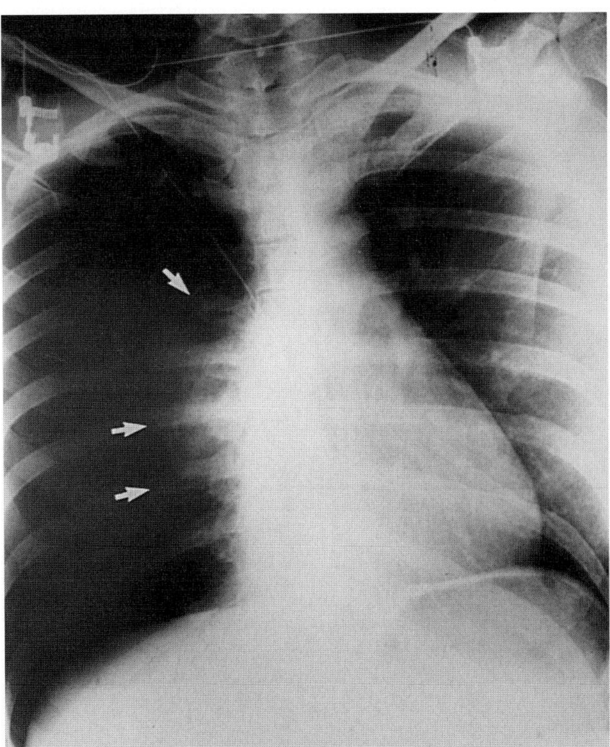

FIGURE 42–3 ■ A pneumothorax is identified by finding the location of the visceral pleura.

lung with contralateral shift of the heart and mediastinum and inversion of the hemidiaphragm (Fig. 42–4).

Quantification of the size of a pneumothorax may be useful for making a therapeutic decision. Unfortunately, the methods used for this quantification vary greatly and lack standardization (Axel, 1981). In 1954, Kirchner and Swartzel suggested measurements of the collapsed lung and of the hemithorax on a standard PA radiograph. In 1982, Rhea and coworkers proposed averaging the interpleural distance by measuring this distance at the apex and at midpoints of both upper and lower lung fields. The average interpleural distance is then reported on a constructive nomogram that provides an estimate of the size of the pneumothorax. In 1993, Light suggested measuring the average diameters of the collapsed lung and involved hemithorax. These diameters were then cubed to estimate the percentage of collapsed lung.

Because the precision of these quantitative methods is limited by their dependence on the constant shape of the lung during its collapse, CT scanning is currently being assessed to improve the estimation of the size of a pneumothorax. CT scanning is also used to better delineate associated parenchymal disease (Fig. 42–5). In a study of CT scanning in the etiologic assessment of pneumothorax, Lesur and coauthors (1990) reported moderate but diffuse centrilobar emphysema in 12 young smokers with primary spontaneous pneumothoraces. In 1992, Mitlehner and colleagues also showed the efficacy of CT examination for the delineation of the anatomic distribution of bullae and blebs in patients with pneumothoraces. A detailed description of the number, size, and location of the blebs from CT scanning also appears to be useful in predicting contralateral occurrences (Warner et al, 1991).

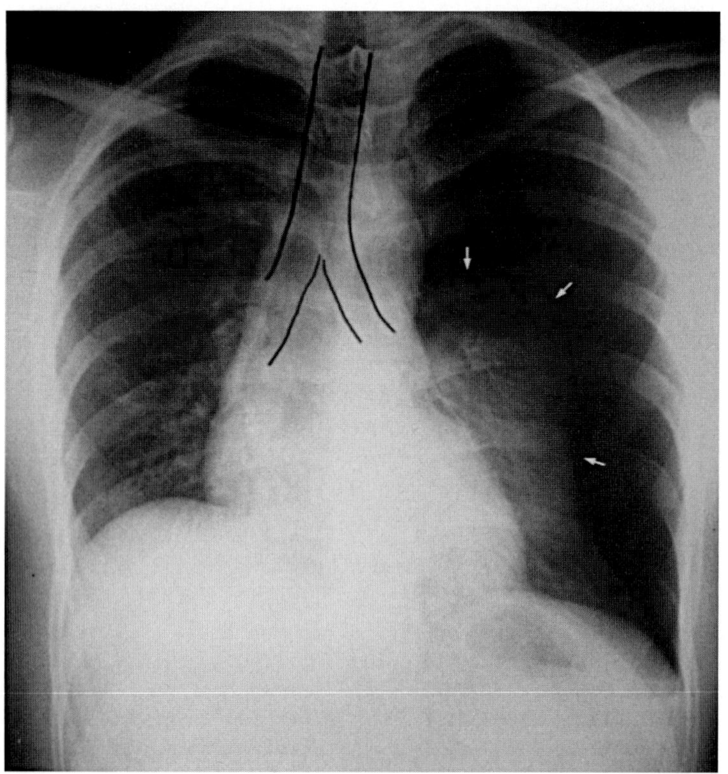

FIGURE 42–4 ■ Chest radiograph showing a tension pneumothorax with mediastinal shift and deviated trachea.

Patients with pneumothoraces can also have abnormal electrocardiographic readings. In patients with left-sided pneumothoraces, for instance, the electrocardiogram may show changes such as a right-sided shift of the QRS axis with a decrease in precordial R wave voltage and QRS amplitude and a precordial T-wave inversion. These findings usually resolve with re-expansion of the lung (Walston et al, 1974). When a large pneumothorax is present, the interposition of air between the heart and the electrode may also lead to a decrease in QRS amplitude as well as that of the R and T waves, simulating an anterior myocardial infarction (Diamond and Estes, 1982).

Complications

Persistent air leak is defined as an air leak that lasts more than 48 hours after initial therapy with chest tube drainage. Although it is common in patients with secondary pneumothoraces, it occasionally occurs in patients with primary spontaneous pneumothoraces (Chee, 1998). When an air leak does not resolve in an apparently well-drained chest cavity or when there is incomplete re-expansion of the lung, a second or a third chest tube may be required or surgery may become necessary.

A tension pneumothorax is a serious complication that occurs when alveolar air continuously enters the pleural space without any possibility for its evacuation. The patient usually shows signs of respiratory distress with tachycardia, anxiety, dyspnea, and pain. Occasionally, the patient rapidly becomes hypotensive with peripheral cyanosis and extreme tracheal deviation, indicating a life-threatening situation. Immediate decompression of the pleural space with a needle, chest drain, or other instrument then becomes imperative (Rivarola, 1990).

Pneumomediastinum is secondary to the dissection of air along the bronchi and vascular sheets of pulmonary vessels. It is generally of no clinical significance, but on occasion injury to major airways or perforation of the esophagus may have to be ruled out. Pneumoperitoneum secondary to a pneumothorax is uncommon, and in this situation one must rule out a perforated abdominal hollow viscus (Maunders et al, 1984). Interstitial emphysema and subcutaneous emphysema, which often accompany secondary pneumothoraces, are usually of no clinical consequence.

Hemopneumothoraces occur in 10% to 12% of cases. Their incidence is 30 times higher in men than in women (Tatebe et al, 1996). The hemorrhage is due to a torn vascular adhesion between the parietal and visceral pleura or less frequently to rupture of vascularized blebs or bullae. The clinical manifestations of spontaneous hemopneumothoraces can be dramatic and are largely dependent on the amount of blood lost. Although lung re-expansion may help tamponade the bleeding site, early surgery is often warranted to stop the bleeding, evacuate the coagulated blood, resect the site of the air leak, and proceed to a pleurectomy or pleural abrasion (Tatebe et al, 1996). Bilateral pneumothoraces occur in 10% to 15% of cases. Although these may be synchronous, more often they are sequential (metachronous). They are relatively uncommon in patients with emphysema (Graf-Dewel and Knoblauch, 1994).

Recurrence is the most frequent complication of primary spontaneous pneumothoraces; it occurs in approximately 25% of cases. Most recurrences are seen within 2 years of the first episode (Sadikot et al, 1997; Singh, 1982) and the majority are ipsilateral (Getz and Beasely, 1983). After a second pneumothorax, the risk of having

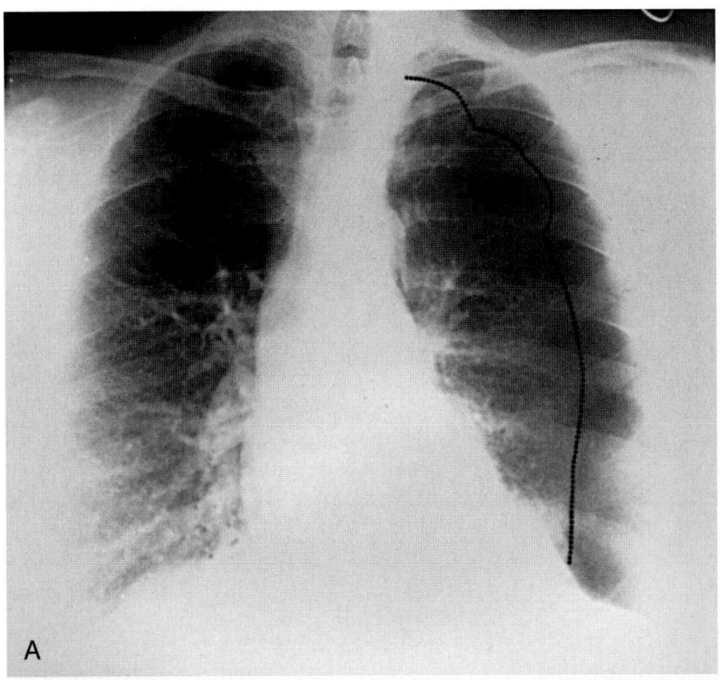

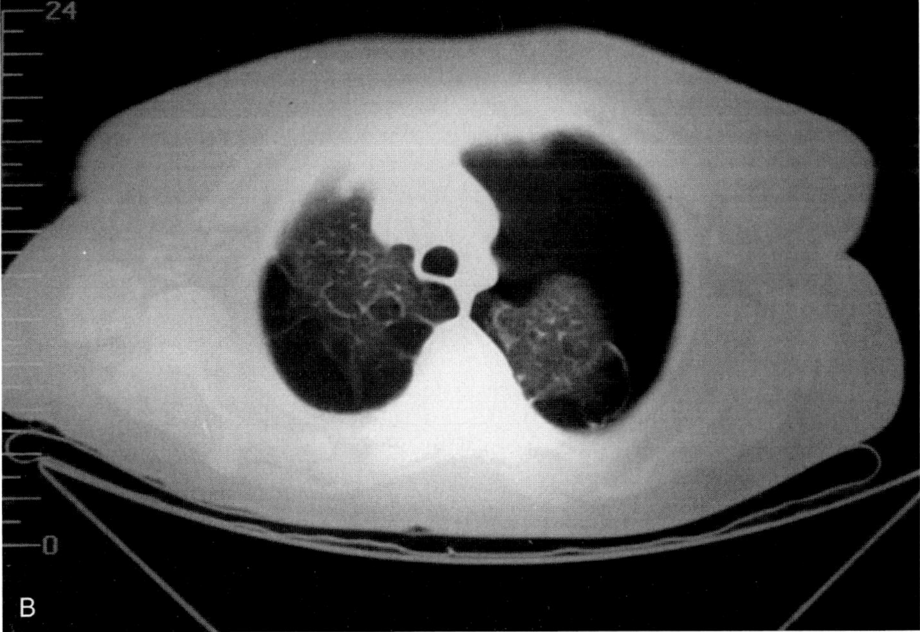

FIGURE 42–5 ■ *A*, Chest radiograph showing left-sided pneumothorax and normal right lung. *B*, A computed tomography scan of the same patient showing ipsilateral and contralateral bullae with left-sided pneumothorax.

a third one increases to more than 50% (Cran and Rumball, 1967; Gobbel et al, 1963). Smoking appears to be a major prognostic factor for recurrences (Sadikot et al, 1997).

Management

Initial Management

At the time of a first episode, different therapeutic strategies may be used depending on the size of the pneumothorax and the absence or presence of symptoms.

Asymptomatic patients in previous good health, with less than 20% pneumothorax, and without evidence of clinical and radiographic progression may be treated expectantly (Clague and El-Ansory, 1984). Air resorption from the pleural space is estimated to be 1.25% of the volume of the pneumothorax per 24 hours (50 to 70 ml/day) (Kircher and Swartzel, 1954). Administration of oxygen, which is reabsorbed faster than room air, is an effective method to enhance the rate of resolution, especially when the pneumothorax is smaller than 30% (Hill et al, 1995). This strategy may reduce morbidity and duration of hospitalization and in certain circumstances avoid the need for a drainage procedure (Chadha and Cohn, 1983).

Because there is a possibility of severe complications, patients who are treated expectantly should be observed very closely, especially if they are sent home. Before hospital discharge, they should be instructed about the potential hazards of developing a tension pneumothorax, and they should be followed with weekly chest radiographs until the pneumothorax has completely resolved. The main inconvenience of this method of treatment is the duration of the pneumothorax, which far exceeds the duration after tube thoracostomy. In addition, one must be cautious with this approach because in 1989 O'Rourke and Yee reported a 5% mortality rate associated with unrecognized tension in 40 patients treated by observation alone. Nevertheless, careful observation remains a valid therapeutic option for patients with small pneumothoraces. Because prolonged observation can lead to the development of an entrapped lung, tube drainage should be carried out when the lung is incompletely re-expanded after 1 week of observation.

Aspiration of pneumothoraces with a 16-gauge intravenous cannula connected to a three-way stopcock and 60-ml syringe is a method of treatment (Bevelaqua and Aranda, 1982) that is successful in approximately 50% of patients (Delius et al, 1989). According to Archer and colleagues (1985), however, the method is successful in only 33% of patients with pre-existing lung disease but in 83% of patients without lung disease, especially if the patient is younger than 50 years and has an estimated pneumothorax of less than 50%. In a study of 61 patients who were admitted for a first episode or a first recurrence of primary spontaneous pneumothorax, Andrivet and coworkers (1995) assigned patients randomly to treatment by tube drainage and simple needle aspiration, and they concluded that needle aspiration was safe as first-line therapy. Because aspiration techniques are limited by a 20% to 50% recurrence rate in spontaneous pneumothoraces (Seremetis 1970), small-caliber catheters are mostly used to decompress pneumothoraces complicating percutaneous lung biopsy or other types of iatrogenic pneumothoraces (Casola et al, 1988; Minami et al, 1992).

Since the introduction of the dart technique for the emergency treatment of pneumothoraces (Sargent and Turner, 1970), several devices have become commercially available. The McSwain dart, for instance, is a 16 French (F), 15-cm-long polyethylene catheter with a winged flange attached to a flutter valve (Wayne and McSwain, 1980), and the thoracic vent is a small-bore 13 F urethane catheter trocar with a one-way valve connected to a suction apparatus or underwater-seal system (Samuelson et al, 1991). Small 9 F chest tubes with or without flutter valves can be used as alternatives to larger tubes (Conces et al, 1988), but problems associated with malfunctioning and occlusion have been reported.

Conventional tube thoracostomy remains the procedure of choice for the management of moderate to large pneumothoraces (Miller and Sahn, 1987). Significant symptoms, radiographic progression, total collapse, tension, contralateral pulmonary disease, and failure of re-expansion after aspiration are all indications for tube thoracostomy. With proper tube drainage, the lung re-expands rapidly, and in the majority of patients, the air leak stops in less than 48 hours. Although underwater-seal drainage is usually sufficient, we prefer the use of negative intrapleural pressure to maintain lung re-expansion during the first 24 hours. In spite of satisfactory lung re-expansion, immediate relapse after removal of the tube is not uncommon (Davis et al, 1994; Seremetis, 1970).

When tube drainage is carried out, Light (1993) recommended maintenance of suction drainage for a period of 5 to 7 days. Schoenenberger and associates (1991) suggested a more aggressive approach, with surgery performed within 48 to 72 hours, in cases of persistent air leak or incomplete re-expansion of the lung. The chest tube should be removed after the air leak has stopped for at least 24 hours and preferably 48 hours (So and Yu, 1982). Tube clamping before removal is not recommended (Miller and Jarvey, 1993). As described by Mahfood and coauthors (1988) and Baumann and Sahn (1993), re-expansion pulmonary edema can occur after thoracostomy drainage, especially if the pneumothorax has been present for a long time (see Chapter 47).

The Heimlich (1968) flutter valve is a passive, one-way, ambulatory, chest tube drainage system. It was shown by Mercier and colleagues (1976) to be safe and efficient in the outpatient treatment of primary spontaneous pneumothorax. In our experience, it should be installed with underwater-seal drainage for several hours to permit a full re-expansion of the lung. If the lung maintains its expansion and if the air leak is minimal, the valve is installed, and the patient is discharged from the hospital. If a large air leak persists or if the lung cannot be re-expanded during the follow-up period, the patient must be admitted for underwater-seal or suction drainage until the air leak stops.

Treatment of Complications and Recurrences

Treatment of complications or recurrences of primary spontaneous pneumothoraces can include thoracotomy, minimally invasive surgical techniques, or chemical pleurodesis.

Surgical Therapy

Indications for Surgery. Surgery is indicated at the time of the first episode if the pneumothorax is complicated by persistent air leak, hemothorax, failure of the lung to re-expand, bilaterality, or tension (Table 42–4).

Rarely, surgery may also be indicated for psychological

TABLE 42–4 ■ Indications for Surgery in Primary Spontaneous Pneumothorax

FIRST EPISODE
Early complications
Prolonged air leak
Nonre-expansion of the lung
Bilaterality
Hemothorax
Tension
Complete pneumothorax
Potential hazards
Occupational hazard
Absence of medical facilities in isolated areas
Associated single large bulla
Psychological
SECOND EPISODE
Ipsilateral recurrence
Contralateral recurrence after a first pneumothorax

reasons such as fear of chest tube drainage or of another episode (Nazari, 1997) or for safety reasons, especially if the patient is at risk for recurrence because of his or her occupation. Some authors suggest that young patients with a very symptomatic or complete collapse during the first episode are selected for definitive treatment. We tend to disagree with these indications because the majority of such patients never have a recurrence and will therefore never require surgery.

Most air leaks that are related to primary spontaneous pneumothorax seal within 24 to 48 hours of tube drainage, and only 3% to 5% of patients have a persistent fistula (Seremetis, 1970). Because it has been shown that continuing drainage for periods of 8 to 10 days results in only minimal increases in pulmonary healing (Schoenenberger et al, 1991), surgery is recommended after 3 to 4 days of tube drainage (Baumann and Strange, 1997; Granke et al, 1986). If the lung only partially re-expands because of a significant air leak or associated pachypleuritis, surgery may also be necessary to decorticate the lung, resect the site of the fistula, and proceed with pleurodesis.

The occurrence of simultaneous bilateral pneumothoraces is uncommon, but when it occurs it should be followed by definitive surgery on one side (Graf-Dewel and Knoblauch, 1994). In patients with significant hemothoraces, surgery may also be urgently required for definitive control of the bleeding site. Secondary large clotted hemothoraces (more than 1000 ml) inadequately drained may lead to late complications, such as empyema and fibrothorax, and therefore should be evacuated.

Patients at risk of developing pneumothoraces in relation to their occupation, such as flight personnel or scuba divers, may be treated by surgery at the time of the first episode (Clark et al, 1972). Patients living in isolated areas or patients who travel frequently, especially those with evidence of bullae on chest radiographs, may also be candidates for early surgery. The management of a pneumothorax that occurs in a pregnant woman during the first trimester or near parturition should be conservative.

Tension occurring during the first episode is an absolute indication to proceed with surgery. Because of the high risk of recurrence in patients in whom a single large bulla is identified on chest radiograph or CT scan, surgery is also recommended (Gaensler et al, 1986). In those patients, when CT scanning clearly identifies multiple subpleural blebs, it is not clear whether surgery should be recommended because nobody has ever reported the incidence of recurrences in such individuals.

Recurrence is the most common indication for surgery in patients with primary spontaneous pneumothoraces. We agree with Murray and colleagues (1993) that a patient who has a recurrence should be spared tube drainage and undergo fairly immediate surgical treatment. When a recurrence occurs during pregnancy, surgical treatment can be carried out safely during the second trimester (Dhalla and Teskey, 1985).

Principles of Surgery. The principles involved in the surgical treatment of spontaneous pneumothoraces include resection of blebs and bullae and obliteration of the pleural space.

In most patients, simple wedge resection of the apical blebs is sufficient to control the disease (Lichter, 1974), although multiple wedge resections may be required when there are blebs at several sites (Brooks, 1973). Anatomic segmentectomies or lobectomies are usually unnecessary. With the exception of Ferguson and coworkers (1981), who recommended bulla resection without pleurodesis, most authors combine blebectomy with some type of procedure to obliterate the pleural space. There is still some debate about whether parietal pleurectomy without blebectomy is sufficient to prevent recurrences (Schramel et al, 1997).

Obliteration of the pleural space can be accomplished by parietal pleurectomy or mechanical abrasion. Both of these methods create an inflammatory surface with secondary "fixation" of the lung to the endothoracic fascia. Gaensler (1956) was the first to describe the use of pleurectomy, and Thomas and Gebauer (1958) were the first to report on its efficacy. Askew (1976) and Deslauriers and colleagues (1980) have shown that a pleurectomy limited to the apex creates sufficient adhesion to prevent recurrences. The morbidity associated with apical pleurectomy is generally low, but some authors (Weeden and Smith, 1983) have reported a significant rate of complications after subtotal pleurectomy. Most authors have reported no operative deaths. In a follow-up study, Gaensler (1956) showed no impairment of respiratory function after pleurectomy, and Singh (1982) and Weeden and Smith (1983) also found no differences in pulmonary function between prepleurectomy and postpleurectomy values. The results of pleurectomy are usually excellent with recurrence rates of 1% to 5% (Caes et al, 1987; Deslauriers et al, 1980; Ferraro et al, 1994).

Pleural abrasion produces effective obliteration of the pleural space (Moores, 1990) and has the added advantages of preserving an extrapleural plane and involving lower postoperative morbidity (Pairolero and Payne, 1986) than does pleurectomy. The recurrence rate of pneumothorax after pleural abrasion was 2.3% in nine reported series reviewed by Weeden and Smith (1983). In 1992, Maggi and associates reported on 94 patients treated by pleural abrasion; 80 patients followed for 7 to 91 months postoperatively had no recurrences. Failure to identify and ablate blebs may, however, result in a significantly higher recurrence rate (Naunheim et al, 1995).

Surgical Approaches. A full posterolateral thoracotomy is seldom necessary for the treatment of spontaneous pneumothoraces because the apex of the lung can be resected, and a pleurectomy or pleural abrasion can easily be done through a less invasive and more cosmetically acceptable axillary incision (Becker and Munro, 1976; Deslauriers et al, 1980; Ferraro et al, 1994; Murray et al, 1993). A minimal thoracotomy through the auscultatory triangle (Donahue et al, 1993; Lau and Shawkat, 1982) has also been described as an alternative to the axillary incision.

At surgery, apical blebs are readily identified and resected. The apical pleurectomy can be started at the site of the incision, and the pleura can be stripped from the endothoracic fascia up to the apex. Bleeding is controlled with hemoclips and electrocautery. If necessary, the remaining parietal pleura can also be abraded with a dry gauze sponge. A single 28 F chest tube is left in the pleural place; this tube can often be removed within 48 hours of the surgery. Most patients are discharged from the hospital by the third postoperative day. Some surgeons advocate the use of a median sternotomy (Ikeda et al, 1988; Kalnins et al, 1973; Neal et al, 1979) when bilateral disease is present, but we think it is seldom indicated and much prefer bilateral staged operations.

Levi and coauthors (1990) were the first to describe the use of VATS for the treatment of primary spontaneous pneumothoraces. Subsequently, Nathanson and colleagues (1991) presented a detailed description of the VATS approach, including anesthesia, the patient's position, trocar placement, insufflation, inspection of the lung, and technique for bleb ligation and pleurectomy.

The procedure is performed using general anesthesia and a double-lumen endotracheal tube. Three ports of entry are usually necessary to introduce a rigid telescope with video attachment and other instruments to perform the blebectomy, pleurectomy, or pleural abrasion (Janssen et al, 1994; Kleinman et al, 1991).

Proper port placement is essential to produce the triangulation that is necessary for full access to all lung zones and to eliminate crisscrossing of instruments. Selection of the appropriate intercostal space for placement of trocars is adjusted according to the patient's morphology. Blebs are best resected with an endoscopic linear stapler followed by pleural abrasion or subtotal parietal pleurectomy (Kleinman et al, 1991). At completion of the procedure, a single chest tube is left in the pleural space; this tube is removed within 2 to 3 days of the operation or when the air leak has stopped. Most patients have minimal early postoperative discomfort, although chronic postoperative pain requiring analgesic medication is always possible after VATS procedures. Operative morbidity is minimal.

Several authors (Mouroux et al 1996; Naunheim et al, 1995; Schramel et al, 1995) have reported the results for large series of treated patients. In 1996, Bertrand and associates reported a series of 163 patients who were treated by stapling of bullae and pleural abrasion. During follow-up, only three patients developed a recurrence that required reoperation, and three other patients had a limited recurrence that was treated conservatively. Similarly, Freixinet and colleagues (1997) reported a series of 132 young patients who were treated by VATS apical blebectomy and pleural abrasion. Although the follow-up was relatively short, the results were comparable with those obtained with open approaches. In the series of Passlick and associates (1998), conversion to lateral thoracotomy was necessary in 9% of patients with primary spontaneous pneumothorax and 10% of patients with secondary spontaneous pneumothorax. Postoperative complications were uncommon, and recurrences occurred in 4.8% with a median follow-up of 29 months. A summary of the VATS experience is shown in Table 42–5.

TABLE 42–5 ■ **Results of Video Thoracoscopic Surgery in the Management of Primary Spontaneous Pneumothorax**

Authors	*No. of Cases*	*Procedure*	*Recurrence Rate (%)*	*Follow-up (mo)*
Inderbitzi et al (1994)	70	R/P	8.3	19.6
Liu et al (1995)	82	R/P	0	22
Naunheim et al (1995)	113	R/P	4	13.1
Schramel et al (1995)	97	R/P	4	24.1
Bertrand et al (1996)	163	R/P	3.8	24.5
Mouroux et al (1996)	97	R/P	3	30
Freixinet et al (1997)	132	R/P	6	—
Passlick et al (1998)	99	R	4.8	29

R, resection of blebs; P, pleurodesis by pleurectomy or abrasion.

Comparison of Video-Assisted Thoracic Surgery Techniques and Axillary Thoracotomy. Some authors have tried to document the superiority of VATS over conventional thoracotomy in the treatment of primary spontaneous pneumothoraces. In a prospective controlled randomized study (Waller et al, 1993), 60 patients with spontaneous pneumothorax were treated by VATS or posterolateral thoracotomy. Patients undergoing VATS had significantly longer operative time, but patients who had a thoracotomy had more severe alterations of their postoperative pulmonary function. No differences were found in duration of tube drainage, treatment failure, recurrence, or operative mortality. The authors concluded that VATS was superior to thoracotomy because of lower postoperative analgesic requirement and decreased duration of hospitalization.

In 1997, Jiménez-Merchan and coworkers reported the results of a retrospective analysis comparing 110 patients with pneumothorax treated by VATS with 627 patients treated by thoracotomy. Decreased postoperative pain, faster recovery, and shorter length of hospital stay were found in the VATS group. Atta and colleagues (1997) also reported that VATS was as safe and effective in the treatment of recurrences as thoracotomy.

In a retrospective study, Cole and associates (1995) compared 89 patients treated by axillary thoracotomy with 30 patients who underwent VATS procedures. The authors failed to demonstrate any advantage of VATS over axillary thoracotomy in terms of hospital stay or morbidity. Kim and colleagues (1996) also showed no advantages of VATS over axillary thoracotomy with regard to operating time, amount of analgesics used during the first postoperative day, duration of tube drainage, and number of postoperative recurrences. Indeed, Horio and coworkers (1998) showed that the recurrence rate after VATS was double that seen after limited axillary thoracotomy. In 1997, Dumont and coauthors compared the result of axillary thoracotomy in 237 patients with thoracoscopic treatment in 101 patients. There were no major differences between the two groups with regard to chest tube duration and hospital stay. The overall morbidity was 16% in the axillary thoracotomy group and 11% in the thoracoscopic group.

With VATS now being easily available, we use a combination of small transaxillary intercostal thoracotomy (5 cm) and one thoracoscopic port incision for a video camera. The resection of the blebs or lung parenchyma and the apical pleurectomy and extensive gauze abrasion of the parietal pleura are done through the open incision under thoracoscopic guidance. Postoperative pain is minimal because the transaxillary incision is never spread open by thoracic retractors. A single chest tube is left through the port site.

Medical Thoracoscopic Approach

In Europe, "medical" thoracoscopy has long been used for the diagnosis and treatment of spontaneous pneumothoraces (Boutin et al, 1991; Swierenga et al, 1974). According to its proponents, the technique allows proper staging of the disease and treatment according to endoscopic findings. In 1988, Verschoof and colleagues even suggested that thoracoscopy should be performed routinely at the time of the first episode to classify patients in one of three categories: (1) no obvious abnormalities, (2) small apical blebs, and (3) more generalized bullous disease. The decision to perform thoracoscopic chemical pleurodesis or open surgery is based on thoracoscopic findings, and patients with generalized bullae or larger blebs are selected for early surgical treatment (Janssen et al, 1994; Vanderschueren, 1990; Wied et al, 1983).

In 1991, Gillet-Juvin and Guérin described thoracoscopic talc poudrage done under local anesthesia for the treatment of pneumothoraces associated with large emphysematous bullae. In their series of 71 patients, the results were good to excellent in 93% of cases, with minimal morbidity. In 1997, Tschopp and associates also reported on 93 patients treated by thoracoscopic talc pleurodesis performed under local anesthesia. The procedure was successful in 95% of patients with a mean follow-up of 5 years.

In 1997, Nezu and coauthors reported the results of thoracoscopic resection of blebs performed with local anesthesia and mild sedation in 34 consecutive patients without preoperative evidence of hemodynamic instability or arterial blood gas abnormalities. Only one patient had a recurrence, 3 months after the procedure. In general, talc poudrage is an accepted technique for patients with COPD or cystic fibrosis, but it is controversial for the management of primary spontaneous pneumothorax (Waller, 1997).

In 1989, Hansen and associates reported on 35 patients with spontaneous pneumothorax who were treated by the application of an aerosol of fibrin glue nebulized over the lung surface under thoracoscopic control. Treatment failed in two patients, and nine additional patients had recurrences. Takevo (1993) also reported a series of 163 patients in whom initial treatment with chest tube drainage had failed. These patients were subsequently treated with nebulization of fibrin glue with a success rate of 80%.

With the development of VATS, electrocautery (Wakabayashi 1989) and endoscopic laser ablation of blebs (LoCicero et al, 1985) have become surgical options in the management of pneumothoraces. Torre and Belloni (1989) were the first to report a significant experience with neodymium:yttrium-aluminum-garnet (Nd:YAG) laser pleurodesis done through a thoracoscope. They reported on 14 patients treated by coagulation of the apical blebs and scarification of the parietal pleura. Thirteen of the 14 patients had no recurrences during a follow-up averaging 29 months. In 1990, Wakabayashi and colleagues described the use of a carbon dioxide laser in the treatment of patients with apical blebs and diffuse bullous emphysema. The procedure was conducted using general anesthesia with a double-lumen endotracheal tube in the presence of a collapsed lung. Two small openings were made over the anterior and posterior axillary lines at the level of the fifth interspace, and these were used to introduce the thoracoscope and one operating instrument. Pleural adhesions were first divided with endoscopic scissors and electrocautery, and then the entire inner surface of the lung was exposed to the carbon dioxide laser.

The use of the argon beam electrocoagulator was evaluated in 1990 by Rusch and coauthors, who considered its effectiveness in controlling blood loss and sealing air leaks. It functions in a noncontact manner and appears to be safe and efficient and causes less tissue injury than does standard electrocautery. In 1993, Wakabayashi presented results obtained for electrocautery obliteration of blebs under thoracoscopic guidance in a series of 10 patients with spontaneous pneumothorax. The technique was effective for blebs but somewhat less so for bullae, with a failure rate of 15%. Takevo (1993) also reported a recurrence rate of 18.6% for thoracoscopic electrocoagulation of blebs in patients with spontaneous pneumothorax.

Nonsurgical Therapy

Some clinicians use chemical pleurodesis as first-line treatment for recurrences. The use of these techniques is, however, much debated, and surgeons have generally been concerned about the liberal use of chemicals in the pleural space for the treatment of benign diseases. Many agents, such as quinacrine (Janssen et al, 1994; Janzing et al, 1993; Larrieu et al, 1979), autologous blood (Robinson, 1987), and bleomycin (Hantiuk et al, 1990) as well as tetracycline and talc, have been used for that purpose.

Because of its low pH and irritating effect, tetracycline has long been used in the management of malignant pleural effusions (Sahn et al, 1979). It was instilled through a chest tube at a dose of 500 mg to 1 g diluted in 250 ml of normal saline. To reduce pleuritic pain, lidocaine (250 mg of 1% solution) or ketamine (Stephenson, 1985) was added to the solution. In 1990, Light and colleagues reported the results of a prospective multicenter randomized and controlled clinical trial in which tetracycline was used intrapleurally to prevent recurrences of pneumothoraces. The results were disappointing, with a 25% recurrence rate at 5 years in the tetracycline-treated group. Intrapleural tetracycline injection is no longer available because the production of this drug has been discontinued (Heffner et al, 1994).

Talc is a powder of hydrous magnesium silicate containing different contaminants, which has been shown to be effective in treating malignant pleural effusions and spontaneous pneumothoraces (Vanderschueren, 1981). Commercially available purified talc is free of asbestos and considered safe for therapeutic use (Selikoff et al, 1987). It is effective in inducing pleural fibrosis and adhesions, but the morbidity associated with its use includes fever, pain, and possible impairment of pulmonary function. Talc can be injected through a chest tube in suspension form (2 g to 5 g diluted in 50 ml to 250 ml of normal saline) (Kennedy and Sahn, 1994) or sprinkled with a syringe over the entire pleural surfaces (Weisberg, 1986). It can also be insufflated in its powder form through a thoracoscope (Gillet-Juvin and Guérin, 1991) or with a talc insufflator (Deslauriers and Piraux, 1990).

The most compelling concern about using talc to treat spontaneous pneumothoraces is the risk of inducing respiratory failure, as noted by Kennedy and associates (1995). Because of this possible complication, it is now recommended that the maximum dose for intrapleural use is 5 g (Kennedy et al, 1994). In a study reported in 1989, Viskum and coauthors found no evidence of impaired pulmonary function in a group of 99 patients, and in a series of patients reported by Lange and colleagues (1988), there was only mild restrictive impairment without clinical significance 22 to 25 years after talc insufflation. The world's experience with the use of talc to treat pneumothoraces was reviewed in 1991 by Boutin and colleagues. In 75 reported series, the recurrence rate was approximately 7%.

Surgeons are generally concerned about the use of chemopleurodesis in patients who may eventually require thoracotomy because it may be associated with higher morbidity rates. At present, chemical pleurodesis should be used only in selected cases in which surgery is too dangerous or impossible.

Rate of Recurrence After Therapy

The rate of recurrence after various therapies was analyzed by Boutin and colleagues (1991) and found to vary from 2% to 30%, depending on the type of treatment. Recurrences are definitely more common when patients are treated by observation, long-term tube thoracostomy, or chemical pleurodesis; better results are achieved by surgery.

In 1997, Schramel and coauthors reviewed several series and reported their own results. For patients treated with bed rest, needle aspiration, and chest tube drainage (series from 1963 to 1995 including 1242 patients), the recurrence rate was 30%. In surgical series from 1957 to 1993 including 977 patients, the recurrence rate after conventional surgical treatment was 1.5% with a follow-up from 5 to 10 years. The authors also reported the results obtained with VATS in series from 1993 to 1995 involving 805 patients, in which the recurrence rate was 4%.

SECONDARY SPONTANEOUS PNEUMOTHORAX

Spontaneous pneumothorax can be secondary to a variety of pulmonary or nonpulmonary disorders (Table 42–6). According to Schoenenberger and coworkers (1991), most patients with secondary pneumothoraces are male, are older than 45 years, and have documented or clinically apparent pulmonary disease. The most common causes of secondary spontaneous pneumothorax are listed in Table 42–6.

Pneumothorax Secondary to Chronic Obstructive Pulmonary Disease

COPD is the most common cause of secondary pneumothorax, which almost always occurs in patients older than 50 years and results from the rupture of emphysematous bullae.

Most patients with COPD and pneumothorax have chest pain and acute respiratory distress with hypoxia, hypercarbia, and acidosis. Because of their limited pulmonary function, these patients often show little tolerance for even a small pneumothorax. The clinical diagnosis may be difficult to establish because the physical findings are those of COPD with hyper-resonance on percussion and diminished breath sounds at auscultation. The cor-

TABLE 42–6 ■ **Common Causes of Secondary Spontaneous Pneumothorax**

AIRWAY AND PULMONARY DISEASE
Chronic obstructive pulmonary disease (bullous or diffuse emphysema)
Asthma
Cystic fibrosis
INTERSTITIAL LUNG DISEASE
Pulmonary fibrosis
Sarcoidosis
INFECTIOUS DISEASE
Tuberculosis and other mycobacterial infections
Bacterial infections
Pneumocystis carinii infections
Parasitic infections
Mycotic infections
AIDS
NEOPLASTIC
Bronchogenic carcinoma
Metastatic (lymphoma or sarcoma)
CATAMENIAL (ENDOMETRIOSIS)
MISCELLANEOUS
Marfan's syndrome
Ehlers-Danlos syndrome
Histiocytosis X
Scleroderma
Lymphangiomyomatosis
Collagen diseases

rect diagnosis is made by chest radiography, which on occasion may be difficult to interpret because of the increased radiolucency of the diseased lung. In those cases, CT scanning is helpful in confirming the diagnosis and localizing the pneumothorax (Bourgouin et al, 1985). Under certain circumstances, a CT scan may also help to distinguish between a large bulla and a pneumothorax.

In 1987, Videm and associates showed that because of decreased lung vascularization, patients with COPD and pneumothorax are more likely to have prolonged air leaks, leading to higher incidences of in-hospital infections and empyema. If the pleural space is adequately drained and the lung is maintained in a re-expanded state by suction drainage, the air leak eventually stops. In some patients, however, a persistent bronchopleural fistula may necessitate open thoracotomy or thoracoscopy. The recurrence rate varies widely. In 1986, Granke and colleagues reported a 22% recurrence rate in patients treated by chest tube drainage but no recurrences in patients who had surgery. Similarly, Seremetis (1970) reported a 49% recurrence rate in patients treated with observation, a 38% recurrence rate in patients treated by tube drainage, and no recurrence after open thoracotomy.

Most often, tube thoracostomy with or without pleurodesis is the first-line treatment for recurrences (Tanaka et al, 1993). Subsequently, the choice of therapy is based on the severity and duration of symptoms, severity of underlying parenchymal disease, number of previous episodes, occupation of the patient, and experience of the surgical team. Although the fear of operative risk tends to justify prolonged conservative treatment, Baumann and Strange (1997) recommended that a surgical decision is made early after tube drainage has been initiated.

If surgery becomes necessary, the procedure must be individualized for each patient and based on the extent of disease and presumed location of the air leak. Ligation or staple resection of bullae followed by subtotal parietal pleurectomy or pleural abrasion is the best surgical option. The operative mortality may reach 10% (Keszler, 1990; Martigne et al, 1984), and the morbidity is also significant (Weeden and Smith, 1983).

The use of VATS was described by Waller and coworkers in 1994. This approach requires one-lung ventilation, which may cause ventilatory problems during surgery. Thus, flexibility in the anesthetic technique is required. Before proceeding with surgery, CT scanning should always be done to locate the bullae and facilitate trocar placement without damaging the lung. For the same reason, digital palpation is necessary before inserting the trocars. After full mobilization of the apex by division of adhesions, an operative decision can be made regarding possible bulla resection and pleurectomy. Some authors (Tanaka et al, 1993) believe that pleural abrasion alone is associated with an unacceptable rate of recurrence.

In 1994, Waller and colleagues reported an operative morbidity of 23%, a mortality rate of 9%, and a mean postoperative stay after surgery of 9 days in a series of 22 patients who had undergone VATS for secondary pneumothoraces. Some authors (Graham et al, 1995) believed that thoracotomy allows better direct oversewing of emphysematous bullae and is therefore a more effective and safer procedure than VATS.

Other surgical procedures such as electrocautery, talc insufflation (Daniel et al, 1993), and use of the carbon dioxide laser or Nd:YAG laser can also be used for the treatment of these patients. In individuals with poor overall physical condition, anesthesia may be risky, and alternative options such as tube chemical pleurodesis (Almassi and Haasler, 1989), autologous blood injection (Robinson, 1987), and permanent drainage with a fistula (Hood et al, 1986) should be considered.

Pneumothorax Secondary to Cystic Fibrosis

Pneumothorax, which occurs in about 10% of patients with cystic fibrosis, may lead to life-threatening situations in patients with poor lung function. Although the outcome of conservative therapy is associated with a high rate of recurrence, the possibility of subsequent lung transplantation has to be considered before making a decision about surgery (Tribble et al, 1986) and pleural abrasion. At present, the best surgical option is a thoracoscopic approach with lung resection and limited pleurodesis (Noyes and Orenstein, 1992). Noppen and coauthors (1994) also reported successful treatment by localized apical thoracoscopic talc poudrage.

Pneumothorax Secondary to Infection

Pneumothorax can be secondary to lung infection (bacterial, viral, mycotic, or parasitic), pleural infection (empyema), or intra-abdominal infection (subphrenic abscess). Cavitary pulmonary infections are particularly prone to rupture with secondary pneumothoraces. Pulmonary tuberculosis, for instance, is known to be associated with pneumothoraces that often require prolonged periods of tube drainage (Wilder et al, 1962). In these patients, surgery should not be undertaken until the patient has received adequate systemic antituberculous therapy.

Pneumothorax and Acquired Immunodeficiency Syndrome

Since the early 1980s, several reports have described the association of spontaneous pneumothorax, pneumomediastinum, and AIDS (Byrnes et al, 1989). These pneumothoraces are usually secondary to *P. carinii* pneumonia (Joe et al, 1986). In 1987, DeLorenzo and associates reported a 6% incidence of pneumothorax in the AIDS population, with pneumothorax occasionally being the initial manifestation of the disease (Kuhlman et al, 1989). In AIDS patients, the pneumothorax may remain small and asymptomatic, but it may also enlarge rapidly and come under tension, causing severe respiratory failure. In this population, there is also an increased incidence of synchronous bilateral pneumothoraces, significant bronchopleural fistulas, and higher rates of both ipsilateral and contralateral recurrences.

The high incidence of pneumothoraces in AIDS patients is probably the result of cystic lesions that are most common at apices and consist of subpleural air spaces filled with eosinophilic exudate, *P. carinii* organisms, fibrous material, and macrophages (Travis et al, 1990).

Histologic studies suggested that such lesions are the result of infection associated with tissue destruction and fibrosis (DeLorenzo et al, 1987).

Whenever possible, the initial management should be conservative; sometimes small pneumothoraces resolve with observation alone. Unfortunately, most patients have large and persistent air leaks that eventually require tube thoracostomy (Byrnes et al, 1989; Fleisher et al, 1988). On occasion, patients may be treated on an outpatient basis with a one-way flutter valve (Driver et al, 1991; Trachiotis et al, 1996).

To prevent recurrences, chemical pleurodesis has been used but without good results (Chechani, 1990; Slabbynck et al, 1994). Surgical resection of the diseased area with pleurectomy remains the most effective mode of therapy. Although significant operative mortality rates have been reported, Beers and coauthors (1990) suggested that AIDS patients can tolerate surgery reasonably well and that most do not require mechanical ventilation during the postoperative period. Treatment with VATS and talc poudrage can also be used to control the pneumothorax and associated air leak (Wait, 1997). When bilateral disease is present, median sternotomy (Byrnes et al, 1989) and bilateral staged axillary thoracotomies (Wait, 1997) are options. Fortunately, the introduction of new medical therapies for AIDS has led to a decrease in the incidence of related pneumothoraces.

Pneumothorax and Neoplasia

Occasionally, bronchial obstruction by a lung cancer may lead to a pneumothorax, which may also develop as the result of pleural space rupture of an ischemic primary tumor or metastasis. Pneumothoraces may also occur during chemotherapy (Lote et al, 1981) or radiotherapy.

Pneumothoraces are commonly associated with metastatic sarcomas (Dines et al, 1973; Karlawish et al, 1995; Smevik and Klepp, 1982) but have also been described with teratomas, Wilms' tumors, melanomas, carcinomas of the kidney and pancreas, gynecologic malignancies (Helmkamp et al, 1982), lymphomas (Yellin and Benfield, 1986), choriocarcinomas (Ouellette and Inculet, 1992), and lymphangiomatosis (Warren et al, 1993).

In these patients, closed-tube drainage is the therapy of choice; surgery is seldom indicated. On occasion, chemical pleurodesis may be used to prevent recurrences (Rammohan et al, 1986).

Catamenial Pneumothorax

Pneumothoraces occurring within 48 to 72 hours of the onset of menstruation were first described by Maurer and Schall (1958) and Lillington and coauthors (1972). According to Nakamura and associates (1986), catamenial pneumothorax may afflict up to 3% to 6% of women between 20 and 30 years of age. Most catamenial pneumothoraces are on the right side, and they may be recurrent over several years before being diagnosed. They are usually small, and patients present with chest pain and dyspnea (Carter and Etten Sohn, 1990).

The pathogenesis of catamenial pneumothorax is still unclear (Fonseca, 1998). Air may reach the pleural space from the cervix and abdomen through congenital diaphragmatic defects (Maurer and Schall, 1958), or there may be focal thoracic endometrial implants on the visceral pleura or in the lung, with air leakage occurring during menstruation. Endometrial implants may also obstruct bronchioles, causing distal hyperinflation and alveolar rupture (Lillington et al, 1972). Increased levels of prostaglandin F_2 tromethamine at the time of menses may also cause bronchial and vascular constriction, leading to alveolar rupture and subsequent pneumothorax. It is likely that several of these mechanisms are involved simultaneously in the development of catamenial pneumothoraces.

Management is similar to that of other types of pneumothoraces; small and asymptomatic episodes may be treated conservatively, and large and symptomatic episodes require chest tube drainage. The management of recurrence is more controversial, and several options are possible according to Carter and Etten Sohn (1990): (1) treatment of each episode with tube thoracostomy, (2) use of oral contraceptives or weak androgens to suppress ovulation, (3) chemical pleurodesis, (4) hysterectomy and bilateral oophorectomy, and (5) thoracotomy with pleural abrasion or pleurectomy.

In 1990, Fleisher and associates proposed a treatment algorithm taking into consideration whether hormonal therapy is contraindicated and pregnancy desired or not. In their opinion, thoracotomy is indicated when pregnancy is desired or when laparoscopic tubal ligation is contraindicated.

Miscellaneous

Other diseases that have sometimes been associated with pneumothorax include Marfan's syndrome (Sensenig and Lamarche, 1980), Ehlers-Danlos syndrome, histiocytosis X, pulmonary infarction, interstitial fibrosis, eosinophilic granuloma, sarcoidosis, and tuberous sclerosis.

PRIMARY SPONTANEOUS PNEUMOMEDIASTINUM

Primary spontaneous pneumomediastinum was first described in 1939 by Hamman. It is an uncommon and benign condition that occurs more frequently in men than in women. In contrast to primary spontaneous pneumothorax, spontaneous pneumomediastinum usually occurs after physical exertion or after an increase in intra-abdominal pressure (McMahon, 1976; Vass and Keszler, 1990). According to Yellin and colleagues (1983), asthmatic patients may also be more prone to develop primary spontaneous pneumomediastinum. Drug inhalation or marijuana, crack, or cocaine usage is also frequently associated with the development of primary spontaneous pneumomediastinum (Panacek et al, 1992).

Spontaneous pneumomediastinum results from the rupture of alveoli and alveolar septa. The interstitial air dissects along the peribronchial and perivascular spaces to reach the mediastinum and eventually the neck through the mediastinocervical fascia (Keszler, 1988).

In most cases of pneumomediastinum, chest pain is a major symptom, although incapacitating dyspnea, dysphagia, and cough may also be present. In 1994, Ralph-Edwards and Pearson reported two patients with spontaneous pneumomediastinum who presented with odynophagia and dysphagia that were suggestive of esophageal perforation. Subsequent investigation, however, showed no evidence of esophageal perforation, and the symptoms resolved rapidly.

In primary spontaneous pneumomediastinum, physical examination often reveals subcutaneous emphysema, which can be felt over the neck or chest wall, and a continuous murmur, which may be heard over the apex of the heart (Hamman's sign). The diagnosis is confirmed by chest radiography, but other investigations may also be required to rule out esophageal or tracheal perforation (Gray and Hanson, 1966).

After other causes of mediastinal emphysema have been ruled out, primary spontaneous pneumomediastinum can be treated expectantly. Only rarely is emergency surgical decompression required. If air dissects into the pleural space and creates a pneumothorax, tube thoracostomy may be necessary (Abolnik et al, 1991).

COMMENTS AND CONTROVERSIES

I agree with the authors on most of their views on the management of spontaneous pneumothoraces. The relative merits of the VATS approach and the limited axillary incision are still debated, although it appears that the results are similar in terms of both operative morbidity and prevention of recurrences. When performing surgery in young people with primary and recurrent spontaneous pneumothorax, it is probably more important to perform an adequate pleurodesis than to remove the blebs, which could recur over time. This pleurodesis should, however, be limited to the apex, and although we still prefer parietal pleurectomy, pleural abrasion is probably just as effective. The use of intrapleural talc or of any other product is not recommended in young people because their long-term effects are still not well documented.

The problems associated with pneumothoraces secondary to COPD are different because all of these patients are older, often have comorbidities, and, in general, present with a much higher risk of recurrence, an event that can be poorly tolerated in individuals with limited pulmonary reserve. This is why we recommend early surgery, often during the first episode if the patient has an acceptable operative risk. In these individuals, the emergence of the VATS approach has considerably changed the magnitude of operation, which can be done with low operative morbidity or mortality even in high-risk cases. In this population, the use of talc is perfectly safe and efficient.

J.D.

KEY REFERENCES

Boutin C, Viallat JR, Aelony Y: Practical Thoracoscopy. Berlin, Springer-Verlag, 1991.

This book has an excellent chapter on the thoracoscopic management of pneumothoraces.

Deslauriers J, Lacquet LK: Surgical management of pleural diseases. In: International Trends in General Thoracic Surgery, Vol. 6. St. Louis, Mosby–Year Book, 1990.

In this volume devoted to the pleural space, there are several good chapters written on the management of different types of pneumothoraces.

Hood MR, Antman K, Boyd A et al.: Surgical Diseases of the Pleura and Chest Wall. Philadelphia, WB Saunders, 1986.

This is a book devoted to the surgical approach of pleural diseases, including a well-written chapter on pneumothoraces.

Killen DA, Gobbel WG: Spontaneous Pneumothorax. Boston, Little, Brown, 1968.

Although published more than 20 years ago, this book remains a classic in the understanding of pneumothoraces and is the most complete review of the history of pneumothoraces.

Light RW: Pleural Diseases, 3rd ed. Philadelphia, Lea & Febiger, 1995.

A complete review of the diagnosis and treatment of pleural diseases is provided with a good chapter on primary and secondary pneumothoraces.

REFERENCES

Abolnik I, Lossos IS, Brewer R: Spontaneous pneumomediastinum: A report of 25 cases. Chest 100:93, 1991.

Adesina AM, Vallyathan V, McQuillen EN et al: Bronchiolar inflammation and fibrosis associated with smoking: A morphologic cross-sectional population analysis. Am Rev Respir Dis 143:144, 1991.

Agostini E: Mechanics of the pleural space. In Fishman AP (ed): Handbook of Physiology, Sect 3, Vol 3. Bethesda, MD, American Physiological Society, 1986, p 531.

Almassi GH, Haasler GB: Chemical pleurodesis in the presence of persistent air leak. Ann Thorac Surg 47:786, 1989.

Andrivet P, Djedaini K, Teboul JL et al: Spontaneous pneumothorax: Comparison of thoracic drainage vs immediate or delayed needle aspiration. Chest 108:335, 1995.

Anthonisen NR: Regional lung function in spontaneous pneumothorax. Am Rev Respir Dis 115:873, 1977.

Archer GJ, Hamilton AAD, Upadhyay R, Finlay M: Results of simple aspiration of pneumothoraces. Br J Dis Chest 19:177, 1985.

Askew AR: Parietal pleurectomy for recurrent pneumothorax. Br J Surg 63:203, 1976.

Atta HM, Latouf O, Moore JE, et al: Thoracotomy versus video-assisted thoracoscopic pleurectomy for spontaneous pneumothorax. Am Surg 63:209, 1997.

Axel L: A simple way to estimate the size of a pneumothorax. Invest Radiol 16:165, 1981.

Baumann MH, Strange C: Treatment of spontaneous pneumothorax: A more aggressive approach? Chest 112:789, 1997.

Baumann MH, Sahn SA: Tension pneumothorax: Diagnostic and therapeutic pitfall. Crit Care Med 21:177, 1993.

Baumann MH, Sahn SA: Hamman's sign revisited: Pneumothorax or pneumomediastinum? Chest 102:1281, 1992.

Becker RM, Munro DD: Transaxillary minithoracotomy: The optimal approach for certain pulmonary and mediastinal lesions. Ann Thorac Surg 22:254, 1976.

Beers MF, John M, Swartz M: Recurrent pneumothorax in AIDS patients with *Pneumocystis* pneumonia. Chest 98:266, 1990.

Bense L, Edlund G, Hedenstierna G, Wiman LG: Nonsmoking, non-alpha, antitrypsin deficiency–induced emphysema in nonsmokers with healed spontaneous pneumothorax, identified by computed tomography of the lungs. Chest 103:433, 1993.

Bense L, Eklund G, Wiman LG: Smoking and the increased risk of contracting spontaneous pneumothorax. Chest 92:1009, 1987.

Bense L: Spontaneous pneumothorax related to falls in atmospheric pressure. Eur J Respir Dis 65:544, 1984.

Bertrand PC, Regnard JF, Spaggiari L et al: Immediate and long-term results after surgical treatment of primary spontaneous pneumothorax by VATS. Ann Thorac Surg 61:1641, 1996.

Bevelaqua FA, Aranda C: Management of spontaneous pneumothorax with small lumen catheter manual aspiration. Chest 81:6, 1982.

Bigger IA: Operative Surgery. St. Louis, CV Mosby, 1937.

Bourgouin P, Cousineau G, Lemire P, Hebert G: Computed tomography used to exclude pneumothorax in bullous lung disease. Can Assoc Radiol J 36:341, 1985.

Boutin C, Viallat JR, Aelony Y: Practical Thoracoscopy. Berlin, Springer-Verlag, 1991.

Brooks JW: Open thoracotomy in the management of spontaneous pneumothorax. Ann Surg 177:798, 1973.

Byrnes TA, Brevig JK, Yeoh CB: Pneumothorax in patients with acquired immunodeficiency syndrome. J Thorac Cardiovasc Surg 98:546, 1989.

Caes F, Cham B, Van den Brande P, Welch W: Transaxillary thoracotomy for treatment of spontaneous pneumothorax. Acta Chir Belg 87:137, 1987.

Carr JJ, Reed JC, Choplin RH et al: Plain and computed radiography for detecting experimentally induced pneumothorax in cadavers: Implications for detection in patients. Radiology 183:193, 1992.

Carter JE, Etten Sohn DB: Catamenial pneumothorax. Chest 98:713, 1990.

Casola G, Vansonnenberg E, Keightley A et al: Pneumothorax: Radiologic treatment with small catheters. Radiology 166:89, 1988.

Chadha TS, Cohn MA: Noninvasive treatment of pneumothorax with oxygen inhalation. Respiration 44:147, 1983.

Chechani V: Tetracycline pleurodesis for persistent air leak. Ann Thorac Surg 49:166, 1990.

Chee CBE: Persistent air-leak in spontaneous pneumothorax: Clinical course and outcome. Respir Med 92:757, 1998.

Clagett OT: The management of spontaneous pneumothorax (Editorial). J Thorac Cardiovasc Surg 56:761, 1968.

Clague H, El-Ansory E: Conservative management of spontaneous pneumothorax. Lancet 1:687, 1984.

Clark TA, Hutchinson DE, Deaner RM et al: Spontaneous pneumothorax. Am J Surg 124:728, 1972.

Cole FH, Cole FH, Khandekar A et al: Video-assisted thoracic surgery: Primary therapy for spontaneous pneumothorax? Ann Thorac Surg 60:931, 1995.

Conces DJ, Tarver RD, Gray C et al: Treatment of pneumothoraces utilizing small caliber chest tubes. Chest 95:55, 1988.

Cormier Y: Gas transfer in the pleural space. In Deslauriers J, Lacquet LK (eds): International Trends in General Thoracic Surgery, Vol 6. St. Louis, Mosby–Year Book, 1990, p 10.

Cran IR, Rumball CA: Surgery of spontaneous pneumothorax in the Royal Air Force. Thorax 22:462, 1967.

Daniel TM, Kern JA, Tribble CG et al: Thoracoscopic surgery for diseases of the lung and pleura. Ann Surg 217:566, 1993.

Davis JW, Mackersie RC, Hoyt DB, Garcia J: Randomized study of algorithms for discontinuing tube thoracostomy drainage. J Am Coll Surg 179:553, 1994.

Delius RE, Obeid FN, Horst HM et al: Catheter aspiration for simple pneumothorax. Arch Surg 124:833, 1989.

DeLorenzo LJ, Huang TC, Maguire JP, Stone DJ: Roentgenographic patterns of *Pneumocystis carinii* pneumonia in 104 patients with AIDS. Chest 91:323, 1987.

Dermksian G, Lamb LE: Spontaneous pneumothorax in apparently healthy flying personnel. Ann Intern Med 51:39, 1959.

Deslauriers J, Piraux M: Diagnosis and management of spontaneous pneumothorax in the young adult: Role of parietal pleurectomy. In Deslauriers J, Lacquet LK (eds): International Trends in General Thoracic Surgery, Vol 6. St. Louis, Mosby–Year Book, 1990, p 119.

Deslauriers J, Beaulieu M, Despres JP et al: Transaxillary thoracotomy for treatment of spontaneous pneumothorax. Ann Thorac Surg 30:35, 1980.

Desmeules M, Deslauriers J, Beauchamp G: Surgical anatomy of the pleura. In Deslauriers J, Lacquet LK (eds): International Trends in General Thoracic Surgery, Vol 6. St. Louis, Mosby–Year Book, 1990, p 13.

Despars JA, Sassoon CSH, Light RW: Significance of iatrogenic pneumothoraces. Chest 105:1147, 1994.

De Vries WC, Wolfe WG: The management of spontaneous pneumothorax in emphysema. Surg Clin North Am 60:851, 1981.

Dhalla SS, Teskey J: Surgical management of recurrent spontaneous pneumothorax during pregnancy. Chest 88:201, 1985.

Diamond JR, Estes MN: ECG changes associated with iatrogenic left pneumothorax simulating anterior myocardial infarction. Am Heart J 103:303, 1982.

Dines DE, Cortese DA, Brennon MD et al: Malignant pulmonary neoplasia predisposing to spontaneous pneumothorax. Mayo Clin Proc 48:541, 1973.

Dines DE, Clagett OT, Payne WS: Spontaneous pneumothorax in emphysema. Mayo Clin Proc 45:481, 1970.

Donahue M, Wright CD, Viale G, Mathisen DJ: Resection of pulmonary blebs and pleurodesis for spontaneous pneumothorax. Chest 104:1767, 1993.

Donovan PJ: Bilateral spontaneous pneumothorax. Ann Emerg Med 16:1277, 1987.

Driver GA, Peden JG, Adams HG, Rumley RL: Heimlich valve, treatment of *Pneumocystis carinii* associated pneumothorax. Chest 100:281, 1991.

Dumont P, Diemont F, Massard G et al: Does a thoracoscopic approach for surgical treatment of spontaneous pneumothorax represent progress? Eur J Cardiothorac Surg 11:27, 1997.

Edge J, Simon G, Reid L: Peri-acinar paraseptal emphysema: Its clinical, radiological, and physiological features. Br J Dis Chest 60:10, 1966.

Emerson CP: Pneumothorax: A historical, clinical and experimental study. Johns Hopkins Rep 11:1, 1903.

Ferguson LJ, Imrie CW, Hutchison J: Excision of bullae without pleurectomy in patients with spontaneous pneumothorax. Br J Surg 68:214, 1981.

Ferraro P, Beauchamp G, Lord F et al: Spontaneous primary and secondary pneumothorax: A 10-year study of management alternatives. Can J Surg 37(3):197, 1994.

Fleisher AG, Clement PB, Nelems B: Catamenial pneumothorax: Pathophysiology and management. In Deslauriers J, Lacquet LK (eds): International Trends in General Thoracic Surgery, Vol 6. St. Louis, Mosby–Year Book, 1990, p 132.

Fleisher AG, McElvaney G, Lawson L et al: Surgical management of spontaneous pneumothorax in patient with acquired immunodeficiency syndrome. Ann Thorac Surg 45:21, 1988.

Fonseca P: Catamenial pneumothorax: A multifactorial etiology. J Thorac Cardiovasc Surg 116:872, 1998.

Freixinet J, Canalis E, Rivas JJ et al: Surgical treatment of primary spontaneous pneumothorax with video-assisted thoracic surgery. Eur Respir J 10:409, 1997.

Fukuda Y, Haraguchi S, Tanaka S, Yamanaka N: Pathogenesis of blebs and bullae of patients with spontaneous pneumothorax: Ultrastructural and immunohistochemical studies. Am J Respir Crit Car Med 149:A1022, 1994.

Gaensler EA, Jederlinic PJ, Fitzgerald MY: Patient work-up for bullectomy. J Thorac Imaging 1:75, 1986.

Gaensler EA: Parietal pleurectomy for recurrent spontaneous pneumothorax. Surg Gynecol Obstet 102:293, 1956.

Getz SB, Beasely WE: Spontaneous pneumothorax. Am J Surg 145:823, 1983.

Gillet-Juvin K, Guérin JC: Le talcage sous thoracoscopie des pneumothorax par rupture de bulles d'emphysème. Rev Mal Respir 8:289, 1991.

Gilmartin JJ, Wright AJ, Gibson GJ: Effects of pneumothorax or pleural effusion on pulmonary function. Thorax 40:60, 1985.

Gobbel WG Jr, Rhea WG Jr, Nelson IA et al: Spontaneous pneumothorax. J Thorac Cardiovasc Surg 46:331, 1963.

Graf-Dewel E, Knoblauch A: Simultaneous bilateral spontaneous pneumothorax. Chest 105:1142, 1994.

Graham ANJ, McManus KG, McGuigan JA: Videothoracoscopy and spontaneous pneumothorax. Ann Thorac Surg 59:257, 1995.

Granke K, Fischer CR, Gago O et al: The efficacy and timing of operative intervention for spontaneous pneumothorax. Ann Thorac Surg 42:540, 1986.

Gray JM, Hanson GG: Mediastinal emphysema: Etiology, diagnosis and treatment. Thorax 21:325, 1966.

Gutsman P, Yerger L, Wanner A: Immediate cardiovascular effects on tension pneumothorax. Am Rev Respir Dis 127:171, 1983.

Hamman L: Spontaneous mediastinal emphysema. Bull Johns Hopkins Hosp 64:1, 1939.

Hansen MK, Kruse-Andersen S, Watt-Boolsen S: Spontaneous pneumothorax and fibrin glue sealant during thoracoscopy. Eur J Cardiothorac Surg 3:512, 1989.

Hantiuk OW, Dillard TA, Oster CN: Bleomycin sclerotherapy for bilateral pneumothoraces in a patient with AIDS. Ann Intern Med 113:988, 1990.

Heffner JE, Standerfer RJ, Torstveit J, Unruh L: Clinical efficacy of doxycycline for pleurodesis. Chest 105:1743, 1994.

Heimlich HJ: Valve drainage of the pleural cavity. Dis Chest 53:282, 1968.

Helmkamp BF, Beecham JB, Wandtke TJ, Keys H: Spontaneous pneumothorax in gynecologic malignancy. Am J Obstet Gynecol 142:706, 1982.

Hill RC, DeCarlo DP, Hill JF et al: Resolution of experimental pneumothorax in rabbits by oxygen therapy. Ann Thorac Surg 59:825, 1995.

Hood MR, Antman K, Boyd A et al: Surgical Disease of the Pleura and Chest Wall. Philadelphia, WB Saunders, 1986.

Horio H, Nomori H, Fuyuno G et al: Limited axillary thoracotomy vs video-assisted thoracoscopic surgery for spontaneous pneumothorax. Surg Endosc 12:1155, 1998.

Hunninghake GW, Crystal RG: Cigarette smoking and lung destruction: Accumulation of neutrophils in the lungs of cigarette smokers. Am Rev Respir Dis 128:833, 1983.

Hurewitz AN, Sidhu EH, Bergofsky B et al: Cardiovascular and respiratory consequences of tension pneumothorax. Bull Eur Physiopathol Respir 22:545, 1986.

Ikeda M, Uno A, Yamane Y, Hagiwara N: Median sternotomy with bilateral bullous resection for unilateral spontaneous pneumothorax, with special reference to operative indications. J Thorac Cardiovasc Surg 96:615, 1988.

Inderbitzi RGC, Leiser A, Furrer M, Althaus U: Three years' experience in video-assisted thoracic surgery (VATS) for spontaneous pneumothorax. J Thorac Cardiovasc Surg 107:1410, 1994.

Janssen JP, Mourik JV, Valentin MC et al: Treatment of patients with spontaneous pneumothorax during videothoracoscopy. Eur Respir J 7:1281, 1994.

Janzing HMJ, Derom A, Derom E et al: Intrapleural quinacrine instillation for recurrent pneumothorax or persistent air leak. Ann Thorac Surg 55:364, 1993.

Jiménez-Merchan R, Garcia-Diaz F, Arenas-Linares C et al: Comparative retrospective study of surgical treatment of spontaneous pneumothorax. Surg Endosc 11:919, 1997.

Joe L, Gorden F, Parker RH: Spontaneous pneumothorax with *Pneumocystis carinii* infection: Occurrence in patients with acquired immunodeficiency syndrome. Arch Intern Med 146:1816, 1986.

Kalnins I, Torda TA, Wright JS: Bilateral simultaneous pleurodesis by median sternotomy for spontaneous pneumothorax. Ann Thor Surg 15:202, 1973.

Karlawish JHT, Smith GW, Gabrielson EW, Liu MC: Spontaneous hemothorax caused by a chest wall chondrosarcoma. Ann Thorac Surg 59:231, 1995.

Kennedy L, Vaughan LM, Steed LL, Sahn SA: Sterilization of talc for pleurodesis. Chest 107:1032, 1995.

Kennedy L, Rusch VW, Strange C et al: Pleurodesis using talc slurry. Chest 106:342, 1994.

Kennedy L, Sahn SA: Talc pleurodesis for the treatment of pneumothorax and pleural effusion. Chest 106:1215, 1994.

Keszler P: Management of pneumothorax in the emphysematous patient. In Deslauriers J, Lacquet LK (eds): International Trends in General Thoracic Surgery, Vol 6. St. Louis, Mosby–Year Book, 1990, p 130.

Keszler P: Surgical pathology of bullae with and without pneumothorax. Eur J Cardiothorac Surg 2:146, 1988.

Killen DA, Gobbel WG: Spontaneous Pneumothorax. Boston, Little, Brown, 1968.

Kim KH, Kim HK, Han JY et al: Transaxillary minithoracotomy versus video-assisted thoracic surgery for spontaneous pneumothorax. Ann Thorac Surg 61:1510–1512, 1996.

Kirchner LT Jr, Swartzel RL: Spontaneous pneumothorax and its treatment. JAMA 155:24, 1954.

Kjaergaard H: Spontaneous pneumothorax in the apparently healthy. Acta Med Scand Suppl 43:159, 1932.

Klassen KP, Meckstroth CV: Treatment of spontaneous pneumothorax: Prompt expansion with controlled thoracotomy tube suction. JAMA 182:1, 1962.

Kleinmann P, Levi JF, Debesse B: La pleurectomie pariétale percutanée par video-endoscopie. Rev Mal Respir 8:459, 1991.

Klingman R, Angellillo V, DeMeester T: Cystic and bullous lung disease. Ann Thorac Surg 52:576, 1990.

Kondo T, Tagami S, Yohioka A et al: Current smoking of elderly men reduces antioxidants in alveolar macrophages. Am Rev Respir Dis 143:144, 1991.

Kuhlman JE, Knowles MC, Fishman EK, Siegelman SS: Premature bullous pulmonary damage in AIDS: CT diagnosis. Radiology 173:23, 1989.

Lange P, Mortensen J, Groth S: Lung function 22–35 years after treatment of idiopathic spontaneous pneumothorax with talc poudrage or simple drainage. Thorax 43:559, 1988.

Larrieu AJ, Tyers GFU, Williams EH et al: Intrapleural instillation of quinacrine for treatment of recurrent spontaneous pneumothorax. Ann Thorac Surg 28:146, 1979.

Lau OJ, Shawkat S: Pleurectomy through the triangle of auscultation. Thorax 37:945, 1982.

Lesur O, Delorme N, Fromaget JM et al: Computed tomography in the etiologic assessment of idiopathic spontaneous pneumothorax. Chest 98:341, 1990.

Levi JF, Kleinmann P, Riquet M, Debesse B: Percutaneous parietal pleurectomy for recurrent spontaneous pneumothorax. Lancet 336:1577, 1990.

Lichter I: Long term follow-up of planned treatment of spontaneous pneumothorax. Thorax 29:32, 1974.

Lichter I, Gwynne JF: Spontaneous pneumothorax in young subjects: A clinical and pathological study. Thorax 26:409, 1971.

Light RW: Management of spontaneous pneumothorax. Am Rev Respir Dis 148:245, 1993.

Light RW, O'Hara VS, Moritz TE et al: Intrapleural tetracycline for the prevention of recurrent spontaneous pneumothorax. JAMA 264:2224, 1990.

Lillington GA, Mitchell SP, Wood GA: Catamenial pneumothorax. JAMA 219:1328, 1972.

Liu HP, Chang CH, Lin PJ, Hsieh MJ: Thoracoscopic loop ligation of parenchymal blebs and bullae: Is it effective and safe? J Thorac Cardiovasc Surg 113:50, 1995.

LoCicero J, Hartz RS, Frederiksen JA et al: New applications of the laser in pulmonary surgery: Hemostasis and sealing of air leaks. Ann Thorac Surg 40:546, 1985.

Lote K, Dahl O, Vigander T: Pneumothorax during combination chemotherapy. Cancer 47:743, 1981.

Maggi G, Ardissone F, Oliaro A et al: Pleural abrasion in the treatment of recurrent or persistent spontaneous pneumothorax, results of 94 consecutive cases. Int Surg 77:99, 1992.

Mahfood S, Hix WR, Aaron BL et al: Reexpansion pulmonary edema. Ann Thorac Surg 45:340, 1988.

Martigne C, Velly JF, Levy F et al: La chirurgie du pneumothorax spontané chez l'insuffisant respiratoire chronique. Bordeaux Med 17:507, 1984.

Maunders RJ, Pierson DJ, Hudson LD: Subcutaneous and mediastinal emphysema. Arch Intern Med 144:1447, 1984.

Maurer ER, Schall JA: Chronic recurrent spontaneous pneumothorax due to endometriosis of the diaphragm. JAMA 168:2013, 1958.

McMahon DJ: Spontaneous pneumomediastinum. Am J Surg 131:550, 1976.

Melton LJ, Hepper NG, Offord KP: Incidence of spontaneous pneumothorax in Olmsted County, Minnesota: 1950 to 1974. Am Rev Respir Dis 120:1379, 1979.

Mercier C, Page A, Verdant A et al: Out-patient management of intercostal tube drainage in spontaneous pneumothorax. Ann Thorac Surg 22:163, 1976.

Miller AC, Jarvey JE: Guidelines for the management of spontaneous pneumothorax. BMJ 307:114, 1993.

Miller KS, Sahn SA: Chest tubes: Indications, technique, management and complications. Chest 91:258, 1987.

Minami H, Saka H, Senda K et al: Small caliber catheter drainage for spontaneous pneumothorax.Am J Med Sci 304:345, 1992.

Mitlehner W, Friedrich M, Dissmann W: Value of computer tomography in the detection of bullae and blebs in patients with primary spontaneous pneumothorax. Respiration 59:221, 1992.

Moores D: Pleurodesis by mechanical pleural abrasion for spontaneous pneumothorax. In Deslauriers J, Lacquet LK (eds): International Trends in General Thoracic Surgery, Vol 6. St. Louis, Mosby–Year Book, 1990, p 126.

Moran JF, Jones RH, Wolfe WG: Regional pulmonary function during experimental unilateral pneumothorax in the awake state. J Thorac Cardiovasc Surg 74:396, 1977.

Mouroux J, Elkaim D, Padovani B, et al: Video-assisted thoracoscopic treatment of spontaneous pneumothorax: Technique and results of one hundred cases. J Thorac Cardiovasc Surg 112:385, 1996.

Muller NL: CT diagnosis of emphysema: It may be accurate, but is it relevant? Chest 103:329, 1993.

Murray KD, Matheny RG, Howanitz EP, Myerowitz PD: A limited

axillary thoracotomy as primary treatment of recurrent spontaneous pneumothorax. Chest 103:137, 1993.

Nakamura H, Konischiike J, Sugamura A et al: Epidemiology of spontaneous pneumothorax in women. Chest 89:378, 1986.

Nathanson LK, Shermi SM, Wood RA, Cuschieri A: Video thoracoscopic ligation of bullae and pleurectomy for spontaneous pneumothorax. Ann Thorac Surg 53:316, 1991.

Naunheim KS, Mack MJ, Hazelrigg SR et al: Safety and efficacy of video-assisted thoracic surgical techniques for the treatment of spontaneous pneumothorax. J Thorac Cardiovasc Surg 109:1198, 1995.

Nazari S: Psychological implications in the surgical treatment of pneumothorax. Ann Thorac Surg 63:1830, 1997.

Neal JF, Vargas G, Smith DE et al: Bilateral bleb excision through median sternotomy. Am J Surg 138:794, 1979.

Nezu K, Kushibe K, Tojo T et al: Thoracoscopic wedge resection of blebs under local anesthesia with sedation for treatment of a spontaneous pneumothorax. Chest 111:230, 1997.

Noppen M, Mahler T, Dab I, Vincken W: Successful management of recurrent pneumothorax in cystic fibrosis by localized apical thoracoscopic talc poudrage. Chest 106:261, 1994.

Norris RM, Jones JG, Bishop JM: Respiratory gas exchange in patients with spontaneous pneumothorax. Thorax 23:427, 1968.

Noyes BE, Orenstein DM: Treatment of pneumothorax in cystic fibrosis in the era of lung transplantation. Chest 101:1187, 1992.

Ohata M, Suzuki H: Pathogenesis of spontaneous pneumothorax with special references to the ultrastructure of emphysematous bullae. Chest 77:771, 1980.

O'Rourke JP, Yee ES: Civilian spontaneous pneumothorax: Treatment options and long-term results. Chest 96:1302, 1989.

Ouellette D, Inculet R: Unsuspected metastatic choriocarcinoma presenting as unilateral spontaneous pneumothorax. Ann Thorac Surg 53:144, 1992.

Pairolero PC, Payne SW: The surgical management of recurrent or persistent pneumothorax: Abrasive pleurodesis. In Kittle FC (ed): Current Controversies in Thoracic Surgery. Philadelphia, WB Saunders, 1986, p 43.

Panacek EA, Singer AJ, Sherman BW et al: Spontaneous pneumomediastinum: Clinical and natural history. Ann Emerg Med 21:1222, 1992.

Passlick B, Born C, Haussinger K, Thetter O: Efficiency of video-assisted thoracic surgery for primary and secondary spontaneous pneumothorax. Ann Thorac Surg 65:324, 1998.

Ralph-Edwards AC, Pearson FG: Atypical presentation of spontaneous pneumomediastinum. Ann Thorac Surg 58:1758, 1994.

Rammohan G, Bonacini M, Dwek JH, Das A: Pleurodesis in metastatic pneumothorax. Chest 90:918, 1986.

Reid L: Emphysema: Classification and clinical significance. Br J Dis Chest 60:57, 1966.

Rhea JT, DeLuca SA, Greene RE: Determining the size of pneumothorax in the upright patient. Radiology 144:733, 1982.

Rivarola CH: Tension pneumothorax. In Deslauriers J, Lacquet LK (eds): International Trends in General Thoracic Surgery, Vol 6. Philadelphia, Mosby–Year Book, 1990, p 153.

Robbins RA, Gossman GL, Nelson KJ et al: Inactivation of chemotactic factor inactivator by cigarette smoke: A potential mechanism of modulating neutrophil recruitment of the lung. Am Rev Respir Dis 142:763, 1990.

Robinson CLN: Autologous blood pleurodesis in recurrent and chronic spontaneous pneumothorax. Can J Surg 30:428, 1987.

Rusch VW, Schmidt R, Shoji Y, Fujimura Y: Use of the argon beam electrocoagulator for performing pulmonary wedge resections. Ann Thorac Surg 49:287, 1990.

Rutherford RB, Hurt HH Jr, Brickman RD et al: The pathophysiology of progressive tension pneumothorax. J Trauma 8:212, 1968.

Sadikot RT, Green T, Meadows K, Arnold AG: Recurrence of primary spontaneous pneumothorax. Thorax 52:805, 1997.

Sahn SA, Good IT Jr, Potts DE: The pH sclerosing agents: A determinant of pleural symphysis. Chest 76:198, 1979.

Samuelson SL, Goldberg EM, Ferguson MK: The thoracic vent, clinical experience with a new device for treating simple pneumothorax. Chest 100:880, 1991.

Sargent EN, Turner AF: Emergency treatment of pneumothorax: A single catheter technique for use in the radiology department. AJR 109:531, 1970.

Schoenenberger RA, Haefeli EW, Weiss P, Ritz RF: Timing of invasive procedure in therapy for primary and secondary spontaneous pneumothorax. Arch Surg 126:764, 1991.

Schramel FMNH, Postmus PE, Vanderschueren RGJRA: Current aspects of spontaneous pneumothorax. Eur Respir J 10:1372, 1997.

Schramel FMNH, Sutedja TG, Janssen JP et al: Prognostic factors in patients with spontaneous pneumothorax treated with video-assisted thoracoscopy. Diagn Ther Endosc 2:1, 1995.

Scott GC, Berger R, McKean HE: The role of atmospheric pressure variation in the development of spontaneous pneumothoraces. Am Rev Respir Dis 139:659, 1989.

Selikoff IJ, Broder RA, Bader ME: Asbestosis and neoplasia. Am J Med 424:87, 1987.

Sensenig DM, Lamarche P: Marfan syndrome and spontaneous pneumothorax. Am J Surg 139:601, 1990.

Seremetis MG: The management of spontaneous pneumothorax. Chest 57:65, 1970.

Singh SV: The surgical treatment of spontaneous pneumothorax by parietal pleurectomy. Scand J Thorac Cardiovasc Surg 16:75, 1982.

Slabbynck H, Kovitz KL, Vialette JP et al: Thoracoscopic findings in spontaneous pneumothorax in AIDS. Chest 106:1582, 1994.

Smevik B, Klepp O: The risk of spontaneous pneumothorax in patients with osteogenic sarcoma and testicular cancer. Cancer 49:1734, 1982.

So S, Yu D: Catheter drainage of spontaneous pneumothorax: Suction or no suction, early or late removal. Thorax 37:46, 1982.

Stephenson LW: Treatment of spontaneous pneumothorax with intrapleural tetracycline. Chest 88:803, 1985.

Sugiyama Y, Maeda H, Yotsumoto H et al: Familial spontaneous pneumothorax. Thorax 41:969, 1986.

Suster B, Ackerman M: Pulmonary manifestations of AIDS: Review of 106 episodes. Radiology 161:87, 1986.

Swierenga J: Atlas of Thoracoscopy. Ingelheim, Boehringer, 1977.

Swierenga J, Wagennar JPM, Gergstein PGM: The value of thoracoscopy in the diagnosis and treatment of diseases affecting the pleura and lung. Pneumologie 151:11, 1974.

Takevo Y: Thoracoscopic treatment of spontaneous pneumothorax. Ann Thorac Surg 56:688, 1993.

Tanaka F, Itoh M, Esaki H et al: Secondary spontaneous pneumothorax. Ann Thorac Surg 55:372, 1993.

Tatebe S, Kanazawa H, Tamazaki Y et al: Spontaneous hemopneumothorax. Ann Thorac Surg 62:1011, 1996.

Tetely TD: Proteinase imbalance: Its role in lung disease. Thorax 48:560, 1993.

Thomas PA, Gebauer PW: Pleurectomy for recurrent spontaneous pneumothorax. J Thorac Surg 35:117, 1958.

Torre M, Belloni P: Nd:YAG laser pleurodesis through thoracoscopy: New curative therapy in spontaneous pneumothorax. Ann Thorac Surg 47:887, 1989.

Trachiotis GD, Vricella LA, Alyono D et al: Management of AIDS-related pneumothorax. Ann Thorac Surg 62:1608, 1996.

Travis WD, Pittaluga S, Lipschik GY et al: Atypical pathologic manifestations of *Pneumocystis carinii* pneumonia in the acquired immune deficiency syndrome Am J Surg Pathol 14:615, 1990.

Tribble CB, Selden RF, Rogers BM: Talc poudrage in the treatment of spontaneous pneumothorax in patients with cystic fibrosis. Ann Surg 677:204, 1986.

Tschopp JM, Brutsche M, Frey JG: Treatment of complicated spontaneous pneumothorax by simple talc pleurodesis under thoracoscopy and local anaesthesia. Thorax 52:329, 1997.

Tueller EE, Crise R, Belton JC, McLaughlin RF: Idiopathic spontaneous pneumothorax: Electron-microscopic study. Chest 71:419, 1977.

Tyson MD, Crandall WB: The surgical treatment of recurrent idiopathic spontaneous pneumothorax. J Thorac Surg 10:566, 1941.

Vanderschueren RG: The role of thoracoscopy in the evaluation and management of pneumothorax. Lung 168(Suppl):1122, 1990.

Vanderschueren RG: Le talcage pleural dans le pneumothorax spontané. Poumon Coeur 37:273, 1981.

Vass G, Keszler P: Primary spontaneous mediastinal emphysema. In Deslauriers J, Lacquet LK (eds): International Trends in General Thoracic Surgery, Vol 6. St. Louis, Mosby–Year Book, 1990, p 159.

Verschoof GPM, Velde T, Greve LH et al: Thoracoscopic pleurodesis in the management of spontaneous pneumothorax. Respiration 53:197, 1988.

Videm V, Pillgram-Larsen J, Ellingsen O et al: Spontaneous pneumothorax in chronic obstructive pulmonary disease: Complications, treatment and recurrences. Eur J Respir Dis 71:365, 1987.

Viskum K, Lange P, Mortensen J: Long term sequelae after talc pleurodesis for spontaneous pneumothorax. Pneumologie 43:105, 1989.

Wait MA: AIDS-related pneumothorax. Ann Thorac Surg 64:285, 1997.

Wait MA, Estrera A: Changing clinical spectrum of spontaneous pneumothorax. Am J Surg 164:528, 1992.

Wakabayashi A: Thoracoscopic technique for management of giant bullous lung disease. Ann thorac Surg 56:708, 1993.

Wakabayashi A, Brenner M, Wilson A et al: Thoracoscopic treatment of spontaneous pneumothorax using carbon dioxide laser. Ann Thorac Surg 50:786, 1990.

Wakabayashi A: Thoracoscopic ablation of blebs in the treatment of recurrent or persistent spontaneous pneumothorax. Ann Thorac Surg 48:651, 1989.

Waller DA: Management of spontaneous pneumothorax. Thorax 52:836, 1997.

Waller DA, Forty J, Soni AK et al: Videothoracoscopic operation for secondary spontaneous pneumothorax. Ann Thorac Surg 57:1612, 1994.

Waller DA, Yoruk Y, Morritt GN: Videothoracoscopy in the treatment of spontaneous pneumothorax: An initial experience. Ann R Coll Surg Engl 75:237, 1993.

Walston A, Brewer DL, Kitchens CS et al: Electrocardiographic manifestation of spontaneous left pneumothorax. Ann Intern Med 80:375, 1974.

Warner BW, Bailey WW, Shipley RT: Value of computed tomography of the lung in the management of primary spontaneous pneumothorax. Am J Surg 162:39, 1991.

Warren SE, Lee D, Martin V, Messink W: Pulmonary lymphangiomyomatosis causing bilateral pneumothorax during pregnancy. Ann Thorac Surg 55:995, 1993.

Wayne M, McSwain NE: Clinical evaluation of a new device for the treatment of tension pneumothorax. Ann Surg 191:760, 1980.

Weeden D, Smith GH: Surgical experience in the management of spontaneous pneumothorax 1972–1982. Thorax 387:37, 1983.

Weisberg D: The surgical management of recurrent or persistent pneumothorax: Pleuroscopy and talc poudrage. In Kittle FC (ed): Current Controversies and Thoracic Surgery. Philadelphia, WB Saunders, 1986, p 46.

Wied U, Halkier E, Hosier-Madsen K et al: Tetracycline versus silver nitrate pleurodesis in spontaneous pneumothorax. J Thorac Cardiovasc Surg 86:591, 1983.

Wilder RJ, Beacham KG, Ravitch MM: Spontaneous pneumothorax complicating cavitary tuberculosis. J Thorac Cardiovasc Surg 43:561, 1962.

Yellin A, Benfield JR: Pneumothorax associated with lymphoma. Am Rev Respir Dis 134:590, 1986.

Yellin A, Gapany-Gapanavicius M, Lieberman Y: Spontaneous pneumomediastinum: Is it a rare cause of chest pain? Thorax 38:383, 1983.

Youmans CR Jr, Williams RD, Monthy RM: Surgical management of spontaneous pneumothorax by bleb ligation and pleural dry sponge abrasion. Am J Surg 120:644, 1970.

CHAPTER **43**

Rare Infections of the Pleural Space

Jorge Nin Vivó
Mario Brandolino

Pleural Hydatidosis

Hydatid pleural disease is always secondary to the rupture of hydatid cysts located in organs that are adjacent to the pleura such as the lung, the liver, or, less commonly, the pericardium, spleen, or chest wall (ribs, spine, or diaphragm). Invasion of the pleural space will result in formation of a new hydatid cyst, which will eventually develop into so-called secondary pleural hydatidosis.

HISTORICAL NOTE

Since the Intercolonial Medical Congress of Australia in 1889, hydatid cystic disease of the lung has been recognized as a surgical pathologic condition. At that meeting, Thomas (Perez Fontana, 1948) reported a mortality rate of 61.4% among 208 patients with hydatid cysts of the lung who had been treated conservatively. He also introduced a surgical technique consisting of pleurotomy, cyst puncture, incision, and marsupialization of the pericyst and evacuation of its contents, leaving a chest tube inside the cyst cavity. He later reported a series of 38 patients who were treated by this technique with 32 good results. Three hydatic cysts of the lung that ruptured in the pleura were treated by pleurotomy.

At about the same time, many cases of hydatidosis were seen in Argentina and Uruguay, where there were two different schools of thought. Some surgeons performed one-stage procedures (Posadas, 1895), with cyst evacuation through the pleural space and pericyst or lung suture to the chest wall with marsupialization, whereas others, such as Lamas and Mondino, performed the surgery in two stages, first inducing pleural adhesions and then evacuating the parasites through these adhesions, thereby avoiding operative pneumothoraces (Fossati, 1943).

In 1937, Déré reported 11 cases of secondary pleural hydatidosis; three of them were complications from surgery. Armand Ugon (1935) also reported cases of secondary pleural hydatidosis and hydatid pneumothoraces. In 1945, he described patients in whom surgery had been performed with good results, and in 1947 he published his technique for the treatment of hydatid cysts of the lung. The technique consisted of enucleation of the hydatid with partial resection and capitonnage of the emergent pericyst layer. In 1947, Barret described a similar technique.

HISTORICAL READINGS

Armand Ugon CV: Técnica de la extirpación del quiste hidático del pulmon. Bol Soc Cir Montevideo XVIII:167, 1947.
Barret NR: The treatment of pulmonary hydatid disease. Thorax 1:21, 1947.
Déré E: L'échinococcose secondaire de la plèvre. J Chir (Paris) 49:497, 1937.
Fossati A: Quistes hidaticos de pulmon: Metodo de Lamas y Mondino/ Tecnica (Personal y breve comentario). An Fac Med (Montevideo) 28:793, 1943.
Lamas A: Quelques details a propos du traitement chirurgical au kyste hydatique du poumon. J Chir (Paris) T.XLI:406, 1933.
Perez Fontana V: Nuevo metodo de operar en el quiste hidatico del pulmon. Arch Pediatr (Uruguay) 19:5, 1948.
Posadas A: Quistes hidatidicos. An Circulo Med Argent 23:613, 1895.
Ugon AV: Equinococosis pleural secundaria. An Dep Cient Salud Publ (Montevideo) 2:389, 1935.

BASIC SCIENCE

Pathology

Pleural Complications of Hydatid Cysts of the Lung

Hydatid cysts of the lung are slowly progressive lesions. Their pericyst layer is weak. They can give rise to two varieties of pleural lesions: parahydatid and hydatid pleural complications (Fig. 43–1).

In parahydatid complications, the cyst itself is not ruptured, and the clinical manifestations are related either to a pneumothorax (periadventitial complication) or to a serofibrinous pleurisy secondary to mechanical or allergic pleural irritation.

Hydatid pleural complications are produced by the rupture of both the hydatid and the pericyst layer, giving rise to a hydatid hydropneumothorax. When a bronchoadventitial pleural fistula is also present, secondary infection of the cavity will produce a hydatid pyopneumothorax. Occasionally, the lung will remain collapsed for some time, and its surface will be covered by a fibrinous coat that gives rise to loculated collections of hydatid fluid, air, or pus. With these types of effusions, scolices will grow to become hydatids. This phenomenon is called *hydatid thorax*. If the bronchopleural fistula closes and the lung re-expands, scolices will remain between the pleural surfaces and eventually grow as independent hydatids. In this form of secondary pleural hydatidosis, which is called hydatid pleural implant (the form most commonly encountered in clinical practice), cysts are mainly located in dependent areas and at the sites of pleural reflections.

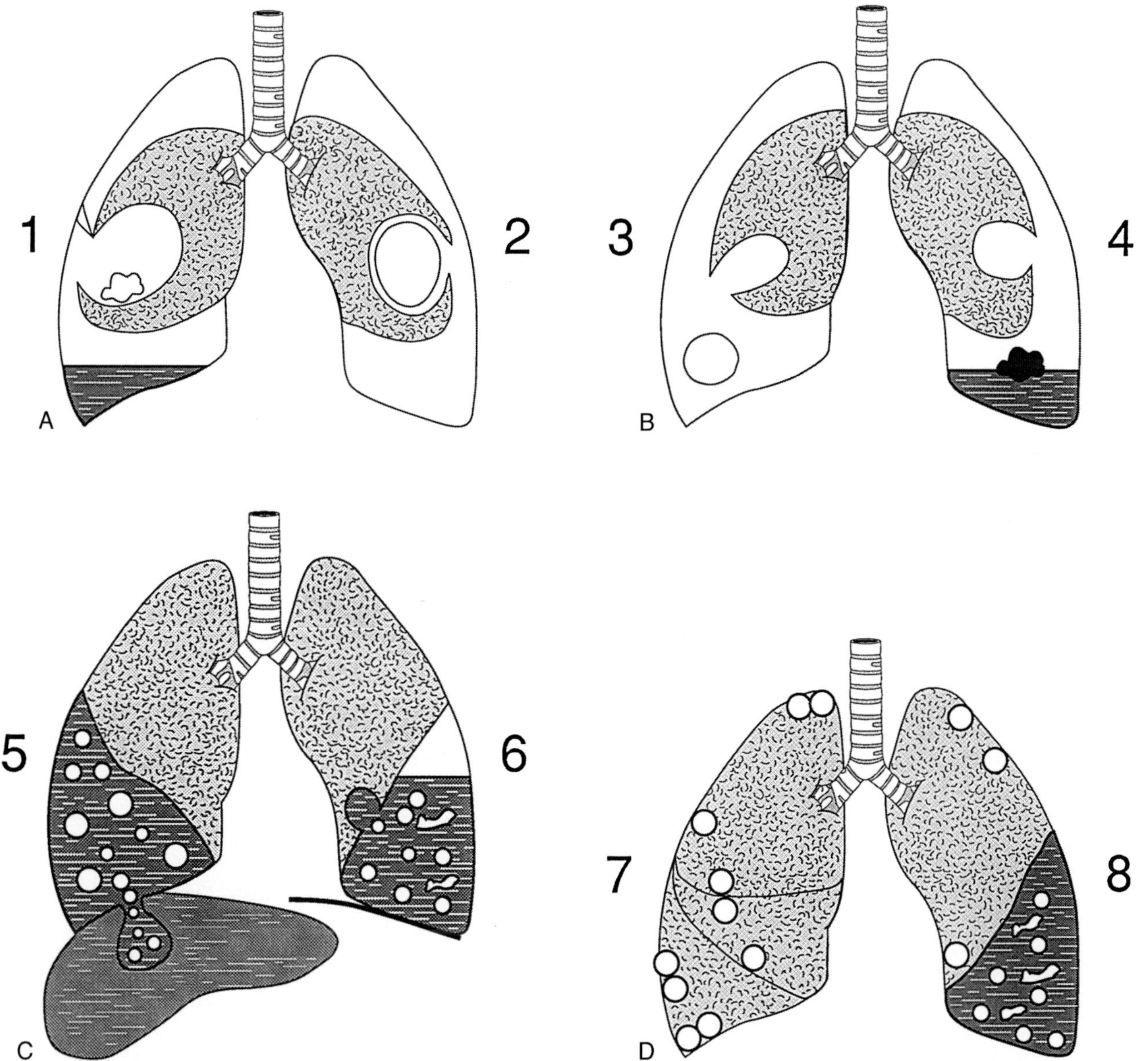

FIGURE 43–1 ■ Different presentations of hydatid pleural disease. *(A)* 1, Pyopneumothorax (membrane retention); 2, pneumothorax. *(B)* 3, Heterotropic pleural primitive hydatidosis; 4, pyopneumothorax (water lily sign). *(C)* 5, Hydatid thorax of hepatic origin; 6, pneumohydatid thorax. *(D)* 7, Hydatid implant; 8, mixed form (hydatid thorax and hydatid pleural implant).

Infrequently, ruptured lung hydatid cysts will simultaneously contaminate both the pleural space and the bronchus, giving rise to secondary pleural hydatidosis and bronchogenic secondary pulmonary hydatidosis, the so-called massive pleuropulmonary hydatidosis (Ugon, 1935). Accidental surgical rupture of a hydatid cyst of the lung may also produce a secondary pleural hydatidosis. Additionally, there is a rare variety of secondary pleural hydatidosis called heterotopic pleural primitive hydatidosis, in which isolated pericyst rupture allows passage of the intact hydatid into the pleural cavity.

Pleural Complications of Hepatic Hydatidosis

Pleural complications of hepatic hydatidosis develop in two different stages: the plastic and the perforative stages. During the plastic stage, the liver cyst, which is normally located posteriorly and superiorly, will grow upward, and the diaphragm will progressively become thinner with areas of relative ischemia. During this process, infection is common, because roughly one third of hepatic hydatid cysts have already ruptured in the biliary tract. During the perforative stage, the pathologic process involves the cyst, the diaphragm, the pleura, and the lung; negative intrapleural pressure elevates the cyst toward the chest, a process helped by the obstructive biliary hypertension. When the diaphragm is perforated (the site of perforation usually does not exceed 2 cm), hydatic collections reach the pleural space, producing a hepatic, thoracic, transdiaphragmatic pleural hydatidosis.

Pleural Complications Originating in Osseous Echinococcosis

In the spine, the parasite can invade the bone, producing necrosis and destruction of trabeculations and generating new spaces in which it will eventually grow in an irregular and asymmetric fashion. If this occurs, the hydatic collection may invade adjacent tissues such as the pleura and become pleural hydatidosis.

DIAGNOSIS

Clinical Features

Initial Pleural Accident

The initial accident is often a dramatic clinical event with sudden and acute thoracic pain, cardiovascular collapse (sometimes leading to shock), and hydatid allergy (urticaria, bronchospasm, and fever.) Often the patient will have a tension hydropneumothorax with mediastinal shift. When the lung cyst is accidentally ruptured during a surgical procedure, there are no symptoms, although occasionally the patient will show signs of allergy. The patient with hepatic, thoracic, transdiaphragmatic hydatidosis may present in an acute condition, with epigastric pain, cough, fever, shortness of breath, bilipthisis, and anaphylactic reactions.

Secondary Pleural Hydatidosis

With secondary pleural hydatidosis, symptoms often appear years after the initial accident (Fig. 43–2). Hydatid pleural implant is often asymptomatic or produces mild symptoms, whereas hydatid cysts located in the thoracic vertex can produce symptoms of mediastinal compression. In the hydatid thorax form, the clinical presentation depends on whether secondary infection is present.

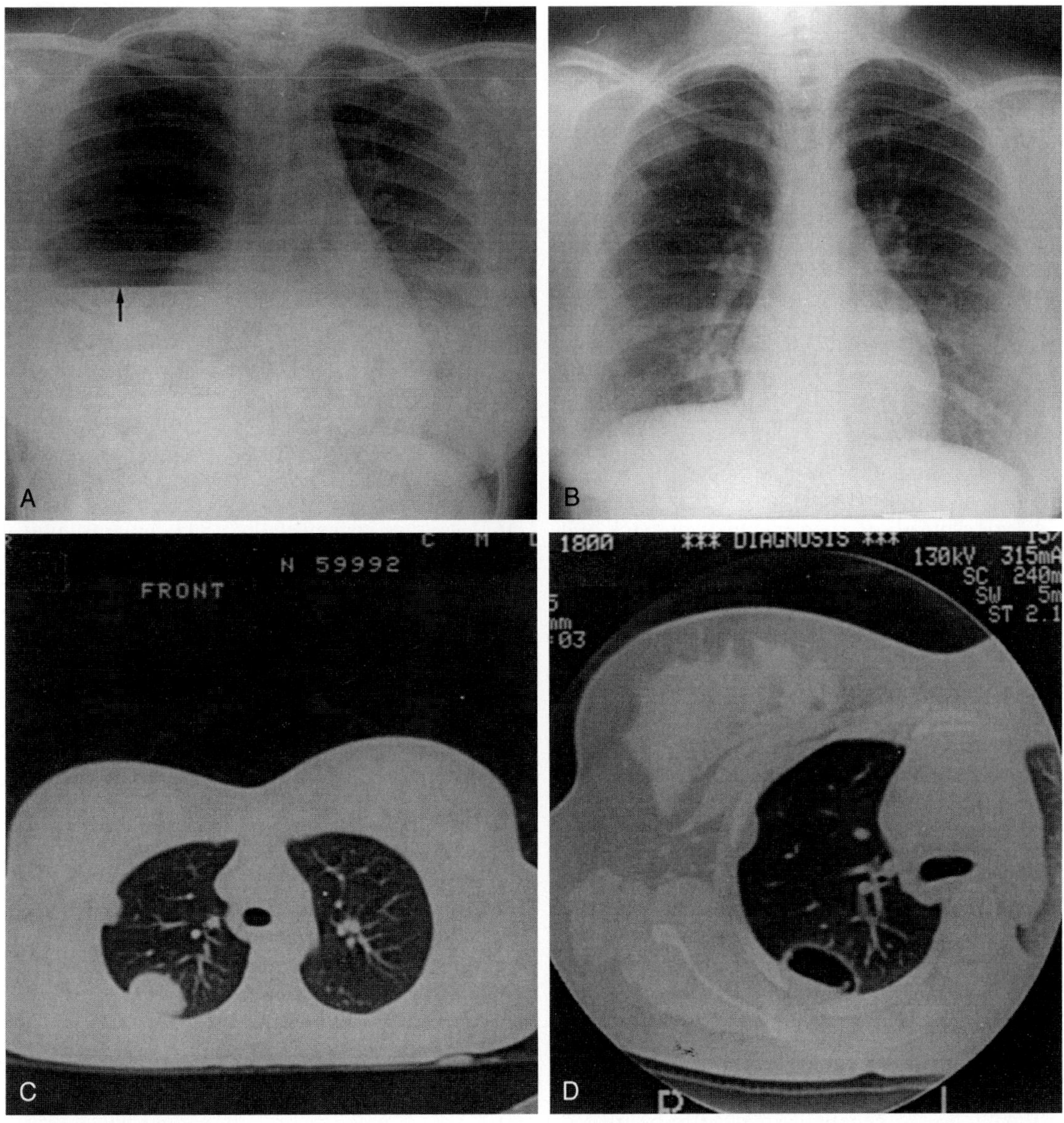

FIGURE 43–2 ■ Secondary pleural hydatidosis. *A*, Standard chest radiograph taken during the initial accident shows a right pyopneumothorax. The patient underwent thoracotomy, pleural drainage, and cavity treatment. Three years later, chest radiograph *(B)* and computed tomography scan *(C)* show hydatid pleural implants. *D*, Computed tomography scan taken after treatment with albendazole. Note that the contents of one cyst were expectorated.

Differential Diagnosis

Clinical and radiologic diagnoses of pleural hydatidosis are usually presumptive, because only the expectoration of hydatid debris or the identification of hydatid elements by thoracentesis is pathognomonic of the disease. The rate of positive finding in immunologic testing (hemagglutination, immunofluorescence, and electrosyneresis) varies between 40% and 85%. Immunoelectrophoresis testing is useful, but Casoni's reaction, Weinberg's test, and the eosinophil count are nonspecific.

Chest radiographs may show a blurred hemidiaphragm or a loculated pleural effusion. In the hydatid pleural implant, the lung may be riddled with multiple rounded opacities projecting into the pleural space. In heterotopic pleural primitive hydatidosis, a hydatid pneumothorax with or without pleural effusion and a "wanderer" cyst changing its location with different radiologic positions can be seen. Ultrasound and computed tomography (CT) scans of the thorax and liver may demonstrate the presence of cystic lesions.

MANAGEMENT

Therapy

Treatment of the initial accident is on an emergency basis, and drainage of the pleural contents is mandatory. Definitive therapy, which should be delayed until the anaphylactic reaction is over, consists of removing the parasites, evacuating all pleural contents, and treating the affected lung by meticulous bronchial suturing and capitonnage of the adventitial cavity. The procedure is always completed by profuse pleural swabbing with hydrogen peroxide.

Hydatid pleural implant is a diffuse pleural process (Fig. 43–3) in which cysts can be few or many and can be localized, widespread, or even included in thick and fibrous areas of pachypleuritis. Often this arrangement makes the exploration of the whole pleural cavity very difficult. Because few of these cysts can be enucleated, most have to be treated by aspiration followed by injection of a parasiticide solution into the cyst.

Thoracotomy alone or with laparotomy is performed electively when the hydatid thorax has originated from a hepatic thoracic transdiaphragmatic hydatidosis. The pleural cavity is first totally evacuated and cleaned. An anterolateral radial diaphragmatic incision is then made in a way that trauma to the vena cava and suprahepatic veins is avoided, but a distance from infected tissues is maintained. The contents of the hydatid hepatic cyst are suctioned away with a trocar, and the hepatic cavity is opened wide, totally evacuated, cleaned, and drained by two large-bore tubes, which are inserted through a separate abdominal incision. If there is an associated obstruction of the common bile duct, it should be decompressed and drained by simultaneous laparotomy or by endoscopic retrograde cholangiography with papillotomy. Only occasionally do the hepatic cysts need to be treated by hepatic resection. Mebendazole and albendazole are useful during the postoperative period to prevent seeded scolices from growing.

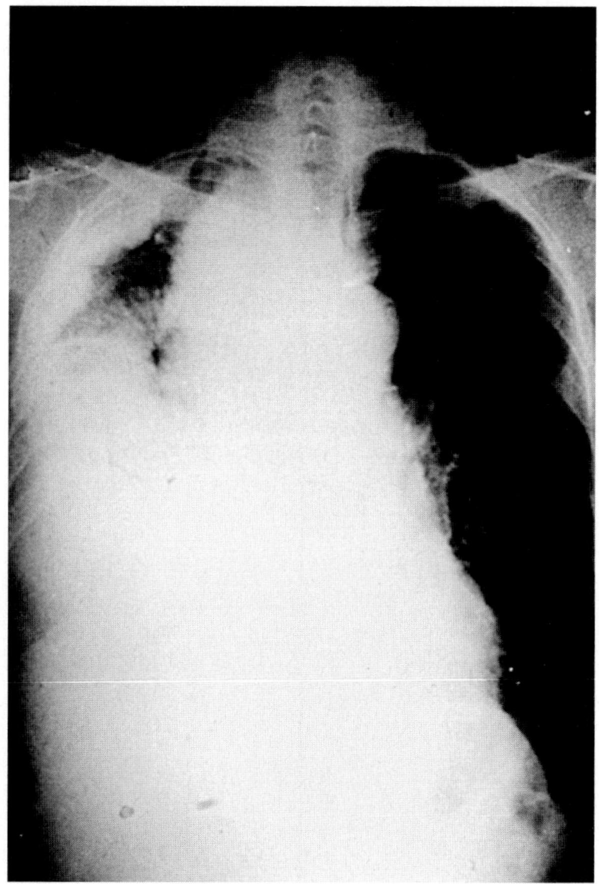

FIGURE 43–3 ■ Standard chest radiograph showing hydatid pleural implant.

Clinical Series

In 1988, we reviewed the 1841 patients who had been operated on in the Saint Bois Thoracic Department in Montevideo since 1947 for thoracic hydatidosis and the 77 with pleural complications who had been seen (Nin Vivó et al, 1990). A subsequent series included patients who were seen between 1970 and 1990. A total of 449 patients were operated on for thoracic hydatidosis, and 46 had pleural complications (Fig. 43–4), which originated in the lung in 23 patients, in an organ located below the diaphragm in 19, in the spine in 2, in the pericardium in 1, and in the diaphragm in 1. Among the 23 patients who previously had hydatid cysts of the lung, 2 developed heterotopic pleural primitive hydatidosis, 10 had pleural complications that never progressed to secondary pleural hydatidosis, and 11 developed true secondary pleural hydatidosis. Among the 19 patients with abdominothoracic, transdiaphragmatic pleural hydatidosis, this complication originated in the liver in 16, in a subphrenic hydatid cyst in 2, and in a splenic cyst in 1. All 19 patients reached the stage of secondary pleural hydatidosis, and the 2 with thoracic vertebral hydatidosis and the 1 with secondary pericardial hydatidosis also developed secondary pleural hydatidosis. The diaphragmatic cyst secondarily produced a parahydatid pleural effusion. Of the 33 patients who eventually developed

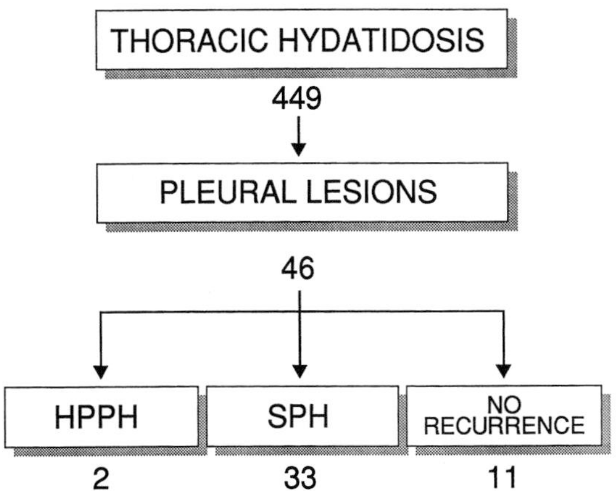

FIGURE 43–4 ■ Pleural hydatidosis. (HPPH, heterotropic pleural primitive hydatidosis; SPH, secondary pleural hydatidosis.)

secondary pleural hydatidosis, 17 had previously undergone surgery.

There was no operative mortality during this period, and early complications, which included empyemas, wound infections, biliary fistulas, and hemorrhage, were all successfully treated. In all patients with prior hydatic pleural disease, it is important that follow-up is done at regular intervals because of the possibility of a recurrence of the hydatid disease. In this series, the two patients with secondary pleural hydatidosis of vertebral origin required laminectomy, cord decompression, and vertebral resection, and one of them ended up with permanent paraplegia.

Currently, the number of new cases is considerably lower, not only because of the efficient work in prevention by the Uruguayan Committee that fights against hydatidosis but also because the Saint Bois Thoracic Department, which was the reference center in this pathology for more than 40 years, has been closed.

Case Study

This clinical case was chosen to illustrate what Ugon (1935) described as massive pleuropulmonary hydatidosis (Fig. 43–5). It is that of a 21-year-old man who had dyspnea of acute onset, right-sided chest pain, cough, fever, and a vomica of foul-smelling liquid. Initial chest radiographs showed a pleural effusion with the so-called water-lily sign, and thoracentesis confirmed the diagnosis of pleural hydatidosis. A chest tube was inserted, and hydatid membranes with pus were evacuated from the pleural space. The patient made a good recovery, but 18 months later, while he was in ostensibly good health, follow-up radiographs showed rounded opacities consistent with the diagnosis of secondary pleural hydatidosis. He then underwent thoracotomy with excision and formolization of 32 hydatid cysts, and 10 days later he had a third-space, anterolateral thoracotomy with extrapleural excision of 20 additional cysts. After 16 months, he had again developed cough, hemoptysis, and abundant expectoration of hydatid membranes, and a mass was noted over the sixth intercostal space. Because of his poor medical status, hydatid debris and pus were evacuated by pleurotomy. However, 2 months later, a right pleuropneumonectomy was required, and the postoperative course was uneventful.

Pleural Amebiasis

BASIC SCIENCE

Pathology

Amebiasis is a parasitic infection produced by an amoeba called *Entamoeba histolytica*. Approximately 500 million people worldwide are infected, and as many as 10% will eventually develop the disease. The expected mortality rate is 0.75 per 100,000 infected persons (Whitton, 1990).

The parasite is mainly transmitted by fecal-oral mechanisms. Once absorbed through the portal system, it migrates to the liver, where it produces abscesses or periportal fibrosis. Amebic liver abscesses contain an acellular, proteinaceous material, and the trophozoites are located in the periphery of the abscess, where they further invade adjacent tissues. Although periportal fibrosis is common, only 5% of patients with symptomatic amebiasis develop true hepatic abscesses. When the abscess ruptures or if it extends to the surrounding tissues, it can produce pleuropulmonary or pericardial complications.

As reported by Ochsner and DeBakey (1943), pleuropulmonary contamination is the most common complication of amebic hepatic abscesses. In their series of over 181 patients with amebiasis-induced hepatic abscesses, 26 had a pleuropulmonary complication (17 pulmonary and 9 pleural), and 1 had a pericardial complication.

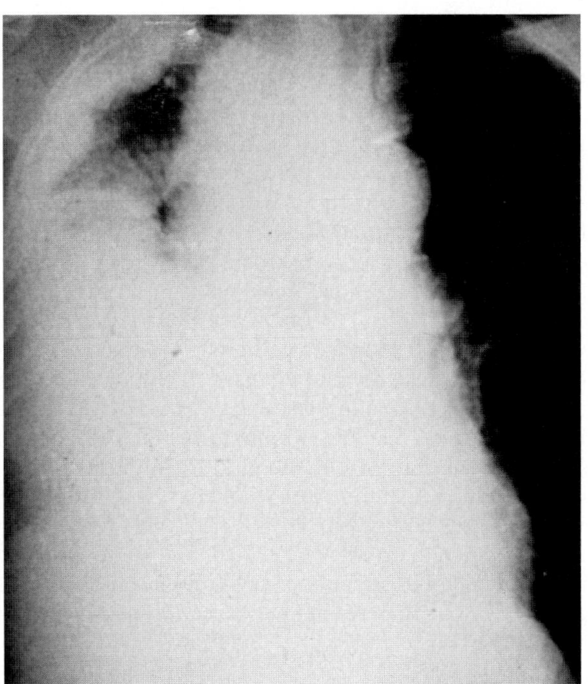

FIGURE 43–5 ■ Standard chest radiograph showing several pulmonary and pleural hydatid cysts. In the vertex and over the mediastinum, there are several hydatid pleural implants.

Most amebic hepatic abscesses develop over the superior and posterior surfaces of the right lobe. As the abscess enlarges, it includes the diaphragm in its wall. If the abscess develops slowly, it may produce a pleural reaction that will generate adhesions at the base of the right lung and sometimes produce a hepatobronchial fistula. However, if the abscess enlarges rapidly, it may rupture in the pleural cavity with consequent empyema. Amebic hepatic abscesses can also rupture in the pericardial cavity, but this is uncommon.

DIAGNOSIS

Clinical Features

The most common symptom of pleural amebiasis is right-sided chest pain with radiation to the shoulder. The cough, initially unproductive, is nearly always followed by production of abundant, purulent expectorations that resemble chocolate sauce and are pathognomonic of an amebic hepatobronchial fistula. At this stage, sputum examination can reveal the parasite and establish the diagnosis. Fever is more pronounced with pleural involvement, and often there is general malaise, weakness, anorexia, and weight loss.

Rupture into the pericardium must be suspected when the patient presents with epigastric pain that radiates to the base of the neck, severe dyspnea, and fever. Occasionally, acute filling of the pericardial sac produces symptoms of cardiac tamponade.

Differential Diagnosis

Characteristically, standard chest radiographs show an elevation of the right hemidiaphragm, a pleural effusion, and in the adjacent lung, areas of consolidation with or without cavitation. CT scan, ultrasound, and magnetic resonance imaging (MRI) are mainly used for the detection of hepatic abscesses.

The pleural fluid is generally exudative, but it can become secondarily infected by other pathogens. Pleural biopsy or needle biopsy of the wall of the hepatic abscess may reveal *E. histolytica*. When there is a pericardial effusion, needle aspiration often yields a fluid that is serofibrinous or contains chocolate-sauce pus.

Serologic techniques are very important in the diagnosis of amebiasis because frequently the parasite cannot be isolated. Serology is positive in most thoracic complications. The most commonly used techniques are the indirect hemagglutination test and enzyme-linked immunosorbent assay (ELISA). Double diffusion and counterimmunoelectrophoresis take longer to complete but may also be useful. Agglutination with latex is a simple test but often gives false-positive results. In most cases erythrocyte sedimentation rate is elevated, and there is a moderate leukocytosis. In pulmonary complications, careful sputum analysis may sometimes reveal the parasite.

MANAGEMENT

The most useful drugs to treat amebiasis are emetine, chloroquine, and metronidazole. Because of its possible cardiotoxicity, emetine must be given with great caution and under electrocardiographic monitoring. Metronidazole is a more effective drug and is less toxic. The usual dosage is 750 mg given three times a day, and when it is combined with drugs such as paromomycin, cures are often seen within 10 days of the beginning of treatment. In hepatobronchial fistulas, postural drainage is useful, and all pleural effusions or empyemas must also be drained. Pericardial effusions may require urgent decompression.

Infections Produced by Higher Bacteria

Actinomycetes are gram-positive and arborescent bacteria that reproduce by fission rather than by sporulation as do the fungi. Their growth is inhibited by antibiotics but not by antifungal drugs. In this group, human disease is produced by (1) *Actinomyces* and related *Arachnia* species, which are anaerobic organisms and produce actinomycosis; and (2) *Nocardia* species, which are aerobes and produce nocardiosis.

ACTINOMYCOSIS

Pleural actinomycosis is mainly caused by *Actinomyces israelii*, but three other species and related *Arachnia propionica* can also cause actinomycosis with pleural involvement. Thoracic actinomycosis has no anatomic boundaries and often involves the lung, pleura, mediastinum, and chest wall. In at least 50% of thoracic actinomycosis cases, there is pleural involvement.

BASIC SCIENCE

Pathology

Actinomycetes are normal inhabitants of the oropharynx, but they are especially abundant in septic dental processes. The point of entry is usually in the area between the skin and the mucosal coating, from where the bacteria travel to the thorax through aspiration, by local contiguous spreading, or via the bloodstream (hematogenously). Once the disease has reached the lung, it propagates by contiguous spread, tending toward externalization through the chest wall or extension to subdiaphragmatic areas.

In 17 cases of thoracic actinomycosis reported by Ming-Jang and colleagues (1993), the chest wall and pleura were involved in seven patients. In eight cases reported by Ibañez-Nolla and colleagues (1993), the pleura was involved in four cases and the chest wall in three additional cases.

DIAGNOSIS

Clinical Features

The symptoms of pleural actinomycosis are entirely nonspecific. Chest pain reflects pleural involvement and can be accompanied by dyspnea, fever, cough, hemoptysis, or weight loss, all symptoms that can wrongly be interpreted as those of tuberculosis. Poor dentition or skin lesions in the area of the jaw or in the neck may suggest the diagnosis of actinomycosis. Unfortunately, previous treatment with antibiotics can change the evolution of the process and complicates diagnosis.

Differential Diagnosis

Chest radiographs and CT scans often show lung masses that may resemble lung cancer or that may be cavitated, with adjacent pleural thickening and pleural effusion. Chest wall involvement, sometimes with destruction of ribs or vertebrae, is common. In most cases, however, the definitive diagnosis can only be made by study of the resected specimen (Dambrin et al, 1957).

Pleural fluid may be either serous or purulent, and typical 1- to 2-mm–diameter sulfur granules can be found. These granules are conglomerates of filamentous organisms with characteristically clubbed peripheral radiations. Actinomycosis organisms must be cultured both aerobically and anaerobically. Sulfur granules can also be isolated from sputum, bronchial washings, or pus from dental abscesses or infected cutaneous tracts. In general, erythrocyte sedimentation rate and leukocytosis are elevated. An eosinophil count of 13% was found in a patient with a hydatid cavity in which lung actinomycosis had developed with secondary actinomycotic empyema (Cazes, 1965).

MANAGEMENT

Treatment consists of penicillin in doses of up to 30 million U/day given for 5 weeks. In the presence of sepsis and empyema, longer periods of treatment may be required. Erythromycin and tetracyclines have also been successfully used in patients with penicillin allergy. When the pleural effusion is only an exudate, there is usually a good response to antibiotic treatment, but when the pleural fluid is infected, pleural drainage must be instituted. Late sequelae consisting of lung abscesses and chest wall fistulas determine the need for lung or chest wall resections.

NOCARDIOSIS

Nocardia species are normal inhabitants of the soil, and in tropical countries they constitute the principal cause of foot mycetoma. *N. asteroides* is the organism responsible for pleuropulmonary infections that are clinically and radiologically similar to actinomycosis. It often invades immunosuppressed patients, and up to 25% of patients with lung nocardiosis also have pleural involvement, with effusion, empyema, or bronchopleural fistula. Hematogenous dissemination from the lung frequently affects the central nervous system and the subcutaneous tissues.

Nocardia species identification is not enough to establish a diagnosis of nocardiosis, because these bacteria can be found in the respiratory tree as saprophytes. Response to treatment with antibiotics is important (Ugedo et al, 1997).

DIAGNOSIS

The diagnosis of nocardiosis may be confirmed by identification of the bacteria in the pleural fluid, sputum, or bronchial washings. Because *N. asteroides* is slightly acid-fast, it can be incorrectly identified as *Mycobacterium tuberculosis*; therefore, acid-alcohol solutions must be used, because with these solutions, acid-fast characteristics are often lost. Definitive identification of *Nocardia* species requires culture under anaerobic conditions (to inhibit actinomycosis) or cultures under aerobic conditions with blood agar in which *Nocardia* species will grow.

MANAGEMENT

Sulfonamides are the drugs of choice. Sulfadiazine is usually used, but trimethoprim-sulfamethoxazole can also be used with similar results. In severe infections and in immunosuppressed patients, use of ampicillin or erythromycin with sulfonamide therapy is also recommended. These drugs should be given for at least 6 weeks and should be continued for 1 year in immunosuppresesd patients. The only role of surgery is to drain the pleural space in cases of empyema.

Pleural Tuberculosis

Tuberculosis, a disease seldom seen in many areas of the world, frequently occurs in underdeveloped countries. The amount of tuberculosis bacilli spilling in the pleura and the delayed hypersensitivity of the pleura seem to play dominant roles in determining which disease pattern will occur.

Tuberculous pleurisy generally results from rupture of a subpleural focus of caseous necrosis of the lung. Less commonly, it is secondary to the spillage of a tuberculous node in the pleura; in this process, the contamination is light but there is a pleural hypersensitivity reaction with a secondary scarce-to-moderate aqueous effusion. Most of the time, the effusion will regress over 1 to 2 months without treatment. It is the most common form of extrapulmonary tuberculosis and usually occurs within 6 months of the primary infection. Tuberculous pleurisy as a manifestation of primary tuberculosis is more common in adults who are between 25 and 45 years of age than it is in older adults, and it is rarely seen in children.

In tuberculous empyema, the pleural contamination is massive, the pleural fluid is purulent, and it is common to find resistant acid-fast bacilli on direct examination or culture of the pleural fluid. Tuberculous empyemas may be pure empyemas or pyopneumothoraces. In mixed tuberculous and pyogenic empyemas, bacterial superinfection is produced by a persistent bronchopleural fistula, or it occurs secondary to thoracentesis or chest tube drainage.

DIAGNOSIS

Clinical Features and Differential Diagnosis

Tuberculous Pleurisy

In two thirds of cases, patients with tuberculous pleurisy have an acute infection with low-grade fever, a nonproductive cough, pleuritic chest pain, and general malaise. When both cough and pleuritic chest pain are present, the pain usually precedes the cough. In the remaining one third of patients, the clinical presentation is more insidious and nonspecific, with asthenia, anorexia, weight loss, and nocturnal sweats as the main symptoms. Respiratory symptoms such as cough and chest pain appear only later.

Peripheral white blood cell count is often normal, but the tuberculin skin test is positive in 70% to 80% of patients. However, a negative skin reaction does not exclude the diagnosis, because during the acute stage of tuberculous pleuritis, circulating adherent cells suppress the specifically sensitized circulating T-lymphocytes. Because those cells are not present in the pleural space (Ellner, 1978), this effect explains why in some cases there is pleural hypersensitivity to the tuberculosis bacillus with cutaneous energy.

Apart from the moderate and usually unilateral pleural effusion, chest radiographs may be normal. Pulmonary foci are frequently not seen because they are small and peripheral; when present, they are always ipsilateral. In those cases with minimal findings, thoracic CT scan (Hulnick et al, 1983) or thoracoscopy may be more useful in demonstrating the pulmonary lesions. In general, the presence of a massive effusion favors a nontuberculous etiology.

Once a pleural effusion has been diagnosed, fluid must be sampled for analysis. In tuberculous pleurisy, the pleural fluid is yellow or sometimes serohemorrhagic with little or no opalescence. The presence of a frankly hemorrhagic effusion eliminates the possibility of tuberculous pleurisy. The fluid is exudative, with a protein content of more than 3 g/dl and frequently over 5 g/dl.

The remainder of the biochemical workup on the pleural fluid is of little help. Fluid with a pH below 7.3 or with a low glucose level is nonspecific and can be seen in other pathologies, including rheumatoid arthritis and carcinoma. High levels of lactic acid are also nonspecific and not very useful in making the diagnosis of tuberculous pleurisy. Piras and colleagues (1978) showed that the more sensitive and useful biochemical markers for tuberculous pleurisy were an increase of the adenosine deaminase level to more than 30 IU/L and an increase in the pleural/serum–lysozyme ratio. Lymphocytes are nearly always predominant in the cell count of the pleural fluid (they usually are in the range of 50% to 70%), although in the first 2 weeks of tuberculous pleurisy, polymorphonuclear leukocytes may predominate (Berger and Mejia, 1973). When lymphocytes are in excess of 50% to 70%, lymphoma should be suspected. Mesothelial cells are seldom above 5%, and if eosinophils are found, they are never in excess of 10%. Acid-fast bacilli are seldom identified by direct analysis of the pleural fluid or by culture. To enhance the chances of isolating acid-fast bacilli, it is advisable to centrifuge all obtained fluid, but even with this technique, only 20% to 30% of patients will have positive fluid. Percutaneous pleural biopsy with the Cope or the Abrams needle is one of the better diagnostic methods because it reveals the presence of granulomas in the parietal pleural fluid in 60% to 80% of patients. Identification of areas of caseous necrosis or of acid-fast bacilli is helpful but is not absolutely necessary to make the diagnosis.

Pleural biopsies should always be complemented by fluid evacuation, but because chest tubes can promote infection, their use should be discouraged. Thoracoscopic biopsies should be considered when other methods have failed. This technique has the advantage of providing visualization of all surfaces so that proper areas can be selected for biopsy. In our personal series of 312 thoracoscopies performed for undiagnosed pleural effusions, only five were related to pleural tuberculosis.

A presumptive diagnosis of tuberculous pleural effusion is often enough to initiate treatment. This diagnosis is based on the combination of a positive tuberculin skin test and a predominantly lymphocytic reaction in the pleural fluid. A biopsy showing caseating or noncaseating epithelioid granulomas is further proof of underlying tuberculosis. However, only direct identification of acid-fast bacilli or culture of these organisms on biopsy specimens provides definitive documentation of tuberculous pleural disease.

Tuberculous Empyema

Tuberculous empyema is less common than tuberculous pleurisy. In 90% of cases, it originates from a focus of tuberculous primary infection, and in the remaining 10%, it is due to reactivation of cavitated or fibrocaseous lesions. Clinically, patients with tuberculous empyemas have a productive cough, fever, and dyspnea—the severity of symptoms being related to the volume of the empyema. Erythrocyte sedimentation rates are classically above 60 mm/min and are accompanied by leukocytosis and moderate anemia. Resistant acid-fast bacilli are found in the sputum and in the pleural fluid in over 70% of patients (Fig. 43–6).

Mixed Empyema

Mixed empyemas are the result of pleural fluid contamination by thoracentesis, chest tube insertion, or bronchopleural fistula. Symptoms are those of the primary tuberculous effusion associated with those of empyema or pyopneumothorax.

MANAGEMENT

Tuberculous Pleurisy

In the therapy of tuberculous pleurisy, the objectives are to prevent tuberculosis from becoming active and to prevent long-term pleural sequelae. In the face of a presumptive diagnosis of pleural tuberculosis with a positive purified protein derivative (PPD) skin test and a predominantly lymphocytic pleural effusion, treatment for 6 to 9 months with a regimen that includes two to four antituberculous drugs is suggested. If the skin test is negative at the start of therapy, the drugs can be stopped after 2 months.

In our clinic, we prefer to document the presence of acid-fast bacilli either in the sputum or in the gastric contents or to identify tuberculous granulomas by pleural biopsy before initiating drug therapy. Antituberculous

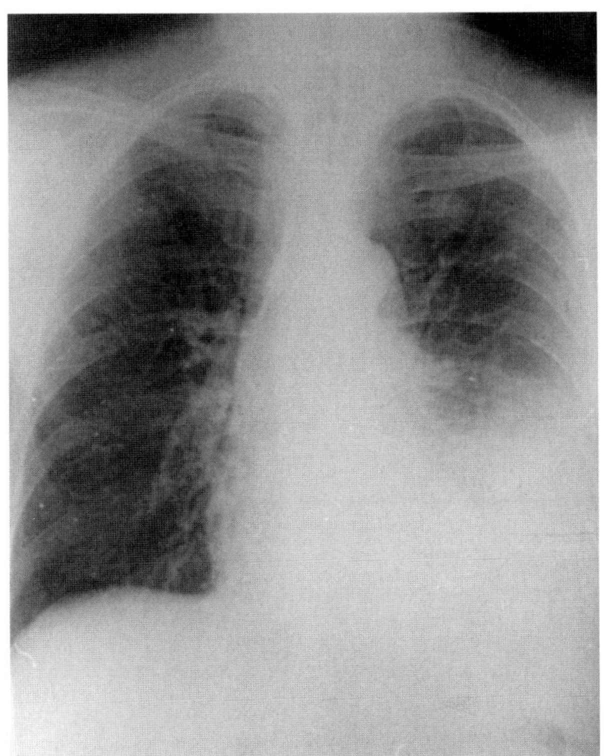

FIGURE 43–6 ■ Standard chest radiograph of a patient with a tuberculous empyema.

treatment is then given for a total of 7 months starting with the four drugs isoniazid, rifampicin, ethambutol, and pyrazinamide during the first 2 months. During the following 5 months, twice weekly doses of isoniazid and rifampicin are given. Patients with persistent large effusions or intense toxic reactions after adequate antituberculous drug treatment and pleural evacuation may need systemic or intrapleural corticotherapy. Lung decortication is seldom needed, because the pleural process usually resolves with adequate treatment.

Mixed and Tuberculous Empyema

Pleural drainage is indicated in tuberculous empyemas with large effusions and in all mixed empyemas, especially if there is a bronchopleural fistula with its inherent risks of contralateral aspiration. Luizy and colleagues (1966) described a pleural irrigation technique consisting of continuous aspiration and washing.

When the lung does not expand after drainage, or if there is a residual fibrothorax, the condition of the underlying lung should be determined before planning decortication because the presence of fibrotic lesions, cavities, or bronchiectasis can make decortication difficult, impossible, or inadvisable. In those cases, pulmonary resection with decortication may be required. A review of all available radiographs is important, because they will often indicate the topography and evolution of pulmonary lesions. CT scanning is also useful to determine the nature and extent of pulmonary lesions and to differentiate them from pleural lesions. If pulmonary resection is contemplated, bronchoscopy is imperative in documenting the presence or absence of active endobronchial tuberculosis.

In a classic study, Hood and associates (1986) divided these patients into two groups. The first group included patients with only pleural involvement, and the second group included those with significant associated parenchymal disease. In the first group, decortication was considered when the constrictive pleuritis extended to 25% to 30% of the pleural space or when 25% of predicted pulmonary function was lost. Occasionally, smaller collections were also treated surgically because they entailed the risks of tuberculous perforation into the bronchus (bronchopleural fistula) in addition to sometimes interfering with pulmonary function. Decortication was performed when there was no longer evidence of clinical toxicity and tuberculosis was medically controlled. Ideally, the sputum was negative for 4 months preoperatively, and if it had always been negative, antituberculous drug treatment was given for approximately 4 to 6 months prior to surgery. In Hood's second group, patients had severe parenchymal lesions in addition to pleural tuberculosis, and to eradicate the disease as well as to prevent reactivation, these patients required pulmonary resection and decortication.

If the empyema is small or loculated, it can be enucleated by the procedure called empyemectomy (Odell, 1990). In most cases, however, pleural decortication is necessary, and it is advisable to decorticate both parietal and visceral surfaces. The diaphragm must also be freed to allow for better mobility, and if the lung does not expand, an individualized thoracoplasty of usually no more than three to five ribs may have to be added to the decortication.

In general, tuberculous lesions predominate in upper lobes, and, therefore, this is the most common type of resection performed in association with decortication. Thoracoplasty may also have to be added if there is any doubt about pulmonary re-expansion. Pleuropneumonectomy is rarely indicated and is generally reserved for patients with destroyed lung, empyema, or bronchopleural fistula. In all those cases, special care must be taken to protect the bronchial stump, and pleural drainage with daily irrigations must be maintained for 1 to 3 weeks postoperatively.

Open thoracostomy is indicated when the empyema cannot be managed by closed thoracostomy and when the patient is medically unstable or, more importantly, is not considered a candidate for resection. The window thoracostomy should be initiated in a dependent position, and in patients without important pulmonary lesions, pleural space obliteration can be achieved in 6 to 9 months. For these individuals, open thoracostomy is more comfortable than a chest tube, with the added advantage of allowing pleural washing to be performed more easily. If there is a bronchopleural fistula, pleural washings should be done carefully, with the patient always in the upright position and the solution introduced slowly (Fig. 43–7).

Calcified fibrothoraces, which sometimes occur as late sequelae of tuberculous empyemas or of prior therapeutic pneumothoraces, must not be operated on unless absolutely necessary. Decortication is usually neither desirable

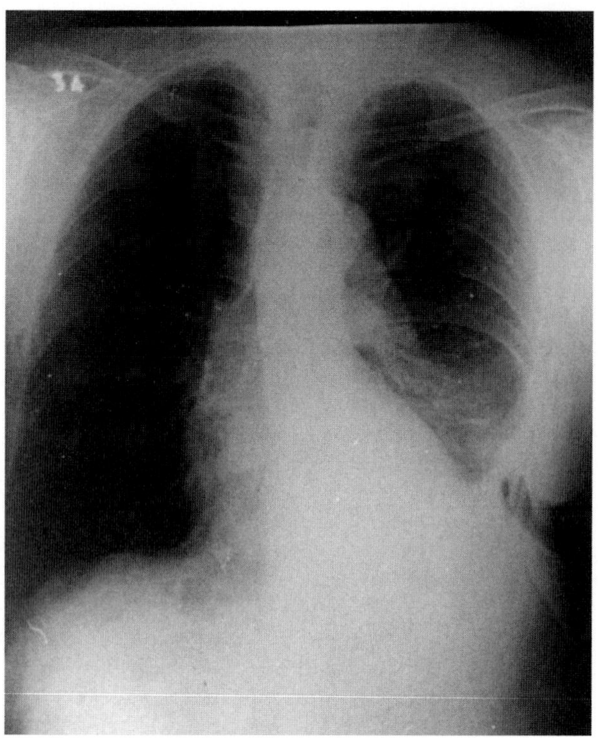

FIGURE 43–7 ■ A tuberculous empyema treated by open thoracostomy.

nor possible, and sometimes these patients will develop secondary pyogenic empyemas with or without bronchopleural fistula years later (Fig. 43–8), for which they may require pleuropneumonectomy (Fig. 43–9).

Nontuberculous Mycobacteriosis

The main causative organisms of nontuberculous mycobacteriosus are *Mycobacterium kansasii*, seen in the urban population, and *M. intracellulare*, seen more often in rural areas. The symptoms are similar to those seen in association with tuberculosis, although they may be somewhat attenuated. The PPD test is negative, but the pleural fluid may have elevated proteins and lymphocytes. Fluid glucose is normal or even decreased, and, occasionally, cultures of the biopsy specimen will identify *Mycobacterium*. Therapy for atypical mycobacterial disease consists of administration of drugs such as rifampicin, ethambutol, and isoniazid until the disappearance of the effusion or until the bacteriology is negative for 6 months.

Cryptococcosis

Cryptococcosis is a disease of universal distribution that is produced by an opportunistic fungus, *Cryptococcus neoformans*. This organism is widely distributed in nature, its principal reservoir being dry pigeon excreta. Cryptococcosis is the most common fungal pulmonary infection in the acquired immunodeficiency syndrome (AIDS), and its site of entry is believed to be the respiratory tract. In the early 1950s, 25% of patients with cryptococcosis had pulmonary lesions. More recently (1987), Wasser and Talavera reported that in five of 11 patients with cryptococcosis and AIDS, pulmonary lesions were the initial manifestation, and that three had a pleural effusion (two with pleural fluid positive for cryptococci). Pleural cryptococcosis is usually produced when a subpleurally located lung nodule extends into the pleura. The main symptoms are fever, cough, pleuritic chest pain, dyspnea, and weight loss.

DIAGNOSIS

Although chest radiographs and CT scans may show pulmonary infiltrates or nodules, mediastinal masses, and pleural effusions, the diagnosis of cryptococcosis can only be made by isolating the organism from pulmonary cavities, pleural fluid, or bronchial secretions. By using staining techniques such as hematoxylin-eosin (H & E), periodic acid–Schiff (PAS), Alcian blue, or Gomori on biopsy specimens, spheroid or ovoid formations of 10-μm average diameter can be seen, surrounded by a clear halo, which is characteristic of cryptococcosis.

MANAGEMENT

Drug treatment consists of amphotericin B and flucytosine. Fluconazole can also be used, with the same effec-

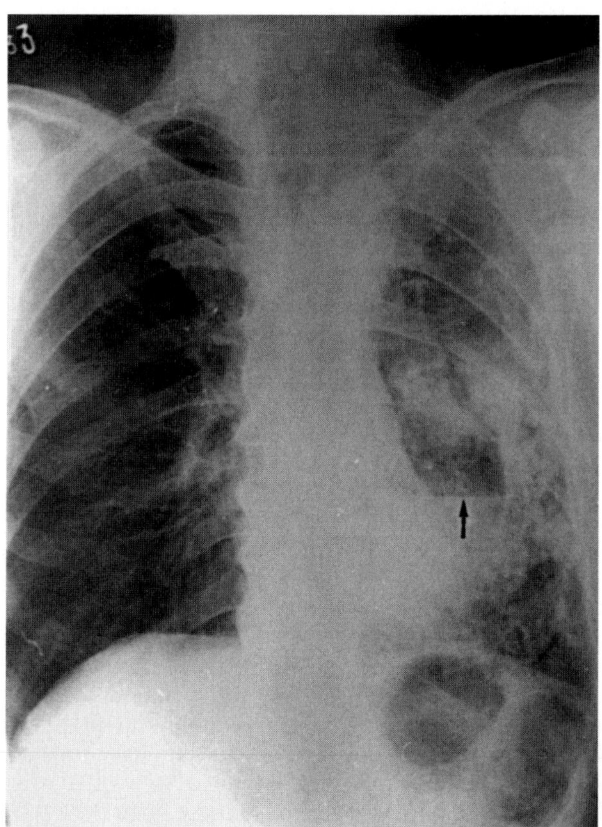

FIGURE 43–8 ■ Standard chest radiograph showing an empyema with a bronchopleural fistula that has developed in an area of calcified pleural sequelae. This patient was treated by open thoracotomy.

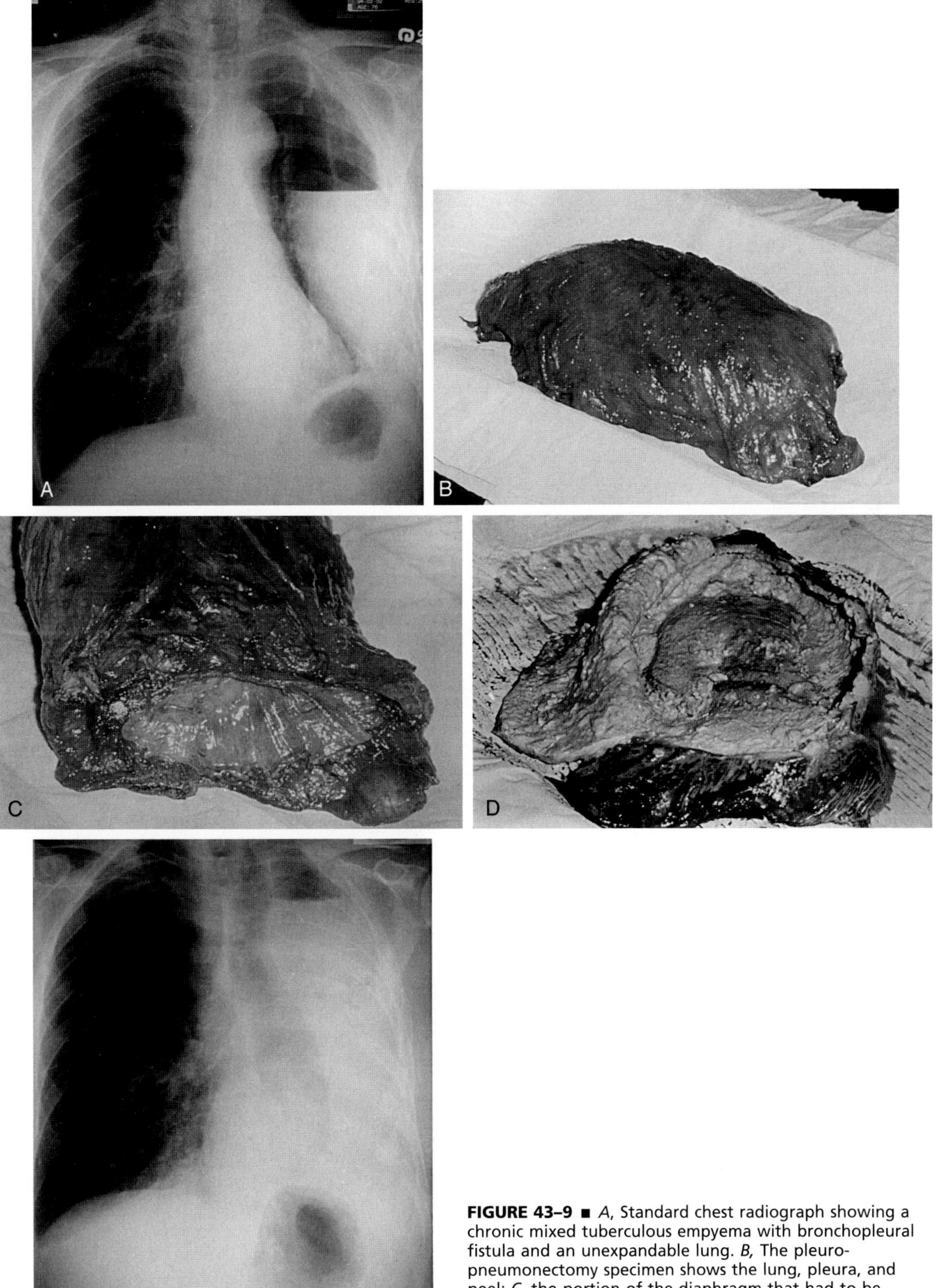

FIGURE 43–9 ■ *A*, Standard chest radiograph showing a chronic mixed tuberculous empyema with bronchopleural fistula and an unexpandable lung. *B*, The pleuropneumonectomy specimen shows the lung, pleura, and peel; *C*, the portion of the diaphragm that had to be resected to avoid contamination of the space; *D*, the inside of the cavity. *E*, Postoperative chest radiograph showing partial filling of the space.

tiveness but with fewer side effects on kidneys, liver, and bone marrow. In immunosuppressed patients, the treatment must be continued for 6 to 12 months to avoid extrapulmonary dissemination. Pleural drainage is generally not necessary. If a previously undiagnosed pulmonary nodule is found at operation to be cryptococcosis, resection must be followed by drug treatment.

Aspergillosis

Aspergillosis is a disease caused by the opportunistic fungus *Aspergillus fumigatus*, which is adaptive to life both in soil and in organic matter. Humans become infected by inhalation of the conidia, which are suspended in the air. *Aspergillus* may initiate several pathologic processes in the lung, such as mycetomas, invasive aspergillosis, and allergic bronchopulmonary aspergillosis. Pleural aspergillosis usually develops over pre-existing pathologies; it may be a sequela of therapeutic pneumothoraces (intrapleural or extrapleural), residual pleural cavities following pleural or pulmonary surgery, or other pleural diseases (e.g., chronic hemothoraces, pneumothoraces, pleural tuberculosis, or pleural hydatidosis) (Bisson, 1990). In those situations, *Aspergillus* pleural contamination is often secondary to a bronchopleural fistula, which initiates suppuration and *Aspergillus* infection of the pleural residual cavity. Sometimes the fungus may be isolated from the pleural fluid or biopsy specimens of the pulmonary tissues. Serologic studies identifying antibodies against *Aspergillus* are also useful for diagnosis except in immunosuppressed patients, in whom these studies are negative.

In 1992, Massard and colleagues reported a series of 77 patients with pleuropulmonary aspergillomas, of whom 16 had pleural aspergillosis. In 10 of the 16 aspergillosis developed following lobectomy; in one it developed in a residual space after exploratory thoracotomy; in three it followed collapse therapy; and, in two it followed a spontaneous bronchopleural fistula. Chest radiographs showed thickening of the pleura in 10 patients and a pleural effusion that turned out to be an empyema in 6 others. Thirteen patients with pleural aspergillosis were treated by surgery; two died. The risk is higher in symptomatic patients.

Patients with pleural aspergillosis must be carefully selected for surgery, and, whenever possible, radical and aggressive operations should be avoided. We prefer to use closed pleural drainage or, preferably, open thoracotomy with or without added thoracoplasty. Amphotericin B should be given for several months when necessary. Nebulized liposomal amphotericin B and oral itraconazole have been used with good results in the treatment of *Aspergillus fumigatus* empyemas (Purcell and Corris, 1995).

Histoplasmosis

Histoplasmosis is the most important fungal disease involving the respiratory system, but pleural involvement is unusual. It is produced by *Histoplasma capsulatum*, a dimorphic fungus living in the soil. Pleural lesions originate from a contiguous pulmonary focus or by hematogenous dissemination (George et al, 1985).

The most common symptoms associated with pleural histoplasmosis are pleuritic pain, fever, malaise, and signs of a pleural effusion. Diagnosis is based on the identification of the fungus either in the pleural fluid or on biopsy specimens. In 1966, Schub reported four patients with pleural histoplasmosis. In two of them *Histoplasma* was identified by open pleural or pulmonary biopsies; in a third *Histoplasma* was cultured in the pleural fluid; and in the fourth the diagnosis was made by a histoplasmin sensitivity test and elevation of antibody titer.

In 1997, Richardson and George reported a patient with empyema, bronchopleural fistula, and a granulomatous process in the lower lobe of the right lung. Cultures demonstrated *H. capsulatum* both in the pleural fluid and in the pulmonary parenchymal process.

Small- or moderate-size effusions do not need specific therapy. Amphotericin B therapy should be reserved for immunosuppressed patients or for patients with chronic pulmonary histoplasmosis and secondary pleural effusion.

Coccidioidomycosis

Coccidioidomycosis is a fungal disease produced by a dimorphic fungus called *Coccidioides immitis*. This fungus, first described in Argentina (Posadas, 1895), grows as a mycelium that eventually develops into arthrospores that are inhaled in the lungs. The incidence of pleural effusion with coccidioidomycosis is about 7% (Salkin et al, 1967).

Pleural effusions may be associated with acute primary coccidioidomycosis. In 1976, Lonky and colleagues reported on a series of 28 patients with coccidioidal pleural effusion. In 90%, it was secondary to direct spread from a contiguous pulmonary infection site. *C. immitis* was identified in the effusion of only three of 15 patients, but in all eight patients who had pleural biopsies, cultures were positive. In acute disease, the prognosis is excellent, often without specific therapy.

Pleural effusion may also be secondary to chronic pulmonary coccidioidomycosis. In these cases, coccidioidal cavities rupture in the pleural space, where they may produce a pneumothorax, an empyema, or a bronchopleural fistula. Rapidly, a pleural peel will develop and entrap the lung. The definitive diagnosis can be made by the identification of the fungus in the pleural fluid, by needle biopsy, or by culture. A serologic diagnosis can also be obtained by precipitin and complement fixation tests, which are accurate and relatively specific (Hood et al, 1986).

When a positive diagnosis of pleural coccidioidomycosis is made, specific drug therapy with amphotericin B is indicated. Surgical management also includes tube drainage of pneumothoraces or empyemas and lung decortication, or it includes pulmonary resection to manage a bronchopleural fistula.

Blastomycosis

Blastomycosis is a fungal infection produced by a dimorphic fungus called *Blastomyces dermatitidis*. This fungus is present in warm and nitrogen-rich soils and has worldwide distribution. Blastomycosis is a less common mycotic infection than either coccidioidomycosis or histoplasmosis. Entry is through inhalation of the conidia into the lungs.

The symptoms are similar to those seen with other acute fungal infections and include cough, fever, myalgia, erythema nodosum, chest pain, and pleural effusion. In the chronic form of the disease, pleural involvement produces a pleural effusion or an empyema, often without specific symptoms.

Diagnosis can be made by the identification of the fungus in bronchial secretions, pleural fluid, or on pleural biopsies. These are frequently positive either on a smear or by culture. Pleural biopsy may also show granulomas, with stains and cultures of the material defining the etiology. Serologic and skin tests are of limited value. Acute blastomycosis with pleural effusion does not generally require specific therapy. Pleural involvement associated with chronic pulmonary infection must be treated with amphotericin B and tube drainage when necessary.

In 1995, Failla and colleagues reported seven cases of pulmonary blastomycosis, two of them with pleural effusions. In 18 children with culture-proven, acute pulmonary blastomycosis reported by Alkrinawi and colleagues (1995), pleural effusions were seen in three patients.

COMMENTS AND CONTROVERSIES

A variety of rare pleural infections that are seldom encountered in North America are discussed in this chapter. Pleural aspergillosis is particularly difficult to manage and carries a significant mortality both with conservative nonsurgical management and after operation. Surgical indications depend largely on the patient's overall medical status, but, whenever possible, the infected space must be obliterated either by muscle transplant or by thoracoplasty. When these procedures are carried out, prolonged postoperative treatment with antifungal drugs is also imperative. If these principles are not followed, the risks of recurrent pleural aspergillosis and death are very significant.

J.D.

REFERENCES

Alkrinawi S, Reed MH, Pasterkamp H: Pulmonary blastomycosis in children: Findings on chest radiographs. AJR Am J Roentgenol 165:651–654, 1995.

Barret NR: The treatment of pulmonary hydatid disease. Thorax 1:21, 1947.

Berger HW, Mejia E: Tuberculous pleurisy. Chest 63:88, 1973.

Bisson A: Pleural aspergillosis. In Deslauriers J, Lacquet LK (eds): International Trends in General Thoracic Surgery, Vol 6: Surgical Management of Pleural Diseases. St. Louis, Mosby–Year Book, 1990.

Cazes M: Actinomicosis pleuropulmonar injertada sobre secuela hidatica. El Torax 14:81, 1965.

Dambrin P, Moreau G, Eschapasse H et al: Les formes pseudocancéreuses de l'actinomycose pulmonaire. Ann Chir 2:223, 1957.

De Miguel J, García JL, Prats E et al: Actinomicosis torácica. Enf Inf y Microb 15:500–501, 1997.

Déré F: L'échinococcose secondaire de la plèvre. J Chir (Paris) 49:497, 1937.

Ellner JJ: Pleural fluid and peripheral blood lymphocyte function in tuberculosis. Ann Intern Med 89:932, 1978.

Failla PJ, Cerise FP, Karam GH, Summer WR: Blastomycosis: Pulmonary and pleural manifestations. South Med J 88:405–410, 1995.

Fossati A: Quistes hidáticas de pulmon. Método de Lamas y Mondino. An Fac Med Montevideo 28:793, 1943.

George RB, Penn RL, Kinasewitz GT: Mycobacterial, fungal, actinomycotic and nocardial infections of the pleura. Clin Chest Med 6:63, 1985.

Hood RM, Antman K, Boyd A et al: Surgical Diseases of the Pleura and Chest Wall. Philadelphia, WB Saunders, 1986.

Hulnick DH, Naidich DP, McCauley DI: Pleural tuberculosis evaluated by computed tomography. Radiology 149:759, 1983.

Ibañez-Nolla J, Carratalá J et al: Actinomicosis torácica. Enf Inf y Microb Clin 11:433–436, 1993.

Lamas A: Quelques details a propos du traitement chirurgical au kyste hydatique du poumon. J Chir (Paris) T.XLI:406, 1933.

Lonky SA, Catanzaro A, Moser KM et al: Acute coccidioidal pleural effusion. Am Rev Resp Dis 114:681, 1976.

Luizy J, Mathey JP, Le Brigand H et al: Technique d'irrigation pleurale sous depression continue dans le traitement des pyothorax. Rev Tuberc 30:393 1966.

Massard G, Roeslin N, Wihlm JM et al: Pleuropulmonary aspergilloma: Clinical spectrum and results of surgical treatment. Ann Thorac Surg 54:1159, 1992.

Ming-Jang H, Hui Ping L et al: Thoracic actinomycosis. Chest 104:366–370, 1993.

Nin Vivó J, Brandolino MV, Pomi JA et al: Hydatid pleural disease. In Deslauriers J, Lacquet LK (eds): International Trends in General Thoracic Surgery, Vol 6: Surgical Management of Pleural Diseases. St. Louis, Mosby–Year Book, 1990.

Ochsner A, DeBakey M: Amebic hepatitis abscess. Surgery 13:460, 1943.

Odell JA: Pleural tuberculosis. In Deslauriers J, Lacquet LK (eds): International Trends in General Thoracic Surgery, Vol 6: Surgical Management of Pleural Diseases. St. Louis, Mosby–Year Book, 1990.

Perez Fontana V: Nuevo metodo de operar en el quisto hidatico del pulmon. Arch Pediatr Uruguay 19:5, 1948.

Piras MA, Gakis C, Budroni M et al: Adenosine deaminase activity in pleural effusions: An aid to differential diagnosis. BMJ 4:1751, 1978.

Posadas A: Quistes hidatidicos. An Circulo Med Argent 23:613, 1895.

Purcell IF, Corris PA: Use of nebulized liposomal amphotericin B in the treatment of *Aspergillus fumigatus* empyema. Thorax 50:1321–1323, 1995.

Richardson JV, George RB: Bronchopleural fistulae and lymphocyte empyema due to *Histoplasma capsulatum*. Chest 112:1130–1132, 1997.

Salkin D, Birswer TW, Tarr AD et al: Roentgen analysis of coccidioidomycosis. In Ajello ED (ed): Coccidioidomycosis. Tucson, University of Arizona Press, 1967.

Schub HM, Spivey CG, Baird GD: Pleural involvement in histoplasmosis. Am Rev Resp Dis 94:225, 1966.

Ugedo J, Pérez A et al: Nocardiosis pulmonar: Presentación de 3 casos clínicos. Enf Inf Microb Clin 15:19–21, 1997.

Armand Ugon CV: Equinococosis pleural secundaria. An Dep Cient Salud Publ (Montevideo) 2:389, 1935.

Wasser L, Talavera W: Pulmonary cryptococcosis in AIDS. Chest 92:692, 1987.

Whitton I: Pleural amebiasis. In Deslauriers J, Lacquet LK (eds): International Trends in General Thoracic Surgery, Vol 6: Surgical Management of Pleural Diseases. St. Louis, Mosby–Year Book, 1990, p 452.

CHAPTER **44**

The Thoracic Duct and Chylothorax

Richard A. Malthaner

Richard I. Inculet

Thoracic Duct

HISTORICAL NOTE

Aristotle and the anatomists Herophilos and Erasistratos are said to have described the lymphatic system in approximately 300 BC. In the 16th century, Vesalius, professor of anatomy and surgery at Padua, named the thoracic duct the vena alba thoracis because of the milky white fluid that it contained. In Aselli's 1627 illustration of the lymphatic channels in the mesentery of the dog, he traced these vessels into the abdominal receptaculum chyli but mistakenly believed that they ended in the liver. In 1651, Pecquet of Paris observed the intestinal lacteal channels that empty into the receptaculum chyli, then into the thoracic duct, and eventually into "the whirlpool of the heart." He confirmed these observations in an autopsy of the body of a criminal who had eaten a large final meal. In 1653, Bartholin named these vessels "lymphatics." In 1784, William Hunter, with his assistants at the Hunterian School, Hewson and Cruikshank, recognized that the lymphatic vessels are the same as the lacteal vessels and "that these altogether with the thoracic duct constitute one great and general system dispersed through the whole body for absorption."

In 1878, Claude Bernard's conception of the mammalian milieu intérieur and Starling's work (1896) on hydrostatic and colloid osmotic pressure further illuminated the role of the lymphatic channels. Drinker and Field (1931) measured protein flux from the capillaries to the tissues. They confirmed the notion that the lymphatic channels and the thoracic duct act as vessels that return protein molecules to the central circulation.

Reports on the chylothorax were rare before the 19th century. From the medical literature dating back to 1691, Bargebuhr (1894) compiled a review of 40 patients with nontraumatic chylothorax. All had neoplasms of the abdomen and thorax. Although the first traumatic chylothorax was reported by Quinke (1875), Zesas' review (1912) stated that Longelot in 1663 was probably the first to describe a traumatic chylothorax. In this collected series of 24 patients, 12 died.

On the basis of his review of the literature and personal experimental work on ligation of the thoracic duct, Lee (1922) concluded that injuries should be treated by direct repair when possible and, if not, by ligation. This represented the first challenge to the accepted dogma that the duct was essential to life. Blalock and colleagues (1936) noted chylothorax after ligation of the superior vena cava. Their attempts at complete lymphatic blockage by duct ligation were successful in only 3 of 72 animals, because collateral lymph channels developed rapidly and relieved the obstruction.

Heppner (1934) first pointed out that progressive obliteration of the pleural space around the opening rather than healing of the injured duct was the mechanism of spontaneous resolution of thoracic duct fistulas. Daily thoracenteses were advocated, and many attempts at pleurodesis subsequently failed. Intravenous injection of aspirated chyle was tried in the early 1900s by Oeken but was abandoned after several anaphylactic reactions (Whitcomb and Scoville, 1942). Readministering chyle by mouth or rectum was also found to be unhelpful. Phrenic nerve sectioning also proved to be unsuccessful.

Although Crandall and coworkers (1943) successfully treated a thoracic duct fistula in the neck by direct thoracic duct ligation, it was Lampson (1948) who ligated the thoracic duct in the chest and marked the turning point in the therapy of chylothorax. The mortality rate at that time was nearly 100% in nontraumatic chylothorax and 50% in traumatic chylothorax, with the latter figure suggesting that one half closed spontaneously.

Schumacker and Moore (1951) suggested feeding cream to infants preoperatively to help localize the duct. Klepser and Berry (1954) introduced intraoperative visualization of the duct with lipophilic dyes and early ligation. Their approach through the right chest at the level of the diaphragm regardless of the side of injury has become one of the most commonly used approaches today for thoracic duct injuries.

■ *HISTORICAL READINGS*

Aselli G: De Factibus Sive Lacteis Verris, Quarto Vasorum Mesdarai Corum Genere Novo Invento. Milan, JB Bieldellium Mediolani, 1627.

Bernard C: Leçons sur les Phénomènes de la vie Communs aux Animaux et aux Végétaux, Vol 1. Paris, JB Bailliere et Fils, 1878.

Blalock A, Cunningham RS, Robinson CS: Experimental production of chylothorax by occlusion of the superior vena cave. Ann Surg 104:359, 1936.

Lampson RS: Traumatic chylothorax: A review of the literature and report of a case treated by mediastinal ligation of the thoracic duct. J Thorac Cardiovasc Surg 17:778, 1948.

Lee FC: The establishment of collateral circulation following ligation of the thoracic duct. Bull Johns Hopkins Hosp 33:21, 1922.

BASIC SCIENCE

Anatomy

Davis (1915) characterized the anatomy of the thoracic duct as "constant only in its variability." The thoracic duct is the left main collecting vessel of the lymphatic system and is far larger than the right terminal lymphatic duct (Fig. 44–1). The duct originates from the cisterna chyli in the abdomen but may be absent in 1 of 50 people. The cisterna chyli is a globular structure that is 3 to 4 cm long and 2 to 3 cm in diameter. It is found along the vertebral column at the level of L2, but it may be found anywhere between T10 and L3 on the right side of the aorta. From the cisterna chyli, the thoracic duct ascends along the spine to enter the thorax through the aortic hiatus at the level of T10 to T12, just to the right of the aorta. It ascends extrapleurally along the right anterior surface of the vertebral bodies, posterior to the esophagus, between the aorta and the azygos vein, and anterior to the right intercostal arteries.

At the level of T5 to T7, the duct crosses behind the aorta to the left posterior side of the mediastinum and ascends on the left side of the esophagus beneath the pleural reflection and posterior to the left subclavian artery. In this region, the duct is vulnerable during operations involving the aortic arch, left subclavian artery, or

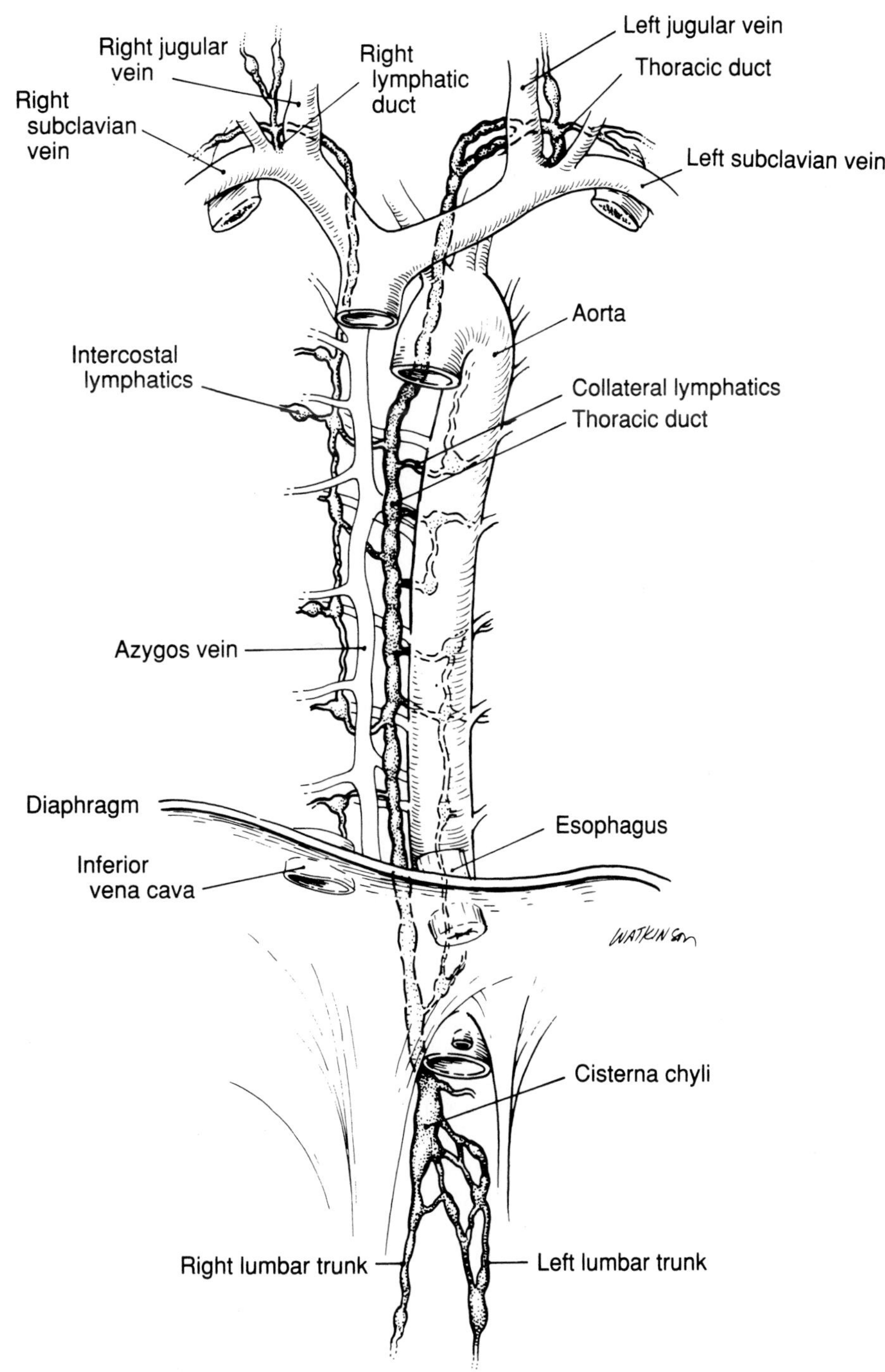

FIGURE 44–1 ■ Surgical anatomy of the thoracic duct.

esophagus. At 4 cm above the clavicle, the duct turns laterally behind the carotid sheath and jugular vein, anterior to the inferior thyroid and vertebral arteries, subclavian artery, and phrenic nerve. At the medial margin of the anterior scalene muscle, it turns inferiorly, entering the venous system at the subclavian–internal jugular vein junction on the left, although it may empty into the left innominate, left internal jugular, left vertebral, or even the right internal jugular vein. The duct contains a variable number of valves throughout its course with one consistent bicuspid valve at the lymphaticovenous junction that protects it against the reflux of blood (Pflug et al, 1968).

Van Pernis (1949) and Kausel and colleagues (1957) noted that variability is common, with 40% to 60% of individuals having anomalous collaterals communicating with the azygos, intercostal, and lumbar veins. Meade and coworkers (1950) found that 25% to 33% of individuals have multiple ducts at the level of the diaphragm, which has implications if an operation is considered.

The right duct is small (2 cm in length) and is rarely visualized. It drains lymph from the right side of the head, neck, and chest wall through the jugular trunk and from the right lung, heart, and lower half of the left lung through the bronchomediastinal trunk. Lymph from the dome of the liver, the right diaphragm, and the right upper anterior chest drains through the right internal mammary trunk to the right duct.

These anatomic relationships explain why injury to the duct below the level of T5 to T6 usually results in a right chylothorax, and injury above this level results in a left chylothorax. The collateral communications also explain why the duct can be ligated at any point in the chest or neck without impairing the delivery of lymph to the central circulation.

Embryology

The thoracic duct is a bilateral structure, and it may have many varied anatomic patterns. The lymphatic system begins to develop at the end of the fifth week, about 2 weeks later than the cardiovascular system. Sabin (1916) showed that the original lymph sacs arose from the endothelium of the adjacent veins. She described six original lymph spaces (Fig. 44–2). The two jugular sacs arise from the anterior cardinal vein, and the two iliac sacs arise near the junction of the iliac veins and the posterior cardinal veins. The single retroperitoneal sac is situated in the root of the mesentery on the posterior abdominal wall, and the primitive cisterna chyli arises from the mesonephric vein and the veins at the dorsomedial edge of the wolffian bodies. The cisterna chyli is then formed by the union of two lumbar lymphatic trunks and the intestinal trunk within the abdomen. Lymphatic buds appear from the original sacs and follow the tissue planes of least resistance, principally along veins, toward the periphery.

The thoracic duct is formed from a downward growth of the left jugular sac and an upward growth of the right thoracic duct from the cisterna chyli. Initially, the duct is represented by a bilateral symmetric plexus of lymph vessels, each side attached to the jugular sac and each

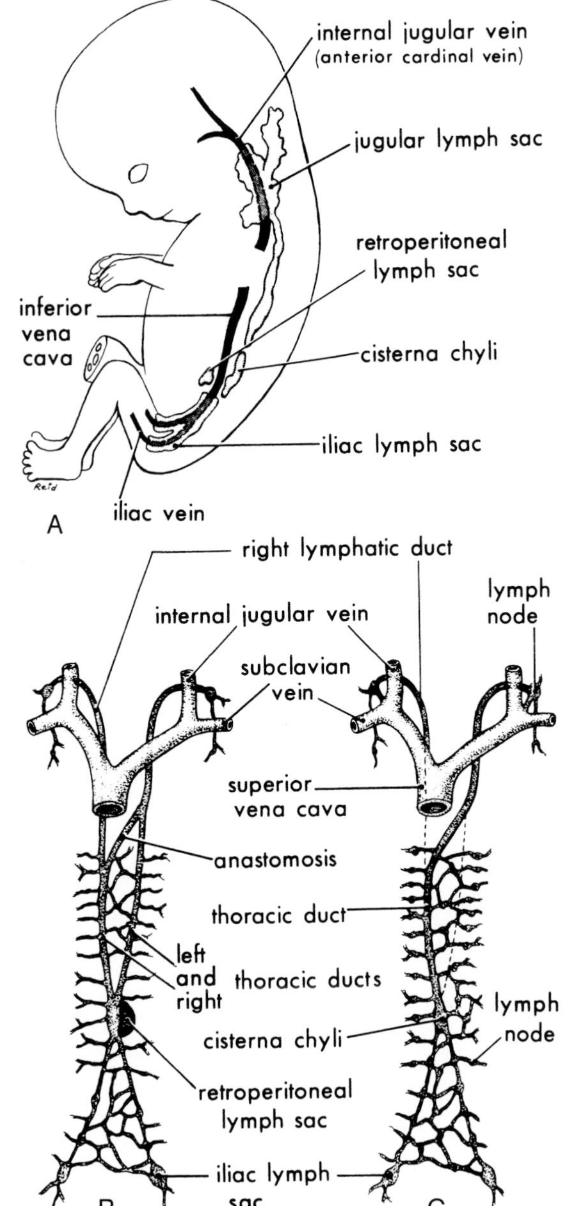

FIGURE 44–2 ■ Embryologic origin of the lymphatic channels and the thoracic duct in the human embryo. *A*, Left side of a 7-week-old embryo with the six lymph sacs. *B*, Ventral view at 9 weeks showing the paired thoracic ducts. *C*, Later stage showing the formation of the adult thoracic duct and the right lymphatic duct. (From Moore KL, Persaud TVN: The Developing Human, 5th ed. Philadelphia, WB Saunders, 1993.)

with several anastomoses between them. The azygos and the intercostal veins also contribute to the formation of a major portion of the duct. This explains the multiple connections between the duct and these vessels that allow chyle to be carried into the bloodstream when the duct is ligated. With maturation, the upper one third of the right duct and the lower two thirds of the left duct are obliterated, but the main communication between them persists to give the adult thoracic duct configuration. If the upper portion on the right side is not obliterated, a right lymphatic duct prevails.

Histology

Lymphatic capillaries consist of single layers of flat endothelial cells, slightly larger and thinner than blood capillary cells. The basement membrane is absent or vestigial, which allows large molecules to permeate the walls easily. The lymphatic capillaries can be distinguished from blood capillaries by the absence of the basement membrane and blind endings, and the lack of arterial and venous connections. Lymphatic capillaries do not have associated pericytes, but they do have anchoring filaments that attach to the surface of the endothelial cells and extend out into the connective tissue around the capillary. These filaments seem to hold the capillaries open during times when the surrounding edematous pressure might cause them to collapse.

The thoracic duct, however, contains a well-developed basement membrane and has three layers within the wall: intima, media, and adventitia. The intima contains elastic fibers. The media is well developed, consisting of smooth muscle fibers supported by connective tissue containing elastic fibers. It is this well-developed layer that contracts rhythmically to aid in lymph flow. The adventitia is supplied by the vasa vasorum and contains smooth muscle fibers running both longitudinally and obliquely.

The thoracic duct and all lymphatic channels, except the smallest ones, have valves. The valves have two leaflets, consisting of folds of intima with delicate connective tissue in the middle covered with endothelium. They are more numerous and closer together than the valves of veins. The valves are so close together that a distended lymphatic vessel appears beaded because of the dilated sections between the valves.

Physiology

The principal function of the thoracic duct is the transport of digestive fat to the venous system. According to Frazer (1951), small fatty acids with less than 10 carbon atoms are absorbed directly into the portal system, whereas larger lipids are absorbed into the intestinal lymphatic vessels as micelles. The transport time of absorbed fat from the mouth until it appears in the venous blood is less than 1 hour after ingestion, with the peak absorption 6 hours after ingestion.

The volume of lymph flow is estimated to be 1.38 ml/kg of body weight per hour. Volumes up to 2500 ml of chyle in 24 hours have been collected from the cannulated human thoracic duct. Crandall and colleagues (1943) found the flow of lymph in the thoracic duct to range from 0.38 ml/min at rest to 3.9 ml/min after a meal or during abdominal massage. It was found that 95% of the volume comes from the liver and intestinal lymphatic channels, although the amount from the extremities is negligible. Lymphatic flow in amphibians, reptiles, and some birds is propelled by lymph hearts, whereas mammals have more complex mechanisms. The forward flow of chyle from the abdomen in humans is influenced by four factors.

1. Vis a tergo, from the Latin "force exerted from the back," is the transmission of pressure to the cisterna chyli from the intestinal lacteal vessels by the absorption of lymph. This force comes from the inflow of chyle into the lacteal system produced by the intake of food and liquid meals and intestinal movement. It is proportional to the volume of the food and independent of the external pressure or wall pressure.

2. There is a pressure gradient. Negative intrathoracic pressure and positive intra-abdominal pressure create a gradient favoring flow of lymph toward the central circulation.

3. Muscular contractions by the duct itself are probably the most important factor in propelling lymph forward; the valves within the duct prevent retrograde flow. Kinmonth and Taylor (1956) observed that contractions occur every 10 to 15 seconds that are independent of respiratory movements. The intraductal pressure ranges from 10 to 25 cm H_2O and may rise to 50 cm H_2O with obstruction, as observed by Shafiroff and Kau (1959). Acetylcholine produced by fibers of the vagus nerve constricts the duct; epinephrine dilates it (Acevedo, 1943).

4. Birt and Connolly (1951) believed that there is a Bernoulli suction effect produced by the flow of blood past the lymphaticovenous junction, creating a vacuum.

The lymphatic vessels perform the vital functions of collecting and transporting tissue fluid, extravasated plasma proteins, absorbed lipids, and other large molecules from the interstitial space to the intravascular space. Most of the body's lymphocytes are circulated through the duct.

Chylothorax

DEFINITION

Chylothorax is the accumulation of excess lymphatic fluid in the pleural space, usually as a result of a leak from the thoracic duct or one of its major branches. The term *chyle* comes from the Latin "chylus," meaning "juice," and usually connotes the milky appearance of intestinal lymph caused by the presence of emulsified fats. (Note that chyme is the semifluid mass of partly digested food found in the small intestine.)

BASIC SCIENCE

Etiology

The prevalence of chylothorax ranges from 0.5% to 2.0% in selected series, according to Sachs and coauthors (1991). Chylothorax is thought to result from either an obstruction or laceration of the thoracic duct. The most common causes are neoplasms, trauma, tuberculosis, and venous thrombosis (Randolph and Gross, 1957; Roy et al, 1967). A classification adapted from DeMeester (1983) is shown in the box on page 1232.

Congenital chylothorax is the leading cause of pleural effusion in the neonate according to Randolph and Gross (1957). Fifty percent of newborns with chylothorax develop symptoms in the first 24 hours. The fluid is initially clear, but it quickly turns turbid when milk feeding begins. The cause is not always clear, but birth trauma or congenital defects in the duct or both may be precipi-

ETIOLOGY OF CHYLOTHORAX

- Congenital
  - Atresia of thoracic duct
  - Thoracic duct–pleural space fistula
  - Birth trauma
- Traumatic
  - Blunt
  - Penetrating
- Surgical
  - Cervical
    - Excision of lymph nodes
    - Radical neck dissection
  - Thoracic
    - Ligation of patent ductus arteriosus
    - Excision of coarctation
    - Esophagectomy
    - Resection of thoracic aortic aneurysm
    - Resection of mediastinal tumor
    - Pneumonectomy or lobectomy
    - Left subclavian artery operations
    - Sympathectomy
  - Abdominal
    - Sympathectomy
    - Radical lymph node dissection
- Diagnostic procedures
  - Lumbar arteriography
  - Subclavian vein catheterization
  - Left-sided heart catheterization
- Neoplasms
  - Benign
  - Malignant
- Infections
  - Tuberculous lymphadenitis
  - Nonspecific mediastinitis
  - Ascending lymphangiitis
  - Filariasis
- Miscellaneous
  - Venous thrombosis
    - Left subclavian or jugular vein
    - Superior vena cava
  - Secondary to chylous ascites
  - Pancreatitis
  - Spontaneous

From DeMeester TR: The pleura. In Sabiston DC, Spencer FC (eds): Surgery of the Chest, 4th ed. Philadelphia, WB Saunders, 1983.

tating factors. Increased venous pressure during a difficult delivery may cause rupture of the thin walls of the thoracic duct.

Chylothorax has been associated with a variety of syndromes including Noonan's syndrome, Down's syndrome, Gorham's syndrome, Adams-Oliver syndrome, hereditary lymphedema (Nonne-Milroy-Meige syndrome), yellow nail syndrome, Behçet's disease, and tracheoesophageal fistula (Farrell et al, 1993; Konishi et al, 1988; Smeltzer et al, 1986; Tie et al, 1994; Valmary et al, 1988; Zbranca et al, 1990). Malformations of the lymphatic system are rare causes of congenital chylothorax. The anomalous duct may be absent or atretic, or it may have multiple dilated lymphatic channels with abnormal communications between the duct and pleural space. Anomalies of the thoracic duct may be associated with polyhydramnios or lymphedema.

Traumatic Chylothorax

Traumatic injury to the thoracic duct may occur with blunt or penetrating trauma or during surgery (Cevese et al, 1975b). Injury may occur at any point along the course of the duct, making localization difficult. The most common mechanism of nonpenetrating injury is sudden hyperextension of the spine, resulting in rupture of the duct just above the diaphragm. Birt and Connolly (1951) thought that this is caused by a shearing of the duct by the right crus of the diaphragm or by sudden stretching over the vertebral bodies. Costal fractures are not necessary to produce this injury, especially after a meal.

Penetration by gunshot or stab wounds is rare. These injuries are usually overshadowed by life-threatening damage to other structures. Ductal injury, however, should be considered during the evaluation of a thoracotomy for trauma.

Surgical injury to the thoracic duct has been reported after almost every thoracic surgical procedure, especially those performed in the upper part of the left side of the chest. Surgical injury is possible during procedures involving the heart, lungs, aorta, esophagus, sympathetic chain, and subclavian vessels. The duct is most vulnerable in the upper part of the left chest during mobilization of the aortic arch, the left subclavian artery, or the esophagus (Higgins and Mulder, 1971).

Injury has also been reported after radical neck dissection and scalene node biopsy. Operations in the abdomen, such as sympathectomy and radical lymph node dissection, also result in damage to the thoracic duct. Diagnostic procedures, such as translumbar aortography and central venous line placement in the jugular or subclavian vein, also cause thoracic duct injuries.

Neoplasms

The thoracic duct can be involved with benign and malignant tumors, lymphatic permeation, direct invasion, or tumor embolus. The most frequently found tumors include lymphomas, lymphosarcomas, and primary lung carcinomas. Unilateral or bilateral chylothorax results from the rupture of distended tributaries or erosion into the duct.

Benign lesions of the thoracic duct include lymphangiomas, mediastinal hygromas, and pulmonary lymphangiomyomatosis. Lymphangiomyomatosis, reported by Corrin (1975) and Silverstein (1974) and their colleagues, occurs in young women and is associated with pneumothorax and hemoptysis. It is characterized by proliferation of smooth muscle in the peribronchial, perivascular, and perilymphatic regions of the lung, resulting in obstruction of the lymphatic channels. Dyspnea is the major symptom, and these women usually die of pulmonary insufficiency within 10 years of diagnosis (Bradley et al, 1980).

Tumors cause more than 50% of chylothoraces in adults. Roy and associates (1967) reported that lymphomas were found 75% of the time. A chylous effusion should always be evaluated as a possible signal for an unsuspected mediastinal or retroperitoneal malignancy.

Malignant obstruction may occasionally cause leakage of chyle into the pericardium, producing signs and symptoms of cardiac tamponade.

Infections

Infectious causes of chylothorax include tuberculosis, fungal diseases, lymphangiitis, filariasis, and nonspecific mediastinitis, which result in lymph node enlargement and obstruction (Yater, 1935).

Other Causes of Chylothorax

Vomiting or violent coughing can cause a "spontaneous rupture," especially when the duct is full after a fatty meal. When rupture does occur after such minor trauma, the possibility of an underlying malignancy must be considered. Thrombosis of the great veins into which the thoracic duct drains can produce a chylous effusion (Ross, 1961).

Chylous effusions in the chest can be the result of chylous ascites, which is usually caused by a malignancy, commonly lymphoma. Primary fistulas and lymphatic disease in children can cause intraperitoneal chylous accumulation. Exudative enteropathy caused by congenital intestinal lymphatic and chylous leaks from the lumen of the bowel is another cause. Amyloidosis can be complicated by chylothorax when the disease process causes ductal obstruction. Chylous ascites also occurs after various abdominal operations and with pancreatitis (Traquair, 1945).

COMPOSITION OF CHYLE

Thoracic duct lymph is not pure chyle but a mixture of lymph originating in the lungs, the intestine, the liver, the abdominal wall, and the extremities. Most chyle is produced in the intestine, and the amount of lymph originating from the extremities is negligible under normal circumstances. Chyle is characteristically milky white, odorless, and alkaline. The ductal lymph is clear during fasting and becomes milky after a fatty meal, as observed by Munk and Rosenstein (1891). It is strongly bacteriostatic and contains lipids, proteins, electrolytes, lymphocytes, and various other elements. The normal composition of chyle is shown in Table 44–1.

Lipids

The main component of chyle is fat. Chyle contains from 14 to 210 mmol/L total fat, including neutral fat, free fatty acids, sphingomyelin, phospholipids, cholesterol, and cholesterol esters. Sixty to seventy percent of ingested fat is absorbed by the intestinal lymphatic channels and conveyed to the blood by the thoracic duct.

TABLE 44–1 ■ **Normal Characteristics and Composition of Chyle**

Characteristics and Composition	*Normal Plasma Concentrations*
CHARACTERISTICS	
Milky appearance with a creamy layer that clears when fat is extracted by alkali or ether	
pH 7.4–7.8 (alkaline)	
Odorless	
Specific gravity 1.012–1.025	
Sterile and bacteriostatic	
Fat globules staining with Sudan III	
Lymphocytes 400 to 6800 × 10^6/L	1500–4000 × 10^6/L
Erythrocytes 0.050 to 0.6 × 10^9/L	4500–6500 × 10^9/L
COMPOSITION	
Total protein 21–59 g/L	65–80 g/L
Albumin 12–41.6 g/L	40–50 g/L
Globulin 11–30.8 g/L	25–35 g/L
Fibrinogen 0.16–0.24 g/L	1.5–3.5 g/L
Antithrombin globulin >25% plasma concentrate	
Prothrombin >25% plasma concentrate	
Fibrinogen >25% plasma concentrate	
Total fat 14–210 mmol/L	
Triglycerides—above plasma value	0.84–2.0 mmol/L
Cholesterol—plasma value or lower	4.4–6.5 mmol/L
Glucose 2.7–11.1 mmol/L	2.5–4.2 mmol/L
Urea 1.4–3.0 mmol/L	3.0–7.0 mmol/L
Electrolytes—similar to plasma	
Pancreatic exocrine enzymes present	
Lipoprotein electrophoresis—chylomicron band	
Cholesterol/triglyceride ratio <1	

Ross (1961) reported that neutral fat in lymph is transported as chylomicrons measuring 0.5 mm in diameter. Fatty acids with less than 10 carbon atoms are absorbed directly by the portal venous system. This is the basis for using medium-chain triglycerides as the oral diet in the medical management of chylothorax. The triglyceride content greatly exceeds the cholesterol content.

Protein

The lymphatic vessels are the main pathways for the return of extravascular proteins to the vascular space. Nix and coworkers (1957) and Ross (1961) found that the protein content is approximately one half the plasma concentration, ranging from 21 to 59 g/L. The albumin concentration ranges between 12 and 41.6 g/L and the globulin concentration is between 11 and 30.8 g/L.

Electrolytes

The electrolyte composition of chyle is similar to that found in plasma; the glucose concentration ranges from 2.7 to 11.1 mmol/L. The predominant ions include sodium, potassium, chloride, calcium, and inorganic phosphorus.

Cellular Elements

Lymphocytes are the main cellular elements in the thoracic duct lymph and arise from the peripheral lymphatic channels and lymphoid organs. Hyde and coworkers (1974) found that 90% of the lymphocytes are T lymphocytes, and they react differently to antigenic stimulation compared with blood lymphocytes. There is a continuous circulation of cells from blood to lymph and back again. Prolonged drainage can deplete the lymphocytes and impair the immune system. In clear lymph there are 0.05×10^9 erythrocytes per liter, but this may rise to 0.6×10^9 in postabsorptive states, as reported by Shafiroff and Kau (1959).

Miscellaneous Elements

Other components of chyle include fat-soluble vitamins, antibodies, urea nitrogen, and enzymes, including pancreatic lipase, alkaline phosphatase, aspartate transaminase, and alanine transaminase.

Pathophysiology

Chylothorax results from a tear or rupture in the thoracic duct. It can cause cardiopulmonary abnormalities and metabolic and immunologic deficiencies. Lymph commonly accumulates in the posterior mediastinum until the mediastinal pleura ruptures, usually on the right side at the base of the pulmonary ligament. The accumulation of chyle in the chest can compress the underlying lung and compromise pulmonary function, resulting in shortness of breath and respiratory distress.

Empyema is a rare complication of chylothorax because of the bacteriostatic actions of lecithin and fatty acids. Sterile chyle is nonirritating and therefore does not cause pleuritic pain or a fibrotic inflammatory reaction.

Although fat is the most conspicuous constituent of chyle, the loss of protein and vitamins is more important in terms of serious metabolic and nutritional defects. Shafiroff and Kau (1959) emphasized that loss of protein, fat-soluble vitamins, lymphocytes, and antibodies from a persistent chyle leak can lead to immunodeficiency, coagulopathy, malnutrition, inanition, and death.

DIAGNOSIS

Clinical Features

The onset of chylothorax is usually insidious, and rapid accumulation, tachypnea, tachycardia, and hypotension can occur. There is often a latent interval of 2 to 10 days before the chylothorax becomes clinically evident because many injured or postsurgical patients receive a restricted diet. Clinical manifestations of chylothorax are initially the result of the mechanical compression of the ipsilateral lung and mediastinum, causing dyspnea, fatigue, and heaviness. The problems of protein, fat-soluble vitamin, and antibody loss can be accentuated by repeated thoracenteses or chronic tube drainage. Fluid losses can reach 2500 ml of chyle per day and result in cardiovascular instability if they are not replaced. Death is inevitable when supportive treatment fails unless the fistula closes spontaneously or is ligated surgically.

History

A pleural effusion in a patient with any of the diagnoses associated with chylothorax should always be evaluated for chyle. A history of trauma after a heavy meal or a recent surgical procedure in the distribution of the thoracic duct should raise the suspicion of chylothorax.

Laboratory Studies

Laboratory studies of blood chemistry and hematologic parameters are often normal immediately after traumatic injury to the duct. Chronic effusion or chylothorax in infancy may cause hypoproteinemia, decreased triglyceride levels, and lymphocytopenia.

Radiologic Studies

There are no valid radiologic findings to differentiate chylothorax from other pleural effusions. As reported by Sachs and coauthors (1991), bipedal lymphangiograms were found to be useful in diagnosing thoracic duct laceration (Fig. 44–3). In this procedure, 10 ml of ethiodized oil is injected into lymphatic vessels on the dorsum of the foot, followed 1 to 2 hours later by radiography of the abdomen and chest. This technique, however, may

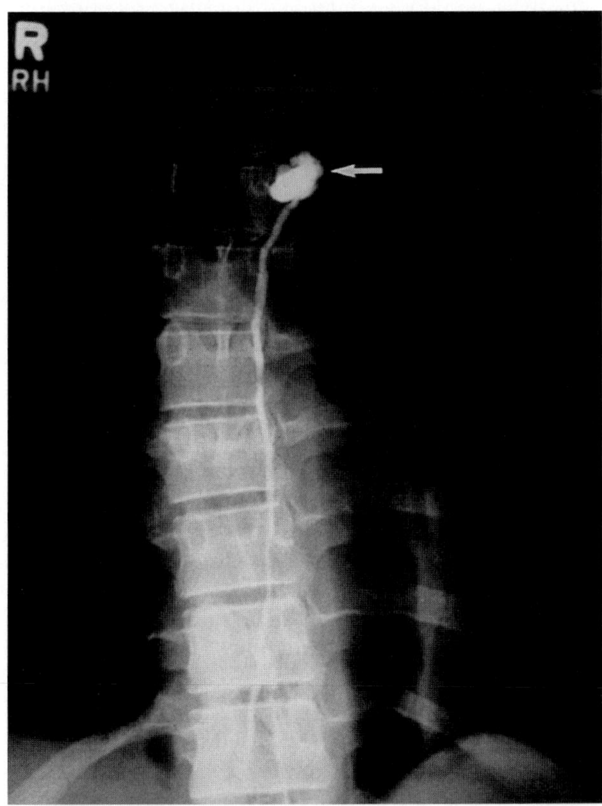

FIGURE 44–3 ■ Bipedal lymphangiogram showing the site of a chylous leak with resulting chyloma *(arrow)*. (Courtesy of B.R. Boulanger, MD.)

cause pulmonary edema, lymphangiitis, or rarely cerebral oil embolism. Radionuclide imaging with ^{99m}Tc antimony sulfide colloid injected subcutaneously yields images within 3 hours. The radionuclide technique can demonstrate obstruction, but it is limited in localizing the site of leakage (Freundlich, 1975). Computed tomography also has limited use in localizing the site of leakage but may demonstrate a mediastinal mass, enlarged lymph nodes, or a primary lung carcinoma.

Fluid Analysis

Chylothorax is suggested by the presence of nonclotting milky fluid obtained from the pleural space at thoracentesis or chest tube drainage. The characteristics of chyle are listed in Table 44–1. The diagnosis is confirmed by finding free microscopic fat, a fat content that is higher than that of the plasma, and a protein content that is less than one half the plasma level. The fat globules clear with alkali or ether and stain with Sudan III. Chyle may be mistaken for pus, but there is no odor, and cultures are negative. Gram's staining is helpful because the cells in chyle are lymphocytes rather than polymorphonuclear leukocytes, and no bacteria are seen.

It is important to recognize that chyle is milky white only when fat is being transported from the gut. A finding of clear or bloody fluid does not rule out a chylous leak. Traumatic injury to the duct in the fasting state may yield chyle, which initially appears blood stained. It may eventually become clear and serous. Lymphocytes are the predominant cells in chyle, and a 90% lymphocyte count is virtually diagnostic. In traumatic effusions, there is an admixture of erythrocytes and other blood elements.

The diagnosis may be delayed in patients receiving parenteral nutrition and nasogastric suction. Before an effusion is evident, patients may show a widening of the superior mediastinum caused by a chyloma or accumulation of chyle within the mediastinal pleural envelope. The chyloma may drain into the pleural space and develop into chylothorax, and there is often a decrease in the leukocyte count as a result of a selective decrease in the lymphocytes. Another useful hint is the rate of fluid accumulation in the chest. A disproportionately high volume of fluid drainage from the chest, averaging 700 to 1200 ml/day in a patient who has suffered a hyperextension injury or has undergone esophagectomy or thoracic aortic surgery, should be evaluated for a chylous leak.

Staats and coauthors (1980) stated that chyle has a cholesterol/triglyceride ratio of less than 1, whereas nonchylous effusions have a ratio greater than 1. If the fluid has a triglyceride level that is greater than 1.24 mmol/L, there is a 99% chance that the fluid is chyle. If the triglyceride content is less than 0.56 mmol/L, there is only a 5% chance that the fluid is chyle (Staats et al, 1980). An intermediate value requires lipoprotein electrophoresis, and the presence of chylomicrons is specific for the diagnosis of chylothorax (Seriff et al, 1977).

Methylene blue dye may be injected into the lymphatic channel to help visualize the duct and fistula at surgery. Ductal visualization can also be enhanced by preoperative ingestion of cream or instillation of methylene blue into the stomach (Engevik, 1976; Murphy and Piper, 1977).

DIAGNOSTIC TESTS

Gram's stain
pH
Sudan III stain
Cholesterol/triglyceride ratio <1
Triglyceride level >1.24 mmol/L
Chylomicrons on electrophoresis

Differential Diagnosis

In the differential diagnosis of milky effusions, pseudochylothorax and cholesterol pleural effusions need to be considered. Long-standing chronic pleural effusions may have a chylous appearance. These cholesterol effusions are seen in tuberculosis or rheumatoid arthritis and are related to the high cholesterol content of the fluid, as reported by Bower (1968). They do not contain fat globules or chylomicrons on electrophoresis. The presence of cholesterol crystals on smears of the sediment is diagnostic of pseudochylothorax (Coe and Aikawa, 1961).

Boyd (1986) reported that pseudochyle occurs with the thickened or calcified pleura seen with malignant tumors or infections and is milky because of the presence of a lecithin globulin complex. There is only a trace of fat, and fat globules cannot be seen with Sudan III. It contains less cholesterol and protein than does chyle.

A complex pleural effusion exists when a thoracic duct leak is present in addition to some other cause of pleural effusion (e.g., congestive heart failure, infections, tumors, or trauma). The analysis may be misleading because of a dilutional effect.

In summary, thoracentesis and fluid analysis for cell count, Gram's staining, and lipid levels should be diagnostic in the majority of cases.

MANAGEMENT

The management of chylothorax depends on judgment, and opinion varies about the aggressiveness and timing of surgery. The dangers of chylothorax include dehydration, malnutrition, and immune deficiency, all related to the large losses of lymphatic fluid. The modalities used in the management of chylothorax are listed in the following. Lampson (1948) introduced thoracic duct ligation, which decreased the mortality rate from 50% to 15%. Nontraumatic chylothorax at that time had a nearly 100% mortality rate.

Prevention is important, and injuries need to be recognized or anticipated intraoperatively. Ductal ligation at the aortic hiatus is easily accomplished at the time of esophageal or thoracic aortic dissection. Many surgeons routinely ligate the thoracic duct if an extensive lymphadenectomy or posterior mediastinal node dissection is carried out. Surgical intervention to ligate the thoracic duct should be performed before the debilitating complications of thoracic duct leakage or its therapy are manifested. Although the repair of a ductal fistula has been accomplished by thoracoscopy (Shirai et al, 1991), the open procedure for ligating the duct through a small

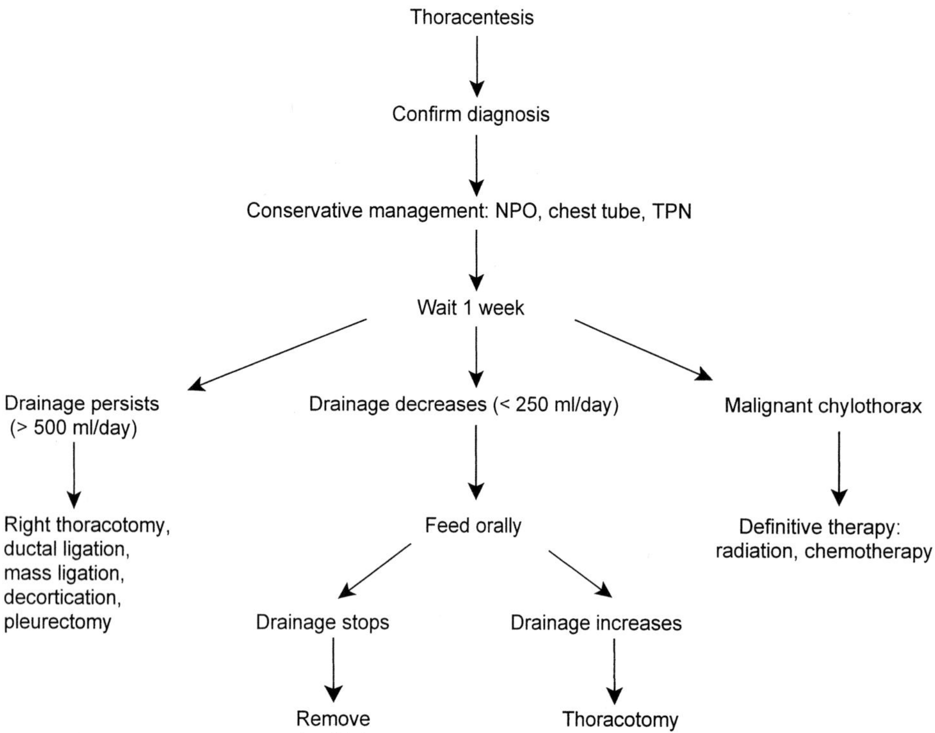

FIGURE 44–4 ■ Algorithm for the treatment of chylothorax. (NPO, nothing by mouth; TPN, total parenteral nutrition.)

right thoracotomy remains the standard. It is often easier for the patient than is a prolonged course of hyperalimentation. This is particularly true in infants and children, in whom central lines are associated with significant morbidity rates. Our approach is summarized in Figure 44–4.

Conservative

The diagnosis is established by analysis of the pleural fluid, as described earlier. Patients with congenital, postoperative, or traumatic chylothorax in whom immediate thoracotomy for the control of an associated lesion is not required should be managed initially by conservative treatment. The goals of treatment are re-expansion of the lung by drainage of the chylothorax, prevention of dehydration, maintenance of nutrition, and reduction of chyle formation. Drainage of the pleural space can be achieved by thoracentesis, tube thoracostomy, or pleuroperitoneal shunt. Repeated thoracenteses rarely achieve complete pleural evacuation and can result in hemothorax, pneumothorax, or empyema. Tube thoracostomy allows rapid continuous drainage, achieves lung re-expansion, and is the most widely used method.

The most important aspects of chylothorax management are maintaining adequate nutrition and correcting fluid and electrolyte imbalance (Bessone et al, 1971). Intravenous injection of chyle was used in the 1930s and then abandoned in the 1940s because of anaphylactic reactions (Peet and Campbell, 1943; Whitcomb and Scoville, 1942). Thomson and Simms (1993) have successfully reinfused chyle using a 40-μm blood filter and a volumetric pump. They recommended a small test dose to avoid anaphylaxis.

Enteral formulas with a low fat content supplemented with medium-chain triglycerides have been recommended but rarely work. In 1951, Frazer discovered that long-chain fatty acids (more than 10 carbon atoms) undergo a second esterification and pass into the lymph as chylomicrons. Medium-chain fatty acids, however, pass directly into the portal vein bound to albumin. Despite this preferential uptake of medium-chain triglycerides directly into the portal circulation, intestinal triglycerides derive from endogenous as well as exogenous sources. Eighty percent of chylous triglycerides have been found to be non–medium-chain triglycerides despite a medium-chain diet (Jensen et al, 1989). Any oral intake increases chyle production (Robinson, 1985). Total parenteral nutrition and nothing by mouth are, therefore, the most effective methods for decreasing chyle production (Hashim et al, 1964).

Surgical

There is no consensus on the length of time that attempts to manage conservatively should be made before initiating surgical therapy. Williams and Burford (1963) and Selle and colleagues (1973) recommended 14 days as the maximum limit of conservative management before proceeding with surgical ligation. Twenty-five to fifty percent of leaks close spontaneously during this interval, and the other 50% to 75% require surgical intervention. We favor a shorter course of nonsurgical management, especially in neonates or debilitated patients severely compromised by the lymphocyte, antibody, and protein loss from an active thoracic duct fistula.

If spontaneous closure is thought to have occurred, a high-fat challenge meal should be given before removing

THERAPY OF CHYLOTHORAX

- Medical
  - Nothing by mouth
  - Central hyperalimentation
  - Drainage of pleural space
    - Thoracentesis
    - Closed chest tube thoracostomy
- Complete expansion of the lung
- Surgical
  - Direct ligation of thoracic duct
  - Mass ligation of thoracic duct tissue
  - Pleuroperitoneal shunting
  - Pleurectomy
  - Fibrin glue
  - Thoracoscopy
- Radiation therapy
- Chemotherapy

the chest tube. If the chest tube drainage is consistently greater than 500 ml/day for more than 1 week, surgical intervention is definitely indicated. Surgery should, however, be avoided in patients in whom the risk is outweighed by other considerations, such as vertebral fractures, unresectable tumors, or multiple organ injuries. If a lung is entrapped, malignancy is suspected or multiple loculations are present, and early surgical intervention is appropriate (Brewer, 1955; Goorwitch, 1955).

Operative Techniques

Several surgical techniques for repairing chylothorax have been described: (1) direct ligation of the thoracic duct, (2) supradiaphragmatic mass ligation of the thoracic duct, (3) pleuroperitoneal shunting, (4) pleurodesis and pleurectomy, (5) suture ligation of leaking mediastinal pleura, (6) anastomosis of the duct to the azygos vein, (7) decortication, (8) fibrin glue, and (9) thoracoscopy (Cevese et al, 1975a).

Thoracic duct ligation at the time of the initial thoracotomy should be done whenever an extensive mediastinal dissection is performed or if a chyle leak is suspected because of a continuous accumulation of watery fluid in the thorax. If the site of the chyle leak can be identified, many surgeons prefer to perform thoracotomy on the side of the chylothorax to ligate the site of the suspected leak with suture material. The use of tissue or felt pledgets often helps with the fixation ligatures. If the leak cannot be found, extensive dissection should be avoided. Mass ligation of all tissue between the aorta and azygos vein should be performed above the diaphragm as reported by Lampson (1948), Klepser and Berry (1954), Selle and coauthors (1973), and Murphy and Piper (1977) and championed by Patterson (1981) and Milsom (1985) and their coworkers. Van Pernis (1949) reported that the duct is a single structure from T12 to T8 in more than 60% of patients; therefore, there is an almost 40% incidence of duplication of the mediastinal thoracic duct in its caudal portion. Mass ligation is important to avoid missing a major channel.

Duct ligation can be performed through either a right or left thoracotomy. On the right side, a short posterolateral thoracotomy incision is used. The fibrin deposits on the pleura are removed, and the inferior pulmonary ligament is released. Thickened pleura or enlarged nodes should undergo a biopsy to rule out a malignant process causing the chylothorax. All the tissue between the azygos vein and the aorta is ligated by using nonabsorbable suture material. No attempt is made to close the fistula directly (Fig. 44–5). On the left side, the lower 10 cm of esophagus is mobilized to the left. The tissue to the right of the aorta is dissected until the azygos vein is identified. Mass ligation of all tissue between the aorta and azygos vein is then performed. The minor lymphaticovenous anastomoses between the duct and the azygos, intercostal, and lumbar veins quickly compensate for this localized interruption. Even if the duct cannot be found, mass ligation is successful in 80% of patients (Patterson et al, 1981). In infants, a transient edema of the legs and ascites may be seen for several days and usually then resolves.

It is helpful to detect preoperatively whether the aorta is ectatic in its location above the diaphragm. A supradiaphragmatic aorta that is located to the right of the vertebral body makes access to the thoracic duct by way of a right thoracotomy difficult. In this case, a left-sided approach is preferred.

Ross (1961) suggested instilling 100 to 200 ml of olive oil 2 to 3 hours before the operation through the nasogastric tube. This causes filling of the duct with a milky chyle and allows its easy recognition. Any residual oil is aspirated from the stomach before the induction of anesthesia. An alternative method is injection of 1% aqueous Evans blue dye into the leg. The dye stains the duct within 5 minutes and lasts about 12 minutes. The disadvantage is that other tissues may also be stained. Preoperative administration of 2 oz of cream 30 minutes before thoracotomy has been recommended by Schumacker and Moore (1951). Filling the thorax with saline intraoperatively may help in the detection of milky chyle leaking from the duct.

Some believe that the best method for chylothorax repair is to find the leak and close it with nonabsorbable sutures and Teflon pledgets, allowing the main portion of the duct to remain patent, as discussed by Miller (1989). Reimplantations of the divided duct into a vein or other anastomoses are complicated and unnecessary. A parietal pleurectomy may be performed to achieve pleurodesis in addition to duct ligation or may be used alone if the duct is not accessible. If the lung is trapped, it may require decortication.

Stenzl and coauthors (1983) reported the successful use of fibrin glue in one patient, and intrapleural fibrin glue was used by Akaogi and associates (1989) with thoracoscopy. Thoracoscopic ligation of the duct has been reported by Kent and Pinson (1993). The fistula can be located by lymphangiography or by direct visualization. As our experience with thoracoscopy increases, less invasive methods should become the standard in the future.

Postoperative Chylothorax

Chylothorax is uncommon after thoracic surgical procedures (Cerfolio et al, 1996). The incidence appears to be

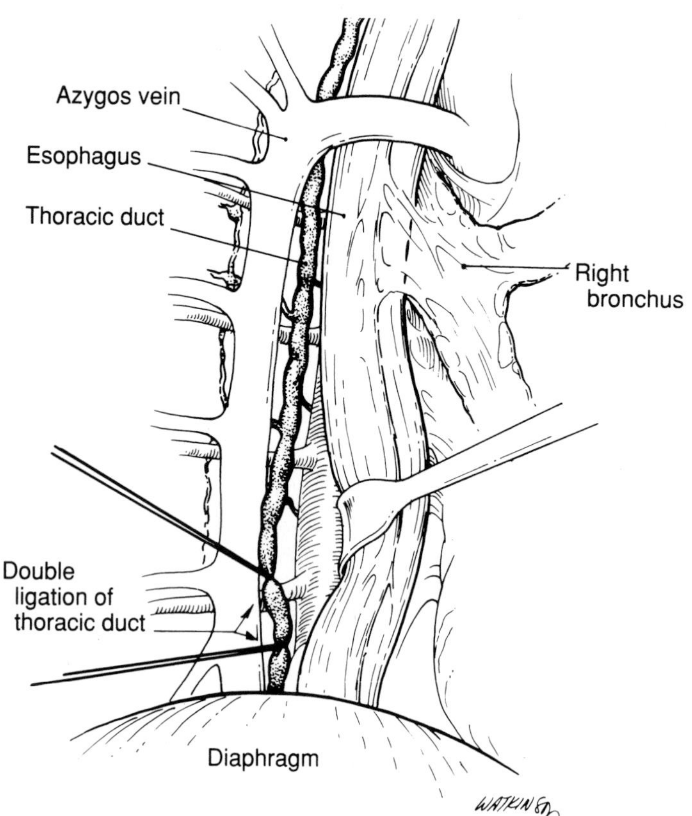

FIGURE 44–5 ■ Therapy for chylothorax using mass ligation of the supradiaphragmatic thoracic duct. (From Moore KL, Persaud TVN: The Developing Human, 5th ed. Philadelphia, WB Saunders, 1993.)

higher after esophagectomy with mediastinal lymphadenectomy than after pulmonary resections (3% and 0.4%, respectively), and surgical ligation is often required. Conservative management with drainage, hyperalimentation, and lung re-expansion should seal the leak after lobectomy. Chylothorax after pneumonectomy is difficult to diagnose. It is suggested by rapid filling of the pneumonectomy space and confirmed by analysis of fluid obtained by thoracentesis. Most cases remain undiagnosed unless the patient develops hemodynamic problems.

Stable patients with no mediastinal shift can be simply observed. Rapid opacification of the pneumonectomy space accompanied by a mediastinal shift to the contralateral side, however, requires urgent tube thoracostomy drainage (Sarsam et al, 1994). Subsequent management is controversial but should be guided by the response to conservative therapy and the size of the leak (Vallieres et al, 1993). Persistent chyle drainage for more than 1 week should be surgically explored, and the duct should be ligated.

Pediatric Chylothorax

Bond and colleagues (1993) reviewed 26 postoperative chylothoraces in pediatric patients and found a spontaneous cessation rate of 73% with drainage and hyperalimentation. Failure of conservative management was associated with venous hypertension resulting from elevated right-sided cardiac pressures or central venous thrombosis. The authors suggested that the elevated pressure is transmitted to the lymphatic system and hinders closure and recommended thoracotomy on the affected side with duct ligation when conservative treatment fails.

Other Techniques

In nontraumatic chylothorax, the cause must be determined and appropriately treated. Chylous fistulas that result from obstruction by malignancies respond poorly to surgical ligation unless the underlying disease can be treated effectively. For lymphomas or other malignancies, radiation or chemotherapy may be needed. This may not be totally successful. Pleuroperitoneal shunting with the double-valve Denver shunt has been reported by Milsom and coauthors (1985), Weese and Schouten (1984), and Miller (1989) in high-risk patients. Success rates of 75% to 90% have been reported in pediatric chylothorax (Murphy et al, 1989; Rheuban et al, 1992; Sade and Wiles, 1990). The shunt is relatively simple to place and reduces the nutritional, fluid, and cellular losses seen with external drainage. To compress the pump chamber periodically, however, requires the patient's compliance. Shunt occlusion with fibrin requiring shunt replacement occurs in 10%. Chylous ascites does not appear to be a significant problem, but its presence remains a contraindication to shunt placement.

Neoplastic chylothorax usually responds to irradiation or chemotherapy directed at the primary disease. Miller (1996) has also used 20 Gy of radiation in successful treatment of postoperative chylothoraces in four patients.

Pleurodesis with talc, nitrogen mustard, quinacrine, or bleomycin may help temporarily when there is a contraindication to surgery. The combination of ductal ligation with pleurodesis or parietal pleurectomy in addition to chemotherapy and radiation may be advisable for persistent chylothorax that is associated with malignant disease.

CONCLUSIONS

Chylothorax is an infrequent but important cause of pleural effusion. The diagnosis is often complicated by the superimposition of other causes of pleural effusion. Early recognition and therapy prevent the nutritional depletion that can result from a continuous chylous leak. Thoracentesis is used for diagnosis, and a chest tube is inserted for drainage and pulmonary expansion. This intervention, combined with the elimination of oral feeding and parenteral nutrition, may obliterate the leak if there is no underlying obstruction of lymphatic flow into the central circulation.

Chylothorax in the neonate may respond to drainage, but prompt ligation should be considered if there is continued drainage with high volumes of fluid, cells, and nutrients. When nontraumatic chylothorax is associated with venous or lymphatic obstruction, specific treatment of the underlying process is required for success. If widespread disease is present, chemical pleurodesis is a reasonable choice before operative intervention is considered. Traumatic leaks may be managed with drainage and parenteral support. Thoracoscopic ligation is feasible. Surgical repair is best accomplished by supradiaphragmatic ligation of the thoracic duct through a right thoracotomy. This should be done early before complications set in.

COMMENTS AND CONTROVERSIES

Although chylothorax is more common after surgery of the thoracic aorta, correction of cardiovascular malformations, or resection of the esophagus and lung, injuries to the thoracic duct can complicate any type of intrathoracic operations. With more extensive types of pulmonary resections, often involving radical lymph node excisions, the incidence of postoperative chylothoraces is increasing and is currently in the range of 0.3% to 0.5%.

Knowledge of the anatomy of the thoracic duct is the key to understanding how this structure can be damaged and how to prevent damage. In most cases of pulmonary resection for lung cancer, intraoperative trauma to the thoracic duct or to collecting trunks occurs during nodal staging or radical node dissection. On the right side, leaks are usually in the posterior mediastinum just below the carina; on the left, most are secondary to extensive dissections above the aortic arch. As mentioned in this chapter, many surgeons, such as Wong, routinely ligate the thoracic duct if an extensive lymphadenectomy is carried out.

Because of reduced lymph flow and pressure, chylous leaks are difficult to reco[illegible]ntraoperatively if they are not specifically investig[illegible]stoperatively, the diagnosis is usually made within 48 to 72 hours when the patient resumes a normal diet and the drainage from the chest tube becomes milky. These patients should be started immediately on total parenteral nutrition because oral preparations containing medium-chain triglycerides are generally ineffective. In fact, patients should not be allowed to eat or drink anything because even the smallest amount of water increases lymph flow.

When reoperation becomes necessary, I prefer direct ligation of the fistula site after the patient has been given 300 ml of 30% cream 2 to 3 hours preoperatively. This is done because it is possible that even after ligation of the main duct, lymph will continue flowing through abnormal or secondary ducts.

J.D.

KEY REFERENCES

Bessone LN, Ferguson TB, Burford TH: Chylothorax. Ann Thorac Surg 12:527, 1971.

This is a classic in-depth review of the anatomy, pathophysiology, and management of chylothorax. It contains 133 references, and it still remains the most complete review of the subject.

Cevese PG, Vecchioni R, Cordiano C et al: Surgical techniques for operations on the thoracic duct. Surg Gynecol Obstet 140:958, 1975.

This is an excellent compilation of the surgical approaches and techniques related to thoracic duct pathologic conditions. Although simpler methods have been advised, the background is an essential element in the armamentarium of the thoracic surgeon.

DePalma RG: Disorders of the lymphatic system. In Sabiston DC (ed): Textbook of Surgery, 13th ed. Philadelphia, WB Saunders, 1987, p 1479.

This chapter summarizes the lymphatic system with respect to the historical and the basic science aspects. It is concise and well written and has 124 references.

REFERENCES

Acevedo D: Motor control of thoracic duct. Am J Physiol 139:600, 1943.

Akaogi E, Mitsui K, Sohara Y et al: Treatment of postoperative chylothorax with intrapleural fibrin glue. Ann Thorac Surg 48:116–118, 1989.

Aselli G: De Factibus Sive Laceteis Verris, Quarto Vasorum Mesarai Corum Genere Novo Invento. Milano, 1627.

Bargebuhr A: Chylose und chyliforme Ergusse im Pleura und Pericardialraum. Dtsch Arch Klin Med 54:410, 1894.

Bernard C: Leçons sur les Phenomenes de la vie Communs aux Animaux et aux Vegetaux. Paris, JB Bailliere et Fils, 1878.

Bessone LN, Ferguson TB, Burford TH: Chylothorax. Ann Thorac Surg 12:527–550, 1971.

Birt AB, Connolly NK: Traumatic chylothorax: A report of a case and a survey of the literature. Br J Surg 39:564, 1951.

Blalock A, Cunningham RS, Robinson CS: Experimental production of chylothorax by occlusion of the superior vena cava. Ann Surg 104:359, 1936.

Bond SJ, Guzzetta PC, Snyder ML, Randolph JG: Management of pediatric postoperative chylothorax. Ann Thorac Surg 56:469–472, 1993.

Bower GC: Chyliform pleural effusion in rheumatoid arthritis. Am Rev Respir Dis 97:455–459, 1968.

Boyd A: Surgical Diseases of the Pleura and Chest Wall, 1st ed. Philadelphia, WB Saunders, 1986.

Bradley SL, Dines DE, Soule EH, Muhm JR: Pulmonary lymphangiomyomatosis. Lung 158:69–80, 1980.

Brewer LA: Surgical management of lesions of the thoracic duct. Am J Surg 90:210, 1955.

Cerfolio RJ, Allen MS, Deschamps C et al: Postoperative chylothorax. J Thorac Cardiovasc Surg 112:1361–1365, 1996.

Cevese PG, Vecchioni R, Cordiano C et al: Surgical techniques for operations on the thoracic duct. Surg Gynecol Obstet 140:957–965, 1975a.

Cevese PG, Vecchioni R, D'Amico DF et al: Postoperative chylothorax: Six cases in 2,500 operations, with a survey of the world literature. J Thorac Cardiovasc Surg 69:966–971, 1975b.

Coe JE, Aikawa JK: Cholesterol of pleural effusion. Arch Intern Med 108:163–174, 1961.

Corrin B, Liebow AA, Friedman PJ: Pulmonary lymphangiomyomatosis: A review. Am J Pathol 79:348–382, 1975.

Crandall L Jr, Barker SB, Graham DC: A study of the lymph from a patient with thoracic duct fistula. Gastroenterology 1:1040, 1943.

Davis MK: A statistical study of the thoracic duct in man. Am J Anat 171:212, 1915.

DeMeester TR: The pleura. In Sabiston DC, Spencer FC (eds): Surgery of the Chest, 4th ed. Philadelphia, WB Saunders, 1983.

Drinker CK, Field ME: The protein content of mammalian lymph and the relation of lymph to tissue fluid. Am J Physiol 9:32, 1931.

Engevik L: Traumatic chylothorax. Scand J Thorac Cardiovasc Surg 10:77–78, 1976.

Farrell SA, Warda LJ, LaFlair P, Szymonowicz W: Adams-Oliver syndrome: A case with juvenile chronic myelogenous leukemia and chylothorax. Am J Med Genet 47:1175–1179, 1993.

Frazer AC: The mechanism of fat absorption. Biochem Soc Symp 9:5, 1951.

Freundlich IM: The role of lymphangiography in chylothorax: A report of six nontraumatic cases. Am J Roentgenol Radium Ther Nucl Med 125:617–627, 1975.

Goorwitch J: Traumatic chylothorax and thoracic duct ligation. J Thorac Cardiovasc Surg 29:467, 1955.

Hashim SA, Roholt RB, Babayan UK et al: Treatment of chyluria and chylothorax with medium chain triglycerides. N Engl J Med 270:756, 1964.

Heppner GJ: Bilateral chylothorax and chyloperitoneum. JAMA 102:1294, 1934.

Higgins CB, Mulder DG: Chylothorax after surgery for congenital heart disease. J Thorac Cardiovasc Surg 61:411–418, 1971.

Hunter W: Two Introductory Lectures in His Last Course of Anatomic Lectures at His Theatre in Windmill Street, 1st ed. London, J Johnston, 1784.

Hyde PV, Jersky J, Gishen P: Traumatic chylothorax. S Afr J Surg 12:57–59, 1974.

Jensen GL, Mascioli EA, Meyer LP et al: Dietary modification of chyle composition in chylothorax. Gastroenterology 97:761–765, 1989.

Kausel WH, Reeve TS, Stain AA et al: Anatomic and pathologic studies of the thoracic duct. J Thorac Cardiovasc Surg 34:631, 1957.

Kent RB, Pinson TW: Thoracoscopic ligation of the thoracic duct. Surg Endosc 7:52–53, 1993.

Kinmonth JB, Taylor GW: Spontaneous rhythmic contractility in human lymphatics. J Physiol (Lond) 133:3, 1956.

Klepser RG, Berry JF: The diagnosis and surgical management of chylothorax with the aid of lipophilic dyes. Dis Chest 24:409, 1954.

Konishi T, Takeuchi H, Iwata J, Nakano T: Behçet's disease with chylothorax: Case report. Angiology 39:68–71, 1988.

Lampson RS: Traumatic chylothorax: A review of the literature and report of a case treated my mediastinal ligation of the thoracic duct. J Thorac Cardiovasc Surg 17:778, 1948.

Lee FC: The establishment of collateral circulation following ligation of the thoracic duct. Bull Johns Hopkins Hosp 33:21, 1922.

Meade RH Jr, Head JR, Moen CW: The management of chylothorax. J Thorac Cardiovasc Surg 19:709, 1950.

Miller JI: Chylothorax and anatomy of the thoracic duct. In Shields TW (ed): General Thoracic Surgery, 3rd ed. Philadelphia, Lea & Febiger, 1989, pp 625–632.

Miller JI: Discussion of postoperative chylothorax. J Thorac Cardiovasc Surg 112:1365–1366, 1996.

Milsom JW, Kron IL, Rheuban KS, Rodgers BM: Chylothorax: An assessment of current surgical management. J Thorac Cardiovasc Surg 89:221–227, 1985.

Moore KL: The circulatory system: The cardiovascular and lymphatic systems. In The Developing Human, 2nd ed. Toronto, WB Saunders, 1977, pp 284–286.

Munk I, Rosenstein A: Zur Lehre von der Resorption im Dark nach Untersuchungen an einer Lymph (chylus) fistel beim Menschen. Virchows Arch A Pathol Anat Histopathol 123:484, 1891.

Murphy MC, Newman BM, Rodgers BM: Pleuroperitoneal shunts in the management of persistent chylothorax. Ann Thorac Surg 48:195–200, 1989.

Murphy TO, Piper CA: Surgical management of chylothorax. Am Surg 43:715–718, 1977.

Nix JT, Albert M, Dugas JE et al: Chylothorax and chyloascites: A study of 302 selected cases. Am J Gastroenterol 28:40, 1957.

Patterson GA, Todd TR, Delarue NC et al: Supradiaphragmatic ligation of the thoracic duct in intractable chylous fistula. Ann Thorac Surg 32:44–49, 1981.

Peet MM, Campbell KN: Massive chylothorax following splanchnicectomy. Hosp Bull Ann Arbor 9:2, 1943.

Pflug J, Calnan J: The valves of the thoracic duct at the angulus venosus. Br J Surg 55:911, 1968.

Quinke H: Über fetthaltige Transudate: Hydros chylosus und Hydrops adiposus. Dtsch Arch Klin Med 16:121, 1875.

Randolph JG, Gross RE: Congenital chylothorax. Arch Surg 74:405, 1957.

Rheuban KS, Kron IL, Carpenter MA et al: Pleuroperitoneal shunts for refractory chylothorax after operation for congenital heart disease. Ann Thorac Surg 53:85–87, 1992.

Robinson CL: The management of chylothorax. Ann Thorac Surg 39:90–95, 1985.

Ross JK: A review of the surgery of the thoracic duct. Thorax 16:12, 1961.

Roy PH, Carr DT, Payne WS: The problem of chylothorax. Mayo Clin Proc 42:457, 1967.

Sabin FR: The origin and development of the lymphatic system. Rep Johns Hopkins Hosp 17:347, 1916.

Sachs PB, Zelch MG, Rice TW et al: Diagnosis and localization of laceration of the thoracic duct: Usefulness of lymphangiography and CT. AJR Am J Roentgenol 157:703–705, 1991.

Sade RM, Wiles HB: Pleuroperitoneal shunt for persistent pleural drainage after Fontan procedure. J Thorac Cardiovasc Surg 100: 621–623, 1990.

Sarsam MA, Rahman AN, Deiraniya AK: Postpneumonectomy chylothorax. Ann Thorac Surg 57:689–690, 1994.

Schumacker HB, Moore TC: Surgical management of traumatic chylothorax. Surg Gynecol Obstet 93:46, 1951.

Selle JG, Snyder WH, Schreiber JT: Chylothorax: Indications for surgery. Ann Surg 177:245–249, 1973.

Seriff NS, Cohen ML, Samuel P, Schulster PL: Chylothorax: Diagnosis by lipoprotein electrophoresis of serum and pleural fluid. Thorax 32:98–100, 1977.

Shafiroff GP, Kau QY: Cannulation of the human thoracic lymph duct. Surgery 45:814, 1959.

Shirai T, Amano J, Takabe K: Thoracoscopic diagnosis and treatment of chylothorax after pneumonectomy. Ann Thorac Surg 52:306–307, 1991.

Silverstein EF, Ellis K, Wolff M, Jaretzki A: Pulmonary lymphangiomyomatosis. Am J Roentgenol Radium Ther Nucl Med 120:832–850, 1974.

Smeltzer DM, Stickler GB, Fleming RE: Primary lymphatic dysplasia in children: Chylothorax, chylous ascites, and generalized lymphatic dysplasia. Eur J Pediatr 145:286–292, 1986.

Staats BA, Ellefson RD, Budahn LL et al: The lipoprotein profile of chylous and nonchylous pleural effusions. Mayo Clin Proc 55:700–704, 1980.

Starling EH: On the absorption of fluid from the connective tissue spaces. J Physiol (Lond) 19:312, 1896.

Stenzl W, Rigler B, Tscheliessnigg KH, et al: Treatment of postsurgical chylothorax with fibrin glue. Thorac Cardiovasc Surg 31:35–36, 1983.

Thomson IA, Simms MH: Postoperative chylothorax: A case for recycling? Cardiovasc Surg 1:384–385, 1993.

Tie ML, Poland GA, Rosenow EC: Chylothorax in Gorham's syndrome: A common complication of a rare disease. Chest 105:208–213, 1994.

Traquair K: Chylothorax following traumatic pseudocyst of the pancreas. Br J Surg 33:297, 1945.

Vallieres E, Shamji FM, Todd TR: Postpneumonectomy chylothorax. Ann Thorac Surg 55:1006–1008, 1993.

Valmary J, Delbrouck P, Herning R et al: Syndrome des ongles jaunes avec epanchements chyleux [Yellow nail syndrome with chylous effusions]. Rev Med Interne 9:425–428, 1988.

Van Pernis PA: Variation of the thoracic duct. Surgery 26:308, 1949.

Weese JL, Schouten JT: Internal drainage of intractable malignant pleural effusions. Wis Med J 83:21–23, 1984.

Whitcomb BB, Scoville WB: Postoperative chylothorax: Sudden death following infusion of aspirated chyle. Arch Surg 45:747, 1942.

Williams KR, Burford TH: The management of chylothorax related to trauma. J Trauma 3:317, 1963.

Yater WM: Non-traumatic chylothorax and chylopericardium: Review and report of a case due to carcinomatous thromboangiitis obliterans of the thoracic duct and upper great veins. Ann Intern Med 9:600, 1935.

Zbranca V, Arama A, Mihaescu T, Covic M: Limfedem ereditar (boala Nonne-Milroy-Meige) asociat cu chilotorax: Consideratii pe marginea a doua cazuri [Hereditary lymphedema (Nonne-Milroy-Meige syndrome) associated with chylothorax: Comments on 2 cases]. Rev Med Chir Soc Med Nat Iasi 94:189–192, 1990.

Zesas DG: Die nicht operative entstandenen Verletzungen des Ductus Thoracicus. Dtsch Z Chir 115:49, 1912.

CHAPTER **45**

Mesothelioma and Less Common Pleural Tumors

Valerie W. Rusch

HISTORICAL NOTE

Pleural mesothelioma is a uncommon neoplasm with an estimated annual incidence in the United States of 2000 to 3000 cases. The first report of a primary pleural tumor is attributed to Lieutaud in 1767 (Scharifker and Kenko, 1979), but an accurate pathologic description did not become available until 1937 when Klemperer and Rabin classified mesotheliomas as either localized or diffuse (Klemperer and Rabin, 1937). Cell culture experiments by Stout and Murray (1942) defined the histopathologic origin of these tumors. The epidemiology of diffuse malignant mesothelioma was first elucidated in 1960 when Wagner and associates reported 33 cases of malignant pleural mesothelioma in asbestos mine workers from the North Western Cape Province of South Africa (Wagner et al, 1960). Subsequent studies, especially by Selikoff in the United States, confirmed that asbestos exposure was the major risk factor for malignant mesothelioma (Selikoff et al, 1965; Whitwell and Rawcliffe, 1971).

The biology of mesothelioma is still poorly understood, and the clinical management of this disease remains controversial. Pleural mesotheliomas were previously classified as benign or malignant. However, "benign mesotheliomas" are now termed *fibrous tumors of the pleura* in recognition of their being pathologically and clinically distinct from diffuse malignant mesothelioma.

FIBROUS TUMORS OF THE PLEURA

Fibrous tumors of the pleura are rare, with approximately 600 cases reported. They are not associated with asbestos exposure, they are as common in women as in men, and they occur predominantly during the sixth and seventh decades of life.

Fibrous tumors of the pleura usually present clinically as discrete, encapsulated tumors, but they have a variable histologic appearance. The "patternless pattern" originally described by Stout and Murray, characterized by a random mixture of fibroblast-like cells and connective tissue, is the most common histologic appearance (Stout and Murray, 1942). A hemangiopericytoma-like pattern is the second most common appearance, but leiomyoma-like or neurofibroma-like patterns are also seen. A mixture of histologic patterns is common and occurs in approximately 40% of cases (Moran et al, 1992). In contrast to diffuse malignant mesotheliomas, fibrous tumors do not have epithelial features histologically, do not stain for keratins on immunohistochemical analysis, and do not have long branching microvilli on electron microscopy (Said et al, 1984). Localized mesotheliomas are thought to arise from the primitive submesothelial mesenchymal cell rather than from the mesothelial cell itself (Briselli et al, 1981).

Fibrous tumors of the pleura can be either benign or malignant. The pathologic features that distinguish these two entities are shown in Table 45–1. Benign fibrous tumors are usually pedunculated, arise from the visceral pleura, measure less than 10 cm, are relatively acellular, and have few mitoses (Fig. 45–1). Occasionally they grow to a huge size and fill the entire hemithorax (McNicholas et al, 1980; Watts et al, 1989). Malignant fibrous tumors are usually larger, nonpedunculated tumors that arise from the parietal, mediastinal, or diaphragmatic pleura and have a greater tendency toward increased cellularity, pleomorphism, and frequent mitoses (Fig. 45–2).

Most patients with fibrous tumors of the pleura present with an asymptomatic mass incidentally diagnosed on chest radiography. Among the 30% to 40% of patients who have symptoms, cough, chest pain, and dyspnea are the most common complaints, but fever, hypertrophic pulmonary osteoarthropathy, and hemoptysis can also occur (Okike et al, 1978; Scharifker and Kenko, 1979). The relative incidence of these symptoms in 360 cases of

TABLE 45–1 ■ **Pathologic Features That Distinguish Benign from Malignant Localized Fibrous Tumors of Pleura**

	Benign (N = 141)		*Malignant* (N = 82)*	
Feature*	*No.*	*(%)*	*No.*	*(%)*
Gross				
Pedunculated	73	(52)	21	(26)
Atypical location†	67	(48)	55	(67)
Size (>10 cm)	34	(24)	45	(55)
Necrosis and hemorrhage	21	(15)	53	(65)
Microscopic				
Increased cellularity	18	(13)	62	(76)
Pleomorphism‡	14	(10)	69	(84)
Mitosis (> 4 mf/10 hpf)	2	(1)	63	(77)

*For all features, the differences between benign and malignant tumors are statistically significant by the chi-square test ($P < .05$).

†Tumor attached to parietal pleura, fissure, or mediastinum or inverted into peripheral lung.

‡Pleomorphism expressed as increased nuclear grades.

Reprinted with permission from England DM, Hochholzer L, McCarthy MJ: Localized benign and malignant fibrous tumors of the pleura: A clinico-pathologic review of 223 cases. Am J Surg Pathol 13:647, 1989.

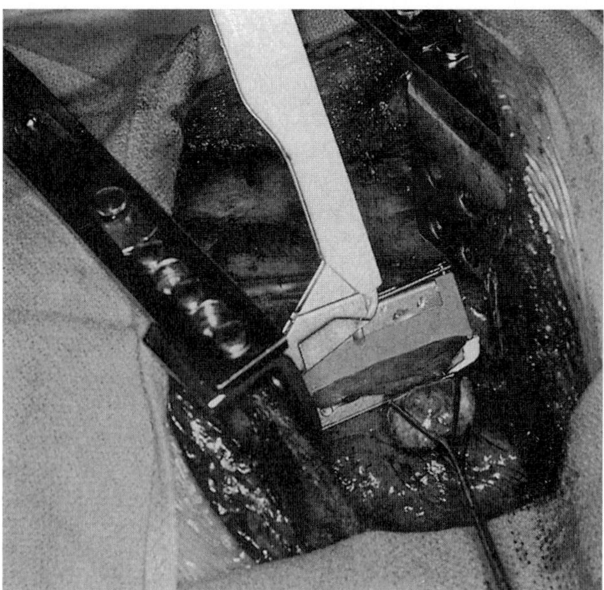

FIGURE 45–1 ■ Intraoperative photograph of a benign mesothelioma. The stapler is placed across the pulmonary parenchyma just beyond the base of this pedunculated tumor.

localized mesothelioma is shown in Table 45–2. Hypoglycemia has been reported in approximately 4% of patients and is almost always associated with tumors larger than 10 cm. Hypoglycemia is caused by secretion of an insulin-like growth factor (IGF II) and resolves after the tumor is resected (Cole et al, 1990; Immerman et al, 1982). Pleural effusion, clubbing of the fingers, hemoptysis, and pulmonary osteoarthropathy are also reported to occur sometimes in association with fibrous tumors (Briselli et al, 1981; England et al, 1989).

Signs and symptoms occur more often with malignant than with benign fibrous tumors. However, neither the pathologic features nor the clinical presentation fully predicts the behavior and long-term outcome of these tumors. Overall survival is directly related to whether the tumor can be completely resected. Pedunculated masses, no matter what their size or histologic characteristics, are more easily removed than sessile tumors involving the diaphragm, chest wall, or mediastinum. With rare exceptions, pedunculated tumors are completely cured by surgical resection. If they recur, they do so locally. Sessile tumors are potentially curable by complete resection. When incompletely resected, they recur locally, metastasize, and are usually fatal within 2 to 5 years. There is no indication currently that any adjuvant treatment is beneficial, and surgical resection remains the mainstay of therapy (de Perrot et al, 1999; Okike et al, 1978; Scharifker and Kenko, 1979; Suter et al, 1998).

DIFFUSE MALIGNANT PLEURAL MESOTHELIOMA

Incidence and Epidemiology

Malignant pleural mesothelioma (MPM) is by definition a diffuse process that involves all pleural surfaces. It is far more common and clinically important than fibrous tumors of the pleura. The incidence of this disease has risen steadily since 1970, and there are currently an estimated 2300 new cases annually in the United States. The incidence in women has remained relatively stable at 3 per million population, whereas the number of cases in men has increased to 15 per million population per year. This trend reflects the impact of occupational asbestos exposure (McDonald and McDonald, 1987). The latency period between asbestos exposure and the development of disease is at least 20 years, and, therefore, the recent surge in the number of cases reflects the widespread industrial use of asbestos from the 1940s to the 1960s. In the United States, the incidence of MPM is expected to decline after the year 2000 (Price, 1997). However, in other countries such as Great Britain, where asbestos remained a significant occupational hazard during the 1970s, the incidence of MPM is still increasing and constitutes a significant public health problem (Peto et al, 1995).

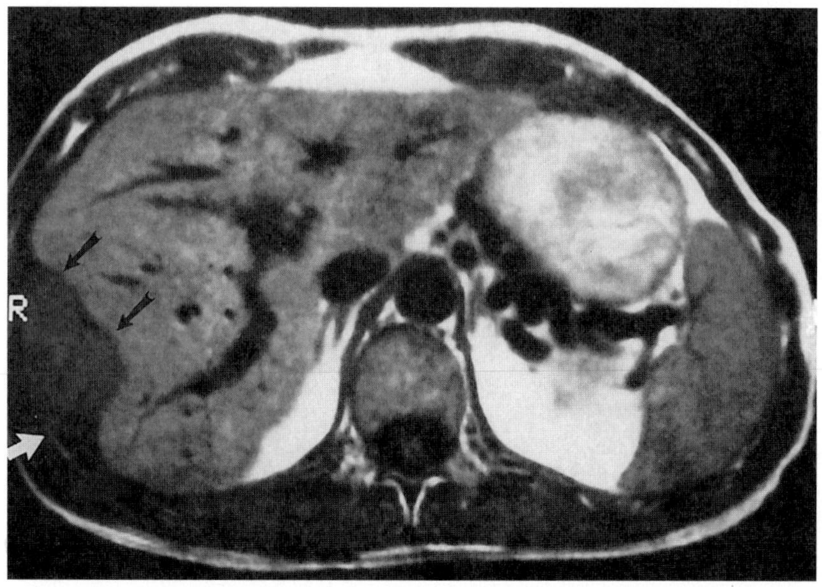

FIGURE 45–2 ■ Magnetic resonance scan of a localized malignant fibrosarcomatous mesothelioma (*white arrow*), which originated from the parietal pleura in the right costophrenic angle. The scan shows a distinct plane (*black arrows*) between the mass and the liver. At thoracotomy, the tumor did not traverse the diaphragm, and the remainder of the pleura was normal. The patient remained disease-free 2.5 years after wide resection with reconstruction of the chest wall and diaphragm.

TABLE 45–2 ■ **Summary of Reported Features in 360 Cases of Solitary Fibrous Tumor of the Pleura**

Years	*No. Patients*	*Age Range (y)*	*Sex: Male/Female*	*Symptomatic Patients (% of total)*	*Prevalence of Various Symptoms (%)*						*Pleural Laterality: Right/Left*	*Clinical Origin: Visceral/Parietal*	*Behavior: Benign/Lethal*
					Cough	Chest Pain	Dyspnea	Pulmonary Osteoarthropathy	Fever	Other			
1942–1972	190	12–82	84/106 (mean 50)	72	39	40	26	47	24	37	61/60	51/28	147/20
1973–1980	170	5–87	81/89 (mean 53)	54	54	51	49	22	25	25	78/68	90/23	142/18
Total	360	5–87	165/195 (mean 51)	64	46	44	37	35	24	32	139/128	141/51	289/38

Reprinted with permission from Briselli M, Mark EJ, Dickersin GR: Solitary fibrous tumors of the pleura: Eight new cases and review of 360 cases in the literature. Cancer 47:2687, 1981.

The type of asbestos fiber plays a critical role in this causal relationship. Asbestos fibers are divided into two mineralogic groups: amphibole and serpentine. Chrysotile asbestos is the only member of the serpentine group, whereas crocidolite, amosite, tremolite, anthophyllite, and actinolite asbestos belong to the amphibole group. These silicate minerals differ considerably in structure. Serpentine fibers are large curly fibers that do not travel beyond the major airways; amphibole fibers are narrow and straight fibers that pass into pulmonary parenchyma and are taken up in the lymphatic vessels (Pooley, 1987). The amphibole fibers, especially crocidolite asbestos, are the ones most clearly associated with MPM. Crocidolite asbestos is found in South Africa and, until recently, was also mined in Western Australia (Musk et al, 1989). Chrysotile accounts for 97% of the world asbestos production and is mined principally in the Ural mountains in Russia, Quebec Province in Canada, Zimbabwe and Swaziland in southern Africa, the Italian Alps, and Cyprus (Wagner, 1986). Whether chrysotile itself causes MPM is controversial. However, it is often contaminated with amphibole fibers such as tremolite or amosite (Churg and DePaoli, 1988). Chrysotile appears to be a far greater risk factor for the development of lung cancer, particularly in patients who are smokers (McDonald et al, 1989).

Individuals can be exposed to asbestos in many situations because it has more than 1000 industrial applications. The areas of the world that have the highest incidence of MPM are those with asbestos mines or asbestos industries, or industries that use large amounts of asbestos, such as shipyards, insulation, or fireproofing (Andersson and Olsen, 1985). In North America, the highest incidence areas include the provinces of Quebec and British Columbia in Canada, which have asbestos mines, and Seattle, Hawaii, San Francisco-Oakland, New York-New Jersey, and New Orleans in the United States, which have either large shipyards or asbestos industries (McDonald and McDonald, 1987). It is difficult to document a relationship between the duration or intensity of asbestos exposure and the development of MPM. Sometimes the form of exposure is not easily recognized by patients or physicians. For instance, during the 1950s, the filters used in Kent cigarettes contained crocidolite asbestos and probably led to significant asbestos exposure in millions of smokers (Longo et al, 1995). Patients with peritoneal MPM usually have a history of very heavy exposure, whereas patients with pleural disease may have had brief or indirect exposure (Levine, 1981).

MPM is also caused by other naturally occurring and synthetic fibers that share the physical properties of amphibole asbestos fibers (i.e., have a diameter of less than 0.25 μm and a length greater than 5.0 μm). The most notable example of this is erionite (Wagner, 1986), a zeolite fiber that is found in volcanic deposits of central Turkey and is the major building material of homes in that area. In Karain, a village with a population of 575, MPM was the single most common cause of death, with 36 cases recorded over the 6-year period from 1970 to 1976 (Baris et al, 1978).

There are other less common causes of MPM. Radiation exposure for periods ranging from 10 to 31 years before the development of MPM is the best documented cause and is seen primarily as a late complication of treatment for Hodgkin's disease or breast cancer (Cavazza et al, 1996). Extravasation of radioactive thorium dioxide during radiologic procedures and exposure to isoniazid in utero have also been anecdotally reported causes (Anderson et al, 1985; Lerman et al, 1991). Various other substances (Malker et al, 1985; Peterson et al, 1984), some of which are listed in Table 45–3, have been implicated as possible risk factors for MPM, based on epidemiologic or experimental studies. However, smoking does not appear to be a risk factor for MPM. This is in distinct contrast to lung cancer, for which asbestos and smoking act as synergistic carcinogens (McDonald et al, 1989).

The peak incidence for the majority of individuals who develop MPM is in the sixth decade of life. MPM is

TABLE 45–3 ■ Nonasbestos Causes of Mesothelioma

Agent	Species Tumor Observed in or Induced in*
Naturally occurring mineral fibers	
Zeolites (eronite)	Human, rat
Minerals	
Nickel	Rat
Silica powder	Rat
Beryllium	Rat, ?human
Radiation	Human, rat
Organic chemicals	
Polyurethane, polysilicone	Rat
Sterigmatocystin (aflatoxin B1-related compound)	Rat
Ethylene oxide	Rat
N-methyl-*N*-Nitrosourea	Guinea pig
N-methyl-*N*-Nitrosourethane	Mouse
3-Methylcholanthrene	Mouse
Methyl nitrosamine	Rat
1-Nitroso-5, 6-Dihydrouracil	Rat
Diethylstilbesterol	Monkey
Stilbesterol	Dog
3, 4, 5-Trimethyloxycinnamaldehyde	Rat
Mineral oil	Human
Liquid paraffin	Human
Viruses	
MC 29 avian leukosis virus	Chicken
SV 40	Hamster
Chronic inflammation	
Recurrent lung infections	Human
Tuberculous pleuritis	Human
Recurrent diverticulitis	Human
Familial Mediterranean fever	Human
Nonspecific industrial exposure	
Shoe industry workers	Human
Petrochemical-oil industry workers	Human
Stone cutters	Human
Leather factory or textile workers	Human
Occupations involving exposure to copper, nickel, fiberglass, rubber or glass dust	Human
Cocarcinogens	
3-Methylcholanthrene-asbestos	Rat
Radiation-asbestos	Rat
N-methyl-*N*-Nitrosourea-asbestos	Rat
Hereditary predisposition	Human

*Note: In some instances the tumors induced in animals by various agents may represent sarcomas and not mesotheliomas.

Reprinted with permission from Hammar SP, Bolen JW: Pleural neoplasms. In Dail DH, Hammar SP (eds): Pulmonary Pathology. New York, Springer-Verlag, 1988, p 979.

predominantly a disease of adults because of the long latency period between exposure to causative agents and the development of cancer, but it occasionally occurs in childhood (Fraire et al, 1988). In that setting, it seems to be idiopathic. MPM sometimes develops in young adults because of exposure to risk factors during childhood (Kane et al, 1990).

Pathology and Molecular Biology

MPMs arise from multipotential mesothelial or subserosal cells that can develop into either an epithelial or a sarcomatoid neoplasm. In contrast to fibrous tumors of the pleura, MPMs always have an epithelial component. However, they exhibit a wide array of histologic patterns (Table 45–4) and often have a mixture of epithelial and sarcomatoid features (Hammar and Bolen, 1988). In a review of 819 cases, Hillerdal (1983) reported that 50% were of epithelial type, 34% were of mixed type, and 16% were of the sarcomatoid type. The histologic appearance of MPM is easily confused with that of other neoplasms, and there is often disagreement among pathologists when light microscopy is used as the sole method of diagnosis. The reclassification rate of tumors originally diagnosed by morphology alone as MPM ranges from 30% to 84% when these specimens are reviewed by panels of reference pathologists. The most frequent challenge for the pathologist is to distinguish pure epithelial MPMs from metastatic adenocarcinoma. Very early stage MPM can also be difficult to distinguish from benign mesothelial hyperplasia, and the rare desmoplastic form of MPM often resembles benign fibrosis because of its predominantly fibroblastic cell type and sparsely cellular appearance (Cantin et al, 1982; Hammar and Bolen, 1988). Some histochemical stains may distinguish MPM from other tumors. Pulmonary adenocarcinomas usually stain positively with mucicarmine, whereas MPM does not. About 20% of epithelial MPMs produce an acidic mucosubstance, hyaluronic acid, which can be seen either within or between cells with an alcian blue or colloidal iron stain (Hammar and Bolen, 1988).

However, immunohistochemistry and electron microscopy have become the standard approach to diagnosis.

TABLE 45–4 ■ Histologic Classification of Malignant Pleural Mesothelioma

Epithelial
Tubulopapillary
Epithelioid
Glandular
Large cell/giant cell
Small cell
Adenoid-cystic
Signet ring
Sarcomatoid (fibrous, sarcomatous, mesenchymal)
Mixed epithelial-sarcomatoid (biphasic)
Transitional
Desmoplastic
Localized fibrous mesothelioma

Reprinted with permission from Hammar SP, Bolen JW: Pleural neoplasms. In Dail DH, Hammar SP (eds): Pulmonary Pathology. New York, Springer-Verlag, 1988, p 979.

Useful immunohistochemical stains include antibodies to cytokeratin, vimentin, carcinoembryonic antigen (CEA), and calretinin. MPMs stain positively for low molecular weight cytokeratins, a feature that distinguishes them from sarcomas; and they rarely stain for CEA and usually stain positively for calretinin, features that distinguish them from adenocarcinoma (Ordóñez, 1998; Wirth et al, 1991). If immunohistochemical stains yield equivocal results, electron microscopy will usually lead to a definitive diagnosis. The most prominent feature of MPMs on electron microscopy is that they have numerous, long, sinuous microvilli, whereas adenocarcinomas have short, straight microvilli that are covered by a fuzzy glycocalyx (Burns et al, 1985; Hammar and Bolen, 1988).

The biology of MPM is still poorly understood. Flow cytometric examination of MPMs surprisingly shows them to be predominantly diploid (approximately 65% of cases), with intermediate or low proliferative rates (Burmer et al, 1989). Like most solid tumors, MPMs develop as a result of a multistep process involving activation of oncogenes and growth factors and inactivation of tumor-suppressor genes. However, the currently identified molecular abnormalities in MPM differ from those known to occur in lung cancer (Fig. 45–3) (Lechner et al, 1997). Losses of chromosomes 6p, 1p, and 22q may be among the earliest events (Cheng et al, 1994; Lee et al, 1996; Taguchi et al, 1993; Tiainen et al, 1992). Allelic losses at one or both arms of chromosome 4 are also frequent, as are deletions of 15q (Balsara et al, 1999; Shivapurkar et al, 1999). Polysomies of chromosomes 5, 7, 12, and 20 have also been reported (Tiainen et al, 1989). Corresponding to these chromosomal abnormalities, deletions of the genes p16, WT1, and NF2 are known to be common in MPM (Kumar-Singh et al, 1997; Sekido et al, 1995). In contrast to lung cancer, abnormalities of p53 and Rb are uncommon, and it is thought that the pathways involving these important tumor-suppressor genes may be perturbed by abnormalities in other related genes such as p16 (Xiao et al, 1995). The SV40 virus has also been identified in some MPMs, particularly in North America, and this may inactivate p53 (Carbone et al, 1997; Mulatero et al, 1999; Testa et al, 1998).

Activated oncogenes include *C-jun*, *C-fos*, and *C-myc* (Tiainen et al, 1992). The epithelial growth factor receptor and its ligands, which are frequently overexpressed in non–small cell lung cancers, are not usually altered in MPM. However, platelet-derived growth factor-a, platelet-derived growth factor-b, and insulin-like growth factor-1 are frequently overexpressed and probably play important roles in tumor initiation and growth (Langerak et al, 1995; Lee et al, 1993). Cytokine expression, especially interleukin-6, is also common and may participate in tumor growth and progression (Monti et al, 1994). Interleukin-6 is probably responsible for signs and symptoms such as fever and thrombocytosis that are characteristic of MPM. Increased telomerase activity is common in MPM and is likely important in tumorigenesis (Dhaene et al, 1998). Figure 45–1 displays the possible steps in the genesis of MPM, but this sequence of progressive genetic abnormalities remains hypothetical. Further study is needed to define which abnormalities occur in the various stages and tumor histologies of MPM.

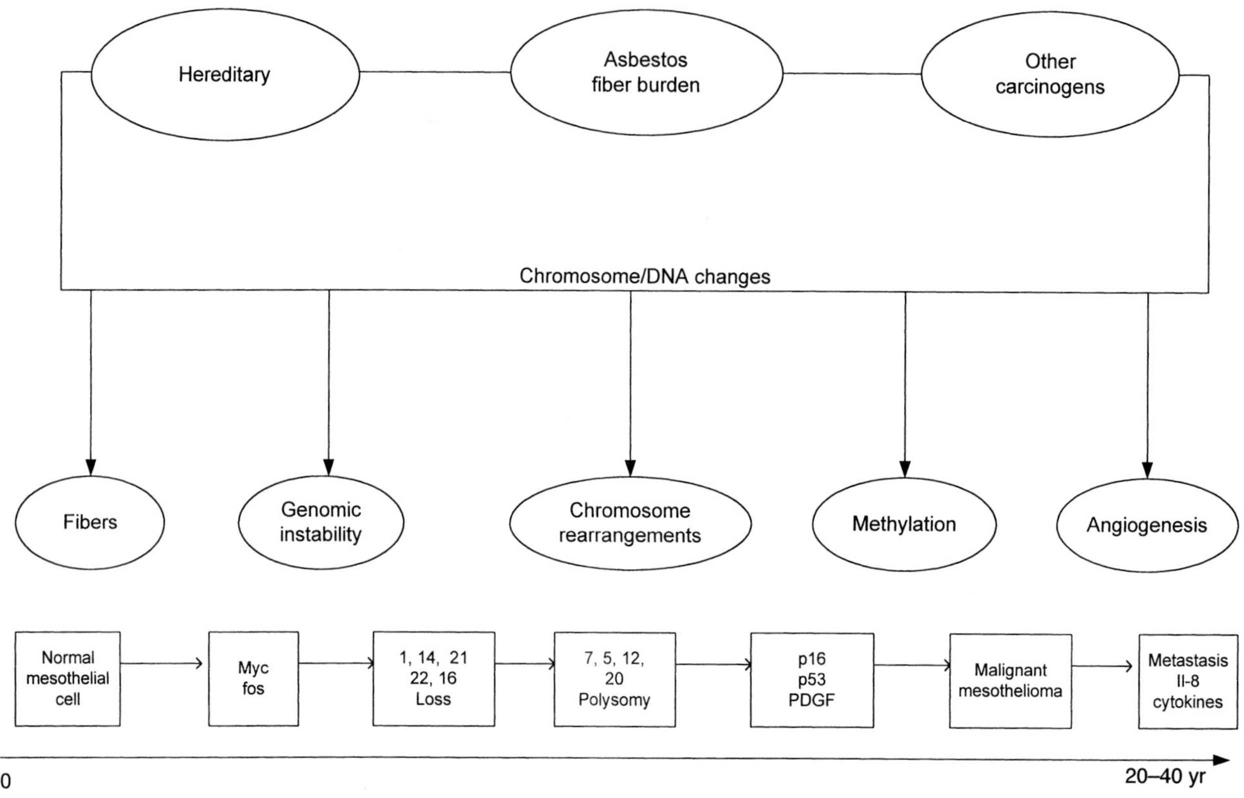

FIGURE 45–3 ■ Possible steps in the genesis of mesothelioma. PDGF, platelet-derived growth factor. (From Lechner JF, Tesfaigzi J, Gerwin BI: Oncogenes and tumor-suppressor genes in mesothelioma: A synopsis. Environ Health Perspect 105 (Suppl 5):1061, 1997.)

Clinical Presentation and Diagnosis

The clinical presentation of MPM is insidious and nonspecific. Because of this, the interval between the onset of symptoms and diagnosis is often 3 to 6 months. Dyspnea and chest pain are the most common symptoms, occurring in 90% of patients. Weight loss is seen in about 30% of patients. Less common signs and symptoms include cough, weakness, anorexia, and fever. Hemoptysis, hoarseness, dysphagia, Horner's syndrome, and dyspnea from a spontaneous pneumothorax occur rarely. The physical examination is usually unrevealing, demonstrating only dullness to percussion and diminished breath sounds over the affected hemithorax. Patients who have locally advanced disease may have a palpable chest wall mass, diffuse infiltration of the chest wall by tumor, and, rarely, palpable supraclavicular lymph nodes (Elmes and Simpson, 1976; Ruffie et al, 1989; Sheard et al, 1991).

Paraneoplastic syndromes are uncommon, but autoimmune hemolytic anemia, hypercalcemia, hypoglycemia, the syndrome of inappropriate secretion of antidiuretic hormone, and hypercoagulability not related to thrombocytosis have been reported (Gerwin et al, 1987). Thrombocytosis, defined as a platelet count of more than 400,000/μL, occurs in about 40% of patients and can be associated with a leukemoid reaction (Olesen and Thorshauge, 1988).

Patients with MPM often have abnormal electrocardiographic (ECG) and echocardiographic findings. In a review of 64 patients, Wadler and colleagues (1986) found that 55 patients (89%) had an abnormal ECG. Sinus tachycardia was seen in 42%, and non–life-threatening ventricular or atrial arrhythmias occurred in 17% of patients. More than 33% of patients had some form of bundle branch block. Although pericardial invasion or myocardial involvement was a common finding at autopsy in these patients, most ECG abnormalities occurred more than 6 months before death, suggesting that these abnormalities are not solely related to the presence of advanced disease. Echocardiography was somewhat insensitive but highly specific for involvement of the pericardium or myocardium by tumor. Three patients who had pericardial effusions diagnosed by echocardiogram had pericardial and myocardial involvement at autopsy, whereas 5 patients who had pericardial tumor at autopsy had a normal echocardiogram premortem.

There are no tumor markers that are routinely used for MPM. The serum hyaluronan concentration may be elevated in some patients, not a surprising finding given the positive staining for hyaluronic acid seen in many epithelial MPMs. In one study of 37 patients, a rise in the serum hyaluronan level had a sensitivity of 65% and a specificity of 85% as a predictor of progressive disease. Hyaluronan can be measured using a commercial kit, but it is not readily available in most hospitals (Dahl et al, 1989). CA-125 is elevated in approximately 20% of patients, but the utility of this as a marker has not been investigated in large numbers of patients (Rusch et al, 1994).

MPM is classically portrayed as a massive tumor involving all pleural surfaces, encasing the lung and chest wall, and producing severe unremitting pain. In fact, this appearance is characteristic only of locally advanced MPM. In the earliest stage of disease, tumor is confined to the parietal pleura, and pleural effusion is the dominant feature. This is responsible for the dyspnea that often leads patients to seek medical attention. As the tumor grows it spreads to involve the visceral pleura, and the pleural effusion becomes loculated. Subsequently, the pleural tumor becomes confluent, obliterating the pleural space. At this stage, patients experience vague sensations of chest discomfort along with mild shortness of breath. The massive pleural rind characteristic of locally advanced disease produces both dyspnea because of restrictive lung disease and pain from encasement of the chest wall and infiltration of the intercostal spaces and nerves (Law et al, 1982b).

The radiologic appearance of MPM is variable and nonspecific. In early-stage MPM, a large pleural effusion is often the only sign of disease (Fig. 45–4). Multiple discrete pleural-based masses may be seen on computed tomography (CT) (Fig. 45–5). Subsequently, pleural-based masses become evident and are often intermixed with multiloculated effusions (Gotfried et al, 1983). Rarely, a dominant pleural-based mass may be the initial presentation, but ultimately the involvement of the pleura is always diffuse. Eventually, a thick irregular pleural rind develops with encasement of the lung and obliteration of the pleural space (Fig. 45–6). Mediastinal adenopathy, direct extension of the tumor into the mediastinum, involvement of the pericardium with pericardial effusion, and extension into the chest wall or through the diaphragm are seen in very locally advanced tumor (Fig. 45–7). CT permits a far better appreciation of the extent of the disease than does plain radiography, which cannot demonstrate many of these abnormalities (Alexander et al, 1981; Law et al, 1982a; Mirvis et al, 1983; Rabinowitz et al, 1982). CT is currently the most accurate noninvasive way to stage cancer, to gauge the response to therapy,

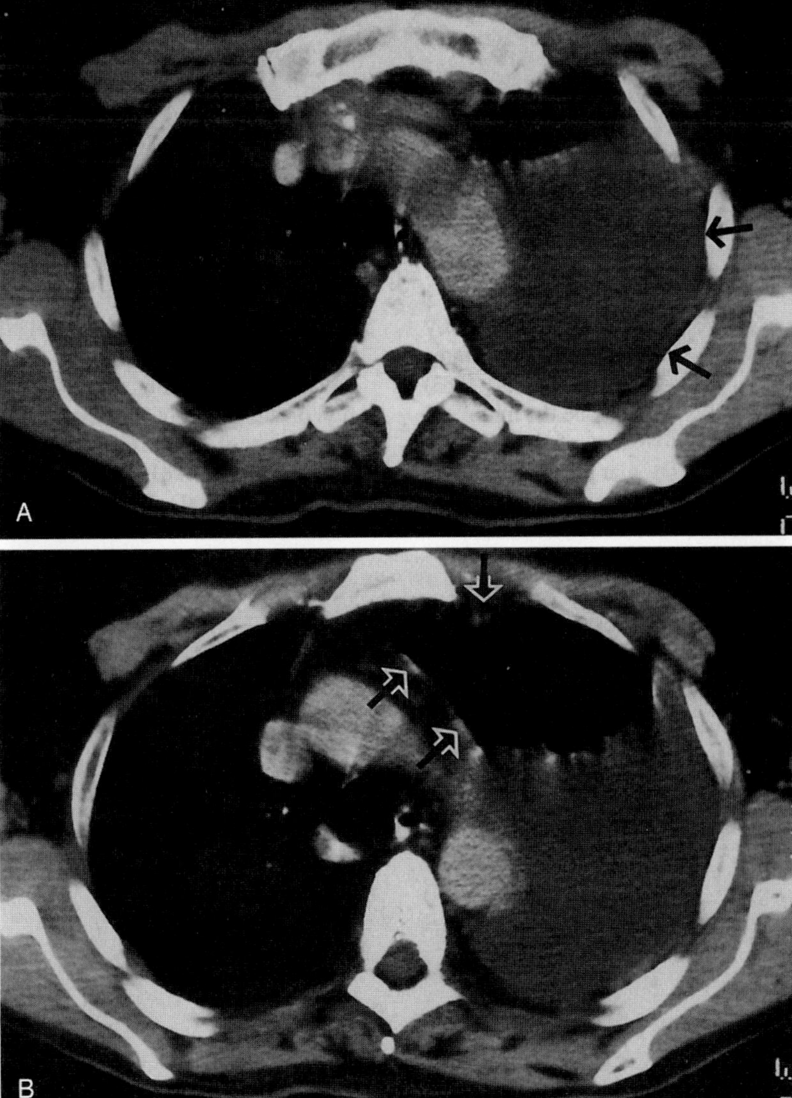

FIGURE 45–4 ■ A computer tomography (CT) scan of early-stage diffuse mesothelioma. *A*, The CT cut at the level of the aortic arch shows a large left pleural effusion (*arrows*) with no evidence of pleural disease. *B*, The CT cut at the level of the aortopulmonary window shows mild pleural thickening and irregularity (*arrows*) in addition to the effusion. At thoracotomy there was diffuse studding of the pleura with tumor nodules that were 1 to 2 mm in diameter.

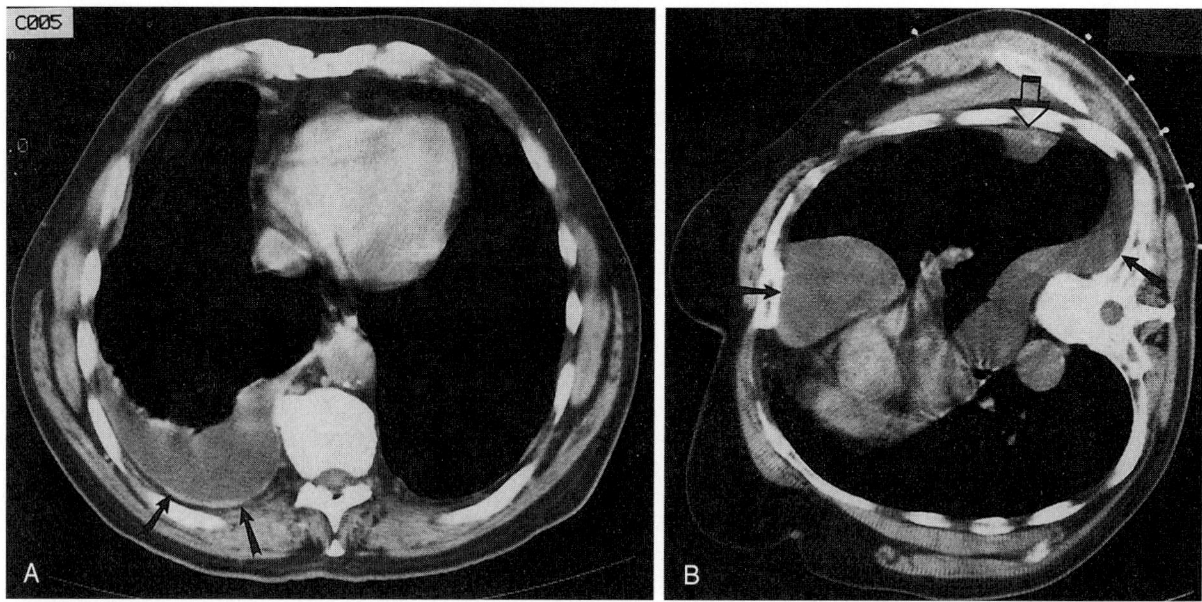

FIGURE 45–5 ■ A computed tomography (CT) scan of another early-stage mesothelioma. *A*, There is a large pleural effusion with diffuse mild pleural thickening and irregularity (*arrows*). *B*, A CT cut obtained with the patient in the lateral position shows a dominant chest wall mass (*large arrow*) and a freely flowing effusion (*small arrow*).

and to detect recurrent disease postoperatively, but it is often inaccurate in diagnosing chest wall involvement or extension through the diaphragm (Rusch et al, 1988). It was hoped that magnetic resonance imaging would be more accurate in this regard. However, a prospective trial comparing these two imaging modalities failed to show that magnetic resonance imaging was consistently superior to CT in staging MPM preoperatively (Heelan et al, 1999). Positron emission tomography is reported to show increased uptake in virtually all MPMs (Bénard et al, 1998), but its role in staging the disease needs to be defined.

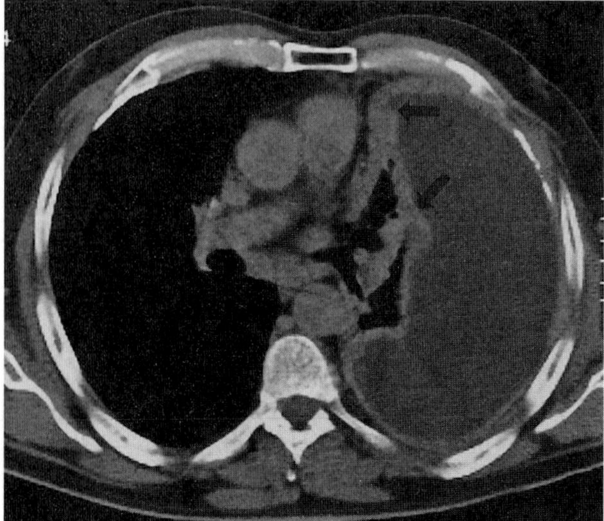

FIGURE 45–6 ■ A computed tomography scan of a more locally advanced mesothelioma. There is a thick confluent pleural peel along the chest wall (*large arrows*) that encases the collapsed lung and extends into the fissure.

Thoracentesis is usually the initial diagnostic procedure because most patients present with a pleural effusion. Pleural fluid cytology is positive for malignancy in only 30% to 50% of patients. Percutaneous pleural biopsy yields a diagnosis of malignancy in up to one third of cases, but it usually does not provide the pathologist a large enough specimen on which to perform the immunohistochemical or electron microscopic studies that are so critical to a definitive diagnosis (Lewis et al, 1981; Ruffie et al, 1989). Video-assisted thoracoscopy (VATS) is the optimal diagnostic procedure because it uniformly yields a diagnosis but does not commit the patient to a major surgical procedure (Boutin and Rey, 1993). The appearance of the pleural space is variable and depends on the extent of disease and the cell type. In the earliest stages of MPM, involvement of the pleura is microscopic and the only visible finding is a large pleural effusion. As the disease progresses, the thoracoscopic appearance evolves from pleural studding with a free pleural space and a large pleural effusion, to larger but still discrete masses with multiloculated pleural effusions, to a confluent irregular sheet of tumor with obliteration of the pleural space. The tumor ranges from being soft, friable, and hypervascular to being densely fibrotic, depending on the mixture of cell types. No clinical findings are pathognomonic of MPM.

VATS is not technically feasible in the patient whose pleural space is obliterated by locally advanced tumor. A small incision (4 to 5 cm in length) is then used for open pleural biopsy. This incision should be placed in line with a possible subsequent thoracotomy incision, so that it can be excised at the time of the definitive operation. MPM has a notorious propensity to implant in the chest wall, and placing thoracoscopy or biopsy incisions in a random manner complicates the local management of this disease by potentially causing local chest wall recur-

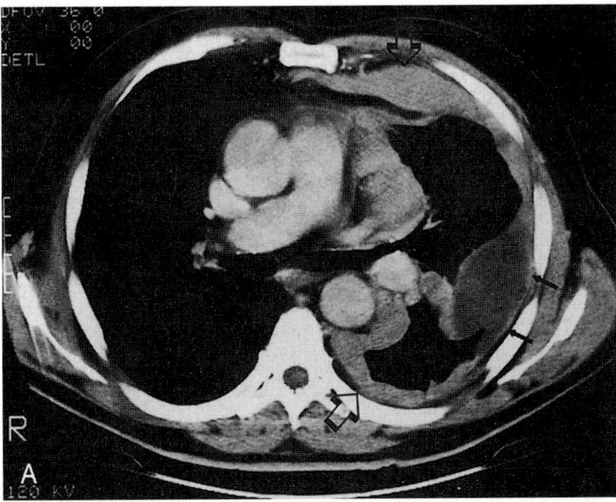

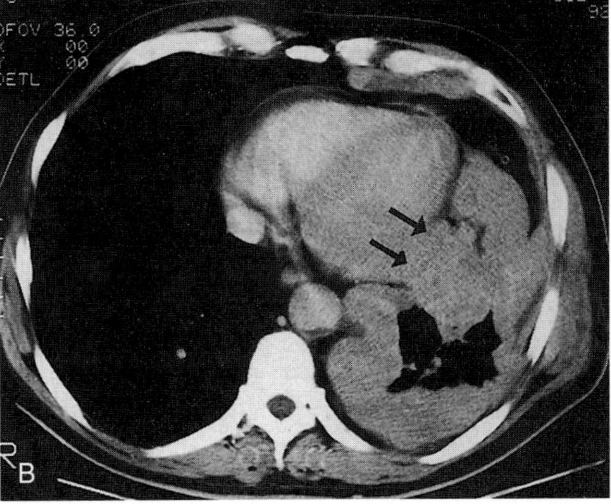

FIGURE 45–7 ■ A computed tomography scan of another locally advanced mesothelioma. *A,* A cut at the level of the pulmonary artery shows a thick irregular confluent pleural peel (*large arrow*) with a loculated pleural effusion (*small arrow*). *B,* A cut at the level of the midheart shows a massive tumor encasing and collapsing the lung and suggesting invasion of the pericardium (*arrows*).

rence. A diagnostic thoracotomy should be avoided because it exposes patients who have metastatic adenocarcinoma to the unnecessary morbidity of a major operation and makes a subsequent therapeutic thoracotomy for MPM technically difficult.

Immunohistochemical staining can now be reliably performed on paraffin-embedded tissue. However, if difficulty is anticipated in reaching a definitive tissue diagnosis, tissue should be submitted fresh to the pathologist, so that it is placed in the appropriate fixatives for electron microscopy.

Natural History and Staging

An understanding of the natural history of a malignancy is pivotal to evaluating treatment results and to developing novel therapies. Previously, our understanding of the natural history and prognostic factors in MPM was poor because it is an uncommon tumor for which there was no accurate, universally accepted staging system. The staging system used most often was one proposed by Butchart and colleagues in 1976 (Butchart et al, 1976), which included imprecise descriptors for the primary tumor and for lymph node involvement (Table 45–5). For example, stage I included tumors that had minimal pleural studding, a free pleural space, and a pleural effusion, as well as locally advanced tumors with a thick, confluent sheet of tumor with obliteration of the pleural space. In addition, the prognostic implications of lymph node metastases were not clearly established, and the inclusion of "lymph node involvement within the chest" in stage II and "lymph node involvement outside the chest" was empirical. Several other staging systems were subsequently proposed, but none of these was well validated or widely accepted (Dimitrov and McMahon, 1987).

Early reports failed to define the natural history of MPM well because patients were assessed only by symptoms, physical examination, and chest radiographs. The inaccuracy of such a clinical assessment with no attempt to classify patients by stage leads to a heterogeneous patient population. Most series also recorded outcome in small numbers of patients, seen over long periods of time and treated in a highly individualized manner. Little wonder that reported survival rates varied widely. For example, Law and co-workers (1984) reported a median survival of 18 months for 64 patients treated with supportive care, with no differences in survival according to cell type. Twelve of the 64 patients survived longer than 5 years, but the diagnosis of MPM in this study was based on histology alone, and fewer than a third of all patients were staged by CT. In contrast, Hulks and associates (1989) reported a median survival of 30 weeks for 68 patients treated with supportive care. They based their pathologic diagnosis on both histologic findings and immunohistochemical results. No CT was performed, and patients were classified mainly according to symptoms. Those who presented with dyspnea lived significantly longer than patients who presented with pain (median survival of 44 versus 22 weeks), probably reflecting the extent of disease at diagnosis. The cell type did not appear to influence overall survival.

TABLE 45–5 ■ **Staging Proposed by Butchart and Colleagues**

Stage I	Tumor confined within the "capsule" of the parietal pleura (i.e., involving only ipsilateral pleura, lung, pericardium, and diaphragm)
Stage II	Tumor invading chest wall or involving mediastinal structures (e.g., esophagus, heart, opposite pleura); lymph node involvement within the chest
Stage III	Tumor penetrating diaphragm to involve peritoneum; involvement of opposite pleura; lymph node involvement outside the chest
Stage IV	Distant blood-borne metastases

Reprinted with permission from Dimitrov NV, McMahon S: Presentation, diagnostic methods, staging and natural history of malignant mesothelioma. In Antman K, Aisner J (eds): Asbestos-Related Malignancy. Orlando, FL, Grune & Stratton, 1987, p 233.

Other authors tried to identify prognostic factors in MPM but have done this through retrospective reviews of patients with different stages of disease, treated with widely varying regimens. Contrary to the data reported by Law and by Hulks and their colleagues, epithelial histology has generally been a favorable prognostic factor. The absence of chest pain and good performance status are also thought to be favorable prognostic factors, but they probably just reflect an early stage of the disease. Other factors including female gender and age younger than 50 years have incidentally been cited as favorable prognostic factors. In several series, a platelet count greater than 400,000/μL appears to have a negative impact on survival (Adams et al, 1986; Antman et al, 1988; Olesen and Thorshauge, 1988; Ruffie et al, 1989).

Although MPM was long thought to be a tumor that remained localized to the chest (Nauta et al, 1982), several autopsy series have now disproved this. Ruffie and associates (1989) found that 45 of 92 (49%) patients had distant metastases at autopsy. The liver was the most common site and the contralateral lung the second most common site of distant disease. However, metastases in sites as widely disseminated as the prostate, brain, and thyroid were also found. Elmes and Simpson (1976) found distant metastases in 48 of 148 (33%) patients at autopsy. The metastases were widely disseminated, but the liver and the contralateral lung were once again the most common sites of disease. Similar findings have been reported by Roberts (1976) and by Whitwell and Rawcliffe (1971). The uncommon but definite occurrence of brain and spine metastases has been emphasized in several reports (Kaye et al, 1986; Ruffie et al, 1989; Walters and Martinez, 1975). Virtually all patients have advanced local or regional disease at death, however. Because the symptoms related to local-regional tumor are usually the most difficult to palliate, they are the most clinically important (Nauta et al, 1982). Patients with MPM face a dual problem: (1) control of the local-regional tumor throughout the course of their disease and (2) prevention of distant metastases as a late manifestation of their cancer.

During the late 20th century several large series better defined the natural history and prognostic factors in MPM, particularly in patients undergoing surgical resection. Boutin and colleagues (1993b) showed that patients with disease limited to the parietal pleural have the earliest stage of MPM and experience a median survival of 32.7 months with supportive care. These tumors are considered stage Ia in the International Mesothelioma Interest Group (IMIG) system. These researchers reported that tumors involving the visceral as well as the parietal pleura (stage Ib) are associated with a median survival of only 7 months. However, subsequent surgical series suggest that stage Ib tumors have a more favorable prognosis, with a median survival of 27 months and a 3-year survival of approximately 40% (Rusch and Venkatraman, 1996). The discrepancy in outcome between these two reports could reflect the inaccuracy of staging by thoracoscopy only, the benefit of surgical resection and various adjuvant therapies, or both.

Several other reports have helped define the relationship between TNM status and outcome (Allen et al, 1994; Pass et al, 1997a; Rusch and Venkatraman, 1996, 1999; Sugarbaker, 1991, 1993, 1999; Tammilehto, 1995), especially in patients undergoing surgical resection. Information from these series led to the development of a new staging system by the IMIG shown in Table 45–6 (Rusch and IMIG, 1995). This system reconciles and updates several previously proposed staging systems. It reflects the important relationship between T status and overall survival and also the adverse prognostic significance conferred by nodal metastases (Pass et al, 1997a; Rusch and Venkatraman, 1999; Sugarbaker et al, 1999). However, the precise significance of N1 versus N2 nodal disease remains unclear, and additional data are needed to refine the T descriptors in this staging system. This system is designed to be applicable to the radiologic and pathologic as well as the surgical staging of MPM (Patz et al, 1996). Although the IMIG staging system will require revision in the future as additional information about the natural history of MPM becomes available, it provides an important basis for the evaluation of treatment results and the design of clinical trials internationally.

Treatment

As for any other cancer, the treatment options for MPM include surgery, irradiation, chemotherapy, immunotherapy, or some combination of these modalities. However, the choice of treatment is influenced by factors that do not apply to some other malignancies, that is, the extensive nature of this tumor, its proximity to intrathoracic organs, and the general medical condition of these patients, who are usually older and often have serious underlying diseases. The assessment of therapeutic regimens for MPM is still hampered by a lack of large prospective clinical trials. Until recently, most patients were treated in a highly individualized manner.

Radiation

It is difficult to evaluate the success of radiation as the only therapy because it has usually been given in conjunction with surgical resection or chemotherapy. The use of radiation therapy is limited by the volume of the primary tumor, which involves the entire hemithorax, and by proximity of the tumor to many vital structures that are intolerant of high doses of radiation. For the most part, radiation doses to the affected hemithorax have been kept at 4500 cGy or less to minimize toxicity to the heart, esophagus, lung, and spinal cord (Ball and Cruickshank, 1990; Brady, 1981; Gordon et al, 1982). Maasilta (1991) has documented the severe pulmonary toxicity caused by higher-dose hemithoracic radiation: the radiographic changes and the deterioration in pulmonary function and in oxygenation that develop over the year after radiation are compatible with a total loss of lung function on the radiated side. In several studies, the toxicity of radiation may also be potentiated by the administration of chemotherapy, including drugs such as doxorubicin (Sinoff et al, 1982). Therefore, radiation is not used as a primary form of treatment but is generally reserved for palliation of a symptomatic area of tumor invading the chest wall or mediastinum. Radiation ap-

TABLE 45–6 ■ IMIG Staging System for Diffuse Malignant Pleural Mesothelioma

T—Tumor		
T1	T1a	Tumor limited to the ipsilateral parietal ± mediastinal ± diaphragmatic pleura *No involvement of the visceral pleura*
	T1b	Tumor involving the ipsilateral parietal ± mediastinal ± diaphragmatic pleura *Tumor also involving the visceral pleura*
T2	Tumor involving each of the ipsilateral pleural surfaces (parietal, mediastinal, diaphragmatic, and visceral pleurae) with at least one of the following features: Involvement of diaphragmatic muscle Extension of tumor from visceral pleura into the underlying pulmonary parenchyma	
T3	Describes locally advanced but *potentially resectable* tumor Tumor involving all of the ipsilateral pleural surfaces (parietal, mediastinal, diaphragmatic, and visceral pleurae) with at least one of the following features: Involvement of the endothoracic fascia Extension into the mediastinal fat Solitary, completely resectable focus of tumor extending into the soft tissues of the chest wall Nontransmural involvement of the pericardium	
T4	Describes locally advanced *technically unresectable* tumor Tumor involving all of the ipsilateral pleural surfaces (parietal, mediastinal, diaphragmatic, and visceral pleurae) with at least one of the following features: Diffuse extension or multifocal masses of tumor in the chest wall, with or without associated rib destruction Direct transdiaphragmatic extension of tumor to the peritoneum Direct extension of tumor to the contralateral pleura Direct extension of tumor to mediastinal organs Direct extension of tumor into the spine Tumor extending through to the internal surface of the pericardium with or without a pericardial effusion; or tumor involving the myocardium	
N—Lymph nodes		
NX	Regional lymph nodes cannot be assessed	
N0	No regional lymph node metastases	
N1	Metastases in the ipsilateral bronchopulmonary or hilar lymph nodes	
N2	Metastases in the subcarinal or the ipsilateral mediastinal lymph nodes including the ipsilateral internal mammary nodes	
N3	Metastases in the contralateral mediastinal, contralateral internal mammary, ipsilateral or contralateral supraclavicular lymph nodes	
M—Metastases		
MX	Presence of distant metastases cannot be assessed	
M0	No distant metastasis	
M1	Distant metastasis present	

Staging			
Stage I			
Ia	T1a	N0	M0
Ib	T1b	N0	M0
Stage II	T2	N0	M0
Stage III	Any T3	Any N1 Any N2	M0
Stage IV	Any T4	Any N3	Any M1

pears to be more effective as an adjuvant treatment postoperatively, and this is discussed in more detail later.

Chemotherapy

Numerous phase II studies of chemotherapeutic agents have been performed in MPM, and these are well summarized in a recent review (Table 45–7). Response rates as high as 30% to 40% have been reported in small single-institution studies but are usually in the 15% to 20% range. The results of these studies are influenced by the inclusion of patients with varying stages of disease and different MPM cell types and by the lack of use of CT to assess response. Previously, active agents included doxorubicin, cyclophosphamide, cisplatin, carboplatin, methotrexate, edatrexate, 5-azacytidine, and 5-fluorouracil (Chahinian et al, 1978; Dabouis et al, 1981; Dimitrov et al, 1982; Raghavan et al, 1990; Umsawasdi et al, 1991). Combination therapy has usually not proven to be superior to single-agent treatment. In a randomized phase II trial comparing the combination of cisplatin and doxorubicin to that of cisplatin and mitomycin, the Cancer and Leukemia Group B initially reported a 13% response rate for cisplatin and doxorubicin versus a 28% response rate for cisplatin and mitomycin, but there was no difference in overall survival between these regimens (Chahinian et al, 1993).

More recent chemotherapy trials suggest that several newer drugs may be more effective in MPM. A response rate of 44% was reported with a combination of mitomycin, bleomycin, cisplatin, and doxorubicin administered in conjunction with hyaluronidase (Breau et al, 1993). Perhaps the most promising results are those reported by Byrne and associates (1999). In a phase II trial of cisplatin and gemcitabine, the overall response rate in 21 patients was 48%. If confirmed by larger multicenter trials, this well-tolerated regimen could also be applied as preopera-

TABLE 45–7 ■ **Series of ≥ 15 Patients with Malignant Mesothelioma Treated with Single-Agent Chemotherapy**

Agent	*First Author/Year*	*No. Patients*	*Responders*		*95% Confidence Interval (%)*
			No.	%	
Doxorubicin	Lerner/1983	51	7	14	7–26
Doxorubicin	Sorenson/1985	15	0	0	0–20
Detorubicin	Colbert/1985	35	9	26	14–42
Pirarubicin	Kaukel/1987	35	8	22	11–38
Epirubicin	Magri/1991	21	1	5	1–23
Epirubicin	Mattson/1992	48	7	15	6–28
Mitoxantrone	Eisenhauer/1986	28	2	7	2–22
Mitoxantrone	van Breukelen/1991	34	1	3	0–27
Cisplatin	Mintzer/1985	24	3	13	4–31
Cisplatin	Zidar/1988	35	5	14	6–29
Carboplatin	Mbidde/1986	17	2	12	0–27
Carboplatin	Raghavan/1990	31	5	16	5–34
Carboplatin	Vogelzang/1990	40	3	7	2–21
Vindesine	Kelsen/1983	17	1	6	0–17
Vindesine	Boutin/1987	21	0	0	0–15
Vincristine	Martensson/1989	23	0	0	0–14
Vinblastine	Cowan/1988	20	0	0	0–16
Paclitaxel	Vogelzang/1994	15	2	13	4–38
Cyclophosphamide	Sorenson/1985	16	0	0	0–19
Ifosfamide	Alberts/1988	17	4	24	10–48
Ifosfamide	Zidar/1992	26	2	8	1–25
Ifosfamide	Falkson/1992	40	1	3	1–14
Mitomycin	Bajorin/1987	19	4	21	8–43
Methotrexate	Solheim/1992	60	22	37	26–50
Trimetrexate	Vogelzang/1994	51	6	12	2–33
Edatrexate	Belani/1994	20	5	25	9–49
Edatrexate + leucovorin	Belani/1994	17	3	18	6–41
CB3717	Cantwell/1986	18	1	6	0–27
5-FU	Harvey/1984	20	1	5	1–24
DHAC	Harmon/1991	42	7	17	9–31
Amsacrine	Falkson/1980	19	1	5	1–24
Diaziquone	Eagan/1986	20	0	0	0–17
BCG	Webster/1982	30	NA	NA	NA
Acivcin	Alberts/1988	19	0	0	0–17
Interferon alfa-2a	Christmas/1993	25	3	12	4–30
Interleukin-2	Eggermont/1991	17	4	24	10–48
Interferon gamma	Boutin/1991	22	5	23	10–44

Reprinted with permission from Ong ST, Vogelzang NJ: Chemotherapy in malignant pleural mesothelioma: A review. J Clin Oncol 14:1007–1017, 1996.

tive or postoperative treatment to patients undergoing surgical resection.

Several additional drugs are currently in clinical trials. These include the new antifolate drugs MTA and PDX and several antiangiogenesis compounds. Given these promising results, chemotherapy is likely to play a greater role in both the primary and combined modality therapy of MPM during the next few years.

Immunotherapy

Interferons are known to facilitate cell differentiation and to have a direct antiproliferative effect on MPM cell lines. Studies performed on MPM xenografts in nude mice have shown the efficacy of recombinant human interferon alfa-2a combined with mitomycin C (Sklarin, 1988). These experimental data prompted the development of clinical trials using interferon, either alone or in combination with other agents.

Boutin and associates (1994) tested the use of intrapleural interferon gamma (IFN-γ) in 89 patients at a dose of 40×10^6 IU for 6 hours twice a week for 8 weeks. The response was directly linked to disease stage and ranged from 44.8% for stage I tumors to only 6% for stage II tumors. The mean duration of partial responses as assessed by CT and serial thoracoscopy was 19 months.

A phase II trial of interferon alfa-2a and carboplatin was performed at Memorial Sloan-Kettering Cancer Center in patients with locally advanced or metastatic disease. Only one partial response was seen in 15 patients entered on this trial, and most patients had early disease progression. This combination did not have significant antitumor activity (O'Reilly et al, 1999).

Interleukin-2 (IL-2) has also been tested in patients with MPM and has led to several objective responses (Goey et al, 1995). The rationale for using IL-2 is that it activates lymphokine activated killer (LAK) cells and induces a cytolytic response (Yasumoto et al, 1987). In vitro studies indicate that human natural killer (NK) cell activity is suppressed by asbestos fibers but restored by IL-2 (Robinson, 1989). Human MPM cell lines are lysed by NK and LAK cells (Manning et al, 1989). In a trial by Astoul and associates (1998), 22 patients were treated with intrapleural IL-2, and one complete and 11 partial responses were seen. As with intrapleural IFN-γ, these responses were related to early stage, minimal tumor thickness, and epithelioid tumor histology.

The results of these trials suggest that IFN-γ and IL-2 have activity in MPM, particularly in early-stage tumors. However, the precise ways in which they could be combined with other treatment modalities require further investigation.

Surgery

The limitations of radiation and chemotherapy have made surgery the mainstay of treatment for MPM. Operations for MPM can be divided into two categories—those performed for palliation and those performed with curative intent. With respect to palliative procedures, VATS with talc pleurodesis is an effective way to control pleural effusions in patients who are not candidates for further surgical resection. Thoracotomy and partial pleurectomy is necessary only in situations in which the pleural effusion has loculated and cannot be evacuated by VATS.

The operations performed with curative intent are extrapleural pneumonectomy and pleurectomy/decortication.

Surgical Technique

Extrapleural pneumonectomy is an en bloc resection of the pleura, the lung, ipsilateral hemidiaphragm, and pericardium. It is performed via an extended S-shaped posterolateral thoracotomy incision that extends to the costal margin (Fig. 45–8*A*). The sixth rib is excised to facilitate exposure to the extrapleural plane (Fig. 45–8*B*). This approach is slightly lower than for a standard pulmonary resection because the greatest bulk of tumor is usually in the lower half of the hemithorax. Blunt dissection is begun in the extrapleural plane between the parietal pleura and the endothoracic fascia and is continued with a sweeping motion of the hand up to the apex of the chest (Fig. 45–8*C*). A similar dissection is then performed inferiorly from the intercostal incision down to the diaphragm. The dissection is carried anteriorly to the pericardium and posteriorly to the spine. It is important to pack each section of the chest sequentially as this dissection is performed because otherwise there can be a substantial blood loss. The Argon Beam Electrocoagulator (Electro Medical Systems Division, Birtcher Corporation, Englewood, CO) is very helpful in controlling this diffuse chest wall bleeding.

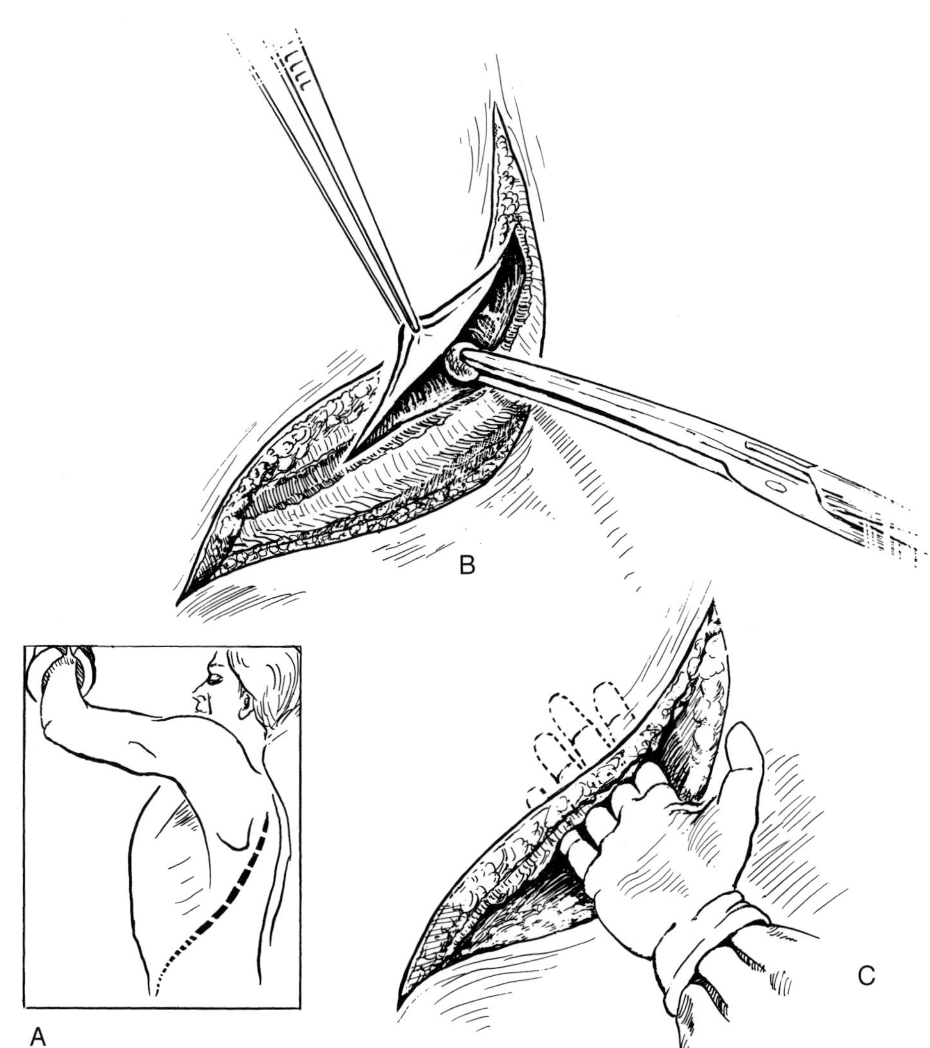

FIGURE 45–8 ■ *A*, Initial approach for a pleurectomy or an extrapleural pneumonectomy. An extended posterolateral thoracotomy or thoracoabdominal incision is performed. A parallel counterincision in the tenth intercostal space, with or without a separate skin incision, can be added to improve exposure to the diaphragm. *B*, The extrapleural plane is opened after resection of the sixth rib, and the parietal pleura is bluntly dissected away from the endothoracic fascia, *C*.

When the parietal pleura has been mobilized away from the chest wall, a chest retractor is inserted. Dissection is continued under direct vision, mobilizing the pleura away from the mediastinum superiorly, anteriorly, and posteriorly (Fig. 45–9). On the left side, care must be taken to identify the esophagus, the plane between the adventitia of the aorta and the tumor, and the origins of the intercostal vessels. On the right side, dissection along the superior vena cava must be performed very gently. After this portion of the dissection, the pleura and lung will have been completely mobilized in the upper half of the chest, exposing the superior and posterior aspects of the hilum.

A standard en bloc dissection of the subcarinal lymph nodes is performed for staging purposes and to expose the mainstem bronchus. The lymph nodes are submitted separately to the pathologist, appropriately labeled. In some patients, there is a clean plane of dissection between the mediastinal pleura and the pericardium, also allowing exposure of the anterior aspect of the hilum. In other patients, this plane is obliterated and the anterior mediastinal pleura has to be resected en bloc with the pericardium later in the operation.

Attention is then turned to the resection of the diaphragm. There is always a palpable "edge" between the tumor and normal diaphragmatic muscle or peritoneum. This plane can be entered and the tumor mobilized along the diaphragmatic surface by blunt dissection in much the way that one would perform a Kocher maneuver. Once the tumor is mobilized from the posterior costophrenic angle, it is rotated up into the thoracotomy incision, rolled back on itself and placing strong traction on the diaphragm. This part of the resection varies considerably from one patient to the next. If the involvement of the diaphragm is extensive, the entire thickness of the diaphragm will be removed, peeled away from the peritoneum. If the involvement of the diaphragm is superficial, dissection can be carried through the diaphragmatic muscle using the electrocautery (Fig. 45–10). Every effort is made not to enter the peritoneum because of the propensity of MPM to produce tumor implants. The most difficult place to avoid entering the abdomen is at the level at the central tendon, and often a small opening in the peritoneum is unavoidable but should be immediately closed.

The diaphragmatic portion of the tumor is completely

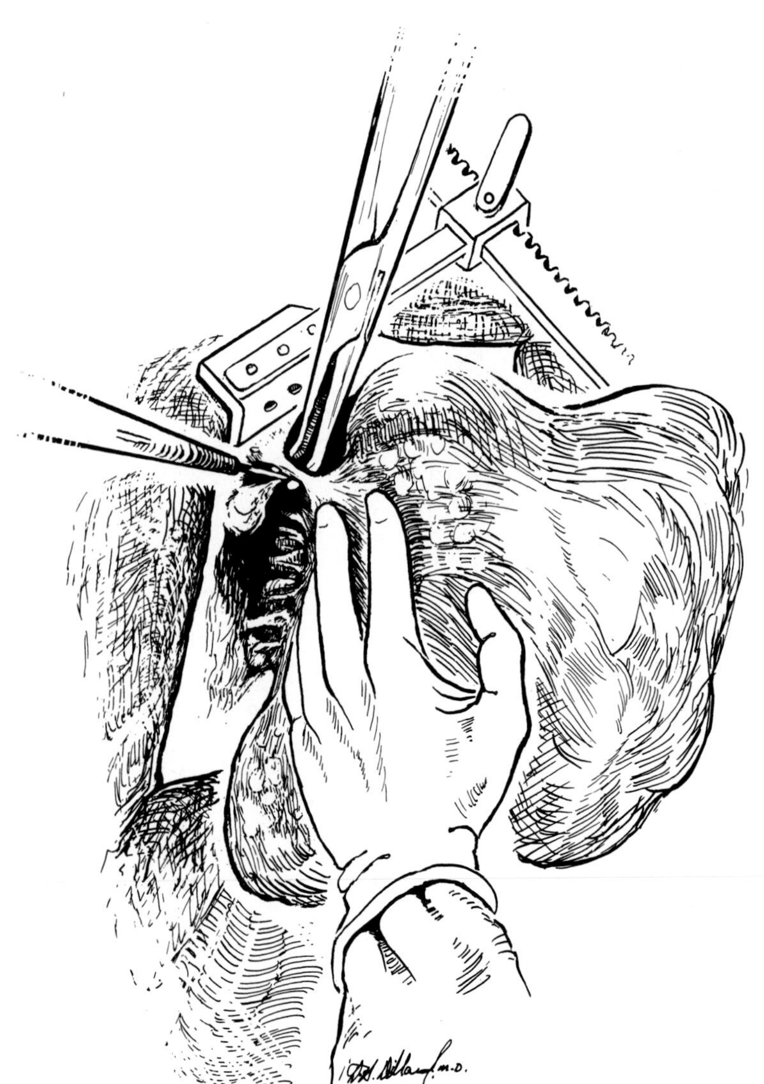

FIGURE 45–9 ■ After the parietal pleura has been mobilized from the chest wall, a chest retractor is inserted, and the mediastinal pleura is freed from the mediastinal structures under direct vision using a combination of sharp and blunt dissection.

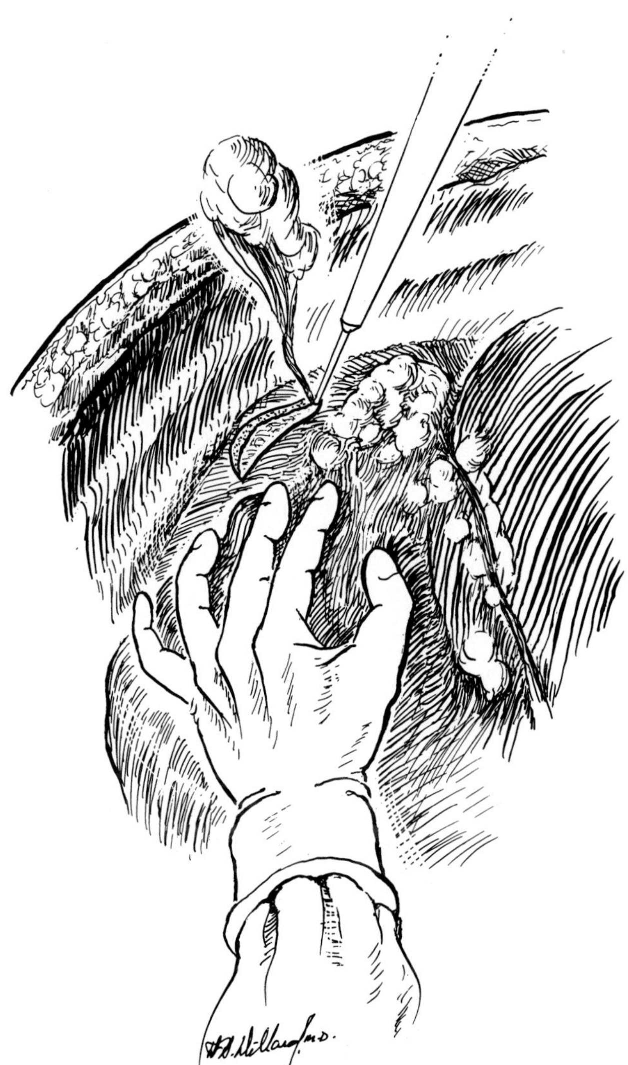

FIGURE 45–10 ■ The tumor has been bluntly mobilized out of the costophrenic sulcus. Strong traction is placed on the pleural tumor and underlying lung, and cautery is used to dissect the diaphragmatic surface of the tumor away from the diaphragmatic muscle or peritoneum.

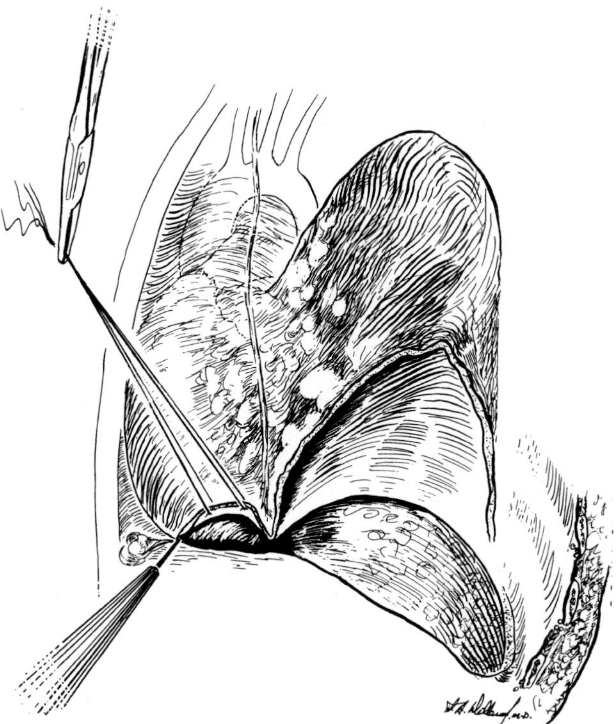

FIGURE 45–11 ■ The pericardium is opened after the tumor has been completely mobilized from all other directions, including the diaphragm.

mobilized back to the pericardium medially. If resection of the pericardium is required, the pericardium is entered only when the tumor has been mobilized as fully as possible from all other directions because traction on the pericardium causes arrhythmias and hemodynamic instability (Fig. 45–11). The hilar structures are divided in whatever sequence is technically easiest and requires the least manipulation of the large tumor mass. Usually, this means dividing the mainstem bronchus first, then the inferior pulmonary vein, the superior pulmonary vein, and lastly the main pulmonary artery. If the pericardium is being resected, it is gradually opened as this portion of the dissection is carried out. Traction sutures are placed on the pericardium to prevent it from retracting toward the opposite hemithorax. The traction sutures also minimize changes in the position of the heart and reduce hemodynamic instability (Fig. 45–12). The specimen consisting of pleura, lung, and diaphragm, with or without pericardium, is removed en bloc. Sampling or

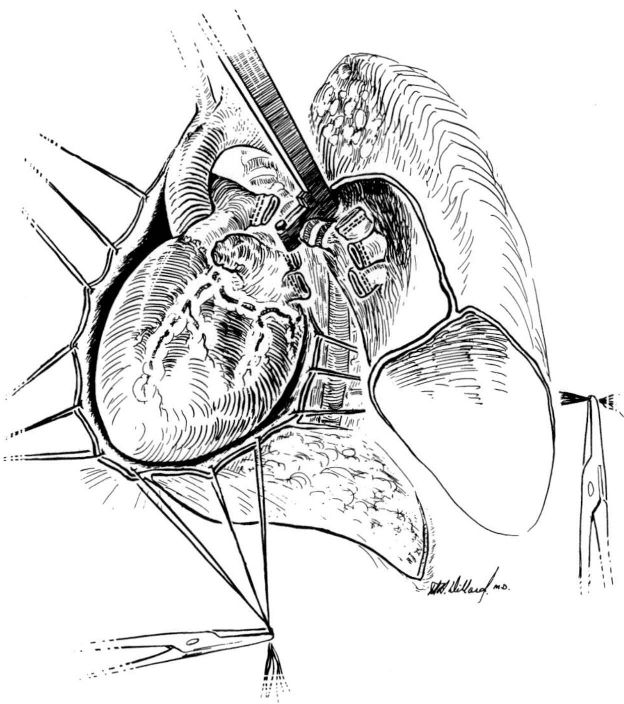

FIGURE 45–12 ■ The hilar vessels have been divided intrapericardially. Traction sutures have been placed on the edge of the pericardium as it was opened to prevent it from retracting into the contralateral hemithorax.

dissection of the paratracheal lymph nodes if the operation is on the right, or of the aortopulmonary window nodes if the operation is on the left, is performed for staging purposes. Again, these nodes are submitted separately to the pathologist, appropriately labeled.

Reconstruction of the diaphragm is then performed (Fig. 45–13). On the right side Dexon mesh is used because the underlying liver assists in preventing herniation of the intra-abdominal contents. On the left side, Gore-Tex is used because a heavier, nonabsorbable material is required to prevent herniation. If the diaphragmatic muscle has been completely resected back to its costal insertion, the prosthesis is secured by placing sutures around the ribs laterally (Fig. 45–14). Posteriorly, it is sutured to the crus or gently tacked with fine sutures to the wall of the esophagus. Medially, it is sewn to the edge of the pericardium. If the pericardium has been resected, it is reconstructed with Dexon mesh. This prevents cardiac herniation into the empty hemithorax and facilitates postoperative radiation to the hemithorax by maintaining the heart in a central position. Meticulous attention is given to obtaining hemostasis throughout the operation and particularly before closure of the chest. The thoracotomy incision is closed in the usual manner.

A similar approach is used for the initial portion of the operation for a pleurectomy/decortication. As for an extrapleural pneumonectomy, the intent of a pleurectomy/decortication is to remove all gross tumor, the only difference being that the lung is left in place (Rusch, 1993). Mobilization of the parietal and mediastinal pleurae and of the diaphragmatic surface is the same as for an extrapleural pneumonectomy. If the pericardium cannot be easily separated from the pleura, it is also resected and reconstructed as previously described.

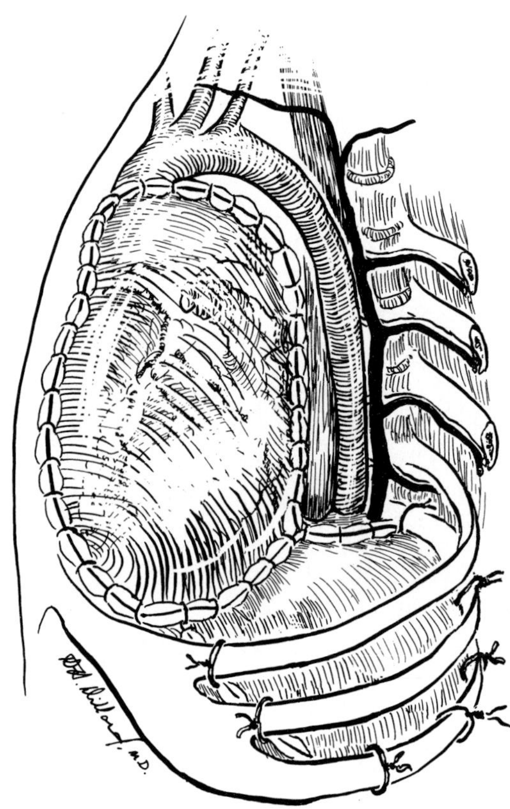

FIGURE 45–14 ■ The completed pericardial and diaphragmatic reconstruction. If the diaphragm was detached from its costal insertion, the prosthetic material can be secured by sutures that are placed around the ribs laterally.

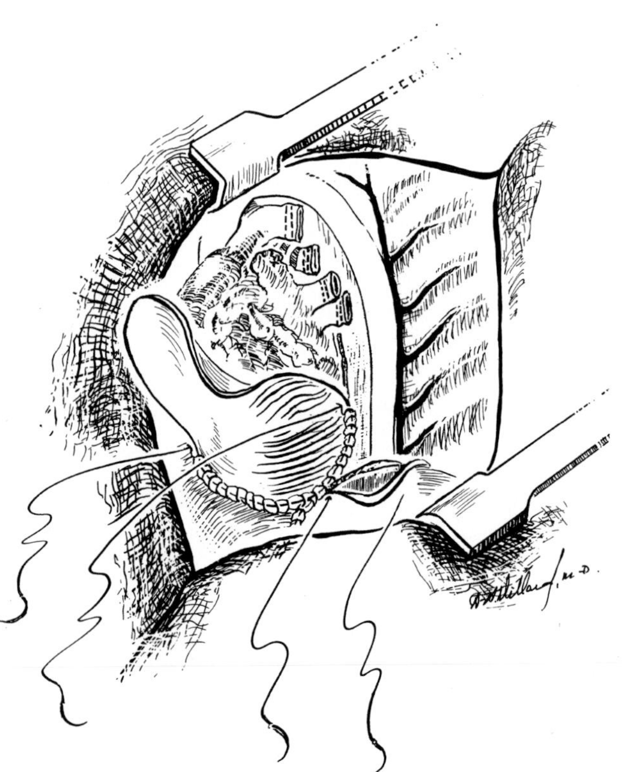

FIGURE 45–13 ■ The pericardial and diaphragmatic defects are reconstructed with prosthetic material. Reconstruction of the diaphragm is not always necessary, especially on the right side.

When all of this dissection has been completed, the parietal pleura is opened, and the decortication begun (Fig. 45–15). The degree to which the parietal and visceral pleurae are separable and to which the visceral pleural tumor can be peeled cleanly away from the lung is extremely variable. Sometimes it is necessary to remove large sections of the visceral pleura, leaving the raw pulmonary parenchyma exposed. This is accomplished by a combination of sharp dissection with the electrocautery and very gentle dissection with a peanut sponge. Although air leaks from the lung surface are large initially, they seal quickly—usually within 72 hours—as long as the lung re-expands fully after the operation. This portion of the operation can be very tedious but if properly performed will result in the removal of all gross tumor. The parietal pleura is progressively resected in sections as the pleural surfaces are separated and the decortication is performed. Care is taken to remove all tumor from the fissures where it is often extensive.

When all gross tumor has been removed, attention is turned to the diaphragmatic reconstruction. If the diaphragm has been partially resected it can sometimes be closed primarily by plication as described previously (Fig. 45–16). If it has been completely resected, it is recon-

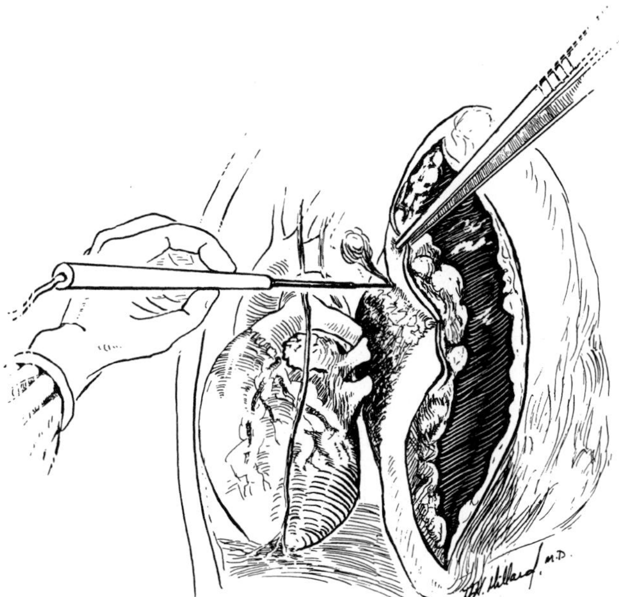

FIGURE 45–15 ■ Technique of pleurectomy and decortication. The initial dissection shown in Figures 45–8 to 45–10 is identical for a pleurectomy and an extrapleural pneumonectomy. Resection of the pericardium may not be necessary. After the lung and overlying parietal and diaphragmatic pleura have been mobilized, the pleural space is entered, and the visceral pleural tumor is separated from the underlying lung by a combination of blunt dissection and sharp dissection with cautery.

structed with Dexon mesh or with Gore-Tex, just as is done after an extrapleural pneumonectomy. However, when the lung is left in place, it is important to make this reconstruction taut to prevent the "diaphragm" from rising and causing lower lobe atelectasis. After obtaining careful hemostasis, three chest tubes are inserted, one placed anteriorly up to the apex, another placed posteriorly, and a right-angle chest tube inserted on the diaphragm. This ensures complete re-expansion of the lung and drainage of the pleural space, which is critical in the first few days postoperatively.

The use of a double-lumen endotracheal tube is important for both of these operations, especially for a pleurectomy/decortication. During the decortication, the lung may be inflated or deflated depending on what facilitates the dissection technically in each particular case. Deflation minimizes the blood loss, whereas inflation exposes the plane of dissection between the tumor peel and the lung or visceral pleura. Patients are monitored intraoperatively with an arterial line and pulse oximeter as they would be for any other major thoracotomy. The anesthesiologist should be aware that blood loss for these operations, even when performed carefully, can be as high as 2000 to 3000 ml because of diffuse bleeding from the chest wall, and the patient should be transfused accordingly. Because of this, a central venous line is useful for perioperative monitoring.

Results of Surgical Resection

Until recently, the value of extrapleural pneumonectomy compared with pleurectomy/decortication was controversial because of the difference in mortality between these two operations. In an initial report by Butchart and coworkers (1976), extrapleural pneumonectomy carried an operative mortality of 30%. During the 1980s, operative mortality remained high. In 1991, a prospective multi-institutional study reported a mortality rate of 15% (Rusch et al, 1991). However, recent data show a substantial reduction in this mortality, reflecting better patient selection and improved perioperative care. Preoperative CT scanning, accurate assessment of pulmonary function, echocardiography, and radionuclide stress tests now allow the selection of patients who have completely resectable tumors and adequate cardiopulmonary reserve to undergo the operation safely. In this regard, a quantitative ventilation-perfusion lung scan and complete pulmonary function tests, especially measurement of the diffusion capacity, are very important in determining whether patients can tolerate a pneumonectomy. The diffusion capacity is often diminished because of underlying interstitial lung disease from asbestosis. Intraoperative monitoring and anesthetic management are also vastly improved compared with 20 years ago. Operative mortality rates are now consistently in the range of 5% when patients are carefully selected and operated on by a surgeon specializing in this area (Allen et al, 1994; DeLaria et al, 1978; DeValle et al, 1986; Rusch and Venkatraman, 1999; Sugarbaker et al, 1999). The operative mortality and overall survival after extrapleural pneumonectomy as reported in several series are shown in Table 45–8.

By contrast, pleurectomy/decortication is associated with a mortality of 3.5% or less (McCormack et al, 1982; Rusch and Venkatraman, 1999). These figures parallel those reported for pulmonary resections for lung cancer

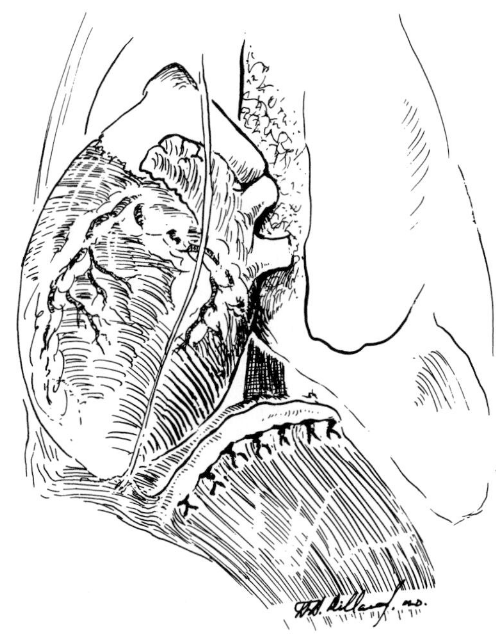

FIGURE 45–16 ■ If most of the diaphragm has been left intact, it is plicated after the tumor has been removed. This is an important maneuver because, even if the phrenic nerve is anatomically intact, the diaphragm has often been defunctionalized and will rise, causing lower lobe atelectasis postoperatively.

TABLE 45-8 ■ **Results of Extrapleural Pneumonectomy**

Author	No. Patients	Operative Mortality	2-Year Survival
Worn, 1974	62	Not Stated	37%
Butchart et al, 1976	29	31%	10%
Devalle et al, 1986	33	9%	24%
Vogt Moykopf, 1987	55	5.5%	16%
Rusch (LCSG), 1991	20	15%	33%
Allen et al, 1994	40	7.5%	25%
Sugarbaker et al, 1999	183	3.8%	38%
Rusch, 1999	115	5.2%	35%

and merely confirm that operative mortality is related to the extent of pulmonary resection, which is 5% to 8% for a standard pneumonectomy. Both operations, and particularly extrapleural pneumonectomy, are complex and are not performed frequently by most surgeons. Therefore, patients will benefit by referral to centers dedicated to the treatment of MPM.

The focus of the controversy with regard to surgical therapy has been the relative survival benefit of an extrapleural pneumonectomy compared with a pleurectomy/decortication. One problem is that extrapleural pneumonectomy cannot be performed in all patients because underlying cardiopulmonary disease and other medical problems may preclude pneumonectomy in these patients (Rusch et al, 1991). However, these patients can often tolerate pleurectomy/decortication. On the other hand, extrapleural pneumonectomy allows more complete tumor resection and facilitates postoperative radiation, which can be administered to a much higher total dose after pneumonectomy than after pleurectomy/decortication. In addition, some patients do not have a tumor that is technically resectable by pleurectomy/decortication. A confluent sheet of tumor encasing the lung with obliteration of the pleural space is resectable only by extrapleural pneumonectomy. This situation can often be recognized by the preoperative CT scan (see Figs. 45–9 and 45–10) and by a preoperative ventilation/perfusion lung scan showing decreased function on the affected side. A recent analysis of 231 patients who underwent either extrapleural pneumonectomy or pleurectomy/decortication indicates that survival is influenced by tumor stage and histology and not by which of these two operations was performed (Rusch and Venkatraman, 1999). Therefore, the choice of operation should be based on the extent of the tumor and the patient's cardiopulmonary reserve.

Combined Modality Treatment

Extrapleural pneumonectomy and pleurectomy/decortication are by definition cytoreductive operations. Both procedures permit a complete resection of all gross tumor (R1 resection). However, the location and extent of tumor in MPM and its proximity to vital intrathoracic organs do not allow obtaining wide resection margins as is possible for other solid tumors such as lung, colon, or breast cancers. Patients treated with surgery alone relapse rapidly (Rusch et al, 1991). Therefore, most treatment regimens have focused on combined modality treatment. It has been difficult to evaluate the results of combined modality treatment because most series report small numbers of patients treated in a highly individualized manner over long periods of time (Achatzy et al, 1989; Alberts et al, 1988; Chahinian et al, 1982). The approaches to combined modality treatment can be categorized into those designed to enhance only local control and those aimed at preventing both local and systemic relapse.

Approaches to Enhancing Local Control

The approaches to enhancing local control have focused on adding irradiation, photodynamic therapy, or gene therapy to surgical resection. The initial large experience with this strategy was reported by the Memorial Sloan-Kettering Cancer Center. From 1976 to 1988, 105 patients underwent pleurectomy/decortication. Any gross tumor present at completion of the thoracotomy was treated with iodine-125 or iridium-192 implants. Patients then received external-beam irradiation to the entire hemithorax using a mixed photon-electron beam to a total dose of 4500 cGy (Hilaris et al, 1983; Kutcher et al, 1987). The median survival for all 105 patients was 12.6 months, and the 1- and 2-year actuarial survivals were 52% and 23%. However, the 27 patients who had an epithelial histology and minimal gross residual disease that required only external-beam irradiation without brachytherapy had a median survival of 15 months and 1- and 2-year survivals of 68% and 35%. There were 20 complications, including 12 cases of radiation pneumonitis and 8 patients with pericarditis and tamponade. Local failure occurred in 64 of the 105 patients (63%) (Mychalczak et al, 1989). This experience indicates that a low-dose mixed photon-electron beam technique, although theoretically attractive, often does not succeed in sparing the underlying pulmonary parenchyma and fails to provide long-term local control for most patients (Soubra et al, 1990).

The successful use of fast neutron therapy has been described in one report (Blake et al, 1985). Small series have reported the use of radioactive colloidal compounds including radioactive gold (^{198}Au) and chromic phosphate (^{32}P), but these appear ineffective in treating any substantial tumor bulk within the pleural cavity (Brady, 1981).

External-beam radiation is more easily administered after extrapleural pneumonectomy when it is no longer necessary to protect the lung. At the Dana Farber Cancer Institute, 35 patients received adjuvant hemithoracic radiation after extrapleural pneumonectomy in doses ranging from 20 to 41.1 Gy (median dose of 30.6 Gy). There were no significant radiation-related complications, but 67% of the patients who developed recurrent disease experienced relapse in the ipsilateral hemithorax, suggesting that low-dose adjuvant radiation was not sufficient for local control (Baldini et al, 1997).

These experiences suggested that postoperative irradiation was safer after extrapleural pneumonectomy than after pleurectomy/decortication and that low-dose irradiation was not effective adjuvant therapy. To test the potential benefit of higher-dose adjuvant irradiation, a prospective trial was recently completed at Memorial Sloan-Kettering Cancer Center. From 1993 to 1998, 57 patients received postoperative hemithoracic irradiation at a dose of 54 Gy after extrapleural pneumonectomy. As expected, survival was related to tumor stage and ranged from a median of 33.8 months for stages I and II to 10 months for stage III. However, only 8.7% of recurrences in this study were local (Rusch et al, 2000). The results of this trial strongly suggest that adjuvant high-dose hemithoracic radiation is feasible and effective in achieving local control. Systemic relapse has now become the major challenge in this setting.

The use of photodynamic therapy has been tested both experimentally and clinically. In vitro and animal model studies suggest that photodynamic therapy, either with hematoporphyrin derivative or with chlorin sensitizers, allows effective targeted tumor destruction (Keller et al, 1990; Ris et al, 1991, 1997). The feasibility of this approach using Photofrin (Quadra Logic Technologies, Vancouver, BC) and light energy from an argon dye laser as adjuvant therapy after surgical resection has been shown in two clinical trials (Pass et al, 1997b; Takita and Dougherty, 1995). However, this modality does not appear to improve local control or survival (Pass et al, 1997b). Only preliminary studies have been performed testing the use of intrapleural gene therapy, specifically the introduction of toxic or "suicide" genes into tumor cells to facilitate their destruction. A large body of experimental work supports the feasibility of this approach, but initial clinical trials of intrapleural gene therapy have been disappointing. Further work is required to determine the feasibility and efficacy of this treatment modality (Sterman et al, 1998).

Approaches to Enhancing Local Control and Decreasing Systemic Relapse

Several approaches have been tested to enhance local control and decrease systemic relapse, including intrapleural and systemic chemotherapy and adjuvant chemotherapy in conjunction with radiation. In a phase II trial performed at Memorial Sloan-Kettering Cancer Center, patients received a single dose of intrapleural cisplatin (75 mg/m^2) and mitomycin (8 mg/m^2) after complete resection of all gross tumor by pleurectomy/decortication. Additional chemotherapy was then administered systemically starting 1 month postoperatively using two cycles of cisplatin 50 mg/m^2 per week $\times$ 4 and mitomycin 8 mg/m^2 $\times$ 1. This approach of surgical resection and brief, but very intensive, chemotherapy sought to address the dual problem of local control and eventual distant metastases experienced by most MPM patients. It was based on the well-established use of intraperitoneal chemotherapy in ovarian cancer and on a smaller but successful experience with intracavitary chemotherapy in both pleural and peritoneal MPM (Lederman et al, 1987; Markman et al, 1986; Mintzer et al, 1985). From 1989 to 1992, 28 patients were treated in this manner. Two patients developed grade 4 renal toxicity. The median survival was 17 months, and the 2-year survival was 40%. However, local-regional relapse was the most common form of recurrence. Although this combined-modality regimen was feasible, it was ineffective in achieving local control and did not appear to enhance survival significantly. The results of this trial led to the high-dose adjuvant radiation trial described earlier (Rusch et al, 1994). Another study of adjuvant intrapleural and systemic chemotherapy essentially confirms these results (Rice et al, 1994).

At the Dana Farber Cancer Institute, adjuvant CAP (cyclophosphamide, doxorubicin [Adriamycin], and cisplatin) chemotherapy and hemithoracic radiation have been administered to 183 patients after extrapleural pneumonectomy. This large trial has confirmed the prognostic importance of epithelial histology, nodal metastases, and complete resection. It has also shown the feasibility of a trimodality approach, although total irradiation and chemotherapy doses have varied. The precise impact of the individual adjuvant therapies (i.e., chemotherapy versus radiation) is unclear, because neither of these has been studied prospectively or individually (Sugarbaker et al, 1999).

Taken as a whole, these studies suggest that excellent local control of MPM can be achieved through a combination of complete surgical resection and high-dose hemithoracic irradiation. The contribution of chemotherapy requires further study, through the use of newer, more effective chemotherapy regimens administered either preoperatively or postoperatively.

MPM has long been regarded as an uncommon cancer characterized by a relentless progression of disease. By and large, treatment has been haphazard and empiric. Only in the past 10 years has there been an effort to develop a better staging system and to perform carefully designed prospective clinical trials. Innovative strategies to control both local and distant disease are being tested, and a rational approach to the management of MPM is finally beginning to emerge.

OTHER, LESS COMMON TUMORS OF THE PLEURA

Primary tumors of the pleura other than MPM are exceedingly rare and include lipomas, endotheliomas, angiomas, and cysts. Most of these are thought to arise from the subpleural tissues rather than from the pleura itself (Le Roux, 1962). Lipomas are the most common among these rare tumors, but a review of the 7751 CT examinations of the chest found pleural lipomas to be present incidentally in only 0.14% of cases (Christmas et al, 1991). Lipomas have a characteristic appearance on chest radiograph, being smooth, well-defined masses flattened against the chest wall. Pleural cysts usually arise at the pleuropericardial angle and are seen on chest radiograph as discrete, unilocular masses (Le Roux, 1962).

In the past, these uncommon pleural-based tumors have been excised mainly for diagnostic purposes because they rarely become symptomatic. VATS now allows the diagnosis and excision of these lesions, thereby obviating the need for exploratory thoracotomy.

COMMENTS AND CONTROVERSIES

This chapter provides a complete analysis of all available information concerning malignant pleural mesotheliomas (MPMs). Of particular importance to surgeons is the fact that these tumors are often difficult to diagnose by thoracentesis alone. Thoracoscopic biopsy is therefore important, and specimens should be sent for immunohistochemical staining and electron microscopy to differentiate MPM from metastatic adenocarcinoma. No more than 50% of patients with MPM have a definite history of asbestos exposure.

Despite the claim that extrapleural pneumonectomy followed by extensive high-dose radiation therapy to the involved hemithorax is the treatment of choice in early-stage disease, management of MPM is still controversial, and it ranges from supportive care to extensive operations. As pointed out by Rusch, extrapleural pneumonectomy is a formidable operation that should be done only in specialized centers if one is to keep the operative mortality at an acceptable level (i.e., below 10%). This factor alone makes this treatment option impractical other than in very selected cases. The same limitation applies to parietal pleurectomy, in which complete excision of the tumor is generally not possible if the neoplasm involves the visceral or the mediastinal pleura. When selecting treatment of MPM, it is important to remember that 10% to 15% of patients will have a very slow course and will still be alive at 5 years without any treatment.

If one elects to perform an extrapleural pneumonectomy, we suggest using the latissimus dorsi to replace the diaphragm. This muscle is readily available, and its usage avoids the necessity of using a prosthetic graft.

J. D.

REFERENCES

Achatzy R, Beba W, Ritschler R et al: The diagnosis, therapy and prognosis of diffuse malignant mesothelioma. Eur J Cardiothorac Surg 3:445, 1989.

Adams VI, Unni KK, Muhm JR et al: Diffuse malignant mesothelioma of pleura: Diagnosis and survival in 92 cases. Cancer 58:1540, 1986.

Alberts AS, Falkson G, Goedhals L et al: Malignant pleural mesothelioma: A disease unaffected by current therapeutic maneuvers. J Clin Oncol 6:527, 1988.

Alexander E, Clark RA, Colley DP et al: CT of malignant pleural mesothelioma. AJR Am J Roentgenol 137:287, 1981.

Allen KB, Faber LP, Warren WH: Malignant pleural mesothelioma: Extrapleural pneumonectomy and pleurectomy. Chest Surg Clin North Am 4:113, 1994.

Anderson KA, Hurley WC, Hurley BT et al: Malignant pleural mesothelioma following radiotherapy in a 16-year-old boy. Cancer 56:273, 1985.

Andersson M, Olsen JH: Trend and distribution of mesothelioma in Denmark. Br J Cancer 51:699, 1985.

Antman KH, Shemin R, Ryan L et al: Malignant mesothelioma: Prognostic variables in a registry of 180 patients, the Dana-Farber Cancer Institute and Brigham and Women's Hospital experience over two decades, 1965–1985. J Clin Oncol 6:147, 1988.

Astoul P, Picat-Joossen D, Viallat J-R, Boutin C: Intrapleural administration of interleukin-2 for the treatment of patients with malignant pleural mesothelioma: A phase II study. Cancer 83:2099, 1998.

Baldini EH, Recht A, Strauss GM et al: Patterns of failure after trimodality therapy for malignant pleural mesothelioma. Ann Thorac Surg 63:334, 1997.

Ball DL, Cruickshank DG: The treatment of malignant mesothelioma of the pleura: Review of a 5-year experience, with special reference to radiotherapy. Am J Clin Oncol 13:4, 1990.

Balsara BR, Bell DW, Sonoda G et al: Comparative genomic hybridization and loss of heterozygosity analyses identify a common region of deletion at 15q11.1–15 in human malignant mesothelioma. Cancer Res 59:450, 1999.

Baris YI, Sahin AA, Ozesmi M et al: An outbreak of pleural mesothelioma and chronic fibrosing pleurisy in the village of Karain/Ugrup in Anatolia. Thorax 33:181, 1978.

Bénard F, Sterman D, Smith RJ et al: Metabolic imaging of malignant pleural mesothelioma with fluorodeoxyglucose positron emission tomography. Chest 114:713, 1998.

Blake PR, Catterall M, Emerson PA: Pleural mesothelioma treated by fast neutron therapy. Thorax 40:72, 1985.

Boutin C, Nussbaum E, Monnet I et al: Intrapleural treatment with recombinant gamma-interferon in early stage malignant pleural mesothelioma. Cancer 75:2460, 1994.

Boutin C, Rey F: Thoracoscopy in pleural malignant mesothelioma: A prospective study of 188 consecutive patients. I: Diagnosis. Cancer 72:389, 1993.

Boutin C, Rey F, Gouvernet J et al: Thoracoscopy in pleural malignant mesothelioma: A prospective study of 188 consecutive patients. II: Prognosis and staging. Cancer 72:394, 1993.

Brady LW: Mesothelioma—the role for radiation therapy. Semin Oncol 8:329, 1981.

Breau JL, Boaziz C, Morère JF et al: Chemotherapy with cisplatin, adriamycin, bleomycin and mitomycin C, combined with systemic and intrapleural hyaluronidase in stage II and III mesothelioma. Eur Respir Rev 3:223, 1993.

Briselli M, Mark EJ, Dickersin R: Solitary fibrous tumors of the pleura: Eight new cases and review of 360 cases in the literature. Cancer 47:2678, 1981.

Burmer GC, Rabinovitch PS, Kulander BG et al: Flow cytometric analysis of malignant pleural mesotheliomas. Hum Pathol 20:777, 1989.

Burns TR, Greenberg SD, Mace ML et al: Ultrastructural diagnosis of epithelial malignant mesothelioma. Cancer 56:2036, 1985.

Butchart EG, Ashcroft T, Barnsley WC et al: Pleuropneumonectomy in the management of diffuse malignant mesothelioma of the pleura: Experience with 29 patients. Thorax 31:15, 1976.

Byrne MJ, Davidson JA, Musk AW et al: Cisplatin and gemcitabine treatment for malignant mesothelioma: A phase II study. J Clin Oncol 17:25, 1999.

Cantin R, Al-Jabi M, McCaughey WTE: Desmoplastic diffuse mesothelioma. Am J Surg Pathol 6(3):215, 1982.

Carbone M, Rizzo P, Grimley PM et al: Simian virus-40 large-T antigen binds p53 in human mesotheliomas. Nat Med 3:908, 1997.

Cavazza A, Travis LB, Travis WD et al: Post-irradiation malignant mesothelioma. Cancer 77:1379, 1996.

Chahinian AP, Antman K, Goutsou M et al: Randomized phase II trial of cisplatin with mitomycin or doxorubicin for malignant mesothelioma by the Cancer and Leukemia Group B. J Clin Oncol 11:1559, 1993.

Chahinian AP, Pajak TF, Holland JF et al: Diffuse malignant mesothelioma. Prospective evaluation of 69 patients. Ann Intern Med 96:746, 1982.

Chahinian AP, Suzuki Y, Mandel EM et al: Diffuse pulmonary malignant mesothelioma: Response to doxorubicin and 5-azacytidine. Cancer 42:1687, 1978.

Cheng JQ, Jhanwar SC, Klein WM et al: *p16* alterations and deletion mapping of 9p21–p22 in malignant mesothelioma. Cancer Res 54:5547, 1994.

Christmas TI, Manning LS, Davis MR et al: HLA antigen expression and malignant mesothelioma. Am J Respir Cell Mol Biol 5:213, 1991.

Churg A, DePaoli L: Environmental pleural plaques in residents of a Quebec chrysotile mining town. Chest 94:58, 1988.

Cole FH Jr, Ellis RA, Goodman RC et al: Benign fibrous pleural tumor with elevation of insulin-like growth factor and hypoglycemia. South Med J 83:690, 1990.

Dabouis G, LeMevel B, Corroller J: Treatment of diffuse pleural malignant mesothelioma by *cis*-dichlorodiammine platinum (CDDP) in nine patients. Cancer Chemother Pharmacol 5:209, 1981.

Dahl IMS, Solheim OP, Erikstein B et al: A longitudinal study of the hyaluronan level in the serum of patients with malignant mesothelioma under treatment: Hyaluronan as an indicator of progressive disease. Cancer 64:68, 1989.

de Perrot M, Kurt A-M, Robert JH et al: Clinical behavior of solitary fibrous tumors of the pleura. Ann Thorac Surg 67:1456, 1999.

DeLaria GA, Jensik R, Faber LP et al: Surgical management of malignant mesothelioma. Ann Thorac Surg 26:375, 1978.

DeValle MJ, Faber LP, Kittle CF et al: Extrapleural pneumonectomy for diffuse, malignant mesothelioma. Ann Thorac Surg 42:612, 1986.

Dhaene K, Van Marck E, Kumar-Singh S et al: Telomerase activity in human pleural mesothelioma. Thorax 53:915, 1998.

Dimitrov NV, Egner J, Balcueva E et al: High-dose methotrexate with citrovorum factor and vincristine in the treatment of malignant mesothelioma. Cancer 50:1245, 1982.

Dimitrov NV, McMahon S: Presentation, diagnostic methods, staging, and natural history of malignant mesothelioma. *In* Antman K, Aisner J (eds): Asbestos-Related Malignancy. Orlando, FL, Grune & Stratton, 1987, pp 225–238.

Elmes PC, Simpson MJC: The clinical aspects of mesothelioma. Q J Med New Series 45(179):427, 1976.

England DM, Hochholzer L, McCarthy MJ: Localized benign and malignant fibrous tumors of the pleura: A clinicopathologic review of 223 cases. Am J Surg Pathol 13:640, 1989.

Fraire AE, Cooper S, Greenberg SD et al: Mesothelioma of childhood. Cancer 62:838, 1988.

Gerwin BI, Lechner JF, Reddel RR et al: Comparison of production of transforming growth factor-β and platelet-derived growth factor by normal human mesothelial cells and mesothelioma cell lines. Cancer Res 47:6180, 1987.

Goey SH, Eggermont AMM, Punt CJA et al: Intrapleural administration of interleukin 2 in pleural mesothelioma: A phase I–II study. Br J Cancer 72:1283, 1995.

Gordon W Jr, Antman KH, Greenberger JS et al: Radiation therapy in the management of patients with mesothelioma. Int J Radiat Oncol Biol Phys 8:19, 1982.

Gotfried MH, Quan SF, Sobonya RE: Diffuse epithelial pleural mesothelioma presenting as a solitary lung mass. Chest 84:99, 1983.

Hammar SP, Bolen JW: Pleural neoplasms. In Dail DH, Hammar SP (eds): Pulmonary Pathology. New York, Springer-Verlag, 1988, pp 973–1028.

Heelan RT, Rusch VW, Begg CB et al: Staging of malignant pleural mesothelioma: Comparison of CT and MR imaging. Am J Radiol 172:1039, 1999.

Hilaris BS, Nori D, Beattie EJ Jr, et al: Value of perioperative brachytherapy in the management of non-oat cell carcinoma of the lung. Int J Radiat Oncol Biol Phys 9:1161, 1983.

Hillerdal G: Malignant mesothelioma 1982: Review of 4710 published cases. Br J Dis Chest 77:321, 1983.

Hulks G, Thomas JStJ, Waclawski E: Malignant pleural mesothelioma in western Glasgow 1980–1986. Thorax 44:496, 1989.

Immerman SC, Sener SF, Khandekar JD: Causes and evaluation of tumor-induced hypoglycemia. Arch Surg 117:905, 1982.

Kane MJ, Chahinian AP, Holland JF: Malignant mesothelioma in young adults. Cancer 65:1449, 1990.

Kaye JA, Wang A-M, Joachim CL et al: Malignant mesothelioma with brain metastases. Am J Med 80:95, 1986.

Keller SM, Taylor DD, and Weese JL: In vitro killing of human malignant mesothelioma by photodynamic therapy. J Surg Res 48:337, 1990.

Klemperer P, Rabin CB: Primary neoplasms of the pleura: A report of five cases. Arch Pathol 11:385, 1937.

Kumar-Singh S, Segers K, Rodeck U et al: *WT1* mutation in malignant mesothelioma and WT1 immunoreactivity in relation to *p53* and growth factor receptor expression, cell type transition, and prognosis. J Pathol 181:67, 1997.

Kutcher GJ, Kestler C, Greenblatt D et al: Technique for external beam treatment for mesothelioma. Int J Radiat Oncol Biol Phys 13:1747, 1987.

Langerak AW, Williamson KA, Miyagawa K et al: Expression of the Wilms' tumor gene *WT1* in human malignant mesothelioma cell lines and relationship to platelet-derived growth factor A and insulin-like growth factor 2 expression. Genes Chrom Cancer 12:87, 1995.

Law MR, Gregor A, Hodson ME et al: Malignant mesothelioma of the pleura: A study of 52 treated and 64 untreated patients. Thorax 39:255, 1984.

Law MR, Gregor A, Husband JE et al: Computed tomography in the assessment of malignant mesothelioma of the pleura. Clin Radiol 33:67, 1982a.

Law MR, Hodson ME, Heard BE: Malignant mesothelioma of the pleura: Relation between histological type and clinical behaviour. Thorax 37:810, 1982b.

Le Roux BT: Pleural tumors. Thorax 17:111, 1962.

Lechner JF, Tesfaigzi J, Gerwin BI: Oncogenes and tumor-suppressor genes in mesothelioma—a synopsis. Environ Health Perspect 105(Suppl 5):1061, 1997.

Lederman GS, Recht A, Herman T et al: Long-term survival in peritoneal mesothelioma: The role of radiotherapy and combined modality treatment. Cancer 59:1882, 1987.

Lee TC, Zhang Y, Aston C et al: Normal human mesothelial cells and mesothelioma cell lines express insulin-like growth factor I and associated molecules. Cancer Res 53:2858, 1993.

Lee W-C, Balsara B, Liu Z et al: Loss of heterozygosity analysis defines a critical region in chromosome 1p22 commonly deleted in human malignant mesothelioma. Cancer Res 56:4297, 1996.

Lerman Y, Learman Y, Schachter P et al: Radiation associated malignant pleural mesothelioma. Thorax 46:463, 1991.

Levine RL: Asbestos: An Information Resource (NIH publication No. 81–1681). Bethesda, MD, National Institutes of Health, 1981.

Lewis RJ, Sisler GE, Mackenzie JW: Diffuse, mixed malignant pleural mesothelioma. Ann Thorac Surg 31:53, 1981.

Longo WE, Rigler MW, Slade J: Crocidolite asbestos fibers in smoke from original Kent cigarettes. Cancer Res 55:2232, 1995.

Maasilta P: Deterioration in lung function following hemithorax irradiation for pleural mesothelioma. Int J Radiat Oncol Biol Phys 20:433, 1991.

Malker HSR, McLaughlin JK, Malker BK et al: Occupational risks for pleural mesothelioma in Sweden, 1961–79. J Natl Cancer Inst 74:61, 1985.

Manning LS, Bowman RV, Darby SB et al: Lysis of human malignant mesothelioma cells by natural killer (NK) and lymphokine-activated killer (LAK) cells. Am Rev Respir Dis 139:1369, 1989.

Markman M, Cleary S, Pfeifle CE et al: Cisplatin administered by the intracavitary route as treatment for malignant mesothelioma. Cancer 58:18, 1986.

McCormack PM, Nagasaki F, Hilaris BS et al: Surgical treatment of pleural mesothelioma. J Thorac Cardiovasc Surg 84:834, 1982.

McDonald AD, McDonald JC: Epidemiology of malignant mesothelioma. In Antman K, Aisner J (eds): Asbestos-Related Malignancy. Orlando, FL, Grune & Stratton, 1987, pp 31–55.

McDonald JC, Armstrong B, Case B et al: Mesothelioma and asbestos fiber type: Evidence from lung tissue analyses. Cancer 63:1544, 1989.

McNicholas KW, Rose EA, Edie RN et al: Resection of giant benign fibrous mesothelioma of pleura. NY State J Med March:626, 1980.

Mintzer DM, Kelsen D, Frimmer D et al: Phase II trial of high-dose cisplatin in patients with malignant mesothelioma. Cancer Treat Rep 69:711, 1985.

Mirvis S, Dutcher JP, Haney PJ et al: CT of malignant pleural mesothelioma. AJR Am J Roentgenol 140:655, 1983.

Monti G, Jaurand M-C, Monnet I et al: Intrapleural production of interleukin 6 during mesothelioma and its modulation by γ-interferon treatment. Cancer Res 54:4419, 1994.

Moran CA, Suster S, Koss MN: The spectrum of histologic growth patterns in benign and malignant fibrous tumors of the pleura. Semin Diagn Pathol 9(2):169, 1992.

Mulatero C, Surentheran T, Breuer J et al: Simian virus 40 and human pleural mesothelioma. Thorax 54:60, 1999.

Musk AW, Dolin PJ, Armstrong BK et al: The incidence of malignant mesothelioma in Australia, 1947–1980. Med J Aust 150:242, 1989.

Mychalczak BR, Nori D, Armstrong JG, et al: Results of treatment of malignant pleural mesothelioma with surgery, brachytherapy, and external beam irradiation. Endocurie Hypertherm Oncol 5:245, 1989.

Nauta RJ, Osteen RT, Antman KH et al: Clinical staging and the tendency of malignant pleural mesotheliomas to remain localized. Ann Thorac Surg 34:66, 1982.

O'Reilly EM, Ilson DH, Saltz LB et al: A phase II trial of interferon alpha-2a and carboplatin in patients with advanced malignant mesothelioma. Cancer Invest 17:195, 1999.

Okike N, Bernatz PE, Woolner LB: Localized mesothelioma of the pleura: Benign and malignant variants. J Thorac Cardiovasc Surg 75:363, 1978.

Olesen LL, Thorshauge H: Thrombocytosis in patients with malignant pleural mesothelioma. Cancer 62:1194, 1988.

Ordóñez NG: In search of a positive immunohistochemical marker for mesothelioma: An update. Adv Anatom Pathol 5:53, 1998.

Pass HI, Kranda K, Temeck BK et al: Surgically debulked malignant pleural mesothelioma: Results and prognostic factors. Ann Surg Oncol 4:215, 1997a.

Pass HI, Temeck BK, Kranda K et al: Phase III randomized trial of surgery with or without intraoperative photodynamic therapy and postoperative immunochemotherapy for malignant pleural mesothelioma. Ann Surg Oncol 4:628, 1997b.

Patz EF Jr, Rusch VW, Heelan R: The proposed new international TNM staging system for malignant pleural mesothelioma: Application to imaging. AJR Am J Roentgenol 166:323, 1996.

Peterson JT, Greenberg SD, Buffler PA: Non–asbestos-related malignant mesothelioma: A review. Cancer 54:951, 1984.

Peto J, Hodgson JT, Matthews FE et al: Continuing increase in mesothelioma mortality in Britain. Lancet 345:535, 1995.

Pooley FD: Asbestos mineralogy. In Antman K, Aisner J (eds): Asbestos-Related Malignancy. Orlando, FL, Grune & Stratton, 1987, pp 3–27.

Price B: Analysis of current trends in United States mesothelioma incidence. Am J Epidemiol 145:211, 1997.

Rabinowitz JG, Efremidis SC, Cohen B et al: A comparative study of mesothelioma and asbestosis using computed tomography and conventional chest radiography. Radiology 144:453, 1982.

Raghavan D, Gianoutsos P, Bishop J et al: Phase II trial of carboplatin in the management of malignant mesothelioma. J Clin Oncol 8(1):151, 1990.

Rice TW, Adelstein DJ, Kirby TJ et al: Aggressive multimodality therapy for malignant pleural mesothelioma. Ann Thorac Surg 58:24, 1994.

Ris HB, Altermatt JH, Inderbitzi R et al: Photodynamic therapy with chlorins for diffuse malignant mesothelioma: Initial clinical results. Br J Cancer 64:1116, 1991.

Ris HB, Giger A, Hof VI et al: Experimental assessment of photodynamic therapy with chlorins for malignant mesothelioma. Eur J Cardiothorac Surg 12:542, 1997.

Roberts GH: Distant visceral metastases in pleural mesothelioma. Br J Dis Chest 70:246, 1976.

Robinson BWS: Asbestos and cancer: Human natural killer cell activity is suppressed by asbestos fibers but can be restored by recombinant interleukin-2. Am Rev Respir Dis 139:897, 1989.

Ruffie R, Feld R, Minkin S et al: Diffuse malignant mesothelioma of the pleura in Ontario and Quebec: A retrospective study of 332 patients. J Clin Oncol 7:1157, 1989.

Rusch VW: Pleurectomy/decortication and adjuvant therapy for malignant mesothelioma. Chest 103(Suppl):382S, 1993.

Rusch VW, Godwin JD, Shuman WP: The role of computed tomography scanning in the initial assessment and the follow-up of malignant pleural mesothelioma. J Thorac Cardiovasc Surg 96:171, 1988.

Rusch VW, Piantadosi S, Holmes EC: The role of extrapleural pneumonectomy in malignant pleural mesothelioma. J Thorac Cardiovasc Surg 102:1, 1991.

Rusch VW, Rosenzweig K, Venkatraman ES et al: A prospective trial of surgical resection and high dose hemithoracic radiation for malignant pleural mesothelioma. Proc ASCO 19:578a, 2000.

Rusch VW, Saltz L, Venkatraman E et al: A phase II trial of pleurectomy/decortication followed by intrapleural and systemic chemotherapy for malignant pleural mesothelioma. J Clin Oncol 12:1156, 1994.

Rusch VW: The International Mesothelioma Interest Group: A proposed new international TNM staging system for malignant pleural mesothelioma. Chest 108:1122, 1995.

Rusch VW, Venkatraman E: The importance of surgical staging in the treatment of malignant pleural mesothelioma. J Thorac Cardiovasc Surg 111:815, 1996.

Rusch VW, Venkatraman ES: Important prognostic factors in patients with malignant pleural mesothelioma, managed surgically. Ann Thorac Surg 68:1799, 1999.

Said JW, Nash G, Banks-Schlegel S et al: Localized fibrous mesothelioma: An immunohistochemical and electron microscopic study. Hum Pathol 15:440, 1984.

Scharifker D, Kenko M: Localized fibrous "mesothelioma" of pleura (submesothelial fibroma): A clinicopathologic study of 18 cases. Cancer 43:627, 1979.

Sekido Y, Pass HI, Bader S et al: Neurofibromatosis type 2 (*NF2*) gene is somatically mutated in mesothelioma but not in lung cancer. Cancer Res 55:1227, 1995.

Selikoff IJ, Churg J, Hammond EC: Relation between exposure to asbestos and mesothelioma. N Engl J Med 272:560, 1965.

Sheard JDH, Taylor W, Soorae A et al: Pneumothorax and malignant mesothelioma in patients over the age of 40. Thorax 46:584, 1991.

Shivapurkar N, Virmani AK, Wistuba II et al: Deletions of chromosome 4 at multiple sites are frequent in malignant mesothelioma and small cell lung carcinoma. Clin Cancer Res 5:17, 1999.

Sinoff C, Falkson G, Sandison AG et al: Combined doxorubicin and radiation therapy in malignant pleural mesothelioma. Cancer Treat Rep 66:1605, 1982.

Sklarin NT, Chahinian AP, Feuer EJ et al: Augmentation of activity of *cis*-diamminedichloroplatinum (II) and mitomycin C by interferon in human malignant mesothelioma xenografts in nude mice. Cancer Res 48:64, 1988.

Soubra M, Dunscombe PB, Hodson DI et al: Physical aspects of external beam radiotherapy for the treatment of malignant pleural mesothelioma. Int J Radiat Oncol Biol Phys 18:1521, 1990.

Sterman DH, Kaiser LR, Albelda SM: Gene therapy for malignant pleural mesothelioma. Hematol Oncol Clin North Am 12:553, 1998.

Stout AP, Murray MR: Localized pleural mesothelioma. Arch Pathol 34:951, 1942.

Sugarbaker DJ, Flores RM, Jaklitsch MT et al: Resection margins, extrapleural nodal status, and cell type determine postoperative long-term survival in trimodality therapy of malignant pleural mesothelioma: Results of 183 patients. J Thorac Cardiovasc Surg 117:54, 1999.

Sugarbaker DJ, Heher EC, Lee TH et al: Extrapleural pneumonectomy, chemotherapy, and radiotherapy in the treatment of diffuse malignant pleural mesothelioma. J Thorac Cardiovasc Surg 102:10, 1991.

Sugarbaker DJ, Strauss GM, Lynch TJ et al: Node status has prognostic significance in the multimodality therapy of diffuse, malignant mesothelioma. J Clin Oncol 11:1172, 1993.

Suter M, Gebhard S, Boumghar M et al: Localized fibrous tumours of the pleura: 15 new cases and review of the literature. Eur J Cardiothorac Surg 14:453, 1998.

Taguchi T, Jhanwar SC, Siegfried JM et al: Recurrent deletions of specific chromosomal sites in 1p, 3p, 6q, and 9p in human malignant mesothelioma. Cancer Res 53:4349, 1993.

Takita H, Dougherty TJ: Intracavitary photodynamic therapy for malignant pleural mesothelioma. Semin Surg Oncol 11:368, 1995.

Tammilehto L, Kivisaari L, Salminen US et al: Evaluation of the clinical TNM staging system for malignant pleural mesothelioma: An assessment in 88 patients. Lung Cancer 12:25, 1995.

Testa JR, Carbone M, Hirvonen A et al: A multi-institutional study confirms the presence and expression of simian virus 40 in human malignant mesotheliomas. Cancer Res 58:4505, 1998.

Tiainen M, Kere J, Tammilehto L et al: Abnormalities of chromosomes 7 and 22 in human malignant pleural mesothelioma: Correlation between Southern blot and cytogenetic analyses. Genes Chrom Cancer 4:176, 1992.

Tiainen M, Tammilehto L, Rautonen J et al: Chromosomal abnormalities and their correlations with asbestos exposure and survival in patients with mesothelioma. Br J Cancer 60:618, 1989.

Umsawasdi T, Dhingra HM, Charnsangavej C et al: A case report of malignant pleural mesothelioma with long-term disease control after chemotherapy. Cancer 67:48, 1991.

Wadler S, Chahinian AP, Slater W et al: Cardiac abnormalities in patients with diffuse malignant pleural mesothelioma. Cancer 58:2744, 1986.

Wagner JC: Mesothelioma and mineral fibers. Cancer 57:1905, 1986.

Wagner JC, Slegg CA, Marchand P: Diffuse pleural mesotheliomas and asbestos exposure in Northwestern Cape Province. Br J Ind Med 17:260, 1960.

Walters KL, Martinez AJ: Malignant fibrous mesothelioma: Metastatic to brain and liver. Acta Neuropathol (Berlin) 33:173, 1975.

Watts DM, Jones GP, Bowman GA et al: Giant benign mesothelioma. Ann Thorac Surg 48:590, 1989.

Whitwell F, Rawcliffe RM: Diffuse malignant pleural mesothelioma and asbestos exposure. Thorax 26:6, 1971.

Wirth PR, Legier J, Wright GL Jr: Immunohistochemical evaluation of seven monoclonal antibodies for differentiation of pleural mesothelioma from lung adenocarcinoma. Cancer 67:655, 1991.

Xiao S, Li D, Vijg J et al: Codeletion of *p15* and *p16* in primary malignant mesothelioma. Oncogene 11:511, 1995.

Yasumoto K, Miyazaki K, Nagashima A et al: Induction of lymphokine-activated killer cells by intrapleural instillations of recombinant interleukin-2 in patients with malignant pleurisy due to lung cancer. Cancer Res 47:2184, 1987.

CHAPTER **46**

Fibrothorax and Decortication

Jean Deslauriers
Francisco Paris
Vicente Tarrazona

Under normal conditions, the pleural space is a virtual cavity interposed between the chest wall and the lung. The visceral and parietal linings of this cavity are 1 to 2 mm thick and serve as permeable membranes for transport of cells and fluid. Under pathologic conditions, these relationships may be altered, leading to the development of chronic infections, trapped lung, and severely impaired respiration. Although infrequently encountered, these pathologies must be well understood, not only because they are of historical interest but also because they present challenging management problems.

HISTORICAL NOTE

Between the years 1892 and 1894, Delorme in France and Fowler in America described an operation designed to substitute for the mutilating thoracoplasty of Schede (1890). The purpose of the operation was to promote lung re-expansion instead of letting the chest wall collapse to fill in the space. This procedure was called *decortication*. The exact sequence of these descriptions is still somewhat controversial despite some clarifications offered by Violet (1904).

In a sealed letter deposited at the French Academy of Medicine in 1892 and at a surgical meeting in 1893, Delorme, Professeur au Val-de-Grâce, described his method for the treatment of chronic empyemas. In a patient with a large chest wall abscess, he performed a scalpel and scissors dissection of the wall of the abscess, which was 1 cm thick and covered the left lung and pericardium. He concluded that he had freed the lung from this "fausse membrane." The apparent success of this procedure and further autopsy work, in which he was able to decorticate encased lung ("décortiquer une membrane résistante comme du cuir") and subsequently re-expand healthy lung ("poumon sain, crépitant et extensible"), further confirmed his belief that this procedure could be useful for patients with large, residual, infected intrathoracic spaces.

In 1894, Delorme performed the first planned decortication, and 4 days later he reported the case at the Academy. At a French surgical meeting in 1896, he presented 26 cases of pulmonary decortication and concluded that: (1) it is possible to free a lung from the membrane that holds it down even long after an operation for an empyema; (2) the method is applicable not only on the right but also on the left side; and (3) it is better than the Estlander operation because it expands and tends to restore the function of an otherwise useless lung (Lund, 1911).

In 1893, Fowler also described the operation of decortication, which he had performed for the first time that year on a 35-year-old woman who had had an empyema with a fistula for 10 years. He dissected out the scar tissue surrounding the fistulous tract and removed the entire mass of fibrous tissue from the diaphragm and lung. He was surprised to discover that the lung began to re-expand as soon as the thick scar tissue was peeled from it (Mayo and Beckman, 1914). His method was applicable to the treatment of chronic empyemas, in which he thought that failure of the lung to re-expand was mostly due to encasement by an inexpandable fibrous peel. According to Lund (1911), the credit for the operation belongs to Delorme because he apparently had a definite plan to accomplish what he was after, as opposed to Fowler, who had no special plan, apparently, of allowing the lung to expand by removal of the tough, fibrous covering over the lung. According to Mayo and Beckman (1914), Fowler was indeed "surprised to discover that the lung began to re-expand as soon as this thick scar tissue was peeled from it." In 1906, Ransahoff advised making multiple incisions at right angles to each other through this thickened pleura down to the lung thus allowing the lung to re-expand at numerous points.

During the early 20th century and until some years after World War I, the procedure was used sporadically, and finally, because it carried a high fatality rate that results did not appear to justify, it encountered increasing disapproval. Several factors accounted for this lack of enthusiasm, including inadequacy of anesthesia, lack of antimicrobial agents in the face of infection, lack of blood transfusion ability, and lack of technical expertise (Milfield et al, 1978). It was often a prolonged and shocking operation. Expansion soon after operation was frequently lost owing to wound breakdown from infection. Re-expansion did not always follow successful decortication because of underlying defects such as parenchymal fibrosis, fistulas, or other active diseases (Himmelstein et al, 1948).

In 1911, Lund reported the experience of Lloyd (1908), who had stated that in the treatment of old empyemas, it was not necessary to remove the pulmonary pleura but simply to break up the adhesions at the borders of the cavity between the parietal and visceral pleurae. Lund presented the cases of seven patients and described the operation performed in the first case: "On splitting this membrane with the scissors and separating it carefully from the surface of the lung, the lung began to expand, and when the child coughed at the close of the operation, the red, velvety lung blew up like a soap bubble and came up against the chest wall, where it remained."

In 1915, Lilienthal also treated nontuberculous suppurations with decortication. He reported on 23 such patients, among whom there was an operative mortality of 17% (4 of 23) and a good result in all survivors. He insisted on the importance of full lung mobilization and called attention to the dangerous hemorrhage that may follow the tearing away of tough adhesions between the lung and the chest wall.

Other early contributions were those of Mayo and Beckman (1914) and Eggers (1923), who reported shortly after World War I on 146 patients who had undergone decortication for chronic empyemas. He correctly identified the objective of decortication as excision of the peel holding the lung rather than removal of the visceral pleura itself.

The advances in management of thoracic trauma that occurred during and after World War II placed further emphasis on decortication of the lung following clotted traumatic hemothorax. Impressive results and new applications of the procedure were reported by Samson and Burford (1946, 1947), who formulated the newer concept of early and total decortication of the lung. Samson and associates (1946) showed that complete pulmonary mobilization (decortication) should not be deferred for the length of time usually necessary to transfer the patient to a specialty center (in the "interior" zone in military situations). In those cases, early decortication results in immediate pulmonary re-expansion and prevents the development of fibrothoraces. Other investigators such as Patton and colleagues (1952) showed that decorticated lungs actually regained function if the underlying parenchyma was free of disease.

■ *HISTORICAL READINGS*

Burford TH, Parker EF, Samson PC: Early decortication in the treatment of post-traumatic empyema. Ann Surg 122:163, 1945.

Delorme E: Nouveau traitement des empyèmes chroniques. Gaz Hôp 67:94, 1894.

Eggers C: Radical operation for chronic empyema. Ann Surg 77:327, 1923.

Estlander JA: Sur la résection des côtes dans l'empyème chronique. Rev Mens 8:885, 1897.

Fowler GR: A case of thoracoplasty for removal of a large cicatricial fibrous growth from the interior of the chest, the result of an old empyema. Med Rec 44:838, 1893.

Himmelstein A, Miscall L, Kirschner PA: Decortication in tuberculosis. Surg Clin North Am 28:1601, 1948.

Lilienthal H: Empyema: Exploration of the thorax with primary mobilization of the lung. Ann Surg 62:309, 1915.

Lund FB: The advantages of the so-called decortication of the lung in old empyema. JAMA 57:693, 1911.

Mayo CH, Beckman EH: Visceral pleurectomy for chronic empyema. Am Surg 59:884, 1914.

Milfield DJ, Mattox KL, Beal AC: Early evacuation of clotted hemothorax. Am J Surg 136:686, 1978.

Patton WE, Watson TR, Gaensler EA: Pulmonary function before and at intervals after surgical decortication of the lung. Surg Gynecol Obstet 95:477, 1952.

Ransahoff J: Discussion of the pleura in the treatment of chronic empyema. Ann Surg 43:502, 1906.

Samson PC, Burford TH: Total pulmonary decortication: Its evolution and present concepts of indications and operative technique. J Thorac Surg 16:127, 1947.

Samson PC, Burford TH, Brewer LA, Burbank B: The management of war wounds of the chest in a base center: The role of early pulmonary decortication. J Thorac Surg 15:1, 1946.

Schede M: Die Behandlung der Empyeme. Proceedings of the Ninth Congress of Internal Medicine. Wiesbaden, Germany. Vol 9, 1890, p 41.

Violet D: De la décortication pulmonaire dans l'empyème chronique. Arch Gen Med 81:657, 1904.

BASIC SCIENCE

Fibrothorax is characterized by the presence of abnormal fibrous tissue within the pleural space, a feature that usually complicates clotted hemothoraces, pleural tuberculosis, or chronic empyemas. As a result of this fibrosis, the lung becomes entrapped and the hemithorax contracts, resulting in reduced mobility. Eventually, there is a marked loss of function in the collapsed lung.

Over the years, several terms (listed in Table 46–1) have been used in reference to fibrothoraces. In some cases, the visceral peel has been wrongly thought to be thickened pleura (Mayo and Beckman, 1914), and this has contributed to perpetuation of some misunderstandings about this disease. The so-called lung en cuirasse seen in restrictive pleurisy associated with asbestos exposure (Sterling and Herbert, 1980) should also be distinguished from the "peel" seen in fibrothoraces, because the latter does not represent thickened pleura.

Decortication, a term derived from Latin, literally means stripping or peeling off of the "bark" from the lung (Lund, 1911). It is a surgical procedure that consists of removing a restricting fibrotic membrane from the visceral pleural surface of the lung. Its purpose is to free the trapped lung as well as to obliterate the pleural space. It is a different operation from the early thoracotomy done for deloculation of the pleural space in cases of fibrinopurulent empyemas (Mayo, 1985; Morin et al, 1972) or hemothoraces (Beall et al, 1966). Deloculation consists of cleaning out a cavity littered with fibrous membranes to improve on closed drainage. It is not a decortication in the true sense of the word, because a mature peel has not yet formed over the lung.

Decortication is also different from empyemectomy, which is the complete excision of the empyema and its contents without entering the cavity itself, the purpose being to avoid soiling the interior of the hemithorax (LeRoux et al, 1986). Finally, decortication is different from the limited decortication described for the management of pediatric empyema (Kosloke and Cartwright,

TABLE 46–1 ■ **Commonly Used Terminology Referring to Fibrothorax**

Trapped lung
Encased lung
Unexpanded lung
Restrictive pleurisy
Constrictive pleurisy/pleuritis/peel
Organizing hemothorax/empyema
Frozen chest
Lung en cuirasse
Pleural constriction

TABLE 46–2 ■ **Causes of Fibrothorax**

Common Causes
Traumatic or nontraumatic hemothorax
Chronic empyema
Chronic pneumothorax
Sequelae of tuberculosis
Therapeutic pneumothoraces
Tuberculous pleurisy or empyema
Neglected pleural effusion
Uncommon bacterial and parasitic diseases of the pleural space

Rare Causes
Chylothorax
Pancreatic diseases
Talc poudrage

1988). This procedure is similar to early deloculation and is used to remove pleural contents that are believed to be in the fibrinopurulent stage and have not yet organized.

Causes of Fibrothorax

The causes of fibrothorax are listed in Table 46–2. In the early 20th century, most fibrothoraces were seen in association with tuberculosis, and they resulted from therapeutic pneumothoraces in which the lung became unexpandable or from untreated or unresponsive tuberculous pleurisy or empyema. In recent years, classic examples have been those of a trapped lung secondary to chronic empyema, clotted hemothorax, or neglected pleural effusion. In each of these situations, the pleural collections of pus, blood, or fluid precipitate into fibrin, which eventually becomes fibrous tissue and is deposited over the pleural surfaces and the diaphragm.

Rare causes of fibrothoraces include uncommon bacterial and parasitic diseases of the pleural space, chylothoraces (Fairfax et al, 1986), and pleural complications of pancreatitis (Shapiro et al, 1970). In some patients with fibrothoraces, no specific cause can be identified either by clinical history or at the time of thoracotomy.

Pathophysiology

Although it was originally thought that the fibroblastic reaction in the pleural space was a specific response to the presence of blood, it became apparent that any insult to the pleura would result in the same reaction (Samson et al, 1958).

Any undrained or untreated pleural collection of fluid, pus, blood, or chyle is always followed by precipitation of fibrin on the exposed surfaces. As the process evolves into the stage of organization, fibroblasts and angioblasts proliferate and the exudate eventually becomes a mature peel, which is composed of adult tissue rich in collagen but relatively poor in blood supply, cells, and elastic fibers. As the peel further thickens, the underlying lung is covered and entrapped, and its normal expansion is impeded. Wachsmuth and Schautz (1961) and Rudström and Thoren (1955) have shown that the fully developed parietal peel consists of three poorly defined layers: (1) a layer of comparatively vascular, loosely organized tissue nearest the parietal pleura; (2) a layer of connective tissue containing few vessels and cells, which forms the main bulk of the peel; and (3) an inner layer bounding the central cavity and consisting of necrotic tissues, fibrinoid masses, and detritus with or without bacteria. As the peel ages even more, the fibrotic component increases, and the loose layer nearest the pleura becomes thinner and finally disappears. In addition to the peel, there are almost always dense adhesions between the lung, chest wall, pericardium, diaphragm, and mediastinum. As shown by Williams (1950), these adhesions restrain the lung and are important in the production of the pulmonary collapse associated with fibrothorax. Pleurolysis is, therefore, an essential part of decortication.

The parietal peel is always thicker than the visceral peel, possibly 2 cm or more. Calcifications are common over the inner surface of the peel, and they are usually associated with chronic exudative effusions, hemothoraces, or tuberculous empyemas. Unless the lung has been damaged by tuberculosis or other parenchymal disease, neither the visceral nor parietal pleura becomes thickened, and both remain largely normal membranes.

In patients with small hemothoraces (<200 ml), the continuous movement of the heart and lungs may defibrinate the blood, which will be reabsorbed in a fluid state by the pleural lymphatics. If, however, the hemothorax is larger, if there is continued bleeding, or if air (Drummond and Craig, 1967) or bacteria are also present, a clot with multiple pockets containing air or fluid will form, and eventually this clot will become organized into a peel that will encase the lung.

In empyemas, the rapidity of organization varies according to factors such as proper antibiotic treatment, immunologic status of the host, and type of bacteria (Kosloske and Cartwright, 1988). Ultimately, the lung is compressed by the pleural contents, imprisoned by the peel, and restrained by the pleural adhesions (Williams, 1950). Although these factors are not equally important in maintaining the lung in its collapsed state, to be successful the decortication operation must evacuate the pleural contents, remove the peel, and completely mobilize the lung by freeing the adhesions.

Physiologic Consequences

There are many functional consequences of a fibrothorax. Several authors have shown that loss of pulmonary function bears no relationship to the degree of pleural thickening as seen on chest radiographs. In other words, a thick pleural peel does not necessarily imply reduced ventilation and perfusion any more than a thin peel (Fraser and Pare, 1979). Other authors have also demonstrated that even a relatively localized pleural restriction may be associated with profound alterations in ventilation and blood flow to the entire lung (Autio, 1959; Hughes et al, 1975; Robin et al, 1966). In 1959, Autio showed that localized costophrenic pleuritis could decrease ventilation to the affected lung by an average of 23%, and when the disease was clearly visible, ventilation was reduced well over 50%.

The physiologic aberrations in pulmonary function seen in patients with fibrothoraces are those of a restriction producing decreased lung volumes, diffusion capacity, and expiratory flows. Patton and colleagues (1952) studied pulmonary function before and at intervals after surgical decortication of the lung. In eight patients, the average maximum breathing capacity was reduced to 68% of the predicted normal and the average vital capacity to 65%. The almost equal reduction of maximum breathing capacity and vital capacity indicated that the ventilatory defect was of the restrictive type. Bronchospirometric observations showed the ventilatory insufficiency to be almost entirely owing to extensive collapse of the involved lung. Similar abnormalities in pulmonary function have been reported by Carroll and colleagues (1951) and Siebens and colleagues (1956).

Diffusion on the affected side is invariably low. This is likely due to a reduction in the available alveolocapillary gas exchange surface. Because of mechanical limitations of pulmonary vasculature and of hypoxic vasoconstriction, ipsilateral lung perfusion is also decreased. Characteristically, perfusion is decreased disproportionately to ventilation (Grossman, 1979); this reduction is adaptive to the reduced ventilation and is not accompanied by structural arterial changes. This adjustment in the pulmonary blood flow prevents the arterial hypoxia that would otherwise develop (Wright et al, 1949). In patients studied with ^{133}Xe, Davidson and Glazier (1972) also provided some evidence that the mechanical function of both lungs could be affected in unilateral disease. In 1966, Robin and associates reported four patients in whom severe pulmonary hypertension was associated with chronic constrictive pleuritis, and they speculated about a possible pulmonary vasoconstrictive substance originating in lung tissue, which markedly reduced but still maintained perfusion.

Bolliger and de Kock (1988) have shown that when the movement of the chest wall is impaired by fibrothorax and the lung tissue is not involved, the flow-volume curve has a relatively characteristic pattern, which can be differentiated from that of pure restrictive lung disease. Another difference between fibrothorax and restrictive parenchymal disease that is revealed in pulmonary function studies is the lack of elevation of maximal static pulmonary recoil pressure observed in patients with fibrothorax (Fraser and Pare, 1979).

DIAGNOSIS

Clinical Features

The clinical presentation of a fibrothorax may vary according to the cause and extent of the process and the presence or absence of underlying parenchymal disease and associated conditions. The most common complaint is that of dyspnea upon exertion, which is typically progressive over a protracted period of time. Occasionally, the patient may experience pain. Right ventricular failure with clinical signs of cor pulmonale may also occur in extreme cases. Physical examination reveals a unilateral fixation of the chest with limited respiratory excursion and atrophy of the overlying musculature. Palpation shows decreased fremitus with dullness to percussion, and auscultation identifies diminished or absent breath sounds.

Fibrothoraces due to tuberculosis may represent a complication of parenchymal disease. Those caused by chronic empyema may be associated with their own complications, such as empyema necessitatis, chondritis, rib osteomyelitis, bronchopleural fistula, pericarditis, or mediastinal abscesses. In those cases, signs and symptoms of infections may dominate the clinical picture, and the patient may present with fever, toxicity, and weight loss.

Investigative Techniques

The diagnosis and pathogenesis of a given fibrothorax should always be substantiated by careful review of past medical history and by comparison of old and current chest films and computed tomography (CT) scans. Pulmonary and pleural malignancies must be ruled out, because they often mimic benign fibrothoraces. Diagnostic techniques such as bronchoscopy, ultrasound, nuclear magnetic resonance (NMR) imaging, angiography, percutaneous pleural biopsy, and thoracoscopy will usually serve that purpose.

Standard chest radiographs with posteroanterior and lateral views often provide clues to the presence of a fibrothorax. The pleura may appear uniformly thickened, initially over the diaphragmatic and lateral surfaces. This may be visible as a markedly increased water density surrounding the lung in an antigravity distribution (Guenter and Welch, 1982). Later in the process, the entire pleural surface may be obliterated, and other signs of advanced fibrothorax, such as narrowing of the intercostal spaces, diminished size of the involved hemithorax, and ipsilateral displacement of the mediastinum may be present. Mottled calcifications may be seen over the inner aspect of the parietal peel. These may be used to determine the actual thickness of the parietal peel.

Radiography may contribute to the identification of the causative process in addition to giving clues as to the status of both the involved and the contralateral lung. This evaluation is important, because functional improvement after decortication does not occur if extensive parenchymal disease is present. Morton and colleagues (1970) have demonstrated that absence of underlying parenchymal disease is the best assurance that there will be significant improvement in pulmonary function after operation.

CT scanning is essential in assessing the extent and anatomic characteristics of the fibrothorax. Important information concerning the underlying parenchyma may also be obtained by CT scanning, which can identify tuberculous lesions, bronchiectasis, fibrosis, or other conditions that could affect the result of decortication. NMR imaging has not shown any advantage over CT scanning and has no precise role in the evaluation of fibrothoraces.

Bronchoscopy, either flexible or rigid, must be performed to ensure the integrity on the bronchus in the entrapped lung (Scannell, 1990). A concomitant carcinoma must be ruled out, and the bronchus of the lung to be decorticated must be free of both active endobronchial tuberculosis and cicatricial post-tuberculous bronchial stricture.

Pulmonary function studies, including spirometry, diffusion studies, and exercise tolerance testing are useful in quantifying the degree of respiratory impairment. They also provide for postoperative comparison. Isotope perfusion lung scanning is helpful in determining the contribution of each lung to overall function. In general, anatomic and functional evaluation is useful in predicting whether or not decortication will improve dyspnea, whether or not the decorticated lung will re-expand, and whether or not the re-expanded lung will function in a satisfactory manner.

Nutritional assessment may finally be necessary to identify chronic hypovolemia, anemia, and hypoalbuminemia and institute appropriate supportive measures.

TABLE 46–3 ■ **Indications for Decortication**

Space Deloculation (1 to 3 weeks)
Inadequately drained multiloculated empyema
Early clotted hemothorax
Early decortication (4 to 12 weeks)
Organizing hemothorax
Unresolving pleural effusion
Empyema
Late Decortication (>3 months)
Post-traumatic fibrothorax
Chronic empyema
Idiopathic fibrothorax
Pleural tuberculosis

MANAGEMENT

Fibrothorax is best treated by prevention. When the potential for pleural effusion is recognized, the patient should be treated by early and complete drainage of the pleural space. In one series of 478 patients treated for traumatic hemothorax (Pomerantz, 1979), only eight eventually required decortication and in each there had been some error in management. Villalba and colleagues (1979) also recognized that decortication can be prevented by early recognition of hemothorax or pneumothorax; early tube thoracostomy with complete evacuation of blood and expansion of the lung; careful daily monitoring of subsequent fluid accumulation; and prompt evacuation when such fluid accumulates.

Decortication

The objectives of decortication are two-fold: first, to re-expand the trapped lung and restore lung, diaphragm, and chest wall function; and second, to obliterate the space and control the infection. In some patients with tuberculosis or chronic empyemas, functional recovery may be a secondary consideration to space obliteration (Ackman and Madore, 1951), because a lung that is re-expanded after a long period of compression may have impaired ventilation but still be able to fill the space (Okano and Walkup, 1962). In those cases, decortication may obviate the need for more extensive procedures such as thoracoplasty or pleuropneumonectomy. If decortication is performed for an organizing hemothorax, the objectives are to recover function and prevent late suppurative complications.

Mayo and associates (1982) have described three conditions that are critical to the optimal success of decortication: it should be the primary surgical procedure; it should be performed at the earliest opportunity; and all elements of the intrathoracic peel should be removed to ensure complete lung re-expansion and both chest wall and diaphragmatic mobility.

Surgery

Indications for and optimal timing of surgery are described in Table 46–3.

Indications for Early Deloculation

Early deloculation is indicated in cases of multiloculated empyemas or of hemothoraces when lung expansion cannot be promoted by closed tube thoracostomy alone. Van Way and colleagues (1988) reported 40 patients with class III complicated empyemas with multiple loculations. Limited thoracotomy for drainage and placement of tubes was performed in 22 patients, all of whom had resolution of the empyema with no additional procedures. They recommended limited thoracotomy immediately or during the first week of treatment for all multiloculated and complex empyemas (Figs. 46–1 and 46–2). Similarly, Fishman and Ellertson (1977) advocated early decortication for empyemas in immunosuppressed patients. Their approach was based on the following therapeutic principles: (1) early, thorough evacuation of the abscess cavity; (2) obliteration of the cavity by removal of the peel, allowing the restricted lung to inflate; and (3) avoidance of a chest wall sinus tract. Mayo and colleagues (1982) reported 21 pediatric patients who had acute or mature empyemas and were treated by open thoracotomy and decortication. There were no deaths or complications, and the authors concluded that early thoracotomy and decortication yielded uniformly good results. It is, therefore, appropriate to recommend early space deloculation in empyema patients in whom closed thoracostomy does not bring about adequate drainage and lung re-expansion. Personne (1990) also recommended that thoracotomy is avoided beyond the third week because at this stage the empyema is not well organized and the peeling of the lung will lead to tearing, bleeding, and prolonged air leaks. He suggested waiting at least 3 months and then proceeding with full decortication.

Culinear and colleagues (1959), Beall and colleagues (1996), and Milfield and colleagues (1978) have shown that early evacuation of clotted hemothoraces decreases mortality, morbidity, and hospital stay and prevents the development of post-traumatic empyema. In the series of Milfield and colleagues, 10 patients underwent evacuation of a clotted hemothorax within 5 days of admission, with no mortality and an average hospital stay of 10 days. Among the 41 patients who underwent decortication more than 5 days after injury, there was one death (2.4% mortality), and the average period of hospitalization was 25 days. At an early stage, simple removal of clots is all that is required, whereas if organization is allowed to occur, formal decortication becomes necessary (Beall et al, 1966). In a study of 452 patients with traumatic hemothorax, Wilson and associates (1979) concluded

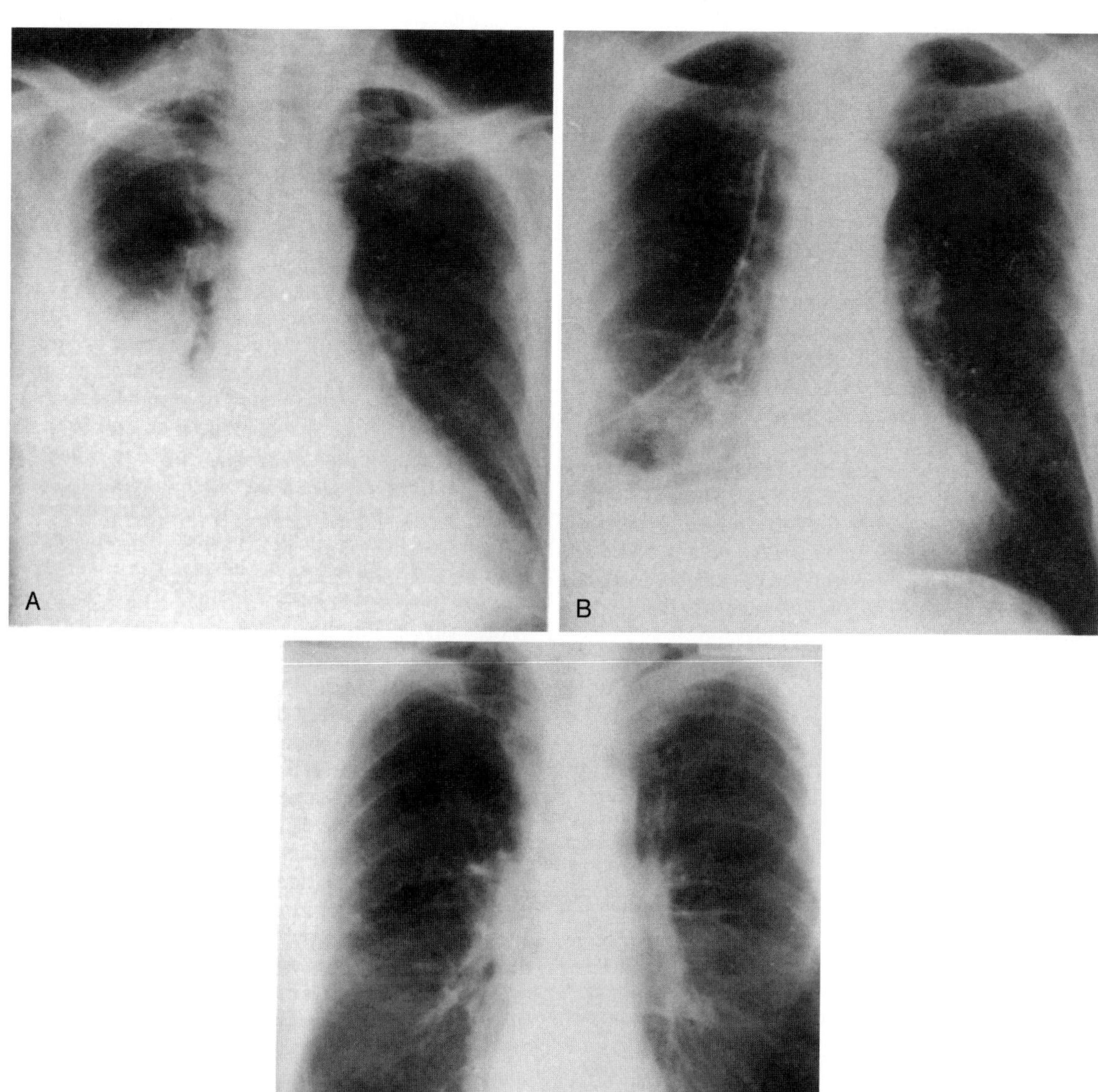

FIGURE 46–1 ■ Deloculation for an acute empyema. *A*, Chest radiograph of a 52-year-old man admitted for fever, cough, and right-sided chest pain. *B*, Chest radiograph following a minithoracotomy for deloculation of the empyema. *C*, Chest radiograph taken 1 year later and showing complete lung re-expansion and obliteration of the space.

that early open operative intervention to remove residual blood clot is usually not necessary and that the emphasis of therapy should be on prompt and adequate pleural drainage.

Indications for Decortication

The decision to proceed with decortication in patients with organized fibrothoraces depends on several factors. Because many conditions associated with acute pleural swelling may resolve spontaneously, decortication should only be considered if the pleural thickening has been present for several weeks or months, if the patient's lifestyle is significantly compromised by exertional dyspnea, and if there is evidence of reversible physiologic impairment of the underlying lung. Samson and colleagues (1946) found that patients with chronic hemothoraces for whom surgery is indicated are those in whom there is at least 50% compression of the lung, especially if the apex is collapsed; those in whom aspiration has been unsuccessful; and those in whom there has been no

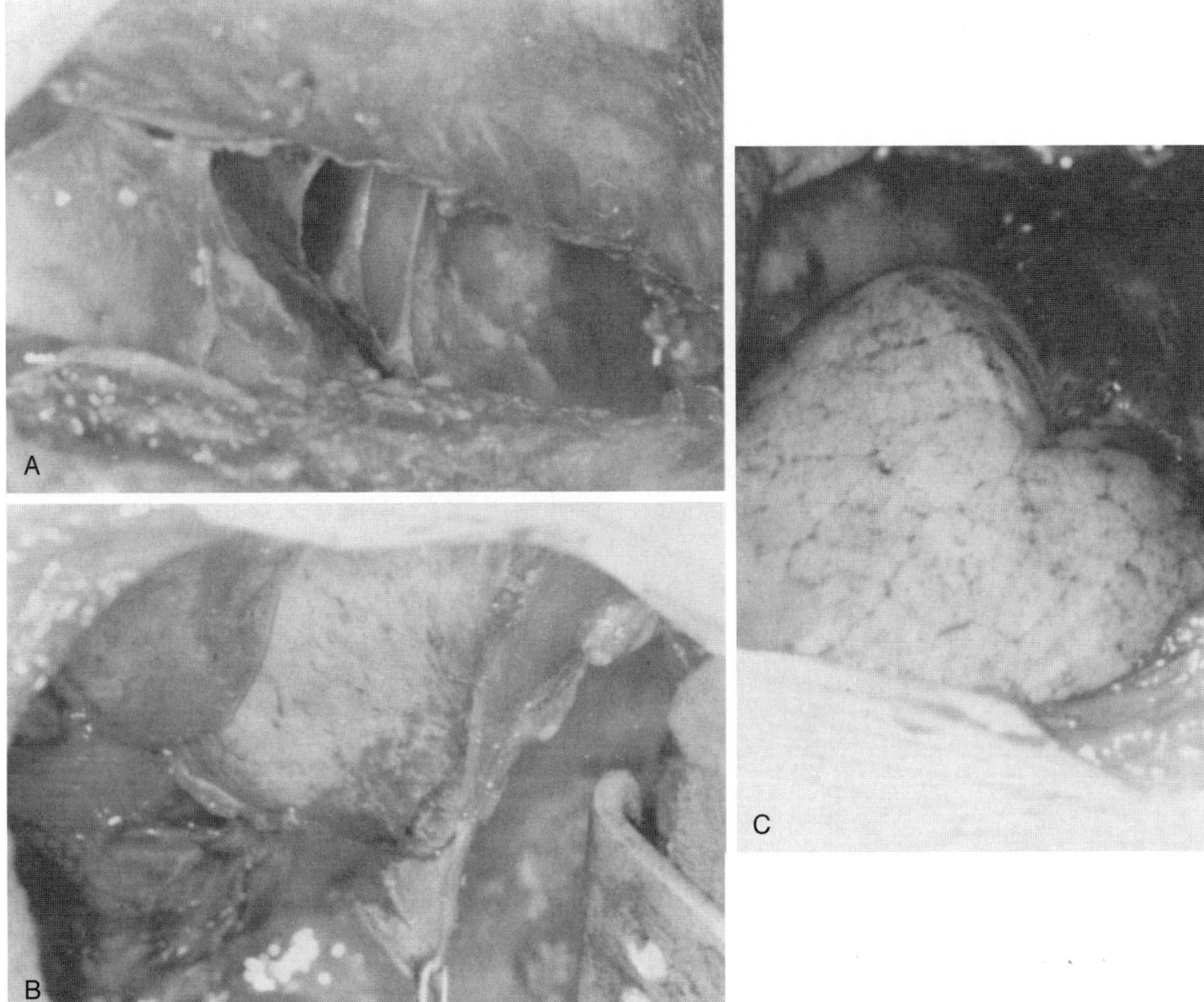

FIGURE 46–2 ■ Operative photographs showing a multiloculated empyema with multiple pockets of fluid and fibrin *(A)*; inflammatory peel being removed from the visceral pleura *(B)*; and complete re-expansion of the lung *(C)*. (Courtesy of Jean Morin, MD.)

appreciable pulmonary expansion at the end of 4 to 6 weeks following injury. In those cases, one can expect full recovery of function because the lung parenchyma is less likely to have been involved in the disease process. It is important to decorticate early (3 to 5 weeks) in patients with hemothoraces, because in time fibrosis may extend into the lung and limit re-expandability. It is also possible that with time, the plane between the visceral pleura and peel will be lost.

In patients with chronic empyemas, the therapeutic aims are: (1) to release and expand the collapsed lung if there is marked restriction. The amount of pulmonary restriction that constitutes an indication for decortication is variable, but Petro and colleagues (1982) considered that this operation should not be done unless there is a reduction of the vital capacity in the order of 30%; (2) to re-establish the intrathoracic spatial relationship so that false re-expansion, characterized by overdistention of the contralateral lung with mediastinal shift, elevation of the diaphragm, and contraction of the chest wall, does not occur; and (3) to control infection by evacuation and obliteration of the pleural space (Fig. 46–3). Villalba and colleagues (1979) recommended that once a post-traumatic empyema becomes well established and refractory to standard modalities, decortication with evacuation of the empyema cavity should be performed as soon as possible.

It is worth noting again that most patients with hemothoraces, pleural effusions, or empyemas will never need decortication if they are properly treated at the onset of disease. In a series of 19 patients, Young and colleagues (1972) reported that in each patient an error in management had been made or a complication had occurred during therapy. They concluded that strict adherence to the principle of complete drainage may require insertion of several chest tubes but is necessary if the incidence of trapped lung is to be decreased.

In pleural tuberculosis, therapy is primarily medical, and surgical treatment is only used to eliminate or correct those residues of disease that cannot be further altered by antibiotherapy (Langston et al, 1967). In those cases, decortication is performed when evidence of toxicity is no longer present, when thoracentesis fails to yield fluid, or when fluid removal fails to alter the radiographic

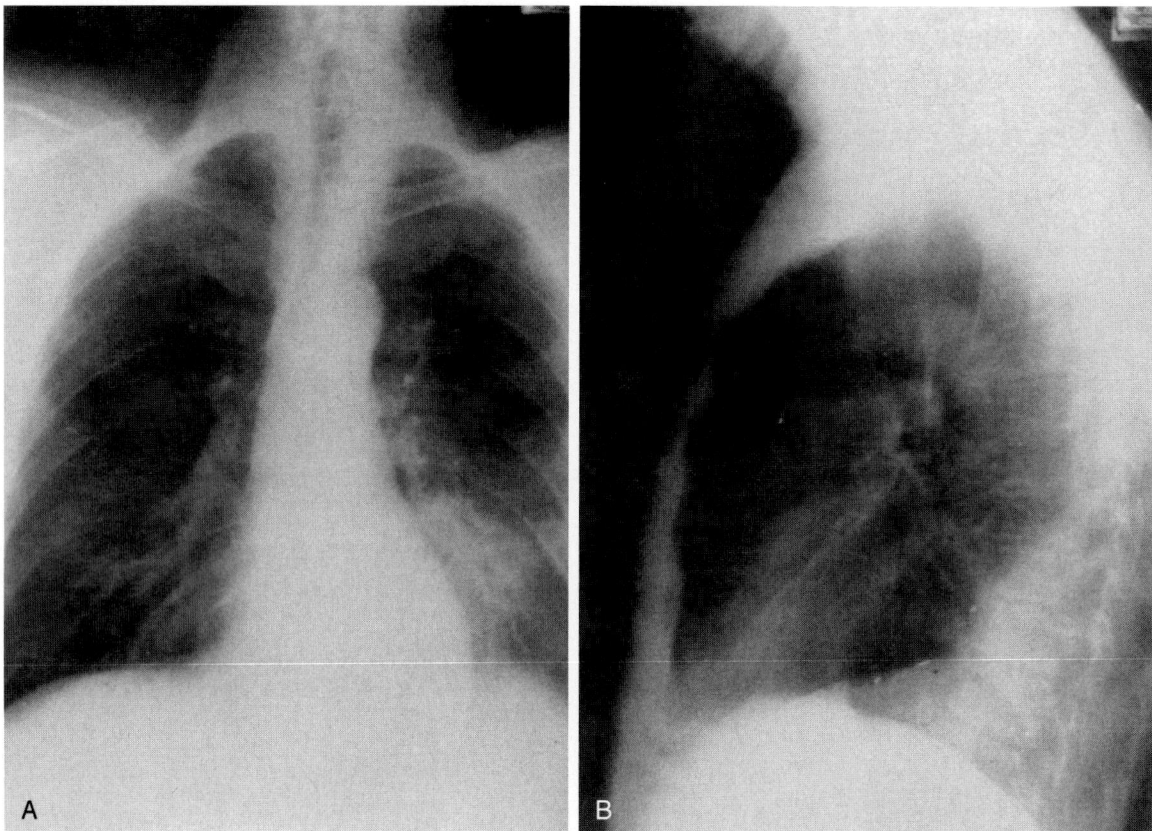

FIGURE 46–3 ■ Decortication for a chronic empyema. Standard posteroanterior *(A)* and lateral *(B)* chest radiographs of a 49-year-old man admitted for cough, hemoptysis, and purulent sputum of 4 months' duration. Note on the lateral radiograph the inverted D-shaped density typical of a chronic empyema. This patient was treated by complete lung decortication.

appearance. The extent of pleural involvement should also be taken into consideration and should be equivalent to one third to one fourth of the hemithorax and cast a clearly discernible shadow on the lateral projection (Langston et al, 1967). Decortication may finally be indicated for patients with mixed tuberculous empyemas and for patients with unexpandable lungs secondary to therapeutic pneumothoraces (Mulvihill and Klopstock, 1948; Weinberg et al, 1948; Weinberg and Davis, 1949).

Contraindications

Although extensive disease or fibrosis of the lung represents a major obstacle to successful decortication and may contraindicate its use (Table 46–4), the only absolute contraindication to the procedure is stenosis of a major bronchus feeding the lobe or lung to be decorticated (Savage and Fleming, 1955). O'Rourke and colleagues (1949) have shown that major pulmonary lesions, especially those of tuberculous nature, are also contraindications to decortication, owing to their detrimental effect on re-expansion of the lung and to the risk of a flare-up of the original process. According to Thurer (1996) and Magdeleinat and colleagues (1999), absent or greatly diminished perfusion to the involved lung contraindicates decortication.

Other relatively absolute contraindications include uncontrolled invasive infection in the lung or pleura, significant operative risk, and debilitation. It may also be inappropriate to decorticate a lung when there is significant contralateral disease. Relative contraindications include asymptomatic or minimally symptomatic patients and patients with little evidence of physiologic impairment.

Operative Technique

With few exceptions, the operative technique described by Samson and Burford (1947), Samson (1955), and Williams (1950) is still being followed. For an excellent description of the procedure, the readers should refer to

TABLE 46–4 ■ **Contraindications for Decortication**

Absolute
Extensive disease in the collapsed lung
Bronchial stenosis
Relatively absolute
Uncontrolled invasive infection
Significant operative risk
Debilitation
Contralateral disease
Relative
Minimal symptoms
Little evidence of physiologic impairment

the classic article written by Witz and Whilm in 1991. The operation requires establishment of a plane between the peel and the visceral pleura, freeing of the lung from all adhesions, and decortication of the diaphragm.

Decortication is performed through a sixth or seventh interspace posterolateral thoracotomy because incision at this lower level offers better exposure of the diaphragm where adhesions are often denser than those encountered elsewhere (Williams, 1950) or worse than preoperatively assessed on chest radiographs. Excision of the sixth rib is not always necessary but may improve exposure, especially when the intercostal spaces have been narrowed by the contractile process of the thickened pleura.

After the intercostal space has been entered, the parietal pleura is separated for a distance of several centimeters on each side of the incision so that a rib spreader can be inserted. If a space is present, it is opened, and its contents are thoroughly evacuated. If the contents are purulent, contamination of the operating field will be unavoidable, but this is of little consequence if adequate lung re-expansion is later achieved. When there is no free space, the peel must first be freed from the parietal pleura, starting over the mediastinal surface, where it is usually free from adhesions (Fig. 46–4).

As the next step, the peel is elevated from the visceral pleura. This is done by incising it with a scalpel until the visceral pleura, which is thin and pliable, is reached. The edges of the peel are then grasped with forceps and separated from the visceral pleura by gentle, blunt dissection with either a "pusher" or a gauze-covered finger. The initial incision in the peel may be vertical or horizontal or several incisions may be made to start the decortication. Gentle re-expansion of the lung by the anesthetist often facilitates separation of the peel, which must be removed over the entire surface of the lung, including the interlobar fissures. If thick adhesions to the visceral pleura are encountered, they may be left in situ to avoid trauma to the lung or the opening of old tuberculous foci.

The ease of stripping is unpredictable, and a number of tears to the underlying lung will be made. Large tears can be oversewn, whereas most small tears will heal easily once the lung has achieved complete re-expansion. Sometimes, sealants mixed with antibiotics to reduce the risks of local infection can also be used to help reduce air leakage from the decorticated lung (Bayfield and Spotnitz, 1996). More recently, Macchiarini and colleagues (1999) have reported the use of a new synthetic absorbable sealant, polymerizing polyethylene glycol (Focal Inc., Lexington, KY) to avoid the immunogenicity and risks of disease transmission inherent to fibrin or collagen-based products.

If the formation of the peel is secondary to an inflammatory process in the lung, separation almost always presents greater difficulties, because the loose subendothelial layer of the visceral pleura is replaced by fibrous, organized granulation tissue (Rudström and Thoren, 1955; Zenker et al, 1954). In extreme cases, it is necessary to remove the visceral pleura to achieve complete lung re-expansion (Fig. 46–5). Unfortunately, this excision leaves a hemorrhagic and air-leaking lung surface, which greatly increases postoperative discomfort and the duration of chest tube drainage.

Complete pleurolysis with mobilization of the lung from the diaphragm, pericardium, chest wall, and mediastinum is done next. The diaphragm must be decorticated down to the costophrenic angles, which can prove difficult because fibrosis can be very dense at that level and a plane for dissection is seldom found. Although it is important to restore the mobility of the diaphragm, it is sometimes better to leave plaques of thickened pleura than to damage the muscle.

The removal of the parietal peel is controversial. Arguments against performing this step include the possibility that heavy bleeding may occur because the endothoracic fascia may be very vascular and the fact that complete pulmonary re-expansion achieved by visceral decortica-

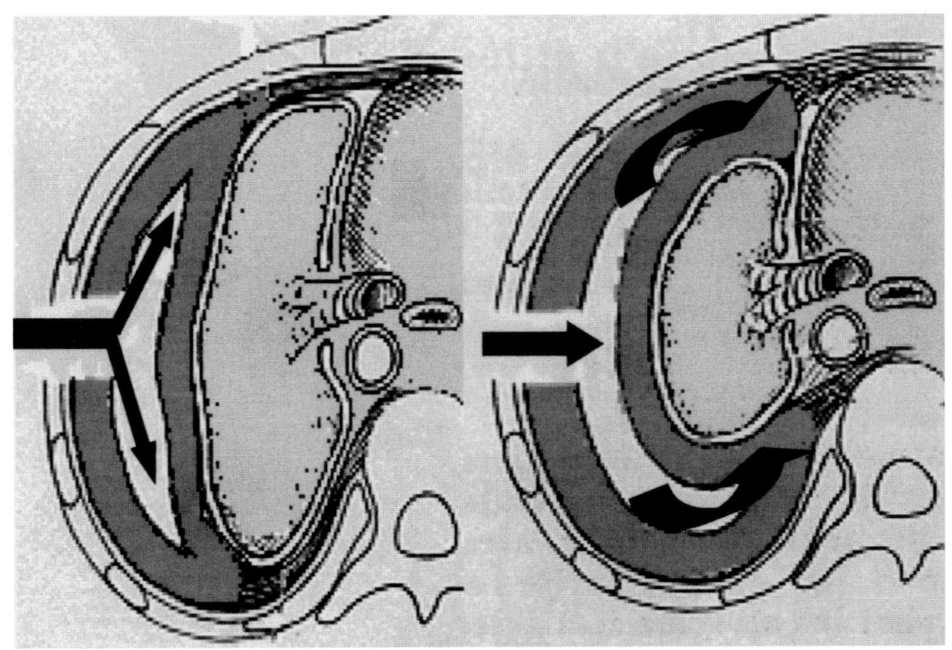

FIGURE 46–4 ■ A schematic drawing showing the regions where decortication should be started in cases of partial *(left)* or total *(right)* lung collapse. Often it is easier to start freeing the lung at the reflection between the mediastinal and the parietal pleura where there is less inflammatory reaction. (Modified from Lebrigand H: Nouveau Triaté de Technique Chirurgicale: Appareil Respiratoire, Médiastin, Paroi Thoracique, Vol 3. Paris, Masson, 1973, p 404.)

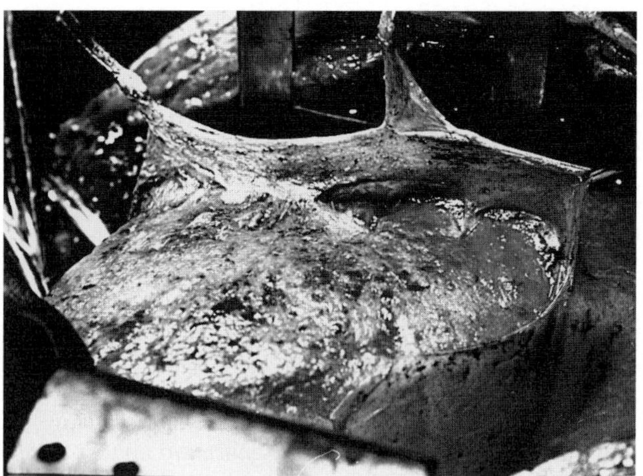

FIGURE 46–5 ■ An operative photograph showing the surface of the lung after excision of the visceral pleura. Note the hemorrhagic and air-leaking lung surface.

tion may set the stage for resorption of even the thickest of parietal peels. Proponents of removing the parietal peel argue that this is important to restore the full motion of the thoracic cage (Waterman et al, 1957) and achieve the best functional results. The parietal peel can be excised at the beginning of the operation or after visceral decortication has been completed. When this is done, the plane of dissection is between the parietal pleura and the endothoracic fascia (the parietal pleura cannot be freed from the peel), and in addition to an increased blood loss, technical difficulties can be encountered over the lung apex and mediastinum. At the apex, dense adhesions between the upper lobe and the first two ribs may be present, so that pleurolysis or parietal decortication may be difficult. In some cases, cavities may have penetrated beyond the pleural layer so that to excise them a resection of the costal chest wall, in part at least, may be required (Langston et al, 1967). Care must be taken not to injure the lower trunk of the brachial plexus, the vagus nerve and subclavian artery on the left side, and the sympathetic chain. Over the mediastinum, the dissection is usually considerably easier, but care must be taken to avoid injury to the esophagus, thoracic duct, phrenic and recurrent nerves, and hilar blood vessels. It is remarkable that not even old and thick peels are bound to large vessels, which usually are surrounded by a layer of loose tissue (Rudström and Thoren, 1955). At the end of the procedure, two properly placed chest tubes must be left in the pleural space.

In Williams' technique of decortication (1950), complete pleurolysis is first performed, mobilizing the lung from the diagram, pericardium, chest wall, and mediastinum. Once pleurolysis has been completed, the lung is inflated by the anesthetist with the peel still in place, and the decortication is carried out as described earlier (Fig. 46–6). According to Williams (1950), this technique facilitates removal of the peel, which is done in a vertical rather than a horizontal plane. Occasionally, selective decortication can be achieved leaving a plaque of peel over some areas of lung disease. Leaving small islands of densely attached pleura may also help to reduce postoperative air leaks (Scannell, 1990).

If there is a pulmonary lesion (a situation commonly seen with tuberculosis or its sequelae), resection of lung parenchyma may be necessary in addition to decortication. In such cases, complete filling of the residual space with the remaining lung must be ensured. If this is not possible, addition of a small tailoring thoracoplasty with preservation of the intercostal muscles or collapse of the parietal wall without rib resection may obliterate the space (Ilioka et al, 1985). This has also been used to provide closure of permanent thoracic sinuses (Dowd, 1909). Muscle flaps, such as the latissimus dorsi flap mobilized at the time of decortication, may also be used, thus avoiding the need for thoracoplasty (Ali and Unruh, 1990). Obviously, the addition of these procedures is likely to negate the gain in pulmonary function that may have otherwise been obtained.

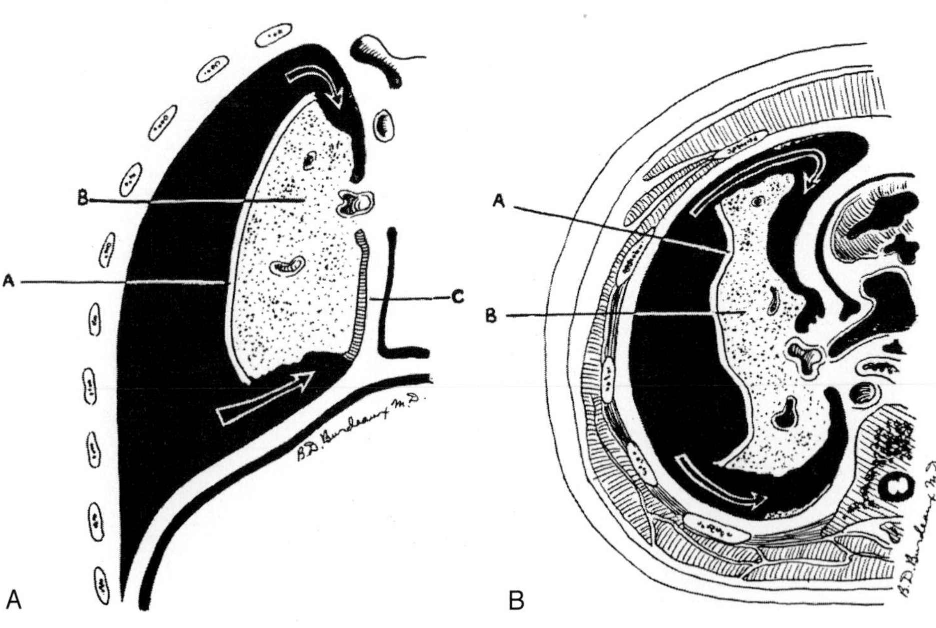

FIGURE 46–6 ■ The step of pleurolysis is illustrated in the central section *(A)* and the cross-section *(B)*. The visceral peel has been divided at its periphery, and the lung is being fully mobilized. *B*, All the adhesions have been divided, and the lung is ready for inflation and decortication. (From Williams MH: The technique of pulmonary decortication and pleurolysis. J Thorac Surg 20:652, 1950.)

Thoracoscopy and Decortication

The use of thoracoscopy (video-assisted thoracic surgery [VATS]) for deloculation of early-stage empyemas is no longer a matter of debate. Hutter and colleagues (1985) reported the use of thoracoscopy for deloculation and débridement of 12 empyemic cavities. Following lavage of the cavity, the thoracoscope helped in the placement of irrigation drains under direct vision; this resulted in the complete cure of 11 of the 12 patients within an average of 20 days after the procedure. One patient required a second thoracoscopy and drainage course but also eventually healed. In 1991, the same group (Ridley and Braimbridge, 1991) reported on a total of 30 patients with a cure rate of 60%.

VATS is particularly useful in the management of empyemas seen in early stages (Deslauriers and Mehran, 1993), wherein the cavity can be deloculated under direct vision; the lung can be re-expanded; and chest drains can be properly placed at dependent sites. It is also useful for deloculation of postpneumonectomy empyemas, because the whole cavity can be explored and débrided and chest tubes can be placed at appropriate sites for lavage and attempted sterilization of the space.

In cases of organized stage 3 empyemas, it may be difficult to obtain a good endothoracic image, and true VATS decortication of the lung is hazardous, traumatic, and of limited value. Furthermore, the pulmonary decortication that is often required in these situations may not be in the field of expertise of most clinicians performing thoracoscopies. Decortication using the VATS technique has been reported, although no details about the operative techniques have been given (Coltharp et al, 1992; Lewis et al, 1992; Mack et al, 1992).

Results of Decortication

Operative Morbidity and Mortality

In most series, the operative mortality varies between 0% and 5%. Major postoperative complications include sepsis from a residual empyema or from wound infection, bronchopleural fistula, or peripheral bronchoalveolar air leaks and hemorrhage. The incidence of these complications can be lessened by meticulous surgical technique with intraoperative control of air leaks and hemorrhage, achievement of optimal pulmonary re-expansion, and proper tube drainage. The incidence of major complications is substantially increased in patients who require combined pulmonary resection and decortication. Diaphragmatic avulsion during decortication has been reported by Mayo and associates (1982). In patients with tuberculosis, dissemination of tuberculosis or development of tuberculous sinuses is uncommon if patients are given antituberculous drugs.

Functional Results

Re-expansion of the lung with obliteration of the space is almost always achieved if the underlying parenchyma is normal. This result is usually permanent and is accompanied by subjective improvement, particularly if decortication takes place early in the process of traumatic hemothorax or empyema (Morin et al, 1972; Villalba et al, 1979).

Wright and associates (1949) were the first to report elaborate preoperative and postoperative studies in two patients who underwent decortication. Preoperative respiratory deficiency was shown by marked diminution of maximum breathing capacity and vital capacity, and bronchospirometry demonstrated that the abnormal findings occurred because of a lack of participation of the involved lung. Postoperative studies showed almost normal overall function. In 1958, Samson and colleagues reported the results of decortication for the pleural complications of pulmonary tuberculosis. Among 104 patients in whom decortication was the main operation, 4 (3.8%) died; 79 (77%) had a good to excellent result, with prompt pulmonary re-expansion, clear costophrenic sulcus, adequate motion of diaphragm and thoracic cage, and satisfactory improvement in pulmonary function; and 21 (20%) had a fair to poor result, in almost every case owing to prior disease involving fibrosis of the lung. More recently, LeMense and colleagues (1994) reported excellent results in 21 of 22 patients with an empyema. In that series, there was no associated mortality and minimal morbidity.

Although some authors have reported no or minimal improvement in individual cases (Gordon and Welles, 1949; Toomes et al, 1983), decortication is usually followed by improved ventilation and increased lung volumes, measured as improvements in vital capacity, total lung capacity, and maximum breathing capacity. Partial recovery of normal pulmonary blood flow to the diseased side may also be seen (Morton et al, 1970). In Toomes and colleagues' series (1983), in which the indication for decortication was an empyema, the procedure was not followed by significant improvement in pulmonary function. The authors only noted a mean increase of 13.8% in vital capacity for patients who had preoperative reduction of more than 40%. In Gordon and Welles' series (1949) of patients who underwent decortication for pleural tuberculosis, complete studies of pulmonary function before and after operation were given in four cases of re-expansion and little or no improvement was shown. Of note, three of these four patients had been subjected to thoracoplasty before decortication.

Swoboda and colleagues (1990) studied pulmonary function and scintigraphic lung perfusion before and after decortication in nine patients treated for chronic pleural empyema. Preoperatively, vital capacity ranged between 40% and 78% of predicted (mean of 60%), forced expiratory volume in one second (FEV_1) averaged 65% of predicted value and perfusion of the affected side was reduced by 22% (range of 10% to 42%). Following decortication (3 months to 4 years), all parameters were improved. The vital capacity improved by 78.5% (range of 60% to 95%), the FEV_1 by 60% to 95% (mean of 79.5%), and the postoperative lung perfusion of the affected side increased by 26% to 48% (mean of 37.8%). Magdeleinat and colleagues (1999) reviewed 25 patients submitted to decortication for empyema (mean follow-up time of 54 months). In eight patients studied preoperatively and postoperatively, vital capacity improved by 40% (15% to 66%). Vital capacity remained stable in six patients, and in one patient it showed a 25% reduction (this last patient was a smoker with chronic bronchitis). The authors concluded that pulmonary decortication is an effective (23 of 24 patients with complete lung re-expansion) but relatively major operation to treat chronic encysted empyemas.

In 1952, Patton and coworkers reported the pulmonary function of 14 patients with unilateral constrictive disease, who were studied before and at intervals up to 3 years after surgical decortication.

Restoration of function was closely related to the presence or absence of pre-existing disease, and there was a progressive gain in function during the entire period of observation. The ultimate gain of pre-existing disease, and there was a progressive gain in function, was not influenced by the preoperative duration of collapse or by the presence or absence of infection in the pleural fluid, but it bore a close relationship to the amount of re-expansion seen in the chest films. Patients in whom visceral decortication was performed showed improvement comparable with that seen in patients who underwent complete visceral and parietal decortication (Patton et al, 1952). Other investigators such as Barker and associates (1965) and Carroll and colleagues (1951) have shown similar results—rises in vital capacity and maximum breathing capacity and improved oxygen uptake being observed postoperatively. Barker and colleagues (1965) documented apparent improvement in ventilatory function in the uninvolved lung following contralateral simple decortication. However, contrary to the data and opinion of Patton and associates (1952), several investigators have shown that the best results seen after decortication are obtained in patients with pleural disease of short duration (Carroll et al, 1951; Morton et al, 1970; Thomas and Jarvis, 1956). Long-term results of decortication in children with empyema showed no limitations of function at intervals of 12 to 18 years after the procedure (Mayo et al, 1982).

After elaborate studies of pulmonary function, Patton and colleagues (1952) observed that pulmonary function seldom returns to the predicted normal postoperatively. This is partly due to loss of parietal elasticity, which persists to some degree even after the most satisfactory decortication. It also relates to other irreversible changes such as overdistention of the good lung, shift of the mediastinum, elevation of the diaphragm, and decrease in size of the hemithorax.

Causes of Failure

Failure of decortication leads to a recurrence of the empyema with or without bronchopleural fistula and to possible deterioration of pulmonary function. In all such cases, it is likely that further surgery will be required. The main causes of failure after decortication are listed in Table 46–5. They are numerous, but most are avoidable with adequate preoperative selection and meticulous surgical technique.

The importance of underlying parenchymal disease (Figs. 46–7 and 46–8), especially in cases of decortication performed for tuberculous pleural disease, has been well identified by Gurd (1947), who stated, "When it comes to applying the principles of decortication to typical pulmonary tuberculosis associated with a draining empyema of tuberculous associated with a draining empyema of tuberculous or mixed infection, I would like to sound a note of warning. The prognosis depends chiefly on the extent and severity of the underlying intrapulmonary disease, and is frequently hopeless" (Fig. 46–9). Mulvihill and Klopstock (1948) also described a case of failure to re-expand owing to marked fibrosis of the lung (Fig. 46–10). In the 1952 series of Patton and colleagues, patients with advanced parenchymal disease had a maximum breathing capacity that was 6% less and a vital capacity that was 16% less than before decortication. By

TABLE 46–5 ■ Causes of Failure after Decortication

Underlying parenchymal disease
Tuberculosis (active, fibrosis, bronchiectasis, bronchial stricture)
Other parenchymal diseases limiting re-expansion
Long duration of lung collapse
Technical difficulties
Difficulties in removing the peel
Air leakage
Poor re-expansion of the lung
Inadequate postoperative space drainage
Associated pulmonary resection
Trauma to the phrenic nerve
Others
Parietal peel not removed over the diaphragm or chest wall
Postoperative complications

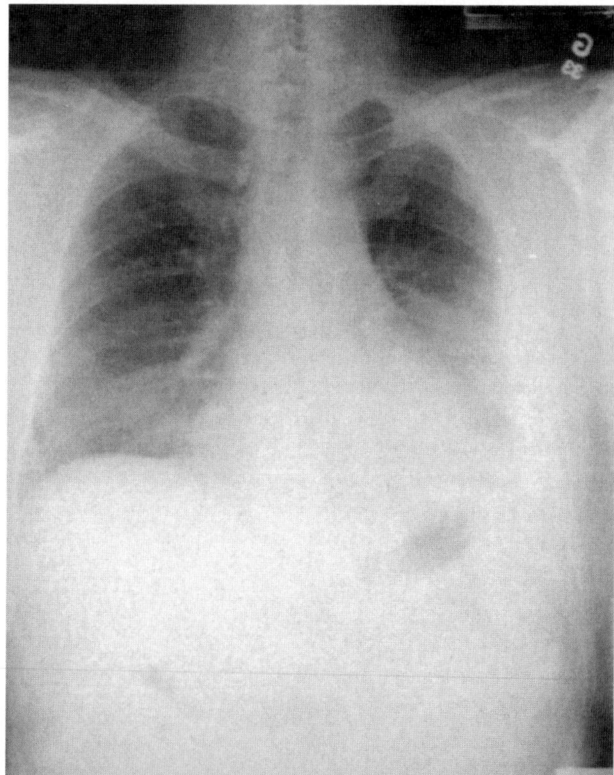

FIGURE 46–7 ■ Fibrothorax. Standard posteroanterior chest radiograph showing an organized left-sided fibrothorax secondary to undrained pleural bleeding following an aortocoronary bypass. Note the trapping of the left lung, which appears otherwise normal.

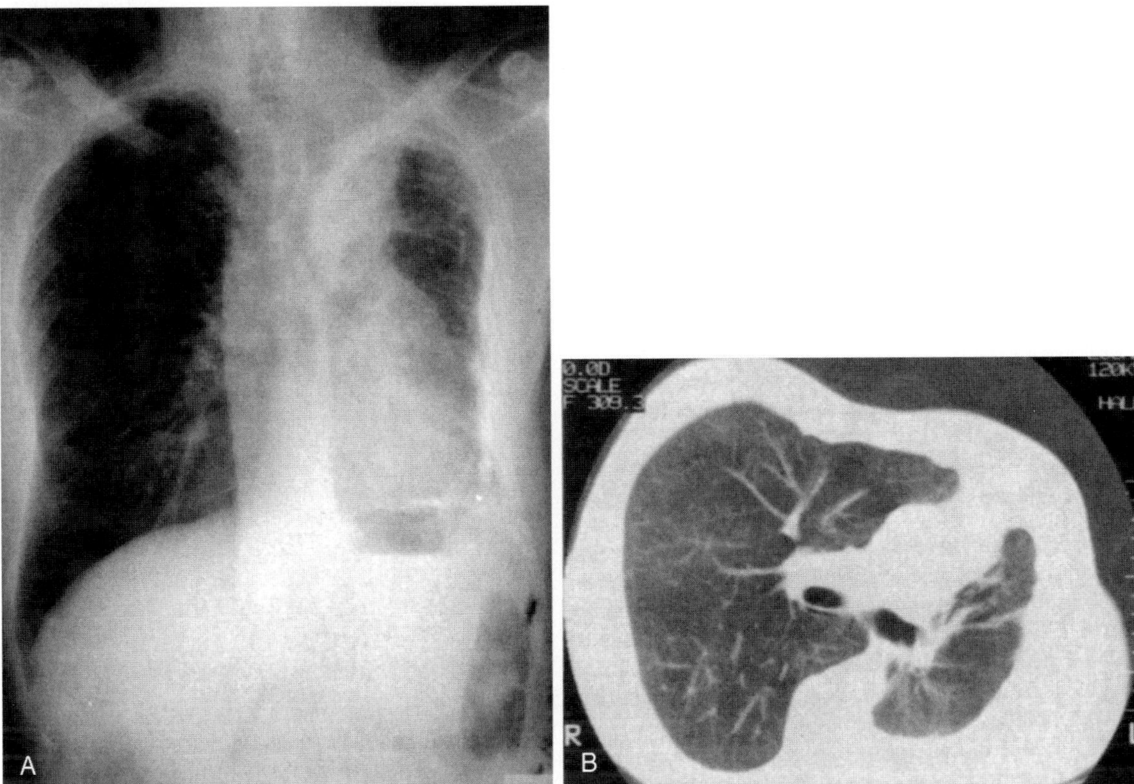

FIGURE 46–8 ■ Severe fibrothorax with the destroyed lung. Chest radiograph *(A)* and computed tomography scan *(B)* of a patient with extensive post-tuberculous fibrothorax. Note the severe trapping of the left lung and the absence of peripheral blood vessels, indicative of low perfusion.

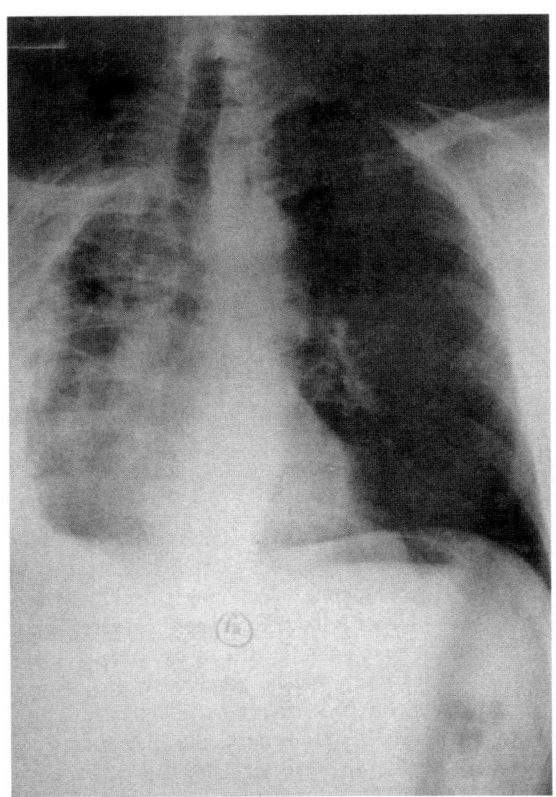

FIGURE 46–9 ■ A standard posteroanterior chest radiograph of a patient with a markedly thickened and calcified pleural peel secondary to tuberculous pleurisy.

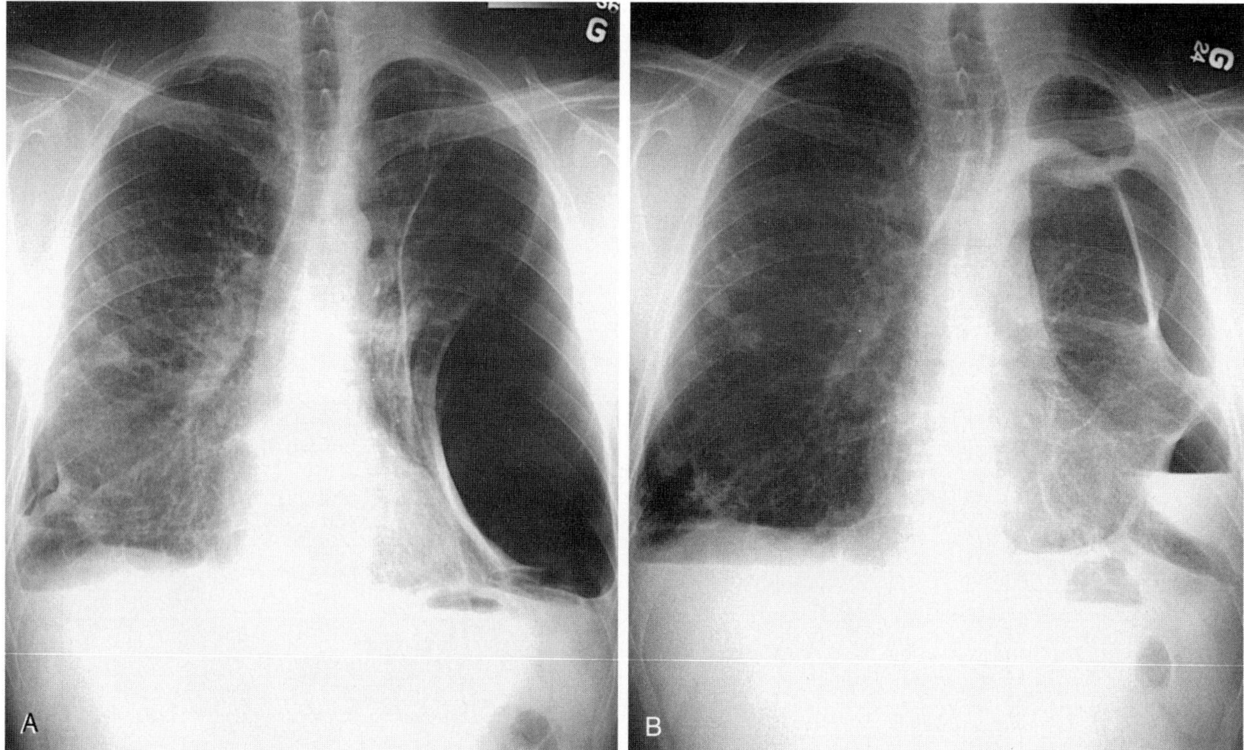

FIGURE 46–10 ■ *A*, A standard posteroanterior chest radiograph of a young patient with bilateral collapsed lungs secondary to a chronic empyema. Note the pulmonary nodules due to rheumatoid arthritis. *B*, Chest film taken 1 month after decortication of the left lung showing minimal gain in lung re-expansion.

contrast, patients with little parenchymal disease ultimately showed a mean increase of 47% in maximum breathing capacity and a 31% increase in vital capacity. Siebens and colleagues (1956) have also shown that in the absence of extensive parenchymal disease, a lung that contributes negligibly to respiration preoperatively may show striking improvement postoperatively.

The duration of lung collapse can also play a role in the failure of decortication, and it is generally acknowledged that decortication should be done at the earliest possible time. In a group of 141 patients who underwent lung decortication, Morton and colleagues (1970) concluded that patients with pleural disease of short duration demonstrated more improvement after decortication than did those who had had thickened pleura for prolonged periods of time. This is due to the pleural fibrosis that eventually extends into the lung, thus limiting further its expandibility.

Technical difficulties are probably the most common cause of failure after decortication. Sometimes there is inflammatory thickening of the visceral pleura, which makes peel removal very difficult. This condition is likely to be seen in tuberculous lungs or in lungs that have been the site of pneumonic processes. In those cases, there will be several sites of air leakage and of bleeding on the lung surface, which may compromise lung expansion. If this occurs, the lung must be decorticated very gently; all large tears must be repaired; and the lung must be fully mobilized from all adhesions so that it can re-expand. Bleeding from the surface of the lung is seldom a major problem, but if the lung does not re-expand or if the pleural space is inadequately drained, collections of fluid may occur in the space, with secondary formation of a new fibrothorax.

In all cases, the phrenic nerve must be identified so that diaphragmatic function is preserved. This is usually fairly easy because the mediastinum is almost always free of adhesions. Associated pulmonary resections are also a cause of failure, not only because they indicate the presence of lung disease but also because they increase the magnitude of the procedure and reduce the amount of parenchyma available for space filling. In Okano and Walkup's series (1962), major complications occurred in 35% of patients treated by combined decortication and pulmonary resection.

Other factors considered to be potential factors for failure of decortication are non-removal of the parietal peel over the diaphragm and thoracic wall, which may impair the mechanics of breathing, and the occurrence of postoperative complications such as empyemas or bronchopleural fistulae. Okano and Walkup (1962) reported significant ventilatory functional improvement and no complications in most of their patients who underwent decortication. On the other hand, patients who had postoperative bronchopleural fistula and empyema requiring thoracoplasty had variable changes, and some had a diminution in function.

■ *KEY REFERENCES*

Patton WE, Watson TR, Gaensler EA: Pulmonary function before and at intervals after surgical decortication of the lung. J Thorac Surg 95:477, 1952.

The authors provide an excellent review of the mechanisms involved in improving pulmonary function after decortication.

Scannell JG: The captive lung: Indications for and techniques of decortication. In Deslauriers J, Lacquet LK (eds): International Trends in General Thoracic Surgery, Vol 6: The Pleural Space. St. Louis, Mosby–Year Book, 1990.

This is an excellent overview of the indications and techniques of decortication.

Williams MH: The technique of pulmonary decortication and pleurolysis. J Thorac Surg 20:652, 1950.

This article describes the technique of decortication and emphasizes the importance of pleural adhesions in the production of the pulmonary collapse.

Witz JP, Whilm JM: Problèmes chirurgicaux posés par les pleurésies purulentes. In Techniques chirurgicales. Thorax. Paris, Encycl Med Chir, 1991.

Excellent description of the technique of decortication.

■ REFERENCES

Ackman FD, Madore P: Decortication preceding thoracoplasty for the elimination of long-standing tuberculous empyema. J Thorac Cardiovasc Surg 22:358, 1951.

Ali I, Unruh H: Management of empyema thoracis. Ann Thorac Surg 50:335, 1990.

Autio V: The reduction of respiratory function by parenchymal and pleural lesions: A bronchospirometric study of patients with unilateral involvement. Acta Tuberc Scan 37:112, 1959.

Barker WL, Neuhaus H, Langston HT: Ventilatory improvement following decortication in pulmonary tuberculosis. Ann Thorac Surg 1:532, 1965.

Bayfield MS, Spotnitz WD: Fibrin sealant in thoracic surgery: Pulmonary applications, including management of bronchopleural fistula. Chest Surg Clin North Am 6:567, 1996.

Beall AC, Crawford HW, DeBakey ME: Considerations in the management of acute traumatic hemothorax. J Thorac Cardiovasc Surg 52:353, 1966.

Bollinger CT, de Kock MA: Influence of a fibrothorax on the flow volume curve. Respiration 54:197, 1988.

Burford TH, Parker EF, Samson PC: Early decortication in the treatment of post-traumatic empyema. Ann Surg 122:163, 1945.

Carroll D, McClement J, Himmelstein A, Cournand A: Pulmonary function following decortication of the lung. Am Rev Tuberc 63:231, 1951.

Coltharp WH, Arnold JH, Alford WC et al: Videothoracoscopy: Improved technique and expanded indications. Ann Thorac Surg 53:775, 1992.

Culinear MM, Roc BB, Grimes OF: The early effective surgical approach to the treatment of traumatic hemothorax. J Thorac Cardiovasc Surg 38:780, 1959.

Davidson FF, Glazier JB: Unilateral pleuritis and regional lung function. Ann Intern Med 77:37, 1972.

Delorme E: Nouveau traitement des empyèmes chroniques. Gaz Hôp 67:94, 1894.

Deslauriers J, Mehran RJ: Role of thoracoscopy in the diagnosis and management of pleural diseases. Semin Thorac Cardiovasc Surg 5:284, 1993.

Dowd CN: Persistent thoracic sinus following empyema: A report of fifteen cases treated by decortication of lung and thoracoplasty. JAMA 53:1281, 1909.

Drummond DS, Craig RH: Traumatic hemothorax: Complications and management. Am Surg 33:403, 1967.

Eggers C: Radical operation for chronic empyema. Ann Surg 77:327, 1923.

Estlander JA: Sur la résection des côtes dans l'empyème chronique. Rev Mens 8:885, 1897.

Fairfax AJ, McNabb WR, Sprio SG: Chylothorax: A review of 18 cases. Thorax 41:880, 1986.

Fishman VH, Ellertson DG: Early pleural decortication for thoracic empyema in immunosuppressed patients. J Thorac Cardiovasc Surg 74:537, 1977.

Fowler GR: A case of thoracoplasty for removal of a large cicatricial fibrous growth from the interior of the chest, the result of an old empyema. Med Rec 44:838, 1893.

Fraser RG, Pare JA: Diagnosis of Diseases of the Chest, Vol 3, 2nd ed. Philadelphia, WB Saunders, 1979, p 1780.

Gordon J, Welles ES: Decortication in pulmonary tuberculosis including studies of respiratory physiology. J Thorac Surg 18:337, 1949.

Grossman GD: Fibrothorax. In Cherniak RM (ed): Current Therapy of Respiratory Disease, Vol 3. Philadelphia, Mosby–Year Book, 1979.

Guenter CA, Welch MH: Pleural Disease in Pulmonary Medicine, 2nd ed. Philadelphia, JB Lippincott, 1982, p 597.

Gurd FB: Decortication in chronic empyema of tuberculous origin. J Thorac Cardiovasc Surg 16:587, 1947.

Himmelstein A, Miscall L, Kirschner PA: Decortication in tuberculosis. Surg Clin North Am 28:1601, 1948.

Hughes RL, Jensik RJ, Faber LP, Bliss K: Evaluation of unilateral decortication. Ann Thorac Surg 19:704, 1975.

Hutter JA, Harari D, Braimbridge MV: The management of empyema thoracis by thoracoscopy and irrigation. Ann Thorac Surg 39:517, 1985.

Ilioka S, Sawanura K, Mori T et al: Surgical treatment of chronic empyema: A new one stage operation. J Thorac Cardiovasc Surg 90:179, 1985.

Kosloke AM, Cartwright KC: The controversial role of decortication in the management of pediatric empyema. J Thorac Cardiovasc Surg 96:166, 1988.

Langston AT, Barker WL, Graham AA: Pleural tuberculosis. J Thorac Cardiovasc Surg 54:511, 1967.

Lebrigand H: Décortication pulmonaire, ablation isolée des poches de pyothorax. In Lebrigand H (ed): Nouveau Traité de Technique Chirurgicale: Appareil Respiratoire, Médiastin, Paroi Thoracique. Paris, Masson, 1973.

LeMense GF, Strange CH, Sahn S: Empyema thoracis: Therapeutic management and outcome. Chest 107:1532, 1994.

LeRoux BT, Mohlala ML, Odell JA, Whitton ID: Suppurative diseases of the lung and pleural space. I: Empyema, thoracic and lung abscess. Curr Probl Surg 23:27, 1986.

Lewis RJ, Caccavale RJ, Sissler GE, Mackenzie JW: One hundred consecutive patients undergoing video-assisted thoracic operations. Ann Thorac Surg 54:421, 1992.

Lilienthal H: Empyema: Exploration of the thorax with primary mobilization of the lung. Ann Surg 62:309, 1915.

Lund FB: The advantages of the so-called decortication of the lung in old empyema. JAMA 57:693, 1911.

Macchiarini P, Wain JW, Almy S, Dartevelle P: Experimental and clinical evaluation of a new, synthetic, absorbable sealant to reduce air leaks in thoracic operations. J Thorac Cardiovasc Surg 117:751, 1999.

Mack MJ, Aronoff RJ, Acuff TE et al: Present role of thoracoscopy in the diagnosis and treatment of diseases of the chest. Ann Thorac Surg 54:403, 1992.

Magdeleinat P, Icard P, Pouzet B et al: Indications actuelles et résultats des décortications pulmonaires pour pleurésies purulentes non tuberculeuses. Ann Chir 53:41, 1999.

Mayo CH, Beckman EH: Visceral pleurectomy for chronic empyema. Am Surg 59:884, 1914.

Mayo P: Early thoracotomy and decortication for nontuberculous empyema in adults with and without underlying disease. Am Surg 51:230, 1985.

Mayo WP, Saha SP, McElvein RB: Diaphragmatic avulsion following decortication. Ala J Med Sci 19:81, 1982.

Milfield DJ, Mattox KL, Beal AC: Early evacuation of clotted hemothorax. Am J Surg 136:686, 1978.

Morin JE, Munro DD, MacLean LD: Early thoracotomy for empyema. J Thorac Cardiovasc Surg 64:530, 1972.

Morton JR, Boushy SF, Guinn GA: Physiological evaluation of results of pulmonary decortication. Ann Thorac Surg 4:321, 1970.

Mulvihill DA, Klopstock R: Decortication of the nonexpandable post-pneumothorax tuberculous lung. J Thorac Cardiovasc Surg 17:723, 1948.

Okano T, Walkup HE: Chronic purulent tuberculous empyema and pulmonary tuberculosis treated by decortication and resections. J Thorac Cardiovasc Surg 43:752, 1962.

O'Rourke P, O'Brien E, Tuttle W: Decortication of the lung in patients with pulmonary tuberculosis. Am Rev Respir Dis 59:30, 1949.

Patton WE, Watson TR, Gaensler EA: Pulmonary function before and at intervals after surgical decortication of the lung. Surg Gynecol Obstet 95:477, 1952.

Personne C: Role of early thoracotomy in the treatment of acute empyema. In Deslauriers J, Lacquet LK (eds): International Trends in General Thoracic Surgery, Vol 6: The Pleural Space. St. Louis, Mosby–Year Book, 1990.

Petro W, Maassen W, Greschuchna D et al: Regional and global lung function in unilateral fibrothorax after conservative therapy and decortication. Thorac Cardiovasc Surg 30:137, 1982.

Petty TL, Filley GF, Mitchell RS: Objective functional improvement by decortication after twenty years of artificial pneumothorax for pulmonary tuberculosis: Report of a case and review of the literature. Am Rev Respir Dis 84:572, 1961.

Pomerantz M: Discussion of Wilson JM et al: Traumatic hemothorax: Is decortication necessary? J Thorac Cardiovasc Surg 77:494, 1979.

Ransahoff J: Discussion of the pleura in the treatment of chronic empyema. Ann Surg 43:502, 1906.

Ridley PD, Braimbridge MV: Thoracoscopic debridement and pleural irrigation in the management of empyema thoracis. Ann Thorac Surg 51:461, 1991.

Robin ED, Cross CE, Kroetz F et al: Pulmonary hypertension and unilateral pleural construction with speculations on pulmonary vasoconstrictive substance. Arch Intern Med 118:391, 1966.

Rudström P, Thoren L: Decortication of the lung. Acta Chir Scand 110:437, 1955.

Samson PC, Burford TH: Total pulmonary decortication: Its evolution and present concepts of indications and operative technique. J Thorac Surg 16:127, 1947.

Samson PC, Burford TH, Brewer LA, Burbank G: The management of war wounds of the chest in a base center: The role of early decortication. J Thorac Surg 15:1, 1946.

Samson PC, Merrill DL, Dugan DJ et al: Technical considerations in decortication for the pleural complications of pulmonary tuberculosis. J Thorac Surg Cardiovasc 36:431, 1958.

Savage T, Flemin JA: Decortication of the lung in tuberculous disease. Thorax 10:293, 1955.

Scannell JG: The captive lung: Indications for and techniques of decortication. In Deslauriers J, Lacquet LK (eds): International Trends in General Thoracic Surgery, Vol 6: The Pleural Space. St. Louis, Mosby–Year Book, 1990.

Schede M: Die Behandlung der Empyeme. Proceedings of the Ninth Congress of Internal Medicine. Wiesbaden, Germany, 1890, Vol 9, p 41.

Shapiro DH, Anagnostopoulos CE, Dineen JP: Decortication and pleurectomy for the pleuropulmonary complications of pancreatitis. Ann Thorac Surg 9:76, 1970.

Siebens AA, Storey CF, Newman MM et al: The physiologic effects of fibrothorax and the functional results of surgical treatment. J Thorac Surg 32:43, 1956.

Sterling GM, Herbert A: Lung in cuirasse: Restrictive pleurisy associated with asbestos exposure. Thorax 35:715, 1990.

Swoboda L, Laule K, Blatmann H, Hasse J: Decortication in chronic pleural empyema: Investigation of lung function based on perfusion scintigraphy. Thorac Cardiovasc Surg 38:359, 1990.

Thomas GI, Jarvis FJ: Decortication in primary tuberculous pleuritis and empyema with a study of functional recovery. J Thorac Surg 32:178, 1956.

Thurer J: Decortication in thoracic empyema: Indications and surgical technique. Chest Surg Clin North Am 6:491, 1996.

Toomes H, Vogt-Moykopf I, Ahrend T: Decortication of the lung. Thorac Cardiovasc Surg 31:338, 1983.

Van Way C, Narrod J, Hopeman A: The role of early thoracotomy in the treatment of empyema. J Thorac Cardiovasc Surg 96:436, 1988.

Villalba M, Lucas CE, Ledgerwood AM, Asfaw I: The etiology of post-traumatic empyema and the role of decortication. J Trauma 19:414, 1979.

Violet D: De la décortication pulmonaire dans l'empyème chronique. Arch Gen Med 81:657, 1904.

Wachsmuth W, Schautz R: Untersuchungen über die Lungen—Pleura-Grenzschicht beider extrapleuralen Dekortikation. Chirurg 22:337, 1961.

Waterman DH, Domm SE, Rogers WK: A clinical evaluation of decortication. J Thorac Cardiovasc Surg 33:1, 1957.

Weinberg J, Davis JD: Pleural decortication in pulmonary tuberculosis. Am Rev Respir Dis 60:288, 1949.

Weinberg J, Horner JC, Davis JD: Decortication of the unexpanded tuberculous lung following induced pneumothorax. Surg Clin North Am 28:1591, 1948.

Williams MH: The technique of pulmonary decortication and pleurolysis. J Thorac Surg 20:652, 1950.

Wilson JM, Boren CH, Peterson Sr, Thoams AN: Traumatic hemothorax: Is decortication necessary? J Thorac Cardiovasc Surg 77:489, 1979.

Witz JP, Whilm JM: Problèmes chirurgicaux posés par les pleurésies purulentes. In Techniques chirurgicales. Paris, Encycl Med Chir, 1991.

Wright GW, Yee LB, Filley GF, Stranaham A: Physiologic observations concerning decortication of the lung. J Thorac Cardiovasc Surg 18:372, 1949.

Young D, Simon J, Pomerantz M: Current indications for and status of decortication for "trapped lung." Ann Thorac Surg 14:631, 1972.

Zenker R, Heberer G, Lohr H: Die Lungenresektionen. Berlin, Springer-Verlag, 1954, p 200.

CHAPTER **47**

Surgical Techniques in the Pleura

CLOSED DRAINAGE AND SUCTION SYSTEMS

Jocelyn Grégoire
Jean Deslauriers

The first attempts to drain the pleural space with a tube are credited to Playfair (1875) and Hewett (1876), who both reported, over a century ago, on an underwater seal drainage system for the management of empyemas. Since then, the concept of pleural space drainage has evolved considerably, not only because of a better understanding of pleural space physiology but also because of improved technology and the changing needs of physicians.

Despite the claims of many manufacturers, no currently available thoracic drainage system is ideal. Each available system has desirable features, but each also has deficiencies. Two features are particularly important for surgeons: (1) The system must meet the physiologic and therapeutic needs of the patient, and (2) its design must be straightforward so that its functioning can be thoroughly understood by the entire surgical team.

HISTORICAL NOTE

Although Hippocrates (Hippocrates, 1952) may have been the first to consider drainage of the pleural space when he described incisions, cautery, and metal tubes to drain empyemas (Miller and Sahn, 1987), the concept of closed pleural drainage originated in England in the 1870s. In 1891, Bülau also described a method of siphon drainage for the management of empyemas (Fig. 47–1). According to his understanding of pleural mechanics and physiology, this method was safer and less complicated than the more radical and then more popular procedure involving resection of the overlying ribs and open drainage of the space. In his original paper, written in German and reported by Meyer (1989), Bülau wrote: "I have always believed that the principal advantage of siphon-drainage is that it lowers the pressure within the pleural space, thereby bringing about re-expansion of the lung."

The importance of closed-tube drainage of empyemas was not recognized until the release of a 1918 survey by the Surgeon General of the U.S. Army, which reported mortality rates for rib resection and open drainage of empyemas to be averaging 30% (Graham and Bell, 1918). Because of the creation of an open pneumothorax, death frequently occurred within one-half hour of the operation (Churchill, 1958). The Surgeon General appointed the Empyema Commission, headed by Major Evarts A. Graham, which recommended closed drainage in the early stages of empyema. Immediately after adoption of these changes, the mortality of empyema drainage decreased to approximately 3%.

The use of chest tubes in postoperative thoracic care was reported by Lilienthal in 1922 and Brunn in 1929. Today, tube thoracostomy is an integral part of therapy for a variety of pleural disorders.

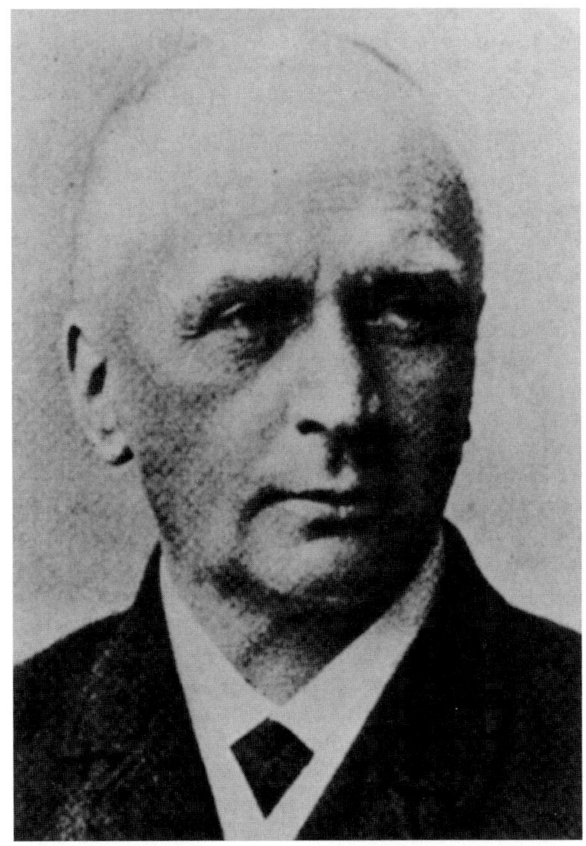

FIGURE 47–1 ■ Gotthard Bülau (1836–1900) of Hamburg, Germany, originator of the method of closed water-seal drainage of the chest. (From Nissen R, Wilson RHL: Pages in the history of Chest Surgery. Springfield, IL, Charles C Thomas, 1960.)

■ *HISTORICAL READINGS*

Brunn H: Surgical principles underlying one-stage lobectomy. Arch Surg 18:490, 1929.

Bülau G: Für die Heber-Drainage bei Behandlung des Empyems. Z Klin Med 18:31, 1891.

Churchill ED: Wound surgery encounters a dilemma. J Thorac Surg 35:279, 1958.

Graham EA, Bell RD: Open pneumothorax: Its relation to the treatment of empyema. Am J Med Sci 156:839, 1918.

Hewett CF: Thoracenthesis: The plan of continuous aspiration. Br Med J 1:317, 1876.

Hippocrates: Writings. In Hutchins RA (ed): Great Books of the Western World, Vol 29. Chicago, Encyclopedia Britannica, 1952, p 142.

Lilienthal H: Resection of the lung for suppurative infections with a report based on 31 consecutive operative cases in which resection was done or intended. Ann Surg 75:257, 1922.

Meyer JA: Gotthard Bülau and closed water-seal drainage for empyema, 1875–1891. Ann Thorac Surg 48:597, 1989.

Playfair GE: Case of empyema treated by aspiration and subsequently by drainage: Recovery. Br Med J 1:45, 1875.

TABLE 47–1 ■ **Indications for Tube Drainage**

Pneumothorax
Spontaneous (primary, secondary)
Open pneumothorax
Tension pneumothorax
Traumatic
Iatrogenic (central venous access procedure, thoracentesis, pleural biopsy, needle biopsy of lung, positive-pressure ventilation)
Hemothorax
Empyema
Parapneumonic effusions
Frank empyemas
Pleural Effusion
Chylothorax
Postoperative Drainage
Thoracic procedures
Cardiac surgery

BASIC SCIENCE

Physiology of the Pleural Space

The pleura is a thin and slippery membrane originating from the internal coelom. The parietal segment completely lines the inner surfaces of the ribs, diaphragm, and mediastinum; the visceral pleura, in continuity with the parietal pleural, begins at the pulmonary hilum and covers all lung surfaces, including the fissures. The two pleural leaflets are separated by a virtual space containing 5 to 15 ml of lubricating fluid. This arrangement provides a smooth and efficient mechanical coupling between the lung, a passive elastic structure, and the chest wall, a dynamic structure activated by respiratory muscles. There are no communications between the left and right pleural spaces.

During quiet breathing, the elastic forces of the lung and chest wall pull in opposite directions, thereby creating a negative intrapleural pressure, which keeps the two pleural surfaces apposed and the lung expanded. Normal intrapleural pressures vary between −8 cm H_2O during inspiration and −2 cm H_2O during expiration. With forced inspiration and forced expiration, these pressures may exceed −54 cm H_2O and +70 cm H_2O, respectively (Kam et al, 1993; Munnell, 1997). In patients with abnormal accumulations of air, blood, or other fluids in the pleural space, the negative pressure is lost and the lung recoils inward, causing hypoxemia and alveolar hypoventilation. Ultimately, this pressure buildup can be large enough to displace the mediastinum to the other side and compromise both the ventilation of the opposite lung and the venous return.

The purpose of thoracic drainage is to promote air or fluid evacuation, lung re-expansion, and restoration of intrapleural negative pressure. Because air has a low density, it tends to accumulate in the upper half of the pleural space; fluids with a higher density tend to collect in the lower half, inferiorly in the sitting position and posteriorly in the supine position.

Indications for Tube Drainage

In patients with spontaneous pneumothorax, tube drainage is the treatment of choice, not only because it allows for rapid evacuation of air but also because it helps to re-expand the lung (Table 47–1). Both tension pneumothorax and open pneumothorax are immediately life-threatening conditions and require emergency pleural drainage. In blunt trauma, pneumothoraces are often the consequence of a fractured rib puncturing the underlying lung; these pneumothoraces should be drained unless they are small, asymptomatic, and nonprogressive. Most iatrogenic pneumothoraces are secondary to central venous access (Dalbec and Krome, 1986; Herbst, 1978), and they should also be drained. The same policy applies to patients who develop a pneumothorax while receiving mechanical ventilation. The use of prophylactic tube thoracostomy during administration of positive end-expiratory pressure (PEEP) or continuous positive-pressure breathing is still debated (Hayes and Lucas, 1976) because complications related to the technique have been well described, including possible tension pneumothorax (Burge, 1992).

In general, patients with traumatic hemothoraces should have a chest tube to monitor the rate of bleeding, re-expand the lung, and prevent chronic lung entrapment and late empyema. The general issue of how to treat parapneumonic effusions is controversial (Deslauriers et al, 1987). It has been suggested that pleural drainage be considered if pleural fluid pH is lower than 7.2, glucose level is lower than 40 mg/dl, and lactate dehydrogenase is greater than 1000 U, or if microorganisms are identified from Gram's stain or culture (Klein, 1999; Light, 1985). Many surgeons believe that the only absolute indication for tube drainage is the positive identification of bacteria in the effusion. Frank empyemas always require tube drainage whether the tube is inserted under local anesthesia or during thoracoscopy.

Malignant pleural effusions should be drained if they are recurrent and symptomatic, or if sclerotherapy is contemplated. If the effusion is loculated, it is drained more efficiently with the use of imaging modalities, such as fluoroscopy, ultrasound, and computed tomography (CT) scan (Collins et al, 1992). Chylothoraces should nearly always be drained. A thoracostomy tube should always be left in the pleural space after any intrathoracic procedure regardless of its magnitude (Watkins, 1961).

This is even more important following partial lung resection, which requires that air and fluid be properly evacuated so that lung re-expansion and sealing of peripheral air leaks can be achieved. After pulmonary surgery, pleural drainage is also helpful to avoid such complications as bronchopleural fistulas and empyemas (Storey, 1968). After a lobectomy or a lesser pulmonary resection, a single chest tube is usually sufficient to drain the space, but two tubes—one anterior at the apex and one posterior at the base—may be necessary if excessive air leakage or bleeding is anticipated (Harris and Graham, 1991).

Contraindications to Tube Drainage

There are virtually no contraindications to tube drainage, although one has to be cautious when inserting a chest tube in a patient with a bleeding disorder, or in a patient receiving anticoagulants. The presence of pleural adhesions may sometimes complicate the procedure, and the drainage of multiloculated effusions often requires precise preoperative localization of the collections. Other relative contraindications include patients with giant bullae in whom there is a danger of perforating the bullae, and patients with a mainstem bronchial occlusion with complete atelectasis of the lung, which suggests a large pleural effusion on the chest radiograph. In these latter cases, the associated mediastinal shift and diaphragmatic elevation may complicate or even contraindicate tube drainage (Iberti and Stern, 1992). Hepatic hydrothorax is a relative contraindication to tube drainage because continuous evacuation of the effusion may lead to massive protein and electrolyte depletion, and ultimately to the death of the patient (Runyon et al, 1986). A chest tube should be inserted with extreme caution in a trauma patient with suspected diaphragmatic injury. In such cases, it is recommended that diaphragmatic rupture be ruled out before tube drainage is performed.

TUBE THORACOSTOMY

Chest Tube Sizes

Most chest tubes currently used in North America are made of transparent plastic (Silastic). They have multiple side holes, a radiopaque stripe, and outer diameters ranging from No. 6 French gauge (pediatric) to No. 40 French gauge. As pointed out by Couraud and co-workers (1990), these tubes are firm yet pliable. They induce minimal skin or pleural reaction, and they are inexpensive.

Rubber tubes are used only by a handful of surgeons and for the sole purpose of postoperative drainage. There is no clear evidence that the material of a chest tube (rubber or Silastic) has any impact on the recurrence rate of spontaneous pneumothoraces, although Hood and colleagues (1966) have demonstrated a relative lack of tissue reaction associated with polyvinyl as compared with rubber tubes. They suggested that this lack of tissue reaction may reduce pleural surface adhesions and prolong air leaks. However, the more irritating rubber tubes could be helpful in promoting the formation of fibrous tracks; therefore, they may be more suited for the drainage of chronic empyemas (Kam et al, 1993).

Foley catheters can be used for thoracic drainage, but they have a relatively small lumen and are not radiopaque (Lawrence, 1983). They do have, however, the advantage of permitting withdrawal to the inner chest wall, where a partially inflated balloon restrains them from further removal. Tinckler (1976) has also described a self-retaining chest drainage tube that uses an inflatable balloon.

In patients with pneumothoraces, smaller tubes (20 to 24 French) directed toward the apex are sufficient for evacuating air from the pleural space. Very small caliber catheters (16 French) have also been used successfully for the drainage of small pneumothoraces or to provide relief of tension pneumothoraces (Wayne and McSwain, 1980). They can be connected to standard drainage systems, although a Heimlich valve is often used in an outpatient setting (Conces et al, 1988; Iberti and Stern, 1992; Minami et al, 1992; Sargent and Turner, 1970). For patients with hemothoraces, malignant effusions, or empyemas, larger tubes (28 to 40 French) are preferred because the hemorrhagic fluid or the intense fibrinous reaction tends to occlude tubes of smaller diameter (Deslauriers, 1990).

Most currently used chest tubes are straight, although curved chest catheters have been recommended for optimal drainage of malignant pleural effusions (Ishikawa et al, 1998). These are also used in cardiac surgery patients to circumvent the transcostal route, thus minimizing postoperative pain (Jakob et al, 1997).

CHEST TUBE INSERTION

Preoperative Management

A complete history and physical examination should always be done prior to tube thoracostomy. The patient's chest radiographs should be examined compulsively and be readily available at the patient's bedside (Harris and Graham, 1991). Likewise, CT scans and ultrasound results should be reviewed, and the exact site of the collection well documented. In cases of pleural effusion, the results of thoracentesis should be available and the exact nature of the effusion known before tube drainage is undertaken. Indeed, some of these effusions may not require drainage at all.

Patients should be informed not only about the indication for tube thoracostomy but also about the technique of tube insertion. Fearful and anxious patients often nervously anticipate this apparently simple operation, a feature that may immensely complicate the procedure. When air or fluid is drained, sudden re-expansion of the lung may cause cough and shoulder and chest pain. The patient may also experience bradycardia, hypotension, and even faintness (Iberti and Stern, 1992). As was emphasized by Hiebert (1995), thorough explanations, adequate local anesthesia, and light sedation should reassure the patient and alleviate some of these unpleasant symptoms.

Insertion Site

For tube drainage, the patient should be positioned with the involved side slightly elevated and supported by a

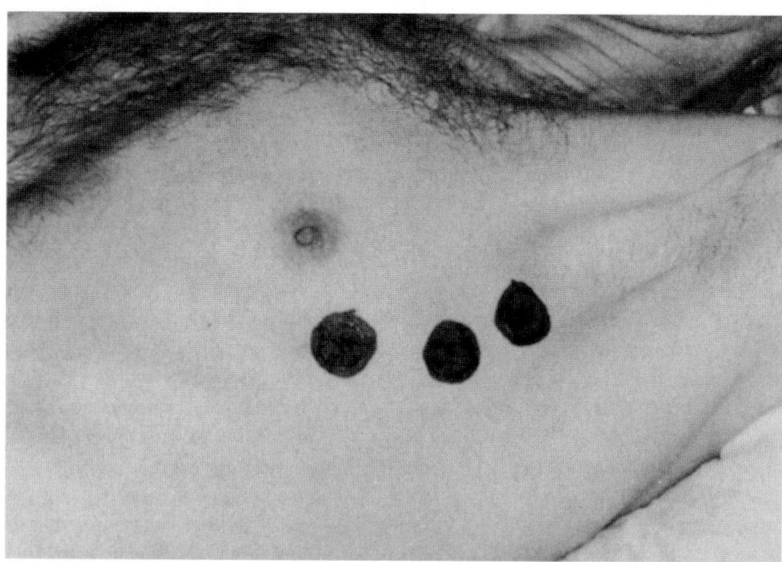

FIGURE 47–2 ■ The ideal site of tube insertion is the anterior or midaxillary line behind the pectoralis major fold. The dots shown on this picture are acceptable locations for chest tube placement.

pillow. The arm can be elevated over the head, or it can be resting at the edge of the bed. The operator should wear a mask and be gowned and gloved.

For closed thoracostomy, whether for the drainage of a pneumothorax or of pleural fluid, the ideal site of tube insertion is the third or fourth intercostal space in the anterior or midaxillary line, immediately behind the pectoralis major fold (Kovarik and Brown, 1969) (Fig. 47–2). In this location, the scar is hardly visible and the technique of tube insertion is easier because there are no muscles other than the intercostals to traverse. If, in addition, the tube has to be left in the pleural space for any length of time, it is more comfortable and less restrictive for such activities as eating, sleeping, or receiving chest physiotherapy. Finally, proper positioning at the apex is easier when the drain is inserted from the axilla because of its natural tendency to slide upward along the curve of the lateral chest wall (Fig. 47–3). The only exception to axillary tube insertion occurs with drainage of loculated pleural fluid; in this situation, the chest tube has to be inserted in a specific location, which is shown by chest films and ultrasound.

The second interspace in the midclavicular line is often mentioned (Miller and Sahn, 1987; Richards, 1978) but seldom used because chest tube placement in this position necessitates dissection through the pectoralis muscle, which may cause troublesome bleeding. It may also leave a highly visible scar. In addition, the tube may be difficult to direct to the apex or at the base, and these maneuvers may be quite painful (Harris and Graham, 1991; Tomlinson and Treasure, 1997). Posterior apical tube placement with an incision in the second or third intercostal space medial to the inner border of the scapula has also been suggested (Aslam et al, 1970; Galvin et al, 1990). Riquet and associates (1998) have recently reported their experience in using a posterior approach (Monaldi catheters No. 16 F, 18 F) to drain apical spaces. The technique was used in 50 cases, obviating the need for thoracoplasty or intrathoracic transposition of extrathoracic skeletal muscles in these patients. The authors of this chapter are of the opinion that this technique is almost never indicated, not only because of the difficulties associated with inserting the tube, but also because of the awkward position of the catheter.

Insertion Technique

Chest tubes are usually inserted under local anesthesia after proper cleansing of the skin with an antiseptic solution (Iberti and Stern, 1992). The parietal pleura

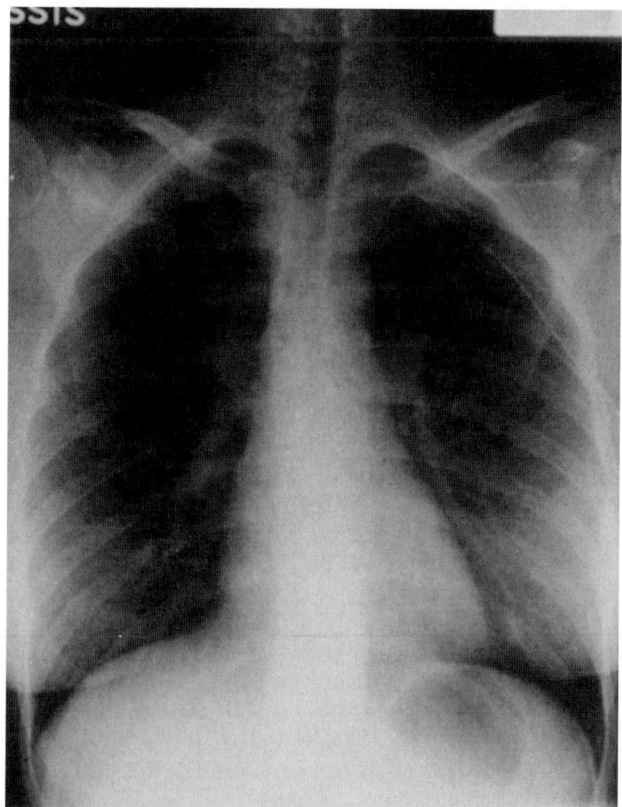

FIGURE 47–3 ■ Chest radiograph showing a well-positioned tube at the apex.

should be infiltrated generously. Often the effect of the local anesthetic is improved if one waits a few minutes before incising the skin to allow diffusion of the drug (Munnell, 1997). Aspiration of air or fluid through a needle and syringe is used to confirm the proper location of the drainage site. A 2-cm incision is then made in the interspace, and to avoid injury to the neurovascular bundle, blunt dissection is carried out over the superior border of the rib. It is generally recommended that the skin incision be made one space below the interspace to be used, so that an upward diagonal tunnel can be created. This arrangement provides a better seal when the tube is removed.

Chest tubes can be inserted by the trocar method or by the technique of blunt dissection. The trocar is a sharp-tipped metal rod used to guide the chest tube through the chest wall and parietal pleura. The technique is simple, but because the trocar is often introduced forcefully into the pleural space, there is risk of injury to the underlying lung or any other intrathoracic structure (Iberti and Stern, 1992). Trocar insertion should be reserved for patients with a large space, although Neptune (1977) and others have found that the trocar, when correctly used is an efficient, safe, and practical means of inserting a chest tube, especially in the management of spontaneous pneumothorax.

The authors prefer and recommend blunt dissection of a tunnel through intercostal muscles and parietal pleura using a curved Kelly clamp (Fig. 47–4). When this technique is used, the pleural space can first be inspected with the index finger, and the tube then simply advanced into its proper position. Although forceful trocar insertion is ill advised, some authors feel that chest tubes can be better guided and positioned with the help of a trocar (Harris and Graham, 1991; Ishikawa et al, 1998). In this situation, the trocar should be withdrawn a few millimeters after the parietal pleura is penetrated and the tube advanced into the space. As the tube is positioned, the trocar can be fully retracted (Munnell, 1997; Tomlinson and Treasure, 1997).

When the tube is in place, air condensation is easily noted over the walls of the catheter with each expiration, indicating proper placement within the pleural space (Iberti and Stern, 1992).

To facilitate tube insertion with a Kelly hemostat, Ring and Shapiro (1989) and others (Davis, 1987) advocate the use of a tunnel-tip catheter (Fig. 47–5). With this technique, there is less dissection of the muscles of the chest wall, and the tip of the tube advances more easily into the pleural space. Ring and Shapiro (1989) have also observed that there is less air leakage around the catheter because the thoracostomy tract is not as large as with regular catheters. Tunnel-tip thoracic catheters are available (Sherwood Medical, St. Louis, MO) in straight and right-angled forms. Dilators (Thal and Quick, 1988) and guidewires (Guyton et al, 1988; Mellor, 1996; Semrad, 1988) that facilitate tube insertion have also been described.

In the early 1990s, Galloway and colleagues (1993) and Kang and associates (1994) suggested the use of the disposable surgiport trocar-cannula for tube insertion, and in 1999, Waksman and co-workers reported their experience with the endoscopic trocar-cannula, which was used in more than 112 patients with trauma, spontaneous pneumothoraces, and pleural effusions. In that series, the authors had a less than 1% complication rate

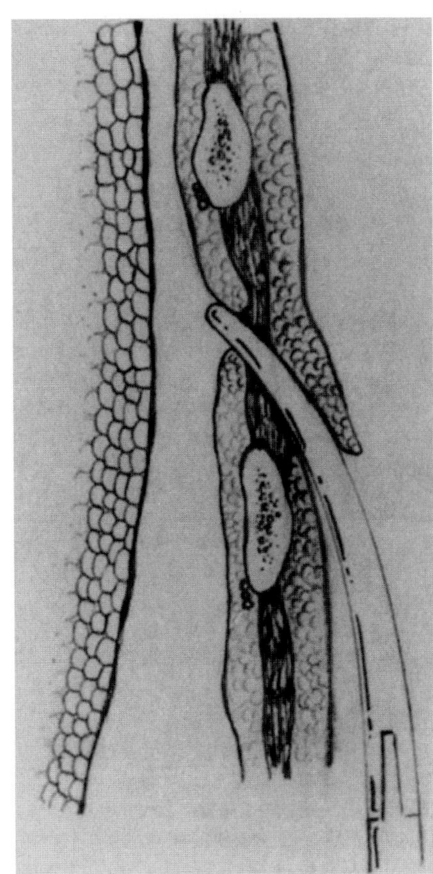

FIGURE 47–4 ■ Blunt dissection through intercostal muscles with a curved Kelly clamp. Note the upward diagonal tunnel and the dissection, which is carried out over the superior border of the rib.

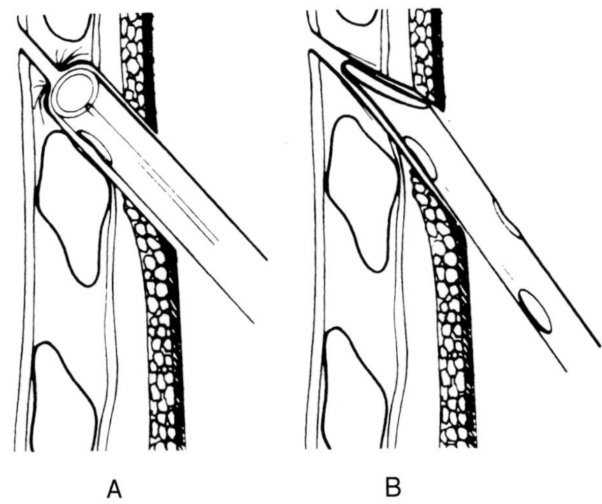

FIGURE 47–5 ■ Tube thoracostomy facilitated by using *B*, a tunnel-tip, rather than *A*, a blunt-tip chest tube. (From Ring EM, Shapiro MJ: The tunnel tip thoracic catheter. Surg Gynecol Obstet 169:553, 1989.)

(lung perforation). An expansible cannula is also available for tube insertion, and in the series of Gill and associates (1992), there were no complications in the 22 reported patients. The McSwain dart technique was designed to treat tension pneumothoraces more efficiently (Wayne and McSwain, 1980) but its use has been discouraged (Bayne, 1982) because of potential lung injuries.

To prevent postoperative dislodgment of the tube, it should be sutured to the skin with heavy silk mattress sutures (Iberti and Stern, 1992). Black (1999) even recommends that such anchoring sutures be tied flush with the chest tube, thus approximating the skin against the tube, and preventing air or fluid leak at the skin level. Recently, Boyle (1999) recommended using a 1-cm cylinder of connecting tube to anchor the chest tube to the suture, thus preventing drain migration.

Characteristics of Connecting Tubing

The best tube connectors are made of plastic and have serrated ends. It is most important that these connectors have a large internal diameter (1/4 inch, 6 mm) and that their ends not be tapered so that the flow of hemorrhagic fluids is not impaired. When more than one chest tube is required, the tubes can be connected to the same unit through a Y connector. Taping the ends of the connector to the connecting tubing does not ensure air tightness but only aids in preventing accidental separation at the site (Miller and Sahn, 1987).

Connecting tubes are made either of clear plastic or of latex. They usually are 5 to 6 feet long with an internal diameter of 12 mm. Plastic tubes have the advantage of water-clear transparency so that the fluctuation of fluid can easily be observed. With latex tubing, samples of fluid can be directly obtained from the tube through a No. 18 or 20 needle.

When the size of chest tubes, connectors, and tubing is selected, gas and fluid dynamics must be considered. Batchelder and Morris (1962), in a study of critical factors determining adequate pleural drainage, have shown that gas moving through tubing displays laminar flow and obeys Poiseuille's equation,

$$V = r^4P/8lv$$

where V is the volume flow rate, l is the length of the tube, v is the viscosity, r is the tube's internal radius, and P is the pressure drop. In this equation, the volume of gas in laminar flow through the tube is inversely related to the length of the tube and directly proportional to the fourth power of its radius. Tubes with an internal diameter of 1/4 inch (6 mm) allow a minimum flow rate of 15 L of air per minute, and tubes of 1/2-inch (12 mm) internal diameter are capable of handling flows of 50 to 60 L/min.

It has also been shown by Swenson and Birath (1957) that moist air has turbulent flow characteristics, which are expressed by the Fanning equation for turbulent flow,

$$v = \pi^2r^5P/fl$$

where f is a friction factor. In this relation, the flow rate is proportional to an even higher power of the radius of the lumen.

Tube Management

A chest radiograph should always be obtained immediately after tube insertion so that lung re-expansion and tube position can be assessed (Table 47–2). Thereafter, daily chest radiographs should be done for as long as the chest tube is in place (Martino et al, 1999; Mattox, 1989). Stark and colleagues (1983) have shown that sometimes both frontal and lateral radiographs are necessary to evaluate thoracostomy tube placement. In their study, eight of nine malpositioned chest tubes were documented only on a lateral film. By contrast, Kurihara and co-workers (1996) found that improper position of a chest tube within a fissure could easily be determined from the frontal chest radiograph alone. Placement of a chest tube in a lung fissure, for instance, can result in inadequate drainage (Maurer et al, 1982; Webb and Laberge, 1983), although Curtin and associates (1994) have shown that the location of a tube, even if it is within a lobar fissure, is not a critical factor in the drainage of fluid or air in the traumatized patient. This suggests that as long as the tube functions well, it should not be repositioned or replaced just because it is located in an interlobar fissure. Careful monitoring of the nature and volume of fluid drainage is recommended until after the tube has been removed.

Drainage tubes should not be allowed to hang as dependent loops (Fig. 47–6) because fluids and clots accumulating in the tubing increase the resistance of the system (Kam et al, 1993; Morgan and Orcutt, 1972; Munnell, 1997; Sim, 1996). In an experimental model, Gordon and colleagues (1997) demonstrated very nicely that with a dependent-loop position, pressure on the "lung" side of the tube increased significantly, and drainage dropped to zero. Drainage was improved, however, by lifting intermittently (every 15 minutes) the dependent-loop tubing.

Tubes should almost never be clamped, although Munnell and Thomas (1975), in a survey of 328 thoracic surgeons, have shown that close to 75% of experienced thoracic surgeons did in fact clamp tubes at some time during the postoperative period. Chest tubes were clamped to transport patients (35%), to rule out an air leak (21%), to change a bottle or connecting tube (18%), or to treat patients in whom a tube was used following

TABLE 47–2 ■ **Principles of Tube Management**

- Monitoring
  - Early and daily chest radiographs
  - Nature and volume of air leak and fluid drainage
- Clamping of the chest tube
- Functional status of the tube
- Maintenance of patency
  - Milking and stripping
  - Irrigation
- Avoidance of dependent loops
- Airtightness of the system

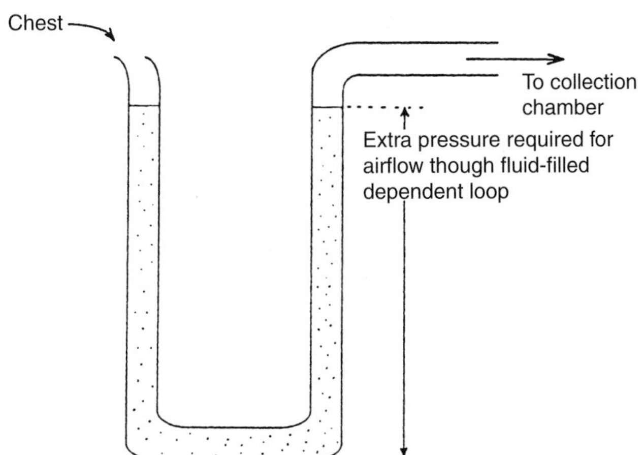

FIGURE 47–6 ■ Effect of fluid-filled dependent loop in a pleural drainage system. (From Kam AC, O'Brien M, Kam PCA: Pleural drainage systems. Anesthesia 48:155, 1993.)

pneumonectomy (7%). Clamping during patient transportation, especially if the patient has an air leak, can be catastrophic because of potential lung collapse, subcutaneous emphysema, or tension pneumothorax (Harris and Graham, 1991; Hyde et al, 1997; Sim, 1996). If a chest tube becomes accidentally disconnected from the drainage system, it should simply be reconnected without previous clamping (Morgan and Orcutt, 1972). If the drainage system completely breaks (in the case of a glass bottle), a one-way flutter valve, if available, may also be connected while a new system is prepared (Sim, 1996).

When the functional status of a tube is in question, observation of fluid oscillation in the water seal or in the tubing is important. Oscillations that are synchronous with respiratory movements (tidaling) indicate tube patency. If there are no oscillations, the tube may be obstructed, or this may result from complete re-expansion of the lung (Kam et al, 1993). Increased oscillations are a sign of high negative intrapleural pressures, often associated with atelectasis or incomplete lung re-expansion.

Air tightness of the system should be assessed on a daily basis and one has to be very suspicious of a *continuous* air leak that does not vary with the respiratory cycle. In such cases, sequential clamping of each of the components of the system may unveil a defect in the tubing or drainage system, which should be corrected immediately (Iberti and Stern, 1992). Indeed a continuous air leak associated with a break in the tubing may be the cause of a persistent pneumothorax or residual air space.

Whether or not a chest tube should be milked or stripped to dislodge clots and debris and maintain patency is a question of controversy (Iberti and Stern, 1992; Lim-Levy et al, 1986; Oakes et al, 1993; Teplitz, 1991). When a chest tube is milked or stripped, clots, which may have been attached to the sides of the tube, are mechanically pressed toward the collecting chamber or back into the pleural space (Von Hippel, 1970). In a study conducted after open heart surgery, Lim-Levy and co-workers (1986) showed that chest tubes remained patent with or without milking or stripping. Duncan and Erickson (1982) have also shown that by stripping the entire length of the chest tube, negative intrapleural pressures exceeding 400 cm H_2O can be obtained. Whether these high pressures can cause injury to the lung or to other intrathoracic structures is unknown.

Taping drain connections has been advocated by many to prevent accidental disconnection. One has to remember, however, that taped tubing may disconnect without being noticed, thereby creating a false sense of security about the system (Godden and Hiley, 1998).

If the system becomes occluded, some authors have suggested use of saline (Miller and Sahn, 1987) or even of fibrinolytic agents (Miller et al, 1951) to irrigate the tube. Others have suggested the use of a sterile suction catheter introduced into the chest tube through a sterile cap (Halejian et al, 1988). In accordance with Munnell (1997), the authors do not recommend these procedures because each manipulation increases the risk of contamination of the pleural space. When a drainage collection system is replaced, the tube should be clamped for a short time and the procedure should be simple, standardized, efficient, and well taught to the house and nursing staffs. This often prevents undesirable complications, such as tension pneumothorax, or infection, which could be secondary to clumsy manipulation of the tubing system (Macey and Landstrom, 1993).

Chest Tube Removal

Chest tubes can be removed when there is no longer fluctuation in the fluid column of the tube (indicating complete lung re-expansion or tube occlusion), when daily fluid drainage is minimal (<100 ml in 24 hours), and when the air leak has stopped. The proper timing of tube removal is subject to some controversy. Sharma and associates (1988), for example, showed that in 40 patients subjected to tube thoracostomy for spontaneous pneumothorax, removal of the tube within 6 hours of re-expansion led to recollapse of the lung in 25% of cases. None of the patients suffered recollapse when the tube was withdrawn after 48 hours of lung re-expansion. In a randomized study of algorithms for discontinuing tube thoracostomy drainage, Davis and colleagues (1994) showed that a 24-hour period with no air leak, or less than 2 ml/kg/day of fluid drainage, constituted safe circumstances for tube removal because of the low (2.5%) risk of recurrence under these circumstances. Keeping suction until the tube is removed, as opposed to a trial period of water-seal drainage, seems to decrease the overall chest tube drainage period in trauma patients (Davis et al, 1994). In another prospective, randomized trial on thoracostomy removal algorithms, Martino and coworkers (1999) concluded that a short period of water-seal drainage observation (6–8 hours), without suction, resulted in a significantly decreased incidence of pneumothorax requiring tube reinsertion, when compared with tube removal immediately after low-pressure wall suction is discontinued. There were, however, no differences between the two groups in hospital lengths of stay or chest tube duration. Russo and associates (1998) also published their experience on early chest tube removal (within 90 minutes) after video-assisted thoracoscopic wedge resection of parenchymal lung disease. They believe that this practice is safe and cost effective, providing strict criteria are met.

Many surgeons favor clamping the tube for 12 to 24 hours before removal (Munnell and Thomas, 1975) because clamping allows for identification of a persistent air leak or reaccumulation of fluid. So and Yu (1982) also believe that once the lung has re-expanded and there is no further air leak, the catheter should be clamped for 24 hours before being removed. The authors think that trial clamping before removal is seldom necessary, although it may be useful in cases in which an air leak has been persistent over several days (Harris and Graham, 1991).

Although some authors have suggested that chest tubes should be removed at end-expiration (Miller and Sahn, 1987) or when a Valsalva maneuver is performed (Roe, 1965; Tomlinson and Treasure, 1997), the authors and others believe that this should occur at end-inspiration. This opinion is based on the observation that patients experiencing an acute pain, like that which may occur on tube removal (Gift et al, 1991), tend to inhale rather than exhale, thereby increasing the chances of air entry at the drainage site. Chest tube removal should be carried out by two people, one swiftly pulling out the tube while the other ties down the ligature (Daly et al, 1985).

Several techniques can be used to seal the thoracotomy incision at the time of tube removal. Probably the most common method used is the tying down of a U stitch across the wound as the tube is withdrawn. Other methods involve the use of petroleum jelly (Vaseline) gauze, skin staples, or adhesives to cover the wound (Lo and Mirza, 1984; Prats, 1990). Whatever method is preferred, the incision should be sealed rapidly to prevent any air entry into the pleural space.

A chest radiograph should be obtained 12 to 24 hours after tube removal for observation of possible reaccumulation of air or fluid in the pleural space. Panicek and colleagues (1987) and Gilsanz and Cleveland (1978) have shown that chest tube tracks, which are parallel lines corresponding to the prior position of the tube, may persist for some time after the tube is removed. These lines, which represent local pleural thickening due to the proliferation of mesothelial cells and deposition of fibrin along the course of the tube, have no clinical significance.

DRAINAGE SYSTEMS

Passive Drainage Systems

Passive drainage systems (Table 47–3) (Couraud et al, 1990) provide one-way drainage that allows the outflow of gas or fluid during expiration but prevents their return into the pleural space during inspiration. These systems are often sufficient to evacuate the pleural space because the slightly positive pressure that prevails during expiration or cough forces out both air and fluid (Von Hippel, 1970, 1975).

The most basic of these drainage systems is the one-way flutter valve (Heimlich, 1968), a device particularly useful in emergency situations or for drainage of uncomplicated pneumothoraces (Fig. 47–7, Heimlich valve, Becton-Dickinson, Franklin Lake, NJ). This flutter valve consists of a piece of rubber tubing, one end of which is compressed and retains its flattened shape. It allows fluid and air to flow out of the chest while preventing their reflux back into the pleural cavity. Several authors (Mercier et al, 1976; Niemi et al, 1999; Ponn et al, 1997) have shown that outpatient management of individuals with spontaneous pneumothoraces through the use of a flutter valve is safe, efficient, and economical. Heimlich valves have also been shown to be useful in the management of pneumothoraces secondary to metastatic lung disease (Van Hengel and Van de Bergh, 1994) and *Pneumocystis carinii* infection (Driver et al, 1991). In 1996, McKenna and associates reported the successful use of a flutter valve to shorten hospital stay after lung volume reduction surgery, even if patients have large residual apical spaces.

One possible complication of the Heimlich valve relates to improper attachment of the valve to the chest tube. In several reported cases (Maimimi and Johnson, 1990; Spouge and Thomas, 1991), the valve was inadvertently attached backward, resulting in a tension pneumothorax. As has been described by Spouge and Thomas (1991), the design of the valve can predispose to such errors because the chest tube can be attached to either end of the valve.

Tension pneumothorax has also been reported in a patient with a valve connected to a Foley catheter drain-

TABLE 47–3 ■ Pleural Space Drainage Systems

Passive Drainage Systems
Commercially available one-way flutter valves (Heimlich valves)
Thoracic vent
Portex ambulatory chest drainage systems
PLEURX pleural catheter
Portable chest drainage device
Homemade emergency one-way valves
Underwater seal units
One-bottle units
Two-bottle units
Active Drainage Systems
Three-bottle units
Homemade systems
Disposable and commercially available units
Units with mechanical manometers (dry suction)
High-pressure systems
Balanced drainage system
Drainage of the pneumonectomy space
Drainage following repair of diaphragmatic hernia
Pleuroperitoneal shunt

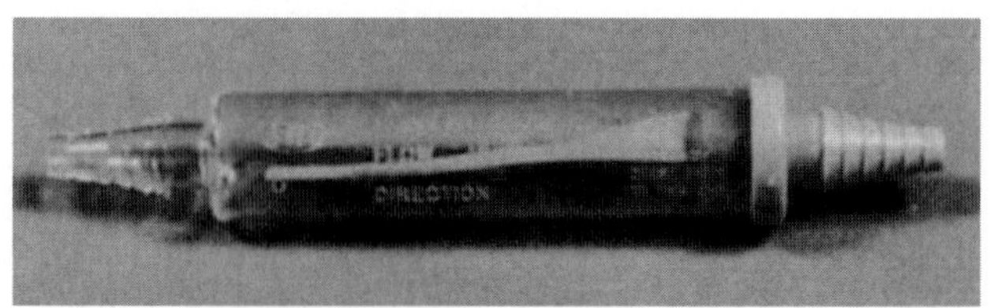

FIGURE 47–7 ■ Heimlich one-way flutter valve.

age bag that had been deliberately punctured to permit venting. Inadvertent covering with adhesive tape of the site of penetration of the valve in the bag led to inadequate drainage and predictably to a tension pneumothorax (Mariani and Sharma, 1994). The valve can also be subjected to patient tampering, as was described by Crocker and Ruffin (1998), who reported a case of tension pneumothorax secondary to insertion of a drinking straw in the Heimlich flutter valve assembly!

If one of these commercially made valves is not available, a homemade system can be fashioned by attaching a surgical glove to the end of the chest tube and puncturing the end of any of its fingers (Sim, 1996).

Modified urinary collecting bags have been used with few complications (Adegboye et al, 1996; Bar-El et al, 1992; Cerfolio, 2000) for prolonged, passive closed-chest drainage. Several authors (Graham et al, 1992; Joshi, 1996; McManus et al, 1998; Waller et al, 1999) have also reported on the use of a portable one-way flutter valve (Fig. 47–8) drainage bag (Portex Limited, Hythe, UK) to manage pneumothoraces and postoperative patients. More recently, Lodi and Stefani (2000) have reported their experience with a portable chest drainage device that provides a one-way valve connected to the chest tube for drainage of air and fluid, a reservoir for collecting fluid, and a one-way exhaust valve to evacuate air from the bag. These authors believe that ambulatory management of patients with moderate to large pleural fluid drainage is troublesome with the Heimlich valve and that their device is more effective. An indwelling pleural catheter (PLEURX pleural catheter, Scientific Medics, Denver Biomaterials Inc., Golden, CO) has also been recently reported for the management of recurrent malignant effusions. This apparatus was safely used in 47 patients and provided good patient care at reduced hospital cost (Putnam et al, 1998). One of the main advantages of the PLEURX system is that the patient can go home shortly after tube insertion (often on the same day) as compared with patients who must stay in the hospital for several days after chemical pleurodesis. The main disadvantage of the system is the required change of drainage bottles, which leads to increased costs.

Indwelling small pleural catheter needle thoracentesis (No. 7 French, Turkel Safety Thoracentesis System, Sherwood-Davis & Geck, Wayne, NJ) and subcutaneous access ports with fenestrated catheters have also been reported to be effective and economical means for managing recurrent pleural effusions (Grodzin and Balk, 1997; Reed et al, 1999).

Although some authors are cautious about recommending widespread acceptance of these devices (Sarniak, 1992), others such as Samelson and colleagues (1991) and Röggla and co-workers (1996b) have reported good results with the use of the thoracic vent (Truclose, Thoracic vent, Davis & Geck, Wayne, NJ) in patients with uncomplicated pneumothoraces or small pleural effusions. These authors claim that these systems are as efficient and safe as conventional thoracostomy units, and that they can be used safely in an outpatient setting. One possible disadvantage is that further tube drainage might be required should the device become dislodged owing to suboptimal fixation to the thoracic wall (Röggla et al, 1996b).

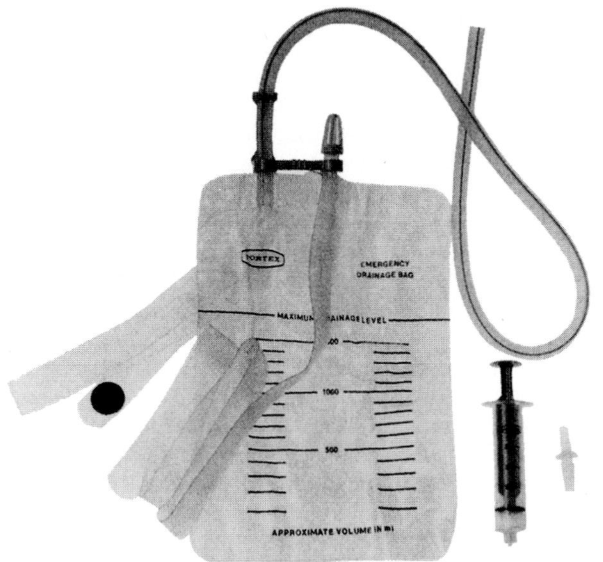

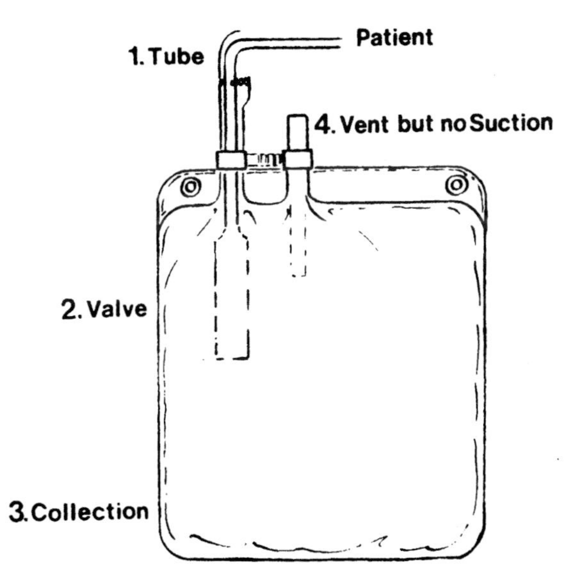

FIGURE 47–8 ■ Ambulatory chest drainage system (Portex Limited, Hythe, UK) that incorporates a "non-stick," vertically orientated flutter valve device within a drainage bag (From McManus K, Spence G, McGuigan J: Outpatient chest tubes [Letter]. Ann Thorac Surg 66:296, 1998.)

With the underwater seal drainage system, water acts as a seal to prevent air from going back up the drain during inspiration. Drainage by means of a single bottle is the simplest of all systems; this single bottle serves as both the collection chamber and the water seal. Drainage is effected by connecting the end of the tubing to a long plastic or glass tube, which reaches from the bottom of the bottle containing water to a height of about 2 cm. The extremity of the tube must be at a point below the water level, and the bottle itself must be located below the patient's chest for the pleural fluid to drain by gravity. Thus, this system employs both the mechanics of respiration (positive expiratory pressure) and gravity to bring about drainage. As air or fluids are evacuated, the pleural surfaces are brought together and the intrapleural pressure becomes negative again. A vent is used to provide for the escape of air from the drainage bottle into the atmosphere.

The use of the one-bottle underwater seal drainage unit may be limited, however, by the mounting level of fluid in the bottle, which imposes an increased resistance to drainage. In addition, froth can occur as a result of the mixing of air and blood in the same bottle, making measurement of fluid drainage difficult. Foaming of serosanguineous fluid can be minimized intermittently by adding 30 ml of alcohol to the drainage bottle.

To circumvent these problems, a two-bottle system (Fig. 47–9) can be fashioned by interposing a collection bottle, which traps fluids and passes air onward, thereby ensuring that the underwater seal is kept at a fixed constant level (Kam et al, 1993). Although this system allows for easier inspection and quantification of drainage, a potential drawback is the additional volume of tubing and dead space, which may sometimes allow reversal of airflow during inspiration (air may flow back into the pleural space). This extra dead space can also create an air lock, which can prevent complete re-expansion of the lung. It is also added to the patient's own respiratory dead space, thereby increasing respiratory work (Kam et al, 1993). Applying negative pressure to the system increases the pressure difference between the pleural space and collection chamber, thus enhancing drainage efficiency.

Active Drainage Systems

Active drainage by the use of continuous suction (Enerson and McIntyre, 1966; Pickard and Beall, 1983; Roe, 1958) is often necessary to achieve and maintain complete re-expansion of the lung and apposition of the visceral and parietal pleural surfaces. This is particularly important when the amount of air leakage exceeds the underwater seal capacity of the system, or when the underlying lung is noncompliant and is generating high negative intrapleural pressures exceeding the maximum negative pressure of the unit. Most authors recommend active suction with negative pressures in the neighborhood of -20 cm H_2O. Others, such as Pecora (1981) and Storey (1968), recommend use of higher negative pressures, especially for drainage after thoracotomy. In a prospective study, Johansson and associates (1998) showed, however, that passive underwater chest drainage was just as effective as active drainage after elective esophagectomy.

An ideal active drainage system must be able to evacuate efficiently and thoroughly the contents of the pleural space, whether these are fluids, clots, pus, or air. It must not limit airflow and must be able to reach constant negative suction pressures in the vicinity of -60 cm H_2O (Kam et al, 1993). It must be compact, unbreakable, easy to set up and use, fail-safe in operation, and easy for any member of the management team to understand. It must also have a collection chamber that can be readily emptied. Insofar as possible, active drainage units must also be inexpensive.

Three-Bottle Units

To provide active suction, a third bottle, used for suction control, can be added to the two-bottle water-seal drainage system (Howe, 1952; Kam et al, 1993; Sweet, 1954) (Fig. 47–10). When a built-in wall suction is used as vacuum (unregulated vacuum), this third bottle regulates the amount of suction applied throughout the entire system. If the vacuum is greater than the desired level of negative pressure (the depth of a central vent below the water level determines the amount of negative pressure), air is drawn from the atmosphere. Bubbling in the suction-control bottle indicates that the suction source is applying the right amount of negative pressure, usually -15 to -20 cm H_2O. The advantage of the three-bottle units resides in their safety because negative pressures greater than -15 to -20 cm H_2O can never be reached, a feature that may be important if a large bronchopleural fistula develops. The main deficiency of these units is that they may provide inadequate airflow in the event of a large air leak. Additional negative pressure can be added to the three-bottle unit by having a higher column of water in the third bottle, by using mercury instead of water in the suction-control bottle (McGrath and Kruger, 1962), or by adding a fourth bottle to the system (Julian and Pennell, 1987). These higher negative pressures are, however, seldom required in a normal thoracic surgical

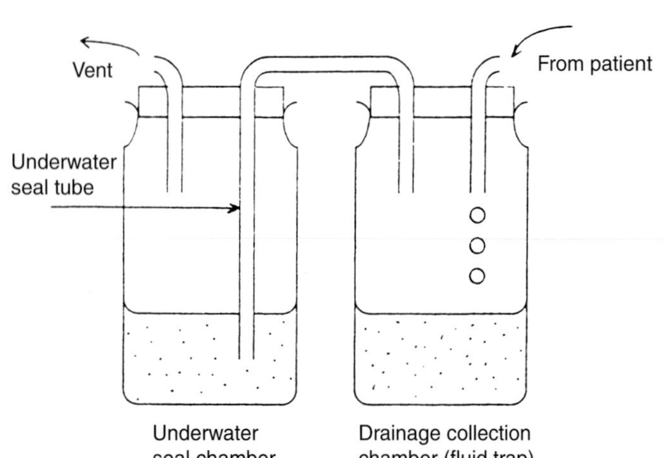

FIGURE 47–9 ■ Two-bottle system. (From Kam AC, O'Brien M, Kam PCA: Pleural drainage systems. Anesthesia 48:154, 1993.)

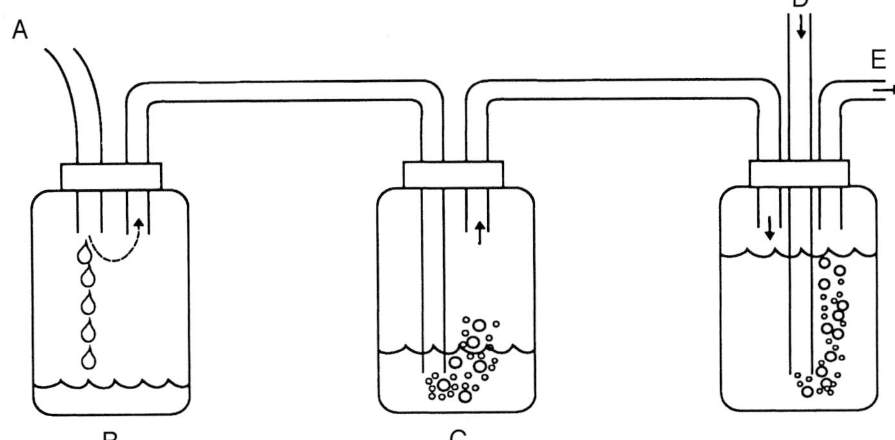

FIGURE 47–10 ■ Three-bottle water-seal unit in which the third bottle is used to regulate the amount of suction applied through the entire system, *A*, from the patient. *B*, Collecting bottle; *C*, Water-seal; *D*, Vent tube; *E*, To wall suction.

setting. Interestingly, adding a fourth, differently mounted bottle can act as a safety underwater seal chamber, thus venting the entire system or relieving any pressure buildup, should there be a failure of suction (Kam et al, 1993).

Disposable units using the same three-bottle suction drainage principles are now used in most institutions. These units are compact, light, and easy to assemble and operate. All are advertised as ideal systems, and each unit is alleged to be superior to the previous one. Most have safety devices or other components often considered useful by the manufacturer but unnecessary by the surgeon. In fact, some of these devices can make the system so complicated that its functioning is difficult for the surgeon, let alone the staff, to understand. All are relatively expensive.

Disposable plastic units that duplicate the three-bottle drainage system include the improved Thora Seal III, Aquaseal and Sentinel Seal (Kendall, Sherwood-Davis & Geck, St. Louis, MO), the Decknatel-Snowden-Pencere Pleur-Evac and Thora-Klex (Tucker, GA), and the Atrium Compact (Atrium Medical Corp., Hudson, NH). All these disposable plastic units have a collection chamber, a water seal, and a suction-control bottle. The Thora-Seal III also has a separate collection bottle (2500 ml), which can be replaced when required. Most manufacturers include an optional attached container so that blood drained from the pleural space can be salvaged for autotransfusion.

Dry Mechanical Suction Systems

New drainage units with mechanical manometers are now commercially available. Instead of a third bottle to maintain a constant level of suction, these units have a mechanical suction regulator, which allows for changes in suction level without adding or removing water. In the Decknatel Pleur-Evac unit, the desired level of suction can be reached by adjusting the suction source until the fluorescent indicator appears in the window on the face of the unit (Decknatel advertisement). With this system, higher negative pressures (up to -40 cm H_2O) can be safely applied to the system and to the pleural space.

The Thora-Klex chest drainage system has a rubber diaphragm flutter valve, which is incorporated in the suction port. With this system, fluid drops into the collection chamber and air passes into the air leak indicator and then flows through the one-way valve into the suction source. A potential problem of the flutter valve active drainage unit is that the slit could be held open by clots or debris, thereby allowing to-and-fro air movement.

These dry suction units with mechanical manometers eliminate the noise of bubbling in the third bottle, a feature considered annoying by many. Their problem, however, is the apparent difficulty in maintaining a constant negative pressure when a large air leak is present. In addition, the noise of bubbling in the third bottle may be a desirable feature because it indicates proper functioning of the unit.

High-Volume Systems

When high suction is required to achieve effective evacuation of the pleural space, high-volume systems such as the Emerson pump (J.H. Emerson Co., Cambridge, MA) can be used (Fig. 47–11). These are capable of reaching negative pressures in the order of -60 cm H_2O with airflows of more than 20 L/min. Rusch and colleagues (1988) and Capps and co-workers (1985) have shown that any pleural drainage unit is effective for the management of small air leaks when it functions with -20 cm H_2O of suction. Increasing the suction further to -40 cm H_2O does not significantly alter the flow via the chest tube. When a major air leak is present, the high-pressure, high-volume Emerson pump is the only unit capable of absorbing this airflow, with flows up to 35.5 L/min. Mobile suction units are also available for transportation of patients requiring continuous thoracic suction (Enerson and McIntyre, 1966). These high-volume systems can certainly handle large air leaks, but one should not forget that the lowest level of chest tube suction that is required to maintain adequate lung expansion is desirable (Munnell, 1997). Too much suction may potentially increase the magnitude of an air leak (Powner et al, 1985); may encourage air steal, which may lead to hypoxia (Pierson, 1982); or may unexpectedly trap lung parenchyma in chest tube holes (Stahley and Tench, 1977).

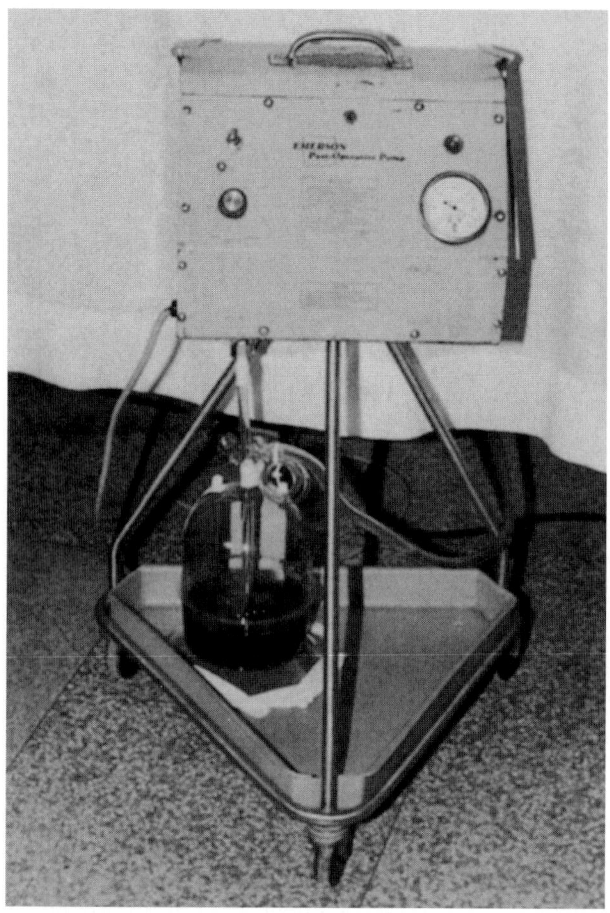

FIGURE 47–11 ■ Emerson pump.

Balanced Drainage Systems

Drainage of the Pneumonectomy Space

Following pneumonectomy, most surgeons do not advocate routine drainage of the pleural space. Air can be removed simply by needle and syringe aspiration at the end of the procedure, or by leaving a small thoracic catheter, which is withdrawn in the recovery room. Potential advantages of draining the pneumonectomy space are the possible immediate recognition of hemorrhage and the prevention of catastrophic tension pneumothorax should the suture line acutely break down. When a tube is used, it is usually connected to an underwater seal system and is kept clamped at all times. It is only unclamped to monitor or evacuate pleural collections or to readjust pleural pressure (Harris and Graham, 1991; Kam et al, 1993). Most chest tubes are removed within 48 hours of the pneumonectomy (Deslauriers and Grégoire, 1999; Harris and Graham, 1991).

Balanced drainage of the pneumonectomy space was described by Storey and Laforet (1953) and Laforet and Boyd (1964) as a method to maintain optimal physiologic position of the mediastinum. Appropriate arrangement of the bottles is as shown in Figure 47–12. The first bottle serves as a trap, and the other two bottles serve as pressure regulators. The second, or positive-pressure regulator, bottle is a simple water seal, so arranged that any pressure within the system (pleural space) exceeding 1 cm H_2O will be vented. The third bottle is a negative-pressure regulator bottle. It is a reverse water seal, so constructed that any pressure more negative than -10 to -15 cm H_2O that may develop in the system will automatically be reduced to this level by a compensatory ingress of air. Most balanced drainage units are homemade, although Decknatel Incorporated has one such unit commercially available.

One possible disadvantage of the balanced pneumonectomy drainage system is that extensive subcutaneous emphysema may occur when air is pushed into the soft tissues of the chest wall as a result of coughing. This emphysema tends to increase as additional air is made available from the drainage system. To limit the extent of this problem, Laforet and Boyd (1964) suggest tight and meticulous closure of the pleura, and Pecora and Cooper (1955) also suggest the use of a tight dressing over the incision. Another possible disadvantage of the balanced drainage system is that room air has access to the pleural space, with secondary risk of infection. This may be alleviated by interposing an air filter over the vent of the negative-pressure regulator bottle. Balanced drainage systems can also be useful for draining contaminated pneumonectomy spaces (Miller et al, 1975) or for drain-

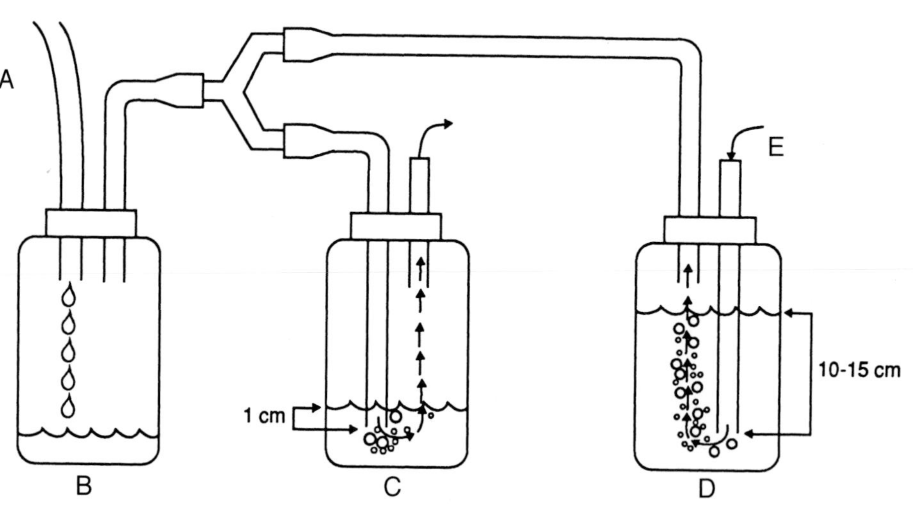

FIGURE 47–12 ■ Balanced drainage unit for pneumonectomy space drainage: *A*, Connecting tube from patient; *B*, Collecting bottle; *C*, Positive pressure regulator; *D*, Negative pressure regulator; and *E*, Air entering system from atmosphere. (Adapted from Laforet EG, Boyd TF: Balanced drainage of the pneumonectomy space. Surg Gynecol Obstet 118:1051, 1964, with permission.)

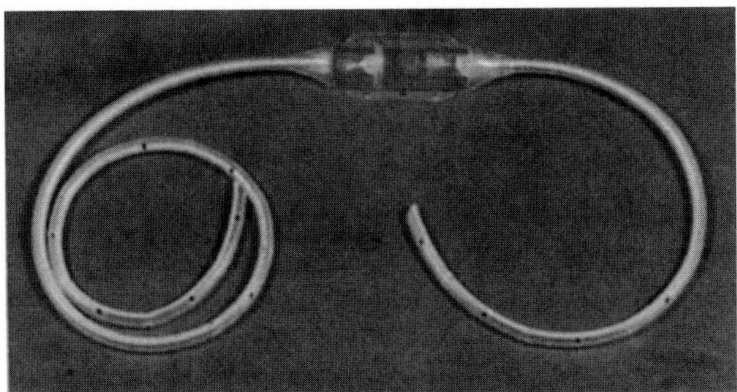

FIGURE 47–13 ■ Denver pleuroperitoneal shunt.

ing the rare patient with a postpneumonectomy chylothorax (Vallières et al, 1999).

Drainage Following Repair of Diaphragmatic Hernia

Overdistention of the hypoplastic lung is a major cause of pulmonary injury and death following surgical repair of congenital diaphragmatic hernia in newborns. Tyson and colleagues (1985) have shown that, by maintaining physiologic intrathoracic pressures, balanced thoracic drainage can minimize the risks of further pulmonary injury despite rapidly changing ventilatory or intrathoracic conditions.

Pleuroperitoneal Shunt

The Denver pleuroperitoneal shunt (Denver Biomaterials Inc., Evergreen, CO) is a single-unit medical-grade silicone conduit consisting of a unidirectionally valved pumping chamber located between fenestrated pleural and peritoneal catheters (Fig. 47–13). A barium sulfate stripe in the wall of the proximal and distal catheters permits visualization by chest radiograph or fluoroscopy. Manual compression of the shunt is required 150 to 200 times per day, and each compression transports about 1.5 ml of fluid from the pleural space to the peritoneum. The technique of pumping is neither painful nor difficult to master.

The technique of shunt placement is straightforward and has been well described by Ponn and associates (1991). A short inframammary incision is made over the sixth intercostal space, and a guidewire is passed posteriorly into the pleural space. A contiguous subcutaneous pocket large enough to contain the pump apparatus is then developed inferior to this incision. The pocket needs to be located over the anterolateral costal margin to provide a stable base for external shunt compression. A second, upper quadrant, muscle-splitting incision provides access to the peritoneal cavity. The pleural limb of the shunt is then passed into the pleural space through an introducer, and the distal catheter is directed toward the pelvis.

Malignant pleural effusions and chylothoraces are two of the most common indications for pleuroperitoneal shunting. Much has been written about shunting for intractable pleural effusions, the advantages of shunting over the more conventional forms of sclerotherapy being the simplicity of the procedure, the early hospital discharge, and the predictable excellent results. The disadvantages of the technique are the cost of the device, the need for manual pumping, the potential contamination of the peritoneum by malignant cells, and the possible occlusion of the conduit (15%) (Little et al, 1988). In a series of 17 patients in whom pleuroperitoneal shunts were implanted for pleural effusions, Ponn and colleagues (1991) reported palliation of dyspnea at rest in all patients. Four shunts became occluded between 1 and 10 months after placement, and two of these had to be replaced. Other series present similar data (Cimochowski et al, 1986; Little et al, 1986; Tsang et al, 1990; Weese and Schouten, 1984). Whether pleuroperitoneal shunting should be the first line of treatment for malignant effusions or whether it should be used only after other methods have failed remains controversial.

Pleuroperitoneal shunting may be useful in the management of persistent chylothorax. In 1989, Murphy and colleagues reported on 16 pediatric patients with refractory chylothoraces due to a variety of causes, in each of whom the chylothorax had been unresponsive to thoracentesis, tube thoracostomy, and dietary manipulation. Of the 16 patients, 12 had excellent results, with complete elimination of the chylothorax and resolution of symptoms following insertion of a pleuroperitoneal shunt.

COMPLICATIONS OF TUBE THORACOSTOMY

A variety of complications have been described in relation to tube thoracostomy, and the morbidity rate varies between 9% and 21% (Daly et al, 1985; Etoch et al, 1995) (Table 47–4). As for most other intrathoracic procedures, the incidence of complications is minimal when the procedure is indicated, well planned, and done with care, and when the operator has experience with the technique and is familiar with the local anatomy of the intercostal space (Moore, 1982). In a retrospective study, Etoch and colleagues (1995) showed that the overall complication

TABLE 47–4 ■ **Possible Complications of Tube Thoracostomy**

- Misplacement of the chest tube
  - Tube in the soft tissues of the chest wall
  - Tube in the wrong pleural space
  - Injury to intrathoracic structures: lung, diaphragm
  - Abdominal placement of the tube
- Hemorrhage
  - Cutaneous
  - Intercostal arteries
  - Injury to superior vena cava, inferior vena cava, heart
- Surgical emphysema
- Empyema
- Re-expansion pulmonary edema
- Intercostal neuralgia and thoracostomy lung herniation
- Miscellaneous rare complications
  - Horner's syndrome
  - Diaphragmatic paralysis
  - Necrotizing fasciitis
  - Chylothorax
  - Aortic obstruction

rate of tube thoracostomy done in trauma patients was higher if the technique was performed by emergency physicians as opposed to surgeons (13% versus 6%, respectively). These results emphasize that only well-trained personnel should execute these techniques.

In a questionnaire survey on chest tube management sent to junior medical practitioners in the Singapore area, up to 90% of respondents never attended a lecture on the subject, and only 25% gave appropriate answers to the questionnaire (Sim, 1996). Obviously, the potential for serious complications is higher in such settings, and Harris and Graham (1991) suggest that junior staff members should always be supervised when performing this technique.

Misplacement of Thoracostomy Tubes

An effort should always be made to avoid misplacement of chest tubes. One must make sure that the last hole of the tube is well inside the pleural space; obviously, a chest tube inserted in the wrong pleural space can have catastrophic consequences (Iberti and Stern, 1992). Careful review of the clinical history and radiographs should help in avoiding such complications. When the tube is not advanced far enough, it may cause a false air leak or the development of surgical emphysema (Fig. 47–14), or it may have physiologic consequences similar to those associated with an open pneumothorax. A tube advanced too far in can press against the parietal pleura, causing chest or shoulder pain (Iberti and Stern, 1992). The tube can also be kinked, thereby hindering optimal pleural drainage. Tube drainage will obviously be less than optimal if half or all of the chest tube is located in the soft tissues of the chest wall. Similar problems can result from inadequate suturing of the tube to the thoracostomy incision, accidental pullback by the patient, or loosening of the skin after prolonged drainage (Harris and Graham, 1991). Under these circumstances, it is often safer to reinsert another tube through a separate incision rather than risk infection by mobilizing the displaced catheter.

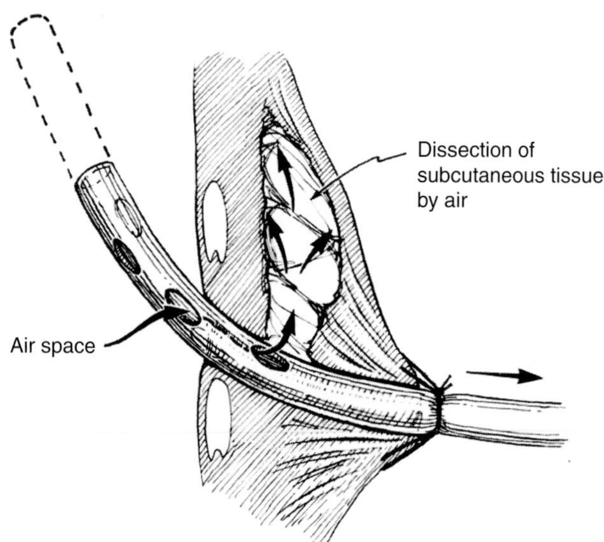

FIGURE 47–14 ■ Tube pullback in the soft tissues of the chest wall generating subcutaneous emphysema. (From Fishman NH: Thoracic drainage: A manual of procedures. Chicago–London, Mosby–Year Book, 1983.)

A number of intrathoracic organs are at risk of being injured when there is unchecked passage of chest tubes, usually with the trocar method (Temple, 1975). Lung perforation, for example, has been recognized both in children and adults, and its occurrence is said to be related to pre-existing intrinsic lung disease (Moessinger et al, 1978; Wilson and Krous, 1974), pleural adhesions, and the use of the trocar catheter. In 1988, Fraser suggested that the true incidence of this complication may be greater than appreciated because clear-cut clinical and radiologic evidences of perforation are usually absent. Prophylaxis against lung injury includes the use of clamp dissection and finger exploration of the pleural space before tube insertion. If lung injury is suspected, one should pull the tube back 1 to 4 cm and then wait until the air leak stops. Occasionally, the tube will be inserted into a large bulla that has been misinterpreted as a pneumothorax. When this is recognized, surgery may be required, or it may be decided to leave the tube as it is and wait until the air leak stops. Prophylaxis against this complication includes a high index of suspicion and use of CT scanning before chest drainage.

Diaphragmatic and intra-abdominal injuries are complications bound to happen when the diaphragm is elevated (fourth or fifth interspace), which occurs in obese individuals, in patients with diaphragmatic palsy (Foresti et al, 1992), in patients in supine position (Iberti and Stern, 1992), or after surgical procedures such as pneumonectomies. Although every organ in the upper abdomen is in jeopardy, the spleen, liver, and stomach are most often injured (Millikan et al, 1980; Robinson and Brodman, 1981). Shapira and colleagues (1993) have also described delayed perforation of a normal esophagus by a closed thoracostomy tube. In such cases, the clinical manifestations depend on the organ involved, its vascularity, and the existence of abdominal peritoneal adhesions (Robinson and Brodman, 1981). Some injuries may be apparent immediately; others may not become evident until after the tubes have been removed. Most injuries involving diaphragmatic perforation by the chest tube can be prevented by high placement of the intercostal tube and finger exploration of the thoracic space prior to tube insertion.

Hemorrhage

Minimal bleeding related to the thoracostomy incision is usually of no consequence. Intercostal artery injury with resulting massive bleeding is uncommon and is often related to placement of the tube close to the inferior border of the rib. It usually occurs in older patients, whose intercostal arteries are more tortuous (Carney and Ravin, 1979; Iberti and Stern, 1992). The internal mammary artery has also been severed during percutaneous thoracic interventions (Glassberg and Sussman, 1990). Left coronary artery and diaphragmatic artery lacerations with secondary cardiac hemorrhage and hemoperitoneum have also been described after thoracentesis (Heffner and Sahns, 1981; Sellier et al, 1994).

Massive hemorrhage can be secondary to injury to one of the cavae (Eriksson, 1982), the suprahepatic vein (Pagé and Verdant 1988; Weissberg and Fintsi, 1982), the right atrium (Casillas and de la Fuente, 1983; Meisel et al, 1990), the left ventricle (de la Fuente et al, 1994), the right ventricle, the main pulmonary artery (Van Kralingen et al, 1991), or the aorta (Koutras et al, 1969). These complications are rare and are almost always due to inadequate forceful trocar insertion of the chest tube. One known predisposing factor is the extreme mediastinal shift sometimes seen after pneumonectomy or in association with postlobectomy atelectasis. In such circumstances, the right ventricle is located underneath the anterolateral chest wall and is susceptible to tube injury, especially if the pericardium has been opened during prior pulmonary resection. If this type of penetration occurs, the tube should be clamped and the patient brought back to the operating room for immediate repair. At operation, the chest tube track is followed and the laceration repaired with a pledgeted suture. Occasionally, one may have to convert to a median sternotomy with pump standby to obtain good control of the injured vascular structure in the chest (Moore, 1979; Pagé and Verdant, 1988). If a major cardiac or vascular injury is suspected, one should never remove the tube in the patient's room, as exsanguinating hemorrhage is likely to follow. Van Kralingen and associates (1991) have even suggested leaving the trocar in, thereby preventing major blood losses. If the trocar has been removed, the tube should be clamped swiftly, and the patient rushed to the operating room for proper repair (Reuben, 1991; Weissberg and Fintsi, 1982).

Surgical Emphysema

Surgical emphysema can occur shortly after chest tube placement or during the days following tube insertion. It is always secondary to inadequate drainage of the pleural space as air reaches the subcutaneous tissues through the perforated pleura at the thoracostomy site. The problem may be due to improper location of the tube in the pleural space, as is seen when pleural adhesions are numerous; to occlusion of the tube or of the connecting tubes; to a large air leak, with inadequate absorption by the drainage unit; or to tube pullback in the soft tissues of the chest wall. When any of these occurs, the drainage system and thoracostomy site should first be thoroughly checked. If the whole system is airtight and the tube is functioning, the level of suction should be increased. If this does not solve the problem, the tube should be pulled back or another tube inserted.

Empyema

Because the incidence of empyema is low after tube drainage of a sterile collection, prophylactic antibiotic administration is not usually indicated. In a 1971 study, Neugebauer and colleagues examined the value of routine prophylactic antibiotic therapy following pleural space intubation. Those patients who received prophylactic antibiotic therapy had a higher rate of complications and a longer hospitalization period than those patients who did not receive antibiotics. In 1992, Hornick and co-workers reported no bacterial contamination of pleural fluid drainage in 38 postoperative patients, up to 6 days after tube insertion. They concluded that the underwater seal drainage system can be left in place close to 1 week postoperatively, without fear of contamination. However, all patients received prophylactic antibiotics for as long as the tubes were in place.

The incidence of empyema in acute trauma patients ranges from 1% to 16%, with an average of less than 3% (Etoch et al, 1995; Helling et al, 1989). In those patients, tube thoracostomy may contribute to infectious complications by providing a route for contamination, although most empyemas are probably the result of the injury itself or of inadequate drainage with incomplete re-expansion of the lung. In a study by Eddy and associates (1989), 6 of 12 patients with incomplete evacuation of the pleural space developed empyema, and none of the 105 patients with complete evacuation of the pleural space developed this complication. They recommended that if the pleural space cannot be completely evacuated with simple measures such as tube thoracostomy, early limited thoracotomy should be considered. The precise indication for antibiotics in the trauma setting needs further definition (Millikan et al, 1980), although LoCurto and colleagues (1986) have suggested that patients requiring tube thoracostomy for trauma, whether blunt or penetrating, should receive the benefit of systemic prophylactic antibiotic therapy. Davis and co-workers (1994), however, found no case of empyema in their series of 80 chest trauma patients, with no prophylactic antibiotic protocol.

Re-expansion Pulmonary Edema

Unilateral pulmonary edema and re-expansion hypotension are rare but potentially lethal complications. They occur when air or fluid is evacuated too rapidly in a patient with lung collapse that has persisted for longer than 3 days (Mahfood et al, 1988; Rozenman et al, 1996). Possible factors implicated in the pathogenesis of this complication include increased pulmonary vascular permeability, airway obstruction, loss of surfactant, and pulmonary artery pressure changes (Pavlin et al, 1986). The increased pulmonary vascular permeability is a particularly important etiologic factor, with the rapid re-expansion of a collapsed lung causing a rapid increase in pulmonary capillary pressure and blood flow (Ziskind et al, 1965). This in turn leads to fluid transportation across the capillary and alveolar membranes and results in an increase in pulmonary extravascular water (Sewell et al, 1978). Damage to the capillary and alveolar membranes may also be due to oxygen-derived free radicals found when hypoxic areas of the lung are reperfused and reventilated (Mahfood et al, 1988; Woodring, 1997).

Patients with this problem usually present with uncontrolled and progressive cough that may produce pink, frothy sputum, or even frank hemoptysis. They may also have tachypnea, tachycardia, diaphoresis, and pleuritic chest pain (Woodring, 1997). On auscultation, rales may be heard, and chest radiographs disclose unilateral pulmonary edema, usually within 1 to 24 hours after drainage (Iberti and Stern 1992; Woodring, 1997). It has been reported that some patients may be asymptomatic, and that radiologic edema may develop only in the portion of the lung that was collapsed before drainage (Woodring, 1997). According to Mahfood and associates (1988), this complication is fatal in about 20% of patients, although the edema is usually self-limited and resolves over a period of a few days in most (Woodring, 1997). To prevent its occurrence, the tube should be clamped and unclamped intermittently until resolution of the pneumothorax or drainage of the effusion is complete.

Intercostal Neuralgia and Thoracostomy Herniation

Placement of a chest tube may result in trauma or even transsection of the intercostal nerve, which can cause persistent postoperative pain. As was described in the 1966 edition of *Gray's Anatomy of the Human Body* (Goss, 1966) and by Moore (1982), the main branch of the intercostal nerves (T2 to T11) lies between the ribs rather than in the costal groove, and it may be traumatized during chest tube insertion. When this occurs, the patient experiences intercostal pain radiating anteriorly; this pain persists for some time after the tube has been withdrawn. Although these neuralgias can be quite painful on occasion, most are mild and self-limiting. Therapy consists of analgesia and reassurance; intercostal blocks are almost never required.

Damage to the long thoracic nerve can also occur with consecutive loss of innervation of the serratus anterior muscle, causing a winged scapula. Fortunately, this complication is rarely seen and can be avoided by careful blunt dissection beneath the skin (Iberti and Stern, 1992).

Intercostal herniation of pleural fluid or lung at the site of drainage is exceedingly rare, and management is generally conservative.

Miscellaneous Rare Complications

Horner's syndrome has been reported to occur following tube thoracostomy (Bourque and Paulus, 1986; Campbell et al, 1989; Dutro and Phillips, 1985; Fleishman et al, 1983; Kahn and Brandt, 1985). This syndrome may be permanent (Pearce et al, 1995), but is usually transient and is related to direct injury to preganglionic sympathetic fibers coursing near the apex of the lung. Hematoma or pressure ischemia over the sympathetic chain has also been implicated in the pathogenesis of this syndrome. Prophylaxis against this complication involves placement of the extremity of the tube below the level of the second or third rib. If Horner's syndrome is recognized after tube insertion, the tube should be pulled back or reinserted at another site.

Necrotizing fasciitis following tube insertion has been reported by Pingleton and Jeter (1983). In their case, the fasciitis followed drainage of an empyema containing anaerobic organisms, and the patient eventually died from multi-organ failure. Intrathoracic silicosis was described secondary to thoracostomy in the presence of mammary implants (Rice et al, 1995). Mediastinal perforation with contralateral pneumothorax (Gerard et al, 1993) and hemothorax (Rashid et al, 1998) have also been seen. In 1998, Olivier and colleagues reported on two sedated patients who experienced ulnar nerve palsy from a chest tube lying beneath their elbow.

Even though chest wall implantation of lung cancer has seldom been described after fine-needle aspiration biopsy, Sugi and co-workers (1997) reported a case of chest wall seeding at the drainage tube site after a right lower lobectomy for lung adenocarcinoma. Another exceedingly rare complication of tube thoracostomy in the form of a chest wall–to–lung arteriovenous fistula has also been reported (Cox et al, 1967).

In children, reported complications include diaphragmatic paralysis due to injury to the intrathoracic segment of the phrenic nerve (Odita et al, 1992; Palomeque et al, 1990), chylothorax secondary to trauma of the thoracic duct (Kumar and Belik, 1984), and aortic obstruction due to medially deployed thoracostomy tubes (Gooding et al, 1981).

COMMENTS AND CONTROVERSIES

Insertion of a chest catheter looks beguilingly simple but is fraught with the potential for major troubles. Missing the target of fluid or air is one thing, but spearing a bordering viscus is always serious and may convert what ought to be a small operation into an unexpectedly complicated one. Injury to the spleen or liver usually results from excessive enthusiasm to position the tube "in a dependent position," the operator forgetting that these organs lie underneath the ribs and ignoring the fact that the intubated patient is most likely to be supine anyway.

Less dramatic but important is the bleeding that may result from an undetected or forgotten coagulopathy, the most common being that induced by aspirin or warfarin. If a bleb is perforated, an air leak may be worsened or a new one created. Additionally, infection of the chest wall, residual numbness, and the memory of a painful insertion are unwelcome concerns.

More egregious errors include the insertion of a chest tube without review of the patient's history, physical findings, and chest films. Asking the radiologist to place a radiopaque marker near the target is no substitute for personal verification of the optimal site of the thoracostomy, let alone the need for it in the first place.

For most people, the prospect of a tube thrust deep into the chest is a matter of gravity. The prescription for allaying apprehension consists of one part sedation, two parts local anesthesia, and a heaping measure of quiet explanation. There is no excuse for allowing the patient to view the tray of surgical instruments.

The first step is to inject lidocaine hydrochloride (Xylocaine) around the intercostal nerve and wait several minutes for deep anesthesia to set in before proceeding. It should be remembered that the pleura may still be sensitive; additional infiltration takes only a few seconds. The same needle employed for anesthesia or a slightly larger one may then be used to probe for air or fluid and thus to verify the correctness of the chosen site. A hemostat applied to the needle at the point of penetration serves to steady it and to calibrate the interval from skin to cavity.

If the tube is being placed to evacuate a pneumothorax, the patient should be alerted to expect a paroxysm of coughing as the lung re-expands.

Once the tube is in position and is draining well, it must be secured so that it does not dislodge when the patient moves or is moved. Nurses need to be reminded that tubes should be fixed to bed linen with rubber bands and safety pins to ensure a straight lie. "Were an imaginary marble placed in the tube, it should roll continuously downhill." A sagging, fluid-filled tube works as well as a clamped tube.

Chest tubes should be removed in the morning, lest inadvertent introduction of air or recurrent pneumothorax stress nighttime services. Gloves should be worn! The patient has a right to know what to expect in the way of discomfort.

Most of the mentioned problems would be avoided if the invitation to "put in a chest tube" triggered the same sequence of reflection and concerned attention that is part of the routine for major thoracic surgery: Verify the diagnosis. Know the patient. Operate carefully. And do no harm.

C.A.H.

■ *KEY REFERENCES*

Fishman NH: Thoracic Drainage. A Manual of Procedures. Chicago, Year Book Medical Publishers, 1983.

A comprehensive and well-illustrated overview of drainage procedures.

Miller KS, Sahn SA: Chest tubes. Indications, techniques, management and complications. Chest 91:258, 1987.

Excellent review article on chest drainage and suction systems.

Munnell ER: Thoracic drainage. Ann Thorac Surg 63:1497, 1997.

Meticulous collective review on closed drainage and thoracic drainage systems.

Munnell ER, Thomas EK: Current concepts in thoracic drainage systems. Ann Thorac Surg 19:261, 1975.

Results of a survey done among thoracic surgeons about their views on pleural space drainage. Looks at tubes and drainage systems.

Rusch VW, Capps JS, Tyler ML, Pierson DL: The performance of four pleural drainage systems in an animal model of bronchopleural fistula. Chest 93:859, 1988.

Results of a carefully done analysis of the performance of four pleural drainage systems. Discussion on which unit is the best to drain high-volume or high-pressure leaks.

■ *REFERENCES*

Adegboye VO, Adebo OA, Osinowo O et al: Closed chest drainage without an underwater seal. Afr J Med Sci 25:353, 1996.

Aslam PA, Eastridge CE, Hughes FA: Insertion of apical chest tube. Surg Gynecol Obstet 130:1097, 1970.

Bar-El Y, Lieberman Y, Yellin A: Modified urinary collecting bags for prolonged underwater chest drainage. Ann Thorac Surg 54:995, 1992.

Batchelder TL, Morris KA: Critical factors in determining adequate pleural drainage in both the operated and non-operated chest. Am Surg 28:296, 1962.

Bayne CG: Pulmonary complications of the McSwain dart. Ann Emerg Med 11:136, 1982.

Black JJM: Securing intercostal drains (Letter to the editor). J Accid Emerg Med 16:462, 1999.

Bourque PR, Paulus EM: Chest-tube thoracostomy causing Horner's syndrome. Can J Surg 29:202, 1986.

Boyle A: Securing intercostal drains. J Accid Emerg Med 16:239, 1999.

Brunn H: Surgical principles underlying one-stage lobectomy. Arch Surg 18:490, 1929.

Bülau G: Für die Heber-Drainage bei Behandlung des Empyems. Z Klin Med 18:31, 1891.

Burge TS: Complications for prophylactic intercostal tube drainage including tension pneumothorax. J R Army Med Corps 138:138, 1992.

Campbell P, Neil T, Wake PN: Horner's syndrome caused by an intercostal chest drain. Thorax 44:305, 1989.

Capps JS, Tyler ML, Rusch VW, Pierson DJ: Potential of chest drainage units to evacuate broncho-pleural air leaks. Chest 88(Suppl):57, 1985.

Carney M, Ravin CE: Intercostal artery laceration during thoracentesis. Chest 75:520, 1979.

Casillas J, de la Fuente A: Right atrium perforation by a pleural drain. Report of a case with survival. Thorac Cardiovasc Surg 31:247, 1983.

Cerfolio RJ: Invited commentary. A new portable chest drainage device. Ann Thorac Surg 69:1001, 2000.

Churchill ED: Wound surgery encounters a dilemma. J Thorac Surg 35:279, 1958.

Cimochowski GE, Joyner LR, Fardin R et al: Pleuroperitoneal shunting for recalcitrant pleural effusions. J Thorac Cardiovasc Surg 92:866, 1986.

Collins JD, Shaver ML, Disher AC et al: Fluoroscopic chest tube insertion and patient care. J Natl Med Assoc 84:869, 1992.

Conces DJ, Tarver RD, Gray WC et al: Treatment of pneumothoraces utilizing small caliber chest tubes. Chest 94:55, 1988.

Couraud LL, Velly JF, N'Diaye M: Principles and techniques of chest drainage and suction. In Delarue NC, Eschapasse H (eds): Thoracic Surgery: Surgical Management of Pleural Diseases. In Deslauriers J, Lacquet LK (eds): International Trends in General Thoracic Surgery, Vol 6. St. Louis, CV Mosby, 1990, p 103.

Cox P, Keshishian J, Blades B: Traumatic arteriovenous fistula of the chest wall and lung. J Thorac Cardiovasc Surg 54:109, 1967.

Crocker HL, Ruffin RE: Patient induced complications of a Heimlich flutter valve. Chest 113:838, 1998.

Curtin JJ, Goodman LR, Quebbeman EJ et al: Thoracostomy tubes after acute chest injury: Relationship between location in a pleural fissure and function. AJR Am J Roentgenol 163:1339, 1994.

Dalbec DL, Krome RL: Thoracostomy. Emerg Med Clin North Am 4:441; 1986.

Daly RC, Mucha P, Pairolero PC et al: The risk of percutaneous chest tube thoracostomy for blunt thoracic trauma. Ann Emerg Med 14:865, 1985.

Davis JW, Mackersie RC, Hoyt DB et al: Randomized study of algorithms for discontinuing tube thoracostomy drainage. J Am Col Surg 179:553, 1994.

Davis LL: Easier chest tube insertion [Letter]. Ann Thorac Surg 43:688, 1987.

De la Fuente A, Sanchez R, Suarez J et al: Left ventricular perforation by a pleural tube. Texas Heart Inst J 21:175, 1994.

Deslauriers J: More about chest tubes and suction systems. In Delarue NC, Eschapasse H (eds): Thoracic Surgery: Surgical Management of Pleural Diseases. In Deslauriers J, Lacquet LK (eds): International Trends in General Thoracic Surgery, Vol 6. St. Louis, CV Mosby, 1990.

Deslauriers J, Grégoire J: Techniques of pneumonectomy. Drainage after pneumonectomy. Part I, Pneumonectomy. Chest Surg Clin N Am 2:437, 1999.

Deslauriers J, Liu G, Mousset X et al: On the use of chest tubes [Letter]. Chest 92:959, 1987.

Driver AG, Peden JG, Adams HG et al: Heimlich valve treatment of *Pneumocystis carinii*–associated pneumothorax. Chest 100:281, 1991.

Duncan C, Erickson R: Pressures associated with chest tube stripping. Heart Lung 11:166, 1982.

Dutro JA, Phillips LG: Ipsilateral Horner's syndrome as a rare complication of tube thoracostomy [Letter]. N Engl J Med 313:121, 1985.

Eddy AC, Luna GK, Copass M: Empyema thoracis in patients undergoing emergent closed tube thoracostomy for thoracic trauma. Am J Surg 157:494, 1989.

Enerson DM, McIntyre J: A comparative study of the physiology and physics of pleural drainage systems. Thorac Cardiovasc Surg 52:40, 1966.

Eriksson A: Fatal iatrogenic exsanguination from pleural drain insertion into the inferior cava. Thorac Cardiovasc Surg 30:191, 1982.

Etoch SW, Bar-Natan MF, Miller FB et al: Tube thoracostomy. factors related to complications. Arch Surg 130:521, 1995.

Fishman NH: Thoracic Drainage. A Manual of Procedures. Chicago, Year Book Medical Publishers, 1983.

Fleishman JA, Bullock JD, Rosset JS, Beck RW: Iatrogenic Horner's syndrome secondary to chest tube thoracostomy. J Clin Neuroophthalmol 3:205, 1983.

Foresti V, Villa A, Casati O et al: Abdominal placement of tube thoracostomy due to lack of recognition of paralysis of hemidiaphragm. Chest 102:292, 1992.

Fraser RS: Lung perforation complicating tube thoracostomy: Pathologic description of three cases. Hum Pathol 19:518, 1988.

Galloway PJ, King PM, Freeland P et al: Use of autosuture surgiport for pleural drain insertion. Injury 24:538, 1993.

Galvin IF, Gibbons JRP, Magout M et al: Placement of an apical chest tube by a posterior approach. Br J Hosp Med 44:330, 1990.

Gerard PS, Kaldawi E, Litani V et al: Right-sided pneumothorax as a result of a left-sided chest tube. Chest 103:1602, 1993.

Gift AG, Bolgiano CS, Cunningham J: Sensation during chest tube removal. Heart Lung 20:131, 1991.

Gill SS, Nkere UU, Walesby RK: An expansible cannula: A new technique for chest drain insertion. Thorax 47:657, 1992.

Gilsanz V, Cleveland RH: Pleural reaction to thoracostomy tube. Chest 74:167, 1978.

Glassberg R, Sussman S: Life-threatening hemorrhage due to percutaneous transthoracic intervention. Importance of the internal mammary artery. AJR Am J Roentgenol 154:47, 1990.

Godden J, Hiley C: Managing the patient with a chest drain: A review. Nurs Stand 12:35, 1998.

Gooding CA, Kerlan RC, Brasch RC et al: Medially deployed thoracostomy tubes: Cause of aortic obstruction in newborns. AJR Am J Roentgenol 136:511, 1981.

Gordon PA, Norton JM, Guerra JM et al: Positioning of chest tubes: Effects on pressure and drainage. Am J Crit Care 6:33, 1997.

Goss CM (ed): Gray's Anatomy of the Human Body, 28th ed. Philadelphia, Lea & Febiger, 1966.

Graham ANJ, Cosgrove AP, Gibbons JRP et al: Randomized clinical trial of chest drainage systems. Thorax 47:461, 1992.

Graham EA, Bell RD: Open pneumothorax: Its relation to the treatment of empyema. Am J Med Sci 156:839, 1918.

Grodzin CJ, Balk RA: Indwelling small pleural catheter needle thoracentesis in the management of large pleural effusions. Chest 111:981, 1997.

Grover FL, Richardson JD, Fewel JG et al: Prophylactic antibiotics in the treatment of penetrating chest wounds. J Thorac Cardiovasc Surg 74:528, 1977.

Guyton SN, Paull DL, Anderson RP: Introducer insertion of minithoracostomy tubes. Am J Surg 155:693, 1988.

Halejian BA, Badach MJ, Trilles F: Maintaining chest tube patency. Surg Gynecol Obstet 167:521, 1988.

Harris DR, Graham TR: Management of intercostal drains. Br J Hosp Med 45:383, 1991.

Hayes DF, Lucas CE: Bilateral tube thoracostomy to preclude fatal tension pneumothorax in patients with acute respiratory insufficiency. Am Surg 42:330, 1976.

Heffner JE, Sahns A: Abdominal hemorrhage after perforation of a diaphragmatic artery during thoracentesis. Arch Intern Med 141:1238, 1981.

Heimlich HJ: Valve drainage of the pleural cavity. Chest 53:282, 1968.

Helling TS, Gyles NR, Eisenstein CL et al: Complications following blunt and penetrating injuries in 216 victims of chest trauma requiring tube thoracostomy. J Trauma 29:1367, 1989.

Herbst CA: Indications, management, and complications of percutaneous subclavian catheters. An audit. Arch Surg 113:1421, 1978.

Hewett CF: Thoracenthesis: The plan of continuous aspiration. Br Med J 1:317, 1876.

Hiebert CH: Comments and controversies: Closed drainage and suction systems. In Pearson G, Deslauriers J, Ginsberg RJ et al (eds): Thoracic Surgery. New York, Churchill Livingstone, 1995, p 1133.

Hippocrates: Writings. In Hutchins RA (ed): Great Books of the Western World, Vol 29. Chicago, Encyclopedia Brittanica, 1952, p 142.

Hood RH, Dooling JA, Beddingfield GW et al: Drainage of the pleural space. Drainage tube composition in relation to complications. Ann Thorac Surg 2:94, 1966.

Hornick P, John LCH, Wallis J et al: Contamination of underwater seal drainage systems in thoracic surgery. Ann R Coll Surg Engl 74:26, 1992.

Howe B: Evaluation of chest suction with artificial thorax. Surg Forum 2:1, 1952.

Hyde J, Sykes T, Graham T: Reducing morbidity from chest drains [Editorials]. BMJ 314:914, 1997.

Iberti TJ, Stern PM: Chest tube thoracostomy. Crit Care Clin 8:879, 1992.

Ishikawa H, Satoh H, Yamashita T et al: Curved chest tube for drainage of malignant pleural effusion. Respir Med 92:633, 1998.

Jakob H, Kamler M, Hagl S: Doubly angled pleural drain circumventing the transcostal route relieves pain after cardiac surgery. Thor Cardiovasc Surg 45:263, 1997.

Johansson J, Lindberg CG, Johnsson F et al: Active or passive chest drainage after oesophagectomy in 101 patients: A prospective randomized study. Br J Surg 85:1143, 1998.

Joshi JM: Intercostal tube drainage of pleura: Urosac as chest drainage bag. J Assoc Physicians India 44:381, 1996.

Julian JS, Pennell TC: A review of the basics of closed thoracic drainage. NC Med J 48:127, 1987.

Kahn SA, Brandt LJ: Iatrogenic Horner's syndrome: A complication of thoracostomy tube replacement [Letter]. N Engl J Med 312:245, 1985.

Kam AC, O'Brien M, Kam PCA: Pleural drainage systems. Anesthesia 48:154, 1993.

Kang SS: Use of the disposable laparascopic trocar-cannula for chest tube insertion. J Am Coll Surg 179:230, 1994.

Klein J: Interventional techniques in the thorax. Clin Chest Med 20:805, 1999.

Koutras P, Kwon V, Holland RH, Webb WR: An unusual cause of perforation of the aorta. Ann Thorac Surg 8:575, 1969.

Kovarik JL, Brown RK: Tube and trocar thoracostomy. Surg Clin North Am 49:1455, 1969.

Kumar SP, Belik J: Chylothorax—a complication of chest tube placement in a neonate. Crit Care Med 12:411, 1984.

Kurihara Y, Galvin JR, Thompson BH et al: The utility of the frontal chest radiograph in the evaluation of chest drain placement. Clin Radiol 51:350, 1996.

Laforet EG, Boyd TF: Balanced drainage of the pneumonectomy space. Surg Gynecol Obstet 118:1051, 1964.

Lawrence GH: Closed chest tube drainage for pleural space problems. The primary therapeutic modality. Major Probl Clin Surg 28:13, 1983.

Light RW: Para-pneumonic effusions and empyema. Clin Chest Med 6:55, 1985.

Lilienthal H: Resection of the lung for suppurative infections with a report based on 31 consecutive operative cases in which resection was done or intended. Ann Surg 75:257, 1922.

Lim-Levy F, Babler SA, De Groot-Kosolcharoen J et al: Is milking and stripping chest tubes really necessary? Ann Thorac Surg 42:77, 1986.

Little AG, Ferguson MK, Golomb HM et al: Pleuro-peritoneal shunting for malignant pleural effusions. Cancer 58:2740, 1986.

Little AG, Kadowaki M, Ferguson MK et al: Pleural peritoneal shunting: Alternative therapy for pleural effusions. Ann Surg 208:443, 1988.

Lo LF, Mirza FA: Removal of chest tube using stomadhesive. Surg Gynecol Obstet 158:497, 1984.

LoCurto JJ, Tischler CD, Swan KG et al: Tube thoracostomy and trauma—antibiotics or not? J Trauma 26:1067, 1986.

Lodi R, Stefani A: A new portable chest drainage device. Ann Thorac Surg 69:998, 2000.

Macey BA, Landstrom LL: Replacing a chest-tube drainage-collection device. Am J Nurs 93:95, 1993.

Mahfood S, Hix WR, Aaron BL et al: Reexpansion pulmonary edema. Ann Thorac Surg 45:340, 1988.

Maimimi SE, Johnson FE: Tension pneumothorax complicating small-caliber chest tube insertion. Chest 97:759, 1990.

Mariani PJ, Sharma S: Iatrogenic tension pneumothorax complicating out patient Heimlich valve chest drainage. J Emerg Med 12:477, 1994.

Martino K, Merrit S, Boyakye K et al: Prospective randomized trial of thoracostomy removal algorithms. J Trauma 46:369, 1999.

Mattox KL: Prehospital care of the patient with an injured chest. Surg Clin North Am 69:21, 1989.
Maurer JR, Friedman PJ, Wing VW: Thoracostomy tube in an interlobar fissure: Radiologic recognition of a potential problem. AJR Am J Roentgenol 139:1155, 1982.
McGrath D, Kruger BK: Chest suction. Using mercury instead of water. Am J Nurs 62:72, 1962.
McKenna RJ, Fischel RJ, Brenner M, Gelb AF: Use of the Heimlich valve to shorten hospital stay after lung reduction surgery for emphysema. Ann Thorac Surg 61:1115, 1996.
McManus KG, Spence GM, McGuigan JA: Outpatient chest tubes [Personal communication]. Ann Thorac Surg 66:296, 1998.
Meisel S, Ram Z, Priel I et al: Another complication of thoracostomy—perforation of the right atrium. Chest 98:772, 1990.
Mellor DJ: A new method of chest drain insertion. Anesthesia 51:713, 1996.
Mercier C, Page A, Verdant A et al: Outpatient management of intercostal tube drainage in spontaneous pneumothorax. Ann Thorac Surg 22:163, 1976.
Meyer JA: Gotthard Bülau and closed water-seal drainage for empyema, 1875–1891. Ann Thorac Surg 48:597, 1989.
Miller J, Fleming WH, Hatcher CR: Balanced drainage of the contaminated pneumonectomy space. Ann Thorac Surg 19:585, 1975.
Miller JM, Ginsberg M, Lipin RJ et al: Clinical experience with streptokinase and streptodornase JAMA 145:620, 1951.
Miller KS, Sahn SA: Chest tubes. Indications, techniques, management and complications. Chest 91:258, 1987.
Millikan JS, Moore EE, Steiner E: Complications of tube thoracostomy for acute trauma. Am J Surg 140:738, 1980.
Minami H, Saka H, Kazuyoshi S et al: Small caliber catheter drainage for spontaneous pneumothorax. Am J Med Sci 304:345, 1992.
Moessinger AC, Driscoll JM, Wigger HJ: High incidence of lung perforation by chest tube in neonatal pneumothorax. J Pediatr 92:635, 1978.
Moore DC: Anatomy of the intercostal nerve: Its importance during thoracic surgery. Am J Surg 144:371, 1982.
Moore HV: Complications of thoracentesis and thoracostomy. In Cordell AR, Ellison RG (eds): Complications of Intrathoracic Surgery. Boston, Little Brown, 1979, p 351.
Morgan CV, Orcutt TW: The care and feeding of chest tubes. Am J Nurs 72:305, 1972.
Munnell E: Thoracic drainage. Ann Thorac Surg 63:1497, 1997.
Munnell ER, Thomas EK: Current concepts in thoracic drainage systems. Ann Thorac Surg 19:261, 1975.
Murphy MC, Newman BM, Rodgers BM: Pleuroperitoneal shunts in the management of persistent chylothorax. Ann Thorac Surg 48:195, 1989.
Neptune WB: Trocar for thoracostomy [Letter]. Ann Thorac Surg 23:195, 1977.
Neugebauer MK, Forsburg RG, Trummer MJ: Routine antibiotic therapy following pleural space intubation. J Thorac Cardiovasc Surg 61:882, 1971.
Niemi T, Hannukainen J, Aarnio P: Use of the Heimlich valve for treating pneumothorax. Ann Chir Gynaecol 88:36, 1999.
Nissen R, Wilson RHL: Pages in the History of Chest Surgery. Springfield, IL, Charles C Thomas, 1960.
Oakes LL, Hinds P, Rao B et al: Chest tube stripping in pediatric oncology patients: An experimental study. Am J Crit Care 2:293, 1993.
Odita J, Khan A, Dincsoy M et al: Neonatal phrenic nerve paralysis resulting from intercostal drainage of pneumothorax. Pediatr Radiol 22:379, 1992.
Olivier L, Peillon P, David G et al: Paralysie cubitale secondaire à un drainage thoracique prolongé. Ann Fr Anesth Réanim 17:55, 1998.
Pagé A, Verdant A: Suprahepatic vein perforation secondary to chest tube insertion [Personal communication], 1988.
Palomeque A, Canadell D, Pastor X: Acute diaphragmatic paralysis after chest tube placement [Letter]. Intensive Care Med 16:138, 1990.
Panicek DM, Randall PA, Witanowski LS et al: Chest tube tracks. Radiographics 7:321, 1987.
Pavlin DJ, Raghu G, Rogers TR et al: Reexpansion hypotension. A complication of rapid evacuation of prolonged pneumothorax. Chest 89:70, 1986.
Pearce SH, Rees CJ, Smith RH: Horner's syndrome: An unusual iatrogenic complication of pneumothorax. Br J Clin Pract 49:48, 1995.
Pecora DV: Post-thoracotomy suction [Letter]. Chest 79:613, 1981.
Pecora DV, Cooper P: Pleural drainage following pneumonectomy: Description of apparatus. Surgery 37:251, 1955.
Pickard LR, Beall AC: Portable suction device for use in patients with postoperative pleural air leaks. Ann Thorac Surg 36:103, 1983.
Pierson D: Persistent bronchopleural air during mechanical ventilation: A review. Respir Care Clin N Am 27:408, 1982.
Pingleton SK, Jeter J: Necrotizing fasciitis as a complication of tube thoracostomy. Chest 83:925, 1983.
Playfair GE: Case of empyema treated by aspiration and subsequently by drainage: Recovery. Br Med J 1:45, 1875.
Ponn RB, Blancaflor J, D'Agostino RS et al: Pleuroperitoneal shunting for intractable pleural effusions. Ann Thorac Surg 51:605, 1991.
Ponn RB, Silverman HJ, Federico JA: Outpatient chest tube management. Ann Thorac Surg 64:1437, 1997.
Powner D, Cline C, Rodman C: Effect of chest tube suction on gas flow through a bronchopleural fistula. Crit Care Med 13:99, 1985.
Prats I: Simplified chest tube removal: A new technique. Curr Surg 47:110; 1990.
Putnam JB, Roth JA, Walsh GL et al: Early cost comparison between tube thoracostomy vs. chronic indwelling pleural catheter (PLEURX) for treatment of malignant pleural effusion. Abstract presented at the Southern Thoracic Surgical Congress, Orlando, Florida, November 1998.
Rashid MA, Wilkström T, Örtenwall P: Mediastinal perforation and contralateral hemothorax by a chest tube. Thorac Cardiovasc Surg 46:375, 1998.
Reed DN, Vyskobil JJ, Rao V: Subcutaneous access ports with fenestrated catheters for improved management of recurrent pleural effusions. Am J Surg 177:145, 1999.
Reuben CF: Complications of thoracostomy [Letter to the editor]. Chest 100:886, 1991.
Rice DC, Agasthian T, Clay RP et al: Silicone thorax: A complication of tube thoracostomy in the presence of mammary implants. Ann Thorac Surg 60:1417, 1995.
Richards V: Procedures in family practice. Tube thoracostomy. J Fam Pract 6:629, 1978.
Ring EM, Shapiro MJ: The tunnel tip thoracic catheter. Surg Gynecol Obstet 169:553, 1989.
Riquet M, Chehab A, Souilamas R et al: Elective drainage of the apical chest by posterior approach. Ann Thorac Surg 66:1824, 1998.
Robinson G, Brodman R: Going down the tube [Editorial]. Ann Thorac Surg 31:400, 1981.
Roe BB: Physiologic principles of drainage of the pleural space with special reference to high flow, high vacuum suction. Am J Surg 96:246, 1958.
Roe BB: Improved technique for closure of thoracostomy incision. Surg Gynecol Obstet 121:845, 1965.
Röggla M, Röggla G, Muellner M et al: The cost of treatment of spontaneous pneumothorax with the thoracic vent compared with conventional thoracic drainage [Letter to the editor]. Chest 110:303, 1996a.
Röggla M, Wagner A, Brunner C et al: The management of pneumothorax with the thoracic vent versus conventional intercostal tube drainage. Wien Klin Wochenschr 108:330, 1996b.
Rozenman J, Yellin A, Simansky D: Re-expansion pulmonary oedema following spontaneous pneumothorax. Respir Med 90:235, 1996.
Runyon BA, Greenblatt M, Ming RHC: Hepatic chylothorax is a relative contraindication to chest tube insertion. Am J Gastroenterol 81:566, 1986.
Rusch VW, Capps JS, Tyler ML, Pierson DL: The performance of four pleural drainage systems in an animal model of bronchopleural fistula. Chest 93:859, 1988.
Russo L, Wiechmann R, Magovern J et al: Early chest tube removal after video-assisted thoracoscopic wedge resection of the lung. Ann Thorac Surg 88:1751, 1998.
Samelson SL, Goldberg EM, Ferguson MK: The thoracic vent: Clinical experience with a new device for treating simple pneumothorax. Chest 100:880, 1991.
Sargent E, Turner A: Emergency treatment of pneumothorax: A simple catheter technique for use in the radiology department. AJR Am J Roentgenol 109:531, 1970.
Sarniak RM: Randomized clinical trial of chest drainage systems [Letters to the editor]. Thorax 47:1086, 1992.
Sellier E, Billaud-Debarré C, Baron O et al: Une cause inhabituelle

d'épanchement péricardique au cours d'un drainage pleural. Ann Fr Anesth Réanim 13:421, 1994.
Semrad N: A new technique for closed thoracostomy insertion of chest tube. Surg Gynecol Obstet 166:171, 1988.
Sewell RW, Fewel JG, Grover FL, Arom KV: Experimental evaluation of reexpansion pulmonary oedema. Ann Thorac Surg 26:126, 1978.
Shapira OM, Aldea GS, Kupferschmid J et al: Delayed perforation of the esophagus by a closed thoracostomy tube. Chest 104:1897, 1993.
Sharma TN, Agnihotri SP, Jain NK et al: Intercostal tube thoracostomy in pneumothorax—factors influencing re-expansion of lung. Indian J Chest Dis Allied Sci 30:32, 1988.
Sim KM: A questionnaire survey on practice of chest tube management. Singapore Med J 37:572, 1996.
So SY, Yu DYC: Catheter drainage of spontaneous pneumothorax: Suction or no suction, early or late removal? Thorax 37:46, 1982.
Spouge AR, Thomas HA: Tension pneumothorax after reversal of a Heimlich valve. AJR Am J Roentgenol 158:763, 1991.
Stahley T, Tench W: Lung entrapment and infarction by chest tube suction. Radiology 122:307, 1977.
Stark DD, Federle MP, Goodman PC: CT and radiographic assessment of tube thoracostomy. AJR Am J Roentgenol 141:253, 1983.
Storey CF: Intrapleural suction. Is it being used to best advantage? [Editorial]. Ann Thorac Surg 6:196, 1968.
Storey CF, Laforet EG: The surgical management of bronchiectasis: A review based on the analysis of 100 consecutive resections. US Armed Forces Med J 4:469, 1953.
Sugi K, Nawata K, Veda K et al: Chest wall implantation of lung cancer at the drainage site: Report of a case. Surg Today 27:666, 1997.
Sweet RH: Thoracic Surgery. Philadelphia, WB Saunders, 1954, p 52.
Swenson EW, Birath G: Resistance to air flow in bronchospirometric catheters. J Thorac Surg 33:275, 1957.
Temple LJ: Hazards of Argyll trocar catheter [Letter]. Br Med J 1:334, 1975.
Teplitz L: Update: Are milking and stripping chest tubes necessary? Focus Crit Care 18:506, 1991.
Thal AP, Quick KL: A guided chest tube for safe thoracostomy. Surg Gynecol Obstet 167:517, 1988.
Tinckler LF: Self-retaining chest drainage tubes. Br J Surg 63:141, 1976.
Tomlinson MA, Treasure T: Insertion of a chest drain: How to do it. Br J Hosp Med 58:248, 1997.
Tsang V, Fernando HC, Goldstraw P: Pleuroperitoneal shunt for recurrent malignant pleural effusions. Thorax 45:369, 1990.
Tyson KRT, Schwartz MZ, Marr CC: "Balanced" thoracic drainage is the method of choice to control intrathoracic pressure following repair of diaphragmatic hernia. J Pediatr Surg 20:415, 1985.
Vallières E, Karmy-Jones R, Wood D: Early complications. Chylothorax. Part 2, Pneumonectomy. Chest Surg Clin N Am 9:609, 1999.
Van Hengel P, Van de Bergh JHAM: Heimlich valve treatment and outpatient management of bilateral metastatic pneumothorax. Chest 105:1586, 1994.
Van Kralingen KW, Stam J, Rauwerda J: Complications of thoracostomy [Letter to the editor]. Chest 100:3, 1991.
Von Hippel A: Chest Tubes and Chest Bottles. Springfield, IL, Charles C Thomas, 1970.
Von Hippel A: Correspondence. Ann Thorac Surg 20:721, 1975.
Waksman I, Bickel A, Szabo A et al: Use of endoscopic trocar-cannula for chest drain insertion in trauma patients and others. J Trauma 46:941, 1999.
Waller DA, Edwards JG, Rajesh PB: A physiological comparison of flutter valve drainage bags and underwater seal systems for postoperative air leaks. Thorax 54:442, 1999.
Watkins E: Principles of postoperative management in thoracic surgery. Surg Clin North Am 41:603, 1961.
Wayne MA, McSwain NE: Clinical evaluation of a new device for the treatment of tension pneumothorax. Ann Surg 191:760, 1980.
Webb WR, Laberge J: Major fissure tube placement [Letter]. AJR Am J Roentgenol 140:1039, 1983.
Weese JL, Schouten JT: Internal drainage of intractable malignant pleural effusions. Wis Med J 83:21, 1984.
Weissberg D, Fintsi Y: Unintentional placement of pleural drain in the hepatic vein. Thorac Cardiovasc Surg 30:412, 1982.
Wilson AJ, Krous HF: Lung perforation during chest tube placement in the stiff lung syndrome. J Pediatr Surg 9:213, 1974.
Woodring JH: Focal reexpansion pulmonary edema after drainage of large pleural effusions: Clinical evidence suggesting hypoxic injury to the lungs as the cause of edema. South Med J 90:1176, 1997.
Ziskind MM, Weill H, George RA: Acute pulmonary edema following the treatment of spontaneous pneumothorax with excessive negative intra-pleural pressure. Am Rev Respir Dis 62:632, 1965.

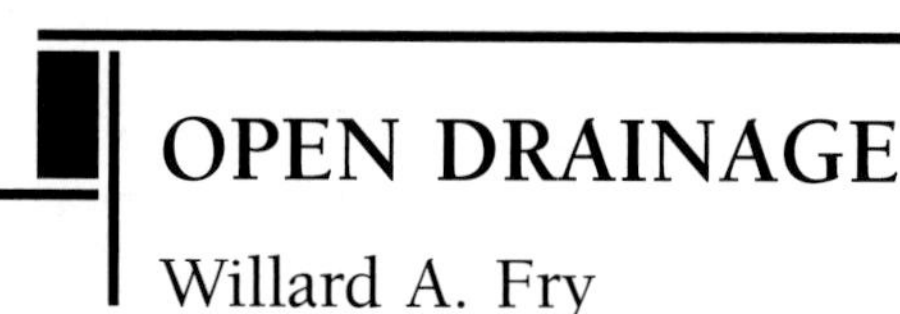

OPEN DRAINAGE

Willard A. Fry

Open drainage is an old-fashioned operation for an old-fashioned disease. It is usually accomplished with rib resection involving one or more ribs. Whereas it was once one of the very common operative procedures of the thoracic surgeon, it is currently used infrequently because other means of therapy, such as early tube thoracostomy and video-assisted thoracic surgical (VATS) débridement, have rendered it of limited use in the treatment of complicated parapneumonic effusions. However, this procedure should be in the surgical repertoire of the fully trained thoracic surgeon and used when indicated.

In general, there are three instances (Table 47–5) in which classic rib resection with open drainage is indicated: (1) Postpneumonectomy empyema, wherein the surgeon needs to have prolonged, adequate, and dependent drainage of the pneumonectomy space; (2) recurrent focal empyema for which an open procedure such as decortication does not seem indicated (usually the patient is in poor general condition and is not a good candidate for general anesthesia); and (3) focal empyema for which closed tube drainage or VATS débridement does not seem like a good surgical option. This would apply to a large posterior empyema for which tube drainage would be

TABLE 47–5 ■ **Indications for Rib Resection and Open Drainage**

Postpneumonectomy empyema
Recurrent focal empyema in a high-risk patient
Focal empyema with desire to avoid tube thoracostomy

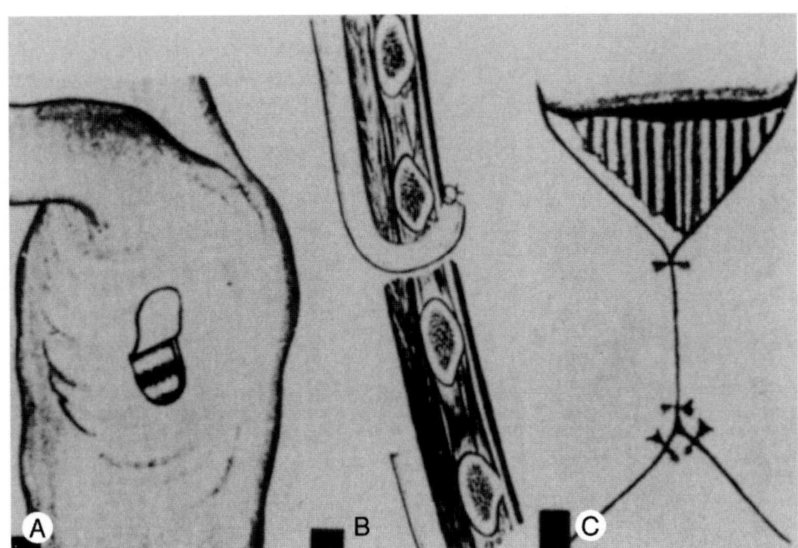

FIGURE 47–15 ■ Original Eloesser flap. This is not an open drainage in the sense of this chapter. It was an attempt to provide a one-way valve. In his paper, Eloesser promised follow-up information, but there was no additional publication. (From Eloesser LA: An operation for tuberculous empyema. Surg Gynecol Obstet 60:1096, 1935.)

uncomfortable and perhaps would preclude transfer to an extended care facility.

HISTORICAL NOTE

Surgeons in general are historically oriented, and it is the belief of the author that thoracic surgeons have a particular interest in surgical history. Certainly, it is hard for the thoracic resident to avoid knowing that in the fifth century BC, Hippocrates described incision and drainage of pointing thoracic abscesses. In a recent publication, Somers and Faber (1996) gave an excellent account of the history of open drainage for thoracic empyema. Earlier, Meade's (1961) *History of Thoracic Surgery* gave additional details in the development of the many and various treatments. Majno (1975) also includes interesting direct quotes from antiquity, such as "When the pus becomes as thin as water, slippery to the finger, and scanty, put into the wound a hollow tin drain."

With the development of chest radiography at the beginning of the 20th century, an earlier diagnosis of empyema became possible. During the great influenza epidemic of 1918, the traditional treatment of empyema, by rib resection and open drainage, led to an alarming treatment mortality. Bacterial pneumonia was often a complication of those influenza cases, and many pneumonias had complicated parapneumonic effusions that progressed to thoracic empyema. Rib resection and open drainage were often applied before loculations and adhesions had developed. Because the lung would not "hold up," an open pneumothorax was added to the clinical setting, and that contributed greatly to the disease mortality.

The Empyema Commission headed by Graham and Bell (1918) pointed out this problem and the resulting need to provide some form of initial closed drainage until adhesions were formed to hold the lung against the chest wall. Classically, when the pleural fluid from such a patient included more than 50% as a sediment overnight, one could empirically proceed to open drainage with the assurance that "the lung would stay up." This was true even in patients with a bronchopleural fistula. Those principles still apply today.

As a part of our thoracic surgical core, there is one confirmed story (Rasmussen, 2000) of a patient with open drainage complicated by chronic bronchopleural fistula, who appeared in Ripley's "Believe it or not" exposition of the Chicago World's Fair of 1933. This patient could keep his head immersed in a bucket of water for longer than 5 minutes. He kept his shirt on and maintained his respiration through the open drainage hole with its bronchopleurocutaneous fistula. The patient subsequently performed in various carnival shows in Michigan in the late 1930s and 1940s.

Open drainage is often called an Eloesser flap, although the procedure as originally described by Leo Eloesser (1935) was quite different (Fig. 47–15). His basic idea was to use a skin flap to function as a one-way valve for draining a chronic pleural effusion, often tuberculous, into the dressings. It is in reality quite different from the classic open drainage described in this chapter. In 1971, Symbas and associates described a U-shaped skin incision that was sutured to the pleura to maintain an open tract; that U-shaped incision subsequently became synonymous with an "Eloesser flap" (Fig. 47–16). The U-shaped incision works, but the author's opinion is that it has no advantage over the more standard oblique incision described here.

Rib resection with open drainage remains a safe, quick way to manage a focal empyema in a high-risk patient. The operation can be performed under local anesthesia, and it satisfies the three criteria for abscess drainage in that it is adequate and dependent, and it can be prolonged until the abscess cavity is obliterated (Table 47–6).

TABLE 47–6 ■ **Criteria for Empyema Drainage**

Adequate
Dependent
Prolonged

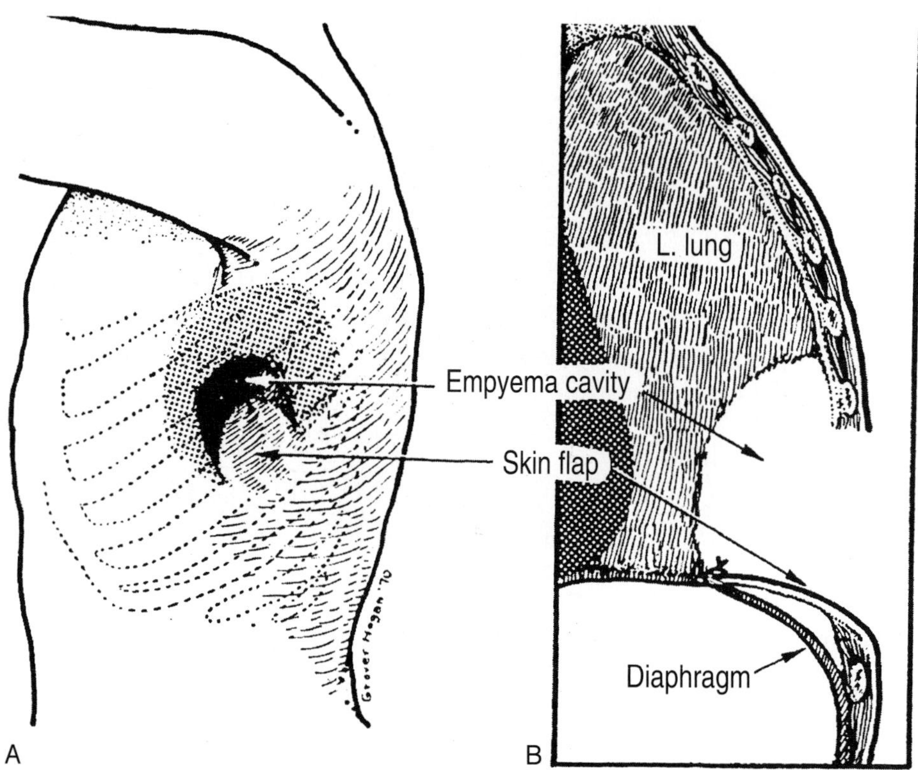

FIGURE 47–16 ■ Symbas' modification of the Eloesser flap. This was a paradigm for open drainage for many years, and it works. The putative benefit of the U-shaped incision is open for discussion (From Symbas PN, Nugent JT, Abbott OA et al: Nontuberculous empyema in adults. Ann Thorac Surg 12:69, 1971.)

In the postpneumonectomy state, total cavity obliteration does not occur spontaneously (Ali et al, 1996).

In tuberculous empyema patients, contraction and obliteration occur with time, even in advanced cases.

■ *HISTORICAL READINGS*

Ali SM, Siddiqui AA, McLaughlin JS: Open drainage of massive tuberculous empyema with progressive reexpansion of the lung: An old concept revisited. Ann Thorac Surg 62:218, 1996.

Eloesser LA: An operation for tuberculous empyema. Surg Gynecol Obstet 60:1096, 1935.

Graham EA, Bell RD: Open pneumothorax: Its relation to the treatment of acute empyema. Am J Med Sci 156:839, 1918.

Majno G: The Healing Hand. Cambridge, Harvard University Press, 1975, p 157.

Meade RJ: History of Thoracic Surgery. Springfield, IL, Charles C Thomas, 1961, pp 234–256.

Rasmussen RA: Personal communication, Grand Rapids, Michigan, February 13, 2000.

Somers J, Faber LP: Historical developments in the management of empyema. Chest Surg Clin North Am 6:403, 1996.

Symbas PN, Nugent JT, Abbott OA et al: Nontuberculous pleural empyema in adults. Ann Thorac Surg 12:69, 1971.

TECHNIQUE

The typical patient for an open drainage is an elderly patient in poor general condition with a recurrent or chronic, focal, posterior empyema cavity. It is also often a patient for whom general anesthesia is not recommended and who can be returned home or to an extended care facility once tube drainage is discontinued (Fig. 47–17).

Computed tomography (CT) scanning should always be done preoperatively as it helps to define the extent of disease, to demonstrate loculations, if there be any, and to reveal the exact location that is best for the incision (Fig. 47–18). With the patient appropriately positioned, an 8- to 12-cm incision is made parallel to the ribs and placed as closely as possible over the lower aspect of the empyema cavity. As has previously been discussed, the procedure can be carried out under local or general anesthesia. It is the opinion of the author that the U-shaped incision described by Symbas and colleagues (1971) provides no special benefit (Fig. 47–19). Other authors (Jacques and Deslauriers, 1995) have described an H-

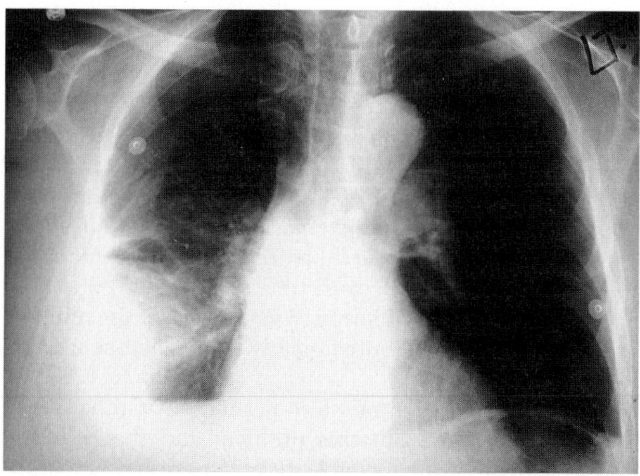

FIGURE 47–17 ■ Posteroanterior chest radiograph of a patient with recurrent empyema after unsuccessful videoassisted thoracic surgery treatment of a traumatic hemothorax. The patient had many medical co-morbidities and was a poor candidate for general anesthesia and time-consuming decortication.

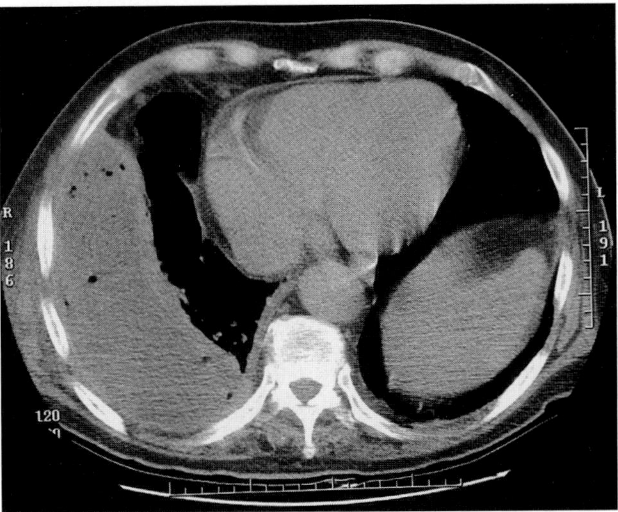

FIGURE 47–18 ■ A computed tomography of the patient in Figure 47–17. The empyema pocket is well localized and posterior. A chest tube would be very uncomfortable.

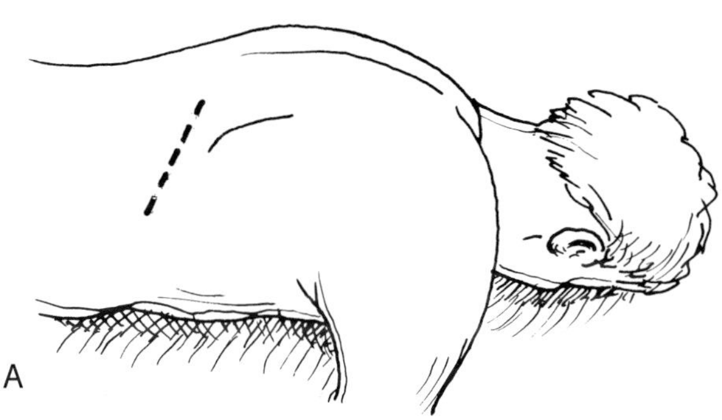

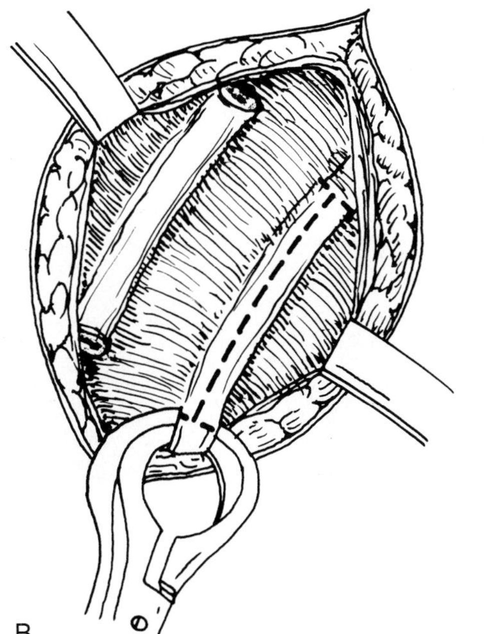

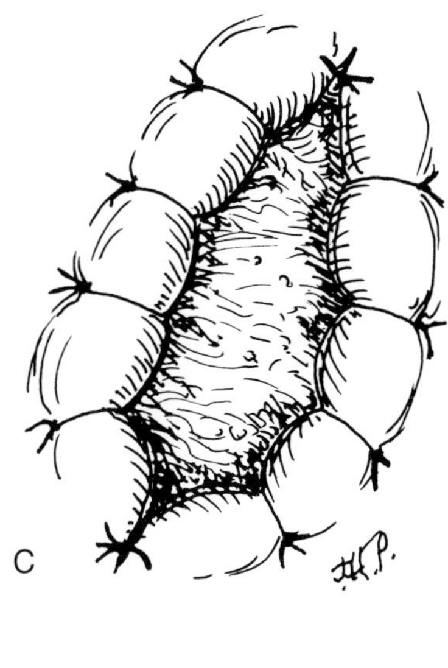

FIGURE 47–19 ■ Operative technique of open drainage. An incision is made in line with the ribs. Two ribs are resected, and the skin is sutured to the parietal pleura with absorbable suture to marsupialize the incision. (N.B.: The original artwork for this figure can be obtained directly from Dr. Willard Fry.)

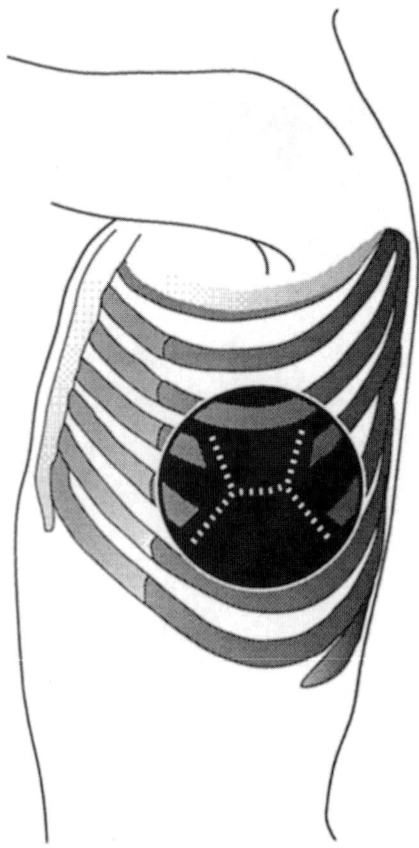

FIGURE 47–20 ■ The H-shaped incision that is recommended by some for open drainage but not by this author.

shaped incision that this author believes also offers no advantages (Fig. 47–20).

The electrosurgical unit is used for musculofascial dissection and hemostasis, and an 8- to 10-cm section of rib is removed subperiosteally. The pleural space is then entered and explored. In general, a second segment of rib is also removed to ensure that open drainage is truly adequate. The author believes that in most cases, two ribs need to be resected because as healing occurs, the skin opening can quickly contract down, leaving an inadequate aperture for drainage. This is also the reason why adequate lengths of ribs must be resected (Table 47–7).

Whether the second rib to be removed is above or below the originally resected rib is decided by the surgeon after careful inspection and palpation of the cavity, and keeping in mind that one wants to achieve optimal dependent drainage. The intercostal muscles with their neurovascular bundles should be ligated at each end with absorbable suture material. The midportion can then be removed, ensuring a large opening in the parietal wall. Nonabsorbable suture material such as silk should be avoided as this can become a nidus for infection. For the record, the size of the space is evaluated by noting the amount of irrigating fluid in milliliters that is needed to fill it.

Marsupialization of the open drainage is accomplished by suturing the skin to the parietal pleural edges with interrupted heavy absorbable sutures. These sutures can be removed at a later date, but in the event that there is a delay, or that the sutures are difficult to remove, they will not remain as permanent foreign bodies. The cavity is then loosely packed with absorbable gauze such as Kerlex, and dressings are applied.

An immediate chest radiograph following completion of the operation is essential to ensure that "the lung is up" and is adherent to the chest wall surrounding the drained cavity (Fig. 47–21). Traditionally, the initial packing was done with iodoform gauze or with gauze soaked in povidone-iodine, 5% or 10% (half or full strength), although the author is unaware of any clinical study that has shown such material to be superior to saline-soaked gauze. Indeed, those iodine-containing solutions are radiopaque; therefore, if they are used, the postoperative film can disturb the unfeathered (Fig. 47–22).

If there is a pneumothorax on the postoperative film, closed drainage must be instituted. Classically, a rubber glove was fashioned to cover the opening, the tip of one finger was cut, a chest tube draining the cavity was brought out through the opening in the finger and connected to an underwater seal, and the rubber glove was cut partially open and taped to the edges of the incision to make it "airtight." Nowadays, an airtight dressing can be fashioned from one of the currently used plastic adherent dressings.

After several days, a repeat chest radiograph can be taken with the patient off water-seal drainage, and if the lung is "held up," open drainage can be reinstituted. Because open drainage is done for chronic empyemas with established adhesions and not for an acute fibrinopurulent process, this complication should be a very rare event.

TABLE 47–7 ■ **Key Points in Rib Resection and Open Drainage**

Provide adequate incision
Resect two or more ribs
Ligate and remove intercostal muscle and bundles
Marsupialize with absorbable sutures

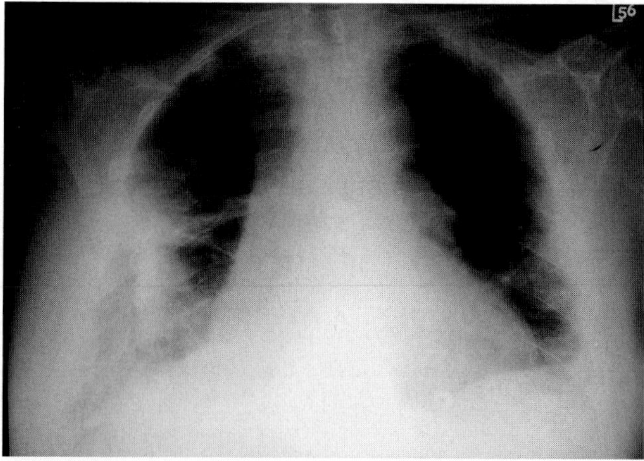

FIGURE 47–21 ■ Postoperative chest radiograph showing that the lung is expanded with no pneumothorax.

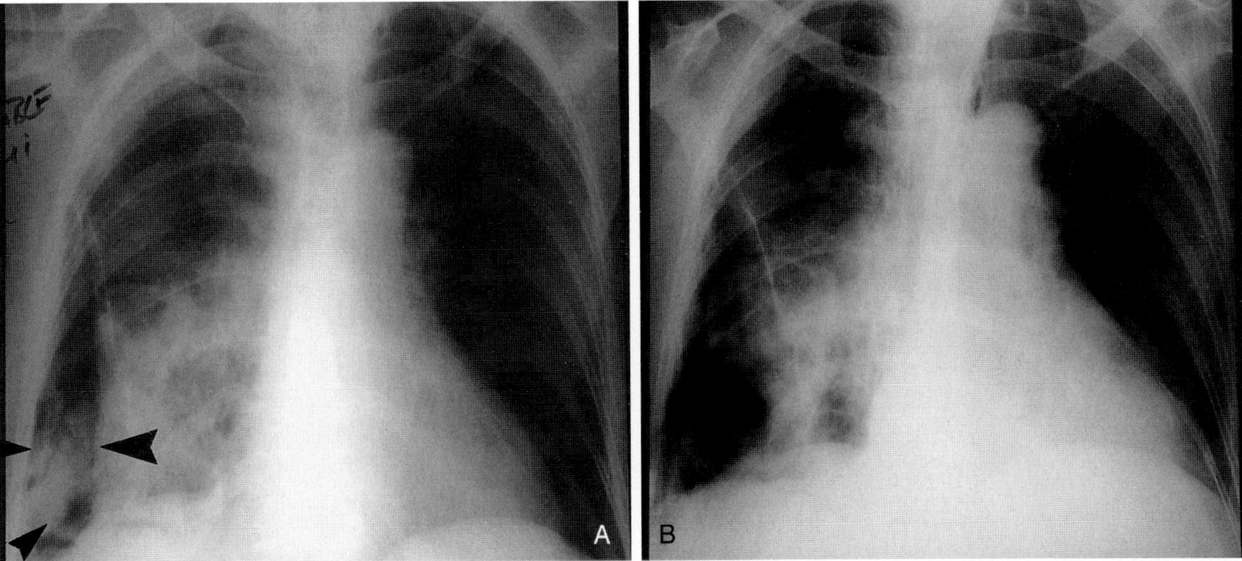

FIGURE 47–22 ■ The effect of iodine on chest radiograph when the drained cavity is packed with iodoform gauze or povidone-iodine soaked gauze. *A*, Note the "infiltrate" *(arrows)* in the drained empyema space. *B*, Chest film taken the day after the iodoform pack was removed and replaced with saline-soaked gauze.

POSTOPERATIVE CARE

Dressings are changed as needed but at least daily and are repacked initially with saline-soaked gauze. If these dressing changes are done gently, they are well tolerated, even initially. Periodically, the volume of the space can be measured by recording the number of milliliters of water or saline needed to fill it (Fig. 47–23). After several weeks, the skin sutures used for marsupialization can be removed, if they are still present.

Initially, the patient and relatives will need to be reassured that the cavity will contract and close, but over many weeks. The initial viewing by the patient and family can also be a surprise if the surgeon has not taken care to discuss the issue in advance. Once the patient is mobile, he or she can get into the shower or bath, and if a hose and nozzle are available, the cavity can be irrigated with ordinary tap water.

Loose dressings are needed to absorb the expected drainage. Initially, adhesive tape dressings can be used for the dressings. but over time they irritate the skin, so that Montgomery straps with laces may be more appropriate. The author's preference is to wrap the patient with 6- or 8-inch elastic wraps, as these do not irritate the skin and can be laundered with ease at home. Follow-up chest radiographs are taken at appropriate intervals, usually every 4 to 6 weeks until cavity obliteration has occurred (Fig. 47–24). Over time, which can be weeks or months, the skin will heal with a slight dimple as the cavity contracts (Fig. 47–25). Should the final healing dimple be cosmetically undesirable to the patient, the scar can be excised and revised under local anesthesia.

In the overall management of these patients, the im-

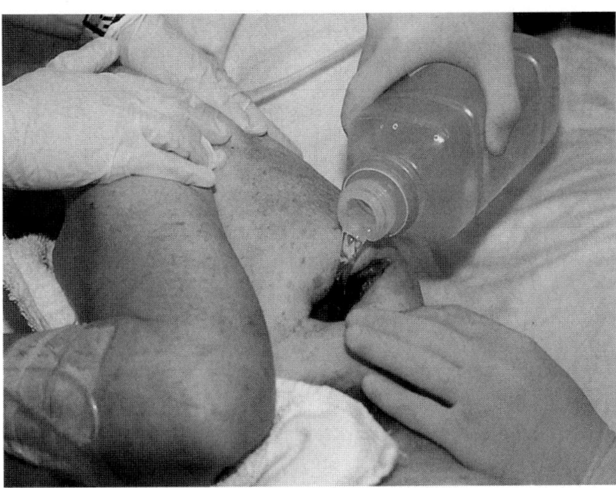

FIGURE 47–23 ■ Measuring the volume of the space. Water or saline is poured in the cavity, and the amount is noted.

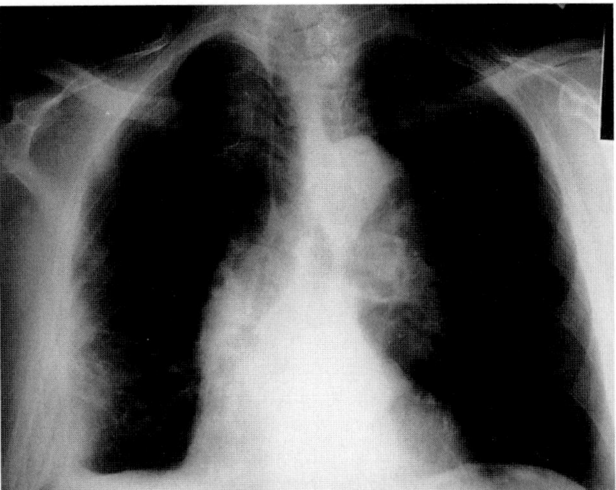

FIGURE 47–24 ■ Posteroanterior chest radiograph of the patient in Figures 47–17 and 47–18 after open drainage and showing complete obliteration of the space.

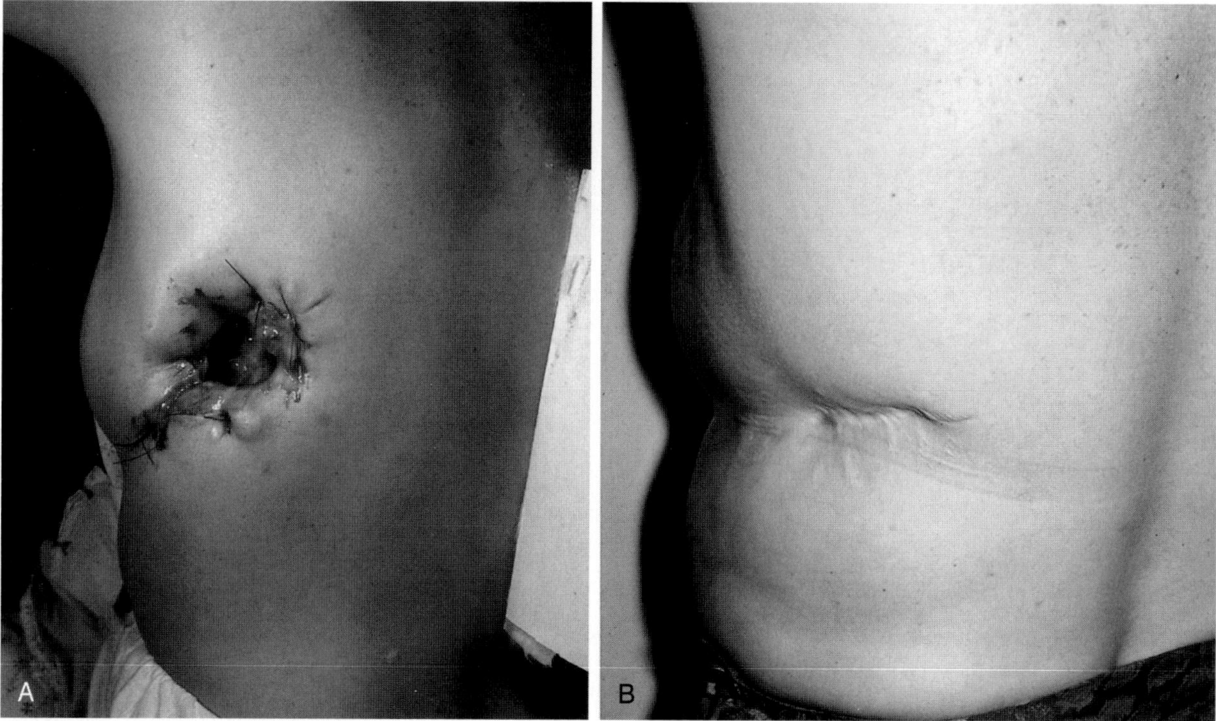

FIGURE 47–25 ■ *A*, Open drainage freshly done. Note the size of the drainage hole. *B*, After weeks, there remains only a cosmetically acceptable depressed scar.

portance of adequate nutrition is obvious and cannot be overemphasized.

COMMENTS AND CONTROVERSIES

Although we agree with Fry that open window thoracostomy (OWT) can be done under local anesthesia, it is much easier and safer to carry it out under general anesthesia with which an appropriate number of ribs can be removed in an unhurried manner. As has been pointed out by Fry, open window thoracostomies have a tendency to contract down so that at least two ribs, and preferably three, should be removed to avoid the risk that the skin opening will get too small and will have to be revised. I prefer the use of an H-type incision when performing an OWT because it allows the making of larger skin flaps, which then are used to marsupialize the undersurface of the window.

After the OWT has been done, I use petroleum jelly gauzes for the first packing of the space. This is done because the first dressing change is not undertaken until 3 to 4 days postoperatively (to avoid bleeding), and such gauzes are easier and less painful to remove after that length of time. After the first dressing change, which is always done by the surgeon, subsequent changes are carried out by nurses on a daily basis, or more often if necessary. For the first few weeks, I recommend dry dressings or dressings slightly moistened with physiologic saline solution or Dakin's solution (strength of 1/32).

When the space is packed, gauzes are tied to each other so that they are easier to remove and one is certain that none is forgotten inside the space. In some cases, a forgotten gauze inside the space can be the source of chronic purulent drainage which will stop with the removal of the gauze.

If one is careful with the timing of OWT, a pneumothorax should never occur, and I have never been obliged to use the technique described by Fry for such an event. Obviously, an OWT should never be carried out when one is unsure whether the underlying lung is fixed to the chest wall by dense adhesions. I agree with Fry that given time, most OWTs become completely obliterated through lung re-expansion, wall contraction, and skin re-epithelialization.

Overall, OWT is well tolerated despite the inconveniences of daily wound care. It is an infrequently used procedure but for patients in poor medical condition, it is very useful for achieving optimal drainage of chronic empyemas.

In 1971, Symbas and colleagues reported the results of OWT for the treatment of empyema in 34 patients. Complete healing of the empyema cavity occurred in all patients within a median time of $3\frac{1}{2}$ months after the operation. All patients had good long-term results, and only two required revision of the stoma because of early closure.

J.D.

KEY REFERENCES

Hurvitz RJ, Tucker BL: The Eloesser flap: Past and present. J Thorac Cardiovasc Surg 92:958, 1986.

Describes the modifications in both concept and design that have happened to the Eloesser flap over the years. Excellent description of the history of the flap.

Symbas PN, Nugent JT, Abbott OA et al: Nontuberculous empyema in adults. Ann Thorac Surg 12:69, 1971.

This is an excellent case series of patients who underwent open drainage for a variety of conditions.

■ *REFERENCES*

Ali SM, Siddiqui AA, McLaughlin JS: Open drainage of massive tuberculous empyema with progressive reexpansion of the lung: An old concept revisited. Ann Thorac Surg 62:218, 1996.

Eloesser LA: An operation for tuberculous empyema. Surg Gynaecol Obstet 60:1096, 1935.

Graham EA, Bell RD: Open pneumothorax: Its relation to the treatment of acute empyema. Am J Med Soc 156:839, 1918.

Hurvitz RJ, Tucker BL: The Eloesser flap: Past and present. J Thorac Cardiovasc Surg 92:958, 1986.

Jacques LF, Deslauriers J: Open drainage. In Pearson FG, Deslauriers J, Ginsberg RJ et al (eds): Thoracic Surgery. New York, Churchill Livingstone, 1995, pp 1136–1140.

Majno G: The Healing Hand. Cambridge, Harvard University Press, 1975, p 157.

Meade RJ: History of Thoracic Surgery. Springfield, IL, Charles C Thomas, 1961, pp 234-256.

Rasmussen RA: Personal communication, Grand Rapids, Michigan, February 13, 2000.

Somers J, Faber LP: Historical developments in the management of empyema. Chest Surg Clin N Am 6:403, 1996.

Symbas PN, Nugent JT, Abbott OA et al: Nontuberculous pleural empyema in adults. Ann Thorac Surg 12:69, 1971.

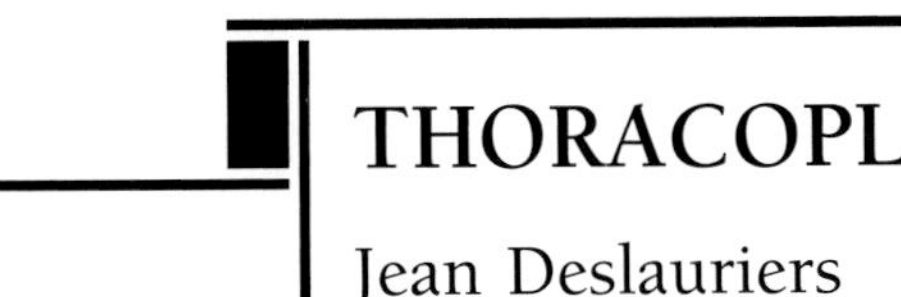

THORACOPLASTY

Jean Deslauriers
Jocelyn Grégoire

Thoracoplasty is a surgical procedure originally designed to permanently collapse the cavities of pulmonary tuberculosis by removing the ribs from the chest wall. Until supplanted by effective chemotherapy, it was one of several methods used to put the lung to rest with the hope of inactivating the disease. Other methods such as artificial pneumothoraces, intercostal neurectomy, scalenotomy, and phrenic nerve interruption were also used with variable results for the same purpose.

Thoracoplasty is currently being used for the treatment of patients with chronic pleural space infection in whom the lung cannot be expanded. Since the early 1960s, however, it has lost much of its popularity not only because it is considered a mutilating procedure but also because of the advent of better techniques of muscle transfer to fill infected spaces.

In spite of this "bad press," there remain a few patients with chronic empyemas with no remaining lung or with a lung that cannot be expanded because of intrinsic disease, who are potential candidates for thoracoplasty. In this chapter, we describe the important technical points to consider while one is performing a thoracoplasty. We also attempt to define the role of this procedure in the context of contemporary thoracic surgery.

HISTORICAL NOTE

Estlander (1879) was the first surgeon to use the term *thoracoplasty* to denote removal of ribs for the purpose of bringing the chest wall down to the lung (Young and Moor, 1976). In 1885, De Cerenville of Lausanne also described a technique in which short segments of two or more ribs were resected with the goal of collapsing the chest wall over areas of apical cavitary tuberculosis.

The thoracoplasty described by Schede in 1890 was an operation that included not only multiple rib resections but also the removal of the periosteum, intercostal muscles and nerves, and parietal pleura. In 1896, Paget (Langston, 1991) provided a description of the technique of thoracoplasty as described by Schede at the medical conference in Vienna in 1890:

> "Using a large U-shaped incision carried to rib level, a flap of skin and extracostal soft tissue is created and raised. All the ribs over the cavity are resected subperiosteally, from a point a little beyond their angles posteriorly to the costochondral junction anteriorly. The ribs are divided at about their midpoint with bone forceps. The cut ends are drawn apart and broken up. Anteriorly, they break at the costochondral junction, and posteriorly, they always break at or close to the tubercule."

According to Kergin (1953), the Schede thoracoplasty was formulated on the basis of accurate knowledge of the pathology of chronic empyemas but it had serious disadvantages: It was shocking and mutilating; it involved the resection of intercostal nerves with resulting cutaneous anesthesia; and it left a large open wound, which required a long period of packing and dressing.

In 1907, Friedrich, following Rudolph Brauer's (an internist) suggestion that thoracoplasty must collapse the diseased lung (Young and Moor, 1976), resected full lengths of the second to the ninth rib with an operative mortality of 43% (four of seven patients survived the operation). Subsequently, Wilms (1913) and Sauerbruch (1925) resected the posterior segments of the first 11 ribs during an operation that became known as the *paravertebral thoracoplasty*. They pointed out that resection of the posterior ribs would bring about a greater collapse of the underlying lung than would resection of the more anterior segments.

All these procedures evolved into the classical three-stage thoracoplasty popularized in 1925 by John Alexander (1925, 1937), which involved resecting the posterior segments of the ribs and sometimes portions of the transverse processes, but leaving the periosteum, to ensure that new bone formation would maintain long-term collapse of the lung. The following outline of the first stage of Alexander's thoracoplasty (1937) is given by Langston (1991):

"A periscapular incision permitted elevation of the scapula. The upper digitations of the serratus anterior muscle were separated. The third and second ribs were resected subperiosteally from the level of the transverse process to approximately the mid and anterior axillary lines, respectively. The first rib and its cartilage was resected, along with the tip of the transverse process, to the sternum. The second and third transverse processes with the underlying rib were resected to the level of the lamina of the vertebra. The periosteal beds were dried and rubbed with 10% formalin to delay regeneration. The wound was closed without drainage."

The second and third stages followed at 3-week intervals, and using this technique, Alexander was able to achieve cavity closure in 93% of survivors with an operative mortality of 10%.

In 1934, Semb described an important addition to the technique of thoracoplasty, which he called *extrafascial apicolysis*. His method consisted of extrapleural division of all adhesions between the pleural dome at the apex and the soft tissues around the base of the neck and cervical spine. This dissection, carried out outside the plane of the endothoracic fascia, provided more complete collapse of the lung without requiring resection of the transverse processes of the vertebrae.

Because conventional thoracoplasty was considered cosmetically unacceptable, other surgeons described plombage thoracoplasty, introduced by Tuffier in 1891 as a method of extrapleural pneumolysis. By means of this procedure, air was insufflated extrapleurally to maintain lung collapse. Subsequent variations included the use of omentum (Tuffier, 1914) or paraffin extrapleurally or of other products such as lucite balls between the freed periosteum and the ribs.

In contemporary thoracic surgery, thoracoplasty is seldom used; indeed most young surgeons have never seen a single case, let alone performed the procedure.

■ *HISTORICAL READINGS*

Alexander J: The Surgery of Pulmonary Tuberculosis. Philadelphia, Lea & Febiger, 1925.

Alexander J: The Collapse Therapy of Pulmonary Tuberculosis. Springfield, IL, Charles C Thomas, 1927.

de Cerenville EB: De l'intervention dans les maladies du poumon. Rev Med Suisse Normande 5:441, 1885.

Estlander JA: Résection des côtes dans l'empyème chronique. Rev Med Chir (Paris) 3:157, 1879.

Friedrich PL: Die operative beeinflubsung einseitiger lungphtliser lurch totale brustwandmobilisierung. Arch Klin Chir 27:588, 1908.

Kergin FG: An operation for chronic pleural empyema. J Thorac Surg 26:430, 1953.

Langston HT: Thoracoplasty: The how and why. Ann Thorac Surg 52:1351, 1991.

Paget S: The Surgery of the Chest. Bristol, England, John Wright and Co, 1896. (As reproduced for Classics of Surgery by Grypron Editions, Birmingham, England, 1990, pp 275–279.)

Sauerbruch E: Die chirurgie der brustorgane, Vol 12. Berlin, Springer-Verlag, 1925 p 876.

Schede M: Die behandlung der empyeme. Verh Long Innere Med Wiesbaden 9:41, 1890.

Semb C: Technique of plastic operation of apicolysis. Acta Chir Scand 74:478, 1934.

Tuffier T: État actuel de la chirurgie intrathoracique. Paris, Masson, 1914, pp 90, 163.

Wilms M: Die pfeilerresektion der Rippen Zur Verengerung des thorax bei lungentuberculose. Ther Gegenhwart 54:17, 1913.

Young WG, Moor GF: The surgical treatment of pulmonary tuberculosis. In Sabiston DC, Spencer FC (eds): Gibbon's Surgery of the Chest, 3rd ed. Philadelphia, WB Saunders, 1976, p 567.

BASIC SCIENCE

Although the techniques of thoracoplasty in current use are numerous and varied in their details (Peppas et al, 1993), the principles involved in the operation remain as described by Alexander (Young and Ungerleider, 1990):

1. There is a better chance that thoracoplasty will be successful in patients whose empyema is not postresectional.
2. A tailoring thoracoplasty performed concomitantly with pulmonary resection has a high likelihood of failure because of poor chest wall mechanics during the postoperative period.
3. The chances for a successful response to thoracoplasty are characteristically increased if the procedure is preceded by large open-window drainage for which the tube has been inserted through a hole created by resection of a portion of rib.
4. It is especially critical that the first rib be resected for apical space obliteration, as well as a portion of the transverse process if the space is posterior.
5. Preoperative preparation is especially important, including complete control of tuberculous infection and the use of at least one additional antitubercle drug to cover potential activation during the surgical procedure.
6. Thoracoplasty of any type should not be used in "undefined desperation cases" in which uncontrolled sepsis is present, cancer persists, or unidentified sites of hemorrhage exist.

Types of Thoracoplasty

The various types of thoracoplasty are shown in Table 47–8.

A thoracoplasty is total if the posterior segments of the first eleven ribs are removed, and partial if only eight or nine ribs are resected. An extended thoracoplasty removes, in addition to the posterior segments of the ribs, the anterior extremities of the upper ribs (Fey et al, 1955). Most thoracoplasties are done subperiosteally because the ribs can regenerate when the periosteum is left in place. When both rib and periosteum are removed, the procedure is called an *extraperiosteal thoracoplasty.*

A pedicled myoplasty may be added to the thoracoplasty (thoracomyoplasty) when the space to be obliterated is large, or when it appears that an associated bronchopleural fistula is unlikely to close with collapse alone (Barker et al, 1971; Jaretzki, 1991; Pairolero and Trastek, 1990).

TABLE 47–8 ■ Types of Thoracoplasty

INTRAPLEURAL THORACOPLASTY	
Schede (1890):	Resection of ribs, parietal pleura, intercostal muscles, and neurovascular bundles
Heller (1934):	Preservation of intercostal muscles
Kergin (1953):	Excision of parietal pleura and fibrous tissue from intercostal muscles
Horrigan and Snow (1990):	Limited rib resection
EXTRAPLEURAL THORACOPLASTY	
Alexander (1937):	Resection of ribs but retention of periosteum, intercostal muscles, and parietal pleura
Semb (1935):	Extrafascial pneumolysis
Björk (1954):	Osteoplastic thoracoplasty
PLOMBAGE THORACOPLASTY	
Tuffier (1891):	Extrapleural plombage
Modern version (1949–50):	Extrafascial and extraperiosteal plombage
Andrews' thoracomyoplasty (1961)	
Sawamura's technique (1985)	
LIMITED AND TAILORING THORACOPLASTIES	

Intrapleural Thoracoplasty

As has been described by Schede (1890), intrapleural thoracoplasty involves multiple rib excisions, as well as resection of the parietal pleura, periosteum, intercostal muscles, and intercostal neurovascular bundles. Only the skin and thoracic muscles remain to collapse over the residual lung or space; a large open wound is left, with packing to fill the space. To prevent bleeding from the posterior intercostal arteries, Schede compressed each vessel between "thumb and forefinger first" before cutting and ligating it afterward (Langston, 1991).

The Schede thoracoplasty was performed mostly in those patients in whom the walls of the space were so thick that rib resection alone would be insufficient to appropriately collapse the cavity. The procedure, which is no longer done, was considered a mutilating operation; this was further compounded by severe cutaneous anesthesia and abdominal wall paresis, which eventually led to chest wall instability, paradox, and even cardiac exposure in some instances (Barker, 1994).

Modifications of the technique were therefore proposed by Heller (1934) and Wangensteen (1935). These surgeons described an operation in which, after removal of the ribs overlying the cavity, the rib beds were incised to create a series of ribbons, each consisting of an intercostal muscle with the accompanying vessels, nerve, parietal pleura, and fibrous tissue (Kergin, 1953). These ribbons were dropped into the cavity to act as space fillers.

Grow (1946) and Kergin himself (1953) described an operation by which they excised the parietal pleura and fibrous tissue from those ribbons so that they became more flexible in adapting to all corners of the empyema cavity (Fig. 47–26). The main advantages of the Kergin thoracoplasty were that the intercostal nerves were preserved and the ribs were able to regenerate, thereby giving stability to the chest wall. In addition, the space was filled with living tissue with an excellent vascular supply. Horrigan and Snow (1990) used a similar technique but confined the rib removal below the third rib to the more posterior aspect of the chest. They used adjacent trapezius, latissimus, serratus, or rhomboid muscle to reinforce the fistula closure and fill the space. The results were good and severe deformity was avoided in most patients.

Extrapleural Thoracoplasty

The extrapleural thoracoplasty was popularized by Alexander (1937) as a procedure that retains the periosteum of the ribs, the intercostal muscles, and the parietal pleura. It provides lateral collapse of the lung. Because the apex is often held up at the level of the cervical spine by strong muscular and fibrous bands, Semb (1935)

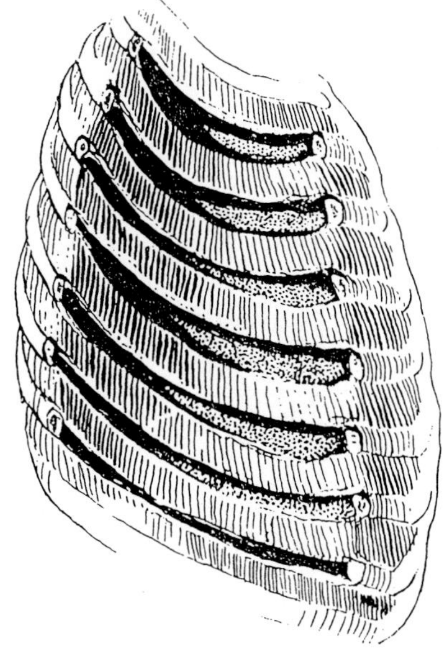

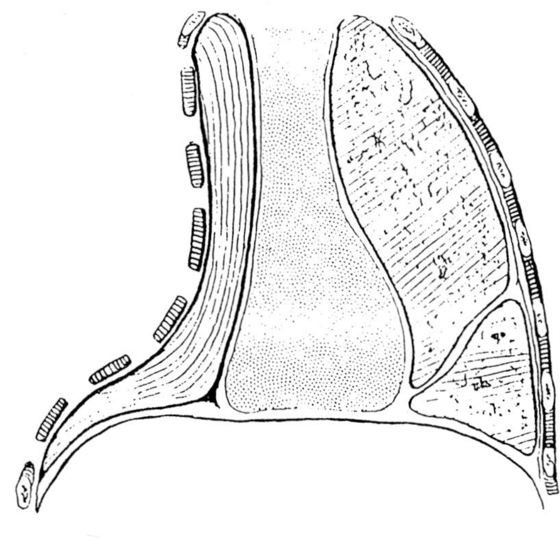

FIGURE 47–26 ■ After resection of the parietal wall, the muscle bundles are laid in the cavity. (From Kergin FG: An operation for chronic pleural empyema. J Thorac Surg 26:430, 1953.)

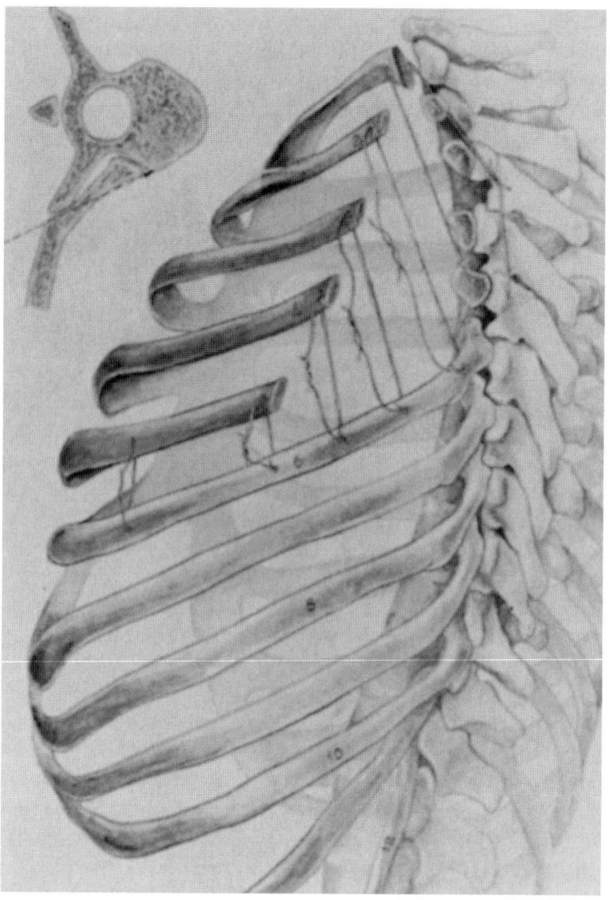

FIGURE 47–27 ■ The posterior ends of the upper five ribs are resected in increasing lengths. (From Björk VO: Thoracoplasty: A new osteoplastic technique. J Thorac Surg 28:194, 1954.)

proposed the operation of extrafascial apicolysis, by which vertical relaxation was obtained to complement lateral relaxation. The difficulties inherent in this technique are that the fibrous bands that must be divided to free the apex often surround the subclavian artery and vein along with the lower trunk of the brachial plexus.

In 1954, Björk described his osteoplastic technique of thoracoplasty, whereby a new roof of the thorax was obtained by resection of posterior portions of the ribs in increasing lengths from above downward. The ribs were then bent into the costal cartilages and fixed to the posterior end of the uppermost intact rib with stainless steel sutures (Fig. 47–27). With this technique, a stable chest wall was obtained and the lung was prevented from re-expanding above the new roof. A similar technique was described by Barclay and Welch (1957).

Plombage Thoracoplasty

Plombage thoracoplasty was initiated in 1891 by Tuffier, who described the merits of performing and maintaining an extrapleural pneumothorax to collapse the lung (Tuffier, 1914). The method was simple, and initially Tuffier left the extrapleural space empty. He later inserted air, omentum, or "fresh lipomas" for this purpose (Horowitz et al, 1992). Unfortunately, material placed in this plane often eroded into the underlying lung parenchyma and either was expectorated or created a bronchopleurocutaneous fistula.

In the late 1940s and early 1950s, several articles appeared reporting the same operation but with an extrafascial (outside the endothoracic fascia) and extraperiosteal, rather than an extrapleural, pneumothorax. Initially, the collapse was maintained by paraffin (paraffin plombage thoracoplasty), which was associated with an infection rate of 15% and an extrusion rate of 30% (Barker, 1994). Subsequently, at least 29 different materials (Horowitz et al, 1992; Walkup and Murphy, 1949) were used to maintain collapse of affected areas of the lung, including gauze sponge, silk, wax, various oils and gelatin, rubber balloons, drawing crayons, and lead bullets (Horowitz et al, 1992). These products were inserted between the endothoracic fascia and periosteum on one side and the ribs on the other.

In 1946, Wilson reported his experience using balls made of polymethyl-methacrylate (Lucite) for plombage (Fig. 47–28). These plombage operations had the advantage of providing good selective collapse without paradoxical respiration, but the disadvantage of making the patient more prone to infection. Advantages of the lucite balls over other products included that they were relatively nonirritating and were of light weight and radiolucent (Wilson et al, 1956). Plombage is no longer used by thoracic surgeons, and the last report appears to be the one by Mayer and associates (1973), who described the use of a silicone mammary prosthesis in a patient with

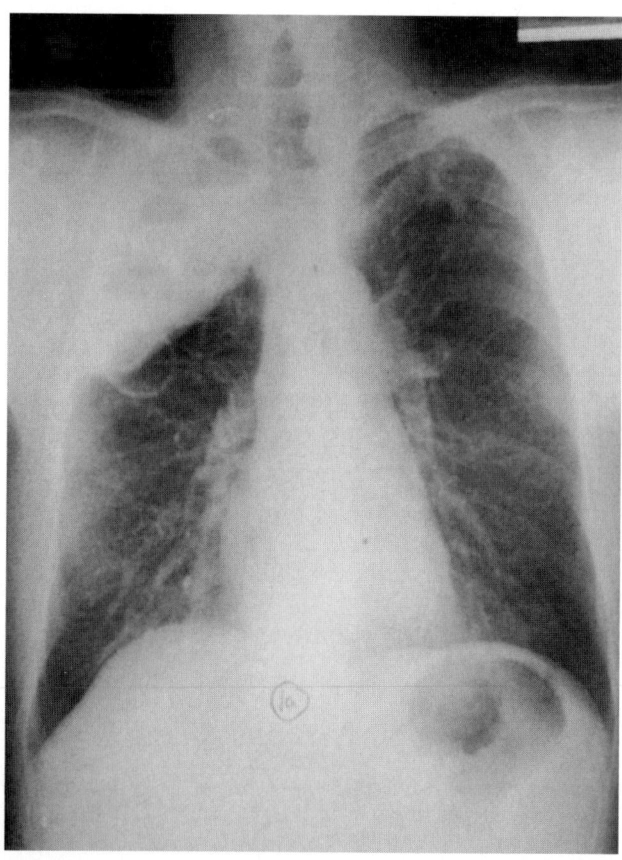

FIGURE 47–28 ■ Plombage thoracoplasty with Lucite balls. No ribs have been resected.

hemoptysis and tuberculosis. In recent years, several articles have reported late complications occasionally seen after plombage thoracoplasty (Ashour et al, 1985; Horowitz et al, 1992; Schmid and DeHaller, 1986; Wood and Watson, 1988).

In 1985, Iioka and colleagues described a technique whereby the parietal pleura, periosteum, and intercostal muscles are collapsed without rib resection (technique of Sawamura), thereby obliterating the empyema cavity. This collapse created an extraperiosteal space, which filled with the patient's own blood and serum. Ultimately, this exudate, which serves as an extraperiosteal filler, reabsorbs. In their paper, the authors reported a good result in 60 of 65 patients treated with this technique. They recommended that the procedure be reserved for individuals who, because of their general condition, cannot sustain a more formidable decortication or extended thoracoplasty. They also noted that their technique tends to better preserve pulmonary function and precludes deformity.

Thoracomyoplasty was described by Andrews in 1961 as a method for treating tuberculous empyemas often complicated by bronchopleural fistula. The technique involves the following steps (Fig. 47–29): (1) Rib resection over the empyema space strictly adjusted to the size of the cavity without resection of the head and neck of the rib and the transverse process of the spine; (2) opening of the cavity through an incision overlying a rib bed; (3) evacuation of the contents of the space and cartilage of the parietal wall until it becomes pliable and can be collapsed over the peel covering the lung or mediastinum; and (4) placement of the pleuromusculoperiosteal flap in juxtaposition to the lung (this is secured using absorbable sutures to obliterate the space). Associated bronchopleural fistulas are separately closed by means of primary suturing or by covering the site of the fistula with an intercostal muscle that has been freed from the parietal wall. The subscapular extramusculoperiosteal space is drained temporarily, but the drains are removed as quickly as possible. No chest drain is left inside the collapsed chest wall.

The results of this procedure are presented in Table 47–9.

Limited and Tailoring Thoracoplasties

A limited thoracoplasty is a procedure that is restricted to the removal of only a few ribs for the purpose of eliminating an infected space. A limited tailored thoracoplasty or tailoring thoracoplasty is done in association with a pulmonary resection in which a space problem is anticipated. In 1959, Melloy and co-workers reported the effectiveness of preresection upper rib limited thoracoplasty in reducing the overall incidence of postresection empyemas. According to Barker (1994), preresection tailoring thoracoplasty is seldom indicated in contemporary thoracic surgery and should be used only in patients in whom it is felt after careful evaluation that the amount of lung left after resection will be too small to fill the space.

Even under those circumstances, reduction of pleural space boundaries by means of simple maneuvers such as pleural tent or pneumoperitoneum is nearly always sufficient to prevent postoperative spaces. These procedures can be done at the time of resection, and they are not associated with paradoxical respiration. Therapeutic pneumoperitoneum can also be initiated postoperatively if a residual space is likely to become infected.

INDICATIONS FOR THORACOPLASTY

Despite the decline in the popularity of thoracoplasty, four recent studies have shown that it is an excellent therapeutic option for selected patients. In the series of Hopkins and associates (1985), 30 patients were treated with thoracoplasty over a 14-year period. The surgery was performed to close a persistent pleural space in 28 patients, and to adapt the thoracic cavity for diminished lung volume concomitantly with pulmonary resection in the other 2 patients. Among the 28 patients with persistent infected spaces, 24 had an associated bronchopleural fistula, and in 19, infection had occurred following an operation. In the authors' own series (Grégoire et al, 1987), 17 patients underwent thoracoplasty for a postpneumonectomy empyema, and 7 had an associated bronchopleural fistula. In 1990, Horrigan and Snow reported a series of 13 patients who underwent thoracoplasty between 1976 and 1989. Five of these patients had chronic apical empyema spaces without prior resection of lung, and all had extensive destruction of upper lobe tissue. Eight patients had undergone prior pulmonary resection and had infected postoperative residual spaces. In the series of Peppas and colleagues (1993), 19 patients underwent the operation to control complications of resection for lung cancer, and 18 patients had the operation during the course of management of disease not related to lung cancer.

Current indications for thoracoplasty are summarized in Table 47–10. It is worth noting that, contrary to what can be achieved with infected apical spaces, thoracoplasty is almost never indicated for the treatment of basal spaces such as those sometimes seen after right and middle lower lobectomies. These lower spaces are better managed with open thoracic window drainage or by filling of the space with muscle flaps. In patients with postpneumonectomy empyemas, thoracoplasty presents specific advantages over space-filling or space-sterilization meth-

TABLE 47–9 ■ **Results of Andrews Thoracomyopleuroplasty**

Author (yr)	*No. of Patients*	*Operative Mortality*	*Cure, Immediate*	*Cure, Late*	*Failure*
Andrews (1961)	35	1 (3%)	28	5	1
Cornet et al (1980)	73	4 (5.4%)	58	9	2
Icard et al (1999)	29	1 (3.5%)	21	4	3

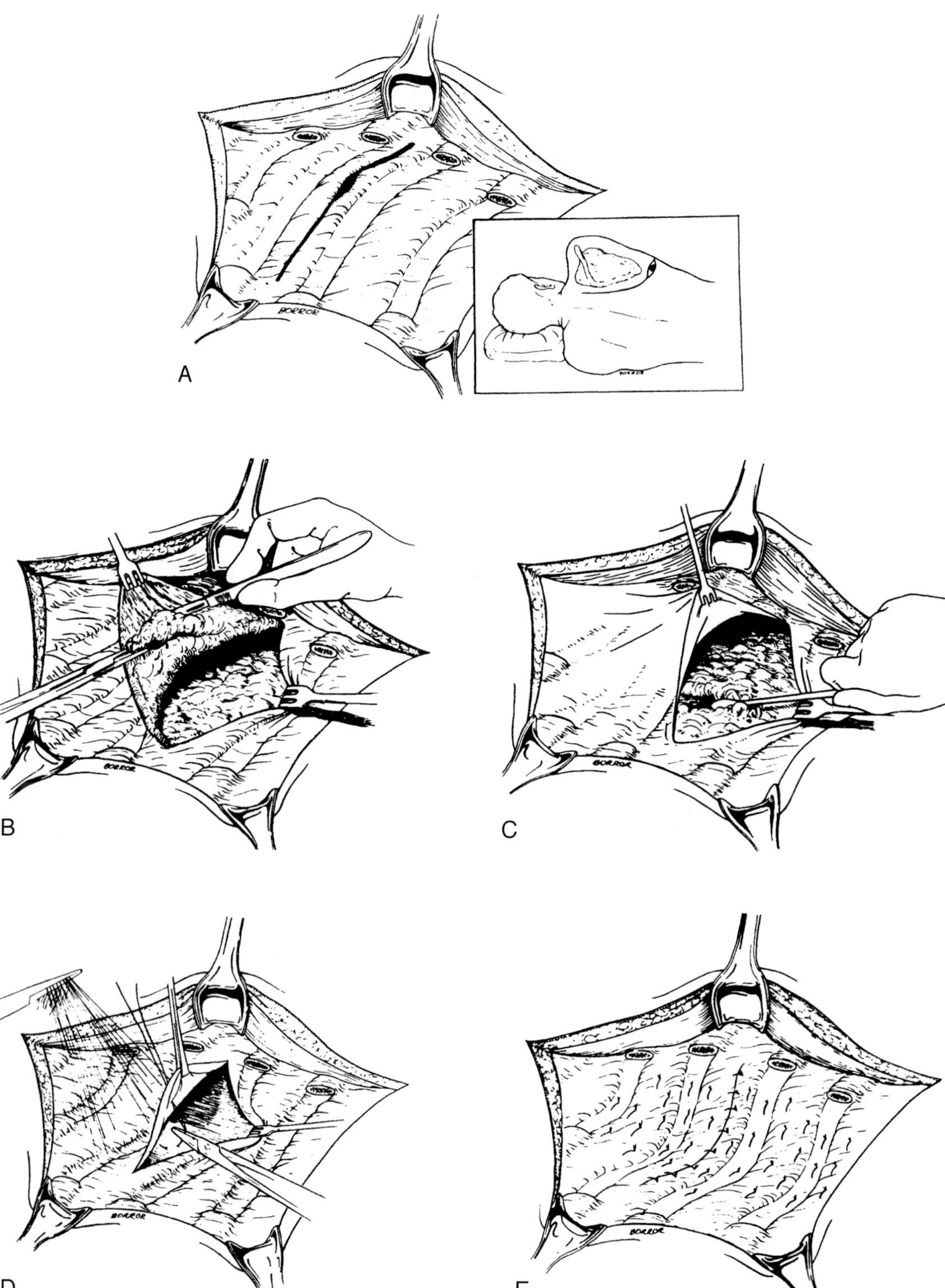

FIGURE 47–29 ■ *A*, First step of Andrews' thoracomyopleuroplasty: rib resection over the cavity. *B*, The cavity is entered through a costal bed and curetted. *C*, Curettage of the visceral and mediastinal pleura. *D*, U type of stitch used to obliterate the cavity. *E*, All stitches are tied up. (From Andrews NC: Thoraco-mediastinal plicature: A surgical technique for chronic empyema. J Thorac Surg 41:806, 1961.)

TABLE 47–10 ■ Current Indications for Thoracoplasty

Persistent spaces after lung resection or other thoracic procedures
- Infected apical spaces after upper or upper and middle lobectomies
- Postpneumonectomy empyema

Unresolving chronic empyemas unrelated to resection
- Apical empyemas
- Empyema in a space following previous therapeutic pneumothorax
- Pleural aspergillosis

Tailoring thoracoplasty done before or concomitantly with lung resection

ods (Claggett and Geraci, 1963), and treatment failures are uncommon (Grégoire et al, 1987). In nonresectional apical empyemas with destroyed upper lobes, or in an empyema that has developed in an apical space following previous therapeutic pneumothorax, decortication is inadvisable and will almost inevitably result in failure because of the underlying lung disease (see Chapter 46). In these situations, thoracoplasty may be indicated to collapse the space. Thoracoplasty may also be indicated in the management of complicated pleuropulmonary aspergillosis (Al-Zeerah and Jeyasingham, 1989) (Fig. 47–30). Finally, tailoring thoracoplasty may be indicated after pulmonary resection when it appears that the remaining lobe or lobes will be unable to completely fill the space.

TECHNIQUE

Incisions and Surgical Access

All thoracoplasties are performed under one-lung anesthesia maintained with a double-lumen tube. The use of this type of tube is very important for preventing aspiration of the empyema contents into the contralateral lung.

Thoracoplasty can be done through a posterior or a posterolateral approach or through an axillary incision. The posterior approach was commonly used during the early years of thoracoplasty, but it has now been largely abandoned because it involves division of both the trapezius (superficial layer) and the rhomboid (deep layer) muscles, which unite the spine with the lateral border of the scapula. These muscles are important for elevating the scapula and preventing it from free floating. To prevent this problem, Brock (1946) and others have shown that the muscles have to be divided close to the spine, thereby preventing injury to either the spinal nerve or the posterior spinal artery.

In recent years, most thoracoplasties are performed through a standard posterolateral thoracotomy, which can be extended vertically upward to enable adequate access to the upper ribs (Peppas et al, 1993). The posterior division of the latissimus dorsi and the division of the serratus anterior muscles completely free the scapula, which can then be elevated to expose the ribs. Maintenance of this exposure is achieved by inserting a chest retractor (Finochietto) between a lower rib and the tip of the scapula.

The axillary incision can be used for limited thoracoplasties. It has the advantage of providing good and easy access to the rib cage; its disadvantages are that the scapula cannot be mobilized, and access to the most posterior portion of the ribs is difficult to attain.

Conventional Posterolateral Thoracoplasty (Alexander Type)

This procedure consists of extramusculoperiosteal resection of a sufficient number of ribs to enable complete collapse of the space. As was originally described by Alexander (1937), it involved the resection of 10 or 11 ribs, and it was done in three stages to prevent paradoxical respiration. Today, most spaces requiring thoracoplasty are the result of postoperative infections; these can be treated in one stage and with the use of a more limited number of rib resections. If the operation is done in stages, the interval between stages varies from 10 to 30 days.

The second to the eighth ribs are usually resected (Fig. 47–31); it is best to start with the third rib, next resect the second, and then resect the fourth to the seventh or eighth ribs. The extent of resection is regulated by the pathologic extent of disease; as a rule of thumb, one should extend rib resection to one rib below the most inferior area of disease. Sloping resection of the anterior portion of the ribs with progressively less anterior rib being removed preserves the normal configuration of the anterolateral thoracic wall. This maneuver also helps to decrease the paradox and prevent collapse of the healthy lung, which is usually located anteriorly. Posteriorly, the ribs should be taken through their neck or head, or should even be completely disarticulated from the costovertebral joint. To maximize paravertebral collapse and accentuate transverse compression of the lung, part or all of the transverse processes may also have to be resected. If the sixth rib is resected, the tip of the scapula may be moving onto and off of the seventh rib, producing unpleasant sensations. When this is anticipated, the problem can be prevented by resecting either the seventh rib or the lower third of the scapula.

There is some controversy as to whether the first rib should be resected. Jaretzki (1991) summarized well the changing attitudes toward resection of the first rib:

> "When the classic ten-rib Alexander thoracoplasty was performed in the treatment of tuberculosis, removal of the first rib was necessary to obtain adequate collapse therapy (Fig. 47–32). However, in performing a limited thoracoplasty to assist in the elimination of an infected space, or a limited tailored thoracoplasty in association with a pulmonary resection where a space problem is anticipated, the first rib should not be removed."

As was shown by Grégoire and associates (1987), Mansour (1991), and others, preserving the first rib is important for maintaining the integrity of the neck, shoulder girdle, and upper thorax (Fig. 47–33).

Whether or not the first rib is resected, apicolysis is a most important step in the operation of thoracoplasty. It can be done extrapleurally, as described by Holst and colleagues (1935), or extrafascially (Semb, 1935) (Fig. 47–34). The purpose of apicolysis is to bring the apex of the lung and other soft tissues downward to obliterate the space. It involves division of upper intercostal muscle

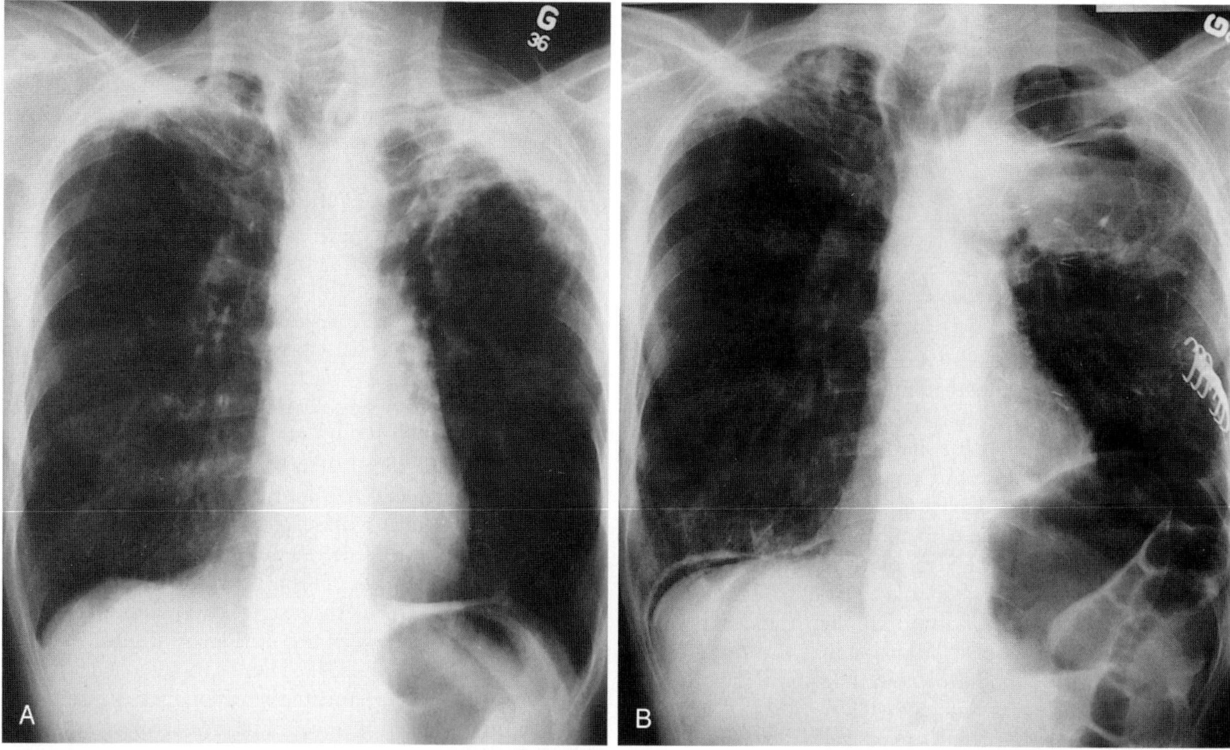

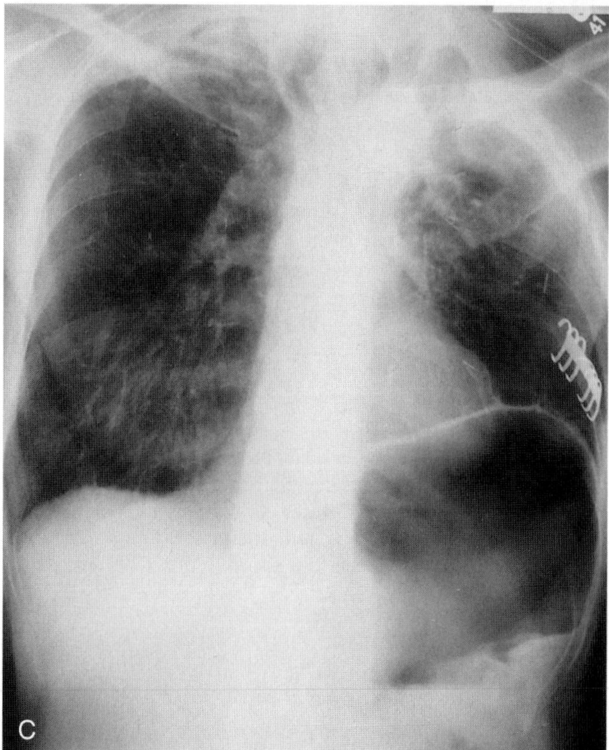

FIGURE 47–30 ■ *A*, Standard posteroanterior chest radiograph of a 60-year-old man with bilateral aspergillomas and massive hemoptysis. *B*, After left upper lobectomy and apical segmental resection of the lower lobe, the patient had a residual apical space with positive culture for aspergillosis (pleural aspergillosis). *C*, Standard posteroanterior chest radiograph following axillary thoracoplasty that shows complete obliteration of the space.

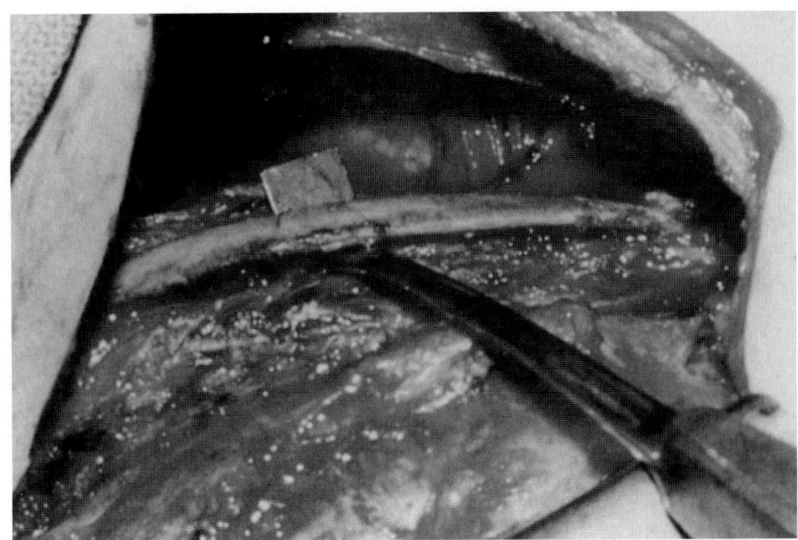

FIGURE 47–31 ■ Operative photograph showing rib resection and collapse of the space during thoracoplasty.

bundles and fibrous tissue close to the spine, as well as separation of all apical attachments to the chest wall. If the apicolysis is done extrapleurally with the first rib intact, the periosteum over the rib is incised with the use of diathermy and is stripped from its superior surface. Once the rib is freed, the space is collapsed by digital pressure and scissor division of fibrous tissue posteriorly.

There is also some controversy as to whether a bronchopleural fistula, when present, should be closed. It has been the authors' policy (Grégoire et al, 1987) not to close small bronchopleural fistulas (<2 mm) because collapse of the space nearly always results in spontaneous closure. If a large fistula is present, a posteriorly pedicled intercostal muscle flap is brought down through the space to cover the bronchial stump. Peppas and co-workers (1993) and others have suggested that all fistulas, whether small or large, should be closed by direct suture or by opposition of a myoplastic flap.

Adequate postoperative intra- and extrapleural drainage is mandatory. The intrapleural drain, which is usually in place before the thoracoplasty takes place, is left until complete obliteration of the space is achieved. The extrapleural drain, located in the noninfected extrapleural space, can be removed within 4 to 5 days of surgery.

RESULTS

Morbidity and Mortality

In most recent series, the operative mortality associated with thoracoplasty ranges between 0% and 10%. Postoperative complications include failure to heal, failure to obliterate the space, failure to control infection, failure to close the bronchopleural fistula, and respiratory failure. Late results show successful collapse and obliteration of the spaces in 80% to 90% of patients.

Complications Related to Specific Types of Thoracoplasties

Most thoracoplasties produce some degree of chest wall and shoulder deformity. Progressive scoliosis (Fig. 47–35) may develop if the transverse processes of the spine and the first rib have been resected. Patients may also have chronic postoperative chest pain and hyperanesthesia of the chest wall. With intrapleural types of thoracoplasties such as the Schede, patients have a greater number of thoracic deformities, in addition to having cutaneous anesthesia and paresthesias over the lower thoracic and upper abdominal walls. Patients may demonstrate restric-

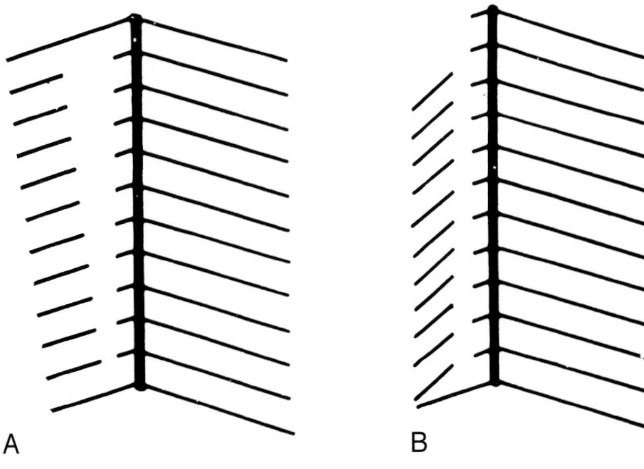

FIGURE 47–32 ■ Alexander's version of the suspensory role of the first rib in thoracoplasty. *A*, All ribs have been removed except the first, and the collapse is incomplete. *B*, The first rib has been removed, with more adequate collapse. (From Alexander J: The Collapse Theory of Pulmonary Tuberculosis. Springfield, IL, Charles C. Thomas, 1937.)

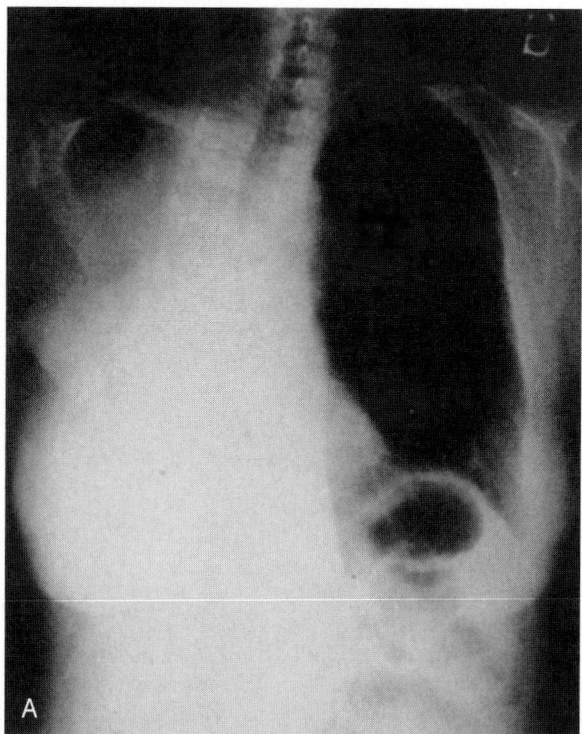

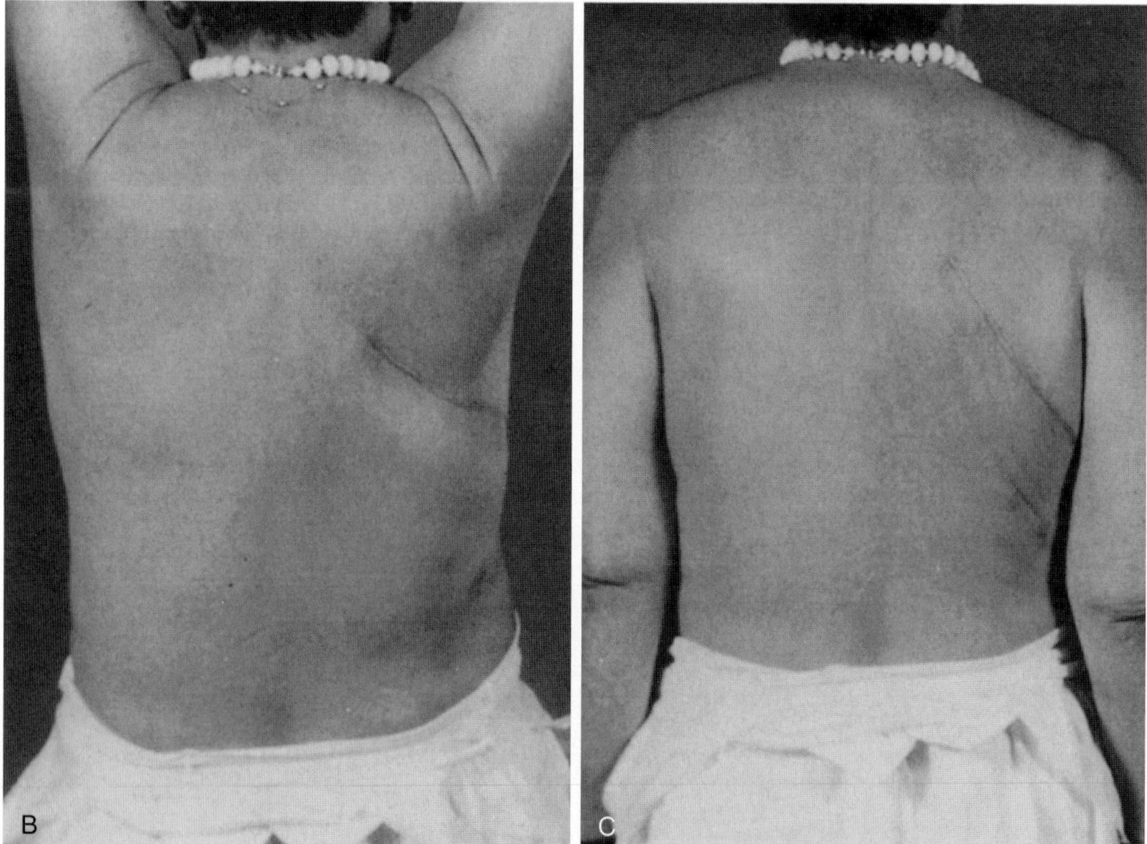

FIGURE 47–33 ■ *A*, Chest radiograph film and, *B & C*, photographs of a 53-year-old woman 6 months after right-sided thoracoplasty for a postpneumonectomy empyema. Structural integrity of neck and shoulder girdle is maintained by retaining first rib.

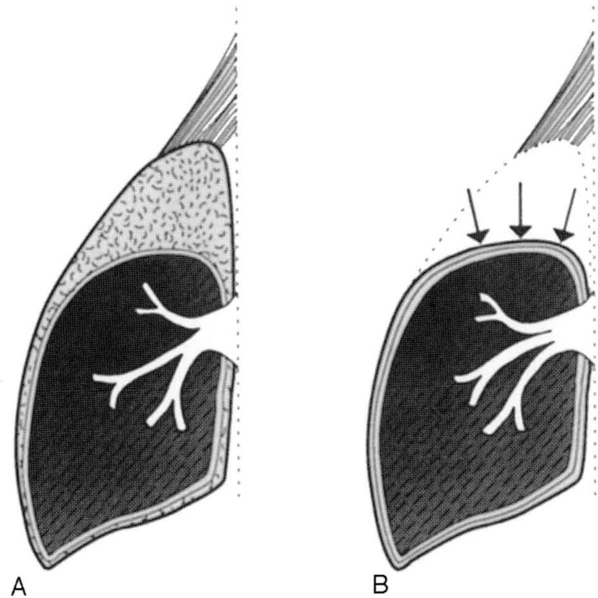

FIGURE 47–34 ■ *A*, Extrapleural apicolysis and, *B*, extrafascial apicolysis. (Adapted from Fey B, Mocquot P, Oberlin S et al: Traité de Technique Chirurgicale, Vol 4. Paris, Masson, 1955.)

tion of shoulder motion on the involved side because the scapula becomes adherent to the chest wall (Horrigan and Snow, 1990), especially if a portion of that bone has been resected; the appearance is that of a frozen shoulder. Gaensler and Struder (1951) have shown that some patients will develop progressive respiratory failure. These authors reported permanent functional loss of approximately 27% of the preoperative vital capacity and 21% of maximal voluntary ventilation of the contralateral lung. In a study of 24 patients after thoracoplasty that was done 3 to 27 years before, Powers and Himmelstein (1951) also presented evidence that the development of scoliosis after thoracoplasty resulted in a marked decrease in ventilatory function. These authors attributed the scoliosis to the detachment of muscles that normally act in opposition in the two hemithoraces. After thoracoplasty, the muscles on the opposite side are unopposed and may undergo contracture with a resulting rotoscoliosis. Most of these problems can be avoided by limiting the size of the thoracoplasty and avoiding resection of the first rib; meticulous surgical technique and early postoperative rehabilitation are also helpful.

■ KEY REFERENCES

Barker WL: Thoracoplasty. Chest Surg Clin N Am 4:593, 1994.

This is a complete review of indications, techniques, and results of thoracoplasty.

Hopkins RA, Ungerleider RM, Staub EW, Young WG: The modern use of thoracoplasty. Ann Thorac Surg 40:181, 1985.

Excellent review describing modern indications and results of thoracoplasty. Describes the Alexander principles of thoracoplasty.

Peppas G, Molnar TF, Jeyasingham K, Kirk AB: Thoracoplasty in the

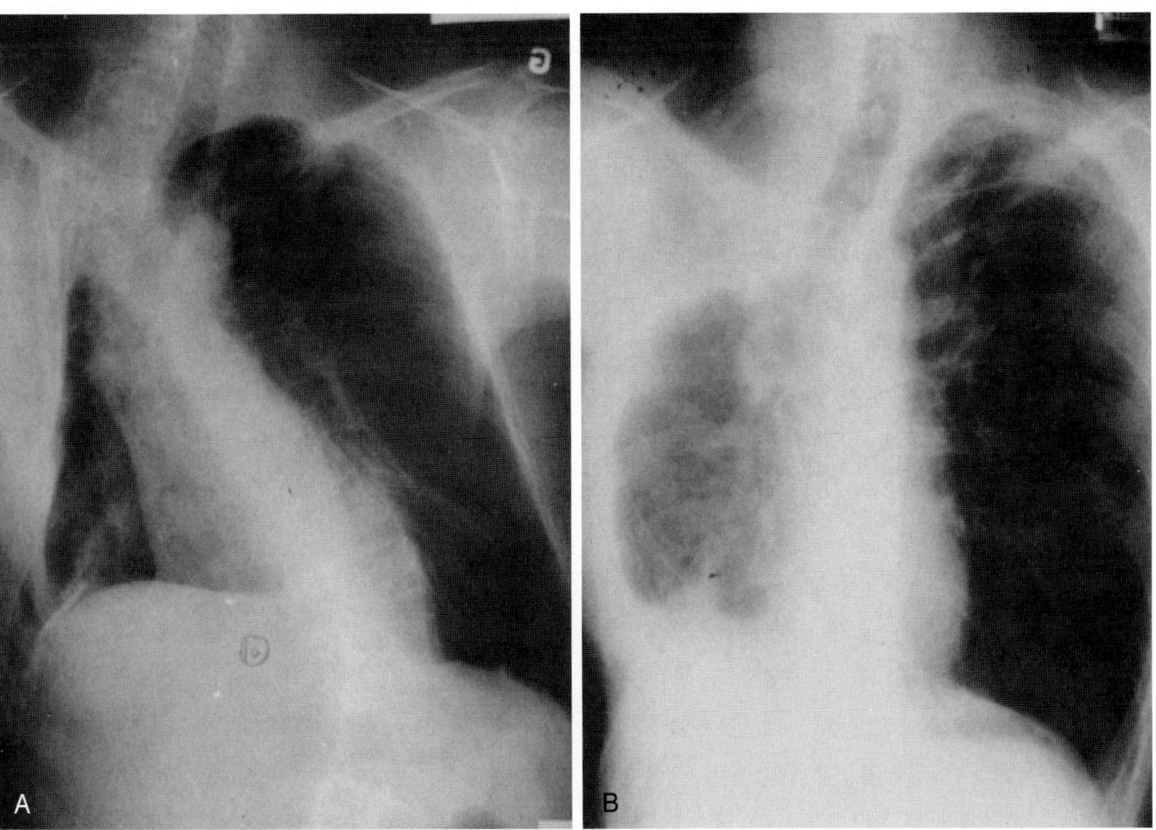

FIGURE 47–35 ■ *A*, Severe scoliosis seen after extensive six-rib thoracoplasty. Note that the first rib has been removed. *B*, Less extensive scoliosis, with first-rib preservation.

context of current surgical practice. Ann Thorac Surg 56:903, 1993.

This is a review of 37 patients who underwent thoracoplasty between 1975 and 1991. Presents a good discussion of the various types of thoracoplasty and their indications.

■ *REFERENCES*

Alexander J: The Surgery of Pulmonary Tuberculosis. Philadelphia, Lea & Febiger, 1925.

Alexander J: The Collapse Therapy of Pulmonary Tuberculosis. Springfield, IL, Charles C Thomas, 1937.

Al-Zeerah M, Jeyasingham K: Limited thoracoplasty in the management of complicated pulmonary aspergillomas. Thorax 44:1027, 1989.

Andrews NC: Thoraco-mediastinal plicature (a surgical technique for chronic empyema). J Thorac Surg 41:806, 1961.

Ashour M, Campbell IA, Umachandran V, Butchart EG: Late complications of plombage thoracoplasty. Thorax 40:394, 1985.

Barclay RS, Welch TM: Thoracoplasty with apical fixation. Scott Med J 2:20, 1957.

Barker WL: Thoracoplasty. Chest Surg Clin N Am 4:593, 1994.

Barker WL, Faber LP, Ostermiller WE et al: Management of persistent bronchopleural fistula. J Thorac Cardiovasc Surg 62:393, 1971.

Björk VO: Thoracoplasty. A new osteoplastic technique. J Thorac Surg 28:194, 1954.

Brantigan OC, Rigdov HL: Extrapleural pneumolysis with lucite ball plombage. Dis Chest 18:277, 1950.

Brock RC: Musculo-plastic incision for posterior thoracoplasty. J Thorac Surg 15:182, 1946.

Claggett OT, Geraci JE: A procedure for the management of postpneumonectomy empyema. J Thorac Cardiovasc Surg 45:141, 1963.

Cornet E, Dupon H, Michaud JL et al: Résultats éloignés de la thoracoplastie selon la technique d'Andrews. À propos de 73 observations. Ann Chir Thorac Cardiovasc 34:636, 1980.

De Cerenville EB: De l'intervention dans les maladies du poumon. Rev Med Suisse Romande 5:441, 1885.

Estlander JA: Résection des côtes dans l'empyème chronique. Rev Med Chir (Paris) 3:157, 1879.

Fey B, Mocquot P, Oberlin S et al: Traité de Technique Chirurgicale, Vol 4. Paris, Masson, 1955, p 212.

Friedrich PL: Die operative Beeinflussung einseitiger Lungphthise durch totale Brustwandmobilisierung. Arch Klin Chir 27:588, 1908.

Gaensler EA, Struder JW: Progressive changes in pulmonary function after pneumonectomy: The influence of thoracoplasty, pneumothorax, oleothorax, and plastic sponge plombage on the side of the pneumonectomy. J Thorac Surg 22:1, 1951.

Grégoire R, Deslauriers J, Beaulieu M, Piraux M: Thoracoplasty: Its forgotten role in the management of nontuberculous postpneumonectomy empyema. Can J Surg 30:343, 1987.

Grow JB: Chronic pleural empyema. Dis Chest 12:26, 1946.

Heller H: Ueber Verhutung und Behandlung der Emphysemresthohlen. Chirurg 6:297, 1934.

Holst J, Semb C, Frimann-Dahl J: On surgical treatment of pulmonary tuberculosis. Acta Chir Scand 76:1, 1935.

Horowitz MD, Otero M, Thurer RJ, Bolooki H: Late complications of plombage. Ann Thorac Surg 53:803, 1992.

Horrigan TP, Snow TJ: Thoracoplasty: Current application to the infected pleural space. Ann Thorac Surg 50:695, 1990.

Icard P, LeRochais JP, Rabut B et al: La thoracopleuroplastie d'Andrews: Un traitement efficace des empyèmes tuberculeux et des empyèmes post-pneumonectomie: À propos de 29 cas. J Chir Thorac Cardiovasc 3:131, 1999.

Iioka S, Sawamura K, Mori T et al: Surgical treatment of chronic empyema. A new one-stage operation. J Thorac Cardiovasc Surg 90:179, 1985.

Jaretzki A: Role of thoracoplasty in the treatment of chronic empyema [Letter]. Ann Thorac Surg 52:584, 1991.

Kergin FG: An operation for chronic pleural empyema. J Thorac Surg 26:430, 1953.

Langston HT: Thoracoplasty: The how and why. Ann Thorac Surg 52:1351, 1991.

Mansour KA: Reply to the editor. Ann Thorac Surg 52:585, 1991.

Mayer JH III, Moire JD, Gayo O: Silicone elastoner plombage for severe hemoptysis. Arch Surg 107:101, 1973.

Melloy FJ, Kalden A, Langston HT: Space problems in extensive resection for pulmonary tuberculosis: The use of tailoring thoracoplasty. J Thorac Surg 37:442, 1959.

Paget S: The Surgery of the Chest. Bristol, England, John Wright and Co, 1896. (As reproduced for the Classics of Surgery by Gryphon Editions, Birmingham, England, 1990, pp 275–279.)

Pairolero PC, Trastek VF: Surgical management of chronic empyema: The role of thoracoplasty. Ann Thorac Surg 50:689, 1990.

Powers SR, Himmelstein A: Late changes in ventilatory function following thoracoplasty. J Thorac Surg 22:45, 1951.

Sauerbruch F: Die Chirurgie der Brustorgane, Vol 2. Berlin, Springer-Verlag, 1925, p 876.

Schede M: Die Behandlung der Empyeme. Verh Cong Innere Med Wiesbaden 9:41, 1890.

Schmid FG, DeHaller R: Late exudative complication of collapse therapy for pulmonary tuberculosis. Chest 89:822, 1986.

Semb C: Technique of plastic operation of apicolysis. Acta Chir Scand 74:478, 1934.

Semb C: Thoracoplasty with Apicolysis. Oslo, NationaltryKKehut, 1935.

Tuffier T: État Actuel de la Chirurgie Intrathoracique. Paris, Masson, 1914, pp 90, 163.

Tuffier T: Du décollement pariétal en chirurgie pulmonaire. Arch Med Chir Appl Respir 1:32, 1926.

Walkup HE, Murphy JD: Extrapleural pneumolysis with plombage. Am J Surg 78:245, 1949.

Wangensteen OH: The pedicle muscle flap in the closure of persistent bronchopleural fistula. J Thorac Surg 5:27, 1935.

Wilms M: Die Pfeilerresektion der Rippen zur Verengerung des Thorax bei Lungentuberculose. Ther Gegenwart 54:17, 1913.

Wilson DA: The use of methylmethacrylate plombage in the surgical treatment of pulmonary tuberculosis. Surg Clin North Am 26:1060, 1946.

Wilson NJ, Arnada O, Vindzberg WV, O'Brien WB: Extra periosteal plombage thoracoplasty. Operative technique and results with 161 cases with unilateral surgical problems. J Thorac Surg 32:797, 1956.

Wood JB, Watson DCT: Suptum wax-worms after plombage. Br J Dis Chest 82:321, 1988.

Young WG, Moor GF: The surgical treatment of pulmonary tuberculosis. In Sabiston DC, Spencer FC (eds): Gibbon's Surgery of the Chest, 3rd ed. Philadelphia, WB Saunders, 1976, p 567.

Young WG, Ungerleider RM: Surgical approach to the chronic empyema: Thoracoplasty in thoracic surgery. Surgical management of pleural diseases. In Deslauriers J, Lacquet LK (eds): Trends in General Thoracic Surgery, Vol 6. St. Louis, CV Mosby, 1990.

THERAPEUTIC THORACOSCOPY FOR PLEURAL DISEASE

Joseph B. Shrager
Larry R. Kaiser

Video-assisted thoracoscopic surgery (VATS) has had a significant impact on the practice of general thoracic surgery over the past 10 years. The development of a light-sensitive chip that could be placed on the end of a thoracoscope brought video imaging to the operating room. The projection of an image of the thorax onto a video monitor allows the surgeon to work with an assistant, freeing his hands to carry out more complex procedures than could be performed through the previously available rigid pleuroscope. Thus, a technique that was formerly useful only for the most basic diagnostic procedures has now burgeoned to allow the performance of both diagnostic and complex therapeutic procedures on the lungs and pleura. This chapter focuses on the therapeutic uses of VATS in the treatment of pleural disease.

EMPYEMA

The mode of successful management of empyema is highly dependent on the timing of the therapy in the course of the disease. In the early, exudative phase, while the effusion is still free flowing and full expansion of the lung is not restricted, tube thoracostomy usually provides adequate management. Late in the disease, when a well-defined fibrotic peel prevents lung re-expansion, even following removal of pus from the pleural space, it is generally agreed that a thoracotomy with formal decortication is required.

It is in the intermediate, fibrinopurulent phase of empyema that VATS has played a major role (Cassina et al, 1999; Silen and Naunheim, 1996). This phase, which may occur over a wide range of time between a few days to up to 3 weeks following the onset of illness, is characterized by the development of thickening pleural fluid and loculations. At this point, drainage by a even a large-bore chest tube is not effective, but formal thoracotomy is not yet required because a frank, fibrous peel has not yet formed on the lung surface. Thoracoscopic débridement (called *decortication* by some authors, although the authors of this chapter prefer to reserve this term for formal removal of a peel, which can in most cases be performed only at thoracotomy) allows loculations to be broken up and gelatinous, organizing pleural material and pus to be completely removed, allowing the still largely unrestricted lung to expand (Striffeler et al, 1998). At this stage, the VATS approach yields results comparable with those of thoracotomy but is associated with more rapid recovery and a shorter hospital stay (Angelillo Mackinlay et al, 1996). In cases that straddle the fibrinopurulent and early fibrotic stages at the time of presentation, VATS can also be successful, as some amount of peel can often be removed by a patient VATS surgeon (Fig. 47–36). In most cases, however, the authors of this chapter have found it best to proceed to thoracotomy to ensure complete decortication.

A reasonable algorithm for the treatment of bacterial empyema is as follows: A patient with a free-flowing effusion should have a large-bore chest tube placed in a dependent position. If the chest radiograph does not show complete evacuation of fluid within approximately 2 days of tube placement, the patient should undergo VATS débridement. A patient whose effusion is demonstrably loculated by chest radiograph or computed tomography (CT) and in whom the time since the onset of illness is less than 3 weeks is best served by undergoing VATS directly. In a patient with a loculated empyema presenting beyond 3 weeks from the onset of illness, most would proceed immediately to thoracotomy, although some would argue that there is nothing lost by a preliminary attempt at thoracoscopy.

Some mention should be made of intrapleural administration of fibrinolytic agents to promote complete drainage of empyema in the fibrinopurulent phase. This has been reported by some groups to be effective in a high proportion of loculated empyemas (Robinson et al, 1994), although others have noted failure in up to 31% of patients (Temes et al, 1996). The personal experience

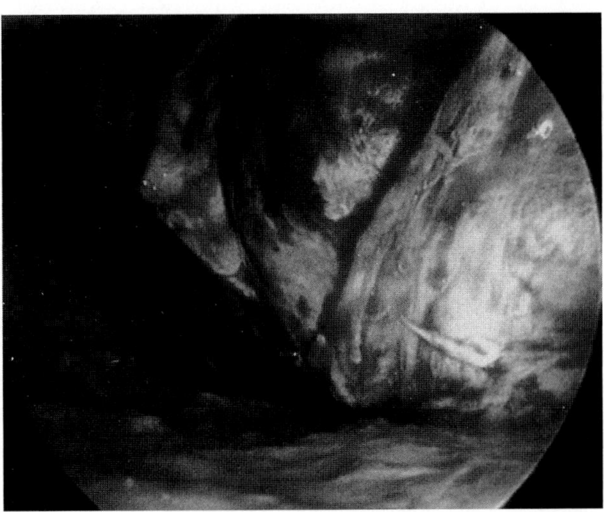

FIGURE 47–36 ■ Stripping a fibrous peel away from the lung during a video-assisted thoracic surgery (VATS) débridement/decortication for empyema.

of the authors with this approach has been discouraging. A small, randomized study of primary VATS treatment versus intrapleural fibrinolytic therapy found the VATS approach to be more efficacious, more efficient, and less costly (Wait et al, 1997).

Most VATS procedures for empyema require a three-port approach, with the incisions placed to optimize access to the collection, as demonstrated on preoperative studies. A finger should be placed into the chest at each port site to perform preliminary deloculation to create a working space in which the video camera and instruments can be maneuvered. Fluid and debris are removed, and fibrinous bands are broken down, allowing progressive enlargement of the working area and clearance of the pleural space. Once all gross debris has been removed, the chest is irrigated extensively with saline. The lung is then examined for re-expansion under positive pressure. If there is incomplete expansion, attempts are made to decorticate using VATS. As in open procedures, this is often best done on a moderately expanded lung. Inability to completely decorticate by VATS should lead to thoracotomy to complete the procedure. Chest tubes are left to suction for at least 48 hours, but after this time, they may be removed when drainage is less than 150 ml per 24 hours.

HEMOTHORAX

Several retrospective reports have documented the safety and efficacy of VATS intervention for retained hemothoraces. Hemothorax may occur iatrogenically but most commonly follows thoracic trauma. Initial management when bleeding is not massive and thus does not require urgent surgery is placement of a large-bore chest tube. In patients in whom this tube does not appear to have completely drained the pleural space, management decisions become more complex because after the initial presentation, it becomes increasingly difficult to fully drain what has become clotted blood through a tube of limited size. Before the advent of VATS, the typical therapy in this situation was placement of an additional tube or tubes in the effort to avoid thoracotomy. The result was a high rate of undrained collections causing trapped lungs, reduced vital capacity, and the potential for empyema. Later thoracotomy was often required.

With the availability of VATS, most surgeons now favor early evacuation of retained hemothoraces (Fig. 47–37). This often can be done through only two port sites (one in addition to the previous chest tube site), resulting in minimal additional morbidity. The algorithm followed by the authors and others begins with prompt placement of a large chest tube in a patient with thoracic trauma and a pleural effusion. If chest radiograph within 24 hours does not demonstrate complete resolution of the fluid, the authors proceed directly to VATS evacuation of the hemothorax.

A recent paper clearly demonstrates the efficacy of this approach (Meyer et al, 1997). These authors prospectively randomized 39 patients with retained hemothoraces to either a second chest tube or VATS. Patients in the VATS group had a shorter duration of chest tube drainage, a shorter hospital stay, and lower costs, and no patient required conversion to thoracotomy. Ten of 24 patients who underwent placement of a second chest tube remained incompletely drained and required operative intervention.

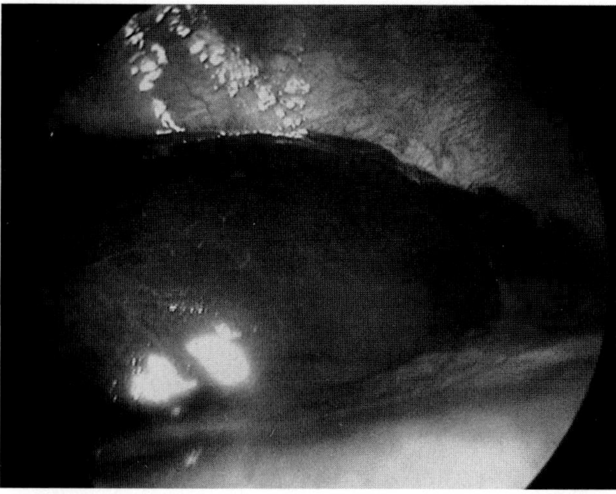

FIGURE 47–37 ■ Retained clot as viewed at VATS after chest tube drainage failed to completely resolve a post-traumatic hemothorax.

Another interesting study that may have an impact on the care of these patients examined the role of chest CT in the selection of candidates for VATS (Velmahos et al, 1999). These investigators obtained CT scans on post-trauma Day 1 in all patients who had undergone chest tube placement for hemothorax and in whom chest radiograph continued to show opacification of more than the costophrenic angle. They found that interventions that would have been instituted on the basis of the chest radiograph findings alone were felt to be unnecessary in 31% of patients following CT. The presence of contusion in the lung is the most common finding identifiable by CT that, on chest radiograph, may be indistinguishable from hemothorax. Twenty-one percent of patients nevertheless required VATS evacuation. The cost effectiveness of obtaining a routine chest CT in patients with this clinical scenario remains to be demonstrated.

MALIGNANT PLEURAL EFFUSION

Video thoracoscopic methods of managing patients with the common problem of malignant pleural effusion have also been advanced. Traditional management for this disease process has consisted of chest tube placement, followed by chemical pleurodesis if the lung expands well to fill the hemithorax after the fluid has been evacuated. Talc appears to be the most effective of the several materials that have been used for this purpose (Zimmer et al, 1997); reported success rates with talc slurry pleurodesis are in the range of 60% to 95%. When the lung has become entrapped by chronic effusion, thoracic surgeons have usually preferred to avoid thoracotomy and decortication because of the usually limited life span of the patient. The remaining option is placement of a pleuroperitoneal shunt, but this too is fairly unattractive as a shunt requires frequent pumping by a sometimes debilitated patient and is prone to occlusion.

Thoracoscopic management of malignant effusions has been offered in a variety of forms. For free-flowing malignant pleural effusion without trapped lung, some favor VATS through one or two ports for evacuation of fluid and insufflation of talc in its powdered form over chest tube placement and talc slurry. Advocates of this approach claim that the talc can be more reliably distributed throughout the pleural space in this manner, resulting in a more effective pleurodesis. A prospective, randomized study of chest tube slurry versus VATS talc, however, did not bear this out (Yim et al, 1996). A larger, multi-institutional study of the same issue is ongoing. Certainly, in patients in whom a diagnosis of malignancy has been unobtainable by fluid cytology and who for this reason are undergoing diagnostic VATS, talc should be insufflated at the time of the procedure, once a diagnosis of malignancy is obtained (Fig. 47–38).

In patients with loculated malignant effusions that cannot be drained by placement of a single chest tube, VATS for deloculation and talc insufflation is the appropriate procedure with the best chance for a good pleurodesis and the least morbidity. Some have reported successfully performing limited VATS decortication with pleurodesis for malignant effusion with trapped lung, but it has been the authors' experience that complete decortication in these circumstances is often quite difficult. These patients are generally best managed, if severely symptomatic, with a pleuroperitoneal shunt, or, if robust and with an anticipated long survival, with thoracotomy and formal decortication.

CHYLOTHORAX

Chylothorax is another vexing problem for which many surgical approaches have been put forward. Conservative treatment with drainage and total parenteral nutrition often fails to control the fistula. In this circumstance, options prior to the advent of VATS had been few but included chemical pleurodesis, pleuroperitoneal shunt placement, and thoracotomy and supradiaphragmatic thoracic duct ligation. The latter was clearly the most successful of these approaches (Robinson, 1985), but it was often delayed to a point at which the patient suffered significant immunologic compromise because of the fear of the morbidity associated with thoracotomy.

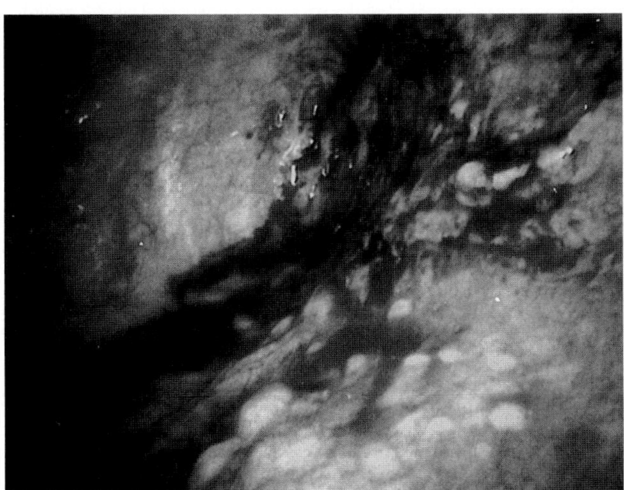

FIGURE 47–38 ■ Metastatic adenocarcinoma to the pleura in a patient with pleural effusion undergoing VATS for diagnosis and subsequent talc pleurodesis.

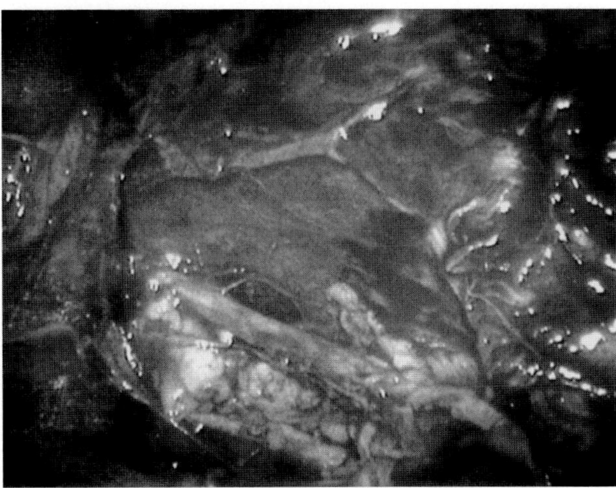

FIGURE 47–39 ■ VATS view of the thoracic duct a few centimeters above the right hemidiaphragm prior to placement of clips to ligate the duct in a patient with post-traumatic chylothorax.

The VATS approach allows supradiaphragmatic thoracic duct interruption to be performed in essentially the same manner as via thoracotomy with less postoperative pain (Fig. 47–39). The ability to perform the procedure without the morbidity of thoracotomy has encouraged many to undertake ligation earlier, ostensibly resulting in shorter hospital stays and decreased morbidity related to prolonged thoracic duct leakage. Although the technique has been reported only anecdotally in the literature, the authors' personal experience has been that of immediate closure of chyle fistulas in 10 of 12 patients treated by VATS thoracic duct clipping.

BENIGN PLEURAL TUMORS

This therapeutic application of VATS, though simple conceptually, is quite rare owing to the rare occurrence of these tumors. Benign fibrous tumors of the pleura are localized tumors arising from the visceral pleura in 70% and the parietal pleura in 30%. One half of patients are asymptomatic at presentation, with discovery on routine chest radiograph showing a solitary, sharply defined, discrete mass at the periphery of the lung. Interestingly, hypertrophic pulmonary osteoarthropathy occurs in approximately 20% of patients, and up to 40% present with symptomatic hypoglycemia. CT suggests the diagnosis when a large, noninvasive, enhancing pleural mass is identified.

When this diagnosis is being considered, as with most other suspected pleural diseases that require a tissue diagnosis, VATS should be undertaken. The gross appearance of the tumor at thoracoscopy confirms the diagnosis (Fig. 47–40); complete resection by VATS can then be undertaken with a three-port approach. There is typically a discrete plane of separation or stalk between the tumor

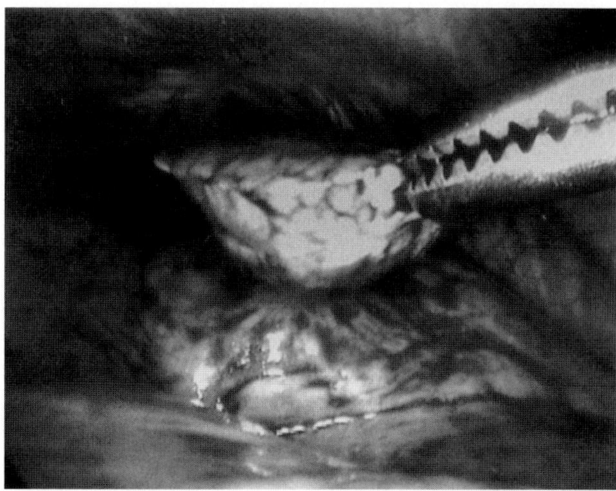

FIGURE 47–40 ■ A benign fibrous tumor of the pleura as viewed through the thoracoscope before the stalk was divided with a linear endoscopic stapler.

and the underlying lung. Larger tumors may require extension of the most anterior port incision, where the intercostal space is naturally widest, to allow removal from the chest.

SPONTANEOUS PNEUMOTHORAX

Although resulting from parenchymal lung disease, spontaneous pneumothorax is discussed in this chapter on VATS treatment of pleural disease. The first presentation of primary spontaneous pneumothorax (i.e., pneumothorax with no known predisposing lung disease) has traditionally been managed nonoperatively because the likelihood of recurrence is only approximately 30% (Clark et al, 1972). Operative therapy for first-time pneumothoraces has classically been reserved for those patients with persistent air leaks, those whose work requires them to undergo extremes of atmospheric pressure, and those who live in isolated areas without easy access to medical care. Otherwise, surgery has been indicated following an ipsilateral recurrence or for the patient who has suffered bilateral pneumothoraces.

The traditional operative management of primary spontaneous pneumothorax consists of thoracotomy (either posterolateral or axillary) with excision of blebs and some form of pleurectomy or pleurodesis (Brooks, 1973; Deslauriers et al, 1980). Thoracoscopic management of spontaneous pneumothorax allows the same procedures to be achieved through a minimally invasive approach, which decreases operative morbidity.

The prototype VATS procedure for primary spontaneous pneumothorax is performed through three port sites. The sites are positioned slightly more craniad on the chest than for other VATS procedures because the pathology tends to be found at the apex of the lung or in the superior segment of the lower lobe. Blebs are easily visualized (Fig. 47–41) and excised with the linear endoscopic stapler. Following this, some form of pleurectomy or pleurodesis is performed. It remains controversial whether true apical pleurectomy is required, although it can certainly be performed by a VATS approach if it is believed necessary. Most thoracic surgeons create a mechanical pleurodesis by abrading the parietal pleura to the point of punctate bleeding with gauze or a cautery "scratch-pad," or they create a chemical pleurodesis with doxycycline or talc. If no blebs are identified, the authors of this chapter and others favor excising a wedge of lung from the apex of the upper lobe to rule out underlying pulmonary pathology that might otherwise remain obscure.

Results with this approach have been excellent. In a randomized comparison of VATS and open blebectomy with pleurectomy, Waller and associates (1994) found that those patients with primary spontaneous pneumothorax undergoing VATS benefited from decreased postoperative pain, shorter hospital stay, and less pulmonary dysfunction. No patient in either the VATS or the thoracotomy groups suffered treatment failures. Although long-term follow-up is not yet available, recent retrospective studies with mean follow-up times of 13 to 30

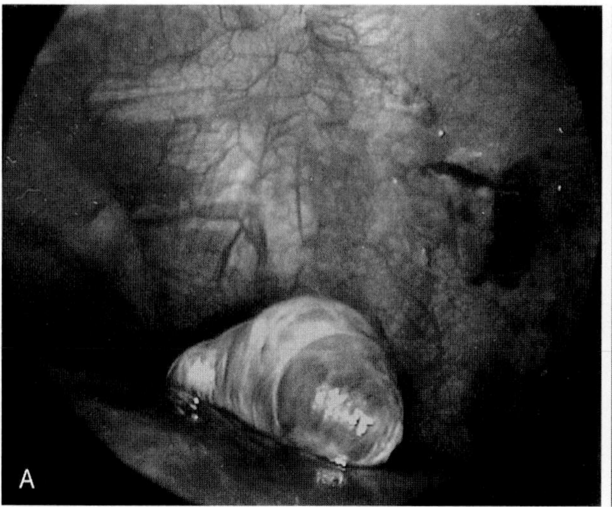

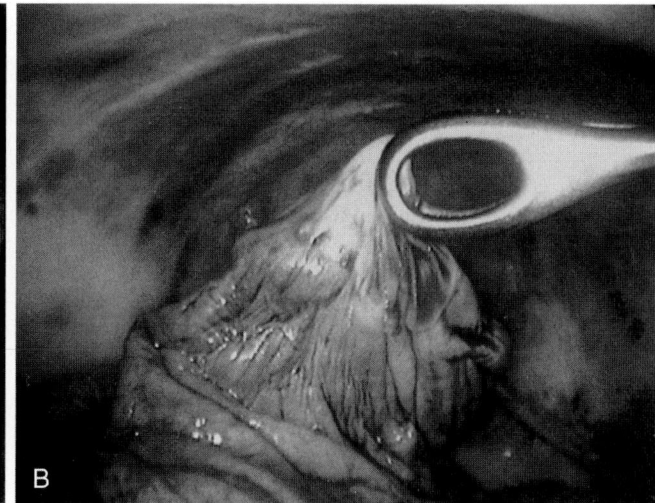

FIGURE 47–41 ■ Apical blebs identified by VATS in patients with primary, spontaneous pneumothorax undergoing bleb excision and mechanical pleurodesis: *A*, Intact bleb. *B*, Ruptured bleb.

months (Bertrand et al, 1996; Mouroux et al, 1996; Naunheim et al, 1995; Passlick et al, 1998) document recurrence rates of 3% to 6%. This compares favorably with results following thoracotomy, although certainly longer follow-up will be required before definite conclusions can be drawn. Other important pieces of information that are becoming clear from these and other reports are that (1) VATS is probably not indicated for *secondary* spontaneous pneumothorax, as rates of conversion to thoracotomy and failure have been reported to be much higher following VATS attempts in these patients, and (2) failure to identify and ablate a bleb at operation is probably associated with a higher rate of recurrence.

With the availability of VATS technology, some have advocated changing the operative indications for primary spontaneous pneumothorax and operating at the time of the initial occurrence. Although more data are necessary before this question can be answered, one retrospective study compared patients treated for first-time or recurrent spontaneous pneumothorax by conservative therapy (pleural drainage or observation) versus VATS (Schramel et al, 1996). These investigators found that drainage and hospitalization times were longer, and complication and recurrence rates were higher, when conservative therapy was used. Their data also suggest that VATS may be cost effective when used for initial occurrences. Only large-scale, prospective, randomized studies can eliminate the bias inherent in this type of study and determine whether this is an appropriate approach.

■ *KEY REFERENCES*

Kaiser LR, Daniel TM: Thoracoscopic Surgery. Boston, Little, Brown, 1993.

The original, comprehensive textbook/atlas of thoracoscopic surgery.

Waller DA, Forty J, Morritt GN: Video-assisted thoracoscopic surgery versus thoracotomy for spontaneous pneumothorax. Ann Thorac Surg 58:372, 1994.

The first prospective, randomized study to demonstrate an advantage of VATS over the open approach for a specific disease process with respect to pain, hospital stay, and postoperative pulmonary function.

■ *REFERENCES*

Angelillo Mackinlay TA, Lyons G, Chimondeguy DJ et al: VATS débridement versus thoracotomy in the treatment of loculated postpneumonia empyema. Ann Thorac Surg 61:1626, 1996.

Bertrand PC, Regnard JF, Spaggiari L et al: Immediate and long-term results after surgical treatment of primary spontaneous pneumothorax by VATS. Ann Thorac Surg 61:1641, 1996.

Brooks JW: Open thoracotomy in the management of spontaneous pneumothorax. Ann Surg 177:798, 1973.

Cassina PC, Hauser M, Hillejan L et al: Video-assisted thoracoscopy in the treatment of pleural empyema: Stage-based management and outcome. J Thorac Cardiovasc Surg 117:234, 1999.

Clark TA, Hutchinson DE, Deaner RM et al: Spontaneous pneumothorax. Am J Surg 124:728, 1972.

Deslauriers J, Beaulieu M, Depres JP et al: Transaxillary pleurectomy for treatment of spontaneous pneumothorax. Ann Thorac Surg 30:569, 1980.

Meyer DM, Jessen ME, Wait MA et al: Early evacuation of traumatic retained hemothoraces using thoracoscopy: A prospective, randomized trial. Ann Thorac Surg 64:1396, 1997.

Mouroux J, Elkaim D, Padovani B et al: Video-assisted thoracoscopic treatment of spontaneous pneumothorax: Technique and results of one-hundred cases. J Thorac Cardiovasc Surg 112:385, 1996.

Naunheim KS, Mack MJ, Hazelrigg SR et al: Safety and efficacy of video-assisted thoracic surgical techniques for the treatment of spontaneous pneumothorax. J Thorac Cardiovasc Surg 109:1198, 1995.

Passlick B, Born C, Haussinger K et al: Efficiency of video-assisted thoracic surgery for primary and secondary spontaneous pneumothorax. Ann Thorac Surg 65:324, 1998.

Robinson CLN: The management of chylothorax. Ann Thorac Surg 39:90, 1985.

Robinson LA, Moulton AL, Fleming WH et al: Intrapleural fibrinolytic treatment of multiloculated thoracic empyemas. Ann Thorac Surg 57:803, 1994

Schramel FM, Sutedja TG, Braber JC et al: Cost-effectiveness of video-assisted thoracoscopic surgery versus conservative treatment for first time or recurrent spontaneous pneumothorax. Eur Respir J 9:1821, 1996.

Silen ML, Naunheim KS: Thoracoscopic approach to the management of empyema thoracis: Indications and results. Chest Surg Clin N Am 6:491, 1996.

Striffeler H, Gugger M, Hof VI et al: Video assisted thoracoscopic surgery for fibrinopurulent pleural empyema in 67 patients. Ann Thorac Surg 65:319, 1998.

Temes RT, Follis F, Kessler RM et al: Intrapleural fibrinolytics in management of empyema thoracis. Chest 110:102, 1996.

Velmahos GC, Demetriades D, Chan L et al: Predicting the need for thoracoscopic evacuation of residual traumatic hemothorax: Chest radiograph is insufficient. J Trauma 46:65, 1999.

Wait MA, Sharma S, Hohn J et al: A randomized trial of empyema therapy. Chest 111:1548, 1997.

Waller DA, Forty J, Morritt GN: Video-assisted thoracoscopic surgery versus thoracotomy for spontaneous pneumothorax. Ann Thorac Surg 58:372, 1994.

Yim AP, Chan AT, Lee TX et al: Thoracoscopic talc insufflation versus talc slurry for symptomatic malignant pleural effusion. Ann Thorac Surg 62:1655, 1996.

Zimmer PW, Hill M, Casey K et al: Prospective randomized trial of talc slurry vs bleomycin in pleurodesis for symptomatic malignant pleural effusions. Chest 112:430, 1997.

Chest Wall and Sternum

CHAPTER 48

Anatomy and Physiology of the Chest Wall and Sternum

Geoffrey M. Graeber
Michael F. Szwerc

The anatomy and physiology of the chest wall are completely intertwined. The musculoskeletal structure of the chest wall has evolved as a mobile but firm encasement of the lungs and thoracic viscera, which provides for functional utility while affording some protection for vital organs. Certain muscles of the upper extremities and the trunk assist the chest wall in performing its physiologic functions under usual circumstances. An appreciation of the embryology of the chest wall helps in understanding its function.

EMBRYOLOGY

The primordial structures that form the chest wall are derived from both the axial and the appendicular skeleton (Arey, 1965; Graeber, 1986; Moore and Persaud, 1993; Ravitch, 1977). The sternum arises from the appendicular skeleton; the ribs and costal cartilages are derived from the axial skeleton. Each starts independently, but fusion occurs around the seventh week of gestation, when the primitive ribs and costal cartilages reach the emerging sternum.

The sternum arises from three distinct precursors of the appendicular skeleton. The largest are the two lateral mesenchymal bands, which arise laterally in the body wall in proximity to the emerging pectoralis major muscles at 5 to 6 weeks' gestation. The mesenchymal bands migrate medially and anteriorly to reach the ventral midline, where fusion occurs. The union starts in the cephalad end during the seventh week of gestation and proceeds caudad. The primitive manubrium is formed by fusion of the cephalad medial mesenchymal mass, which most probably corresponds with the presternum of lower animals, with two variable lateral suprasternal elements. Fusion progresses in a craniocaudad fashion until union is complete at 9 weeks.

The ribs, costal cartilages, and associated musculature arise from the posterior common vertebral mass in the axial skeleton at the same time that the lateral sternal bars appear (Arey, 1965; Graeber, 1986; Ravitch, 1977). These primordia grow laterally, anteriorly, and then medially to create the contour of the emerging body wall. By 9 weeks, the costal cartilages of ribs one through seven have fused with the sternum. Subsequently, the emerging costal cartilages of ribs eight through ten fuse with each other and the sternum to complete skeletal development of the chest wall.

PHYSIOLOGY AND ANATOMY

Chest wall integrity is mandatory for adequate ventilation (Graeber, 1986; Guyton, 1991; Netter, 1996; West, 1977, 1979, 1991). The best model for conceptual visualization of ventilation is a piston moving up and down in a fixed column. The fixed column is the chest wall; the piston is the diaphragm. When the diaphragm contracts, it draws the central tendon downward in the chest, creating a negative intrathoracic pressure. Because the lung is in contact with the chest wall in the normal physiologic state, contraction of the diaphragm with subsequent migration downward causes the lung to expand. When inspiration is complete, the diaphragm relaxes and the elastic components of the lung allow it to contract to its volume prior to the inspiratory effort. During quiet respiration, the excursion of the diaphragm is all the change in volume necessary to effect adequate ventilation. For the most part, the chest wall does not move during quiet respiration. Obviously, the chest wall must maintain its position for the lungs to expand properly. The negative pressure created in the chest by the excursion of the diaphragm causes air to come in through the tracheobronchial tree and be distributed to the respective lungs. Deeper inspiration and expiration must be facilitated by movement of the chest wall.

Because the lung follows the chest wall and diaphragm in their movements, the logical way to increase inspiration after the diaphragm has reached maximum contraction is to increase the diameter of the cylinder. By using the same piston model, we can see that if we increase the diameter of the cylinder in which the piston is moving up and down, the volume in the cylinder will increase in proportion to the increase in diameter. The ribs and sternum move in an upward and outward fashion so as to increase the intrathoracic distances, and thereby increase expansion of the lung. The sternum has been compared to a handle on a water pump in that it has an upward and downward motion by which it is fixed at the top and is most mobile distally. The manubrium articulates with the first rib and the clavicles. Its major motion is upward and anterior with the axis of rotation running through the two heads of the clavicles. The body of the sternum follows the manubrium in an upward and anterior direction. The ribs move much like the handle on a bucket (Fig. 48–1). They are relatively fixed anteriorly and posteriorly in that they articulate with the sternum and the spinal column, respectively. When they are moved upward and outward, they increase the volume within the thorax. The posterior articulation with the spinal column is most fixed, whereas the anterior point of articulation with the sternum does move cephalad and anteriorly with the sternum (Figs. 48–1 and 48–2). Contraction of intercostal muscles also plays a role in this movement as do muscle fibers of the diaphragm that are perpendicular to the costal margin. Maximum inspiration is achieved when the sternum is elevated anteriorly as far as possible

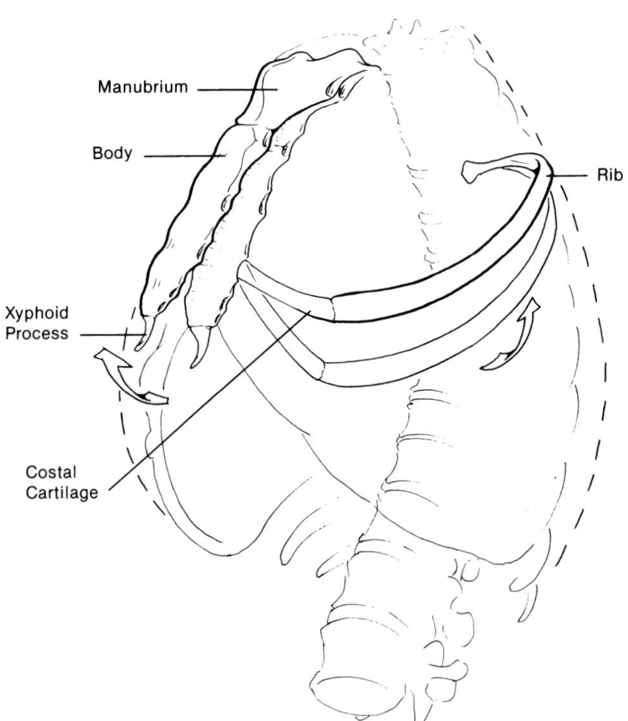

FIGURE 48–2 ■ The expansion and contraction of the chest wall are governed by the motion of the individual ribs, costal cartilages, and sternum. The sternum works as a handle on a water pump. As it is moved upward, the xiphoid process and body go more anteriorly and cephalad, whereas the manubrium articulates with the first rib and clavicle and rotates anteriorly and cephalad. The bucket handle motion of the ribs and costal cartilages is facilitated by articulations both posteriorly and anteriorly. The posterior articulations of the rib, with the head, the vertebral body, and the articular facet, move against the transverse process of the vertebral body below. The costal cartilage articulates with the sternum and moves upward on forced inspiration and downward on forced expiration.

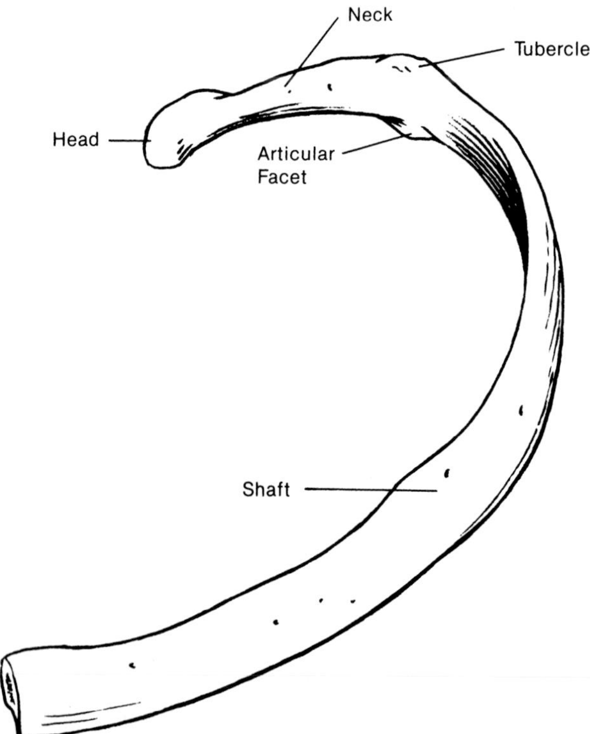

FIGURE 48–1 ■ The anatomy of a rib. The head abuts on the vertebral body. The articular facet in the region of the tubercle articulates with the transverse process on the vertebral body below. The neck, after it extends to the region of the tubercle and the facet, blends with the elongated shaft. The anterior surface abuts on the corresponding costal cartilage.

and the ribs are elevated in a similar fashion laterally and cephalad (Figs. 48–3 and 48–4). The accessory muscles of inspiration are responsible for moving the ribs and sternum upward and outward to achieve maximal expansion of the thorax and hence of the lungs (Fig. 48–5).

Maximal expiration is achieved by relaxation of the diaphragm and by downward and inward displacement of the sternum and ribs (Graeber, 1986; Guyton, 1991; Netter, 1996; West, 1977, 1979, 1991). The downward movement of the sternum causes the posterior and inferior rotation of the manubrium and the posterior and inferior rotation of the sternal body. The ribs are brought downward and inward so that the internal diameters of the chest are reduced to a minimum. The accessory muscles of expiration are responsible for these movements. The summation of their actions causes a decrease in the volume of the thorax and achieves maximal expiration (Fig. 48–6). These same muscles also press inward on the abdominal viscera and force the relaxed diaphragm upward.

BLOOD SUPPLY AND INNERVATION

The arterial supply to the chest wall arises from the subclavian arteries and the aorta itself. The intercostal

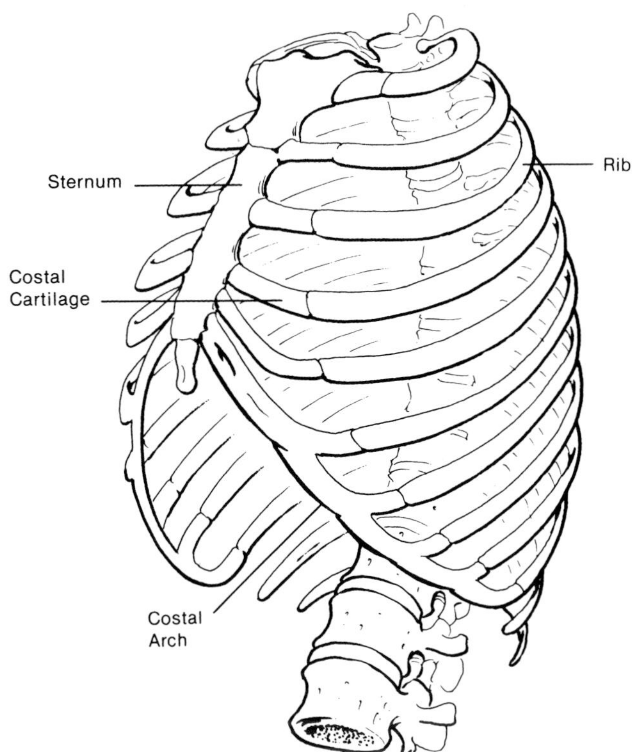

FIGURE 48–3 ■ The entire bony and cartilaginous thorax is depicted in this left anterior oblique projection. The costal cartilages articulate with the sternum and the individual ribs. In the lower aspects of the costal margin, individual costal cartilages blend. Note that the eleventh and twelfth ribs are completely free of attachment in any way to the sternum. The spine forms the posterior articular aspects for each of the ribs.

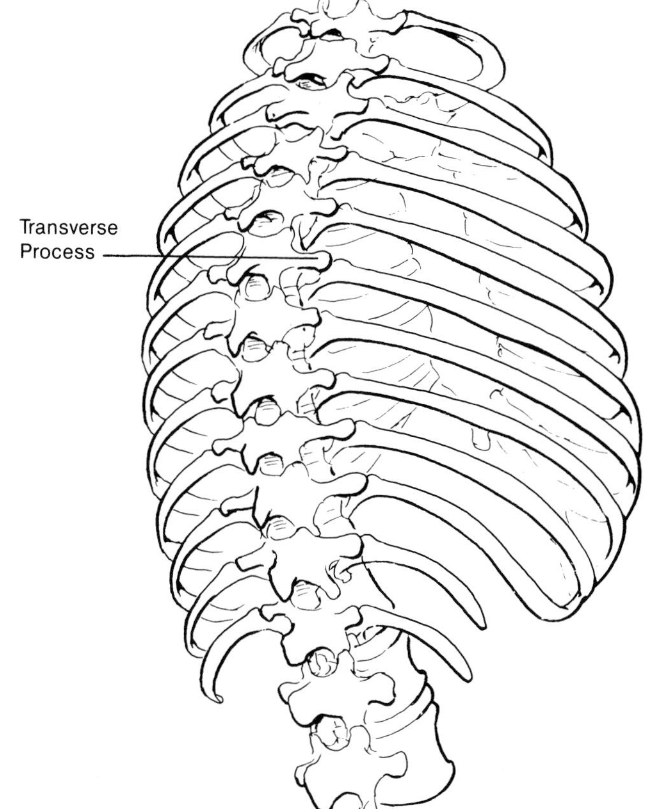

FIGURE 48–4 ■ This right posterior oblique projection shows the relationship of each individual rib to the vertebral bodies and their transverse processes. Note that the head of each rib articulates with the vertebral bodies, whereas the articular processes of each rib articulate with the transverse processes.

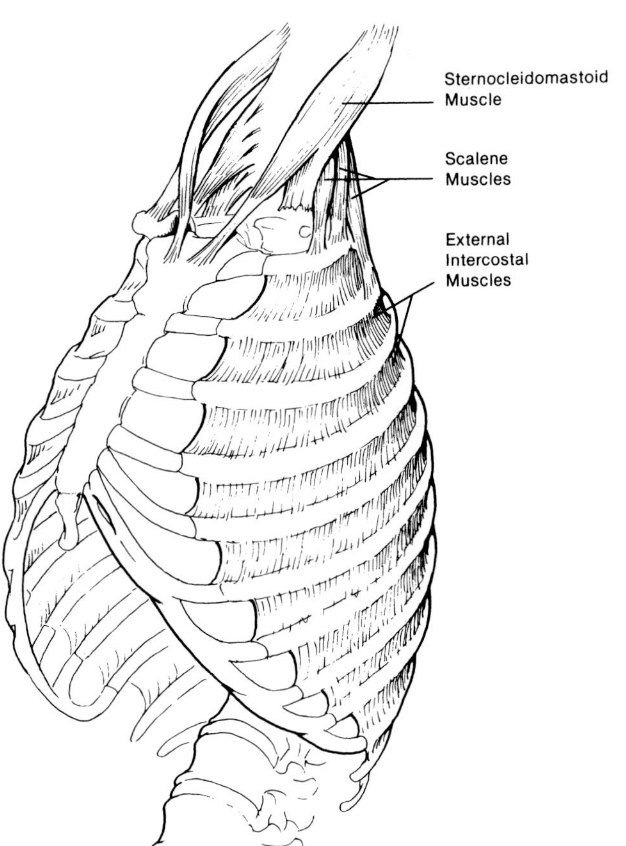

FIGURE 48–5. ■ Accessory muscles of inspiration. Note that all of this musculature is directed at raising the fibromuscular skeleton and extending it anteriorly. This coordinated motion increases the intrathoracic diameters and allows further expansion of the lungs.

arteries, which run under each rib, supply the posterior and lateral aspects of the chest wall (Clemente, 1985b). The internal thoracic artery and the intercostal arteries combine to provide the arterial supply to the anterior portion of the chest wall. The internal thoracic and the highest two intercostals generally arise from the subclavian artery. The lower ten intercostal arteries arise from the descending thoracic aorta and course anteriorly underneath the ribs in the neurovascular bundle (Fig. 48–7). The intercostal arteries course anteriorly to anastomose with the internal thoracic at the lateral margin of the sternum. Each of these arteries sends out numerous twigs to the intercostal muscles, the pleura, and the periosteum of the ribs (see Fig. 48–7).

Major contributors to the blood supply of the anterior chest wall, and particularly the sternum, are the paired internal thoracic arteries (Fig. 48–8). Each of these vessels arises from the subclavian artery and courses distally along the internal peristernal aspect of the chest (Clemente, 1985b). Distally, the internal thoracic artery bifurcates into two major branches: the direct extension, which becomes the superior epigastric artery after it exits the thoracic cavity through the space between the sternal and costal slips of the diaphragm; and the lateral branch, which is the musculophrenic artery. The superior epigastric artery arises from the direct extension of the internal thoracic artery once the internal mammary has gone through the potential foramen of Morgagni and has entered the posterior aspect of the rectus sheath. The superior epigastric further communicates with intercostals coming down from above and with the inferior epigastric artery in the distal end of the rectus sheath. The musculophrenic artery courses laterally toward the costophrenic sinus, where it continues on in the diaphragmatic musculature to anastomose with the distal ends of the intercostal arteries in the lower chest wall. Each internal thoracic artery is the collateral supply for the other. Each one has a major portion of its arterial supply devoted to the sternum. Perforating branches from the anteromedial aspect of each of the internal thoracic arteries supply the respective sides of the sternum. Perforating vessels also go through the intercostal muscles to join with the intercostal arteries underneath each rib and to become the secondary blood supply to the pectoralis major muscle, which lies anteriorly. Another small but important branch of the internal thoracic artery is the pericardiophrenic artery. This artery arises in the proximal portion of the internal thoracic and courses laterally and posteriorly to the phrenic nerve, where it joins the nerve to supply arterial blood to the nerve and to a small portion of the diaphragm; the phrenic nerve perforates this structure before innervating its musculature (see Fig. 48–8).

The venous drainage of the chest wall consists of numerous intercostal veins, which course with the intercostal arteries underneath the respective ribs (Fig. 48–9). These vessels drain to the hemiazygous and azygous systems, depending on their anatomic position (Clemente, 1985c). The internal thoracic arteries have corres-

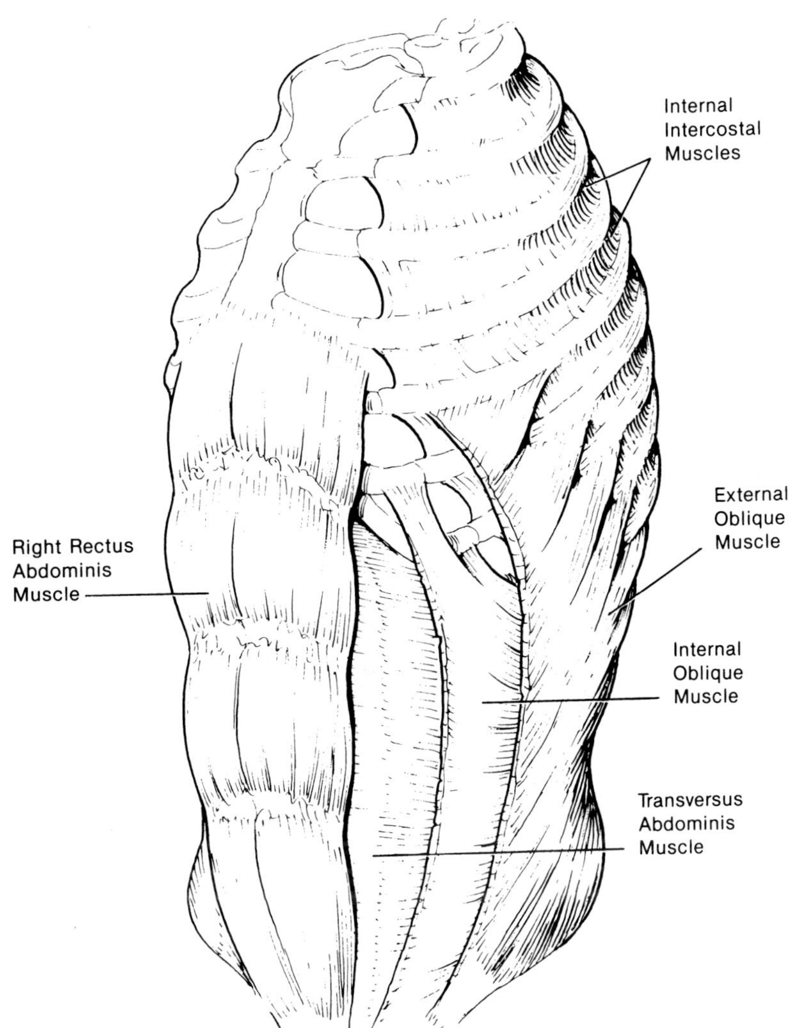

FIGURE 48–6 ■ All the accessory muscles of expiration are shown in this left anterior oblique projection. The internal intercostal muscles, the rectus abdominus, and the three flat muscles of the abdomen all draw the ribs, costal cartilages, and the sternum downward and inward to decrease the volume in the entire thoracic cavity.

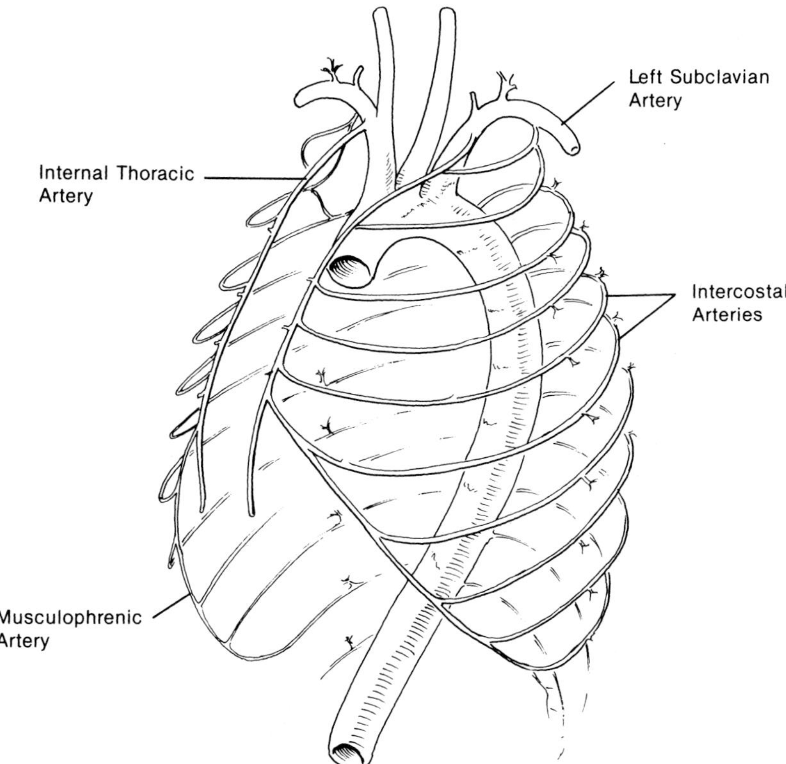

FIGURE 48–7 ■ The arterial supply of the chest wall is shown in this left anterior oblique projection. Note that the intercostal arteries arise from the aorta posteriorly for the lower 10 intercostal spaces. The highest intercostal arteries branch off from the subclavian. The paired internal thoracic arteries arise from the subclavian and course down along the posterolateral aspect of the sternum. They give rise to a major branch, the musculophrenic artery, which goes along the costal cartilages to anastomose with the intercostal arteries. The continuation of the internal thoracic artery becomes the superior epigastric artery.

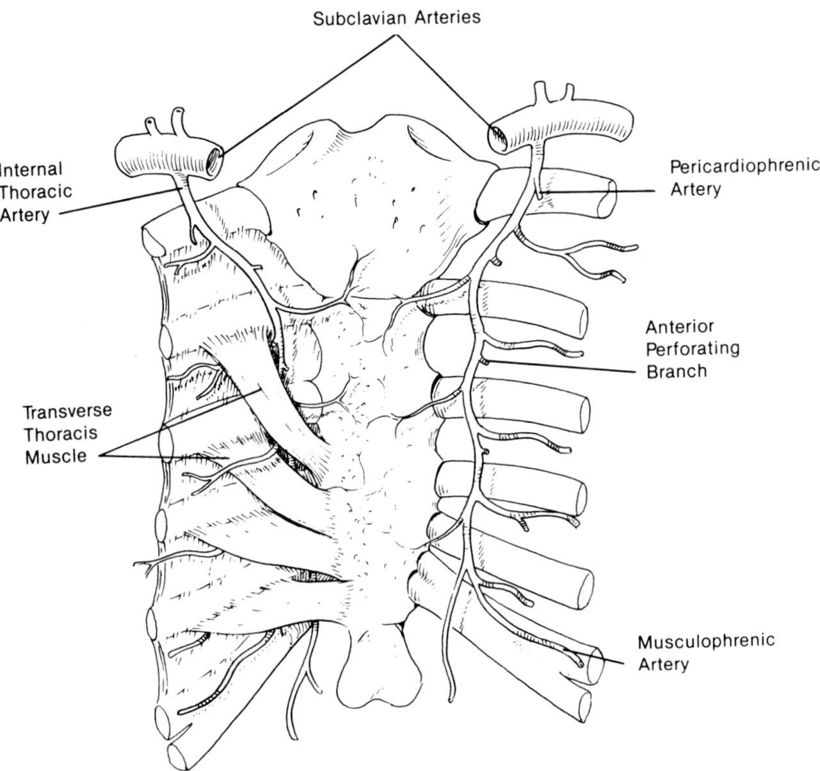

FIGURE 48–8 ■ Illustrated is the detail of the internal thoracic artery and its major branches. The pericardiophrenic arteries arise from the proximal portion of the internal thoracic arteries. They join with the pericardiophrenic veins, which are usually paired, and progress to the diaphragm with the phrenic nerve. The perforators arising from each internal thoracic are shown, as are the communications with the intercostal vessels. The internal thoracic arteries provide the major blood supply to the sternum. The distal arteries arising from the internal thoracic include the musculophrenic, which goes laterally into the costophrenic sinus at the edge of the diaphragm, and the superior epigastric, which penetrates the diaphragm between the costal and sternal portions of the musculature.

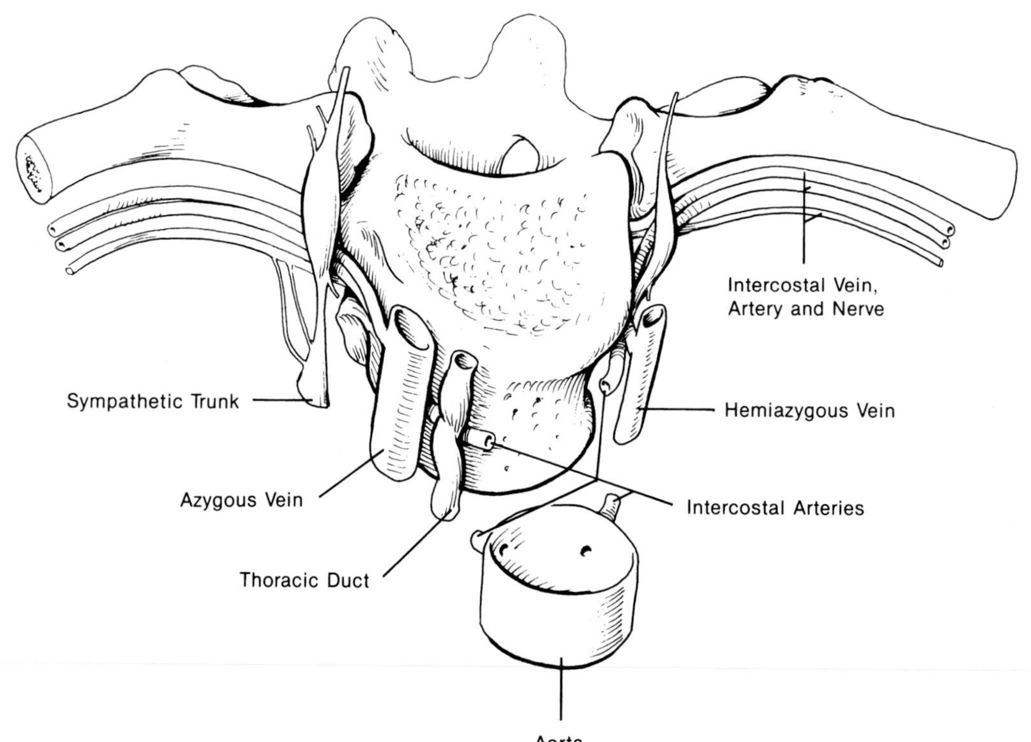

FIGURE 48–9 ■ The relationship of the intercostal arteries, veins, and nerves is shown. Note that the intercostal arteries are directly caudad to each rib. Sequentially below these are the intercostal artery and nerve. The veins drain into the azygos system on the right and into the hemiazygos system on the left. The intercostal nerves arise from the spinal cord, exit the spinal canal, and are joined by communicating branches from the sympathetic trunks.

ponding paired veins, which drain to the subclavian veins. The veins have anastomotic junctions with the corresponding superior epigastric and musculophrenic veins. Perforating veins from the chest wall also go into the internal mammary veins to drain the anterior portion of the intercostal muscles.

The intercostal nerves provide the primary motor and sensory innervation of the entire chest wall (Clemente, 1985d). They arise within the spinal canal, exit through the intervertebral foramina, and course anteriorly underneath the inferior margin of each of the ribs (see Fig. 48–9). Several important anatomic features of these nerves need to be mentioned. The sympathetic trunk conveys sympathetic fibers to the nerves just after the nerves exit the spinal canal (see Fig. 48–9). The nerves also lie most distal of the three structures of the neurovascular bundle underneath each rib (see Fig. 48–9). The intercostal vein is most cephalad, followed progressively by the intercostal artery and finally the intercostal nerve. The first six to seven intrathoracic nerves supply the sensory innervation and dermatomes ranging from the posterior aspect of the back around to the midline of the sternum. The eighth intercostal nerve supplies the anterior wall for sensory fibers around the region of the xiphoid process. The ninth intercostal nerve supplies the upper portion of the epigastrium just distal to the xiphoid, and the tenth intercostal is responsible for sensation at the level of the umbilicus. These relationships are important because intrathoracic processes (such as Boerhaave's syndrome) may affect the intrathoracic portions of each of these nerves and may create symptoms compatible with an intra-abdominal process. Hence, irritation of these nerves posteriorly can create many signs of acute abdomen.

UPPER EXTREMITY MUSCULATURE

A number of upper extremity and abdominal muscles have their origins on the chest wall. Anteriorly, the pectoralis major, the pectoralis minor, and the serratus anterior muscles originate and insert onto the upper extremity (Clemente, 1985a). The pectoralis major arises from the lower costal cartilages and ribs, the sternum, and the clavicle to form a unified muscle, which inserts on the intertubercular sulcus of the humerus. The pectoralis major muscles are supplied by medial and lateral pectoral nerves from the brachial plexus. These muscles function to adduct and rotate the arm medially. In addition, they may elevate it or depress it. The pectoralis minor lies beneath the pectoralis major and has origins on the second through fourth ribs. Its insertion is on the coracoid process of the clavicle. The serratus anterior muscle arises from major muscular slips near the anterior axillary line on the anterior aspect of the ribs and inserts on the scapula (Fig. 48–10). Each of these muscles has obvious importance, not only for governing the motion of the upper extremity but also for thoracic surgical incisions. Each of these muscles receives its primary blood supply and innervation from the cephalad aspect of the chest near the axilla.

A number of muscles from the upper extremity have their origins on the posterior aspect of the chest. These are particularly important in creating and reconstructing thoracic surgical incisions (Fig. 48–11). The two most

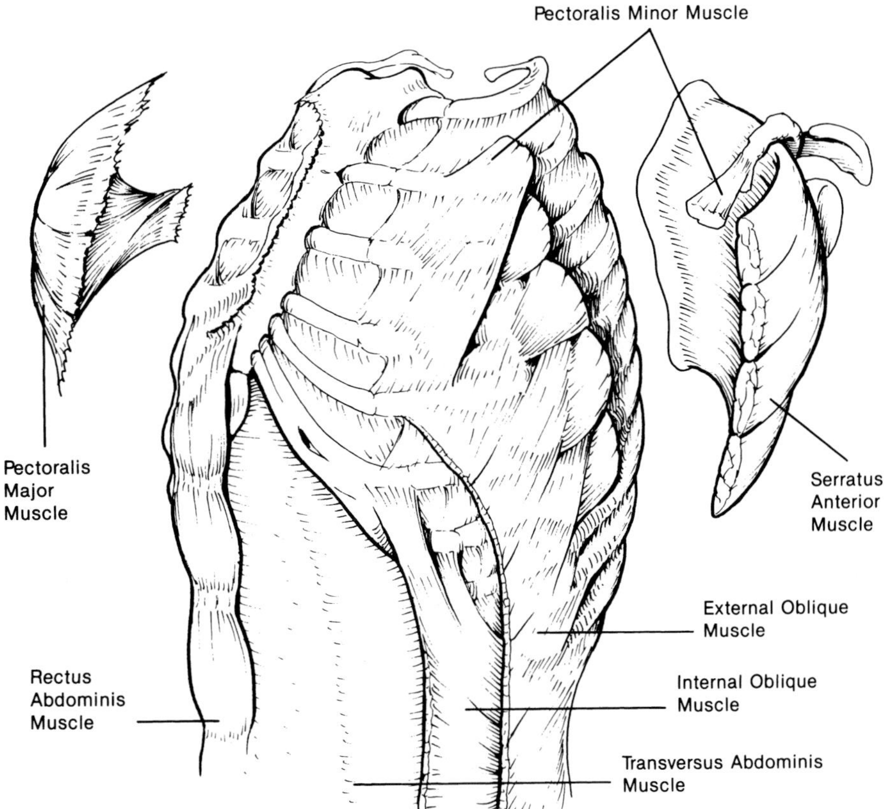

FIGURE 48–10 ■ The relationship of the major anterior muscles of the pectoral girdle is shown in this left anterior oblique projection. On the *right side* the pectoralis major muscle is shown elevated away from the chest wall. Its cut origins along the medial aspect of the sternum and costal cartilage on the right side are apparent. The pectoralis major and serratus anterior have been transected on the *left side* and are placed away from the chest wall for clarity.

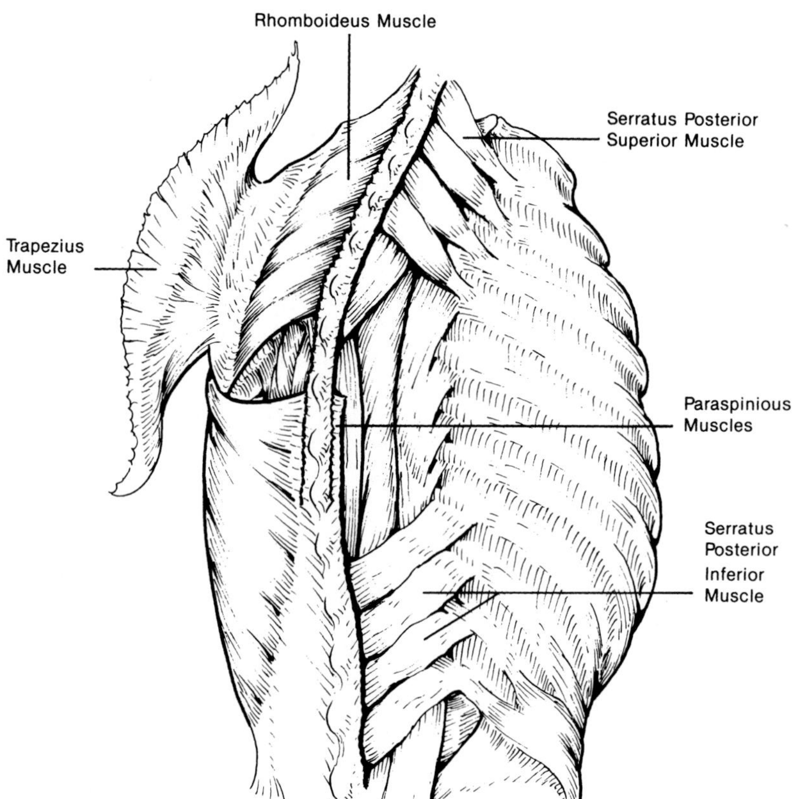

FIGURE 48–11 ■ This right posterior oblique view of the torso shows the major musculature on the posterior aspects of the chest wall. Note that the trapezius muscle on the left side has been cut to expose the rhomboid muscles beneath it. The rhomboid major is below and the rhomboid minor is above. These connect the scapula with the spinal column. Beneath the rhomboids are the serratus posterior superior muscles. The latissimus dorsi has been left intact on the left side but has been cut away on the right side to show the serratus posterior inferior muscles. The paraspinus muscles run longitudinally along the spine and connect the spinal column to the individual ribs.

superficial muscles are the trapezius and the latissimus dorsi. The latissimus dorsi arises from the lumbodorsal fascia and the fascia of the paraspinous muscles, as well as the aponeurosis going to the iliac crest, and inserts on the humerus. Its blood supply and innervation come from the axilla and proceed downward to the posterolateral aspect of the chest. Thoracotomy incisions that divide this muscle cause a significant alteration in its physiology. When the neuromuscular bundle is divided, the distal portion of the muscle depends on its secondary blood supply for viability. When the distal portion of the muscle has become dependent on the perforating arteries of the lumbodorsal fascia, rotation of this muscle as a flap for closure of intrathoracic fistulas or chest wall defects is contraindicated, as this would cause the distal portion of the muscle to die. The proximal portion in these circumstances still maintains the thoracodorsal artery as its primary blood supply. The distal portion of the muscle is no longer dependent on the blood supply arising from above but rather on the secondary supply. Rotation of the entire muscle under these circumstances generally results in necrosis of the distal portion of the muscle. When this is used to close a fistula or to reconstruct a portion of the chest, it causes a severe subsequent complication in that the distal flap generally necroses.

The trapezius muscle, infrequently used in chest wall reconstruction, is more superficial and cephalad; it originates in the paraspinous area and courses laterally to insert on the scapula. The rhomboid muscles lie directly beneath the trapezius and course laterally to insert on the scapula. Directly beneath the rhomboids are the serratus posterior superior muscles, which arise on the spinous processes of the vertebral column and insert on the upper four ribs. The paraspinous muscles, which run the entire length of the spinal column, constitute the deepest layer of the musculature of the back. They run up and down along the spine and connect the vertebral column to the inferior aspects of the ribs. The serratus posterior inferior muscles join the inferior aspects of the lowest four ribs to the lumbar vertebrae. In general, most thoracic incisions do not encounter these muscles because they are placed very low on the thoracic skeleton. Deep to these muscles lie the lower portions of the paraspinous muscles (see Fig. 48–11).

ANATOMY OF SUPERIOR AND INFERIOR APERTURES

The inferior thoracic aperture lies at the boundary between the chest and the abdomen. The anatomy of the diaphragm and the inferior rim of the musculoskeletal thorax is discussed in Chapter 56 on the diaphragm and is not considered here. The superior thoracic aperture has unique anatomic features, which govern surgical procedures in this region. The main muscles of this region are the sternocleidomastoid and scalene muscles (Clemente, 1985a). The sternocleidomastoid muscle originates on the temporal bone of the skull and courses inferiorly and anteriorly to insert on the manubrium of the sternum and on the medial third of the clavicle (Fig. 48–12). Its action is to rotate the skull to the opposite side. It also functions as an accessory muscle of respiration in that it elevates the head of the sternum and causes minimal elevation of the clavicle. The three scalene

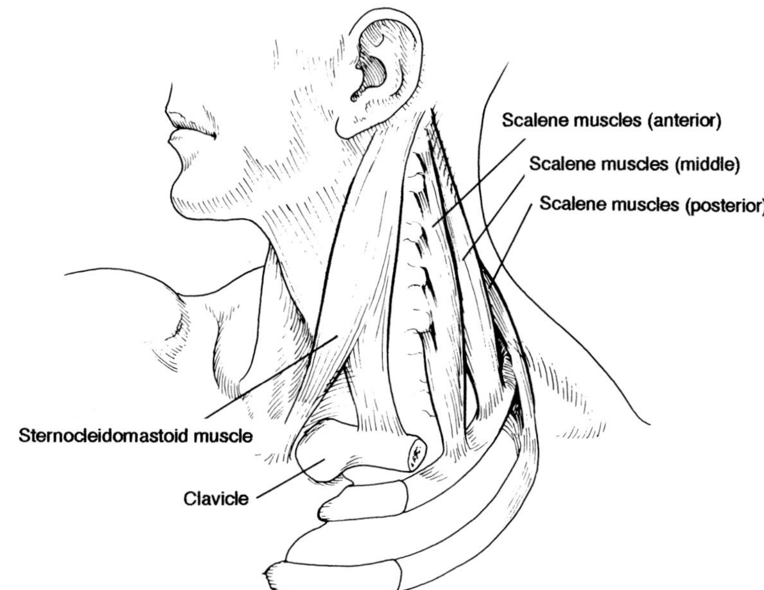

FIGURE 48–12 ■ The muscles of the superior thoracic inlet are shown here. The sternocleidomastoid muscle has two major heads, one going to the manubrium of the sternum and the second to the clavicle. The scalene muscles—anterior, middle, and posterior—originate from the anterior cervical spine and progress anteriorly and caudad until they insert on the first and second ribs. The anterior and middle scalene muscles join on the first rib; the posterior inserts on the superior aspect of the second rib.

muscles—anterior, middle, and posterior—are also accessory muscles of respiration in that they elevate the first and second ribs and raise them somewhat anteriorly through the bucket handle mechanism. These three muscles originate on the cervical vertebrae and insert on the first two ribs. The anterior and middle scalene muscles insert on the cephalad aspect of the first rib. The posterior scalene muscle inserts on the cephalad aspect of the dorsal third of the second rib.

The major vessels of the head and upper extremities, as well as the trachea and esophagus, exit the thorax through the superior thoracic aperture. In Figure 48–13, the clavicles and musculature have been removed to show the relationship of the major vessels to the skeletal thorax and to the trachea and esophagus. The subclavian vein, which is the most anterior vascular structure, lies directly behind the clavicle (Clemente, 1985b). The axillary vein becomes the subclavian vein as soon as it transverses the angle between the first rib and the clavicle. The subclavian vein combines with the internal jugular vein to

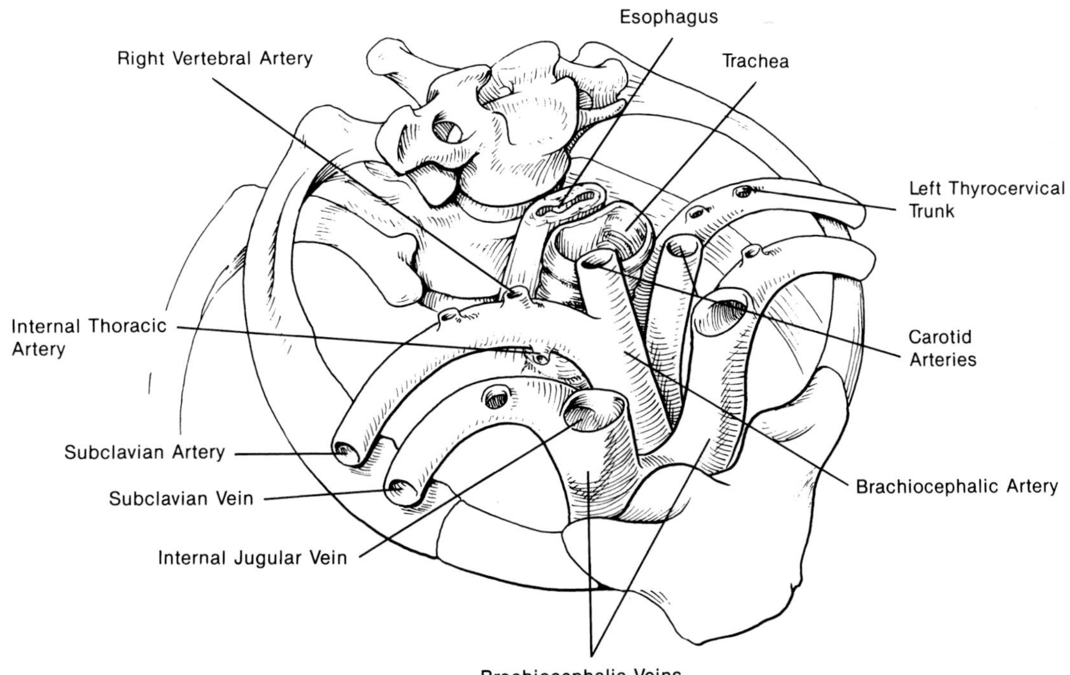

FIGURE 48–13 ■ The major vascular structures that exit through the superior thoracic aperture are shown in relation to the bony skeleton, the trachea, and the esophagus. Note that the great veins are anterior to the arteries, the arteries are between the great veins and the trachea, and the esophagus lies between the trachea and the spinal column. The clavicles have been removed from this picture for clarity.

create the brachiocephalic vein. The subclavian vein also is the point of termination for the thyrocervical trunk, internal thoracic veins, and pericardiophrenic veins. The insertions of these smaller veins onto the larger vessels are somewhat variable. The confluence of the two brachiocephalic veins creates the superior vena cava. As may be noted in Figure 48–13, the left brachiocephalic vein courses behind the manubrium along its posterior aspect to join the right brachiocephalic vein at the right posterolateral aspect of the manubrium to form the vena cava.

The three great arteries exit the chest through the superior thoracic aperture (Clemente, 1985b). The first is the innominate artery (brachiocephalic artery), which gives rise to the right carotid artery and the right subclavian artery. The second branch of the aortic arch exiting through the superior thoracic aperture is the left carotid artery. The left subclavian artery, the third great vessel to arise from the aortic arch, courses medially and cephalad to the apex of the chest and exits over the left first rib just under the clavicle. The paired subclavian arteries each give rise to a vertebral artery, a thyrocervical trunk, and the internal thoracic artery. The first two intercostal arteries generally originate on the inferior aspect of the subclavians. The innominate artery lies directly anterior to the trachea, as is apparent to anyone performing a cervical mediastinoscopy. The proximity of this vessel to the anterolateral wall of the trachea is important because tracheostomy tubes placed with undue tension on the tube and excessive inflation of the occlusive cuff can result in a trachea–innominate artery fistula. The brachial plexus, although not a true thoracic structure, lies in proximity to the apex of the pleura posteriorly near the first rib. The major trunks of the brachial plexus course posterior to the subclavian artery and travel over the first rib to reach the upper extremity.

Acknowledgments

We would like to express my gratitude to Ms. Monica Krupinski for her dedication and excellent preparation of this manuscript. Also, we would like to thank Gary G. Wind, M.D., for his creation of the line drawings for this chapter.

■ KEY REFERENCES

Arey LB: Developmental Anatomy: A Textbook and Laboratory Manual of Embryology, 7th ed. Philadelphia, WB Saunders, 1965.

This is a classic work on developmental anatomy. The various aspects of embryologic development are treated in a realistic fashion. A number of specific drawings outline the development of the embryo and are informative regarding the actual relationships of one structure to another.

Clemente CD: Gray's Anatomy, 30th American ed. Philadelphia, Lea & Febiger, 1985.

This has for generations been the standard textbook describing the anatomy of the human body. It has thorough descriptions of all structures and appropriate illustrations and correlations of structure with function. It is strongly recommended that this text be consulted concerning the musculature of the chest wall, the bony skeleton of the thorax, and any other anatomic features in the region.

Graeber GM: Embryology, anatomy, and physiology of the chest wall. In Seyfer AK, Graeber GM, Wind GG (eds): Atlas of Chest Wall Reconstruction. Rockville, MD, Aspen Publishers, 1986, p 11.

This chapter outlines the embryology, anatomy, and physiology of the chest wall and the important aspects of chest wall anatomy and physiology used in developing flaps for reconstruction of chest wall defects. Other chapters describe methods for maturing various flaps and their use in repairing chest wall defects.

Guyton AC: Pulmonary ventilation. In Texbook of Medical Physiology, 8th ed. Philadelphia, WB Saunders, 1991, p 402.

A thorough and concise treatment of pulmonary physiology. The roles of the diaphragm, chest wall, and accessory muscles are clearly outlined. An essential preliminary description of respiratory physiology, which serves as an excellent introduction to the topic, is presented.

Moore KL, Persaud TVN: The Developing Human: Clinically Oriented Embryology, 5th ed. Philadelphia, WB Saunders, 1993.

This text traces the human embryo from conception through birth and details all aspects of development and maturation with respect to gestational time. Clinical correlation is provided for developmental defects that cause disease in the fully developed child and subsequent adult.

Netter FM: The Ciba Collection of Medical Illustrations, Vol 7, Respiratory System, Section II, Physiology. Summit, NJ, Ciba-Geigy Corporation, 1996.

The illustrations of Frank Netter combined with the accompanying text present a dynamic and insightful view of respiratory physiology. The illustrations are particularly excellent, and they demonstrate major principles well. This reference is strongly recommended because the visual images significantly increase understanding of respiratory physiology.

Ravitch MM: Congenital Deformities of the Chest Wall and Their Operative Correction. Philadelphia, WB Saunders, 1977.

This is a classic monograph on chest wall abnormalities and their correction, written by one of the true experts in congenital abnormalities of the thorax. The book is richly illustrated with clinical pictures and drawings, which delineate proper reconstruction of the abnormalities.

West JB: Pulmonary Pathophysiology—The Essentials, 2nd ed. Baltimore, Williams & Wilkins, 1977.

West is particularly adept at describing the pathophysiologic problems of the pulmonary system and how they may present clinically. The illustrations are superlative. His text and illustrations lead to a higher understanding of pulmonary problems and their clinical correlates.

West JB: Respiratory Physiology—The Essentials, 2nd ed. Baltimore, Williams & Wilkins, 1979.

West has a particularly informative and flowing style of writing, which allows him to convey the essentials of respiratory physiology in a particularly lucid fashion. The illustrations clearly illustrate the major points and increase understanding.

West JB: Mechanics of breathing. In West JB (ed): Best and Taylor's Physiologic Basis of Medical Practice, 12th ed. Baltimore, Williams & Wilkins, 1991, p 560.

This reference describes both basic and more advanced pulmonary physiology. It gives dimension and depth to the topic while presenting the material in a straightforward and cogent fashion.

■ REFERENCES

Arey LB: Developmental Anatomy: A Textbook and Laboratory Manual of Embryology, 7th ed. Philadelphia, WB Saunders, 1965.

Clemente CD: Muscles and fasciae. In Clemente CD (ed): Gray's Anatomy, 30th American ed. Philadelphia, Lea & Febiger, 1985a.

Clemente CD: The arteries. In Clemente CD (ed): Gray's Anatomy, 30th American ed. Philadelphia, Lea & Febiger, 1985b.

Clemente CD: The veins. In Clemente CD (ed): Gray's Anatomy, 30th American ed. Philadelphia, Lea & Febiger, 1985c.

Clemente CD: The peripheral nervous system. In Clemente CD (ed): Gray's Anatomy, 30th American ed. Philadelphia, Lea & Febiger, 1985d.

Graeber GM: Embryology, anatomy, and physiology of the chest wall. In Seyfer AK, Graeber GM, Wind GG (eds): Atlas of Chest Wall Reconstruction. Rockville, MD, Aspen Publishers, 1986, p 11.

Guyton AC: Pulmonary ventilation. In Texbook of Medical Physiology, 8th ed. Philadelphia, WB Saunders, 1991, p 402.

Moore KL, Persaud TVN: The Developing Human: Clinically Oriented Embryology, 5th ed. Philadelphia, WB Saunders, 1993.

Netter FM: The Ciba Collection of Medical Illustrations, Vol 7, Respiratory System, Section II, Physiology. Summit, NJ, Ciba-Geigy Corporation, 1996.

Ravitch MM: Congenital Deformities of the Chest Wall and Their Operative Correction. Philadelphia, WB Saunders, 1977.

West JB: Pulmonary Pathophysiology—The Essentials, 2nd ed. Baltimore, Williams & Wilkins, 1977.

West JB: Respiratory Physiology—The Essentials, 2nd ed. Baltimore, Williams & Wilkins, 1979.

West JB: Mechanics of breathing. In West JB (ed): Best and Taylor's Physiologic Basis of Medical Practice, 12th ed. Baltimore, Williams & Wilkins, 1991, p 560.

CHAPTER **49**

Diagnostic Modalities of the Chest Wall and Sternum

Geoffrey M. Graeber

Pathologic processes that involve the chest wall present numerous perplexing problems to the pulmonologist, the radiologist, and the thoracic surgeon. The detection, evaluation, and characterization of these processes requires many different diagnostic modalities. The recent expansion of cross-sectional imaging techniques has allowed more precise anatomic definition of chest wall pathologic conditions than was previously available (Schaefer and Burton, 1989). Certain lesions that were difficult, if not impossible, to evaluate two decades ago are now assessed with precision and accuracy (Kuhlman et al, 1994). The challenge to delineate the full extent of the chest wall pathologic process remains because many vital structures lie in close proximity to the ribs, costal cartilages, and sternum. In this chapter, most of the methods used to evaluate chest wall disease are discussed, but the focus is on imaging techniques because their importance is paramount. Diagnostic biopsy by both surgical and needle techniques is covered in the chapter on primary chest wall neoplasms (see Chapter 53).

The discussion that follows provides a logical approach to evaluating the patient with a chest wall pathologic condition. Each patient should undergo a thorough initial evaluation, which includes standard radiographic techniques. Some traditional imaging modalities still yield valuable information in the assessment of chest wall disease, despite the availability of more sophisticated techniques (Schaefer and Burton, 1989). Axial imaging techniques, such as computed tomography (CT) and magnetic resonance imaging (MRI), have expanded our ability to evaluate chest wall pathologic conditions. The assets and limitations of CT and MRI are compared. The potentially confusing presence of healing rib fractures and metastatic neoplasms in the evaluation of chest wall disease is discussed. Chest wall neoplasms may be benign or malignant; they can also result from extension of tumors from adjacent organs and overlying skeletal structures. The pertinent findings associated with chest wall infection are also presented. Finally, the salient features of important congenital chest wall deformities are chronicled. Selected images, mostly taken from the author's recent experience, are used to illustrate major points.

INITIAL EVALUATION AND CONSULTATION

A careful history and physical examination are mandatory in the evaluation of the patient with a suspected chest wall pathologic condition because metastatic neoplasms and healing rib fractures are the most common maladies found in the chest wall (Graeber et al, 1982). In most instances, a careful history and review of systems reveal signs and symptoms that suggest the presence of neoplastic disease. Similarly, careful questioning evokes any history of trauma, no matter how slight, which could alert the physician to the possibility of healing rib fractures. The physical examination denotes the characteristics of the pathologic type and focuses the physician's thinking toward specific diagnoses. Standard chest radiographs obtained in the posteroanterior and lateral projections often give additional information concerning the nature of the pathologic condition (Schaefer and Burton, 1989). When this basic information has been obtained, it is wise to consult with the radiologist concerning which imaging modalities will yield the most information with the least cost.

TRADITIONAL RADIOGRAPHIC TECHNIQUES

Routine chest radiographs taken in the posteroanterior and lateral projections reveal chest wall pathologic findings in many instances. These standard films document the presence of disease and help determine which more sophisticated imaging techniques are required. Most importantly, they provide a set of baseline films to which all subsequent radiographs may be compared. Plain films, moreover, may be helpful in defining whether a tumor is extrapleural (Schaefer and Burton, 1989). The characteristics of subpleural lesions that extend into the pleural cavity include a clearly defined, smooth contour that is convex toward the lung, tapering peripheral margins, and broad-based attachment to the chest wall (Felson, 1973) (Fig. 49–1).

Routine tomography plays a very limited role in the evaluation of chest wall pathologic conditions since CT and MRI have assumed increasing capabilities (Schaefer and Burton, 1989). The newer imaging techniques have surpassed standard tomography in the information they can provide on chest wall disease. Induced pneumothorax, when combined with standard radiographs, may have a limited role in the evaluation of some chest wall pathologic conditions. The induced pneumothorax allows the lung to recede from the chest wall. In many cases, when no adhesions are present, the precise origin of the mass may be defined accurately (Schaefer and Burton, 1989) (Fig. 49–2).

Induced pneumothorax may also be combined with

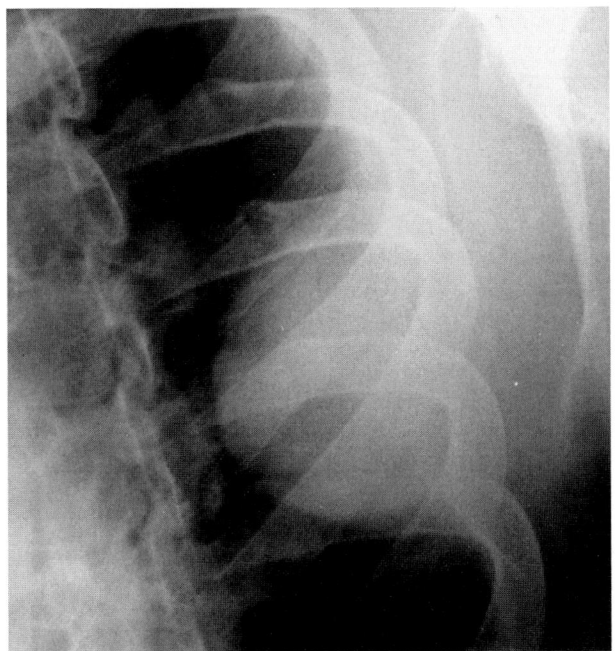

FIGURE 49–1 ■ This selected radiograph of a neural sheath tumor growing inside the ribs shows the characteristics that define an extrapleural lesion. Note that the mass has a sharp, smooth contour, tapering margins along its base on the chest wall, and a broad-based attachment to the chest wall. (From Schaefer PS, Burton BS: Radiographic evaluation of chest wall lesions. Surg Clin North Am 69:911, 1989.)

CT to detect the origin of tumors and whether primary pulmonary malignancies have invaded the chest wall or mediastinum. In one study, the authors used induced pneumothorax combined with CT in 12 patients who had already had initial CT scans that were indeterminate to establish the origin or define the invasion of intrathoracic masses (Watanabe et al, 1991). In 11 of the 12 patients investigated, correct information, confirmed by surgical exploration, was obtained. In the one patient who had a false-positive reading for mediastinal invasion by lung cancer, adhesions from a previous inflammatory process prevented the lung from receding from the mediastinum. At surgery, the adhesions were transected, and the malignancy was found to be free of the mediastinum. Yokoi and colleagues (1991) have been even stronger advocates of CT in association with induced pneumothorax in the evaluation of invasion of lung cancer into the mediastinum and chest wall. In their experience with 43 patients, CT in conjunction with pneumothorax was 100% accurate for chest wall and 76% accurate for mediastinal invasion.

Two other standard techniques that may be used in the evaluation of the extent of thoracic involvement by disease processes that primarily afflict the chest wall are fluoroscopy and decubitus films (Schaefer and Burton, 1989). The integrity of the phrenic nerve and diaphragm to function may be evaluated by fluoroscopy while the patient performs rapid, short inspirations. Decubitus films are also helpful to detect free pleural effusions because the fluid, if not loculated, flows to the most dependent aspect of the chest.

ASSETS AND LIMITATIONS OF COMPUTED TOMOGRAPHY AND MAGNETIC RESONANCE IMAGING

The use of CT and MRI in the evaluation of patients with cancer has yielded more information than plain radiography, but neither modality has provided the diagnostic accuracy that was anticipated (Kuhlman et al, 1994). In fact, CT and MRI have fallen short of anticipated goals in the detection of mediastinal or chest wall involvement by pulmonary malignancies (Miller et al, 1992; Webb et al, 1991). There is no substantial difference between the two modalities in their ability to predict chest wall invasion (Webb et al, 1991). They should be considered to be complementary to one another in the evaluation of chest wall pathologic conditions (Kuhlman et al, 1994; Schaefer and Burton, 1989). Both continue to undergo evaluation to define their role in the assessment of chest wall disease. Because MRI is newer and has more possible variables to apply, the potential for growth in knowledge is greater with this technique (Templeton et al, 1990).

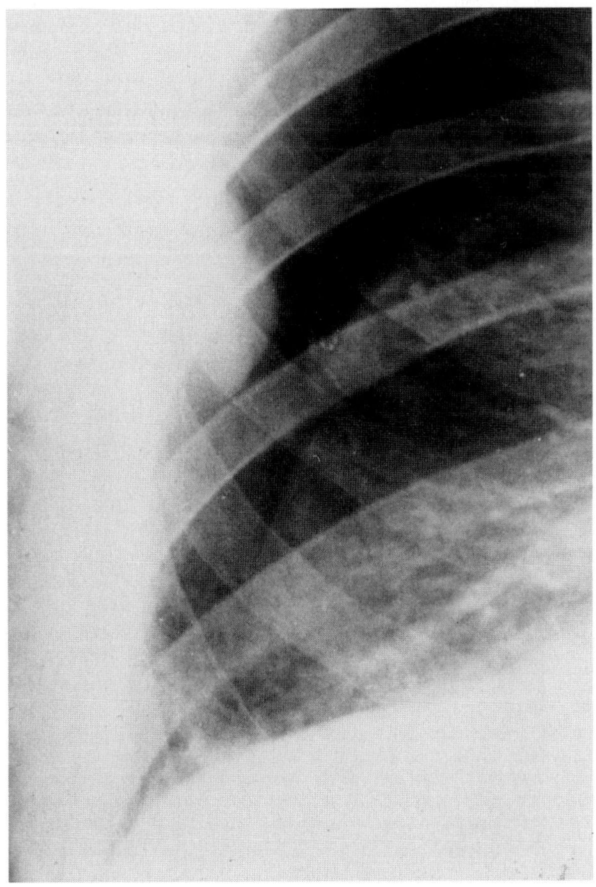

FIGURE 49–2 ■ This patient underwent induced pneumothorax and chest radiography to determine whether a chest wall mass had its origin in the lung. The lesion (a perineural fibroblastoma) was suspected to be extrapleural, as determined by the characteristics noted in Figure 49–1. The parietal pleura is stretched over the neoplasm. The *medial line* represents the receding visceral pleura on the lung surface. (From Schaefer PS, Burton BS: Radiographic evaluation of chest wall lesions. Surg Clin North Am 69:911, 1989.)

Axial imaging with CT does have some advantages (Kuhlman et al, 1994). CT has a good capacity to assess cortical bone destruction by neoplastic masses and infection. The changes must be definitive, however, or a firm diagnosis of tumor invasion or osteomyelitis cannot be substantiated (Libshitz, 1990). Pearlberg and colleagues (1987) found that definite bony destruction was the only truly reliable finding to substantiate chest wall invasion by a tumor. In some studies, local pain has been as effective as CT in the prediction of chest wall invasion (Gamsu, 1986; Glaser et al, 1985).

The utility of CT has been extended by specialized techniques to yield somewhat improved results. Mention has already been made of the combination of CT with induced pneumothorax to evaluate tumor invasion of the chest wall and mediastinum (Watanabe et al, 1991; Yokoi et al, 1991). CT has also been used in conjunction with progressive expiration in an attempt to determine chest wall invasion by lung cancer (Murata et al, 1994). Based on a small number of patients, it appeared that expiratory CT was highly successful in the evaluation of chest wall invasion. Confirmation of these findings awaits a larger series of patients.

CT has also been compared with ultrasound (US) to assess chest wall invasion by lung cancer (Suzuki et al, 1993). In a series of 120 patients evaluated by both CT and US, 19 had chest wall invasion. The authors found that the sensitivity of US was 100% and its specificity was 98%. The sensitivity of CT was only 68%, and its specificity was 66%. The accuracy of US was 98%; that of CT was 67%. The results of this interesting study await the publication of a larger series and confirmation by other authors.

MRI has some distinct advantages over CT to evaluate primary chest wall neoplasms or the extent of chest wall involvement associated with malignancies of other organs that may extend into the chest wall (Kuhlman et al, 1994). MRI can image in several planes (coronal, sagittal, and axial) to obtain better definition of neoplastic masses and their relationship to adjacent structures (Kuhlman et al, 1994; Libshitz, 1990; Templeton et al, 1990). Because MRI can be adjusted, it is more useful to highlight infiltration of bone marrow and soft tissue invasion (Kuhlman et al, 1994). Because of these mentioned abilities, MRI is used preferentially to evaluate superior sulcus tumors (Kuhlman et al, 1994; Libshitz, 1990; Templeton et al, 1990).

In summary, these imaging techniques should be considered to be complementary modalities, which should be used judiciously and selectively in the evaluation of chest wall pathologic conditions as part of a thorough and comprehensive workup (Kuhlman et al, 1994; Libshitz, 1990; Templeton et al, 1990). Most thoracic surgeons perform standard radiographs and obtain a CT scan, if indicated, as a guide to surgical therapy (Libshitz, 1990; Templeton et al, 1990). If further delineation of disease is necessary, MRI may be considered to guide definitive therapy (Templeton et al, 1990). Neither modality by itself or in confirmation with the findings of other diagnostic modalities should be considered absolute

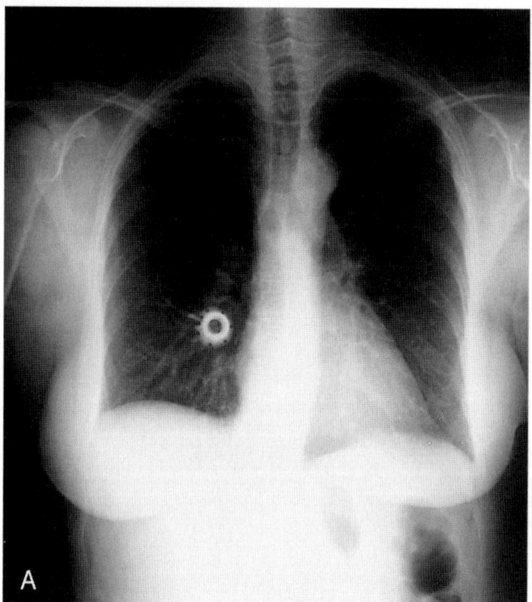

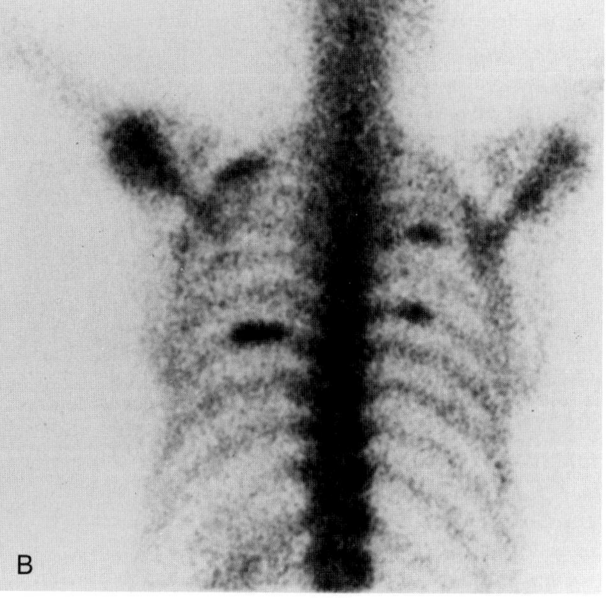

FIGURE 49–3 ■ *A*, This posteroanterior radiograph of a 42-year-old woman with known breast cancer shows minimal irregularities in the posterior aspects of the left eighth rib. Because the patient had some posterior tenderness and this irregularity of the eighth rib was detected, the patient was scheduled for a bone scan. It should also be noted that the patient fell and landed on her left shoulder approximately 6 months prior to this radiograph. *B*, A posterior projection from the bone scan conducted on the patient whose radiograph is presented in *A*. Note that the left eighth rib concentrates the radiopharmaceutical most actively. Three other ribs also concentrate the radiopharmaceutical, as does the head of the left humerus. The patient underwent needle biopsy of the left eighth rib, which showed nonspecific inflammatory changes. An excisional biopsy was performed of the eighth rib, which showed a healing rib fracture.

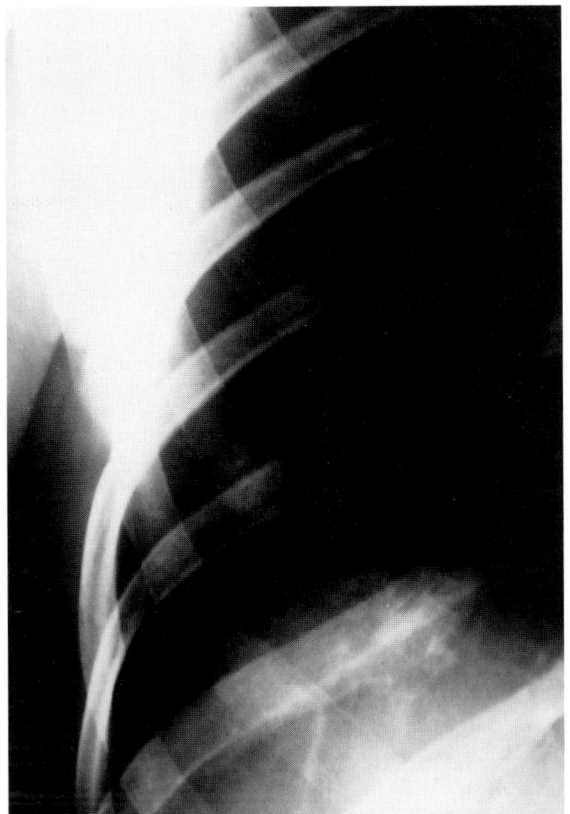

FIGURE 49–4 ■ This selected radiograph of the ribs demonstrates a mass lesion anteriorly near the costochondral junction. Despite an extensive workup, no other lesions were found. The patient denied any history of significant trauma. The lesion underwent biopsy and was found to be a healing rib fracture.

or definitive enough to withhold surgical therapy based on images alone (Libshitz, 1990). Indeed, the presence and extent of disease is still determined by tissue biopsy and pathologic examination.

METASTASES TO THE CHEST WALL AND HEALING RIB FRACTURES

As already mentioned, metastases from distant cancers and healing rib fractures are far more common than primary chest wall neoplasms (Graeber et al, 1982). Because many such lesions may be found on routine chest radiographs, they become an important problem. Differentiation of metastases from healing rib fractures or primary chest wall neoplasms can be impossible with imaging techniques alone (Graeber et al, 1982; Schaefer and Burton, 1989) (Figs. 49–3 and 49–4). Radiographs and images taken of the chest at some prior time may be most helpful to determine the nature of a mass found in the chest wall on a routine radiograph (Schaefer and Burton, 1989). In the absence of previous images, a biopsy may need to be performed to ascertain the exact nature of the pathologic finding. Despite active direct questioning, the patient may deny trauma or minimize its extent such that a biopsy will become necessary.

In the event that the lesion is a metastasis, a biopsy is required to substantiate the disease finding and to direct appropriate therapy (Graeber et al, 1982). The most common offenders that cause metastases in the chest wall are primary malignancies of the breast, lung, kidney, and thyroid, although exceptions occur with reasonable frequency (Fig. 49–5). MRI may be particularly helpful to determine the amount of soft tissue involvement (Fig. 49–6).

Observation of a chest wall lesion is only warranted if its presence has been established on prior radiographic examination and the lesion has been stable for a considerable period (Graeber et al, 1982). Primary neoplasms and metastases need histologic confirmation and appropriate therapy as soon as possible. Although infectious processes can occur as a mass, constitutional symptoms (such as fever and leukocytosis) usually reveal the cause. Because neoplasia, active healing, and infection all arouse active inflammation, masses caused by all three etiologic factors yield a positive bone scan (see Fig. 49–3). If there

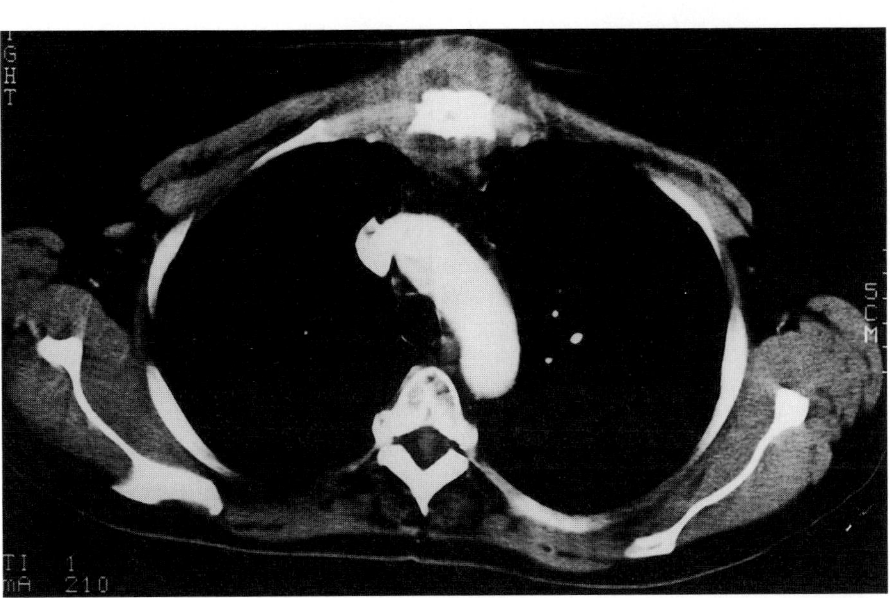

FIGURE 49–5 ■ A 42-year-old man with a recent onset of a painful enlarging mass of his sternum. Radiographically, the tumor appeared to be a primary sarcoma of the sternum. An extensive workup did not reveal any other similar lesions or any suggestion of a primary. Biopsy detected a metastatic adenocarcinoma, most likely of colonic origin. Although the primary was never found, several other areas of metastasis developed, and the patient died of disseminated disease. This figure shows a representative computed tomography axial image of the chest that demonstrates how the metastatic tumor had enveloped the sternum.

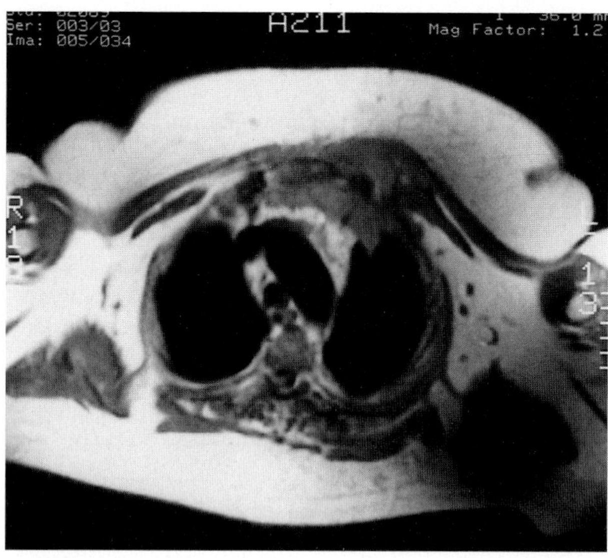

FIGURE 49–6 ■ Magnetic resonance imaging may be used to delineate soft-tissue involvement by metastatic neoplasms, such as in this patient who has a history of metastatic carcinoma of an unknown primary. This is a thin-density T_1-weighted axial image through the upper thorax that shows a mass involving the chest wall with involvement of the pectoralis major and minor, direct extension into the sternum, and involvement of the anterior mediastinum.

is concern or doubt over the nature of a given lesion or its cause, surgical biopsy is indicated because needle biopsy of chest wall lesions is often imprecise (Graeber et al, 1982) (see Fig. 49–3).

BENIGN PRIMARY CHEST WALL NEOPLASMS

In most series, approximately one half of all primary chest wall neoplasms are benign (Graeber et al, 1982; Ryan et al, 1989). Most of these benign neoplasms are of cartilaginous origin. Enchondromas, juxtacortical chondromas, and osteochondromas are some of the more commonly occurring neoplasms (Fig. 49–7). Most often these lesions are incidental, asymptomatic findings on routine radiographs or on radiographs conducted to assess other conditions. Many of these neoplasms have radiographic characteristics on plain films that identify them. At times other radiographic techniques, such as CT or MRI, are required to determine the most likely diagnosis. Once the presence of one of these neoplasms has been documented, the treating physician may elect to observe the tumor. If this course is taken, the surveillance must be precise and continuous because malignant degeneration, although rare, does occur (Graeber et al, 1982). This is particularly true in chondromatous lesions. Observation of such neoplasms must be exceptionally thorough in patients who have certain inherited syndromes, such as multiple hereditary osteochondromatosis or enchondromatosis, because malignant degeneration may occur in 5% to 20% of benign neoplasms in these patients (Resnick and Niwayama, 1981). Change in any lesion, particularly expansion accompanied by discomfort, should arouse the physician's serious suspicion of malignant degeneration.

Fibrous dysplasia in some series represented 20% to

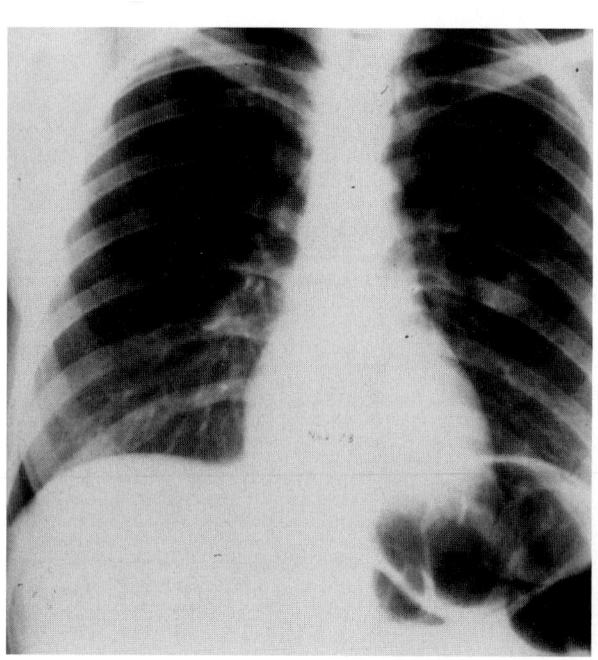

FIGURE 49–7 ■ Radiograph of an osteochondroma arising in the region near the posterior aspect of the left sixth rib. Note that the ribs in the area appear to have intact cortices and that there is no erosion. The lesion is rounded, has a sharp margin, and does not appear to encroach on any other structures.

30% of all benign neoplastic processes found in the chest wall (Teitelbaum, 1972). In reality, the condition probably is not a true neoplasm but rather a developmental abnormality of the bone-forming mesenchyme, which is characterized by filling of the medullary cavity with fibrous tissue and random formation of poor trabeculae (Resnick and Niwayama, 1981). Characteristically, the abnormality is often a painless, lytic lesion of the posterior aspect of a rib. Areas of bone expansion may be present. Over time, the lesion may progress through increasing density to a ground-glass appearance. Continuation of this process may finally result in a homogeneous sclerosis (Schaefer and Burton, 1989).

Other true, benign neoplasms of the musculoskeletal thorax are less common. These neoplasms, plus other benign conditions that may mimic a neoplasm, are important because, in some instances, they may have radiographic characteristics that suggest malignancy. One characteristic that may particularly suggest malignancy is presentation as a lytic area in a rib. Most commonly, however, these lesions are clearly circumscribed lesions that are discernible on standard chest radiographs. Among these lesions are eosinophilic granulomas, chondroblastomas, giant cell tumors, hemangiomas, aneurysmal bone cysts, and osteoblastomas (Fig. 49–8). CT may be indicated in any of these conditions to define the true extent of the malignancy if there is any suggestion of a soft tissue mass or evidence of cortical breakthrough (Schaefer and Burton, 1989).

Probably the most common benign neoplasm of the tissues that are intimate to the musculoskeletal thorax is the lipoma (Stout and Lattes, 1967). Many arise just outside the parietal pleura. Some have both an intrathoracic and an extrathoracic component, which are joined by an isthmus that extends between two ribs (Schaefer and Burton, 1989). If the lipoma is of sufficient size, it may be detectable on plain radiographs. A lipoma usually appears as a mass of relatively lucent tissue because fat is less dense compared with the other structures of the chest wall. CT can be diagnostic of lipomas in the chest wall because of their low density. CT scanning can generally differentiate between lipomas and liposarcomas because the sarcomas almost always have areas of higher density (Goodwin, 1984).

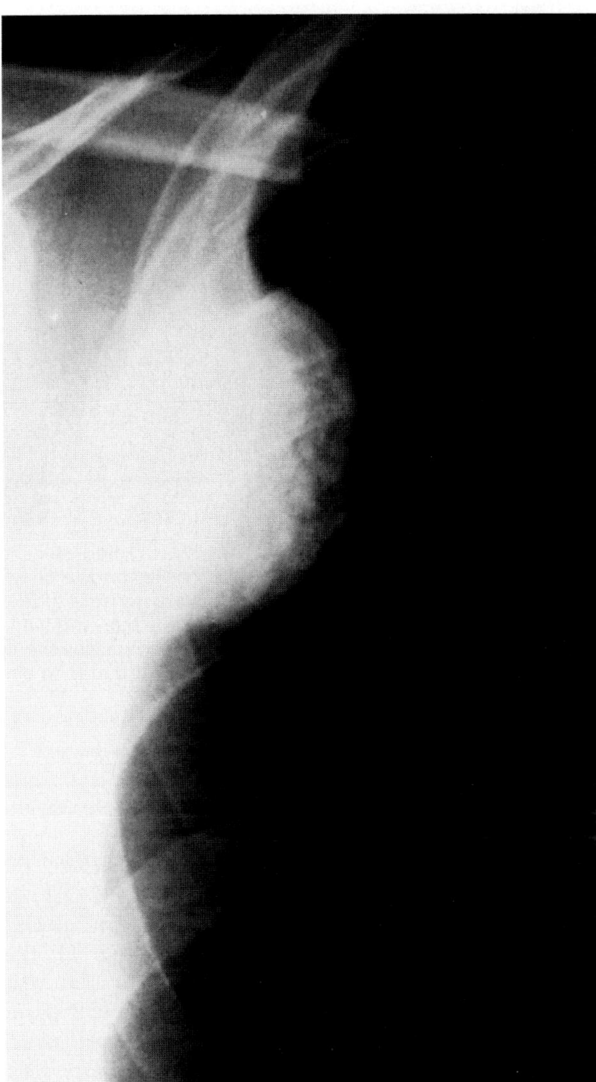

FIGURE 49–8 ■ A plain chest radiograph of an asymptomatic 44-year-old man revealing a 6-cm mass growing off the right third rib. The flocculent chondroid calcifications are notable. This broad-based lesion with the chondroid calcifications demonstrates all the characteristics of a chondroblastoma. As with all chondromatous lesions, the true nature can only be confirmed after a thorough histologic examination by a pathologist. By the size criteria noted in the text, the lesion should be regarded as a chondrosarcoma until proved otherwise.

MALIGNANT PRIMARY CHEST WALL NEOPLASMS

Although certain malignant primary chest wall neoplasms have radiographic characteristics that strongly suggest their type, none has an imaging signature that is unequivocally diagnostic (Graeber et al, 1982; Schaefer and Burton, 1989). Two malignant primary chest wall neoplasms that have imaging characteristics that are strongly suggestive of their respective histologic types are osteogenic and Ewing's sarcomas. Both lesions are relatively rare and tend to arise in younger individuals. Ewing's arises principally in the pediatric population and osteogenic sarcoma, usually in young adults. Ewing's sarcoma has a radiographic appearance that suggests multiple layering as a result of its physical characteristics. It may be a lytic or an expansile lesion of a rib or clavicle that is surrounded by periosteal new bone formation and a soft tissue mass (Franken et al, 1977). Unfortunately, Ewing's sarcoma is not only the most common malignant primary chest wall neoplasm in children, it is one of the more frequent malignancies to metastasize to the bony thorax (Larsson and Lorentzon, 1974; Schaefer and Burton, 1989). Osteogenic sarcomas often have a "sunburst" appearance when they originate from components of the thoracic skeleton. Exceptions to these radiographic characteristics obviously occur.

Among the other malignant primary chest wall neoplasms, general tendencies can be identified, but exceptions are frequent. An obvious example is the chest wall plasmacytoma (Graeber et al, 1982; Schaefer and Burton,

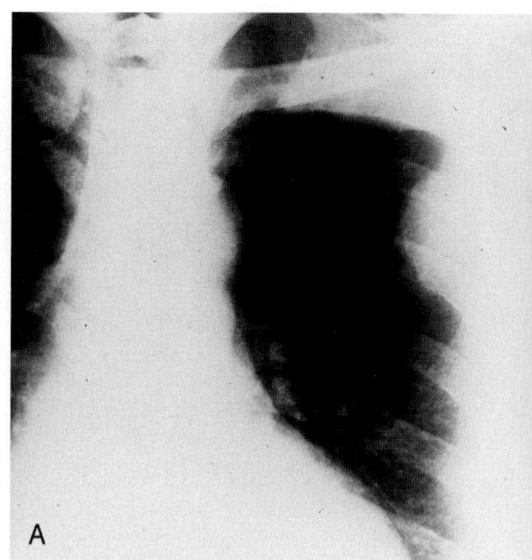

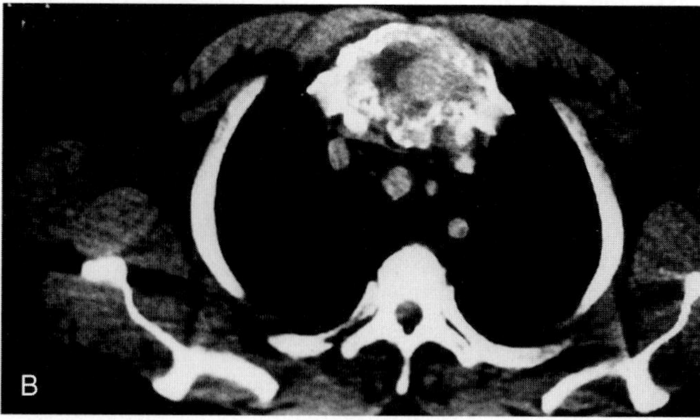

FIGURE 49–9 ■ *A,* Posteroanterior chest radiograph showing a mass in the chest wall on the lateral aspect of the left pleura. Note that the mass encroaches on the pleural space. It is contiguous with the chest wall structures. Even though the mass had radiographic characteristics suggestive of a chondrosarcoma, on excision it was found to be a plasmocytoma. *B,* Computed tomography scan showing a large irregular mass that has replaced the entire manubrium of the sternum. Note that it displaces the great vessels posteriorly. This mass, which was a rapidly enlarging neoplasm of the sternum, was thought to be a chondrosarcoma. Pathologic examination confirmed that it was a plasmacytoma.

1989). The solitary chest wall plasmacytoma is often the first sign of systemic myeloma. In a number of instances, the chest wall lesion occurs several years before the systemic disease is apparent (Graeber et al, 1982). When systemic myeloma has first become apparent in another area, the disease frequently involves several or all ribs and the sternum (Omell et al, 1973). The CT scan may show subtle lytic lesions in the bone or small soft tissue masses when plain film findings of the chest wall structures are negative (Edelstein et al, 1985). Solitary plasmacytoma may also present as soft tissue masses or as lytic lesions of the sternum (Fig. 49–9).

Chondrosarcoma, which has frequently been cited as the most common malignant primary chest wall neoplasm, is generally a large, lobulated, excrescent mass of the chest wall that shows scattered flocculent calcifications in a characteristic cartilaginous matrix (Schaefer and Burton, 1989). Such a lesion may be particularly indistinguishable from its close relatives, the benign osteochondroma or the enchondroma. Larger lesions, especially those that are greater than 4 cm in greatest extent, are considered malignant until proved otherwise (Marcove, 1971).

Fibrosarcomas are some of the most common chest wall tumors and may be reported as the most frequent primary chest wall malignancies in some series (Graeber et al, 1982; Threlkel and Adkins, 1971). As discussed, the broad classification of sarcoma in some instances may include other tumors with "spindle cell" histologic types, such as malignant fibrous histiocytoma, malignant schwannoma, and synovial sarcoma (Enzinger and Weiss, 1983). Radiographically, all of these spindle cell tumors appear in virtually identical fashion in that all appear as masses of soft tissue density (Schaefer and Burton, 1989). Necrotic, low-density areas may be present; these are likely to represent necrosis. If focal areas of calcification are present, they are generally noted on the CT scan.

LUNG CANCER THAT INVOLVES THE CHEST WALL

MRI and CT scans have their advantages and disadvantages when they are used to assess the amount of chest wall involvement, as has already been described. Two instances that occur infrequently in patients with lung cancer can be more accurately assessed by MRI than by CT because of MRI's multiplanar imaging capacities (Haggar et al, 1987; Musset et al, 1986). Tumors of the lung apex can be evaluated to determine involvement of apical thoracic structures and tumors of the lung base, to determine the presence or absence of diaphragmatic invasion. Because superior sulcus neoplasms occur more frequently than do tumors that extend into the diaphragm, they have received more attention.

One group investigated 10 patients with superior sulcus tumors with MRI to assess the extent of apical tumor invasion (McCloud et al, 1989). Five of the 10 patients had chest wall invasion or extension into the base of the neck that was demonstrated by the contrast between the bright signal intensity of the tumor and the low signal intensity of muscle on T_2-weighted images. MRI clearly depicted direct invasion of the mediastinum in three patients because of the inherent contrast between mediastinal fat and neoplastic tissue. In all of the cases studied by these authors, MRI clearly defined the relationship of the tumor to the subclavian artery and the brachial plexus. In two patients, MRI projections confirmed encasement of the artery, and brachial plexus involvement was confirmed in three. One problem noted by these authors was that MRI did not detect evidence of rib destruction in five patients who had rib involvement, confirmed by other studies. Other authors have confirmed the ability of MRI to assess tumor involvement of apical structures and to detect the presence of spinal canal extension (Kuhlman et al, 1994). In our own experience, we found MRI to be particularly useful to evaluate the extent of tumor involvement of soft tissues of the mediastinum and the base of the neck, the subclavian vessels, and the spinal column (Figs. 49–10 and 49–11). MRI has been particularly helpful to determine the status of a tumor in the spinal canal and its relationship to the spinal cord (Figs. 49–10 and 49–11).

BREAST CANCER THAT INVOLVES THE CHEST WALL

Some studies estimate that 5% to 25% of patients treated for breast cancer have local or regional recurrence (Donegan, 1979; Lindfors et al, 1985). CT scan has been particularly helpful to assess recurrences, document

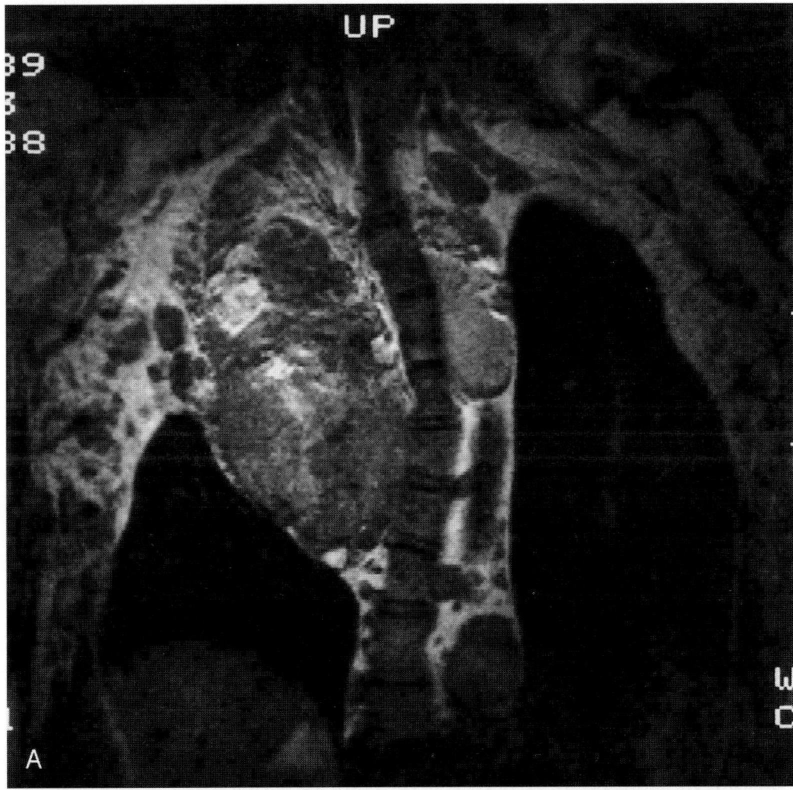

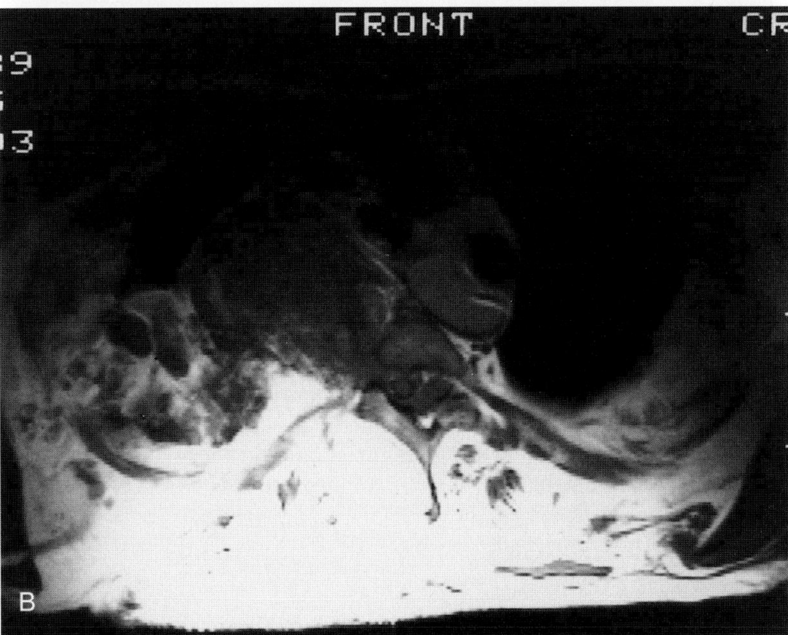

FIGURE 49–10 ■ *A*, A T_1-weighted magnetic resonance image (MRI) through the thorax from a patient with invasive angiolipomatosis. A heterogeneous mass is seen involving the chest wall with extension into the posterior mediastinum adjacent to the spinal column. *B*, An axial T_1-weighted image through the thorax in the same patient as in *A*. Note that the image clearly shows a large chest-wall mass with mediastinal involvement and evidence for invasion of the spinal canal with spinal cord impingement. The multiple planes available with MRI helped to define the extent of this process.

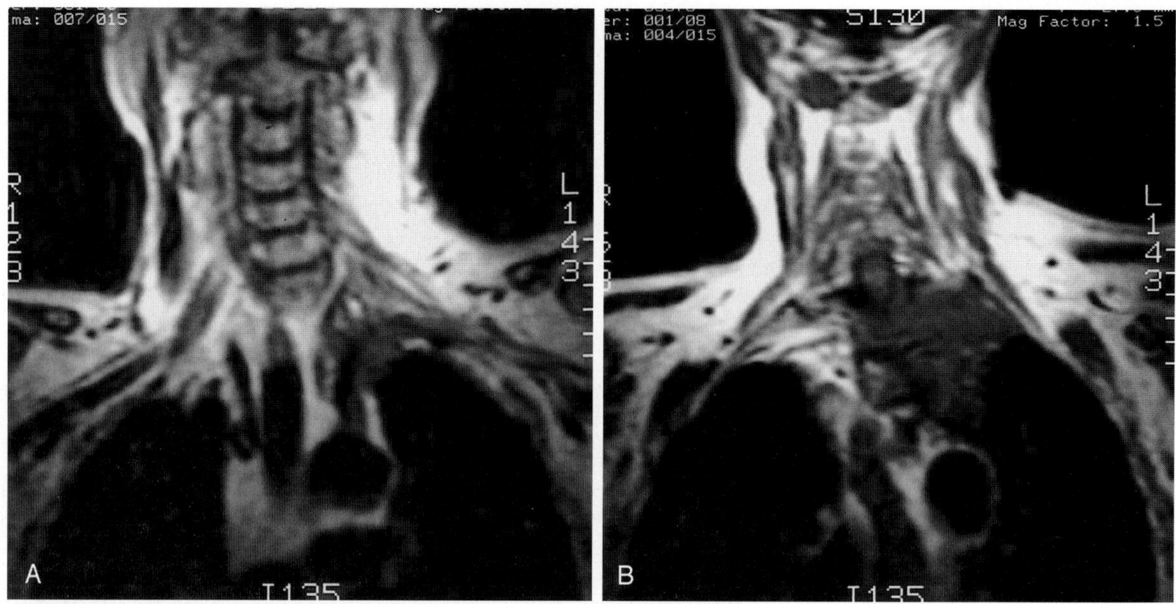

FIGURE 49–11 ■ *A*, Magnetic resonance imaging is most useful to define the structures involved by a superior sulcus tumor. This T_1-weighted coronal image through the lower neck and upper thorax demonstrates a mass at the left lung apex with superior sulcus involvement and encasement of the left subclavian artery. *B*, A T_1-weighted image demonstrating the mass with involvement of the spinal cord and extension into the region of the brachial plexus.

changes in the chest wall anatomy, and follow the progression of breast disease in the chest wall when it is under therapy (Schaefer and Burton, 1989). In several clinical series, it has been shown to be more accurate than physical examination in the assessment of the extent of recurrent disease. Many times CT identifies additional sites of recurrent disease that have not been suspected clinically (Lindfors et al, 1985; Villari et al, 1985).

The most common findings of recurrent or residual breast cancer in the chest wall are masses of soft tissue density (Shea et al, 1987) (Fig. 49–12). Breast cancer may also appear as lytic lesions in the ribs or other bones of the thoracic and axial skeleton. MRI has been particularly helpful to assess recurrent breast disease in the chest wall when CT scanning is not completely able to delineate the extent of recurrent or residual disease. Great care must be taken to confirm the histologic character of the lesions when they have been found. In our experience, the patient who is being treated for breast cancer can have other conditions, which can mimic recurrent disease (Fig. 49–13). Besides healing rib fractures, we must be constantly aware that therapeutic modalities can produce their own problems. One of these problems, which we have seen in several patients, is the destruction of bone by radiotherapy. The lesion presents as a lytic area in bone in the field of previous radiotherapy. The question arises after CT and MRI have been conducted as to whether the lytic area represents recurrent disease (Fig. 49–13). In all instances, the absolute histologic type of the offending lesion should be confirmed before any changes in therapy are instituted.

PYOGENIC INFECTIONS OF THE CHEST WALL

Pyogenic infections of the chest wall can be caused by processes in the chest wall itself or by extensions of intrathoracic problems that arise in the pleura or the underlying lung. In many instances the pyogenic infections may be due to trauma or to a surgical procedure. The diagnosis of early pyogenic infections can be difficult because it is usually 1 to 2 weeks after the onset of symptoms before the characteristic bony changes may be apparent on standard radiographs (Resnick and Niwayama, 1981). The characteristic "moth-eaten" appearance of bones afflicted by osteomyelitis generally occurs after the infection is established and the bone has been thoroughly invaded. Early detection combines careful physical diagnostic procedures to denote the extent of tenderness in the chest wall, the extent of erythema present in the soft tissues, and any evidence of tissue edema. These physical findings, when associated with bone scans, usually allow the clinician to estimate the extent of disease. In fact, radionuclide bone scanning may be particularly helpful when it is combined with a standard ^{99m}T-MPD bone scan with an ^{111}In-labeled leukocyte or ^{67}Ga scan (Schaefer and Burton, 1989). The combination of these modalities may be diagnostic of osteomyelitis several days or weeks before any conventional or radiographic changes appear on standard radiographs.

CT scan has been particularly helpful to delineate infections of the chest wall because its actual axial projections are extremely sensitive to the changes associated with osteomyelitis. It is particularly effective to localize the infection, identify the limits of the soft tissue process that surrounds the osteomyelitis, and allow a direct guide for drainage (Schaefer and Burton, 1989). The characteristic findings of infection include a bone that has an adjacent soft tissue mass of recent onset, loss of deep soft tissue planes that are normally present, and periosteal elevation on the afflicted bone. These findings are particularly important when they are correlated with the clinical findings.

The most common cause of pyogenic infection of the

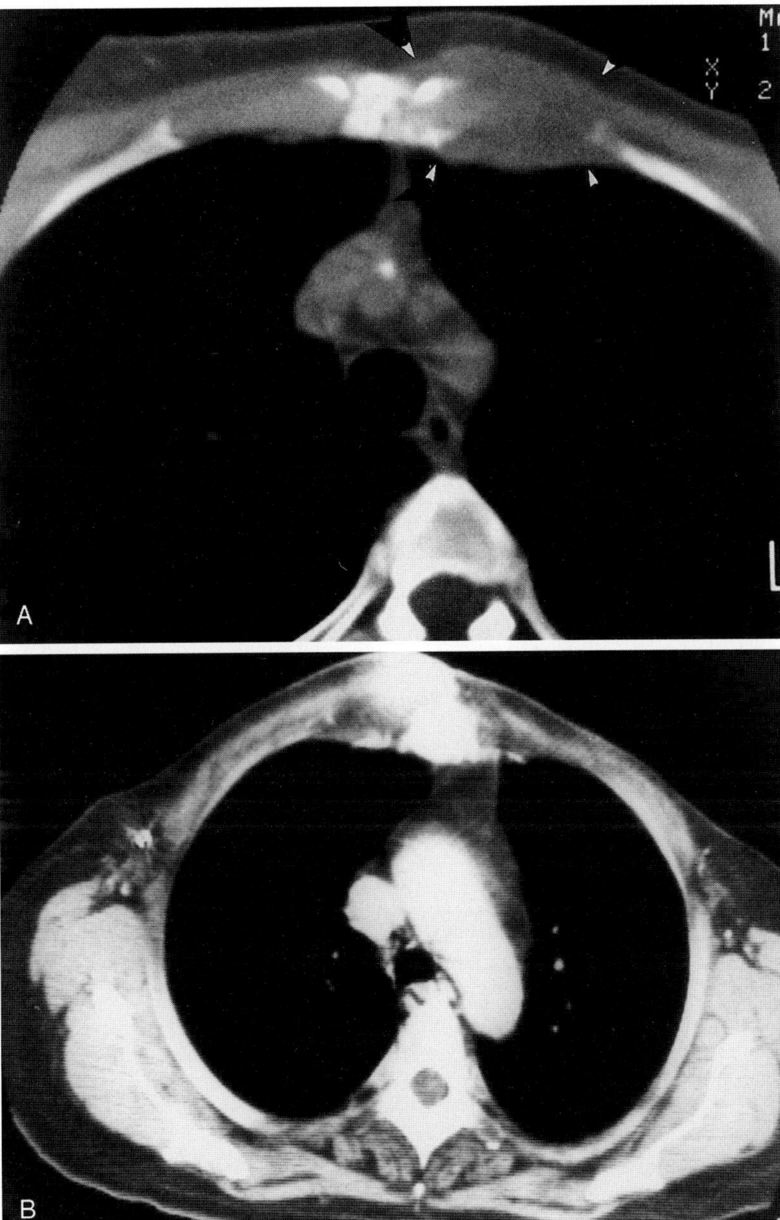

FIGURE 49–12 ■ An axial computed tomography (CT) image demonstrating asymmetry of the sternocostochondral junction. There is an apparent soft tissue mass on the left side (*arrows*). Biopsy revealed a clinically unsuspected residual carcinoma of the breast. *B*, An axial CT image taken after bilateral mastectomies demonstrates the presence of a soft tissue mass in the right peristernal region. In this patient, biopsy yielded the diagnosis of recurrent adenocarcinoma of the breast. (From Schaefer PS, Burton BS: Radiographic evaluation of chest wall lesions. Surg Clin North Am 69:911, 1989.)

chest wall at the current time is the dehisced median sternotomy. Plain radiographs may be particularly helpful to suggest this problem because air may be readily apparent between the two halves of the sternum early in a sternal dehiscence. This characteristic dark stripe between the two halves of the sternum not only suggests the nonunion of bone but also reflects the air that is between the separated sternal halves (Fig. 49–14). In such instances the CT scan may be particularly helpful to show where air is present within the mediastinum, what fluid pockets are present, and where a clot is present. The CT scan is also particularly helpful to follow the progression of therapy because subsequent images will delineate loculated pockets within the pericardium or the mediastinum (Fig. 49–15).

CHEST WALL TUBERCULOSIS

The radiographic picture of chest wall involvement by tuberculosis may vary, as does the radiographic appearance of this disease when it afflicts soft tissues (Schaefer and Barton, 1989). Tuberculosis may cause lytic lesions of chest wall structures, such as a rib and the sternum. Interestingly, tuberculosis is the most common inflammatory disease to afflict the ribs, and it is second only to metastatic cancer (including myeloma) as a cause of true destruction of ribs (Tatelman and Drouillard, 1953). Tuberculous infection of the sternum and ribs commonly results in sharply demarcated areas of destruction, which may at times have an expansile, cystic appearance (Schaefer and Burton, 1989). Multicystic lesions can occur; sclerotic margins may also be apparent. Although associated soft tissue masses are relatively common, pathologic fractures are rare (Feigin and Madewell, 1981). The formation of sinus tracts and chest wall abscesses can be demonstrated in approximately 25% of patients who present with chest wall involvement (Sinoff and Segal, 1975).

Tuberculosis may afflict the chest wall by extension of

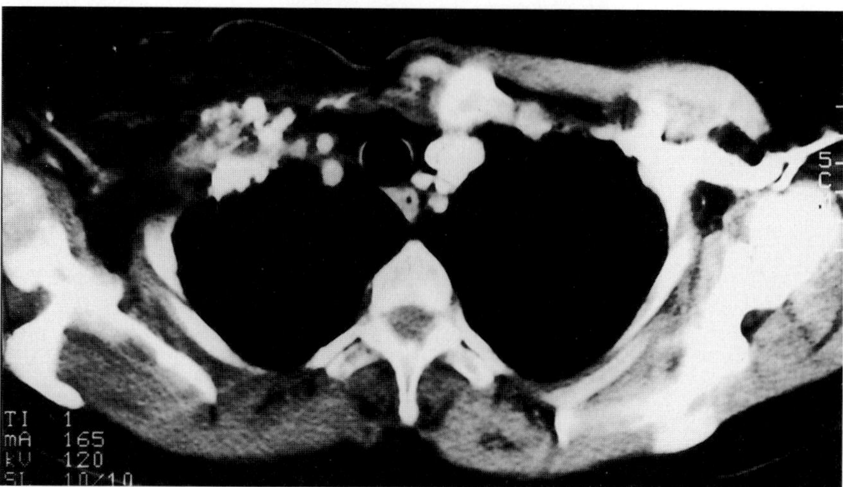

FIGURE 49–13 ■ This 58-year-old woman underwent a mastectomy for carcinoma of the right breast 4 years prior to this examination. She had a reconstruction of the chest wall with an ipsilateral latissimus dorsi flap and had received substantial radiotherapy to the chest wall. Images taken of the chest wall revealed a lytic lesion in the right clavicle, suggestive of recurrent breast carcinoma. A major operative procedure to resect a portion of the chest wall and perform a secondary reconstruction was contemplated. Fortunately, the excisional biopsy of the lytic area revealed radiation necrosis of the clavicle. There was no evidence of recurrent breast carcinoma. Although radiation-induced chondrosarcomas do occur in heavily radiated bones, there was no evidence of such a sarcoma in this patient.

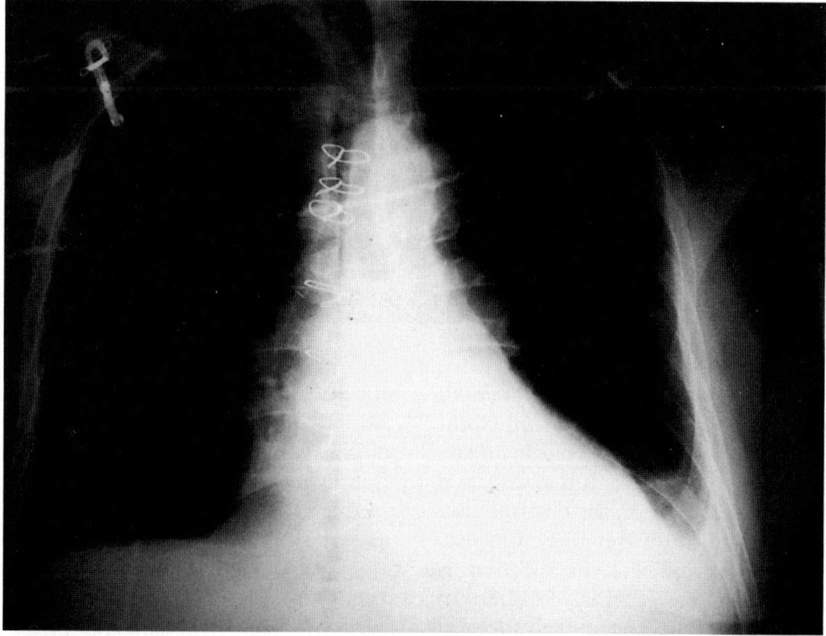

FIGURE 49–14 ■ An upright portable chest radiograph of a patient 9 days after a myocardial revascularization through a median sternotomy showing an air stripe between the two halves of the sternum. Note also that the sternal wires have either broken or pulled through. The air was introduced in between the two halves of the sternum when fluid drained from the inferior portion of the incision. The patient subsequently underwent rewiring and had aggressive therapy with both topical and systemic antibiotics. The wound healed successfully.

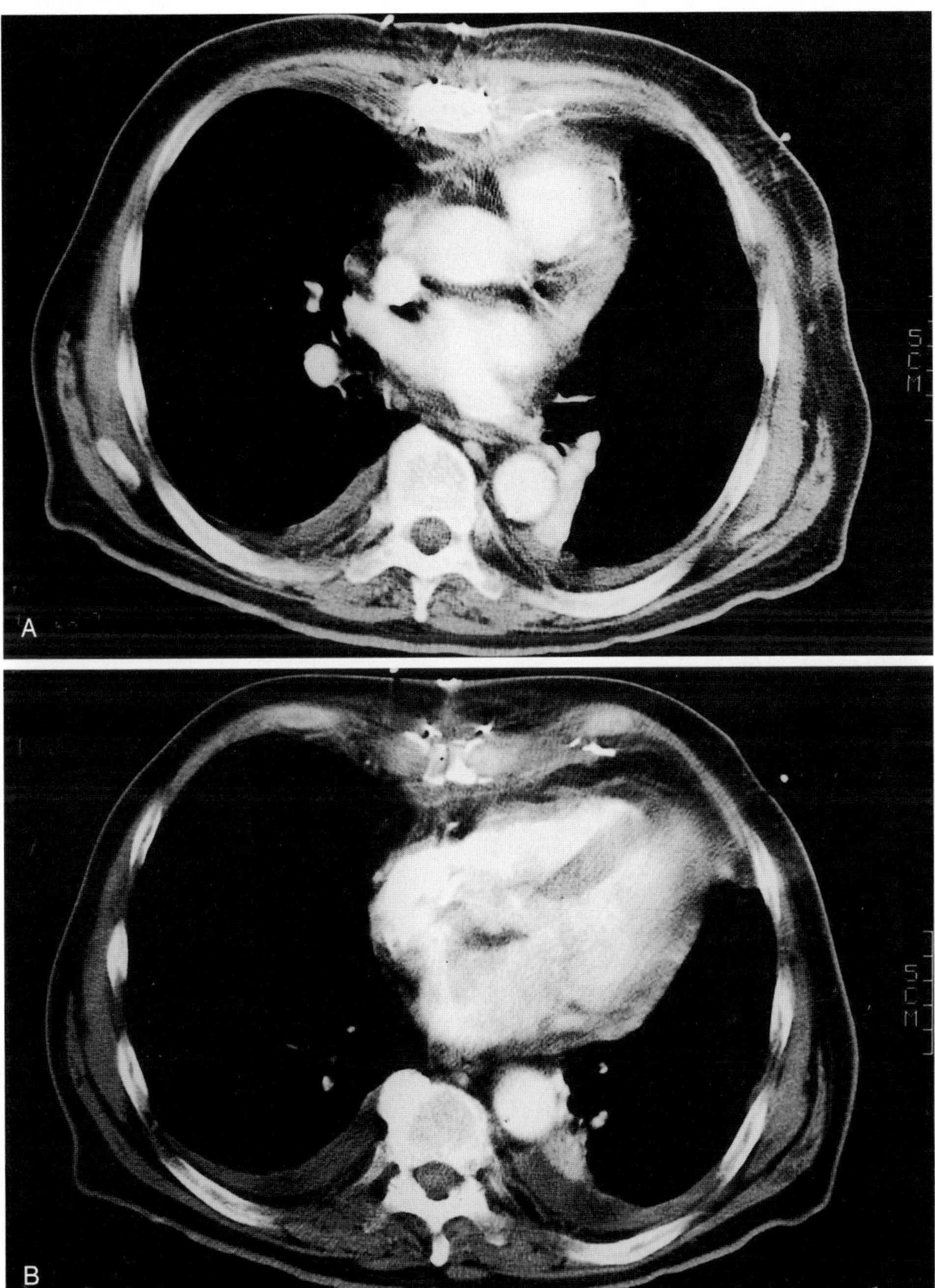

FIGURE 49–15 ■ Selected axial computed tomography images of the patient shown in Figure 49–14. These images were taken just prior to the wound draining. Careful examination of images shows air around the healing sternum. *A*, This image shows air around the sternum and some fluid around the great vessels within the pericardial sack. Note that the sternum has an irregular appearance. *B*, This image shows that there is air around the sternum and malalignment of the two sternal halves. Fluid is also apparent within the pericardial cavity directly behind the sternum.

infection from an adjacent lung or pleura. More commonly, the disease may seed a rib hematogenously without evidence of active pulmonary disease (Schaefer and Burton, 1989). Whatever the method of infection, chest wall tuberculosis should be suspected in patients who are prone to this disease. Today such infection should arouse suspicion of an immunocompromised patient. Appropriate precautions and thorough diagnostic evaluation should be undertaken in such patients.

CT has particular efficacy in the evaluation of the lesions associated with tuberculosis of the chest wall. In one published series based on four patients who were not immunocompromised, the authors concluded that chest wall tuberculosis could result in bone or costal cartilage destruction and soft tissue masses, which have peripheral calcification and rim enhancement with or without evidence of underlying lung or pleural disease (Adler et al, 1993). In their series, two patients had rib involvement, and one had costal cartilage disease. In the fourth, the sternoclavicular joint was involved. CT demonstrated osseous and cartilaginous destruction in all four, soft tissue masses with calcification in two, and rib enhancement after intravenous contrast administration in two.

FUNGAL INFECTIONS OF THE CHEST WALL

Fungal infections may occasionally afflict the chest wall. These include blastomycosis, candidiasis, coccidioidomycosis, cryptococcosis, and nocardiosis (Smilack and Gentry, 1976). Actinomycosis, which usually arises from infected underlying lung and pleura, is more common. It has a well-recognized indolent course, which may result in chest wall fistulas. Imaging techniques are important to define the extent of chest wall disease, and direct aspirations and biopsies are necessary to document the presence of fungal infection. CT scans and chest radiographs are useful to follow the extent of disease and its response to treatment (Snape, 1993). A study of three patients with *Aspergillus* chest wall involvement in chronic granulomatous disease suggests that CT and MRI may be complementary and allow progressive assessment of the process as it responds to therapy (Kawashima et al, 1991).

CONGENITAL ABNORMALITIES OF THE CHEST WALL

In many instances, conventional radiographs document the presence of congenital chest wall disease (Schaefer and Burton, 1989). Abnormalities, such as the absence, hypoplasia, or fusion of ribs; cervical ribs; and ankylosed vertebral bodies, are well delineated on standard plain radiographs. The abnormalities generally associated with Poland syndrome are apparent on plain films (Fig. 49–16). In some instances, CT and MRI may be particularly helpful to identify skeletal abnormalities and their relationship to underlying viscera. Compression of the heart may be apparent on axial CT images and may suggest

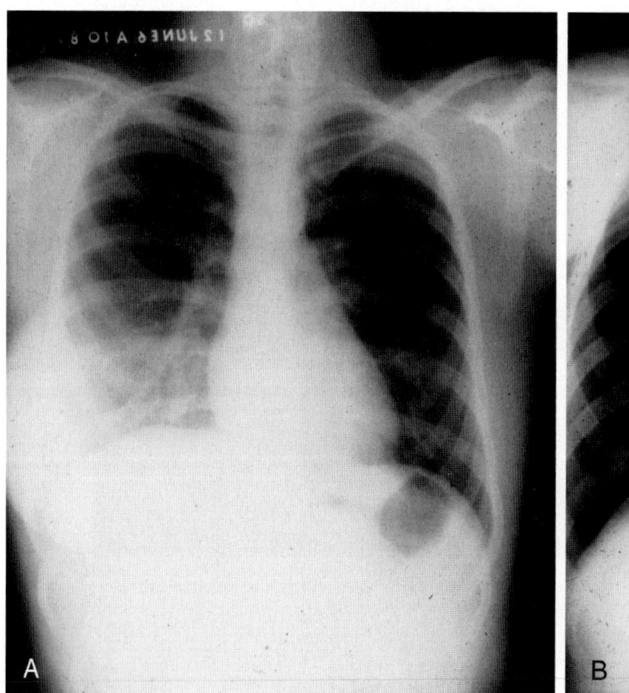

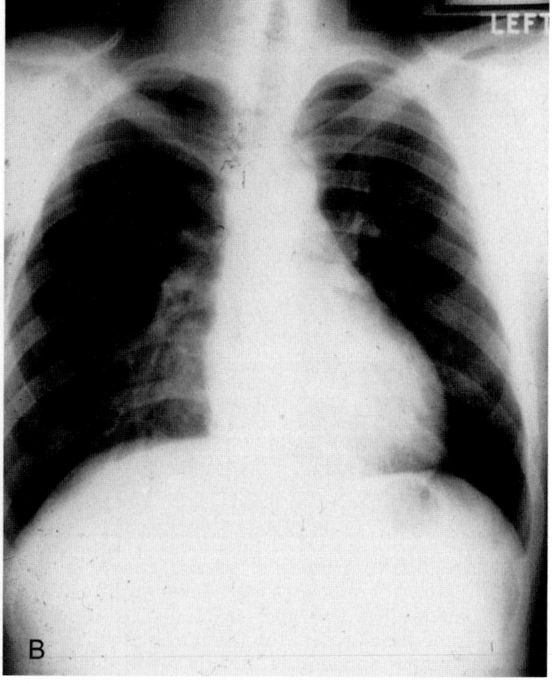

FIGURE 49–16 ■ *A*, A posteroanterior radiograph of a young man with Poland's syndrome. Note that the ends of ribs 2, 3, and 4 on the right side are either hypoplastic or absent. The corresponding costal cartilages were absent. The pectoralis major and minor and soft tissues in the region were also absent. The absence of these structures caused the hyperlucency seen over the apex of the right lung field. *B*, Although Poland syndrome occurs more often on the right, this 16-year-old woman had a left-sided Poland's syndrome. Note that she has absence of the left breast along with hypoplasia or absence of the anterior segments of ribs 2, 3, and 4. The corresponding pectoralis major and minor were nonexistent. The absence of the normal tissues over the left hemithorax causes the relative hyperlucency of the left lung.

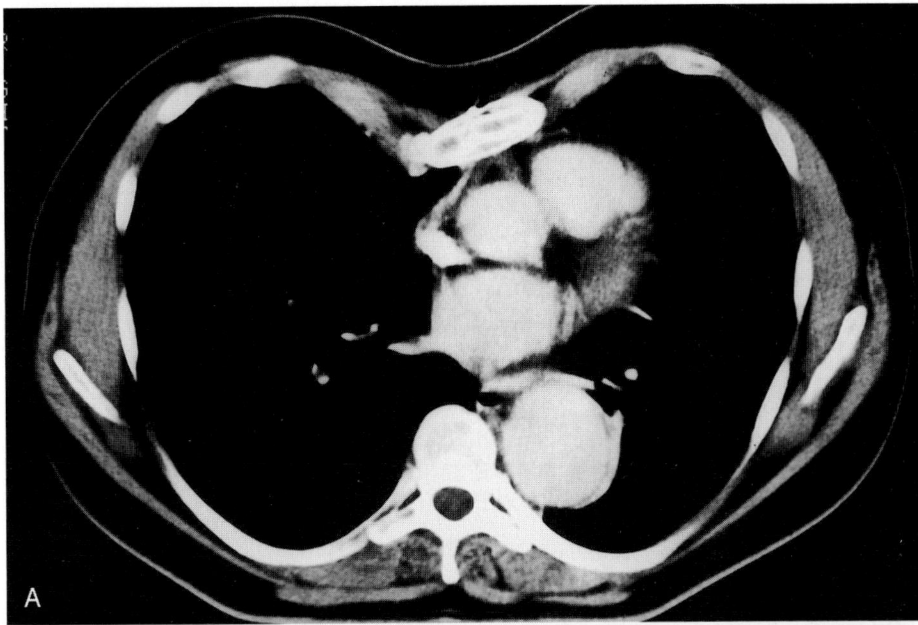

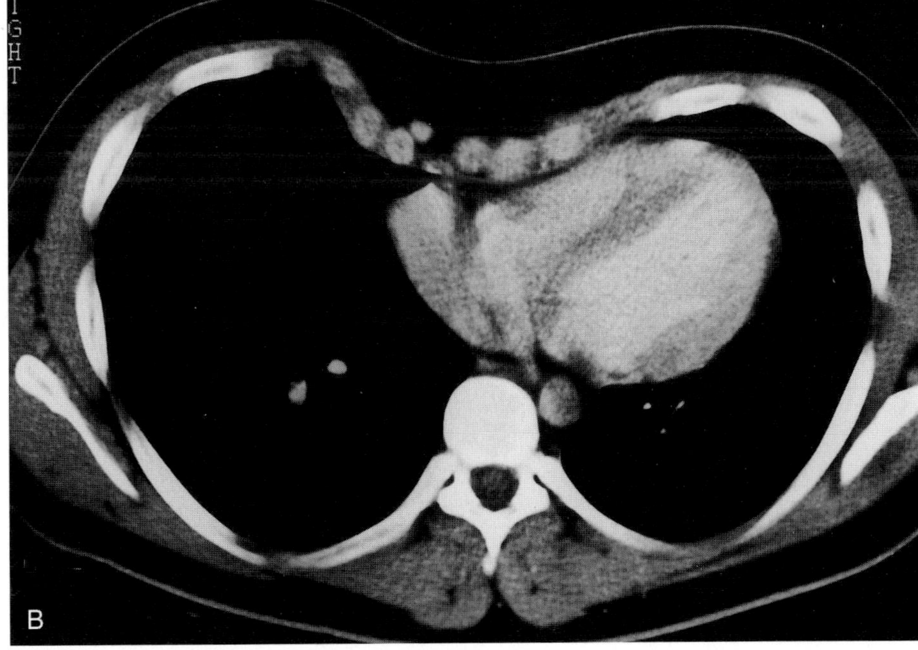

FIGURE 49–17 ■ An axial computed tomography (CT) image of an 18-year-old man showing a marked pectus deformity and its relationship to the cardiac silhouette. The patient had no symptoms at the time of the examination but had elected to refrain from vigorous activity because of Marfan's syndrome. *B*, An axial CT image showing persistent pectus in a 46-year-old man with Marfan's syndrome and a repaired ascending aorta. Two years after ascending aortic repair, the patient had incurred an acute, type I dissection.

embarrassment of diastolic filling (Fig. 49–17). CT and MRI may also be helpful to assess visceral conditions that may be associated with chest wall abnormalities (see Fig. 49–17). An example of this is Marfan's syndrome in which the major arteries of the body may be followed by axial imaging in conjunction with chest wall abnormalities.

■ *KEY REFERENCES*

Kuhlman JE, Bouchardy L, Fishman EK, Zerhouni EA: CT and MR imaging evaluation of chest wall disorders. Radiographics 14:571, 1994.

This article discusses the positive and negative aspects of both CT and MR imaging in a number of chest wall disorders. The article is richly illustrated with excellent radiographic material. The authors offer guidelines for detecting different types of suspected chest wall pathologic processes.

Schaefer PS, Burton BS: Radiographic evaluation of chest-wall lesions. Surg Clin North Am 69:911, 1989.

This article presents a thorough discussion of the different imaging techniques as they are used to evaluate chest wall pathologic conditions. There are a number of illustrations that demonstrate the major points the authors make. The list of references cited is thorough.

Webb WR, Gatsonis C, Zerhouni EA et al: CT and MR imaging in staging non-small cell bronchogenic carcinoma: Report of the Radiologic Diagnostic Oncology Group. Radiology 178:705, 1991.

This report gives a thorough evaluation of the use of CT and MRI in staging non-small cell bronchogenic carcinoma. It gives good guidelines as to the capabilities and drawbacks of both CT and MRI in the evaluation of non-small cell bronchogenic carcinoma.

■ *REFERENCES*

Adler BD, Padley SPG, Miller NL: Tuberculosis of the chest wall: CT findings. J Comput Assist Tomogr 17:271, 1993.

Donegan WL: Cancer of the breast: Local and regional recurrence. Major Probl Clin Surg 5:484, 1979.

Edelstein G, Levitt RG, Slaker DP et al: CT observation of rib abnormalities: Spectrum of findings. J Comput Assist Tomogr 9:65, 1989.

Enzinger FM, Weiss SW: Soft Tissue Tumors. St. Louis, CV Mosby, 1983.

Feigin DS, Madewell JE: Disorders of the chest wall. In Teplick JG, Haskin ME (eds): Surgical Radiology. Philadelphia, WB Saunders, 1981.

Felson B: Chest Roentgenology. Philadelphia, WB Saunders, 1973.

Franken EA, Smith JA, Smith WL: Tumors of the chest wall in infants and children. Pediatr Radiol 6:13, 1977.

Gamsu G: Magnetic resonance imaging in lung cancer. Chest 89:242S, 1986.

Glaser HS, Duncan-Meyer J, Aronberg DJ et al: Pleural and chest wall invasion in bronchogenic carcinoma. Radiology 157:191, 1985.

Goodwin JD: Computed Tomography of the Chest. Philadelphia, JB Lippincott, 1984.

Graeber GM, Snyder RJ, Flemming AW et al: Initial and long-term results in the management of primary chest wall neoplasms. Ann Thorac Surg 34:664, 1982.

Haggar AM, Pearlberg JL, Froelich JW et al: Chest wall invasion by carcinoma of the lung: Detection by MR imaging. AJR Am J Roentgenol 148:1075, 1987.

Kawashima A, Kuhlman JE, Fishman EK et al: Pulmonary Aspergillus chest wall involvement in chronic granulomatous disease: CT and MRI findings. Skeletal Radiol 20:487, 1991.

Larsson SE, Lorentzon R: The incidence of malignant primary bone tumors in relation to age, sex, and site. J Bone Joint Surg [Br] 56:534, 1974.

Libshitz HI: Computed tomography in bronchogenic carcinoma. Semin Roentgenol 25:64, 1990.

Lindfors KK, Meyer JE, Busse PM et al: CT evaluation of local and regional breast cancer recurrence. AJR Am J Roentgenol 145:833, 1985.

Marcove RC: Cartilaginous tumors of the ribs. Cancer 27:794, 1971.

McCloud TC, Filion RB, Edelman RR, Shepard JA: MR imaging of superior sulcus carcinoma. J Comput Assist Tomogr 13:233, 1989.

Miller JD, Gorenstein LA, Patterson GA: Staging: The key to rational management of lung cancer. Ann Thorac Surg 53:170, 1992.

Murata K, Takahashi M, Mori M et al: Chest wall and mediastinal invasion by lung cancer: Evaluation with multisection expiratory dynamic CT. Radiology 191:251, 1994.

Musset D, Grenier P, Carette MF et al: Primary lung cancer staging: Prospective comparative study of MR imaging with CT. Radiology 160:607, 1986.

Omell GH, Anderson LS, Bramson RT: Chest wall tumors. Radiol Clin North Am 11:197, 1973.

Pearlberg JL, Sandler MA, Beute GM et al: Limitations of CT in evaluation of neoplasm involving the chest wall. J Comput Assist Tomogr 11:29, 1987.

Resnick DM, Niwayama G (eds): Diagnosis of Bone and Joint Disorders. Philadelphia, WB Saunders, 1981.

Ryan MB, McMurtrey MJ, Roth JA: Current management of chest-wall tumors. Surg Clin North Am 69:1061, 1989.

Shea WJ, deGneer G, Webb WR: Chest wall after mastectomy. Radiology 162:162, 1987.

Sinoff CL, Segal I: Tuberculous osteomyelitis of the rib. S Afr Med J 49:685, 1975.

Smilack JD, Gentry LO: Candida costochondral osteomyelitis. J Bone Joint Surg Am 58:888, 1976.

Snape PS: Thoracic Actinomyces: An unusual childhood infection. South Med J 86:222, 1993.

Stout AP, Lattes R: Tumors of the soft tissue. In Atlas of Tumor Pathology. Series 2. Fascicle 1. Washington, DC, Armed Forces Institute of Pathology, 1967.

Suzuki N, Saitoh T, Kitamura S: Tumor invasion of the chest wall in lung cancer: Diagnosis with ultrasound (US). Radiology 187:39, 1993.

Tatelman M, Drouillard JP: Tuberculosis of the rib. AJR Am J Roentgenol 70:923, 1953.

Teitelbaum S: Twenty years' experience with intrinsic tumors of the bony thorax at a large institution. J Thorac Cardiovasc Surg 63:776, 1972.

Templeton PA, Caskey CI, Zerhouni EA: Current uses of CT and MR imaging in staging of lung cancer. Radiol Clin North Am 28:631, 1990.

Threlkel JB, Adkins PB: Primary chest wall tumors. Ann Thorac Surg 11:450, 1971.

Villari, Fargnoli R, Mungai R: CT evaluation of chest wall recurrence in breast cancer. Eur J Radiol 5:206, 1985.

Watanabe A, Shimokata K, Salsa H et al: Chest CT combined with artificial pneumothorax: Value in determining origin and extent of tumor. AJR Am J Roentgenol 156:707, 1991.

Yokoi K, Mori K, Miyazawa N et al: Tumor invasion of the chest wall and mediastinum in lung cancer: Evaluation with pneumothorax CT. Radiology 181:147, 1991.

CHAPTER **50**

Congenital Deformities of the Chest Wall and Sternum

Robert C. Shamberger

W. Hardy Hendren III

Pectus Excavatum

Congenital anterior thoracic deformities can be divided into four groups: (1) pectus excavatum; (2) pectus carinatum; (3) Poland's syndrome; and (4) sternal clefts and defects, including ectopia cordis. Pectus excavatum (often called "funnel chest" in English or "Trichterbrust" in German) is a depression of the sternum and the lower costal cartilages. The first and second ribs and their costal cartilages as well as the manubrium are usually normal (Fig. 50–1). The extent of sternal and cartilaginous deformity is variable. Numerous methods of grading and defining these deformities have been proposed, but none has been universally accepted. Asymmetry is frequently present but may be unappreciated until the time of surgical correction. The right side is often more depressed than the left side, and the sternum is rotated.

HISTORICAL NOTE

Surgical repair of this deformity was first achieved by Meyer and Sauerbruch in 1911 and 1913, respectively. The method of repair has evolved as experience has increased, and the primary components of the deformity have been identified. Ochsner and DeBakey summarized their experience with repair in 1939. Ravitch, in 1949, reported a technique that involved excision of all deformed costal cartilages with the perichondrium, division of the xiphoid from the sternum, division of the intercostal bundles from the sternum, and transverse sternal osteotomy, displacing the sternum anteriorly with Kirschner wires in the first two patients and silk sutures in patients treated later. In 1957 and 1958, Baronofsky and Welch reported a technique for the satisfactory and safe correction of pectus excavatum that emphasized total preservation of the perichondrial sheaths of the costal cartilage, preservation of the upper intercostal bundles, and osteotomy of the sternum. The technique that we use today remains essentially unchanged, more than 700 cases later, with the addition of a supporting strut to maintain the anterior correction of the defect.

■ *HISTORICAL READINGS*

Baronofsky ID: Technique for the correction of pectus excavatum. Surgery 42:884–890, 1957.

Meyer L: Zur chirurgischen Behandlung der angeborenen Trichterbrust. Verh Berl Med Ges 42:364, 1911.

Ochsner A, DeBakey M: Chonechondrosternon: Report of a case and review of the literature. J Thorac Surg 8:469, 1939.

Ravitch MM: The operative treatment of pectus excavatum. Ann Surg 129:429, 1949.

Sauerbruch F: Die Chirurgie der Brustorgane. Berlin, J Springer, 1920.

Welch KJ: Satisfactory surgical correction of pectus excavatum deformity in childhood: A limited opportunity. J Thorac Surg 36:697, 1958.

BASIC SCIENCE

Etiology

Pectus excavatum may be as common as 1 in 300 to 400 live births (Ravitch, 1977). It is usually noticed at birth or within the first year of life in 86% of cases and appears in adolescence in less than 5% of cases (Shamberger and Welch, 1988a). Transient deformity with vigorous breathing or crying is common in infants. Therefore, correction of pectus excavatum should never be performed on patients younger than 2 years of age. There is a family history of some form of anterior thoracic deformity in 37% of patients. Scoliosis has been identified in 26% of recent patients with pectus excavatum or carinatum, and in 11% of these patients there is a family history of scoliosis.

Patients with Marfan's syndrome have a high incidence of severe chest wall deformities, usually accompanied by scoliosis (Fig. 50–2). Patients with abdominal musculature deficiency syndrome (prune belly syndrome) commonly have pectus excavatum; this was the case with 8 of 43 patients in a series by Welch and Kearney (1974).

The cause of pectus excavatum is unknown. Early investigators (Lester, 1957) attributed its development to an abnormality of the diaphragm, but there is little evidence to support this theory except for the reported occurrence of pectus excavatum in patients with congenital diaphragmatic hernia (Greig and Azmy, 1990).

Pathophysiology

Pectus excavatum is well tolerated in infancy. Older children may complain of pain in the area of the deformed cartilages or of precordial pain after sustained exercise. A few patients have palpitations or syncope, presumably owing to transient atrial arrhythmias. These patients may have mitral valve prolapse, which is associated with atrial arrhythmias and has been identified in patients with pectus excavatum (Shamberger et al, 1987a).

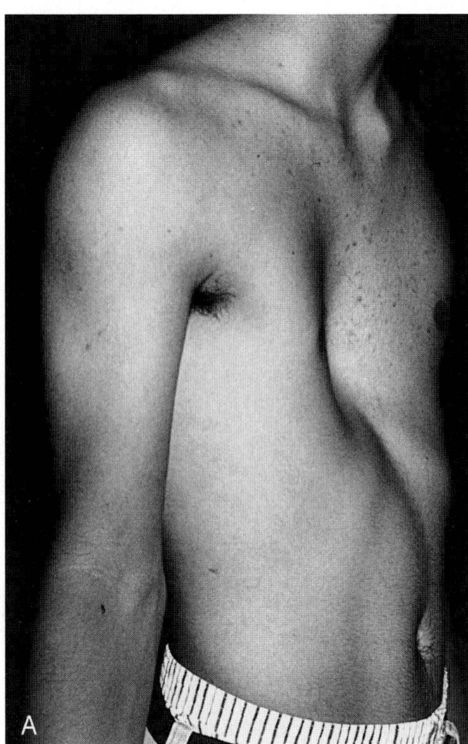

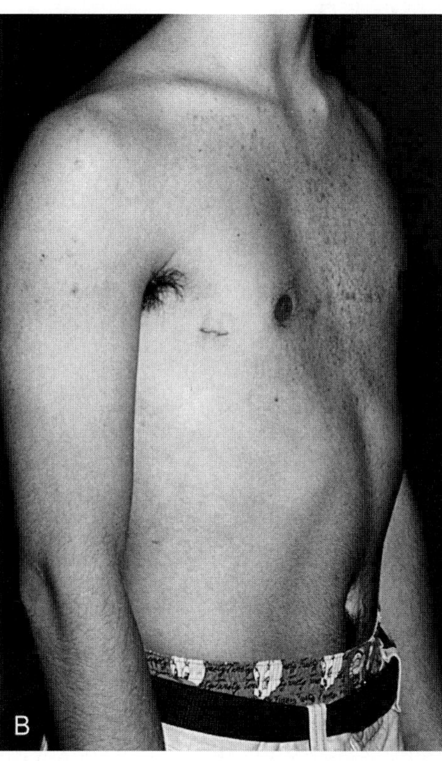

FIGURE 50–1 ■ *A*, Preoperative photograph of a 14-year-old boy with a symmetric pectus excavatum deformity. *B*, The excellent postoperative result is seen after repair with a retrosternal strut.

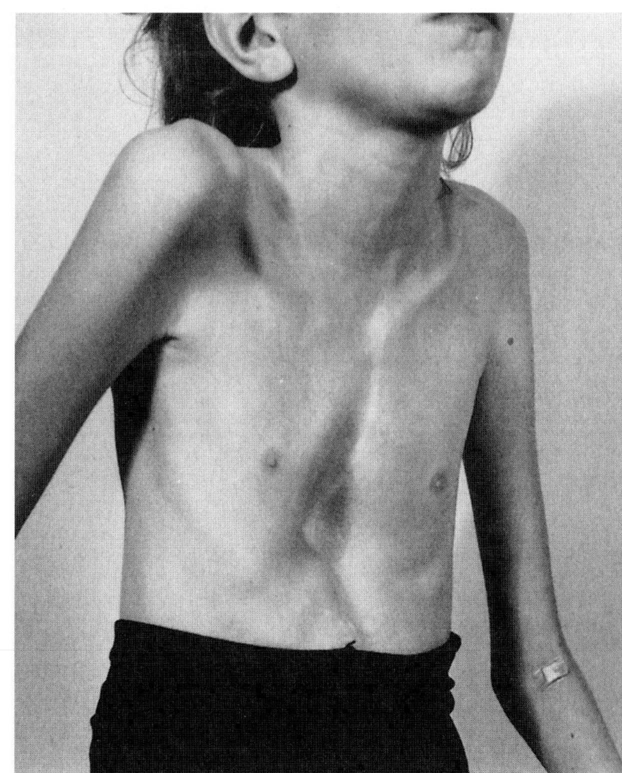

FIGURE 50–2 ■ An 8-year-old girl with Marfan's syndrome. She demonstrated all the characteristic findings of Marfan's syndrome, namely extreme laxity of the joints, posterior dislocation of her optic lenses, and cardiac valvular disease. She required mitral valve repair in infancy. A severe excavatum deformity is noted, as well as a sternotomy scar.

Some authors have said that no cardiovascular or pulmonary impairment results from pectus excavatum deformity (Haller et al, 1970). This opinion contrasts, however, with the general clinical impression that many patients have increased stamina following surgical repair. A summary of clinical studies of these patients has been reported (Shamberger and Welch, 1988b).

The symptomatic improvement in patients following surgery for pectus excavatum has been attributed to improved pulmonary function. Seven patients with pectus excavatum, four of whom were symptomatic with exercise, were evaluated in a study by Castile and associates (1982). The mean total lung capacity (TLC) in the excavatum patients was 79% of that predicted. The measured oxygen uptake exceeded predicted values as the workloads approached maximum. This pattern of oxygen uptake differed from that of normal subjects, who had a linear response. The mean oxygen uptake at maximal effort exceeded the predicted values by 25.4% in the symptomatic patients. The three asymptomatic patients, however, demonstrated a normal pattern of linear increase in oxygen uptake during progressive exercise. This increased oxygen uptake in the symptomatic patients suggests that their breathing work was increased, although their vital capacities were only mildly reduced or normal. Cahill and associates (1984) studied 14 patients with pectus excavatum; maximal voluntary ventilation was significantly improved after repair in all. Exercise tolerance was also improved, as measured by total exercise time and maximal oxygen uptake. Furthermore, there was a consistent decrease in heart rate at a given power output postoperatively, with no change in oxygen consumption. In another report by Blickman and colleagues (1985), ^{133}Xe perfusion and ventilation scintigraphy were used to study 17 patients. Of 12 patients with regional ventilatory deficits, primarily in the left lower lung, seven had normal ventilation scans after surgery. Of 10 patients with decreased regional perfusion abnormalities, also primarily in the left lower lung, six had normal perfusion scans after surgery. Abnormal ventilation/perfusion ratios became normal in 6 of 10 patients following surgery. Derveaux and colleagues (1989) evaluated 88 patients with pectus excavatum and carinatum with pulmonary function tests, before and 1 to 20 years after repair (mean, 8 years), by a technique that involved a fairly extensive chest wall dissection. Preoperative studies were within the normal range (>80% of predicted lung function) except in those subjects with both scoliosis and pectus excavatum. The postoperative values for forced expiratory volume in 1 second and vital capacity (VC) were decreased in all groups when expressed as a percentage of that predicted, although the absolute values at follow-up may have been greater than at the preoperative evaluation. Radiologic evaluation of these individuals confirmed improved chest wall configuration, suggesting that the relative deterioration in pulmonary function was not the result of recurrence of the pectus deformity. An inverse relationship was found between the preoperative and the postoperative function. Those individuals with less than 75% of predicted function had improved function after operation, whereas results were worse after operation if the preoperative values were greater than 75% of predicted. Similar results were found in a study by Morshuis and colleagues (1994a), who evaluated 152 patients before and at a mean follow-up of 8 years after operation for pectus excavatum. These physiologic results were in contrast to the subjective improvement in symptoms from the subjects and the improved chest wall configuration. The decline in pulmonary function in the postoperative studies was attributed to the operation, because the preoperative defect appeared to be stable regardless of the age at initial repair. Both of these studies were marred by the obvious lack of an age- and severity-matched control group without surgery.

Derveaux and colleagues (1988) evaluated transpulmonary and transdiaphragmatic pressures at TLC in 17 individuals with pectus excavatum. Preoperative and long-term follow-up evaluations were performed at mean intervals of 12 years. Reduced transpulmonary and transdiaphragmatic pressures suggested that the increased restrictive defect was produced by extrapulmonary rather than pulmonary factors or that surgery produced increased rigidity of the chest wall.

Wynn and colleagues (1992) assessed 12 children with pectus excavatum by pulmonary function tests and exercise testing. Eight underwent repair and were evaluated before and after operation. Four patients had two sets of evaluation but no surgery. A decline in the TLC was identified in the repaired group compared with stable values in the control group. Cardiac output and stroke volume increased appropriately with exercise before and after operation in both groups, and operation was believed to have produced no physiologically significant effect on the response to exercise.

Kaguraoka and colleagues (1992) evaluated pulmonary function in 138 patients before and after operation for pectus excavatum. A decrease in the VC occurred during the initial 2 months after operation with recovery to preoperative levels by 1 year after surgery. At 42 months, the values remained at baseline despite a significant improvement in the chest wall configuration. Tanaka and colleagues (1993) found similar results in patients who had the more extensive sternal turnover technique. These patients experienced a more significant and long-term decrease in the VC. Morshuis and colleagues (1994b) evaluated 35 patients with pectus excavatum who underwent repair as teenagers or young adults (aged 17.9 ± 5.6 years). Preoperative evaluations were performed and repeated 1 year after operation. Preoperative TLC (86% ± 14.4% of predicted) and VC (79.7% ± 16.2%) were significantly decreased from predicted values and decreased further after operation (−9.2% ± 9.2% and −6.6% ± 10.7%, respectively). The efficiency of breathing at maximal exercise improved significantly after operation. Ventilatory limitation of exercise occurred in 43% of the patients before operation, and most of them improved after operation. However, the group with no ventilatory limitation initially demonstrated a limitation after operation by a significant increase in oxygen consumption.

Taken together, these studies of pulmonary function over the last 4 decades have failed to document consistent improvement in pulmonary function resulting from surgical repair. Recent studies, in fact, have demonstrated deterioration in pulmonary function at long-term evaluation. This has been attributed to increased chest wall rigidity after operation. Despite this finding, workload studies have shown improvement in exercise tolerance following repair.

Beiser and colleagues (1972) performed cardiac catheterization in six patients with moderate degrees of pectus excavatum. Normal pressures were obtained in patients at rest and in the supine position. The cardiac index was normal in patients at rest in the supine position, and the response to moderate exercise was within the normal range. The response to upright exercise was below the predicted normal in two patients and at the lower limit of normal in three. Postoperative studies were performed in three patients, two of whom achieved a higher level of exercise tolerance following surgery. The cardiac index was increased by 38%; the heart rates were unchanged, and the increase resulted from an enhanced stroke volume following surgery.

Peterson and colleagues (1985) used first-pass radionuclide angiocardiography to evaluate 13 patients who were upright, both at rest and during bicycle exercise. Although no changes were seen in patients at rest or during exercise in left ventricular ejection fraction or cardiac output, substantial increases were observed in both right and left ventricular volumes postoperatively, which suggests relief of cardiac compression by displacement of the sternum anteriorly. Workload studies were also performed on these patients. Of the 13, 10 were able to reach the target heart rate before surgical repair, four without symptoms. After operation, all except one patient reached the target heart rate during the exercise protocol, and 9 of 13 reached the target without becoming symptomatic.

SURGICAL REPAIR

Baronofsky (1957) and Welch (1958) reported similar techniques that achieved safe and satisfactory correction of pectus excavatum. They emphasized total preservation of the perichondrial sheaths of the costal cartilage, preservation of the upper intercostal bundles, and anterior fixation of the sternum with silk sutures. This technique has been used at The Children's Hospital in Boston for more than 700 cases in the past 3 decades. Others (Adkins and Blades, 1961; Rehbein and Wernicke, 1957) have used internal fixation with Kirschner wires or metallic struts, but there is no proof that such methods provide better long-term results than those achieved without metal fixation. Willital (1981) reported 92% satisfactory results using struts in a large series of 1112 patients, whereas Hecker and associates (1981) reported 91% satisfactory results in 392 patients using a modification of the Ravitch procedure without struts. Oelsnitz (1981) and Hecker and associates (1981) reached the same conclusion—that internal fixation did not provide a major benefit in their large series, in which satisfactory repairs were achieved in 90% to 95% of patients. Nevertheless, we prefer to use the struts devised by Rehbein (W.H.H.) or Adkins and Blades (R.C.S.) to hold the sternum in an anterior position. It provides stability and greater patient comfort and less chance for early recurrence of sternal depression. The struts are removed in the ambulatory operating room 6 to 12 months after repair. We have not seen problems related to the struts.

Three other variations of repair deserve mention. Haller and associates (1976) add three-point "tripod" fixation by placing an osteotomy and creating oblique chondrotomies of the upper costal cartilages. The medial posterior portion of the costal cartilage is then anterior to the lateral portion of the cartilages and helps support the sternum anteriorly.

In the French literature, Judet and Judet (1956) and Jung and associates (1964) propose a "sternal turnover" technique. It has been used primarily in Japan by Wada and associates (1970), who reported a large series. In this technique, a "free graft" of sternum that is rotated 180 degrees and secured back to the costal cartilages is used. This method is radical for children with pectus excavatum, because major complications can be encountered if infection occurs and the alternatives are generally successful. Recent technical modifications to maintain the perfusion of the rotated sternum still fail to justify general use of this method. A method of elevation of the sternum with a retrosternal bar without resection or division of the costal cartilages has been reported by Nuss and associates (1998), but confirmation of the safety and efficacy of this method await its replication by other centers.

Our operative technique is illustrated in Figure 50–3. In females, particular attention is taken to place the incision within the inframammary fold, thus avoiding the complications of breast deformity and abnormal development. Skin flaps are mobilized primarily in the midline to the angle of Louis superiorly and to the xiphoid inferiorly. Use of Bovie electrocautery minimizes blood loss. Starting medially, the pectoral muscles are detached and retracted to expose the depressed costal cartilages. The lateral extent of muscle elevation is the costochondral junction of the third to fifth ribs and rarely the second. Particular attention is taken to avoid injury to the intercostal bundles, which can result in significant bleeding. Subperichondrial resection of the costal cartilages is performed with removal of the entire third, fourth, and fifth cartilages to the costochondral junctions. Longer (5- to 6-cm) segments of the sixth and seventh cartilages are resected to the point where they flatten to join the costal arch. There are often bridges joining the fifth and sixth costal cartilages lateral to the sternum.

Transverse osteotomy of the anterior table of the sternum is performed with the Hall drill (Zimmer USA, Warsaw, IN). This allows the lower sternum to be brought forward. The posterior table of the sternum is fractured behind the osteotomy, which must be of adequate size so that the sternum comes forward easily. The rectus muscles may be detached from the lower sternum and xiphoid to allow blunt dissection behind the sternum. The xiphoid often projects forward and should be removed in these cases. The osteotomy is then closed with heavy silk sutures while the surgeon holds the sternum forward in a deliberately overcorrected position. Alternatively, struts can be used to hold the sternum forward. Struts are especially helpful when there is extensive sternal rotation or a severe depression. Fixation with struts is also required in patients with Marfan's syndrome or other con-

Text continues on page 1360

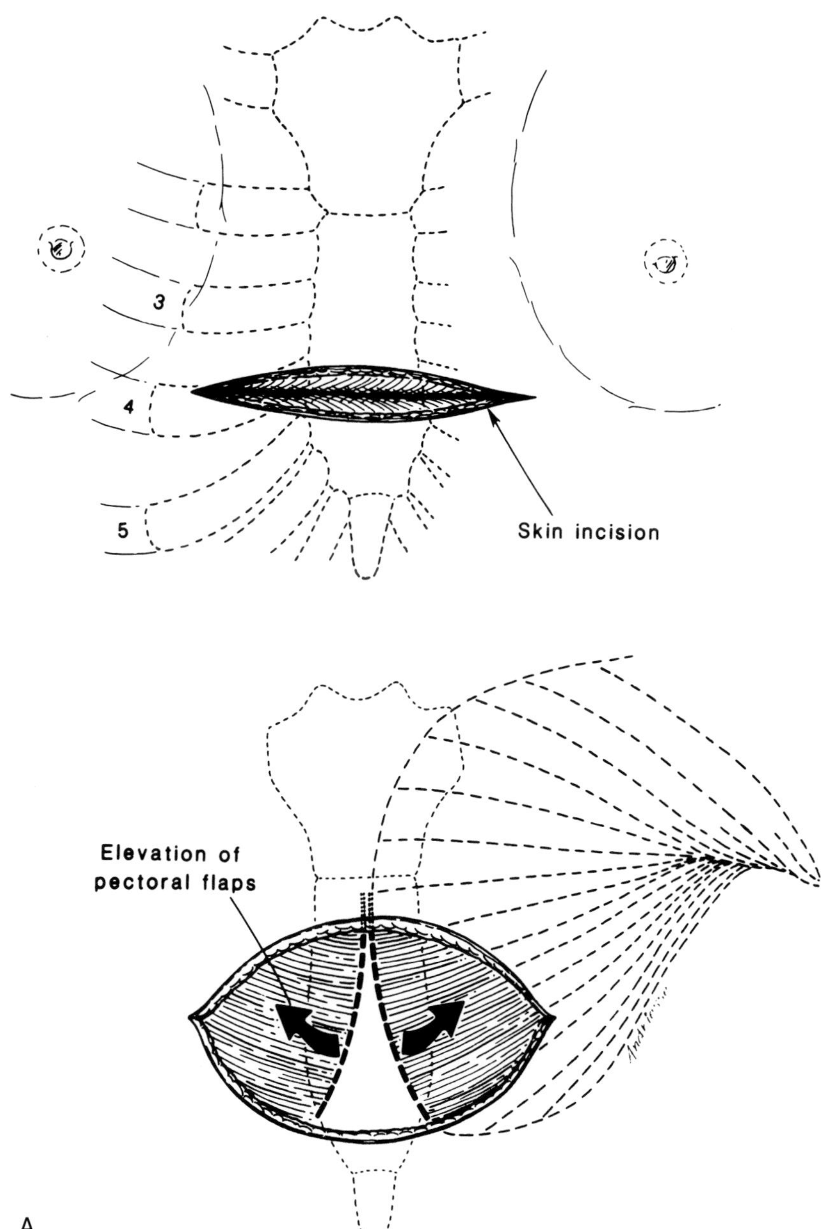

FIGURE 50–3 ■ *A*, A transverse incision is placed below and well within the nipples at the site of the future inframammary crease. The pectoralis major muscle is detached from the sternum along with portions of the pectoralis minor and serratus anterior muscles and retracted forward and laterally to expose the depressed costal cartilages (usually the third to seventh).

Illustration continued on following page

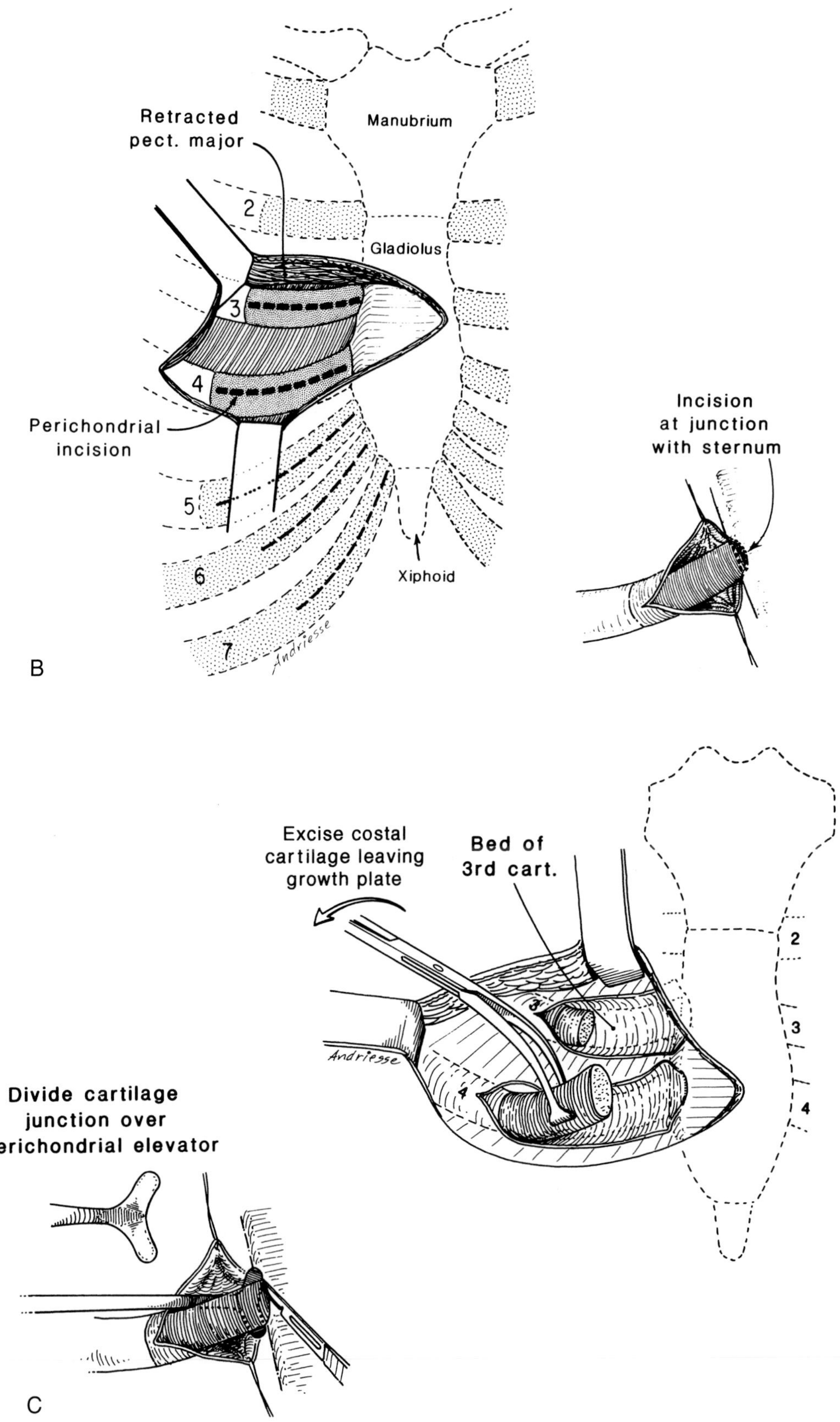

FIGURE 50–3 ■ *Continued. B*, Subperichondrial resection of the costal cartilages is achieved by incising the perichondrium anteriorly. It is then dissected from the costal cartilages in the bloodless plane between the perichondrium and the costal cartilage. Cutting the perichondrium 90 degrees in each direction at its junction with the sternum *(inset)* facilitates visualization of the back wall of the costal cartilage. *C*, The cartilages are divided at the sternal junction using a Welch perichondrial elevator held posteriorly to elevate the cartilage and protect the mediastinum *(inset)*. The divided cartilage is then held with an Allis clamp and elevated; the costal cartilage is then excised, preserving a margin on the rib to protect the costochondral junction and the longitudinal growth plate.

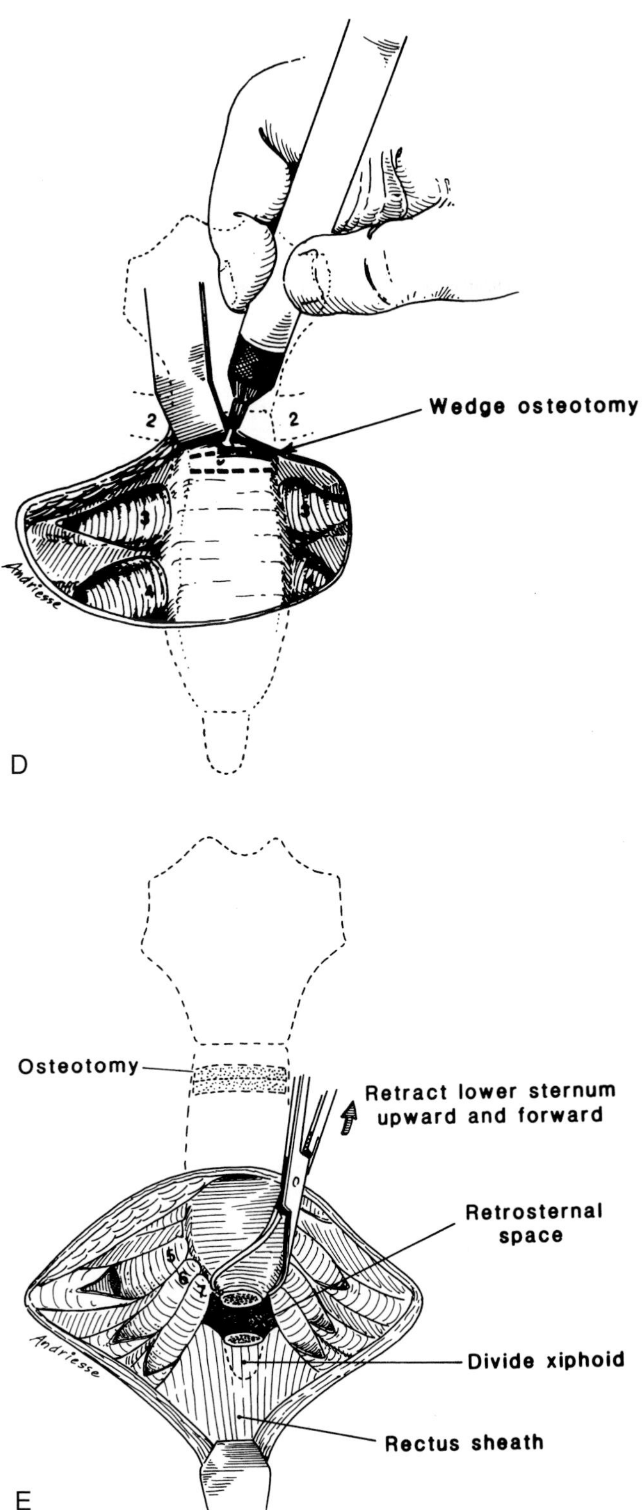

FIGURE 50–3 ■ *Continued. D,* The sternal osteotomy is created above the level of the last deformed cartilage and the posterior angulation of the sternum, generally the third cartilage, but occasionally the second. Two transverse sternal osteotomies are created 2 to 4 mm apart through the anterior cortex using a Hall air drill. *E,* The base of the sternum and the rectus muscle flap are elevated with two towel clips, and the xiphoid can be divided from the sternum with electrocautery, allowing entry into the retrosternal space. This step is not necessary with the use of a retrosternal strut. Preservation of the attachment of the sheaths and xiphoid avoids an unsightly depression, which can occur below the sternum.

Illustration continued on following page

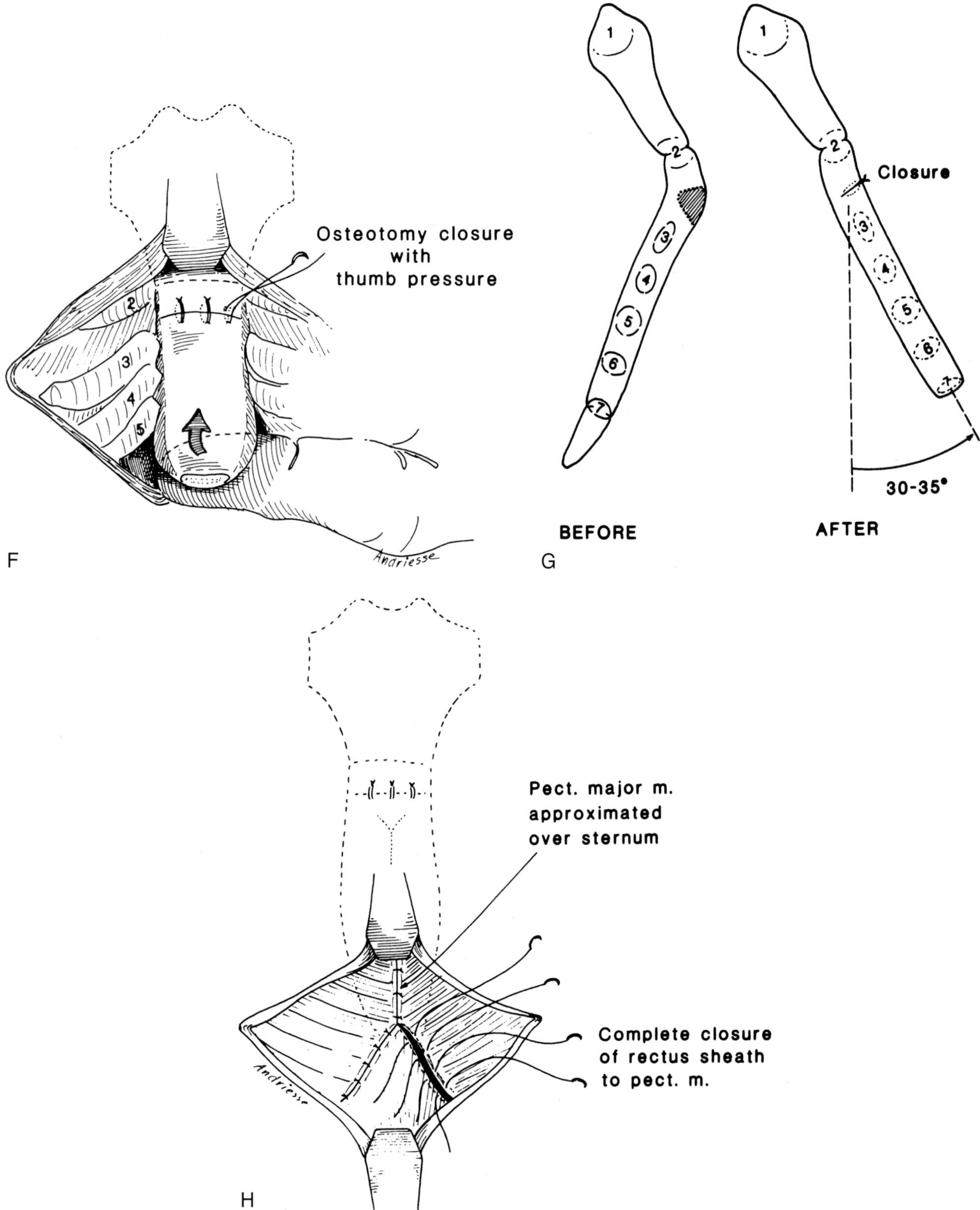

FIGURE 50–3 ■ *Continued. F,* The osteotomy is closed with several heavy silk sutures as the sternum is being elevated with the assistant's thumb if a strut is not used. *G,* Correction of the abnormal position of the sternum is achieved by creation of a wedge-shaped osteotomy, which is then closed, bringing the sternum anteriorly into an overcorrected position. *H,* The pectoral muscle flaps are secured to the midline of the sternum while being advanced to provide coverage of the entire sternum. The rectus muscle flap is then joined to the pectoral muscle flaps.

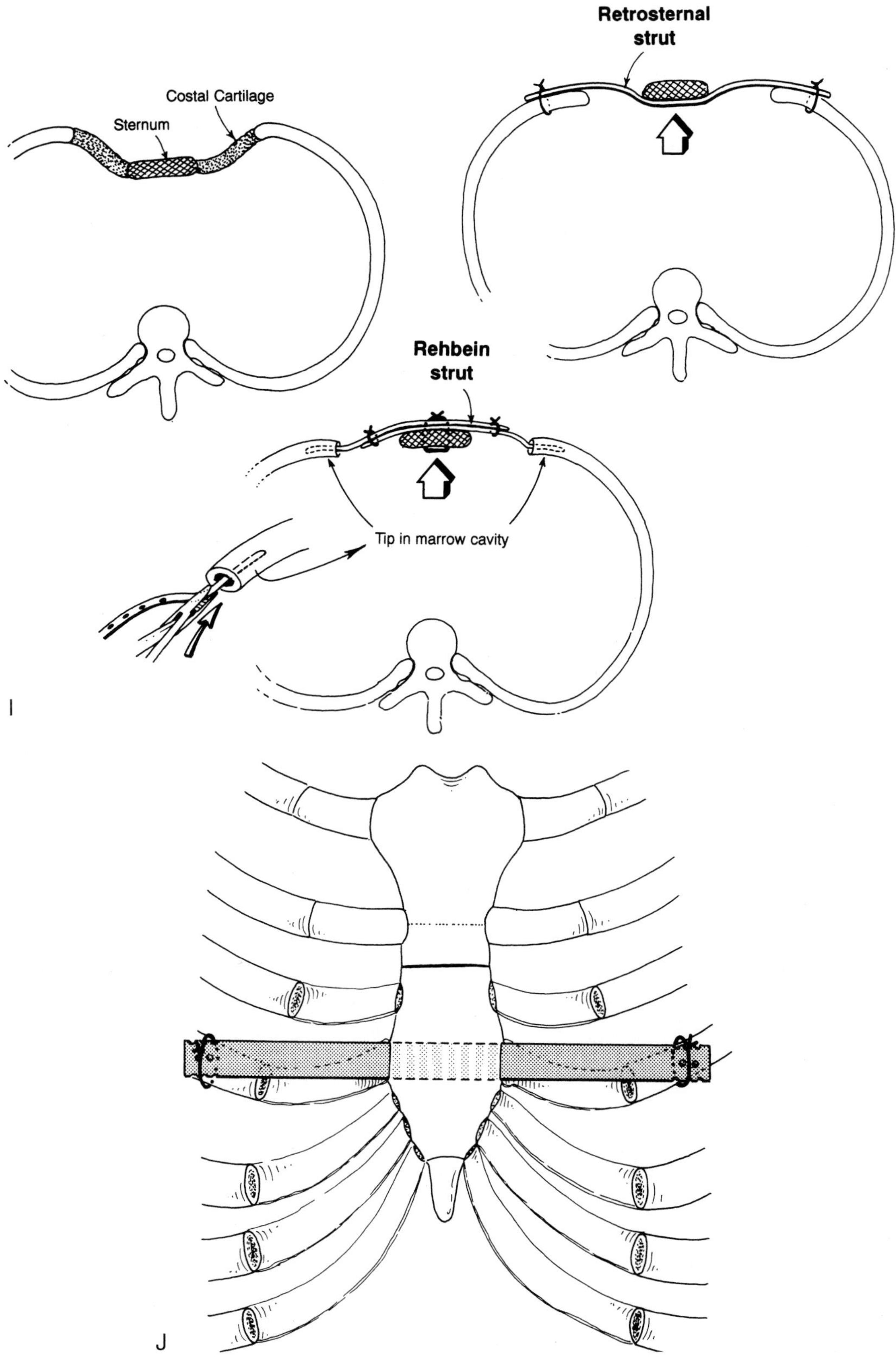

FIGURE 50–3 ■ *Continued. I*, Demonstration of the use of both retrosternal struts and Rehbein struts. The Rehbein struts are inserted into the marrow cavity *(inset)* of the third and fourth ribs and are then joined to each other medially to create a metal arch anterior to the sternum. The sternum is sewn to the arch to secure it in its new forward position. The retrosternal strut is placed behind the sternum and is secured to the rib ends laterally to prevent migration. *J*, Anterior depiction of the retrosternal struts (V. Mueller). The perichondrial sheath to either the third or fourth rib is divided from its junction with the sternum, and the retrosternal space is bluntly dissected to allow passage of the strut behind the sternum. It is secured with two pericostal sutures laterally to prevent migration. (*A–H*, From Shamberger RC, Welch KJ: Surgical repair of pectus excavatum. J Pediatr Surg 23:615, 1988. *I–J*, From Shamberger RC: Chest wall deformities. In Shields TW [ed]: General Thoracic Surgery, 4th ed. Baltimore, Williams & Wilkins, 1994.)

nective tissue disorders in whom risk of recurrence is higher (Scherer et al, 1988). In some cases, the lowest one or two sets of intercostal bundles (sixth and seventh) are divided from the sternum if required to bring it forward without excessive tension. We limit the number of perichondrial bundles divided, however, to minimize an unsightly local depression inferior to the tip of the sternum.

The technique described previously provides a precise resection of costal cartilages with preservation of perichondrial sheaths, without injury to mediastinal structures, and usually without pleural or pericardial entry. If the pleura is entered, the hole should be made large enough to prevent tension pneumothorax intraoperatively, and the lungs should be ventilated with enough positive pressure to maintain inflation. Any pleural air present is aspirated through a temporary catheter, which is withdrawn when the defect is covered by the pectoralis muscle closure. The wound is flooded with warm saline and cefazolin to remove clots. A single-limb medium Hemovac drain (Snyder Laboratories, New Philadelphia, OH) is brought through the inferior skin flap with the suction ports in a parasternal position to the level of the highest costal cartilage resection. The pectoralis muscle flaps are sutured to the sternum with advancement of the muscles medially and inferiorly to cover the underlying sternum with muscle. The rectus muscles are then reattached to the lower sternum medially and to the pectoralis muscles laterally. A postoperative chest radiograph is obtained in the recovery room. Perioperative antibiotics are administered, including one dose of cefazolin immediately prior to surgery and three postoperative doses. Blood loss is well below transfusion requirement in patients of all ages. A review of this technique in 704 patients at our institution disclosed no deaths and few complications (4.4%) (Shamberger and Welch, 1988a). Safe and effective repair is possible at any age.

Complications

Complications of pectus excavatum repair should be few and minor. In 2% of patients, a limited pneumothorax required aspiration or was simply observed. Tube thoracostomy has not been required in the past decade and was needed by only four patients in our series. Wound infection was rare with the use of perioperative antibiotic coverage.

The most distressing complication following surgical correction of pectus excavatum is the major recurrence of the deformity years after the original repair (17 of 704 patients). It is difficult to predict which unfortunate patients will have a major recurrence, but they often seem to have an asthenic or "marfanoid" habitus, with poor muscle development and a narrow anteroposterior chest wall diameter.

Impaired chest wall growth is a recently identified complication. Martinez and colleagues (1990) first described a deficiency in thoracic growth in children following repair of pectus excavatum, which was most noticeable in children repaired early during the preschool years. Haller (1996) reported on 12 children who have presented in their teens with apparent limited growth of the ribs following resection of the costal cartilages at an early age, producing a band-like narrowing of the midchest (Fig. 50–4). In some cases, the first and second ribs in which the costal cartilages have not been resected have

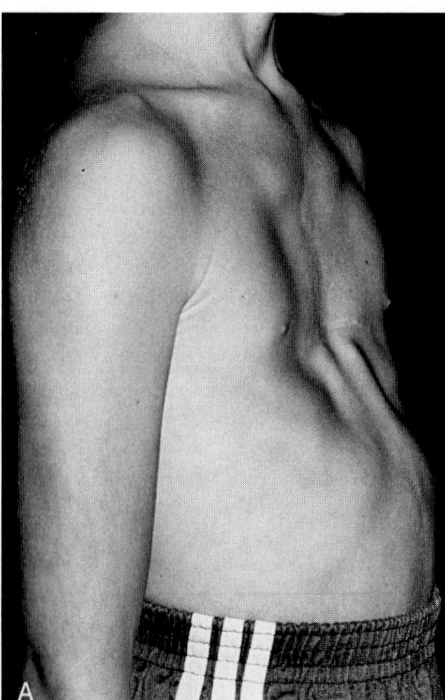

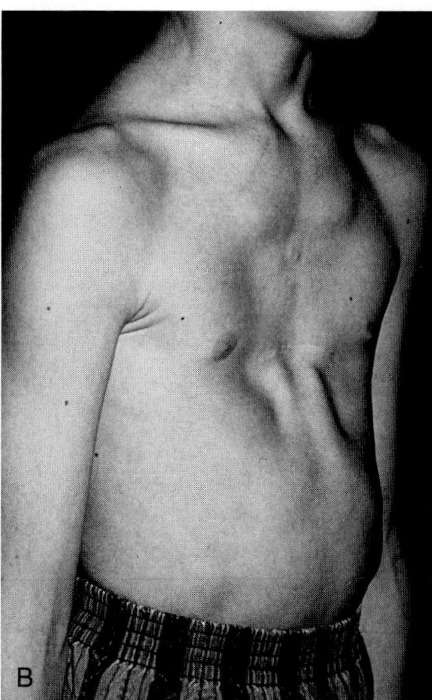

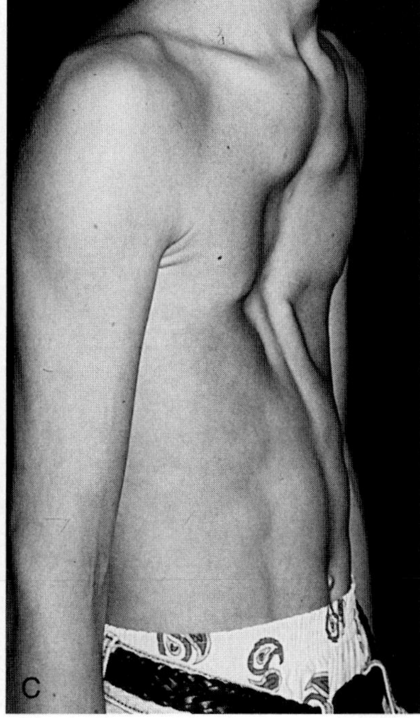

FIGURE 50–4 ■ Sequence of figures demonstrating deterioration in the quality of a repair, which can occur with time. This boy initially had excellent result from a Welch repair with suture fixation of the sternum at 4 years and 3 months of age. The follow-up photographs at 7 years and 6 months *(A)*, at 9 years and 3 months *(B)*, and at 14 years and 3 months *(C)*, demonstrate progressive depression of the sternum and costal cartilages and relative overgrowth of the upper chest.

apparent relative overgrowth, producing anterior protrusion of the upper sternum. This occurrence has been attributed by Haller to injury of the costochondral junctions, which are the longitudinal growth centers for the ribs, and to decreased growth of the sternum resulting from injury to its growth centers or vascular supply.

Martinez demonstrated experimentally in 6-week-old rabbits that resection of the costal cartilages produced a marked impairment in chest growth, particularly the anterioposterior diameter, during a 5.5-month period of observation. Less severe impairment occurred if only the medial three quarters of the costal cartilage was resected leaving the growth centers at the costochondral junction. This impairment was attributed to fibrosis and scarring within the perichondrial sheaths. Perichondrial sheaths, bone, or other prosthetic tissues that cannot grow also should not be joined posterior to the sternum, because they will form a band-like stricture across the chest. This complication of delayed thoracic growth was described primarily in children repaired in early childhood and can be avoided by delaying surgery until the children are older. Preservation of the costochondral junction leaving a segment of the cartilage on the osseous portion of the rib may also minimize growth impairment. We delay surgery until the children have begun their pubertal growth spurt.

Pectus Carinatum

Pectus carinatum is the most accepted term for anterior protrusion deformities of the chest wall. Protrusion deformities are much less frequent in our experience than the depression deformities (constituting 16.7% of the total group). The most frequent form of pectus carinatum consists of symmetric anterior displacement of the sternum with concavity of the costal cartilages laterally, a chondrogladiolar defect (Fig. 50–5). Asymmetric deformities with anterior displacement of the costal cartilages on one side, normal cartilages on the contralateral side, and a normally positioned or oblique sternum are much less common. "Mixed" lesions have a carinate deformity on one side and a depression or excavatum deformity on the contralateral side. The upper or chondromanubrial deformities, the so-called pouter pigeon deformities, are the most unusual, with protrusion of the manubrium and second and third costal cartilages and relative depression of the short body of the sternum (Fig. 50–6).

HISTORICAL NOTE

Surgical repair of carinate deformities has had a colorful history, starting with the first reported correction of the upper or chondromanubrial deformity by Ravitch in 1952. He resected several costal cartilages and performed a double sternal osteotomy. In 1953, Lester reported two methods of repair for chondrogladiolar deformity. The first, involving resection of the anterior portion of the sternum, was abandoned because of excessive blood loss and unsatisfactory results. The second (not a less radical technique) used subperiosteal resection of the entire sternum. Chin (1957) advanced the transected xiphoid and attached rectus muscles to a higher site on the sternum. This operation, the xiphosternopexy, produced posterior displacement of the sternum in younger patients with a flexible chest wall. Howard (1958) combined this method with subperichondrial costal cartilage resection and a sternal osteotomy. In 1973, Welch and Vos reported an approach to these deformities that we continue to use today.

■ *HISTORICAL READINGS*

Chin EF: Surgery of funnel chest and congenital sternal prominence. Br J Surg 44:360, 1957.

Howard R: Pigeon chest (protrusion deformity of the sternum). Med J Aust 2:664, 1958.

Lester CW: Pigeon breast (pectus carinatum) and other protrusion deformities of the chest of developmental origin. Ann Surg 137:482, 1953.

Ravitch MM: Unusual sternal deformity with cardiac symptoms—operative correction. J Thorac Surg 23:138, 1952.

Welch KJ, Vos A: Surgical correction of pectus carinatum (pigeon breast). J Pediatr Surg 8:659, 1973.

BASIC SCIENCE

Etiology

The cause of pectus carinatum is not better understood than that of pectus excavatum. It appears as an overgrowth of the costal cartilages with forward buckling and anterior displacement of the sternum. Again, there is a clear-cut family incidence, which suggests a genetic basis. In a review of 152 patients, 26% had a family history of chest wall deformity (Shamberger and Welch, 1987b), and a family history of scoliosis was obtained in 12% of the patients. Pectus carinatum is much more frequent in boys (119 of Shamberger and Welch's patients) than in girls (33 patients). Scoliosis and other deformities of the spine are the most common associated musculoskeletal deformities.

Pectus carinatum usually appears in childhood, and in almost half of the patients the deformity has not been identified until after the 11th birthday. The deformity may appear in a mild form at birth and often progresses, particularly during the period of rapid growth at puberty. The chondromanubrial deformity, linked by Currarino and Silverman (1958) with an increased risk of congenital heart disease, is noted at birth and is associated with a short truncated sternum, with absent sternal segmentation or premature obliteration of sternal sutures. In a prospective review by Lees and Caldicott (1975), 135 patients with sternal fusion anomalies were identified, and 18% of these had documented congenital heart disease.

Pathophysiology

Unlike pectus excavatum, cardiopulmonary impairment has not been demonstrated in patients with pectus carinatum. Pain from local trauma to the protuberant mass or inability to sleep prone are the most frequent symptoms reported by patients.

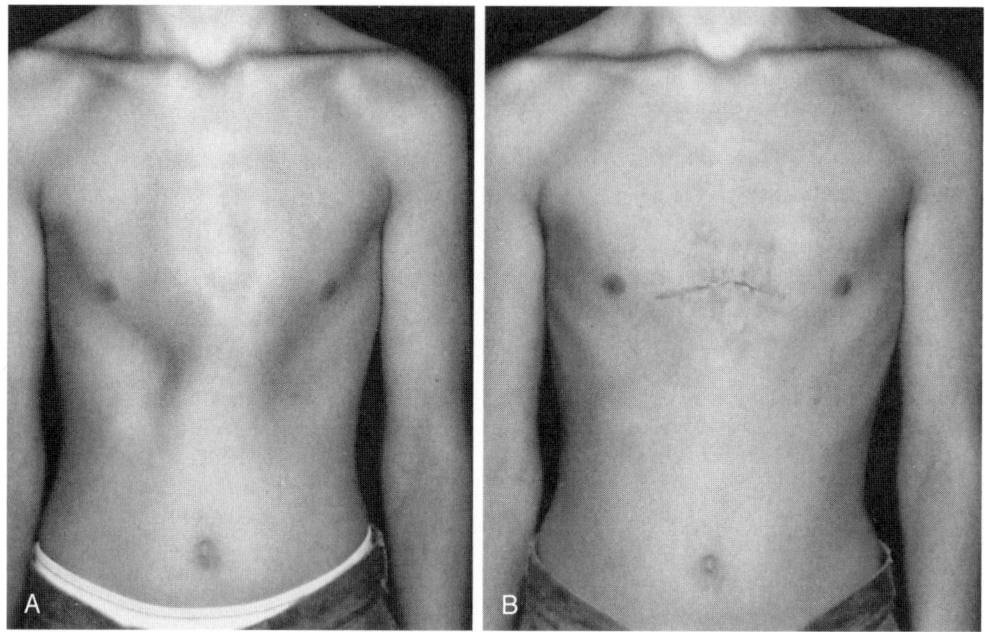

FIGURE 50–5 ■ *A*, Preoperative photograph of a patient with a symmetric pectus carinatum deformity demonstrating symmetric anterior protrusion of the body of the sternum and the costal cartilages. *B*, The postoperative result shows marked improvement in the chest wall contour.

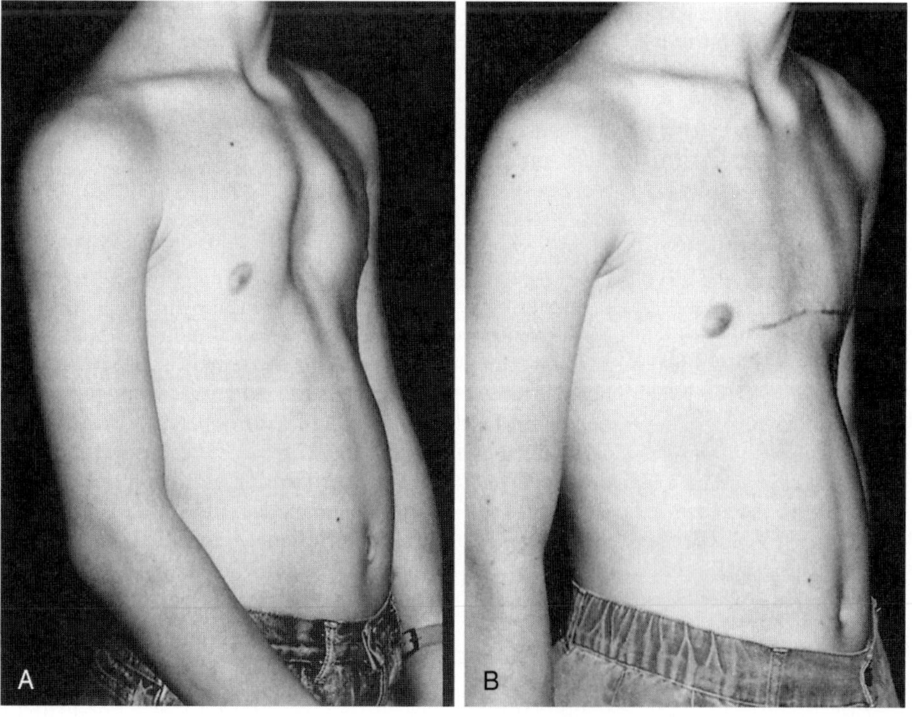

FIGURE 50–6 ■ *A*, Preoperative photograph of a patient with the upper form of a pectus carinatum deformity, with marked anterior protrusion of the manubrium and second and third costal cartilages along with depression of the body of the sternum—the "pouter pigeon" deformity. *B*, The postoperative result shows correction of both the depression and superior protrusion components of the deformity.

SURGICAL REPAIR

A transverse incision is made just below and within the nipples similar to the repair of pectus excavatum, with identical mobilization of the pectoral muscle flaps and subperichondrial resection of the deformed costal cartilages. A sternal osteotomy is created with the Hall air drill, allowing the sternum to be fractured and displaced posteriorly into an orthotopic position (Fig. 50–7*A*). Occasionally, a second osteotomy is required to displace the lower portion of the body of the sternum posteriorly. The upper or chondromanubrial deformity must be managed in a special manner, as described by Shamberger and Welch (1988c). In this situation, the costal cartilages must be resected from the second cartilage inferiorly. A generous wedge osteotomy is then performed at the point of maximal protrusion of the sternum. The superior segment of the sternum can then be displaced posteriorly as the osteotomy is closed, advancing the inferior segment anteriorly (see Fig. 50–7*B*). This method corrects both components of the deformity. Mixed pectus carinatum-excavatum deformities are managed with a transverse, wedge-shaped osteotomy, which allows anterior displacement and rotation of the sternum (see Fig. 50–7*C*). Closure and postoperative drainage are performed as in patients who have pectus excavatum.

Operative Results

Surgical correction of pectus carinatum is very successful. In a review of 152 cases by Shamberger and Welch (1987b) postoperative recovery was generally uneventful.

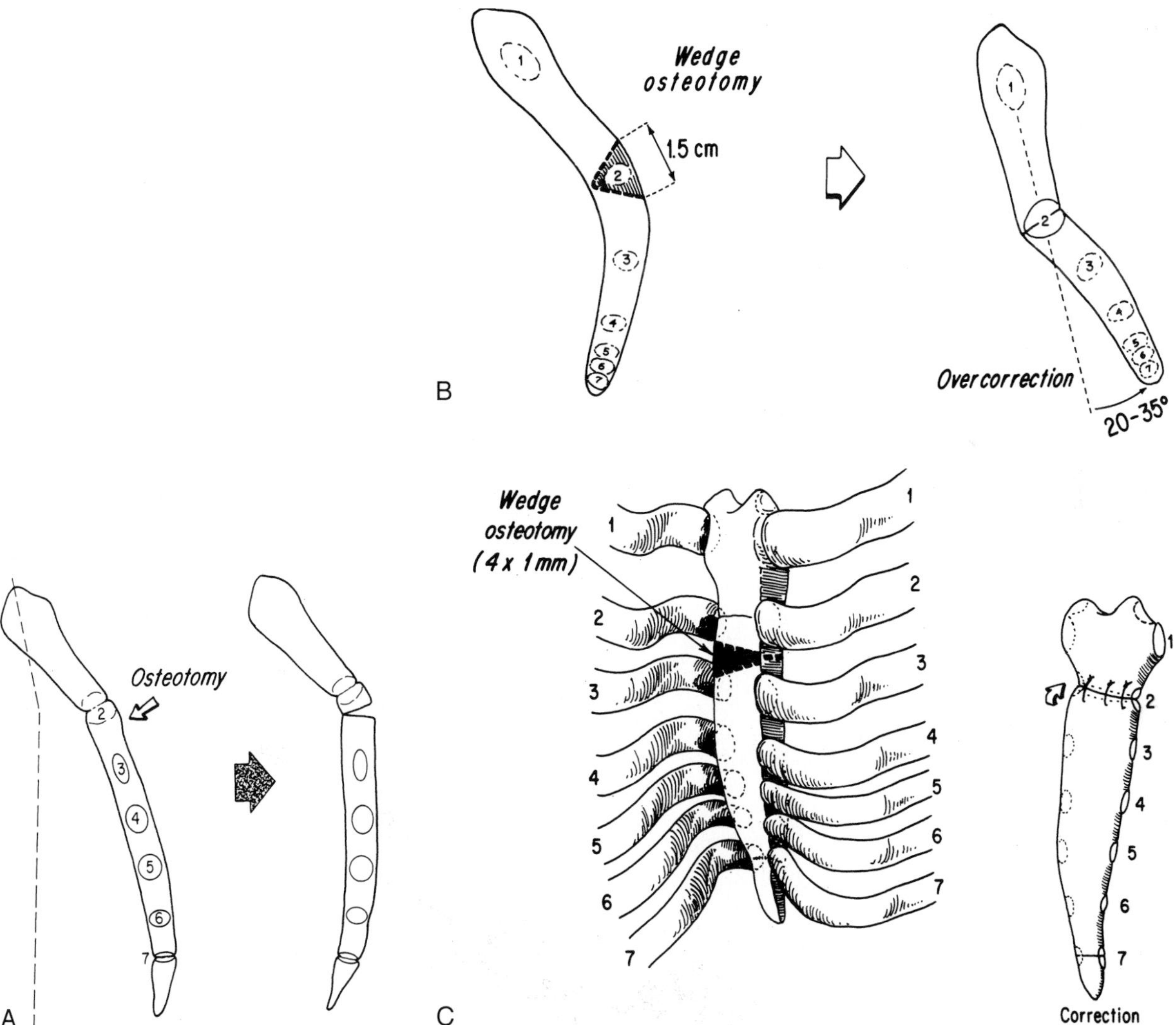

FIGURE 50–7 ■ *A*, Chondrogladiolar deformity (90.8% of all carinate deformities) is managed with a single or double osteotomy after resection of the costal cartilages. This allows posterior displacement of the sternum to an orthotopic position. *B*, Chondromanubrial deformity is rare. The broad superior osteotomy achieves anterior displacement of the body of the sternum and posterior displacement of the manubrium. *C*, The mixed pectus deformity is corrected by symmetric resection of the third to seventh costal cartilages followed by a transverse, offset (0- to 10-degree), wedge-shaped, sternal osteotomy. Closure of this defect achieves both anterior displacement and rotation of the sternum. (*B*, From Shamberger RC, Welch KJ: Surgical correction of chondromanubrial deformity [Currarino-Silverman syndrome]. J Pediatr Surg 23:319, 1988. *C*, From Shamberger RC, Welch KJ: Surgical correction of pectus carinatum. J Pediatr Surg 22:48, 1987.)

Blood transfusions are rarely required, with none given since the early 1980s. There is a 3.9% rate of complications, which have included pneumothorax, wound infection, recurrence, and postoperative pneumonitis. Only three patients have required revision, each having additional lower costal cartilages resected for persistent unilateral malformation of the costal arch.

Poland's Syndrome

In 1841, Alfred Poland described congenital absence of the pectoralis major and minor muscles associated with syndactyly. It has become apparent that this entity is a spectrum, often involving chest wall and breast deformities as well. The extent of thoracic involvement may range from hypoplasia of the sternal head of the pectoralis major muscle and the pectoralis minor muscle with normal underlying ribs to severe hypoplasia of the ribs with complete absence of the anterior portions of the second to fourth ribs and cartilages (Fig. 50–8). The extent of chest wall involvement is depicted in Figure 50–9, and the findings in our series of 75 patients are shown in Table 50–1 (Shamberger et al, 1989). Breast involvement is frequent and ranges from mild hypoplasia to complete absence of the breast (amastia) and nipple (athelia). Minimal subcutaneous fat and absence of axillary hair are often found on the involved side. Hand deformities are frequent, as occurred in the patient described by Poland, and may include hypoplasia (brachydactyly), fused fingers (syndactyly), and mitten or claw deformity (ectromelia). There is no correlation between the extent of hand, breast, and thoracic deformity.

HISTORICAL NOTE

Poland's syndrome is a classic example of the wrong eponym being attached to a syndrome. In 1841, Alfred

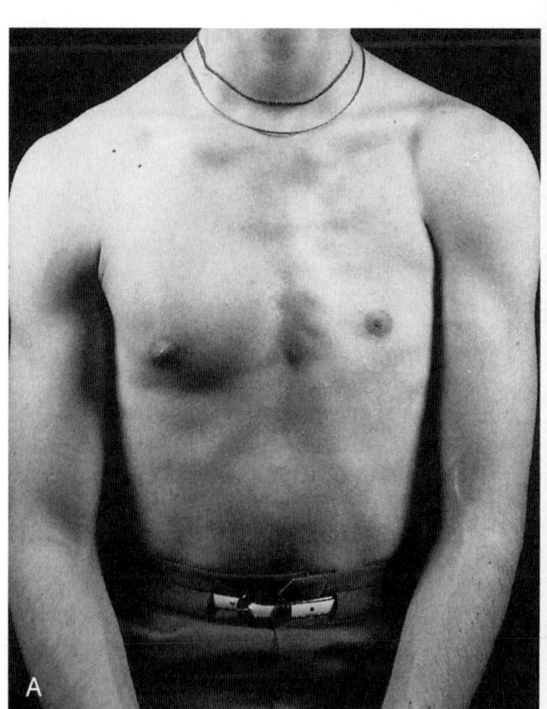

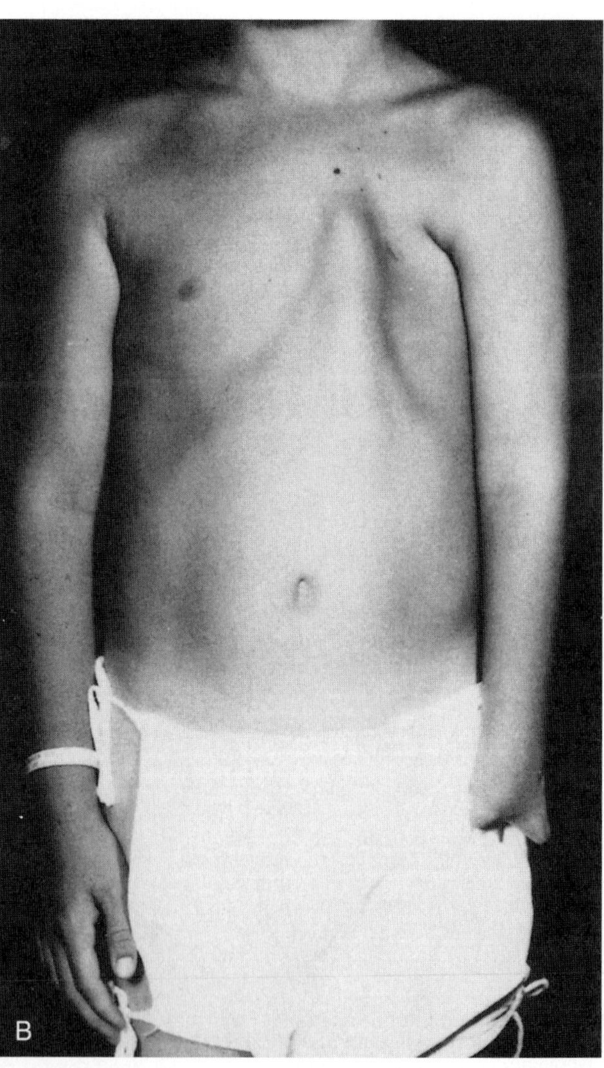

FIGURE 50–8 ■ *A*, A 16-year-old boy with Poland's syndrome with absent pectoralis major and pectoralis minor muscles. Ribs are intact and in a normal contour. *B*, A 10-year-old boy with Poland's syndrome in whom the anterior third to fifth left ribs are hypoplastic and do not reach the sternum. The left nipple is also hypoplastic and displaced superiorly. This child also had a severe hand deformity with absence of most of the bony elements of the hand and wrist. (From Shamberger RC, Welch KJ, Upton J III: Surgical treatment of thoracic deformity in Poland's syndrome. J Pediatr Surg 24:760, 1989.)

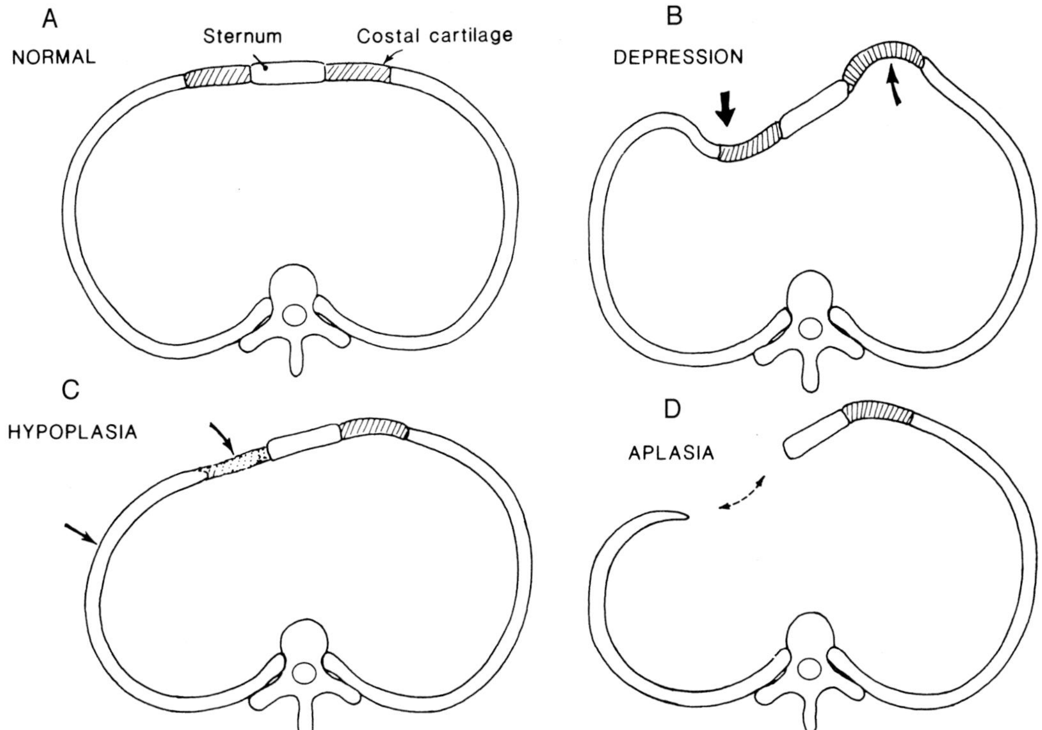

FIGURE 50–9 ■ The spectrum of rib cage abnormality seen in Poland's syndrome. *A*, Most frequently an entirely normal rib cage is seen with only pectoral muscles absent. *B*, Depression of the involved side of the chest wall with rotation and often depression of the sternum. A carinate protrusion of the contralateral side is frequently present. *C*, Hypoplasia of the ribs on the involved side, without significant depression. This usually does not require surgical correction. *D*, Aplasia of one or more ribs is usually associated with depression of adjacent ribs on the involved side and rotation of the sternum. (From Shamberger RC, Welch KJ, Upton J III: Surgical treatment of thoracic deformity in Poland's syndrome. J Pediatr Surg 24:760, 1989.)

Poland reported results of an anatomic dissection that he performed while he was still a medical student. He found a constellation of anomalies, including absence of the pectoralis major and minor muscles and syndactyly. The syndrome had, however, been previously described by Lallemand (1826) and Froriep (1839) in the French and German literature, respectively. The full spectrum of anomalies was first summarized by Thomson in 1895 prior to Clarkson attributing the syndrome to Poland in 1962.

■ *HISTORICAL READINGS*

Clarkson P: Poland's syndactyly. Guy's Hosp Rep 111:335, 1962.

Froriep R: Beobachtung eines Falles von Mangel der Brustdruse. Notizen Geb Nat Heilk 10:9, 1839.

Lallemand LM: Absence de trots cotes simulant un enforcement accidental. Ephérmérides Médicales de Montpellier 1:144, 1826.

Poland A: Deficiency of the pectoralis muscles. Guy's Hosp Rep 6:191, 1841.

Thomson J: On a form of congenital thoracic deformity. Teratologia 2:1, 1895.

TABLE 50–1 ■ **Chest Wall Deformities in 75 Patients with Poland's Syndrome**

Condition	*No. of Patients*
Normal chest wall	41
Hypoplasia of ribs without depression	10
Depression deformity of ribs	
Major	11
Minor	5
Aplasia of ribs	8
Total	75

BASIC SCIENCE

Poland's syndrome is present from birth and has an estimated incidence of 1 in 30,000 to 1 in 32,000 live births (Freire-Maia et al, 1975; McGillivray and Lowry, 1977). Abnormalities in the breast can be identified at birth by notation of the absence of the underlying breast bud and hypoplasia or aplasia of the often superiorly displaced nipple. The etiology is unknown, and cases are sporadic in their occurrence.

SURGICAL REPAIR

Assessment of the extent of involvement of the various musculoskeletal components is critical for optimal thoracic reconstruction in Poland's syndrome. If involvement is limited to the sternal component of the pectoralis major and minor muscles, there is little functional deficit, and repair is not necessary except for breast augmentation in girls, which should be performed at full growth. If the underlying costal cartilages are depressed or absent, repair of the chest wall must be considered to minimize the concavity, to eliminate the paradoxic motion of the chest wall, and, in girls, to provide an optimal base for breast reconstruction. Ravitch (1966) reported correction of posteriorly displaced costal cartilages by unilateral resection of the cartilages, a wedge osteotomy of the sternum allowing rotation of the sternum, and fixation with Rehbein struts and Steinmann pins. We have found that suitable repair can often be achieved with bilateral costal cartilage resection and an oblique osteotomy, such as in the patients with the mixed pectus carinatum-excavatum deformity (Shamberger et al, 1989). This allows correction of the rotational deformity (Fig. 50–10). The sternum is displaced anteriorly, which corrects the posterior displacement of the costal cartilages. An unappreciated carinate deformity is often present on the contralateral side, accentuating the ipsilateral concavity.

Absence of the medial portion of the ribs can be managed with split rib grafts taken from the contralateral side (see Fig. 50–10*E*). These must be secured to the sternum medially and to the hypoplastic rib ends laterally. The grafts can be covered with a prosthetic mesh, if needed, for further support. In these cases, it must be remembered that there is little tissue present between the endothoracic fascia and the fascial remnants of the pectoral muscles. Coverage of this area can be augmented by transfer of a latissimus dorsi muscle flap. This is particularly helpful in girls, who will require breast augmentation (Urschel et al, 1984; 2000). Latissimus transfer is seldom, if ever, required in boys and has the disadvantage of adding a second thoracic scar as well as removing one of the major functional muscles of the shoulder and arm (Haller et al, 1984).

Sternal Defects

CLEFT STERNUM

Deformities involving failure of ventral fusion of the thoracic wall can be divided into three groups: (1) cleft sternum without ectopia cordis, (2) thoracic ectopia cordis, and (3) thoracoabdominal ectopia cordis. Cleft sternum with an orthotopic heart is the simplest of these deformities. The cleft may be complete or incomplete and results from failure of ventral fusion of the sternal bars, which occurs at the eighth week of gestation. In cleft sternum, the midline sternal separation is covered, and the pericardium, pleura, and diaphragm are intact. Omphaloceles do not occur in this entity, but an unexplained association with hemangiomas has been recognized. Crying or a Valsalva maneuver produces a dramatic increase in the apparent severity of the deformity. Intrinsic congenital heart disease is rare.

Treatment in the newborn period is recommended, when the malformation can be closed primarily without prosthetic materials or cardiac compression. Primary closure in older patients produces excessive cardiac compression. Reconstruction of the anterior chest wall using multiple oblique chondrotomies, as reported by Sabiston (1958), lengthens the costal cartilages and decreases cardiac compression in the older patients with a less flexible chest wall. Autologous grafts, including costal cartilages, split ribs, and resection of the costal arch complex, have been described, but repair in the newborn period is optimal and avoids the need for these methods (Fig. 50–11).

THORACIC ECTOPIA CORDIS

Although management of an isolated cleft sternum is uniformly successful, only a limited number of patients survive surgical treatment of thoracic and thoracoabdominal ectopia cordis. These patients have a high incidence of associated intrinsic cardiac anomalies in addition to the abnormal cardiac position and overlying somatic structures. In thoracic ectopia cordis, nothing covers the heart, which is external to the thorax, protruding at the upper to midthoracic level (Fig. 50–12). The apex of the heart points anteriorly. Attempts to return the heart to the thorax occlude the great vessels and are not tolerated. Only a few infants have undergone successful repair, and they generally lack associated cardiac anomalies (Shamberger and Welch, 1990).

THORACOABDOMINAL ECTOPIA CORDIS (CANTRELL'S PENTALOGY)

The features of the Cantrell pentalogy (Cantrell et al, 1958) are a cleft lower sternum, an anterior diaphragmatic defect due to failure of development of the septum transversum, absence of the parietal pericardium, an adjacent or completely separate omphalocele, and, in most patients, a cardiac anomaly, frequently the tetralogy of Fallot.

Immediate neonatal intervention to close the abdominal wall is required in patients with an omphalocele and lower sternal cleft (Fig. 50–13). An aggressive approach should be taken with these infants if salvage is to be achieved. After somatic closure, repair of the cardiac defect can be performed.

Thoracic Deformities in Diffuse Skeletal Disorders

ASPHYXIATING THORACIC DYSTROPHY (JEUNE'S SYNDROME)

In 1954, Jeune and associates first described a newborn with a narrow, rigid chest and multiple cartilage anomalies, who died early in the perinatal period because of respiratory insufficiency. Other authors have further characterized this form of osteochondrodystrophy, which has variable skeletal involvement. It is inherited in an autosomal recessive pattern and is not associated with chromosome abnormalities (Tahernia and Stamps, 1977). Its most prominent feature is a narrow "bell-shaped" thorax and protuberant abdomen. The thorax is narrow in both the transverse and sagittal axes and has little respiratory motion owing to the horizontal direction of the ribs (Fig. 50–14). The ribs are short and wide, and the splayed costochondral junctions barely reach the anterior axillary line. The costal cartilage is abundant and irregular like a rachitic rosary. Microscopic examination of the costo-

Text continues on page 1372

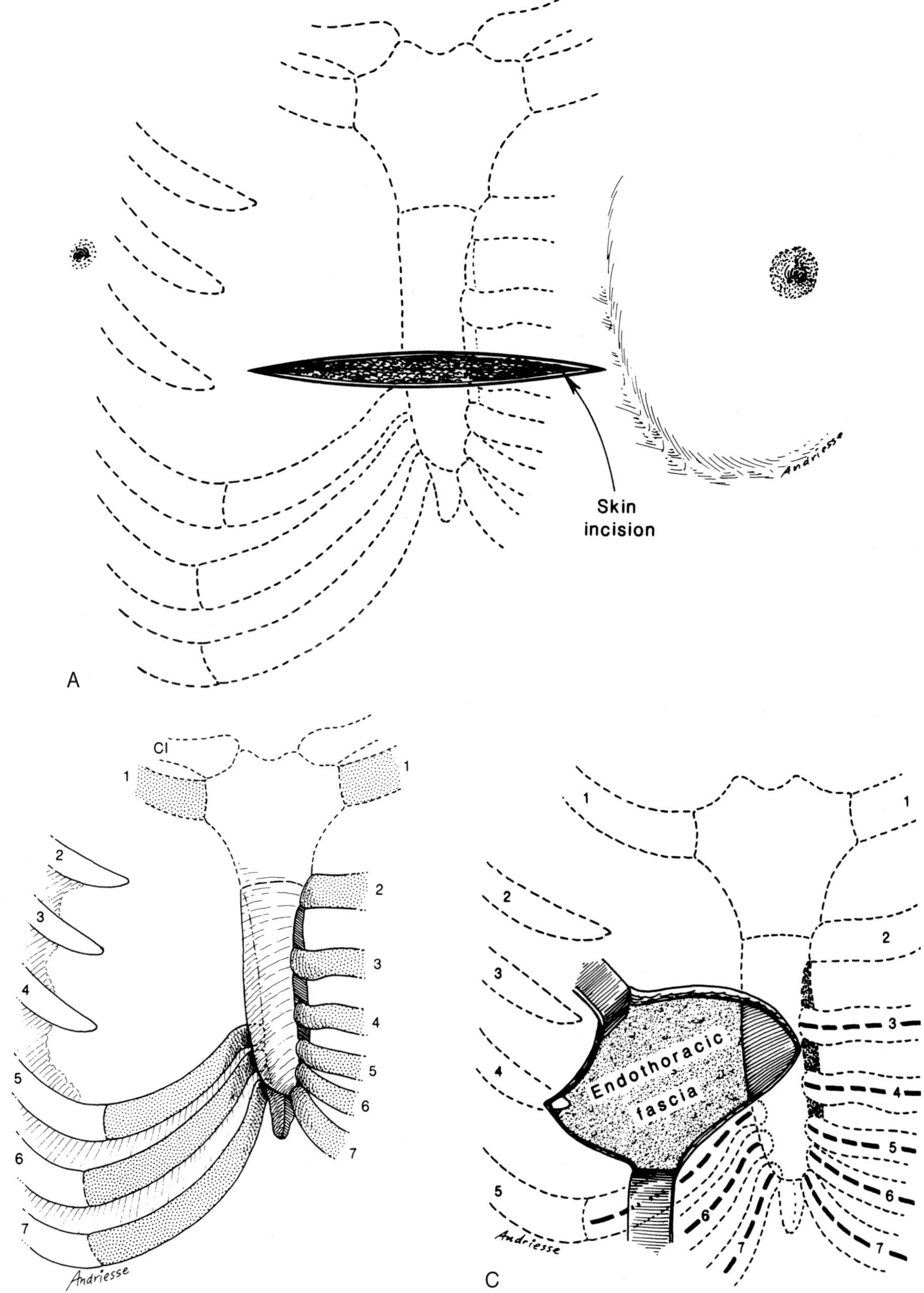

FIGURE 50–10 ■ *A*, A transverse incision is placed below the nipple lines, and in females in the site of the future inframammary crease. *B*, Schematic depiction of the deformity with rotation of the sternum, depression of the cartilages of the involved side, and carinate protrusion of the contralateral side. *C*, In cases with aplasia of the ribs, the endothoracic fascia is encountered directly below the attenuated subcutaneous tissue and pectoral fascia. The pectoral muscle flap is elevated on the contralateral side and the pectoral fascia, if present, on the involved side. Subperichondrial resection of the costal cartilages is then carried out as shown by the *dashed lines*. Rarely, this must be carried to the level of the second costal cartilage.

Illustration continued on following page

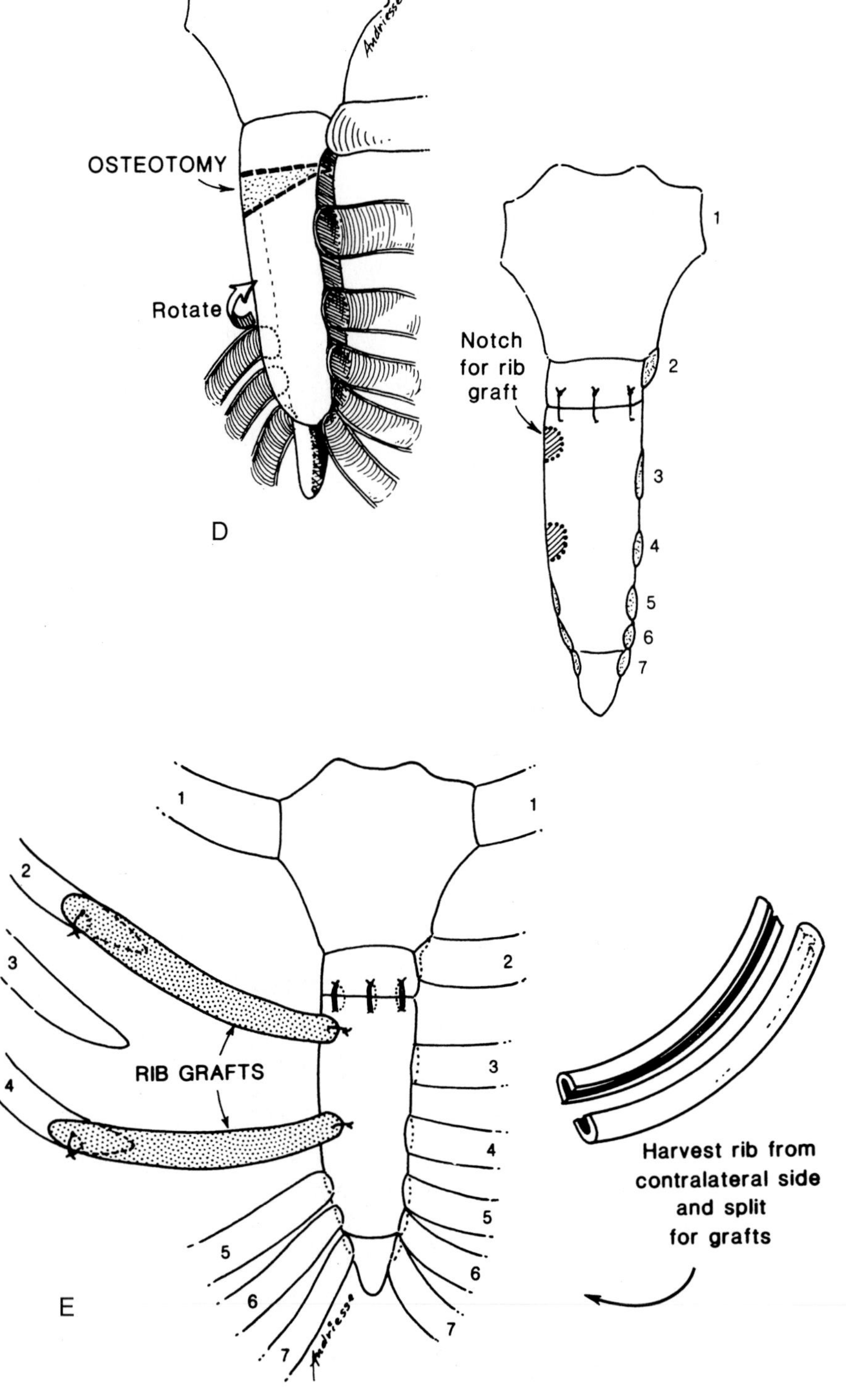

FIGURE 50–10 ■ *Continued. D,* A transverse, offset, wedge-shaped osteotomy is then created below the second costal cartilage. Closure of this defect with heavy silk sutures or by elevation of the sternum with a strut corrects both the posterior displacement and the rotation of the sternum. *E,* In patients with rib aplasia, split rib grafts are harvested from the contralateral fifth or sixth ribs and then secured medially with wire sutures into previously created sternal notches and laterally with wire to the native ribs. Ribs are split as shown along their short axis to maintain maximum mechanical strength. (From Shamberger RC, Welch KJ, Upton J III: Surgical treatment of thoracic deformity in Poland's syndrome. J Pediatr Surg 24:760, 1989.)

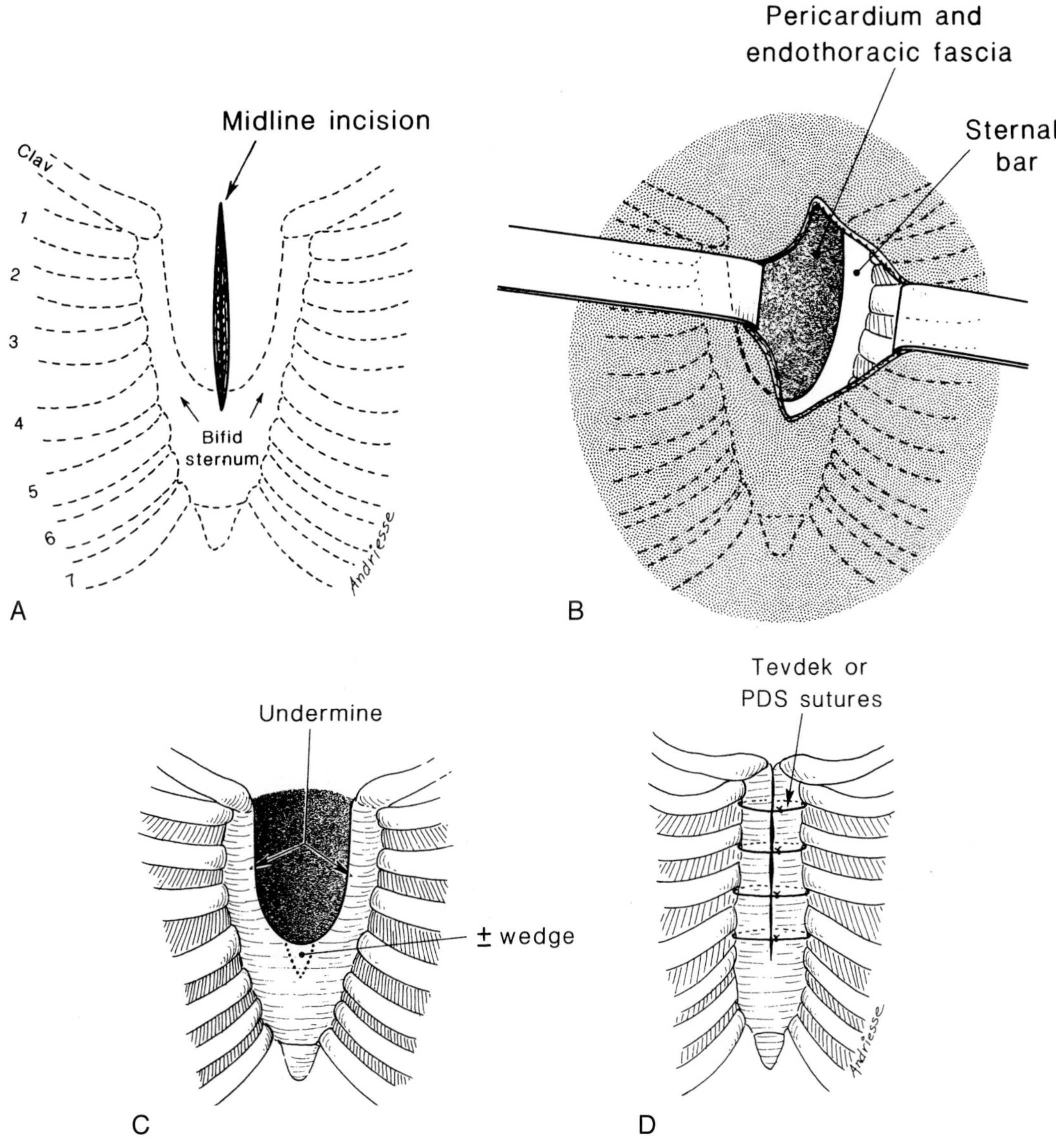

FIGURE 50–11 ■ *A*, Repair of a bifid sternum is best performed through a longitudinal incision extending the length of the defect. *B*, The sternal bars are encountered directly beneath the subcutaneous tissues; pectoral muscles are present lateral to the bars. The endothoracic fascia and pericardium are located just below these structures. *C*, The endothoracic fascia is mobilized off the sternal bars posteriorly with blunt dissection to allow safe placement of the sutures. Approximation of the sternal bars may be facilitated by excising a wedge of cartilage inferiorly. Repair is best accomplished in the neonatal period because of the flexibility of the chest wall. *D*, The defect is closed with permanent sutures. (From Shamberger RC, Welch KJ: Sternal defects. Pediatr Surg Int 5:156, 1990.)

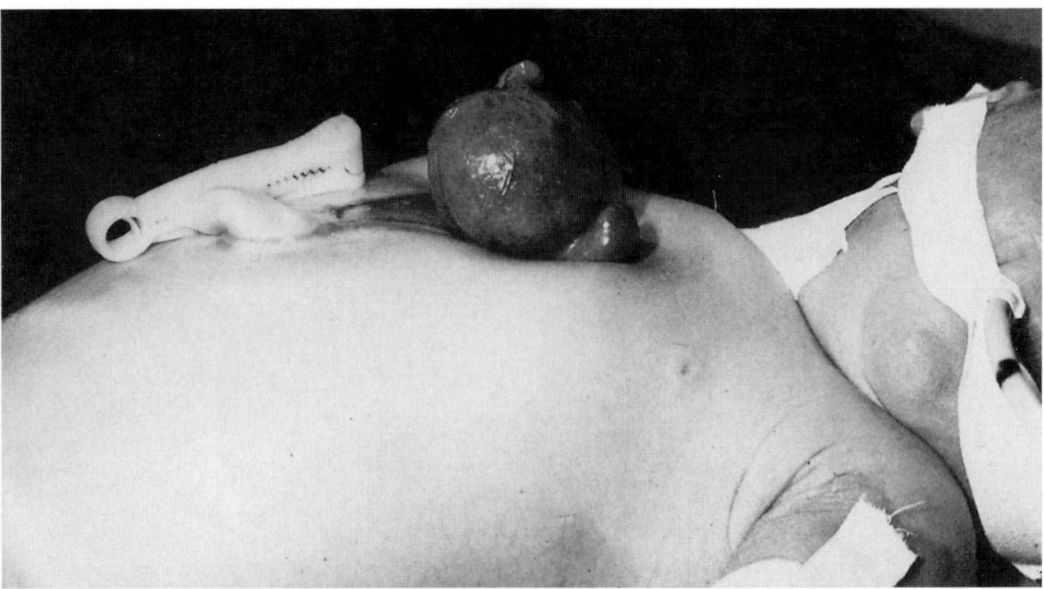

FIGURE 50–12 ■ Infant with thoracic ectopia cordis with no significant abdominal wall defect present. Note characteristic high insertion of the umbilicus.

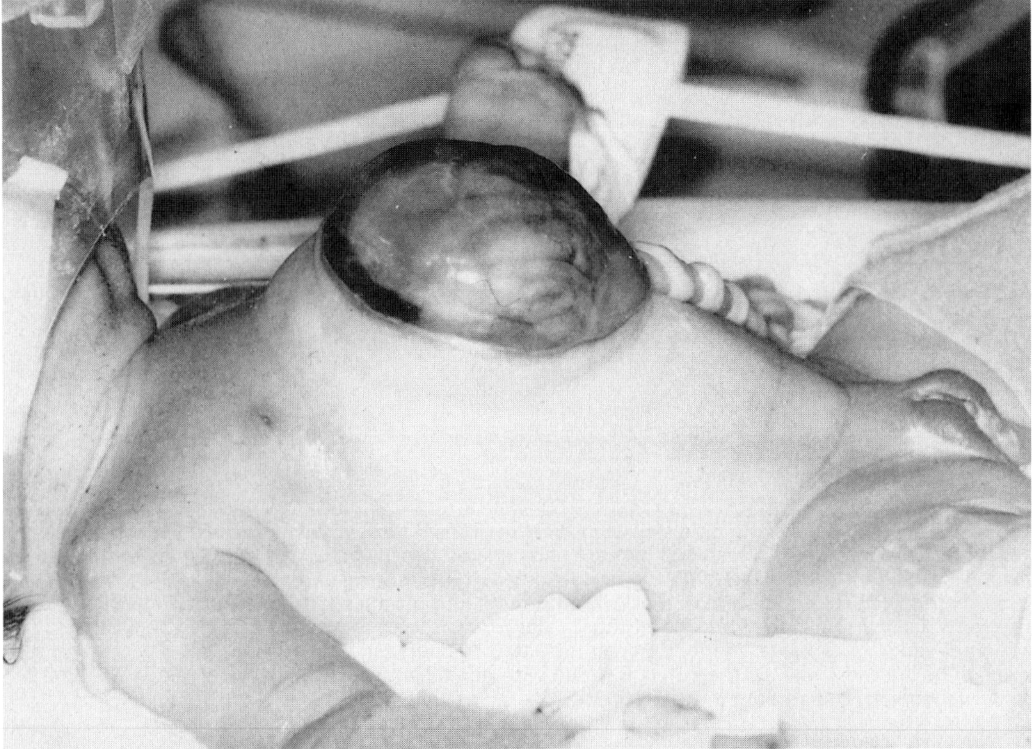

FIGURE 50–13 ■ Infant with thoracoabdominal ectopia cordis demonstrating a high abdominal wall defect and an omphalocele below the costal arch. The infant's head is to the left, and the heart was palpable just below the skin superior to the defect.

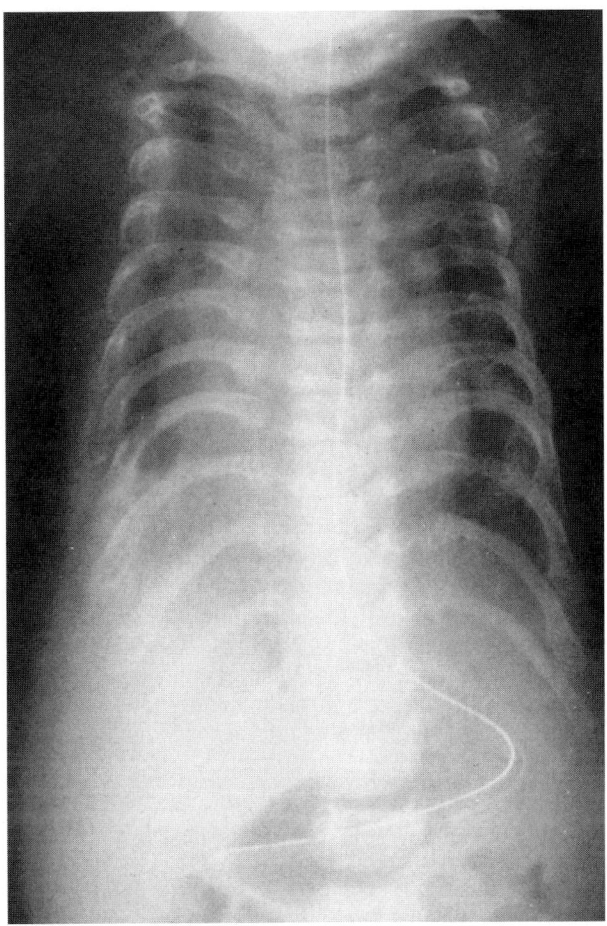

FIGURE 50–14 ■ Infant with asphyxiating thoracic dystrophy (Jeune's syndrome). Radiograph shows the short horizontal ribs and narrow thorax with limited lung volumes.

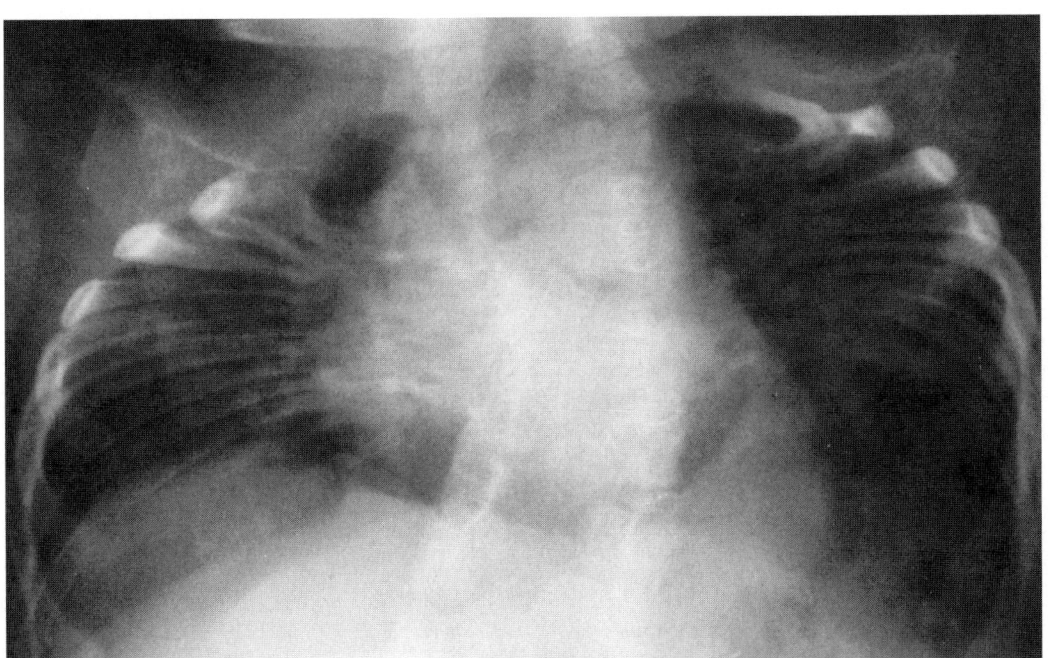

FIGURE 50–15 ■ Radiograph of an infant with spondylothoracic dysplasia (Jarcho-Levin syndrome). Severe abnormality of the spine is apparent, with multiple hemivertebrae and "crab-like" ribs, with close approximation posteriorly and splaying out anteriorly.

chondral junction reveals disordered and poorly progressing endochondral ossification, resulting in decreased rib length.

Associated skeletal abnormalities include short and stubby extremities with relatively short and wide bones. The clavicles are in a fixed and elevated position, and the pelvis is small and hypoplastic with square iliac bones.

The syndrome has variable expression and degree of pulmonary impairment. Although the initial cases reported resulted in neonatal death, subsequent reports have documented a wide range of survival of patients with this syndrome (Kozlowski and Masel, 1976). The pathologic findings in autopsy cases also vary and show a range of abnormal pulmonary development; however, in most cases the bronchial development is normal, and there is variable decrease in alveolar divisions (Williams et al, 1984).

Surgical interventions for this condition have had very limited success. All have involved splitting the sternum longitudinally and widening the distance between the two sternal halves to increase the intrathoracic volume. Rib grafts, stainless steel struts, iliac bone grafts with metal plate fixation, and polymethylmethacrylate prostheses have all been used to maintain sternal separation. Results of these surgical attempts depend on the degree of underlying pulmonary hypoplasia.

SPONDYLOTHORACIC DYSPLASIA (JARCHO-LEVIN SYNDROME)

Spondylothoracic dysplasia is an autosomal recessive deformity in which there are multiple vertebral and rib malformations. Death occurs in early infancy from respiratory failure and pneumonia (Jarcho and Levin, 1983). Patients have multiple alternating hemivertebrae, which affect most, if not all, of the thoracic and lumbar spine. The vertebral ossification centers rarely cross the midline. Multiple posterior fusions of the ribs as well as remarkable shortening of the thoracic spine results in a "crab-like" radiographic appearance of the chest (Fig. 50–15). One third of patients with this syndrome have associated malformations, including congenital heart disease and renal anomalies. Its occurrence has been reported by Heilbronner and Renshaw (1984), primarily in Puerto Rican families (15 of 18 cases). Bone formation is normal in these patients.

Thoracic deformity is secondary to the spine anomaly, which results in close posterior approximation of the origin of the ribs. Although most infants with this entity succumb before 15 months of age, no surgical efforts have been proposed or attempted (Roberts et al, 1988).

COMMENTS AND CONTROVERSIES

The advantages of early repair of pectus excavatum or carinatum are that it can minimize pathophysiologic abnormalities, cardiac/pulmonary displacement, and psychological damage secondary to significant deformities as the individual enters puberty and adolescence. Disadvantages of early repair (e.g., at 2 years) revolve around the high recurrence rate because of continuation of growth, particularly of the rib cartilages, which may produce further deformity or recurrence of deformity. From this point of view, the best time for repair would be after the main growth has stopped (i.e., after adolescence—in the late teens or early 20s). Although the operation is more traumatic at this time, the results are far better, with minimal recurrence.

For pectus excavatum and carinatum repair after removing the abnormal costal cartilages, some surgeons place a stainless steel rod through the sternum at the appropriate angle to stabilize it in the correct position. This is removed after an interval of time. Other surgeons reverse the sternum and fix it in a number of different ways. This has not been particularly appealing in our experience.

H.C.U.

KEY REFERENCES

Shamberger RC, Welch KJ: Cardiopulmonary function in pectus excavatum. Surg Gynecol Obstet 166:383, 1988b.

This comprehensive summary of articles that evaluate cardiopulmonary function in patients with pectus excavatum presents a comparison of these studies and attempts to clarify the conflicting reports in the literature.

Shamberger RC, Welch KJ: Sternal defects. Pediatr Surg Int 5:156, 1990.

A summary of world literature on sternal defects including bifid sternum, Cantrell's pentalogy, and thoracic ectopia cordis.

REFERENCES

Adkins PC, Blades B: A stainless steel strut for correction of pectus excavatum. Surg Gynecol Obstet 113:111, 1961.

Baronofsky ID: Technique for the correction of pectus excavatum. Surgery 42:884, 1957.

Beiser GD, Epstein SE, Stampfer M et al: Impairment of cardiac function in patients with pectus excavatum, with improvement after operative correction. N Engl J Med 287:267, 1972.

Blickman JG, Rosen PR, Welch KJ et al: Pectus excavatum in children: Pulmonary scintigraphy before and after corrective surgery. Radiology 156:781, 1985.

Cahill JL, Lees GM, Robertson HT: A summary of preoperative and postoperative cardiorespiratory performance in patients undergoing pectus excavatum and carinatum repair. J Pediatr Surg 19:430, 1984.

Cantrell JR, Haller JA, Ravitch MM: A syndrome of congenital defects involving the abdominal wall, sternum, diaphragm, pericardium and heart. Surg Gynecol Obstet 107:602, 1958.

Castile RG, Staats SA, Westbrook PR: Symptomatic pectus deformities of the chest. Am Rev Respir Dis 126:564, 1982.

Chin EF: Surgery of funnel chest and congenital sternal prominence. Br J Surg 44:360, 1957.

Clarkson P: Poland's syndactyly. Guy's Hosp Rep 111:335, 1962.

Currarino G, Silverman FN: Premature obliteration of the sternal sutures and pigeon-breast deformity. Radiology 70:532, 1958.

Derveaux L, Clarysse I, Ivanoff I, Demedts M: Preoperative and postoperative abnormalities in chest x-ray indices and in lung function in pectus deformities. Chest 95:850, 1989.

Derveaux L, Ivanoff I, Rochette F, Demedts M: Mechanism of pulmonary function changes after surgical correction for funnel chest. Eur Resp J 1:823, 1988.

Freire-Maia N, Chautard EA, Opitz JM et al: The Poland syndrome—clinical and genealogical data, dermatoglyphic analysis, and incidence. Hum Hered 23:97, 1973.

Froriep R: Beobachtung eines Falles von Mangel der Brustdruse. Notizen Geb Nat Heilk 10:9, 1839.

Greig JD, Azmy AF: Thoracic cage deformity: A late complication following repair of an agenesis of diaphragm. J Pediatr Surg 25:1234, 1990.

Haller JA, Colombani PM, Humphries CT et al: Chest wall construction after too extensive and too early operations for pectus excavatum. Ann Thorac Surg 61:1618, 1996.

Haller JA Jr, Colombani PM, Miller D et al: Early reconstruction of Poland's syndrome using autologous rib grafts combined with a latissimus muscle flap. J Pediatr Surg 19:423, 1984.

Haller JA Jr, Katlic BA, Shermeta DW et al: Operative correction of pectus excavatum: An evolving perspective. Ann Surg 184:554, 1976.

Haller JA, Peters GN, Mazur D et al: Pectus excavatum: A 20 year surgical experience. J Thorac Cardiovasc Surg 60:375, 1970.

Hecker WC, Procher G, Dietz HG: Results of operative correction of pigeon and funnel chest following a modified procedure of Ravitch and Haller. Z Kinderchir 34:220, 1981.

Heilbronner DM, Renshaw TS: Spondylothoracic dysplasia. J Bone Joint Surg [Am] 66:302, 1984.

Howard R: Pigeon chest (protrusion deformity of the sternum). Med J Aust 2:664, 1958.

Jarcho S, Levin PM: Hereditary malformation of the vertebral bodies. Johns Hopkins Med J 62:216, 1938.

Jeune M, Carron R, Beraud CL et al: Polychondrodystrophie avec blocage thoracique d'évolution fatale. Pediatrie 9:390, 1954.

Judet J, Judet R: Sternum en entonnoir par résection et retournement. Mem Acad Chir 82:250, 1956.

Jung A, Wiest E, Vierling J-P: Traitement par le "retournement pédiculé" de la cuvette sterno-chondrale: Résultats éloignés. Rev Chir Orthop 50:446, 1964.

Kaguraoka H, Ohnuki T, Itaoka T et al: Degree of severity of pectus excavatum and pulmonary function in preoperative and postoperative periods. J Thorac Cardiovasc Surg 104:1483, 1992.

Kozlowski K, Masel J: Asphyxiating thoracic dystrophy without respiratory disease: Report of two cases of the latent form. Pediatr Radiol 5:30, 1976.

Lallemand LM: Absence detrois côtes simulant un enforcement accidental. Ephérmérides Médicales de Montpellier 1:144, 1826.

Lees RF, Caldicott WJH: Sternal anomalies and congenital heart disease. AJR Am J Roentgenol 124:423, 1975.

Lester CW: The etiology and pathogenesis of funnel chest, pigeon breast, and related deformities of the anterior chest wall. J Thorac Surg 34:1, 1957.

Lester CW: Pigeon breast (pectus carinatum) and other protrusion deformities of the chest of developmental origin. Ann Surg 137:482, 1953.

Martinez D, Juame J, Stein T et al: The effect of costal cartilage resection on chest wall development. Pediatr Surg Int 5:170, 1990.

McGillivray BC, Lowry RB: Poland syndrome in British Columbia: Incidence and reproductive experience of affected persons. Am J Med Genet 1:65, 1977.

Meyer L: Zur chirurgischen Behandlung der angeborenen Trichterbrust. Verh Ber Med Ges 42:364, 1911.

Morshuis W, Folgering H, Barentsz J et al: Pulmonary function before surgery for pectus excavatum and at long-term follow-up. Chest 105:1646, 1994a.

Morshuis W, Folgering HT, Barentsz J et al: Exercise cardiorespiratory function before and one year after operation for pectus excavatum. J Thorac Cardiovasc Surg 107:1403, 1994b.

Ochsner A, DeBakey M: Chonechondrosternon: Report of a case and review of the literature. J Thorac Surg 8:469, 1939.

Oelsnitz G: Fehlbildungen des Brustkorbes. Z Kinderchir 33:229, 1981.

Peterson RJ, Young WG Jr, Godwin JD et al: Noninvasive assessment of exercise cardiac function before and after pectus excavatum repair. J Thorac Cardiovasc Surg 90:251, 1985.

Poland A: Deficiency of the pectoralis muscles. Guy's Hosp Rep 6:191, 1841.

Ravitch MM: Atypical deformities of the chest wall-absence and deformities of the ribs and costal cartilages. Surgery 59:438, 1966.

Ravitch MM: Congenital Deformities of the Chest Wall and Their Operative Correction. Philadelphia, WB Saunders, 1977, p 78.

Ravitch MM: The operative treatment of pectus excavatum. Ann Surg 129:429, 1949.

Ravitch MM: Unusual sternal deformity with cardiac symptoms-operative correction. J Thorac Surg 23:138, 1952.

Rehbein F, Wernicke HH: The operative treatment of the funnel chest. Arch Dis Child 32:5, 1957.

Roberts AP, Conner AN, Tolmie JL et al: Spondylothoracic and spondylocostal dysostosis: Hereditary forms of spinal deformity. J Bone Joint Surg Br 70:123, 1988.

Sabiston DC Jr: The surgical management of congenital bifid sternum with partial ectopia cordis. J Thorac Surg 35:118, 1958.

Sauerbruch F: Die Chirurgie der Brustorgane. Berlin, J Springer, 1920, p. 437.

Scherer LR, Arn PH, Dressel DA et al: Surgical management of children and young adults with Marfan syndrome and pectus excavatum. J Pediatr Surg 23:1169, 1988.

Shamberger RC, Welch KJ: Surgical correction of chondromanubrial deformity (Currarino-Silverman syndrome). J Pediatr Surg 23:319, 1988c.

Shamberger RC, Welch KJ: Surgical correction of pectus carinatum. J Pediatr Surg 22:48, 1987b.

Shamberger RC, Welch KJ: Surgical correction of pectus excavatum. J Pediatr Surg 23:615, 1988a.

Shamberger RC, Welch KJ, Sanders SP: Mitral valve prolapse associated with pectus excavatum. J Pediatr 111:404, 1987a.

Shamberger RC, Welch KJ, Upton J III: Surgical treatment of thoracic deformity in Poland's syndrome. J Pediatr Surg 24:760, 1989.

Tahernia AC, Stamps P: "Jeune syndrome" (asphyxiating thoracic dystrophy): Report of a case, a review of the literature, and an editor's commentary. Clin Pediatr (Phila) 16:903, 1977.

Tanaka F, Kitano M, Shindo T et al: Postoperative lung function in patients with funnel chest. J Jap Assoc Thorac Surg 41:2161, 1993.

Thomson J: On a form of congenital thoracic deformity. Teratologia 2:1, 1895.

Urschel HC, Byrd HS, Sethi SM, Razzuk MA: Poland's syndrome: Improved surgical management. Ann Thorac Surg 37:204, 1984.

Urschel HC Jr: Poland's syndrome. Chest Surg Clin North Am 10:393, 2000.

Wada J, Ikeda K, Ishida T, Hasegawa T: Results of 271 funnel chest operations. Ann Thorac Surg 10:526, 1970.

Welch KJ: Satisfactory surgical correction of pectus excavatum deformity in childhood: A limited opportunity. J Thorac Surg 36:697, 1958.

Welch KJ, Kearney GP: Abdominal musculature deficiency syndrome: Prune belly. J Urol 111:693, 1974.

Welch KJ, Vos A: Surgical correction of pectus carinatum (pigeon breast). J Pediatr Surg 8:659, 1973.

Williams AJ, Vawter G, Reid LM: Lung structure in asphyxiating thoracic dystrophy. Arch Pathol Lab Med 108:658, 1984.

Willital GH: Operationsindikation-Operationstechnik bei Brustkorbdeformierungen. Z Kinderchir 33:244, 1981.

Wynn SR, Driscoll DJ, Ostrom NK et al: Exercise cardiorespiratory function in adolescents with pectus excavatum. J Thorac Cardiovasc Surg 99:41, 1990.

CHAPTER **51**

Complications of Midline Sternotomy

Francis Robicsek

At the dawn of cardiac surgery, different areas of the heart were exposed through either a conventional anterolateral or a posterolateral thoracotomy. As cardiac interventions became more complex, these incisions were commonly extended across the sternum, often into the contralateral pleural cavity. Midline axial sternotomy, first described by Milton in 1887, was recommended in 1957 by Julian and colleagues (1957) for a more extended exposure of the heart. This approach soon replaced the then popular "clamshell" incision. Although changes in cardiac surgery, such as the "off-pump" and other types of minimally invasive methods, revived some of the old forms of exposure and introduced new ones (Fig. 51–1), midline axial sternotomy still remains the most popular technique of cardiac exposure because of its quick and easy performance, minimal blood loss, and little if any functional impairment. Despite these unsurpassed advantages, however, there is a potential for complications that may result in significant morbidity and mortality and increased costs for patients undergoing cardiac surgery (Cremer et al, 1997). The purpose of this chapter is to discuss the mechanism, the predisposing conditions, and the diagnosis and management of clinical problems associated with midline sternotomy.

The sternotomy complications are discussed in three principal categories: *noninfectious complications without sternal instability, sternal instability,* and *sternal wound infection.*

NONINFECTIOUS COMPLICATIONS WITHOUT STERNAL INSTABILITY

Superficial wound problems such as skin separation and hematomas are to be handled according to general rules of surgical practice. Because of their potential to involve the sternum, however, every effort should be made to reduce their occurrence, including strict observance of sterile and atraumatic techniques, meticulous hemostasis, discriminate use of electrocautery, and protection of the subcutaneous tissues from protracted exposure.

Chronic pain frequently occurs in and around sternotomy incisions. In contrast to recurrent angina, poststernotomy pain is typically associated with tenderness around the surgical incision and is often induced by the action of different muscles of the chest wall and the shoulder girdle. It can typically be handled with common pain medications and seldom requires special measures.

After sternotomy, however, there are several types of stubborn pain syndromes, whose pathogenetic mechanisms are distinctly different and may require special attention. *Postcardiotomy syndrome*, which is considered an inflammatory reaction of the pericardiac tissues, usually responds to nonsteroidal anti-inflammatory agents. The proposed mechanism of *poststernotomy brachial plexopathy*, which occurs in about 5% of the cases, may be hyperabduction of the arm during anesthesia or overstretching of the sternum with retractors (Hanson et al, 1983; Vander Salm et al, 1982). The severity of plexopathy might vary from a simple dysesthesia and numbness to a radiculopathy in the C8-T1 area and the entire arm. Motor signs range from mild clumsiness of the hands to marked weakness of the intrinsic muscles. Plexopathy usually responds to physiotherapy and pain relievers. Brachial plexus injury in connection with open heart surgery may also occur during cannulation of the internal jugular vein. *Poststernotomy neuralgia* is caused by scar-entrapped neuromas of the anterior terminal branches of the intercostal nerves and may be treated by local injection of analgesics such as bupivacaine, aqueous phenol, or alcohol (Defalque and Bromley, 1989).

In *post-traumatic osteochondritis*, the tenderness and sometimes swelling in the parasternal area are localized to one or two costal cartilages. The condition is often associated with sternochondral separation, in which case the patient experiences a feeling of "clicks" and pain that is more intense during deep inspiration or when the shoulder is moved. Mobility of the separated chondral ends may be felt by the examiner and occasionally also by the patient. Confirmation by radiography is usually difficult and sometimes impossible. Initial treatment consists of infiltration of the tender area with local anesthetics or steroids. If symptoms persist, especially if there is continued mobility of the separated edges, removal of 3 to 4 cm of the involved cartilage including the separated end portion almost always leads to cessation of pain and discomfort by eliminating the rubbing together of the costal ends.

Because the costal cartilage has neither intrinsic nor segmental blood supply but is nourished by diffusion from the perichondrium, it is especially vulnerable to aseptic necrosis after surgical stripping or blunt trauma. Such *aseptic chondral necrosis* may less frequently involve the rib as well. In acute and subacute forms of this disease, microscopic examination shows accumulation of neutrophils, lymphocytes, and monocytes. Hemorrhage is frequently present. Clinically, the area may be indurated and is painful on palpation. Chronic forms of aseptic necrosis can lead to fistula formation, and because the

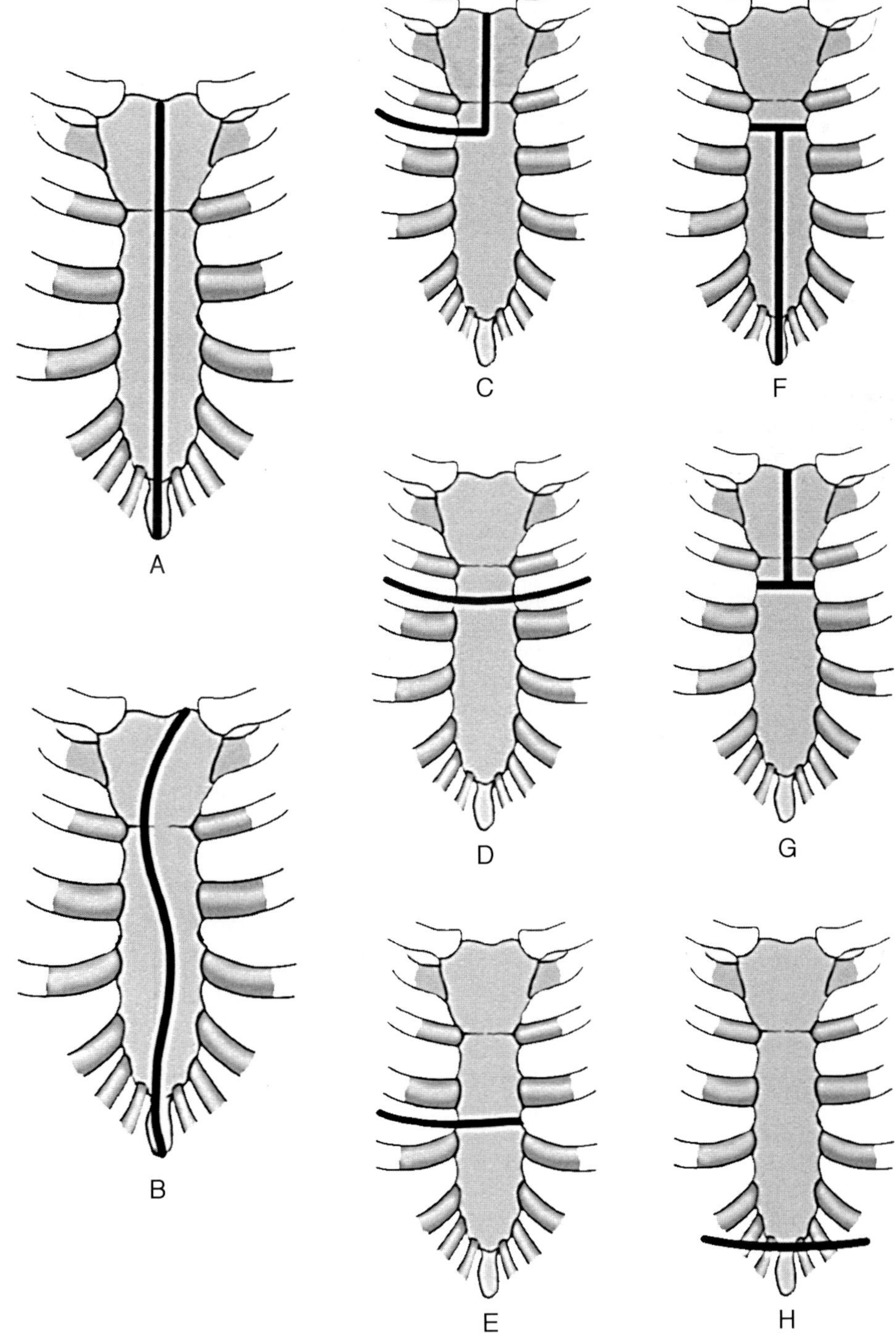

FIGURE 51–1 ■ Different types of sternotomy incisions used to expose the heart. *A*, Midline axial sternotomy; *B*, Slightly curved midline sternotomy for better alignment; *C*, Modified trap door; *D*, Clamshell; *E*, Anterior thoracotomy with transverse sternotomy; *F*, T-shaped lower sternotomy; *G*, Manubriotomy; *H*, Transxiphoid exposure.

necrotic portion of the rib acts as a foreign body, healing occurs only after the sequestered bone or cartilage is extruded spontaneously or removed surgically.

Sternal wire sutures may cause chest wall pain if a tied knot or a broken end lies against the skin. Another type of chronic chest wall pain that is attributed to sternal wires may occur 2 months to several years after the sternotomy; it is described as sharp, stabbing, or a deep-seated ache and is caused by an exaggerated fibrous *tissue reaction to wire sutures*. That biologic sensitivity to stainless steel occasionally becomes a surgical problem has been documented in the past with pacemakers and orthopedic implants (Ancalmo et al, 1993). Nickel has been implicated most frequently, although chromium and cobalt have also been shown to cause hypersensitivity reactions. It has been observed that the culprit wires had elevated electrical potentials, and iron ions collect at the anodic point of corrosion. Removal of these wires relieves the symptoms of pain and tenderness. Serial sections of the fibrous tissue usually reveal entrapment of sensory nerve fibers (Eastridge et al, 1991). A particular symptom of sensitivity to wire alloy is *persistent itching* in the sternotomy scar. If chest wall pain continues, other causes should be looked for, including myocardial ischemia.

Development of *mammary arteriovenous fistulas* may be caused by either direct injury by needle or by erosion of a wire suture (Silva et al, 1989; Scovotti et al, 1991). It is treated by direct ligation or by selective catheter embolization (Bentivegna and Humphrey, 1989; Frank et al, 1998) or by selective catheter embolization (Sapoval et al, 1993).

Other chronic complications of sternotomy that are occasionally seen are stubborn *seromas* and *incisional hernias* occurring in the subxiphoid portion of the incision. Unsightly *keloids* may require attention of a plastic surgeon.

STERNAL INSTABILITY

The term "unstable" sternum is applied to abnormal mobility of the breastbone related to either fracture, sternocostal separation, or disruption of a suture line reuniting the surgically divided sternum. Trauma to the chest and radical resection of sternal tumors may also create sternal instability. Most such patients that a cardiovascular surgeon sees in daily practice have complications from cardiac surgery.

Biomedical studies that analyze disruption of the sternotomy suture line are scarce and involve primarily comparative analysis of different suture materials (Cheng et al, 1993; McGregor et al, 1999; Otaki et al, 1998). Although their conclusions appear to be valid, their practical value is limited.

The only *cohesive force* acting on the reunited sternum in the postoperative period is the holding power of the sternal sutures. The particulars of this force are the strength, the number, and the location of the sutures as well as their tightness and the applied stress (force/area) exerted. Counterforces leading to sternal disruption include the action of the respiratory muscles and the respiratory volume changes of the thorax.

Logically, given the same number of wires, the tighter the wires and the smaller the area on which they act, the stronger the closure is. Besides the holding force of the wires in the long run, one has to deal with the stress-load and sturdiness of the sternum, because the tauter and narrower the wires are, the more likely they are to cut into the bone. Although this is of little significance at the time of tying, if the wires cut into the sternum after they are tied, the sutures loosen, the sternum halves first moderately separate, and later with the respiratory motion of the chest wall, the loose wires literally saw the sternum into segments. Coughing and sneezing could exacerbate this process.

The strongest force tending to disrupt the sternotomy suture line is that of the pectoralis muscles. Among the respiratory muscles, they are the largest, and, by pulling in exactly the opposite direction to the wire sutures, are the most disruptive at any strength.

The force of inspiratory expansion of the thoracic cage acts in the lateral direction; however, it also has an anteroposterior bending component pivoted at the sternotomy suture line. Mobility of one sternal half in relation to the other in the axial direction may be induced by the rectus abdominis muscles but only if one of them is detached from the sternum and the other is not, an unlikely situation (Fig. 51–2).

The strength and the vectors of these forces on the chest wall of embalmed cadavers were studied by McGregor and colleagues (1999). Upon applying four types of distracting forces within physiologic levels (<400 N) in the lateral, anteroposterior, and rostral-caudal directions as well as by simulated Valsalva force, they found, as expected from clinical observations, that sternum separation occurred as a result of wires cutting into the bone rather than as a result of wire fractures. They confirmed that the least force needed to cause disruption was that which occurred with a vector in the lateral direction (McGregor et al, 1999).

Clinical Consequences of Sternal Instability

Sternal instability that occurs shortly after surgery is called *sternal dehiscence* or *disruption*; in the late postoperative period it is called *nonunion*. The separation of the sternal halves may be *total*, involving the entire sternal suture line, or *partial*, limited to a portion (usually the lower portion) of the sternotomy.

The early sequelae of sternal instability are relatively modest. As the sternal edges are now separated or held slackly together by broken or loose wire sutures, they rub against each other, and there is a feeling of pain as well as of abnormal motion and a click. If nothing is done, the unbroken wires either fracture or eventually cut through the sternum (Fig. 51–3). This process may take several days. If the skin remains intact, there is ample time for intervention, the cornerstone of which is to correct sternal disruption before the skin breaks and the wound potentially becomes infected. Such an event may also be heralded by an increasing amount of serous drainage, usually from the lower edge of the incision.

Sternal disruption *per se* causes neither flail chest nor paradox breathing. The latter occurs only when the

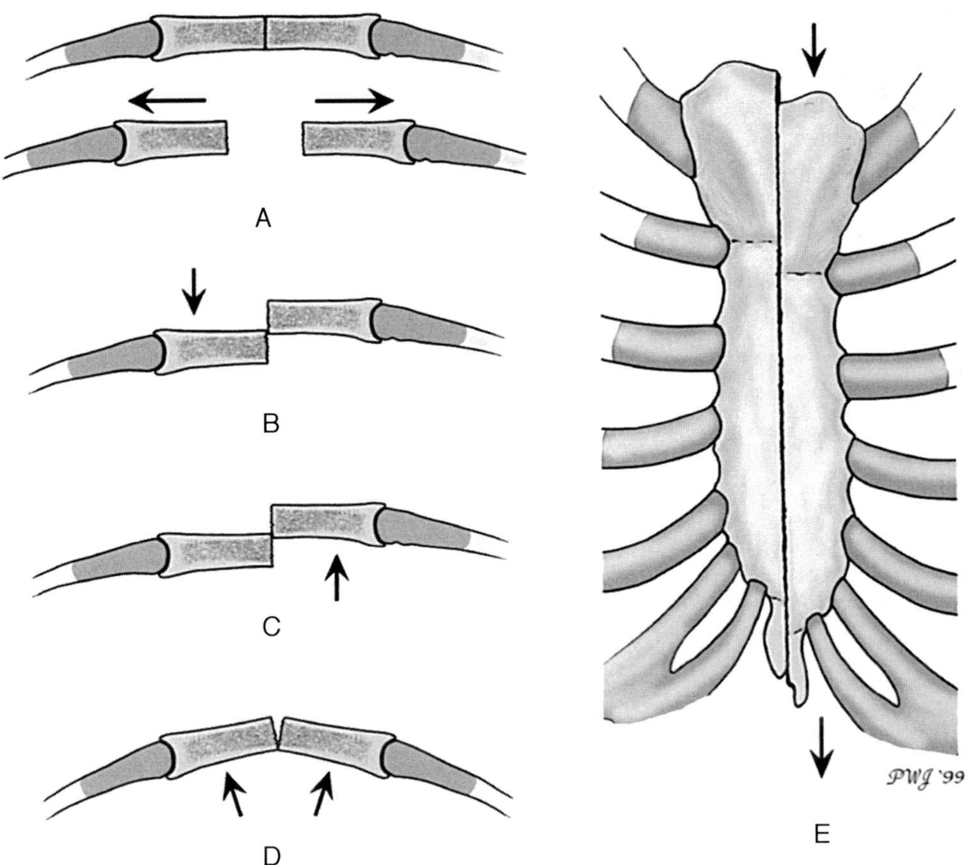

FIGURE 51–2 ■ Disruptive forces acting on the sternotomy. *A*, Lateral pull by the pectoralis muscles; *B* to *D*, Forces that may be generated by Valsalva action; *E*, The rectus abdominis muscle exerting uneven pull.

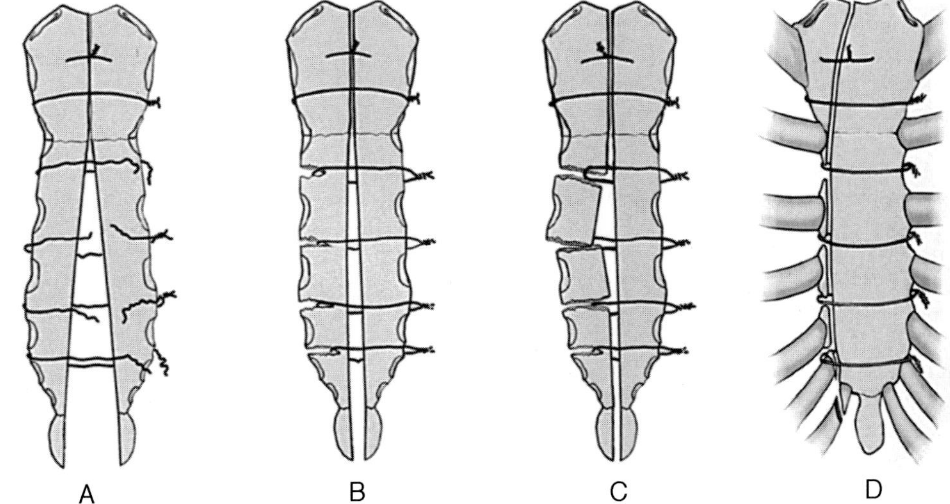

FIGURE 51–3 ■ The different types of sternal disruptions. *A*, Broken wires; *B*, Wires cutting into the bone; *C*, Sternal fragmentation; *D*, Off-side sternotomy.

integrity of the sternocostal cage is interrupted along at least two vertical lines instead of only one, as occurs in the sternotomy. Respiratory embarrassment, however, may still develop because of the vicious cycle of pain, rapid and shallow breathing, and inadequate air exchange.

Sternal nonunion is seen in the late postoperative period and is characterized by chronic discomfort as well as clicking and a feeling of abnormal motion (Hendrickson et al, 1996). It usually involves the lower portion of the sternotomy incision, or less frequently is caused by separation of costal cartilages at the sternocostal junction. Although the consequences are certainly not life threatening, pain associated with the bony surfaces rubbing against each other may be most uncomfortable.

Predisposing Conditions and Prevention

Sternal disruption occurs in 2% to 8% of the patients who undergo cardiac surgery (Opie and Phillips, 1974). *Predisposing conditions* include old age, smoking (Bryan et al, 1992), osteoporosis, obesity, very large breasts, chronic obstructive pulmonary disease (COPD), immunosuppressed state, renal failure, history of radiation, nutritional status, and medications such as prednisone that may hinder osseous healing.

Introaperative events that may increase the likelihood of sternal instability are related to how the sternum is divided and spread as well as the way it is reunited. What the sternum is divided with—that is, Lebsche knife; oscillating, rotating, or reciprocating saws—seems to have little, if any, significance; however, how the sternotomy is done is a salient risk factor for sternal disruption (Culliford et al, 1976; Serry et al, 1980; Shafir et al, 1989). Before the sternum is divided, the midaxial line should be clearly marked by electrocautery, and the sternotomy should be done precisely as guided. Deviation from the midline, especially if the sternum is narrow, as is often the case in women of small stature, may further enfeeble the corresponding sternal half to such a degree that it will not hold sutures (Shafir et al, 1989). Such a faulty technique should be avoided at any cost.

It takes only a peek into the microscope to see the array of ova and insect legs to make any surgeon shudder and reconsider the use of bone wax. Our studies showed not only that the application of wax to the exposed sternal edges fails to reduce blood loss but also that most of the wax rubbed into the bone marrow embolizes into the lungs (Robicsek et al, 1981). It also increases the possibility of infection and probably hinders bone healing. The use of fibrin glue appears to be a much more attractive technique to control bleeding from the divided bone (Watanabe et al, 1997).

Spreading the sternum should be done gently and gradually. Spreaders with one pair of narrow blades may exert undue pressure on the friable bone and cause sternal fragmentation. Their use should be abandoned in favor of instruments with wider blades that distribute the spreading force along most of the sternal length. If retractors with one pair of blades are used, they should be inserted into the lower end of the divided sternum, never into the central part (Cooley DA, personal communication). "Overspreading" of the sternum should be avoided regardless of the type of retractor applied (Fig. 51–4).

When it is time to *close the divided sternum*, most surgeons use interrupted transverse guidewires either passed through the bone by needles, awls, gimlets, or drills or preferably encircling the sternal body (Yokoyama et al, 1988). The sutures most commonly used are different varieties of stainless steel, which are among the strongest and most inert metals and are standards against which other materials used to suture bones are measured.

By definition, stainless steel contains at least 50% iron and 11% chromium. Other elements may be added to impart particular characteristics such as resistance to corrosion to the resulting alloy. If stainless steel is implanted in live tissue and exposed to the strain of excess bending, twisting, and knotting, however, the body can become a hostile environment ready to attack it with a vigor generally reserved for less noble metals. Therefore, proper handling of the wires is important to preserve their integrity in the long run. Care should be taken that knotting occurs only at the point where desired (Brantigan et al, 1979) and that knots are not tied under tension. This may be achieved by asking the assistant to "cross and pull" the untied wire sutures temporarily both above and below the suture to be secured or to hold the sternum halves tight together with large towel clips or different "approximators" while the wires are tied. Studies have also shown that twists are stronger than knots or bends and that commercial devices provide firmer and more reproducible twists than do ordinary pliers (Breyer et al, 1991). The approximator of Timmes and coworkers (1973) not only ensures closeness of the sternal edges but also a tight union of the wire ends.

Besides the material of which it is made, the thickness of the wire is also important (Schultz et al, 1985). In a test of three sizes of stainless steel surgical wires with a noncyclic tensile load, not surprisingly, the load failure level increased with wire diameter and thicker wires held better than thinner ones. Because it is more difficult to make a tight twist with heavier wires and their bulkiness may create wound problems, one must find an acceptable compromise by applying medium-strength (No. 5 to 6) guidewire sutures.

The number of sternal sutures applied and how they are spaced are also of consequence. One should use a minimum of six or seven evenly spaced wires to close the sternum of an adult, probably more for heavyset persons. The axiom that one wire should be placed per 10 kg body weight (Stoney et al, 1978) is a sound one. Suture materials other than steel, such as Tevdek (Deknatel, Falls River, NJ), Ethiflex (Ethicon, Sommerville, NJ), and Mersilene (Ethicon, Sommerville, NJ) (Okies et al, 1974) have also been applied for sternal closure without any evident advantages.

Application of *bands* instead of wires to hold the sternum together is an idea that is certainly mechanically sound. The smaller the surface on which the cohesive force of the taut sutures acts, the more likely it is that they will cut into the bone. Spreading this force through a larger area as occurs with a wider band decreases the applied stress and possible damage to the bone.

The first bands used to close the sternum were made

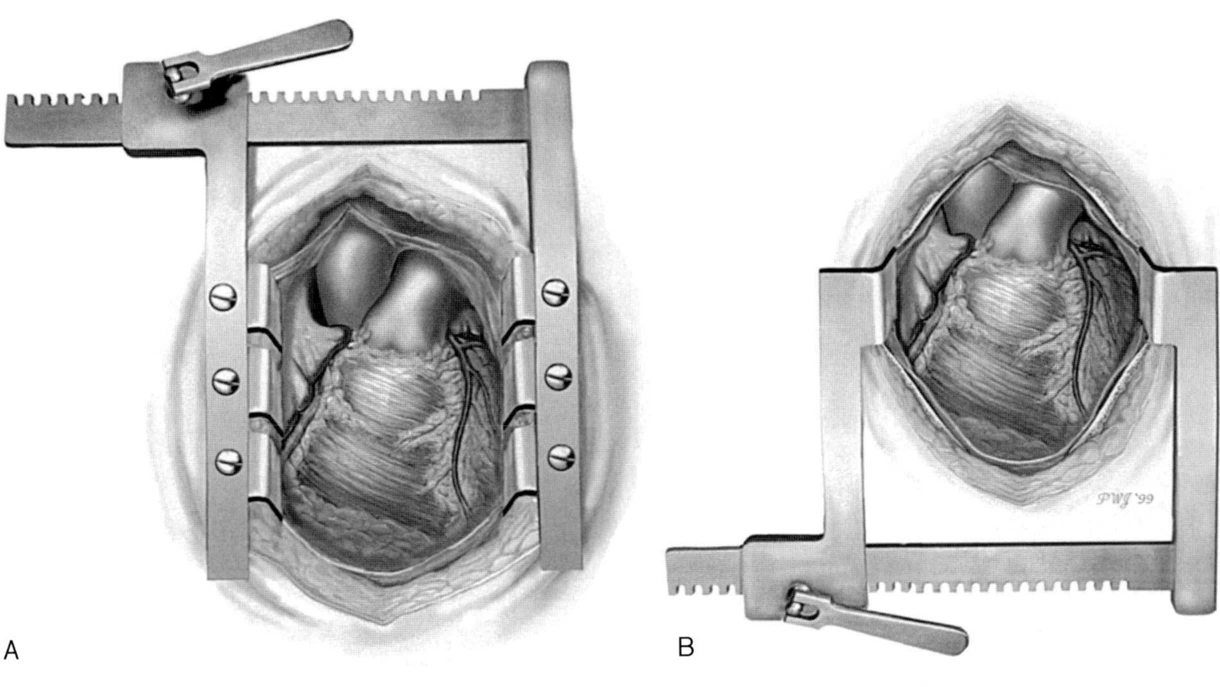

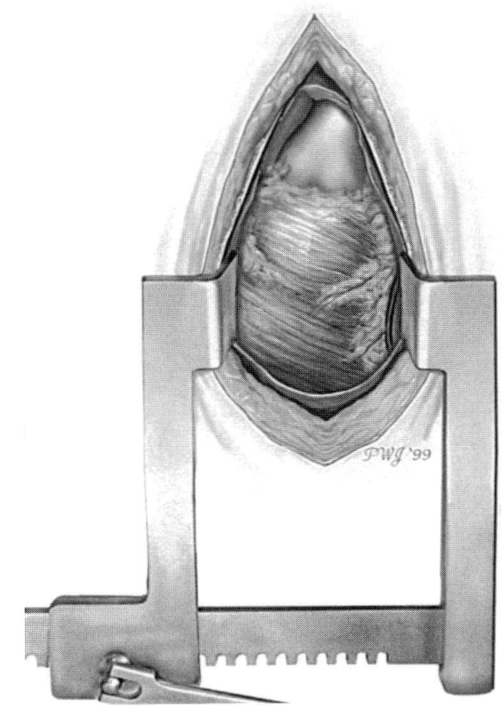

FIGURE 51–4 ■ Application of sternal retractors. *A*, Wide-grip retractor distributes the spreading force over a wide area. *B*, Improperly applied single-pair retractor may break the sternum if applied in the midriff of the sternum. *C*, Placement in the lower third prevents damage.

of nylon (DuPont Chemical Corp., Wilmington, DE) (Leveen and Piccone, 1968) and were associated with a large number of complications consisting of infection, dehiscence, draining sinuses, and chronic pain (Sanfelippo and Danielson, 1972). Bands of Mersilene (Ethicon, Sommerville, NJ) or metal (Badellino et al, 1988) fared better, but because of the difficulty in handling them and their higher cost they did not achieve wider acceptance.

Another idea that did not become popular was replacing metal sutures with *absorbable materials* such as polyglycolic and polydioxanone sutures (Greve et al, 1986; Kreitman et al, 1992). The aim was to eliminate the continued presence of palpable and painful knots that are sometimes observed in thin individuals, especially pediatric patients. Because of data indicating that, at least in some cases, sternal healing is delayed and the sole force holding the sternal halves together is the stainless steel wire, absorbable materials are not recommended for sternal closure. A number of publications have also advocated more complex methods of approximation, such as *plates*, *screws*, and other *orthopedic paraphernalia* for routine sternal closure (Brown et al, 1996; Hendrickson et al, 1996). None of these techniques has shown any statistically significant benefits over properly applied simple wire sutures (Ozaki et al, 1998).

A common technical shortcoming in closing the divided sternum is *misalignment of the sternal halves*. In a study of patients by sternal scanning in the early postoperative period, good alignment as well as proper contact of the sternal layers was an exception rather than the rule. Dislocation of the sternum in the anteroposterior or the longitudinal dimension was common, as was sternal spacing. In only 15% was the sternal approximation judged "perfect" when wires were used and in none when the sternum was united with bands (Vanleeuw et al, 1991).

Although closing the sternum with multiple individual wire sutures is a safe and effective procedure, in a group of patients, especially those who have a friable sternum, are overweight, or have severe COPD, it is often not enough to ensure a good and permanent union. In such patients it is wise to go one step further and use special measures of prevention. Because studies of embalmed cadavers (McGregor et al, 1999) and clinical experience suggest that in most cases the wire suture would cut through the bone before breaking or unwinding because of increased stress, it is logical to direct our efforts toward making the sternum nonpenetrable rather than inventing a new suture material. This can best be done by "parasternal weaving," a technique we found most effective in both the prophylaxis and the repair of sternal disruption (Robicsek, 1976; Robicsek et al, 1977). It also is wise to place *retention sutures* in obese people, especially women with pendulous breasts (Copeland et al, 1994). In extreme cases, there may be such significant tension on the soft tissues and skin that sternal closure (preferably weaving) may be combined with bilateral breast reduction (De Fontaine et al, 1996).

Postoperatively, our ability to prevent disruption is limited. We should try to decrease the strain of coughing and sneezing, treat dyspnea, or in special cases maintain the patient with assisted respiration. Hugging a pillow or other soft object (teddy bear preferred) while coughing may be of benefit, but we discourage wearing special halters as they may interfere with deep respiratory movements. Especially in heavier patients, crossing the arms in a "self-hugging" posture while being turned or moved may take the stress off the sternal suture line.

REPAIR OF STERNAL DEHISCENCE

Instability of the sternum is self-perpetuating, and even if sternal separation is moderate, more often than not the loose wires either break or work themselves through the bone. Fluid accumulates, the skin dehisces, and a situation that initially could have been handled easily ends in a surgical disaster. Therefore, if, in the early postoperative period, abnormal mobility of the sternum is detected, it should be addressed surgically in a most expeditious fashion.

Even if there are no clinical signs of infection, all cases of sternal disruption after the first 3 to 4 postoperative days should be regarded as potentially contaminated. To determine whether infection indeed exists, one should consider whether the patient has a septic course, there is drainage of pus or serum that yields a positive bacterial culture, or the wound appears to be grossly infected.

If the answer to any of these questions is affirmative, the reader is referred to Postoperative Sternomediastinitis later in this chapter. Even if none of these conditions is present, however, a Gram stain should be obtained in the operating room, and only if it shows no bacteria can the wound be tentatively regarded as "noninfected." Cultures and sensitivity swabs should still be obtained and the results considered in further planning.

There are cases in which the wound is reopened and the wires are found to be broken, but the disrupted sternum is without visible damage. In such a situation, instead of simply rewiring the sternum, the surgeon should first consider why the wires broke or came untied. Unless there has been an obvious technical fault in the closure, reuniting the sternum as before may not be sufficient to prevent re-disruption. Instead of reinserting the same sutures at the same places and tying them in the same way, a more extended procedure should be performed to minimize the possibility of a second episode of disruption. The safest and easiest way to accomplish this is to buttress the sternal edges with wire weave; thus, instead of tying wire over bone, the surgeon is wrapping wire over wire. Since we presented this technique more than 20 years ago (Robicsek et al, 1977), it has been used successfully in thousands of patients.

Parasternal Weaving

In the course of this procedure, which we termed *parasternal weaving*, continuous returning No. 6 guidewire suture lines are placed parallel to and on both sides of the sternum. Each suture begins at the level of the second lowest chondrosternal junction and is passed alternatingly anterior and posterior to the costal cartilages up to the level of the second costosternal junction. The suture is then reversed and led caudally, posterior to where it had been anterior and vice versa, and then tied. After both sides of the sternum have been so reinforced, seven or eight interrupted transverse sutures encircling the sternum are placed in the usual manner and tied taut (Figs. 51–5 and 51–6). Attention is given to placing these sutures lateral to the weaving-suture line and avoiding injury to the mammary vessels.

A special problem exists when the line of sternotomy is off center but a narrow strip of bone is left on one side or, in extreme cases, the costal cartilages are completely sheared off. In such cases, on the respective side, we direct the initial part of the weaving suture cranially not around but through the costal cartilages and then do the weaving in the caudal direction as well as on the contralateral side as described before (Fig. 51–7).

Pectoralis Muscle Advancement

In connection with parasternal weaving, we also recommend routine application of *pectoralis muscle advancement*, a technique also referred to as "presternal padding," which consists of bilaterally detaching the sternal insertion of the pectoralis major muscles and suturing them together presternally (Robicsek and Hamilton, 1989). In the course of the procedure, the muscles are separated from the sternal edges by electrocautery and then, using blunt rather than sharp technique, dissected from the rib cage bilaterally not more than a length of 4 to 6 cm, just enough to allow tension-free presternal approximation. The muscle should not be separated from the subcutaneous layers. If the mammary artery has been used for grafting, the muscle detachment on that side should be sparing. The sutures uniting the muscles should be strategically placed to bury the knots (Fig. 51–8).

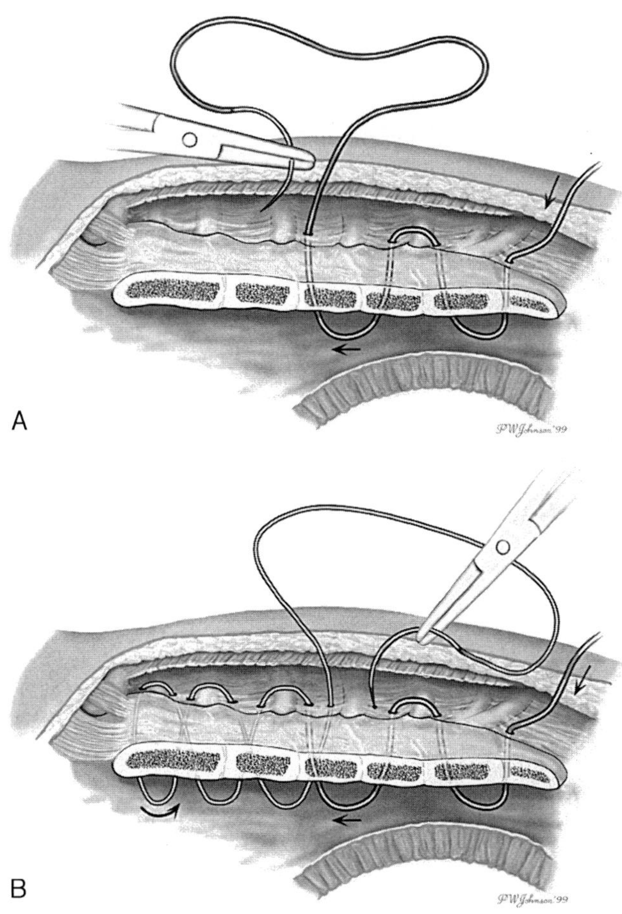

FIGURE 51–5 ■ Parasternal weaving I. *A*, The suture begins at the level of the second lowest sternochondral junction and is passed anterior–posterior up to the level of the second costosternal junction. *B*, The suture is then reversed and led caudally, posterior to where it had been anterior and vice versa, then tied.

This simple maneuver, which we used previously in cases of repair of pectus deformities (Robicsek et al, 1968), takes a few minutes to perform and yields important benefits. First, recall that the main disrupting force on the sternotomy suture line is the diverse pull of the two pectoralis muscles. By detaching the muscles of the sternum, one may not only neutralize this force but also, by suturing the two muscles together, reverses the direction and convert them from a disruptive force into a cohesive one.

The second, probably even more important advantage of pectoralis muscle advancement is that it covers the sternotomy incision with well-vascularized muscle tissue. This is beneficial for both healing and prevention or elimination of infection and in thin invidivuals with scarce subcutaneous tissues puts a nice pad of muscle between the sternotomy and the skin. It not only removes the sternotomy suture line from the immediate vicinity of the potentially colonized area of the skin but also covers otherwise palpable wire sutures. This padding of the sternotomy incision by the pectoralis muscles could be used as an adjunct to routine sternotomy closure as well as parasternal weaving (Robicsek and Hamilton, 1989).

Weaving may also be applied in the repair of *partial sternal nonunions*. In such cases, the manubrium is usually healed and holds steadfast but the sutures intended to hold the body of the sternum are broken, and the sternum is spaced in the form of an upturned letter Y (⅄). Instead of pulling together the separated halves under tension or reopening the previous sternotomy in its entire length, the surgeon should mobilize the right half of the separated lower sternum by cutting through it in a transverse fashion at the highest level of the separation. This allows easy approximation of the two halves, which can now be united by three or four circular transverse wire sutures buttressed over parasternal weaving (Robicsek et al, 1998) (Fig. 51–9).

Besides weaving, other *methods of buttressing* have also been recommended using wires (Chlosta and Elefteriades, 1995), intrasternal clips, and different orthopedic devices, especially Kirschner wires. We found most of these techniques to be inferior to weaving, and some of them are also dangerous because of the possibility of the device dislodging and entering vital organs such as the heart, lung, or aorta (Liu et al, 1992). There are also reports of limited individual experiences in which metal plates, bone, autografts (Geiger et al, 1996), and homografts (Chiu et al, 1997) were used to stabilize the disrupted sternum.

After sternal repair, the old broken sternal wires should be removed if feasible because they might migrate into vital structures.

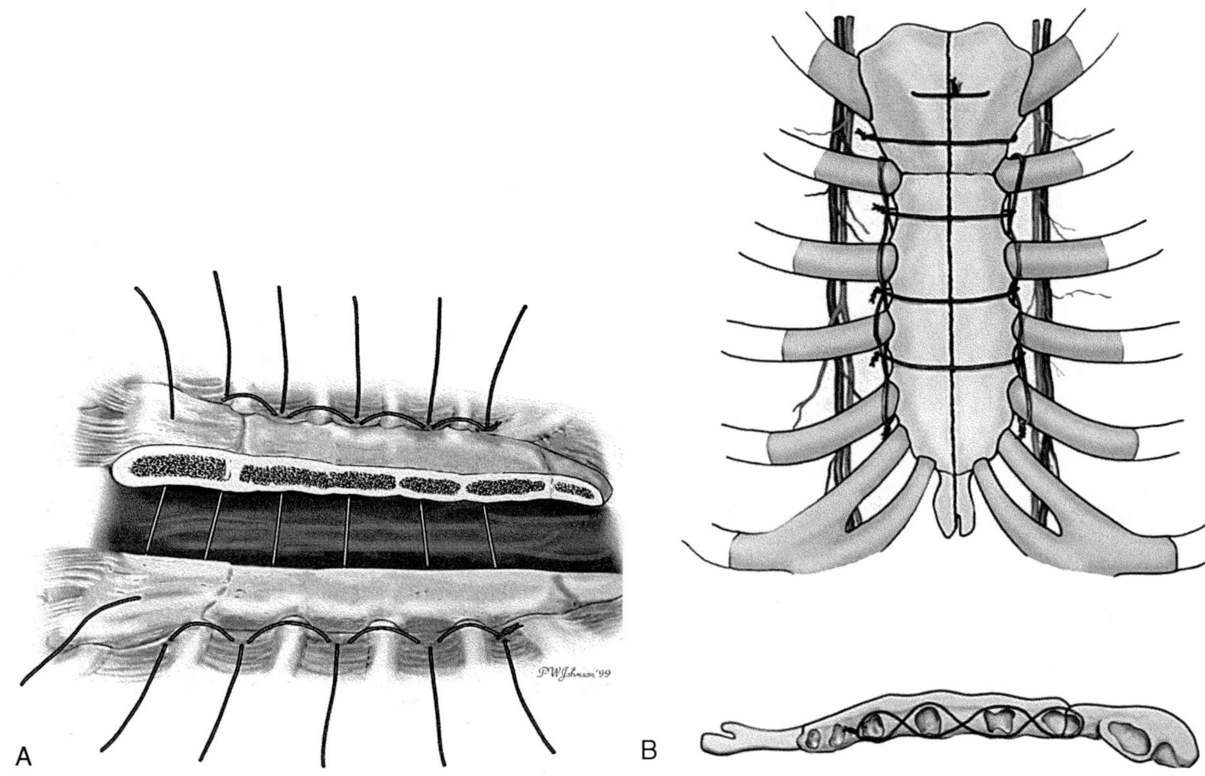

FIGURE 51–6 ■ Parasternal weaving II. *A*, After the weaving is completed, transverse, encircling sutures are placed lateral to the weave, then tied *(B)*.

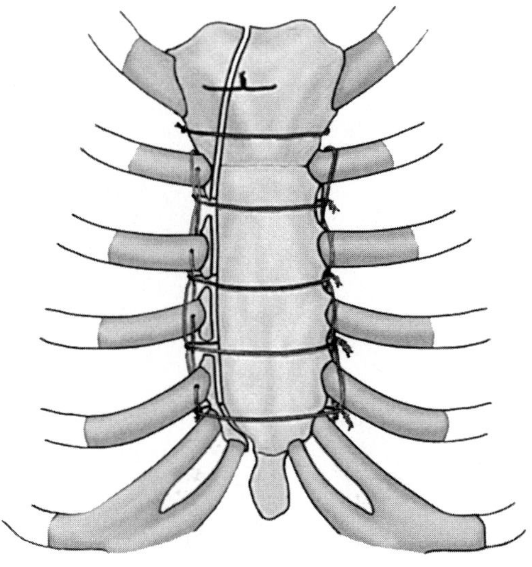

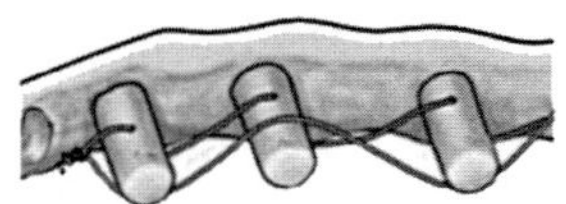

FIGURE 51–7 ■ If the line of sternotomy is far off center, the initial part of the weaving suture is directed, not around, but through the costal cartilages; at the contralateral side, it is done as described in Figures 51–5 and 51–6.

A special problem in sternal reconstruction is the patient with severe *pectus excavatum* who is in need of heart surgery. We recommend that in such situations simultaneous repair of the cardiac as well as the sternal defect is performed by using transverse instead of axial sternotomy; bilateral resection; and retrosternal application of a Marlex mesh "hammock" (Robicsek, 1988, 1989, 1998).

INFECTIOUS COMPLICATIONS OF THE STERNOTOMY

Superficial wound infections may be treated by removing a few skin sutures, dressing changes, and administering appropriate antibiotics. More extensive involvement may require reopening part of the entire wound, packing with moist gauze, and then allowing spontaneous healing by granulation. Continued fever, malaise, and elevated white cell count after initial wound care suggest deeper penetration, as do abnormal mobility of the sternum, pericardial drainage through the sternotomy incision, a "sucking" wound or appearance of bubbles in the incision. Such events require special and immediate measures.

Postoperative Sternomediastinitis

The anterior mediastinum is a unique area that thwarts standard surgical approaches to treating infections (Colen et al, 1989). It has a tendency to form blind pockets. The blood supply is poor. Suture lines, prosthetic materials, tissue fragments, or parts of devascularized bone add other dimensions to the problem.

Sternomediastinitis, which now occurs in about 0.75% to 1.40% of all cardiac operations, most often arises in the early postoperative period, usually within a week or two, and is associated with morbidity and mortality rates that range from 7% to 45% (Sanfelippo, and Danielson, 1972). It is often accompanied by incisional erythema, wound drainage, spiking high temperatures, and leukocytosis. Pathogens commonly encountered are *Staphylococcus aureus* and gram-negative bacteria such as *Escherichia coli*. *Pseudomonas*, *Enterococcus*, *Enterobacter*, and *Staphylococcus epidermidis* are also often seen. If the sternum is not disrupted initially, it soon will be, because the infected bone will not hold the wire sutures and the closure will dehisce. For this reason, patients with sternomediastinitis should be treated for sternal instability as well.

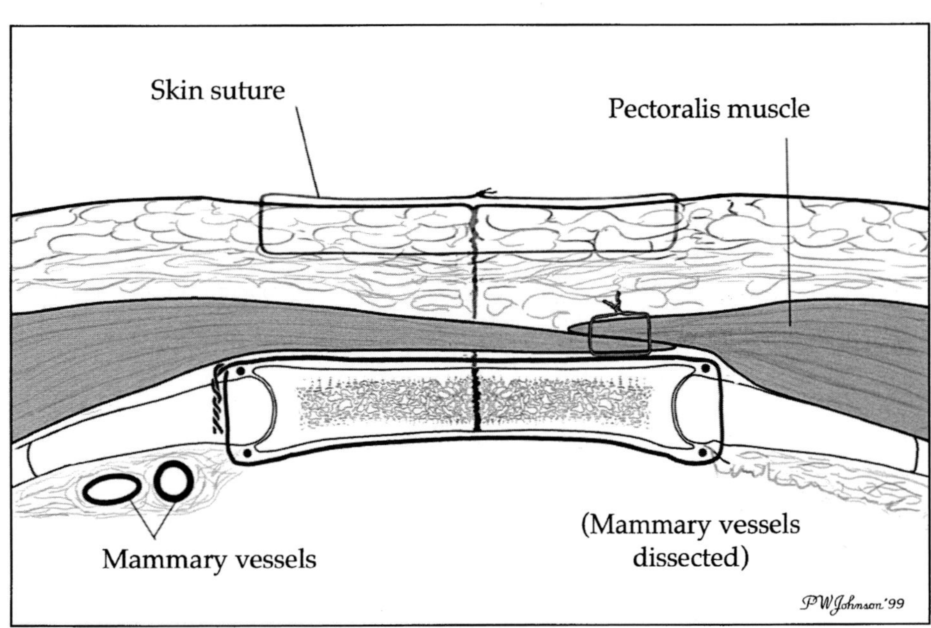

FIGURE 51–8 ■ Cross-sectional view of presternal suturing of the advanced pectoralis major muscles. Note that the advancement is more sparing on the side where the mammary vessels have been dissected.

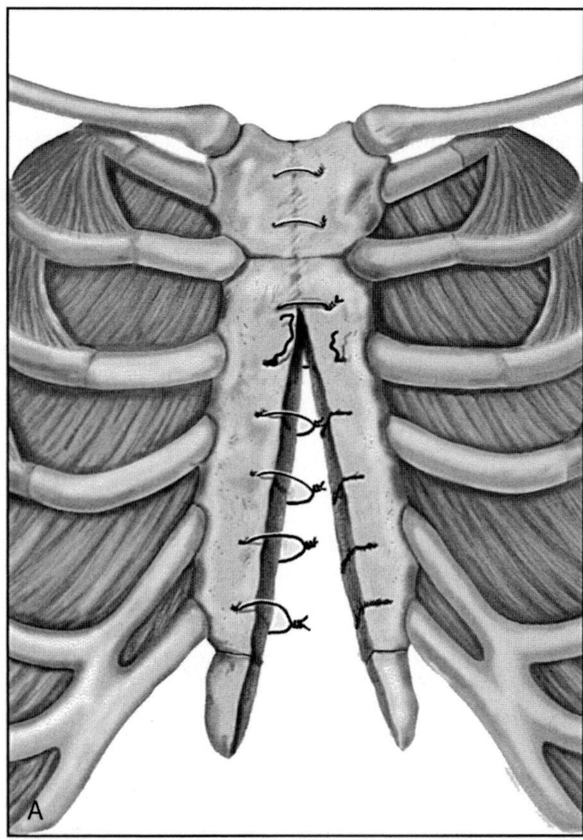

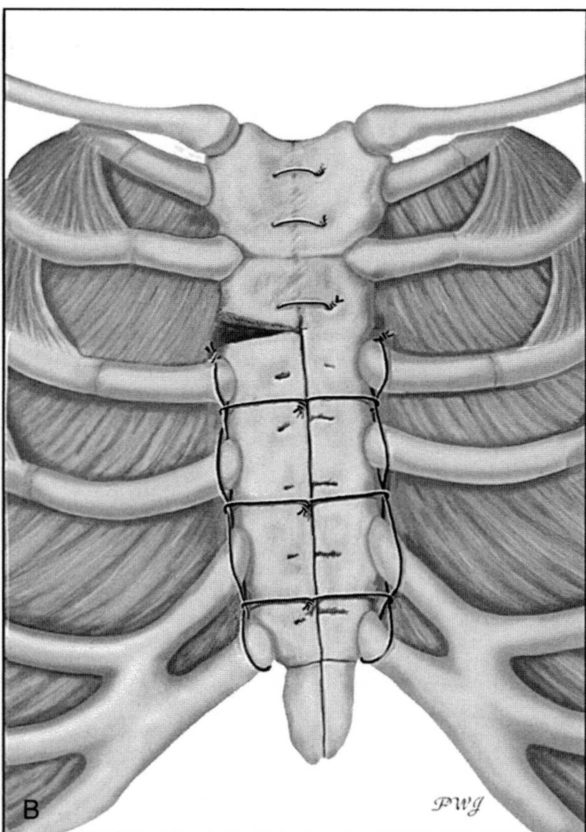

FIGURE 51–9 ■ Chronic partial sternal separation, *A*. Repair is accomplished by mobilizing the right half of the sternum by cutting through it in a transverse fashion at the highest level of separation. This will allow easy approximation and suture over parasternal weaving *(B)*.

Predisposing Conditions and Prevention

The importance of *meticulous sterile technique* cannot be emphasized enough. The environment should be kept painstakingly clean, and infection control measures should be kept up to date. The patient's preoperative stay should be short. Preparation for surgery should include showering with chlorhexidine. Body hair should be removed with a clipper or depilatory cream rather than with a razor. Because of the complex nature of open heart operations, there are multiple possibilities for breaks in sterile technique and contamination of the operative field. These occurrences need to be eliminated. By tightening the rules of operating room asepsis, the infection rate may be reduced from 7.5% to 0.8% (Bryan et al, 1992; DeGeest et al, 1996).

Prophylactic antibiotics are routinely applied in cardiac surgery; however, their value has not been fully proved scientifically. Cefazolin, cefamandole, ceforanide, and ceftriaxone have all proved efficacious (Beam, 1987). The ideal agent, the dosage, and the length of administration, however, have yet to be defined. In the selection of antibiotics, individual institutions should consider the pathogens that most commonly cause infections in their own environment.

Factors predisposing to sternomediastinitis grouped according to time period are as follows.

Preoperatively, one should try to eliminate infections at other sites, improve diminished left ventricular function, and treat alcoholism, renal failure, and diabetes. Operative urgency should also be considered.

In relation to *surgical planning and technique*, atraumatic management of the sternotomy wound and discriminate use of electrocautery are important in preventing infections. Also of significance are the length of cardiopulmonary bypass and the duration of the operation (Blanchard et al, 1995). The proven survival benefits of grafting a single *mammary artery* led to an increase in the use of both mammary arteries in an attempt to avoid late graft closure and improve event-free survival. The observation that there is an appreciable decrease of blood flow to the sternum after dissection of the mammary artery, especially if done bilaterally, raises concern, however (Carrier et al, 1992; Seyfer et al, 1988). If the mammary artery is harvested by skeletonization, the ischemia of the sternum is significantly less than if it is dissected wide and more extensively as a pedicle (Parish et al, 1992).

The degree to which the application of the mammary arteries as bypass grafts may influence the chances of sternotomy disruption or sternal infection is a subject of controversy. Studies in the late 1980s suggested that bilateral mammary artery grafting is indeed a risk factor in patients with diabetes, especially those who are overweight (Cosgrove et al, 1988). Later studies on the same subject gave variable results. However, it is reasonable to avoid bilateral mammary artery grafting in patients with diabetes and in morbidly obese patients, especially if there is a combination of both. Clinical data also suggest that for patients who are older than 75 years and have impaired respiratory function or require emergent revascularization, bilateral mammary artery grafting should not be done so that sternal complications may be kept to a minimum (Uva et al, 1998).

Efforts to bring live vascularized tissue close to the reunited sternotomy are reasonable. For this purpose, shifting the fat pedicle of the mediastinum to the back side of the sternotomy suture line has been proposed (Kerjiwal and Paterson, 1997; Wehrens et al, 1996). As stated before, a simple and certainly more effective measure is to advance the pectoralis muscles and unite them in the front of the sternal suture line (Robicsek and Hamilton, 1989). During the course of surgery, the exposed edges of the sternum should be protected with moist pads or with laps soaked in povidone-iodine.

Postoperative risk factors include reoperation for bleeding, concomitant infections, cardiopulmonary resuscitation (Wehrens et al, 1996), and mechanical ventilation for more than 2 days (Blanchard et al, 1995). An important event is sternal instability itself. Instability begets infection; thus, all conditions listed as risk factors for sternal instability are risk factors for sternal infection as well.

Diagnosis of Sternomediastinitis

Cardiothoracic surgeons traditionally rely on physical examination of the wound and on appropriate conventional laboratory and radiographic studies to establish the presence and to judge the extent of sternotomy infections. To these methods computed tomography, radiolabeled imaging of white cells, and thermography have been added.

Computed tomography can be used both for the diagnosis and the follow-up of surgical treatment of sternomediastinitis (Maddern et al, 1993). It may demonstrate fluid accumulation and different pathologies of the soft tissue, but the presumption that computed tomography would be the "gold standard" for diagnosing poststernotomy sternal wound infections has not been validated. It is occasionally useful and has a good overall sensitivity of 93% and a lower specificity of 90% (Gur et al, 1998).

Radiolabeled white blood cell imaging is a complementary physiologic approach to the identification and localization of the infections and other inflammatory processes. Leukocytes tagged with radioactive substances such as indium-111 yield a sensitivity, specificity, and accuracy of 86%, 97%, and 95%, respectively (Oates and Payne, 1994). Another "high-technology" method of diagnosing sternal wound infection is the application of ^{99m}Tc-labeled *monoclonal granulocyte antibody scintigraphy.* Proponents of this method claim nearly 100% accuracy of the diagnosis and that it can show the extent of sternal wound infections.

In cases of low-grade, smoldering mediastinal infections in which signs of infection are vague or absent, *thermography* can be extremely useful. In a large prospective series, we found that thermographic demonstration of temperature rise at the sternotomy site more than 2 weeks after surgery yielded 100% sensitivity and specificity in differentiating infections from postpericardiotomy syndrome–like situations (Fig. 51–10). The method also proved to be useful in monitoring the efficiency of both surgical treatment and antibiotic therapy in already diagnosed infections (Robicsek et al, 1984).

The most important confirmation of the diagnosis is *microbiologic proof* of bacterial seeding. In all patients with continued temperature elevation in whom obvious sources cannot be identified, the sternal wound should be aspirated. One may be surprised how often gross pus or infected fluid may be found in wounds that appear to be healing normally (Colen et al, 1989). If simple aspirations fail, a computed tomography–directed retrosternal tap may be attempted. In an effort to obtain microbiologic proof, we found cultures of epicardial pacing wires rewarding. Whenever the pacer wires are removed from a patient who is suspected of having or considered to be at higher than usual risk for mediastinal infection, tips of the wires should be cultured. This easy test may not only confirm the diagnosis of infection but also facilitate early and specific antimicrobial therapy (Hastings and Robicsek, 1993). In a comparison of the value of computed tomography, indium-111, leukocyte scanning, and epicardial pacer wire cultures, the last proved to be the most reliable (Browdie et al, 1991).

Surgical Management of Sternomediastinitis

Several aspects of postoperative sternomediastinitis still remain controversial (Molina, 1993); however, there is agreement that the goals for the surgical management of sternomediastinitis are twofold: (1) to bring the infectious process under control in the shortest possible time, and (2) to ensure sternal stability and provide the best possible cosmetic results.

Historically, cardiac surgeons first tried to handle sternomediastinitis with the *open technique* as the definite method. This involved reopening the sternum, packing, and waiting for spontaneous closure by granulation, which usually required 40 to 60 days. Because of the associated high mortality, this open method was largely replaced in the early 1970s with initial drainage followed by *primary closure of the sternum and irrigation* (Culliford et al, 1976; Molina, 1993), applying fenestrated drainage and infusion catheters (Bryan et al, 1992), and use of antibiotic or antiseptic solutions (Thiel and Bircks, 1990) with either passive drainage or suction (Fig. 51–11).

The advantage of the closed technique over the open method was that it discouraged additional bacterial colonization and did not interfere much with respiratory function. The mortality rate with the application of the closed method improved but still remained high (12.5%) (Klutsal et al, 1991). Its shortcomings, such as creation of potential dead spaces, the possibility of catheter erosion into vital organs, and the chance of systemic absorption of irrigation fluids (Cohen et al, 1997), made surgeons look for alternative treatment methods.

The modern treatment of postoperative sternomediastinitis is based on *Pairolero's categorization* (Pairolero et al, 1991).

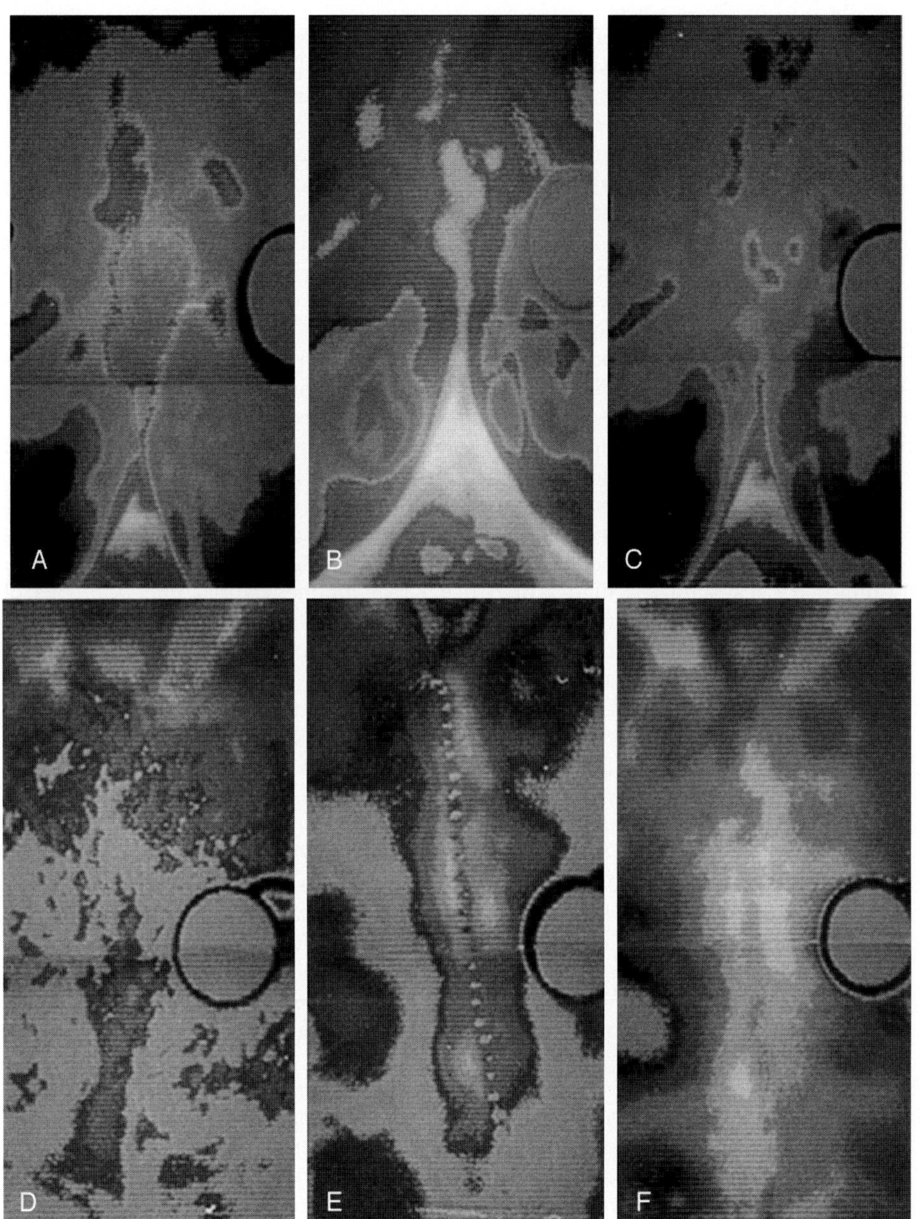

FIGURE 51–10 ■ Thermographic picture of a normally healing *(A, B, C)* and an infected *(D, E, F)* sternotomy. *A*, Preoperative thermography shows a "cool" chest. *B*, One week after surgery, the incision is "warm" owing to the healing process. *C*, Two weeks after surgery, the normally healing incision is "cool" again. The skin of the patient with sternomediastinitis remains "hot." Also note the continual increase in temperature if the sternotomy is infected *(F)*.

Type I sternomediastinitis refers to serosanguineous drainage within a few days after sternotomy; pus, osteomyelitis, and chondritis are notably absent. Mediastinal tissues are still soft and pliable. Bacterial cultures are initially negative or yield staphylococci. In such cases the sternotomy should be reopened, all "blind pockets" eliminated, and the mediastinum irrigated. This type of infection is then best managed by reinsertion of drainage tubes, reclosure of the sternum over parasternal weaving, and aggressive antibiotic treatment.

Type II sternomediastinitis is a fulminant mediastinitis that occurs 1 to 3 weeks after surgery. Besides reopening drainage and irrigation, these patients also require débridement of necrotic soft tissue, bone, and cartilage. This may be done when the wound is reopened, but it should be delayed if the patient is septic or his or her general condition is critical for other reasons. An effort should be made to remove all foreign material such as felt pledgets or pacer wires. Exposed suture lines should be reinforced with autogenous tissue, such as fascia lata, or covered with muscle flaps. The wound is then kept open and treated with daily dressing change, irrigation with normal saline, and antibiotic or povidone-iodine solution. After the drainage ceases and septicemia subsides, the sternotomy wound is closed using omental or muscle flaps covered with subcutaneous tissue and skin.

Type III sternomediastinitis occurs a month to a year after surgery. The patient typically has chronic draining sinus tracts that lead to the infected sternum, cartilages, or retained foreign bodies. Repair requires wide exposure, extensive débridement, often total sternectomy, and flap coverage using autogenous tissues.

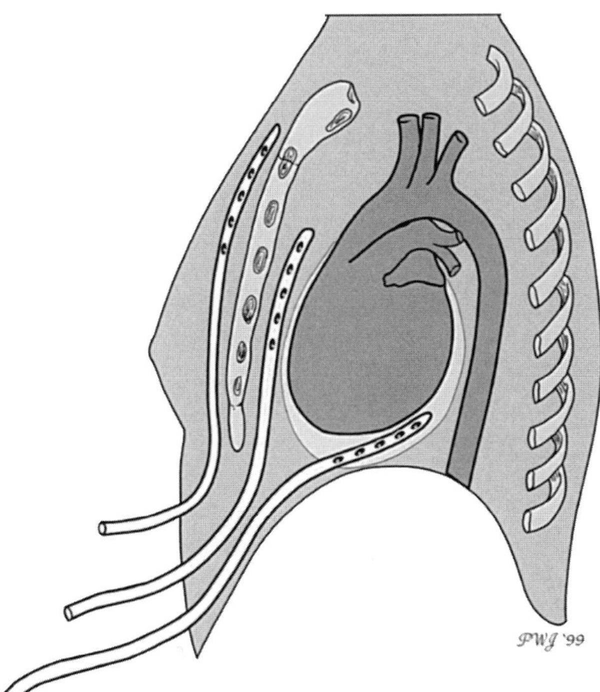

FIGURE 51–11 ■ The position of irrigation and drainage catheters during "closed" treatment of sternomediastinitis (Blanchard et al, 1995).

Autogenous tissues most commonly used in mediastinal reconstruction are omentum and muscle flaps, both of which are eminently suitable to cover surfaces and fill up space with living, well-vascularized tissue.

The omentum has a long and distinguished history in sepsis control in cardiovascular surgery and was first recommended as a mediastinal flap by Lee and colleagues (1976) (Fig. 51–12). Transfer of omental pedicles with or without muscle flaps is the technique preferred by many surgeons, especially when synthetic or homograft material is exposed.

Muscle flaps were first used by Jurkiewicz and coworkers (1980) to obliterate potentially infected hollows of the mediastinum and to cover the damaged sternum. This method, which was perfected by Pairolero and associates (1991), combined with adequate débridement of the anterior chest wall, irrigation, appropriate antibiotics, and good supportive care, improved the clinical results significantly and at the same time decreased the length and cost of hospitalization.

The pectoralis major is the preferred muscle for creating mediastinal flaps because of its excellent blood supply from the thoracoacromial vessels and its length, which easily covers the upper two thirds of the sternum (Fig. 51–13). It can be applied as a single flap, or, if necessary, both pectoralis muscles can be used. To cover more extensive resections, pectoralis flaps may be combined with the rectus abdominis. The latissimus dorsi is usually used as a myocutaneous flap to ensure tension-free skin closure (Banic et al, 1995) (Fig. 51–14). The sternocleidomastoid may occasionally be applied to fill gaps in the upper mediastinum. An interesting proposition is the so-called bipedicle flap (Montandon, 1991; Solomon and Granick, 1998) (Fig. 51–15), which consists of the superiorly based pectoralis muscle left in continuity with the inferiorly based rectus abdominis. In cases of very large, pendulous breasts, the application of muscle flaps may have to be combined with reduction mammoplasty (De Fontaine et al, 1996). Repeated débridements and revision of flaps are often necessary (Pairolero et al, 1991). In cases of larger skin defects, the muscle flaps may be covered with split-thickness skin or the problem may be addressed by creating myocutaneous "island" flaps (Neale et al, 1981).

Twenty years ago, the management of sternomediastinitis was associated with a mortality approaching 50% in some series (Jones et al, 1997). When the management was changed to a few days of open treatment followed by radical sternal débridement and closure with omentum or muscle flaps, the mortality dropped to less than 10% (Grossi et al, 1991; Jones et al, 1997). This method, however, is not without potential problems.

A definite drawback of sternal débridement and flap repair is that about half of the patients note discomfort above the levels that one may expect long after a routine sternotomy. This discomfort is probably due to intercostal nerve irritation. Interestingly, the extent of sternal resection does not necessarily correlate with the patients' complaints (Ringelman et al, 1994). One may also wonder how successful muscle flaps are in providing long-term stable wound closure. Half of these patients continue to experience abnormal sternal motion, usually manifested as a clicking or rubbing sensation on coughing or sneezing (Ringelman et al, 1994). The shoulder girdle muscles seem not to be affected (Colen et al, 1989), but abdominal wall muscle function has been shown to be decreased (Nahai et al, 1989). In addition, when omentum or rectus abdominis flaps were used, there was a significant incidence of hernias and bulges of the abdominal wall (Lejour and Dome, 1991). The latter could be prevented using different synthetic materials; unfortunately, these cannot be applied to a contaminated environment. A disadvantage of omental flaps is the potential for herniation of parts of the gastrointestinal system, especially the colon, into the mediastinum (Boiskin et al, 1995).

Concern has also been raised regarding possible deterioration of respiratory function, which in most of these patients has already been compromised before surgery. In the study of Kohman and coworkers (1990), postoperative pulmonary function tests were found to be unchanged compared with preoperative tests, and only patients who were dyspneic before cardiac surgery because of a pre-existing medical condition were short-winded after flap repair. Others found that muscle flap repair resulted in only mild restrictive impairment of lung function and the results favored a pectoralis major as compared with a rectus abdominis muscle flap.

Leaving the sternum flap covered, but not united, does not create flail chest per se, but the potential for remote complications exists. There are reports of severe respiratory failure resulting in flail chest in a patient with a non-united sternum who later suffered simple acute rib fracture (Adams et al, 1987).

Another late complication of treated sternotomy infections is localized septic costochronditis and osteomyelitis with sinus tract formation, which occurred in about 25%

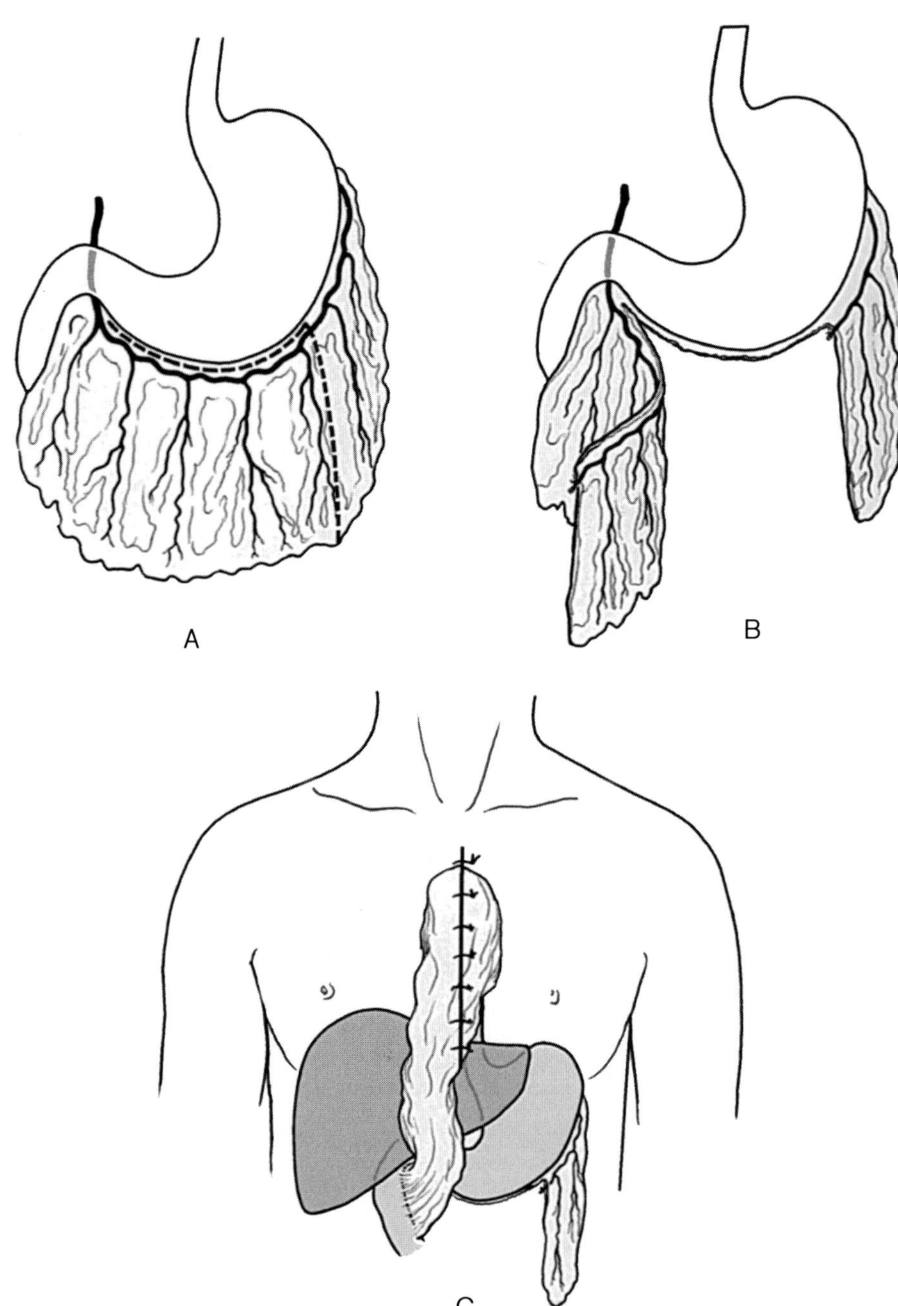

FIGURE 51–12 ■ *A–C*, Creation of a retrosternal omental flap. (Modified from Maddern IR, Goodman LR, Almassi GH et al: CT after reconstructive repair of the sternum and chest wall. Radiology 50:1019–1023, 1993.)

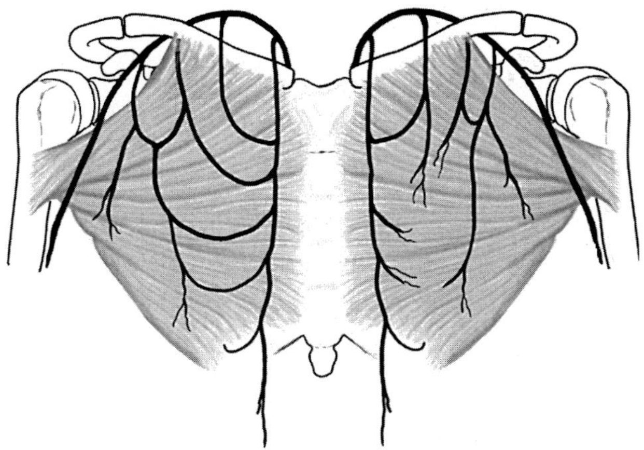

FIGURE 51–13 ■ The blood supply to the pectoralis major muscles.

of patients (Pairolero et al, 1991). When the sinus tract is explored, all infected or necrotic bone and soft tissue must be removed. If the sinus tract leads into the mediastinum, there is usually retained foreign material, which also should be extricated. After débridement, the wound should be left open and a delayed closure should be performed, usually with muscle flaps with preference for the pectoralis muscles (Pairolero et al, 1991).

Late mycotic pseudoaneurysm formation from suture lines of the heart and aorta is rare, but it does occur and may cause severe, sometimes exsanguinating hemorrhage (O'Connell et al, 1995).

The effect of sternomediastinitis on the patency of aortocoronary grafts has not been completely clarified; however, generally mediastinal infections do not adversely affect aortocoronary graft vein patency (Macmanus and Okies, 1976).

THE HANUMAN SYNDROME

Closure of the sternotomy incision may be delayed for hemodynamic reasons, for packing of otherwise uncontrollable coagulopathy, or to accommodate temporary cardiac assist devices. Most commonly, the mediastinum is kept open for drainage, irrigation, and delayed débridement as part of the management of florid sternomediastinitis. In such cases, the sternotomy either is left open or needs to be reopened later.

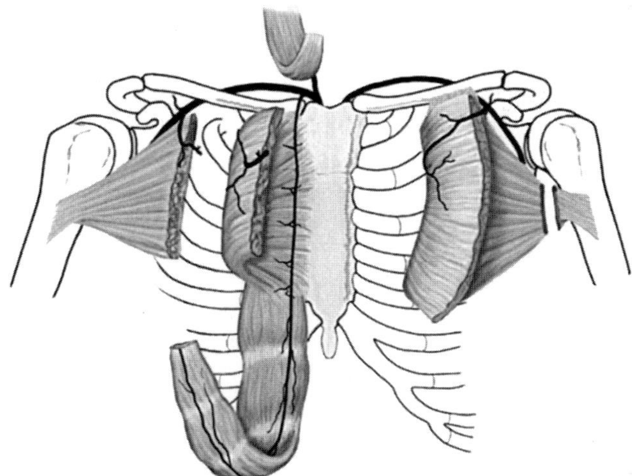

FIGURE 51–14 ■ Creation of pectoralis and rectus abdominis muscle flaps. (Modified from Maddern IR, Goodman LR, Almassi GH et al: CT after reconstructive repair of the sternum and chest wall. Radiology 50:1019–1023, 1993.)

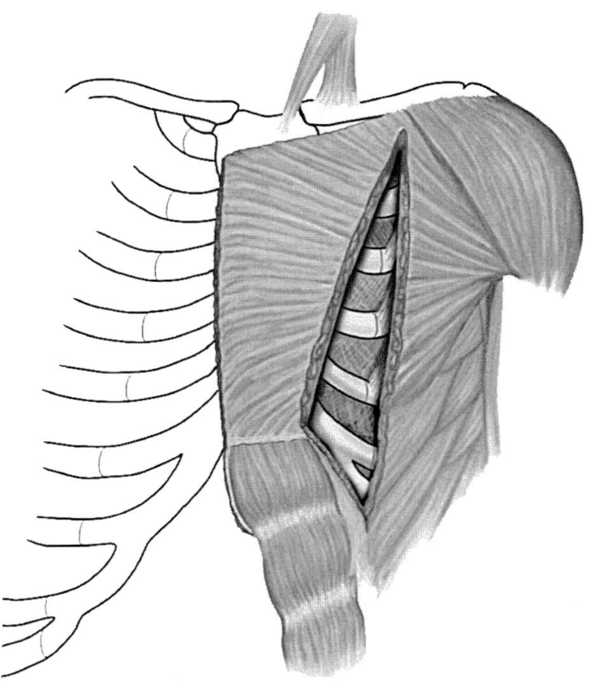

FIGURE 51–15 ■ The pectoralis-rectus abdominis bipedicular flap. (Modified from Solomon NP, Granick MS: Bipedicle muscle flaps in sternal wound repair. Plast Reconstr Surg 101:356–360, 1998.)

This situation, characterized by a gaping sternotomy with the heart exposed, is referred to as the *Hanuman syndrome* after Hanuman, the monkey king of Indo-Siamese mythology, who, to demonstrate his good will, opened his chest to show his heart to the god Rama (Fig. 51–16). The cardinal issues in the management of patients with the Hanuman syndrome are (1) prevention of contamination if the field is sterile; (2) management of infection, if present; (3) minimization of additional bacterial colonization; and (4) prevention of additional complications, primarily hemorrhage from the exposed heart (Robicsek, 1997).

If the field is not contaminated, every effort should be made to keep it sterile. Even if the sternum is left open, the skin edges should be approximated whenever the situation allows. Drains and other tubes should be placed through separate stab wounds. The mediastinum may be packed with sponges soaked in normal saline solution or in povidone-iodine. Tourniquets should be made short and left entirely intramediastinal. The edges of the sternum should be covered with wet sponges or laps soaked in povidone-iodine, and finally the entire field should be shielded with antiseptic film adhesive.

To ensure drainage and at the same time prevent compression of the heart in hemodynamically compromised cases, the sternal edges should not overly approximate. This may be achieved with packing or by using commer-

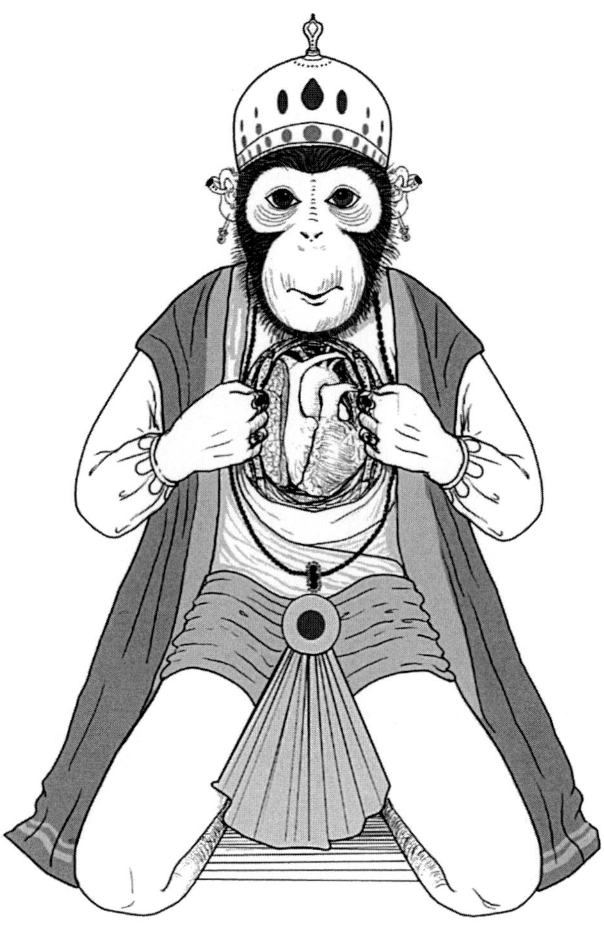

FIGURE 51–16 ■ Hanuman, the monkey king of Indo-Siamese mythology.

cially available (Thiel and Bircks, 1990) or improvised (Sato et al, 1998) stents. Methylmethacrylate plates (Yokoyama et al, 1988) were also applied successfully as indwelling stents to spread the sternal edges. In nonseptic pediatric cases in which the sternum could not be closed for hemodynamic reasons or because a conduit was inserted, different materials including plates made of ceramic or of hydroxyapatite (coral) were recommended as permanent sternal inserts (Baumgart et al, 1991).

Some patients can maintain a reasonable respiratory state on their own; however, in the acute stage (first 1 to 2 weeks) the patient should be heavily sedated, intubated, and also paralyzed. The principal reason for this is to prevent the occurrence of exsanguinating hemorrhage from the heart, which is the most dreaded complication of the open method of treating sternal infection. Although such a hemorrhage may also be caused by direct injury by left-in wires, by the jagged edges of the sternum, or by the infectious process attacking exposed suture lines, there is a special form of life-threatening bleeding that is particular to the Hanuman syndrome. While the patient is at rest, the heart more or less "stays away" from the unopened sternotomy site. If, however, the patient coughs or strains, the heart is forced against the window of the open sternotomy incision. Where the heart meets the edge of the sternum, the bone may cut deeply into the myocardium and cause severe, often fatal, hemorrhage. The occurrence of such a Valsalva maneuver–like situation can be eliminated only by paralyzing the patient and instituting controlled ventilation (Robicsek, 1997) (Fig. 51–17).

If bleeding occurs, pressure is applied for initial control, and then the patient should immediately be returned to the operating room with available cardiopulmonary bypass. The latter is best instituted through the femoral vessels. If the bleeding is caused by a tear on the heart, usually on the right ventricle, it may be closed with sutures with autogenous tissue pledgets and then covered with a patch of pericardium attached with biologic or cyanoacrylate glue (Robicsek et al, 1994). Bleeding from suture lines is always infectious in origin and to be handled by additional sutures and simultaneous muscle flap coverage. Small "signal" hemorrhages often precede a major one. Therefore, any bleeding from the exposed mediastinum, however small, should be taken most seriously.

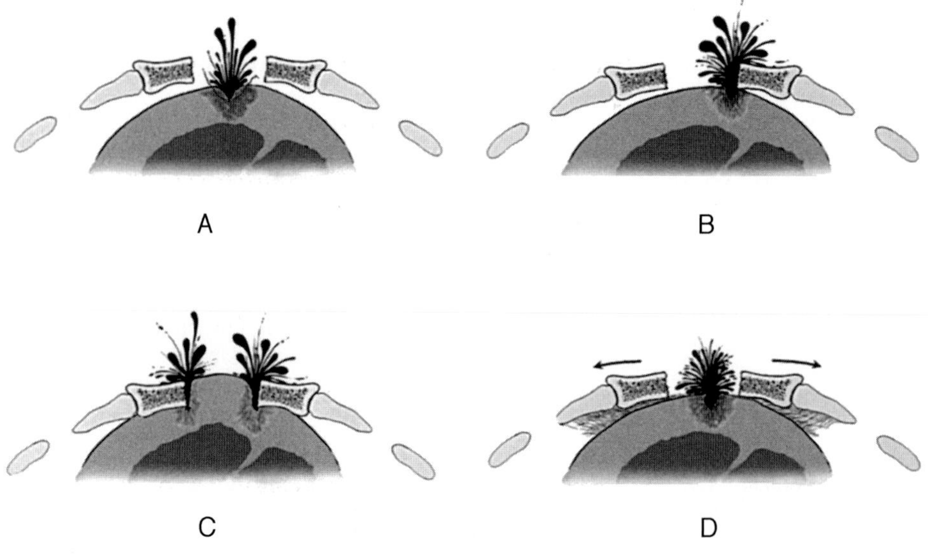

FIGURE 51–17 ■ Illustration of how hemorrhage may occur in the exposed heart in the course of open management. *A*, Direct extension of the infectious process. *B*, Injury by the jagged edge of the sternum. *C*, Increased intrathoracic pressure forcing the heart against the sternal "window." *D*, Tear on the heart caused by dense adhesions to the anterior chest wall.

To prevent the devastating complication of hemorrhage from the exposed heart, every effort should be made to keep the period during which the mediastinum is exposed as short as possible. Whenever the condition, either hemodynamic or infectious, that made the exposure necessary has been brought under reasonable control, the mediastinum should be closed without undue delay. If the sternum was left open for hemodynamic reasons, it can usually be closed primarily. If the Hanuman syndrome was created to treat sternomediastinitis, the closure should be effected using muscle flaps.

COMMENTS AND CONTROVERSIES

Dr. Robicsek's ingenuity and creativity markedly improve our understanding and repair of this potentially disastrous complication. The usual association of coronary bypass grafts in the field increases the morbidity, because infection and sternal instability increase the incidence of bypass occlusion. Prompt recognition of the problem with simple and safe reconstruction is extremely important. Dr. Robicsek's technique of sternal weaving has been used extensively and is a "tried and true" technique.

H. C. U.

REFERENCES

Adams JW, Hazard PB, Gooch JB: Flail chest injury in a patient with surgical absence of the sternum. Chest 92:185–186, 1987.

Ancalmo N, Perniciaro C, Ochsner J: Hypersensitivity reaction to sternal wires: A possible cause of persistent postoperative pain. Cardiovasc Surg 1:439–441, 1993.

Badellino M, Cavarocchi NC, Kolff J et al: Sternotomy closure with Parham bands. J Card Surg 3:235–236, 1988.

Banic A, Ris HB, Erni D, Striffeler H: Free latissimus dorsi flap for chest wall repair after complete resection of infected sternum. Ann Thorac Surg 60:1028–1032, 1995.

Baumgart D, Herbon G, Borowski A, de Vivie ER: Primary closure of median sternotomy with interposition of hydroxyapatite blocks: A new approach in pediatric cardiac surgery. Eur J Cardiothorac Surg 5:383–385, 1991.

Beam TR Jr: Preventing infection in open heart surgery. Chemioterapia 6:208–214, 1987.

Bentivegna PE, Humphrey CB: Arteriovenous fistula of internal mammary artery after median sternotomy. J Cardiovasc Surg (Torino) 30:375–377, 1989.

Blanchard A, Hurni M, Ruchat P et al: Incidence of deep and superficial sternal infection after open heart surgery: A ten year retrospective study from 1981 to 1991. Eur J Cardiothorac Surg 9:153–157, 1995.

Boiskin I, Karna A, Demos TC, Blakeman B: Herniation of the transverse colon: An unusual compication of pedicled omentoplasty. Can Assoc Radiol J 46:223–225, 1995.

Brantigan CO, Brown RK, Brantigan OC: The broken wire suture. Am Surg 45(1):38–41, 1979.

Breyer RH, Mills SA, Hudspeth AS et al: A prospective study of sternal wound complications. Ann Thorac Surg 37:412–416, 1984.

Browdie DA, Bernstein RW, Agnew R et al: Diagnosis of poststernotomy infection: Comparison of three means of assessment. Ann Thorac Surg 51:290–292, 1991.

Brown RP, Esmore DS, Lawson C: Improved sternal fixation in the transsternal bilateral thoracotomy incision. J Thorac Cardiovasc Surg 112:137–141, 1996.

Bryan AJ, Lamarra M, Angeline GD et al: Median sternotomy wound dehiscence: A retrospective case control study of risk factors and outcome. J R Coll Surg Edinb 37:305–308, 1992.

Carrier M, Grégoire J, Tronc F et al: Effect of internal mammary artery dissection on sternal vascularization. Ann Thorac Surg 53:115–119, 1992.

Cheng W, Cameron DE, Warden KE et al: Biomechanical study of sternal closure techniques. Ann Thorac Surg 55:737–740, 1993.

Chiu WC, D'Amelio LF, Hammond JS: Sternal fractures in blunt chest trauma: A practical algorithm for management. Am J Emerg Med 15:252–255, 1997.

Chlosta WF, Elefteriades JA: Simplified method of reinforced sternal closure. Ann Thorac Surg 60:1428–1429, 1995.

Cohen M, Yaniv Y, Weiss J, et al: Median sternotomy wound complication: The effect of reconstruction on lung function. Ann Plast Surg 39:36–43, 1997.

Colen LB, Huntsman WT, Morain WD: The integrated approach to suppurative mediastinitis: Rewiring the sternum over transposed omentum. Plast Reconstr Surg 84:936–940, 1989.

Copeland M, Senkowski C, Ulcickas M et al: Breast size as a risk factor for sternal wound complications following cardiac surgery. Arch Surg 129:757–759, 1994.

Cosgrove DM, Lyte BW, Loop FD et al: Does bilateral internal mammary artery grafting increase surgical risk? J Thorac Cardiovasc Surg 95:850–856, 1988.

Cremer J, Gerber I, Mehler D, Haverich A: Sternal infections following open heart surgery: A cost analysis. Langenbecks Arch Chir Suppl Kongressbd 114:1356–1357, 1997.

Culliford AT, Cunningham JN, Zeff RH et al: Sternal and costochondral infections following open-heart surgery: A review of 2,594 cases. J Thorac Cardiovsac Surg 72:714–726, 1976.

Defalque RJ, Bromley JJ: Poststernotomy neuralgia: A new pain syndrome. Anesth Analg 69:81–82, 1989.

De Fontaine S, Devos S, Goldschmidt D: Reduction mammaplasty combined with pectoralis major muscle flaps for median sternotomy wound closure. Br J Plast Surg 49:220–222, 1996.

DeGeest S, Kesteloot K, Adraenssen G et al: Clinical and cost comparison of three postoperative skin preparation protocols in CABG patients. Prog Cardiovasc Nurs 11:4–16, 1996.

Eastridge CE, Mahfood SS, Walker WA, Cole FH: Delayed chest wall pain due to sternal wire sutures. Ann Thorac Surg 51:56–59, 1991.

Frank MW, Alexander JC, Pineless GR et al: False aneurysm of the right internal mammary artery: Late rupture after sternotomy. Tex Heart Inst J 25:86–87, 1998.

Geiger JP, Tabak CA, Aronstam EM: Primary sternal closure and mediastinal decompression by inlay autologous rib grafts. Ann Thorac Surg 61:215–216, 1996.

Greve H, Clajus P, Dittrich H: Closure of median sternotomy with resorbable synthetic sutures. Langenbecks Arch Chir 368:65–71, 1986.

Grossi EA, Esposito R, Harris LJ et al: Sternal wound infections and use of internal mammary artery grafts. J Thorac Cardiovasc Surg 102:342–347, 1991.

Gur E, Stern D, Weiss J et al: Clinical-radiological evaluation of poststernotomy wound infection. Plast Reconstr Surg 101:348–355, 1998.

Hanson MR, Breuer AC, Furlan AJ et al: Mechanism and frequency of brachial plexus injury in open-heart surgery: A prospective analysis. Ann Thorac Surg 36:675–679, 1983.

Hastings JC, Robicsek F: Clinical significance of epicardial pacing wire cultures. J Thorac Cardiovasc Surg 105:165–167, 1993.

Hendrickson SC, Koger KE, Morea CJ et al: Sternal plating for the treatment of sternal nonunion. Ann Thorac Surg 62:512–518, 1996.

Jones G, Jurkiewicz MJ, Bostwick J et al: Management of the infected median sternotomy wound with muscle flaps: The Emory 20-year experience. Ann Surg 225:766–778, 1997.

Julian OC, Lopez-Belio M, Dye WS et al: The median sternal incision in intracardiac surgery with extracorporeal circulation: A general evaluation of its use in heart surgery. Surgery 21:172–173, 1957.

Jurkiewicz MJ, Bostwick J 3d, Hester TR et al: Infected median sternotomy wound: Successful treatment by muscle flaps. Ann Surg 191:738–740, 1980.

Klutsal A, Ibrisim E, Catav Z et al: Mediastinitis after open heart surgery: Analysis of risk factors and management. J Cardiovasc Surg (Torino) 32:38–41, 1991.

Kohman LJ, Coleman MJ, Parker FB: Bacteremia and sternal infection after coronary artery bypass grafting. Ann Thorac Surg 49:454–457, 1990.

Lee AB, Schimert G, Shatkin S: Total excision of the sternum and thoracic pedicle transposition of the greater omentum, useful stratagerns in managing severe mediastinal infection following open heart surgery. Surgery 80:433–436, 1976.

Lejour M, Dome M: Abdominal wall function after rectus abdominis transfer. Plast Reconstr Surg 87:1054–1068, 1991.

Leveen HL, Piccone VA: Nylon-band chest closure. Arch Surg 96:36–39, 1968.

Liu HP, Chang CH, Lin PJ et al: Migration of Kirschner wire from the right sternoclavicular joint into the main pulmonary artery: A case report. Chang Keng I Hsueh 15:49–53, 1992.

Macmanus Q, Okies JE: Mediastinal wound infection and aortocoronary graft patency. Am J Surg 132:558–561, 1976.

Maddern IR, Goodman LR, Almassi GH et al: CT after reconstructive repair of the sternum and chest wall. Radiology 50:1019–1023, 1993.

McGregor WE, Trumble DR, Magovern JA: Mechanical analysis of midline sternotomy wound closure. J Thorac Cardiovasc Surg 117:1144–1150, 1999.

Milton AF cited by Kirschner M: Tratadad de tecnica operatoria general y especial (Editorial). Labor S A Barcelona 4:756–760, 1944.

Molina JE: Primary closure for infected dehiscence of the sternum. Ann Thorac Surg 55:459–463, 1993.

Montandon D: The infected sternotomy. Helv Chir Acta 58:95–98, 1991.

Nahai F, Rand RP, Hester TR et al: Primary treatment of the infected sternotomy wound with muscle flaps: A review of 211 consecutive cases. Plast Reconstr Surg 84:434–441, 1989.

Neale HW, Kreilein JG, Schreiber JT, Gregory RO: Complete sternectomy for chronic osteomyelitis with reconstruction using a rectus abdominis myocutaneous island flap. Ann Plast Surg 6:305–314, 1981.

Oates E, Payne DD: Postoperative cardiothoracic infection: Diagnostic value of indium-111 white blood cell imaging. Ann Thorac Surg 58:1442–1446, 1994.

O'Connell JB, Newton CG, Sandberg GW: Mycotic pseudoaneurysm complication flap closure of an infected median sternotomy. Ann Plast Surg 35:420–422, 1995.

Okies JE, Phillips SJ: Sternal approximation (Letter). Ann Thorac Surg 4:423–424, 1974.

Ozaki W, Buchman SR, Iannettoni MD, Frankenburg EP: Biomechanical study of closure using rigid fixation techniques in human cadavers. Ann Thorac Surg 65:1660–1665, 1998.

Pairolero PC, Arnold PG, Harris JB: Long-term results of pectoralis major muscle transposition for infected sternotomy wounds. Ann Surg 213:583–590, 1991.

Parish MA, Asai T, Grossi EA et al: The effects of different techniques of internal mammary harvesting on sternal blood flow. J Thorac Cardiovasc Surg 104:1303–1307, 1992.

Ringelman PR, Vander Kolk CA, Cameron D et al: Long-term results of flap reconstruction in median sternotomy wound infections. Plast Reconstr Surg 93:1208–1216, 1994.

Robicsek F: Discussion of article: Sternal and costochondral infections following open heart surgery, by Culliford AT, Cunningham JN, Zeff KH et al. Thorac Cardiovascular Surg 72:714–726, 1976.

Robicsek F: Pectus carinatum. Collected works of the International Thoracic Congress, Tokyo, 1988, pp 235–256.

Robicsek F: Pectus excavatum and carinatum. In Hermes C. Grillo (ed): Current Therapy in Cardiothoracic Surgery. Toronto, BC Decker, 1989, pp 87–90.

Robicsek F: Prevention of secondary hemorrhage in Hanuman syndrome (open mediastinal drainage). J Cardiovasc Surg (Torino) 38:601–603, 1997.

Robicsek F: Surgical repair of pectus excavatum and carinatum deformities. J Cardiovasc Surg (Torino) 39(Suppl 1):155–159, 1998.

Robicsek F, Hamilton DA: Presternal muscle padding following midline sternotomy. J Card Surg 4:299–301, 1989.

Robicsek F, Sanger P, Daugherty H: The repair of recurrent pectus excavatum. J Thorac Cardiovasc Surg 56:141–143, 1968.

Robicsek F, Daugherty HK, Cook JW: The prevention and treatment of sternum separation following open-heart surgery. J Thorac Cardiovasc Surg 73:267–268, 1977.

Robicsek F, Daugherty HK, Cook JW, et al: *Mycobacterium fortuitum* epidemics afoer open-heart surgery. J Thorac Cardiovasc Surg 75:91–96, 1978.

Robicsek F, Masters TN, Littman L, Born GVR: The embolization of bone wax from sternotomy incisions. Ann Thorac Surg 31:357–359, 1981.

Robicsek F, Masters TN, Daugherty HK et al: The value of thermography in the early diagnosis of postoperative sternal wound infections. Thorac Cardiovasc Surg 32:260–265, 1984.

Robicsek F, Hoffman PC, Masters TN, et al: Rapidly growing nontuberculous mycobacteria: A new enemy of the cardiac surgeon. Ann Thorac Surg 46:703–710, 1988.

Robicsek F, Rielly J, Marroum M: The use of cyanoacrylate adhesive (Krazy Glue) in cardiac surgery. J Card Surg 9:353–356, 1994.

Robicsek F, Cook JW, Rizzoni W: Sternoplasty for incomplete sternum separation. J Thorac Cardiovasc Surg 116:361–362, 1998.

Sanfelippo PM, Danielson GK: Complications associated with median sternotomy. J Thorac Cardiovasc Surg 63:419–423, 1972.

Sato T, Isomura T, Hisatomi K, Nayashida N: Bilateral thoracotomy for coronary artery bypass grafting in a patient with unfavorable median sternotomy. J Cardiovasc Surg (Torino) 39:229–232, 1998.

Schultz RS, Boger JW, Dunn HK: Strength of stainless steel surgical wire in various fixation modes. Clin Orthop 198:304–307, 1985.

Scovotti CA, Ponzone CA, Leyro-Diaz RM: Reinforced sternal closure. Ann Thorac Surg 51:844–845, 1991.

Serry C, Bleck PC, Javid H et al: Sternal wound complications: Management and results. J Thorac Cardiovasc Surg 80:861–867, 1980.

Seyfer AE, Shriver CD, Miller TR, Graeber GM: Sternal blood flow after median sternotomy and mobilization of the internal mammary arteries. Surgery 104:899–904, 1988.

Shafir R, Weiss J, Herman O, Elami A: The danger in skin grafting the bare mediastinum after sternectomy for postcoronary bypass dehiscence. Ann Thorac Surg 48:584–586, 1989.

Silva J, Gonzalez-Santos J, Perez M et al: Iatrogenic mammary arteriovenous fistula caused by sternal wire. Ann Thorac Surg 66:1398–1399, 1998.

Solomon MP, Granick MS: Bipedicle muscle flaps in sternal wound repair. Plast Reconstr Surg 101:356–360, 1998.

Stoney WS, Alford WC, Burrus GR et al: Median sternotomy dehiscence. Ann Thorac Surg 26:421–426, 1978.

Thiel R, Bircks W: Arteriovenous fistulas after median sternotomy: Report of 2 cases and review of the literature. Thorac Cardiovasc Surg 38:195–197, 1990.

Timmes JJ, Wolvek S, Fernando M et al: A new method of sternal approximation. Ann Thorac Surg 5:544–546, 1973.

Uva MS, Braunberger E, Fisher M et al: Doss bilateral internal thoracic artery grafting increase surgical risk in diabetic patients? Ann Thorac Surg 65:2051–2055, 1998.

Vander Salm TJ, Cutler BS, Okike ON: Brachial plexus injury following median sternotomy: Part II. J Thorac Cardiovasc Surg 83:914–917, 1982.

Vanleeuw P, Roux D, Fournial G et al: Early postoperative sternal approximation after ITA harvesting: Computed tomographic evaluation. Ann Thorac Surg 52:518–522, 1991.

Watanabe G, Misaki T, Kotoh K: Microfibrillar collagen (Avitene) and antibiotic-containing fibrin-glue after median sternotomy. J Card Surg 12:110–111, 1997.

Wehrens XH, Doevendans PA, van Dantzig JM et al: Infected sternal fracture hematoma after cardiopulmonary resuscitation initially seen as pericarditis. Am Heart J 132:685–686, 1996.

Yokoyama M, Wada J, Chino K, Ade WR: New wire suture for sternal fixation. J Cardiovasc Surg (Torino) 29:146–147, 1988.

CHAPTER **52**

Thoracic Outlet Syndromes

Susan Mackinnon
G. Alexander Patterson
Harold C. Urschel, Jr.

DEFINITION

Thoracic outlet syndrome, a term coined by Rob and Standover (1958), refers to compression on the subclavian vessels and brachial plexus at the superior aperture of the chest. It was previously designated as the scalenus anticus, costoclavicular, hyperabduction, cervical rib, or first thoracic rib syndrome, depending on the presumed cause. The various syndromes are similar, and the compression mechanism is often difficult to identify. Most compressive factors operate against the first rib (Clagett, 1962; Urschel et al, 1968) (Fig. 52–1).

HISTORICAL NOTE

Until 1927 the cervical rib was commonly thought to be the cause of symptoms of the thoracic outlet syndrome. Galen and Vesalius first described the presence of a cervical rib (Borchardt, 1901). Hunauld, who published an article in 1742, is credited by Keen (1907) as being the first to describe the importance of the cervical rib in causing symptoms. In 1818, Cooper treated symptoms of cervical rib with some success (Adson and Coffey, 1927); and in 1861, Coote performed the first cervical rib removal. Sir James Paget, in 1875 in London, and von Schroetter, in 1884 in Vienna, described the syndrome of thrombosis of the axillary-subclavian vein (Paget-Schroetter syndrome). Halsted (1916) stimulated interest in dilatation of the subclavian artery distal to cervical ribs, and Law (1920) reported the role of adventitious ligaments in the cervical rib syndrome. Naffziger and Grant (1938) and Ochsner and associates (1935) popularized section of the scalenus anticus muscle. Falconer and Weddell (1943) and Brintnall and associates (1956) incriminated the costoclavicular membrane in the production of neurovascular compression. Wright (1945) described the hyperabduction syndrome with compression in the costoclavicular area by the tendon of the pectoralis minor.

Rosati and Lord (1961) added claviculectomy to anterior exploration, scalenotomy, resection of the cervical rib (when one was present), and section of the pectoralis minor and subclavian muscles as well as of the costoclavicular membrane. The role of the first rib in causing symptoms of neurovascular compression was recognized by Bramwell in 1903. Murphy (1910) is credited with the first resection of the first rib and in 1916 provided a collective review of 112 articles related to compression from the cervical ribs. Brinckner and Milch (1925), Brinckner (1927), Telford and Stopford (1937), and Telford and Mottershead (1948) suggested that the first rib was the culprit. Clagett (1962) emphasized the first rib and its resection through the posterior thoracoplasty approach to relieve neurovascular compression. Falconer and Li (1962) reported the anterior approach for first rib resection, whereas Roos (1966) introduced the transaxillary route for first rib resection and extirpation. Krusen (1968) and Caldwell and co-workers (1971) introduced the measurement of motor conduction velocities across the thoracic outlet in diagnosing thoracic outlet syndrome. Urschel and associates (1976) popularized reoperation for recurrent thoracic outlet syndrome and thrombolysis with prompt transaxillary rib resection for Paget-Schroetter syndrome. Wilborn (1999) emphasized the controversial nature of neurogenic thoracic outlet syndrome without intrinsic muscle wasting. Mackinnon and Novak (1994, 1996, 1999) stressed the merits of appropriate physical therapy and recognition of associated distal entrapment neuropathies in the management of the patient with thoracic outlet syndrome.

■ *HISTORICAL READINGS*

Clagett OT: Presidential address: Research and prosearch. J Thorac Cardiovasc Surg 44:153, 1962.
Paget J: Clinical Lectures and Essays. London, Longmans-Green, 1875.
Sanders RJ: Thoracic Outlet Syndrome: A Common Sequela of Neck Injuries. Philadelphia, JB Lippincott, 1991.
Urschel HC Jr, Razzuk MA, Albers JE, et al: Reoperation for recurrent thoracic outlet syndrome. Ann Thorac Surg 21:19, 1976.
Von Schroetter L: Erkrankungen der Gefèsse. In Nothnagel (ed): Handbuch der Pathologie und Therapie. Vienna, Holder, 1884.

BASIC SCIENCE

Surgical Anatomy

At the superior aperture of the thorax, the subclavian vessels and the brachial plexus traverse the cervicoaxillary canal to reach the upper extremity (Ravitch and Steichen, 1988). The cervicoaxillary canal is divided by the first rib into two sections: the proximal one, composed of the scalene triangle and the costoclavicular space (the space bounded by the clavicle and the first rib), and the distal one, composed of the axilla (Fig. 52–2). The proximal division is the more critical for neurovascular compression. It is bounded superiorly by the clavicle, inferiorly by the first rib, anteromedially by

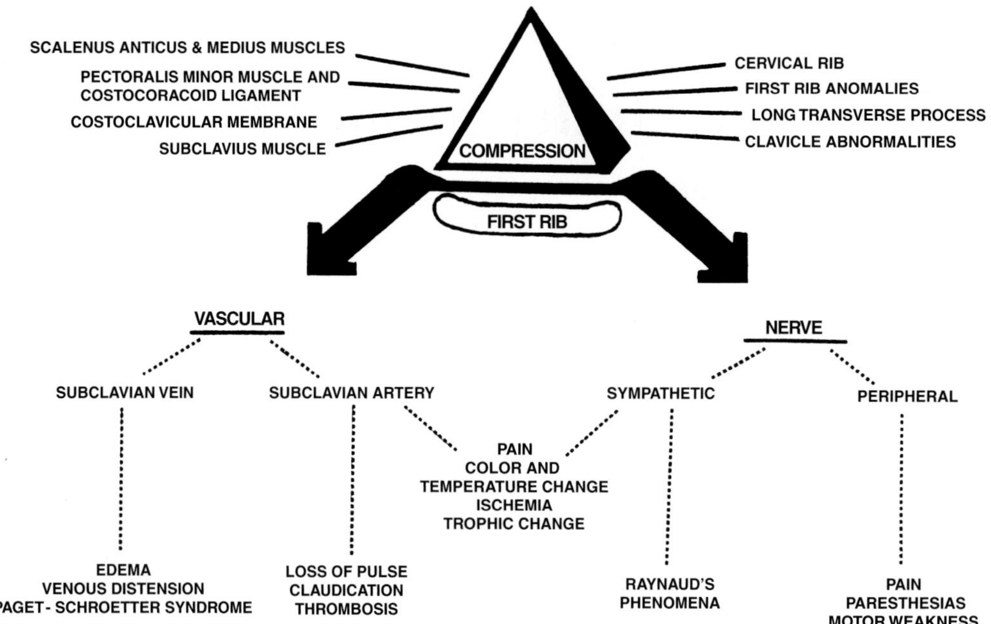

FIGURE 52–1 ■ The relation of muscle, ligament, and bone abnormalities in the thoracic outlet that may compress neurovascular structures against the first rib.

the costoclavicular ligament, and posterolaterally by the scalenus medius muscle and the long thoracic nerve. The scalenus anticus muscle, which inserts on the scalene tubercle of the first rib, divides the costoclavicular space into two compartments: the anteromedial compartment, which contains the subclavian artery and the brachial plexus; and the scalene triangle, which is bounded by the scalenus anticus anteriorly, the scalenus medius posteriorly, and the first rib inferiorly. This region of neurovascular compression is in reality the thoracic inlet and not the thoracic outlet (Ranney, 1996).

Functional Anatomy

The cervicoaxillary canal, particularly its proximal segment, the costoclavicular area, normally has ample space for passage of the neurovascular bundle with compression. This space narrows during functional maneuvers. It narrows during abduction of the arm because the clavicle rotates backward toward the first rib and the insertion of the scalenus anticus muscle. In hyperabduction, the neurovascular bundle is pulled around the pectoralis minor tendon, the coracoid process, and the head of the humerus. During this maneuver, the coracoid process tilts downward and thus exaggerates the tension on the bundle. The sternoclavicular joint, which ordinarily forms an angle of 15 to 20 degrees, forms a smaller angle when the outer end of the clavicle descends (as in drooping of the shoulders in poor posture), and narrowing of the costoclavicular space may occur (Rosati and Lord, 1961). Normally, during inspiration the scalenus anticus muscle raises the first rib and thus narrows the costoclavicular space. This muscle may cause an abnormal lift of the first rib, as in cases of severe emphysema or excessive muscular development, which is typically seen in young male adults.

The scalene triangle, which is normally located between the scalenus anticus anteriorly, the scalenus medius posteriorly, and the first rib inferiorly, permits the passage of the subclavian artery and the brachial plexus, which are in direct contact with the first rib. The triangle is 1.2 cm at its base and approximately 6.7 cm in height. There is little space between the neurovascular bundle and this triangular space. Anatomic variations may narrow the superior angle of the triangle, cause impingement on the upper components of the brachial plexus, and produce the upper type of scalenus anticus syndrome, which involves the trunk-containing elements of C5 and C6. If the base of the triangle is raised, compression of the subclavian artery and the trunk-containing components of C7, C8, and Tl results in the lower type of scalenus anticus syndrome. Both types have been described by Swank and Simeone (1944).

Compression Factors

Many factors may cause compression of the neurovascular bundle at the thoracic outlet, but the basic factor is displaced anatomy, to which congenital, traumatic, and occasionally atherosclerotic factors may contribute (Rosati and Lord, 1961) (see box). Bony abnormalities are present in approximately 10% of patients, in the form of a cervical rib, a bifid first rib, fusion of first and second ribs, or clavicular deformities or as the result of previous thoracoplasties. These abnormalities can be visualized on the plain posteroanterior chest film, but special radiographic views of the lower cervical spine may be required in some cases of cervical ribs.

Histopathology of Chronic Human Nerve Compression

Nerve compression is treated with surgical release rather than with surgical excision. Thus, there are very few

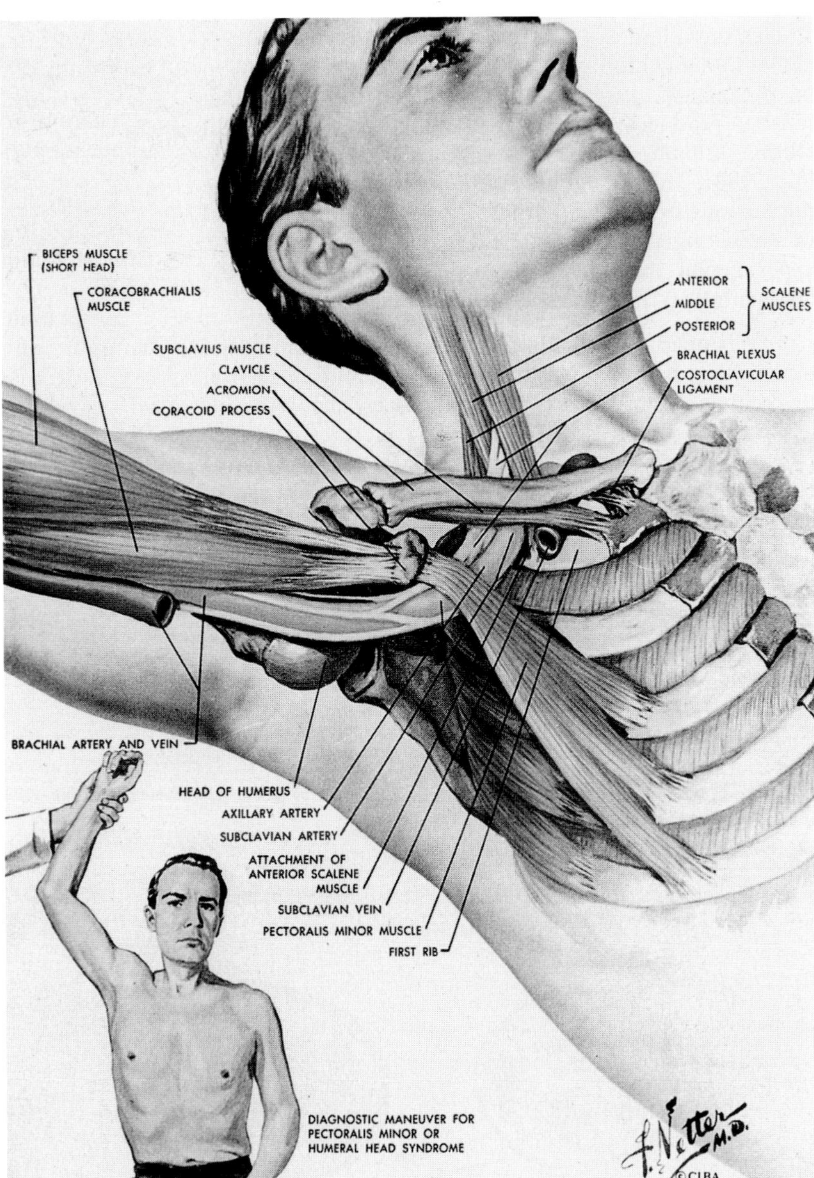

FIGURE 52–2 ■ Hyperabduction of the right arm with anatomic structures as noted.

NEUROVASCULAR COMPRESSION FACTORS

- Anatomic
  - Potential sites of neurovascular compression
    - Interscalene triangle
    - Costoclavicular space
    - Subcoracoid area
- Congenital
  - Cervical rib and its fascial remnants
  - Rudimentary first thoracic rib
  - Scalene muscles
    - Anterior
    - Middle
    - Minimus
  - Adventitious fibrous bands
  - Bifid clavicle
  - Exostosis of first thoracic rib
  - Enlarged transverse process of C7
  - Omohyoid muscle
  - Anomalous course of transverse cervical artery
  - Brachial plexus postfixed
  - Flat clavicle
- Traumatic
  - Fracture of clavicle
  - Dislocation of head of humerus
  - Crushing injury of upper thorax
  - Sudden, unaccustomed muscular efforts involving shoulder girdle muscles
  - Cervical spondylosis and injuries to cervical spine
- Atherosclerosis

studies providing any documentation of the histopathology of human chronic nerve compression. An experimental rodent and primate model has been developed that reliably produces changes mimicking those seen with chronic human nerve compression (Mackinnon and Dellon, 1988). This model has been useful in demonstrating the histopathology of chronic nerve compression and in evaluating current treatment modalities. From these experimental studies, several key points relating to the histopathology have been determined:

1. Histopathology spans a broad spectrum from initial blood-nerve barrier changes to epineural and perineural thickening to segmental demyelination and finally to wallerian degeneration (Fig. 52–3).
2. These changes are slowly progressive and influenced by the degree of compression and the duration of nerve compression.
3. Within the compressed nerve, histologic changes vary from fascicle to fascicle (Figs. 52–4 and 52–5).

These histopathologic findings have significant clinical implications:

1. Just as the histopathology spans a broad spectrum from mild to severe changes, the patient's symptoms and clinical findings vary along a similar continuum (Fig. 52–6).
2. As long as factors that contribute to chronic nerve compression (e.g., provoking occupation or activity, systemic disease) continue unmodified, the patient will develop progressive problems with nerve compression.
3. The fact that one fascicle within a compressed nerve may be normal while another demonstrates significant histologic changes corresponds with the situa-

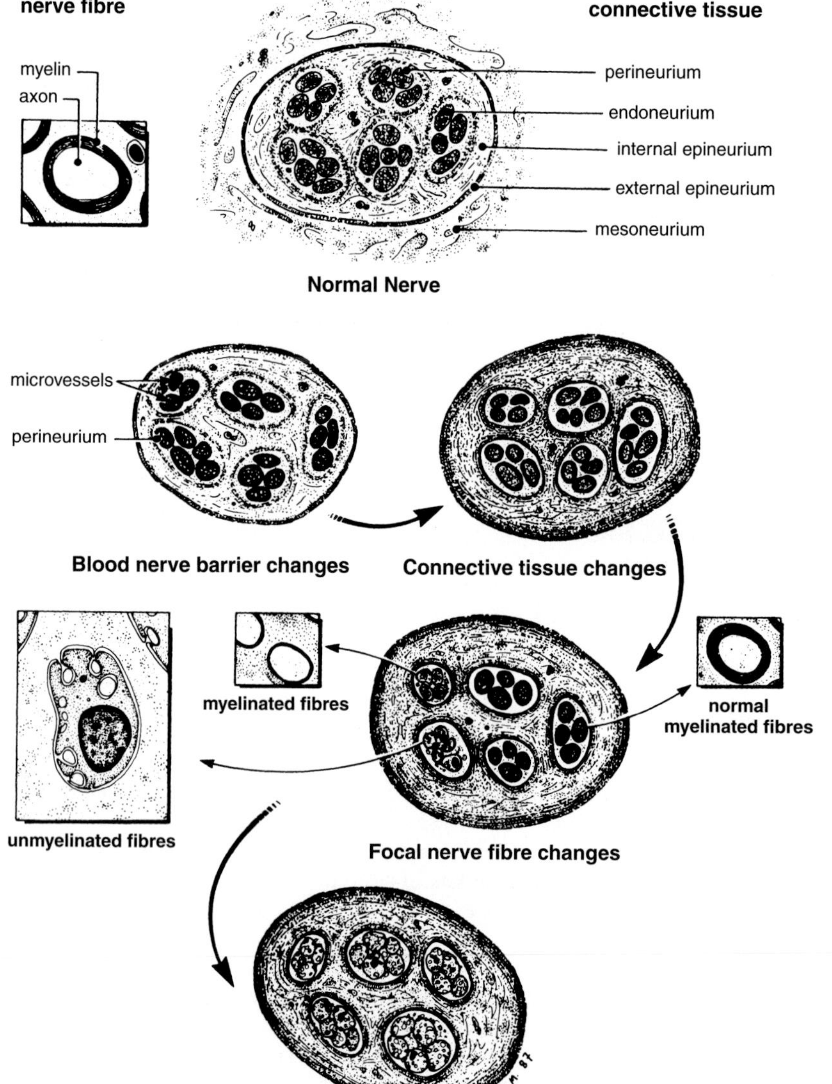

FIGURE 52–3 ■ The histopathology of chronic nerve compression progresses across a broad spectrum from blood-nerve barrier changes to connective tissue changes to focal nerve fiber changes and finally to wallerian degeneration. (From Mackinnon SE, Dellon AL: Surgery of the Peripheral Nerve. New York, Thieme, 1988.)

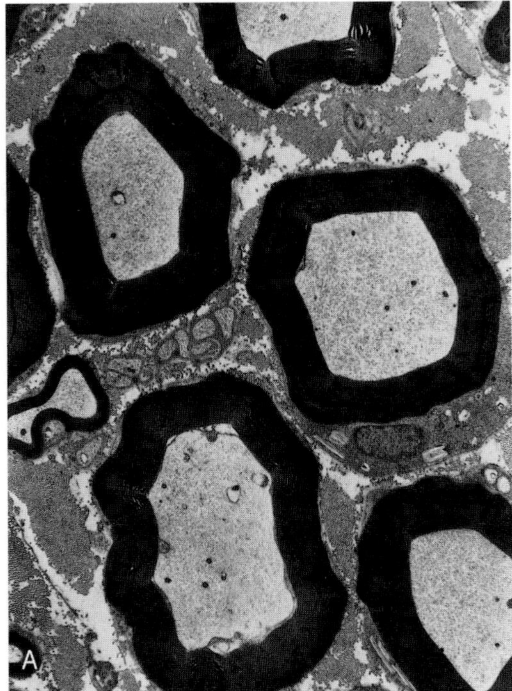

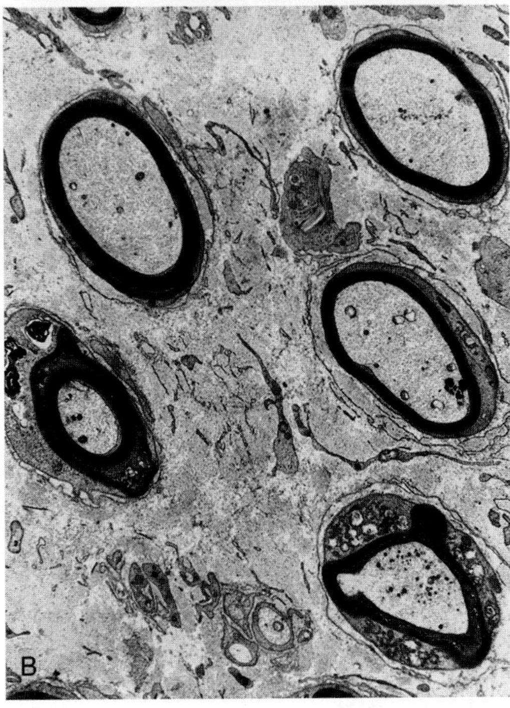

FIGURE 52–4 ■ *A*, A normal myelinated fiber population. *B*, With chronic nerve decompression, segmental demyelination occurs. The large myelinated fibers are associated with only a thin ring of myelin (From Mackinnon SE, Dellon AL: Chronic human nerve compression: A histological assessment. Neuropathol Appl Neurobiol 12:547, 1986.)

tion in which the unaffected fascicles are reflected in normal electrical studies while the patient's symptomatology is related to the fascicles demonstrating nerve damage.

In a fresh cadaver study the roots (C5 through Tl) and trunks of the brachial plexus were sampled. We noted in C8, T1, and the lower trunk the same histomorphologic changes of chronic nerve compression (epineurial thickening, demyelination, a loss of large myelinated fibers and Renaut's bodies) as were noted in other human and experimental studies of chronic nerve compression (Figs. 52–7 and 52–8).

Double and Multiple Crush Syndromes

In their report of the double crush syndrome in 1973, Upton and McComas stated that a proximal source of nerve compression will render the distal nerve segment more susceptible to a second site of compression. They hypothesized that one site alone would not cause clinical disturbance but that the summation of two sites would produce symptomatology. This hypothesis is directly applicable to brachial plexus compression in that several anatomic structures may compress the brachial plexus by amounts that on their own would not be enough to cause symptoms. Similarly, the recognized association between the carpal and cubital tunnel syndromes and the thoracic outlet syndrome is supported by the double crush hypothesis (Fig. 52–9). In our series of patients with thoracic outlet syndrome who were receiving workers' compensation, all patients had clinical evidence of either carpal or cubital tunnel syndrome, but only 24% had electrical evidence of these syndromes.

A clinical entity associated with an increase in occupations requiring repetitive activity (assembly lines, keyboarding) and previously termed *cumulative trauma disorder* or *repetitive stress disorder* is now termed *work-related upper extremity musculoskeletal disorder*. A significant component of this disorder relates to multilevel nerve compression. Specific anatomic structures and particular positions of the extremity will increase the pressure around the nerve and ultimately produce symptomatic nerve compression. (If the wrist is in other than a neutral position, pressures increase around the median nerve in the carpal tunnel; elbow flexion produces increased pressure around the ulnar nerve in the cubital tunnel; and elevation of the arms overhead theoretically increases pressure around the lower trunk of the brachial plexus.) Patients with cumulative trauma disorders will frequently have bilateral multilevel nerve compression.

Hand surgeons who are trained to focus on the distal portion of the extremity are encouraged to evaluate their patients for concomitant thoracic outlet syndrome. Similarly, cardiothoracic surgeons treating patients with thoracic outlet syndrome will find a significant association between this syndrome and carpal and cubital tunnel syndromes. We now recognize that both upper extremities work together as a single functional unit and that problems in one extremity can be associated with complaints in the opposite extremity secondary to compensatory overuse. (Similarly, physicians recognize that pathology at an ankle joint can eventually result in pathology at the contralateral hip joint.) The patient should be evaluated for pathology at all points in the "circle" (wrist, elbow, shoulder, and neck), all components of which

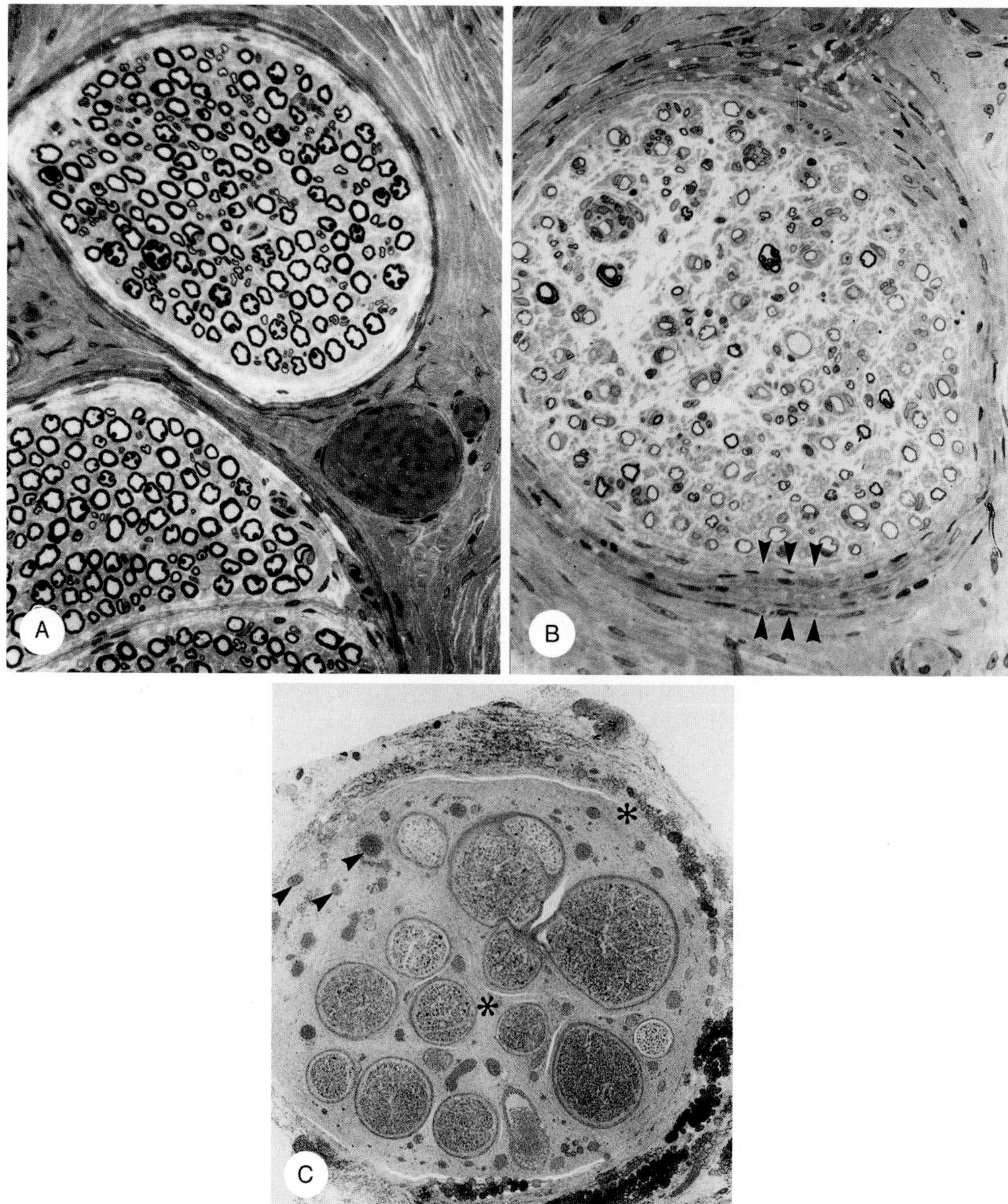

FIGURE 52–5 ■ *A*, The cross section of the compressed median nerve in a primate demonstrates increased vascularity and increased epineural connective tissue. *B*, A fascicle demonstrating wallerian degeneration and severe histologic changes is noted (*arrows* indicate perineurial thickening). *C*, Fascicles adjacent to those seen in Figure 52–4*B* show a more normal histologic pattern. (From Mackinnon SE, Dellon AL, Hudson AR: A primate model for chronic nerve compression. J Reconstr Microsurg 1:185, 1985).

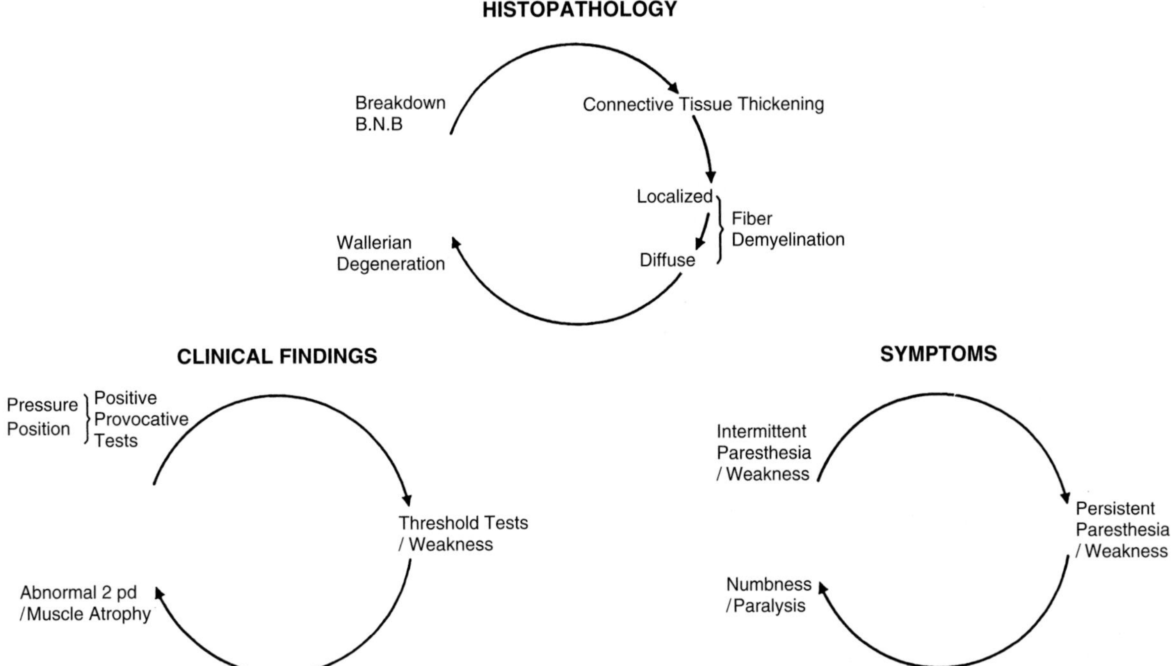

FIGURE 52–6 ■ The continuum of chronic nerve compression is illustrated. The histopathologic changes begin with breakdown of the blood-nerve barrier (B. N. B.) and conclude with wallerian degeneration. The patient's presentation, including subjective symptoms and clinical evaluation, will parallel the histopathology of the nerve.

are now recognized as interrelated (Fig. 52–10). Initial conservative management can be directed at several components of this circle. Surgery directed at distal problems in the extremity can result in an improvement in overall function without necessitating proximal surgical intervention. However, if significant pathology exists in the neck or the region of the thoracic outlet, distal procedures may improve but will not completely relieve the patient's symptoms (Mackinnon and Novak, 1994).

DIAGNOSIS

Symptoms and Signs

The symptomatology of thoracic outlet syndrome depends on whether the nerves and/or blood vessels are compressed in the cervicoaxillary canal. Neurogenic manifestations are observed more frequently than vascular ones. Symptoms consist of pain and paresthesias, which are present in approximately 95% of cases, as well as motor weakness and occasionally atrophy of the intrinsic hand muscles, which occur in less than 5%. The symptoms occur most commonly in areas supplied by the lower brachial plexus (C8–T1), which include the medial aspects of the arm and hand and the fourth and fifth fingers. The onset of pain is usually insidious and commonly involves the neck, shoulder, arm, and hand. The paresthesias may be precipitated by strenuous physical exercises or sustained physical efforts with the arm in an elevated position. Symptoms may be initiated by raising the arms above the head. In other cases, trauma to the upper extremities or the cervical spine is a precipitating factor. Physical findings usually consist of hypesthesia along the medial aspects of the forearm and hand. Atrophy is rarely present; when it is evident, it is present in the intrinsic muscles and is associated with clawing of the fourth and fifth fingers. If pure ulnar nerve atrophy is present (hypothenar, interosseous muscles) without wasting of the thenar muscles, compression of the ulnar nerve at the elbow (cubital tunnel syndrome) is suspected. When both median and ulnar innervated muscles are involved, this localizes proximally to the lower brachial plexus or cervical disk level. In the upper type of thoracic outlet syndrome, in which components of C5 and C6 nerves are involved in compression, pain is usually in the deltoid area and the lateral aspects of the arm. The presence of this pain indicates testing to exclude a herniated cervical disk (Rosati and Lord, 1961). In these cases Spurling's test will be positive. Similarly, rotator cuff tendinitis should be excluded in patients with shoulder and lateral arm pain. Components of the C5–T1 nerves can occur at the thoracic outlet because of a cervical rib and can produce symptoms of various degrees in the distribution of these nerves.

In some patients the pain is atypical, involving the anterior chest wall or parascapular area, and is termed *pseudoangina* because it simulates angina pectoris. These patients may have normal coronary arteriograms. The shoulder, arm, and hand symptoms that usually provide the clue for the diagnosis of thoracic outlet syndrome initially may be absent or minimal as compared with the severity of the chest pain. The diagnosis of thoracic outlet syndrome is frequently overlooked; many of these patients are committed to becoming "cardiac cripples" without an appropriate diagnosis, or they may develop severe psychological depression when told that their coronary arteries are normal and that they have no significant cause for their pain (Urschel et al, 1973).

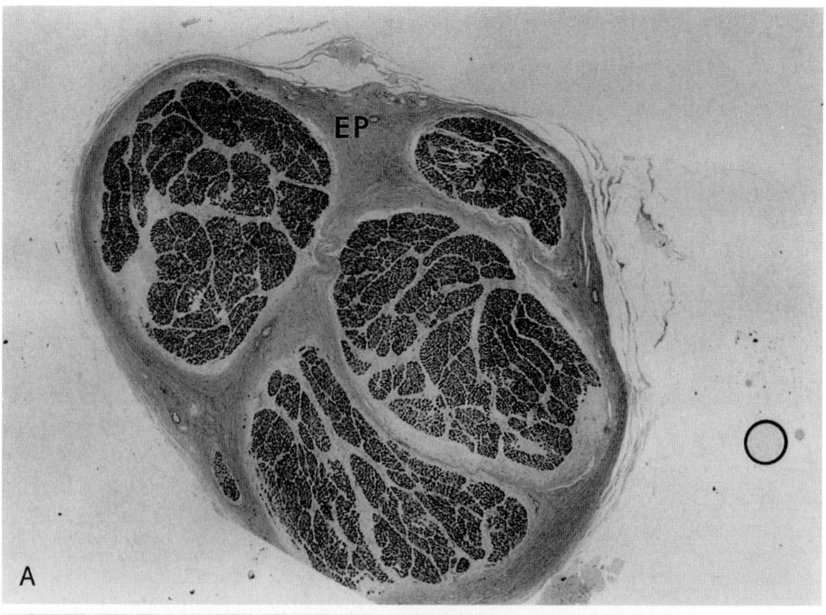

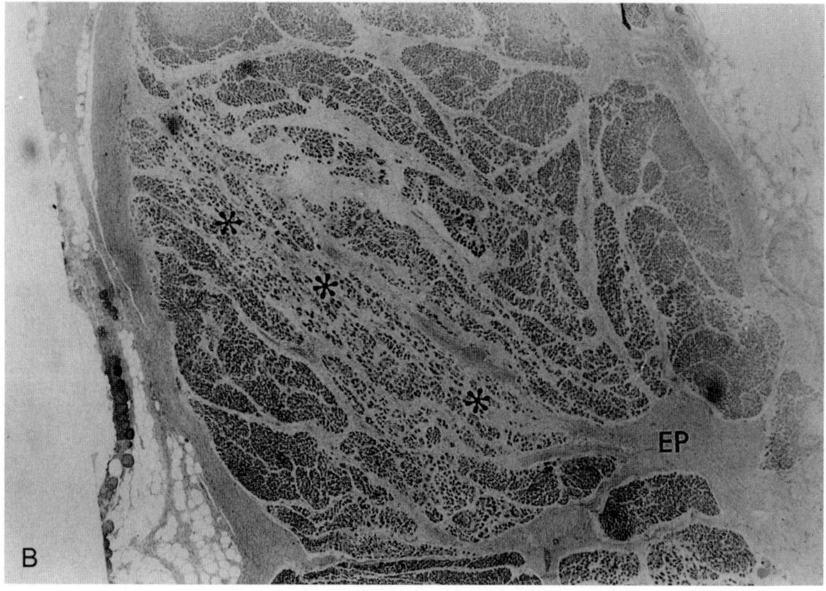

FIGURE 52–7 ■ Photomicrographs of cross section of C5 root (*A*) and T1 (*B*), noting increased epineural (*EP*) thickening, especially in T1 and fiber fallout in T1 (*asterisks*). (Toluidine blue, × 88.)

Symptoms of arterial compression include coldness, weakness, and easy fatigability of the arm and hand, and pain that is usually diffuse (Urschel et al, 1968; Urschel and Razzuk, 1972). Raynaud's phenomenon is noted in approximately 7.5% of patients with thoracic outlet syndrome (Urschel et al, 1968). Unlike Raynaud's disease, which is usually bilateral and symmetric and elicited by cold or emotion, Raynaud's phenomenon in neurovascular compression is usually unilateral and is more likely to be precipitated by hyperabduction of the involved arm, turning of the head, or carrying of heavy objects. Sensitivity to cold may also be present. Symptoms include sudden onset of coldness and blanching of one or more fingers, followed slowly by cyanosis and persistent rubor. Vascular symptoms in neurovascular compression may be precursors of permanent arterial thrombosis (Rosati and Lord, 1961). Arterial occlusion, usually of the subclavian artery when present, is manifested by persistent coldness, cyanosis or pallor of the fingers, and, in some cases, ulceration or gangrene. Palpation in the parascapular area may reveal prominent pulsation, which indicates poststenotic dilatation or aneurysm of the subclavian artery.

Less frequently, the symptoms are those of venous obstruction or occlusion, commonly recognized as effort thrombosis or Paget-Schroetter syndrome. The condition characteristically results in edema, discoloration of the arm, distention of the superficial veins of the limb and shoulder, and some degree of aches and pains. In some patients the condition is observed on waking; in others it follows sustained efforts with the arm in abduction. Sudden backward and downward bracing of the shoulders, heavy lifting, or strenuous physical activity involving the arm may constrict the vein and initiate venospasm, with or without subsequent thrombosis. In cases of definite venous thrombosis there is usually moderate tenderness over the axillary vein on examination, and a cord-like structure may be felt corresponding to the

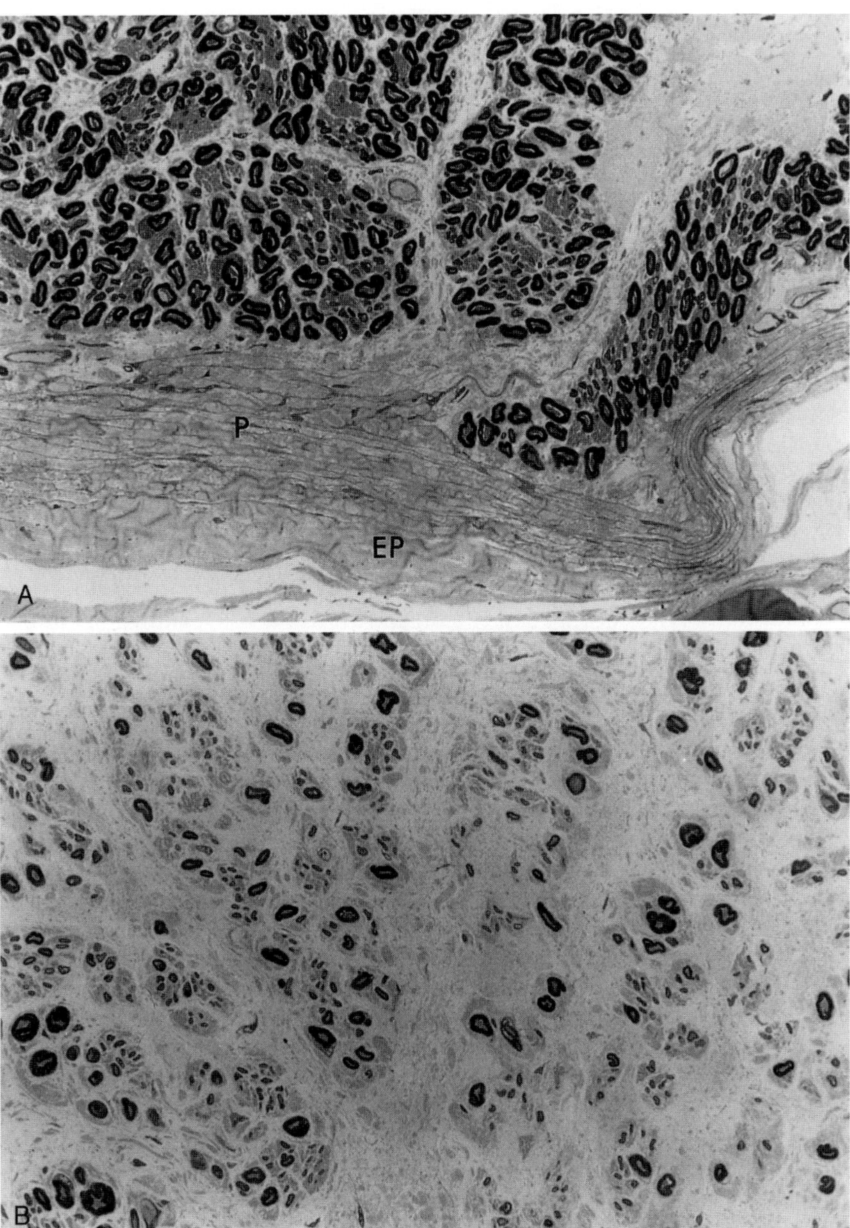

FIGURE 52–8 ■ Higher power micrograph of C5 (*A*) and T1 (*B*). Note perineurial (*P*) thickening in C5 and marked fiber fallout in T1. (Toluidine blue × 140.)

course of the vein. The acute symptoms may subside in a few weeks or days as the collateral circulation develops. Recurrence follows when the collateral circulation is inadequate (Rosati and Lord, 1961).

Objective physical findings are more common in patients with primarily vascular rather than neural compression. Loss or diminution of radial pulse and reproduction of symptoms can be elicited by the three classic clinical maneuvers: the Adson or scalene test (Adson, 1947), the costoclavicular test, and the hyperabduction test (Urschel and Razzuk, 1997).

Diagnostic Methods

The diagnosis of thoracic outlet syndrome includes history, physical and neurologic examination, films of the chest and cervical spine, electromyogram, and nerve conduction studies. In some cases with atypical manifestations, other diagnostic procedures such as cervical myelography, peripheral (Rosenberg, 1966) or coronary arteriography, or phlebography (Adams et al, 1968) should be considered. A detailed history and physical and neurologic examinations can often result in a tentative diagnosis of neurovascular compression. This diagnosis is strengthened when one or more of the classic clinical maneuvers is positive (Urschel and Razzuk, 1972).

Clinical Maneuvers

The clinical evaluation is best based on the physical findings of reproduction of symptoms, which can be elicited by the three classic maneuvers, the modified Roos test, and the Mackinnon-Patterson-Novak arm elevation test.

1. The Adson or scalene test (Adson, 1927) (Fig. 52–11*A*) consists of a maneuver that tightens the anterior

and middle scalene muscles and thus decreases the interspace and magnifies any pre-existing compression of the subclavian artery and brachial plexus. The patient is instructed to take and hold a deep breath, extend the neck fully, and turn the head toward the side. Obliteration or decrease of the radial pulse suggests compression (Rosati and Lord, 1961; Urschel and Razzuk, 1973b).

2. In the costoclavicular (Halstead) test (Fig. 52–11*B*), the shoulders are drawn downward and backward (military position). This maneuver narrows the costoclavicular space by approximating the clavicle to the first rib and thus tends to compress the neurovascular bundle. Changes in the radial pulse with production of symptoms indicate compression (Rosati and Lord, 1961; Urschel and Razzuk, 1973b).

3. In the hyperabduction test (Wright) (Fig. 52–11*C*), the arm is hyperabducted to 180 degrees, which pulls the components of the neurovascular bundle around the pectoralis minor tendon, the coracoid process, and the head of the humerus. If the radial pulse is decreased, compression should be suspected (Rosati and Lord, 1961; Urschel and Razzuk, 1973).

4. Roos (1966) has described a test of 90 degrees of abduction with external rotation of the shoulder to reproduce symptoms. He has modified this by incorporation of a 3-minute stress test of rapidly closing and opening the hand (Fig. 52–11*D*).

5. Mackinnon, Patterson, and Novak emphasize reproduction of symptoms in 1 minute with arm elevation. The elbow is kept extended to avoid testing for associated cubital tunnel syndrome. The wrist is kept in neutral to avoid eliciting symptoms from an associated carpal tunnel syndrome. Digital pressure on the brachial plexus will decrease the time of onset of symptoms.

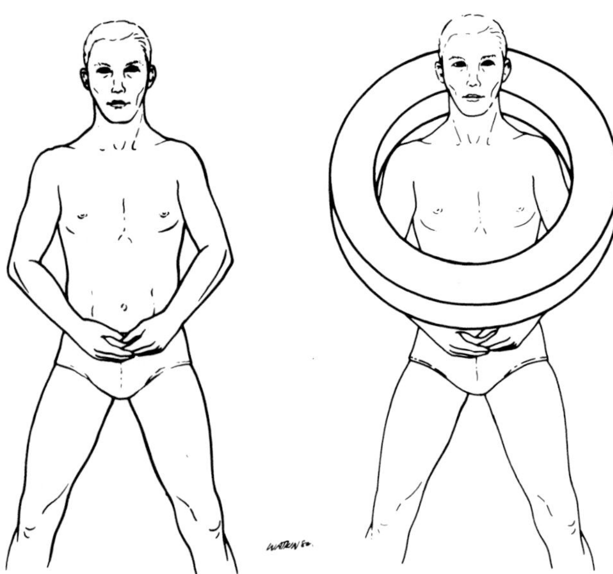

FIGURE 52–10 ■ The upper extremities and the cervical thoracic region work as a single unit. Pathology anywhere along this "ring" or "circle" will predispose some other area for overuse. The over-compensation can produce symptoms at new sites. Evaluation of patients with upper extremity complaints should include examination for problems at all points on the circle.

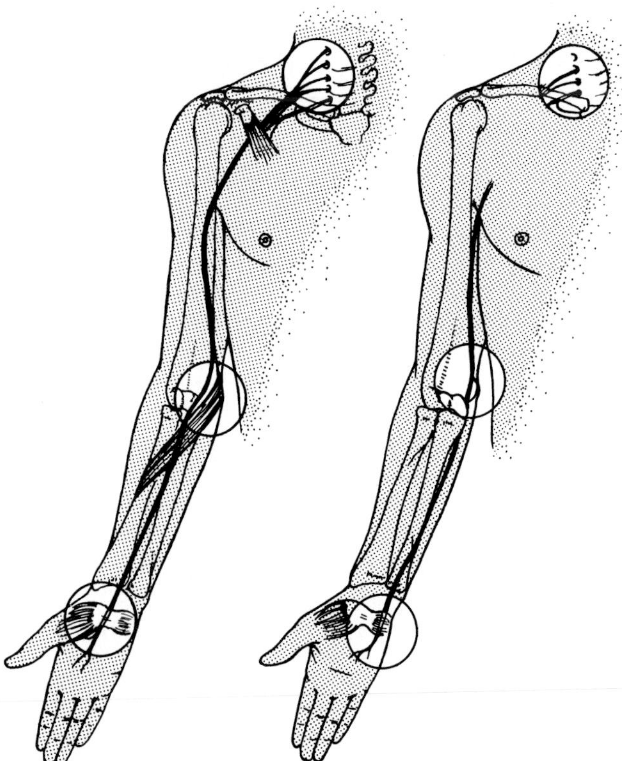

FIGURE 52–9 ■ The double crush hypothesis can be extrapolated to a multiple crush hypothesis. At the left, carpal tunnel is associated with median nerve compression in the forearm and cervical disk disease. At the right, thoracic outlet is associated with cubital tunnel and ulnar nerve compression in Guyon's canal.

Radiographic Findings

Films of the chest and cervical spine are helpful in revealing bony abnormalities, particularly cervical ribs, prolonged transverse processes, and bony degenerative changes. If osteophytic changes and intervertebral space narrowing are present on plain cervical films, cervical computed tomography (CT) or magnetic resonance imaging (MRI) should be performed to rule out bony encroachment and narrowing of the spinal canal and the intervertebral foramina (Rapoport, 1988).

Electrodiagnostic Testing

Sensory Testing

Just as the histopathology of chronic nerve compression spans a broad spectrum, so will the patient's clinical findings. Initially, patients may be completely asymptomatic at rest and become symptomatic only with positional or pressure provocative maneuvers. With time, patients may have persistent subtle abnormalities in the sensory system, which can be detected only with sensitive tests that determine the threshold of the system by vibratory or pressure threshold measurements. Eventually, there will be nerve injury and loss of nerve fibers, with loss of discriminatory function as measured with two-point discrimination.

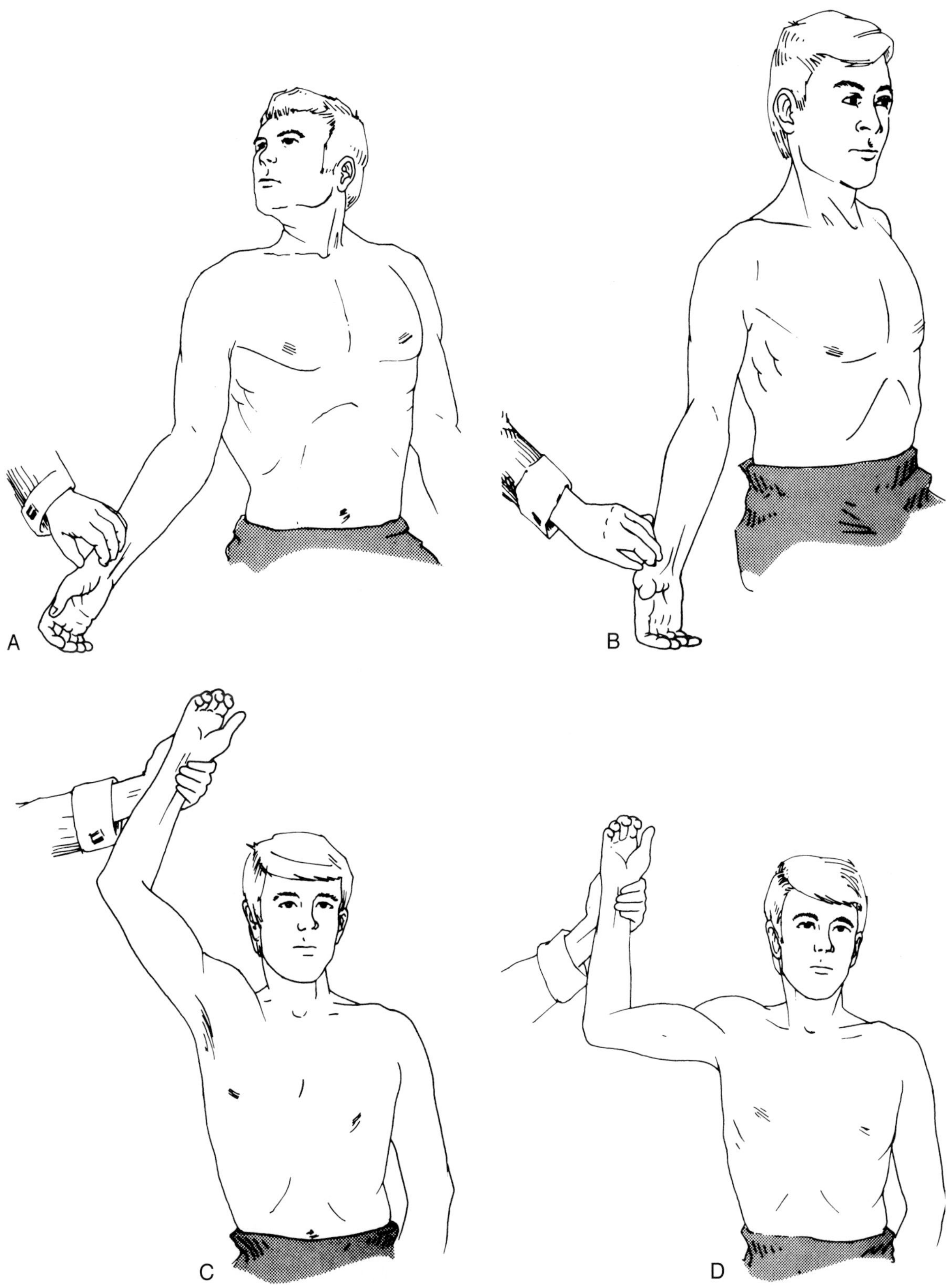

FIGURE 52–11 ■ *A*, The Adson maneuver occludes the pulse when the head is turned toward the affected side and the patient inspires deeply. Others have modified this test by turning the head to the unaffected side and requiring reproduction of the patient's symptoms. *B*, The Halstead maneuver puts the patient in a military position with the shoulders braced down to the side to obliterate the pulse. The test is now considered positive if the symptoms are reproduced. *C*, Wright described a hyperabduction maneuver to obliterate the pulse, with reproduction of the patient's symptoms being considered a positive test result. Wright suggested that the elbows are flexed. We have modified this test to keep the elbows extended, as elbow flexion will reproduce symptomatology with ulnar nerve compression in the cubital tunnel. We consider reproduction of the patient's symptoms after 1 minute of arm elevation to be a positive test result. We can decrease the time necessary for a positive test by placing digital pressure over the brachial plexus in the supraclavicular fossa. *D*, Roos' test has been modified by Roos to add a 3-minute stress test of rapidly opening and closing the hand. The test is positive if the patient's symptoms are reproduced. (From Luoma A, Nelems B: Thoracic outlet syndrome. thoracic surgery perspective. Neurosurg Clin N Am 2:187, 1991.)

Recent efforts have been directed toward developing tests to evaluate sensory function in the hand. The accepted tests and the correlation between these tests and the fiber receptor system are understood.

Provocative tests are used to elicit symptoms from a patient who is asymptomatic at rest. These include percussion of the nerve (Tinel's sign) and pressure and positional provocative tests. In patients with thoracic outlet syndrome, these tests are performed at the common nerve entrapment sites in the upper extremity (carpal tunnel, median nerve in the forearm, cubital tunnel, and brachial plexus). The examiner percusses over the nerve with four to six taps, and the presence or absence of a tingling sensation within the distribution of that nerve is recorded (Tinel's sign). Movement and pressure provocative tests are applied for a total of 60 seconds and are considered positive if paresthesia, numbness, or pain occurs in the appropriate nerve distribution. Movement provocative tests include arm elevation, elbow flexion, and wrist flexion (Phalen's sign). The pressure provocative tests include direct pressure with the examiner's fingertips on the brachial plexus, the ulnar nerve in the cubital tunnel, and the median nerve in the proximal forearm and just proximal to the carpal tunnel (Fig. 52–12). A rest period of approximately 1 minute is permitted between each test to allow return to the asymptomatic state.

Several instruments can be used to measure vibration thresholds (Fig. 52–13*A*,*B*). The threshold of the rapidly adapting fiber receptor system can be assessed both qualitatively with a tuning fork and quantitatively with a vibrometer. The "wrong end" of a 256-cps tuning fork is held against the skin. This end of the tuning fork is used to provide adequate amplitude for perception of the stimulus. A fixed-frequency (120-cps) variable-amplitude Vibratron II (Sensortek, Clifton, NJ) can be used to quantify the threshold of the quickly adapting fibers. The vibrating portion of the Vibratron II is placed against the skin, and the smallest stimulus perceived is identified as the baseline vibration threshold and recorded in micrometers of motion. (Variable-frequency, variable-amplitude vibrometers are also available and provide a "vibrogram" of the patient's response to a number of frequencies of vibration. Because the higher frequencies of vibration are the most sensitive to nerve compression, such an instrument is potentially of interest in evaluating patients with thoracic outlet syndrome.)

Pressure thresholds can be assessed quantitatively with Semmes-Weinstein monofilaments. These nylon monofilaments are applied perpendicular to the cutaneous surface, and pressure is increased until bending of the monofilament is observed. Probes of increasing weight are used, with the lightest monofilament marked 1.65 and the heaviest marked 6.65. The number of the probe on the filament represents the logarithm of 10 times the force in tenths of a milligram that is required to bow the monofilament. The number of the lightest probe that will elicit perception and localization of pressure is recorded (Fig. 52–13*C*).

Assessment of innervation density provides an indication of the number of innervated receptors. The innervation density of the slowly adapting receptors is measured by a static two-point discrimination test, and that of the rapidly adapting receptors is measured by a moving two-point discrimination test. Moving and static two-point discrimination are assessed with a Disk-Criminator (Neuroregen, Baltimore, MD). The moving discrimination test is carried out by slowly moving the prongs of the Disk-Criminator longitudinally with just enough pressure to elicit a response. The subject is then asked to identify if one or two prongs are felt. The smallest spacing at which the subject is able to correctly identify two of three trials is recorded in millimeters (Fig. 52–14). The simple analogy shown in Figure 52–15 helps to describe and understand the relationship between innervation density and threshold and the tests used to measure sensibility. Measurement of two-point discrimination is the standard accepted measurement of sensibility by hand surgeons and hand therapists.

In a prospective study we evaluated 50 patients whom

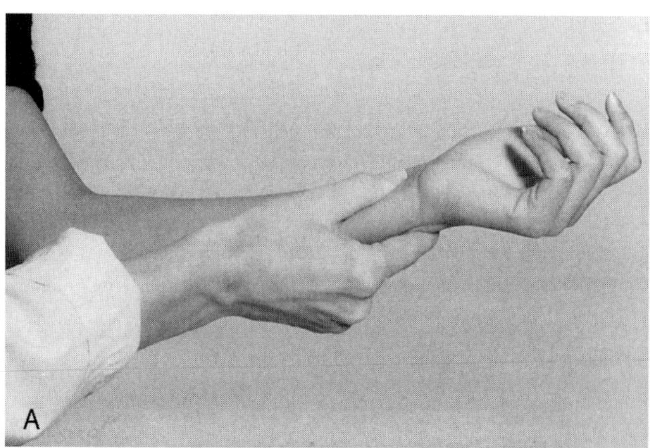

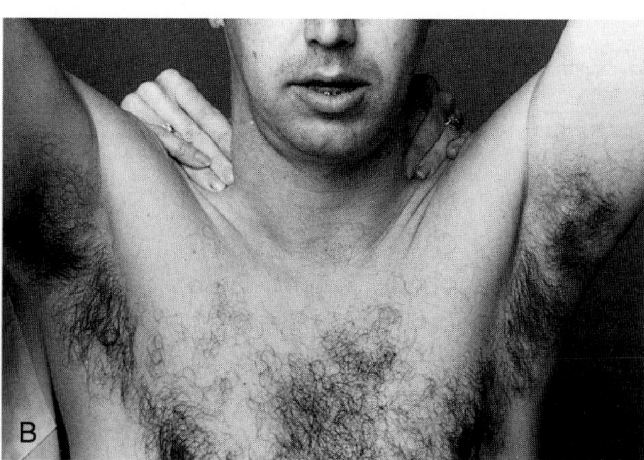

FIGURE 52–12 ■ *A*, Pressure provocative tests can be used to reproduce symptomatology; in particular, pressure over the median nerve just proximal to the carpal tunnel will produce paresthesia in the distribution of the median nerve within just a few seconds if the carpal tunnel syndrome is present. This similar test can be used to evaluate cubital tunnel syndrome with pressure over the ulnar nerve in the cubital tunnel. *B*, Pressure over the brachial plexus and supraclavicular fossa will produce paresthesia in the hand in patients with thoracic outlet syndrome. Symptoms can be accelerated by combining this with elevation of the upper extremities above the head.

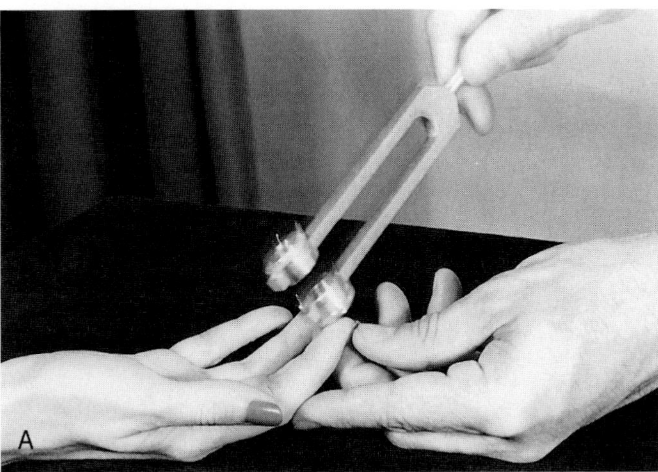

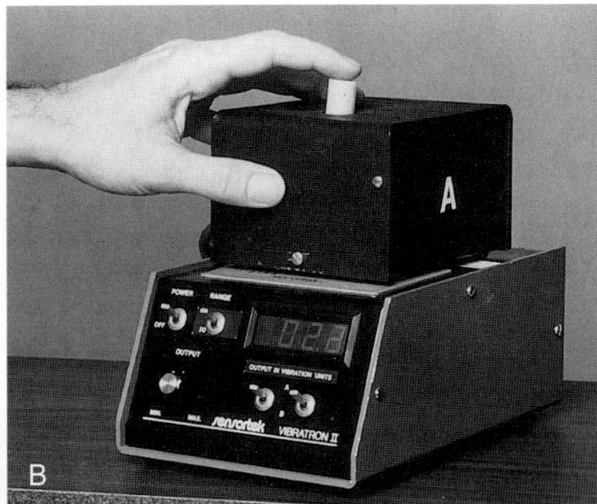

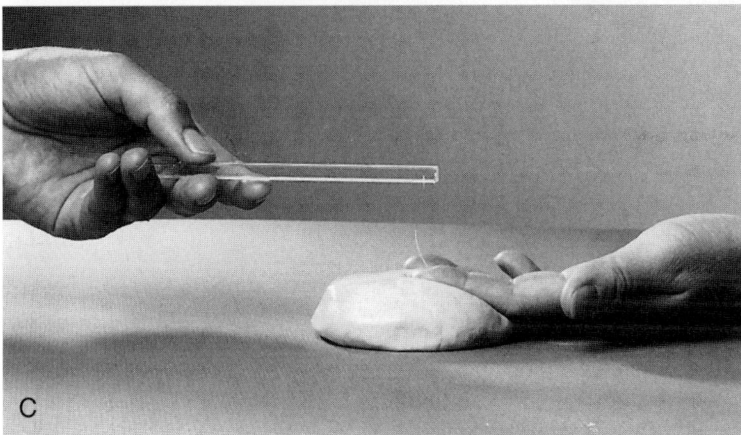

FIGURE 52–13 ■ *A*, Threshold testing includes vibration and pressure assessment. Response to vibration can be measured qualitatively with a tuning fork. *B*, Vibration thresholds can be measured quantitatively with a fixed-frequency variable-amplitude vibrometer. *C*, Pressure thresholds are measured with Semmes-Weinstein monofilaments. (From Mackinnon SE, Dellon AL: Surgery of the Peripheral Nerve. New York, Thieme, 1988.)

we believed to have thoracic outlet syndrome. The physical examination included provocative tests (positional, percussion [Tinel], and compressive) and sensory evaluation (baseline and postprovocative vibration thresholds and two-point discrimination). In 47 (94%) of these patients, provocative position and compression tests were positive (see clinical test No. 5 listed earlier) (Fig. 52–16), and two-point discrimination was normal in 49 (98%). Measurements of sensory thresholds during provocation of symptoms were significantly elevated as compared with thresholds measured at rest.

Somatosensory Potentials

Somatosensory evoked potentials (SSEPs) have been suggested in the diagnosis of thoracic outlet syndrome to

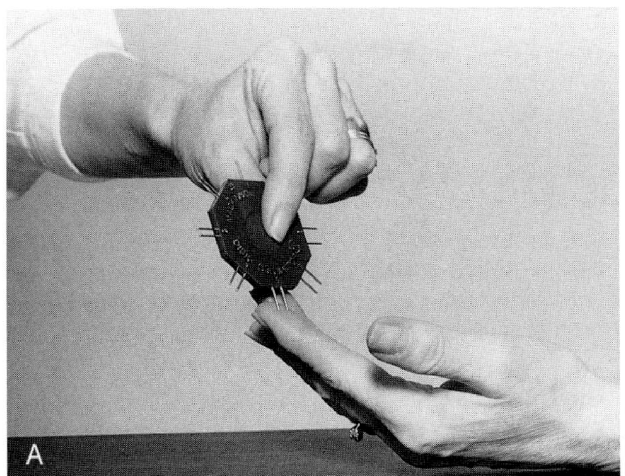

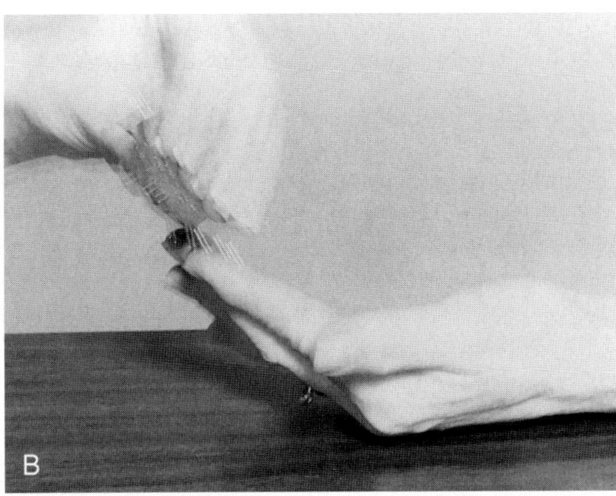

FIGURE 52–14 ■ *A*, Two-point discrimination is measured with a Disk-Criminator. *B*, Moving two-point discrimination is measured by moving the two prongs of the Disk-Criminator across the surface of the skin. (From Mackinnon SE, Delon AL: Surgery of the Peripheral Nerve. New York, Thieme, 1988.)

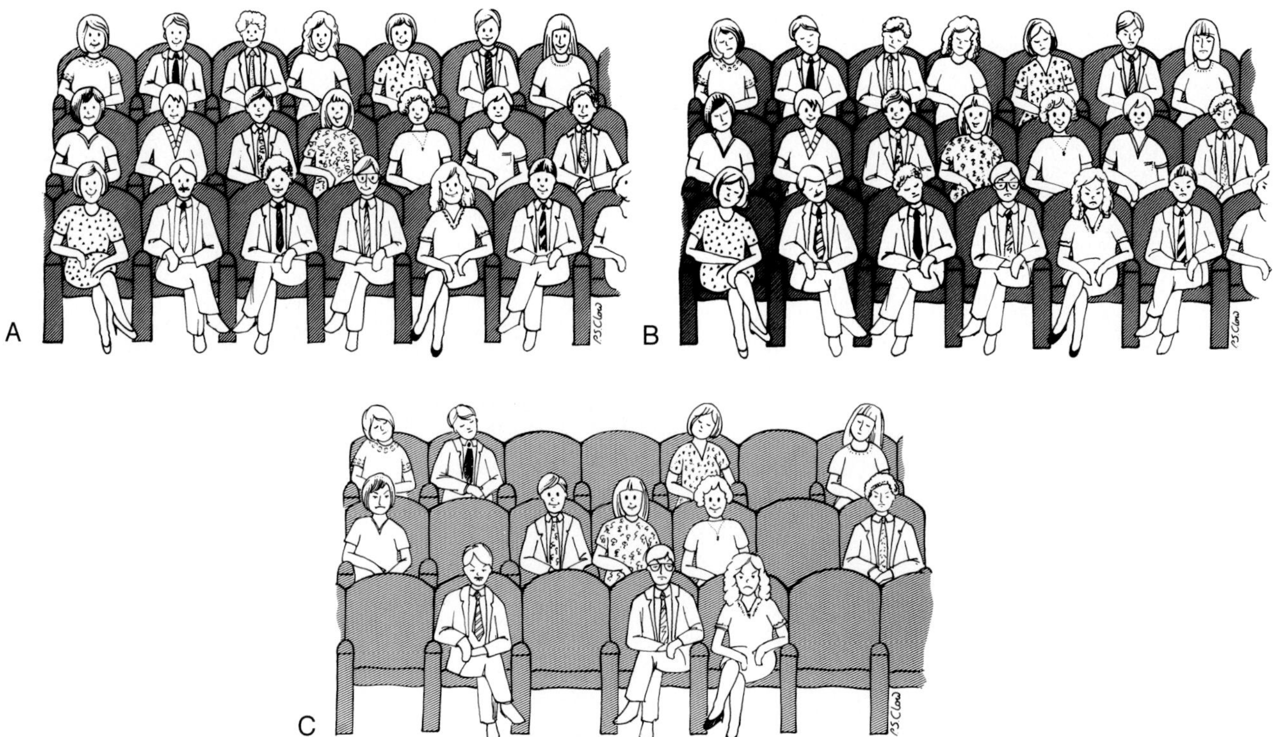

FIGURE 52–15 ■ *A,* A simple analogy helps to describe the relationship between innervation density and threshold. If each person in the audience is considered as a single-fiber sensory receptor unit, the number of people present in the audience can be considered the innervation density. A test of threshold will evaluate the "status, health, or wellbeing" of the individual. If all the seats in the auditorium are full and the individuals in the audience are "awake and content," all testing for fiber receptor function (both innervation density and threshold tests) will be normal. *B,* Threshold testing will be abnormal (vibration and Semmes-Weinstein monofilaments) if the individuals are not "awake and content" but are "asleep or unhappy." It will take more effort (i.e., greater pressure, larger amplitude) to "wake up" these sleepy receptors. Moving and static two-point discrimination will be normal because all members of the audience are present and eventually will respond to stimulation. *C,* If individuals in the audience vacate the auditorium, the innervation density testing (two-point discrimination) will be abnormal. If the remaining individuals are other than happy and content, the threshold tests will be abnormal as well. (From Mackinnon SE: Peripheral nerve injuries in the hand. In Vistnes LM (ed): How They Do It: Procedures in Plastic and Reconstructive Surgery. Boston, Little, Brown, 1991, p. 321.)

deal with the proximal location of the compressive problem. Machleder and associates (1987) demonstrated in a group of 80 patients with thoracic outlet syndrome that 74% had abnormal SSEPs. Similarly, Yiannikas and Walsh (1983) found SSEPs to be useful in the diagnosis. By contrast, Borg and colleagues (1988) found SSEPs to be abnormal only in patients with positive clinical signs. Both Borg and colleagues and Machleder and associates stressed the dynamic nature of this compressive neuropathy by suggesting SSEP assessment in first neutral and then stressed positions. We have evaluated patients with thoracic outlet syndrome and found SSEPs not to be useful in this patient population (Komanetsky, 1996).

Nerve Conduction Velocities

Determination of nerve conduction velocities is a widely used test in differential diagnosis of the etiologies of arm pain, tingling, and numbness with or without motor weakness of the hand. Such symptoms may result from compression at various sites: in the spine; at the thoracic outlet; around the elbow, where it causes ulnar nerve palsy; or on the volar aspect of the wrist, where it produces carpal tunnel syndrome. One author (HCU) relies on the ulnar nerve conduction velocity; the other two authors (SEM, GAP) do not. For completeness it is reviewed in detail. For diagnosis and localization of the site of compression, cathodal stimulation is applied at various points along the course of the nerve (Razzuk et al, in press). Motor conduction velocities of the ulnar, median, radial, and musculocutaneous nerves can be measured reliably (Jebsen, 1967). Caldwell and associates (1971) have improved the technique of measuring ulnar nerve conduction velocity for evaluation of patients with thoracic outlet compression. Conduction velocities over proximal and distal segments of the ulnar nerve are determined by recording the acting potentials generated in the hypothenar or first dorsal interosseous muscle. The points of stimulation are the supraclavicular fossa, middle upper arm, below the elbow, and at the wrist (Urschel and Razzuk, 1972). Electromyography is usually normal in thoracic outlet syndrome.

Measuring Equipment. Electromyographic examination of each upper extremity and determination of conduction velocities are performed with the Meditron 201 AD or 312 electromyograph; a coaxial cable with three needles or surface electrodes is used to record muscle potentials, which appear on the fluorescent screen.

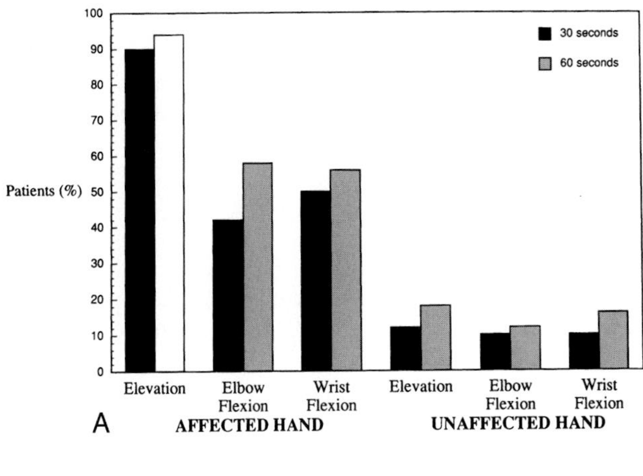

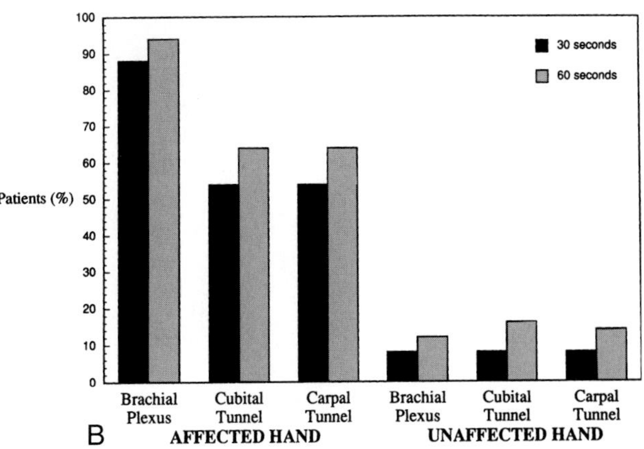

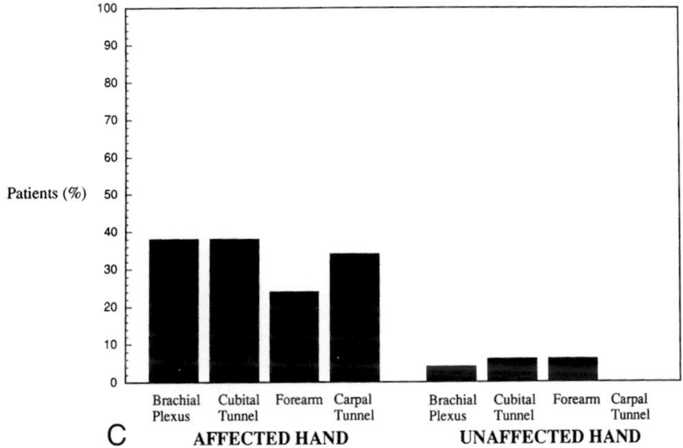

FIGURE 52–16 ■ *A*, Distribution of positive provocative movement, showing the percentage of patients represented with positive signs with each provocative movement (arm elevation to reproduce thoracic outlet symptoms, elbow flexion to reproduce cubital tunnel symptoms, and wrist flexion to reproduce carpal tunnel symptoms) within 30 seconds and the total number within 60 seconds. Both affected and unaffected hands are illustrated. *B*, Distribution of positive pressure provocative movement, showing the percentage of patients with positive signs provoked with pressure of common nerve entrapment sites within 30 seconds and the total number within 60 seconds. *C*, Distribution of positive Tinel's sign, showing the percentage of patients with a positive Tinel's sign at entrapment sites in the upper extremity (carpal tunnel, forearm, cubital tunnel, and brachial plexus). (From Novak CB, Mackinnon SE, Patterson GA et al: Evaluation of patients for thoracic outlet decompression. J Hand Surg [Am] 18:292, 1992, with permission.)

Technique. The conduction velocity is determined by the Krusen-Caldwell technique (Caldwell et al, 1971). The patient is placed on the examination table with the arm fully extended at the elbow and in about 20 degrees of abduction at the shoulder to facilitate stimulation over the course of the ulnar nerve.

The ulnar nerve is stimulated at four points by a special stimulation unit, which imparts a 350-V electrical stimulus, which is approximately equivalent to 300 V in view of the patient's skin resistance of 5000 ohms. Supramaximal stimulation is used at all points to obtain maximal response. The duration of the stimulus is 0.2 msec, except for muscular individuals, for whom it is 0.5 msec. The times of stimulation, conduction delay, and muscle response appear on the electromyograph screen; time markers occur each millisecond on the sweep.

The latency period to stimulation from the four stimulation points to the recording electrode is obtained from the TECA digital recorder or calculated from the tracing on the screen.

Calculation of Velocities. After the latencies (which are expressed in milliseconds) are obtained, the distance in millimeters between two adjacent sites of stimulation is measured with a steel tape. The velocities, which are expressed in meters per second, are calculated by subtracting the distal latency from the proximal latency and dividing the distance between two points of stimulation by the latency difference (Fig. 52–17) according to the formula

$$\text{Velocity (m/sec)} = \text{distance between two adjacent stimulation points (mm)} \div \text{difference in latency (ms)}$$

Normal Ulnar Nerve Conduction Velocities. The normal values of the ulnar nerve conduction velocities according to the Krusen-Caldwell technique (Caldwell et al, 1971) are 72 m/sec or more across the outlet; 55 m/sec or more around the elbow; and 59 m/sec or more in the forearm. Wrist delay is 2.5 to 3.5 msec. Decreased velocity in a segment of increased delay at the wrist indicates compression, injury, neuropathy, or neurologic disorders. Decreased velocity across the outlet is consistent with thoracic outlet syndrome, and decreased velocity around the elbow signifies ulnar nerve entrapment or neuropathy.

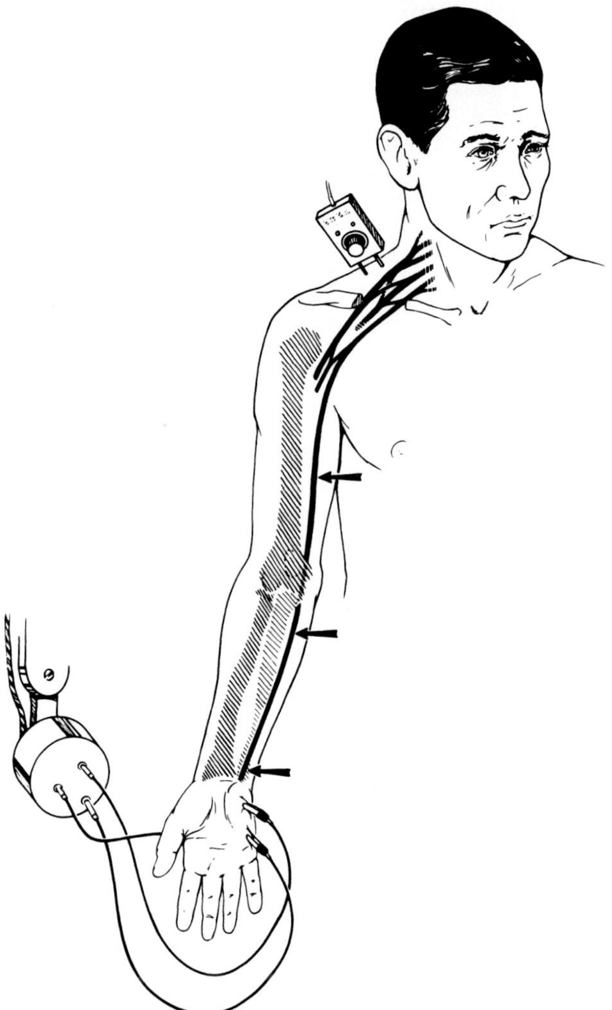

FIGURE 52–17 ■ Technique for stimulating and recording during the evaluation of nerve conduction velocities.

Increased delay at the wrist is encountered in carpal tunnel syndrome.

Grading of Compression. The clinical picture of thoracic outlet syndrome correlates fairly well with the conduction velocity across the outlet. Any value less than 70 m/sec indicates neurovascular compression. The severity is graded according to decrease of velocity across the thoracic outlet: compression is called slight when the velocity is 66 to 69 m/sec, mild when the velocity is 60 to 65 m/sec, moderate when the velocity is 55 to 59 m/sec, and severe when the velocity is 54 m/sec or less.

Angiography

Simple clinical observations usually suffice to determine the degree of vascular impairment in the upper extremity. Peripheral angiography (Lang, 1962; Rosenberg, 1966) is indicated in some cases, as in the presence of a paraclavicular pulsating mass, the absence of radial pulse, or the presence of supraclavicular or infraclavicular bruits. Retrograde or antegrade arteriograms of the subclavian and brachial arteries should be obtained to demonstrate or localize the pathology (Figs. 52–18 and 52–19). In cases of venous stenosis or obstruction, as in Paget-Schroetter syndrome, phlebograms are used to determine the extent of thrombosis and the status of the collateral circulation.

Differential Diagnoses

The thoracic outlet syndrome should be differentiated from various neurologic, vascular, cardiac, pulmonary, and esophageal conditions (Rosati and Lord, 1961; Urschel et al, 1973).

Neurologic causes of pain in the shoulder and arm are more difficult to recognize and may arise from involvement of the nerve roots, the brachial plexus, or the peripheral nerves. A common neurologic cause of pain in the upper extremities is a herniated cervical intervertebral disk. The herniation almost invariably occurs at the interspace between the fifth and sixth or the sixth and seventh cervical vertebrae and produces characteristic symptoms. Onset of pain and stiffness of the neck is manifested with varying frequency. The pain radiates along the medial border of the scapula into the shoulder, occasionally into the anterior chest wall, and down the lateral aspect of the arm, into the fingers. Numbness and paresthesias in the fingers may be present. The segmental distribution of pain is a prominent feature. A herniated disk between the C5 and C6 vertebrae, which compresses the C6 nerve root, causes pain or numbness primarily in the thumb and to a lesser extent in the index finger. The biceps muscle and the radial wrist extensor may be weak, and the reflex of the biceps muscle is reduced or abol-

DIFFERENTIAL DIAGNOSES

Neurologic Phenomena

Cervical spine: ruptured intervertebral disk, degenerative disease, osteoarthritis, spinal cord tumors

Brachial plexus: superior sulcus tumors, trauma-postural palsy

Peripheral nerves: entrapment neuropathy, carpal tunnel-median nerve, ulnar nerve-elbow, radial nerve, suprascapular nerve, medical neuropathies, trauma, tumor

Vascular Phenomena

Arterial: arteriosclerosis-aneurysm (occlusive), thromboangiitis obliterans, embolism, functional (Raynaud's disease), reflex (vasomotor dystrophy), causalgia, vasculitis, collagen disease, panniculitis

Venous: thrombophlebitis, mediastinal venous obstruction (malignant or benign)

Other Diseases

Angina pectoris

Esophageal

Pulmonary

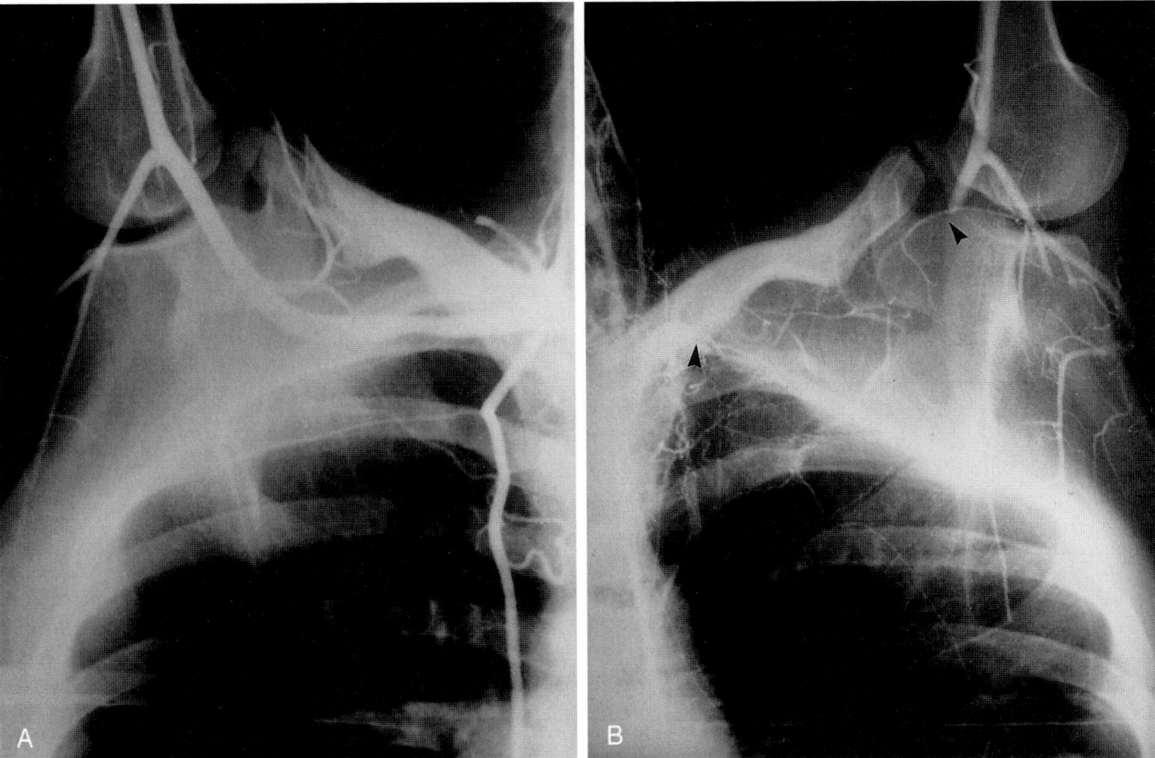

FIGURE 52–18 ■ In a patient with symptoms of vascular compression in the left upper extremity, an arteriogram with both arms elevated demonstrated a patent subclavian artery in the right arm (*A*) and occlusion of the subclavian in the left arm (*B*) (*arrows*). (Courtesy of P. M. Weeks, MD, Washington University School of Medicine, St. Louis.)

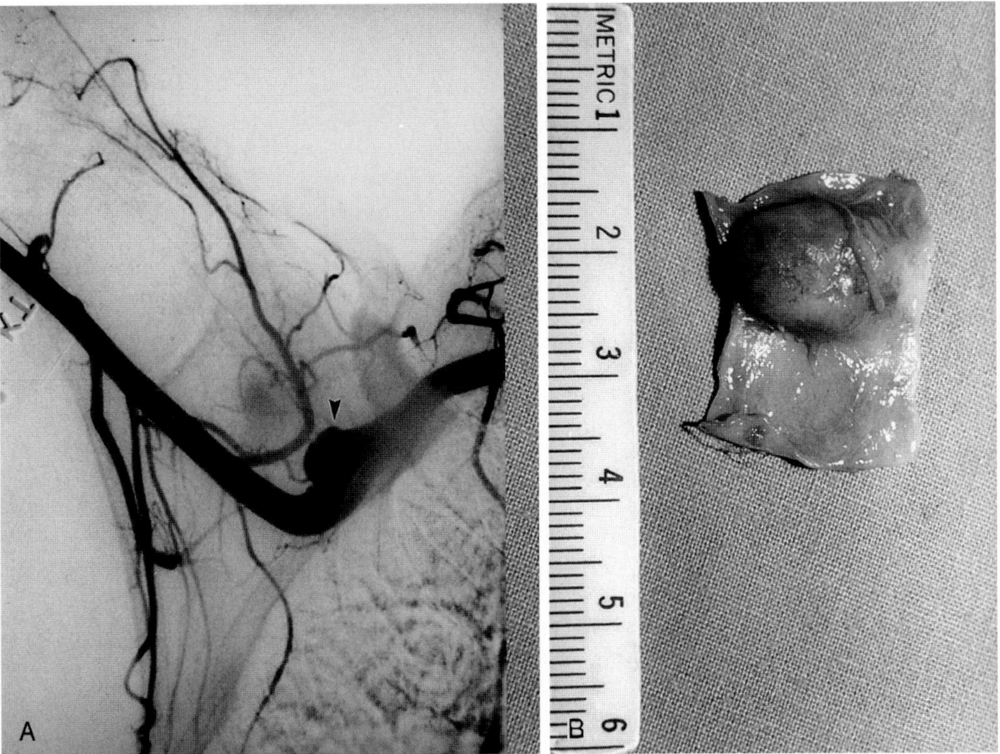

FIGURE 52–19 ■ Evaluation of vascular thoracic outlet syndrome using an arteriogram may demonstrate unusual findings such as this aneurysm (*A*) (*arrow*), which was excised at surgery (*B*). (Courtesy of J. J. McDonough, MD, Cincinnati.)

ished. A herniated disk between the C6 and C7 vertebrae, which compresses the C7 nerve root, produces pain or numbness in the index finger and weakness of index finger flexion and ulnar wrist extension; the triceps muscle is weak, and its reflex is reduced or abolished. Any of these herniated disks may cause numbness along the ulnar border of the arm and hand due to spasm of the scalenus anticus muscle. Rarely, pain and paresthesias in the ulnar distribution may be related to herniation between the C7 and T1 vertebrae, which causes compression of the C8 nerve root. Compression of the C8 and T1 nerve roots produces weakness of intrinsic hand muscles (Krusen, 1968; Rosati and Lord, 1961). Although rupture of the fifth and sixth disks produces hypesthesia in this area, only rupture of the seventh disk produces pain down the medial aspect of the arm (Rosati and Lord, 1961).

The diagnosis of a ruptured cervical disk is based primarily on the history and physical findings; lateral films of the cervical spine reveal loss or reversal of cervical curvature, with the apex of the reversal of curvature at the level of the disk involved. Electromyography can localize the site and extent of the nerve root irritation. When a herniated disk is suspected, cervical myelography should be done to confirm the diagnosis (Krusen, 1968; Rosati and Lord, 1961).

Another condition that causes upper extremity pain is cervical spondylosis, a degenerative disease of the intervertebral disk and the adjacent vertebral margin that causes spur formation and the production of ridges into the spinal canal or intervertebral foramina. Radiographs, a CT scan of the cervical spine, and electromyography help in making the diagnosis of this condition.

Several arterial and venous conditions can be confused with thoracic outlet syndrome; the differentiation can often be made clinically (Rosati and Lord, 1961).

In atypical patients who present with chest pain alone, it is important to suspect the thoracic outlet syndrome in addition to angina pectoris. Exercise stress testing and coronary angiography may exclude coronary artery disease when there is a high index of suspicion of angina pectoris (Urschel et al, 1973; Urschel and Razzuk, 1973b).

MANAGEMENT

Principles of Management

The initial method of management in the majority of patients with thoracic outlet syndrome is nonoperative. Patients are instructed that overhead activity aggravates their symptoms. Modifications in their job or even a job change should be attempted. Work that requires overhead activity, heavy lifting, repetitive motions, or use of vibratory tools will aggravate the thoracic outlet syndrome and discourage a good long-term surgical result. Rest periods with the arms down are recommended at intervals during the day. Particularly at night, patients tend to sleep with arms above the head, aggravating the thoracic outlet syndrome; with elbows flexed, aggravating the cubital tunnel syndrome; or with wrists off the neutral position, provoking carpal tunnel symptoms. These sleeping patterns are described to patients and their partners, and patients are encouraged to develop sleeping patterns with arms by the sides (Fig. 52–20). If patients have concomitant carpal or cubital tunnel syndrome, conservative management is directed toward these problems. In particular, night resting wrist splints to maintain the wrist in a neutral position and soft elbow pads to cushion the ulnar nerve and block extreme elbow flexion are recommended. A soft cervical collar made from two rolls of stockinette stuffed with soft gauze pads can be used. Obesity and hypertrophic breasts will aggravate thoracic outlet syndrome, and weight loss plans are recommended. Occasionally, breast reduction is indicated, and it has dramatically improved the patient's symptoms (Fig. 52–21).

Physical Therapy

Many of the symptoms of thoracic outlet syndrome are a consequence of muscle imbalance in the cervicothoracic region. A relaxed forward posture with the head anteriorly displaced in relation to the thorax will result in a shortening of the flexor muscles, weakness of the extensor muscles, and subsequent loss of the cervical lordosis. We follow Mackenzie's approach (1983) and recognize

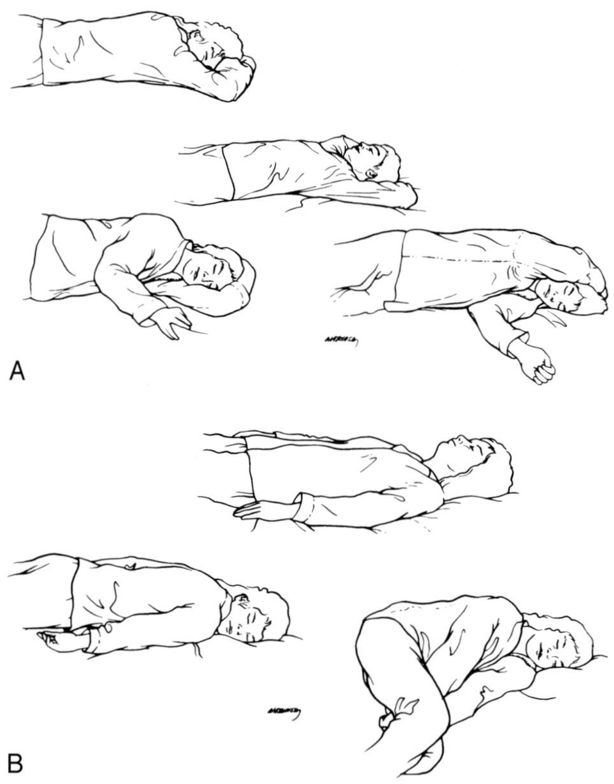

FIGURE 52–20 ■ *A*, Certain positions of the extremities put particular nerves at risk for increased pressure. Especially at night, patients assume these postures. Flexion or extension of the wrist aggravates carpal tunnel syndrome, elbow flexion aggravates cubital tunnel syndrome, and elevation of the arms above the head aggravates thoracic outlet symptoms. The sleeping positions illustrated put the nerves at risk for compression. *B*, Patients should be advised to train themselves to sleep with their arms by their sides and their wrists in neutral.

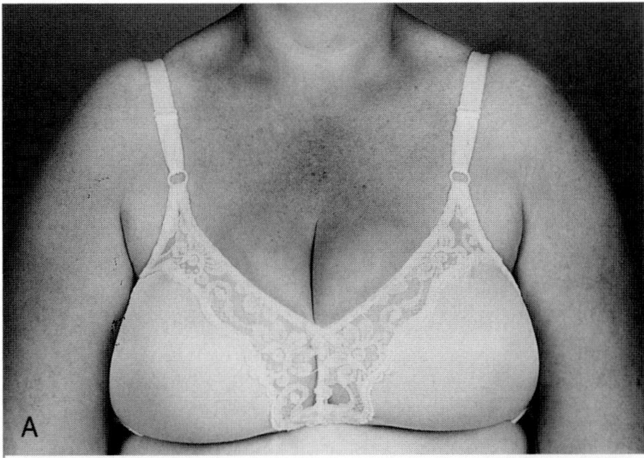

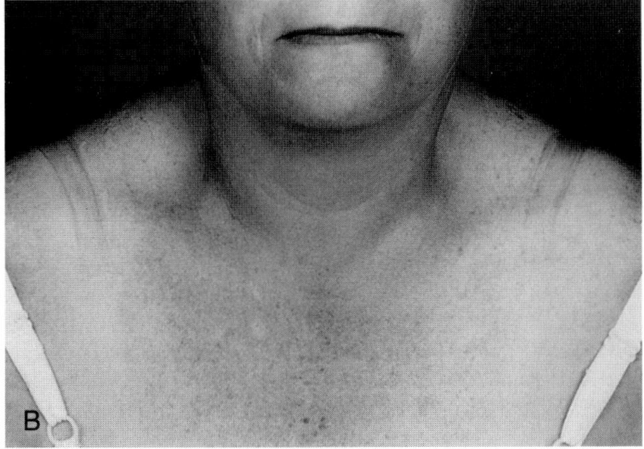

FIGURE 52–21 ■ *A*, Occasionally, breast hypertrophy can be a factor in producing thoracic outlet syndrome. In some patients breast reduction can dramatically reduce symptoms. *B*, Note the strap marks on the patient's shoulders, which, although not directly over the brachial plexus, offer evidence for chronic downward pressure on the shoulders.

three factors that predispose to pain in this region, namely, faulty posture, an increased frequency of cervical flexion, and loss of extension. Exercises are recommended to increase neck retraction and correct the cervical lordosis. In addition to postural abnormalities, muscle imbalance is addressed. Muscular assessment will identify muscle imbalance patterns (weakness versus tightness) and also identify referred pain patterns via trigger points. Muscle imbalance occurs when some muscles become tight while others become weak.

Janda (1988) has described a proximal crossed syndrome in the upper extremity in patients with thoracic outlet syndrome in which the pectoralis major and minor, upper trapezius, scalene, and sternocleidomastoid muscles become tight. Weakness occurs in the scapular stabilizers, including the middle and lower trapezius, rhomboid, and serratus anterior muscles. Tightness of the scalene muscles is well recognized as a major contributor to nerve compression of the brachial plexus. Muscles that exhibit decreased range of motion or strength can be evaluated for the presence of hyperirritable fossae (myofascial trigger points).

Patients with very tight and tender scalenes may benefit from local anesthetic or botulism toxin block of the scalene muscles at their insertion at the first rib. Travell and Simons (1983) have described a technique for the treatment of trigger points, including stretching and spraying with Fluori-Methane. With a decrease in the irritability of the lesion, more aggressive stretching can be implemented, including hold-relaxed techniques (maximal contraction followed by maximal relaxation). Once control of pain and improved range of motion are achieved, a progressive strengthening program is instituted, which is directed toward the scapular stabilizers, the upper back, and the posture muscles of the cervical spine (middle and lower trapezius, rhomboids, and serratus anterior). During these strengthening exercises, the stretching and range of motion program is maintained. A successful, conservative physical therapy program for thoracic outlet syndrome requires that patients incorporate these exercises into their daily routine and become responsible for their home program.

Abnormal posture patterns are demonstrated to the patients, and efforts are made to correct these. As mentioned earlier, a soft cervical collar made from two rolls of stockinette stuffed with soft gauze pads can be used, weight loss plans are recommended for obese patients, and occasionally breast reduction is indicated for patients with hypertrophic breasts.

Patients with thoracic outlet syndrome should be given physical therapy when the diagnosis is made. Proper physical therapy includes stretching of the scalenus muscles, strengthening of the middle and lower trapezius muscle and the serratus anterior muscle, and posture instruction.

If symptoms of neurovascular compression continue after physical therapy and conservative management of any associated distal entrapments, surgery can be considered. Surgical correction of associated distal entrapments is frequently preferable to first rib resection because of fewer potential complications. Surgical resection of the first rib and the cervical rib, when present, should be considered (Urschel et al, 1968, 1971; Urschel and Razzuk, 1972) when conservative management and surgical treatment of distal entrapments fail. Clagett (1962) popularized the high posterior thoracoplasty approach for first rib resection; Falconer and Li (1962) emphasized the anterior approach; and Roos (1966) introduced the transaxillary route.

Paget-Schroetter Syndrome (Effort Thrombosis)

Effort thrombosis of the axillary subclavian vein (Paget-Schroetter syndrome) is usually secondary to unusual or excessive use of the arm, in addition to the presence of one or more compressive elements in the thoracic outlet (Adams and DeWeese, 1971; Johnston, 1989).

Sir James Paget in 1875 in London and von Schroetter in 1884 in Vienna described this syndrome of thrombosis of the axillary subclavian vein. The word "effort" (Aziz et al, 1986) was added to "thrombosis" because of the frequent association with exertion, producing either direct or indirect compression of the vein. The thrombosis is caused by trauma (Cikrit et al, 1990; Coon and Willis, 1966) or unusual occupations requiring repetitive muscular activity, as has been observed in professional athletes, linotype operators, painters, and beauticians. Cold and traumatic factors such as carrying skis over the shoulder tend to increase the proclivity for thrombosis (Daskalakis and Bouhoutsos, 1980). Elements of increased thrombogenicity also increase the incidence of the problem and exacerbate its symptoms on a long-term basis.

Adams and DeWeese (1971) and DeWeese and coworkers (1970) reported long-term results in patients treated conservatively with elevation and warfarin (Coumadin). There was a 12% incidence of pulmonary embolism. Occasional venous distention developed in 18%, and late residual arm symptoms of swelling, pain, and superficial thrombophlebitis were noted in 68% of the patients (deep venous thrombosis with postphlebitic syndrome). Phlegmasia cerulea dolens was present in one patient.

For many years therapy included elevation of the arm and use of anticoagulants, with subsequent return to work. If symptoms recurred, the patient was considered for a first rib resection, with or without thrombectomy (Cooley and Wukasch, 1979; DeWeese et al, 1970), as well as resection of the scalenus anterior muscle and removal of any other compressive element in the thoracic outlet, such as the cervical rib or abnormal bands (Inahara, 1968; Prescott and Tikoff, 1979; Roos, 1989).

Recent availability of thrombolytic agents (Rubenstein and Greger, 1980; Sundqvist et al, 1981) combined with prompt surgical decompression of the neurovascular compressive elements in the thoracic outlet (Taylor et al, 1985), have reduced morbidity and the necessity for thrombectomy and have substantially improved clinical results, including the ability to return to work (Urschel and Razzuk, 2000).

One advantage of urokinase over streptokinase is the direct action of urokinase on the thrombosis distal to the catheter, producing a local thrombolytic effect (Becker et al, 1983; Drury et al, 1984; Eisenbud et al, 1990). Streptokinase produces a systemic effect involving potential complications. Heparin decreases the need for thrombectomy after use of the thrombolytic agent followed by aggressive surgical intervention; this is another advantage, because some of the long-term disability is related to morbidity from thrombectomy as well as to recurrent thrombosis (Campbell et al, 1977; Drapanas and Curran, 1966; Painter and Karpf, 1984).

The natural history of Paget-Schroetter syndrome suggests moderate morbidity (Tilney et al, 1970) with conservative treatment alone. Bypass with vein or other conduits (Hansen et al, 1985; Hashmonai et al, 1976; Jacobson and Haimov, 1977) has limited application. Causes other than thoracic outlet syndrome must be treated individually (Loring, 1952). Intermittent obstruction of the subclavian vein (McLaughlin, 1939) can lead to thrombosis, and decompression should be employed prophylactically (Hashmonai et al, 1976; Jacobson and Haimov, 1977).

Surgical Management

Several routes have been described to remove the first rib, including posterior, transaxillary, supraclavicular, infraclavicular, transthoracic, and through the bed of the resected clavicle.

Surgical Results

A definitive review of the surgical management of thoracic outlet syndrome has been published by Sanders (1991). Sanders concludes that transaxillary first rib resection, scalenotomy, and supraclavicular first rib resection with scalenotomy give essentially the same results (Fig. 52–22). This is contradicted by Urschel and Razzuk's (1998) study and other long-term follow-up studies (longer than 10 years) of scalenectomy alone, which demonstrate a 65% recurrence rate.

Urschel's results after 20 years show 79% good results with complete rib resection and only 33% good results with scalenectomy. Failure to completely remove the most posterior aspect of the first rib is the most likely cause for recurrence and best explains poor long-term results (Martinez, 1979).

Reoperation for Recurrent Thoracic Outlet Syndrome

Extirpation of the first rib frequently relieves symptoms in patients with thoracic outlet syndrome not relieved by

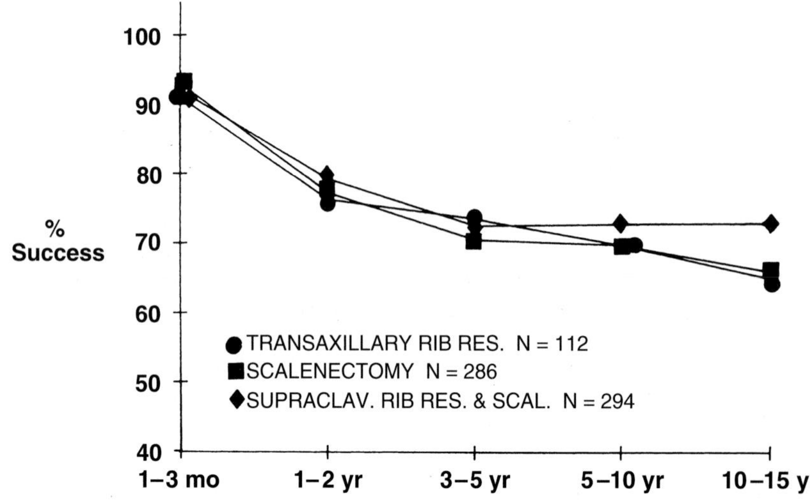

FIGURE 52–22 ■ Results of the three primary operations for thoracic outlet syndrome. (From Sanders RJ: Thoracic Outlet Syndrome: A Common Sequela of Neck Injuries. Philadelphia, JB Lippincott, 1991.)

physical therapy. Of the surgically treated patients, 10% develop various degrees of shoulder, arm, and hand pain and paresthesias; these are usually mild and short-lasting and respond well to a brief course of physical therapy and muscle relaxants. In some patients, symptoms persist, become progressively more severe, and often involve a wider area of distribution. Symptoms may recur 1 month to 7 years after rib resection but usually within the first 6 months. Symptoms consist of an aching or burning type of pain, often associated with paresthesias, involving the neck, shoulder, parascapular area, anterior chest wall, arm, and hand. Vascular lesions are uncommon and consist of an occasional injury of the subclavian artery, with subsequent false aneurysm formation caused by the sharp edge of a remaining posterior stump of an incompletely resected first rib. Recurrence is diagnosed on the basis of history, physical examination, and decreased nerve conduction velocity across the outlet. Diagnostic evaluation should also include thorough neurologic evaluation, chest and cervical spine radiography, cervical myelography, and subclavian artery angiography, when indicated.

Two groups of patients who require reoperation can be identified. "Pseudorecurrence" has been noted in patients who did not have relief of symptoms after the initial operation. These patients can be identified etiologically as those in whom the second rib was mistakenly resected, leaving a rudimentary first rib. True recurrence has occurred in patients whose symptoms were relieved after the first operation but who retained a significant posterior segment of the first rib and showed excessive scar formation around the brachial plexus.

Physical therapy and pain management should be given to all patients with symptoms of neurovascular compression after first rib resection. If the symptoms persist and a psychological profile is normal, reoperation can be considered.

Reoperation for thoracic outlet syndrome can be performed via the posterior thoracoplasty approach to provide better exposure of the nerve roots and brachial plexus, which reduces the danger of injury to these structures and provides adequate exposure of the subclavian artery and vein. This incision also provides a wider field for resection of any bony abnormalities or fibrous bands and allows extensive neurolysis of the nerve roots and brachial plexus, which is not always possible with the limited exposure of the transaxillary approach. The anterior or supraclavicular approach is inadequate for reoperation.

The basic elements of reoperation include resection of persistent or recurrent bony remnants of a cervical or first rib, neurolysis of the brachial plexus and nerve roots, and dorsal sympathectomy. Sympathectomy removes T1, T2, and T3 thoracic ganglia (Smithwick, 1936; Urschel and Razzuk, 1985). Care is taken to avoid damage to the C8 ganglion (upper aspect of the stellate ganglion), which produces Horner's syndrome. The reoperation provides paresthesias in the supraclavicular and infraclavicular areas. The incidence of so-called postsympathetic syndrome has been negligible in this group of patients. A nerve stimulator is used to differentiate scar from nerve root to avoid damage from reoperation in these patients.

The results of reoperation are good if an accurate diagnosis is made and the proper procedure is used (Urschel and Razzuk, 1986b). More than 800 patients have been followed for 6 months to 15 years (Urschel 1986). All patients improved initially after reoperation, and in 79% the improvement was maintained for more than 5 years. In 14% of the patients, symptoms were managed with physical therapy, but 7% required a second reoperation, in every case because of rescarring. There were no deaths, and only one patient had an infection that required drainage.

SUMMARY

Thoracic outlet syndrome is recognized in approximately 8% of the population. Its manifestations may be neurologic, vascular, or both, depending on the component of the neurovascular bundle predominantly compressed. The diagnosis is suspected by reproduction of symptoms with arm elevation and the exclusion of other causes. Treatment is initially conservative, but persistence of significant symptoms, which occur in only 5% of patients with diagnosed thoracic outlet syndromes, is an indication for first rib resection. Symptoms of various degrees may recur after first rib resection in approximately 10% of patients. Most patients improve with physical therapy, and only 1.6% require reoperation. Reoperation for recurrent symptoms is done through a high posterior thoracoplasty incision in carefully selected patients (Urschel and Razzuk, 1986b, 1998).

COMMENTS AND CONTROVERSIES

Although there has been much discussion regarding the efficacy of nerve conduction velocity studies across the thoracic outlet, in my experience with over 15,000 patients, I have found that it is extremely difficult to manage patients with neurogenic thoracic outlet syndrome and pain, both primary and recurrent, without this objective diagnosis. It is absolutely essential in our practice to learn to use these techniques. It is as important as the measurement of nerve conduction velocity across the carpal tunnel.

The surgical approach selected for management of thoracic outlet syndrome varies with the experience, expertise, and skill of the operator. Our preference is to employ the supraclavicular approach for arterial reconstruction (endarterectomy and bypass) combined with the infraclavicular approach for the distal anastomosis. To use the supraclavicular approach for primary neurogenic and venous compression, the brachial plexus and vascular structures must be retracted to expose the first rib and to perform the dorsal sympathectomy that is often needed. Although certain authors have an excellent record with this approach, the standard of care shows that nerve injury is much higher with this approach than with any other approaches because of the required retraction of the brachial plexus with the "average" operator. Cosmetically, the supraclavicular approach is not as good because 80% of these patients are women.

Our preferred approach for primary neurogenic and

venous compression is the transaxillary route, in which the rib is proximal to the operator and requires no retraction of the brachial plexus or the blood vessels.

For patients with recurrent thoracic outlet syndrome who need re-operation, the supraclavicular approach may be used by skillful surgeons; however, in our experience, the easiest and safest is the posterior, high thoracoplasty, muscle-splitting incision. This allows easy resection of the posterior rib remnant that is usually present, regeneration and formation of fibrocartilage over the brachial plexus, and neurolysis of the brachial plexus as well as a dorsal sympathectomy.

H. C. U.

■ KEY REFERENCES

Clagett OT: Presidential address: Research and prosearch. J Thorac Cardiovasc Surg 44:153, 1962.

This is the classic reference explaining the anatomic and pathophysiologic basis for first rib resection to alleviate neurovascular compression in the thoracic outlet. The incision is the high posterior thoracoplasty approach.

Roos DB: Transaxillary approach for first rib resection to relieve thoracic outlet syndrome. Ann Surg 163:354, 1966.

The transaxillary approach was initially described by Atkins (1949, 1954) and popularized by Roos. The technical aspects of this approach and the pathophysiology are described.

Rosati LM, Lord JW: Neurovascular Compression Syndromes of the Shoulder Girdle. Modern Surgical Monographs. Orlando, FL, Grune & Stratton, 1961.

Frank Netter's drawings appeared first in this classic monograph demonstrating neurovascular compression. It is the preferred method for diagnosis and management of neurovascular compression syndromes.

Urschel HC Jr, Razzuk MA: Neurovascular compression in the thoracic outlet: Changing management over 50 years. Ann Surg 228:609, 1998.

Fifty years' experience with over 15,000 patients is presented with a description of improved methods of diagnosis, therapy, and outcomes.

Urschel HC Jr, Razzuk MA: Paget-Schroetter syndrome: What is the best management? Ann Thorac Surg 69:1663, 2000.

This report of the largest series of axillary subclavian vein thromboses describes the current management with urokinase thrombolysis followed by prompt first rib resection.

Urschel HC Jr, Razzuk MA, Wood RE, Paulson DL: Objective diagnosis (ulnar nerve conduction velocity) and current therapy of the thoracic outlet syndrome. Ann Thorac Surg 12:608, 1971.

The first positive objective technique for diagnosing neurologic thoracic outlet syndrome compression is detailed.

■ REFERENCES

Adams JT, DeWeese JA: Effort thrombosis of the axillary and subclavian veins. J Trauma 11:923, 1971.

Adams JT, DeWeese JA, Mahoney EB, Rob CG: Intermittent subclavian vein obstruction without thrombosis. Surgery 63:147, 1968.

Adson AW: Surgical treatment for symptoms produced by cervical ribs and the scalenus anticus muscle. Surg Gynecol Obstet 85:687, 1947.

Adson AW, Coffey IR: Cervical rib: a method of anterior approach for relief of symptoms by division of the scaleneus anticus. Ann Surg 85:839, 1927.

Atkins HJB: Peraxillary approach to the stellate and upper thoracic sympathetic ganglia. Lancet 2:1152, 1949.

Atkins HJB: Sympathectomy by the axillary approach. Lancet 1:538, 1954.

Aziz K, Straenley CJ, Whelan TJ: Effort-related axilla-subclavian vein thrombosis. Am J Surg 152:57, 1986.

Becker GJ, Holden RW, Robe FE et al: Local thrombolytic therapy for subclavian and axillary vein thrombosis. Radiology 149:419, 1983.

Borchardt M: Symptomatologie und Therapie der Halsrippen. Berl Klin Wochenschr 38:1265, 1901.

Bramwell E: Lesion of the first dorsal nerve root. Rev Neurol Psychiatr 1:236, 1903.

Brinckner WM: Brachial plexus pressure by the normal first rib. Ann Surg 85:858, 1927.

Brinckner WM, Milch H: First dorsal vertebra simulating cervical rib by maldevelopment or by pressure symptoms. Surg Gynecol Obstet 40:38, 1925.

Brintnall ES, Hyndman OR, Van Allen WM: Costoclavicular compression associated with cervical rib. Ann Surg 144:921, 1956.

Caldwell JW, Crane CR, Krusen EM: Nerve conduction studies in the diagnosis of the thoracic outlet syndrome. South Med J 64:210, 1971.

Campbell BE, Chandler JG, Tegtmeyer CJ: Axillary, subclavian and brachiocephalic vein obstruction. Surgery 82:816, 1977.

Cikrit DF, Dalsing MC, Bryahd BJ et al: An experience with upper extremity vascular trauma. Am J Surg 160:229, 1990.

Clagett OT: Presidential address: Research and prosearch. J Thorac Cardiovasc Surg 44:153, 1962.

Cooley DA, Wukasch DC: Techniques in Vascular Surgery. Philadelphia, WB Saunders, 1979.

Coon WW, Willis PW: Thrombosis of axillary subclavian veins. Arch Surg 94:657, 1966.

Coote H: Pressure on the axillary vessels and nerve by an exostosis from a cervical rib; interference with the circulation of the arm; removal of the rib and exostosis, recovery. Med Times Gaz 2:108, 1861.

Daskalakis E, Bouhoutsos J: Subclavian and axillary vein compression of musculoskeletal origin. Br J Surg 67:573, 1980.

DeWeese JA, Adams JT, Gaiser DI: Subclavian venous thrombectomy. Circulation 16(Suppl 2):158, 1970.

Drapanas T, Curran W: Thrombectomy in the treatment of "effort" thrombosis of the axillary and subclavian veins. J Trauma 6:107, 1966.

Drury EM, Trout HH, Giordono JM et al: Lytic therapy in the treatment of axillary and subclavian vein thrombosis. J Vasc Surg 2:821, 1984.

Eisenbud DE, Brener BJ, Shoenfeld R et al: Treatment of acute vascular occlusions with intra-arterial urokinase. Am J Surg 160:160, 1990.

Falconer MA, Li FWP: Resection of the first rib in costoclavicular compression of the brachial plexus. Lancet 1:59, 1962.

Falconer MA, Weddell G: Costoclavicular compression of the subclavian artery and vein: Relation to scalenus syndrome. Lancet 2:539, 1943.

Galbraith NF, Urschel HC Jr, Wood RE et al: Fracture of first rib associated with laceration of subclavian artery: Report of a case and review of literature. J Thorac Cardiovasc Surg 65:4, 1973.

Ganong WF: Review of Medical Physiology, 3rd ed. East Norwalk, CT, Appleton & Lange, 1967.

Halsted WS: An experimental study of circumscribed dilation of an artery immediately distal to a partially occluding band, and its bearing on the dilation of the subclavian artery observed in certain cases of cervical rib. J Exp Med 24:271, 1916.

Hansen B, Feins RS, Detman DE: Simple extra-anatomic jugular vein bypass for subclavian vein thrombosis. J Vasc Surg 2:291, 1985.

Hashmonai M, Schramek A, Farbstein J: Cephalic vein cross-over bypass for subclavian vein thrombosis: A case report. Surgery 80:563, 1976.

Inahara T: Surgical treatment of "effort" thrombosis of the axillary and subclavian veins. Am Surg 34:479, 1968.

Jacobson JH, Haimov M: Venous revascularization of the arm: Report of three cases. Surgery 81:599, 1977.

Janda V: Muscles and cervicogenic pain syndromes. In Grant R (ed): Physical Therapy of the Cervical and Thoracic Spine. New York, Churchill Livingstone, 1988.

Jebsen RH: Motor conduction velocities in the median and ulnar nerves. Arch Phys Med Rehabil 48:185, 1967.

Johnston KW: Neurovascular conditions involving the upper extremity. In Rutherford RB (ed): Vascular Surgery, 3rd ed. Philadelphia, WB Saunders, 1989, p 801.

Keen WW: The symptomatology, diagnosis and surgical treatment of cervical ribs. Am J Sci 133:173, 1907.

Komanetsky RM, Novak CB, Mackinnon SE et al: Somatosensory

evoked potentials fail to diagnose thoracic outlet syndrome. J Hand Surg [Am] 21:622, 1996.
Krusen EM: Cervical pain syndromes. Arch Phys Med Rehabil 49:376, 1968.
Kuntz A: Distribution of the sympathetic rami to the brachial plexus. Arch Surg 15:871, 1927.
Lang EK: Roentgenographic diagnosis of the neurovascular compression syndromes. Audiology 79:58, 1962.
Law AA: Adventitious ligaments simulating cervical ribs. Ann Surg 72:497, 1920.
Litwin MS: Postsympathectomy neuralgia. Arch Surg 84:591, 1962.
Lord JW, Urschel HC: Total claviculectomy. Surg Rounds 11:17, 1988.
Loring WE: Venous thrombosis in the upper extremity as a complication of myocardial failure. Am J Med 397, 1952.
Machleder HI, Moll F, Nuwer M, Jordan S: Somatosensory evoked potentials in the assessment of thoracic outlet syndrome. J Vasc Surg 6:177, 1987.
Mackenzie RA: Treat Your Own Neck. Waikanes, New Zealand, Spinal Publications, 1983.
Mackinnon SE: Thoracic outlet syndrome: Introduction. Semin Thorac Cardiovasc Surg 8:175, 1996.
Mackinnon SE: Thoracic outlet syndrome. Chest Surg Clin North Am 9:701, 1999.
Mackinnon SE, Dellon AL: Surgery of the Peripheral Nerve. New York, Thieme, 1988.
Mackinnon SE, Novak CB: Clinical commentary: Pathogenesis of cumulative trauma disorder. J Hand Surg [Am] 19A:873, 1994.
Martinez NS: Posterior first rib resection for total thoracic outlet syndrome decompression. Contemp Surg 15:13, 1979.
McLaughlin CW, Popma AM: Intermittent obstruction of the subclavian vein. JAMA 113:1960, 1939.
Murphy JB: Cervical rib excision: Collective review on surgery of cervical rib. Clin John B Murphy 5:227, 1916.
Murphy T: Brachial neuritis caused by pressure of first rib. Aust Med J 15:582, 1910.
Naffziger HC, Grant WT: Neuritics of the brachial plexus—mechanical in origin: The scalenus syndrome. Surg Gynecol Obstet 67:722, 1938.
Ochsner A, Gage M, DeBakey M: Scalenous anticus (Naffziger) syndrome. Am J Surg 28:699, 1935.
Paget J: Clinical Lectures and Essays. London, Longmans Green, 1875.
Painter TD, Karpf M: Deep venous thrombosis of the upper extremity: 5 years' experience at a university hospital. Angiology 35:743, 1984.
Palumbo LT: Upper dorsal sympathectomy without Horner's syndrome. Arch Surg 71:743, 1955.
Palumbo LT: Anterior transthoracic approach for upper extremity thoracic sympathectomy. Arch Surg 72:659, 1956.
Prescott SM, Tikoff G: Deep venous thrombosis of the upper extremity: A reappraisal. Circulation 59:350, 1979.
Ranney D: Thoracic outlet: An anatomical redefinition that makes clinical sense. Clin Anat 9:50, 1996.
Rapoport S, Blair DN, McCarthy SM et al: Brachial plexus: Correlation of MR imaging and CT pathologic findings. Radiology 167:161, 1988.
Ravitch MM, Steichen FM: Atlas of General Thoracic Surgery. Philadelphia, WB Saunders, 1988.
Razzuk MA, Krusen EM, Caldwell JW, Urschel HC Jr: The clinical value and technique of measuring nerve conduction velocities for thoracic outlet syndrome. In Greep JC, Lemmen HAJ, Roos DB, Urschel HC Jr (eds): Pain in Shoulder and Arm. The Hague, Martinus Nijhoff, 1979.
Rob CG, Standover A: Arterial occlusion complicating thoracic outlet compression syndrome. BMJ 2:709, 1958.
Roos DB: Transaxillary approach for first rib resection to relieve thoracic outlet syndrome. Ann Surg 163:354, 1966.
Roos DB: Thoracic outlet nerve compression. In Rutherford RB (ed): Vascular Surgery, 3rd ed. Philadelphia, WB Saunders, 1989, p 858.
Roos DB, Owens JC: Thoracic outlet syndrome. Arch Surg 93:71, 1966.
Rosati LM, Lord JW: Neurovascular Compression Syndromes of the Shoulder Girdle. Modern Surgical Monographs. Orlando, FL, Grune & Stratton, 1961.
Rosenberg JC: Arteriography demonstrations of compression syndromes of the thoracic outlet. South Med J 59:400, 1966.
Rubenstein M, Greger WP: Successful streptokinase therapy for catheter induced subclavian vein thrombosis. Arch Intern Med 140:1370, 1980.
Sanders RJ: Thoracic Outlet Syndrome: A Common Sequela of Neck Injuries. Philadelphia, JB Lippincott, 1991.
Smithwick RH: Modified dorsal sympathectomy for vascular spasm (Raynaud's disease) of the upper extremity. Ann Surg 104:339, 1936.
Stoney WS, Addlestone RB, Alford WC Jr et al: The incidence of venous thrombosis following long-term transvenous pacing. Ann Thorac Surg 22:166, 1976.
Sundqvist SB, Hedner U, Kullenberg KHE et al: Deep venous thrombosis of the arm: A study of coagulation and fibrinolysis. BMJ 283:265, 1981.
Swank WL, Simeone FA: The scalenus anticus syndrome. Arch Neurol Psychiatry 51:432, 1944.
Taylor LM, McAllister WR, Dennis DL et al: Thrombolytic therapy followed by first rib resection for spontaneous subclavian vein thrombosis. Am J Surg 149:644, 1985.
Telford ED, Mottershead S: Pressure of the cervicobrachial junction. J Bone Joint Surg Am 30:249, 1948.
Telford ED, Stopford JSB: The vascular complications of the cervical rib. Br J Surg 18:559, 1937.
Tilney NL, Griffiths HFG, Edwards EA: Natural history of major venous thrombosis of the upper extremity. Arch Surg 101:792, 1970.
Travell JG, Simons DG: Myofascial Pain and Dysfunction: The Trigger Point Manual. Baltimore, Williams & Wilkins, 1983.
Upton ARM, McComas AJ: The double crush in nerve entrapment syndromes. Lancet 2:259, 1973.
Urschel HC Jr: Reoperation for thoracic outlet syndrome. In International Trends in General Thoracic Surgery, vol 2. St. Louis, CV Mosby, 1986.
Urschel HC Jr: Thoracic outlet syndrome. In Gibbons Surgery of the Chest, 5th ed. Philadelphia, WB Saunders, 1989.
Urschel HC Jr, Cooper J: Atlas of Thoracic Surgery. New York, Churchill Livingstone, 1995.
Urschel HC Jr, Paulson DL, McNamara JJ: Thoracic outlet syndrome. Ann Thorac Surg 6:1, 1968.
Urschel HC Jr, Razzuk MA: Current management of thoracic outlet syndrome. N Engl J Med 286:21, 1972.
Urschel HC Jr, Razzuk MA: Thoracic outlet syndrome. Surg Annu 5:229, 1973.
Urschel HC Jr, Razzuk MA: Thoracic outlet syndrome. In Shields TW (ed): General Thoracic Surgery, 2nd ed. Philadelphia, Lea & Febiger, 1983.
Urschel HC Jr, Razzuk MA: Posterior thoracic sympathectomy. In Malt RA (ed): Surgical Techniques Illustrated: A Comparative Atlas. Philadelphia, WB Saunders, 1985.
Urschel HC Jr, Razzuk MA: Upper plexus thoracic outlet syndrome: Optimal therapy. Ann Thorac Surg 63:935, 1997.
Urschel HC Jr, Razzuk MA: The failed operation for thoracic outlet syndrome: The difficulty of diagnosis and management. Ann Thorac Surg 42:523, 1986b.
Urschel HC, Razzuk MA: Neurovascular compression in the thoracic outlet: Changing management over 50 years. Ann Surg 228:609, 1998.
Urschel HC Jr, Razzuk MA: Paget-Schroetter syndrome: What is the best management? Ann Thorac Surg 69:1663, 2000.
Urschel HC Jr, Razzuk MA, Albers JE et al: Reoperation for recurrent thoracic outlet syndrome. Ann Thorac Surg 21:19, 1976.
Urschel HC Jr, Razzuk MA, Hyland JW et al: Thoracic outlet syndrome masquerading as coronary artery disease. Ann Thorac Surg 16:239, 1973.
Urschel HC Jr, Razzuk MA, Wood RE, Paulson DL: Objective diagnosis (ulnar nerve conduction velocity) and current therapy of the thoracic outlet syndrome. Ann Thorac Surg 12:608, 1971.
Von Schroetter L: Erkrankungen der Gefässe. In Nothnagel (ed): Handbuch der Pathologie und Therapie. Vienna, Holder, 1884.
White JC, Smithwick RH, Simeone FA: The Autonomic Nervous System: Anatomy, Physiology and Surgical Application, 3rd ed. New York, Macmillan, 1952.
Wilborn AJ: Thoracic outlet syndrome: A neurologist's perspective. Chest Surg Clin North Am 1999.
Wright IS: The neurovascular syndrome produced by hyperabduction of the arm. Am Heart J 29:1, 1945.
Yiannikas C, Walsh JC: Somatosensory evoked responses in the diagnosis of thoracic outlet syndrome. J Neurol Neurosurg Psychiatry 46:234, 1983.

CHAPTER **53**

Primary Neoplasms

Geoffrey M. Graeber
David R. Jones
Peter C. Pairolero

DEFINITION

Chest wall tumors encompass a kaleidoscopic panorama of bone and soft tissue pathologic conditions. Included are primary and metastatic neoplasms of both the bony skeleton and soft tissues and the primary neoplasms that invade the thorax from adjacent structures such as the breast, lung, pleura, and mediastinum. Nearly all of these neoplasms have at one time or another been irradiated, and it is fairly common for these patients to present with postradiation necrotic ulceration. The thoracic surgeon is asked to evaluate all of these patients. Most are seen to establish a diagnosis, some to treat for cure, and a few to manage necrotic, foul-smelling, chest wall malignant ulcers. Primary chest wall neoplasms previously considered unresectable because of their size or extension into adjacent structures are now being resected, and the chest wall is reconstructed with little morbidity. In many patients, surgical extirpation is often the only remaining modality of therapy. This may be compromised by an incorrect diagnosis or an inability to reconstruct large chest wall defects (Pairolero and Arnold, 1985).

HISTORICAL NOTE

Because primary chest wall neoplasms are uncommon, relatively few series have previously been reported. Moreover, most reports have included only patients with bone tumors (Groff and Adkins, 1967; Pascuzzi et al, 1957; Stelzer and Gay, 1980). When bone neoplasms are combined with primary soft tissue tumors, however, the soft tissues become a major source of chest wall neoplasms and account for nearly one half of these tumors treated surgically (Graeber et al, 1982; King et al, 1986; Pairolero and Arnold, 1985). The incidence of malignancy in these tumors is variable and has been reported to range from 50% to 80%. The higher malignancy rates are found in those series that include soft tissue tumors. When combined, malignant fibrous histiocytoma (fibrosarcoma), chondrosarcoma, and rhabdomyosarcoma are the most frequent primary malignant neoplasms that the thoracic surgeon is asked to manage. Cartilaginous tumors (osteochondroma and chondroma) and desmoid tumors are the most common primary benign tumors.

■ *HISTORICAL READINGS*

Groff DB, Adkins PC: Chest wall tumors. Ann Thorac Surg 4:260, 1967.
Pascuzzi CA, Dahlia DC, Clagett OT: Primary tumors of the ribs and sternum. Surg Gynecol Obstet 104:390, 1957.
Stelzer P, Gay WA Jr: Tumors of the chest wall. Surg Clin North Am 60:779, 1980.

CLINICAL FEATURES

The mean age of presentation for a patient with a benign tumor of the chest wall is approximately 15 years younger than for those with primary malignancies. The average patient age for benign tumors is 26 years old; for malignant tumors, the average age is 40 years old (Pass, 1989). The male to female ratio is approximately 2:1 (Gordon et al, 1991; Graeber et al, 1982; Sabanathan et al, 1985) for most tumors, with the exception of the desmoid tumors, which have a 1:2 male to female preponderance (Gordon et al, 1991; McKinnon et al, 1989). Chest wall tumors generally present as slowly enlarging masses. Most are initially asymptomatic, but with continued growth, pain invariably occurs. At first, the pain is generalized, and the patient is frequently treated for a neuritis or musculoskeletal complaint. The incidence of a chest wall mass is 70%, and pain is seen in 25% to 50% of patients (Gordon et al, 1991; King et al, 1986). These

PRIMARY CHEST WALL NEOPLASMS

- Malignant
  - Myeloma
  - Malignant fibrous histiocytoma
  - Chondrosarcoma
  - Rhabdomyosarcoma
  - Ewing's sarcoma
  - Liposarcoma
  - Neurofibrosarcoma
  - Osteosarcoma
  - Hemangiosarcoma
  - Leiomyosarcoma
  - Lymphoma
- Benign
  - Osteochondroma
  - Chondroma
  - Desmoid
  - Lipoma
  - Fibroma
  - Neurilemmoma

chest wall masses may be large and have been present for long periods. The size of these tumors may rarely prevent the patient from dressing and thus cause the patient to seek therapy. Pain is more common in malignant tumors but cannot be used to exclude the diagnosis of benignity because one third of patients with benign chest wall neoplasms have associated pain. Less common symptoms include weight loss, fever, lymphadenopathy, and brachial plexus neuropathy.

DIAGNOSIS

The evaluation of patients with suspected chest wall tumors should include a careful history and physical and laboratory examination followed by conventional plain and tomographic chest radiography. Old chest radiographs are important to determine the growth rate. Computed tomographic scans (CT) should be obtained to delineate soft tissue, pleural, mediastinal, and pulmonary involvement. The role of magnetic resonance imaging (MRI) is not yet fully known, but preliminary evaluation indicates still further enhancement of tissue pathologic findings, which may make it the diagnostic modality of choice in the future. A bone survey should be done if metastases are suspected. Pulmonary function testing should also be obtained.

Most primary chest wall neoplasms should be diagnosed by excisional biopsy. The reasons for excisional biopsy include (1) removal of the entire mass, (2) adequate tissue sampling to establish the tumor's histologic type, and (3) earlier administration of adjuvant therapy if necessary. Cavanaugh and others (1986) recommended a limited incisional biopsy to establish the diagnosis and allow appropriate management plans to be made that are based on the histologic type. In this series, 73% of the lesions were benign, and no further surgery was performed. In most series, however, the rate of malignancy is 50% to 80%, and all require en bloc resection (Graeber et al, 1982; King et al, 1986; Pairolero and Arnold, 1985). Incisional biopsies may confuse the histologic diagnosis because certain tumors, particularly chondrosarcomas, have areas that histologically appear benign and other areas in which frank malignancy is present (Graeber et al, 1982). Clinical decisions based on the wrong pathologic diagnosis may be catastrophic. If an incisional biopsy is performed, it should be made in such a way that the definitive excision will not be compromised. No flaps or extensive dissection should be used to prevent tumor cell seeding. Needle biopsy of a lesion in a patient with a known prior malignancy may be helpful. Ayala and Zornosa (1983) demonstrated a 79% accuracy rate in the diagnosis of primary bone tumors with percutaneous needle biopsy. Most thoracic surgeons still prefer excisional biopsy whenever possible.

Laboratory analysis and diagnostic studies should include liver function tests, alkaline phosphatase levels, and a CT or MRI of the chest. Many of these tumors metastasize to the lungs or involve the lung. Involvement of the underlying lung does not preclude resection, but it is associated with a worse prognosis, particularly in a patient with high-grade sarcomas (King et al, 1986; Perry et al, 1990). Ultrasound of chest wall tumors helps to localize the tumor's relationship to the pleura and lung parenchyma (Saito et al, 1988). If the tumor is confined to the chest wall, its movement during respiration is synchronous with the chest wall movement and not with the lung parenchyma.

BENIGN TUMORS

Benign chest wall tumors require diagnostic studies similar to those for malignant tumors. Radiographic studies may suggest the diagnosis of benignity, but histologic evidence is necessary. The more common benign chest wall tumors are discussed earlier. Less common benign tumors include lipomas, osteomyelitis, mesenchymomas, fibroxanthomas, hemangioendotheliomas, and some neural tumors.

Chondroma

Chondroma is the most common benign tumor of the chest wall (Graeber et al, 1982; Ryan et al, 1989; Sabanathan et al, 1985). They usually arise in the ribs near the costochondral junction anteriorly. These patients present with a mass that may be painful. Radiographically, the lesion has a lobulated radiodense appearance, which frequently displaces the bony cortex but does not penetrate it (Fig. 53–1). Calcification may be diffuse or focal with a stippled pattern. Histologically, there is mature hyaline cartilage with foci of myxoid degeneration and calcification. These lesions may grow to enormous size if untreated, and the therapy of choice is wide local excision with 2-cm margins.

Fibrous Dysplasia

Fibrous dysplasia occurs in young adults and presents as a painless, asymptomatic mass. It can arise anywhere on the chest wall but occurs frequently in the posterior ribs (Boyd, 1986). There is an association with trauma. Radiographs show a central, fusiform, expanded mass with thinning of the cortex and absence of calcification (Sabanathan et al, 1985). Cortical bone erosion is not uncommon. Histologically, there is a characteristic fishhook configuration of the trabeculae and lack of transformation of the coarse bony fibers to lamellar bone. This suggests that fibrous dysplasia represents a maturation defect. Excision of this lesion is curative.

Osteochondromas

Osteochondroma is a rare chest wall tumor that occurs in the first or second decade of life. The radiographic appearance is typical. The lesion, which is usually located in the metaphysis, grows in a direction opposite to that of the adjacent joint (Fig. 53–2). Infrequently, it has a focal radiolucent area surrounded by osteosclerotic tissue (Sabanathan et al, 1985). Grossly, the tumor consists of mature bone trabeculae covered by a cartilaginous cap. Most lesions are greater than 4 cm in diameter but may become larger if untreated. Solitary osteochondromas are benign and rarely may degenerate into malignancy. Multi-

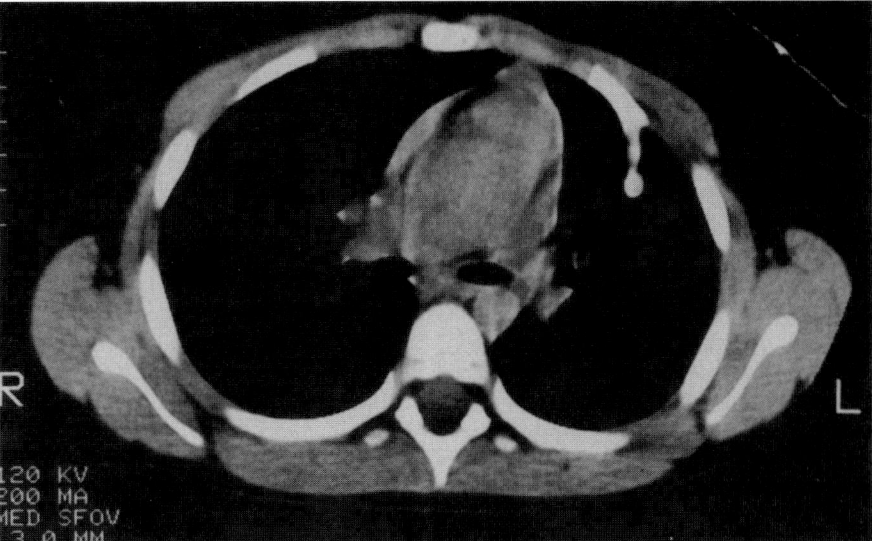

FIGURE 53–1 ■ A computed tomography image in a 42-year-old man of a lobulated chondroma arising near the costochondral junction in the left fourth rib. The therapy was resection with adequate margins of excision.

ple osteochondromas have a higher incidence of malignancy (Boyd, 1986). The therapy is wide local excision.

Eosinophilic Granuloma

Eosinophilic granuloma is a disease of the lymphoreticular system and not a true bone tumor. It may be solitary or multifocal and is a unifying feature of the conditions designated as histiocytosis X. Microscopically, there is an abundance of Langerhans cells, giant cells, eosinophils, and neutrophils. The peak incidence is between 5 and 15 years. It occurs in either the metaphysis or diaphysis of the bone and has no malignant potential. These lesions show osteolytic activity with adjacent osteosclerosis by radiography. They are frequently confused with Ewing's sarcoma or osteomyelitis. The therapy consists of either resection or radiotherapy.

Desmoid Tumor

Desmoid tumors occur most commonly in the third to fourth decades of life and have a 2:1 female to male predominance. The desmoid tumor is frequently difficult to differentiate from the low-grade fibrosarcoma. Histologically, the desmoid tumor contains sheets of fibroblasts with well-differentiated abundant collagen, which lacks encapsulation. The fibrosarcoma is usually well encapsulated with a herringbone pattern and distinct mitoses (McKinnon et al, 1989). Although one third of patients with Gardner syndrome have desmoid tumors, only 2% of patients with a desmoid tumor have Gardner syndrome (Hayery and Scheinin, 1988). Desmoids have also been reported to occur after trauma and to be associated with estrogen-induced growth (Hayery and Scheinin, 1988; McKinnon et al, 1989).

The clinical presentation is usually one of a dull, aching mass, which may be fixed to the underlying tissues but not to the skin (Graeber et al, 1985). The growth of the mass is slow, and it does not metastasize. There are no characteristic radiographic findings, and the diagnosis should be made by excisional biopsy.

The therapy is wide local excision with margins of at least 4 cm. Because desmoids may spread along fascial

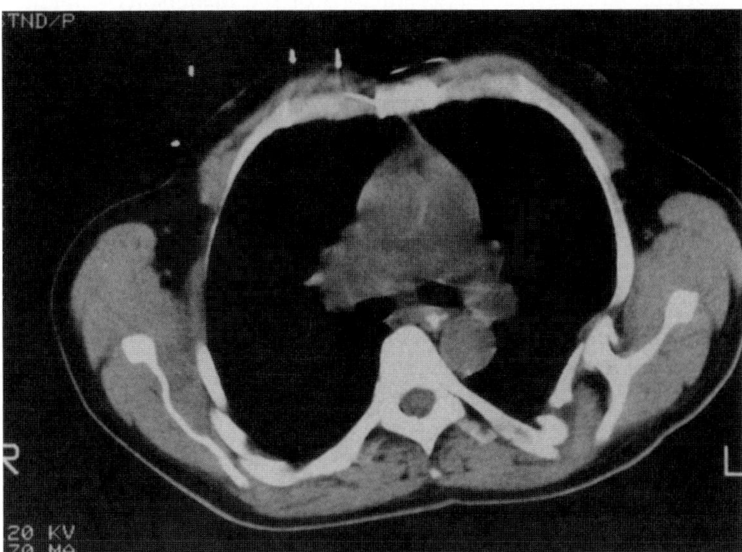

FIGURE 53–2 ■ A representative computed tomography scan of a solitary osteochondroma of the posterior left scapula with displacement of the third rib anteriorly. This produced dull posterior chest wall pain in the patient.

planes well beyond the primary, the wider resection margins are recommended. The recurrence rates for desmoid tumors after excision range from 4% to as high as 50% (McKinnon et al, 1989; Posner et al, 1989). The recurrence rates were directly related to resection margin status in a study by McKinnon and coworkers (1989), and 45% of patients with positive resection margins had recurrences. Only 4% with negative resection margins had relapses. In patients with recurrence or gross residual disease, radiotherapy is effective for local control (Leibel et al, 1983; Sherman et al, 1990). The recommended radiation doses of 50 to 60 Gy at 1:8 Gy/fraction prevent the dose-related complications of radiotherapy (Sherman et al, 1990). Chemotherapy plays no role in the therapy of desmoid tumors. Because of the hormonal influence on the desmoid's growth, tamoxifen has been reported to decrease both the size and symptoms of these tumors (Kinzbrunner et al, 1983).

The actual survival rates after wide local excision are 90% at 10 years, with a cause-specific survival rate of 100% (Graeber, 1989). Local recurrence remains the most difficult challenge for this locally aggressive, benign tumor.

MALIGNANT TUMORS

Malignant primary chest wall tumors can be cured if certain surgical principles are followed. These tumors may require extensive chest wall resection, but with the aid of muscle flaps, chest wall reconstruction is successful. Adjuvant therapy has become increasingly important in the management of these tumors. The most common primary malignant chest wall tumors were shown previously. Less common malignant tumors include neurofibrosarcomas, malignant hemangioendotheliomas, and leiomyosarcomas. The survival rates after therapy for these tumors vary, but all histologic subtypes have some long-term survivors (Fig. 53–3).

Chondrosarcoma

Chondrosarcoma is the most common primary chest wall malignant tumor. It accounts for 50% of the malignant neoplasms and 25% of all primary chest wall tumors (Sabanathan et al, 1985). Eighty percent of these tumors arise in the ribs, and 20% arise in the sternum (McAfee et al, 1985).

Most of these tumors are solitary and have been present an average of 18 months prior to presentation (McAfee et al, 1985).

The conventional radiographic findings of a chondrosarcoma include a lobulated mass that arises in the medullary portion of the rib or sternum, often with cortical bone destruction. Calcification of the tumor is missed in 45% of chest radiographs but detected on chest CT scan. A stippled calcification pattern is most common, but rings and arcs of calcification may be present (Aoki et al, 1989).

The diagnosis of these tumors should be made by an excisional biopsy. The incisional biopsy has no place in the diagnosis of these lesions because the histologic findings vary from a poorly differentiated cellular appearance to an extremely well-differentiated lesion that is indistinguishable from a benign chondroma (Fig. 53–4) (McAfee et al, 1985; Sabanathan et al, 1985). The incidence of chondrosarcomatous change in a solitary osteochondroma is reportedly 1% to 2% (Lichtenstin, 1977). The natural history of these tumors is one of slow growth, with frequent local recurrence and late metastasis. Chondrosarcomas have been related to previous chest wall trauma in 12.5% of patients (McAfee et al, 1985).

The therapy of choice is wide local excision, including several partial ribs above and below the lesion, with surgical margins of at least 4 cm. If the lesion originates in the sternum, a sternotomy with a corresponding resection of the costal arches bilaterally should be performed (Arnold and Pairolero, 1978). Chest wall reconstruction is frequently necessary.

Chondrosarcomas are extremely radioresistant and chemoresistant. The prognostic factors include the tumor's grade, diameter, and location. Tumors less than 6 cm and sternal tumors have a better patient prognosis. The 10-year survival rates are 96% with wide local excision, 65% with local excision, and 14% with palliative excision (McAfee et al, 1985). The local recurrence rate is higher with local excision (50%) than wide local excision

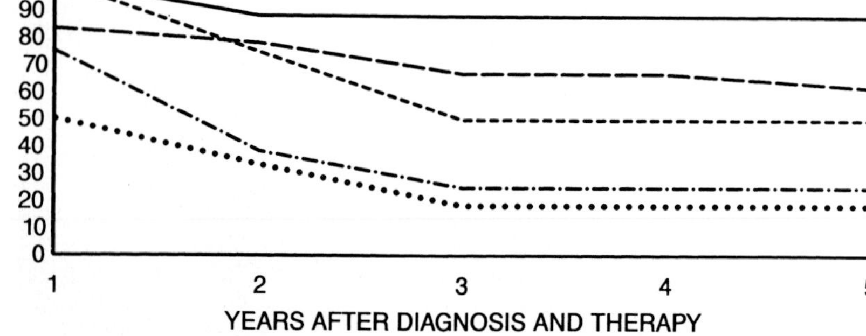

FIGURE 53–3 ■ Survival rates in patients with malignant neoplasms of the chest wall. The total number of patients used to generate this graph was 44 rather than 47 because 2 patients with fibrosarcomas were lost to follow-up and an 84-year-old man with a massive chondrosarcoma of the chest wall was not considered a candidate for resection.

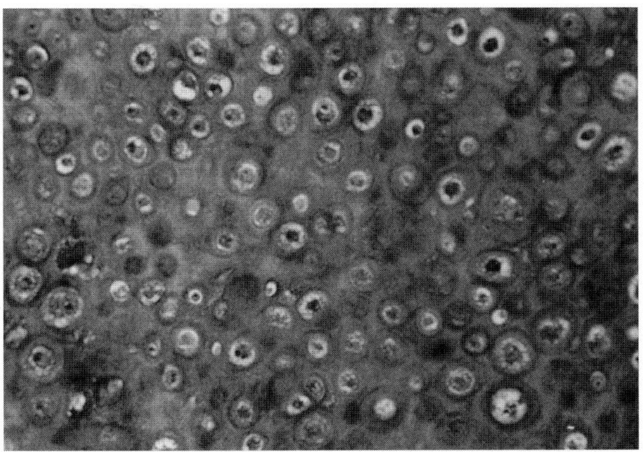

FIGURE 53–4 ■ This photomicrograph presents a characteristic field from a histologic section of a chondrosarcoma. The histologic characteristics of this tumor include a cartilaginous neoplasm, which has anaplastic cells with one or more bizarre, hyperchromatic nuclei. This malignant neoplasm is also known to have frequent variations in the grade of tumor cells present throughout the presenting mass (H & E, × 200).

(17%). The possibility of late local recurrences of chondrosarcomas necessitates long-term follow-up of these patients (Graeber et al, 1982).

Ewing's Sarcoma and Askin's Tumor

Ewing's sarcoma is a small, round tumor with characteristics of a primitive neuroectodermal tumor (PNET) and a neural histogenesis, as indicated by experimental studies (Cavazanna et al, 1987). It is the most common primary chest wall malignancy in children and occurs in 8% to 22% of malignant chest wall lesions in adults (Graeber et al, 1982; King et al, 1986; Sabanathan et al, 1985; Shamberger et al, 1989). The differential diagnosis of small, round cell malignant tumors includes neuroblastomas, embryonal rhabdomyosarcomas, and lymphomas in addition to Ewing's sarcomas (Stefanco et al, 1988). A highly malignant alternative to Ewing's sarcoma is the PNET, which was first described by Askin and colleagues (1979). PNET is considered similar to Ewing's sarcoma because of a common neuroectodermal differentiation and a frequently seen translocation between the long arms of chromosomes 11 and 22 [t(11:22)(q24:q12)] (Turc-Cavel et al, 1983; Whang-Peng et al, 1984). PNET and Ewing's sarcoma are grouped together because the diagnosis and therapy of each are similar.

Most patients are between 5 and 30 years old and present with progressive chest wall pain with or without the presence of a mass. Some patients have a modest leukocytosis and elevated erythrocyte sedimentation rate. The typical radiographic picture is the characteristic onion-peel appearance, which is produced by multiple layers of periosteal new bone formation (Sabanathan et al, 1985). Bony destruction, sclerosis of the widened cortex, and a widened medulla are also common radiographic findings. The tumor may involve several ribs but usually is confined to one rib. The diagnosis may be made with percutaneous needle biopsy (Ayala and Zornosa, 1983), but as with other primary chest wall malignancies, an excisional biopsy is best (Fig. 53–5). The preoperative workup should include standard chest imaging and bone marrow aspiration.

These patients are best treated through a multimodality approach. The entire marrow cavity of the rib is considered to be at risk for malignancy; therefore, the entire involved rib is removed along with a partial rib resection above and below the lesion (Shamberger et al, 1989). Postoperative external beam irradiation to the tumor bed provides excellent local control. If complete surgical resection and irradiation are performed, local control rates of 93% have been reported (Thomas et al, 1983).

Chemotherapy is used to control distant disease and has been shown to decrease the incidence of distant metastases and improve survival rates (Hayes et al, 1983; Thomas et al, 1983). Doxorubicin, dactinomycin, cyclophosphamide, and vincristine are the four drugs used in combination most frequently. Failure to include doxorubicin in this combination has detrimental results (Perez et al, 1981). Preoperative chemotherapy has been reported to facilitate subsequent local therapy, but its use is not well established (Brown et al, 1987; Shamberger et al, 1989). The survival rate was improved with multimodality therapy to 52% at 5 years in one study (Hayery and Scheinin, 1988). Patients with distant metastasis rarely survive 5 years.

The complications of extensive chest wall resections in children with Ewing's sarcoma include scoliosis and restrictive pulmonary disease (Grosfeld et al, 1988; Malangoni et al, 1980). Harrington rod fusion may be necessary for severe scoliosis. The restrictive pulmonary function usually does not result in any long-term respiratory difficulties.

Osteosarcoma

Osteosarcomas occur between the ages of 10 and 25 years and again after age 40 years in association with several other disease processes. They frequently present as a

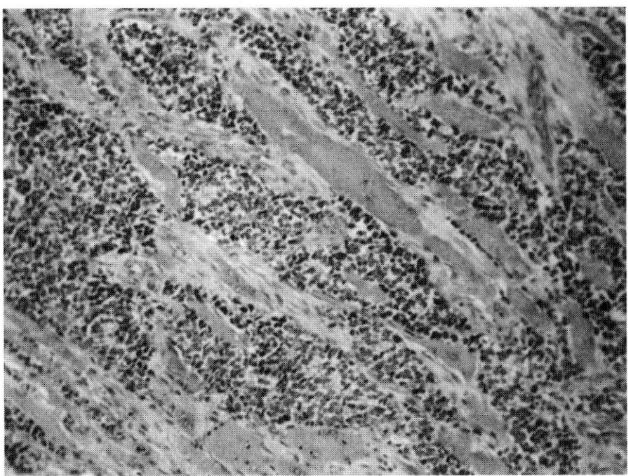

FIGURE 53–5 ■ This photomicrograph shows a characteristic sample taken from a Ewing sarcoma. The histologic characteristics of this tumor include closely packed, small, round cells, which are infiltrating muscle fibers (H & E, × 200).

painful mass with a duration of symptoms prior to presentation that lasts from weeks to months. Most osteosarcomas arise de novo and are located in the metaphysial portion of the long bones, such as the femur, the tibia, and the humerus. They do, however, account for a small but significant number of rib-based malignancies (Fig. 53–6) (Graeber et al, 1982). There is an association between the development of osteosarcomas and previous irradiation, Paget's disease, and chemotherapy (Huvos, 1986; Souba et al, 1986; Tucker et al, 1987). The latency period for the development of osteosarcoma after irradiation is approximately 10 years (Huvos et al, 1985).

The preoperative evaluation of a patient considered to have an osteosarcoma should include an excisional biopsy to confirm the diagnosis. An elevated serum alkaline phosphatase level may be present by laboratory analysis, but this is nonspecific. One study showed that tumors associated with a serum elevation of this enzyme had increased metastatic rates (Raymond et al, 1987). Radiographically, the classic "sunburst" pattern of new periosteal bone formation is frequently seen (Boyd, 1986; Pass, 1989). Triangular elevation of the periosteum secondary to reactive new bone formation may be seen radiographically and is known as Codman's triangle sign. Histologically, we see eosinophilic staining and a glassy appearance with irregular contours of the osteoid. Interspersed with the osteoblastic cells are foci of fibroblastic and chondroblastic cells, which help divide osteosarcomas into those three subtypes (Fig. 53–7) (Rosai, 1989).

The therapy for osteosarcoma of the chest is preoperative chemotherapy, which usually consists of a combination of doxorubicin, high-dose methotrexate, and cisplatin (Winkler et al, 1984). This is done to shrink the tumor prior to resection and to evaluate the tumor's response to chemotherapy. Tumors with a significant amount of tumor necrosis postchemotherapy are associated with better patient survival rates (Raymond et al, 1987). Preoperative intra-arterial chemotherapy with cisplatin has produced significant disease-free survival rates in patients who have a complete or partial response (Jaffe et al, 1989). Radiotherapy is usually ineffective for osteosarcomas.

The prognostic factors include the response to preoperative chemotherapy, an association with Paget's disease (worse prognosis), and unifocal osteosarcoma. The addition of multidrug chemotherapy to the therapy of osteosarcoma has increased 5-year disease-free survival rates to greater than 50% (Lane et al, 1986).

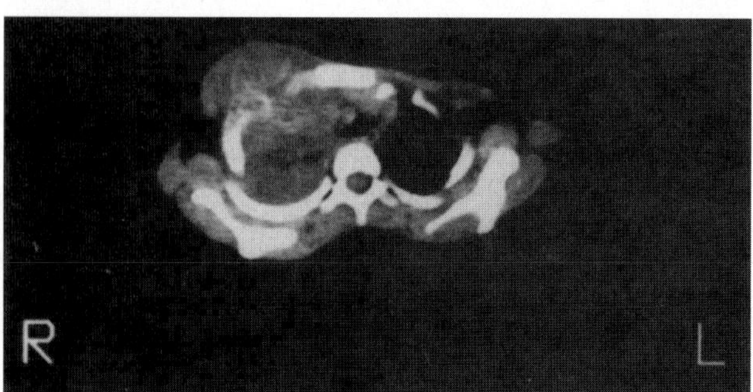

FIGURE 53–6 ■ Osteosarcoma. A computed tomography scan of a right third rib–based osteosarcoma with destruction of the bone is shown here. The diagnosis was confirmed by an excisional biopsy.

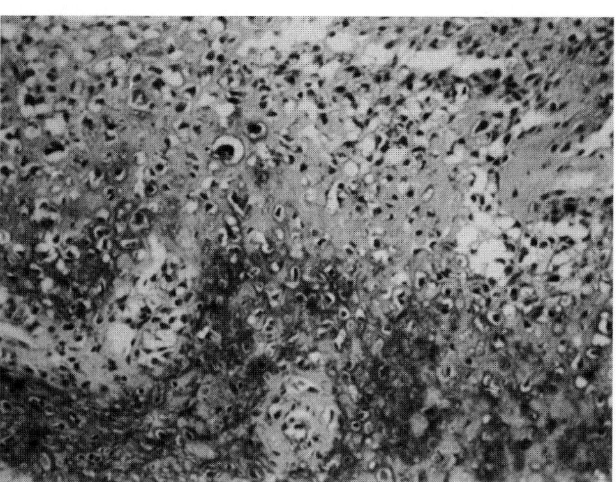

FIGURE 53–7 ■ This photomicrograph shows a characteristic section taken from an osteosarcoma. The histologic characteristics include anaplastic osteoblasts in an osteoid matrix with atypical calcification (H & E, × 200).

Plasmacytoma

Solitary plasmacytomas that arise in bone account for 10% to 30% of primary chest wall malignancies (Graeber et al, 1982; Pass, 1989). They are more common in male patients and usually occur later in life, with a mean age of 60 years (Graeber et al, 1982). The most common chest wall location is the ribs, followed by the clavicle and sternum. Soft tissue invasion from bone lesions may occur. The radiographic appearance of the plasmacytoma demonstrates an osteolytic process with several paracostal opacities frequently present (Galluccio et al, 1989).

Confirmation that the plasmacytoma is localized to the chest wall requires several studies. The patient should undergo a bone marrow aspiration, skeletal radiographs, and immunoelectrophoretic examination of the serum and urine. A patient with a solitary plasmacytoma usually has a normal calcium level and is not anemic. Evidence of monoclonality of one of the immunoglobulins with normal levels of the other circulating immunoglobulins strongly suggests that the plasmacytoma is solitary. Serum β_2-microglobulin levels are usually normal in the solitary plasmacytoma. Most bone lesions show a predominance of immunoglobulin reactivity; upper respiratory tract lesions are predominantly immunoglobulin (Rosai, 1989). The diagnosis of a solitary plasmacytoma should be made only if all studies for disseminated disease have negative findings.

Microscopically, plasmacytomas are composed of sheets of plasma cells and are often hypervascular. The nucleoli are prominent and have a characteristic pinwheel appearance. Amyloid may be present in 25% of the lesions (Fig. 53–8) (Meis et al, 1987).

The role of surgery is to establish the diagnosis by excisional biopsy. High-dose radiotherapy (5000 to 6000 cGy) has been shown to be successful for the local con-

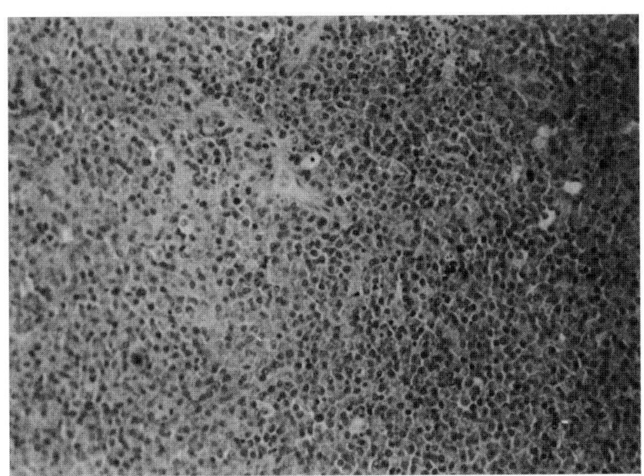

FIGURE 53–8 ■ This is a representative photomicrograph taken from a plasmacytoma. The characteristic features of this neoplasm include a large field of well-differentiated plasma cells that have eccentric nuclei that are surrounded by an adjacent "halo" (H & E, × 200).

trol of solitary plasmacytomas (Mill and Griffith, 1980). If the lesion is refractory to radiotherapy, then a more extensive surgical excision can be done. Systematic chemotherapy should only be given for evidence of disease progression (Pass, 1989). Local recurrence is uncommon for plasmacytomas. Spontaneous regression of a chest wall plasmacytoma has been reported, but this is rare (Arunabh et al, 1988). After they are treated for a solitary plasmacytoma, in approximately 35% to 55% of patients, multiple myeloma develops, often 10 to 12 years after the initial diagnosis (Meis et al, 1987). The presence of nuclear immaturity with prominent nucleoli may have a positive predictive value for the development of multiple myeloma. The presence of a monoclonal protein in the serum or urine has no predictive value for the development of multiple myeloma (Rosai, 1989).

The 10-year survival rate for all bony locations of solitary plasmacytoma is 68% (Bataille and Sany, 1981). A 25% to 37% 5-year survival rate after therapy for primary chest wall plasmacytomas is expected (Gordon et al, 1991; Graeber et al, 1982). Close follow-up of these patients with frequent urine and serum electrophoretic studies is necessary because the development of multiple myeloma is fairly common.

Soft Tissue Sarcoma

Primary soft tissue sarcomas of the chest wall are uncommon, and few centers have treated extensive series of these tumors. The more common tumors include fibrosarcomas, liposarcomas, malignant fibrous histiocytomas, rhabdomyosarcomas, dermatofibrosarcomas protuberans, and angiosarcomas (Gordon et al, 1991; Graeber et al, 1987). These tumors compromise nearly 50% of all primary chest wall sarcomas (Ryan et al, 1989; Souba et al, 1986). The factors that may predispose the patient to the development of soft tissue sarcomas include a history of previous irradiation and syndromes such as von Recklinghausen's disease (neurofibromatosis), Gardner's syndrome, and Werner's syndrome (Lynch et al, 1973; Seyer, 1988).

Fibrosarcomas are large, painful masses that occur in all age groups and often involve adjacent structures (Fig. 53–9) (Boyd, 1986). The radiographic findings show a large irregular mass with frequent destruction of the bone. The therapy includes wide local excision, with tumor-free margins for low-grade sarcomas and the addition of chemotherapy for high-grade lesions (Gordon et al, 1991). The difficulty in treating this neoplasm is related to the significant incidence of local recurrence and a propensity for the tumor to metastasize to the lungs (Graeber et al, 1982). The 5-year survival rate is 53% to 86% after surgery, with or without adjuvant therapy (Graeber et al, 1982).

Rhabdomyosarcoma is a rare primary chest wall tumor. It accounts for 4% to 26% of primary malignant tumors. These tumors arise from undifferentiated mesoderm and are usually diagnosed after an incisional biopsy. Microscopically, the tumor cells are small and spindle shaped (Fig. 53–10). There are highly cellular regions that surround blood vessels and alternate with abundant parvicellular regions of muscle intercellular material. Immunocytochemical analysis of the tissue has been very useful in the diagnosis of rhabdomyosarcoma. The markers used include myoglobin, desmin, myosin, actin, and antiskeletal muscle antibody from myasthenic patients. The therapy is wide surgical excision and multidrug chemotherapy. Radiotherapy is usually not effective in this tumor.

Malignant fibrous histiocytoma (MFH) is an uncommon primary tumor to the chest wall. These tumors arise from tissue histiocytes and have the potential to produce collagen (Fig. 53–11) (Ozzello et al, 1963). CT scanning aids in the operative planning and in the evaluation of metastatic disease. The therapy is by wide local excision for primary and locally recurrent tumors (Venn et al, 1986). MFH frequently has local recurrence and distant metastasis. However, MFH is generally resistant to chemotherapy. Adjuvant brachytherapy for soft tissue sarco-

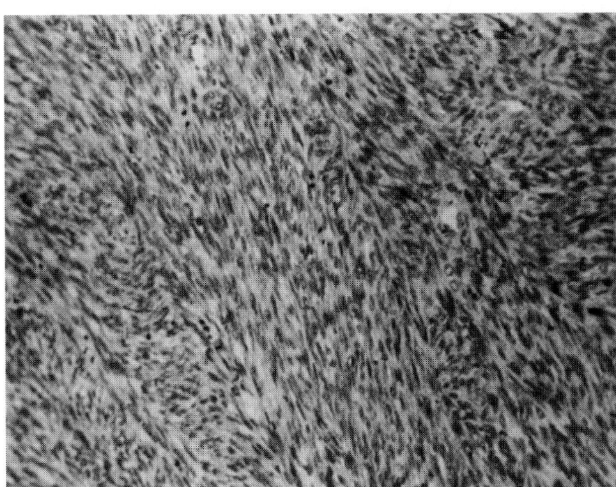

FIGURE 53–9 ■ This photomicrograph shows a representative sample of a fibrosarcoma. The histologic characteristics of this tumor show malignant spindle cells, which are arranged in a "herring bone" fashion. This alignment is characteristic of the tumor (H & E, × 200).

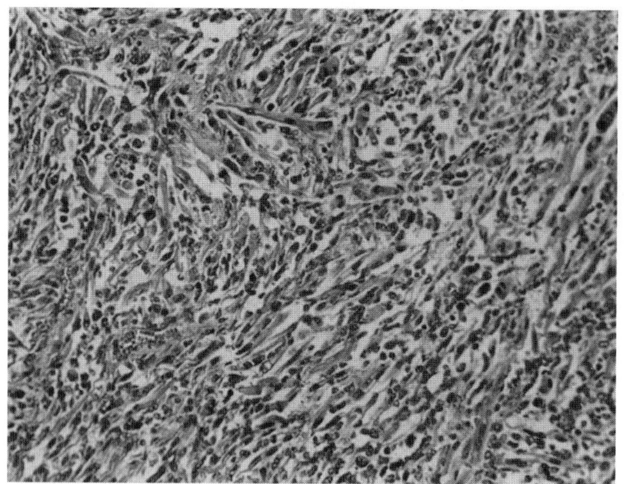

FIGURE 53–10 ■ This photomicrograph depicts some of the histologic characteristics associated with a rhabdomyosarcoma. Included in the field are large, elongated tumor cells that have abundant eosinophilic cytoplasm, racket cells, and more primitive rhabdomyoblasts (H & E, × 200).

mas has been shown to be beneficial if the patients are undergoing resection for locoregional recurrence in a previously irradiated site (Wallner et al, 1991). Postoperative external beam radiation may be effective, particularly if the resection margins are inadequate (Venn et al, 1986; Wallner et al, 1991).

Liposarcoma accounts for 15% of primary chest wall soft tissue sarcomas (Gordon et al, 1991). Most (70%) are low grade, and en bloc resection is the therapy of choice. Local recurrence was found in 33% of patients in the study by Greager and colleagues (1987), and was treated by wide local excision alone. The presence of local recurrence has no significant effect on the overall survival rate (Gordon et al, 1991). Radiotherapy may be effective in the control of local recurrence, but its role is unclear. The 5-year survival rate is 83% (Graeber et al, 1982).

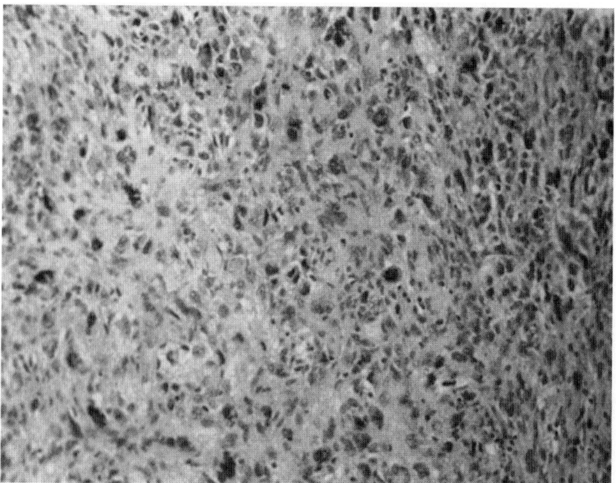

FIGURE 53–11 ■ This photomicrograph shows a representative field from a malignant fibrous histiocytoma. The characteristics of this neoplasm include a pleomorphic tumor, which has many large, bizarre-shaped cells in a fibrous stroma (H & E, × 200).

The prognostic indicators for primary tissue sarcomas include the tumor grade, presence of distant metastases, and positive surgical resection margins (Gordon et al, 1991; Graeber et al, 1982; Perry et al, 1990). Tumors that are low grade are associated with a 90% 5-year survival rate; high-grade sarcomas have a 49% 5-year survival rate (Souba et al, 1986). Positive resection margins negatively affect both the disease-free survival and overall survival rates in high-grade sarcomas, which emphasizes the importance of negative margins (Perry et al, 1990). Radiotherapy and chemotherapy have no prognostic value for high-grade sarcomas in the adult patient. Because sarcomas tend to metastasize to the lungs, CT scans of the chest should be performed. However, up to 50% of lung parenchyma nodules discovered at surgery are not seen on preoperative CT scans (Jablons et al, 1989). The presence of these synchronous pulmonary metastases is associated with a worse prognosis (Perry et al, 1990).

SURGERY

Chest Wall Resection

Wide resection of primary malignant chest wall neoplasm is essential to successful management. However, the extent of resection should not be compromised because of an inability to close a large chest wall defect (Arnold and Pairolero, 1979, 1984a; Pairolero and Arnold, 1985, 1986a, b). Opinions differ as to what constitutes wide resection. In a recent report from the Mayo Clinic (King et al, 1986), in which the effect of the extent of resection on the long-term survival of patients with primary malignant chest wall tumors was analyzed, 56% of patients with a 4-cm or greater margin of resection remained free from recurrent cancer at 5 years compared with only 29% for patients with a 2-cm margin (Fig. 53–12). For many surgeons, a resection margin of 2 cm would be considered adequate. Although this margin may be adequate for chest wall metastases, benign tumors and certain low-grade malignant primary neoplasms, such as chondrosarcoma, a 2-cm resection margin is inadequate for more malignant neoplasms, such as osteogenic sarcoma and malignant fibrous histiocytoma, which have the potential to spread within the marrow cavity or along tissue planes, such as the periosteum or parietal pleura. Consequently, all primary malignant neoplasms initially diagnosed by excisional biopsy should undergo further resection to include at least a 4-cm margin of normal tissue on all sides. High-grade malignancies should also have the entire involved bone resected. For neoplasms of the rib cage, this would include removal of the involved ribs, the corresponding anterior costal arches if the tumor is located anteriorly, and several partial ribs above and below the neoplasm. For tumor of the sternum and manubrium, resection of the entire involved bone and corresponding costal arches bilaterally is indicated. Any attached structures, such as the lung, thymus, pericardium, or chest wall muscles, should also be excised.

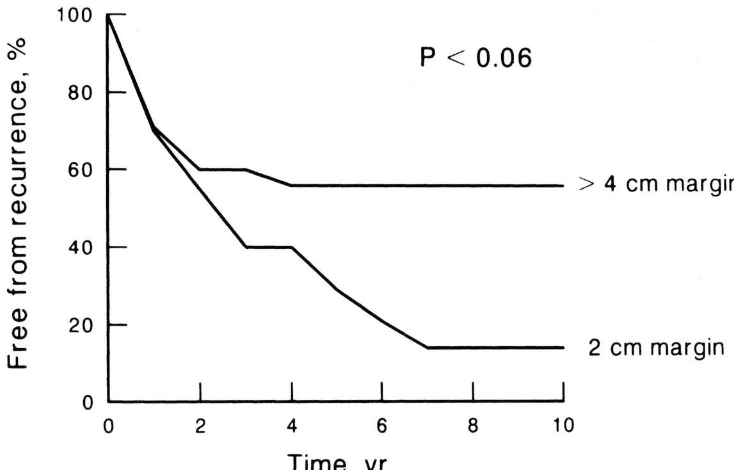

FIGURE 53–12 ■ Percentage of patients with malignant chest wall tumors free from recurrent tumors by extent of resection margin. Zero time on the abscissa represents the day of the chest wall resection. (From King RM, Pairolero PC, Trastek VH et al: Primary wall tumors: Factors affecting survival. Ann Thorac Surg 41:597, 1986.)

Chest Wall Reconstruction

The ability to close large chest wall defects is of prime importance in the surgical therapy of chest wall neoplasms. The critical questions of whether the reconstructed thorax will support respiration and protect the underlying organs must be answered when we consider that both the extent of resection and dependable reconstruction are the mandatory ingredients for successful therapy. These two important items are accomplished most safely by the joint efforts of a thoracic and a plastic surgeon (Arnold and Pairolero, 1984a).

Reconstruction of chest wall defects involves a consideration of many factors. The location and size of the defect are of the utmost importance, but the medical history and local conditions of the wound may drastically alter a reconstructive choice. Primary closure remains the best option available if possible. If full-thickness reconstruction is required, which is usually the situation in most primary neoplasms that have not been previously treated, consideration must be given to both the structural stability of the thorax and the soft tissue coverage.

CONSIDERATION FOR RECONSTRUCTION OF CHEST WALL DEFECTS

- Location
- Size
- Depth
  - Partial thickness
  - Full thickness
- Duration
- Condition of local tissue
  - Irradiation
  - Infection
  - Residual tumor
  - Scarring
- General condition of patient
  - Chemotherapy
  - Corticosteroid
  - Chronic infection
- Lifestyle and type of work
- Prognosis

Skeletal Reconstruction

Reconstruction of the bony thorax is controversial. Differences of opinion exist both as to which patients should undergo reconstruction and what type of reconstruction should be done. The decision not to reconstruct the skeleton depends on the size and location of the defect and whether the wound is infected. In general, infected wounds should not be reconstructed simultaneously. Similarly, defects less than 5 cm in greatest diameter anywhere on the thorax are usually not reconstructed. Likewise, high posterior defects less than 10 cm do not require reconstruction because the overlying scapula provides support. However, if the defect is located near the tip of the scapula, the defect, even if 5 cm or less in size, should be closed to avoid impingement of the tip of the scapula into the chest with movement of the arm. Alternatively, the lower half of the scapula could be resected. Finally, all larger defects located anywhere on the chest should be reconstructed, and either autogenous tissue or prosthetic material may be used.

Stabilization of the bony thorax is best accomplished with prosthetic material, such as Prolene mesh (Ethicon, Somerville, NJ) or 2-mm-thick Gore-Tex (polytetrafluroethylene) soft tissue patch. When either of these materials is placed under tension, the rigidity of the prosthesis is improved in all directions. Currently, the Gore-Tex soft tissue patch is superior because this material has the added advantage of preventing movement of fluid and air across the reconstructed chest wall. Marlex mesh (Daval, Providence, RI) is used less frequently because when it is placed under tension, this material is rigid in one direction only. Reconstruction with rigid material, such as methylmethacrylate-impregnated meshes is not necessary.

All large, full-thickness skeletal defects that result from the resection of a neoplasm in both the sternum and lateral chest wall should be reconstructed if the wound is not contaminated. If the wound is contaminated from previous radiation necrosis or nectrotic neoplasm, reconstruction with prosthetic material is not advised because the prosthesis may subsequently become infected, which would result in obligatory removal. In this situation, reconstruction with a musculocutaneous flap alone is preferred. Similarly, resection of full-thickness bony thorax in a patient who has been previously irradiated may not require skeletal reconstruction because the lung is frequently adherent to the underlying parietal pleura and pneumothorax may not occur with chest wall resection.

> **AUTOGENOUS TISSUE AVAILABLE FOR CHEST WALL RECONSTRUCTION**
>
> Muscle
> - Latissimus dorsi
> - Pectoralis major
> - Rectus abdominis
> - Serratus anterior
> - External oblique
> - Trapezius
>
> Omentum

Soft Tissue Reconstruction

Both muscle and omentum can be used to reconstruct soft tissue chest wall defects. Muscle can be transposed as muscle alone or as a musculocutaneous flap and is the tissue of choice for closure of most full-thickness soft tissue defects. All major chest wall muscles can be mobilized on a single axis of rotation and transposed to another location of the chest wall (McGraw and Arnold, 1986). If muscle is not available because of previous radiation damage or an operation, free muscle flaps from another location can be reimplanted with the expectation of dependable long-term coverage. The omentum should be reserved for partial-thickness reconstruction or as a back-up procedure when muscle is either not available or has failed in a previous full-thickness repair.

Latissimus Dorsi

The latissimus dorsi is the largest flat muscle in the thorax. Its dominant thoracodorsal neurovascular leash has an arc of rotation that allows coverage of the lateral and central back and the anterolateral and central front of the thorax (Bostwick et al, 1979; Campbell, 1950). Its dependable, musculocutaneous vascular connections permit it to be used also as a reliable musculocutaneous flap. This muscle flap can cover huge chest wall defects because virtually one half of the back can be elevated on the blood supply of a single latissimus dorsi in the uninjured, nonirradiated patient. The donor site posteriorly may require skin grafting when large musculocutaneous flaps are elevated, but this represents a minor disadvantage when we consider that large, robust flaps can be transposed to either the anterior or the posterior chest for full-thickness reconstruction. If the dominant blood supply has been compromised by previous trauma or surgery, the muscle can still be transposed dependably on the branch of the adjacent serratus anterior (Fisher et al, 1983).

Pectoralis Major

The pectoralis major is the second largest flat muscle on the chest wall and in many respects is the mirror image of the latissimus dorsi. Its dominant thoracoacromial neurovascular leash, which enters posteriorly about midclavicle, allows both elevation and rotation centrally of the muscle as either a muscle or a musculocutaneous flap (Arnold and Pairolero, 1979). The pectoralis major flap is as reliable as the latissimus dorsi flap. It is of major benefit in the reconstruction of anterior chest wall defects, such as those that result from sternal tumor excisions (Arnold and Pairolero, 1978; Pairolero and Arnold, 1984, 1986). Generally, only the muscle without the overlying soft tissue and skin is transposed, which thus avoids the distortion created by a centralization of the breast. Reconstruction in this manner is more symmetric and more aesthetically acceptable. If sternal skin must be excised, the symmetry of the breast can still be maintained because the transposed muscle readily accepts and supports a skin graft. If necessary, the muscle may also be transposed on its secondary blood supply through the perforators from the internal mammary vessels.

Rectus Abdominis

Use of the rectus abdominis for chest wall reconstruction is based on the internal mammary neurovascular leash. The inferior epigastric vessels must be divided to allow rotation to the chest wall. This muscle can be mobilized and moved either as a muscle or as a musculocutaneous flap, with the skin component oriented either horizontally, vertically, or both. The vertical skin flap, however, is more reliable because it is oriented along the long axis of the muscle and thus maintains more musculocutaneous perforators. The donor site is usually closed primarily.

The rectus abdominis is most useful in the reconstruction of lower sternal wounds. Either muscle can be used because their arc of rotation is identical. Care must be taken to choose the muscle that has patent and uninjured internal mammary vessels. Angiographic demonstration of vessel patency may be helpful to determine which musculocutaneous unit would be the most reliable, particularly in previously irradiated patients or in patients who had prior coronary artery bypass surgery.

Serratus Anterior

The serratus anterior is a smaller, flat muscle that is located along the midaxillary chest wall. Its blood supply comes from the serratus branch of the thoracodorsal vessels and from the long thoracic artery and vein. Although this muscle can be used alone, it is more commonly utilized in chest wall reconstruction as an adjunctive muscle in tandem with either the pectoralis major or the latissimus dorsi to close larger defects. The muscle also augments the skin-carrying ability of either adjacent muscle (Arnold and Pairolero, 1984b). This muscle is particularly useful as an intrathoracic muscle flap (Arnold and Pairolero, 1984b; Pairolero et al, 1983).

External Oblique

The external oblique muscle may also be transposed as either a muscle or a musculocutaneous flap, and it is most useful in closing defects of the upper abdomen and lower thorax. It reaches the inframammary fold without tension but does not readily extend higher (Hodgkinson and Arnold, 1980). The primary blood supply is from the lower thoracic intercostal vessels. The advantage of this muscle is that lower chest wall defects can be closed without a distortion of the breast.

Trapezius

The trapezius muscle is useful to close defects at the base of the neck or the thoracic outlet, but it is not a consistently useful muscle as far as the remainder of chest wall reconstruction is concerned. Its primary blood supply is the dorsal scapular vessels.

Omentum

Omental transposition has been useful in the reconstruction of the partial-thickness chest wall defects that may occur with certain soft tissue neoplasms or radiation necrosis (Arnold and Pairolero, 1986; Jurkiewicz and Arnold, 1977). In the latter situation, the skin and soft tissue are débrided down to what remains of the thoracic skeleton, which may be either bone or cartilage but frequently is only irradiated ischemic scar. The transposed omentum, with its excellent blood supply from the gastroepiploic vessels, adheres to the irradiated wound and readily accepts and supports an overlying skin graft. Because the omentum has no structural stability on its own, it is not useful in full-thickness defects because additional support with fascia lata, bone, or prosthetic material would be necessary.

Omental transposition is exceedingly helpful in situations in which planned muscle flaps have been used but have failed because of partial necrosis. Generally, this results in only a soft tissue defect, and a pleural seal with respiratory stability is not required, which thus allows a most threatening situation to be salvaged.

Late Results

During the past 10 years, more than 60 chest wall resections for primary neoplasms were performed at the Mayo Clinic by one team of surgeons (unpublished data). Nearly two thirds of these neoplasms were malignant. Malignant fibrous histiocytoma and chondrosarcoma were the most common malignant neoplasms, and desmoid tumor was the most common benign tumor. The patients' ages ranged from 12 to 80 years (median, 43.5 years). An average of 3.9 ribs were resected. Total or partial sternectomies were performed in 13 patients. Skeletal defects were closed with prosthetic material in 2 patients and with autogenous ribs in 5. Fifty-four patients underwent 68 muscle transpositions; these included 24 pectoralis major, 23 latissimus dorsi, 6 serratus anterior, 3 external oblique, 2 rectus abdominis, 2 trapezius, and 8 other. The omentum was transposed in eight patients. The median hospitalization was 9 days. There were no 30-day operative deaths. The patients were generally extubated during the evening of the operation or on the following morning. Two patients required tracheostomy. Most other patients had only minor changes in pulmonary function (Meadows et al, 1985).

The long-term survival of patients with primary chest wall malignant neoplasms is dependent on the cell type and the extent of chest wall resection. In the Mayo Clinic series, the overall 5-year survival rate was 57% (King et al, 1986). Wide resection for chondrosarcoma resulted in a 5-year survival rate of 96% (McAfee et al, 1985) compared with only 70% for patients who had local excision (Fig. 53–13). The 5-year overall survival rate for patients with either chondrosarcoma or rhabdomyosarcoma was 70% (King et al, 1986), in contrast to a rate of only 38% for patients with malignant fibrous histiocytomas (Fig. 53–14). Recurrent neoplasm, however, was an ominous sign; only 17% of patients in whom recurrence developed survived 5 years.

TABLE 53–1 ■ **Estimates of Number of New Cases of Primary Malignant Chest Wall Tumors in the United States in 1993**

Tumor	*All Sites (No.)*	*Chest Wall (No.)*
Soft tissue sarcoma	6,000	360
Chondrosarcoma	400	60
Ewing's sarcoma	300	45
Solitary plasmacytoma	125	25
Osteosarcoma	600	18
Total	7,425	508

SUMMARY

The key to successful therapy of primary chest wall neoplasms remains early diagnosis and aggressive surgical resection. This procedure can generally be performed in one operation, with minimal respiratory insufficiency and with low operation mortality rates. When combined with current methods of reconstruction, potential cure is likely for most patients with primary chest wall neoplasms.

COMMENTS AND CONTROVERSIES

As documented by Drs. Graeber, Jones, and Pairolero, primary malignant tumors of the chest wall are relatively uncommon. Because almost all primary malignant chest wall neoplasms can be classified as either soft tissue sarcomas or malignant neoplasms of bone or cartilage, estimates can be made of the number of tumors expected to be diagnosed in the United States in 2000. Approximately 500 new cases of primary malignant chest wall tumors will be diagnosed yearly in the United States. Because it is estimated that there will be 1,170,000 new cases of cancer diagnosed in the United States yearly, primary malignant tumors of the chest wall comprised only 0.04% of all new cancers. Because primary malignant tumors of the chest wall are relatively uncommon, data to support therapy options are sparse, but nicely outlined in this chapter.

There is only one area of disagreement, and that is the classification by the authors that chest wall desmoid tumors are benign. Many pathologists currently accept the desmoid tumor as a low-grade fibrosarcoma and not a benign disease (Brodsky et al, 1992; Posner et al, 1989).

M. E. B.

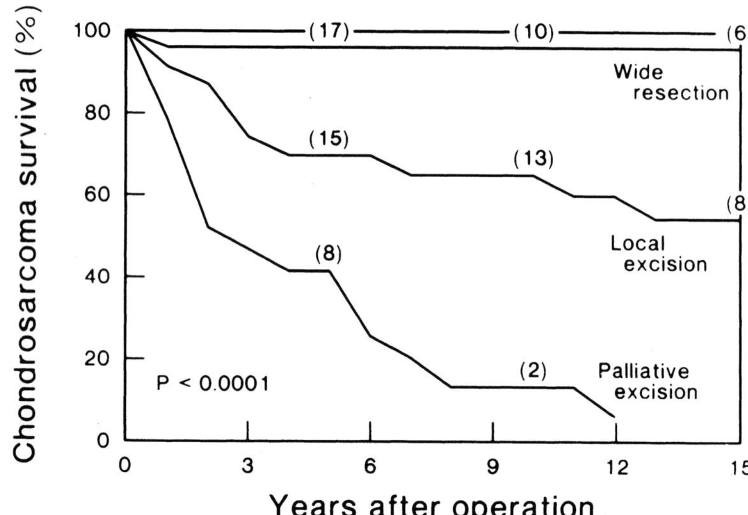

FIGURE 53–13 ■ Survival of patients with chest wall chondrosarcomas by extent of operation. Zero time on the abscissa represents the day of chest wall resection. (From McAfee MK, Pairolero PC, Bergstrahl EJ et al: Chondrosarcoma of the chest wall: Factors affecting survival. Ann Thorac Surg 40:535, 1985.)

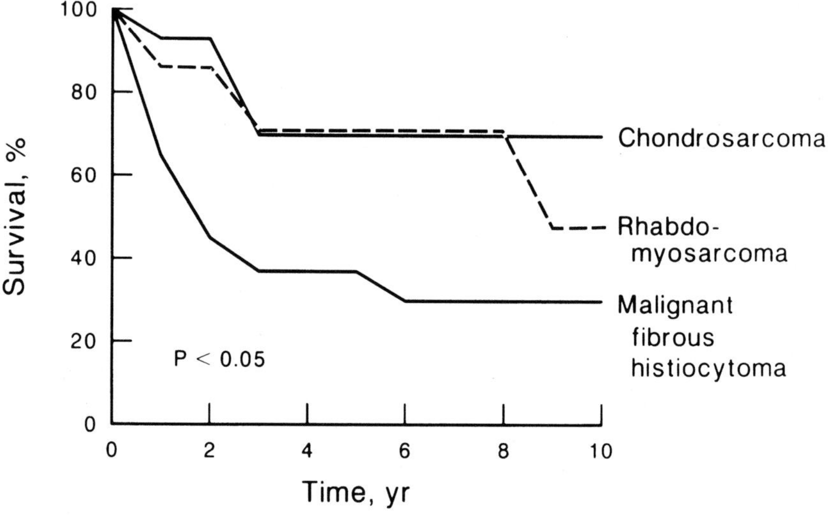

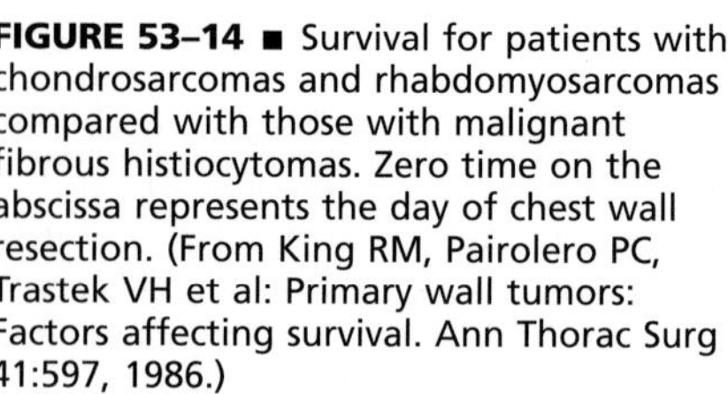
FIGURE 53–14 ■ Survival for patients with chondrosarcomas and rhabdomyosarcomas compared with those with malignant fibrous histiocytomas. Zero time on the abscissa represents the day of chest wall resection. (From King RM, Pairolero PC, Trastek VH et al: Primary wall tumors: Factors affecting survival. Ann Thorac Surg 41:597, 1986.)

■ *KEY REFERENCES*

Graeber GM, Snyder RJ, Fleming AW et al: Initial and long-term results in the management of primary chest wall neoplasms. Ann Thorac Surg 34:664, 1982.

These authors present the Armed Forces Institute of Pathology's experience with 110 patients with primary chest wall neoplasms. Included are both soft tissue and bone neoplasms. The roles of chemotherapy and radiotherapy for each type of malignant neoplasm are discussed.

King RM, Pairolero PC, Trastek VF et al: Primary chest wall tumors: Factors affecting survival. Ann Thorac Surg 41:597, 1986.

This series represents a 20-year experience of chest wall tumors treated at the Mayo Clinic from 1955 to 1975 and includes both soft tissue and bony tumors. Both chondrosarcoma and rhabdomyosarcoma had a better prognosis than did malignant fibrous histiocytoma.

McAfee MK, Pairolero PC, Bergstralh EJ et al: Chondrosarcoma of the chest wall: Factors affecting survival. Ann Thorac Surg 40:535, 1985.

These authors present a single institution's experience (96 patients) with chondrosarcoma of the chest wall. This series is the largest series of chest wall chondrosarcoma reported to date and clearly demonstrates that the natural history of chondrosarcoma is one of slow growth and local recurrence.

McGraw JB, Arnold PG: McGraw and Arnold's Atlas of Muscle and Musculocutaneous Flaps. Hampton Press, 1986.

The anatomy, indications for, and technique of commonly used muscle flaps in all areas of the body are each summarized, illustrated by color photographs of fresh cadaver dissections, and then supplemented by appropriate intraoperative color photographs of clinical cases. This atlas should be read by every surgeon interested in the reconstruction of the chest wall.

Pairolero PC, Arnold PG: Chest wall tumors: Experience with 100 consecutive patients. J Thorac Cardiovasc Surg 90:367, 1985.

This series represents a single team of surgeons' experience in the management of 100 consecutive patients with chest wall tumors. This series of patients demonstrates that aggressive resection for a chest wall tumor with reliable reconstruction can be accomplished safely and that early wide resection is potentially curative therapy.

■ *REFERENCES*

Aoki J, Moser RP Jr, Kransdorf MJ: Chondrosarcoma of the sternum: CT features. J Comput Assist Tomogr 13:535, 1989.

Arnold PG, Pairolero PC: Surgical management of the radiated chest wall. Plast Reconstr Surg 77:605, 1986.

Arnold PG, Pairolero PC: The serratus anterior muscle: Intrathoracic and extrathoracic utilization. Plast Reconstr Surg 73:240, 1984.

Arnold PG, Pairolero PC: Chest wall reconstruction: Experience with 100 consecutive patients. Ann Surg 199:725, 1984.

Arnold PG, Pairolero PC: Use of pectoralis major muscle flaps to repair defects of anterior chest wall. Plast Reconstr Surg 63:205, 1979.

Arnold PG, Pairolero PC: Chondrosarcoma of the manubrium: Resection and reconstruction with pectoralis major muscle. Mayo Clinic Proc 53:54, 1978.

Arunabh, Gupta SD, Bal S et al: Spontaneous regression of extramedullary plasmacytoma: A case report. Jpn J Surg 18:455, 1988.

Askin FB, Rosai J, Sibley K et al: Malignant small cell tumor of the thoracopulmonary region in childhood. Cancer 43:2438, 1979.

Ayala AG, Zornosa J: Primary bone tumors: Percutaneous needle biopsy. Radiology 149:675, 1983.

Bataille R, Sany J: Solitary myeloma: Clinical and prognostic features of a review of 114 cases. Cancer 48:845, 1981.

Boring CC, Squires TS, Tong T, Montgomery S: Cancer Statistics, 1994. CA J Clin 44:7, 1994.

Bostwick J III, Nahai F, Wallace JG, Vasconez LO: Sixty latissimus dorsi flaps. Plast Reconstr Surg 63:31, 1979.

Boyd A: Tumors of the chest wall. In Hood RM, Antman K, Boyd A et al (eds): Surgical Diseases of Pleura and Chest Wall. Philadelphia, WB Saunders, 1986.

Brodsky JT, Gordon MS, Hajdu SI, Burt M: Desmoid tumors of the chest wall: A locally recurrent problem. J Thor Cardiovasc Surg 104:900, 1992.

Brown AP, Fixen JA, Plowman PN: Local control of Ewing's sarcoma: An analysis of 67 patients. Br J Radiol 60:261, 1987.

Burt M: Primary malignant tumors: The Memorial Sloan-Kettering Cancer Center Experience. Chest Surg Clin N Am 4:137, 1994.

Campbell DA: Reconstruction of the anterior thoracic wall. J Thorac Surg 19:456, 1950.

Cavanaugh DG, Cabellon S Jr, Peake JB: A logical approach to chest wall neoplasms. Ann Thorac Surg 41:436, 1986.

Cavazzana AO, Miser JS, Ferrerson J, Triche TJ: Experimental evidence for a neural origin of Ewing's sarcoma of bone. Am J Surg Pathol 127:507, 1987.

Fisher J, Bostwick J, Powell RW: Latissimus dorsi blood supply after thoracodorsal vessel division: The serratus collateral. Plast Reconstr Surg 72:502, 1983.

Galluccio G, Conti L, Fiorucci F, Li Bianchi E: Solitary plasmacytoma of the chest wall. Panminerva Med 31:189, 1989.

Gordon MS, Hajdu SE, Bains MS, Burt ME: Soft tissue sarcomas of the chest wall. J Thorac Cardiovasc Surg 101:843, 1991.

Graeber GM, Seyfer AE, Shriver CD, Awan M: Desmoid tumor of the paraspinous muscle involving the chest wall. Mil Med 150:458, 1985.

Greager JA, Patel MK, Briele HA et al: Soft tissue sarcomas of the adult thoracic wall. Cancer 59:370, 1987.

Groff DB, Adkins PC: Chest wall tumors. Ann Thorac Surg 4:260, 1967.

Grosfeld JL, Rescoria FJ, West KW et al: Chest wall resection and reconstruction for malignant conditions in childhood. J Pediatr Surg 23:667, 1988.

Hayery P, Reitamo JJ, Tofferman S et al: The desmoid tumor II. Am J Clin Pathol 77:674, 1982.

Hayery P, Scheinin TM: The desmoid (Reitamo) syndrome: Etiology, manifestation, pathogenesis, and treatment. Curr Probl Surg 25:4, 1988.

Hayes FA, Thompson EI, Hustu HO et al: The response of Ewing's sarcoma to sequential cyclophosphamide and adriamycin induction therapy. J Clin Oncol 1:45, 1983.

Hodgkinson DJ, Arnold PG: Chest-wall reconstruction using the external oblique muscle. Br J Plast Surg 33:316, 1980.

Huvos AG: Osteogenic sarcoma of bones and soft tissues in older person. Cancer 57:1442, 1986.

Huvos AG, Woodard HQ, Cahan WG et al: Postradiation osteogenic sarcoma of bone and soft tissues. Cancer 55:1244, 1985.

Jablons D, Steinberg SM, Roth J et al: Metastasectomy for soft tissue sarcoma: further evidence for efficacy and prognostic indicators. J Thorac Cardiovasc Surg 97:695, 1989.

Jaffe N, Raymond AK, Ayala A et al: Effect of cumulative courses of intraarterial cis-diamminedichloroplatin-II on the primary tumor in osteosarcoma. Cancer 63:63, 1989.

Jurkiewicz MJ, Arnold PG: The omentum: An account of its use in the reconstruction of the chest wall. Ann Surg 185:548, 1977.

Kinzbrunner B, Ritter S, Domingo J, Rosenthal CJ: Remission of rapidly growing desmoid tumors after tamoxifen therapy. Cancer 52:2201, 1983.

Lane JM, Hurson B, Boland PJ, Glasser DB: Osteogenic sarcoma. Clin Orthop 204:93, 1986.

Leibel SA, Wara WM, Hill DR et al: Desmoid tumors: Local control and patterns of relapse following radiation therapy. Int J Radiat Oncol Biol Phys 9:1167, 1983.

Lichtenstein L: Bone Tumors. St. Louis, CV Mosby, 1977.

Lynch HT, Krush AJ, Harlan WL, Sharp EA: Association of soft tissue sarcoma, leukemia, and brain tumors in families affected with breast cancer. Am Surg 39:199, 1973.

Malangoni MA, Ofstein LC, Grosfeld JL et al: Survival and pulmonary function following chest wall resection and reconstruction in children. J Pediatr Surg 15:906, 1980.

McKinnon JG, Neifeld JP, Kay S et al: Management of desmoid tumors. Surg Gynecol Obstet 169:104, 1989.

Meadows JA III, Staats BA, Pairolero PC et al: Effect of resection of the sternum and manubrium in conjunction with muscle transposition on pulmonary function. Mayo Clin Proc 60:604, 1985.

Meis JM, Butler JJ, Osborne BM, Ordonez NG: Solitary plasmacytomas of the bone and extramedullary plasmacytomas: A clinicopathologic and immunohistochemical study. Cancer 59:1475, 1987.

Mill WB, Griffith R: The role of radiation therapy in the management of plasma cell tumors. Cancer 45:647, 1980.

Ozzello L, Stout AP, Murray RM: Cultural characteristics of malignant histiocytomas and fibrous xanthomas. Cancer 16:331, 1963.

Pairolero PC, Arnold PG: Primary tumors of the anterior chest wall. Surg Rounds 9:19, 1986a.

Pairolero PC, Arnold PG: Thoracic wall defects: Surgical management of 205 consecutive patients. Mayo Clin Proc 61:557, 1986b.

Pairolero PC, Arnold PG: Management of recalcitrant median sternotomy wounds. J Thorac Cardiovasc Surg 88:357, 1984.

Pairolero PC, Arnold PG, Piehler JM: Intrathoracic transposition of extrathoracic skeletal muscle. J Thorac Cardiovasc Surg 86:809, 1983.

Pascuzzi CA, Dahlin DC, Clagett OT: Primary tumors of the ribs and sternum. Surg Gynecol Obstet 104:390, 1957.

Pass HI: Primary and metastatic chest wall tumors. In Roth JA, Ruckdeschel JC, Weisenburger TH (eds): Thoracic Oncology. Philadelphia, WB Saunders, 1989.

Perez CA, Tefft M, Nesbit M et al: The role of radiation therapy in the management of non-metastatic Ewing's sarcoma of bone: Report of the Intergroup Ewing's Sarcoma Study. Int J Radiat Oncol Biol Phys 7:141, 1981.

Perry RR, Venzon D, Roth JA, Pass HI: Survival after surgical resection for high-grade chest wall sarcomas. Ann Thorac Surg 49:363, 1990.

Posner MC, Shiu MH, Newsome JL et al: The desmoid tumor: Not a benign disease. Arch Surg 124:191, 1989.

Raymond AK, Chawla SP, Carrasco CH et al: Osteosarcoma chemotherapy effect: A prognostic factor. Semin Diagn Pathol 4:212, 1987.

Rosai J: Ackerman's Surgical Pathology. St. Louis, CV Mosby, 1989.

Ryan MB, McMurtrey MJ, Roth JA: Current management of chest-wall tumors. Surg Clin North Am 69:1061, 1989.

Sabanathan S, Salama FD, Morgan WE, Harvey JA: Primary chest wall tumors. Ann Thorac Surg 39:4, 1985.

Saito T, Kobayashi H, Kitamura S: Ultrasonographic approach to diagnosing chest wall tumors. Chest 94:1271, 1988.

Seyer AE: Radiation-associated lesions of the chest wall. Surg Gynecol Obstet 167:129, 1988.

Shamberger RC, Grier HE, Weinstein HJ et al: Chest wall tumors in infancy and childhood. Cancer 63:774, 1989.

Sherman NE, Romsdahl M, Evans H et al: Desmoid tumors: A 20-year radiotherapy experience. Int J Radiat Oncol Biol Phys 19:37, 1990.

Souba WW, McKenna RJ Jr, Meis J et al: Radiation-induced sarcomas of the chest wall. Cancer 57:610, 1986.

Stefanko J, Turnbull AD, Helson L et al: Primitive neuroectodermal tumors of the chest wall. J Surg Oncol 37:33, 1988.

Stelzer P, Gay WA Jr: Tumors of the chest wall. Surg Clin North Am 60:779, 1980.

Thomas PRM, Foulkes MA, Gilula LA et al: Primary Ewing's sarcoma of the ribs: A report from the Intragroup Ewing's Sarcoma Study. Cancer 51:1021, 1983.

Tucker MA, D'Angio GJ, Boice JD Jr et al: Bone sarcomas linked to radiotherapy and chemotherapy in children. N Engl J Med 317:588, 1987.

Turc-Cavel C, Philip I, Berger M et al: Chromosomal translocations in Ewing's sarcoma. N Engl J Med 309:497, 1983.

Venn GE, Gellister J, DaCosta PE, Goldstraw P: Malignant fibrous histiocytoma in thoracic surgical practice. J Thorac Cardiovasc Surg 91:234, 1986.

Wallner KE, Nori D, Burt M et al: Adjuvant brachytherapy for treatment of chest wall sarcomas. J Thorac Cardiovasc Surg 101:888, 1991.

Whang-Peng J, Triche TJ, Knutsen T et al: Chromosome translocation in peripheral neuroepithelioma. N Engl J Med 311:584, 1984.

Winkler K, Beron G, Kotz R et al: Neoadjuvant chemotherapy for osteogenic sarcoma: Results of a cooperative German/Austrian study. J Clin Oncol 2:617, 1984.

CHAPTER **54**

Radionecrosis and Infection of the Chest Wall and Sternum

Robert B. Lee
Joseph I. Miller, Jr.

Injury to the chest wall is generally a result of neoplasm, trauma, radionecrosis, or infection. Congenital deformity may cause a severe defect with resulting physiologic derangement, but it is not considered damage inflicted to the body by external force. Neoplastic, traumatic, and congenital diseases of the chest wall have been dealt with elsewhere in this text. This discussion focuses on two entities: radionecrosis of the chest wall and infection of soft tissues and supporting structures of the chest wall.

Most of our knowledge and management techniques for radiation-induced injury comes from the experience gained by resection of chest wall tumors and defects related to radionecrosis (Arnold and Pairolero, 1989; Bostwick et al, 1984; Larson et al, 1982; Miller, 1986; Seyfer, 1988). The principles of wide excision of obviously necrotic and questionably viable tissue followed by immediate reconstruction with omentum, muscle, or musculocutaneous flaps are essential to success. The preoperative considerations, techniques of resection and reconstruction, postoperative management, and clinical experience are examined in detail in this chapter.

Chest wall infection involves the skin and soft tissues, the cartilaginous and bony undercarriage, or, frequently, a combination of the two. The cause of the infection may be de novo and thus primary in nature or secondary and resulting from a previously existing disease or procedure. The management may be simple and require parenteral or intravenous antibiotics or complex and necessitate radical débridement and reconstruction. The causes of chest wall infections are emphasized as are many of the techniques of resection and reconstruction that have been examined in relation to radiation-induced injury.

HISTORICAL NOTE

The historical development of the management of both radionecrosis and infection of the chest wall is based on the two basic techniques: (1) adequate débridement of devitalized defunctionalized necrotic tissue, and (2) reconstruction of the structural and physiologic integrity of the chest wall. Halstead established the principles and techniques of débridement. Although new devices, such as the electrocautery and laser scalpels, have come into use, the surgical principles are unchanged. Reconstruction of the chest wall, however, has undergone remarkable evolution during the last 100 years. The management of chest wall radiation injury has paralleled the advancement of reconstruction techniques of the chest wall. Pare remarked that "gangrene and mortification as complications of treatment give more evil to surgeons and patients than the maladies in which they occur" (Woods et al, 1979). This is certainly the case with radiotherapy, a two-edged sword that not only results in the cessation of primary and recurrent neoplastic growth, but may also induce neoplastic growth in the radiated site (Bostwick et al, 1984; Larson and McMurtry, 1984; Seyfer, 1988; Woods et al, 1979). Some changes have occurred in the techniques of radiotherapy that have reduced the severity of the ionizing effects. However, the frequency of injury may actually become increasingly more evident as patients choose breast-conservation procedures and radiotherapy for primary breast malignancies (Lenene et al, 1977).

Radiation-caused injury was recognized clinically and described histologically in the early 1900s by Wolback (1909). During the late 1960s, it became customary to treat the internal mammary lymph node chain prophylactically when a primary breast carcinoma occurred in the inner quadrant. The axilla was also irradiated (Haagensen et al, 1969). Some decrease in the severity of injury has been seen with the use of megavoltage compared with the earlier use of orthovoltage. The severity of injury is still less with the newer techniques of cobalt–beam therapy and supervoltage (Latham, 1966). Electron linear acceleration may further decrease the toxic effects as the ionizing beam becomes more focused. Although these changes have somewhat lessened the severity of the malady of radionecrosis, the most significant advances have come in the reconstruction of the chest wall after resection of the injury. Resection of the chest wall was attempted and described in 1898 by Parham (1898), who echoed the woes of his predecessors when he iatrogenically produced a pneumothorax: "Suddenly was presented to our anxious view one of the most startling clinical pictures that the surgeon can ever be called upon to witness . . . no wonder the old surgeons discountenanced such operations . . . so sudden in my case was the pneumothorax and so striking were the manifestations of profound shock, threatening almost instant dissolution before our eyes, that I resolved to acquaint myself more thoroughly with the dangers of thoracic surgery. . . ." Significant advancement did not occur until the advent of endotracheal intubation, positive pressure ventilation, closed chest drainage, and antibiotic therapy (Arnold and Pairolero, 1984).

Reconstruction of the chest wall began in earnest in 1947 when fascia lata grafts were used for closure of the chest wall by Watson and James (1947). Simultaneously, Maier (1947) was using large cutaneous flaps, which included the opposite breast in patients with defects caused by mastectomies, to close the resulting anterior chest wall defects. He also used and reported this technique for the management of chest wall radiation-caused injury. Many autogenous tissues, such as bone, cartilage, and ribs were tried to provide structural support. Prosthetic materials were introduced and tried in the 1940s and 1950s (Sando and Jurkiewicz, 1986). Different cutaneous flaps were proposed. Not a new concept, cutaneous flaps were described in 600 BC in the Sushruta Samhita (Kittle, 1986). Campbell (1949) popularized the use of the latissimus dorsi muscular flap, originally described by Tansaii (1906) for chest wall coverage. The use of Marlex was popularized by Usher and Wallace (1959) when they successfully used this more pliable prosthetic material for reconstruction; it was extensively used for the support of the chest wall both as a single layer and with acrylic reinforcement (Kittle, 1986; Usher and Wallace, 1959).

During this period, most reconstructions were multistaged, complicated undertakings. Kiricuta (1963) of Rumania performed and described transposition of pedicle omentum for the management of partial-thickness radiation-induced injury in 1963. He previously introduced the techniques in 1956 for the therapy of vesicovaginal fistulas (Arnold and Pairolero, 1989; Kiricuta, 1963). The use of the latissimus dorsi muscle flap, as described by Camel in 1950, was unfortunately essentially unnoticed and ignored for 20 years until the mid-1970s, although many other skin flaps, muscle flaps, and prosthetic materials were tried (Pairolero and Arnold, 1986). Modern management of the sequelae of chest wall radiotherapy is founded on the aforementioned principles of aggressive resection of necrotic and questionably viable tissue with immediate reconstruction that uses healthy oxygen- and nutrient-carrying muscles. These principles were established by Bostwick and Jurkiewicz at Emory University–affiliated hospitals (Bostwick et al, 1984), Larson and McMurtry (1984) at M. D. Anderson, and Arnold and Pairolero at the Mayo Clinic (Arnold and Pairolero, 1984, 1986, 1989; Pairolero and Arnold, 1986). Their philosophies, techniques, and results have been widely accepted and used by plastic and thoracic surgeons and form the basis of the following discussion.

■ *HISTORICAL READINGS*

Arnold PG, Pairolero PC: Chest wall reconstruction, experience with 100 consecutive patients. Ann Surg 199:725, 1984.

Arnold PG, Pairolero PC: Reconstruction of the radiation-damaged chest wall. Surg Clin 69:1081, 1989.

Arnold PG, Pairolero PC: Surgical management of the radiated chest wall. Plast Reconstr Surg 77:605, 1986.

Bostwick J, Stevenson TR, Nahai F et al: Radiation to the breast, complications amenable to surgical treatment. Ann Surg 200:543, 1984.

Campbell AA: Reconstruction of the anterior thoracic wall. J Thorac Cardiovasc Surg 19:456, 1949.

Haagensen CD, Bhonjlay SB, Guttmann RJ et al: Metastasis of carcinoma of the breast to the periphery of the regional lymph node filter. Ann Surg 169:174, 1969.

Kiricuta I: C'empoli du grand epiplasm dans la churzie du sein cancereux. Presse Med 71:15, 1963.

Kittle FC: Muscle flaps and thoracic problems. Kittle FC (ed): In Current Controversies in Thoracic Surgery. Philadelphia, WB Saunders, 1986.

Larson DL, McMurtry MJ: Musculocutaneous flap reconstruction of chest wall defects: An experience with 50 patients. Plast Reconstr Surg 73:734, 1984.

Latham WD: Operative treatment for post-radiation defects of the chest wall. Am Surg 32:700, 1966.

Lenene MB, Harris JR, Hellman S: Treatment of carcinoma of the breast by radiation therapy. Cancer 39:28840, 1977.

Maier HC: Surgical management of large defects of the thoracic wall. Surgery 22:169, 1947.

Pairolero PC, Arnold PG: Muscle flaps and thoracic problems: Chest wall defects: reconstruction with antogenous tissue. In Kittle FC (ed): Current Controversies in Thoracic Surgery. Philadelphia, WB Saunders, 1986.

Parham FW: Thoracic resection for tumors growing from the bony wall of the chest. Trans South Surg Gynecol Assoc 11:223, 1898.

Sando W, Jurkiewicz MJ: An approach to repairs of radiation necrosis of chest wall and mammary gland. World J Surg 10:206, 1986.

Seyfer AE: Radiation-associated lesions of the chest wall. Surg Gynecol Obstet 167:129, 1988.

Usher FC, Wallace SA: Tissue reaction to plastics. Arch Surg 76:997, 1959.

Watson WC, James AG: Fascia lata grafts for chest wall defects. J Thorac Cardiovasc Surg 16:399, 1947.

Wolbach SR: Pathologic history of chronic x-ray dermatitis and early x-ray carcinoma. J Med Res 21:415, 1909.

Woods JE, Arnold PG, Masson JK et al: Management of radiation necrosis and advanced cancer of the chest wall in patients with breast malignancy. Plast Reconstr Surg 63:235, 1979.

Radionecrosis

ETIOLOGY

Radiotherapy has been shown to be effective in controlling certain malignancies of the chest, which include Hodgkin's lymphoma, bronchogenic carcinoma, and mammary carcinoma. The ionizing radiation may control not only a primary malignancy, but it also may eventually induce a secondary malignancy years later (Bostwick et al, 1984; Latham, 1966; Pizzarello and Witcofoki, 1975). Furthermore, the ionizing radiation is not limited to the neoplastic cells but also affects the undiseased mediastinum and chest wall structures. There are numerous reports of accelerated coronary atherosclerosis (Arsenian, 1991), cardiac valvular disease (Carlson et al, 1991), and cardiac arrhythmias (Seama et al, 1991) caused by radiation effects in the literature.

Ionizing rays affect rapidly dividing cells by releasing free radicals and peroxidase and thus splitting DNA; such radiation is lethal to the dividing neoplastic cells. Concurrent transmission of radiation to surrounding vascular structures damages the endothelial cells of small arteries and arterioles, which results in luminal obliteration by myointimal fibrosis and myxoid degeneration of the intima. The resulting occlusion leads to relative tissue anoxemia, which eventually causes ischemic fibrosis. As expected, the less well-vascularized tissues, such as cartilage, tendon, and bone, are particularly vulnerable. The ultimate result is soft tissue ulceration with underlying osteoradionecrosis and chondroradionecrosis (Arnold and Pairolero, 1986; Latham, 1966; MacMillan et al, 1986; Smith et al, 1982).

A dose-response relationship appears to exist (Bostwick et al, 1984). Standard doses of 4500 to 5000 cGy that are given over 5 to 6 weeks in 200-cGy increments appear to be associated with fewer complications (Meyer, 1978; Pantoja et al, 1978). However, doses as low as 2200 cGy may cause significant skeletal damage (Parker and Berry, 1976; Smith et al, 1982). Originally, orthovoltage was used for radiotherapy. As technology advanced, megavoltage was developed. Although the amount of radiation administered was increased, there was believed to be no significant increase in complications (Smith et al, 1982). Subsequently, it was shown that megavoltage induces damage to deeper tissues, which may lead to lethal changes. Thus, there is no modality that is free of possible ill effects. Even when "safe doses" are given, incorrect dosage calculations, improper machine calibrations, inaccurate field marking, or overlapping of the portals may result in serious radiation-induced injury (Larson et al, 1982; Pantoja et al, 1978).

After either low radiation doses or the initial dose, skin erythema may occur; this is called radiodermatitis. The skin may become tender, edematous, and firm from the endothelial injury to arterioles, capillaries, and lymphatic vessels. Higher doses or prolonged administration may result in blistering of the skin, with varying degrees of necrosis. The body's natural repair mechanisms may reverse these superficial changes in a short period of days to weeks. However, because of the vascular injury and induced endarteritis obliterans, the deeper tissue changes persist and progress. The inflammatory response and anoxemia produce fibrosis and scarring. As the subcutaneous tissues undergo fibrosis, the epithelium, now friable, is disrupted, frequently ulcerates, and becomes chronically infected. The underlying structural support of bone and cartilage may become necrotic (Robinson, 1975). Thus, full-thickness injury may occur, which produces devastating tissue loss and a significant challenge for the surgeon.

MANAGEMENT

Preoperative Assessment and Planning

In-depth preoperative assessment and planning is essential for success in this patient population. The typical patient with a chest wall defect from radionecrosis is a 40- to 50-year-old woman who has undergone radical or modified mastectomy followed by postoperative radiotherapy for residual microscopic disease. They generally have large, malodorous, necrotic wounds that do not heal and are surrounded by significant fibrosis. Pain is a prominent component, and these patients require greater than average doses of opioids for relief (Bostwick et al, 1984; Latham, 1966). Frequently, these patients are chronically depressed as a result of their original disease process, the therapy thereof, and the resulting complications. All too often they have been told that "this is the price to be paid for the cure of the cancer," "recurrent tumor is the cause of the problem," or worse, "there is no hope." These patients should be encouraged and given accurate facts and options, thereby allowing them to participate in their own care (Bostwick et al, 1984; Latham, 1966; Seyfer, 1988).

PREOPERATIVE EVALUATION

- History and physical evaluation
  - Original primary lesion
  - Amount, type, and portals of radiotherapy
  - Co-morbid disease processes (i.e., diabetes mellitus)
  - Area and depth of destruction
  - Involvement of bone, cartilage, or lung
  - Limitation of motion of upper extremities
  - Exercise tolerance and nutritional status
- Radiologic evaluation
  - Posteroanterior and lateral chest radiograph with rib detail
  - Computed tomographic chest scan
  - Bone scan
  - Magnetic resonance imaging scan (if spinal column involvement is suspected)
- Physiologic evaluation
  - Thallium stress test
  - Pulmonary function test
  - Nutritional status (i.e., concentrations of albumin, prealbumin, and transferrin, and skin testing for anergy)
  - Biopsy of lesion to determine presence or absence of residual or recurrent tumor

The assessment should include a physical and psychological profile. The history should be ascertained in regard to the amount and type of radiation, recent bleeding from the site, and possible recent changes in cardiac or pulmonary status. Recent sudden or profound bleeding may indicate underlying involvement of the internal mammary vessels, intercostal vessels, or great vessel involvement. Knowledge of coexisting cardiac, pulmonary, renal, and endocrine disease may influence the operative plan. Diabetes, steroid dependency, recent chemotherapy, and obesity may influence the postoperative healing and the choice of flaps (Larson and McMurtry, 1984; Sando and Jurkiewicz, 1986).

The location on the chest wall determines which flaps are available for reconstruction (Larson and McMurtry, 1984; Sando and Jurkiewicz, 1986). The size and depth of the wound determine whether partial- or full-thickness chest wall resection will be required and what amount of tissue will be necessary for the reconstruction. The presence of chronic infection may require preoperative antibiotic therapy and local wound care prior to the surgical intervention. Every effort should be made to determine the presence or absence of malignancy in the wound. The presence of malignancy obviously requires more extensive resection. If malignancy is found, further studies may be necessary to evaluate the extent of invasion (Arnold and Pairolero, 1989; Bostwick et al, 1984; Larson et al, 1982; Larson and McMurtry, 1984; Seyfer, 1988).

Plain radiographs may reveal necrosis of bone, which alerts the surgeon to resect deeper tissues. When malignancy is identified or suspected preoperatively, computed tomography or magnetic resonance imaging scans may be performed to assess the depth of invasion or involvement of underlying lung or mediastinal structures (Arnold and Pairolero, 1989). It may be necessary to resect underlying lung. Pulmonary function testing provides data to guide the extent of resection. Frequently, the underlying lung is fibrotic from prior radiotherapy and may not contribute to overall pulmonary function. Larson and McMurtry (1984) showed that chest wall resection for tumor and radionecrosis may be asociated with no change and even an improvement in the forced expiratory volume in 1 second and vital capacity. The dipyridamole thallium stress test accurately predicts which patients undergoing thoracic procedures are at risk for a cardiac event (Miller, 1992).

Perhaps the most important assessment involves the patient's life-style, ability to work, and prognosis. These patients are generally debilitated and unable to work either because of the therapy of the primary malignancy or because of complications of the postoperative radiotherapy. The prognosis for patients with breast cancer that is recurrent in the local chest wall tissues is poor; most die of distant metastasis within 14 months (Larson et al, 1982; Larson and McMurtry, 1984; Seyfer, 1988). Similarly, postradiation sarcomas are lethal (Larson and McMurtry, 1984). Given this, many surgeons would not undertake extensive resections. However, Woods and colleagues (1979) noted that, in their series, several of the patients undergoing resection and reconstruction died just a few months afterward, but prior to death, they stated that they had great improvement in the quality of their lives after the removal of the foul-smelling, gangrenous, ulcerating malignant lesions, which indicated that the extensive procedure was indeed worthwhile.

Resection Techniques

Larsen and coworkers (1982) succinctly described the purpose of resection as follows: "to rid the patient of the disease process, maintaining chest wall and pleural continuity with a single-stage reconstruction, minimizing donor morbidity and thus rehabilitating the patient as quickly as possible." Virtually all authors advocate aggressive resection of the radionecrotic and questionably viable tissue (Arnold and Pairolero, 1989; Bostwick et al, 1984; Larson and McMurtry, 1984; Latham, 1966; Seyfer, 1988). Simple excision and primary closure are usually not satisfactory (Woods et al, 1979). To be successful, the resection must encompass all soft tissues, cartilage, and bone of poor quality, turgor, color, and vascularity (Seyfer, 1988). Occasionally, partial-thickness resections can be performed, but more often, full-thickness resection is required to remove all necrotic tissue (Arnold and Pairolero, 1986; Bostwick et al, 1984; Larson et al, 1982; Seyfer, 1988). Full-thickness resection of the lesion may require additional resection of normal rib, approximately 2 inches, to allow a comfortable route of entry for the muscle flaps chosen to close the residual space. No residual space should be left, and there must be sufficient transposed tissue to close any intrathoracic space (Miller, 1986).

Full-thickness resection is generally the rule. The surgeon must be prepared to resect underlying vascular structures and pulmonary parenchyma, if necessary, and not to leave nonviable cartilage and bone, which might produce chronic draining fistulas, regardless of the needed coverage. If the pleural space is entered or the pulmonary parenchyma is resected, pneumothorax may not occur because the lung is frequently stiff and has undergone fibrosis, and the pleural space has been obliterated as a result of the adhesions produced by prior radiotherapy. After all nonviable tissue has been completely resected, reconstruction may proceed.

Reconstruction of Partial-Thickness Defects

Devitalized skin or small ulcerations that are not associated with underlying soft tissue, cartilage, or bony necrosis may be amenable to partial-thickness resection. This usually is not the case, and full-thickness resections are generally required (Arnold and Pairolero, 1984, 1989; Larson et al, 1982; Pairolero and Arnold, 1986). However, if a partial-thickness resection results in procurement of healthy viable tissue, primary closure of a small superficial wound is preferable (Larson et al, 1982; Sando and Jurkiewicz, 1986). Primary closure is usually not an option and often compromises resection attempts, thus eventually failing (Larson and McMurtry, 1984; Miller, 1986). Irradiated tissues appear to respond differently to débridement; therefore, what appears to be adequate at the time of the operation may be necrotic the next day. When the primary wound breaks down, more aggressive resection is indicated. Topical antibiotics, such as Sefomylon or silver sulfadiazine, may be used to improve wound characteristics in anticipation of a meshed split-thickness skin graft (Sando and Jurkiewicz, 1986).

More often, partial-thickness resection requires reconstruction with transposed tissue. After viable tissues are obtained, omentum may be harvested as a graft on a pedicle and may be brought into the area. Based on the right or left gastric epiploic artery or both, omentum is healthy, well vascularized tissue that is capable of angiogenesis (Bostwick et al, 1984; Fix and Vasconez, 1989). The omentum may be used alone or with a split-thickness skin graft (Bostwick et al, 1984; Larson et al, 1982; Sando and Jurkiewicz, 1986; Woods et al, 1979). The techniques for omental usage and harvest have been well documented by Alday (Alday and Goldsmith, 1972).

Bostwick and colleagues (1984) described the use of the omental free graft for the management of radiation-induced injury. As a free graft, the omentum may be used to cover partial chest wall defects, to wrap the brachial plexus after neurolysis, or to treat radiation-induced hemifacial atrophy (Arnold and Irons, 1981; Bostwick et al, 1984). Most authors now use omentum for partial-thickness defect reconstruction or as a back-up when flaps fail in the therapy of full-thickness reconstructions (Bostwick et al, 1984; Larson et al, 1982; Seyfer, 1988; Woods et al, 1979).

MacMillan and colleagues (1986) recently introduced the concept of tissue expanders for the management of the partial-thickness injury. The expander is placed in a nearby area of nonirradiated skin. An advancement flap of sufficient size, which includes skin and subcutaneous tissues, can be "stretched to sufficient size to cover the partial defect" (MacMillan et al, 1986).

TABLE 54–1 ■ **Choice of Flaps for Reconstruction of Full-Thickness Defects of the Chest Wall**

Muscle	*Neurovascular Supply*	*Origin*	*Insertion*
Latissimus dorsi	Primary: thoracodorsal nerve, artery, and vein Secondary: artery to serratus anterior	T6–S3, posterior crest of ileum	Intratubular groove of the humerus
Pectoralis major	Primary: thoracoabdominal nerve, artery, and vein Secondary: internal mammary and intercostal arteries	Sternum, clavicle, ribs 1–7	Tricipital groove of humerus
Rectus abdominis	Primary: superior and inferior epigastric arteries	Pubic crest	Rib cartilage of ribs 5–7, xiphoid
Serratus anterior	Primary: serratus branch of thoracodorsal artery Secondary: long thoracic artery	Outer surface and superior border of ribs 8–10; intercostal fascia	Scapula tip
External oblique	Primary: lower thoracic intercostal artery, nerve, and vein	External surface and inferior border of ribs 4–12	Iliac crest, lower abdominal process
Trapezius	Primary: transverse cervical artery, nerve, and vein Secondary: occipital branches and intercostal perforators	Occipital bone, C7–T12 spinous processes	Posterior and lateral third of clavicle, acromion, superior lip of scapular spine

Reconstruction of Full-Thickness Defects

Full-thickness resection of soft tissue, cartilage, and bone destroyed by radionecrosis is required more often than is partial-thickness resection. Radical resection results in defects that can be a reconstructive challenge for the surgeon. Skeletal and supporting elements may need to be supplemented. The surgeon is presented with a wide variety of choices of muscle and myocutaneous flaps (Table 54–1 and Fig. 54–1) (Seyfer et al, 1986).

Skeletal reconstruction is controversial, and each patient should be assessed individually, based on the site and extent of resection. The preoperative cardiopulmonary status provides data that is important when choosing which patients may need skeletal support. Larger anterior full-thickness resections (more than 5 cm) and complete sternal resections (which have the potential for paradox) may require structural support. A true rib resection laterally or a posterior resection in an area protected by the scapula is usually well tolerated and does not require support (Bostwick et al, 1984; Pairolero and Arnold, 1986). The chest wall and underlying parenchyma are often fibrotic after radiotherapy, which provides further stability to the chest.

Prolene and Marlex meshes alone or in combination with methyl methacrylate provide excellent stabilization after chest wall resection (Eschapasse et al, 1981; McCor-

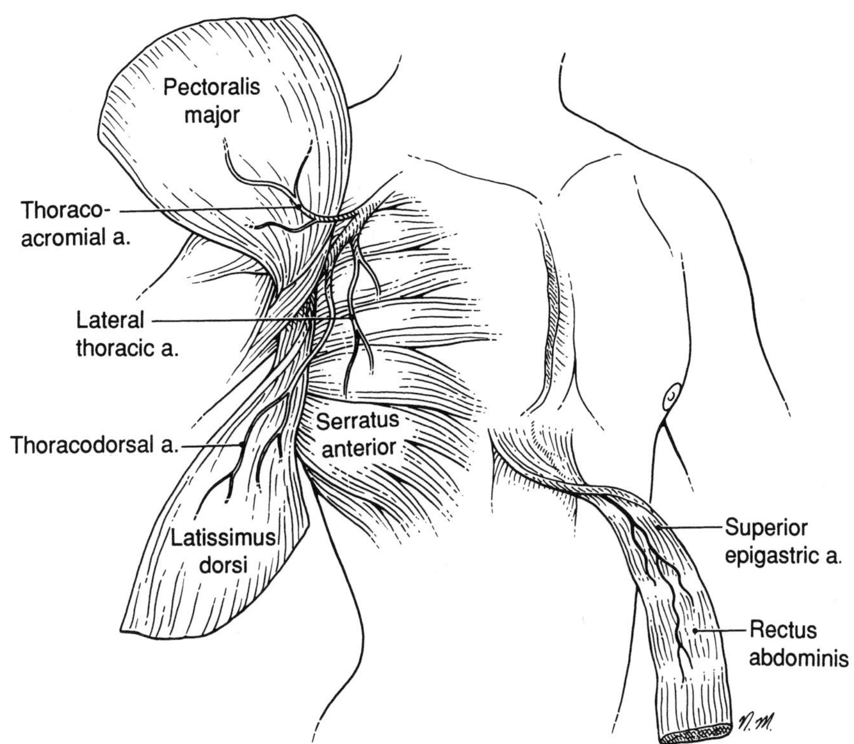

FIGURE 54–1 ■ Available muscle and musculocutaneous flaps for chest-wall reconstruction. Note vascular pedicles.

mack et al, 1981). However, their use should be avoided at all costs in the presence of a contaminated wound, which frequently is associated with osteoradionecrosis. The use of such substances in this setting is associated with high failure rates because of the subsequent infection of the prosthesis. Most authors now believe the use of larger muscle or musculocutaneous flaps results in adequate structural support after full-thickness resection of the chest wall (Arnold and Pairolero, 1984; Bostwick et al, 1984; Seyfer, 1988; Woods et al, 1979).

Our preference for reconstruction of the full-thickness defect is the muscular or musculocutaneous flap, most frequently the latissimus dorsi flap (Bostwick et al, 1984; Sando and Jurkiewicz, 1986). As described earlier, the size, location, and depth determine which muscle is the most appropriate. Figure 54–2 is a schematic representation of the possible defects and suggested muscle for reconstruction. Each of the possible muscles is briefly described (see Table 54–1).

Latissimus Dorsi. The most frequently used flap for lateral and anterior defects is the latissmus dorsi, which is supplied by the thoracodorsal neurovascular bundle. It also receives a blood supply from the branches that supply the serratus anterior and can be based on this vascular pedicle. Excellent musculocutaneous collaterals allow significant skin to be taken with the muscle. It is the largest extrathoracic flap (25 × 35 cm) with a skin area of 30 × 40 cm. It has a large pedicle and a wide arc of rotation. Its origin is T6 to T12, L1 to L4, S1 to S3, and the posterior crest of the ileum. Its insertion is the intertubular groove of the humerus. The donor site rarely causes morbidity but may require a skin graft (Bostwick et al, 1984; Harashina et al, 1983; Larson and McMurtry, 1984; Pairolero and Arnold, 1986; Sando and Jurkiewicz, 1986; Seyfer, 1988; Seyfer et al, 1986).

Pectoralis Major. The pectoralis major is the second most frequently used flap. It is appropriate for anterior and midline defects. Its primary blood supply is the thoracoacromial neurovascular bundle, which arises at midclavicle. Its secondary blood supply is from the internal mammary artery, the lateral intercostal arteries, and the lateral thoracic perforators. The pectoralis major is the second largest muscle (15 × 23 cm) with a potential skin area of 20 × 28 cm. Its origin is the sternum, the clavicle, and the first seven ribs. Its insertion is the bicipital groove of the humerus. It may be used as a graft with a pedicle if the flap is based on the primary blood supply or a "turn-over flap" if the secondary supply is used. The harvest must take into account the possible displacement of the breast and the loss of adduction and medial rotation of the arm. This flap has excellent reliability (Arnold and Pairolero, 1984; Bostwick et al 1984; Larson et al, 1982; Nahai et al, 1986; Sando and Jurkiewicz, 1986; Seyfer et al, 1986).

Rectus Abdominis. The third most frequently used flap is the rectus abdominis. It is appropriate for lower anterior chest wall repairs. Two dominant vascular pedicles exist: the superior epigastric artery supply and the deep inferior epigastric. If it is based on the superior epigastric artery, the inferior epigastric artery must be divided. Therefore, adequate flow through the superior epigastric artery through the internal mammary artery must be ensured. Anterior chest wall irradiation may damage the internal mammary artery; therefore, angiography is suggested. The rectus abdominis is a smaller muscle (surface

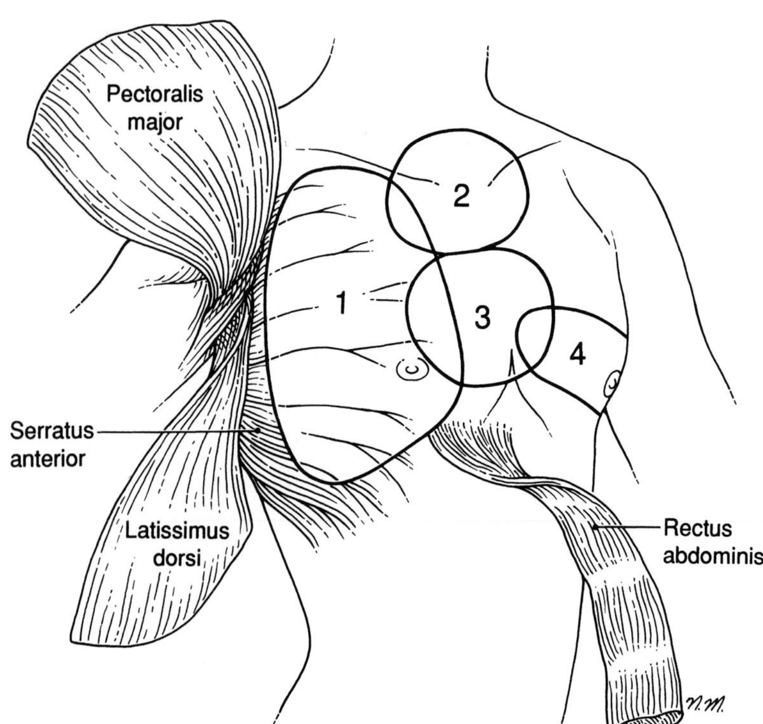

FIGURE 54–2 ■ Common sites of chest wall defects and available myocutaneous flaps for reconstruction.

area, 6 × 25 cm), with a potential skin area of 21 × 14 cm. It has a longitudinal pedicle, and the skin flap may be oriented vertically or horizontally. Vertical orientation preserves more musculocutaneous perforators and therefore is safer. Its origin is the pubic crest. Its insertion is rib cartilage of ribs five, six, and seven and the xiphoid. Increased donor site morbidity occurs in obese and diabetic patients as a result of ventral hernia and infection. The relative reliability of the flap is fair, but atrophy occurs because of loss of the innervation that is prerequisite in the harvest (Bostwick et al, 1984; Larson and McMurtry, 1984; Pairolero and Arnold, 1986; Robinson, 1975; Sando and Jurkiewicz, 1986).

Serratus Anterior. The serratus anterior is less often used for extrathoracic reconstruction. It is located between the latissimus dorsi and the pectoralis in the midaxillary line. It is a small muscle that is best suited as an intrathoracic flap. The serratus anterior may be used in combination with the latissimus dorsi or the pectoralis to supplement the blood supply of the cutaneous segments of these larger musculocutaneous flaps. Its primary blood supply is the serratus branch of the thoracodorsal pedicle, and its secondary blood supply is the long thoracic artery. Its origin is the outer surfaces and superior borders of the upper eighth, ninth, and tenth ribs and the intercostal fascia. Its insertion is the tip of the scapula. The blood supply of this flap is reliable, but the bulk of the muscle is small. Therefore, this limits its usefulness as an extrathoracic flap to areas of the axilla (Arnold and Pairolero, 1984; Arnold et al, 1983; Larson and McMurtry, 1984; Sando and Jurkiewicz, 1986; Seyfer et al, 1986).

External Oblique. The external oblique is infrequently used. It may be used for upper abdomen and lower thoracic defects as far as the inframammary fold. The primary blood supply is the lower thoracic intercostal vessels. Its origin is the external surface and inferior border of the lower eight ribs. Its insertion is the iliac crest and lower abdominal fascia (Arnold and Pairolero, 1989; Seyfer et al, 1986).

Trapezius. The trapezius is infrequently used. Occasionally, it is used for upper chest and neck defects. It is most useful for the base of the neck and thoracic outlet defects. Its major pedicle is the transverse cervical artery by the thyrocervical trunk. Its secondary blood supply includes the occipital branches and intercostal perforators. The trapezius is of moderate size and bulk (34 × 18 cm) with potential skin island of 20 × 8 cm. Its origin is the occipital bone, C7, and all thoracic vertebral spinous processes. Its insertion is the posterior and lateral third of the clavicle, the acromian, and the superior lip of the spine of the scapula (Arnold and Pairolero, 1989; Sando and Jurkiewicz, 1986; Seyfer et al, 1986).

Omentum. Omentum was frequently used early in the history of reconstruction of full-thickness defects. Now it is used for partial-thickness defects and salvage of failed muscle flaps. Its major pedicle is the right and left gastroepiploic arteries. The right pedicle is longer. Its advantages include abundant vascularity, wide arc of rotation, large surface area, and minimal bulk. Its disadvantage is that it requires a laparotomy for harvest (Pairolero and Arnold, 1986; Sando and Jurkiewicz, 1986).

Others. A combination of muscle flaps may be used—for example, latissimus dorsi and pectoralis, or pectoralis and serratus anterior, or pectoralis and rectus abdominis. Three muscle flaps have been used on occasion (generally when primary flaps fail). Latissimus dorsi free flaps and gluteal muscle free flaps have also been used for salvage (Sando and Jurkiewicz, 1986; Woods et al, 1979).

Postoperative Management

Although these patients generally require major chest wall resection and reconstruction the postoperative morbidity and mortality rates are low (Larson et al, 1982; Larson and McMurtry, 1984; Seyfer, 1988; Woods et al, 1979). Complications are usually due to infection and partial graft failure; total graft failure is uncommon (Arnold and Pairolero, 1986; Larson et al, 1982; Woods et al, 1979). After major anterolateral chest wall resection, there may be a brief period of paradoxic chest movement, but large muscle flaps offer good stability for the chest wall. Few patients require prolonged ventilation postoperatively if they do not have significant underlying pulmonary disease (Arnold and Pairolero, 1986; Larson and McMurtry, 1984). Tracheostomy was used routinely in early series but is performed uncommonly now (Seyfer, 1988). Chest tubes and suction catheters should be left in place for 7 to 10 days, and antibiotic therapy should be guided by cultures of the wound (Miller, 1986). The hospital stay averages 11 to 21 days; most authors report means of 12 to 14 days (Arnold and Pairolero, 1984; Larson et al, 1982; Woods et al, 1979).

Recurrent breast cancer in the chest wall and recurrent malignancy in radionecrotic wounds is associated with a particularly poor outcome and virtually no long-term survivors (Larson et al, 1982; Seyfer, 1988; Woods et al, 1979). Therefore, most surgeons believe it is ill advised to put the patient through such a major operative procedure; however, the patients feel great relief and improved well-being when the painful, malodorous lesions have been removed.

CONCLUSION

Many authors have shown the feasibility and advisability of chest wall resection to remove lesions caused by radionecrosis (Arnold and Pairolero, 1989; Bostwick et al, 1984; Larson et al, 1982). The muscular or musculocutaneous flap is preferred for reconstruction. These procedures can be performed in a well-planned, one-stage operation with minimal morbidity and mortality rates. The quality of life for these patients is significantly improved after surgery.

Chest Wall Infections

Chest wall infections secondary to previous procedures, such as median sternotomy and thoracotomy, occur in less than 1.5% to 2% of the cases. This has been discussed adequately elsewhere. Primary chest wall infections are also uncommon. The true incidence is difficult to establish because of the sporadic nature of the problem and lack of reporting. The management has changed greatly since the antibiotic revolution. Most infections can be treated successfully with the administration of topical or intravenous antibiotics. Some infectious maladies require radical resection. We divide this discussion into (1) skin and soft tissue infections, and (2) cartilage and bony structure infections.

SKIN AND SOFT TISSUE

Soft tissue infections of superficial abrasions, furuncles, carbuncles, and so on occur in the chest wall with a similar incidence as in other body areas. Herpes zoster ("shingles") occurs in older people who have been previously exposed to herpes simplex type II virus. It occurs along dermatomal paths and is generally self-limited, except in the immunocompromised host. The therapy consists of analgesics, nonsteroidal anti-inflammatory medications, and, occasionally, acyclovir applied topically. Infrequently when systemic dissemination occurs in the immunocompromised host, systemic acyclovir is indicated.

Soft tissue infections may occur when infectious material is drained by a thoracostomy tube through the chest wall. As reported by Pingleton and Jeter (1983), *Bacteroides melaninogenicus* and *Streptococcus viridans* cause a synergistic gangrene after tube thoracostomy drainage of an empyema, which eventually leads to the patient's death. LoCicero and Vanelko (1985) reported a clostridial myonecrosis at the site of a tube thoracostomy in a patient with Boerhaave's syndrome. Infrequently seen but reported cases of anthrax (Navacharoen et al, 1985), actinomycosis (Golden et al, 1985), and hydatid cysts (Rami et al, 1985) can occur as pseudotumors or infections of the chest wall.

Mondor's disease is thrombophlebitis of the superficial veins of the breast and anterior chest wall. It is frequently treated as a chest wall infection, but this disease entity results from sclerosing endophlebitis of the affected vein with complete or partial obliteration of the vessel lumen (Farrow, 1955). A spontaneous, self-limited condition, it occurs as a hard cord in the subcutaneous tissue of the axilla or anterior chest wall, and it is fairly common after mastectomy and breast augmentation (Green and Dowden, 1988; Kikano et al, 1991). The skin "puckering" produced may be mistaken for inflammatory breast carcinoma, which should be ruled out. Patients may be treated symptomatically with nonsteroidal anti-inflammatory agents. Excision of the affected veins is rarely required.

CARTILAGE AND BONY STRUCTURES

Once frequently seen as a result of the tuberculous bacillus, cartilage and bone infection of the chest wall is now uncommon. The use of prophylactic antibiotics during cardiac and thoracic procedures has virtually eliminated many of the perioperative pathogens. Sternal wound infection following median sternotomy is discussed elsewhere in this text. Costochondritis, when it occurs apart from surgical procedures, may be due to a wide variety of organisms: staphylococci, streptococci, *Pseudomonas aeruginosa*, *Escherichia coli*, *Mycobacterium tuberculosis*, and others. Because the cartilages are fused and continual, a local infection tends to spread that involves all confluent cartilages. These infections are often insidious and indolent and manifest as local pain, swelling, and, frequently, a draining sinus. The cartilage is avascular and thus is remote, from systemic antibiotics. The therapy of choice is radical débridement with reconstruction, as previously discussed.

A particular malady of the chest wall often discussed in the literature is Tietze's syndrome. A benign, self-limited entity, it is characterized by nonsupportive, tender, swelling of the costal cartilage (usually the second or third). The cause is unknown (Jurik and Graudal, 1988). Some authors have associated the syndrome with seronegative rheumatologic disease (Aeschlimann and Kahn, 1990). The therapy should be conservative with analgesics and nonsteroidal anti-inflammatory agents.

Control of tuberculosis and the sophisticated use of systemic antibiotics has virtually eliminated osteomyelitis of the rib cage that is unassociated with sternal infections. It is occasionally seen associated with open drainage of chronic empyema by the Eloesser technique. When persistent infection occurs, radical débridement is usually required for elimination.

CONCLUSION

Because of the increasing sophistication of antibiotic therapy and refinement in surgical technique, chest wall infections are becoming increasingly uncommon. When they do occur, infections of the cartilage and bone require radical excision and débridement for elimination. Perhaps the most commonly seen chest wall conditions are Mondor's disease and Tietze's syndrome. These two entities are not infections in nature and require only relief of symptoms for resolution.

COMMENTS AND CONTROVERSIES

The most common infection of the chest wall is that of the sternum following median sternotomy for coronary artery bypass or other cardiac surgical procedures. The primary therapy in these cases is resection of necrotic tissue, use of local and systemic antibiotics, and reconstruction with omentum or muscle flaps. If no tissue is necrotic, then débridement, antibiotics, and Robicsek weaving of the sternum provide stability and healing.

When there is extensive necrotic infection of the costal cartilages that cannot be treated by simple débridement and reconstruction or other conventional methods because of the poor blood supply, resection of normal cartilage in a perimeter is carried out. This is called "prairie fire containment" by Dr. Robert Shaw and involves cutting out healthy cartilage at the perimeter of the infection to stop the spread of infection, with subsequent reconstruction with omentum or muscle flaps (see Chapter 51).

H.C.U.

■ KEY REFERENCES

Aeschlimann A, Kahn MF: Tietze's syndrome: A critical review. Clin Exp Rheumatol 8:407, 1990.

Drs. Aeschlimann and Kahn have written an excellent review of a frequently underdiagnosed chest wall malady. The article provides guidance for diagnosing and treating Tietze's syndrome.

Arnold PG, Pairolero PC: Reconstruction of the radiation-damaged chest wall. Surg Clin 69:1081, 1989.

Drs. Pairolero and Arnold describe the techniques of surgical resection and reconstruction of osteoradionecrosis.

Arnold PG, Pairolero PC: Chest wall reconstruction: Experience with 100 consecutive patients. Ann Surg 199:725, 1984.

Drs. Pairolero and Arnold describe their vast experience with 100 patients who have required chest wall reconstruction following resection of various chest wall lesions.

Larson DL, McMurtry MJ: Musculocutaneous flap reconstruction of chest wall defects: An experience with 50 patients. Plast Reconstr Surg 73:734, 1984.

Drs. McMurtry and Larson describe the resection of lesions secondary to osteoradionecrosis with immediate reconstruction, which was done in one of America's foremost cancer institutes.

Seyfer A, Graeber G, Wind G: Atlas of Chest Wall Reconstruction. Rockville, MD, Aspen, 1986.

This is a beautifully illustrated atlas of chest wall reconstructions. It serves as an excellent reference for those who perform reconstructive procedures that require muscle and myocutaneous flaps.

■ REFERENCES

Alday ES, Goldsmith HS: Surgical technique for omental lengthening based on arterial anatomy. Surg Gynecol Obstet 135:103, 1972.

Arnold PG, Irons GB: The greater omentum: Extension in transposition and free transfer. Plast Reconstr Surg 67:169, 1981.

Arnold PG, Pairolero PC: Chest wall reconstruction: An account of 500 consecutive patients. Plastic Reconstr Surg 98:804, 1996.

Arnold PG, Pairolero PC: Surgical management of the radiated chest wall. Plast Reconstr Surg 77:605, 1986.

Arnold PG, Pairolero PC, Waldorf JC: The serratus anterior muscle: Intrathoracic and extrathoracic utilization. Plast Reconstr Surg 73:240, 1983.

Arsenian MA: Cardiovascular sequelae of therapeutic thoracic radiation. Prog Cardiovasc Dis 33:299, 1991.

Bostwick J, Stevenson TR, Nahai F et al: Radiation to the breast, complications amenable to surgical treatment. Ann Surg 200:543, 1984.

Campbell AA: Reconstruction of the anterior thoracic wall. J Thorac Cardiovasc Surg 19:456, 1949.

Carlson RG, Mayfield WR, Normann S et al: Radiation-associated vascular disease. Chest 99:538, 1991.

Chapelier AR, Bacha EA, DeMontpreville VT et al: Radical resection of radiation-induced sarcoma of the chest wall: Report of 15 cases. Ann Thorac Surg 63:214, 1997.

Cohen RM: Reconstruction of complex chest wall defects. Am J Surg 172:35, 1996.

Eschapasse H, Gailland J, Henry F et al: Repair of large chest wall defects: Experience with 23 patients. Ann Thorac Surg 32:329, 1981.

Farrow JH: Thrombophlebitis of the superficial veins of the breast and anterior chest wall (Mondor's disease). Surg Gynecol Obstet 101:63, 1955.

Fix RJ, Vasconez LO: Use of omentum in chest wall reconstruction. Surg Clin 69:1029, 1989.

Golden N, Cohen H, Weissbrot J et al: Thoracic actinomycosis in childhood. Clin Pediatr 24:646, 1985.

Granick MS, Larson DL, Solomon MP: Radiation-related wounds of the chest wall. Clin Plast Surg 20:559, 1993.

Green RA, Dowden RV: Mondor's disease in plastic surgery patients. Ann Plast Surg 20:231, 1988.

Haagensen CD, Bhonjlay SB, Guttmann RJ et al: Metastasis of carcinoma of the breast to the periphery of the regional lymph node filter. Ann Surg 169:174, 1969.

Harashina T, Takayama S, Yaji I et al: Reconstruction of chest wall radiation ulcer with free latissimus dorsi muscle flap and meshed skin graft. Plast Reconstr Surg 71:805, 1983.

Jurik AG, Graudal H: Sternocostal joint swelling—clinical Tietze's syndrome. Scand J Rheumatol 17:33, 1988.

Kikano GE, Caceres VM, Sebas JA: Superficial thrombophlebitis of the anterior chest wall (Mondor's disease). J Fam Pract 33:643, 1991.

Kiricuta I: C'empoli du grand epiplasm dans la chuurzie du sein cancereux. Presse Med 71:15, 1963.

Kittle FC: Muscle flaps and thoracic problems. In Kittle FC (ed): Current Controversies in Thoracic Surgery. Philadelphia, WB Saunders, 1986.

Lardinols D, Muller M, Furrer M et al: Functional assessment of chest wall integrity after methylmethacrylate reconstruction. Ann Thorac Surg 69:919, 2000.

Larson DL, McMurtry MJ, Howe HJ et al: Major chest wall reconstruction after chest wall irradiation. Cancer 49:1286, 1982.

Latham WD: Operative treatment for post-radiation defects of the chest wall. Am Surg 32:700, 1966.

Lenene MB, Harris JR, Hellman S: Treatment of carcinoma of the breast by radiation therapy. Cancer 39:28840, 1977.

LoCicero J, Vanelko RM: Clostridial myonecrosis of the chest wall complicating spontaneous esophageal rupture. Ann Thorac Surg 40:396, 1985.

MacMillan RW, Arias JA, Stayman JW: Management of radiation necrosis of the chest wall following mastectomy: A new treatment option. Plast Reconstr Surg 77:832, 1986.

Maier HC: Surgical management of large defects of the thoracic wall. Surgery 22:169, 1947.

McCormack P, Boins MS, Beattie EJ et al: New trends in skeletal reconstruction after resection of chest wall tumor. Ann Thorac Surg 31:45, 1981.

Meyer JE: Thoracic effects of therapeutic irradiation for breast carcinoma. AJR Am J Roentgenol 130:877, 1978.

Miller JI: Thallium imaging in preoperative evaluation of the pulmonary resection candidate. Ann Thorac Surg 54:249, 1992.

Miller JI: Muscle flaps and thoracic problems: Applicability and utilizations for various conditions. In Kittle FC (ed): Current Controversies in Thoracic Surgery. Philadelphia, WB Saunders, 1986.

Nahai F, Morales L, Bone DK et al: Pectoralis major muscle turnover flaps for closure of the infected median sternotomy wound with preservation of form and function. Plast Reconstr Surg 70:471, 1986.

Navacharoen N, Sirisanthana T, Navacharoen W et al: Oropharyageal anthrax. J Laryngol Otol 99:1293, 1985.

Pairolero PC, Arnold PG: Muscle flaps and thoracic problems: Chest wall defects: Reconstruction with autogenous tissue. In Kittle FC (ed): Current Controversies in Thoracic Surgery. Philadelphia, WB Saunders, 1986.

Pantoja E, Fede T, Kunchaia S: Complications of postoperative radiation in breast cancer. Breast 4:4, 1978.

Parham FW: Thoracic resection for tumors growing from the bony wall of the chest. Trans South Surg Gynecol Assoc 11:223, 1898.

Parker RG, Berry HC: Late effects of therapeutic irradiation on the skeleton and bone marrow. Cancer 37:1162, 1976.

Pingleton SK, Jeter J: Necrotizing fasciitis as a complication of tube thoracostomy. Chest 83:925, 1983.

Pizzarello PJ, Witcofoki RL: Basic Radiation Biology. Philadelphia, Lea & Febiger, 1975.

Rami P, Porta R, Bravo-Bravo JL et al: Tumours and pseudotumours of the chest wall. Scand J Thorac Cardiovasc Surg 19:97, 1985.

Robinson DW: Surgical problems in the excision and repair of radiated tissue. Plast Reconstr Surg 55:41, 1975.

Sando W, Jurkiewicz MJ: An approach to repairs of radiation necrosis of chest wall and mammary gland. World J Surg 10:206, 1986.

Schwartz RE, Burt M: Radiation-associated malignant tumors of the chest wall. Ann Surg Oncol 3:387, 1996.

Seama MS, LeGulardeo D, Seberg C et al: Complete arterioventricular block following mediastinal irradiation: A report of six cases. PACE Pacing Clin Electrophysical 14:1112, 1991.

Seyfer AE: Radiation-associated lesions of the chest wall. Surg Gyaecol Obstet 167:129, 1988.

Smith R, Davidson JK, Flatman GE: Skeletal effects of orthovoltage and megavoltage therapy following treatment of nephroblastoma. Clin Radiol 33:601, 1982.

Usher FC, Wallace SA: Tissue reaction to plastics. Arch Surg 76:997, 1959.

Watson WC, James AG: Fascia lata grafts for chest wall defects. J Thorac Cardiovasc Surg 16:399, 1947.

Wolbach SR: Pathologic history of chronic x-ray dermatitis and early x-ray carcinoma. J Med Res 21:415, 1909.

Woods JE, Arnold PG, Masson JK et al.: Management of radiation necrosis and advanced cancer of the chest wall in patients with breast malignancy. Plast Reconstr Surg 63:235, 1979.

CHAPTER **55**

Surgical Techniques for the Chest Wall and Sternum

CHEST WALL RESECTION

Geoffrey M. Graeber

Chest wall resection is usually performed for one of four reasons: removal of neoplasms, eradication of entrenched infection, excision of radiation injuries, and débridement of traumatic wounds. These indications for chest wall resection are not mutually exclusive, since infection can be a major complication for each of the other three. Recurrent tumor and infection together can complicate radiation injuries. The following discussion delineates the essential surgical principles governing chest wall resection for each of the four major indications. Before any major resection, the surgeon should make a thorough and accurate assessment of the patient in order to avoid major complications (Azarow et al, 1989; Seyfer et al, 1986b). In the trauma patient the resection may have to proceed even in victims who are poor operative risks, since allowing devitalized material to remain invites catastrophic infection (Seyfer et al, 1986c).

RESECTION FOR NEOPLASMS

Before embarking on a biopsy of any chest wall neoplasm, the surgeon must take a complete history and conduct a thorough physical examination with the intent of identifying any history of chest wall trauma and of uncovering any malignancy that could spawn a chest wall metastasis. Metastatic lesions and healing rib fractures are far more prevalent than all primary chest wall neoplasms combined (El-Tamer et al, 1989; Graeber et al, 1982). Either a healing rib fracture or a chest wall metastasis may have many of the same radiographic features as a primary chest wall neoplasm (see Chapter 53). The age of the patient, the presentation of the tumor, its physical location and characteristics on the chest wall, and its radiographic appearance will strongly suggest the true character of the neoplasm (see Chapter 53).

The evaluation of a suspected primary chest wall tumor includes standard chest radiographs plus a computed tomographic (CT) scan of the thorax that completely images all ribs, the totality of both leaves of the diaphragm, and the entire base of the neck. The treating surgeon should seek several consultations before embarking on a biopsy (Graeber et al, 1982; Seyfer et al, 1986d). The first consultation should be with a radiologist who specializes in imaging of the thorax. After the chest radiographs and CT scan have been reviewed by the surgeon and radiologist together, they should determine whether specialized diagnostic imaging techniques could be useful in providing more information about the neoplasm. These specialized studies should be undertaken before any diagnostic biopsy is conducted. The surgeon should also consult with a medical oncologist and a radiation therapist to see if any specialized studies need to be conducted on tissue obtained at the time of biopsy. Finally, a pathologist who regularly reads pathologic specimens containing musculoskeletal neoplasms should be consulted. The pathologist usually suggests how much tissue is necessary to perform the tests required to achieve a proper diagnosis. Continuing consultation with the pathologist at the time of surgery is mandatory. Frozen sections are generally of limited value in assessing chest wall neoplasms since so many of them have bony or cartilaginous components. The surgeon and the pathologist should work together to obtain enough appropriate material at the time of biopsy to ensure an accurate diagnosis.

The question of how much tumor needs to be biopsied remains controversial (El-Tamer et al, 1989; Graeber et al, 1982). The technique of biopsy and how much tumor is removed depends on the suspected type of tumor and the pathologist. At one extreme is the needle biopsy, a technique that has proved particularly effective for the group at the University of Texas M. D. Anderson Cancer Center in evaluating children with Ewing's sarcoma of the chest wall (Ryan et al, 1989). In one study of primary bone tumors, needle biopsy accurately diagnosed 83% of malignant and 64% of benign neoplasms (Ayala and Zornosa, 1983). Incisional biopsy is indicated if the needle biopsy is not diagnostic or if the pathologist needs more tissue to make a definitive diagnosis. Conduct of the incisional biopsy should be governed by the anticipation of possible radical resection if the tumor proves malignant. The surgeon should bear in mind that 5 cm of clear skin from the margin of the biopsy site should be resected with radical surgical extirpation (Seyfer et al, 1986d). Meticulous surgical technique is mandatory since hematoma within the wound predisposes to tumor extension. The biopsy site ideally should be closed without a

I wish to thank Mrs. Karen DeShong for her expert preparation of the manuscript.

drain because a drain increases the chance of infection, which would complicate definitive resection and reconstruction. Excisional biopsy is indicated for smaller lesions (2 to 3 cm) and also for chondromatous lesions, since these neoplasms may well include benign as well as malignant areas within the same neoplastic mass (Graeber et al, 1982). Wide excision of osteochondromas and neurofibromas is also indicated, particularly in patients suffering from the familiar syndromes of multiple osteochondromas and neurofibromatosis, as malignant degeneration has been recorded in both entities (Martini et al, 1969).

Once the true nature of the primary chest wall neoplasm has been established, definitive therapy can be undertaken. Proper resection of benign neoplasms consists of surgical excision with preservation of the overlying skin and surrounding musculature. In the event that the benign neoplasm falls into one of the categories of chondromatous lesions noted previously, wider excision should be conducted (Ryan et al, 1989).

Although there has been some variance in reporting, the generally accepted rate of malignancy for primary chest wall neoplasms is 50% (Graeber et al, 1982; Groff and Adkins, 1967; Stelzer and Gay, 1980). The most common malignancies in most series are the chondrosarcomas, with the incidence of fibrosarcoma not far behind. Adjuvant chemotherapy and radiation therapy have a role in treating some primary chest wall malignancies. For this reason preoperative consultation with a radiation therapist and a medical oncologist is indicated before conducting a radical chest wall resection in any patient suffering from a chest wall neoplasm.

The most common primary chest wall malignancy, chondrosarcoma, is resistant to both chemotherapy and radiotherapy (Ryan et al, 1989). Appropriate radical resection with tumor-free margins of at least 5 cm has yielded excellent results (Graeber et al, 1982; Arnold and Pairolero, 1978; Pairolero and Arnold, 1985; King et al, 1986; McAfee et al, 1985). Survival is related to the tumor's histologic grade and size and the adequacy of resection (Fig. 55–1). In one series, patients with grade I lesions had a 10-year survival rate of 70%, and patients with a tumor less than 6 cm in greatest dimension had an 87% 10-year survival (McAfee et al, 1985). On the other hand, the same series noted that patients with grade III or dedifferentiated chondrosarcomas had very poor survival.

Primary fibrosarcomas of the chest wall are usually treated with aggressive surgical resection (Graeber et al, 1982; Martini et al, 1969). Most chemotherapeutic agents have relatively little effect on these malignancies. Some success has been reported with the use of radiotherapy for lower-grade fibrosarcomas (desmoids) of the chest wall (Ryan et al, 1989).

Preoperative and postoperative chemotherapy appears to be beneficial in treating primary chest wall osteosarcomas (Ryan et al, 1989). Although most series are small, primary radical surgical resection can yield long-term survivors (Graeber et al, 1982). Preoperative chemotherapy causes a degree of necrosis in the primary, which may aid in selecting postoperative agents (Martini et al, 1969). Cisplatin and doxorubicin, either alone or in combination with other agents, appear to be effective (Ryan et al, 1989).

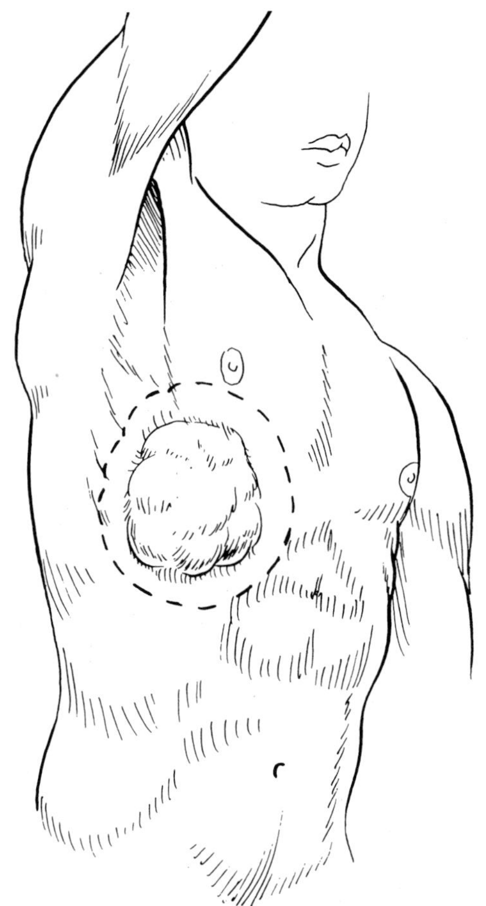

FIGURE 55–1 ■ Large anterior lateral chest wall neoplastic mass, such as would be seen with a chondrosarcoma. The tumor has obvious physical margins. The *dotted line* represents the planned area of resection around the tumor, which includes resection of an adequate, approximately 5-cm margin of healthy tissue around the tumor itself. This is the best way to eliminate local recurrence, which is the most common cause of treatment failure in chondrosarcomas. (From Seyfer AE, Graeber GM, Wind GG: Planning the reconstruction. In Seyfer AE (ed): Atlas of Chest Wall Reconstruction. Rockville, MD, Aspen, 1986e.)

Ewing's sarcoma generally presents in the second decade of life and is unusual in the ribs (Ryan et al, 1989). When it presents as a chest wall tumor, it generally has a worse prognosis than when it is a primary in a long bone of an extremity, since metastases to the lungs occur in about half of the cases (Ryan et al, 1989). When Ewing's sarcoma is localized to the chest wall, the patient is treated with CyVADIC (cyclophosphamide-vincristine-Adriamycin-imidazole carboxamide) induction chemotherapy for 2 to 5 cycles before undertaking resection of the primary. In general, the goals of the resection are to excise the primary with minimal soft tissue margins and with the entirety of the affected rib(s) (Ryan et al, 1989). CyVADIC is then continued for 7 to 8 cycles postoperatively without administration of radiation therapy (Ryan et al, 1989). Although some few survivors have been reported with surgery alone, the prudent use of neoadjuvant and adjuvant chemotherapy for treating primary Ewing's sarcoma of the chest wall is strongly indicated (Graeber et al, 1982; Ryan et al, 1989). Radiotherapy is reserved only for patients who have residual disease after definitive therapy (Rao et al, 1988; Ryan et al, 1989).

Primary solitary plasmacytomas are infrequent chest wall neoplasms, which can be treated by radiotherapy or by resection (Graeber et al, 1982). In general, the Walter Reed group has favored primary resection with adequate margins for several reasons (Graeber et al, 1982). Most patients who present with primary chest wall plasmocytomas return with multiple myeloma within 10 years. If the primary has been eradicated by radiotherapy, the amount of subsequent radiotherapy that may be available for the patient may be small or nonexistent. Hence, the patient may present later with severe pain due to myeloma of the thoracic spine and be unable to undergo more radiotherapy because of having already received a maximal dose of radiotherapy to the thorax. Resection is indicated also for larger lesions, since radiotherapy alone often does not eradicate the disease entirely. The patient then presents with a partially treated neoplasm, which has an open necrotic ulcer and infection. Resection and reconstruction in such cases is much more difficult and more likely to have complications.

Wide surgical excision remains the treatment of choice for patients suffering from malignant fibrous histiocytoma (Ryan et al, 1989; Venn et al, 1986). Aggressive surgical resection has been successful in selected cases in eliminating locally recurrent disease. These tumors are relatively resistant to radiotherapy and chemotherapy. Consequently, radiotherapy is reserved for residual tumor remaining in margins of resection where total resection was not possible anatomically (Ryan et al, 1989).

Rhabdomyosarcomas of the chest wall are usually found in the pediatric population. They are responsive to chemotherapy in most cases (Ryan et al, 1989). Management generally consists of chemotherapy, complete surgical resection, and long-term postoperative chemotherapy. Since radiotherapy is not particularly effective against these tumors, it is employed only in treating lesions for which complete surgical extirpation is not possible or in which the margins of surgical resection are questionable (Ryan et al, 1989).

Chest wall resection for breast cancer today is most often conducted for recurrent local disease after failure of other forms of therapy (Ryan et al, 1989; Seyfer et al, 1986d). Systemic recurrence is common, and chest wall resection is directed at palliating pain, removing friable, ulcerating tumor, and reducing odor. Patients must be selected carefully in the light of survival expectancy. Chemotherapy is beneficial prior to resection and as part of continuing therapy after chest wall resection. The resection should be conducted with the aim of removing all radiation-damaged chest wall, since allowing irradiated tissue to remain often compromises healing. With appropriate chest wall stabilization and rotation of pedicled flap(s) into the resected area, chest wall stability and durability can be achieved. The most gratifying aspect of these resections is the improved quality of life that this resection affords, since pain and tenderness are almost always relieved. The patient's need for analgesics and narcotics is always diminished if not relieved entirely.

Extension of primary lung tumors into the chest wall requires resection in many cases, but chest wall reconstruction is indicated only infrequently (El-Tamer et al, 1989; Seyfer et al, 1986d). Patients with primary lung cancers invading the chest wall must be screened carefully before resection to confirm that systemic disease that would preclude meaningful long-term survival is not present. A 5-cm margin of uninvolved chest wall should be resected en bloc with the primary. Entrance into the chest is planned so that neither the tumor itself nor the margin of resection is violated. Tumors that have extended through the chest wall and overlying musculature to invade or ulcerate the skin are found infrequently, since the disease is lethal systematically prior to such local extension. Hence, in most cases the overlying muscles of the upper extremity, subcutaneous tissues, and skin remain intact over the site of chest wall resection, and with so much intact tissue remaining, the need for chest wall stabilization and flap reconstruction is quite rare.

RESECTION FOR INFECTION

Currently the most common indication for chest wall resection is probably infection due to a dehisced median sternotomy incision. With the increase in cardiac surgery and the use of a median sternotomy incision for access to the heart, the absolute number of median sternotomy dehiscences has increased, although the incidence of this occurrence ranges from 1% to 3% (Miller and Nahai, 1989). Experimental work in the laboratory on the blood flow to the sternum has shown a marked, precipitous decrease in perfusion of the ipsilateral hemisternum immediately after harvesting of the internal mammary artery (Seyfer et al, 1988). This is one of many predisposing factors that can increase the incidence of median sternotomy dehiscence. The association of internal mammary artery harvesting with median sternotomy dehiscence remains a clinical problem of continuing concern (Graeber, 1992). The reconstruction of the dehisced median sternotomy incision continues to be an area of interest for numerous investigators (Arnold and Pairolero, 1984; Miller and Nahai 1989; Pairolero and Arnold, 1986; Seyfer et al, 1986h).

Initial evaluation of the patient with a dehisced median sternotomy incision consists of a precise physical examination, which focuses on the median sternotomy wound and its characteristics (Arnold and Pairolero, 1984; Miller and Nahai, 1986; Pairolero and Arnold, 1986; Seyfer et al, 1986h). Tenderness and erythema generally delineate the margins of the infected tissue. Once these margins have been determined by careful palpation, the anticipated margin of necessary resection to achieve a clean wound and ensure a satisfactory reconstruction is established. The wound is checked for fluctuance, and any fluid that may be expressed from the wound is sent for culture and sensitivities. Crepitus, which may present to varying degrees, usually does not represent clostridial infection but rather reflects air that has entered the wound through the incision itself. When the patient coughs or the ventilator cycles, the sternum is generally unstable. This is heralded by a palpable click, which may be present over varying amounts of the sternum. Determination of exactly how much bone remains unstable within the wound is important, since preservation of as much sternum as possible is beneficial for stabilizing respiratory mechanics.

Several different radiologic techniques have been shown to be of benefit in evaluating these patients (Schaefer and Burton, 1989). Standard posteroanterior and lateral radiographs of the chest will generally show air in the mediastinum and between the two halves of the sternum. Occasionally, air may be seen lateral to the primary incision. When this occurs, the evaluating surgeon can usually suspect either a separation of the bony and cartilaginous elements or the presence of pockets behind the sternum. CT of the chest is helpful in delineating any abscess pockets, recesses, and extensions of the infectious process into the mediastinum. Although a CT scan is not always necessary, it may be helpful in determining where fluid collections may be extravasated. Leaving any fluid collections, especially if they are infected, complicates the subsequent reconstruction of the wound.

Fluid and clot sequestrations may also be delineated by echocardiography, which is also beneficial in evaluating ventricular function and whether or not any of the fluid collection present in the mediastinum embarrasses cardiac function in any way. Magnetic resonance imaging (MRI) may in some cases be of assistance in evaluating these wounds. It appears to be most helpful in delineating where fluid collections may be separated from major vascular structures. The risks and benefits of this examination must be considered in the light of the patient's general condition. The presence of wires within the wound also causes a scattering effect on both the CT and MRI procedures. One particularly helpful nuclear medicine test is the bone scan. Because of its ability to delineate active areas of inflammation, it may be very useful in denoting areas of persistent osteomyelitis and chondritis within a chronically infected median sternotomy incision.

Antibiotic therapy in these patients is directed at the specific culture sensitivities and results (Miller and Nahai, 1989). The most commonly offending organisms are *Staphylococcus aureus* and *Staphylococcus epidermidis*. Enterobacteriaceae and *Pseudomonas* species are the most common gram-negative bacilli that populate these wounds (Miller and Nahai, 1989). Antibiotic therapy should be directed at these species, as well as any pathogens that may be specifically delineated on the culture results. The patient should receive systemic antibiotics 6 hours prior to the intended resection, with continuing therapy throughout the time of resection and for 2 days immediately thereafter. The antibiotics are started early so that adequate levels may be maintained in the healthy tissue surrounding the intended area of resection. Postoperative antibiotic coverage is directed at minimizing seeding of other areas within the body associated with bacteremia.

In the operating room several important considerations must be addressed during the positioning and preparation of the patient (Seyfer et al, 1986h). The patient should be placed in the supine position on the operating table so that the entire anterior thorax is accessible to the operating surgeon for débridement and for possible repair of any cardiovascular injury that may occur during the procedure. Full monitoring is instituted, just as it would be for any patient undergoing a major cardiovascular procedure. This precaution is taken so that if the patient does need to go on cardiopulmonary bypass (a rare occurrence), the surgeon and anesthesiologist are not compromised in their options. One or both groins are prepared for placement of arterial and venous cannulas from a cardiopulmonary bypass machine should bypass be needed. Most surgeons prefer to avoid cannulation through the infected incision, since when tissues are inflamed, they may well be friable, and the repair of the cannulation sites can be extremely difficult. A portion of at least one leg is also prepared in case a segment of saphenous vein should be needed to repair a bypass graft or a major vascular structure.

Once the resection is undertaken, the wound should be actively débrided of all dead tissue (Bellamy and Zajtchuk, 1991b). All nonvital prosthetic tissue and sutures are removed when the wound is opened. Portions of the sternum that show no evidence of bleeding from either the periosteum or the marrow are resected until healthy bleeding is encountered. Any musculature of the chest wall that appears to be compromised is also débrided. In the event that costal cartilages become exposed, the cartilages are resected subperichondrally, since the blood supply to the cartilages is so poor. Once the cartilages are exposed, they should be regarded as infected throughout their entirety. The blood supply to the viable musculature of the chest wall and to any remaining tissues should be preserved scrupulously. Care should be taken to preserve any internal mammary arteries that may be present, since they are the primary blood supply to the rectus abdominis muscles. If one of these muscles is needed as a flap for reconstruction, its arc of rotation is seriously compromised, if not precluded, when the ipsilateral internal mammary artery has been resected or has been used as a cardiac conduit. The ultimate goal of the resection is to remove all tissue that does not have vital capabilities and does not bleed well. Once the resection has been conducted to healthy tissue margins, reconstruction may be contemplated.

In some few cases the margins of resection after débridement of a dehisced median sternotomy may be questionable. In such a case, the wound may be packed with povidone-iodine–soaked gauze and treated as an open wound for 48 hours (Seyfer et al, 1986h). After the wound has been repacked several times by the surgical team and the patient has been stabilized, the patient may be returned for a secondary débridement and reconstruction. The goal of the secondary débridement is to remove any other tissue that is questionable so that only a healthy margin remains. By use of secondary débridement, persistently infected, recalcitrant median sternotomy infections may be treated successfully. Obviously, retention of any tissue, bone, or cartilage that is devascularized compromises subsequent reconstruction.

RESECTION FOR RADIATION INJURY

Resection for radiation injuries of the chest wall is usually conducted for palliation. In most such patients there are several concurrent indications for chest wall resection. Many patients have concurrent infection as well as recurrent tumor in the irradiated field. Complete and thorough evaluation of the patient is necessary, since the benefits and detriments of the resection and reconstruction need to be viewed in the light of the patient's predicted survival. The palliation that is afforded by the resection in terms of decreased pain, improved cosmesis, and decrease in odor must be weighed against the total survival of the patient. Although a number of chest wall tumors may be irradiated, the malignancy most often associated with chest wall radiation is carcinoma of the breast (Seyfer, 1988). Extensive experiences have been recorded by several institutions in dealing with the irradiated chest wall (Arnold and Pairolero, 1986, 1989; Pairolero and Arnold, 1986; Seyfer, 1988).

Preoperative evaluation of these patients starts with thorough metastatic evaluation. Biopsies are taken from any portions of the irradiated field that are suspected of having recurrent tumor. The chest wall should be evaluated to determine the margins of viable tissue. When doing this, it is very important to consider the contralateral chest as an example of healthy tissue for the region. Once the tissue becomes discolored, the epidermis appears thin, and the vascularity appears abnormal, the tissue should be regarded as tenuous. Evaluation should always be conducted with an eye toward conserving as much healthy tissue as possible, yet not leaving any of the radiation-damaged chest wall behind. Radiation-damaged tissue provides an unstable margin for reconstruction. In planning the resection, the entire margin of irradiated tissue should be removed (Fig. 55–2).

The same principles that govern surgical resection for infection govern resection for radiation injury, since infection is often present at the time of surgery. Preparation of the patient is similar to that for resection of infection, as described in the previous section. In the case of infection localized to one area of ulceration, I and my colleagues use a double preparation technique. The first step is to prepare the ulcerated, irradiated tissue with a separate instrument set and to isolate this area from the remaining surgical area with a povidone-iodine-impregnated gauze sponge, which is placed in the wound and then covered with a piece of plastic sheeting or rubber glove (Fig. 55–3). A second preparation is then conducted throughout the entire operative field on the patient so that there is no contamination from the infected ulcer. Resection is then carried out to healthy tissue margins (Seyfer, 1988).

Even though the resection may be extensive, it is necessary to achieve healthy margins throughout the wound so that good tissue healing may occur. Radiation-damaged tissue does not heal well, and it offers further chance for breakdown at the margins of the wound. Such tissue offers poor structural support to the chest wall and is inadequate to allow firm fixation of any stabilization material. If marginal tissue is retained at the edges of resection, the chances for poor healing between any flaps that may be rotated into the wound and the surgical edges of resection are considerable.

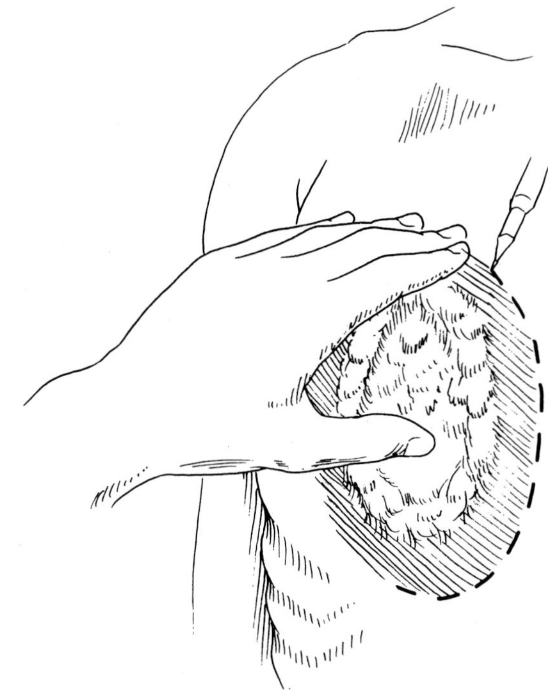

FIGURE 55–2 ■ Method for determining resection of recurrent cancer in an irradiated field. Note that the line of resection, denoted by the *heavy dotted line*, is drawn at the margin of skin showing any radiation change. The chest wall excision should include all tissue that is apparently damaged even though the defect may be large. Healing will be better if the flaps are approximated to healthy tissues. (From Seyfer AE, Graeber GM, Wind GG: The rectus abdominis muscle and musculocutaneous flaps. In Seyfer AE (ed): Atlas of Chest Wall Reconstruction. Rockville, MD, Aspen, 1986e.)

RESECTION FOR TRAUMA

Traumatic injuries of the chest wall may be broadly categorized as either blunt or penetrating (Pate, 1989). In most cases penetrating wounds are the ones most often responsible for serious chest wall injury requiring surgical repair. Since there has been a tremendous increase in domestic trauma, particularly related to criminal activity, the need for understanding these wounds and treating them appropriately is great (LoCicero and Mattox, 1989). Military weapons, including handguns, shoulder weapons, automatic rifles, and assault weapons, are all being used with greater frequency in domestic violence today. Patients who suffer blast injuries to the chest from detonated ordinance rarely live to reach an emergency center.

Early attempts at treating chest wall injuries were rudimentary at best. In the first part of the 20th century, during World War I, most chest wounds were left open to granulate. If the patient survived, it was purely owing to luck and personal fortitude (Fig. 55–4). Few patients with significant injuries of the chest ever survived during this period. By the time of World War II, there were some organized efforts at treating wounds of the chest effectively. After thorough débridement, local flaps of

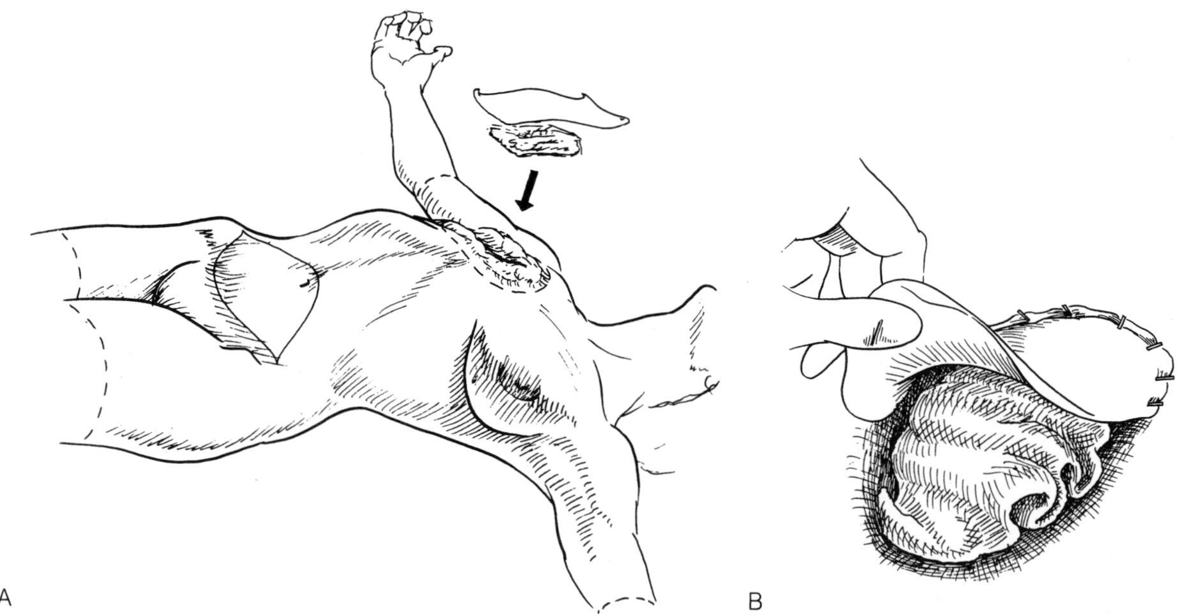

FIGURE 55–3 ■ *A*, The patient has been placed in a supine position on the operating table, and the anticipated margins of resection have been drawn on the chest wall. The *dotted lines* on the extremities show the preparation of the patient. In this case, a transverse musculocutaneous rectus abdominis (TRAM) flap based on the left rectus muscle will be used to reconstruct the defect. The *solid line* on the lower abdomen depicts the skin island that will be taken with the flap. Preparation of the patient for resection includes a double preparation, the first of which is directed at cleaning the ulcerated wound on the chest. Once this has been closed and covered with a gauze sponge impregnated with providone-iodine solution, which is covered with a piece of plastic or a section of rubber after being placed in the wound, a second preparation can be conducted over the entire area. *B*, Close-up of the way the ulcer is filled with the gauze sponge in the defect. Note that the rubber patch, a portion of the glove, or a piece of sterile impermeable drape is stapled in placed so that the entirety of the ulcer is excluded from the field during the second preparation. (*A*, From Seyfer AE, Graeber GM, Wind GG: The rectus abdominis muscle and musculocutaneous flaps. In Seyfer AE (ed): Atlas of Chest Wall Reconstruction. Rockville, MD, Aspen, 1986a. *B*, From Seyfer AE, Graeber GM, Wind GG: The omentum. In Seyfer AE (ed): Atlas of Chest Wall Reconstruction. Rockville, MD, Aspen, 1986i.)

tissue were advanced to attempt coverage of the wound (Fig. 55–5). Currently, effective management consists of thorough débridement and stabilization of the wound followed by flap reconstruction. Since all the wounds are severely infected, chest wall stabilization with synthetic materials is not recommended.

The devastating nature of military and civilian weapons has been well documented (Bellamy and Zajtchuk, 1991a, 1991b). Detonation of antipersonnel devices such as grenades, mines, and heavy ordinance are rarely encountered in civilian practice; however, in today's world some few patients suffering blast injuries may come to a thoracic surgeon for treatment. The critical effects of blasts have recently been well documented by several authors in military publications (Phillips and Zajtchuk, 1991; Stuhmiller et al, 1991). Frequently, weapons of civilian origin also cause significant injuries to the chest wall that need resection. The most common weapon of this type is the shotgun, which causes a devastating soft tissue loss of the chest wall while penetrating the lung and underlying viscera.

Preoperative preparation is directed at stabilizing the patient and giving broad-spectrum antibiotics to cover the bacteremia, which is always present with such wounds. The patient is given vigorous fluid resuscitation to restore cardiodynamic integrity and is transported to the operating room as soon as possible. Surgery is directed at stabilizing the life-threatening injuries within the thorax and at débridement of the chest wall. It is necessary to emphasize that the lung should be managed in a conservative fashion because of its tremendous regenerative capacity. The need for total lobectomy and/or pneumonectomy remains infrequent, since the major vessels and bronchi may be closed on the surface of the lung without radical extirpation. Once the lung has been stabilized, it should be ventilated and expanded to its greatest extent. Pleural abrasion is very helpful in securing fixation of the lung to the remaining chest wall. Chest tubes should be placed so that they are not exposed in the open defect but rather drain the inferior as well as the superior portion of the chest of all possible fluid and air that may remain in the pleural cavity (Fig. 55–6).

The resection of the chest wall itself is most important, since removal of all devitalized tissue, foreign material, portions of clothing, dead skin, and hair should be conducted vigorously. The resection should be conducted so that healthy muscle is seen throughout the margin of the wound and there is active bleeding throughout all remaining tissues. The four major qualities consistent with a high degree of viability are color, consistency, contractility, and circulation (Bellamy and Zajtchuk, 1991b). The lung is expanded to the margins of resection and the defect is closed with an impregnated providone-iodine gauze to secure an airtight seal on the chest wall. The chest tubes evacuate any blood or air that accumulate in the pleural cavity and maintain expansion of the lung

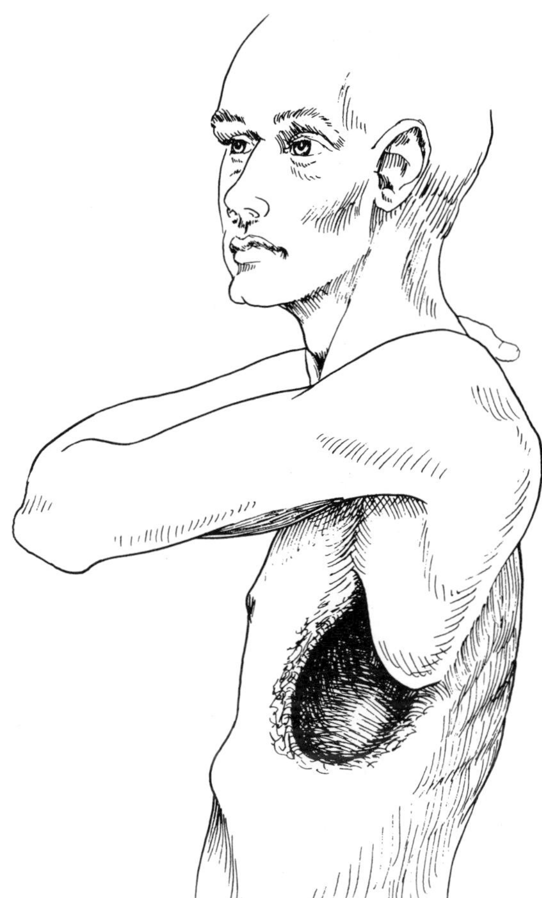

FIGURE 55–4 ■ Patient with severe chest wall wound that has been treated in accordance with the principles of military medicine as dictated in the early part of the 20th century. Note that the wound has been débrided widely and allowed to granulate. Some patients treated in this manner, including soldiers wounded in World War I, survived despite their wounds. The wound continued to granulate and remain superficially infected, causing severe nutritional depletion of the patient. Hence, the patient looked quite cachectic, because depletion occurred slowly over time. Few of these individuals survived the long term. (From Seyfer AE, Graeber GM, Wind GG: Some historical aspects of chest wall reconstruction. In Seyfer AE (ed): Atlas of Chest Wall Reconstruction. Rockville, MD, Aspen, 1986c.)

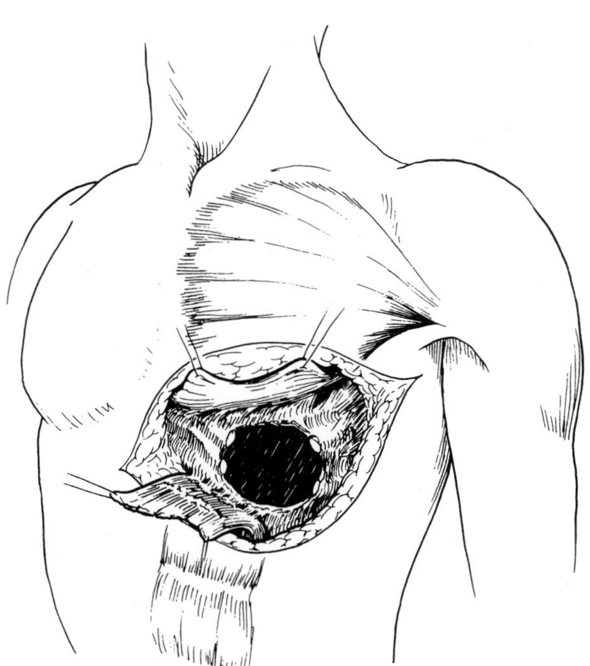

FIGURE 55–5 ■ Closure of wounds in World War II usually consisted of mobilization of local slips of muscle for closure over the previously débrided defect. This drawing depicts one of the attempts at closure, which was conducted on a patient suffering an anterior thoracic wall wound during World War II. Note that the area had been débrided widely and that closure was attempted only when all evidence of infection had receded. (From Seyfer AE, Graeber GM, Wind GG: Some historical aspects of chest wall reconstruction. In Seyfer AE (ed): Atlas of Chest Wall Reconstruction. Rockville, MD, Aspen, 1986c.)

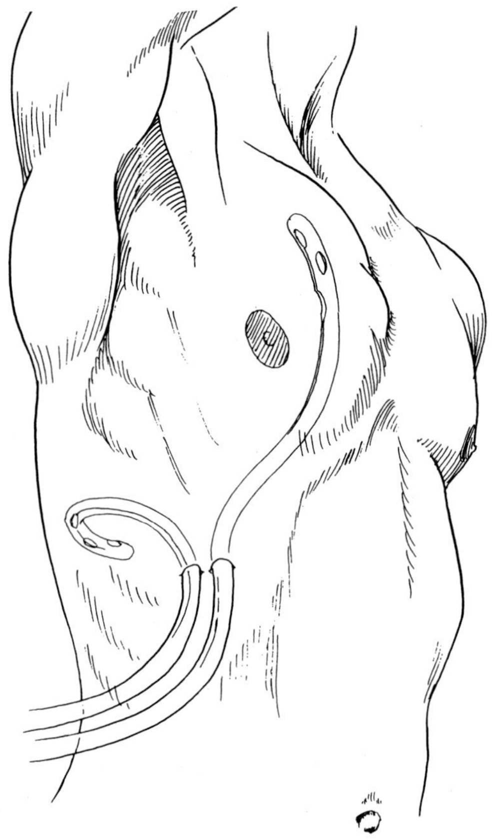

FIGURE 55–6 ■ Placement of chest tubes as they would be situated for an anterolateral thoracic wound. In placing the tubes, care is taken to remain away from the wound site itself so that the tubes do not traverse the area of the open chest wall. One tube is placed over the apex of the chest to drain any air that may be remaining within the pleural cavity; the other tube is placed low and posterior so that it will evacuate any blood or tissue fluids that may collect in the posterior costophrenic sinus. (From Seyfer AE, Graeber GM, Wind GG: Resection and débridement of the chest wall. In Seyfer AE (ed): Atlas of Chest Wall Reconstruction. Rockville, MD, Aspen, 1986d.)

against the remaining chest wall. A second débridement is often necessary 24 and 48 hours after the initial injury since additional tissue may lose viability in this time. The necessity for close observation of the wound and subsequent débridement cannot be underestimated. Retention of foreign material and devitalized tissue within the margins of the wound can lead to clostridial infection and rapid demise of the patient. Fortunately, with adequate initial débridement this is rare.

In the final analysis, the viability of the patient depends on the individual surgeon's persistence, skill, and creativity. The patient must be observed constantly for any evidence of pending sepsis and evaluated for evidence of crepitus within the margins of the wound. Creativity must be constantly exhibited, since the wound will have to be tailored when it has become stabilized. Constant attention to patients is mandatory since they can deteriorate and die very quickly.

■ KEY REFERENCES

McCraw JB, Arnold PG: McCraw and Arnold's Atlas of Muscle and Musculocutaneous Flaps. Norfolk, VA, Hampton Press, 1986.

This excellent atlas depicts the major muscular and musculocutaneous flaps that may be harvested throughout the human body. Copiously illustrated, this provides an excellent guide for the anatomic dissection of most existing muscular and musculocutaneous flaps. It should be considered an excellent reference for chest wall reconstruction since it depicts both pedicled and free flaps.

Seyfer AE, Graeber GM (eds): Chest wall reconstruction, Surg Clin North Am 69(5):142–145, 1989.

This monograph specifically addresses chest wall reconstruction in all its major aspects. Major authorities in the field of chest wall reconstructions discuss each of the major flaps that may be used. Specific problems encountered in chest wall reconstruction, such as the dehisced median sternotomy and radiation injuries of the chest wall, are covered in depth. The monograph provides an excellent review of the entire field since each of the articles has an extensive list of references.

Seyfer AE, Graeber GM, Wind GG: Atlas of Chest Wall Reconstruction. Rockville, MD, Aspen Publishers, 1986a.

This atlas specifically delineates the methods used in chest wall reconstruction. It covers most aspects of chest wall reconstruction, starting from the evaluation of the patient and continuing through postoperative care. Major emphasis is placed on pedicled flap reconstruction and on specific problems afflicting the chest wall. The illustrations depict all the major steps necessary in each of the reconstructions cited.

■ REFERENCES

Arnold PG, Pairolero PC: Chondrosarcoma of the manubrium. Resection and reconstruction with pectoralis major muscle. Mayo Clin Proc 53:54, 1978.

Arnold PG, Pairolero PC: Chest wall reconstruction: Experience with 100 consecutive patients. Ann Surg 199:725, 1984.

Arnold PG, Pairolero PC: Surgical management of the radiated chest wall. Plast Reconstr Surg 77:605, 1986.

Arnold PG, Pairolero PC: Reconstruction of the radiation-damaged chest wall. Surg Clin North Am 69:1081, 1989.

Ayala AG, Zornosa J: Primary bone tumors: Percutaneous needle biopsy. Radiology 149:675, 1983.

Azarow KS, Mallow M, Seyfer AE, Graeber GM: Preoperative evaluation and general preparation for chest wall operations. Surg Clin North Am 69:899, 1989.

Bellamy RF, Zajtchuk R: The weapons of conventional land warfare. In Bellamy RF, Zajtchuk R (eds): Conventional Warfare: Ballistic, Blast, and Burn Injuries. In Textbook of Military Medicine. Part I: Warfare Weaponry and the Casualty. Vol 5. Washington, DC, Office of the Surgeon General. U.S. Army, 1991a.

Bellamy RF, Zajtchuk R: Assessing the effectiveness of conventional weapons. In Bellamy RF, Zajtchuk R (eds): Conventional Warfare: Ballistic, Blast, and Burn Injuries. In Textbook of Military Medicine. Part I: Warfare Weaponry and the Casualty. Vol 5. Washington, DC, Office of the Surgeon General. U.S. Army, 1991b.

Bellamy RF, Zajtchuk R: The physics and biophysics of wound ballistics. In Bellamy RF, Zajtchuk R (eds): Conventional Warfare: Ballistic, Blast, and Burn Injuries. In Textbook of Military Medicine. Part I: Warfare Weaponry and the Casualty. Vol 5. Washington, DC, Office of the Surgeon General. U.S. Army, 1991c.

Bellamy RF, Zajtchuk R: The management of ballistic wounds of soft tissue. In Bellamy RF, Zajtchuk R (eds): Conventional Warfare: Ballistic, Blast, and Burn Injuries. In Textbook of Military Medicine Part I: Warfare Weaponry and the Casualty. Vol 5 Washington, DC, Office of the Surgeon General. U.S. Army, 1991d.

El-Tamer M, Chaglassian T, Martini N: Resection and debridement of chest-wall tumors and general aspects of reconstruction. Surg Clin North Am 69:947, 1989.

Graeber GM: Harvesting of the internal mammary artery and the healing median sternotomy (Editorial). Ann Thorac Surg 53:7, 1992.

Graeber GM: Snyder RJ, Fleming AW et al: Initial and long-term results in the management of primary chest wall neoplasms. Ann Thorac Surg 34:664, 1982.

Groff DB, Adkins PC: Chest wall tumors. Ann Thorac Surg 4:260, 1967.

King RM, Pairolero PC, Trastek VF et al: Primary chest wall tumors: Factors affecting survival. Ann Thorac Surg 41:597, 1986.

LoCicero J, Mattox KL: Epidemiology of chest trauma. Surg Clin North Am 69:15, 1989.

Martini N, Starzynski TE, Beattie EJ: Problems in chest wall resection. Surg Clin North Am 49:313, 1969.

McAfee MK, Pairolero PC, Bergstrahl EJ et al: Chondrosarcoma of the chest wall: Factors affecting survival. Ann Thorac Surg 140:535, 1985.

Miller JI, Nahai F: Repair of the dehisced median sternotomy incision. Surg Clin North Am 69:1091, 1989.

Pairolero PC, Arnold PG: Management of recalcitrant median sternotomy wounds. J Thorac Cardiovasc Surg 88:357, 1984.

Pairolero PC, Arnold PG: Chest wall tumors: Experience with 100 consecutive patients. J Thorac Cardiovasc Surg 90:367, 1985.

Pairolero PC, Arnold PG: Thoracic wall defects: Surgical management of 205 consecutive patients. Mayo Clin Proc 61:557, 1986.

Pate JW: Chest wall injuries. Surg Clin North Am 69:59, 1989.

Phillips YY, Zajtchuk JT: The management of primary blast injury. In Bellamy RF, Zajtchuk R (eds): Conventional Warfare: Ballistic, Blast, and Burn Injuries. In Textbook of Military Medicine. Part I: Warfare Weaponry and the Casualty. Vol. 5. Washington, DC, Office of the Surgeon General. United States Army, 1991.

Rao BN, Hayes FA, Thompson EI et al: Chest wall resection for Ewing's sarcoma of the rib: An unnecessary procedure. Ann Thorac Surg 46:40, 1988.

Ryan MB, McMurtrey MJ, Roth JA: Current management of chest-wall tumors. Surg Clin North Am 69:1061, 1989.

Schaefer PS, Burton BS: Radiographic evaluation of chest-wall lesions. Surg Clin North Am 69:911, 1989.

Seyfer AE: Radiation-associated lesions of the chest wall. Surg Gynecol Obstet 167:129, 1988.

Seyfer AE, Graeber GM, Wind GG: Preoperative care and considerations. In Seyfer AE (ed): Atlas of Chest Wall Reconstruction. Rockville, MD, Aspen Publishers, 1986b.

Seyfer AE, Graeber GM, Wind GG: Some historical aspects of chest wall reconstruction. In Seyfer AE (ed): Atlas of Chest Wall Reconstruction. Rockville, MD, Aspen Publishers, 1986c.

Seyfer AE, Graeber GM, Wind GG: Resection and debridement of the chest wall. In Seyfer AE (ed): Atlas of Chest Wall Reconstruction. Rockville, MD, Aspen Publishers, 1986d.

Seyfer AE, Graeber GM, Wind GG: Planning the reconstruction. In Seyfer AE (ed): Atlas of Chest Wall Reconstruction. Rockville, MD, Aspen Publishers, 1986e.

Seyfer AE, Graeber GM, Wind GG: The rectus abdominis muscle and musculocutaneous flaps. In Seyfer AE (ed): Atlas of Chest Wall Reconstruction. Rockville, MD, Aspen Publishers, 1986f.

Seyfer AE, Graeber GM, Wind GG: The pectoralis major muscle and musculocutaneous flaps. In Seyfer AE (ed): Atlas of the Chest Wall Reconstruction. Rockville, MD, Aspen Publishers, 1986g.

Seyfer AE, Graeber GM, Wind GG: The dehisced median sternotomy incision. In Seyfer AE (ed): Atlas of Chest Wall Reconstruction. Rockville, MD, Aspen Publishers, 1986h.

Seyfer AE, Shriver CD, Miller TR, Graeber GM: Sternal blood flow after median sternotomy and mobilization of the internal mammary arteries. Surgery 104:899, 1988.

Stelzer D, Gay WA: Tumors of the chest wall. Surg Clin North Am 60:779, 1980.

Stuhmiller JH, Phillips YY, Richmond DR: The physics and mechanisms of primary blast injury. In Bellamy RF, Zajtchuk R (eds): Conventional Warfare: Ballistic, Blast, and Burn Injuries. In Textbook of Military Medicine Part I: Warfare Weaponry and the Casualty. Vol 5. Washington, DC, Office of the Surgeon General. U.S. Army, 1991.

Venn GE, Gellister J, DaCosta PE et al: Malignant fibrous histiocytoma in thoracic surgery practice. J Thorac Cardiovasc Surg 91:234, 1986.

CHEST WALL STABILIZATION

Geoffrey M. Graeber

The first step in chest wall reconstruction is preservation of function through stabilization. In some cases the resection itself does not sufficiently compromise chest wall function and thereby also respiratory mechanics to warrant stabilization. If stabilization is necessary, a number of materials have been used successfully to preserve chest wall integrity and respiratory mechanics. Some have remained useful and have earned a secure place in chest wall reconstruction, while others have proved marginally or minimally successful and have been abandoned. The indications for chest wall stabilization as a part of an integrated reconstruction are reviewed; the materials, both biologic and synthetic, that have been used in this capacity are listed; and the most popular methods used by surgeons today are summarized.

INDICATIONS FOR STABILIZATION

Chest wall reconstruction is generally viewed as a procedure with two aspects, chest wall stabilization and soft tissue reconstruction. In some cases the consistency of the soft tissue reconstruction affords satisfactory stabilization to preserve respiratory mechanics (Seyfer et al, 1986a, 1986b), whereas in others, the flaps used in providing soft tissue coverage have little intrinsic consistency (e.g., omentum flaps) and usually need stabilization (Fix and Vasconez, 1989; Seyfer et al, 1986c). Each case must be assessed and handled individually since respiratory mechanics must be preserved. The final decision of whether chest wall stabilization is necessary involves consideration of multiple factors, the most important of which are the general condition and respiratory capabilities of the patient, the size and location of the resection performed, the integrity and quality of the structures overlying the defect, and the intrinsic qualities of the flaps used for soft tissue coverage. The final goal is to provide a reconstruction that has minimal if any paradoxical chest wall motion during respiration so that the patient can be weaned from ventilatory support as soon as possible after reconstruction (McCormack, 1989; Seyfer et al, 1986a, 1986b). Satisfactory cosmesis is an important secondary goal that merits careful consideration (Seyfer et al, 1986a, 1986b).

The general condition and respiratory capabilities of the patient are major factors in determining whether chest wall stabilization is required as a part of chest wall reconstruction (Seyfer et al, 1986d). The operating surgeon must evaluate the patient who will undergo chest wall resection carefully to determine just how much respiratory embarrassment the patient can tolerate and yet still be able to be weaned from a respirator early in the postoperative period. A reasonable guiding principle is that any patient who is able to tolerate a pulmonary lobectomy based on pulmonary function studies, arterial blood gas determination, and exercise testing will also be able to tolerate a major chest wall resection (Seyfer et al, 1986e). Special consideration should be given to the unusual patient who needs a pulmonary resection in conjunction with a major chest wall resection and reconstruction. Obviously, a younger, more robust patient with excellent nutrition will tolerate a large resection and reconstruction better than a frail, elderly patient who suffers from cachexia.

The location and size of the chest wall resection are major determinants of whether chest wall stabilization is required as a part of successful reconstruction. Small defects (5 to 7 cm in greatest diameter) seldom need stabilization, since the amount of paradoxical motion is small and can be tolerated by most patients (McCormack, 1989; Pairolero and Arnold, 1986). Larger defects almost always need some form of chest wall stabilization to preserve respiratory function (Pairolero and Arnold, 1986; Seyfer et al, 1986e). Location of the resection is important, since major structures of the ipsilateral upper extremity may provide the necessary overlying support. The scapula is an example of such a structure posteriorly, but its relation to the defect may impinge on the margin requiring partial resection of the inferior scapular pole (Pairolero and Arnold, 1986). Anteriorly the pectoralis major muscle, if it and its overlying skin and subcutaneous tissues are left intact, may provide sufficient support that chest wall stabilization is not necessary. Resections that are lateral and inferoanterior generally require stabilization, since major muscles and bones do not overlie the chest wall in these regions.

The size of the flap employed in soft tissue reconstruction and its intrinsic consistency have direct bearing on whether chest wall stabilization is required. As noted previously, the omentum usually is very flaccid, with little intrinsic rigidity; hence stabilization is almost always required when the omentum is used. In contrast, a large musculocutaneous flap (such as a latissimus dorsi) has an intrinsic robust quality, which may allow coverage of a defect without stabilization. All flaps, like any other surgically manipulated tissues, generate edema within 48 hours of the procedure. Because edema tends to make tissues more rigid, the flap has less paradoxical motion on the second through fourth postoperative days. The flap becomes less robust as the edema fluid is mobilized later in the postoperative period, but usually the patient has been weaned from the ventilator by this time.

MATERIALS USED IN CHEST WALL STABILIZATION

A host of materials have been used to stabilize the chest wall and preserve respiratory mechanics since the inception of chest wall resection and reconstruction. An excellent review by McCormack (1989) has summarized most of these and should be consulted. The following discussion is based on experiences recorded in the literature by other authors and on personal observations recorded during major reconstructions performed on patients by myself and colleagues at our respective university institutions. This section presents a classification of materials that have been used to stabilize the chest wall. The last section of this review highlights the major methods used in chest wall stabilization which are practiced regularly because of ease in handling, durability, relative radiographic permeability, and superior performance.

The first major category is biologic implants. The assets of autogenous tissues are availability and biocompatibility. Their liabilities include poor resistance to infection, increased operating time, substantially increased patient discomfort, and relative flaccidity when compared with synthetic materials (McCormack, 1989; Seyfer et al, 1986a). Their presence in a wound can be disastrous if infection supervenes. Fascia lata is devascularized tissue, which acts as a perfect culture medium for bacteria. Bone chips added to fascia lata provide no stabilization since they are resorbed (McCormack, 1989). Their presence on fascia lata compounds the problem of infection, since they act as yet another source of devascularized tissue on which microorganisms can thrive. For all the aforementioned reasons, fascia lata alone or in conjunction with bone chips has fallen into disfavor.

BIOLOGIC MATERIALS USED FOR CHEST WALL STABILIZATION

- Human tissues
  - Autogenous
    - Fascia lata
    - Bone grafts
      - Ribs, whole and longitudinally split
      - Tibia
      - Fibula
      - Iliac crest
    - Composite
  - Preserved
    - Dura mater
    - Fascia
    - Pericardium
- Preserved animal tissues
  - Dura mater
  - Pericardium
  - Os fascia

Bone grafts can be used judiciously in selected instances for chest wall stabilization. Although portions of tibia, fibula, and iliac crest have been used successfully, their harvesting adds another operative site, with its associated discomfort and potential for complications (McCormack, 1989; Seyfer, et al, 1986a). Rib grafts have the advantage of being more likely to follow the natural curvature of the chest wall, but they have significant liabilities. If they are harvested in a subperiosteal fashion, the resultant chest wall instability may be consequential and the rib may regenerate from the remaining periosteum poorly or not at all. Ribs that are partially resected by using a longitudinal line of resection leave a compromised rib in place at the donor site while providing a graft that is particularly frail. The result is suboptimal stabilization at both the donor and recipient sites.

The use of rib grafts by my colleagues and me has been limited to carefully selected patients who need protection for vital intrathoracic structures (such as the heart and great vessels) while maintaining an acceptable cosmetic contour to the reconstruction. The patient must have relatively good pulmonary function, since the discomfort from the donor site, when compounded with that of the reconstruction, can produce a serious decrease in respiratory function. Placement of an epidural catheter to maintain regional anesthesia in the immediate postoperative period has decreased patient discomfort in our experience, so that early weaning from the ventilator is the rule. If rib grafts are placed properly, marrow from the intact ribs at the margins of the resection grow into and vascularize the marrow of the graft, ensuring its prolonged viability (Seyfer et al, 1986a) (Fig. 55–7). Rib grafts in any position are dependent on surrounding tissues, particularly on the rib to which they are attached, for postoperative viability (Graeber et al, 1985). If a rib graft or any bone graft does not receive a new blood supply, the graft is resorbed by the body, leaving only a fibrous remnant (Graeber et al, 1985; McCormack, 1989).

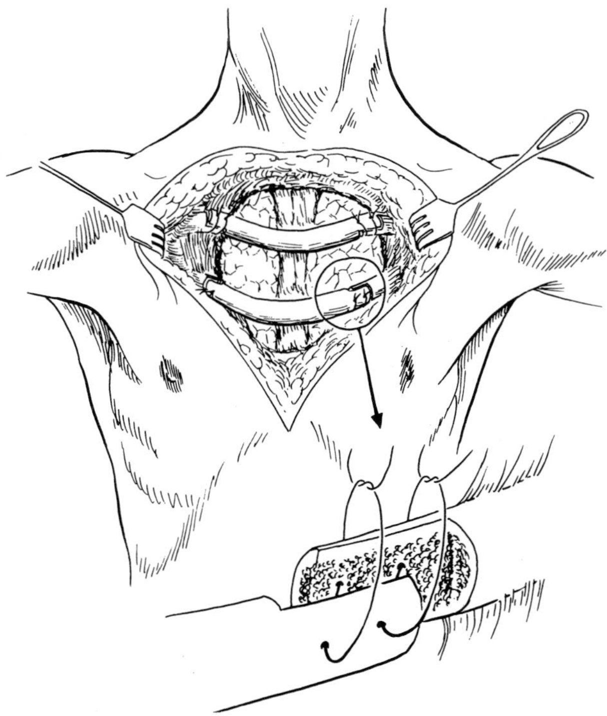

FIGURE 55–7 ■ Use of rib grafts in anterior chest wall stabilization. Note that the grafts, as well as the ribs, are notched so that they can be secured with transfixing permanent sutures. Notching also allows a greater area of interface between the rib and the graft marrow cavities. The greater interface of the two marrows increases the likelihood that the bone graft will survive, because the marrow of the graft is dependent on the ingrowth of cellular material from the end of the rib. (From Seyfer AE, Graeber GM, Wind GG: Planning the reconstruction. In Seyfer AE (ed): Atlas of Chest Wall Reconstruction. Rockville, MD, Aspen, 1986a.)

Preserved tissues, human or animal, were mostly used before synthetic cloth and sheeting became available and proved so successful (McCormack, 1989; Seyfer et al, 1986a). There have been some recent proponents of these tissues for chest wall stabilization (Kuakowski and Ruka, 1987). Although these membranes may provide substantial initial stability, they may become flaccid with time owing to peripheral stress on anchoring tissues as well as to intrinsic weakening of structural proteins. The patient's body reacts to these materials as it does to any foreign body, with an intense fibrous reaction. These facts, plus the relatively inferior resistance of biologic materials to infection, has led to a decrease in their use.

The rise in the use of synthetic materials for chest wall stabilization has been fostered by their variety and availability, their perceived inert nature, and their general ease of handling (McCormack, 1989; Seyfer et al, 1986a). At the outset, any surgeon should realize that absolutely no material is completely inert when placed in a patient. The patient's natural healing process will at least respond to any foreign material with a fibrous reaction to form a pseudocapsule.

Rigid materials have had some popularity in chest wall reconstruction, but they have some liabilities, which have limited their application (McCormack, 1989; Seyfer et al, 1986a). Since the chest wall is a dynamic structure, which is constantly active in respiration, rigid materials have a tendency to migrate and fracture. Migration, when it is external, finally causes dermal erosion, which exposes the rigid material. Infection of the entire capsule surrounding the rigid support ensues quickly, requiring removal of the foreign material. If the rigid bar or strut erodes internally, major viscera (such as the lung) and great vessels may be entered serious if not lethal hemorrhage producing (McCormack, 1989). Metallic struts are for the most part currently limited to stabilization of the sternum after repair of a severe pectus deformity (Garcia et al, 1989; Seyfer et al, 1986f). In most cases these struts are not permanent but are removed after the chest wall has become stable (Fig. 55–8).

Most synthetic materials used for human implantation are produced as sheets or as meshes. Many of these have been employed, with varying degrees of success, as stabilizing membranes in chest wall reconstruction (Boyd et al, 1981; McCormack, 1989; Pairolero and Arnold, 1985, 1986). Each has its assets and liabilities. For example, Marlex mesh can be stretched along one axis while it is rigid along the perpendicular axis. Prolene mesh is a double-stitch knit, which is rigid along all axes. Gore-Tex, which is very malleable as a soft tissue patch, is impervious to air and water but is most difficult to contour and sew in place tightly. Although each of these materials is relatively inert, they all provoke an intense fibrous reaction when placed in the chest wall. Even polypropylene, which has been touted as quite unreac-

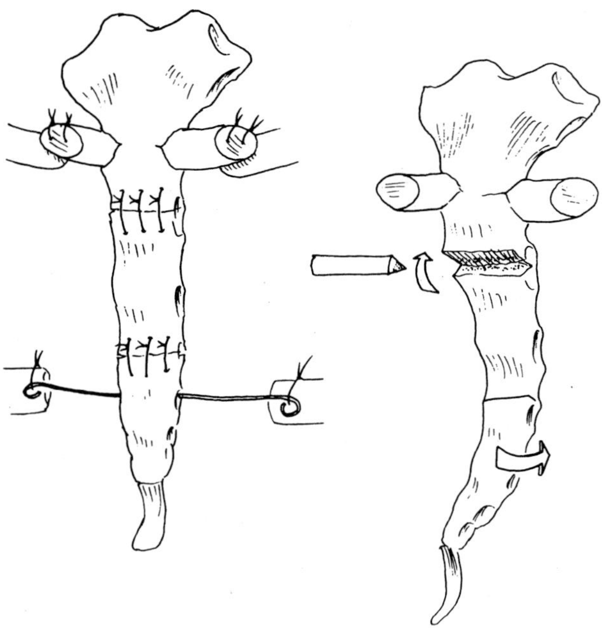

FIGURE 55–8 ■ Use of a Steinmann pin in stabilizing a repaired sternum as part of a correction for pectus excavatum. The pin is secured to the ribs lateral to the repair. It will be removed in most cases after the repair has healed. (From Seyfer AE, Graeber GM, Wind GG: Congenital defects: Poland's syndrome, pectus deformities and sternal clefts. In Seyfer AE (ed): Atlas of Chest Wall Reconstruction. Rockville, MD, Aspen, 1986f.)

tive, was found to provoke an intense fibrous reaction from the lung and pleura in one experimental model (Graeber et al, 1985).

ALLOPLASTIC AND SYNTHETIC MATERIALS USED IN CHEST WALL STABILIZATION

- Plates and struts
  - Metal
    - Tantulum steel
    - Stainless steel
  - Other materials
    - Lucite
    - Fiberglass
- Synthetic materials
  - Sheets and meshes
  - Polytetrafluorethylene (Teflon) sheeting and patch
  - Nylon
  - Polypropylene
  - Prolene mesh
  - Vicryl mesh
- Solid and firm prosthetics
  - Acrylic
  - Teflon
  - Silastic
  - Silicone
- Composite
  - Marlex mesh combined } prosthesis
  - Methyl methacrylate }

A number of synthetic materials can be produced with variable degrees of firmness. Success has been reported with acrylic, silicone, Silastic, and methyl methacrylate prostheses (Eschaposse et al, 1977; Mendelson and Masson, 1977; Allen and Douglas, 1979; Marcove et al, 1977). They may be used alone or in composites as prosthetics in chest wall reconstruction (Hochberg et al, 1994). Although such techniques have been available since well before the early 1980s, recent concerns about silicone, particularly as it has been used in mammary implants, indicate extreme caution in its use (Lavey et al, 1982; deCamara et al, 1993). Current U.S. Food and Drug Administration guidelines for implanting silicone should be consulted before embarking on such a reconstruction. In current practice, customized prostheses are used for both chest wall stabilization and partial chest wall reconstruction only in selected cases in which standard stabilization and flap reconstruction either has failed or offers exceptionally limited options (Hochberg et al, 1994). Such individualized prostheses may be created to reconstruct complex defects with rounded contours; however, they are difficult to secure to the chest wall, require sophisticated, computerized techniques to generate the prosthetic, and are subject to all the recognized liabilities of a firm foreign body in the dynamic chest wall. Excellent long-term results have been recorded in carefully selected patients with very special reconstructive needs (Hochberg et al, 1994).

McCormack and others have had particularly beneficial experience with composite prostheses generated in the operating room from Marlex mesh and methyl methacrylate monomer (McCormack et al, 1981; McCormack, 1989). A customized prosthesis is made by measuring the size of the defect on the patient, laying a piece of Marlex mesh over a surface of similar contour, applying the methyl methacrylate to the Marlex to match the size and shape of the defect as determined by the previously measured pattern, and then applying another layer of Marlex over the still soft methyl methacrylate so that the Marlex bonds to it. The resulting prosthesis has a firm, contoured center of polymethyl-methacrylate, which lies between two layers of Marlex. The 5-cm rim of Marlex that extends beyond the hard central polymethyl-methacrylate prosthesis acts as a sewing ring for securing it to the chest wall defect. The prosthesis has several assets: it has an absolutely rigid center, conforms well to the anticipated curve of the chest wall, and has a pliable sewing ring. One of its true liabilities arises with its creation: the reaction leading to the hardening of the methyl methacrylate is extremely exothermic, often reaching temperatures near 140°F. Appropriate curvature may be obtained by shaping the prosthesis over a chest tube collection bottle or over the patient's thigh, which can be protected with towels to prevent the exothermic reaction from causing thermal tissue injury. Once in place, the prosthesis is subject to all the problems, as noted previously, attendant on rigid prostheses in a dynamic environment.

Investigators working at the National Cancer Institute have identified another problem associated with methyl methacrylate prostheses (Pass, 1989). In their method for creating the prosthesis, the lung is dropped away from the defect in the chest wall and the prosthesis is actually created on the patient from Marlex, steel mesh, and methyl methacrylate. After the prosthesis has been created, the lung is re-expanded against the prosthesis. A metabolic acidosis, which is secondary to anion replacement with methyl methacrylate, ensues. This has to be corrected during the reconstruction.

METHODS OF IMPLANTATION

Chest wall stabilization is necessary to provide a firm surface on which to set the soft tissue flaps that complete the reconstruction. The key point to remember is that stabilization is directed at reducing paradoxical motion of the chest wall and maintaining its contour. Technical aspects of the three most popular methods of stabilization are discussed subsequently. It should be remembered that creativity is necessary in all aspects of chest wall reconstruction, including achievement of a desired cosmetic result.

There are several important points to consider in implanting the polymethyl-methacrylate "sandwich." The prosthesis has a central rigid area, which follows the chest contour and is extremely rigid. The sewing ring, which consists of the 5-cm rim of Marlex around the central hard prosthesis, is used to join the prosthesis to the chest wall. If sutures have to be placed through the central, hard portion of the prosthesis, a tunnel has to be created with a drill to allow passage of the needle since the methyl methacrylate sets to the same consistency as a football helmet.

Stabilization with either mesh or screening requires creative tailoring to suture the material to the chest wall (Fig. 55–9). The margin of resection should be palpated to determine the most stable point, which is usually a rib or a remaining portion of the sternum. A horizontal mattress suture of braided, permanent synthetic material is placed through the edge of the patch or the screening and through the periosteum of the bone and is tied in place. A second suture is placed through the synthetic material so that it can be secured firmly to the most stable point 180 degrees opposite to the original suture. Another set of sutures is placed through the prosthetic material at the edge of the resection so that the material is drawn tight and secured to the periosteum along an axis perpendicular to the line between the first two sutures. Sutures are then placed in a radial fashion so that the material is drawn tightly across the wound. Once the entirety of the prosthesis has been adjusted in place, any excess margins are trimmed.

An alternative method is to start with the firmest point on the margin of resection and secure the prosthesis to the periosteum. Sutures are then placed sequentially in a radial fashion around the defect, drawing the synthetic material progressively tighter. Tailoring cuts are made in the prosthetic material after each suture so that the material will tuck underneath the edges of the margin neatly. If the sutures are placed appropriately by either method, a firm, taut surface for accepting the soft tissue flaps is created.

In some patients with very difficult reconstructive problems, a customized prosthesis can be made to achieve chest wall stabilization and replace the soft tissue defect (Fig. 55–10). In such cases there has to be soft tissue coverage of the prosthesis after it is in place. Usually, the soft tissue placed over the prosthesis is the native tissue remaining at the site, but in some cases a musculocutaneous flap is necessary for sufficient coverage. The customized prosthesis is generated via computer modeling: the opposite side of the patient's chest wall is surveyed, measurements are taken, a mirror image of the chest wall is created through a computer model, the dimensions of the model are printed, and a plaster model is created (Hochberg et al, 1994).

In the case illustrated in Figure 55–10, the patient also needed a breast prosthesis. A silica gel prosthesis was

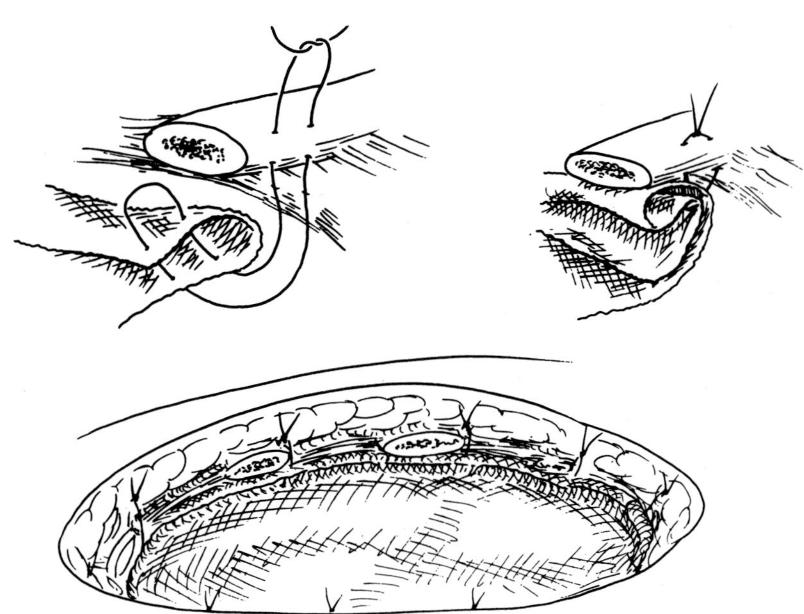

FIGURE 55–9 ■ A successful method for securing synthetic mesh or sheeting to a chest wall defect to achieve stabilization. Note that the sutures are placed on the cephalad aspect of the ribs to avoid the neurovascular bundles that course along the caudad surfaces of the ribs. Sutures are placed starting at one point in the defect and are placed sequentially and radically to achieve a relatively taut surface on which to place the flap(s) used to reconstruct the soft tissue defect. (From Seyfer AE, Graeber GM, Wind GG: Planning the reconstruction. In Seyfer AE (ed): Atlas of Chest Wall Reconstruction. Rockville, MD, Aspen, 1986a.)

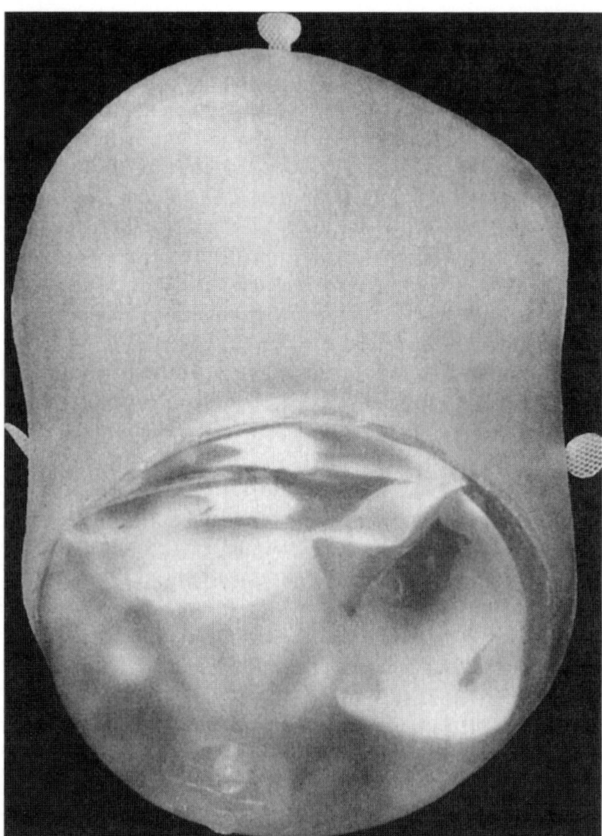

FIGURE 55–10 ■ Composite prosthesis with two components: a hard Silastic posterior segment, which replaces the upper anterior thoracic wall, and a soft gel prosthesis, which gives contour and shape to the absent breast. Note that there are three integral plastic tabs on the margins of the prosthesis. These plastic tabs are used to secure the prosthesis to bones on the thoracic wall and thereby prevent migration. (From Hochberg J, Ardenghy M, Graeber GM, Murray GF: Complex reconstruction of the chest wall and breast utilizing a customized silicone implant. Ann Plast Surg 32:524, 1994.)

added to the heavy Silastic contoured model of the chest wall. The composite model is custom manufactured, and the prosthesis is sterilized by the manufacturer and delivered to the surgeon for implantation in the patient. Implantation of this model is dependent on integral plastic tabs, which may be seen in Figure 55–10. These tabs are sutured to stable skeletal structures so that the prosthesis does not migrate. In the case cited, the three tabs were secured respectively to the sternum medially, the clavicle superiorly, and the ribs laterally. Heavy, braided synthetic sutures were placed through the plastic tabs and through the periosteum of the bony structures noted. In some situations, as with the clavicle or the sternum, the sutures may actually be placed around the entire structure to provide added security.

One final point cannot be overemphasized. Each reconstruction must be individualized and creative in order to achieve an excellent contour and reduce paradoxical motion in the chest wall to a minimum.

■ *REFERENCES*

Allen RG, Douglas M: Cosmetic improvement of thoracic wall defects using a rapid setting silastic mold: A special technique. J Pediatr Surg 14:745, 1979.

Boyd AD, Shaw WW, McCarthy JG et al: Immediate reconstruction of full-thickness chest wall defects. Ann Thorac Surg 32:337, 1981.

deCamara D, Sheridan JM, Kammer BA: Rupture and aging of silicone gel breast implants. Plast Reconstr Surg 91:828, 1993.

Eschaposse M, Gaillard J, Fournial G et al: Use of acrylic prosthesis for the repair of large defects of the chest wall. Acta Chir Belg 76:281, 1977.

Fix RJ, Vasconez LO: Use of the omentum in chest-wall reconstruction. Surg Clin North Am 69:1029, 1989.

Garcia VF, Seyfer AE, Graeber GM: Reconstruction of congenital chest-wall deformities. Surg Clin North Am 69:1103, 1989.

Graeber GM, Cohen DJ, Patrick DR et al: Rib fracture healing in experimental flail chest. J Trauma 25:903, 1985.

Hochberg J, Ardenghy M, Graeber GM, Murray GF: Complex reconstruction of the chest wall and breast utilizing a customized silicone implant. Ann Plast Surg 32:524, 1994.

Kuakowski A, Ruka W: Dura mater (Lyodural) in reconstruction of the abdominal and chest wall defects after radical excision of soft tissue neoplasms: case reports. Eur J Surg Oncol 23:63, 1987.

Lavey E, Aplelberg DB, Lash H et al: Customized silicone implants of the breast and chest. Plast Reconstr Surg 69:646, 1982.

Marcove RC, Egwele R, Searfoss R et al: Chest wall reconstruction with methyl methacrylate implantation. Compr Ther 3(12):5, 1977.

McCormack PM: Use of prosthetic materials in chest-wall reconstruction: Assets and liabilities. Surg Clin North Am 69:965, 1989.

McCormack PM, Bains MS, Beattie EJ et al: New trends in skeletal reconstruction after resection of chest wall tumors. Ann Thorac Surg 31:45, 1981.

Mendelson B, Masson JK: Silicone implants for contour deformities of the trunk. Plast Reconstr Surg 59:538, 1977.

Pairolero PC, Arnold PG: Chest wall tumors: Experience with 100 consecutive patients. J Thorac Cardiovasc Surg 90:367, 1985.

Pairolero PC, Arnold PG: Thoracic wall defects: Surgical management of 205 consecutive patients. Mayo Clin Proc 61:557, 1986.

Pass HI: Primary and metastatic chest wall tumors. In Roth JA, Ruchdeschel JC, Weisenferges TH (ed): Thoracic Oncology. Philadelphia, WB Saunders, 1989.

Seyfer AE, Graeber GM, Wind GG: Planning the reconstruction. In Seyfer AE (ed): Atlas of Chest Wall Reconstruction. Rockville, MD, Aspen Publishers, 1986a.

Seyfer AE, Graeber GM, Wind GG: Postoperative care. In Seyfer AE (ed): Atlas of Chest Wall Reconstruction. Rockville, MD, Aspen Publishers, 1986b.

Seyfer AE, Graeber GM, Wind GG: The omentum. In Seyfer AE (ed): Atlas of Chest Wall Reconstruction, Rockville, MD, Aspen Publishers, 1986c.

Seyfer AE, Graeber GM, Wind GG: Embryology, anatomy and physiology of the chest wall. In Seyfer AE (ed): Atlas of Chest Wall Reconstruction, Rockville, MD, Aspen Publishers, 1986d.

Seyfer AE, Graeber GM, Wind GG: Preoperative care and considerations. In Seyfer AE (ed):Atlas of Chest Wall Reconstruction. Rockville, MD, Aspen Publishers, 1986e.

Seyfer AE, Graeber GM, Wind GG: Congenital defects: Poland's syndrome, pectus deformities and sternal clefts. In Seyfer AE (ed): Atlas of Chest Wall Reconstruction. Rockville, MD, Aspen Publishers, 1986f.

SOFT TISSUE RECONSTRUCTION

Geoffrey M. Graeber

Soft tissue reconstruction of the chest wall has been revived and expanded since the early 1970s. The concept of pedicled flap reconstruction has been the mainstay of this movement since its inception. Tissue reconstruction has continued to grow, with delineation of new applications of pedicled flaps to repair increasingly complex defects. Free flap transfer has had some limited applications in carefully selected cases. The following discussion presents the major considerations in planning soft tissue coverage of a chest wall defect, the salient characteristics of the pedicled flaps, and the complications associated with specific reconstructions. Several major works have focused on this field, with comprehensive treatments of all aspects of chest wall reconstruction (McCraw and Arnold, 1986; Seyfer et al, 1986a; Seyfer and Graeber, 1989). Surgeons contemplating chest wall reconstruction should consult these texts for a thorough understanding of the complexities associated with successful thoracic reconstruction.

PLANNING THE RECONSTRUCTION

Pedicled reconstruction of chest wall defects may be conducted on any anatomic region of the chest wall. Certain areas have more options for reconstruction than others. Selection of appropriate flaps is mandatory, because tension on a flap's margin or its pedicle spells disaster. Designation of secondary flaps in each instance is essential, since one flap may not cover the entire defect without introduction of supplemental tissue, and rotation of replacement flaps may become necessary if the primary flap proves unsuitable (Azarow et al, 1989; Seyfer et al, 1986b).

Coverage of the anterior and anterolateral chest wall offers the most options because several pedicled flaps may be rotated successfully (Azarow et al, 1989; Seyfer et al, 1986b). Major pedicled flaps that may be used in this area include the pectoralis major, rectus abdominis, and latissimus dorsi muscular and musculocutaneous flaps as well as the omentum (Fig. 55–11). The serratus anterior muscular flap may be used in some limited applications.

The lateral chest wall has more limited options for pedicled reconstruction (Azarow et al, 1989; Seyfer et al, 1986b). The latissimus dorsi muscular and musculocutaneous flap is the first choice (Fig. 55–12). The rectus abdominis muscular or musculocutaneous flap is the second choice for these areas, and the omentum is the third choice. The serratus anterior flap and abdominal wall flaps have limited roles in this region, but they may be used if the main options have been exhausted or if their rotation is not possible (McCraw and Arnold, 1986).

Reconstruction of the chest wall posteriorly is more difficult because of limited options (Fig. 55–13). The latissimus dorsi muscular and musculocutaneous flap is clearly the best choice for cephalad rotation. On the upper

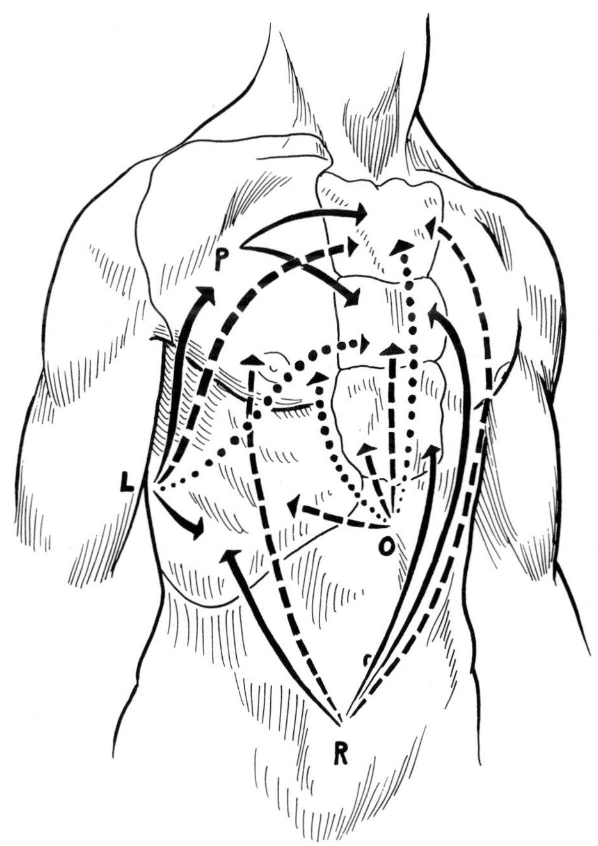

FIGURE 55–11 ■ Anterior and anterolateral areas of the chest wall and the pedicled flaps that may be used to reconstruct these areas. The sternum has been divided into upper, middle, and lower sections. The area over the pectoralis major muscle has been designated by a *solid line* extending from the shoulder around the clavicle to the sternum and to just below the breast; this is the upper lateral region. The lower lateral region is directly below this area and covers the rest of the thoracic cage from the anterior axillary line to the sternum. The areas of transfer for each muscle are shown by arrows: the first choice for coverage of a given area is designated by a *solid arrow*, the second choices by *dashed arrows*, and the third choices by *dotted arrows*. Each of the flaps is designated by a letter: L, latissimus dorsi; O, omentum; P, pectoralis major; R, rectus abdominis. (From Seyfer AE, Graeber GM, Wind GG: Planning the reconstruction. In Seyfer AE (ed): Atlas of Chest Wall Reconstruction. Rockville, MD, Aspen, 1986b.)

I wish to thank Ms. Karen DeShong for her assistance in the preparation of this manuscript.

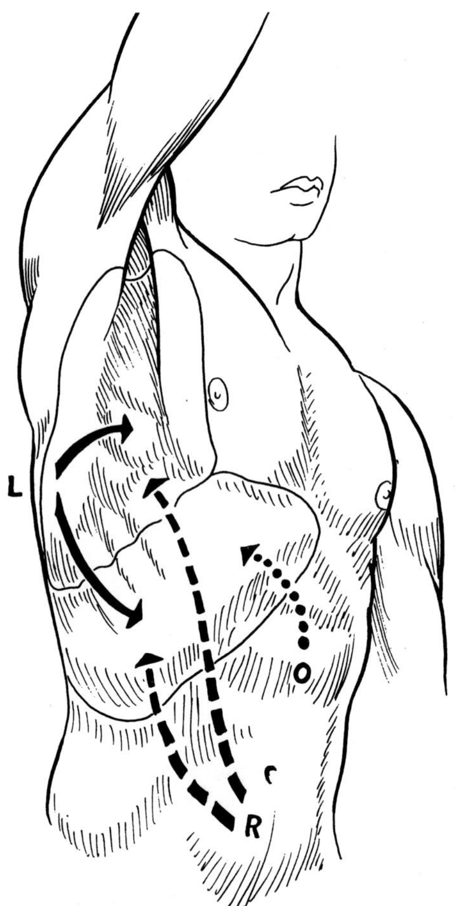

FIGURE 55–12 ■ The lateral areas of the chest wall may be reconstructed with either latissimus dorsi or rectus abdominis muscular or musculocutaneous flaps or the omentum. The two distinct areas, which are outlined by *solid lines*, represent an upper and a lower region. Note that the latissimus dorsi (designated by L) is the primary pedicled flap for reconstruction in both areas, the rectus abdominis (designated by R) is the secondary flap, and the omentum (designated by O) is the tertiary flap for reconstructing these areas. The *heavy black line* designates the latissimus as the primary flap for reconstruction in both areas, the *dashed arrows* indicate the rectus as the secondary flap, and the *dotted line*, associated with the omentum, indicates that it is the third choice. (From Seyfer AE, Graeber GM, Wind GG: Planning the reconstruction. In Seyfer AE (ed): Atlas of Chest Wall Reconstruction. Rockville, MD, Aspen, 1986b.)

chest, the trapezius muscle may be rotated to cover spinal and paraspinal defects. In extreme cases, free flap transfer may be used as long as suitable arterial and venous supply is maintained, the pedicle is not placed under tension, and the margins of the flap are not overextended.

Occasionally, a defect may be so large that more than one flap may be necessary to provide for adequate soft tissue coverage (Azarow et al, 1989; Seyfer et al, 1986b). In such cases secondary and tertiary flaps may be rotated to achieve satisfactory soft tissue coverage without tension on the pedicle(s) or on the margins of the flaps. In some extreme circumstances, the pedicles of the flaps may be dissected maximally, and the size of the flap may extend to its extreme to achieve coverage. Such reconstructions using combined latissimus dorsi and rectus abdominis flaps to close large contralateral defects have been reported (Matsuo et al, 1991).

FLAPS FOR RECONSTRUCTION

Each of the flaps used in reconstruction of the chest wall has assets and liabilities as well as a defined are of rotation. Transposition of any of the flaps requires precise understanding of the blood supply. Successful rotation of any flap depends on preservation of the blood supply and prevention of any tension on the pedicle and on the margins of the flap. Previous surgical procedures and pathologic conditions may preclude successful rotation of specific flaps.

Pectoralis Major Muscle

One of the most frequently used muscular and musculocutaneous flaps is the pectoralis major. The utility and durability of this flap has been shown in several series

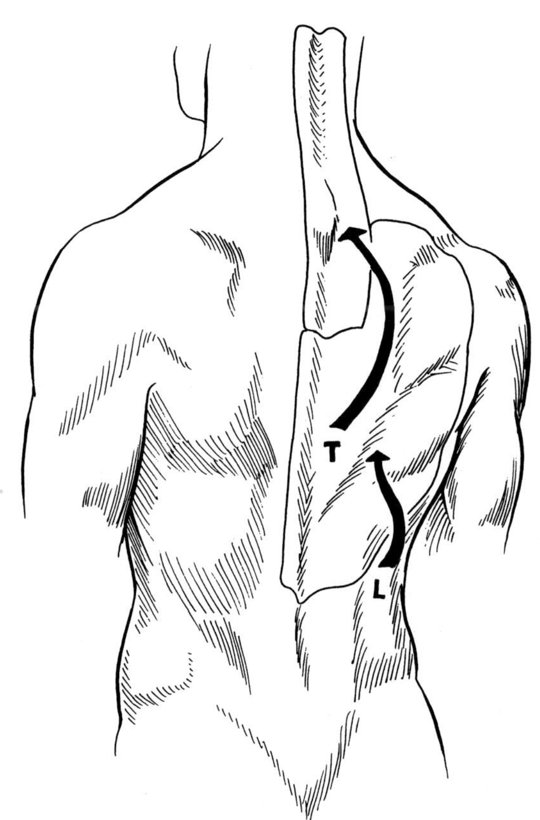

FIGURE 55–13 ■ The limited options for reconstruction of the posterior aspect of the chest wall are delineated. Note that there are two areas for reconstruction: the upper spinous and the paraspinous area and the lower, larger area that encompasses most of the back. The primary flap for reconstruction of the upper area is the trapezius muscle (designated by T). The latissimus dorsi (designated by L) is the muscle and musculocutaneous flap that can be used most effectively to cover most of the back. (From Seyfer AE, Graeber GM, Wind GG: Planning the reconstruction. In Seyfer AE (ed): Atlas of Chest Wall Reconstruction. Rockville, MD, Aspen, 1986b.)

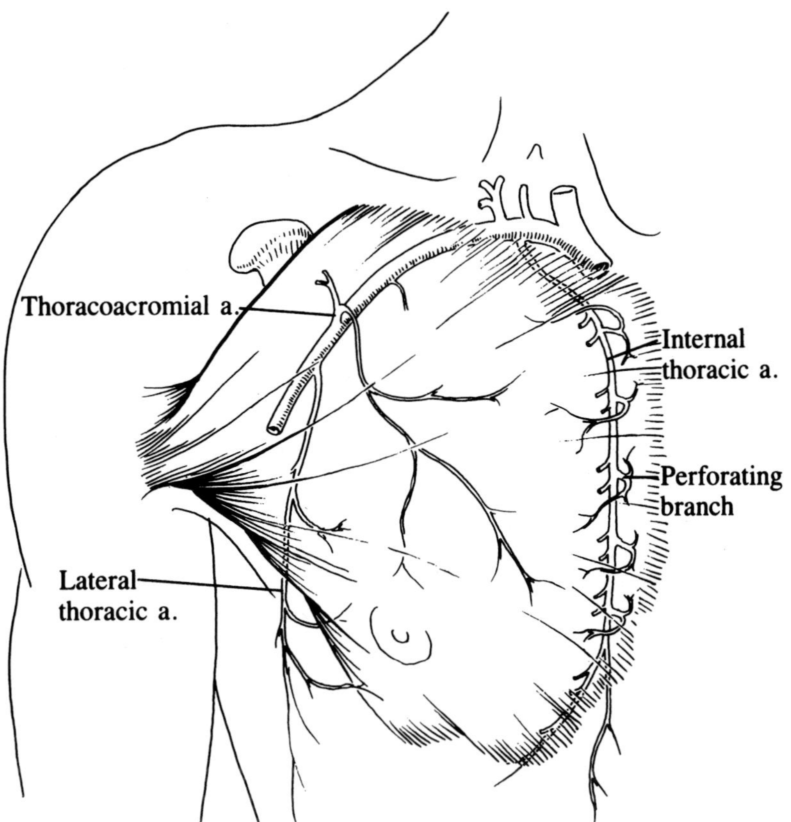

FIGURE 55–14 ■ The primary and secondary blood supply for the right pectoralis major muscle. Note that the thoracoacromial artery and vein constitute the primary supply, with the major vessel directed from cephalad to caudad. The next most abundant vascular supply to the muscle consists of the internal thoracic artery and vein, which course along the lateral aspect of the sternum to give rise to perforators, which penetrate the intercostal spaces and give blood to the pectoralis major muscle. The tertiary supply consists of some random branches of the lateral thoracic artery and of the intercostal arteries as they give rise to small vessels that perforate the muscle. Pedicled flaps have been described that are based on the thoracoacromial neurovascular bundle and on the internal thoracic artery and its penetrating branches that supply the medial aspect of the pectoralis major muscle. (From Seyfer AE, Graeber GM, Wind GG: The pectoralis major muscle and musculocutaneous flaps. In Seyfer AE (ed): Atlas of Chest Wall Reconstruction: Rockville, MD, Aspen, 1986c.)

(Arnold and Pairolero 1984; Graeber et al, 1982; Pairolero and Arnold, 1986b). Because of its primary and secondary blood supply, it can be transferred as a pedicled flap based on the thoracoacromial neurovascular bundle or on the perforators arising from the ipsilateral internal mammary artery (Seyfer et al, 1986b; Tobin, 1989) (Fig. 55–14). It is particularly well suited for use in repairing defects of the upper anterior chest wall and in the upper part of the ipsilateral pleural space (Arnold and Pairolero 1978, 1979) (Fig. 55–15).

Major assets of the pectoralis major muscle and musculocutaneous flap are its ability to be based on two different blood supplies and thus allow successful transfer and its intrinsic ability to be divided into segments so that structure and function may be preserved while maintaining the natural contour of the thoracic wall. It may be moved into the upper portion of the pleural space, into a dehisced median sternotomy incision, or into the head and neck for reconstruction depending on the pathology present (Seyfer et al, 1986c; Tobin, 1989).

It has relatively few problems, which can be addressed successfully if they are appreciated prior to reconstruction (Seyfer et al, 1986c; Tobin, 1989). One is elimination of a pedicle due to trauma or removal of the primary blood supply for a pedicle. These complications are quite rare for the primary pedicle, the thoracoacromial neurovascular bundle. They are not uncommon, unfortunately, for the secondary pedicle, the internal thoracic (mammary) artery. If the ipsilateral internal thoracic artery has been harvested for revascularization of the myocardium, rotation of the pectoralis based on the secondary pedicle (ipsilateral internal thoracic artery) is contraindicated, since the muscle pedicle would be based on the tertiary blood supply, the intercostal vessels. Under these conditions, the viability of the flap would be extremely questionable. The blood supply to the flap can also be compromised by a sternal wire that perforates the internal thoracic vessels. Hence, closure of a dehisced median sternotomy incision with pectoralis major muscular flaps based on the ipsilateral internal thoracic artery and vein must be undertaken only after thorough evaluation of the integrity of these vessels.

One of the most common indications for use of the pectoralis major muscular flap is the reconstruction of the dehisced median sternotomy (Miller and Nahai, 1989; Pairolero and Arnold, 1984, 1986a). One method describes advancement of the pectoralis major muscular flaps into the wound based on their primary pedicles, the thoracoacromial neurovascular bundles. In such cases both muscles in their entirety are dissected free of their origins and insertions and are advanced into the wound together to reconstruct the wound closure (Seyfer et al, 1986c) (Fig. 55–16). An alternative is to base the flaps on the perforators arising from the respective internal thoracic arteries, divide the thoracoacromial vessels, and turn the flaps over into the dehisced median sternotomy wound (Morain et al, 1981; Nahai et al, 1982) (Fig. 55–17). Variations of these two approaches based on the segmental anatomy of the pectoralis major muscle have been described, in which the first method is used on one side and a variation of the second is used on the contralateral side (Miller and Nahai, 1989; Tobin, 1989).

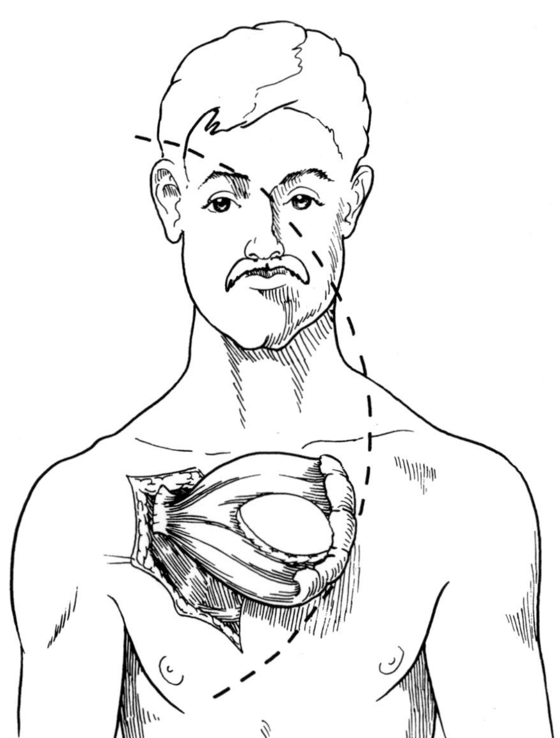

FIGURE 55–15 ■ The arc of rotation of the pectoralis major muscular and musculocutaneous flap when based on the thoracoacromial neurovascular bundle. Note that the origin and the insertion of the muscle have been cut and have retracted toward the center. The muscle may be rotated over the entire anterolateral chest wall and into the head and neck region. (From Seyfer AE, Graeber GM, Wind GG: The pectoralis major muscle and musculocutaneous flaps. In Seyfer AE (ed): Atlas of Chest Wall Reconstruction. Rockville, MD, Aspen, 1986c.)

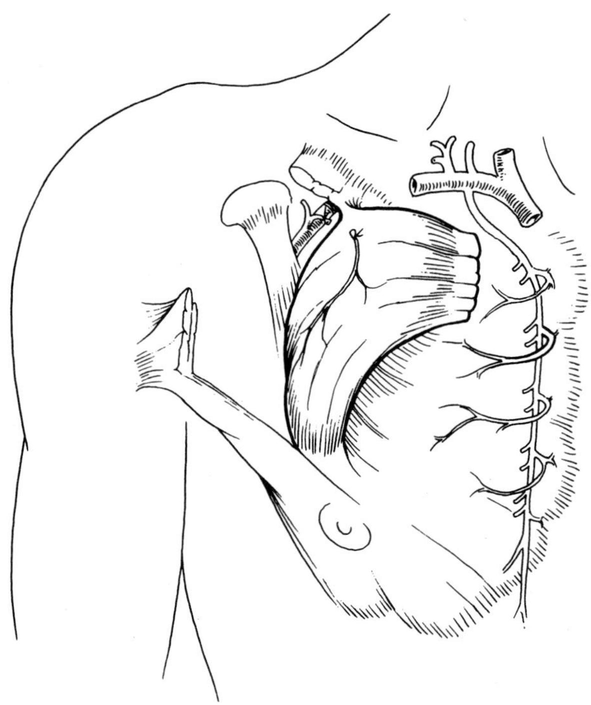

FIGURE 55–17 ■ The pectoralis major muscular flap may be based on the internal thoracic perforators arising along the origin of the muscle just lateral to the sternum. In this dissection, the inferior part of the muscle is saved to preserve function and cosmesis. (From Seyfer AE, Graeber GM, Wind GG: The pectoralis major muscle and musculocutaneous flaps. In Seyfer AE (ed): Atlas of Chest Wall Reconstruction. Rockville, MD, Aspen, 1986c.)

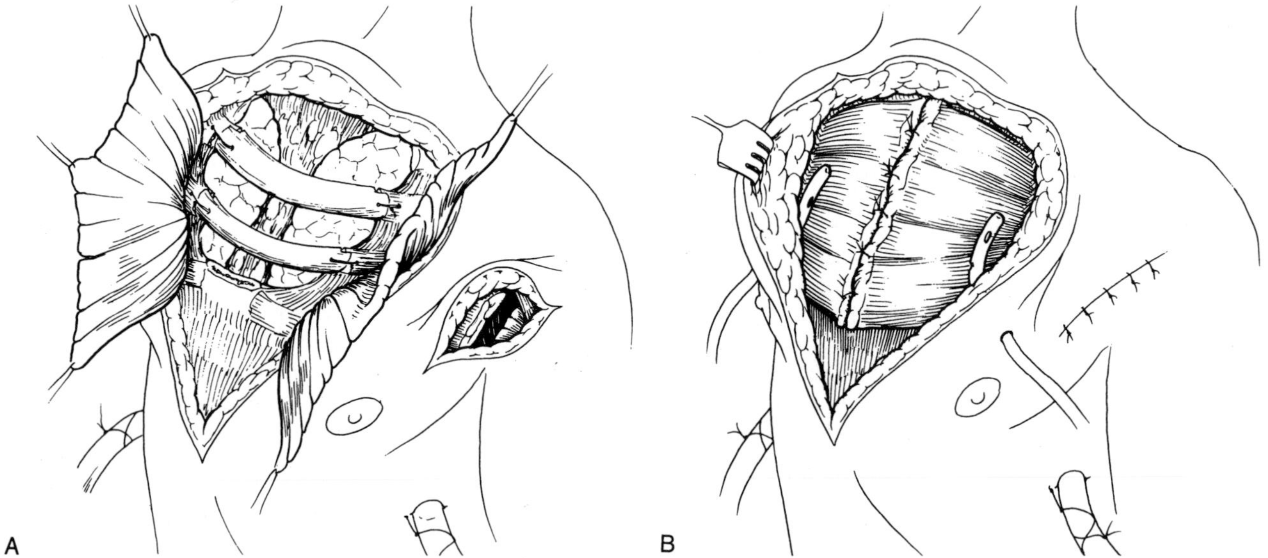

FIGURE 55–16 ■ *A*, Mobilization of the pectoralis major flaps for reconstruction of the upper anterior thorax. Both muscles have been pedicled on their respective thoracoacromial arteries and veins. Note that the origins of both muscles as well as the insertions have been transected. *B*, Muscles reconstructed over the sternal defect. Note that the pectoralis major muscles join together in the midline to add support to the wound. (From Seyfer AE, Graebar GM, Wind GG: The pectoralis major muscle and musculocutaneous flaps. In Seyfer AE (ed): Atlas of Chest Wall Reconstruction. Rockville, MD, Aspen, 1986c.)

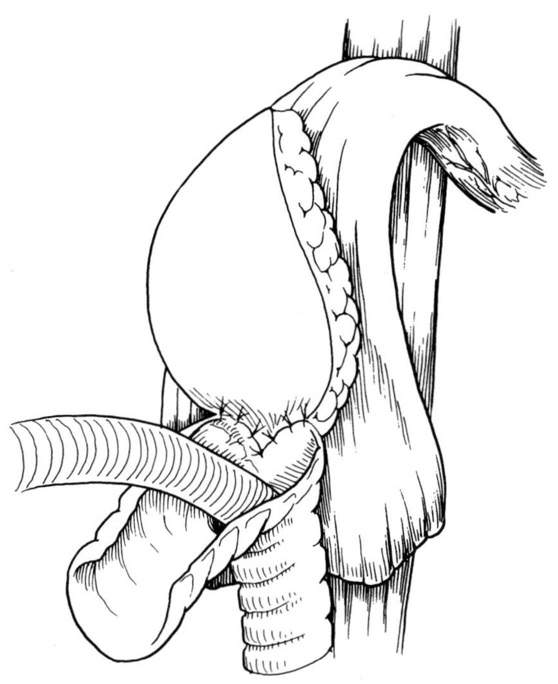

FIGURE 55–18 ■ The pectoralis major musculocutaneous flap has been placed over the repaired esophagus, which is posterior. The skin island is being joined to the open area of the trachea so that the membranous portion is being replaced. Any exposed portion of the muscle that remains after the reconstruction will be covered with meshed, split-thickness skin grafts. (From Seyfer AE, Graeber GM, Wind GG: Tracheoesophageal and bronchopleural/cutaneous fistulas. In Seyfer AE (ed): Atlas of Chest Wall Reconstruction. Rockville MD, Aspen, 1986d.)

In addition to reconstruction of the anterior chest wall after tumor resection and reconstruction of the dehisced median sternotomy, the pectoralis major muscular and musculocutaneous flap has been useful in reconstruction of the radiation-damaged chest wall, in treating bronchopleural fistulas and their associated empyemas, and in repairing tracheoesophageal fistulas. In the experience at the Mayo Clinic, the pectoralis major and latissimus dorsi flaps have been the most commonly used in treating patients with radiation damage of the chest wall (Arnold and Pairolero, 1989). The pectoralis major muscular flap has been successful in treating high bronchopleural fistulas and their associated empyemas (Pairolero and Arnold, 1989). For this application the flap has been based on the thoracoacromial neurovascular bundle in most cases (Pairolero and Arnold, 1989). Reconstruction of tracheoesophageal fistulas has also been successfully performed by using this flap (Seyfer et al, 1986d). A skin island appended to the flap may be used to reconstruct the membranous trachea, or alternatively, a meshed, split-thickness skin graft may be used for this purpose and for epithelializing any exposed portions of the muscle (Fig. 55–18).

Rectus Abdominis Muscle

The rectus abdominis muscle has been important in chest wall reconstruction both as a muscular and as a musculocutaneous flap. It is a large muscle, with the capacity to carry substantial islands of tissue to repair defects on the chest wall and in the thorax. It can have both a longitudinal and a transverse cutaneous island. Its blood supply is particularly favorable in that it usually has a balance between the superior and inferior epigastric arteries. The intercostals, which end in the rectus sheaths along the abdominal wall, are the tertiary blood supply. Flaps may be constructed based on the superior or inferior epigastric artery. In some cases involving particularly large defects of the chest wall, flaps have been rotated based on both rectus muscles and both internal thoracic arteries (Glafkides and Toth, 1991). Accurate, comprehensive descriptions of the methodologies for rotating these muscular and musculocutaneous flaps are available (Coleman and Bostwick, 1989; Seyfer et al, 1986e). This muscle, and particularly its musculocutaneous flap, has been quite useful in reconstruction of the breast, with several authors presenting extensive experiences with this muscle for breast reconstruction (Bunkis et al, 1983; Dinner et al, 1982; Hartrampf et al, 1982; Jacobsen et al, 1994).

The rectus abdominis muscle has a large arc of rotation, which allows it or its musculocutaneous flap to be rotated onto most of the anterior, anterolateral, and lateral thoracic wall (Seyfer et al, 1986e). The domain of the flap for chest wall reconstruction is extensive and covers virtually all of the anterior and lateral thorax (Fig. 55–19). Besides its significant use in reconstruction of the breast, it has been particularly effective in repair of the dehisced median sternotomy. It must be used carefully in this capacity since its blood supply is dependent on the integrity of the internal thoracic artery (see later). Because of the amount of tissue that can be transferred, the rectus abdominis muscular and musculocutaneous flap has been particularly useful in the reconstruction of anterior and lateral chest wall defects after resection of malignant tumors. These flaps have also been used extensively in reconstruction of the chest wall after radiation injuries, particularly those associated with breast cancer therapy.

The blood supply to the rectus abdominis muscle allows rotation of the entire muscle and an associated subcutaneous and cutaneous island along with the flap onto the greater part of the chest wall (Seyfer et al, 1986f). The superior epigastric vessels, which are the direct extensions of the internal thoracic artery and vein, are the principal vessels in the pedicle on which this muscular and musculocutaneous flap is based for rotation onto the anterior and lateral thoracic wall (Brown et al, 1975; Miller et al, 1988). Because of the rich vascular plexus within the muscle, the entire length of the rectus abdominis may be transferred cephalad with the superior epigastric vessels used as the sole pedicle (Figs. 55–20 and 55–21). In some very rare cases, both rectus abdominis muscles and a large associated subcutaneous and cutaneous island may be rotated onto the anterior thorax based on both pairs of epigastric vessels (Ishii et al, 1985). This flap must be rotated with great care, since the blood supply must be preserved.

Obviously, previous abdominal incisions can have a deleterious effect on the blood supply to the muscle and hence to the flap. Incisions that may modify or preclude the use of this flap include the paramedian, midline, and upper transverse incisions (Fig. 55–22). The upper

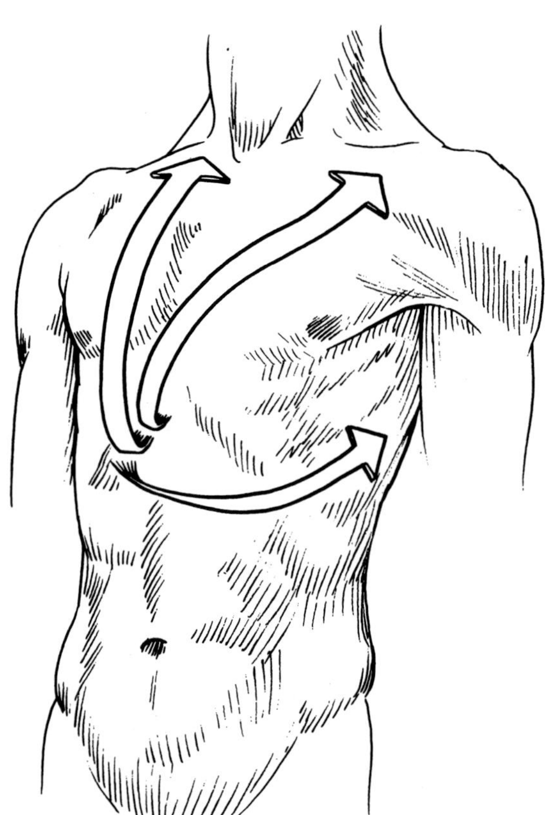

FIGURE 55–19 ■ The rectus abdominis muscle and musculocutaneous flap are particularly useful in reconstruction of the anterior and lateral chest wall. In all instances of this application, the pedicle is based on the superior epigastric vessels, which are continuations of the internal thoracic (mammary) artery and vein. (From Seyfer AE, Graeber GM, Wind GG: The rectus abdominis muscle and musculocutaneous flaps. In Seyfer AE (ed): Atlas of Chest Wall Reconstruction. Rockville, MD, Aspen, 1986e.)

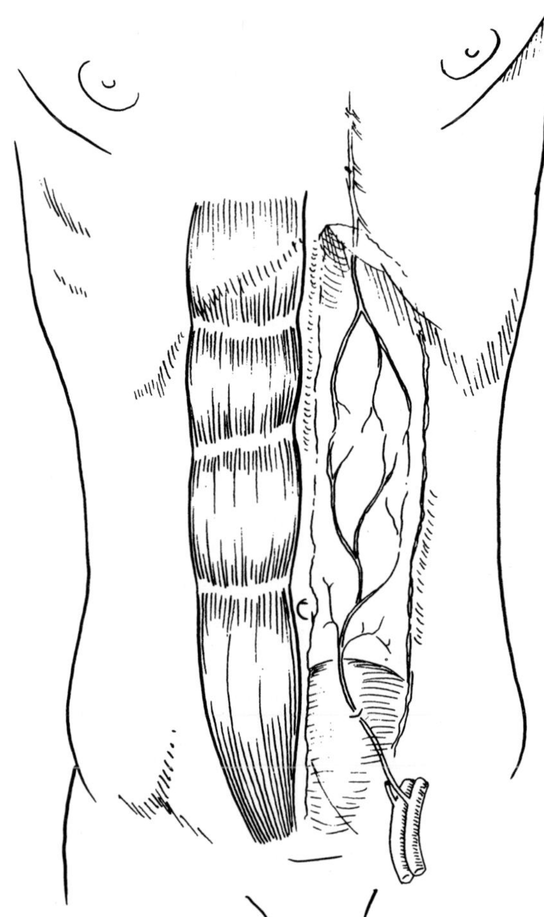

FIGURE 55–20 ■ The rectus abdominis muscle may be based on either the superior or the inferior epigastric vascular pedicles. The rich anastomosis between the vessels, which is in the center portion of the muscle, ensures the viability of the distal portion of the flap when it is based on either pedicle. (From Seyfer AE, Graeber GM, Wind GG: Blood supply to the skin of the chest wall. In Seyfer AE (ed): Atlas of Chest Wall Reconstruction. Rockville MD, Aspen, 1986f.)

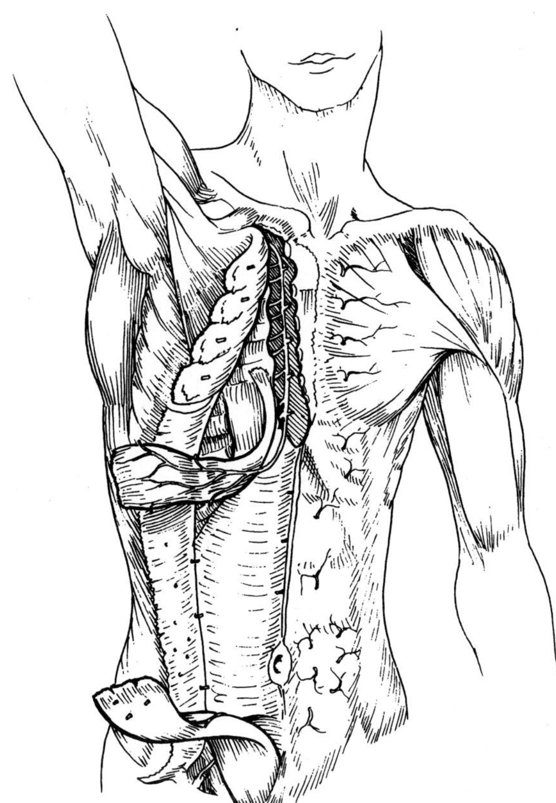

FIGURE 55–21 ■ This anatomic dissection shows the direct dependence of the superior epigastric vessels on the extension of the internal thoracic artery and vein. The rectus abdominis has been divided in its midportion to show the rich plexus of penetrating vessels, which allow viability of the skin when transferred with the muscular flap. (From Seyfer AE, Graeber GM, Wind GG: Blood supply to the skin of the chest wall. In Seyfer AE (ed): Atlas of Chest Wall Reconstruction. Rockville, MD, Aspen, 1986f.)

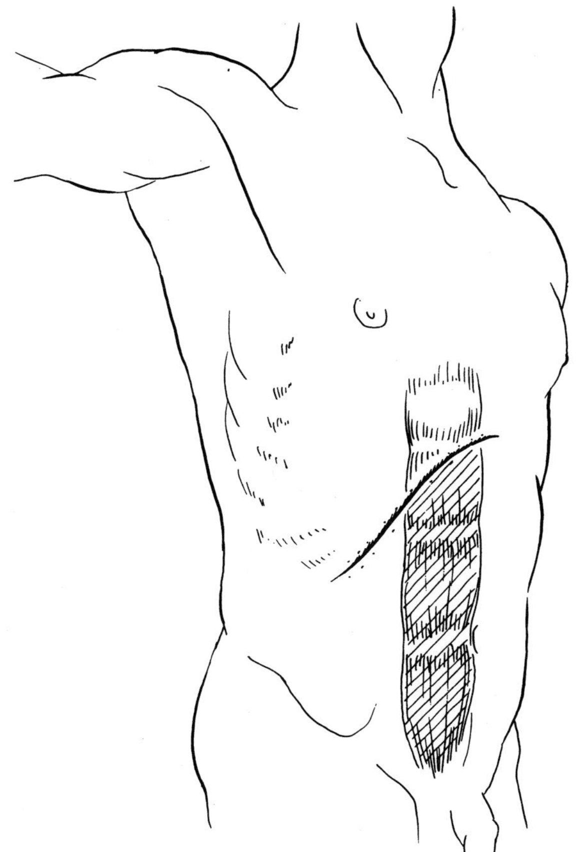

FIGURE 55–22 ■ Whenever the rectus abdominis muscle is contemplated for reconstruction of the thorax, the surgeon must analyze the previous incisions on the abdomen. In this instance, an upper right subcostal incision precludes the use of the rectus based on the superior epigastric vessels. If a flap based on these vessels were to be rotated, any tissue distal to the line of incision would die, because all this tissue has become dependent on the inferior epigastric vessels after the transverse incision. (From Seyfer AE, Graeber GM, Wind GG: Planning the reconstruction. In Seyfer AE (ed): Atlas of Chest Wall Reconstruction. Rockville, MD, Aspen, 1986b.)

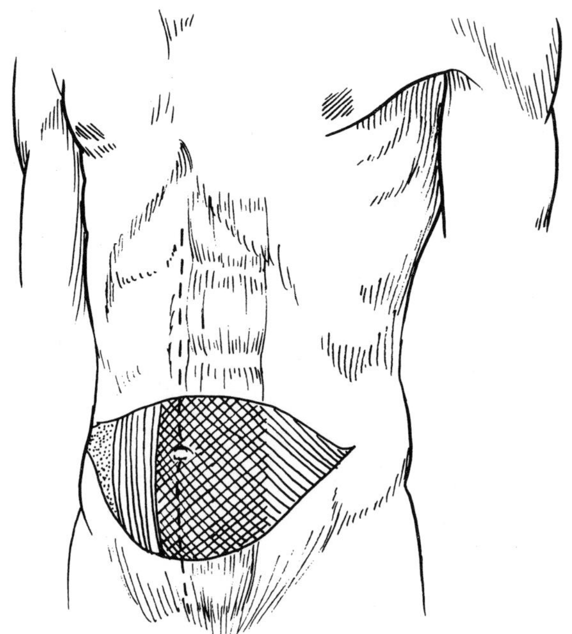

FIGURE 55–23 ■ The potential viability of skin and subcutaneous tissues when transferred with the rectus abdominis as a transverse musculocutaneous rectus abdominis (TRAM) flap is depicted. The skin and subcutaneous tissues directly overlying the rectus muscle have the highest probability of viability after transfer. These are denoted by the *cross-hatched area*. Other areas that are directly juxtaposed to this well-vascularized tissue may remain viable but can still suffer necrosis under certain conditions. These areas are denoted by the *vertical* and the *oblique lines*. The soft tissue that is far distal to the main flap is of questionable viability and should not be used; this area is represented by the *stippled area* on the right anterior abdominal wall. This drawing depicts a left rectus flap; if a right rectus flap were contemplated, the areas of tissue viability would be the mirror image of that shown here. (From Seyfer AE, Graeber GM, Wind GG: Blood supply to the skin of the chest wall. In Seyfer AE (ed): Atlas of Chest Wall Reconstruction. Rockville, MD, Aspen, 1986f.)

transverse incisions, which cross either rectus abdominis muscle, almost always interrupt the superior epigastric vessels so that the muscle distal to the incision becomes dependent on the inferior epigastric vessels for its viability. Cephalad rotation based on the superior epigastric vessels is therefore not indicated, since the distal portion of the muscle will die under these circumstances. A midline incision limits the amount of subcutaneous tissue and skin that may be transferred on the distal portion of the flap, since the subcutaneous and cutaneous blood supply will be interrupted lateral to the midline incision. Under these circumstances, any soft tissue that is lateral to the midline incision and is transferred with the flap will most likely succumb. Paramedian incisions generally disrupt the entire vascular plexus and preclude successful rotation.

There are several methods for using this muscular and musculocutaneous flap in chest wall reconstruction. The muscle itself may be transposed to fill a dehisced median sternotomy incision. The muscle itself may also be rotated to close a particularly low fistula within the thorax. Most frequently, the rectus is rotated into the chest as a musculocutaneous flap with either a transverse or a longitudinal orientation. The transverse rectus abdominis musculocutaneous (TRAM) flap is very popular for reconstruction of the breast and of radiation injuries of the anterior chest wall (Bunkis et al, 1983; Dinner et al, 1982; Hartrampf et al, 1982; Jacobsen et al, 1994) (Figs. 55–23 and 55–24). The TRAM flap has been used in many creative ways to reconstruct absent breasts (Figs. 55–25 and 55–26). The longitudinal musculocutaneous flap is particularly beneficial in repairing a severely dehisced median sternotomy incision. The longitudinal island may be rotated with the flap to completely fill a severe defect associated with the severe dehiscence of a median sternotomy wound, such as those more frequently seen in diabetic patients (Fig. 55–27). If one of the internal mammary arteries has been harvested for myocardial revascularization, the rectus abdominis musculocutaneous flap used for repair of a dehisced median sternotomy should be rotated based on the opposite superior epigastric vessel. If both mammaries have been harvested for myocardial revascularization, the rectus abdominis should not be rotated into the wound, since the muscular or musculocutaneous flap will most likely die in this situation.

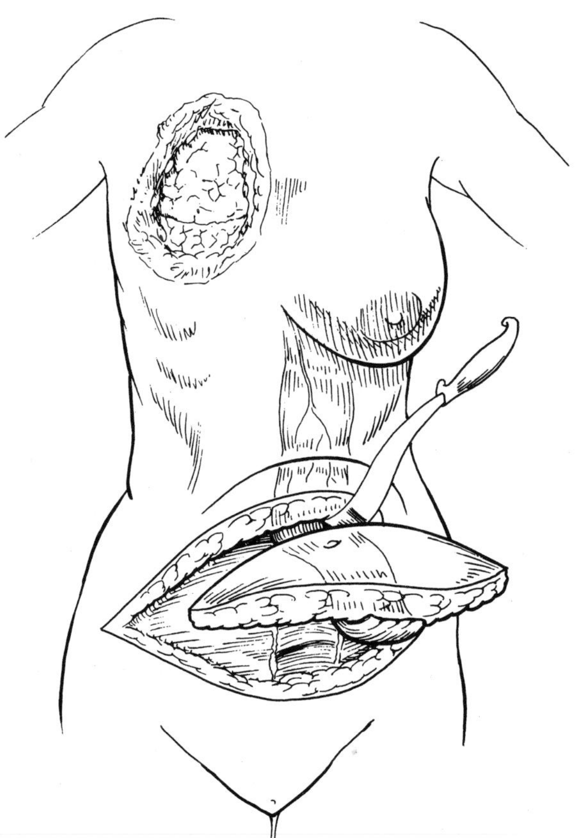

FIGURE 55–24 ■ A TRAM flap being harvested to repair a radiation defect of the right anterior chest wall. Note that the flap is based on the left rectus abdominis muscle and that the distal transverse subcutaneous and cutaneous skin island is being transferred in continuity with the rectus muscle. (From Seyfer AE, Graeber GM, Wind GG: Blood supply to the skin of the chest wall. In Seyfer AE (ed): Atlas of Chest Wall Reconstruction. Rockville, MD, Aspen, 1986f.)

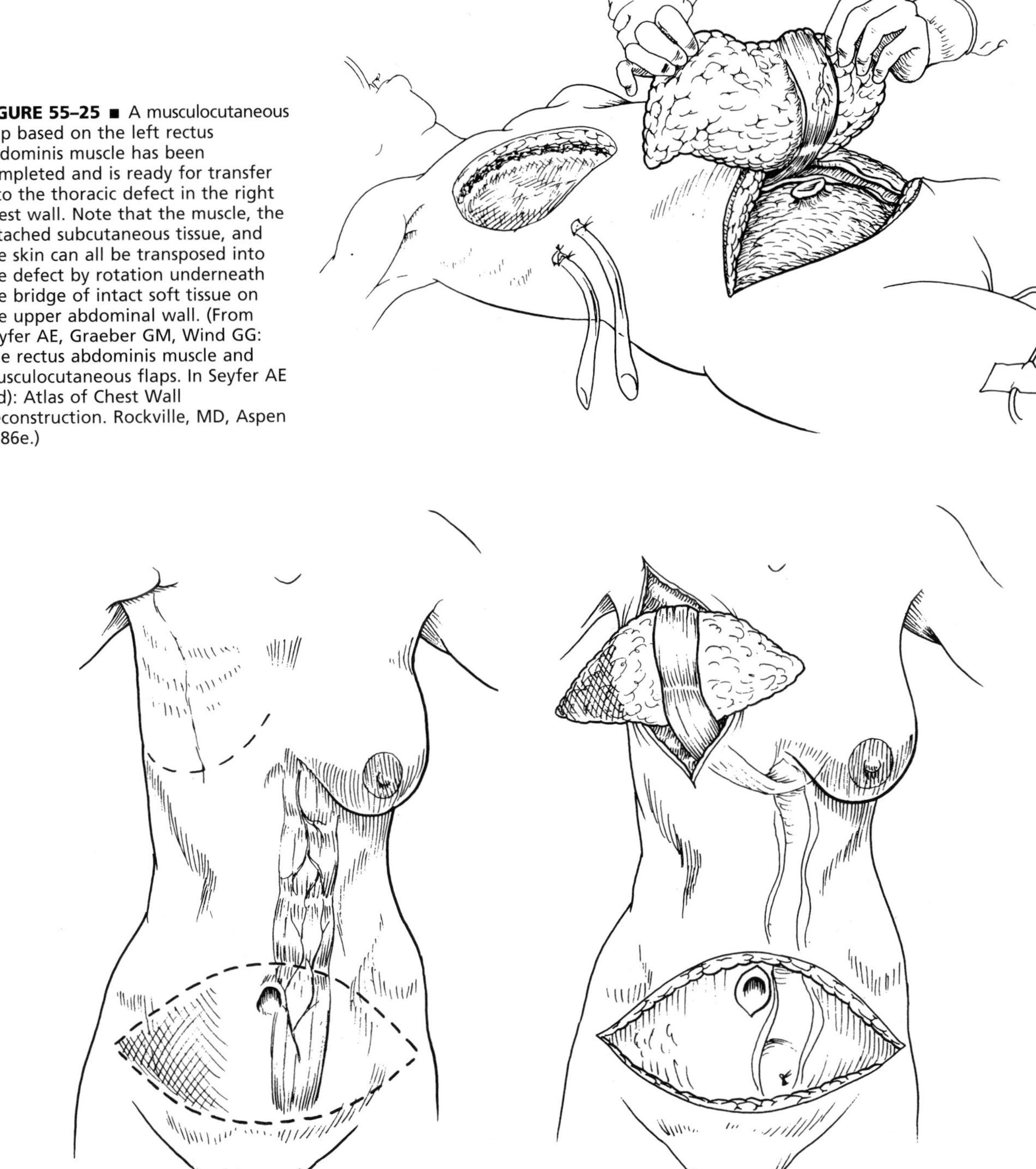

FIGURE 55–25 ■ A musculocutaneous flap based on the left rectus abdominis muscle has been completed and is ready for transfer into the thoracic defect in the right chest wall. Note that the muscle, the attached subcutaneous tissue, and the skin can all be transposed into the defect by rotation underneath the bridge of intact soft tissue on the upper abdominal wall. (From Seyfer AE, Graeber GM, Wind GG: The rectus abdominis muscle and musculocutaneous flaps. In Seyfer AE (ed): Atlas of Chest Wall Reconstruction. Rockville, MD, Aspen 1986e.)

FIGURE 55–26 ■ *A*, Planned reconstruction of the right breast using a left rectus abdominis TRAM flap. There is no associated radiation ulcer of the chest wall. *B*, The completed left rectus abdominis TRAM flap rotated up into the thoracic defect. The lower abdominal incision can then be closed with preservation of the umbilicus. The flap may be tailored to provide for adequate reconstruction of the breast. (From Seyfer AE, Graeber GM, Wind GG: Reconstruction of the breast following mastectomy. In Seyfer AE (ed): Atlas of Chest Wall Reconstruction. Rockville, MD, Aspen, 1986g.)

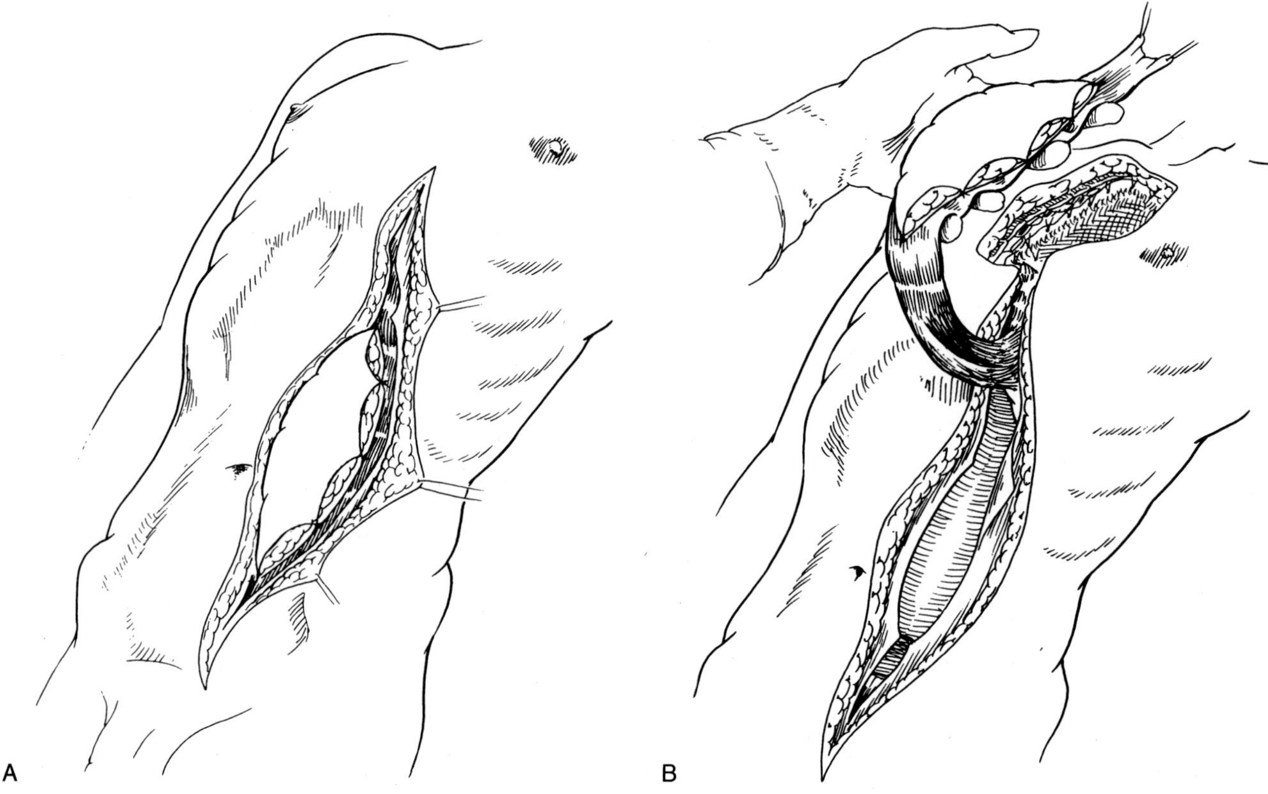

FIGURE 55–27 ■ *A*, The rectus abdominis myocutaneous flap may be used in reconstructing defects of the sternum and the dehisced median sternotomy as long as the ipsilateral internal thoracic vessels are intact. A longitudinal musculocutaneous flap has been fashioned for anterior wall reconstruction in this drawing. *B*, The completed longitudinal musculocutaneous flap ready to be rotated based on the superior epigastric vessels. The longitudinal flap will be laid into the defect and adjusted to the edges. The blood supply to the musculocutaneous flap must be scrupulously maintained. The viability of the internal thoracic artery for this type of reconstruction is absolutely mandatory. (From Seyfer AE, Graeber GM, Wind GG: The rectus abdominis muscle and musculocutaneous flaps. In Seyfer AE (ed): Atlas of Chest Wall Reconstruction. Rockville, MD, Aspen, 1986e.)

The use of the rectus abdominis has been extended by free transfer and by creative vascular anastomoses. Free flap transfers of the rectus abdominis muscle, the omentum, and the latissimus dorsi have been reported in the management of complex intrathoracic problems (Hammond et al, 1993). These free flaps have been most useful in repairing bronchopleural-cutaneous fistulas. The rectus itself may have its blood supply enhanced and its vertical configuration of tissue transfer enlarged by anastomosing the inferior epigastric artery and vein to their axillary counterparts (Yamamoto et al, 1994). Flaps enhanced in this manner have been particularly useful in filling large anterior wall defects.

The Latissimus Dorsi Muscle

Pedicled muscular and musculocutaneous flaps based on the latissimus dorsi muscle have found wide application in chest wall reconstruction, since this muscle has an extensive arc of rotation when the pedicle is based on the thoracodorsal neurovascular bundle (Moelleken et al, 1989; Seyfer et al, 1986h) (Fig. 55–28). When a latissimus dorsi muscular or musculocutaneous flap has been based on its primary blood supply, the flap can be used to cover defects on the anterior, lateral, and posterior aspects of the thorax (McCraw et al, 1978). When the pedicle of a latissimus dorsi flap is based on its secondary blood supply (the ipsilateral ninth through eleventh intercostal arteries and their perforators), the flap's arc of rotation is more limited, and the flap is best suited for posterior intrathoracic applications (Moelleken et al, 1989).

The primary blood supply to this large, flat muscle located on the posterolateral aspect of the chest wall is the thoracodorsal artery and its associated veins (Rowsell et al, 1984). In the vast majority of cases, the axillary artery gives rise to the subscapular artery, which divides to create the thoracodorsal artery and the artery or arteries to the serratus anterior muscle (Rowsell et al, 1984). In 74% of cadavers studied by Rowsell and co-workers (1984), the artery to the serratus anterior was single; in 24% it was represented by two or more branches. The thoracodorsal artery, which is a direct extension of the subscapular artery in most cases, descends to the body of the latissimus dorsi, where it most commonly divides into two branches (Fig. 55–29). The more anterior branch descends parallel to the lateral border of the muscle; the medial branch usually traverses more horizontally in the body of the muscle. Both branches form collaterals with the secondary blood supply (the ninth through the eleventh intercostal arteries and their perforators) in the body of the muscle.

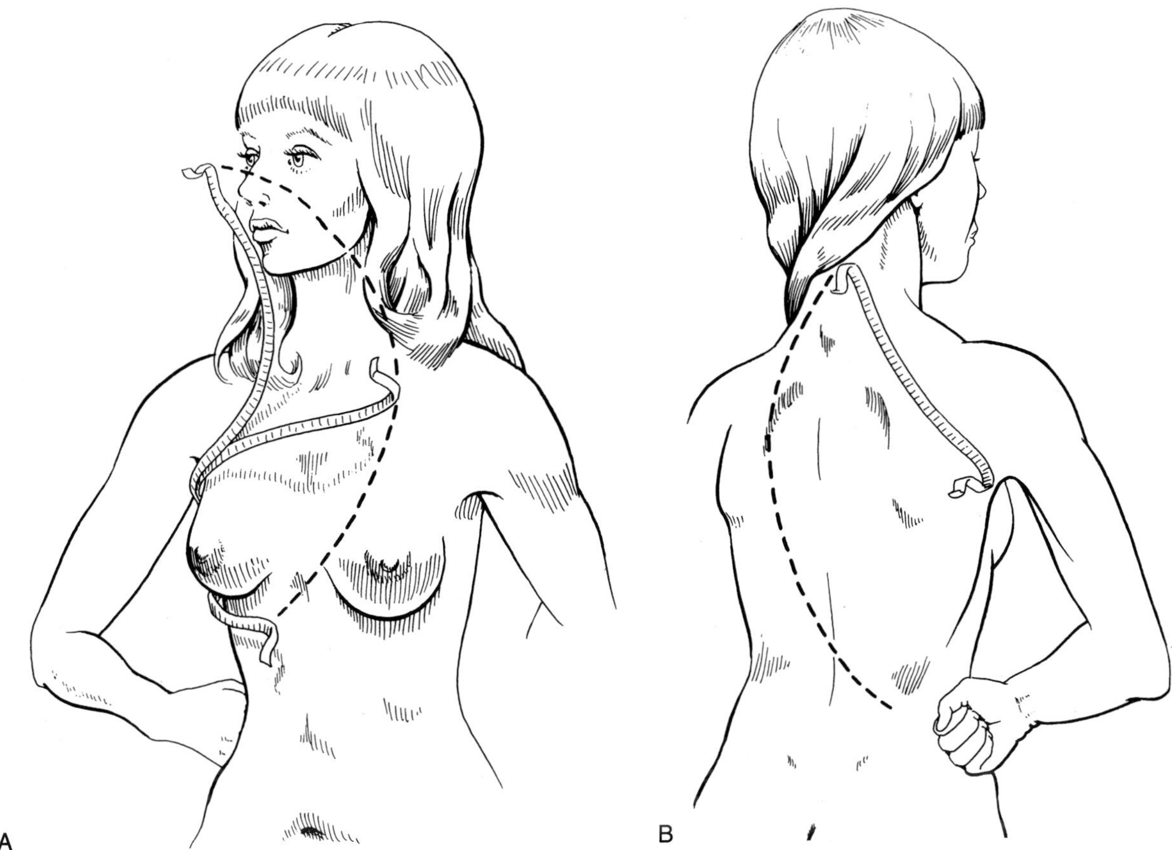

FIGURE 55–28 ■ *A*, Arc of rotation over the anterior chest for latissimus dorsi muscular and musculocutaneous flaps based on the thoracodorsal neurovascular pedicle. The *tape measure* depicts the length of the flap and its rotation when the posterior aspect of the tape is held against the anticipated pedicle. Note that this flap has a great ability to reconstruct defects in the lateral, anterior, and superior aspects of the chest wall. This flap is not recommended for covering defects in the region of the distal sternum and xiphoid process. *B*, The arc of rotation of the latissimus dorsi muscle when it is pedicled on the thoracodorsal neurovascular bundle. This muscular and musculocutaneous pedicle is the most useful one for covering defects of the posterior thoracic wall. (From Seyfer AE, Graeber GM, Wind GG: The latissimus dorsi muscle and musculocutaneous flaps. In Seyfer AE (ed): Atlas of Chest Wall Reconstruction. Rockville, MD, Aspen, 1986h.)

The blood supply to the latissimus dorsi has allowed some creativity with the primary pedicle. When the subscapular artery has been divided by previous surgery, a latissimus dorsi muscular or musculocutaneous flap may still be rotated by basing it on the continuity of the arteries from the serratus anterior muscle to the thoracodorsal (Fisher et al, 1983; Moelleken et al, 1989). When the pedicle for rotation has been created in this fashion, the integrity of the arteries from the serratus anterior must be maintained scrupulously. As might be expected, the arc of rotation in this situation is more limited by the need to preserve the vessels to the serratus anterior.

Some serious limitations to the use of latissimus dorsi muscular and musculocutaneous flaps based on the thoracodorsal pedicle have been found to exist (Moelleken et al, 1989; Seyfer et al, 1986h). Previous radiation to the axilla can cause constriction of the thoracodorsal vessels, which limits blood supply and rotation. Probably the most common cause of this problem has been radiation to the chest wall and axilla during therapy for breast carcinoma (Moelleken et al, 1989). Another serious problem with use of latissimus dorsi arises when a full posterolateral thoracotomy has been performed (Moelleken et al, 1989; Seyfer et al, 1986h). Division of the muscle and the thoracodorsal vessels causes the distal part of the muscle to become dependent on the secondary blood supply. If the entire muscle is raised as a flap based on the thoracodorsal vessels, the tissues distal to the scar undergo necrosis. Hence, the entire muscle can no longer be transferred to reconstruct chest wall defects or to repair intrathoracic problems such as bronchopleural-cutaneous fistulas (Fig. 55–30).

A number of authors have favored the use of muscle-sparing thoracotomies so that the blood supply to the latissimus dorsi and the serratus anterior is preserved. The necessity for muscle-sparing incisions is particularly apparent in the pediatric population (Malczyewski et al, 1994; Soucy et al, 1991).

Despite these limitations, the latissimus dorsi pedicled muscular and musculocutaneous flaps have found wide appreciation for reconstruction of all types of chest wall defects (Moelleken et al, 1989; Seyfer et al, 1986h). The use of these flaps in repairing posterior and spinal defects is well recognized (McCraw et al, 1978). Even though radiation may have been applied to the axilla in treating mammary or other malignancies, these flaps may still be

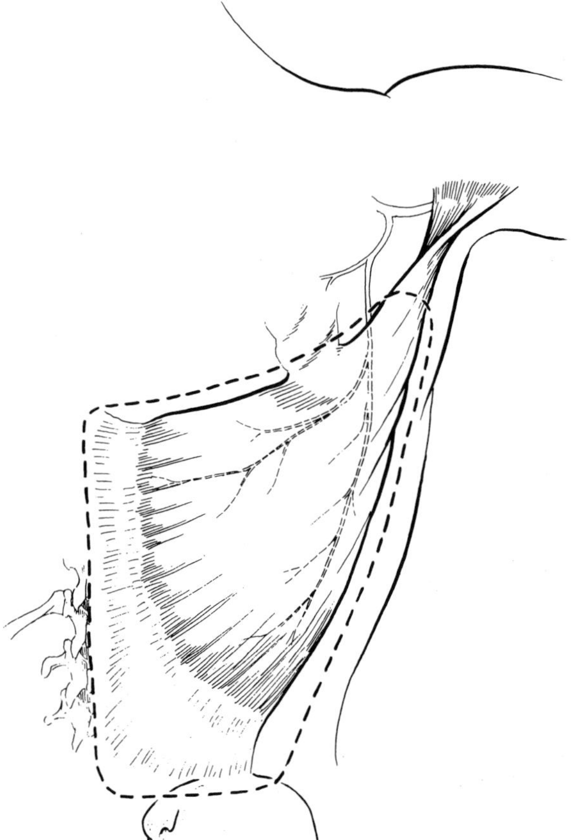

FIGURE 55–29 ■ Arterial supply to the latissimus dorsi based on the thoracodorsal artery. Note that the subscapular artery originates from the axillary artery. The subscapular artery divides into two branches: a branch that courses medially to the serratus anterior, and the thoracodorsal artery, which is the direct extension of the subscapular artery. Once the subscapular artery enters the latissimus dorsi muscle, it divides into a lateral and a medial branch. The *dotted line* represents the maximal domain of the cutaneous island that may be carried with this muscle. (From Seyfer AE, Graeber GM, Wind GG: The latissimus dorsi muscle and musculocutaneous flaps. In Seyfer AE (ed): Atlas of Chest Wall Reconstruction. Rockville, MD, Aspen, 1986h.)

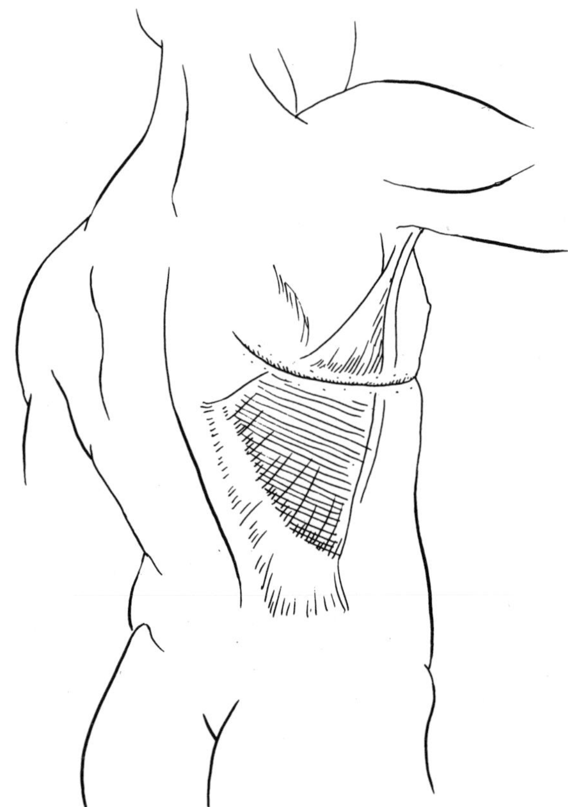

FIGURE 55–30 ■ If the patient has had a previous posterolateral thoracotomy incision, the distal portion of the latissimus dorsi muscle and any cutaneous elements that may overlie the muscle receive their blood supply from the secondary vessels that penetrate the lumbodorsal fascia. If the entire muscle were raised on a pedicle based on the thoracodorsal vessels, the distal portion of the muscle beyond the incision would undergo necrosis. Rotation of the entire muscle based on the thoracodorsal pedicle after a posterolateral thoracotomy incision is contraindicated. (From Seyfer AE, Graeber GM, Wind GG: Planning the reconstruction. In Seyfer AE (ed): Atlas of Chest Wall Reconstruction. Rockville, MD, Aspen, 1986b.)

used quite effectively in breast reconstruction, closure of defects secondary to resection of radiation-induced chest wall necrotic tissue, and reconstruction of the axilla (Seyfer, 1988). This musculocutaneous flap may have its capacity for closing defects enhanced by tissue expansion (Slavin, 1994).

Omentum

The omentum may be used in chest wall reconstruction. It has tremendous ability to reach all portions of the anterior and lateral chest wall as well as both pleural spaces (Fix and Vasconez, 1989; Seyfer et al, 1986i). Indeed, the omentum has been lengthened so that it has been used to repair cervical and cranial defects as well (Fig. 55–31). It has the distinct asset of being able to contain infection well. Since the omentum has no dermal covering, it must be covered to achieve cutaneous continuity; probably the most efficacious method of doing so is application of a meshed, split-thickness skin graft. When the mesh remains small, the continuity of the skin graft follows promptly and provides for a smooth surface.

The blood supply of the omentum is based on the right and left gastroepiploic arteries and veins (Powers et al, 1976). These vessels create a continuous arcade, which runs along the greater curvature of the stomach. A pedicled flap may be created that is based on either the right or the left gastroepiploic artery or on both. The caliber of the right and left gastroepiploic arteries may vary from individual to individual. One artery may be larger than the other and therefore may be more suitable as a pedicle on which to base an omental flap. The omentum in any given individual is subject to variation of the blood supply.

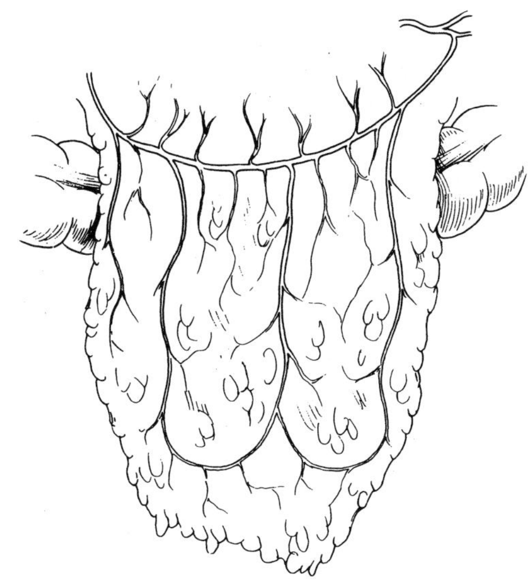

FIGURE 55–32 ■ The omentum enjoys a dual blood supply, which is based on the right and left gastroepiploic vessels. This drawing represents the arcades that are usually found in the omentum. The main arterial arcade runs along the greater curvature of the stomach and is continuous between the right and left gastroepiploic arteries. There are usually two secondary arterial arcades that descend into the omentum. (From Seyfer AE, Graeber GM, Wind GG: The omentum. In Seyfer AE (ed): Atlas of Chest Wall Reconstruction. Rockville, MD, Aspen, 1986i.)

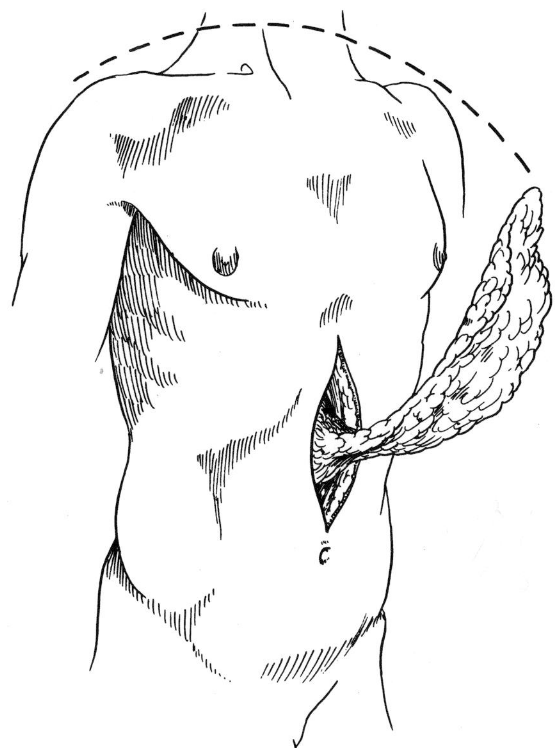

FIGURE 55–31 ■ The arc of rotation of the omentum is quite large when the pedicle is based on the epiploic vessels. This shows the potential realm of application for the omentum in reconstruction of chest wall defects. The omentum is particularly useful in treating contaminated and infected defects of the anterior and lateral chest wall. (From Seyfer AE, Graeber GM, Wind GG: The omentum. In Seyfer AE (ed): Atlas of Chest Wall Reconstruction. Rockville, MD, Aspen, 1986i.)

The most common anatomic variation has two arcades that are continuous with one another (Fig. 55–32). The omentum may be lengthened by judicious division of the arcades (Alday and Goldsmith, 1972) (Fig. 55–33). Great care should be taken to maintain pulses distally in the omentum when the arcades are divided. Appropriate blood supply may be maintained by testing with a Doppler ultrasound device prior to the division of any of the arcades. The point of division of each of the arcades should be occluded by soft vascular clamps prior to the actual division. If the pulse remains good distal to the anticipated points of division, there is a high probability that the distal portion of the omentum will remain viable.

The blood supply to the omentum also allows free flap transfer to new positions to achieve soft tissue coverage and repair. The omentum has been used as a free flap to cover defects on the extremities or on the head and neck and to repair intrathoracic problems such as bronchopleural fistulas (Arnold and Irons, 1981; Jurkiewicz and Nahai, 1982). Unique aspects of the omental blood supply, its ability to contain infection, and its malleable nature have allowed creative transfer and sculpting to fill complex defects.

A number of liabilities may be associated with pedicled omental flaps when they are used for chest wall recon-

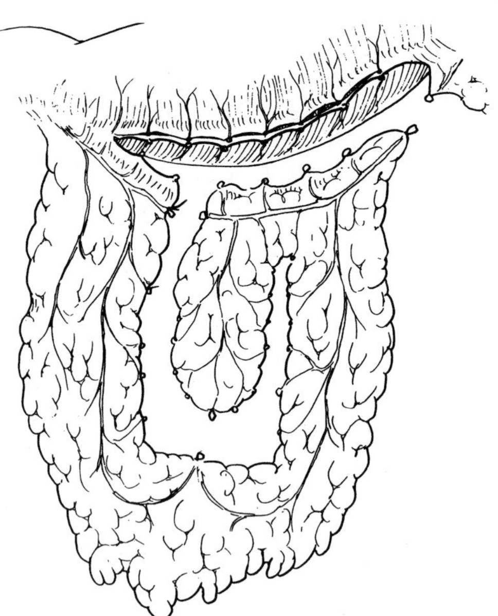

FIGURE 55–33 ■ One of the most beneficial aspects of the omentum is that it may be tailored to fit irregular defects and lengthened on the basis of the vascular supply. This drawing depicts one of the possible lengthening procedures based on the right gastroepiploic artery. Note that the entire omental arcade has been dissected from the stomach, which is cephalad. The secondary arcades have been divided so that there is continuity of blood flow throughout the omentum. Obviously, because there is variation in the arcades, a continuous pulse must be ascertained before dividing any one of the arcades. Use of fine vascular clamps and Doppler ultrasound allows precise division of these arcades with ensurance of good distal arterial supply. (From Seyfer AE, Graeber GM, Wind GG: The omentum. In Seyfer AE (ed): Atlas of Chest Wall Reconstruction. Rockville, MD, Aspen, 1986i.)

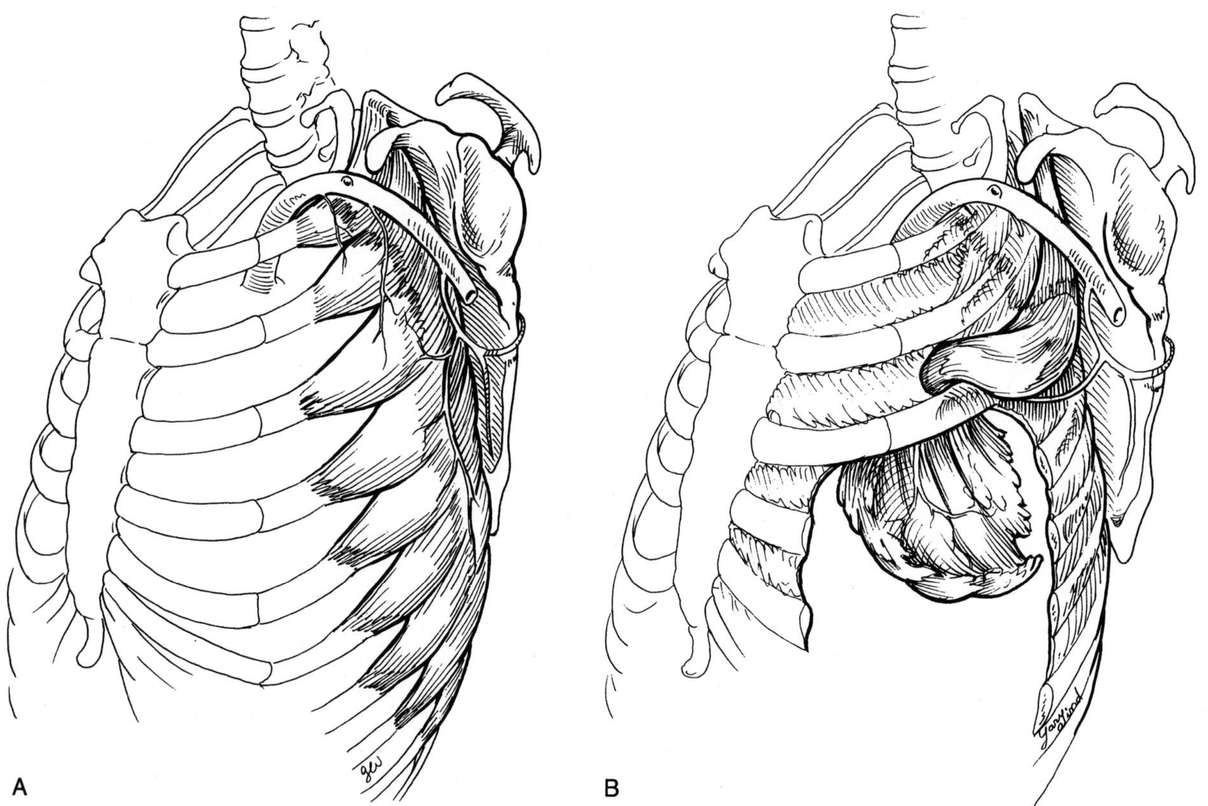

FIGURE 55–34 ■ *A*, Arterial supply to the left serratus anterior muscle. The major arterial pedicle comes from the subscapular artery at the origin of the thoracodorsal. Other arteries enter the cephalad aspect of the muscle from the axillary artery. *B*, Because the serratus anterior is often spared in performing a posterolateral thoracotomy, this muscle may be used effectively in repairing bronchopleural fistulas after pulmonary resection. This line drawing depicts the use of the muscle developed on its primary blood supply arising from the subscapular artery. The muscle has been introduced into the chest through the second intercostal space. Portions of the second and/or third rib may be resected to facilitate transposition of the muscle into the pleural space. As with all muscle transpositions, there should be no tension on the muscle itself or its primary blood supply.

struction (Mathiesen et al, 1988; Seyfer et al, 1986i). Previous abdominal surgery or abdominal infection may preclude use of the omentum. Gastric surgery, in particular, may have interrupted the arcades and may eliminate many possibilities for omental transfer. Previous infection may have caused so many adhesions that the omentum cannot be harvested without jeopardizing portions of it. The omentum can also be a channel for spreading infection from the chest to the abdomen; although this complication is rare, it has been documented. Finally, there is the ever-present complication of chest wall or diaphragmatic hernia associated with thoracic reconstruction using the omentum. The omentum has to be brought to the anterior chest wall through an epigastric hernia. Most often, an iatrogenic anterior defect has to be created in the diaphragm to allow the omentum to pass into either pleural space. Such defects offer the potential for herniation of abdominal viscera into the thoracic cavity. Obviously, an epigastric hernia may be filled with more than omentum as the healing process progresses.

Despite its liabilities, the greater omentum has been used to cover virtually all possible types of chest wall defects (Mathiesen et al, 1988). It has been particularly helpful in repairing dehisced median sternotomies and in repairing radiation injuries to the chest wall (Miller and Nahai, 1989; Seyfer, 1988). In such applications its ability to contain infection and to fill irregular defects has proved most useful.

Serratus Anterior

The serratus anterior muscle has found some specific applications in thoracic reconstruction. The most common one is transposition into the thoracic cavity for control of bronchopleural fistulas (Pairolero and Arnold, 1989). Since this muscle is often spared with a lateral or posterolateral thoracotomy, it may be transposed intact with its cephalad blood supply to close chest wall or intrathoracic defects. It has a rather limited arc of rotation since the pedicle must be based on the artery to the serratus anterior, which arises from the subscapular artery (Fig. 55–34). When the serratus anterior is introduced into the chest, the secondary blood supply, which consists of small arteries arising from the axillary artery and some perforators from the intercostals, must be transected. The muscle may be brought through an intercostal space; however, a portion of the second or third rib may be resected to facilitate intrathoracic transposition (Fig. 55–34).

Trapezius

Although posterior defects are generally infrequent, the trapezius muscle offers an option for closure of such defects. The muscle may be used in conjunction with the pedicled latissimus dorsi flap or may be used alone to cover selected defects. This musculocutaneous flap is most useful in covering defects around the shoulder, the suprascapsular region, and the perispinous region. It is usually rotated on the descending branch of the transverse scapular artery (Seyfer et al, 1986i). The muscle

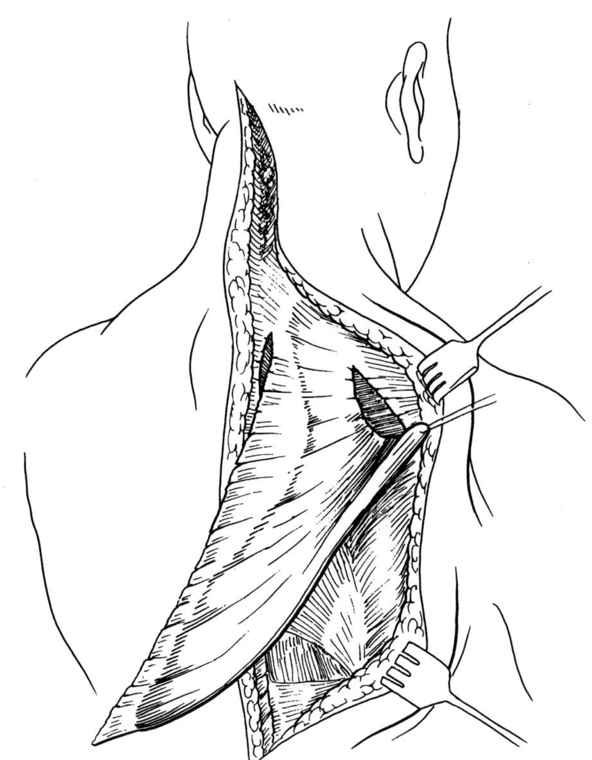

FIGURE 55–35 ■ The trapezius muscle may be used to reconstruct defects in the region of the shoulder or the spine. Its limited domain of rotation includes the area of the scapula, the apex of the shoulder, and the vertebral region. It is an excellent muscle for closing small defects in these areas. It may be used alone or in addition to a latissimus dorsi flap. (From Seyfer AE, Graeber GM, Wind GG: The trapezius muscle and musculocutaneous flap. In Seyfer AE (ed): Atlas of Chest Wall Reconstruction. Rockville, MD Aspen, 1986j.)

also finds some limited use in correcting defects at the extreme apex of the pleural space (Fig. 55–35).

■ *KEY REFERENCES*

McCraw JB, Arnold PG: McCraw and Arnold's Atlas of Muscle and Musculocutaneous Flaps. Norfolk, VA, Hampton Press Publishing, 1986.

This is an excellent atlas that depicts the development and use of all the major pedicled flaps. Excellent dissections are provided to show the major aspects of constructing each flap, and the text is supplemented by clear photographic illustrations of all the flaps. Since most of the flaps were constructed on cadavers, the anatomic landmarks, blood supply, and individual characteristics of each flap are clearly depicted.

Seyfer AE, Graeber GM (eds): Chest Wall Reconstruction. Surg Clin North Am 69:1989.

This monograph addresses all the major aspects of chest wall reconstruction. A number of authors who have contributed much to the field of thoracic reconstruction have written major chapters. The entire monograph is richly illustrated; the reference lists are extensive; and the text is clear and conveys all major points concerning chest wall reconstruction in a sequential fashion.

Seyfer AE, Graeber GM, Wind GG: Atlas of Chest Wall Reconstruction. Rockville, MD, Aspen Publishers, 1986a.

This atlas is based on the large experience of the authors at Walter Reed Army Medical Center in Washington, DC. Each of the flaps is precisely illustrated, and the techniques of developing each one are carefully described. The drawings are particularly helpful, since the artist is also a surgeon.

■ REFERENCES

Alday ES, Goldsmith HS: Surgical technique for omental lengthening. Surg Gynecol Obstet 135:103, 1972.

Arnold PG, Irons GB: The greater omentum: Extensions in transposition and free transfer. Plast Reconstr Surg 67:169, 1981.

Arnold PG, Pairolero PC: Chondrosarcoma of the manubrium. Resection and reconstruction with pectoralis major muscle. Mayo Clin Proc 53:54, 1978.

Arnold PG, Pairolero PC: Use of the pectoralis major muscle flaps to repair defects of the anterior chest wall. Plast Reconstr Surg 63:205, 1979.

Arnold PG, Pairolero PC: Chest wall reconstruction: Experience with 100 consecutive patients. Ann Surg 199:725, 1984.

Arnold PG, Pairolero PC: Reconstruction of the radiation-damaged chest wall. Surg Clin North Am 69:1081, 1989.

Azarow KS, Malloy M, Seyfer AE, Graeber GM: Preoperative evaluation and general preparation for chest wall operations. Surg Clin North Am 69:899, 1989.

Brown R, Vasconez L, Jurkiewicz M: Transverse abdominal flaps and the deep epigastric arcade. Plast Reconstr Surg 55:416, 1975.

Bunkis J, Walton R, Mathes S et al: Experience with the transverse lower rectus abdominis operation for breast reconstruction. Plast Reconstr Surg 72:819, 1983.

Coleman JJ, Bostwick J: Rectus abdominis muscle—musculocutaneous flap in chest-wall reconstruction. Surg Clin North Am 69:1007, 1989.

Das SK: The size of the human omentum and methods of lengthening it for transplantation. Br J Plast Surg 29:170, 1976.

Dinner M, Labandter H, Dowden R: The role of the rectus abdominis myocutaneous flap in breast reconstruction. Plast Reconstr Surg 69:209, 1982.

Fisher J, Bostwick J, Powell RW: Latissimus dorsi blood supply after thoracodorsal vessel division: The serratus collateral. Plast Reconstr Surg 72:502, 1983.

Fix RJ, Vasconez LO: The use of the omentum in chest-wall reconstruction. Surg Clin North Am 69:1029, 1989.

Glafkides MC, Toth BA: Split bipedicle transverse rectus abdominis flaps: Expanding their uses in breast reconstruction. Ann Plast Surg 27:9, 1991.

Graeber GM, Snyder RJ, Flemming AW et al: Initial and long-term results in the management of primary chest wall neoplasms. Ann Thorac Surg 34:664, 1982.

Hammond DC, Fisher J, Meland NB: Intrathoracic free flaps. Plast Reconstr Surg 91:1259, 1993.

Hartrampf C, Scheflan M, Black P: Breast reconstruction with a transverse abdominal island flap. Plast Reconstr Surg 69:216, 1982.

Ishii C, Bostwick J, Raine T et al: Double-pedicle transverse rectus abdominis myocutaneous flap for unilateral breast and chest wall reconstruction. Plast Reconstr Surg 76:901, 1985.

Jacobsen WM, Meland NB, Woods JE: Autologous breast reconstruction with use of transverse rectus abdominis musculocutaneous flap: Mayo Clinic experience with 47 cases. Mayo Clin Proc 69:635, 1994.

Jurkiewicz MJ, Nahai F: The omentum: Its use as a free vascularized graft for reconstruction of the head and neck. Ann Surg 195:756, 1982.

Malczyewski MC, Colony L, Cobb LM: Latissimus-sparing thoracotomy in the pediatric patient: A valuable asset for thoracic reconstruction. J Pediatr Surg 29:396, 1994.

Mathiesen DJ, Grillo HC, Vlahakes GJ et al: The omentum in the management of complicated cardiothoracic problems. J Thorac Cardiovasc Surg 95:677, 1988.

Matsuo K, Hirose T, Hayashi R, Kiyono M: Reconstruction of large chest wall defects using a combination of a contralateral latissimus dorsi and a rectus abdominis musculocutaneous flap. Br J Plast Surg 44:102, 1991.

McCraw JB, Penix JO, Baker JW: Repair of major defects of the chest wall and spine with a latissimus dorsi myocutaneous flap. Plast Reconstr Surg 62:97, 1978.

Miller JI, Nahai F: Repair of the dehisced median sternotomy incision. Surg Clin North Am 69:1091, 1989.

Miller L, Bostwick J, Hartrampf C et al: The superiorly based rectus abdominis flap: Predicting and enhancing its blood supply based on an anatomic and clinical study. Plast Reconstr Surg 81:713, 1988.

Moelleken BRW, Mathes SA, Chang N: Latissimus dorsi muscle-musculocutaneous flap in chest-wall reconstruction. Surg Clin North Am 69:977, 1989.

Morain WD, Cohen LV, Hutchings JC: The segmental pectoralis major muscle flap: A function-preserving procedure. Plast Reconstr Surg 67:753, 1981.

Nahai F, Morales L Jr, Bone DK et al: Pectoralis major muscle turnover flap for closure of the infected sternotomy wound with preservation of form and function. Plast Reconstr Surg 70:471, 1982.

Pairolero PC, Arnold PG: Bronchopleural fistula: Treatment by transposition of pectoralis major muscle. J Thorac Cardiovasc Surg 79:142, 1980.

Pairolero PC, Arnold PG: Management of recalcitrant median sternotomy wounds. J Thorac Cardiovasc Surg 88:357, 1984.

Pairolero PC, Arnold PG: Management of infected median sternotomy wounds. Ann Thorac Surg 42:1, 1986a.

Pairolero PC, Arnold PG: Thoracic wall defects: Surgical management of 205 consecutive patients. Mayo Clin Proc 61:557, 1986b.

Pairolero PC, Arnold PG: Intrathoracic transfer of flaps for fistulas, exposed prosthetic devices and reinforcement of suture lines. Surg Clin North Am 69:1047, 1989.

Powers JC, Fitzgerald JF, McAlvanah MJ: The anatomic basis for the surgical detachment of the greater omentum from the transverse colon. Surg Gynecol Obstet 143:105, 1976.

Rowsell AR, Davies DM, Eisenberg N et al: The anatomy of the subscapular-thoracodorsal arterial system: Study of 100 cadaver dissections. Br J Plast Surg 37:574, 1984.

Seyfer AE: Radiation-associated lesions of the chest wall: Longitudinal experience with 31 patients. Surg Gynecol Obstet 167:129, 1988.

Seyfer AE, Graeber GM, Wind GG: Planning the reconstruction. In Seyfer AE (ed): Atlas of Chest Wall Reconstruction. Rockville, MD, Aspen Publishers, 1986b.

Seyfer AE, Graeber GM, Wind GG: The pectoralis major muscle and musculocutaneous flaps. In Seyfer AE (ed): Atlas of Chest Wall Reconstruction. Rockville, MD, Aspen Publishers, 1986c.

Seyfer AE, Graeber GM, Wind GG: Tracheoesophageal and bronchopleural/cutaneous fistulas. In Seyfer AE (ed): Atlas of Chest Wall Reconstruction. Rockville, MD, Aspen Publishers, 1986d, p 217.

Seyfer AE, Graeber GM, Wind GG: The rectus abdominis muscle and musculocutaneous flaps. In Seyfer AE (ed): Atlas of Chest Wall Reconstruction. Rockville, MD, Aspen Publishers, 1986e, p 159.

Seyfer AE, Graeber GM, Wind GG: Blood supply to the skin of the chest wall. In Seyfer AE (ed): Atlas of Chest Wall Reconstruction. Rockville, MD, Aspen Publishers, 1986f.

Seyfer AE, Graeber GM, Wind GG: Reconstruction of the breast following mastectomy. In Seyfer AE (ed): Atlas of Chest Wall Reconstruction. Aspen Publishers, Rockville, MD, 1986g

Seyfer AE, Graeber GM, Wind GG: The latissimus dorsi muscle and musculocutaneous flaps. In Seyfer AE (ed): Atlas of Chest Wall Reconstruction. Rockville, MD, Aspen Publishers, 1986h.

Seyfer AE, Graeber GM, Wind GG: The omentum. In Seyfer AE (ed): Atlas of Chest Wall Reconstruction. Rockville, MD, Aspen Publishers, 1986i.

Seyfer AE, Graeber GM, Wind GG: The trapezius muscle and musculocutaneous flap. In Seyfer AE (ed): Atlas of Chest Wall Reconstruction. Rockville, MD, Aspen Publishers, 1986j

Slavin SA: Improving the latissimus dorsi myocutaneous flap with tissue expansion. Plast Reconstr Surg 93:811, 1994.

Soucy P, Bass J, Evans M: The muscle-sparing thoracotomy in infants and children. J Pediatr Surg 26:1323, 1991.

Tobin GR: Pectoralis major muscle-musculocutaneous flap for chest-wall reconstruction. Surg Clin North Am 69:991, 1989.

Yamamoto Y, Nohira K, Shintomi Y et al: Turbo-charging the vertical rectus abdominis myocutaneous (turbo-VRAM) flap for reconstruction of extensive chest wall defects. Br J Plast Surg 47:103, 1994.

SUPRACLAVICULAR APPROACH FOR THORACIC OUTLET SYNDROME

Susan Mackinnon

G. Alexander Patterson

The supraclavicular approach to relieve thoracic outlet syndrome by decompression of the brachial plexus and excision of the first rib releases structures that compress soft tissue in the region of the interscalene portion of the brachial plexus. The lower nerve trunk and C8 and T1 nerve roots can be completely identified and protected as the most posterior aspect of the first rib is resected under direct vision. Any cervical ribs or prolonged transverse processes are easily removed by this supraclavicular approach. This operative procedure is detailed in Figure 55–36.

Loupe magnification (4.5×) and microbipolar cautery are used, and a portable nerve stimulator (Concept 2, Clearwater, FL) is frequently applied throughout the procedure. A sandbag is placed between the scapula and the neck and extended to the nonoperative side. Long-acting paralytic agents are avoided. An incision in a neck crease, parallel to and 2 cm above the clavicle, is made in the supraclavicular fossa.

The supraclavicular nerves are identified just beneath the platysma and mobilized to allow vessel loop retraction. The omohyoid is divided and the supraclavicular fat pad is elevated, after which the scalene muscles and the brachial plexus are easily palpated. The lateral portion of the clavicular head of the sternocleidomastoid is divided, and at the end of the procedure is repaired. The phrenic nerve is seen on the anterior surface of the anterior scalene muscle, and similarly, the long thoracic nerve is noted on the posterior aspect of the middle scalene muscle.

The anterior scalene muscle is divided from the first rib. The subclavian artery is noted immediately behind this, and an umbilical tape is placed around the subclavian artery. The phrenic nerve is not mobilized, but rather is simply avoided. The upper, middle, and lower trunks of the brachial plexus are easily visualized and gently mobilized. The middle scalene muscle is now divided from the first rib. It has a broad attachment to the first rib, and care must be taken to avoid injury to the long thoracic nerve, which in this position may have multiple branches and may pass through and posterior to the middle scalene muscle. With division of the middle scalene muscle, the brachial plexus is easily visualized and mobilized, and the lower trunk and the C8 and T1 nerve roots are identified above and below the first rib. Congenital bands and thickening in Sibson's fascia are divided.

The first rib is then encircled and divided where it is easily visible with bone-cutting instruments, and its posterior segment is removed back to its spinal attachments by rongeur technique. By using a fine elevator, the soft tissue attachments to the first rib are separated. Finally, the posterior edge of the first rib is grasped firmly with a rongeur, and then a rocking and twisting motion is used to remove the entire aspect of the rib, so that the cartilaginous components of its articular facets with both the costovertebral and costotransverse joints can be identified on the specimen. The anterior portion of the first rib is removed in a similar fashion in order to decompress the neurovascular elements.

Cervical ribs or long transverse processes are removed by the same technique (Fig. 55–37). We use a technique described by Nelems to open the pleura, facilitating drainage of any postoperative blood collection into the chest cavity rather than allowing the blood to collect in the operative site around the brachial plexus. When the pleura is opened, care is taken to protect the intercostal brachial nerve, which is noted on the dome of the pleura. The wound is closed in a subcuticular fashion, and a simple suction drain is placed and sealed after wound closure and maximal inflation of the lungs by the anesthetist.

COMMENTS AND CONTROVERSIES

The surgical approach selected for management of thoracic outlet varies with the experience, expertise, and the skill of the operator. Our preference is to use the supraclavicular approach for arterial reconstruction (endarterectomy and bypass) combined with the infraclavicular approach for the distal anastamosis. To use the supraclavicular approach for primary neurogenic and venous compression, the surgeon must retract the brachial plexus and vascular structures to expose the first rib and to perform the dorsal sympathectomy that is often needed. Although some authors have an excellent record with this approach, the standard of care shows that nerve injury is much higher with this than with any other approach because of the level of skill required to properly retract the brachial plexus. Cosmetically, the supraclavicular approach is not as desirable, because 80% of these patients are women.

H. C. U.

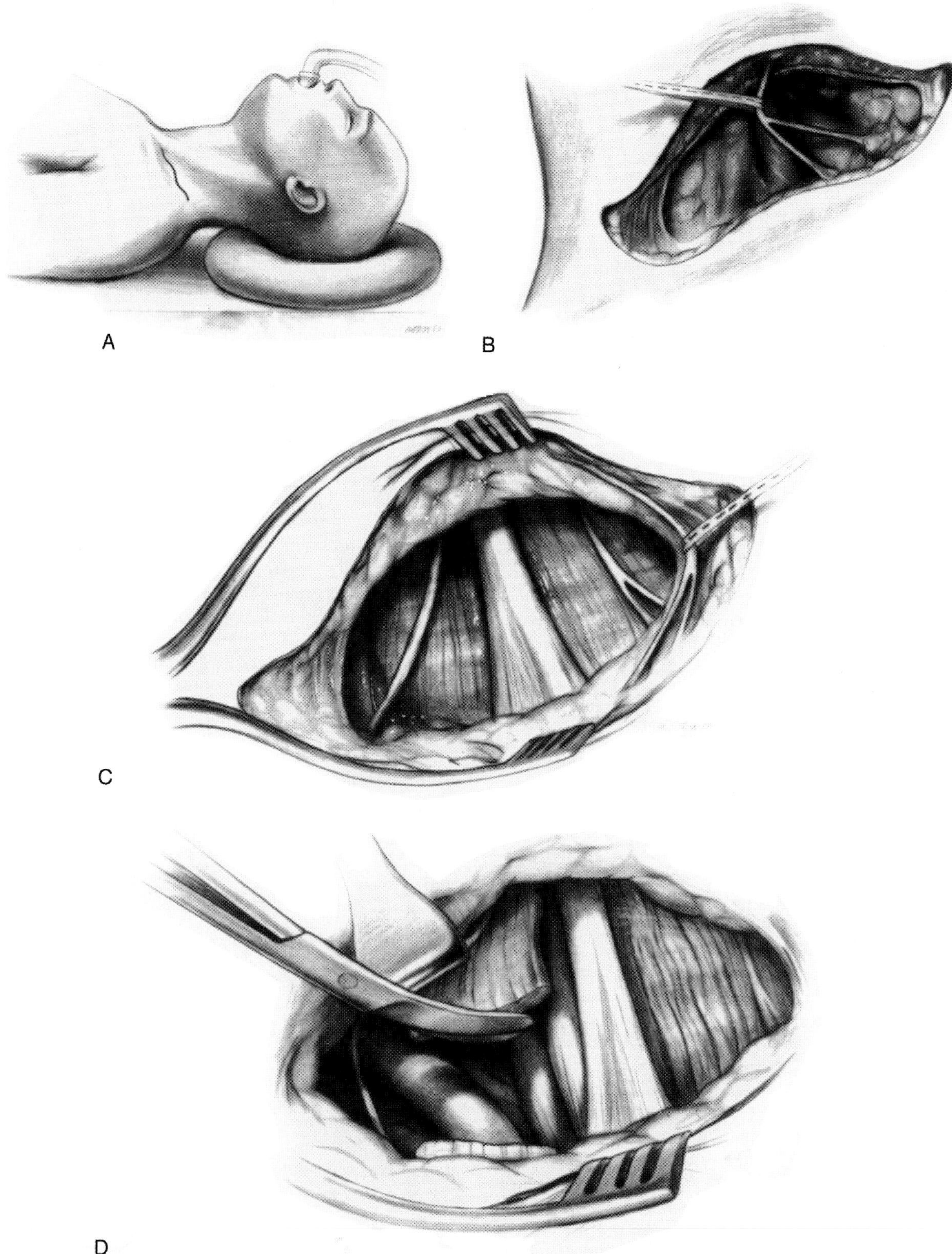

FIGURE 55–36 ■ *A*, The surgical incision is parallel to the clavicle. *B*, The supraclavicular nerves are protected. *C*, The fat pad has been retracted to identify the phrenic nerve on the scalene anticus muscle and the long thoracic nerve exiting from the posterior border of the scalene medius muscle, with the brachial plexus noted in the interscalene position. *D*, The phrenic nerve is protected, and the scalene anticus is divided. The subclavian artery can now be seen in its location behind the scalene anticus muscle.

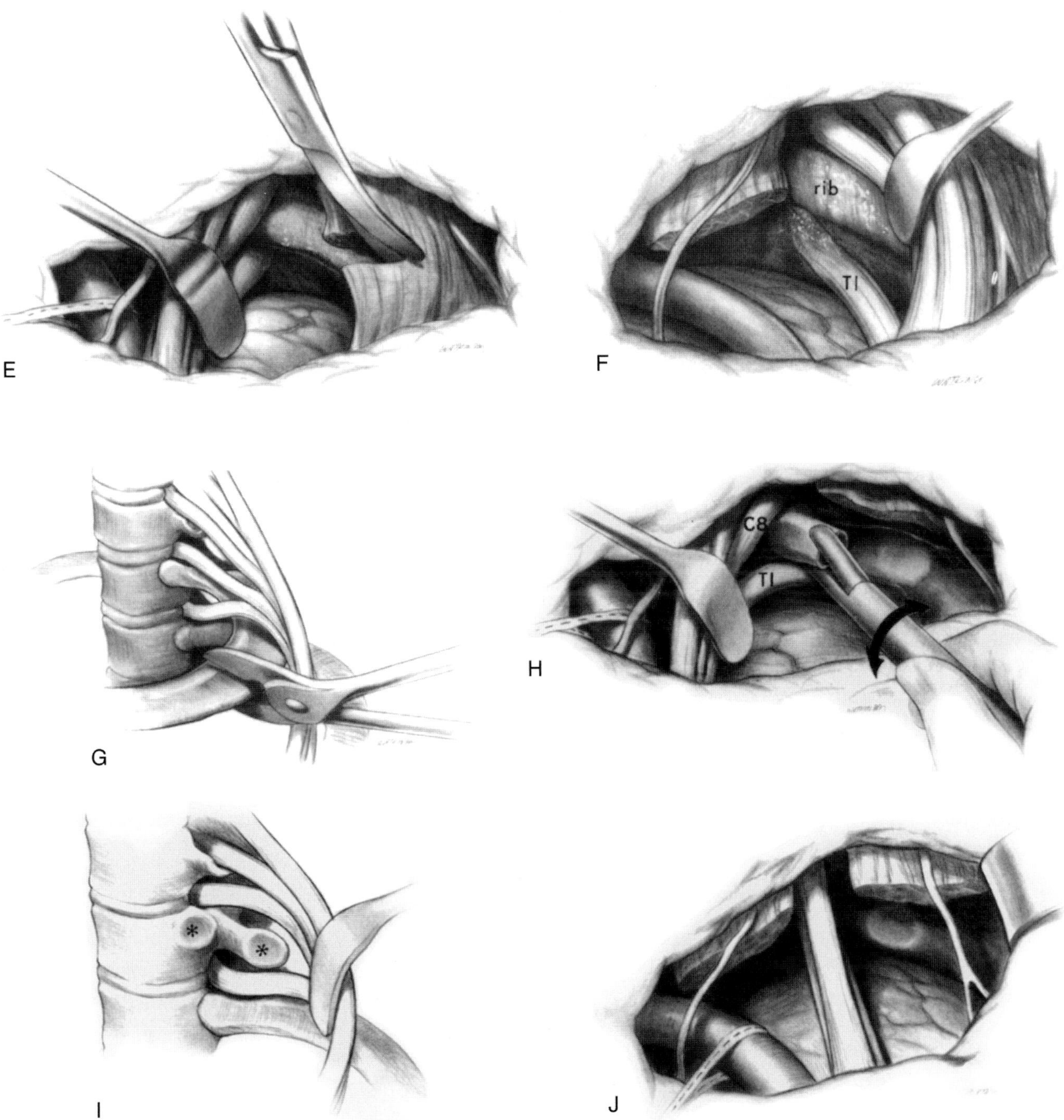

FIGURE 55–36 ■ (*Continued*). *E*, The scalene medius muscle is divided from the first rib with care to protect the long thoracic nerve. *F*, The upper portion of the brachial plexus is retracted to identify the first rib. T1 can be seen below the first rib. *G*, The first rib is divided where it is easily visualized, and then the posterior and anterior aspects of the rib are removed. The relationship of T1 and C8 to the head of the first rib can be seen. *H*, The nerve roots are reflected anteriorly, and with a twisting motion using rongeurs, the posterior aspect of the first rib is removed. *I*, The entire posterior portion of the first rib is removed so that no residual first rib remains to produce new bone formation and subsequent recurrence of symptoms. The articular facets of the costovertebral and costotransverse joints are noted (*asterisks*). *J*, The brachial plexus has been completely decompressed. The phrenic and long thoracic nerves have been protected.

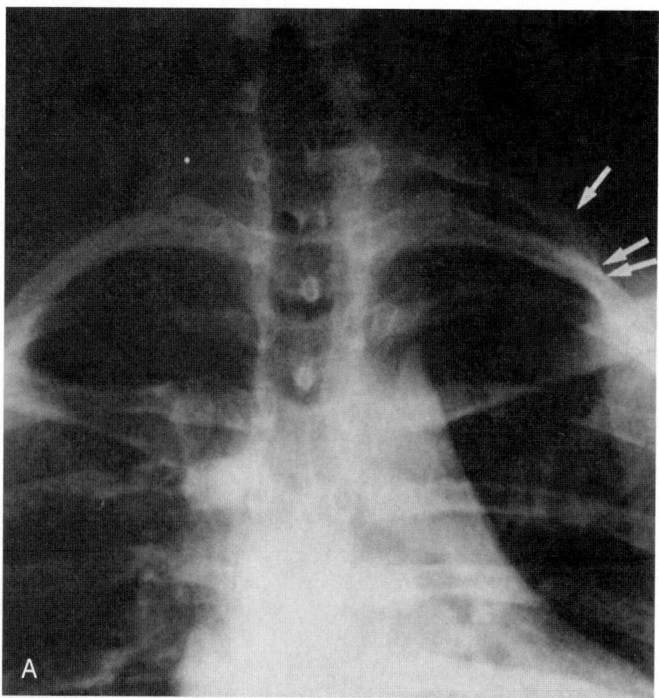

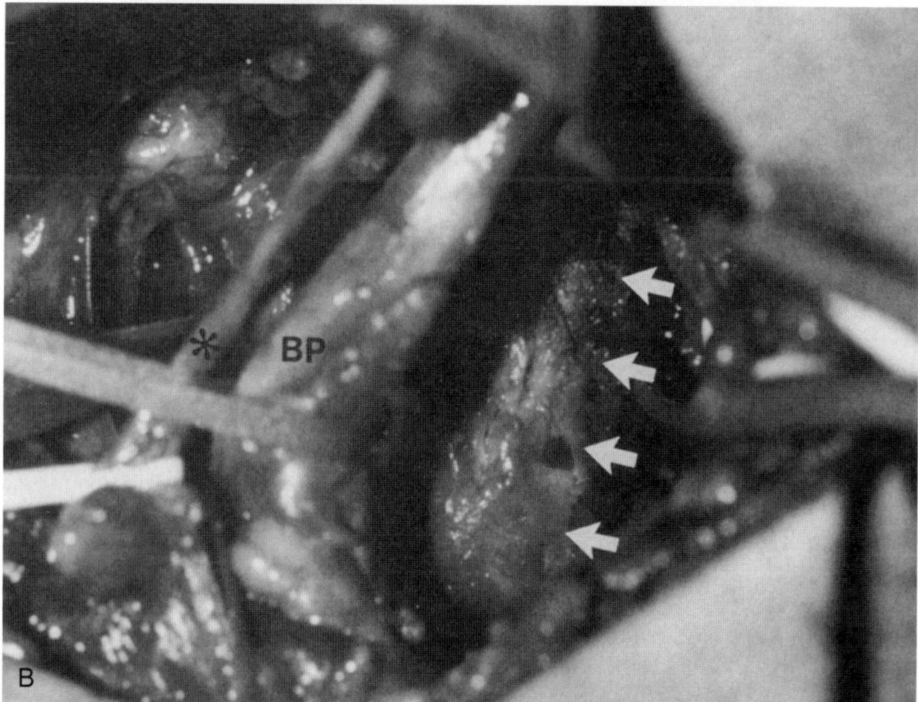

FIGURE 55–37 ■ *A*, Radiograph demonstrating a prominent transverse process on the right (*asterisk*) and a large cervical rib on the left. The pseudojoint noted in the cervical rib (*single arrow*) is a frequent finding. The cervical rib can be seen to articulate with the first rib (*double arrow*). *B*, Operative photograph corresponding to radiograph, demonstrating the relationship between the branchial plexus (BP) and the cervical rib (*arrows*). Note supraclavicular nerve retracted (*asterisk*).

TRANSAXILLARY APPROACH WITH DORSAL SYMPATHECTOMY FOR THORACIC OUTLET SYNDROME

Harold C. Urschel, Jr.

In surgery to relieve thoracic outlet syndrome, the transaxillary route is an expedient approach for complete removal of the first rib with neurovascular decompression and dorsal sympathectomy when indicated. First rib or cervical rib resection can be performed without the need for major muscle division, as in the posterior approach (Clagett, 1962); without the need for retraction of the brachial plexus, as in the anterior supraclavicular approach (Falconer and Li, 1962); and without the difficulty of removing only the posterior segment of the rib, as in the infraclavicular approach. In addition, transaxillary first rib resection shortens postoperative disability and provides better cosmetic results than the anterior and posterior approaches, particularly because 80% of patients are female (Roos, 1966; Urschel and Razzuk, 1972; Urschel et al, 1968, 1971, 1993, 1995, 1998).

The patient is placed in the lateral position with the involved extremity abducted to 90 degrees by traction straps wrapped around the forearm and attached to an overhead pulley. An appropriate weight, usually 2 lb, is used to maintain this position without undue traction (Urschel and Razzuk, 1972).

A transverse incision is made below the axillary hairline between the pectoralis major and the latissimus dorsi muscles and is deepened to the external thoracic fascia (Fig. 55–38). Care should be taken to prevent injury to the intercostobrachial cutaneous nerve, which passes from the chest wall to the subcutaneous tissue in the center of the operative field.

The dissection is extended cephalad along the external thoracic fascia to the first rib. With gentle dissection, the neurovascular bundle and its relation to the first rib and both scalenus muscles are clearly outlined to avoid injury to its components. The insertion of the scalenus anticus muscle is identified, skeletonized, and divided. The scalenus anticus muscle is resected into the neck so it will not reattach to Sibson's fascia. The first rib is dissected with a periosteal elevator and separated carefully from the underlying pleura to avoid pneumothorax. A triangular segment of the middle portion of the rib is resected with the vortex of the triangle at the scalene tubercle. After the costoclavicular ligament is divided, the anterior portion of the rib is resected to the costochondral junction. The posterior segment of the rib is resected at the articulation with the transverse process. The scalenus medius muscle should carefully be stripped with a periosteal elevator to avoid injury to the long thoracic nerve that lies on its posterior margin.

The head and neck of the first rib are removed completely with a long, reinforced Urschel double-action pituitary rongeur. The C8 and T1 nerve roots are carefully protected. If a cervical rib is present, its anterior portion, which usually articulates with the first rib, should be resected at a point at which the middle portion of the first rib is removed. The remaining segment of the cervical rib should be removed after removal of the posterior segments of the first rib.

A No. 20 chest tube is used for drainage. Only the subcutaneous tissues and skin require closure because no large muscles have been divided. The patient is encouraged to use the arm for self-care but to avoid heavy lifting until at least 3 months after the operation.

It is preferable to remove the first rib entirely, including the head and neck, to avoid future regeneration and recurrent symptoms.

■ *KEY REFERENCES*

Clagett OT: Presidential Address: Research and prosearch. J Thorac Cardiovasc Surg 44:153, 1962.

Roos DB: Transaxillary approach for first rib resection to relieve thoracic outlet syndrome. Ann Surg 163:354, 1966.

The transaxillary approach to first rib resection was initially described by Atkins and popularized by Roos.

Urschel HC Jr, Cooper JD: Atlas of Thoracic Surgery, New York, Churchill Livingstone, 1995.

Urschel HC Jr, Paulson DL, McNamara JJ: Thoracic outlet syndrome. Ann Thorac Surg 6:2, 1968.

Urschel HC Jr, Razzuk MA: Neurovascular compression in the thoracic outlet: Changing management over 50 years. Ann Surg 228:609, 1998.

■ *REFERENCES*

Falconer MA, Li FWP: Resection of the first rib in costoclavicular compression of the brachial plexus. Lancet 1:59, 1962.

Urschel HC Jr, Razzuk MA: Current management of thoracic outlet syndrome. N Engl J Med 286:21, 1972.

Urschel HC Jr, Razzuk MA, Wood RE, Paulson DL: Objective diagnosis (ulnar nerve conduction velocity) and current therapy of the thoracic outlet syndrome. Ann Thorac Surg 12:608, 1971.

Urschel HC Jr: Video-assisted sympathectomy and thoracic outlet syndrome. Chest Surg Clin North Am 3:299, 1993.

COMMENTS AND CONTROVERSIES

Our preferred approach for primary neurogenic and venous compression is the transaxillary route wherein the rib is proximal to the operator, and retraction of the brachial plexus or blood vessels is not required.

H. C. U.

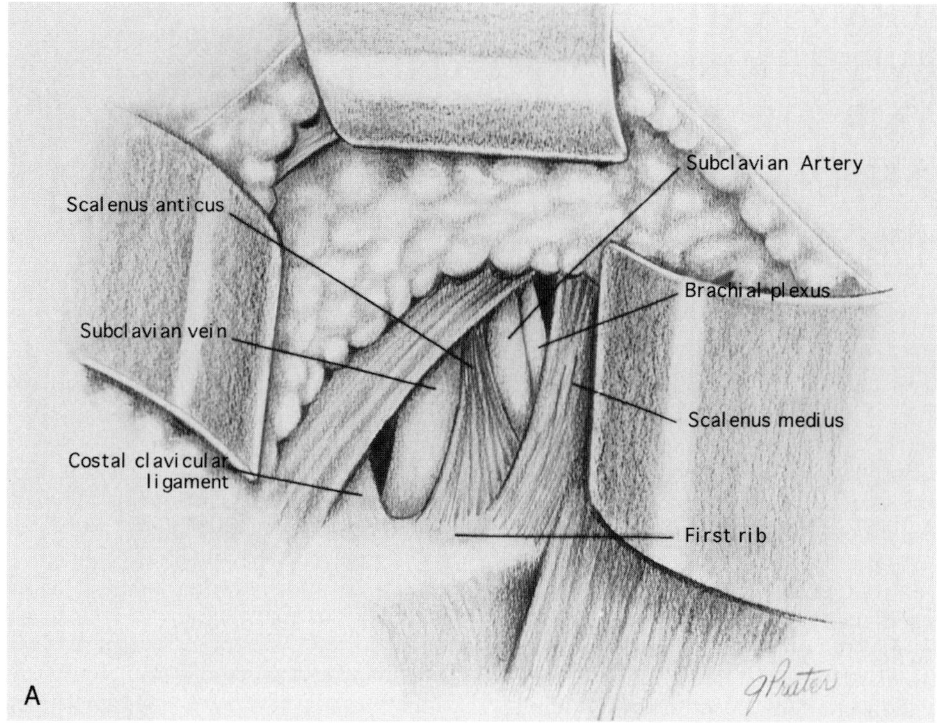

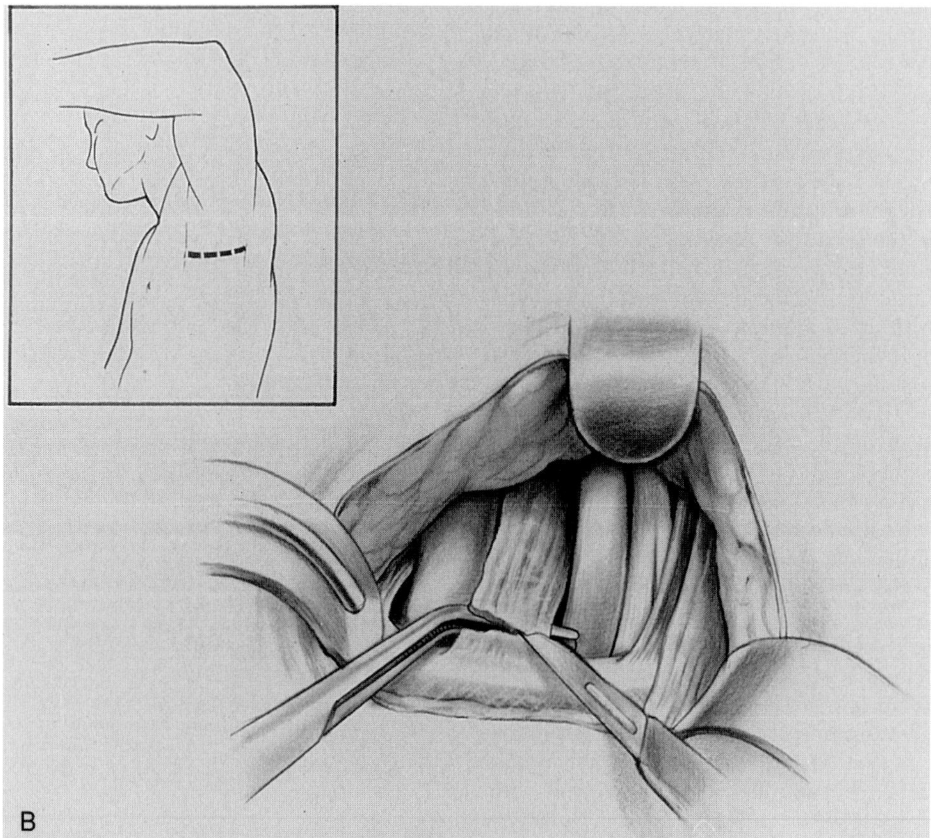

FIGURE 55–38 ■ *A*, A schematic drawing illustrating the relationship of the neurovascular bundle to the scalene muscles, first rib, costoclavicular ligament, and subclavius muscle. *B*, *Inset*: A transaxillary incision below the axillary hairline between the pectoralis major and the latissimus dorsi muscles. The scalenus anticus muscle is isolated and divided at its insertion in the first rib.

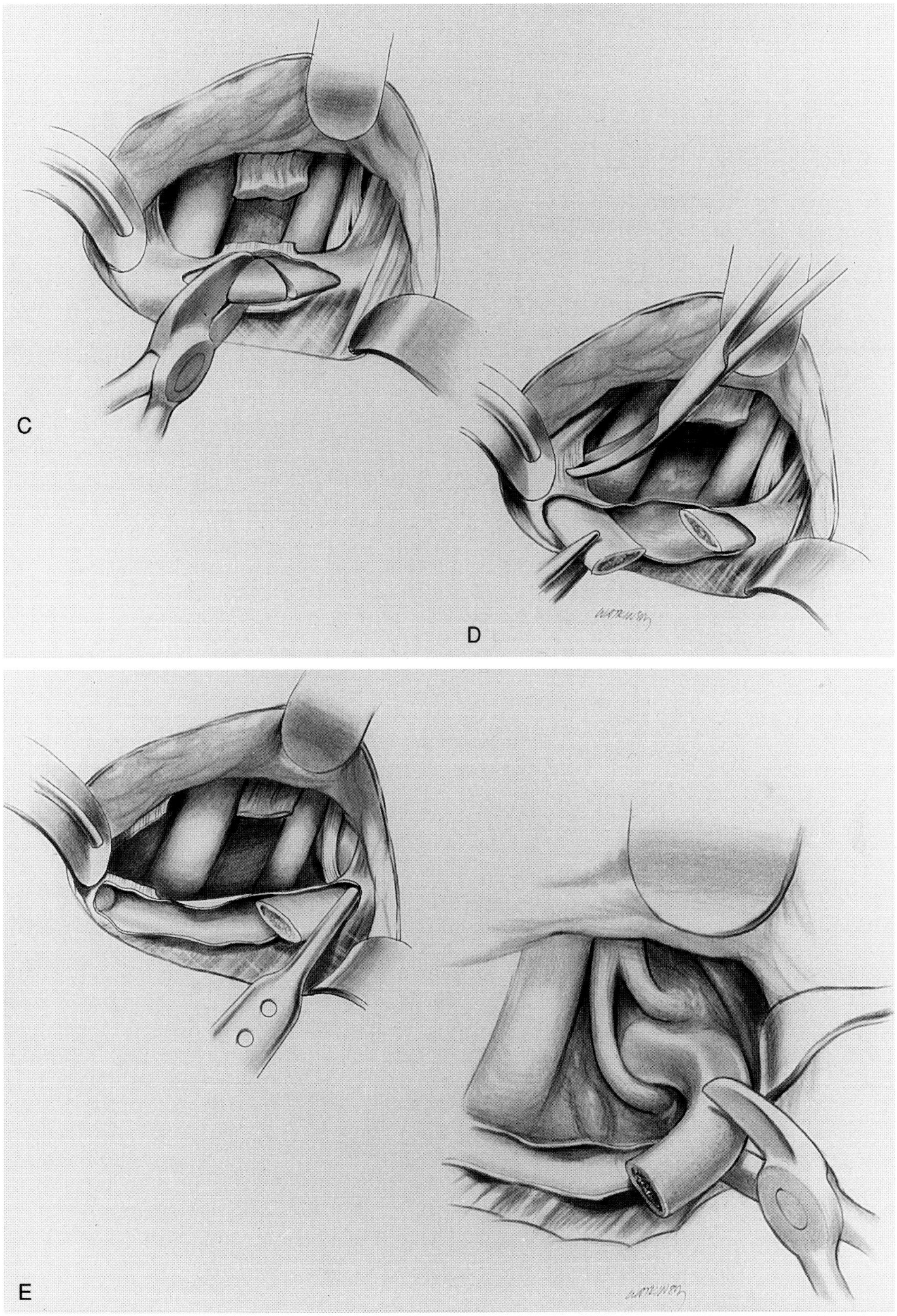

C

D

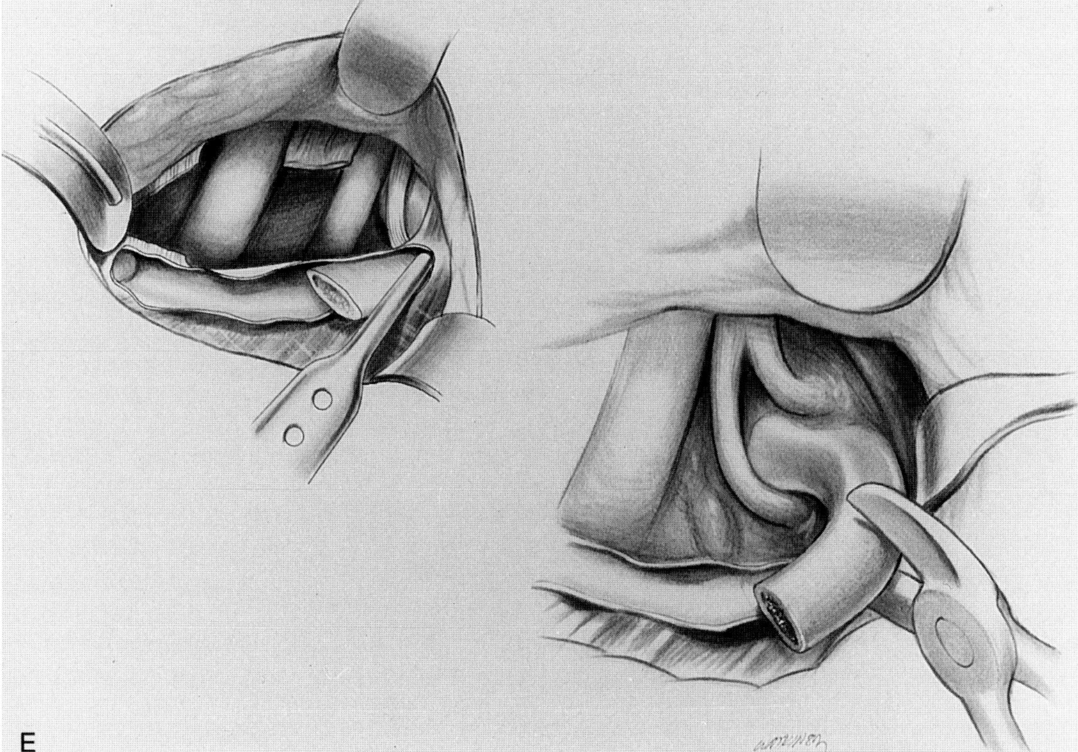

FIGURE 55–38 ■ *Continued. C,* The triangular portion of the rib is removed with the vortex of the triangle at the scalene tubercle. The scalenus anticus muscle is resected back up into the neck. *D,* The costoclavicular ligament is divided and the anterior part of the rib is resected to the costocartilage of the sternum. *E,* The axillary subclavian vein and artery are decompressed. The posterior part of the rib is resected to the transverse process of the vertebrae and divided.

Illustration continued on following page

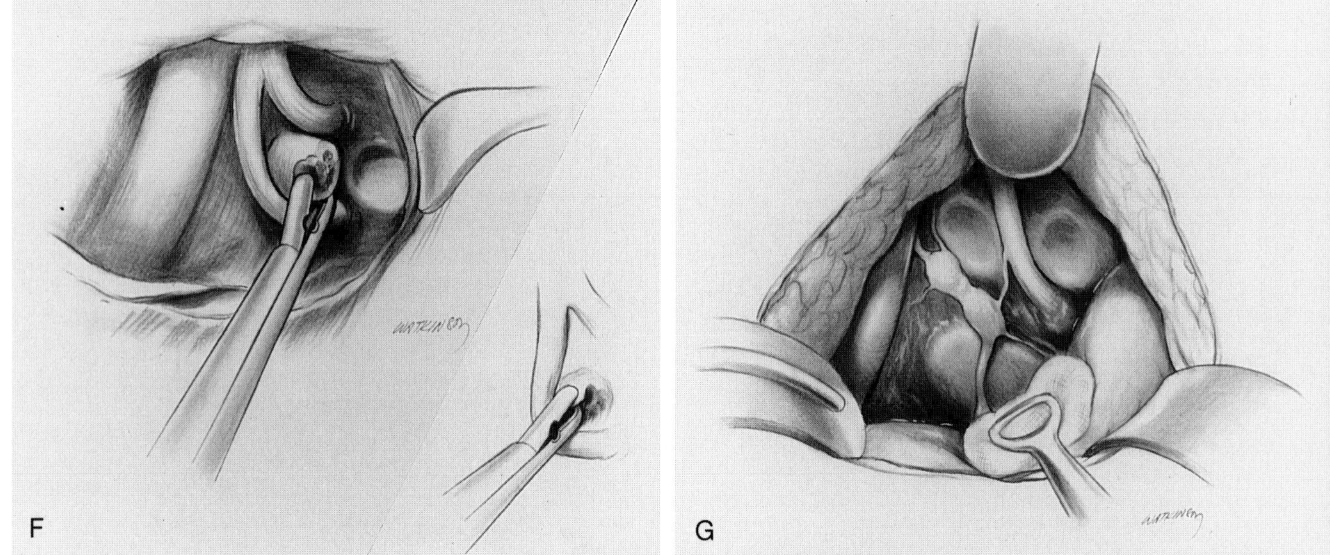

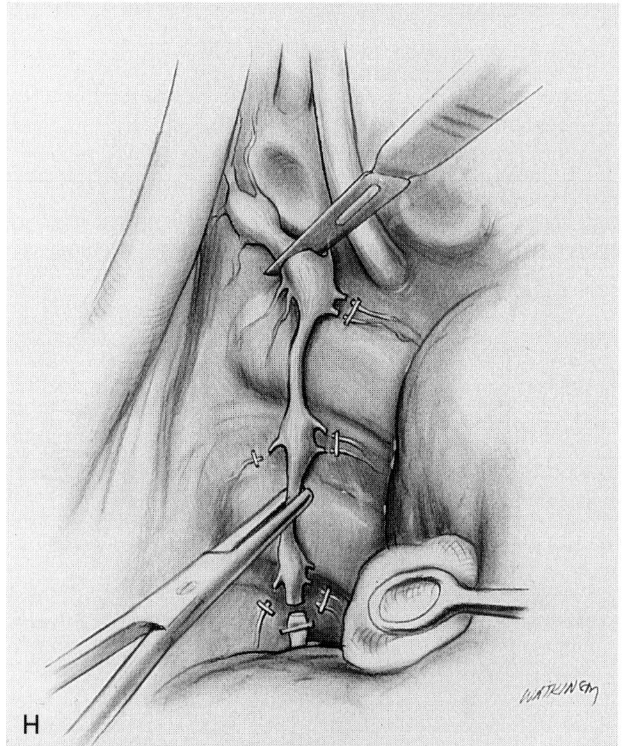

FIGURE 55–38 ■ *(Continued). F,* The head and neck of the rib are removed with a special reinforced Urschel pituitary rongeur, with care taken to avoid injury to the C8 and T1 nerve roots. The complete rib is thus excised. *G,* The dorsal sympathetic chain is identified by sweeping the pleura inferiorly from the T1 nerve root. *H,* The T1, T2, and T3 ganglions are removed along with the chain.

RECURRENT REOPERATION THROUGH THE POSTERIOR THORACOPLASTY APPROACH WITH DORSAL SYMPATHECTOMY FOR THORACIC OUTLET SYNDROME

Harold C. Urschel Jr.

Recurrent thoracic outlet syndrome occurs infrequently. It is most commonly observed in patients in whom the first rib was not removed completely at the first procedure. A segment of rib allows osteoblasts to grow from the end, producing a fibrocartilage that can compress the neurovascular structures. If the initial operation was performed through the supraclavicular or transaxillary approach, it is far safer to perform the reoperation through the posterior high thoracoplasty approach (Figs. 55–39 to 55–44). This provides a virgin field and allows careful neurolysis of the nerve roots and brachial plexus as well as release of the vascular structures when indicated. A dorsal sympathectomy is usually performed because the sympathetic-maintained pain syndrome and causalgia are present in most cases of recurrent thoracic outlet syndrome. Reoperation is indicated when conservative management has failed (Urschel et al, 1995, 1998).

■ REFERENCES

Urschel HC Jr, Cooper JD: Atlas of Thoracic Surgery. New York, Churchill Livingstone, 1995.

Urschel HC Jr, Razzuk MA: Neurovascular compression in the thoracic outlet: Changing management over 50 years. Ann Surg 228:609, 1998.

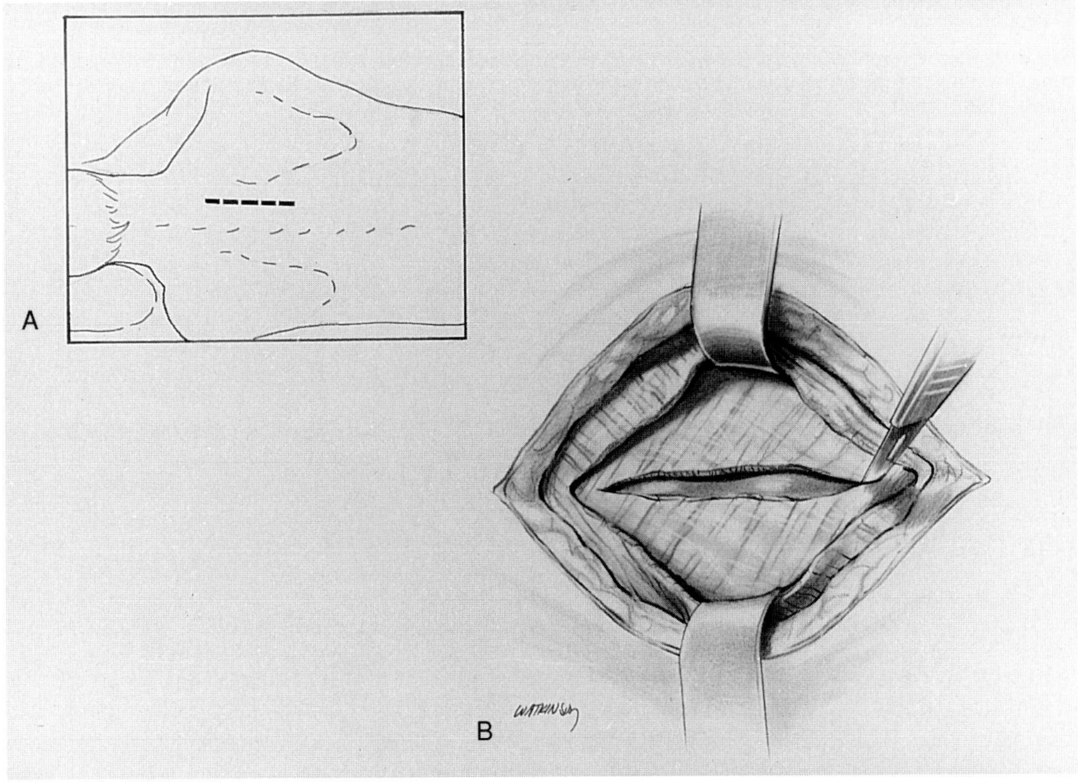

FIGURE 55–39 ■ *A, Inset*: A high thorocoplasty incision is performed halfway between the angle of the scapula and the spine and extends about 4 cm above and 2 cm below the angle of scapula. *B*, The incision is carried through the skin and the subcutaneous tissue to the trapezius muscle. The trapezius and rhomboid muscles are split along their fiber lines.

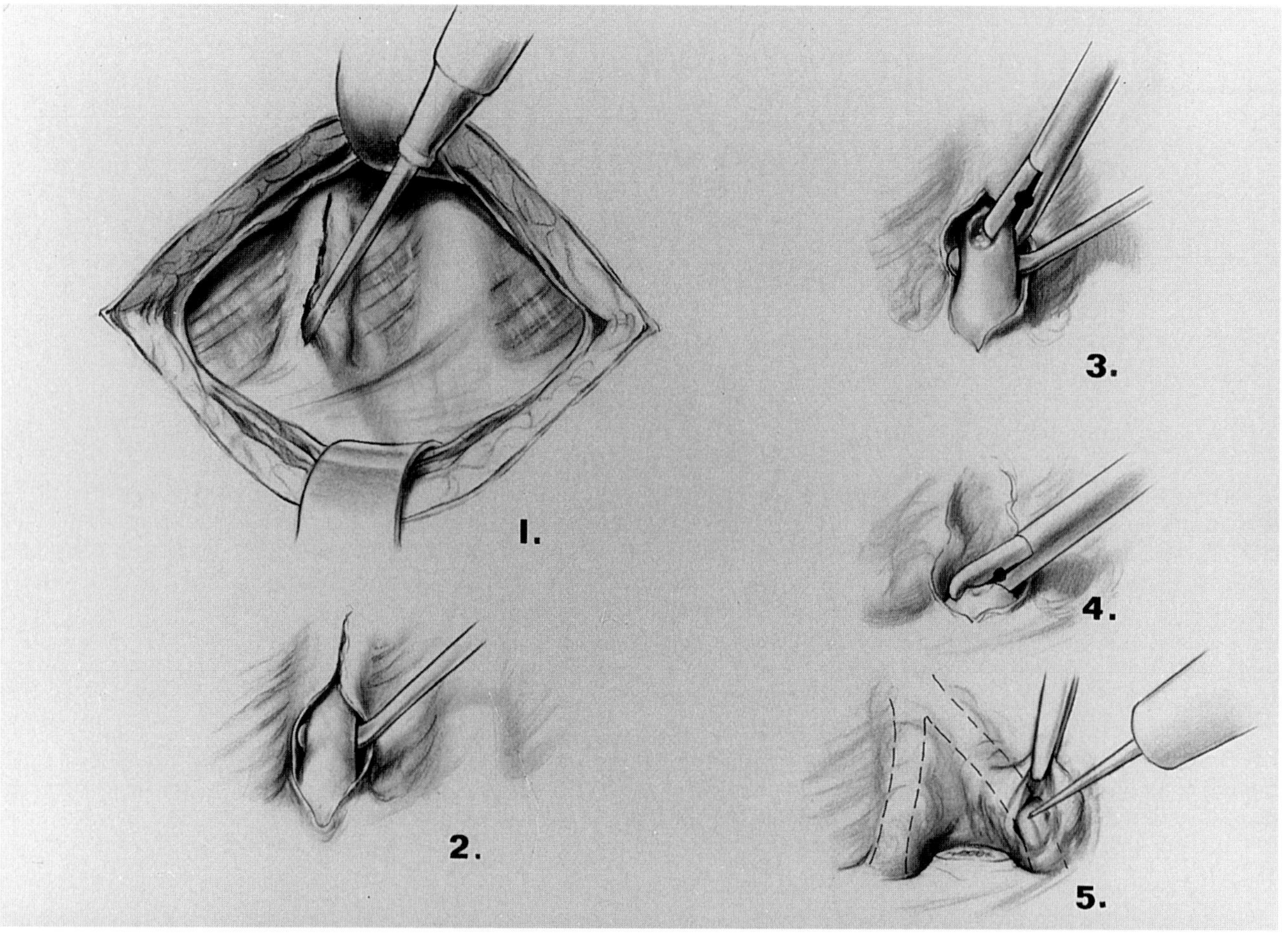

FIGURE 55–40 ■ *1*, The rib remnant or recurrent piece of the first rib is identified, and a cautery is used to incise the periosteum. *2*, The rib stump is removed subperiostially. *3*, The rongeur is used to remove the rib at its head and neck part. *4*, The T1 nerve root is identified and touched with a nerve stimulator.

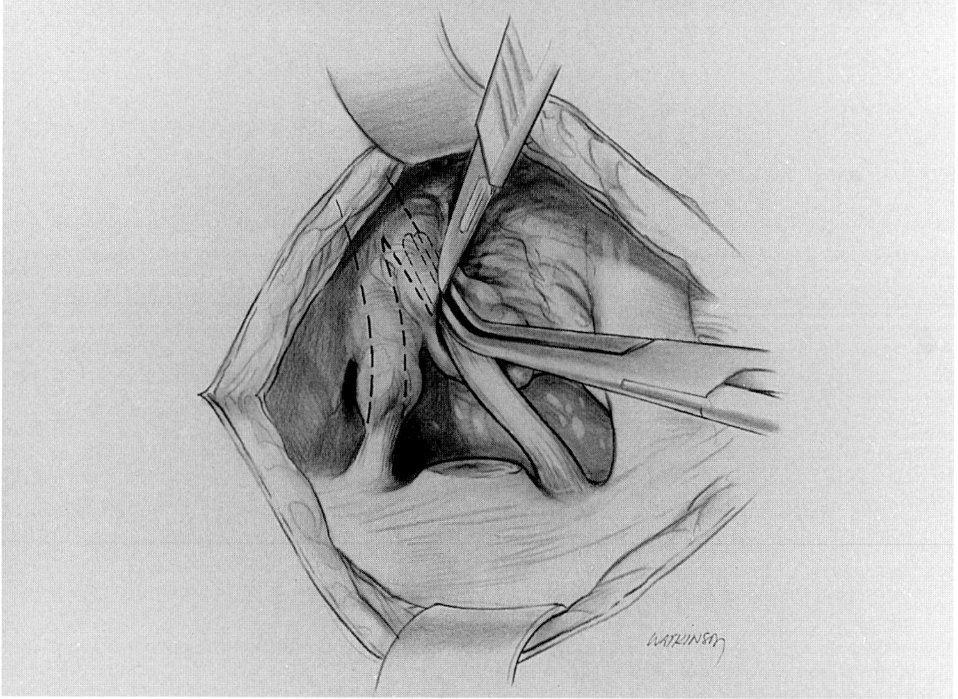

FIGURE 55–41 ■ Neurolysis of the scar over the T1 nerve root is carefully performed with magnification so that the nerve sheath is not injured.

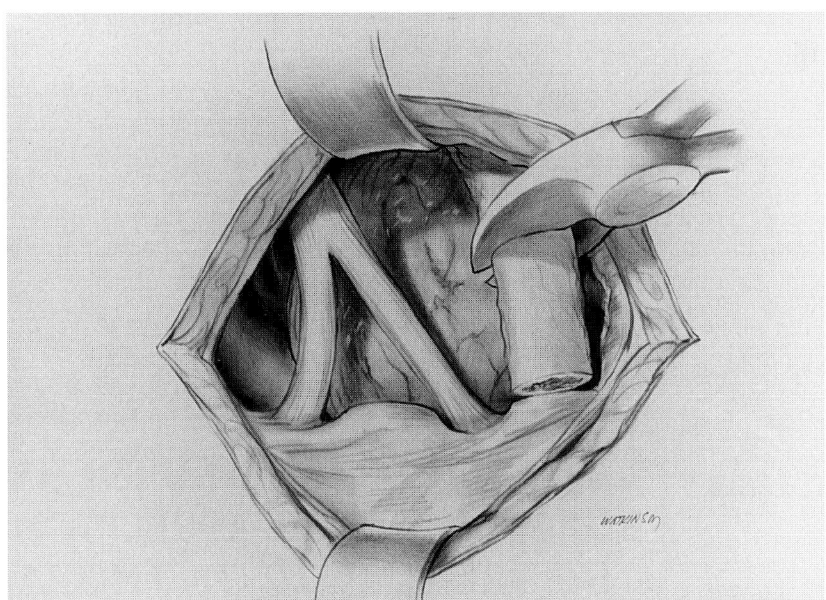

FIGURE 55–42 ■ The neurolysis is completed on the C8 and T1 nerve roots, and a piece of the second rib is removed posteriorly.

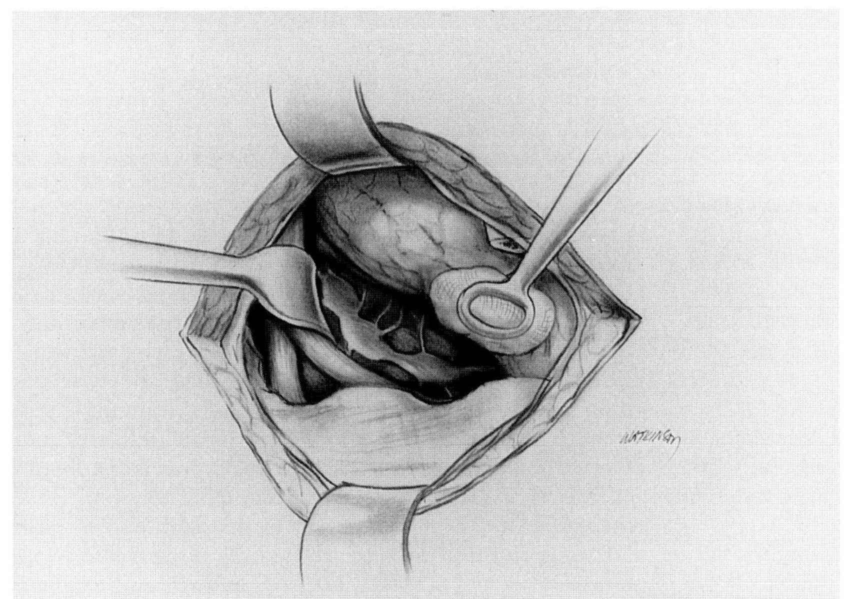

FIGURE 55–43 ■ The dorsal sympathetic chain and the stellate ganglion are identified.

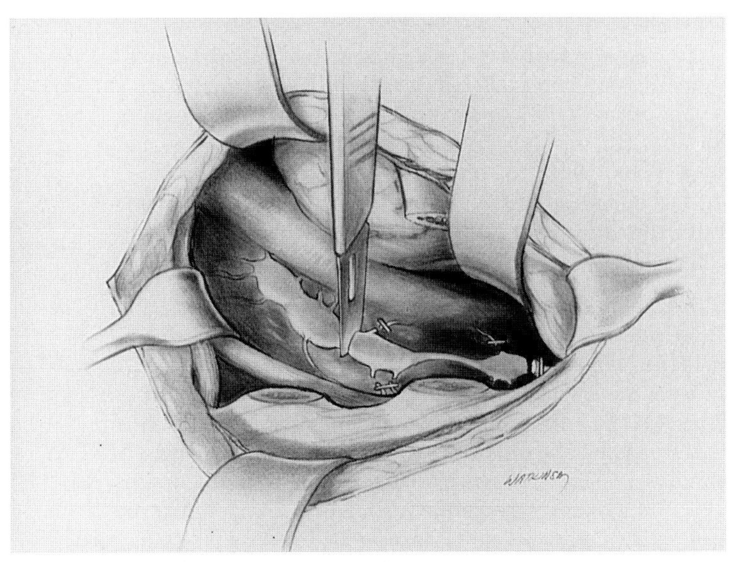

FIGURE 55–44 ■ The T1, T2, and T3 ganglia are removed with the dorsal sympathectomy.

COMMENTS AND CONTROVERSIES

Recurrent thoracic outlet syndrome, in our opinion, is best operated on posteriorly with a high thoracoplasty approach and a muscle-splitting incision, because this method gives excellent exposure in virgin territory. The usual rib remnant and fibrocartilage impinging on the brachial plexus is easier to remove posteriorly. This approach also allows expeditious neurolysis of the brachial plexus and dorsal sympathectomy. The supraclavicular approach may also be used for neurolysis of the brachial plexus; however, it is difficult to remove the rib stump posteriorly without retracting the brachial plexus, and doing so requires great skill and experience.

H. C. U.

COMBINED EXPOSURE OF THE FIRST RIB: A MODIFIED APPROACH FOR THE TREATMENT OF THORACIC OUTLET SYNDROME

Francis Robicsek

Since its first description, much controversy has existed over the condition known as "thoracic outlet syndrome." Urschel and associates (1968) give credit to Bramwell, who, in 1903, recognized the first rib as the possible cause of neurovascular compression in the thoracic inlet, and Murphy, who was the first to resect it in 1910 to relieve the symptoms associated with this condition. It is generally recognized that first-rib resection—with or without scalenotomy—is a requisite in the treatment of most, if not all, cases of thoracic outlet syndrome (Clagett, 1962; Ferguson et al, 1958; Roos, 1966; Urschel et al, 1968).

Even with over a century of experience, surgeons have yet to define the ideal method for the treatment of thoracic outlet syndrome. Different authors recommend various approaches. The three principal methods applied are:

1. The *posterior approach,* that is, the "old-fashioned" thoracoplasty exposure (Clagett, 1962).
2. The *axillary approach,* which allows the removal of the first rib through a small, cosmetically pleasing incision (Roos, 1966).
3. The *anterior approach,* which exposes the thoracic inlet through a supraclavicular incision (Nelson and Davis, 1969).

All three types of exposure have their virtues and shortcomings. Although the posterior and axillary approaches appropriately expose the first rib, they do not provide satisfactory exposure of other important structures that are important in the pathophysiology of the thoracic inlet: the subclavian vessels, the nerves, and the anterior scalene muscle. When the symptoms of neurovascular compression are induced by bony spurs or anomalous ligaments, the posterior and axillary approaches may leave them undetected, and thus, untreated (Stoney and Cheng, 1995). An additional advantage of the supraclavicular approach is that it allows easy division of the anterior scalene muscle, an important component in the development of thoracic outlet narrowing. The disadvantage of the anterior supraclavicular approach, however, is that it provides only a limited exposure to the first rib, making its removal difficult and, more often than not, incomplete. For these reasons, recurrences are frequent. An additional shortcoming of the procedure is that it requires the insertion of sharp instruments, such as rongeurs, blindly under the clavicle to resect the anterior portion of the first rib, and, through necessity, the subclavian artery may be left overlying ragged bony edge.

The difficulties of the anterior approach were realized by Quarfordt and colleagues (1984) who used the anterior approach for radical scalenotomy but in addition removed the first rib through a separate transaxillary incision. In cases of "effort" subclavian vein thrombosis, Thompson and colleagues (1992) suggested simultaneous separate supraclavicular and infraclavicular incisions to remove the first rib. Gol's technique involved the resection of the entire first rib using an infraclavicular incision (Gol et al, 1968).

In our view, the "ideal" operation for adequate decompression of the thoracic inlet should include the following:

1. Adequate exposure, through a single skin incision, of *all* potentially compromised neurovascular structures.
2. Easy access to both radical scalenotomy and removal of the entire first rib.

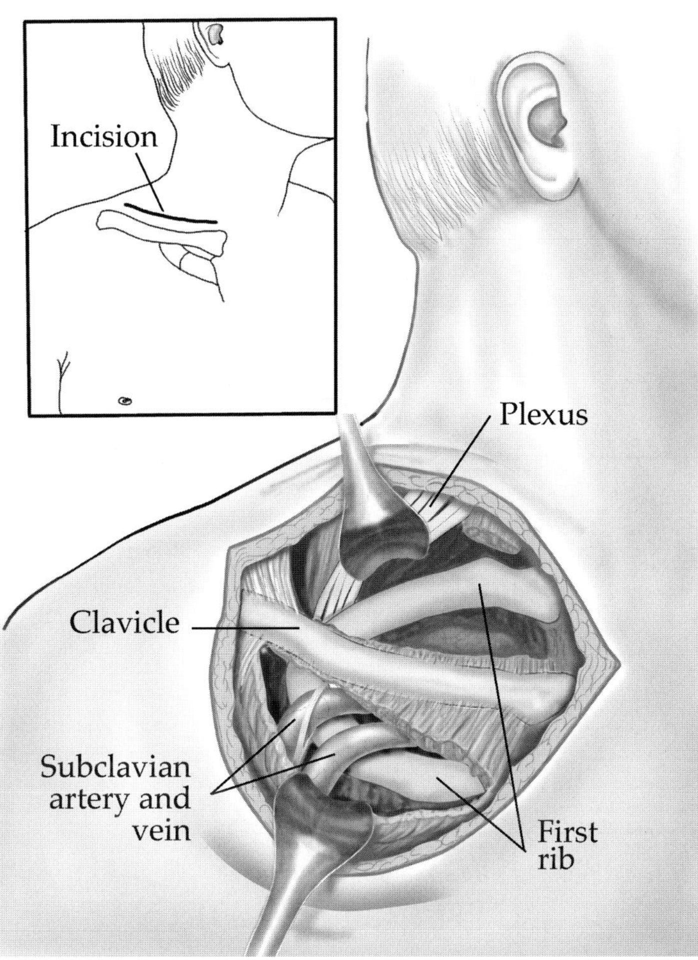

FIGURE 55–45 ■ Exposure of the first rib with the "above-under" approach.

To accomplish these goals, we now recommend the following approach (Robicsek and Eastman, 1997). A single 6- to 9-cm–long skin incision is made 1 cm above and parallel with the clavicle. The subcutaneous fat and the platysma are divided while the phrenic nerve is carefully protected. The anterior scalene muscle is divided using electrocautery. The brachial plexus and the subclavian vessels are exposed and retracted laterally and downward, respectively. The dorsal aspect of the first rib is cleared of its periosteum, and the rib is divided with a rongeur at approximately 2 cm distal of its junction with the costotransversal process. The divided rib is elevated, freed of all of its soft tissue connections, followed under the clavicle, and transected with a rongeur just behind the subclavian vessels (Fig. 55–45 and 55–46). After the mobilized proximal half of the first rib is removed, an incision is made under the retroactive inferior skin-flap across the clavicular attachment of the pectoralis msucle. Using sharp and blunt dissection, the remaining anterior portion of the first rib is exposed and grabbed with an alligator forceps, and its attachment to the sternocostal cartilage is divided. The first rib is then removed in its entirety. The pectoralis muscle is re-attached to the clavicle, and the subcutaneous tissues, as well as the skin, are closed. If the pleural cavity is inadvertently entered, a Robinson catheter is inserted through the incision, placed on water-sealed drainage for a few hours, then removed.

We have found this modified approach very useful in decompressing the thoracic inlet. The technique allows both supraclavicular and infraclavicular exposure of the first rib through a single skin incision, and it provides excellent visualization of the important structures of the thoracic inlet, thus ensuring both safety and radical intervention.

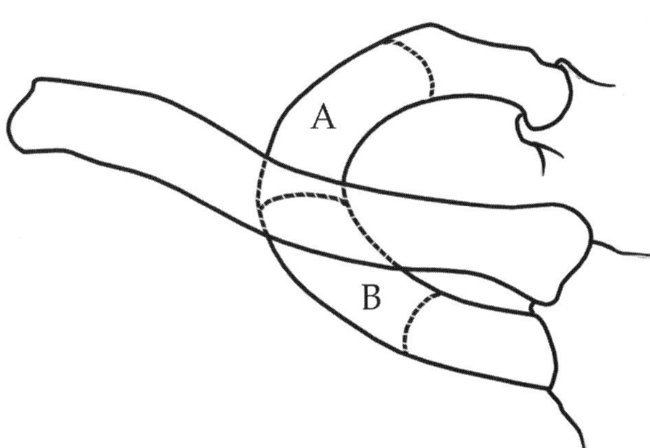

FIGURE 55–46 ■ The posterior portion of the first rib, *A*, is removed supra, and the sternal portion, *B*, is removed infraclavicularly. *Dotted lines* represent lines of rib transection.

COMMENTS AND CONTROVERSIES

This approach is an optional one and is rarely used in the treatment of thoracic outlet syndrome. It requires significant retraction of the various structures, as does the supraclavicular approach, evidenced by the multiple retractors shown in the illustration. It is an acceptable approach for arterial bypass, as is the supraclavicular and infraclavicular approach, however it is not the preferred approach for treatment of nerve or venous compression or for re-operation.

H. C. U.

REFERENCES

Bramwell E: Lesion of the first dorsal nerve root. Rev Neurol Psychiatry 1:236, 1903.

Clagett CT: Research and prosearch. J Thorac Cardiovasc Surg 44:153–166, 1962.

Ferguson TB, Burford TH, Roper CL: Neurovascular compression at the superior thoracic operature: Surgical management. Ann Surg 167:573–579, 1958.

Gol A, Patrick DW, McNeal DP: Relief of the costoclavicular syndrome by infraclavicular removal of the first rib: Technical note. J Neurosurg 28:81, 1968.

Murphy T: Brachial neuritis caused by compression of the first rib. Aust Med J 15:582, 1910.

Nelson RM, Davis RW: Thoracic outlet compression syndrome. Ann Thorac Surg 48:437–451, 1969.

Qvarfordt PG, Ehrenfeldt WK, Stoney RJ: Supraclavicular radical scalenectomy and transaxillary first rib resection for the thoracic outlet syndrome. A combined approach. Am J Surg 148:111–116, 1984.

Robicsek F, Eastman D: "Above-under" exposure of the first rib: A modified approach for the treatment of thoracic outlet syndrome. Ann Vasc Surg 11:304–306, 1997.

Roos DB: Transaxillary approach for first rib resection to relieve thoracic outlet syndrome. Ann Surg 163:354–358, 1966.

Stoney JR, Cheng SWK: Neurogenic thoracic outlet syndrome. In Rutherford RB (ed): Vascular Surgery, 4th ed. Philadelphia, WB Saunders, 1995, pp 976–992.

Thompson RW, Schenider PA, Nelken NA et al: Circumferential venolysis and paraclavicular thoracic outlet decompression for "effort thrombosis" of the subclavian vein. J Vasc Surg 16:723–732, 1992.

Urschel HC Jr, Paulson DL, McNamara JJ: Thoracic outlet syndrome. Ann Thorac Surg 6:1–10, 1968.

THORACOSCOPIC FIRST RIB RESECTION FOR THORACIC OUTLET SYNDROME

Randall K. Wolf

Alvin H. Crawford

Beverly Hahn

Resection of the first rib is performed for surgical treatment of thoracic outlet syndrome (TOS). Thoracic outlet syndrome refers to compression of the subclavian vessels or the brachial plexus by the first rib and adjacent structures at the superior aperture of the chest (MacKinnon et al, 1995).

The anatomy, clinical presentation, and evaluation of the patient with thoracic outlet syndrome has been extensively reviewed by Urschel (1989, 1990, 1995), and the reader is referred to Urschel's atlas (1995) for clear, concise, and exhaustive information concerning the history, anatomy, presentation, testing and accepted management of TOS. This chapter presents a new minimally invasive thoracoscopic surgical technique for excision of the first rib for treatment of thoracic outlet syndrome.

ANATOMY

On thoracoscopic examination, the first rib can be easily identified in the "roof" of the thorax. The first rib is a wide, flat rib that forms a "C" in the apex of the chest cavity. It is clearly visualized endoscopically and can be "palpated" indirectly using an endoscopic Kitner. Care should be taken to note the relationship of the internal mammary artery anteriorly and the sympathetic chain posteriorly to the borders of the first rib. On the left, the subclavian artery is also easily visualized on thoracoscopic examination (Fig. 55–47).

PROCEDURE

Room setup is depicted in Figure 55–48. The surgeon positions himself or herself on the anterior or posterior side of the patient. The patient is placed in the lateral position after induction of general anesthesia with a double-lumen tube. Three 10-mm thoracic ports are used for the operation: the two highest ports, in the anterior third or fourth and lateral fifth intercostal spaces for the working instruments, and a lower port on the lateral wall in the sixth intercostal space for a rigid 30-degree scope (Fig. 55–49). The thoracoscopic approach to first rib resection has been presented by Wolf and his co-workers

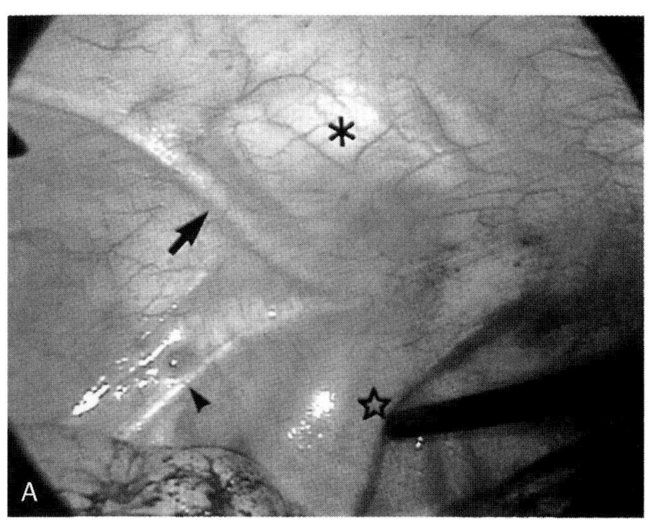

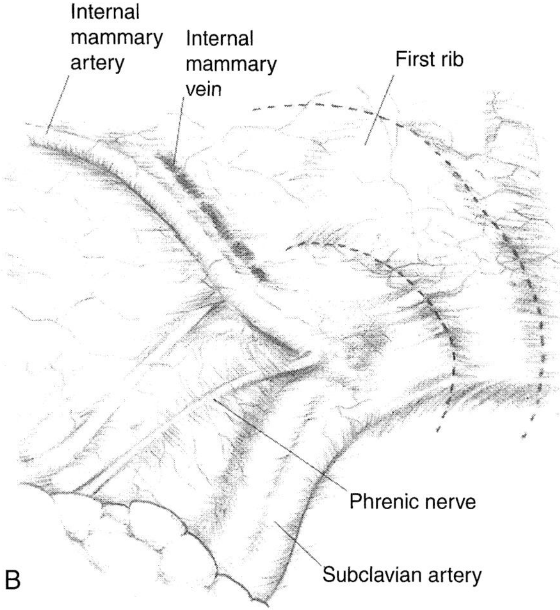

FIGURE 55–47 ■ *A*, The anatomy of the left superior thorax as seen through the thoracoscope—*asterisk*, left first rib; *large arrow*, internal mammary artery; *star*, left subclavian artery; *small arrow*, phrenic nerve. *B*, An accompanying artist's rendition. (From Wolf RK, Crawford AH, Hahn B: Thoracoscopic first rib resection for thoracic outlet syndrome. In Yim APC, Hazelrigg SR, Issat MB et al [eds]: Minimal Access Cardiothoracic Surgery. WB Saunders, Philadelphia, 2000.)

(1999). Endoscopic instruments including endoscopic elevators, curets, and rongeurs (Sofamor Danek, Tenn) were altered from the regular orthopedic tools by extension and modification to pass through 10-mm endoscopic ports (Regan, 1995). In the initial report by Ohtsuka and associates (in press), an endoscopic drill (Midas Rex, Pneumatic Tools Inc, Tex) capable of pulverizing bone through ports with a coarse ball tip revolving at high speed was also used. The Harmonic Scalpel (Ethicon Endo-Surgery, Cincinnati, Ohio), which operates with ultrasonic energy producing less smoke and lower heat than regular electrocautery, was developed to facilitate endoscopic dissection (Amaral, 1994).

After double-lumen endotracheal intubation, the patient is placed in the lateral decubitus position. The kidney rest is raised to slightly open the ribs, and selective ventilation is initiated. Three 10-mm ports are placed (see Procedure): two are flexible ports (Flexipath, Ethicon Endo-Surgery, Cincinnati, Ohio), and one is a rigid port. A 10-mm, 30-degree endoscope with three-chip camera is placed through the rigid inferior port. The flexible ports are used for placement of the orthopedic instruments. The anatomy is carefully evaluated. The thoracoscopic rib resection begins by dissecting the parietal pleura as well as intercostal muscles from the costal edge of the first rib using the Harmonic Scalpel (Figs. 55–50 and 55–51). The subclavian vein and artery and brachial plexus, lying from anterior to posterior in each groove of the first rib, are freed from the bone bluntly using an endoscopic Cobb elevator and endoscopic curets (Fig. 55–52). Next, cautious dissection with a spinous process elevator frees the ribs circumferentially. Recently, special angled elevators have been manufactured to facilitate this maneuver. To divide the rib in two cases, an endoscopic drill was then used. The subclavian vessels and nerves were protected from the revolving drill by placing an endoscopic elevator behind the rib. The powdered tissue was evacuated by suction. Currently, the drill has been replaced by an endoscopic rib cutter (Fig. 55–53). The endoscopic rib cutter is simpler, easier to use, and safer than the drill. The endoscopic rib cutter is employed to divide the first rib both anteriorly and posteriorly in its midportion. The divided rib is then removed through one of the port incisions (Fig. 55–54). Endoscopic orthopedic rongeurs are then used to trim the resected ends of the rib back to the transverse process posteriorly, and anteriorly to the manubrium (Fig. 55–55). Final assessment should include palpation of the transverse process posteriorly, as well as the costochondral junction anteriorly. This allows for complete excision of the first rib, a point emphasized by Urschel.

A few technical points of the thoracoscopic first rib resection are worth emphasizing. Care must be taken in developing the plane of dissection, and it is recommended to dissect anterior to the vein initially. After transection of the rib, any additional muscle attachments, such as scalenus anticus or medius, can be divided under direct vision. The rib can be delivered easily through one of the port sites after removing the port. During this dissection, the mammary artery anteriorly and the sympathetic chain posteriorly are clearly observed and preserved. Port sites are best placed at some distance from the target to allow adequate manipulation of the instruments in a comfortable arc. After complete thoracoscopic first rib excision, the contents of the neurovascular bundle drape gently across the apex of the pleural cavity. The extent of rib resection and its immediate effect on the structures of the thoracic outlet are clearly visualized.

RESULTS

In seven cases performed by Wolf and colleagues (1999), the first rib was removed by this technique to decompress

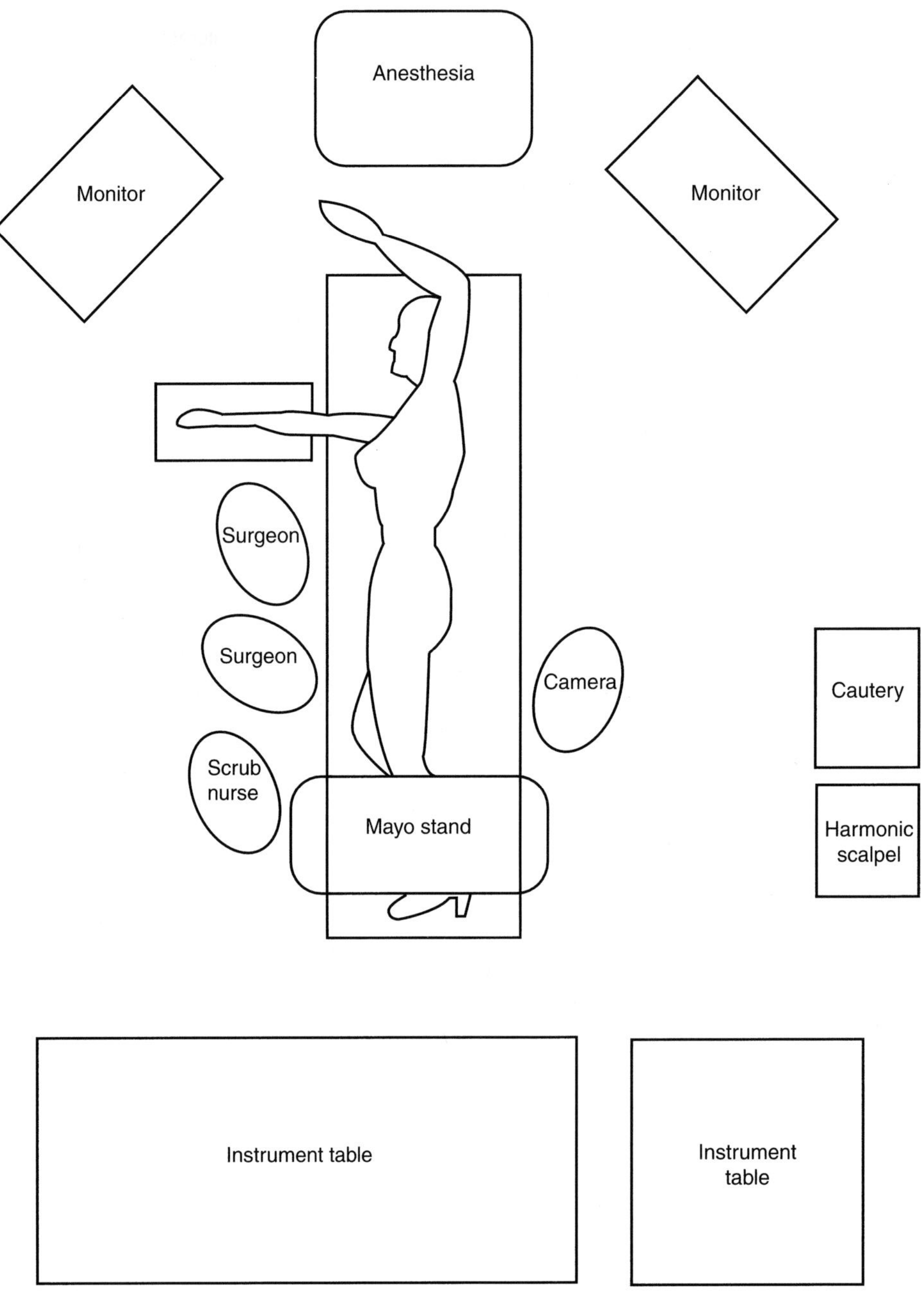

FIGURE 55–48 ■ Room setup for thoracoscopic first rib resection. (From Wolf RK, Crawford AH, Hahn B: Thoracoscopic first rib resection for thoracic outlet syndrome. In Yim APC, Hazelrigg SR, Issat MB et al [eds]: Minimal Access Cardiothoracic Surgery. WB Saunders, Philadelphia, 2000.)

the subclavian vessels and brachial plexus lying on the first rib. In the first patient, who presented with right subclavian vein thrombosis, the symptoms on the right side resolved completely after the procedure. He subsequently developed symptoms in the left arm and underwent the same procedure on the left side. The duration of the initial operation was 110 minutes. However, the operation times were reduced with experience to 100 minutes for the second case and 75 minutes for the third. Blood loss was minimal in each case, and hospital stay was 3, 2 and 1 day in the first, second, and third cases, respectively. Currently, a 1-day stay in the hospital is routine. Three years after surgery, the patient with Paget-Schroetter syndrome remains asymptomatic. More recently, in the last three patients the endoscopic rib cutter has been used to transect the first rib. The rib cutter appears to add safety to the division maneuver and is relatively easy to use compared with the drill. Richard Fischel (Personal communication) has completed six cases of first rib resection with histories including trauma, sudden onset of numbness, and long-standing pain and weakness secondary to an overhead lifting job. These patients had all failed conservative treatments. All had good improvement with relief of pain and numbness.

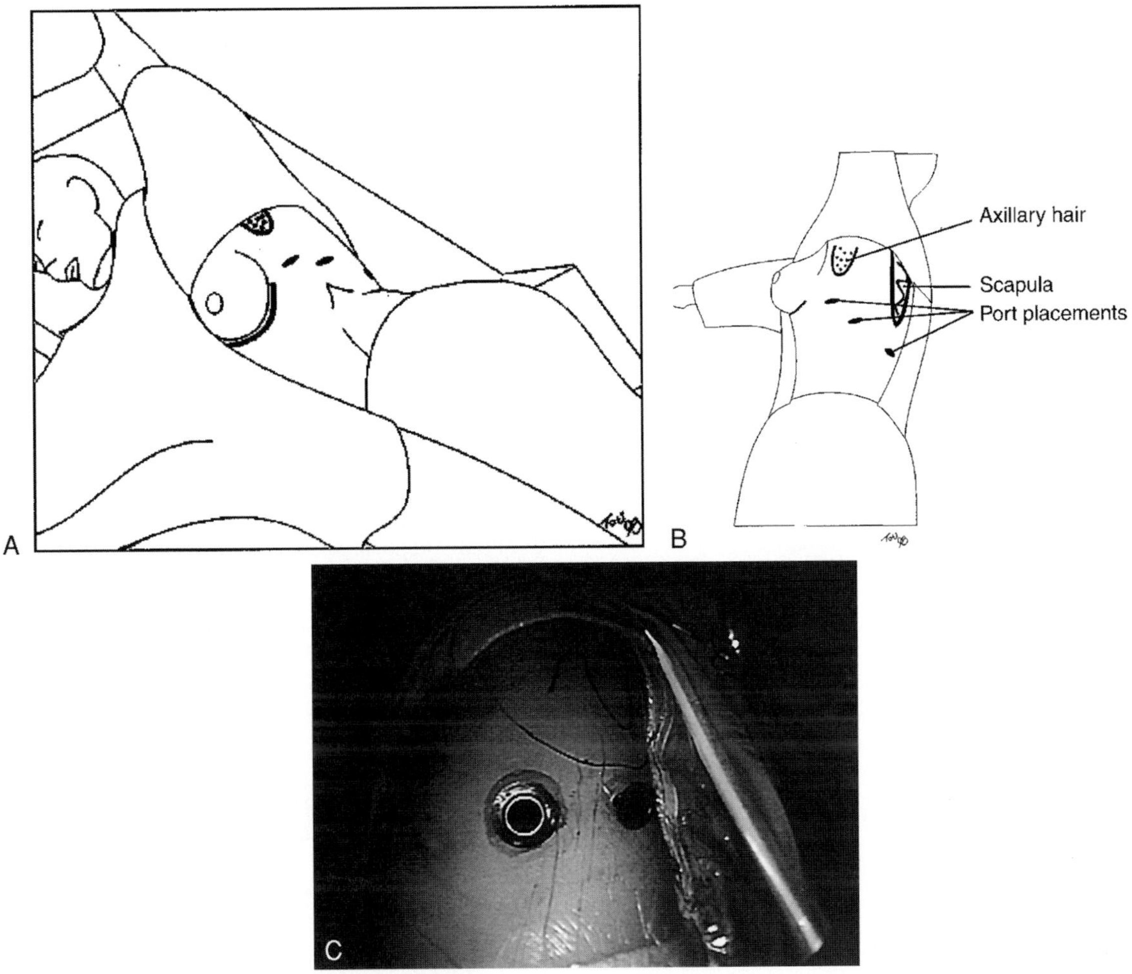

A B

Axillary hair
Scapula
Port placements

C

FIGURE 55–49 ■ *A*, Topical anatomy, and *B* and *C*, port sites for thoracoscopic first rib resection. (*A* and *B*, From Wolf RK, Crawford AH, Hahn B: Thoracoscopic first rib resection for thoracic outlet syndrome. In Yim APC, Hazelrigg SR, Issat MB et al [eds]: Minimal Access Cardiothoracic Surgery. WB Saunders, Philadelphia, 2000.)

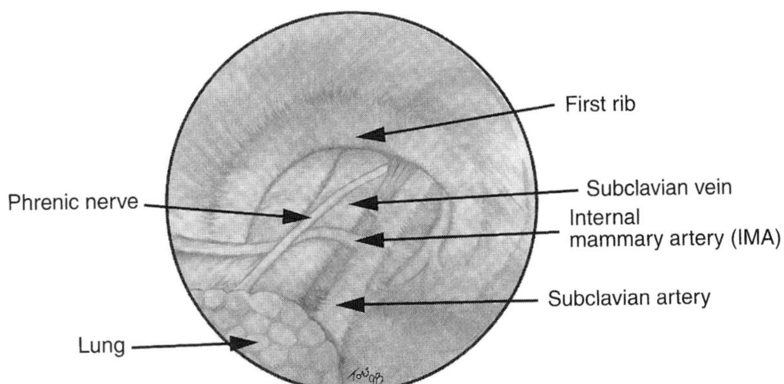

FIGURE 55–50 ■ Thoracoscopic view of the left first rib. (From Wolf RK, Crawford AH, Hahn B: Thoracoscopic first rib resection for thoracic outlet syndrome. In Yim APC, Hazelrigg SR, Issat MB et al [eds]: Minimal Access Cardiothoracic Surgery. WB Saunders, Philadelphia, 2000.)

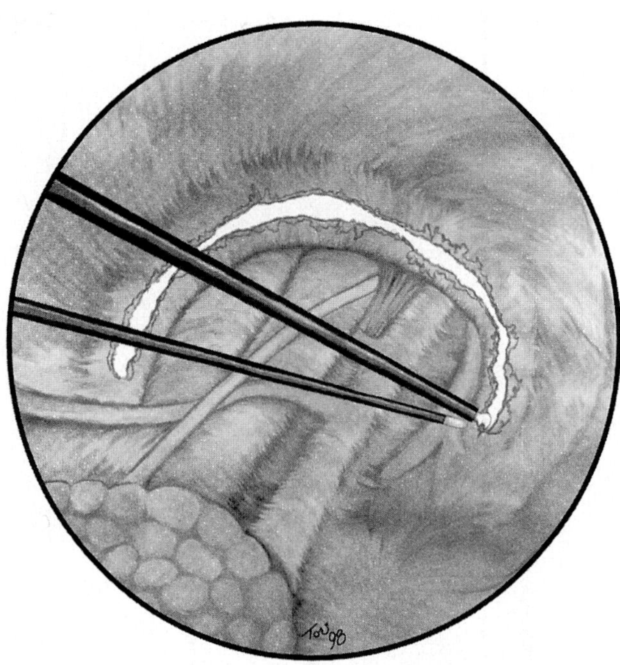

FIGURE 55–51 ■ Initial dissection of the pleura overlying the first rib as performed with the harmonic scalpel. (From Wolf RK, Crawford AH, Hahn B: Thoracoscopic first rib resection for thoracic outlet syndrome. In Yim APC, Hazelrigg SR, Issat MB et al [eds]: Minimal Access Cardiothoracic Surgery. WB Saunders, Philadelphia, 2000.)

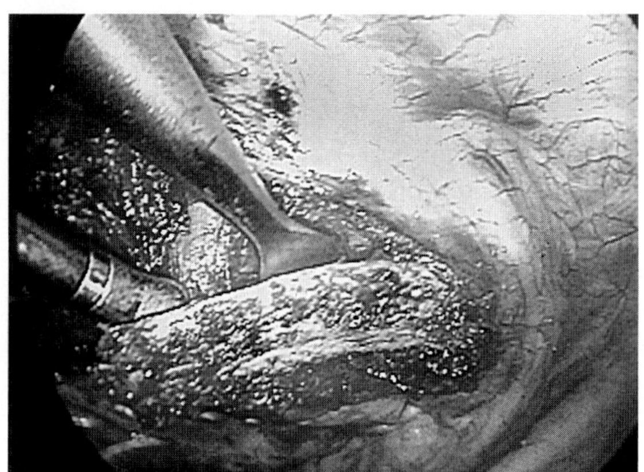

FIGURE 55–52 ■ The right rib is freed from its muscular attachments with an elevator.

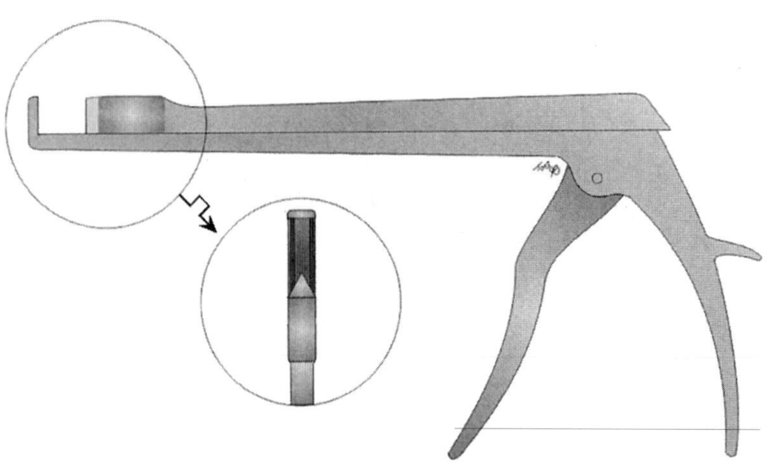

FIGURE 55–53 ■ Thoracoscopic rib cutter (Sofamor Danek, Medthronic, Minneapolis, MN) used on subsequent cases. (From Wolf RK, Crawford AH, Hahn B: Thoracoscopic first rib resection for thoracic outlet syndrome. In Yim APC, Hazelrigg SR, Issat MB et al [eds]: Minimal Access Cardiothoracic Surgery. WB Saunders, Philadelphia, 2000).

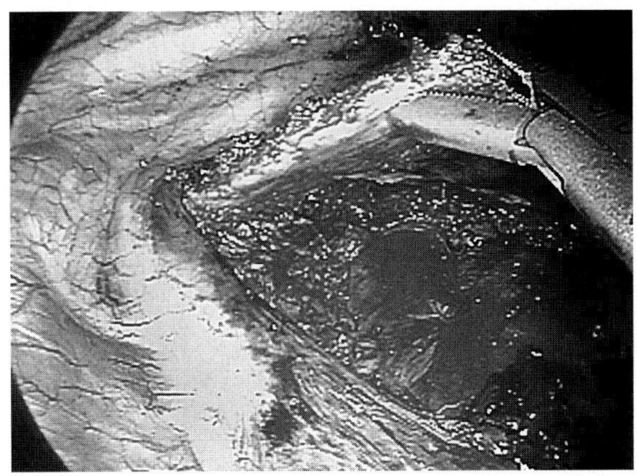

FIGURE 55–54 ■ The resected right first rib is shown before removal.

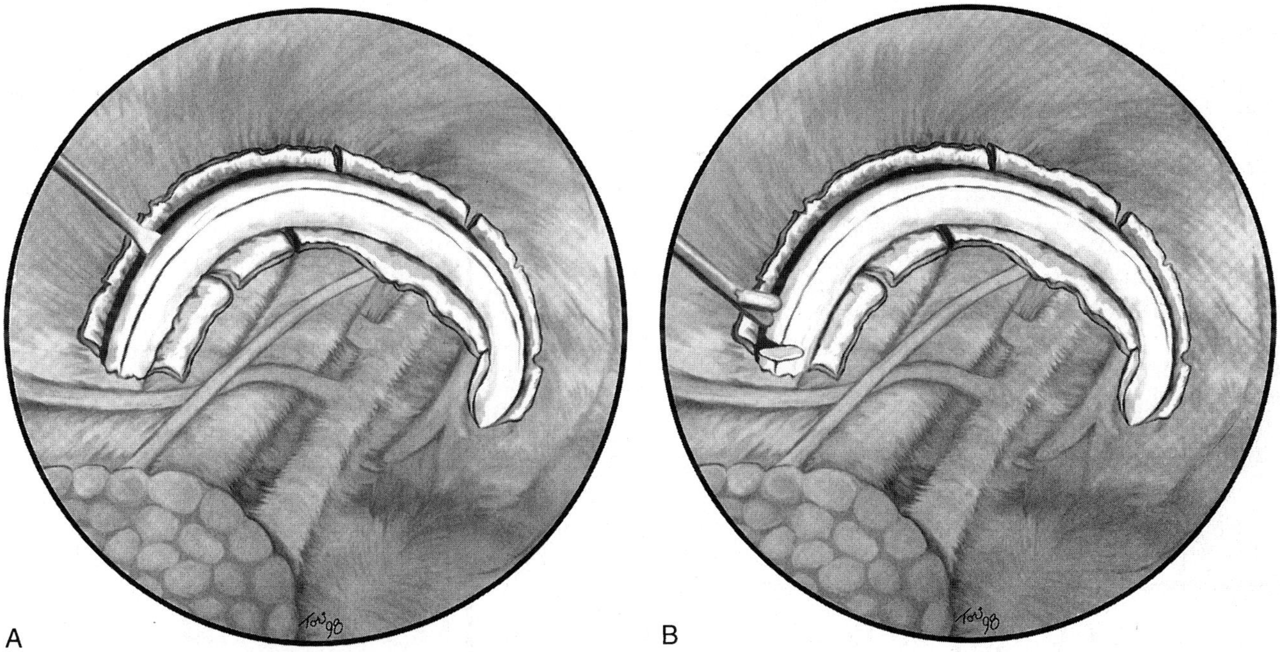

A

B

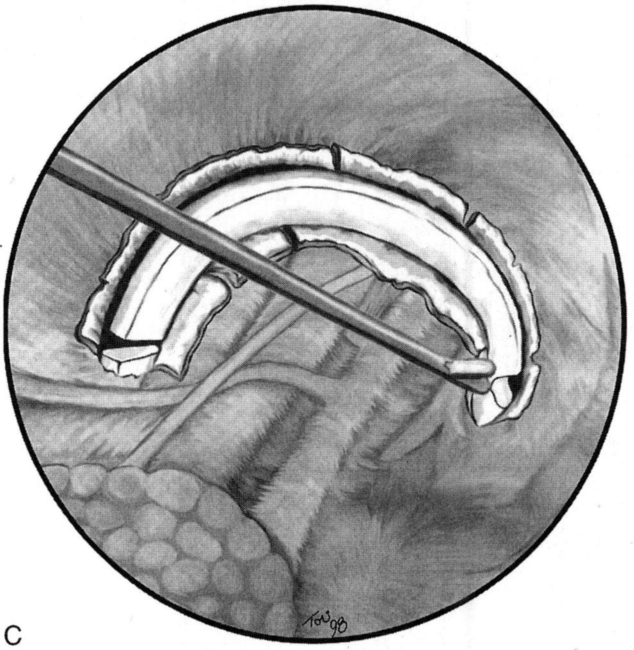

C

FIGURE 55–55 ■ *A through C,* Further thoracoscopic dissection and division of the first rib. (From Wolf RK, Crawford AH, Hahn B: Thoracoscopic first rib resection for thoracic outlet syndrome. In Yim APC, Hazelrigg SR, Issat MB et al [eds]: Minimal Access Cardiothoracic Surgery. WB Saunders, Philadelphia, 2000.)

COMMENTS AND CONTROVERSIES

The use of the thoracoscope for resection of the first rib from inside the chest cavity is a novel and creative one. It allows direct access to the rib without retraction of any of the structures, similar to the exposure of the transaxillary approach. It also has the advantage of minimal invasion as far as the length of an incision (although the transaxillary incision is not painful and does not require prolonged hospitalization).

It must be remembered that this thoracoscopic, intrathoracic technique is experimental and very new as can be evidenced by the small number of cases presented. However, I think that with development of better instruments, this may become a standard approach in the future.

A major risk of this approach is injury to the nerves or blood vessels that are on the other side of the rib and difficult to visualize. Care must be taken with this procedure and experience with thoracoscopy is critical.

H. C. U.

■ REFERENCES

Amaral JF: The experimental development of an ultrasonically activated scalpel for laparoscopic use. Surg Laparosc Endosc 4:92–99, 1994.

Atkins HJB: Sympathectomy by the axillary approach. Cancer 1:538, 1954.

Lindgren KA, Oksala I: Long-term outcome of surgery for thoracic outlet syndrome. Am J Surg 169:358–360, 1995.

MacKinnon SE: Thoracic outlet syndrome. Ann Thorac Surg 58:287–289, 1994.

MacKinnon SE, Patterson GA, Urschel HC: Thoracic outlet syndromes. In Pearson FG, Deslauriers J, Ginsburg RJ et al (eds): Thoracic Surgery. New York, Churchill Livingstone, 1995.

Ohtsuka T, Wolf RK, Dunsker SB: Port-access first rib resection with new instruments: A report of two cases. J Surg Endosc, in press.

Poole GV, Thomae KR: Thoracic outlet syndrome reconsidered. Am Surg 62:287–291, 1996.

Regan JJ: Equipment and instrumentation for endoscopic spine surgery. In Regan JJ, McAfee PC, Mack MJ (eds): Atlas of Endoscopic Spine Surgery. New York, Quality Medical Publishing, 1995.

Roos DB: Transaxillary approach for first rib resection to relieve thoracic outlet syndrome. Ann Surg 163:354–358, 1996.

Urschel Hc Jr, Cooper JD: Atlas of Thoracic Surgery. New York, Churchill Livingstone, 1995.

Urschel HC: Thoracic outlet syndrome. In Shields (ed): General Thoracic Surgery. Philadelphia, Lea & Febiger, 1989.

Urschel HC: Thoracic outlet syndrome. In Sabiston S (ed): Surgery of the Chest. Philadelphia, WB Saunders, 1990.

Wilson, et al. Thoracic outlet disorders, Vascular Surgery, Principles and Practice. McGraw-Hill, 1987.

Wolf RK, Crawford AH, Hahn BY: Thoracoscopic First Rib Resection for Thoracic Outlet Syndrome. In Yim Y et al (eds): Minimal Access Cardiothoracic Surgery. Philadelphia, WB Saunders, 1999.

SURGERY OF THE CLAVICLE

Harold C. Urschel Jr.
Jere W. Lord

Total claviculectomy, although rarely performed, is a valuable clinical procedure for a variety of pathologic conditions. It can be performed bilaterally without significant limitation of function or cosmetic deformity and should be part of the armamentarium of general, vascular, and thoracic surgeons.

FUNCTIONAL ANATOMY

The sternoclavicular joint plays a considerable part in the combined movements of the shoulder-girdle complex. It possesses an intra-articular disk that adapts the shoulder girth to a wider range of motion. The motion is gliding, with the center of motion outside the joint. The fulcrum of motion is the clavicular insertion of the costoclavicular ligament, which not only contributes greatly to joint stability but also lies close to the joint and gives greater angular value to the excursions in comparison with the gliding distance.

The upward and downward movement around the sagittal axis has an excursion range of 60 degrees, the forward and backward movement around the perpendicular axis has an excursion range of 30 degrees, and the length rotation movement around the frontal axis has an excursion range of 30 degrees.

The acromioclavicular joint, the articulation between the clavicle and acromion, is a weak, simple, arthrodial or gliding joint with synovial cavity, capsule, and reinforcing extracapsular ligaments, namely, the superior and inferior acromioclavicular ligaments. The acromioclavicular joint provides mobility between the clavicle and the scapula. Its construction is reinforced by the powerful coracoclavicular ligament, providing a stronger union between the two bones.

The subclavian artery leaves the thorax by arching over the first rib behind the scalenus anticus muscle and in front of the scalenus medius. It then passes under the subclavius muscle and clavicle and enters the axilla beneath the pectoralis minor muscle.

Except that it passes anterior, rather than posterior, to the scalenus anticus muscle, the subclavian vein has an identical course. The vein passes under the clavicle through a tunnel bounded medically by the costoclavicular ligament, laterally by the scalenus anticus muscle, superiorly by the subclavius muscle and clavicle, and inferiorly by the first rib. The brachial plexus follows the route of the subclavian artery, but it lies a little more posteriorly and laterally.

From its origin at the root of the neck to the lowermost boundary of the axilla, the neurovascular supply of the upper limb is closely confined within rather rigid spaces by an overlying myofascial layer (Fig. 55–56). From above downward, this consists of the fascia of the omohyoid (so-called muscular fascial division of the enveloping layer of the deep cervical fascia); the posterior belly of the omohyoid, which is enclosed in this fascia; below the omohyoid, this fascia splits to envelop the subclavius muscle; it then joins again to form the clavipectoral fascia, whose thickened lateral portion forms the costocoracoid membrane; this fascial layer is prolonged inferiorly and splits again to enclose the pectoralis minor; finally, it rejoins again to form the suspensory ligament of the axilla.

PATHOPHYSIOLOGY

Deformities of the clavicle may occur secondary to malignant or benign tumors (primary or metastatic); trauma with callous formation or fracture nonunion; or congenital defects. The pressure may involve one or more of the structures passing below the clavicle in the thoracic out-

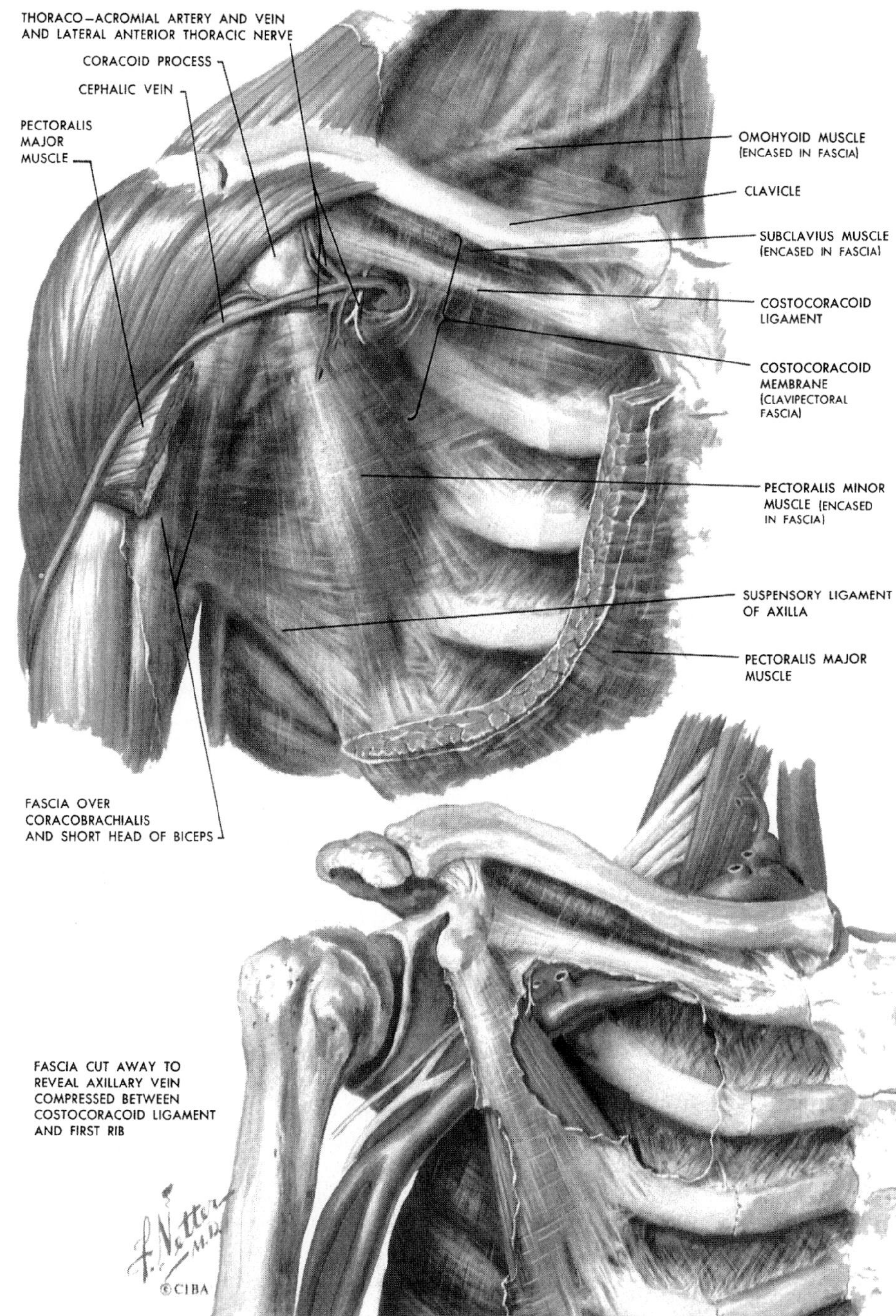

FIGURE 55–56 ■ From its origin at the root of the neck to the lower-most boundary of axilla, the neurovascular supply of the upper limb is closely confined within rigid spaces by an overlying myofascial layer. This consists of the fascia of the omohyoid, the posterior belly of the omohyoid, the subclavius muscle, the clavipectoral fascia, the costocoracoid membrane, the pectoralis minor, and the suspensory ligament of the axilla. (From Lord JW Jr, Rosati LM: Thoracic-outlet syndromes. Clin Symp 23:1, 1971. Illustrated by Frank H. Netter, MD, 1971, CIBA-Geigy Corp.)

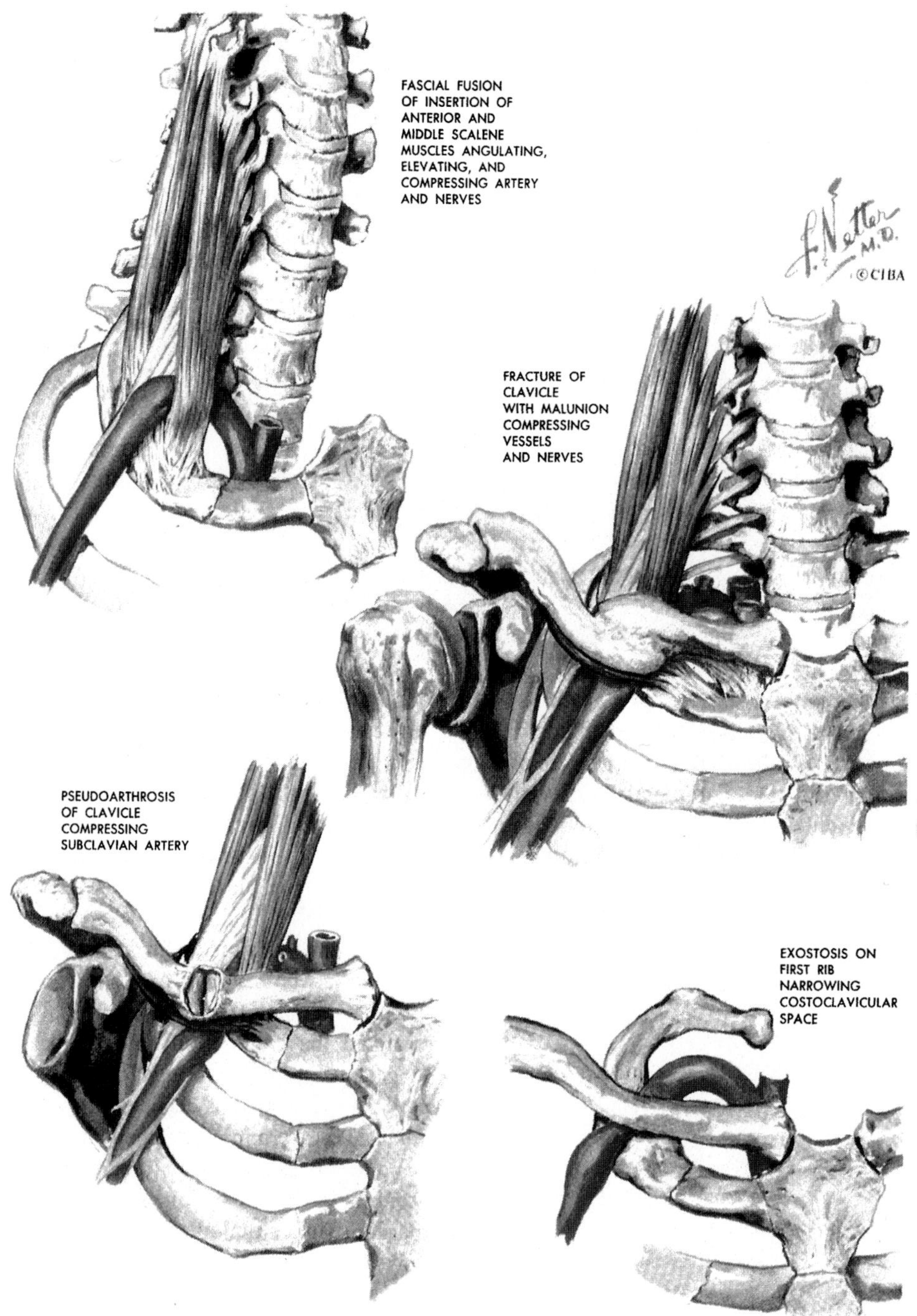

FIGURE 55–57 ■ The various structural abnormalities that cause compression. (From Lord JW Jr, Rosati LM: Thoracic-outlet syndromes. Clin Symp 23:1, 1971. Illustrated by Frank H. Netter, MD, 1971, CIBA-Geigy Corp.)

let, such as the axillary-subclavian vein, artery, or nerve (brachial plexus, peripheral asympathetic) (Fig. 55–57).

The Paget-Schroetter syndrome, or effort thrombosis of the vein may be secondary to any of the aforementioned pathologic conditions superimposed on a congenital lateral insertion of the costoclavicular ligament; weightlifting, which increases the size of the scalenus anticus muscle; or trauma.

The subclavian artery may develop post–stenotic dilation aneurysm or occlusion or severe intermittent spasm secondary to any of the previously mentioned forces operating in the thoracic outlet, requiring clavicular resection.

Total claviculectomy with excision of the periosteum provides excellent exposure for safe removal of aneurysms of the second and third portions of the subclavian artery and, in selected patients, for reconstruction of occlusions in this area.

DIAGNOSIS

Diagnosis is established clinically in patients with deformities of the clavicle secondary to tumors, bony abnormalities, or nonunion secondary to trauma or birth defects. Diagnosis can be confirmed by special radiographic views of the clavicle. Computed tomography (CT) or magnetic resonance imaging (MRI) scans are helpful if the tumor is medial. One patient presented as having an intrathoracic mass initially thought to be in the lung until location in the clavicle was confirmed by CT scan. Careful clinical assessment should be made of arterial pulses, the venous and sympathetic nervous systems, as well as sensory and motor neurologic evaluation of the extremity. A defined pain history is also critical.

Examination of the radial pulse in the various positions of compression may be helpful (e.g., hyperabduction, hyperextension, and the military position). Assessment of arterial bruits and venous hums by auscultation or Doppler scan in both the supraclavicular and intraclavicular positions is important for vascular lesions. Venograms and arteriograms, both prograde and retrograde, may be helpful for specific lesions and may demonstrate the location of collateral circulation, which is important to preserve in most patients. Stellate ganglion blocks may be helpful for sympathetic-maintained pain syndrome.

In patients with predominant pain and paresthesia who have nerve compression, electromyography is usually normal except that the conduction velocity is prolonged over the thoracic outlet (Miller, 1981; Urschel and Razzuk, 1972, 1986, 1995, 1996). Preoperative needle biopsy of clavicle tumors is valuable in determining whether or not the tumor is malignant. A malignant tumor requires a wider excision and a greater margin than a simple benign tumor, and it may be difficult to diagnose by frozen section.

INDICATIONS FOR SURGERY

Indications for operation in the 11 cases with pathologic clavicles were obvious; the other resections in 26 extremities were primarily for diagnosis of thoracic outlet syndrome that did not respond to conservative medical management or physical therapy. In one of these patients, a transaxillary first rib resection had been unsuccessful in managing symptoms; claviculectomy was successful (Fig. 55–58). In the past claviculectomy for thoracic outlet syndrome was performed for severe symptomatology prior to the popularization of the transaxillary or posterior resection of the first rib.

OPERATIVE TECHNIQUE

The operation is carried out by an incision over the length of the clavicle with subperiosteal resection of the bone. The periosteum is completely and carefully removed, avoiding injury to the subclavian vein (Fig. 55–59). The scalenus anticus muscle is sectioned at its insertion into the first rib. Any anomalous bands are excised. Following careful hemostasis, the incision is closed without drainage in most cases. Occasionally, for a large mass or bony abnormality, a round Jackson-Pratt suction catheter is brought out through a subcutaneous tunnel. Antibiotic solution is used, and antibiotics are given prophylactically.

ANATOMIC AND FUNCTIONAL RESULTS

Removal of the clavicle eliminates angulation and pressure on the subclavian artery and vein by the scalenus anticus muscle. When the clavicle is removed and the scalenus muscle divided, the vessels roll down and forward. Thus, the vessels are displaced anteriorly along with the subclavian muscle. The elimination of the clavicle allows the shoulder to move anteriorly and medially, relaxing the pectoralis minor tendon, thereby functionally lengthening the artery, vein, and brachial plexus (Fig. 55–60).

Cosmetically the appearance is satisfactory, and postoperative function of the extremity is excellent. Bilateral claviculectomy allows the shoulders to be brought together in the midline; however, there are no adverse consequences, and function is excellent.

INDICATIONS AND CLINICAL STUDY

From 1950 through 1996, 37 clavicles were resected in 30 patients suffering from arterial, venous, and neurologic symptoms involving the upper extremity. The patients ranged in age from 17 to 78 years; there were 17 males and 13 females. Eleven clavicles were pathologic: posttraumatic nonunion (4), congenital nonunion (2), posttraumatic abnormal bony union (2), neoplastic (2), and post–radiation necrosis (1) (see Fig. 55–57). The subclavian artery was occluded in 8 extremities and intermittently obstructed in 21. The subclavian vein was occluded in 6 extremities (Paget-Schroetter syndrome) (Urschel and Razzuk, 2000) and intermittently obstructed in three. Neurologic involvement occurred in 8 extremities involving sensory or motor symptoms of thoracic outlet syndrome. These generally occurred in the ulnar nerve distribution, but they also presented, though less frequently, in the medial nerve distribution. Several patients had more than one system involved.

Mean follow-up for the 30 patients was 8 years. One patient who failed to improve with transaxillary resection of the first rib was completely relieved by claviculectomy for large callous formation. Results in 37 clavicles were classified as excellent in 19 extremities, good in 13, fair in 4, and poor in 1 (Table 55–1). There was no mortality and only one complication, leakage from the thoracic duct, which was easily controlled without operation.

CASE REPORT

A 42-year-old woman had sustained bilateral fractures of the clavicle 17 years prior to admission. Six weeks following the clavicular fractures, overriding was noted, and bilateral open reduction with fixation of the fragments by kangaroo tendon was performed. A satisfactory functional result was obtained on the right, but there was intermit-

TABLE 55–1 ■ **Results of 37 Claviculectomies**

Excellent	19 extremities
Good	13 extremities
Fair	4 extremities
Poor	1 extremity
Follow-up	
Mean	8 yr
Range	1–33 yr

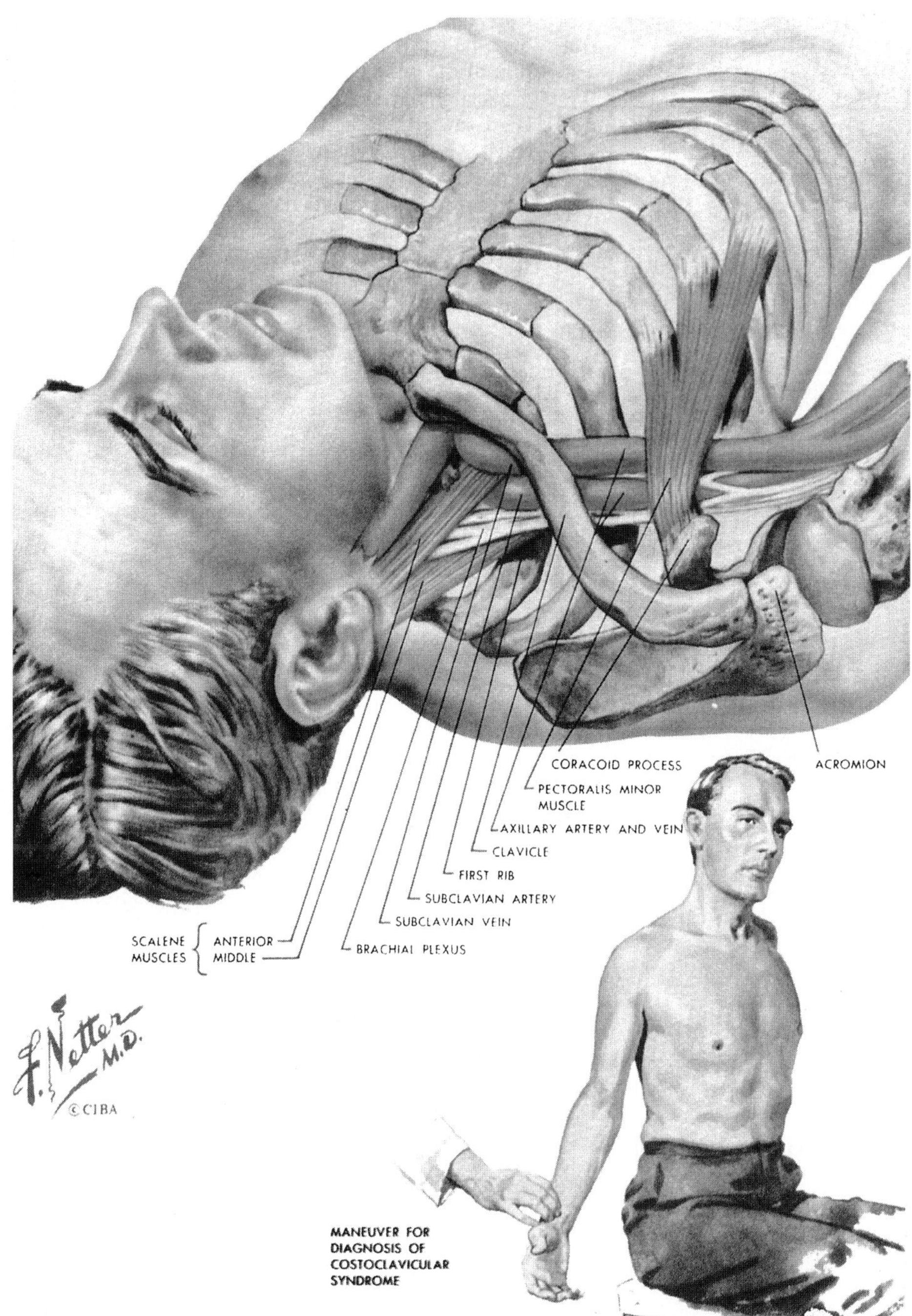

FIGURE 55–58 ■ The exaggerated military position, with the shoulders drawn downward and backward, is used to detect compression in the costoclavicular interval. The subclavian vein lies in the inner medial angle, between the insertion of the anterior scalene muscle posteriorly and the inner end of the clavicle, with its underlying tendon of insertion of the subclavius muscle and the costocoracoid ligament inserting into the first rib anteriorly. (From Lord JW Jr, Rosati LM: Thoracic-outlet syndromes. Clin Symp 23:1, 1971. Illustrated by Frank H. Netter, MD, 1971, CIBA-Geigy Corp.)

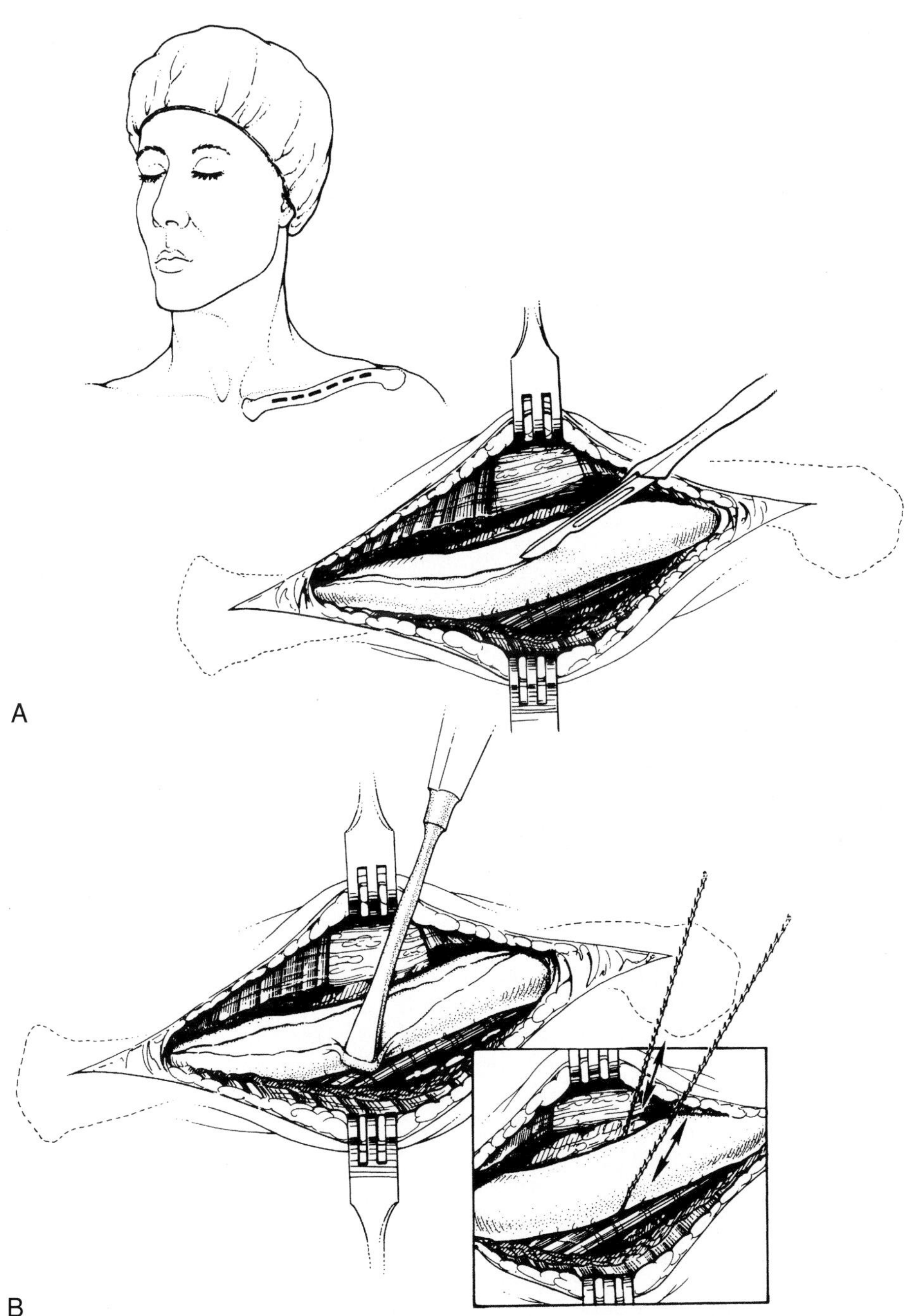

FIGURE 55–59 ■ The operation is carried out by an incision over the length of the clavicle with subperiosteal resection of the bone (*A*), Reflecting periosteum from the clavicle. *Insert* shows a section of the clavicle that was hit with a Gigli saw (*B*). (Illustrations by Robin Markovits Jensen, adapted from The New York Academy of Medicine, Diseases of the Circulatory System, Macmillan, 1952.)

Illustration continued on following page

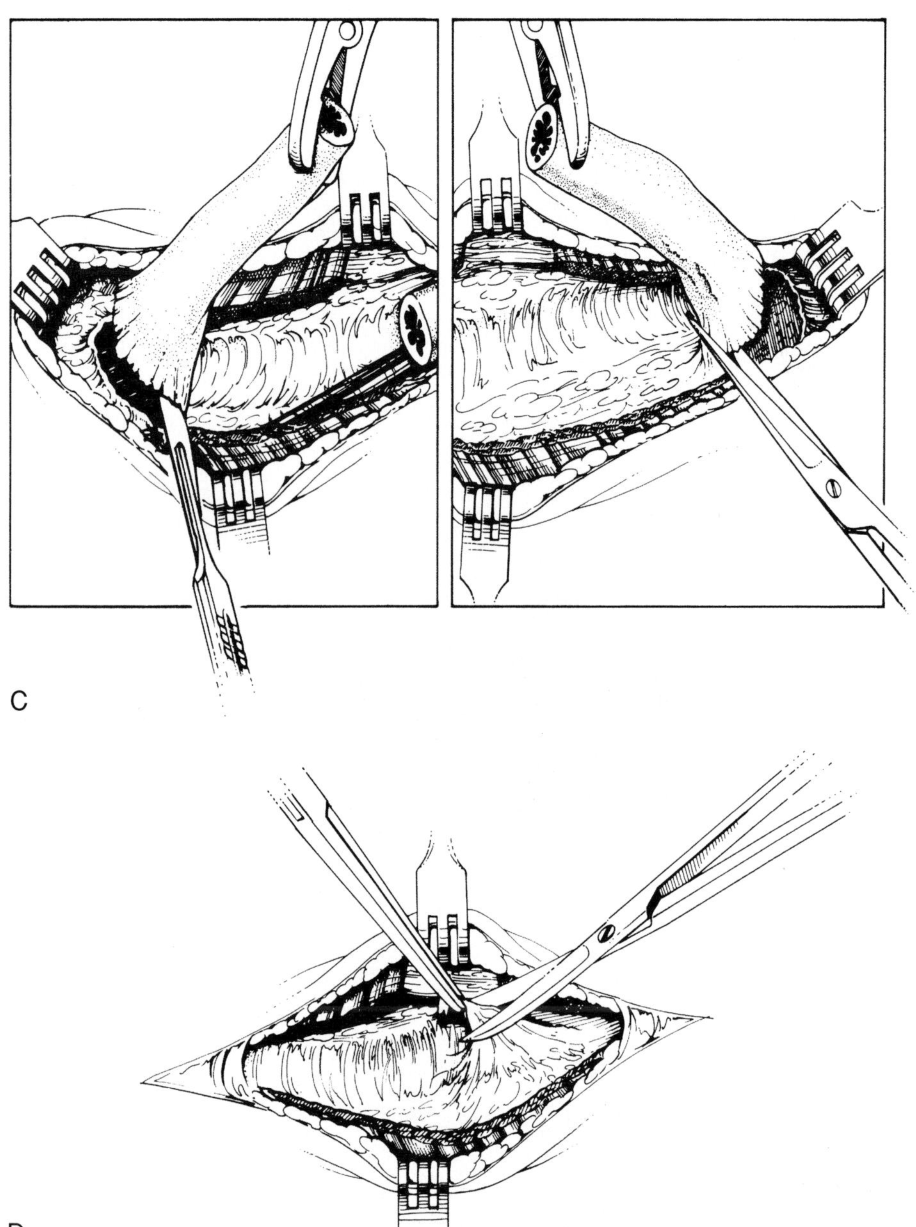

FIGURE 55–59 ■ *(Continued)* Removal of the medial segment of the clavicle is seen on the left; removal of the lateral segment of the clavicle is seen on the right (*C*). The periosteum is excised from the clavicular bed (*D*). (Illustrations by Robin Markovits Jensen, adapted from The New York Academy of Medicine, Diseases of the Circulatory System, Macmillan, 1952.)

tent discomfort in the region of the clavicle and shoulder on the left side.

Four months prior to admission, the patient noted that her left arm was larger than the right and that this arm fatigued more readily than the right. There was no swelling of the forearm or hand, and no paresthesias were noted. The swelling and weakness gradually increased until 4 days prior to admission when, following a swim, the whole left arm became markedly swollen. There was extreme weakness of the extremity and a subjective sensation of coolness.

Examination revealed a malunited fracture of the left clavicle. Dilated superficial veins extended from the left arm and shoulder to the pectoral region. The entire left upper extremity was moderately swollen. Skin temperature of the arms was equal on gross testing. With the patient recumbent and the left arm at her side, the radial pulse was strong. However, on sitting, which produced a modified costoclavicular maneuver, the radial pulse was obliterated by deep inspiration. Turning the head to either side, or abduction of the left arm to 45 degrees, also obliterated the pulse. Radiography of the clavicle revealed a malunited fracture on the left, with significant overriding of the medial fragment (Fig. 55–61).

At operation, the patient was found to have a large number of venous collateral channels in the retroclavicular space, and the subclavian vein was thrombosed. The inner tip of the lateral clavicular fragment was pressing on the subclavian artery and apparently was responsible for the intermittent compression of this vessel on deep inspiration or hyperabduction. The clavicular fragments, including the periosteum, were resected. Immediately after the operation, the patient could hyperabduct the left arm to 180 degrees without obliterating the radial pulse.

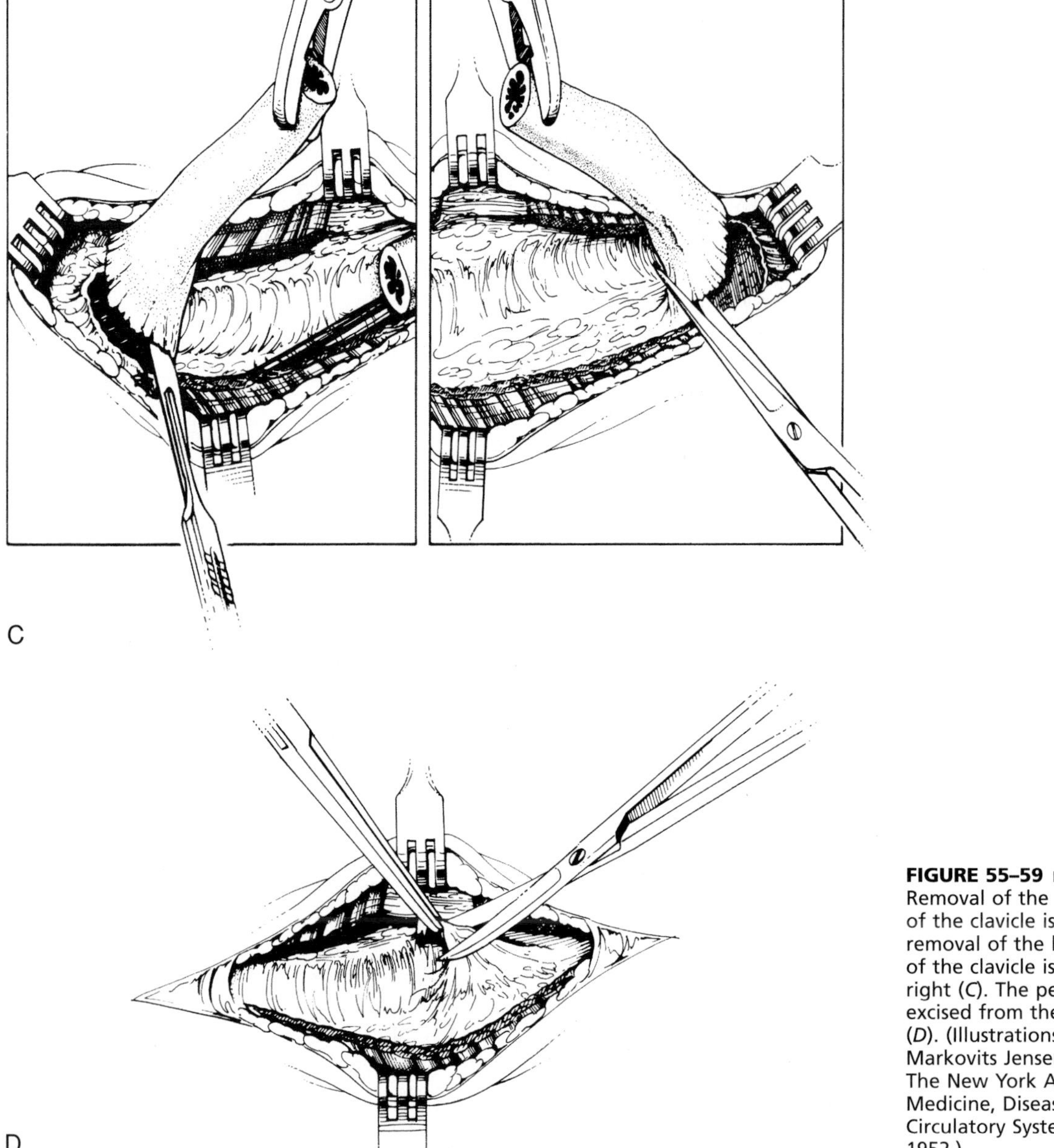

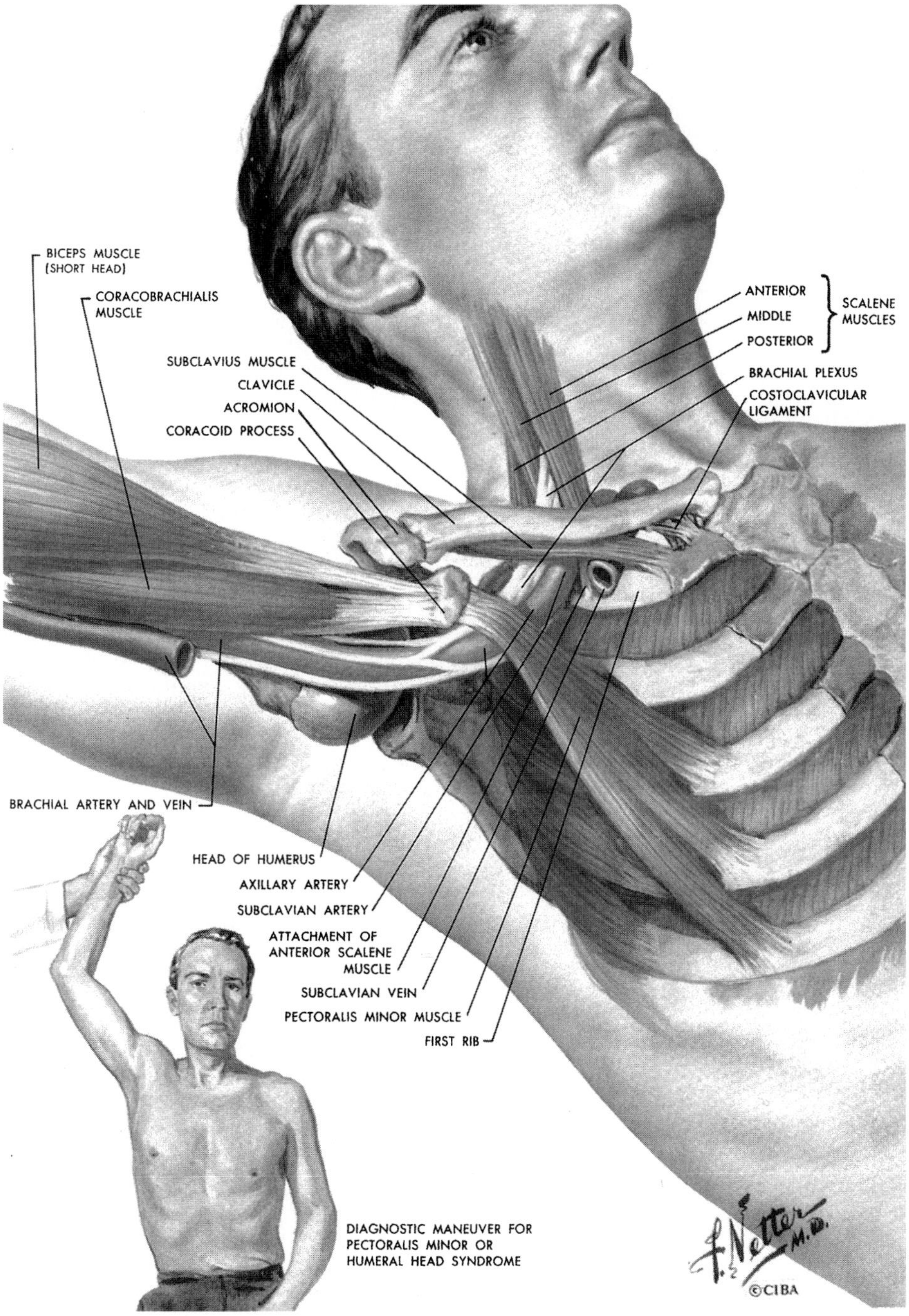

FIGURE 55–60 ■ The elimination of the clavicle allows the shoulder to move anteriorly and medially, relaxing the pectoralis minor tendon and thus functionally lengthening the artery, the vein, and the brachial plexus.

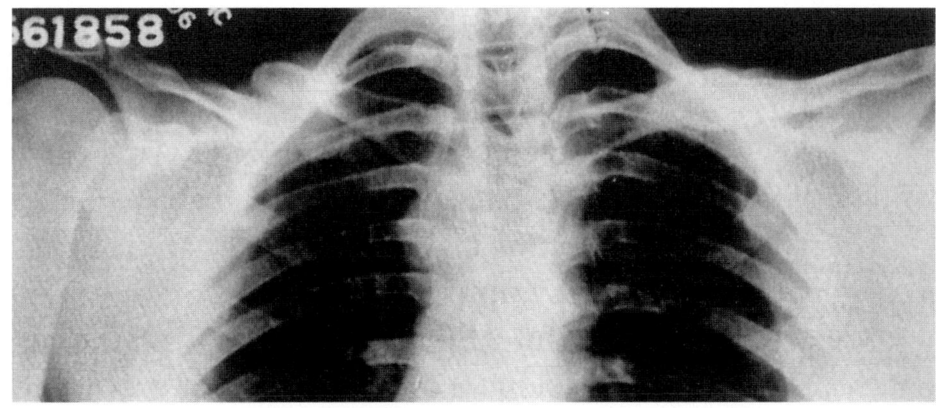

FIGURE 55–61 ■ Radiograph of the clavicle reveals a malunited fracture of the left, with significant overriding of the medial fragment.

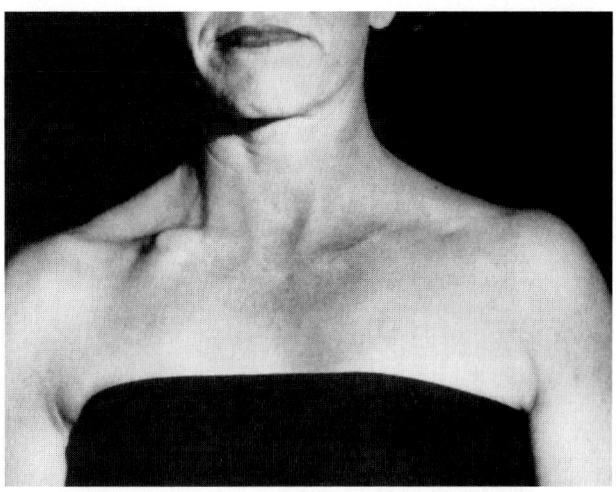

FIGURE 55–62 ■ Four years postoperatively, the left arm was slightly larger than the right, but turning of the head, depressing the shoulder, deep inspiration, and hyperabduction did not dampen the left radial pulse.

The postoperative course was uncomplicated. The patient maintained her arm in a position of elevation, and anticoagulant therapy was instituted and maintained for approximately 1 month. At the time of discharge, 7 days after the operation, the left upper arm was 2 inches larger in circumference than the right. There was no difference in size between the left and right forearms and hands. The patient was fitted with an elastic sleeve.

Four years postoperatively (Fig. 55–62), the left arm remained slightly larger than the right. Turning the head, depressing the shoulders, deep inspiration, and hyperabduction did not dampen the left radial pulse.

During the 21-year follow-up, the patient has had no pain in the clavicular or shoulder region and has noted no fatigue or paresthesias in the left upper extremity. It is her impression that the collateral veins over the left shoulder have become slightly more prominent. There has been no evidence of clavicular regeneration.

DISCUSSION

The initial incentive to consider total claviculectomy was for relief of neurovascular compression in the shoulder girdle, later referred to as the thoracic outlet syndrome. It came in part from the work of Fraser B. Gurd (1947), who described several bones in the body, including the clavicle, that could be removed without functional impairment. Irving Wright, whose interest in the field has been well documented (1945), encouraged the senior author (J.L.) to develop the operation of total claviculectomy, removal of the periosteum, and section of the scalenus anticus muscle in patients with compression syndromes unresponsive to conscientious conservative therapy. (Lord, 1953).

Partial claviculectomy has been recommended for exposure of the subclavian vessels by Elkin and Cooper (1946), Shumacker (1947), and recently by Aziz and associates (1986). This procedure has a potential for complications. We resected the middle two-fourths of the clavicle with relief of neurovascular compression in two patients only to have complaints of "lightning-like" pain down the arms when the shoulders were hunched forward, causing the inner end of the lateral fragment to impinge on the brachial plexus. Relief followed total claviculectomy with removal of the periosteum.

In recent years, transaxillary resection of the first rib, developed by Roos and Owens in 1966, has been the procedure favored by many surgeons to relieve symptoms due to pressure on the brachial plexus (thoracic outlet syndrome) (Miller, 1981; Urschel and Razzuk, 1972, 1986, 1995, 1998). Other approaches for first rib resection include supraclavicular, posterior (thoracoplasty), or combined (supraclavicular and thoracoplasty). It should be emphasized that for the occasional operator, total claviculectomy combined with scalenectomy is the safest surgical approach (Lord and Urschel, 1988).

Following the initial success of total claviculectomy as the preferred treatment for intractable thoracic outlet syndrome in the early 1950s, excellent functional result and adequate cosmetic appearance have justified its use for other problems involving the clavicle and shoulder. To know that one does not lose significant shoulder function by resection of the clavicle on one side is valuable, but to know that if both clavicles are resected, the patient is not significantly debilitated is even more helpful when planning any kind of treatment.

■ *REFERENCES*

Aziz S, Straehley CJ, Whelan TJ Jr: Effort-related axillo-subclavian vein thrombosis: A new theory of pathogenesis and a plea for direct surgical intervention. Am J Surg 152:57, 1986.

Elkin DC, Cooper FW: Resection of the clavicle in vascular surgery. J Bone Joint Surg 28:117, 1946.

Gurd FB: Surplus parts of the skeleton: A recommendation for the excision of certain portions as a means of shortening the period of disability following trauma. Am J Surg 74:705, 1947.

Lord JW Jr: Surgical management of shoulder girdle syndromes: New operative procedures for hyperabduction, costoclavicular, cervical rib, and scalenus anticus syndromes. Arch Surg 66:69, 1953.

Lord JW, Urschel HC Jr: Total claviculectomy. Surg Rounds 11:17, 1988.

Miller DS: Review of Greep JM, Lemmens HAJ et al: Pain in shoulder and arm: An integrated view. Int Surg 66:373, 1981.

Roos DB, Owens JC: Thoracic outlet syndrome. Arch Surg 93:71, 1966.

Schumacker HB Jr: Resection of the clavicle, with particular reference to the use of bone chips in the periosteal bed. Surg Gynecol Obstet 84:245, 1947.

Urschel HC Jr, Razzuk MA: Current concepts: Management of the thoracic outlet syndrome. N Engl J Med 286:1140, 1972.

Urschel HC Jr, Razzuk MA: The failed operation for thoracic outlet syndrome: The difficulty of diagnosis and management. Ann Thorac Surg 42:523, 1986.

Urschel HC Jr: Thoracic Outlet Syndrome: Atlas of Thoracic Surgery. NY, Churchill-Livingstone, 1995.

Urschel HC Jr, Razzuk MA: Neurovascular decompression in the thoracic outlet: Changing management over 50 years. Ann Thorac Surg 609:617, 1998.

Urschel HC Jr, Razzuk MA: Paget-Schroetter syndrome: What is the best management? Ann Thorac Surg 69:1663, 2000.

Wright IS: The neurovascular syndrome produced by hyperabduction of the arms: Immediate changes produced in 150 normal controls and effects on some persons of prolonged hyperabduction of the arms, as in sleeping and in certain occupations. Am Heart J 29:1, 1945.

Diaphragm

CHAPTER **56**

The Diaphragm

ANATOMY, EMBRYOLOGY, PATHOPHYSIOLOGY, AND SURGERY OF THE PHRENIC NERVE AND DIAPHRAGM

Konstadinos A. Plestis
Stanley C. Fell

The diaphragm is the major muscle of ventilation. It is a dome-shaped, musculofibrous sheet that separates the thoracic cavity from the abdominal cavity. Its periphery consists of three groups of muscular fibers that converge into a central tendon. These muscular fibers originate from the lower six ribs bilaterally, from small slips arising from the posterior aspect of the xiphoid process, from the medial and lateral arcuate ligaments, and from the lumbar vertebrae by two pillars or crura. The medial and lateral arcuate ligaments are tendinous bands that extend the vertebral attachments of the diaphragm across the upper portion of the psoas major and quadratus lumborum muscles. The right crus, broader and longer than the left, arises from the upper three lumbar vertebrae, while the left crus arises from the corresponding upper two lumbar vertebrae. The medial margins of the two crura meet in the midline to form a poorly defined arch above the aorta, the median arcuate ligament. The right crus forms the esophageal hiatus in 64% of individuals; however, it is not uncommon (34% of individuals) that fibers of the left crus take part in the formation of the right side of the esophageal orifice. Also, in 2% of individuals the left crus makes up the major part of the esophageal hiatus (Collis, 1968). The central tendon is a roughly trifoliate aponeurosis. Its two lateral leaves relate to the parietal pleura superiorlyand the peritoneum inferiorly, while the middle leaf is fused to the pericardium superiorly and relates to the triangular ligament of the liver in the abdomen.

Embryologically, the diaphragm arises from five morphologic elements: the central tendon, two ventrolateral parts, and two dorsal parts. The central tendon is formed from the transverse septum, the ventrolateral portions arise from the ventrolongitudinal muscle layer of the body, and the dorsal portions are derived from the paravertebral musculature. These five segments fuse and leave a pleuroperitoneal foramen posteriorly in each side of the thoracic cavity. These two foramina close early in fetal life. The openings through which congenital and acquired diaphragmatic hernias occur are the pleuroperitoneal openings posteriorly; two small passages anteriorly, just behind the sternum; and the esophageal hiatus between the two dorsal divisions of the diaphragm.

Contraction of the costal portion of the diaphragm causes the lower ribs to elevate with concomitant flattening of the diaphragmatic convexity, thus enlarging the thoracic cavity. Similarly, contraction of the crural portion adds downward displacement of the diaphragm with a lesser effect on overall ventilation. Diaphragmatic contraction occurs during the early phases of expiration during quiet breathing.

During expiration, the anterior and inferior margins of the lung do not extend as far forward and inferiorly as the corresponding portions of the pleural space. These portions of the pleural cavity that are entered by the lung only during inspiration are termed pleural recesses; therefore, penetrating wounds or inaccurately placed thoracic drainage tubes do not enter the pleural space (Robinson and Brodman, 1981).

The arterial supply to the diaphragm is largely via the right and left inferior phrenic arteries, the intercostal arteries, and the musculophrenic branches of the internal thoracic artery. There are minor contributions from the pericardiophrenic arteries that run with the phrenic nerves, entering the diaphragm where the nerve penetrates. Venous drainage of the diaphragm is via the inferior phrenic veins, which drain into the inferior vena

*Supported by the Feldesman Fund for Thoracic Surgery at Montefiore Medical Center.

cava. In the thorax venous drainage is via the azygos and hemiazygos vein system. Necrosis of the diaphragm because of vascular insufficiency has not been reported. Motor and sensory innervation of the diaphragm is via the phrenic nerves. The lower six or seven intercostal nerves distribute some sensory fibers to the peripheral portion of the diaphragm.

The diaphragm has three major apertures: the aortic, the esophageal, and the inferior vena cava. It also has a number of smaller ones. The esophageal hiatus, elliptical in shape, is located at the level of T10, just left of the midline and anterior to the aortic hiatus. It transmits the esophagus, the vagi and sympathetic trunks, esophageal branches of the left gastric vessels, and lymphatic vessels. The fascia on the inferior surface of the diaphragm extends upward into the opening in a conical fashion to attach to the wall of the esophagus about 2 cm above the gastroesophageal junction. This fascial expansion limiting the upward displacement of the esophagus is known as the phrenoesophageal ligament. The vena cava traverses the right leaf of the central tendon of the diaphragm at the level of the T8-T9 intervertebral disk. The inferior vena cava orifice is stretched during diaphragmatic contraction, thus facilitating the flow of venous blood into the thorax during inspiration. Small branches of the right phrenic nerve and a few lymphatics also traverse the vena cava orifice. The aortic aperture, strictly speaking, is an osseoaponeurotic opening, located anterior to the lower border of T12, between the crura and behind the median arcuate ligament. The aortic aperture also transmits the azygos vein, the thoracic duct, and lymphatic vessels that ascend from the cisterna chyli to the thorax.

There are also two lesser apertures in each crus, one transmitting the greater splanchnic nerve and the other, the lesser splanchnic nerve. Other structures that pass between the abdomen and the thorax through the diaphragm or posterior to it are the superior epigastric vessels between the sternal and costal origins of the diaphragm, the musculophrenic vessels between the diaphragmatic origins at the level of the T7-T8 cartilages, the lower five intercostal nerves at the level of the T7 cartilage inferiorly, the sympathetic trunk deep to the medial arcuate ligament, and the inferior hemiazygos vein.

There may be a triangular gap between the sternal and costal origins of the diaphragm bilaterally, where the pleura and the peritoneum are separated merely by loose areolar tissue. Similarly, the muscular fibers of the diaphragm may be deficient between the costal portion of the diaphragm and the portion arising from the lateral arcuate ligament bilaterally. These potential spaces are not as common as the parasternal spaces, and when they exist the superior surface of the kidney is separated from the pleura only by areolar tissue. It is through these potential spaces that congenital diaphragmatic hernia may occur in the adult. In contrast to the acute, often life-threatening symptoms of congenital diaphragmatic hernia in the neonate, this entity is almost always asymptomatic in the adult population (MacDougal et al, 1963). On routine chest radiographs, congenital diaphragmatic hernia may easily be misinterpreted as mediastinal or pulmonary tumors (Raymond et al, 1996). The most common finding on a chest radiograph is a well-defined, usually rounded, homogeneous mass in the lower right lung field, occupying the cardiophrenic angle on the posteroanterior view. The frequent use of computed tomography (CT) scans has led to an increase in the diagnosis of congenital diaphragmatic hernia in asymptomatic adults (Figs. 56–1 and 56–2).

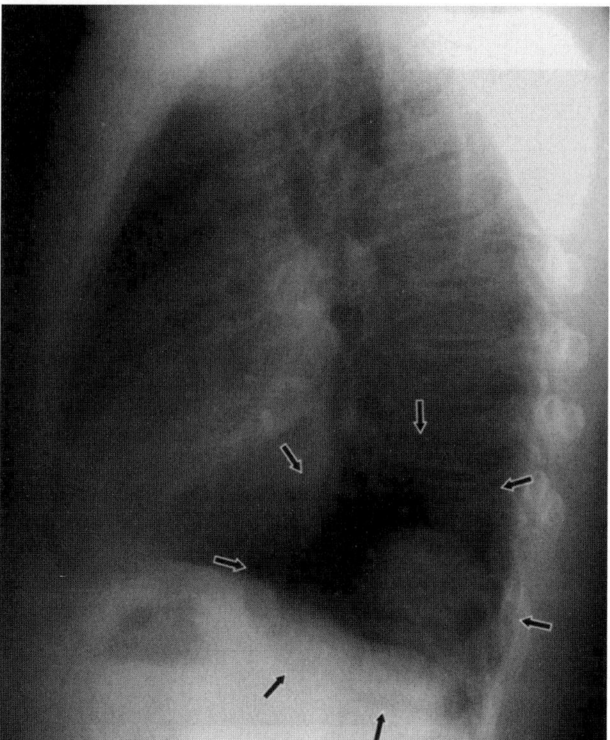

FIGURE 56–1 ■ Lateral chest film demonstrating intrathoracic tumor in an asymptomatic patient.

Morgagni's hernia is rare; a cumulative 3.6% incidence of Morgagni's hernia has been found among all patients with congenital diaphragmatic hernias (Berandi et al, 1997). It is more common in adults than in children. It

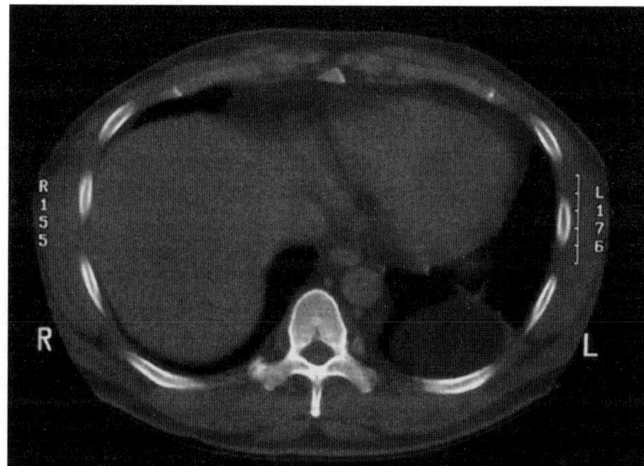

FIGURE 56–2 ■ A computed tomography (CT) scan demonstrates a Bochdalek hernia containing retroperitoneal fat. Surgical repair was not performed.

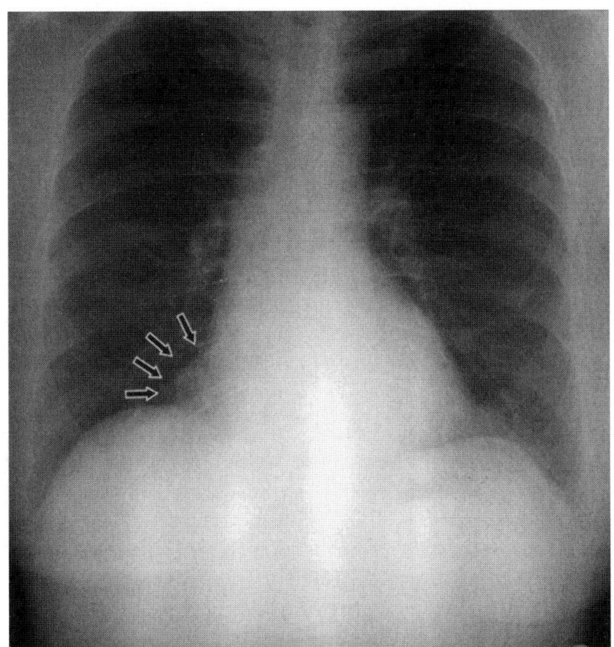

FIGURE 56–3 ■ A chest film of elderly female, interpreted as demonstrating a juxtapericardial fat pad.

occurs parasternally through a defect between the costal and sternal origins of the diaphragm, as previously described. Morgagni's hernia is almost always asymptomatic (Figs. 56–3 and 56–4). When present, symptoms are usually gastrointestinal, such as epigastric discomfort or bloating. Rarely, intestinal obstruction may occur. These hernias are more common on the right hemidiaphragm because the pericardium protects the left side of the diaphragm; occasionally they occur bilaterally. Obese, elderly females are most usually affected. A sac is almost always present, and omentum and colon are the usual contents. Surgical repair, when indicated, is best performed via a subcostal transperitoneal approach. The contents are reduced, the sac is excised, and the diaphragmatic defect is closed by suturing the edge of the defect to the posterior rectus sheath, and to the lower ribs, if required. Laparoscopic repair and repair via video-assisted thoracoscopic surgery (VATS) have been described in symptomatic patients, the former being technically easier than the latter (Hussong et al, 1997; Newman et al, 1995). The hernia sac should not be removed during laparoscopic repair, as this may result in massive pneumomediastinum with potential cardiorespiratory complications.

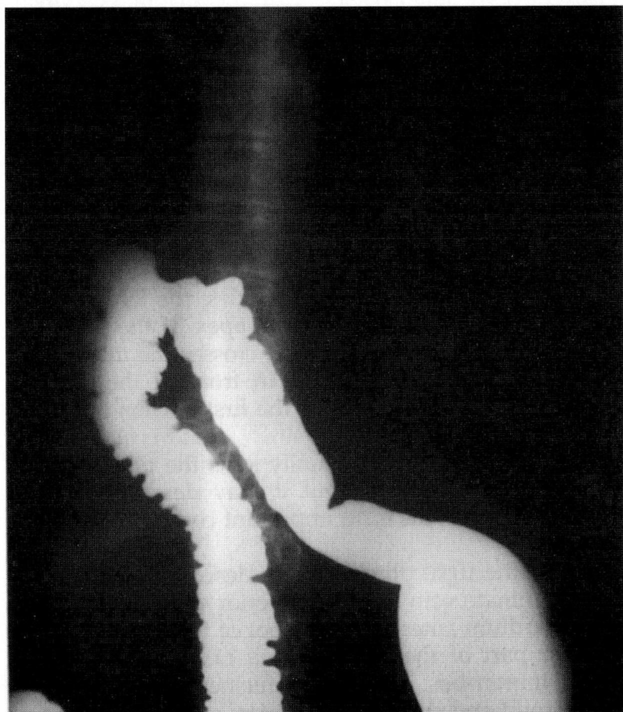

FIGURE 56–4 ■ A barium enema, in the same patient as that in Figure 56–3, performed to investigate sigmoid colon, demonstrates a Morgagni hernia. Surgery was not indicated in this case.

Bochdalek's hernia has been reported in up to 6% of the adult population (Gale, 1985). These hernias may contain retroperitoneal fat, omentum, colon, and stomach (Kirkland, 1959). Right hemidiaphragm occurrence has been reported (Campbell and Lilly, 1982). Symptoms caused by intestinal obstruction or respiratory compromise may be episodic due to spontaneous reduction of herniated viscera. The diagnosis of a Bochdaleck hernia in a patient with intermittent symptoms may prove a challenge despite the most sophisticated diagnostic testing. Repair in the adult is best performed via the transthoracic approach. Large defects may require a prosthetic patch or advancement of the diaphragm to a higher rib for adequate repair. VATS has also been employed in the management of this condition with promising results (Silen et al, 1995).

POROUS DIAPHRAGM SYNDROMES

Porous diaphragm syndrome is defined as the phenomenon of peritoneopleural transphrenic passage of fluids, blood, gases, tissue, and exudates by way of a common pathophysiologic feature, a hole in the diaphragm. Kirschner (1998) was the first to clearly define the various porous diaphragm syndromes (Table 56–1). The defects are usually located in the tendinous portions of the diaphragm between the interlacing tendinous or muscle fibers, and less commonly in the muscular portions of the diaphragm. They may be single, multiple, or even cribriform. Ranging in size from a tiny pinhole to a centimeter or more in diameter, they definitely favor the right hemidiaphragm. Some defects may be congenital; however, the majority are acquired. Kirschner noted that acquired defects occur as a result of challenges to the integrity of the diaphragm by various space-occupying intraperitoneal substances that increase intra-abdominal pressure or produce necrosis of the diaphragm. Clinically, patients usually present with thoracic findings such as pleural effusion, pneumothorax, hemothorax, and empyema secondary to abdominal pathology.

THE PHRENIC NERVE

The phrenic nerve arises chiefly from the C4 nerve root with contributions from the C3 and C5 nerve roots. It

TABLE 56–1 ■ Porous Diaphragm Syndromes

FLUIDS

Spontaneous ascites
Cirrhosis of the liver
Meigs' syndrome
Pancreatic ascites
Chylous ascites
Iatrogenic ascites
Peritoneal dialysis
Hemoperitoneum
Abdominal/tubal pregnancy
Ruptured spleen
Ruptured aortic aneurysm
Operative hemorrhage
Endometriosis

GASES

Pneumoperitoneun
Catamenial pneumothorax
Therapeutic pneumoperitoneum
Spontaneous pneumoperitoneum
Laparoscopic pneumoperitoneum
Diagnostic pneumoperitoneum

TISSUE

Endometriosis
Catamenial pneumothorax
Pleural endometriosis

EXUDATES/SECRETIONS

Subphrenic abscess
Liver abscess
Pancreatic pseudocyst
Bilothorax

INTESTINAL CONTENTS

Perforated peptic ulcer disease

From Kirschner PA: Porous diaphragm syndromes. Chest Surg Clin North Am 8:449–472, 1998; with permission.

originates on the scalenus medius, at the lateral border of the scalenus anterior under the sternomastoid muscle, at the level of the upper border of the thyroid cartilage. It descends on this muscle beneath a tough fascial investment, crossing the muscle from its lateral to its medial border on the way to the thoracic outlet. At the root of the neck, the phrenic nerve is crossed by the transverse cervical and suprascapular arteries; the left phrenic nerve is crossed also by the thoracic duct. At the apex of the thorax the right phrenic nerve lies behind the innominate vein and crosses the internal mammary artery laterally to medially, usually in front of the artery. The left phrenic nerve descends on the front of the first portion of the subclavian artery to enter the thorax. The C5 nerve root usually joins the phrenic nerve trunk on the surface of the scalenus anterior. However, it may descend into the thorax before it joins the main nerve. This is an important consideration in diaphragmatic pacing. In the thorax the right phrenic nerve descends along the right side of the innominate vein and the superior vena cava, and then along the side of the pericardium anterior to the hilum of the lung. It then passes along the upper border of the inferior vena cava to just above the diaphragm where it branches. The left phrenic nerve descends between the left common carotid and subclavian arteries crossing in front of the left vagus nerve, then passing lateral to the arch of the aorta continuing down the side of the pericardium where it branches.

Merendino and associates (1956) clearly established the anatomic and physiologic distribution of the phrenic nerves at the diaphragm, and they also developed the strategy for diaphragmatic incisions. Their findings are freely quoted or paraphrased. The right phrenic nerve reaches the diaphragm just lateral to the inferior vena cava, while the left phrenic nerve enters the diaphragm lateral to the left border of the heart, in a slightly more anterior plane than the right phrenic nerve. Both nerves divide at the level of the diaphragm or just above it into several terminal branches, the right phrenic nerve being the mirror image of the left. Two or three of these terminal branches are usually very fine and are distributed to the serosal surfaces of the diaphragm. Three muscular branches arise directly from the phrenic nerve; one is directed anteromedially toward the sternum, another is directed laterally anterior to the lateral leaf of the central tendon, and the third one is directed posteriorly. The last-mentioned ramus divides into a branch that runs posterior to the lateral leaf of the tendon, and a branch that runs posteriorly and medially to the region of the crus. These four branches are named the sternal or anterior branch, the anterolateral branch, the posterolateral branch, and the crural or posterior branch (Fig. 56–5). They are usually located deep within the muscle rather than lying exposed on the undersurface of the diaphragm as it is described in anatomic texts. Because of the rapid diminution in the size of the phrenic nerve rami, it is impractical to delineate areas in the diaphragm where incisions can be made safely. However, circumferential incisions anywhere in the periphery of the diaphragm result in little, if any, loss of diaphragmatic function (Fig. 56–6). Similarly, incisions in the central tendon and lateral or transverse incisions from the midaxillary line medially do not result in diaphragmatic paralysis (Sicular, 1992). Prior to Merendino's seminal work, radial incisions in the diaphragm were customarily employed. The radial incision in the diaphragm from the costal margin to the esophageal hiatus results in almost total diaphragmatic paralysis, and it should be condemned (Fig. 56–7). The radial incision was a major cause of postoperative morbidity and mortality in patients subjected to thoracolaparotomy; it resulted in ineffective cough, lower lobe atelectasis, and associated pneumonia. Nevertheless, it is still described in the literature (Heitmiller, 1992).

Technique for Diaphragmatic Incision

A circumferential incision is made with electrocautery 3 cm from the costal margin. The cut edges of the diaphragm are grasped with Allis clamps and elevated, facilitating further incision. Bleeders are managed with electrocautery, but large branches of the phrenic artery are best controlled with suture ligatures. When a diaphragmatic incision is made in association with antireflux procedures, it is best to use only the anterolateral two thirds of the diaphragm. Stay sutures are placed in the diaphragmatic flap and elevated over the rib spreader, as described

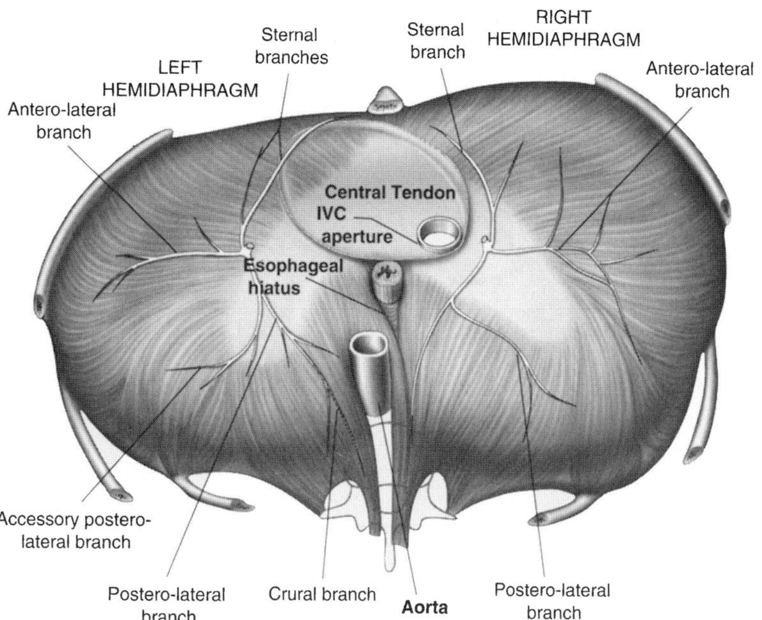

FIGURE 56–5 ■ Branches of the phrenic nerve at the diaphragm. (Adapted from Meredino KA, Johnson RS, Skinner HH et al: The intradiaphragmatic distribution of the phrenic nerve with particular reference to the placement of diaphragmatic incisions and controlled segmental paralysis. Surgery 39:189, 1956.)

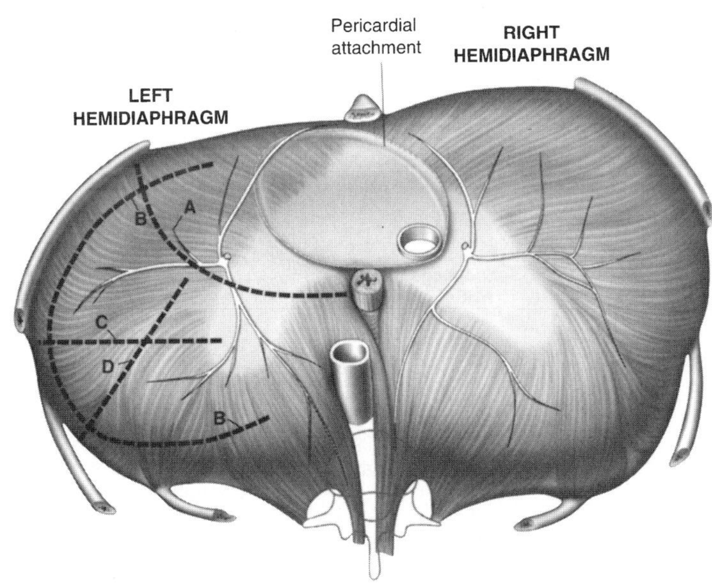

FIGURE 56–6 ■ Diaphragm incisions. (*A,* radial incision; *B,* circumferential incision; *C* and *D,* incisions in safe areas.) (Adapted from Meredino KA, Johnson RS, Skinner HH et al: The intradiaphragmatic distribution of the phrenic nerve with particular reference to the placement of diaphragmatic incisions and controlled segmental paralysis. Surgery 39:189, 1956.)

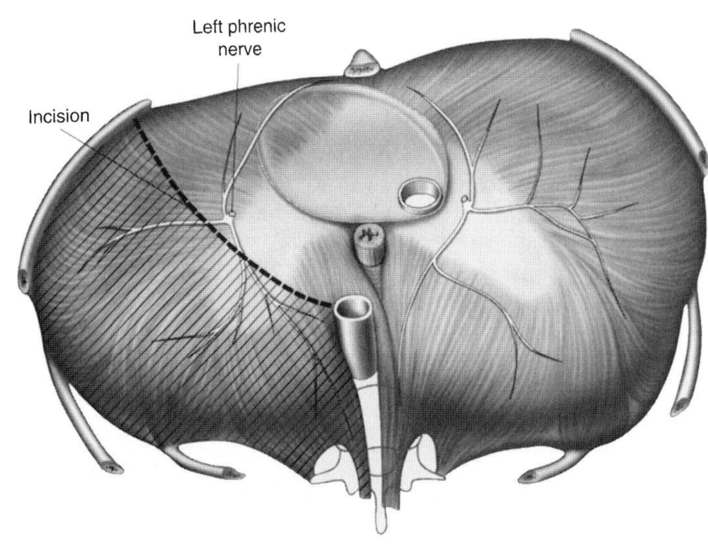

FIGURE 56–7 ■ A radial incision that can cause paralysis of a major portion of phrenic nerve. (Adapted from Meredino KA, Johnson RS, Skinner HH et al: The intradiaphragmatic distribution of the phrenic nerve with particular reference to the placement of diaphragmatic incisions and controlled segmental paralysis. Surgery 39:189, 1956.)

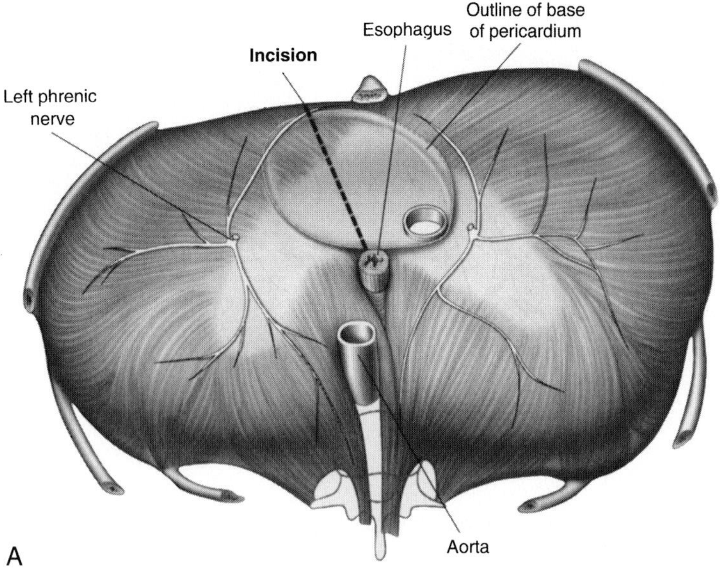

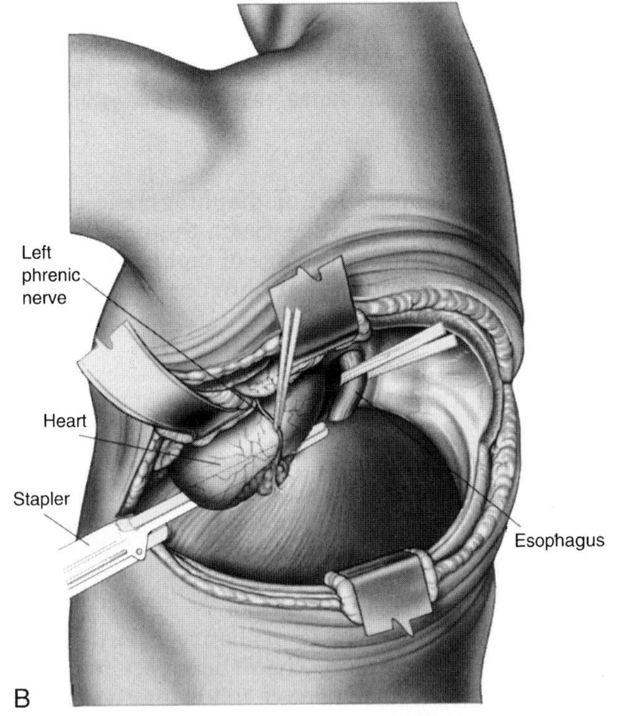

FIGURE 56–8 ■ Septum transversum incision for transdiaphragmatic exposure of the cardia. *A*, Cross-section view; *B*, side view. (Adapted from Meredino KA, Johnson RS, Skinner HH et al: The intradiaphragmatic distribution of the phrenic nerve with particular reference to the placement of diaphragmatic incisions and controlled segmental paralysis. Surgery 39:189, 1956; and Sicular A: Direct septum transversum incision to replace circumferential diaphragmatic incision in operations of the cardia. Am J Surg 164:167, 1992.)

by Collis (1968). This maneuver gives ample exposure to the "attic of the abdomen" and simplifies management of the vasa brevia and the gastrohepatic ligament. By retracting the stay sutures caudally, the operator can dissect the intrathoracic aspect of the diaphragmatic attachment to the esophagogastric junction with two fingers inserted in the abdomen while dissecting the chest, allowing for repair of the crura in the abdomen and performance of a fundoplication before closure of the diaphragmatic incision. For left transthoracic esophagogastric resections, the circumferential incision may be carried down to the esophageal hiatus. If the tumor is adherent to the diaphragm, wide resection of the diaphragm can be easily performed using this technique. The diaphragmatic incision through the central tendon described by Sicular (1992) is shorter compared with the circumferential incision and has the advantage of rapid performance (Fig. 56–8). However, it does impose some risk of trauma to the left phrenic nerve. Incisions in the diaphragm should be closed with two layers of nonabsorbable sutures. A first layer of interrupted mattress sutures is followed by a layer of continuous polypropylene sutures. This technique obviates the risk of diaphragmatic disruption, which is a known complication of diaphragmatic closure with absorbable sutures.

Phrenic Nerve Injury

Causes of phrenic nerve injury are listed in Table 56–2. Cardiac procedures in both the pediatric and adult popu-

TABLE 56–2 ■ Causes of Phrenic Nerve Injury

Cervical
Birth injury
Blunt-penetrating trauma: spine or soft tissue
Operative injury
Neck surgery: thyroid, neck dissection, splenectomy
Jugular vein cannulation
Deliberate: crush, exeresis for tuberculosis
Thoracic
Trauma
Operative injury
Thymectomy/mediastinal tumor
Pulmonary resection
Deliberate: pneumonectomy, hiatal hernia repair
Blalock-Taussig shunt
Pericardiectomy
Aortic arch aneurysms
CABG: pericardial traction, topical hypothermia, ITA harvest
Neoplastic
Lung cancer
Malignant mediastinal tumor
Lymphoma
Infectious
Typhoid, pneumonias
Viral: polio, herpes zoster, rubella
Idiopathic
(Probable undiagnosed viral infection)

CABG, coronary artery bypass graft; ITA, internal thoracic artery.

lations are the most common cause of phrenic nerve injury with resultant paralysis of the hemidiaphragm. Phrenic nerve injury during cardiac procedures may result from transection, contusion, and stretch or thermal injury. Thermal injury may be due to heat caused by the injudicious application of electrocautery or due to cold following topical cardiac hypothermia. In a series of 831 closed cardiac surgical procedures in infants and children, Zhao and co-workers (1985) noted an incidence of phrenic nerve injury in 2.1% of cases. This injury is most commonly noted following systemic–pulmonary artery anastomosis, atrial septectomy, or combined pulmonary artery banding and ligation of a patent ductus arteriosus. The most frequent cause of phrenic nerve injury during operations for acquired heart disease is from the intrapericardial application of saline slush as a means of myocardial preservation. The incidence of this complication has been reported to be as high as 73%. However, it was reduced to 17% with the use of an insulating pad to protect the phrenic nerves (Esposito and Spencer, 1987). Typically the left hemidiaphragm is most commonly affected, although bilateral injuries are occasionally noted. The proximity of the phrenic nerves to the internal mammary artery puts them at risk during harvest of the artery for coronary artery bypass procedures. Nerve injury in these cases is usually caused by thermal injury from cautery dissection or due to stretch injury (Markland et al, 1985). Phrenic nerve paralysis was formerly employed as an adjunct to collapse therapy for tuberculosis. Resection of the phrenic nerve was performed to ensure total and permanent paralysis (Fig. 56–9), while in other instances phrenic nerve crush was used. After the latter procedure, diaphragmatic function usually returned in 6 months; however, it was permanent in 20% of cases (Iverson et al, 1966). Notably, in 50% of these patients there was delayed evidence of diminished diaphragmatic function resulting in ventilatory loss. Currently, temporary paralysis of the phrenic nerve can be instituted during thoracotomy by local anesthetic injection. This technique is used occasionally to diminish the pleural space following pulmonary resections. Pneumoperitoneum is instituted concomitantly to facilitate elevation of the diaphragm.

In the postoperative patient who is supine and on ventilatory support, diaphragmatic paralysis may not be suspected because positive-pressure ventilation tends to mask abnormal findings. In the spontaneously breathing patient, left pleural effusion, lower lobe atelectasis, and elevation of the left hemidiaphragm are, unfortunately, common sequelae of cardiac surgery and may mask phrenic nerve injury. Similarly, diaphragmatic paralysis is difficult to diagnose by either chest radiography or fluoroscopy. In cases with a high index of suspicion, phrenic nerve conduction studies are required (Russel et al, 1991). Measurement of phrenic nerve conduction time allows direct evaluation of phrenic nerve function and integrity. An electrical stimulus is applied over the phrenic nerve in the neck and a diaphragmatic electromyogram from T7 and T8 intercostal spaces is displayed on a storage oscilloscope. Prolongation of the phrenic latency by more than 2 msec is considered indicative of phrenic nerve paralysis. This test can establish the diagnosis at the bedside, and if it is serially performed, may prognosticate recovery. In cases in which recovery of phrenic nerve function is expected, prolonged ventilatory support is indicated.

In the nonacute situation, elevation of the hemidiaphragm on chest radiograph may suggest paralysis. Flu-

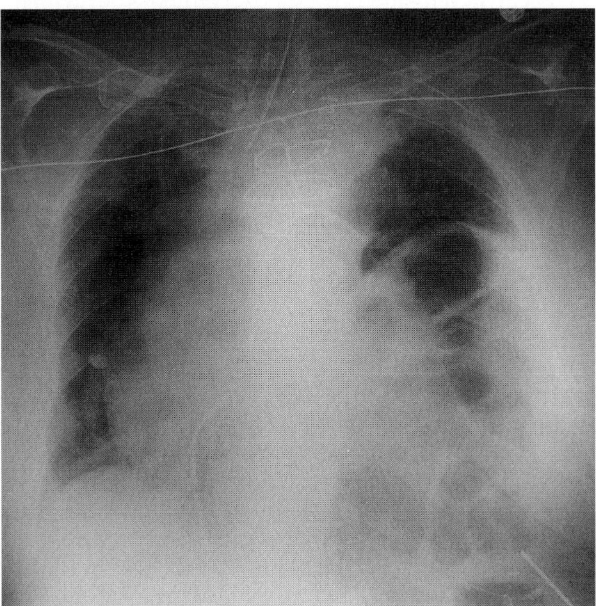

FIGURE 56–9 ■ Chest film of 70-year-old female who had phrenicectomy for treatment of pulmonary tuberculosis 40 years prior to her coronary artery bypass.

oroscopy is considered the most reliable method to document diaphragmatic paralysis. The diagnosis is established by the "sniff test," which demonstrates paradoxical motion of the diaphragm on fluoroscopy. The paradoxical excursion should involve the entire hemidiaphragm and should exceed 2 cm for establishment of the diagnosis of diaphragmatic paralysis (Alexander, 1996). However, paradoxical movement of the diaphragm has been noted in 6% of normal subjects during the sniff test (Shim, 1980).

Pathophysiology of Diaphragmatic Paralysis

Infants are more likely to have respiratory difficulties from diaphragmatic paralysis than older children and adults. The intercostal and accessory muscles of respiration in infants do not contribute significantly to respiratory mechanics; thus unilateral diaphragmatic paralysis may produce a 50% loss in pulmonary function (Mickell et al, 1978). Because infants are customarily maintained in the recumbent position, there is further reduction in vital capacity. Also, the mobile mediastinum of the infant is shifted to the nonaffected side, further diminishing pulmonary function. Further, the narrow airway in infants predisposes to bronchial obstruction from retained secretions that cannot be readily evacuated by crying or cough.

In normal adults, diaphragmatic excursion may contribute 30% to 60% of total tidal volume. With unilateral diaphragmatic paralysis, there is a decrease of 20% to 30% of vital capacity and maximum voluntary ventilation, and a 20% decrease in oxygen uptake on the involved side, as well as decreased residual volume and total lung capacity (Zhao et al, 1985). Hypoxemia and hypercapnia result. These numbers increase when patients are supine. Disabling gastroesophageal reflux may occur in left-sided paresis. These findings are increased with the patient supine. Disabling gastroesophageal reflux may occur in left-sided paresis. Nevertheless, in patients with sufficient respiratory reserve, unilateral diaphragmatic paralysis may not be symptomatic despite the ventilatory losses previously noted.

Treatment of Diaphragmatic Paralysis

A few cases of repair of a transected phrenic nerve have been reported, without documentation of success by electrophysiologic testing (Merav et al, 1983; Shoemaker et al, 1981). The management of phrenic nerve injury and diaphragmatic paralysis in infants following cardiac surgery is still controversial. Some authors have used ventilatory support in excess of 1 month for managing this problem and rarely do they employ diaphragmatic plication (Zhao et al, 1985). In Mickell and co-workers's series (1978) 19 of 32 patients demonstrated complete resolution of diaphragmatic paralysis, 9 were asymptomatic with persistent defect, and 1 patient was treated with surgical plication. Shoemaker and co-workers (1981) demonstrated reduction in the duration of ventilatory support, extubating his patients within 6 days following diaphragmatic plication. It is clear that intraoperative recognition of phrenic nerve injury in the neonate is an indication for immediate diaphragmatic plication; however, when this injury is noted in a child older than 3 months, it can usually be managed successfully with continuous positive airway pressure through a nasotracheal tube. In 34 cases of diaphragmatic paralysis following pediatric cardiac surgery, it was noted that no patient older than 3 years of age required intubation for longer than 2 weeks (Lynn et al, 1982). Patients younger than 3 years of age who still required intubation and continuous positive airway pressure 3 to 4 weeks following surgery were candidates for diaphragmatic plication because of the potential complications of long-term intubation (pulmonary and systemic infection) and difficulties in maintaining adequate caloric intake. Shoemaker and associates report (1981) confirmed the need for diaphragm plication in infants less than 5 months old.

Most adults with unilateral diaphragmatic paralysis are asymptomatic; those having troublesome dyspnea on exertion or orthopnea may benefit from diaphragmatic plication. Graham and associates (1990) reported 10-year follow-up of 17 patients treated with diaphragmatic plication. All patients were less dyspneic with objective improvement in spirometry and oxygenation. Diaphragmatic plication has also been successfully employed in adults following phrenic nerve injury associated with cardiac surgery and after pneumonectomy with deliberate sacrifice of the phrenic nerve (Glassman et al, 1994; Takeda et al, 1994).

■ *REFERENCES*

Alexander C: Diaphragm movements and a diagnosis of diaphragmatic paralysis. Clin Radiol 17:79–83, 1966.

Berandi RS, Tenquist J, Sauter D et al: An update on the surgical aspects of Morgagni's hernia. Surg Rounds 370–376, 1997.

Campbell DN, Lilly JR: The clinical spectrum of right Bochdalek's hernia. Arch Surg 117:341–344, 1982.

Collis JL: Surgical control of reflux in hiatus hernia. Am J Surg 115:465–471, 1968.

Collis JL, Kelly TD, Wiley AM: Anatomy of the crura of the diaphragm and the surgery of hiatus hernia. Thorax 9:175–189, 1954.

Eposito JA, Spencer FC: The effect of pericardial insulation on hypothermic phrenic nerve injury during open heart surgery. Ann Thorac Surg 43:303–308, 1987.

Gale ME: Bochdaleck hernias: Prevalence and CT characteristics. Radiology 156:449–452, 1985.

Glassman LR, Spencer FC, Bauman G et al: Successful plication for postoperative diaphragmatic paralysis in an adult. Ann Thorac Surg 58:1754–1755, 1994.

Graham ER, Kaplan D, Evans CC et al: Diaphragmatic plication for unilateral diaphragmatic paralysis: A ten-year experience. Ann Thorac Surg 49:248–252, 1990.

Heitmiller R: Results of standard left thoracoabdominal esophagogastrectomy. Semin Thorac Cardiovasc Surg 4:314–319, 1992.

Hussong R, Landreneau R, Cole F: Diagnosis and repair of Morgagni hernia with video assisted thoracic surgery. Ann Thorac Surg 63:1474–1475, 1997.

Iverson LI, Mittal A, Dugan D et al: Injuries to the phrenic nerve resulting in diaphragmatic paralysis with special reference to stretch trauma. Am J Surg 132:263–266, 1966.

Kirkland JA: Congenital posterolateral diaphragmatic hernia in the adult. Br J Surg 47:16–22, 1959.

Kirschner PA: Porous diaphragm syndromes. Chest Surg Clin North Am 8:449–472, 1998.

Lynn A, Jenkins J, Edmonds J: Diaphragmatic paralysis after pediatric cardiac surgery: A retrospective analysis of 34 cases. Crit Care Med 11:280–282, 1982.

MacDougal J, Abbott A, Goodhand T: Herniation through congenital diaphragmatic defects in adults. Can J Surg 6:301–316, 1963.

Markand O, Moorthy S, Mahomed Y: Postoperative phrenic nerve palsy

in patients with open heart surgery. Ann Thorac Surg 39:68–73, 1985.
Merav A, Attai L, Condit D: Successful repair of a transected phrenic nerve with restoration of diaphragmatic function. Chest 84:642–644, 1983.
Merendino KA, Johnson RJ, Skinner HH et al: The intradiaphragmatic distribution of the phrenic nerve with particular reference to the placement of diaphragmatic incisions and controlled segmental paralysis. Surgery 39:189–198, 1956.
Mickell J, Oh K, Siewers R et al: Clinical implications of postoperative unilateral phrenic nerve paralysis. J Thorac Cardiovasc Surg 76:297–304, 1978.
Newman L, Eubanks S, Bridges WM et al: Laparoscopic diagnosis and treatment of Morgagni hernia. Surg Laparosc Endosc 5:27–31, 1995.
Raymond GS, Miller RM, Muller NL, Logan PM: Congenital thoracic lesions that mimic neoplastic disease on chest radiographs of adults. AJR Am J Roentgenol 168:763–769, 1996
Robinson G, Brodman R: Going down the tube. Ann Thorac Surg 31:400–401, 1981.
Russel R, Molvey D, LaRoche C et al: Bedside assessment of phrenic nerve function in infants and children. J Thorac Cardiovasc Surg 101:143–147, 1991.
Shim C: Motor disturbances of the diaphragm. Clin Chest Med 1:125–129, 1980.
Shoemaker R, Palmer G, Brown J et al: Aggressive treatment of acquired phrenic nerve paralysis in infants and small children. Ann Thorac Surg 32:252–259, 1981.
Sicular A: Direct septum transversum incision to replace circumferential diaphragmatic incision in operations on the cardia. Am J Surg 164:167–170, 1992.
Silen ML, Canvasser DA, Kurkchubasce AG et al: Video-assisted thoracic surgical repair of a foramen of Bochdalek hernia. Ann Thorac Surg 60:448–450, 1995.
Takeda S, Nakahara K, Fujii Y et al: Plication of paralyzed hemidiaphragm after right sleeve pneumonectomy. Ann Thorac Surg 58:1755–1778, 1994.
Zhao H, D'Agostino R, Pitlick P et al: Phrenic nerve injury complicating closed cardiovascular surgical procedures for congenital heart disease. Ann Thorac Surg 39:445–449, 1985.

IMAGING OF THE DIAPHRAGM

David S. Gierada
Richard M. Slone
Matthew J. Fleishman

Diagnostic imaging of the diaphragm is challenging due to its thin structure and complex shape. Abnormalities that affect the diaphragm are often first detected on chest radiographs as an alteration in position or shape. Cross-sectional imaging studies, primarily computed tomography (CT) and occasionally magnetic resonance imaging (MRI), can depict structural defects and intrinsic and adjacent pathology in greater detail. Fluoroscopy is the primary radiologic means of evaluating diaphragm motion, although MRI and ultrasound can also image this function. This chapter illustrates the normal appearance of the diaphragm; the evaluation of abnormalities in shape, position, and structure; and the role of imaging in specific conditions, including congenital and acquired hernias, diaphragm paralysis, and diaphragm masses.

THE NORMAL DIAPHRAGM

Radiography

On chest radiographs, the superior margin of each hemidiaphragm with overlying parietal pleura forms a dome-shaped interface separating aerated lung from the opaque soft tissues of the abdomen. The heart with subjacent pericardium and fat forms a relative depression between the two hemidiaphragms, obscuring the central and anteromedial portions of the diaphragm. Intraperitoneal free air outlining the inferior surface of the diaphragm reveals its thinness (Fig. 56–10). A smooth scalloped or polyarcuate contour of the diaphragm is a normal variation, and most frequently involves the right hemidiaphragm. The lumbar portions of the diaphragm occasionally may be seen on the frontal view and the sternocostal insertions are visible on the lateral view when there is adequate x-ray penetration and adjacent fat on both sides.

Several signs help distinguish the right from left hemidiaphragm on the lateral radiograph (Fig. 56–11). The entire anteroposterior (AP) extent of the right hemidiaphragm is usually visible because of its interface with the lung, while a variable segment of the anterior left hemidiaphragm is usually obscured by the adjacent heart and mediastinal fat. Gas in the stomach or splenic flexure of the colon beneath the left hemidiaphragm can be used to identify this side on the lateral projection; interposition of the colon between the liver and right hemidiaphragm is seen in less than 1% of patients (Prassopoulos et al, 1996). Finally, in a left lateral radiograph (left side of the patient is in contact with the film cassette), the right ribs are more magnified than the left ribs. Therefore, the hemidiaphragm that inserts along the margin of the larger ribs can be identified as the right, and vice versa.

Cross-Sectional Imaging

The muscular diaphragm can be seen on cross-sectional imaging studies; however, due to its shape, thinness, and

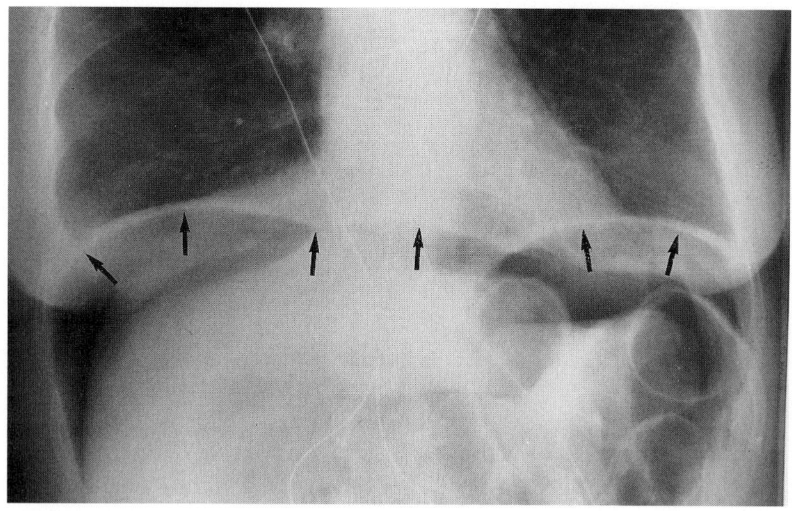

FIGURE 56–10 ■ Normal diaphragm thickness. Erect radiograph reveals the shape and thickness of the diaphragm (*arrows*) in a patient with a large amount of intraperitoneal free air secondary to a bowel perforation. The superior margins of the central, anterior aspect of the diaphragm are obscured by the heart and mediastinal fat. (From Gierada DS, Slone RM, Fleishman MJ: Imaging evaluation of the diaphragm. Chest Surg Clin North Am 8:237, 1998.)

close contact with the liver and spleen, portions are often obscured. On CT, the diaphragm has the attenuation of skeletal muscle, and is best seen where it is surrounded by lower attenuation fat (Fig. 56–12*A*). However, some segments of the diaphragm in contact with the liver or spleen may be visible because the diaphragm enhances to a lesser degree with intravenous contrast (Fig. 56–12*B*). Nodular infoldings of the diaphragm near costal insertions are often seen (Fig. 56–13), particularly in elderly individuals, and these may indent the liver or spleen to simulate focal lesions (Fig. 56–14) or simulate peritoneal implants. The domes of the diaphragm are best depicted using volumetric (helical) CT and coronal or sagittal reformations (Brink et al, 1994).

The direct multiplanar imaging capability of MRI can improve depiction of the diaphragm, which is clinically useful in selected cases. On MRI, the muscular diaphragm has signal intensity similar to skeletal muscle, liver, and spleen on all pulse sequences, and similar to CT, it is best depicted where it is separated from these structures by high signal intensity abdominal or mediastinal fat (Gierada et al, 1996). As on CT studies, the greater enhancement of the liver after intravenous gadolinium administration can improve depiction of the diaphragm with MRI (Kanematsu et al, 1995). Occasionally, short segments are sufficiently thick to allow distinction from the adjacent liver without contrast (Gierada et al, 1996).

The diaphragmatic crura arise from the anterior aspects of the L1-L3 vertebral bodies on the right and the L1 and L2 vertebral bodies on the left (Williams et al, 1989). The right crus is larger, and its medial fibers decussate around the esophagus to form the esophageal hiatus, which may be seen on CT or MRI scans when appropriately oriented in the axial plane (Fig. 56–14*A*). The crura form the boundary of the retrocrural space (Fig. 56–14*B* and *C*). The aortic hiatus, which lies posterior to the esophageal hiatus, and the inferior vena caval hiatus, which passes through the central tendon, are not well depicted in the axial plane, but they may be seen in coronal or sagittal planes.

Lymph nodes along the anterior aspect of the central diaphragm drain the diaphragm, anterior mediastinum, and adjacent liver (Rouviere, 1938). These anterior diaphragmatic (also referred to as pericardial and cardiophrenic angle) lymph nodes are located anterior to the diaphragm and posterior to the xiphoid and adjacent costal cartilages in the cardiophrenic angles (Fig. 56–15). One or two lymph nodes, usually smaller than 5 mm in diameter, are normally visible on CT scans (Aronberg et al, 1986). The inferior pulmonary ligaments (Cooper et al, 1983; Godwin et al, 1983; Rost and Proto, 1983) and phrenic nerves and vessels (Berkmen et al, 1989; Ujita et al, 1993) are sometimes visible along the domes of the diaphragm on CT.

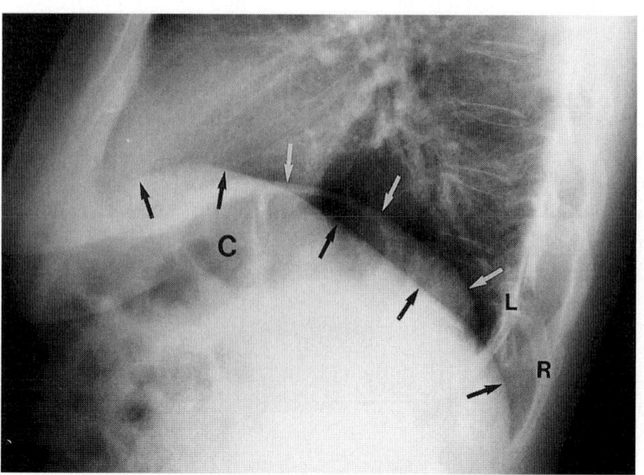

FIGURE 56–11 ■ Distinguishing the hemidiaphragms on the lateral chest radiograph. The right hemidiaphragm (*black arrows*) is visible to the anterior chest wall and extends posteriorly to the margin of the more magnified right ribs (R) on this standard lateral film obtained with the left side of the chest in contact with the film cassette. The left hemidiaphragm (*white arrows*) is obscured anteriorly by the subjacent heart, extends posteriorly to the less magnified left ribs (L), and lies above air-filled colon (C). (From Gierada DS, Slone RM, Fleishman MJ: Imaging evaluation of the diaphragm. Chest Surg Clin North Am 8:237, 1998.)

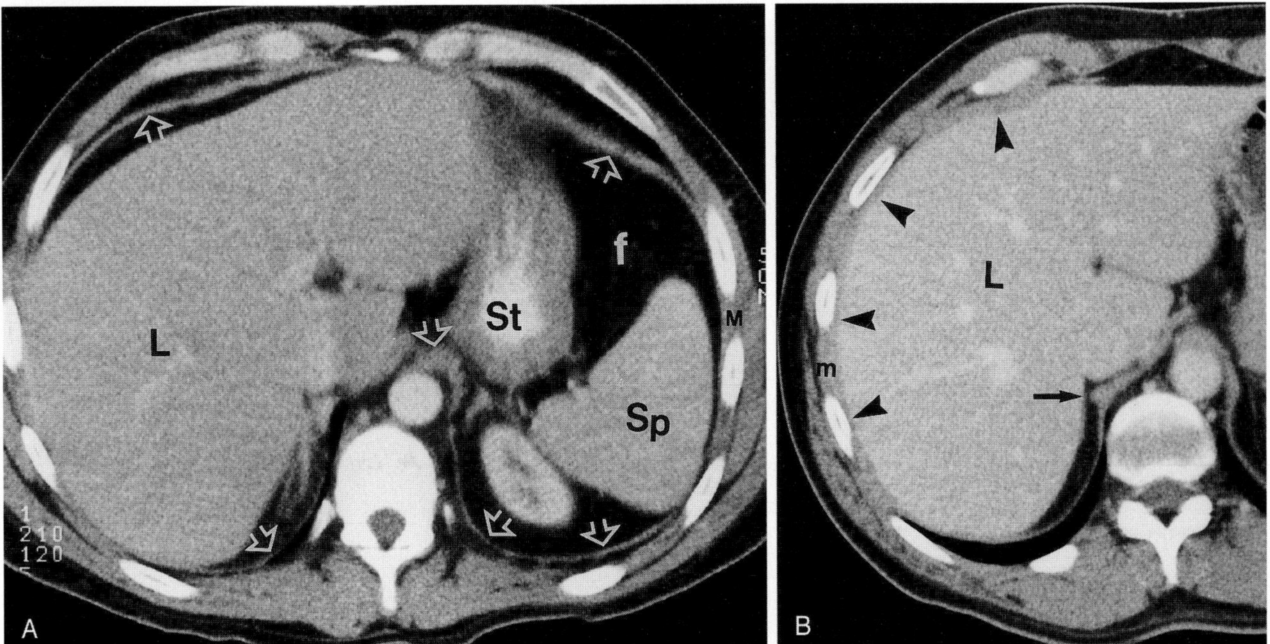

FIGURE 56–12 ■ Normal diaphragm on a contrast enhanced computed tomography scan. *A*, A scan through the upper abdomen in a 30-year-old man reveals portions of the diaphragm (*open arrows*) that have adjacent low attenuation fat (f) or aerated lung. Segments of the diaphragm in contact with structures having similar attenuation such as the liver (L), spleen (Sp), or skeletal muscle (M) are not separately visible. St, stomach. *B*, In this 78-year-old man, the diaphragm (*arrowheads*) enhances less than the liver (L), but the same as skeletal muscle (m) and can be distinguished. Note the normal nodular appearance of the right crus (*black arrow*). (From Gierada DS, Slone RM, Fleishman MJ: Imaging evaluation of the diaphragm. Chest Surg Clin North Am 8:237, 1998.)

The diaphragm can also be seen using ultrasound. Although of similar echogenicity to the liver, the diaphragm can be distinguished because the acoustic impedance of these structures differs, resulting in specular reflections that delineate the interface between them. However, the field of view with ultrasound is limited, and the diaphragm is more difficult to see in obese patients, in whom liver is positioned higher up under the rib cage, and in areas where the sound waves are blocked by air in the stomach or intestines. Hence, ultrasound is used infrequently in clinical evaluation.

Abnormalities Affecting the Diaphragm

ABNORMALITIES OF DIAPHRAGM POSITION

Alterations in diaphragm position or contour seen on chest radiographs may be due to intrathoracic or intra-abdominal processes, or they may be intrinsically related to the diaphragm. Normally, the dome of the right hemidiaphragm projects at about the level of the anterior 6th

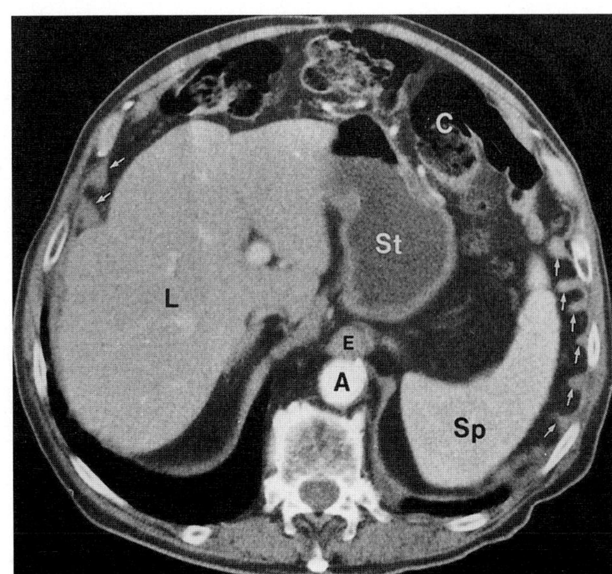

FIGURE 56–13 ■ Nodular diaphragm folds. Image in a 76-year-old man demonstrates multiple normal nodular infoldings of the right and left hemidiaphragm (*arrows*). (A, aorta; C, colon; E, esophagus; L, liver; Sp, spleen; St, stomach.) (From Gierada DS, Slone RM, Fleishman MJ: Imaging evaluation of the diaphragm. Chest Surg Clin North Am 8:237, 1998.)

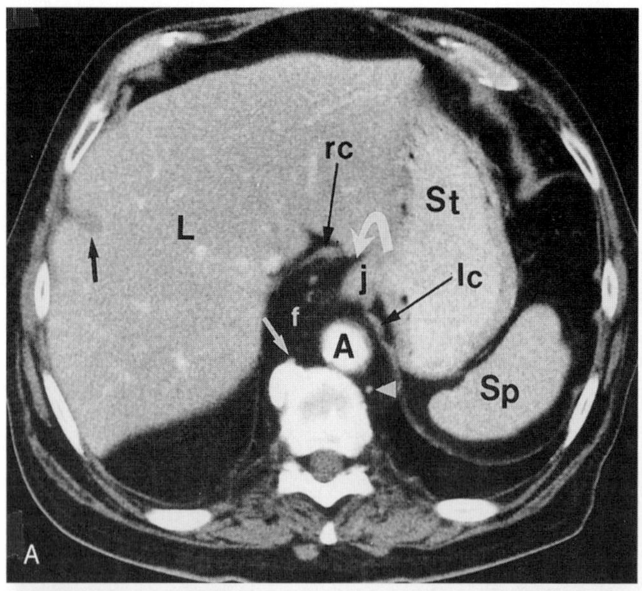

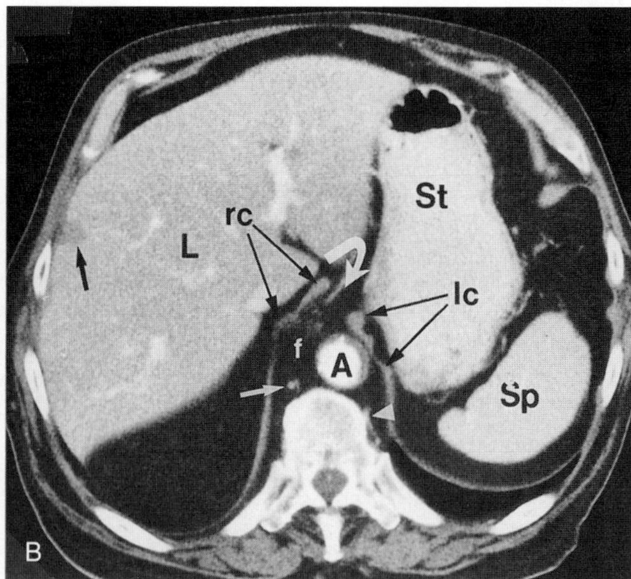

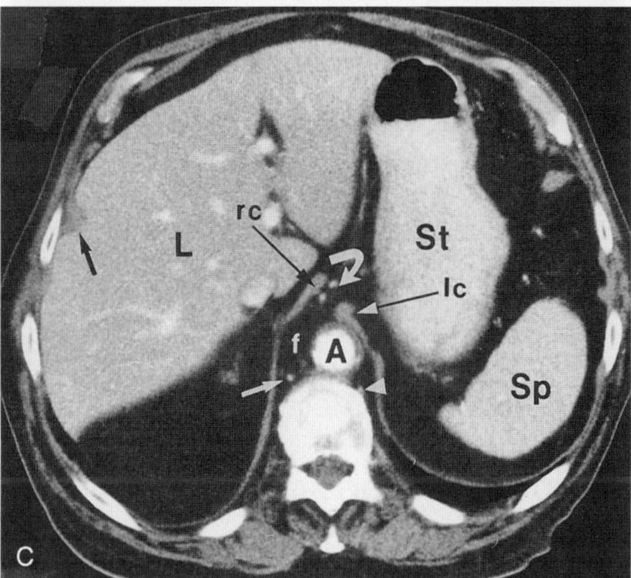

FIGURE 56–14 ■ Normal variation of costal diaphragm slips and normal retrocrural space. *A*, A computed tomography scan through the upper abdomen reveals a nodular, low attenuation focus surrounded by hepatic parenchyma (*black arrow*). *B* and *C*, On successive caudal images, the nodular focus is seen to be contiguous with a thickened portion of the diaphragm near its costal attachment. Also note the esophageal hiatus (*curved arrow*) bordered by the right (rc) and left (lc) crura. The crura outline the retrocrural space, which contains the aorta (A), lower posterior mediastinal fat (f), azygos (*white arrow*) and hemiazygos (*arrowhead*) veins. Smaller structures adjacent to the azygos vein likely represent the thoracic duct and tiny lymph nodes. (A, aorta; j, gastroesophageal junction; L, liver; Sp, spleen; St, stomach.) (From Gierada DS, Slone RM, Fleishman MJ: Imaging evaluation of the diaphragm. Chest Surg Clin North Am 8:237, 1998.)

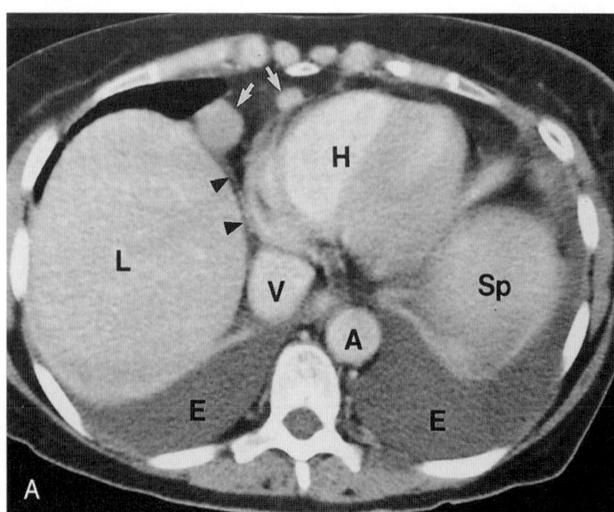

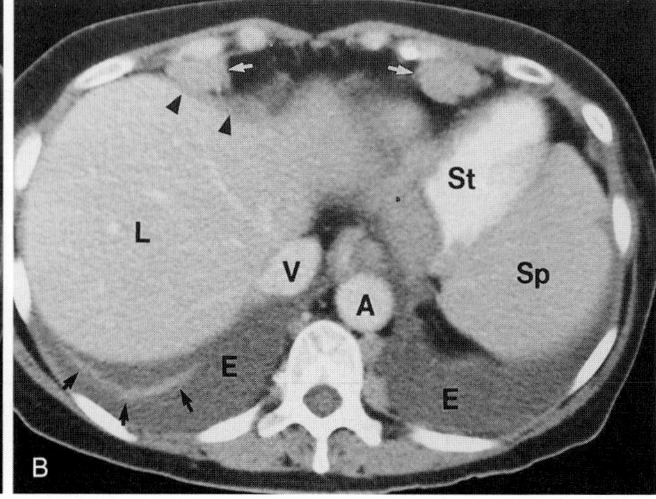

FIGURE 56–15 ■ Anterior diaphragmatic lymphadenopathy in a patient with lymphoma. *A* and *B*, A computed tomography scan shows enlarged lymph nodes (*white arrows*) in the pericardial fat, anterior to the diaphragm (*arrowheads*). Note the thin enhancing caudal tip of atelectatic lung (*black arrows*), not to be mistaken for the diaphragm. (A, aorta; E, pleural effusion; H, heart; L, liver; Sp, spleen; St, stomach; V, inferior vena cava.)

rib and posterior 10th rib on erect PA chest radiographs obtained in full inspiration (Juhl, 1987; Lennon and Simon, 1965). It may be slightly higher (one-half rib level) in obese individuals and lower in thin persons. The left hemidiaphragm is usually positioned up to one rib interspace, or several centimeters, below the right hemidiaphragm (Armstrong et al, 1995; Juhl, 1987; Tarver et al, 1989), although in about 10% of normal subjects it is at the same level or slightly higher (Felson, 1973).

CT usually helps in further assessment of diaphragm position or contour abnormalities, and sometimes it reveals unsuspected abnormalities when it is performed for other indications. The primary indication for MRI of the diaphragm is assessment of congenital or acquired hernias. Suspected diaphragm paralysis is assessed using fluoroscopy.

Unilateral Elevation

Lung volume loss is one of the most common causes of unilateral hemidiaphragm elevation (Table 56–3); it can be due to atelectasis, partial lung resection, radiation or post-inflammatory fibrosis, or congenital hypoplasia. Additional signs of volume loss that may be present include ipsilateral shifting of mediastinal structures and narrowing of the intercostal spaces. Malignant mesothelioma can encase the lung and cause restrictive disease with resultant ipsilateral volume loss and hemidiaphragm elevation (Fraser et al, 1994; Kawashima and Libshitz, 1990; Rabinowitz et al, 1982).

TABLE 56–3 ■ Hemidiaphragm Elevation

UNILATERAL

- Lung volume loss (atelectasis, lobar collapse, partial lung resection, radiation fibrosis, congenital pulmonary hypoplasia, encasement by tumor)
- Eventration
- Abdominal disease (dilated stomach or colon, hepatomegaly, splenomegaly, subphremic abscess)
- Phrenic nerve paralysis
- Splinting (rib fracture, pneumonia, infarction, abscess, peritonitis)
- Mimics (subpulmonic pleural effusion, large pleural mass, diaphragmatic hernia)
- After single lung transplant for pulmonary fibrosis
- Phrenoplasty

BILATERAL

- Lung volume loss (suboptimal inspiration, supine positioning, atelectasis, lung resection, pulmonary fibrosis)
- Abdominal mass effect (obesity, pregnancy, marked bowel dilation, ascites, hepatosplenomegaly, large abdominal tumors)
- Eventration
- Subpulmonic pleural effusions
- Neuromuscular disease (quadriplegia, multiple sclerosis, amyotrophic lateral sclerosis, Guillain-Barré syndrome, myasthenia gravis, Eaton-Lambert syndrome, muscular dystrophy, steroid or alcohol myopathy, rhabdomyolysis)
- Connective tissue disease (fibrosis in rheumatoid arthritis, sclerodema, and ankylosing spondylitis; weakness in systemic lupus erythematosus, polymyositis)
- Endocrine and metabolic disorders (hypothyroidism, hyperthyroidism, Cushing's disease, hypokalemia, hypophosphatemia, hypomagnesemia, metabolic alkalosis)
- Phrenic nerve paralysis

Eventration is a frequently encountered cause of hemidiaphragm elevation. The abnormally thin portions of the diaphragm are more easily stretched and displaced upward by the liver and abdominal viscera (Hesselink et al, 1978; Vogl and Small, 1955). This may be of congenital etiology due to incomplete muscularization of the pericardioperitoneal membrane (Tarver et al, 1989), but the increased incidence with age suggests that eventration of the right hemidiaphragm is often acquired (Okuda et al, 1979). Eventration is usually unilateral and incomplete, but it may involve the entire hemidiaphragm. The anteromedial right hemidiaphragm is most commonly affected by partial eventration (Armstrong et al, 1995; Vogl and Small, 1955), while complete eventration usually occurs on the left hemidiaphragm and in males (Tarver et al, 1989). Partial eventration is seen as a focal, broad-based, mass-like, upward bulge of the hemidiaphragm (Fig. 56–16). Complete eventration results in smooth elevation of the hemidiaphragm on radiographs, with slight paradoxical, little, or no movement during inspiration on fluoroscopy, which may be indistinguishable from phrenic nerve paralysis (Armstrong et al, 1995; Tarver et al, 1989). CT, MR, ultrasound, and liver scintigraphy can be used to determine the contents of the eventration. If small, distinction from a localized herniation may be difficult (Fig. 56–17).

Unilateral hemidiaphragm elevation may be related to abdominal disease. Large abdominal tumors (Fig. 56–18) or fluid collections, such as subphrenic abscesses (Fig. 56–19) are potential causes. Hemidiaphragm elevation may also be associated with dilatation of the stomach or colon.

Phrenic nerve paralysis, discussed subsequently in greater detail, is often first suspected when hemidiaphragm elevation is noted on a chest radiograph (Fig. 56–20). Impaired inspiratory excursion of the diaphragm and rib cage due to pain from a rib fracture or pleurisy ("splinting") can also produce hemidiaphragm elevation. Additional causes of splinting include acute lower lobe pneumonia or infarction, and acute intra-abdominal inflammatory processes such as subphrenic abscess, cholecystitis, and peritonitis (Fraser et al, 1994).

Subpulmonic accumulation of pleural fluid can mimic hemidiaphragm elevation. This is suspected primarily when the dome of the apparent hemidiaphragm margin is positioned more laterally than usual (Fig. 56–21) (Fleischner, 1963; Hessén, 1951; Peterson, 1960). On the left, the distance between the gastric air bubble and the apparent hemidiaphragm margin may be increased (Armstrong et al, 1995; Fleischner, 1963; Fraser et al, 1994; Hessén, 1951; Peterson, 1960), but this can be seen in the absence of subpulmonic fluid if the gastric air bubble is positioned anterior and inferior to the hemidiaphragm dome (Felson, 1973). Subpulmonic fluid, if not loculated, can be confirmed by lateral decubitus radiographs (see Fig. 56–21). A large basilar pleural mass may also mimic hemidiaphragm elevation.

Phrenoplasty to minimize the pleural dead space following pulmonary resection by dissecting the ipsilateral hemidiaphragm away from the pericardium and increasing the hemidiaphragm surface area allows the hemidi-

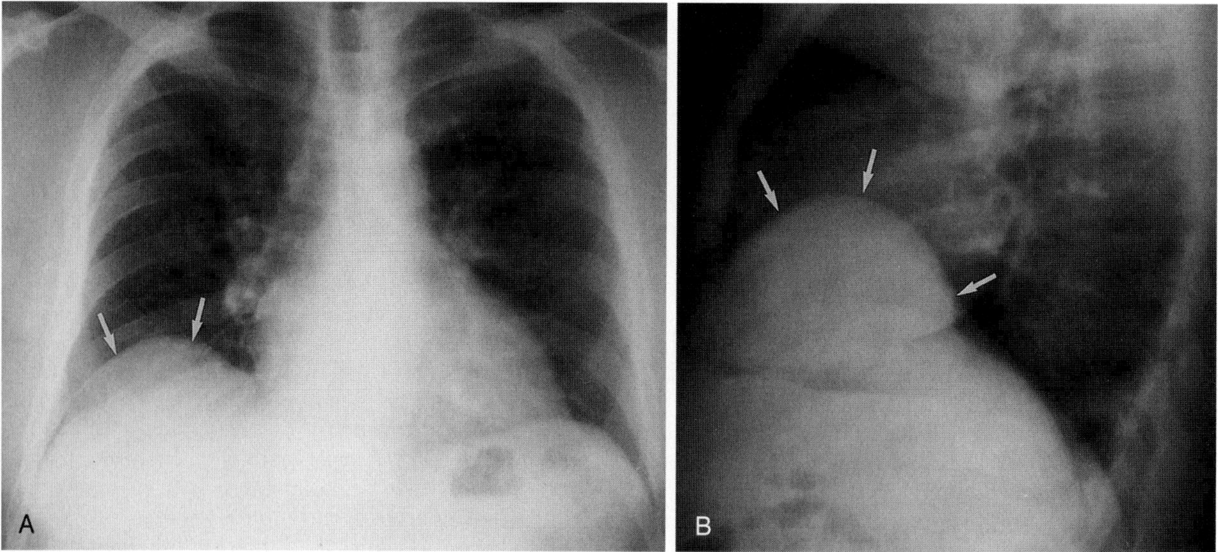

FIGURE 56–16 ■ Partial eventration. Posteroanterior (*A*) and lateral (*B*) radiographs in a 42-year-old man reveal a broad, upwardly bulging segment (*arrows*) of the anteromedial right hemidiaphragm.

aphragm to rise higher, resulting in unilateral elevation (Brewer and Gazzaniga, 1968). This technique minimizes the size of fluid collections accumulating in the lobectomy space when the remaining lung is too small to fill the thoracic cavity.

Bilateral Elevation

The most frequently encountered cause of bilateral hemidiaphragm elevation (see Table 56–3) is obesity. The hemidiaphragms of pregnant women are also typically positioned higher than usual. A large amount of ascites, diffuse bowel dilatation due to ileus or mechanical obstruction, marked hepatosplenomegaly, and intra-abdominal tumors are additional causes of bilateral elevation (Felson, 1973).

Lung volume loss is the most common intrathoracic cause of bilateral elevation. Etiologies include bilateral atelectasis, diseases causing bilateral pulmonary fibrosis, and bilateral partial lung resection. Lung volume may

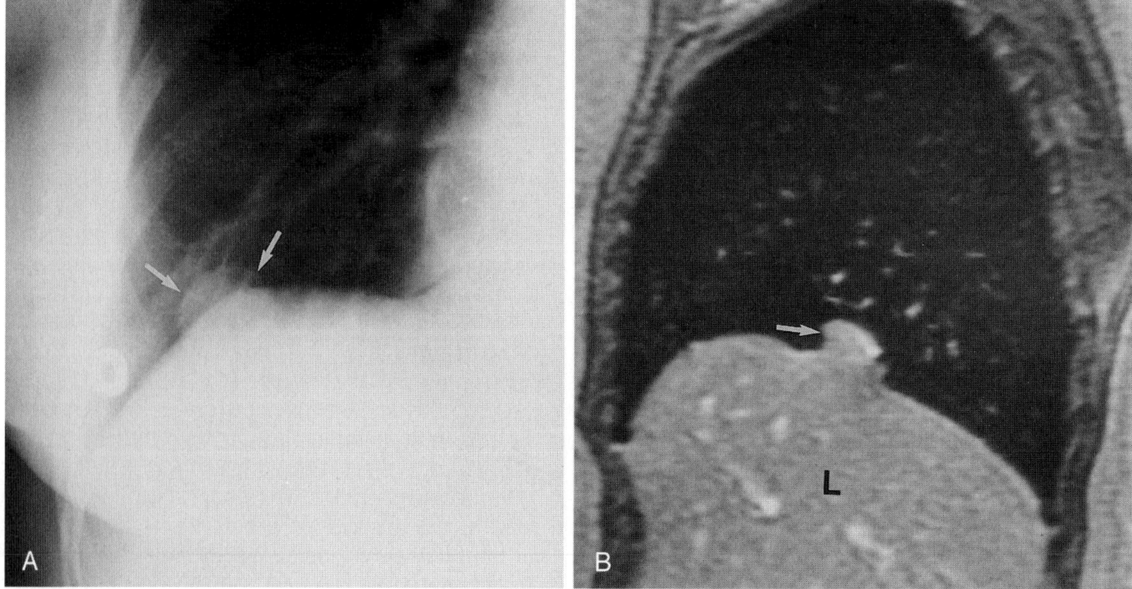

FIGURE 56–17 ■ Multiplanar magnetic resonance image (MRI) of focal diaphragm defect. *A*, Radiograph in a patient with breast cancer reveals a rounded "mass" (*arrows*) in the right lung base, suspicious for a lung nodule. *B*, Postcontrast sagittal MRI that the "mass" (*arrow*) represents a focal bulge of the liver (L). The enhancement and signal characteristics on this and other pulse sequences were identical to the liver, consistent with a small, focal eventration or herniation. (From Slone RM, Gierada DS: Pleura, Chest Wall, and Diaphragm. In Lee JKT, Sagel SS, Stanley RJ, Heiken JP (eds): Computed Body Tomography with MRI Correlation, Vol 1, 3rd ed. Philadelphia, Lippincott-Raven, 1998.)

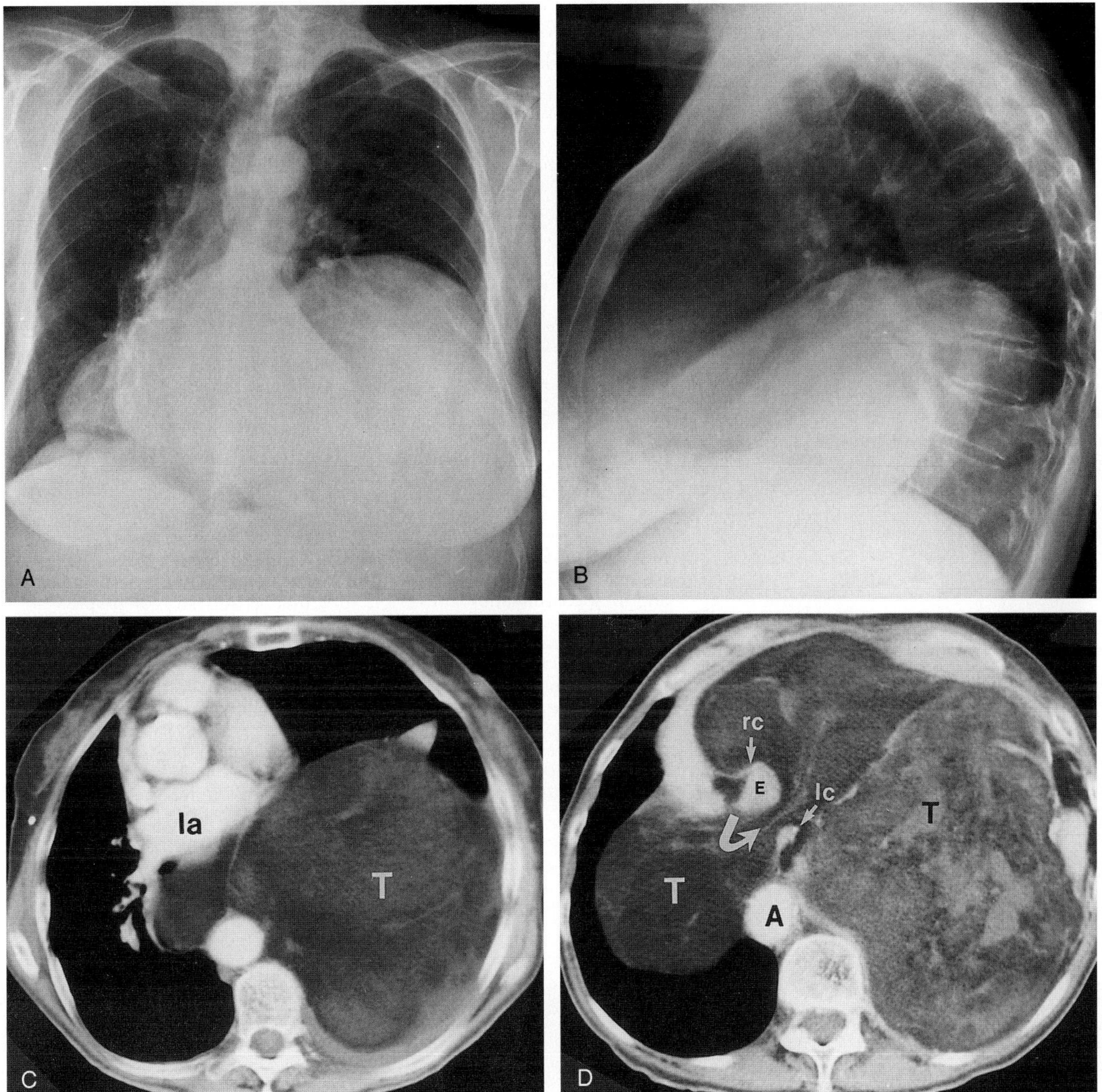

FIGURE 56–18 ■ Abdominal liposarcoma. Posteroanterior (*A*) and lateral (*B*) radiographs show left hemidiaphragm elevation and retrocardiac mass. *C* and *D*, Computed tomography images reveal that radiographic findings are due to a large tumor (T) of mixed fat and soft tissue attenuation, which extends through the esophageal hiatus (*curved arrow in D*). (A, aorta; E, esophagus; la, left atrium; lc, left crus of diaphragm; rc, right crus of diaphragm.)

also be diminished in the absence of pulmonary disease due to suboptimal patient inspiratory effort, as it may be on supine portable radiographs since supine positioning lowers functional residual capacity (Blair and Hickam, 1955).

Bilateral phrenic nerve paralysis results in bilateral hemidiaphragm elevation. Bilateral subpulmonic pleural effusions can simulate bilateral hemidiaphragm elevation. Numerous neuromuscular, endocrine, and metabolic diseases are rare etiologies of bilateral hemidiaphragm elevation due to diaphragm weakness or paralysis (Reid, 1995; Wilcox and Pardy, 1989). Connective tissue diseases such as polymyositis and systemic lupus erythematosus may cause diaphragm elevation on the basis of weakness, while other diseases such as rheumatoid arthritis, scleroderma, and ankylosing spondylitis may cause diaphragm elevation when they result in pulmonary fibrosis (Reid, 1995; Wilcox and Pardy, 1989).

Unilateral Depression

Unilateral hemidiaphragm depression (Table 56–4) is a relatively infrequent finding. One cause is a tension pneumothorax, in which there may be ipsilateral hemidiaphragm depression accompanying contralateral mediastinal shift. In supine patients, a pneumothorax of substantial size may collect anteriorly (preferentially in the base of the hemithorax, the least dependent position)

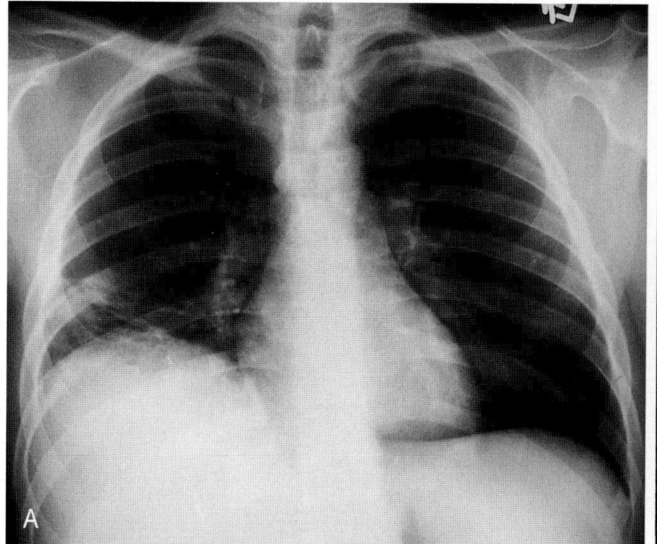

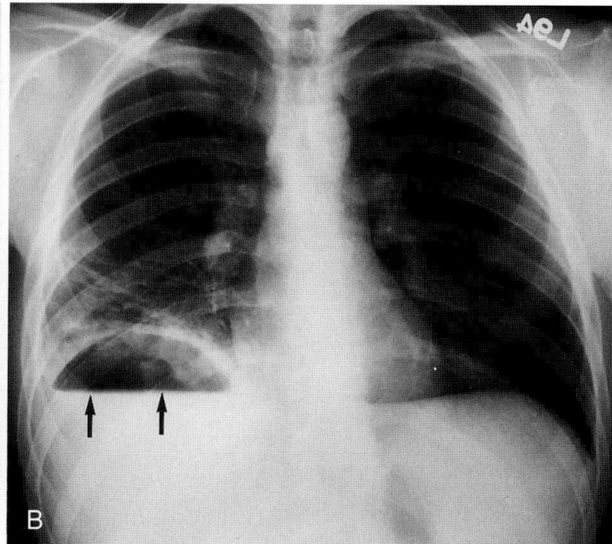

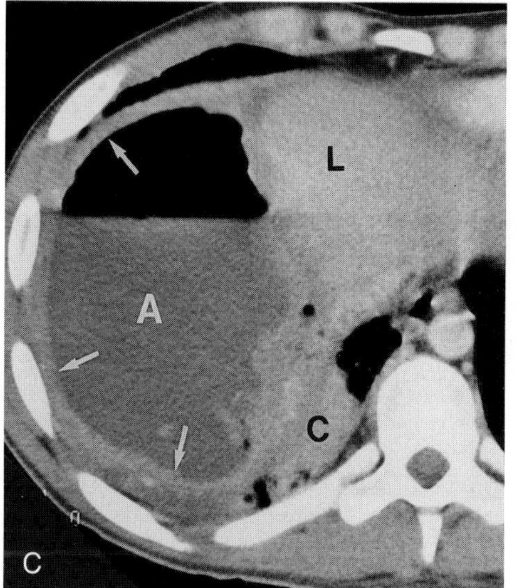

FIGURE 56–19 ■ Subphrenic abscess. *A*, A radiograph in a febrile 29-year-old man demonstrates elevation of the right hemidiaphragm with atelectasis and focal consolidation in the right lung base. *B*, A chest radiograph obtained 3 weeks later reveals an air-fluid level (*arrows*) in the right subphrenic space, consistent with an abscess. *C*, A computed tomography scan confirms that the abscess (A) is within the abdomen, internal to the hemidiaphragm (*arrows*) and adjacent to the liver (L). Consolidation (C) is present in the medial right lung base. The patient had sustained a liver laceration in a motor vehicle accident 9 months previously and developed a biloma that required percutaneous catheter drainage; the drains had been removed 4 months previously. (From Gierada DS, Slone RM, Fleishman MJ: Imaging evaluation of the diaphragm. Chest Surg Clin North Am 8:237, 1998.)

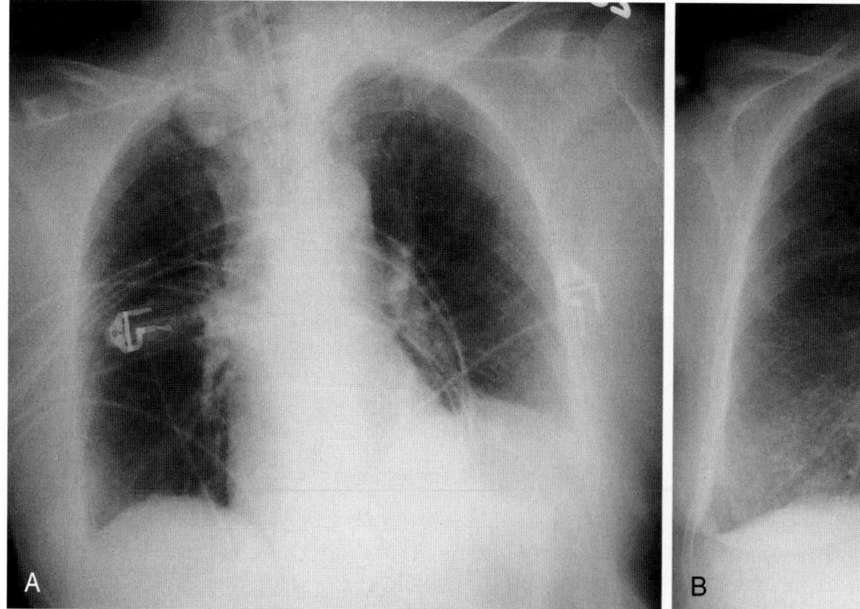

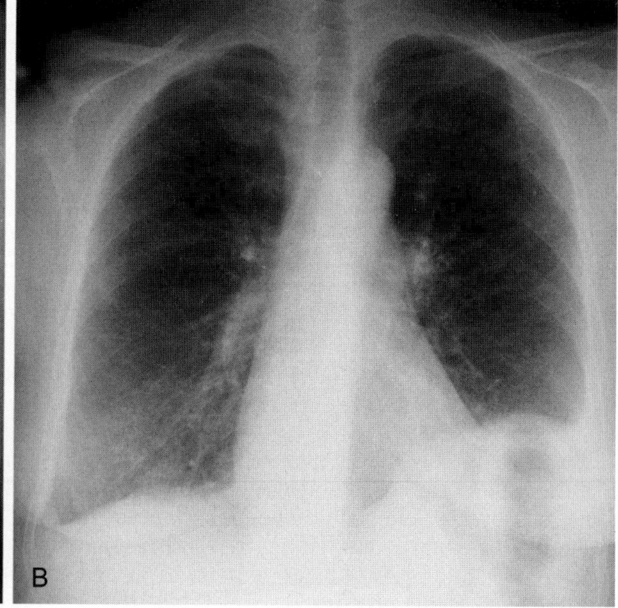

FIGURE 56–20 ■ Paralyzed hemidiaphragm. *A*, Postoperative chest radiograph obtained after left carotid endarterectomy demonstrates an elevated left hemidiaphragm. Note the skin staples in left lower neck. *B*, A radiograph obtained 1 month later shows no change. Fluoroscopy revealed left hemidiaphragm paralysis.

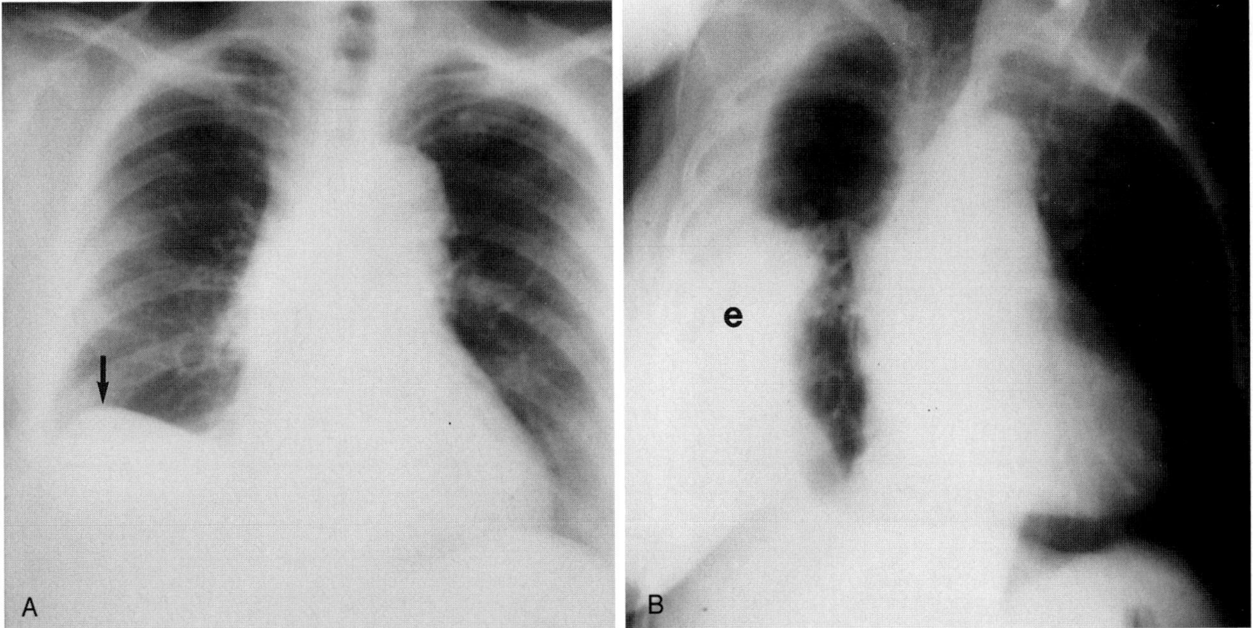

FIGURE 56–21 ■ Subpulmonic pleural effusion. *A*, Apparent elevation of the right hemidiaphragm with a laterally positioned dome (*arrow*) suggests the presence of a subpulmonic pleural effusion. *B*, Right lateral decubitus view (*right side down*) confirms a mobile pleural effusion (e) of moderate size. (Courtesy of Harvey S. Glazer, MD, St. Louis, MO.) (From Gierada DS, Slone RM, Fleishman MJ: Imaging evaluation of the diaphragm. Chest Surg Clin North Am 8:237, 1998.)

without significant separation of the lateral and apical visceral pleural margins. Hemidiaphragm depression therefore can be an indirect sign of a pneumothorax in the supine patient. Erect or lateral decubitus views with the abnormal side up can resolve difficult cases.

Asymmetric bullous emphysema can be associated with relatively greater hemidiaphragm depression on the more severely affected side (Fig. 56–22). After single lung transplantation for emphysema, the hemidiaphragm on the transplanted side assumes a more normal position, and unilateral depression is seen on the side of the native lung.

A large pleural effusion may invert a hemidiaphragm (Mulvey, 1965; Swingle et al, 1969); in such cases, drainage of pleural fluid by thoracentesis may result in little apparent change in the position of the pleural fluid margin on radiographs (Felson, 1973). However, detection of hemidiaphragm inversion on radiography may be difficult because the normal diaphragm-lung interface is obscured by the fluid. Hemidiaphragm inversion is more readily recognized on the left, since depression of the stomach or colon may be seen (Armstrong et al, 1995). On axial CT images, pleural fluid inverting the right hemidiaphragm may resemble a cystic intrahepatic mass (Hertzanu and Solomon, 1986).

TABLE 56–4 ■ **Hemidiaphragm Depression**

UNILATERAL
Large pneumothorax
Asymmetric bullous emphysema
Large pleural effusion
Foreign body aspiration
Congenital lobar emphysema
Single lung transplant for emphysema
BILATERAL
Chronic obstructive pulmonary disease (emphysema, asthma)
Deep inspiration (young, thin person)
Bilateral large pneumothorax
Mechanical ventilation at high pressures
Cystic fibrosis
Pulmonary histiocytosis X
Lymphangioleiomyomatosis
Tuberous sclerosis

In children, unilateral hemidiaphragm depression raises the suspicion of congenital lobar emphysema or an aspirated foreign body. In congenital lobar emphysema, there is marked hyperinflation of the affected lobe with depression of the ipsilateral hemidiaphragm and contralateral shift of the mediastinum, and often compressive atelectasis of the other lobes. Uncommonly, the enlarged lobe may be completely opacified due to impairment of fluid drainage by bronchial obstruction. Aspiration of foreign bodies, particularly in children, is a reported etiology of obstructive overinflation. However, this effect may simply be related to air trapping, since full inspiratory radiographs can be difficult to obtain in children (Fraser et al, 1994).

Bilateral Depression

Bilateral hemidiaphragm depression (see Table 56–4) is seen most often with hyperinflation in patients with chronic obstructive pulmonary disease (Fig. 56–23). In emphysema, the hemidiaphragms are often flat and may be inverted; in asthma, they may be slightly less curved but are rarely flat (Armstrong et al, 1995). With the marked hyperinflation sometimes seen in advanced em-

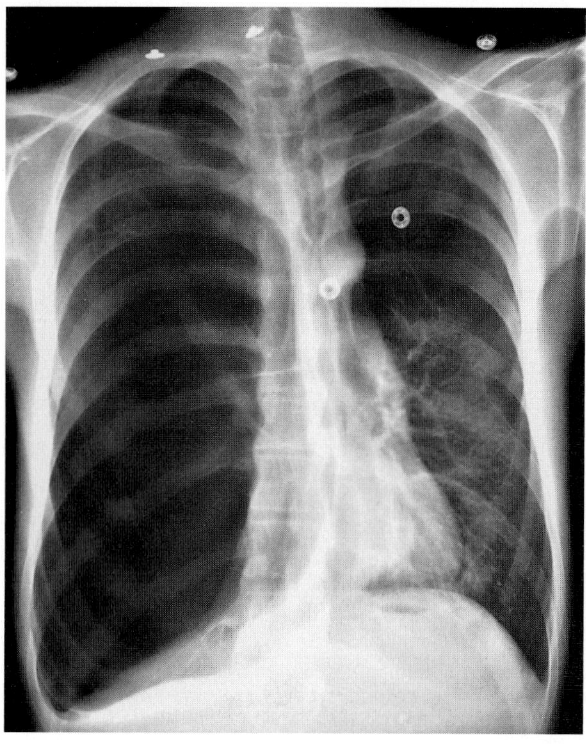

FIGURE 56–22 ■ Asymmetric bullous emphysema. Severe bullous emphysema in a 36-year-old man is more severe on the right, resulting in right hemidiaphragm depression and contralateral mediastinal shift.

physema, the costal insertions of the diaphragm may be visible on radiographs (see Fig. 56–23) (Fraser et al, 1994; Slone and Gierada, 1996). Healthy normal individuals, particularly those who are young and thin, may occasionally have a relatively low diaphragm. Mechanical ventilation at high pressure and bilateral tension pneumothorax can produce bilateral hemidiaphragm depression. Finally, cystic fibrosis typically results in hyperin-

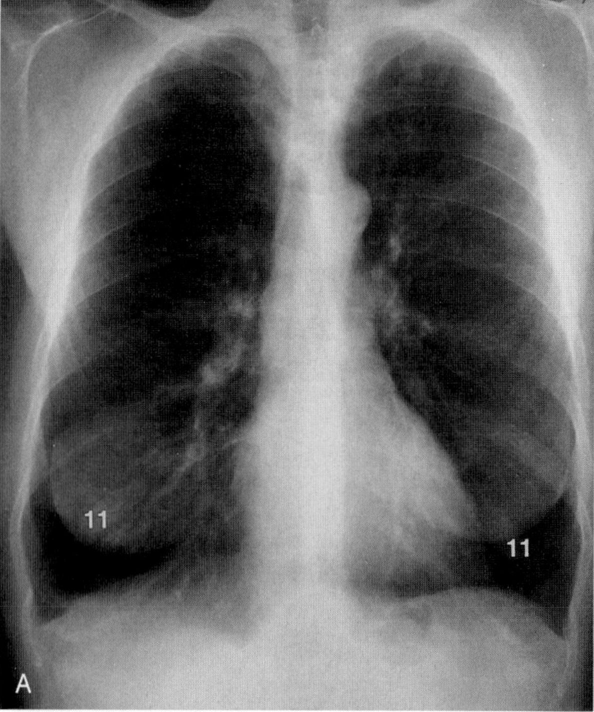

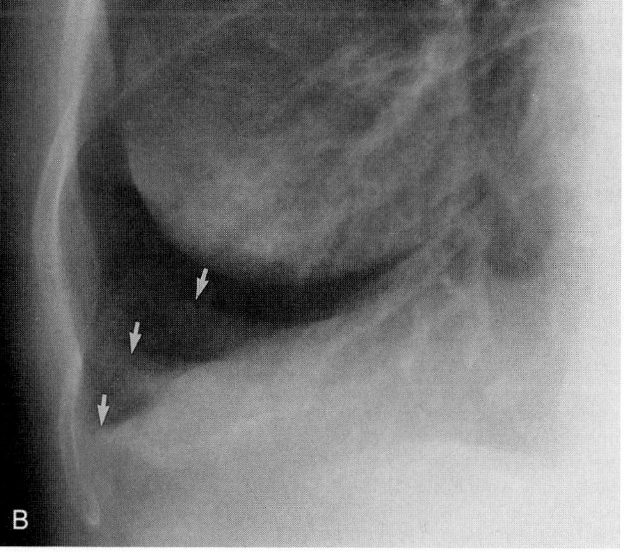

FIGURE 56–23 ■ Severe emphysema. *A*, A radiograph in a 65-year-old woman with severe emphysema demonstrates hyperinflation with depression of the hemidiaphragm to below the 11th posterior ribs (11) and flattening of the diaphragm contour. *B*, Close-up view of the right hemidiaphragm reveals its costal insertions (*arrows*). (From Gierada DS, Slone RM, Fleishman MJ: Imaging evaluation of the diaphragm. Chest Surg Clin North Am 8:237, 1998.)

flation, and interstitial lung disease in association with normal or increased lung volumes can be seen in histiocytosis X, lymphangioleiomyomatosis, and tuberous sclerosis.

CONGENITAL HERNIAS OF THE DIAPHRAGM

Bochdalek's Hernia

Bochdalek's hernia results from incomplete closure of the embryonic pleuroperitoneal membrane. Despite the name, it typically occurs through posterolateral defects in the diaphragm separate from the foramen of Bochdalek (White and Suzuki, 1972). The defect is usually located laterally, but it also occurs medially and may be small or large (Fraser et al, 1994). This hernia is seen far more commonly on the left than right diaphragm, an observation that has been attributed to earlier closure of the right pleuroperitoneal membrane (Tarver et al, 1989) and the protection of right-sided defects by the liver (Fraser et al, 1994). A small defect may contain only retroperitoneal fat, while larger defects can contain abdominal viscera such as the stomach, intestine, spleen or kidney on the left, and the liver on the right (Panicek et al, 1988; Tarver et al, 1989).

In the neonatal period, a large Bochdalek hernia (congenital diaphragmatic hernia) is a surgical emergency (Kirks and Caron, 1991). Newborns present with severe respiratory distress and a scaphoid abdomen. The initial chest radiograph usually reveals opacification of the hemithorax and contralateral shift of the mediastinum due to herniation of the abdominal contents into the chest (Fig. 56–24). As air is swallowed, bowel loops in the chest become filled with gas and produce multiple lucencies. Morbidity and mortality are related to the degree of underlying pulmonary hypoplasia. Prenatal diagnosis is possible using fetal ultrasound (Bencerraf and Greene, 1986).

In the adult, a Bochdalek hernia is seen on the chest radiograph as a soft tissue mass of variable size bulging upward through the posterior aspect of a hemidiaphragm. The hernia contents usually can be defined without difficulty on CT, which can also demonstrate the diaphragmatic defect (Fig. 56–25). Other radiologic studies can be used to demonstrate the hernia contents; barium studies may reveal herniated bowel loops, intravenous urography may reveal a herniated kidney, and ^{99m}Tc sulfur colloid scintigraphy may demonstrate herniation of the liver or spleen. Small, focal diaphragmatic defects or discontinuity, with or without herniated fat or viscera, are seen in more than 10% of adults on CT (Fig. 56–26) (Caskey et al, 1989; Gale, 1985). Their increasing incidence with age, obesity, and emphysema strongly suggests that the majority of such abnormalities are acquired, and are not true Bochdalek hernias (Caskey et al, 1989).

Morgagni's Hernia

Foramen of Morgagni hernias are related to maldevelopment of the embryologic septum transversum with failure of fusion of the sternal and costal fibrotendinous elements of the diaphragm (Panicek et al, 1988; Tarver et al, 1989). In contrast to the true Bochdalek hernia, a hernia sac of peritoneum and pleura surrounds the contents of a Morgagni hernia (Fraser et al, 1994). Morgagni's hernia is most often right sided, probably because left-sided defects are covered by the heart and pericardium, and it is often associated with obesity. The hernia sac usually contains omentum, but it may contain transverse colon or rarely stomach, small bowel, or liver (Tarver et al, 1989). Most Morgagni's hernias are asymptomatic

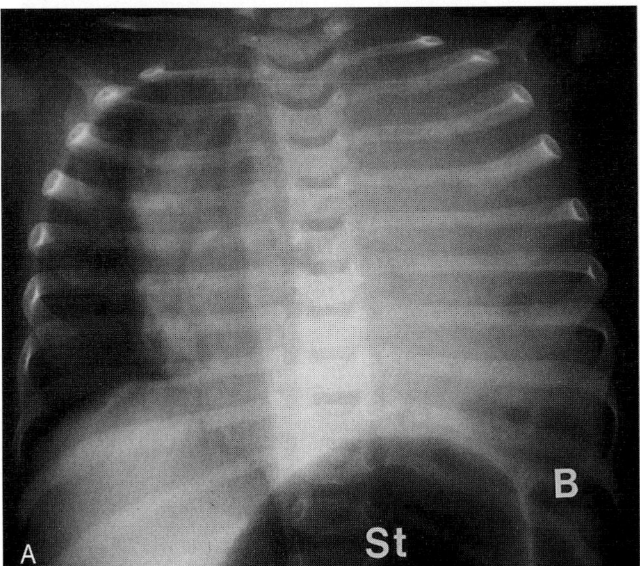

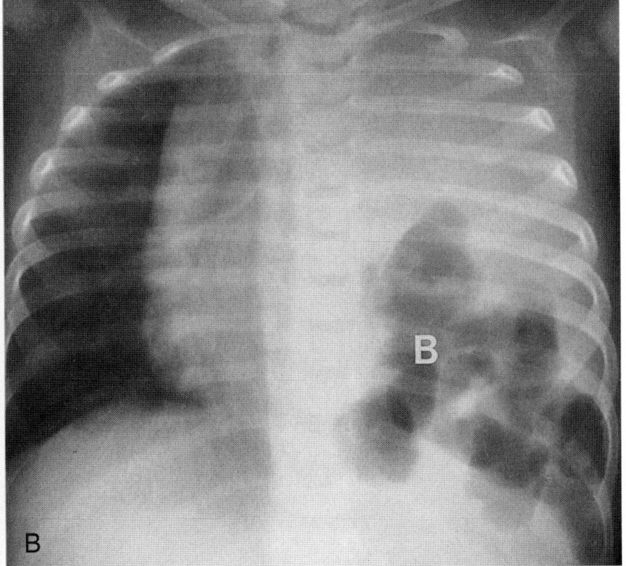

FIGURE 56–24 ■ Congenital diaphragmatic hernia. *A*, a radiograph obtained in an infant shortly after birth reveals partial opacification of the left hemithorax; a dilated, air-filled stomach (St); and upper abdominal bowel gas (B). *B*, Hours later, air has passed into bowel loops (B) in the left hemithorax, confirming a large congenital hernia. (Courtesy of Marilyn J. Siegel, MD, St. Louis, MO.) (From Gierada DS, Slone RM, Fleishman MJ: Imaging evaluation of the diaphragm. Chest Surg Clin North Am 8:237, 1998.)

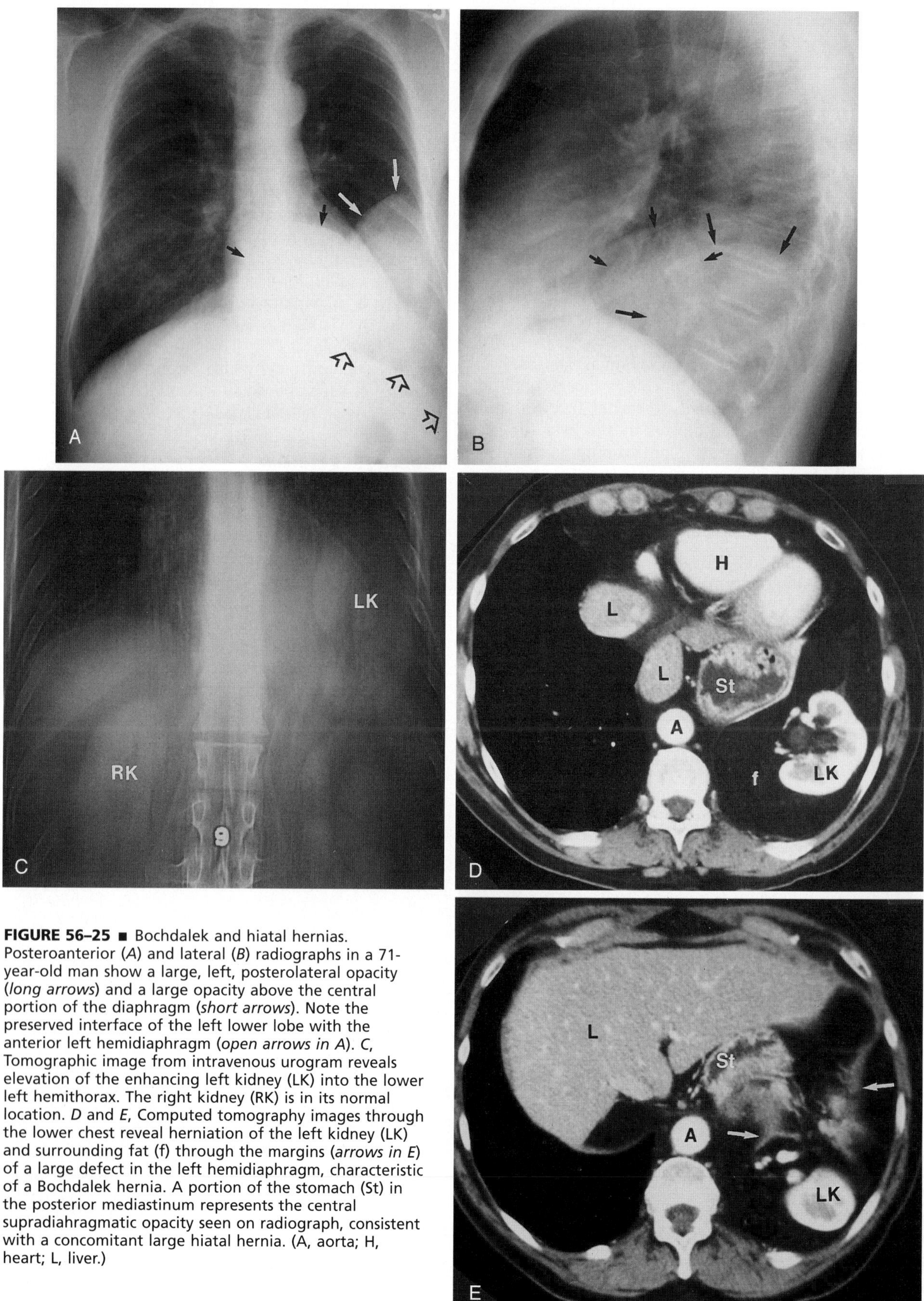

FIGURE 56–25 ■ Bochdalek and hiatal hernias. Posteroanterior (*A*) and lateral (*B*) radiographs in a 71-year-old man show a large, left, posterolateral opacity (*long arrows*) and a large opacity above the central portion of the diaphragm (*short arrows*). Note the preserved interface of the left lower lobe with the anterior left hemidiaphragm (*open arrows in A*). *C*, Tomographic image from intravenous urogram reveals elevation of the enhancing left kidney (LK) into the lower left hemithorax. The right kidney (RK) is in its normal location. *D* and *E*, Computed tomography images through the lower chest reveal herniation of the left kidney (LK) and surrounding fat (f) through the margins (*arrows in E*) of a large defect in the left hemidiaphragm, characteristic of a Bochdalek hernia. A portion of the stomach (St) in the posterior mediastinum represents the central supradiahragmatic opacity seen on radiograph, consistent with a concomitant large hiatal hernia. (A, aorta; H, heart; L, liver.)

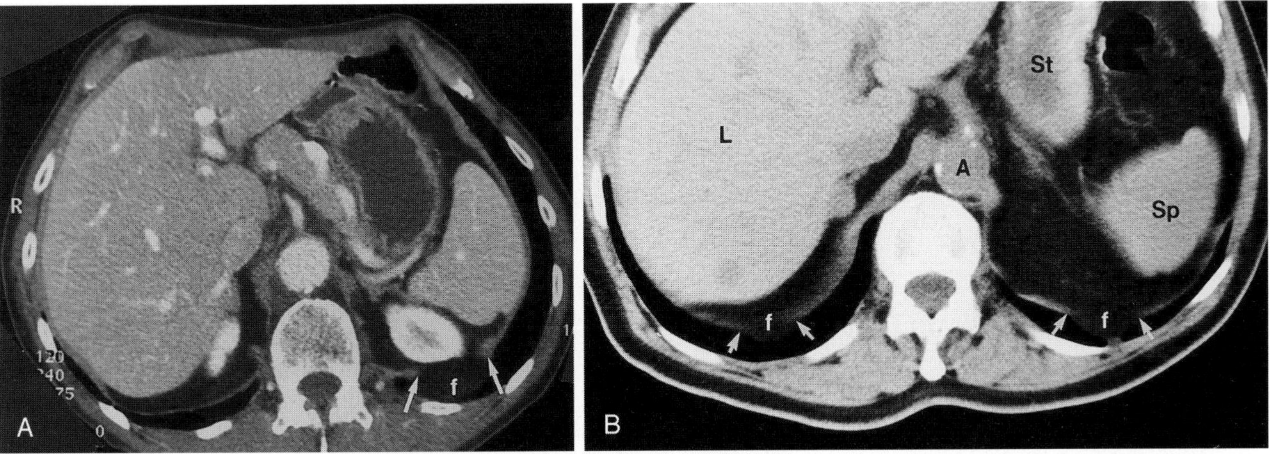

FIGURE 56–26 ■ Posterior diaphragm defects. *A* and *B*, Computed tomography images in two different patients reveal herniation of abdominal fat (f) through the margins (*arrows*) of posterior diaphragm defects, which could be either congenital or acquired with aging. (*A*, aorta; L, liver; Sp, spleen; St, stomach.) (*B*, from Slone RM, Gierada DS: Pleura, Chest Wall, and Diaphragm. In Lee JKT, Sagel SS, Stanley RJ, Heiken JP [eds]: Computed Body Tomography with MRI Correlation, Vol 1, 3rd ed. Philadelphia, Lippincott-Raven, 1998.)

although some produce epigastric pressure or discomfort, and rarely strangulation of contained portions of the gastrointestinal tract (Fraser et al, 1994).

Morgagni's hernias usually come to clinical attention as asymptomatic right cardiophrenic angle masses detected on chest radiographs (Fig. 56–27). Gas-filled intestinal loops may be present, facilitating radiographic diagnosis. CT permits distinction from other causes of cardiophrenic angle masses such as pericardial cysts, pericardial fat pads, and pleural or parenchymal masses by revealing omental fat, omental vessels, and abdominal viscera peripheral to the diaphragm in the lower anterior chest (see Fig. 56–27). The actual diaphragmatic defect may be difficult to identify owing to its typically small size. As with the Bochdalek hernia, liver scintigraphy or multiplanar MRI are occasionally useful.

ACQUIRED HERNIAS OF THE DIAPHRAGM

Hiatal Hernia

Hiatal hernia is the most frequently encountered type of diaphragmatic hernia in adults. Acquired enlargement of the esophageal hiatus and laxity of the phrenoesophageal ligament are etiologic factors, often associated with conditions resulting in increased intra-abdominal pressure,

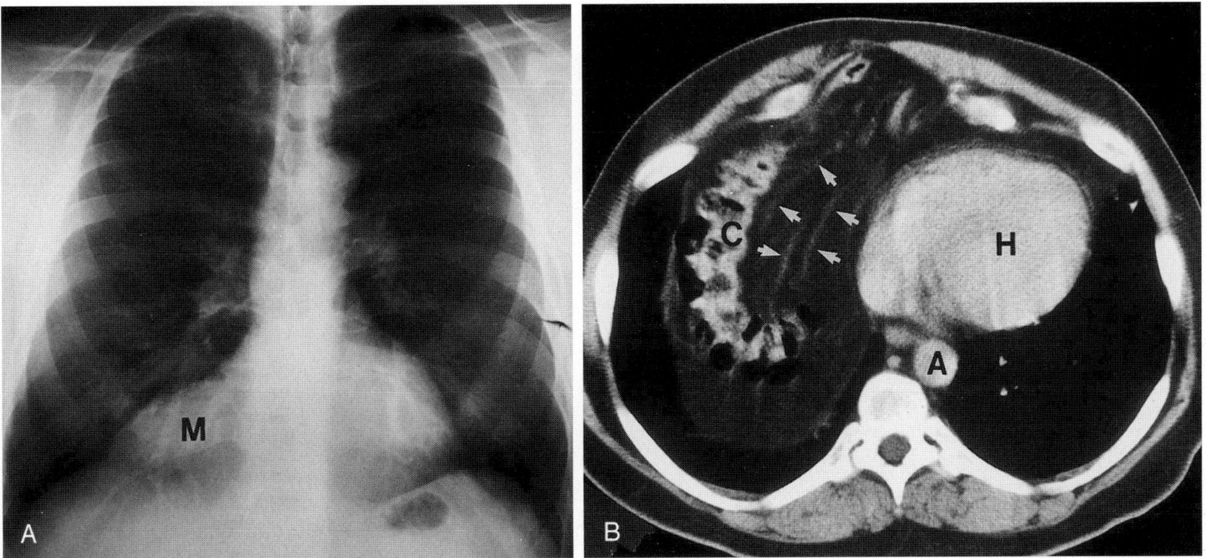

FIGURE 56–27 ■ Morgagni hernia. *A*, Posteroanterior radiograph in a 50-year-old man demonstrates a right cardiophrenic angle mass (M). *B*, A computed tomography scan through the lower chest reveals transverse colon (C) surrounded by omental and mesenteric fat in the right lower chest. Mesenteric vessels (*arrows*) are seen coursing from the right parasternal region. The diaphragm defect was not depicted. (A, aorta; H, heart.) (*B*, from Slone RM, Gierada DS: Pleura, Chest Wall, and Diaphragm. In Lee JKT, Sagel SS Stanley RJ, Heiken JP [eds]: Computed Body Tomography with MRI Correlation, Vol 1, 3rd ed. Philadelphia, Lippincott-Raven, 1998.)

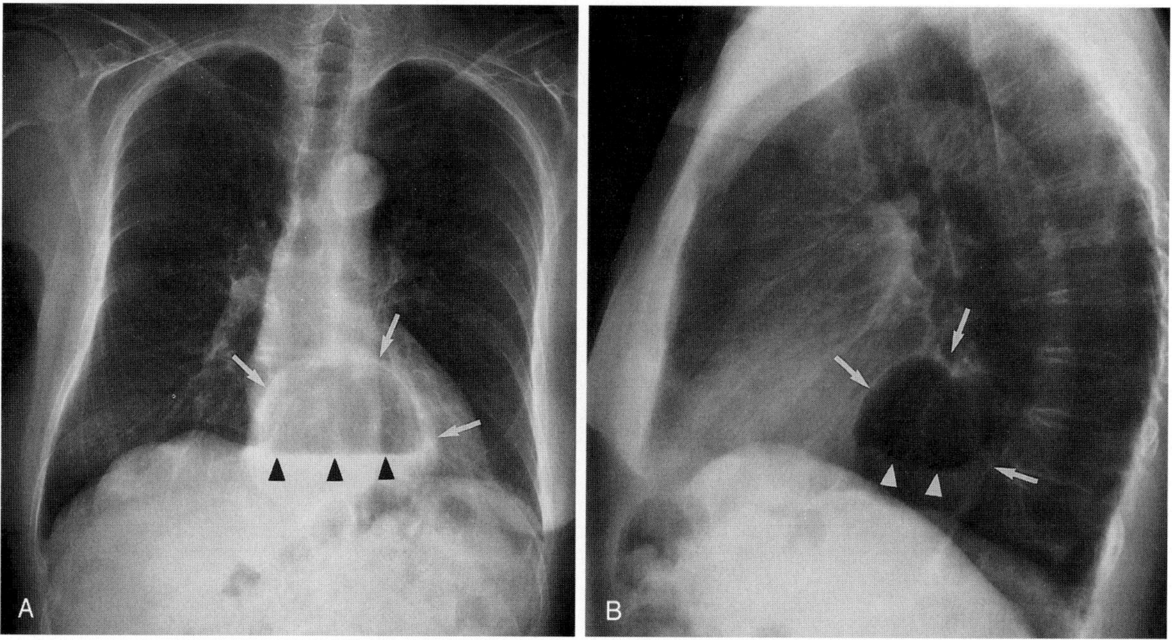

FIGURE 56–28 ■ Hiatal hernia. Posteroanterior (*A*) and lateral (*B*) radiographs in an 83-year-old man reveal a large, retrocardiac mass containing an air-fluid level (*arrowheads*) representing the herniated intrathoracic portion of the stomach (*arrows*).

such as obesity and pregnancy (Fraser et al, 1994; Tarver et al, 1989). Sliding hiatal hernias (Fig. 56–28) are much more common than the periesophageal variety, in which the stomach herniates up alongside the lower esophagus.

On chest radiography, hiatal hernias are depicted as lower posterior mediastinal, retrocardiac soft tissue masses, often containing air and fluid (see Fig. 56–28). The diagnosis is easily confirmed by a barium esophagogram, although this is rarely necessary. Very large hernias can become incarcerated or undergo volvulus (Pearson et al, 1983). Hiatal hernias are frequent incidental findings on CT scans. Extension of a portion of the proximal stomach into the lower mediastinum is seen, and an abnormally wide esophageal hiatus may be identified if it is appropriately oriented in the transverse plane (Fig. 56–29). When marked ascites is present in a patient with a hiatal hernia, CT may show fluid extending into the lower posterior mediastinum mimicing a mediastinal abscess, necrotic tumor, or foregut cyst (Godwin and MacGregor, 1987).

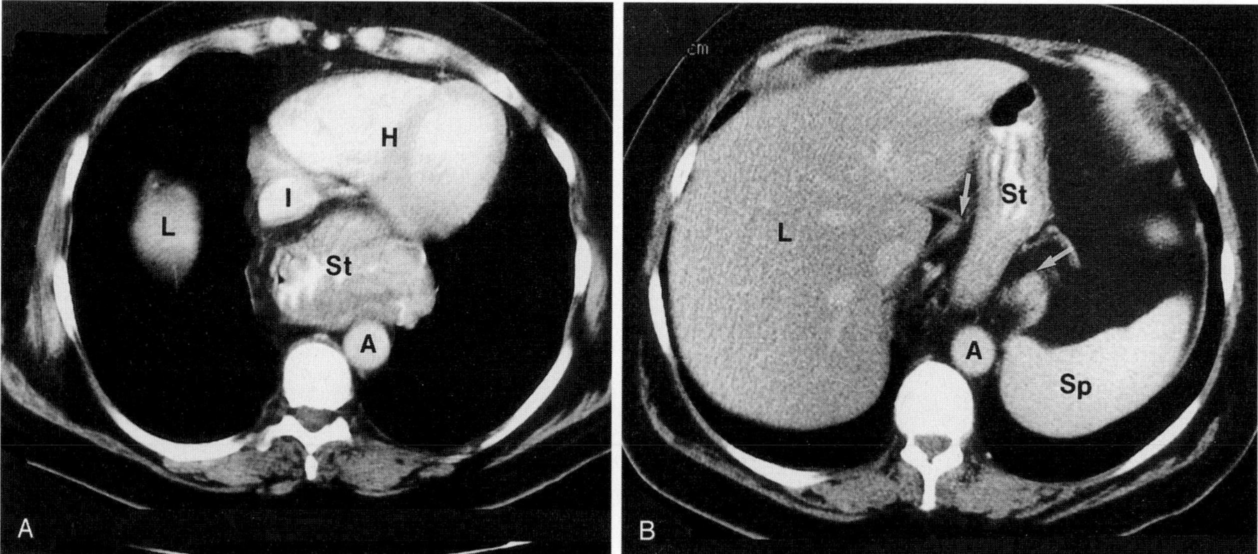

FIGURE 56–29 ■ Hiatal hernia. *A*, A computed tomography scan through the lower chest demonstrates herniation of a portion of the stomach (St) into the lower mediastinum. *B*, Image obtained several centimeters caudad demonstrates widening of the esophageal hiatus (*arrows*) and herniation of the stomach (St). (A, aorta; H, heart; I, inferior vena cava; L, liver; Sp, spleen.) (*A*, from Gierada DS, Slone RM, Fleishman MJ: Imaging evaluation of the diaphragm. Chest Surg Clin North Am 8:237, 1998.)

Traumatic Hernia

Traumatic diaphragmatic hernia can result from either penetrating or blunt injury. Diaphragmatic rupture is recognized in 0.5% to 6% of blunt trauma survivors in various series (Guth et al, 1995; Rodriguez-Morales et al, 1986; Voeller et al, 1990; Ward et al, 1981). It more often affects the left hemidiaphragm, possibly because of the protection of the right hemidiaphragm by the liver or because of the inherently greater weakness of the left hemidiaphragm; infrequently, bilateral rupture occurs (Chen and Wilson, 1991; Gelman et al, 1991; Guth et al, 1995; Kearney et al, 1989; Rodriguez-Morales et al, 1986; Voeller et al, 1990; Ward et al, 1981). Penetrating trauma due to stab wounds most often affects the left hemidiaphragm, since most people are right-handed, while gunshot wounds affect both sides with equal frequency (Chen and Wilson, 1991). Blunt traumatic tears can involve any portion of the diaphragm (Boulanger et al, 1993), although they usually involve the posterior central aspect of a hemidiaphragm and extend radially, or they result in disruption of the posterolateral attachments (Hood, 1971; Ward et al, 1981). Blunt traumatic defects are usually large, often more than 10 cm in length (Chen and Wilson, 1991; Panicek et al, 1988; Voeller et al, 1990; Wise et al, 1973). Penetrating wounds are usually less than 2 cm in length (Wise et al, 1973).

Herniation through a traumatic defect most frequently involves the stomach on the left and the liver on the right, but it can also involve the large or small bowel, omentum, liver, or spleen (Rodriguez-Morales et al, 1986; Voeller et al, 1990; Ward et al, 1981). In virtually all cases, traumatic rupture of the diaphragm is associated with multisystem injuries that more directly determine survival in the acute setting (Boulanger et al, 1993; Chen and Wilson, 1991; Guth et al, 1995; Voeller et al, 1990; Ward et al, 1981), and there are no reliable clinical signs or symptoms (Rodriguez-Morales et al, 1986). In addition, conservative management of patients whose abdominal injures can now be followed by CT or ultrasound precludes the identification of diaphragmatic tears that would have been detected during exploratory laparotomy. The diagnosis of diaphragm rupture therefore may be overlooked and requires a high degree of suspicion (Desforges et al, 1957; Guth et al, 1995). Early diagnosis is important since the pleuroperitoneal pressure gradient can cause defects to enlarge over time (Chen and Wilson, 1991; Marchand, 1957) with eventual bowel incarceration, strangulation, and obstruction (Andrus and Morton, 1970; Boulanger et al, 1993; Desforges et al, 1957; Gourin and Garzon, 1974; Probert and Havard, 1961).

Numerous studies have found the chest radiograph to be the most valuable test in the preoperative diagnosis of diaphragmatic rupture. However, the range of reported sensitivities is wide, from 20% to 71% (Chen and Wilson, 1991; Gelman et al, 1991; Guth et al, 1995; Rodriguez-Morales et al, 1986; Voeller et al, 1990; Ward et al, 1981). Herniation of hollow viscera into the chest (Fig. 56–30) or identification of a nasogastric tube in the intrathoracic

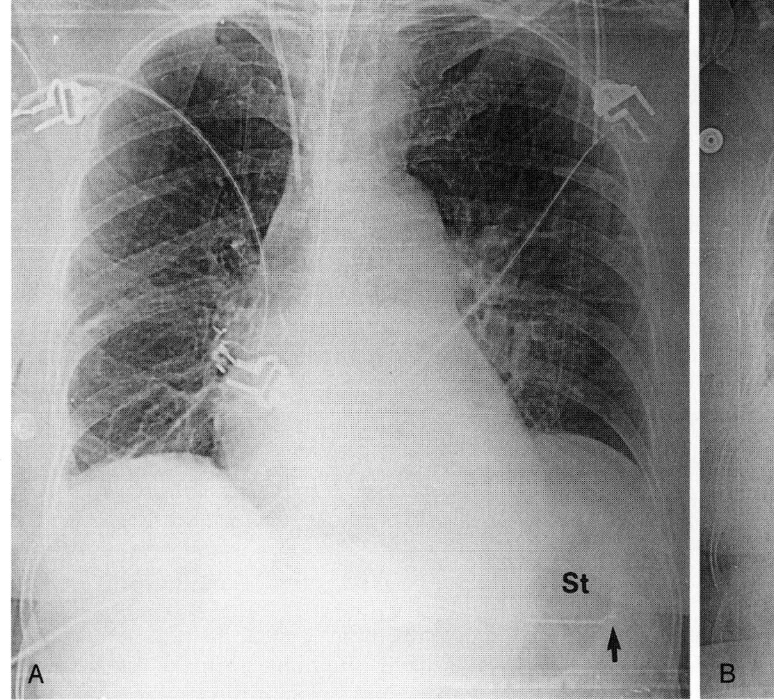

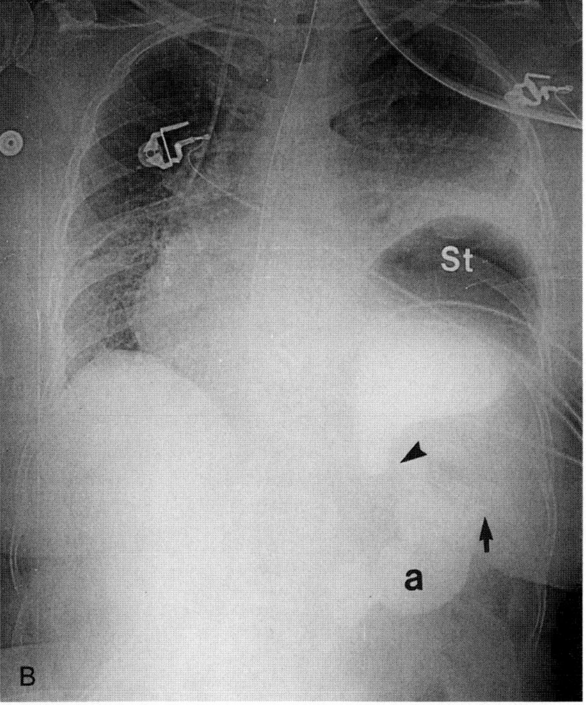

FIGURE 56–30 ■ Diaphragmatic hernia caused by surgical trauma. *A*, Portable radiograph obtained immediately following surgical repair of an abdominal aortic aneurysm reveals a normal position of the diaphragm and a nasogastric tube tip (*arrow*) positioned in the proximal stomach (St). *B*, Portable radiograph 2 days later, after injection of an oral contrast agent through the nasogastric tube, demonstrates marked upward displacement of a dilated stomach (St). The position of the nasogastric tube tip (*arrowhead*) is unchanged, but there is focal narrowing (*arrowhead*) of the body of the stomach where the stomach has herniated through the diaphragm into the chest, resulting in gastric obstruction and dilatation of the fundus. (a, gastric antrum.) (*A*, from Gierada DS, Slone RM, Fleishman MJ: Imaging evaluation of the diaphragm. Chest Surg Clin North Am 8:237, 1998.)

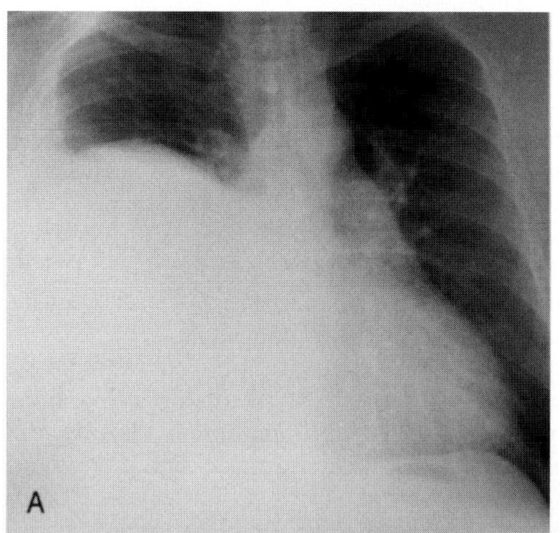

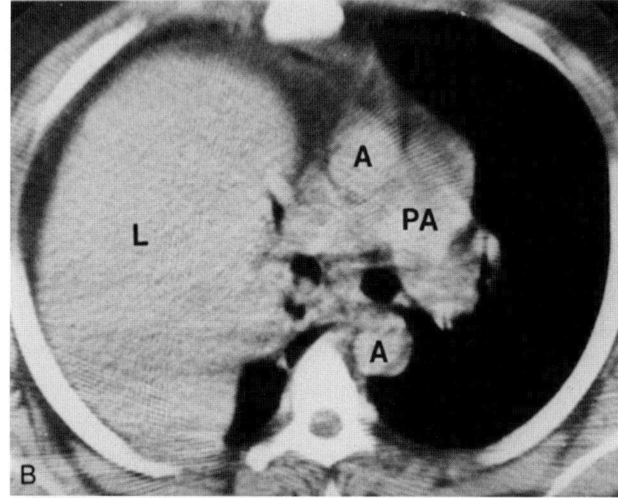

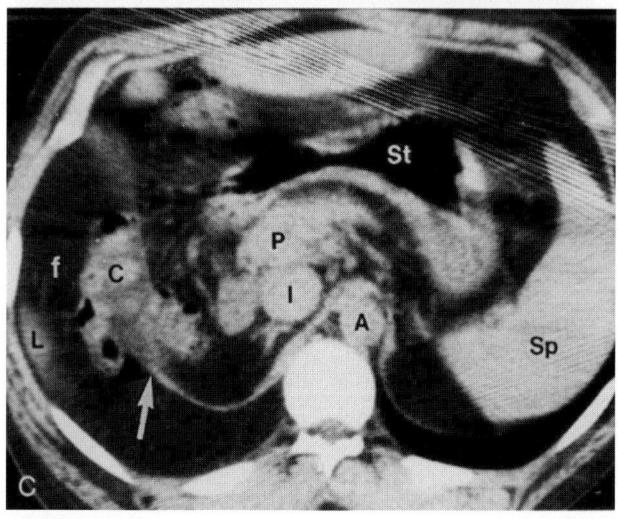

FIGURE 56–31 ■ Traumatic diaphragm rupture. *A*, A radiograph showing apparent elevation of the right hemidiaphragm in a 28-year-old man complaining of increasing shortness of breath. *B*, A computed tomography scan (CT) at the level of the main pulmonary artery (PA) reveals the cause—herniation of the liver (L) into the thorax. *C*, CT through the upper abdomen demonstrates the free edge of the torn right hemidiaphragm (*arrow*), with herniation of omental fat (f) and colon (C); the caudal tip of the herniated liver (L) is also seen. The patient reported involvement in an automobile accident 9 years previously. (A, aorta; I, inferior vena cava; P, pancreas; PA, pulmonary artery; Sp, spleen; St, stomach.) (From Slone RM, Gierada DS: Pleura, Chest Wall, and Diaphragm. In Lee JKT, Sagel SS, Stanley RJ, Heiken JP [eds]: Computed Body Tomography with MRI Correlation, Vol 1, 3rd ed. Philadelphia, Lippincott-Raven, 1998.)

stomach are the most specific radiographic signs. Diaphragm rupture should be suspected whenever radiographs reveal apparent elevation of a hemidiaphragm, although this can be due to atelectasis, eventration, posttraumatic paralysis, or subpulmonic pleural effusion. Because nonspecific apparent elevation of the hemidiaphragm is usually the only sign of right hemidiaphragm rupture (Fig. 56–31), right-sided rupture is more difficult to detect. Evidence of rupture may not be present on the initial film, but it may develop on subsequent films; therefore, serial radiographs can be helpful in diagnosis (Desforges et al, 1957; Rodriguez-Morales et al, 1986; Voeller et al, 1990). Other plain radiographic findings of diaphragm injury include hemothorax, basal lung opacity, or abnormal contour of a hemidiaphragm. Rarely, herniated omental fat can simulate pleural fluid on chest radiographs (Gurney et al, 1985). Radiographic findings are absent or nonspecific in most penetrating injuries, and early diagnosis typically requires direct inspection (Shackleton et al, 1998).

Diaphragm tears are often documented on CT, with several findings indicative of traumatic disruption (Demos et al, 1989; Heiberg et al, 1980; Holland and Quint, 1991; Worthy et al, 1995). Abrupt discontinuity of the diaphragm may be visible with or without visceral herniation (see Fig. 56–31). Inability to identify the diaphragm (absent diaphragm sign) in an area where it does not contact another organ and should normally be seen may be noted. Identification of abdominal structures external to the diaphragm indicates intrathoracic herniation. Finally, as on barium studies, focal constriction of the stomach (collar or hourglass sign) at the site of herniation occasionally is demonstrated on CT.

Retrospective analyses indicate that most diaphragmatic tears are detectable by CT (Murray et al, 1996; Worthy et al, 1995), but several studies have found CT to be of limited value in prospectively making the diagnosis (Chen and Wilson, 1991; Gelman et al, 1991; Voeller et al, 1990). If hemidiaphragm elevation is only mild and a defect is not seen on CT, further imaging may be indicated. In problematic cases, direct coronal or sagittal imaging with MR (Carter et al, 1996; Dosios et al, 1993; Gelman et al, 1991; Mirvis et al, 1988; Shanmuganathan et al, 1996), or spiral CT with coronal and sagittal reformatting (Fig. 56–32) (Israel et al, 1996), can be definitive. These imaging planes can be of particular value in depicting the secondary sign of a focal bulge or mushrooming in the diaphragmatic contour, particularly on the right hemidiaphragm where diagnosis can be difficult.

Other imaging studies are sometimes useful when radiographic or CT examinations are equivocal. Ultrasound may be of particular value in assessing the right hemidiaphragm by depicting the free edge of the hemidiaphragm as a flap within pleural fluid or demonstrating liver herniated into the chest (Somers et al, 1990). Scintigraphy can also demonstrate traumatic herniation of the liver or spleen. Contrast studies of the upper or lower gastrointestinal tract may be useful, particularly in delayed presentation.

PARALYSIS OF THE DIAPHRAGM

Paralysis of the diaphragm can be due to an abnormality at any point along its neuromuscular axis. It may be unilateral or bilateral and has numerous potential causes (Fraser et al, 1994; Ingram, 1987; Reid, 1995; Tarver et al, 1989). Phrenic nerve trauma related to surgery (stretch, crush, or transection) (see Fig. 56–20) and invasion by a malignant neoplasm (Fig. 56–33) are the most common causes, although many cases are idiopathic. Central nervous system etiologies such as multiple sclerosis, Arnold-Chiari malformation, syringomyelia, and high cervical quadriplegia are associated with bilateral hemidiaphragm paralysis. Hypothermic injury of the phenic nerve related to the use of cold topical cardioplegia during coronary artery bypass surgery can lead to unilateral (usually left) or bilateral hemidiaphragm paralysis. Numerous other causes have been implicated, including mediastinal masses such as lymphadenopathy, aortic aneurysm, and substernal goiter, and diabetes, vasculitis,

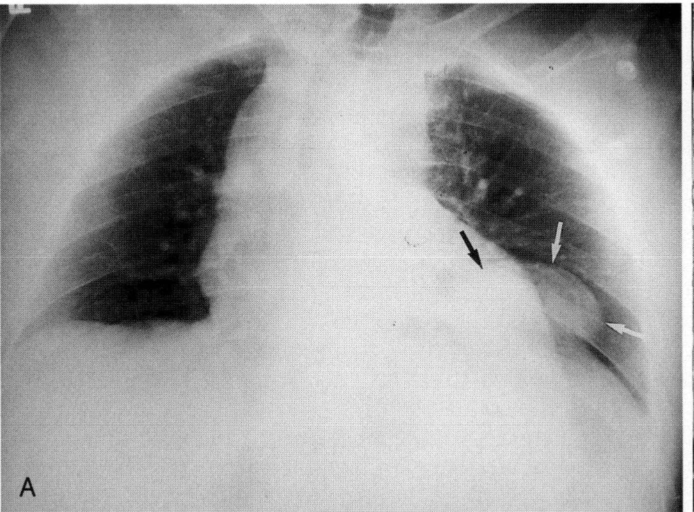

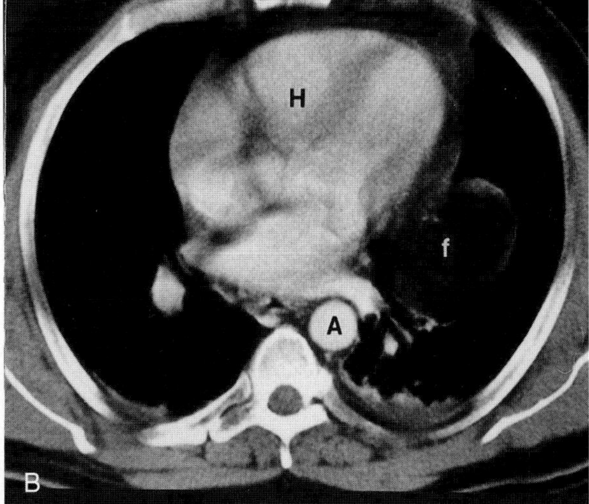

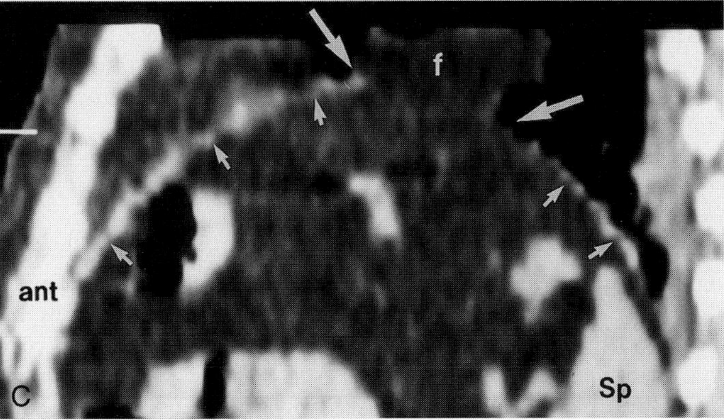

FIGURE 56–32 ■ Traumatic diaphragm rupture. *A*, A radiograph in a 53-year-old man obtained following a motor vehicle accident reveals a soft tissue bulge (*arrows*) along the left hemidiaphragm. Transaxial computed tomography (CT) image (*B*) and sagittal image reconstructed from the transaxial CT images (*C*) reveal herniation of abdominal fat (f) into the chest. The sagittal image demonstrates a defect (*arrows*) in the left hemidiaphragm (*small arrows*). There was no visceral herniation. (A, aorta; ant, anterior; H, heart; Sp, spleen.) (From Gierada DS, Slone RM, Fleishman MJ: Imaging evaluation of the diaphragm. Chest Surg Clin North Am 8:237, 1998.)

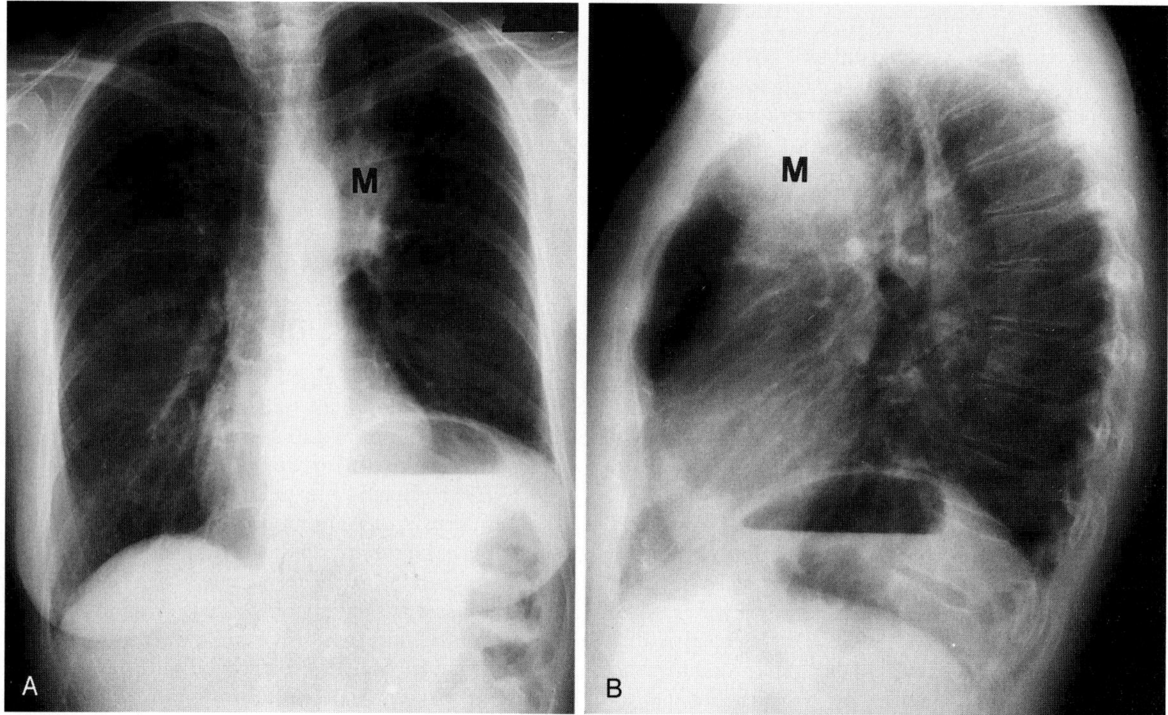

FIGURE 56–33 ■ Paralyzed hemidiaphragm. Radiograph demonstrates an elevated left hemidiaphragm and a large left paramediastinal mass (M) representing bronchogenic carcinoma involving the expected location of the phrenic nerve. Fluoroscopic examination confirmed hemidiaphragm paralysis, consistent with phrenic nerve invasion. (From Gierada DS, Slone RM, Fleishman MJ: Imaging evaluation of the diaphragm. Chest Surg Clin North Am 8:237, 1998.)

herpes zoster, and birth injury. As noted previously, diaphragm weakness without paralysis can be found in numerous conditions, including myopathies, connective tissue diseases, and various endocrine and metabolic disorders (see Table 56–3).

Fluoroscopy is the simplest, quickest, and most practical method of assessing diaphragm movement. Diaphragm movement can also be assessed by ultrasound, MRI, and by comparing radiographs obtained in full inspiration and expiration. In most studies, the average maximal excursion of the domes of the diaphragm is 3 to 5 cm (range, 2 to 10 cm) (Alexander, 1966; Gierada et al, 1995; Harris et al, 1983; Simon et al, 1969). Normal excursion is usually greater than 2.5 cm, but excursion of less than 3 cm is fairly frequent (Armstrong et al, 1995; Fraser et al, 1994; Simon et al, 1969; Young and Simon, 1972) and can be seen in healthy persons with a normal vital capacity (Young and Simon, 1972). Unequal excursion of the hemidiaphragms is common, generally differing by less than 1.5 cm, and it may be greater on either side (Gierada et al, 1995; Young and Simon, 1972). Asynchronous motion of the hemidiaphragms is not unusual (Felson, 1973; Gierada et al, 1995; Juhl, 1987).

Depicting motion by MRI requires scanner hardware that can produce strong magnetic field gradients to acquire repeated images every 1 second or less in a single plane during breathing. Relative advantages of MRI include a large field of view, easily obtained measurements due to the inherent digital spatial calibration and lack of image magnification, and the ability to view motion of segments of the diaphragm in multiple planes rather than just the highest points of the diaphragm as with fluoroscopy, which provides a projection view only. Relative disadvantages include limited temporal resolution (currently 3 to 5 images per second), restriction to horizontal patient positioning, and greater time and expense. We have used dynamic MRI to assess diaphragm motion in patients undergoing lung volume reduction surgery and have observed improved diaphragm excursion and better coordination of chest wall and diaphragm movement postoperatively (Fig. 56–34) (Slone and Gierada, 1996). Ultrasound has the advantage of portability so that it can be performed at the bedside if necessary, but it has the disadvantages of a limited field of view and potential difficulty in imaging the left hemidiaphragm due to gas in the stomach or intestine. These modalities may be of value in assessing motion when the diaphragm margin is obscured on fluoroscopy by a pleural effusion or consolidation.

Fluoroscopy is the most efficient and reliable radiologic means of assessing for diaphragm paralysis. The examination is typically performed with the patient erect; however, supine positioning stresses the diaphragm by removing the aid of gravity during inspiration and may increase the sensitivity of the test. In most adults, the fluoroscopic field of view in the frontal projection is large enough to view only an entire hemidiaphragm or the medial aspects of both hemidiaphragms. With oblique or lateral positioning, both hemidiaphragms are completely included in the field of view and can be assessed simultaneously.

In unilateral paralysis, a paralyzed hemidiaphragm paradoxically moves upward on inspiration and downward on expiration (Fig. 56–35), passively following changes in intrapleural and intra-abdominal pressure (Juhl, 1987; Tarver et al, 1989). In bilateral paralysis, both hemidiaphragms move upward on inspiration, con-

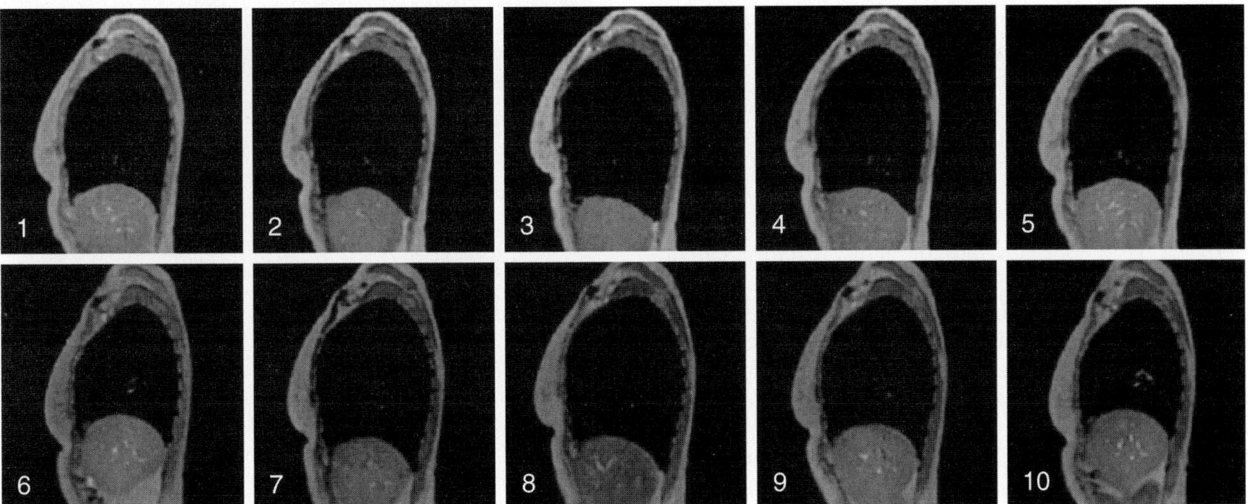

FIGURE 56–34 ■ Dynamic magnetic resonance image of diaphragm motion. These sequential right midsagittal images were obtained during slow, deep breathing in a 56-year-old woman with severe emphysema before (*1–5, top row*) and 6 months after (*6–10, bottom row*) lung volume reduction surgery. Five of the 30 images obtained in each sequence are shown. Comparison of the end-expiratory images (*1 with 6, 5 with 10*) and end-inspiratory images (*3 with 8*) reveals improved curvature of the diaphragm and increased diaphragm excursion postoperatively. (From Gierada DS, Slone RM, Fleishman MJ: Imaging evaluation of the diaphragm. Chest Surg Clin North Am 8:237, 1998.)

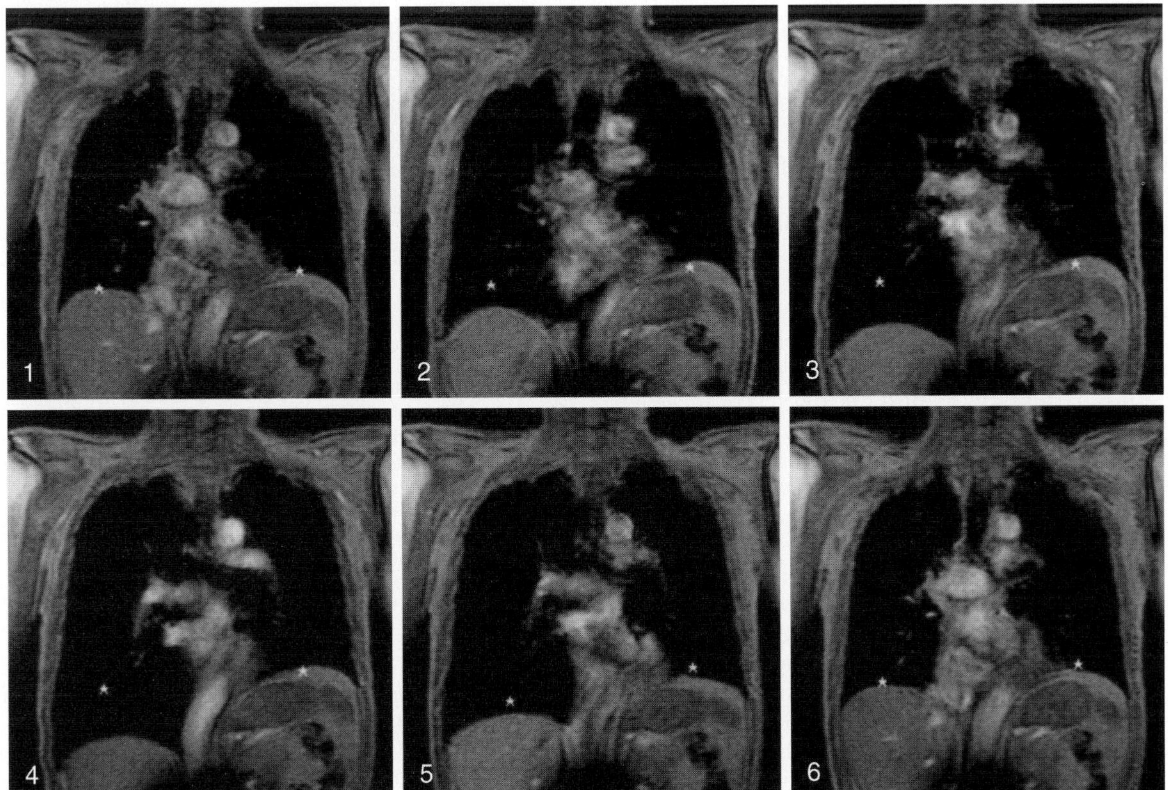

FIGURE 56–35 ■ Left hemidiaphragm paralysis following lung volume reduction surgery. Sequence of coronal magnetic resonance images obtained during slow, deep inspiration (*1–4*) and expiration (*4–6*), with stars marking the end expiratory position of the hemidiaphragm domes, reveals normal, full excursion of the right hemidiaphragm but slight paradoxical motion of the left hemidiaphragm. Paradoxical movement during a subsequent fluoroscopic sniff test was also consistent with left hemidiaphragm paralysis. (From Gierada DS, Slone RM, Fleishman MJ: Imaging evaluation of the diaphragm. Chest Surg Clin North Am 8:237, 1998.)

comitant with inward rather than normal outward movement of the abdominal wall (Higgenbottam et al, 1977). However, a paralyzed hemidiaphragm may show a slight descent on slow, deep inspiration due to passive stretching as the rib cage expands.

The sniff test is therefore necessary to confirm that abnormal hemidiaphragm excursion is due to paralysis rather than unilateral weakness. For the stiff test, the patient inhales rapidly and forcefully through the nose with the mouth closed. This normally produces a sharp, brief descent of both hemidiaphragms. Paradoxical upward motion greater than 2 cm of an entire hemidiaphragm, as seen in oblique or lateral projection, is consistent with hemidiaphragm paralysis (Alexander, 1966).

Several potential difficulties may limit the fluoroscopic assessment of diaphragm paralysis. Diaphragm motion may be diminished due to inflammatory processes such as pneumonia, pleuritis, pleural effusion, peritonitis, and subphrenic abscess, so fluoroscopic assessment is best delayed until such reversible conditions that may affect the diaphragm have resolved. Complete eventration may be difficult or impossible to distinguish from diaphragm paralysis (Fraser et al, 1994), and severe weakness or fatigue may appear identical to bilateral paralysis on fluoroscopy (Tarver et al, 1989). Although some patients with bilateral paralysis show the typical paradoxical upward motion of both hemidiaphragms during a deep inspiration or sniff maneuver, normal inspiratory descent of the diaphragm can be mimicked in those patients who perform the compensatory maneuver of actively exhaling below functional residual capacity using their abdominal muscles, then inhaling by relaxation of the abdominal muscles, which causes passive descent of the diaphragm (Kreitzer et al, 1978). This effect can be detected by carefully observing abdominal motion during breathing (Malagari and Fraser, 1995), and it is minimized by performing the examination with the patient in the recumbent position, which eliminates the assistance of gravity and allows the paradoxical or absent motion to be detected (Ch'en and Armstrong, 1993).

In some patients with phrenic nerve injury, even though fluoroscopy demonstrates paralysis, the paralysis may not be permanent. Regeneration of phrenic nerve fibers may lead to partial or complete recovery of diaphragm function over time, usually within 1 year based on the normal rate of peripheral nerve regeneration (Wilcox et al, 1990). The diagnosis of diaphragm paralysis can also be difficult in patients with severe hyperinflation due to chronic obstructive pulmonary disease, in whom the normal hemidiaphragm moves very little; or in weak, debilitated patients who cannot produce a strong inspiratory effort or forceful sniff. Care must be taken not to mistake the jerking upward motion of the entire thorax produced by some patients in their attempt to sniff forcefully for paradoxical upward diaphragm motion. Definitive diagnosis of phrenic nerve paralysis can be obtained using cervical phrenic nerve stimulation with electromyographic measurement of phrenic nerve latency (Gandevia, 1987; Shochina et al, 1983) or with concomitant fluoroscopic or ultrasound monitoring of the diaphragm to look for diaphragm contraction (McGauley and Labib, 1984).

Several studies have reported that the sonographic assessment of diaphragm motion or thickness is equivalent to fluoroscopy in making the diagnosis of diaphragm dysfunction (Diament et al, 1985; Gottesman and McCool, 1997; Houston et al, 1995). Dynamic MRI of diaphragm movement can reveal abnormal motion due to hemidiaphragm paralysis (see Fig. 56–35), but the accuracy of this technique has not been studied.

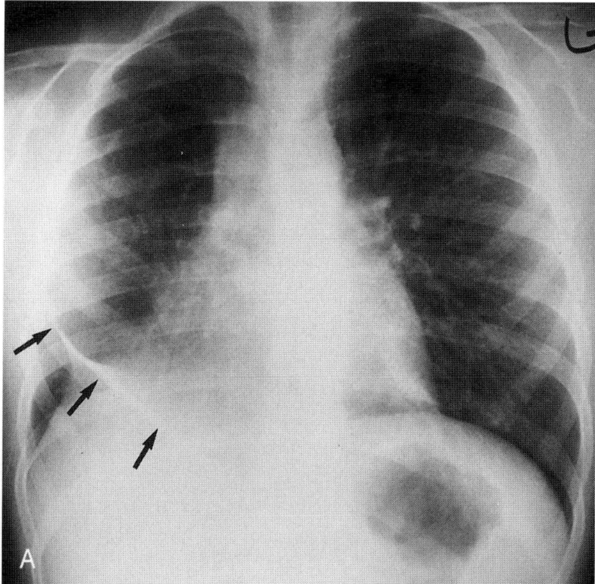

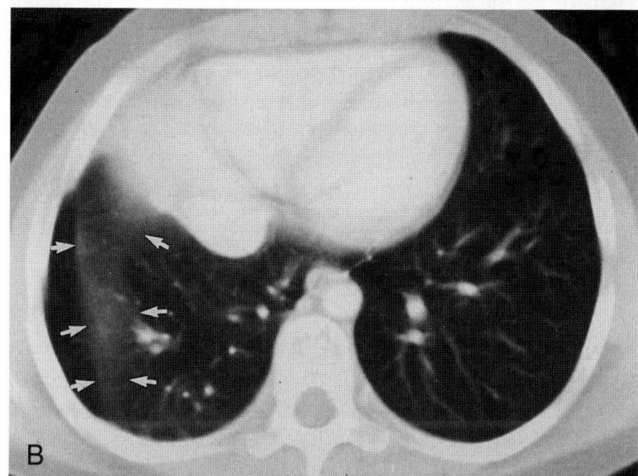

FIGURE 56–36 ■ Accessory hemidiaphragm. *A*, A radiograph obtained in a 7-year-old girl demonstrates a small right hemithorax, a hazy increase in opacity obscuring the right heart border, and a curvilinear band of tissue (*arrows*) extending laterally from the right hemidiaphragm. *B*, A computed tomography scan reveals a thin band of tissue (*open arrows*) coursing through the right lower lobe parenchyma to a posterior rib. Partial anomalous pulmonary venous return to the right atrium was evident on other images. The thin tissue band with these associated findings is characteristic of a rare accessory hemidiaphragm; no pathologic proof was obtained. (Courtesy of Marilyn J. Siegel, MD, St. Louis, MO.) (From Gierada DS, Slone RM, Fleishman MJ: Imaging evaluation of the diaphragm. Chest Surg Clin North Am 8:237, 1998.)

ACCESSORY DIAPHRAGM

An accessory, or duplicated, diaphragm is a rare congenital anomaly in which a thin, fibromuscular membrane is attached to the diaphragm anteriorly and courses posteriorly and cephalad to attach to the posterior rib cage

(Davis and Allen, 1968; Hopkins and Davis, 1988; Wille et al, 1975). Most reported cases occur on the right side. The accessory diaphragm may follow a fissure or divide the lower lobe. There is a frequent association with other congenital anomalies, particularly pulmonary hypoplasia, partial anomalous arterial supply or venous drainage, congenital heart disease (Davis and Allen, 1968; Kenanoglu and Tuncbilek, 1978), and congenital pulmonary venolobar ("scimitar") syndrome (Woodring et al, 1994). The diagnosis is most frequently made during childhood due to repeated respiratory infections or respiratory distress, but it may occur incidentally in an asymptomatic patient.

On frontal radiographs, the affected hemithorax is usually small due to the accompanying pulmonary hypoplasia, and the mediastinal border is indistinct and blurred by a hazy increase in opacity (Fig. 56–36). The lateral radiograph reveals a retrosternal band of increased opacity produced by loose areolar connective tissue filling the space between the anterior chest wall and the small lung (Davis and Allen, 1968). The findings closely resemble those of right upper and middle lobe atelectasis or left upper lobe atelectasis or, alternatively, primary pulmonary hypoplasia (Currarino and Williams, 1985; Davis and Allen, 1968; Kenanoglu and Tuncbilek, 1978; Wille et al, 1975). A thickened, oblique septum may be seen extending posteriorly and cephalad from the diaphragm to the posterior chest wall. CT (see Fig. 56–36) or MRI may be helpful in suggesting the diagnosis (Becmeur et al, 1995).

TUMORS OF THE DIAPHRAGM

Primary tumors of the diaphragm are very rare. Benign tumors are most common, with lipomas (Castillo and Shirkhoda, 1985) and cystic masses such as bronchogenic (Gourlay and Aspinall, 1966), mesothelial, and teratoid (Muller, 1986) cysts reported most frequently (Olaffson et al, 1971). Most malignant tumors are sarcomas of fibrous or muscular origin (Olaffson et al, 1971). Numerous other tumors have been reported, including schwannoma (Koyama et al, 1996), chondroma (Itakura et al, 1990), pheochromocytoma (Buckley et al, 1995), and endometriosis (Posniak et al, 1990).

Tumors of the diaphragm large enough for radiographic detection produce a focal bulge or contour abnormality and can resemble a diaphragmatic hernia, eventration, or a pleural lesion. Since the diaphragm is a thin structure, the diaphragmatic origin of a mass may be difficult to confirm as separate from the lung, pleura, or abdominal viscera, even on CT, MRI, or ultrasound. Small masses of fat density are occasionally seen on CT within the diaphragm muscle, which may represent lipomas that are too small for clinical or radiographic detection, or the density may be age-associated fat containing diaphragmatic defects (Caskey et al, 1989). The CT appearance of nonlipomatous soft tissue tumors generally is not specific.

Pleural plaques related to prior asbestos exposure or prior pleural inflammatory disease may produce calcified (Fig. 56–37) or noncalcified diaphragmatic masses. Calcified plaques can be detected on chest radiography, but CT is more sensitive for detection of both calcified and noncalcified pleural plaques. Features helpful in distinguishing asbestos-related diaphragmatic plaques from pleural metastases, mesothelioma, or the rare primary diaphragmatic tumor include bilateral occurrence, calcification, sharp margins, and flattened contour.

Thoracic and abdominal tumors may secondarily involve the diaphragm by direct extension. Such tumors include bronchogenic carcinoma; mesothelioma and other primary or secondary pleural or chest wall malig-

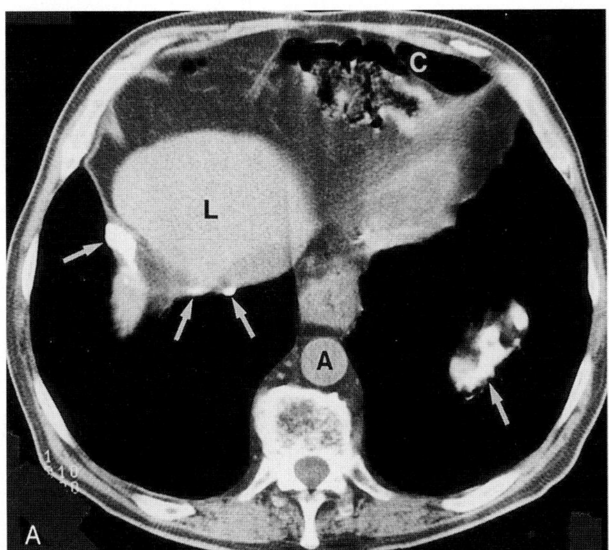

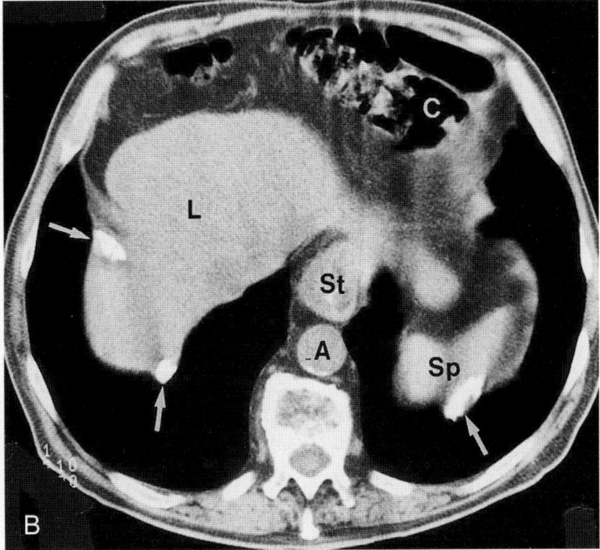

FIGURE 56–37 ■ Calcified pleural plaques. Computed tomography scans at (*A*) and just below (*B*) the left hemidiaphragm dome demonstrate irregular calcified plaques (*arrows*) along the diaphragmatic pleura bilaterally in a 74-year-old man, characteristic of prior asbestos exposure. Note the small hiatal hernia containing proximal stomach (St). (*A*, aorta; C, colon; L, liver; Sp, spleen.) (From Gierada DS, Slone RM, Fleishman MJ: Imaging evaluation of the diaphragm. Chest Surg Clin North Am 8:237, 1998.)

nancies; tumors of the stomach, kidney, adrenal gland, colon, or retroperitoneum; lymphoma; and peritoneal carcinomatosis (Tarver et al, 1989). However, when thoracic or abdominal masses abut the diaphragm without traversing it on imaging studies, definitive diagnosis of invasion cannot be made.

CONCLUSION

The diaphragm performs most of the physiologic work of inspiration and forms an anatomic barrier between the thoracic and abdominal cavities. Disorders of the diaphragm can be related to impairment in either of these functions, with most having radiologic manifestations. Both intrathoracic and intra-abdominal disease processes can alter the normal radiologic appearance of the diaphragm. Abnormalities are usually first detected on chest radiographs, often incidentally in asymptomatic patients, and many require further characterization by other imaging studies for definitive diagnosis. CT, MRI, and fluoroscopy are the most frequently useful additional studies, while ultrasound, barium contrast studies, and liver-spleen scintigraphy are occasionally helpful. Selection of the most appropriate radiologic examination in a given clinical situation can facilitate the diagnosis of diaphragm abnormalities.

COMMENTS AND CONTROVERSIES

Diaphragmatic imaging is a subject that is not frequently considered in the practice of general thoracic surgery. Nonetheless, in recent years standard imaging techniques have been augmented considerably to provide superb imaging by CT and MRI. In addition, dynamic MRI enables real-time imaging of diaphragmatic function and pathology. Drs. Gierada and Slone have written a clear and extremely detailed chapter discussing the issues of diaphragmatic imaging. The illustrations clearly depict the points under discussion.

G.A.P.

■ REFERENCES

Alexander C: Diaphragm movements and the diagnosis of diaphragmatic paralysis. Clin Radiol 17:79, 1966.

Andrus CH, Morton JH: Rupture of the diaphragm after blunt trauma. Am J Surg 119:686, 1970.

Armstrong P, Wilson AG, Dee P, Hansell DM: Imaging of Diseases of the Chest, 2nd ed. St. Louis, CV Mosby, 1995.

Aronberg DJ, Peterson RR, Glazer HS, Sagel SS: Superior diaphragmatic lymph nodes: CT assessment. J Comput Assist Tomogr 10:937, 1986.

Becmeur F, Horta P, Donato L et al: Accessory diaphragm—review of 31 cases in the literature. Eur J Pediatr Surg 5:43, 1995.

Bencerraf BR, Greene MF: Congenital diaphragmatic hernia: US diagnosis prior to 22 weeks' gestation. Radiology 158:809, 1986.

Berkmen YM, Davis SD, Kazam E et al: Right phrenic nerve: Anatomy, CT appearance, and differentiation from the pulmonary ligament. Radiology 173:43, 1989.

Blair E, Hickam JB: The effect of change in body position on lung volume and intrapulmonary gas mixing in normal subjects. J Clin Invest 34:383, 1955.

Boulanger BR, Milzman DP, Rosati C, Rodriguez A: A comparison of right and left blunt traumatic diaphragmatic rupture. J Trauma 35:255, 1993.

Brewer LAD, Gazzaniga AB: Phrenoplasty, a new operation for the management of pleural dead space following pulmonary resection. Ann Thorac Surg 6:119, 1968.

Brink JA, Heiken JP, Semenkovich J et al: Abnormalities of the diaphragm and adjacent structures: Findings on multiplanar spiral CT scans. AJR Am J Roentgenol 163:307, 1994.

Buckley KM, Whitman GJ, Chew FS: Diaphragmatic pheochromocytoma. AJR Am J Roentgenol 165:260, 1995.

Carter EA, Cleverley JR, Delany DJ, Lea RE: Case report: Cine MRI in the diagnosis of a ruptured right hemidiaphragm. Clin Radiol 51:137, 1996.

Caskey CI, Zerhouni EA, Fishman EK, Rahmouni AD: Aging of the diaphragm: a CT study. Radiology 171:385, 1989.

Castillo M, Shirkhoda A: Computed tomography of diaphragmatic lipoma. J Comput Tomogr 9:167, 1985.

Ch'en IY, Armstrong JDI: Value of fluoroscopy in patients with suspected bilateral hemidiaphragmatic paralysis. AJR Am J Roentgenol 160:29, 1993.

Chen JC, Wilson SE: Diaphragmatic injuries: Recognition and management in sixty-two patients. Am Surg 57:810, 1991.

Cooper C, Moss AA, Buy JN et al: CT appearance of the normal inferior pulmonary ligament. AJR Am J Roentgenol 141:237, 1983.

Currarino G, Williams B: Causes of congenital unilateral pulmonary hypoplasia: A study of 33 cases. Pediatr Radiol 15:15, 1985.

Davis WS, Allen RP: Accessory diaphragm. Duplication of the diaphragm. Radiol Clin North Am 6:253, 1968.

Demos TC, Solomon C, Posniak HV, Flisak MJ: Computed tomography in traumatic defects of the diaphragm. Clin Imag 13:62, 1989.

Desforges G, Strieder JW, Lynch JP et al: Traumatic rupture of the diaphragm. J Thorac Surg 34:780, 1957.

Diament MJ, Boechat MI, Kangarloo H: Real-time sector ultrasound in the evaluation of suspected abnormalities of diaphragmatic motion. J Clin Ultrasound 13:539, 1985.

Dosios T, Papachristos IC, Chrysicopoulos H: Magnetic resonance imaging of blunt traumatic rupture of the right hemidiaphragm. Eur J Cardiothorac Surg 7:553, 1993.

Felson B: Chest Roentgenology. Philadelphia, WB Saunders, 1973.

Fleischner FG: Atypical arrangement of free pleural effusion. Radiol Clin North Am 1:347, 1963.

Fraser RS, Paré JAP, Fraser RG, Paré PD: Synopsis of Diseases of the Chest, 2nd ed. Philadelphia, WB Saunders, 1994.

Gale ME: Bochdalek hernia: Prevalence and CT characteristics. Radiology 156:449, 1985.

Gandevia SC: Assessment of hemidiaphragmatic "paralysis." Am Rev Respir Dis 135:1214, 1987.

Gelman R, Mirvis SE, Gens D: Diaphragmatic rupture due to blunt trauma: Sensitivity of plain chest radiographs. AJR Am J Roentgenol 156:51, 1991.

Gierada DS, Curtin JJ, Erickson SJ et al: Diaphragmatic motion: Fast gradient-recalled-echo MR imaging in healthy subjects. Radiology 194:879, 1995.

Gierada DS, Curtin JJ, Erickson SJ et al: Fast gradient echo magnetic resonance imaging of the normal diaphragm. J Thorac Imaging 12:70, 1996.

Godwin JD, MacGregor JM: Extension of ascites into the chest with hiatal hernia: Visualization on CT. AJR Am J Roentgenol 148:31, 1987.

Godwin JD, Vock P, Osborne DR: CT of the pulmonary ligament. AJR Am J Roentgenol 141:231, 1983.

Gottesman E, McCool FD: Ultrasound evaluation of the paralyzed diaphragm. Am J Respir Crit Care Med 155:1570, 1997.

Gourin A, Garzon AA: Diagnostic problems in traumatic diaphragmatic hernia. J Trauma 14:20, 1974.

Gourlay RH, Aspinall RJ: Bronchogenic cyst of the diaphragm: A case report. Can J Surg 9:169, 1966.

Gurney J, Harrison WL, Anderson JC: Omental fat simulating pleural fluid in traumatic diaphragmatic hernia. J Comput Assist Tomogr 9:1112, 1985.

Guth AA, Pachter HL, Kim U: Pitfalls in the diagnosis of blunt diaphragmatic injury. Am J Surg 170:5, 1995.

Harris RS, Giovanetti M, Kim BK: Normal ventilatory movement of the right hemidiaphragm studied by ultrasonography and pneumotachography. Radiology 1983:141, 1983.

Heiberg E, Wolverson MK, Hurd RN et al: CT recognition of traumatic rupture of the diaphragm. AJR Am J Roentgenol 135:369, 1980.

Hertzanu Y, Solomon A: Inversion of the right diaphragm: A thoracoabdominal CT pitfall. Gastrointest Radiol 11:200, 1986.

Hesselink JR, Chung KJ, Peters ME, Crummy AB: Congenital partial eventration of the left diaphragm. AJR Am J Roentgenol 131:417, 1978.

Hessén I: Roentgen examination of pleural effusion. A study of the localization of free effusion, the potentialities of diagnosing minimal quantities of fluid and its existence under physiological conditions. Acta Radiol Suppl 86:7, 1951.

Higgenbottam T, Allen D, Loh L, Clark JTH: Abdominal wall movement in normals and in patients with hemidiaphragmatic and bilateral diaphragmatic palsy. Thorax 32:589, 1977.

Holland DG, Quint LE: Traumatic rupture of the diaphragm without visceral herniation: CT diagnosis. AJR Am J Roentgenol 157:17, 1991.

Hood RM: Traumatic diaphragmatic hernia. Ann Thorac Surg 12:311, 1971.

Hopkins RL, Davis SH: Haziness of the right hemithorax in a newborn. Chest 94:662, 1988.

Houston JG, Fleet M, Cowan MD, McMillan NC: Comparison of ultrasound with fluoroscopy in the assessment of suspected hemidiaphragmatic movement abnormality. Clin Radiol 50:95, 1995.

Ingram RH: Disease of the pleura, mediastinum, and diaphragm, In Braunwald E, Isselbacher KJ, Petersdorf RG et al (eds): Harrison's Principles of Internal Medicine, 11th ed. New York, McGraw-Hill, 1987.

Israel RS, Mayberry JC, Primack SL: Diaphragmatic rupture: Use of helical CT scanning with multiplanar reformations. AJR Am J Roentgenol 167:1201, 1996.

Itakura M, Shiraishi K, Kadosaka T, Matsuzaki S: Chondroma of the diaphragm—report of a case. Endoscopy 22:276, 1990.

Juhl JH: Diseases of the pleura, mediastinum, and diaphragm. In Juhl JH, Crummy AB (eds): Paul and Juhl's Essentials of Radiologic Imaging, 5th ed. Philadelphia, JB Lippincott, 1987.

Kanematsu M, Imaeda T, Mochizuki R et al: Dynamic MRI of the diaphragm. J Comput Assist Tomogr 19:67, 1995.

Kawashima A, Libshitz HI: Malignant pleural mesothelioma: CT manifestations in 50 cases. AJR Am J Roentgenol 155:965, 1990.

Kearney PA, Rouhana SW, Burney RE: Blunt rupture of the diaphragm: Mechanism, diagnosis, and treatment. Ann Emerg Med 18:1326, 1989.

Kenanoglu A, Tuncbilek E: Accessory diaphragm in the left side. Pediatr Radiol 7:172, 1978.

Kirks DR, Caron KH: Gastrointestinal tract. In Kirks DR (ed): Practical Pediatric Imaging, 2nd ed. Boston, Little, Brown, 1991.

Koyama S, Araki M, Suzuki K et al: Primary diaphragmatic schwannoma with a typical target appearance: Correlation of CT and MR imagings and histologic findings. J Gastroenterol 31:268, 1996.

Kreitzer SM, Feldmon NT, Saunders NA, Ingram RH: Bilateral diaphragmatic paralysis with hypercapneic respiratory failure. A physiologic assessment. Am J Med 65:89, 1978.

Lennon EA, Simon G: The height of the diaphragm in the chest radiograph of normal adults. Br J Radiol 38:937, 1965.

Malagari K, Fraser RG: Imaging of the chest wall and diaphragm. In Roussos C (ed): The Thorax. Part C: Disease. New York, Marcel Dekker, 1995, pp 1763–1837.

Marchand P: A study of the forces productive of gastroesophageal regurgitation and herniation through the diaphragmatic hiatus. Thorax 12:189, 1957.

McGauley RGK, Labib KB: Diaphragmatic paralysis evaluated by phrenic nerve stimulation during fluoroscopy or real-time ultrasound. Radiology 153:33, 1984.

Mirvis SE, Keramati B, Buckman R, Rodriguez A: MR imaging of traumatic diaphragmatic rupture. J Comput Assist Tomogr 12:147, 1988.

Muller NL: CT features of cystic teratoma of the diaphragm. J Comput Assist Tomogr 10:325, 1986.

Mulvey RB: The effect of pleural fluid on the diaphragm. AJR Am J Roentgenol 84:1080, 1965.

Murray JG, Caoili E, Gruden JF, et al: Acute rupture of the diaphragm due to blunt trauma: Diagnostic sensitivity and specificity of CT. AJR Am J Roentgenol 166:1035, 1996.

Okuda K, Nomura F, Kawai M et al: Age-related gross changes of the liver and right diaphragm, with special reference to partial eventration. Br J Radiol 52:870, 1979.

Olaffson G, Rausing A, Holen O: Primary tumors of the diaphragm. Chest 59:568, 1971.

Panicek DM, Benson CB, Gottlieb RH, Heitzman ER: The diaphragm: Anatomic, pathologic, and radiologic considerations. Radiographics 8:385, 1988.

Pearson FG, Cooper JD, Ilves et al: Massive hiatal hernia with incarceration: A report of 53 cases. Ann Thorac Surg 35:45, 1983.

Peterson JA: Recognition of infrapulmonary pleural effusion. Radiology 74:34, 1960.

Posniak HV, Keshavarzian A, Jabamoni R: Diaphragmatic endometriosis: CT and MR findings. Gastrointest Radiol 15:349, 1990.

Prassopoulos PK, Raissaki MT, Gourtsoyiannis NC: Hepatodiaphragmatic interposition of the colon in the upright and supine position. J Comput Assist Tomogr 20:151, 1996.

Probert WR, Havard C: Traumatic diaphragmatic hernia. Thorax 16:99, 1961.

Rabinowitz JG, Efremidis SC, Cohen B et al: A comparative study of mesothelioma and asbestosis using computed tomography and conventional chest radiography. Radiology 144:453, 1982.

Reid WD: Respiratory muscle pathology. In Roussos C (ed): The Thorax. Part C: Disease. New York, Marcel Dekker, 1995.

Rodriguez-Morales G, Rodriguez A, Shatney CH: Acute rupture of the diaphragm in blunt trauma: Analysis of 60 patients. J Trauma 26:438, 1986.

Rost RC, Proto AV: Inferior pulmonary ligament: Computed tomographic appearance. Radiology 148:479, 1983.

Rouviere H: Anatomy of the Lymphatic System. Ann Arbor, MI, Edwards Brothers, 1938.

Shackleton KL, Steward ET, Taylor AJ: Traumatic diaphragmatic injuries: Spectrum of radiographic findings. Radiographics 18:49, 1998.

Shanmuganathan K, Mirvis SE, White CS, Pomerantz SM: MR imaging evaluation of hemidiaphragms in acute blunt trauma: Experience with 16 patients. AJR Am J Roentgenol 167:397, 1996.

Shochina M, Ferber I, Wolf E: Evaluation of the phrenic nerve in patients with neuromuscular disorders. Int J Rehabil Res 6:455, 1983.

Simon G, Bonnell J, Kazantzis G, Waller RE: Some radiological observations on the range of movement of the diaphragm. Clin Radiol 20:231, 1969.

Slone RM, Gierada DS: Radiology of pulmonary emphysema and lung volume reduction surgery. Semin Thorac Cardiovasc Surg 8:61, 1996.

Somers JM, Gleeson FV, Flower CD: Rupture of the right hemidiaphragm following blunt trauma: The use of ultrasound in diagnosis. Clin Radiol 42:97, 1990.

Swingle JD, Logan R, Juhl JH: Inversion of the left hemidiaphragm. JAMA 208:863, 1969.

Tarver RD, Conces DJJ, Cory DA, Vix VA: Imaging the diaphragm and its disorders. J Thorac Imag 4:1, 1989.

Ujita M, Ojiri H, Ariizumi M, Tada S: Appearance of the inferior phrenic artery and vein on CT scans of the chest: A CT and cadaveric study. AJR Am J Roentgenol 160:745, 1993.

Voeller GR, Reisser JR, Fabian TC et al: Blunt diaphragm injuries. A five-year experience. Am Surg 56:28, 1990.

Vogl A, Small A: Partial eventration of the right diaphragm (congenital diaphragmatic herniation of liver). Ann Intern Med 43:61, 1955.

Ward RE, Flynn TC, Clark WP: Diaphragmatic disruption secondary to blunt abdominal trauma. J Trauma 21:35, 1981.

White JJ, Suzuki H: Hernia through the foramen of Bochdalek: A misnomer. J Pediatr Surg 7:61, 1972.

Wilcox PG, Pardy RL: Diaphragmatic weakness and paralysis. Lung 167:323, 1989.

Wilcox PG, Pare PD, Pardy RL: Recovery after unilateral phrenic injury associated with coronary artery revascularization. Chest 98:661, 1990.

Wille L, Holthusen W, Willich E: Accessory diaphragm. Report of 6 cases and a review of the literature. Pediatr Radiol 4:14, 1975.

Williams P, Warwick R, Dyson M, Bannister L: Gray's Anatomy, 37th ed. Edinburgh, Churchill Livingstone, 1989.

Wise L, Connors J, Hwang YH, Anderson C: Traumatic injuries to the diaphragm. J Trauma 13:946, 1973.

Woodring JH, Howard TA, Kanga JF: Congenital pulmonary venolobar syndrome revisited. Radiographics 14:349, 1994.

Worthy SA, Kang EY, Hartman TE et al: Diaphragmatic rupture: CT findings in 11 patients. Radiology 194:885, 1995.

Young DA, Simon G: Certain movements measured on inspiration-expiration chest radiographs correlated with pulmonary function studies. Clin Radiol 23:37, 1972.

CONGENITAL DIAPHRAGMATIC HERNIAS

Geoffrey M. Graeber
Jacob Davtyan
Joseph I. Miller, Jr.

Congenital diaphragmatic hernias are classified as (1) posterolateral (Bochdalek), (2) retrosternal anterior (Morgagni), (3) septum transversum (central), or (4) esophageal hiatal. The first three are discussed in this chapter. Hiatal hernias are discussed in *Esophageal Surgery*, Section IV.

Posterolateral Hiatal Hernia of Bochdalek

HISTORICAL NOTE

Although Vincent Bochdalek's 1848 description was that of bowel herniation through a dorsal diaphragmatic split the lumbocostal triangle, the coagenital posterolateral diaphragmatic hernia (CPLDH) carries his name. In 1946, Cross performed the first successful repair of CPLDH in a newborn. Bartlett and co-workers (1976) reported successful application of extracorporeal membrane oxygenation (ECMO) in infancy. German and co-workers (1977) reported the first survivor of ECMO in the treatment of CPLDH.

CPLDH occurs in 1:2000 to 1:5000 live births (Harrison and de Lorimier, 1981) and is a result of failure of the pleuroperitoneal canal to close at the eighth week of gestation (Gray and Skandalakis, 1972). Of these hernias, 80% occur on the left side. Bilateral hernias are extremely rare (Levy et al, 1969), and very few of these newborns survive (Sokal et al, 1990). In only 10% of cases is there a true hernia sac. The abdominal organs herniate into the chest through the diaphragmatic defect, compressing and retarding the growth and development of the ipsilateral lung. The mediastinum may be shifted to the opposite side, affecting the contralateral lung as well. The morphology of the diaphragmatic muscle is normal (Dietz and Pongratz, 1991). The morphologic and biochemical development of the lungs is retarded in most cases, particularly on the ipsilateral side (Nakamura et al, 1991). The susceptibility of these babies to bronchopulmonary dysplasia during artificial ventilation is probably related to a defective antioxidant system and defective surfactant production (Molenaar et al, 1991). Pulmonary hypoplasia is also evident in pulmonary function studies. Nakayama and associates (1991) showed restrictive lung defects in infants who survived neonatal repair of CPLDH, and Geggel and colleagues (1985) reported decrease of the cross-sectional area of the pulmonary arterial bed in infants dying after repair of CPLDH. Associated major anomalies occur in up to 40% of live births (Cunniff et al, 1990). Thorpe-Beeston (1989) reported prenatal diagnosis of major abnormalities in 48% of fetuses, including chromosomal defects in 31% and major malformations in 17% Trisomy 18 and trisomy 13 are the most common chromosomal abnormalities. Cardiac, neural, and genitourinary anomalies are frequent (Adzick et al, 1989). Malrotation of the bowel is always present.

■ *HISTORICAL READINGS*

Bartlett RH, Gazzaniga AB, Jeffries MR et al: Extracorporeal membrane oxygenation (ECMO): Cardiopulmonary support in infancy. Trans Am Soc Artif Intern Organs 22:80, 1976.

Cunniff C, Jones KL, Jones MC: Patterns of malformation in children with congenital diaphragmatic defects. J Pediatr 116:258, 1990.

Dietz HG, Pongratz D: Morphology of the diaphragmatic muscle in CDH. Eur J Pediatr Surg 1:85, 1991.

Geggel RL, Murphy JD, Langleben D et al: Congenital diaphragmatic hernia: Arterial structural changes and persistent pulmonary hypertension after surgical repair. J Pediatr 107:457, 1985.

German JC, Gazzaniga AB, Amlie R et al: Management of pulmonary insufficiency in diaphragmatic hernia using extracorporeal circulation with a membrane oxygenator (ECMO). J Pediatr Surg 12:905, 1977.

Gray SW, Skandalakis JE: The diaphragm. In Embryology for Surgeons: The Embryological Basis for the Treatment of Congenital Defects. Philadelphia, WB Saunders, 1972 p 359.

Gross RE: Congenital hernia of the diaphragm. Am J Dis Child 71:580, 1946.

Harrison MR, de Lorimier AA: Congenital diaphragmatic hernia. Surg Clin North Am 61:1023, 1981.

Levy JL Jr, Guyner WA, Louis JE et al: Bilateral congenital diaphragmatic hernias through the foramina of Bochdalek. J Pediatr Surg 4:557, 1969.

Molenaar JC, Bos AP, Hazelbrock FWJ, et al: Congenital diaphragmatic hernia, what defect? J Pediatr Surg 26:248, 1991.

Nakamura Y, Yamamoto I, Fukuda S et al: Pulmonary acinar development in diaphragmatic hernia. Arch Pathol Lab Med 115:372, 1991.

Nakayama DK, Motoyama EK, Mutich RL et al: Pulmonary function in newborns after repair of congenital diaphragmatic hernia. Pediatr Pulmonol 11:49, 1991.

Sokal MM, Yellin PB, Mestel AL et al: Survival after bilateral congenital diaphragmatic hernia. Clin Pediatr (Phila) 29:677, 1990.

Thorpe-Beeston JG, Gosden CM, Nicolaides KH: Prenatal diagnosis of congenital diaphragmatic hernia: Associated malformations and chromosomal defects. Fetal Ther 4:21, 1989.

BASIC SCIENCE

Pathophysiology

The pathophysiology of CPLDH depends on the interplay of pulmonary hypoplasia and pulmonary hypertension.

Hypoplastic lungs result in various degrees of hypoxia. In addition, such lungs have increased sensitivity to the stimuli increasing pulmonary vascular resistance, namely hypoxia, acidosis, hypercarbia, and hypothermia (Shochat, 1987). The resulting pulmonary hypertension reverses the flow through the patent ductus arteriosus and opens the foramen ovale with right-to-left shunting. Thus, the syndrome of persistent fetal circulation (Gersony et al, 1969) is established, resulting in the vicious circle of hypoxia, acidosis, even higher pulmonary resistance, and increasing right-to-left shunting, which ultimately culminates in the death of these babies.

DIAGNOSIS

The clinical presentation depends on the degree of respiratory compromise, which may vary from severe distress at birth to delayed presentation in infancy or early childhood. The age of the patient at presentation is one of the determining factors of morbidity and mortality (Reynolds et al, 1984). The newborn with CPLDH is usually dyspneic, tachycardic, and frequently cyanotic with a striking scaphoid abdomen. The trachea and the heart are shifted to the contralateral side. Breath sounds are decreased or absent on the ipsilateral side. Chest radiography may be diagnostic, with bowel loops in the affected hemithorax and contralateral mediastinal shift. The gastric tube may be seen in the chest, and paucity of gas is noted in the abdomen. On the right the defect may be blocked by the liver, with less extensive herniation and milder respiratory compromise.

The clinical presentation of the infant suffering from foramen of Bochdalek hernia is dependent on the size of the defect and the amount of visceral migration that occurs from the peritoneal cavity to the ipsilateral pleural space. In small hernias the amount of migration of abdominal viscera into the thoracic cavity is minimal. These patients do not present until later in infancy or even childhood. Symptoms range from discomfort to feeding abnormalities and colicky symptoms with poor progression of growth. Radiographs of the chest generally define these hernias because air is located in one of the viscera that has herniated through the foramen.

Correction of small hernias presenting after the perinatal period is generally conducted through an ipsilateral thoracotomy. The hernia sac, if present, is generally identified, the abdominal viscera are reduced into the peritoneal cavity, the sac is excised, and the defect is closed. Closure is usually performed by horizontal mattress sutures placed over pledgets. Occasionally the repair is reinforced with a running suture line placed superficial to the horizontal mattress sutures. Prosthetic patch reconstruction is seldom necessary. In infants and children presenting in this manner, morbidity and mortality from the condition and its operative correction are minimal. The condition can be severe, however, because severe respiratory distress and even death have been reported with rapid expansion of abdominal viscera into the chest.

Infants who present with large congenital defects of the diaphragm usually have respiratory distress very early in the immediate perinatal period. Auscultation of the chest at that time reveals bowel sounds in the chest on the side of the hernia. In the usual presentation of an infant with this type of hernia, the bowel sounds are in the left chest, and the heart sounds are displaced toward the right side of the chest. The abdomen is scaphoid because the viscera are in the chest. Compression of the ipsilateral lung also causes a severe decrease in or absence of breath sounds on the ipsilateral side. The mediastinum is shifted to the contralateral side, and in severe cases the contralateral lung is also compressed by the shift of the thoracic viscera secondary to the migration of the abdominal viscera into the pleural space. Auscultation of the abdomen demonstrates a relative absence of bowel sounds, which is consistent with the migration of the bowels into the left chest. Confirmation of the diagnosis is usually obtained radiographically. If a nasogastric or orogastric tube has been placed prior to radiography, the tip of the tube is seen above the diaphragm, particularly with left-sided hernias. This defines the stomach as being in the left pleural space. The radiograph also demonstrates bowels in the affected pleural space (Fig. 56–38). The infant should not have mask ventilation at this time, since mask ventilation promotes deposition of air in the gastrointestinal tract, which causes further distention of the stomach. The infant should be intubated, an umbilical line should be established, and he or she should be prepared for immediate surgical correction.

MANAGEMENT

Preoperative Management

The clinical suspicion of CPLDH in a newborn with respiratory distress mandates endotracheal intubation, assisted ventilation, and orogastric tube decompression of the gastrointestinal tract to prevent further bowel distention and worsening of respiratory compromise. These babies are maintained with an inspired oxygen fraction (FIO_2) of 1.0, peak inspiratory pressure below 30 cmH_2O, positive end-expiratory pressure (PEEP) of less than 5 cmH_2O, and hyperventilation. High-frequency ventilation may be used. Preductal and postductal arterial blood gases are monitored by right radial and umbilical arterial catheters, respectively. Ideally, postductal arterial oxygen tension (PaO_2) is maintained above 100 mm Hg, arterial carbon dioxide tension ($PaCO_2$) below 30 mm Hg, and pH above 7.50 to prevent and alleviate pulmonary vasospasm. Sodium bicarbonate and tromethamine (THAM) may be used to treat acidosis. Venous access and maintenance of systolic blood pressure higher than 50 mm Hg are basic. Fluids are kept to a minimum. Babies should be paralyzed with pancuronium and anesthetized with fentanyl. Fentanyl use is thought to be associated with decreased frequency and severity of episodes of pulmonary hypertension (Vacanti, 1989; Vacanti et al, 1984) as well as decreased incidence of pneumothorax, a catastrophic complication (Hansen et al, 1984).

Multiple attempts have been made to define the predictive factors of mortality of patients with CPLDH (Raphaely and Downes 1973; Boix-Ochoa et al, 1974; Boix-Ochoa et al 1977; Manthei et al, 1983; Mishalany et al, 1979; Ruff et al 1980; Wilson et al, 1991). 1983; Wilson et al, 1991; Ruff et al, 1980). Admission or preoperative

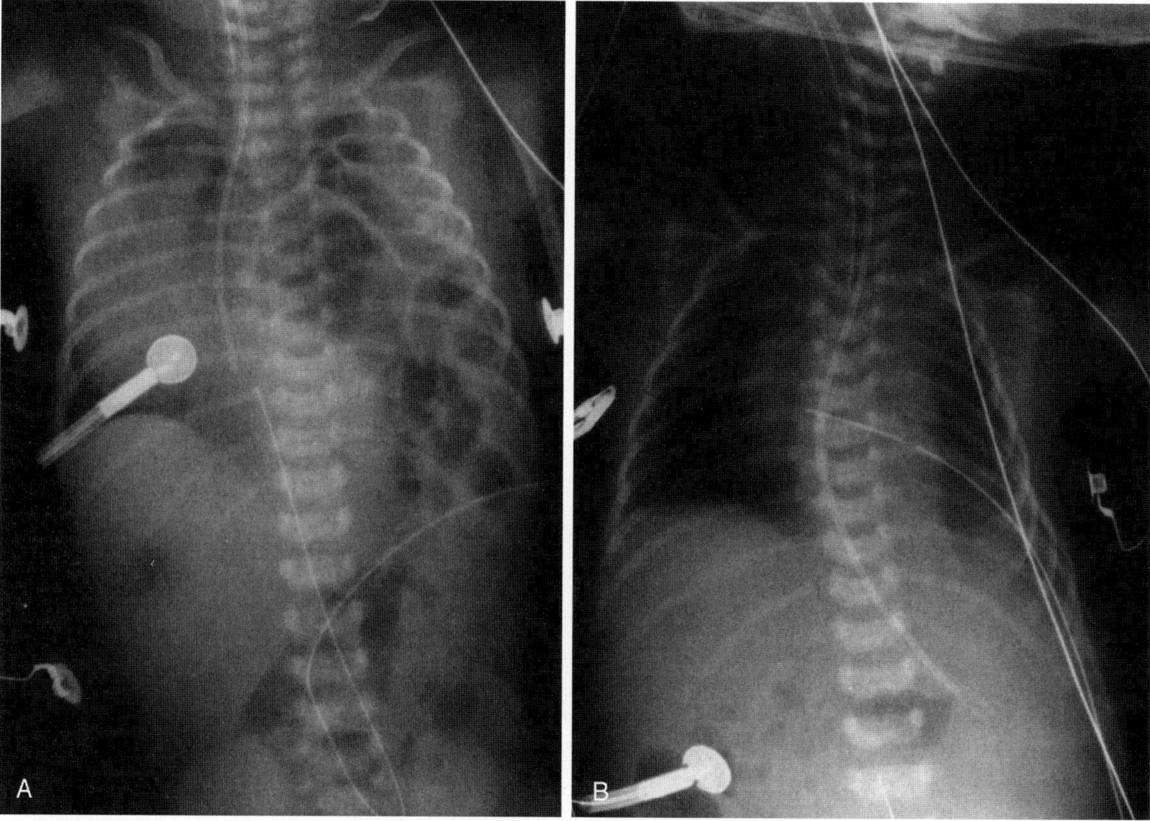

FIGURE 56–38 ■ *A*, This radiograph demonstrates typical findings in a newborn infant who has a foramen of Bochdalek hernia. Note that the abdominal viscera have migrated through the diaphragm and are occupying the left pleural space. The mediastinal contents, great vessels, and tracheobronchial tree are all shifted to the right. Note that the cardiac silhouette blends with the compressed pulmonary parenchyma on the right side and that the stomach, colon, and small bowel are all in the left chest. The child has been intubated and is being prepared for emergency surgical correction. *B*, This postoperative chest radiograph shows that the hernia has been corrected and that a chest tube is in place in the left pleural space. Note that the left lung does not totally fill the left pleural space. This is consistent with severe hypoplasia in the lung; the chest tube has been properly placed but does not establish complete expansion of the lung. The tracheal air column, the cardiac silhouette, the great vessels, and the rest of the mediastinal structures have returned to their normal position. Note also that the right lung is fully expanded and is no longer compressed by the displacement of the mediastinal structures.

blood gas values, specifically, a pH higher than 7.2, a PaCO_2 below 35 mm Hg, and a PaO_2 above 100 mm Hg are associated with an excellent prognosis. Patients with a pH below 7.0, PaCO_2 above 50 mm Hg, and PaO_2 below 80 mm Hg fare poorly. Vacanti and co-workers (1984) termed the infants achieving a postductal PaO_2 above 100 mm Hg with standard therapy *responders* and those who were unable to achieve a postductal PaO_2 of 100 mm Hg with maximum therapy *nonresponders* The responders most often survived without ECMO. Nonresponders had more severe pulmonary hyperplasia and pulmonary hypertension not responsive to medical and ventilatory interventions; in the past all these babies died without ECMO (Vacanti, 1989). Bohn (1987) compared preductal PaCO_2 levels with ventilatory index (VI). Among those with a PaCO_2 of 40 mm Hg and a VI over 1000 there was 100% survival. Preoperative alveolar-arterial oxygen difference ($\text{PA}_2 - \text{Pa}\text{O}_2$) calculated from preductal (right radial) arterial blood gas is another predictor of outcome. Survivors have $\text{PA}_2 - \text{PaQ}_2$ below 200 mm Hg; those with $\text{PA}_2 - \text{PaQ}_2$ above 200 mm Hg rarely survive (Bohn, 1987).

Operative Repair

Traditionally, newborns with CPLDH are taken to the operating room emergently after expeditious resuscitation. Neck lines should be avoided, preserving the vessels for possible ECMO. A transabdominal subcostal approach is preferred by most for left-sided lesions, whereas a transthoracic approach may be more useful for right-sided hernias. Herniated organs are returned to the peritoneal cavity, and the seldom-present hernia sac is excised. The lung is inspected, but no attempt should be made to expand the hypoplastic lung. Extralobar pulmonary sequestration, occasionally present, should be excised. The edges of the defect are defined. Frequently, a significant span of the posterior diaphragm can be unrolled after incision of the posterior peritoneum.

Most of the defects can be closed primarily with interrupted nonabsorbable sutures. In rare cases of absent posterior rim, the sutures can be passed around the ribs. Large defects can be closed with a prosthetic patch. The left pleural space is drained with a 12 French chest tube, which should be placed to an underwater seal but never to suction. A contralateral chest tube is also placed. If the patient's condition permits, the malrotation should be corrected. The abdomen is closed by using techniques developed for closure of abdominal wall defects, and digital stretching of the anterior wall is performed. If primary fascial closure is impossible, only the skin can be closed, leaving ventral hernia to be closed later. Occasionally the "silo" technique has to be used.

Surgical correction of a severe foramen of Bochdalek hernia presenting in the perinatal period is conducted through an upper abdominal approach. After the peritoneal cavity has been opened, the abdominal viscera are reduced from the pleural cavity. If a peritoneal sac is present, it is resected following the removal of the abdominal viscera from the defect. A 10 French chest tube is placed in the pleural cavity to evacuate fluids, to aid in the re-expansion, and to ensure that no pressure occurs in the affected pleural space. Although the chest tube in many cases may not completely re-expand the ipsilateral lung, the equalization of pressure allows return of the mediastinum to the midline and removes any pressure on the contralateral lung. Before the defect is repaired, any extralobar pulmonary sequestration that may be present should be surgically removed. If the defect is relatively small, it may be closed by the direct suture technique as outlined previously. If the defect is substantial and can only be closed with tension, synthetic patch reconstruction should be performed. The patch should be sewn to the margin of the defect with permanent horizontal mattress sutures. Some surgeons believe that this suture line should be reinforced with a running, fine Prolene suture superficial to the original layer of horizontal mattress sutures. The peritoneal cavity should then be inspected for obstructing duodenal bands and malrotation of the midgut, which are often present. These conditions should be corrected before closure is started.

Closure of the abdomen can sometimes be difficult, since the abdominal viscera have not matured in the peritoneal cavity. With return of the abdominal viscera into the peritoneal cavity, compression of the diaphragm can occur with a tight abdominal wall closure. Such compression would impede good excursion of the diaphragm and ventilation of the patient. In order to avoid this serious complication, a ventral epigastric hernia may be created. In such cases the fascia and musculature are left open, and only the skin is closed. If sufficient relaxing incisions cannot be made by mobilizing only the skin and subcutaneous tissues to close the defect, a surgical gastroschisis is created. In such cases the peritoneal cavity is not large enough to hold the viscera without causing serious encroachment on the diaphragm. The surgical gastroschisis repair is made by using synthetic material to fashion a pouch along the anterior abdominal wall that contains a portion of the viscera. The abdominal viscera are gradually returned to the enlarging peritoneal cavity by gentle, progressive compression of the pouch without causing undue embarrassment of respiratory function.

The management of the chest tube during the operation and in the immediate postoperative period has been a source of some controversy. Some surgeons prefer to leave the chest tube to water seal, whereas others advocate placing a one-way valve in the tube and allowing for manual pressure equalization. Still others advocate gentle negative pressure generated through a water seal system to promote expansion of the lung and relief of pressure in the chest. In general, the majority feel that water seal drainage or gentle suction across a water seal drainage is most beneficial.

Timing of the Operation

As stated earlier, most newborns with CPLDH are operated on emergently. Recently, however, there have been several reports of comparable or even better results with delayed repair after various periods of medical stabilization (Breaux et al, 1991; Cartlidge et al, 1986; Charlton et al, 1991; Haugen et al, 1991; Hazelbrock et al, 1988; Langer et al, 1988). To answer these and many other questions regarding the proper management of newborns with CPLDH, a large, multicenter, prospective randomized study is necessary.

A recent development in the treatment of CPLDH is antenatal surgical therapy (Harrison and deLorimier, 1981; Harrison et al, 1990a,b). There is an ongoing debate over the feasibility of this experimental therapy (Stolar, 1990). It imposes a risk to the mother as well as to the fetus with potentially fatal results for both. The proper indications for this procedure are yet to be defined (Wenstrom et al, 1991).

Long-Term Results

Although some respiratory abnormalities can be found in survivors of CPLDH, they generally have a normal life and carry on normal physical activity (Frenckner and Freyschuss, 1988). Most of these studies were performed in the follow-up of patients operated on in the pre-ECMO era. As more severely affected babies survive the modern therapy, their prognosis may be different (Falconer et al, 1990).

Retrosternal Anterior Diaphragmatic Hernia (Morgagni)

BASIC SCIENCE

Retrosternal anterior diaphragmatic hernia was described by Morgagni in 1769. It is much less frequent than posterolateral hernia, accounting for only 1% to 6% of all congenital defects of the diaphragm (Cullen et al, 1985). The herniation occurs between the xiphoid and costochondral attachments of the diaphragm, more frequently on the right side (Gray and Skandalakis, 1972).

In rare cases, foramen of Morgagni hernias arise in the potential spaces between the sternum and the costal muscular portions of the diaphragm. These spaces, through which the internal thoracic vessels exit the thorax to become the superior epigastric vessels as they enter the rectus sheath, exist just lateral to the posterior table of the sternum. On the left side this potential space is partially protected by the pericardium. For this reason herniation through this foramen is more common on the right side. The visceral peritoneum is

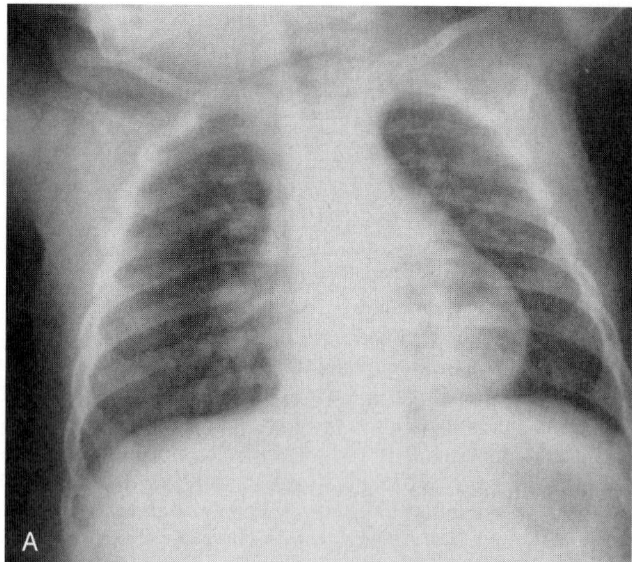

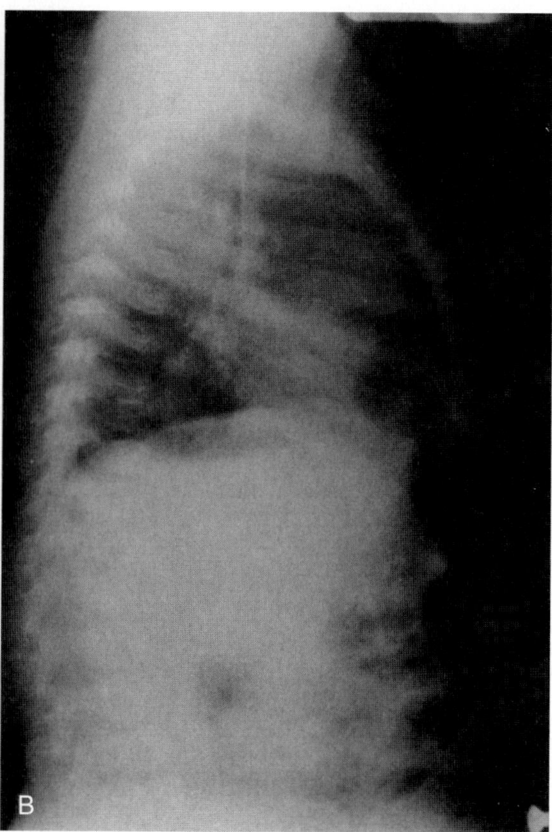

FIGURE 56–39 ■ *A* and *B*, These radiographs demonstrate a loop of colon filled with air that protrudes into a foramen of Morgagni hernia. The bowel was not strangulated or obstructed when the examination was performed. The patient suffered from fullness and cramping abdominal pain. An abdominal approach was used in correcting the hernia. The child had an uneventful postoperative course.

usually completely adjacent to both potential spaces. Hence, a foramen of Morgagni hernia usually has a true hernia sac when the abdominal viscera protrude into this space. Any one of the abdominal viscera that has a mesentery may protrude into either one of these potential spaces.

The most frequent organs to protrude into a foramen of Morgagni hernia are the colon, omentum, stomach, and small bowel. Such hernias infrequently present in childhood; more commonly this rare entity presents in the adult with varying symptoms. Obese individuals are more commonly affected than slender patients, and women are more commonly affected than men. Many foramen of Morgagni hernias may be missed because the radiographic indication of a fat pad to the right of the pericardium is mistaken for a pericardial fat pad or a pleuropericardial cyst. Colicky pain is a relatively infrequent finding, as is vascular compromise of the organs herniated into the space. Colonic, gastric, and intestinal volvulus has been reported, although the volvulus is seldom total; rather, the volvulus is relenting in nature, causing the patient to have intermittent symptoms of partial gastric, colonic, or intestinal obstruction. Complete obstruction of any one of these viscera can occur but is extremely rare.

DIAGNOSIS

A strong suspicion of the foramen of Morgagni hernia may be generated by plain posterior, anterior, and lateral radiographs. An excessively large density in the region of the fat pad on the pericardium should suggest the diagnosis, which can occasionally be confirmed by plain films alone. Computed tomography (CT), magnetic resonance imaging (MRI), and ultrasound may confirm the diagnosis, depending on what abdominal viscera are in the sac. Occasionally, upper gastrointestinal or colonic contrast radiography are necessary to confirm the diagnosis by identification of the stomach, small bowel, or colon above the diaphragm in the peristernal position (Fig. 56–39). Often CT scans or MRI make this diagnosis without contrast since loops of bowel are found in a demonstrable hernia sac. If the patient has only omentum in the hernial sac or the diagnosis is equivocal for any reason, a diagnostic pneumoperitoneum may be conducted to outline the hernia sac. In such cases the hernia sac is outlined by the air entering the hernia and defining the omentum or other structures.

MANAGEMENT

Surgical Repair

An abdominal approach for repair of this hernia is indicated in most instances. An upper abdominal incision based on the patient's body habitus, the size of the hernial contents, and the extent of the hernia sac allows excellent visualization. Foramen of Morgagni hernias have been repaired through subcostal, paramedian, and midline incisions. Once the peritoneal cavity is entered, the abdominal viscera are withdrawn from the hernia sac and reduced to their normal anatomic positions. All adhesions are taken down. The hernia sac is then defined, introduced into the peritoneal cavity, and resected. The repair of the defect may be effected by several means.

When the defect is small and the edges are relatively mobile, horizontal mattress sutures of 0-gauge braided permanent material may be placed to close the defect. Some surgeons prefer using polypropylene. In some instances the edges may be oversewn with a running suture superficial to the horizontal mattress suture to further secure closure. Under no circumstances should the edges of the defect be closed under tension because the hernia has a distinct tendency to recur. Many surgeons prefer to close the defect with synthetic patch material if the defect is too large for the edges to come together without tension. In such cases the prosthetic material is joined to the edges of the diaphragmatic defect or the chest wall by permanent synthetic horizontal mattress sutures, which are tied individually. Some surgeons prefer to oversew the suture line with a running polypropylene suture after the horizontal mattress suture layer has been placed. Prosthetic materials that have found favor include polytetrafluoroethylene (Teflon) sheeting, woven Dacron, and various synthetic meshes. Most surgeons now prefer Teflon sheeting since it has a relatively low adhesion rate, is pliable, and sutures well to both muscle and the chest wall.

When the foramen of Morgagni hernia is identified through a thoracic incision, the principles of repair are much the same. The hernial sac is entered, the visceral contents are dissected and reduced into the abdomen, the sac is resected, and repair is performed. Under no circumstances should closure be completed under tension. If horizontal mattress sutures cannot close the defect appropriately, a soft tissue patch, such as Teflon sheeting, may be used for this purpose. In such instances horizontal mattress sutures of permanent material are placed around the edges. Some practitioners prefer using pledgets on the diaphragmatic surface. Along the chest wall, the sutures may be placed around a rib or costal cartilage to secure the closure. Occasionally sutures have to be placed through the periosteum of the sternum to effect an adequate repair. The primary suture line may then be reinforced, if necessary, with a continuous running suture.

Postoperative Management

Postoperative care is the same as with any other patient who has had major abdominal surgery. The patient is kept NPO until bowel sounds return and flatus is passed per rectum. Judicious intravenous fluid replacement therapy is maintained. Antibiotics are used appropriately if any one of the abdominal viscera has been opened. If the hernia has been repaired through a thoracic incision, chest tubes are placed to maintain the expansion of the lung. In most cases the patient enjoys a benign postoperative course and should be discharged within 6 to 10 days after the repair.

Septum Transversum (Central) Diaphragmatic hernia

BASIC SCIENCE

Septum transversum diaphragmatic hernias are extremely rare. They are among the midline congenital defects that may also include omphalocele, sternal defect, and pentalogy of Cantrell (Cantrell et al, 1958; Milne et al, 1990). A high incidence of gastrointestinal anomalies, absent pericardium, and herniation of the heart through the defect occurs (Lee et al, 1991; Wesselhoeft and DeLuca, 1984).

DIAGNOSIS AND MANAGEMENT

Diagnostic workup may include plain radiographs of the chest and abdomen, ultrasound, contrast studies of the gastrointestinal tract, and nuclear scan. A cardiac workup may be required to delineate the congenital heart defects.

Surgical repair is best done through the abdomen to enable correction of intra-abdominal pathology. The first priority is to reduce the herniated organs into their respective cavities and to close the diaphragmatic defect (Touloukian, 1984). Only then is the omphalocele, if present, dealt with. Congenital heart defects may require repair as well.

■ KEY REFERENCES

Connors RH, Weber TR, Randolph JG: The diaphragm: Developmental, traumatic, and neoplastic disorders. In Baue AE, Geha AS, Hammond GL et al (eds): Glenn's Thoracic and Cardiovascular Surgery, 5th ed. East Norwalk, CT, Appleton & Lange, 1991, p 531.

A good reference to general disorders of the diaphragm.

O'Rourke PP, Lillehei CW, Crone RK et al: The effect of extracorporeal membrane oxygenation on the survival of neonates with high-risk congenital diaphragmatic hernia: 45 cases from a single institution. J Pediatr Surg 26:147, 1991.

Excellent review article on the role of ECMO in congenital diaphragmatic hernia.

■ REFERENCES

Adzick NS, Vacanti JP, Lillehei CW et al: Fetal diaphragmatic hernia: Ultrasound diagnosis and clinical outcome in 38 cases. J Pediatr Surg 24:654, 1989.

Bartlett RH, Gazzaniga AB, Jeffries MR et al: Extracorporeal membrane oxygenation (ECMO): Cardiopulmonary support in infancy. Trans Am Soc Artif Intern Organs 22:80, 1976.

Bohn D: Blood gas and ventilatory parameters in predicting survival in congenital diaphragmatic hernia. Pediatr Surg Int 2:336, 1978.

Boix-Ochoa J, Natal A, Canal J et al: The important influence of arterial blood gases on the prognosis of congenital diaphragmatic hernia. World J Surg 1:783, 1977.

Boix-Ochoa J, Peguero G, Seijo G et al: Acid-base balance and blood gases in prognosis and therapy of congenital diaphragmatic hernia. J Pediatr Surg 19:49, 1974.

Breaux CW Jr, Rouse TM, Cain WS et al: Improvement in survival of patients with congenital diaphragmatic hernia utilizing a strategy of delayed repair after medical and/or extracorporeal membrane oxygenation stabilization. J Pediatr Surg 26:333, 1991.

Cantrell JR, Haller JA, Ravitch MM: A syndrome of congenital defects involving the abdominal wall, sternum, diaphragm, pericardium, and heart. Surg Gynecol Obstet 107:602, 1958.

Cartlidge PHT, Mann NP, Kapila L: Preoperative stabilization in congenital diaphragmatic hernia. Arch Dis Child 61:1226, 1986.

Charlton AJ, Bruce J, Davenport M: Timing of surgery in congenital diaphragmatic hernia. Low mortality after preoperative stabilization. Anaesthesia 46:820, 1991.

Cullen ML, Klein MD, Phillippart AI: Congenital diaphragmatic hernia. Surg Clin North Am 65:1115, 1985.

Cunniff C, Jones KL, Jones MC: Patterns of malformation in children with congenital diaphragmatic defects. J Pediatr 116:258, 1990.

Dietz HG, Pongratz D: Morphology of the diaphragmatic muscle in CDH. Eur J Pediatr Surg 1:85, 1991.

Falconer AR, Brown RA, Helms P et al: Pulmonary sequelae in survivors of congenital diaphragmatic hernia. Thorax 45:126, 1990.

Frenckner B, Freyschuss U: Pulmonary function after repair of congenital diaphragmatic hernia—a short review. Pediatr Surg Int 3:11, 1988.

Geggel RL, Murphy JD, Langleben D et al: Congenital diaphragmatic hernia: Arterial structural changes and persistent pulmonary hypertension after surgical repair. J Pediatr 107:457, 1985.

German JC, Gazzaniga AB, Amlie R et al: Management of pulmonary insufficiency in diaphragmatic hernia using extracorporeal circulation with a membrane oxygenator (ECMO). J Pediatr Surg 12:905, 1977.

Gersony WM, Duc CV, Sinclair JD: "PFC" syndrome (persistence of fetal circulation). Circulation 39 (Suppl III):87, 1969.

Gray SW, Skandalakis JE: The diaphragm. In Embryology for Surgeons. The Embryological Basis for the Treatment of Congenital Defects. Philadelphia, WB Saunders, 1972, p 359.

Gross RE: Congenital hernia of the diaphragm. Am J Dis Child 71:580, 1946.

Hansen J, Jones S, Burrington J et al: The decreasing incidence of pneumothorax and improving survival in infants with congenital diaphragmatic hernia. J Pediatr Surg 19:385, 1984.

Harrison MR, Adzick NS, Longaker MT et al: Successful repair in utero of a fetal diaphragmatic hernia after removal of herniated viscera from the left thorax. N Engl J Med 322:1582, 1990a.

Harrison MR, de Lorimier AA: Congenital diaphragmatic hernia. Surg Clin North Am 61:1023, 1981.

Harrison MR, Langer JC, Adzick NS et al: Correction of congenital diaphragmatic hernia in utero. V. Initial clinical experience. J Pediatr Surg 25:47, 1990b.

Haugen SE, Linker D, Eik-Nes S et al: Congenital diaphragmatic hernia: determination of the optimal time for operation by echocar-diographic monitoring of the pulmonary arterial pressure. J Pediatr Surg 26:560, 1991.

Hazelbrock FWJ, Tibboel D, Bos AP et al: Congenital diaphragmatic hernia: impact of preoperative stabilization. A prospective pilot study in 13 patients. J Pediatr Surg 23:1139, 1988.

Langer JC, Filler RM, Bohn DJ et al: Timing of surgery for congenital diaphragmatic hernia: is emergency operation necessary? J Pediatr Surg 23:731, 1988.

Lee P, Franks R, Sreeram N: Diaphragmatic hernia with extrathoracic heart. Int J Cardiol 33:176, 1991.

Levy JL Jr, Guyer WA, Louis JE et al: Bilateral congenital diaphragmatic hernias through the foramina of Bochdalek. J Pediatr Surg 4:557, 1969.

Manthei U, Vaucher Y, Crowe CP: Congenital diaphragmatic hernia. Immediate preoperative and postoperative oxygen gradients identify patients requiring prolonged respiratory support. Surgery 93:83, 1983.

Milne LW, Morosin AM, Campbell JR et al: Pars sternalis diaphragmatic hernia with omphalocele: a report of two cases. J Pediatr Surg 25:726, 1990.

Mishalany HG, Nakkada K, Wooley MM: Congenital diaphragmatic hernias: eleven years experience. Arch Surg 114:1118, 1979.

Molenaar JC, Bos AP, Hazelbrock FWJ et al: Congenital diaphragmatic hernia, what defect? J Pediatr Surg 26:248, 1991.

Morgagni GB, Alexander B (transl): Seats and Causes of Disease Investigated by Anatomy. Vol. 3. Miller & Cadell, London 1769, p. 205.

Nakamura Y, Yamamoto I, Fukuda S et al: Pulmonary acinar development in diaphragmatic hernia. Arch Pathol Lab Med 115:372, 1991.

Nakayama DK, Motoyama EK, Mutich RL et al: Pulmonary function in newborns after repair of congenital diaphragmatic hernia. Pediatr Pulmonol 11:49, 1991.

Raphaely RC, Downes JJ Jr: Congenital diaphragmatic hernia: prediction of survival. J Pediatr Surg 8:815, 1973.

Reynolds M, Luck SR, Lappen R: The "critical" neonate with diaphragmatic hernia: a 21-year perspective. J Pediatr Surg 19:364, 1984.

Ruff SJ, Campbell JR, Harrison MW et al: Pediatric diaphragmatic hernias. Am J Surg 139:641, 1980.

Shochat SJ: Pulmonary vascular pathology in congenital diaphragmatic hernia. Pediatr Surg Int 2:331, 1987.

Sokal MM, Yellin PB, Meswtel AI et al: Survival after bilateral congenital diaphragmatic hernia. Clin Pediatr (Phila) 29:677, 1990.

Stolar CJH: Repair in utero of a fetal diaphragmatic hernia (letter; comment). N Engl J Med 323:1279, 1990.

Thorpe-Beeston JG, Gosden CM, Nicolaides KH: Prenatal diagnosis of congenital diaphragmatic hernia: associated malformations and chromosomal defects. Fetal Ther 4:21, 1989.

Touloukian RJ: Discussion of Wesselhoeft CW, DeLuca FG: Am J Surg 147:481, 1984.

Vacanti JP: Congenital diaphragmatic hernia. In Grillo HC, Austen WG, Wilkins EW et al. (eds): Current Therapy in Cardiothoracic Surgery. DC Decker, Philadelphia, 1989, p. 68.

Vacanti JP, Crone RK, Murphy JD et al: The pulmonary hemodynamic response to perioperative anesthesia in the treatment of high-risk infants with congenital diaphragmatic hernia. J Pediatr Surg 19:672, 1984.

Wenstrom KD, Weiner CP, Hanson JW: A five year statewide experience with congenital diaphragmatic hernia. Am J Obstet Gynecol 165:838, 1991.

Wesselhoeft CW, DeLuca FG: Neonatal septum transversum diaphragmatic defects. Am J Surg 147:481, 1984

Wilson JM, Lund DP, Lillehei CW et al: Congenital diaphragmatic hernia: predictors of severity in the ECMO era. J Pediatr Surg 26:1028, 1991.

CONGENITAL EVENTRATION AND ACQUIRED ELEVATION OF THE DIAPHRAGM

Éric Fréchette
Raymond Cloutier
Jean Deslauriers

Eventration ("e," out of; "venter," the belly) is a condition in which all or a portion of one hemidiaphragm is permanently elevated yet retains its continuity and normal attachments to the costal margins. This congenital anomaly has a left-sided predominance with a marked decrease in muscular fibers (Wright et al, 1985). Eventration is differentiated from a hernia by the unbroken continuity of the diaphragm in the former. By contrast, diaphragmatic paralysis is an acquired condition in which the diaphragm, even if somewhat atrophic, is still muscular. Diaphragmatic paralysis is generally related to pathologic involvement of the phrenic nerve. Although different, eventration and diaphragmatic paralysis often produce the same radiographic appearance and lead to the same physiologic disturbances.

In this chapter, we discuss the etiology, diagnosis, indications for surgery, techniques of repair, and results for both of these conditions. We also describe the methods used for distinguishing eventration from diaphragmatic paralysis.

HISTORICAL NOTE

Eventration of the diaphragm was first recognized in 1774 by Jean-Louis Petit in his *Oeuvres médicales posthumes* (Petit, 1760) It was in 1829, however, that Béclard first introduced the term "eventration of the diaphragm" (cited in Cruveilhier, 1829). About one century later, Wood (1916) (cited in Thomas, 1970) "expanded further on eventration and made a plea that one should not confuse this with diaphragmatic herniation. He further suggested that surgical plication could be done if symptoms were sufficiently disabling and distressing (cited in Laxdal et al, 1954). The term eventration is still currently used, although numerous other definitions such as idiopathic high-lying diaphragm, relaxatio diaphragmatica, relaxed diaphragm, insufficiency of the diaphragm, and neurogenic muscular aplasia (Bovornkitti et al, 1960) have been mentioned over the years. Clopton (1923) and Beck (1950) speculated that eventration is a congenital anomaly that is likely the result of a failure of muscularization of the diaphragm.

Before the use of radiography, the diagnosis of eventration of the diaphragm was difficult to make, and Korns in 1921 was able to collect only 65 cases in the world literature. In 1935, only 183 cases had been published (Reed and Borden, 1935). In 1951, a report by Nylander and Elfving identified localized eventration that was sometimes encountered on mass chest surveys. Bilateral eventration in infants and children has since been reported by Avnet (1962) and Lindstrom and Allen (1966).

In 1923, Morrison performed the first successful repair of an eventration, and he described the surgical principles that are still used today. He plicated the diaphragm of a 10-year-old girl with immediate relief of symptoms (Morrison, 1923a). In infants, there were only 11 cases of eventration described prior to the first successful repair made by Bisgard (1947) in a 6-week-old male. In addition to giving a good description of the technique, he provided the presently accepted definition of eventration as an abnormally high or elevated position of one leaf of the intact diaphragm (cited in Thomas, 1970).

Eventration of the diaphragm still remains a rare condition for which surgery is seldom indicated. In a 1954 review article by Arnheim, 300 surgical cases had been reported, but only a few patients were operated on (Laxdal et al, 1954). The value of plication was even questioned by Svanberg (1956), who doubted whether any functional benefit would result from fixing the diaphragm in a lower position.

■ *HISTORICAL READINGS*

Arnheim EE: Congenital eventration of the diaphragm in infancy. Surgery 35:809, 1954.

Avnet NL: Roentgenologic features of congenital bilateral anterior diaphragmatic eventration. Am J Roentgenol 88:743, 1962.

Beck WC: Etiologic significance of eventration of the diaphragm. Arch Surg 60:1154, 1950.

Bisgard JD: Congenital eventration of the diaphragm. J Thorac Surg 16:484, 1947.

Bovornkitti S, Kangsadal P, Sangvichien S, Chatikavanij K: Neurogenic muscular aplasia (eventration) of the diaphragm. Am Rev Respir Dis 82:876, 1960.

Clopton MB: Eventration of the diaphragm. Ann Surg 78:154, 1923.

Cruveilhier J: Atlas d'anatomiepathologique, Vol 1, Book 17, Plate V. Paris, Baillière, 1829, p 2.

Korns HM: The diagnosis of eventration of the diaphragm. Arch Intern Med 28:192, 1921.

Laxdal OE, McDougall H, Mellin GW: Congenital eventration of the diaphragm. New Engl J Med 250:401, 1954.

Lindstrom CH, Allen RP: Bilateral congenital eventration of the diaphragm. Am J Roentgenol 97:216, 1966.

Morrison JMW: Elevation of one diaphragm, unilateral phrenic paralysis: A radiological study with special reference to differential diagnosis. Arch Radiol Electrother 27:353, 1923a.

Nylander PEA, Elfving G: Partial eventration of the diaphragm. Ann Chir et Gynec Fenniae 40:1, 1951.

Petit JL: Traité des maladies chirurgicales et des opérations qui leur conviennent: Ouvrage posthume de J. L. Petit Vol 2 (revised ed). Paris, Meguignon, 1760, p. 233.
Reed JA, Borden DL: Eventration of the diaphragm. Arch Surg 31:30, 1935.
Svanberg L: Clinical value of analysis lung function in some intrathoracic diseases: Spirometric, bronchospirometric and angiopneumographic investigation. Acta Chir Scand 111:1196, 1956.
Thomas TV: Congenital eventration of the diaphragm. Ann Thorac Surg 10:180, 1970.
Wood HG: Eventration of the diaphragm. Surg Gynecol Obstet 23:344, 1916.

BASIC SCIENCE

Terminology: Eventration and Paralysis of the Diaphragm

According to most authors (Chin and Lynn, 1956; Simoneau et al, 1983; Wright et al, 1985), true eventrations are always derived from a congenital defect in the musculature of one portion or the entire central part of the diaphragm. It results from an incomplete migration of myoblasts from the cervical somites into the pleuroperitoneal membrane during the fourth week of embryologic development (Moore, 1988). McNamara and colleagues (1968a) even suggested that the anomaly involved a defect similar to that observed in a Bochdalek hernia, but it occurred at a slightly later stage. According to Thomas (1970), a premature return of the viscera to the abdominal cavity after their rotation and the absence of ingrowth striated muscles to the pleuroperitoneal membrane from the septum transversum may be factors involved in the development of eventration. Based on this theory, the premature return of the viscera to the peritoneal cavity might prevent complete development of the diaphragm by stretching it out. This concept is further supported by the observation that both eventration and Bochdalek's hernia occur more frequently on the left side, most often in males, and generally have an intact anterior muscular rim (Kirklin and Hodgson, 1947; McNamara et al, 1968a, b; Reed and Borden, 1935).

TABLE 56–5 ■ Anatomic Classification of Eventration

Total	Bilateral
Partial (localized)	Partial
Anterior	Complete
Posterolateral	
Medial	

From Thomas TV: Non-paralytic eventration of the diaphragm. J Thorac Cardiovasc Surg 55:586, 1968.

Macroscopically, the eventrated diaphragm is thin with a membranous appearance, whereas the more peripheral portion is still muscular with normal attachments of the muscle to the sternum, lower ribs, and dorsolumbar spine. Indeed, Wright and associates (1985) pointed out that there is little difficulty at thoracotomoy in distinguishing eventration with its membranous appearance from diaphragmatic paralysis, in which the diaphragm, even if somewhat atrophic, is still partly muscular.

Histologically, the attenuated portion of the eventrated diaphragm is composed of fibroelastic tissue (Shah-Mirany et al, 1968) with muscle fibers and nerve bundles seldom seen and no evidence of degeneration of the phrenic nerve. Based on their location, eventrations can be further divided into three types (Thomas, 1968, 1970) Table 56–5): (1) anterior (Fig. 56–40), (2) posterolateral, and (3) medial. Bilateral eventrations are mostly seen

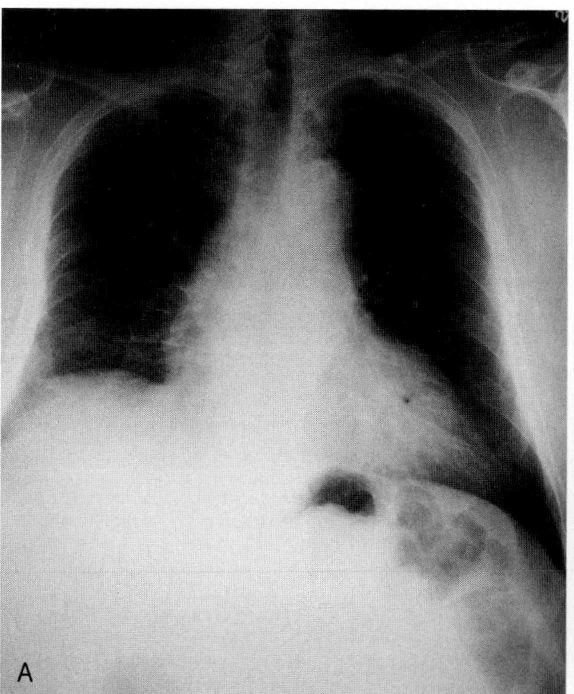

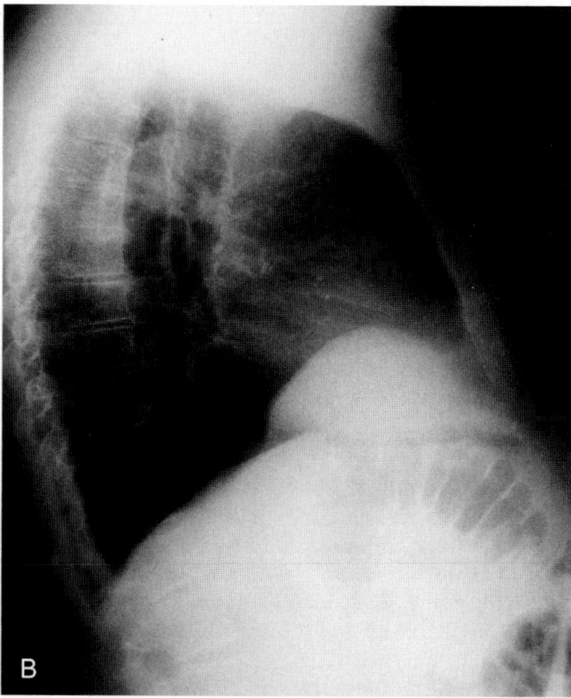

FIGURE 56–40 ■ *A*, Standard posteroanterior chest radiograph showing an asymptomatic congenital eventration of the right hemidiaphragm diagnosed in an adult moderate right diaphragm eventration. *B*, Lateral view showing the incomplete anterior nature of the eventration.

TABLE 56–6 ■ **Acquired Elevation of the Diaphragm**

Intact phrenic nerve
- Mechanical factors or blunt trauma
- Idiopathic

Abnormal phrenic nerve
- Post-traumatic or postoperative
- Sequelae of neuromuscular or infectious disorders
- Malignancies of lung or mediastinum
- Idiopathic

within the context of polymalformations (Elberg et al, 1989).

In a carefully analyzed review, Revillon and Fekete (1982) showed that cases of true eventrations could occur in any location over the dome of the diaphragm, such as underneath the heart (6 patients), partially central (15 patients), partially peripheral (13 patients), and complete (6 patients). These authors also showed that microscopically the abnormal area always contained some muscular fibers, although these were fewer in number and dispersed in every direction. Often, muscular fibers were replaced by fibrous tissue rich in collagen and leucocytic infiltrate.

Occasionally, eventrations have been reported to be associated with other developmental defects such as hypoplastic aorta, cleft palate, transposition of the abdominal organs, or undecended testicle. In Smith and coworkers' series (1986) of 10 infants with congenital eventrations, 7 had significant associated problems, including congenital heart disease in 4. Eventration of the diaphragm can also be associated with prenatal cytomegalovirus infections and maternal exposure to drugs such as thiopental (Becroft, 1979; Elberg et al, 1989). In complete eventration, the ipsilateral lung is nearly always hypoplastic, similar to what is seen with diaphragmatic hernias (Fig. 56–41).

At birth, breech deliveries or difficult and prolonged forceps deliveries can result in phrenic nerve injuries, often associated with vocal cord paralysis or brachial plexus injuries (Cavrot and Richard, 1956). These injuries are usually the result of a pull on the C3-C5 nerve root, but in severe cases, they may be produced by an actual tearing off of these nerve roots (Stauffer and Rickham, 1972). If there are no associated injuries, these lesions can be difficult to differentiate from congenital eventration.

Acquired elevation of the diaphragm (often inappropriately termed eventration) can be associated with an intact or an abnormal phrenic nerve (Fig. 56–42, Table 56–6). In both cases, loss of contractility progressively leads to muscular atrophy and distention of the dome. Ultimately, the physiologic disturbances associated with eventration and acquired elevation of the diaphragm are similar. Table 56–7 outlines the main differences between the two conditions.

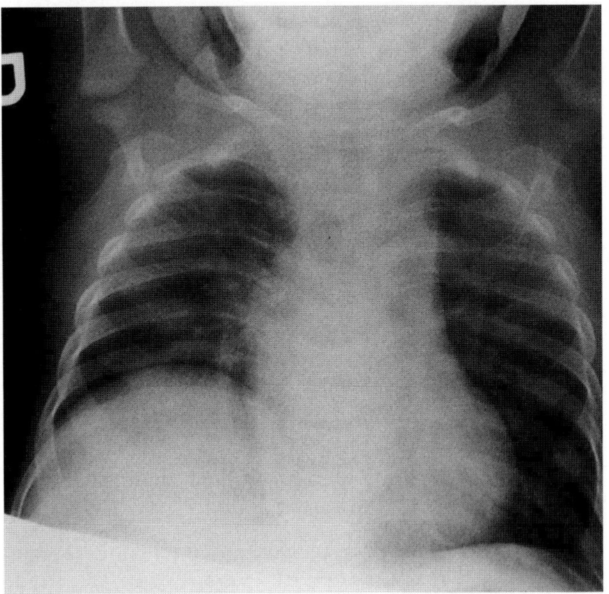

FIGURE 56–41 ■ Standard posteroanterior chest radiograph of a 10-month-old child with complete eventration of the right hemidiaphragm.

Physiologic Consequences of an Elevated Diaphragm

The most significant physiologic derangements associated with a high hemidiaphragm relate to the respiratory system because the diaphragm contributes to a large proportion of the tidal volume in normal individuals (Agostini and Sant'Ambrogio, 1970; Clague and Hall, 1979). Consequently, several authors have been able to document a restrictive pattern characterized by a reduction in lung volumes and mild hypoxemia, all changes made worse when measurements are obtained with the patient in a supine position (Graham et al, 1990). In the group of patients reported by Wright and colleagues (1985), there was moderate hypoxia, and the total lung capacity (TLC), vital capacity (VC), and expiratory reserve volume were

TABLE 56–7 ■ **Differences Between True Congenital Eventration and Acquired Elevation of the Diaphragm**

Feature	*Eventration*	*Paralysis*
Incidence	Rare	Common
Etiology	Congenital anomaly in formation of the diaphragm	Acquired lesion
Associated congenital anomalies	Yes	No
Phrenic nerve	Intact	Often abnormal
Appearance of the diaphragm	Marked decrease in muscular fibers Membranous appearance	Atrophic but still muscular
Sniff test	Decreased motion but not paradoxical	Paradoxical motion

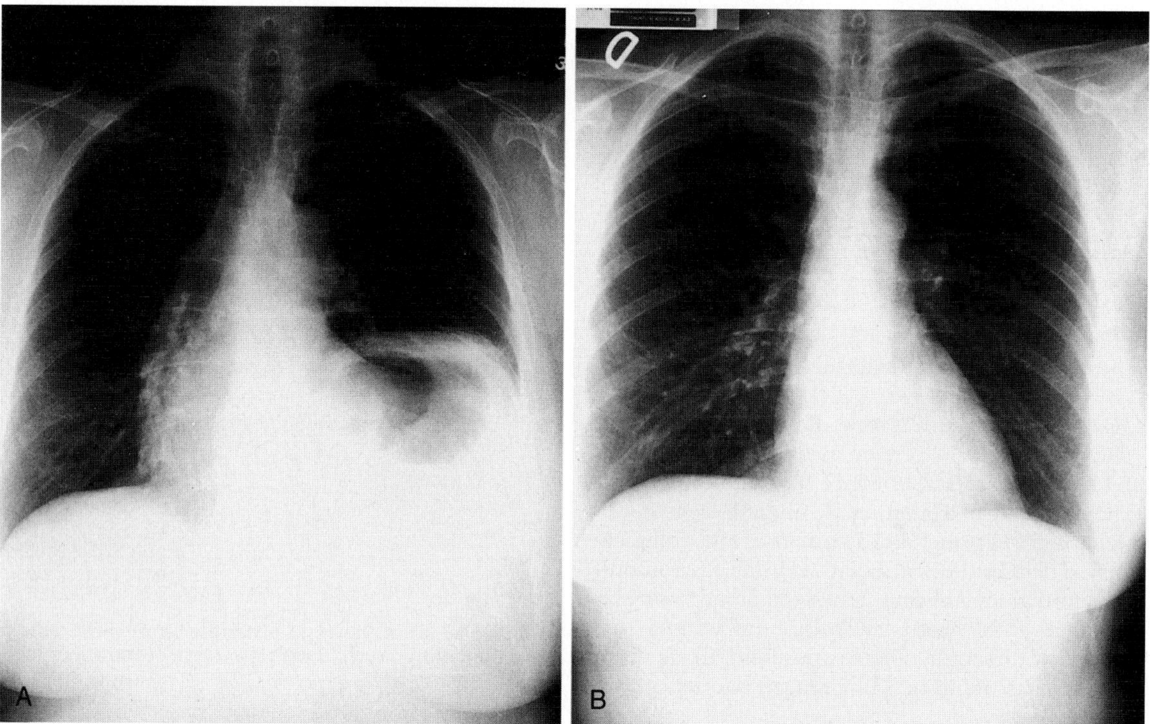

FIGURE 56–42 ■ *A*, Standard posteroanterior chest radiograph of a 55-year-old woman with an idiopathic elevation (often called eventration) of the left diaphragm. At fluoroscopy, the diagram moves very little but there was no paradoxical motion. No cause could be found to explain the anomaly. Spirometric studies showed a restrictive pattern with a vital capacity of 72% of predicted. *B*, Standard chest radiograph taken 4 years before *A* and considered normal.

lower than predicted with the patients seated, falling further away from predicted values with the patients in the supine position. Obviously, this restrictive pattern is more severe in cases of paralysis and complete eventration, while it can be nonexistent in cases of partial or mild eventrations. Thus some patients with diaphragmatic elevation have few or no respiratory symptoms, whereas others may present with shortness of breath, poor exercise tolerance, orthopnea, or even frank respiratory failure if the patient has an underlying lung disease. In addition to this restrictive defect, many authors (Easton et al, 1983; McCredie et al, 1962; Ridyard and Stewart, 1976) have shown various degrees of compressive atelectasis with decreased ventilation and perfusion in the involved lung base.

In 1979, Clague and Hall studied the effect of posture on lung volume, airway closure, and gas exchange in eight patients with diaphragmatic paralysis. They showed that the mean VC in the sitting position was 81% of the predicted normal value; in the supine position it fell by a further 19% in right-sided paralysis and 10% in left-sided paralysis. The mean PO_2 was also less than predicted in the sitting position and fell significantly on lying. All of these findings were attributed to the inability of the paralyzed hemidiaphragm to resist movements of the abdominal contents into the chest on lying down, when gravitational forces must be overcome.

One other important respiratory consequence commonly seen in newborns with an abnormal diaphragm is the phenomenon of paradoxical respiration, in which the normal lung is compressed by the mediastinum during forceful or even quiet inspiration. Thus, there is paradoxical deflation of the lung on the involved side during inspiration and paradoxical inflation during expiration resulting in rebreathing of dead space air (Rodgers and McGahren, 1989). This paradoxical respiration is explained by the negative intrapleural pressure created by the normal diaphragm that is not counterbalanced by the paralyzed diaphragm on the affected side. Because of weak intercostals, soft thoracic cage, and very mobile mediastinum, this phenomenon is often worse in newborns than in children or adults. Indeed, paradoxical respiration is often aggravated by the increased abdominal pressure associated with the supine position of newborns and by the small caliber of their bronchial tree (Arnheim, 1954; Ribet and Linder, 1992; Stone et al, 1987), which results in higher airway resistance and greater tendency toward airway obstruction caused by secretions. Coexisting cardiac or pulmonary malformations may further aggravate the situation. In a series of nine patients with eventration seen during the first 19 months of life reported by Paris and associates (1973), severe respiratory symptoms were present in five of nine patients. In Jarry et al's series (1982), four of seven patients required assisted ventilation prior to correctional surgery.

Elevation of the diaphragm can also be the cause of digestive symptoms related to the rotation of the gastric fundus underneath the diaphragm, or even to complete volvulus of the stomach with outlet obstruction. According to Laxdal and others (1954), the stomach may lie in any one of the following positions, all of which are the result of its being drawn up into the chest: (1) normal position, except that the fundus rises unusually high under the diaphragm (Buckstein, 1948); (2) inversion with the greater curvature lying adjacent to the undersurfaces of the diaphragm (Fichardt, 1946; Malenchini and Roca, 1946); and (3) inversion with partial or complete volvulus (Ferrière, 1948).

CONGENITAL EVENTRATION OF THE DIAPHRAGM

The true incidence of eventration of the diaphragm is unknown, but Chin and Lynn (1956) reported that the Southampton and Portsmouth mass radiography units had diagnosed only 32 cases of elevation of the diaphragm in 412,000 subjects during a 5-year period (1949–1954) for an incidence of approximately 1:1400. In that series, it occurred nine times more often on the left side than on the right side. In another series reported by Christensen (1959), 38 cases out of 107,778 persons examined were found, for a frequency four times greater than in the Chin and Lynn report. In neonates and young children, the true incidence of eventration is even harder to pinpoint. In a review of 2500 chest radiographs of neonates, Beck and Motsay (1952) found some diaphragmatic weakness in 4% of 2500 chest radiographs in newborns, but only 3 patients had severe symptoms, indicating that the incidence may have been overestimated. In another study, Kinser and Cook (1944) identified an abnormally elevated diaphragm in 31 of 412,149 radiographs.

Overall, males are affected more often than females, and the left hemidiaphragm is involved more frequently than the right (Chin and Lynn, 1956; Wayne et al, 1974).

Clinical Presentation and Diagnosis

As many infants with unilateral eventration have few or no symptoms, especially if the defect is focal, congenital eventration is often undiagnosed until later in life when weight gain and reduction of cardiopulmonary reserve may generate pulmonary symptoms.

When eventration is symptomatic, the spectrum of clinical presentation ranges from mild respiratory insufficiency to cyanosis, or even respiratory failure necessitating intubation (Kizilcan et al, 1993; McIntyre et al, 1994; Sarihan et al, 1996). Most often, however, difficulty in feeding, repeated attacks of pneumonitis, and dyspnea are the prominent symptoms. The symptoms of congenital eventration can also develop very insidiously with intermittent vomiting, necessitating small feedings given in an upright position. Interestingly, the clinical course of eventration in children does not always correlate with the severity of involvement, as sometimes patients are asymptomatic with large or complete eventrations.

According to Michelson (1961), one of the most valuable signs of eventration is the Hoover sign (Hoover, 1920), or accentuated outward excursion of the costal margin from the midline on inspiration owing to failure of the diaphragmatic action to oppose that of the intercostals. Diminished breath sounds, contralateral tracheal shift, and depression of the abdomen of the involved side are other clinical signs that may be found on physical examination (Huault et al, 1982; Rodgers and McGabren, 1989). In such cases, it is also important to look for signs of birth trauma that could indicate diaphragmatic paralysis rather than eventration.

The diagnosis of congenital eventration is usually suggested on chest radiographs (see Fig. 56–41), and the classic appearance is that of an elevated hemidiaphragm often associated with loss of volume of the ipsilateral lung and displacement of the mediastinum toward the contralateral side. The lateral film is useful to determine the degree of involvement as well as the type of eventration. On fluoroscopy, complete eventration results in smooth elevation of the hemidiaphragm with little or slightly paradoxical movement during inspiration, often indistinguishable from phrenic nerve paralysis (Gierada et al, 1998). In an attempt to clearly outline diaphragmatic contours and rule out possible diaphragmatic hernia, some authors (Avnet, 1962; Buchwald, 1965; Zeitlin, 1930) have described the use of peritoneography and pneumoperitoneography, but these have now been replaced by the less invasive techniques of ultrasound and computed tomography (CT) scanning. Ultrasound is particularly useful because it can be carried out at bedside in neonatal units and can be used to assess diaphragmatic motion and thickness as well as detect cysts or masses that may on occasion mimic diaphragmatic elevation (Othersen and Lorenzo, 1977). Prenatal ultrasound has also been described as an aid to the diagnosis of eventration (Rodgers and McGahren, 1989). Occasionally, CT, magnetic resonance imaging (MRI), liver isotope scan, and gastrointestinal studies are useful to determine the contents of the eventration.

Management

In all cases of newborns or infants with severe respiratory difficulties, initial treatment must aim at supporting oxygenation and achieving gastric decompression. In severe cases, the child may have to be intubated and placed on a mechanical ventilator. Once the patient is stabilized, the diagnosis is confirmed and surgical plication, often a life-saving procedure, is carried out in a timely fashion. Before proceeding with operation, it is particularly important to ensure that the respiratory symptoms are due to the eventration and not to associated cardiac malformations or pulmonary anomalies.

If the eventration is only partial, if the child is asymptomatic, or if he or she responds well to conservative management, most surgeons agree that operation can be delayed or even totally avoided. This approach is somewhat controversial in the pediatric literature because some investigators recommend to proceed with early surgery even in mildly symptomatic patients in order to maximize development of the underlying lung (Gaultier, 1976; Revillon and Fekete, 1982) (Fig. 56–43). This is especially true if the eventration limits expansion of the thoracic cage or is the cause of repeated pulmonary infections.

The operation is usually carried out through a posterolateral thoracotomy, and simple plication is recommended because it is faster, can be done with minimal blood loss,

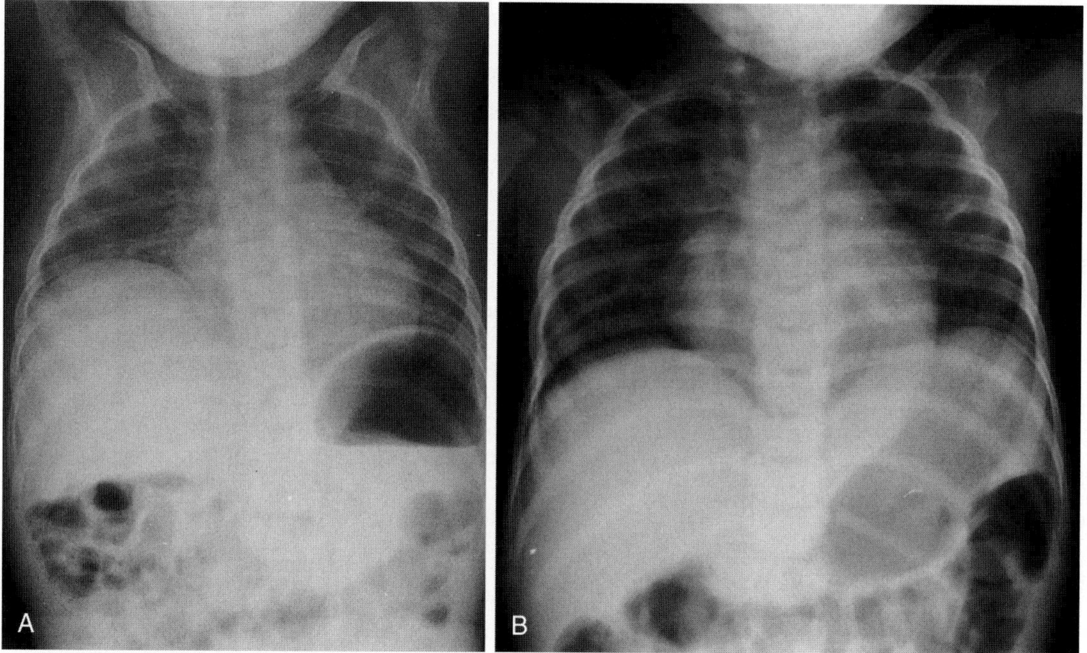

FIGURE 56–43 ■ Preoperative (*A*) and postoperative (*B*) chest radiograph of a child with incomplete eventration of the right hemidiaphragm. Surgical plication was carried out to maximize development of the underlying lung.

and involves no entry into the peritoneal cavity where the spleen, liver, or other digestive organs can be injured (Table 56–8) (Jewett and Thomson, 1964; Paris et al, 1973; Schwartz and Filler, 1978; Stone et al, 1987). To plicate the diaphragm, most surgeons use the technique (or modifications of the technique) described by Schwartz and Filler (1978) in which the slack of the diaphragm is pulled in a radial direction, and pleats are created by the placement of full-thickness horizontal mattress nonabsorbable sutures or staples (Maxson et al, 1993) in the anteromedial to posteromedial direction, while avoiding injury to branches of the phrenic nerve. This type of plication gives the diaphragm an "accordion" appearance. In this manner, the diaphragm can be plicated with as many rows of sutures as necessary for it to become taut. During this type of plication, one should aim at replacing the diaphragm one or two intercostal spaces below where it should ultimately be located. Graham (1990) and co-workers also suggested buttressing the final layers of suture with polytetra fluroethylene (Leflon) pledgets in order to prevent tearing out of sutures. Central diaphragmatic pleating with two circular purse-string sutures, and circumferential pleating directly on the thoracic wall, have also been described, but they are used less frequently (Affatato et al, 1988; Shoemaker et al, 1981).

TABLE 56–8 ■ **Surgical Techniques for Repair of Congenital Eventration**

Advantages
Plication
Easier and faster operation
Minimal blood loss
No entry in peritoneal cavity
Excision and plication
Possible reapproximation of normal muscle with recovery of functions
Avoids inadvertent injury to abdominal organs

The alternative technique of plication (Bishop and Koop, 1958; Thomas, 1970) is to open and resect the excess aponeurotic portion of the diaphragm, followed by a two-layer overlapping approximation of normal peripheral muscle while avoiding inadvertent injury to underlying abdominal viscera. With this technique, it is possible to anticipate a better functional recovery of the diaphragm, although it is associated with increased blood loss, phrenic nerve injury, and diaphragmatic dehiscence (Revillon and Fekete, 1982).

As part of the plication procedure, the diaphragm can be sutured anteriorly to the ribs (State, 1949; Stauffer and Rickham, 1972) and posteriorly to the crurae. If the medial component of the diaphragm is lacking, it is recommended to use the diaphragmatic portion of the pericardium or other autologous tissue or meshes for reinforcement (Thomas, 1968, 1970). If the abdominal cavity is not large enough to accommodate the return of intrathoracic organs, the creation of a temporary ventral hernia may be necessary (Thomas, 1970).

Patients who have bilateral eventration or those with infracardiac involvement are best managed through an abdominal approach. In such cases, an upper transverse incision with liver mobilization allows the surgeon access to both right and left hemidiaphragms. The abdominal approach also allows for the creation of a transverse abdominal muscle flap that can be used to reinforce the repair (Rogers and McGahren, 1989). If a gastric volvulus is present, a gastrostomy with gastropexy may be necessary.

TABLE 56–9 ■ **Results of Plication for Congenital Eventration of the Diaphragm in the Pediatric Population**

Author	No. of Patients	Operative Mortality	Length of Follow-up	Improvement		
				Clinical	Radiographic	Functional
Stauffer and Rickham, 1972	8	0%	Up to 11 yr	100%	100%	—
Revillon and Fekete, 1982	28	4%	Unknown	—	95%	—
Stone et al, 1987	11	36% (4/11)	1–7 yr	—	100%	—
Kizilcan et al, 1993	25	0%	1.5–11 yr	92%	75%	5/6
Total	**83**	**6% (5/83)**		**97%**	**91%**	**83%**

Results

The results of surgical plication for congenital eventration of the diaphragm are shown in Table 56–9. In one series (Kizilcan et al, 1993), assessment of long-term function of plicated diaphragms was done by fluoroscopic, ultrasound, and spirometric studies. The absence of paradoxical motion with normal localization of the diaphragm was documented in all patients, while satisfactory motion of the diaphragm was also documented by fluoroscopy in 9 of 12 patients. Additionally, normal pulmonary function test values were obtained in five of six patients of suitable age for spirometric assessment. In another study (Revillon and Fekete, 1982), good anatomic results as seen on chest radiographs were obtained in 25 of 27 children who had plication of the diaphragm while not in respiratory failure.

Several authors have noted that most ventilator-dependent patients can be extubated within 1 week of plication Revillon and Fekete, 1982; Smith et al, 1986; Symbas et al, 1977).

In general, the surgical correction of bilateral eventration is associated with a higher operative mortality because of associated malformations and more severe hypoplasia of the lung (Watanabe et al, 1987).

ACQUIRED ELEVATION OF THE DIAPHRAGM

Etiology

In the adult, diaphragmatic elevation is often found on routine chest radiographs done in asymptomatic or mildly symptomatic patients. In some of these patients, the diagnosis is clearly that of a congenital eventration (true eventration) that had gone unnoticed during childhood only to become symptomatic with decreased pulmonary function caused by obesity, chronic obstructive lung disease, or any other pulmonary disorder. In most other adult patients with an elevated diaphragm, the disorder is acquired and it can be associated with an intact or an abnormal phrenic nerve (see Table 56–6). Often the cause of diaphragmatic elevation is difficult to determine and in Donzeau-Gouge and associates series (1982) of 20 patients, no clear etiology for the elevation of the diaphragm could be found even after full surgical exploration. In those cases, diaphragmatic elevation may be the early manifestation of a malignant disease or a disabling neuromuscular disorder. In 1982, Piehler and others reported an interesting study of 247 patients who were seen at the Mayo Clinic between 1960 and 1980. In 142 of 247 patients, initial evaluation failed to suggest a cause for the elevated hemidiaphragm. In this cohort, a cause for diaphragmatic paralysis was found in only six patients (five tumors, one neurogenic) during follow-up ranging from 5 months to 20 years. The authors concluded that patients with unexplained diaphragmatic elevation are unlikely to have an underlying occult malignant process, but that recovery of diaphragmatic function is also unlikely.

Most cases of diaphragmatic elevation with an intact phrenic nerve are related to mechanical factors, such as seen with loss of volume of the thoracic cage and increased intrapleural negative pressure. Indeed, most of these situations are associated with normal diaphragmatic function or temporary paralysis with full recovery expected. When pneumonectomy has been carried out, the diaphragm is always elevated, but it seldom produces symptoms requiring specific therapy (Fig. 56–44). An abnormally thin and elevated diaphragm with a macroscopic aspect of eventration has been described following blunt trauma (Holgersen and Schnaufer, 1973).

Diaphragmatic elevation related to involvement of the phrenic nerve can be classified as post-traumatic, secondary to neuromuscular or infectious diseases, neoplastic, or idiopathic (Table 56–10). Injuries to the phrenic nerve can occur after any type of operation in the thorax or in the neck, but they are more commonly reported after the correction of congenital cardiovascular anomalies (Mok et al, 1991) resulting from the use of electrocautery (Allen et al, 1979) or following dissection (Affatato et al, 1988) near the zone where the phrenic nerve runs. In a large series of children undergoing operation for congenital heart disease, Mickell and collaborators (1978) found the incidence of postoperative symptomatic diaphragmatic paralysis to be 1.7%. In the adult patient undergoing open heart surgery, the use of ice or slush topical hypothermia is associated with a higher rate of diaphrag-

TABLE 56–10 ■ **Causes of Phrenic Nerve Paralysis**

Traumatic	Surgical, obstetric, chest tube
Infectious diseases	Poliomyelitis, herpes zoster, diphtheria, influenza, syphilis, tuberculosis, echinococcus infections
Neoplastic diseases	Mediastinal tumors, N2 diseases
Others	Dystrophia myotoxica, pericarditis, subphrenic abscess, lead poisoning
Idiopathic	

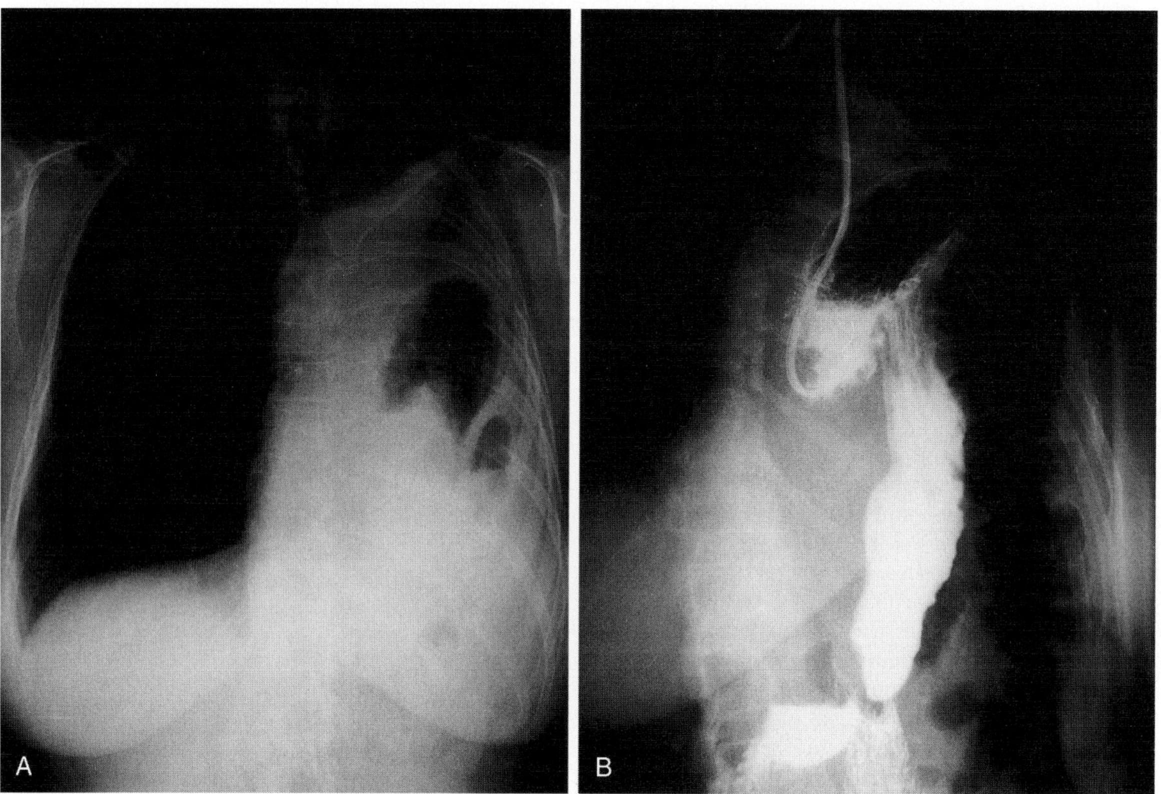

FIGURE 56–44 ■ *A*, Standard posteroanterior chest film. *B*, Barium swallow showing a severe degree of elevation of the diaphragm after pneumonectomy with volvulus of the stomach and outlet obstruction. Note that the gastric fundus is above the level of the carina.

matic paralysis (Efthimiou et al, 1991), but many patients with these injuries are expected to fully recover. Phrenic nerve palsy after insertion of a chest tube has also been reported (Arya et al, 1991; Ayalon et al, 1979; Marinelli et al, 1981). A number of neuromuscular or infectious disorders affecting the phrenic nerve or diaphragm have been reported to be associated with an elevated diaphragm; these include poliomyelitis, herpes zoster (Anderson, 1970; Brostoff, 1966), dystrophia myotoxica (Chin and Lynn, 1956), diphtheria, influenza, syphilis, lead poisoning (Wynn-Williams, 1954), pericarditis, subphrenic abscesses (Hoover, 1913), and echinococcus infection of the liver (Meyler and Huizinga, 1950). Perhaps the most publicized cases have been those associated with the epidemic of polymyelitis in the early 1950s. In 52 surviving adults submitted to follow-up examination by Sötrup (cited in Christensen, 1959), seven cases of permanent eventration were found: four right-sided, two left-sided, and one bilateral.

Neoplastic involvement of the phrenic nerve is often the cause of diaphragmatic elevation, and in patients with bronchogenic carcinomas, phrenic nerve paralysis is usually secondary to mediastinal node disease. Phrenic nerve paralysis can also be associated with malignant mediastinal masses such as thymomas, lymphomas, and germ cell tumors.

Acquired diaphragmatic elevation can also be classified according to the location of the disorder that is responsible for the anomaly (Table 56–11). When both hemidiaphragms are elevated, neuromuscular, connective tissue, or metabolic disorders must be suspected although the most common causes are obesity and pregnancy (Gierada et al, 1998).

Clinical Presentation and Diagnosis

In the adult population, symptoms associated with acquired elevation of the diaphragm are predominantly respiratory. Most patients complain of dyspnea and sometimes cough and retrosternal or epigastric pain. Other complaints include a variety of digestive symptoms, ranging from gas bloat, nausea; vomiting, heartburn, frequent and uncontrollable belching to loud, abnormal noises originating from air moving along the gastrointestinal tract.

TABLE 56–11 ■ **Common Causes of Acquired Diaphragmatic Elevation**

Supradiaphragmatic	Atelectasis Pulmonary resection Radiation fibrosis Restrictive pleural disease (diffuse mesothelioma) Phrenic nerve paralysis
Diaphragmatic	Idiopathic elevation Post-traumatic
Infradiaphragmatic	Hepatomegaly, splenomegaly Subphrenic abscess Abdominal mass Colon or stomach distention

The diagnosis of acquired elevation of the diaphragm can usually be made on standard PA and lateral chest films. The diaphragm is clearly elevated and forms a round, unbroken line arching from the mediastinum to the costal arch (Laxdal et al, 1954). The stomach is drawn up into the chest, and it may be normally positioned with a high fundus or it may be inverted with a partial or complete volvulus. If there is involvement of the phrenic nerve, true paradoxical motion of the diaphragm is seen on fluoroscopy. Fluoroscopic examination may also be useful in ruling out pericardial cysts or excess mediastinal fat located at the cardiophrenic angle that may simulate eventration. Diagnostic pneumoperitoneum might be useful to distinguish between an elevated diaphragm and frank herniation, although in chronic hernias adhesions would prevent air from reaching the pleural space. The original technique described by Zeitlin (1930) involved the introduction of air, nitrous oxide, or carbon dioxide into the peritoneal cavity, followed by an upright chest radiograph to outline the diaphragmatic continuity. Unfortunately, CT scanning and ultrasound are not very helpful in differentiating between elevated diaphragm and true herniation (Yamashita et al, 1993). Michelson (1961) has also shown that faradic stimulation of the phrenic nerve at the time of thoracotomy may be helpful to document the integrity of the phrenic nerve. Electromyographic studies can also be used preoperatively to document the integrity of the phrenic nerve (Witz et al, 1982).

Two other issues in the investigation of an elevated hemidiaphragm in adults must be addressed during the workup of these patients. The first involves the ruling out of a malignancy by CT scanning and if necessary by bronchoscopy and the second is to document the consequences of the disorder on pulmonary function through spirometric and exercise studies.

Management

Most cases of eventration occurring in adult life should be treated conservatively unless severe dyspnea interfering with normal activities, orthopnea, or gastrointestinal symptoms are clearly related to the high position of the diaphragm. In infants with phrenic nerve paralysis secondary to open heart surgery, aggressive treatment by plication of the diaphragm is recommended by many authors if the child is symptomatic or cannot be weaned off the respirator. In the report of Shoemaker et al (1981), six of seven patients treated by plication of the diaphragm survived, the one death occurring in a premature infant with multiple congenital cardiac defects. Children older than 2 years of age are usually asymptomatic or have only minor respiratory problems and as a rule they do not require surgery (Tonz et al, 1996).

Although Wood (1916) was the first to suggest plication if symptoms were sufficiently distressing, Morrison (1923b) is credited with being the first surgeon who actually performed a successful plication of the diaphragm. The operation is usually carried out through a posterolateral approach, and the repair can be done with a simple plication without opening the diaphragm, or through the excision of a central ellipse of aponeurotic diaphragm followed by double breast suturing. In all cases, the objectives of surgery are to immobilize the diaphragm in a lower flat position, to reduce its paradoxical movement and compression of the ipsilateral lung and mediastinum, and possibily to recover function if there is adequate residual muscle under the costal arch. An abdominal approach is recommended for the repair of bilateral eventrations, if there is infracardiac involvement (Othersen and Lorenzo, 1977) or if there is a gastric volvulus that requires repositioning.

More recently, plication done through a video-assisted thoracic surgery approach was described by Mouroux and co-workers (1996) (Fig. 56–45). With this technique, the eventrated diaphragm is pushed down by endoscopic long clamps and then plicated by the use of two superimposed transverse continuous sutures. The first line of sutures holds the diaphragm down and keeps the excess tissue within the abdomen, while the second suture line completes the repair by placing the desired tension over the dome. One obvious advantage of the technique is the minimal access type of surgery, which facilitates postoperative recovery and respiratory re-education.

Surgical repair of a transected phrenic nerve with restoration of diaphragmatic function has been reported in patients with operative trauma to the phrenic nerve, even 4 months after the injury (Brouillette et al, 1986; Merav et al, 1983). In such cases, sural or intercostal nerve grafts can be used to bridge the gap between the severed segments. Nerve regenerates at a rate of 1 mm per day, so several months of observation are required before restoration of motor function to the diaphragm. Good results can be expected in approximately 75% of cases (Fig. 56–46) (Millesi, 1981).

Results

Indications for surgery in adults are uncommon, and the clinician must be very careful before recommending plication for respiratory or digestive symptoms thought to be related to elevation of the diaphragm. Table 56–12 summarizes the results obtained after surgical correction of an elevated diaphragm. In Graham and co-workers' series (1990) of 17 patients with a mean age of 53.7 years who underwent plication of the diaphragm, all patients showed both subjective and objective improvement (Table 56–13). Six patients were reassessed 5 or more years after plication (range, 5 to 7 years) and the improvement was maintained. In that series, the main considerations before surgery were that the patient had dyspnea interfering with normal activities and orthopnea as well as respiratory function tests typical of diaphragmatic paralysis. In a very interesting paper reported by Wright and colleagues (1985), seven adult patients underwent plication of the diaphragm for dyspnea resulting from unilateral diaphragmatic paralysis. There were no postoperative complications and all patients' symptoms were improved after surgery. After plication, significant increases were noted in PaO_2 and all lung volumes except residual volume. The authors concluded that diaphragmatic plication is a safe and effective procedure for adult patients with dyspnea resulting from unilateral diaphragmatic paralysis. Similarly, Ribet and Linder (1992) reported good results in 11 adults followed up for a mean

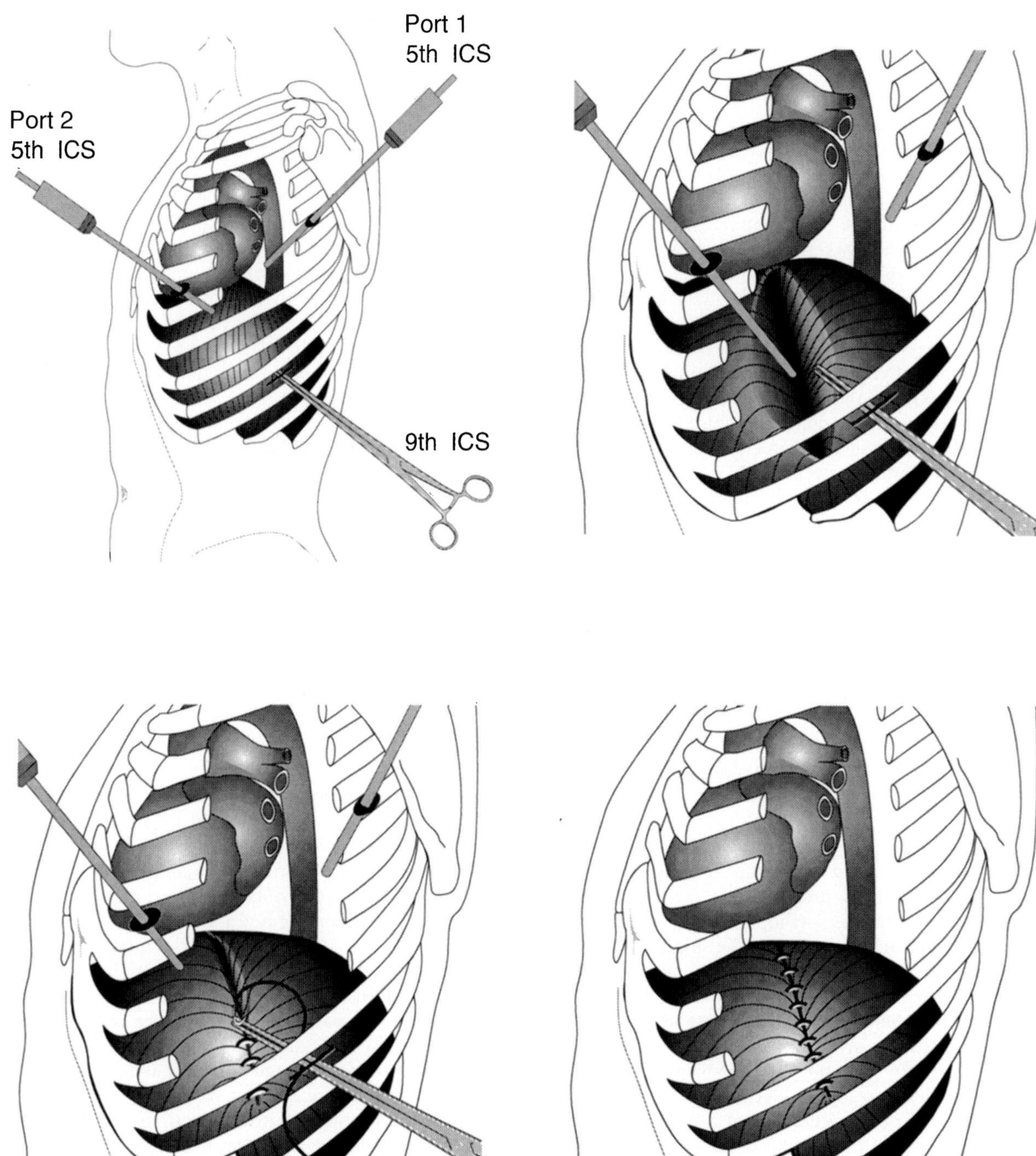

FIGURE 56–45 ■ *A*, Position of the two thoracoscopic ports. A minithoracotomy is made over the ninth intercostal space for the suturing of the diaphragm. *B*, With the use of Duval forceps, the apex of the eventration is pushed down toward the abdomen. *C*, The newly created transverse fold of diaphragm is sutured with nonabsorbable material. *D*, Completed operation. ICS, intercostal space. (From Mouroux J, Padovani B, Poirier NC et al: Technique for the repair of diaphragmatic eventration. Ann Thorac Surg 62:905, 1996.)

TABLE 56–12 ■ **Results of Plication for Diaphragmatic Elevation in the Adult Population**

Author	*No. of Patients*	*Operative Mortality (%)*	*Length of Follow-up (yr)*	*Improvement*		
				Clinical	*Radiographic*	*Functional*
Graham et al, 1990	17	0	5–7	6/6	6/6	6/6
Wright et al, 1985	7	0	0.3–4	7/7	7/7	7/7
Ribet and Linder, 1992	11	0	8.5 (mean)	10/11	—	—
Pastor et al, 1982	15	0	1–15	13/15	15/15	—
Donzeau-Gouge et al, 1982	9	10	0.4–10	7/8	—	—
McNamara et al, 1968a	13	0	1–5	12/13	—	—
Total	**72**	**1.3%**		**92%**	**100%**	**100%**

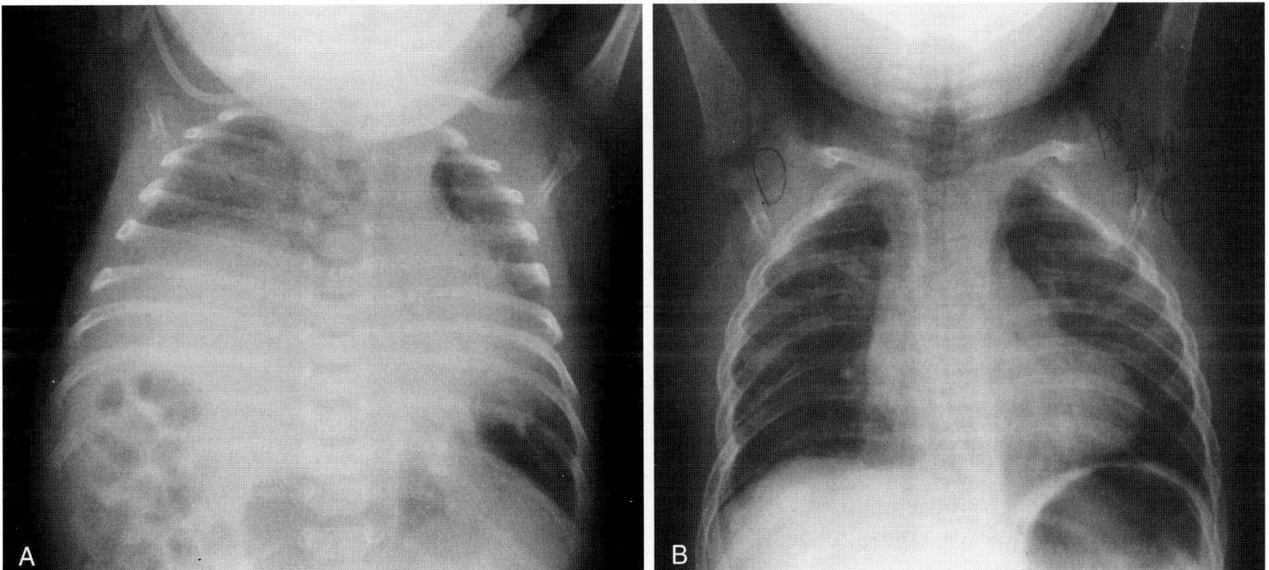

FIGURE 56–46 ■ *A*, Preoperative chest radiograph of a neonate with acquired elevation of the right hemidiaphragm secondary to transection of the phrenic nerve, which occurred during chest tube insertion for pneumothorax. *B*, Chest radiograph done 12 months after plication and primary repair of the phrenic nerve.

TABLE 56–13 ■ **Dyspnea Scores and Physiologic Measurements Before and After Unilateral Diaphragmatic Plication**

	Before Operation	*After Operation*	*P* **value**
Dyspnea Score	7.4 ± 0.8	3.3 ± 0.9	<0.001
FVC			
Sitting	2.7 ± 0.7	3.2 ± 0.5	<0.001
Lying	1.9 ± 0.5	2.7 ± 0.6	<0.001
TLC			
Sitting	4.1 ± 1.6	4.5 ± 1.7	<0.002
Lying	3.4 ± 0.8	4.2 ± 1.7	<0.002
FRC	2.5 ± 0.2	2.9 ± 0.2	<0.01
ERV	0.6 ± 0.2	0.9 ± 0.2	<0.01
RV	1.9 ± 0.2	2.0 ± 0.7	NS
DLCO (% predicted)	85 ± 4.5	100 ± 6.9	<0.05
Pa_{O_2}	73.1 ± 10.9	85.6 ± 13.2	<0.001
Pa_{CO_2}	39.8 ± 6.7	38.4 ± 6.1	<0.001

DLCO, diffusion coefficient; ERV, expiratory reserve volume; FRC, Functional residual capacity; FVC, forced vital capacity; NS, not significant; RV, residual volume; TLC, total lung capacity.

From Graham DR, Kaplan D, Evans CC, et al: Diaphragmatic plication for unilateral diaphragmatic paralysis: A 10-year experience. Ann Thorac Surg 49:249, 1990.

period of 8.5 years after plication of the diaphragm. In that series, the authors recommended surgery when there were symptoms that could not be related to another cause after complete thoracic and abdominal examinations.

CONCLUSION

Although there are few papers reporting the results of surgical plication of the diaphragm for congenital eventration, the operation can be life-saving in newborns and infants. In these cases, the indication for surgery is nearly always respiratory failure, and the results show that operative treatment should be undertaken promptly. In adults, great caution is recommended before plicating the diaphragm for acquired elevation. In these cases, it is important to rule out other possible causes of dyspnea and sometimes small measures such as rehabilitation, conditioning, proper respiratory hygiene, and weight loss lessen dyspnea and orthopnea and help to avoid unnecessary surgery. If the patient has predominantly digestive symptoms, one has to be even more careful in recommending surgery before an appropriate period of observation and medical treatment.

COMMENTS AND CONTROVERSIES

The subject of diaphragmatic paralysis and eventration is a puzzling one. This is a problem not frequently encountered by the adult thoracic surgeon. In their subchapter, Dr. Deslauriers and his colleagues have made a significant contribution in clarifying the circumstances of diaphragmatic paralysis and eventration. They point out the severe physiologic and often life-threatening impairment in the pediatric population and the need for early diaphragmatic plication. Of greater interest to the adult thoracic surgeon is the significant improvement that can be obtained by diaphragmatic plication in symptomatic adult patients. There is a growing literature clearly documenting improved lung function after diaphragmatic plication.

G.A.P.

KEY REFERENCES

Wayne ER, Campbell JB, Burrington JD and Davis WS: Eventration of the diaphragm. J of Pediatr Surg 9:643, 1974.

Excellent description of both congenital and acquired eventration seen in children.

Wright CD, Williams JG, Ogilvie CM and Connelly RJ: Results of diaphragmatic plication for unilateral diaphragmatic paralysis. J Thorac Cardiovasc Surg 90:195, 1985.

Shows that diaphragmatic plication is a safe and effective procedure for adult patient with dyspnea resulting from unilateral diaphragmatic paralysis.

McNamara JJ, Paulson DL, Urschel HC, Razzuk MA: Eventration of the diaphragm. Surgery 64:1013, 1968b.

Outlines symptomatology, diagnosis, indications for surgery, surgical treatment, and results of surgery.

Symbas PN, Hatcher CR, Waldo W: Diaphragmatic eventration in infancy and childhood. Ann Thorac Surg 24:113, 1977.

Describes experience with diagnosis and management of eventration in infancy and childhood.

REFERENCES

Affatato A, Villagra F, De Leon JP et al: Phrenic nerve paralysis following pediatric cardiac surgery: Role of diaphragmatic plication. J Cardiovasc Surg (Turino) 29:606, 1988.

Agostini E, Sant'Ambrogio G: The diaphragm. In Campbell E, Agostini E, Newson DJ (eds): The Respiratory Muscles, Mechanics and Neurological control. England, Lloyd-Luke, 1970, pp 145–160.

Allen RG, Haller JA, Pickard LR et al: Discussion of management of diaphragmatic paralysis in infants with special emphasis on selection of patients for operative plication. J Pediatr Surg 14:779, 1979.

Anderson JP: Paralysis in herpes zoster (Letter). BMJ 5:587, 1970.

Arnheim EE: Congenital eventration of the diaphragm in infancy. Surgery 35:809, 1954.

Arya H, Williams J, Ponsford SN, Bissenden JG: Neonatal diaphragmatic paralysis caused by chest drains. Arch Dis Child 66:441, 1991.

Avnet NL: Roentgenologic features of congenital bilateral anterior diaphragmatic eventration. Am J Roentgenol 88:743, 1962.

Beck WC: Etiologic significance of eventration of the diaphragm. Arch Surg 60:1154, 1950.

Beck WC, Motsay DS: Eventration of the diaphragm. Arch Surg 65:557, 1952.

Becroft DMO: Prenatal cytomegalovirus infection and muscular deficiency (eventration) of the diaphragm. J Pediatr 94:74, 1979.

Bisgard JD: Congenital eventration of the diaphragm. J Thorac Surg 16:484, 1947.

Bishop HC, Koop CE: Acquired eventration of the diaphragm in infancy. Pediatrics 22:1088, 1958.

Bovornkitti S, Kangsadal P, Sangvichien S, Chatikavanij K: Neurogenic muscular aplasia (eventration) of the diaphragm. Am Rev Respir Dis 82:876, 1960.

Brostoff J: Diaphragmatic paralysis after herpes zoster. BMJ 2:1571, 1966.

Brouillette RT, Hahn YS, Noah ZL et al: Successful reinnervation of the diaphragm after phrenic nerve transsection. J Pediatr Surg 21:63, 1986.

Buchwald W: Die verwendung schnell rebobierbarer gase bei diagnostichen gainsufflationen. Kritische Stellungnahne zum problem der gasembolie. Fortschr Roentgenstr 103:187, 1965.

Buckstein J: The Digestive Tract in Roentgenology. Philadelphia, JB Lippincott, 1948, p 743.

Cavrot E, Richard J: Paralysie diaphragmatique obstétricale. Bull Soc R Belge Gynecol Obstet 8:26, 1956.

Chin EF, Lynn RB: Surgery of the eventration of the diaphragm. J Thorac Surg 32:6, 1956.

Christensen P: Eventration of the diaphragm. Thorax 14:311, 1959.

Clague HW, Hall DR: Effect of posture on lung volume: Airway closure and gas exchange in hemidiaphragm paralysis. Thorax 34:523, 1979.

Clopton MB: Eventration of the diaphragm. Ann Surg 78:154, 1923.

Cruveilhier J: Atlas d'anatomie pathologique, Vol I, Book 17, Plate V. Paris, 1829, p 2.

Donzeau-Gouge GP, Personne C, Lechien J et al: Éventrations diaphragmatiques de l'adulte. À propos de vingt cas. Ann Chir Thorac Cardiovasc 36:87, 1982.

Easton PA, Fleetham JA, de la Rocha A et al: Respiratory function after paralysis of the right hemidiaphragm. Am Rev Respir Dis 127:125, 1983.

Efthimiou J, Butler J, Woodham C et al: Diaphragm paralysis following cardiac surgery: Role of phrenic nerve cold injury. Ann Thorac Surg 52:1005, 1991.

Elberg JJ, Brok KE, Pedersen SA, Friskock KE: Congenital bilateral eventration of the diaphragm in a pair of male twins. J Pediatr Surg 24:1140, 1989.

Ferrière A: Splénomégalie congestive avec éventration diaphragmatique et volvulus gastrique. Acta Clin Belg 3:103, 1948.

Fichardt T: Eventration of the diaphragm associated with inversion of the stomach. Clin Proc 5:328, 1946.

Gaultier C: Développement post-natal du poumon humain: Ses rapports avec la fonction pulmonaire et la pathologie respiratoire. Ann Pediatr 23:447, 1976.

Gierada DS, Slone RM, Fleishman MJ: Imaging evaluation of the diaphragm. Chest Surg Clin North Am 8:237, 1998.

Graham DR, Kaplan D, Evans CC et al: Diaphragm plication for unilateral diaphragmatic paralysis: A 10-year experience. Ann Thorac Surg 49:248, 1990.

Holgersen LO, Schnaufer L: Hernia and eventration of the diaphragm secondary to blunt trauma. J Pediatr Surg 8:433, 1973.

Hoover CF: The functions of the diaphragm and their diagnostic significance. Arch Intern Med 12:214, 1913.

Hoover CF: The diagnostic significance of inspiratory movements of the costal margins. Am J Med Sci 159:633, 1920.

Huault G, Checoury A, Binet JP: Paralysie et éventration diaphragmatique. Ann Chir Thorac Cardiovasc 36:79, 1982.

Jarry JM, Aubert JV, Camboulives J et al: Traitement chirurgical de la paralysie et de l'éventration diaphragmatique symptomatique durant les trois premiers mois de la vie. Ann Chir 36:74, 1982.

Jewett TC, Thomson NB: Iatrogenic eventration of the diaphragm in infancy. J Thorac Cardiovasc Surg 48:861, 1964.

Kinser RE, Cook JC: Lesions of diaphragm with eventration. AJR Am J Roentgenol 52:611, 1944.

Kirklin BR, Hodgson JR: Roentgenologic characteristics of diaphragmatic hernia. Am J Roentgenol 58:77, 1947.

Kizilcan F, Tanyel FC, Hicsonmez A, Buyukpamukcu N: The long-term results of diaphragmatic plication. J Pediatr Surg 28:42, 1993.

Korns HM: The diagnosis of eventration of the diaphragm. Arch Int Med 28:192, 1921.

Laxdal OE, McDougall H, Mellin GW: Congenital eventration of the diaphragm. New Engl J Med 250:401, 1954.

Lindstrom CH, Allen RP: Bilateral congenital eventration of the diaphragm. Amer J Roentgen 97:216, 1966.

Malenchini M, Roca J: Hernia y eventraticion diafragmatica. Dia Med 18:767, 1946.

Marinelli PV, Ortiz A, Alden ER: Acquired eventration of the diaphragm. A complication of chest tube placement in neonatal pneumothorax. Pediatrics 67:552, 1981.

Maxson T, Robertson R, Wagner CW: An improved method of diaphragmatic plication. Surg Gynec and Obstet 177:620, 1993.

McCredie M, Lovejoy FW, Kaltreider NL: Pulmonary function in diaphragmatic paralysis. Thorax 17:213, 1962.

McIntyre RC, Bensard DD, Karrer FM et al: The pediatric diaphragm in acute gastric volvulus. J Am Coll Surg 178:234, 1994.

McNamara JJ, Eraklis AJ, Gross RE: Congenital posterolateral diaphragmatic hernia in the newborn. J Thorac Cardiovasc Surg 55:55, 1968a.

McNamara JJ, Paulson DL, Urschel HC, Razzuk MA: Eventration of the diaphragm. Surgery 64:1013, 1968b.

Merav AD, Attai LA, Condit DD: Successful repair of a transected phrenic nerve with restoration of diaphragmatic function. Chest 84:642, 1983.

Meyler L, Huizinga E: Temporary high position of the diaphragm. J Thorac Surg 19:283, 1950.

Michelson E: Eventration of the diaphragm. Surgery 49:410, 1961.

Mickell JJ, Oh KS, Siewers RD et al: Clinical implications of postoperative unilateral phrenic nerve paralysis. J Thorac Cardiovasc Surg 76:297, 1978.

Millesi H: Reappraisal of nerve repair. Surg Clin North Am 61:321, 1981.

Mok Q, Ross-Russell R, Mulvey D et al: Phrenic nerve injury in infants and children undergoing cardiac surgery. Br Heart J 65:287, 1991.

Moore KL: The developing human. In Clinically Orientated Embryology, 4th ed. Philadelphia, WB Saunders, 1988, pp 164–169.

Morrison JMW: Elevation of one diaphragm, unilateral phrenic paralysis: A radiological study with special reference to differential diagnosis. Arch Radiol Electrother 27:353, 1923a.

Morrison JMW: Eventration of the diaphragm due to unilateral phrenic nerve paralysis. Arch Radiol Electrother 28:72, 1923b.

Mouroux J, Padovani B, Poirier NC et al: Technique for the repair of diaphragmatic eventration. Ann Thorac Surg 62:905, 1996.

Nylander PEA, Elfving G: Partial eventration of the diaphragm. Ann Chir Gynec Fenniae 40:1, 1951.

Othersen HB, Lorenzo RL: Diaphragmatic paralysis and eventration: Newer approaches to diagnosis and operative correction. J Pediatr Surg 12:309, 1977.

Paris F, Blasco E, Canto A et al: Diaphragmatic eventration in infants. Thorax 28:66, 1973.

Pastor J, Blasco E, Garcia-Zarza A et al: Éventrations diaphragmatiques de l'adulte traitées par plicature. Ann Chir Thorac Cardiovasc 36:84, 1982.

Petit JL: Traité des maladies chirurgicales et des opérations qui leur conviennent: Ouvrage posthume de J. L. Petit, Vol II. (revised ed). Paris, Meguignon 1760, p 233.

Piehler JM, Pairolero PC, Gracey DR, Bernatz PE: Unexplained diaphragmatic paralysis: A harbinger of malignant disease? J Thorac Cardiovasc Surg 84:861, 1982.

Reed JA, Borden DL: Eventration of the diaphragm. Arch Surg 31:30, 1935.

Revillon Y, Fekete CN: Éventration diaphragmatique chez l'enfant. Étude de trente-six cas de 1951 à 1980. Ann Chir Thorac Cardiovasc 36:71, 1982.

Ribet M, Linder JL: Plication of the diaphragm for unilateral eventration or paralysis. Eur J Cardiothorac Surg 6:357, 1992.

Ridyard JB, Stewart RM: Regional lung function in unilateral diaphragmatic paralysis. Thorax 31:438, 1976.

Rodgers BM, McGahren ED: Congenital eventration of the diaphragm. Mod Probl Paediatr 24:117, 1989.

Sarihan H, Cay A, Akyazici R et al: Congenital diaphragmatic eventration: Treatment and postoperative evaluation. J Cardiovasc Surg 37:173, 1996.

Schwartz MZ, Filler RM: Plication of the diaphragm for symptomatic phrenic nerve paralysis. J Pediatr Surg 13:259, 1978.

Shah-Mirany J, Schmitz GL, Watson RR: Eventration of the diaphragm. Physiologic and surgical significance. Arch Surg 96:844, 1968.

Shoemaker R, Palmer G, Brown JW, King H: Aggressive treatment of acquired phrenic nerve paralysis in infants and small children. Ann Thorac Surg 32:251, 1981.

Simoneau G, Sartene R, Girard P et al: Les dysfonctions diaphragmatiques. Revue du Praticien 33:2155, 1983.

Smith CD, Sade RM, Crawford FA, Othersen HB: Diaphragmatic paralysis and eventration in infants. J Thorac Cardiovasc Surg 91:490, 1986.

State D: The surgical correction of congenital eventration of the diaphragm in infancy. Surgery 25:461, 1949.

Stauffer UG, Rickham PP: Acquired eventration of the diaphragm in the newborn. J Pediatr Surg 7:635, 1972.

Stone KS, Brown JW, Canal DF, King H: Long-term fate of the diaphragm surgically plicated during infancy and early childhood. Ann Thorac Surg 44:62, 1987.

Svanberg L: Clinical value of analysis lung function in some intrathoracic diseases: Spirometric, bronchospirometric and angiopneumographic investigation. Acta Chir Scand 111:1196, 1956.

Symbas PN, Hatcher CR, Waldo W: Diaphragmatic eventration in infancy and childhood. Ann Thorac Surg 24:113, 1977.

Thomas TV: Congenital eventration of the diaphragm. Ann Thorac Surg 10:180, 1970.

Thomas TV: Nonparalytic eventration of the diaphragm. J Thorac Cardiovasc Surg 55:586, 1968.

Tonz M, van Segesser LK, Mihaljevic T et al: Clinical complications of phrenic nerve injury after pediatric cardiac surgery. J Pediatr Surg 31:1265, 1996.

Watanabe T, Trusler GA, Williams WG et al: Phrenic nerve paralysis after pediatric cardiac surgery. Retrospective study of 125 cases. J Thorac Cardiovasc Surg 94:383, 1987.

Wayne ER, Campbell JB, Burrington JD, Davis WS: Eventration of the diaphragm. J Pediatr Surg 9:643, 1974.

Witz JP, Jesel M, Roeslin N et al: Les éventrations diaphragmatiques de l'adulte. Apport dé l'électromyographie. Ann Chir Thorac Cardiovasc Surg 36:91, 1982.

Wood HG: Eventration of the diaphragm. Surg Gynecol Obstet 23:344, 1916.

Wright CD, Williams JG, Ogilvie CM, Donnelly RJ: Results of diaphragmatic plication for unilateral diaphragmatic paralysis. J Thorac Cardiovasc Surg 90:195, 1985.

Wynn-Williams N: Hemidiaphragmatic paralysis and paresis of unknown aetiology without any marked rise in level. Thorax 9:299, 1954.

Yamashita K, Minemori K, Matsuda H et al: MR imaging in the diagnosis of partial eventration of the diaphragm (Letter). Chest 104:328, 1993.

Zeitlin NS: Diagnostic pneumoperitoneum in diaphragmatic pathology. Radiology 14:152, 1930.

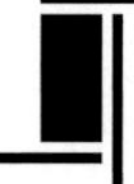

PHRENIC NERVE PACING

Jacquelyn A. Quin
John A. Elefteriades

The process of breathing, though seemingly simple, requires several components, all of which must function and appropriately interact in order to achieve adequate ventilation. Included are upper and lower motor neurons, the diaphragm and other muscles of ventilation, and the lungs themselves. Injury or involvement of any singular component with disease may completely or permanently interfere with the process of ventilation. Selected individuals with respiratory failure, who would otherwise have been dependent on mechanical ventilation, have regained independence through diaphragm pacing. The purpose of this chapter is to review diaphragmatic pacing including diseases that respond to pacing, the process itself, and results of pacing.

DIAPHRAGMATIC STRUCTURE AND FUNCTION

As elucidated by West (1995), respiration is controlled via respiratory centers, which are collections of upper motor neurons located within the pons and medulla. Three respiratory centers exist: (1) The medullary respiratory center, located in the reticular formation of the medulla, consists of inspiratory and expiratory areas, which together influence the rhythm of breathing; (2) the apneustic center, located in the lower pons, is believed to prolong the inspiratory phase of breathing, while (3) the pneumotaxic center, located in the upper pons, inhibits inspiration and participates in the "fine tuning" of respiration. Although it is considered an involuntary function, voluntary control of breathing may supersede the brainstem reflex.

Input for regulation is provided by central and peripherally located chemoreceptors. Central chemoreceptors, located near the medullary respiratory control center, respond to changes in surrounding cerebral spinal fluid (CSF) pH. During states of decreased ventilation, higher partial pressures of carbon dioxide (P_{CO_2}) result in increased CO_2 diffusion across the blood-brain barrier. The subsequent decrease in CSF pH and corresponding increase in free $[H^+]$ ions stimulate increased respiration (Fig. 56–47). Peripheral chemoreceptors, located in the carotid bodies, respond to decreased arterial partial pressures of oxygen (Pa_{O_2}); less of a response is seen with changes in pH and P_{CO_2} (Fig. 56–47*B*).

Of the muscles that effect ventilation, the diaphragm is the most important. This muscular sheet has two distinct components: The thinner, costal muscle inserts on the ribs and sternum and causes the diaphragm to flatten and displace caudally. A thicker, crural component inserts

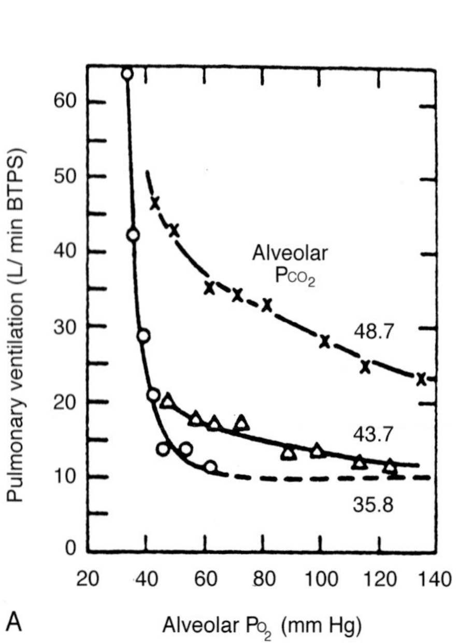

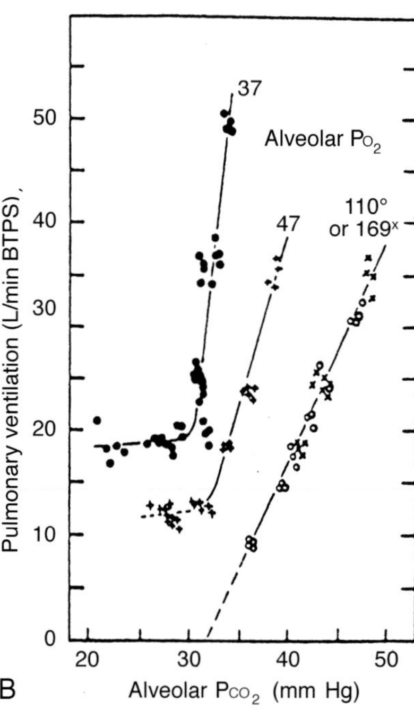

FIGURE 56–47 ■ *A*, Ventilatory response to increasing CO_2 at different curve concentrations of alveolar P_{O_2}. *B*, Ventilatory response to hypoxia at different concentrations of alveolar P_{CO_2}. (BTPS, body temperature, ambient pressure, saturated with water vapor.) (From West JB: Respiratory Physiology: The essentials. Baltimore, Williams & Wilkins, 1995.)

on the lumbar vertebrae. In addition to diaphragm contraction, crural fibers increase thoracic diameter during inspiration by elevating the lower ribs (DeTrover, 1982).

Three types of muscle fibers comprise the diaphragm. Approximately 55% of diaphragm fibers are type 1, slow-twitch, highly oxidative fibers that resist fatigue. Type IIA fibers (21%) are fast-twitch, highly oxidative fibers that resist fatigue to an intermediate degree. Type IIB fibers (24%), by contrast, are fast-twitch, glycolytic fibers that are prone to fatigue (Lieberman et al, 1973). This ratio of different fiber types allows the diaphragm versatility in meeting the metabolic demands of routine and strenuous activity. During normal respiration, only a fraction of the total number of fibers are stimulated during any given respiration; this allows a proportion of fibers to recover metabolically even as the diaphragm performs continuous work.

The phrenic nerve, arising from the C3-C5 nerve roots, carries lower motor innervation to the diaphragm. In as many as 76% of patients, contribution of the C5 nerve root does not occur until the nerve trunk is in the thorax, several centimeters below the level of the clavicle (Kelley, 1950). This anatomic variant is important when considering placement of the nerve electrode; a cervically placed electrode may not capture all of the phrenic nerve fibers. Although the nerve is comprised mostly of motor fibers, a small number of sensory fibers innervates both the thoracic and peritoneal surfaces of the muscle.

INJURY AND DISEASE

Injury may occur to any of the components of respiration: diaphragm, phrenic nerve, or the central respiratory upper motor neuron; however, the change in respiration may be imperceptible if the insult is slight. Symptomatic injury is managed according to the affected ventilatory component. In this regard, accurate assessment of the level of injury is paramount, as this knowledge influences the likelihood of successful phrenic nerve pacing.

Diaphragm

The diaphragm may be involved in a number of pathologic states, systemic diseases, and drug toxicities, as outlined extensively by Syabbalo (1998). In general, phrenic pacing is ineffective in these circumstances. Medical or surgical management of the underlying disease is appropriate. A different situation is encountered in quadriplegic patients with diaphragm atrophy resulting from chronic disuse. Provided it is otherwise normal with an intact phrenic nerve, the diaphragm is expected to respond favorably to diaphragmatic pacing.

Lower Motor Neuron and Phrenic Nerve

Iatrogenic phrenic nerve injury as a result of topical cardiac hypothermia during cardiac surgery is well described; the overall incidence ranges from less than 10% to over 70%, depending on the method of diagnosis (Dajee et al, 1983; Chroni et al, 1995; DeVita, 1993). Injury more commonly occurs to the left phrenic nerve secondary to an increased risk of hypothermia exposure (Dimopoulou et al, 1998). In this regard, placement of an insulation pad within the pericardial well has been shown to offer significant protection to the phrenic nerve. In Wheeler and co-workers' (1985) study of 120 patients, the incidence of injury was reduced from 60% to 8%. Laub and associates (1991) demonstrated a reduction in phrenic injury from 18% in the control group to 0% in the protected group.

Injury to the phrenic nerve may occur during the harvest of the left internal mammary artery owing to the close proximity of the nerve to the origin of the artery (Fig. 56–48) (Setina et al, 1993). Direct or thermal injury may occur during dissection of the artery; injury may also result from reduced perfusion of the nerve as the proximal branches of the corresponding mammary artery are divided (O'Brien et al, 1991). Iatrogenic injury to the phrenic nerve during various congenital heart procedures has been reported (Watanabe et al, 1997). Anecdotal causes of phrenic nerve injury may occur as a result of trauma (Merev et al, 1983) or during noncardiac procedures (Sheridan et al, 1995). The phrenic nerve may be directly involved in malignancy, infection, or other metabolic disorders.

As with diaphragm injury, lower motor neuron injury essentially precludes diaphragmatic pacing. Most cases of

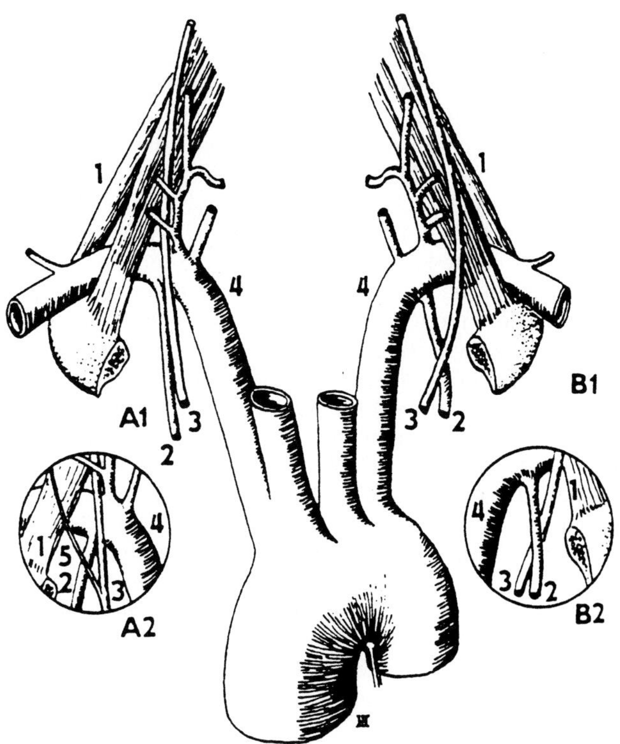

FIGURE 56–48 ■ Interrelationships between the internal mammary nerve and phrenic nerve. *A*, Right side. *B*, Left side. Anatomic structures: 1, scalenus anticus muscle; 2, internal mammary artery; 3, phrenic nerve; 4, subclavian artery; 5, accessory phrenic nerve. (From Setina M, Carry S, Grim M, Pirk J: Anatomical interrelation between the phrenic nerve and the internal mammary artery as seen by the surgeon. J Cardiovasc Surg (Torino) 34:449, 1993.)

lower motor injury are well tolerated and temporary; conservative management usually suffices. However, prolonged or bilateral paralysis may occur with significant mortality and morbidity due to repeated pneumonia, ventilatory failure with repeated incubation, and prolonged mechanical ventilation (Diehl et al, 1994; Tonz et al, 1996).

Upper Motor Neuron Disease

Upper motor neuron injury may occur secondary to tumor involvement, infection, trauma, or stroke. Idiopathic nerve dysfunction may occur. Upper motor neuron injuries are amenable to phrenic nerve pacing provided the phrenic nerve is intact. The majority of phrenic nerve patients fall into one of two categories of upper motor neuron disease: central alveolar hypoventilation or quadriplegic.

Central alveolar hypoventilation (CAH) or central sleep apnea falls under the category of sleep apnea disorders. In general, sleep apnea represents a spectrum of disturbed sleep patterns characterized by episodes of failed respiration lasting greater than 10 seconds. The number of apnea episodes varies: from 5 to greater than 20 episodes per hour may be seen in afflicted patients. The exact prevalence is unknown; however, the reported incidence varies from 0.3% to 15% of the population (Davies and Stradling, 1995).

Central alveolar hypoventilation is also commonly known as Ondine's curse. The history of this term is outlined both by Goldblatt (1995) and Fodstad (1995). The term originates from the Latin word for wave, *unda*. Swiss philosopher von Hohenheim used the appellation "undine" in his 1807 rendition of nature in which the earth is represented by four types of spirits. In this scheme, gnomes symbolize the earth and sylphs represent the air. Salamanders depict fire and undines, or female nymphs, epitomize water. In 1811, German playwright de la Motte Fouqué published *Undine*, a fictional story of a mortal, Knight Huldbrand, who marries Undine, an underwater spirit with an evil uncle, Kühleborn. Following a disagreement with Huldbrand, Undine is forced to return to water, to the service of her uncle. She returns on the wedding night of Huldbrand's remarriage to another mortal to claim his life on behalf of Kühleborn. Several variations of the original story followed, including the French play *Ondine*, by Jean Giraudoux, translated into English by Valency in 1954. In this variation, Ondine's husband Hans is fatally cursed for unfaithfulness by forgetting to breathe. The term *Ondine's curse* was subsequently borrowed by Severinghaus and Mitchell (1962) to describe three patients with failure of nocturnal hypoventilation.

CAH is caused by a diminished response of the receptors in the medulla to increased P_{CO_2} (Mellins et al, 1970). The normal increase in ventilation that occurs in response to increasing arterial P_{CO_2} is diminished or absent in individuals with CAH; the ventilatory response to decreases in P_{O_2} is also blunted. Although the respiratory impairment is continuous, affected individuals may consciously augment ventilation while awake. At night, with the loss of this voluntary contribution, episodic apnea may ensue. However, because the condition is not truly nocturnal, the term "central alveolar hypoventilation" is preferred over sleep apnea. Adults may present with CAH secondary to medullary involvement with tumor or infection. In the pediatric population, congenital CAH is often diagnosed in association with other congenital diseases including Hirshsprung's disease, metabolic disorders, and other neuropathic conditions and tumors (Del Carmen Sanchez et al, 1996).

Patients with central alveolar hypoventilation, or *central* sleep apnea, must be distinguished from those with *obstructive* sleep apnea. Patients with either affliction may present with nocturnal episodes of apnea and complaints of daytime somnolence (Mendelson, 1997); however, patients with obstructive sleep apnea have a normal ventilatory response to hypoxia and hypercarbia. Sleep apnea is caused by mechanical airway obstruction secondary to obesity, abnormal pharyngeal anatomy, exaggerated relaxation of the pharyngeal musculature with sleep, or by space-occupying pharyngeal tumors.

The diagnosis of sleep apnea and the distinction between the two entities is usually performed using polysomnography in an overnight sleep laboratory. The process is an involved one in which several parameters including sleep, oxygenation, breathing airflow patterns, and body movement are studied (Douglas, 1995). The diagnosis is made in children similarly (Guilleminault et al, 1996). Yen and colleagues (1997) have suggested a simpler method of distinguishing between the two entities using measurements of airway impedance. Though obstructive and central sleep apneas are considered two distinct diseases, individuals may demonstrate characteristics of both components. In such cases, if the obstructive component is present less than 50% of the time, the apnea is considered central in origin (Mendelson, 1997).

Distinction between the two entities is necessary for proper patient management. Patients with CAH are considered for phrenic nerve pacing; patients with obstructive sleep apnea are encouraged to undergo weight loss if necessary, and they are supported at night with the use of continuous positive airway pressure (CPAP). In more advanced cases, patients with obstructive sleep apnea may undergo uvulopalatopharyngoplasty, the removal of redundant upper airway soft tissue to reduce upper airway impedance. In extreme cases, tracheostomy may be necessary to secure an airway during sleep (Yen et al, 1997).

The other common condition that is treatable by phrenic nerve pacing is cervical spinal cord injury. The worldwide incidence of spinal cord injury varies from less than 20 per million to over 40 per million population; the incidence in industrialized countries appears slightly higher (Karamenhetoglu, 1995; Lan et al, 1993; Otom et al, 1997). In the United States, the estimated incidence is 45 per million population (Johnson et al, 1997). Most injuries are related to motor vehicle crashes (Burney et al, 1993; Shingu et al, 1994; Thurman et al, 1995) with a high degree of cervical injury and associated quadriplegia or quadriparesis (Price et al, 1994). Among the adolescent population, preventable sport-related causes of cervical injury are seen with a disturbingly high frequency (Scher 1998; Tator et al, 1997; Tyroch et al,

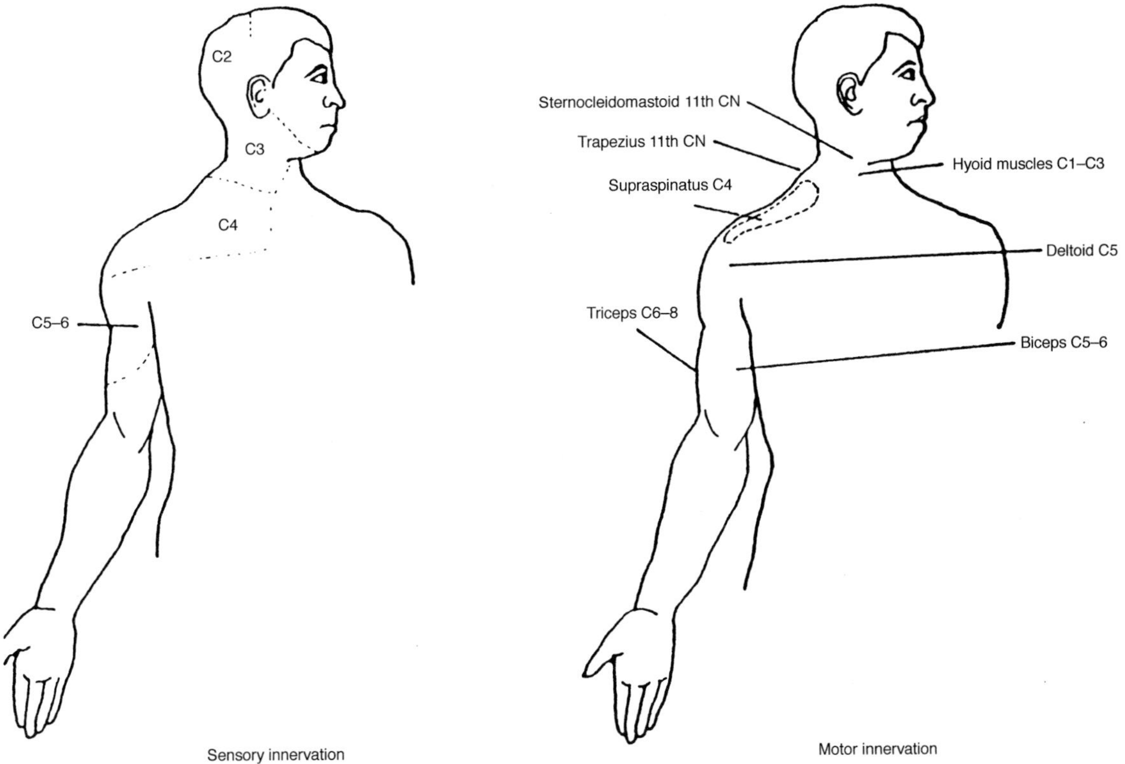

FIGURE 56–49 ■ Sensory and motor findings that distinguish "high" quadriplegia. Quadriplegia at C2-3 is amenable to diaphragm pacing. (From Shields TW: General Thoracic Surgery, 4th ed. Baltimore, Williams & Wilkins, 1994.)

1997). In the elderly, cervical injuries from falls predominate (Alander et al, 1994; Spivak et al, 1994).

In general, patients with high cervical injury, that is, above the C3 level, are most likely to benefit from pacing since the nerve roots of C3-C5 and the integrity of the phrenic nerve are maintained. The necrologic examination in these patients demonstrates intact sensation to the clavicles, and motor function of the trapezius and sternocleidomastoid muscles only (Fig. 56–49). Patients whose cord injury involves any part of the C3-C5 nerve roots have a compromised phrenic nerve, which may interfere with pacing. Patients with cord injury below the C5 level have an intact and functional phrenic nerve, and they should be able to breathe independently although it may not be apparent at the immediate time of injury. In order to make this determination, a waiting period of approximately 3 months is advised.

Diaphragmatic pacing has been attempted in two additional clinical situations: chronic obstructive pulmonary disease (COPD) (Glenn, 1978) and intractable hiccups. As patients with COPD become accustomed to chronic hypercarbia, they become dependent on "hypoxic drive" instead. If supplemental oxygen is required, episodic respiratory failure may occur, which may be treated using phrenic nerve pacing. Fortunately, in practice, few patients have such advanced COPD. Similarly, intractable hiccups have been treated with diaphragm pacing; however, the discomfort of pacing has often led to voluntary cessation. Reports of phrenic nerve pacing in various other diseases are not considered standard practice.

HISTORICAL BACKGROUND OF PACING

Although full-time, simultaneous bilaterally diaphragmatic pacing has been in practice only for the last 2 to 3 decades, the concept of diaphragmatic contraction and artificial respiration through electrical stimulation of the phrenic nerve can be traced back to the late 1700s, beginning with Cavallo in 1777 (Beard and Rockwell, 1875). In 1818, phrenic nerve stimulation was carried out by Ure, who described his experimentation in a criminal who had just recently been hanged: "The chest heaved and fell; the belly was protruded and again collapsed, with the relaxing and retiring diaphragm" (Ure, 1819).

Clinical applications of phrenic nerve stimulation followed thereafter. Guillaume Duchenne de Boulogne used phrenic nerve pacing to treat cholera patients who developed secondary asphyxia during a cholera epidemic in 1849 (Erdmann, 1858). Israel (1927) reported on the successful use of phrenic nerve stimulation to support ventilation in six asphyxiated newborns. In 1950, Sarnoff and co-workers reported the use of phrenic nerve stimulation in the management of patients with bulbar poliomyelitis.

Long-term, continuous pacing of the conditioned diaphragm as it exists today was largely pioneered by Glenn and his associates at Yale. Applying their background knowledge of cardiac pacemakers, they first reported on continuous phrenic nerve stimulation in an animal model (Glenn et al, 1964), followed by its clinical application in a patient with primary hypoventilation (Judson and

Glenn, 1968). The next step in the development of phrenic nerve pacing systems should logically focus on the refinement of a commercially available, totally implantable pacing system with automatic rate adjustment, based on the patient's end-tidal Pa_{CO_2}. While such advances have been realized experimentally Hogan et al, 1989; Lanmüller et al, 1997; the clinical application and availability of such devices continue to be hindered by the relatively small patient population who use such devices and subsequent lack of interest in their commercial development.

However, experimentation continues in the development of artificial and assisted ventilation. Investigations include the use of intercostal nerve stimulation as a sole or supplementary source of artificial respiration (DiMarco et al, 1989, 1994) and in combination with phrenic nerve pacing (Supinski et al, 1991). Attempts to restore disrupted phrenic nerve function have been reported, including phrenic nerve grafting (Baldissera et al, 1993; Krieger et al, 1994) and intradiaphragmatic phrenic nerve stimulation (Peterson et al, 1994a, b). Other avenues of research involve the study of diaphragm mechanics (Coirault et al, 1995), strength and fatigue (Golgeli, 1995; Mador, 1996; Rochester, 1985), histology (Bisschop et al, 1997), and gene expression (Gosselin et al, 1995). The diaphragmatic response to pharmacologic agents (Fujii et al, 1995; Van Lunteren and Moyer, 1996; Van Lunteren et al, 1995), free radical scavengers (Supinski et al, 1997; Travaline et al, 1997), and steroids (Dekhuijzen et al, 1995) are under study.

PREREQUISITES FOR PACING

It must be emphasized that phrenic nerve pacing is reserved for patients with an intact phrenic nerve and functional diaphragm. Accurate assessment of both is imperative. New and modified techniques for assessment of diaphragm strength and contraction have been described (Maclean, 1981; Markland, 1984; McCauley, 1984; Syabbalo, 1998); however, established screening tests for phrenic nerve function often suffice. These include observational assessment of the diaphragm during transcutaneous phrenic nerve stimulation, fluoroscopy, and phrenic nerve conduction studies.

Initial testing of the nerve is carried out by percutaneous stimulation in the neck, using a technique similar to electromyography (Sarnoff et al, 1950; Shaw et al, 1975). The lateral edge of the clavicular head of the sternocleidomastoid muscle is displaced medially. A thimble electrode is placed at this level and a current is directed posteriorly toward the presumed location of the nerve (Fig. 56–50). Simple observation often suffices in assess-

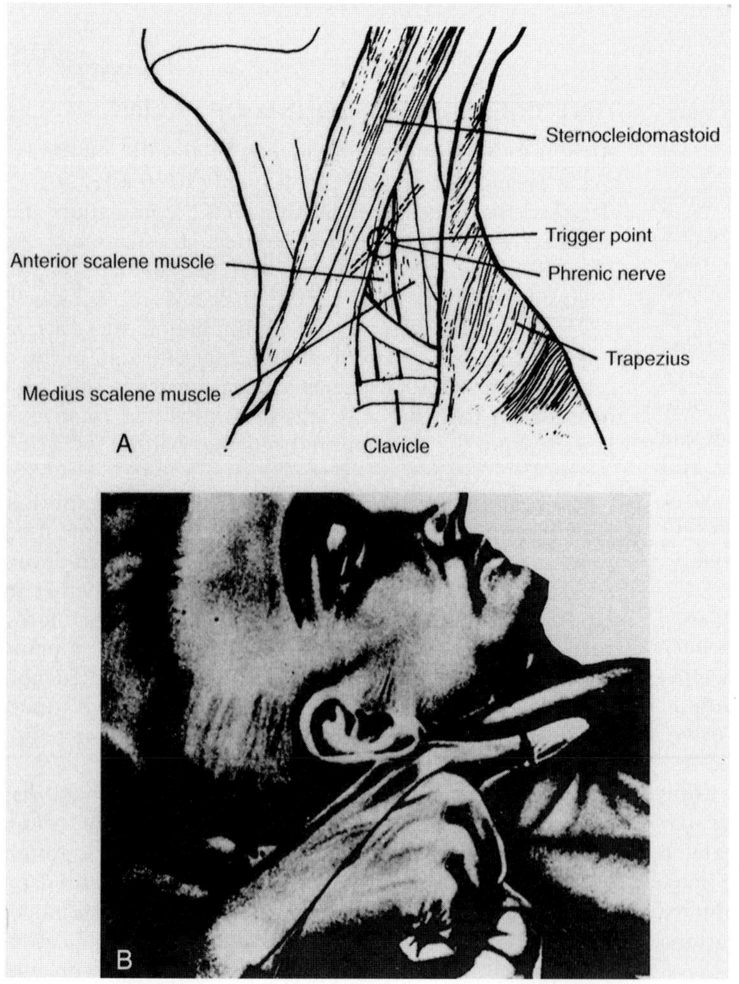

FIGURE 56–50 ■ Access of the phrenic nerve for stimulation studies. *A*, The phrenic nerve "trigger point" is identified at the lateral border of the sternocleidomastoid muscle where the nerve crosses the scalene muscles. *B*, Application of the thimble electrode. (From Sarnoff SJ et al: Electrophrenic respiration. VII. The motor point of the phrenic nerve in relation to external stimulation. Surg Gynecol Obstet 93:190, 1975.)

ment of diaphragm function; significant and obvious contraction of the diaphragm should ensue if the nerve is intact. Failure to elicit this response implies nerve compromise, as the accuracy of the test approximates 100% (Mier et al, 1987; Shaw et al, 1980). Phrenic nerve conduction time is also assessed, using two surface electrodes (placed over the anterior and posterior axillary line at the T8-T9 intercostal level) and an oscilloscope. The interval time from cervical stimulation of the phrenic nerve until a diaphragm action potential is recorded. The average value in normal volunteers is 8.4 + 0.78 msec. A prolonged latency (10 to 14 msec) is abnormal; however, this does not necessarily preclude successful pacing (Glenn and Sairenji, 1985).

Quantitative diaphragm function is evaluated fluoroscopically. A ruler with radiographically opaque numbers is placed behind the pacing candidate such that the dome of the unstimulated diaphragm lies over the numeral 1. Maximal diaphragmatic descent on inspiration or phrenic nerve stimulation is measured. In normal individuals, the diaphragm descends approximately 8 to 10 cm; excursion of at least 5 cm is desired for pacing (Glenn, 1985). Phrenic nerve paralysis is suspected by elevation of the affected hemidiaphragm on chest radiography or fluoroscopy. This is confirmed with a positive sniff test in which a paradoxical, rapid upward movement of the diaphragm is seen when the supine patient sniffs briskly through the nose with the mouth closed. A functional phrenic nerve should provide a brisk downward deflection of the diaphragm on nerve stimulation. The current required to produce minimal contraction of the diaphragm is defined as the threshold current; the maximal current is defined as the least amount of current that produces maximal excursion of the diaphragm.

Cervical magnetic stimulation (CMS) offers an alternative method to assess phrenic nerve conduction and diaphragm function. A magnetic coil, placed over the C3-C5 nerve roots, causes depolarization of these roots. The test is relatively painless and well tolerated. Because depolarization is applied to the roots comprising the phrenic nerve rather than the nerve per se, cross-stimulation of the other muscles of respiration that are supplied by the same nerve roots may occur; therefore, the test is not specific for the phrenic nerve itself. The nerve roots may be tested unilaterally (Mills et al, 1995) or bilaterally (Similowski et al, 1998). Clinical applications using CMS have included detection of diaphram fatigue (Laghi et al, 1996; Similowski et al, 1998), and the selection of phrenic nerve pacing candidates (Similowski et al, 1996); however, experience with this mode of phrenic nerve assessment is limited.

Transdiaphragmatic pressure may also be used for phrenic nerve and diaphragm assessment. Indwelling midesophageal and stomach balloon catheters indirectly measure pleural and abdominal pressures, respectively. The transdiaphragmatic pressure (Pdi) is calculated as the difference in pressure between the two catheters. A value of approximately 10 cm H_2O is seen with phrenic nerve stimulation in normal individuals (Moxham and Shneerson, 1993). Diaphragm atrophy as well as phrenic nerve dysfunction may cause lower values; thus, careful interpretation of results is required.

In addition to a functional phrenic nerve and diaphragm, phrenic pacing patients should have adequate pulmonary function parameters and normal chest morphology. Patients with CAH should demonstrate arterial blood gas improvement with hyperventilation. All patients must be knowledgeable and cooperative and have adequate medical and psychological support, including a team of health care providers who can be made well versed in phrenic nerve pacing, and a supportive network of family members and friends. Patients with underlying pulmonary disease, chest wall deformities, and neuromuscular disorders involving the diaphragm are poor candidates for diaphragm pacing. Similarly, patients who lack adequate nursing and emotional support often fail pacing.

PACING PHYSIOLOGY

Unlike the heart, which is an electrical syncytium and contracts with a single stimulus, the diaphragm requires a series of stimuli to effect contraction. This form of pacing, termed "pulse train stimulation," has several associated definitions (Fig. 56–51). The pulse width defines the duration of an individual stimulus within a pulse train. The pulse interval, which defines the duration of time between individual stimuli, may be alternatively expressed as its reciprocal, frequency (frequency = 1000 per pulse interval). The pulse train duration defines the total duration of a given series of pulse currents; this corresponds to the actual duration of diaphragm contractions. The amplitude of the pulse current measures the voltage of the pulse train stimuli; this determines the strength of diaphragmatic contraction as reflected by the resulting tidal volume.

Unlike normal physiologic excitation, stimulation of the phrenic nerve with a unipolar electrode causes simul-

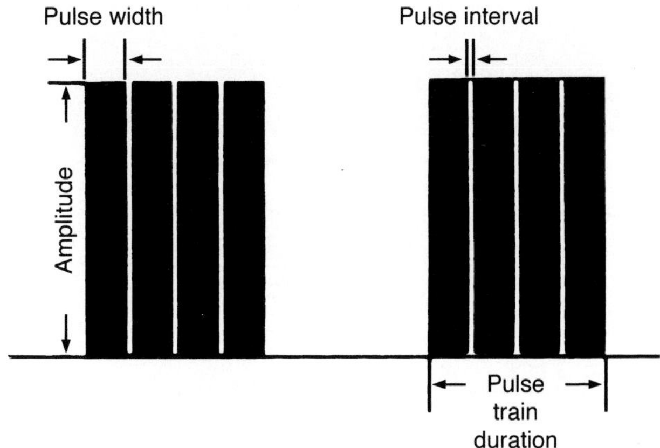

FIGURE 56–51 ■ Pulse-train stimulation, associated parameters, and units of measurements: amplitude (volts), voltage of each stimulus within the pulse train; pulse width (msec), duration of an individual pulse; pulse interval (msec), duration between pulses within a train; pulse train duration (msec), overall duration of one train of pulses. Frequency refers to the timing of stimuli within a pulse train (i.e., frequency [Hz] = 1000/pulse interval). Rate is defined as the number of pulse trains delivered in one minute. (From Shields TW: General Thoracic Surgery, 4th ed. Baltimore, Williams & Wilkins, 1994.)

taneous depolarization of the entire nerve including all associated motor units. Because the composition of the native diaphragm includes fibers that are relatively prone to fatigue, continuous, full-time pacing requires conditioning of the diaphragm to electrical stimulation over a period of weeks. As this occurs, the histology of the diaphragm evolves from the existing composition of fast (glycolytic) and slow (oxidative) fibers to one exclusively of slow fibers. The vascular supply increases, enzyme patterns change, and mitochrondria are increased (Mannion and Stephenson, 1985; Salmons and Hendriksson, 1981). These changes reflect the diaphragm's "plasticity" and its inherent ability to sustain continuous mechanical work.

PACING EQUIPMENT AND COMMERCIAL DEVICES

Currently, three phrenic pacing systems are in clinical use: the Avery model (Avery, Glen Cove, NY, USA), the Jukka Astrostim (Atrotech OY, Tampere, Finland) and the "Vienna phrenic pacemaker" (MedImplant, Vienna, Austria). Although each model varies slightly in design, all subscribe to the same concept of phrenic nerve pacing (Fig. 56–52): an extracorporeal generator and antenna are used to encode pulse trains into radiofrequency signals which are transmitted across intact skin to a subcutaneously implanted radio receiver. The receiver translates the radiofrequency signal into direct current, which is delivered through an electrode to the phrenic nerve. All three systems use increasing amplitude within each pulse train to generate a smooth, gradual contraction of the diaphragm. At present, there is no totally implanted phrenic nerve pacing system available for clinical use.

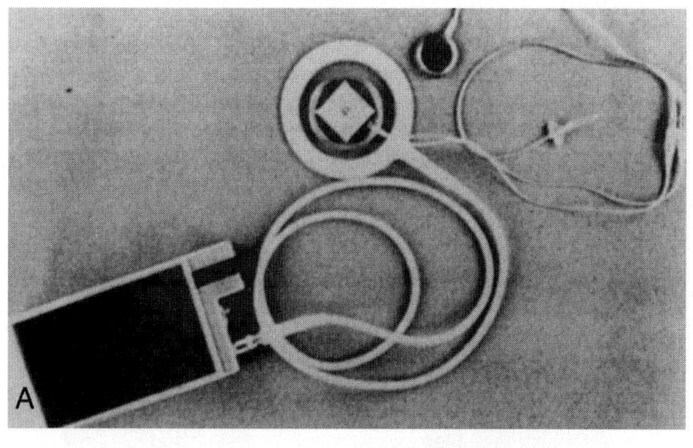

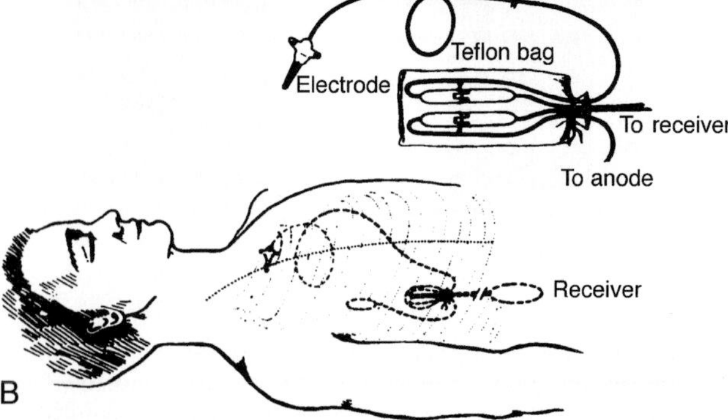

FIGURE 56–52 ■ Components of the diaphragm pacer. *A*, The external generator and antenna (*shown overlying the receiver*) and the implanted receiver and electrode. *B*, Electrode and receiver as placed in patient. The phrenic nerve is placed at the level of the upper thorax. The receiver is positioned over a flat portion of the lower chest wall. (From Shields TW: General Thoracic Surgery, 4th ed. Baltimore, Williams & Wilkins, 1994.)

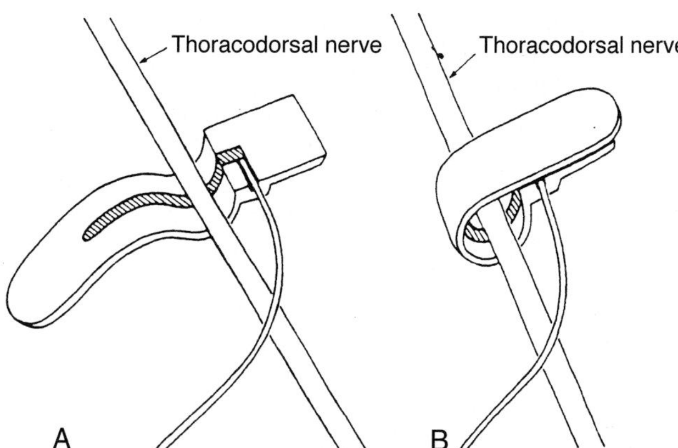

FIGURE 56–53 ■ The two nerve-cuff electrode configurations for phrenic nerve stimulation. *A*, 180-degree or "half cuff" electrode configuration; *B*, 360-degree or "full cuff" configuration. (From Letsou GV, Hogan JF, Lee P et al: Comparison of 180-degree and 360 degree skeletal muscle nerve cuff electrodes. Ann Thorac Surg 54:925, 1992.)

The Avery model uses the prototypic design of Glenn and associates at Yale. The stationary extracorporeal generator is approximately the size of a clock radio. A handheld, portable generator is also available. The antenna coil is taped securely to the patient's skin, directly over the subcutaneously implanted receiver. The receiver, about the size of a pocket watch, is placed subcutaneously over the lower, anterolateral aspect of the rib cage. The unipolar electrode stimulates the entire phrenic nerve with every impulse. A bipolar electrode is available for patients in whom a competing device, such as a cardiac pacemaker, is a consideration. The electrode is preferentially placed beneath the nerve as a half-cuff or 180-degree configuration, as opposed to the cirumferential full-cuff or 360-degree configuration (Fig. 56–53), to avoid the potential complication of circumferential scar tissue that may occur with the latter (Letsou et al, 1992).

The Jukka Astrostim unit has a quadripolar electrode made of two strips of polytetrafluoroethylene (Teflon) with two electrode contacts on each strip. One strip is placed in front of the nerve and the other behind it. In theory, at any given time only *partial* recruitment of motor units occurs, using one of the four electrode contacts as a cathode, while the opposite side serves as the anode (see Fig. 56–53*A*). Unstimulated motor units are allowed time for metabolic recovery. This pattern of nerve stimulation, which is designed to mimic the pattern of metabolic recovery during natural ventilation, is believed to alleviate diaphragm fatigue. At regular intervals, the stimulation threshold may be increased to achieve a larger tidal volume. These "sighs" condition additional diaphragm muscle mass in the event that recruitment of these "reserve" muscle fibers are needed to meet increased

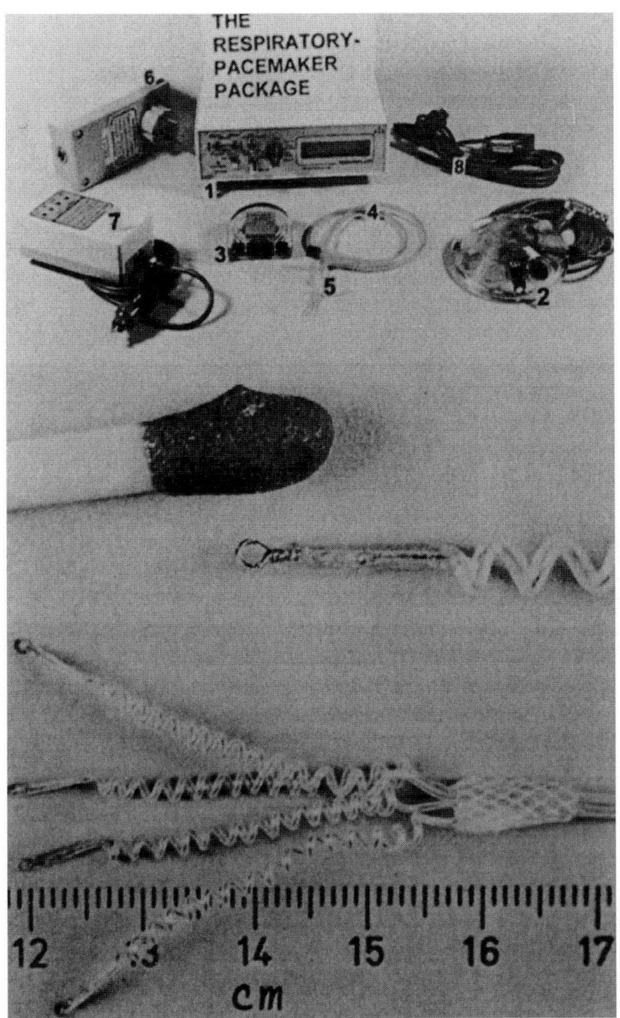

FIGURE 56–54 ■ Quadrapolar electrodes. *A*, Atrotech electrode. *B*, Single prong of the Vienna Pacemaker electrode, enlarged to show sewing ring. Matchstick placed for comparison. *C*, Full, 4-pronged Vienna Pacemaker electrode. (From Creasey G, Elefteriades J, Dimarco A et al: Electrical stimulation to restore respiration. J Rehab Res Dev 33:123, 1996.)

metabolic demands (Talonen et al, 1990). Similarly, the MedImplant model stimulates the nerve in a partial, staggered fashion using multiple electrode contacts. After each breath, the cathode-anode combination is alternated bilaterally to avoid diaphragm fatigue. Each electrode has four contact prongs that are sutured to the phrenic nerve epineurium using 8–0 suture (Fig. 56–54).

SURGICAL PLACEMENT

In placing the phrenic nerve electrode, the operator must use extreme caution in handling the nerve because injury essentially precludes pacing or spontaneous breathing. Muscle relaxants are avoided intraoperatively as they can obfuscate pacing assessment. The prophylactic use of antibiotics and careful aseptic surgical technique are of paramount importance to avoid the disastrous complication of infection.

Electrode placement for the Avery of Atrotech model is carried out through a limited anterior thoracotomy in the T2 or T3 intercostal space (Fig. 56–55). The internal mammary artery and vein are divided to avoid injury or disruption. The phrenic nerve is identified as it courses anterior to the hilum, and a location is chosen to allow flat, tension-free placement of the electrode. Two parallel incisions are made in the mediastinal pleura on either side of the phrenic neurovascular bundle. The electrode is gently slipped behind the nerve and vessels such that the phrenic nerve bundle is in contact with the electrode without tension or distortion. Minor bleeding encountered during the dissection is anticipated to stop spontaneously; cautery, with potential injury to the phrenic nerve, is best avoided.

Extra electrode length is left in the thorax to safeguard against tension on the phrenic nerve by the electrode with lung re-expansion. An intercostal segment of chest tube is used to facilitate passage of the electrode wire through the chest wall. After the electrode wire is connected to the receiver unit, excess wire is placed into a Teflon bag for easy, safe access later. The receiver and bag are placed in a subcutaneous pocket with the receiver closer to the skin surface to optimize signal transmission. The subcutaneous tissues are closed tightly to avoid receiver migration within the pocket, with the skin incision well away from the underlying receiver. Chest closure is standard. Before undraping the patient, the system is tested under sterile conditions. A stimulation threshold of 1.0 to 2.9 mA indicates a functional unit. Failure to achieve this necessitates re-evaluation of electrode placement and component parts. If indicated, the contralateral unit is placed approximately 2 weeks after the first implantation. It is anticipated that thoracosopic electrode placement may eventually supersede the open technique. However, one must always adhere to the principle of minimal nerve trauma, regardless of the method of placement.

Cervical electrode placement remains somewhat controversial. Advantages of this approach include the avoidance of bilateral thoracotomy, which may be advantageous in patients with pulmonary parenchymal disease or chest wall deformity. Bilateral concurrent implantation may be performed in the neck. The major disadvantage of cervical electrode placement is failure to provide complete phrenic nerve stimulation in individuals with an accessory or bifurcated phrenic nerve; these components often do not consolidate until the phrenic nerve is in the thorax. Other anatomic variations of the nerve in the neck, including an intramuscular segment within the scalenus anticus, or proximity to the brachial plexus (Fodstad 1987), may preclude effective pacing. The electrode may also migrate with excessive neck movement.

In the event that cervical electrode placement is performed, temporary endotracheal intubation, removal of the tracheostomy, and occlusion of the tracheostomy site may be used to decrease the risk of electrode contamination during placement. Exposure is obtained using a supraclavicular incision. The lateral border of the sternocleidomastoid muscle is identified and retracted medially. The nerve is almost always found overlying the scalenus anticus muscle at this level, crossing from the lateral to medial aspect of the muscle, just deep to the scalene

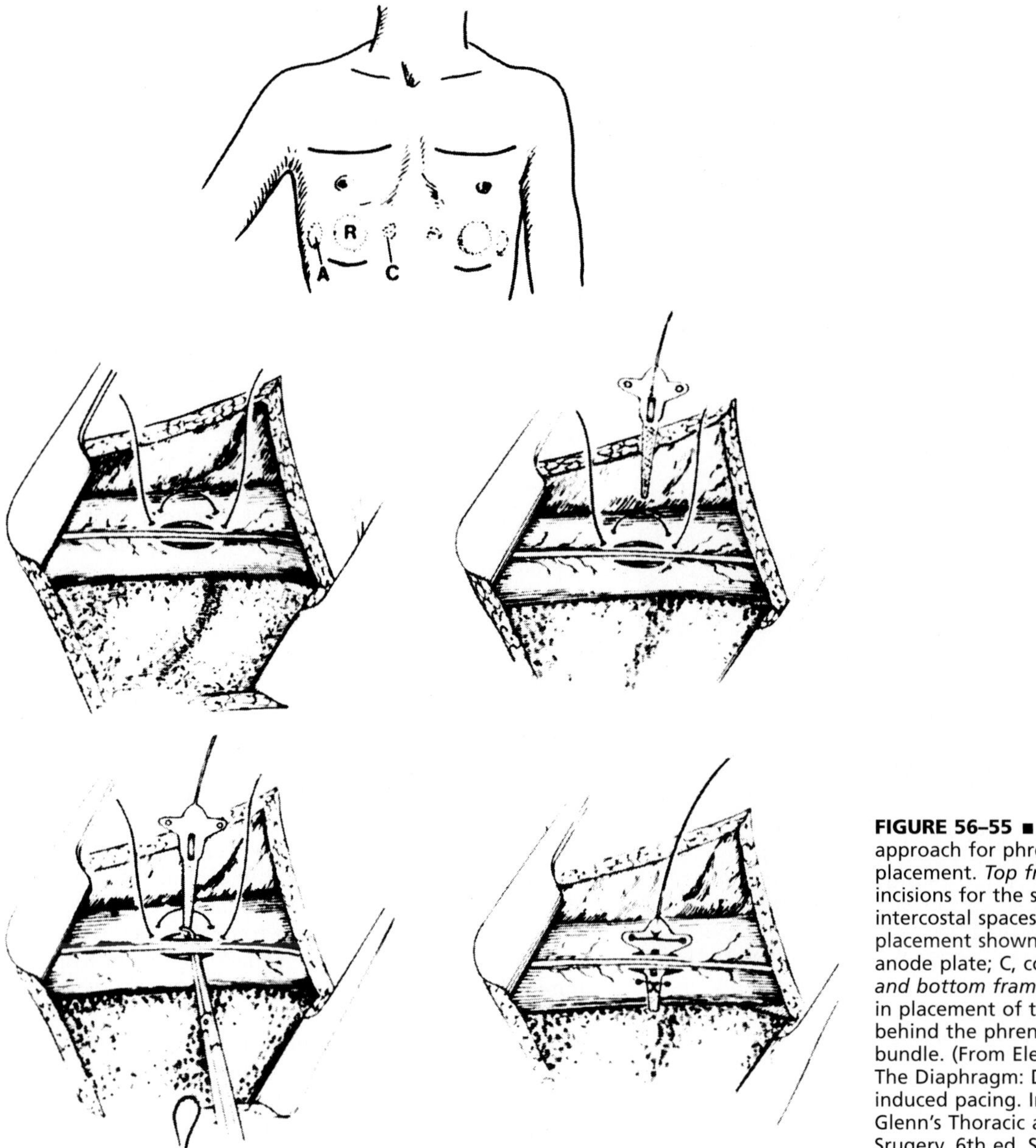

FIGURE 56–55 ■ Transthoracic approach for phrenic nerve electrode placement. *Top frame*: separate incisions for the second to third intercostal spaces and for receiver placement shown (R, receiver; A, anode plate; C, connectors.) *Middle and bottom frames*: sequential steps in placement of the electrode behind the phrenic neurovascular bundle. (From Elefteriades JA et al: The Diaphragm: Dysfunction and induced pacing. In Baue CL (ed): Glenn's Thoracic and Cardiovascular Srugery, 6th ed. Stamford, CT, Appleton & Lange, 1996.)

fascia. A stimulation probe is placed in this area, and 2 to 10 mA of current is applied. Diaphragm contraction confirms correct identification of the nerve. Placement of the nerve electrode and radio receiver is similar to that in the chest. The subcutaneous pocket is placed inferior to the clavicle, using the existing supraclavicular incision.

The MedImplant system is placed through a median sternotomy with bilateral simultaneous electrode placement. The electrode prongs are sutured to the phrenic nerve epineurium using fine polypropylene suture and the surgical microscope. The receiver is placed underneath the rectus abdominis fascia.

A permanent tracheostomy is present in most, if not all, patients in whom phrenic nerve pacing is undertaken. This provides a secure airway in the event of pacemaker malfunction, and it should be maintained, even after full-time continuous pacing is achieved. The conventional tracheostomy may be replaced by a Teflon tracheal button to maintain the airway with improved cosmesis and less tracheal irritation.

CONDUCT OF PACING

Approximately 2 weeks of recovery are allowed after device implantation before pacing is initiated, as attempts to pace earlier may cause bloody pleural effusion, thought secondary to disruption of immature pleural adhesions. Low-frequency, continuous, bilateral simultaneous pacing is preferred in individuals totally dependent on diaphragmatic pacing; in adults with central alveolar hypoventilation, unilateral pacing may suffice. Pacemaker settings preset from the manufacturer (Avery) include inspiratory duration (1.3 seconds for adults, 0.6 second for children) and pulse width (150 msec). Settings for current are placed just above the maximum threshold level. The respiratory rate is individualized for each patient. Rates of 6 to 10 breaths/min usually suffice for patients who pace bilaterally; higher rates are required for children and for patients who pace unilaterally (Weese-Mayer, 1989).

Quadriplegia patients with diaphragm atrophy require conditioning of the diaphragm prior to continuous, bilateral stimulation. The usual conditioning regimen starts with 15 minutes of pacing during each waking hour. The number of minutes of each hour and the number of hours paced each day are gradually increased until continuous pacing is achieved. Patients are monitored during pacing sessions using measurements of tidal volume, minute ventilation, end-tidal CO_2, oxygen saturation, and occasionally, blood gas measurements. A fall in tidal volume with a corresponding rise in end-tidal CO_2 is an indication that the diaphragm may be beginning to fatigue. The patient is rested on mechanical ventilation overnight or longer if necessary, and on resuming the pacing schedule, a shorter pacing period is set. Advances in the pacing schedule are made every 7 to 14 days (or less) as tolerated by the patient. The conditioning phase usually lasts 3 to 6 months; however, this process may be longer in quadriplegic patients with severe diaphragm atrophy. Once continuous pacing is achieved, the frequency of stimuli within each pulse train and the number of breaths per minute are decreased to minimize diaphragm fatigue. Patients who require only intermittent pacing may initiate the full pacing schedule without conditioning, as diaphragm fatigue is unlikely. In children, bilateral pacing should be performed to avoid mediastinal shifts, which may occur with unilateral pacing. A faster respiratory rate and shorter inspiratory duration (0.6 second) are preferred in the pediatric population. Children over the age of 8 to 10 may essentially pace as adults.

Unlike cardiac pacemakers, which are essentially maintenance free, phrenic pacemakers require constant vigilance and a thorough understanding of the pacing device, its limitations, and associated caveats to avert potential complications including infection, respiratory insufficiency, nerve injury, and diaphragmatic fatigue. Pacemaker failure may occur from receiver or electrode malfunction or from interference by another pacing device such as a cardiac pacemaker.

RESULTS

Given the relatively low numbers of phrenic nerve pacemakers implanted worldwide, the number of institutions with reported series of patients are few. The largest series of patients with follow-up was that reported by Glenn and associates, in 1988, of 165 patients who underwent device implantation at one of six centers: Yale-New Haven Medical Center, Children's Memorial Hospital (Chicago), Toronto Western Hospital, Umea University Hospital (Sweden), Mayo Clinic, and Children's Hospital of Los Angeles. Sixty-five patients underwent unilateral electrode placement; the remaining 100 patients underwent bilateral placement. Twenty-seven percent of patients paced full time; 61% paced part time. Pacing successfully met the ventilatory requirements of 47%, and was partially successful in an additional 36%. The majority of patients in the study had paced for less than 5 years (108 patients, 68%). Thirty-one patients (20%) paced for 5 to 10 years, 16 patients (10%) paced for 10 to 15 years, and 4 patients (16%) paced for 15 to 20 years.

More recently, Weese-Mayer and associates (1996) reported results with the quadripolar electrode, using both physician questionnaire and the Atrotech registry. Sixty-four individuals (35 children, 29 adults) from 13 countries underwent device implantation. Thirty-three children and 27 adults paced bilaterally. At a mean follow-up of 2.0 ± 1.0 years, 94% of 35 children paced successfully. Of the 29 adults, 86% adults paced successfully at a mean follow-up of 2.2 ± 1.1 years. Thirteen (45%) of the adults paced full time. Twelve (41%) adults paced part time; two of these patients paced less than 5 hours daily. Nine (26%) of the children paced full time; 66% of the children paced part time (at least 5 hours daily). Complication-free pacing rates were lower (60% of pediatric and 52% of adult patients, at follow-up periods of 2.0 ± 1.0 and 2.2 ± 1.1 years, respectively). Complications included electrode dysfunction (19%), electrode failure requiring replacement (3.1%), receiver failure (5.9%), infection (2.9%), and iatrogenic nerve injury (3.8%).

Several series provide data on long-term follow-up after pacemaker implantation. Fodstad (1995) reports experience with device implantation in 42 patients (33 bilateral, 9 unilateral) with a mean follow-up of 62 months. Nineteen patients continued to pace full time, 5 patients paced intermittently, and 8 patients did not pace. Seven patients had died after pacing for periods ranging from 4 months to 11 years. Three patients died before achieving pacing. Of the 8 patients who did not pace at the time of follow-up, six patients with partial phrenic nerve damage (C3-C5 injury) stopped pacing after periods ranging from 1 month to 3 years. The two remaining patients, both of whom underwent pacemaker implantation for hiccups, stopped pacing voluntarily, shortly after device implantation. Mayr and associates (1993) reported on experience using the Vienna pacemaker in 15 patients with high cervical quadriplegia and complete ventilatory insufficiency. Three patients were undergoing conditioning. Eleven patients who achieved conditioned diaphragm pacing, at time of follow-up, had paced a mean of 43.3 months (range, 5 to 83 months); included were 4 patients who died after pacing 7, 31, 58 and 60 months. One patient was able to pace intermittently for 2 to 3 hours at a time. Experience with the Vienna pacemaker in eight pediatric patients, with ages ranging from 2 to 13 years (mean age, 9 ± 3), was reported by Girsch (1996). At the time of follow-up, one patient continued to undergo diaphragm conditioning. Continuous phrenic nerve pacing was achieved in four patients after a mean conditioning period of 13 months; these four patients had paced for periods of 10, 28, 38, and 48 months. Two of these patients subsequently died of complications of pneumonia. Two patients paced intermittently for 24 and 36 months, respectively; at the time of follow up, both had died from complications of pneumonia. One patient refused to pace after device implantation and was ventilated mechanically.

Of 14 quadriplegia patients conditioned at Yale for

bilateral full-time pacing, seven paced full time at a mean follow-up of 7.6 years, when first reported by the senior author (Elefteriades et al, 1992). Five patients continue to pace full time and have all done so for over 10 years; the longest paced patient has done so for 17 years (Elefteriades, unpublished data, 1997). Three patients are deceased, two of whom previously paced for 10.5 years and 6 months, respectively. Six patients did not achieve or maintain pacing for multiple reasons, including medical complications of quadriplegia, insufficient nursing care, patient preference, and insufficient finances to support pacing.

DIAPHRAGM PACING: ADVANTAGES AND CAVEATS

When applied to carefully selected patients, the success of long-term phrenic nerve pacing has been shown unequivocally by patients who pace for several years without interruption. For quadriplegia patients this diaphragm pacing represents their *only* source of ventilation. Patients who may otherwise face institutionalization and mechanical ventilation have greater autonomy with phrenic pacing, often with great psychological benefit. With proper supportive care, patients live independently and carry out productive lives including full-time employment, travel, and leisure. Children who are paced have greater ventilatory capacity and are able to participate in sports and other strenuous activities. Diaphragm pacing more closely mimics physiologic negative pressure ventilation and may pose less lung barotrauma, may decrease pulmonary vascular resistance and may increase systemic blood flow (Ishii et al, 1990). No randomized studies directly compare phrenic nerve pacing with mechanical ventilation; however, Esclarín and co-workers' (1994) retrospective study comparing the two modalities suggest that patients managed with phrenic nerve-pacing phonate optimally, are more mobile, achieve a higher rate of hospital discharge, and are managed at lower cost.

However, emphasis must be placed on the importance of proper selection for pacing candidates. Patients with equivocal indications, who fail to meet the prerequisites for pacing, often fail during pacing, after having invested considerable emotional, physical, and financial effort and resources. Conversely, patients with the proper indications and with adequate medical and social support may enjoy the benefits of successful pacing both in terms of quality of life, medical condition, and financial costs and may do so for extended periods.

■ *REFERENCES*

Alander DH, Andreychik DA, Stauffer ES: Early outcome in cervical spinal cord injured patients older than 50 years of age. Spine 19:2299, 1994.

Baldissera F, Cavallari P, Marini G, Tredici G: Diaphragm reinnervation by laryngeal motoneurons. J Appl Physiol 75:639, 1993.

Beard GM, Rockwell AD: Practical Treatise on the Medical and Surgical Uses of Electricity, 2nd ed. London, Lewis, 1875.

Bisschop A, Gayan-Ramirez G, Rollier H et al: Intermittent inspiratory muscle training induces fiber hypertrophy in rat diaphragm. Am J Respir Crit Care Med 155:1583, 1997.

Brouillette RT, Ilbawi MN, Hunt CE: Phrenic nerve pacing in infants and children: A review of the experience and report on the usefulness of phrenic nerve stimulation studies. J Pediatr 102:32, 1983.

Burney RE, Maio RF, Maynard F, Karunas R: Incidence, characteristics, and outcome of spinal cord injury at trauma centers in North America. Arch Surg 238:596, 1993.

Chroni E, Patel RL, Taub N et al: A comprehensive electrophysiological evaluation of phrenic nerve injury related to open-heart surgery. Acta Neurol Scand 91:255, 1995.

Coirault C, Riou B, Bard M et al: Contraction, relaxation and economy of force generation in isolated human diaphragm muscle. Am J Respir Crit Care Med 152 (4 Pt 1): 1275, 1995.

Dajee A, Pellegrini J, Cooper G, Karison K: Phrenic nerve palsy after topical cardiac hypothermia. Int Surg 68:345, 1983.

Davies R, Stradling JR: The epidemiology of sleep apnoea. Am J Respir Crit Care Med 152:711, 1995.

Dekhuijzen PN, Gayan-Ramirez G, Bisschop A et al: Corticosteroid treatment and nutritional deprivation cause a different pattern of atrophy in rat diaphragm. J Appl Physiol 78:629, 1995.

Del Carmen Sanchez M, Lopez-Herce J, Carrillo A et al: Late onset central hypoventilation syndrome. Pediatr Pulmonol 21:189, 1996.

DeTroyer A, Sampson M, Sigrist S, Macklem PT: Action of costal and crural parts of the diaphragm on the rib cage in dog. J Appl Physiol 53:30, 1982.

DeVita MA, Robinson LR, Rehder J et al: Incidence and natural history of phrenic neuropathy occurring during open heart surgery. Chest 103:850, 1993.

Diehl J, Lofaso F, Delueze P et al: Clinically relevant diaphragmatic dysfunction after cardiac operations. J Thorac Cardiovasc Surg 107:487, 1994.

DiMarco AF, Budzinska K, Supinski GS: Artificial ventilation by means of electrical activation of the intercostal/accessory muscles alone in anesthetized dogs. Am Rev Respir Dis 139:961, 1989.

Dimarco AF, Supinski GS, Petro JA, Takaoka Y: Evaluation of intercostal pacing to provide artificial ventilation in quadriplegics. Am J Respir Crit Care Med 150:934, 1994.

Dimopoulou I, Daganou M, Dafni U et al: Phrenic nerve dysfunction after cardiac operations. Electrophysiologic evaluation of risk factors. Chest 113:8, 1998.

Doblas A, Herrera M, Venegas J et al: Failure in phrenic pacing induced by varicella (Letter). Pacing Clin Electro Physiol 12:1961, 1989.

Douglas NJ: Sleep-related breathing disorders. How to reach a diagnosis in patients who may have the sleep apnea/hypopnea syndrome. Thorax 50:883, 1995.

Edwards RHT, Faulkner JA: Structure and functions of the respiratory muscle. The Thorax: Part A. In Lenfant C (ed): Lung Biology in Health and Disease, Vol 29. New York, Marcel Dekker, 1985, pp 297–326.

Elefteriades JA, Hogan JF, Handler A, Loke JS: Long-term follow-up of bilateral pacing of the diaphragm in quadriplegia. N Engl J Med 326:1433, 1992.

Erdmann BA: Die ortiche Anwendung der elektricitat in der Physiologie, Pathologie und Therapie, 2nd ed. Leipzig, Barth, 1858, p 240.

Esclarín A, Bravo P, Arroyo O et al: Tracheostomy ventilation vs. diaphragmatic pacemaker ventilation in high spinal cord injury. Paraplegia 32:687, 1994.

Fodstad H: Phrenicodiaphragmatic pacing. In Roussos C (ed): The Thorax. New York, Marcel Dekker, 1995.

Fodstad H: The Swedish experience in phrenic nerve stimulation. Pacing Clin Electrophysiol 10:240, 1987.

Fujii Y, Toyooka H, Amaha K: Amrinone improves contractility of fatigued diaphragm in dogs. Can J Anesth 42:80, 1995.

Giraudoux J: Ondine. Translated by Maurice Valency. New York, Random House, 1954.

Girch W, Koller R, Holle J et al: Vienna phrenic pacemaker: Experience with diaphragm pacing in children. Eur J Pediatr Surg 6:140, 1996.

Glenn WWL, Bouillette RT, Dentz B et al: Fundamental consideration in pacing of the diaphragm for chronic ventilatory insufficiency: A multi-center study: Part II. Pacing Clin Electrophysiol 11:2121, 1988.

Glenn WWL, Gee JBL, Schachter EN: Diaphragm pacing. Application to a patient with chronic obstructive pulmonary disease. J Thorac Cardiovasc Surg 75:273, 1978.

Glenn WWL, Hageman JH, Mauro A et al: Electrical stimulation of excitable tissue by radio-frequency transmission. Ann Surg 160:338, 1964.

Glenn WWL, Sairenji H: Diaphragm pacing in the treatment of chronic ventilatory insufficiency. In Roussos C, Macklem PT (eds): The Thorax. New York, Marcel Dekker, 1985, pp 1407–1449.

Goldblatt D: Historical note: Qndine's curse. Semin Neurol 15:218, 1995.

Golgeli A, Ozesmi C, Ozesmi M: Dependence of fatigue properties on the pattern of stimulation in the rat diaphragm muscle. Indian J Physiol Pharmacol 39:315, 1995.

Gosselin LE, Sieck GC, Aleff RA et al: Changes in diaphragm muscle collagen gene expression after acute unilateral denervation. J Appl Physiol 79:1249, 1995.

Guilleminault C, Pelayo R, Leger D et al: Recognition of sleep-disordered breathing in children. Pediatrics 98:871, 1996.

Hogan JF, Koda H, Glenn WWL: Electrical techniques for stimulation of the phrenic nerve to pace the diaphragm: Inductive coupling and battery powered total implant in asynchronous and demand modes. Pacing Clin Electrophysiol 12:847, 1989.

Ishii K, Kurosawa H, Koyanagi H et al: Effects of bilateral transvenous diaphragm pacing on hemodynamic function in patients after cardiac operations: Experimental and clinical study. J Thorac Cardiovasc Surg 100:108, 1990.

Israel F: Ueber die Wiederbelebung schientoter Neugeborener mit Hilfe des elektrischen Stromes. Zentralblatt Geburtschilfe Gynäkologie 91:602, 1927.

Johnson RL, Gabella BA, Gerhart KA et al: Evaluating sources of traumatic spinal cord injury surveillance data in Colorado. Am J Epidemiol 146:266, 1997.

Judson JP, Glenn WWL: Radiofrequency electrophrenic respiration: Long-term application to a patient with primary hypoventilation. JAMA 203:1033, 1968.

Karamenhetoglu SS, Unal S, Karacan I et al: Traumatic spinal cord injuries in Istanbul, Turkey. An epidemiological study. Paraplegia 33:469, 1995.

Kelley WO: Phrenic nerve paralysis: Special consideration of the accessory phrenic nerve. J Thorac Surg 19:923, 1950.

Krieger AJ, Gropper MR, Adler RJ: Electrophrenic respiration after intercostal to phrenic nerve anastomosis in a patient with anterior spinal artery syndrome: A technical case report. Neurosurgery 35:760, 1994.

Laghi F, Harrison MJ, Tobin MJ: Comparison of magnetic and electrical phrenic nerve stimulation in assessment of diaphragmatic contractility. J Appl Physiol 80:1731, 1996.

Lan C, Lai JS, Chang KH, Lamb et al, 1991 et al: Traumatic spinal cord injuries in the rural region of Taiwan: An epidemiological study in Hualien county 1986–1990. Paraplegia 31:398, 1993.

Lanmüller H, Bijak M, Mayr W et al: Useful applications and limits of battery powered implants in functional electrical stimulations. Artif Organs 21:210, 1997.

Laub GW, Muralidharan S, Chen C et al: Phrenic nerve injury. A prospective study. Chest 100:376, 1991.

Letsou GV, Hogan JF, Lee P et al: Comparison of the 180 degree and 360 degree skeletal muscle nerve cuff electrodes. Ann Thorac Surg 54:925, 1992.

Lieberman DA, Faulkner JA, Craig AB Jr, Maxwell LC: Performance and histochemical composition of guinea pig and human diaphragm. J Appl Physiol 34:233, 1973.

MacLean JC, Mattioni TA: Phrenic nerve conduction studies: A new technique and its application in quadriplegic patients. Arch Phys Med Rehabil 62:70, 1981.

Mador JM, Rodis A, Diaz J: Diaphragmatic fatigue following voluntary hyperpnea. Am J Respir Crit Care Med 154:63, 1996.

Mannion JD, Stephenson LW: Potential uses of skeletal muscle for myocardial assistance. Surg Clin North Am 65:67, 1985.

Markland ON, Kincaid JC, Pourmand RA et al: Electrophysiologic evaluation of diaphragm by transcutaneous phrenic nerve stimulation. Neurology 34:604, 1984.

Mayr W, Fijak M, Girsch W et al: Multichannel stimulation of phrenic nerves by epineural electrodes: Clinical experience and future developments. ASAIO J 39:M729, 1993.

McCauley RGK, Habib KB: Diaphragmatic paralysis evaluated by phrenic nerve stimulation during fluoroscopy or real-time ultrasound. Radiology 153:33, 1984.

Mellins RB, Balfour HH, Turino GM, Winters RW: Failure of autonomic control of ventilation (Ondine's curse). Medicine 49:487, 1970.

Mendelson WB: Experiences of a sleep disorders center: 1700 patients later. Cleve Clin J Med 64:46, 1997.

Merav AD, Attai LA, Condit DD: Successful repair of the transected phrenic nerve with restoration of diaphragmatic function. Chest 84:642, 1983.

Mier A, Brophy C, Moxham J, Green M: Phrenic nerve stimulation in normal subject and in patients with diaphragmatic weakness. Thorax 42:885, 1987.

Mills GH, Kyroussis D, Hamnegard CH et al: Unilateral magnetic stimulation of the phrenic nerve. Thorax 50:1162, 1995.

Moxham J, Shneeerson JM: Diaphragmatic pacing. Am Rev Respir Dis 148:533, 1993.

O'Brien JW, Johnson SH, VanSteyn SJ et al: Effects of internal mammary artery dissection on phrenic nerve perfusion and function. Ann Thorac Surg 52:182, 1991.

Otom AS, Doughan AM, Kawar JS, Hatter EZ: Traumatic spinal cord injuries in Jordan—an epidemiological study. Spinal Cord 35:253, 1997.

Peterson DK, Nochomovitz ML, Stellato TA, Mortimer JT: Long-term intramuscular electrical activation of the phrenic nerve: Safety and reliability. IEEE Trans Biomed Engineer 41:1115, 1994a.

Peterson DK, Nochomovitz ML, Stellato TA, Mortimer JT: Long-term intramuscular electrical activation of the phrenic nerve: Efficacy as a ventilatory prosthesis. IEEE Trans Biomed Engineer 41:1127, 1994b.

Price C, Makintubee S, Herndon W, Istre GR: Epidemiology of traumatic spinal cord injury and acute hospitalization and rehabilitation charges for spinal cord injuries in Okalahoma, 1988–90. Am J Epidemiol 139:37, 1994.

Rochester DF: The diaphragm: Contractile properties and fatigue. J Clin Invest 75:1397, 1985.

Russel RI, Mulvey D, Laroche C: Bedside assessment of phrenic nerve function in infants and children. J Thorac Cardiovasc Surg 10:143, 1991.

Sagner A: En bask kritiker-Paracelsus. In Livets Tjanare, Fjarde upplagan. Malmoe, Bengt Forsbergs Forlag AB, 1980, pp 138–140.

Salmons S, Hendriksson J: The adaptive response of skeletal muscle to increased use. Muscle Nerve 4:94, 1981.

Sarnoff SJ, Maloney JV, Sarnoff FC et al: Electrophrenic respiration in acute bulbar poliomyelitis. JAMA 143:1383, 1950.

Scher AT: Rugby injuries to the cervical spine and spinal cord: A 10-year review. Clin Sports Med 17:195, 1998.

Setina M, Cerny S, Grim M, Pirk J: Anatomical interrelation between the phrenic nerve and the internal mammary artery as seen by the surgeon. J Cardiovasc Surg (Torino) 24:499, 1993.

Severinghaus JS, Mitchell RA: Ondine's curse—failure of respiratory center automaticity while awake. J Clin Res 10:122, 1962.

Shaw REK, Glenn WWL, Holcomb WG: Phrenic nerve conduction studies in patients with diaphragm pacing. Surg Forum 26:195, 1975.

Shaw RK, Glenn WWL, Hogan JF, Phelps ML: Electrophysiologic evaluation of phrenic nerve function in candidates for diaphragm pacing. J Neurosurg 53:345, 1980.

Sheridan PH Jr, Cheriyan A, Doud J et al: Incidence of phrenic neuropathy after isolated lung transplantation. J Heart Lung Transplant 14:684, 1995.

Shingu H, Ikata T, Katoh S, Akatsu T: Spinal cord injuries in Japan: A nationwide epidemiological survey in 1990. Paraplegia 32:3, 1994.

Shingu H, Ohama M, Ikata T et al: A nationwide epidemiological survey of spinal cord injuries in Japan from January 1990 to December 1992. Paraplegia 33:183, 1995.

Shneerson J: Sleep apneas. In Disorders of Ventilation. Oxford, England, Blackwell Scientific, 1988.

Similowski T, Mehiri S, Duguet A et al: Comparison of magnetic and electrical phrenic nerve stimulation in assessment of phrenic nerve conduction time. J Appl Physiol 82:1190, 1997.

Similowski T, Straus C, Attali V et al: Assessment of the motor pathway to the diaphragm using cortical and cervical magnetic stimulation in the decision making process of phrenic pacing. Chest 110:1441, 1996.

Similowski T, Straus C, Attali V et al: Cervical magnetic stimulation as a method to discriminate between diaphragm and rib cage muscle fatigue. J Appl Physiol 84:1692, 1998.

Spivak JM, Weiss MA, Cotler JM, Call M: Cervical spine injuries in patients 65 and older. Spine 19:2303, 1994.

Supinski GS: Effect of synchronizing intercostal muscle and diaphragm contraction on inspired volume production (Abstract). Am Rev Respir Dis 143:A566, 1991.

Supinski G, Nethery D, Stofan D, DiMarco A: Effect of free radical scavengers on diaphragmatic fatigue. Am J Respir Crit Care Med 155:622, 1997.

Syabbalo N: Assessment of respiratory muscle function and strength. Postgrad Med J 74:208, 1998.

Synder RW, Kukora JS, Bothwell WN, Torres GR: Phrenic nerve injury following stretch trauma: Case reports. J Trauma 36:734, 1994.

Talonen PP, Baer GA, Häkkinen V, Ojala JK: Neurophysiological and technical considerations for the design of an implantable phrenic nerve stimulator. Med Biol Eng Comput 28:31, 1990.

Tator CH, Carson JD, Edmonds VE: New spinal injuries in hockey. Clin J Sport Med 7:17, 1997.

Thurman DJ, Burnett CL, Beaudoin DE et al: Risk factors and mechanisms of occurrence in motor vehicle–related spinal cord injuries: Utah Accident Analysis and Prevention 27:411, 1995.

Tibballs J: Diaphragmatic pacing: An alternative to long-term mechanical ventilation. Anaesth Intens Care 19:597, 1991.

Tonz M, von Segesser KL, Milhalijevic T et al: Clinical implications of phrenic nerve injury after pediatric cardiac surgery. J Pediatr Surg 31:1265, 1996.

Travaline JM, Sudarshan S, Roy BG et al: Effect of *N*-acetylcysteine on human diaphragm strength and fatigability. Am J Respir Crit Care Med 156:1567, 1997.

Tyroch AH, Davis JW, Kaups KL, Lorenzo M: Spinal cord injury. A preventable public burden. Arch Surg 132:778, 1997.

Ure A: An account of some experiments made on the body of a criminal immediately after execution, with physiological and practical observations. Journal of Science and Arts 6:283, 1819.

Van Lunteren E, Moyer M: Effect of DAP on diaphragm force and fatigue, including fatigue due to neurotransmission failure. J Appl Physiol 81:2214, 1996.

Van Lunteren E, Moyer M, Torres A: Effect of K^+ channel blockade on fatigue in rat diaphragm muscle. J Appl Physiol 79:783, 1995.

Watanabe T, Trusler GA, Williams WG et al: Phrenic nerve paralysis after pediatric surgery. J Thorac Cardiovasc Surg 94:383, 1997.

Weese Mayer DE, Morrow AS, Brouillette RT et al: Diaphragm pacing in infants and children: A life-table analysis of implanted components. Am Rev Respir Dis 139:974, 1989.

Weese-Mayer DE, Silvestri JM, Kenny AS et al: Diaphragm pacing with a quadrapolar phrenic nerve electrode: An international study. Pacing Clin Electrophysiol 19:1311, 1996.

West JB: Respiratory Physiology—The Essentials. Baltimore, Williams & Wilkins, 1995, pp 117–132.

Wheeler WE, Rubis LJ, Jones CW, Harrah JD: Etiology and prevention of topical cardiac hypothermia-induced phrenic nerve injury and left lower lobe atelectasis during cardiac surgery. Chest 88:680, 1985.

Yen F, Hehbehani K, Lucas EA, Axe JR: A noninvasive technique for detecting obstructive and central sleep apnea. IEEE Transactions on Biomedical Engineering 44:1262, 1997.

Mediastinum

CHAPTER 57

Anatomy and Surgical Access of the Mediastinum

Paul A. Kirschner

This chapter on the anatomy of the mediastinum is presented from a meaningful, functional, surgical aspect rather than in terms of "traditional," often artificial, static diagrams of "compartments" and the recital of the gamuts of their contents. The true anatomic relationships of the various structures, organs, and other processes (i.e., infections) are emphasized on the basis of fascial continuity, whether in the mediastinum itself or between it and the neck above and the abdomen below. Such a presentation deals with anatomically determined routes of surgical access and structural localization. It serves as an anatomic basis for the diagnosis and management of the many aspects of mediastinal pathology that are presented elsewhere in more detail in this volume. The terms describing the topography of the mediastinum (i.e., superior, inferior, anterior, middle, and posterior) are ingrained and are used for gross orientation rather than precise anatomic localization.

BASIC TOPOGRAPHY

The mediastinum is a bulkhead-like median partition of the thorax that separates the lungs in their respective pleural cavities. It is a three-dimensional, interpleural space shaped roughly like a squat irregular pyramid (Fig. 57–1). It ranges in thickness from a membranous anterosuperior commissure above, just under the manubrium where the right and left mediastinal pleurae coapt, to a broad almost amorphous space below. It contains all of the thoracic organs except for the lungs. It can be regarded as the "third space" of the thorax or, as Wilson (1884) has said, "The space between the spaces." Its contour and extent vary, particularly posteriorly, depending on how the "posterior" mediastinum is defined (see later). The density and character of the contents of the mediastinum vary from solid (parenchymal organs) to liquid (blood, lymph, swallowed saliva, serous pericardial fluid) to gaseous (trachea and main bronchi and intermittently the esophagus). Dynamically, it reflects the intrapleural subatmospheric pressure with respiratory variations that can be displayed by an intraesophageal recording device. The mediastinum is bounded on either side by the mediastinal pleurae, which are intact except for where they are pierced by the pulmonary hila. Other than this, there is no mediastinopleural continuity.

Superiorly, the mediastinum is in free communication with the neck via three distinct fascial planes (see later). The superior "aperture" of the mediastinum is obliquely disposed, being higher posteriorly than anteriorly, corresponding to the obliquity of the first rib. There is no precise structural line of demarcation between the mediastinum and the neck. Rather, it is a zone that varies as much as 2.5 to 5.0 cm depending on the degree of flexion or extension of the neck. Even organs, such as a low-lying thyroid gland or a hyperplastic thymus, may bob up and down between the neck and mediastinum within their fascial planes, especially with changes of position of the head and strong respiratory efforts. This superior

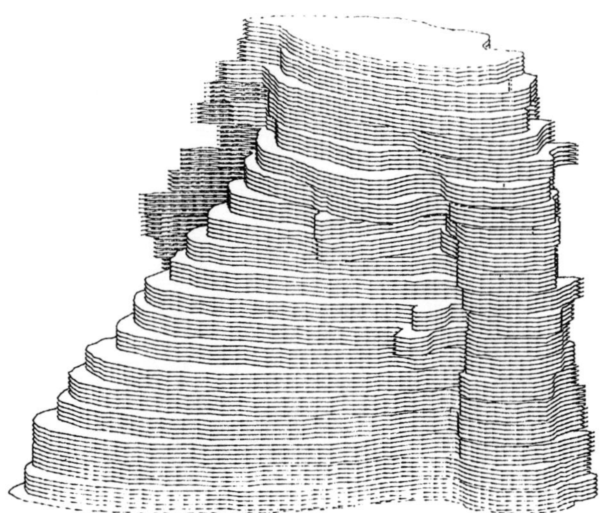

FIGURE 57–1 ■ Three-dimensional reconstruction of a normal mediastinum derived from a computed tomography scan.

aperture has been called the critical space of Grawitz because enlarging unyielding masses or displaced organs (such as those mentioned) may exert pressure on the surrounding normal structures and conduits traversing this space.

Inferiorly, the mediastinum is sharply delimited by the diaphragm. The foramina for the inferior vena cava and the aorta are well sealed. However, within the esophageal hiatus, there is a looseness that provides a pathway of communication and dissection between the abdomen below and the posterior mediastinum above. Anteriorly, the lower part of the anterior mediastinum can be accessed from just under the xiphoid process, and the anteroinferior aspect of the pericardium lies just beyond this.

Posteriorly, there is no unified concept of this area of the mediastinum. Traditionally, it is delimited by the anterior spinal ligament of the vertebral column, but in a reappraisal by Shields (1991) the posterior extent includes the paravertebral sulci, thus giving the mediastinum a bilateral wing-like (alar) configuration (Fig. 57–2).

CONTENTS OF THE MEDIASTINUM

The mediastinum is tightly packed with intertwined organs and conduits that include (1) cardiovascular structures (heart and great vessels), (2) airways (trachea and main bronchi), (3) alimentary tract (esophagus), (4) neural tissue (nerves and ganglia), and (5) lymphatic tissue (lymph nodes, thoracic duct, and thymus gland). It contains a serous cavity—the pericardium. The intervening tissue, combining tougher fibrous tissue and looser areolar tissue, defines fascial planes in the mediastinum proper and its communication with the neck and abdomen.

COMPARTMENTS

It has been customary for anatomists, surgeons, and radiologists to divide the mediastinum arbitrarily into "spaces" or "compartments." This artifice is used to aid in the localization of structures and organs and lesions derived from them (i.e., cysts, tumors, displaced organs, and anomalies along with abscesses and spread of infections). However, several different "compartmental models" have been proposed, some with only scant reference to basic anatomy.

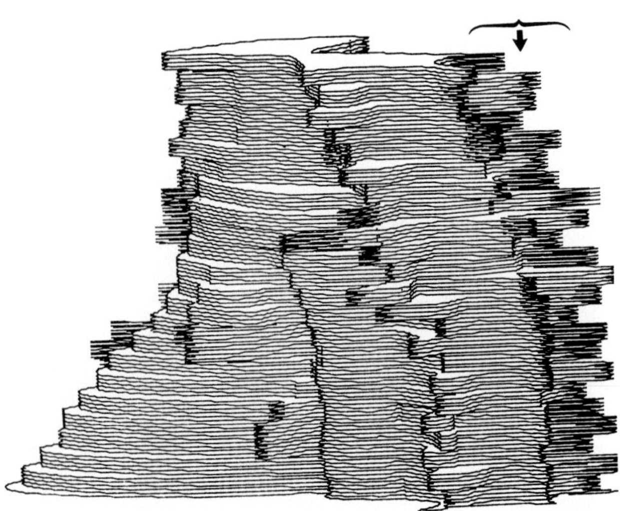

FIGURE 57–2 ■ Three-dimensional reconstruction of a normal mediastinum including the paravertebral sulci *(bracket and arrow).*

In 1889, even before the discovery of x-rays, Hare commented that "anatomists divide this region into an anterior, middle, and posterior space, although, as usual in such instances the lines of demarcation between each of the spaces are not rigidly marked."

Even after the advent of x-rays in 1895, the demarcations and "partitions" of the mediastinum remained largely artificial. Because the mediastinal structures are mainly "stacked" in the anteroposterior axis, it has been customary to display them on the lateral view of the chest radiograph. However, the demarcation of these compartments was based to a great extent on imaginary lines and planes superimposed on the x-ray picture. There has been no universal agreement about the topography of the mediastinum, and hence several different compartment models have been created. These vary from three-compartment models, including the newer one proposed by Shields (1991), to a six-compartment model described by the radiologist Heitzman (1977). An extreme example of a nonanatomic demarcation is one suggested by Felson (1969), a noted chest radiologist, who stated: "The divisions of the mediastinum defined by the anatomists are not suitable for the roentgen diagnosis of mediastinal lesions . . . with gall born of desperation I have ignored the great anatomic teachings of the past and use a new anatomic classification based on roentgen projection rather than anatomic dissection." An extreme example of Felson's nonanatomic "desperation" is his characterization of the "boundary" between the "middle" and "posterior" compartments as a "line" connecting a point on each thoracic vertebra 1 cm behind its anterior margin!

Traditional Four-Compartment Model

Most dictionaries and anatomy textbooks use a four-compartment model of the mediastinum (Fig. 57–3). Based on the lateral radiograph, these compartments are demarcated by dividing the mediastinum as a whole into a superior and an inferior division, with the latter being divided into anterior, middle, and posterior compartments.

The "superior" mediastinum is the area above an imaginary plane extending from the manubriosternal junction (angle of Louis) posteriorly to the inferior border of the T4 vertebra. This plane corresponds roughly to the aortic arch and the tracheal bifurcation. It contains all of the structures passing through the superior inlet (i.e., the great vessels, trachea, esophagus, veins, lymphatics, lymph nodes, thoracic duct, and thymus). No mention is made of the three distinct anatomic cervicomediastinal fascial planes that exist in this compartment: the prevascular plane, retrovascular (postvascular) pretracheal plane, and posterior peri-pharyngoesophageal plane.

The rest of the mediastinum is divided into three more compartments—the anterior, middle, and posterior. The

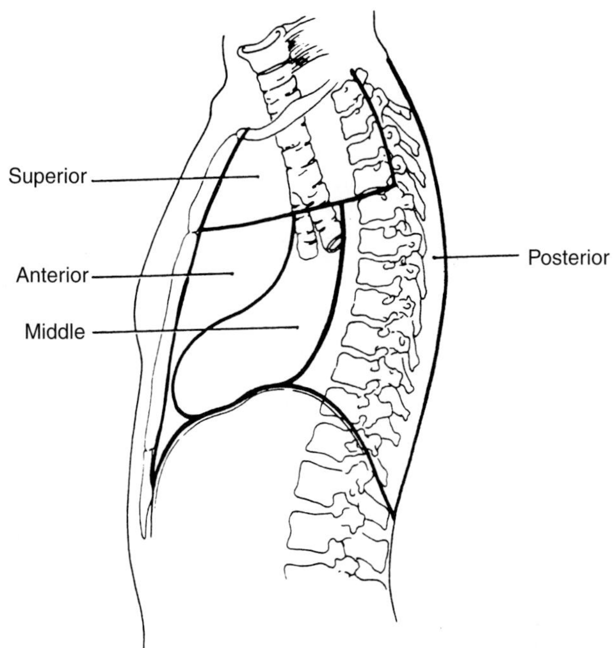

FIGURE 57–3 ■ Traditional four-compartment model of the mediastinum. (From Dresler CM: Anatomy and classification. In Pearson FG (ed): Thoracic Surgery. New York, Churchill Livingstone, 1995, p 1326.)

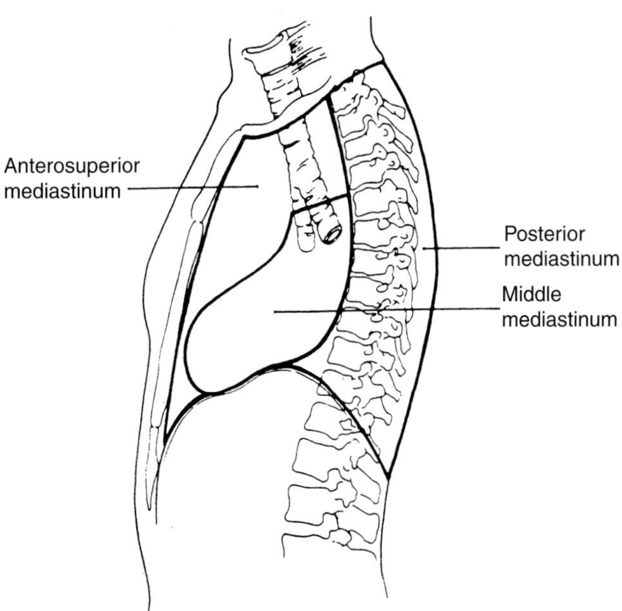

FIGURE 57–4 ■ Traditional three-compartment model of the mediastinum. (From Dresler CM: Anatomy and classification. In Pearson FG (ed): Thoracic Surgery. New York, Churchill Livingstone, 1995, p 1326.)

"anterior" mediastinum is located between the back of the sternal body (gladiolus) and the anterior surface of the pericardium. It contains the main body of the thymus and preaortic lymph nodes (stations 5 and 6) embedded in fibrofatty tissue.

The "middle" mediastinum, located between the anterior and posterior, is occupied by the pericardium and its contents—the carina, the proximal main bronchi, and the tracheobronchial lymph nodes (stations 2R and L, 4 R and L, and 7).

The "posterior" mediastinum, located between the back of the pericardium and the anterior spinal ligament, contains the esophagus, the aorta, the nerves, the ganglia, and the thoracic duct.

Traditional Three-Compartment Model

This designation (Fig. 57–4) combines the anterior two thirds of the superior mediastinum and the entire anterior mediastinum; the middle includes the heart and pericardium and the posterior extends the entire length of the spine. This model also ignores anatomic cervicomediastinal fascial planes.

Shields' Three-Compartment Model

This description of the mediastinum (Fig. 57–5) is the most truly anatomic of all. In the words of Shields (1991), "it consists of an anterior compartment, a visceral compartment, and the paravertebral sulci *bilaterally*." Each compartment extends from the thoracic inlet to the diaphragm. At their cervical aspect, these three compartments correspond to true anatomic dissection zones. The anterior compartment, located between the undersurface of the sternum and the anterior surface of the great vessels, can be called the "prevascular" zone. The visceral compartment, located behind the great vessels between them and the trachea, can be called the "retrovascular" (postvascular, pretracheal) zone. Posterior to these two zones is a retrovisceral zone (periesophageal), which Shields has combined with the paravertebral sulci, the latter being the only paired component of the mediastinum. Note that the words superior, anterior, middle, and posterior are not used at all.

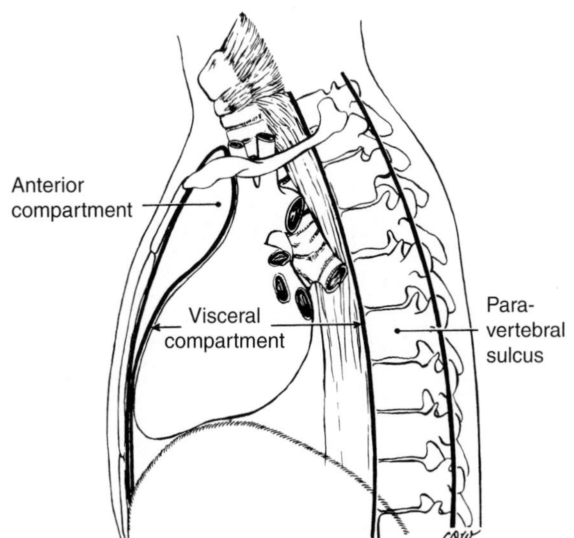

FIGURE 57–5 ■ Shields' three-compartment model of the mediastinum. (From Dresler CM: Anatomy and classification. In Pearson FG (ed): Thoracic Surgery. New York, Churchill Livingstone, 1995, p 1326.)

PRACTICAL APPLIED SURGICAL ANATOMY

The "true" anatomy of the mediastinum emerges when there is disease (i.e., tumors, anomalies, displaced organs, and infections) that requires diagnosis and treatment. As Neuhof and Jemerin (1943) put it, "This customary anatomical classification [i.e., the traditional "compartments"] is artificial and gives no impression of the continuity which exists not only between the superior and inferior mediastinum but also between the superior mediastinum and the neck." This continuity is defined by cervicomediastinal fascial planes that delineate the *true anatomic compartments*. Such anatomic information was derived in the past from (1) a study of pathways of "descending" cervicomediastinal infections and (2) a study of cross-sectional anatomy in the cadaver (Eycleshymer and Shoemaker, 1911). Today, the availability of computerized imaging techniques in multiple planes and parameters facilitates the acquisition of such critical cross-sectional anatomic information. However, the compartment concept is so ingrained in our thinking that it serves a useful purpose for a means of expression.

SURGICAL ACCESS TO THE MEDIASTINUM

Prevascular Zone (Anterior Compartment)

Cervical Approach (Extended Mediastinoscopy)

A transverse incision in the suprasternal notch traverses the superficial layer of the deep cervical fascia including the strap muscles (Fig. 57–6). Just beneath these, the cervical cornua of the thymus can be identified in the prevascular plane. Downward dissection allows transcervical thymectomy and exposure to other tumors in this plane along with lymph nodes in stations 5 and 6. Exploration of this zone is called "extended" mediastinoscopy (Kirschner, 1991) (see Fig. 57–6).

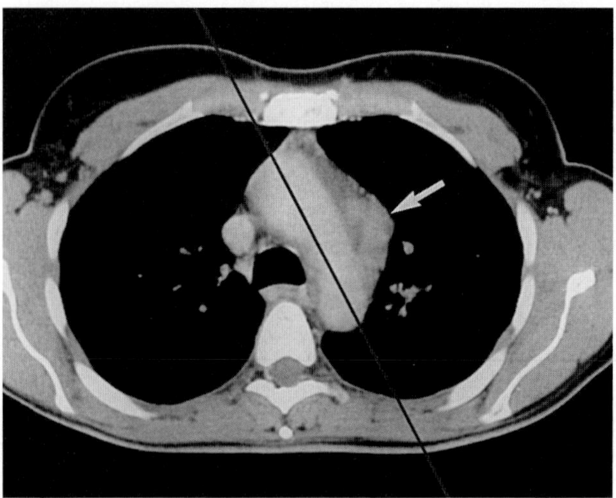

FIGURE 57–6 ■ A computed tomography scan showing adenopathy in the "prevascular" zone *(anterior compartment)*. (From Kirschner PA: Cervical mediastinoscopy. Chest Surg Clin North Am 6:9, 1996.)

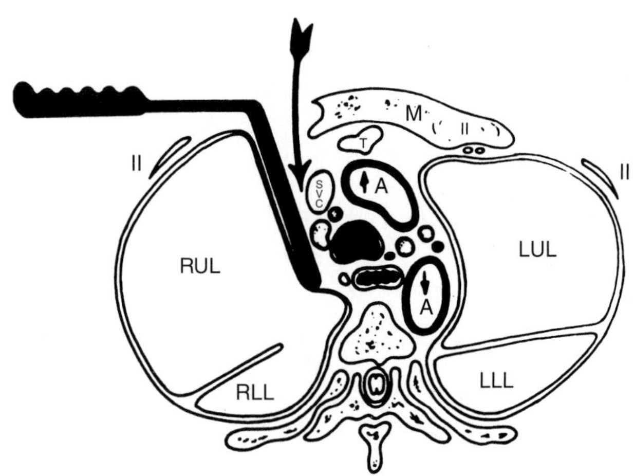

FIGURE 57–7 ■ "Chamberlain" procedure. (A, aorta; II, 2nd costal cartilage and rib; LLL, left lower lobe; LUL, left upper lobe; M, manubrium; RLL, right lower lobe; RUL, right upper lobe; SVC, superior vena cava.) (From McNeill TM, Chamberlain JM: Diagnostic anterior mediastinotomy. Ann Thorac Surg 2:532, 1961.)

Parasternal Approach (Anterior Mediastinotomy)

This approach is commonly known as the Chamberlain procedure (McNeill and Chamberlain, 1966) and consists of entering the prevascular substernal zone on either side via a parasternal incision carried through the interchondral interspace or through the space of the excised second costal cartilage. It is particularly useful for biopsies of preaortic lymph nodes in stations 5 and 6. Although a left-sided Chamberlain procedure is the best route to these preaortic nodes, either side of the sternum can be used to gain access to other tumors and other pathology (Fig. 57–7).

Postvascular (Pretracheal) Zone (Visceral Compartment)

By deepening the suprasternal notch incision beyond the great vessels and traversing the next layer of deep cervical fascia, the pretracheal layer, it is now possible to enter the "retrovascular pretracheal" plane (the "visceral" compartment of Shields) (Fig. 57–8). This is the plane of classic cervical mediastinoscopy (Carlens, 1959; Kirschner, 1996) (Fig. 57–9). By digital blunt dissection between the innominate artery and the trachea and with the aid of the mediastinoscope, access is obtained to the pretracheal and paratracheal areas, the subcarinal area, and the two main bronchi. Lymph nodes of stations 2 R and L, 4 R and L, and 7 are located in these areas. Other neoplastic lesions may be encountered as well.

Posterior (Prevertebral Periesophageal) Zone (Posterior Longitudinal Sulci)

This zone is the deepest of the three compartments that are accessible through the neck and is best approached from either side rather than from the midline. It is this zone that is considered by most to be the "posterior" mediastinum. It is here that deep infections of the neck are located. In this zone, also, so-called descending necro-

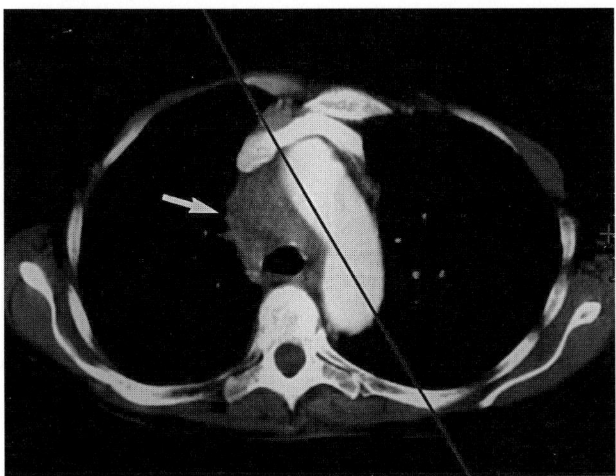

FIGURE 57–8 ■ A computed tomography scan showing adenopathy in the "postvascular" zone *(visceral compartment)*. (From Kirschner PA: Cervical mediastinoscopy. Chest Surg Clin North Am 6:9, 1996.)

tizing mediastinitis occurs (Ris et al, 1996; Seybold et al, 1950; Wheatley et al, 1990).

Cervical Approach

Depending on the localization (left or right) of a posterior mediastinal abscess, the cervical incision is made along the anterior border of the sternocleidomastoid muscle, deepening it by ligating and dividing the middle thyroid vein and traversing the buccopharyngeal fascia to enter the peripharyngoesophageal space. This exposure often suffices for superiorly located abscesses (Fig. 57–10).

Paravertebral Approach

In some instances, exposure via the neck may be inadequate (Wheatley et al, 1990) and a lower paravertebral approach is necessary, resecting posterior segments of one or more ribs and entering the retropleural plane leading to the posterior mediastinum (Seybold et al, 1950).

"Extended" Approach to Posterior Mediastinum (Various Forms of Thoracotomy)

The virulence of mediastinal infections, especially those secondary to esophageal perforations or other anaerobic infections, results in extensive and rapid spread up and down the mediastinum from the neck down to the retroperitoneum and even into either or both pleural cavities (Fig. 57–11). Localized small incisions, notwithstanding their anatomic correctness, often do not suffice. It may be necessary to perform a wide-open, transpleural thoracotomy, possibly including a "clamshell" incision to control the infection (Ris et al, 1996).

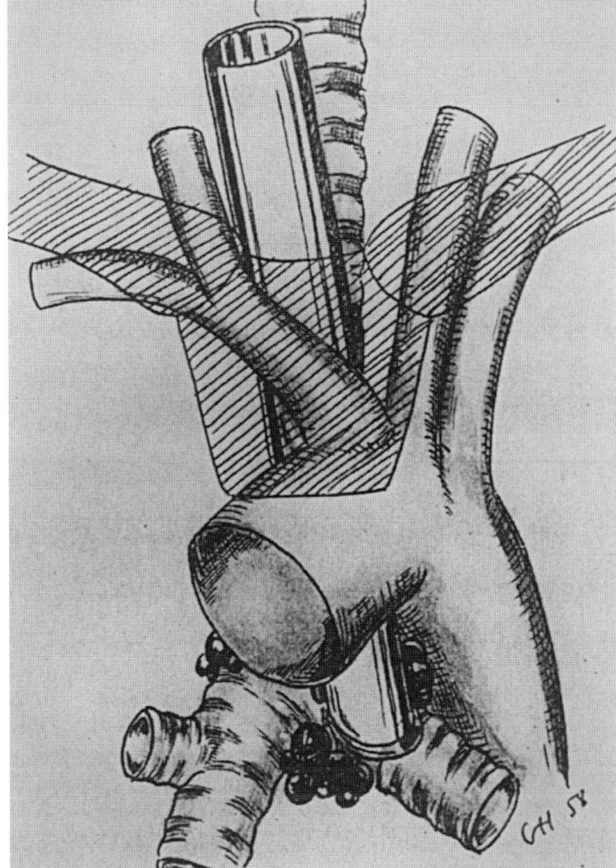

FIGURE 57–9 ■ Classic Carlens' mediastinoscopy showing the scope in the "postvascular" zone *(visceral compartment)*. (From Carlens E: Mediastinoscopy: A method for inspection and tissue biopsy in the superior mediastinum. Dis Chest 36:343, 1959.)

Inferior Access to the Posterior Mediastinum

The inferior part of the posterior mediastinum is accessible transabdominally through the esophageal hiatus. Such

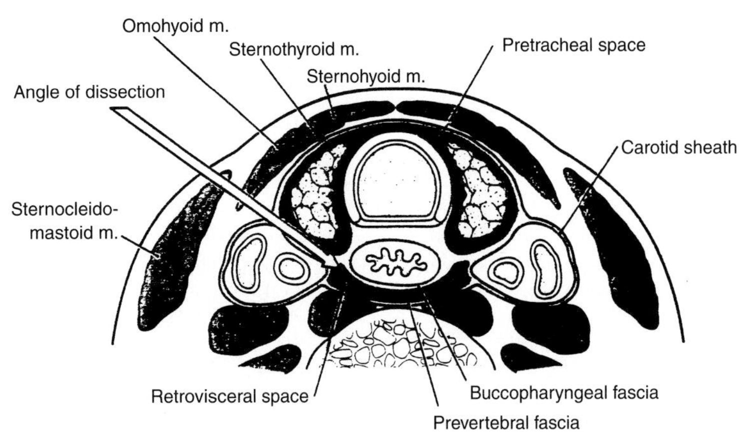

FIGURE 57–10 ■ Cervical approach to the prevertebral peripharyngoesophageal plane. The different fascial planes in the neck by which infections may spread inferiorly into the mediastinum are shown. The *arrow* demonstrates the standard surgical approach to the prevertebral fascia medial to the sternocleidomastoid muscle and carotid sheath and lateral to the strap muscles and thyroid gland. (From Wheatley MJ, Stirling MC, Kirsh MM et al: Descending necrotizing mediastinitis: Transcervical drainage is not enough. Ann Thorac Surg 49:780, 1990.)

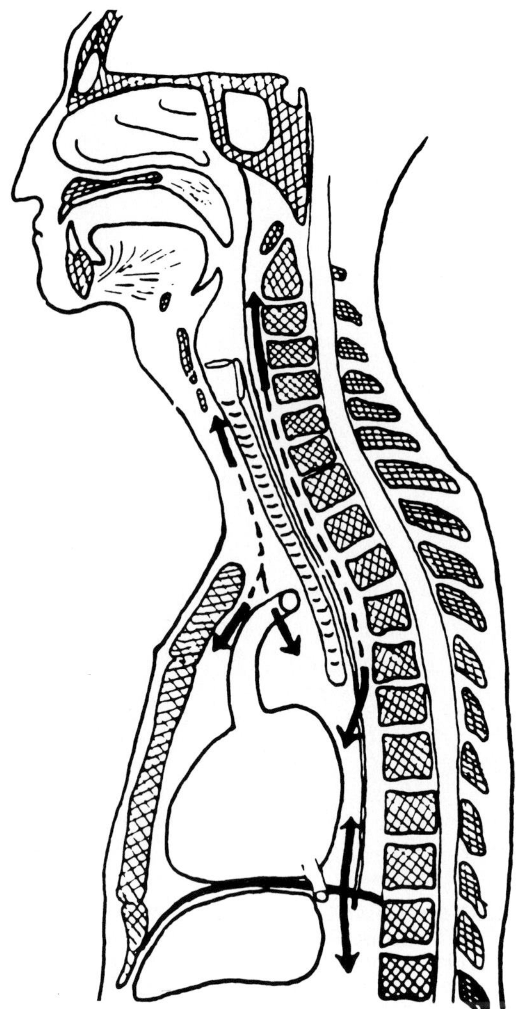

FIGURE 57–11 ■ Spread of virulent infection throughout the mediastinal planes. (From Kornblum K, Osmond LH: Mediastinitis. AJR Am J Roentgenol 32:33, 1934.)

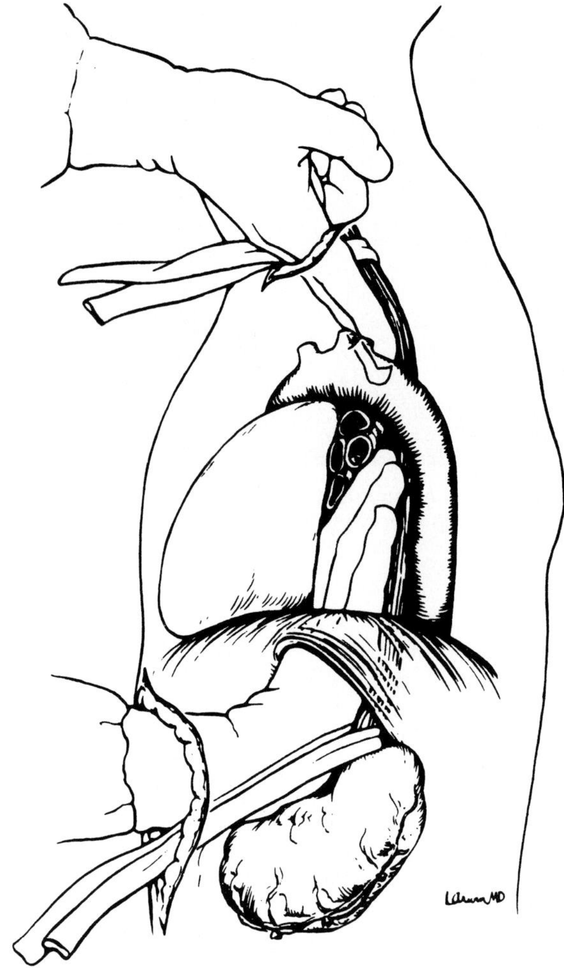

FIGURE 57–12 ■ Esophageal mobilization for transhiatal esophagectomy. (From Orringer MB: Transhiatal esophagectomy without Thoracotomy. New York, Churchill Livingstone, 1995, p 689.)

procedures include various antireflux operations and hiatal hernia repairs as well as the inferior mobilization of almost the entire esophagus in the operation of transhiatal esophagectomy (Fig. 57–12). Such inferior mobilization combined with an appropriate corresponding cervical incision and mobilization from above provides the opportunity for removing the esophagus extrapleurally without traversing the pleural cavities or bony thorax. It can be used as a bed to transplant the stomach, colon, or small bowel to restore alimentary continuity.

Knowledge of the anatomy of the mediastinum based on fascial planes facilitates precise and efficient access to the many tumors and other pathologic processes affecting this complex thoracic space.

■ *REFERENCES*

Carlens E: Mediastinoscopy: A method for inspection and tissue biopsy in the superior mediastinum. Dis Chest 36:343, 1959.

Eycleshymer AC, Shoemaker DM: A Cross-section Anatomy. New York, Appleton-Century-Crofts, 1911.

Felson B: The mediastinum. Semin Roentgenol 4:41–58, 1969.

Hare HA: The Pathology, Clinical History and Diagnosis of Affections of the Mediastinum. Philadelphia, Blakiston, 1889.

Heitzman ER: The Mediastinum: Radiologic Correlations with Anatomy and Pathology. St. Louis, CV Mosby, 1977.

Kirschner PA: Cervical substernal "extended" mediastinoscopy. In Shields TW (ed): Mediastinal Surgery. Philadelphia, Lea & Febiger, 1991.

Kirschner PA: Cervical mediastinoscopy. Chest Surg Clin North Am 6:1–20, 1996.

McNeill TM, Chamberlain JM: Diagnostic anterior mediastinotomy. Ann Thorac Surg 2:532–539, 1966.

Neuhof H, Jemerin EE: Acute Infections of the Mediastinum. Baltimore, Williams & Wilkins, 1943, p 294.

Ris H-B, Banic A, Furrer M et al: Descending necrotizing mediastinitis: Surgical treatment via clamshell approach. Ann Thorac Surg 62:1650, 1996.

Seybold WD, Johnson MA III, Leary WV: Perforation of the esophagus: An analysis of 50 cases and an account of experimental studies. Surg Clin North Am 30:1155–1183, 1950.

Shields TW (ed): Mediastinal Surgery. Philadelphia, Lea & Febiger, 1991.

Wheatley MJ, Stirling MC, Kirsh MM et Al: Descending necrotizing mediastinitis: Transcervical drainage is not enough. Ann Thorac Surg 49:780–784, 1990.

Wilson JC: On the diagnosis of tumors of the anterior mediastinum. JAMA 3:113, 1884.

CHAPTER **58**

Imaging of the Mediastinum

Gordon L. Weisbrod

Stephen Herman

The mediastinum can be divided into anterior, middle, and posterior compartments. The anterior mediastinal compartment is bounded anteriorly by the sternum and posteriorly by the pericardium, aorta, and brachiocephalic vessels. It contains the thymus gland or its remnants, branches of the internal mammary artery and vein, lymph nodes, and variable amounts of fat. The middle mediastinal compartment contains the pericardium and its contents, the ascending and transverse portions of the aorta, the superior and inferior venae cavae, the brachiocephalic artery and vein, the phrenic nerves and upper portion of the vagus nerves, the trachea and main bronchi and their contiguous lymph nodes, and the pulmonary arteries and veins. The posterior mediastinal compartment is bounded anteriorly by the pericardium and extends posteriorly to the chest wall, including the paravertebral gutters. It contains the descending thoracic aorta, esophagus, thoracic duct, azygos and hemiazygos veins, nerves, fat, and lymph nodes (Fraser et al, 1989).

When a mediastinal abnormality is identified on conventional radiographs and the cause is not immediately apparent, the most productive procedure to perform is computed tomography (CT) (Baron et al, 1981a). CT can differentiate cystic and solid mediastinal masses, localize such masses relative to other mediastinal structures, determine their tissue composition (adipose tissue, calcium, water), assess whether mediastinal widening is pathologic or simply an anatomic variation (i.e., physiologic fat deposition), and differentiate a solid mass from a vascular anomaly or aneurysm.

Helical CT offers many advantages over conventional CT. Smaller collimation and a larger number of axial sections may be attained during the period of optimal vascular enhancement because of the rapid imaging time for helical scanning. In addition, the entire study may be performed during one or two breath-holds, reducing misregistration artifacts. Multiplanar and three-dimensional reconstructions, which are created from the helical CT data set, may add useful information, particularly for the surgeons in planning the operation (Quint et al, 1996).

Magnetic resonance imaging (MRI) has the advantages of no ionizing radiation, no intravenous contrast, and multiplanar reconstruction. Its excellent demonstration of vascular structures is also a decided advantage in showing vascular anomalies or vascular compromise. The initial enthusiasm about the ability of MRI to differentiate a tumor mass from post-treatment fibrosis has not been supported clinically. Because of its inherent contrast resolution, MRI can be useful in showing the relationship of large complex mediastinal masses to adjacent structures.

Mediastinal tumors or masses usually show a strong predilection for one of the three mediastinal compartments. Thus, it is logical to classify these masses on the basis of anatomic location. However, overlap from one compartment to another commonly occurs, in which case the predominant compartment affected should be indicated. A 1971 review of the literature documented 34 previous reports of mediastinal tumors in a total of 3364 patients (Ingels et al, 1971). Excluding metastatic pulmonary carcinoma and inflammatory conditions, the frequency of tumors was as follows: neurogenic neoplasms, 19.4%; lymphoma, 15.8%; bronchial and pericardial cysts, 14.2%; germ cell tumors, 12.8%; thymoma, 11.5%; and thyroid tumors, 6%, with a variety of miscellaneous tumors making up the remainder. Almost half of all patients with mediastinal masses are asymptomatic, the abnormalities being discovered on a screening chest radiograph (Wychulis et al, 1971).

ANTERIOR MEDIASTINAL MASSES

Thymic Lesions

Normal Thymus

Before discussing the various diseases that may affect the thymus gland and their radiographic manifestations, it is necessary to review the normal CT appearance of the gland. Baron and colleagues (1982b) measured the size and shape of the normal thymus gland in 154 patients in all age groups. The findings were described in terms of the width and thickness of each of the lobes of the gland and were summarized in tabular form for each age group. They found that there was a decrease in the thickness and width of the gland with increasing age, with less variation in the gland thickness within each group. Generally speaking, in those older than 20 years the upper limit of normal (as defined by the mean thickness plus 2 standard deviations) was always less than 1.1 cm (1.18 cm for the right lobe in the age group 20 to 29 years). In younger patients the gland had the same density as muscle, but with time there was gradual fatty replacement; islands of thymic tissue could be seen within this fat (Fig. 58–1).

Heiberg and associates (1982) described the appearance on CT of the thymus gland in 40 patients who were younger than 20, of whom 34 had a normal gland and 6 had a thymoma. The normal gland had smooth lateral margins, which tended to be convex in the very young

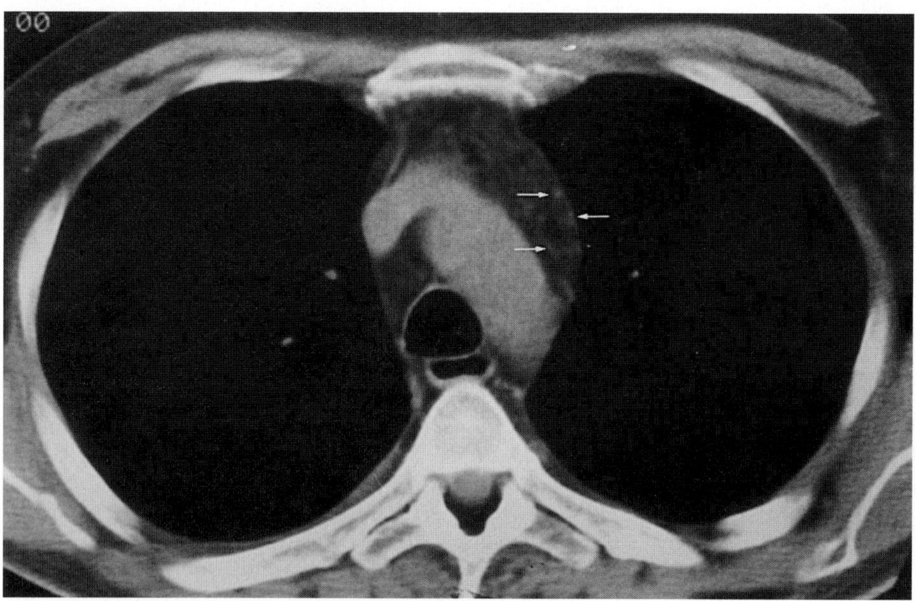

FIGURE 58–1 ■ A computed tomography scan of a 43-year-old man with involution of the thymus gland and fatty replacement. The thymus gland has been almost completely replaced by fat. There are only tiny islands of soft tissue density *(arrows)* scattered about the gland.

but became straight or concave with increasing age. The lateral aspect sometimes exhibited a sharp angular contour. This group found higher values for the thickness of the gland than did Baron and colleagues (1982b) in the patients aged 10 to 19; both groups claimed that their own values were valid, and no cause for the discrepancy was evident.

A third study described the appearance on CT of the thymus in 64 patients in whom the status of the gland was determined by thymectomy or by biopsy at mediastinal exploration (Moore et al, 1983). The normal gland had a bi-lobed, arrowhead-shaped appearance. The density was that of soft tissue, and this was gradually replaced by fatty infiltration beginning at age 20. The rate of replacement was most rapid between the ages of 31 and 40, and in most patients who were older than 40 years, most or all of the gland had been completely replaced by fat. The gland retained its size and shape as fatty involution occurred. A thymoma appeared as a mass, which usually caused a convexity at the mediastinal margin. It was not difficult to recognize it as such in patients who were older than 40 (in whom all of the thymomas in this study occurred), but it could be difficult to distinguish from an island of residual thymic tissue in persons aged 20 to 40 years.

In another study (Francis et al, 1985), the gland was homogeneous in density in patients who were younger than 10 years and had a quadrilateral shape with convex (or occasionally straight or concave) margins. The gland enlarged and became more triangular in shape until puberty, after which it became more inhomogeneous in density as fatty infiltration developed. Over 50% of patients who were older than 40 had total fatty replacement. When thymic tissue did remain, it was in the form of linear or oval soft tissue densities that were less than 7 mm in the short axis; some round tissue was occasionally present in this age group but was never larger than 7 mm, and there was never any alteration in contour of mediastinal fat.

In a study in which the thymus was examined by MRI (de Geer et al, 1986), the gland appeared to be larger than it was seen on CT. This observation was believed to be due to the fact that the MRI aided in distinguishing between thymic fat and mediastinal fat. The size of the thymus that was determined with MRI correlated better with the true anatomic size than did the CT size (the anatomic size was assessed by published values, not by direct correlation with the patients in this study). Thymic fat differed from mediastinal fat in its hydrogen density, and the T_1 relaxation times of the thymus were much longer than those of fat, but this difference decreased with age. The T_2 values of the thymus were basically equal to those of fat, and they did not change with age.

Thymoma

Thymomas are neoplasms of the epithelial elements of the thymus and have variable amounts of infiltration by reactive lymphocytes. They are most common in middle-aged adults, being quite rare in those who are younger than 20 years of age. They occur approximately equally in men and women. These tumors are usually well encapsulated and are either spherical or lobulated. The diagnosis of benignity or malignancy is usually not made by microscopic examination of the thymus but rather by the operative findings. Cases in which the surgeon notes local invasion through the capsule at the time of sternotomy are considered malignant. It should be noted, however, that the tumor can be adherent to adjacent structures without actual tissue invasion. Within the thorax, thymoma usually spreads by direct extension into mediastinal fat and to the pleura. Distant metastases are uncommon.

Patients with thymomas may be asymptomatic, but approximately one third have symptoms that are related to compression or invasion of adjacent mediastinal structures. These symptoms include dyspnea, chest pain, and cough; however, the most common symptom is weakness that is caused by associated myasthenia gravis, which occurs in about 35% to 50% of patients with thymoma.

Other associated abnormalities include pure red cell aplasia, hypogammaglobulinemia, and other rarer conditions.

Patients with myasthenia gravis have approximately a 15% chance of having a thymoma. About 60% have thymic lymphoid hyperplasia, and the gland is atrophic in about 25% of patients. These prevalences vary with the age and sex of the patient. Hyperplasia is much more common in females than it is in males, and it is rare in patients who are older than 50 years of age. Surgical removal of hyperplastic glands results in excellent symptomatic improvement of the myasthenia in most patients. Patients who are older than 50 years of age have either a thymoma or thymic atrophy, the latter being much more common in men. Surgery is indicated for thymoma but not for atrophy because symptoms are not improved by resecting an atrophic gland.

Radiographically, a thymoma appears as a mediastinal mass in the anterior superior mediastinum, near the junction of the heart with the great vessels (Ellis and Gregg, 1964; Good, 1947) (Fig. 58–2). Occasionally, thymomas are located adjacent to the heart laterally. They are usually well defined and protrude to one or possibly both sides of the mediastinum. Calcification, either peripheral or scattered throughout the mass, is occasionally seen. Thymomas can be missed on plain film examination, but

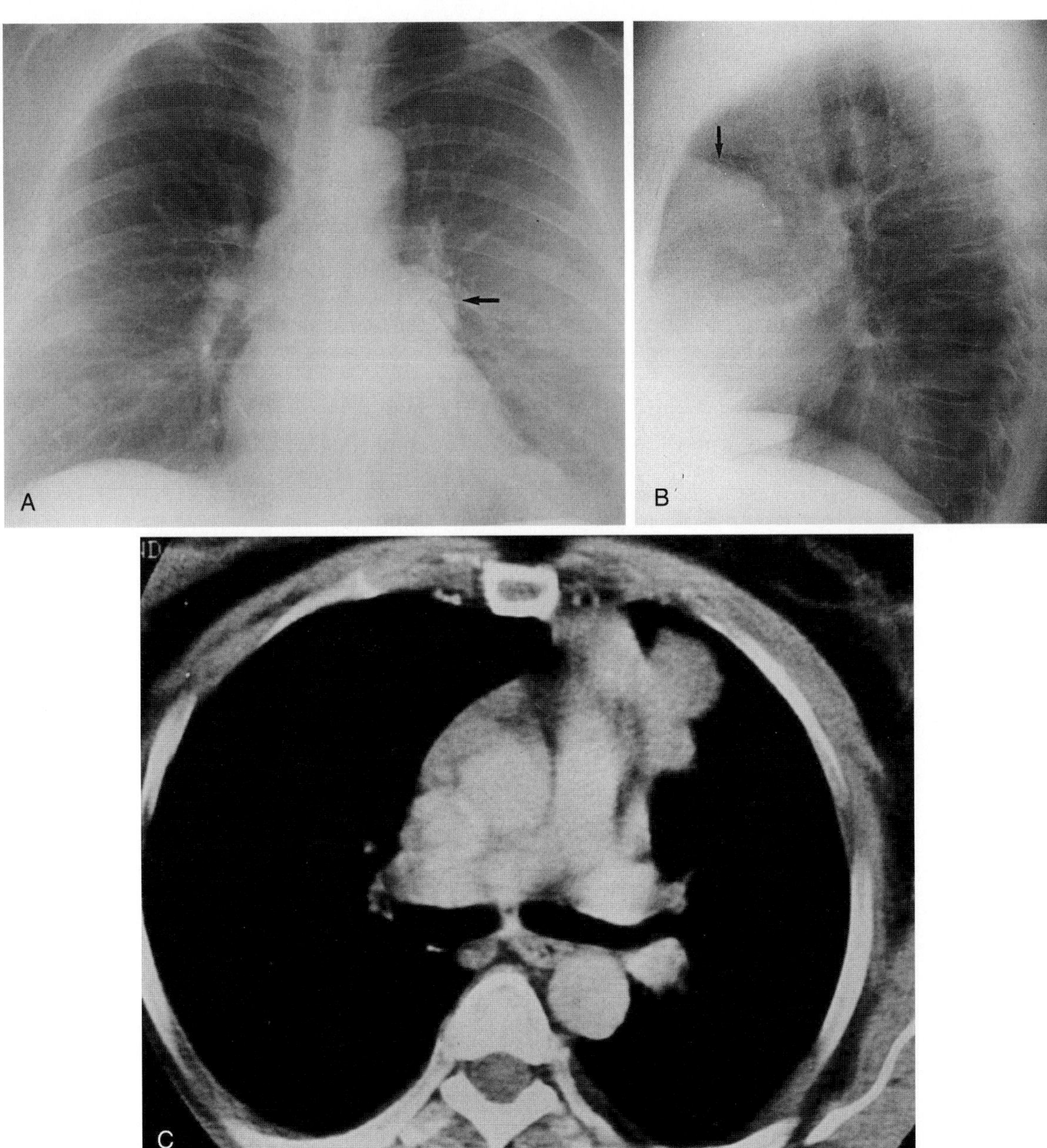

FIGURE 58–2 ■ Chest radiograph of a 55-year-old woman with malignant thymoma. *A*, Posteroanterior and *B*, lateral. An anterior mediastinal mass *(arrows)* projects to the left of midline. *C*, Computed tomography scan shows an ill-defined anterior mediastinal mass with an intact fat plane between the mass and the main pulmonary artery but with extension of the tumor into the left anterior lung. At surgery, this tumor was growing through the pleura into the lingula, requiring a wedge resection of lung with the mass.

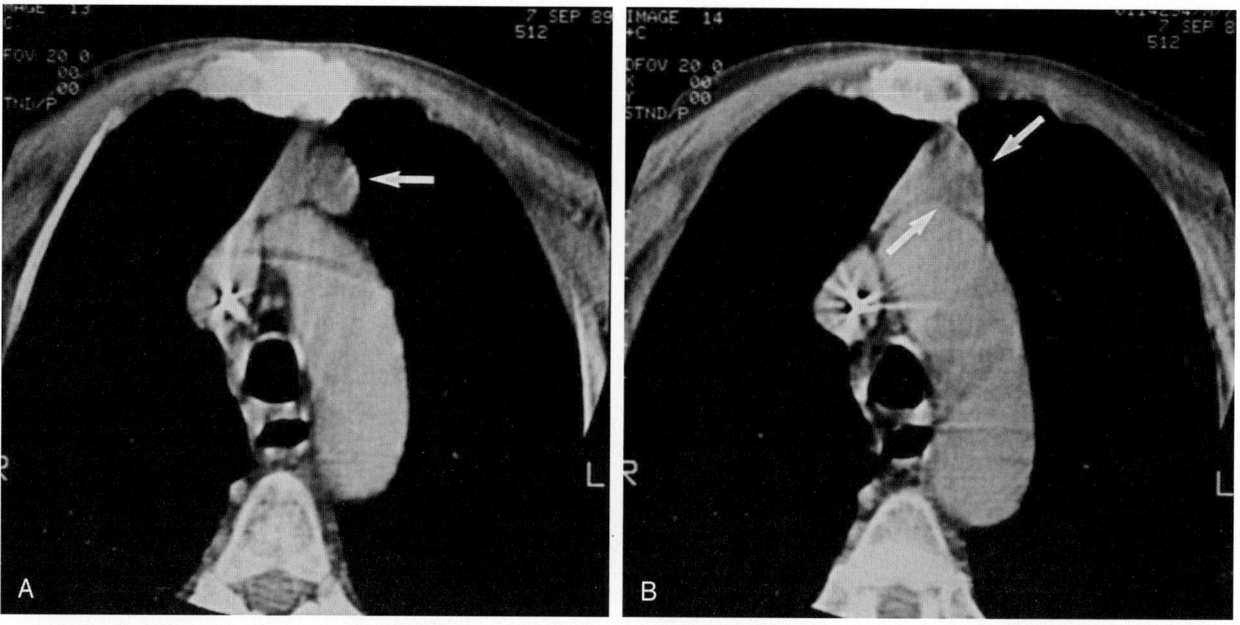

FIGURE 58–3 ■ Seventy-six-year-old man with myasthenia gravis and a thymoma within a hyperplastic thymus gland. *A*, Computed tomography scan shows a mass *(arrow)* within the left lobe of the thymus gland bulging its margins. *B*, Computed tomography scan 5 mm inferior to *A*. Increased thickness *(between arrows)* of the left lobe in a person of this age suggests hyperplasia (proven pathologically).

may be detected retrospectively when they enlarge or when a patient with myasthenia gravis proceeds to CT examination. Reasons for diagnostic error include minimal protrusion of a small convexity into the adjacent lung and confusion about whether a visible convexity represents a normal vascular structure or the cardiac margin (Brown et al, 1980).

Although thymomas may be first detected by chest radiography, they are best assessed by CT. This technique can suggest whether the tumor is invasive and, in a patient with myasthenia gravis, may reveal a thymoma that is not seen on chest radiography. When a thymoma is present, it appears as a rounded or lobulated mass of soft tissue density that causes the margins of the thymus gland to bulge (Fig. 58–3). The mass may be completely separated from adjacent structures by an intact fat plane (Fig. 58–4), or it may be less well-defined and in intimate contact with adjacent structures (Fig. 58–5). CT may demonstrate extension of the mass along fascial planes and into the pleural space or lung (see Fig. 58–2), features that suggest malignancy. Areas of low density are occasionally noted within the tumor mass, indicating

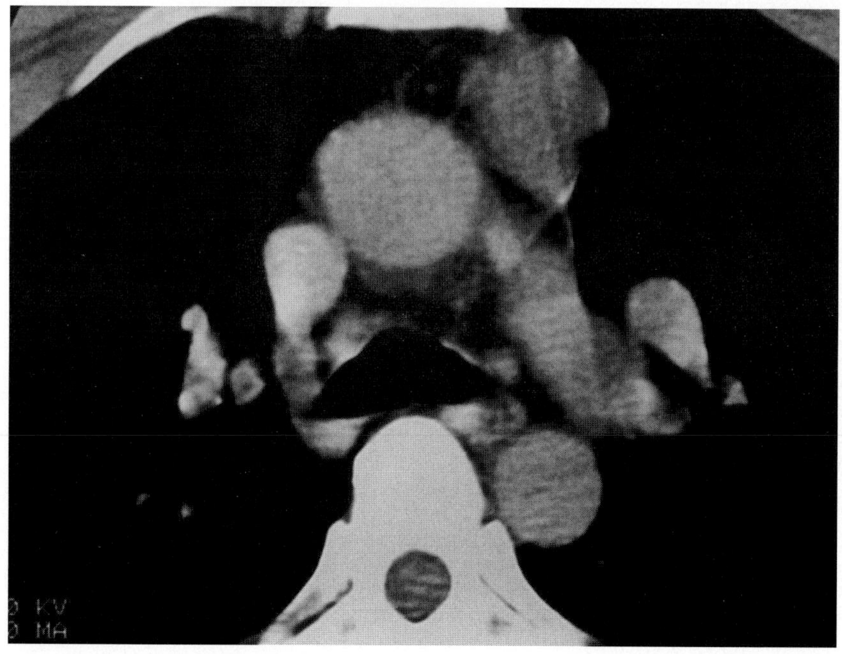

FIGURE 58–4 ■ A 44-year-old man with myasthenia gravis and benign thymoma. A computed tomography scan shows a slightly lobulated left anterior mediastinal mass. The fat plane between the mass and the adjacent ascending aorta is intact.

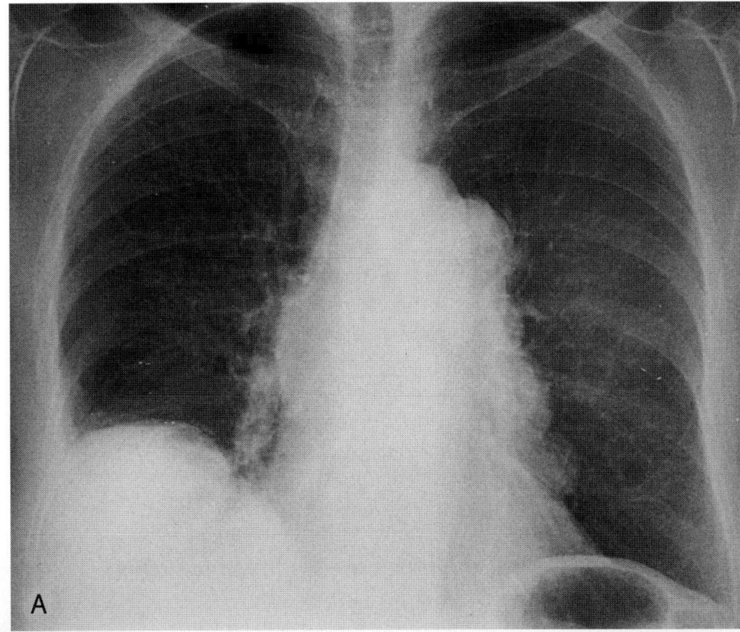

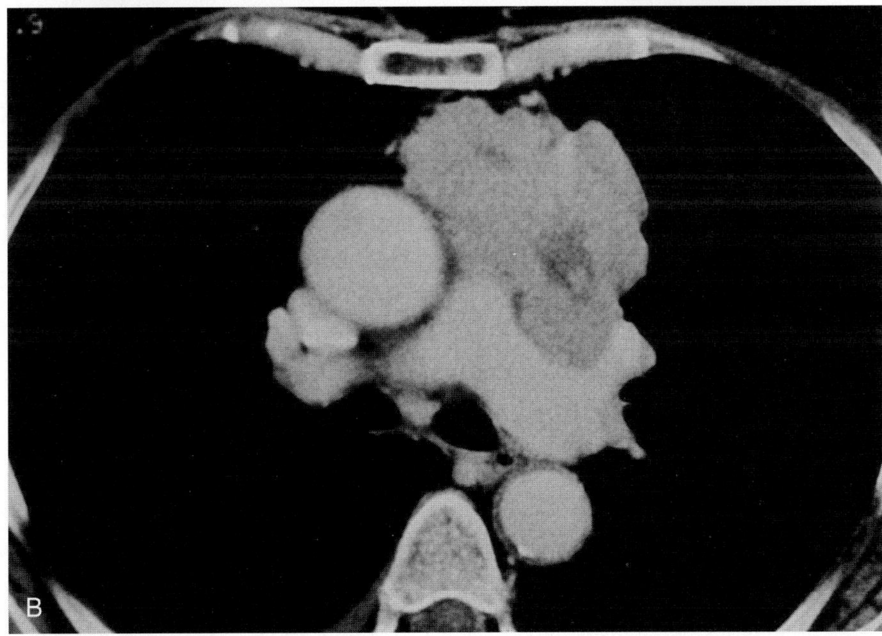

FIGURE 58–5 ■ A 70-year-old woman with malignant thymoma. *A*, A posteroanterior chest radiograph shows a long lobulated left-sided mediastinal mass. The large, right lower lobe mass is a coincident adenocarcinoma. *B*, A computed tomography scan shows a large, lobulated, ill-defined mass in the anterior mediastinum located predominantly left of the midline. Areas of low density are noted within the mass, which presumably represent necrosis. An intact fat plane is seen between the mass and the ascending aorta, but there is loss of this plane between the mass and the main artery and between the mass and the left pulmonary artery.

necrosis. Occasionally, calcification is present, but it may also occur in other anterior mediastinal masses (germ cell neoplasms, thyroid masses). Lymphoma rarely calcifies, especially before treatment. Calcification occurs equally in benign and malignant thymomas.

In a series of eight patients, Baron and coworkers (1982a) were able to visualize all eight thymomas by CT but only six by chest radiography. Similarly, Moore and associates (1982) noted that CT detected four of four thymomas, one of which was not seen by chest radiography. However, of 19 normal or hyperplastic glands, 2 were classified as thymoma on CT and 3 on chest radiography. In a study by Brown and colleagues (1983), all six thymomas were diagnosed correctly, but there were five false positives (cysts, hyperplasia, hemangioma). In a later study (Ellis et al, 1988), 17 of 20 thymomas were correctly diagnosed by CT and 12 were seen with chest radiography; there was only one false positive with CT. Three of three malignant thymomas were classified as malignant with CT, but one benign tumor was also called malignant because of its large size. In a study using MRI, two of two thymomas were diagnosed by chest radiography, CT, and MRI, but MRI was considered to be inferior to CT in studying thymic pathology because of its poorer spatial resolution, longer scan time, and lack of visualization of calcium (Batra et al, 1987).

In our own group's study of 69 patients with thymic resections, we were able to detect 33 of 34 thymomas (97%) by CT (Chen et al, 1988). In addition, by assessing the presence or absence of the fat plane between the tumor and adjacent mediastinal structure, we attempted to determine whether the tumor was malignant. Of 13 patients with completely preserved fat planes, 12 had no invasion and 1 had focal microscopic capsular invasion. Three patients had complete obliteration of the fat planes, and all of these had malignant tumors. There were 15 tumors with some preserved and some obliterated planes; 7 of these were benign and 8 were malignant.

Thymic Hyperplasia

Thymic lymphoid hyperplasia refers to the presence of germinal centers in the thymus as seen pathologically. It is the most common thymic disease associated with myasthenia gravis, being seen in about 60% of cases. It usually, but not always, causes enlargement of the gland.

The thymus gland may atrophy in response to stress or after steroid therapy or chemotherapy; withdrawal of these stimuli may cause so-called rebound thymic hyperplasia (Carmosino et al, 1985; Choyke et al, 1987; Kissin et al, 1987; Shin and Ho, 1983b). This condition is especially frequent in children and young adults. In a study of patients receiving chemotherapy for a variety of neoplasms, a significant volume decrease was observed in almost all patients after administration of chemotherapy (Choyke et al, 1987). After this, thymic rebound (defined as a greater than 50% increase in thymic size above baseline as assessed by CT) was noted in 5 of 22 patients. In a study of 120 patients who were receiving chemotherapy for malignant testicular teratomas, thymic enlargement was seen on CT in 14 patients (11.6%) (Kissin et al, 1987).

Thymic lymphoid hyperplasia may be visible as an anterior mediastinal mass on chest radiography, but it is best assessed by CT. In pathologically proven cases, the thymus appears abnormally large (best determined by an increase in the thickness of the gland) in about 70% of cases (see Fig. 58–3*B*). Rebound thymic hyperplasia may cause thymic enlargement, which may be visualized on chest radiography or CT.

In a study by Baron and colleagues (1982a), using their own data from normal individuals (Baron et al, 1982b), six of eight hyperplastic glands were more than 2 standard deviations (SD) above normal thickness. Thorvinger and coworkers (1987) were able to diagnose six of eight hyperplastic glands by CT. However, Batra and coauthors (1987) noted that six of seven hyperplastic glands appeared normal in size on CT and MRI. In our group's study (Chen et al, 1988), using the normal criteria of Baron and colleagues (1982b) and designating as abnormal more than 1.5 SD above the mean for each age group, we correctly detected 20 of 28 cases of hyperplasia (71%). One normal gland was falsely identified as hyperplastic.

Thymolipomas

Thymolipomas are rare tumors, mentioned here because of their striking radiographic appearance. Because they are soft and pliable, they do not affect adjacent structures and may therefore grow to a very large size before being diagnosed. Radiographically, they are seen as huge mediastinal masses that tend to fall away from the superior mediastinum and become most evident in the lower chest, where they drape the heart and may mimic cardiomegaly (Yeh et al, 1983) (Fig. 58–6). CT reveals a huge mass of fat density with islands of soft tissue density representing thymic tissue.

Thymic Cysts

Thymic cysts are uncommon lesions that are usually asymptomatic and are discovered by routine radiography. Most often they are simple cysts of no consequence, but they must be distinguished from thymomas, which may contain cystic elements. Occasionally, the main portion of the tumor mass is cystic in nature, with only a thin rim of neoplastic tissue (Fig. 58–7). Furthermore, Hodgkin's disease involving the thymus may be partially cystic; the cystic component may become especially prominent after therapy (Baron et al, 1981b; Lindfors et al, 1985). A

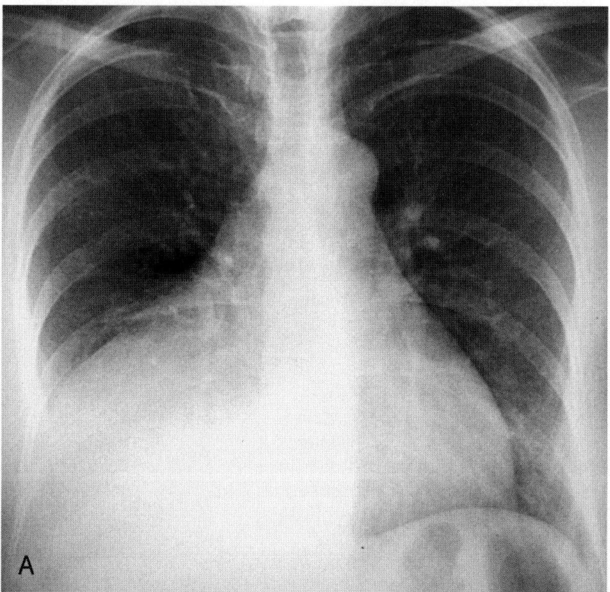

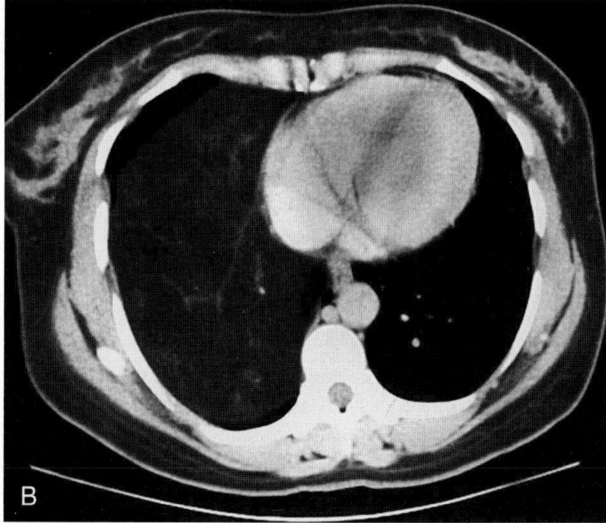

FIGURE 58–6 ■ A 39-year-old woman with thymolipoma. *A*, A posteroanterior chest radiograph shows a large mass occupying the right mediastinum and simulating cardiomegaly. *B*, A computed tomography scan shows the mass to be of fatty attenuation. A large thymolipoma weighing 852 g was resected.

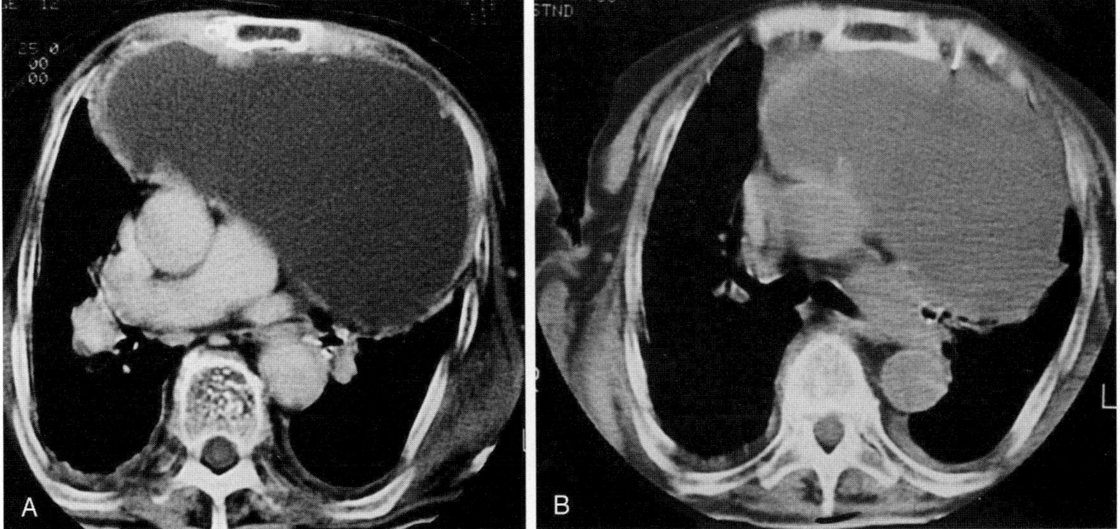

FIGURE 58–7 ■ *A*, A computed tomography (CT) scan of a 93-year-old woman with benign thymoma shows a large anterior mediastinal mass that is almost entirely cystic with only a very thin rim of soft tissue. There is significant displacement of the mediastinal vascular structures posteriorly and to the right. *B*, CT shows the tip of a needle within the soft tissue component of this mass at CT-guided transthoracic needle biopsy (at which time the diagnosis of thymoma was made).

thymic cyst appears as a nonspecific anterior mediastinal mass on chest radiography. Although the water density of these cysts is usually evident on CT, occasionally they are soft tissue in density, suggesting either a solid tumor or a complication such as hemorrhage into the cyst (Brown et al, 1983; Dunne and Weksberg, 1983).

Thymic Carcinoid

Carcinoid tumors sometimes occur in the thymus gland, usually in young men. They may be encapsulated or may invade adjacent structures. Like other mediastinal masses, they may be asymptomatic or may cause symptoms because of compression of adjacent mediastinal structures. In addition, however, they may be part of a multiple endocrine neoplasia (MEN) syndrome. The most common associated endocrine dysfunction is Cushing's syndrome, which is caused by ectopic production of adrenocorticotropic hormone (ACTH). This tumor appears as an anterior mediastinal mass on chest radiography and CT (Birnberg et al, 1982) but is frequently missed on chest radiography. A mediastinal CT scan should be obtained early in the course of the investigation of patients with suspected ectopic ACTH production (Brown et al, 1982).

Germ Cell Neoplasms

In large series, germ cell tumors are almost as common as thymomas, but unlike thymomas, most occur in adolescence or young adulthood. Males tend to develop malignant germ cell neoplasms, whereas females tend to develop benign thymic tumors. In most series, the benign teratoma is the most common of this group, occurring in approximately 70% of cases. The most common malignant neoplasm is the seminoma; the other malignant neoplasms include embryonal carcinoma, malignant teratoma, choriocarcinoma, and endodermal sinus tumor. Multiple cell types may be present within the same tumor.

Radiologically, the benign tumors tend to be spherical masses that grow slowly. They are most commonly seen in the superior mediastinum. There may be calcification, but it is usually not helpful in diagnosis because it can be seen in other anterior mediastinal masses, including thymoma and thyroid goiter. Occasionally, benign teratomas are recognized by the visibility of mature bone or a tooth in the neoplasm. In general, malignant tumors tend to be larger than benign ones, tend to be lobulated, and grow more rapidly (Fig. 58–8). CT may reveal evidence of mediastinal invasion or lymphadenopathy as well as metastatic disease in lungs, pleurae, or chest wall.

In a report of five benign teratomas of the mediastinum (Brown et al, 1987), all appeared as large (5 to 25 cm in diameter) masses on chest radiography. Four of these were located in the anterior mediastinum, and one was in the right hemithorax. On CT, three were predominantly cystic in nature, containing only small soft tissue components (Fig. 58–9); one contained approximately equal amounts of cystic and soft tissue components; and the fifth had a whorled, low-density appearance. The density of the cystic regions was higher than that of water. Three of the masses contained a single, dense calcific focus in the periphery of the mass. Similarly, three of six mediastinal teratomas in another report (Suzuki et al, 1983) had a cystic component, and two of the six contained dense "ossification." In a third study (Mori et al, 1987), six benign germ cell tumors had a thick wall with homogeneous contents that were slightly higher in density than water. A fat-fluid level has been reported in mediastinal cystic teratomas (Fulcher et al, 1990). A cystic anterior mediastinal lesion in a patient younger than 20 years, especially if it contains a dense calcific focus peripherally, should be considered a cystic teratoma. In this age group thymic cysts and thymomas

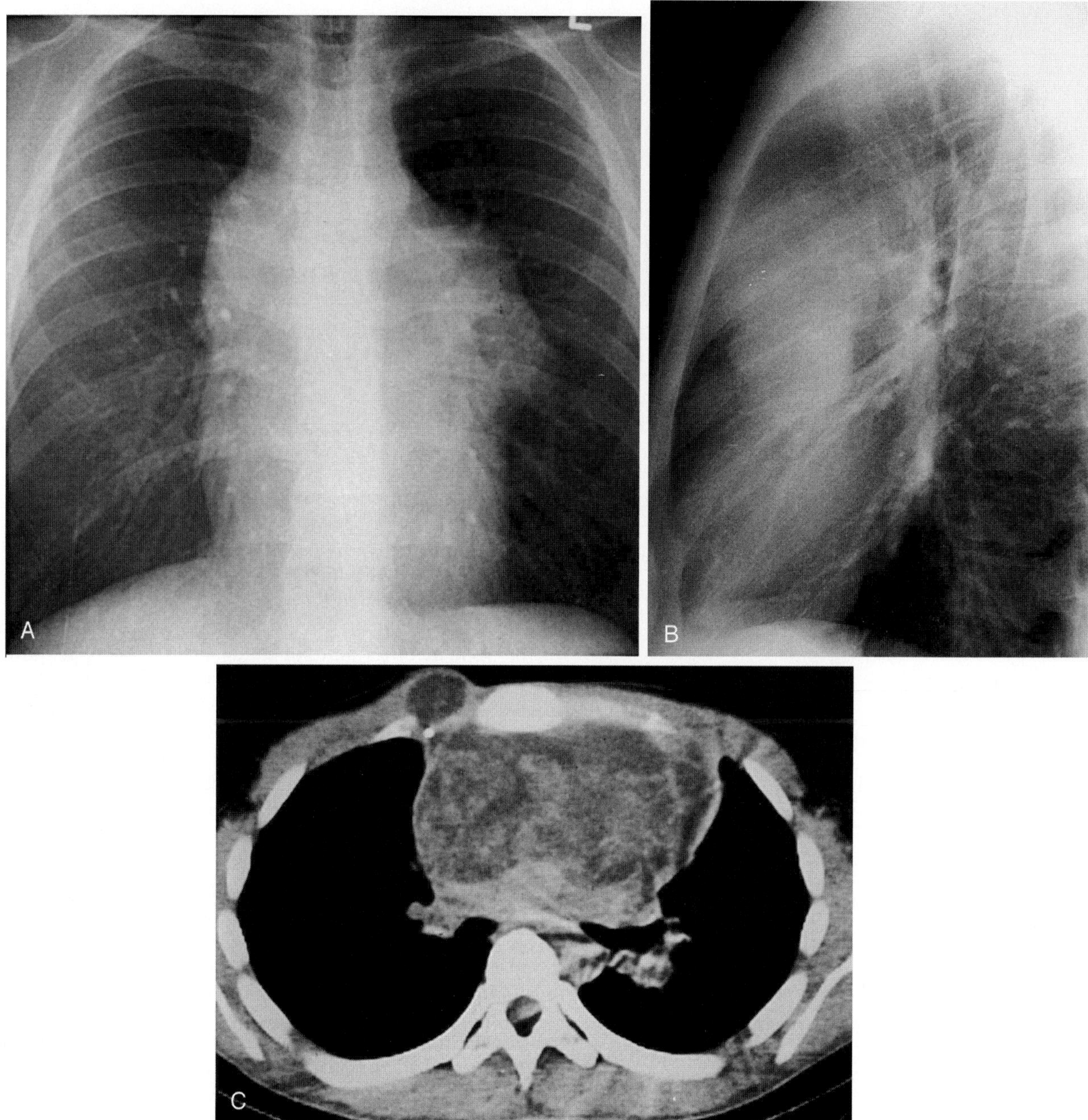

FIGURE 58–8 ■ A 23-year-old man with malignant nonseminomatous germ cell tumor. Chest radiographs, posteroanterior *(A)* and lateral *(B)*, show a very large, lobulated, anterior mediastinal mass projecting to both sides of the mediastinum. *C*, A computed tomography scan shows a very large inhomogeneous anterior mediastinal mass containing large areas of necrosis. The fat plane between the mass and the great vessels is obliterated, and the mediastinal structures are displaced posteriorly. Note the extension of the tumor anteriorly into the right chest wall.

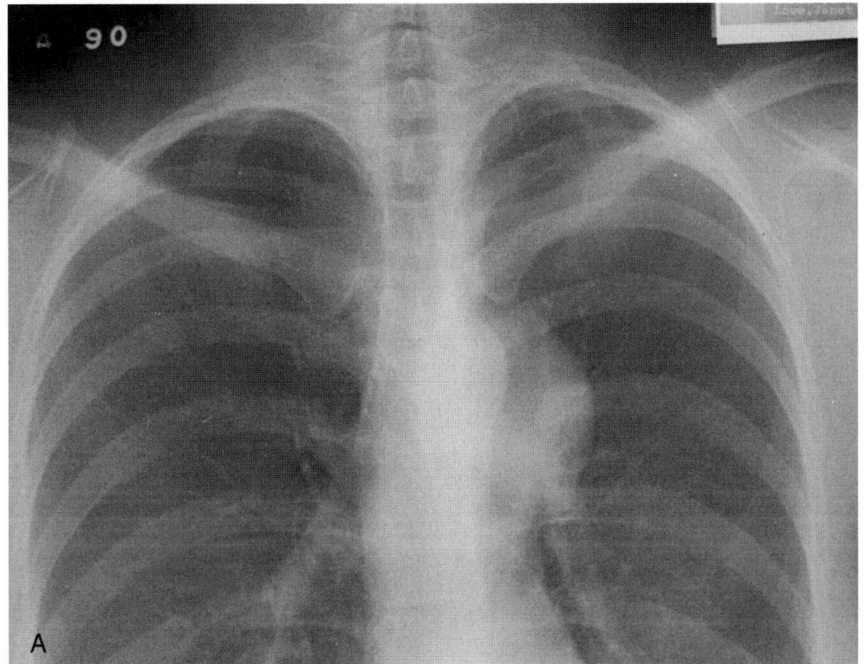

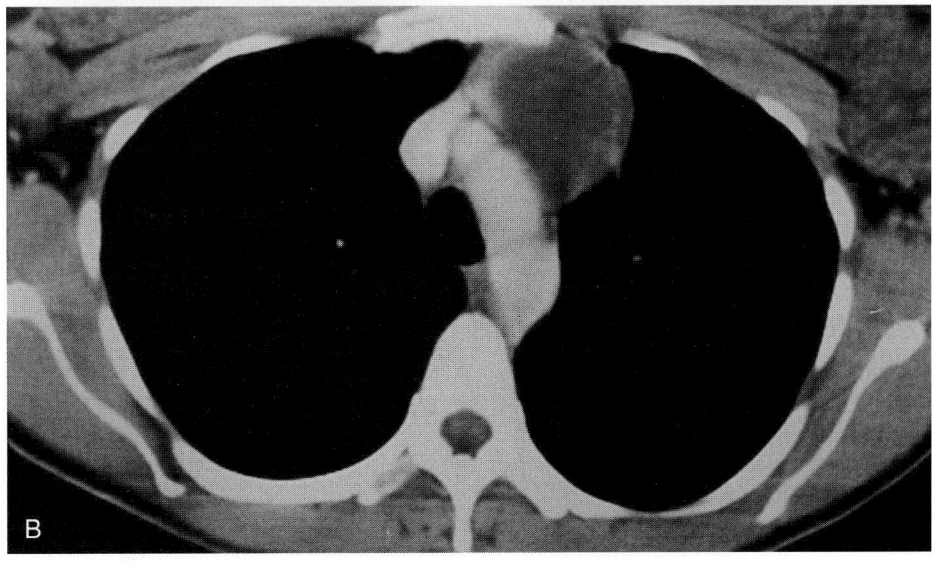

FIGURE 58–9 ■ *A*, Posteroanterior chest radiograph of a 29-year-old woman with a dermoid cyst shows a well-defined, left mediastinal mass, which was noted to be in the anterior mediastinum on the lateral view (not shown). *B*, A computed tomography scan shows a left anterior mediastinal mass whose attenuation is slightly greater than water, indicating its cystic nature. A small amount of soft tissue is noted on the right side of the mass.

are uncommon; bronchogenic cysts rarely occur in the anterior mediastinum.

In one report of four patients with malignant germ cell tumors (Levitt et al, 1984), all neoplasms were very large, obliterated fat planes between the mass and adjacent vessels, and tended to extend predominantly along the left side of the mediastinum. All three nonseminomatous tumors contained areas of density that was near that of water that were presumed to represent areas of necrosis and hemorrhage. The single seminoma was homogeneous in density. In a report of 13 patients with malignant germ cell tumors of the mediastinum (Lee et al, 1989), four of five seminomas exhibited obliteration of fat planes and two invaded the chest wall. There were two pleural effusions and one pericardial effusion. Four of the tumors exhibited small areas of low density. Six of eight nonseminomas had spiculated margins, and fat planes were obliterated in seven. More than 50% of the mass was of low density in five cases, with these areas having a septate internal architecture. Five of the eight had pleural and three had pericardial effusions. In another report of two seminomas (Shin and Ho, 1983a), both were very large with sharply defined margins but with loss of the fat planes between the mass and adjacent structures. Both tumors were homogeneous in density.

In a report of seven endodermal sinus tumors (Fox and Vix, 1980), all appeared radiographically as large, lobulated, uncalcified anterior mediastinal masses. Similar radiographic findings were reported in two other patients with this tumor, who also presented with large, lobulated anterior mediastinal masses (Blomlie et al, 1988). In these patients, CT revealed mixed areas of low and high attenuation and mediastinal fat planes were obliterated. One patient also had pleural and pericardial effusions and invasion of the anterior chest wall.

Thyroid Enlargement

Mediastinal thyroid enlargement is usually due to a nodular goiter; carcinoma is the cause in about 3% of cases (Katlic et al, 1985). The nodular goiters can become quite large and may contain areas of calcification, hemorrhage, and cyst formation. They tend to arise from the inferior aspect of the thyroid gland and extend into the anterior mediastinum anterior to the trachea, but occasionally they occur in a retrotracheal location. Most often they are asymptomatic and discovered on routine radiography, although if large enough they may cause dyspnea, hoarseness, dysphagia, and even the superior vena cava syndrome. On chest radiography, these goiters appear as well-defined, occasionally calcified, lobulated masses in the superior mediastinum. They tend to cause tracheal displacement and, occasionally, narrowing (Fig. 58–10).

Thyroid scintigraphy has been shown to be useful in demonstrating that a superior mediastinal mass is due to thyroid tissue and should probably be the next imaging procedure performed when a chest radiograph has revealed a mass that may represent a goiter (Park et al, 1987). In one study, 93% (39 of 42) of intrathoracic goiters took up radiolabeled agent (^{123}I, ^{131}I, ^{99m}Tc pertechnetate), whereas 100% (12 of 12) of nonthyroid masses did not (Park et al, 1987).

The CT features of mediastinal thyroid have been well described (Bashist et al, 1983; Glazer et al, 1982; Silverman et al., 1984). These include (1) well-defined borders; (2) definite continuity with the cervical thyroid gland; (3) pretreatment attenuation that is greater than that of adjacent muscles; (4) an increase in attenuation after injection of intravenous contrast agent; (5) focal, punctate nodular, or curvilinear calcifications; (6) discrete, nonenhancing areas of low attenuation; and (7) insinuation of the mass between the trachea and the great vessels, displacing the latter laterally (rarely, medial vascular displacement can be seen). With significant caudal extension, the mass usually remains posterior to the great vessels and aortic arch; however, it rarely comes to be located anterior to the aortic arch (Bashist et al, 1983; Glazer et al, 1982). It is not always possible to distinguish benign from malignant thyroid masses, but CT features suggesting malignancy include (1) ill-defined areas of low attenuation within the gland; (2) adjacent lymphadenopathy; (3) ill-defined margins, with loss of the fat planes between the mass and adjacent mediastinal structures; and (4) destruction of adjacent structures (Pearlberg et al, 1989; Silverman et al, 1984) (Fig. 58–11).

MRI has been shown to provide images of the thyroid that exhibit excellent correlation with pathologic findings (Gefter et al, 1987; Higgins et al, 1986; Noma et al, 1987, 1988). Tumors generally, but not always, had ill-defined margins and exhibited prolonged T_1 and T_2 values as compared with normal thyroid tissue. Enlarged lymph nodes were clearly visualized, as was the intrathoracic extent of the tumor, with coronal and sagittal views being especially helpful in evaluating the latter.

Although CT and ultrasound have been shown to be of equal value in most patients with thyroid abnormalities, ultrasound was able to detect some small nodules that were not imaged by CT, but CT was better at assessing intrathoracic extension of the gland (Radecki et al, 1984).

Lymphadenopathy

Lymph node enlargement in the anterior mediastinum is usually caused by lymphoma (Fig. 58–12) or metastatic disease (Fig. 58–13). Other rare causes include Castleman's disease, granulomatous diseases, and angioimmunoblastic lymphadenopathy.

In patients with newly diagnosed Hodgkin's disease, intrathoracic involvement was noted in 67%, with 90% of these having superior mediastinal adenopathy (Filly et al, 1976). Similarly, patients with non-Hodgkin's lymphoma had thoracic involvement on the initial chest radiograph in 43% of cases, with superior mediastinal adenopathy in 46% of these. On the chest radiograph, this lymphadenopathy appears as an otherwise typical anterior mediastinal mass. On CT, discrete enlarged nodes may be visible, or one may note the presence of a large soft tissue mass with ill-defined margins and with loss of the fat plane adjacent to other mediastinal structures (Blank and Castellino, 1987). The mass frequently contains areas of low density representing necrosis; this necrosis does not correlate with the size of the nodal mass and has no prognostic significance in patients with

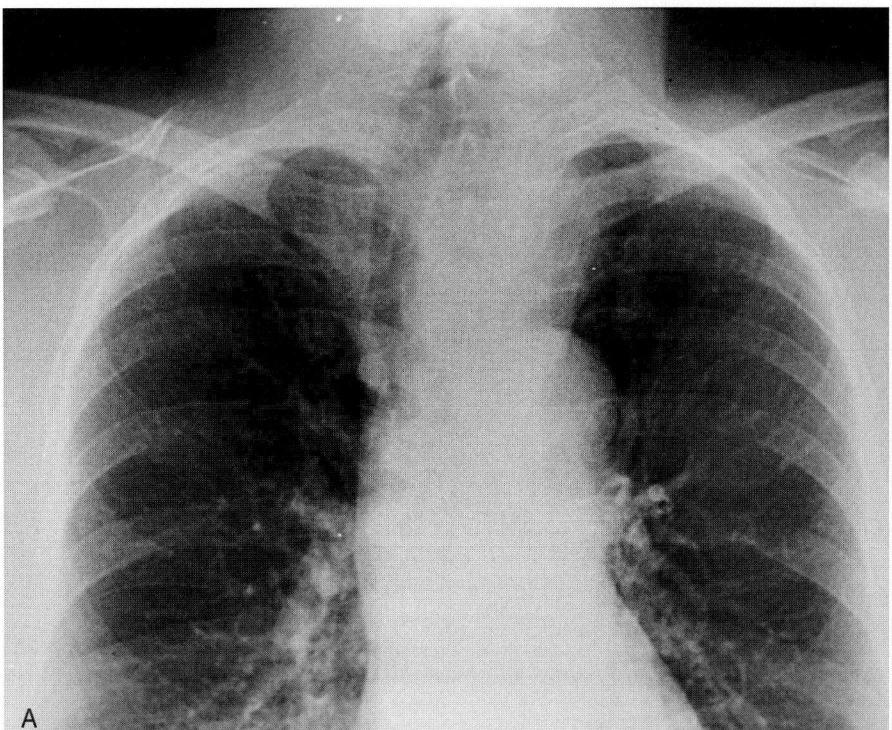

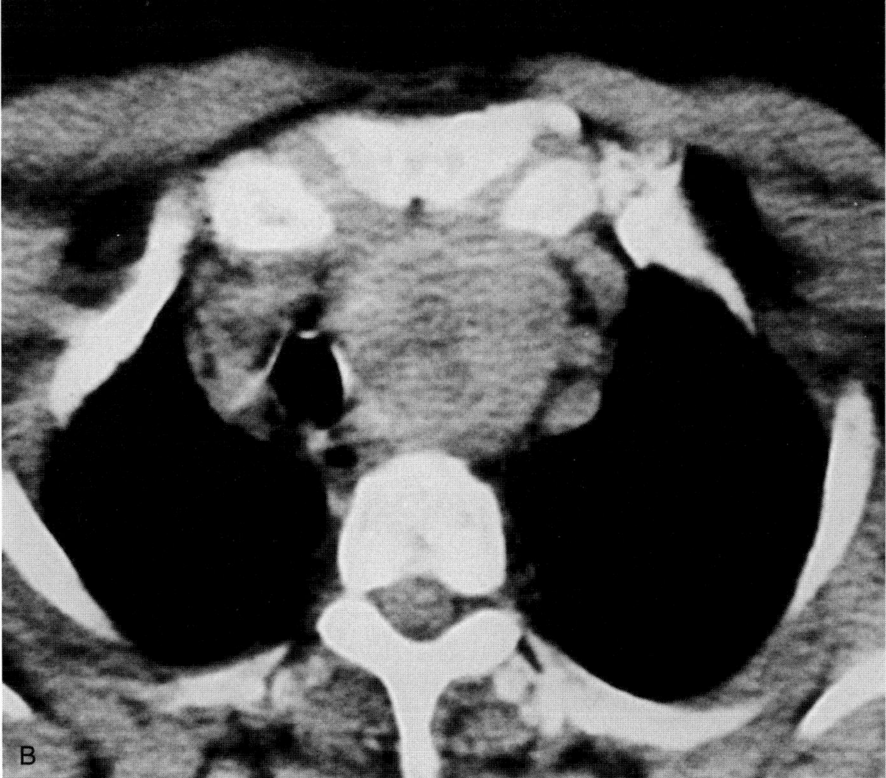

FIGURE 58–10 ■ Benign goiter in a 70-year-old woman. *A*, Posteroanterior chest radiograph shows a large, left paratracheal mass that is causing significant displacement of the trachea to the right. *B*, A computed tomography scan shows a well-defined, left paratracheal mass containing areas of low density centrally. Note the intact fat plane between this mass and the adjacent great vessels, which are displaced laterally.

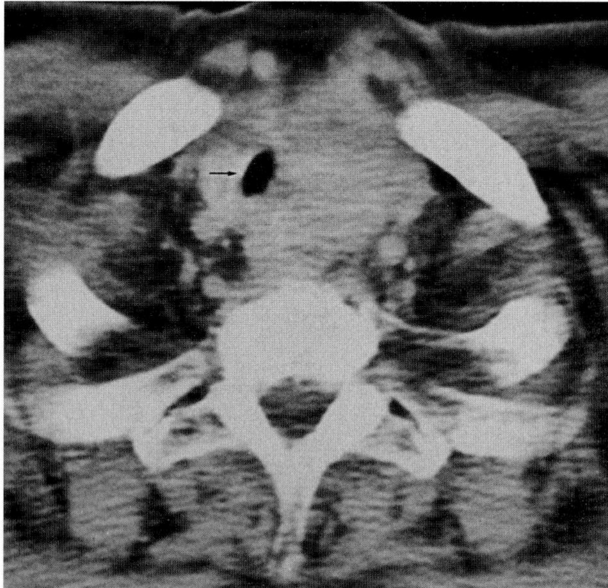

FIGURE 58–11 ■ A computed tomography scan of an 85-year-old man with thyroid carcinoma. There is an ill-defined, left paratracheal mass displacing the trachea to the right. There is loss of the fat plane between the mass and the adjacent structures, including the great vessels, and lack of a sharp demarcation between the mass and the adjacent mediastinal fat. The tracheal cartilage has been destroyed by the tumor (note the presence of calcium in the intact tracheal cartilage on the right *[arrow]*).

newly diagnosed Hodgkin's disease (Hopper et al, 1990). These lymphomatous masses can directly invade the chest wall (Gouliamos et al, 1980; Press et al, 1985) and rarely calcify, especially if untreated (Lautin et al, 1990). A different pattern of involvement is the so-called permeating continuum, which refers to a large mass lesion with no discernible borders that blends imperceptibly with other mediastinal structures.

A cystic form of Hodgkin's disease, which appears as a mass containing large areas with the density of water that obliterates adjacent fat planes, may mimic germ cell tumors and thymomas (Federle and Callen, 1979). Thymic cysts have been described after successful irradiation for Hodgkin's disease; these appear as smooth, thin-walled structures that contain homogeneous material of water density and should not be confused with recurrent tumor (Baron et al, 1981b).

Miscellaneous Lesions

Not uncommonly, a chest radiograph can suggest the presence of a mass lesion but no such mass is seen with CT. This may be due to increased amounts of anterior mediastinal fat (Fig. 58–14). A number of other rare causes of anterior mediastinal masses have been described. One of these, which must always be kept in mind, especially if a biopsy of the mass is contemplated, is an aortic aneurysm. On the chest radiograph an aneurysm of the ascending aorta, which is usually congenital or mycotic in etiology, most often projects to the right of the midline. On CT it can be recognized by the fact that it rapidly takes up intravenous contrast material, although some or most of the aneurysm may be filled with thrombus. Other causes of mass lesions in this location include parathyroid adenoma, cystic hygroma, paraganglioma, hemangioma, lipoma, and liposarcoma.

MIDDLE MEDIASTINAL MASSES

The middle mediastinal compartment contains the heart and pericardium and all the major vessels leaving and entering this organ, the trachea and main bronchi, paratracheal and tracheobronchial lymph nodes, phrenic nerves, and the upper portion of the vagus nerves.

Lymph Node Enlargement

Lymph node enlargement is the most common cause of a mediastinal mass and can be caused by lymphoma, metastatic carcinoma, sarcoidosis, and infection (particularly with *Histoplasma capsulatum* and *Mycobacterium tuberculosis*). Uncommon causes include Castleman's disease (giant lymph node hyperplasia) (Hammond, 1979) (Fig. 58–15), granulomatous mediastinitis (Weinstein et al, 1983) (Fig. 58–16), and amyloidosis.

Primary Tracheal Neoplasms

Primary tracheal neoplasms are uncommon. Squamous cell carcinoma is the most common, followed by adenoid cystic carcinoma. These may lead to a subtle alteration in the tracheal air column on routine chest radiography or, if more extensive, may cause widening of the upper middle mediastinal soft tissues. In any patient with dyspnea, wheezing, or stridor, the tracheal air column should be carefully scrutinized on conventional radiographs to exclude a subtle mass (Fig. 58–17). CT is superior in showing the extent of tumor involvement (Fig. 58–18). Adenoid cystic carcinomas tend to be infiltrative tumors, often underestimated in extent even by CT (Spizarny et al, 1986).

Bronchogenic Cysts

Most mediastinal bronchogenic cysts arise near the tracheal carina in relationship to the major airways (Davis and Simonton, 1956). They rarely communicate with the tracheobronchial tree. Radiologically, they appear as round or oval masses of homogeneous soft tissue density located just inferior to the carina and often protruding posteriorly and slightly to the right (Reed and Sobonya, 1974) (Fig. 58–19). Calcification of the cyst wall is uncommon (Ziter et al, 1969). CT may show a cyst of water density. The attenuation is commonly higher than one would associate with a cyst because of the content of thick mucoid material (Mendelson et al, 1983). Calcium in the cyst contents may also produce high CT numbers (Yernault et al, 1986). MRI shows the cyst to be hypointense on T_1-weighted images and markedly hyperintense on T_2-weighted images (Marin et al, 1991). This combination of findings including hypoattenuation on CT is strongly suggestive of a bronchogenic cyst (Fig. 58–20). Transthoracic and transbronchial needle aspirations are

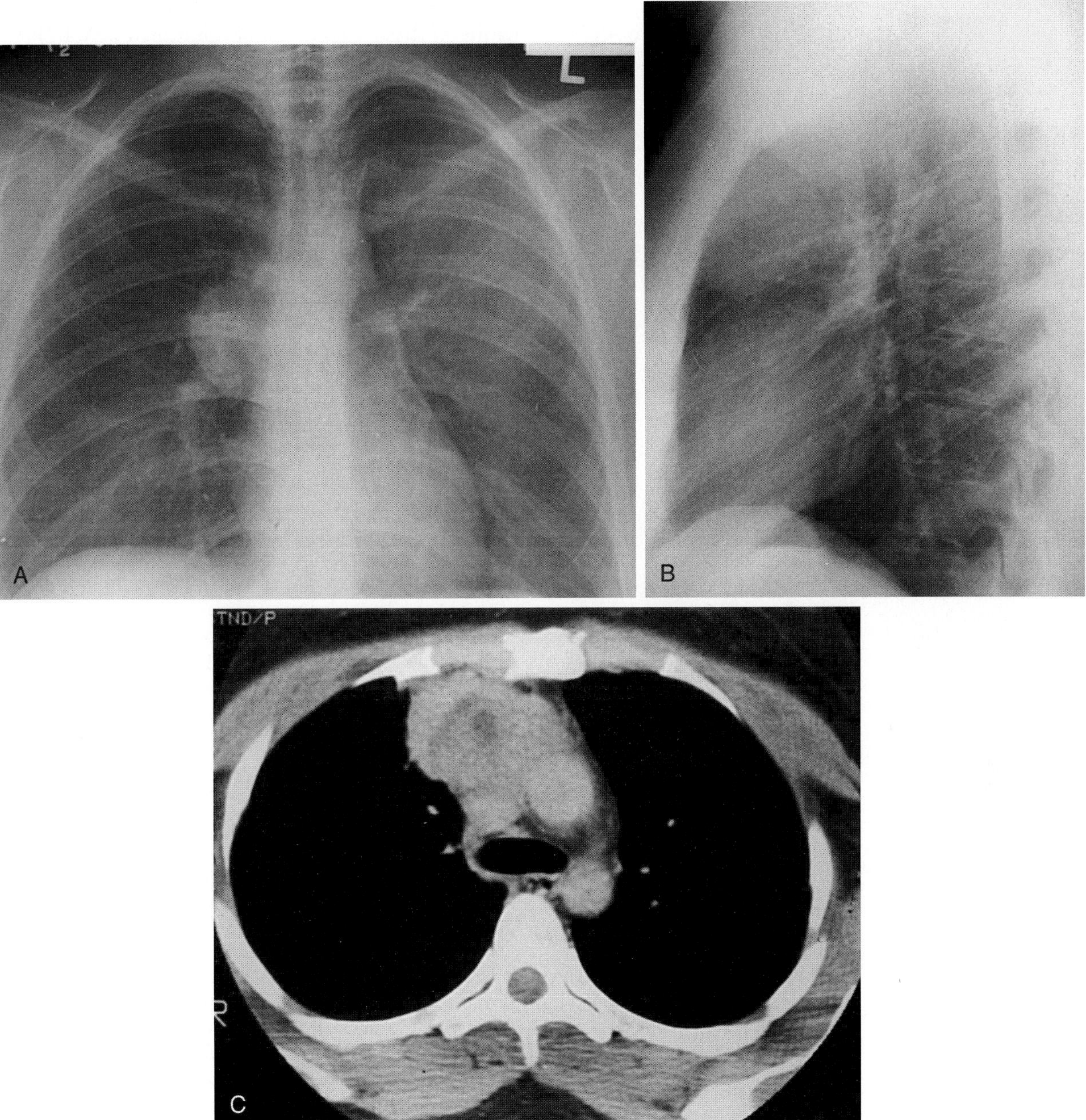

FIGURE 58–12 ■ A 25-year-old asymptomatic woman with Hodgkin's disease. Chest radiographs, posteroanterior *(A)* and lateral *(B)*, show a right anterior mediastinal mass. *C*, A computed tomography scan shows an ill-defined mass in the anterior mediastinum containing areas of decreased attenuation that presumably represent necrosis. Note the loss of fat plane between the posterior aspect of the mass, the superior vena cava, and ascending aorta.

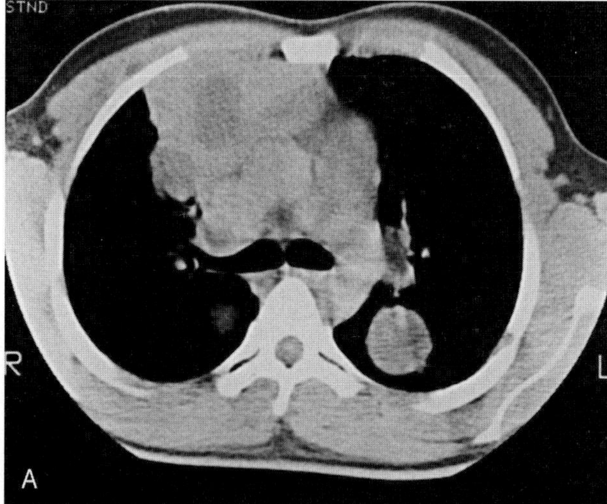

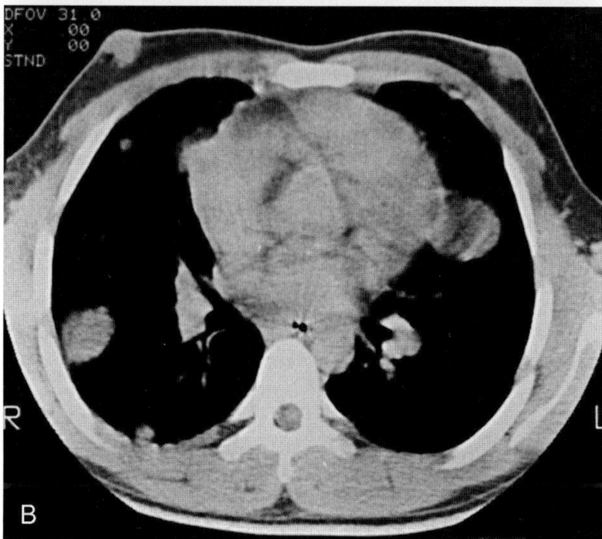

FIGURE 58–13 ■ *A*, A computed tomography (CT) scan of a 22-year-old man with testicular choriocarcinoma metastatic to the lungs and anterior mediastinum shows a large, lobulated, right anterior mediastinal mass. There are areas of low density within this mass, most likely representing necrosis. It is ill-defined where it contacts the adjacent mediastinal structures. *B*, CT scan taken 3 cm below *A*. There are bilateral pulmonary metastases. Note the bilateral gynecomastia owing to the very high levels (> 300,000 U) of β-HCG (human chorionic gonadotropin).

useful procedures, both diagnostically and therapeutically (Kuhlman et al, 1988). Mucoid material of varying color and consistency may be aspirated.

MASSES IN THE ANTERIOR CARDIOPHRENIC ANGLE

Masses in the anterior cardiophrenic angle can arise from lung parenchyma, pleura, mediastinum, or diaphragm or from beneath the diaphragm. CT is useful in the differential diagnosis of these lesions (Modic and Janicki, 1980). The most common lesions include a large pleuropericardial fat pad (Paling, 1987), pericardial cyst, and hernia through the foramen of Bochdalek.

Pericardial Cysts

Pericardial cysts are congenital mesothelial cysts and are usually smooth, round or oval masses in the right anterior cardiophrenic angle (Feigin et al, 1977) (Fig. 58–21). The lateral radiograph may show a teardrop configuration as the cyst extends into the interlobar fissure. The cystic nature of these masses can be confirmed by CT (Pugatch et al, 1978) or ultrasound. Calcification is rare. Percutaneous fine-needle aspiration shows the contained clear or straw-colored fluid and can be therapeutic as well (see Fig. 58–21).

Dilatation of the Major Mediastinal Arteries and Veins

Dilatation of the superior vena cava as a result of increased central venous pressure may cause a smooth widening of the right superior mediastinal soft tissues. Dilatation of the azygos vein may cause a round or oval mass in the right tracheobronchial angle. A dilated vein can be differentiated from a true mass by demonstrating an increase in the size of the structure in the supine position as compared with its size in the erect position. The superior vena caval syndrome is characterized by edema of the face, neck, upper extremities, and thorax and dilated chest wall veins. It is caused by obstruction of the superior vena cava, most commonly by bronchogenic carcinoma. Lymphoma, metastatic carcinoma, and chronic sclerosing mediastinitis are uncommon causes. A mass in the right superior mediastinum is usually present. The obstruction of the vein can be confirmed by CT or venography (Bechtold et al, 1985).

Aneurysms of the aorta or its major branches may produce a middle (Fig. 58–22) or posterior mediastinal mass. Spiral CT angiography with bolus injection of contrast material is the method of choice in diagnosis of all types of aortic aneurysms. CT angiography is a new minimally invasive vascular imaging modality. Its advantages over conventional angiography are high-quality, thin axial sections that demonstrate mural changes; high contrast resolution and high sensitivity for detecting calcified lesions; multiplanar or three-dimensional display of vascular structures (Fig. 58–23); demonstration of extrinsic causes of vascular compromise; demonstration of spatial relationships with adjacent organs; and lower skin surface dose (Chung et al, 1996). For any patient with a middle or posterior mediastinal mass that could be related to the aorta, CT should be performed before invasive procedures such as percutaneous needle biopsy. The aneurysm is frequently occluded by thrombus so that little if any opacification of the lumen may occur with contrast material. MRI is also useful and makes aortography unnecessary.

Congenital anomalies of the aorta may appear with a middle mediastinal mass (Fig. 58–24). A right aortic arch is the most common anomaly and is seen as a right upper paratracheal mass that displaces the tracheal air column to the left and anteriorly (Fig. 58–25) (Shuford et al, 1970). Usually the diagnosis is evident from plain chest radiographs. CT, aortography, or MRI is diagnostic.

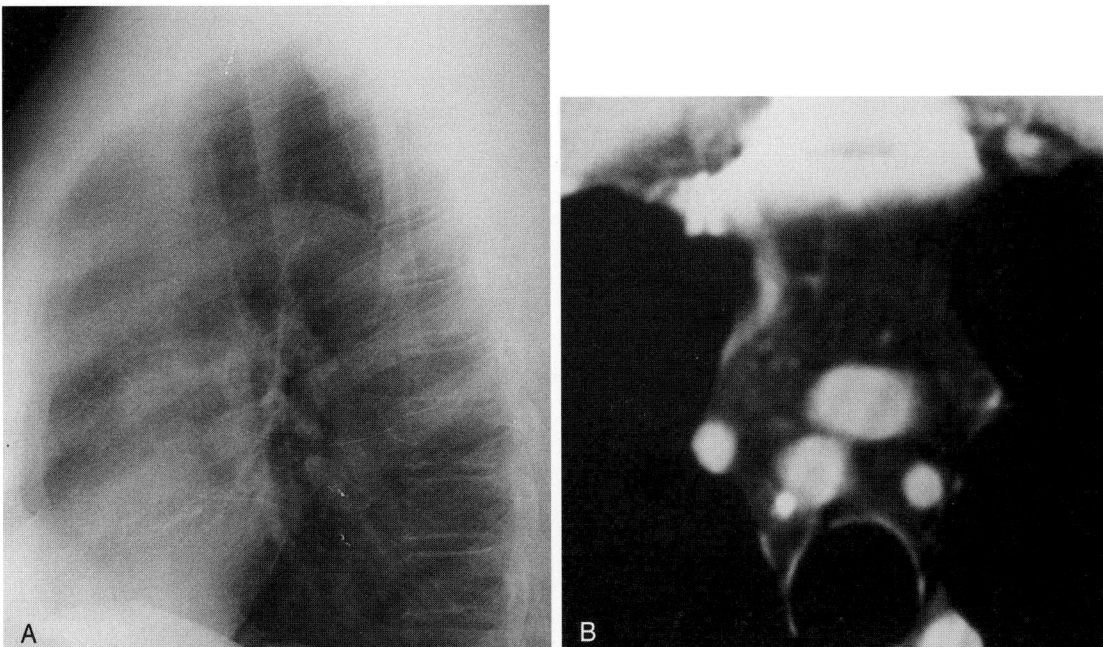

FIGURE 58–14 ■ A 63-year-old man with mediastinal lipomatosis and myasthenia gravis. *A*, Lateral chest radiograph shows fullness in the anterior mediastinum, suggesting the presence of a mass. *B*, A computed tomography scan indicates that increased amounts of anterior mediastinal fat are causing the plain film findings.

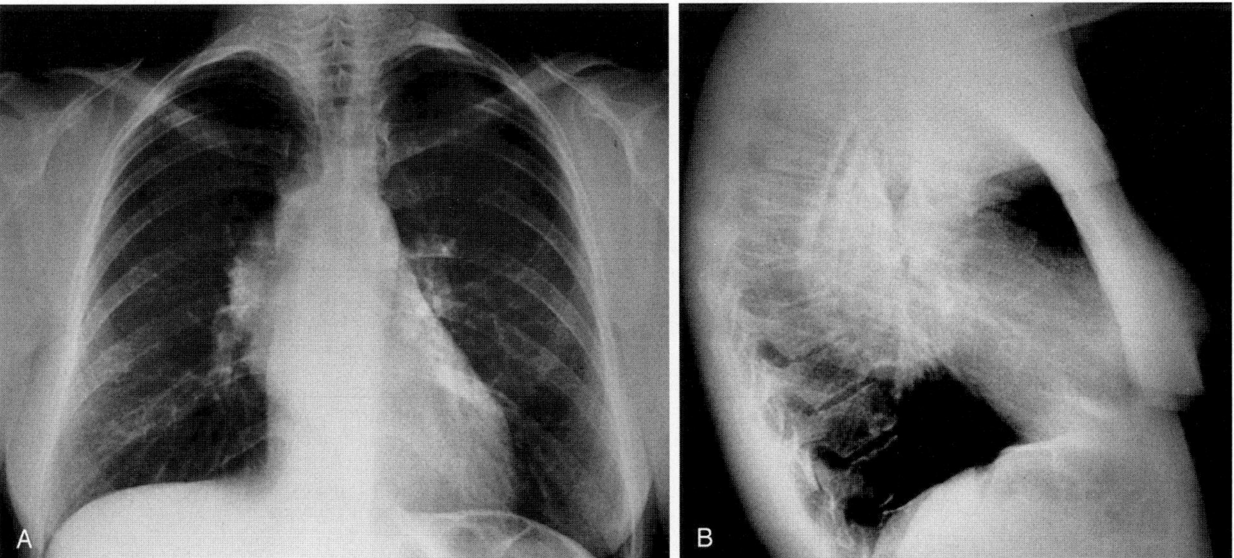

FIGURE 58–15 ■ A 21-year-old woman was found to have a mediastinal mass on a chest radiograph taken because of an upper respiratory tract infection. Posteroanterior *(A)* and lateral *(B)* chest radiographs show a large mass arising in the mediastinum just posterior to the distal trachea and upper posterior heart. Thoracotomy revealed a very vascular mass that could not be removed entirely because of bleeding. Biopsy showed giant lymph node hyperplasia (hyaline vascular type).

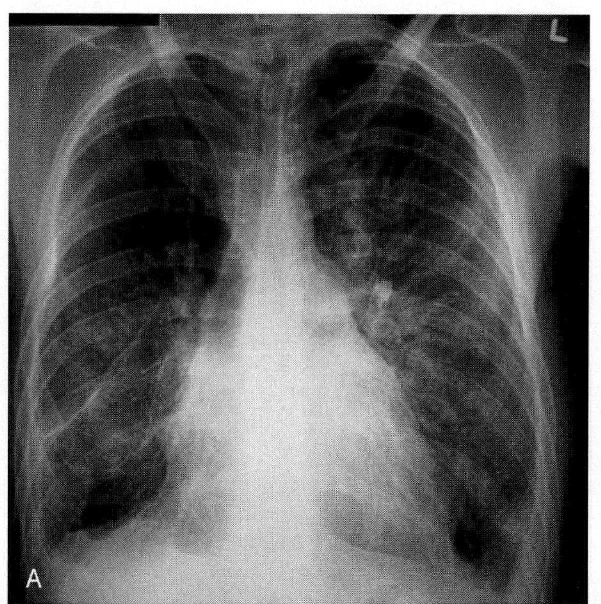

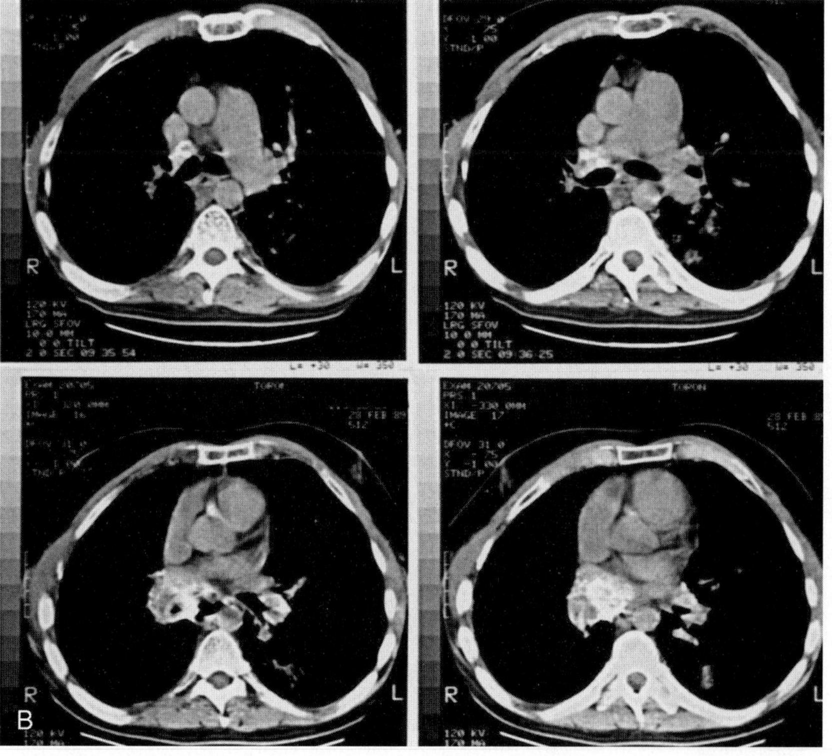

FIGURE 58–16 ■ A 43-year-old man with a 20-year history of granulomatous mediastinitis. Right thoracotomy and open biopsy of a mediastinal mass in the past showed "burned-out histoplasmosis." At presentation he was severely dyspneic and hypoxemic with pulmonary arterial hypertension. *A*, Posteroanterior chest radiograph shows evidence of a previous right thoracotomy with resection of the fifth rib. Increased density is present in the right and left lower lung zones. The right and left lateral costophrenic sulci are blunted by pleural effusions. *B*, A computed tomography scan shows calcified nodal tissue in the right tracheobronchial angle. A large, retrocardiac, right periesophageal mass is present, containing a large amount of calcification. The main pulmonary artery and central pulmonary arteries are dilated. There is complete obstruction of the bronchus intermedius and the origin of the right middle lobe and right lower lobe bronchi. A pulmonary angiogram showed complete obstruction of the right pulmonary artery. The patient died shortly after a left lung transplant. At autopsy, a diagnosis of sclerosing mediastinitis was confirmed. There was encasement of bronchovascular structures at the hila of both lungs, resulting in obstruction of the right pulmonary artery and stenosis of the left pulmonary artery, both pulmonary veins, and main bronchi. Patchy pulmonary congestion, edema, hemosiderosis, and chronic interstitial fibrosis were present.

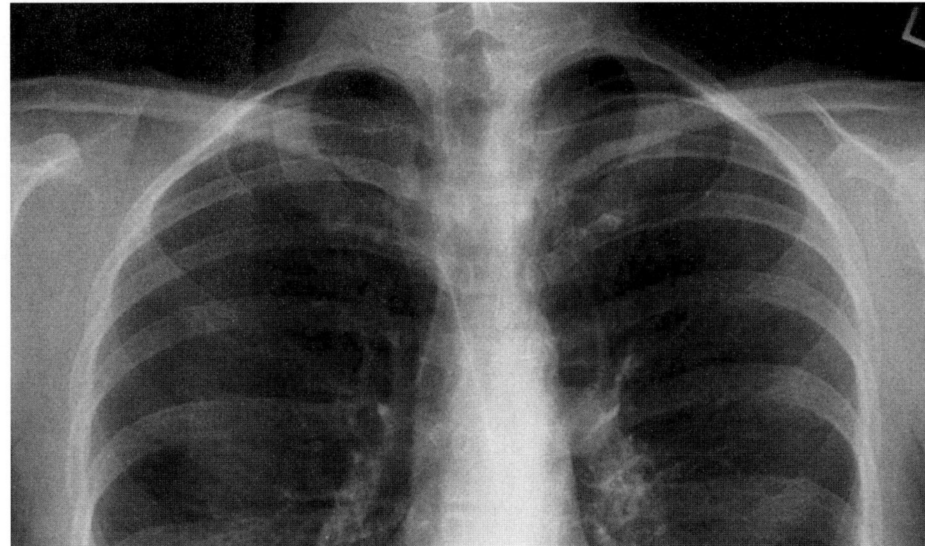

FIGURE 58–17 ■ A 31-year-old woman with cough and stridor for 1 year. This posteroanterior chest radiograph shows increased density in the midtrachea, with loss of the tracheal outline. This was caused by an adenoid cystic carcinoma.

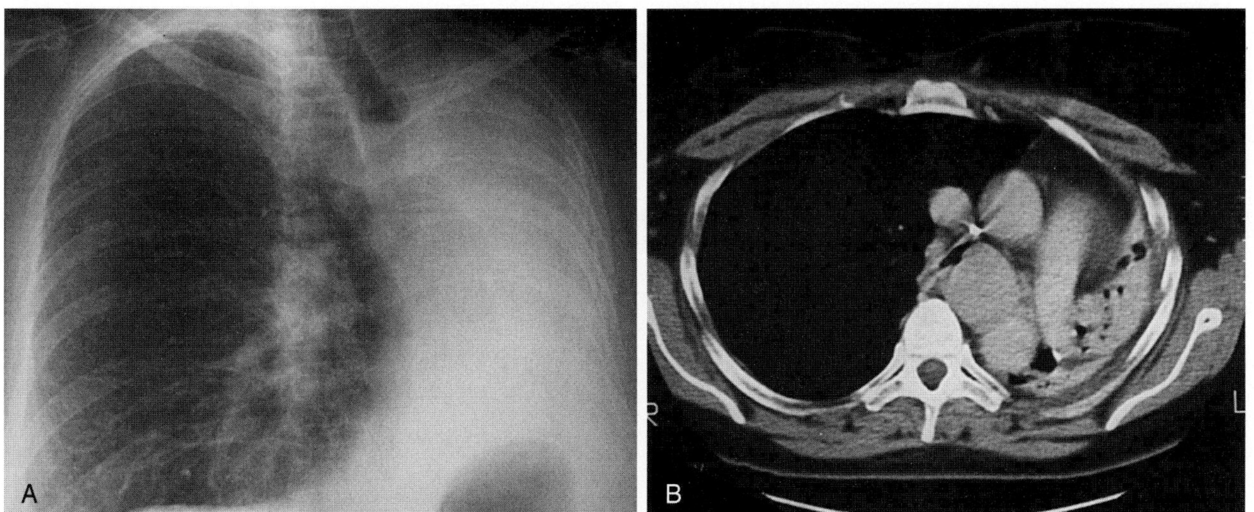

FIGURE 58–18 ■ A 55-year-old woman with adenoid cystic carcinoma. She had dyspnea for 2 years and recent hemoptysis. *A*, This posteroanterior chest radiograph shows total atelectasis of the left lung. *B*, A computed tomography scan shows a large mass that is severely narrowing the distal trachea and completely obstructing the left main bronchus. The extent of tumor involvement is well shown. The left lung is totally atelectatic. Bronchoscopy with a biopsy showed adenoid cystic carcinoma.

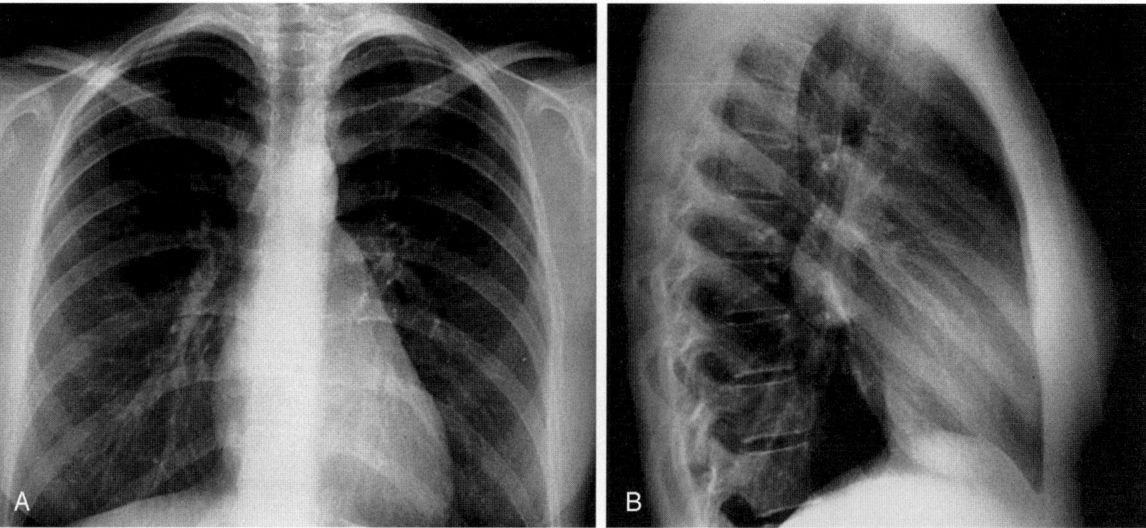

FIGURE 58–19 ■ A 17-year-old girl with dysphasia was noted to have a middle mediastinal mass. Posteroanterior *(A)* and lateral *(B)* chest radiographs reveal an oval, well-defined mass occurring in a typical location for a bronchogenic cyst, inferior to the carina and projecting posteriorly and to the right. Percutaneous needle aspiration revealed mucus, respiratory epithelial cells, and microcalcifications consistent with a bronchogenic cyst.

POSTERIOR MEDIASTINAL MASSES

Neurogenic Tumors

Neurogenic tumors are a common cause of a posterior mediastinal mass, accounting for almost 20% of mediastinal tumors (Ingels et al, 1971). Neurogenic tumors arising from peripheral nerves include neurofibroma, neurilemmoma (schwannoma), and neurogenic sarcoma (malignant schwannoma) (Fig. 58–26). These usually arise from intercostal nerves; vagus and phrenic neurofibromas are rare. Radiologically, these tumors are seen as well-defined, round or oval masses in the paravertebral region (Fig. 58–27). Calcification is rare. CT may show expansion of the intervertebral foramen. MRI is useful in showing any spinal canal component. Percutaneous fine-needle aspiration biopsy may reveal no diagnostic cells or spindle cells that are indicative of a spindle cell neoplasm. Cytologically, the differential diagnosis is that of a spindle cell tumor, but this, when combined with typical radiology, can be diagnostic of a neurogenic tumor.

Neurogenic tumors originating from sympathetic ganglia include ganglioneuroma, ganglioneuroblastoma, neuroblastoma, and paraganglioma (chemodectoma, pheochromocytoma). Radiologically, these tumors are similar to those of the peripheral nerve group. However, they tend to be more elongated in the cephalocaudal direction, meeting the mediastinum at an obtuse rather than an acute angle (Theros, 1969). Consequently, they are often less easily seen on a lateral view (Reed et al, 1978) (Fig. 58–28). Calcifications are not uncommon; however, bony changes are unusual. Percutaneous fine-needle aspiration biopsy may reveal no diagnostic cells, nondiagnostic spindle cells, or a combination of spindle cells and ganglion cells, which are diagnostic of a ganglioneuroma.

Gastroenteric (Duplication) Cysts

Duplication cysts may cause a middle or posterior mediastinal mass, particularly in the young (Kuhlman et al, 1985). Histologically, these cysts can be lined by nonkeratinizing squamous, ciliated columnar, gastric, or small intestinal epithelium. They may occur within or adjacent to the wall of the esophagus. Communication with the upper gastrointestinal tract is uncommon (Dresler et al, 1990) (Fig. 58–29). Neurenteric cysts have a connection to the meninges and are associated with congenital defects of the thoracic spine.

Diseases of the Esophagus

Esophageal neoplasm, diverticulum, hiatus hernia, megaesophagus, and esophageal varices (Fig. 58–30) (Jonsson and Rian, 1970) may cause posterior mediastinal masses in relation to the esophagus. Plain chest radiography is frequently normal in patients with esophageal carcinoma. Abnormalities may be subtle and include a retrocardiac mass (Fig. 58–31*A*), abnormal azygoesophageal recess interface, widened mediastinum, widened retrotracheal stripe, and esophageal air-fluid level (Lindell et al, 1979). CT is useful in staging esophageal carcinoma, and it is highly accurate in predicting tumor size and assessing invasion of mediastinum and tracheobronchial tree as well as spread to the liver, adrenals, and upper abdominal lymph nodes (Picus et al, 1983) (Fig. 58–31*B*).

Paravertebral Masses

Primary or metastatic tumors of the thoracic spine may appear with a posterior mediastinal paravertebral mass. The bony lesion should be evident radiologically. Lymphomas, particularly Hodgkin's disease, may involve the posterior parietal group of lymph nodes and produce a fusiform paravertebral soft tissue mass. Infections (e.g., tuberculosis) and post-traumatic hematomas may also cause a paravertebral mass. Rare causes of posterior mediastinal masses include mediastinal extension of a pancre-

Text continued on page 1597

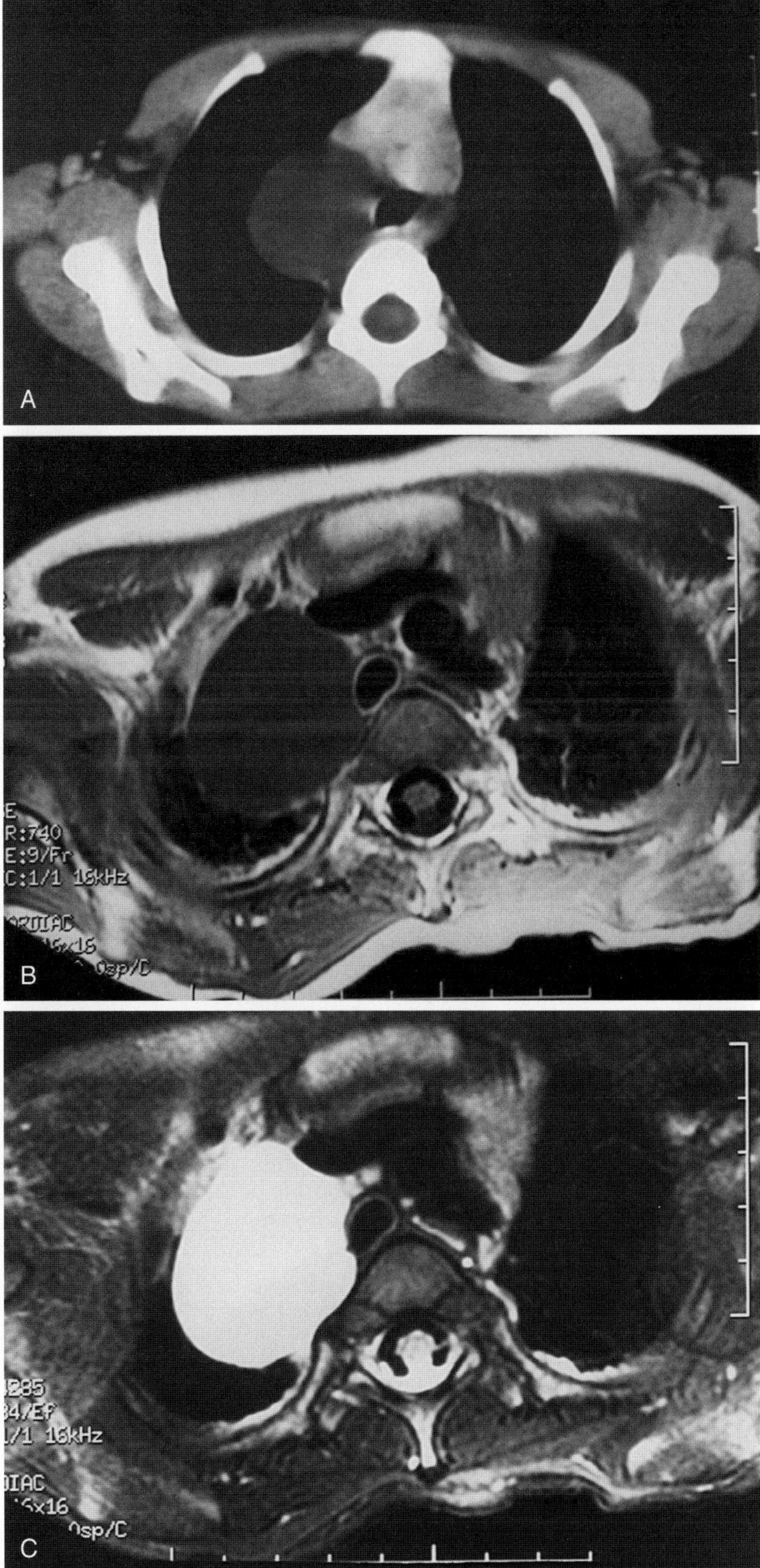

FIGURE 58–20 ■ A 5-year-old girl with a bronchogenic cyst. *A*, A computed tomography scan shows a cystic mass in the right paratracheal area. *B*, A magnetic resonance image (MRI) (T_1) shows low signal intensity in the mass. *C*, MRI (T_2) shows high signal intensity.

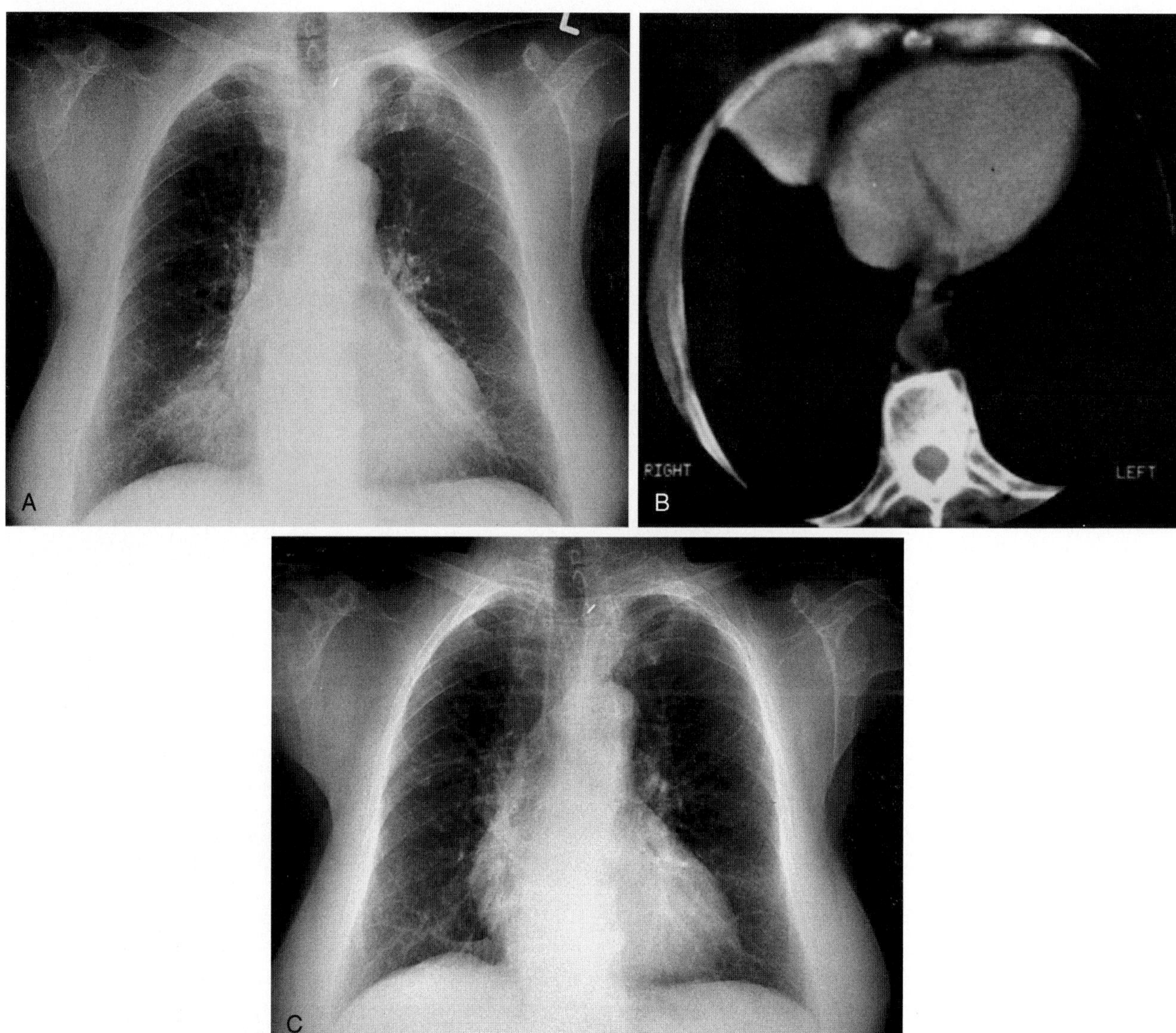

FIGURE 58–21 ■ *A*, A 64-year-old asymptomatic woman has a mass in the right, anterior, cardiophrenic angle. *B*, A computed tomography scan shows a mass of water density in this angle. *C*, Posteroanterior film taken after aspiration of clear serous fluid shows a decrease in the size of the mass and development of an air-fluid level.

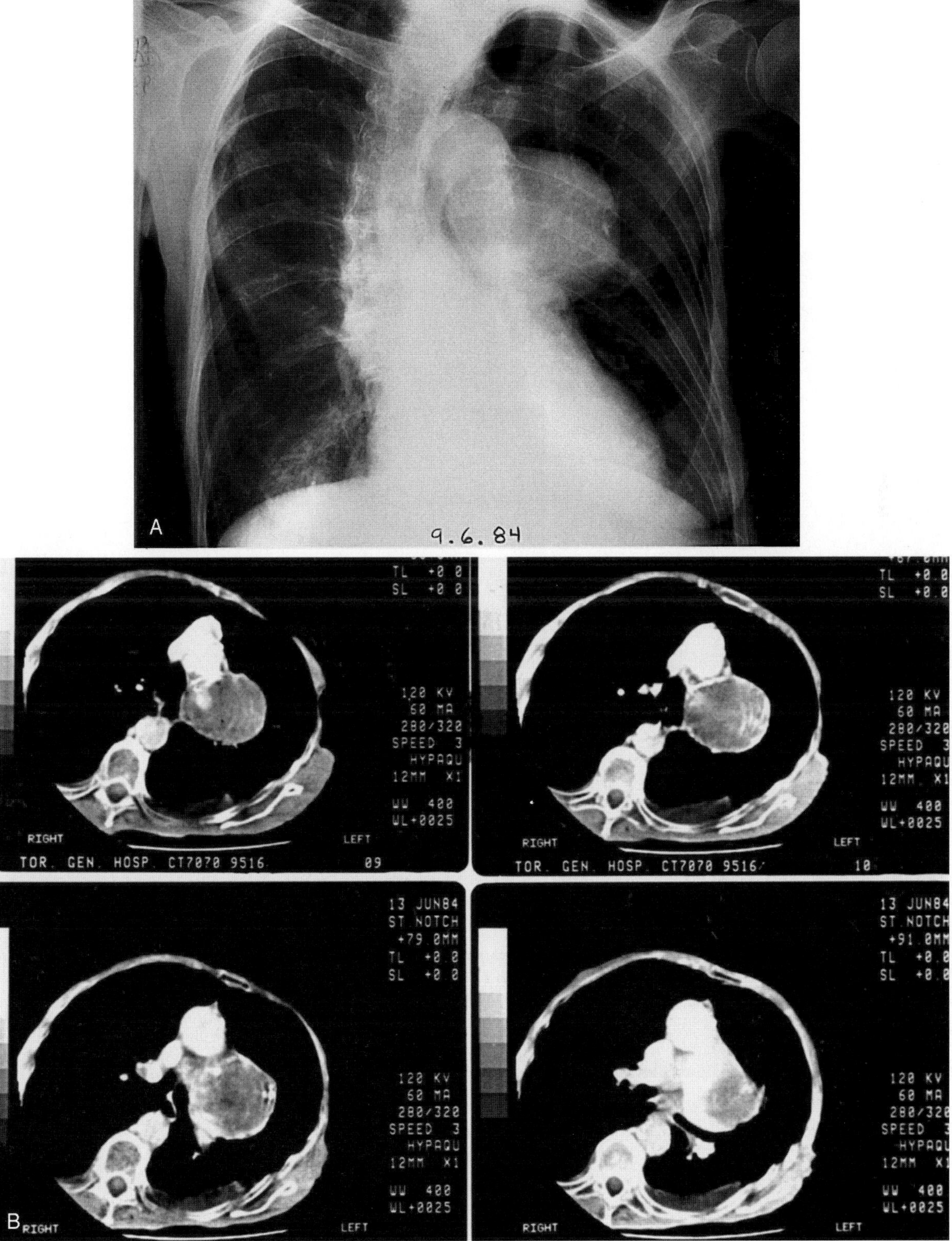

FIGURE 58–22 ■ A 73-year-old woman with an aortic aneurysm. *A*, A posteroanterior chest radiograph shows a large, round mass occupying the left aorticopulmonary window. Spotty calcification is seen within the mass laterally. *B*, A computed tomography scan shows a small, opacified lumen, with most of the mass occupied by a thrombus. The findings were confirmed at autopsy.

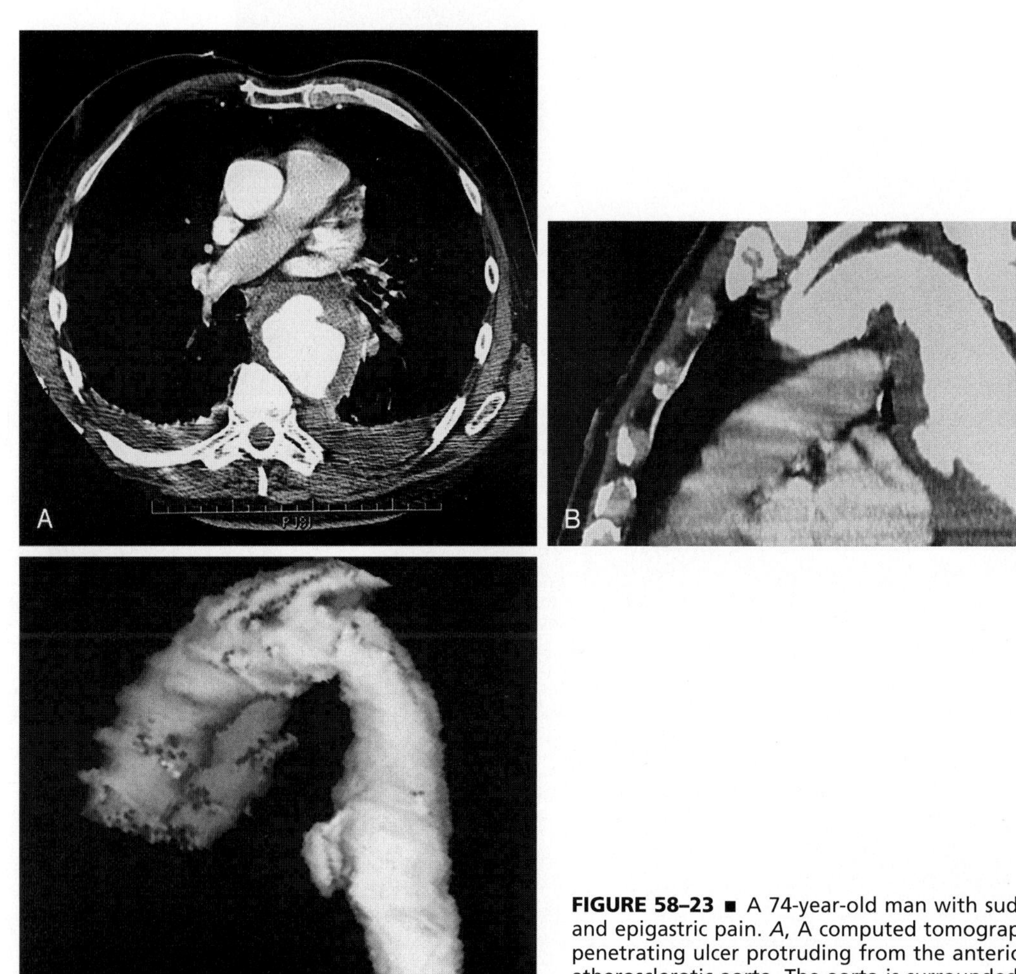

FIGURE 58–23 ■ A 74-year-old man with sudden onset of midback and epigastric pain. *A*, A computed tomography scan shows a penetrating ulcer protruding from the anterior wall of a dilated atherosclerotic aorta. The aorta is surrounded by hematoma. Bilateral pleural effusions are present. *B*, A multiplanar reconstructed image shows the anterior penetrating ulcer. *C*, The shaded surface displays the image. The diagnosis was confirmed by surgery.

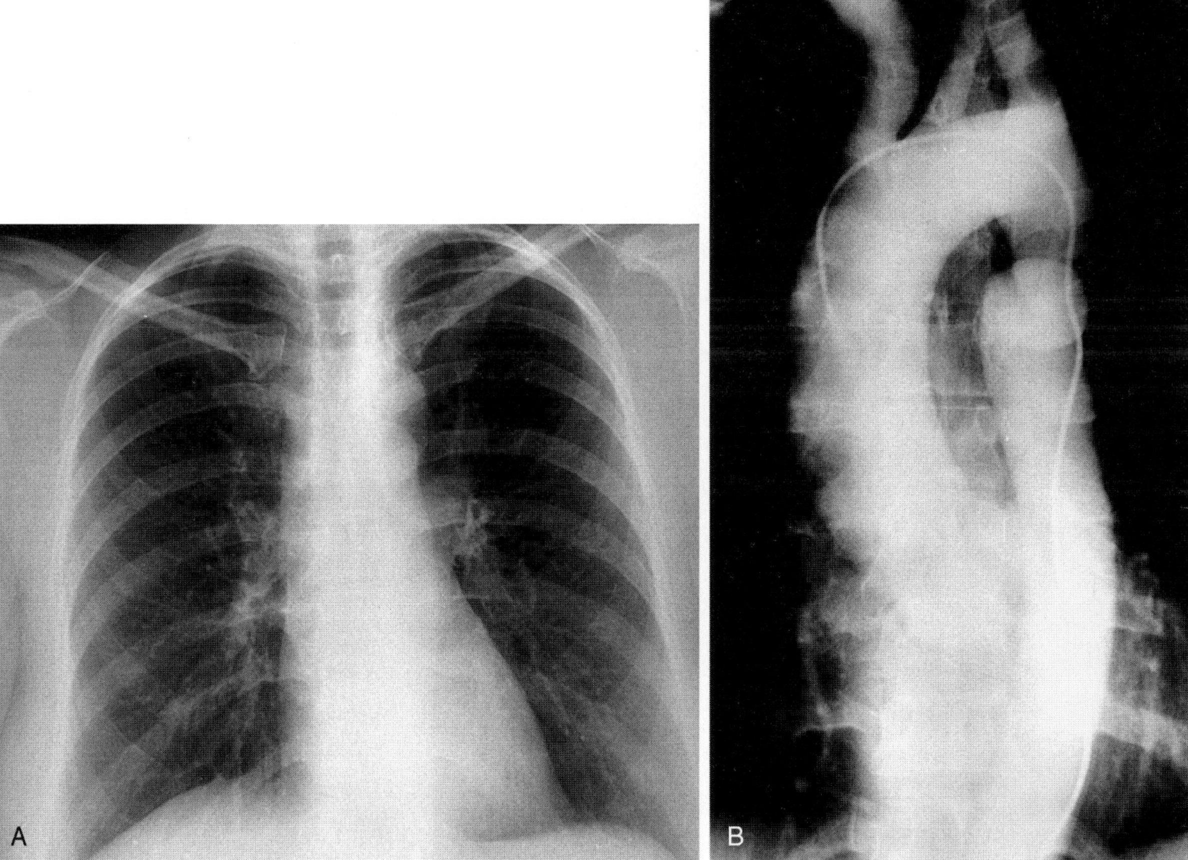

FIGURE 58–24 ■ *A*, A posteroanterior radiograph of a 39-year-old woman shows a left upper middle mediastinal mass. *B*, An aortogram shows a pseudocoarctation with elongation and bucking distal to the left subclavian artery.

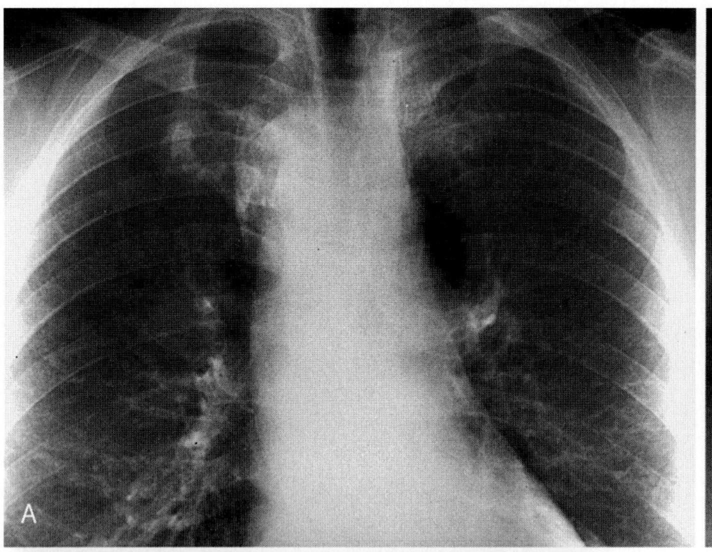

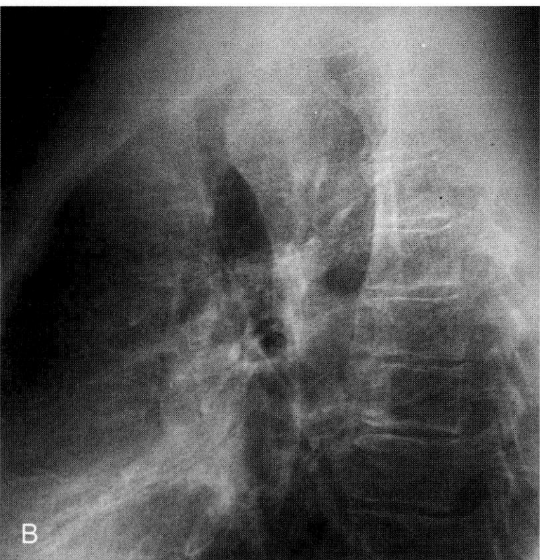

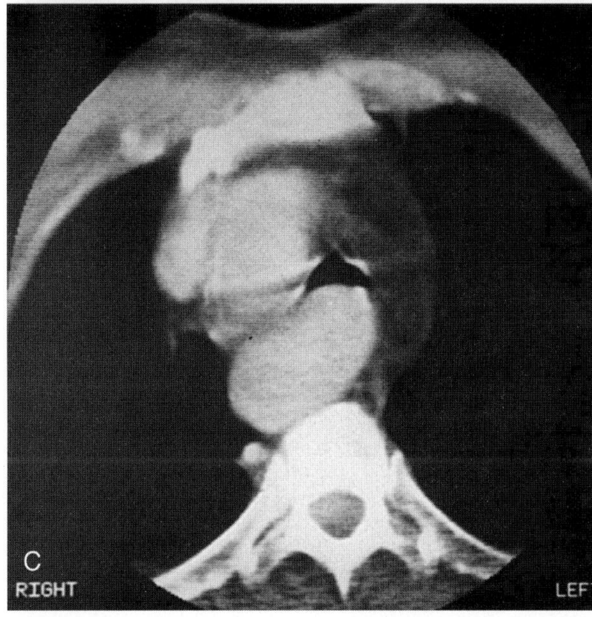

FIGURE 58–25 ■ A 52-year-old man with right aortic arch. Posteroanterior *(A)* and lateral *(B)* chest radiographs show the right aortic arch indenting the right lateral and posterior wall of the trachea. *C*, A computed tomography scan shows the right arch. The posterior wall of the trachea is indented by the arch and the dilated origin of an aberrant left subclavian artery.

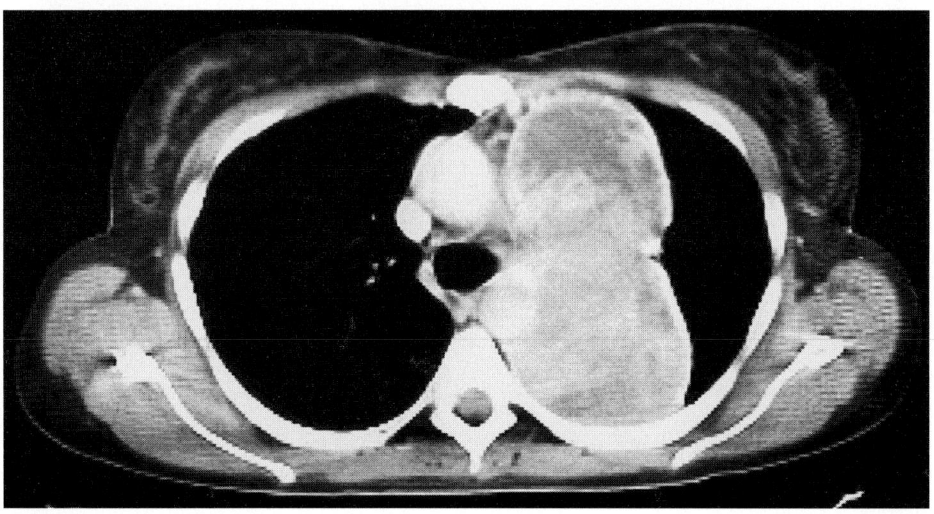

FIGURE 58–26 ■ A computed tomography scan of a 41-year-old woman with left chest pain and cough shows a large tumor mass of inhomogeneous density (necrosis) occupying the left side of the mediastinum. Other scans showed separate pleural nodules. Left thoracotomy revealed an unresectable neurogenic sarcoma.

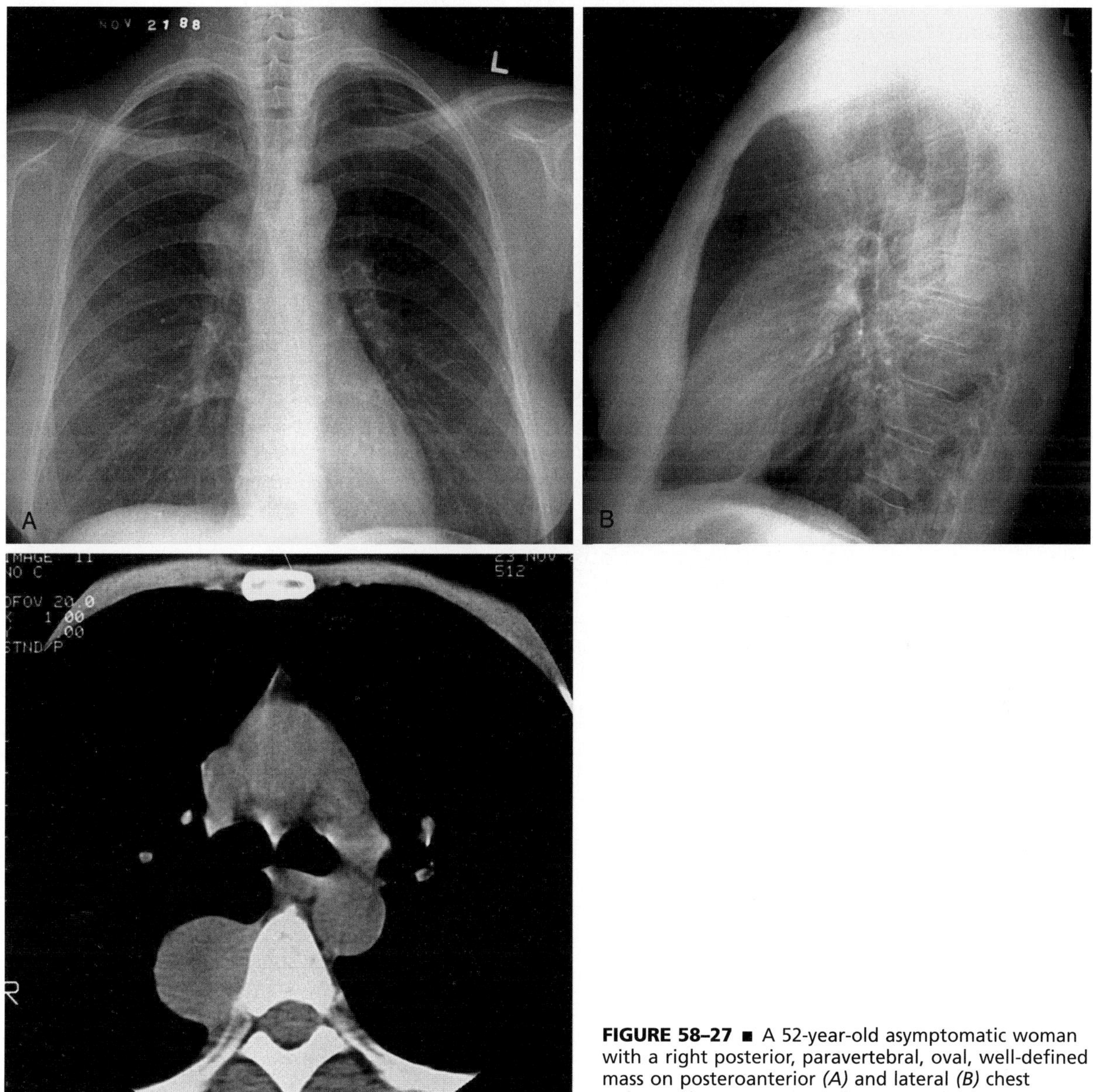

FIGURE 58–27 ■ A 52-year-old asymptomatic woman with a right posterior, paravertebral, oval, well-defined mass on posteroanterior *(A)* and lateral *(B)* chest radiographs. *C*, A computed tomography scan shows the typical location of the neurofibroma.

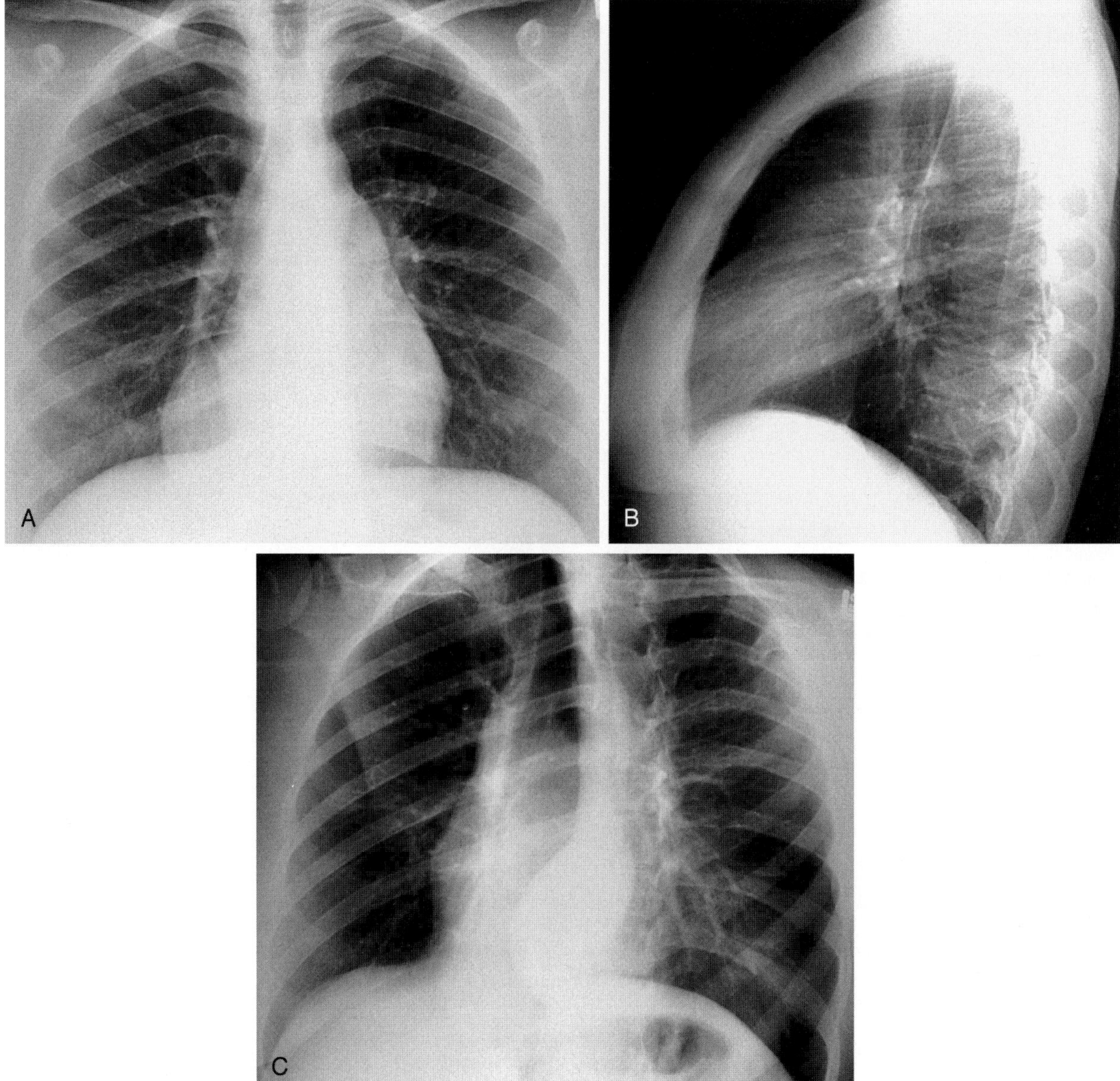

FIGURE 58–28 ■ *A*, A posteroanterior chest radiograph of a 20-year-old asymptomatic woman with a right, lower posterior, paravertebral mediastinal mass. *B*, The mass is poorly seen on the lateral radiograph. *C*, Left anterior oblique radiograph shows the typical, well-defined, elongated shape of the mass making obtuse angles with the mediastinum.

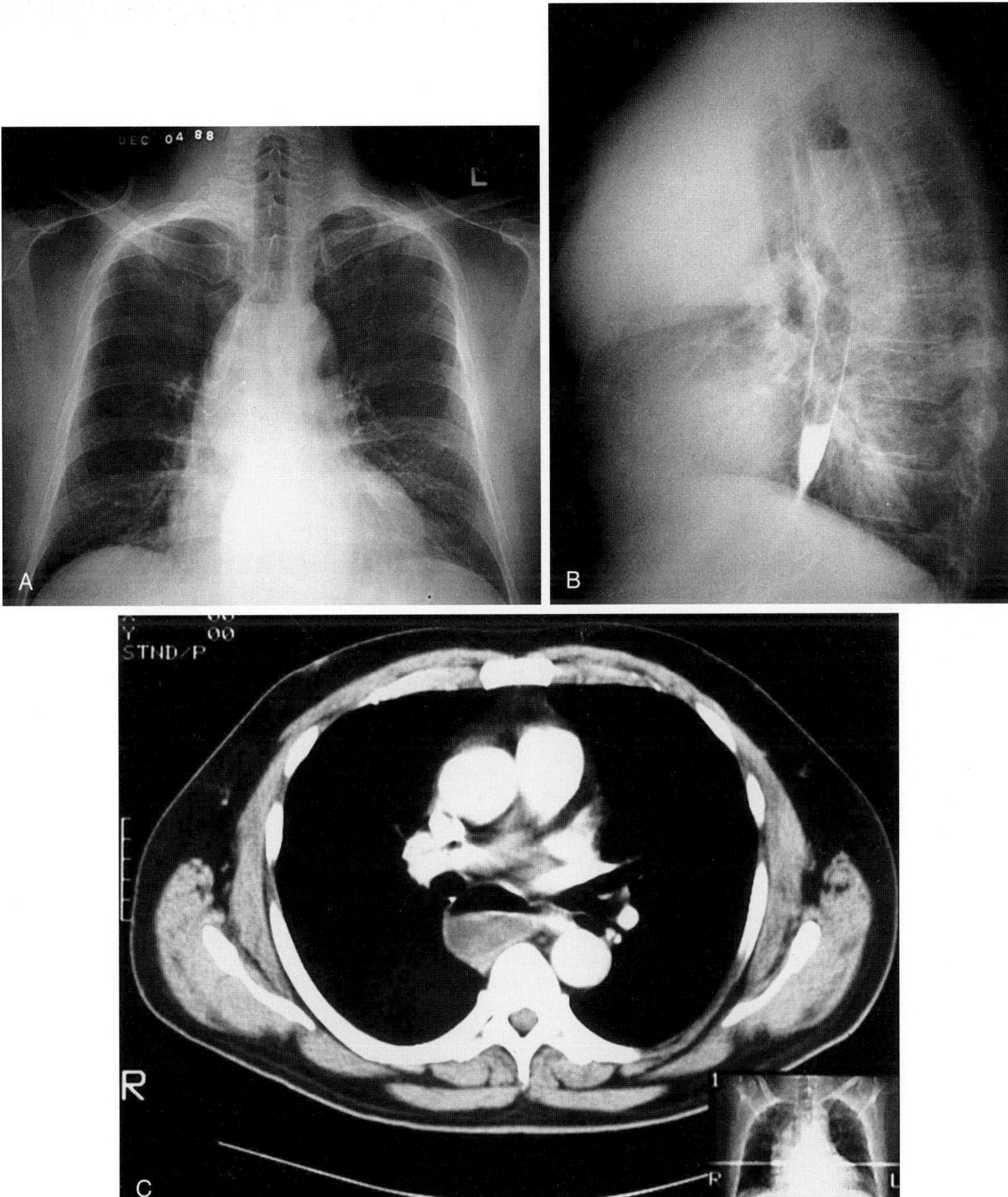

FIGURE 58–29 ■ A 53-year-old man with iron deficiency anemia. Posteroanterior *(A)* and lateral *(B)* chest radiographs show a posterior mediastinal mass adjacent to the barium sulfate–filled esophagus. A short air-fluid level is noted in its upper portion. *C*, A computed tomography scan shows the cystic mass with air-fluid level, which extended the entire length of the posterior mediastinum into the upper abdomen. Barium examination of the upper gastrointestinal tract showed a communication with the second portion of the duodenum, where a diverticulum-like structure was present. Right thoracotomy and laparotomy removed a duplication cyst running from the neck down to the second portion of the duodenum. The cyst was lined by esophageal epithelium in the chest and gastric epithelium in the abdomen. Ulceration was present, likely producing the iron deficiency anemia.

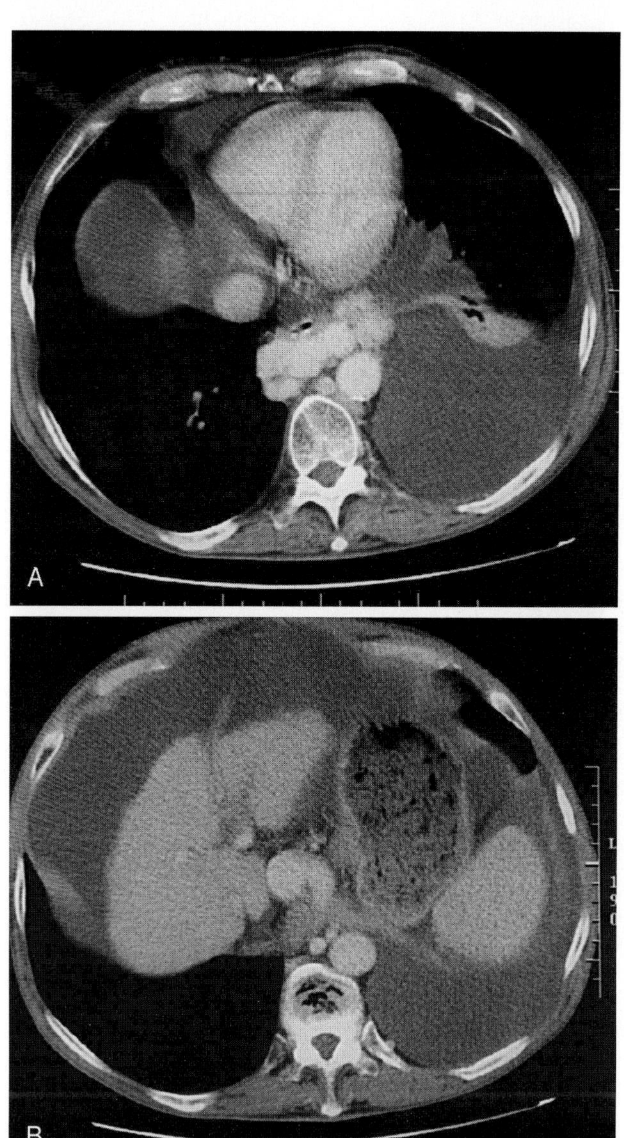

FIGURE 58–30 ■ A 63-year-old man with cirrhosis. *A*, A computed tomography (CT) scan shows enhanced vessels around the lower esophagus indicating paraesophageal varices. Left pleural effusion is present. *B*, The CT scan shows a small cirrhotic liver with ascites.

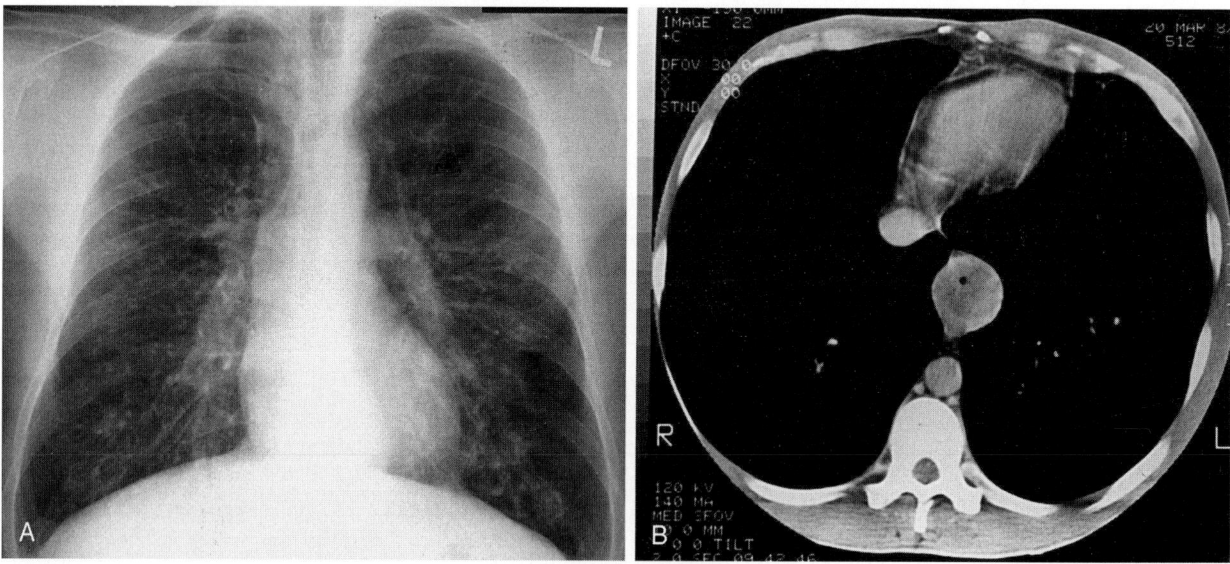

FIGURE 58–31 ■ *A*, A posteroanterior chest radiograph shows a left lower mediastinal retrocardiac mass. *B*, A computed tomography scan shows a well-defined mass in the lower esophagus without invasion of adjacent structures. This proved to be a carcinoma of the lower esophagus.

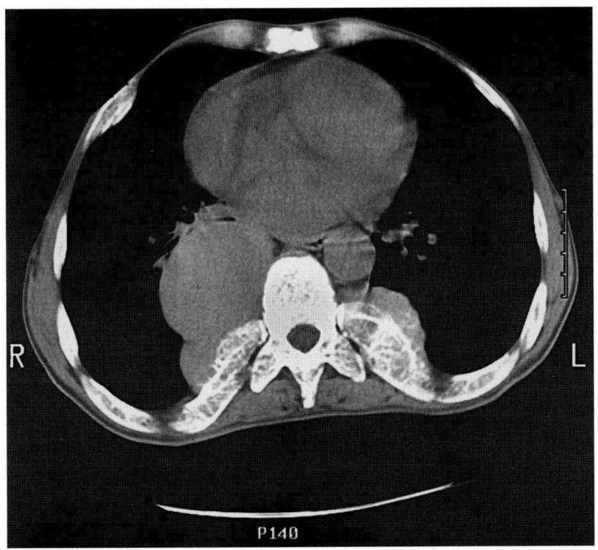

FIGURE 58–32 ■ A 40-year-old man with β-thalassemia and extramedullary hemopoiesis (EMH). A computed tomography scan shows lobulated right and left paravertebral paraosseous masses. The posterior ribs are markedly expanded and osteopenic. These are typical signs of EMH.

atic pseudocyst (Johnston et al, 1986), extramedullary hematopoiesis (Fig. 58–32) (Ross and Logan, 1969), and meningocele (Edeiken et al, 1969).

COMMENTS AND CONTROVERSIES

Weisbrod and Herman have provided an excellent review of imaging capability in evaluating mediastinal masses. The lack of commentary regarding positron emission tomography (PET) imaging reflects the lack of experience with this modality in their institution. PET imaging is covered in detail in Chapter 21. Ultrasound has been of some value in the evaluation of anterior mediastinal lesions, particularly for the purpose of needle biopsy guidance.

This commentator would disagree with a number of points made by Weisbrod and Herman in the discussion of thymoma. Traditionally it has been felt that malignancy of thymoma was judged by the operative findings. However, it has become obvious that a number of patients with Masaoka stage II lesions have that descriptor assigned on the basis of pathologic examination of the resected specimen demonstrating microscopic invasion of the thymic capsule. In our experience, far fewer than one third of patients with thymoma have symptoms of local compression or invasion of adjacent structures. Such symptoms are exceedingly uncommon. Patients with thymoma having no evidence of myasthenia gravis are usually asymptomatic.

G. A. P.

REFERENCES

Baron RL, Lee JKT, Sagel SS et al: Computed tomography of the abnormal thymus. Radiology 142:127, 1982a.

Baron RL, Lee JKT, Sagel SS et al: Computed tomography of the normal thymus. Radiology 142:121, 1982b.

Baron RL, Levitt RG, Sagel SS et al: Computed tomography in the evaluation of mediastinal widening. Radiology 138:107, 1981a.

Baron RL, Sagel SS, Baglan RJ: Thymic cysts following radiation therapy for Hodgkin's disease. Radiology 141:593, 1981b.

Bashist B, Ellis K, Gold RP: Computed tomography of intrathoracic goiters. AJR Am J Roentgenol 140:455, 1983.

Batra P, Herrman C, Mulder D: Mediastinal imaging in myasthenia gravis: Correlation of chest radiography, CT, MR, and surgical findings. AJR Am J Roentgenol 148:515, 1987.

Bechtold RE, Wolfman NT, Karstaedt N et al: Superior vena caval obstruction: Detection using CT. Radiology 157:485, 1985.

Birnberg FA, Webb WR, Selch MT et al: Thymic carcinoid tumors with hyperparathyroidism. AJR Am J Roentgenol 139:1001, 1982.

Blank N, Castellino RA: The mediastinum in Hodgkin's and nonHodgkin's lymphomas. J Thorac Imaging 2:66, 1987.

Blomlie V, Lien HH, Fossa SD et al: Computed tomography in primary nonseminomatous germ cell tumors of the mediastinum. Acta Radiol 29:289, 1988.

Brown LR, Aughenbaugh GL, Wick MR et al: Roentgenologic diagnosis of primary corticotropin-producing carcinoid tumors of the mediastinum. Radiology 142:143, 1982.

Brown LR, Muhm JR, Aughenbaugh GL et al: Computed tomography of benign mature teratomas of the mediastinum. J Thorac Imaging 2:66, 1987.

Brown LR, Muhm JR, Gray JE: Radiographic detection of thymoma. AJR Am J Roentgenol 134:1181, 1980.

Brown LR, Muhm JR, Sheedy PF et al: The value of computed tomography in myasthenia gravis. AJR Am J Roentgenol 140:31, 1983.

Carmosino L, Dibenedetto A, Feffer S: Thymic hyperplasia following successful chemotherapy: A report of two cases and review of the literature. Cancer 56:1526, 1985.

Chen J, Weisbrod GL, Herman SJ: Computed tomography and pathologic correlations of thymic lesions. J Thorac Imaging 3:61, 1988.

Choyke PL, Zeman RK, Gootenberg JE et al: Thymic atrophy and regrowth in response to chemotherapy: CT evaluation. AJR Am J Roentgenol 149:269, 1987.

Chung JW, Park JH, Im J-G et al: Spiral CT angiography of the thoracic aorta. Radiographics 16:811, 1996.

Davis JG, Simonton JH: Mediastinal carinal bronchogenic cysts. Radiology 67:391, 1956.

de Geer G, Webb WR, Gamsu G: Normal thymus: Assessment with MR and CT. Radiology 158:313, 1986.

Dresler CM, Patterson GA, Taylor BR et al: Complete foregut duplication. Ann Thorac Surg 50:306, 1990.

Dunne MG, Weksberg AP: Thymic cyst: Computed tomography and ultrasound correlation. J Comput Assist Tomogr 7:351, 1983.

Edeiken J, Lee KF, Libshitz H: Intrathoracic meningocele. AJR Am J Roentgenol 106:381, 1969.

Ellis K, Austin JHM, Jaretzki A: Radiologic detection of thymoma in patients with myasthenia gravis. AJR Am J Roentgenol 151:873, 1988.

Ellis K, Gregg HG: Thymomas-roentgen considerations. AJR Am J Roentgenol 91:105, 1964.

Federle MP, Callen PW: Cystic Hodgkin's lymphoma of the thymus: Computed tomography appearance. J Comput Assist Tomogr 3:542, 1979.

Feigin DS, Fenoglio JJ, McAllister HA et al: Pericardial cysts: A radiologic-pathologic correlation and review. Radiology 125:15, 1977.

Filly R, Blank N, Castellino RA: Radiographic distribution of intrathoracic disease in previously untreated patients with Hodgkin's and non-Hodgkin's lymphoma. Radiology 120:277, 1976.

Fox MA, Vix VA: Endodermal sinus (yolk sac) tumors of the anterior mediastinum. AJR Am J Roentgenol 135:291, 1980.

Francis IR, Glazer GM, Bookstein GL, et al: The thymus: Reexamination of age-related changes in size and shape. AJR Am J Roentgenol 145:249, 1985.

Fraser RG, Pare JAP, Pare PD et al: Diagnosis of Diseases of the Chest, 3rd ed. Philadelphia, WB Saunders, 1989.

Fulcher AS, Proto AV, Jolles H: Cystic teratoma of the mediastinum: Demonstration of fat/fluid level. AJR Am J Roentgenol 154:259, 1990.

Gefter WB, Spritzer CE, Eisenberg B et al: Thyroid imaging with high-field-strength surface-coil MR. Radiology 164:483, 1987.

Glazer GM, Axel L, Moss AA: CT diagnosis of mediastinal thyroid. AJR Am J Roentgenol 138:495, 1982.

Good CA: Roentgenologic findings in myasthenia gravis associated with thymic tumor. AJR Am J Roentgenol 57:305, 1947.

Gouliamos AD, Carter BL, Emami B: Computed tomography of the chest wall. Radiology 134:433, 1980.

Hammond DI: Giant lymph node hyperplasia of the posterior mediastinum. J Can Assoc Radiol 30:256, 1979.

Heiberg E, Wolverson MK, Sunaram M, et al: Normal thymus: CT characteristics in subjects under age 20. AJR Am J Roentgenol 138:491, 1982.

Higgins CB, McNamara MT, Fisher MR et al: MR imaging of the thyroid. AJR Am J Roentgenol 147:1255, 1986.

Hopper KD, Diehl LF, Cole BA et al: The significance of necrotic mediastinal lymph nodes on CT in patients with newly diagnosed Hodgkin's disease. AJR Am J Roentgenol 155:267, 1990.

Ingels GW, Campbell DC Jr, Giampetro AM et al: Malignant schwannomas of the mediastinum: Report of 2 cases and review of the literature. Cancer 27:1190, 1971.

Johnston RH Jr, Owensby LC, Vargas GM et al: Pancreatic pseudocyst of the mediastinum. Ann Thorac Surg 41:210, 1986.

Jonsson K, Rian RL: Pseudotumoral esophageal varices associated with portal hypertension. Radiology 97:593, 1970.

Katlic MR, Wang C, Grillo HC: Substernal goiter. Ann Thorac Surg 39:391, 1985.

Kissin CM, Husband JE, Nicholas D et al: Benign thymic enlargement in adults after chemotherapy: CT demonstration. Radiology 163:67, 1987.

Kuhlman JE, Fishman EK, Wang KP et al: Mediastinal cysts: Diagnosis by CT and needle aspiration. AJR Am J Roentgenol 150:75, 1988.

Kuhlman JE, Fishman EK, Wang KP et al: Esophageal duplication cyst: CT and transesophageal needle aspiration. AJR Am J Roentgenol 145:531, 1985.

Lautin EM, Rosenblatt M, Friedman AC et al: Calcification in nonHodgkin's lymphoma occurring before therapy: Identification on plain films and CT. AJR Am J Roentgenol 155:739, 1990.

Lee KS, Im J, Han CH et al: Malignant primary germ cell tumors of the mediastinum: CT features. AJR Am J Roentgenol 153:947, 1989.

Levitt RG, Husband JE, Glazer HS: CT of primary germ-cell tumors of the mediastinum. AJR Am J Roentgenol 142:73, 1984.

Lindell MM Jr, Hill CA, Libshitz HI: Oesophageal cancer: Radiographic chest findings and their prognostic significance. AJR Am J Roentgenol 133:461, 1979.

Lindfors KK, Meyer JE, Dedrick CG et al: Thymic cysts in mediastinal Hodgkin disease. Radiology 156:37, 1985.

Marin ML, Romney BM, Franco K et al: Bronchogenic cyst: A case report emphasizing the role of magnetic resonance imaging. J Thorac Imaging 6:43, 1991.

Mendelson DS, Rose JS, Efremidis SC et al: Bronchogenic cysts with high CT numbers. AJR Am J Roentgenol 140:463, 1983.

Modic MT, Janicki PC: Computed tomography of mass lesions of the right cardiophrenic angle. J Comput Assist Tomogr 4:521, 1980.

Moore AV, Korobkin M, Olanow W et al: Age-related changes in the thymus gland: CT-pathologic correlation. AJR Am J Roentgenol 141:241, 1983.

Moore AV, Korobkin M, Powers B et al: Thymoma detection by mediastinal CT: Patients with myasthenia gravis. AJR Am J Roentgenol 138:217, 1982.

Mori K, Eguchi K, Moriyama H et al: Computed tomography of anterior mediastinal tumors: Differentiation between thymoma and germ cell tumor. Acta Radiol 28:395, 1987.

Noma S, Kanaoka M, Minami S et al: Thyroid masses: MR imaging and pathologic correlation. Radiology 168:759, 1988.

Noma S, Nishimura K, Togashi K et al: Thyroid gland: MR imaging. Radiology 164:495, 1987.

Paling MR, Williamson BRJ: Epipericardial fat pad: CT findings. Radiology 165:335, 1987.

Park H, Tarver RD, Siddiqui AR et al: Efficacy of thyroid scintigraphy in the diagnosis of intrathoracic goiter. AJR Am J Roentgenol 148:527, 1987.

Pearlberg JL, Sandler MA, Talpos GB et al: Computed tomographic evaluation of intrathoracic thyroid malignancy. Comput Med Imaging Graph 13:411, 1989.

Picus D, Balfe DM, Koehler RE et al: Computed tomography in the staging of esophageal carcinoma. Radiology 146:433, 1983.

Press GA, Glazer HS, Wasserman TH et al: Thoracic wall involvement by Hodgkin's disease and non-Hodgkin lymphoma: CT evaluation. Radiology 157:195, 1985.

Pugatch RD, Braver JH, Robbins AH et al: CT diagnosis of pericardial cysts. AJR Am J Roentgenol 131:515, 1978.

Quint LE, Francis IR, Williams DM et al: Evaluation of thoracic aortic disease with the use of helical CT and multiplanar reconstructions: Comparison with surgical findings. Radiology 201:37, 1996.

Radecki PD, Arger PH, Arenson RL et al: Thyroid imaging: Comparison of high-resolution real-time ultrasound and computed tomography. Radiology 153:145, 1984.

Reed JC, Hallet KK, Feigin DS: Neural tumors of the thorax: Subject review from the AFIP. Radiology 126:9, 1978.

Reed JC, Sobonya RE: Morphologic analysis of foregut cysts in the thorax. AJR Am J Roentgenol 120:851, 1974.

Ross P, Logan W: Roentgen findings in extramedullary hematopoiesis. AJR Am J Roentgenol 106:604, 1969.

Shin MS, Ho K: Computed tomography of primary mediastinal seminomas. J Comput Assist Tomogr 7:990, 1983a.

Shin MS, Ho K: Diffuse thymic hyperplasia following chemotherapy for nodular sclerosing Hodgkin's disease: An immunologic rebound phenomenon? Cancer 51:30, 1983b.

Shuford WH, Sybers RG, Edwards FK: The three types of right aortic arch. AJR Am J Roentgenol 109:67, 1970.

Silverman PM, Newman GE, Korobkin M et al: Computed tomography in the evaluation of thyroid disease. AJR Am J Roentgenol 141:897, 1984.

Spizarny DL, Shepard JO, McLoud TC: CT of adenoid cystic carcinoma of the trachea. AJR Am J Roentgenol 146:1129, 1986.

Suzuki M, Takashima T, Itoh H et al: Computed tomography of mediastinal teratomas. J Comput Assist Tomogr 7:74, 1983.

Theros KG: RPC of the month from the AFIP. Radiology 93:677, 1969.

Thorvinger B, Lyttkens K, Samuelsson L: Computed tomography of the thymus gland in myasthenia gravis. Acta Radiol 28:399, 1987.

Weinstein JB, Aronberg DJ, Sagel SS: CT of fibrosing mediastinitis: Findings and their utility. AJR Am J Roentgenol 141:247, 1983.

Wychulis AR, Payne WS, Clagett OT et al: Surgical treatment of mediastinal tumors: A 40 year experience. J Thorac Cardiovasc Surg 62:379, 1971.

Yeh H, Gordon A, Kirschner PA et al: Computed tomography and sonography of thymolipoma. AJR Am J Roentgenol 140:1131, 1983.

Yernault J-C, Kuhn G, Dumortier P et al: "Solid" mediastinal bronchogenic cyst: Mineralogic analysis. AJR Am J Roentgenol 146:73, 1986.

Ziter FM Jr, Bramwit DN, Holloman KR et al: Calcified mediastinal bronchogenic cysts. Radiology 93:1025, 1969.

CHAPTER **59**

Infections of the Mediastinum

Maruf A. Razzuk*
Linda M. Razzuk
Susan J. Hoover
Tyron Hoover
Tada Butler
Harold C. Urschel

Infections of the mediastinum evoke an inflammatory response that initially affects the soft tissue components and lymph nodes of the mediastinum.

An inflammatory response caused by gram-stained bacteria could resolve completely at the cellulitic phase or evolve into a destructive exudative process. Infection caused by acid-fast bacteria or certain fungi (when the hilar and mediastinal lymph nodes are involved) induces a granulomatous response that may progress to dense cicatrix, which can cause encroachment and occlusion of visceral structures.

Mediastinitis encompasses a group of acute and chronic entities with heterogeneous clinical and pathologic manifestations. It can be primary, but on the whole, it is secondary to infections originating from a variety of pathologic conditions affecting the esophagus, sternum, oropharynx, neck, spine, lungs, or abdomen. The infecting organisms, in a general way, relate to the etiologic source of mediastinitis. In acute mediastinitis, signs and symptoms usually appear promptly and consist of substernal pain, fever, leukocytosis, subcutaneous emphysema, dysphagia, and dyspnea. If the condition goes untreated, overwhelming sepsis follows, producing prostration and collapse. Early diagnosis and well-directed therapeutic measures, including antimicrobial drugs and appropriate surgical intervention, are paramount in circumventing the morbid outcome. Symptoms of the chronic granulomatous, sclerosing form vary according to the compromised structure, whether superior vena cava, esophagus, airway, or pulmonary vessels.

HISTORICAL NOTE

Since Boerhaave's 1724 report of a fulminant and fateful case of acute mediastinitis (Boerhaave, 1955), this morbid disorder has gained recognition because of its aggressive, bewildering, and often fatal course. The severe, often fatal, mediastinal infections descending via the neck from oropharyngeal abscesses triggered early, diligent research to understand how the infection was spread. The first experiments to study the neck compartments were undertaken in the 19th century in Europe, as has been reviewed by Pearse (1938); early researchers included Bichat in 1801; Henke in 1872; Soltmann, Konig, and Riedle in 1882; Paulsen in 1882; and Schmitt in 1893. Essential facts about cervical fascia and the manner of spread of infection were learned from these experiments. In North America, significant contributions to the delineation of the paths of spread of oropharyngeal and cervical infections to the mediastinum were made by Mosher (1929), Iglauer (1935), Coller and Yglesias (1937), Furstenberg and Yglesias (1937), Pearse (1938), and Grodinsky (1938). Much was learned from those investigations, including the importance of early recognition of the morbid pathology caused by the infection and the value of well-directed surgical intervention to reduce the severity of the outcome by bringing improvement and even cure.

In the preantibiotic era, the acute and chronic forms of mediastinitis were both fairly frequent and associated with enormous complications and a high mortality rate. Keefer (1938) reported the breakdown of a tuberculous lymph node to be the most frequent cause of mediastinitis. Tuberculosis, peritonsillar abscess (quinsy), and Ludwig's angina were listed by Pearse (1938) as the most common forerunners of mediastinitis. Hemolytic streptococci, staphylococci, and tubercle bacilli were the most frequent offending organisms (Howell et al, 1976). Chronic granulomatous fibrous mediastinitis was most commonly caused by tuberculosis, syphilis, actinomycosis, and paragonimiasis (Keefer, 1938). The first reference to mediastinal granulomatous fibrosis was made by Tonnele in 1829, who reported a symptomatic case of mediastinal granuloma and a "fibrous mass." Oulmont in 1856 described mediastinal fibrosis. Olser in 1903 reported the disorder in conjunction with superior vena cava obstruction (Goodwin et al, 1972).

Medical advances in therapeutics have changed the panorama of infectious disease. After Alexander Fleming demonstrated the bactericidal effect of penicillin in 1928, Florey, Chain, and Abraham worked to usher in the era of antibiotics; the crude material of penicillin became available in May 1940 (Ackerknecht, 1973; Mandell and Sande, 1990). Thereafter streptomycin (1944), chloromycetin (1948), and later generations of potent antibiotics and microbicidals were added to the therapeutic armamentarium. This wide spectrum of drugs has altered both

*Deceased.

the incidence and the bacteriologic makeup of mediastinitis. Syphilis is no longer listed as a cause of granulomatous sclerosing mediastinitis (Fry and Shields, 1991). The incidence of tuberculous mediastinitis is down, although a resurgence is appearing in the wake of the acquired immunodeficiency syndrome (AIDS) epidemic (FitzGerald et al, 1991; Nelems, 1995). Medical technology introduced the so-called "altered host"—a patient who receives cytotoxic and immunosuppressive therapy for cancer and organ transplants. These patients have become vulnerable to opportunistic microbes that are usually innocuous or dormant in normal individuals (Lichtenberg, 1989). Fungi that lead to opportunistic infection, such as *Aspergillus fumigatus, Mucor, Candida albicans,* and *Cryptococcus neoformans* (although a primary pathogen), have appeared on the list of etiologic organisms of mediastinitis (Fry and Shields, 1991; Williams et al, 1973).

Technologic advances with the invention of esophageal endoscopy, bougienage, and dilatation have introduced the iatrogenic perforation of the esophagus as a causative factor of acute mediastinitis. The introduction of the flexible endoscope may have made esophagoscopy safer; however, the overall rate of esophageal perforation by instrumentation has remained basically unchanged. Esophagoscopic perforation accounts for less than 0.01% of instrumental perforation, whereas the majority is due to balloon dilatation for achalasia (6%) and bougienage for stricture (1%) (Pett, 1995; Vessal et al, 1975).

The development of both cardiopulmonary bypass and a multitude of cardiac surgical procedures has also contributed to the incidence of mediastinitis resulting from deep sternotomy wound infections.

In an ever-changing medical world, the journey of mediastinitis shall continue to be turbulent, especially as genetic diversification leads to the emergence of antibiotic-resistant bacterial strains.

ANATOMIC CONSIDERATIONS

Knowledge of the anatomy of the fascial spaces connecting the pharynx and neck to the mediastinum is of significant clinical importance. Infection travels along these spaces and should be intercepted and drained there. The spaces lie between layers of fascia and the investing fascia of the muscles, glands, and blood vessels as well. Because the system of fascia and spaces is so intricate, this chapter limits the discussion to the anatomic aspects that relate to the spread of infection.

The Fascia

1. The *superficial fascia.* This area deep to the subcutaneous fascia encircles the neck completely and invests the platysma and sternocleidomastoid and trapezius muscles, then inserts on the spinous processes. Superior to the sternal notch, it splits to form the suprasternal space of Burns.
2. The *middle fascia.* The middle fascia has three layers:
   a) The outer layer, which invests the sternohyoid and omohyoid muscles
   b) The middle layer, which invests the sternothyroid muscle
   c) The visceral layer, which completely surrounds the thyroid gland, trachea, and esophagus

   The two outermost layers invest the strap muscles and fuse laterally with the superficial fascia, which invests the sternocleidomastoid muscle, opposite the carotid sheath.
3. The *posterior fascia.* This is the deepest subdivision of the deep cervical fascia. It consists of two layers:
   a) The alar fascia, which lies posterior to the visceral fascial compartment; it attaches laterally to the transverse processes and then continues laterally to form the carotid sheath
   b) The prevertebral fascia, which fuses laterally with the alar fascia at the transverse processes from the base of the skull down to the coccyx (Grodinsky, 1938) (Fig. 59–1)

Fascial Spaces

The spaces formed by these fasciae include:

1. A cleft between the superficial fascia and the outer layer of the middle fascia (the sternohyoid-omohyoid layer), termed *space 2* by Grodinsky.

2. A second cleft between the outer layer (sternohyoid-omohyoid layer) and the middle layer (sternothyroid layer) of the middle fascia, termed *space 2* by Grodinsky and the *fascial cleft* by Gray (1966) (see Fig. 59–1). The latter clefts are potential spaces and do not communicate with the mediastinum.

3. A space that is well defined for the most part, lying between the sternothyroid fascial layer and the visceral fascia, termed *space 3* by Grodinsky, the *perivisceral fascial cleft* by Gray, and the *previsceral space* by Pearse (1938). This space is the plane used to expose the thyroid gland during surgery. It lies beneath the strap muscles. Anteriorly, this space extends from the thyroid cartilage to the upper border of the aortic arch (level of fourth thoracic vertebra), where it terminates by adhesions extending from the fibrous pericardium to the posterior surface of the manubrium sterni. These fibrous adhesions form a relative barrier to the downward gravitational spread of infection into the anterior mediastinum (Furstenberg, 1939). Posteriorly, it stretches from the base of the skull down to a level between the sixth cervical and fourth thoracic vertebrae, where it ends (Fig. 59–2). Anteriorly, it is continuous across the midline but terminates laterally by adhesions between the alar fascia and the visceral fascia around the inferior thyroid arteries. Posteriorly, the space becomes attenuated by adhesions between the visceral and alar fasciae (Grodinsky, 1938) (see Fig. 59–1).

The visceral compartment, called the *visceral* or *tracheoesophageal space* or *compartment,* contains the thyroid gland, trachea, and esophagus, each with its own thin fascial capsule. All are enclosed by the visceral fascia. The compartment extends from the larynx to the tracheal bifurcation (level of T4 vertebrae) (see Fig. 59–2). The pretracheal space is a potential space. It is open during mediastinoscopy, thyroid surgery, and tracheostomy, and in perforating wounds of the trachea. Should an infection occur or reach these spaces, it is likely to gravitate into the mediastinum.

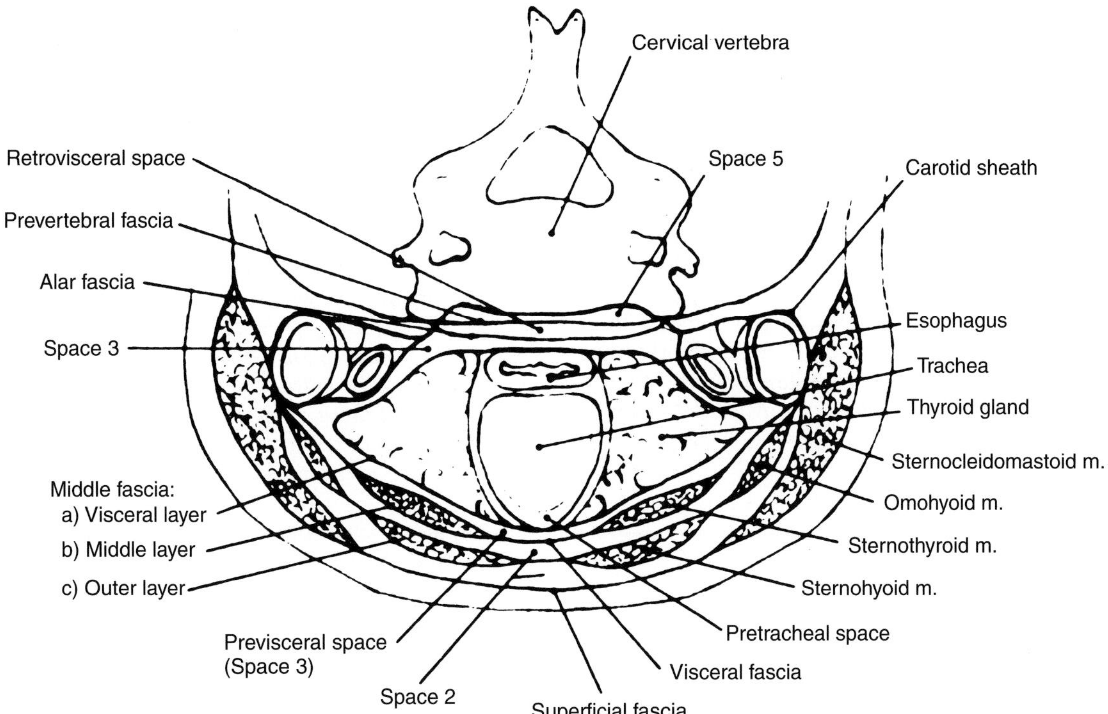

FIGURE 59–1 ■ Diagram of the fasciae of the neck. Transverse section at the level of the sixth cervical vertebra. (From Grodinsky M, Holyoke EA: The fasciae and fascial spaces of the head, neck and adjacent regions. Am J Anat 63:367, 1938.)

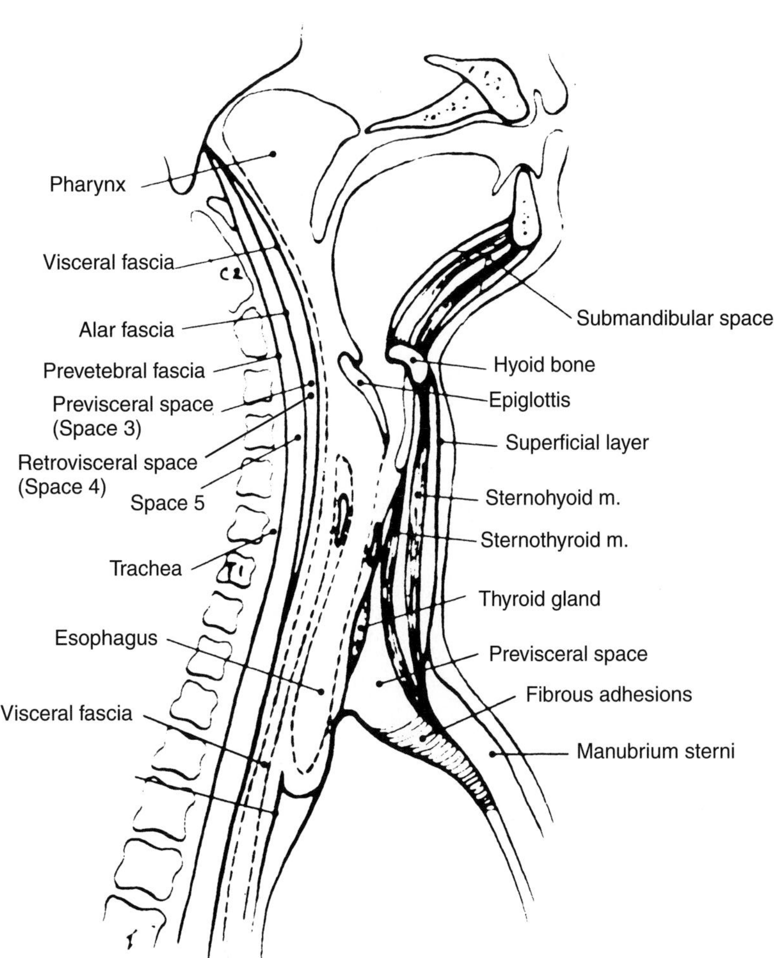

FIGURE 59–2 ■ Diagram of the fasciae and spaces of the head, neck, and mediastinum in midsagittal section. (From Grodinsky M, Holyoke EA: The fasciae and fascial spaces of the head, neck and adjacent regions. Am J Anat 63:367, 1938.)

lies an important space referred to as the "danger space" because of its relation to the posterior mediastinum. It has been termed *space 4* by Grodinsky, *the retrovisceral space* by Pearse, and *the retropharyngeal fascial* cleft by Gray. It extends from the base of the skull through the neck and posterior mediastinum down to the diaphragm. It seals off laterally at the transverse processes (see Figs. 59–1 and 59–2).

5. Between the prevertebral fascia and the vertebral bodies lies a potential space *(space 5)* that extends from the base of the skull to the coccyx laterally and to the transverse processes bilaterally (Grodinsky, 1938) (see Figs. 59–1 and 59–2). Vertebral infections can involve this space.

Spaces of the Oropharynx

The pertinent spaces include:

1. *Lateral pharyngeal space.* This space is bounded by the tonsil and pharynx medially, the parotid gland posterolaterally, the mandible anterolaterally, the carotid sheath posteriorly, and the submaxillary gland anteriorly (Fig. 59–3). It does not communicate with the carotid sheath, as was reported by Coller and Yglesias (1937). It does, however, communicate with the submandibular space on one side and the previsceral space (space 3) on the other side (Grodinsky, 1938).
2. *Submandibular space.* This space includes the region of the submental and submaxillary triangles lying between the floor of the mouth and the superficial layer of the deep fascia. The spaces between the layers of the investing fasciae of the muscles of this region (the sublingual and submaxillary spaces) make up the submandibular space, which communicates with the lateral pharyngeal space (Grodinsky, 1938) (see Fig. 59–3).

The Fascial Anatomy and the Spread of Infection

The fascial planes fail to confine certain infections with virulent organisms, which can freely spread along fascial spaces and through fascial planes (Stuteville, 1958). Although the fascial planes do not pose an inviolate barrier to the spread of infection, nonetheless they influence the early spread of infection and are important to an understanding of both the evolution of signs and symptoms and the planning of treatment (Payne and Larson, 1969).

The lateral pharyngeal space is a relay for infections originating in the dental and alveolar borders of the mandible, parotid gland, tonsils (peritonsillar abscess or "quinsy"), and cellulitis of the sublingual and submaxillary spaces (Ludwig's angina). Infections in these areas can make their way to the lateral pharyngeal space and the connecting previsceral space. Infection in the previsceral space may spread down the neck and into the anterior mediastinum, or may break through the alar fascia to reach the danger space (the retrovisceral space) that leads to the posterior mediastinum and retroperitoneum (see Figs. 59–1 and 59–2).

CLASSIFICATION

A classification of mediastinal infections was previously advanced by Neuhof (1936). He grouped them into nonsuppurative and suppurative, with the latter subdivided into a localized form, given the term "mediastinal ab-

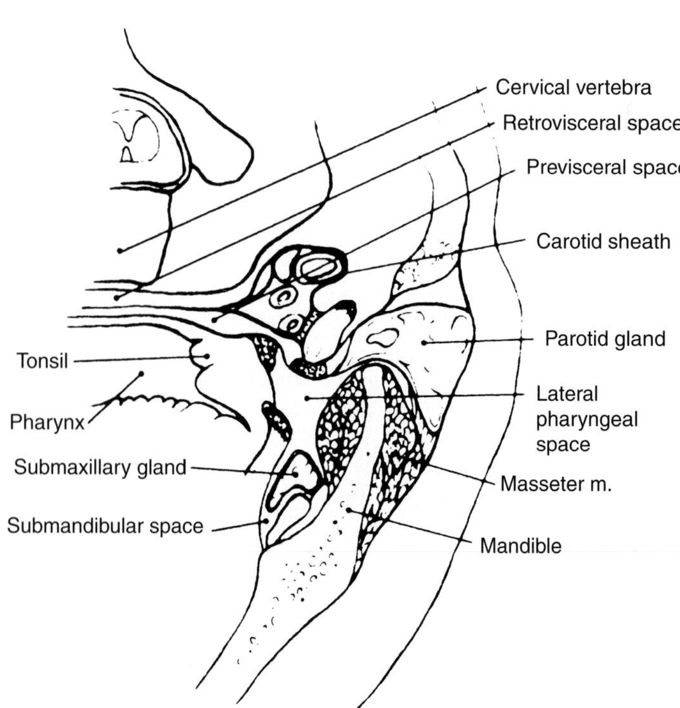

FIGURE 59–3 ■ Transverse section through the tongue and the palatine tonsil. (From Grodinsky M, Holyoke EA: The fasciae and fascial spaces of the head, neck and adjacent regions. Am J Anat 63:367, 1938.)

scess," and a diffuse form termed "phlegmonous mediastinitis." Additional descriptive terms—necrotizing mediastinitis (Cogan, 1973) and descending necrotizing mediastinitis (Estrera et al, 1983)—alluded to a form of suppurative infection of the mediastinum originating from primary infection in the oropharynx.

It is difficult to classify acute mediastinitis morphologically. The morphologic changes associated with acute mediastinitis are neither fully characteristic of the disorder nor diagnostic of the specific etiology. In contrast to the diversity of microorganisms that may evoke mediastinitis, the patterns of tissue response to these organisms are limited. At the microscopic level, many pathogens produce identical morphologic patterns, and only a few features are unique to each organism. Although pyogenic organisms produce suppurative inflammation, organisms that secrete strong toxins induce necrotizing inflammation, wherein cellular necrosis is the dominant feature and exudate is relatively limited.

In chronic mediastinitis, morphologic patterns of granulomatous lesions can be distinctive in *Mycobacterium tuberculosis*, *Histoplasma capsulatum*, and *Coccidioides immitis*. However, in the scarring stage, the morphologic changes are nonspecific.

Mediastinitis can be classified into:

I. Infectious
   A. Acute
      1. Suppurative
         a. Localized (abscess formation)
         b. Compartmentalized
      2. "Synergistic necrotizing"
   B. Chronic
      1. Granulomatous—fibrosing
      2. End-stage sclerosing fibrosis
II. Idiopathic, seen in association with retroperitoneal fibrosis, Riedel's struma, or sclerosing cholangitis (Ewing and Hardy, 1991)
III. Pharmacologic, seen in response to methysergide (a serotonin antagonist used in the treatment of migraine) (Ewing and Hardy, 1991)

The diagnosis of mediastinitis in its acute form is made on the basis of the clinical course, the gross pathologic findings, the extent of involvement of the mediastinal compartments, and the bacteriologic makeup. In granulomatous mediastinitis, morphologic changes and serologic findings can be helpful in establishing a diagnosis. In this presentation, only the infectious categories of mediastinitis are discussed.

ACUTE MEDIASTINITIS

Acute mediastinitis can be primary or secondary. However, the overwhelming majority of cases are secondary to infections originating from other sources.

Primary mediastinitis is quite rare (Pett, 1995). It can occur spontaneously (Feldman and Gromisch, 1971) or in association with pharyngitis (Enquist et al, 1976), epiglottitis (Thaler et al, 1986), pneumonia (Feldman and Gromisch, 1971; Pane et al, 1983), or bronchitis and pericarditis (Pearse, 1938). The infection can become self-limited and heal with complete resolution. In some cases, however, it may ascend into the neck, dissect the broad ligament of the lung, move beneath the visceral pleura, or move into the substance of the lung and through the bronchus (Feldman and Gromisch, 1971).

Secondary mediastinitis constitutes the statistical majority of mediastinal infections.

Incidence

In the preantibiotic era (prior to 1940), acute mediastinitis was not uncommon. An incidence of 15% was reported.

Current literature describes the frequency of acute mediastinitis as "uncommon," without statistical data to vouch for this conclusion. Advances in medical therapeutics and health care have decreased the frequency of some etiologies of mediastinitis, such as tuberculosis and oropharyngeal infection. On the other hand, however, technologic advances have increased the incidence of sternal wound infection and mediastinitis as the result of the proliferation of cardiac operations performed with cardiopulmonary bypass. AIDS and immunosuppression have revived tuberculosis and certain fungal infections. How these opposing trends of medical advances fare with the incidence of mediastinitis and what the overall incidence is remain undetermined.

Etiologic Factors

Secondary infection of the mediastinum may originate from many different sources, including esophageal disruption; infections of sternotomy wound, oropharynx and neck, lung and pleura, subphrenic abscess, or rib and vertebra; blunt and penetrating trauma; and metastatic infections from distant sources (Ewing and Hardy, 1991; Payne and Larson, 1969; Pett, 1995) (Table 59–1).

Although esophageal disruption accounts for the majority of mediastinal infections, not every esophageal perforation leads to mediastinitis. Puncture perforations usually heal spontaneously. Large tears require surgical intervention (Pett, 1995). Leaks secondary to slow esophageal erosion by a foreign body are likely to get walled off by an inflammatory reaction, without the development of invasive mediastinitis (Nashef et al, 1992). The lack of an investing serosal layer of the esophageal wall aggravates the extravasation of bacteria, bile, digestive juices, and enzymes into the mediastinum in cases of esophageal perforation (Kim-Deobald and Kozarek, 1992).

The median sternotomy incision initially proposed by Julian and associates in 1957 for use in open intracardiac procedures has become the incision of choice for most such procedures. A collective review by McClelland (1998) on deep sternotomy wound infection and mediastinitis between 1984 and 1996 showed an incidence ranging from 0.3% to 5%. In one series of this review with an incidence of deep sternotomy wound infection of 0.46%, the mortality rate was 11%.

The incidence of major upper and lower respiratory tract infections has declined as a result of antibiotics and mouth hygiene awareness. Consequently, respiratory tract infections have become rare causes of mediastinitis (Payne and Larson, 1969). Oropharyngeal infections such

TABLE 59–1 ■ Etiologic Factors in Acute Mediastinitis

Esophageal Perforation
Iatrogenic
Balloon dilatation (for achalasia)
Bougienage (for peptic stricture)
Esophagoscopy
Sclerotherapy (for variceal bleeding)
Spontaneous
Postemetic (Boerhaave's syndrome)
Straining during:
Elimination
Weight lifting
Seizure
Pregnancy
Childbirth
Ingestion of Foreign Bodies
Trauma
Blunt
Penetrating
Postsurgical
Infection
Anastomotic leak
Erosion by cancer
Deep Sternotomy Wound Infection
Oropharynx and Neck Infections
Ludwig's Angina
Quinsy
Retropharyngeal Abscess
Cellulitis and Suppurative Lymphadenitis of Neck
Infections of Lung and Pleura
Subphrenic Abscess
Rib or Vertebral Osteomyelitis
Hematogenous or Metastatic Abscesses

as Ludwig's angina, quinsy, and retropharyngeal abscess arouse considerable anxiety. The seriousness of these infections stems from their tendency to spread along the fascial planes and invade the mediastinum, causing morbid necrotizing mediastinitis.

Currently, subphrenic and retroperitoneal infections, osteomyelitis of spine or ribs, and metastatic infections seldom play a role in the causation of mediastinitis.

Immunosuppression and AIDS are promoting a new combination of infectious processes. Acute mediastinitis secondary to a chest wall pyogenic infection has been reported in young heroin addicts seropositive for human immunodeficiency virus (HIV) (Dreyfuss et al, 1992).

The Classification of Acute Mediastinitis

Acute mediastinitis is subdivided into:

1. Suppurative
   a. Localized (abscess formation)
   b. Compartmentalized
2. "Synergistic necrotizing"

The difference between the two subdivisions is relative and a matter of degree, especially in the clinical features, course, and therapeutic approaches. However, the pathologic changes, the pathogenesis, and the bacteriologic makeup exhibit differential features.

Pathology and Pathogenesis

The pathologic changes of acute mediastinitis are mandated by the makeup and virulence of the infecting organisms, the host's immune status, and associated risk factors.

The pathogens evoke identical reaction patterns, and few of the features are unique to or pathognomonic of each organism. For this reason, at the microscopic level, no specific features clearly distinguish between the suppurative and necrotizing forms of acute mediastinitis. Qualitatively, the gross pathologic changes induced by the infection are somewhat similar. Both forms exhibit tissue destruction, manifesting as a combination of exudate and necrosis. However, the basic difference is quantitative. In suppurative mediastinitis, there is an abundance of purulent exudate and significant liquefactive necrosis, which is equivalent to pus. In the necrotizing form, necrosis is the dominant feature, with a relatively small exudative component. The latter findings have also been observed by Cogan (1973). The extent of tissue destruction and host response depends on the organisms involved, the host resistance, and risk factors (Samuelson, 1999).

Poststernotomy mediastinitis is an example of suppurative mediastinitis. It is characterized by the presence of abundant amounts of pus. It tends to remain compartmentally localized. Necrosis of tissue does occur, but it is liquefaction necrosis that turns the tissue into pus. Pyogenic staphylococci are preponderant, although *E. coli, Serratia,* and *Candida* can be present.

Mediastinitis secondary to esophageal perforation is pathologically and bacteriologically similar to that resulting from a descending oropharyngeal infection. In both, the infection does not remain limited to a compartment; rather, the tissue planes are violated by a rapid necrotizing process, wherein there is extensive necrosis that quantitatively supersedes the purulent component. The morbidity of the descending infection is featured by the spread of the infection to the danger space, the retrovisceral space. Esophageal perforation as well may lead to mediastinal infection that also can violate fascial planes and spaces and reach the retrovisceral space. Moreover, in both conditions, the bacterial makeup has similarities: both have gram-positive aerobic and anaerobic bacteria. The coexistence of these two bacterial components initiates synergistic infection, which is essential for the rapid necrotizing process (Stone and Martin, 1972). We offer the term "synergistic necrotizing mediastinitis" to describe both etiologies of mediastinitis—that is, the descending source and the esophageal source.

The mediastinal infection can localize as an abscess or it can become diffuse, or both may coexist at times (Neuhof, 1936). Abscesses can involve the anterior mediastinum, the posterior mediastinum, or both depending on the source of the infection, its virulence, the mixture of organisms, and synergism.

The anterior mediastinal abscess, if uncontrolled, tends to extend upward, projecting in the space of Burns, or it may gravitate downward, causing tenderness in the xiphoid area (Keefer, 1938). The most common cause of anterior mediastinal abscess is deep sternotomy wound infection; a less frequent cause is extension of pharyngeal and neck infections.

Abscess in the posterior mediastinum is more frequent than in the anterior space, with esophageal perforation being the most common cause. Other causes of posterior mediastinal abscess include extension of infection from the oropharynx, spine, lung pleura, or abdominal cavity. The abscess may extend and expand, predisposing patients to symptomatic compression of the mediastinal structure. The most common symptoms of posterior mediastinal abscess are pain, dysphagia, cough, and dyspnea. The pain occurs most often on swallowing and coughing, and is felt posteriorly in the interscapular region or may radiate anteriorly. The symptoms are due to encroachment on the esophagus and trachea in the upper part of the chest (Keefer, 1938). In diffuse mediastinitis involving the posterior mediastinum, there is an increased coexistence of pericarditis and bilateral exudative pleuritis (Neuhof, 1936).

Bacteriology

The etiologic source of acute mediastinitis relates in a general way to the floral makeup of the infecting organisms. In the preantibiotic era, hemolytic streptococci, staphylococci, and tubercle bacilli were the most frequently cultured organisms in cases of mediastinitis (Keefer, 1938). In recent times, however, there has been increased awareness of the frequency of anaerobic infections and the role of anaerobic bacteria in causing "synergistic necrotizing cellulitis." This cellulitic response is produced by symbiosis between aerobic and anaerobic bacteria. The condition is associated with extensive muscle necrosis in the absence of comparable cutaneous damage or major vascular embarrassment (Stone and Martin, 1972).

Necrotizing fasciitis (Wilson, 1952) is a rapid necrotizing process known also as Meleney's streptococcal gangrene, or Meleney's cellulitis (Meleney, 1924). It is characterized by extensive necrosis, undermining of skin and subcutaneous tissue, and necrosis of the latter tissues if the condition is not treated. Necrosis of skin and subcutaneous tissue is due to thrombosis of the nutrient vessels as they pass through the zone of the involved fascia (Crosthwait et al, 1963). These changes may occur in the neck in cases of necrotizing mediastinitis resulting from a descending infection of the oropharynx. Contrary to Meleney's traditional concept of a single organism responsible for the disease, Meade and Mueller (1968) reported a combination of organisms, both aerobic and anaerobic, that interact synergistically to cause this process. Stone and Martin in 1972 emphasized the concept of synergism in this process, which they termed "synergistic necrotizing cellulitis." The responsible organisms are gram-positive cocci, an anaerobic streptococcus, and a hemolytic *Staphylococcus aureus* (Stone and Martin, 1972). Animal experiments demonstrated that tissue destruction could not be produced by either organism alone (Meade and Mueller, 1968). The pathology can be reproduced also by a combination of microaerophilic streptococci plus enteric organisms (Altemier, 1942; Arndt, 1965). In necrotizing fasciitis, a combination of these organisms (hemolytic streptococci with *Staphylococcus aureus* or enteric organisms) was reported by Crosthwait and colleagues (1963).

Mediastinal infections resulting from esophageal perforations cover a wide range of both gram-positive and gram-negative aerobic and anaerobic bacteria. Included in these flora are *Streptococcus, Pseudomonas, Candida, Escherichia coli, Enterobacter, Enterococcus, Staphylococcus, Bacteroides, Klebsiella, Proteus,* and *Serratia.* The most common strains are *Streptococcus, Pseudomonas,* and *Candida* (Burnett et al, 1990).

In poststernotomy deep wound infection (mediastinitis), the infecting organisms include *Staphylococcus albus, Klebsiella, Candida albicans, E. coli, Pseudomonas, Streptococcus faecalis, Proteus mirabilis, Citrobacter,* and *Serratia; S. albus, Klebsiella, C. albicans,* and *E. coli* were the most common single and multiple organisms isolated from the mediastinum (Engleman et al, 1973).

Mediastinitis secondary to oropharyngeal infection was caused by multiple organisms, which included gram-positive aerobic cocci (β-hemolytic *Streptococci,* α-hemolytic *Streptococci,* and other staphylococci); gram-positive anaerobic cocci (anaerobic *Streptococci* and *Peptostreptococci);* gram-positive aerobic rods *(Corynebacterium diphtheriae);* gram-negative aerobic rods (*Pseudomonas*); gram-negative anaerobic rods *(Bacteroides, Fusobacterium);* and facultative gram-negative rods *(E. coli).* The most common organisms were β-hemolytic *Streptococci, Bacteroides,* α-hemolytic *Streptococci,* and *E. coli* (Estrera et al, 1983).

Primary (idiopathic) staphylococcal mediastinitis and primary β-hemolytic streptococcal mediastinitis are seen in rare cases in infants and children, respectively. Mediastinitis secondary to rare vertebral osteomyelitis has been described in cases of tuberculosis and fungal infection (Ewing and Hardy, 1991).

Diagnosis

Early diagnosis of acute mediastinitis is paramount in circumventing the lethal consequences of the disorder. Awareness of the clinical presentation and of diagnostic aids provides early recognition for administering the appropriate antibiotics and undertaking timed surgical measures.

Clinical Presentation

The manifestations of acute mediastinitis vary with the site of infection, the toxicity of the infecting organism, and the extent of the pathologic changes.

The symptoms generally include fever, pain, dysphagia, and respiratory distress. In a general way, the pain reflects the site of mediastinal involvement (Payne and Larson, 1969). In anterior mediastinal abscess, the pain is a conspicuous feature and is usually substernal and throbbing. In posterior mediastinitis, the pain is generally between the scapulae and may radiate anteriorly along the course of the intercostal nerves. When the trachea is encroached on, cough or swallowing may elicit upper chest pain. Dysphagia may occur as a result of compression by a collection of pus, especially in the upper part of the chest

(Keefer, 1938), but it is characteristic in acute mediastinitis due to esophageal perforation. The pain and discomfort are often localized to the site of esophageal perforation (Payne and Larson, 1969). Pain in the neck or upper chest is usually associated with perforation at the level of the cricopharyngeus muscle (Sabiston and Oldham, 1976). Respiratory distress usually indicates pleurisy with effusion, and if it is associated with esophageal perforation, its lateralization is helpful in defining the site of perforation. Severe dyspnea or evidence of systemic arterial desaturation may indicate the development of airway compression (Payne and Larson, 1969). In infants, acute mediastinitis should be included in the differential diagnosis of disorders that constitute respiratory emergencies (Feldman and Gromisch, 1971).

Physical examination is usually not diagnostic. Cervical cellulitis and tenderness occur with extending pharyngeal infection into the neck and mediastinum, or with perforation of the cervical esophagus (Marchevsky and Knack, 1991). Cervical crepitus is common with injury of the cervical esophagus (Pett, 1995). Although cervical tenderness is commonly seen with cervical esophageal perforation, lower esophageal perforations can produce signs indistinguishable from those of acute abdomen (Payne and Larson, 1969).

Diagnostic Aids

Blood

The total leukocyte count and sedimentation rate are usually elevated. The count is a useful diagnostic sign. Serial determination of neutrophils and band count provides prognostic information during the course of infection.

Fibrinogen significance is often overlooked in the infectious processes. It plays an important role in hemostasis and thrombosis. The clotting system and inflammation are intimately connected processes. Bacterial endotoxin and other toxins activate macrophages to secrete interleukin-1 (IL-1) and tumor necrosis factor (TNF), which induce the acute-phase responses associated with infection, including the hemodynamic effects of septic shock and procoagulant activity. The clotting system is activated through a cascade wherein factor I is converted to active factor Ia in the common pathway. Factor Xa converts prothrombin to thrombin, which then converts fibrinogen to fibrin. In conjunction with activated factor XIII, the fibrin is converted into an insoluble fibrin clot (Pierce, 1999). The increased fibrinogenesis requires an increase in fibrinogen, which is synthesized by the liver. Fibrinogen levels as high as 1000 to 1200 mg/dl (normal levels approximately 150 to 400 mg/dl) have been observed in acute mediastinitis. Elevated fibrinogen in platelet aggregation is an ominous sign in an environment of sepsis potentially primed for thrombosis (Pierce, 1999). Hyperfibrinogenemia in acute mediastinitis should be sought and carefully treated. Active factor X in the presence of sepsis binds to effector cell receptor 1 causing an increase in vascular permeability and leukocyte exudate (Collins, 1999).

Radiologic Evaluations

Radiographs of the neck and chest can be helpful in diagnosing mediastinitis. They generally show pleural effusion, pneumomediastinum in the tissue, air-fluid level, or widening of the mediastinum, particularly if an abscess is present. If gas is present in the neck or mediastinum, the presence of anaerobic bacteria must be considered (Howell et al, 1976).

If the diagnosis remains uncertain or the extent of the infection is unclear, a computed tomographic (CT) scan of the neck and chest should be obtained (Fig. 59–4).

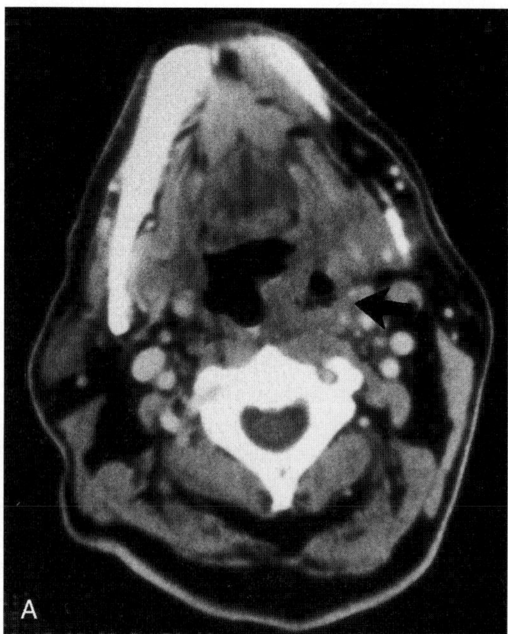

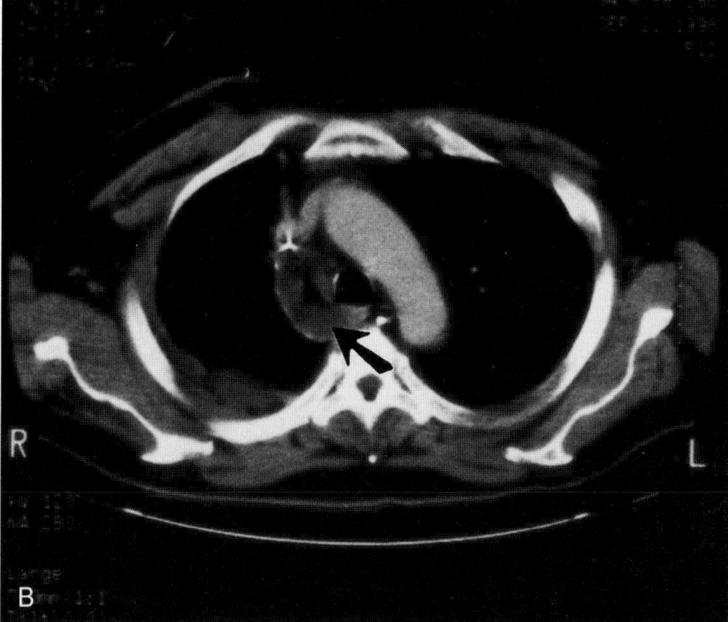

FIGURE 59–4 ■ A computed tomography scan from a patient with acute synergistic necrotizing mediastinitis. *A,* A left peritonsillar abscess with tissue induration and free air in the tissue *(arrow)*. *B,* A posterior mediastinal abscess secondary to infection that descended from the peritonsillar abscess *(arrow)*. An asssociated right pleural effusion is also present.

Chest CT is particularly helpful in diagnosing postoperative deep median sternotomy wound infection (mediastinitis) because the clinical parameters (i.e., fever, leukocytosis, tachycardia, dyspnea) may not be present in certain postoperative settings or may be falsely attributed to atelectasis or primary cardiac disease.

CT evidence of imperfect sternal closure (communication between presternal and retrosternal spaces) is not helpful in differentiating deep from superficial infection. Dots of air in the retrosternal space up to 7 days postoperatively may be considered normal. Well-circumscribed focal masses with high CT numbers (greater than 28 HU) probably represent hematoma. However, loss of the integrity of the retrosternal soft tissue fat planes implies mediastinitis. Amorphous masses or diffuse retrosternal haziness obliterating the mediastinal fat also indicates mediastinitis (Kay et al, 1983).

Management

Acute mediastinitis calls for urgent initiation of treatment. A compromised airway should be secured. Hypovolemia secondary to sepsis should be corrected. Serum fibrinogen levels above 600 mg/dl should be treated to prevent vascular thrombosis. Dextran 40 (Rheomacrodex) given intravenously is helpful in reducing platelet aggregation and blood viscosity caused by high concentrations of fibrinogen. If, however, fibrinogen levels remain elevated, low-molecular-weight heparin should be administered and continued until serum fibrinogen falls to a level below 500 mg/dl (Pierce, 1999).

Pleural effusion seen with increasing frequency in synergistic necrotizing mediastinitis is almost always an exudate rather than a transudate. This is determined by an analysis of the fluid that shows a pH <7.1, glucose <70 mg/dl, a white blood cell count (WBC) of 2200 to 29000 cells/mm, and the presence of fibrinogen. In the early course of mediastinitis, the fluid is thin and represents an early stage in the continuum of empyema thoracis. Failure of effective evacuation of the fluid, preferably by closed thoracostomy tube drainage, may result in deposition of fibrin with formation of multiple intrapleural loculations, fibrosis, and entrapment of the lung. The latter may require decortication by thoracoscopy or open thoracotomy. Recurrence of the empyema and entrapment of the lung necessitating reoperation can occur (Pierce, 1999).

Intrapleural instillation of thrombolytic agents has been used to treat empyema thoracis. It helps prevent intrapleural fibrinogenesis, facilitates drainage of intrapleural fluid collections, and may obviate the need for surgical intervention (Jerjes-Sanchez et al, 1996; Taylor et al, 1994); it is also safe and efficacious (Chin and Lim, 1997; Temes et al, 1996). It has no associated systemic fibrinolytic action. Streptokinase is the most commonly used agent in this therapeutic modality. Urokinase has low antigenicity, but because it is expensive its use will remain occasional (Bouros et al, 1994). Aliquots of 250,000 units of streptokinase in 10 ml normal saline are instilled into the pleural cavity via the chest tube, which is then clamped for 3 hours. The mean number of instillations is about 6 (1 per day for 6 days) (Bouros et al, 1994). After decortication, intrapleural streptokinase therapy should be used to prevent recurrence of empyema thoracis (Pierce, 1999).

Antibiotic therapy based on the likely etiologic organisms should be started immediately and adjusted later according to culture results. The infecting agents are related in a general way to the etiology of mediastinitis (Ewing and Hardy, 1991). Infections resulting from esophageal perforation grow gram-positive cocci (aerobic and anaerobic), gram-negative rods (aerobic [*Pseudomonas, Serratia*] and anaerobic [*Bacteroides, E. coli*]), and *Candida* (Burnett et al, 1990). Mediastinal infections originating in the oropharynx include a wide variety of gram-positive cocci, both aerobic *(Streptococcus, Staphylococcus)* and anaerobic (anaerobic *Streptococcus),* as well as gram-negative rods—aerobic *(Pseudomonas),* anaerobic *(Bacteroides, Fusobacterium),* and facultative *(E. coli)* (Estrera et al, 1983). In poststernotomy deep wound infection with mediastinitis, *Staphylococcus, Klebsiella, Candida,* and *E. coli* are the most common organisms (Engleman et al, 1973). Mediastinal infections secondary to esophageal perforation and oropharyngeal infection basically have a similar flora of organisms. Knowledge of the bacterial makeup of the different causative pathologies of acute mediastinitis is helpful in the choice of initial antibiotics.

The ravages of anaerobic infection should prompt a laboratory search for the causative organisms. The suspicion of their presence is heightened when gas is observed in the neck and mediastinal tissues, or when foul-smelling pus is found in drainage of an abscess. An immediate Gram stain should be obtained as a guide to preliminary antibiotic therapy. Anaerobic bacteria require special culture techniques, including prompt placement of the specimen on special culture media and longer incubation periods (Howell et al, 1976).

Identification of the primary etiology of acute mediastinitis not only aids in the selection of initial antibiotics, but more importantly, it helps in undertaking the appropriate surgical measures to prevent the continued soiling of the mediastinum from sources such as esophageal perforation or active oropharyngeal abscess.

There is a growing interest in conservative approaches to the treatment of small esophageal perforations, which are usually caused by esophageal dilatation for strictures. These perforations are usually associated with limited contamination confined to the immediate periesophageal area by adhesion and chronic fibrous tissue reaction. Such lesions have been successfully treated with antibiotics and conservative measures. However, they should be carefully monitored because of the potential of progression to severe mediastinitis (Ewing and Hardy, 1991). In general, however, perforations accompanied by mediastinal contamination—the extent of which can be determined by the radiologic findings as observed by plain chest films, Gastrografin swallow, and cine esophagogram—are best treated surgically to avoid or control mediastinitis, unless medical conditions preclude aggressive surgical intervention (Burnett et al, 1990; Kim-Deobald and Kozarek, 1992; Payne and Larson, 1969).

In all patients with esophageal perforation, immediate supportive therapy should be started. This includes insurance of adequate airway; intravenous hydration; high doses of broad-spectrum intravenous antibiotics; parenteral hyperalimentation; gastric decompression; pharyngeal aspiration; and chest physiotherapy. This treatment can be used in patients with small, contained, uncomplicated perforations that drain back into the esophagus.

Complicated perforations, major leaks, and mediastinal suppuration require urgent surgical intervention. Direct repair of the esophagus is subject to the underlying pathology and the degree of local inflammation, which can progress rapidly to preclude repair of the esophagus within a period of 12 to 36 hours. Repair of a previously normal esophagus within 24 to 36 hours of rupture is usually successful (Bladergroen et al, 1986; Pett, 1995). Buttressing the repair with a pedicle flap of intercostal muscle, a pleural flap, or pericardial fat is recommended (Pate et al, 1989). Perforations associated with achalasia (5%) can be directly repaired when combined with myotomy (Skinner et al, 1980). For perforations associated with stricture and gastroesophageal reflux, direct repair of the esophagus and the antireflux procedure have been used successfully (Richardson et al, 1985). Perforations more than 24 to 36 hours old are not amenable to direct repair and present considerable problems and poor prognosis. The preferred approach in these cases is wide mediastinal drainage, esophageal diversion and exclusion (Urschel et al, 1974), or stenting across the perforation to eliminate ongoing mediastinal contamination. Wide mediastinal drainage alone is inadequate. Extirpative treatment of esophageal perforation is directed primarily toward extensive esophageal devitalization (Burnett et al, 1990). Total esophagectomy with staged reconstruction is indicated (DeMeester, 1986; Skinner et al, 1980).

The diagnosis of postoperative mediastinitis following median sternotomy is difficult. Purulent wound drainage is, frequently, attributed to superficial wound infection when, in fact, it may represent an early manifestation of mediastinitis. CT scanning seems to be helpful in diagnosing and staging median sternotomy infection. Postoperative sternal wound complications have been classified according to the type of therapy that must be initiated:

1. Superficial wound infection without retrosternal involvement requires only local drainage.
2. Retrosternal infection or sternal dehiscence requires immediate reoperation for mediastinal drainage or sternal rewiring (Kay et al, 1983).

Deep sternotomy wound infection is treated with thorough débridement of the involved mediastinal tissue, sternal edges, and costal cartilages; placement of drainage tubes for postoperative mediastinal irrigation; closure of the sternum; and appropriate antibiotics (Serry et al, 1980). Serious infections may necessitate débridement of the entire sternum and costal arches. In such cases, the wound is left open, and secondary closure is performed later (Culliford et al, 1976).

Postoperative pain control in these gravely ill patients is mandatory to prevent postsurgical pulmonary atelectasis or pneumonia. The administration of epidural analgesia or epidural block in the immediate postoperative period is extremely effective in pain control. Concomitantly, morphine sulfate or meperidine hydrochloride (Demerol) should be given via patient-controlled pump. Ketorolac tromethamine (Toradol) administered intravenously is very effective in producing pain relief.

SCLEROSING FIBROSIS OF THE MEDIASTINUM

Sclerosing fibrosis of the mediastinum refers to a fibrous proliferative inflammatory process that usually involves the superior mediastinum. The fibrosis encases the mediastinal structures, causing entrapment and compression. Primarily low-pressure structures such as the superior vena cava, azygous vein, innominate veins, pulmonary veins, and pulmonary arteries are involved, although the esophagus and trachea can be affected (Urschel et al, 1990).

Similar fibrotic changes have been reported in other sites, referred to as retroperitoneal fibrosis, sclerosing cholangitis, and Riedel's fibrosing thyroiditis.

Etiology

Many etiologic factors have been cited in the causation of fibrosing mediastinitis, including fungal infection (histoplasmosis, aspergillosis, mucormycosis, and cryptococcosis, with histoplasmosis being most common), bacterial infection (tuberculosis, nocardiosis, and actinomycosis), autoimmune disease, sarcoidosis, and drugs (Marchevsky and Kaneko, 1992).

Pathogenesis

Sclerosing fibrosis of the mediastinum is an end-stage and chronic granulomatous inflammation that begins in the lymph nodes and continues as a low-grade smoldering response that may lead ultimately to the scarring stage. A delayed hypersensitivity reaction was proposed to be the central process that leads to the development of progressive fibrosis in granulomatous mediastinitis evoked by tubercle bacilli and *Histoplasma* (Goodwin et al, 1972).

This type of inflammatory response can be evoked by a variety of agents, including tubercle bacilli and certain fungi, particularly *Histoplasma capsulatum*. The agents induce delayed-type hypersensitivity reactions that are cell mediated and specifically initiated by sensitized T lymphocytes. The reactions are characterized by the accumulation of lymphocytes around small veins and venules, producing perivascular "cuffing" and increased microvascular permeability that causes tissue induration. In fully developed lesions, the lymphocyte-cuffed venules exhibit marked endothelial hypertrophy and, in some cases, hyperplasia. Immunoperoxidase staining of the lesions reveals a preponderance of $CD4^+$ (helper) T lymphocytes. With certain persistent nondegradable antigens, such as tubercle bacilli, the initial perivascular lymphocytic infiltrate is replaced by macrophages. The accumulated macrophages often undergo a morphologic transformation into epithelium-like cells referred to as epithelioid cells. An aggregation of epithelioid cells surrounded by a collar of lymphocytes is called a granuloma. A granuloma caused by insoluble particles that are capable of inducing a cell-mediated immune response is referred to as an immune granuloma (Collins, 1999). This type of granuloma differs from foreign body granulomas. Typically, the latter form when inert materials such as talc particles or sutures are large enough to preclude phagocytosis by a single macrophage and so do not incite an inflammatory or immune response. Epithelioid cells and giant cells become apposed to the surface of the foreign body, thus encompassing it (Cotran et al, 1999).

The cell-mediated inflammation induced by insoluble particles or nondegradable antigens that is characteristic of type IV hypersensitivity begins with the first exposure of the individual to the agent (e.g., tubercle bacillus). Naive $CD4^+$ T cells recognize peptides derived from the bacillus in association with class II molecules on the surface of monocytes. This initial encounter drives the differentiation of naive $CD4^+$ T cells to T_H1 cells. The T_H1 cells are important because the expression of the delayed hypersensitivity depends largely on cytokines secreted by them.

Why certain antigens preferentially induce the T_H1 response is not entirely clear. Cytokines relevant to the delayed hypersensitivity reaction include interleukin-12 (IL-12) produced by macrophages. IL-12 is critical for the induction of T_H1 response, and hence delayed hypersensitivity. On initial encounter with a microbe, the resting macrophages attempt to phagocytose and kill the organism. The resting macrophages are not particularly adept at these functions. Nonetheless, this interaction leads to the production of IL-12, which, in turn, drives the differentiation of naive $CD4^+$ helper cells to T_H1 cells, which produce IL-2, TNF, and interferon-γ (IFN-γ).

IFN-γ is an important mediator of delayed-type hypersensitivity. It is a powerful activator of macrophages, causing them to further secrete IL-12. Activated macrophages have an augmented ability to phagocytose and kill microorganisms. They express more class II molecules on the surface, thus facilitating further antigen presentation. Their capacity to kill tumor cells is enhanced. They secrete several polypeptide growth factors, such as platelet-derived growth factor and transforming growth factor-β (TGF-β), that stimulate fibroblast proliferation and augment collagen synthesis. Thus activated, macrophages serve to eliminate the offending antigen, and if the activation is sustained, fibrosis results (Cotran et al, 1999). The sustained fibrosis is the phase of the granulomatous inflammation encountered in the mediastinum. The delayed hypersensitivity is a major mechanism of defense against a variety of intracellular pathogens, including mycobacteria and fungi.

Pathology

With healing of the acute pulmonary infection, fibrocaseous granulomas develop in the lymph nodes connected to the lymphatic channels from the lungs. These include the hilar and subcarinal lymph nodes that drain into the right paratracheal nodes. As the inflammation evolves, more fibrosis develops in the infected areas. Extensive fibrosis within the right paratracheal area involves the superior vena cava and the azygous vein. Subcarinal fibrosis with anterior extension involves the pulmonary veins; with posterior extension, the esophagus; and with lateral extension, the main bronchi and pulmonary arteries (Goodwin et al, 1972). In a study reported by Goodwin and associates (1972), 29% of patients with mediastinal fibrosis had symptoms of bronchial obstruction; 23% had superior vena cava obstruction; 15% had pulmonary vein obstruction with a clinical picture of advanced mitral stenosis; 14% had pulmonary artery obstruction with symptoms of cor pulmonale; and 8% had esophageal obstruction, the great majority of whom also had dysphagia.

The degree of fibrosis determines the clinical significance of the mediastinal lesions. The fibrosis seems to invade the adjacent structures, a phenomenon not observed in retroperitoneal fibrosis, in which a zone of demarcation exists, with no invasion, between the area of fibrosis and the structure compressed (most commonly the ureters) (Goodwin et al, 1972).

Remnants of the offending organisms have been reported to persist in healed caseous lesions (Goodwin et al, 1972). Grossly, the fibrotic reaction creates a picture that resembles concrete. These uncleared remnants act as the stimulus for the persistence of the inflammatory response, which leads to more fibroblastic proliferation and scar formation.

Granulomatous lesions with mild fibrosis are indistinguishable grossly, whether due to *Mycobacterium* infection or to histoplasmosis. However, lesions with excessive to massive fibrosis are usually due to histoplasmosis (Goodwin et al, 1972). Microscopically, the tissues show dense collagen bands with fibroblastic activity and inflammatory cellular infiltrate composed mainly of mature lymphocytes and plasma cells. The collagen bands are interspersed with areas of hyalinization. A striking feature is the presence of arteriolar obliteration caused by intimal hyperplasia and medial thickening, and not due to vasculitis, as evidenced by the absence of necrosis and inflammatory cell infiltrate in the vessel wall (Urschel et al, 1990) (Fig. 59–5).

Diagnosis

The diagnosis of sclerosing mediastinitis should be considered in the differential diagnosis of patients presenting

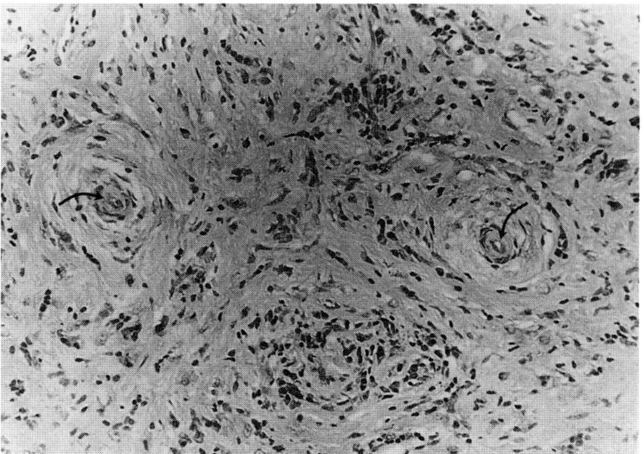

FIGURE 59–5 ■ A photomicrograph showing collagen bands interspersed with areas of hyalinization. Arterioles with luminal obliteration can be seen *(arrows)*.

with signs of superior vena cava (SVC) syndrome, dysphagia, dyspnea, or findings suggestive of cor pulmonale or mitral stenosis, particularly when no specific etiology is found to explain these manifestations. A good medical history review and physical examination, standard radiographs, and CT scans of neck, chest, and upper abdomen are recommended. In patients with SVC obstruction, simultaneous bilateral brachial phlebograms should be performed. Esophagoscopy is performed in patients with a history of dysphagia. Bronchoscopy and either cervical or second space mediastinoscopy should be done in all cases. Care should be exercised during the mediastinal exploration to prevent bleeding due to the increased collateral circulation. Bronchial washings and mediastinal tissue biopsy specimens should be obtained and sent for microscopy; stains and cultures should be done for tuberculosis and for certain fungi such as *Histoplasma, Coccidioides, Blastomyces, Nocardia,* and *Actinomyces*. Complement fixation studies should be performed for histoplasmosis, coccidioidomycosis, and blastomycosis. Titers of 1:32 or higher strongly suggest histoplasmosis (Urschel et al, 1990).

Clinical Manifestations

Sclerosing fibrosis of the mediastinum can affect any age group. It is more common among young whites, particularly women. Most patients present with nonspecific symptoms such as cough, dyspnea, chest pain, fever, wheezing, dysphagia, or hemoptysis. Approximately 40% of patients are asymptomatic, and the mediastinal fibrosing disorder is discovered as an incidental radiologic finding related to asymmetric widening of the mediastinum with distortion of tissue planes (Fry and Shields, 1991; Marchevsky and Kaneko, 1992).

Entrapment and compression of the visceral mediastinal structures and the severity of the pathology can lead to an incapacitating morbid clinical picture. The thin-walled, low-pressure structures, especially the SVC, are involved most frequently (Howell et al, 1976; Urschel et al, 1990). The luminal compromise of the SVC results in SVC syndrome. Symptoms of this syndrome include swelling and edema of the upper extremities, face, and anterior chest wall, as well as an increase in dilated superficial veins and flushing in these areas (Urschel et al, 1990). Symptoms of SVC obstruction may show regression as collateral circulation develops. The SVC syndrome was observed in 59% (Urschel et al, 1990) and 23% (Goodwin et al, 1972) of cases with mediastinal structure involvement. Other compression symptoms occur less frequently. Central nervous system symptoms include headache, nausea, and dizziness with visual disturbance. Dysphagia due to esophageal compression; intermittent stridor and dyspnea secondary to tracheal compression; cardiac tamponade due to pericardial effusion; and cor pulmonale and mitral stenosis–like symptoms secondary to pulmonary vessel compression are observed in this disorder (Urschel et al, 1990). Pulmonary vein obstruction is a serious condition and can end fatally (Goodwin et al, 1972).

Radiographic Findings

On standard radiographs, most patients show a widening of the superior mediastinum with a mass-like effect and obliteration of normal tissue planes. Calcified lymph nodes may be evident (Fry and Shields, 1991).

CT study may further delineate the pathologic changes and degree of compression of the involved structures. It can be helpful in identifying the mediastinal changes, especially when the plain radiographs appear to be within normal limits. Magnetic resonance imaging is useful in demonstrating the extent of involvement of the great vein, especially if there is a history of hypersensitivity to contrast materials (Fry and Shields, 1991). CT with contrast may be helpful in delineating the nature of the compression in cases of unusual venous obstruction.

Phlebograms should be obtained to assess the venous anatomy and the location of the site of obstruction, as well as the collateral circulation, and the status of the azygous vein. The latter can be anastomosed to the inferior vena cava to palliate SVC obstruction symptoms (Urschel et al, 1990). Pulmonary arteriography may be helpful in demonstrating pulmonary vessel obstruction in suspected cases of sclerosing mediastinitis (Fry and Shields, 1991; Wieder, 1982). In rare instances, pulmonary infarct due to arterial or venous thrombosis may occur (Katzenstein and Mazur, 1980). Pulmonary interstitial fibrosis, which can follow a course similar to that of the usual interstitial pneumonitis, has been reported (Wieder and Rabinowitz, 1977).

Treatment

There is no universally accepted therapeutic modality for the treatment of mediastinal granuloma and fibrosing mediastinitis. Surgical intervention is initially indicated in most patients to establish a diagnosis and particularly to rule out neoplasia. Surgery consists of bronchoscopy and either cervical or second space exploration. Bronchial washings and mediastinal biopsy specimens should be obtained for cytologic and microbial testing (Urschel et al, 1990). If the disease presents as a noncalcified mass, which shows no neoplasia on biopsy, concomitant thoracotomy can be performed to debulk the mass by removing as much granuloma as is technically feasible (Dines et al, 1970). In approximately 25% of patients with localized granulomas, complete excision of the lesion can be achieved. In some cases, excision of local granulomas prevented the development of subsequent progressive fibrosis (Marchevsky and Kaneko, 1992).

In a few patients, surgical intervention is necessary to alleviate airway obstruction, esophageal obstruction, vascular obstruction, or cardiac tamponade. Reconstructive surgery for SVC obstruction has been recommended (Doty et al, 1990; Urschel et al, 1990). A SVC bypass graft using a reconstructed spiral saphenous vein graft or azygous vein transposition has been used by the authors. Urschel and associates (1990) suggested administering a prolonged course of oral ketoconazole, and repeating it if necessary, if the histoplasma complement fixation titer is high.

Pneumonectomy may be required for pulmonary complications resulting from the obstruction (Fry and Shields, 1991).

The effect for administering corticosteroid or antifungal therapy when no evidence of active infection is present is controversial (Marchevesky and Kaneko, 1992).

Prognosis

The prognosis for fibrosing mediastinitis, generally speaking, is good. However, the health of many surviving patients becomes compromised as a result of disease progression. Also, those patients with occlusion of a major airway or of a pulmonary artery or vein have a poor prognosis. In a series of 71 patients reported by Loyd and associates (1988), 30% of patients died. Death was due to cor pulmonale or persistent respiratory compromise. The interval between onset of symptoms and death was about 6 years.

SUMMARY

Mediastinitis in both its acute and chronic forms can be disabling or lethal.

Acute mediastinitis can be primary, but is usually secondary to other etiologies, such as esophageal perforation, poststernotomy deep wound infection, and descending oropharyngeal infection. It may become self-contained and heal uneventfully, or it may progress to a fulminant suppurative or necrotizing form. The clinicopathologic evolution of such ravaging infection is determined by bacteriologic makeup, bacterial synergism, and host resistance. Although early diagnosis can be challenging owing to the nonspecific nature of the early clinical picture, a good history and physical examination with appropriate laboratory assessment and radiologic evaluation, including CT scan of the neck and chest, may prompt timely diagnosis of mediastinitis and the underlying etiology.

An early diagnosis of acute mediastinitis and urgent commencement of supportive measures, intravenous wide-spectrum antibiotics, and surgical intervention may favorably alter the morbid outcome.

Chronic sclerosing mediastinitis is an end stage of a delayed hypersensitivity granulomatous process incited by certain fungi and bacteria. Failure of the reacting cells to clear the infecting agent evokes this cell-mediated response. The fibrosing process of this disorder is responsible for the morbid and disabling obstruction of visceral structures of the mediastinum, namely, the great veins, the pulmonary vessels, the esophagus, and the airways. Diagnosis is established by the clinical picture, radiologic evaluation, serologic assessment, and tissue biopsy. Surgery is necessary to alleviate significant vascular, esophageal, and airway obstruction. Medical therapy should be administered in cases of positive identification of the microbe or in cases of rising serologic titer.

COMMENTS AND CONTROVERSIES

This chapter provides a detailed review of the anatomic relationships and fascial planes of the mediastinum. Understanding of these various compartments is critical in planning appropriate drainage and débridement for severe mediastinal infections.

The authors have raised a number of controversial points. They have advocated esophageal diversion for all delayed esophageal perforations. In this commentator's experience, it is often possible to salvage a delayed perforation by mediastinal débridement and primary closure of the inflamed but well-vascularized esophageal mucosa. Postrepair leak is common following primary closure of delayed perforations. However, if drains are precisely located near the site of repair, subsequent leaks can always be well controlled, and most will heal, providing a satisfactory long-term result and avoiding the need for major reconstructive surgery.

The authors also recommend surgical intervention for patients with mediastinal granulomatosis. In our experience, patients who have isolated problems such as broncholiths or bronchoesophageal fistulas benefit from direct operative intervention. However, we have not had much success with resectional or reconstructive strategies for patients with more diffuse mediastinal fibrosis. Our preference is to treat these patients with palliative measures such as periodic dilatation and stenting.

G.A.P.

REFERENCES

Ackerknecht EH: Therapeutics from the Primitives to the 20th Century. New York, Hafner Press, 1973, p 141.

Altemier WA: Pathogenicity of the bacteria of appendicitis peritonitis. Surgery 11:374, 1942.

Arndt WF Jr: Synergistic infections. In Maibach HI (ed): Skin Bacteria and Infection. San Francisco, McGraw-Hill, 1965, Chap 10.

Bladergroen MR, Lowe JE, Postlethwait RW: Diagnosis and recommended management of esophageal perforation and rupture. Ann Thorac Surg 42:235–239, 1986.

Boerhaave H: Atrocis, nec descripti prius, morbi historia. (1724). Verbatim English translation (Derbes V, Mitchell R). Bull Am Library A 43:216, 1955.

Bouros D, Schiza S, Panagou P et al: Role of streptokinase in the treatment of acute loculated parapneumonic pleural effusions and empyema. Thorax 49:852, 1994.

Burnett CM, Rosemurgy AS, Pfeiffer EA: Life-threatening acute posterior mediastinitis due to esophageal perforation. Ann Thorac Surg 49:979–983, 1990.

Chin NK, Lim TK: Controlled trial of intrapleural streptokinase in the treatment of pleural empyema and complicated parapneumonic effusions. Chest 111:275, 1997.

Cogan MIC: Necrotizing mediastinitis secondary to descending cervical cellulitis. Oral Surg 36:307, 1973.

Coller FA, Yglesias L: The relation of the spread of infection to fascial planes in the neck and thorax. Surgery 1:323, 1937.

Collins T: Acute and chronic inflammation. In Cotran RS, Kumar V, Collins T (eds): Robbins Pathologic Basis of Disease, 6th ed. Philadelphia, WB Saunders, 1999, p 50.

Cotran RS, Kumar V, Collins T (eds): Robbins Pathologic Basis of Disease, 6th ed. Philadelphia, WB Saunders, 1999.

Crosthwait RW Jr, Crosthwait RW, Jordan GL: Necrotizing fascitis. J Trauma 4:148, 1963.

Culliford AT, Cunningham JN Jr, Zeff RH et al: Sternal and costochondral infections following open-heart surgery. J Thorac Cardiovasc Surg 72:714–726, 1976.

Davies RJO, Traill ZC, Gleeson FV: Randomized controlled trial of intrapleural streptokinase in community acquired pleural infection. Thorax 52:416, 1997.

DeMeester TR: Perforation of the esophagus. Ann Thorac Surg 42:231–232, 1986.

Dines D, Payne W, Bernatz P, Pairolero P: Mediastinal granuloma and fibrosing mediastinitis. Chest 75:3, 1970.

Doty D, Doty J, Jones K: Bypass of superior vena cava. J Thorac Cardiovasc Surg 99:889, 1990.

Dreyfuss D, Djedaini K, Bidault-Lapomme C et al: Nontraumatic acute anterior mediastinitis in two HIV-positive heroin addicts. Chest 101:583–585, 1992.

Engleman RM, Williams CD, Gouge TH et al: Mediastinitis following open-heart surgery: Review of 2 years' experience. Arch Surg 107:772–778, 1973.

Enquist RW, Blanck RR, Butler RH: Nontraumatic mediastinitis. JAMA 236:1048–1049, 1976.

Estrera AS, Landay MJ, Grisham JM et al: Descending necrotizing mediastinitis. Surg Gynecol Obstet 157:545–552, 1983.

Ewing HP, Hardy JD: The mediastinum. In Baue AE, Geha AS, Hammond GL et al (eds): Glenn's Thoracic and Cardiovascular Surgery, 5th ed, vol 1. Norwalk, Appleton & Lange, 1991, p 569.

Feldman R, Gromisch DS: Acute suppurative mediastinitis. Am J Dis Child 121:79–81, 1971.

FitzGerald JM, Grzybowski S, Allen EA: The impact of human immunodeficiency virus infection on tuberculosis and its control. Chest 100:191–200, 1991.

Fry WA, Shields TW: Acute and chronic mediastinal infections. In Shield TW (ed): Mediastinal Surgery. Philadelphia, Lea & Febiger, 1991, pp 101–108.

Furstenberg AC: Acute mediastinal suppuration. Trans Am Laryngol Rhinol Otol Soc 35:210, 1939.

Furstenberg AC, Yglesias L: A clinical study with practical anatomic considerations of neck and mediastinum. Arch Otolaryngol 25:539, 1937.

Goodwin RA, Nickell JA, Des Prez RM: Mediastinal fibrosis complicating healed primary histoplasmosis and tuberculosis. Medicine 51:227, 1972.

Gray H: Anatomy of the Human Body, 28th ed. Philadelphia, Lea & Febiger, 1966, p 396.

Grodinsky M, Holyoke EA: The fasciae and fascial spaces of the head, neck and adjacent regions. Am J Anat 63:367, 1938.

Grodinsky M: Ludwig's angina, retropharyngeal abscess and other deep abscesses of the head and neck. JAMA 114:18–22, 1940.

Howell HS, Prinz RA, Pickleman JR: Anaerobic mediastinitis. Surg Gynecol Obstet 43:353–359, 1976.

Iglauer S: Surgical approaches to deep suppuration in the neck and posterior mediastinum. Arch Otolaryngol 21:707, 1935.

Jerjes-Sanchez C, Ramirez-Rivera A, Elizaldel JJ et al: Intrapleural fibrinolysis with streptokinase as an adjunctive treatment in hemothorax and empyema. Chest 109:1514, 1996.

Julian OC, Lopez-Belio M, Dye WS et al: The median incision in intracardiac surgery with extracorporeal circulation. Surgery 42:753, 1957.

Katzenstein KA, Mazur MT: Pulmonary infarct: An unusual manifestation of fibrosing mediastinitis. Chest 77:521, 1980.

Kay HR, Goodman LR, Teplick SK et al: Use of computed tomography to assess mediastinal complications after median sternotomy. Ann Thorac Surg 36:706–714, 1983.

Keefer CS: Acute and chronic mediastinitis. Arch Intern Med 62:109, 1938.

Kim-Deobald J, Kozarek RA: Esophageal perforation: An 8-year review of a multispecialty clinic's experience. Am J Gasteroenterol 87:1112–1119, 1992.

Lichtenberg FV: Infectious disease. In Robbins SL, Cotran VK, Robbins RS (eds): Pathologic Basis of Disease, 4th ed. Philadelphia, WB Saunders, 1989, pp 307–433.

Loyd JE, Tillman BF, Atkinson JB: Mediastinal fibrosis complicating histoplasmosis. Medicine 67:295, 1988.

Mandell GL, Sande M: Antimicrobial agents. In Gilman AG, Rall TW, Nies AS, Taylor P (eds): Goodman and Gilman's The Pharmacological Basis of Therapeutics, 8th ed. New York, McGraw-Hill, 1990, p 1065.

Marchevsky AM, Kaneko M: Surgical Pathology of the Mediastinum, 2nd ed. New York, Raven Press, 1992.

McCafferty EL, Lyons C: Suppurative fasciitis as the essential feature of hemolytic streptococcus gangrene. Surgery 24:438, 1948.

McClelland RN: Non-cardiac thoracic surgery. SRGS 25:55, 1998.

Meade JW, Mueller CB: Necrotizing infections of subcutaneous tissue and fascia. Ann Surg 168:274–280, 1968.

Meleney FL: Hemolytic streptococcus gangrene. Arch Surg 9:317, 1924.

Moncada R, Warpeha R, Pickleman J et al: Mediastinitis from odontogenic and deep cervical infection: Anatomic pathways of propagation. Chest 73:497–500, 1978.

Mosher HP: The submaxillary fossa approach to deep pus in the neck. Trans Am Acad Ophthalmol 34:19, 1929.

Nashef SA, Klein C, Martigne C et al: Foreign body perforation of the normal oesophagus. Eur J Cardiothorac Surg 6:565–567, 1992.

Nelems B: Mediastinal infections. In Pearson FG, Deslauriers J, Ginsberg RJ, Hiebert CA et al (eds): Thoracic Surgery. Philadelphia, Churchill Livingstone, 1995.

Neuhof H: Acute infection of the mediastinum with special reference to mediastinal suppuration. J Thorac Cardiovasc Surg 6:184, 1936.

Pane GA, Hamilton GC, Call E: Nontraumatic suppurative mediastinitis presenting as acute mediastinal widening. Ann Emerg Med 12:777–779, 1983.

Pate JW, Walder WA, Cole FH Jr et al: Spontaneous rupture of the esophagus: A 30-year experience. Ann Thorac Surg 47:689–692, 1989.

Payne WS, Larson RH: Acute mediastinitis. Surg Clin North Am 49:999–1009, 1969.

Pearse HE Jr: Mediastinitis following cervical suppuration. Ann Surg 108:588, 1938.

Pett S: Mediastinal infections. In Fry DE (ed): Surgical Infections. Boston, Little, Brown, 1995, p 383.

Pierce TB, Razzuk L, Luterman D et al: Acute mediastinitis. Baylor University Medical Center Proceedings 13:31–33, 2000.

Pierce TB, Razzuk MA, Razzuk LM, Hoover SJ: A comprehensive review of the physiology of hemostasis and antithrombotic agents. Baylor University Medical Center Proceedings 12:39–49, 1999.

Richardson JD, Martin LF, Borzotta AP et al: Unifying concepts in treatment of esophageal leaks. Am J Surg 149:157–162, 1985.

Sabiston DC, Oldham HN: The mediastinum. In Sabiston DC, Spencer FC (eds): Gibbon's Surgery of the Chest, 3rd ed. Philadelphia, WB Saunders, 1976.

Samuelson J: Infectious disease. In Cotran RS, Kumar V, Tucker C (eds): Pathologic Basis of Disease, 6th ed. Philadelphia, WB Saunders, 1999.

Serry C, Bleck PC, Javid H et al: Sternal wound complications: Management and results. J Thorac Cardiovasc Surg 80:861–867, 1980.

Skinner DB, Little AG, DeMeester TR: Management of esophageal perforation. Am J Surg 139:760–764, 1980.

Stone HH, Martin JD Jr: Synergistic necrotizing cellulitis. Ann Surg 175:702–711, 1972.

Stuteville OH: Spread of infections in the head and neck. J Int Coll Surg 29:750, 1958.

Taylor RFH, Rubens MB, Pearson MC, Barnes NC: Intrapleural streptokinase in the management of empyema. Thorax 49:856, 1994.

Temes RT, Follis F, Kessler RM et al: Intrapleural fibrinolytics in management of empyema thoracis. Chest 110:102–106, 1996.

Thaler F, Maurel C, Monteil JP et al: Acute epiglottitis in adults. N Engl J Med 315:1163–1164, 1986.

Urschel HC Jr, Razzuk MA, Netto GJ et al: Sclerosing mediastinitis: Improved management with histoplasmosis titer and ketoconazole. Ann Thorac Surg 50:215–221, 1990.

Urschel HC, Razzuk MA, Wood RE: Improved management of esophageal performation. Exclusion and diversion in continuity. Ann Surg 179:587, 1974.

Vessal K, Montali RJ, Larson SM et al: Evaluation of barium and gastrografin as contrast media for the diagnosis of esophageal ruptures or perforation. Am J Roentgenol Radium Nucl Med 123:307–319, 1975.

Wieder S, Rabinowitz JG: Fibrous mediastinitis: A late manifestation of mediastinal histoplasmosis. Radiology 125:305, 1977.

Wieder S, White TS, Salayar J: Pulmonary artery occlusion due to histoplasmosis. Am J Roentgenol 138:243, 1982.

Williams CD, Cunningham JN, Falk EA et al: Chronic infection of the costal cartilages after thoracic surgical procedures. J Thorac Cardiovasc Surg 66:592–598, 1973.

Wilson B: Necrotizing fascitis. Am Surg 18:416, 1952.

CHAPTER **60**

Pericardial Disease

William G. Jones II

The pericardium is a serous sac that surrounds, supports, and protects the heart. The smooth pericardial surface adjacent to the heart and the small amount of pericardial fluid normally present within the pericardial sac provide a frictionless chamber for cardiac motion, thus improving the efficiency of myocardial contractions. The pericardium, however, is subject to disease, including inflammation, infection, trauma, and malignancy. Impairment of pericardial compliance or intrapericardial fluid accumulation, resulting in reduction of the relative volume of the pericardial space secondary to disease processes, may lead to pathophysiologic and hemodynamically significant restriction of cardiac function. Prompt recognition and treatment of pericardial disease is often lifesaving.

HISTORICAL NOTE

Hippocrates is credited with the first description of the human pericardium in 460 BC. Three hundred years later Galen first described inflammatory changes and effusions in animals with pericarditis. Similar studies of pericardial disease in humans, however, did not occur until the 17th and 18th centuries, when Lower (1669) first described cardiac tamponade secondary to the accumulation of pericardial fluid and Lancisi and Morgani wrote of the diminution of cardiac function resulting from constrictive pericarditis.

The classic pathologic description of the "bread and butter" appearance of acute pericarditis by Laennec (1819) was later followed by characterization of the pathology of chronic pericarditis associated with hepatic disease by Pick (1886). Knowledge of the pathophysiology of pericardial disease was advanced by the hemodynamic observations of Kussmaul (1873), including the description of pulsus paradoxus in association with tamponade. Modern experimental studies by Beck and Griswald (1930) subsequently contributed to our understanding of pericardial disease and led to advances in its treatment.

Early reports of symptomatic relief produced by pericardiocentesis by Karaeneff (1840) introduced the era of treatment of pericardial disease. Rehn (1913) and Sauerbruch (1925) independently described methods for pericardial resection, followed by modifications by Schmieder and Fischer (1926). Based on the successes of these reports, Churchill (1936) performed the first pericardiectomy in the United States for constrictive disease in 1929.

HISTORICAL READINGS

Beck CS, Griswald RA: Pericardiectomy in the treatment of the Pick syndrome: Experimental and clinical observations. Arch Surg 21:1064, 1930.

Churchill ED: Pericardial resection in chronic constrictive pericarditis. Ann Surg 104:516, 1936.

Karanaeff P: Paracentese des Brustkastens und des Pericardiums. Med Z 9:251, 1840.

Kussmaul A: Ueber schwielige Mediatino-perikarditis und dem Paradoxen Puls. Berl Klin Wochenschr 10:433, 1873.

Laennec RTH: Traité d'Auscultation Médicale et des Maladies du Poumon et du Coeur. Paris, Brosson & JS Chaude, 1819.

Lower R: Tractatus de Corde. London, 1669, p 104.

Pick F: Ueber chronische, unter dem Bilde der Lebercirrhose Verlaufen der Pericarditis (Pericarditis pseudolebercirrhose) nebst Bemerkungen ueber Zuckergussleber. Z Klin Med 29:385, 1886.

Rehn L: Zurexperimentellen pathologic des herzbeutels. Verh Dtsch Ges Chir 42:339, 1913.

Sauerbruch F: Die Chirurgie der Brestorgane, vol II. Berlin, 1925.

Schmieder V, Fischer H: Die Herzbeutelentzunchung und ihre Folgezustande. Ergeb Chir Orthop 19:98, 1926.

BASIC SCIENCE

Embryology

The pericardium is derived from membranous partitions, which begin to form between the pleural and peritoneal cavities during the third week of fetal development. By the seventh gestational week, these membranes grow to envelop the fetal heart, ultimately fusing to form the complete pericardial sac. Because of their common origins during development, the pericardium remains intimately associated with and in some areas contiguous with the pleurae and diaphragm.

Anatomy

The parietal pericardium consists of a tough fibrous outer layer, with an inner serosal surface that is composed of cuboidal cells. The serosa of the pericardium is organized into microvilli and cilia, which produce and reabsorb the pericardial fluid. The serosal layer is then reflected into the epicardial surface to form the visceral pericardium and becomes contiguous with the adventitia of the great vessels superiorly. The pericardium is further anchored anteriorly to the sternum by the superior and inferior pericardiosternal ligaments and inferiorly to the diaphragm. The phrenic nerves and associated blood vessels lie within the anterolateral portion of the pericardial fat pad bilaterally.

Physiology

The smooth serosal surface of the pericardial sac provides a frictionless chamber, facilitating cardiac contraction, whereas the fibrous outer layer provides protection against the spread of infection from the adjacent mediastinum and pleural cavities. The fixed pericardium also supports the heart and prevents cardiac torsion by maintaining the heart in a relatively fixed position despite body motion. The pericardium contributes to the maintenance of a functionally optimal cardiac shape, preventing acute overdilatation, which may damage the myocardium. Negative pressure within the pericardium may also enhance atrial filling to a small degree.

Normally 15 to 20 ml of clear, straw-colored fluid is present within the pericardial space. Pericardial fluid is produced by the serosal cells and is an ultrafiltrate of plasma (Gibbon and Segal, 1940). Microvilli on the serosal surface both produce and reabsorb pericardial fluid. Although membrane characteristics of these cuboidal serosal cells favor absorption rather than production of fluid (Pegram and Bishop, 1981), the net turnover of pericardial fluid is determined by a number of factors, including intravascular and interstitial oncotic pressure, volume, and composition and the adequacy of the lymphatic drainage of the pericardium.

Histologic section of the fibrous portion of the pericardium reveals that the collagen bundles are arranged in a wavy, "herringbone" pattern (Elias and Boyd, 1960). This configuration gives the pericardium compliance, allowing it to be stretched to where the collagen strands become straightened and aligned. The size of the pericardial sac when the collagen fibers are maximally stretched represents the limiting volume of the pericardial space and the point beyond which further distention is impossible (Ferguson and Willerson, 1991; Holt, 1970). However, chronic stretching of the pericardium over time results in pericardial hypertrophy and increased pericardial compliance, thus producing a rightward shift in the limiting volume. However, adherence of the pericardium on the epicardial surface of the heart diminishes pericardial compliance, reduces the ability of the pericardium to stretch by even small amounts, and may ultimately restrict cardiac filling.

The normal pressure within the pericardium is less than atmospheric and is equal to the intrapleural pressure. The normal volume of the pericardial sac exceeds the size of the heart by approximately 20% (Shabetai, 1987), allowing physiologic enlargement of the heart to occur without restriction. Additionally, the compliance or distensibility of the normal pericardium allows relatively large increases to occur in either pericardial fluid volume or cardiac size without an increase in intrapericardial pressure, particularly when such increases occur over time. As pericardial distention approaches the limiting volume, however, intrapericardial pressure begins to rise. Tamponade occurs when the intrapericardial pressure exceeds right ventricular filling pressure. The slope of the pericardial pressure-volume curve and the point at which tamponade occurs thus depend on the rate of pericardial fluid accumulation, pericardial compliance, and the intravascular volume status, which determines right ventricular filling pressure (Holt, 1970; Shabetai et al, 1970).

DISEASE CONDITIONS

Acute Pericarditis

Etiology and Pathophysiology

Acute pericarditis may often be the early manifestation of a systemic illness such as connective tissue disease or myocardial infarction. As many as half of all cases of acute pericarditis, however, are due to neoplastic disease, are uremic or infectious in origin, or result from unclear processes and are thus termed *idiopathic* or *nonspecific* (Shabetai, 1990). Other less common causes of acute pericarditis are listed in Table 60–1.

Symptoms in acute pericarditis result from inflammation of the pericardium as well as from irritation of adjacent tissues. Pathologic examination of the pericardium during acute pericarditis demonstrates inflammatory cell infiltration and fibrin deposition leading to a characteristic "bread and butter" appearance of the serosal surface.

Diagnosis

Acute pericarditis is often preceded by a prodrome of fever, myalgias, and malaise that may last for 3 to 7 days. As the inflammation in the pericardium worsens, chest pain and leukocytosis ensue. The substernal pain associated with acute pericarditis is excruciating and may be confused with angina, although pain associated with pericarditis is usually more pleuritic, increased by supination or deep inspiration. Dyspnea is common and accompanied by a nonproductive cough with clear lung fields. The classic friction rub associated with acute pericarditis has been described as resembling the "squeak of leather on a new saddle" (Collin, 1955).

The cardiac silhouette may appear enlarged on a chest radiograph, especially when pericarditis is complicated by a large effusion. Electrocardiographic (ECG) changes in pericarditis, consisting of ST segment elevation without Q waves or T wave inversion, may be helpful in differentiating pericarditis from an acute myocardial infarction, particularly because pericarditis may rarely result in an elevation of the creatine kinase MB fraction (Shabetai et al, 1990). An echocardiogram should be obtained in most cases of acute pericarditis to determine the size of the associated effusion and to examine for signs of tamponade when indicated. It may also be useful in the detection of intrapericardial lymphoma or metastatic disease. If the etiology of acute pericarditis is un-

TABLE 60–1 ■ **Less Common Causes of Acute Pericarditis**

- Drug/hypersensitivity reactions
  - Procainamide
  - Warfarin
  - Hydralazine
  - Phenytoin
  - Others
- Aortic aneurysms and dissections
- Connective tissue diseases
  - Arteritis
  - Rheumatoid arthritis
  - Systemic lupus erythematosus
  - Rheumatic fever
  - Sarcoidosis
- Secondary to or postmyocardial infarct or cardiac surgery
- Secondary to or postradiation
- Secondary to or post-trauma
- Myxedema
- Amyloidosis

clear, minimal workup should include cultures for an infectious etiology, a renal profile, and antibody titers for collagen-vascular disease.

Management

In general, acute pericarditis that is not complicated by tamponade should be treated by bed rest and pain control. Narcotic analgesia is usually required in the early phase and should be supplemented with nonsteroidal anti-inflammatory agents. Severe and persistent pain may require corticosteroids for control. Persistent fevers despite therapy warrant pericardiocentesis to ensure the proper diagnosis and to examine the pericardial fluid for purulence or signs of an infectious etiology. Other indications for pericardiocentesis are to relieve tamponade and to evaluate the etiology in cases in which the effusion persists beyond 2 to 3 weeks.

Infectious pericarditis may result from direct contamination of the pericardial space by penetrating trauma or surgery, from seeding of the pericardium and pericardial fluid during bacteremia, or from rupture of an adjacent infected collection into the pericardial space. Treatment of infectious pericarditis requires control of the primary source of the infection and drainage of the pericardial space. In infectious pericarditis, the effusion develops quickly and is often thick and purulent and associated with multiple intrapericardial loculations. Pericardiocentesis, although helpful in establishing the diagnosis, may provide inadequate drainage, and early pericardiotomy with careful exploration to open all loculated areas may be required, especially in children with *Haemophilus influenzae* infection (Moores and Dziuban, 1995).

Tuberculous pericarditis necessitates triple-drug therapy for at least 9 months (Fowler, 1991). Although controversial, addition of corticosteroids to the antituberculous regimen has also been reported to decrease the need for repeated pericardiocentesis procedures to control the associated effusion (Strang et al, 1988). Early operative intervention should also be considered in tuberculous pericarditis, because the dense fibrous pericardial reaction may prevent concentration of antituberculous drugs to eradicate the infection. Furthermore, this fibrous reaction will ultimately produce a thickened, constrictive pericardium (Larrieu et al, 1980).

Acute pericarditis has been reported to complicate 5% to 15% of all patients infected with the human immunodeficiency virus (HIV) at some time during the course of the illness (Acierno, 1989). Most cases of pericardial effusion in HIV-positive patients are asymptomatic, and the etiology remains unidentified. In those patients with symptomatic pericardial effusions, two thirds are either infectious or neoplastic in origin and therapy should be directed at the primary cause (Estok and Wallach, 1998).

Uremic pericarditis occurs most often in patients with renal failure who are undergoing hemodialysis. Specific symptoms may be absent until tamponade develops and pericardiocentesis or pericardiotomy is required. Uremic pericarditis without tamponade may respond to more frequent hemodialysis or to a change to peritoneal dialysis (Shabetai, 1990). Intrapericardial instillation of corticosteroids has also been reported to be successful in selected patients (Buselmier et al, 1976).

Acute pericarditis develops in 10% to 15% of patients who are receiving radiation therapy and may occur months to years after therapy (Applefield et al, 1981). Radiation-induced pericarditis produces both pericardial effusions and fibrosis and should be treated with systemic corticosteroids. Symptoms of constriction may require pericardiectomy, although great care should be taken to attempt to differentiate constrictive pericarditis from radiation-induced myocardial fibrosis in these patients (Schneider and Edwards, 1979).

Idiopathic acute pericarditis will recur with relapsing episodes in 15% to 30% of all cases. Although recurrences are often numerous and may occur over more than 10 to 15 years, the risk of tamponade in recurrent pericarditis is lower than in acute pericarditis (Fowler and Harbin, 1986). Therapy is similar to that for the initial episode, consisting of bed rest and pain control. Corticosteroids are often useful in producing remission, and some patients require long-term therapy to prevent recurrence. Colchicine has also been reported to be useful in preventing recurrences (Guindo et al, 1990). Pericardiectomy will relieve symptoms in 50% to 80% of cases (Fowler and Harbin, 1986; Hatcher et al, 1971) but should be reserved for those patients who develop complications from their corticosteroid therapy or who have failed to obtain a lasting remission.

Constrictive Pericarditis

Etiology and Pathophysiology

Constrictive pericarditis usually results from acute pericarditis that has progressed to chronic scarring and fibrosis, leading to a thickened and noncompliant pericardium. The most common causes of constrictive pericarditis are neoplastic disease and the effects of mediastinal radiation therapy, chest surgery, or trauma (Ferguson and Willerson, 1991). Tuberculous pericarditis, formerly the most common cause of constrictive pericarditis, is now less common in the United States but remains problematic in other areas of the world. Less commonly, constrictive pericarditis may be secondary to uremia and collagen-vascular disorders or may follow acute bacterial pericarditis. It is estimated that between 0.02% and 0.3% of all cardiac surgical procedures are complicated by pericardial constriction (Kutcher et al, 1982; Marsa et al, 1979; Miller et al, 1982). The development of constrictive pericarditis secondary to cardiac surgery may be related to complete closure of the pericardium after the procedure and to irrigation of the pericardial cavity with irritating solutions (Ribeiro, 1984).

Constriction occurs when a chronically diseased pericardium restricts cardiac function by limitation of diastolic filling. Thickening, fibrosis, and calcification of the pericardium diminish pericardial compliance and result in a fixed, often somewhat contracted intrapericardial volume. As the pericardium becomes more rigid and nondistensible, the limiting volume or ultimate limit of pericardial distention decreases. This leads to an abrupt cessation of the early rapid phase of diastolic filling when the limiting volume of the pericardium is reached. Most commonly the fibrotic process affects most of the pericardial surface and produces a uniform restriction of filling of all heart chambers, resulting in both pulmonary and systemic venous congestion, decreased cardiac output, a fall in systemic blood pressure, and exertional intolerance. Localized constriction and compression may also occur if the disease process in the pericardium is limited.

Diagnosis

Physical examination in constrictive pericarditis reveals evidence of right-sided heart failure, including jugular venous distention, peripheral edema, hepatosplenomegaly, and ascites. Kussmaul's sign, an inspiratory increase in jugular venous pressure, may be present, but pulsus paradoxus does not usually occur. An early diastolic pericardial knock by auscultation and occasionally by palpation is present and corresponds to the cessation of rapid ventricular filling caused by the diminished limiting volume of the constricted pericardium.

Pericardial calcification may be prominent on chest radiography, especially in the lateral view (Fig. 60–1). The ECG may display nonspecific ST segment changes but is often only remarkable for low QRS voltages. Other diagnostic studies may be helpful in determining the extent of pericardial disease and the degree of impairment of cardiac function. Echocardiography can document thickening of the pericardium and may demonstrate the abnormal diastolic function in association with normal ventricular systolic function that is characteristic of constriction. Computed tomography (CT) and magnetic resonance imaging (MRI) allow measurement of pericardial thickness and assessment of dilatation of the inferior and superior venae cavae and the hepatic veins and are superior to echocardiography at delineating the extent of neoplastic pericardial disease (Smith et al, 1998). MRI is more sensitive at detecting pericardial thickening than CT (Jarad et al, 1993), and Gd-DTPA enhanced MRI may be particularly useful in differentiating pericardial thickening from an associated effusion in early effusive-constrictive pericarditis (Watanabe et al, 1998). Angiography with intrachamber pressure monitoring will demonstrate the abrupt cessation of ventricular diastolic filling and equalization of left and right ventricular diastolic pressure. Angiography may also be helpful in operative planning in older patients if concurrent significant coronary artery disease is suspected.

It may be difficult to differentiate between cardiac dysfunction resulting from constrictive pericarditis and that resulting from a restrictive cardiomyopathy, especially in the patient with disease resulting from prior mediastinal irradiation. Differentiation, however, is crucial, because resection of the constrictive pericardium can be expected to produce a marked resolution of symptoms, whereas removal of the pericardium in patients in whom the primary problem is restrictive cardiomyopathy will be unsuccessful and poorly tolerated (Hatle et al, 1989). Restrictive cardiomyopathy results from an infiltrative process in the myocardium, such as amyloidosis or radiation-induced fibrosis, that produces diastolic dysfunction. The resulting hemodynamic pattern may be indistinguishable from constrictive pericarditis. Restrictive car-

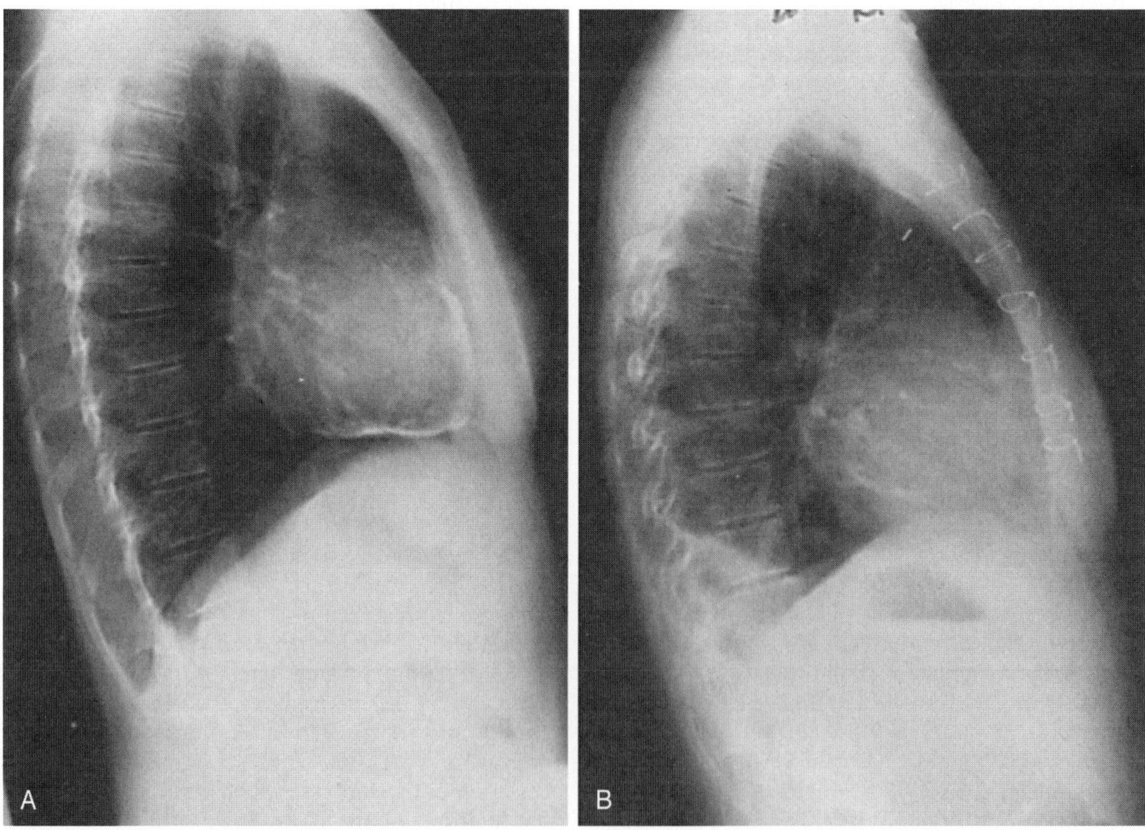

FIGURE 60–1 ■ *A*, Lateral chest radiograph of a patient with constrictive pericarditis, demonstrating extensive calcification of the pericardium; *B*, The same patient following pericardiectomy.

diomyopathy may, however, affect the left ventricle more than the right and may be associated with signs of other organ involvement in systemic diseases, such as amyloidosis. At angiography, restrictive cardiomyopathy may be distinguished from constrictive pericarditis by the presence of right ventricular systolic hypertension. Restrictive cardiomyopathy also results in impaired function throughout diastole, whereas only the latter portion of the rapid filling phase is affected in constrictive pericarditis. Noninvasive techniques such as cine MRI have also demonstrated value in the differentiation of constrictive pericarditis from restrictive cardiomyopathy (White, 1995).

Management

Thickening, fibrosis, and calcification of the pericardium in constrictive pericarditis are not reversible and therefore necessitate operative intervention if significant. Adequate resection of the pericardium in these cases leads to both immediate relief of symptoms and a later improvement in exercise tolerance (Copeland et al, 1975; Pugliese et al, 1984; Seifert et al, 1985; McCaughan et al, 1985). However, pericardiectomy may be a difficult procedure because the pericardium is often firmly adherent to the epicardial surface, obscuring planes of dissection. Operative mortality of up to 5% has been reported (DeValeria et al, 1991). Failure to improve after pericardiectomy may result from inadequate resection of the visceral portion of the pericardium, leading to continued constriction, or from underlying myocardial disease, atrophy, or fibrosis (Culliford et al, 1980; Ni et al, 1990).

Timing of operative intervention remains controversial. Early pericardiectomy, even before the onset of symptoms, has been recommended in pericardial disease processes in which the likelihood that constriction will develop is high, as in tuberculous pericarditis (Larrieu et al, 1980). For most other disease processes, surgery may be delayed until the patient actually begins to demonstrate signs of early constriction. Serial echocardiograms may be helpful in following these patients and planning intervention. Median sternotomy is the standard surgical approach, although some surgeons perform pericardiectomy through a left anterior thoracotomy if the disease process is limited to the anterior pericardium. However, complete resection of the pericardium from beyond the right phrenic nerve to the left pulmonary vessels with preservation of the phrenic bundles bilaterally is to be recommended to decrease the risk of recurrent constriction, because reoperation for additional pericardial resection carries a significantly higher morbidity and mortality (Culliford et al, 1980). Careful removal of the visceral portion of the pericardium is also crucial in preventing recurrence. Cardiopulmonary bypass should be available at the time of operation in case it is needed to obtain an adequate pericardial resection, but it should probably be avoided if possible to obviate the need for systemic heparinization with its attendant higher risk of bleeding.

Pericardial Effusive Disease and Cardiac Tamponade

Etiology and Pathophysiology

Pericardial effusions result when the net rate of pericardial fluid production exceeds the rate of fluid resorption. The pericardial effusion fluid may be serous, purulent, or hemorrhagic or a combination of the three types. More than 75% of pericardial effusions are secondary to malignancy, most commonly of the lung or breast or lymphoma (Press and Livingston, 1987). Benign causes of pericardial effusive disease include acute pericarditis, especially if viral and idiopathic in origin or after cardiac surgery; trauma; rupture of an ascending aorta aneurysm or dissection; radiation therapy; and myocardial infarction, particularly in association with anticoagulation.

Irritation and inflammation of the pericardial serosa produce an exudative reaction resulting in increased pericardial fluid. Likewise, implantation of metastatic disease in the serosa leads to exudation of fluid into the pericardial space. When the resorptive capacity of the pericardial serosa is exceeded or inflammatory or neoplastic processes begin to obstruct the venous and lymphatic drainage of the pericardium, a significant effusion develops that may result in cardiac tamponade when the limiting volume of the pericardium is reached.

The normal function of the heart and circulation is compromised when the presence of fluid under increased pressure within the pericardial space compromises diastolic filling. Because the normally compliant pericardium allows some distensibility, the rate of pericardial fluid accumulation may be as important as the total amount of fluid present in determining the point at which cardiac function will be compromised. Mild cardiac compression may only produce an elevated central venous pressure with normal systemic blood pressure, because impaired diastolic function may be adequately compensated by a normal heart and circulation. Severe compression leads to further compromise of diastolic filling beyond the compensatory capabilities of the heart and results in tamponade and ultimately in cardiogenic shock.

Diagnosis

Pericardial effusive disease without significant cardiac compromise or tamponade is often asymptomatic. Because the development of a pericardial effusion may not diminish the quality of friction rubs or cause ECG changes in acute pericarditis, a high index of suspicion must be maintained for early diagnosis to be made. A pericardial effusion should be suspected when patients with pericarditis, metastatic neoplasms, or uremia and renal failure requiring hemodialysis develop diminished QRS voltages on ECG or an enlarged cardiac silhouette on chest radiography (Fig. 60–2), especially in association with clear lung fields or an unexplained increase in venous pressure.

Acute cardiac tamponade occurs when a pericardial effusion rapidly develops, such as after blunt or penetrating chest trauma, postinfarction ventricular rupture, or intrapericardial rupture of an aortic dissection or from bleeding after cardiac surgery. The central venous pressure markedly increases in association with systemic hypotension. Beck's triad of distended neck veins, muffled heart sounds, and hypotension is characteristic, and pulsus paradoxus may be detectable. Recognition of tamponade in this setting is crucial and should prompt rapid volume infusion to further raise venous pressure to pro-

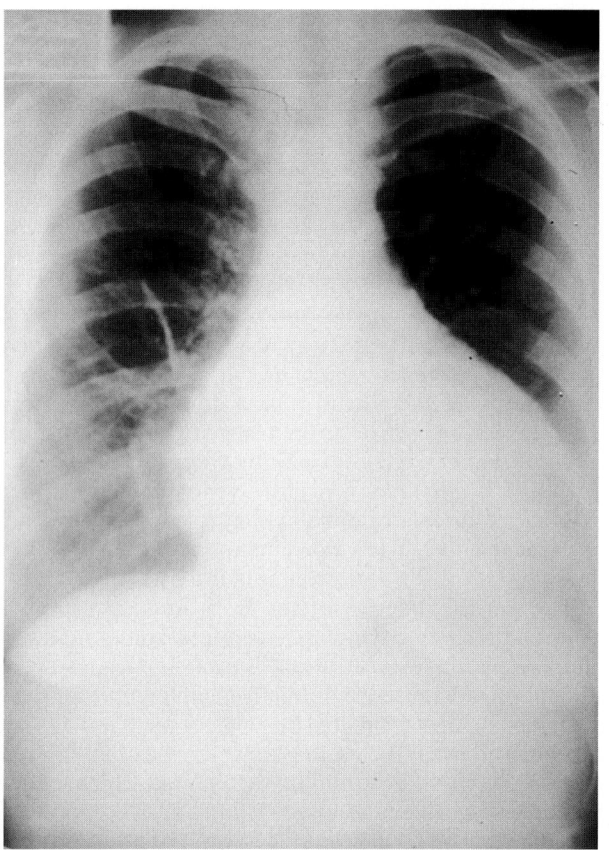

FIGURE 60–2 ■ Chest radiograph demonstrating an enlarged, smooth-bordered cardiac silhouette in a patient with a large pericardial effusion and impending cardiac tamponade.

mote diastolic filling, as well as emergent pericardiocentesis for decompression. Definitive identification and correction of the primary abnormality may then be pursued.

Subacute tamponade presents as progressive dyspnea on even minimal activity and should be suspected in hemodynamically compromised patients who have pericarditis, aortic dissections, or known or suggested intrathoracic or metastatic neoplasms or who are recovering from chest trauma or cardiac surgery. Hypotension may be present, but the systemic blood pressure may be maintained by elevated peripheral vascular resistance. A narrow pulse pressure accompanied by pulsus paradoxus, distant heart sounds, and an elevated central venous pressure is characteristic. Tachycardia results as a compensatory mechanism to maintain cardiac output, whereas rales are uncommon. Chest radiographs confirm the presence of an enlarged cardiac silhouette with clear lung fields, whereas the ECG demonstrates low QRS voltages and ST segment alterations. Electrical alternans, or QRS voltages that vary from beat to beat, may also be present; this reflects swinging of the heart in the pericardial fluid during contractions.

Proper diagnosis of tamponade requires demonstration of a pericardial effusion, demonstration of hemodynamic abnormalities attributable to pericardial fluid under pressure, and improvement of these hemodynamic abnormalities after drainage of the pericardial fluid (Burstow et al, 1989). Echocardiography (Fig. 60–3) has proven to be the most helpful adjunct in the diagnosis of pericardial effusive disease and tamponade in the subacute setting. M-mode echocardiography allows diagnosis of pericardial effusion by the demonstration of an echo-free space between the heart and pericardium. The heart may be seen to swing freely in the effusion in association with electrical alternans (Vignolo et al, 1976). The effusion may be characterized as small if present only behind the left ventricle, moderate if also present in front of the right ventricle, and massive if the echo-free area surrounds the heart during all phases of the cardiac cycle (Horowitz et al, 1977; Martin et al, 1978). Furthermore, two-dimensional echocardiograms can quantify the amount and location of the effusion, identify loculations and adhesions, and suggest impending tamponade (Martin et al, 1980).

Hemodynamic compromise and cardiac tamponade may be demonstrated echocardiographically by a decreased right ventricular diameter with compression of the right atrium. Paradoxical septal motion and systolic collapse with inward motion of the right atrial and ventricular walls in early systole suggest severe compromise requiring emergent decompression. Other echocardiographic findings of tamponade may include persistent full distention of the inferior vena cava throughout the entire cardiac cycle and an exaggerated respiratory variation in the velocity of flow through the mitral and tricuspid valves (D'Cruz et al, 1975).

Management

Treatment of pericardial effusive disease without evidence of hemodynamic compromise may be directed toward the cause of the effusion alone if the underlying condition is self-limited or responsive to therapy, the effusion does not appear to be enlarging, the patient can be followed for signs of increased effusion or evolving tamponade, and fluid is not necessary to establish a primary diagnosis. The indications for pericardiocentesis in the absence

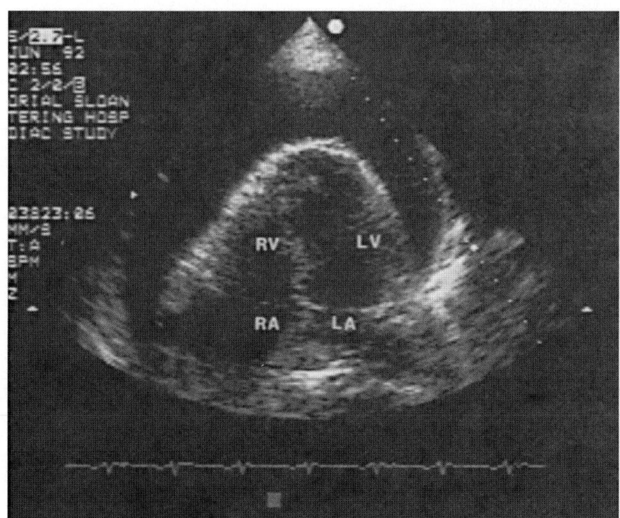

FIGURE 60–3 ■ Echocardiogram demonstrating a large pericardial effusion in a patient with metastatic breast cancer that is compressing the right atrium and ventricle at end diastole.

of tamponade are to eliminate the possibility of a purulent effusion that requires operative drainage, to differentiate a neoplastic effusion in patients with malignancy from a reactive effusion after irradiation or chemotherapy, and to obtain fluid for proper diagnosis when the etiology of the effusion is unclear or when an exact diagnosis is necessary in choosing therapy (Mueller et al, 1997; Wenger, 1991).

Signs of impending tamponade on examination or echocardiography are an indication for emergent pericardial decompression by pericardiocentesis or open drainage. While being prepared for drainage, the patient should be treated by volume expansion with saline solutions despite elevated venous pressures. Volume infusion will increase right atrial pressure without affecting intrapericardial pressure, thus promoting diastolic filling. Infusion of dobutamine may also be helpful in the interim management of these patients before drainage by decreasing heart size through improved inotropy and systemic vasodilatation. However, it cannot be overemphasized that emergent decompression of the pericardial space is the only maneuver in impending tamponade that is lifesaving.

The choice of pericardiocentesis versus open drainage procedures for tamponade remains controversial and depends on the etiology of the effusion, the condition of the patient, and the available facilities and physician experience. Pericardiocentesis is less expensive than open drainage and requires fewer resources. Placement of a catheter into the pericardial space permits an exact hemodynamic diagnosis and allows pressure monitoring for evaluating the effects of drainage on hemodynamics. Sclerosis may be subsequently performed for treatment of malignant effusions. Pericardiocentesis is associated with morbidity and occasional mortality from errant catheter placement into the heart or inferior vena cava and from bleeding due to laceration of an epicardial or coronary vessel. Although decompression may be obtained, complete drainage of the effusion, especially if loculated or purulent, may be difficult, necessitating repeated taps or open drainage.

Pericardiotomy may be performed through either a subxiphoid or a left anterior thoracotomy approach. Open drainage through such incisions is performed under direct vision, allows for exploration of the pericardial space, and permits pericardial biopsy if indicated. The incision may be extended if necessary, and pericardiectomy may be performed. Open drainage has the disadvantages that a fully equipped and staffed operating room is necessary and accurate intraoperative pericardial pressure measurements are difficult to obtain. Furthermore, general anesthesia is necessary, at least for the anterior thoracotomy approach, and anesthetic induction in these hemodynamically compromised patients may be hazardous.

OTHER DISEASES OF THE PERICARDIUM

Congenital Anomalies

Partial or complete absence of the pericardium is rare and usually asymptomatic. An incomplete defect on the left side is the most common finding and is often associated with other congenital cardiac malformations, including patent ductus arteriosus, atrial septal defect, mitral valve stenosis and prolapse, and tetralogy of Fallot (Nasser, 1970). No significant pathophysiology accompanies a pericardial defect unless it is large enough to allow herniation of the left side of the heart or torsion of the great vessels.

Pericardial cysts and diverticula are smooth and rounded structures usually first found on a routine chest radiograph (Klatte and Young, 1972). They most commonly occur in the right cardiophrenic angle anteriorly (Craddock, 1950; Loehr, 1952). The diverticula differ from the cysts by the persistence of a connection to the coelomic cavity (Bates and Lever, 1951). Both uncomplicated cysts and diverticula are asymptomatic but when discovered should be differentiated from neoplasms by CT or occasionally by surgical exploration (Fig. 60–4).

Pericardial Neoplasms

Although metastatic disease of the pericardium is common, primary neoplasms of the pericardium are rare. Mesothelioma is the most common primary pericardial neoplasm; and as with primary pleural mesothelioma, effective therapy producing long-term control is lacking at present. Pericardial resection may be necessary to control pericardial effusions. Treatment with doxorubicin, cyclophosphamide, and cisplatin has also met with limited success (Artman, 1980). Other reported primary pericardial neoplasms include lymphagiomas, hemangiomas, teratomas, rhabdomyosarcomas, and lipomas.

Metastatic neoplasms are far more common than primary pericardial tumors. Metastases spread to the pericardium by hematogenous or lymphatic routes or through direct invasion of the pericardium. Common primary tumors that metastasize to or involve the pericardium include lung, breast, colon, esophagus, kidney, ovary, prostate, and stomach neoplasms, leukemia and lymphoma, melanoma, and soft tissue sarcomas (Press and

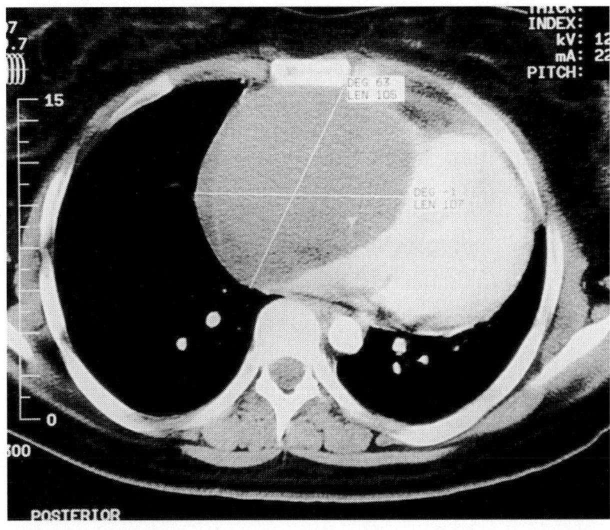

FIGURE 60–4 ■ Computed tomography scan of the chest in a patient with a large congenital cyst of the visceral pericardium overlying the right ventricle.

Livingston, 1987). The most common presentation of tumor involving the pericardium is a pericardial effusion, and metastatic disease is the most common cause of pericardial effusions. The presence of the pericardial effusion almost invariably indicates unresectability for cure. Treatment should be directed toward systemic chemotherapy and effective palliation and control of the effusion by pericardial drainage (Davis et al, 1978; Hawkins and Vacek, 1989). Sclerosis of the pericardial cavity with doxycycline, talc, or bleomycin may be indicated if the effusion is recurrent, enlarging, or hemodynamically significant (Shepard et al, 1987).

Postpericardiotomy Syndrome

As many as 25% to 30% of patients undergoing surgical procedures in which the pericardium is opened experience symptoms that are associated with the postpericardiotomy syndrome. Studies have demonstrated elevated antiheart and viral antibody titers in some of these patients (Engle et al, 1974), but the etiology and pathophysiology of the syndrome remain poorly understood. Symptoms resemble those of acute pericarditis with pleuritic chest pain and dyspnea, a pericardial friction rub, and, less frequently, fevers and leukocytosis. Most patients are well controlled by administration of nonsteroidal anti-inflammatory agents until symptoms have resolved, although rarely a patient may require pulse corticosteroid therapy to control symptoms. Some patients relapse with recurrence of symptoms after cessation of therapy and require more prolonged therapy.

PERICARDIOCENTESIS AND PERICARDIAL SURGERY

Preoperative and Anesthetic Considerations

Patients undergoing procedures for decompression of the pericardial space for impending tamponade should be volume loaded with saline solutions as preparations for the procedure are being made. Volume expansion is crucial, even with already elevated venous pressures, to maintain hemodynamic stability and promote diastolic filling by increasing right atrial pressure above intrapericardial pressure. A careful history for corticosteroid therapy within the past year for pericarditis or underlying disease should be sought; and if it is found, stress corticosteroid therapy should be administered.

Arterial and central venous pressure monitoring is essential for open procedures and highly recommended during pericardiocentesis. Safe anesthetic induction in hemodynamically compromised patients is difficult and necessitates close cooperation between the surgeon and the anesthesiologist. Sudden loss of vascular tone due to anesthetic administration in patients with impending tamponade will result in hypotension, further hemodynamic compromise, and cardiac arrest if it is not anticipated and proper precautionary actions are not taken. Induction and intubation should not be begun until after the patient is properly positioned on the surgical table with the head elevated. The patient should be prepared and draped awake, and the surgical team should be prepared to commence the operation as the rapid sequence induction is initiated. Pericardiocentesis and partial decompression before open drainage may also improve hemodynamic stability and response to anesthesia and surgery.

Pericardiocentesis

Pericardiocentesis is indicated to establish the diagnosis of pericardial disease by examination of effusion fluid, to treat acute or impending tamponade, to differentiate from constriction in the etiology of elevated venous pressures in association with pericardial disease, and as an interim treatment before surgical drainage for tamponade to aid anesthetic management (Miller and Hatcher, 1990).

The patient is placed in a semiupright position, and the midanterior chest is prepared and draped. A parasternal placement of the catheter through the fourth or fifth intercostal space may be chosen, but the subxiphoid approach is generally easier and safer. An entry point is chosen 2 cm inferior to the xiphoid and to the left of the midline. A 21-gauge spinal needle is directed at a 45-degree angle aimed toward the left shoulder. The direction of the needle may also be guided by ECG monitoring, with a watch for deflection as the needle contacts the epicardial surface (Bishop et al, 1956); by echocardiography (Callahan et al, 1985); or by fluoroscopy with pressure monitoring in an angiography suite. The needle is continuously aspirated as it is advanced, and once fluid is encountered, the needle may be changed over a guidewire to a flexible Silastic catheter. Returned bloody fluid should be examined carefully for clotting to rule out inadvertent cardiac puncture. A pneumopericardium, produced by insufflation of air into the pericardial space, was often used in the past, after completion of drainage of the pericardial fluid, to permit determination of pericardial thickness or the presence of masses by plain chest radiography (Hancock, 1979). This technique has largely been supplanted by the widespread use of echocardiography (Martin et al, 1980). The catheter may also be left in place for subsequent fluid drainage or sclerosis of the pericardial space.

Bleeding is the most common complication of pericardiocentesis and may result from inadvertent cardiac entry, cardiac or epicardial laceration, or injury to a coronary artery (Scannell, 1989). The risk of cardiac injury and significant hemorrhage is increased in patients with thrombocytopenia, coagulopathies, or small or loculated effusions and when a presumptive effusion is drained without echocardiographic confirmation (Wong et al, 1979). Vasodilatation secondary to rapid decompression of the pericardial space may also occur and should be treated by volume administration. Failure to adequately drain the effusion or the recurrence of fluid may lead to later tamponade.

The choice of pericardiocentensis over an open surgical drainage procedure depends on the disease process being treated, the availability of facilities, and the experience of the physician performing the procedure. Open drainage should be favored when the accessibility of the effusion by pericardiocentesis is questionable, in the presence of a coagulopathy or other condition that increases the risk of bleeding, or when constrictive pericarditis, which will need resection, is concomitantly present. Suspicion of the presence of partially clotted blood or purulent fluid within the pericardial space should also prompt an open procedure to ensure adequate drainage.

Pericardiotomy

Open pericardial drainage and pericardiotomy are indicated for pericardial effusions containing clotted blood; for effusions associated with a likely cardiac bleeding site, such as a traumatic injury; for suspected purulent or loculated effusion; for effusions that are recurrent or likely to recur, as in uremic pericarditis; or when pericardial biopsy is required for diagnosis.

Pericardiotomy may be performed by using either a subxiphoid or left anterior thoracotomy incision. The subxiphoid approach may be used with the patient under local anesthesia. A 3- to 4-cm vertical incision is made in the midline just above and inferior to the xiphoid process. Dissection is continued posteriorly and superiorly to the reflection of the pericardium onto the diaphragm. The pericardial space is entered at that point, and the effusion is drained. The pericardial space is carefully explored to ensure adequate drainage and open loculations. Substernal pericardial tubes are then placed for continued drainage and sclerosis if required.

Use of a left anterior thoracotomy approach allows improved visualization, greater exploration of the pericardial space, and a wider resection of the pericardium, establishing a drainage pathway into the left pleural space. The incision may be extended to perform a pericardiectomy if indicated. General anesthesia is required for the anterior thoracotomy, which is also more painful postoperatively than the subxiphoid procedure. Use of video-assisted thoracic surgery (VATS) instrumentation is now allowing many of the benefits of the thoracotomy approach with reduced postoperative pain and morbidity. Pericardiotomy and partial pericardial resection can easily be performed by a surgeon who is skilled in these techniques, although the ability to explore the pericardial space remains limited.

Pericardiectomy

Pericardiectomy is indicated for constrictive pericarditis and for selected cases of recurrent pericarditis or recurrent pericardial effusive disease that is unresponsive to medical therapy. A median sternotomy approach is preferred, although some surgeons still favor a left anterior thoracotomy incision. Resection of both the parietal and the visceral pericardium are necessary for adequate treatment of constrictive pericarditis, whereas it is less crucial to remove the visceral layer in the treatment of recurrent effusions.

The extent of resection for constrictive disease is usually from the right phrenic nerve to the level of the left pulmonary vasculature anteriorly, to the reflection onto the great vessels superiorly, and to the posterior diaphragm inferiorly. The phrenic nerves and associated blood vessels are preserved bilaterally as 1-cm tissue bridges. The visceral pericardium may then be "teased" from the surface of the epicardium with care taken to remain in the proper plane of dissection (Fig. 60–5). The pericardium over the left ventricle is resected when possible before that over the right ventricle to minimize early blood loss, because the latter is the more easily injured of the two chambers. This sequence also theoretically avoids pulmonary congestion, which might occur if right ventricular output were allowed to increase while the left ventricle remained constricted. After the resection, both pleural cavities should be widely opened to allow improved postoperative drainage of blood and exudative fluid.

Complications may occur in 10% to 30% of cases (Culliford et al, 1980; DeValeria et al, 1991). Bleeding may be profuse and can occur from the raw epicardial surface or from laceration of the right atrium, right ventricle, or coronary vessels. Arrhythmias are common and

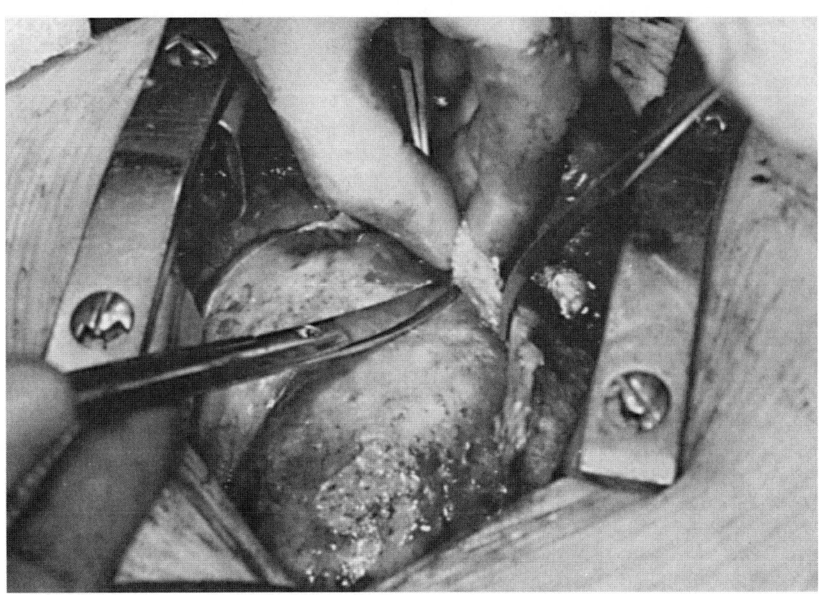

FIGURE 60–5 ■ Surgical technique of "teasing" the visceral pericardium from the epicardial surface during pericardiectomy for constrictive pericarditis.

are due to atrial irritability, manipulation of the heart, or injury to branches of the coronary arteries. Some surgeons have recommended the use of cardiopulmonary bypass during pericardiectomy to facilitate control of cardiac lacerations and hemorrhage and to allow safer manipulation of the heart for more complete resection (Copeland et al, 1975; Culliford et al, 1980; Pugliese et al, 1984). However, systemic heparinization may make control of bleeding from the raw epicardial surface more difficult and actually increase operative morbidity. Although the routine use of cardiopulmonary bypass is not indicated, it should be available on a standby basis for all pericardial resections for constrictive disease.

COMMENTS AND CONTROVERSIES

Dr. Jones has concisely outlined the challenge of differentiating constrictive pericarditis from restrictive cardiomyopathy. Although pericardiectomy will often benefit those patients with constrictive pericarditis, such a major operative procedure is poorly tolerated and often fatal in a patient with restrictive cardiomyopathy.

The surgical options for diagnostic and therapeutic evacuation of pericardial effusion are clearly presented. Pericardial centesis is underemployed as a means to avoid operative intervention. Of the operative approaches—subxiphoid, left anterolateral thoracotomy or video-assisted thoracostomy—our preference is to accomplish a pericardial window by means of a subxiphoid approach. This approach provides easiest access with the minimum amount of preoperative preparation. Arterial lines and single-lung ventilation are not necessary. The subxiphoid approach can be accomplished under local anesthesia, a definite advantage in the patient who is hemodynamically unstable.

In the discussion of congenital anomalies, it is suggested that pericardial cysts may occasionally require resection for diagnostic purposes. With currently available imaging modalities, including computed tomography, magnetic resonance imaging, and echocardiography, the diagnosis of pericardial cysts should never be in doubt, and surgical resection should never be performed on an asymptomatic patient.

G. A. P.

KEY REFERENCES

Culliford AT, Lipton M, Spencer FC: Operation for chronic constrictive pericarditis: Do the surgical approach and degree of pericardial resection influence the outcome significantly? Ann Thorac Surg 29:146, 1980.

This excellent study and subsequent discussion of surgical treatment of constrictive pericarditis weighs the controversies regarding adequate therapy and surgical technique.

Press OW, Livingston R: Management of malignant pericardial effusion and tamponade. JAMA 257:1088, 1987.

A well-organized review of etiology and management of malignant pericardial disease includes both medical and surgical treatment options.

Shabetai R, Fowler ND, Gunthenok WG: The hemodynamics of cardiac tamponade and constrictive pericarditis. Am J Cardiol 26:480, 1970.

Pericardial pressure-volume relationships and the hemodynamic consequences of pericardial tamponade and constrictive pericarditis are thoroughly discussed.

REFERENCES

Acierno LJ: Cardiac complications in acquired immunodeficiency syndrome (AIDS): A review. J Am Coll Cardiol 13:1144, 1989.

Applefield MM, Slawson RG, Hall-Craigs M et al: Delayed pericardial disease after radiotherapy. Am J Cardiol 47:210, 1981.

Artman K: Current concepts: Malignant mesothelioma. N Engl J Med 303:200, 1980.

Bates JC, Lever FY: Pericardial coelomic cysts: Presentation of 5 new cases and 5 similar cases illustrating difficulty of diagnosis. Radiology 57:300, 1951.

Beck CS, Griswald RA: Pericardiectomy in the treatment of the Pick syndrome: Experimental and clinical observations. Arch Surg 21:1064, 1930.

Bishop LH, Estes EH, McIntosh HD: Electrocardiograms as a safeguard in pericardiocentesis. JAMA 162:264, 1956.

Burstow DJ, Oh JK, Bailey KR et al: Cardiac tamponade: Characteristic Doppler observations. Mayo Clin Proc 64:312, 1989.

Buselmier TJ, Simmons RL, Najarian JS et al: Uremic pericardial effusion. Nephron 16:371, 1976.

Callahan JA, Seward JB, Nishimura RA et al: Two-dimensional echocardiographically guided pericardiocentesis: Experience with 117 consecutive patients. Am J Cardiol 55:476, 1985.

Churchill ED: Pericardial resection in chronic constrictive pericarditis. Am Surg 104:516, 1936.

Collin V, as quoted in Boyd LJ, Elias H: Contributions to disease of the heart and pericardium. Bull NY Med Coll 18:1, 1955.

Copeland JG, Stinson EB, Griepp RB, Shumway NE: Surgical treatment of chronic constrictive pericarditis using cardiopulmonary bypass. J Thorac Cardiovasc Surg 69:236, 1975.

Craddock WL: Cysts of the pericardium. Am Heart J 40:619, 1950.

Culliford AT, Lipton M, Spencer FC: Operation for chronic constrictive pericarditis: Do the surgical approach and degree of pericardial resection influence the outcome significantly? Ann Thorac Surg 29:146, 1980.

D'Cruz IA, Cohen HC, Parbhu R et al: Diagnosis of cardiac tamponade by echocardiography: Changes in mitral valve motion and ventricular dimensions, with special reference to paradoxical pulse. Circulation 52:460, 1975.

Davis S, Sharma SM, Blumberg ED et al: Intrapericardial tetracycline for the management of cardiac tamponade secondary to malignant pericardial effusion. N Engl J Med 299:1113, 1978.

DeValeria PA, Baumgartner WA, Casale AS et al: Current indications, risks and outcome after pericardiectomy. Ann Thorac Surg 52:219, 1991.

Elias H, Boyd LJ: Notes on the anatomy, embryology and histology of the pericardium. J NY Med Coll 2:50, 1960.

Engle MA, McCabe JC, Ebert PA, Zabriskie J: The postpericardiotomy syndrome and antiheart antibodies. Circulation 49:401, 1974.

Estok L, Wallach F: Cardiac tamponade in a patient with AIDS: A review of pericardial disease in patients with HIV infection. Mt Sinai J Med 65:33, 1998.

Ferguson JJ, Willerson JT: Constrictive pericarditis. In Hurst JW (ed): Current Therapy in Cardiovascular Disease, 3rd ed. Philadelphia, BC Decker, 1991, p 269.

Fowler NO: Acute and recurrent pericarditis. In Hurst JW (ed): Current Therapy in Cardiovascular Disease, 3rd ed. Philadelphia, BC Decker, 1991, p 260.

Fowler NO, Harbin AD: Recurrent pericarditis: Follow-up study of 31 patients. J Am Coll Cardiol 7:300, 1986.

Gibbon AT, Segal MB: A study of the composition of pericardial fluid with special reference to the probable mechanism of fluid formation. J Physiol 277:635, 1940.

Guindo J, Rodriguez de la Seina A, Ramiero J et al: Recurrent pericarditis: Relief with colchicine. Circulation 82:1117, 1990.

Hancock EW: Management of pericardial disease. Mod Concepts Cardiovasc Dis 47:1, 1979.

Hatcher CR, Logue RB, Logan WD et al: Pericardiectomy for recurrent pericarditis. J Thorac Cardiovasc Surg 62:371, 1971.

Hatle LK, Appleton CP, Popp RL: Differentiation of constrictive pericarditis and restrictive cardiomyopathy by Doppler echocardiography. Circulation 79:357, 1989.

Hawkins JW, Vacek JL: What constitutes definitive treatment of malignant pericardial effusion? "Medical" versus surgical treatment. Am Heart J 118:428, 1989.

Holt JP: The normal pericardium. Am J Cardiol 26:455, 1970.

Horowitz MS, Schultz CS, Stinson EB et al: Sensitivity and specificity of echocardiographic diagnosis of pericardial effusion. Circulation 72:744, 1977.

Jarad NA, Underwood SR, Rudd RM: Asbestos-related pericardial thickening detected by magnetic resonance imaging. Respir Med 87:309, 1993.

Karaeneff P: Paracentese des Brustkastens und des Pericardiums. Med Z 9:251, 1840.

Klatte EC, Young HY: Diagnosis and treatment of pericardial cysts. Radiology 104:541, 1972.

Kussmaul A: Ueber schwielige Mediatino-perikarditis und dem paradoxen Puls. Berl Klin Wochenschr 10:433, 1873.

Kutcher MA, King SB, Alimurung BN et al: Constrictive pericarditis as a complication of cardiac surgery: Recognition of an entity. Am J Cardiol 50:742, 1982.

Laennec RTH: Traité d'Auscultation Médicale et des Maladies du Poumon et du Coeur. Paris, Brosson & JS Chaude, 1819.

Larrieu AJ, Tyers FO, Walthams EH, Derrick JC: Recent experience with tuberculous pericarditis. Ann Thorac Surg 29:464, 1980.

Loehr WM: Pericardial cysts. AJR Am J Roentgenol 68:584, 1952.

Lower R: Tractatus de Corde. London, 1669, p 104.

Marsa R, Mehta S, Willis W, Bailey L: Constrictive pericarditis after myocardial revascularization: Report of three cases. Am J Cardiol 44:177, 1979.

Martin RP, Bowden R, Filly K et al: Intrapericardial abnormalities in patients with pericardial effusion: Findings by two-dimensional echocardiography. Circulation 61:568, 1980.

Martin RP, Rakowski H, French J et al: Localization of pericardial effusion with wide angle phased array echocardiography. Am J Cardiol 42:904, 1978.

McCaughan BC, Schaff HV, Piehler JM et al: Early and late results of pericardiectomy for constrictive pericarditis. J Thorac Cardiovasc Surg 89:340, 1985.

Miller JI, Hatcher CR: Surgical management of pericardial disease. In Hurst JW (ed): The Heart, Vol 1. New York, McGraw-Hill, 1990, p 2185.

Miller JI, Mansour KA, Hatcher CR: Pericardiectomy: Current indications, concepts and results in a university center. Ann Thorac Surg 34:40, 1982.

Moores DW, Dziuban SW: Pericardial drainage procedures. Chest Clin North Am 5:359, 1995.

Mueller XM, Tevaearai HT, Hurni M, et al: Etiologic diagnosis of pericardial disease: The value of routine tests during surgical procedures. J Am Coll Surg 184:645, 1997.

Nasser WK: Congenital absence of the left pericardium. Am J Cardiol 26:470, 1970.

Ni Y, von Seegesser LK, Turina M: Futility of pericardiectomy for postirradiation pericarditis? Ann Thorac Surg 49:445, 1990.

Pegram BL, Bishop VS: An evaluation of the pericardial sac as a safety factor during cardiac tamponade. Cardiovasc Res 48:701, 1981.

Pick F: Ueber chronische, unter dem Bilde der Lebercirrhose Verlaufen der Pericarditis (Pericarditis pseudolebercirrhose) nebst Bemerkungen ueber Zuckergussleber. Z Klin Med 29:385, 1886.

Press OW, Livingston R: Management of malignant pericardial effusion and tamponade. JAMA 257:1088, 1987.

Pugliese P, Bernabei M, Eufrate S: Total pericardiectomy for chronic constrictive pericarditis using femero-femoral bypass. Int Surg 69:39, 1984.

Rehn L: Zurexperimentellen pathologic des Herzbeutels. Verh Dtsh Ges Chir 42:339, 1913.

Ribeiro P: Constrictive pericarditis as a complication of coronary artery bypass surgery. Br Heart J 51:205, 1984.

Sauerbruch F: Die Chirurgie der Brestorgane, Vol II. Berlin, 1925.

Scannell JG: Malignant pericardial effusion. In Grillo HC, Austin WG, Wilkins EW et al (eds): Current Therapy in Cardiothoracic Surgery. Toronto, BC Decker, 1989, p 295.

Schmieder V, Fischer H: Die Herzbeutelentzunchung und irhe Folgezustande. Ergeb Chir Orthop 19:98, 1926.

Schneider JS, Edwards JE: Irradiation induced pericarditis. Chest 75:560, 1979.

Seifert FC, Miller DC, Osterle SN et al: Surgical treatment of constrictive pericarditis: Analysis of outcome and diagnostic error. Circulation 72:264, 1985.

Shabetai R: Pericardial and cardiac pressure. Circulation 77:1, 1987.

Shabetai R: Diseases of the pericardium. In Hurst JW (ed): The Heart, Vol 1. New York, McGraw-Hill, 1990, p 1348.

Shabetai R, Fowler ND, Gunthenok WG: The hemodynamics of cardiac tamponade and constrictive pericarditis. Am J Cardiol 26:480, 1970.

Shepard FA, Morgan C, Evans WK et al: Medical management of malignant pericardial effusion by tetracycline sclerosis. Am J Cardiol 60:1161, 1987.

Smith DN, Shaffer K, Patz EF: Imaging features of nonmyxomatous neoplasms of the heart and pericardium. Clin Imaging 22:15, 1998.

Strang JIG, Gibson DG, Mitchison DA et al: Controlled clinical trial of complete open surgical drainage and of prednisolone in the treatment of tuberculous pericardial effusion in Transkei. Lancet 2:759, 1988.

Vignolo PA, Pohost GM, Curfrued GD, Myers G: Correlation of echocardiographic and clinical findings in patients with pericardial effusion. Arch Intern Med 136:979, 1976.

Watanabe A, Hara Y, Hamada M, et al: A case of effusive pericarditis: An efficacy of Gd-DTPA enhanced magnetic resonance imaging to detect a pericardial thickening. Magn Reson Imaging 16:347, 1998.

Wenger NK: Pericardial effusion. In Hurst JW (ed): Current Therapy in Cardiovascular Disease, 3rd ed. Philadelphia, BC Decker, 1991, p 264.

White CS: MR evaluation of the pericardium. Topics Magn Reson Imaging 7:258, 1995.

Won G, Murphy J, Chang CJ: The risk of pericardiocentesis. Am J Cardiol 44:1110, 1979.

CHAPTER **61**

Surgery of Myasthenia Gravis

Michael G. Wood

Jeffrey A. Hagen

Myasthenia gravis is a neurologic disorder that is defined clinically on the basis of weakness or fatigability that follows repetitive exercise and resolves with rest. It is an autoimmune disorder of neuromuscular transmission in which antibodies reduce the number of functional acetylcholine receptors at the neuromuscular junction. The clinical course in patients with myasthenia gravis is unpredictable, with frequent spontaneous remissions followed by relapses. The response to therapy is also unpredictable, and specifically with regard to thymectomy, it may be delayed.

The initiating events and the factors that sustain this autoimmune attack on the neuromuscular junction are unknown. The thymus gland is believed to play an important role for several reasons. First, it has been observed, especially in young patients, that the thymus gland either is hyperplastic or contains a thymoma in up to 80% of cases (Buckberg et al, 1967). Second, antibodies to acetylcholine receptors (Almon et al, 1974) and antibodies to other striated muscle antigens (Williams and Lennon, 1986) have been demonstrated in the thymus of patients with myasthenia. It is believed that the myoid cells that are present in the thymus may serve as the antigenic source of these autoantibodies. Finally, the importance of the thymus gland in the pathogenesis of myasthenia is supported by the beneficial effect observed after thymectomy.

Myasthenia gravis is a relatively uncommon disorder, occurring in 0.5 to 5 per 100,000 population. It can occur at virtually any age; the peak age of onset is of 20 to 30 years in women and older than 50 years in men. Overall, it is more common in women; there is a female predominance of 3:2. The disease is nonfamilial in most cases. In young patients, a genetic predisposition for myasthenia gravis has been associated with the histocompatibility antigens human leukocyte antigen (HLA)-B8 and HLA-Drw3, and in older patients with thymoma an association between histocompatibility antigens HLA-A2 and HLA-A3 and myasthenia has been observed (Seybold and Lindstrom, 1982). The disease is more common in patients with other autoimmune disorders, such as Graves' disease, Hashimoto's thyroiditis, rheumatoid arthritis, systemic lupus erythematosus, and pernicious anemia (Seybold, 1983). There are no known racial or geographic predilections.

Although the incidence in the general population is low, myasthenia gravis is one of the more common disorders of neuromuscular transmission and one of the most clearly understood physiologically. There remains a great deal of controversy, however, in regard to the diagnosis and therapy of this disorder. Much of this controversy is related specifically to the role of thymectomy in these patients.

HISTORICAL NOTE

Clinical recognition of the disorder that is now known as myasthenia gravis dates back to 1877, when Wilks reported on a patient with progressive weakness who ultimately died of respiratory paralysis. Autopsy revealed no evidence of a central nervous system cause. Over the next several years, similar case reports appeared in the literature of patients who died of respiratory paralysis without central nervous system causes. Goldflam (1893) summarized these case reports, along with his own collected series of patients. He described the clinical findings that were common in these patients; these findings became known as the Erb-Goldflam symptom complex. Two years later, in his classic description of the decremental response to repetitive tetanic stimulation in these patients, Jolly (1895) coined the term *myasthenia gravis pseudoparalytica*.

The treatment of these patients dates back to 1934, when Walker first used anticholinesterase drug therapy. After her subsequent report in 1935, neostigmine (Prostigmin) remained the drug of choice until Osserman and colleagues (1954) reported on the use of pyridostigmine bromide, which remains the standard therapeutic agent to this day. The idea of surgical therapy for patients with myasthenia gravis began with the recognition by Weigert (1901) of a thymoma in a patient who died of myasthenia gravis. Subsequently, Bell (1917) reported on a series of cases collected at autopsy, which revealed thymic abnormalities in 27 of 57 patients who died of myasthenia gravis. During the same period, the first thymectomy operations were being developed. Originally performed by the transcervical route, thymectomy was most often performed in patients with thyrotoxicosis. Von Haberer (1917) reported on 40 such operations, including one performed on a patient with myasthenia gravis. After thymectomy, the patient's myasthenic symptoms improved. Blalock and associates (1939) first intentionally removed the thymus in a young woman who had a thymoma and myasthenia gravis. The thymus was removed because of the tumor, not as specific therapy for her myasthenia. She experienced improvement in her myasthenic symptoms, which encouraged the performance of six more thymectomies in patients without thymomas reported by Blalock and associates (1941). By 1944, Blalock had accumulated a total of 20 patients who had undergone thymectomy for myasthenia gravis. He emphasized that the results were best in patients with a short duration of myasthenia and he cited the importance of complete thymectomy, two observations that remain important to this day.

Although the initial surgical approach was transcervical, the work of Blalock and that of Keynes (1955), who reported on 260 cases, led to the adoption of the median sternotomy approach. Akakura (1965), Crile (1966), and Carlens and coworkers (1967) reintroduced the transcervical method of thymectomy. This technique became attractive because it minimized surgical morbidity and increased patients' acceptance. A potential limitation of this approach was proposed by Henze (1984) and Jaretzki (1988) and their colleagues, who noted that removal of as little as 3 g of residual thymic tissue after thymectomy by standard or transcervical approaches led to substantial improvement in patients with persistent myasthenic symptoms. Modifications of the transcervical approach, as reported by Cooper and colleagues (1988), have resulted in improved exposure and more complete thymectomy with this technique, potentially reducing the amount of residual thymic tissue. Subsequently, minimally invasive approaches to thymectomy using video-assisted thoracic surgery (VATS) were advocated (Mack et al, 1996; Mineo et al, 1996; Novellino et al, 1994; Sugarbaker, 1993; Yim et al, 1995). This newly described technique awaits confirmation of efficacy by larger clinical trials that include adequate long-term follow-up.

■ *HISTORICAL READINGS*

Blalock A: Thymectomy in the treatment of myasthenia gravis: Report of twenty cases. J Thorac Cardiovasc Surg 13:316, 1944.

Goldflam S: Ueber einen scheinbar heilbaren bulbar paralytischen symptomen Complex mit Beteiligung der Extremitaten. Dtsch Z Nervenheilkd 4:312, 1893.

Keynes G: Investigations into thymic disease and tumor formation. Br J Surg 62:449, 1955.

Walker MB: Treatment of myasthenia gravis with physostigmine. Lancet 1:1200, 1934.

BASIC SCIENCE

To appreciate the important aspects of diagnosis and therapy for patients with myasthenia gravis, it is important to have an understanding of a few fundamentals of the normal physiology of neuromuscular transmission. In contrast to the complex integration of impulses at other synapses, neuromuscular transmission involves a relatively simple process of relays between motor neuron terminals and the postsynaptic receptors on the muscle cell. In response to nerve stimulation and calcium entry into the motor neuron, acetylcholine is released. The acetylcholine diffuses across the synaptic cleft, where it binds to receptors on the muscle cell (Fig. 61–1). Binding to the receptor creates an ion channel that allows the influx of positively charged ions, principally sodium, down the normal electrochemical gradient. This influx of positively charged ions results in localized depolarization of the muscle cell membrane, which is referred to as a miniature endplate potential. If the sum of several of these miniature endplate potentials is of sufficient amplitude, which depends on the amount of acetylcholine bound to receptors, the threshold for activation of the muscle cell is reached. This results in the generation of an action potential and calcium influx by activation of membrane calcium channels, which causes muscle contraction (Keesey, 1989).

Under normal circumstances, more acetylcholine is released from the motor neuron than is necessary to create an action potential in the muscle cell. In addition, many times more acetylcholine receptors are present on the motor endplate than are needed. These two factors provide a safety factor (Waud and Waud, 1975), which ensures neuromuscular transmission under normal circumstances. Alterations in this safety factor cause disorders of neuromuscular transmission, such as myasthenia gravis.

The autoimmune nature of myasthenia gravis was first suggested by Seybold (1983), who identified antibodies to acetylcholine receptors in up to 80% of patients with myasthenia gravis. Pestronk and colleagues (1985) localized these antibodies to the neuromuscular junction in patients with myasthenia gravis, which further supports the autoimmune hypothesis. It has also been shown that the number of acetylcholine receptors is reduced in these patients. Although normal amounts of acetylcholine are released from the motor neuron, the number of resultant miniature endplate potentials is decreased because of the reduced number of functional acetylcholine receptors. As a result, the endplate potentials generated may not reach the threshold for action potential generation, leading to failed neuromuscular transmission. Drachman and coworkers (1980) proposed three mechanisms for this antibody-mediated interference with neuromuscular transmission. First, cross-linking of receptors may result in accelerated degradation of acetylcholine receptors. Second, antibodies may bind to receptor sites, which would render them unavailable for acetylcholine binding. Third, binding of antibodies may produce complement activation, which would result in degradation of the acetylcholine binding site.

This process of binding to or destruction of acetylcholine receptors is not uniform. As a result, two or more muscle fibers that are innervated by a single motor neuron may show variation in the number of miniature endplate potentials that occur in response to acetylcholine binding and hence in the timing of action potential generation. This variability in action potential formation is manifested on single-fiber electromyography (EMG) as "jitter," which is characteristic of myasthenia gravis. When this variability in response between muscle cells reaches 80 to 100 msec, one of the pair of muscle cells innervated by the motor neuron may not generate an action potential. This phenomenon, known as "blocking," is the cellular cause of the decremental response to repetitive stimulation seen on standard EMG, and it results in the fatigue seen after repetitive exercise in patients with myasthenia.

Pathologically, abnormalities of the thymus gland are well recognized in patients with myasthenia gravis. The most common abnormality seen is follicular lymphoid hyperplasia (Fig. 61–2), which is present in up to 60% of patients. These lymphoid follicles have been shown by

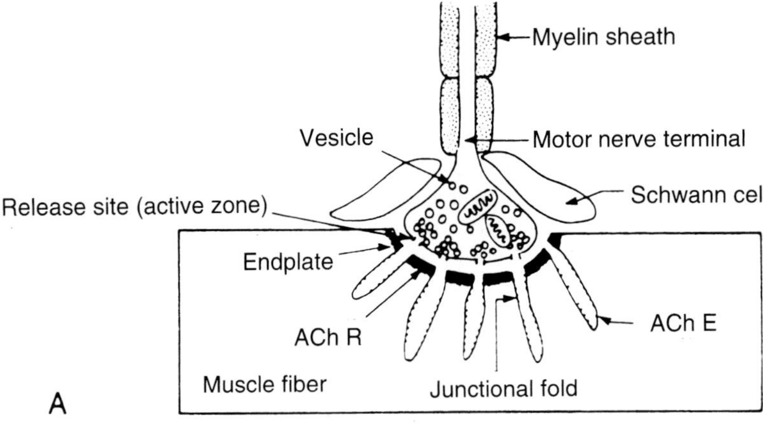

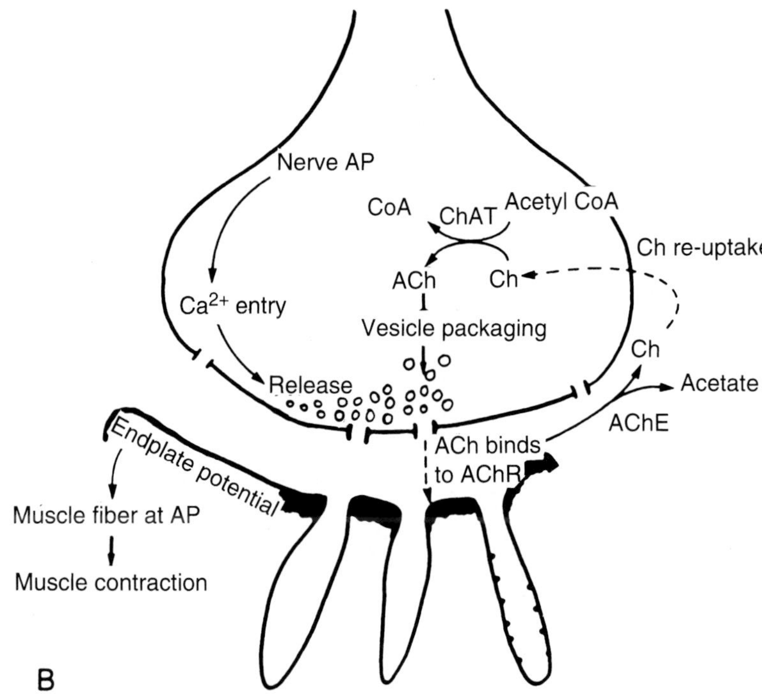

FIGURE 61–1 ■ *A*, Schematic representation of the neuromuscular junction. *B*, Magnification showing details of the mechanisms of acetylcholine release, degradation, and binding to receptors, leading to muscle contraction. (From Pascuzzi RM: Introduction to the neuromuscular junction and neuromuscular transmission. Semin Neurol 10:1, 1990.)

Pahwa and coworkers (1979) to contain B lymphocytes, which produce antibodies to acetylcholine receptors. Thymomas are present in 10% to 25% of patients with myasthenia gravis (Rivner and Swift, 1990). In addition, myasthenia gravis has been shown to occur in 30% to 60% of patients with thymoma. Given the association between myasthenia gravis and thymoma, all patients who are diagnosed with myasthenia gravis should have a computed tomographic (CT) scan of the chest at the time of diagnosis. The thymus gland in a typical patient is depicted in Figure 61–3, which shows uniform enlargement of the thymus without focal nodularity, suggesting a thymoma. The pathologic features of thymoma and the anatomic features of the thymus gland are considered in Chapters 58 and 59.

DIAGNOSIS

The diagnosis of myasthenia gravis is suspected on the basis of clinical findings of fluctuating weakness and early fatigue after repetitive exercise that improves with rest. The muscle groups involved and the degree of their involvement vary considerably over time. The ocular muscles are the most frequently involved, with approximately one half of the patients showing ocular muscle weakness at the time of diagnosis. Ocular muscles are ultimately involved in 90% of patients as the disease progresses, resulting in ptosis and diplopia. Involvement of other cranial nerves can result in dysphagia, choking, flattened smile, or nasal regurgitation.

Over time, 85% of patients develop generalized skeletal muscle involvement. The proximal muscles, diaphragm, and neck extensors tend to be involved. The weakness is often asymmetric and more commonly involves the upper extremities without loss of reflexes or alteration of sensation or coordination. The clinical severity of the myasthenia, commonly graded functionally and regionally on a scale proposed by Osserman and Genkins (1971), is depicted in Table 61–1.

The natural history of myasthenia gravis is not well

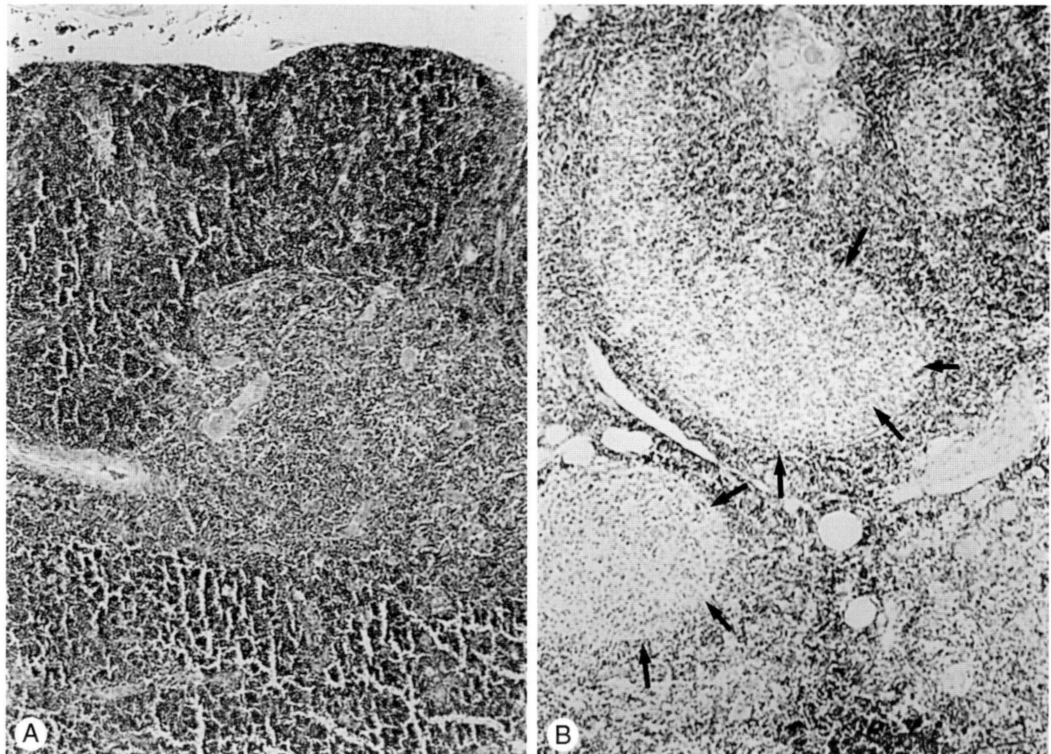

FIGURE 61–2 ■ *A*, Photomicrograph of a normal thymus. Note the absence of lymphoid follicles (H & E, × 80). *B*, Photomicrograph from a patient with myasthenia gravis. Note the prominent pale staining germinal centers *(arrows)* that represent follicular lymphoid hyperplasia (H & E, × 80).

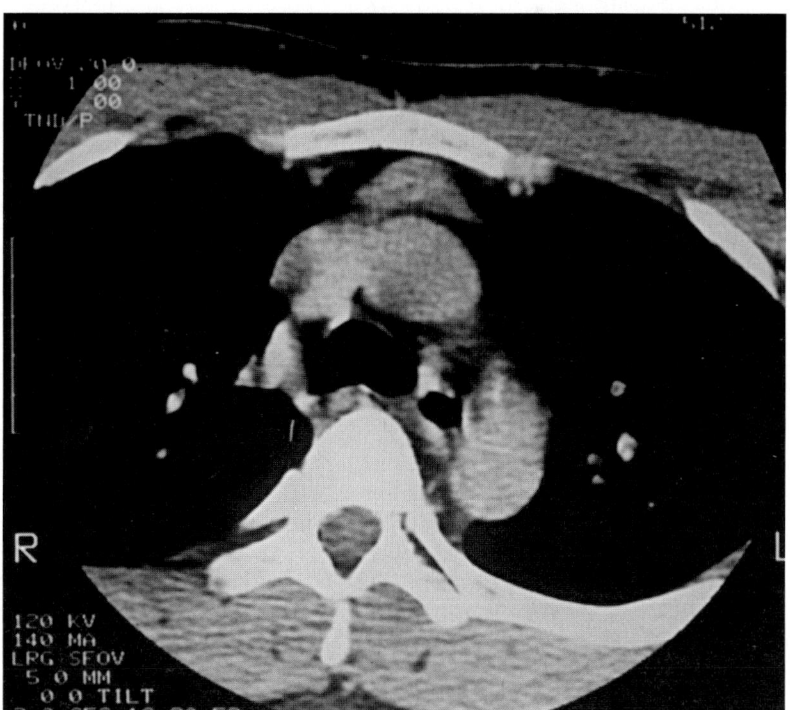

FIGURE 61–3 ■ Computed tomography scan with contrast revealing uniform enlargement of the thymus in a patient with myasthenia gravis.

TABLE 61–1 ■ Summary of Osserman and Genkins Classification System for Severity of Myasthenia Gravis

NEONATAL MG (1%)	
	Occurs in offspring of myasthenic mothers
	Self-limited (<6 wk)
	Due to placental transfer of antibodies
	Progression to juvenile or adult forms is rare
JUVENILE MG (9%)	
	Onset from birth to puberty
	Tends to be permanent
	Differentiated from neonatal form by permanency and lack of maternal disease
	Subclassified by nature and degree of defect as in adult forms
ADULT MG	
I	Ocular MG (20%)
	Disease limited to ocular involvement
	Carries excellent prognosis
	Rarely progresses after 2 yr of isolated ocular symptoms
IIA	Mild generalized MG (30%)
	Initial ocular symptoms progress gradually to generalized symptoms
	Respiratory muscles are spared
	Good response to medical therapy
IIB	Moderate generalized MG (20%)
	More severe generalized involvement
	Bulbar symptoms are common
	Relative sparing of respiratory muscles
	Less responsive to medical therapy
III	Acute fulminating MG (11%)
	Rapid onset of severe generalized weakness
	Prominent respiratory symptoms
	Highest association with thymoma
	High mortality rate
	Poor response to therapy
IV	Late severe MG (9%)
	Patients with severe symptoms developing more than 2 yr after onset of ocular or mild myasthenia gravis
	Thymoma common
	Poor response to therapy

MG, myasthenia gravis.

From Osserman KE, Genkins G: Studies in myasthenia gravis: Review of twenty year experience in over 1200 patients. Mt Sinai J Med 38:497, 1971.

documented; early studies suggested a mortality rate of 30% to 60% (Kennedy and Moersch, 1937). However, these studies were performed before the existence of intensive care units and the use of mechanical ventilation. Later data in regard to the natural history are lacking, because medical therapy with cholinesterase inhibitors became commonplace in 1934, and thymectomy has been used with increasing frequency since 1939.

A large retrospective series reported by Grob and associates (1987) highlights some features of the natural history of this disease. They found that ocular complaints were the most common initial symptoms; they occurred in 53% of patients. Bulbar dysfunction occurred as the presenting symptom in 11%, leg weakness in 10%, and generalized muscle weakness in 9%. Within 1 month, only 40% of patients had purely ocular symptoms; generalized muscle weakness was present in 40% of patients. In the long term, only 14% continued to have only ocular symptoms. The rate of progression to generalized weakness varied; 87% of patients had progression within the first year. They reported a spontaneous remission rate of 10%.

Bever and coauthors (1983) reported similar findings concerning the natural history of myasthenia gravis. Ocular symptoms were present in 84%, and roughly one half of patients had only ocular symptoms. Forty-nine percent of those who presented with ocular symptoms progressed to generalized weakness, with 85% doing so in the first 2 years. They also noted that in 17 of 20 patients in whom myasthenic crisis developed, it did so within 2 years of the onset of disease. The rate of spontaneous remission was 17%; 30% of remissions occurred in the first year. However, spontaneous remission occurred as late as 13 years after the onset of illness.

Although the diagnosis of myasthenia gravis may be suspected on the basis of clinical symptoms, confirmatory laboratory testing is essential. The following order of testing is recommended: anticholinesterase test, repetitive nerve stimulation, acetylcholine receptor antibody assay, and single-fiber electromyography (if necessary) (Drachman, 1994).

Edrophonium chloride (Tensilon) is commonly used for the anticholinesterase test because of the rapid onset (30 seconds) and short duration (about 5 minutes) of its effect. Although the exact sensitivity and specificity are unknown, Phillips and Melnick (1990) estimated a sensitivity of 85% for ocular myasthenia gravis and 95% for generalized myasthenia.

The diagnosis of myasthenia gravis can also be confirmed on the basis of elevated acetylcholine antibody titers. First detected by Almon and colleagues (1974), the presence of elevated titers of acetylcholine antibodies is highly specific for myasthenia gravis. The sensitivity ranges from 64% in patients with ocular disease to as high as 89% in patients with generalized disease (Phillips and Melnick, 1990).

Finally, since the first description of the classic decremental response on EMG by Harvey and Masland (1941), the techniques of EMG have been refined, improving the accuracy of this test in myasthenia gravis. Phillips and Melnick (1990) reviewed the diagnostic tests applicable for patients with myasthenia gravis. For all patients with myasthenia, they found a sensitivity of 34% for standard EMG; the sensitivity was 76% for patients with generalized disease. A technique of single-fiber EMG has been developed that, by the detection of jitter or blocking, may allow the identification of subclinical cases of myasthenia gravis. Single-fiber EMG may also improve the sensitivity and specificity of EMG testing. The findings have been shown to be abnormal in approximately 90% of patients with mild generalized myasthenia and in virtually 100% of those with moderate to severe disease (Massey, 1990). In patients with isolated ocular myasthenia, single-fiber EMG gives positive results in 60% to 75% (Stalberg and Sanders, 1981).

Myasthenia gravis must be differentiated from a variety of conditions that affect both muscle function and neuromuscular transmission. All types of muscular dystrophy, amyotrophic lateral sclerosis, a variety of ophthalmoplegias, and the weakness associated with psychoneurosis or hyperthyroidism can cause symptoms similar to those seen in myasthenia gravis. A thorough physical examination, including a detailed neurologic evaluation, usually differentiates these disorders from myasthenia gravis. The use of edrophonium as a diagnostic test also excludes these disorders, as no improvement in symptoms occurs with its administration.

The differential diagnosis of myasthenia gravis includes drug-induced myasthenia, botulism, Lambert-Eaton syndrome, congenital myasthenic syndromes, organophosphate intoxication, and certain snakebites. Drugs that induce myasthenia can be divided into two groups—those inducing an autoimmune disorder and those directly affecting neuromuscular transmission.

In the autoimmune-induced syndrome, most frequently seen with D-penicillamine, patients have elevated serum acetylcholine receptor antibodies, and the process usually remits within weeks of discontinuation of the medication. Other drugs such as curare, procainamide, quinines, and aminoglycosides affect synaptic transmission and can cause weakness in normal patients or exacerbate weakness in myasthenic patients. These effects are dose related and resolve after removal of the drug.

Botulism is a disease of neuromuscular transmission caused by the toxin of the bacterium *Clostridium botulinum*. The bacteria can either be ingested in contaminated food or produced in anaerobically infected wounds. This toxin causes a descending paralysis involving the eye muscles first, then the other muscles of the head and neck, followed by generalized skeletal muscle weakness. The defect in neuromuscular transmission involves impaired acetylcholine release from the motor neurons (Simpson, 1986), in contrast to the impaired binding to receptors seen in myasthenia gravis. As a result, EMG reveals an incremental response to repetitive testing.

The Lambert-Eaton syndrome is a myasthenic syndrome involving fluctuating weakness of the proximal muscle groups. The weakness may involve the facial muscles but to a lesser extent than in myasthenia gravis. This syndrome, also presumed to be autoimmune, is associated with an underlying malignancy in the majority of cases. Small cell cancer of the lung is the most common underlying malignancy, occurring in 70% of patients (Lambert, 1986). In contrast to patients with myasthenia gravis, patients with Lambert-Eaton syndrome having diminished deep tendon reflexes and autonomic symptoms are not uncommon. EMG shows an incremental response to repetitive stimulation compared with the decremental response seen in myasthenia gravis.

Finally, patients presenting with isolated ocular symptoms must be differentiated from those with intracranial mass lesions affecting the cranial nerves and from those suffering from progressive external ophthalmoplegia. In patients with purely ocular symptoms, the clinical distinction between myasthenia gravis and a mass lesion may be difficult. These patients should be carefully evaluated for intracranial lesions with a CT scan or by magnetic resonance imaging (MRI) if warranted (Moorthy et al, 1989). Progressive external ophthalmoplegia is a rare condition that is characterized by weakness of the extraocular muscles, and occasionally the proximal extremity muscles, that is associated with mitochondrial abnormalities in most patients (Moraes et al, 1989). This diagnosis can be confirmed by skeletal muscle biopsy.

MANAGEMENT

Therapeutic options for patients with myasthenia gravis include medical therapy with cholinesterase inhibitors or immunosuppressive medications, plasmapheresis or intravenous immunoglobulin (IVIg), and surgical treatment by thymectomy. There is considerable controversy with regard to the various combinations of these therapies and their sequence of use. Much of this controversy centers on difficulties in classifying the extent of disease to allow a comparison of various modes of therapy. In addition, the variable natural history of this disease, with its remissions and relapses, makes the benefits of any therapeutic modality difficult to discern.

Drug Therapy

Although it has no direct effect on the underlying disease, anticholinesterase therapy can lead to substantial improvement in symptoms in patients with myasthenia gravis. These drugs work by decreasing the hydrolysis of acetylcholine at the motor endplate. Pyridostigmine (Mestinon) has a relatively long duration of action and is the most commonly used agent. Neostigmine, with its more rapid onset and shorter duration of action, may be more useful in the perioperative period. Edrophonium, with its rapid onset and short duration of action, is used mostly as a diagnostic test. The optimal doses of these preparations vary widely from patient to patient and require careful adjustment to achieve the maximal response while minimizing the muscarinic side effects of abdominal cramping, diarrhea, excessive salivation, diaphoresis, and bradycardia.

A particularly feared complication of cholinesterase inhibition therapy is the development of a so-called cholinergic crisis. The mechanism for this profound weakness is unknown, but it may be due to excessive accumulation of acetylcholine at the neuromuscular junction, which results in a depolarizing blockade. Differentiation of this drug-induced cholinergic crisis from myasthenic crisis on clinical grounds alone can be difficult. This differentiation can be made by administration of the short-acting drug edrophonium, which results in an improvement in strength in patients who have a myasthenic crisis but no improvement in those with a cholinergic crisis.

Corticosteroid therapy has been reported to result in improvement in up to 80% of patients with myasthenia gravis (Pascuzzi et al, 1984), although no controlled trials exist to document this benefit. Usually reserved for patients who do not respond to anticholinesterase therapy or for those in whom intolerable side effects develop, steroids have also been used in the preparation of patients for thymectomy. The side effects of long-term corticosteroid therapy limit their usefulness, and relapses are common after discontinuation. Patients with moderate to severe symptoms may develop a transient steroid-induced exacerbation of their weakness at the initiation of steroid therapy and should have their dose gradually increased in a hospital setting.

Immunosuppression with azathioprine (Imuran) has also been advocated as an alternative for patients who do not respond to, or are intolerant of, anticholinesterase therapy. Again, there are relatively few controlled studies to document the usefulness of azathioprine, although response rates in retrospective studies ranged from 71% (Matell, 1987) to 83% (Witte et al, 1984). Side effects are common and lead to a dosage reduction or discontinuation of therapy in many patients.

Immunotherapy

Plasmapheresis removes antibodies from the circulation and has been reported to result in short-term clinical improvement in patients with myasthenia gravis. The proposed indications for plasmapheresis include short-term intervention in preparation for thymectomy in patients with severe weakness, relief of acute myasthenic weakness threatening respiration or swallowing, and control of symptoms before immunosuppressive therapy has become effective. Typically, five exchanges of 3 to 4 L each performed over 10 days are sufficient, reducing the immunoglobulin G (IgG) levels to less than 10% of the baseline value (Shumak and Rock, 1984).

Complications of plasmapheresis are related to the removal of plasma constituents other than the autoantibodies to acetylcholine receptors. Nonspecific reduction of immunoglobulins may predispose these patients to infection and has led many physicians to administer human pooled gamma globulin after a course of plasma exchange. Theoretically, loss of coagulation factors during exchange may predispose to hemorrhage, and antithrombin III removal may predispose to thrombosis. In addition, complement levels and platelet counts are reduced (Keller et al, 1979; Thorlacius et al, 1988). Actual complications are rare, however. The cost of plasmapheresis and the transient nature of the benefit limit the usefulness of the technique in the long-term treatment of myasthenic patients.

The indications for IVIg are similar to those for plasmapheresis: rapid improvement of symptoms of myasthenia for a limited period of time. IVIg is usually given at a dose of 400 mg/kg/day for 5 days. Arsura (1989) showed a response in 70% of patients with a mean duration of response of 30 days. The mechanism of action of IVIg is currently unknown, although levels of acetylcholine receptor antibodies are unchanged after treatment. The limitations of IVIg include the side effects of headache, fluid overload, a transient period of weakness at the onset of treatment, and the risks associated with pooled human blood products. As with plasmapheresis, the cost and the transient nature of IVIg therapy limit its usefulness in the long-term management of myasthenia gravis.

Thymectomy

Since Blalock's report in 1941, many series have been reported that demonstrate a favorable response to thymectomy in patients with myasthenia gravis. Thymectomy removes both a source of acetylcholine receptor antigen (expressed on the thymic myoid cells) and activated lymphocytes. Although it is generally agreed that thymectomy is of benefit to many patients, there are no prospective randomized studies comparing the roles of surgery and medical therapy in the treatment of patients with myasthenia gravis. Support for the concept of thymectomy for myasthenia gravis comes from a study by Buckingham and associates (1976). In this study, patients were retrospectively computer matched on the basis of age, sex, and severity and duration of disease between those treated medically and those who underwent thymectomy. Complete remission was found in 35% of surgical patients versus 8% of those medically treated. In addition, more patients were classified as clinically improved, and long-term survival was better in the surgical group.

The generally accepted indications for thymectomy include all patients with thymomas and patients with severe generalized myasthenia gravis who are between the ages of puberty and approximately 60 years (Rowland, 1987). In addition, many surgeons consider surgery for patients who are experiencing early generalized symptoms of these conditions. This concept is based on the observation, made initially by Blalock and subsequently by Masaoka (1996), DeFilippi (1994), and Papatestas (1987) and their colleagues, that patients with a short duration of illness are most likely to benefit from thymectomy.

The indications for thymectomy in patients with isolated ocular symptoms are less clear. Schumm and coauthors (1985) reported a series of 18 patients with isolated ocular symptoms; they noted clinical improvement after thymectomy in 80% and a complete remission rate of 17%. Papatestas and colleagues (1987), in reporting the results for more than 2000 patients treated for myasthenia gravis, agreed with the concept of thymectomy for isolated ocular symptoms, noting that results after 10 years were not significantly different from the remission rates noted after thymectomy in patients with mild generalized disease. More important, thymectomy prevented progression to generalized disease in these patients. They also showed that the results of thymectomy are best if the procedure is performed early in the course of the disease, before progression to severe generalized symptoms. Because the morbidity associated with the transcervical operation is minimal, an approach employing early thymectomy would avoid the risk of side effects from immunosuppressive drugs and may provide improved remission rates.

Before the operation, the patient's symptoms should be controlled medically, usually by anticholinesterase therapy. In some cases, steroids are administered, although these are to be avoided if possible by using preoperative plasmapheresis instead. Particular attention should be paid to pulmonary mechanics, especially if a sternotomy is contemplated. A CT scan is performed in all cases to rule out the presence of thymoma.

The surgical options currently available range from transcervical thymectomy and variations of the classic transsternal thymectomy to VATS. Advocates of the transcervical and VATS procedures emphasize the decreased morbidity associated with the less invasive procedures, which still achieve satisfactory remission and response rates. The minimal morbidity of these procedures may also facilitate acceptance of thymectomy early in the course of the disease, even if symptoms are well controlled with medication. Advocates of a more extensive dissection (Ashour, 1995; Jaretzki, 1997) emphasize the importance of total thymectomy, citing the common finding of aberrant thymic tissue in these patients. They have also shown that in patients with persistent myasthenic symptoms after lesser thymectomy, removal of as little as 3 g of thymic tissue may result in remission. On this basis, a combined cervical and transsternal approach for "maximal thymectomy" has been advocated. Although proponents of each procedure disagree on the optimal approach, all agree that the ultimate goal should be total removal of the thymus.

Transsternal Thymectomy

The technique of transsternal thymectomy involves the performance of a standard median sternotomy. The mediastinal extension of the deep cervical fascia is identified on the undersurface of the sternothyroid muscle. This fascia layer is incised at the midline to expose the thymus gland. Each lower pole is then dissected bluntly from the undersurface of this fascia, from the pericardium posteriorly, and from the extrapleural fascia laterally. As the dissection proceeds superiorly, one or two arterial branches to the thymus that arise from the internal mammary arteries are identified and divided. When the dissection is continued superiorly, with downward traction on the gland, the superior poles can be brought into the wound. At the apex of each superior pole, there is usually an arterial branch, which arises from the inferior thyroid artery. Finally, blunt dissection posterior to the gland separates the thymus from the innominate vein. It is here that the venous drainage, that is, one or two branches that drain directly into the innominate vein, can be ligated. The anterior mediastinum is drained (as are the pleural spaces if they are entered), and the wound is closed with sternal wires and appropriate subcutaneous and skin sutures.

Maximal Thymectomy

The maximal thymectomy approach described by Jaretzki and coauthors (1988) combines a horizontal cervical incision with a median sternotomy to allow "removal of all thymic tissue predictably." This approach was based on their observations concerning the variability of the anatomy of the thymus (Jaretzki et al, 1977). In this operation, all mediastinal tissue anterior to the pericardium and great vessels is removed. The dissection extends laterally to a point located posterior to the phrenic nerves. The resection includes removal of the mediastinal pleura. In the neck, the upper poles are removed en bloc with the adjacent fatty tissue.

Transcervical Thymectomy

The transcervical approach, because of its less invasive nature, has continued to be of interest. As mentioned, this was the initial approach historically until it was replaced by the transsternal approach by Blalock (1944) and others. Interest in the transcervical approach was rekindled by articles by Carlens and coworkers (1967), Crile (1966), and Akakura (1965). Kirshner and associates (1969) reported on 40 patients treated by transcervical thymectomy, and this was soon followed by a report by Papatestas and colleagues (1987) that involved more than 700 cases of myasthenia treated by transcervical thymectomy. The technique was further enhanced by a report by Cooper and coworkers (1988) of the use of a specially designed retractor that facilitates exposure to ensure a more complete transcervical thymectomy.

The operative technique is as follows. The patient is placed supine with the shoulders elevated on an inflatable bag and the head resting at the top of the operating table in a "donut." An intravenous line is placed in the right arm, and the blood pressure is measured in the patient's left arm. The patient should be prepared as if a sternotomy is to be performed, should it become necessary. The skin incision is made along a skin crease approximately 2 cm above the sternal notch; this is extended laterally to each sternocleidomastoid muscle. Flaps are raised superiorly to the level of the thyroid gland and inferiorly to the level of the sternum, in a plane beneath the platysma. The strap muscles are split vertically at the midline, and the thymus gland is identified immediately beneath the sternothyroid muscle. The uppermost aspect of the left upper pole is identified near the inferior thyroid vein, where it is ligated. The ligature is left attached for purposes of traction. The right upper pole is similarly dissected and ligated before division. The upper poles are then bluntly dissected free to the level of the sternal notch, where they typically fuse anterior to the innominate vein. A finger is inserted into the mediastinum anterior to the gland to dissect it from the undersurface of the sternum. When the superior poles are retracted anteriorly at this point, the veins that drain to the innominate vein are easily identified, ligated, and divided.

At this point, a specially designed narrow right-angle retractor is placed beneath the sternum (Cooper Thymectomy Retractor, Pilling Company, Ft. Washington, PA) and attached to a Poly-Tract (Pilling Company) overhead bar (Fig. 61–4). After the sternum is lifted with this apparatus, the inflatable pillow beneath the shoulders is deflated; this allows the shoulders to fall backward and improves the exposure. When this technique is used, the entire mediastinal portion of the thymus can be dissected under direct vision. The dissection begins on the right lateral aspect of the gland and extends inferiorly to the limits of the right lower pole. The gland is then swept off the anterior surface of the aorta and pericardium, which mobilizes the left lower pole and includes the tail of tissue that often extends downward toward the aortopulmonary window. After the gland has been removed entirely (Fig. 61–5), the remaining mediastinal fat is removed on both sides extending to the mediastinal pleura. The wound is then closed in layers over a red rubber catheter. This catheter is removed as the platysma is closed with the lungs held in static inflation. With this technique, a chest tube is rarely required, even if one or both pleural spaces were entered.

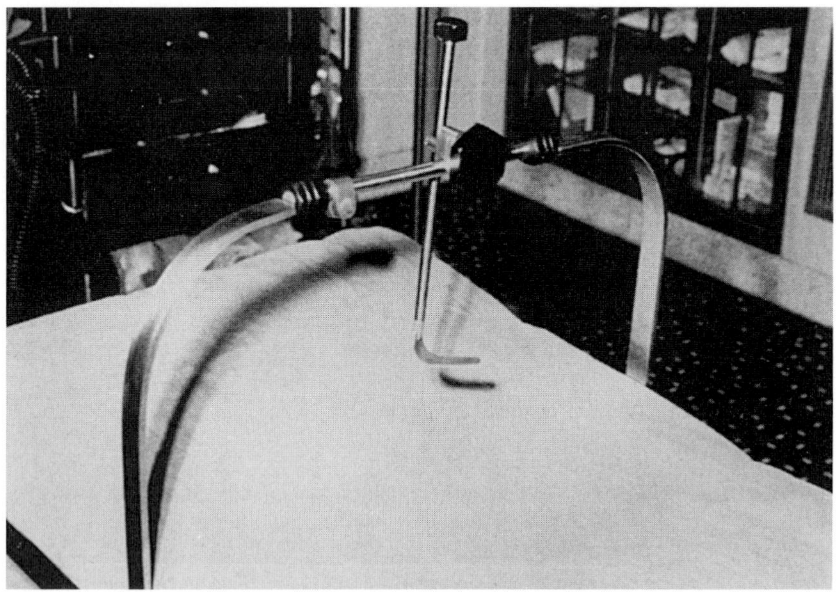

FIGURE 61–4 ■ Specially designed, right-angle retractor attached to an overhead bar. The retractor is placed behind the manubrium to provide upward lift on the sternum. (From Cooper JD, Al-Silaihana AN, Pearson FG et al: An improved technique to facilitate transcervical thymectomy for myasthenia gravis. Ann Thorac Surg 45:242, 1988.)

Video-Assisted Thoracoscopic Thymectomy

Video-assisted thoracoscopy techniques have been advocated for thymectomy in patients with myasthenia gravis. The arguments for and against VATS are similar to those made regarding transcervical thymectomy. Proponents of VATS approaches believe that an adequate thymectomy can be performed under direct vision and that the morbidity is comparable with that of the transcervical approach. Opponents argue that the increased operating room time and the use of a double-lumen endotracheal tube add their own morbidity, and that VATS procedures provide limited exposure of important mediastinal structures. Because the thymus is a midline structure, some surgeons (Mineo et al, 1998) use a left-sided approach and others (Mack et al, 1996; Yim et al, 1995) use a right-sided approach. Novellino and coworkers (1994) advocated a video-assisted thoracoscopic extended thymectomy (VATET) using a bilateral VATS approach combined with a cervical incision. Although the procedure is technically feasible, data on the remission rates after VATS thymectomy in larger series of patients with long-term follow-up are required to determine the success of these new procedures.

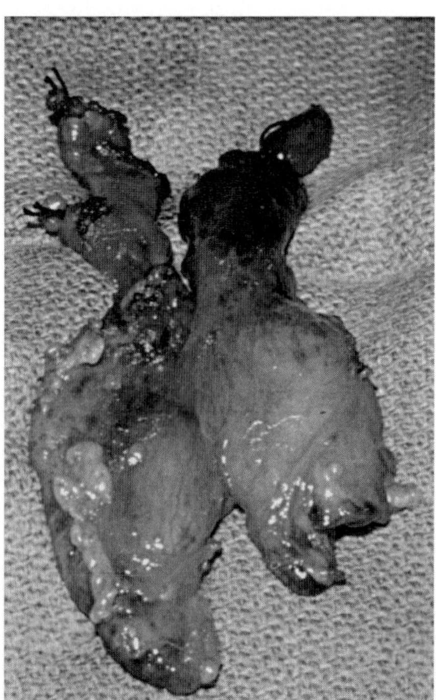

FIGURE 61–5 ■ Photograph of a thymectomy specimen, from the patient in Figure 61–3, that was removed by transcervical thymectomy.

Postoperative Care

The essentials of postoperative care center on early extubation, aggressive attention to the patient's pulmonary status, and early ambulation, whether a transmediastinal or transcervical approach has been used. Care should be used with narcotics because of their potential for respiratory depression and the possibility that cholinesterase inhibitors may potentiate the analgesic effects of morphine, hydromorphine, codeine, and opium alkaloids (Howard, 1990). Anticholinesterase medication is resumed when the patient is extubated. Attempts to wean patients from medical therapy are delayed for several weeks after the procedure. Early postoperative results with this approach have been satisfying, with mortality rates in the range of 0% to 2% and morbidity rates between 2% and 15% of patients in the reported series.

Results of Surgery

Although thymectomy has been performed for myasthenia gravis since 1941, slight variations in surgical technique, heterogeneous groups of patients, lack of uniform clinical staging, and varying length of follow-up make interpretation of the reported results difficult. In addition, the unpredictable nature of myasthenia gravis with spontaneous remissions and relapses and the often delayed response to surgery make it difficult to compare results

TABLE 61–2 ■ **Thymectomy for Myasthenia Gravis**

Author	Patients	Type of Procedure	Remission Rates (%) 2 Year	5 Year	10 Year	15 Year	Morbidity (%)	Mortality (%)
Jaretzki et al (1988)	72	Maximal thymectomy	24	50	N/A	N/A	7	0
Masaoka et al (1996)	375	Extended transsternal	22	45.8	55.7	67.2	N/A	0
Cooper et al (1988)	65	Transcervical	28	40	N/A	N/A	2	0
Papatestas et al (1987)	962	Transcervical	12	23	40	N/A	N/A	0
Mack et al (1996)	33	VATS	22.2	N/A	N/A	N/A	3	0

N/A, not applicable; VATS, video-assisted thoracic surgery.

of different surgical series. The commonly agreed upon end point of surgical success is remission of symptoms without the use of any medications.

When comparing the different surgical groups, most authors agree that the maximal thymectomy is the benchmark against which other procedures should be measured (Cooper et al, 1989). Outcomes in reported series are summarized in Table 61–2. In the only VATS series published to date with a symptomatic outcome, Mack and coauthors (1996) reported a 2-year remission rate that is similar to that in the other reported series. Proponents of the transcervical and VATS procedures argue that although the remission rates are slightly less, patients are more likely to seek earlier surgical intervention, and that the response to surgery is greater when patients are treated early in the disease course. They also note that the morbidity and hospital costs are less with their techniques. The proponents of transsternal procedures believe that the best remission rates possible should be obtained, regardless of the added morbidity associated with sternotomy, which they claim is minimal. The observation that reoperation and removal of residual thymus resulted in remission in a number of patients with persistent symptoms after lesser thymectomy techniques (Jaretzki et al, 1988; Masaoka et al, 1982) suggests the feasibility of a minimally invasive transcervical or VATS approach initially, with transsternal maximal thymectomy for those with persistent symptoms.

Specific predictors of improvement after thymectomy were addressed by Frist and colleagues (1994). Age younger than 45 years was found to be an independent predictor of improved outcome after thymectomy. However, in other series, such as those of Olanow (1987) and Papatestas (1987) and their coworkers, no association was found between age and outcome. Female gender was also identified in this series as an independent predictor of a favorable response to surgery. This finding was also observed by Hatton and associates (1989) but not by Jaretzki (1988) or Papatestas (1987) and their colleagues. Frist also found that an earlier stage of disease at the time of thymectomy predicted a favorable outcome. The duration of symptoms alone, however, does not appear to be an independent predictor of outcome (Frist et al, 1994; Huang et al, 1988; Jaretzki et al, 1988). The presence of a thymoma is a generally agreed upon predictor of a worse outcome.

COMMENTS AND CONTROVERSIES

This chapter is a concise review of the etiology and autoimmune pathogenesis of myasthenia gravis. The standard techniques of thymectomy are presented in detail. It is interesting that the three standard approaches to thymectomy for myasthenia gravis (transsternal, maximal, and transcervical) have been in use for many years, yet there does not appear to be any significant difference in outcome according to a large number of retrospective reviews from various centers, each advocating its own preferred approach.

With the introduction of the VATS technique, yet another technical approach is available. However, without a cervical extension of the VATS technique, the upper poles cannot easily be excised. In addition, in the opinion of this commentator, the VATS technique adds a significant degree of technical complexity that is avoided by a simpler transcervical approach. In Chapter 64, Keshavjee addresses yet another technical modification of video-assisted transcervical thymectomy.

It is often argued that these less invasive techniques would be more readily accepted by referring neurologists and their younger patients with thymic hyperplasia. This might lead to earlier referral and thymectomy for suitable patients. Consensus opinion suggests that results are superior when thymectomy is undertaken earlier in the course of disease.

G.A.P.

KEY REFERENCES

Finley JC, Pascuzzi RM: Rational therapy of myasthenia gravis. Semin Neurol 10:70, 1990.

This is a thorough discussion of the natural history of, and therapeutic options available for, myasthenia gravis. It includes an extensive list of references that cover all available therapeutic modalities.

Keesey JC: Electrodiagnostic approach to defects in neuromuscular transmission. Muscle Nerve 12:613, 1989.

This is a comprehensive reference that summarizes the rationale behind the use of single-fiber EMG and repetitive nerve stimulation in diseases of neuromuscular transmission.

Osserman KE, Genkins G: Studies in myasthenia gravis: Review of a twenty year experience in over 1200 patients. Mt Sinai J Med 38:497, 1971.

This classic reference includes observations in regard to the important aspects of diagnosis and therapy of patients with myasthenia gravis from the myasthenia gravis clinic at Mount Sinai Hospital. A classification system is described, and the results of therapy are outlined based on the largest reported series of myasthenic patients.

Pascuzzi RM: Introduction to the neuromuscular junction and neuromuscular transmission. Semin Neurol 10:1, 1990.

This is a concise informative overview of the mechanisms of neuromuscular transmission. It includes a discussion of the principles of EMG.

Phillips LH, Melnick PA: Diagnosis of myasthenia gravis in the 1990s. Semin Neurol 10:62, 1990.

A concise summary of the diagnostic tests available for myasthenia gravis, this article includes the rationale behind their application, an interesting analysis of the clinical decision-making process, and a proposed decision-making strategy.

■ REFERENCES

Akakura I: Mediastinoscopy. Presented at the XI International Congress of Bronchoesophagology, Hakone, Japan, 6, 1965.

Almon RR, Andrew AG, Appel SH: Serum globulin in myasthenia gravis: Inhibition of L-bungarotoxin to acetylcholine receptors. Science 186:55, 1974.

Arsura E: Experience with intravenous immunoglobulin in myasthenia gravis. Clin Immunol Immunopathol 53:S170, 1989.

Ashour M: Prevalence of ectopic thymic tissue in myasthenia gravis and its clinical significance. J Thorac Cardiovasc Surg 109:632,1995.

Bell ET: Tumors of the thymus in myasthenia gravis. J Nerv Ment Dis 45: 130, 1917.

Bever CT Jr, Aquino AV, Penn AS et al: Prognosis of ocular myasthenia. Ann Neurol 14:516, 1983.

Blalock A: Thymectomy in the treatment of myasthenia gravis: Report of twenty cases. J Thorac Cardiovasc Surg 13:316, 1944.

Blalock A, Harvey AM, Ford RF, Lilienthal JL Jr: The treatment of myasthenia gravis by removal of the thymus gland. JAMA 117:1529, 1941.

Blalock A, Mason MF, Morgan HJ, Riven SS: Myasthenia gravis and tumors of the thymic region: Report of a case in which the tumor was removed. Ann Surg 110:544, 1939.

Buckberg GD, Herrmann C, Dillon JR, Mulder DG: A further evaluation of thymectomy for myasthenia gravis. J Thorac Cardiovasc Surg 53:401, 1967.

Buckingham JM, Howard FM Jr, Bernatz PE et al: The value of thymectomy in myasthenia gravis: A computer assisted matched study. Ann Surg 184:453, 1976.

Carlens E, Johansson L, Olsson P: Mediastinoscopy auxiliary to thymectomy by the cervical route. Bronches 17:408, 1967.

Cooper JD, Al-Jilaihawa AN, Pearson FG et al: An improved technique to facilitate transcervical thymectomy for myasthenia gravis. Ann Thorac Surg 45:242, 1988.

Cooper JD, Jaretzki A III, Mulder DG, Papatestas AS: Symposium: Thymectomy for myasthenia gravis. Contemp Surg 34:65, 1989.

Crile G Jr: Thymectomy through the neck. Surgery 59:213, 1966.

DeFilippi VJ, Richman DP, Ferguson MK: Transcervical thymectomy for myasthenia gravis. Ann Thorac Surg 57:194, 1994.

Drachman DB: Myasthenia gravis. N Engl J Med 330:1797, 1994.

Drachman DB, Adams RN, Stanley EF, Pestronk A: Mechanisms of acetylcholine receptor loss in myasthenia gravis. J Neurol Neurosurg Psychiatry 43:601, 1980.

Frist WH, Thirumalai S, Doehring CB et al: Thymectomy for the myasthenia gravis patient: Factors influencing outcome. Ann Thorac Surg 57:334, 1994.

Goldflam S: Ueber einen scheinbar heilbaren bulbar paralytischen symptomen Complex mit Beteiligung der Extremitaten. Dtsch Z Nervenheilkd 4:312, 1893.

Grob D, Arsura EL, Brunner NG, Namba T: The course of myasthenia gravis and therapies affecting outcome. Ann N Y Acad Sci 505:472, 1987.

Harvey AM, Masland RL: The electromyogram in myasthenia gravis. Bull Johns Hopkins Hosp 69:1, 1941.

Hatton PD, Diehl JP, Daly BDP et al: Transsternal radical thymectomy for myasthenia gravis: A 15 year review. Ann Thorac Surg 47:838, 1989.

Henze A, Biberfeld P, Christensson B et al: Failing transcervical thymectomy in myasthenia gravis: An evaluation of transsternal reexploration. Scand J Thorac Cardiovasc Surg 18:235, 1984.

Howard JF: Adverse drug effects on neuromuscular transmission. Semin Neurol 10:89, 1990.

Huang M, King K, Ksu W et al: The outcome of thymectomy in nonthymomatous myasthenia gravis. Surg Gynecol Obstet 166:436, 1988.

Jaretzki A III: Thymectomy for myasthenia gravis: Analysis of the controversies regarding technique and results. Neurology 48(Suppl 5):S52, 1997.

Jaretzki A, Bethea M, Wolff M et al: A rational approach to total thymectomy in the treatment of myasthenia gravis. Ann Thorac Surg 24:120, 1977.

Jaretzki A, Penn AS, Younger DS et al: "Maximal" thymectomy for myasthenia gravis. J Thorac Cardiovasc Surg 95:747, 1988.

Jolly F: Ueber Myasthenia gravis pseudoparalytica. Klin Wochenschr 32:1, 1895.

Keller AJ, Chirnside A, Urbaniak SJ: Coagulation abnormalities produced by plasma exchange on the cell separator with special reference to fibrinogen and platelet levels. Br J Haematol 42:593, 1979.

Kennedy FS, Moersch FP: Myasthenia gravis: A clinical review of 87 cases observed between 1915 and the early part of 1932. Can Med Assoc J 37:217, 1937.

Keynes G: Investigations into thymic disease and tumor formation. Br J Surg 62:449, 1955.

Kirschner PA, Osserman KE, Kark AK: Studies in myasthenia gravis: Transcervical total thymectomy. JAMA 209:906, 1969.

Lambert EH: The Lambert-Eaton myasthenic syndrome: Clinical features and pathophysiology. Presented at the Seventh International Conference on Myasthenia Gravis, New York Academy of Sciences, New York, March 6, 1986.

Mack MJ, Landreneau RJ, Yim AP et al: Results of video-assisted thymectomy in patients with myasthenia gravis. J Thorac Cardiovasc Surg 112:1352, 1996.

Masaoka A, Monden Y, Seike Y et al: Reoperation after transcervical thymectomy for myasthenia gravis. Neurology 32:83, 1982.

Masaoka A, Yamakawa Y, Niwa H et al: Extended thymectomy for myasthenia gravis: A 20-year review. Ann Thorac Surg 62:853, 1996.

Massey JM: Electromyography in disorders of neuromuscular transmission. Semin Neurol 10:6, 1990.

Matell G: Immunosuppressive drugs: Azathioprine in the treatment of myasthenia gravis. Ann N Y Acad Sci 505:588, 1987.

Mineo CT, Pompeo E, Ambrogi V et al: Adjuvant pneumomediastinum in thoracoscopic thymectomy for myasthenia gravis. Ann Thorac Surg 62:1210, 1996.

Mineo CT, Pompeo E, Ambrogi V et al: Video-assisted completion thymectomy in refractory myasthenia gravis. J Thorac Cardiovasc Surg 115:252, 1998.

Moorthy G, Behrens NM, Drachman DB, et al: Ocular pseudomyasthenia or myasthenia 'plus': A warning to clinicians. Neurology 39:1150, 1989.

Moraes CT, DiMauro MS, Zeviani M et al: Mitochondrial DNA deletions in progressive external ophthalmoplegia and Kearns-Sayre syndrome. N Engl J Med 320:1293, 1989.

Novellino L, Longoni M, Spinelli L et al: "Extended" thymectomy, without sternotomy, performed by cervicotomy and thoracoscopic technique in the treatment of myasthenia gravis. Int Surg 79:378, 1994.

Olanow CW, Wechsler AS, Siratkin-Roses M et al: Thymectomy as primary therapy in myasthenia gravis. Ann N Y Acad Sci 505:595, 1987.

Osserman KE, Teng P, Kaplan LI: Studies in myasthenia gravis: Preliminary report on therapy with Mestinon bromide. JAMA 155:961, 1954.

Pahwa R, Ikehara S, Pahwa SG, Good RA: Thymic function in man. Thymus 1:27, 1979.

Papatestas AK, Genkins G, Kornfeld P et al: Effects of thymectomy in myasthenia gravis. Ann Surg 206:79, 1987.

Pascuzzi RM, Coslett HB, Johns TR: Long-term corticosteroid treatment of myasthenia gravis: Report of 116 patients. Ann Neurol 15:291, 1984.

Pestronk A, Drachman DB, Self SG: Measurement of junctional acetylcholine receptors in myasthenia gravis: Clinical correlates. Muscle Nerve 8:245, 1985.

Rivner MH, Swift TR: Thymoma: Diagnosis and management. Semin Neurol 10:83, 1990.

Rowland LP: General discussion on therapy in myasthenia gravis. Ann N Y Acad Sci 505:607, 1987.

Schumm JF, Wietholter H, Fateh-Moghadam A, Dichgans J: Thymectomy in myasthenia with pure ocular symptoms. J Neurol Neurosurg Psychiatry 48:332, 1985.

Seybold ME: Myasthenia gravis: A clinical and basic science review. JAMA 250:2516, 1983.

Seybold ME, Lindstrom JM: Immunopathology of acetylcholine receptors in myasthenia gravis. Springer Semin Immunopathol 5:389, 1982.

Shumak KH, Rock GA: Therapeutic plasma exchange. N Engl J Med 310:762, 1984.

Simpson LL: Molecular pharmacology of botulinum toxin and tetanus toxin. Annu Rev Pharmacol Toxicol 26:427, 1986.

Stalberg E, Sanders DB: Electrophysiologic tests of neuromuscular transmission. In Stalberg E, Young RR (eds): Clinical Neurophysiology. London, Butterworth, 1981.

Sugarbaker DJ: Thoracoscopy in the management of anterior mediastinal masses. Ann Thorac Surg 56:653, 1993.

Thorlacius S, Mollnes TE, Garred P et al: Plasma exchange in myasthenia gravis: Changes in serum complement and immunoglobulins. Acta Neurol Scand 78:221, 1988.

Von Haberer A: Zur klinischen Bedeutung der Thymus Drüse. Arch Klin Chir 109:193, 1917.

Walker MB: Treatment of myasthenia gravis with physostigmine. Lancet 1:1200, 1934.

Waud DR, Waud BE: In vitro measurement of margin of safety of neuromuscular transmission. Am J Physiol 229:1632, 1975.

Weigert C: Pathologisch-anatomischer Beitrag zur Erb-schen Krankheit (myasthenia gravis). Neurol Zentralbl 20:597 1901.

Wilks S: On cerebritis, hysteria and bulbar paralysis. Guy's Hosp Rep 22:7, 1877.

Williams CL, Lennon VA: Thymic B lymphocyte clones from patients with myasthenia gravis secrete monoclonal striational antibodies reacting with myosin, alpha actin, or actin. J Exp Med 164:1043, 1986.

Witte AS, Cornblath DR, Parry GJ et al: Azathioprine in the treatment of myasthenia gravis. Ann Neurol 15:602, 1984.

Yim PC, Kay LC, Ho KS: Video-assisted thoracoscopic thymectomy for myasthenia gravis. Chest 108:1440, 1995.

CHAPTER **62**

Cysts

CYSTS AND DUPLICATIONS IN INFANTS AND CHILDREN

Robert C. Shamberger

W. Hardy Hendren III

Cystic masses within the mediastinum are an infrequent problem in infants and children. They are of both neoplastic and congenital origin. Accurate anatomic localization of these cysts often provides a strong indication of both their organ of origin and etiology (Fig. 62–1). Cystic lesions in the anterior mediastinum consist primarily of teratomas or lymphangiomas; less frequently, thymic cysts involve the mediastinum, and rarely, Hodgkin's disease presents as a cystic mass of the thymus. Cystic lesions in the middle mediastinum are primarily bronchogenic cysts, and lesions in the posterior mediastinum are primarily esophageal duplications or neurenteric cysts. These lesions are grouped for presentation by their anatomic location within the mediastinum to facilitate discussion of their symptoms at presentation, differential diagnosis, and therapy (Table 62–1).

ANTERIOR MEDIASTINUM

Teratomas

Mediastinal teratomas are generally benign and may present at any age (Gottschalk et al, 1980). By definition, teratomas contain derivatives of all three germ cell layers and are frequently cystic. Teratomas are the second most common tumor of the anterior mediastinum, the most common being Hodgkin's disease, which almost invariably occurs as a solid tumor. Teratomas may contain components of either a yolk sac tumor or choriocarcinoma. Serum alpha-fetoprotein and beta–human chorionic gonadotropin (HCG) levels, which are excellent markers for yolk sac tumors and choriocarcinoma, respectively, should be obtained before resection of a suspected teratoma.

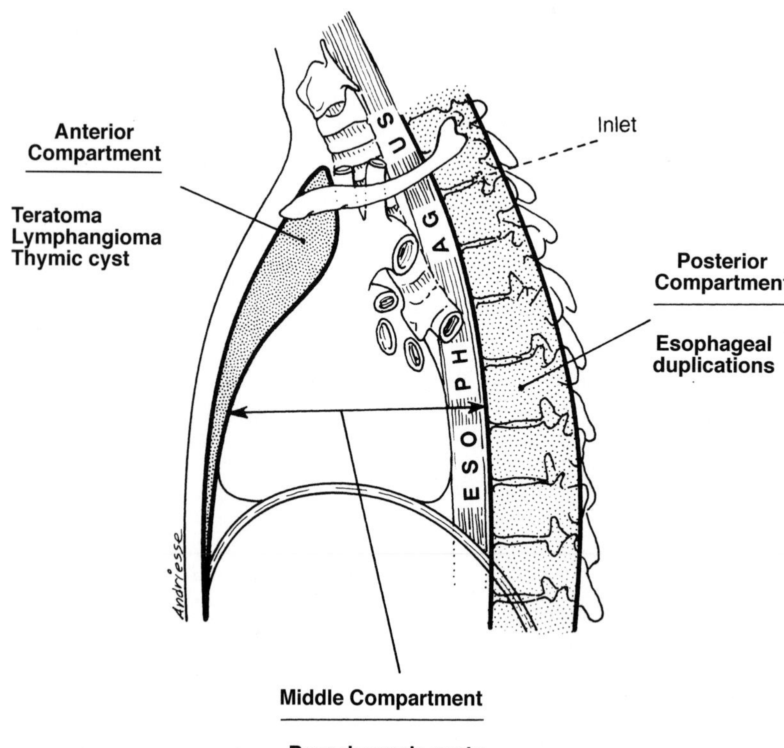

FIGURE 62–1 ■ Shown are the three compartments of the mediastinum. The most frequently occurring cystic lesions in the anterior mediastinum are teratomas, lymphangiomas, and thymic cysts. Rarely, Hodgkin's disease involving the thymus occurs as a cystic mass. The middle compartment is most frequently involved with bronchogenic cysts or lymphangiomas that extend from the anterior mediastinum. The posterior mediastinum most frequently contains esophageal duplications.

TABLE 62–1 ■ **Summary of Cystic Lesions of the Mediastinum Reported in Six Pediatric Series**

Lesion	*No. (%)*
Teratoma	52 (34)
Lymphangioma	18 (12)
Thymic cyst	9 (6)
Pericardial cyst	2 (1)
Bronchogenic cyst	35 (23)
Esophageal duplication	36 (24)
Total	152

Symptoms at presentation are respiratory in nature, the most frequent being cough. Teratomas may become very large, and they occasionally produce dyspnea. Because of their cystic nature, tracheal compression and airway compromise rarely occur. Mediastinal teratomas may become infected or may rupture into the bronchus, pleura, or pericardium, causing acute inflammatory symptoms (Thompson and Moore, 1969). Computed tomography (CT) scan best defines the extent of the lesion and demonstrates tracheal compression if it is present. If the calculated tracheal area is less than 50% of expected, or the peak expiratory flow rate is less than 50% of predicted, acute respiratory obstruction may occur on induction of general anesthesia (Shamberger et al, 1991, 1995). Tissue of varying densities and calcifications within the mass suggests the diagnosis of teratoma (Fig. 62–2).

Surgical resection is usually curative, and local recurrence of benign tumors is rare. Teratomas may be resected through either a midline sternotomy or a thoracotomy if the mass extends primarily into one chest cavity. The patient with malignant elements requires chemotherapy in addition to resection to prevent local or distance relapse.

Lymphangiomas (Cystic Hygromas)

Lymphangioma is a multilocular, thin-walled cystic mass of lymphatic origin. It develops from lymphatic tissues that become sequestered from the developing lymphatic system during early embryonic life (Childress et al, 1956). The cyst is filled with serous fluid and is lined by a thin, almost transparent membrane. Histologically, it consists of a single layer of flattened endothelium with varying amounts of fibrous tissue. It may occur in the anterior mediastinum, and involvement of this site should be considered in all patients with cervical or upper thoracic lymphangiomas (cystic hygromas). Routine chest radiographs should be obtained for any patient who has a lymphangioma in the neck or axilla, to define the extent of mediastinal involvement, which occurs in up to 10% of these patients (Fig. 62–3). Rarely, as has been described by Perkes and associates (1979), a lymphangioma is entirely confined to the mediastinum (Fig. 62–4).

Therapy for lymphangioma of the mediastinum is surgical resection. These lesions may extend from the base of the neck to the diaphragm; although they primarily involve the anterior mediastinum, the middle mediastinum may be involved as well. At resection, the lymphangioma is often less discrete than it appears radiographically. Extension of small branches of the lesion in all directions along fascial planes and into vital structures may make complete excision impossible. Resection is performed to the greatest extent possible without injury of vital structures and should remove the bulk of the mass that is producing respiratory symptoms or compression of vital structures. Resection of these masses may be

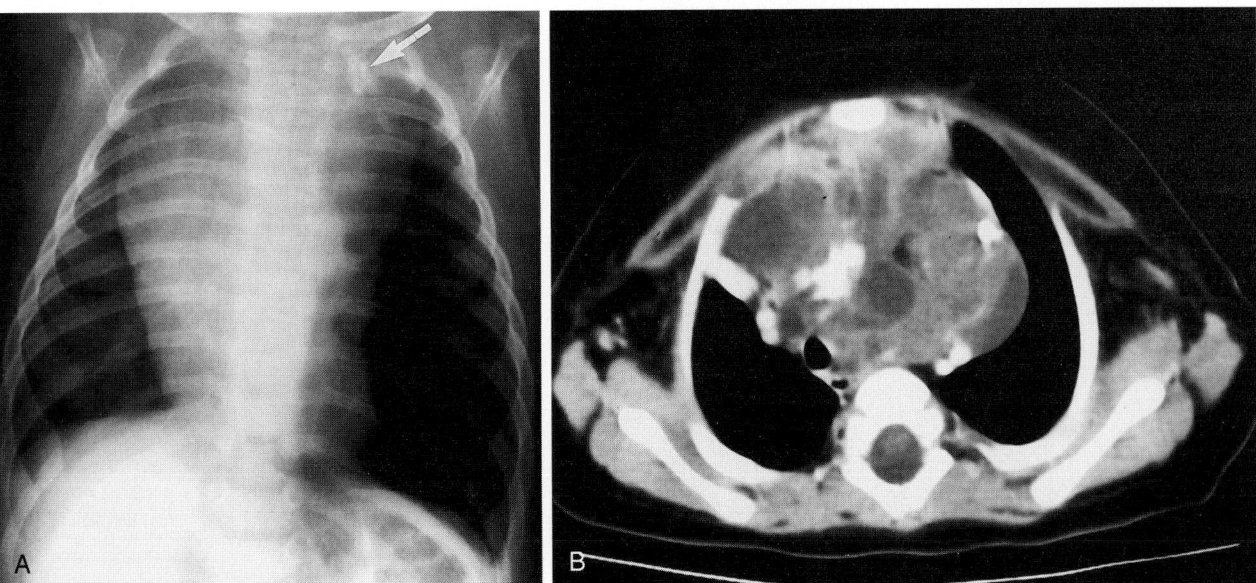

FIGURE 62–2 ■ *A,* A chest radiograph of a 4-month-old boy with a 2-month history of progressive cough and wheezing. The study revealed a large anterior mediastinal mass. Note calcification within the mass *(arrow)*. *B,* A computed tomography scan of the boy in *A* demonstrated a solid, cystic mass of various densities that markedly displaced the trachea and the esophagus to the right. Areas of calcification are again well seen.

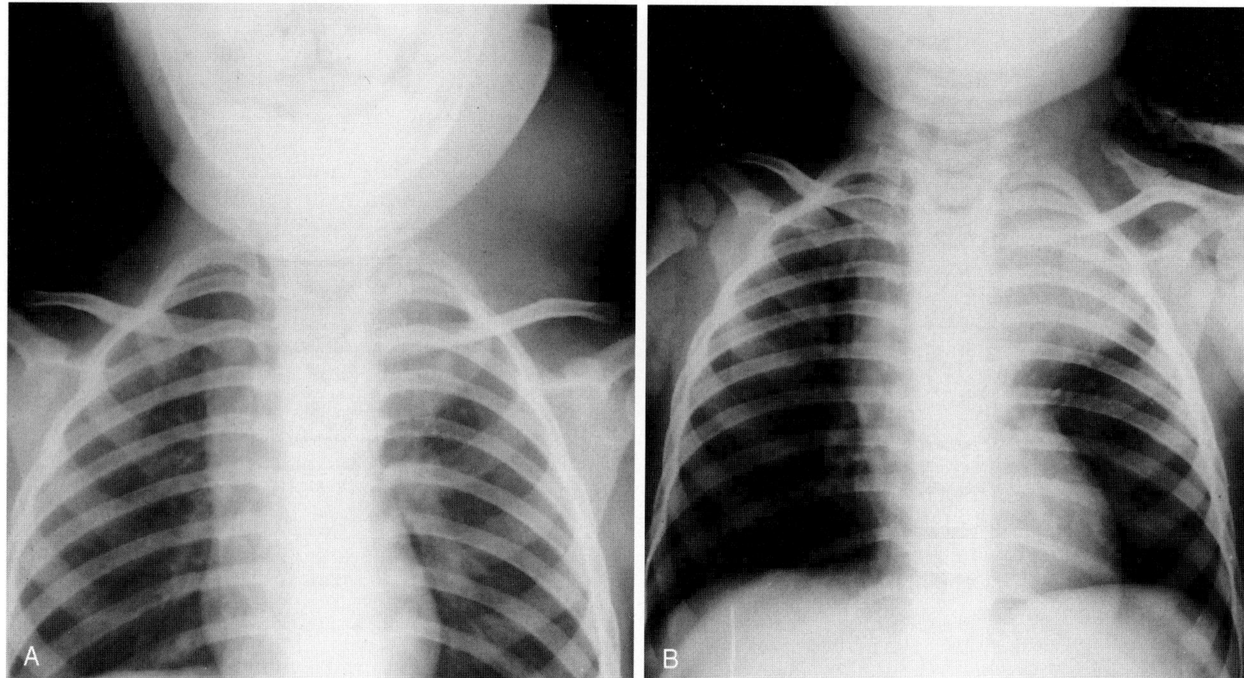

FIGURE 62–3 ■ *A*, A chest radiograph of an infant with a lymphangioma of the left neck. Extension of the lesion into the left upper anterior mediastinum is demonstrated. *B*, This radiograph, obtained with manual compression of the cervical mass, is presented to condemn this practice. Pressure applied to the cervical mass increases the size of the mediastinal component, which can cause acute airway obstruction and consequent respiratory distress.

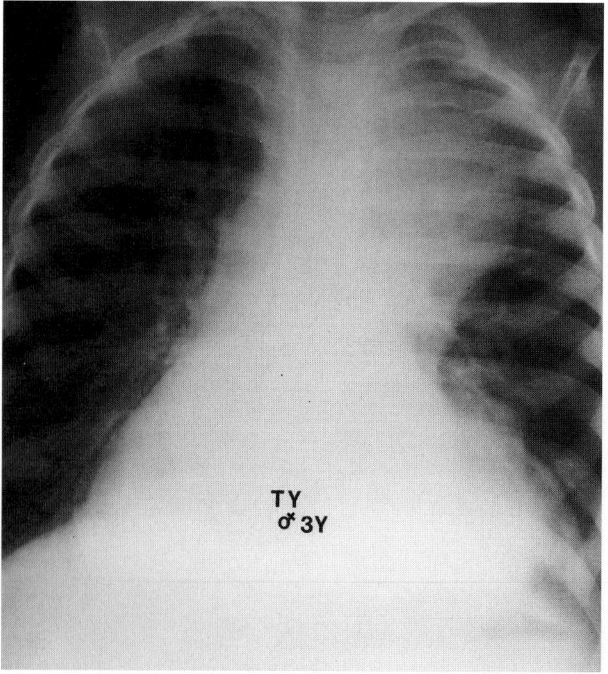

FIGURE 62–4 ■ A chest radiograph of a 3-year-old boy with mild stridor. The radiograph demonstrated a large anterior mediastinal mass; no cervical component was present on physical examination. At resection, a large, soft, spongy, cystic lesion was resected and was histologically found to be a lymphangioma.

approached through the neck by excising the external lesion and extending the resection into the anterior mediastinum. Extensive mediastinal involvement requires either a posterolateral thoracotomy or a sternotomy for resection, as does the entire mediastinal lymphangioma. Efforts to ligate all communicating lymphatics decrease either the frequency of chylothorax or its severity following resection.

Thymic Cysts

Thymic cysts are much rarer than teratomas. They can present as lesions at the base of the neck, or they may be entirely intrathoracic. These cysts are lined by epithelium that is often ciliated. The lining of the wall may contain lymphocytes as well as cholesterol crystals and granulomas. Thymic tissue is always present and is relatively normal in appearance (Lamesch et al, 1974). Thymic cysts are often asymptomatic and may become fairly large before they produce any symptoms.

Rapid expansion of thymic cysts, which may result from hemorrhage or respiratory infection, produces respiratory symptoms (Fig. 62–5). Many thymic cysts, however, are identified as incidental findings on chest radiographs. They are best defined by CT scan performed with intravenous contrast. The cysts are of homogeneous density and contiguous with the thymus, often protruding into one hemithorax (Welch et al, 1979). Resection is curative as malignant thymomas rarely occur in children or present as cystic lesions. Thymic cysts presenting at the base of the neck often can be resected through a transverse cervical incision and do not require thoracotomy (Bower et al, 1977).

Pericardial Cysts

Pericardial cysts (simple cysts, springwater cysts, coelomic cysts) are benign, unilocular lesions found at the cardiophrenic angle, most frequently on the right side. These cysts are invariably asymptomatic and are identified on radiographs as incidental findings. They are thin-walled cysts, lined by flattened mesothelium, and they contain clear fluid. Rarely do they communicate with the pericardium. They may be easily removed, and the primary reason for excision is to confirm the diagnosis.

Hodgkin's Disease

Hodgkin's disease generally presents as a solid mass in the anterior mediastinum. Rarely, primary involvement of the thymus may occur (Fig. 62–6), and in these cases it may present as a cystic mass (Nogués et al, 1987). The diagnosis is often established only after resection of the cystic mass. Chemotherapy or radiotherapy, depending on the stage of the disease, is required for definitive treatment.

MIDDLE MEDIASTINUM

Bronchogenic Cysts

Most cystic lesions in the middle mediastinum are of bronchopulmonary origin. They are found in close proximity to the tracheobronchial tree, often in a perihilar or subcarinal location. However, they may be found entirely within the lung adjacent to a bronchus. They may produce severe respiratory symptoms, primarily in the infant or young child. Bronchogenic cysts in a subcarinal location are often very difficult to diagnose on standard

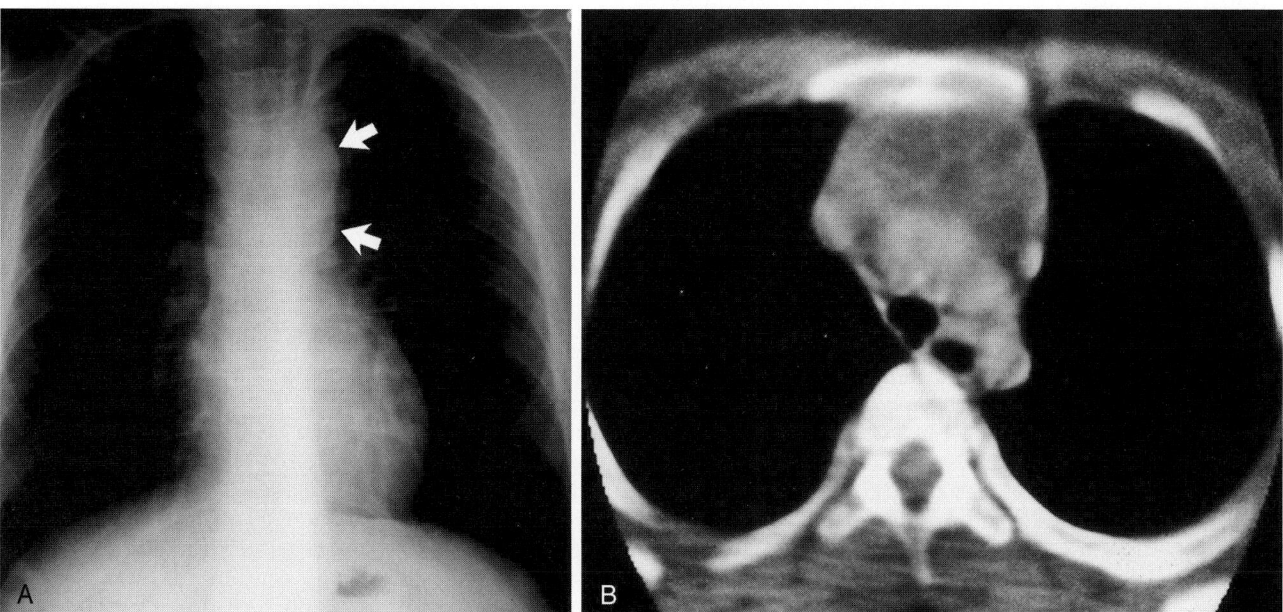

FIGURE 62–5 ■ *A*, A chest radiograph of an 11-year-old boy with upper respiratory symptoms and wheezing that demonstrates a mass in the superior mediastinum *(arrows)*. *B*, A computed tomography scan shows a multilocular, nonenhancing mass that extends from below the thyroid to the region of the great vessels. A multilocular thymic cyst was removed several days later, and the respiratory symptoms entirely resolved.

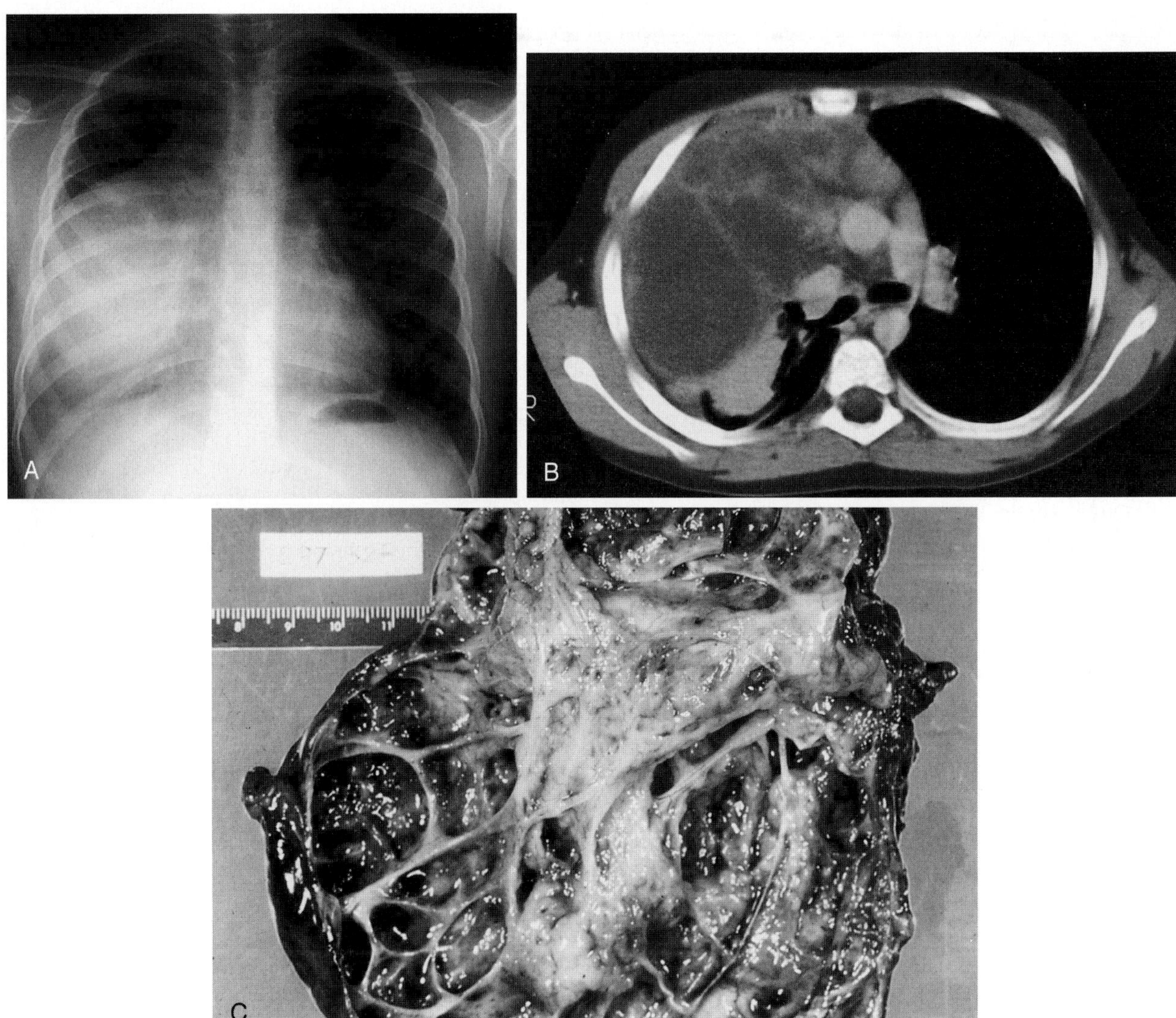

FIGURE 62–6 ■ *A*, A chest radiograph of a 10-year-old boy who had a brief episode of right pleural chest pain. On evaluation, the absence of breath sounds on the right led to the study, which demonstrated a large, right, thoracic mass. The patient had had an entirely normal chest radiograph 18 months before this study. *B*, A computed tomography scan shows a cystic mass with multiple septation. *C*, Resection of the cystic mass was performed through a right thoracotomy. The mass arose from the thymus and extended into the right pleural space. The walls of the mass were thick and irregular with areas of nodularity, which raised concern about malignancy. Pathologic gross examination of the open specimen shown here revealed a thymic cyst with extensive involvement by Hodgkin's disease.

radiographs (Ribet et al, 1995). They are hidden by the cardiac silhouette, and airway compression may be difficult to identify. Their presence may be suggested only by unilateral emphysema produced by air trapping in one lung, or by partial collapse of a lung, depending on the degree of bronchial obstruction (Fig. 62–7).

Opsahl and Berman (1962) reviewed 31 infants with bronchogenic cysts. Twenty-five infants had respiratory symptoms, but the lesion was seen on a standard radiograph in only 14; it was successfully removed in 12 of these patients. The critical nature of bronchogenic cysts in infants was best demonstrated in the 11 symptomatic children for whom there were no radiographic findings or surgical resection, as all died. Eraklis and associates (1969) reported similar findings in 10 infants with bronchogenic cysts, 7 of whom had severe or moderate respiratory distress (Fig. 62–8). The cyst was identified only at autopsy in four infants in whom a mediastinal mass was not recognized radiographically or at operation, and in two additional infants who died without operation.

The laryngotracheal groove appears at the end of the third week of gestation in the embryonic foregut. The dorsal portion of the foregut subsequently elongates to form the esophagus, and the ventral portion ultimately differentiates into the respiratory tract, with ciliated epithelium lining both the fetal esophagus and the trachea (Moore and Parson, 1993; Skandalakis et al, 1994). Bronchogenic cysts and esophageal duplications may arise during this embryonic process, when the primitive foregut divides into the laryngotracheal ridge anteriorly and the esophagus posteriorly. Outpouchings from these structures may become separated and give rise to cystic remnants (Grafe et al, 1966). The embryonic tissues associated with the development of the trachea and

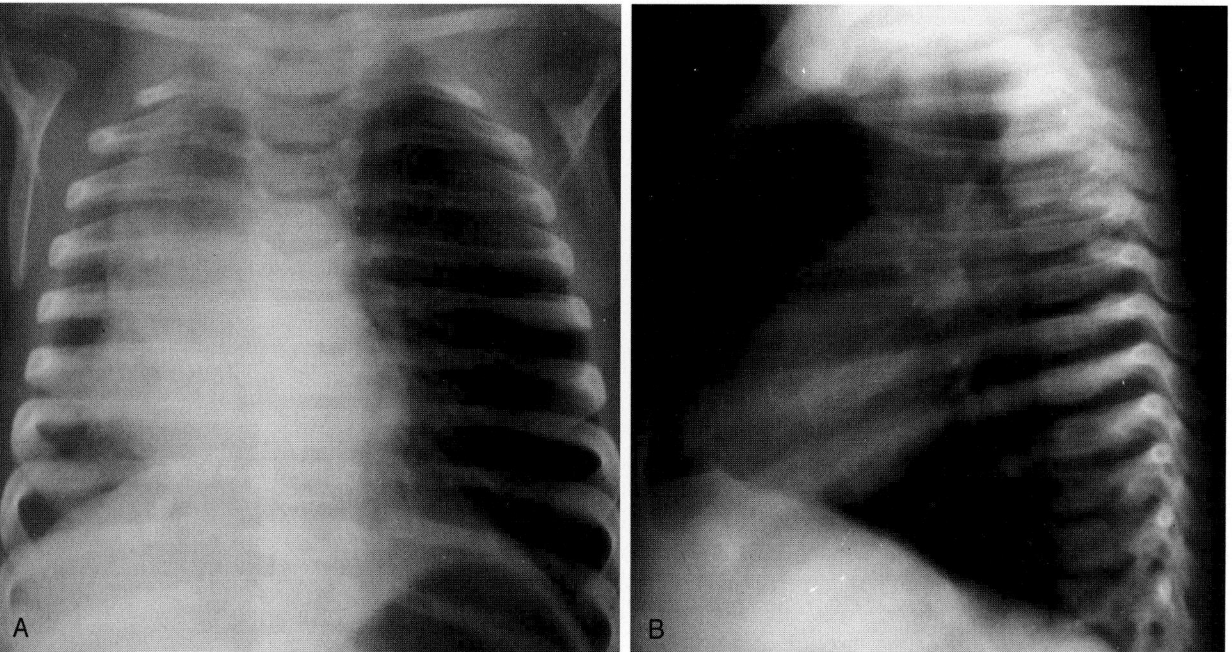

FIGURE 62–7 ■ *A*, Chest radiographs of a 3-month-old-girl who had experienced cyanotic attacks for 2 months. The infant had always had distinct wheezing. She was extremely dyspneic and had a severe respiratory grunt. Hyperresonance was present on the left side of the chest, and heart sounds were displaced to the right. Radiographs show gross hyperinflation of the left lung, but no mass lesion was identified on the PA, *A*, or lateral view, *B*. A bronchoscopy was performed to investigate the possibility of a foreign body. Extrinsic compression of the left bronchus was seen. The child died shortly thereafter before a thoracotomy could be performed. Autopsy demonstrated a large subcarinal bronchogenic cyst that was compressing the left mainstem bronchus. It measured 1.5 cm in diameter and had been completely concealed by the heart on plain radiographs. A barium swallow, something that was rarely performed in 1927, presumably would have demonstrated compression. PA, posteroanterior.

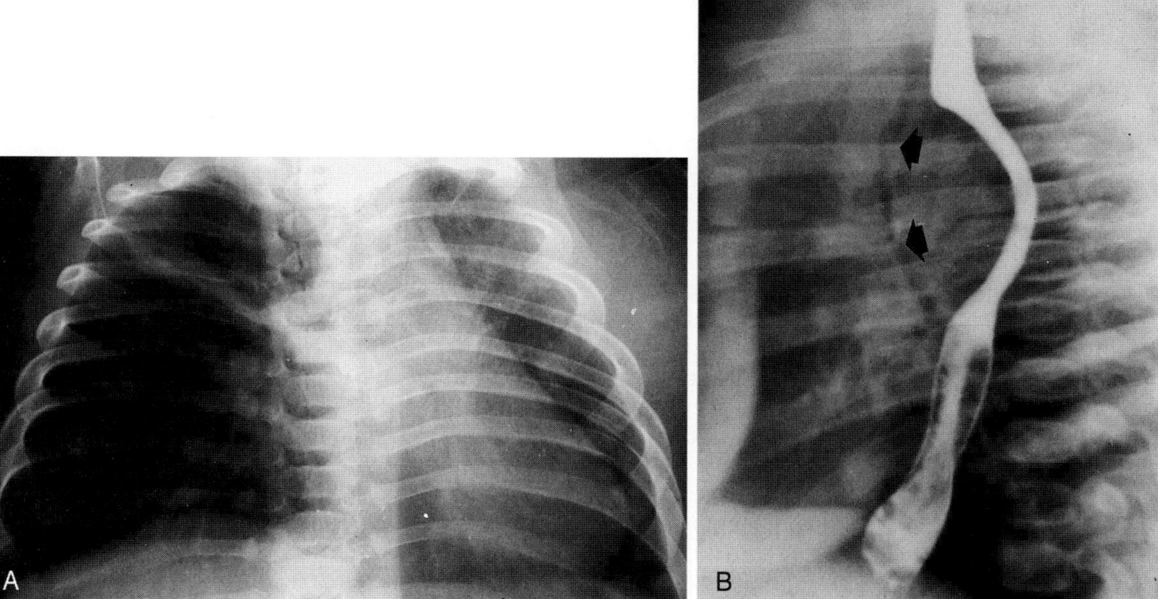

FIGURE 62–8 ■ *A*, A chest radiograph of a 6-month-old infant who was admitted with a history of stridor and labored respiration. Tachypnea with sternal and substernal retractions were first noted at birth. Acute exacerbation of substernal retraction, wheezing, and rhonchi led to evaluation. A chest radiograph revealed hyperinflation of the right lung. *B*, A barium swallow demonstrated a mass that was compressing and displacing the trachea anteriorly *(arrows)* and the esophagus posteriorly. A left posterolateral thoracotomy was performed, and a 3.5-cm bronchogenic cyst that was found densely adherent to the posterior wall of the carina was resected. No communication to the trachea was present. Recovery was uneventful.

esophagus have the capacity to develop into respiratory or gastrointestinal structures, which explains why the histologic appearance of these cysts is so variable. We believe that bronchogenic cysts and esophageal duplications are best defined by their proximity to the trachea and bronchus, or to the esophagus (Nobuhara et al, 1997), rather than by their histologic appearance, as proposed by Reed and Sobonya (1974).

Bronchogenic cysts are usually lined by ciliated, pseudostratified epithelium characteristic of the respiratory tract, although they occasionally may be lined by esophageal or gastric mucosa despite their anatomic location in close proximity to the trachea or bronchus (Nobuhara et al, 1997). Cartilage and smooth muscle may also be found within the walls. Communication with the trachea or bronchus is rare. The mucosal lining of these cysts produces mucus, thereby increasing the size of the cyst. Rarely, these cysts occur within the pericardial sac (Dabbs et al, 1957). The ability to obtain CT scans has greatly facilitated identification of occult bronchogenic cysts (Snyder et al, 1985). Determination of their precise location to facilitate surgical resection is critical. In older children, bronchogenic cysts are often asymptomatic and are identified on radiographs obtained for unrelated symptoms.

Surgical resection by thoracotomy or video-associated thoracoscopy is the therapy of choice for bronchogenic cysts (Cioffi et al, 1998). The primary indications for resection are the concern that progressive fluid collection will produce respiratory symptoms if they are not already present, or that the cyst may become infected. A secondary indication for resection is the occurrence of malignant degeneration within the cysts, including embryonal rhabdomyosarcoma reported by Krous and Sexauer (1981), squamous cell carcinoma discussed by Cuypers and colleagues (1996), and adenocarcinoma described by Suen and co-workers (1993). Complete resection of the mucosal lining is important for preventing recurrence of the cyst (Gharagozloo et al, 1995; Metersky et al, 1995).

POSTERIOR MEDIASTINUM

Esophageal Duplications

Esophageal duplications, also called enterogenous cysts, gastrogenous cysts, enteric cysts, or neurenteric cysts, account for the bulk of the cystic lesions in the posterior mediastinum. They may produce a variety of symptoms, including respiratory distress or dysphagia, if their size is adequate to cause tracheobronchial or esophageal compression. Severe respiratory distress has been reported from tracheal compression of a cervical esophageal duplication (Winslow et al, 1984). Neurologic symptoms from associated abnormalities of the spine and spinal cord also lead to identification of esophageal duplications. Rarely, bleeding or perforation may produce acute symptoms of pleuritic pain or hemorrhage.

Esophageal duplications are generally in contact with the esophagus but rarely communicate with its lumen. They are identified more frequently in the left hemithorax than on the right. Barium swallow may demonstrate extrinsic compression of the esophagus (Fig. 62–9). CT or magnetic resonance imaging (MRI) readily demonstrates the cystic nature of these lesions and distinguishes them from the more frequent neurogenic tumors arising in the posterior sulcus of the chest (Fig. 62–10). The lining of these duplication cysts is usually respiratory, but may also consist of squamous epithelium (Nobuhara et al, 1997). A surprisingly high frequency of heterotopic gastric mucosa (Fig. 62–11) has been reported, varying from 2 of 6 lesions in the series by Ildstad and associates (1988) to 9 of 15 in that of Superina and colleagues (1984). Two of the lesions in the latter series actually presented with acute perforation. A preoperative technetium pertechnetate scan demonstrates the gastric lining of the cyst (Ferguson et al, 1973), but this study is not required unless the cyst is to be observed without resection.

Esophageal duplications are generally isolated, but they may occur in association with esophageal atresia (Hemalatha et al, 1980); in up to 25%, a second duplication in the abdominal cavity will be identified (Holcomb et al, 1989). Vertebral anomalies, including hemivertebrae, spina bifida, and vertebral fusions, occur with a frequency varying from 3 of 16 (Bower et al, 1977) to 14 of 19 patients (Superina et al, 1984). In the latter series, six patients presented with neurologic symptoms. Back pain, sensory or motor deficits, or gate disturbances may be the first symptoms of an esophageal duplication occurring in conjunction with anomalies of the spine.

This association of vertebral anomalies with duplication cysts supports the notochord theory of Veeneklaas (1952) for the origin of these mediastinal duplications. The notochord first appears during the third week of embryologic life, wedging itself between cells forming the endoderm and the ectoderm. The theory postulates that, if there is an incomplete separation of the notochord from the endoderm, traction may be exerted on the primitive gut in such a manner that the outpouching is drawn toward the vertebral bodies. Loss of continuity between the pouch and the primitive gut from which it arose may result in a separate duplication. Rarely, a long, tubular esophageal duplication extends through the diaphragm to end in close proximity to, or even in communication with, the stomach, pancreas, duodenum, or jejunum. Those duplications not associated with vertebral anomalies presumably arise during separation of the primitive foregut, as was discussed earlier for bronchogenic cysts. This again explains the marked variety of epithelium, glands, and cartilage that occurs within the cyst.

All patients with vertebral anomalies or neurologic symptoms and posterior cystic lesions should have the spinal canal evaluated prior to surgery. In the past, myelograms were used, but now, MRI scans easily demonstrate the extent of protrusion of the cyst into the spinal canal, as well as any associated anomalies of the spinal cord.

Surgical resection is the therapy of choice for all esophageal duplications. This is required for four reasons. First, the cyst may progressively increase in size with accumulation of secretions, which may compress the trachea, bronchus, or esophagus. Second, the cyst may become infected by a hematogenous route. Third, malignant lesions may occur in these cysts, including squamous cell carcinoma (Tapia and White, 1985) and adenocarcinoma

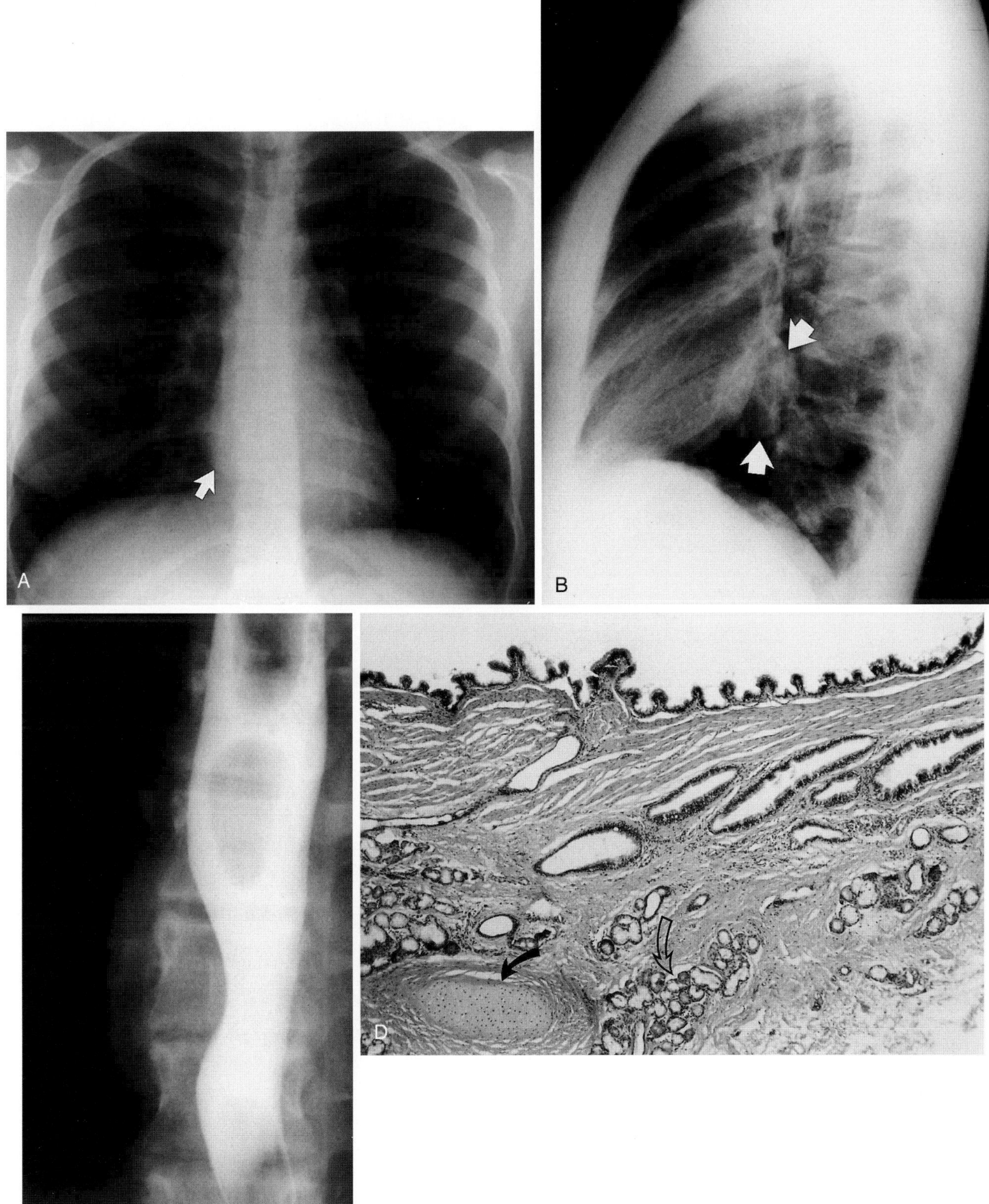

FIGURE 62–9 ■ *A*, A chest radiograph of a 13-year-old girl with mild dysphagia, that demonstrates a spherical mass protruding at the margin of the right side of the heart *(arrow)*, which is best demonstrated on *B*, the lateral radiograph *(arrows)*. *C*, Barium swallow demonstrates compression of the esophagus. At resection, the cyst was enveloped by esophageal muscles. It was resected in a submucosal fashion, where it was adjacent to the esophagus. The cyst was filled with mucus. *D*, Pathologic examination demonstrated pseudostratified epithelium and walls with cartilage *(solid arrow)* and mucous glands *(open arrow)*, which are more characteristic of respiratory lining.

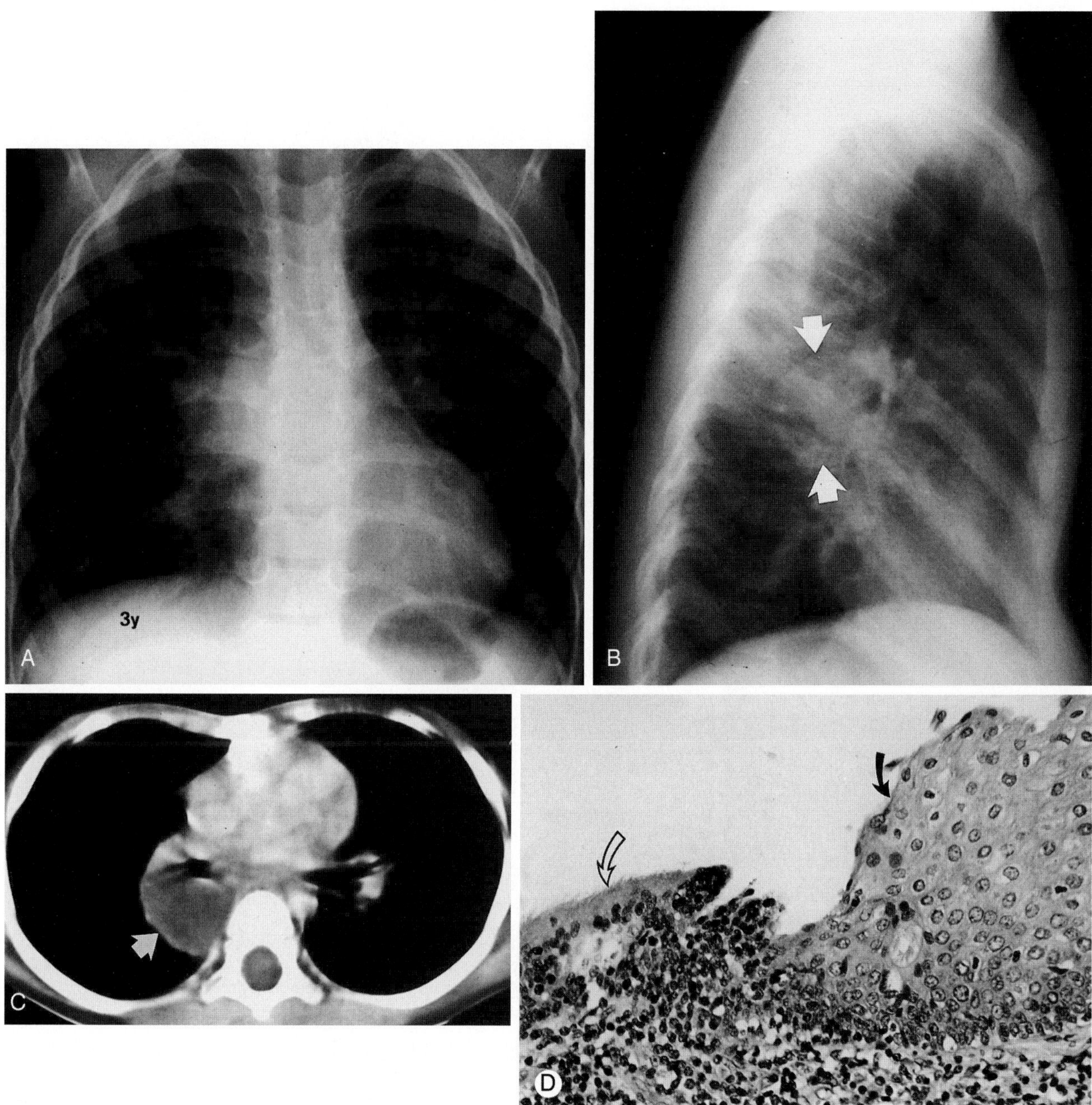

FIGURE 62–10 ■ *A*, A chest radiograph of a 3-year-old boy that was obtained because of mild pectus excavatum. The radiograph demonstrates a right-sided retrohilar mass, also seen on *B*, the lateral view *(arrows)*. Barium swallow showed that the mass was indenting the esophagus. *C*, A computed tomography scan shows a cystic mass *(arrow)* that was not enhanced with intravenous contrast administered posterior to the right bronchus and adjacent to the esophagus. At resection, the mass was closely adherent to the right bronchus, but it was also intimately associated with the esophagus, with esophageal muscle coming up onto the posterior aspect of the mass. This case demonstrates the close association and overlap between a bronchogenic cyst and esophageal duplication, because their mechanism of origin is probably identical. *D*, Histologically, the common origin of the cyst is demonstrated as well. The cyst contained both nonkeratinizing stratified squamous epithelium *(solid arrow)* and ciliated pseudostratified columnar epithelium *(open arrow)*.

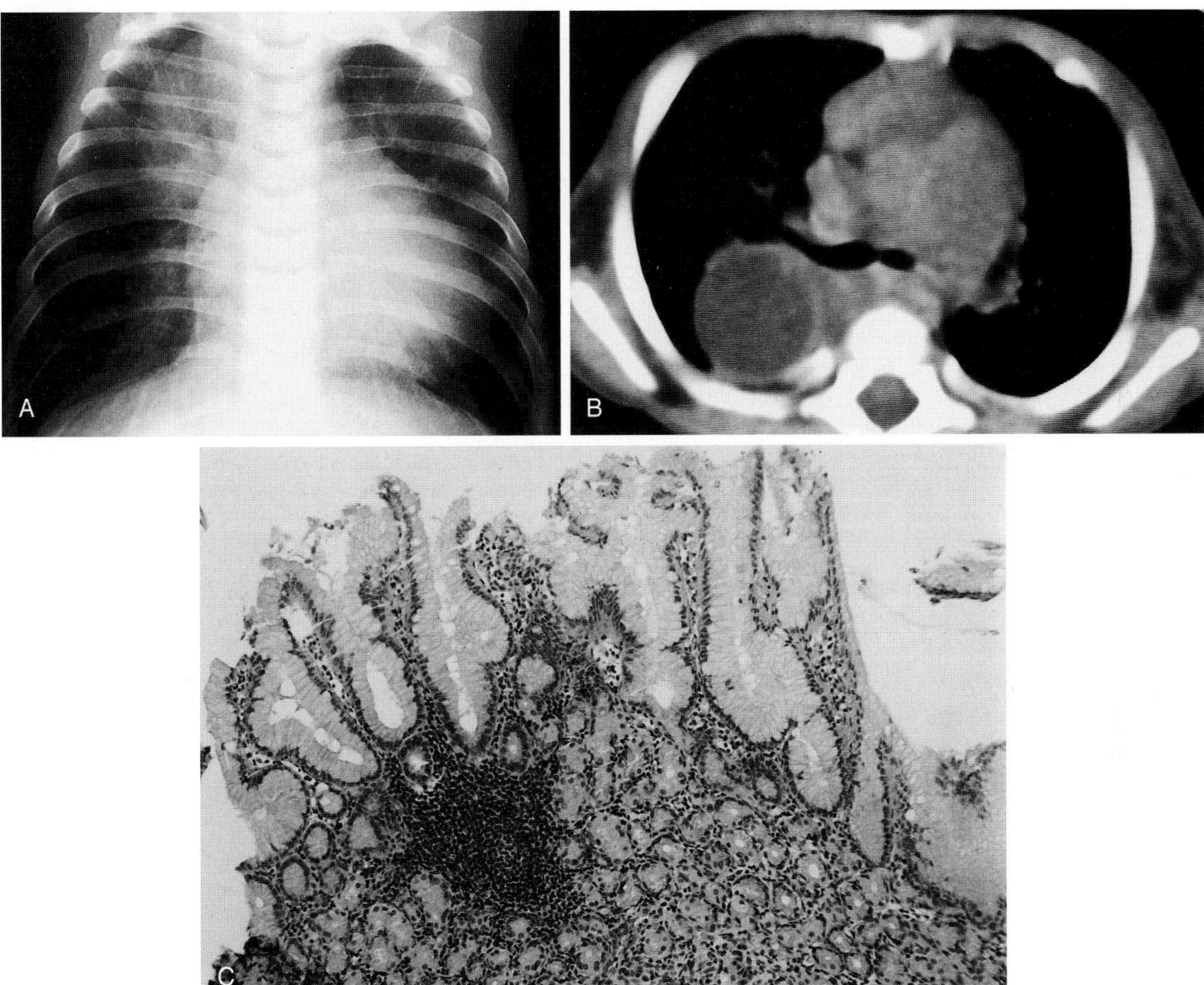

FIGURE 62–11 ■ *A*, A chest radiograph of a 7-month-old boy, who was born with trisomy 21, complete atrioventricular canal, and duodenal stenosis, shows a right-sided thoracic mass in the right posterior mediastinum. *B*, A computed tomography scan demonstrates a cystic mass in the posterior sulcus, which did not enhance with intravenous contrast. At resection, edema was found around the cyst. The cyst was adjacent to the esophagus but not surrounded by esophageal muscles. Anatomically, it lay to the right of the esophagus and posterior to the trachea, and the right mainstem bronchus was draped over its inferior portion. The cyst was not densely adherent, however, to any of these structures. *C*, Pathologic examination revealed gastric antral-type mucosa surrounded by loose connective tissue and smooth muscles.

(Chuang et al, 1981). Fourth, the cysts, as previously indicated, are frequently lined by gastric mucosa, and hemorrhage or perforation can occur.

Esophageal duplications frequently share a common muscular wall with the esophagus. Resection of only the mucosal portion of the cyst in the area of its contact with the esophagus prevents entry into the esophageal lumen. Rarely is there a communication between the cyst and the esophagus unless it results from erosion and ulceration from ectopic gastric mucosa, which may cause hemorrhage.

The occasional thoracoabdominal cysts are recognized by their large size and their tubular nature, suggesting abdominal extension, in contrast with the more common esophageal duplications limited to the thorax. Successful resection of these lesions was first reported by Gross in 1948. Complete resection to their site of origin at the stomach, duodenum, jejunum, or pancreas is vital. In the collected series reported by Pokorny and Goldstein (1984), the cysts communicated with the gastrointestinal tract in 17 of 25 patients. Patients with these large thoracoabdominal duplications may present with respiratory symptoms secondary to their large size (12 of 25 patients), anemia (10 of 25), melena (8 of 25), emesis (8 of 25), pain (5 of 25), failure to thrive (4 of 25), or hemoptysis from peptic ulceration from ectopic gastric mucosa (1 of 25). Younger children and infants present more frequently with respiratory symptoms, and older children with anemia, melena, hematemesis, or pain. Either a thoracoabdominal incision or separate thoracic and abdominal incisions may be required for resection, depending on the extent of proximal communication of the lesion (Fig. 62–12).

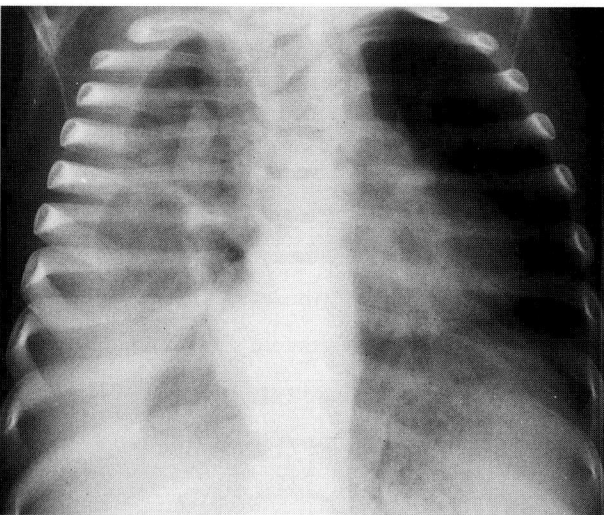

FIGURE 62–12 ■ A chest radiograph of 1-year-old infant who developed respiratory difficulty with a large, right pleural effusion. Thoracentesis revealed serosanguinous fluid with no bacteria but a high amylase level. The chest film also showed vertebral anomalies in the upper thoracic vertebrae. This was a major clue to the presence of a duplication cyst. A soft tissue mass was suggested, with bulging from T6 to T10 along the right parasternal region. A barium swallow and aortogram showed that the esophagus and the aorta were displaced to the left. At thoracotomy, the cyst was found to have ruptured into the right cavity. It was resected from its extent up to the inferior cervical vertebral bodies. The cyst was lined by respiratory epithelium, mucous glands, hyaline cartilage, and gastric mucosa.

COMMENTS AND CONTROVERSIES

Drs. Shamberger and Hendren have provided an excellent perspective on the diagnosis and management of mediastinal cysts and duplications in the pediatric population. With the advent of current imaging modalities, including computed tomography, magnetic resonance imaging, and endoscopic ultrasound, diagnosis of these lesions should seldom be in doubt. This is particularly true for pericardial cysts and bronchogenic cysts for which excision for diagnostic purposes should never be required. In the adult population, it is common practice to follow the asymptomatic bronchogenic cyst or esophageal duplication cyst because these rarely cause problems and can be very easily monitored by serial follow-up imaging studies. However, from the pediatric perspective, Drs. Shamberger and Hendren argue that over the long passage of time, increase in size so as to produce symptoms and infection with its attendant complications and small risk of malignancy justify early intervention at the time of diagnosis. From this commentator's perspective, this represents a legitimate difference in management perspective between adult and pediatric populations.

G.A.P.

REFERENCES

Bower RJ, Sieber WK, Kiesewetter WB: Alimentary tract duplications in children. Ann Surg 188:669, 1977.

Childress ME, Baker CP, Samson PC: Lymphangioma of the mediastinum. J Thorac Cardiovasc Surg 31:338, 1956.

Chuang MT, Barba FA, Kaneko M, Teirstein AS: Adenocarcinoma arising in an intrathoracic duplication cyst of foregut origin: A case report with review of the literature. Cancer 47:1887, 1981.

Cioffi U, Bonavina L, De Simone M et al: Presentation and surgical management of bronchogenic and esophageal duplication cysts in adults. Chest 113:1492, 1998.

Cuypers P, De Leyn P, Cappelle L et al: Bronchogenic cysts: A review of 20 cases. Eur J Cardiothorac Surg 10:393, 1996.

Dabbs CH, Berg R Jr, Pierce EC II: Intrapericardial bronchogenic cysts: Report of two cases and probable embryologic explanation. J Thorac Surg 34:718, 1957.

Eraklis AJ, Griscom NT, McGovern JB: Bronchogenic cysts of the mediastinum in infancy. N Engl J Med 281:1150, 1969.

Ferguson CC, Young LN, Sutherland JB et al: Intrathoracic gastrogenic cyst: Preoperative diagnosis by technetium pertechnetate scan. J Pediatr Surg 8:827, 1973.

Gharagozloo F, Dasumann MJ, McReynolds SD et al: Recurrent bronchogenic pseudocyst 24 years after incomplete excision. Chest 108:880, 1995.

Gottschalk E, Lichey C, Friedich U: Thorakale Teratome bei Kindern. Z Kinderchir 29:303, 1980.

Grafe WR, Goldsmith EI, Redo SF: Bronchogenic cysts of the mediastinum in children. J Pediatr Surg 1:384, 1966.

Hemalatha V, Batcup G, Brereton RJ et al: Intrathoracic foregut cyst (foregut duplication) associated with esophageal atresia. J Pediatr Surg 15:178, 1980.

Holcomb GW III, Gheissari A, O'Neill JA et al: Surgical management of alimentary tract duplications. Ann Surg 209:167, 1989.

Ildstad ST, Tollerud DJ, Weiss RG et al: Duplications of the alimentary tract: Clinical characteristics, preferred treatment, and associated malformations. Ann Surg 208:184, 1988.

Krous HF, Sexauer CL: Embryonal rhabdomyosarcoma arising within a congenital bronchogenic cyst in a child. J Pediatr Surg 16:506, 1981.

Lamesch A, Capesius C, Theisen-Aspesberro MC: Cervical thymic cysts in infants and children. Z Kinderchir 14:213, 1974.

Metersky ML, Moskowitz H, Thayer JO: Recurrent mediastinal bronchogenic cyst. Respiration 62:234, 1995.

Moore KL, Parson TVN: The developing human. In Clinically Oriented Embryology, 6th ed. Philadelphia, WB Saunders, 1993, p 261.

Nobuhara KK, Gorski YC, La Quaglia MP et al: Bronchogenic cysts and esophageal duplications: Common origins and treatment. J Pediatr Surg 32:1408, 1997.

Nogués A, Tovar JA, Suñol M et al: Hodgkin's disease of the thymus: A rare mediastinal cystic mass. J Pediatr Surg 22:996, 1987.

Ochsner JL, Ochsner SF: Congenital cysts of the mediastinum: 20 year experience with 42 cases. Ann Surg 136:909, 1966.

Opsahl T, Berman EJ: Bronchogenic mediastinal cysts in infants: Case report and review of the literature. Pediatrics 30:372, 1962.

Perkes EA, Haller JO, Kassner EG et al: Mediastinal cystic hygroma in infants: Two cases with no extension into the neck. Clin Pediatr (Phila) 18:168, 1979.

Pokorny WJ, Goldstein IR: Enteric thoracoabdominal duplications in children. J Thorac Cardiovasc Surg 87:821, 1984.

Reed JC, Sobonya RE: Morphologic analysis of foregut cysts in the thorax. AJR Am J Roentgenol 120:851, 1974.

Ribet ME, Copin MC, Gosselin B: Bronchogenic cysts of the mediastinum. J Thorac Cardiovasc Surg 109:1003, 1995.

Shamberger RC, Holzman RS, Griscom NT et al: CT quantitation of tracheal cross-sectional area as a guide to the surgical and anesthetic management of children with anterior mediastinal masses. J Pediatr Surg 26:138, 1991.

Shamberger RC, Holzman RS, Griscom NT et al: Prospective evaluation by computed tomography and pulmonary function tests of children with mediastinal masses. Surgery 118:468, 1995.

Skandalakis JE, Gray SW, Ricketts R: The esophagus. In Skandalakis JE, Gray SW (eds): Embryology for Surgeons, 2nd ed. Baltimore, Williams and Wilkins, 1994.

Snyder ME, Luck SR, Hernandez R et al: Diagnostic dilemmas of mediastinal cysts. J Pediatr Surg 20:810, 1985.

Suen HC, Mathisen DJ, Grillo HC et al: Surgical management and radiological characteristics of bronchogenic cysts. Ann Thorac Surg 55:476, 1993.

Superina RA, Ein SH, Humphreys RP: Cystic duplications of the esophagus and neurenteric cysts. J Pediatr Surg 19:527, 1984.

Tapia RH, White VA: Squamous cell carcinoma arising in a duplication cyst of the esophagus. Am J Gastroenterol 80:325, 1985.

Thompson DP, Moore TC: Acute thoracic distress in childhood due to spontaneous rupture of a large mediastinal teratoma. J Pediatr Surg 4:416, 1969.

Veeneklaas GMH: Pathogenesis of intrathoracic gastrogenic cysts. Am J Dis Child 83:500, 1952.

Welch KJ, Tapper D, Vawter GP: Surgical treatment of thymic cysts and neoplasms in children. J Pediatr Surg 14:691, 1979.

Winslow RE, Dykstra G, Scholten DJ et al: Duplication of the cervical esophagus: An unrecognized cause of respiratory distress in infants. Am Surg 50:506, 1984.

CYSTS AND DUPLICATIONS IN ADULTS

Mark S. Allen

Cysts are among the most common masses seen in the mediastinum. In Davis's and Cohen's reports of 630 patients with surgically treated mediastinal masses, 60% had a benign mediastinal mass or cyst (Cohen et al, 1991; Davis et al, 1987). In 1971, Oldham collected a series of 1000 mediastinal tumors and cysts from five authors and found that 21% of the masses were cysts (Oldham, 1971). This collection of 214 mediastinal cysts comprised 41% bronchogenic, 35% pericardial, 10% enteric, and 14% nonspecific cysts. Even though cysts are a relatively common mediastinal mass, they are still only occasionally seen by the general thoracic surgeon. In support of this relative rarity, a report from a hospital with more than 54,000 admissions annually indicated that only six patients with mediastinal cysts were seen over a 4-year period (Allen and Payne, 1992). Coselli reported that bronchogenic cysts were seen in only one of 42,000 admissions (Coselli et al, 1987).

The terminology used to describe mediastinal cysts has varied with time. The terms *duplication, bronchogenic, enteric,* and *esophageal cysts* have all been used. Similarly, there have been many different ways to classify these lesions. In 1948, Maier used the lesions' anatomic location to organize this group of lesions (Maier, 1948). In 1954, Fallon and associates used the embryologic origin, along with the anatomic location, to classify these cysts (Fallon et al, 1954). Others have used the histology of the epithelial lining as the defining characteristic. The classification system devised by Fallon, Gordon, and Lendrum uses location, embryologic origin, and predominant epithelial lining in its scheme (Fallon et al, 1954).

Many different types of cysts are found in the mediastinum. This chapter discusses bronchogenic cysts, esophageal cysts, neurenteric cysts, thymic cysts, mesothelial (pleural and pericardial) cysts, pancreatic cysts, and thoracic duct cysts. Each of these is discussed separately but because the embryologic origin of these lesions is an important concept in all, it will be discussed in general for all of these lesions.

EMBRYOLOGY

When the embryo is only 18 days old, the notochord (the beginning of the nervous system) begins to form when the ectoderm forms the primitive pit and develops into the primitive streak. The vertebral bodies form around the notochord. If, during this infolding, some endoderm is trapped in the ectoderm, a split in the notochord develops, known as the split notochord syndrome. This malformation is thought to be the cause of a neurenteric cyst. As is detailed later, this type of mediastinal cyst is often associated with a defect in the vertebral body, which makes sense embryologically because the defect originates at the time of vertebral body formation.

The esophageal and respiratory systems begin to develop in the 26-day-old embryo. This commences with the appearance of a laryngeal groove in the ventral wall of the primitive pharynx. This groove deepens and is surrounded by mesenchymal tissue. The groove begins to form buds, elongates, and branches to eventually form the trachea, bronchi, and alveoli. If one of these buds, which are lined with endoderm, separates, it can give rise to a cyst that is lined with respiratory epithelium and is known a bronchogenic cyst.

As the lung bud elongates, a septum develops that divides the pouch into two separate diverticula. As this division enlarges and matures, it partitions the lung pouch from the esophageal pouch. The esophagus rapidly elongates and reaches its final relative length of growth by 7 weeks. As this is occurring, the endoderm of the esophagus proliferates and nearly occludes the lumen. At 6 weeks, microcysts form in this tube and begin to coalesce. These cysts or vacuoles start to fuse and gradually form the esophageal lumen. If one of these vacuoles persists, it can result in an esophageal cyst in the wall or adjacent to the esophagus.

BRONCHOGENIC CYSTS

Cystic lesions of the lung have been reported since the 17th century, but the first report in the American literature of a mediastinal bronchogenic cyst was by Mixter and Clifford in 1929 (Mixter and Clifford, 1929). Since this first report, several series have demonstrated that bronchogenic cysts are the most common mediastinal cyst, accounting for about 60% of mediastinal masses (Rice, 1992). Because the lesion originates from an abnormality in lung development, the cyst may be located anywhere along the course of lung development. If a lung bud that is destined to become a bronchogenic cyst breaks off early in development, it ends up in the mediastinum; if it breaks off late in development, it ends up in the lung parenchyma (Flinner and Hammond, 1989; Rodgers and Osmer, 1964). When bronchogenic cysts develop in the mediastinum, the most common location is the subcarinal area. However, they can occur anywhere in the body and have been reported in association with the esophagus, pericardium, or sternum (Bagwell and Schiffman, 1988; Gomes and Hufnagel, 1975). They can be dumbbell-shaped on either side of the diaphragm (Amendola et al, 1982). They also have been reported in the skin as a blind sinus tract.

As was mentioned above, bronchogenic cysts are the most common mediastinal foregut cysts but they still account for only about 5% of all mediastinal masses (Wychulis et al, 1971). In other series, the incidence of primary cysts varied from 11% to 25% (Davis et al, 1987). There seems to be a relative decrease in the number of benign cysts in recent reports; however, this may be the result of a relative increase in the number of malignant tumors found in the mediastinum. Bronchogenic cysts are usually an isolated finding, but they have been reported in association with pulmonary sequestration, Down syndrome, and accessory pulmonary lobes (Black et al, 1988; Ramenofsky et al, 1979; Schenck, 1936).

Many authors have reported that bronchogenic cysts usually present as an asymptomatic finding (Jeffries, 1987; Kirwan et al, 1973; Maier, 1948; Whitaker et al, 1980). Support for this comes from a series of young military patients (who are more likely to undergo screening chest roentgenography) in which 78% of bronchogenic cysts were found incidentally (Fontenelle et al, 1971). Other reports contradict this finding (Di Lorenzo et al, 1989; Eraklis et al, 1969; Ramenofsky et al, 1979; Schmidt and Drapanas, 1972; Sirivella et al, 1985). In Di Lorenzo's series, only 7 patients of 26 were asymptomatic (Di Lorenzo et al, 1989). In a recent series of a mixed-aged population, 75% of patients presented with symptoms (Cartmill and Hughes, 1989). In another series, even if the patients did not initially present with symptoms, most (67%) eventually became symptomatic with long-term follow-up (Rice, 1992).

Symptoms from a mediastinal bronchogenic cyst are usually the result of pressure on adjacent structures or infection in the cyst. When symptoms are caused by compression, the specific symptom varies according to what structure is compressed. In children, compression symptoms are more acute and often can be life-threatening. In adults, the symptoms are less acute but can be quite pronounced. If the cyst compresses a mainstem bronchus, distal pneumonia, hyperinflation, or wheezing can occur. Dysphagia can occur from compression of the esophagus. Superior vena caval syndrome and left atrial compression have been reported from an enlarging mediastinal cyst (Gomes and Hufnagel, 1975; Miller et al, 1978; Volpi et al, 1988). Interestingly, sometimes symptoms are positional in nature, and symptoms may be made worse by recumbency. This odd symptom complex should alert the physician to look for a mediastinal mass.

If the cyst becomes infected, which is postulated to occur via an occult communication with the bronchial tree, a different type of symptom occurs. An infected bronchogenic cyst may cause fatigue, chest pain, or fever with or without leukocytosis (Estrera et al, 1987). Patients may also cough up material from the cyst if there is a large enough communication with the bronchial tree. Cysts may also become infected after mediastinoscopy and biopsy, or following transtracheal aspiration. If the infected cyst fuses with the pleura, it is also possible for an empyema to develop if the cyst ruptures into the pleural space (Latimer, 1967; Ramenofsky et al, 1979).

Physical examination is usually unrevealing. Fever or tachycardia may be present if the cyst is infected, and occasional positional wheezing may be heard.

Diagnosis

Mediastinal cysts are best imaged by chest computed tomography (CT), but a standard chest roentgenogram is still useful. A chest radiograph usually shows a smooth, round mass in the mediastinum (Figs. 62–13 and 62–14). The size is variable; it can fill an entire thorax or be occult (Holesh, 1973). In one series, the average size was 3.6 cm (Salyer et al, 1977). Calcification is not common,

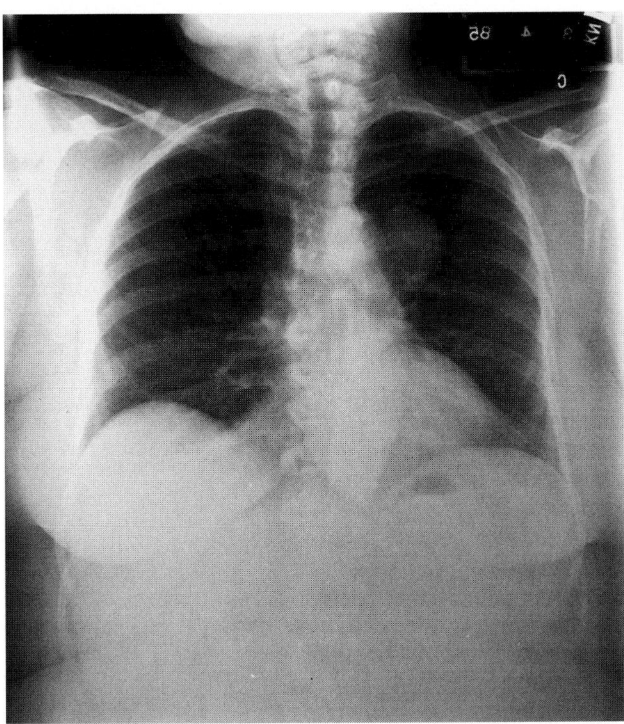

FIGURE 62–13 ■ Posteroanterior and lateral chest radiograph of an adult with a bronchogenic cyst that is adjacent to the aortic arch. It is clearly seen as a smooth, round mass in the medial portion of the left chest.

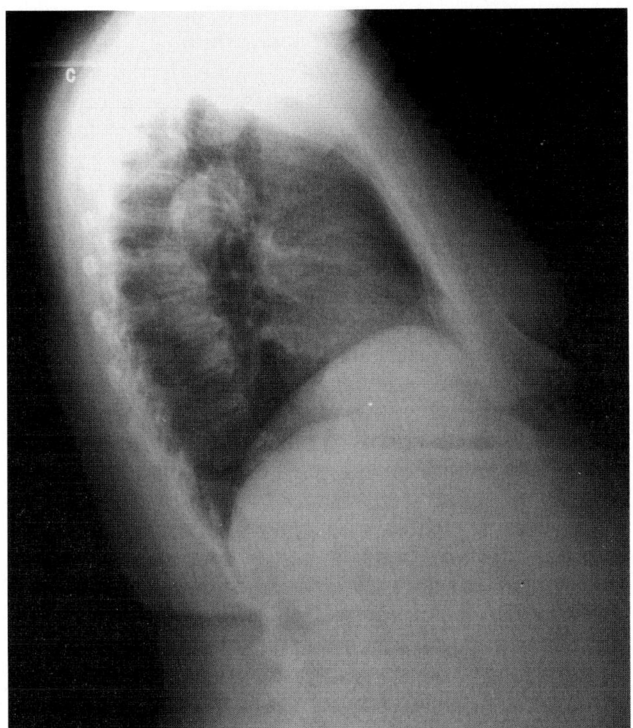

FIGURE 62–14 ■ Lateral chest radiograph of the patient in Figure 62–13 showing the mass in the mediastinum. It is a smooth-bordered, rounded mass immediately superior to the hilum.

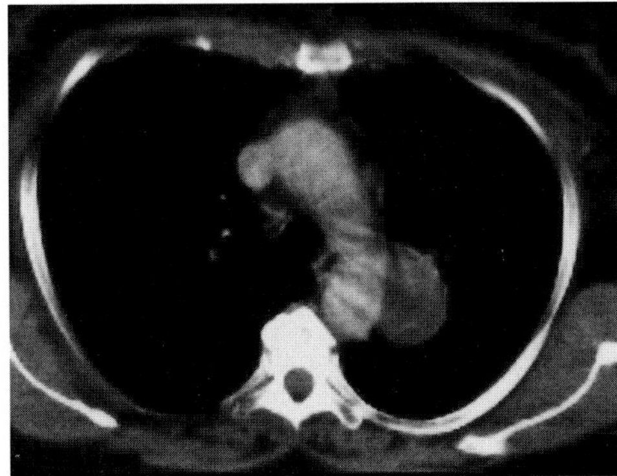

FIGURE 62–15 ■ A computed tomography of the patient in Figure 62–13 with a left-sided bronchogenic cyst. This is adjacent to the descending aorta, immediately distal to the aortic arch. Computed tomography provides excellent localization of bronchogenic cysts.

but cysts filled with calcium milk have been described (Cubillo and Rockoff, 1971; Hogg, 1986).

CT is very useful for pinpointing the location of the cyst (Figs. 62–15 and 62–16). The cyst usually has a homogeneous density and an attenuation value in a range consistent with fluid (0–20 Hounsfield units). If the cyst is infected, it appears more dense and inhomogeneous on CT, so homogeneity is not a reliable finding. Magnetic resonance imaging (MRI) allows differentiation of a bronchogenic cyst from a vascular lesion, but these two lesions are rarely confused (Figs. 62–17 through 62–20). MRI is a longer and more uncomfortable examination (especially for patients with claustrophobia), so it is rarely useful in patients with a bronchogenic cyst (Rice, 1992). Barium swallow can demonstrate compression of the esophagus by an adjacent cyst. In the fetus, prenatal ultrasonography has been used to make an antenatal diagnosis (Young et al, 1989). Bronchography, often used in the past to delineate airway compression or bronchial communication, is only of historic interest today.

Pathology

The typical bronchogenic cyst is a smooth, rounded lesion that, in the absence of infection, can be shelled out of its mediastinal location with little difficulty. The content of the cyst is usually a clear, thin fluid but it can be

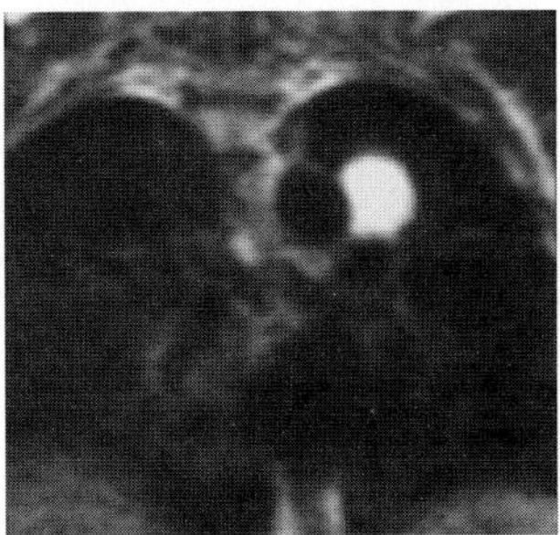

FIGURE 62–16 ■ Coronal section of a magnetic resonance image of the patient in Figure 62–13 with the bronchogenic cyst in the left periaortic area. The lesion appears as a *white nodule* that is adjacent to the *black void* in the aorta.

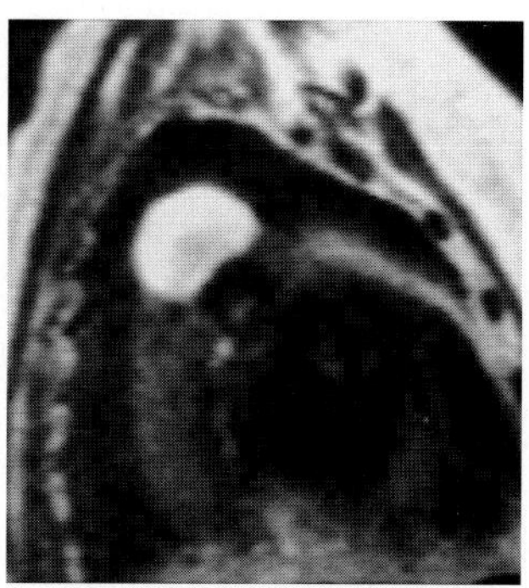

FIGURE 62–17 ■ A magnetic resonance imaging sagittal view of the patient in Figure 62–13. Again, the mass appears as a *white mass* adjacent to a *black void*, which is the vascular structure.

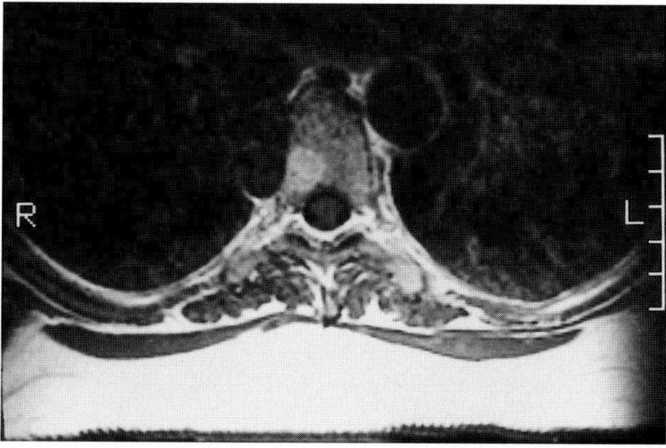

FIGURE 62–19 ■ A magnetic resonance image of the patient in Figure 62–13 with a right paravertebral bronchogenic cyst.

yellow, white, or viscous. Grossly, the inside of the cyst can be uniloculated or trabeculated. Microscopically, the lining can be ciliated columnar respiratory epithelium, squamous cell epithelium, or a flattened type of epithelium (Allen and Payne, 1992). Glands may be present; rarely, cartilage, smooth muscle, or fibrous tissue is present.

Treatment

If a certain preoperative diagnosis cannot be made of a mediastinal mass, then it usually should be removed to obtain a tissue diagnosis. However, what about the patient in whom you are fairly sure that a simple bronchogenic cyst is present? Does this always have to be excised? The answers to these questions come from examining the surgical problems of removal. The procedure for removing a simple bronchogenic cyst is relatively easy with minimal morbidity to the patient. With the advent of video-assisted thoracic surgical (VATS) techniques, a simple cyst can usually be removed through several small incisions, which requires only overnight hospitalization and a brief period of disability (Hazelrigg et al, 1993). Removal via the mediastinoscope has also been described (Ginsberg et al, 1972; Smythe et al, 1998).

However, waiting until the cyst becomes symptomatic or infectious makes the surgical procedure more difficult for both the surgeon and the patient. Therefore, unless there is a compelling medical reason not to proceed with surgery, most of these cysts should be removed. Another danger in observing a bronchogenic cyst is that it may contain malignant tissue. Bennheim described a leiomyosarcoma that arose from a bronchogenic cyst, and Bauer reported on a sarcoma that was present in one (Bauer, 1961; Bennheim et al, 1980). At our institution, we have seen two patients who developed an invasive epithelial carcinoma within a bronchogenic cyst. Additionally, hemorrhage into a bronchogenic cyst has been reported (Gatinsky et al, 1978).

The cyst is usually approached through the right chest with either VATS or a small thoracotomy. Of course, the location, as determined by the CT, should dictate the incision used. Complete excision is the goal, and the cyst should be removed intact if possible. If the cyst was infected and dense adhesions to a vital structure have developed, then the cyst can be opened and at least the lining removed. No secreting mucosal surface should be left behind. When these goals are accomplished, the outcome is uniformly excellent. Recurrence is extremely rare, and the patient's symptoms are relieved.

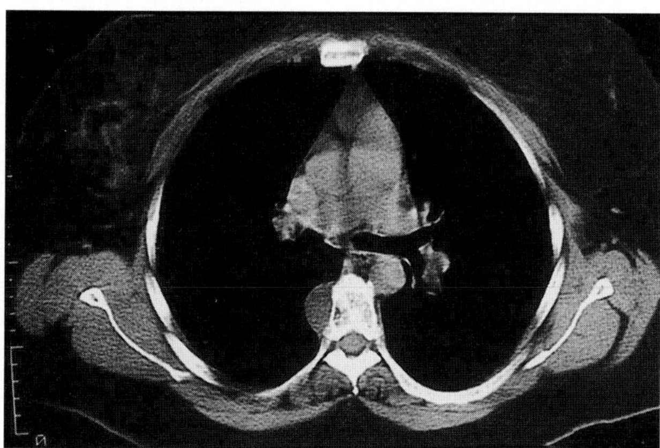

FIGURE 62–18 ■ A computed tomography scan showing a bronchogenic cyst along the right posterior gutter.

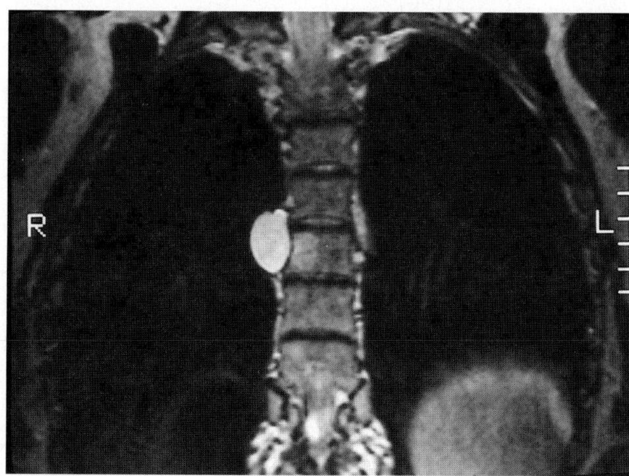

FIGURE 62–20 ■ A coronal view of a magnetic resonance image in a patient with a bronchogenic cyst along the right paravertebral area. The mass is clearly outlined in this view.

ESOPHAGEAL CYSTS

Esophageal cysts are similar to bronchogenic cysts, so much so that some authors classify them as a single lesion and use the term enterogenous cysts to refer to them. In 1952, Palmer proposed three criteria for calling a cyst an esophageal one: (1) attachment to the esophagus, (2) epithelium that represented some level of the gastrointestinal tract, and (3) presence of two layers of muscularis propria (Palmer, 1952). The most reliable method for identifying an esophageal cyst is to use the term only when referring to a cyst that has its embryologic origin from the esophagus and, thus, has an enteric histology. There are difficulties in differentiating esophageal cysts from bronchogenic cysts; however, the differentiation is not all that important because the treatment of either is the same (i.e., complete excision).

Esophageal cysts are much less common than bronchogenic cysts. They account for only 5% to 14% of mediastinal cysts (Salyer et al, 1977; Wychulis et al, 1971). They are the third most common cause of a benign mass arising from the esophagus, after leiomyomas and benign polyps. Most of these cystic lesions occur in the lower third of the esophagus. Of 246 benign masses in a series from the Mayo Clinic, only 55 were cystic. Patients under the age of 16 make up about 70% to 75% of patients with esophageal cysts, and of all alimentary tract cysts, only 10% to 15% are removed from the esophagus.

Symptoms

The usual presentation of an esophageal cyst is an asymptomatic finding on a computed tomography for another reason. Some patients do, however, present with symptoms. In children, respiratory symptoms predominate from pressure on surrounding structures (Fig. 62–21). In adults, dysphagia and pain are more likely to be the presenting symptoms, if they are symptomatic. Nausea, vomiting, weight loss, anorexia, and wheezing have all been reported. The cysts can become infected, as with bronchogenic cysts, in which case the symptoms are related to the infection. Spontaneous hemorrhage into the cyst can also occur, and if this ruptures into the esophageal lumen or the bronchial tree, hematemesis or hemoptysis can occur. Waterston has stated that when a child has hemoptysis, the diagnosis is a foregut cystic malformation until proven otherwise (Postlethwait, 1983; Waterston, 1972). Of course, the cyst may also rupture into the pleural cavity, causing an empyema if the cyst was infected or a hemothorax if it was filled with blood.

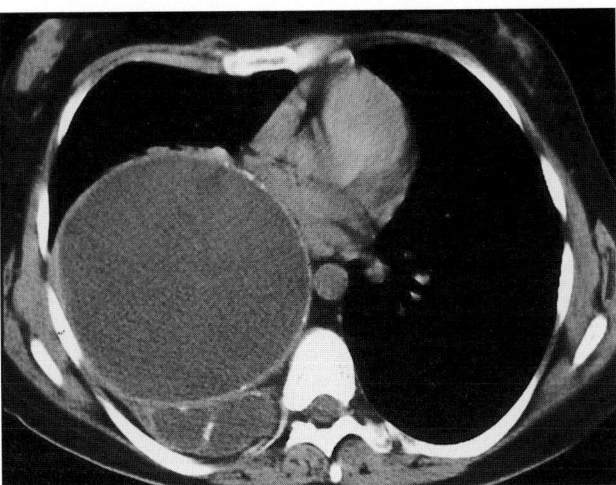

FIGURE 62–21 ■ A computed tomography scan of a patient with a large esophageal duplication cyst. This mass is almost filling the right hemithorax, and it compresses the left atrium.

Diagnosis

The chest roentgenogram shows a round mass with smooth borders. However, CT provides much better visualization and localization. The cyst has a low attenuation number unless hemorrhage or infection is present. Magnetic resonance imaging (MRI) has been reported to be helpful in characterizing the nature of the fluid within the cyst (Lupetin and Dash, 1987). Gastric mucosa is in the lining of an esophageal cyst about 50% of the time, so a ^{99m}TC pertechnetate scan may be able to demonstrate the gastric epithelium. Calcium may also be present, and if the cyst is in communication with the aerodigestive tract, an air-fluid level can be present. A barium swallow may show external compression by the mass. Mansour has suggested that the absence of a sharp-step effect on the superior and inferior margins of the defect is indicative of a cyst rather than a leiomyoma (Mansour et al, 1977). However, differentiation of the two lesions is not difficult because a CT usually shows a cyst to be of low density and a leiomyoma to be of muscle density. Because cysts may become filled with material other than water, it is safe to say that a definitive diagnosis cannot be made by radiographic means alone.

Esophagoscopy is useful. It shows a smooth, soft, compressible mass and no mucosal abnormality. The lesion should not be needled or biopsied with the endoscope, for infection will result in making the removal more difficult. The addition of esophageal ultrasound helps to determine if the lesion is cystic or solid and can determine which layers of the esophagus are involved.

Pathology

Esophageal cysts are filled with mucoid material and are usually unilocular. The epithelium is variable and can be squamous, columnar, ciliated columnar, or a combination of all these. Glands may be present, and there is often a mild inflammatory reaction seen even though there is not an overt infection. The wall of the cyst has a two-layer muscularis, often with a myenteric plexus, which is thought by some to be diagnostic of an esophageal cyst. The cyst is usually located in the wall of the native esophagus, and many are just under the submucosal layer.

Treatment

As with bronchogenic cysts, complete excision is the recommended treatment. This can usually be accomplished with little morbidity and no mortality. Cysts that are found incidentally should also be removed electively unless there are serious medical contraindications. If observed, these cysts often get infected or hemorrhage and can harbor malignancy. A small thoracotomy is the preferred approach because resection of many of these cysts leaves a small defect in the esophagus, which needs to be carefully closed. Ideally, the cyst can be removed intact and any defects in the wall of the esophagus closed over an indwelling dilator to prevent esophageal narrowing. VATS is a possible option but only for those who are skillful at intrathoracic suturing. The surgeon should have a low threshold for conversion to an open procedure. Aspiration and decompression through a bronchoscope or esophagoscope have been reported (Gourin et al, 1976). This technique increases the risk of infection; because it does not remove the lining of the cyst, recurrence seems very likely if not certain. Therefore, it cannot be recommended as optimal therapy.

NEURENTERIC CYSTS

This type of mediastinal cyst is considerably different from a bronchogenic or esophageal cyst. As has been mentioned earlier, these are thought to form very early in embryologic development. They are quite rare. In a series from Heimburger and Battersly in 1965, only two were found (Heimburger and Battersly, 1965). In a series of intrathoracic foregut cysts from England, only 6 of 41 were of this type (Rescorla and Grosfeld, 1991). Because the lesion is generally associated with a spinal cord defect (recall that this cyst is thought to be formed by a defect in the primitive spinal cord and vertebral bodies), the symptoms usually are evident in childhood or at birth. Most present in the first year of life with respiratory symptoms from an enlarging mass lesion in the mediastinum. Occasionally, the mass is quiescent until adolescence, but the cyst is rarely an asymptomatic finding. The triad of a mediastinal mass, a vertebral body abnormality, and respiratory symptoms was found in 70% of patients by Ahmed and associates (Ahmed et al, 1972).

If the cyst compresses the esophagus, dysphagia, nausea, and vomiting can occur. The cyst may secrete acid from gastric glands in the epithelium, and peptic ulceration or bleeding can occur. Neurologic symptoms may be present and include back pain, motor disturbances, sensory loss, or paraplegia.

The diagnosis of a neurenteric cyst can be made by chest roentgenogram, but this only rarely demonstrates the mediastinal cyst and the vertebral abnormality. CT is usually necessary to demonstrate the cyst and the vertebral abnormality. The vertebral defect is often rostral to the cyst because the cyst migrates caudally during development. Roentgenograms of the spine may show hemivertebrae, fusion, or other anomalies. Ideally, MRI demonstrates the relationship between the cyst and the vertebral anomaly. Myelography can be helpful in further defining the neurologic defect. If gastric mucosa is present, ^{99m}Tc pertechnetate can demonstrate it, but this test is not routinely indicated or reliable.

The epithelium of this type of cyst can be squamous, pseudostratifed, columnar, or cuboidal. As was mentioned earlier, these cysts can have gastric or small bowel–appearing mucosa. The intraspinal component tends to be a thin-walled, single layer of columnar epithelium (D'Almeida and Stewart, 1981; Rhaney and Barclay, 1959).

As with the other cysts described earlier, complete excision is the optimal treatment. If the cyst is related to the vertebral body by only a fibrous tether, it can be removed via a thoracotomy. If it protrudes through the diaphragm, then a thoracoabdominal approach may be necessary. If the vertebral abnormality is severe, this portion of the defect should be addressed first by a neurosurgeon or orthopedic surgeon. The mediastinal cyst can then be completely resected once its attachments to the spinal cord have been severed. With complete resection, most patients do well. Scoliosis, chest wall deformities, and recurrence after partial resection have all occurred.

PERICARDIAL CYSTS

Pericardial cysts are also known as springwater cysts, mesothelial cysts, and pericardial coelomic cysts (Oldham, 1971). They are formed by a failure of the primitive pericardial lacunae to fuse, or from abdominal folds in the embryonic pleura (Kindral, 1950). The usual location is the right cardiophrenic angle or along the diaphragm. In separate series reported by Grundmann and colleagues and Feigin and co-workers, the location was in the mediastinum, unrelated to the diaphragm in 11% and 8%, respectively (Feigin et al, 1977; Grundmann et al, 1955) (Fig. 62–22). Usually, this aberrant location is along the right or left heart border but occasionally, it can be in the superior mediastinum (Stoller et al, 1986). Radiographically, these cysts can be confused with a foramen of Morgagni hernia or a pericardial fat pad. They can be large enough to fill the hemithorax and may contain several liters of fluid, but they are usually much smaller. Symptoms are rare, and discovery is usually the result of a routine chest roentgenogram or an echocardiogram. CT, with needle aspiration confirmation, can often definitively diagnose these lesions. Resection is usually not necessary because they have no malignant potential; resection is necessary only when the diagnosis is in doubt.

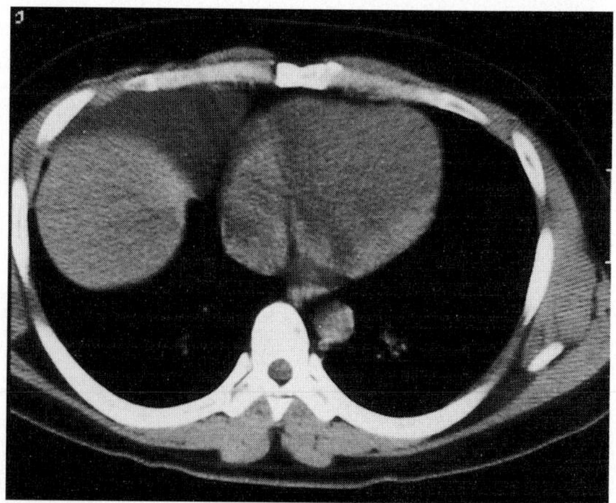

FIGURE 62–22 ■ A computed tomography scan of a patient with a right pericardial cyst. The *low attenuation* in the anterior portion of the right chest is the cyst. The *lighter attenuated round structure* is the top of the right diaphragm.

Percutaneous aspiration of a pericardial cyst has been reported with no recurrence, although long-term follow-up is not yet available (Friday, 1973; Funch and Wenger, 1955; Klatte and Yune, 1972; Unverferth and Wooley, 1979; Westcott, 1981).

THYMIC CYSTS

True cysts of the thymus are uncommon in adults (Graeber et al, 1984). When cystic teratomas and cystic thymomas are excluded from this category, most thymic cysts occur in children. They are usually located in the anterior mediastinum but occasionally can be found in the neck. They can achieve enormous size and extend down to the diaphragm (le Roux et al, 1984). CT scanning and ultrasonography are excellent means of visualizing these lesions. Rarely, calcium is present in the cyst wall. Because the thymus is derived from the brachial pouches, thymic cysts may share a common etiologic mechanism with cysts of the head and neck. An inflammatory process causes cysts to form in ductal epithelial formations from the brachial pouch, and this may be the cause of thymic cysts. Alternatively, they may arise from cystic degeneration of Hassall's corpuscles. Thymic cysts that occur in association with syphilis are thought to have an infectious etiology and are termed "DuBois" abscesses (Allee et al, 1973). The cysts may be unilocular or multiloculated, and can contain fluid that is clear yellow or a thick brown gelatinous soup. The appropriate therapy is excision to prove they are not cystic variants of a thymoma or lymphoma (Rice, 1992).

THORACIC DUCT CYSTS

Thoracic duct cysts in the mediastinum are very rare. Most are found in the posterior mediastinum. Only rarely have anterior cysts been reported (Den Otter, 1979; Tsuchiya et al, 1980). Most patients have presented with compression of the trachea or esophagus. Symptoms may become worse after ingestion of a fatty meal because the cyst may enlarge with an increase in chyle flow. This change in size has been shown radiographically (Fromang et al, 1975). Diagnosis can be made by lymphangiography, but usually the lesion is diagnosed at surgery for an unknown type of mediastinal tumor. These cysts should be excised to eliminate symptoms (Rice, 1992; Sambrook, 1978). Operation is usually complicated by a chylothorax because the cyst usually arises from the thoracic duct (Rodriguez-Perez and Ramirez de Arellano, 1991).

PANCREATIC CYSTS

Pancreatic pseudocysts can extend into the diaphragm. They usually traverse the aortic or esophageal hiatus to get into the mediastinum but may present through a foramen of Morgagni or directly erode the diaphragm. When they pass through the foramen of Morgagni, they are located anterior to the heart, but the posterior mediastinum is a more common location. Diagnosis is usually obtained by CT, which demonstrates a cystic mass transgressing the diaphragm. Endoscopic retrograde cholangiopancreatography (ERCP) can demonstrate the pancreatic ductal communication if the lesion is not loculated. The mass can rupture, causing a pleural effusion that contains a high level of amylase. The preferred surgical approach is transabdominal, not thoracic.

■ *REFERENCES*

Ahmed S, Jolleys A, Park JF: Thoracic enteric cysts and diverticula. Br J Surg 59:963, 1972.

Allee G, Logue B, Mansour K: Thymic cyst simulating multiple cardiovascular abnormalities and presenting with pericarditis and pericardial tamponade. Am J Cardiol 31:377, 1973.

Allen MS, Payne WS: Cystic foregut malformations in the mediastinum. Chest Surg Clin North Am 2:89, 1992.

Amendola MA, Shirazi KK, Brooks J, et al: Transdiaphragmatic bronchopulmonary foregut anomaly: "Dumbbell" bronchogenic cyst. Am J Roentgenol 138:1165, 1982.

Bagwell CE, Schiffman RJ: Subcutaneous bronchogenic cysts. J Pediatr Surg 23:993, 1988.

Bauer S: Carcinoma arising in a congenital lung cyst. Report of a case. Dis Chest 40:552, 1961.

Bennheim J, Griffel B, Versano S, et al: Mediastinal leiomyosarcoma in the wall of a bronchogenic cyst (letter). Arch Pathol Lab Med 104:221, 1980.

Black TL, Fernandes ET, Wrenn EL Jr, et al: Extralobar pulmonary sequestration and mediastinal bronchogenic cyst. J Pediatr Surg 23:999, 1988.

Cartmill JA, Hughes CF: Bronchogenic cysts: A persistent dilemma. Aust N Z J Surg 59:253, 1989.

Cohen AJ, Thompson L, Edwards FH, et al: Primary cysts and tumors of the mediastinum. Ann Thorac Surg 51:378, 1991.

Coselli MP, de Ipolyi P, Bloss RS, et al: Bronchogenic cysts above and below the diaphragm: Report of eight cases. Ann Thorac Surg 44:491, 1987.

Cubillo E, Rockoff SD: Milk of calcium fluid in an intrapulmonary bronchogenic cyst. Chest 60:608, 1971.

D'Almeida AC, Stewart DH Jr: Neuroenteric cysts: Case report and literature review. Neurosurgery 8:596, 1981.

Davis RD, Oldham HN, Sabiston DC: Primary cysts and neoplasms of the mediastinum: Recent changes in clinical presentation, methods of diagnosis, management, and results. Ann Thorac Surg 44:229, 1987.

Den Otter G: Thoracic duct cyst in the anterior mediastinum. Arch Chir Ned 31:107, 1979.

Di Lorenzo M, Collin P-P, Vaillancourt R, et al: Bronchogenic cysts. J Pediatr Surg 24:988, 1989.

Eraklis AJ, Griscom NT, McGovern JB: Bronchogenic cysts of the mediastinum in infancy. N Engl J Med 281:1150, 1969.

Estrera AS, Landay MJ, Pass LJ: Mediastinal carinal bronchogenic cyst: Is its mere presence an indication for surgical excision? South Med J 80:1523, 1987

Fallon M, Gordon ARG, Lendrum AC: Mediastinal cysts of foregut origin associated with vertebral abnormalities. Br J Surg 41:520, 1954.

Feigin DS, Fenoglio JJ, McAllister HA, et al: Pericardial cysts: A radiologic-pathologic correlation and review. Radiology 15:125, 1977.

Flinner RL, Hammond EH: Cysts. In Pathology of the Mediastinum. Chicago, ACSP Press, 1989, p 116.

Fontenelle LJ, Armstrong RG, Stanford W, et al: The asymptomatic mediastinal mass. Arch Surg 102:98, 1971.

Friday RO: Paracardiac cysts: Diagnosis by ultrasound and puncture (Letter). JAMA 226:82, 1973.

Fromang DR, Seltzer MB, Tobias JA: Thoracic duct cyst causing mediastinal compression and acute respiratory insufficiency. Chest 67:725, 1975.

Funch RB, Wenger DS: Preoperative diagnosis of pericardial coelomic cysts: A case report. Am J Roentgenol 73:584, 1955.

Gatinsky P, Fasth S, Hansson G: Intramural oesophageal cyst with massive mediastinal bleeding. A case report. Scand J Thorac Cardiovasc Surg 12:143, 1978.

Ginsberg RJ, Atkins RW, Paulson DL: A bronchogenic cyst successfully treated by mediastinoscopy. Ann Thorac Surg 13:266, 1972.

Gomes MN, Hufnagel CA: Intrapericardial bronchogenic cysts. Am J Cardiol 36:317, 1975.

Gourin A, Garzon AA, Rosen Y, et al: Bronchogenic cysts: Broad spectrum of presentation. NY State J Med 76:714, 1976.

Graeber GM, Thompson LD, Cohen DJ: Cystic lesion of the thymus. J Thorac Cardiovasc Surg 87:295, 1984.

Grundmann G, Fischer R, Grusser G: Kongenitale herbeutelzysten. Thorax-Chirurgie 2:492, 1955.

Hazelrigg SR, Landreneau RJ, Mack MJ, et al: Thoracoscopic resection of mediastinal cysts. Ann Thorac Surg 56:659, 1993.

Heimburger IL, Battersly JS: Primary mediastinal tumors of childhood. J Thorac Cardiovasc Surg 50:92, 1965.

Hogg JIC: Bronchogenic and enteric cysts presenting as asymptomatic mediastinal masses at routine chest radiography. J R Nav Med Serv 72:153, 1986.

Holesh S: Mediastinal tumors. In Shanks SC, Kerley PHK (eds): A Textbook of X-Ray Diagnosis, 4th ed. London, HK Lewis and Co, 1973, p 528.

Jeffries JM III: Asymptomatic bronchogenic cyst of the mediastinum. Postgrad Med 81:235, 1987.

Kindral JE. Quoted by Drash EC and Hyer HJ: Mesothelial mediastinal cysts. J Thorac Surg 19:755, 1950.

Kirwan WO, Walbaum PR, McCormack RJM: Cystic intrathoracic derivatives of the foregut and their complications. Thorax 28:424, 1973.

Klatte EC, Yune HY: Diagnosis and treatment of pericardial cysts. Radiology 104:541, 1972.

Latimer RD: Enterogenous cysts of the oesophagus. Br J Dis Chest 61:136, 1967.

le Roux BT, Kallichurum S, Shama DM. Mediastinal cysts and tumors. Curr Probl Surg 21:5, 1984.

Lupetin AR, Dash N: MRI appearance of esophageal duplication cyst. Gastrointest Radiol 12:7, 1987.

Maier HC: Bronchogenic cysts of the mediastinum. Ann Surg 127:476, 1948.

Mansour KA, Hatcher CV, Harm CC: Benign tumors of the esophagus: Experience with 20 cases. South Med J 70:461, 1977.

Miller DC, Walter JP, Guthaner DF, et al: Recurrent mediastinal bronchogenic cyst: Cause of bronchial obstruction and compression of superior vena cava and pulmonary artery. Chest 74:218, 1978.

Mixter CG, Clifford SH: Congenital mediastinal cysts of gastrogenic and bronchogenic origin. Ann Surg 90:714, 1929.

Oldham HN Jr: Mediastinal tumors and cysts. Ann Thorac Surg 11:246, 1971.

Palmer ED: The Diseases of the Esophagus. New York, Paul B. Hoeber, 1952.

Postlethwait RW: Benign tumors and cysts of the esophagus. Surg Clin North Am 63:925, 1983.

Ramenofsky ML, Leape LL, McCauley RGK: Bronchogenic cyst. J Pediatr Surg 14:219, 1979.

Rescorla FJ, Grosfeld JL: Gastroenteric cysts and neurenteric cysts in infants and children. In Shields TW (ed): Mediastinal Surgery. Malvern, PA, Lea & Febiger, 1991, p 317.

Rhaney K, Barclay CPT: Enterogenous cysts and congenital diverticula of the alimentary canal with abnormalities of the vertebral column and spinal cord. J Pathol Bacteriol 77:457, 1959.

Rice TW: Benign neoplasms and cysts of the mediastinum. Sem Thorac Cardiovasc Surg 4:25, 1992.

Rodgers LF, Osmer JC: Bronchogenic cysts: A review of 46 cases. Am J Roentgenol 91:273, 1964.

Rodriguez-Perez D, Ramirez de Arellano GA: Chylous cysts of the mediastinum: Report of a case and review of the literature. Bol Asoc Med P Rico 83:333, 1991.

Salyer DC, Salyer WR, Eggleston JC: Benign developmental cysts of the mediastinum. Arch Pathol Lab Med 101:136, 1977.

Sambrook Gowar FJ: Mediastinal thoracic duct cyst. Thorax 33:800, 1978.

Schenck SG: Congenital cystic disease of the lungs. Am J Roentgenol 35:604, 1936.

Schmidt FE, Drapanas T: Congenital cystic lesions of the bronchi and lungs. Ann Thorac Surg 14:650, 1972.

Sirivella S, Ford WB, Zikria EA, et al: Foregut cysts of the mediastinum: Results in 20 consecutive surgically treated cases. J Thorac Cardiovasc Surg 90:776, 1985.

Smythe WR, Bavaria JE, Kaiser LR: Mediastinoscopic subtotal removal of mediastinal cysts. Chest 114:614, 1998.

Stoller JK, Shaw C, Matthay RA: Enlarging, atypically located pericardial cyst. Recent experience and literature review. Chest 89:402, 1986.

Tsuchiya R, Sugiura Y, Ogata T, et al: Thoracic duct cyst of the mediastinum. J Thorac Cardiovasc Surg 79:856, 1980.

Unverferth DV, Wooley CF: The differential diagnosis of paracardiac lesions: Pericardial cysts. Cathet Cardiovasc Diagn 5:31, 1979.

Volpi A, Cavalli A, Maggioni AP, et al: Left atrial compression by a mediastinal bronchogenic cyst presenting with paroxysmal atrial fibrillation. Thorax 43:216, 1988.

Waterston D: Oesophageal diseases in infancy and childhood, excluding oesophagotracheal fistula. In Smith RA, Smith RE (eds): Conventry Conference on Surgery of the Oesophagus. New York, Appleton-Century-Crofts, 1972.

Westcott JL: Percutaneous needle aspiration of hilar and mediastinal masses. Radiology 141:323, 1981.

Whitaker JA, Deffenbaugh LD, Cooke AR: Esophageal duplication cyst. Am J Gastroenterol 73:329, 1980.

Wychulis AR, Payne WS, Clagett OT, et al: Surgical treatment of mediastinal tumors: A 40-year experience. J Thorac Cardiovasc Surg 62:379, 1971.

Young G, L'Heureux PRL, Krueckeberg ST, et al: Mediastinal bronchogenic cyst: Prenatal sonographic diagnosis. Am J Roentgenol 152:125, 1989.

CHAPTER **63**

Tumors and Masses

DIAGNOSTIC STRATEGIES IN MEDIASTINAL TUMORS AND MASSES

Jean Deslauriers
Louis Létourneau
Giuseppe Giubilei

The mediastinum lies between the two lungs, extending from the cervicothoracic inlet superiorly to the diaphragm inferiorly and from the sternum anteriorly to the vertebral column and paravertebral thoracic sulci posteriorly. Mediastinal tumors and masses arise from structures normally located in this area as well as from adjacent tissues that may have migrated there. Also included are occasional lesions originating from organs transiting through the mediastinum, such as the trachea, esophagus, or great vessels.

To provide adequate treatment to patients with mediastinal masses, the clinician should establish a clear diagnosis in all cases including patients with a benign-appearing lesion on standard radiographs or computed tomography (CT) scanning. A diagnosis is even more important in cases in which primary treatment is unlikely to be surgical. Barring exceptional circumstances, it is inadvisable to begin chemotherapy or radiation therapy or to plan extensive resection without a positive histologic diagnosis.

Occasionally, the diagnosis of a mediastinal tumor can be obtained through the use of simple methods. In the majority of cases, however, a more complex investigation is necessary and, to be successful, the investigation should involve a close collaboration among surgeons, radiologists, pathologists, and other medical specialists. All diagnostic tests should be carried out within a simple, structured, and cost-effective framework of investigation.

In this chapter, we review all currently available modalities used to investigate mediastinal masses. We also discuss the integrated use of these modalities based on the location of the mediastinal mass and its likely diagnosis.

HISTORICAL NOTE

Mediastinal structures are densely packed, but they lend themselves to anatomic localization (Kirschner, 1998). The cardiac silhouette obscures some masses on the posteroanterior (PA) chest radiograph, but the lateral view unrolls the mediastinum, showing a "geographic" location of the mass—superior, anterior, middle, or posterior—which correlates nicely with the nature of the tumor (Fraser and Paré, 1988; Heitzman, 1977). This correlation has led to dividing the mediastinum into compartments with pseudoanatomic boundaries. According to Shields (1991), these boundaries are defined differently by the many authors who have written on the subject and as a consequence, confusion abounds in the literature relative to these divisions. In 1972, Shields proposed a more simple anteroposterior division of the space. It includes an "anterior" (prevascular) compartment bounded anteriorly by the sternum and posteriorly by the great vessels and pericardium; a "visceral" (retrovascular) compartment extending from the posterior limit of the anterior compartment to the back of the esophagus and anterior surface of the spine, and the bilateral "paravertebral sulci" which lie alongside the spine and under the neck of the ribs.

Historically, noninvasive methods used to evaluate mediastinal masses have had varied success. In early years, PA and lateral chest films and tomograms were helpful to determining the site, volume, and density of mediastinal masses, as well as detecting their homogeneity and the presence of calcifications. In recent years, diagnostic capabilities have been expanded with the availability of CT scanning. In 1979, Livesay and co-workers studied 30 patients with suspected mediastinal masses using CT and concluded that "this technique can yield valuable diagnostic information, influence the clinical management and relate to the prognosis in patients with suspected mediastinal tumors." Eschapasse (1979), an acknowledged leader in the field of thoracic surgery, stated that "CT scanning and ultrasonography are new methods which are likely to be of interest in some cases." The use of reliably sensitive tumor markers for germ cell tumors (Benfield and Sawyer, 1992; Wright et al, 1990) has also changed our approach to the diagnosis and follow-up of these tumors.

Perhaps the most significant advance in the diagnosis of mediastinal masses relates to the use of direct biopsy by surgical techniques, such as mediastinoscopy, described by Carlens (1959) and Pearson (1995), and anterior mediastinostomy, initially reported by McNeil and

Chamberlain (1966) as a method to assess the lymphatics draining the left upper lobe of the lung. Until these procedures gained acceptance, patients had to be subjected to formal posterolateral thoracotomy or sternotomy (Ferguson et al, 1987). More recently, mediastinal tumors have even been biopsied by video thoracoscopy (Kern et al, 1993), and accurate tissue diagnosis has been obtained in most patients.

Unfortunately, classification of mediastinal tumors through the use of fine-needle aspiration as described by Nordenström (1967), Linder and co-workers (1986), and Moinuddin and associates (1984) has never achieved universal acceptance.

■ *HISTORICAL READINGS*

Benfield JR, Sawyer RW: Tumor markers. Chest Surg Clin North Am 2:213, 1992.

Carlens E: Mediastinoscopy: A method for inspection and tissue biopsy in the superior mediastinum. Chest 36:343, 1959.

Eschapasse H: Pathologie du médiastin. Encycl Med Chir Paris. Poumon 6047 A 05, 4–1979.

Ferguson MK, Lee E, Skinner DB, Little AG: Selective operative approach for diagnosis and treatment of anterior mediastinal masses. Ann Thorac Surg 44:583, 1987.

Fraser FG, Paré JAP et al: Diagnosis of Diseases of the Chest, 3rd ed. Philadelphia, WB Saunders, 1988.

Heitzman ER: The Mediastinum: Radiologic Correlations with Anatomy and Pathology. St. Louis, CV Mosby, 1977.

Kern JA, Daniel TA, Tribble LG et al: Thoracoscopic diagnosis and treatment of mediastinal masses. Ann Thorac Surg 56:92, 1993.

Kirschner PA: Classification, diagnosis and management of mediastinal tumor. Proceedings of the New York Thoracic Society postgraduate course. 1998.

Linder J, Olsen GA, Johnston WW: Fine-needle aspiration biopsy of the mediastinum. Am J Med 81:1005, 1986.

Livesay JJ, Mink JH, Fee HJ et al: The use of computed tomography to evaluate suspected mediastinal tumors. Ann Thorac Surg 27:305, 1979.

McNeil TM, Chamberlain JM: Diagnostic anterior mediastinotomy. Ann Thorac Surg 2:532, 1966.

Moinuddin SM, Lee LH, Montgomery JH: Mediastinal needle biopsy. AJR Am J Roentgenol 143:531, 1984.

Nordenström B: Paraxiphoid approach to the mediastinum for mediastinoscopy and mediastinal needle biopsy: A preliminary report. Invest Radiol 2:141, 1967.

Pearson FG: Mediastinoscopy: A method of biopsy of the superior mediastinum. J Thorac Cardiovasc Surg 49:11, 1965.

Shields TW: Primary tumors and cysts of the mediastinum. In Shields TW (ed): General Thoracic Surgery, 1st ed. Philadelphia, Lea & Febiger, 1972, p 908.

Shields TW: The mediastinum and its compartments. In Shields TW (ed): Mediastinal Surgery, 1st ed. Philadelphia, Lea & Febiger, 1991.

Wright CD, Kesler KA, Nichols CR et al: Primary mediastinal nonseminomatous germ cell tumors: Results of a multimodality approach. J Thorac Cardiovasc Surg 99:210, 1990.

BASIC SCIENCE

Anatomic Divisions of the Mediastinum

Anatomically, the mediastinum is defined as the area located between the mediastinal pleura and bordered anteriorly by the sternum and costal cartilages, posteriorly by the spine and necks of the ribs, inferiorly by the diaphragm, and superiorly by the upper thoracic aperture.

Because specific lesions have a predilection for certain sites, dividing the mediastinum into different compartments is helpful when a mediastinal mass is discovered. Classically, the mediastinum is separated into superior and inferior compartments by an imaginary line extending from the sternal angle to the fourth intervertebral disk. The inferior compartment is further subdivided into anterior, middle, and posterior compartments (Fig. 63–1). The anterior mediastinum extends from the back of the sternum to the front of the ascending aorta and pericardium, while the posterior mediastinum is situated between the posterior pericardium and the spine. The middle mediastinum, located between the anterior and posterior mediastinum, contains the pericardium and heart, the ascending and transverse portions of the aorta, the vena cava, the phrenic and vagus nerves, and the trachea, mainstem bronchi, adjacent nodes, and central pulmonary arteries and veins (Fraser et al, 1988).

In 1973, Felson proposed a simplified method of dividing the mediastinum based on easily identifiable landmarks as seen on a lateral chest film (Fig. 63–2). In his classification, a line drawn from the diaphragm to the thoracic inlet along the back of the heart and anterior to the trachea divides the anterior and middle mediastinum, while a line drawn 1 cm behind the anterior margin of

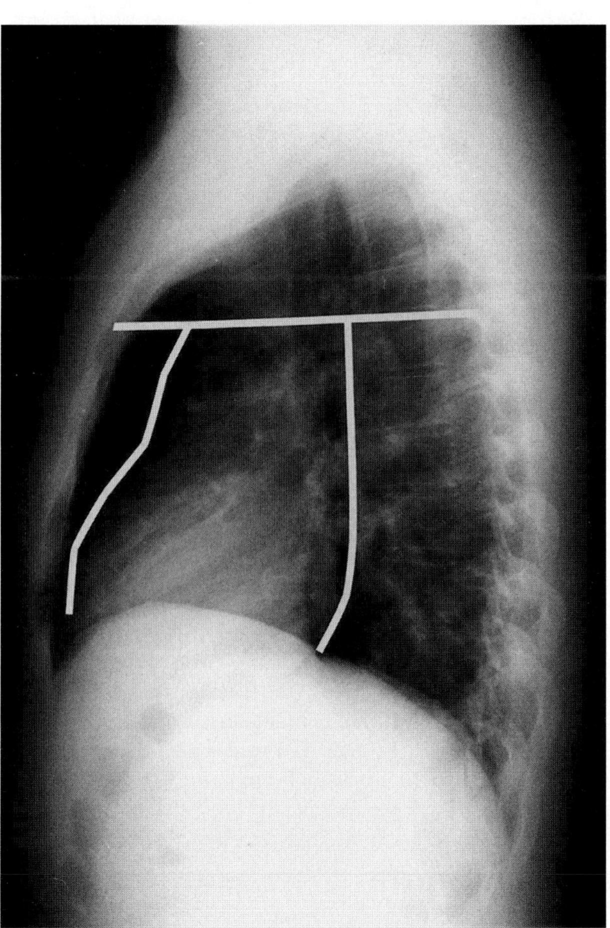

FIGURE 63–1 ■ Classic mediastinal compartments. The mediastinum is divided into a superior and an inferior compartment by a *line* drawn from the sternal angle to the fourth intervertebral disk. The inferior compartment is further subdivided into anterior (prevascular), middle (cardiovascular), and posterior (postvascular) compartments.

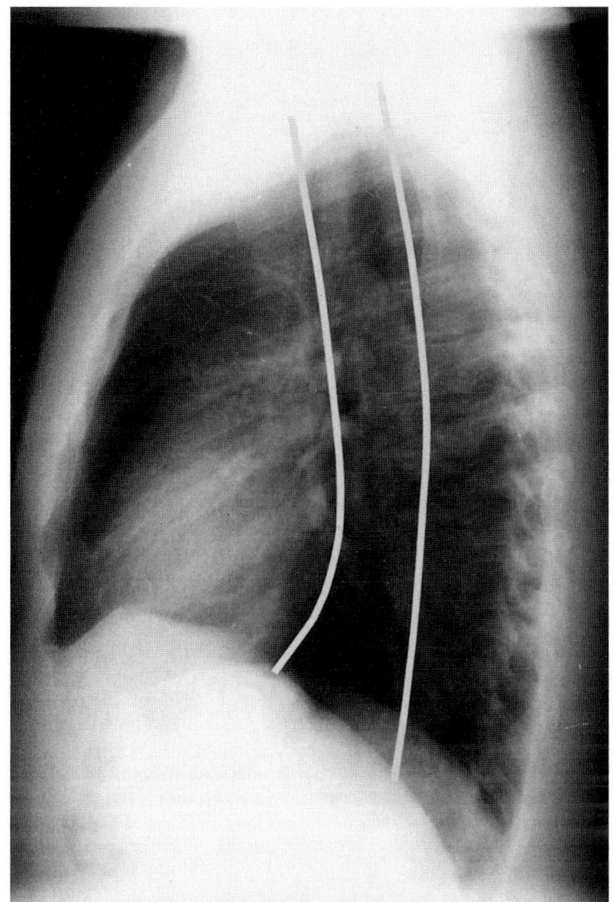

FIGURE 63–2 ■ Mediastinal compartments according to Felson (1973). The anterior and middle mediastinum are divided by a *line* extending along the back of the heart and the front of the trachea. The middle and posterior mediastinum are separated by a *line* connecting each thoracic vertebra 1 cm behind its anterior margin.

the thoracic vertebral bodies separates the middle and posterior mediastinum.

Although encroachment of a mediastinal mass into a different space is common, the differential diagnosis of a mediastinal mass is highly dependent on its location (Table 63–1).

As discussed previously, in 1972 Shields proposed a more simple anteroposterior division of the mediastinum. In his schema, there are two mediastinal compartments (anterior and visceral) and bilateral paravertebral sulci which lie alongside the spine (Fig. 63–3). Thymic lesions are characteristically found in the anterior compartment, bronchogenic cysts in the visceral compartment, and neurogenic tumors in the paravertebral sulci. Lesions of lymphoid origin are largely found in the paratracheal areas of the visceral compartment, although they may also occur in the anterior compartment. Connective tissue tumors including lipomas, fibromas, and hemangiomas are more commonly located in the anterior compartment.

Plan of Investigation

According to Trastek (1987), several questions must be answered while developing a strategy for the evaluation of mediastinal masses: (1) Is the abnormal shadow located in the mediastinum and if it is, is it a true mediastinal tumor? (2) Does the lesion appear to be benign or malignant, and does it need to be biopsied or resected, or both? (3) If biopsy is necessary, which approach should be used, and if surgery is eventually required, what difficulties can the clinician expect to encounter?

The problem of whether a shadow is located in the mediastinum may arise when the opacity is located at the periphery of the mediastinal boundaries. At the upper border of the mediastinum, normal cervical structures such as the thyroid and parathyroid glands may migrate into the mediastinum. Goiters, for instance, may extend downward along the trachea and follow a prevascular or postvascular route. In the majority of cases, a goiter maintains its cervical blood supply, an important fact in helping to determine cervical or transthoracic incisions for operation. Parathyroids, having a common embryology with the thymus, may be found intrathymically but occasionally in other mediastinal compartments as well. Beyond the lateral borders of the mediastinum, it may be difficult to differentiate between a lung or pleural tumor and a true mediastinal mass. Inferiorly, contents of diaphragmatic hernias, specifically Morgagni's hernia, paraesophageal (rolling) hernia, and posterolateral hernia of Bochdalek, may present as mediastinal masses. Morgagni's hernia, for example, projects into the anterior compartment and has the same location, density, and shape as a pericardial cyst. Pancreatic pseudocyst may traverse upward from the pancreatic tail transdiaphragmatically into the posterior mediastinum.

A variety of pseudomediastinal shadows may at times simulate primary mediastinal masses (Table 63–2). Many of these lesions originate from the digestive tract or relate to abnormalities of the vascular system. Meningoceles and vertebral anomalies, cardiovascular pseudotumors, and inflammatory or infectious collections may all simulate primary mediastinal masses. A variety of esophageal

TABLE 63–1 ■ **Common Mediastinal Masses by Location (Excluding Vascular Lesions)**

Anterior	*Middle*	*Posterior*
Thymic tumors	Lymphomas	Neurogenic tumors
Germ cell tumors	Foregut cysts (bronchogenic)	Meningocele
Lymphomas	Pericardial cysts	Foregut cysts (enteric)
Substernal goiters		
Mesenchymal tumors		

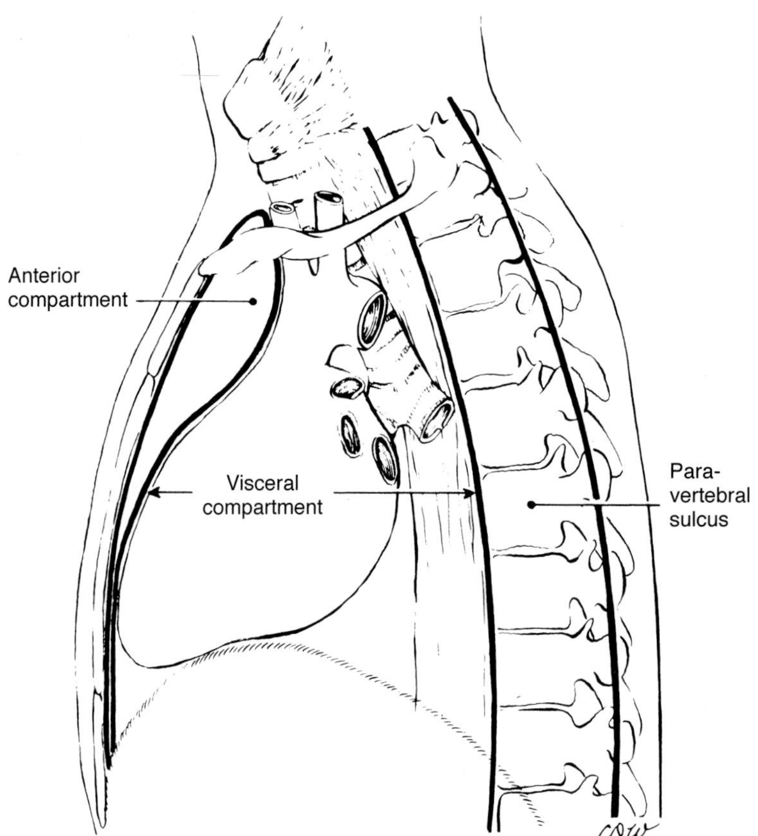

FIGURE 63–3 ■ Proposed anatomic subdivision of the mediastinum by Shields. (From Shields TW: Mediastinal Surgery, 1st ed. Philadelphia, Lea & Febiger, 1991).

lesions such as neoplasms, megaesophagus secondary to achalasia, or esophageal diverticulum can also present as abnormal mediastinal masses.

If the mass represents a vascular structure (10% of all mediastinal masses reported by Lyons et al [1959]), the evaluation and treatment obviously are different from that of other primary mediastinal masses. In the past, the investigation of suspected pseudotumors of vascular origin was done through the use of fluoroscopy and angiography (Kelley et al, 1978), but currently CT scanning with bolus injection of intravenous contrast has all but eliminated the need for angiography (Baron et al, 1981). Systemic venous abnormalities or abnormalities of pulmonary vessels (Bartter et al, 1988) presenting as mediastinal masses are also easily analyzed on CT with contrast injection (Moore, 1992). For vascular lesions, magnetic resonance imaging (MRI) provides similar or better information than CT (Berquist and Brown, 1984; Dooms and Higgins, 1986).

If the tumor is clearly mediastinal, the next question concerns the indication for biopsy. Clearly, not all mediastinal masses require biopsy, and indeed some of them can be resected without a preoperative diagnosis. This approach is preferred for small and well-delineated lesions that on CT examination appear to be amenable to complete resection. The same strategy applies to cystic lesions, localized thymomas, and neurogenic tumors. Overall, biopsies are unnecessary for tumors that are likely to be treated surgically. Indeed in certain tumors, such as thymomas, cells shed from the tumor might implant in the pleural space or mediastinum.

For large tumors or tumors suspected to invade major mediastinal structures, or tumors in which primary treatment is likely to be nonsurgical, a diagnosis should al-

TABLE 63–2 ■ **Common False Tumors of the Mediastinum**

Previsceral Compartment (Anterior)	***Visceral Compartment***	***Paravertebral Sulci (Posterior)***
Aneurysm of ascending aorta, innominate artery, or subclavian artery	Aneurysm of the heart or aortic arch	Diaphragmatic hernias
Abnormal dilatation of superior vena cava or azygos vein	Pericarditis	Aneurysm of descending aorta
Sternal or chondrosternal tumors	Enlarged lymph nodes	Tumor of the esophagus
Lymphangiomas	Mediastinitis	Megaesophagus
	Aneurysm of pulmonary artery	Extralobar sequestration
		Pott's abscess
		Meningocele
		Extramedullary hematopoiesis

ways be obtained prior to any consideration of a surgical approach. This applies to invasive thymomas, all malignant germ cell tumors, and suspected lymphomas. Fine-needle aspiration (FNA) or core needle biopsy can be tried, but they are often inadequate due to the complex histologic nature of many of these neoplasms. Mediastinoscopy and anterior mediastinotomy and more recently video-assisted thoracic surgery (VATS) are acceptable open techniques to obtain tissue for diagnosis.

Of equal importance to establishing a diagnosis, preoperative evaluation must include techniques that provide a clear understanding of possible difficulties that may be encountered during operation or even of possible contraindications to surgery. Classic examples are a thymoma invading the superior vena cava, in which planning must be done for possible venous reconstruction, and a neurogenic tumor extending into the spinal canal, in which a neurosurgeon must be available for the laminectomy and simultaneous excision of the intraspinal portion of the tumor.

Methods of Investigation

Clinical Considerations and Statistical Analysis

In the adult population, at least 50% of mediastinal tumors are asymptomatic and are detected incidentally by chest radiograph. Often, the mediastinal location and nature of the tumor are age dependent, and it should be noted that only 8% of mediastinal tumors occur in children who are less than 15 years of age, whereas 92% occur in adults (Burt, 1995). Incidence by age and location of the most common mediastinal tumors in adults and in children is listed in Table 63–3.

In children, posterior mediastinal tumors are the most common, while in adults, the anterior mediastinum is more frequently affected due to the high incidence of thymomas, which are seldom seen in children. In a collective review of primary anterior mediastinal tumors in children and adults, Mullen and Richardson (1986) analyzed the incidence of specific tumors located in that compartment (Table 63–4). Thymic lesions are the most common in adults, followed by lymphomas, while in children, lymphomas are the most common primary anterior mediastinal tumors.

Approximately 25% of all mediastinal tumors are malignant, in both adults and children. Roughly two thirds of children are symptomatic at presentation, whereas only one third of adults have symptoms. The thorax has a pyramidal shape, so tumors located in the upper half are more likely to be symptomatic, because in that area, several organs are distributed in a narrow and rigid anteroposterior space. Symptoms also depend on whether the mass is benign or malignant, size of tumor, and presence or absence of infection. Most authors agree that malignant lesions are more likely to be symptomatic than benign lesions (King et al, 1982; Silverman and Sabiston, 1977). In Cohen and associates' series (1991), 77.3% of patients with malignant disease were symptomatic. In that series, size of the tumor was also a predictor of malignancy ($P < .005$).

As a corollary, the absence of symptoms correlates very closely with benign neoplasms. In Davis and co-workers' series (1987), 83% of patients who were asymptomatic at presentation had a benign neoplasm. Because of increased use of chest radiography, more aggressive approach to tumor screening, and increased imaging sensitivity, more asymptomatic patients with malignant tumors are seen today than 10 or 20 years ago.

Most symptoms are related to mediastinal structures that are either compressed or invaded. In nearly all series, respiratory symptoms such as cough, stridor, dyspnea, and occasional hemoptysis are the most common, followed by chest pain related to invasion of the chest wall, diaphragm, or mediastinal pleura. Because the mediastinal pleura is innervated by rami originating from the phrenic nerve, pain related to mediastinal tumors may mimic that of angina. Other possible symptoms and signs include dysphagia due to compression of the esophagus, vena cava syndrome, invasion of the pericardium causing signs of tamponade, hoarseness due to recurrent nerve palsy, involvement of the stellate ganglion with Horner's syndrome, and extension into an intervertebral foramen causing reticular pain. In 30 patients with mediastinal masses reviewed by Harris and colleagues (1987), the most common symptom was pain noted in 53% of patients and indicative of malignancy in 88% of this group. Next were weight loss, cough, and fever associated with an 82%, 86%, and 100% incidence of malignancy, respectively. The symptoms and signs in patients with primary mediastinal cysts and tumors in the series from Walter Reed Army Medical Center (Azarow et al, 1993; Cohen et al, 1991) are listed in Table 63–5.

On occasion, patients present with symptoms and signs related to an endocrine-secreting tumor such as a parathyroid adenoma (hypercalcemia) or a pheochromo-

TABLE 63–4 ■ **Relative Frequency of Common Primary Anterior Mediastinal Tumors in Adults and Children**

	Children (n = 702)	*Adults (n = 179)*
Thymic	17%	47%
Germ cell	25%	15%
Lymphoma	45%	23%
Mesenchymal	15%	—
Endocrine	—	16%

From Mullen B, Richardson JR: Primary anterior mediastinal tumors in children and adults. Ann Thorac Surg 42:338, 1986.

TABLE 63–3 ■ **Incidence of Mediastinal Tumors by Age and Location**

	Pediatric	*Adult*
Neurogenic	35%	21%
Thymoma	Rare	19%
Lymphoma	25%	13%
Cysts	16%	18%
Germ cell	10%	10%
Mesenchymal	10%	6%
Endocrine	Rare	6%

TABLE 63–5 ■ **Symptoms and Signs in Patients with Primary Mediastinal Cysts and Tumors**

Symptom	*Benign (n = 146)*	*Malignant (n = 84)*	*Total (N = 230)*
Asymptomatic	82	19	101
Respiratory symptoms	23	17	40
Chest pain	23	20	43
Dysphagia	4	0	4
Superior vena cava syndrome	0	4	4
Sign			
Normal	122	57	179
Weight loss	3	3	6
SVC signs	0	8	8
Neurologic	5	2	7

SVC, superior vena cava.
From Cohen AJ, Thompson L, Edwards FF et al: Primary cysts and tumors of the mediastinum. Ann Thorac Surg 51:378, 1991.

cytoma (high blood pressure). When a patient has an anterior mediastinal mass and myasthenia gravis, the diagnosis of thymoma is virtually certain. Similarly, a posterior mediastinal mass associated with the cutaneous manifestations of von Recklinghausen's disease is always neurogenic. Other systemic manifestations include fever and anemia (lymphoma) and rarely gynecomastia and Klinefelter's syndrome (germ cell tumor).

In all cases of suspected germ cell tumors, careful examination of the testis should be carried out and, if necessary, ultrasound or CT examination should be added to rule out a primary testicular tumor with mediastinal metastases. These examinations are important because testicular tumors can be very small and still give rise to large mediastinal metastases. In one series (Economou et al, 1982), patients were considered to have a primary germ cell tumor of the mediastinum only with absence of clinically detectable testicular masses at any time during the course of the disease.

Imaging

PA and lateral radiographs of the chest continue to be the most valuable technique for the initial evaluation of mediastinal masses (Brown et al, 1990). On the PA view, the clinician can determine if the mass is superior or inferior and if it is unilateral or bilateral. On the lateral film, he or she can determine if the tumor is in the anterior or visceral compartment or paravertebral sulci, thereby starting a differential diagnosis based on location of the mass. Indeed, good knowledge of normal and abnormal anatomy of the mediastinum as seen on PA and lateral chest radiographs is essential because the majority of mediastinal masses are first suspected on standard films. Often the lesion is visible in only one projection not only because its margins are in contact with other structures of the same density but also because it does not present a border tangential to the x-ray beam. In general, characteristic features of mediastinal lesions include sharply defined borders, obtuse angle with the mediastinum, and mass effect on mediastinal structures.

If a spina bifida is associated with a posterior mediastinal mass, the lesion is nearly always a neuroenteric cyst. Similarly, a lesion that extends from the neck through the thoracic inlet and deviates the trachea strongly suggests a retrosternal goiter.

Older techniques that may be useful include fluoroscopic examination of the mass and barium swallow. Under fluoroscopy, the clinician can assess the volume, contours, and transparency of the mediastinal mass. Synchronous movements with respiration and cough are signs that the mass is attached to the tracheobronchial tree. Similarly, deformity of the mass during deep respiratory movements is pathognomonic of a cyst (Robbins, 1943). Barium examination of the esophagus should always be done in posterior mediastinum lesions and often in tumors of the middle mediastinum that extend posteriorly. It is an excellent method to document signs of esophageal compression as well as intrinsic lesions of the esophagus that may indeed be responsible for the mass.

CT is now the examination of choice in virtually all cases of suspected mediastinal masses (Brown et al, 1990; Webb, 1983). Brown and co-workers (1990) have shown that CT is more useful in evaluating the mediastinum than any other region in the thorax. One of the first published experiences with CT evaluation of mediastinal masses is that of Livesay and associates (1979). In their study of 30 patients with suspected mediastinal tumors, these authors concluded that CT scan was useful in (1) yielding information not available by conventional techniques, (2) defining the anatomic location and extent of mediastinal tumors, (3) detecting pulmonary metastasis and involvement of mediastinal nodes in cases of malignancies, and (4) establishing the diagnosis of benign fatty masses.

CT scan can distinguish between fatty, cystic (Graeber et al, 1986), and soft tissue masses, while contrast CT has a 92% accuracy rate in distinguishing vascular from nonvascular etiologies (Baron et al, 1981). In Graeber and co-workers' study, the results suggested that mediastinal masses could be evaluated with a high degree of accuracy for predicting the nature, size, location, and involvement of other organs by the mass. CT scan can further define the soft tissue component of the mass and presence or absence of calcifications. It can also help in determining the most suitable approach for the biopsy of the lesion under investigation.

The presence of significant contrast enhancement (Fig. 63–4) is helpful to further narrow the differential diagnosis of mediastinal masses (Moore, 1992) as well as to document the effect of the abnormality on adjacent blood vessels (Fig. 63–5), information that may affect the resectability of some of these tumors.

MRI is not routinely used in the investigation of mediastinal masses (Gefter, 1988), although "the lack of ionizing radiation, the availability of cross-sectional images in multiple imaging planes, and the ability to distinguish vascular structures without using intravenous contrast has made MR a potentially valuable alternative to CT" (Brown et al, 1990). In general, CT is superior to MRI in spatial resolution, detection of bony destruction, and evaluation of the lung parenchyma, while MRI is superior to CT in evaluating the brachial plexus, neural foramina,

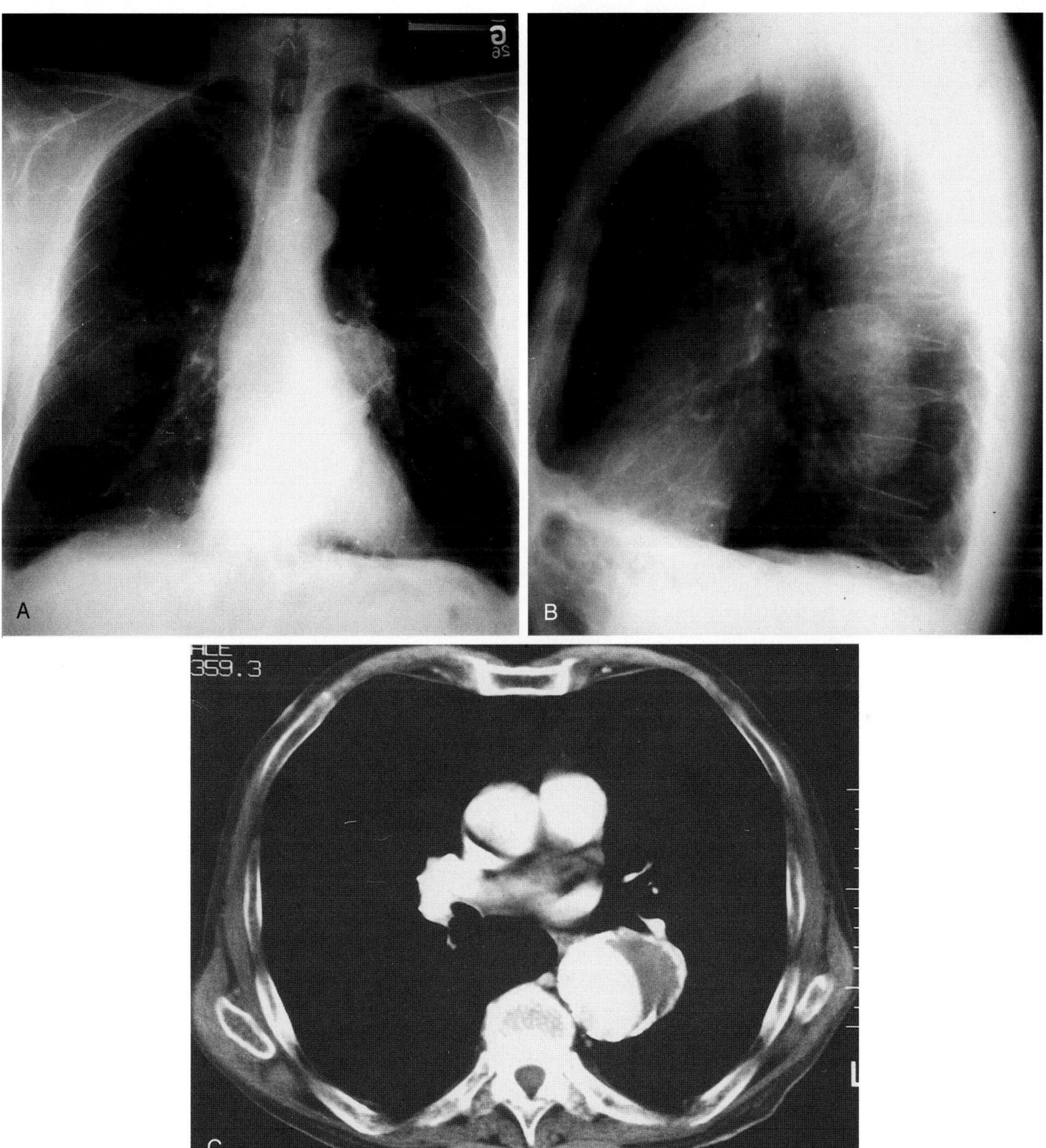

FIGURE 63–4 ■ Aneurysm of the descending thoracic aorta. Posteroanterior *(A)* and lateral *(B)* chest radiographs showing a well-circumscribed mediastinal mass abutting the descending aorta. A contrast-enhanced computed tomography scan *(C)* shows a focal, calcified, and saccular aneurysm of the descending aorta containing a large mural thrombus.

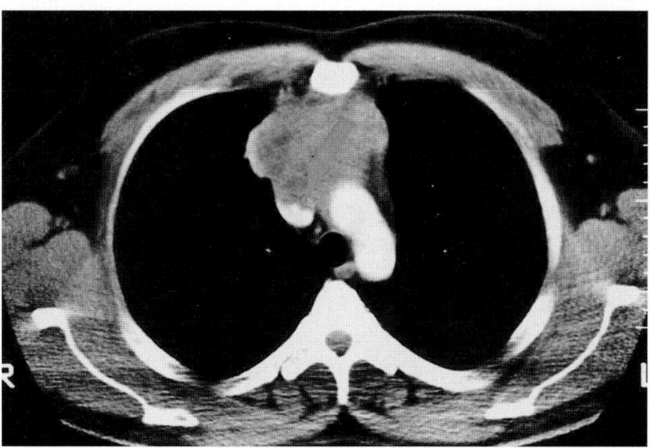

FIGURE 63–5 ■ A contrast-enhanced computed tomography scan showing a lobulated anterior mediastinal mass with involvement of the superior vena cava *(arrow)*. In this case, the superior vena cava had to be resected to completely remove the tumor.

diaphragm, and, possibly, direct mediastinal invasion (Table 63–6). Neurogenic tumors involving the intervertebral foramen or with intraspinal extension are best assessed by MRI. Invasion or encasement of major vascular structures may also be best demonstrated by MRI. In one of the earlier studies on the use of MRI to evaluate mediastinal masses, von Schulthess and associates (1986) were able to demonstrate that MRI provided better insight into the composition of the mass.

In the past, myelography was employed in the evaluation of dumbbell tumors (Akwari et al, 1978), and it could accurately describe the length of tumor extension in the neural canal. Currently this examination is no longer performed because CT and MRI can provide a clearer delineation of the neural foramina and possible intraspinal extension of the tumor (Ribet and Cardot, 1994; Ricci et al, 1990a; Yüksel et al, 1996). Sometimes angiography is useful to differentiate a vascular from a nonvascular lesion (Table 63–7) as well as to document superior vena cava obstruction.

Other possible uses of preoperative angiography in the evaluation of mediastinal masses include the localization of functioning parathyroid adenomas or abnormal parathyroid tissue (Bilezikian et al, 1973; Brennan et al, 1978) or the documentation of possible involvement of the artery of Adamkiewicz by neurogenic tumors. In an interesting study, Davis and associates (1987) showed that angiography was used in 10% to 20% of patients in the period prior to CT scanning, but during the last 5 years of the study period (1981–1986), angiography was not performed.

The use of gallium scans has been recommended by Ferguson and collaborators (1987) in the evaluation of anterior mediastinal masses. These authors and others (Bekerman et al, 1984) report that gallium is avidly taken up by lymphomas, and it is usually positive in bronchogenic carcinomas and in pathologic processes involving active inflammation. By contrast, gallium uptake by carcinoid and germ cell tumors is unpredictable, and thymomas rarely take up gallium.

Tumor Markers and Hormones

Tumor markers and hormones are measurable biologic substances that indicate the presence of a neoplasm (Table 63–8). These include anti-acetylcholine receptor (anti-AChR) antibodies useful in the diagnosis of thymoma and myasthenia gravis (Kirschner, 1992) and tumor markers, such as human chorionic gonadotropin β (β-HCG) and α-fetoprotein (AFP) useful in the diagnosis of nonseminomatous germ cell tumors. About 90% of patients with nonseminomatous tumors have elevation of at least one of these tumor markers (Wright et al, 1990). Changes in the titer of the markers roughly parallel the increase or decrease of tumor activity (Sham et al, 1989), and these are invaluable for estimating prognosis as well as selecting therapy and following its effect (Javadpour, 1979; Kay et al, 1987).

Hormones are common tumor markers, but their measurement is seldom useful in the diagnosis of mediastinal tumors. Occasionally, neuroendocrine tumors of the thymus secrete corticotropin-releasing hormone, and more rarely, neurogenic tumors may secrete insulin and cause hypoglycemia (Odell, 1992).

TABLE 63–6 ■ **Computed Tomography (CT) and Magnetic Resonance Imaging (MRI) in the Evaluation of Mediastinal Masses**

CT Superior	*MRI Superior*	*CT and MRI Equal*
Spatial resolution	Multiplanar imaging capability and no contrast needed	Detection of pure fluid collections
Detection of bony destruction	Identification of complex fluid collection	Detection of chest wall invasion
Detection of calcification	Soft tissue differentiation	Evaluation of vascular obstruction (contrast CT)
Detection of lung nodules	Tumor vs. fibrosis	
Evaluation of lung parenchyma	Tumor vs. obstructive pneumonitis	
Single study of screening for lung, liver, adrenals	Evaluation of	
	Brachial plexus	
	Neural foramina	
	Diaphragm	
	Bone marrow	
	Mediastinal tissue invasion	

From Moore EH: Radiologic evaluation of mediastinal masses. Chest Surg Clin North Am 2:1, 1992.

TABLE 63-7 ■ **Common Vascular Lesions of the Mediastinum**

	Anterior Mediastinum	*Visceral Compartment*	*Paravertebral Sulci*
Venous system	Aneurysm of innominate vein Left superior vena cava	Dilatation of superior vena cava or azygos vein	
Pulmonary artery	Aneurysm of ductus arteriosus	Stenosis of pulmonary valve Idiopathic dilatation of pulmonary artery Congenital absence of pulmonary valve Pulmonary artery hypertension	
Pulmonary vein	Anomalies of venous return (to innominate vein or superior vena cava)	Pulmonary vein varices	
Arterial system	Aortic valve stenosis Aortic aneurysm Tortuosity of innominate artery Coarctation of aorta	Aneurysm of right ascending aorta Aortic valve stenosis	Aneurysm of descending aorta

Biopsy

Biopsy of mediastinal tumors is performed when the diagnosis remains unclear after extensive imaging and other diagnostic studies. Biopsy may be by needle aspiration or core needle biopsy or through more invasive techniques such as mediastinoscopy, anterior mediastinotomy, or video thoracoscopy. Biopsy is mandatory when primary treatment is likely to be nonsurgical, and most lymphomas and germ cell tumors fall into this category. In Ferguson and co-workers' series (1987), 61% of anterior mediastinal masses were treated nonsurgically, re-emphasizing the importance of obtaining tissue diagnosis by less invasive methods than open thoracotomy. In patients in whom cytologic or histologic material has been obtained, specimens must be submitted for immunohistochemical staining and electronic microscopy because cytology or histology alone may be insufficient to distinguish between thymomas and lymphomas (Herman et al, 1991; Yu et al, 1997) or to subclassify non-Hodgkin's lymphomas.

TABLE 63-8 ■ **Tumor Markers and Hormones Commonly Used to Diagnose Mediastinal Tumor**

Neoplasm	*Tumor Marker-Hormone*
Germ cell tumors	
Seminoma	Low titer of β-HCG
Endodermal sinus—yolk sac tumors	AFP
Choriocarcinoma	β-HCG
Embryonal carcinoma, teratocarcinoma	AFP, β-HCG
Thymoma	Anti-AChR antibodies, antimuscle antibodies
Neuroendocrine tumor of thymus	CRH
Parathyroid	Calcitonin
Neurogenic tumors	Insulin

AFP, α-fetoprotein; anti-AChR antibodies, anti–acetylcholine receptor antibodies; β-HCG, human chorionic gonadotropin β; CRH, corticotropin-releasing hormone.

Although the use of FNA biopsy has increased the accuracy of preoperative diagnosis, needle biopsy does not usually provide enough material to serve this purpose in patients with mediastinal lymphomas. Ricci and associates (1990b) state that the diagnosis of lymphoproliferative diseases should be based on histologic and immunohistochemical procedures that necessitate an amount of tissue that can be obtained only by open biopsy of the mediastinum. Yellin and associates (1987) also state that FNA-biopsy can be used as a screening test in patients with mediastinal lymphoma, but that larger specimens only obtainable by open methods are required to establish a firm diagnosis as well as make a distinction between the subclasses of the various lymphomas. In 1991, Herman and co-workers reported that in patients with anterior mediastinal masses, FNA was greater than 90% specific in diagnosing most tumors, but the sensitivity in diagnosing lymphomas was less than 50%.

The same restriction about the use of FNA applies to the diagnosis of germ cell tumors and thymomas. In one series of 56 patients with malignant germ cell tumors of the mediastinum (Knapp et al, 1985) a single germ cell element was present in 66% of tumors, and various combinations of germ cell elements were present in the remaining 34%. The authors concluded that it is imperative to take multiple tissue sections to define all elements, which can only be done through open exploration. In contrast to these reports, Kesler and associates (1999) from the Indiana University School of Medicine presented a series of 91 patients with primary mediastinal nonseminomatous germ cell tumors in whom the diagnosis was confirmed and categorized pathologically by FNA biopsy. If larger cutting needles are used (Moinuddin et al, 1984), the biopsy route must be planned carefully in order to avoid vascular trauma, and the use of ultrasonographic guidance for this purpose has been reported in cases of anterior mediastinal tumors (Wernecke et al, 1989).

Cervical mediastinoscopy, described by Carlens in 1959, is a useful and safe procedure to access the visceral compartment, particularly the paratracheal and subcarinal spaces. In cases of lymphoma, sufficient tissue can be obtained for accurate diagnosis and typing. Cervical mediastinoscopy can also be used for the biopsy of anterior mediastinal masses that extend into the visceral compartment or in patients with superior vena cava obstruction (Little et al, 1985). Mediastinotomy (McNeill and Chamberlain, 1966) is carried out through a short transverse incision over the second costal cartilage and affords access for adequate biopsy of all anterior mediastinal masses. Both of these procedures are associated with few complications and indeed when they are combined, nearly all tumors located in the anterior mediastinum or visceral compartment are accessible to biopsy.

More recently, thoracoscopic biopsy of mediastinal masses has been used instead of mediastinoscopy or anterior mediastinotomy (Kern et al, 1993; Solaini et al, 1998). In Kern and co-workers' series (1993), thoracoscopy provided an accurate tissue diagnosis in 19 of 22 patients without the need for additional open diagnostic procedures. The authors concluded that VATS is minimally invasive and that all areas of the mediastinum can be approached with equal safety and efficacy. One added advantage of VATS is that certain benign lesions can be completely excised during the procedure.

It is important to note that large mediastinal tumors can be associated with significant impairment of cardiopulmonary function, which may in turn lead to catastrophic complications during general anesthesia (Neuman et al, 1984; Pullerits and Holzman, 1989). These issues need to be addressed preoperatively by the surgeon and anesthesiologist, and adequate evaluation and preparation of the patient is of foremost importance. In general, the degree of tracheal compression documented by CT scan (Arizkhan et al, 1985), flow-volume loops, or flexible bronchoscopy (Mackie CB and Watson, 1984) is a good predictor of whether anesthetic difficulties with the airway will be encountered. If the patient has severe airway compromise and cannot tolerate general anesthesia, empiric therapy can be given based on the presumed diagnosis of the mediastinal tumor (Loeffler et al, 1986) or a biopsy can be performed under local anesthesia.

DIAGNOSTIC STRATEGIES

Anterior Mediastinal Tumors

Common anterior mediastinal tumors include thymic neoplasms, germ cell tumors, lymphomas, and mesenchymal tumors, while non-neoplastic conditions include substernal goiters and lymphangiomas.

Thymomas are the most common anterior mediastinal tumor in adults. The average age at presentation is 40 to 60 years (Strollo et al, 1997), and there is no sex predilection. Approximately 50% of patients with thymoma are asymptomatic (Shamji et al, 1984), and 30% of patients with a known thymoma have associated myasthenia gravis. In addition to myasthenia gravis, approximately 5% to 10% of patients present with other paraneoplastic syndromes such as red cell aplasia, hypogammaglobulinemia (10% of patients) (Souadjian et al, 1974), systemic lupus erythematosus, Cushing's syndrome, and inappropriate antidiuretic hormone (ADH) secretion. Because of the high incidence of myasthenia gravis associated with thymoma, all patients with clinically suspected thymic tumors should have a serum anti-ACLR antibody test even if they are asymptomatic (Lennon et al, 1983; Strollo et al, 1997). Chest radiographs and CT scan usually demonstrate a rounded or lobulated soft tissue mass in the anterior mediastinum (Fig. 63–6) with possible areas of cystic degeneration or hemorrhage (Rosado de Christensen et al, 1992). If present, lymphadenopathy should lead to a more likely diagnosis of lymphoma (Wright, 1999). Contrast CT is the best examination to demonstrate local extension into mediastinal fat, pleura and lung, pericardium, and great vessels.

According to Baron and investigators (1982), well-circumscribed thymic tumors are almost always benign, whereas neoplasms showing infiltration into the adjacent mediastinal fat are usually malignant. This distinction is significant because patients with invasive tumors on CT may not be suitable candidates for immediate surgery, and preoperative biopsy by anterior mediastinotomy (Shamji et al, 1984) on the side of the tumor is appropriate. The role of FNA biopsy is still debated, but in a series from the Memorial Sloan-Kettering Cancer Center (Blumberg et al, 1995), preoperative biopsy was performed in 48 thymoma patients by open methods ($n = 26$) or FNA ($n = 22$). Diagnosis was accurate by FNA biopsy in 59% of patients ($n = 13$) as compared to 81% of patients ($n = 21$) with open biopsy. In most patients with suspected thymomas, surgical excision provides the precise histology and stage, and it should be performed without preoperative biopsy. This approach is justified because it has been reported that tumor cells may shed from the surface of the tumor into the pleural space (Weissberg et al, 1973) during biopsy.

Primary germ cell tumors of the mediastinum are relatively rare, accounting for approximately 2% of all germ cell tumors. Benign teratomas occur more frequently in young adults (Lewis et al, 1983), and they are equally distributed between men and women. CT is usually highly suggestive with a well-demarcated fatty and cystic lesion (Fig. 63–7), often with calcifications. Cough productive of hair or sebum is a pathognomonic sign of rupture in the tracheobronchial tree. When a benign teratoma is suspected, surgical excision is recommended without biopsy.

Mediastinal seminomatous germ cell tumors occur in men in their third decade (Sham et al, 1990), and most are symptomatic. Approximately 10% of patients have an elevated β-HCG level but never an elevated AFP level (Strollo et al, 1997). Indeed an elevation of AFP associated with a seminoma is indicative of the presence of nonseminomatous elements (Economou et al, 1982). Radiologically, seminomas present as bulky lobulated homogeneous anterior mediastinal masses (Aygun et al, 1984). Because most of these tumors are infiltrative and their treatment is primarily nonsurgical, a biopsy should be obtained and the patient referred for chemoradiotherapy. In many cases, open biopsy is also necessary to distinguish between mixed and pure seminomas. This distinction is important because pure seminomas are highly radiosensitive and have a good prognosis, whereas mixed tumors have a much poorer prognosis (Sterchi and Cordell, 1975). Symptoms suggestive of metastasis should also be evaluated with proper studies.

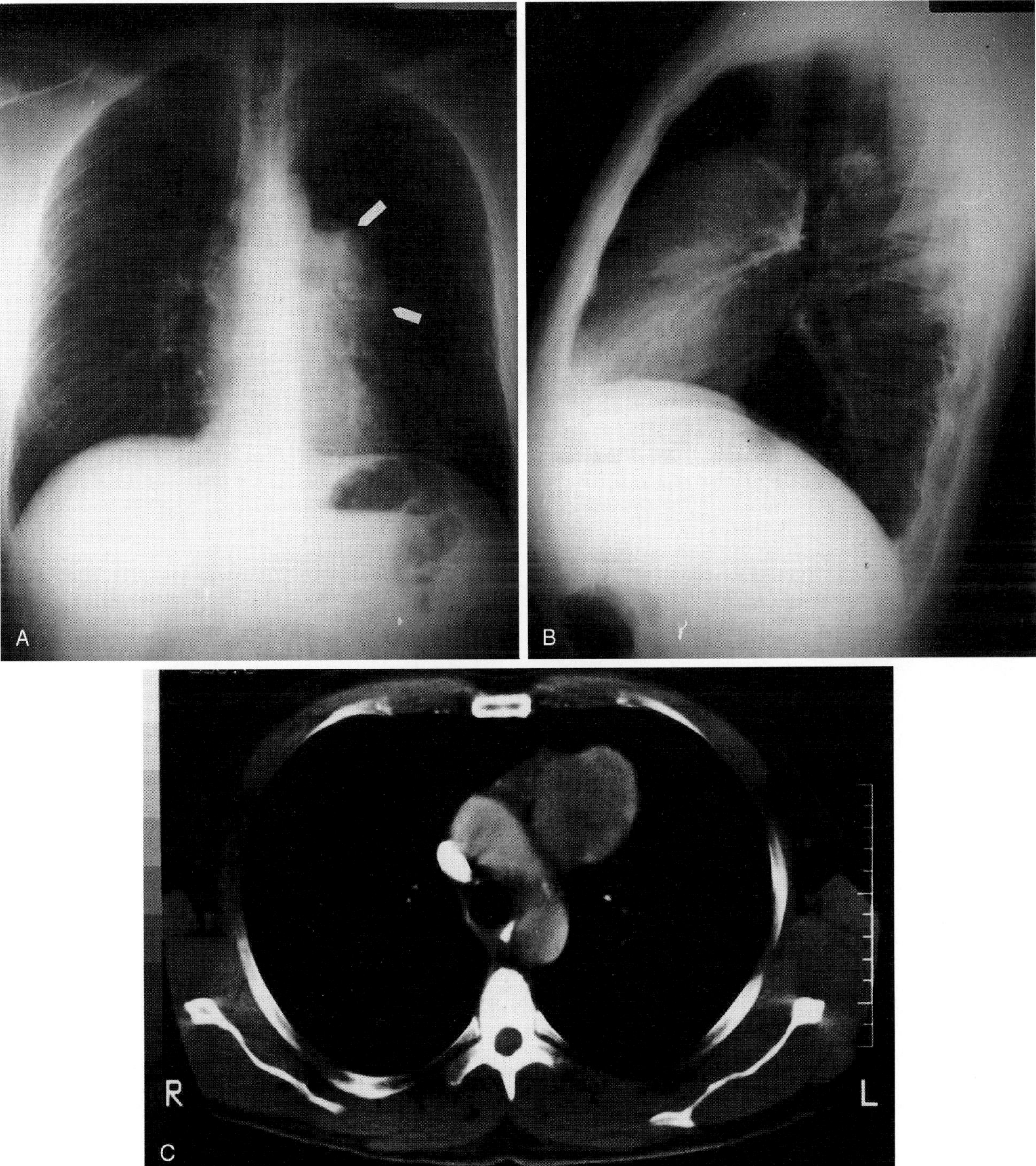

FIGURE 63–6 ■ Localized (noninvasive) thymoma. *A*, Posteroanterior chest radiograph of a 37-year-old woman showing a sharply defined soft tissue mass protruding in the left hemithorax at the level of the hilum and aortopulmonary window. *B*, On the lateral chest radiograph, the mass is located in the anterior mediastinum in front of the ascending aorta. *C*, A computed tomography scan showing a solid mass eccentric to the thymus on the left side of the ascending aorta.

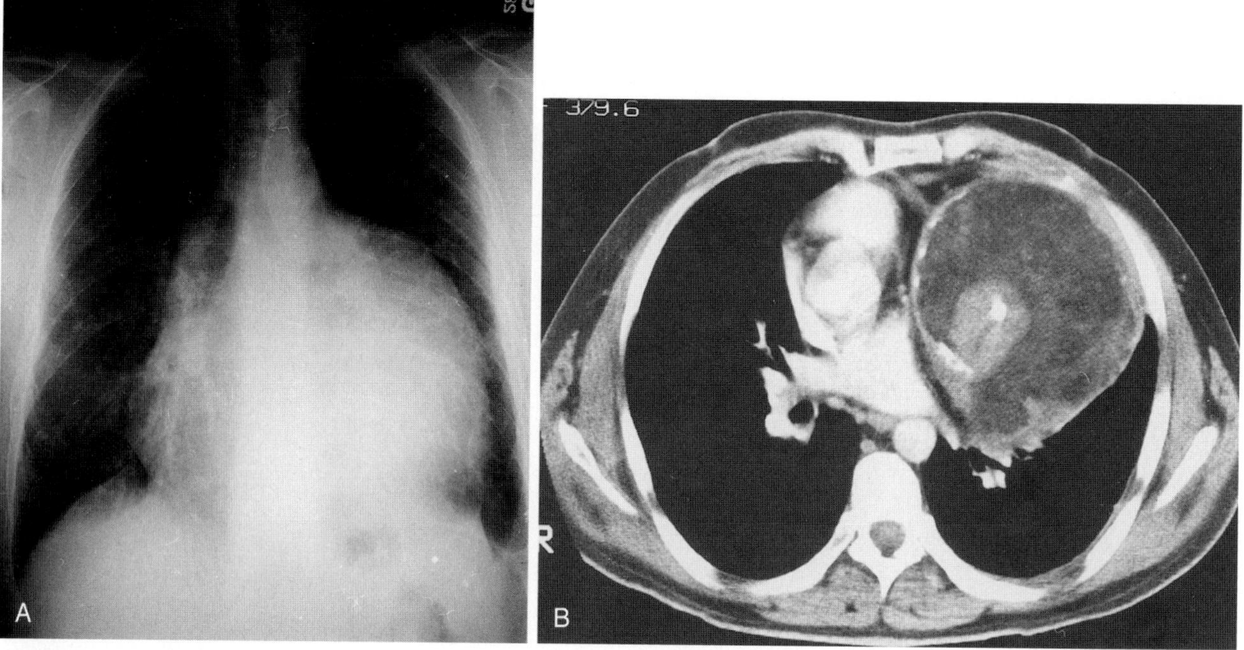

FIGURE 63–7 ■ Benign mature teratoma. *A*, A posteroanterior chest radiograph of a 44-year-old man demonstrating a mediastinal mass obscuring the left border of the cardiac silhouette. *B*, A computed tomography scan shows the mass with predominant fat attenuation and localized areas of calcification. These findings are typical of a benign teratoma.

Nonseminomatous germ cell tumors are rapidly growing neoplasms, and approximately 80% have at least one site of metastatic disease at the time of diagnosis. Almost all patients are young men less than 30 years of age, and most are symptomatic at the time of presentation. Radiologically, the tumors present as large and irregular anterior mediastinal masses with extensive areas of necrosis and hemorrhage (Lee et al, 1989). Measurements of serum levels of β-HCG and AFP are indispensable in the diagnosis and management of these tumors, and in about 90% of cases one or both markers are elevated. In Wright and co-workers' series (1990) of 44 patients with primary nonseminomatous germ cell tumors of the mediastinum, 92% had either one or both serum tumor markers elevated at the time of diagnosis. These are simple measurements that should be done routinely in all patients presenting with presumed malignant anterior mediastinal masses. It is generally agreed that despite positive tumor markers, all patients should have tissue confirmation before treatment (Knapp et al, 1985).

The majority of patients with either Hodgkin's or non-Hodgkin's lymphoma in the mediastinum also have systemic disease, while about 50% of patients with Hodgkin's disease and 20% of patients with non-Hodgkin's lymphoma (Manoharan et al, 1979) have mediastinal disease. Mediastinal involvement usually presents as enlarged lymph nodes in the anterior or middle mediastinum, often identified on the initial chest radiograph (Fig. 63–8). CT is used to confirm (Filly et al, 1976) the involvement as well as to detect additional sites of disease not demonstrated on standard radiographs (Brown et al, 1990). When CT shows enlarged nodes located in the visceral compartment, the differential diagnosis must include sarcoidosis, other inflammatory nodal conditions, and metastatic bronchogenic carcinomas. In these cases, cervical mediastinoscopy provides enough tissue for diagnosis. Approximately 5% to 10% of patients present with primary anterior mediastinal lymphomas in which the differential diagnosis includes thymomas, germ cell tumors, and more uncommonly, mesenchymal tumors.

Mediastinal lymphomas often produce symptoms related to respiratory compression or pleuropericardial involvement. Superior vena cava syndrome is not an uncommon finding when the disease is extensive either in the anterior mediastinum or in the right paratracheal area. The surgeon's role in suspected lymphoma is primarily a diagnostic one, and he or she must ensure that enough material is obtained not only to establish diagnosis but also to type the tumor. Frozen sections of lymphomas are notoriously difficult to interpret, and in Yellin and co-workers' series (1987), these were examined in over 90% of patients, but they sufficed for firm diagnosis in only 10%. Frozen sections should nevertheless be obtained to ascertain whether the pathologist has enough tissue for diagnosis. If the patient is at risk for general anesthesia, FNA biopsy can be done or an anterior mediastinotomy can be carried out under local anesthesia with the patient in the semiupright position (Wright, 1999). Ricci and associates (1990b) concluded that in patients with presumed mediastinal lymphoma, it is necessary to select a surgical approach that is not preclusive of subsequent resection should the tumor turn out to be a thymoma or another tumor that must be eventually treated by resection.

Castleman's disease is characterized by massive enlargement of lymph nodes (angiofollicular lymph node hyperplasia), and it may exist in any of the divisions of the mediastinum. Typically it presents as a well-circumscribed, solitary nodal mass that enhances substantially on CT after contrast injection (Serour et al, 1989). En-

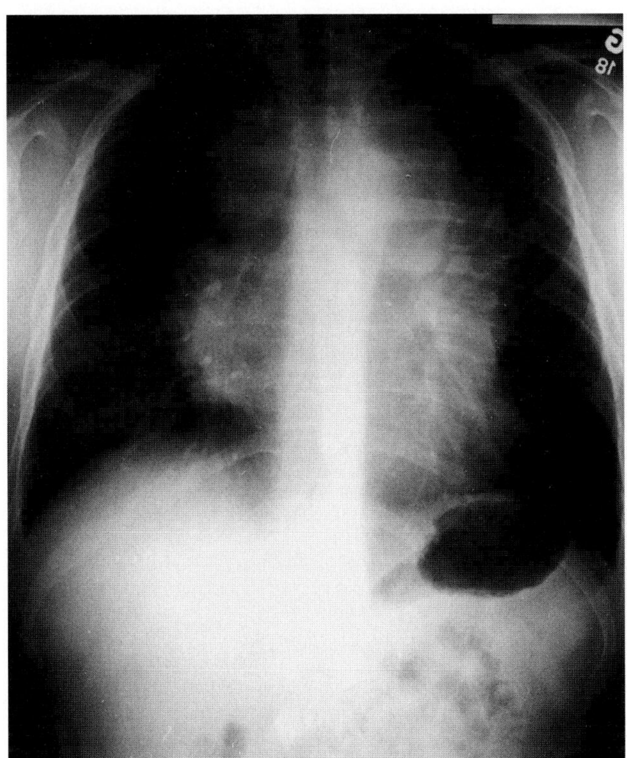

FIGURE 63–8 ■ Hodgkin's disease of the mediastinum. A posteroanterior chest radiograph of a 19-year-old man with extensive Hodgkin's disease involving lymph nodes located in both paratracheal and hilar regions as well as in the aortopulmonary window.

hancement is due to major arterial feeders, which have also been demonstrated by Walter and co-workers (1978) through angiography. Mesenchymal tumors such as lipomas, hemangiomas, fibromas, and lymphangiomas and their malignant counterparts are uncommon, and most are found in the anterior mediastinum. Preoperative diagnosis is usually not possible, and resection is indicated because the presence of malignant components cannot be determined preoperatively.

The vast majority of intrathoracic goiters are continuous with an enlarged cervical thyroid gland and have a typical CT appearance (Fig. 63–9). They have smooth borders, are multinodular, and may include coarse calcifications and low-density cystic areas (Moore, 1992). They are usually located in the anterosuperior mediastinum, although they can extend posteriorly behind the trachea. In 1983, Bashist and associates studied 10 patients with intrathoracic goiters and concluded that CT showed additional features helpful in making the correct diagnosis. These features include clear continuity with the cervical gland (8 of 10 patients); well-defined borders (9 of 10); punctate, coarse, or ring-like calcifications (8 of 10); and nonhomogeneity (9 of 10), often with discrete nonenhancing low-density areas. As demonstrated by Glazer and co-workers (1982), most mediastinal thyroids also have prolonged enhancement with contrast administration. Only 2% of goiters are primary intrathoracic tumors, with their blood supply coming from the chest rather than from the neck.

Approximately 10% to 20% of parathyroid adenomas or hyperplastic parathyroid glands are found within the anterior mediastinum where they present as small, rounded, or oval masses of soft tissue density with variable contrast enhancement (Cates et al, 1988; Krudy et al, 1981).

Tumors of the Visceral Compartment

Common lesions arising in the visceral compartment include pericardial cysts, most bronchogenic cysts, paragangliomas located in the aortopulmonary window, and lesions arising from lymph nodes. Most systemic arterial abnormalities are also located in this compartment, and they can be recognized by CT with contrast injection (see Table 63–7).

Pericardial cysts (Fig. 63–10) are characteristically located at the right cardiophrenic angle (60%), where they present as smooth, round, and homogeneous soft tissue masses contiguous with the hemidiaphragm (Brown et al, 1990). CT shows a mass with an attenuation coefficient consistent with a cystic lesion (Pugatch et al, 1978), and if FNA biopsy is carried out, it yields clear fluid with negative cytologic results.

Most bronchogenic cysts are located in sites adjacent to the tracheobronchial tree (Fig. 63–11) (St-Georges et al, 1991). Many of these cysts are asymptomatic, but if left unattended, complications eventually develop, and they become symptomatic. On standard chest radiograph, bronchogenic cysts tend to present as rounded, sharply demarcated homogeneous masses in close association with the trachea or carina. On CT, bronchogenic cysts have usually low Hounsfield units indicating clear fluid, but they may be infected or contain sufficient mucoid material to give a high CT number (Marvasti et al, 1980; Mendelson et al, 1983). Bronchogenic cysts can be readily recognized by VATS, and occasionally complete cyst excision can be carried out (Lewis et al, 1992) during the procedure.

Paragangliomas (chemodectomas) are rare tumors located in the aortopulmonary window or in the costovertebral sulci. They present as soft tissue masses with increased vascularity as demonstrated by dynamic scanning during bolus injection (Drucker et al, 1987). The exact diagnosis is generally made at surgery, which can be dangerous because of the extreme vascularity of the tumor. The differential diagnosis of such well-vascularized masses includes Castleman's disease and hemangiomas. The use of ^{131}I metaiodobenzylguanidine scintigraphy has been reported to be helpful in identifying these tumors (Shapiro et al, 1984).

By far, the most common masses located in the visceral compartment are in relation to enlarged lymph nodes distributed around the tracheobronchial tree. As previously indicated, the differential diagnosis of these nodes includes sarcoidosis, lymphoma, and metastatic disease originating from the lung. Cervical mediastinoscopy is very useful to biopsy these nodes and correctly diagnose the underlying process. Inflammatory masses due to sequelae of tuberculosis or histoplasmosis may show necrosis or calcifications on CT scan.

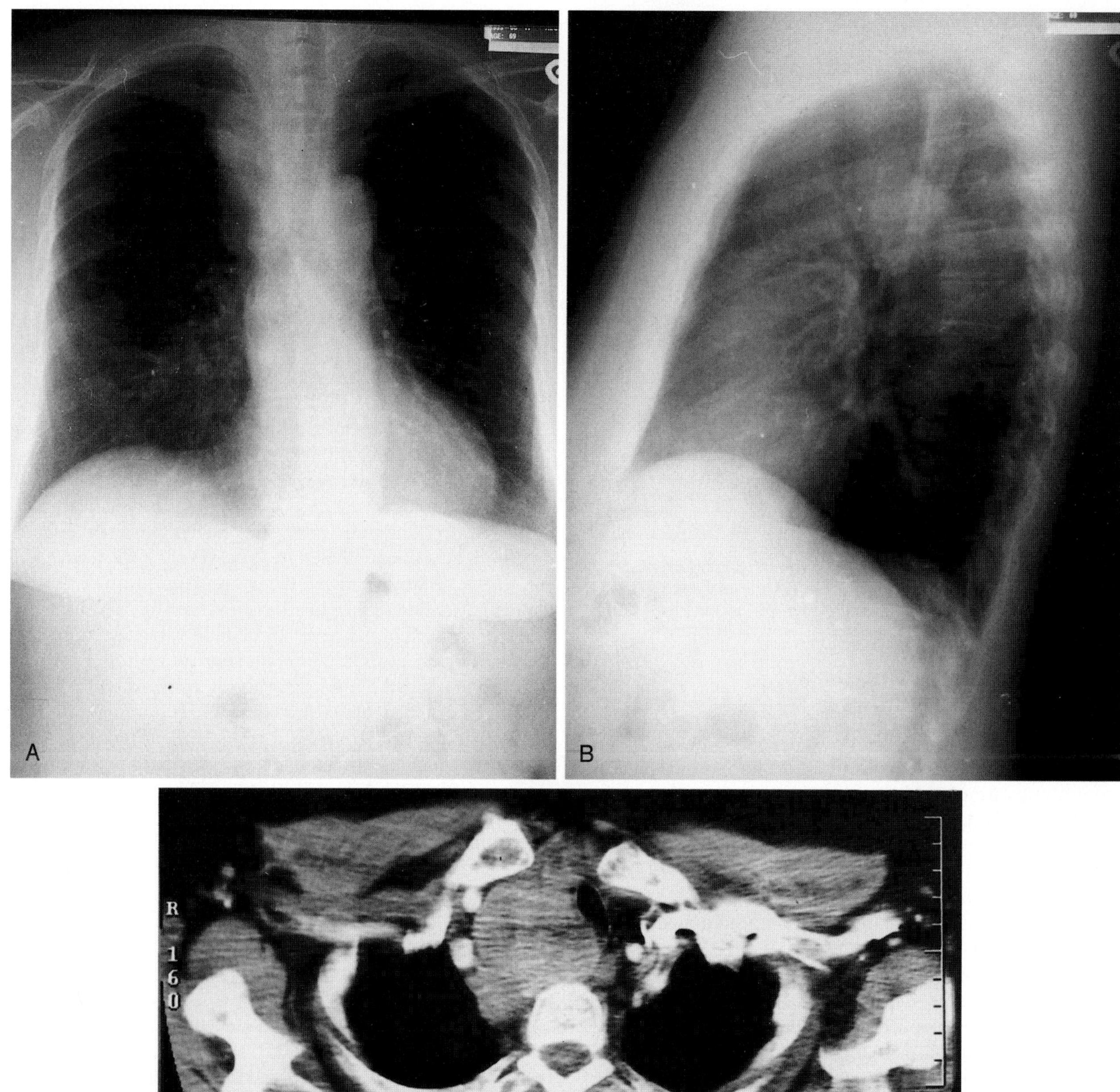

FIGURE 63–9 ■ Intrathoracic goiter. Posteroanterior *(A)* and lateral *(B)* chest radiographs of a 69-year-old woman demonstrating extrinsic compression and smooth displacement of the trachea by a soft tissue mass extending from the neck on the right side of the mediastinum. *C*, A computed tomography scan showing the characteristic appearance of a multinodular goiter with "mass effect" on the trachea.

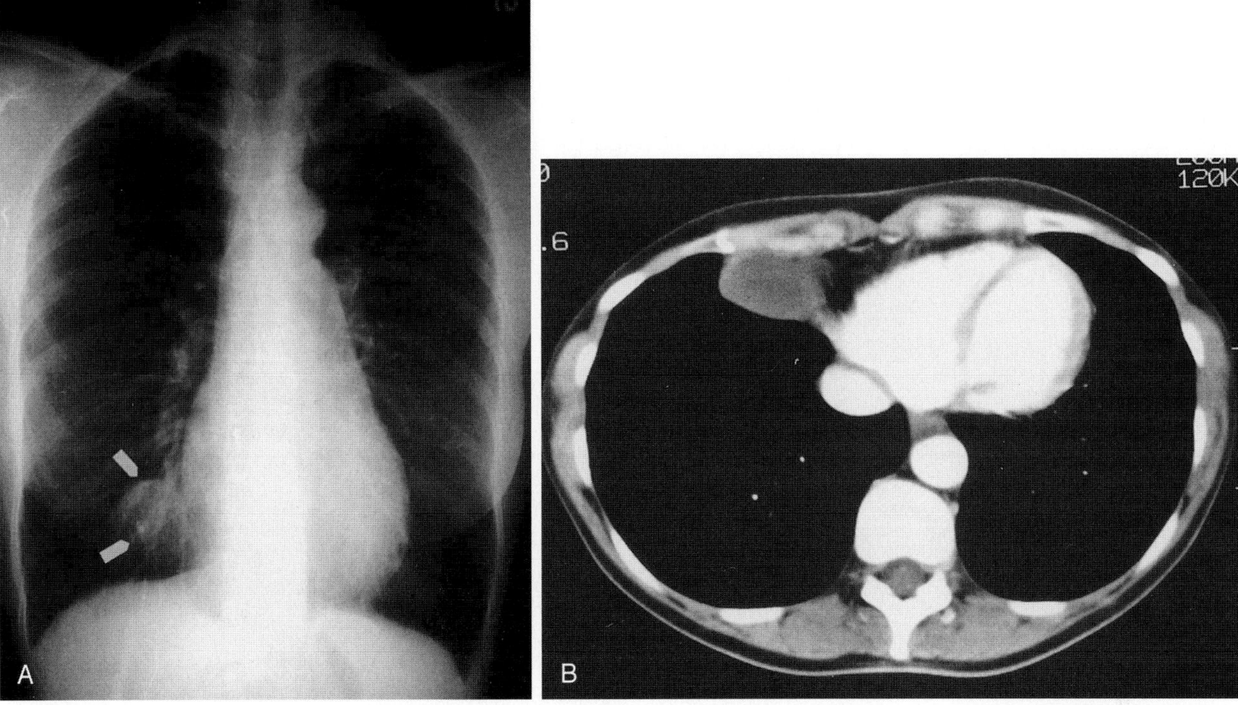

FIGURE 63–10 ■ Pericardial cyst. *A,* Posteroanterior chest radiograph of a 49-year-old asymptomatic woman demonstrating a well-defined mass located at the right cardiophrenic angle *(arrows)*. *B,* Contrast-enhanced computed tomography scan demonstrating a water density cyst with a pedunculated stalk connecting the cyst to the pericardium. The diagnosis of pericardial cyst was confirmed at thoracotomy.

Tumors of the Paravertebral Sulci

Mediastinal masses located in the paravertebral sulci include neurogenic tumors (Fig. 63–12) and some foregut cysts, such as esophageal duplications and neuroenteric cysts. Neurogenic tumors arise from peripheral nerves or sympathetic ganglia. Almost all of these tumors are benign (90%) and slow growing, and the majority are asymptomatic. Neuroblastomas and ganglioneuroblastomas occur in infants and children, while ganglioneuromas occur in young adults. In the adult population, the most common neurogenic tumors are schwannomas and neurofibromas. According to Shields and Reynolds (1988), von Recklinghausen's neurofibromatosis can be identified in 30% of patients with neurofibromas. Radiographically, neurogenic tumors present as rounded masses arising in the costovertebral angle (paravertebral sulcus). Calcifications are rare, but when present they follow one of two patterns: (1) a homogeneous rim of calcium along the margin of areas of cystic change in nerve sheath tumors or (2) a speckled distribution in large ganglioneuromas (Wain, 1992). Erosion, destruction, or spreading of the ribs may occur as may vertebral abnormalities and intraspinal extension (dumbbell tumors). These features are best examined by MRI, which accurately describes the existence and longitudinal extension of the spinal component of the tumor (Hasuo et al, 1993; Ricci et al, 1990a). Grillo and Ojemann (1989) have described three steps in the evaluation of neurogenic tumors: (1) the intervertebral foramen near the tumor location should be scanned for widening and expansion with thin-slice CT; (2) if widening or expansion is detected, MRI or myelography and CT should be performed; (3) if a major spinal artery is at risk from the surgery, its course should be identified with angiography. The artery of Adamkiewicz which supplies the anterior spinal artery originates from the left T9-L2 intercostal artery, but in 15% of the population, it originates from T5-T8 (Doppman et al, 1969). Preoperative biopsy of neurogenic tumors is unnecessary.

Esophageal duplications are rare foregut cysts that result from abnormalities occurring during the recanalization of the primitive esophagus. They are located adjacent or within the esophageal wall, and occasionally they communicate with the esophageal lumen. Neuroenteric cysts are located against the spine and are always associated with vertebral anomalies, the most common being spina bifida.

SUMMARY

Mediastinal masses must be investigated in depth not only to establish a positive diagnosis prior to therapy but also to make sure that the degree of local invasiveness is well documented preoperatively. The classic example is a neurogenic tumor in which intraspinal extension mandates a very different surgical procedure from the one carried out for patients without spinal extension. Fortunately, modern imaging techniques facilitate the investigation and workup of patients being prepared for surgery.

For most tumors that are not well delineated on CT or for which primary treatment is likely to be nonsurgical, a biopsy should be obtained. Although the best method of biopsy is still debated, open techniques are preferable if one is to obtain adequate tissue sampling.

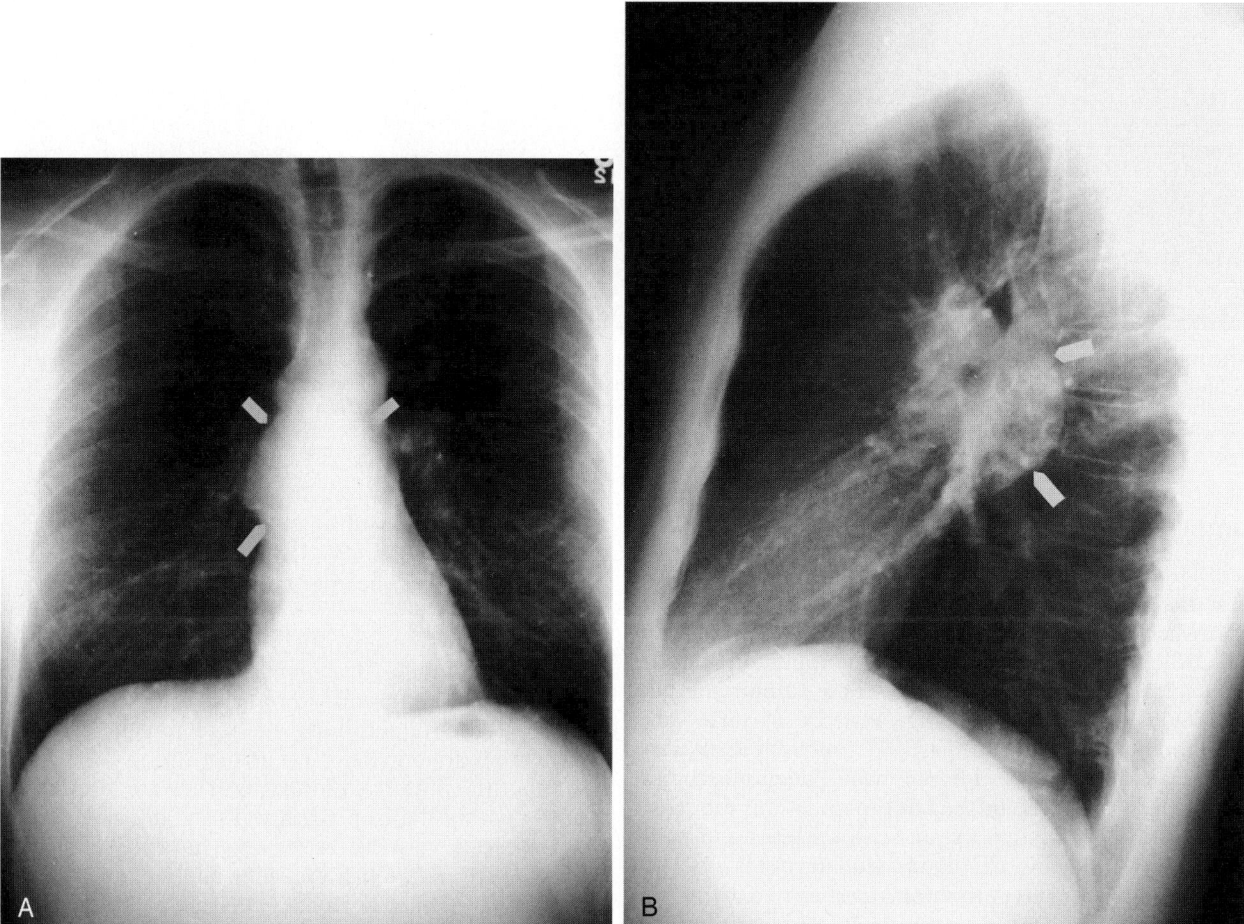

FIGURE 63–11 ■ Bronchogenic cyst. Posteroanterior *(A)* and lateral *(B)* chest radiographs of a 44-year-old woman demonstrating a mediastinal mass located in the subcarinal space *(arrows)*. These images are highly suggestive of a bronchogenic cyst.

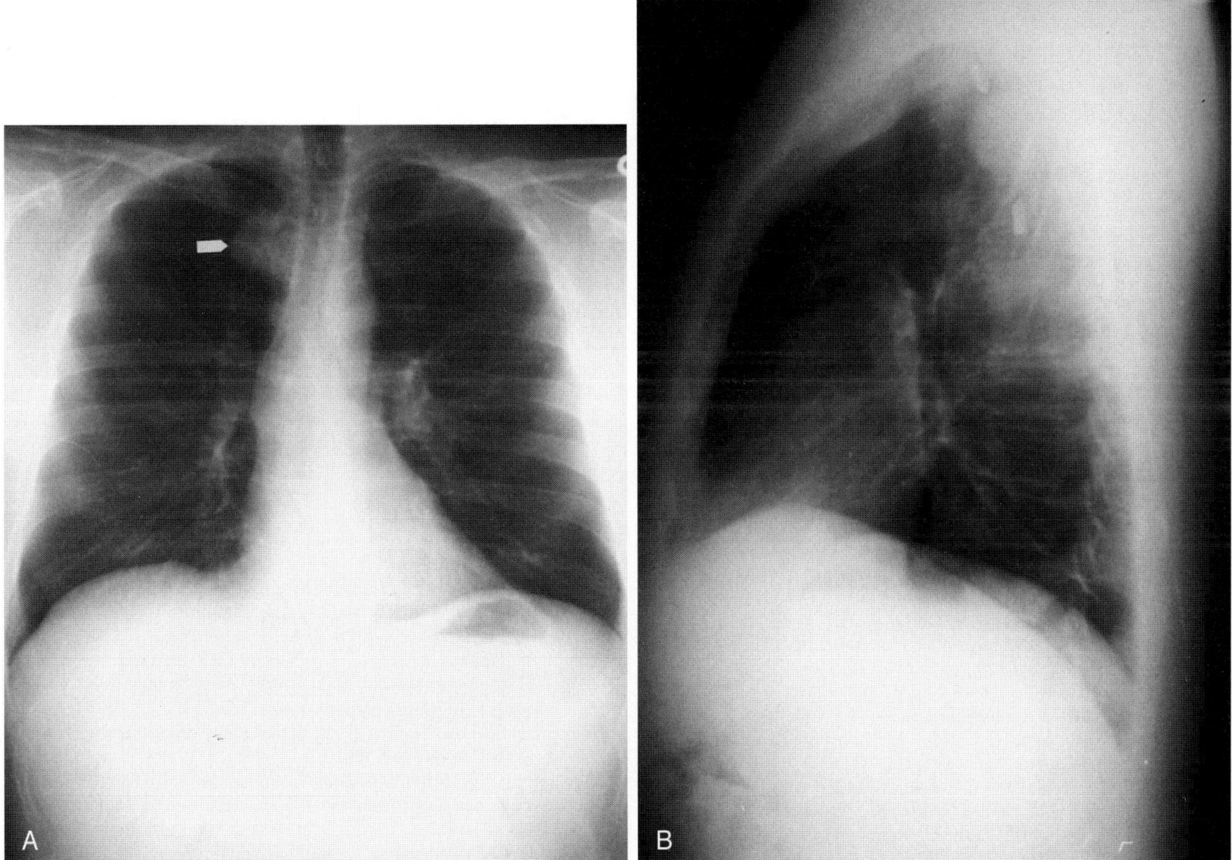

FIGURE 63–12 ■ Schwannoma. Posteroanterior *(A)* and lateral *(B)* chest radiographs showing a typical benign neurogenic tumor located in the right paravertebral sulcus *(arrows)*.

KEY REFERENCES

Brown K, Aberle DR, Batra P, Steckel RJ: Current use of imaging in the evaluation of primary mediastinal masses. Chest 98:466, 1990.

This article provides an excellent review of imaging techniques used in the evaluation of primary mediastinal masses.

Kelley MJ, Mannes EJ, Ravin CE: Mediastinal masses of vascular origin. A review. J Thorac Cardiovasc Surg 76:559, 1978.

In this article, the authors review all vascular lesions that must be considered in the differential diagnosis of mediastinal masses.

Mullen B, Richardson JR: Primary anterior mediastinal tumors in children and adults. Ann Thorac Surg 42:338, 1986.

This is a collective review that details pertinent anatomic, radiologic, pathologic, and clinical information regarding primary anterior mediastinal tumors.

Strollo DC, Rosado de Christensen ML, Jett JR: Primary mediastinal tumors. Part 1: Tumors of the anterior mediastinum. Chest 112:511, 1997.

In this article, the clinical, radiographic, and therapeutic aspects of the most common anterior mediastinal masses are reviewed.

Wain JC: Neurogenic tumors of the mediastinum. Chest Surg Clin North Am 2:121, 1992.

In this article, the authors review all techniques used for the evaluation and diagnosis of neurogenic tumors.

REFERENCES

Akwari OE, Payne WS, Onofrio BM et al: Dumbbell neurogenic tumors of the mediastinum: Diagnosis and management. Mayo Clin Proc 53:353, 1978.

Arizkhan RG, Dudgeon DL, Buck JR et al: Life-threatening airway obstruction as a complication to the management of mediastinal mass in children. J Pediatr Surg 20:816, 1985.

Aygun C, Slawson RG, Bajaj K et al: Primary mediastinal seminoma. Urology 23:109, 1984.

Azarow KS, Pearl RJ, Zurcher R et al: Primary mediastinal masses: A comparison of acute and pediatric population. J Thorac Cardiovasc Surg 106:67, 1993.

Baron RL, Gutierrez FR, Sagel SS et al: CT of anomalies of the mediastinal vessels. AJR Am J Roentgenol 137:571, 1981.

Baron RL, Lee JKT, Sagee SS, Levitt RG: Computed tomography of the abnormal thymus. Radiology 142:127, 1982.

Baron RL, Lewitt RG, Sagel SS, Stanley RJ: Computed tomography in the evaluation of mediastinal widening. Radiology 138:107, 1981.

Bartter T, Irwin RS, Nash G: Aneurysms of the pulmonary arteries. Chest 94:1065, 1988.

Bashist B, Ellis K, Gold RP: Computed tomography of intrathoracic goiters. AJR Am J Roentgenol 140:455, 1983.

Bekerman C, Hoffer PM, Bitran JD: The role of gallium-67 in the clinical evaluation of cancer. Semin Nucl Med 14:296, 1984.

Benfield JR, Sawyer RW: Tumor markers. Chest Surg Clin North Am. 2:213, 1992.

Berquist TH, Brown LR: Nuclear magnetic resonance imaging of the hilum and mediastinum: A comparison with CT and hilar tomography. Radiographics 4:151, 1984.

Bilezikian JP, Doppman JL, Shimkin PM et al: Preoperative localization of abnormal parathyroid tissue: Cumulative experience with venous sampling and arteriography. Am J Med 55:505, 1973.

Blumberg D, Port JL, Weksler B et al: Thymoma: A multivariate analysis of factors predicting survival. Ann Thorac Surg 60:908, 1995.

Brennan MF, Doppman JL, Marx SJ et al: Reoperative parathyroid surgery for persistent hyperparathyroidism. Surgery 83:669, 1978.

Brown K, Aberle DR, Batra R, Steckel RJ: Current use of imaging in the evaluation of primary mediastinal masses. Chest 98:466, 1990.

Burt M: Mediastinal tumors: Current status. Proceedings of the New York Society for Thoracic Surgery postgraduate medical education course, January 1995.

Carlens E: Mediastinoscopy: A method for inspection and tissue biopsy in the superior mediastinum. Chest 36:343, 1959.

Cates JD, Thorsen MK, Lawson TL et al: CT evaluation of parathyroid adenomas: Diagnostic criteria and pitfalls. J Comput Assist Tomogr 12:626, 1988.

Cohen AJ, Thompson L, Edwards FF, Bellamy RF: Primary cysts and tumors of the mediastinum. Ann Thorac Surg 51:378, 1991.

Davis RD, Oldham HN, Sabiston DC: Primary cysts and neoplasms of the mediastinum: Recent changes in clinical presentation, methods of diagnosis, management, and results. Ann Thorac Surg 44:229, 1987.

Dooms GC, Higgins CB: The potential of magnetic resonance imaging for the evaluation of thoracic arterial diseases. J Thorac Cardiovasc Surg 92:1088, 1986.

Doppman JL, Dichino G, Omya KK: Selective Arteriography of the Spinal Cord. St. Louis, WH Green, 1969, pp 35–40.

Drucker EA, McLoud TC, Dechick CG et al: Mediastinal paraganglioma: Radiologic evaluation of an unusual vascular tumor. AJR Am J Roentgenol 148:521, 1987.

Economou JS, Trump DL, Holmes EC, Eggleston JE: Management of primary germ cell tumors of the mediastinum. J Thorac Cardiovasc Surg 83:643, 1982.

Eschapasse H: Pathologie du médiastin. Encycl Med Chir Paris. Poumon 6047 A 05, 4–1979.

Felson B: Chest Roentgenology. Philadelphia, WB Saunders, 1973.

Ferguson MK, Lee E, Skinner DB, Little AG: Selective operative approach for diagnosis and treatment of anterior mediastinal masses. Ann Thorac Surg 44:583, 1987.

Filly R, Blank N, Castellino RA: Radiographic distribution of intrathoracic disease in previously untreated patients with Hodgkin's disease and non-Hodgkin's lymphoma. Radiology 120:227, 1976.

Fraser RG, Paré JAP, Paré PD et al: Diagnosis of Diseases of the Chest, 3rd ed. Philadelphia, WB Saunders, 1988.

Gefter WB: Chest applications of magnetic resonance imaging: An update. Radiol Clin North Am 26:573, 1988.

Glazer GM, Axel L, Moss AA: CT diagnosis of mediastinal thyroid. AJR Am J Roentgenol 138:495, 1982.

Grillo HC, Ojemann RG: Mediastinal and intraspinal dumbbell neurogenic tumors. In Martini N, Vogt Moykoff I (eds): Thoracic Surgery: Frontier and Uncommon Neoplasms. Toronto, CV Mosby, 1989, pp 205–210.

Graeber GM, Shriver CD, Albus RA et al: The use of computed tomography in the evaluation of mediastinal masses. J Thorac Cardiovasc Surg 91:662, 1986.

Harris GJ, Harman PK, Trinkle JK, Grover FL: Standard biplane roentgenography is highly sensitive in documenting mediastinal masses. Ann Thorac Surg 44:238, 1987.

Hasuo K, Uchino A, Matsumoto S et al: MR imaging compared with CT, angiography and myelography supplemented by CT in the diagnosis of spinal tumors. Radiol Med 11:177, 1993.

Heitzman ER: The Mediastinum: Radiologic Correlations with Anatomy and Pathology. St. Louis, CV Mosby, 1977.

Herman SJ, Holub RV, Weissbrod GL, Chamberlain DW: Anterior mediastinal masses: Utility of transthoracic needle biopsy. Radiology 180:167, 1991.

Javadpour N: The value of biologic markers in the diagnosis and treatment of testicular cancer. Semin Oncol 6:37, 1979.

Kay PH, Wills FC, Goldstraw P: A multidisciplinary approach to primary nonseminomatous germ cell tumors of the mediastinum. Ann Thorac Surg 44:578, 1987.

Kelley MJ, Mannes EJ, Ravin CE: Mediastinal masses of vascular origin: A review. J Thorac Cardiovasc Surg 76:559, 1978.

Kern JA, Daniel TA, Tribble LG et al: Thoracoscopic diagnosis and treatment of mediastinal masses. Ann Thorac Surg 56:92, 1993.

Kesler KA, Rieger KM, Ganjoo KN et al: Primary mediastinal nonseminomatous germ cell tumors: The influence of postchemotherapy pathology on long-term survival after surgery. J Thorac Cardiovasc Surg 118:692, 1999.

King RM, Telander RL, Smithson WA et al: Primary mediastinal tumors in children. J Pediatr Surg 17:512, 1982.

Kirschner PA: Myasthenia gravis and other parathymic syndromes. Chest Surg Clin North Am 2:183, 1992.

Kirschner PA: Classification, diagnosis and management of mediastinal tumor. Proceedings of the New York Thoracic Society postgraduate course. 1998.

Knapp RH, Hurt RD, Payne WS et al: Malignant germ cell tumors of the mediastinum. J Thorac Cardiovasc Surg 89:82, 1985.

Krudy AG, Doppman JL, Brennan MF et al: The detection of mediastinal parathyroid glands by computed tomography, selective arteriography, and venous sampling. Radiology 140:739, 1981.

Lee KS, Im JG, Han CH et al: Malignant primary germ cell tumors of the mediastinum: CT features. AJR AM J Roentgenol 153:947, 1989.

Lennon VA, Janes G, Howard F et al: Auto-antibodies to acetylcholine receptors in myasthenia gravis. N Engl J Med 308:402, 1983.

Lewis BD, Hurt RD, Payne S et al: Benign teratomas of the mediastinum. J Thorac Cardiovasc Surg 86:727, 1983.

Lewis RJ, Caccavale RJ, Sisler GE: Imaged thoracoscopic surgery: A new thoracic technique for resection of mediastinal cysts. Ann Thorac Surg 53:318, 1992.

Linder J, Olsen GA, Johnston WW: Fine-needle aspiration biopsy of the mediastinum. Am J Med 81:1005, 1986.

Little AG, Golomb HM, Ferguson MK et al: Malignant superior vena cava obstruction reconsidered: The role of diagnostic surgical intervention. Ann Thorac Surg 40:285, 1985.

Livesay JJ, Mink JH, Fee HJ: The use of computed tomography to evaluate suspected mediastinal tumors. Ann Thorac Surg 27:305, 1979.

Loeffler JS, Leopold KA, Recht A et al: Emergency pre-biopsy radiation for mediastinal masses: Impact on subsequent pathologic diagnosis and outcome. J Clin Oncol 4:716, 1986.

Lyons HA, Calvy FL, Sammons BP: The diagnosis and classification of mediastinal masses. A study of 782 cases. Ann Intern Med 51:897, 1959.

Mackie AM, Watson CB: Anesthesia and mediastinal masses. A case report and review of the literature. Anaesthesia 39:899, 1984.

Manoharan A, Pitney WR, Schonell ME, Bader LV: Intrathoracic manifestations in non-Hodgkin's lymphoma. Thorax 34:29, 1979.

Marvasti MA, Mitchell GE, Burke WA, Meyer JA: Misleading density of mediastinal cysts on computerized tomography. Ann Thorac Surg 31:167, 1980.

McNeill TM, Chamberlain JM: Diagnostic anterior mediastinotomy. Ann Thorac Surg 2:532, 1966.

Mendelson DS, Rose JS, Efremidis SC et al: Bronchogenic cysts with high CT numbers. AJR Am J Roentgenol 140:463, 1983.

Moinuddin SM, Lee LH, Montgomery JH: Mediastinal needle biopsy. AJR Am J Roentgenol 143:531, 1984.

Moore EH: Radiologic evaluation of mediastinal masses. Chest Surg Clin North Am 2:1, 1992.

Mullen B, Richardson JR: Primary anterior mediastinal tumors in children and adults. Ann Thorac Surg 42:338, 1986.

Neuman GG, Weingarten AE, Abramowitz RM et al: The anesthetic management of the patient with an anterior mediastinal mass. Anesthesiology 60:144, 1984.

Nordenström B: Paraxiphoid approach to the mediastinum for mediastinoscopy and mediastinal needle biopsy: A preliminary report. Invest Radiol 2:141, 1967.

Odell WD: Humoral-endocrine manifestations of tumors of the mediastinum. Chest Surg Clin North Am 2:165, 1992.

Pearson FG: Mediastinoscopy: A method of biopsy of the superior mediastinum. J Thorac Cardiovasc Surg 49:11, 1995.

Pugatch RD, Braver JH, Robbins AH, Faling LJ: CT diagnosis of pericardial cysts. AJR Am J Roentgenol 131:515, 1978.

Pullerits J, Holzman R: Anesthesia for patients with mediastinal masses. Can J Anesth 36:681, 1989.

Ribet ME, Cardot GR: Neurogenic tumors of the thorax. Ann Thorac Surg 58:1091, 1994.

Ricci C, Rendina EA, Venuta F et al: Diagnostic imaging and surgical treatment of dumbbell tumors of the mediastinum. Ann Thorac Surg 50:586, 1990a.

Ricci C, Rendina EA, Venuta F et al: Surgical approach to isolated mediastinal lymphoma. J Thorac Cardiovasc Surg 99:691, 1990b.

Robbins LL: The roentgenologic appearance of bronchogenic cysts. AJR Am J Roentgenol 50:321, 1943.

Rosado de Christensen ML, Galobardes J, Moran CA: Thymoma: Radiologic-pathologic correlation. Radiographics 12:151, 1992.

Serour F, Lieberman Y, Rosenman J et al: Castleman's disease of the mediastinum. Misleading clinical and radiological characteristics. Respir Med 83:509, 1989.

Sham JS, Fu KH, Choi PH et al: Primary mediastinal seminoma. Oncology 47:124, 1990.

Sham JS, Fu KH, Chiu CS et al: Experience with the management of primary endodermal sinus tumor of the mediastinum. Cancer 64:756, 1989.

Shamji F, Pearson FG, Todd TR et al: Results of surgical treatment for thymoma. J Thorac Cardiovasc Surg 76:43, 1984.

Shapiro B, Sisson J, Kalff V et al: The location of middle mediastinal pheochromocytomas. J Thorac Cardiovasc Surg 87:814, 1984.

Shields TW: Primary tumors and cysts of the mediastinum. In Shields TW (ed): General Thoracic Surgery, 1st ed. Philadelphia, Lea & Febiger, 1972, p 908.

Shields TW: The mediastinum and its compartments. In Shields TW (ed): Mediastinal Surgery, 1st ed. Philadelphia, Lea & Febiger, 1991, p 4.

Shields TW, Reynolds M: Neurogenic tumors of the thorax. Surg Clin North Am 68:645, 1988.

Silverman NA, Sabiston DC Jr: Primary tumors and cysts of the mediastinum. Curr Prob Cancer 2:1, 1977.

Solaini L, Bagioni P, Campanini A, Poddie BD: Diagnostic role of videothoracoscopy in mediastinal diseases. Eur J Cardiothorac Surg 13:491, 1998.

Souadjian JV, Enriquez P, Silverstein MN et al: The spectrum of diseases associated with thymoma. Arch Intern Med 134:374, 1974.

Sterchi M, Cordell AR: Seminoma of the anterior mediastinum. Ann Thorac Surg 19:371, 1975.

St-Georges R, Deslauriers J, Duranceau A et al: Clinical spectrum of bronchogenic cysts of the mediastinum and lung in the adult. Ann Thorac Surg 52:6, 1991.

Strollo DC, Rosado de Christensen ML, Jett JR: Primary mediastinal tumors. Part 1: Tumors of the anterior mediastinum. Chest 112:511, 1997.

Trastek VF: Management of mediastinal tumors. Ann Thorac Surg 44:227, 1987.

von Schulthess GK, McMurdo K, Tsholakoff D et al: Mediastinal masses: MR imaging. Radiology 158:289, 1986.

Wain JC: Neurogenic tumors of the mediastinum. Chest Surg Clin North Am 2:121, 1992.

Walter JF, Rottenberg RW, Cannon WB et al: Giant mediastinal lymphoma hyperplasia (Castleman's disease): Angiographic and clinical features. AJR Am J Roentgenol 130:447, 1978.

Webb WR: Advances in computed tomography of the thorax. Radiol Clin North Am 21:723, 1983.

Weissberg D, Goldberg M, Pearson FG: Thymoma. Ann Thorac Surg 16:141, 1973.

Wernecke K, Vassalo P, Peters PE, van Bassewitz DB: Mediastinal tumors: Biopsy under US guidance. Radiology 172:473, 1989.

Wright CD, Kesler KA, Nichols CR et al: Primary mediastinal nonseminomatous germ cell tumors. Results of a multimodality approach. J Thorac Cardiovasc Surg 99:210, 1990.

Wright CD: Surgical management of mediastinal tumors and fibrosis. Semin Respir Crit Care Med 20:473, 1999.

Yellin A, Park HY, Burke JS, Benfield JR: Surgical management of lymphomas involving the chest. Ann Thorac Surg 44:363, 1987.

Yu GH, Sallany KE, Gokaslan ST et al: Thymic epithelial cells as a diagnostic pitfall in the fine-needle aspiration diagnosis of primary mediastinal lymphoma. Diagn Cytopathol 16:460, 1997.

Yüksel M, Panir N, Özer F et al: The principles of surgical management in dumbbell tumors. Eur J Cardiothorac Surg 10:569, 1996.

BIOLOGIC MARKERS OF THE MEDIASTINUM

Karen M. McGinnis
Celeste N. Powers
F. Deaver Thomas
Leslie J. Kohman

The mediastinum can be involved in a wide variety of disease processes, many of which present with a mediastinal mass. As these tumors often reside in relatively inaccessible locations within the mediastinum, diagnosis is often a challenge. Better understanding of the basic biology of many of these lesions has led to the development of several diagnostic techniques. These techniques include radionuclide imaging, serum biologic marker detection, and advances in tissue analysis using tissue tumor markers and cytologic techniques. This chapter explains the development and utility of these procedures, and the reader will gain an appreciation for the increasing need for collaboration among radiologist, pathologist, and clinician to provide accurate and specific preoperative diagnosis.

HISTORICAL NOTE

Although some solitary mediastinal masses are biologically inert, others represent ectopic tissue that secretes or takes up various biochemical compounds. While advances in radiologic examination of the mediastinum have allowed for greater elucidation of the anatomy of a lesion, advances in radionuclide imaging have served a complementary role that takes advantage of the tumor's biochemical characteristics. Graham and colleagues (1989) describe the events that led to modern nuclear medicine: the discovery of radioactivity by Becquerel in 1896, the development of the tracer principle, the widespread production of radionuclides during World War II, refinements in image scanning technology from the early point-counting technique to the rectilinear scanner in 1949, and the development of radiopharmaceuticals during the 1950s. The introduction of the scintillation camera in the 1970s had the greatest importance. More recently, single photon emission computed tomography and positron emission tomography technology have found application in mediastinal scanning, particularly in the infant technology of monoclonal antibody scanning.

Diagnostic histopathology has been practiced for well over a century, but it perhaps truly began with the publication of *Cellularpathologie* by Virchow in 1858. Although methods of tissue fixation, processing, and histochemical stains have advanced, the majority of diagnoses still rely on the subjective interpretation of the pathologist using light microscopy. However, after Coons and coworkers (1941) developed and applied the technique of immunofluorescence in the 1940s, the concept of using additional special techniques or stains to confirm the diagnosis became an important aspect of diagnostic histopathology. By the mid-1970s, new techniques such as immunohistochemistry, flow cytometry, and image analysis were developed and refined for diagnostic use.

Immunohistochemistry was first developed as a technique for use on tissue obtained by surgical biopsy, but today it is used with other cellular preparations, such as material derived from fine-needle aspiration and other body fluids. The usefulness of cytologic techniques has resulted in the development of a tremendous selection of antibodies directed against a variety of cellular components and products. Several antibodies apply specifically to the refinement of the diagnosis of mediastinal masses. Beginning in the 1960s (Nordenstrom, 1967), the mediastinum became ever more accessible to needle aspiration for cytologic analysis. Today many patients who would have required a surgical biopsy can receive a diagnosis through minimally invasive means.

■ *HISTORICAL READINGS*

Coons AH, Creeh HJ, Jones RN: Immunologic properties of an antibody containing a fluorescent group. Proc Soc Exp Biol 47:200, 1941.

Graham LS, Keriakes JG, Harris C, Cohen MB: Nuclear medicine from Becquerel to the present. Radiographics 9:1189, 1989.

Nordenström B: Paraxiphoid approach to the mediastinum for mediastinography and mediastinal needle biopsy: A preliminary report. Invest Radiol 2:141, 1967.

Virchow R: Cellular Pathology: As Based Upon Physiological and Pathological Histology. Translated and edited by Frank Chance. Classics in Medicine Library. Birmingham, AL, Division of Gryphon Editions Ltd., 1978.

THE BIOLOGIC BASIS FOR IMAGING OF MEDIASTINAL MASSES

SPECT Imaging

A variety of radiopharmaceuticals and imaging studies are used for imaging of mediastinal masses (Table 63–9). These studies are enhanced by the use of single photon emission computed tomography (SPECT) technology, which gives improved image contrast and three-dimensional (3-D) localization. SPECT has generally replaced conventional planar (two-dimensional) nuclear imaging.

TABLE 63–9 ■ **Nuclear Imaging Relevant to the Mediastinum**

Radiopharmaceutical, Radionuclide, or Radiochemical	*Label*	*Disease of Interest*
Iodine	^{131}I, ^{123}I	Retrosternal goiter, thyroid cancer
Monoclonal antibodies	^{111}In, ^{99m}Tc	Non-SCLC, colon and breast cancer, prostate cancer metastases
Octreotide	^{111}In	APUD tumors: carcinoid, gastrinoma, insulinoma, small cell lung, pheochromocytoma, glucagonoma, medullary thyroid carcinoma, paraganglioma
Gallium	^{67}Ga	Lymphoma, non-SCLC, melanoma
Sestamibi	^{99m}Tc	Medullary thyroid carcinoma, nonfunctional papillary or follicular thyroid carcinoma, Hürthle cell thyroid carcinoma, parathyroid adenoma or carcinoma
Thallium	^{201}Tl	See sestamibi
MIBG	^{131}I, ^{123}I	Pheochromocytoma, neuroblastoma; see also octreotide
Fluorodeoxyglucose	^{18}F	General oncologic imaging, breast and colon cancer, melanoma

MIBG, metaiodobenzylguanidine; non-SCLC, non–small cell lung cancer.

Although it is more time-consuming than the planar technique, SPECT has greater sensitivity, making it more cost and time effective. A typical SPECT chest examination takes 30 to 60 minutes, and image reconstruction requires another 5 to 10 minutes. The resultant study consists of orthogonal slices in the transverse, sagittal, and coronal axes as well as 3-D reconstruction of the chest and mediastinum. The transverse image set can be directly compared to other 3-D techniques such as computed tomography (CT) and magnetic resonance imaging (MRI).

Positron Emission Tomography Imaging

SPECT studies use single-photon emitters such as ^{99m}Tc, ^{111}In, and ^{67}Ga. In positron emission tomography (PET), dual-photon or positron emitters are used for very short lived radionuclides such as ^{11}C, ^{13}N, ^{15}O, and ^{18}F. Fluorine can be made remotely (at a regional cyclotron) and shipped to a local site, which is practical with its 110-minute half-life. The other radionuclides must be made in an on-site cyclotron because their half-lives are 20, 10, and 2 minutes, respectively.

Fluorodeoxyglucose F 18 (FDG-PET) is the major radionuclide in use for oncologic imaging; FDG-PET takes advantage of the increased glucose utilization of most malignancies (Coleman, 1991; Strauss, 1991). The development of regional distribution cyclotron sites around the world has produced a substantial increase in the availability of PET imaging, especially for oncologic work. Medical centers can expect to have PET imaging capabilities with capital investments of $1 to $2 million without requiring a similar investment in a local cyclotron. A U.S. Food and Drug Administration (FDA) approval of FDG-PET evaluation of single pulmonary nodules speaks to the efficacy of this approach in noninvasive techniques. It is expected that similar approval will be forthcoming for breast and lung cancer staging with FDG-PET.

Monoclonal Antibody Imaging

The FDA approval of labeled monoclonal antibodies (MoAb) specific to surface antigens of colon, ovarian, non–small cell lung (non-SCL), and prostate cancers has had a similar beneficial effect on SPECT in oncologic imaging (Fischman, 1989; Goldenberg, 1992). The standard radiolabels are ^{111}In, ^{123}I, and ^{99m}Tc with half-lives of 67, 12, and 6 hours, respectively. ^{111}In is the preferred radionuclide with intact MoAb agents that require a longer clearance time from the bloodstream. ^{99m}Tc or ^{123}I labels are chosen with MoAb fragments and their attendant shorter clearance times.

Receptor-Specific Imaging

In addition to MoAb development, a new field of imaging using receptor-specific agents has developed. Typical is the somatostatin analog octreotide, which, with the ^{111}In label, has an impressive affinity for the APUDomas (Krenning et al, 1993). These neuroectodermal neoplasms include carcinoids, insulinomas, gastrinomas, pheochromocytomas, small cell lung carcinomas, paragangliomas, glucagonomas, and medullary thyroid carcinomas. The presence of abundant somatostatin receptors in these tumors allows the detection of quite small primaries and metastases with this technique. The usual caveat with high sensitivity is the low specificity to be expected: Somatostatin receptors are also found in many other lesions such as non-SCLC, Hodgkin's disease, sarcoidosis, Wegener's granulomatosis, and tuberculosis, all of which demonstrate high sensitivity with the technique. In a patient with a clinical syndrome suggesting a neuroectodermal lesion, however, this agent can have great value. Not only is octreotide useful for localization and staging, it can also predict the efficacy of therapy with somatostatin (Sandostatin) with a positive imaging study. Pheochromocytomas and neuroblastomas are also readily detected with metaiodobenzylguanidine (MIBG), an epinephrine precursor, labeled with ^{131}I or ^{123}I (Spies, 1991).

Imaging of Thyroid Diseases Involving the Mediastinum

Retrosternal goiters present as anterior mediastinal masses that can be identified by functional imaging. CT imaging can delineate the anatomic characteristics, but radioiodine gives unequivocal identification. Most of these goiters have very poor iodine uptake due to compromise of the vascular supply that descends with the thyroid mass through the thoracic inlet. This produces necrosis, cystic degeneration, and irregular calcification mixed with islands of preserved functional tissue. Planar imaging with radioiodine is the standard imaging method, but SPECT imaging provides superior results (Chen, 1988). The best radioiodine isotope is ^{123}I, but it is not always readily available and several hours of delay after administration are required for optimal uptake (Park et al, 1984; Sandler et al, 1984). The more attractive alternatives are ^{99m}Tc as labels to pertechnetate or to sestamibi. ^{99m}Tc sestamibi imaging has the advantage of not requiring a normal level of hormonogenesis to image the thyroid, allowing its use in thyroid-stimulating hormone (TSH)–suppressed patients or those with recent iodine-containing contrast agent injections. Pertechnetate does not have the concentration characteristics of iodine (generally about one tenth of iodine's, but it can be given in much larger doses that produce a better image with SPECT. Both agents give optimal imaging within 15 minutes of administration, providing a substantial time advantage.

Thyroid malignancies may involve the mediastinum, either by direct extension from the neck or by metastatic nodal disease. The most common tumor is papillary carcinoma, which has a high frequency of local cervical nodal metastases and may involve mediastinal nodes in its more aggressive forms. In a case of near-total thyroidectomy, these metastases can be found with ^{131}I imaging and treated with the same radionuclide. The serum marker thyroglobulin is usually elevated with significant tumor residual and may additionally detect either nonfunctional metastases that do not concentrate iodine or micrometastases not yet visible on radioiodine imaging. Radioiodine therapy of micrometastases may still be of value, as evidenced by reduction of the thyroglobulin serum levels following treatment (Black and Sheppard, 1991; Lubin et al, 1994; Schlumberger et al, 1980). Nonfunctional metastases are usually found with sestamibi imaging and these may be surgically accessible. Follicular carcinoma is more aggressive and vascularly invasive, having a tendency for bone metastases, but frequently also lung metastases. It too responds to radioiodine therapy. Its nonfunctional and even more aggressive variant, Hürthle cell carcinoma, cannot be imaged or treated with radioiodine, but it is readily imaged with sestamibi. The least differentiated form, anaplastic carcinoma, carries the worst prognosis, with patient survival typically less than 6 months after diagnosis (Nel et al, 1985). This tumor usually arises from inadequately treated differentiated papillary or follicular cancers of long-standing, and while the still-differentiated components may concentrate iodine, the lethal spindle and giant cells do not. There is usually mediastinal involvement as a result of extension of tumor down the trachea. External-beam radiation therapy should be the first therapeutic modality following surgery, but the outlook is dismal despite aggressive management. Medullary thyroid carcinoma is not of follicular origin but arises from parafollicular (C cell) elements (Williams, 1989). This tumor has its own serum marker (calcitonin) and imaging requirements (sestamibi or octreotide; see Receptor-Specific Imaging). Mediastinal involvement with metastatic nodes is the rule when extrathyroidal disease ensues. Surgical removal of localized tumor is curative, but metastatic disease may be responsive to somatostatin therapy.

Gallium Imaging

Gallium citrate Ga 67 is the standby for lymphoma imaging in the chest and mediastinum. Larger doses (9 mCi) and SPECT have raised the sensitivity to levels that allow confident assessment of residual or recurrent disease when anatomic imaging may be confounded by nodal fibrosis post-therapy (Kostakoglu et al, 1992; Tumeh et al, 1987). Gallium is very dependable for Hodgkin's disease, and most differentiated lymphomas can also be detected. Less differentiated lymphomas may require thailium 201 or ^{99m}Tc sestamibi imaging. Gallium is also quite useful for non-SCLC staging, detection of melanoma metastases, and detection of hepatomas.

Parathyroid Imaging

Earlier techniques to detect parathyroid adenomas or carcinomas used two radionuclides: ^{201}Tl for the parathyroid and thyroid tissue and ^{99m}Tc pertechnetate for the thyroid alone. Image subtraction (Tl minus Tc) gave the resultant parathyroid tissue (Young et al, 1983). The frequent pitfall was maintaining the patient's neck position through both studies, with errors in subtraction producing false-negative or false-positive results (Broughan et al, 1987). The current technique uses a single injection of sestamibi with sequential images obtained 15 minutes and 2 hours after injection (Taillefer et al, 1992). The thyroid gland "washes out" the sestamibi more rapidly than the parathyroid tissue, allowing differentiation of the adenoma. The differential diagnosis of a confounding thyroid adenoma (which can mimic parathyroid kinetics) can be done by a second study using ^{99m}Tc pertechnetate, which concentrates in the thyroid adenoma but not the parathyroid adenoma. Ectopic parathyroid tumors in the mediastinum are usually detected using SPECT and the sestamibi agent alone. There is sufficient concentration of sestamibi to allow a hand-held surgical gamma probe to assist in the surgical removal of these tumors from the neck or chest. (Sestamibi has generally superseded thallium in the detection of malignancies because its imaging characteristics are better.)

Serum Biochemical Markers

Neoplastic cells often produce biologic products that distinguish them from normal cells. These biologic products, called "tumor markers," may be the expression of new gene products, altered amounts of normal gene products, alterations in chromosomal DNA, or many other structural or functional cellular properties (Fenoglio-Prieser and Willman, 1987; Robinson and Radosevich, 1991; Sano et al, 1991). The biologic properties may be readily detected through analysis of serum, urine, cyst fluid, or tissue. Radioimmunoassay (RIA) or enzyme immunoassay (EIA) technologies use monoclonal antibodies to help detect products released into the serum. In most mediastinal tumors, the serum markers resemble tissue markers (Robinson and Radosevich, 1991). Markers relevant to the mediastinum include α-fetoprotein (AFP), human chorionic gonadotropin β (β-HCG), catecholamines and their degradation products, parathyroid hormone (PTH), and lactate dehydrogenase (LDH). The pattern of increased serum levels of these proteins can specifically diagnose certain tumors, particularly in the case of mediastinal germ cell tumors.

AFP and β-HCG are useful tumor markers in the diagnosis and differentiation of germ cell tumors. Pure seminomas have no AFP and little (≤ 100 ng/ml) or no β-HCG (Hainsworth and Greco, 1991a). The small amount of β-HCG (present in approximately 10% of seminomas) originates in syncytiotrophoblasts scattered throughout the tumor. Higher levels suggest the additional presence of nonseminomatous elements (Hainsworth and Greco, 1991a). More than 90% of malignant nonseminomatous germ cell tumors produce either β-HCG or AFP. Eighty percent to 90% of patients with nonseminomatous germ cell tumors also have elevated serum levels of LDH, directly proportional to tumor volume (Brindley and Francis, 1963; Friedman et al, 1980). Patients with yolk sac tumor (endodermal sinus tumor), embryonal carcinoma, or teratocarcinoma have elevated levels of AFP, while those with choriocarcinomas have increased β-HCG. Levels of AFP or β-HCG greater than 500 ng/ml are diagnostic of malignant nonseminomatous germ cell tumor, and these patients may receive chemotherapy without biopsy confirmation (Hainsworth and Greco, 1991a). There are no serum tumor markers of use in patients with benign teratoma (Nichols, 1991).

In addition to facilitating the diagnosis of germ cell tumors, these tumor markers have been described as a useful tool in the detection of recurrence of these tumors (Chan et al, 1996). An interesting phenomenon is a growing mass seen following successful chemotherapy with normalization of tumor markers. This is referred to as the growing teratoma syndrome, and it has been reviewed by Afifi and co-workers (1997).

Carcinoembryonic antigen (CEA), an oncofetal antigen useful in the diagnosis of gastrointestinal, breast, and lung malignancies, does not play a part in the diagnosis of malignant mediastinal germ cell tumors (Robinson and Radosevich, 1991). There is an isolated report of an increase in serum CEA in a patient with a teratoma, but the serum elevation was much less significant than the dramatic elevation of CEA in the cyst fluid (Ono, 1996). Placental alkaline phosphatase (PLAP), a nonspecific marker, typically contributes little to the diagnosis.

Antidiuretic hormone (ADH), a biologic product more commonly associated with lung malignancies, has been reported to be produced by thymic neuroblastomas (Argani et al, 1997). The syndrome of ADH secretion by this tumor was confirmed by immunohistochemical analysis of the tumor cells. Additional serum studies that may help to substantiate various clinical impressions include PTH (parathyroid tumor), catecholamine levels (pheochromocytoma), and ferritin (neuroblastoma or ganglioneuroblastoma).

Thyroid markers have been described earlier in this subchapter. Thyroglobulin can function as a tumor marker, particularly for differentiated, nonmedullary thyroid carcinoma (Van Herle and Uller, 1975). Anaplastic thyroid carcinomas and oxyphilic cells present in differentiated thyroid carcinoma may lack the capacity to synthesize thyroglobulin (Müller-Gärtner and Schneider, 1988). Tumors with papillary characteristics, metastatic nodes in the neck or mediastinum, or small tumor volumes present similar problems. Müller-Gärtner and Schneider addressed these problems by recommending that the evaluation of a mediastinal mass suspected of representing a metastasis from such a tumor should include a determination of the serum thyroglobulin concentrations under endogenous TSH stimulation, as well as high-resolution ultrasonography of the neck and other imaging studies of the mediastinum (Müller-Gärtner and Schneider, 1988).

If analysis of radionuclide examinations and serum markers fails to make a diagnosis of a mediastinal tumor, tissue obtained either by cyst aspiration or fine-needle aspiration may assist in the analysis. Finally, surgical biopsy may be required for the final diagnostic maneuver (Ferguson et al, 1987; Shields, 1991).

Immunohistochemical Tumor Markers

Although serum studies can prove useful in the diagnostic workup, examination of tissue from the mediastinal mass remains a vital part of definitive diagnosis. Pathologists now routinely supplement standard histologic examination with immunofluorescence and immunohistochemistry, both of which rely on the localization of specific antigens by antibodies marked with a visualizable compound. Immunofluorescence uses a fluorochrome responsive to excitation by ultraviolet light. Immunohistochemistry uses various chromagens induced through enzymatic reactions, and by virtue of its easier methodology has become a standard diagnostic technique available to most practicing pathologists. It has a high degree of sensitivity and specificity and can be used successfully on formalin-fixed, paraffin-embedded tissue (Hsu et al, 1981; Taylor, 1978).

The first stage in the diagnosis of any neoplasm involves the determination of what broad category it belongs to, that is, epithelial, mesenchymal, or hematopoietic. Light microscopy alone can often accomplish this; however, if the tumor is poorly differentiated, an immunohistochemical panel of antibodies directed against various cellular proteins assists in the classification (Table 63–10). The antibodies selected for these screening panels may vary; four common choices are leukocyte common antigen (LCA) for lymphoma, cytokeratins for carcinoma, vimentin for sarcoma, and S-100, a calcium-binding protein useful in the identification of melanomas and neural lesions (Battifora et al, 1980; Taylor, 1978).

More specific antibody panels can further subclassify neoplasms. A panel using AFP and β-HCG can often distinguish between the various types of germ cell tumors and indicate the presence of one or more unsuspected components within these tumors (Table 63–11). A lymphocyte typing panel can likewise subclassify the lym-

TABLE 63–10 ■ **Antibodies Useful in the Diagnosis of Mediastinal Masses**

Antibody	*Antigen Type*	*Usefulness*
S-100	Ca^{2+} binding protein	Melanoma; neural tumors
LCA	Membrane glycoprotein	Lymphoma
Cytokeratin	Intracellular proteins	Epithelial differentiation
Vimentin	Intermediate filament	Mesenchymal lesions
Immunoglobulins	Proteins	Subtyping lymphomas
Leu-M1	Protein: monocyte/granulocyte	Hodgkin's disease
β-HCG	Hormone secreted by syncytiotrophoblasts	Germ cell tumors, especially choriocarcinoma
AFP	Plasma glycoprotein	Embryonal carcinoma

AFP, α-fetoprotein; β-HCG, human chorionic gonadotropin β; LCA, leukocyte common antigen.

phomas. This panel consists of a variety of surface antigens to distinguish T cells and the various heavy and light chains to further characterize B cell lymphomas. These immunoglobulin (Ig) components may include γ and α heavy chains, IgG, IgA, and the κ and λ light chains.

Although immunohistochemical techniques have improved the field of diagnostic pathology, these techniques also have pitfalls. For instance, staining for neuron-specific enolase no longer plays a significant part in tumor identification. Certain isoenzymes of this glycolytic enzyme seem to occur preferentially in neurons and certain endocrine cells. Unfortunately, it has a wide distribution in many types of tissue. This lack of specificity makes this marker of little use in the diagnosis of neuroectodermal and neuroendocrine neoplasms. A thorough knowledge of the various artifacts associated with immunohistochemistry, careful attention to the actual performance of the technique, and the use of appropriate controls can avert most of these problems.

Electron Microscopy

Electron microscopy can also provide supplemental information in the workup of neoplasms of the mediastinum (Davis et al, 1987), although its use has decreased since the advent of immunohistochemistry (Berkman et al, 1983; Dabbs and Silverman, 1988; Dardick et al, 1991; Neill and Silverman, 1992; Rosai and Rodriguez, 1968). This technique can usually classify undifferentiated tumors into one of four major categories: carcinoma, malignant lymphoma, malignant melanoma, and sarcoma. Distinctive cytoplasmic structures observed only at the ultrastructural level may indicate differentiation of the lesion beyond that suspected by light microscopy. For example, light microscopy may reveal a tumor composed of large pleomorphic cells with a high nuclear-to-cytoplasmic ratio but no other distinctive features that suggest a specific classification. Ultrastructural examination may reveal premelanosomes indicating melanoma, or well-defined junctional complexes (desmosomes) and scattered tonofibrils suggesting a carcinoma. This technique may also help to further classify small round cell tumors, neuroendocrine neoplasms, and mesotheliomas (Dardick et al, 1991; Rosai and Rodriguez, 1968; Taccagni et al, 1988). Electron microscopy cannot, however, aid in the diagnosis of germ cell tumors, as they do not have any diagnostic ultrastructural features (Hainsworth and Greco, 1991b).

TABLE 63–11 ■ **Tumor Markers in Various Germ Cell Tumors**

Germ Cell Tumor	*AFP*	*β-HCG*
Embryonal carcinoma	+	−
Embryonal carcinoma with syncytiotrophoblasts	+	+
Choriocarcinoma	−	+
Yolk sac tumor	+	+
Teratoma	−	−
Teratoma with embryonal carcinoma	+	−
Seminoma	−	−
Seminoma with syncytiotrophoblasts	−	+

AFP, α-fetoprotein; β-HCG, human chorionic gonadotropin β.

Cytologic Needle Biopsy

Most tumors of the mediastinum require cytologic or histologic confirmation of the clinical diagnosis prior to specific therapy. Methods of obtaining tissue range from fine-needle aspiration (FNA) to excisional biopsy. The choice of a particular method depends in large measure on the clinical and radiologic impression, the location of the mass, and the medical condition of the patient.

FNA provides a safe, cost-effective, and rapid means to diagnosis. Clinical indications for this modality have recently expanded due to the development of specific cytologic criteria, and the use of ancillary immunohistochemical, flow cytometric, and molecular diagnostic techniques that result in accurate diagnoses from cytologic material. The diagnostic accuracy of FNA varies with the experience of those who perform it, as well as the expertise of those who interpret the material obtained. In general, accuracy rates range between 85% and 95% (Ikezoe et al, 1984, 1990; Powers et al, 1996; Rosenberger and Adler, 1978; Sterrett et al, 1983; Weisbrod et al, 1984; Westcott, 1981). Maximum benefit from the technique requires close communication among pathologist, radiologist, and clinician. In the vast majority of mediastinal lesions, FNA takes place with radiologic guidance, most commonly CT (Colquhoun et al, 1991; Moinuddin et al, 1984; Nordenstrom, 1967; van Sonnenberg et al, 1988; Weisbrod et al, 1984). Ultrasonically guided needle biopsy, either aspiration or cutting, may offer advantages in some cases (Ikezoe et al, 1984, 1990; Pedersen et al, 1986; Saito et al, 1988; Sawhney et al, 1991; Yang et al, 1992; Yu et al, 1991). Recently, endoscopic ultrasound (EUS)–guided FNA biopsy has been used with increasing frequency (Bentz et al, 1998; Gupta et al, 1998). Ultrasound often gives better definition of some masses than fluoroscopy, avoids the cost of CT, and allows real-time observation of the needle within the mass. However, it cannot be used for lesions in the middle mediastinum or masses that do not abut the chest wall because aerated lung hinders the signal.

Most mediastinal lesions have well-documented diagnostic criteria (Cristallini et al, 1992; Koss et al, 1984; Powers, 1998; Sterrett, 1983; Todd et al, 1981). FNA can often provide an immediate differential diagnosis of these mediastinal lesions based on cytomorphology alone (Table 63–12) (Geisinger, 1995). Often the clinical presentation, radiologic findings, and specific cytomorphologic patterns result in an initial classification of the mass as metastatic carcinoma, malignant lymphoma, thymoma, germ cell tumor, or neural lesion. Certain lesions such as seminoma, malignant lymphoma, or metastatic small cell carcinoma have characteristic patterns on aspiration smears that make an immediate diagnosis possible. Other more difficult lesions may require further study, which typically includes ancillary techniques (Geisinger, 1995; Nadji, 1980; Powers, 1994; Slagel et al, 1997; Taylor, 1986). Occasionally, errors occur in subclassifications based only on light microscopy. These problems usually arise in cases of insufficient material for supplementary analysis. For example, with no tissue available for marker studies, large malignant cells with no further distinguishing features could represent poorly differentiated carcinoma or a germ cell tumor, such as embryonal carcinoma (Koss et al, 1984; Singh et al, 1997).

A core needle biopsy, processed as a histologic specimen, may provide better diagnostic material than FNA when the lesion is fibrotic or if the FNA yields scant material.

One of the most controversial areas in FNA revolves around malignant lymphomas. Several studies indicate that malignant lymphomas can be diagnosed as well as subtyped by FNA (Al-Sharabati et al, 1991; Das et al, 1991; Erwin et al, 1986; Koo et al, 1989; Pontifex and Klimo, 1984; Silverman et al, 1993; Sneige et al, 1990; Wittich et al, 1992). FNA usually yields adequate material for immunohistochemistry or flow cytometry. Flow cytometry allows rapid measurement of one or more parameters of individual cells. With appropriate staining, that is, "marking," a lymphoma may be typed just as accurately as with immunohistochemistry. This method, however, requires a substantial number of cells. Usually, a dedicated pass with the fine needle yields sufficient cells to allow processing by flow cytometry (Diamond et al, 1982; Koss et al, 1989). These methods document monoclonality and also subtype the lymphoma as T cell or B cell. Either procedure can further characterize B cell lymphoma into specific heavy and light chain type.

The diagnosis of Hodgkin's disease (HD) by FNA also provides a challenge, although specific cytologic criteria, similar to histologic criteria, have been delineated (Friedman et al, 1980; Kardos et al, 1986). Reed-Sternberg cells or their variants, when present, are quite useful and either alone or in conjunction with immunohistochemistry permit a diagnosis of HD. However, Reed-Sternberg cells are infrequent in aspirates from certain types of HD, and in addition, nodular sclerosing HD often yields scant material because of the dense sclerotic stroma. Although aspirates in these situations may be suspicious for HD, definitive diagnosis requires open biopsy.

Thymoma presents another type of challenge for the pathologist interpreting mediastinal FNAs (Ali and Erozan, 1998; Shin and Katz, 1998). Depending on tumor type, the aspirate may contain varying numbers of bland epithelial cells and small lymphocytes. Although lymphocytes may predominate in a grade 1 lesion, they are usually small with regular round nuclei and easily distinguished from the larger lymphocytes with convoluted nuclei often seen in malignant large cell lymphomas (Ali and Erozan, 1998; Battifora et al, 1980; Hoda et al, 1991; Powers, 1998).

Aspirates of germ cell tumors usually show large, discohesive malignant cells with variable numbers of mature lymphocytes scattered throughout the tumor (Collins et al, 1995). Although the cytomorphology of these cells may allow correct categorization as a germ cell tumor, immunochemistry often permits a more specific classification (Battifora et al, 1984; Miettinem et al, 1985; Suster et al, 1998).

Tumors of peripheral nerve origin, such as those occurring in the posterior mediastinum, may also cause problems in FNA diagnosis. Because these neurogenic tumors often have a firm consistency, the aspirate fre-

TABLE 63–12 ■ **Differential Diagnosis Based on Cytomorphology**

Lymphocytes
Malignant lymphoma
Thymoma
Seminoma
Lymphocyte-predominant Hodgkin's disease
Lymphoid hyperplasia
Castleman's disease
Spindle Cells
Spindle cell thymoma
Schwannoma
Atypical carcinoid tumor
Melanoma, spindle cell type
Nodular sclerosing Hodgkin's disease
Mesenchymal spindle cell lesions
Small Cells
Small cell carcinoma
Malignant lymphoma
Carcinoid tumor
Thymoma
Neuroblastoma
Large Cells
Metastatic pleomorphic carcinoma
Ganglioneuroblastoma
Thymic carcinoma
Malignant lymphoma
Melanoma
Hodgkin's disease

quently yields limited material. In addition, cytology alone may not allow distinction between schwannoma and neurofibroma, and between ganglioneuroma and ganglioneuroblastoma. Frequently patients with these differential diagnoses go on to surgical excision without the need for a more specific preoperative diagnosis.

Diagnosis by FNA may fail for several reasons. Sometimes the patient cannot achieve or maintain the appropriate position, or he or she may not cooperate. Technical problems include air drying of the specimen, excessive blood diluting the sample, or difficulty in targeting the lesion. Experience obviates most of these problems as well as most interpretive dilemmas.

FNA often provides a reliable diagnosis, with less cost and complications than surgical biopsy of the mediastinum, particularly since many of these lesions require nonsurgical treatment. Rapid staining techniques allow the cytopathologist to render an interpretation of the aspiration specimen within minutes after a radiologically guided FNA. Such rapid assessments can indicate the need for additional material, or to proceed as appropriate to glutaraldehyde staining for electron microscopy, saline for flow cytometry, or tissue culture medium for immunohistochemistry and cytogenetics.

Cytogenetic Markers

Hainsworth and Greco (1991a) forecast an increasing role for analysis of specific genetic abnormalities in the diagnosis of poorly differentiated neoplasms. High-resolution chromosomal analysis has detected three specific chromosomal abnormalities, correlated with different histologic subtypes, in tissue from non-Hodgkin's lymphoma (Yunis et al, 1982). Bloomfield and associates (1983) found recurring chromosomal abnormalities in lymphoma samples, and they concluded that all lymphomas have cytogenetic abnormalities. Detection of gene rearrangements can help to establish a diagnosis of lymphoma in a puzzling neoplasm and to correctly classify T and B cell lymphomas (Arnold et al, 1983). Germ cell tumors also exhibit cytogenetic abnormalities (Bosl et al, 1989, Dmitrovsky et al, 1990). These characteristics may aid in the classification of mediastinal malignancies of uncertain origin. Some of these patients respond to chemotherapeutic regimens designed for germ cell tumors (Hainsworth and Greco, 1991b; Motzer et al, 1991); as genetic analysis becomes more sophisticated and clinically applicable, some of these tumors may be reclassified as germ cell neoplasms. Samaniego and colleagues (1990) reported on a large series of germ cell tumors studied by cytogenetics, including for the first time a series of primary mediastinal tumors. They found distinctive abnormalities of chromosome 12 as well as cytologic evidence of gene amplification. In the future, cytogenetic analysis will certainly contribute to diagnostic accuracy of many mediastinal malignancies.

COMMENTARY AND CONTROVERSIES

The use of FNA aspiration biopsy has increased in recent years due to two main factors. First, cytologic technique has advanced to the point at which explicit cytologic criteria now allow a wide variety of specific diagnoses, both benign and malignant. Second, this minimally invasive and cost-effective procedure has gained the enthusiastic support of patients, physicians, and hospitals. More pathologists now receive specific training in the performance and interpretation of the procedure. Many medical centers have now established FNA services, headed by someone who has special training and motivation in this modality. This professional works collaboratively with clinician, radiologist, and pathologist to achieve the best and quickest diagnosis.

The diagnosis and typing of lymphoma by cytology remains a controversial area. Dogma has long held that an entire lymph node must be examined to achieve a diagnosis because precise classification depends on architectural features. Also, pathologists without specific training in cytologic procedures and their interpretation feel more comfortable with tissue than with cells when making a diagnosis. The original classification of lymphoma types did indeed rely on architecture, but now a pathologist with specific training in these techniques should be able to provide general classification of lymphomas into categories of large cell, small lymphocytic cell, lymphoblastic, and HD. Most patients can receive treatment based on such a categorization.

C. P.

REFERENCES

Afifi HY, Bosl GJ, Burt ME: Mediastinal growing teratoma syndrome. Ann Thorac Surg 64:359–362, 1997.

Ali SZ, Erozan YS: Thymoma. Cytopathologic features and differential diagnosis on fine needle aspiration. Acta Cytol 42:845–854, 1998.

Al-Sharabati M, Chittal S, Duga-Neulat I et al: Primary anterior mediastinal B-cell lymphoma. Cancer 67:2579, 1991.

Argani P, Erlandson RA, Rosai J: Thymic neuroblastoma in adults: Report of three cases with special emphasis on its association with the syndrome of inappropriate secretion of antidiuretic hormone. Am J Clin Pathol 108:537–543, 1997.

Arnold A, Crossman J, Bakhshi A et al: Immunoglobulin-gene rearrangements as unique clonal markers in human lymphoid neoplasms. N Engl J Med 309:1593, 1983.

Battifora H, Sheibini K, Tubbs RR et al: Antikeratin antibodies in tumor diagnosis: Distinction between seminoma and embryonal carcinoma. Cancer 54:843, 1984.

Battifora H, Sun TT, Bahu RM: The use of antikeratin antiserum as a diagnostic tool: thymoma vs lymphoma. Hum Pathol 11:635, 1980.

Bentz JS, Kochman ML, Faigel DO et al: Endoscopic ultrasound-guided real-time-fine-needle aspiration: Clinicopathologic features of 60 patients. Diagn Cytopathol 18:98–190, 1998.

Berkman WA, Chowdhury L, Brown NL, Padleckas R: Value of electron microscopy in cytologic diagnosis of fine-needle biopsy. AJR Am J Roentgenol 140:1253, 1983.

Black EG, Sheppard MC: Serum thyroglobulin measurements in thyroid cancer: Evaluation of "false positive" results. Clin Endocrinol 35:519, 1991.

Bloomfield CD, Arthur DC, Frizzera G et al: Nonrandom chromosome abnormalities in lymphoma. Cancer Res 43:2975, 1983.

Bosl GJ, Dmitrovsky E, Reuter V et al: i(12p): A specific karyotypic abnormality in germ cell tumors (Abstract). Proc Am Soc Clin Oncol 8:131, 1989.

Brindley LO, Francis FL: Serum lactate dehydrogenase and glutamine-oxalacetic transaminase correlations with measurements of tumor markers during therapy. Cancer Res 23:112, 1963.

Broughan TA, O'Donnell JK, Kropilak MD, Esselstyn CB Jr: Use of thallium-technetium parathyroid scans. Cleve Clin J Med 54:179, 1987.

Chan AT, Ho S, Yim AP et al: Primary mediastinal malignant germ cell tumor: Single institution experience in Chinese patients and correlation with specific alpha-fetoprotein bands. Acta Oncol 35:221–227, 1996.

Chen JJ, LaFrance ND et al: Iodine-123 SPECT of the thyroid in multinodular goiter. J Nucl Med 29:110, 1988.

Coleman RE: Single photon emission computed tomography and positron emission tomography in cancer imaging. Cancer 67:1261, 1991.

Collins KA, Geisinger KR, Wakely PE Jr et al: Extragonadal germ cell tumors: A fine-needle aspiration biopsy study. Diagn Cytopathol 12:223–229, 1995.

Colquhoun SD, Rosenthal DL, Morton DL: Role of percutaneous fine-needle aspiration biopsy in suspected intrathoracic malignancy. Ann Thorac Surg 51:390, 1991.

Coons AH, Creeh HJ, Jones RN: Immunologic properties of an antibody containing a fluorescent group. Proc Soc Exp Biol 47:200, 1941.

Cristallini EG, Ascani S, Farabi R et al: Fine needle aspiration biopsy in the diagnosis of intrathoracic masses. Acta Cytol 36:416, 1992.

Dabbs DJ, Silverman JF: Selective use of electron microscopy in fine needle aspiration cytology. Acta Cytol 32:880, 1988.

Dardick I, Yazdi HM, Brosko RT et al: A quantitative comparison of light and electron microscopic diagnoses in specimens obtained by fine-needle aspiration biopsy. Ultrastruct Pathol 15:105, 1991.

Das DK, Gupta SK, Datta BN, Sharma SC: FNA cytodiagnosis of non-Hodgkin's lymphoma and its subtyping under working formulation of 175 cases. Diagn Cytopathol 7:487, 1991.

Davis RD Jr, Oldham HN Jr, Sabiston DC Jr: Primary cysts and neoplasms of the mediastinum: Recent changes in clinical presentation, methods of diagnosis, management, and results. Ann Thorae Surg 44:229, 1987.

Diamond LW, Nathwani BN, Rappaport H: Flow cytometry in the diagnosis and classifications of malignant lymphomas and leukemia. Cancer 50:1122, 1982.

Dmitrovsky E, Murty VVVS, Moy D et al: Isochromosome 12p in non-seminoma cell lines: Karyologic amplification of c-ki-ras$_2$ without point-mutational activation. Oncogene 5:543, 1990.

Erwin BC, Brynes RK, Chan WC et al: Percutaneous needle biopsy in the diagnosis and classification of lymphoma. Cancer 57:1074, 1986.

Fenoglio-Preiser CM, Willman CL: Molecular biology and the pathologist. Arch Pathol Lab Med 111:601, 1987.

Ferguson MK, Lee E, Skinner DB, Little AG: Selective operative approach for diagnosis and treatment of anterior mediastinal masses. Ann Thorac Surg 44:583, 1987.

Fischman AJ, Khaw BA, Strauss HW: Quo vadis radioimmune imaging. J Nucl Med 30:1911, 1989.

Friedman A, Vugrin D, Golvey R et al: Prognostic significance of serum tumor biomarkers (TM) alfa fetoprotein (AFP), beta subunit chorionic gonadotropin (βHCG) and lactate dehydrogenase (LDH) in non-seminomatous germ cell tumors (Abstract). Proc Am Soc Clin Oncol 21:223, 1980.

Friedman M, Kim U, Shimaoka K et al: Appraisal of aspiration cytology in management of Hodgkin's disease. Cancer 45:1653, 1980.

Geisinger KR: Differential diagnostic considerations and potential pitfalls in fine-needle aspiration biopsies of the mediastinum. Diagn Cytopathol 13:436, 1995.

Goldenberg DM, Larson SM: Radioimmunodetection in cancer identification. J Nucl Med 33:803, 1992.

Graham LS, Keriakes JG, Harris C, Cohen MB: Nuclear medicine from Becquerel to the present. Radiographics 9:1189, 1989.

Gupta S, Gulati M, Rajwanshi A et al: Sonographically guided fine-needle aspiration biopsy of superior mediastinal lesions by the suprasternal route. AJR Am Roentgenol 171:1303, 1998.

Hainsworth JD, Greco FA: General features of malignant germ cell tumors and primary seminomas of the mediastinum. In Shields TW (ed): Mediastinal Surgery. Malvern, PA, Lea & Febiger, 1991a.

Hainsworth JD, Greco FA: Poorly differentiated carcinoma and germ cell tumors. Hematol Oncol Clin North Am 5:1223, 1991b.

Hoda SA, Warren GP, Zaman MB: Extrathoracic metastatic malignant thymoma: Diagnosis by aspiration cytology. Arch Pathol Lab Med 115:399, 1991.

Hsu SM, Raine L, Fanger H: Use of avidin-biotin-peroxidase complex (ABC) in immunoperoxidase techniques. J Histochem Cytochem 29:577, 1981.

Ikezoe J, Morimoto S, Arisawa J et al: Percutaneous biopsy of thoracic lesions. AJR Am J Roentgenol 154:1181, 1990.

Ikezoe J, Sone S, Higashihara T et al: Sonographically guided needle biopsy for diagnosis of thoracic lesions. AJR Am J Roentgenol 143:229, 1984.

Kardos TF, Vinson JH, Behm FG et al: Hodgkin's disease: Diagnosis by fine-needle aspiration biopsy. Am J Clin Pathol 86:286, 1986.

Koo CH, Rappaport H, Sheibani K et al: Imprint cytology of non-Hodgkin's lymphomas. Hum Pathol 20 (Suppl):1, 1989.

Koss LG, Czerniak B, Herz F, Wersto RP: Flow cytometric measurements of DNA and other cell components in human tumors: A critical appraisal. Hum Pathol 20:528, 1989.

Koss LG, Woyke S, Olszewski W: Aspiration Biopsy: Cytologic Interpretation and Histologic Basis. New York, Igaku-Shoin, 1984.

Kostakoglu L, Yeh SDJ, Portlock C et al: Validation of gallium-67-citrate single-photon emission computed tomography in biopsy-confirmed residual Hodgkin's disease in the mediastinum. J Nucl Med 33:345, 1992.

Krenning EP, Kwekkeboom DJ, Bakker WH et al: Somatostatin receptor scintigraphy with [^{111}In-DTPA-D-Phe^{1}]– and [^{123}I-Tyr-3-]-octreotide: The Rotterdam experience with more than 1000 patients. Eur J Nucl Med 20:716, 1993.

Lubin E, Mechlis-Frish S, Zatz S: Serum thyroglobulin and iodine-131 whole-body scan in the diagnosis and assessment of treatment for metastatic differentiated thyroid carcinoma. J Nucl Med 35:257, 1994.

McKitrick WL, Park HM, Kosegi JE: Parallax error in pinhole thyroid scintigraphy: A critical consideration in the evaluation of substernal goiters. J Nucl Med 26:418, 1985.

Miettinem M, Virtanen I, Talerman A: Intermediate filament proteins in human testes and testicular germ cell tumors. Am J Pathol 120:402, 1985.

Millar J, Allen R, Wakefield JS et al: Diagnosis of thymoma by fine-needle aspiration cytology: Light and electron microscopic study of a case. Diagn Cytopathol 3:166, 1987.

Moinuddin SM, Lee LH, Montgomery JH: Mediastinal needle biopsy. AJR Am J Roentgenol 143:531, 1984.

Motzer RJ, Rodriguez E, Reuter VE et al: Genetic analysis as an aid in diagnosis for patients with midline carcinomas of uncertain histologies. J Natl Cancer Inst 83:341, 1991.

Müller-Gärtner H-W, Schneider C: Clinical evaluation of tumor characteristics predisposing serum thyroglobulin to be undetectable in patients with differentiated thyroid cancer. Cancer 61:976, 1988.

Myers JD: Development and application of immunocytochemical staining techniques. Diagn Cytopathol 5:318, 1989.

Nadji M: The potential value of immunoperoxidase techniques in diagnostic cytology. Acta Cytol 2405:442, 1980.

Neill J, Silverman JF: Electron microscopy of fine-needle aspiration biopsies of the mediastinum. Diagn Cytopathol 8:272, 1992.

Nel CJ, van Heerden JA, Goellner JR et al: Anaplastic carcinoma of the thyroid: a clinicopathologic study of 82 cases. Mayo Clin Proc 60:51, 1985.

Nichols CR: Mediastinal germ cell tumors: Clinical features and biologic correlates. Chest 99:472, 1991.

Nordenström B: Paraxiphoid approach to the mediastinum for mediastinography and mediastinal needle biopsy: A preliminary report. Invest Radiol 2:141, 1967.

Ono Y, Sawa Y, Yokoyama H et al: Matured mediastinal teratoma with high levels of tumor markers in cystic fluid. Nihon Kyobu 34:1359, 1996.

Park H-M, Tarver RD, Siddiqui AR et al: Efficacy of thyroid scintigraphy in the diagnosis of intrathoracic goiter. AJR Am J Roentgenol 148:527, 1984.

Pedersen OM, Aasen TB, Gulsvic A: Fine-needle aspiration biopsy of mediastinal and peripheral pulmonary masses guided by real-time sonography. Chest 89:504, 1986.

Pontifex AH, Klimo P: Application of aspiration biopsy cytology to lymphomas. Cancer 53:553, 1984.

Powers CN: Mediastinal fine-needle aspiration. In Atkinson BF, Silverman JF (eds): Atlas of Difficult Diagnoses in Cytopathology. Philadelphia, WB Saunders, 1998.

Powers CN, Silverman JF, Geisinger RR, Frable WJ: Fine-needle aspiration biopsy of the mediastinum: A multi-institutional study. Am J Clin Pathol 105:168, 1996.

Powers CN, Verardo MD, Frable WJ: Fine-needle aspiration biopsy:

Pitfalls in the diagnosis of spindle-cell lesions. Diagn Cytopathol 10:232, 1994.

Robinson PG, Radosevich JA: Mediastinal tumor markers. In Shields TW (ed): Mediastinal Surgery. Malvern PA, Lea & Febiger, 1991.

Rosai J, Rodriguez HA: Application of electron microscopy to the differential diagnosis of tumors. Am J Clin Pathol 50:555, 1968.

Rosenberger A, Adler O: Fine needle aspiration biopsy in the diagnosis of mediastinal lesions. AJR Am J Roentgenol 131:239, 1978.

Saito T, Kobayashi H, Sugama Y et al: Ultrasonically guided needle biopsy in the diagnosis of mediastinal masses. Am Rev Respir Dis 138:679, 1988.

Samaniego F, Rodriquez E, Houldsworth J et al: Cytogenetic and molecular analysis of human male germ cell tumors: Chromosome 12 abnormalities and gene amplification. Genes Chromosomes Cancer 1:289, 1990.

Sandler MP, Patton JA, Sacks GA et al: Evaluation of intrathoracic goiter with I-123 scintigraphy and nuclear magnetic resonance imaging. J Nucl Med 25:874, 1984.

Sano T, Kuramochi S, Takahashi M et al: A case of thymic cyst with elevated sialylated Lewis X-i, carbohydrate antigen 19–9 and tissue polypeptide antigen in the cystic fluid with no elevation of serum tumor markers. Jpn J Clin Oncol 21:388, 1991.

Sawhney S, Jain R, Berry M: Tru-Cut biopsy of mediastinal masses guided by real-time sonography. Clin Radiol 44:16, 1991.

Schlumberger M, Charbord P, Fragu P et al: Circulating thyroglobulin and thyroid hormones in patients with metastases of differentiated thyroid carcinoma. J Clin Endocrinol Metab 51:513, 1980.

Shields TW: Primary mediastinal tumors and cysts and their diagnostic investigation. In Shields TW (ed): Mediastinal Surgery. Malvern, PA, Lea & Febiger, 1991.

Shin HJ, Katz RL: Thymic neoplasia as represented by fine needle aspiration biopsy of anterior mediastinal mases: A practical approach to the differential diagnosis. Acta Cytol 42:855, 1998.

Silverman JF, Raab SS, Park HK: Fine-needle aspiration cytology of primary large cell lymphoma of the mediastinum: Cytomorphologic findings with potential pitfalls in diagnosis. Diagn Cytopathol 9:209, 1993.

Singh HK, Silverman JF, Powers CN et al: Diagnostic pitfalls in fine-needle aspiration biopsy of the mediastinum. Diagn Cytopathol 17:121, 1997.

Slagel DD, Powers CN, Melaragno MJ et al: Spindle cell lesions of the mediastinum: Diagnosis by fine needle aspiration biopsy. Diagn Cytopathol 17:167, 1997.

Sneige N, Dekmezian R, Katz RL et al: Morphologic and immunocytochemical evaluation of 220 fine needle aspirates of malignant lymphoma and lymphoid hyperplasia. Acta Cytol 34:311, 1990.

Spies WG: Radionuclide studies of the mediastinum. In Shields TW (ed): Mediastinal Surgery. Malvern PA, Lea & Febiger, 1991.

Sterrett G, Whitaker D, Shilkin KB, Walters MN: The fine-needle aspiration cytology of mediastinal lesions. Cancer 51:127, 1983.

Strauss LG, Conti PS: The applications of PET in clinical oncology. J Nucl Med 32:623, 1991.

Suster S, Moran CA, Domingues-Malagon H, Quevedo-Blanco P: Germ cell tumors of the mediastinum and testis: A comparative immunohistochemical study of 120 cases. Hum Pathol 29:737, 1998.

Taccagni G, Cantaboni A, Dell'Antonio G, et al: Electron microscopy of fine needle aspiration biopsies of mediastinal and paramediastinal lesions. Acta Cytol 32:868, 1988.

Taillefer R, Boncher Y, Potvin C, Lambert R: Detection and localization of parathyroid adenomas in patients with hyperparathyroidism using a single radionuclide imaging procedure with technetium-99m-sestamibi (double-phase study). J Nucl Med 33:1801, 1993.

Taylor CR: Immunoperoxidase techniques. Arch Pathol Lab Med 102:113, 1978.

Taylor CR: Immunomicroscopy: A Diagnostic Tool for the Surgical Pathologist. Philadelphia, WB Saunders, 1986.

Todd TRJ, Weisbrod G, Tao LC et al: Aspiration needle biopsy of thoracic lesions. Ann Thorac Surg 32:154, 1981.

Tumeh SS et al: Lymphoma—evaluation with Ga-67 SPECT. Radiology 164:111, 1987.

Van Herle AJ, Uller RP: Elevated serum thyroglobulin: A marker of metastases in differentiated thyroid carcinomas. J Clin Invest 56:272, 1975.

van Sonnenberg E, Casola G, Ho M et al: Difficult thoracic lesions: CT-guided biopsy experience in 150 cases. Radiology 167:457, 1988.

Virchow R: Cellular Pathology: As Based Upon Physiological and Pathological Histology. Translated and edited by Frank Chance. Classics in Medicine Library. Birmingham, AL, Division of Gryphon Editions Ltd., 1978.

Weisbrod GL, Lyons DJ, Tao LC et al: Percutaneous fine-needle aspiration biopsy of mediastinal lesions. AJR Am J Roentgenol 143:525, 1984.

Westcott JL: Percutaneous needle aspiration of hilar and mediastinal masses. Radiology 141:323, 1981.

Williams ED: Medullary carcinoma of the thyroid. In DeGroot LJ (ed): Endocrinology. Philadelphia, WB Saunders, 1989.

Wittich GR, Nowels KW, Korn RL et al: Coaxial transthoracic fine-needle biopsy in patients with a history of malignant lymphoma. Radiology 183:175, 1992.

Yang PC, Chang DB, Lee YC et al: Mediastinal malignancy: Ultrasound guided biopsy through the supraclavicular approach. Thorax 47:377, 1992.

Young AE, Gaunt JL, Croft D et al: Location of parathyroid adenomas by thallium-201 and technetium-99m subtraction imaging. Br Med J (Clin Res Ed) 286:1384, 1983.

Yu C-J, Yang P-C, Chang D-B et al: Evaluation of ultrasonically guided biopsies of mediastinal masses. Chest 100:399, 1991.

Yunis JJ, Oken MM, Kaplan ME et al: Distinctive chromosomal abnormalities in histologic subtypes of non-Hodgkin's lymphoma. N Engl J Med 307:1231, 1982.

THYMIC TUMORS

Mark I. Block

Thymomas are the most familiar thymic tumors, and this familiarity often seduces us into using the thymoma as a paradigm for thymic tumors in general. Indeed, other thymic tumors are occasionally mislabeled as "thymomas" despite their histologic or biologic differences. But yielding to this temptation does a disservice to our patients and to ourselves. Thymic neoplasms are a diverse group of tumors with unique features. This diversity reflects the embryology and biology of the organ of adaptive immunity, and covers the spectrum from benign to malignant. This chapter discusses tumors that exhibit features distinctive of thymic origin—thymoma, thymic carcinoma, thymic carcinoid, thymolipoma, and thymic cyst. Lymphomas and germ cell tumors can also arise from the thymus, but these neoplasms are not unique to the gland and are discussed elsewhere.

HISTORICAL NOTE

Interest in anterior mediastinal tumors paralleled early investigations into the nature of myasthenia gravis. The first indication of a link between myasthenia gravis and the thymus was suggested by the independent observations of Hoppe (1892) and Weigert (1901) at the end of the 19th century. Each reported finding a thymic tumor in patients who died of myasthenia gravis. Shortly thereafter, in 1911, Sauerbruch performed the first thymectomy (Sauerbruch and Roth, 1913). Using a transcervical approach, he removed a hypertrophic 49-g thymus from a patient with myasthenia gravis. The patient improved substantially but not completely. Sauerbruch's two subsequent patients died from postoperative complications, but in 1914 von Haberer successfully removed a normal thymus from a 27-year-old man with myasthenia gravis. Three years later, von Haberer published his accomplishment and reported that the patient was better (von Haberer, 1917). Also in 1917, Bell, from the University of Minnesota, published a series in which he reported finding either a thymic tumor or thymic hyperplasia in 27 of 56 patients who died from myasthenia gravis. The accumulating evidence suggested to Blalock that thymectomy might be therapeutic for patients with myasthenia gravis, and in 1936 he removed a thymoma from a 19-year-old myasthenic woman (Blalock, 1939). Safe conduct of the operation was made possible by the introduction of the anticholinesterase inhibitor neostigmine bromide. Within 1 year the patient experienced a near complete remission. Although von Haberer had accomplished a similar feat more than 20 years before, Blalock is considered the pioneer of this operation because he used the median sternotomy to gain access to the thymus. After publication of this result in 1939, Blalock undertook a series of thymectomy for myasthenia gravis in 20 patients (Blalock, 1944).

These efforts were essential to the development of surgical therapy for thymic tumors because even though several types of thymic neoplasms were well recognized by the early 1930s, resection was not considered a viable option. In 1932 Crosby published a review of 166 cases of "sarcomas" and "carcinomas" of the thymus collected from the literature and concluded that "in early diagnosis and x-ray treatment lies the only hope for the patient." The lack of consideration given to surgery was due in large part to the hazards associated with operating in the mediastinum. Although endotracheal intubation and positive-pressure ventilation anesthesia had been developed many years earlier, surgeons were reluctant to employ the technique. As a result, entry into the pleural space during resection of a large mediastinal tumor was a potentially fatal maneuver. The value of endotracheal anesthesia was demonstrated by an early remarkable report by Andrus and Foot (1937). In 1936 they resected a 2235-g thymolipoma from a 13-year-old boy. The tumor occupied most of the left hemithorax and was removed through an extended left anterior thoracotomy. After spending 3 days in an oxygen tent the boy recovered uneventfully and was discharged from the hospital on postoperative day 27. It was the largest thymic tumor that had yet been resected, and the case was one of the few documented procedures in which the patient survived for more than a few days. Increasing recognition of the benefits of positive-pressure ventilation in the years surrounding World War II paralleled advances made by surgeons who sought to treat patients with myasthenia gravis. Together, these two developments pioneered the surgical management of thymic tumors.

■ *HISTORICAL READINGS*

Andrus WD, Foot NC: Report of a large thymic tumor successfully removed by operation. J Thorac Surg 6:648, 1937.

Bell ET: Tumors of the thymus in myasthenia gravis. J Nerv Ment Dis 45:130, 1917.

Blalock A: Thymectomy in the treatment of myasthenia gravis: Report of twenty cases. J Thorac Cardiovasc Surg 13:316, 1944.

Blalock A, Mason M, Morgan H, et al: Myasthenia gravis and tumors of the thymic region: Report of a case in which the tumor was removed. Ann Surg 110:544, 1939.

Crosby E: Malignant tumors of the thymus gland. Am J Cancer 16:461, 1932.

Hoppe HH: Ein beitrag zur Kenntnis der bulbärparalyse. Berl Klin Wochenschr 29:332, 1892.

Sauerbruch D, Roth D: Thymektomie bei einem Fall von Marbus Basedowi mit Myasthenie. Mitt Grenzgeb Med Chir 25:746, 1913.

von Haberer A: Zur klinischen Bedeutung der Thymus Drüse. Arch Klin Chir 109:193, 1917.

Weigert C: Pathologisch-anatomischer beitag zur erb'schen krankheit (myasthenia gravis). Neurol Zentralb 13:597, 1901.

EMBRYOLOGY AND HISTOLOGY OF THE THYMUS

The thymus gland, along with the lower pair of parathyroid glands, is derived from the third pair of pharyngeal pouches (thymus III). Beginning in the sixth week of gestation, pouch epithelium proliferates to form a dorsal bulbar component, destined to become a parathyroid gland, and an elongated ventral portion, destined to become one lobe of the thymus. These thymic primordia migrate medially, where they fuse in the midline, and then descend into the mediastinum. In some cases thymic tissue may also derive from the fourth pair of pharyngeal pouches (thymus IV), but this tissue does not contribute substantially to the intrathoracic gland and is unlikely to persist.

The thymus is formed by tubes of epithelium that develop and proliferate into a branching array. The epithelial cells then disperse away from the central cord, forming thymic lobules, the principal structural and functional units of the gland. These cells remain connected in a loose network called an epithelial reticulum—the scaffolding on which lymphocytes proliferate and mature. Other epithelial cells congregate into small groups called Hassall's corpuscles. The epithelial cells can be recognized by ultrastructural details such as desmosomes and cytoplasmic tonofilaments.

Each lobule is divided into cortical and medullary regions (Fig. 63–13). These regions are easily distinguished by light microscopy because the cortex is rich in lymphocytes and has few epithelial cells, while the medulla has many epithelial cells and few lymphocytes. As a result the cortex is darker on histologic section. This polarity reflects the stages of lymphocyte maturation. Prothymocytes proliferate exuberantly in the subcortical

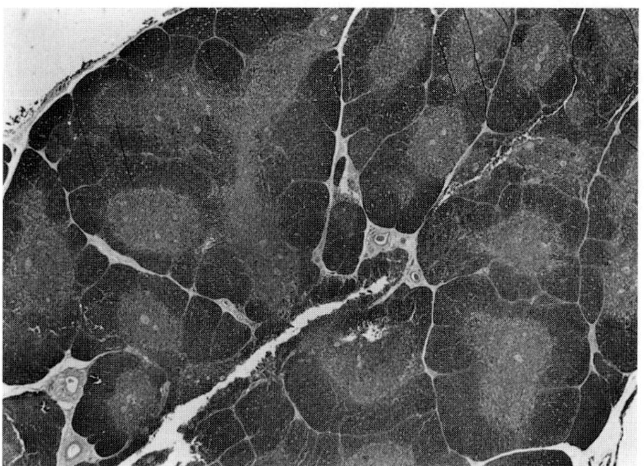

FIGURE 63–13 ■ Normal juvenile thymus. Histologic section from the thymus of a 1-year-old girl. Multiple thymic lobules are separated by fibrofatty septa. Each lobule consists of a pale medulla surrounded by abundant lymphocytes that form the dark-staining cortex.

region, producing large numbers of immature T cells. As lymphocytes migrate through the cortex and into the medulla, T cell receptor rearrangement and positive and negative selection occur. It is estimated that only 1% of lymphocytes survive this process to become mature T cells that are capable of recognizing self–major histocompatibility complex (MHC; positive selection) but are not self-reactive (negative selection, central tolerance) (Shimosato and Mukai, 1997). Mature lymphocytes, recognizable as "single-positive" T cells ($CD3^+/CD4^+/CD8^-$ and $CD3^+/CD4^-/CD8^+$), emerge in the medulla, from where they exit the gland and enter the peripheral lymphatic compartment.

The vast majority of cells within the thymus are T lymphocytes and epithelial cells, but occasional lymphoid follicles with B cells and germinal centers can also be found. These follicles are rare in the normal gland, but they can be relatively prominent in association with disorders such as myasthenia gravis. Also found in the normal thymus are rare "myoid" cells. Thymic myoid cells exhibit many characteristics reminiscent of skeletal muscle cells, including expression of the acetylcholine receptor. These cells are thought to play a pivotal role in the development of myasthenia gravis.

The thymus is relatively large at birth, continues to grow until puberty, and can reach a maximum weight of 50 g. After puberty, fibrofatty tissue begins to replace thymic parenchyma (Fig. 63–14). This gradual process of involution and atrophy leaves the gland barely identifiable in the elderly. Surprisingly, despite the pivotal role that the thymus plays in T cell development and central tolerance, thymectomy at a young age and even in newborn children (as is commonly done during surgery for congenital heart disease) has not been associated with identifiable immunologic defects. In contrast, profound deficiencies in T cell number and function are seen in patients with congenital thymic aplasia (DiGeorge's syndrome).

ANATOMY

The thymus is a bilobed structure that normally lies within the anterior mediastinum, posterior to the sternum and anterior to the great vessels and pericardium (Fig. 63–15). The two lobes are asymmetric and are fused at their midportion, creating a roughly H-shaped gland. The uppermost portion of each lobe usually lies anterior to the brachiocephalic vein and extends into the low neck immediately posterior to the strap muscles. Rarely, one or both lobes can be found posterior to the brachiocephalic vein. Other less common variations include partial or complete failure of thymic descent, and deposition of ectopic thymic tissue in the pulmonary parenchyma or hilum. Blood supply to the thymus is diffuse and comes from multiple small vessels that arise from the inferior thyroid and internal mammary arteries. Venous drainage is relatively constant, with tributaries coalescing in the midline to form one or two major thymic veins. These veins ascend between the lobes to drain into the left brachiocephalic vein or occasionally into the superior vena cava.

CLASSIFICATION OF THYMIC TUMORS

The classification of thymic tumors has spawned at least 21 different proposals since 1916, and continues to generate vigorous debate today (Harris and Müller-Hermelink, 1999; Shimosato and Mukai, 1997). To varying degrees, all classifications have considered histology, embryology, and biology in an attempt to establish a nomenclature that is both developmentally consistent and clinically useful. An important step forward is the 1999 publication of the World Health Organization's (WHO) *Histological Typing of Tumours of the Thymus* (Rosai, 1999), representing the consensus of pathologists who have been most actively engaged in this area over the past several decades (Table 63–13). This system emphasizes the cellular origins of the various neoplasms and reflects well a synthesis of the most widely used classifications.

A brief historical review should help clarify two important areas of confusion: the relationship between thymomas and thymic carcinomas, and the classification of thymomas as either "benign" or "malignant." Thymic carcinomas and thymomas were not recognized as distinct types of thymic epithelial cell neoplasms until the

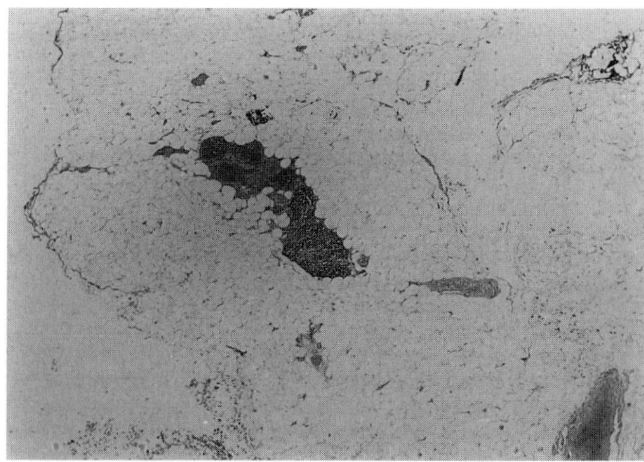

FIGURE 63–14 ■ Normal involuted thymus. Histologic section from the thymus of a 65-year-old man. Note that fat has replaced almost the entire gland.

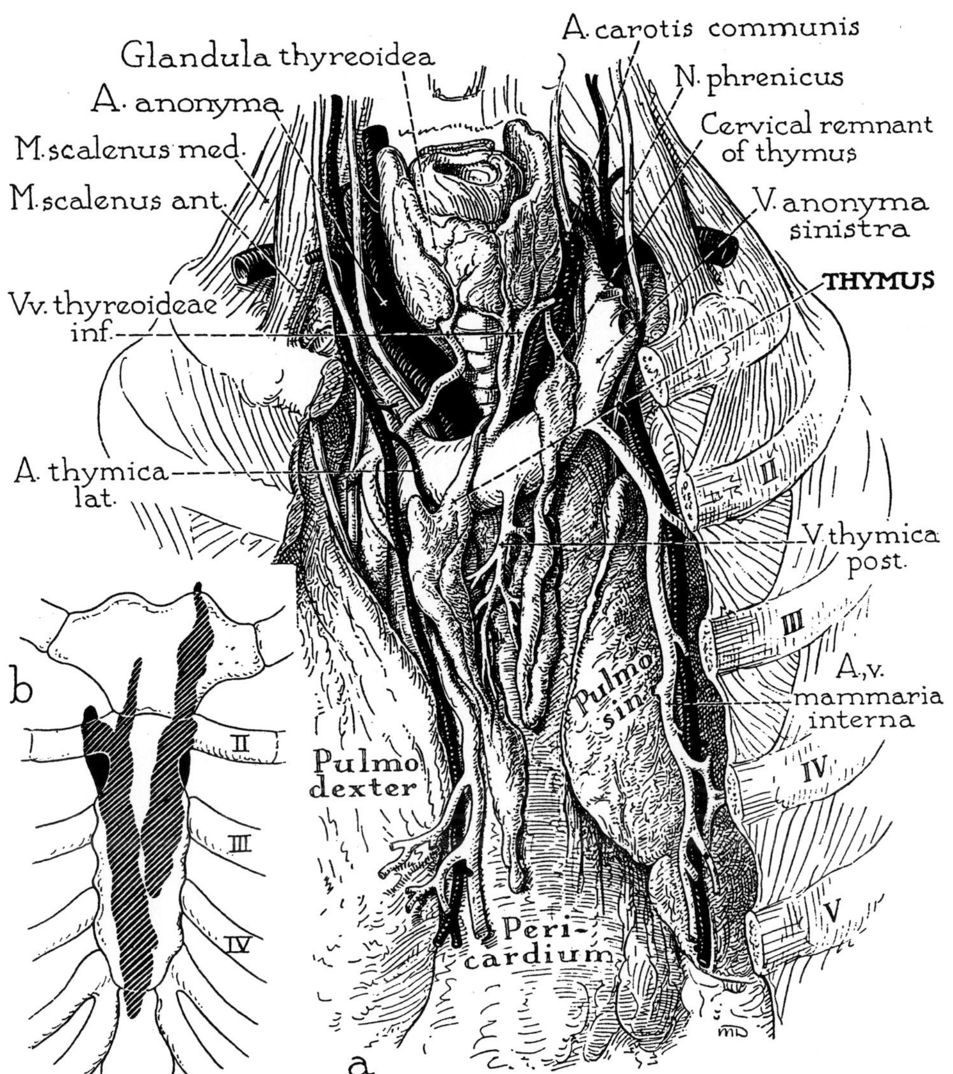

FIGURE 63–15 ■ Anatomy of the thymus in an adult. *a*, The elongated lobes of the normal thymus form a roughly H-shaped gland located in the center of the anterior mediastinum. The central portion of the gland is retracted to demonstrate the venous drainage to the innominate vein. The arterial blood supply is shown arising from the internal mammary arteries. *b*, Surface anatomy of the thymus. (From Bell, Knapp, Anson, and Larson: Q Bull Northwestern Univ Med School 28:156, 1954.)

late 1970s. In the second series of the Armed Forces Institute of Pathology's *Atlas of Tumor Pathology*, published in 1976, Rosai and Levine proposed a system in which thymic carcinomas were not explicitly segregated. A follow-up classification, published 2 years later, divided thymomas into "circumscribed" (benign) and "malignant" types (Levine and Rosai, 1978). Malignant thymomas were further divided into type I (invasive thymoma with no or minimal atypia) and type II (cytologically malignant, thymic carcinoma). This system has had a lasting influence and explains why thymic carcinomas are occasionally called "type II thymomas." In the 1980s Wick and colleagues (1982b) and Lewis and colleagues (1987) introduced the current practice of segregating thymic epithelial cell neoplasms into thymomas and thymic carcinomas. This distinction is now well accepted as biologically meaningful. These classifications also eliminated subtyping thymomas as "benign" and "malignant" in favor of the descriptive terms "encapsulated" and "invasive." Since then, all other classifications have also rejected as histologically inaccurate the division of thymomas into "benign" and "malignant" subtypes. Some authors have suggested eliminating the designations "encapsulated" and "invasive" altogether, preferring instead to subtype thymomas based only on their cytologic appearance (Marino and Müller-Hermelink, 1985). Unfortunately, thymomas continue to be classified as "benign" and "malignant" both in conversation and in the literature. The histologic subtyping of thymomas and thymic carcinomas is complex, and it is discussed in greater detail in the respective sections of this chapter.

PRESENTATION

Most thymic tumors are discovered incidentally when a chest radiograph or chest computed tomography (CT)

TABLE 63–13 ■ Classification of Thymic Tumors

Epithelial tumors
- Thymoma
- Thymic carcinoma

Neuroendocrine tumors
- Carcinoid
- Small cell carcinoma
- Large cell neuroendocrine carcinoma

Germ cell tumors

Lymphoid tumors (lymphomas)

Stromal tumors
- Thymolipoma
- Thymoliposarcoma
- Solitary fibrous tumor
- Rhabdoid tumor

Tumor-like lesions
- True thymic hyperplasia
- Lymphoid hyperplasia
- Multilocular thymic cyst
- Langerhans' cell histiocytosis

Neck tumors of thymic or related branchial pouch derivation
- Ectopic hamartomatous thymoma
- Ectopic cervical thymoma
- Spindle epithelial tumor with thymus-like differentiation (SETTLE)
- Carcinoma showing thymus-like differentiation (CASTLE)

Metastatic tumors

Unclassified tumors

From Rosai J: Histological typing of tumours of the thymus. In World Health Organization: International Histological Classification of Tumours, 2nd ed. Berlin, Springer-Verlag, 1999, pp 5–7. Reprinted with permission.

scan is obtained for apparently unrelated reasons. Presentation with symptoms related to local effects such as chest pain or heaviness, cough, phrenic nerve paralysis, or superior vena cava (SVC) syndrome is unusual and typically is associated with malignancy. Occasionally, a thymic tumor is discovered because of systemic symptoms associated with a clinical syndrome. The most common of these associations is myasthenia gravis and thymoma, but a variety of other syndromes are also associated with thymoma, and other thymic tumors can present with systemic symptoms. Clinical syndromes associated with thymic tumors are covered in greater detail in the sections of this chapter devoted to each of the different thymic tumors.

DIAGNOSIS

Several basic principles guide the diagnostic workup of the patient with a presumed thymic tumor and indicate whether a tissue diagnosis is needed prior to initiating therapy.

1. A thymic tumor in an adult is most likely to be a thymoma, whereas in children or young adults thymomas are rare.
2. Thymectomy is both curative and of low morbidity for most small (<5 cm diameter) thymic tumors.
3. Combined modality therapy with preoperative chemotherapy should be considered for patients with advanced stage thymoma and may be of value for patients with thymic carcinoma.
4. Biopsy of an early-stage thymoma will violate its capsule, with the theoretical risk of dissemination of a previously contained tumor.

Based on these principles, the goals of the diagnostic evaluation should be

1. To avoid biopsy of an early-stage thymoma.
2. To establish the diagnosis if the tumor is an advanced stage thymoma so that preoperative therapy can be considered.
3. To minimize the likelihood of undertaking extensive or potentially morbid resections for lymphomas or germ cell tumors, or for tumors that are widely metastatic.

The essential first steps are an accurate history and a good physical examination. Because thymoma is the most common anterior mediastinal tumor in adults but is rare in children, the age of the patient is critical for determining the direction of further investigations. The most common anterior mediastinal tumors in children are thymic hyperplasia and lymphoma, while in young adults, especially men, germ cell tumors are the most common. A minority of patients also have symptoms or signs of an associated clinical syndrome that further aid in diagnosis.

DIAGNOSTIC EVALUATIONS

Imaging

Imaging is an essential part of the workup of an anterior mediastinal mass and, in conjunction with the history and physical examination, is often the only investigation needed before starting treatment. Following identification of an anterior mediastinal mass on chest radiograph (Fig. 63–16), a chest CT should be obtained (Fig. 63–17). CT clearly demonstrates the precise anatomy of the lesion and its relationships to adjacent structures, and it reveals important characteristics such as whether the lesion is solid or cystic, heterogeneous or homogeneous, or contains fat, fluid, or calcium. CT can also demonstrate features that are suggestive of a benign or malignant diagnosis, such as preservation of tissue planes and evidence of local invasion. Although magnetic resonance imaging (MRI) is usually superfluous, it may be useful for demonstrating vascular invasion or prominent tumor vascularity, especially in patients for whom intravenous contrast is contraindicated (Brown, 1991). Ultrasonography is rarely used to image anterior mediastinal masses.

Nuclear Medicine

Routine use of nuclear medicine to evaluate thymic tumors is not indicated, but some techniques may be very helpful in certain circumstances. The thallium-technetium scan may identify an intrathymic parathyroid adenoma, and ^{111}In pentetreotide scintigraphy (OctreoScan) can identify a neuroendocrine tumor such as a thymic carcinoid, but neither of these studies should be performed unless there is a strong suspicion of the diagnosis. Positron emission tomography with fluorodeoxyglucose (FDG-PET) is a promising tool for evaluating suspected malignancies elsewhere in the body, and it may prove useful for evaluating thymic lesions as well. Isolated

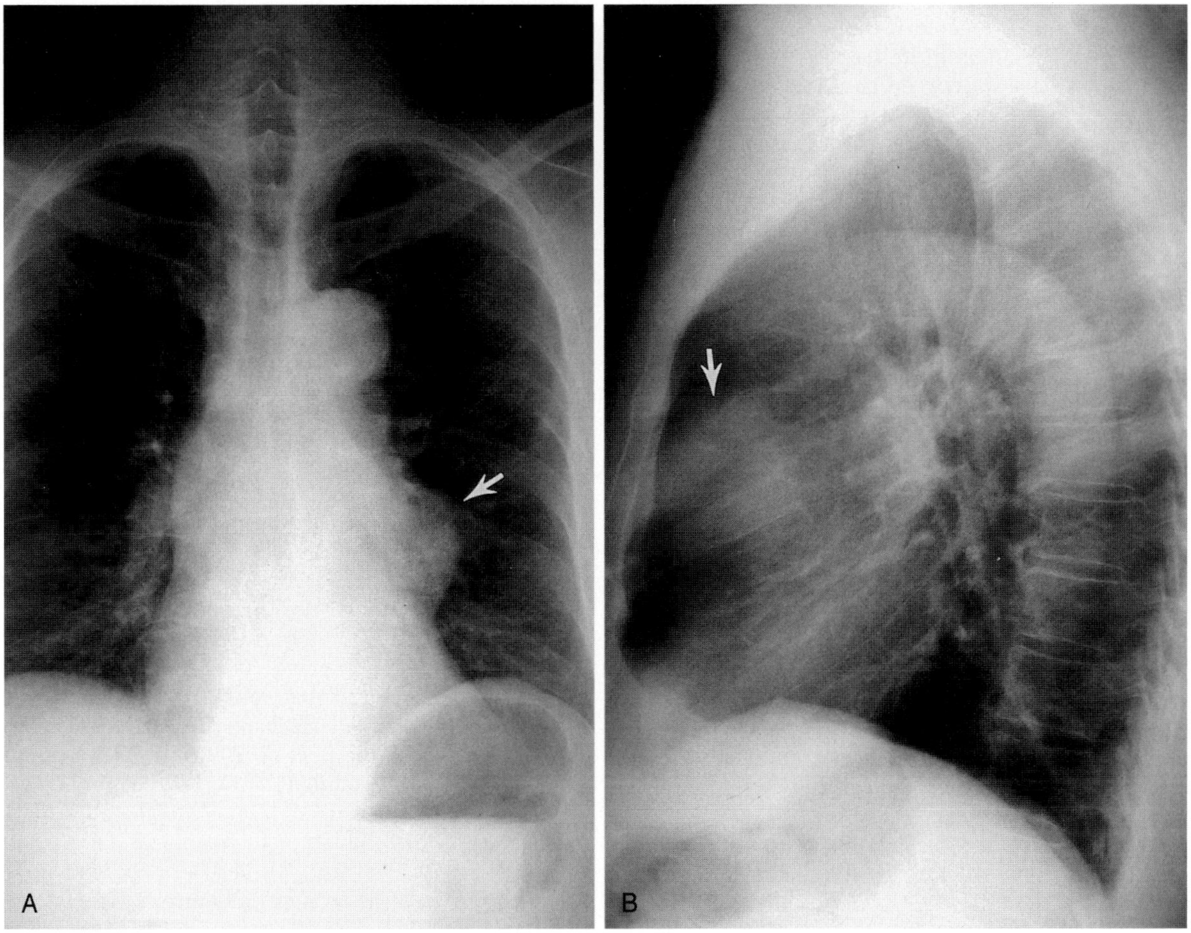

FIGURE 63–16 ■ Anterior mediastinal mass. Chest radiograph of a 58-year-old man who presented with a 1-week history of a nonproductive cough. The mass is visible *(arrows)* on the posteroanterior view *(A)* as a prominence along the left cardiac border, and on the lateral view *(B)* as opacification of the normally radiolucent retrosternal space. Histology confirmed thymoma.

reports and small series in the literature suggest that FDG-PET can distinguish invasive thymomas and thymic carcinomas from benign lesions (Kubota et al, 1996; Liu et al, 1995; Sasaki et al, 1999).

Biopsy

Tissue diagnosis is often, but not always, required before proceeding with therapy. History (presence of myasthenia gravis), imaging (benign teratoma), and tumor markers may be diagnostic. In many circumstances resection is indicated as primary therapy regardless of the diagnosis. Tumor size is an important factor in determining the need for biopsy. Small (<5 cm diameter) tumors are usually encapsulated, amenable to complete resection with minimal morbidity, and associated with a good long-term prognosis. In contrast, large tumors can require

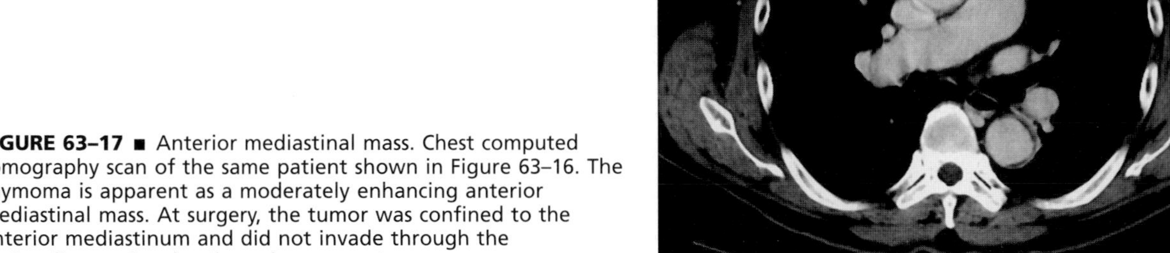

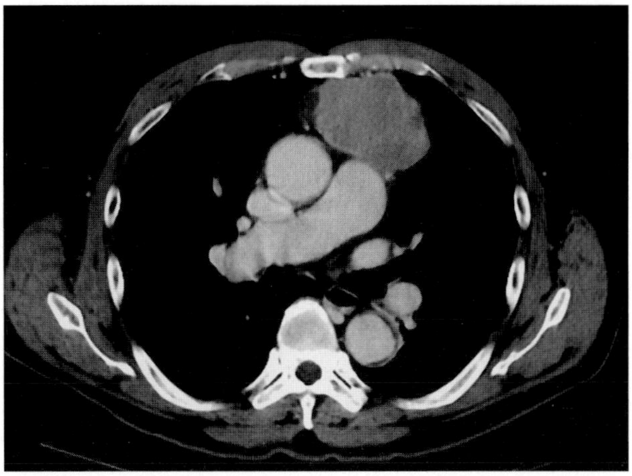

FIGURE 63–17 ■ Anterior mediastinal mass. Chest computed tomography scan of the same patient shown in Figure 63–16. The thymoma is apparent as a moderately enhancing anterior mediastinal mass. At surgery, the tumor was confined to the anterior mediastinum and did not invade through the pericardium to involve the pulmonary artery.

extensive procedures to achieve complete resection, and thymomas greater than 5 cm in diameter are likely to be invasive and to have a poor prognosis (Blumberg et al, 1995). In this circumstance, biopsy does not risk worsening prognosis and avoids the possibility of undertaking extensive resection for a tumor that may be best treated nonoperatively. Preoperative chemotherapy may be indicated if a definitive diagnosis of invasive thymoma or thymic carcinoma is made.

The available techniques for biopsy include fine-needle aspiration (FNA) cytology, core needle biopsy, mediastinotomy, and thoracoscopy. FNA is preferred as the least invasive and often simplest approach. Recent series report a diagnostic accuracy of 80% to 90% (Powers et al, 1996; Shabb et al, 1998; Singh et al, 1997; Zafar and Moinuddin, 1995) and an accuracy at distinguishing benign from malignant of close to 100% (Powers et al, 1996). However, it may not be possible to establish the diagnosis of thymoma or thymic carcinoma with certainty, and thymomas with an extensive lymphocytic component may be difficult to distinguish from lymphoma (Shimosato and Mukai, 1997). Furthermore, FNA may be insufficient for the diagnosis and subtyping of lymphoma. If a definitive diagnosis is needed in this setting, core needle or open biopsy should be used to obtain more tissue. Access to the anterior mediastinum is difficult with cervical mediastinoscopy; therefore, open biopsy of thymic lesions is accomplished via anterior mediastinotomy. Thoracoscopy is an alternative, but it requires more incisions and single-lung ventilation anesthesia (Gossot et al, 1996).

THYMOMA

Thymomas are the most common neoplasms of the anterior mediastinum and are the most common mediastinal lesions in adults. They are rare in children. Approximately half are incidental discoveries. Thymomas are slow-growing tumors that tend to recur locally, but they are unlikely to metastasize hematogenously or to regional lymphatics. Complete resection is the cornerstone of therapy and the most important determinant of long-term survival. Early-stage, encapsulated tumors are associated with an excellent prognosis, but advanced, locally invasive tumors have a relatively poor prognosis. Recent evidence suggests that patients with a locally invasive tumor may benefit from preoperative chemotherapy.

Histology

Although many thymic tumors are called thymomas, the term is specific and appropriate only for those tumors of thymic epithelial cell origin in which the neoplastic epithelial cells have bland cytologic features. Thymomas also contain lymphocytes, but the lymphocytes are not neoplastic and are not considered tumor cells. Interestingly, most lymphocytes found in a thymoma are immature and mirror the population found in the normal thymus, whereas lymphocytes in other solid tumors are mostly mature and are derived from the peripheral lymphatic compartment (Shimosato and Mukai, 1997). This feature is a hallmark of thymomas and suggests that the neoplastic thymic epithelial cells retain some of their normal function as shepherds of T cell development. The histologic differential diagnosis of thymoma includes thymic carcinoma, lymphoma (Hodgkin's disease, diffuse lymphoblastic lymphoma, diffuse small cell lymphoma) and atypical carcinoid tumor (Shimosato and Mukai, 1997).

Subtyping thymomas is an important, confusing, and controversial subject (Harris and Müller-Hermelink, 1999; Shimosato, 1994). Two very different approaches have been taken: one based on the relative abundance of epithelial cells and lymphocytes, and the other based on the histologic appearance of the epithelial cell (Table 63–14). In 1961 Bernatz and colleagues from the Mayo Clinic proposed using the lymphocyte-to-epithelial cell ratio to divide thymomas into lymphocytic, mixed, epithelial, and spindle subtypes (the spindle cell is derived from thymic epithelium). Many subsequent authors modified this system, including Rosai and Levine (1976), and until recently it has been the dominant classification. Epithelial thymomas tend to be more aggressive, and some reports suggest that they are associated with a worse prognosis (Gripp et al, 1998; Shimizu et al, 1992). But others have found that epithelial histology either has no impact on survival (Jackson and Ball, 1991; Mornex et al, 1995; Pescarmona et al, 1990), or that its impact is due entirely to the tendency of epithelial tumors to present at a more advanced stage (Nakahara et al, 1988; Regnard et al, 1996).

In 1985, Marino and Müller-Hermelink suggested a new classification in which thymomas were divided into cortical, medullary, and mixed subtypes. These designations were based on similarities between the neoplastic epithelial cells and epithelial cells in the different regions of the normal thymic lobule. In cortical thymomas, the epithelial cells are large and round or polygonal, with clear round nuclei, conspicuous nucleoli, and poorly defined cytoplasm. In contrast, the epithelial cells found in medullary thymomas are smaller and spindle-shaped, with irregular or fusiform nuclei and inconspicuous nucleoli. The histologic features of cortical thymomas suggest a more malignant phenotype, and indeed they are more aggressive. In a series of 80 patients, Pescarmona and colleagues (1990) found that the Müller-Hermelink classification reliably predicted prognosis: most medullary thymomas were well encapsulated and all were clinically benign, while most cortical thymomas were invasive and clinically malignant. No medullary thymo-

TABLE 63–14 ■ **Histologic Subtyping of Thymoma**

Author	*Histologic Subtype*
Bernatz et al, 1961	Lymphocytic Mixed Epithelial Spindle
Marino and Müller-Hermelink, 1985	Medullary Mixed Cortical

mas had advanced beyond stage II. The authors also found that classification of the same tumors according to the system of Salyer and Eggleston (1976)—an adaptation of the Bernatz system (lymphocytic, epithelial, mixed)—was of no prognostic value (Fig. 63–18).

Although variations of both classifications are currently in use in the literature, the Müller-Hermelink system has gained acceptance in some circles as more clinically meaningful (Ciernik et al, 1994; Quintanilla-Martinez et al, 1994). With the recognition that thymomas fundamentally are tumors of the thymic epithelial cell, it follows that classification based on the appearance of the neoplastic epithelial cell may be the most biologically meaningful. The system published in 1999 by the WHO represents a synthesis of these concepts and is the first attempt to establish an international standard (Rosai, 1999).

Demographics

Twenty percent of all mediastinal lesions are thymomas. They are the most common tumors of the anterior mediastinum and of the mediastinum as a whole. The incidence of thymoma in the general population is not well documented and is probably less than 2000 per year in the United States (SEER, 1999). Thymomas can occur in patients of any age, but the mean is between 40 and 50 years, and most patients are between the ages of 40 and 60 years. Although in most series there is a difference between the number of male and female patients, in the aggregate this difference is not significant and men and women are equally affected.

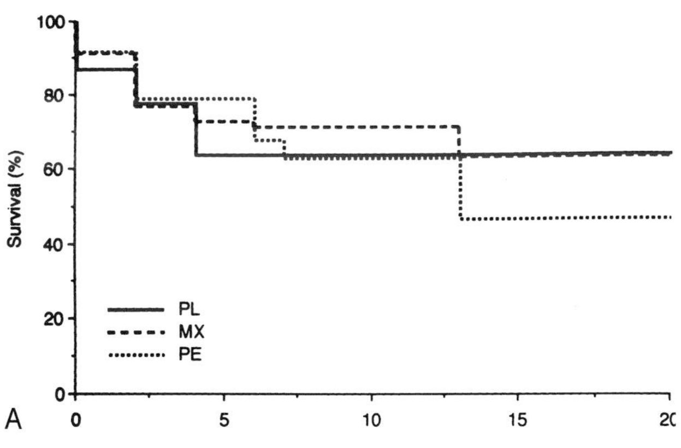

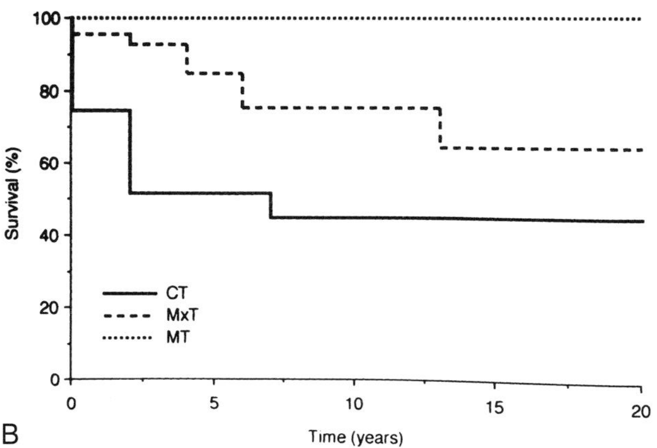

FIGURE 63–18 ■ Prognosis of thymoma by histologic subtype. *A*, Survival curves for patients with thymomas histologically classified according to Salyer and Eggleston (1976) (MX, mixed; PE, epithelial; PL, lymphocytic). *B*, Survival curves for patients with thymomas histologically classified according to Marino and Müller-Hermelink (1985) (CT, cortical; MT, medullary, MxT, mixed). (From Pescarmona E, Rendina EA, Venuta F et al: The prognostic implication of thymoma histologic subtyping: A study of 80 consecutive cases. Am J Clin Pathol 93:190, 1990.)

Presentation

Approximately half of thymomas are found incidentally and are asymptomatic. The other half cause symptoms from local mass effects or from associated systemic syndromes. The most common symptoms of regional tumor growth are chest pain or discomfort, cough, and dyspnea. Aggressive tumors can cause venous obstruction and phrenic nerve paralysis, but these findings are unusual. Tumors that cause one or more local symptoms are more likely to exhibit malignant behavior, while the absence of symptoms is suggestive of a clinically benign lesion. Ectopic primary thymomas are rare and can be found in the neck (Oh et al, 1998), along the pleura (Fushimi et al, 1998; Higashiyama et al, 1996), inside the pericardial sac (Mirra et al, 1997), or within the lung parenchyma (Marchevsky, 1995).

Thymomas are associated with a variety of systemic and autoimmune disorders (Table 63–15). By far the most common of these paraneoplastic syndromes is myasthenia gravis. Approximately 40% of patients with a thymoma have myasthenia gravis (Table 63–16), and myasthenia gravis in a patient with an anterior mediastinal mass is essentially diagnostic of thymoma. In contrast, only 21% of myasthenic patients have a thymoma (Table 63–17). Myasthenia gravis has been reported in association with thymolipoma, but CT or MRI can easily distinguish this tumor from a thymoma. A variety of other hematologic and autoimmune disorders are seen less often in association with thymoma. They include red and white blood cell aplasia, pancytopenia, hypogammaglobulinemia, systemic lupus erythematosus, dermatomyositis, rheumatoid arthritis, thyroiditis, and myocarditis.

Imaging

Most thymomas can be seen on standard chest x-ray (see Fig. 63–16). The posteroanterior (PA) view usually reveals a smooth, lobulated mass in the mid to upper portion of the chest. Often, the tumor lies predominantly to one side of the midline, appearing in silhouette against the lung on the right or in front of the aortic arch on the left. On the lateral view, the tumor is visible as radiodense tissue in the usually radiolucent region between the sternum and anterior pericardium. Smaller thymomas are seen more easily on the lateral than the PA chest radiograph because the lateral view projects the anterior mediastinum against the air-filled lungs, while the PA view projects it against the fluid-filled heart and great vessels.

CT is the best technique for evaluating a suspected or known thymoma (see Fig. 63–17). Younger patients may

TABLE 63–15 ■ **Syndromes Associated with Thymoma**

Neuromuscular syndrome	Collagen diseases and autoimmune disorders
Myasthenia gravis	Systemic lupus erythematosus
Myotonic dystrophy	Rheumatoid arthritis
Eaton-Lambert syndrome	Polymyositis
Myositis	Myocarditis
Hematologic syndromes	Sjögren's syndrome
Red cell hypoplasia	Scleroderma
Erythrocytosis	Endocrine disorders
Pancytopenia	Hyperparathyroidism
Megakaryocytopenia	Hashimoto's thyroiditis
T cell lymphocytosis	Addison's disease
Acute leukemia	Chemodectoma
Multiple myeloma	Renal diseases
Immune deficiency syndromes	Nephrotic syndrome
Hypogammaglobulinemia	Minimal change nephropathy
T cell deficiency syndrome	Dermatologic diseases
Bone disorders	Pemphigus (vulgaris, erythematosus)
Hypertrophic osteoarthropathy	Chronic mucocutaneous candidiasis

From Marchevsky AM, Kaneko M (eds): Surgical Pathology of the Mediastinum. New York, Raven Press, 1984, p 61. Reprinted with permission from Lippincott Williams & Wilkins.

still have a sizable normal thymus, apparent as an enhancing soft tissue mass of intermediate density in the anterior mediastinum, but the anterior mediastinum in most adult patients consists of a thin strip of fat sandwiched between the right and left lungs. In either case a thymic mass stands out as an abnormal soft tissue density, and tumors too small to appreciate by plain chest radiograph are readily visible by CT. There are no features diagnostic of thymoma, but thymomas are usually homogeneous and enhance with intravenous contrast; they may contain calcification, cystic components, or areas of low density and necrosis (Brown and Aughenbaugh, 1991; Do et al, 1995; Laurent et al, 1998; Parish et al, 1984). CT delineates the size and extent of the tumor, and the presence or absence of local invasion or metastases—features that are essential for determining if further workup is necessary and for planning surgery if indicated. Because CT can clearly identify even small thymic tumors, all patients with myasthenia gravis should be screened at least once with a chest CT in addition to regular screening chest radiographs. MRI is of little additional value, and should not be substituted for CT except under special circumstances (Brown and Aughenbaugh, 1991).

TABLE 63–16 ■ **Incidence of Myasthenia Gravis in Patients with Thymoma**

Study	*N*	*Number with Myasthenia Gravis*	*%*
Shamji et al, 1984	52	25	48
Cohen et al, 1984	23	4	17
Nakahara et al, 1988	142	81	57
Curran et al, 1988	103	37	36
Maggi et al, 1991	241	60	66
Shimizu et al, 1992	96	23	24
Wang et al, 1992	61	23	38
Ciernik et al, 1994	31	4	13
Cowen et al, 1995	149	21	14
Blumberg et al, 1995	118	12	10
Yagi et al, 1996	41	14	34
Regnard et al, 1996	307	195	64
Venuta et al, 1997	65	24	37
Gripp et al, 1998	70	12	17
Total	**1499**	**635**	**42**

From Block MI: Mediastinum. In Norton JA, Bollinger RR, Chang AE et al (eds): Surgery: Basic Science and Clinical Evidence. New York, Springer-Verlag, 2001, p 1300. Reprinted with permission.

There is some experience with FDG-PET for imaging thymomas, but it is confined to a few small anecdotal series (Kubota et al, 1996; Liu et al, 1995; Sasaki et al, 1999). Because distinguishing between early- and advanced-stage thymomas is based on clinical findings, and not cellular or histologic characteristics, FDG-PET is less helpful for determining the "malignancy" of thymoma. Additionally, FDG-PET cannot distinguish between a thymoma and other thymic neoplasms. There is evidence, however, that thymic carcinomas and invasive thymomas are more FDG-avid than are clinically benign thymomas (Kubota et al, 1996; Sasaki et al, 1999).

Staging

There is no standard staging system for thymoma, but the one proposed by Masaoka and colleagues in 1981 has gained universal acceptance because it reflects the prognostic significance of capsular invasion (Table 63–18). Most thymomas are well encapsulated and clinically benign. However, evidence of either gross or microscopic capsular invasion portends malignant behavior and a less favorable prognosis. These tumors can be locally aggressive, invading adjacent mediastinal structures and lung. Metastases occur late and are predominantly pericardial and pleural. Hematogenous metastasis to the lung is seen occasionally, but lymphogenous spread through regional lymph nodes is unusual. As a result, the general perception is that little prognostic value is gained by switching from the Masaoka system to a more standardized tumor-node-metastasis (TNM) staging system. Such a system was proposed by Masaoka's group in 1991 (Yamakawa, 1991), but it has not been widely adopted.

Determining the malignancy of a thymoma is difficult,

TABLE 63-17 ■ **Incidence of Thymoma in Patients with Myasthenia Gravis**

Study	*All Patients* *N*	*Thymoma*	*%*	*Thymectomy* *N*	*Thymoma*	*%*
Mulder et al, 1983				249	51	20
Jaretzki et al, 1988				95	15	16
Maggi et al, 1989				662	162	24
Hatton et al, 1989				52	7	13
Mulder et al, 1989				84	11	13
Molnar and Szobor, 1990				425	54	13
Frist et al, 1994				46	4	9
Masaoka et al, 1996				375	89	24
Bramis et al, 1997				76	20	26
Papatestas et al, 1987	2062	226	11	962	174	18
Cosi et al, 1997	438	92	21	280	92	33
Beekman et al, 1997	100	12	12	56	12	21
Robertson et al, 1998	100	12	12	34	12	35
Total	**2700**	**342**	**13**	**3396**	**703**	**21**

From Block MI: Mediastinum. In Norton JA, Bollinger RR, Chang AE et al (eds): Surgery: Basic Science and Clinical Evidence. New York, Springer-Verlag, 2001, p 1297. Reprinted with permission.

even to the point of controversy. Pathologists have been in general agreement that despite the ability to identify histologic subtypes associated with varying degrees of malignant behavior, microscopic examination of the neoplastic epithelial cell does not provide an easy assessment of the malignant potential of a given tumor. As discussed earlier, thymomas that are well encapsulated are often called benign thymomas. However, as observed by Marchevsky and Kaneko (1984), "most encapsulated, benign thymomas have identical histologic and cytologic features to invasive malignant thymoma." Thus, the classification of encapsulated thymomas as benign likely misrepresents the true nature of these tumors and ignores the potential for continued growth, capsular invasion, and metastases. More accurately, these tumors should be referred to as Masaoka stage I thymomas.

Prognostic Significance of Myasthenia Gravis

An early report from the Massachusetts General Hospital suggested that myasthenia gravis was an important negative prognostic factor for patients with thymoma (Wilkins et al, 1966). The authors observed that 10-year survival rates for myasthenic and nonmyasthenic patients were 32% and 67%, respectively. This profound impact on survival was due primarily to deaths from myasthenic crisis, and in a report published 25 years later the same group concluded that myasthenia was no longer a significant risk factor (Wilkins et al, 1991). This conclusion is now well supported by results from other series that demonstrate either no difference in survival (Blumberg et al, 1995; Cowen et al, 1995; Gripp et al, 1998; Lewis et al, 1987; Regnard et al, 1996; Shamji et al, 1984) or even improved survival for patients with myasthenia compared to those without it (Crucitti et al, 1992; Maggi et al, 1991; Nakahara et al, 1988; Wang et al, 1992). One hypothesis to explain the possible favorable impact on prognosis is that presentation with myasthenia gravis prompts discovery of the thymoma at an earlier stage, perhaps even incidentally when therapeutic thymectomy is performed (Maggi et al, 1991; Nakahara et al, 1988). Associated autoimmune disorders other than myasthenia gravis are linked to a worse prognosis. Both Maggi and colleagues (1991) and Blumberg and colleagues (1995) found that patients with red cell aplasia, hypogammaglobulinemia, or lupus had lower survival rates.

TABLE 63-18 ■ **Masaoka Staging System for Thymoma**

Stage	*Definition*
I	Macroscopically—completely encapsulated Microscopically—no capsular invasion
II	Macroscopic invasion into surrounding fatty tissue or mediastinal pleura Microscopic invasion into capsule
III	Macroscopic invasion into neighboring organ (i.e., pericardium, great vessels, or lung)
IVA	Pleural or pericardial dissemination
IVB	Lymphogenous or hematogenous metastasis

From Masaoka A, Monden Y, Nakahara K et al: Follow-up study of thymomas with special reference to their clinical stages. CANCER, Vol. 48, No. 11, 1981, page 2485. Copyright © 1981 American Cancer Society. Reprinted by permission of Wiley-Liss, Inc., a subsidiary of John Wiley & Sons, Inc.

Therapy

Except in cases of widely metastatic disease, surgical removal is the cornerstone of therapy, and complete resection of even extensively invasive tumor is the critical factor in determining long-term survival. Between 40% and 70% of thymomas are encapsulated (Bergh et al, 1978; Lewis et al, 1987; Maggi et al, 1991; Masaoka et al, 1981), for which complete resection is curative. However, microscopic invasion is present in 20% of grossly encapsulated tumors (Kornstein et al, 1988), and up to 12% of tumors without either gross or microscopic evidence of invasion recur locally (Fechner, 1969; Lewis et al, 1987; Masaoka et al, 1981; Monden et al, 1985). Consequently, a large proportion of patients may benefit from additional regional or systemic therapy. With few exceptions, postoperative radiation therapy has been advocated following resection of locally invasive tumors. In addition, recent evidence from trials of combined modality therapy suggests that neoadjuvant or adjuvant chemotherapy may further improve long-term survival for patients with advanced stage disease. Therefore, although biopsy of a thymoma is generally to be avoided, if stage III or IV disease is suspected neoadjuvant therapy may be indicated, and biopsy confirmation of thymoma should be sought.

Surgery

The basic principles underlying successful surgical therapy are (1) operative access via a complete median sternotomy; (2) wide opening of both pleural spaces; (3) total thymectomy, including all normal thymic tissue; (4) extended en bloc resection of invasive (stage III) tumors, including pericardium, lung, brachiocephalic vein, or superior vena cava; and (5) excision of all pleural implants (stage IVa) and lung metastases. For a tumor confined to the anterior mediastinum, wide excision should be performed, extending from phrenic nerve to phrenic nerve and brachiocephalic vein to diaphragm. Lesser resections, even for small and seemingly well-encapsulated tumors, are not appropriate. For large and invasive tumors, preoperative chemotherapy may facilitate complete resection (see Chemotherapy). Metastatic disease to lung and pleura is an indication for resection with metastasectomy.

Many incisions are appropriate for thymic surgery. The purely cervical approach, which in skilled hands provides acceptable exposure of the nonthymomatous gland, has no role in surgery for thymic tumors. It is seldom necessary as an extension of the median sternotomy unless the tumor extends well into the neck. The partial sternotomy, which provides excellent exposure for nonthymomatous thymectomy for myasthenia gravis, is not adequate for full assessment of the posterolateral extent of a thymoma or of transpleural implantation or involvement of the phrenic nerves. Total median sternotomy carries little additional morbidity compared with partial sternotomy and, when combined with bilateral pleurotomy, affords maximal exposure.

Lateral thoracotomy, although it permits easy access to an encapsulated tumor lying in one lobe of the thymus, makes total thymectomy more difficult. In contrast, the bilateral subcostal incision with transverse sternotomy (clamshell) provides wide exposure to the entire mediastinum and both pleural cavities. Neither of these approaches is appropriate for the vast majority of cases, and their use should be confined only to specific circumstances, such as extension of tumor to the posterior mediastinum or reoperation for tumor recurrence.

Thoracoscopic thymectomy for thymoma is technically feasible and has been described by Landreneau and colleagues (1992) as well as others (Yim, 1995). This approach is more time-consuming than median sternotomy and offers no advantage in terms of morbidity or hospital length of stay. The sole advantage of thoracoscopy is cosmetic, and although the importance of this consideration to the patient should not be minimized, it should not outweigh the principal imperative of maximizing the likelihood of a curative resection. Most importantly, although thoracoscopy may provide excellent exposure of the mediastinum, the limited access with this technique raises concerns about the ability to adequately assess subtle signs of local invasion and to perform a complete anterior mediastinal dissection. Given that thymomas are slow growing, determining the success or failure of the thoracoscopic approach depends on long-term rather than short-term follow-up. For this reason validation of this approach awaits more mature results than are currently available.

Technical Considerations. The goal of surgery is complete resection of all tumor, including both invasive and metastatic disease. Extension of tumor beyond the thymus may not be apparent before surgery, and the surgeon should be prepared to make intraoperative decisions regarding the extent of resection.

Pericardium. Removal of the anterior pericardium is not routine, but adhesions between the thymus and the pericardium may make it difficult to exclude direct invasion even in the setting of an encapsulated tumor. Excision of the anterior pericardium can be done with relative impunity, and any adherent portions should be resected. Reconstruction of the resulting defect is optional.

Phrenic nerve. Sacrifice of one but not both phrenic nerves is indicated if doing so yields a complete resection. This maneuver is contraindicated in patients with limited pulmonary function and should be undertaken only with extreme caution in the myasthenic patient. If both phrenic nerves are involved, or if only one is involved but complete resection is prevented by other considerations, then debulking should be performed with preservation of both phrenic nerves.

Vascular structures. Both the superior vena cava and the brachiocephalic vein can be resected and reconstructed, but only if doing so achieves complete resection.

Lung, pleura, and diaphragm. Direct invasion into the lung should be resected as permitted by the limitations of pulmonary function. Stapled wedge excision is most often appropriate; however, segmental resection or anatomic lobectomy may be necessary. Rarely, pneumonectomy or extrapleural pneumonectomy is required to completely resect disease that involves the pulmonary hilum or pleura. This should be undertaken only in a young, otherwise healthy and physiologically uncompromised patient. Parietal pleural implants can be removed by pleural stripping. Diaphragmatic implants are best removed by full-thickness excision of diaphragm.

Results. Operative morbidity and mortality are low. Hospital stays for nonmyasthenic patients are usually less than 3 or 4 days, and mortality following resection of even stage III or IV tumors is less than 3%. Long-term

(10-year) survival following complete resection for stage I disease is 80% to 90%, and for stage II thymomas it is 70% to 80%. For patients with stage III or IV tumors, complete resection is either difficult or impossible. In most large series with extended follow-up, patients received adjuvant radiotherapy after debulking or complete resection; survival rates in these reports are highly variable, but in most cases they were approximately 40% to 60% at 5 years and 30% to 40% at 10 years (Cowen et al, 1995; Park et al, 1994; Regnard et al, 1996; Shimizu et al, 1992).

In a series of 307 patients with thymomas of all stages, Regnard and colleagues (1996) reported that overall 10-year survival was 76% following complete resection and was only 28% following incomplete resection. Using multivariate analysis, these authors concluded that complete resection was the only important prognostic factor, eliminating even the independent impact of Masaoka stage. Jackson and Ball (1991) evaluated 28 patients with stage III or IV thymoma who were treated with surgery and adjuvant radiation therapy. Half had complete resection and half had partial resection or biopsy. Ten-year survival was 62% following complete resection and 29% following partial resection or biopsy. In a recent review of 194 patients, Okumura and colleagues (1999) also concluded that complete resection was associated with better long-term survival. However, for all patients with invasive disease (stage III, n = 56), multivariate analysis indicated that, independent of completeness of resection, involvement of the great vessels (defined as the brachiocephalic veins, the superior vena cava, and the aorta) was the sole statistically significant predictor of survival.

Radiation Therapy

Thymomas are radiosensitive. Radiation therapy is indicated for patients with unresectable disease or residual disease following partial resection or biopsy. It has been so widely accepted in this setting (stage III or IV thymoma) that definitive evidence of its efficacy is hard to find: there are no prospective trials, and results from retrospective series are usually compromised by a small number of patients in the nonradiated group. The retrospective series reported by Wang and Huang (1992) is a good example. They found that, among patients who had mostly stage III or IV disease, 5-year survival with and without adjuvant radiation therapy was 67% (n = 52) and 24% (n = 9), respectively. By themselves, results from a single retrospective series such as this one are inconclusive, but combined with similar results from essentially all published series (Curran et al, 1988; Gripp et al, 1998; Mornex et al, 1995; Nakahara et al, 1988), these findings indicate that radiation therapy is effective against residual or unresectable disease.

The responsiveness of thymomas to radiation therapy suggested to Shamji and colleagues (1984) that it might be useful preoperatively to facilitate resection of bulky tumors. However, more recent data suggest that chemotherapy is more effective than radiation as an induction agent, and that radiation therapy should be reserved for use postoperatively. This approach achieves higher preoperative response rates, eliminates the need to operate in a radiated field, and optimizes radiation therapy's biologic effect by avoiding dose interruption.

Is radiation therapy of benefit for patients with *completely resected* invasive thymoma (stage II or III)? The risk of recurrence in this population may be as high as 40%, suggesting that adjuvant radiotherapy may have a role, but few authors specifically address this question. Regnard and colleagues (1996) found that 10-year disease-free survival rates with and without postoperative radiation were 70% and 55%, respectively. By 15 years the disease-free survival rates were nearly identical (59% and 55%, respectively) and the difference between the overall survival curves was not statistically significant ($P = .45$), but the authors remained advocates of adjuvant radiation therapy. Curran and colleagues (1988) reported a more dramatic difference, although with shorter follow-up. They found that 5-year disease-free survival for patients who received postoperative radiotherapy was 100% (5 of 5), but for those who did not, it was only 43% (9 of 21). The small number of patients in the adjuvant therapy group diminishes the impact of this observation, but the difference in local control is particularly striking because the patients in the adjuvant therapy group were at higher risk for recurrence—80% (4 of 5) had stage III disease, compared with only 14% (3 of 21) with stage III disease in the nonradiated group. None of the patients in this series received chemotherapy, suggesting that radiation therapy was responsible for improved local control. Although these reports support the use of adjuvant radiotherapy, others have been unable to demonstrate a benefit. Haniuda and colleagues (1992) reported that adjuvant radiotherapy had no impact on local control. For patients with stage II disease, the recurrence rates with and without adjuvant radiotherapy were 23% (3 of 13) and 25% (5 of 20), respectively, and for patients with stage III disease they were 30% (3 of 10) and 25% (2 of 8), respectively. (Length of follow-up was not provided, but the shortest seems to have been 3 years, and the longest was greater than 15 years.) Cohen and colleagues (1984) and others (Jackson and Ball, 1991; Park et al, 1994) have also concluded that adjuvant radiation therapy provided no additional benefit beyond complete resection. The conflicting data on this issue are difficult to reconcile because these reports are all retrospective, but overall the "preponderance of evidence" (Kohman, 1997) supports the use of adjuvant radiation therapy for patients with invasive thymoma, regardless of whether or not the tumor has been completely resected. Most authors advocate this approach (Cowen et al, 1995; Masaoka et al, 1981; Nakahara et al, 1988), and current protocols incorporate this philosophy (Venuta et al, 1997).

For patients with encapsulated (stage I) thymomas, the role of adjuvant radiation therapy has not been defined. Monden and colleagues (1985) were early proponents, but other authors have not echoed this sentiment. Surgery alone is associated with an excellent prognosis, and there have been little data to suggest that long-term survival could be improved with the addition of postoperative radiation therapy. Long-term survival for these patients, however, is not 100%, and the ability to better identify important prognostic factors may facilitate selection of patients for whom postoperative therapy would be of benefit. Based on their belief that cortical thymomas are more aggressive tumors, Venuta and colleagues (1997) implemented a multimodality protocol in which patients with stage I cortical thymomas received both chemotherapy and radiation therapy postoperatively. Results were compared with historical controls who did not receive any uniform regimen of adjuvant therapy. At 6 years' follow-up, survival in both groups was 95%; only one patient in the multimodality therapy group was available for evaluation at 8 years, and therefore determination of any potential long-term benefit with this approach awaits additional follow-up.

Chemotherapy

Thymomas respond to chemotherapy, and cisplatin-based regimens have been used for many years to treat patients with unresectable or recurrent disease. Looking forward, these regimens will be used increasingly as part of multimodality therapy for patients with all but early-stage, well-encapsulated tumors. Most importantly, the use of preoperative chemotherapy has shown promise for improving both resectability and long-term survival.

Retrospective Studies. A variety of retrospective reports suggest that cisplatin-based regimens are effective therapy for patients with unresectable or recurrent disease. Fornasiero and colleagues (1991) reported an overall response rate of 90% in a series of 38 patients with stage III (n = 12) or stage IV (n = 26) disease who were treated with cisplatin, doxorubicin, vincristine, and cyclophosphamide. Ten patients went on to resection, and median survival was 1.3 years. Five-year survival for patients with stage III disease was 42%, and for patients with stage IV disease it was 19%. Although these rates may seem low, all patients in this series had active and growing disease and therefore had a very poor prognosis. Cowen and colleagues (1995) compared 31 patients treated with surgery and radiation therapy to 59 similar patients who also received adjuvant chemotherapy (cisplatin, doxorubicin, and cyclophosphamide). All patients had either stage III or IV disease. The overall response rate was not reported, but the addition of postoperative chemotherapy was associated with an increase in the 5-year disease-free survival rate from 15% to 45%. Mornex and colleagues (1995) reported similar results. In a group of 90 patients with stage III or IV disease, they found that 5-year survival rates with and without adjuvant chemotherapy were 55% and 32%, respectively; 10-year survival rates were 41% and 24%, respectively.

Prospective Studies. Several prospective studies published during the past decade report high response rates with chemotherapy and demonstrate an associated survival benefit (Table 63–19). Although cisplatin alone has minimal activity against thymoma (Bonomi et al, 1993), cisplatin combined with other agents is effective against unresectable or recurrent disease. Giaccone and colleagues (1996) reported that etoposide and cisplatin produced a response rate of 56% and was associated with a 5-year survival rate of 50%. The combination of doxorubicin and cyclophosphamide with cisplatin is also effective. Loehrer and colleagues (1997) reported that this regimen, together with radiation therapy, produced a 70% response rate and a 53% 5-year survival rate.

Prospective trials of multimodality therapy for patients with advanced disease indicate that neoadjuvant chemotherapy may improve resectability of locally invasive tumors. Combined with consolidation therapy postoperatively, it may also improve long-term survival. Macchiarini and colleagues (1991) first demonstrated the feasibility of this approach. Seven patients with stage III disease were treated with preoperative chemotherapy (cisplatin, etoposide, and epirubicin) and radiation therapy. The response rate was 100%, all seven patients went on to surgery, and complete resection was achieved in four. Long-term survival was not reported. A subsequent report by Rea and colleagues (1993) included 16 patients with stage III (n = 13) or stage IV (n = 3) disease. Induction chemotherapy with cisplatin, doxorubicin, cyclophosphamide, and vincristine produced a 100% response rate. Five patients (31%) had complete resections and received additional chemotherapy postoperatively; 11 patients had incomplete resection and received radiation therapy postoperatively. Median survival was 5.5 years and 5-year survival rates for patients with stage III or IV disease were 53% and 33%, respectively.

Recent reports by Shin and co-workers (1998) and Venuta and associates (1997) provide the strongest evidence in support of multimodality therapy. Shin and colleagues administered preoperative chemotherapy (cis-

TABLE 63–19 ■ **Prospective Trials of Chemotherapy for Unresectable or Recurrent Thymoma**

Author	*N*	*Treatment*	*RR (%)*	*Survival (yr)* Median	3-Year	5-Year
Bonomi et al, 1993	20	Cisplatin	10	1.5	39	
Giaccone et al, 1996	16	Cisplatin + etoposide	56	4.3	69	50
Loehrer et al, 1994	30	Cisplatin + doxorubicin + cyclophosphamide	50	3.1		32
Loehrer et al, 1997	23	Cisplatin + doxorubicin + cyclophosphamide → XRT	70*	7.8	60	53

*RR for chemotherapy only; for the combination of chemotherapy followed by radiation therapy the response rate was 87%.
RR, response rate; XRT, radiation therapy.

TABLE 63–20 ■ Clinicopathologic Staging of Thymoma for Multimodality Therapy

Masaoka Stage	*Müller-Hermelink Histologic Subtype*		
	Medullary	*Mixed*	*Cortical*
I	Group 1	Group 1	Group 2
II	Group 1	Group 2	Group 3
III			Group 3
IV			Group 3

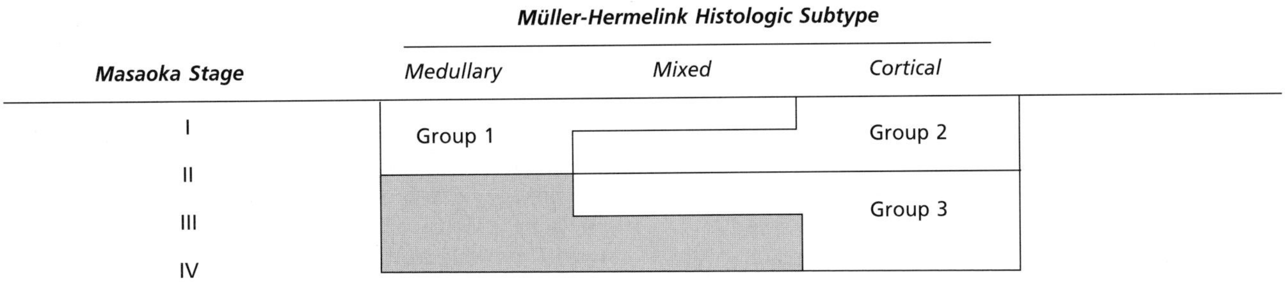

Treament Protocol			
Group 1		Surgery	
Group 2		Surgery →	Chemotherapy + Radiation therapy
Group 3	Chemotherapy →	Surgery →	Chemotherapy + Radiation therapy

From Venuta F, Rendina EA, Pescarmona EO et al: Multimodality treatment of thymoma: A prospective study. Ann Thorac Surg 64:1585, 1997.

platin, doxorubicin, prednisone, and cyclophosphamide) to 12 patients with stage III (n = 4) or stage IV (n = 8) disease. The response rate was 92%, and all patients went on to resection followed by chemotherapy and radiation therapy. With a mean follow-up of 3.6 years, survival was 100%. In a larger report with longer follow-up, Venuta and colleagues described their results with a prospective trial of multimodality therapy for all patients with thymoma. Patients were stratified into three groups based on clinical-pathologic stage so that those with cortical thymomas were treated more aggressively than were those with medullary thymomas (Table 63–20). Results were reported with a mean follow-up of 4.4 years (range, 0.1–8.4) and were compared to historical controls from the same institution. Preoperative chemotherapy induced a partial or complete response in all patients and increased the rate of complete resection compared with controls. Most importantly, survival rates for patients with stage II, III, and IV disease were all higher (Fig. 63–19). These results demonstrate that multimodality therapy improves prognosis for patients with invasive thymomas. Longer follow-up is necessary to determine if adjuvant therapy is worthwhile for patients with stage I cortical thymomas.

Surgery for Extensive, Recurrent, or Metastatic Disease

Because thymomas tend to grow slowly and not to metastasize hematogenously, surgery plays an important role in the management of patients with unresectable, metastatic, or recurrent disease. Most series report that partial resection and debulking are associated with improved survival compared with biopsy. In a review of 90 patients with stage III or IV disease, Mornex and colleagues (1995) found that biopsy was associated with 5- and 10-year survival rates of 39% and 31%, respectively, whereas partial resection was associated with survival rates of 64% and 43%, respectively. All patients received radiation therapy, and most were also given chemotherapy. Cowen and colleagues (1995), Maggi and colleagues (1991), and Nakahara and colleagues (1988) also reported similar improvements in survival with partial resection compared with biopsy. However, some series report that debulking may not be of benefit. Both Regnard and colleagues (1996) and Wang and colleagues (1992) found no difference in survival rates between patients who had partial resection or biopsy, and Ciernik and colleagues (1994) concluded that biopsy with adjuvant radiotherapy was equivalent to partial resection. The debatable importance of partial resection relative to biopsy, particularly with recent improvements in adjuvant chemotherapy, underscores the importance of minimizing the risk of operative morbidity when complete resection cannot be achieved.

Resection of recurrent or metastatic disease may improve survival. Maggi and colleagues (1991) found that among 23 patients with recurrent disease, 5-year survival was better for the 12 patients who underwent resection than for the 11 patients treated medically (71% vs. 41%). Similar favorable results were reported by Blumberg and colleagues (1995) from Memorial Sloan-Kettering Cancer Center. Initial stage of disease and disease-free interval were similar for 25 patients who had either re-resection (n = 13) or medical therapy (n = 12), but at 2 years' follow-up, 90% of patients in the re-resected group were alive compared with only 30% in the medically treated group (P = .0004). Overall 5-year survival for the re-resected group was similar to overall 5-year survival for patients whose disease did not recur (80%). These results are difficult to interpret, however, because 40% of the patients in this series had thymic carcinoma and not thymoma. Additional data to support a role for re-resection were reported by Regnard and colleagues (1996), who found that 10-year survival was 53% if the recurrent disease could be completely resected, but only 11% if a partial resection had been done (n = 11 and 7 respectively; P = .01). In an update of this series published the following year, the authors noted that the benefit of complete re-resection was seen regardless of whether the recurrent disease was local or pleuropericardial (Regnard et al, 1997).

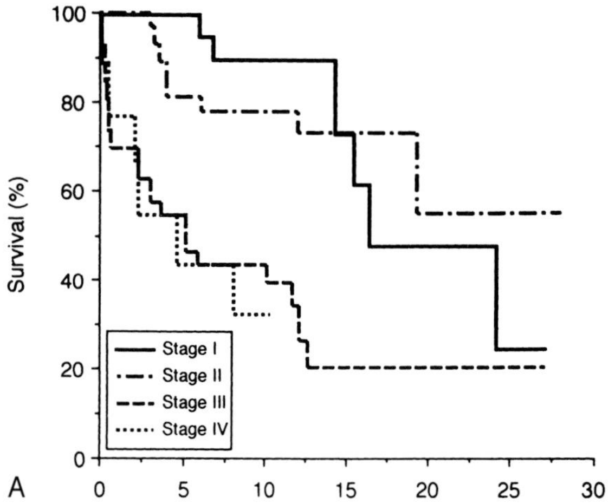

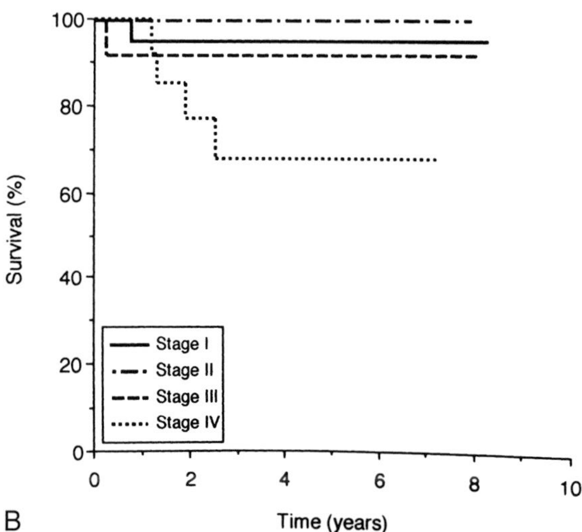

FIGURE 63–19 ■ Multimodality therapy for thymoma. Survival curves by Masaoka stage. *A*, Historical controls (patients treated before 1989). *B*, Patients treated between 1989 and 1995 according to the protocol outlined in Table 63–20. (From Venuta F, Rendina EA, Pescarmona EO et al: Multimodality treatment of thymoma: A prospective study. Ann Thorac Surg 64:1588, 1997.)

THYMIC CARCINOMA

Thymic carcinomas are often considered together with thymomas, and like thymomas they are tumors of thymic epithelial cell origin. However, thymic carcinomas are not thymomas—histologically they are distinguishable by malignant cytologic features and clinically they are characterized by a more malignant behavior. Thymic carcinomas have a high degree of histologic anaplasia, obvious cellular atypia, and increased proliferative activity. The infiltrating lymphocytes are mostly mature. Thymic carcinomas are usually invasive and are refractory to both surgical and medical therapy. They usually recur, frequently with metastases to distant sites such as lymph nodes, lung, liver, and bone. Prognosis is poor, with overall median survival approximately 20 months and long-term survival less than 40%.

Because thymic carcinomas are uncommon, the approach to therapy is varied and generally based on the larger experience with thymoma. There is no recognized standard therapeutic strategy nor is there a universally accepted staging system. The most common approach is surgical resection followed by radiotherapy, chemotherapy, or both. Unfortunately, most tumors are not resectable, and even if complete resection is achieved, the impact of surgery on survival is unclear. Radiation therapy can achieve response rates close to 80%. Chemotherapy, which is usually cisplatin based, has had limited success. Durable responses are unusual and most patients relapse with both local and distant disease. Given these poor results, it is likely that future approaches will explore the efficacy of combined modality and neoadjuvant strategies.

Histology

The defining feature of a thymic carcinoma is the obvious cytologic atypia of the thymic epithelial cell (Shimosato and Mukai, 1997). While the thymic epithelium in a thymoma retains relatively normal structural and even functional characteristics, the thymic epithelial cells in a carcinoma are larger and exhibit prominent nucleoli, high nuclear-to-cytoplasmic ratio, and abundant mitoses. Multifocal and confluent areas of necrosis are also found. Unlike the lymphocytes associated with thymomas, which are largely immature, lymphocytes associated with thymic carcinomas are mostly mature infiltrating T cells. This finding indicates that while the epithelial cell in a thymoma retains both relatively normal form and function, the epithelial cell in a thymic carcinoma loses function as it undergoes malignant degeneration. Some authors argue that the coexistence of a paraneoplastic syndrome, such as myasthenia gravis, indicates that functional epithelium is present and is therefore inconsistent with the diagnosis of thymic carcinoma (Kirschner, 1998; Shimosato and Mukai, 1997; Truong et al, 1990; Yoneda et al, 1999).

Several distinct subtypes of thymic carcinoma have been described. In the largest series yet published, Suster and Rosai (1991b) proposed a classification system based on degree of differentiation (Table 63–21) and found that it correlated well with prognosis. Low-grade tumors, of which squamous cell carcinomas are the most common,

TABLE 63–21 ■ **Histologic Classification of Thymic Carcinomas**

Low-grade histology
Well-differentiated (keratinizing) squamous cell carcinoma
Well-differentiated mucoepidermoid carcinoma
Basaloid carcinoma
High-grade histology
Lymphoepithelioma-like carcinoma
Small cell/neuroendocrine carcinoma
Undifferentiated/anaplastic carcinoma
Sarcomatoid carcinoma
Clear cell carcinoma

From Suster S, Rosai J: Thymic carcinoma: A clinicopathologic study of 60 cases. Cancer 67:1027, 1991. Copyright © 1991 American Cancer Society. Reprinted by permission of Wiley-Liss, Inc., a subsidiary of John Wiley & Sons, Inc.

were associated with a favorable prognosis. With a mean follow-up of 6.6 years, there were no tumor-related deaths among 21 patients. In contrast, high-grade tumors, of which lymphoepithelioma-like carcinomas are the most common, had a very poor prognosis. Among 39 patients in this group, median survival was only 15 months and all but 6 patients succumbed to their disease. Other published reports generally confirm the prognostic relevance of histologic grade (Hsu et al, 1994; Kuo et al, 1990; Truong et al, 1990; Wick et al, 1982b).

Etiology

Rarely, islands of thymomatous cells can be found within a thymic carcinoma, or a patient with a remote history of thymoma presents with a thymic carcinoma (Shimosato and Mukai, 1997; Suster and Rosai, 1991b). As a result, some authors postulate that thymic carcinomas arise from thymomas that undergo malignant degeneration (Suster and Moran, 1999). Lymphoepithelioma-like thymic carcinomas may be related to Epstein-Barr virus (EBV) infection (Dimery et al, 1988; Leyvraz et al, 1985). These tumors are histologically indistinguishable from nasopharyngeal undifferentiated carcinomas, which have been linked to EBV infection. Furthermore, immunohistochemical and in situ hybridization studies have demonstrated EBV-derived genetic material in tumor specimens (Shimosato and Mukai, 1997). These findings suggest that lymphoepithelioma-like thymic carcinomas might be a unique pathologic entity distinct from thymic carcinomas of other histologic subtypes.

Clinical Features

Thymic carcinomas account for approximately 20% of all thymic epithelial tumors and afflict men slightly more often than they do women (ratio of 1.5:1). They have been found in patients of all ages—the youngest reported patient was 4 years old (Wick et al, 1982b) and the oldest was 71 years of age (Suster and Rosai, 1991b)—but most patients are between the ages of 30 and 60 years, and the median age in most series is close to 50 years. Ninety percent of patients with thymic carcinoma present with symptoms. The most common are cough and chest pain, which are caused by local effects of the tumor. SVC syndrome is seen in approximately 20% of patients (Blumberg et al, 1998; Kuo et al, 1990; Truong et al, 1990; Wick et al, 1982b). Generalized symptoms such as fever, weight loss, anorexia, and fatigue may also be present. Ten percent of patients have distant metastases at presentation (Blumberg et al, 1998; Suster and Rosai, 1991b). The most common sites of metastasis are lymph nodes (mediastinal, cervical, and axillary) and bone, followed by lung, liver, and brain. Paraneoplastic syndromes are rare. In the series of 60 cases reported by Suster and Rosai (1991b), no patients had a paraneoplastic syndrome. In the series of 13 cases reported by Marino and Müller (1985), one patient (who had a squamous cell tumor) also had myasthenia gravis. In Blumberg and colleagues' (1998) review of 43 cases from Memorial Sloan-Kettering Cancer Center, 10 patients had myasthenia gravis, 9 of whom had tumors that were classified as well differentiated. The incidence of associated myasthenia gravis in this report is by far the highest in the literature and has been a source of criticism, suggesting to some that several patients in the series may have had thymoma and not thymic carcinoma (Kirschner, 1998).

Differential Diagnosis

Radiographically, thymic carcinomas and thymomas are indistinguishable (Fig. 63–20). Although the presence of symptoms is suggestive of the former, and some argue that the presence of a paraneoplastic syndrome is diagnostic of the latter, tissue is required to make the distinction definitively. If a biopsy is desired prior to resection, FNA is usually performed. Identification of malignant cytologic features and immunohistochemical studies that demonstrate predominantly mature T cells usually are sufficient for diagnosis (Shimosato and Mukai, 1997). However, cytology alone may be inadequate for distinguishing a thymic carcinoma from other anterior mediastinal neoplasms such as atypical carcinoid, dysgerminoma, embryonal cell carcinoma, and diffuse large cell lymphoma. In these cases core needle biopsy, mediastinotomy, or thoracoscopy is indicated. Lastly, metastatic carcinoma to the thymus, particularly from a lung primary, must be excluded. This is an unusual circumstance and is almost always readily apparent.

Staging

No system for staging thymic carcinomas is universally accepted. Most authors use the Masaoka system, even though it was intended only for staging thymomas and its applicability to thymic carcinomas has never been

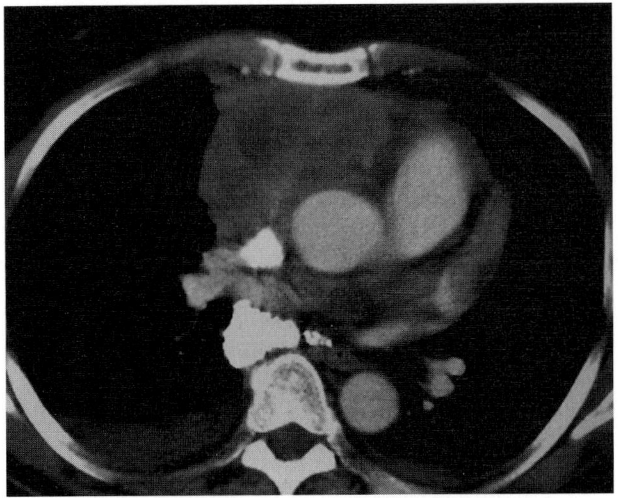

FIGURE 63–20 ■ Thymic carcinoma. Chest computed tomography scan of a 63-year-old man with a thymic carcinoma. The imaging characteristics of the tumor are similar to those of an invasive thymoma. Local invasion is suggested, with compression of the superior vena cava, and the tumor has marked areas of heterogeneity suspicious for malignancy. There are bilateral pleural effusions. Fine-needle aspiration biopsy confirmed thymic carcinoma. Despite induction chemotherapy, this tumor proved unresectable due to invasion into the myocardium.

validated. Suster and Rosai (1991b) found that Masaoka stage had some prognostic significance, but others have been unable to show a correlation (Blumberg et al, 1998; Hsu et al, 1994). In the recent series from Memorial Sloan-Kettering Cancer Center, multivariate analysis indicated that only the presence or absence of brachiocephalic vein invasion had any prognostic value (Blumberg et al, 1998). Yamakawa and colleagues (1991) proposed a TNM system for thymic epithelial tumors, and Tsuchiya and colleagues (1994) suggested its application to thymic carcinomas (Table 63–22). This strategy appropriately reflects the propensity for thymic carcinomas to metastasize by lymphogenous and hematogenous routes and is more consistent with the staging of other carcinomas. In their series of 16 patients, Tsuchiya and colleagues found that TNM stage correlated well with prognosis. Although it has yet to achieve universal acceptance and adoption by the World Health Organization, TNM staging is gaining support as an appropriate and useful system (Shimosato and Mukai, 1997).

Prognosis

The prognosis for patients with thymic carcinoma is poor, and most die from locally progressive or metastatic disease. Suster and Rosai (1991b) reported overall 5- and 10-year survival rates of 50% and 35%, respectively. These results are similar to those reported by others (Blumberg et al, 1998; Hsu et al, 1994) and are considerably worse than for patients with thymoma. In Suster and Rosai's series, tumor encapsulation emerged as an important predictor of long-term survival: "Good circumscription" was associated with a 16% disease-related mortality (4 of 24 patients), while "poor circumscription" was associated with an 88% (22 of 25 patients) disease-related mortality. Histologic subtype was also found to affect prognosis. There were no disease-related deaths among 21 patients with low-grade carcinomas (mostly squamous cell carcinomas), but there was an 85% disease-related mortality rate among 39 patients with high-grade carcinomas (mostly lymphoepithelioma-like carcinomas) (Fig. 63–21). Hsu and colleagues (1994), as well as others, have confirmed the prognostic significance of histologic subtype. In a series of 18 cases, Truong and colleagues (1990) found that all five deaths were in patients with poorly differentiated tumors. Similarly, Kuo and colleagues (1990) found that all seven long-term survivors in their series of 13 patients had squamous cell tumors.

Blumberg and colleagues (1998) challenged the prognostic significance of histologic grade. Although they found a survival difference favoring patients with well-differentiated tumors compared to patients with type II malignant thymomas (recall the classification ambiguities discussed earlier in this subchapter), the difference was not statistically significant. This result highlights two important problems inherent in all survival analyses of patients with thymic carcinoma. First, the rarity of this disease makes subset analyses and comparisons difficult. Even though these authors compiled one of the largest series in the literature, with 43 patients, the study is underpowered to confirm the null hypothesis and conclusively establish that no difference exists (type II error). Second, the confused nomenclature and the use of different classifications by different authors make comparisons between studies nearly impossible. Ultimately, histology probably does affect prognosis. Indeed, Shimosato and Mukai (1997) argue that histologic subtype is the most important prognostic factor and that prognosis correlates well with degree of differentiation and cytologic atypia. Consistently, squamous cell carcinomas are associated with the best long-term survival, and lymphoepithelioma-like carcinomas are associated with the worst.

TABLE 63–22 ■ **Proposed TNM Staging for Thymic Epithelial Tumors**

Tumor	
T1	Completely encapsulated tumor
T2	Tumor breaking through capsule, invading thymus or fatty tissue (may be adherent to mediastinal pleura but not invading neighboring organs)
T3	Tumor breaking through the mediastinal pleura or pericardium, or invading neighboring organs, such as great vessels and lung
T4	Tumor with pleural or pericardial implantation
Nodes	
N0	No lymph node metastasis
N1	Metastasis in anterior mediastinal lymph nodes
N2	Metastasis in intrathoracic lymph nodes excluding anterior mediastinal lymph nodes
N3	Metastasis in extrathoracic lymph nodes
Metastasis	
M0	No distant organ metastasis
M1	With distant organ metastasis

Stage Grouping			
Stage I	T1, T2	N0	M0
Stage II	T1, T2	N1	M0
Stage III	T3	N0, N1	M0
Stage IVa	T4	N0, N1	M0
IVb	any T	N2, N3	M0
IVc	any T	any N	M1

From Tsuchiya R, Koga K, Matsuno Y et al: Thymic carcinoma: Proposal for pathological and TNM staging. Pathol Int 44:505, 1994. Reprinted with permission from Blackwell Science Asia.

Therapy

Because thymic carcinoma is uncommon, our ability to objectively evaluate therapy is limited. Interpretation of published results is difficult because all reports are retrospective and most are small case series, because all classification of histologic subtypes and the distinction between thymoma and low-grade thymic carcinoma are inconsistent, and because treatment regimens used between centers and between patients at any given center are different. In general, treatment for thymic carcinoma has grown out of the experience with thymoma, in which resection of both localized and extensive disease is the principal focus of therapy. This approach has proved inadequate for the majority of patients with thymic carcinoma, and therefore radiation therapy and chemotherapy have assumed considerably more importance.

Surgery

Shimosato and colleagues (1977) are credited with the first published report on thymic carcinoma. In their series

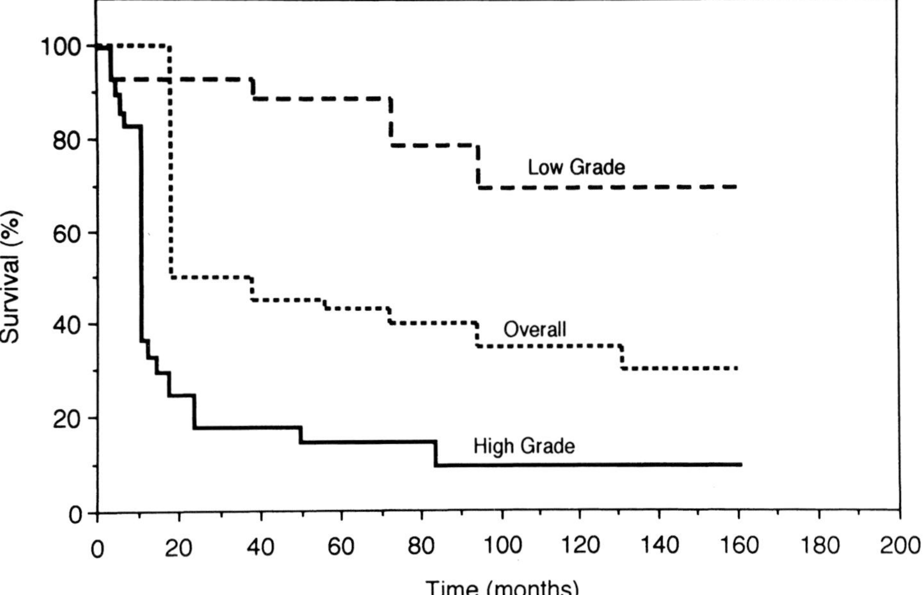

FIGURE 63–21 ▪ Thymic carcinoma. Survival curves for patients with thymic carcinoma by degree of differentiation. (From Suster S, Rosai J: Thymic carcinoma. A clinicopathologic study of 60 cases. Cancer 67:1027, 1991. Copyright © (1991) American Cancer Society. Reprinted by permission of Wiley-Liss, Inc., a subsidiary of John Wiley & Sons, Inc.)

of eight patients, all of whom had squamous cell carcinomas, five underwent complete resection, two had biopsy only, and one did not have surgery. All five patients who had complete resection, and one of the two patients who had biopsy only, were alive at between 1 and 12 years' follow-up. These results suggest that complete resection is an important therapeutic goal. Similar high rates of complete resection were reported by Suster and Rosai (1991b) and Blumberg and colleagues (1998)—80% (48 of 60 patients) and 67% (29 of 43 patients), respectively—but results from other series caution that this goal may not be possible for many patients. In the series published by Truong and colleagues (1990), none of the 13 patients had a complete resection, while in the series reported by Hsu and colleagues (1994), excluding two patients with carcinoid tumors, only 5 of 18 patients had a complete resection.

Although resection is considered primary therapy for patients with thymic carcinoma, the value of surgery is not as clear for this disease as it is for thymoma. Complete resection may be helpful only for those patients with well-encapsulated tumors, and tumor debulking has not translated into any demonstrable survival advantage. Suster and Rosai (1991b) found that tumor "circumscription" was an important prognostic factor (see earlier), but Blumberg and colleagues (1998) found that complete resection had no impact on 5-year survival (68% for complete resection vs. 62% for incomplete resection). Other studies also demonstrate no significant difference in long-term survival between patients who had complete resection and those who had either tumor debulking or biopsy alone (Hsu et al, 1994; Kuo et al, 1990; Shimizu et al, 1994; Truong et al, 1990; Yano et al, 1993). Recognizing the limitations of retrospective analyses based on small sample sizes, we can conclude that complete resection should be attempted in all cases in which the tumor appears well confined. Tumor debulking is of unproved benefit, and en bloc resections that sacrifice vital structures to achieve complete resection are not indicated.

Radiation Therapy

Thymic carcinomas are relatively radiation-sensitive tumors. Yano and colleagues (1993) published a series of eight patients in which seven were treated with radiation as either primary therapy for unresectable disease or as salvage therapy for recurrent disease. All patients also received chemotherapy. Chemotherapy generated only two partial responses, but radiation therapy produced six partial responses and one stable disease. Ultimately, six patients had recurrence of their disease and died, but overall median survival was almost 6 years, which is a good result even considering that most patients in the series had low-grade tumors.

Hasserjian and colleagues (1995) found that radiation therapy was effective against high-grade tumors as well. They reported that, with a mean follow-up of 2.3 years, the only survivors among a group of eight patients were the three who received radiation therapy—two were disease free and the third was alive with disease. Hsu and colleagues (1994) also demonstrated improved survival among patients who received radiation therapy compared to those who did not (39.3 months vs. 15 months). This result is suspect, however, because although the series included 20 patients, only four were not treated with radiation therapy: two had carcinoid tumors, one died from postoperative complications, and the fourth refused therapy.

Chemotherapy

Because patients with thymic carcinoma are few and far between, evaluating the efficacy of chemotherapy is particularly difficult. Most strategies use cisplatin, but the number of different regimens reported in the literature is almost as great as the number of patients who have received them. This finding alone indicates that no combination is clearly effective. Instead, we are left with results from a few small retrospective series and isolated case reports.

Using multivariate analysis, Blumberg and colleagues (1998) concluded that chemotherapy had no impact on survival. However, many different regimens were used in various combinations with surgery and radiation therapy, and therefore it is difficult to conclude anything more than that chemotherapy in general was of no clear benefit. A few smaller series have specifically addressed the role of chemotherapy and seem to suggest otherwise. In the series by Yano and colleagues (1993), four different chemotherapy regimens were used. Only two of the eight patients were treated with a regimen that did not include cisplatin (cyclophosphamide, doxorubicin, and vincristine), but these were the only two who responded to chemotherapy. Of the two patients who received the same regimen plus cisplatin, one progressed and one had stable disease. The authors' tentative conclusion that cisplatin was unhelpful was tempered by the disclosure that they were treating an additional patient with cisplatin and etoposide with "good control." In another small series published the same year, Weide and colleagues (1993) described their experience with five patients who were treated with chemotherapy after undergoing either a tumor debulking procedure or a biopsy. All five patients had poorly differentiated carcinomas. The two patients treated with cisplatin alone did not respond, but the three treated with cisplatin, etoposide, and bleomycin did—one partially and two completely. One of the patients who sustained a complete response ultimately died of progressive disease.

Three case reports in the literature deserve mention. Carlson and colleagues (1990) reported on a patient with thymic carcinoma metastatic to the lungs. Cisplatin, bleomycin, and vinblastine induced a clinical partial response and therefore surgery was performed. This demonstrated a pathologic complete response and the patient continued disease free for at least 5 years. Tweedy and colleagues (1992) treated a 55-year-old patient who presented with SVC syndrome. Carboplatin, etoposide, and radiation therapy induced a complete response and the patient was disease free at 8 months. Finally, Yanagawa and colleagues (1995) treated a young man who had invasive and metastatic disease. Combined radiation therapy and intensive systemic and regional (intrapleural) chemotherapy induced a partial response, but the patient died of recurrent disease within 1 year. Together, these case reports and small series illustrate that it may be possible to identify regimens that produce clinical and pathologic responses, and that at least in some cases, chemotherapy may improve survival.

THYMIC CARCINOID

For many years carcinoid tumors were thought to arise only from the gastrointestinal tract and lung. Tumors of the anterior mediastinum with endocrine features were called variously epithelial thymoma, mediastinal bronchial adenoma, parathyroid adenoma, unclassified mediastinal tumor, or carcinoid tumor of the mediastinum (Shimosato and Mukai, 1997). It was for this reason that in 1970, when Kay and Willson described an adrenocorticotropic hormone (ACTH)–producing thymic tumor in a patient with Cushing's syndrome, they called it a thymoma despite its microscopic similarity to a carcinoid. Two years later Rosai and Higa (1972) published a landmark paper in which they suggested that carcinoid tumors could be of thymic origin. They based their conclusion on a review of 16 patients with thymic endocrine tumors: eight new cases and eight that had been described previously as thymoma. In the same issue of *Cancer* they also described three cases of thymic carcinoid associated with "multiple endocrine adenomatosis" (Rosai et al, 1972). Since then thymic carcinoid tumors have been recognized as a distinct group of thymic neoplasms with a unique biology and a strong association with the multiple endocrine neoplasia (MEN) syndromes, particularly MEN type 1 (MEN-1). They can secrete a variety of hormones and frequently are responsible for ectopic ACTH production and Cushing's syndrome. An association with carcinoid syndrome has not been reported. Unlike their bronchial cousins, thymic carcinoids are aggressive tumors that usually recur and frequently generate widespread metastases. They are almost universally fatal over the long term.

Demographics

Thymic carcinoids are rare. They represent only 4% of all anterior mediastinal tumors (Moran et al, 1999; Valli et al, 1994; Wick et al, 1980), and less than 150 cases have been published in the world's literature. They have been found in patients from 8 (Lin et al, 1999) to 87 years of age (Rosado de Christenson et al, 1999), but most patients are in their fourth, fifth, or sixth decade of life. The average age in all of the larger series is between 43 and 55 years (Fukai et al, 1999; Moran et al, 1999; Rosado de Christenson et al, 1999; Shimosato and Mukai, 1997; Valli, 1994; Wick et al, 1982a). Unlike thymomas or thymic carcinomas, which are equally prevalent in men and women, thymic carcinoids are three times more common in men than they are in women (Economopoulos et al, 1990; Fukai et al, 1999; Rosado de Christenson et al, 1999; Valli et al, 1994; Wick et al, 1982a). This difference is even more pronounced among patients with MEN-1–associated disease.

Association with Multiple Endocrine Neoplasia Syndromes

In 1972 Rosai and Higa described three patients who had both a thymic carcinoid and MEN-1 syndrome. Since then, the association between these two diseases has become a well-recognized phenomenon. Of all patients with MEN-1, approximately 5% have a thymic carcinoid (Birnberg et al, 1982; Rosado de Christenson et al, 1999; Teh et al, 1997; Wick et al, 1982a), while approximately 20% of patients with a thymic carcinoid have MEN-1 (Teh et al, 1997). Thymic carcinoids have not been associated with MEN type 2 (MEN–2). There has been only one documented case (Marchevsky and Dikman, 1979), and one case was reported in a patient with a remote history of medullary thyroid cancer (Economopoulos et al, 1990).

Patients with MEN-1–associated disease are almost exclusively men and tend to be younger than those who present with sporadic disease (thymic carcinoid not associated with MEN-1). In a recent review of the literature, Teh (1998) found 42 male but only 2 female patients, and discovered that, unlike patients with sporadic disease (see later), none of these patients had Cushing's syndrome. At the molecular genetic level, MEN-1–associated parathyroid and pancreatic tumors frequently exhibit loss of heterozygosity at the *MEN-1* locus. Interestingly, Teh and colleagues did not find this abnormality in any of the 20 MEN-1–associated thymic carcinoid tumors that they studied (Teh et al, 1997).

Because thymic carcinoids have a poor prognosis, Teh and colleagues argue that they are an important cause of death among patients with MEN-1 syndrome (Teh, 1998; Teh et al, 1997). Consequently, they and others (Satta et al, 1999) suggest that prophylactic transcervical thymectomy should be considered when patients with MEN-1 undergo parathyroidectomy.

Presentation

The majority of patients with thymic carcinoid present with symptoms either from mass effects of the tumor or from an associated endocrinopathy. In most series that include more than a few patients, less than one third of the tumors were discovered incidentally. The most common symptoms are cough, chest pain, and dyspnea; SVC syndrome is present in 24% of cases (7 of 29 patients) (de Montpréville et al, 1996; Wick et al, 1982a). Approximately one half of patients develop a clinically apparent endocrinopathy. ACTH is the most common endocrine product made by thymic carcinoids (de Montpréville et al, 1996), and 30% to 40% of patients have Cushing's syndrome (Birnberg et al, 1982; Rosado de Christenson et al, 1999; Wang et al, 1994). Cushing's syndrome has been described in an 8-year-old girl, the youngest patient with a thymic carcinoid so far reported (Lin et al, 1999), and was seen as a consequence of metastatic disease in a patient who had not been symptomatic from the primary tumor (de Montpréville et al, 1996).

Other endocrine products that can lead to clinically significant syndromes include antidiuretic hormone (Economopoulos et al, 1990) and parathyroid hormone. Hyperparathyroidism is a relatively common finding because thymic carcinoids occur frequently in patients with MEN-1, but several case reports have demonstrated that the culprit lesion can be the thymic tumor (Birnberg et al, 1982). In one instance, Takayama and colleagues (1993) found a thymic carcinoid that produced not only parathyroid hormone but also calcitonin and human chorionic gonadotropin. Carcinoid syndrome and myasthenia gravis are conspicuously absent from the list of paraneoplastic syndromes. Carcinoid syndrome has never been reported in association with a thymic carcinoid, and myasthenia gravis, a common finding in patients with thymoma, has been described in only one patient with thymic carcinoid. This patient was found to have a completely separate synchronous thymoma (Mizuno et al, 1990).

Invasiveness and Metastatic Potential

In sharp contrast to the generally benign clinical behavior of carcinoid tumors that arise elsewhere in the body, particularly the lung, thymic carcinoid tumors have a propensity for invasion and metastasis. The majority are locally invasive at the time of diagnosis (Economopoulos et al, 1990; Valli et al, 1994; Wang et al, 1994; Wick et al, 1982a) and can involve adjacent structures such as pleura, lung, pericardium, adventitia of the great vessels, brachiocephalic vein, and superior vena cava. In the Mayo Clinic series of 15 patients (Wick et al, 1982a), 8 were found to have locally invasive tumors. In a more recent series, Wang and colleagues (1994) reported that 7 of 8 patients had invasive tumor. Approximately 30% to 50% of patients have metastatic disease at presentation, including the occasional patient with an encapsulated tumor. Similar to thymic carcinomas, thymic carcinoids spread through both lymphogenous and hematogenous routes. Wick and colleagues (1982a) reported that 5 of their 15 patients had metastases at presentation, while de Montpréville and colleagues (1996) and Fukai and colleagues (1999) found metastatic disease in 7 of 14 and 9 of 15 patients, respectively. Mediastinal lymph nodes and bone are the most common sites, followed by lung, liver, and skin. Bone metastases are characteristically osteoblastic.

Ultimately most patients develop widespread disease. Typically the tumor is rapidly progressive, and metastases occur within 1 to 3 years of diagnosis. Takayama and colleagues (1993) reported on a particularly aggressive tumor in a patient who died within 1 year of diagnosis: At autopsy metastases were found in the liver, spleen, pancreas, both kidneys, both adrenal glands, both ovaries, and bone. Occasionally, however, metastases occur relatively late. Wick and colleagues (1982a) reported latency periods of 5 to 8 years in three of their patients, while Shimosato and Mukai (1997) documented a disease-free interval of 12 years in one patient.

Thymic carcinoid tumors that develop in patients with MEN-1 syndrome may be more aggressive than those that occur sporadically. In their series of eight such patients, Teh and colleagues (1997) found that, at presentation, six had invasive tumors and all eight had metastases.

Histogenesis and Histology

In general, carcinoid tumors are thought to arise from neuroendocrine cells of neural crest origin. However, Shimosato and Mukai (1997) argue that thymic carcinoids arise from primitive epithelial cells resident in the thymus, not from cells that migrate into it from the neural crest. Regardless of the progenitor cell's history, it is clear that carcinoid tumors can originate in the thymus. This was not appreciated until 1972, but it should not be unexpected considering that the thymus is derived from the same foregut structures as are the lungs and proximal gastrointestinal tract.

In some respects, thymic carcinoids can be considered a subtype of thymic carcinomas. Their clinical behavior is similar to that of thymic carcinomas: The patterns of metastatic spread and the poor prognoses are similar, and neither tumor is associated with a paraneoplastic autoimmune disorder such as myasthenia gravis. Nevertheless, thymic carcinoids and thymic carcinomas are considered distinct tumor types by most classification schemes, including the one proposed by Shimosato and Mukai (1997). One notable exception is the classification system proposed by Marino and Müller-Hermelink (1985), in which thymic carcinoids are classified as a subtype of thymic carcinoma.

Typically, the cut surface of a thymic carcinoid is pale tan to gray-white, but some pigmented tumors reminiscent of melanomas have been reported (Ho and Ho, 1977; Teh et al, 1997). Thymic carcinoids are usually larger than their bronchial cousins, and they almost always have multiple small foci of necrosis. This finding in a bronchial tumor suggests atypical carcinoid, and for this reason most thymic carcinoids are designated as atypical. The classic thymic carcinoid, similar to classic carcinoids in other tissues, is characterized by "solid nests, rosettes and festoons of small to medium-sized polygonal cells" (Shimosato and Mukai, 1997). The nuclei are centrally located and round, with small nucleoli, and there are few mitoses (2 to 20 per 10 high-power fields). Pathologists have described four other histologic patterns (Moran et al, 1999; Shimosato and Mukai, 1997): an "Indian-file" pattern created by a prominent sclerotic fibrous stroma; a "cribriform" pattern; a "sheet-like" pattern of cells with scant vascular stroma and a vague, organoid cellular arrangement; and a spindle-cell variant. Histologic grade (well, moderately, or poorly differentiated) (Klemm and Moran, 1999) and degree of cellular pleomorphism (Fukai et al, 1999) are new approaches to the classification of thymic carcinoids, but these have yet to be validated or accepted.

Several characteristic features can be demonstrated by additional histologic analysis. Electron microscopy reveals abundant neurosecretory granules and centrally located nuclei with finely dispersed chromatin and inconspicuous nucleoli. Immunohistochemistry shows variable degrees of positive staining for neuron-specific enolase, chromogranin, synaptophysin, and neural cell adhesion molecule. ACTH is very difficult to detect, even in tumors from patients with Cushing's syndrome. This is thought to be a result of rapid secretion following synthesis (Shimosato and Mukai, 1997).

Diagnostic Evaluation

Imaging

Standard imaging with CT or MRI confirms the presence or absence of a thymic tumor, but neither of these modalities demonstrates characteristics that distinguish a thymic carcinoid from the more common thymoma or thymic carcinoma (Fig. 63–22). If there is a high index of suspicion (e.g., a patient with MEN-1 and an anterior mediastinal mass, or a patient with ectopic ACTH production and Cushing's syndrome), nuclear medicine studies may be helpful because they can demonstrate characteristic findings of neuroendocrine metabolism.

Octreotide scintigraphy (^{111}In octreotide) is useful for identifying carcinoid tumors in general, and it has had some success with thymic carcinoids in particular. Teh and colleagues (1997) found that it was positive in all three patients on whom it was used, and Cadigan and colleagues (1996) reported success in a single case. Although octreotide scintigraphy is sensitive, it may not be specific, as both thymomas and thymic carcinomas can accumulate the radiopharmaceutical. Octreotide scintigraphy may be most useful for screening patients with MEN-1 (Cadigan et al, 1996; Satta et al, 1999) and for follow-up of patients who have had a primary tumor resected (Satta et al, 1999; Silva et al, 1999). A negative study, however, is not sufficient to eliminate the possibility of recurrence (Fig. 63–23).

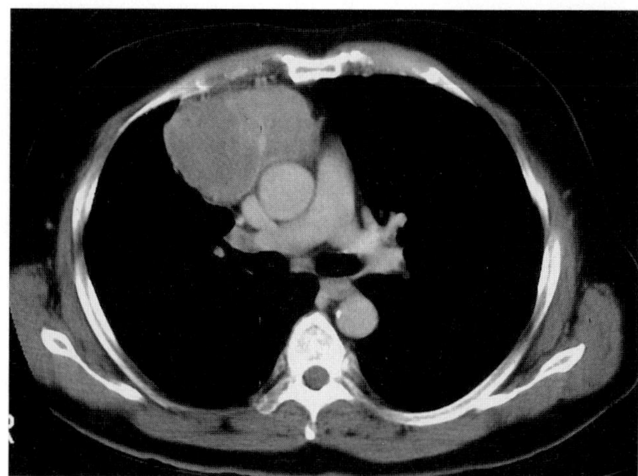

FIGURE 63–22 ■ Thymic carcinoid. Chest computed tomography scan of a 63-year-old man with multiple endocrine neoplasia, type 1 (MEN-1) syndrome. This patient had undergone parathyroidectomy for a parathyroid adenoma and subsequently presented with Zollinger-Ellison syndrome. Evaluation confirmed the presence of a duodenal gastrinoma and also discovered this anterior mediastinal mass. At surgery, this tumor was found to invade pericardium and right lung, but was completely resected. Pathology confirmed thymic carcinoid. Note the similar imaging features to thymoma and thymic carcinoma.

Only a few authors have reported experience with the metaiodobenzylguanidine (MIBG) scan and its utility is questionable. In a study of nine patients with histologically proven carcinoid tumors (five intestinal, three bronchial, and two thymic) Adolph and colleagues (1987) found that while the ^{131}I MIBG scan was positive in all of the patients with intestinal carcinoids, and two of the three with bronchial carcinoids, it was negative in both patients with thymic carcinoids. However, Mey and colleagues (1988) and Hirano and colleagues (1995) reported success in isolated cases. The ^{99m}Tc methoxyisobutylisonitrile scan can localize ectopic ACTH-producing tumors, and Lin and colleagues (1999) reported using it to identify a thymic carcinoid in an 8-year-old girl. Other authors have not reported similar application of the study.

Tissue Biopsy

The decision to obtain a tissue diagnosis should fall within a general algorithm for management of thymic tumors, and a small thymic tumor without evidence of invasion should be resected without preoperative biopsy. If Cushing's syndrome is present, selective venous sampling can confirm that the tumor produces ACTH, facilitating perioperative management of potential adrenal insufficiency (Lin et al, 1999). If the tumor is large, or

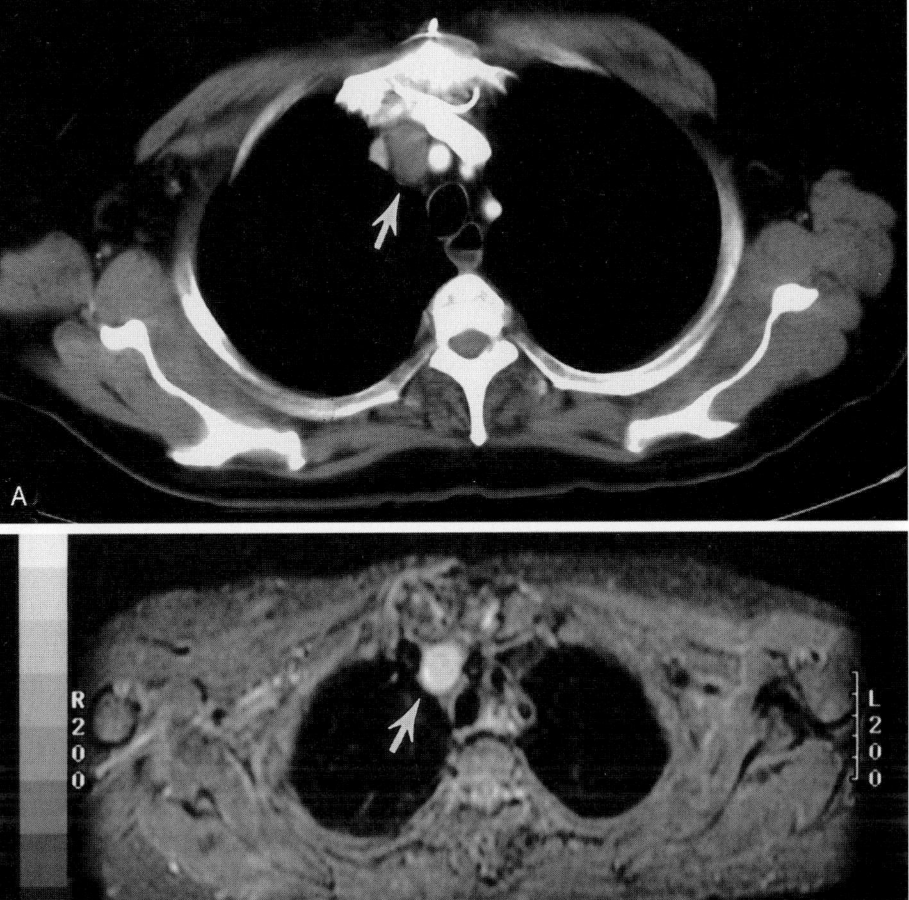

FIGURE 63–23 ■ Recurrent thymic carcinoid. Routine follow-up chest computed tomography scan *(A)* of the patient in Figure 63–22 demonstrates a 2-cm mass posterior to the left brachiocephalic vein, between the right brachiocephalic vein and the brachiocephalic artery *(arrow)*. The recurrent tumor is also demonstrated by magnetic resonance imaging *(B)*, but an octreotide scan was negative. Resection confirmed recurrent thymic carcinoid.

there is evidence of local invasion or metastatic disease, tissue can be retrieved by FNA, core needle biopsy, or open biopsy. The differential diagnosis includes thymoma, poorly differentiated carcinoma, lymphoma, and some germ cell tumors, and therefore adequate material must be obtained. FNA was correct in five of the nine cases reported in the literature (Asbun et al, 1991; Caceres et al, 1998; Georgy et al, 1995; Nichols et al, 1997; Shabb et al, 1998; Wang et al, 1994). Core needle biopsy is of greater diagnostic utility, but a biopsy-site recurrence has been reported (Wang et al, 1995).

Staging

The rarity of thymic carcinoids and their usually advanced stage at the time of diagnosis make it difficult to establish a meaningful staging system. As with thymic carcinoma, the Masaoka system has been used because there is no standard. Recently, Masaoka and his colleagues (Fukai, 1999) advocated using the TNM system that Yamakawa and colleagues proposed for application to all thymic epithelial tumors (Tsuchiya et al, 1994; Yamakawa et al, 1991). This may be the most appropriate approach because even though thymic carcinoids are not usually considered tumors of thymic epithelium, this system reflects the significance of lymphogenous and hematogenous metastases.

Prognosis

Median survival ranges from 2 to 4.5 years (de Montpréville et al, 1996; Economopoulos et al, 1990; Teh, 1998), and long-term survival with this disease is an unusual event. Among patients in four of the larger series, 5-year survival was only 34% (14 of 41 patients) (de Montpréville, 1996; Fukai et al, 1999; Wang et al, 1994; Wick et al, 1982a), and only 4 of the 14 survivors were free of disease. Three patients (9%) survived 10 years—two died of recurrent disease shortly after reaching this mark (Fukai et al, 1999; Wang et al, 1994) and the third was alive and disease free at 15 years (Wick et al, 1982a). Economopolous and colleagues (1990) also reported one long-term survivor (12 years) in their series of seven patients.

The report by Wick and colleagues (1980) identified MEN-1 and Cushing's syndrome as poor prognostic factors. They collected 74 cases from the literature and reported that 10-year survival for patients without either associated syndrome was 71%, while for patients with MEN-1 or Cushing's syndrome, 10-year survival rates were 50% and 35%, respectively. These overall survival statistics are exceptional, and they are inconsistent with more recent reports and with their own experience published 2 years later. However, the negative prognostic impact of MEN-1 and Cushing's syndrome has been confirmed by others (Fukai et al, 1999; Teh, 1998).

Treatment

Surgery is the principal therapeutic modality. In many cases complete resection is possible despite local invasiveness (de Montpréville et al, 1996; Fukai et al, 1999; Herbst et al, 1987; Wang et al, 1994), and some authors argue for aggressive attempts similar to the approach for thymoma. However, given the poor long-term prognosis and the propensity for these lesions to metastasize even when they are not invasive (Teh et al, 1997), sacrifice of vital structures may not be warranted. Nevertheless, there is weak evidence to suggest that complete resection may confer a survival advantage. Based on follow-up of 13 patients, de Montpréville and colleagues (1996) reported that median survival rates following complete resection ($n = 4$), incomplete resection ($n = 5$), or biopsy alone ($n = 4$) were 71, 30, and 5 months, respectively. These findings most likely reflect the extent of disease at presentation and cannot be interpreted as evidence to support a policy of radical attempts at resection. Significantly, no patient survived more than 109 months.

Surgery also plays a role in the management of recurrent and metastatic disease. Although disease may progress rapidly and disseminate widely, the clinical course is often slowly progressive, and some patients live for many years with active disease. In this setting, most centers have pursued resection of foci of disease that are accessible (Economopoulos et al, 1990; Wang et al, 1994; Wick et al, 1982a; Zeiger et al, 1992). Economopoulos and colleagues (1990) performed repeat resections on three patients in their series. One patient underwent four operations (for tumor deposits in lung, chest wall, cervical lymph nodes, and adrenal glands) over a period of 11 years from the date of the initial procedure. The indolent nature of the disease in these circumstances suggests that it may be better for patients to live with their disease than to undergo high-risk procedures that may damage their quality of life.

Radiation therapy is almost always administered, either as primary therapy for unresectable tumors or as an adjuvant to resection. Doses of 50 to 60 Gy are usual. Many authors have reported that radiation therapy can achieve good local control and may help to ameliorate symptoms of paraneoplastic syndromes such as Cushing's (Asbun et al, 1991; Birnberg et al, 1982; Caceres et al, 1998; Chakravarthy et al, 1995; Hallmann et al, 1998). Wang and colleagues (1994), however, found it to be of no help in the three patients for whom it was used as primary therapy.

The experience with chemotherapy is eclectic. There is no standard regimen, and as a result, a wide variety of agents have been employed. Few authors provide any detailed information other than to comment on its lack of efficacy. Birnberg and colleagues (1982) treated one patient at various times with lomustine, doxorubicin, methotrexate, vincristine, cyclophosphamide, 5-fluorouracil, and streptozocin—all without significant benefit. In most cases, experience with carcinoid tumors of intestinal origin guides the choice of agents, consequently 5-fluorouracil and streptozocin are common ingredients. This strategy has also led some authors to the use of α-interferon, but this too has not shown any significant benefit (Caceres et al, 1998; Teh, 1998). Cisplatin, an agent used commonly for thymoma and thymic carcinoma, has seen limited use for thymic carcinoid. Takayama and colleagues (1993) treated one patient with a combination of cisplatin, etoposide, and doxorubicin with only a minimal response, and Hallmann and colleagues (1998) reported on another patient treated with cisplatin and etoposide without benefit. Octreotide therapy is a novel approach to the management of patients with carcinoid tumor. It may help to slow tumor growth, and as is suggested by the ability of octreotide scintigraphy to detect tumors, radiolabeled octreotide may be a vehicle for delivery of targeted cytotoxic therapy (Caplin et al, 1998; Satta et al, 1999). Its use for the treatment of patients with thymic carcinoid has not been reported.

THYMOLIPOMA

A thymolipoma is a benign, slow-growing tumor of the thymus that is composed of both thymic and mature adipose tissue. Lange (1916) is credited with its first description—a report in which he tells of discovering a thymic tumor during autopsy of a patient who died of metastatic uterine cancer. The tumor contained predominantly adipose elements, and therefore he called it a lipoma of the thymus. In 1949 Hall discovered a similar tumor at autopsy of a 47-year-old previously healthy man who died of head trauma. The tumor was a large (1100 g), pedunculated mass that arose from the anterior mediastinum but lay almost entirely in the right pleural cavity. Hall did not reference the report by Lange, but he did identify a 1937 paper by Andrus and Foot in which the authors described a similar "large adipose mass containing small areas of thymic tissue." Because these tumors contained normal thymic elements in addition to mature fat, Hall proposed the term *thymolipoma.* Other terms used to describe this tumor include benign thymoma, thymolipomatous hamartoma, lipothymoma, and mediastinal lipoma with remnants of thymoma (Bigelow and Ehler, 1952; Cicciarelli et al, 1964; Jagadha and Ramaswamy, 1984; Schanher and Hodge, 1949).

Histologic Features

Thymolipomas contain elements derived from both mesenchymal (fat) and endodermal (thymic epithelium) tissues. They are always well encapsulated and soft, with multiple thin septa that divide the tumor grossly into multiple lobules (Moran et al, 1995). Histology is characteristic and reveals "large areas of mature adipose tissue without areas of atypia . . . admixed with [normal] thymic tissue in different proportion" (Moran et al, 1995). Fat usually accounts for 50% or more of the tumor, with one third of tumors having more than 80% fat (Rosado de Christenson et al, 1994). Approximately 80% of the lymphocytes associated with the thymic epithelium are immature double-positive cells ($CD4^+/CD8^+$) (Hull et al, 1995), which is a profile similar to that of the normal thymus.

The differential diagnosis includes mediastinal lipoma, thymic hyperplasia, and liposarcoma. Lipoma is one of the most common benign mesenchymal tumors of the mediastinum. It can occur anywhere within the mediastinum and is composed entirely of adipose tissue without any thymic elements (Shimosato and Mukai, 1997). Thymic hyperplasia is a common finding and can be distinguished histologically by retained normal thymic architecture (Moran et al, 1995). A liposarcoma contains scattered lipoblasts without islands of thymic epithelium (Havlicek and Rosai, 1984).

Histogenesis

The origin of thymolipomas is unclear. Four theories have been proposed based on subtle differences in the features of individual tumors, but none is universally accepted: (1) involution and fatty replacement of a hyperplastic thymus (Rubin and Mishkin, 1954); (2) involution and fatty replacement of a thymoma (Benton and Gerard, 1966); (3) neoplasia of thymic fat that engulfs normal thymic remnants (Dunn and Frkovich, 1956); and (4) hamartomatous change (Jagadha and Ramaswamy, 1984; Moran et al, 1995; Shimosato and Mukai, 1997). Robbins and co-workers (1984) define hamartomatous change as "excessive focal overgrowth of mature normal cells and tissues in an organ composed of identical cellular elements."

Demographics

Thymolipomas account for between 2% and 9% of all thymic tumors (Otto et al, 1982; Ringe et al, 1979; Shimosato and Mukai, 1997), and they can occur in both sexes and at any age. Although it is usually suggested that the ratio of male-to-female patients is roughly 1:1, larger series show a slight male predominance (Moran et al, 1995; Rosado de Christenson et al, 1994). Ringe and colleagues (1979) found that two thirds of 51 patients reported in the literature were men. Compared to patients with other thymic tumors, those with thymolipoma are relatively young. Their mean age is in the late 20s, most present in the second or third decade of life, and 75% of patients are younger than 40 years (Benton and Gerard, 1966; Moran et al, 1995; Ringe et al, 1979; Rosado de Christenson et al, 1994). Because these tumors are benign, they can grow to be quite large without causing significant symptoms. It is not uncommon for them to weigh in excess of 1000 g and to fill much of the anterior mediastinum and one hemithorax. Tumors measuring 36 cm (Rosado de Christenson et al, 1994) in diameter and weighing 6000 g (Benton and Gerard, 1966) have been reported.

Presentation and Diagnosis

The most common symptoms are cough, dyspnea, and chest pressure, but almost 50% of patients are asymptomatic (Benton and Gerard, 1966; Moran et al, 1995; Ringe et al, 1979). An association with myasthenia gravis was first reported in 1978 by Reintgen and colleagues, and subsequent series have suggested that the incidence of this association is approximately 10% (Moran et al, 1995; Pan et al, 1988). Thymolipomas associated with myasthenia gravis tend to be relatively small (Verbist and colleagues [1997] reported the largest one at 340 g), tend to present in patients older than 50 years of age (Le Marc'hadour et al, 1991; Pan et al, 1988), and are occasionally discovered incidentally during therapeutic thymectomy (Takamori et al, 1997). These features suggest that the association between myasthenia gravis and thymolipoma is probably more coincidental than causal. Evidence for an association with other autoimmune disorders is scant. Graves' disease (Benton and Gerard, 1966), aplastic anemia (Barnes and O'Gorman, 1962), and erythrocyte hypoplasia and hypogammaglobulinemia (Otto et al, 1982) have each been described in single case reports.

Small thymolipomas are usually confined to the anterior mediastinum and appear as anterior mediastinal masses, while larger ones slump posteriorly and inferiorly, draping around the mediastinum and growing preferentially into one hemithorax. By chest radiograph, moderate-sized tumors can mimic cardiomegaly, while larger tumors may look like basal atelectasis, pulmonary sequestration, or pleural or pericardial tumors (Fig. 63–24) (Casullo et al, 1992). CT scan and MRI are diagnostic. CT demonstrates a sharply defined mass of predominantly fat density with strands of soft tissue attenuation (Fig. 63–25); these strands correspond to interspersed normal thymic tissue (Brown and Aughenbaugh, 1991; Casullo et al, 1992; Gregory et al, 1997). T_1-weighted spin-echo MRI demonstrates islands of high-attenuation fat with intermixed strands of intermediate signal intensity. On T_2-weighted images the thymic tissue appears bright, while the lobulated areas of fat are of low attenuation (Brown and Aughenbaugh, 1991; Casullo et al, 1992; Gregory et al, 1997; Matsudaira et al, 1994). Diagnosis by FNA has been described (Heimann, 1987), but it is unnecessary, as the diagnosis should be apparent based on CT or MRI studies.

Therapy

Thymolipomas should be resected. Surgery is indicated even in the asymptomatic patient because although thymolipomas are benign tumors, they are slow growing and may cause significant symptoms of dyspnea and chest pressure. Resection is usually straightforward and always curative. There has not been a single report of recurrence following resection, and all accounts in the literature describe a well-encapsulated tumor that does not invade adjacent structures. Because thymolipomas are benign and encapsulated, they may be attractive candidates for thoracoscopic resection provided their size does not prohibit adequate visibility and mobility within the chest.

THYMIC CYST

True thymic cysts are uncommon, accounting for only 1% to 3% of all mediastinal lesions (Brown et al, 1991; Suster and Rosai, 1991a). Typically they are of congenital or developmental origin and are caused by persistence of the thymopharyngeal duct; therefore, they can be found anywhere along the embryologic path of descent of the thymus. Thymic cysts occur equally in both sexes and usually present in childhood (Hendrickson et al, 1998;

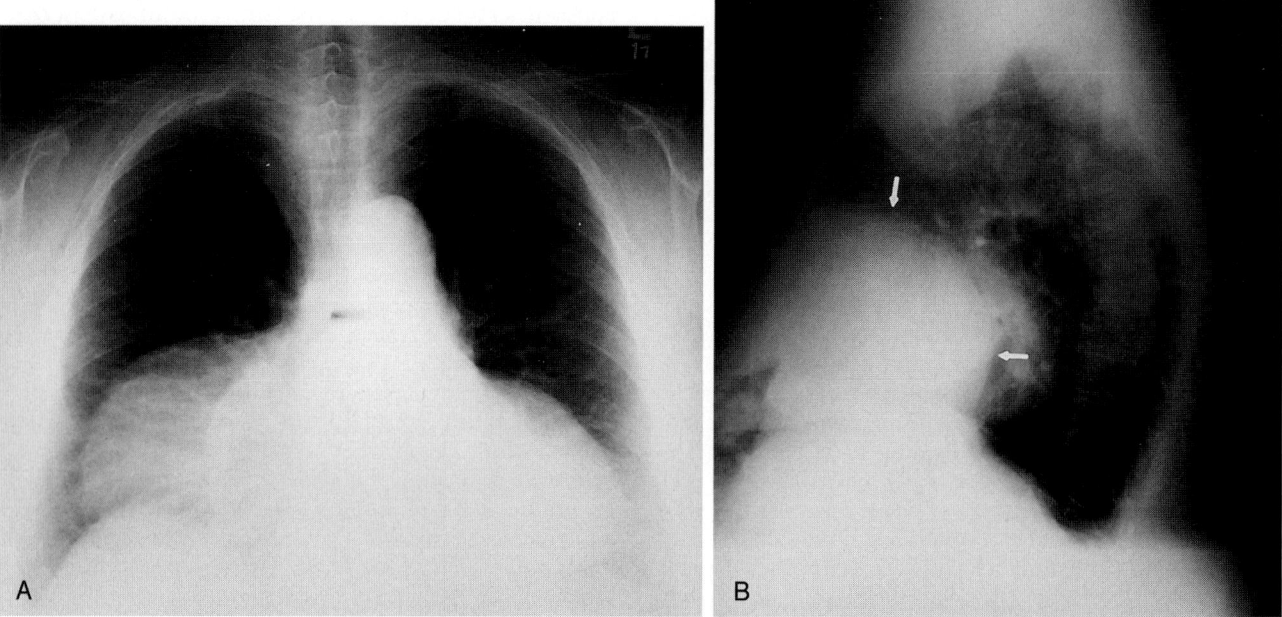

FIGURE 63–24 ■ Thymolipoma. This 63-year-old woman had a vague history of cardiomegaly and was lost to follow-up. She re-presented several years later with this chest radiograph. Posteroanterior and lateral views demonstrate a well-circumscribed large anterior mediastinal mass extending into the right chest.

Shimosato and Mukai, 1997). Approximately one half are cervical and present as neck masses; mediastinal thymic cysts are usually asymptomatic. Like other benign mediastinal lesions such as thymolipoma, thymic cysts can grow to be quite large before being discovered. Cysts as large as 30 cm in greatest dimension have been reported (Gonullu et al, 1996). Hemorrhage into the cyst cavity or calcification of the cyst wall may occur.

Less commonly, thymic cysts are the result of acquired pathology. Many primary thymic neoplasms, such as thymoma, thymic carcinoma, lymphoma, and germ cell tumors, can have cystic components (Suster and Rosai, 1991a; Yamashita et al, 1996), and cystic change in the anterior mediastinum can be seen following medical therapy of any of these lesions. Thymic cysts can also occur many years after mediastinal surgery, and recently they have been found in association with human immunodeficiency virus (HIV) infection (Chhieng et al, 1999; Kontny et al, 1997). It is thought that HIV infection and replication within the thymus cause glandular enlargement, cystic degeneration, and then involution (Kontny et al, 1997; Leonidas et al, 1996).

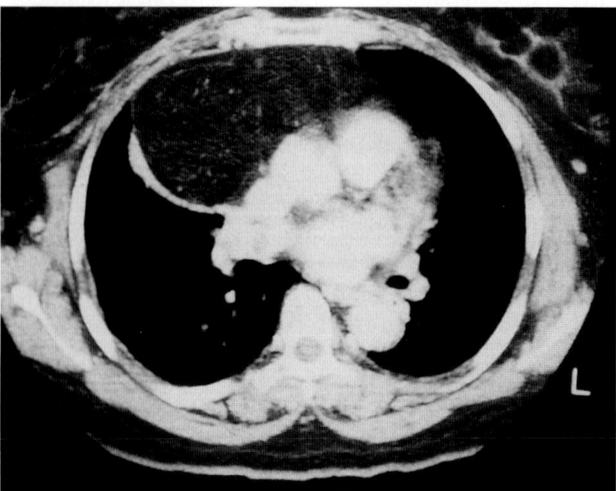

FIGURE 63–25 ■ Thymolipoma. Chest computed tomography scan of the patient shown in Figure 63–24. Note that the anterior mediastinal mass and the subcutaneous fat are of similar attenuation. Higher attenuation strands traverse the tumor. This appearance distinguishes it from a lipoma and is diagnostic of thymolipoma.

Thymic cysts are diagnosed radiographically. Chest radiograph, CT, or MRI demonstrates a cystic mass with a smooth, sharp contour. Cyst contents may have a density that is equivalent to water, or they may have a greater density if hemorrhage has occurred. Cysts that present in the neck are usually tubular, while cysts in the mediastinum are more spherical. They can be unilocular or multilocular. The cyst wall is thin and lined by smooth epithelium, and the wall of a true thymic cyst incorporates normal thymic tissue (Shimosato and Mukai, 1997). Cyst fluid is watery and clear or straw-colored, or in the case of prior hemorrhage, chocolate-colored. Although primary thymic neoplasms may have cystic components, malignant degeneration of a true thymic cyst is rare (Leong and Brown, 1984).

Resection is indicated to alleviate symptoms, to avoid development of symptoms from continued enlargement, and to rule out the presence of malignancy. Thymic cysts are usually easily enucleated, but they may be densely adherent to adjacent structures. In this circumstance, vital structures should not be sacrificed. Instead, as little of the cyst wall as possible should be left attached, and the remaining epithelial lining should be meticulously ablated. Resection can be performed by thoracotomy, by median sternotomy, or with thoracoscopic assistance.

ECTOPIC TUMORS OF THYMIC ORIGIN

A variety of tumors with features suggestive of thymic origin have been found in locations outside the anterior mediastinum. This is not surprising given that the thymus is derived from embryologic foregut structures and migrates from the neck into the mediastinum during development.

Ectopic thymomas have been found in the neck, pericardium (Mirra et al, 1997), lung (Shimosato and Mukai, 1997), and pleura (Fushimi et al, 1998). Ectopic cervical thymomas are the most common, and they are thought to arise from either undescended thymus or from thymic remnants in the neck. Of the few cases that have been described, there is a striking female predominance (Chan et al, 1991). These tumors typically present in the anterolateral neck, deep to the sternocleidomastoid muscle. Their behavior is generally relatively benign, and recurrence or metastases have been reported in only a few cases (Chan and Rosai, 1991; Jung et al, 1999). Ectopic cervical thymic carcinomas have also been described (Dorfman et al, 1998).

Ectopic hamartomatous thymomas are benign tumors that contain a mixture of epithelial tissue, fat, and fibroblasts of thymic origin. They occur in adults, exhibit a marked male predominance (Chan and Rosai, 1991), and are found either superficial or deep to the sternocleidomastoid muscle in the low neck, near the sternoclavicular joint (Fetsch et al, 1990). Their origin is the subject of several theories. Rosai and colleagues (1984) suggested that these tumors may arise from an incompletely descended thymic anlage of the third pharyngeal pouch (thymus III). Fetsch and colleagues (1990) proposed two theories: origin from an unusual thymic anlage of the fourth pharyngeal pouch (thymus IV), or origin from remnants of the sinus of His. The sinus of His is a small pocket of ectoderm that forms between the developing second, third, and fourth branchial pouches, normally regresses, and can give rise to branchial arch cysts. Ectopic hamartomatous thymomas are benign tumors that do not recur following resection. Malignant degeneration has been reported (Michal et al, 1996).

Two other tumors found in the neck exhibit features suggestive of thymic origin and can exhibit a malignant phenotype. The spindle epithelial tumor with thymus-like differentiation (SETTLE) is a malignant tumor that has also been called thyroid spindle cell tumor with mucous cysts, and malignant teratoma of the thyroid. It is found predominantly in children and young adults (Su et al, 1997), and as the alternative names suggest, it presents as an apparent thyroid nodule. This tumor has a "protracted malignant course with [a] propensity to develop delayed distant metastases" (Chan and Rosai, 1991). In one case, metastases appeared 25 years after the primary tumor was resected. The other malignant cervical tumor of probable thymic origin is a carcinoma showing thymus-like differentiation (CASTLE) (Dorfman et al, 1998). It has been called an intrathyroidal epithelial thymoma. Typically, this tumor presents in adults and exhibits an indolent clinical course. Treatment is resection or radiation therapy. Local recurrence has been reported from 5 to 17 years later (Chan and Rosai, 1991), and it is also treated with resection or radiation therapy. Distant metastases have not been reported.

■ *REFERENCES*

Adolph JM, Kimmig BN, Georgi P et al: Carcinoid tumors: CT and I-131 meta-iodo-benzylguanidine scintigraphy. Radiology 164: 199, 1987.

Andrus WD, Foot NC: Report of a large thymic tumor successfully removed by operation. J Thorac Surg 6:648, 1937.

Asbun HJ, Calabria RP, Calmes S et al: Thymic carcinoid. Am Surg 57:442, 1991.

Barnes RDS, O'Gorman P: Two cases of aplastic anaemia associated with tumours of the thymus. J Clin Pathol 15:264, 1962.

Beekman R, Kuks JB, Oosterhuis HJ: Myasthenia gravis: diagnosis and follow-up of 100 consecutive patients. J Neurol 244:112, 1997.

Benton C, Gerard P: Thymolipoma in a patient with Graves' disease: Case report and review of the literature. J Thorac Cardiovasc Surg 51:428, 1966.

Bergh NP, Gatzinsky P, Larsson S et al: Tumors of the thymus and thymic region. I: Clinicopathological studies on thymomas. Ann Thorac Surg 25:91, 1978.

Bernatz PE, Harrison EG, Clagett OT: Thymoma: A clinicopathologic study. J Thorac Cardiovasc Surg 42:424, 1961.

Bigelow NH, Ehler AA: Lipothymoma: An unusual benign tumor of the thymus gland. J Thorac Surg 23:528, 1952.

Birnberg FA, Webb WR, Selch MT et al: Thymic carcinoid tumors with hyperparathyroidism. AJR Am J Roentgenol 139:1001, 1982.

Blumberg D, Burt ME, Bains MS et al: Thymic carcinoma: Current staging does not predict prognosis. J Thorac Cardiovasc Surg 115:303, 1998.

Blumberg D, Port JL, Weksler B et al: Thymoma: A multivariate analysis of factors predicting survival. Ann Thorac Surg 60:908, 1995.

Bonomi PD, Finkelstein D, Aisner S et al: EST 2582 phase II trial of cisplatin in metastatic or recurrent thymoma. Am J Clin Oncol 16:342, 1993.

Bramis J, Pikoulis E, Leppaniemi A et al: Benefits of early thymectomy in patients with myasthenia gravis. Eur J Surg 163:897, 1997.

Brown LR, Aughenbaugh GL: Masses of the anterior mediastinum: CT and MR imaging. AJR Am J Roentgenol 157:1171, 1991.

Caceres W, Baldizon C, Sanchez J: Carcinoid tumor of the thymus: A unique neoplasm of the mediastinum. Am J Clin Oncol 21:82, 1998.

Cadigan DG, Hollett PD, Collingwood PW et al: Imaging of a mediastinal thymic carcinoid tumor with radiolabeled somatostatin analogue. Clin Nucl Med 21:487, 1996.

Caplin ME, Buscombe JR, Hilson AJ et al: Carcinoid tumour. Lancet 352:799, 1998.

Carlson RW, Dorfman RF, Sikic BI: Successful treatment of metastatic thymic carcinoma with cisplatin, vinblastine, bleomycin, and etoposide chemotherapy. Cancer 66:2092, 1990.

Casullo J, Palayew MJ, Lisbona A: General case of the day. Thymolipoma. Radiographics 12:1250, 1992.

Chakravarthy A, Abrams RA: Radiation therapy in the management of patients with malignant carcinoid tumors. Cancer 75:1386, 1995.

Chan JK, Rosai J: Tumors of the neck showing thymic or related branchial pouch differentiation: A unifying concept. Hum Pathol 22:349, 1991.

Chhieng DC, Demaria S, Yee HT et al: Multilocular thymic cyst with follicular lymphoid hyperplasia in a male infected with HIV. A case report with fine needle aspiration cytology. Acta Cytol 43:1119, 1999.

Cicciarelli FE, Soule EH, McGoon DC: Lipoma and liposarcoma of the mediastinum: A report of 14 tumors including one lipoma of the thymus. J Thorac Cardiovasc Surg 47:411, 1964.

Ciernik IF, Meier U, Lutolf UM: Prognostic factors and outcome of incompletely resected invasive thymoma following radiation therapy. J Clin Oncol 12:1484, 1994.

Cohen DJ, Ronnigen LD, Graeber GM et al: Management of patients with malignant thymoma. J Thorac Cardiovasc Surg 87:301, 1984.

Cosi V, Romani A, Lombardi M et al: Prognosis of myasthenia gravis: A retrospective study of 380 patients. J Neurol 244:548, 1997.

Cowen D, Richaud P, Mornex F et al: Thymoma: Results of a multicentric retrospective series of 149 non-metastatic irradiated patients and review of the literature. FNCLCC trialists. Federation Nationale des Centres de Lutte Contre le Cancer. Radiother Oncol 34:9, 1995.

Crucitti F, Doglietto GB, Bellantone R et al: Effects of surgical treatment in thymoma with myasthenia gravis: Our experience in 103 patients. J Surg Oncol 50:43, 1992.

Curran WJ Jr., Kornstein MJ, Brooks JJ et al: Invasive thymoma: The role of mediastinal irradiation following complete or incomplete surgical resection. J Clin Oncol 6:1722, 1988.

de Montpréville VT, Macchiarini P, Dulmet E: Thymic neuroendocrine carcinoma (carcinoid): A clinicopathologic study of fourteen cases. J Thorac Cardiovasc Surg 111:134, 1996.

Dimery IW, Lee JS, Blick M et al: Association of the Epstein-Barr virus with lymphoepithelioma of the thymus. Cancer 61:2475, 1988.

Do YS, Im JG, Lee BH et al: CT findings in malignant tumors of thymic epithelium. J Comput Assist Tomogr 19:192, 1995.

Dorfman DM, Shahsafaei A, Miyauchi A: Immunohistochemical staining for bcl-2 and mcl-1 in intrathyroidal epithelial thymoma (ITET)/ carcinoma showing thymus-like differentiation (CASTLE) and cervical thymic carcinoma. Mod Pathol 11:989, 1998.

Dunn BH, Frkovich G: Lipomas of the thymus gland. Am J Pathol 32:41, 1956.

Economopoulos GC, Lewis JW Jr., Lee MW et al: Carcinoid tumors of the thymus. Ann Thorac Surg 50:58, 1990.

Fechner RE: Recurrence of noninvasive thymomas. Report of four cases and review of literature. Cancer 23:1423, 1969.

Fetsch JF, Weiss SW: Ectopic hamartomatous thymoma: Clinicopathologic, immunohistochemical, and histogenetic considerations in four new cases. Hum Pathol 21:662, 1990.

Fornasiero A, Daniele O, Ghiotto C et al: Chemotherapy for invasive thymoma. A 13-year experience. Cancer 68:30, 1991.

Frist WH, Thirumalai S, Doehring CB et al: Thymectomy for the myasthenia gravis patient: Factors influencing outcome. Ann Thorac Surg 57:334, 1994.

Fukai I, Masaoka A, Fujii Y et al: Thymic neuroendocrine tumor (thymic carcinoid): A clinicopathologic study in 15 patients. Ann Thorac Surg 67:208, 1999.

Fushimi H, Tanio Y, Kotoh K: Ectopic thymoma mimicking diffuse pleural mesothelioma: A case report. Hum Pathol 29:409, 1998.

Georgy BA, Casola G, Hesselink JR: Thymic carcinoid tumors with bone metastases. A report of two cases. Clin Imaging 19:25, 1995.

Giaccone G, Ardizzoni A, Kirkpatrick A et al: Cisplatin and etoposide combination chemotherapy for locally advanced or metastatic thymoma. A phase II study of the European Organization for Research and Treatment of Cancer, Lung Cancer Cooperative Group. J Clin Oncol 14:814, 1996.

Gonullu U, Gungor A, Savas I et al: Huge thymic cysts. J Thorac Cardiovasc Surg 112:835, 1996.

Gossot D, Toledo L, Fritsch S et al: Mediastinoscopy vs thoracoscopy for mediastinal biopsy. Results of a prospective nonrandomized study. Chest 110:1328, 1996.

Gregory AK, Connery CP, Resta-Flarer F et al: A case of massive thymolipoma. J Pediatr Surg 32:1780, 1997.

Gripp S, Hilgers K, Wurm R et al: Thymoma: Prognostic factors and treatment outcomes. Cancer 83:1495, 1998.

Hall GFM: A case of thymolipoma with observations on a possible relationship to intrathoracic lipomata. Br J Surg 36:321, 1949.

Hallmann RS, Schneeweiss LG, Correa E et al: Fine needle aspiration biopsy of thymic carcinoid tumor: A case with immunocytochemical correlation. Acta Cytol 42:1042, 1998.

Haniuda M, Morimoto M, Nishimura H et al: Adjuvant radiotherapy after complete resection of thymoma. Ann Thorac Surg 54:311, 1992.

Harris NL, Müller-Hermelink HK: Thymoma classification. A siren's song of simplicity. Am J Clin Pathol 112:299, 1999.

Hasserjian RP, Klimstra DS, Rosai J: Carcinoma of the thymus with clear-cell features. Report of eight cases and review of the literature. Am J Surg Pathol 19:835, 1995.

Hatton PD, Diehl JT, Daly BD et al: Transsternal radical thymectomy for myasthenia gravis: A 15-year review. Ann Thorac Surg 47:838, 1989.

Havlicek F, Rosai J: A sarcoma of thymic stroma with features of liposarcoma. Am J Clin Pathol 82:217, 1984.

Heimann A, Sneige N, Shirkhoda A et al: Fine needle aspiration cytology of thymolipoma. A case report. Acta Cytol 31:335, 1987.

Hendrickson M, Azarow K, Ein S et al: Congenital thymic cysts in children—mostly misdiagnosed. J Pediatr Surg 33:821, 1998.

Herbst WM, Kummer W, Hofmann W et al: Carcinoid tumors of the thymus. An immunohistochemical study. Cancer 60:2465, 1987.

Higashiyama M, Doi O, Kodama K et al: Ectopic primary pleural thymoma: Report of a case. Surg Today 26:747, 1996.

Hirano T, Otake H, Watanabe N et al: Presurgical diagnosis of a primary carcinoid tumor of the thymus with MIBG. J Nucl Med 36:2243, 1995.

Ho FC, Ho JC: Pigmented carcinoid tumour of the thymus. Histopathology 1:363, 1977.

Hsu CP, Chen CY, Chen CL et al: Thymic carcinoma. Ten years' experience in twenty patients. J Thorac Cardiovasc Surg 107:615, 1994.

Hull MT, Warfel KA, Kotylo P et al: Proliferating thymolipoma: Ultrastructural, immunohistochemical, and flowcytometric study. Ultrastruct Pathol 19:75, 1995.

Jackson MA, Ball DL: Post-operative radiotherapy in invasive thymoma. Radiother Oncol 21:77, 1991.

Jagadha V, Ramaswamy G: An unusual case of thymolipoma with hamartomatous changes. Arch Pathol Lab Med 108:611, 1984.

Jaretzki AD, Penn AS, Younger DS et al: "Maximal" thymectomy for myasthenia gravis. Results. J Thorac Cardiovasc Surg 95:747, 1988.

Jung JI, Kim HH, Park SH et al: Malignant ectopic thymoma in the neck: A case report. AJNR Am J Neuroradiol 20:1747, 1999.

Kay S, Willson MA: Ultrastructural studies of an ACTH-secreting thymic tumor. Cancer 26:445, 1970.

Kirschner PA: Discussion of Blumberg D, Burt ME, Bains MS et al: Thymic carcinoma: Current staging does not predict prognosis. J Thorac Cardiovasc Surg 115:303, 1998.

Klemm KM, Moran CA: Primary neuroendocrine carcinomas of the thymus. Semin Diag Pathol 16:32, 1999.

Kohman LJ: Controversies in the management of malignant thymoma. Chest 112 (Suppl):296S, 1997.

Kontny HU, Sleasman JW, Kingma DW et al: Multilocular thymic cysts in children with human immunodeficiency virus infection: Clinical and pathologic aspects. J Pediatr 131:264, 1997.

Kornstein MJ, Curran WJ Jr., Turrisi AT et al: Cortical versus medullary thymomas: A useful morphologic distinction? Hum Pathol 19:1335, 1988.

Kubota K, Yamada S, Kondo T et al: PET imaging of primary mediastinal tumours. Br J Cancer 73:882, 1996.

Kuo TT, Chang JP, Lin FJ et al: Thymic carcinomas: Histopathological varieties and immunohistochemical study. Am J Surg Pathol 14:24, 1990.

Landreneau RJ, Dowling RD, Castillo WM et al: Thoracoscopic resection of an anterior mediastinal tumor. Ann Thorac Surg 54:142, 1992.

Lange L: Ueber ein lipom des thymus. Zentralbl Allg Pathol 27:97, 1916.

Laurent F, Latrabe V, Lecesne R et al: Mediastinal masses: Diagnostic approach. Eur Radiol 8:1148, 1998.

Le Marc'hadour F, Pinel N, Pasquier B et al: Thymolipoma in association with myasthenia gravis. Am J Surg Pathol 15:802, 1991.

Leong AS, Brown JH: Malignant transformation in a thymic cyst. Am J Surg Pathol 8:471, 1984.

Leonidas JC, Berdon WE, Valderrama E et al: Human immunodeficiency virus infection and multilocular thymic cysts. Radiology 198:377, 1996.

Levine G, Rosai J: Thymic hyperplasia and neoplasia: A review of current concepts. Hum Pathol 9:495, 1978.

Lewis JE, Wick MR, Scheithauer BW et al: Thymoma: A clinicopathologic review. Cancer 60:2727, 1987.

Leyvraz S, Henle W, Chahinian AP et al: Association of Epstein-Barr virus with thymic carcinoma. N Engl J Med 312:1296, 1985.

Lin KL, Chen CY, Hsu HH et al: Ectopic ACTH syndrome due to thymic carcinoid tumor in a girl. J Pediatr Endocrinol Metab 12:573, 1999.

Liu RS, Yeh SH, Huang MH et al: Use of fluorine-18 fluorodeoxyglucose positron emission tomography in the detection of thymoma: A preliminary report. Eur J Nucl Med 22:1402, 1995.

Loehrer PJ Sr, Chen M, Kim K et al: Cisplatin, doxorubicin, and cyclophosphamide plus thoracic radiation therapy for limited-stage unresectable thymoma: An intergroup trial. J Clin Oncol 15:3093, 1997.

Loehrer PJ Sr, Kim K, Aisner SC et al: Cisplatin plus doxorubicin plus cyclophosphamide in metastatic or recurrent thymoma: Final results of an intergroup trial. J Clin Oncol 12:1164, 1994.

Macchiarini P, Chella A, Ducci F et al: Neoadjuvant chemotherapy, surgery, and postoperative radiation therapy for invasive thymoma. Cancer 68:706, 1991.

Maggi G, Casadio C, Cavallo A et al: Thymectomy in myasthenia gravis. Results of 662 cases operated upon in 15 years. Eur J Cardiothorac Surg 3:504, 1989.

Maggi G, Casadio C, Cavallo A et al: Thymoma: Results of 241 operated cases (see comments). Ann Thorac Surg 51:152, 1991.

Marchevsky AM: Lung tumors derived from ectopic tissues. Semin Diag Pathol 12:172, 1995.

Marchevsky AM, Dikman SH: Mediastinal carcinoid with an incomplete Sipple's syndrome. Cancer 43:2497, 1979.

Marchevsky AM, Kaneko M: Surgical Pathology of the Mediastinum. New York, Raven Press, 1984, p 61.

Marino M, Müller-Hermelink HK: Thymoma and thymic carcinoma. Relation of thymoma epithelial cells to the cortical and medullary differentiation of thymus. Virchows Arch A Pathol Anat Histopathol 407:119, 1985.

Masaoka A, Monden Y, Nakahara K et al: Follow-up study of thymomas with special reference to their clinical stages. Cancer 48:2485, 1981.

Masaoka A, Yamakawa Y, Niwa H et al: Extended thymectomy for myasthenia gravis patients: A 20-year review. Ann Thorac Surg 62:853, 1996.

Matsudaira N, Hirano H, Itou S et al: MR imaging of thymolipoma. Magn Reson Imaging 12:959, 1994.

Mey P, George P, Pein F et al: [Thymic carcinoid tumor visualized with I 131-metaiodobenzylguanidine]. Ann Radiol (Paris) 31:181, 1988.

Michal M, Neubauer L, Fakan F: Carcinoma arising in ectopic hamartomatous thymoma. An ultrastructural study. Pathol Res Pract 192:610, 1996.

Mirra M, Zanella M, Bussani R et al: Intrapericardial thymoma: Report of two incidental autopsy cases and review of the literature. Arch Pathol Lab Med 121:59, 1997.

Mizuno T, Masaoka A, Hashimoto T, et al: Coexisting thymic carcinoid tumor and thymoma. Ann Thorac Surg 50:650, 1990.

Molnar J, Szobor A: Myasthenia gravis: Effect of thymectomy in 425 patients. A 15-year experience. Eur J Cardiothorac Surg 4:8, 1990.

Monden Y, Nakahara K, Iioka S et al: Recurrence of thymoma: Clinicopathological features, therapy, and prognosis. Ann Thorac Surg 39:165, 1985.

Moran CA, Rosado de Christenson M, Suster S: Thymolipoma: Clinicopathologic review of 33 cases. Mod Pathol 8:741, 1995.

Moran CA, Suster S: Spindle-cell neuroendocrine carcinomas of the thymus (spindle-cell thymic carcinoid): A clinicopathologic and immunohistochemical study of seven cases. Mod Pathol 12:587, 1999.

Mornex F, Resbeut M, Richaud P et al: Radiotherapy and chemotherapy for invasive thymomas: A multicentric retrospective review of 90 cases. The FNCLCC trialists. Federation Nationale des Centres de Lutte Contre le Cancer. Int J Radiat Oncol Biol Phys 32:651, 1995.

Mulder DG, Graves M, Herrmann C: Thymectomy for myasthenia gravis: Recent observations and comparisons with past experience. Ann Thorac Surg 48:551, 1989.

Mulder DG, Herrmann C Jr, Keesey J et al: Thymectomy for myasthenia gravis. Am J Surg 146:61, 1983.

Nakahara K, Ohno K, Hashimoto J et al: Thymoma: Results with complete resection and adjuvant postoperative irradiation in 141 consecutive patients. J Thorac Cardiovasc Surg 95:1041, 1988.

Nichols GL Jr, Hopkins MB 3rd, Geisinger KR: Thymic carcinoid. Report of a case with diagnosis by fine needle aspiration biopsy. Acta Cytol 41:1839, 1997.

Oh YL, Ko YH, Ree HJ: Aspiration cytology of ectopic cervical thymoma mimicking a thyroid mass. A case report. Acta Cytol 42:1167, 1998.

Okumura M, Miyoshi S, Takeuchi Y et al: Results of surgical treatment of thymomas with special reference to the involved organs. J Thorac Cardiovasc Surg 117:605, 1999.

Otto HF, Loning T, Lachenmaer L et al: Thymolipoma in association with myasthenia gravis. Cancer 50:1623, 1982.

Pan CH, Chiang CY, Chen SS: Thymolipoma in patients with myasthenia gravis: Report of two cases and review. Acta Neurol Scand 78:16, 1988.

Papatestas AE, Genkins G, Kornfeld P et al: Effects of thymectomy in myasthenia gravis. Ann Surg 206:79, 1987.

Parish JM, Rosenow EC 3rd, Muhm JR: Mediastinal masses. Clues to interpretation of radiologic studies. Postgrad Med 76:173, 1984.

Park HS, Shin DM, Lee JS et al: Thymoma. A retrospective study of 87 cases. Cancer 73:2491, 1994.

Pescarmona E, Rendina EA, Venuta F et al: The prognostic implication of thymoma histologic subtyping. A study of 80 consecutive cases. Am J Clin Pathol 93:190, 1990.

Powers CN, Silverman JF, Geisinger KR et al: Fine-needle aspiration biopsy of the mediastinum. A multi-institutional analysis. Am J Clin Pathol 105:168, 1996.

Quintanilla-Martinez L, Wilkins EW Jr, Choi N et al: Thymoma. Histologic subclassification is an independent prognostic factor. Cancer 74:606, 1994.

Rea F, Sartori F, Loy M et al: Chemotherapy and operation for invasive thymoma. J Thorac Cardiovasc Surg 106:543, 1993.

Regnard JF, Magdeleinat P, Dromer C et al: Prognostic factors and long-term results after thymoma resection: A series of 307 patients. J Thorac Cardiovasc Surg 112:376, 1996.

Regnard JF, Zinzindohoue F, Magdeleinat P et al: Results of re-resection for recurrent thymomas. Ann Thorac Surg 64:1593, 1997.

Reintgen D, Fetter BF, Roses A et al: Thymolipoma in association with myasthenia gravis. Arch Pathol Lab Med 102:463, 1978.

Ringe B, Dragojevic D, Frank G et al: Thymolipoma—a rare, benign tumor of the thymus gland: Two case reports and review of the literature. Thorac Cardiovasc Surg 27:369, 1979.

Robbins SL, Cotran RS, Kumar V: Pathologic Basis of Disease, 3rd ed. Philadelphia, WB Saunders, 1984, p 497.

Robertson NP, Deans J, Compston DA: Myasthenia gravis: A population based epidemiological study in Cambridgeshire, England. J Neurol Neurosurg Psychiatry 65:492, 1998.

Rosado de Christenson ML, Abbott GF, Kirejczyk WM et al: Thoracic carcinoids: Radiologic-pathologic correlation. Radiographics 19:707, 1999.

Rosado de Christenson ML, Pugatch RD, Moran CA et al: Thymolipoma: Analysis of 27 cases. Radiology 193:121, 1994.

Rosai J: Histological Typing of Tumors of the Thymus. In World Health Organization: International Histological Classification of Tumours, 2nd ed. Berlin, Springer-Verlag, 1999.

Rosai J, Higa E: Mediastinal endocrine neoplasm, of probable thymic origin, related to carcinoid tumor. Clinicopathologic study of 8 cases. Cancer 29:1061, 1972.

Rosai J, Higa E, Davie J: Mediastinal endocrine neoplasm in patients with multiple endocrine adenomatosis. A previously unrecognized association. Cancer 29:1075, 1972.

Rosai J, Levine G: Tumors of the thymus. In Armed Forces Institute of Pathology: Atlas of Tumor Pathology, Second Series, Fascicle 13. Washington, DC, Armed Forces Institute of Pathology, 1976.

Rosai J, Limas C, Husband EM: Ectopic hamartomatous thymoma. A distinctive benign lesion of lower neck. Am J Surg Pathol 8:501, 1984.

Rubin M, Mishkin S: The relationship between mediastinal lipomas and the thymus. J Thorac Surg 27:494, 1954.

Salyer WR, Eggleston JC: Thymoma: A clinical and pathological study of 65 cases. Cancer 37:229, 1976.

Sasaki M, Kuwabara Y, Ichiya Y et al: Differential diagnosis of thymic tumors using a combination of ^{11}C-methionine PET and FDG PET. J Nucl Med 40:1595, 1999.

Satta J, Ahonen A, Parkkila S et al: Multiple endocrine neoplastic-associated thymic carcinoid tumour in close relatives: Octreotide scan as a new diagnostic and follow-up modality. Two case reports. Scand Cardiovasc J 33:49, 1999.

Schanher PW, Hodge GB: Mediastinal lipoma with inclusion of remnants of thymus gland. Am J Surg 77:376, 1949.

SEER: Surveillance, Epidemiology, and End Results (SEER) cancer incidence public-use database, 1973–1996. Baltimore, MD, National Cancer Institute, DCCPS, Surveillance Research Program, Cancer Statistics Branch, released April 1999.

Shabb NS, Fahl M, Shabb B et al: Fine-needle aspiration of the mediastinum: A clinical, radiologic, cytologic, and histologic study of 42 cases. Diagn Cytopathol 19:428, 1998.

Shamji F, Pearson FG, Todd TR et al: Results of surgical treatment for thymoma. J Thorac Cardiovasc Surg 87:43, 1984.

Shimizu J, Hayashi Y, Morita K et al: Primary thymic carcinoma: A clinicopathological and immunohistochemical study. J Surg Oncol 56:159, 1994.

Shimizu N, Moriyama S, Aoe M et al: The surgical treatment of invasive thymoma. Resection with vascular reconstruction. J Thorac Cardiovasc Surg 103:414, 1992.

Shimosato Y: Controversies surrounding the subclassification of thymoma. Cancer 74:542, 1994.

Shimosato Y, Kameya T, Nagai K et al: Squamous cell carcinoma of the thymus. An analysis of eight cases. Am J Surg Pathol 1:109, 1977.

Shimosato Y, Mukai K: Tumors of the Mediastinum. In Armed Forces Institute of Pathology: Atlas of Tumor Pathology, Third Series, Fascicle 21. Washington, DC, Armed Forces Institute of Pathology, 1997.

Shin DM, Walsh GL, Komaki R et al: A multidisciplinary approach to therapy for unresectable malignant thymoma. Ann Intern Med 129:100, 1998.

Silva F, Vazquez-Selles J, Aguilo F et al: Recurrent ectopic adrenocorticotropic hormone producing thymic carcinoid detected with octreotide imaging. Clin Nucl Med 24:109, 1999.

Singh HK, Silverman JF, Powers CN et al: Diagnostic pitfalls in fine-needle aspiration biopsy of the mediastinum. Diagn Cytopathol 17:121, 1997.

Su L, Beals T, Bernacki EG et al: Spindle epithelial tumor with thymus-like differentiation: A case report with cytologic, histologic, immunohistologic, and ultrastructural findings. Mod Pathol 10:510, 1997.

Suster S, Moran CA: Thymoma, atypical thymoma, and thymic carcinoma. A novel conceptual approach to the classification of thymic epithelial neoplasms. Am J Clin Pathol 111:826, 1999.

Suster S, Rosai J: Multilocular thymic cyst: An acquired reactive process. Study of 18 cases. Am J Surg Pathol 15:388, 1991a.

Suster S, Rosai J: Thymic carcinoma. A clinicopathologic study of 60 cases. Cancer 67:1025, 1991b.

Takamori S, Hayashi A, Tayama K et al: Thymolipoma associated with myasthenia gravis. Scand Cardiovasc J 31:241, 1997.

Takayama T, Kameya T, Inagaki K et al: MEN type 1 associated with mediastinal carcinoid producing parathyroid hormone, calcitonin and chorionic gonadotropin. Pathol Res Pract 189:1090, 1993.

Teh BT: Thymic carcinoids in multiple endocrine neoplasia type 1. J Intern Med 243:501, 1998.

Teh BT, McArdle J, Chan SP et al: Clinicopathologic studies of thymic carcinoids in multiple endocrine neoplasia type 1. Medicine 76:21, 1997.

Truong LD, Mody DR, Cagle PT et al: Thymic carcinoma. A clinicopathologic study of 13 cases. Am J Surg Pathol 14:151, 1990.

Tsuchiya R, Koga K, Matsuno Y et al: Thymic carcinoma: Proposal for pathological TNM and staging. Pathol Int 44:505, 1994.

Tweedy CR, Silverberg DA, Goetowski PG: Successful treatment of thymic carcinoma with high dose carboplatin, etoposide, and radiation. Proc ASCO 11:354, 1992.

Valli M, Fabris GA, Dewar A et al: Atypical carcinoid tumour of the thymus: A study of eight cases. Histopathology 24:371, 1994.

Venuta F, Rendina EA, Pescarmona EO et al: Multimodality treatment of thymoma: A prospective study. Ann Thorac Surg 64:1585, 1997.

Verbist J, Sel R, Van Eyken P et al: Myasthenia gravis associated with thymolipoma: A case report. Acta Chir Belg 97:97, 1997.

Wang DY, Chang DB, Kuo SH et al: Carcinoid tumours of the thymus. Thorax 49:357, 1994.

Wang DY, Kuo SH, Chang DB et al: Fine needle aspiration cytology of thymic carcinoid tumor. Acta Cytol 39:423, 1995.

Wang LS, Huang MH, Lin TS et al: Malignant thymoma. Cancer 70:443, 1992.

Weide LG, Ulbright TM, Loehrer PJ Sr, et al: Thymic carcinoma. A distinct clinical entity responsive to chemotherapy. Cancer 71:1219, 1993.

Wick MR, Carney JA, Bernatz PE et al: Primary mediastinal carcinoid tumors. Am J Surg Pathol 6:195, 1982a.

Wick MR, Scheithauer BW, Weiland LH et al: Primary thymic carcinomas. Am J Surg Pathol 6:613, 1982b.

Wick MR, Scott RE, Li CY et al: Carcinoid tumor of the thymus: A clinicopathologic report of seven cases with a review of the literature. Mayo Clin Proc 55:246, 1980.

Wilkins EW Jr, Edmunds LH Jr, Castleman B: Cases of thymoma at the Massachusetts General Hospital. J Thorac Cardiovasc Surg 52:322, 1966.

Wilkins EW Jr, Grillo HC, Scannell JG et al: J. Maxwell Chamberlain Memorial Paper. Role of staging in prognosis and management of thymoma. Ann Thorac Surg 51:888, 1991.

Yagi K, Hirata T, Fukuse T et al: Surgical treatment for invasive thymoma, especially when the superior vena cava is invaded. Ann Thorac Surg 61:521, 1996.

Yamakawa Y, Masaoka A, Hashimoto T et al: A tentative tumor-node-metastasis classification of thymoma. Cancer 68:1984, 1991.

Yamashita S, Yamazaki H, Kato T et al: Thymic carcinoma which developed in a thymic cyst. Intern Med 35:215, 1996.

Yanagawa H, Bando H, Takishita Y et al: Thymic carcinoma treated with intensive chemotherapy and radiation. Anticancer Res 15:1485, 1995.

Yano T, Hara N, Ichinose Y et al: Treatment and prognosis of primary thymic carcinoma. J Surg Oncol 52:255, 1993.

Yim AP: Video-assisted thoracoscopic management of anterior mediastinal masses. Preliminary experience and results. Surg Endosc 9:1184, 1995.

Yoneda S, Marx A, Heimann S et al: Low-grade metaplastic carcinoma of the thymus. Histopathology 35:19, 1999.

Zafar N, Moinuddin S: Mediastinal needle biopsy. A 15-year experience with 139 cases. Cancer 76:1065, 1995.

Zeiger MA, Swartz SE, MacGillivray DC et al: Thymic carcinoid in association with MEN syndromes. Am Surg 58:430, 1992.

GERM CELL TUMORS OF THE MEDIASTINUM

Cameron D. Wright

INCIDENCE AND EPIDEMIOLOGY

Germ cell tumors are uncommon neoplasms that usually arise in the gonads. About 7000 new cases of germ cell tumors were diagnosed in the United States in 1997 (Bosl and Motzer, 1997). It is estimated that only 1% to 3% of all germ cell tumors arise in the mediastinum (Nichols, 1991). Germ cell tumors also arise in other extragonadal sites, including the retroperitoneum, pineal gland, and sacral area. Mediastinal germ cell tumors represent the most common extragonadal site and account for 50% to 70% of all germ cell tumors in most adult series. Mullen and Richardson (1986) reported that germ cell tumors account for 15% of adult anterior mediastinal tumors (behind thymoma, 47% and lymphoma, 23%) and 24% of pediatric anterior mediastinal tumors (behind lymphoma, 45%). Teratomas are equally present in men and women, with an age range from 1 to 73 years and average age at presentation of 28 years (Lewis et al, 1983). Malignant mediastinal germ cell tumors occur almost exclusively in men (>95%), with an age range from 12 to 46 years and average age at presentation of 28 years (Kessler et al, 1999).

HISTORICAL NOTE

Kantrowitz (1934), Laipply and Shiply (1945), Caes and Cragg (1947), and Friedman (1951) were among the first to report on mediastinal germ cell cancers. Early reports emphasized that these rare tumors affected young men and were usually fatal. Knapp (1985) and Economou (1982) and their co-workers reported two large collective series of malignant mediastinal germ cell tumors before the modern cisplatin chemotherapy era. Patients with nonseminomatous histologies had a uniformly dismal outlook with only rare long-term survival reported. The management of germ cell cancers has changed substantially in the past 20 years because of the ability of cisplatin-based combination chemotherapy to cure advanced disease (Einhorn and Donohue, 1977).

■ *HISTORICAL READINGS*

Caes JH, Cragg RW: Extragenital choriocarcinoma of the male with bilateral gynecomastia—report of a case. US Navy Med Bull 47:1072, 1947.

Economou JS, Trump DL, Homes EC et al: Management of primary germ cell tumors of the mediastinum. J Thorac Cardiovasc Surg 83:643, 1982.

Einhorn LH, Donohue JD: Cis-damminedichloroplatinum, vinblastine, and bleomycin combination chemotherapy in disseminated testicular cancer. Ann Intern Med 87:293, 1977.

Friedman NB: The comparative morphogenesis of extragenital and gonadal teratoid tumors. Cancer 4:265, 1951.

Kantrowitz AR: Extragenital chorioepithelioma in a male. Am J Pathol 10:531, 1934.

Knapp RH, Hurt RD, Payne WS et al: Malignant germ cell tumors of the mediastinum. J Thorac Cardiovasc Surg 89:82, 1985.

Laipply TC, Shiply RA: Extragenital choriocarcinoma in the male. Am J Pathol 21:921, 1945.

EMBRYOLOGY

There is now general acceptance that extragonadal germ cell tumors represent malignant transformation of germ cell elements within these sites without a gonadal primary focus. The initial theory was that these tumors represented an isolated metastasis from an unapparent gonadal primary. Case reports indicated that mediastinal germ cell tumors were occasionally accompanied by carcinoma in situ or scars in the testes of the patients, as reported by Meares and Briggs (1972) and Daugard and colleagues (1987). Luna and Valenzuela-Tamariz (1976) reported an autopsy series of 20 patients with mediastinal germ cell tumors in which only one testicular scar and one testicular primary were found. Autopsy reports in patients with germ cell cancer of the testes by Luna and Johnson (1975) confirmed the rarity of isolated mediastinal metastases.

A theory to account for extragonadal germ cell tumors was proposed by Fine (1962), who suggested that there was an error in migration of primitive germ cells along the urogenital ridge. An alternative hypothesis by Friedman (1987) suggested that there was widespread distribution of germ cells to the liver, brain, thymus, and bone marrow during normal embryogenesis and that later in life these rests may develop into germ cell tumors.

ETIOLOGY

The cause of mediastinal germ cell tumors is unknown. Nichols and coworkers (1987) reported that about 20% of patients with nonseminomatous mediastinal germ cell tumors have Klinefelter's syndrome. This syndrome includes gynecomastia, testicular atrophy, and increased levels of follicle-stimulating hormone. These patients have an abnormal karyotype with an extra X chromosome. The average age of Klinefelter's syndrome patients who develop nonseminomatous germ cell tumors is about 10 years younger than those who do so without the syndrome.

HISTOPATHOLOGY

All histologic variants of gonadal germ cell tumors are found in mediastinal germ cell tumors. Table 63–23

TABLE 63–23 ■ **Histologic Classification of Mediastinal Germ Cell Tumors**

Teratoma
- Mature teratoma—composed of well-differentiated mature elements
- Immature teratoma—with the presence of immature mesenchymal or neuroepithelial elements

Teratomas with malignant elements
1. Teratocarcinoma—with another germ cell tumor (seminoma, embryonal carcinoma, yolk sac tumor)
2. With a non–germ cell epithelial tumor (squamous carcinoma, adenocarcinoma)
3. With a non–germ cell mesenchymal tumor (rhabdomyosarcoma, etc.)

Seminoma

Nonseminomatous tumors
- Embryonal carcinoma
- Yolk sac tumor
- Choriocarcinoma
- Mixed tumors
- Teratocarcinoma

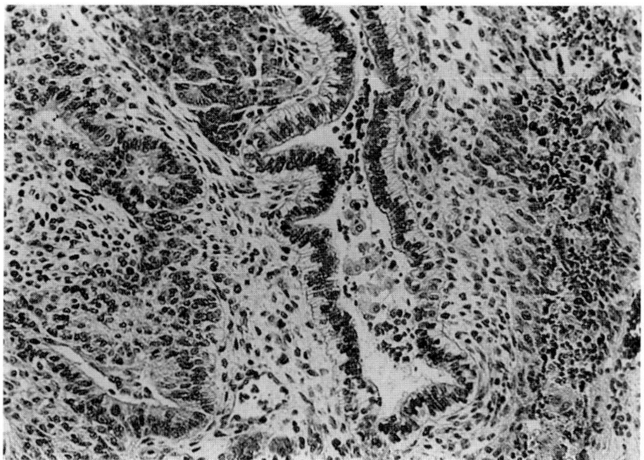

FIGURE 63–27 ■ Histology of a teratocarcinoma.

shows the classification of mediastinal germ cell tumors by histology. About two thirds of all adult mediastinal germ cell tumors are teratomas. Mature teratomas are characterized by the presence of mature tissues representing at least two of the germinal layers (Moran and Suster, 1997). The most commonly encountered mesenchymal elements are cartilage and fat, and the most common epithelial components are squamous and glandular epithelium (Fig. 63–26). Large cystic lesions may occur, which account for the term "dermoid cyst." These cystic tumors may have an unusual expression of the ectodermal component (sometimes including hair and teeth) of the teratoma. Immature teratomas (representing <10% of all teratomas) are characterized by a combination of mature epithelial and connective tissue elements with areas containing immature neuroectodermal and mesenchymal tissue. Teratomas may be associated with additional malignant components. Teratoma with germ cell cancer (teratocarcinoma) demonstrates both benign teratomatous elements and those of a malignant germ cell tumor (yolk sac tumor, embryonal carcinoma, seminoma) (Fig. 63–27). Teratomas may be associated with a non–germ cell tumor of either epithelial (squamous carcinoma, adenocarcinoma) or mesenchymal origin (rhabdomyosarcoma, angiosarcoma, liposarcoma). Seminomas are characterized by sheets of rounded cells with clear cytoplasm (Fig. 63–28). Mitoses are rare, and the nucleoli are prominent. An inflammatory cellular infiltrate is often present at the periphery and in the fibrovascular septum (Moran et al, 1997a). Yolk sac tumors show great variability in their growth patterns (Moran et al, 1997b). Reticular and myxoid patterns are common with small cells with scant cytoplasm embedded in a myxoid or edematous stroma (Fig. 63–29). Numerous microcystic areas are formed, and mitoses are rare. Schiller-Duvall bodies composed of small cells with hyperchromatic nuclei surrounding a vascular core are often seen. Embryonal carcinoma demonstrates a more solid appearance with highly atypical cells containing a moderate amount of eosinophilic cytoplasm and large nuclei. Mitoses are frequent (Fig. 63–30). Choriocarcinomas have a biphasic cellular population with extensive areas of hemorrhage and necrosis. One cell type has round cells with clear cytoplasm

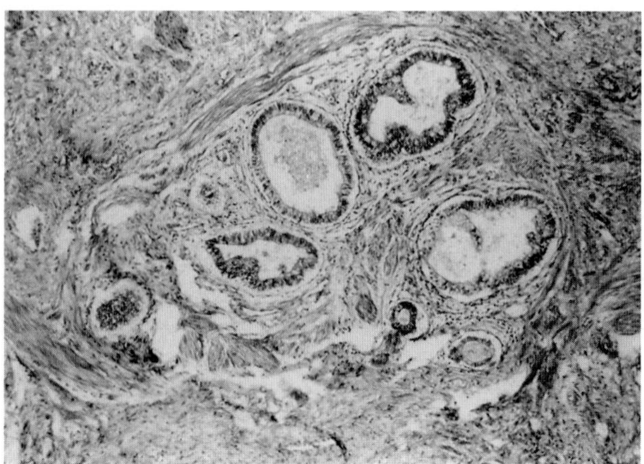

FIGURE 63–26 ■ Histology of a mature teratoma with areas of benign glandular epithelium.

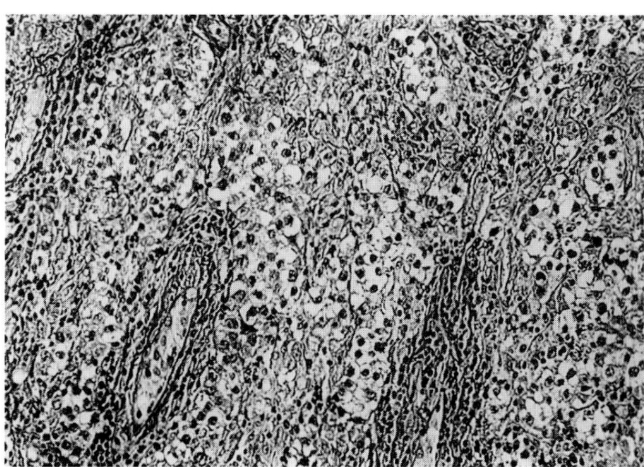

FIGURE 63–28 ■ Histology of a seminoma.

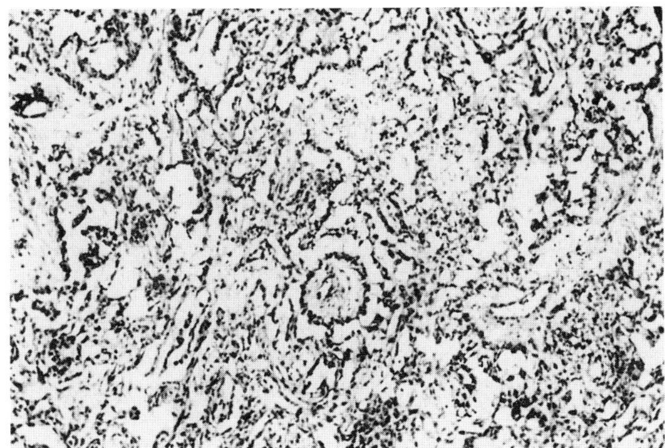

FIGURE 63–29 ■ Histology of a yolk sac tumor.

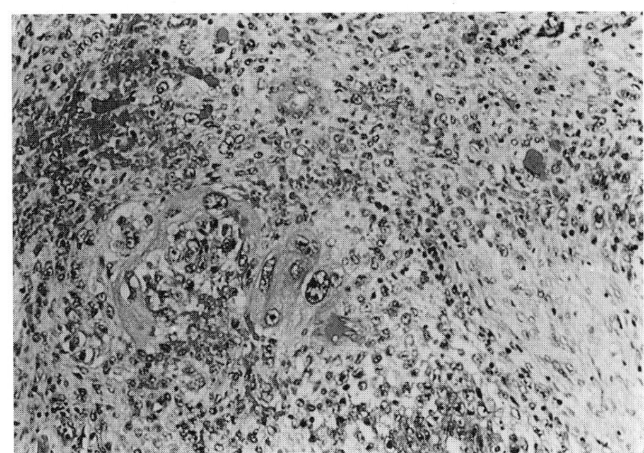

FIGURE 63–31 ■ Histology of a choriocarcinoma.

with round nuclei (cytotrophoblastic cells); the other cell type has malignant, multinucleated giant cells with abundant eosinophilic cytoplasm (syncytiotrophoblastic cells) (Fig. 63–31).

CLINICAL PRESENTATION

The characteristic presentation of these tumors depends on their histology. Benign teratomas are frequently asymptomatic and are discovered on a chest radiograph obtained for unrelated reasons. If symptoms are present, they are usually from a local mass effect and thus may cause cough, dyspnea, or chest pain. Teratomas may rarely cause the superior vena cava syndrome as a result of compression of the superior vena cava. Cough is rarely productive of hair (trichoptysis) and is a pathognomonic symptom. The physical examination is usually negative in patients with a benign teratoma.

Most patients with mediastinal seminoma are symptomatic. These rather large mediastinal masses lead to symptoms of compression including cough, dyspnea, chest pain, or the superior vena cava syndrome. Fever and weight loss are occasionally seen. The physical examination is usually normal, but occasionally stridor, cervical adenopathy, or evidence of the superior vena cava syndrome is present.

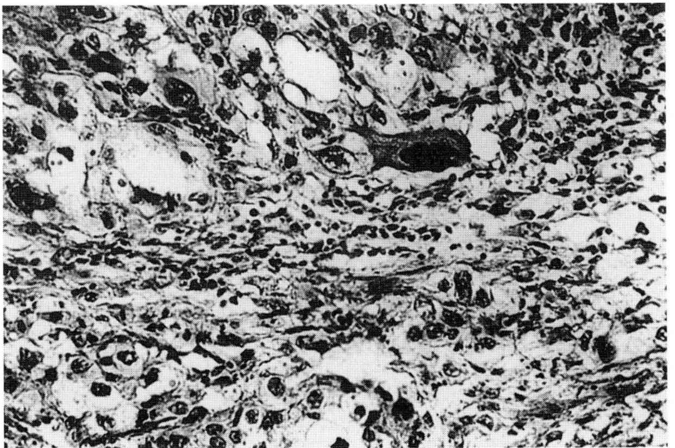

FIGURE 63–30 ■ Histology of an embryonal carcinoma.

Essentially all patients with nonseminomatous germ cell tumors are symptomatic and ill. Symptoms include cough, chest pain, dyspnea, fever, sweats, hemoptysis, superior vena cava syndrome, and symptoms related to metastases. The physical examination is usually abnormal with an ill-appearing young man, often with a resting tachycardia. Cervical adenopathy, evidence of the superior vena cava syndrome, and evidence of a pleural effusion may be observed. All patients with a suspected germ cell tumor should have a careful testicular examination to exclude a primary carcinoma in the testis.

RADIOGRAPHIC FINDINGS

The plain chest radiograph is almost always abnormal with a mediastinal germ cell tumor (Fig. 63–32). The vast majority (over 95%) of these tumors occur in the anterior mediastinum. Benign teratomas may be any size, but malignant mediastinal germ cell tumors are usually large (average size, 10 cm). Computed tomography (CT) with intravenous contrast is the imaging modality of choice with a suspected germ cell tumor. Benign teratomas are usually rounded with sharp margins (Fig. 63–33). They often contain variable amounts of fat, soft tissue density, cystic areas, calcification, and bone or teeth. A fat-fluid level may be seen in cystic teratomas. Seminomas are usually large homogeneous masses with generally smooth margins (Fig. 63–34). Fat planes may be obliterated, and calcification is usually absent. Nonseminomatous tumors are usually large, inhomogeneous masses with areas of necrosis and hemorrhage (Fig. 63–35). Borders are indistinct and infiltration of the pericardium, great vessels, and lung are commonly seen. Compression of vital structures is commonly seen, and mediastinal shift is fairly common. Pleural effusions are common. Magnetic resonance imaging (MRI) does not generally yield additional clinically relevant information over CT.

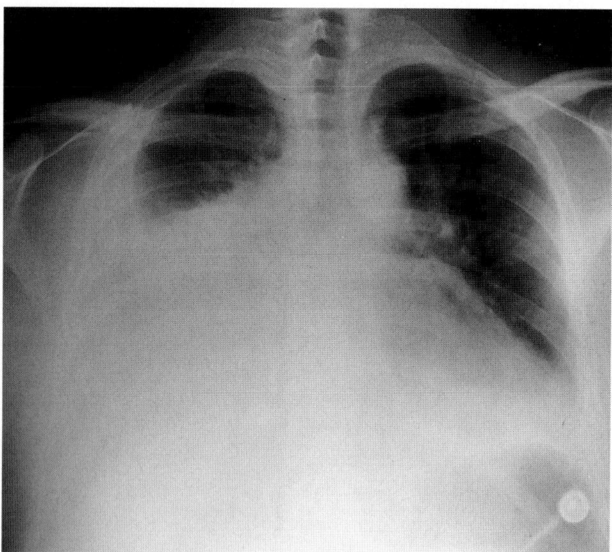

FIGURE 63–32 ■ Chest radiograph of a patient with a nonseminomatous mediastinal germ cell tumor demonstrating a large, right-sided mediastinal mass with compression of the lung and a pleural effusion. The computed tomography scan of this patient is seen in Figure 63–36.

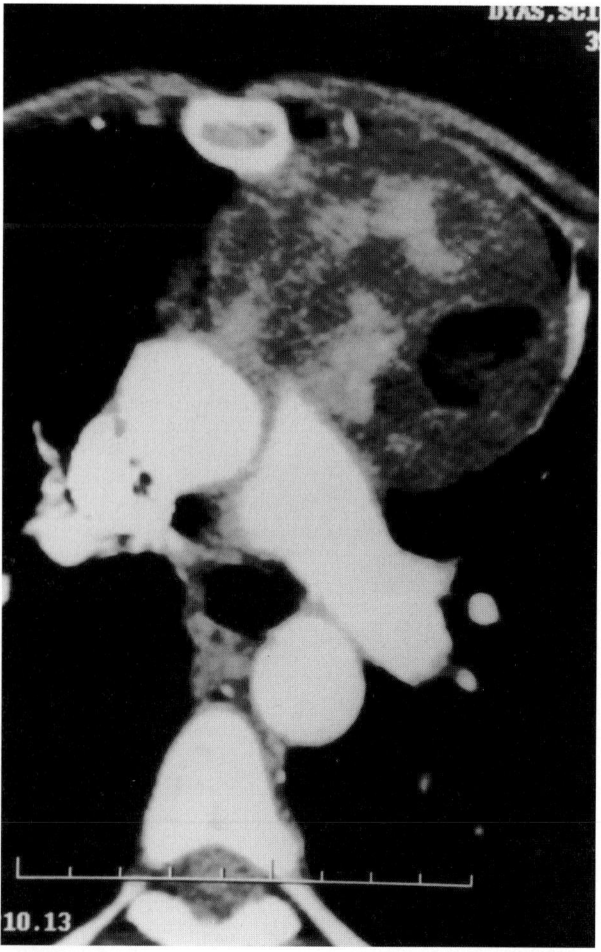

FIGURE 63–33 ■ A computed tomography scan with contrast demonstrating a benign teratoma that appears to be partially cystic and encapsulated.

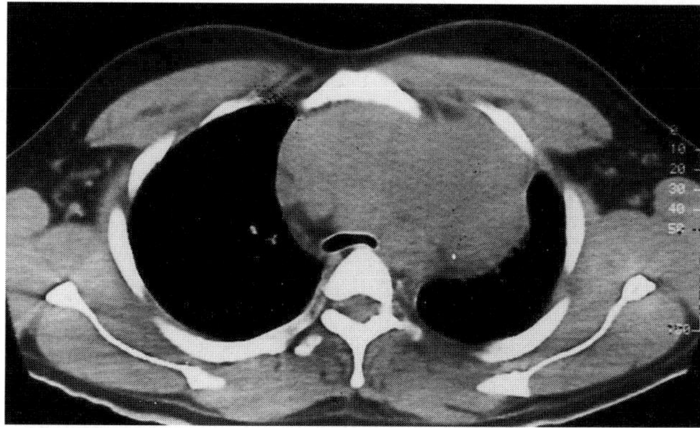

FIGURE 63–34 ■ A computed tomography scan demonstrating a mediastinal seminoma consisting of a large homogeneous mass with fairly distinct margins.

LABORATORY FINDINGS

Measurement of the serum tumor markers human chorionic gonadotropin β (β-HCG) and α-fetoprotein (AFP) is indispensable in the diagnosis and management of malignant mediastinal germ cell tumors (Bosl and Motzer, 1997). Patients with benign teratomas are marker-negative. Mediastinal seminomas can be associated with low-level elevation of β-HCG (usually less than 100 mlU/ml), but any elevation of AFP implies a nonseminomatous element that significantly changes the management of the tumor. About 95% of patients will have at least one elevated tumor marker. About 80% to 95% of patients will have an elevated AFP, and 30% to 50 have an elevated β-HCG. Increased or rising concentrations of AFP or β-HCG imply active disease requiring further therapy. After chemotherapy or surgery the concentrations of the tumor markers should decrease according to their known half-lives. The serum half-life of AFP is 5 to 7 days and that of β-HCG is about 30 hours. A plateau or slow clearance implies residual active disease. Other conditions that may elevate AFP include liver damage, hepatoma, or other gastrointestinal tract cancers. Causes of false-positive β-HCG results include cross-reactivity of the antibody with luteinizing hormone treatment–induced hypogonadism. A third serum marker, lactate dehydrogenase (LDH), is

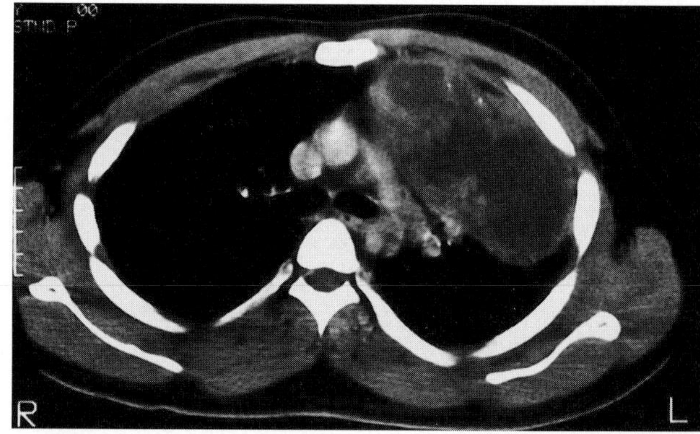

FIGURE 63–35 ■ A computed tomography scan demonstrating a nonseminomatous mediastinal tumor consisting of a large inhomogeneous mass with large areas of necrosis.

less specific but has independent prognostic value in patients with germ cell tumors.

MANAGEMENT

Teratomas

Complete resection of a benign mediastinal teratoma should be curative, and there is no role for adjuvant chemotherapy or radiotherapy (Saabye et al, 1987). The diagnosis is usually made clinically on the basis of the presentation and CT scan, which demonstrates an encapsulated, resectable tumor with characteristic features already mentioned. Preliminary fine-needle aspiration (FNA) is not required and may be difficult to interpret given the large number of possible tissues present. Resection is typically accomplished through a median sternotomy because of the usual anterior location. When tumors project markedly to one side, a lateral thoracotomy may be more appropriate. Adherence to contiguous structures (pericardium, lung, great vessels) has been reported and must be dealt with when encountered. Small, well-encapsulated tumors may be removed by surgeons accomplished in advanced video-assisted thoracic surgery techniques. Lewis and associates (1983) reported no recurrences in 64 long-term survivors of surgical resection of a teratoma.

Mediastinal Seminomas

Therapy of mediastinal seminoma is controversial primarily because of the rarity of the disease. There is no standard staging system for seminoma, and no randomized clinical trials have been carried out in mediastinal seminoma. Complete resection is rarely possible, and the value of subtotal resections is unclear and probably doubtful. As with their testicular counterparts, mediastinal seminomas are very radiosensitive. Doses of 30 to 50 Gy have been used with good local control rates. Seminomas are also very responsive to cisplatin-based chemotherapy with complete response rates close to 100%.

Rarely the diagnosis of a mediastinal seminoma is made by resection of a small, encapsulated mediastinal mass (perhaps thought to be a thymoma). In this case, postoperative adjuvant radiation should be given. Usually the patient presents with a large mass that appears to be focally invasive on the CT. The differential diagnosis also includes a thymoma or lymphoma, and so an incisional biopsy is appropriate. Usually an anterior mediastinotomy (the Chamberlain procedure) gives the best access to the mass, but occasionally mediastinoscopy provides better access to lesions that extend into the middle mediastinum. An advantage of an anterior mediastinotomy approach is that it can be performed under local anesthesia if necessary due to severe compression symptoms (especially tracheal compression). Emergence from general anesthesia and extubation can be very difficult in patients with large masses that compress the airway. In these patients, a very careful approach to the biopsy must be made.

Once the diagnosis of a mediastinal seminoma has been made, both radiation and cisplatin-based chemotherapy as treatment modalities must be considered. As previously mentioned, small, completely resected seminomas (a rarity) probably should be irradiated. Patients with metastatic seminoma obviously require chemotherapy. Common metastatic sites include the regional lymph nodes (cervical, axillary, and periaortic), lung, pleura, and bone. Bulky seminomas are difficult to encompass in a radiation field that spares the lung and have a relatively higher incidence of both metastasis and incomplete response to radiation. Most authors (Gerl et al, 1996; Lemarie et al, 1992; Loehrer et al, 1987) now recommend primary chemotherapy in cases with bulky seminomas. Mediastinal seminomas that are not bulky can be managed either way, although the trend is toward recommending chemotherapy for earlier disease. Certainly, late relapses of patients treated with primary radiation can usually be salvaged with cisplatin-based chemotherapy, as Loehrer and associates (1987) have reported. Table 63–24 lists several series of mediastinal seminomas treated with radiation or chemotherapy. Management of residual mediastinal masses after primary radiation or chemotherapy remains controversial. Small residual masses (<3 cm) are usually dense scar tissue, as noted by Schultz and co-workers (1989). Motzer and colleagues (1987) reported a 25% rate of finding viable seminoma in masses greater than 3 cm. These authors recommend resection of masses greater than 3 cm to ascertain the

TABLE 63–24 ■ **Treatment of Mediastinal Seminoma**

Author	*Year*	*No. of Patients*	*Radiation (RT)*	*Chemotherapy*	*Results*
Bush et al	1981	13	25 to 60 Gy	Salvage only	69% 10-yr survival; 54% relapse-free at 10 yr
Hurt et al	1982	17	13 to 45 Gy	Salvage only	9 Disease-free; 8 dead of disease
Jain et al	1984	15	18 to 46 Gy	7 Primary	RT—4 disease-free; 4 dead of disease Chemo—7 disease-free
Loehrer et al	1987	9		2 Primary 7 Salvage	7 Disease-free; 2 dead of disease
Lemarie et al	1992	23	8 Gy	15 Primary	RT—6 disease-free; 2 relapsed Chemo—13 disease-free; 2 dead of disease
Gerl et al	1996	4	0	4 Primary	4 Disease-free

nature of the residual mass and the need for subsequent treatment. A general treatment scheme is outlined in Figure 63–36.

Nonseminomatous Mediastinal Germ Cell Tumors

Although there is some controversy regarding management of nonmetastatic mediastinal seminomas, all agree that the primary treatment of nonseminomatous tumors is with chemotherapy. Metastases are frequent (25% to 50%) at the time of presentation. Common sites of metastases include the lung, local nodes, pleura, bone, liver, and brain. Patients are usually ill at the time of presentation with a very rapidly dividing tumor. Aggressive subtotal resections are harmful to the patient and serve no role in the modern management of these patients. Confirmation of the serologic diagnosis with FNA biopsy is helpful to confirm the diagnosis and search for non–germ cell elements. An open biopsy is usually not needed if the FNA is suggestive (along with serum tumor markers). Rare, marker-negative tumors usually require an open biopsy to be definitive about the diagnosis. If open biopsy is needed, an anterior mediastinotomy is almost always appropriate unless there are accessible nodal metastases in the neck. Rarely the patient presents critically ill; in these cases serologic confirmation alone is enough to establish the diagnosis so that treatment with chemotherapy can begin. Standard chemotherapy consists of four cycles of cisplatin, etoposide, and bleomycin (BEP), but several alternate regimens exist. It is important that as many of these patients as possible are entered on clinical trials so that improvements can be made in the treatment of this disease. Despite sharing the same histology as their testicular brothers, mediastinal nonseminomatous germ cell tumors have a significantly worse prognosis. Despite this poor prognosis, the overall survival appears to be improving with modern chemotherapy (Table 63–25). Salvage chemotherapy, while benefiting about 30% of testicular patients, rarely leads to durable complete responses in patients with mediastinal tumors (Saxman et al, 1994). Motzer and co-workers (1993) reported promising results in five patients with nonseminomatous mediastinal tumors who received high-dose carboplatin/etoposide chemotherapy with autologous bone marrow transplant. A current Intergroup trial (E3894) randomized patients with high-risk germ cell tumors to either four cycles of BEP or two cycles of BEP followed by two cycles of high-dose carboplatin/etoposide with autologous bone marrow transplant. Walsh and others (1999) reported promising results of a novel rotating chemotherapy regimen with reduced chemotherapy intervals to enhance dose intensity. They reported a 42% 2-year survival in a salvage group of patients with nonseminomatous mediastinal tumors.

The serial CT scans of a young man who recently underwent treatment with four cycles of BEP chemotherapy followed by resection of residual disease are presented in Figure 63–36. A general treatment scheme is outlined in Figure 63–37. Traditional teaching suggested that patients who had persistent serum tumor marker elevation after standard chemotherapy should undergo salvage chemotherapy rather than surgery. More recent findings, especially reports indicating a lack of success with salvage chemotherapy (Kessler et al, 1999), suggest that resection of most residual postchemotherapy masses should be considered. Patients who have progressive disease in the chest or extrathoracic metastases should not undergo resection. All marker-negative residual masses should be resected. Patients who respond to chemotherapy and reduce their serum tumor markers yet have residual, resectable mediastinal disease should probably undergo resection since salvage chemotherapy is currently rarely beneficial. Experienced, careful clinical judgment is required in evaluating these patients for resection. Resection of these residual masses is difficult due to the intense fibrosis enveloping the mass and mediastinal structures. Good exposure is a must. Median sternotomy is the most common approach. A posterolateral thoracotomy is useful for lateral-based masses, especially if they appear to involve the hilum of the lung. Large masses, especially those involving one or both hila of the lung, are best dealt with by a clamshell (bilateral anterior thoracosternotomy) incision, which provides superb exposure. Because most of the patients have received bleomycin, efforts should be made to reduce lung injury during surgery, including efforts to minimize fluid administration, to keep the inspired oxygen concentration as low as possible, and to limit the amount of pulmonary resection to the absolute minimum necessary. Most patients will require a partial pericardiectomy to cleanly remove the tumor, and most will also require a pulmonary resection (usually wedge resection) to remove the tumor. If residual lung nodules are present at the time of operation, they should be removed as well to clarify their histology. Some patients will require resection of a great vein (innominate or superior vena cava) and then require reconstruction of venous drainage. About 25% of tumors involve the phrenic nerve which requires resection. Both phrenic nerves should *not* be sacrificed; if they are involved they should be skeletonized of tumor. During the operation a balance must be achieved between the aggressiveness of the resection and the potential morbidity of the contemplated resection; knowing the histology of the residual mass can help in the decision process. Intraoperative biopsies can be obtained to determine the histology of the residual mass. If teratoma or germ cell cancer is present, continued aggressive resection is in order. If necrosis only is present, enthusiasm for massive en bloc resections should be somewhat tempered.

Postresection histology may include necrosis, benign teratoma, persistent germ cell cancer, or non–germ cell cancer. Patients with teratoma or necrosis need no further therapy and observation only. These patients have a relatively favorable prognosis. If elements of teratoma are left behind, they may grow back significantly in size, compress vital structures again, and simulate return of the malignant nonseminomatous tumor. This is called the "growing teratoma syndrome" which has been well described and recently reviewed by Afifi and associates (1997). Simple resection, not chemotherapy, is the treatment of choice. Patients with persistent germ cell cancer typically receive two additional cycles of chemotherapy and have an intermediate prognosis. Patients with non–

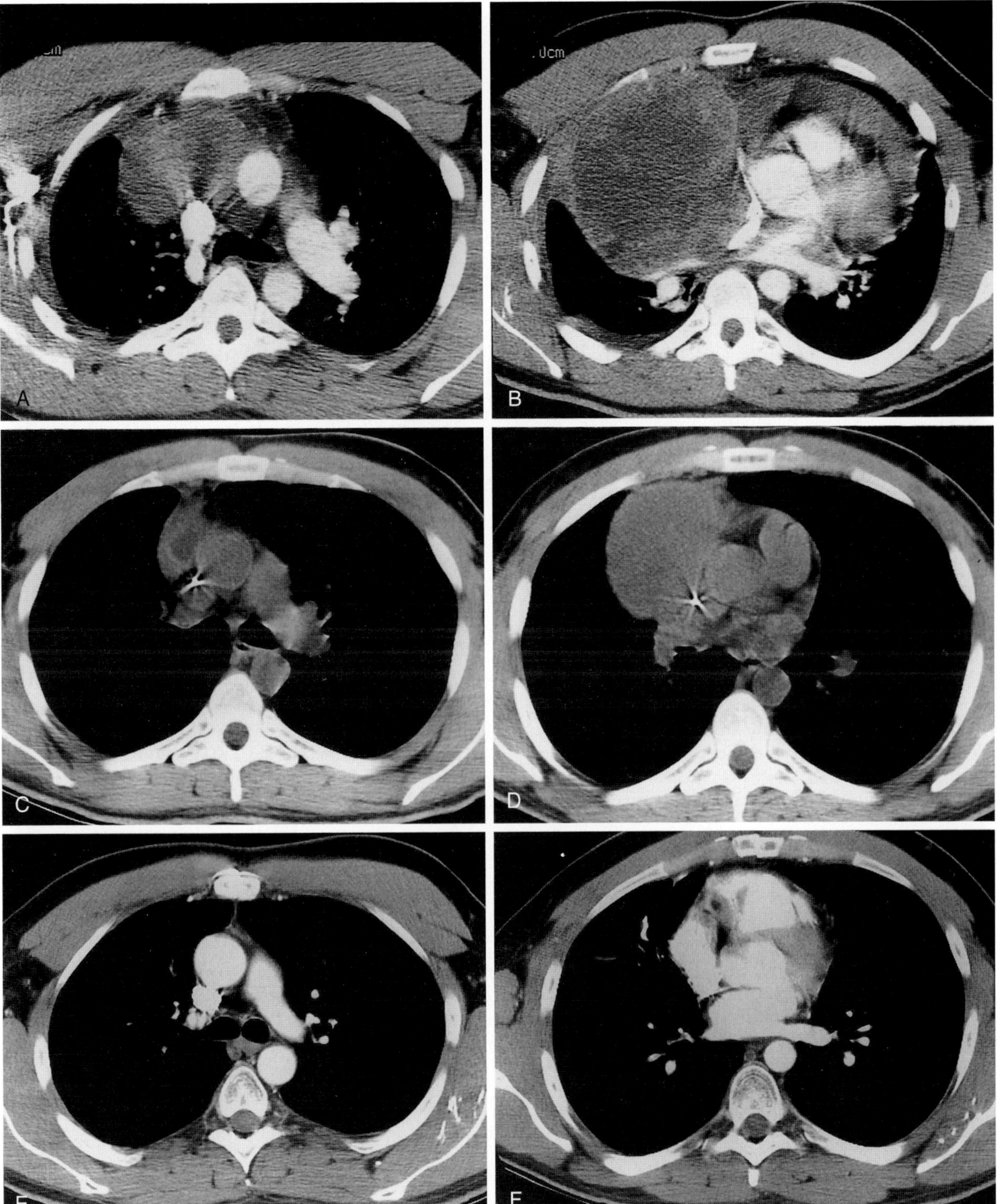

FIGURE 63–36 ■ A computed tomography (CT) scan of a patient with a nonseminomatous mediastinal germ cell tumor before treatment, after cisplatin-based chemotherapy, and after surgical resection of postchemotherapy residual tumor. *A*, Contrast-enhanced CT scan of a young man with a nonseminomatous germ cell tumor. A large anterior mediastinal tumor is present, enveloping the great vessels. *B*, A lower cut of the same CT scan shows a huge tumor compressing the lung and heart. *C*, An unenhanced CT scan at the same level of *A* after three cycles of cisplatin-based chemotherapy. There has been marked reduction in the size of the tumor with a small area of central necrosis. *D*, A lower cut of the same CT scan at the same level as *B* shows marked reduction in size of the tumor and resolution of the mediastinal shift. *E*, Contrast-enhanced CT scan after surgical resection at the same level as *A* demonstrating a normal upper anterior mediastinum. The pathology showed mature teratoma and necrosis only. *F*, A lower cut of the same CT scan at the same level as *B* shows removal of the right-sided mediastinal tumor and a normal heart border. Resection required a pericardectomy and sacrifice of the phrenic nerve.

TABLE 63–25 ■ **Treatment of Nonseminomatous Mediastinal Germ Cell Tumors**

Author	Year	No. of Patients	Chemotherapy	Resected	Results
Parker et al	1983	8	8	6	5 Survivors
Kay et al	1987	12	12	9	5 Survivors
Wright et al	1990	28	28	20	57% Survival at 5 yr
Lemarie et al	1992	64	45	22	45% Survival at 5 yr
Gerl et al	1996	12	12	12	56% Survival at 5 yr
Fizazi et al	1998	38	38	25	40% Survival at 5 yr
Walsh et al	1999	11	11	8	72% Survival at 2 yr
Kessler et al	1999	92	92	79	61% Survival at 4 yr

germ cell cancer (epithelial cancer or sarcoma usually) have a very poor prognosis. These elements have been documented before chemotherapy and hence are not induced by chemotherapy. Chemotherapy against the germ cell elements kills the germ cell cancer but allows the more resistant non–germ cell cancer to proliferate. Ulbright and co-workers (1984) and Manivel and others (1986) have described this problem well. Although it is seen with testicular germ cell cancer, it is more frequent with mediastinal germ cell tumors and is associated with a worse prognosis than its testicular counterpart. Chemotherapy directed against the sarcomatous elements has rarely been successful.

Hematologic malignancies are much more common in patients with mediastinal germ cell tumor than would be expected. Nichols and associates (1985) in a seminal report described three such cases (primarily acute leukemia) among 34 patients with mediastinal germ cell tumors. It is not thought that the leukemias are due to chemotherapy administration, as many cases have been reported prior to chemotherapy and the temporal relationship to chemotherapy has not been characteristic of typical chemotherapy-induced hematologic malignancies. Fizazi and co-workers (1998) recently reported that 17% of their patients developed leukemias and all died. Chromosomal anomalies have been described, especially i(12p), leading to a concept of a common clone shared by the two malignancies in which the progenitor leukemia cells undergo differentiation within the yolk sac component of the mediastinal germ cell tumor.

COMMENTS AND CONTROVERSIES

The diagnosis and management of germ cell tumors are covered in depth in this chapter. Dr. Wright makes a number of important points. It is important to note that the role of needle or surgical biopsy in germ cell tumors differs somewhat from its standard use in other mediastinal tumors. Particularly important to note is the fact

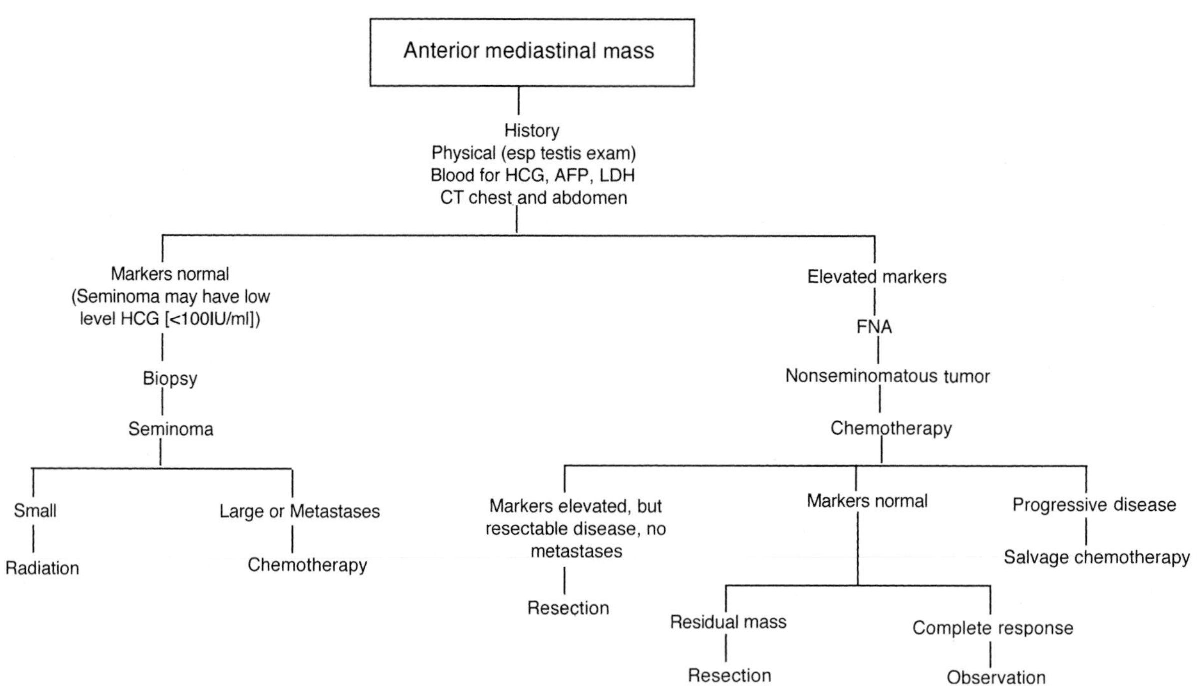

FIGURE 63–37 ■ Treatment algorithm for patients with malignant germ cell tumors. (AFP, alpha-fetoprotein; CT, computed tomography scan; esp, especially; FNA, fine-needle aspiration; HCG, human chorionic gonadotropin; LDH, lactate dehydrogenase.)

that benign teratomas often have a typical radiographic appearance including fat and cartilage. In addition, serum markers β-HCG and AFP are essential for diagnosis and treatment planning. Biopsies should be avoided in serum marker–negative patients who have imaging studies classic for benign teratoma. Also important is the role of surgery and its conduct in patients with residual radiographic "tumor" following chemotherapy for malignant germ cell tumors.

G. A. P.

■ REFERENCES

Afifi HY, Bosl GJ, Burt ME: Mediastinal growing teratoma syndrome. Ann Thorac Surg 64:359, 1997.

Bosl GJ, Motzer RJ: Testicular germ-cell cancer. New Engl J Med 337:242, 1997.

Bush SE, Martinez A, Bagshaw MA: Primary mediastinal seminoma. Cancer 48:1877, 1981.

Caes JH, Cragg RW: Extragenital choriocarcinoma of the male with bilateral gynecomastia—report of a case. US Navy Med Bull 47:1072, 1947.

Daugaard G, von der Maase H, Olsen J et al: Carcinoma-in-situ testis in patients with assumed extragonadal germ-cell tumors. Lancet 2:528, 1987.

Economou JS, Trump DL, Homes EC et al: Management of primary germ cell tumors of the mediastinum. J Thorac Cardiovasc Surg 83:643, 1982.

Einhorn LH, Donohue JD: Cis-diamminedichloroplatinum, vinblastine, and bleomycin combination chemotherapy in disseminated testicular cancer. Ann Intern Med 87:293, 1977.

Fine F, Smith RW Jr, Pachter MR: Primary extragenital choriocarcinoma in the male subject. Case report and review of the literature. Am J Med 32:776, 1962.

Fizazi K, Culine S, Droz JP et al: Primary mediastinal nonseminomatous germ cell tumors: Results of modern therapy including cisplatin-based chemotherapy. J Clin Oncol 16:725, 1998.

Friedman NB: The comparative morphogenesis of extragenital and gonadal teratold tumors. Cancer 4:265, 1951.

Friedman NB: The function of primordial germ cells in extragonadal tissues. Int J Androl 10:43, 1987.

Gerl A, Clemm C, Lamerz R et al: Cisplatin-based chemotherapy of primary extragonadal germ cell tumors: A single institution experience. Cancer 77:526, 1996.

Hurt RD, Bruckman JE, Farrow GM et al: Primary anterior mediastinal seminoma. Cancer 49:1650, 1982.

Jain KK, Bols GH, Bains MS et al: The treatment of extragonadal seminoma. J Clin Oncol 2:820, 1984.

Kantrowitz AR: Extragenital chorionepithelialoma in a male. Am J Pathol 10:531, 1934.

Kay PH, Wells FC, Goldstraw P: A multidisciplinary approach to primary nonseminomatous germ cell tumors of the mediastinum. Ann Thorac Surg 44:578, 1987.

Kessler KA, Rieger KM, Ganjoo KN et al: Primary mediastinal nonseminomatous germ cell tumors: The influence of postchemotherapy pathology on long-term survival after surgery. J Thorac Cardiovasc Surg 118:692, 1999.

Knapp RH, Hurt RD, Payne WS et al: Malignant germ cell tumors of the mediastinum. J Thorac Cardiovasc Surg 89:82, 1985.

Laipply TC, Shiply RA: Extragenital choriocarcinoma in the male. Am J Pathol 21:921, 1945.

Lemarie E, Assouline PS, Diot P et al: Primary mediastinal germ cell tumors: Results of a French retrospective study. Chest 102:1477, 1992.

Lewis B, Hurt R, Payne W et al: Benign teratoma of the mediastinum. J Thorac Cardiovasc Surg 86:727, 1983.

Loehrer PJ, Birch R, Williams SD et al: Chemotherapy of metastatic seminoma: The Southeastern Cancer Study Group experience. J Clin Oncol 5:1212, 1987.

Luna MA, Johnsen DE: Postmortem findings in testicular tumors. In Johnson DE (ed): Testicular Tumors. New York, Medical Examination Publishing, 1975.

Luna MA, Valenzuela-Tamariz J: Germ-cell tumors of the mediastinum: Postmortem findings. Am J Clin Pathol 65:450, 1976.

Manivel C, Wick MR, Abenoza P et al: The occurrence of sarcomatous components in primary mediastinal germ cell tumors. Am J Surg Pathol 10:711, 1986.

Meares EM, Briggs EM: Occult seminoma of the testis masquerading as primary extragonadal germinal neoplasm. Cancer 30:300, 1972.

Moran CA, Suster S: Primary germ cell tumors of the mediastinum: Analysis of 322 cases with special emphasis on teratomatous lesions and a proposal for histopathologic classification and clinical staging. Cancer 80:681, 1997.

Moran CA, Suster S, Przygodzki RM et al: Primary germ cell tumors of the mediastinum: Mediastinal seminomas—a clinicopathologic and immunohistochemical study of 120 cases. Cancer 80:691, 1997a.

Moran CA, Suster S, Koss MN: Primary germ cell tumors of the mediastinum: Yolk sac tumor, embryonal carcinoma, choriocarcinoma, and combined nonteratomatous germ cell tumors of the mediastinum—a clinicopathologic and immunohistochemical study of 64 cases. Cancer 80:699, 1997b.

Motzer R, Bosl G, Heelan R et al: Residual mass: An indication for further therapy in patients with advanced seminoma following systemic chemotherapy. J Clin Oncol 5:1064, 1987.

Motzer RJ, Mazumdar M, Gulati SC et al: Phase II trial of high dose carboplatin and etoposide with autologous bone marrow transplant in first line therapy for patients with poor risk germ cell cancer. J Natl Cancer Inst 85:1828, 1993.

Mullen B, Richardson JD: Primary anterior mediastinal tumors in children and adults. Ann Thorac Surg 42:338, 1986.

Nichols CR: Mediastinal germ cell tumors: Clinical features and biologic correlates. Chest 99:472, 1991.

Nichols CR, Heerema NA, Palmer C et al: Klinefelter's syndrome associated with mediastinal germ cell neoplasms. J Clin Oncol 5:1290, 1987.

Nichols CR, Hoffman R, Einhorn LH et al: Hematologic malignancies associated with primary mediastinal germ-cell tumors. Ann Intern Med 102:603, 1985.

Orazi A, Neiman RS, Ulbright TM et al: Hematopoietic precursor cells within the yolk sac component are the source of secondary hematopoietic malignancies in patients with mediastinal germ cell tumors. Cancer 71:3873, 1993.

Parker D, Holford CP, Begent RHJ et al: Effective treatment for malignant mediastinal teratoma. Thorax 38:897, 1983.

Saabye J, Elbirk A, Andersen K: Teratomas of the mediastinum. Scand J Thorac Cardiovasc Surg 21:271, 1987.

Saxman SB, Nichols CR, Einhorn LH: Salvage chemotherapy in patients with extragonadal nonseminomatous germ cell tumors: The Indiana University experience. J Clin Oncol 12:1390, 1994.

Schultz SM, Einhorn LH, Conces DH et al: Management of postchemotherapy residual mass in patients with advanced seminoma: Indiana University experience. J Clin Oncol 7:1497, 1989.

Ulbright TM, Loehrer PJ, Roth LM et al: The development of non–germ cell malignancies within germ cell tumors: A clinicopathologic study of 11 cases. Cancer 54:1824, 1984.

Walsh GL, Taylor G, Nesbitt JC et al: Intensive chemotherapy and radical resections for primary nonseminomatous mediastinal germ cell tumors. Ann Thorac Surg 69:337, 2000.

Wright CD, Kesler KA, Nichols CR et al: Primary mediastinal nonseminomatous germ cell tumors: Results of a multimodality approach. J Thorac Cardiovasc Surg 99:210, 1990.

LYMPHOMA OF THE MEDIASTINUM

Nancy L. Bartlett
Nina D. Wagner

Lymphomas are malignant neoplasms of lymphocytes and their precursor cells, the principal cellular elements of the immune system (Magrath, 1997a). Historically, lymphomas were classified merely by their histologic appearance, specifically cell size (e.g., small, large, mixed) and architecture (nodular or diffuse). The current classification systems—the Revised European-American Lymphoma (REAL) classification, proposed in 1994 by the International Lymphoma Study Group, and the World Health Organization (WHO) classification—define specific subcategories of lymphoma according to the immunologic and molecular characteristics of the lymphoma cells as well as the morphology (Harris et al, 1994, 1999). Clinicians have slowly accepted this more precise but complex classification system after five expert hematopathologists reclassified 1378 cases of lymphoma according to the REAL classification and validated the diagnostic accuracy and reproducibility of this system, as well as the clinical distinctiveness of the major lymphoma subtypes described (Pileri et al, 1998).

Although every subtype of lymphoma can potentially involve the mediastinum or lungs, only a few ever present as an isolated mediastinal or pulmonary mass. Those with the potential for a primary thoracic presentation are the focus of this chapter, specifically Hodgkin's disease (HD), large cell lymphoma, lymphoblastic lymphoma, and pulmonary mucosa-associated lymphoid tissue (MALT) lymphoma. We discuss the diagnosis, clinical features, staging, treatment, complications of treatment, and prognosis for each of these subtypes when they present in the mediastinum or lung. The final section of the subchapter deals with the clinically challenging problem of residual mediastinal masses, a common finding after treatment for non-Hodgkin's lymphoma (NHL) and HD.

The incidence of NHL continues to rise, and it is estimated that 56,200 new cases of NHL will be diagnosed in the United States in 2001 (Greenlee et al, 2001). The cause of this sustained increase is still not understood. The human immunodeficiency virus (HIV) epidemic and the increase in NHL associated with solid-organ transplantation account for only a minority of these new lymphomas. Primary mediastinal large cell lymphomas represent 2% to 3% of all NHL and 6% to 12% of all diffuse large cell lymphomas (Non-Hodgkin's Lymphoma Classification Project, 1997). Lymphoblastic lymphomas account for approximately 30% of pediatric NHL, but they are much less common in adults, representing less than 5% of all NHL (Skarin and Dorfman, 1997). More than half of patients with lymphoblastic lymphoma present with mediastinal masses (Magrath, 1997c). Primary pulmonary lymphomas are quite rare. Most are low grade and originate from the mucosa-associated lymphoid tissue of the bronchus.

Hodgkin's lymphoma is much less common than NHL, with an estimated 7400 new cases of HD diagnosed in the United States in 2001. In contrast to NHL, there has been no change in the rate of occurrence over the last several decades (Greenlee et al, 2001). The incidence of HD varies significantly with geography, suggesting either an environmental or a genetic association. HD is very rare in Japan, but interestingly, the incidence increases in Japanese Americans, suggesting an important environmental component (Mason and Fraumeni, 1974). HD frequently involves intrathoracic structures, especially mediastinal lymph nodes, but disease limited to intrathoracic sites is uncommon, accounting for approximately 3% of patients diagnosed with HD (Johnson et al, 1983). Presenting symptoms caused by mediastinal adenopathy, such as cough or chest pain, are common. However, during evaluation of these symptoms, a peripheral lymph node is often identified, thereby avoiding the need for a biopsy of mediastinal nodes.

The clinical features of all mediastinal lymphomas have significant overlap. However, subtle differences in presenting signs and symptoms and patient characteristics may make one diagnosis more likely and help guide the evaluation. Symptoms attributable to an enlarging mediastinal mass can include chest pain, cough, dyspnea, wheezing, stridor, hoarseness, dysphagia, and superior vena cava (SVC) syndrome with swelling of the face, neck, and upper extremities. SVC syndrome is more commonly seen in lymphoblastic lymphoma and large cell lymphoma than in HD. Occasionally, cardiac tamponade may ensue from an associated pericardial effusion. Interestingly, patients with bulky mediastinal lymphoma may have no symptoms related to the adenopathy and come to medical attention during evaluation for an enlarged painless peripheral node. Occasionally, patients with isolated mediastinal lymphoma come to medical attention as a result of an incidental finding on a chest radiograph done for unrelated reasons. An asymptomatic presentation is more likely in patients with HD and large cell lymphoma than in patients with lymphoblastic lymphoma. Contrasting clinical features of HD, large cell lymphoma, lymphoblastic lymphoma, and pulmonary lymphoma are discussed in more detail subsequently.

BIOPSY TECHNIQUES AND SPECIMEN HANDLING

Tissue biopsy is essential in the diagnosis and management of patients with primary mediastinal lymphomas.

Recent advances in the immunology and molecular biology of lymphomas, as well as new diagnostic reagents and methods, have resulted in more precise diagnoses (Warnke et al, 1995a). The proper handling of specimens for adjunctive diagnostic tests is critical whenever lymphoma is suspected. Specimens should not be transported on dry towels or surgical sponges; they should be submitted to the pathologist in saline along with the patient's clinical history and differential diagnosis. The pathologist usually reserves fresh cells or frozen tissue for phenotypic or genotypic tests if needed. Most pathologists now perform immunophenotyping, either by flow cytometry or on slides prepared from frozen tissue or paraffin-embedded fixed tissue, on nearly all new cases of NHL or HD. Flow cytometry requires a fresh cell suspension, but it offers the advantage of preservation of antigens. Although fewer antigens are preserved in fixed and embedded tissues, immunohistochemical staining of paraffin-embedded specimens offers correlation with architectural and cellular details (Warnke et al, 1995a). Newer techniques such as microwaving can often unmask antigens after fixation.

Needle Aspiration and Biopsy

Because of the improved diagnostic methods previously discussed, a less invasive procedure such as transthoracic fine-needle aspiration (FNA) or core needle biopsy may lead to a precise diagnosis without the need for surgery in some cases of mediastinal lymphoma (Ben-Yehuda et al, 1996). In addition, the use of computed tomography (CT) scanning has enhanced the accuracy and safety of these techniques in patients with mediastinal lymphoma.

Although FNA is a rapid and cost-effective method, it provides only cytologic material. Cytology alone is less useful for the initial diagnosis of lymphomas because the architectural pattern is often necessary for accurate subclassification. In addition, FNA often does not provide adequate tissue for immunophenotyping, especially when the lymphoma is associated with extensive fibrosis (a common finding in HD and NHL of the mediastinum), limiting the ability to aspirate cells. However, if an adequate number of cells can be aspirated, many pathologists agree that FNA may be adequate in the setting of *relapsed* disease, as it is often easier to confirm a previous diagnosis than to render an initial diagnosis on the basis of limited material.

Due to the lack of fibrosis and a unique cytologic appearance and immunophenotype, lymphoblastic lymphoma (LL) may represent the one setting in which FNA of a mediastinal mass is often diagnostic. This high-grade lymphoma often presents with SVC syndrome or severe dyspnea and progresses extremely rapidly, and the ability of pathologists to provide a preliminary diagnosis within hours on the basis of an FNA may allow earlier initiation of therapy. Wakely and Kornstein (1996) reported their experience with FNA as the initial procedure in the diagnosis of eight children with LL. Six of the children presented with an anterior mediastinal mass. Immunophenotyping established the T cell derivation in all cases, and treatment was initiated based only on FNA results in six cases. Two patients had subsequent surgical biopsies that confirmed the FNA diagnosis of LL.

A multi-institutional study evaluated the utility of FNA biopsy for lesions in the mediastinum by analyzing 189 cases of neoplastic and non-neoplastic lesions (Powers et al, 1996). Of the 189 specimens, 27 were non-neoplastic, 81 were metastatic neoplasms (primarily lung), and 53 were primary mediastinal neoplasms (28 lymphomas, 13 thymomas, 5 germ cell tumors, 3 schwannomas, 1 neuroblastoma, 2 sarcomas, and 2 not otherwise specified). Of the 28 lymphomas, 15 (53%) required surgical biopsies either for confirmation of the diagnosis or subclassification of the lymphoma. Of 16 large cell lymphomas, 2 were misclassified as thymoma and 1 as melanoma on the basis of FNA. In addition, one lesion classified as NHL on FNA was a lymphocyte-predominant thymoma on surgical biopsy. The two most common subtypes of isolated mediastinal lymphoma—that is, large cell lymphoma with sclerosis and nodular sclerosing HD—are both composed of dense bands of fibrosis and often have a paucity of malignant cells, which makes establishing a diagnosis by FNA notably difficult. Large cell lymphomas, undifferentiated carcinomas, and melanomas can be difficult to differentiate cytologically, and artifactual cell clustering and elongation can result in a confusing pattern (Powers et al, 1996).

Other recent series documenting the improved accuracy of peripheral lymph node FNA in establishing an initial diagnosis of lymphoma are probably not generalizable to the specific setting of mediastinal lymphomas. For example, Stewart and collaborators (1998) recently reported that FNA of *palpable* lymph nodes correctly identified 61 of 67 (91%) malignant lymphomas, with 27% of the cases representing recurrent lymphomas. Adjunctive techniques including immunocytochemistry, in situ hybridization for immunoglobulin light chain messenger RNA (mRNA), and polymerase chain reaction (PCR) were applied in many cases. However, no attempt was made to subclassify lymphomas further on FNA cytology, thus limiting the ability to prescribe appropriate treatment on the basis of the initial FNA diagnosis.

The use of core needle biopsies can sometimes overcome the limitations of FNA by retaining the architecture of the tissue and providing serial sections for histochemical and immunocytochemical stains (Pappa et al, 1996). To avoid the risk of pneumothorax, a direct mediastinal approach is chosen over a transthoracic approach, and for patients with anterior mediastinal masses, an anterior parasternal approach is preferred (Herman et al, 1991; Protopapas and Westcott, 1997). If technically feasible, a core biopsy with the largest gauge needle possible, normally 18 gauge, and with multiple passes attempted should always be obtained.

Only limited data are available on the success rate of core needle biopsy specifically for mediastinal lymphomas. A retrospective analysis of 106 image-guided core needle biopsies in 96 patients with lymphoma who had no evidence of peripheral adenopathy included 14 patients with intrathoracic disease (Pappa et al, 1996). Only 14 of the 96 patients had newly suspected NHL, with 82 having a previously established diagnosis of NHL. The biopsies were diagnostic and yielded information on the basis of which treatment was started in 88 patients (83%). The success rate did not depend on the site of disease, disease status, or needle size (14, 18, or 20 gauge). Small sample size and inappropriate tissue were the main causes of failure. Ben-Yehuda and associates (1996) reviewed the impact of 109 CT-guided core biopsies in 100 patients with NHL (n = 71) and HD (n = 29). In 16 of the 100 cases, a mediastinal node was biopsied. Seventeen and 19 patients had previously established diagnoses of NHL and HD, respectively. Eighty-six patients received therapy based on the core needle biopsy results alone, and 14 patients required surgical biopsy owing to uncertain results of the core needle biopsy. Results of the mediastinal biopsies are not reported separately.

Open Biopsy

When a needle aspiration or biopsy is not feasible or does not yield a diagnosis, additional tissue should be obtained by mediastinoscopy or mediastinotomy. Details of these procedures are covered in Chapter 63. Rarely, a thoracoscopy, thoracotomy, or median sternotomy may be needed to establish a diagnosis. When a suspected mediastinal lymphoma is biopsied, a large sample, including the periphery of the tumor, is necessary to distinguish the unique clinical characteristics of the disease. Frozen-section biopsy is necessary to ensure that sufficient tissue is obtained and to guide decisions in obtaining special studies. Surgeons often rely on the results of a frozen-section biopsy to avoid resection when lymphoma is suspected. De Montpreville and co-workers analyzed frozen-section biopsies in 417 patients with mediastinal tumors, including 46 patients with lymphoma. The pathologists obtained sufficient material for a definitive diagnosis (excluding normal or fibrotic lymph nodes) in 351 of 353 cases. In 45 of the 46 cases with lymphoma, the correct diagnosis was suspected on frozen section, permitting avoidance of resection. One patient with HD was incorrectly diagnosed with thymoma on frozen section, leading to the resection of a 5-cm tumor invading a fragment of pericardium.

Pleural Fluid Cytology

Pleural fluid cytology may also provide a diagnosis in patients with large mediastinal masses, especially in patients with lymphoblastic lymphoma. Chaignaud and associates (1998) noted a correlation between pleural effusions and lymphoblastic lymphoma; 10 of 14 (71%) patients with lymphoblastic lymphoma, and only 7 of 60 (12%) patients with HD, had pleural effusions at initial presentation. Subsequently, three children were diagnosed with lymphoblastic lymphoma by performing cytologic and flow cytometric examinations of their pleural fluid. In another study, Dunphy (1996) applied cytology and flow cytometry immunophenotyping techniques to analyze effusion specimens from 30 patients with either suspected (19) or previously diagnosed (11) NHL. Of the 11 patients with previously diagnosed NHL, 5 (50)% had evidence of lymphoma involvement on effusion samples. Sixty-nine percent of the lymphoma-positive effusions represented newly diagnosed NHL, precluding the need for a tissue biopsy in 36% of the cases. Pleural fluid cytology is rarely positive in HD.

Prebiopsy Corticosteroids

Historical teaching dictates that patients with suspected lymphoma should not receive corticosteroids prior to biopsy because of the theoretical risk of obscured results due to rapid tumor response. In reality, except in the rare case of lymphoblastic lymphoma, steroids are unlikely to a have a significant detrimental effect if tissue is obtained within 24 to 48 hours of the first dose. However, the only indication for prebiopsy steroids should be severe, life-threatening airway compromise. While patients with SVC syndrome can be quite symptomatic, these symptoms are not life threatening over the short term, and steroids should not be administered until diagnostic tissue is obtained. If lymphoblastic lymphoma is suspected (see discussion of clinical features later), every effort should be made to obtain tissue within 1 day of presentation and prior to administration of steroids.

HODGKIN'S DISEASE

Pathology

Hodgkin's disease is a neoplastic proliferation of Reed-Sternberg (R-S) cells or R-S variants, large cells with abundant cytoplasm and multiple or multilobed nuclei. R-S cells are surrounded by host inflammatory cells including lymphocytes, plasma cells, neutrophils, and eosinophils (Hudson and Donaldson, 1997; Warnke et al, 1995b). R-S cells are derived, in most cases, from germinal center B cells (Marafioti et al, 2000). R-S cells usually express two cell-surface antigens, CD30 (Ki-1, Ber-H2) and CD15 (Leu-M1). Both the REAL and Rye classification systems still divide HD into four distinct pathologic groups: (1) nodular lymphocyte predominant HD, (2) nodular sclerosing HD, (3) mixed cellularity HD, and (4) lymphocyte-depleted HD. Nodular lymphocyte predominant HD is a distinct clinical and pathologic entity and should be considered separately from the other subtypes, which are often referred to as "classic HD." Nodular sclerosis HD is the most common subtype of primary mediastinal HD and is characterized by dense fibrotic bands that subdivide the abnormal lymphoid tissue into circumscribed nodules.

Clinical and Laboratory Features

Most patients with HD present with asymptomatic peripheral adenopathy. Lymph node involvement is charactrized by contiguous spread with cervical, supraclavicular, and mediastinal nodes being affected most often. There is a bimodal age distribution in most economically developed countries, with a peak at 15 to 40 years of age, and a second peak late in life. Severe, generalized pruritus is common in HD, rare in NHL, and often precedes the diagnosis by months. Alcohol-induced pain in involved lymph nodes is rare but pathognomonic of HD. Approximately two thirds of patients with HD have mediastinal involvement at presentation (Hudson and

Donaldson, 1997). Isolated mediastinal HD occurs most often in young females and usually presents with cough or chest pain. Interestingly, patients who present with cervical or supraclavicular lymphadenopathy are often found to have a bulky asymptomatic mediastinal mass at staging (Fig. 63–38). Systemic symptoms including fever of greater than 38°C for 3 consecutive days, drenching night sweats, or unexplained weight loss of more than 10% of body weight in the preceding 6 months occur in about 25% of patients with HD, but they are uncommon in early-stage disease, including isolated mediastinal disease. Many investigators hypothesize that pruritus, systemic symptoms, and many of the laboratory abnormalities seen in HD are a result of cytokine production by R-S cells.

Nonspecific laboratory abnormalities associated with HD may help in differentiating HD and NHL. Leukocytosis with neutrophilia is common, even in early-stage disease, and is rarely seen in NHL. Thrombocytosis, lymphopenia, eosinophilia, and monocytosis are also seen in a small percentage of patients with HD. Elevated erythrocyte sedimentation rate (ESR) reflects an activated reticuloendothelial system, which, if abnormal at diagnosis, may be useful in following patients after treatment (Hudson and Donaldson, 1997). Serum alkaline phosphatase is elevated in approximately 50% of patients with HD, including those patients without evidence of bony or hepatic involvement. Anemia, low serum albumin, and elevated lactate dehydrogenase (LDH) are usually associated with advanced stage disease.

Staging

The Ann Arbor staging system (Table 63–26) is used to classify both Hodgkin's and non-Hodgkin's lymphomas and is based on the number and location of involved lymph node regions. The absence or presence of systemic symptoms is noted by an A or B, respectively. The designation E applies to involvement of extranodal tissue contiguous with lymph node disease. Multiple E sites including lung, pericardium, pleura, and chest wall are common in patients with bulky mediastinal HD (Bartlett et al, 1995). Pleural fluid cytology is rarely positive in HD. Patients with isolated mediastinal HD have stage I disease if they have no extranodal extension, and stage II_E disease if they have one or more sites of contiguous extranodal involvement.

Clinical staging should include a thorough history and physical examination, placing particular emphasis on assessing adenopathy, sites of extranodal involvement,

TABLE 63–26 ■ Ann Arbor Staging Classification of Hodgkin's and Non-Hodgkin's Lymphoma

Stage I	Involvement of a single lymph node region (I) or a single extralymphatic organ or site (I_E).
Stage II	Involvement of two or more lymph node regions on the same side of the diaphragm (II) or localized involvement of an extralymphatic organ or site and lymph node region(s) on one side of the diaphragm (II_E).
Stage III	Involvement of lymph node regions on both sides of the diaphragm (III) that may include localized involvement of an extralymphatic organ or site (III_E).
Stage IV	Diffuse or disseminated involvement of one or more extralymphatic organs or tissues with or without associated lymph node enlargement. The organs involved are identified by subscripts: H, liver; S, spleen; L, lung; P, pleura; M, marrow; O, bone; D, skin.
Subdivisions	A = No systemic symptoms B = Fevers >38°C, drenching night sweats, or unexplained weight loss >10% of body weight E = Contiguous extranodal site

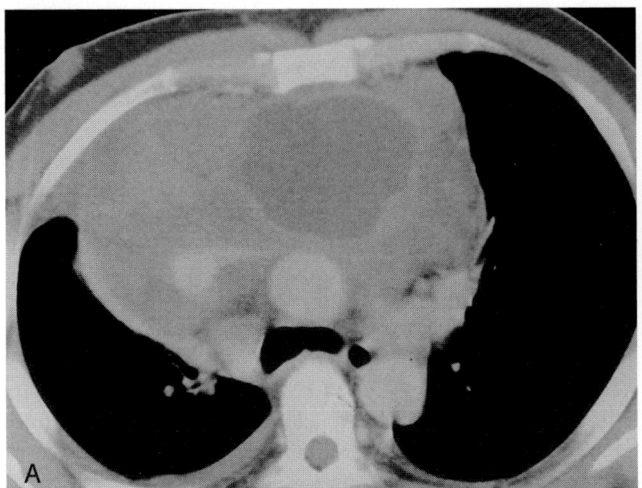

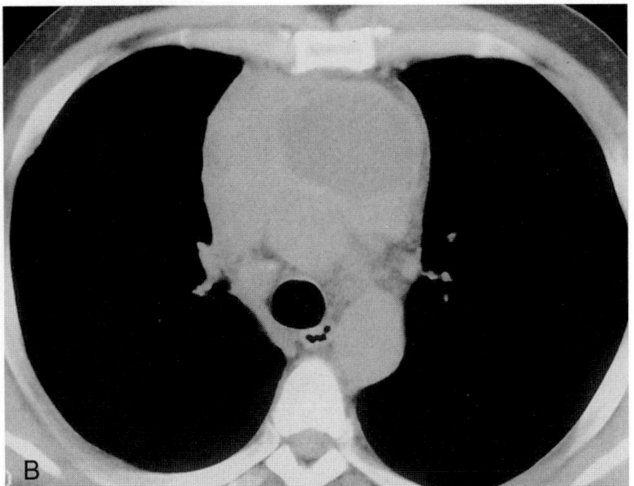

FIGURE 63–38 ■ *A*, Chest computed tomography (CT) scan of a 44-year-old man who presented for evaluation of a 2-cm right supraclavicular mass. Biopsy revealed nodular sclerosing Hodgkin's disease. Staging revealed a large mediastinal mass. He was asymptomatic and specifically denied cough, shortness of breath, or chest pain. *B*, Chest CT scan following treatment with 6 cycles of ABVD (Adriamycin, bleomycin, vinblastine, dacarbazine) chemotherapy and involved field radiotherapy. Gallium scan was negative, and the patient was well with no evidence of relapse 4 years following treatment.

and B symptoms. Identification of a peripheral lymph node in a patient with mediastinal adenopathy may prevent the need for a mediastinal biopsy. Laboratory studies should include a complete blood count (CBC) with differential, ESR, LDH, alkaline phosphatase, albumin, aspartate transaminase, total bilirubin, and calcium. Bilateral bone marrow biopsies should be performed in patients with clinical stage III or IV disease or B symptoms. Patients with stage I or IIA disease are not at risk for bone marrow involvement.

Imaging studies should include a posteroanterior and lateral chest radiograph with calculation of the maximal mediastinal mass ratio (Fig. 63–39) and CT scans of the chest, abdomen, and pelvis. CT is especially useful in designing radiotherapy portals if radiotherapy is planned. Bipedal lymphangiography is only used for staging HD at a few specialized centers. Chest magnetic resonance imaging (MRI) is probably more sensitive than chest CT in evaluating chest wall, pericardial, and pleural involvement, but these results have not had an effect on the outcome of therapy, and thus MRI is not part of standard staging. Gallium scans are relatively insensitive to tumor involvement in the abdomen owing to positive uptake in the liver, intestine, and spleen, and they add little to initial staging evaluation of HD. The value of positron emission tomography (PET) scans for initial staging in HD is currently under investigation. In several small studies, when compared to CT, PET was as least as good as CT in all series, and in one series it upstaged at least 8% of patients (Moog et al, 1997; Stumpe et al, 1998). If additional unresolved PET findings represented true positives, an additional 10% of patients would have been upstaged (Moog et al, 1997). Hoh and associates compared the estimated total cost of conventional staging with that of whole-body PET studies and concluded that fluorodeoxyglucose (FDG)-PET–based staging may be an accurate and cost-effective way for staging and restaging HD and NHL (Hoh et al, 1997).

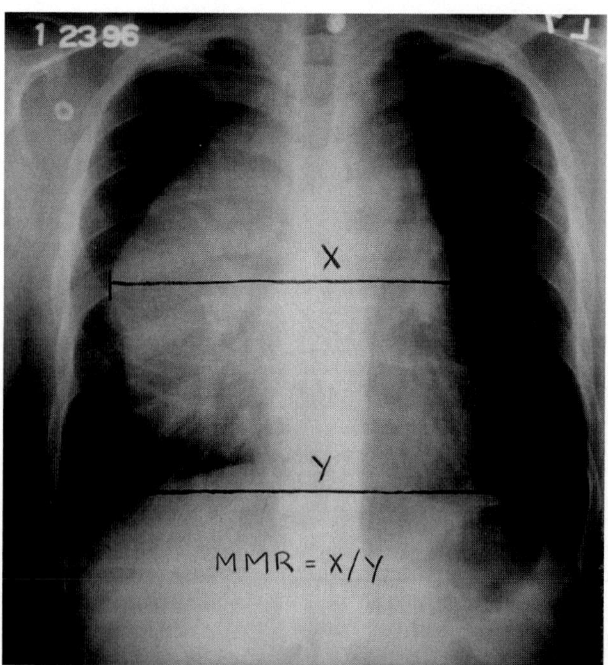

FIGURE 63–39 ■ Chest radiograph of a 44-year-old man with Hodgkin's disease. The mediastinal mass ratio (MMR) is defined as the maximum width of the mediastinal mass (X) divided by the maximum intrathoracic diameter (Y). This patient's MMR was 0.65.

Based on a large randomized trial, the use of diagnostic staging laparotomy and splenectomy for routine staging of patients with early-stage HD has come into question (Carde et al, 1993). In this trial, 6-year progression-free survival and overall survival rates were similar in clinical- and laparotomy-staged patients. Current approaches to the treatment of early-stage HD, most of which incorporate chemotherapy, have also altered our thinking about the necessity of staging laparotomy. Historical series of laparotomy staging have shown a very low risk (<5%) of infradiaphragmatic disease in patients with clinically isolated mediastinal HD, and staging laparatomy is never indicated in this subset of very favorable HD (Johnson et al, 1983; Leibenhaut et al, 1989).

Treatment and Prognosis

Over the last 25 years there has been great success in the treatment of early-stage HD; however, considerable controversy exists in both staging and treatment, primarily because of the increasing incidence of severe, therapy-related late complications occurring more than 10 years after treatment (Cooper, 1999; Mauch, 1994). Historically, following a staging laparotomy, pathologic stage I or II HD, without bulky mediastinal disease, was treated with extended-field radiation therapy, usually subtotal lymphoid irradiation that encompassed all lymph node regions from preauricular to lower para-aortic. The use of mantle irradiation alone may be adequate for patients with pathologically staged I–IIA disease limited to above the carina (Mauch et al, 1995). Given the low incidence of infradiaphragmatic disease in patients with HD limited to intrathoracic sites, patients with nonbulky clinical stage I disease of the mediastinum are also candidates for mantle radiation therapy (RT) (Johnson et al, 1983).

Recent reports of second malignancies and increased cardiovascular mortality related to RT have encouraged evaluation of new therapies, with the hope of maintaining or improving efficacy, while minimizing late effects. These new approaches combine either short-course chemotherapy or a longer course of "mild chemotherapy" with limited RT (lower dose and smaller fields). The availability of effective chemotherapy regimens that do not cause infertility or leukemia have made this approach more attractive (Canellos et al, 1992). Investigators at Stanford compared a relatively mild chemotherapy regimen of vinblastine, methotrexate, and bleomycin (VBM) in combination with regional RT to a regimen of extended-field RT alone in patients with clinical stage I–IIA HD (Horning et al, 1997). This chemotherapy regimen avoided the use of alkylating agents and anthracyclines, both of which have been associated with serious long-term sequelae in a small number of patients. Four-year progression-free survival rates for the combined modality therapy and the RT groups were 87% and 92%, respectively. Although analysis of late toxicities is not available, the responses of the two modalities were comparable. An

Italian trial, for patients with clinical stage I–II HD, tested four cycles of ABVD (doxorubicin [Adriamycin], bleomycin, vinblastine, and dacarbazine) followed either by involved-field RT (IFRT) or subtotal lymphoid irradiation (STLI) (Bonfante et al, 2001). The ABVD regimen is well tolerated and considered first-line therapy for patients with advanced stage HD (Canellos et al, 1992). At 4 years, the progression-free survival and overall survival rates were 94% and 94% for ABVD plus IFRT and 97% and 93% for ABVD plus STLI, indicating that, in the setting of combined modality therapy, the field of RT could be substantially decreased without compromising outcome.

Theoretically, more limited RT fields should significantly reduce the number of radiation-associated second malignancies. In addition, it appears that in combined modality regimens, lower RT doses are equally effective. Consecutive studies by the German Hodgkin's Lymphoma Study group showed no difference in outcome when 20 Gy, 30 Gy, or 40 Gy was administered to nonbulky sites after chemotherapy (Loeffler et al, 1997). As described below, late cardiac toxicities are significantly decreased with mediastinal doses less than 30 Gy (Hancock et al, 1993b). Efforts are also under way to study chemotherapy alone in patients with early-stage disease. A small series of patients treated with six cycles of ABVD had 3-year overall survival and progression-free survival rates of 95% and 84%, respectively (Rueda et al, 1997). Investigators at Memorial Sloan-Kettering Cancer Center are currently comparing six cycles of ABVD to six cycles of ABVD followed by mantle RT in this group of favorable patients.

Patients with clinical stage I or II disease and a bulky mediastinal mass, defined as a mediastinal mass ratio greater than one third (see Fig. 63–39), have a worse prognosis compared with other early-stage patients. Because of high relapse rates in this subset of patients when they are treated with either chemotherapy alone or RT alone, combined modality therapy is recommended (Hughes-Davies et al, 1997). Most patients are treated with four to six cycles of ABVD followed by involved-field RT. An alternative regimen, designed to minimize both acute and long-term toxicities is the Stanford V regimen of 12 weeks of chemotherapy followed by involved-field RT (Bartlett et al, 1995). Cumulative doses of bleomycin and Adriamycin are substantially less with the Stanford V regimen than with ABVD, minimizing the risk of cardiopulmonary toxicity in conjunction with mediastinal RT. Early follow-up shows relapse rates of less than 10% in this subset of patients. Additional efforts to minimize the RT dose in this subset of patients may also be warranted (Loeffler et al, 1997).

Complications of Treatment

Treatment advances have dramatically improved the survival of patients with Hodgkin's disease. Unfortunately, long-term survival frequently goes hand in hand with late-term treatment complications. Consideration of latent side effects should play an integral role in the choice of treatments for this highly curable malignancy.

Investigators at Stanford University performed a retrospective analysis of 2498 patients with HD treated between 1960 and 1995 to determine latent complications of therapy and causes of mortality (Hoppe, 1997). Among 754 patients who died in this group, HD was responsible for 44% of the deaths, other cancers accounted for 21% of the deaths, and cardiovascular disease accounted for 16%. The same group reviewed records of 635 children and adolescents with HD to ascertain the risk of cardiac disease following radiation treatment (Hancock et al, 1993a). No deaths occurred among patients treated without mediastinal radiation or with lower doses of radiation. Mediastinal radiation at doses of 40 to 45 Gy significantly increased the risk of death from heart disease. Deaths occurred 3 to 22 years after the administration of mediastinal RT to individuals 9 to 20 years of age. Similar data exist for mediastinal RT in adults with HD (Hancock et al, 1993b).

Horning and associates (1994) examined pulmonary function in 145 patients to determine the effect of treatment for HD. Patients were stratified into three groups according to prior therapy: mediastinal RT, mediastinal RT plus bleomycin, or bleomycin alone. The analysis revealed that although all treatment arms experienced a decrease in forced vital capacity and DLCO in the first 15 months, followed by recovery within 36 months, mediastinal RT was the only treatment arm that achieved statistical significance. The results of this study were encouraging in that combinations of mantle RT with chemotherapy regimens, such as ABVD, were not associated with permanent pulmonary toxicities. Another prospective evaluation of pulmonary function performed at Memorial Sloan-Kettering Cancer Center demonstrated that ABVD chemotherapy induced acute pulmonary toxicities that further worsened with the addition of RT (Hirsch et al, 1996). Sixty patients received six cycles of ABVD, followed by mantle or mediastinal RT in 30 patients. Fourteen patients (23%) required discontinuation of bleomycin. Patients who received RT experienced a further decline in FVC; however, the functional status of these patients was not significantly affected.

The increased incidence of second malignancies following treatment for HD has been reported in numerous studies. In a cohort of 1641 patients with HD diagnosed before 20 years of age, the cumulative risk of a second malignancy reached 18% at 30 years compared with only 1.9% at 10 years (Sankila et al, 1996). Of 36 malignancies diagnosed in females, 16 were breast cancers. Several other large series have also reported a high risk of breast carcinoma after irradiation of young women with HD (Aisenberg et al, 1997; Hancock et al, 1993c; van Leeuwen et al, 1994). The relative risk of breast carcinoma was significantly higher for individuals who were younger at the time of diagnosis, with a relative risk of 56 for those aged 19 years and younger, 7.0 for those aged 20 to 29 years, and 0.9 for those aged 30 years and older (Aisenberg et al, 1997). Consideration of alternative treatments such as reduced radiation doses, chemotherapy alone, or combined modality therapy with limited RT fields is necessary for younger women with HD.

Another retrospective study evaluated the relative risk of solid tumors in long-term survivors of HD after treatment with conventional RT versus CMT (Salloum et al,

1996). A total of 313 patients were analyzed (116 in the CMT group, 197 in the RT group). The overall relative risk of a secondary solid tumor was 1.5 in the CMT group and 3.3 in the RT group. The actuarial incidence of solid tumors in the RT group was 1.8%, 9.8%, and 15.3% at 10, 15, and 20 years, respectively. A statistically significant risk of lung cancer was seen in the RT group (relative risk, 10.7).

LARGE CELL LYMPHOMA

Pathology

Primary mediastinal large B cell lymphoma (PMLBL) is a distinct form of aggressive lymphoma with characteristic biologic and clinical features. A thymic origin, deriving from medullary thymic B cells, has been described (Addis and Isaacson, 1986; Kanavaros et al, 1995). The tumor is composed of large cells with variable nuclear features, often with abundant pale cytoplasm. Importantly, R-S cells may be present, and immunohistochemistry is essential in differentiating between nodular sclerosing HD and large cell lymphoma of the mediastinum. Many patients have fine, compartmentalizing sclerosis (Harris et al, 1994). Occasionally the tumor cells resemble immunoblasts. Immunohistochemical findings confirm the B cell phenotype by the expression of the B cell–associated antigen (CD20) and absence of the T cell–associated antigen (CD3) (Cazals-Hatem et al, 1996). In contrast to other large B cell lymphomas, the large cells are often surface immunoglobulin negative and exhibit defects in the expression of human leukocyte antigen (HLA)-A, -B, -C, and -DR (Moller et al, 1987). Investigators hypothesize that these HLA-deficient tumor cells may possibly escape immune attack by cytotoxic T cells, accounting for the aggressive behavior of PMLBL.

The unique pattern of molecular genetic alterations also supports classifying PMLBL as a distinct subtype of diffuse large cell lymphoma. Joos and associates (1996) studied genomic imbalances in 26 cases of PMLBL. Gains of chromosomal material were much more common than losses and involved chromosomes 9p, 12q, and Xq and in two cases showed amplification of the proto-oncogene *REL*. This characteristic pattern of chromosomal imbalances suggests a specific pathway of genetic changes for this lymphoma, distinct from other B cell lymphomas.

A provisional entity in the REAL classification, the "anaplastic large-cell lymphoma, Hodgkin's-like" commonly presents with bulky mediastinal disease (Harris et al, 1994; Magrath et al, 1997b). Morphologic features include confluent sheets of tumor cells, often with a sinusoidal growth pattern. The name derives from architectural features that are similar to those of HD, including capsular thickening, nodular growth of tumor cells, and sclerotic bands.

Clinical and Laboratory Features

PMLBL presents at a young age, with a median age in the fourth decade. A higher incidence is noted in females than in males (2:1 ratio). The tumor generally manifests as a locally invasive anterior mediastinal mass originating in the thymus and frequently exhibits contiguous spread to the lung, pleura, pericardium, and chest wall and occasionally to the myocardium or bronchus (Lazzarino et al, 1996). Extrathoracic spread is uncommon at diagnosis; however, at relapse or progression, extranodal involvement is common and tends to involve unusual sites, such as the kidneys, breast, adrenal cortex, ovaries, gastrointestinal tract, and central nervous system (Lazzarino et al, 1997; Todeschini et al, 1990). Similar to other patients with mediastinal masses, patients with PMLBL frequently present with symptoms attributable to the enlarging mediastinal mass, including airway compromise and the SVC syndrome. As with other large cell lymphomas, the most common laboratory abnormality is an elevated LDH, which is an independent poor prognostic factor for response and survival (International Non-Hodgkin's Lymphoma Prognostic Factors Project, 1993).

Staging

The Ann Arbor staging system discussed earlier under Hodgkin's staging (see Table 63–26) is also used to classify non-Hodgkin's lymphomas. As in HD, clinical staging should include a thorough history and physical examination placing particular emphasis on assessing adenopathy, sites of extranodal involvement, and B symptoms. Laboratory studies should include a CBC with differential, LDH, creatinine, calcium, and liver function tests. Bilateral bone marrow biopsies are generally considered part of the routine staging of patients with NHL; however, the low incidence of bone marrow involvement in PMLBL makes the utility of this test questionable. Imaging studies should include a chest radiograph and CT scans of the chest, abdomen, and pelvis. Some investigators recommend a baseline gallium scan in patients with bulky PMLBL in order to more accurately interpret interim and post-treatment gallium scans (Janicek et al, 1997). However, given the sensitivity of current gallium scans using higher doses of gallium and single photon emission computed tomography (SPECT), nearly all patients with a mediastinal mass greater than 1 to 2 cm have a positive pretreatment scan.

Treatment and Prognosis

The standard approach to stage I or II aggressive NHL, including PMLBL, is combined modality therapy. A recent prospective, randomized, multi-institutional study established the superiority of CMT over chemotherapy alone in this setting. Two hundred patients received three cycles of CHOP (cyclophosphamide, Adriamycin, vincristine, and prednisone) chemotherapy followed by involved-field RT, and 201 received eight cycles of CHOP alone (Miller et al, 1998). RT doses ranged from 40 to 55 Gy. Patients with bulky mediastinal masses, defined as a mediastinal mass with a maximal diameter exceeding one third the maximal chest diameter, were excluded. Patients treated with CMT had significantly better 5-year progression-free survival and overall survival rates (77% and 82%, respectively) than patients treated with CHOP alone (64% and 72%, respectively). Cardiac toxicities were more pronounced in the group receiving chemotherapy alone. It is unclear whether these data can be extrapolated to the setting of bulky mediastinal NHL with similar results.

Although a large randomized trial for patients with bulky stage II or stage III–IV disease comparing CHOP chemotherapy to three different third-generation regimens showed no benefit to the newer regimens, several retrospective studies have shown a possible advantage to these newer regimens in PMLBL (Falini et al, 1995; Martelli et al, 1998). The best results have been reported with the 12-week MACOP-B (methotrexate, Adriamycin, cyclophosphamide, vincristine [Oncovin], prednisone, and bleomycin) or VACOP-B (etoposide [VP-16], Adriamycin, cyclophosphamide, vincristine, prednisone, and bleomycin) chemotherapy regimens plus involved-field RT with overall survival of 70% to 90% at 2 to 5 years. Consolidative RT is absolutely essential in the treatment of PMLBL. Recurrence rates of more than 50% have been noted in most series in which patients were treated with chemotherapy alone, regardless of the regimen.

A retrospective study of prognostic features in 57 patients with PMLBL has revealed that the presence of a pleural effusion, more than one involved extranodal site, an LDH greater than three times normal, and a positive post-treatment gallium scan are predictive of disease relapse after chemotherapy (Kirn et al, 1993). Another study of 106 consecutive patients with PMLBL has showed that poor performance status and pericardial effusion are predictive of nonresponse and poor survival (Lazzarino et al, 1997).

LYMPHOBLASTIC LYMPHOMA

Pathology

Lymphoblastic lymphomas are diffuse in histology and composed of a homogeneous population of immature lymphoblastic cells. They are cytologically, histologically, and immunophenotypically identical to acute lymphoblastic leukemia (ALL). In fact, the distinction between lymphoblastic lymphoma and ALL is normally based on marrow involvement, with an arbitrary criterion of greater than 25% to 30% blast cells in the bone marrow used to define a leukemic process. Most lymphoblastic lymphomas are T cell in origin. All lymphoblastic lymphomas express terminal deoxynucleotidyl transferase (TDT), which can be demonstrated in either paraffin or frozen sections. TDT expression is unique to lymphoblastic lymphomas (Yeh et al, 1997).

Clinical and Laboratory Features

Lymphoblastic lymphoma is diagnosed twice as often in men than women and has a bimodal age distribution, with peaks in the second and seventh decades of life (Nathwani et al, 1981). The majority of patients have a large mediastinal mass. Rapid growth of the tumor occasionally causes acute respiratory compromise due to tracheal compression and SVC syndrome and is the most likely NHL to present as a medical emergency (Magrath, 1997c). Pleural effusions occur in as many as 70% of patients, and thoracentesis may be the quickest and least morbid diagnostic procedure. Pericardial effusions are also common. The most common extranodal sites of involvement are bone marrow and the central nervous system (CNS). In contrast to HD and PMLBL, most patients have a markedly elevated LDH.

Staging

The Ann Arbor staging system is used for lymphoblastic lymphoma (see Table 63–26). Most patients present with stage IV disease. Staging evaluation should include posteroanterior and lateral radiograph; CT scan of chest, abdomen and pelvis; bone marrow aspirate and biopsy; a lumbar puncture; and laboratory studies including CBC, electrolytes, LDH, creatinine, uric acid, and liver function tests.

Treatment and Prognosis

Current treatments for lymphoblastic lymphoma are modeled after treatment for acute lymphoblastic leukemia with aggressive multiagent chemotherapy. High-risk stage IV patients with an elevated LDH are considered for autologous or allogeneic stem cell transplantation in first remission (Bouabdallah et al, 1998). The Children's Cancer Group compared two treatment regimens for lymphoblastic NHL, the modified LSA_2L_2 regimen, a 10-drug combination versus the 6-drug regimen, ADCOMP (L-asparaginase, daunorubicin, cyclophosphamide, vincristine, methotrexate, and prednisone) (Tubergen et al, 1995). Toxicity and event-free survival rates were similar for the two regimens. The 5-year event-free survival rate for patients with localized disease was 84%, and for patients with disseminated disease it was 67%. Of 281 eligible and assessable patients, 206 had primary mediastinal masses. Despite treatment with local RT, 34 of 63 treatment failures in the 206 patients with mediastinal disease at presentation occurred in the mediastinum, pleura, or chest wall. All patients with lymphoblastic lymphoma should receive CNS prophylaxis because of the high incidence of CNS relapse. Tumor responses are extremely rapid, often with complete normalization of radiographic studies within a few days (Fig. 63–40). Patients with lymphoblastic lymphoma are at high risk for tumor lysis syndrome, and they should always receive their first dose of chemotherapy as an inpatient with vigorous hydration and prophylactic allopurinol. As discussed previously, patients suspected of having lymphoblastic lymphoma on clinical grounds should not receive corticosteroids prior to a diagnostic biopsy or thoracentesis.

PULMONARY LYMPHOMA

Pathology

The majority of pulmonary lymphomas are low-grade lymphomas, classified as pulmonary mucosa-associated lymphoid tissue (MALT) or bronchus-associated lymphoid tissue (BALT) lymphomas. Historically, many of these were referred to as pseudolymphomas; however, improved immunocytometric and molecular techniques

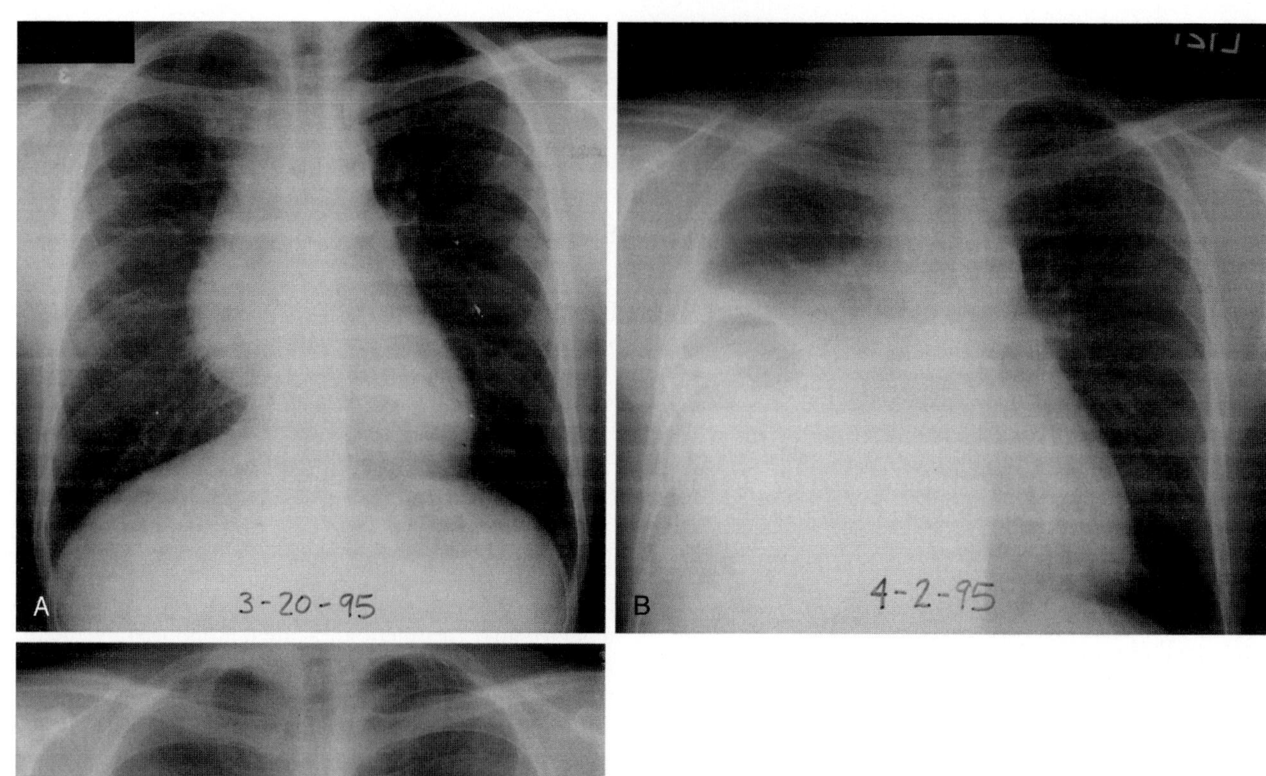

FIGURE 63–40 ■ *A*, Chest radiograph of a 22-year-old man with newly diagnosed lymphoblastic lymphoma. *B*, Chest radiograph 13 days later showing rapid progression of mediastinal adenopathy and development of a malignant pleural effusion. He received his first dose of chemotherapy several hours after this radiograph was taken. *C*, Chest radiograph 5 days after initiating treatment showing complete resolution of all radiographic abnormalities.

now identify these as monoclonal B cell lymphomas (Zaer et al, 1998). They share common morphologic features with other MALT lymphomas including lymphoepithelial lesions, follicular colonization, and presence of plasma cells and Dutcher bodies (Burke, 1999). The lymphoma cells resemble small lymphocytes with round or slightly irregular nuclei that center around reactive follicles with a marginal zone–type distribution (Fiche et al, 1995). A characteristic phenotype includes the presence of the pan–B cell antigen CD20 and lack of the CD5 and CD10 antigens, which is unique among low-grade lymphomas. Approximately 15% to 20% of patients with pulmonary lymphomas have intermediate or high-grade histology, usually diffuse large B cell. At least a portion of these aggressive lymphomas probably represent transformation of a previous BALT lymphoma (Li et al, 1990).

Clinical and Laboratory Features

Pulmonary MALT lymphomas arise in patients between the sixth and seventh decade of life (Li et al, 1990). Respiratory symptoms include dyspnea, cough (with or without sputum), hemoptysis, and chest pain. B symptoms occur in approximately 20% of patients. Interestingly, nearly half of patients are asymptomatic and diagnosed on routine chest radiograph, with Cordier and colleagues (1993) reporting a mean interval of 5.3 years (range, 1.5 to 21 years) between the abnormal chest film and the definitive pathologic diagnosis. Radiographic findings are variable, but they usually consist of a localized mass or infiltrate (O'Donnell et al, 1998). Lobar consolidations and diffuse bilateral infiltrates are seen in some patients. Pleural effusions are uncommon, and mediastinal or hilar adenopathy is noted in less than one third of patients. In one series, 12 of 52 patients with pulmonary MALT lymphoma had a monoclonal gammopathy (Li et al, 1990). The majority of patients with pulmonary MALT lymphomas present with stage IE disease (Burke, 1999). A small number of patients have disseminated disease in other MALT sites such as stomach or salivary glands.

Staging

Disease outside the lung is very uncommon in pulmonary MALT lymphoma. Unless a patient has symptoms referable to an extrathoracic site, chest radiograph, chest CT scan, and serum protein electrophoresis are adequate for pretreatment evaluation. Patients with high-grade histology should have CT scans of the chest, abdomen, and pelvis; bone marrow biopsies; and CBC and LDH determinations.

Treatment and Prognosis

Pulmonary MALT lymphoma is generally managed conservatively with limited resection and mild chemotherapy. In a clinical study of 61 cases of low-grade pulmonary MALT lymphoma, Cordier and co-workers (1993) reported that 42 (69%) patients underwent surgical excision. For 21 patients, surgical excision was the only treatment, while the other 21 received additional therapy; 16 received chemotherapy, 3 received local RT, and 2 received CMT. Of 19 patients not undergoing resection, 16 received chemotherapy and 3 patients received no treatment. Chlorambucil alone, used in 11 patients, was the most effective chemotherapy. More aggressive regimens did not prove more effective, and they were more toxic. Overall survival was 94% at 5 years, and the median survival had not been reached at 10 years. These excellent survival rates are substantiated in two other small series, with 5-year survival rates of 84% and 94% reported (Fiche et al, 1995; Li et al, 1990). Interestingly, in at least one series there was no apparent statistical difference between the survival of these patients and healthy patients of the same age (Li et al, 1990). Patients who present with high-grade pulmonary MALT lymphoma have a significantly worse prognosis than those with the more common low-grade presentation.

RESIDUAL MEDIASTINAL MASSES

Despite improved radiographic techniques over the last two decades, evaluation of residual mediastinal masses following treatment for lymphoma remains a common and difficult problem (see Fig. 63–36). Residual radiographic abnormalities are reported in 64% to 88% of patients with mediastinal HD, and they do not predict for relapse in patients treated with CMT (Jochelson et al, 1985; Radford et al, 1988). Historically, resection or biopsy of these masses was often undertaken, with most showing only residual sclerosis (Chen et al, 1987). Because most patients with mediastinal HD and PMLBL are cured with combined modality therapy, there is rarely an indication for biopsy or resection of residual masses.

One recent retrospective study evaluated the prognostic significance of the size of the residual mass on CT in 28 patients with PMLBL (Smith et al, 1998). Tumor volume (sagittal diameter multiplied by axial diameter, multiplied by coronal diameter, divided by 2) greater than 100 ml after completion of chemotherapy or combined modality therapy predicted for increased risk of relapse. However, because of small patient numbers, these results are inconclusive and not supported by previous studies. Only 4 of 28 patients had a residual volume greater than 100 ml, all of whom had disease relapse. Importantly, 7 of 17 patients with the lowest residual tumor volume, (less than 20 ml) also had relapse, demonstrating the limited usefulness of post-treatment CT.

The usefulness of gallium scans following treatment of HD or NHL has been studied extensively, with mixed conclusions (Front et al, 1995; Kaplan et al, 1990). Many of the older reports described results with suboptimal gallium scan techniques. Few reports are available that evaluate the utility of gallium scans using higher doses of radiogallium (8 to 10 mCi), delayed follow-up imaging (72 to 96 hours), and SPECT. Cooper and co-workers (1993) reported on 48 patients who had post-treatment gallium scans after chemotherapy or combined modality therapy for mediastinal HD. Forty-four of the 48 patients had negative gallium scans following treatment, 12 of whom subsequently had relapse. Two of the four patients with positive post-treatment scans died of progressive disease, and two had their therapy modified and remained in remission at 30 months and 7 years post-treatment, respectively. Only 14 of the gallium scans were performed using SPECT. Similar results were reported by Salloum and co-workers (1997), with 97 of 101 patients having negative gallium scans after treatment for HD. All four patients with positive scans had relapse, and 16 of 97 patients with negative scans had relapse.

Early restaging gallium scans after two to four cycles of chemotherapy may be more predictive of outcome than post-treatment scans in NHL (Janicek et al, 1997). In a study of 30 newly diagnosed patients with large cell NHL, 18 of 20 (94%) patients who had a negative gallium scan after two cycles of chemotherapy remained free of disease at a median follow-up of 31 months. In contrast, only 18% of patients with a positive early restaging gallium scan were disease free.

The usefulness of whole-body FDG-PET for differentiating viable tumor from fibrosis is under investigation, with results of a few small preliminary studies available. Bangerter and co-workers evaluated FDG-PET 2 months after initial treatment of HD or NHL in 36 patients (Bangerter et al, 1998). Of 27 patients with negative FDG-PET scans, 25 remained in complete remission at a median of 25 months (range, 7 to 60 months). Five of nine patients with positive FDG-PET scans had relapse (median, 5 months). In another trial, 34 patients with lymphoma (17 HD, 17 NHL) underwent FDG-PET for a median of 6 weeks following chemotherapy or chemotherapy and radiotherapy (deWit et al, 1997). Thirty-two patients had routine radiographic or physical examination abnormalities. However, none of the patients with negative FDG-PET scans (n = 17) had relapse at a median follow-up of 16 months. Of the 17 patients with positive FDG-PET scans, 4 went on to receive radiotherapy and had no relapse, and 8 of 13 patients who did not receive additional therapy had relapse. Early restaging FDG-PET is also being evaluated (Jerusalem et al, 1997). Twenty patients with high-grade NHL had FDG-PET scans after two or three cycles of chemotherapy. Seven of the 20 patients exhibited increased FDG uptake, and of these 6 had relapse. Eleven of the 13 patients with negative FDG-PET scans remain in complete remission (range, 8 to 36 months from diagnosis). Larger prospective studies are needed to confirm these encouraging results.

A final caveat in evaluating residual mediastinal masses concerns the phenomenon of thymic rebound. Thymic rebound is known to occur in children weeks to months after chemotherapy, but it is also seen in young adults following treatment for HD or NHL. The contour of the mediastinal mass on CT scan should allow differentiation of an enlarged thymus from relapse. Importantly, gallium scans and PET scans may be positive in thymic hyperplasia, and they should not be used to differentiate benign from malignant disease (Burns et al, 1993).

SUMMARY

An isolated intrathoracic presentation of lymphoma is an unusual but challenging diagnostic and therapeutic problem. Adequate diagnostic material must be obtained for precise subclassification of the lymphoma. Despite frequent residual radiographic abnormalities, most patients with primary mediastinal lymphoma or HD are cured. Future challenges include improving treatments to decrease the long-term side effects associated with radiation therapy to the mediastinum and continuing efforts at developing noninvasive methods for detecting residual disease in order to more accurately tailor therapy in the small subset of patients who are destined to relapse.

COMMENTS AND CONTROVERSIES

Mediastinal and pulmonary lymphoma present the thoracic surgeon with an interesting diagnostic challenge. Drs. Bartlett and Wagner have provided a state-of-the-art review of the subject of lymphoma. They outline the typical initial presenting features and the challenges of differential diagnosis. This commentator agrees with the authors' reservation regarding the utility of percutaneous FNA biopsy because subclassification of lymphomas is exceedingly difficult with the small specimens provided by percutaneous aspiration. This diagnostic challenge is made more difficult in those patients who have already undergone chemotherapy and radiation therapy yet have radiographic findings suggestive of residual disease. Establishing proof of recurrence and designing appropriate treatment regimens for these patients are exceedingly difficult.

G.A.P.

■ REFERENCES

Addis BJ, Isaacson PG: Large cell lymphoma of the mediastinum: a B-cell tumor of probable thymic origin. Histopathology 10:370, 1986.

Aisenberg AC, Finkelstein DM, Doppke KP et al: High risk of breast carcinoma after irradiation of young women with Hodgkin's disease. Cancer 79:1203, 1997.

Bangerter M, Kotzerke J, Griesshammer M et al: Role of whole body FDG-PET in predicting relapse in residual masses after treatment of lymphoma. Blood 92:242a, 1998.

Bartlett NL, Rosenberg SA, Hoppe RT et al: Brief chemotherapy, Stanford V, and adjuvant radiotherapy for bulky or advanced-stage Hodgkin's disease: A preliminary report. J Clin Oncol 13:1080, 1995.

Ben-Yehuda D, Polliack A, Okon E et al: Image-guided core needle biopsy in malignant lymphoma: Experience with 100 patients that suggests the technique is reliable. J Clin Oncol 14: 2431, 1996.

Bonfante V, Viviani S, Devizzi L et al: Ten years experience with ABVD plus radiotherapy: Subtotal nodal (STNI) vs. involved field (IFRT) in early-stage Hodgkin's disease (HD) (Abstract). Proc Am Soc Clin Oncol 20:281a, 2001.

Bouabdallah R, Xerri L, Bardou J et al: Role of induction chemotherapy and bone marrow transplantation in adult lymphoblastic lymphoma: A report on 62 patients from a single center. Ann Oncol 9:619, 1998.

Burke JS: Are there site-specific differences among the MALT lymphomas—morphologic, clinical? Am J Clin Pathol 111 (Suppl 1):S133, 1999.

Burns DE, Schiffman FJ: Beguiled by the gallium: Thymic rebound in an adult after chemotherapy for Hodgkin's disease. Chest 104:1916, 1993.

Canellos GP, Anderson JR, Propert KJ et al: Chemotherapy of advanced Hodgkin's disease with MOPP, ABVD, or MOPP alternating with ABVD. N Engl J Med 327:1478, 1992.

Carde P, Hagenbeek A, Hayat M et al: Clinical staging versus laparotomy and combined modality with MOPP versus ABVD in early-stage Hodgkin's disease: The H6 twin randomized trials from the European Organization for Research and Treatment of Cancer Lymphoma Cooperative Group. J Clin Oncol 11:2258, 1993.

Cazals-Hatem D, Lepage E, Brice P et al: Primary mediastinal large B-cell lymphome: A clinicopathologic study of 141 cases compared with 916 nonmediastinal large B-cell lymphomas: A GELA ("Groupe d'Etude des Lymphomes de l'Adulte") study. Am J Surg Pathol 20:877, 1996.

Chaignaud BE, Bonsack TA, Kozakewich HP et al: Pleural effusions in lymphoblastic lymphoma: A diagnostic alternative. J Pediatr Surg 33:1355, 1998.

Chen JL, Osborne BM, Butler JJ: Residual fibrous masses in treated Hodgkin's disease. Cancer 60:407, 1987.

Cooper DL: Treatment of early-stage Hodgkin's disease: Lessons from recent studies. PPO Updates, Principles and Practice of Oncology 13:1, 1999.

Cooper DL, Caride VJ, Zloty M et al: Gallium scans in patients with mediastinal Hodgkin's disease treated with chemotherapy. J Clin Oncol 11:1092, 1993.

Cordier JF, Chailleux E, Lauque D et al: Primary pulmonary lymphomas: A clinical study of 70 cases in nonimmunocompromised patients. Chest 103:201, 1993.

Cossman J, Annunziata CM, Barash S et al: Reed-Sternberg cell genome expression supports a B-cell lineage. Blood 94:411, 1999.

de Montpreville VT, Dulmet EM, Nashashibi N: Frozen section diagnosis and surgical biopsy of lymph nodes, tumors and pseudotumors of the mediastinum. Eur J Cardiothorac Surg 13:190, 1998.

de Wit M, Bumann D, Beyer W et al: Whole-body positron emission tomography (PET) for diagnosis of residual mass in patients with lymphoma. Ann Oncol 8 (Suppl 1):S57, 1997.

Dunphy CH: Combined cytomorphologic and immunophenotypic approach to evaluation of effusions for lymphomatous involvement. Diagn Cytopathol 15:427, 1996.

Falini B, Venturi S, Martelli M et al: Mediastinal large B-cell lymphoma: Clinical and immunohistological findings in 18 patients treated with different third-generation regimens. Br J Haematol 89:780, 1995.

Fiche M, Caprons F, Berger F et al: Primary pulmonary non-Hodgkin's lymphomas. Histopathology 26:529, 1995.

Front D, Israel O: The role of Ga-67 scintigraphy in evaluating the results of therapy of lymphoma patients. Semin Nucl Med 25:60, 1995.

Greenlee RT, Hill-Harmon MB, Murray T et al: Cancer Statistics, 2001. CA Cancer J Clin 51:15, 2001.

Hancock SL, Donaldson SS, Hoppe RT: Cardiac disease following treatment of Hodgkin's disease in children and adolescents. J Clin Oncol 11:1208, 1993a.

Hancock SL, Tucker MA, Hoppe RT: Factors affecting late mortality from heart disease after treatment of Hodgkin's disease. JAMA 270:1949, 1993b.

Hancock SL, Tucker MA, Hoppe RT: Breast cancer after treatment of Hodgkin's disease. J Natl Cancer Inst 85:25, 1993c.

Harris NL, Jaffe ES, Stein H et al: A Revised European-American Classification of lymphoid neoplasms: A proposal from the International Lymphoma Study Group. Blood 84:1361, 1994.

Harris NL, Jaffe ES, Diebold J et al: World Health Organization classification of neoplastic diseases of the hematopoietic and lymphoid tissues: Report of the Clinical Advisory Committee meeting—Airlie House, Virginia, November, 1977. J Clin Oncol 17:3835, 1999.

Herman SJ, Holub RV, Weisbrod GL et al: Anterior mediastinal masses: Utility of transthoracic needle biopsy. Radiology 180:167, 1991.

Hirsch A, Vander Els N, Straus DJ et al: Effect of ABVD chemotherapy with and without mantle or mediastinal irradiation on pulmonary function and symptoms in early-stage Hodgkin's disease. J Clin Oncol 14:1297, 1996.

Hoh CK, Glaspy J, Rosen P et al: Whole-body FDG-PET imaging for staging of Hodgkin's disease and lymphoma. J Nucl Med 38:343, 1997.

Hoppe RT: Hodgkin's disease: Complications of therapy and excess mortality. Ann Oncol 8 (Suppl 1):S115, 1997.

Horning SJ, Adhikari A, Rizk N et al: Effect of treatment for Hodgkin's disease on pulmonary function: Results of a prospective study. J Clin Oncol 12:297, 1994.

Horning SJ, Hoppe RT, Mason J et al: Stanford-Kaiser Permanente G1 study for clinical stage I to IIA Hodgkin's disease: Subtotal lymphoid irradiation versus vinblastine, methotrexate, and bleomycin chemotherapy and regional irradiation. J Clin Oncol 15:1736, 1997.

Hudson MM, Donaldson SS: Hodgkin's disease. Pediatr Clin North Am 44:891, 1997.

Hughes-Davies L, Tarbell NJ, Coleman CN et al: Stage IA-IIB Hodgkin's disease: Management and outcome of extensive thoracic involvement. Int J Radiat Oncol Biol Phys 39:361, 1997.

The International Non-Hodgkin's Lymphoma Prognostic Factors Project: A predictive model for aggressive non-Hodgkin's lymphoma. N Engl J Med 329:987, 1993.

Janicek M, Kaplan W, Neuberg D et al: Early restaging gallium scans predict outcome in poor-prognosis patients with aggressive non-Hodgkin's lymphoma treated with high-dose CHOP chemotherapy. J Clin Oncol 15:1631, 1997.

Jerusalem G, Beguin Y, Fassotte MF et al: Early assessment of response chemotherapy by FDG-PET is highly predictive of outcome in patients with high-grade non-Hodgkin's lymphoma (NHL) (Abstract). Blood 90:388a, 1997.

Jochelson M, Mauch P, Balikian J et al: The significance of the residual mediastinal mass in treated Hodgkin's disease. J Clin Oncol 3:637, 1985.

Johnson DW, Hoppe RT, Cox RS et al: Hodgkin's disease limited to intrathoracic sites. Cancer 52:8, 1983.

Joos S, Otano-Joos MI, Ziegler S et al: Primary mediastinal (thymic) B-cell lymphoma is characterized by gains of chromosomal material including 9p and amplification of the REL gene. Blood 87:1571, 1996.

Kanavaros P, Gaulard P, Charlotte F et al: Discordant expression of immunoglobulin and its associated molecule MB-1/CD79A is frequently found in mediastinal large B-cell lymphomas. Am J Pathol 146:735, 1995.

Kaplan W, Jochelson M, Herman T et al: Gallium-67 imaging: A predictor of residual tumor viability and clinical outcome in patients with diffuse large-cell lymphoma. J Clin Oncol 8:1966, 1990.

Kirn D, Mauch P, Shaffer K et al: Large-cell and immunoblastic lymphoma of the mediastinum: Prognostic features and treatment outcome in 57 patients. J Clin Oncol 11:1336, 1993.

Landis SH, Murray T, Bolden S et al: Cancer statistics, 1999. CA Cancer J Clin 49:8, 1999.

Lazzarino M, Orlandi E, Astori C et al: A low serum β2-microglobulin level despite bulky tumor is a characteristic feature of primary mediastinal (thymic) large B-cell lymphoma: Implications for serologic staging. Eur J Haematol 57:331, 1996.

Lazzarino M, Orlandi E, Paulli M et al: Treatment outcome and prognostic factors for primary mediastinal (thymic) B-cell lymphoma: A multicenter study of 106 patients. J Clin Oncol 15:1646, 1997.

Leibenhaut MH, Hoppe RT, Efron B et al: Prognostic indicators of laparotomy findings in clinical stage I-II supradiaphragmatic Hodgkin's disease. J Clin Oncol 7:81, 1989.

Li G, Hansmann ML, Zwingers T et al: Primary lymphomas of the lung: Morphological, immunohistochemical and clinical features. Histopathology 16:519, 1990.

Loeffler M, Diehl V, Pfreundschuh M at al: Dose-response relationship of complementary radiotherapy following four cycles of combination chemotherapy in intermediate-stage Hodgkin's disease. J Clin Oncol 15:2275, 1997.

Magrath IT: Introduction: Concepts and controversies in lymphoid neoplasia. In Magrath I (ed): The Non-Hodgkin's Lymphomas. New York, Oxford University Press, 1997a, p 3.

Magrath IT: Pathogenesis of Ki-1 + lymphomas. In Magrath I (ed): The Non-Hodgkin's Lymphomas. New York, Oxford University Press, 1997b, p 444.

Magrath IT: Lymphoblastic lymphoma. In Magrath I (ed): The Non-Hodgkin's Lymphomas. New York, Oxford University Press, 1997c, p 817.

Marafioti T, Hummel M, Foss HD et al: Hodgkin and Reed-Sternberg cells represent an expansion of a single clone originating from a germinal center B-cell with functional immunoglobulin gene rearrangements but defective immunoglobulin transcription. Blood 95:1443, 2000.

Martelli MP, Martelli M, Pescarmona E et al: MACOP-B and involved field radiation therapy is an effective therapy for primary mediastinal large B-cell lymphoma with sclerosis. Ann Oncol 9:1027, 1998.

Mason TJ, Fraumeni JF Jr: Hodgkin's disease among Japanese Americans. Lancet 1:215, 1974.

Mauch PM: Controversies in the management of early stage Hodgkin's disease. Blood 83:318, 1994.

Mauch PM, Canellos GP, Shulman LN et al: Mantle irradiation alone for selected patients with laparotomy-staged IA to IIA Hodgkin's disease: Preliminary results of a prospective trial. J Clin Oncol 13:947, 1995.

Miller TP, Dahlberg S, Cassady JR et al: Chemotherapy alone compared with chemotherapy plus radiotherapy for localized intermediate- and high-grade non-Hodgkin's lymphoma. N Engl J Med 339:21, 1998.

Moller P, Moldenhauer G, Momburg F et al: Mediastinal lymphoma of clear cell type is a tumor corresponding to terminal steps of B cell differentiation. Blood 69:1087, 1987.

Moog F, Bangerter M, Diederichs CG et al: Lymphoma: Role of whole-body 2-deoxy-2-[F-18] fluoro-D-glucose (FDG) PET in nodal staging. Radiology 203:795, 1997.

Nathwani BN, Diamond LW, Winberg CD et al: Lymphoblastic lymphoma: A clinicopathologic study of 95 patients. Cancer 48:2347, 1981.

The Non-Hodgkin's Lymphoma Classification Project: A clinical evaluation of the International Lymphoma Study Group classification of non-Hodgkin's lymphoma. Blood 89:3909, 1997.

O'Donnell PG, Jackson SA, Tung KT et al: Radiological appearances of lymphomas arising from mucosa-associated lymphoid tissue (MALT) in the lung. Clin Radiol 53:258, 1998.

Pappa VI, Hussain HK, Reznek RH et al: Role of image-guided core needle biopsy in the management of patients with lymphoma. J Clin Oncol 14:2427, 1996.

Pileri SA, Milani M, Fraternali-Orcioni G et al: From the R.E.A.L. classification to the upcoming WHO scheme: A step toward universal categorization of lymphoma entities? Ann Oncol 9:607, 1998.

Powers CN, Silverman JF, Geisenger KR et al: Fine-needle aspiration biopsy of the mediastinum: A multi-institutional analysis. Am J Clin Pathol 105:168, 1996.

Protopapas Z, Westcott JL: Transthoracic hilar and mediastinal biopsy. J Thorac Imaging 12:250, 1997.

Radford JA, Cowan RA, Flanagan M et al: The significance of residual mediastinal abnormality on the chest radiograph following treatment for Hodgkin's disease. J Clin Oncol 6:940, 1988.

Rueda A, Alba E, Ribelles N et al: Six cycles of ABVD in the treatment of stage I and II Hodgkin's lymphoma: A pilot study. J Clin Oncol 15:1118, 1997.

Salloum E, Brandt DS, Caride VJ et al: Gallium scans in the management of patients with Hodgkin's disease: A study of 101 patients. J Clin Oncol 15:518, 1997.

Salloum E, Doria R, Schubert W et al: Second solid tumors in patients with Hodgkin's disease cured after radiation or chemotherapy plus adjuvant low-dose radiation. J Clin Oncol 14:2435, 1996.

Sankila R, Garwicz S, Olsen JH et al: Risk of subsequent malignant neoplasms among 1,641 Hodgkin's disease patients diagnosed in childhood and adolescence: A population-based cohort study in the five Nordic countries Association of the Nordic Cancer Registries and the Nordic Society of Pediatric Hematology and Oncology. J Clin Oncol 14:1442, 1996.

Skarin AT, Dorfman DM: Non-Hodgkin's lymphomas: Current classification and management. CA Cancer J Clin 47:351, 1997.

Smith D, Shaffer K, Kirn D et al: Mediastinal large cell lymphoma: Prognostic significance of CT findings at presentation and after treatment. Oncology 55:284, 1998.

Stewart CJ, Duncan JA, Farquharson M et al: Fine needle aspiration cytology diagnosis of malignant lymphoma and reactive lymphoid hyperplasia. J Clin Pathol 51:197, 1998.

Stumpe KD, Urbinelli M, Steinert HC et al: Whole-body positron emission tomography using fluorodeoxyglucose for staging of lymphoma: Effectiveness and comparison with computed tomography. Eur J Nucl Med 25:721, 1998.

Todeschini G, Ambrosetti A, Meneghini V et al: Mediastinal large-B-cell lymphoma with sclerosis: A clinical study of 21 patients. J Clin Oncol 8:804, 1990.

Tubergen DG, Krailo MD, Meadows AT et al: Comparison of treatment regimens for pediatric lymphoblastic non-Hodgkin's lymphoma: A Children's Cancer Group study. J Clin Oncol 13:1368, 1995.

van Leeuwen FE, Klokman WJ, Hagenbeek A et al: Second cancer risk following Hodgkin's disease: A 20-year follow-up study. J Clin Oncol 12:312, 1994.

Wakely PE, Kornstein MJ: Aspiration cytopathology of lymphoblastic lymphoma and leukemia: The MCV experience. Pediatr Pathol Lab Med 16:243, 1996.

Warnke RA, Weiss LM, Chan JKC et al: Atlas of Tumor Pathology: Tumors of the Lymph Nodes and Spleen, 3rd ed. Washington, DC, Armed Forces Institute of Pathology, 1995a, pp 15–27.

Warnke RA, Weiss LM, Chan JKC et al: Atlas of Tumor Pathology: Tumors of the Lymph Nodes and Spleen, 3rd ed. Washington, DC, Armed Forces Institute of Pathology, 1995b, p 277.

Yeh KH, Cheng AL, Su IJ et al: Prognostic significance of immunophenotypes in adult lymphoblastic lymphomas. Anticancer Res 17:2269, 1997.

Zaer FS, Braylan RC, Zander DS et al: Multiparametric flow cytometry in the diagnosis and characterization of low-grade pulmonary mucosa-associated lymphoid tissue lymphomas. Mod Pathol 11:525, 1998.

NEUROGENIC TUMORS OF THE MEDIASTINUM

Michael Bousamra

Neurogenic tumors of the mediastinum arise from the cells of the nerve sheath, autonomic ganglia, and paraganglionic tissues, all of which trace their embryologic heritage to the neural crest (Table 63–27). In turn, neurogenic tumors may exhibit a variety of cytologic products and immunohistochemical markers that aid in pathologic diagnosis. The relative incidence of the various cell types and their corresponding risk of malignancy are strongly correlated with age. Children and young adults are more prone to tumors of the autonomic ganglia, two thirds of which are malignant. In adults the vast majority of tumors are of nerve sheath origin, and 98% of these are benign (Davidson et al, 1978; Gale et al, 1974; Oosterwijk and Swierenga, 1968).

TABLE 63–27 ■ **Classification of Neurogenic Tumors of the Mediastinum**

Tumor Origin	*Benign*	*Malignant*
Nerve sheath	Neurilemmoma Neurofibroma Melanotic schwannoma Granular cell tumor	Neurofibrosarcoma
Ganglion cell	Ganglioneuroma	Ganglioneuroblastoma Neuroblastoma
Paraganglionic	Chemodectoma Pheochromocytoma	Malignant chemodectoma Malignant pheochromocytoma

Although neurogenic tumors may arise from neural elements anywhere within the thorax, the posterior mediastinum along the costovertebral sulcus is most common. In this location, intraspinal extension of tumor via the spinal foramen occurs in approximately 10% of cases (Akwari et al, 1978; Ricci et al, 1990). Routine computed tomography (CT) is recommended to screen for this phenomenon and, if present, magnetic resonance imaging (MRI) provides the clearest and most useful images. Patients with von Recklinghausen's neurofibromatosis are the lone identified population at risk for benign and malignant neurogenic tumors (Aughenbaugh, 1984; Wain, 1992). This disease is an autosomal dominant hamartomatous disorder of ectoderm and mesoderm resulting in multiple neurogenic tumors. The benign neurofibroma occurs most frequently in this group, and its malignant counterpart, the neurofibrosarcoma, has been found in 2% to 5% of affected individuals (Ducatman et al, 1986; Sorensen et al, 1986). Lateral meningoceles in the thoracic paravertebral region are also common in patients with neurofibromatosis, and these need to be distinguished from solid tumors. If there is associated scoliosis with convexity toward the mass, it is almost certainly a meningocele (Augenbaugh, 1984). Among von Recklinghausen patients, central nervous system tumors are particularly prevalent and onerous. In addition, a wide spectrum of carcinomas and sarcomas is associated with the disease resulting in a marked reduction in life expectancy (Augenbaugh, 1984; Sorensen et al, 1986).

CLINICAL AND HISTOPATHOLOGIC CHARACTERISTICS

Nerve Sheath Tumors

Benign nerve sheath tumors are the most common neurogenic tumors of the mediastinum. Nerve sheath tumors comprise one fifth of all mediastinal tumors; lymphomas and thymic tumors occur more commonly. More than 95% of these are either neurilemmomas (also known as schwannomas) or neurofibromas (Davidson et al, 1978; Gale et al, 1974; Oosterwijk and Swierenga, 1968). They behave in a clinically similar fashion, appearing as a smooth, rounded density in the costovertebral sulcus with a greater propensity for the upper posterior mediastinum than for the lower. Most nerve sheath tumors are asymptomatic, presenting as an incidental finding on chest radiography. Nerve sheath tumors may cause intercostal nerve irritation, rib displacement, and bone erosion that leads to pleuritic pain or paraspinal discomfort. Tumors arising within the thoracic inlet often involve the stellate ganglion, producing ptosis or complete Horner's syndrome. Because of the narrow confines of the thoracic inlet, larger size may also lead to deviation of the trachea and partial airway obstruction. Cough, dysphagia, and symptoms related to brachial plexus compression have been described (Augenbaugh, 1984; Davidson et al, 1978; Wain, 1992). With significant intraspinal extension, cord compression and paralysis can occur.

Nerve sheath tumors are slow-growing. In the adult patient the smooth to multilobulated contour, relative homogeneity, and characteristic position make a presumptive benign diagnosis an accurate one. Nonetheless, most authorities recommend removal to obviate the risk of malignancy. This risk is generally very small in patients who do not have neurofibromatosis or a history of radiation exposure (see later). It is certainly reasonable to follow asymptomatic, small paravertebral tumors in elderly persons or those with tenuous health. In children, ganglioneuroblastoma and neuroblastoma are more common, and a benign diagnosis cannot be assumed, so these tumors should be addressed promptly.

Neurilemmomas account for three quarters of nerve sheath tumors. They are encapsulated tumors containing two histologic components, Antoni type A and Antoni type B (Fig. 63–41). Antoni type A regions contain compact spindle cells with twisted nuclei and nuclear palisading. Antoni type B regions have loose and myxoid connective tissue harboring a haphazard arrangement of cells. Blood vessel walls tend to be thick, and cystic areas with hyalinization and calcification are noted microscopically (Kornstein, 1995). Neurilemmomas are S-100 positive. Electron microscopic examination demonstrates long cytoplasmic processes with continuous basal lamina that stain positive for vimentin.

Neurofibromas account for approximately 25% of nerve sheath tumors. Thirty percent to 45% of patients with mediastinal neurofibromas have von Recklinghausen's disease. Multiple neurofibromas or a single plexiform neurofibroma (a diffuse tumor of peripheral nerve) is pathognomonic of neurofibromatosis (Figs. 63–42 and 63–43) (Strollo et al, 1997). These tumors are radiographically indistinguishable from neurilemmomas. Histologic features include a disorganized proliferation of all nerve elements (Strollo et al, 1997). Interlacing bundles of spindle cells with wavy nuclei and a stroma of mixed collagenous and mucoid types are characteristic (Fig. 63–44). Neurofibromas may or may not be S-100 positive. Neither the neurilemmoma or the neurofibroma secrete significant amounts of bioactive amines.

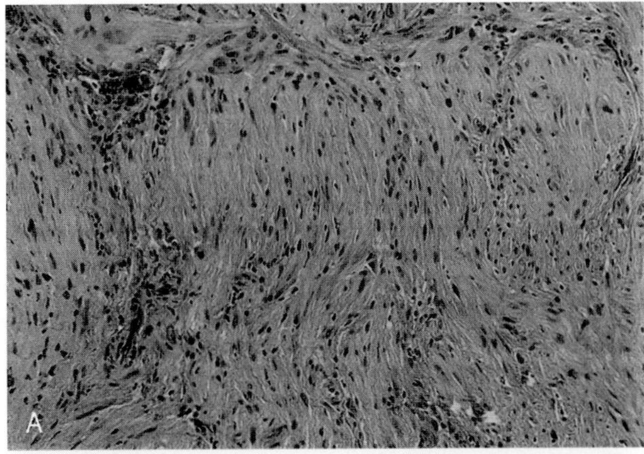

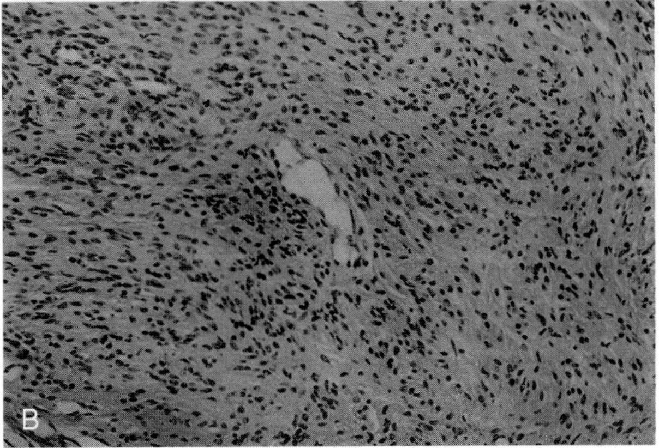

FIGURE 63–41 ■ *A*, Neurilemmoma demonstrating an area of nuclear palisading and elongated nuclei in a compact cellular arrangement consistent with Antoni type A. *B*, The more haphazard and loose arrangement of cells is characteristic of Antoni type B.

Melanotic schwannomas are a pigmented form of neurogenic tumor with melanin present in melanasomes. They have a higher incidence of intraspinal extension (Abbott et al, 1990; Shields, 1994), and approximately 10% are malignant (Carney, 1990). Microscopically, they demonstrate psammomatous calcification. Carney (1990) has described a familial disorder consisting of multiple myxomas, patchy pigmentation, and endocrine hyperactivity (acromegaly, Cushing's syndrome) associated with this entity.

Neurofibrosarcoma (also referred to as neurogenic sarcoma or malignant schwannoma) is a rare malignancy in the general population, but it affects 2% to 5% of patients with neurofibromatosis and arises at an earlier age in these patients (Ducatman et al, 1986; Sorensen et al, 1986). Neurofibrosarcomas are associated with radiation exposure. In 60% of cases, a contiguous neurofibroma is identified, implying sarcomatous degeneration from a previously benign lesion (Ducatman et al, 1986). In con-

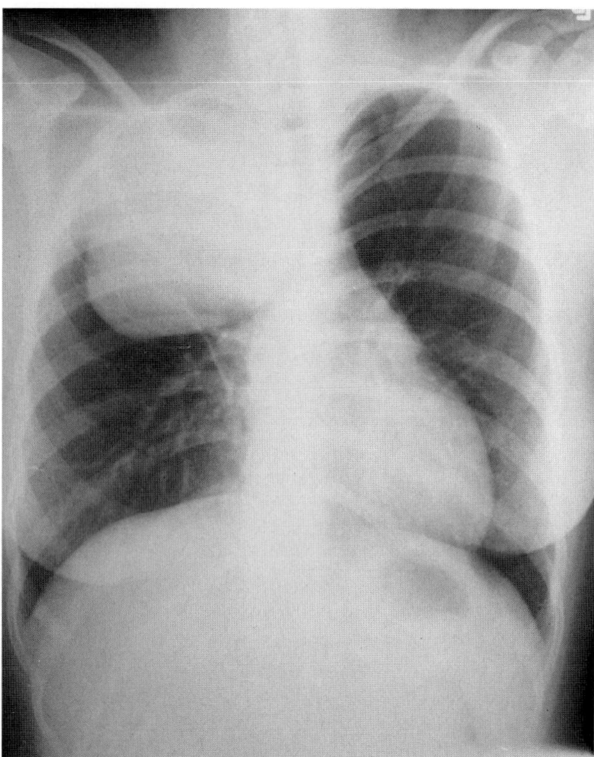

FIGURE 63–42 ■ A 17-year-old woman with neurofibromatosis presented with mild, right-sided chest pain. A large mass is seen in the apex of the right hemothorax that appears to displace both the lung and the mediastinal structures including the trachea. The configuration is suggestive of a pleural or extrapleural mass. Dysplastic changes are noted in the ribs in the area of the lesion. There is also a scoliosis, a finding commonly seen in patients with neurofibromatosis.

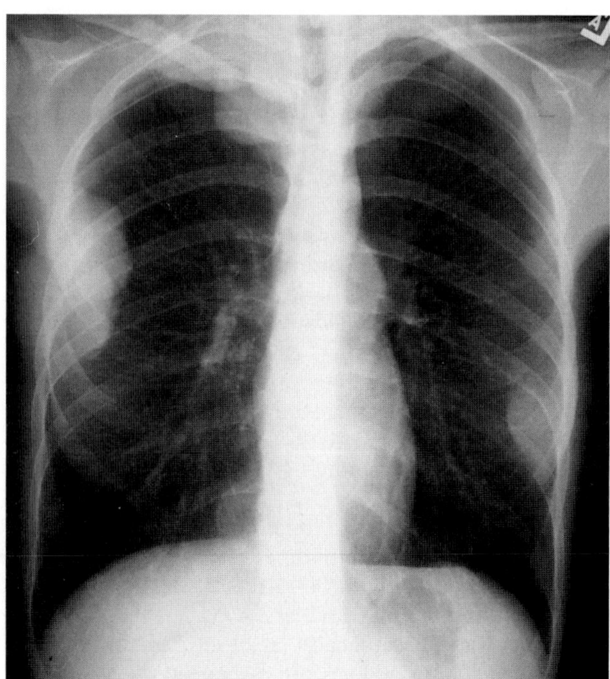

FIGURE 63–43 ■ Multiple neurogenic lesions including intercostal plexiform neuromas diagnostic of neurofibromatosis.

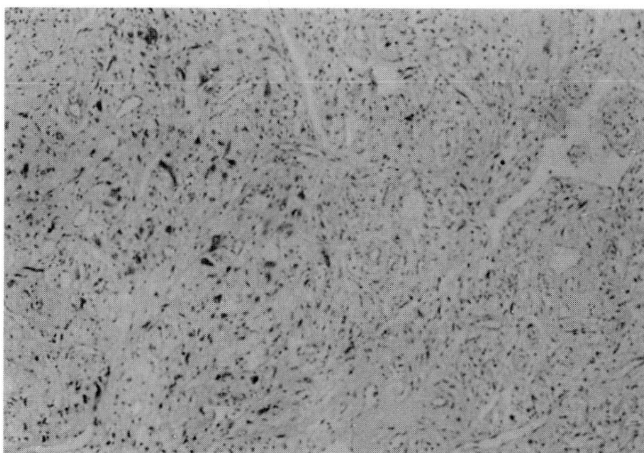

FIGURE 63–44 ■ The disorganized arrangement of connective tissue elements and nerve cells is seen on a background of loose myxoid material in this photomicrograph of a neurofibroma.

trast, neurilemmomas rarely undergo malignant transformation. The sarcomatous lesion can be differentiated from its benign counterparts by a high level of mitotic activity, lack of encapsulation, and absence of Antoni type A and B areas. CT can demonstrate central areas of low attenuation consistent with necrosis, hemorrhage, or cystic degeneration; these are all signs of malignancy (Coleman et al, 1983). Neurofibrosarcomas may undergo divergent differentiation into other sarcomas. Transformation into regions of rhabdomyosarcoma, chondrosarcoma, and osteosarcoma is most frequently observed (Ducatman et al, 1986). Intraneural extension of the tumor within fascicles makes complete resection less probable, and local visceral invasion or hematogenous metastases often prohibits surgical resection. Ducatman and associates (1986) reported a 5-year survival for neurofibrosarcoma of 16% in neurofibromatosis patients and 53% in non-neurofibromatosis patients. Large tumor size (>5 cm) is associated with poorer survival, but large size is also linked with neurofibromatosis. Complete resection is a strong positive prognostic factor, whereas adjuvant chemotherapy and radiation therapy appear to offer little benefit.

Ganglion Cell Tumors

Tumors arising from ganglion cells of the sympathetic chain and adrenal medulla are classified into three histologic types: ganglioneuroma, ganglioneuroblastoma, and neuroblastoma. Together, they occur in infants, children, and young adults. Overlap in their histopathology and clinical behavior forms a continuous spectrum of disease progressing from benign to highly malignant tumors. Ganglioneuroma is the well-differentiated benign manifestation of this group. It accounts for 42% of thoracic tumors arising from sympathetic ganglia (Adam and Hochholzer, 1981; Reed et al, 1978). Roughly half of affected patients are young adults. Most are asymptomatic, although diarrhea related to secretion of vasoactive intestinal peptide by the tumor is recognized (Rosenstein and Engelman, 1963). This tumor is likely to exhibit

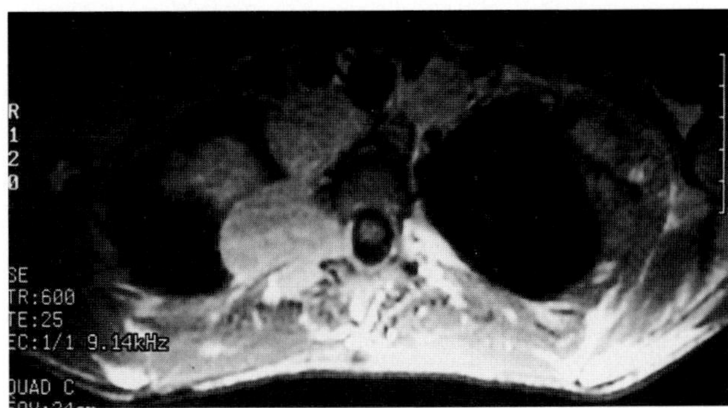

FIGURE 63–45 ■ Magnetic resonance image of a ganglioneuroma with extension across the spinal foramen and encroachment on the spinal cord.

intraspinal canal extension (Fig. 63–45). Davidson and co-workers (1978) reported this histology in seven of eight patients with neurogenic tumors extending through the intervertebral foramen. Ganglioneuromas are encapsulated and on cut section have a whorled pattern. They are recognized histologically by well-differentiated ganglion cells on a background of Schwann cells. The ganglion cells contain abundant cytoplasm, are often multinucleated, and are seen to rest within clear lacunae of the stroma (Fig. 63–46). Complete resection is curative, and local recurrence is uncommon.

Ganglioneuroblastomas contain a mixture of mature ganglion cells and malignant neuroblasts; the latter are characteristic of neuroblastoma. The distribution of neuroblasts within the ganglioneuroblastoma is predictive of clinical behavior. A nodular pattern is associated with a high incidence of metastatic disease, while the diffuse form rarely has metastases (Adam and Hochholzer, 1981). Ganglioneuroblastomas make up approximately one third of autonomic ganglion tumors. Focal calcification is present in regions of the neuroblasts. Grossly, the tumor usually remains encapsulated. Age distribution is similar to neuroblastoma, most arising in infants and children. These tumors are usually resectable, and overall 5-year survival is 88%, as reported by Adam and Hochholzer (1981).

Neuroblastoma occupies the malignant end of the clinical and pathologic spectrum of ganglion cell tumors. It is the most common extracranial solid malignancy in pediatric patients and the most common intrathoracic malignancy of childhood (Green, 1985). Staining of neuroblastoma with H&E reveals that it is composed of nests of blue round cells surrounded by fibrovascular stroma. Homer-Wright rosettes may be present (Fig. 63–47) (Triche and Askin, 1983). The adrenal gland harbors the primary source of neuroblastoma in 38% of all cases; 14% arise within the thorax (Blossom et al, 1997). Extension into the spinal canal and osseous invasion are common. Visceral involvement occurs less commonly in thoracic neuroblastoma; in turn, resection is more often feasible. More than half of neuroblastomas occur in children less than 2 years of age and 90% arise within the first decade of life (Green, 1985), and they are found in boys more frequently than in girls. Tumors arising in neonates and infants may spontaneously differentiate into less malignant forms, or they may involute. Cervical and mediastinal neuroblastomas are associated with heterochromia iridis and Horner's syndrome. Hormonal activity may be manifest in any of the tumors of the autonomic ganglia, but it is characteristic of neuroblastomas. Vasoactive intestinal peptide secretion manifests as diarrhea (Green, 1985; Scheibel et al, 1982). Catecholamine production can be detected by the urinary metabolites vanillylmandelic acid and homovanillic acid. Seeger and colleagues (1982) reported that catecholamines were detected in 95% of neuroblastoma cases. Hormone levels fall after tumor resection and can serve as an indicator of complete resection. Recrudescence of elevated hormone levels is a sign of recurrent disease.

Patients with neuroblastoma are usually symptomatic, and tumors are often extensive at presentation. Local symptoms of cough, chest pain, dyspnea, and Horner's syndrome are common. Thoracic lesions are more commonly associated with myelopathic symptoms resulting from spinal canal invasion. Systemic manifestations include lethargy, fever, and weight loss. Cerebellar ataxia and opsoclonus are thought to result from associated autoimmune phenomena. Jones and co-workers (1984)

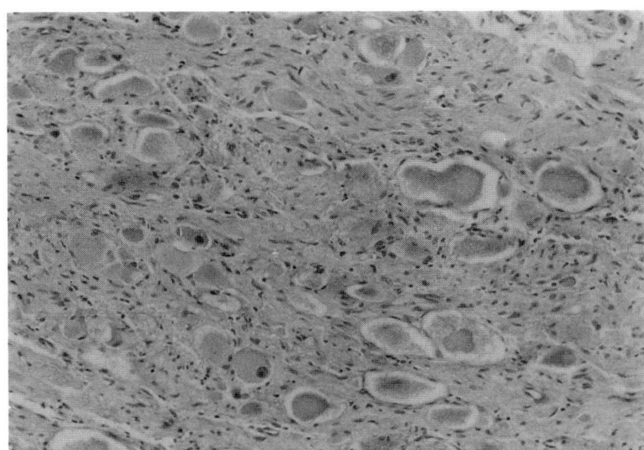

FIGURE 63–46 ■ Ganglioneuromas are characterized by large neuclei of ganglion cells resting in clear lacunae and surrounded by fibrovascular connective tissue.

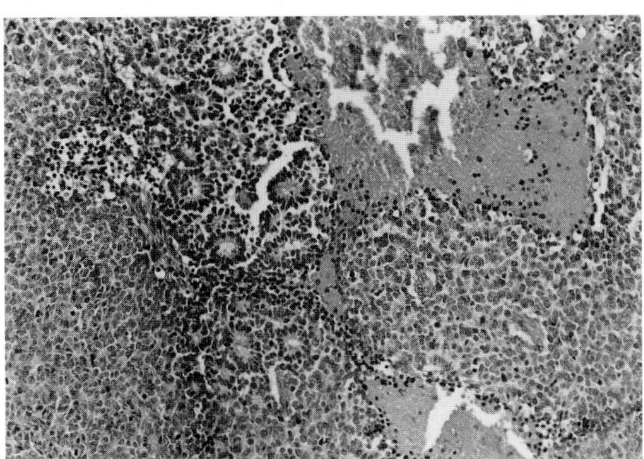

FIGURE 63–47 ■ Pathologic features of neuroblastoma include sheets of small, dark neuroblasts with rosette formation and areas of necrosis.

reported that 8 of 16 infants and children (50%) who presented with cerebellar encephalopathy had neuroblastoma. Flushing, sweating, and tachycardia are related to the catechol excess, but hypertension is uncommon (Weinblatt et al, 1983). Hematogenous metastases are reported in approximately 60% of patients. Involved sites include the liver, bone, bone marrow, lung, and skin. Skeletal pain, periorbital swelling, and ecchymosis are common manifestations of metastatic disease. Tumor deposits within the dermis appear as reddish-purple raised lesions and are amenable to biopsy.

Clinical evaluation of the child with neuroblastoma emphasizes abdominal, thoracic, neurologic, and cutaneous examinations. The color of the iris should be inspected for associated heterochromia. Occasionally, retroperitoneal tumors can be detected only by rectal examination, as they may not be palpable on abdominal examination. The skeletal survey and bone scan are complementary in detecting osseus metastases. Bone marrow biopsy may reveal marrow involvement independent of osseous metastases.

Thoracic lesions are optimally defined by chest CT and MRI. They generally exhibit less calcification on CT than their abdominal counterparts. Intraspinal extension occurs commonly, but it is often asymptomatic. Armstrong and associates (1982) reported symptoms in only 55% of patients subsequently shown to have spinal compression by myelography. Thus, all patients with paraspinal neuroblastoma require MRI with gadolinium contrast to carefully assess for canal invasion.

Various methods of early detection of neuroblastoma are ongoing. Mass screening of infants by detection of urine catecholamine metabolites has been attempted to reduce the fatal impact of the disease in Japan (Nishi et al, 1992; Sawada et al, 1991) and in the province of Quebec, Canada (Woods et al, 1992). Data show that fewer older children harbor the disease and fewer present with metastases. Whether overall mortality is decreased is yet to be determined. In autopsy series, neuroblastoma has been identified in 0.37% to 2.58% of infants younger than 3 months of age who died of other causes, implying that many such tumors undergo involution (Green, 1985). Antenatal diagnosis of neuroblastoma has been made, and infants have done well with subsequent resection of tumors (Ho et al, 1993). The enticing concept of observing these tumors for spontaneous regression has been reported in four infants with antenatal diagnosis of adrenal masses. All four masses resolved by 2.5 to 8 weeks of age (Holgersen et al, 1996).

The staging of neuroblastoma has evolved as factors affecting survival have been elucidated. The extent of primary tumor, lymph node involvement, and the presence of residual disease following resection are the dominant variables affecting prognosis. The International Neuroblastoma Staging System, which reflects these factors, is shown in Table 63–28. Specific genetic and biologic markers also affect survival probability. Multiple copies of the N-*myc* gene appear to be an independent predictor of poor survival (Brodeur et al, 1988; Pelicci et al, 1984). Levels of neuron-specific enolase greater than 100 ng in stage III and IV patients (Zeltzer et al, 1983) and serum lactate dehydrogenase greater than 1000 IU for stage IV disease (Shuster et al, 1992) have been associated with shorter survival in retrospective series.

TABLE 63–28 ■ **International Neuroblastoma Staging System**

Stage	*Description*
Stage I	Localized tumor with complete gross excision, with or without microscopic residual disease; representative ipsilateral lymph nodes negative for tumor microscopically (nodes attached to and removed with the primary tumor may be positive)
Stage IIA	Localized tumor with incomplete gross excision; representative ipsilateral nonadherent lymph nodes negative for tumor microscopically
Stage IIB	Localized tumor with or without complete gross excision, with ipsilateral nonadherent lymph nodes positive for tumor; enlarged contralateral lymph nodes must be negative microscopically
Stage III	Unresectable unilateral tumor infiltrating across the midline (defined as the vertebral column), with or without regional lymph node involvement; or localized unilateral tumor with contralateral lymph node involvement; or midline tumor with bilateral extension by infiltration (unresectable) or by lymph node involvement
Stage IV	Any primary tumor with dissemination to distant lymph nodes, bone, bone marrow, liver, skin, or other organs (except as defined for Stage IVS)
Stage IVS	Localized primary tumor (as defined for Stage I, IIA, or IIB), with dissemination limited to skin, liver, or bone marrow (<10% of nucleated cells identified as malignant; limited to infants younger than 1 year of age)

Surgery plays a dominant role in the treatment of early-stage neuroblastoma. In patients with stage I disease, surgical resection alone produces an 89% relapse-free survival at 4 years (Nitschke et al, 1998). The Children's Hospital Cancer Group (Haase et al, 1995) demonstrated, in more advanced stages, that the extent of postresection residual disease was inversely correlated with survival. Radiation therapy in combination with chemotherapy improves survival in patients with residual disease and in resected patients with nodal disease (Castleberry et al, 1991). Thoracic tumors are not as recalcitrant to medical and surgical therapies. They more commonly exhibit a single copy of the N-*myc* gene, and they usually do not invade thoracic viscera. With the common presentation of metastatic disease, thoracotomy may be required for tissue diagnosis; however, less invasive procedures usually yield adequate tissue for diagnosis. Resection of the primary lesion in stage IV disease may achieve local control, but it does not improve survival in these unfortunate children. Occasionally, resolution of metastatic disease by chemotherapy leaves the patient with a resectable primary mass. Operative removal is indicated, and pathologic examination often demonstrates maturation of the neuroblastoma. Chemotherapy regimens with increasing toxicity have not altered the natural history of patients with advanced disease. Investigations of autologous bone marrow transplantation have yielded highly variable results, with event-free survival after bone marrow transplantation reported to be 6% to 64% (Kushner et al, 1991; Matthay et al, 1994; Sawaguchi et al, 1990).

Paraganglionic Tumors

Thoracic tumors derived from paraganglionic tissues include the hormonally active pheochromocytoma and the hormonally inactive chemodectoma. Thoracic lesions are usually harbored in the costovertebral sulcus, but they may arise in the visceral compartment from the aortic body and within the cardiac atria. Extra-adrenal lesions constitute approximately 10% of pheochromocytomas and, of these, the intrathoracic location is among the rarest. Approximately 10% of intrathoracic pheochromocytomas behave in a malignant fashion, a proportion similar to their retroperitoneal counterparts (Gale et al, 1974). Gale and associates noted multicentric tumors in 4 of 23 thoracic cases. A paravertebral mass in association with paroxysmal or sustained hypertension, hypermetabolism, or diabetes should lead one to suspect pheochromocytoma (Shields, 1994). Confirmation is made by measurement of urinary catecholamines and their metabolites. Identification of middle mediastinal lesions is particularly important because the tumor may be buried in the atria or the great vessels, and failure to remove the catacholamine-producing lesion could lead to life-threatening hemodynamic problems. Localization by ^{131}I metaiodobenzylguanidine scintigraphy and CT has proved to be efficatious (Shapiro et al, 1984). Alternatively, taking advantage of the high vascularity of these lesions, Tanaka and associates (1992) employed MRI to identify them in the costovertebral sulcus; MRI revealed a flow void in the region of the tumor.

Preoperative management stresses pharmacologic blockade of α- and β-adrenergic receptors to prevent malignant hypertension and arrythmias associated with tumor manipulation. The surgeon should also be cognizant that cardiac lesions may derive their blood supply from large vessels arising from the coronary arteries (Shapiro et al, 1984). In general, paraganglionic tumors are highly vascular, and a cautious, circumspect approach to resection is recommended.

Chemodectomas are also highly vascular. Preoperative angioembolization has been advocated, particularly in head and neck regions where vascular control can be problematic (Sessions et al, 1997). Radiation therapy also has an acceptable rate of tumor control and is a rational substitute for surgical extirpation. Chemodectomas, at the base of the skull, where vascular control is difficult, are prime candidates for radiation therapy (Sessions et al, 1997).

SURGICAL TECHNIQUE

Removal of neurogenic tumors arising in the posterior mediastinum is classically achieved through a posterolateral thoracotomy. These tumors are usually tucked snug into the costovertebral sulcus with a broad base. Their lack of mobility can make posterior exposure and separation from the intercostal nerve or sympathetic chain moderately difficult. Incision of the pleural envelope as it reflects over the tumor and blunt dissection generally achieve mobilization and removal. Rough dissection can lead to bleeding from the intercostal vessels. Resection of apical lesions arising from the stellate ganglion or adjacent neural tissue may be complicated by a postoperative Horner's syndrome. This risk can be minimized by maintaining the dissection plane on the capsule of the tumor. Large tumors occupying the thoracic inlet and extending into the base of the neck are optimally removed via a combined cervical and transsternal approach. Through this exposure, the adjacent vascular structures are readily identified, controlled, and separated from the tumor. The recurrent laryngeal nerve, particularly on the right, is to be avoided.

Thoracoscopic resection is now commonly performed for benign neurogenic tumors. Nearly circumferential visualization is provided by the 30-degree thoracoscope. Exposure of the tumor base is facilitated by placing deep sutures within the dense substance of the mass. Retraction on the sutures enables the surgeon to manipulate the position of the tumor. Further advantages of the thoracoscopic approach include less muscle division and small cosmetic incisions. In a retrospective series comparing open and thoracoscopic neurogenic tumor resection, shorter hospitalization and return to work times were observed (Bousamra et al, 1996). When malignancy is suspected or documented, the surgeon should eschew thoracoscopy and suture retraction in favor of standard methods of exposure and resection.

Intraspinal extension of neurogenic tumors requires a combined posterior spinal and thoracic approach for safe resection. The procedure should be performed at a single stage because thoracic manipulation of the tumor can produce hemorrhage, with the spinal component leading to cord compression (Shields, 1994). Various exposures have been described. Grillo and associates (1983) prefer a single incision extending vertically over the spinous processes and continuing laterally beneath the scapular tip. Exposure is gained by hemilaminectomy, enlarging the neural foramen and thoracotomy. Vallieres and colleagues (1995) describe a combined video-assisted thoracoscopic and microneurosurgical removal of a dumbbell tumor.

Benign neurogenic tumors appear to be good candidates for minimally invasive methods of resection, but morbidity from standard techniques of removal has been low (Davidson et al, 1978; Gale et al, 1974). Less invasive procedures need to match or improve the long-standing acceptable outcomes of minimal blood loss, lack of neurologic deficit, and very low incidence of tumor recurrence before they are considered a standard of care.

■ *REFERENCES*

Abbott AE, Hill RC, Flynn MA: Melanotic schwannoma of the sympathetic ganglia: Pathological and clinical characteristics. Ann Thorac Surg 49:1006, 1990.

Adam A, Hochholzer L: Ganglioneuroblastoma of the posterior mediastinum. Cancer 47:373, 1981.

Akwari OE, Payne WS, Onofrio BM: Dumbbell Neurogenic Tumors of the Mediastinum. Mayo Clin Proc 53:353, 1978.

Armstrong EA, Harwood-Nash DC, Ritz CR: CT of neuroblastomas and ganglioneuromas in children. AJR Am J Roentgenol 139:571, 1982.

Aughenbaugh GL: Thoracic manifestations of neurocutaneous diseases. Radiol Clin North Am 22:741, 1984.

Blossom GB, Steiger Z, Stephenson LW: Neoplasms of the mediastinum. In DeVita VT, Hellman S, Rosenberg SA (eds): Cancer—Principles and Practice of Oncology, 5th ed. Philadelphia, Lippincott-Raven, 1997, pp 951–969.

Bousamra M, Haasler GB, Patterson GA: A comparative study of thoracoscopic vs open removal of benign neurogenic mediastinal tumors. Chest 109:1461, 1996.

Brodeur GM, Seeger RC, Barrett A: International criteria for diagnosis, staging, and response to treatment in patients with neuroblastoma. J Clin Oncol 6:1874, 1988.

Carney JA: Psammomatous melanotic schwannoma. Am J Surg Pathol 14:206, 1990.

Castleberry RP, Kun LE, Shuster JJ: Radiotherapy improves the outlook for patients older than 1 year with Pediatric Oncology Group stage C neuroblastoma. J Clin Oncol 9:789, 1991.

Coleman BG, Arger PH, Dalinka MK: CT of sarcomatous degeneration in neurofibromatosis. AJR Am J Roentgenol 140:383, 1983.

Davidson KG, Walbaum PR, McCormack RJ: Intrathoracic neural tumours. Thorax 33:359, 1978.

Ducatman BS, Scheithauer BW, Peipgras DG: Malignant peripheral nerve sheath tumors: A clinicopathologic study of 120 cases. Cancer 57:2006, 1986.

Gale AW, Jelihovsky T, Grant AF: Neurogenic tumors of the mediastinum. Ann Thorac Surg 17:434, 1974.

Green DM: Diagnosis and Management of Malignant Solid Tumors in Infants and Children. Boston, Martinus Nijhoff, 1985, pp 187–256.

Grillo HC, Ojemann RG, Scannell JG: Combined approach to "dumbbell" intrathoracic and intraspinal neurogenic tumors. Ann Thorac Surg 36:402, 1983.

Haase GM, Atkinson JB, Stram DO: Surgical management and outcome of locoregional neuroblastoma: Comparison of the Childrens Cancer Group and the international staging systems. J Pediatr Surg 30:289, 1995.

Ho PT, Estroff JA, Kozakewich H: Prenatal detection of neuroblastoma: A ten-year experience from the Dana-Farber Cancer Institute and Children's Hospital. Pediatrics 92:358, 1993.

Holgersen LO, Subramanian S, Kirpekar M: Spontaneous resolution of antenatally diagnosed adrenal masses. J Pediatr Surg 31:153, 1996.

Jones A, Grooves R, Smithson W: Acute cerebellar encephalopathy (ACE): Its natural history and relationship to neuroblastoma (NB). Proc Am Soc Clin Oncol 3:86, 1984.

Kornstein, MJ: Tumors of neural origin. In Kornstein MJ (ed): Major Problems in Pathology: Pathology of the Thymus and Mediastinum. Philadelphia, WB Saunders, 1995, p 201.

Kushner BH, Gulati SC, Kwon JH: High-Dose melphalan with 6-hydroxydopamine-purged autologous bone marrow transplantation for poor-risk neuroblastoma. Cancer 68:242, 1991.

Look AT, Hayes FA, Nitschke R: Cellular DNA content as a predictor of response to chemotherapy in infants with unresectable neuroblastoma. N Engl J Med 311:231, 1984.

Matthay KK, Seeger RC, Reynolds CP: Allogeneic versus autologous purged bone marrow transplantation for neuroblastoma: A Report From the Children's Cancer Group. J Clin Oncol 12:2382, 1994.

Nishi M, Miyake H, Takeda T: Mass screening of neuroblastoma in Sapporo City, Japan. Am J Pediatr Hematol Oncol 14:327, 1992.

Nitschke R, Smith EI, Shochat S: Localized neuroblastoma treated by surgery: A Pediatric Oncology Group study. J Clin Oncol 6:1271, 1998.

Oosterwijk WM, Swierenga J: Neurogenic tumours with an intrathoracic localization. Thorax 23:374, 1968.

Pelicci PG, Lanfroncone L, Brathwaite MD: Amplification of N-*myc* in untreated human neuroblastomas correlates with advanced disease stage. Science 224:1121, 1984.

Reed JC, Hallet KK, Feigin DS: Neural tumors of the thorax: Subject review from the AFIP. Radiology 126:9, 1978.

Ricci C, Rendina EA, Venuta F: Diagnostic imaging and surgical treatment of dumbbell tumors of the mediastinum. Ann Thorac Surg 50:586, 1990.

Rosenstein BJ, Engelman K: Diarrhea in a child with catecholamine-secreting ganglioneuroma. J Pediatr Surg 63:217, 1963.

Sawada T, Matsumura T, Kawakatsu H: Long-term effects of mass screening for neuroblastoma in infancy. Am J Pediatr Hematol Oncol 13:3, 1991.

Sawaguchi S, Kaneko M, Uchino J: Treatment of advanced neuroblastoma with emphasis on intensive induction chemotherapy. Cancer 66:1879, 1990.

Scheibel E, Rechnitzer C, Fahrenkrug J: Vasoactive intestinal polypeptide (VIP) in children with neural crest tumours. Acta Paediatr Scand 71:721, 1982.

Seeger RC, Siegel SE, Sidell N: Neuroblastoma: Clinical perspectives, monoclonal antibodies, and cetinoic acid. Ann Intern Med 97:873, 1982.

Sessions RB, Harrison LB, Forastiere AA: Tumors of the salivary glands and paragangliomas. In DeVita VT, Hellman S, Rosenberg SA (eds): Cancer—Principles and Practice of Oncology, 5th ed. Philadelphia, Lippincott-Raven, 1997, p 830.

Shapiro B, Sisson J, Kalff V: The location of middle mediastinal pheochromocytomas. J Thorac Cardiovasc Surg 87:814, 1984.

Shields TW: General Thoracic Surgery, 4th ed. Philadelphia, Williams & Wilkins, 1994, pp 1744–1754.

Shuster JJ, McWilliams NB, Castleberry R: Serum lactate dehydrogenase in childhood neuroblastoma. Am J Clin Oncol 15:295, 1992.

Sorensen SA, Mulvihill JJ, Nielsen A: Long-term follow-up of von Recklinghausen neurofibromatosis: Survival and malignant neoplasms. N Engl J Med 314:1010, 1986.

Strollo DC, Rosado-de-Christenson ML, Jett JR: Primary mediastinal tumors. Part II: Tumors of the middle and posterior mediastinum. Chest 112:1344, 1997.

Tanaka F, Kitano M, Tatsumi A: Paraganglioma of the posterior mediastinum: Value of magnetic resonance imaging. Ann Thorac Surg 53:517, 1992.

Triche TJ, Askin FB: Neuroblastoma and the differential diagnosis of small-, round-, blue-cell tumors. Hum Pathol 14:569, 1983.

Vallieres E, Findlay J, Fraser R: Combined microneurosurgical and thoracoscopic removal of neurogenic dumbbell tumors. Ann Thorac Surg 59:469, 1995.

Wain JC: Neurogenic tumors of the mediastinum. Chest Surg Clin North Am 2:121, 1992.

Weinblatt ME, Heisel MA, Siegel SE: Hypertension in children with neurogenic tumors. Pediatrics 71:947, 1983.

Woods WG, Tuchman M, Bernstein ML: Screening for Neuroblastoma in North America. Am J Pediatr Hematol Oncol 14:312, 1992.

Zeltzer PM, Parma AM, Dalton A: Raised neuron-specific enolase in serum of children with metastatic neuroblastoma. Lancet 2:361, 1983.

UNUSUAL MEDIASTINAL TUMORS

Hao Kenith Fang
Sudhir Sundaresan

The category of unusual tumors of the mediastinum encompasses a group of rare lesions that constitute less than 10% of all mediastinal masses. Both the prevalence and malignant potential of these tumors appear to be greater in the pediatric population. The majority of these tumors are mesenchymal in origin. Others include extramedullary hematopoiesis, primary carcinoma of the mediastinum, and giant lymph node hyperplasia (Castleman's disease). Signs and symptoms at presentation are dependent on various factors including tumor size, location, histologic status, as well as the age of the patient. Tumors in the pediatric population appear to be symptomatic more often, perhaps due to their higher frequency of being malignant. Diagnosis usually requires tissue biopsy, although less invasive methods such as fine-needle aspiration have been increasingly used. Treatment continues to center around surgical resection, with chemotherapy and radiation therapy typically being reserved for unresectable tumors, recurrences, and those lesions associated with metastatic disease. Prognosis is highly variable, depending on tumor histology and extent of disease.

HISTORICAL NOTE

Prior to 1963, only scattered case reports existed in the literature documenting the existence of the various mediastinal mesenchymal tumors. However, reviews of the literature were rarely encountered owing to the difficulties inherent in classifying these rare lesions. Case reports were typically subject to poor documentation and composite nomenclature (such as fibroleiomyoma and fibrolipoma). Due to the lack of uniformity of classification, the basis for and results of treatment were sketchy and lacked scientific support. In 1963, Pachter and Lattes from Columbia University College of Physicians and Surgeons published the first paper devoted completely to the review of mediastinal mesenchymal tumors in the journal *Cancer*. In their review, they used a classification system previously developed by Stout from the Armed Forces Institute of Pathology in 1953. Despite the exhaustive nature of their review, only a total of 39 cases were listed in their paper. Since their report, a variety of classification systems with greater uniformity have been proposed by various authors. However, due to the rarity of these lesions, the development of a truly universal system will likely continue to evade us. The classification presented in Table 63–29 is reasonably clear and concise, and is a composite of the various classification systems reported in the literature.

In 1954, Castleman and Towne reported in the *New England Journal of Medicine* what was then believed to be a new disease syndrome. Two years following this initial case report, Castleman and co-workers (1956) described 13 cases of lymph node hyperplasia located within the mediastinum that resembled thymomas both grossly and microscopically. In fact, several of these lesions were originally misdiagnosed as thymomas. The authors speculated that these tumors were neither thymic in origin nor neoplastic growths as originally believed. Their speculations were based on various factors, notably the histologic appearance and also the frequent juxtaposition of these lesions to the tracheobronchial tree (as opposed to thymomas, which are typically located in the midline within the superior anterior mediastinum). Since this initial report, the disease syndrome has been expanded to include lesions outside of the thorax, multiple histologic varieties, and a multicentric form of the disease associated with generalized lymphadenopathy that appears to have a more virulent clinical course.

TABLE 63–29 ■ Classification of Mesenchymal Tumors of the Mediastinum

I. Adipose tissue
   1. Lipoma and lipomatosis
   2. Lipoblastomas and lipoblastomatosis
   3. Liposarcoma
II. Fibrous tissue
   1. Fibroma and fibromatosis
   2. Fibrosarcoma
   3. Malignant fibrous histiocytoma
III. Blood vessels
   1. Hemangioma
   2. Hemangiopericytoma, benign and malignant
   3. Hemangioendothelioma, benign and malignant
IV. Lymphatic vessels
   1. Lymphangioma and lymphangiomatosis
   2. Lymphangiomyomatosis
V. Muscular origin
   1. Striated
      a. Rhabdomyoma
      b. Rhabdomyosarcoma
   2. Smooth
      a. Leiomyoma
      b. Leiomyosarcoma
VI. Skeletal tissue
   1. Osteogenic sarcoma
   2. Chondroma
   3. Chondrosarcoma
VII. Mesenchymoma, benign and malignant
VIII. Others
   1. Fibrous mesothelioma, without pleural or pericardial involvement
   2. Myxoma
   3. Meningioma
   4. Chordoma
   5. Histiocytosis X

■ *HISTORICAL READINGS*

Castleman B, Iverson L, Menendez VP: Localized mediastinal lymph node hyperplasia resembling thymoma. Cancer 9:822, 1956.

Castleman B, Towne VW: Case Records of the Massachusetts General Hospital, Case No. 40011. N Engl J Med 250:26, 1954.

Pachter MR, Lattes R: Mesenchymal tumors of the mediastinum. I: Tumors of fibrous tissue, adipose tissue, smooth muscle and striated muscle. Cancer 16:74, 1963.

Pachter MR, Lattes R: Mesenchymal tumors of the mediastinum. II: Tumors of blood vascular origin. Cancer 16:95, 1963.

Pachter MR, Lattes R: Mesenchymal tumors of the mediastinum. III: Tumors of lymph vascular origin. Cancer 16:108, 1963.

Stout PA: Tumors of the soft tissues. In Armed Forces Institute of Pathology (eds): Atlas of Tumor Pathology, Section 2, Fascicle 5. Washington, DC, Armed Forces Institute of Pathology, 1953.

MESENCHYMAL TUMORS

Mesenchymal tumors arise in virtually all regions of the body. Mesenchymal tumors originating in the mediastinum are very rare; when they occur, they typically demonstrate similar histology to mesenchymal tumors in other locations. The clinical features also generally mimic those of mesenchymal tumors in other locations, but local symptoms and signs can arise secondary to their presence within the mediastinum. These tumors can develop from adipose tissue, connective tissue, blood and lymph vessels, both striated and smooth muscle, or any combination of these. The majority of these (>50%) are vascular or lymphatic in origin.

Mesenchymal tumors make up 6% to 7% of all mediastinal masses, although this frequency has been reported to be as high as 10.7% in the pediatric population. In adults, it has been reported that slightly over one half are malignant. In children, this incidence can be as high as 85%. As a group there appears to be no difference in incidence between males and females. Although many classifications have been suggested, no consensus is agreed on (see Historical Note). The problem with such an undertaking lies in the inherent difficulty in categorizing tumors that involve more than one anatomic region (e.g., thorax, pericardium, or mediastinum), or are composed of many tissue types. Examples include thymolipomas and thymoliposarcomas, which some authors classify among thymic tumors, whereas others group them with tumors of adipose tissue origin. Table 63–29 contains a classification scheme for mesenchymal tumors of the mediastinum. It is a composite of the various classification systems found in the literature that we have found clear and concise. The remainder of this section presents and briefly discusses the various lesions as classified in Table 63–29.

Lipomas/Lipomatosis. In most large series, this lesion represents the most common mediastinal tumor of mesenchymal origin. Lipomas are well-encapsulated lesions (when nonencapsulated and diffuse, this entity is referred to as lipomatosis) with no apparent gender predilection. The age at diagnosis varies from 2 to 60 years. These tumors are reported to achieve extreme size (up to 30 cm) without causing symptoms. This is most likely due to their complete encapsulation and lack of a significant fixation point. They tend to grow along paths of least resistance and predominate in the anterior mediastinum. Three quarters of patients exhibit symptoms at the time of presentation. These symptoms include chest pain, dyspnea, cough, and rare cases of neurologic deficits due to local extension of the tumor into the spinal canal. Lipomas have no documented malignant potential, and although resection is at times challenging because of their enormous size, almost all can be excised for cure.

Lipoblastomas/Lipoblastomatosis. This is a rare type of benign adipose tissue tumor that is found almost exclusively in the pediatric population. Chung and Enzinger (1973) have reported the largest series to date, and they have proposed the nomenclature for the circumscribed form as benign lipoblastoma and for the diffuse form as benign lipoblastomatosis. These lesions can grow to extreme size, similar to lipomas, and also appear to lack any potential for invasion or malignancy. The most common sites of origin of these rare tumors are in the extremities or pelvic region. Their presence in the mediastinum is extremely rare, with only five reported cases in the English literature. These five patients had mediastinal lipoblastomas and all presented with respiratory symptoms (cough, dyspnea, stridor, and hypoxia) due to compression of adjacent structures. Complete local excision appears to be curative.

Liposarcomas. These tumors are very rare in the mediastinum, in contrast to lipomas. Similar to lipomas, there is an equal incidence in men and women. The age at presentation also varies, from young to elderly. However, unlike lipomas, these lesions tend to exhibit extensive local invasion. Almost all patients present with symptoms of severe pain, weight loss, or cough at the time of diagnosis, and these symptoms represent late findings in the course of the disease. Liposarcomas are rarely resectable for cure because of extensive local invasion. Surgery is typically reserved for palliation. Radiation therapy has been used with minimal benefit. Although it has been speculated that lipomas represent precursors to this malignancy, such claims have yet to be substantiated.

Fibroma/Fibromatosis. Tumors of this tissue origin are typically found in the fibromatosis form as an ill-defined lesion with indistinct gross margins. Histologically, the tumor is composed of fibroblasts of uniform shape separated by abundant collagen. Because of its ill-defined border, the tumor often infiltrates into adjacent tissue. These are slow-growing tumors, and thus clinical symptoms are present with only rather advanced lesions. They typically present as incidental findings on chest radiographs or computed tomography (CT) scans. When symptoms arise, they are usually due to compression of adjacent structures such as the vena cava, leading to the development of superior vena cava syndrome. The lesion is benign and does not exhibit metastatic spread. Resection is performed for cure (Fig. 63–48), and if the lesion is incompletely excised, local recurrence occurs. Complete excision is important because these are radioresistant tumors and thus are not amenable to radiation therapy.

Fibrosarcoma. Like other sarcomas in the mediastinum, these are very rare lesions. The last extensive review of

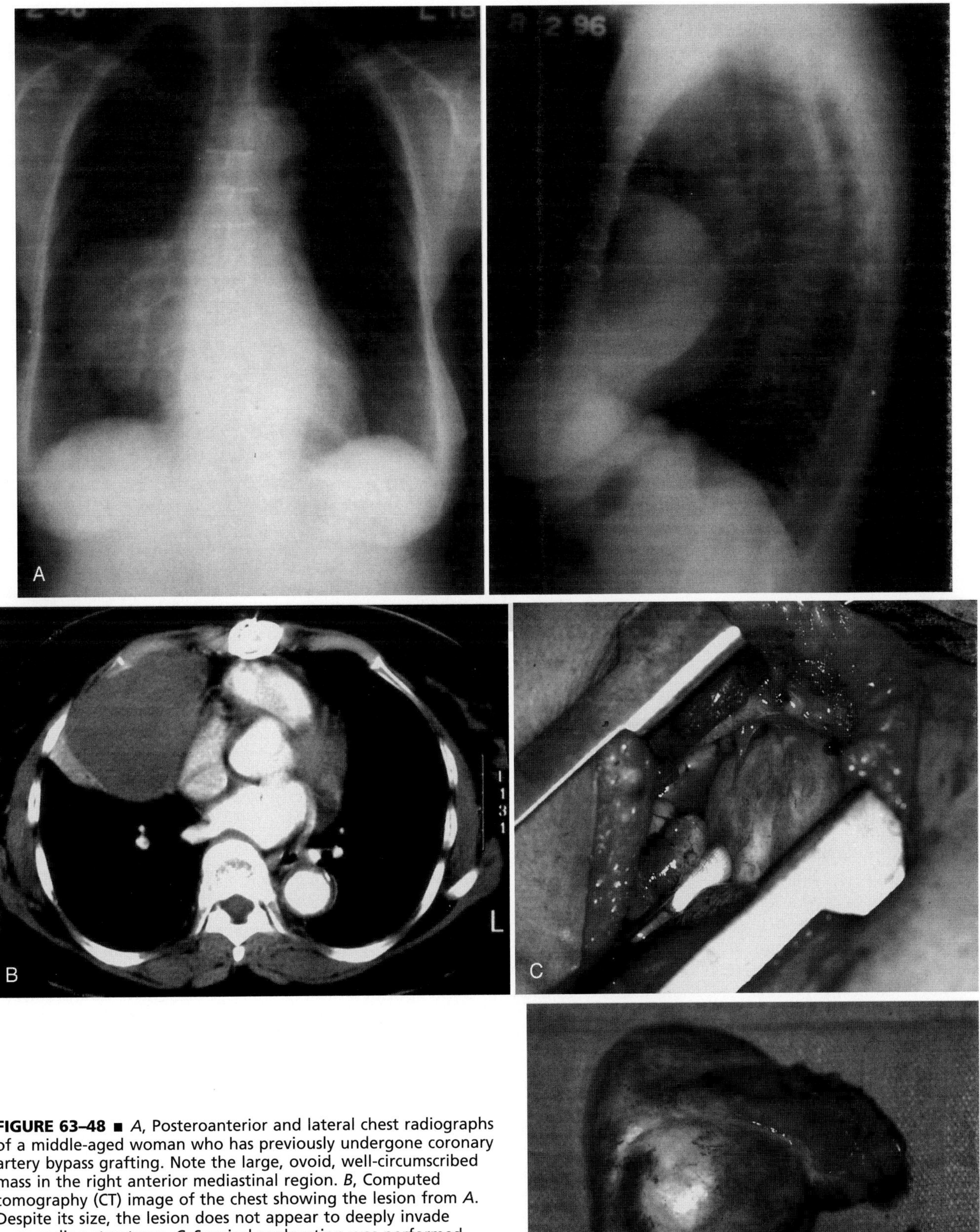

FIGURE 63–48 ■ *A*, Posteroanterior and lateral chest radiographs of a middle-aged woman who has previously undergone coronary artery bypass grafting. Note the large, ovoid, well-circumscribed mass in the right anterior mediastinal region. *B*, Computed tomography (CT) image of the chest showing the lesion from *A*. Despite its size, the lesion does not appear to deeply invade surrounding structures. *C*, Surgical exploration was performed through a right anterolateral thoracotomy and revealed a large ovoid mass with a smooth capsule. *D*, Resected specimen. On histology, the lesion was demonstrated to be a benign fibroma.

the literature by Barua and associates (1979) reported only 36 cases. There appeared to be equal incidence in men and women, with varying ages (13 to 79 years) at the time of presentation. They are lesions that often grow to large size and can infiltrate into adjacent structures. Patients are usually symptomatic at the time of diagnosis. Symptoms may include dyspnea, dysphagia, chest pain, and cough due to local compression and invasion by the tumor. The occurrence of hypoglycemia has been associated with very large tumors, and it can be responsible for some of the presenting symptoms. Although the exact basis of this phenomenon has yet to be determined, the two prevailing theories include increased utilization of glucose by the tumor, and the formation and release by the tumor of metabolites with insulin-like activity. Histologically, fibrosarcomas resemble fibromatosis, but they have frequent mitotic figures and focal areas of necrosis. The tumors can demonstrate aggressive local invasion, but they rarely metastasize distantly. Despite the lack of distant metastasis, these lesions are rarely resectable for cure. Local recurrence is common, and most patients die within a few years as a result of extensive mediastinal invasion. Surgical resection remains the only chance for cure. The benefits of chemotherapy and radiation therapy are unproved.

Malignant Fibrous Histiocytoma (MFH). Although MFH is the most frequently encountered soft tissue sarcoma of late adult life, there have been less than 10 cases of primary mediastinal MFH reported in the English literature. Its rarity is evident by the absence of any mention of this tumor in Pachter and Lattes' large collective series, published in 1963. Tumors of this tissue origin found in the mediastinum usually represent metastatic disease from the extremity or retroperitoneum. Treatment for this lesion is complete excision when possible. However, local recurrence and metastatic spread typify the course of the disease. Weiss and Enzinger (1978), in a review of 200 cases of malignant fibrous histiocytoma found throughout the body, quoted a local recurrence rate of 44% and a distant metastatic incidence of 42%. Although postoperative radiation therapy may have some benefits in reducing local recurrence when resection margins are close or microscopically positive, adjuvant and neoadjuvant therapy has not been shown to improve survival.

Hemangioma. These tumors represent the most common benign vascular tumors of the mediastinum. The majority of patients present with symptoms secondary to local compression of adjacent mediastinal structures by the often extreme size of the tumor. The tumors are most commonly encapsulated, but they may also appear as poorly circumscribed masses that involve adjacent tissues. Although patients can present at varying ages, they tend to be diagnosed in childhood. There are three histologic variants that are classified according to the size and type of the predominant vascular component: cavernous, capillary, and venous variants. Cavernous hemangiomas are by far the most common, with the capillary variant second at approximately 15%. The smooth muscle walls of the vascular spaces can sometimes be quite prominent and therefore can be confused with mesenchymal tumors of smooth muscle origin. This again underscores the inherent difficulty in any attempt to accurately classify these tumors. There has been no evidence of any potential for malignant degeneration. Surgery remains the most effective therapy, but it must be undertaken with great caution due to the extreme size and vascularity of these tumors. Radiotherapy has not been shown to be effective in relieving symptoms.

Hemangiopericytoma. These tumors originate from pericytes that are typically found around capillary arterioles. They are generally solitary encapsulated lesions, unless they arise in the malignant form, in which case they can be poorly circumscribed and locally invasive. Differentiation between benign and malignant forms is thus often based on clinical grounds; histologic differentiation is seldom possible, as both have a similar appearance. Enzinger and colleagues (1983), however, have identified certain histologic findings suggestive of malignancy and therefore a high potential for metastasis. These include four or more mitoses per high-power field, prominent cellular pleomorphism, and areas of hemorrhage and necrosis. Hematologic and lymphatic spread is the typical course of the malignant form. Treatment is excision, but the prognosis cannot be reliably predicted based on intraoperative findings. Radiation therapy and chemotherapy with doxorubicin (Adriamycin) have been tried without demonstrable benefit.

Epithelioid Hemangioendothelioma (Fig. 63–49). These lesions were originally described by Weiss and Enzinger in 1982. In more recent literature, these tumors are believed to be low-grade malignancies derived from endothelial cells. They have histologic features that are intermediate between hemangiomas and angiosarcomas. Similarly, their clinical behavior is also intermediate between the benign hemangiomas and the malignant angiosarcomas. They have been divided into two variants depending on their benign versus malignant histology. The majority display a benign histology, but despite these microscopic findings, approximately 20% metastasize at 5 years. Twenty-five percent of these tumors display a malignant histology with significant atypia, increased mitotic figures, and necrosis. The malignant variant follows a clinical course that is even more virulent than its benign counterpart. Over one half show evidence of metastasis at 5 years, with an accompanying mortality of approximately 30%. Treatment focuses on wide excision that includes regional lymph nodes. Some authors believe that lesions with malignant histology should be treated in a manner similar to other high-grade sarcomas, including radical excision with adjuvant chemotherapy or radiation therapy. However, resection for long-term survival is unfortunately rarely possible. Resection of locally recurrent tumors, as well as metastases to liver and lung, are advocated by many authors. Radiation and chemotherapy can also be applied to distant metastases and to manage local recurrence.

Lymphangioma. Less than 1% of lymphangiomas are confined to the mediastinum. The vast majority that involve the mediastinum are lesions that actually originate in

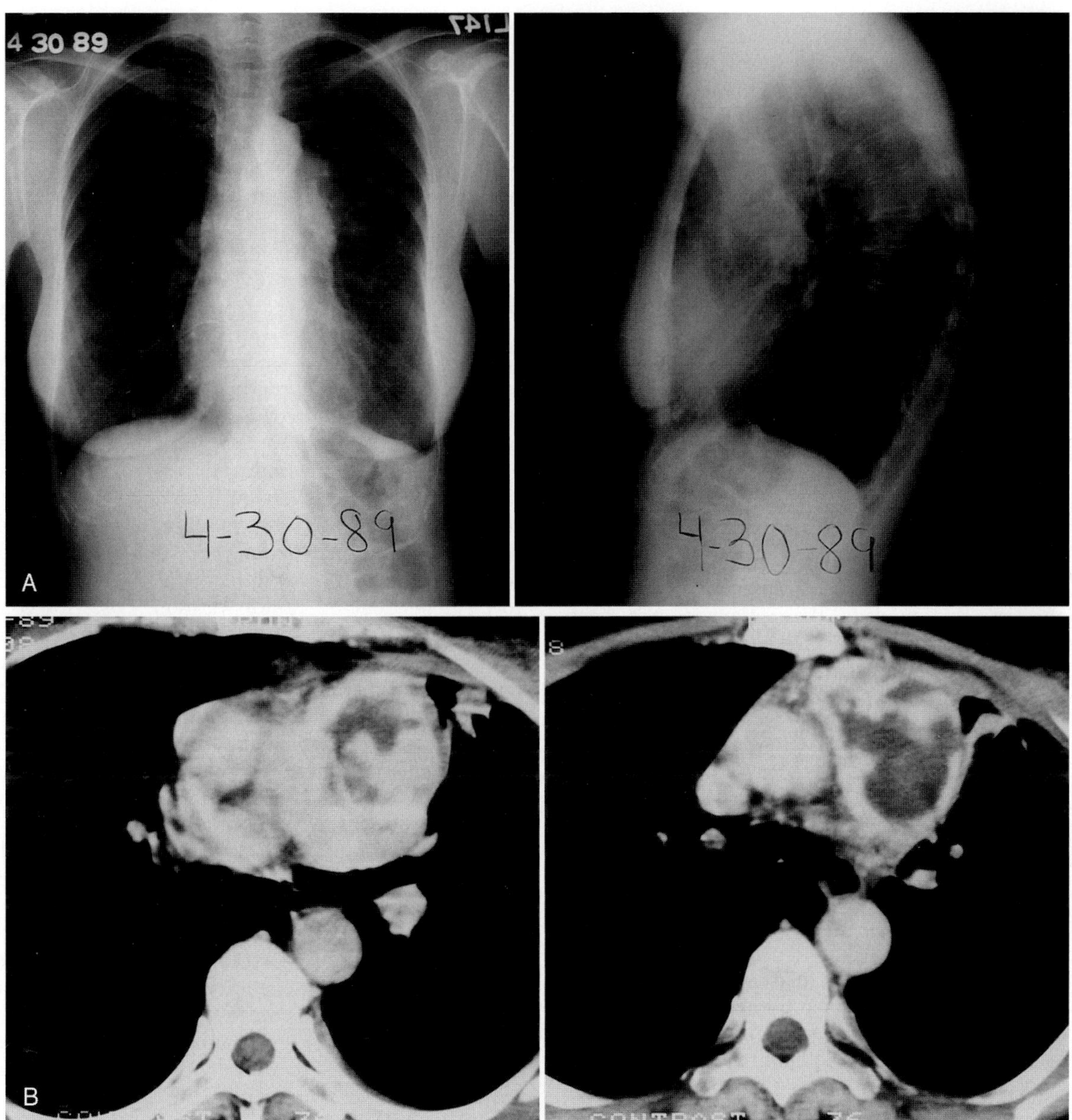

FIGURE 63–49 ■ *A*, Posteroanterior and lateral chest radiographs of a 72-year-old woman with prior history of hyperthyroidism and remote history of ovarian cancer. Note the left anterior mediastinal density. *B*, Chest computed tomography images from the same patient. There is a question of mediastinal infiltration *(see image on left side)*. The lesion shows several areas of low density consistent with necrosis. However, the solid portions of the lesion are brightly enhancing, consistent with significant vascularity. The lesion was resected through a median sternotomy approach, although the left phrenic nerve had to be sacrificed. Pathologic examination showed this to be a hemangioendothelioma.

the cervical region and extend into the anterosuperior mediastinum. Most isolated mediastinal lesions are seen in the adult population. Only one quarter are seen in children, and less than 5% are diagnosed in infants younger than 1 year of age. These tumors can be classified into two morphologic types according to the size of the lymphatic spaces. Lesions featuring large cystic lymphatic spaces are called cystic hygromas, while lesions with smaller spaces grouped into a sponge-like mass are called cavernous lymphangiomas. The pathogenesis involves proliferation of lymphatic vessels that become sequestered from the lymphatic system. Cystic transformation occurs due to accumulation of chyle within the lumen of these vessels, which later fail to communicate with the systemic lymphatic circulation. Differentiation between lymphangiomas and hemangiomas both grossly and microscopically is based on the presence of chyle or blood within the lesions, respectively. However, postsurgical changes can artifactually render lymphangiomas full of blood and mislead the pathologist into misdiagnosing the lesion as a hemangioma. Immunohistochemical staining for intracytoplasmic factor VIII reactivity can aid in the differentiation, as this reactivity is a characteristic of vascular endothelium but is absent in lymphatic vessels. Lymphangiomas are benign lesions that have a clinical behavior similar to hemangiomas. They can grow to a very large size and cause symptoms due to compression or erosion into adjacent structures. They can also present with associated chylothorax, or as an abscess due to secondary infection of the cystic spaces. Treatment is based on surgical resection. Attempts to shrink the lesion with radiotherapy or sclerosing agents are ineffective. In addition, documented cases of malignant transformation by radiotherapy have also been reported, further minimizing the role of this treatment modality. Complete resection is often impossible due to erosion into adjacent structures. However, debulking of the tumor by unroofing the lesion, and resection of as much of the cyst walls as possible, has been recommended.

Rhabdomyoma. These are rare lesions that are divided into two variants, cardiac and extracardiac. In the extracardiac group, there are three recognized subtypes: adult type, fetal type, and genital type. The most common type is the adult, which usually involves the head and neck region. The fetal and genital types are morphologically similar and easily distinguished from the adult subtype. They are typically found in the regions of the head and neck in children and in the female genital tract, respectively. They are benign tumors of striated muscle cell origin. As with many of the mesenchymal tumors, their presence in the mediastinum as a primary tumor is extremely rare. The first documented case of an extracardiac rhabdomyoma originating from the mediastinum was by Miller and associates in 1978. It is believed that these tumors originate from thymic myoid cells, although the histogenesis of these tumors is still unknown. Treatment centers around resection, and local recurrence has been reported due to inadequate resection margins.

Rhabdomyosarcoma. Similar to their benign counterpart, these are extremely rare lesions in the mediastinum, with metastasis from extramediastinal origin being the more common source. The first documented cases were by Pachter and Lattes in 1963. Because of their paucity, our knowledge of their biology, clinical course, and treatment is based primarily on tumors found in soft tissue locations other than the mediastinum. On gross examination rhabdomyosarcomas are rubbery in texture, with a gray-white to pink-tan color on cut sections. Microscopically, there are four subtypes: embryonal, botryoid, alveolar, and pleomorphic. They appear to have a predilection for younger patients, and they have an equal gender distribution. Symptoms arise late in the course of the disease and consist of cough, pain, and dyspnea. Because of extensive local invasion, they are rarely resectable for cure. Radiation and chemotherapy appear to have some benefit. Effective chemotherapeutic agents include doxorubicin, cyclophosphamide, dactinomycin, and vincristine.

Leiomyoma. These tumors most commonly represent extensions of esophageal lesions. Primary tumors without origin from adjacent mediastinal organs are extremely rare. Definitive statements regarding their symptomatology, population dynamics, and clinical course cannot be made because of the paucity of recorded cases. However, the few case reports have documented well-encapsulated tumors in which curative resection was accomplished.

Leiomyosarcoma. These are rare malignant tumors of smooth muscle origin. Most reported cases originate from mediastinal organs such as the superior vena cava, pulmonary vessels, and esophagus. Shields (1991) argued that tumors originating from mediastinal organs are not true mediastinal tumors and should in fact be classified as sarcomas of large vessel origin. True mediastinal leiomyosarcomas not arising from surrounding mediastinal structures are extremely rare. Only 16 cases have been reported to date. The majority are located in the anterosuperior mediastinum, but posterior compartment lesions have also been reported. The origin of these tumors is uncertain, but theories include formation from small vessels within the mediastinum, formation from heterotopic smooth muscle cells derived from splanchnic mesoderm that become displaced during embryologic development, and parasitic tumors from the esophagus that become detached during its growth. Clinical presentation appears to be dependent on tumor location. Posterior compartment lesions are typically asymptomatic, whereas anterior compartment lesions often present with chest discomfort, cough, or malaise. Treatment centers around surgical resection. In contrast to resection of tumors originating from mediastinal organs (superior vena cava, pulmonary vessels, and esophagus), true mediastinal tumors are more easily resected because of their infrequent involvement with adjacent structures. The need for adjuvant therapy is determined by the histologic grade and clinical stage of the tumor, similar to lesions found in other soft tissue locations.

Osteogenic Sarcoma (Extraosseous). The classification of these tumors as extraosseous requires that they be clearly separate from adjacent skeletal structures. As a primary tumor of the mediastinum, they are extremely rare. There appears to be only seven reported cases of extraskeletal osteosarcoma of the mediastinum in the literature. Except for the case reported by Venuta and associates (1993), they have all been located in the anterior mediastinum. The origin of these lesions is uncertain, but the two prevailing theories include metaplasia of the connective tissues, and malignant degeneration of embryonal somatic remnants. Suggested predisposing factors have included prior mediastinal radiation therapy, trauma with subsequent development of myositis ossificans, preexisting soft tissue calcifications, and extravasation of thorium dioxide (Thorotrast). Presenting signs and symptoms have included pain (approximately 33% of patients) and areas of calcification on plain radiographs (50% of patients). These tumors are highly malignant and metastasize early, most commonly to the lungs. Treatment options for extraosseous osteosarcomas have centered around radiation therapy only, resection only, and resection followed by adjuvant therapy. Prognosis is very poor, with a 5-year survival of approximately 13%. The rate of local recurrence has been reported to be 56% within 12 months, and for distant metastases 62% within 24 months. In this regard, primary mediastinal osteosarcomas fare as poorly as primary osteosarcomas of the bony chest wall; this is in contrast to extremity osteosarcomas, in which an aggressive combination of surgical resection combined with adjuvant chemotherapy has improved 5-year survival to almost 50%.

Chondroma. Most chondromas located in the mediastinum arise from either the cartilaginous rings of the trachea or the major bronchi, or from lung parenchyma. They have also been documented to arise from costal cartilage, sternum, vertebral bodies, and joints. However, true soft tissue chondromas of the mediastinum, not attached to the aforementioned structures, are exceedingly rare. Clinical presentation is typically due to airway obstruction by the mass. The benign versus malignant character of these lesions cannot be based on histology alone. Tumors that appear to be malignant histologically can have a benign clinical course, and benign-appearing tumors can recur after resection and even metastasize. Thus, clinical evidence of local tissue invasion despite a benign histology warrants aggressive therapy. Resection remains the only viable method of treatment. Some authors have advocated debulking of malignant tumors that have grown beyond the boundaries of resectability. This is believed to increase the period of disease-free survival.

Chondrosarcoma. These are rare tumors that, when located in the mediastinum, typically arise from the tracheobronchial tree or chest wall. Extraskeletal chondrosarcomas are even less common. When they occur, they are typically found in the muscles of the extremities or the central nervous system and spinal cord. Only a handful of primary tumors of the mediastinum have been reported in the literature. To our knowledge, there has been only one documented case of an extraskeletal mesenchymal chondrosarcoma of the mediastinum. Primary skeletal chondrosarcomas of the mediastinum are similarly rare with only three cases documented in the literature. Therapy is very difficult, and radical surgery remains the most effective treatment. Chemotherapy and radiation therapy have been shown to be more effective in extraskeletal chondrosarcomas, but they still play only a minor palliative role.

Mesenchymoma. These are lesions that consist of two or more soft tissue components within the same tumor. They occur in a diverse age range, and show no predilection for either gender. Both malignant and benign lesions have been described. The benign type is extraordinarily rare and typically well circumscribed, although not encapsulated. Resection is curative. The benign variety has not been shown to be a precursor of the malignant lesion. Malignant tumors, like benign tumors, can occur at any age. They typically show extensive local invasion at the time of diagnosis and, therefore, are rarely resectable. Despite these tumors' unresectability, patients may often survive for many years after the diagnosis.

PRIMARY CARCINOMA OF THE MEDIASTINUM

This diagnosis is applied when a poorly differentiated carcinoma is discovered within the mediastinum such that the pathologic identification of the precise site or tissue of origin is unknown. Unfortunately, this nonspecific diagnosis is at times given because of an inadequate tissue biopsy specimen to allow for clear identification. To minimize the overuse of this designation, a close working relationship between the surgeon and pathologist must be established. The use of more sophisticated pathologic studies such as electron microscopy and immunoperoxidase staining can sometimes help with the identification of the tissue of origin. These tumors present with equal frequency in terms of gender. They make up approximately 4% of all primary mediastinal masses in collective series.

Most are symptomatic at the time of diagnosis due to local mass effect of the tumor. Symptoms arise from compression or invasion of adjacent mediastinal structures such as the esophagus, trachea, recurrent laryngeal nerves, and superior vena cava. Associated symptoms include dysphagia, hoarseness, cough, hemoptysis, dyspnea, superior vena cava syndrome, and chest pain.

In the past, these patients were quite often assumed to have metastatic disease with an unknown primary, and treatment was therefore directed at palliative radiation, or even just symptomatic relief. In short, all patients with the pathologic diagnosis of poorly differentiated carcinoma of the mediastinum should have a thorough workup in an attempt to identify a potential tissue of primary origin.

A complete history and physical examination may direct the search for the primary site. Electron microscopy and immunoperoxidase staining can at times help identify more common mediastinal tumors such as lymphomas, thymomas, and neuroendocrine tumors. Serum human chorionic gonadotropin β and α-fetoprotein, when elevated, may suggest the presence of an extragonadal germ cell tumor. Elderly patients with a history of tobacco use should undergo panendoscopy, including a diligent bronchoscopy and esophagoscopy, to search for a primary site. CT of the chest and abdomen can aid in localizing abnormal growths. Positron emission tomography may also be useful, although there are no published data confirming its utility in this regard.

In cases in which an identifiable tissue of origin cannot be found, and the tumor appears localized to the mediastinum without extensive invasion of adjacent structures, en bloc resection should be attempted. Unfortunately, the percentage of long-term cures in these patients is small. In cases where poorly differentiated carcinomas are unresectable, promising results have been achieved with chemotherapy using cisplatin-based regimens.

EXTRAMEDULLARY HEMATOPOIESIS

These tumors are usually the result of altered hematopoiesis. They are thought to be a compensatory response to a chronic hemolytic state seen in conditions such as hereditary spherocytosis or thalassemia. Alterations in bone marrow function have also been implicated. Intrathoracic extramedullary hematopoiesis is a rare finding, with less than 100 cases reported in the literature. The diagnosis should be sought when a mediastinal mass is found in conjunction with a known history of chronic anemia or disease of the bone marrow. Initial workup employs CT (which demonstrates the mass) and ^{99m}Tc-labeled sulfur colloid scans (the latter usually demonstrates increased uptake by the mass). Definitive diagnosis requires tissue biopsy for histology. Open biopsy is usually recommended. Transthoracic needle biopsy often does not yield a sufficient quantity of tissue for confirmation of the diagnosis, and it can be fraught with hemorrhagic complications that may be avoided or minimized by using an open biopsy technique.

Treatment centers on radiation therapy, which can cause an abrupt reduction in the size of the mass. Asymptomatic patients can usually be followed clinically without intervention. Surgery alone or in combination with radiation therapy is typically reserved for more aggressive tumors that cause local compression or invasion of adjacent mediastinal structures.

GIANT LYMPH NODE HYPERPLASIA (CASTLEMAN'S DISEASE)

Castleman first reported the appearance of giant lymph node hyperplasia in the mediastinum in 1954. Since that time, many descriptive terms have been linked to Castleman's disease. These have included angiofollicular lymph node hyperplasia, giant lymph node hyperplasia, lymph node hamartoma, benign giant lymphoma, and a variety of other terms. The disease can be found wherever lymph nodes are found, but the majority of these tumors originate within the thorax (70%). The exact etiology is still unclear, but theories include reactive lymphoid hyperplasia, hamartomatous change, benign lymphoid tumor, and inflammatory or infectious reactions of the lymph nodes.

There are now three histologically distinct types of Castleman's disease that have been generally agreed on. They are the hyaline vascular variety, the plasma cell variety, and the transitional (mixed cell) variety. Ninety percent of Castleman tumors are of the hyaline vascular variety. These are characterized by the presence of small hyaline follicles with interfollicular capillary proliferation. They are typically asymptomatic and present as isolated lesions found on routine chest radiographs (Fig. 63–50). The plasma cell variety is characterized by the presence of large follicles with interposed sheets of plasma cells. These tumors, in contrast to the hyaline vascular type, typically present with systemic symptoms of fever and night sweats. Consensus is that the plasma cell variety represents a more aggressive form of the disease. The transitional variant is the least common. It is histologically similar to the hyaline vascular variety with foci of numerous plasma cells and some large, normal-appearing germinal centers. Diagnosis is based on tissue histology, but more comprehensive laboratory evaluation may show anemia, hypergammaglobulinemia, and an elevated erythrocyte sedimentation rate.

Although classic Castleman's disease presents as a solitary lesion, in recent years a multicentric form has been shown to exist as generalized lymphadenopathy with the morphologic features of giant lymph node hyperplasia. These patients are typically symptomatic at presentation and can exhibit fever, chills, weight loss, hepatosplenomegaly, and altered immunity. This form of the disease has been associated with human immunodeficiency virus (HIV) infection and the acquired immunodeficiency syndrome (AIDS). Considerable interest is currently being focused on the role of human herpesvirus-8 in this lesion. This recently discovered virus, previously referred to as Kaposi's sarcoma–associated herpesvirus, is generally ab-

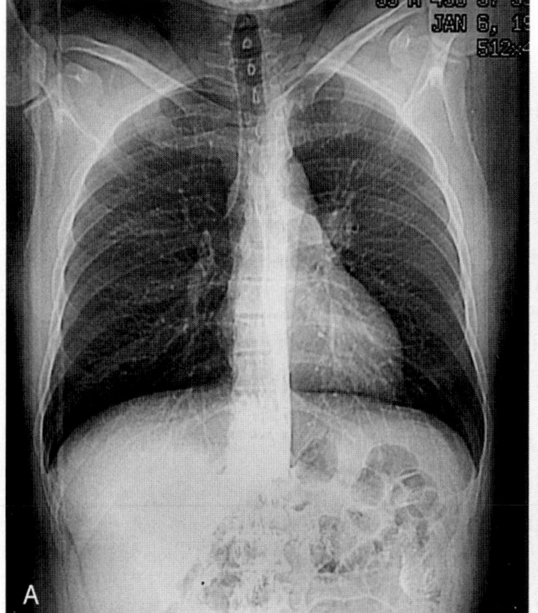

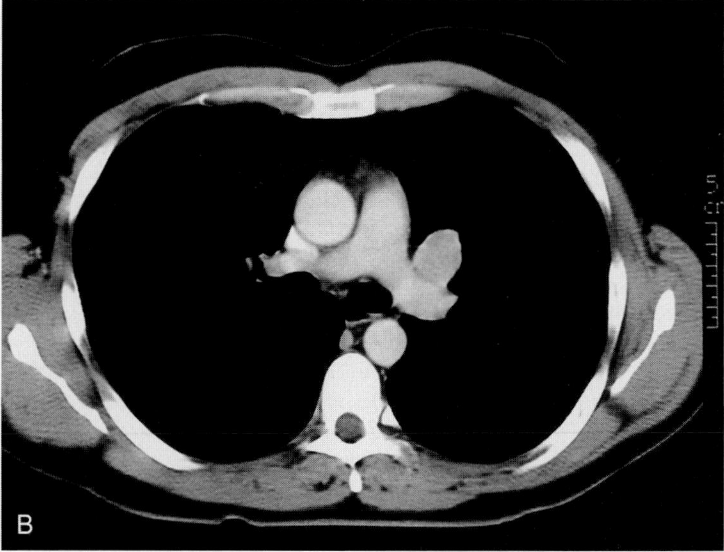

FIGURE 63–50 ■ *A,* Anteroposterior chest radiograph of a healthy 29-year-old man. Note the rounded left paramediastinal density. *B,* Chest computed tomography image from the same patient. The rounded lesion sits apposed to the left pulmonary artery in the subaortic region. It was biopsied through a left anterior mediastinotomy, which revealed features of "typical" Castleman's disease (hyaline vascular variety).

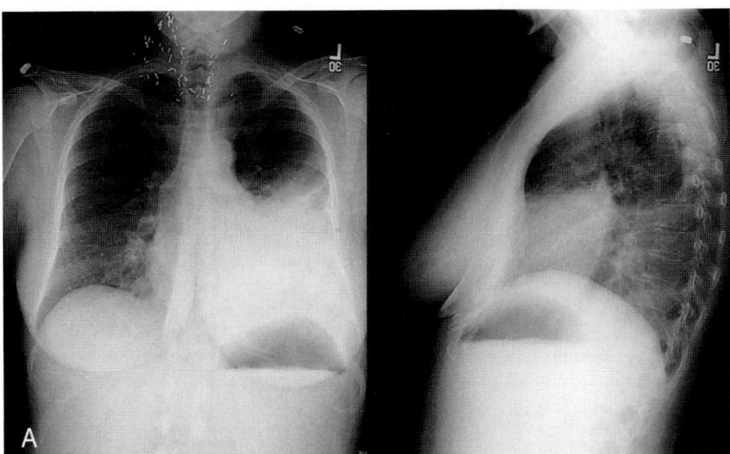

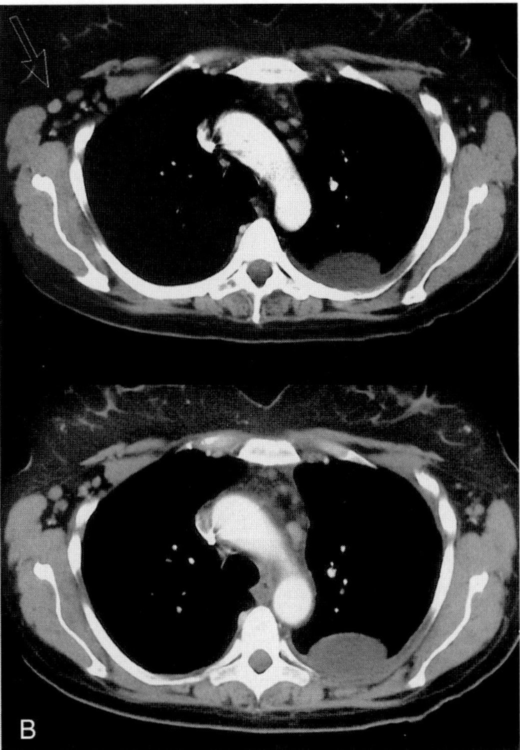

FIGURE 63–51 ■ *A*, Posteroanterior and lateral chest radiographs of a 52-year-old woman with a 1-year history of Castleman's disease (based on biopsy of an upper mediastinal lymph node performed during thyroid cancer resection). She now presents with fever, malaise, and dyspnea. Note the large left pleural effusion. *B*, Chest computed tomography images from the same patient. Thoracentesis revealed a chylothorax. Videothoracoscopy was performed for further evaluation. Biopsy of an enlarged anterior mediastinal lymph node now revealed B-cell lymphoma. Serologic testing revealed the patient to be positive for human herpesvirus (HHV)-8. (*Arrow* indicates axillary lymphadenopathy.)

sent in normal control tissues, inflammatory conditions, and various tumors. However, it is present in most Kaposi's sarcoma lesions (in both HIV-positive and HIV-negative patients); in primary effusion lymphoma (typically an AIDS-related non-Hodgkin's lymphoma in which neoplastic lymphocytes proliferate in serous body cavities and spare solid organs); and in a significant proportion of cases of multicentric Castleman's disease (in patients with or without AIDS), in which it may underlie malignant transformation to lymphoma (Fig. 63–51). The multicentric form of the disease is quite virulent compared with the typically benign course of classic Castleman's disease. Mortality has been reported to be as high as 50%. Although malignant transformation in Castleman's disease is uncommon, when it occurs it usually originates from the multicentric plasma cell type. Mortality for this variety is most commonly due to overwhelming sepsis.

When the diagnosis of Castleman's disease is secure, observation is a reasonable option. However, if symptoms (e.g., from mass effect) are present and severe or disabling, or if malignancy is suspected, surgical resection should be performed and typically offers cure. When resecting a Castleman tumor of the hyaline vascular variety, great care must be taken because of its extreme vascularity. Resection of this variety is often associated with significant intraoperative blood loss. When this tumor is incidentally found during surgery, complete resection should be attempted.

COMMENTS AND CONTROVERSIES

Drs. Fang and Sundaresan have contributed an excellent, concise review of an exceedingly rare group of mediastinal tumors. Each of these individual pathologies occurs with such infrequency that any individual surgeon's experience might comprise only several cases over the course of an entire career. However, in this chapter the authors repeatedly reinforce an extremely important principle: for the majority of these tumors, complete surgical resection is the treatment of choice. Radiation and chemotherapy, as either neoadjuvant or adjuvant strategies, have a limited role. Another important consideration in the diagnosis and management of unusual mediastinal masses is the possibility of metastasis from a distant primary source, most notably renal cell carcinoma.

G.A.P.

REFERENCES

Barua NR, Patel AR, Takita H, Jennings EC: Fibrosarcoma of the mediastinum. J Surg Oncol 12:11, 1979.

Besznyak I, Szende B, Lapis K (eds): Diagnosis and Surgical Treatment of Mediastinal Tumors and Pseudotumors. Basel, Karger, 1984.

Burlew BP, Shames JM: Lymphangiomyomatosis: Hormonal implications in etiology and therapy. South Med J 84:1247, 1991.

Castleman B, Iverson L, Menendez VP: Localized mediastinal lymph node hyperplasia resembling thymoma. Cancer 9:822, 1956.

Castleman B, Towne VW: Case Records of the Massachusetts General Hospital: Case no. 40011. N Engl J Med 250:26, 1954.
Cesarman E, Knowles DM: Kaposi's sarcoma–associated herpesvirus: A lymphotropic human herpesvirus associated with Kaposi's sarcoma, primary effusion lymphoma, and multicentric Castleman's disease. Semin Diagn Pathol 14:54, 1997.
Chetty R: Extraskeletal mesenchymal chondrosarcoma of the mediastinum. Histopathology 17:261, 1990.
Chung EB, Enzinger FM: Benign lipoblastomatosis: An analysis of 35 cases. Cancer 32:482, 1973.
De Nictolis M, Goteri G, Brancorsini D et al: Extraskeletal osteosarcoma of the mediastinum associated with long-term patient survival. A case report. Anticancer Res 15:2785, 1995.
Enzinger FM, Weiss SW: Soft tissue tumors. St. Louis, CV Mosby, 1983.
Feutz EP, Yune HY, Mandelbaum I et al: Intrathoracic cystic hygroma: A report of three cases. Radiology 108:61, 1973.
Greenwood SM, Meschter SC: Extraskeletal osteogenic sarcoma of the mediastinum. Arch Pathol Lab Med 113:340, 1989.
Hoor TT, Hewan-Lowe K, Miller JI et al: A transitional variant of Castleman's disease presenting as a chylous pleural effusion. Chest 115:285, 1999.
Johnson SF, Davey DD, Cibull ML et al: Lymphangioleiomyomatosis. Am Surg 59:395, 1993.
Kim JH, Jun TG, Sung SW et al: Giant lymph node hyperplasia (Castleman's disease) in the chest. Ann Thoras Surg 59:1162, 1995.
King DT, Duffy DM, Hirose FM et al: Lymphangiosarcoma arising from lymphangioma circumscriptum. Arch Dermatol 115:969, 1979.
Loh CK, Alcorta C, McElhinney J: Extramedullary hematopoiesis simulating posterior mediastinal tumors. Ann Thorac Surg 61:1003, 1996.
Marchevsky AM, Kaneko M: Surgical Pathology of the Mediastinum. New York, Raven Press, 1984.
Miller R, Kurtz SM, Powers JM: Mediastinal rhabdomyoma. Cancer 42:1983, 1978.
Montresor E, Abrescia F, Bertrand C et al: Mediastinal chondrosarcoma. Acta Chir Scand 156:733, 1990.
Moran CA, Suster S, Perino G et al: Malignant smooth muscle tumors presenting as mediastinal soft tissue masses. Cancer 74:2251, 1994.
Pachter MR, Lattes R: Mesenchymal tumors of the mediastinum. I: Tumors of fibrous tissue, adipose tissue, smooth muscle and striated muscle. Cancer 16:74, 1963.
Pachter MR, Lattes R: Mesenchymal tumors of the mediastinum. II: Tumors of blood vascular origin. Cancer 16:95, 1963.
Pachter MR, Lattes R: Mesenchymal tumors of the mediastinum. III: Tumors of lymph vascular origin. Cancer 16:108, 1963.
Pescarmona E, Rendina EA, Venuta F et al: Myxoid chondrosarcoma of the mediastinum. Appl Pathol 7:318, 1989.
Irgau I, McNicholas KW: Mediastinal lipoblastoma involving the left innominate vein and the left phrenic nerve. J Pediatr Surg 33:1540, 1998.
Serour F, Lieberman Y, Rosenman J et al: Castleman's disease of the mediastinum: Misleading clinical and radiologic characteristics. Respir Med 83:509, 1989.
Shields TW (ed): Mediastinal Surgery. Philadelphia, Lea & Febiger, 1991.
Stout PA: Tumors of the soft tissues. In Armed Forces Institute of Pathology (ed): Atlas of Tumor Pathology, Section 2, Fascicle 5. Washington, DC, Armed Forces Institute of Pathology, 1953.
Tarr RW, Kerner T, McCook B et al: Primary extraosseous osteogenic sarcoma of the mediastinum: Clinical, pathologic, and radiologic correlation. South Med J 81:1317, 1988.
Taylor JR, Ryu J, Colby TV et al: Brief report: Lymphangioleiomyomatosis—clinical course in 32 patients. N Engl J Med 323:1254, 1990.
Van Schil PE, Colpaert CG, Look RV et al: Primary mediastinal leiomyosarcoma. Thorac Cardiovasc Surg 41:377, 1993.
Vasquez JJ, Fernandez-Cuervo L, Fidalgo B: Lymphangiomyomatosis: Morphogenetic study and ultrastructural confirmation of the histogenesis of the lung lesion. Cancer 37:2321, 1976.
Venuta F, Pescarmona EO, Rendina EA et al: Primary osteogenic sarcoma of the posterior mediastinum. Scand J Thorac Cardiovasc Surg 27:169, 1993.
Weidner N: Atypical tumor of the mediastinum: Epithelioid hemangioendothelioma containing metaplastic bone and osteoclastlike giant cells. Ultrastruct Pathol 15:481, 1991.
Weiss SW, Enzinger FM: Epithelioid hemangioendothelioma: A vascular tumor often mistaken for carcinoma. Cancer 50:970, 1982.
Weiss SW, Enzinger FM: Malignant fibrous histiocytoma. An analysis of 200 cases. Cancer 41:2250, 1978.
Weiss SW, Ishak KG, Dail DH et al: Epithelioid hemangioendothelioma and related lesions. Semin Diagn Pathol 3:259, 1986.
Widdowson DJ, Lewis-Jones HG: Case report: A large soft-tissue chondroma arising from the posterior mediastinum. Clin Radiol 39:333, 1988.
Willis J, Abdul-Karim FW, di Sant' Agnese PA: Extracardiac rhabdomyomas. Semin Diagn Pathol 11:15, 1994.

MEDIASTINAL THYROID TUMORS

Thomas W. Shields

A thyroid mass, most often a nontoxic colloid goiter or occasionally an adenoma, is not an unusual finding below the level of the thoracic inlet. As a result of partial or complete location of the mass within the mediastinum, the substernal thyroid mass is readily mistaken for a primary mediastinal tumor. It has been estimated by Creswell and Wells (1992) that these thyroid masses comprise 5.8% of all mediastinal lesions. In fact, however, almost all such masses descended from their original cervical location in the gland and, as such, are not truly primary tumors of the mediastinum.

HISTORICAL NOTE

The various definitions of substernal thyroid masses were in question during the early part of the 20th century, and many confusing and conflicting classifications were suggested. However, the seminal report of Wakeley and Mulvany (1940), which divided intrathoracic thyroid masses into three types, can be accepted as a reasonable and logical classification. Their three types are (1) "small substernal extension" of a mainly cervical thyroid mass; (2) "partial" intrathoracic, in which the major portion of the mass is situated within the thorax; and (3) "complete," in which all of the mass lies within the thoracic cavity. In these authors' report, all the thyroid masses were colloid goiters, whereas today intrathoracic thyroid masses comprise a variety of thyroid pathologic conditions; this changing pathologic pattern, however, does not invalidate their classification.

Approximately 80% of the substernal thyroid masses in most series are of the small substernal extension type, 15% are partial, and only 2% to 4% are completely within the thorax. According to Sweet (1949), most of these are in the anterior compartment, with only a small percentage located retrotracheally or in the posterior mediastinum. In Wakeley and Mulvany's (1940) series, the overall incidence of all substernal goiters was 8.7%, and the incidences of the three aforementioned types were 81.9%, 15.3%, and 2.7%, respectively. The latter two categories are the ones that the thoracic surgeon is concerned with, and they comprise only 1.6% of all goiters. A similar incidence, 1.4% in 9100 patients with goiter, was reported by DeAndrade (1977). McCort (1949) reported an incidence for the partial and complete lesions of over 3%, but still this represents only a small percentage of patients with thyroid disease.

■ *HISTORICAL READINGS*

DeAndrade MA: A review of 128 cases of posterior mediastinal goiter. World J Surg 1:789, 1977.

McCort JL: Intrathoracic goiter: Its incidence, symptomatology, and roentgen diagnosis. Radiology 53:227, 1949.

Sweet RH: Intrathoracic goiter located in the posterior mediastinum. Surg Gynecol Obstet 89:57, 1949.

Wakeley CPG, Mulvany JH: Intrathoracic goiter. Surg Gynecol Obstet 70:702, 1940.

EMBRYOLOGY

Embryologically the thyroid anlage arises from a midline diverticulum of the floor of the pharynx at a level between the first and second pharyngeal pouches. This site is identified subsequently as the foramen cecum of the tongue. The tissue develops into a bilobed structure, which ends its descent at the level of the laryngeal primordium. In the adult, the lower poles of the thyroid gland usually reach the level of the first tracheal ring, although abnormal descent to the sixth tracheal ring has been recorded. The major ectopic locations of thyroid tissue are from the upper poles of the gland to the base of the tongue. It is possible that tissue from the lower poles may be carried into the anterior compartment along with the thymus and the developing heart. However, in contrast to the presence of ectopic parathyroid tissue in or adjacent to the thymus, there are only rare reports of isolated normal thyroid tissue in such a location. An illustration of an ectopic thyroid follicle located in the parathymic mediastinal fat was published by Meissner and Warren (1969). How common this occurrence is remains unknown. A report of extensive dissection of the anterior mediastinal area by Jaretzki and Wolff (1988) failed to note the identification of thyroid tissue located in the mediastinal fat removed during the operation. Gilmour (1937), in an extensive study of the parathyroid glands in a large series of autopsy specimens, mentioned the occasional difficulty of gross distinction of parathyroid tissue from accessory thyroid nodules, but he failed to describe the anatomic location of these accessory nodules. However, as noted by Meissner and Warren (1969), such nodules are most commonly located adjacent to the normal thyroid gland in the neck; it may be assumed that few, if any, were found in the mediastinum.

ECTOPIC THYROID TISSUE IN THE MEDIASTINUM

From the data available, even though ectopic thyroid tissue can occur in the mediastinum, it is exceedingly rare for a true ectopic thyroid mass to arise in the anterior compartment of the mediastinum. Cove (1988) states that thyroid tissue can be displaced inferiorly during the embryogenesis of the heart, and ectopic thyroid tissue has infrequently been found at the aortic root, in the pericardium, and even within the cardiac muscle or in the esophageal wall. However, such ectopic tissue is rare indeed, although Rogers and Kesten (1962), as well as Willis (1962), have described several examples of ectopic thyroid tissue in these locations. Ectopic thyroid tissue has not been identified paratracheally within the thorax. It is possible that ectopic tissue from the bilateral postbronchial bodies from the rudimentary fifth pharyngeal pouches, which are believed normally to become incorporated and differentiated into normal thyroid, could be carried down into the anterior or visceral compartments. According to Rogers (1978), if these postbronchial bodies fail to be incorporated into the thyroid, differentiation into thyroid tissue does not occur. However, such tissue may give rise to a small cystic structure adjacent to the trachea in the neck or in the visceral compartment of the mediastinum.

The presence of a true ectopic thyroid lesion in the mediastinum has been debated for years. Although Lahey (1945) reported that he had never encountered one in over 24,000 goiter operations, other authors have noted the occurrence of rare true ectopic thyroid lesions in the mediastinum; an incidence of less than 1% usually is stated in the literature. Unfortunately, the documentation of a true ectopic origin of a thyroid mass in the mediastinum is lacking in most cases so reported. The only criteria frequently employed are that the thyroid tissue be completely separated from the gland in the neck and that its blood supply be from vessels arising within the thorax rather than from the inferior thyroid vessels. These criteria are insufficient, and to them must be added the following: (1) the thyroid gland in the neck should be normal or completely absent; (2) no prior surgical removal of the "whole" or portion of the cervical gland should have been done in the past; (3) no invasive malignancy of the thyroid gland should be present or have been present in the past; and (4) no similar pathologic process should be present in both the cervical gland and the ectopic tissue. Following these strict criteria, very few of the case reports of a so-called ectopic thyroid mass can be substantiated. For example, only one case of the several reported by LeRoux (1961), one case of those reported by Salvatore and Gallo (1975), and one case of Sussman and associates (1986) meet these criteria.

Likewise, I have had one such case, initially recorded in 1972 (Shields, 1972). Most cases, including the more recent cases reported by Mishriki (1983) and Hall (1988) and their associates, do not meet the aforementioned criteria and should not be classified as ectopic lesions. The recent case reported by Houck and colleagues (1998) does not meet the aforementioned rigid criteria, but possibly it was aberrant because of its blood supply, so exceptions may exist. However, the ectopic nature of a mediastinal thyroid mass is really the least of the many controversies associated with substernal thyroid masses.

ANATOMIC LOCATION

A major controversy associated with substernal thyroid masses is establishing the true location of the mass. This controversy has been the result of a number of factors, two of which are the presence of numerous different classifications of the mediastinal compartments and the failure to appreciate that the thoracic inlet consists entirely of the superior aspect of the visceral compartment of the mediastinum. The anterior, or prevascular, compartment begins well below the sternal notch and no true posterior compartment exists. The term *superior mediastinum*, unless used specifically to modify the anterior or visceral compartment, only adds to the confusion.

In many series of substernal goiters, such as those of Dahan (1989) and Singh (1994) and their colleagues, the majority of substernal goiters have been reported to be located in the anterior (prevascular) compartment. Most of the thoracic goiters that are classified as being in the anterior compartment are of the small substernal type. These are actually, in most cases, situated anteriorly in the visceral compartment and lie in contact with the undersurface of the manubrium on the cephalad aspect of the great vessels. These vessels may be displaced caudad and even somewhat dorsad. The impression is then gained that the goiter has descended into the prevascular (anterior) mediastinal compartment. However, as a rule the anterior substernal extension remains in the visceral compartment, being confined anteriorly by the pretracheal fascia. The goiter is thus prevented from entering the prevascular space that lies between this fascial layer and the more superficial investing layer of the deep cervical fascia.

However, the descent of a partial or complete intrathoracic goiter into the prevascular space does occur. Fadel and associates (1996) reported that 39% of 63 patients had prevascular goiters and 61% had retrovascular goiters; the size of the goiters and the history of previous thyroid surgery were not noted. Many examples of extension into the prevascular space have been recorded in patients with prior thyroid surgery, in whom the fascial planes sealing this compartment undoubtedly had been violated by the previous procedure. Ellis and associates (1952) reported that all nine patients in their series with goiters in this location had had previous thyroid operations. Examples of a complete substernal thyroid mass in the prevascular compartment visualized by computed tomography (CT) were published by both Glazer (1982) and Bashist (1983) and their associates. In the former report no history was given for the patient, but in the latter report the patient had a definite history of previous goiter removal. An invasive malignant tumor of the thyroid, either a primary or a recurrent lesion, may also invade the anterior compartment. Finally, although this is an infrequent occurrence, a partial or complete intrathoracic goiter on the right that is anterior or partially anterolateral to the trachea may originally enter the mediastinum via the visceral compartment, but once within the thorax, the lower aspect of the mass may pass in front of the ascending arch of the aorta. Thus, its lowermost portion may come to lie in the anterior compartment below the innominate vessels at the thoracic inlet.

In contrast to the occasional location of a partial or complete substernal thyroid mass within the anterior compartment, the majority of such masses are within the visceral compartment. As such, they are located behind and medial to the great vessels as the goiter descends into the thorax in close relationship to the trachea. McCort (1949) initially made this observation and rightly stated that the vessels in the superior portion of the mediastinum were the border-forming structures of the substernal thyroid goiters. His observation has been amply documented by the CT characteristics of these lesions in the studies of Glazer (1982) and Bashist (1983) and their colleagues, as well as by others, including my own similar observations (Shields, 1991) (Fig. 63–52). The vessels, especially the veins, are displaced laterally and may become compressed against the bony structures of the thoracic inlet. In this latter situation the findings of a superior vena cava syndrome may be mimicked.

The vast majority of true partial and completely intrathoracic goiters or other thyroid lesions remain in continuity with the trachea. Of these lesions in the visceral compartment, the majority of goiters are located anterior or lateral to the trachea; the remainder are located posterior to this structure. In the series reported by Fadel and associates (1996), 55% of the lesions in the visceral compartment were located anterior or lateral to the trachea and 45% were located posterior to it. Infrequently, the substernal thyroid mass may become retroesophageal in location. In a much earlier series described by McCort (1949) of 28 partial or complete intrathoracic goiters, 4 were located anterior, 12 anterolateral, 3 bilateral, and 6 posterior to the trachea, with the remaining 3 located posterior to the esophagus. Thus, 9 (32% of the 28 patients had retrotracheal lesions, often referred to as "posterior goiters" in the literature. Dahan and associates (1989) reported that of their 75 posterior substernal goiters, approximately 86% were retrotracheal, almost always on the right side, 4% were retroesophageal, 4% were anterior and to the right of the trachea although arising from the left lobe, and 6% were circumferential ("ring-shaped") about the trachea. In an attempt to simplify the classification of these lesions, Borrelly and associates (1985) suggested a classification of a simple form (SF) and a complex form (CF). The former consists of those substernal goiters located completely in either the pretracheal or the retrotracheal areas, and the latter are those goiters that extend into both spaces in varying combinations. Torre and colleagues (1995), in a series of 237 patients, recorded 59.5% of the goiters to be anterior

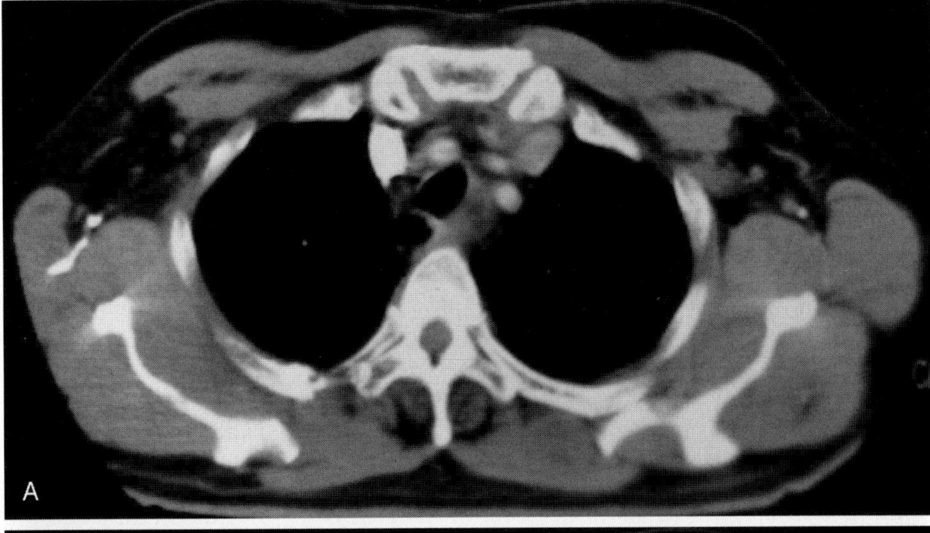

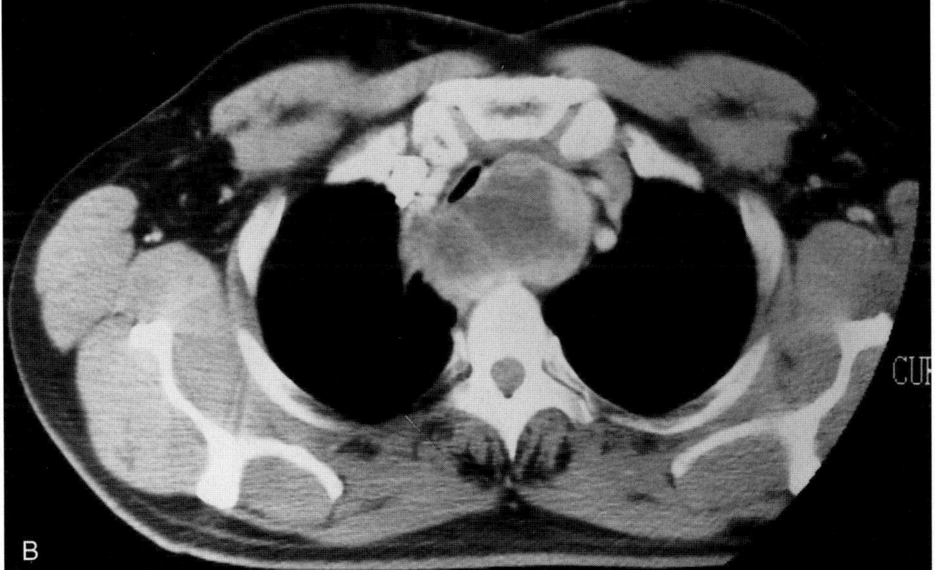

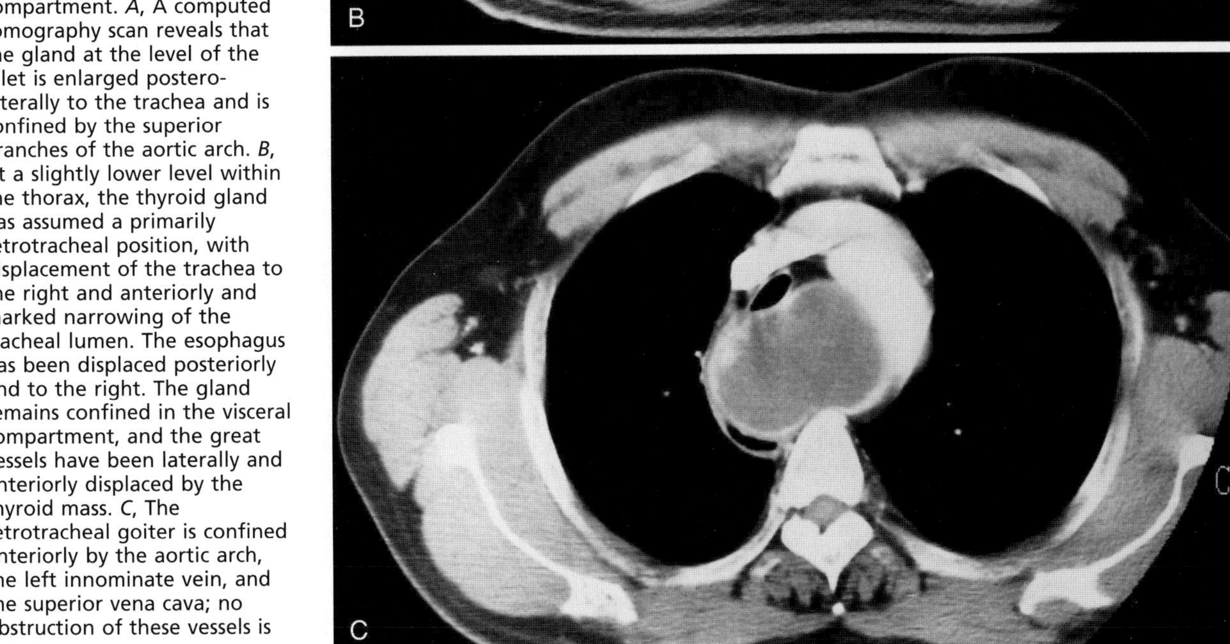

FIGURE 63–52 ■ Typical location of a partial substernal thyroid mass in the visceral compartment. *A*, A computed tomography scan reveals that the gland at the level of the inlet is enlarged postero-laterally to the trachea and is confined by the superior branches of the aortic arch. *B*, At a slightly lower level within the thorax, the thyroid gland has assumed a primarily retrotracheal position, with displacement of the trachea to the right and anteriorly and marked narrowing of the tracheal lumen. The esophagus has been displaced posteriorly and to the right. The gland remains confined in the visceral compartment, and the great vessels have been laterally and anteriorly displaced by the thyroid mass. *C*, The retrotracheal goiter is confined anteriorly by the aortic arch, the left innominate vein, and the superior vena cava; no obstruction of these vessels is present.

to the trachea, 11.4% completely retrotracheal in location, and 29.1% complex forms with varying locations about the trachea.

With goiters in the retrotracheal location (simple or complex), the carotid vessels and recurrent laryngeal nerves are located anterior to the mass rather than in their normal position dorsal to the gland. Consequently, the nerves are difficult to identify, and frequent injury to these nerves during removal of posterior goiters has been reported by Ellis and colleagues (1952), as well as by others.

The greater number of partial and complete goiters, even some of those arising from the left lobe, are located on the right. This is believed to result from the position of the arch of the aorta on the left. Regardless of the lobe of origin, the partial or complete substernal extension is confined, in the majority of cases, within the basket formed by the great vessels anterior to the trachea. Most of the lesions are located above the level of the arch of the aorta, but some may descend to the level of the arch, and a few have even descended to the level of the diaphragm.

The arterial blood supply of almost all the partial and complete intrathoracic goiters arises from the inferior thyroid vessels in the neck. In a few patients with the complete variety, particularly those goiters that have descended beyond the level of the midthorax, and in some patients who have had previous thyroid surgery, the vascular supply from the inferior thyroid vessels may be absent. In these cases, neovascular supply and drainage may be from or to one or more of the great vessels within the thorax. However, this variance in blood supply in itself does not indicate that the site of origin of the goiter was not the original thyroid tissue in the neck.

PATHOLOGY

In most of the early series of substernal thyroid masses, the pathology of the lesion was that of a nontoxic multinodular colloid goiter. Toxic hyperplasia was uncommon, as it still is. However, Higgins (1927) reported 3% of the lesions to be associated with hyperthyroidism, and in addition he noted a 16% incidence of fetal adenomas in his series. Katlick and associates (1985), in a series of 80 patients at the Massachusetts General Hospital, reported an incidence of multinodular goiter of 51%, follicular adenoma, 44%; and Hashimoto's thyroiditis, 5%. Of the follicular adenomas, 23 were classified as simple, 4 as fetal, 2 as colloid, 2 as embryonal, and 3 as Hürthle cell lesions. In two patients an occult papillary carcinoma was identified, for an incidence of malignancy of 2.5%, which is not dissimilar to the incidence reported by Wakeley and Mulvany (1940) but somewhat less than the 5% incidence of malignant lesions reported by Dahan and colleagues (1989). In contrast, Allo and Thompson (1983) reported an incidence of malignancy of 16%, and Sanders and associates (1992) reported one of 21%. However, in the latter series, nine of the malignant lesions, including three cases of lymphoma involving the thyroid, were clinically significant, and in only two patients (4.6%) was an occult tumor discovered at the time of the removal of the substernal thyroid goiter. In a recent review of the literature, Singh and colleagues (1994) found that the incidence of malignancy was 8.3% in 1259 patients with substernal thyroid masses.

CLINICAL FEATURES

Most patients with substernal thyroid masses are in the sixth or a later decade of life. Women are affected two to four times as often as men. A greater or lesser degree of kyphosis is often observed, as is the finding of a short, thick neck. Obesity is common. A variable number of patients report a history of one or more previous thyroid operations. In the series of Katlick (1985) and Sanders (1992) and their co-workers, the incidence was 20% exclusive of those patients with clinically suspicious malignant lesions. Torre and associates (1995) reported an incidence of reoperation of 10.5% in 237 patients.

In patients with small substernal extension of a cervical goiter, there are few, if any, clinical features related to the substernal extension. The clinical features are those of the cervical mass. The majority of patients with partial or complete substernal masses are symptomatic as the result of the substernal mass, although according to Rietz and Werner (1960), Reeve (1962), Lamke (1979), and Katlick (1985) and their colleagues, 15% to 30% of the patients may be asymptomatic. Sanders and colleagues (1992) reported half of their patients to be asymptomatic, whereas Torre and associates (1995) noted that only 5.5% were so.

In the symptomatic patients, a mass of variable size can be palpated in the midline or adjacent to it above the sternal notch. A cervical mass may be lacking in patients with previous thyroid surgery; in those with a so-called plunging goiter (goiter plongeant), which ascends into the lower neck only when the patient strains or coughs; and in those with a complete substernal thyroid lesion.

The majority of patients, however, present with one or more complaints of a cervical mass, a choking sensation, dyspnea, cough, and voice change or hoarseness. Dysphagia is not uncommon when the patient eats solid foods.

In Singh and co-workers' (1994) review of 1444 cases, dyspnea was present in 45%, hoarseness in 11%, and dysphagia in 18%. Wheezing and stridor may be present, and upper airway obstruction, as noted by Torres and colleagues (1983), can occur acutely. This may result as a sequel of an acute respiratory infection or a spontaneous hemorrhage within the mass. LeRoux and colleagues (1984) reported that acute airway obstruction can occur after administration of ^{131}I owing to temporary enlargement of the goiter. Acute airway obstruction can lead to sudden death, as reported by Warren (1979) as well as other authors. Warren recorded one death in four patients who developed acute airway obstruction. The management of this emergent event has been discussed in detail by Shaha and colleagues (1989b). The airway must be promptly established by intubation, and urgent thyroidectomy should be performed.

On physical examination, in addition to a cervical mass that often moves on swallowing, deviation of the trachea away from the mass is common. A cervical scar from previous thyroid surgery is not uncommonly present, in which case a cervical mass may be absent. Facial flushing and distended neck and anterior chest wall veins can be occasionally observed. This superior vena cava–

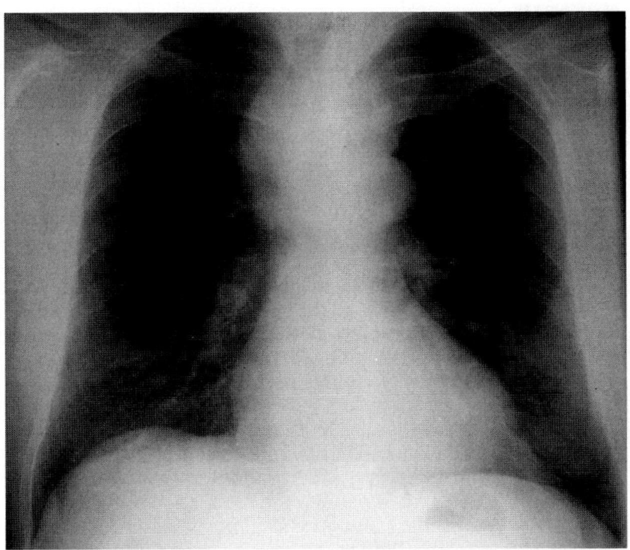

FIGURE 63–53 ■ Large partial substernal mass with deviation of the trachea to the right. The deviation is noted as being above the thoracic inlet.

like venous obstruction is seen in 1% to 5% of patients. Actual obstruction of the superior vena cava is rare, as is the occurrence of pain, pleural effusion, transient ischemic attacks, phrenic nerve palsy (as in the case recently reported by van Doorn and Kranendonk [1996]), or Horner's syndrome.

Most patients are euthyroid, and rarely are signs or symptoms of frank hyperthyroidism present. Shaha and associates (1989a) reported hyperthyroidism in only 1.6% of their patients. However, Allo and Thompson (1983) reported that hyperactivity of the gland was present in 10 (20%) of the 50 patients in their series, and Torre and colleagues (1995) recorded an incidence of 13.1% in their 237 patients. Allo and Thompson (1983) suggested that this hyperactivity probably was the result of autonomously functioning "hot" nodules or the total bulk of functioning thyroid tissue within the mass. In most patients the thyrotoxicosis was manifested by heart failure, cardiac arrhythmia, or a wasting syndrome, the so-called apathetic thyrotoxicosis.

In most series, except those of Allo and Thompson (1983) and Sanders and associates (1992) at the Lahey Clinic, evidence of malignant disease has been absent, and the few tumors discovered have been occult in nature. However, in the series of Sanders and associates, four of the nine patients with malignancy had suspicious lesions clinically, and in the other five the malignant nature of the thyroid mass was readily apparent at the time of operation. Hoarseness due to vocal cord paralysis is a strong indicator of the possibility of a malignant tumor, but it can occur with a benign lesion as well, so that even though it is suggestive of malignancy it is not diagnostic.

DIAGNOSTIC PROCEDURES

Standard Radiographs

Chest and neck radiographs are usually diagnostic for partial substernal thyroid lesions. The mass occupies the superior portion of the chest and extends upward into the neck. Calcifications may be recognized in the mass in a variable number of patients. Lateral deviation of the trachea is almost always present (in 80% to 95% of patients), and in contrast to primary mediastinal masses confined to the mediastinum, the tracheal deviation begins in the neck above the thoracic inlet (Fig. 63–53). In patients with complete substernal thyroid lesions, tracheal deviation may be absent, but when present it is often seen only on the lateral radiographs of the chest, the trachea being displaced in an anterior or a posterior rather than in a lateral direction. In this situation the radiographs are not diagnostic, as they are for a partial substernal thyroid mass.

Contrast Studies

A barium swallow readily demonstrates esophageal displacement and extrinsic compression, particularly in patients with retrotracheal or retroesophageal (posterior) thyroid masses (Fig. 63–54). A venacavogram, although not often indicated, may reveal displacement or even obstruction of the innominate and internal jugular veins

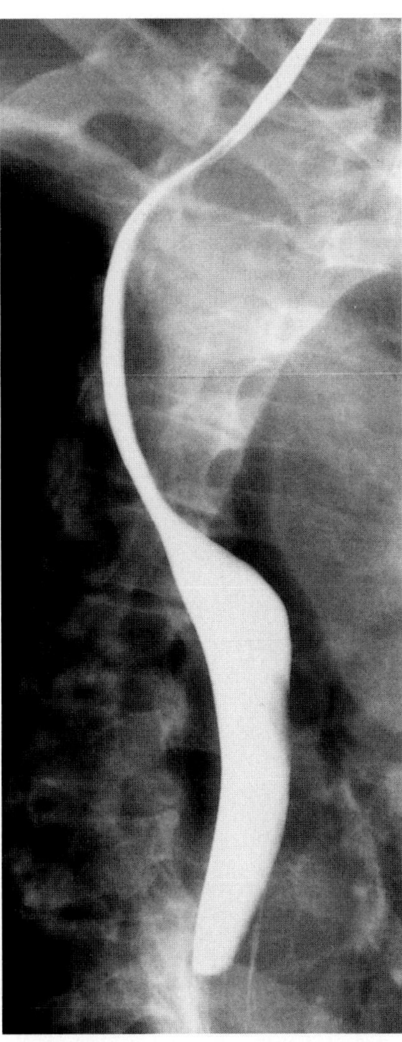

FIGURE 63–54 ■ Barium swallow reveals marked displacement by the substernal mass seen in Figure 63–53.

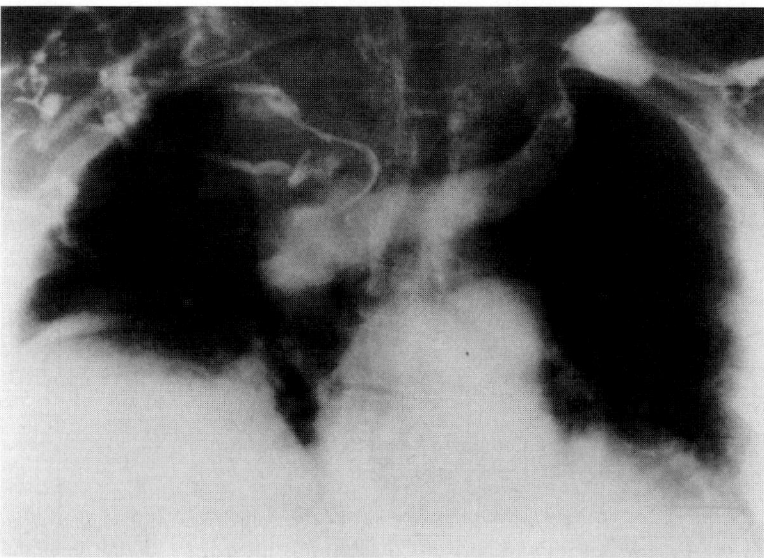

FIGURE 63–55 ■ Intravenous contrast study in a patient with a large partial substernal thyroid mass. Complete obstruction of the right innominate vein with collateral vessels is evident. The distal portion of the left innominate vein is almost completely obstructed at the thoracic inlet, but the major portion of this vein and the superior vena cava, although displaced, are widely patent. (From Silverstein GE et al: Superior vena caval system obstruction caused by benign endothoracic goiter. Chest 56:519, 1969.)

as they are compressed against the thoracic inlet. The superior vena cava, however, remains intact (Fig. 63–55).

Computed Tomography

Computed tomography (CT) scans are obtained routinely, although they are not always required. However, this study confirms the position of the lesion within the visceral compartment of the mediastinum in most cases and its relationship to the great vessels in the thorax, as previously noted (Fig. 63–56). Glazer (1982) and Bashist (1983) and their associates have described the usual CT findings. These consist of (1) a clear continuity of the mediastinal mass with the cervical gland; (2) well-defined borders; (3) the frequent presence of punctuate, coarse, or ring-like calcifications; (4) the nonhomogeneity of the mass; (5) the presence of nonenhancing low-density areas; (6) precontrast attenuation greater than for the adjacent muscles and even greater enhancement after the injection of iodinated contrast medium; and (7) most importantly, the characteristic pattern of lateral and anterior displacement of the vessels in the superior portion of the visceral compartment of the mediastinum with cradling of the mass by the right and left brachiocephalic vessels. The CT scan may be less diagnostic when the mass is complete in nature and is retrotracheal or retroesophageal in location or, infrequently, is present in the anterior compartment.

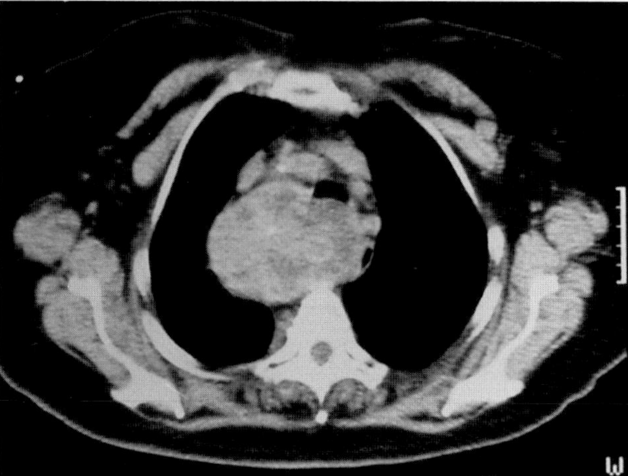

FIGURE 63–56 ■ CT scan of large retrotracheal goiter, showing its position in the visceral compartment and relationship to the adjacent vessels. The mass has well-defined borders, contains a ringlike area of calcification, and is nonhomogeneous in density.

Magnetic Resonance Imaging

Magnetic resonance imaging (MRI) is usually unnecessary, although as reported by von Schulthess and colleagues (1986), it permits excellent delineation of the great vessels and their relationship to the mass. Belardinelli and associates (1995) reported that MRI was a more accurate diagnostic procedure relative to the anatomic-topographic features of a substernal goiter than CT. Otherwise, the findings are similar to those obtained by CT scanning, except for one other important feature—that is, the demonstration of "flow voids" within the mass due to the marked vascularity of the substernal thyroid tissue. This feature should be especially helpful in patients with either the rare complete anterior compartment or posterior retrotracheal or retroesophageal masses (Fig. 63–57).

Thyroid Scintigraphy

Thyroid scintigraphy may be accomplished with ^{99m}Tc-pertechnetate, ^{131}I, or ^{123}I, but it must be done before a CT scan with contrast enhancement has been carried out. As a rule, the procedure is unnecessary except in some complete goiters, the diagnosis of which remains in doubt despite the aforementioned examinations. Unfortunately, the results of the examination are generally less than ideal (less than 50% identification of thyroid tissue in most reports in the literature), although Park and colleagues (1987) report a much higher percentage of posi-

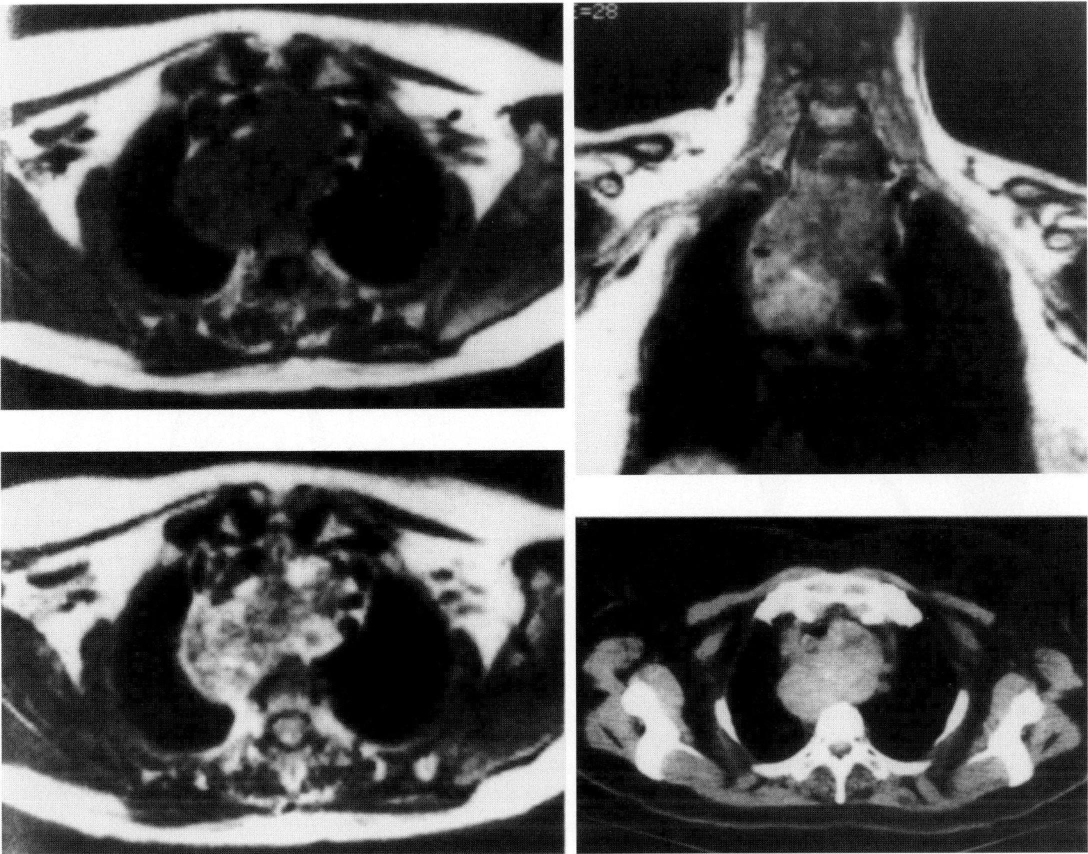

FIGURE 63–57 ■ Series of three magnetic resonance image (MRI) scans of a substernal thyroid mass, compared with a computed tomography scan of the mass (*lower right-hand corner*), reveals the relationship of the mass to the adjacent vessels and the multiple flow void present within the mass on the MRI scan.

tive results if strict attention is paid to the details of the technique used.

Fine-Needle Aspiration Biopsy

Although Lamke and associates (1979) recommended fine-needle aspiration (FNA) biopsy to confirm the nature of the mass, this procedure is unnecessary, may be hazardous according to Newman and Shaha (1995), and is not recommended except under very unusual circumstances. Despite the presence of occult tumor in 1% to 2% of patients, random biopsy is unrewarding in identifying such an occult lesion. Only if a dominant cold nodule is present or if preoperative findings are unequivocally suggestive of a malignancy should a needle biopsy be considered.

Pulmonary Function Studies

Flow-volume loop studies as described by Miller and Hyatt (1973) have been suggested by some investigators to demonstrate the presence of tracheal obstruction. As a rule the presence of obstruction is clearly present on physical examination or is demonstrated by routine chest radiographs so that these studies are superfluous.

MANAGEMENT

The therapy for a partial or complete intrathoracic thyroid mass is surgical resection. The use of radioactive iodine is contraindicated: Not only may it initially aggravate any pre-existing tracheal compression, but as noted by Beierwaltes (1978), radioactive iodine rarely, if ever, alleviates tracheal deviation or compression caused by a large multinodular goiter. L-Thyroxine likewise is of no avail to suppress a thyroid goiter.

Anesthetic management is best accomplished with an endotracheal tube and general anesthesia. The initial surgical incision is a low transverse collar (thyroid) incision, because over 95% of substernal goiters may be removed through this approach. DeAndrade (1977), Katlick (1985), Sanders (1992), and Singh (1994) and their associates reported the necessity of only a cervical incision in 95.3% 97.5%, 94.4% and over 98% of their cases, respectively. Reasons for the cervical approach that are just as or even more compelling are (1) that in almost all patients the blood supply of the intrathoracic mass is from the inferior thyroid arteries, and (2) that injury to the recurrent laryngeal nerve is less likely to occur with this approach.

In those few cases in which additional exposure becomes necessary, a partial sternal splint, initially advocated by Lilienthal (1915), is the procedure used by most thoracic surgeons. However, it is to be noted that, as described by Creswell and Wells (1992), in most cases in which this is necessary, the great vessels are in front of the intrathoracic mass (Fig. 63–58) and not behind it. Gourin and associates (1971) suggested a combined cer-

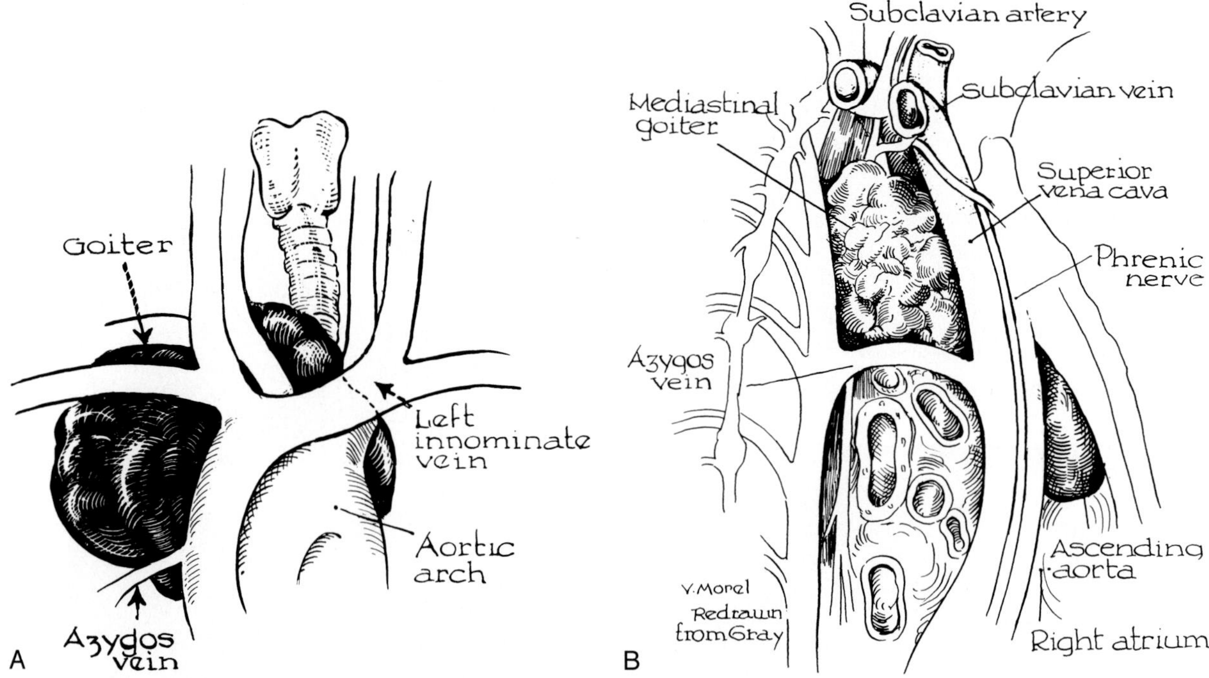

FIGURE 63–58 ■ Schematic illustrations from the frontal *(A)* and lateral *(B)* aspects of a partial intrathoracic goiter lying in the visceral compartment of the mediastinum, resting on the border of the vertebrae behind the superior vena cava and the innominate vessels above the azygos vein (From Johnston JH Jr, Twente GE: Surgical approach to intrathoracic (mediastinal) goiter. Ann Surg 143:572, 1956.)

vicomediastinal approach for all partial and complete intrathoracic goiters. This would seem to be totally unnecessary in view of the aforementioned data. In addition, Le Roux and colleagues (1984) stated that they found the use of a sternal split to be of little help in mobilizing a gland that could not be extracted through the standard cervical approach. Landreneau and associates (1991) have stated that it is important to decompress the intrathoracic negative pressure to facilitate removal of the substernal portion of the gland. They accomplished this decompression by use of a sterile spoon, but I am sure that any blunt instrument would do as well. Actually, the use of a special "goiter spoon" was reported by Kocher in 1901.

Rather than a sternal split, Johnston and Twente (1956) advocated a combined cervicoanterior thoracic approach because they believed that a better exposure of the enlarged gland could be obtained by this method (Fig. 63–59). This approach has also been advocated by DeAndrade (1977). In addition to the better exposure, gentle upward pressure on the goiter to deliver it into the cervical incision is readily accomplished. A posterior lateral thoracotomy approach, as suggested by Sweet (1949) and subsequently reported by Ellis and co-workers (1952), for posterior intrathoracic goiters is to be avoided if at all possible. Appropriate control of the vascular supply from the neck is difficult at best, and a high incidence of recurrent laryngeal nerve injury (approximately 27%) has been recorded by Ellis and associates (1952) and others with the use of this approach. To avoid these problems, Shahian and Rossi (1988) agree with Hilton and Griffin (1968) and Maurer (1955) on the efficiency of a simultaneous cervical and thoracic approach for contralateral retrotracheal or retroesophageal posterior thyroid masses, because this permits control of any mediastinal as well as the cervical vessels and adequately protects the recurrent laryngeal nerve.

In the standard cervical approach, the superior cervical blood supply to the involved lobe is identified and controlled, at least one superior parathyroid gland is identified, and if possible at this time, the vascular supply via the inferior thyroid vessels to the substernal portion of the gland is also controlled and the recurrent laryngeal nerve identified. These latter steps may not be possible until the substernal portion of the gland is removed from the mediastinum. This is accomplished by finger or pledget dissection within the capsule of the goiter to prevent injury to either the nerve or vessels. Infrequently, as noted, it is necessary to provide additional exposure by either a partial upper median sternotomy or a small anterior thoracotomy incision on the appropriate side in the second or third interspace to complete the mobilization. Morcellation of the goiter, as suggested by Lahey (1945), is to be avoided in order to lessen the possibility of bleeding, which may be difficult to control, and because of the possible presence of an occult carcinoma within the gland. After mobilization of the intrathoracic thyroid mass, the inferior thyroid vessels, if not already controlled, are ligated and divided, and the mass is removed.

Collapse of the tracheal wall due to tracheomalacia is frequently feared but rarely observed. When tracheal obstruction does occur, Allo and Thompson (1983) believe this is more likely the result of kinking of the

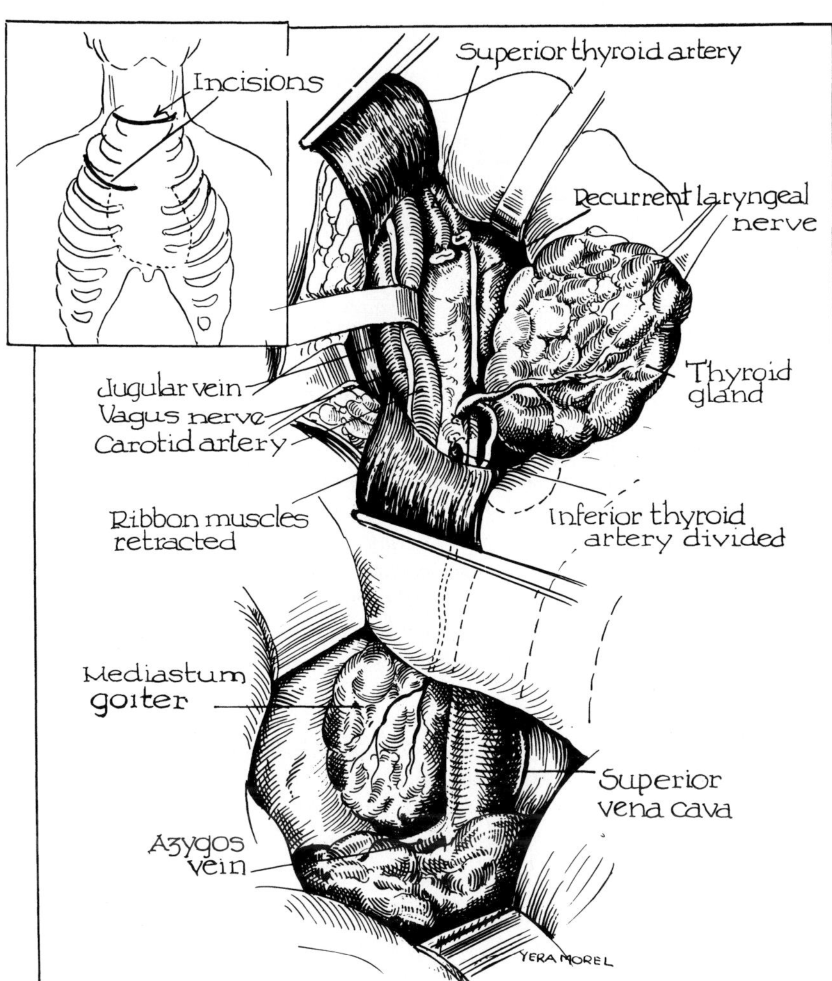

FIGURE 63–59 ■ Schematic illustration of combined cervicoanterior approach to substernal goiters that cannot be removed through a cervical approach alone. (From Johnston JH Jr, Twente GE: Surgical approach to intrathoracic (mediastinal) goiter. Ann Surg 143:572, 1956.)

elongated, distorted trachea. To prevent the occurrence of kinking, they suggest tacking the trachea anteriorly to one of the strap muscles in the neck before closure of the incision. It is a prudent precaution to inspect the tracheal lumen by flexible fiberoptic endoscopy prior to removal of the endotracheal tube; if any narrowing or compromise is suspected, the endotracheal tube should be left in place for 24 to 48 hours postoperatively. Tracheostomy or tracheal stenting may be indicated if airway obstruction persists. The need for the use of Marlex mesh around the trachea, the placement of a tracheal buttress, or the use of a polytetrafluoroethylene graft to support the tracheal wall is rarely indicated. The mediastinal space is drained in all cases to prevent accumulation of fluid within the mediastinal space.

Morbidity and Mortality

Watt-Boolsen and associates (1981) noted permanent unilateral vocal cord paralysis in 10% of their patients, but it was not stated if these were patients who had undergone a lateral thoracotomy. This latter approach, as noted, has a high incidence of recurrent laryngeal nerve injury. Dahan and associates (1989) reported a 6% incidence of recurrent laryngeal nerve paralysis, which is similar to that found by Singh and colleagues (1994) in a review of 1706 cases (77 cases, or 6.9%) collected from the literature. Katlick and associates (1985), on the other hand, reported no instances of vocal cord paralysis. Mediastinal hematoma may occur in a small percentage of patients. Pneumothorax or pneumonia are rare events, as is hypocalcemia.

Postoperative mortality is rare. DeAndrade (1977) reported only 1 death in 128 patients, that is, a 0.7% incidence following the removal of a partial or complete intrathoracic goiter. Dahan and associates (1989) reported a mortality rate of 2.8%. Most authors have reported mortality rates within the range of these two reports; however, in the 322 patients in the series reported by Cho (1986), Shaha (1989b), Katlick (1985), and Sanders (1992) and their associates, as well as by Allo and Thompson (1983), no operative mortality was reported.

Results

Recurrent substernal goiter is uncommon. Unfortunately, a frankly malignant lesion may recur. Thyroid function is usually normal, as is parathyroid function, as was noted by Watt-Boolsen and colleagues (1981) in their long-term follow-up study.

COMMENTS AND CONTROVERSIES

Dr. Shields' excellent chapter summarizes very nicely the current presentation, investigation, and management of patients with mediastinal thyroid. He correctly notes the misconception popularized in the literature that these goiters are frequently prevascular in the anterior mediastinum. In fact, the majority of these lesions are in the posterior mediastinum behind the great vessels. As a result, the vast majority can be resected through a transcervical approach. A transsternal extension to improve exposure is rarely necessary. When sternotomy is required, a full sternotomy rather than upper partial sternotomy is much more expeditious and easily closed. Even for massive posterior lesions, a posterolateral thoracotomy provides excellent exposure of the lower portion of the goiter but completely inadequate exposure of the superior blood supply. This commentator has only used this approach in the very elderly patient in whom it is felt that a combined procedure is not feasible.

The problem of postoperative tracheomalacia is uncommon and usually can be dealt with as Dr. Shields notes, by temporary mechanical ventilation through the endotracheal tube. A reasonable alternative for prolonged malacic problems is endoluminal stenting with currently available expandable stents. Operative correction of malacia should be avoided.

G. A. P.

REFERENCES

Allo MD, Thompson NW: Rationale for operative management of substernal goiters. Surgery 94:969, 1983.

Bashist B, Ellis K, Gold RP: Computed tomography of intrathoracic goiters. AJR Am J Roentgenol 140:455, 1983.

Beierwaltes WH: The treatment of hyperthyroidism with iodine 131. Semin Nucl Med 8:95, 1978.

Belardinelli L, Gualdi G, Ceroni L et al: Comparison between computed tomography and magnetic resonance data and pathologic findings in substernal goiters. Int Surg 80:65, 1995.

Borrelly J, Grosdidier G, Hubert J: Proposition d'une classification affinée des goitres plongeants. A propos d'une série de cent douze cas. Ann Chir 39:153, 1985.

Cho HT, Cohen JP, Som ML: Management of substernal and intrathoracic goiters. Otolaryngol Head Neck Surg 94:282, 1986.

Cove H: The mediastinum. In Coulson WF (ed): Surgical Pathology, 2nd ed. Philadelphia, JB Lippincott, 1988.

Creswell LL, Wells SA Jr: Mediastinal masses originating in the neck. Chest Surg Clin North Am 2:23, 1992.

Dahan M, Gaillard J, Eschapasse H: Surgical treatment of goiters with intrathoracic development. In Delarue NC, Eschapasse H (eds): Thoracic Surgery: Frontiers and Uncommon Neoplasms. International Trends in General Thoracic Surgery, Vol 5. St. Louis, CV Mosby, 1989.

DeAndrade MA: A review of 128 cases of posterior mediastinal goiter. World J Surg 1:789, 1977.

Ellis FH Jr, Good CA, Seybold WD: Intrathoracic goiter. Ann Surg 135:79, 1952.

Fadel E, Chapelier A, Lancelin C, et al: Intrathoracic goiters: 62 surgically treated patients. Presse Med 25:787, 1996.

Gilmour JR: The embryology of the parathyroid glands, the thymus and certain associated rudiments. J Pathol 45:507, 1937.

Glazer GM, Axel L, Moss AA: CT diagnosis of mediastinal thyroid. AJR Am J Roentgenol 138:495, 1982.

Gourin A, Garzon A, Karlson KE: The cervicomediastinal approach to intrathoracic goiter. Surgery 69:651, 1971.

Hall TS, Caslowitz P, Popper C et al: Substernal goiter versus intrathoracic aberrant thyroid: A critical difference. Ann Thorac Surg 46:684, 1988.

Higgins CC: Intrathoracic goiter. Arch Surg 15:895, 1927.

Hilton HD, Griffin WT: Posterior mediastinal goiter. Am J Surg 116:891, 1968.

Houck WV, Kaplan AJ, Reed CE et al: Intrathoracic aberrant thyroid: Identification critical for appropriate operative approach. Am Surg 64:360, 1998.

Jaretzki A III, Wolff M: "Maximal" thymectomy for myasthenia gravis. Surgical anatomy and operative technique. J Thorac Cardiovasc Surg 96:711, 1988.

Johnston JH Jr, Twente GE: Surgical approach to intrathoracic (mediastinal) goiter. Ann Surg 143:572, 1956.

Katlick MR, Grillo HC, Wang C: Substernal goiter: Analysis of 80 patients from Massachusetts General Hospital. Am J Surg 149:283, 1985.

Kocher T: Bericht über ein zweites Tausend Kropfexcisionen. Arch Exp Klin Chir 64:454, 1901.

Lahey FH: Intrathoracic goiters. Surg Clin North Am 25:609, 1945.

Lamke LO, Bergdahl L, Lamke B: Intrathoracic goiter: A review of 29 cases. Acta Chir Scand 145:83, 1979.

Landreneau RJ, Nawarwong W, Boley TM et al: Intrathoracic goiter: approaching the posterior mediastinal mass. Ann Thorac Surg 52:134, 1991.

LeRoux BT: Heterotopic mediastinal thyroid. Thorax 16:192, 1961.

LeRoux BT, Kallichurum S, Shama DM: Mediastinal cysts and tumor. Curr Probl Surg 21:11, 1984.

Lilienthal H: A case of mediastinal thyroid removed by transsternal mediastinotomy. Surg Gynecol Obstet 20:589, 1915.

Maurer ER: The surgical treatment of retrotracheal intrathoracic goiter. Arch Surg 71:357, 1955.

McCort JL: Intrathoracic goiter: Its incidence, symptomatology, and roentgen diagnosis. Radiology 53:227, 1949.

Meissner WA, Warren S: Tumors of the thyroid gland. In Atlas of Tumor Pathology, 2nd Series, Fascicle 4. Washington DC, Armed Forces Institute of Pathology, 1969.

Miller RD, Hyatt RE: Evaluation of obstructing lesions of the trachea and larynx by flow-volume loops. Am Rev Respir Dis 108:475, 1973.

Mishriki YY, Lane BP, Lozowski MS et al: Hürthle-cell tumor arising in the mediastinal ectopic thyroid and diagnosis by fine needle aspiration: Light microscopic and ultrastructural features. Acta Cytol 27:188, 1983.

Newman E, Shaha AR: Substernal goiter. J Surg Oncol 60:207, 1995.

Park HM, Tarver RD, Siddiqui AR et al: Efficacy of thyroid scintigraphy in the diagnosis of intrathoracic goiter. AJR Am J Roentgenol 148:527, 1987.

Reeve TS, Rundle FF, Hales IB et al: The investigation and management of intrathoracic goiter. Surg Gynecol Obstet 115:223, 1962.

Rietz KA, Werner B: Intrathoracic goitre. Acta Chir Scand 119:379, 1960.

Rogers W: Anomalous development of the thyroid. In Werner SC, Ingbar SH (eds): The Thyroid, 5th ed. New York, Harper & Row, 1978.

Rogers WM, Kesten HD: Embryologic bases for thyroid tissue in the heart. Anat Rec 142:323, 1962.

Salvatore M, Gallo A: Accessory thyroid tissue in the anterior mediastinum. J Nucl Med 16:1135, 1975.

Sanders LE, Rossi RL, Shahian DM et al: Mediastinal goiters. The need for an aggressive approach. Arch Surg 127:609, 1992.

Shaha AR, Alfonso AK, Jaffe BM: Operative treatment of substernal goiters. Head Neck 11:325, 1989a.

Shaha AR, Burnett C, Alfonso A, et al: Goiter and airway problems. Am J Surg 158:378, 1989b.

Shahian DM, Rossi RL: Posterior mediastinal goiter. Chest 94:599, 1988.

Shields TW: Lesions masquerading as primary mediastinal tumors or cysts. In Shields TW (ed): Mediastinal Surgery. Philadelphia, Lea & Febiger, 1991, p 118.

Shields TW: Primary tumors and cysts of the mediastinum. In Shields TW (ed): General Thoracic Surgery, 1st ed. Philadelphia, Lea & Febiger, 1972, p 931.

Singh B, Lucente FE, Shaha AR: Substernal goiter: A clinical review. Am J Otolaryngol 15:409, 1994.

Sussman SK, Silverman PM, Donnal JF: CT demonstration of isolated mediastinal goiter. J Comput Assist Tomogr 10:863, 1986.
Sweet RH: Intrathoracic goiter located in the posterior mediastinum. Surg Gynecol Obstet 89:57, 1949.
Torre G, Borgonovo G, Amato A et al: Surgical management of substernal goiter: Analysis of 237 patients. Am Surg 61:826, 1995.
Torres A, Arroyo J, Kastanos N et al: Acute respiratory failure and tracheal obstruction in patients with intrathoracic goiter. Crit Care Med 11:265, 1983.
van Doorn LG, Kranendonk SE: Partial unilateral phrenic nerve paralysis caused by a large intrathoracic goitre. Neth J Med 48:216, 1996.
von Schulthess GK, McMurdo K, Tscholakoff D et al: Mediastinal masses: MR imaging. Radiology 158:289, 1986.
Wakeley CPG, Mulvany JH: Intrathoracic goiter. Surg Gynecol Obstet 70:702, 1940.
Warren CPW: Acute respiratory failure and tracheal obstruction in the elderly with benign goiters. Can Med Assoc J 121:191, 1979.
Watt-Boolsen SW, Blichert-Toft M, Folke K et al: Surgical treatment of benign nontoxic intrathoracic goiter: A long-term observation. Am J Surg 141:721, 1981.
Willis RA: The Borderland of Embryology and Pathology. London, Butterworths, 1962.

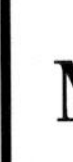

MEDIASTINAL PARATHYROID TUMORS

Carl E. Bredenberg
Clement A. Hiebert

A thoracic surgeon's familiarity with the parathyroid glands is essential for five contingencies:

1. A mediastinal hunt for the elusive quarry may be suggested by an endocrinologist or surgeon following an unsuccessful search for a hyperfunctioning gland or glands in the neck.
2. A mediastinal mass found on routine chest radiography may unexpectedly prove at operation to be a parathyroid cyst or tumor.
3. Failure to identify and reimplant parathyroid tissue during extensive resections of malignant growths of the cervical esophagus may result in life-threatening hypocalcemia. The surgeon needs to be familiar with the appearance and normal location of these lilliputian glands.
4. Hyperparathyroidism may be mimicked by other diseases, including squamous cancers of the lung and esophagus.
5. The thoracic surgeon must be aware that mediastinal parathyroid tumors usually are more accessible through a cervical incision than via a sternotomy or lateral thoracotomy and that the recurrent laryngeal nerve is especially vulnerable when the approach is via a right thoracotomy.

DEFINITION

Primary hyperparathyroidism is a disease caused by a tumor or hyperplasia of the parathyroid glands. Parathyroid hormone (PTH) increases serum ionized calcium, and it is the hypercalcemia that causes most of the symptoms and complications of the disease. Approximately 10% to 20% of abnormal parathyroid glands are found in the mediastinum (Clark 1988; Conn et al, 1991; Hiebert, unpublished data on 191 consecutive parathyroid operations; Russell et al, 1981; Wang, 1986).

HISTORICAL NOTE

The first detailed gross and microscopic description of the parathyroid glands in humans was made in 1877 by a Swedish medical student, Ivar Sandstrom (Thompson, 1990). It took a number of years to establish the physiologic and pathologic role of the parathyroid glands. Halsted at Johns Hopkins in 1906 relieved clinical tetany after thyroidectomy by giving a patient dietary supplements of parathyroid glands harvested from cattle and later confirmed these observations in experimental animals (Halsted, 1961). Also at Johns Hopkins and contemporary with Halsted's work, MacCallum, then a young pathologist, demonstrated experimentally that the parathyroid's major role was control of calcium metabolism and that tetany occurring after total parathyroid excision was caused by hypocalcemia (Halsted, 1961).

The first excision of a parathyroid tumor was for relief of demineralizing bone disease and was performed in 1924 by Felix Mandel in Vienna. Ironically, Mandel's patient had been treated for more than a year with parathyroid extracts and implantation of parathyroid glands in the mistaken belief that the bone disease was a result of parathyroid *insufficiency* (Cady and Rossi, 1991).

Collip, at the University of Alberta, isolated PTH in 1924, and Aub, an endocrinologist at the Massachusetts General Hospital, began using PTH to hasten the elimination of lead from the bones of patients with lead poisoning (Cope, 1966). In so doing, Aub demonstrated the increase in serum calcium, fall in serum phosphate, and increase in urinary elimination of calcium that came to be recognized as characteristic of hyperparathyroidism. This experience allowed Aub in 1926 to diagnose the source of the bone disease in Charles Martel, a sea captain, as a hyperfunctioning parathyroid gland, which led to the first operation in North America for hyperparathyroidism. A total of six neck explorations looking for an enlarged parathyroid gland were made in Captain Martel, beginning in 1926, each without success.

In 1928 Bulger and colleagues at Washington University in St. Louis, stimulated in part by discussions with Aub, diagnosed hyperparathyroidism in a 57-year-old woman with bone disease, and I. Y. Olch was the first surgeon in North America to remove a parathyroid adenoma successfully (Barr et al, 1929).

Persisting and building on the solid endocrinology base of Aub and his medical colleagues Bauer and Albright, Edward Churchill at the Massachusetts General Hospital in 1931 directed Oliver Cope, then his resident, to study the anatomic distribution of parathyroid glands in the autopsy suite. On the basis of the experience obtained in the postmortem dissections, Cope and Churchill in 1932 began a systematic development of surgery for parathyroid disease, and it was these two surgeons who performed the last three of the six unsuccessful cervical explorations in Captain Martel. The relationship of the bone disease and a hyperactive parathyroid gland was so soundly based on the physiologic understanding of their endocrinology colleagues that Cope and Churchill, on the basis of embryologic studies, finally explored the mediastinum of Martel and found the parathyroid tumor "just lateral to the superior vena cava." Its successful removal was the first excision of a *mediastinal* parathyroid adenoma; the patient's calcium promptly fell to tetanic levels (Cope, 1966).

■ *HISTORICAL READINGS*

Barr DP, Bulger HA, Dixon HH: Hyperparathyroidism. JAMA 29:951, 1929.

Cady B, Rossi RL (eds): Surgery of the Thyroid and Parathyroid Glands, 3rd ed. Philadelphia, WB Saunders, 1991.

Cope O: The story of hyperparathyroidism at the Massachusetts General Hospital. N Engl J Med 274:1171, 1966.

Halsted WE: Surgical Papers, Vol 2. Baltimore, Johns Hopkins Press, 1961.

Thompson NW: The history of hyperparathyroidism. Acta Chir Scand 156:5, 1990.

BASIC SCIENCE

Most of the clinical manifestations of primary hyperparathyroidism are caused by hypercalcemia. PTH increases serum calcium by three mechanisms: by stimulating calcium release from bone, by increasing reabsorption of calcium from the renal tubules, and by increasing renal conversion of vitamin D to a metabolically more active form, which in turn increases intestinal absorption of calcium (Cady and Rossi 1991; Clark 1985; Friesen and Thompson, 1990).

PTH also decreases renal tubular reabsorption of phosphorus and bicarbonate. Low serum phosphate is commonly present with primary hyperparathyroidism, and in advanced cases bicarbonate loss may lead to metabolic acidosis. In addition to hyperfunctioning parathyroid glands, other diseases such as sarcoid, hypernephroma, and metastatic cancer may cause hypercalcemia, and some, particularly squamous cell carcinomas of the lung or esophagus, produce a peptide that binds to PTH receptor and mimics some of the actions of PTH.

Pathology

About 85% of patients with primary hyperparathyroidism have a solitary adenoma, 3% have multiple adenomas, and 12% have hyperplasia of all four glands. About 1% have parathyroid cancer (Thompson et al, 1982). The same proportions also apply to mediastinal parathyroids (Clark 1988; Hiebert, unpublished data; Wang et al, 1986). Although histologic criteria have been offered to distinguish between adenoma and hyperplasia—for example, cellular density, amount of interstitial fat, and a rim of "normal" parathyroid around an abnormally dense nodule of parathyroid tissue—none of these histologic findings absolutely distinguishes between the two processes (Bonjer et al, 1992; Wells et al, 1985). Traditionally, the diagnosis of a solitary adenoma required identification by the surgeon of one enlarged parathyroid gland and at least one other normal-sized gland. Classification of multiple gland disease as either multiple adenoma(s) or four-gland hyperplasia is difficult (Bonjer et al, 1992; Wells et al, 1985), and many surgeons advocate routine identification of all four parathyroids (Wells et al, 1985).

The diagnosis of parathyroid cancer is difficult to make on cellular morphology alone and usually requires the identification of invasion of adjacent soft tissue or the finding of metastatic disease (Favia et al, 1998). Parathyroid cysts also occur either in the neck or the mediastinum in the same anatomic distribution as parathyroid tumors. Forty percent to 50% of these are functioning cysts producing PTH and are associated with hypercalcemia (Landau et al, 1997; Shields and Immerman, 1999).

Embryology

The variable position of the parathyroid glands can only be understood on the basis of embryology. The parathyroid glands arise from the third and fourth branchial pouches during the fifth week of embryogenesis (Moore, 1988; Weller, 1933). The superior parathyroids (IV) arise from the fourth branchial pouches contiguous with the lateral components of the thyroid, and they normally come to lie on the posterolateral surface of the thyroid gland above the crossing of the recurrent laryngeal nerve by the inferior parathyroid artery (Fig. 63–60).

The lower parathyroids (III) arise with the thymic primordia in the third pharyngeal pouch and migrate with the future thymus into the lower neck and superior mediastinum (Weller, 1933) (see Fig. 63–60). Parathyroid III thus becomes the lower parathyroid and most often settles at the cephalad end of the thymus immediately below the thyroid's lower pole. This development does not always occur, however, for during the descent of the thymus, anlage scraps of the future lower parathyroids drop off and tumble like pebbles from an advancing glacier. The surgeon must know both the route of the thymus "glacier" and where the randomly displaced parathyroids are likely to have come to rest. It is also important that the thoracic surgeon know "if the search is for parathyroid III or parathyroid IV, so that the most likely "moraine" is searched first (Figs. 63–61 and 63–62).

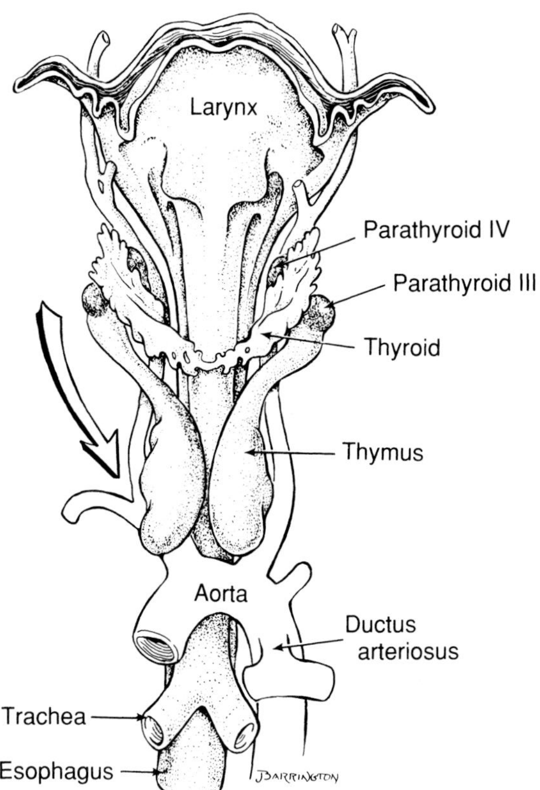

FIGURE 63–60 ■ Drawing of a 23-mm embryo, illustrating embryologic relationships of parathyroids, thyroid, and thymus. Parathyroid IV has come to rest on the posterolateral aspect of the thyroid, which was formed by the union of two lateral components with a midline component. Parathyroid III is still contiguous with the cephalad end of the thymus, and both are in the process of descent into the lower neck and superior mediastinum. Parathyroid III anlage may come to rest anywhere in the thymus itself, on the anterior superior pericardium, or adjacent to the aorta and great arteries and veins of the superior mediastinum. See Figure 63–62 for the same projection in the adult. (Adapted from Weller GL: Development of the thyroid. Parathyroid and thymus glands in man. Contrib Embryol 141:95, 1933.)

Surgical Anatomy

There are normally four parathyroid glands. In 2% to 6% of unselected subjects, there is a fifth gland. In fewer than 3% of otherwise normal individuals only three glands are ever identified (Akerstrom et al, 1984; Wang, 1976). A hyperfunctioning gland or glands are found in the mediastinum in 11% to 22% of patients; fortunately, fewer than 4% of all patients require a thoracotomy for excision (Clark, 1988; Conn et al, 1991; Hiebert, unpublished data; Russell et al, 1981; Wang, 1986).

The locations of ectopic lower parathyroids (embryologically parathyroid III) are shown in Figures 63–61 and 63–62. About one third of normal lower parathyroid glands are found below the lower pole of the thyroid in the cervical tongue of the thymus or in the thyroid-thymic tract of fat, fascia, and vein that extends from the lower pole of the thyroid to the tip of the mediastinal thymus (Akerstrom et al, 1984; Gilmour, 1937, 1938; Wang, 1976). At reoperation for a "missing" parathyroid gland, the thymus itself is a likely site. In one series of mainly cervical reoperations (Wang, 1977), one third of the pathologic glands were found within the thymus, of which 40% were in the cervical thymus and 60% in the mediastinal thymus. Direct surgical re-exploration of the mediastinum through a sternotomy is infrequently required; when it is performed, 50% to 75% of the hyperfunctioning mediastinal parathyroids are found within the thymus (Conn et al, 1991; Norton et al, 1985; Russell et al, 1981; Wang et al, 1986).

Ectopic lower parathyroids that are not within the thymus or the thyroid thymic tract are generally found in one of the following superior mediastinal sites (see Figs. 63–61 and 63–62):

1. Closely related to the thymus anteriorly, or posteriorly between thymus and great vessels and pericardium, or caudad to the thymus on pericardium
2. Related to the left or right innominate vein, or on either side of the superior vena cava
3. Along the ascending aorta, proximal innominate, or right or left common carotid arteries
4. Adjacent to the ascending aorta from the left anterolateral aspect into its concavity and onto the superior or anterior surface of the left pulmonary artery within the mediastinal pleural reflection close to the ligamentum arteriosum (the "aortopulmonary window")

Although the possibility of intrapericardial parathyroids has been mentioned, embryologically this should be impossible (Gilmour, 1937; Norton et al, 1985; Weller, 1933).

Posterior mediastinal glands most usually represent superior parathyroids (embryologically, parathyroid IV). It is thought that the size and weight of the enlarged gland, combined with negative intrathoracic pressure, cause the enlarged gland to fall posteriorly and interiorly toward the esophagus and posterior mediastinum (Wang et al, 1986). These posterior mediastinal glands are found in the retroesophageal space, laterally along the esophagus, or in the tracheal esophageal groove. Almost always they can be extracted via a cervical incision. At reoperation for persistent hyperparathyroidism, one third of missing glands have been found in the retroesophegeal or paraesophageal area, either in the neck or further down in the posterior mediastinum (Wang, 1977).

On rare occasions the middle mediastinum harbors the missing parathyroid (Curley et al, 1988) in the area anterior to the carina or right or left mainstem bronchi, posterior to the ascending aorta, and posterior or superior to the right or left pulmonary artery (Fig. 63–63; see Fig. 63–61).

Finally, a word about supernumerary glands. When four biopsy-proven glands have been uncovered without correcting the hyperparathyroidism, the presence of a fifth gland may be assumed. Two thirds of such elusive tumors are found below the thyroid, associated with the thymus or the thyroid-thymic tract. Most remaining supernumerary glands are found in the neck between the normal locations of the upper and lower parathyroids (Akerstrom et al, 1984; Russell et al, 1982).

DIAGNOSIS

Rarely, abnormal parathyroids may present as an undiagnosed mediastinal mass or cyst. Fifty percent to 60% of

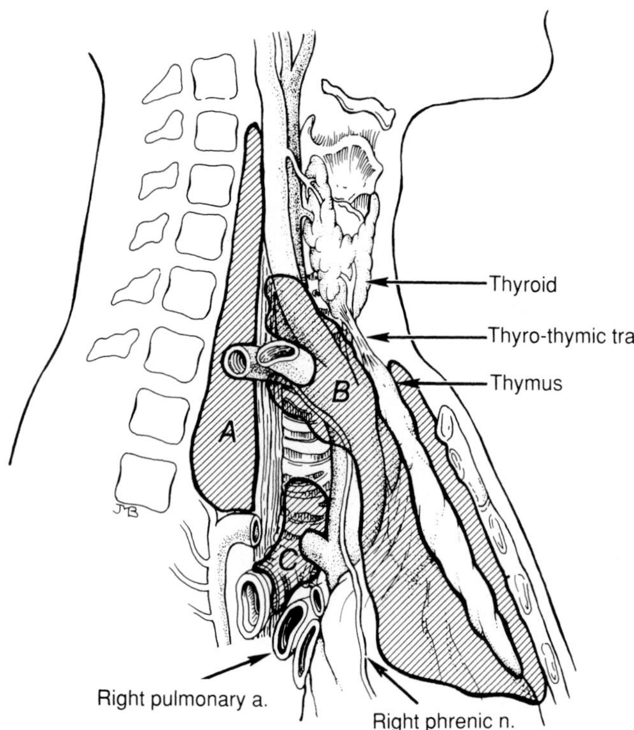

FIGURE 63–61 ■ The three regions in which mediastinal ectopic parathyroid glands are found. A, Retroesophageal and paraesophageal region, which spans both the neck and the upper mediastinum down to the level of the carina (ectopic upper parathyroid IV). B, Anterior mediastinum, including thymus and posteriorly the pericardium, the aortic arch, and the great vessels of the upper mediastinum (ectopic lower parathyroid III). C, Midmediastinal compartment in front of carina and mainstem bronchi. Note the close proximity anteriorly of the right pulmonary artery. This area extends out of view along the left main bronchus underneath the aortic arch into the aortopulmonary window (see Fig. 63–62).

mediastinal parathyroid cysts are nonfunctioning, and in others the hyperfunctioning state may not be clinically evident until serum calcium and PTH levels are drawn (Landau et al 1997; Shields and Immerman, 1999). Even more rarely, acute hemorrhage into a parathyroid adenoma may cause acute chest pain mimicking dissecting aneurysm or other chest pathology (Berry et al, 1974). Usually, however, the thoracic surgeon is consulted when hypercalcemia persists or recurs following one or more unsuccessful surgical explorations of the neck. Because a small percentage of failed operations for abnormal parathyroid glands are the result of disease other than hyperparathyroidism, the original diagnosis should be reconfirmed if there is any doubt.

Hyperparathyroidism is a condition with a wide variety of symptoms and associated diseases. In patients with primary hyperparathyroidism, more severe symptoms are generally associated with higher serum calcium levels and larger glands. Demineralizing bone disease caused by a direct effect of PTH on bone osteoblasts and osteoclasts produces symptoms of bone pain, tenderness, and susceptibility to fractures (Cady and Rossi, 1991). Renal and ureteral calculi were once frequent presenting signs of hyperparathyroidism. Functional abnormalities of the kidney are more frequently found today, arising from renal tubular abnormalities, including decreased reabsorption of bicarbonate and decreased ability to concentrate urine. Thus, dehydration and metabolic acidosis can be part of the clinical presentation of severe hyperparathyroidism. Subtle psychiatric symptoms are common, including difficulty in concentration or mild depression. Mild proximal muscle weakness may also be present. Joint complications, with pain and effusions due to calcification of articular cartilage, as well as true gout and pseudogout, may occur.

Patients with serum calcium levels below 11 mg/dl may be asymptomatic. Patients with calcium levels between 11 and 14.5 mg/dl may have lethargy, anorexia, weight loss, weakness, and fatigue, in addition to any of the foregoing symptoms. Hypercalcemic crisis occurs at serum levels above 14.5 mg/dl and may be associated with anorexia, leading to nausea and vomiting, fatigue, confusion, and ultimately stupor and coma (Cady and Rossi, 1991; Clark, 1985). Hypercalcemic crisis is a life-threatening emergency, therapy of which includes hydration with isotonic saline solution and vigorous diuresis to increase urinary excretion of calcium. Urgent diagnostic workup looking for the etiology of the hypercalcemia must be carried out.

The causes of hypercalcemia, of which malignancy and hyperparathyroidism are the most common, are summarized in Table 63–30. Hyperparathyroidism is more frequently seen in outpatients newly presenting with hypercalcemia, while malignancy is the more common cause of hypercalcemia in hospitalized patients. The hypercalcemia of malignancy may be due to bony metastasis or to tumors, such as some squamous carcinomas, that secrete a PTH-like substance. The most common tumors that cause hypercalcemia are squamous cell carcinomas of the lung, hypernephromas, multiple myelomas, and lymphomas. Chest radiography, urinalysis, intravenous pyelography or kidney ultrasound, complete blood count, and serum electrophoresis are helpful in excluding these malignancies (Clark, 1985). After exclusion of other causes of hypercalcemia, the diagnosis of primary hyperparathyroidism is confirmed by the findings of sustained

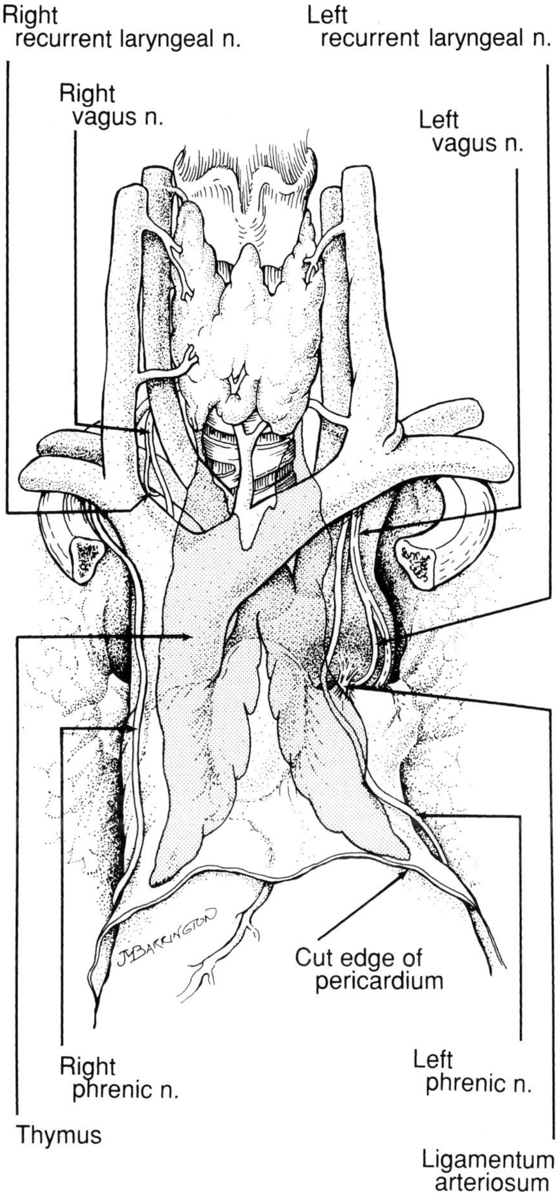

Right recurrent laryngeal n.
Left recurrent laryngeal n.
Right vagus n.
Left vagus n.
Cut edge of pericardium
Right phrenic n.
Left phrenic n.
Thymus
Ligamentum arteriosum

FIGURE 63–62 ■ The moraine of the embryologic descent of the thymic glacier, which includes the sites of the mediastinal ectopic lower parathyroid (III). The pericardium and major vascular structures provide the key landmarks. Note the phrenic, vagus, and recurrent laryngeal nerves, which must be protected on each side. The search may extend onto the anterior surface of the left pulmonary artery or may require division of the ligamentum arteriosum to gain full exposure of the aortopulmonary window. Beneath the aortic arch is the left-sided extension of the "midmediastinal" location of ectopic parathyroids.

elevations in serum calcium and elevated serum PTH levels (Cady and Rossi, 1991; Clark, 1985; Friesen and Thompson, 1990).

Localizing Studies

With the diagnosis of primary hyperparathyroidism secure, the principal diagnostic problem is anatomic localization of the hyperfunctioning parathyroid gland(s). Although localizing studies are not routinely advocated prior to initial cervical exploration for primary hyperparathyroidism, re-exploration of the neck is far more tedious and exposes the patient to greater likelihood of complications, such as recurrent laryngeal nerve injury. Mediastinal exploration is an even larger operation, requiring an extensive and often lengthy search. Hence, preoperative imaging studies aimed at localizing the missing parathyroid are advisable prior to re-exploration.

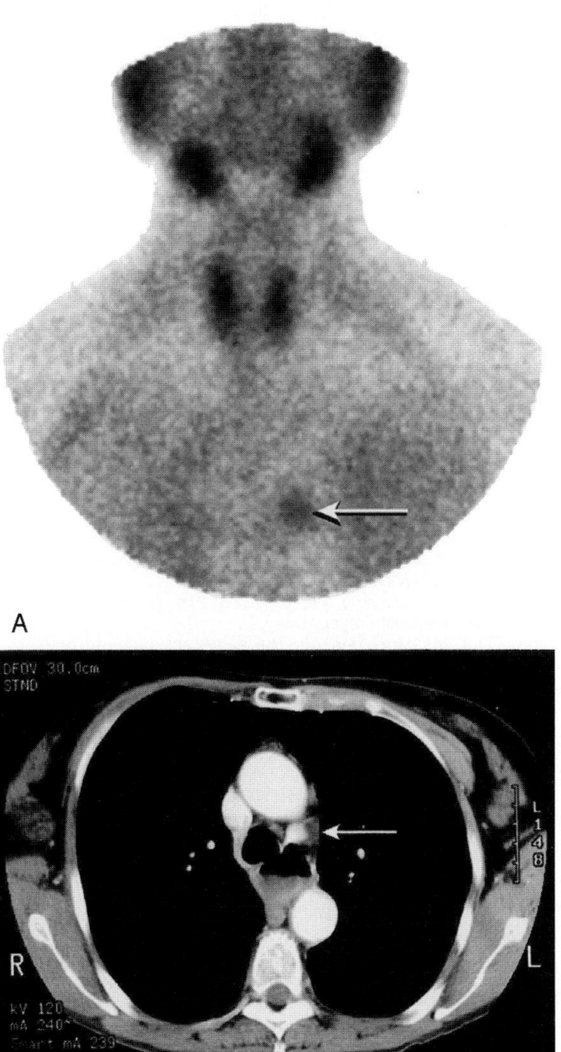

FIGURE 63–63 ■ Images from a patient with persistent hypercalcemia and elevated serum parathyroid hormone following neck exploration in which three normal parathyroid glands were found. *A*, Sestamibi scan. *Arrow* points to midmediastinal parathyroid adenoma. Also illuminated in the neck are the two lobes of the thyroid as well as the salivary glands. *B*, Helical computed tomography scan with IV contrasts and 3-mm thick images of the upper mediastinum. *Arrow* points to a contrast-enhanced 1-cm diameter nodule corresponding to the abnormality seen on the sestamibi scan and located posterior to the ascending aorta on the left anterior lateral aspect of the distal trachea and anterior to a dilated esophagus. This mass was excised via median sternotomy, and histology confirmed a parathyroid adenoma weighing 0.6 g and measuring 1 cm in its greatest dimension.

TABLE 63–30 ■ **Causes of Hypercalcemia**

Condition	*Approximate Frequency (%)*
Malignancy	35
Breast cancer	
Metastatic tumor	
PTH-secreting tumor	
Multiple myeloma	
Acute and chronic leukemia	
Hyperparathyroidism	30
MEA syndrome*	
Artifact (e.g., laboratory error, dirty glassware, cork stopper, tight tourniquet)	10
Increased intake	10
Milk-alkali syndrome	
Vitamin D and A overdose	
Thiazide diuretics	
Lithium	
Aluminum	
Granulomatous disease	5
Sarcoidosis	
Tuberculosis	
Berylliosis	
Other endocrine disorders	5
Hyperthyroidism	
Hypothyroidism	
Addison's disease	
VIP-secreting tumor	
Miscellaneous	5
Immobolization	
Paget's disease	
Idiopathic hypercalcemia of infancy	
Benign familial hypocalciuric hypercalcemia	

*Hyperparathyroidism as a manifestation of MEA syndrome is beyond the scope of this chapter.

MEA, multiple endocrine adenomatosis; PTH, parathyroid hormone; VIP, vasoactive intestinal polypeptide.

From Clark OH, Siperstein AE: The hypercalcemic syndrome: hyperparathyroidism. In Friesen SR, Thompson NW (eds): Surgical Endocrinology, 2nd ed. Philadelphia, JB Lippincott, 1990, with permission.

^{99m}Tc sestamibi is currently the most useful nuclear imaging study for parathyroid adenoma (McHenry et al, 1996; Peeler et al, 1997). The distribution of sestamibi is proportional to blood flow, and it is sequestered primarily in mitochondria, which are abundant in the cells of parathyroid adenomas. Sestamibi also illuminates thyroid and salivary glands, but delayed images or subtraction of radioiodine-labeled images can help distinguish parathyroid from thyroid adenoma (McHenry et al, 1996; Peeler et al, 1997). Success in localization increases with increasing size of the abnormal parathyroid gland. Rates of successful localization range from 60% to 90%. However, sestamibi scanning does not provide precise reference landmarks to direct the surgeon to his quarry. Hence, a second imaging study with more anatomic clarity is recommended, for example, spiral CT scanning with intravenous contrast or magnetic resonance imaging. (The accuracy of both of these imaging techniques also improves with increasing size of the gland.) Twenty-five percent of parathyroid tumors enhance with contrast. The larger the gland, the better the chance of a helpful display (see Fig. 63–63). Overall localization rates for CT or MRI have been 46% to 76% (Peeler et al, 1997).

Ultrasonography is not useful in localizing mediastinal glands (Clark, 1985; Friesen and Thompson, 1990). Highly selective arteriography and selective venous sampling for PTH are seldom used. These tests are less sensitive and even in experienced hands carry significant risks of spinal cord or cerebral infarction (Cady and Rossi, 1991). A 12-minute intraoperative venous assay of PTH has been used to provide intraoperative physiologic confirmation that the excised mass was the offending parathyroid. (Irvin et al, 1994). This test is not routinely available, however.

OPERATIVE MANAGEMENT

The surgeon's goal is to remove either the hyperfunctioning adenoma(s) or, if hyperplasia is the pathologic process, to remove three and a half parathyroid glands. The value of a thorough neck exploration at the first operation is paramount; so is the knowledge that most mediastinal glands can be reached through this initial neck incision. Although 10% to 20% of patients with primary hyperparathyroidism have abnormal glands located in the mediastinum, less than 4% of patients require thoracotomy or sternotomy (Hiebert, unpublished data; Norton et al, 1985; Russell et al, 1981; Wang et al, 1986). Adequate neck exploration includes transcervical thymectomy, retropharyngeal-esophageal exploration, and transcervical exploration of the superior mediastinum, as previously mentioned.

A meticulous and precise identification of parathyroid glands is aided by the use of a head lamp and 2× to 3× optical loupes. In searching the tracheal esophageal groove and paraesophageal space, beware that the recurrent laryngeal nerve may cross a superior parathyroid gland (Fig. 63–64). Be on the lookout for vascular tethers stretching from the thyroid arteries. Be methodical, and above all, don't hurry. Permanent hypoparathyroidism can result from excising or devascularizing too much parathyroid tissue. Take biopsy samples at a distance from the vascular pedicle and avoid grasping the gland with forceps (Friesen and Thompson, 1990; Hiebert, 1993; Thompson et al, 1982; Wang, 1977). The superior parathyroid gland may be found beneath the capsule of the thyroid, which makes it difficult to see until that capsule is incised; 2% to 5% of lower parathyroid glands have been found within the thyroid parenchyma (Thompson et al, 1982; Wang, 1976) and have either been removed by thyroid lobectomy or enucleated after incision of the thyroid parenchyma. At least three or more normal parathyroid glands should have been identified before the neck is ruled out as the source of the missing gland. Following this protocol, Thompson and associates (1982) had a failure rate of initial cervical exploration of only 4%. In one of the authors' (CAH) unpublished series of 191 patients, 21 abnormal glands (11%) were found in the mediastinum at primary operation. Using a cervical incision, mediastinal glands were extracted from the anterior mediastinum within or adjacent to the thymus, from the retroesophageal or paraesophageal posterior mediastinum, from the superior aspect of the aortic arch at the origin of the left common carotid artery, and in one instance from behind the tracheal bifurcation. In these 191 patients, only a single gland

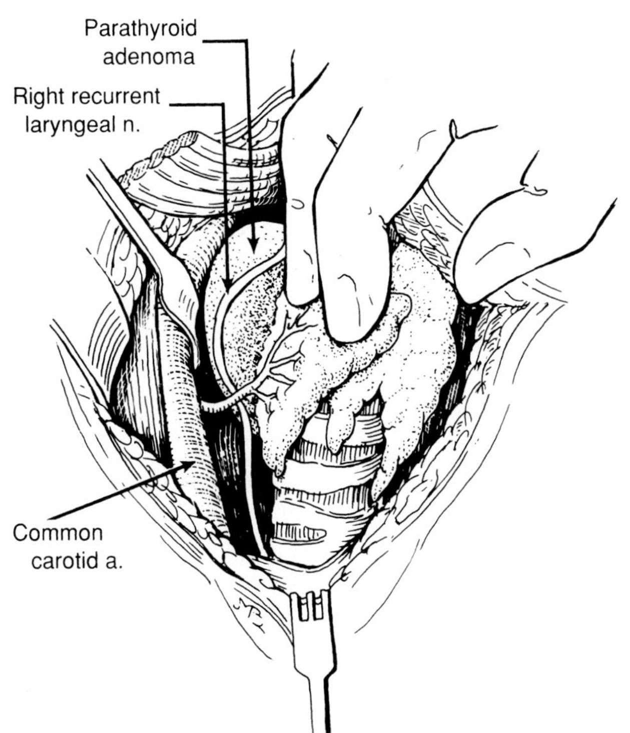

FIGURE 63–64 ■ Drawing of a large superior parathyroid adenoma lying behind the right recurrent laryngeal nerve above the crossing of the inferior thyroid artery and extending back into the retroesophageal space. This space extends caudally into the posterior mediastinum and is a frequent ectopic site of superior parathyroid glands (parathyroid IV). Posterior glands such as these, whether in the neck or lower in the posterior mediastinum, can be removed via a cervical incision. (From Thompson NW, Eckhauser FE, Harnes JK: The anatomy of primary hypoparathyroidism. Surgery 92:814, 1982; and Hiebert CA: unpublished data on 191 connective parathyroid operations, 1993.)

(a fifth supernumerary gland) located on the anterior pericardium caudad to the thymus required subsequent sternotomy for excision. Using a collar incision to remove certain mediastinal parathyroid tumors is analogous to withdrawing a substernal goiter from the neck. Not only is it less traumatic overall to do so, but the recurrent laryngeal nerves may stand a better chance of surviving (see Fig. 63–64).

Even at *re-exploration*, most missing parathyroid glands are found in the neck or can be extracted from the upper mediastinum via a cervical incision; only 20% of reoperations require median sternotomy or other direct thoracic exploration (Clark, 1988; Wang, 1977). Moreover, in one series of sternal explorations (Wang, 1977), two thirds of the glands were found in the upper anterior mediastinum or mediastinal thymus and potentially within reach of cervical exploration.

If thorough neck re-exploration and transcervical exploration of the upper mediastinum give negative results, opinion is divided as to whether to proceed at the same operation to sternotomy and definitive mediastinal exploration or, alternatively, to close and bring the patient back at a later date for reoperation. Most surgeons prefer to close the reoperated neck and return at a later date for mediastinal exploration. The unsuccessful cervical exploration has usually already been tedious and frustrating, which may hamper immediate detailed mediastinal exploration. Other surgeons (Norton et al, 1985) note the improved exposure of the anatomic interface between neck and mediastinum afforded by a combined incision, but a higher wound complication rate has also accompanied this approach.

Unless confident preoperative localization warrants a different approach, median sternotomy offers the most complete exposure. Avoid right lateral thoracotomy, an approach that endangers the recurrent laryngeal nerve (Fig. 63–65). When preoperative studies have identified the anatomic location of the missing parathyroid in the mediastinum, a video-assisted thoracoscopic procedure may be a less traumatic means of excising the gland (Knight et al, 1997).

Outcome

Even in the most experienced hands, mediastinal exploration for missing parathyroids fails to find an abnormal gland in one third of cases (Conn et al, 1991; Russell et al, 1981; Wang et al, 1986). In one series of mediastinal explorations, 85% of patients had an abnormal parathyroid gland removed, but only 70% of these abnormal glands were removed from the mediastinum, the remainder having been found in the neck through a concomitant cervical incision (Norton et al, 1985). In another series of transsternal mediastinal explorations, the missing gland in one third of the failures subsequently was found in a later neck exploration (Wang et al, 1986). In a small number of patients, another etiology for the hypercalcemia is eventually established (Thompson et al, 1982; Wang et al, 1986).

Because mediastinal exploration is a more formidable operation and has a higher failure rate, nonoperative management and simple observation may be chosen in the asymptomatic patient with minimally elevated serum calcium levels (<11 mg/dl) (Wang, 1977; Wang et al, 1986). The rationale is that this mild degree of hyperparathyroidism is rarely life-threatening. Furthermore, with this mild disease the missing gland is generally small and thus more difficult to find at mediastinal exploration or cervical re-exploration.

Postoperative Concerns

Serum calcium levels fall following parathyroidectomy, usually reaching a nadir about 48 to 72 hours following operation. Transient hypocalcemia may occur postoperatively as a consequence of prior suppression of normal parathyroid tissue by hyperfunctioning glands. Also, patients with severe bone disease from hyperparathyroidism can develop "bone hunger" postoperatively, and with the bones taking up calcium and phosphorus, the fall of serum calcium and phosphorus is apt to be rapid (Cady and Rossi, 1991; Clark, 1985).

The clinical manifestations of acute hypocalcemia include numbness around the mouth, paresthesias of fingers and toes, muscle cramps, and carpopedal spasms. Laryngospasm with airway obstruction may also compli-

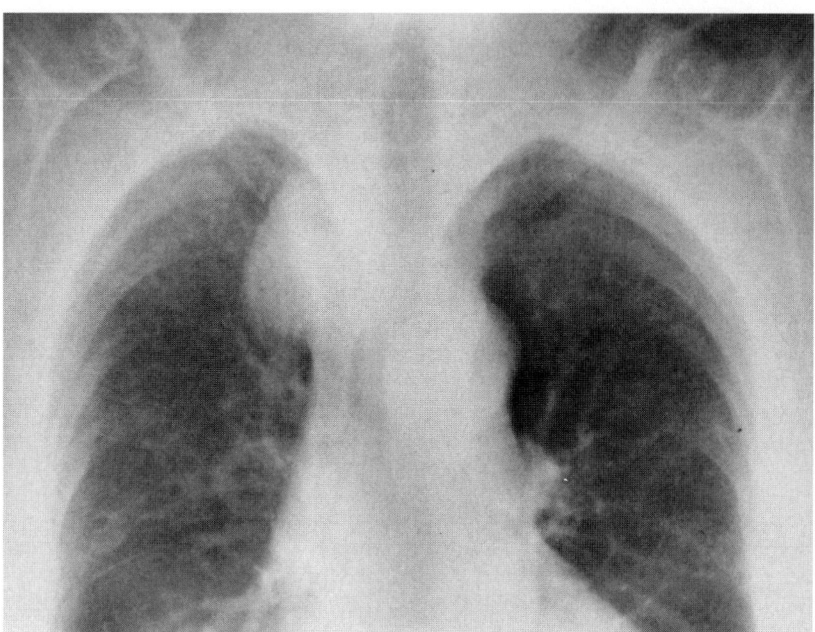

FIGURE 63–65 ■ Chest radiograph of a 57-year-old woman with a 20-year history of nephrolithiasis and a parathyroid tumor in the upper mediastinum. Awkward exposure through a right lateral thoracotomy resulted in inadvertent division of the recurrent laryngeal nerve as it looped around the lower margin of the growth.

cate hypocalcemia. Profound hypocalcemia may lead to tetany (i.e., seizures) and opisthotonos (a form of tetanic spasm of the entire body, in which the head and heels are bent backward and the body bowed forward (Cady and Rossi, 1991; Clark, 1985). Hyperventilation with alkalosis further reduces the ionized calcium and can aggravate symptoms, whereas renal failure with acidosis may mask hypocalcemia temporarily. Chvostek's sign can be elicited by tapping the patient in the preauricular area over the facial nerve and observing a twitching of the ipsilateral corner of the mouth. This test is positive in 10% of normal persons (Cady and Rossi, 1991). Trousseau's sign is the observation of carpal spasms with flexion of the metacarpopharyngeal joints and extension of the interpharyngeal joints after inflation of an arm tourniquet above systolic pressure for 3 minutes. This test may be painful to the patient.

Low serum magnesium levels may also cause tetany, and thus both serum magnesium and calcium levels should be checked. Treatment of mild hypocalcemia (serum calcium, approximately 7.5 mg/dl) can be treated with oral calcium (calcium carbonate, 1 to 2 g three times daily with water). More severe hypocalcemia or tetany is treated with intravenous calcium, usually 10 to 20 ml of 10% calcium chloride or 20 to 30 ml of 10% calcium gluconate, given slowly by intravenous push over 5 minutes. An intravenous calcium drip is then started. Chronic hypoparathyroidism requires the administration of both oral calcium and vitamin D or its active component, calcitriol (Rocaltrol), 0.25 mg twice daily (Cady and Rossi, 1991; Clark, 1985).

A strategy for prevention of permanent hypoparathyroidism when one is uncertain of the adequacy of residual functioning tissue is to transplant parathyroid tissue to an easily accessible site such as the forearm or antecubital fossa, where 1-mm slices can be deposited in small muscle pockets and marked for future excision should recurrent hyperparathyroidism develop (Baumann and Wells, 1993). Parathyroid tissue can also be frozen and cryopreserved for later surgical autotransplantation if necessary (Norton et al, 1985). Autotransplantation of fresh or frozen parathyroid tissue into sternal mastoid muscle or the forearm may also prevent life-threatening hypocalcemia following extensive resections of cervical malignancy including the esophagus (Baumann and Wells, 1993). These techniques are all modern updates of experimental work done at the beginning of the century by Halsted and the subsequent clinical work of Churchill and Cope.

COMMENTS AND CONTROVERSIES

Drs. Bredenberg and Hiebert have provided a detailed summary of the investigation and management of hyperparathyroidism with particular reference to the mediastinal parathyroid. The detailed embryology and anatomic discussions provide full explanation for the anatomic location of most mediastinal parathyroids. They correctly point out that the majority of these lesions can be excised via the transcervical approach. This approach is facilitated by the use of an upper-hand retractor and adequate illumination. Use of a video thoracoscope with the cervical incision may provide further improvement in exposure. Indeed, for lesions in the lower mediastinum or subaortic window, a video-assisted thoracoscopic approach may be the approach of preference for complete excision of these lesions.

G. A. P.

■ KEY REFERENCES

Thompson NW, Eckhauser FE, Harnes JK: The anatomy of primary hyperparathyroidism. Surgery 92:814, 1982.

From one of the world's leading endocrine surgery services, a review of the pathology and anatomic location of abnormal parathyroids in 273 patients with primary hyperparathyroidism. Their 96% success rate of surgical exploration for primary hyperparathyroidism sets a standard.

Wang CA: The anatomic basis of parathyroid surgery. Ann Surg 183:271, 1976.

A well-written and clearly illustrated summary of the location of normal adult parathyroid glands found in the dissection of 160 cadavers. The adult anatomy is clearly related to embryology.

Wang CA: Parathyroid re-exploration: A clinical and pathological study of 112 cases. Ann Surg 186:140, 1977.

A review of 45 years of experience at the Massachusetts General Hospital in reoperation following one or more failed cervical explorations for abnormal hyperfunctioning parathyroids. This study documents the cervical and mediastinal location of abnormal glands found at re-exploration and outlines management principles for reoperative parathyroid surgery.

Wang CA, Gaz RD, Moncure AC: Mediastinal parathyroid exploration: A clinical and pathologic study of 47 cases. World J Surg 10:687, 1986.

A review of nearly 60 years of experience at the Massachusetts General Hospital, going back to the very first mediastinal exploration on Captain Martel in 1926. A clear description of the pathology and most importantly, the anatomic locations of abnormal parathyroids that were found at median sternotomy. Of a total of 1200 patients with hyperparathyroidism surgically treated during that interval, 47 underwent mediastinal exploration.

Weller GL: Development of the thyroid, parathyroid and thymus glands in man. Contrib Embryol 141:95, 1933.

The fundamental study documenting the embryologic development of the parathyroid glands. It includes the embryology of the thyroid and thymus glands and is invaluable for understanding the anatomy of these structures.

■ *REFERENCES*

Akerstrom G, Malmaeus J, Bergstrom R: Surgical anatomy of human parathyroid glands. Surgery 95:14, 1984.

Barr DP, Bulger HA, Dixon HH: Hyperparathyroidism. JAMA 29:951, 1929.

Baumann DS, Wells SA: Parathyroid autotransplantation. Surgery 113:130, 1993.

Berry BE, Carpenter PC, Fulton RE, Danielson GK: Mediastinal hemorrhage from parathyroid adenoma simulating dissecting aneurysm. Arch Surg 108:740, 1974.

Bonjer HJ, Bruining HA, Birkenhager JC: Single and multigland disease in primary hyperparathyroidism: Clinical follow-up, histopathology, and flow cytometric DNA analysis. World J Surg 16:737, 1992.

Cady B, Rossi RL (eds): Surgery of the Thyroid and Parathyroid Glands, 3rd ed. Philadelphia, WB Saunders, 1991.

Clark OH: Endocrine Surgery of the Thyroid and Parathyroid Glands. St. Louis, Mosby, 1985.

Clark OH: Mediastinal parathyroid tumors. Arch Surg 123:1096, 1988.

Conn JM, Goncalves MA, Mansour KA, McGrity WC: The mediastinal parathyroid. Am Surg 57:62, 1991.

Cope O: The story of hyperparathyroidism at the Massachusetts General Hospital. N Engl J Med 274:1171, 1966.

Curley IR, Wheeler MH, Thompson NW et al: The challenge of the middle mediastinal parathyroid. World J Surg 12:818, 1988.

Favia G, Lumachi F, Polistina F, D'Amico DF: Parathyroid carcinoma: Sixteen new cases and suggestions for correct management. World J Surg 22:1225, 1998.

Friesen SR, Thompson NW: Surgical Endocrinology: Clinical Syndromes, 2nd ed. Philadelphia, JB Lippincott, 1990.

Gilmour JR: The embryology of the parathyroid glands, the thymus and certain associated rudiments. J Pathol 45:507, 1937.

Gilmour JR: The gross anatomy of the parathyroid glands. J Pathol 46:133, 1938.

Halsted WS: Surgical Papers, Vol. 2. 3rd Printing. Baltimore, Johns Hopkins Press, 1961.

Irvin GL III, Prudhomme DL, Deriso GT et al: A new approach to parathyroidectomy. Ann Surg 219:574, 1994.

Knight R, Ratzer ER, Fenoglio ME, Moore JT: Thoracoscopic excision of mediastinal parathyroid adenomas: A report of two cases and review of the literature. J Am Coll Surg 185:481, 1997.

Landau O, Chamberlain DW, Kennedy RS et al: Mediastinal parathyroid cysts. Ann Thorac Surg 63:951, 1997.

McHenry CR, Lee K, Saadey J et al: Parathyroid localization with technetium-99m-sestamibi: A prospective evaluation. J Am Coll Surg 183:25, 1996.

Moore KL: The Developing Human: Clinically Oriented Embryology, 4th ed. Philadelphia, JB Lippincott, 1988.

Norton JA, Schneider PD, Brennan MF: Median sternotomy in reoperations for primary hyperparathyroidism. World J Surg 9:807, 1985.

Peeler BP, Martin WH, Sandler MP, Goldstein RE: Sestamibi parathyroid scanning and preoperative localization studies for patients with recurrent/persistent hyperparathyroidism or significant comorbid conditions: Development of an optimal localization strategy. Am Surg 63:37, 1997.

Russell CF, Edis AJ, Scholz DA et al: Mediastinal parathyroid tumors: Experience with 38 tumors requiring mediastinotomy for removal. Ann Surg 193:805, 1981.

Russell CF, Grant CS, Van Heerden JA: Hyperfunctioning supernumerary parathyroid glands. Mayo Clin Proc 57:121, 1982.

Shields TW, Immerman SC: Mediastinal parathyroid cysts revisited. Ann Thorac Surg 67:581, 1999.

Thompson NW: The history of hyperparathyroidism. Acta Chir Scand 156:5, 1990.

Wells SA, Leight GS, Hensley M, Dilley WG: Hyperparathyroidism associated with the enlargement of two or three parathyroid glands. Ann Surg 202:533, 1985.

CHAPTER **64**

Surgical Techniques

VIDEOTHORACOSCOPIC TRANSCERVICAL THYMECTOMY

Stephen D. Cassivi
Shaf Keshavjee

HISTORICAL NOTE

Thymectomy, for myasthenia gravis, was first performed in a nonthymomatous patient in 1911 by Sauerbruch, with postoperative improvement of myasthenic symptoms (Schumacher and Roth, 1913; Viets and Schwab, 1960). It was later, in 1939, that thymectomy was formally suggested as a treatment for myasthenia gravis by Alfred Blalock. He reported his encouraging results in a 19-year-old female with thymoma associated with myasthenia gravis (Blalock et al, 1939). Five years later, he reported the results of a further twenty thymectomies, including patients with nonthymomatous myasthenia (Blalock, 1944).

Since that time, thymectomy has become a mainstay of therapy for patients with myasthenia gravis (Saunders and Scopetta, 1994). Reports of modern case series have demonstrated the overall superiority of thymectomy to medical management alone, achieving a good or complete response in 85% of patients with minimal associated morbidity and mortality (Cooper et al, 1988; Frist et al, 1994; Mulder et al, 1989). For these reasons, myasthenic patients should be considered for thymectomy on presentation with early, generalized symptoms; with isolated ocular disability poorly controlled by medical management with anticholinesterase agents; or when side effects limit the use of these medications. Favorable outcomes after thymectomy have been particularly associated with the following specific factors: age under 45 years, female sex, short history of symptoms, preoperative symptoms not requiring corticosteroids or immunosuppressants, and thymic hyperplasia (Frist et al, 1994). It is our perception that acceptance of the transcervical thymectomy by neurologists and patients alike has led to referrals for surgical therapy earlier in the course of the disease.

PREOPERATIVE MANAGEMENT

Patients undergoing thymectomy should have their medical condition optimized prior to surgery with anticholinesterase medications along with the use of plasmapheresis in selected cases. Corticosteroids are generally avoided preoperatively in order to minimize the perioperative complications associated with steroid use.

There is no role for urgent thymectomy in patients with myasthenic crisis as immediate clinical improvement postoperatively should not be expected. Rather, a period of 3 to 12 months is most often observed before clinical improvement can be seen following thymectomy (Bulkley et al, 1997). Furthermore, surgery in the setting of myasthenic crisis predisposes the patient to a significantly increased risk of postoperative respiratory failure (Gracey et al, 1984).

Preoperative computed tomographic (CT) scanning is essential in all patients to rule out the presence of thymoma. If a thymoma is present, the preferred surgical approach is through a sternotomy or a partial upper sternotomy.

Anesthetic considerations revolve around the use of muscle relaxants. Myasthenic patients tend to be particularly sensitive to nondepolarizing agents. In general, for transcervical thymectomy, no muscle relaxants are required (El-Dawlatly and Ashour, 1994). The cervical incision has minimal postoperative pain, which, in general, is effectively controlled with oral analgesics.

SURGICAL OPTIONS

There are several surgical options for thymectomy. These include a videothoracoscopic transcervical thymectomy (VTCT), which is described in this chapter; a standard sternotomy; and the more radical procedure of "maximal thymectomy" via a median sternotomy combined with a horizontal cervical incision, as described by Jaretzki and associates (1988). Without randomized comparative studies, the decision as to surgical approach must rest on the surgeon's individual experience and facility with each given procedure. The underlying goal for thymectomy for myasthenia gravis remains the same regardless of surgical approach—a safe and complete thymectomy.

We prefer the VTCT approach for the treatment of nonthymomatous myasthenia gravis because, despite being a less invasive procedure, it gives excellent bilateral exposure of the thymus, including the lower poles, and permits, in the vast majority of cases, complete thymectomy. Furthermore, unlike transthoracic video-assisted thymectomies, the transcervical route obviates entry into the pleural spaces, provides enhanced exposure in the neck region, and does not require split lung anesthesia via a double-lumen endotracheal tube.

Transcervical thymectomy was the approach used for the earliest described thymectomies (Schumacher and Roth, 1913; Viets and Schwab, 1960), but it was replaced by the transsternal approach by Blalock and his contemporaries midway through the past century (Blalock, 1944). The transcervical approach was revisited in the 1960s by surgeons such as Crile (1966), Carlens and coworkers (1967), and Kirschner and colleagues (1969). A series of over 700 cases of transcervical thymectomy for myasthenia gravis by Papatestas and associates (1987), along with the technical refinement of improved retraction reported by Cooper and colleagues (1988), further demonstrated the utility of this approach. We have further modified the technique with the addition of the videothoracoscopic technique for improved visualization of the mediastinum through the transcervical approach.

OPERATIVE TECHNIQUE

The patient is intubated with a single-lumen tube in the supine position. The neck is extended, and an inflatable pillow is placed beneath the patient transversely, at the level of the scapulae, to permit further hyperextension of the neck (Fig. 64–1). The neck and full chest are prepared should a sternotomy be required.

A curvilinear incision is made in the skin at the base of the neck, one fingerbreadth above the sternal notch and extending, on each side, one fingerbreadth above the clavicular head to the medial border of the sternocleidomastoid muscle (Fig. 64–2). This incision is extended through the skin and platysma muscle. Flaps are then developed superiorly to the level of the inferior aspect of the thyroid cartilage and inferiorly to the sternal notch. The interclavicular ligament is divided. The strap muscles are then split vertically in the midline and elevated bilaterally to expose the superior poles of the thymus gland, which lie opposed to the posterior surface of the sternothyroid muscles. It is imperative that this be done using careful, sharp dissection with meticulous attention to control of small blood vessels with electrocautery. A bloodless field makes it significantly easier to delineate the upper poles of the thymus gland from fatty tissue in the neck.

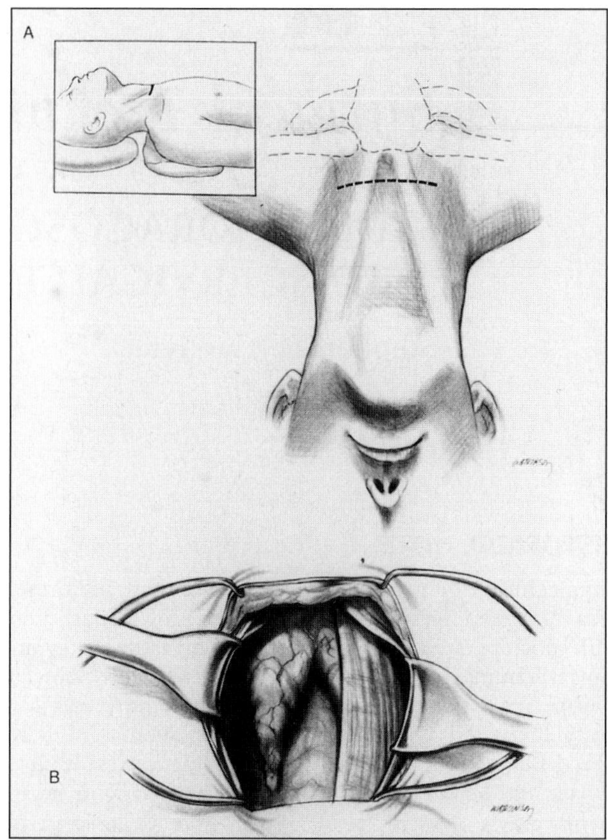

FIGURE 64–2 ■ *A*, Displayed from the surgeon's perspective at the head of the table, the incision is made one fingerbreadth above the sternal notch and clavicular heads, extending laterally to the medial border of the sternocleidomastoid muscle on each side. *B*, Dissection and lateral retraction of the strap muscles reveals the upper poles of the thymic gland.

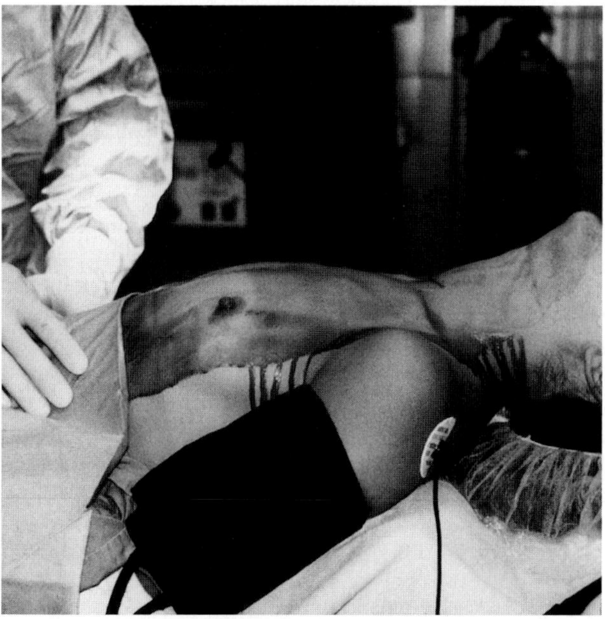

FIGURE 64–1 ■ The patient is positioned supine with the neck extended. An inflatable pillow permits further hyperextension of the neck, as necessary.

Each superior pole of the gland is mobilized near the inferior thyroid vein. The upper pole is divided between ties at the point at which the thymic tissue terminates. A heavy silk suture, cut long, is placed on each upper pole and is used as a "traction" suture to facilitate retraction of the gland. The thymus gland is then dissected inferiorly to the thoracic inlet, using a combination of blunt and sharp dissection (Fig. 64–3). A retrosternal space is cleared with blunt finger dissection. It is important to keep this dissection immediately substernal and to dissect at least 5 to 8 cm inferiorly to accommodate the placement of the Cooper retractor. Otherwise, the thymus will be pulled into the mediastinum by the retractor as it is inserted.

The Upper Hand retractor (Poly-Tract, Pilling Company, Fort Washington, PA), with the Cooper thymectomy re-

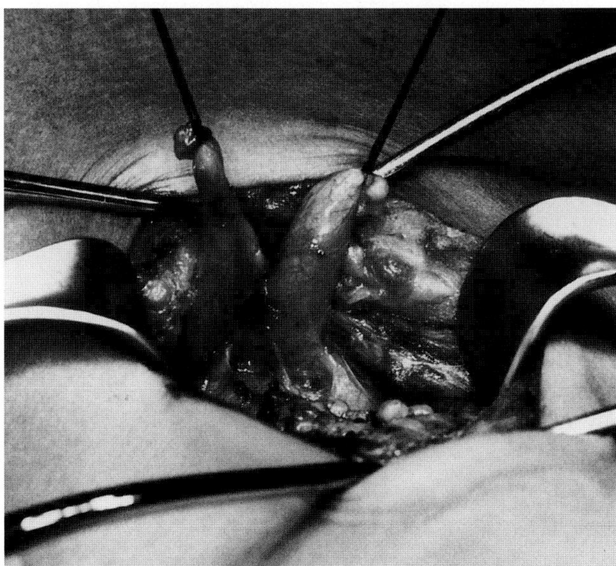

FIGURE 64–3 ■ Both upper poles are drawn anteriorly on traction ligatures.

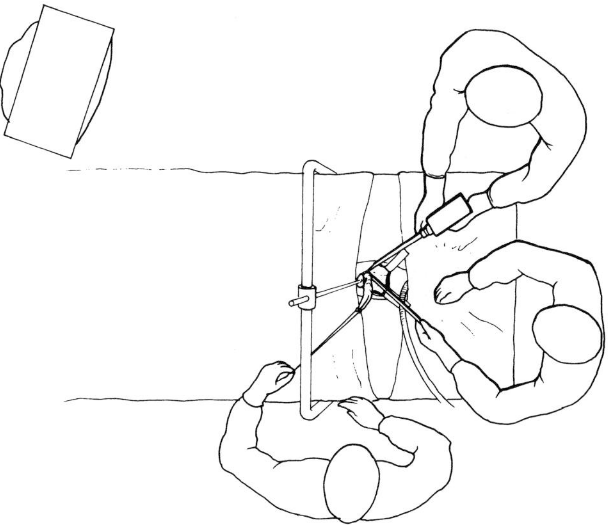

FIGURE 64–5 ■ This positioning of the surgeon and the assistants relative to the patient and the operative field permits optimal use of the 30-degree videoscope.

tractor blade (Pilling Company), is then placed beneath the sternum to elevate it and to open the thoracic inlet farther (Fig. 64–4). The inflatable pillow that was placed at the start of the procedure is deflated at this point to further improve the thoracic inlet exposure. Care should be taken to make sure that the patient's head is not elevated off the operating table pillow by the sternal retraction.

The 30-degree videothoracoscope is then placed at the right lateral aspect of the neck incision to provide light for direct operating and a video-magnified view of the operating field on a monitor for the surgeon and assistants (Fig. 64–5). Pressure is maintained laterally with the thoracoscope in order to keep the telescope out of the line of sight of the operating surgeon as much as possible. The dissection of the gland is carried down into the thorax using primarily blunt dissection. The thymic veins (there are often several), which drain into the innominate vein, are identified posteriorly and divided between stainless steel clips (Fig. 64–6). Two clips are placed on the innominate vein side. The arterial vessels, which enter the gland laterally from the internal thoracic arteries, are also clipped with stainless steel clips. The ventilatory tidal volume and rate can both be decreased in order to facilitate exposure in the mediastinum. The dissection of the gland is carried down alternately on both sides until the inferior poles of the gland are clearly identified, and a dissecting "peanut" on a curved Swedish-Debakey dissector is used to sweep each inferior pole upward (Fig. 64–7). The dissector is placed on the pericardium, distal to the inferior pole of the thymus gland,

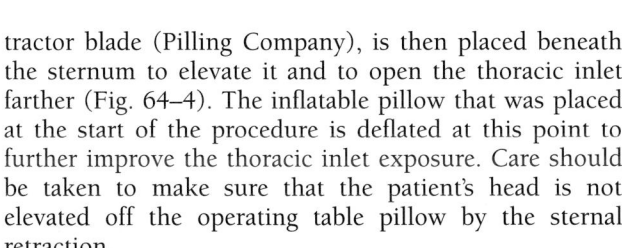

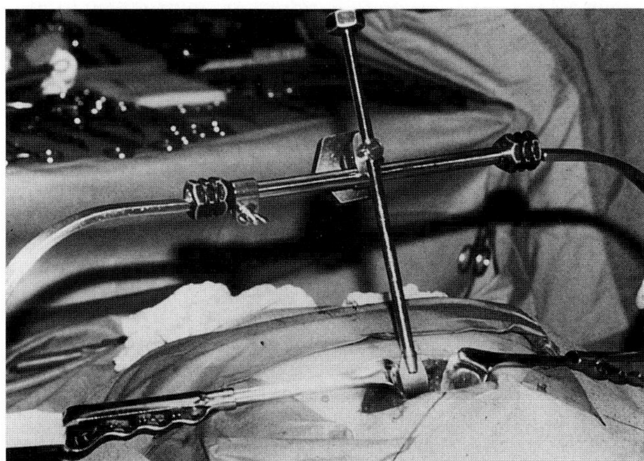

FIGURE 64–4 ■ The upper-hand retractor with the Cooper thymectomy retractor blade is positioned with the blade in the dissected retrosternal space. This allows elevation of the sternum and opening of the thoracic inlet.

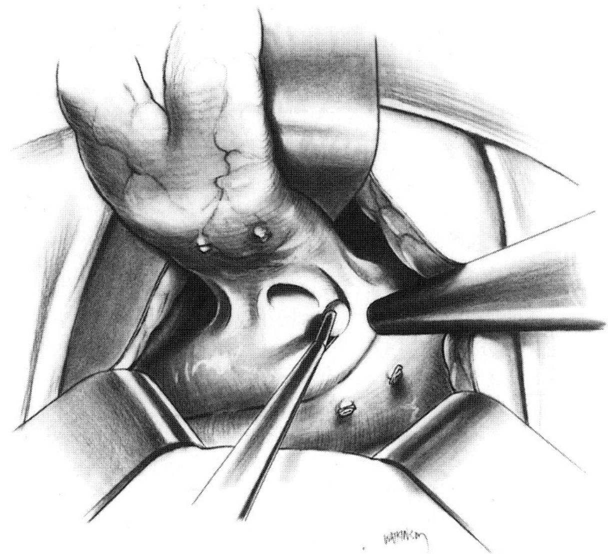

FIGURE 64–6 ■ The thymic veins have been identified posteriorly and divided between surgical clips as they enter the innominate vein.

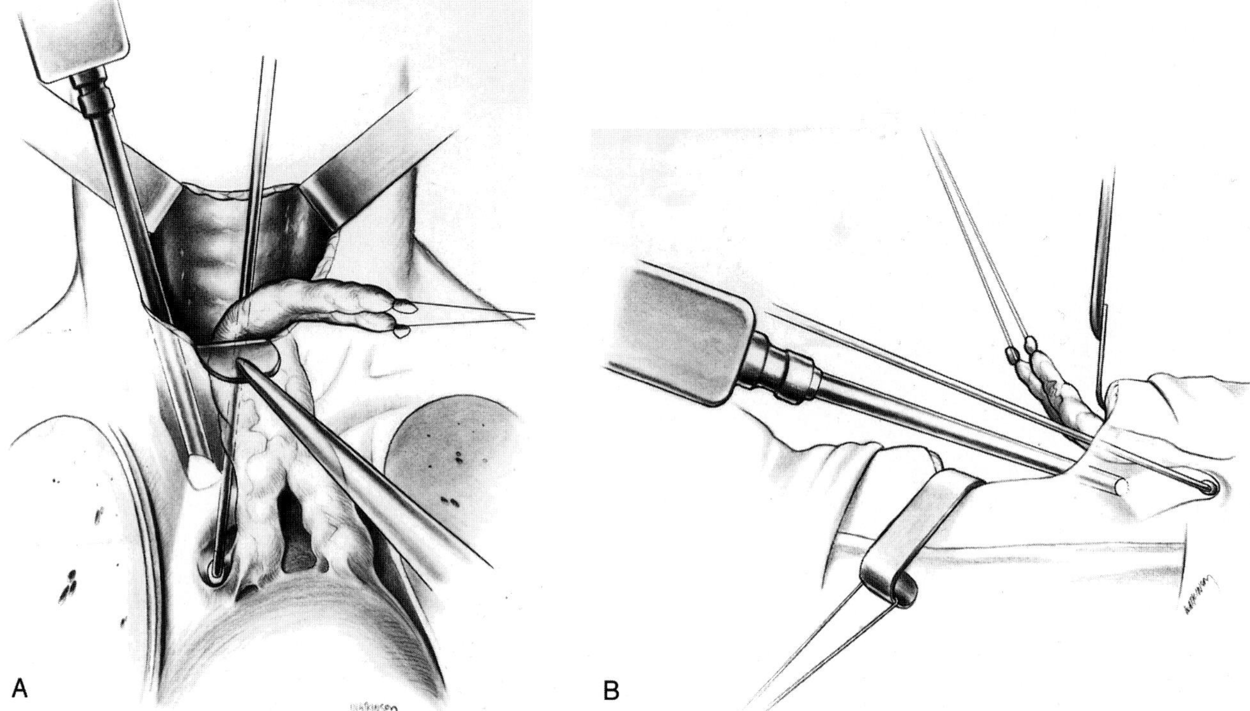

FIGURE 64–7 ■ *A*, Blunt dissection is carried down bilaterally. *B*, This allows progressive mobilization of the gland down to its lower poles, where it can be swept off the pericardium.

and in a sweeping motion the gland is extracted from the inferior mediastinum (Fig. 64–8). After this maneuver, the "socket" in which the inferior pole of the gland resided is clearly visible, as is the underlying pericardium.

This technique can be done under direct vision with the light of the thoracoscope as an aid, or surgeons comfortable with thoracoscopic operating can operate using the thoracoscopic images on the monitor to perform the operation. The assistance of the videothoracoscope routinely provides good visualization of the lower mediastinum, down to the diaphragm if necessary. On occasion, when it would have been impossible to complete the operation through the transcervical route using direct vision only, the videothoracoscope has enabled successful completion of a thymectomy without requiring conversion to a sternotomy.

Once the gland has been excised, if there is any further mediastinal fatty tissue present that is suspicious for being thymic tissue, this is excised or biopsied for frozen section analysis to ensure that residual thymic tissue is not left behind. A No. 7 Jackson-Pratt (JP) drain (Zimmer, Dover, OH) is inserted through a lateral stab wound in the neck and placed down into the mediastinum; the Cooper retractor is removed. The strap muscles are approximated with a single figure-eight Vicryl suture (Davis & Geck, Danbury, CT), and the platysma is closed with a running 3–0 Vicryl suture. The skin is closed with a running 4–0 Vicryl subcuticular stitch.

If it is felt that a safe total thymectomy cannot be completed through the transcervical route, we convert to a partial upper sternotomy. This is usually carried out by the addition of a vertical incision extending down from the cervical incision to just below the manubrium. The incision in the sternal bone is then "J'd" out into the third or fourth intercostal space with the oscillating saw, to create a partial upper sternotomy, which is usually sufficient to complete the operation. This has been necessary in less than 5% of cases, when it was felt that complete excision of the thymus gland was not possible, or when troublesome bleeding was encountered.

POSTOPERATIVE CARE

The patient's respiratory status and requirements for ventilatory support are, by far, the most salient issues in the postoperative period. Patients are extubated in the operating room. They are instructed to take their morning dose of anticholinesterase medication with a sip of water preoperatively, to optimize their strength at the time of extubation. They are given an additional dose of pyridostigmine bromide (Mestinon) in the recovery room.

Their medications are continued at the same dose as was given preoperatively. In general, the JP drain is removed and the patients are discharged home the following morning. Their medications are not altered until 1 month after surgery when they are seen by the surgeon and the neurologist. Some patients may become transiently worse postoperatively; it is this exacerbation of myasthenic symptoms, rather than surgical considerations, that is the usual reason to keep a patient in hospital for longer than 1 day. If symptoms worsen, the medication regimen may have to be altered to include prednisone or azathioprine. An occasional patient may deteriorate considerably. These patients should be expediently

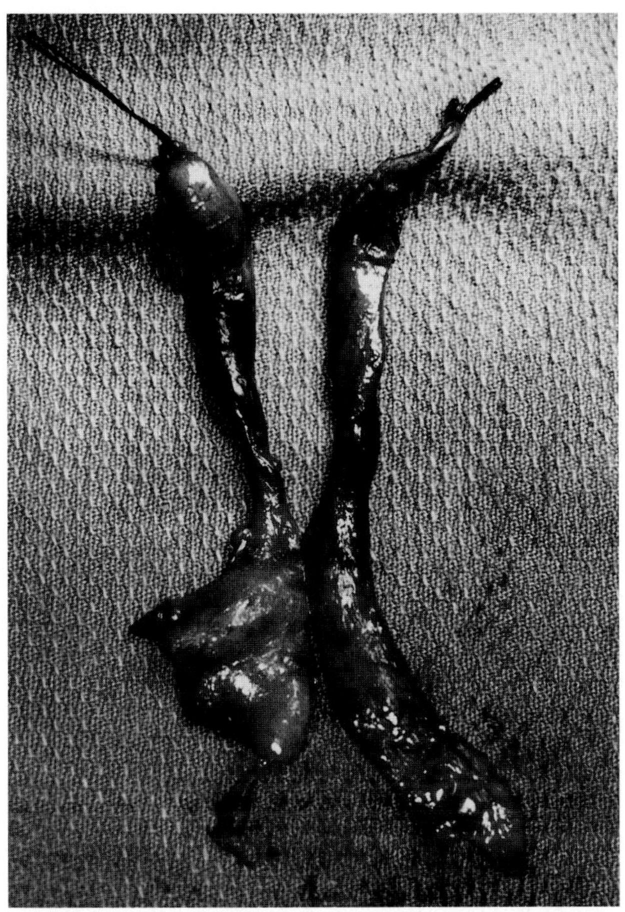

FIGURE 64–8 ■ Photograph of a thymectomy specimen that was removed by videothoracoscopic transcervical thymectomy.

treated with plasmapheresis to prevent deterioration to the point of requiring ventilatory support.

SUMMARY

The transcervical thymectomy is a well-accepted surgical approach to the treatment of myasthenia gravis. We have described the addition of videothoracoscopic assistance to this operation. This provides light for direct operation, enhanced videothoracoscopic operative visualization of the lower mediastinum in difficult cases, and the ability for the teaching surgeon to visualize every detail of the operation being performed, all of which have greatly facilitated the teaching of this operation. In our experience, this has proved to be an effective procedure with low morbidity and short hospital stay; it has been very well accepted by neurologists and patients alike.

COMMENTS AND CONTROVERSIES

Drs. Cassivi and Keshavjee have described an interesting modification of the technique of transcervical thymectomy. The standard exposure and technique of transcervical thymectomy have been augmented by the utilization of video-assisted technology. The advantage of this procedure is that it certainly improves illumination and vision. Perhaps more importantly, it avoids the multiple thoracostomy ports required for video-assisted thymectomy using the video-assisted thoracic surgery (VATS) approach. In the opinion of the authors, this video thoracoscopic addition has avoided the need for transsternal exposure in the occasional patient for whom transcervical exposure alone would have been insufficient. Our own experience with transcervical thymectomy indicates that transsternal exposure is almost never required to achieve a complete thymectomy via the transcervical route. However, with this technique, visualization and illumination do seem to be superior.

G. A. P.

REFERENCES

Blalock A, Mason MF, Morgan HJ, Riven SS: Myasthenia gravis and tumors of the thymic region. Report of a case in which the tumor was removed. Ann Surg 110:544, 1939.

Blalock A: Thymectomy in the treatment of myasthenia gravis. Report of twenty cases. J Thorac Surg 13:316, 1944.

Bulkley GB, Bass KN, Stephenson GR et al: Extended cervicomediastinal thymectomy in the integrated management of myasthenia gravis. Ann Surg 226:324, 1997.

Carlens E, Johansson L, Olsson P: Mediastinoscopy auxiliary to thymectomy by the cervical route. Bronches 17:408, 1967.

Cooper JD, Al-Jilaihawa AN, Pearson FG et al: An improved technique to facilitate transcervical thymectomy for myasthenia gravis. Ann Thorac Surg 45:242, 1988.

Crile G Jr: Thymectomy through the neck. Surgery 59:213, 1966.

El-Dawlatly AA, Ashour MH: Anaesthesia for thymectomy in myasthenia gravis: A non-muscle-relaxant technique. Anaesth Intensive Care 22:458, 1994.

Frist WH, Thirumalai S, Doehring CB et al: Thymectomy for the myasthenia gravis patient: Factors influencing outcome. Ann Thorac Surg 57:334, 1994.

Gracey DR, Divertie MB, Howard FM Jr et al: Postoperative respiratory care after transsternal thymectomy in myasthenia gravis. A 3 year experience in 53 patients. Chest 86:67, 1984.

Jaretzki A, Penn AS, Younger DS et al: "Maximal" thymectomy for myasthenia gravis. J Thorac Cardiovasc Surg 95:747, 1988.

Kirschner PA, Osserman KE, Kark AE: Studies in myasthenia gravis: Transcervical total thymectomy. JAMA 209:906, 1969.

Mulder DG, Graves M, Herrmann C: Thymectomy for myasthenia gravis: Recent observations and comparisons with past experience. Ann Thorac Surg 48:551, 1989.

Papatestas AE, Genkins G, Kornfeld P et al: Effects of thymectomy in myasthenia gravis. Ann Surg 206:79, 1987.

Saunders DB, Scopetta C: The treatment of patients with myasthenia gravis. Neurol Clin N Am 12:343, 1994.

Schumacher, Roth: Thymektomie bei einem Fall von morbus Basedow mit Myasthenia. Mitt Grenzgeb Chir 25, 1913.

Viets HR, Schwab RS: Thymectomy for myasthenia gravis. Springfield, IL, Charles C Thomas, 1960.

RESECTION AND RECONSTRUCTION OF THE SUPERIOR VENA CAVA

Paolo Macchiarini
Philippe Dartevelle

Although resection of the superior vena cava (SVC) has a well-demonstrated benefit in selected patients (Dartevelle et al, 1991; Macchiarini and Dartevelle, 1998; Warren et al, 1998), its reconstruction is essential to ensure upper venous drainage and avoid disastrous neurologic complications. Yet, with SVC reconstruction, significant morbidity may be involved—not only acute cerebral edema related to prolonged cross-clamping time, but also late graft thrombosis and infection, as well as anastomotic pitfalls.

Careful attention to patient selection and technical details at the time of surgery will minimize the risks of most intra- or postoperative complications.

SURGICAL ANATOMY

The SVC originates from the confluence of the two innominate veins at the level of the cartilaginous portion of the first right rib. It descends down into the anterior mediastinum and enters the right atrium. Its trunk has an average length of 7 cm and a transverse diameter of 2 cm. It is confined by the thymus gland and right pleura and lung anteriorly; the right laterotracheal lymphatic chain, pulmonary artery, and superior pulmonary vein posteriorly; the ascending aorta medially; and the right pleura, phrenic nerve, and small superior diaphragmatic vessels laterally (Fig. 64–9).

The caval-atrial junction is within the pericardium. The serous pericardium envelops the antero-external surface of the SVC for a length of 2 cm. The sinus node is located along the anterolateral aspect of the junction between the SVC and the right atrium. It is superficial, lying just beneath the epicardial surface in the crista terminalis, and is approximately 15 × 5 × 1.5 mm. This area should not be surgically manipulated or incised, to minimize the risk of compromising atrial conduction. The medial area, lying between the intrapericardial SVC and the ascending aorta, includes (1) an extrapericardial region in which the origin of the right main bronchus lies, and (2) the anterior aspect of the pulmonary artery, lying behind the SVC and the right orifice of the Thiele sinus.

The four main collateral routes of the SVC in humans include the following (McIntire and Sykes, 1949): (1) the azygous venous system (only collateral draining directly into the posterior surface of the SVC above the right pulmonary artery and main bronchus); (2) the internal thoracic venous system (wherein the blood pours into the inferior vena cava [IVC] from the internal thoracic vein through the superior and inferior epigastric veins and the external and common iliac veins); (3) the vertebral venous system (in which the blood from the sinus venosus and the bilateral brachiocephalic veins flows into the intercostal, lumbar, and sacral veins, and then pours into the IVC—portions of this blood flow into the internal thoracic veins); and (4) the external thoracic venous system (this is the superficial collateral system by which the blood from the subclavian vein and the axillary vein reaches the lateral thoracic vein, and then pours into the femoral vein through the thoracoepigastric and superficial epigastric veins).

HEMODYNAMICS

The first clinical experiences with SVC reconstruction (Jarvis and Kanar, 1956; Salsali, 1966; Thomas, 1959)

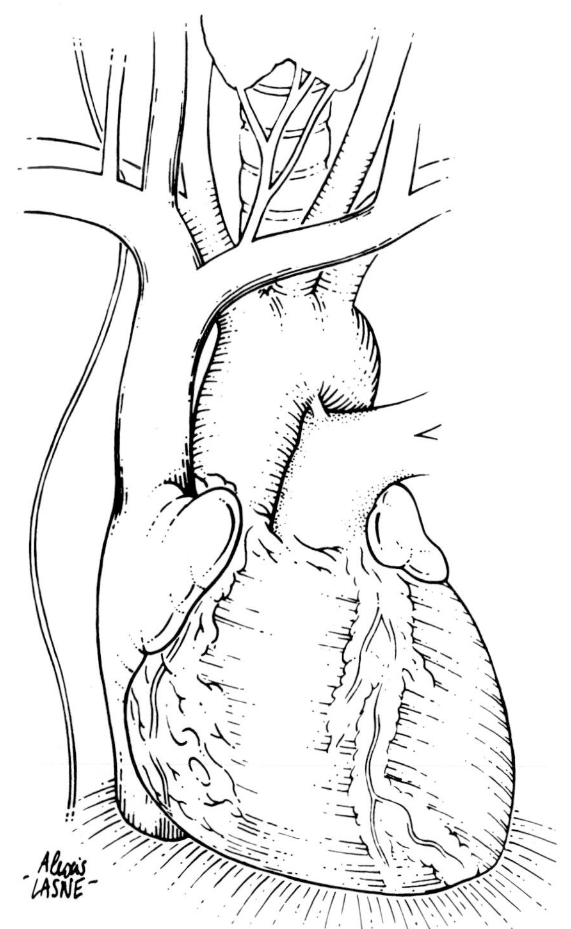

FIGURE 64–9 ■ Surgical anatomy of the superior vena cava.

consistently reported cerebral edema nearly 60 minutes after interruption of the venous flow. Potential triggering factors for this include venous stasis at the level of the cephalic territory, problems with the absorption capacity of the cerebral fluid, and cellular hypoxia and hypercapnia resulting from the vascular stasis. In addition, it is well known that hypercapnia vasodilates, increases the permeability of the cerebral vessels, and thus induces vasogenic cerebral edema.

Recently, however, we (Dartevelle et al, 1995) provided evidence that the hemodynamic consequences of SVC clamping depend on whether or not the SVC is obstructed. For patients whose SVC is completely obstructed or is tightly stenosed, intraoperative venous clamping results in negligible hemodynamic compromise because a functioning collateral venous network already exists, which supplements the flow obstruction to the SVC. For patients whose invaded SVC is unobstructed, even short venous cross-clamping triggers a hemodynamic cascade of events, including on the one hand decreased cardiac inflow, outflow, and cerebral perfusion pressure (the safe physiologic level of which should be above 60 mm Hg [McDowall 1985]), and on the other hand increased venous pressure of the cerebral territory and alterations of the cerebral arterial-venous gradient, leading to irreversible brain damage.

INDICATIONS AND CONTRAINDICATIONS

The SVC is usually subject to easy obstruction owing to its anatomic site, thin wall, low hemodynamic pressure, and encirclement by chains of lymph nodes draining all the thoracic cavity and mediastinal tissues. The main indications and contraindications for SVC resection and reconstruction are outlined in Table 64–1. Major elective SVC reconstructive procedures should be limited to mediastinal tumors and to the less than 1% of operable patients (McCormack, 1995) with right-sided bronchogenic tumors invading the SVC either directly or, more frequently, by superior mediastinal lymph nodes containing metastatic disease (Macchiarini and Dartevelle, 1998). Palliative SVC procedures are very rare and are limited to slow-growing diseases such as mediastinal primary or secondary fibrosis, SVC thrombosis of unknown etiology, or saccular SVC aneurysms.

TABLE 64–1 ■ **Indications and Contraindications for Superior Vena Cava Resections**

Indications	*Contraindications*
Neoplasms	
Non–small cell lung tumors	SVC syndromes related to unresectable tumors
Anterior mediastinal tumors	
Primary SVC tumors	
Vascular	
Primary saccular aneurysms	Obstructed SVC with a rich collateral vein circulation
Primary malformations	
Trauma	
Iatrogenic, blunt, or penetrating	Abnormal walls of the proximal veins

SVC, superior vena cava.

Surgery should not be performed when (1) the cephalic venous bed is obstructed, (2) the proximal veins have abnormal venous walls, or (3) the SVC is chronically obstructed. Under these circumstances, the existing, well-developed, competitive collateral venous circulation reduces blood flow through the graft, exposing it to thrombotic events. In these situations, SVC revascularization could be made using either the jugular or the axillary veins as proximal implantation sites. These revascularizations are, however, at higher thrombotic risk because of the reduced venous blood flow through the graft (preexisting collateral venous network) and the longer prosthesis (passing subcutaneously with major kinking and risk of thrombosis).

PREOPERATIVE ASSESSMENT

A clinical preoperative workup evaluating extension of the primary disease should be made routinely. All patients should have superior vena cavography by simultaneous injection in both arm veins before operation to anatomically delineate the site and extension of the venous obstruction and the presence of possible proximal thrombosis and to anticipate where the proximal graft anastomosis can be made. Systemic venous anatomy is carefully evaluated by angiography to determine the presence of a contralateral SVC (e.g., a persistent left SVC), and an azygous or hemiazygous continuation of the inferior vena cava.

Echocardiography can demonstrate thrombotic extension into the right atrium and the patency of the jugular and axillary veins. Because patients with bronchogenic cancer may present with clinically and radiologically silent SVC invasion, thoracic computed tomography (invasion of the posterior wall of the terminal SVC) and pulmonary angiography (amputation of the right upper mediastinal artery) are key diagnostic tools for anticipating SVC resection. The brain should also be investigated to assess its tolerance to SVC cross-clamping.

INTRAOPERATIVE MONITORING

Appropriate invasive and noninvasive monitoring is essential. Patients should be ventilated through a double-lumen tube to obtain one-lung ventilation. A pulse oximeter is used to continuously monitor systemic oxygen saturation. A radial arterial line should be inserted transcutaneously for continuous pressure monitoring and arterial blood gas determination. A catheter is inserted into the cephalic vein in the forearm, or more proximally in the antecubital fossa or into the right internal jugular vein, to monitor the venous pressure in the cephalic territory. These lines are essential for monitoring the physiologic arterial-venous pressure gradient across the brain.

A Foley catheter is inserted. Electrocardiographic monitoring should be in position to monitor cardiac electrophysiologic alterations during venous clamping because the distal clamp may be too close to the sinus node. At least two venous lines should be placed in the lower limbs to achieve volume expansion during venous clamping. Transesophageal echocardiography and nasogastric tubes are optional.

SURGICAL APPROACH

The usual approaches include a right thoracotomy in the fourth or fifth intercostal space for bronchogenic tumors, and a median sternotomy for tumors originating from the anterior compartment of the mediastinum. Median sternotomy allows excellent exposure of the entire anterior mediastinum, right atrium, both brachiocephalic veins, and the SVC throughout their entire lengths. This incision can be easily extended to the neck for additional exposure if necessary. A right thoracotomy yields the best exposure of the right hilum and excellent visualization of the SVC and right atrium but renders the dissection, control, and revascularization of the left brachiocephalic vein technically demanding.

CHOICE OF MATERIAL

When less than 30% of the circumference of the caval wall is involved, a partial resection of the vein is possible with direct closure, providing acceptable results (Fig. 64–10). An alternative technique for those malignant or benign lesions whose SVC stenosis is limited in circumference and height and is not associated with a thrombosis would be the interposition of an autologous pericardial or venous patch (Fig. 64–11).

If there is greater circumferential involvement, complete replacement and reconstruction of the SVC is mandatory. The currently available materials for SVC reconstruction include autogenous venous (Doty, 1982), pericardial (Warren et al, 1998), and prosthetic (Dartevelle et al, 1991) grafts. Autogenous venous grafts represent the nearest approximation of the ideal blood vessel substitute and are acknowledged to provide the best results for vascular reconstruction. Whatever venous graft—superficial, femoral, jugular, or internal saphenous veins—the diameter of these vessels must be at least as great as that of the brachiocephalic vein. One way to construct an adequately sized autologous venous graft is to make a spiral vein. This requires that the necessary length (l) of the venous graft be used to replace the length of the resected SVC:

$$l = \frac{R}{r} \times L$$

where *R* is the radius of the brachiocephalic vein, *r* the radius of the autologous venous graft, and *L* the length of the resected SVC.

Prosthetic grafts in the venous system are far more likely than arterial grafts to occlude, because of the relative slow venous flow against a hydrostatic pressure gradient, low intraluminal pressure, and presence of competitive flow from venous collaterals. Not surprisingly, prosthetic replacement of the SVC has been usually regarded as an absolute surgical contraindication because of the absence of suitable graft material for reconstruction and the technical fear concerning the effects of SVC clamping, graft thrombosis, and infection. However, the feasibility of reconstructing the SVC has been ameliorated by the efficacy of the presently available graft materials.

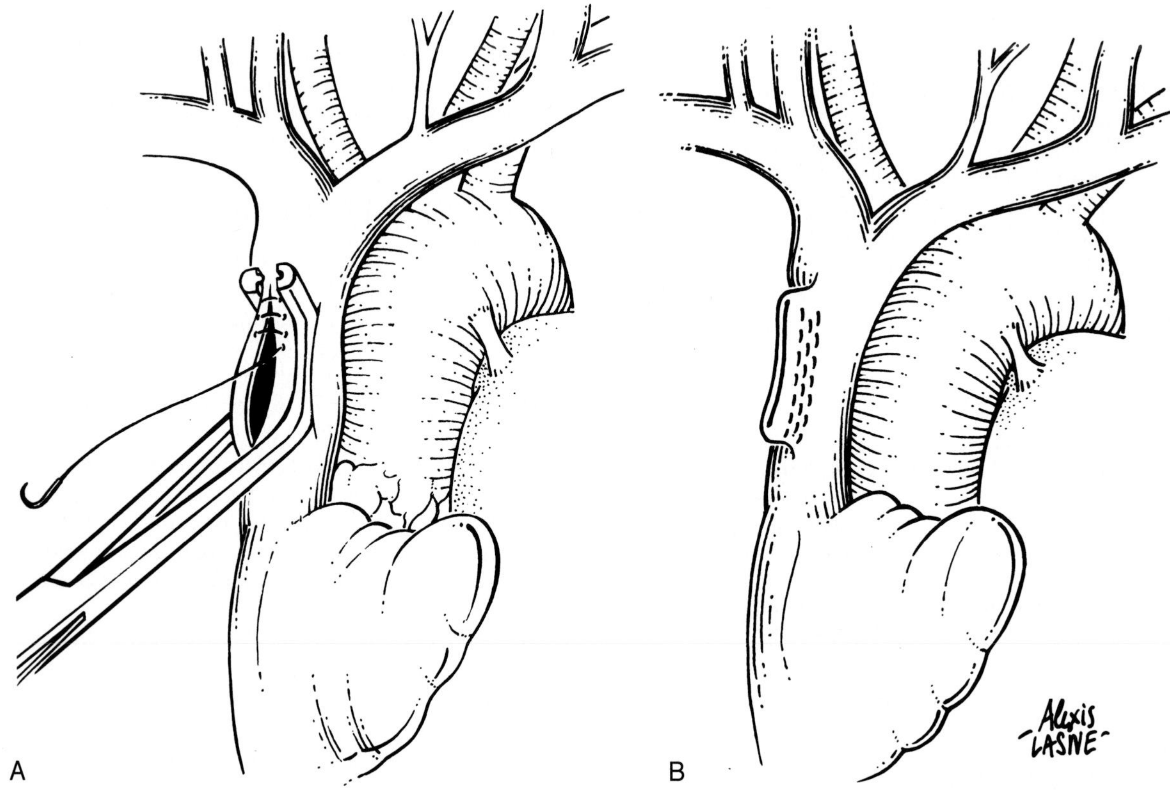

FIGURE 64–10 ■ Invasion of less than 30% of the superior vena cava can be resected and closed directly using a running *(A)* or mechanical *(B)* suture.

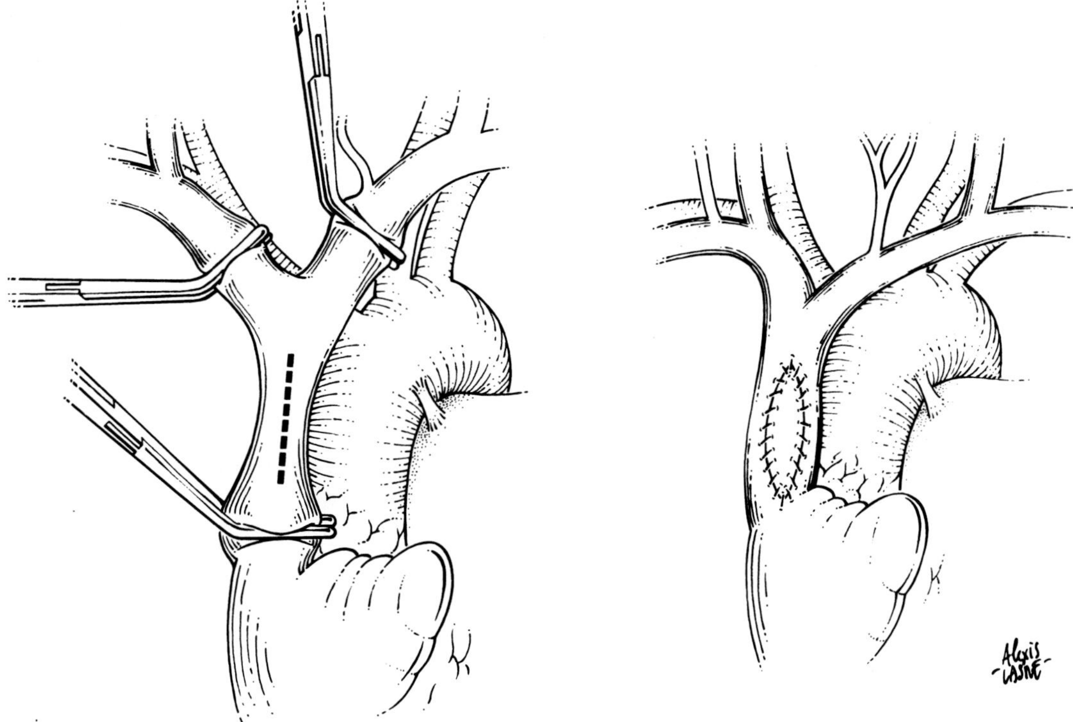

FIGURE 64–11 ■ Enlargement of the superior vena cava (SVC) stenosis that is limited in circumference and height and not associated with a thrombosis can be accomplished by the interposition of an autologous pericardial or venous patch.

The synthetic nontextile polytetrafluoroethylene (PTFE) vascular graft is the material of choice for SVC reconstruction. In effect, it is the only synthetic material remaining patent over the long term; shortly after its implantation, it becomes re-epithelialized with autogenous endothelial cells in human beings. Also, its surgical implantation is associated with a negligible rate of complications. Technically speaking, these grafts do not require preclotting, do not leak, are potentially easier to thrombectomize than vein grafts or Dacron conduits if graft thrombosis occurs, are more resistant to infection, have less platelet deposition and less thrombogenicity of the flow surface compared with Dacron grafts, and cause substantially less complement activation, and therefore less leucocyte infiltration and release of inflammatory mediators (Brewster, 1995).

PREVENTION OF CROSS-CLAMPING EFFECTS

Clamp placement that occludes less than 50% of the circumference of the SVC is usually not associated with significant hemodynamic imbalance. Several technical details may minimize the hemodynamic compromise resulting from the total cross-clamping of an SVC.

Shunt Procedures

Intraluminal shunting of the blood from one of the innominate veins into the right atrium may reduce the hemodynamic consequences of venous cross-clamping in animals (Gonzales-Fajardo et al, 1994) and humans (Warren et al, 1998) for at least 35 minutes. Unfortunately, the mean clamping time of the SVC during excision of lung or mediastinal tumors is usually longer. Whatever the type of shunt used, major drawbacks include the longer operating time, extended incisions and dissections, and their potential thrombosis.

Pharmacologic Agents and Fluid Implementation

These are aimed at increasing venous blood return to the right atrium; they maintain the physiologic arterial-venous gradient within the cerebral territory. The first target is achieved by adequate compensation of all blood losses with the use of blood components and macromolecules. Because the cranial venous pressure may rise up to 40 mm Hg during venous clamping, maintenance of the cerebral arterial-venous gradient requires fluid administration and, eventually, the use of vasoconstrictive agents. Ideally, a mean systemic arterial pressure in the cephalic territory greater than 60 mm Hg should be maintained throughout the clamping period.

Shortening Venous Clamping Time

This target can be obtained through a planned surgical strategy. For right bronchogenic tumors with carinal or proximal pulmonary artery invasion, it is often easier to perform the vascular step first and then the airway procedure. During the latter, all attention should be di-

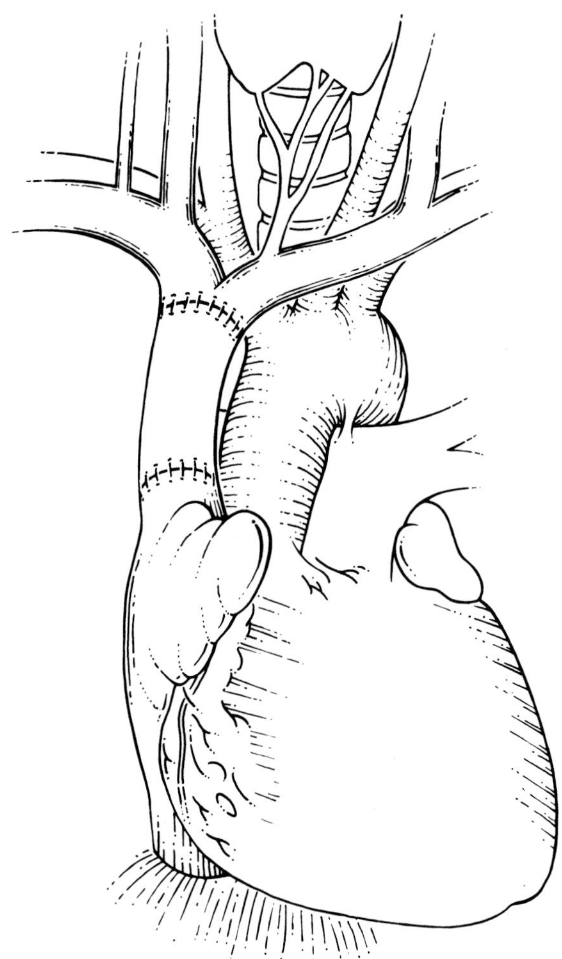

FIGURE 64–12 ■ Truncular superior vena cava revascularization using an unringed, synthetic, nontextile polytetrafluoroethylene vascular graft.

rected toward avoiding bacterial contamination of the prosthesis. For mediastinal tumors involving both upper lobes, operation should be made from the left to the right side. This permits a safe and immediate revascularization between the left innominate vein and the right atrium; the right part of the excision is performed thereafter.

Anticoagulation Therapy

Like other venous replacements, intravenous sodium heparin is given before clamping.

TYPES OF PROSTHETIC RECONSTRUCTION OF THE SUPERIOR VENA CAVA

Truncular Replacement

This requires a tumor-free confluence of both innominate veins. The procedure (Fig. 64–12), commonly associated with a right pneumonectomy, employs a straight unringed PTFE graft (No. 18 or 20) because the proximal and distal SVC stumps are usually healthy. After proximal (innominate vein confluence) and distal (cavoatrial junction) clamping, the invaded segment of the vena cava is completely excised. The proximal anastomosis between the SVC stump and the prosthesis is then performed first using a continuous 5–0 polypropylene (Prolene, Ethicon, Inc., Somerville, NJ) suture, started at the posterior aspect of the prosthesis in an inside-to-outside fashion. Following proximal anastomosis completion, the distal anastomosis is then performed in the same way. Before the distal suture is tightened, the proximal clamp is released and the prosthesis is flushed with saline heparinized solution and extensively de-aired. The distal clamp is then released and the knots tied. To avoid kinking of the prosthesis, the length of the graft should be adapted so that the distal anastomosis rests under tension. At the end of the surgical procedure, the graft should be encircled with a vascularized pedicle of parietal pleura.

Revascularization from the Left Innominate Vein

This procedure (Fig. 64–13), which is always performed through a median sternotomy, requires a ringed PTFE graft (No. 12 or 13). The ringed graft is imperative because after closure of the median sternotomy, the prosthesis may be too long, thus inducing its kinking. Minimal dissection of the left innominate vein is also mandatory to avoid its rotation above the proximal anastomosis.

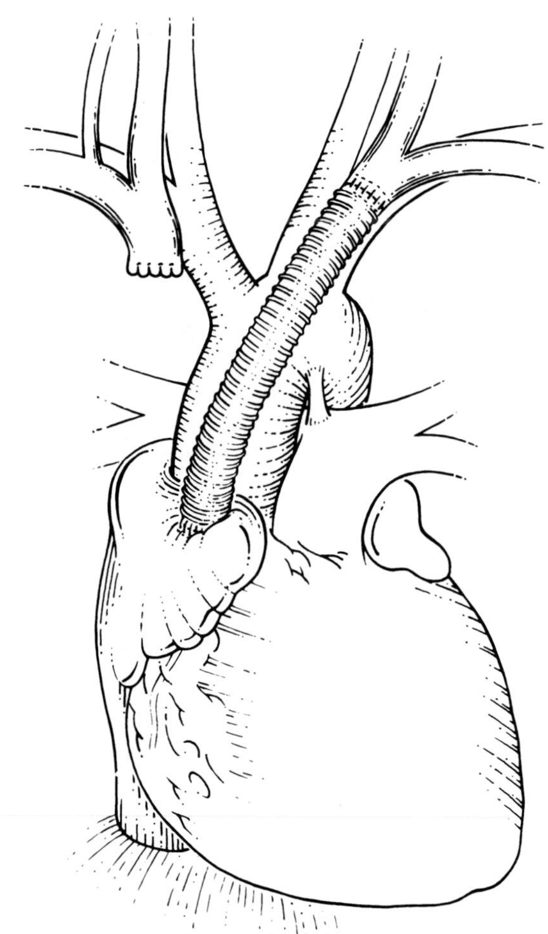

FIGURE 64–13 ■ Revascularization between the left innominate vein and the right atrium using a ringed, synthetic, nontextile polytetrafluoroethylene vascular graft.

The distal anastomosis can be performed on either the right atrium or appendage, or the inferior stump of the SVC; however, it is preferably performed to the right atrium because of the absence of the pectinate muscles lining the right appendage.

Revascularization from the Right Innominate Vein

For this procedure (Fig. 64–14), ringed grafts are preferred (No. 12 or 14), to maintain their patency and to avoid compression by postoperative fibrosclerosis. The risks of kinking are minimal because the direction of the graft is almost vertical. The proximal anastomosis is not always easy to perform because the residual stump of the right innominate vein is often short; it has to be performed first. The distal anastomosis should be made to the SVC stump. This architecture results in the straightest and shortest graft, and represents the revascularization of choice for mediastinal tumors involving the origin of the SVC.

Revascularization from Both Innominate Veins

This technique (Fig. 64–15) should not be performed because the blood flow through each graft is less than that observable after single revascularization.

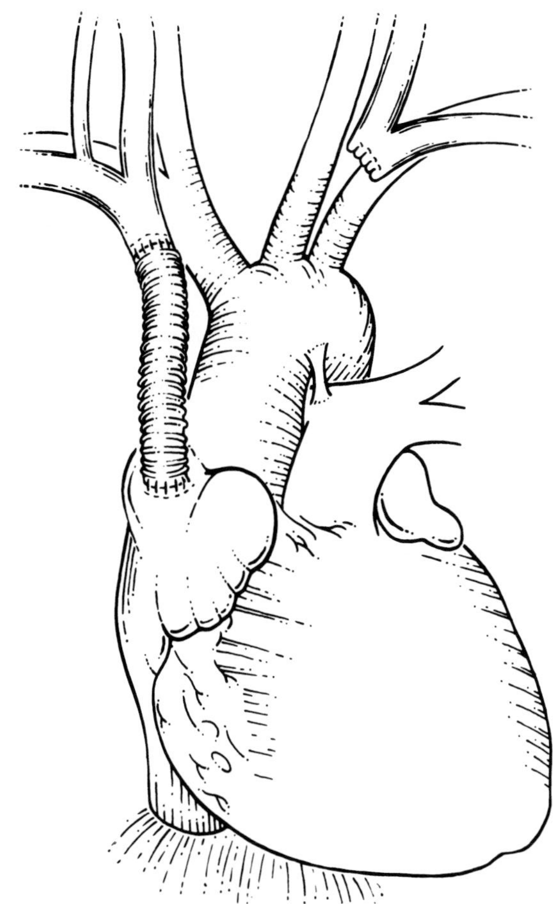

FIGURE 64–14 ■ Revascularization between the right innominate vein and the right atrium using a ringed, synthetic, nontextile polytetrafluoroethylene vascular graft.

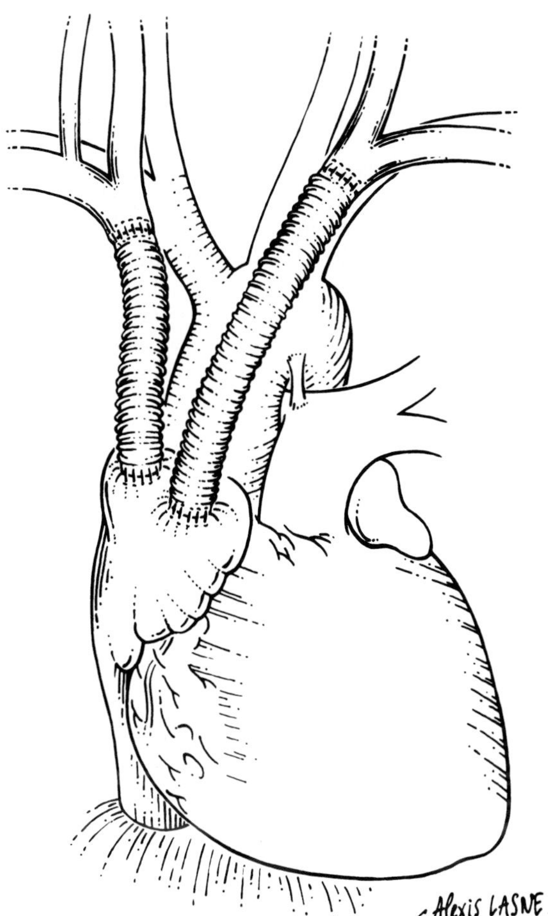

FIGURE 64–15 ■ Revascularization of both innominate veins with polytetrafluoroethylene grafts that are implanted independently on the right atrium.

POSTOPERATIVE CARE

Postoperative hemodynamics and pulmonary status are monitored closely. The administration of maintenance fluids and blood products is minimized to prevent pulmonary edema, especially in patients requiring pneumonectomy. The head and upper body are elevated to reduce the risk of SVC syndrome by providing a hemodynamic advantage for upper body blood return. Intravenous sodium heparin is continued as soon as bleeding is controlled, to reduce the risk of graft thrombosis; a switch is made to warfarin agents or aspirin at the time of hospital discharge.

COMPLICATIONS OF RECONSTRUCTION OF THE SUPERIOR VENA CAVA

With appropriate patient selection, significant early morbidity and mortality after resection and reconstruction of the SVC can be minimized.

Anastomotic Stricture

SVC revascularization requires a perfect technical performance. Postoperative angiographic examination should be routinely performed to correct eventual anastomotic technical failures. Because the vein usually incorporates the graft on its entire transverse diameter, a stenosis at the level of the proximal anastomosis is almost impossible to observe. By contrast, an anastomotic stenosis is more commonly related to an intraoperative excessive dissection of the vein proximal to the anastomosis, which might kink, rotate, or become involved by fibrotic tissue after performance of the prosthetic-venous anastomosis. When excessive venous length or rotation is diagnosed postoperatively, surgical correction is advised. By contrast, a stenosis induced by fibrosis may be corrected with angioplastic dilation or the placement of an intraluminal covered stent.

Graft Thrombosis

Most often, this is an early postoperative complication associated with either mechanical obstruction to the flow through the graft or an inappropriate indication (e.g., implantation on a recanalized vein with major pathologic venous wall sequelae, insufficient proximal vein bed, or a chronic SVC syndrome with a very well developed venous collateral circulation). The major consequence of graft thrombosis is an acute clinical SVC syndrome, leading to reversible brain damage or passage and lodgment of thrombotic clot(s) in the pulmonary circulation.

Graft Infection

Graft infection is a serious risk inherent to all prosthetic vascular replacements; it is more likely to develop when the airway is opened, bronchial suturing and lung parenchymal resections are done, or surgery is performed after induction chemoradiation. Infection can manifest itself by mediastinitis, thoracic empyema, or septicemia, as in infected thrombophlebitis. Treatment depends on the presence or absence of systemic septicemia. In the absence of a severe septic syndrome, the prosthesis might be conserved by using an omentoplasty covering the graft. However, septicemia or a severe septic syndrome necessitates graft excision, which may be badly tolerated in patent grafts.

DISCUSSION

Patients most suitable for elective SVC reconstruction are those with operable anterior mediastinal tumors or right-sided bronchogenic tumors without hemodynamically significant venous outflow obstruction. Intraoperative shunting is almost never necessary when adequate hemodynamic measurements targeting maintenance of the cerebral arterial-venous gradient are taken. Partial (30%) invasion can be surgically managed by resection and either direct closure or patch (autologous veins or pericardium) interposition. Prosthetic caval reconstruction represents the treatment of choice for more extended SVC invasion but it requires great technical expertise. Despite the addition of significant procedural time, the long-term survival and patency of SVC prosthetic reconstruction appear to exceed the related morbidity and operative mortality.

COMMENTS AND CONTROVERSIES

When vena cava resection and possible reconstruction are considered, patient selection is paramount. For those with malignant disease, basic oncologic principles apply and complete resection is mandatory. For those patients who have already established excellent collateral circulation, reconstruction is not required. This chapter clearly outlines the many details important in preoperative planning, including bilateral upper extremity venography, so as to enable precise planning of the intended resection and reconstruction. Also emphasized are the critically important intraoperative patient management protocols necessary for maintaining acceptable cerebral arterial-venous pressure gradients and the important technical details mandatory if satisfactory early and long-term results are to be achieved.

G. A. P.

REFERENCES

Beck SD, Lalke SG: Long-term results after inferior vena caval resection during retroperitoneal lymphadenectomy for metastatic germ cell cancer. J Vasc Surg 28:808, 1998.

Brewster DC: Prosthetic grafts. In Rutherford RB (ed): Vascular Surgery. Philadelphia, WB Saunders, 1995, pp 492–521.

Dartevelle P, Chapelier A, Pastorino U et al: Long-term follow-up after prosthetic replacement of the superior vena cava combined with resection of mediastinal-pulmonary malignant tumors. J Thorac Cardiovasc Surg 102:259, 1991.

Dartevelle P, Macchiarini P, Chapelier A: Superior vena cava resection and reconstruction. In Faber P (ed): Techniques of Pulmonary Resection. Philadelphia, WB Saunders, 1995, pp 345–358.

Doty DB: Bypass of superior vena cava: Six years experience with spiral vein graft for obstruction of superior vena cava due to benign and malignant disease. J Thorac Cardiovasc Surg 83:326, 1982.

Gonzales-Fajardo JA, Garcia-Yuste M, Florez S et al: Hemodynamic and cerebral repercussions from surgical interruption of the superior vena cava. J Thorac Cardiovasc Surg 107:1044, 1994.

Inoue H, Shohtsu A, Koide S et al: Resection of the superior vena cava for primary lung cancer: 5 years' survival. Ann Thorac Surg 50:661, 1990.

Jarvis FJ, Kanar EA: Physiologic changes following obstruction of the superior vena cava. J Thorac Cardiovasc Surg 27:213, 1956.

Macchiarini P, Dartevelle P: Extended resections for lung cancer. In Roth JA, Hong WK, Cox JD (eds): Lung Cancer, 2nd ed. Cambridge, MA, Blackwell Scientific, 1998.

McCormack PM: Extended pulmonary resections. In Pearson FG, Deslauriers J, Ginsberg RJ et al (eds): Thoracic Surgery. New York, Churchill Livingstone, 1995.

McDowall DG: Induced hypotension and brain ischemia. Br J Anaesth 57:110, 1985.

McIntire FT, Sykes EM Jr: Obstruction of the superior vena cava: A review of the literature and report of two personal cases. Ann Intern Med 30:925, 1949.

Salsali M: A safe technique for resection of the nonobstructed superior vena cava. Surg Gynecol Obstet 123:92, 1966.

Thomas CP: Conservative and extensive resection for carcinoma of the lung. Ann R Coll Surg Engl 24:345, 1959.

Tsuchiya R, Asamura H, Kondo H et al: Extended resection of the left atrium, great vessels, or both for lung cancer. Ann Thorac Surg 57:960, 1994.

Warren WH, Piccione W, Faber LP: Superior vena caval reconstruction using autologous pericardium. Ann Thorac Surg 66:291, 1998.

THORACOSCOPIC MEDIASTINAL SURGERY

Keith S. Naunheim

When video-assisted thoracic surgery (VATS) was first introduced, it was used for the assessment of disease processes within the lungs and pleurae. With advances in instrumentation and increasing experience, practitioners found that they were also able to apply these minimally invasive techniques to disease processes within the mediastinum. During the early portion of this experience, VATS was used essentially for diagnostic purposes (Kern et al, 1993). However, as expertise developed, surgeons began to perform truly therapeutic procedures within the mediastinum. Because therapeutic mediastinal procedures using VATS have been undertaken only within the last 6 years, limited data are available providing long-term results; thus, it is difficult to state definitively that this minimally invasive modality is equal or superior to standard operative incisions. However, the feasibility of therapeutic mediastinum procedures has been well documented; it is hoped that the relative value of a thoracoscopic approach, as compared with an open one, will be determined within the coming decade.

OPERATIVE TECHNIQUES

Thoracoscopic mediastinal surgery requires a quiet and clear operative field without impingement by the lungs. Thus, single lung ventilation using a double-lumen endotracheal tube is relatively standard. The choice for using a left- or right-sided approach depends not only on the location of the entity being dealt with but also somewhat on the surgeon's preference. Preoperative imaging studies, such as computed tomography (CT) scans or magnetic resonance imaging (MRI), are useful in determining how a lesion might most easily be approached. It is mandatory that these studies be available in the operating room during the time of the procedure. Very commonly, mediastinal lesions are somewhat off of midline, and CT or MRI scans will indicate whether a left- or a right-sided approach would provide better operative access to the lesion.

Once the operative site has been determined, the patient is put into the appropriate lateral decubitus position. Many practitioners use a kidney rest underneath the midportion of the chest, as this maneuver will "stretch out" the chest wall on the operative side and increase the size of intercostal spaces, thus making manipulation of surgical instruments easier.

With the patient in the lateral thoracotomy position, the lung generally collapses against the mediastinum and obscures the operative field. The operative table can be tilted to the left or right, as well as into a Trendelenburg or reverse Trendelenburg position. Such positioning, in conjunction with gentle lung retraction, allows the lung to fall away from the area of interest and provides appropriate exposure.

The position of the trocar sites varies with the position of the operative lesion being addressed. In general, it is best to place the thoracoscope through a trocar at least 15 to 20 cm distant from the lesion. This allows the trocar to be pulled back for greater panoramic viewing and to be advanced, allowing for magnification of the operative field. It is best that the trocar be faced in the same direction as the operating surgeon so that the view obtained is the same as that available through an open incision. A thoracoscope inserted into the chest so that it provides a view at 180 degrees opposite that of the surgeon provides a mirror image, thus making it much more difficult for the instruments to be manipulated appropriately. The ports for the instrumentation should be placed on either side of the port used for the thoracoscope, thus allowing for a relatively natural manipulation of the instruments with the left and right hands.

When a mediastinal lesion is being excised and there is a question as to its benignity, the specimen must be removed inside a specimen bag to prevent seeding of the trocar sites with malignant cells. If the specimen is so large that it is not removable via a trocar site, the site itself can easily be enlarged or an auxiliary thoracotomy incision can be made, allowing for the removal of larger specimens.

Lesions within the mediastinum are usually classified by location, depending on whether their site of origin is in the anterior, middle, or posterior mediastinal compartment. It is easiest to organize VATS mediastinal surgery using the same classification.

ANTERIOR MEDIASTINAL COMPARTMENT

Diagnosis

Anterior mediastinal masses most often require that a histologic diagnosis be obtained prior to the institution of therapy. In specific cases (e.g., anterior mediastinal mass with elevated β-human chorionic gonadotropin and α-fetoprotein), treatment can be instituted without the need for biopsy. However, in the majority of patients, a tissue diagnosis is required prior to therapeutic intervention. A CT-guided fine-needle aspiration (FNA) occasionally provides diagnostic cytology. Many lesions, especially lymphomas, require the acquisition of a piece of tissue for histologic analysis. Those lesions that are accessible via cervical mediastinoscopy should be approached in this fashion because a small muscle-splitting incision is required with no need for violation of the pleural cavity.

This obviates the need for single lung ventilation and chest tube drainage. Cervical mediastinoscopy has evolved into a simple outpatient procedure.

Anterior mediastinal lesions not accessible to mediastinoscopy can be biopsied either via an anterior mediastinotomy (Chamberlain procedure) approach or via thoracoscopy (Gossot et al, 1996). Both approaches have some disadvantages such as the potential for malignant seeding of the pleural cavity or subcutaneous tissue. VATS is certainly an acceptable alternative in such cases. For those patients in whom concomitant pleural or pulmonary lesions exist, thoracoscopy is a superior approach as it allows for simultaneous inspection and biopsy of the lung, pleural surfaces, and mediastinum.

Therapy

A number of anterior mediastinal lesions have been resected using VATS. Thoracoscopy has been used for the excision of intrathoracic parathyroid adenomas not accessible from the neck. Accurate preoperative localization of such lesions is imperative as they may be difficult to locate in the parathymic fat (DiBisceglie et al, 1998). Cystic lesions within the thymus or adjacent to the pericardium (the so-called springwater cyst) can also be excised in this fashion (Hazelrigg et al, 1993).

There is significant controversy regarding the issue of resection of anterior mediastinal tumors such as thymomas and benign teratomas. Reports by Landreneau, Yim, and Roviaro all report anecdotal cases or small series of patients undergoing resection of such lesions, which appear to be benign both on preoperative imaging studies and at the time of surgical excision (Landreneau et al, 1992; Roviaro et al, 1994; Yim, 1995). Yim has reported thymectomies in 11 such cases, with a median hospital stay of 3 days and no surgical mortality or intraoperative complications. A long-term follow-up is not yet available to demonstrate definitively that no late recurrences will appear. Although these authors have demonstrated the feasibility of this approach, its advisability must still be questioned. Such procedures should be undertaken only by an experienced thoracoscopic surgeon who will participate in careful postoperative surveillance. Any clinical or radiologic indication that an anterior mediastinal tumor is malignant constitutes, at present, an absolute contraindication to a thoracoscopic approach for resection.

The optimal operative approach for thymectomy in the treatment of myasthenia gravis patients (without thymoma) has been a controversial issue for many years. Both the sternotomy and cervical approaches have been touted as optimal by different investigators, with different degrees of radicalism suggested regarding resection. The addition of thoracoscopic thymectomy as an alternate surgical approach certainly does not clarify this situation. The feasibility of a VATS approach has been demonstrated by Mack, Mineo, and Yim (Mack and Scruggs, 1998; Mineo et al, 1997; Yim et al, 1999). Mineo's group tends to favor a left-sided approach using CO_2 insufflation (Mineo et al, 1997). However, Yim and colleagues favor a right-sided approach, stating that the visibility of the superior vena cava allows it to be identified quite easily; then dissection may be continued along the innominate vein where the veins from the thymus can be controlled and divided (Yim et al, 1999). Early results as reported by Mack and Scruggs (1998) are encouraging. At a mean follow-up of 23 months, 88% of all patients were improved, and 22% of patients without thymoma have experienced complete remission.

However, VATS thymectomy is technically a very challenging procedure, the results of which must be compared with those of the sternotomy and transcervical approaches. Low morbidity, short hospital stays, and minimal analgesic requirements are also reported with the alternate approaches. The primary advantage of VATS thymectomy over the other two procedures appears at this point to be aesthetic. Continued follow-up is required to ensure long-term efficacy. Although this appears to be an acceptable alternative in appropriate hands, it is uncertain at present which is the optimal approach.

MIDDLE MEDIASTINUM

Diagnosis

A lymphoma is one of the most common lesions occurring within the middle compartment of the mediastinum; the majority of these can be adequately approached and biopsied via cervical mediastinoscopy. As was noted earlier, this approach is generally preferred over thoracoscopy as it is less invasive and can essentially be performed on an outpatient basis. However, for those patients for whom a concomitant pleural or pulmonary lesion is to be evaluated, thoracoscopy provides an excellent approach for both biopsy of the mass and evaluation of the pleural and pulmonary structures.

VATS has also been used for lymph node staging in patients with both lung cancer (Mentzer et al, 1997) and carcinoma of the esophagus (Krasna, 1997). Nodes at levels 2, 3, 4, and 7 are easily evaluated via cervical mediastinoscopy, and this continues to be the method of choice for most patients with lung cancer. However, certain patients may demonstrate enlarged lymph nodes at level 10, level 8, or level 9; thoracoscopy provides an excellent alternative to thoracotomy for evaluation in such patients. Patients with enlarged nodes at stations 5 and 6 can be evaluated with either an anterior mediastinotomy or a VATS approach. Many surgeons prefer the latter option as it provides excellent visualization of these nodal stations and simultaneously provides an opportunity for evaluation of potential pleural, mediastinal, and chest wall masses and for ruling out any involvement by the primary tumor.

The staging of esophageal cancer via a combined thoracoscopic and laparoscopic approach is feasible and has been reported by Krasna (1997) to be accurate in over 90% of patients. His mediastinal lymph node dissection is usually performed via a right thoracoscopic approach with exposure of the esophagus from thoracic inlet to hiatus. For patients in whom the CT scan or endoscopic ultrasound suggests left-sided disease, a left-sided approach is also undertaken. An in-hospital stay of 2 to 4 days is routinely required. Although these procedures may be appropriate for achieving optimal staging in the setting of neoadjuvant protocols, they have not been widely adopted by the thoracic surgical community. This approach entails additional expense, inconvenience, and discomfort on the part of the patient and a greater investment of surgeon time and effort. If this minimally invasive staging protocol is someday proven to provide significant clinical benefit, it will likely be more widely adopted.

Therapy

The most common lesion in the middle mediastinal compartment that can be managed thoracoscopically is a bronchogenic cyst. Although these lesions are frequently adherent to adjacent structures, in most cases they can be entirely excised using only a VATS approach (Hazelrigg et al, 1993; Lewis et al, 1992; Naunheim and Andrus, 1993). Occasionally, the wall of such a cyst will become adherent to a major vascular structure (Fig. 64–16). In such cases, subtotal excision of the cyst can be undertaken with a portion of the wall left adherent to the vital structure. The lining of the cyst wall is cauterized in such cases to prevent secretion of fluid accumulation.

POSTERIOR MEDIASTINUM

Diagnosis

The majority of masses found in the posterior mediastinum of adults are benign. Unless these lesions are massive, excisional biopsy can often be safely performed via thoracoscopic approach. Occasional lymph nodes present in this compartment, and these can be easily biopsied for histology using VATS.

Therapy

Many small to moderately sized (less than 5 cm) posterior mediastinal masses can be excised thoracoscopically. Esophageal leiomyomas and gastrointestinal stromal tumors are infrequent but are amenable to thoracoscopic excision. These usually present as submucosal masses

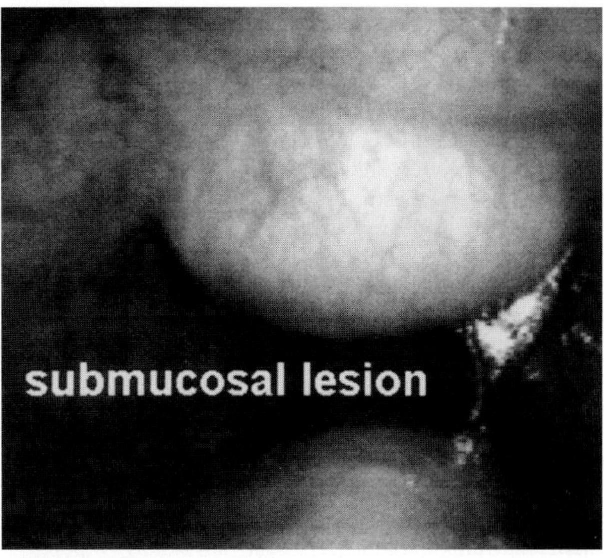

FIGURE 64–17 ■ An endoscopic view of submucosal mass in patient presenting with dysphagia.

(Fig. 64–17) that cause dysphagia. Endoscopic ultrasound confirms the presence of a solid submucosal mass that invades neither the mucosa nor the outermost layer of musculature (Fig. 64–18). VATS resection of esophageal leiomyomas has been reported by several surgeons (Gossot et al, 1993; Roviaro et al, 1998; Tamura et al, 1998). Mafune (1997) suggests that an esophageal balloon dilator placed immediately underneath the leiomyoma defines the edge of the tumor and allows the operator to more easily identify the submucosal plane in which dissection should occur. Although closure of the remaining musculature over the exposed submucosa is not an absolute necessity, one case of the development of a pseudodiverticulum at this site has been reported; thus, closure is encouraged, if possible (Bardini and Asolati, 1997).

Similarly, esophageal duplication or foregut duplication cysts in the posterior mediastinum have been re-

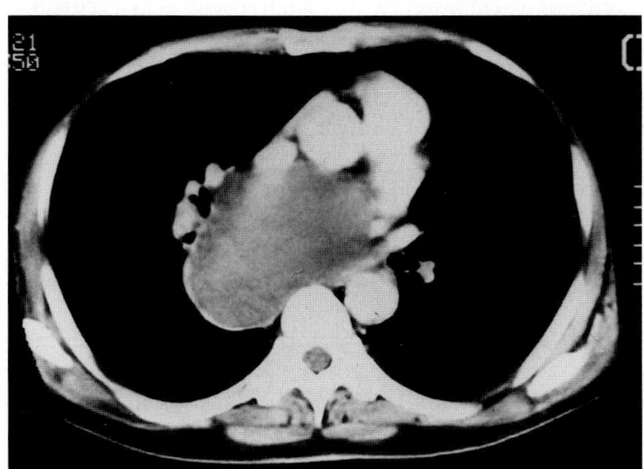

FIGURE 64–16 ■ A large middle mediastinal bronchogenic cyst in subcarinal location. This cyst was densely adherent to the right main pulmonary artery and bronchus.

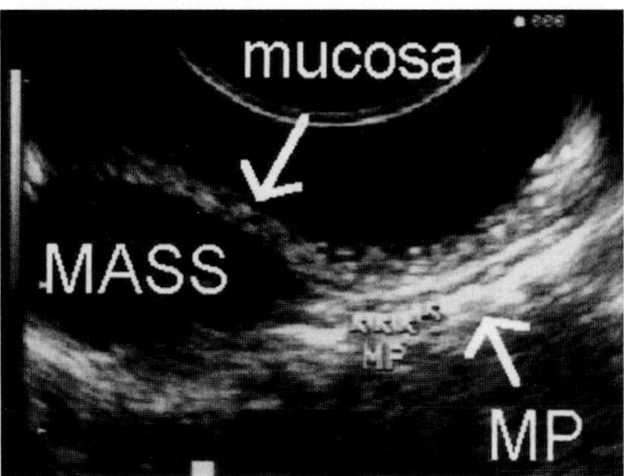

FIGURE 64–18 ■ An endoscopic ultrasound of esophageal leiomyoma demonstrating the extramucosal and intramuscular location. MP, muscularis propria.

sected via the thoracoscopic approach. This technique of surgery is quite similar to that of the leiomyoma in which a submucosal plane must be identified before the dissection is carried out within the plane. Similarly, closure of the muscular defect is advised.

It has been suggested that neurogenic tumors within the posterior mediastinum are usually ideal lesions for thoracoscopic excision as they are nearly all benign with relatively sparse vasculature. CT or MRI examination of these tumors is mandatory for ruling out spinal involvement (Fig. 64–19). One must be aware that up to 10% of these lesions extend through the neural foramen and lie adjacent to the dura overlying the spinal cord. These so-called "dumbbell" tumors must be identified preoperatively and treated with a combined neurosurgical/thoracic surgical approach. Avulsion of the tumor from its intraforaminal extension can lead to hemorrhage within the spinal canal and compression of the cord, with subsequent neurologic damage. There are many reports of thoracoscopic excision of simple neurogenic tumors (Dummy et al, 1998; Riquet et al, 1995); recently, even the dumbbell tumors have been resected with a combined thoracoscopic/neurosurgical approach (Heltzer et al, 1995; McKenna et al, 1995; Vallieres et al, 1995). Contraindications to a thoracoscopic incision include intraspinal extension of the tumor, evidence of malignant nature (infiltration of the surrounding structures), and tumors greater than 5 or 6 cm in diameter. A comparison of hospital stays of patients undergoing neurogenic tumor resection via the VATS and thoracotomy approaches has been published (Bousamra et al, 1996). The authors found that operative time was 50% longer in a thoracoscopy group, but that patients left the hospital on average 2 days earlier and returned to work 3 weeks earlier in the VATS cohort.

One of the most common therapeutic maneuvers undertaken within the posterior mediastinum is ablation of the sympathetic chain. Although this sympathetic denervation is occasionally undertaken for treatment of reflex sympathetic dystrophy, most commonly it is performed in the management of hyperhidrosis or facial blushing. Sympathetic denervation has been achieved in a number of ways, including cauterization of ganglia (Tan and Nam, 1998), division of the main sympathetic trunk (Rex et al, 1998), division of the rami communicantes (Gossot et al, 1997), application of a hemoclip on the trunk (Lin et al, 1998), and resection of the nerve (Krasna et al, 1998). The goal of all these maneuvers is to ablate the sympathetic innervation to the upper trunk or face.

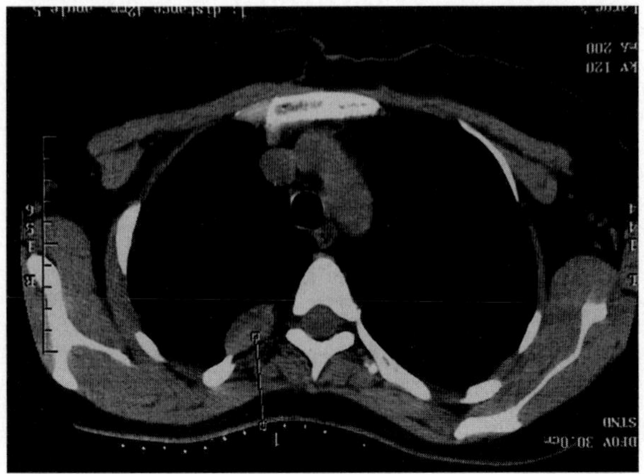

FIGURE 64–19 ■ A posterior mediastinal tumor in paraspinus location with no evidence of intraforaminal involvement.

The most frequent indication for sympathectomy is a palmar or axillary hyperhidrosis. Treatment of palmar hyperhidrosis requires ablation of the T2 sympathetic ganglion, although some investigators ablate the T3 ganglion as well. For axillary hyperhidrosis, many practitioners ablate the T2 through T4 ganglia. Sympathetic ablation at the T2 level has also been successfully used to treat the syndrome of severe episodic facial blushing, which has also been described as "social phobia" (Rex et al, 1998).

Thoracoscopic sympathectomy can be undertaken via one or two incisions in the midaxillary area. Five-millimeter ports are placed in the second, third, or fourth intercostal space, the lung is collapsed, and the sympathetic nerve is identified running along the heads of the thoracic ribs. The pleura is divided over the sympathetic chain, and the method of choice is used to ablate the sympathetic nerve. My own preference is excision of the second and third ganglia for palmar hyperhidrosis and resection of T2 through T4 for axillary hyperhidrosis. Success rates are generally highest for palmar hyperhidrosis and average approximately 95%. Axillary hyperhidrosis is alleviated in 68% to 90% of cases, and facial blushing in approximately 75% of cases (Rex et al, 1998). There are, however, some complications or side effects that may result from thoracoscopic sympathectomy for hyperhidrosis syndromes. Compensatory sweating is noted in the face, trunk, or legs in approximately 25% to 50% of cases. Although this is bothersome, the majority of people remain satisfied with the results. Damage to the stellate ganglion located at the apex of the chest can result in Horner's syndrome, with its resulting significant cosmetic defect. The incidence of this is approximately 1% or less, but it can prove to be a bothersome complication. Finally, gustatory sweating has been reported in approximately 10% of patients.

The majority of patients are quite happy with the results of their surgery, although there is a recurrence rate of approximately 5% (Gossot et al, 1997). Whether this is due to sympathetic regeneration of the nerve or establishment of alternate nerve pathways (nerve of Kuntz) is uncertain. However, the majority of patients do have a satisfactory long-term outcome and are free of hyperhidrosis for periods in excess of 15 years (Zacherl et al, 1998).

SUMMARY

Although it may not be performed frequently, thoracoscopic surgery in the mediastinum is feasible and can provide a minimally invasive approach to many lesions and diseases involving the mediastinum; however, it is paramount that the practitioner remember that the goal is more important than the approach. The mere ability to perform an operation in a minimally invasive fashion should not change the operative indications. Thoracoscopy provides an attractive and sophisticated approach to diseases of the mediastinum; however, it should not be used if there is an easier method for achieving the goal. One such example is the use of a thoracoscopic biopsy when a CT-directed fine-needle biopsy would suffice. Similarly, one should not make compromises or cut corners when performing an operation just so it can be completed thoracoscopically. Conversion to open thoracotomy is not a sin and is to be encouraged when doubt arises as to the safety or efficacy of a thoracoscopic procedure. Finally, it is important that thoracic surgeons realize that many mediastinal procedures require significant expertise and experience to be undertaken safely. This can represent relatively advanced thoracoscopic surgery, and a beginning surgeon should start with simpler pleural or pulmonary procedures prior to attempting a complex operation. If these rules are followed, thoracoscopic mediastinal surgery can yield significant benefit for the thoracic surgical patient population.

COMMENTS AND CONTROVERSIES

This chapter presents a balanced view of the current role of video-assisted thoracoscopy in the evaluation and treatment of mediastinal pathologies. At this point, less than a decade following the initial application of video-assisted thoracoscopic technology, there are a limited number of large case series and even fewer reports with genuine long-term follow-up. This is of particular relevance for a number of conditions, for example, myasthenia gravis. Although a number of authors advocate a video thoracoscopic approach for thymectomy, there are no data to suggest that this approach provides superior results to those obtained by a more conventional transsternal or transcervical approach. Indeed, it could be argued that the transcervical approach represents the least morbid technique for thymectomy.

However, for a number of other conditions such as dorsal sympathectomy or excision of benign neurogenic tumors, the video-assisted technique offers clear advantages. As technology further develops, video-assisted thoracoscopic approaches will become much more widely and successfully applied.

G. A. P.

REFERENCES

Bardini R, Asolati M: Thoracoscopic resection of benign tumours of the esophagus. Int Surg 82:5, 1997.

Bousamra M II, Hostler GB, Patterson GA, Roper CL: A comparative study of thoracoscopic vs open removal of benign neurogenic mediastinal tumors. Chest 109:1461, 1996.

Dummy TL, Krasna ME, Detterbeck FC et al: Multicenter VATS experience with mediastinal tumors. Ann Thorac Surg 66:187, 1998.

DiBisceglie M, Voltolini L, Paladini P et al: Ectopic parathyroid adenoma. Two cases treated with video-assisted thoracoscopic surgery. Scand J Thorac Cardiovasc Surg 32:51, 1998.

Gossot D, Toledo L, Celerier M: The thoracoscope as diagnostic tool for solid mediastinal masses. Surg Endosc 10:504, 1996.

Gossot D, Fourquier P, el Meteini M, Celerier M: Technical aspects of endoscopic removal of benign tumors of the esophagus. Surg Endosc 7:102, 1993.

Gossot D, Toledo L, Fritsch S, Celerier M: Thoracoscopic sympathectomy for upper limb hyperhidrosis: Looking for the right operation. Ann Thorac Surg 64:975, 1997.

Hazelrigg SR, Landreneau RJ, Mack ME, Acuff TE: Thoracoscopic resection of mediastinal cysts. Ann Thorac Surg 56:659, 1993.

Heltzer JM, Krasna ME, Aldrich F, McLaughlin JS: Thoracoscopic excision of a posterior mediastinal "dumbbell" tumor using a combined approach. Ann Thorac Surg 60:431, 1995.

Kern JA, Daniel TM, Tribble CG et al: Thoracoscopic diagnosis and treatment of mediastinal masses. Ann Thorac Surg 56:92, 1993.

Krasna ME: The role of thoracoscopic lymph node staging in esophageal cancer. Int Surg 82:7, 1997.

Krasna ME, Dummy TL, McKenna RJ, Mack ME: Thoracoscopic sympathectomy: The U.S. experience. Eur J Surg S580:19, 1998.

Landreneau RJ, Dowling RD, Castillo WM, Ferson PF: Thoracoscopic resection of an anterior mediastinal tumor. Ann Thorac Surg 54:142, 1992.

Lewis RJ, Caccavale RJ, Sisler GE: Imaged thoracoscopic surgery: A new thoracic technique for resection of mediastinal cysts. Ann Thorac Surg 53:318, 1992.

Lin CC, Mo LR, Lee LS et al: Thoracoscopic T2-sympathetic block by clipping: A better and reversible operation for treatment of hyperhidrosis palmaris: Experience with 326 cases. Eur J Surg S(580):13, 1998.

Mack ME, Scruggs G: Video-assisted thoracic surgery thymectomy for myasthenia gravis. Chest Surg Clin N Am 8:809, 1998.

Mafune K, Tanaka Y: Thorascopic enucleation of an esophageal leiomyoma with balloon dilator assistance. Surg Today 27:189, 1997.

McKenna RJ Jr, Maline D, Pratt G: VATS resection of a mediastinal neurogenic dumbbell tumor. Surg Laparosc Endosc 5:480, 1995.

Mentzer SJ, Swanson SJ, DeCamp MM et al: Mediastinoscopy, thoracoscopy, and video-assisted thoracic surgery in the diagnosis and staging of lung cancer. Chest 112(4S):239S, 1997.

Mineo TC, Pompeo E, Ambrogi V: Video-assisted thoracoscopic thymectomy: From the right or from the left? J Thorac Cardiovasc Surg 114:516, 1997.

Naunheim KS, Andrus CH: Thoracoscopic drainage and resection of giant mediastinal cyst. Ann Thorac Surg 55:156, 1993.

Rex LO, Drott C, Claes G et al: The Boras experience of endoscopic thoracic sympathicotomy for palmar, axillary, facial hyperhidrosis and facial blushing. Eur J Surg S(580):23, 1998.

Riquet M, Mouroux J, Pons F et al: Videothoracoscopic excision of thoracic neurogenic tumors. Ann Thorac Surg 60:943, 1995.

Roviaro G, Rebuffat C, Varoli F et al: Videothoracoscopic excision of mediastinal masses: Indications and technique. Ann Thorac Surg 58:1679, 1994.

Roviaro GC, Maciocco M, Varoli F et al: Video thoracoscopic treatment of esophageal leiomyoma. Thorax 53:190, 1998.

Tamura K, Takamori S, Tayama K et al: Thoracoscopic resection of giant leiomyoma of the esophagus with mediastinal outgrowth. Ann Thorac Cardiovasc Surg 4:351, 1998.

Tan V, Nam H: Results of thoracoscopic sympathectomy for 96 cases of palmar hyperhidrosis. Ann Thorac Cardiovasc Surg 4:244, 1998.

Vallieres E, Findlay JM, Fraser RE: Combined microneurosurgical and thoracoscopic removal of neurogenic dumbbell tumors. Ann Thorac Surg 59:469, 1995.

Yim AP: Video-assisted thoracoscopic management of anterior mediastinal masses. Preliminary experience and results. Surg Endosc 9:1184, 1995.

Yim AP, Kay RL, Izzat MB, Ng SK: Video-assisted thoracoscopic thymectomy for myasthenia gravis. Semin Thorac Cardiovasc Surg 11:65, 1999.

Zacherl J, Huber ER, Imhof M et al: Long-term results of 630 thoracoscopic sympathicotomies for primary hyperhidrosis: The Vienna experience. Eur J Surg S(580):43, 1998.

Trauma

CHAPTER 65

Pathophysiology and Initial Management of Trauma

Joshua H. Burack
Lisa S. Dresner

HISTORICAL NOTE

Successful treatment of injuries to the thorax requires a fundamental base of anatomic and physiologic knowledge, combined with technical skill and creativity. Many milestones in thoracic surgery were first reported on patients with traumatic injury.

The Smith Papyrus, an account of Egyptian civilization in 3000 BC, records three cases of penetrating chest injury. Two substantial chest wall injuries were treated conservatively and a third wound to the cervical esophagus was repaired with suture. Homer, in an account of the siege of Troy in 950 BC, described a multitude of chest wounds, including the infamous death of Sarpedon, who exsanguinated after removal of a spear that had penetrated the heart (Meade, 1961).

Many current advances and observations that are essential to the seminal growth of thoracic surgery occurred on the battlefield. Theodoric promoted the débridement and primary closure of chest wounds in the 13th century. The value of an occlusive thoracic dressing, in the setting of open hemopneumothorax, was inadvertently discovered by the Napoleonic surgeon Larrey in 1767. The mystique surrounding direct suture of the heart was dispelled by the German surgeon Rehn, who performed the first successful cardiorrhaphy for a penetrating injury in 1896 (Hochberg, 1960; Meade, 1961).

Over the past century, mortality rates from military thoracic injury have steadily declined from 63% in the American Civil War to 9% in the Vietnam conflict (Kovaric et al, 1969; Meade, 1961). The modern advances in surgical technique, early transport and resuscitation, pleural drainage, precise diagnostic tests, and direct operative repair, along with advances in antibiotic therapy, transfusion methods, and anesthesia, continue to promote a greater likelihood of survival.

INCIDENCE

In the United States, 150,000 people die each year as a result of trauma. It is the most common cause of death in people younger than 40. Approximately 25% of the deaths can be directly related to thoracic injury (Krantz et al, 1997). Fortunately, devastating multitrauma or massive injury to the heart, lungs, or great vessels is relatively rare and is usually responsible for death moments after injury. In the first hour after hospital admission, thoracic vascular and neurologic trauma are the most common causes of death (Acosta et al, 1998). Overall, thoracic trauma has a mortality rate of approximately 10%, and treatment is usually straightforward and successful. Most patients survive as a result of a prompt resuscitation, efficient diagnostic testing, and simple therapeutic maneuvers. Formal operative treatment is required in less than 10% of blunt and between 15% and 30% of penetrating injuries (Mattox and Wall, 1997; Oglesby 1971; Stewart et al, 1997; Tarantino and Bernhard, 1992). It is the initial management, in the "golden hour" after injury, that is responsible for a substantial survival.

ANATOMIC CONSIDERATIONS

Precise anatomic knowledge is crucial for the initial assessment of injury. In the diagnostic phase, injury must be considered to be multicavity if the superior or inferior extent of the thorax has been violated (Fig. 65–1). The diaphragm, at the inferior margin, is frequently injured in truncal trauma. The skin landmarks for the diaphragm extend between the umbilicus and nipple (fourth intercostal space) anteriorly and the inferior tip of the scapula posteriorly. The bony landmarks for the diaphragm extend from T8 to L1. At the superior margin of the chest lies the thoracic outlet, often referred to as zone 1 of the neck. The zone extends from the cricothyroid membrane to the sternal notch. Particularly in penetrating trauma, injuries at either margin of the chest increase the potential for complex injury. Furthermore, hemothorax may be the result of an extrathoracic injury decompressing into

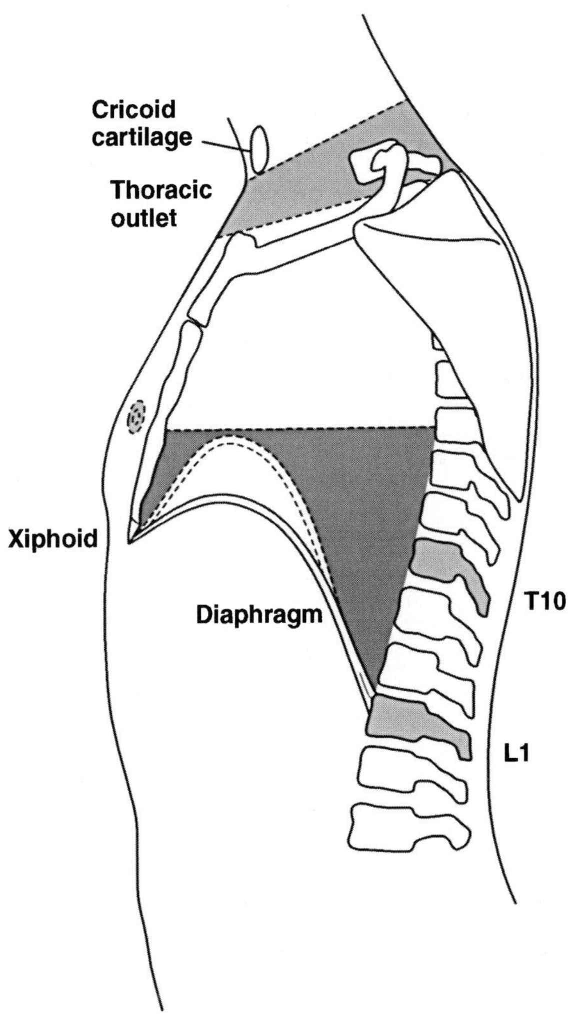

FIGURE 65–1 ■ The boundaries of the thorax: diaphragmatic excursion and the thoracic outlet.

the chest through the diaphragm or from the vessels in the neck.

The thorax is divided into separate body cavities defined by the parietal membrane attachments: the pleural spaces, the pericardium, and the posterior mediastinum. These cavities can readily communicate with the peritoneum or the cervical structures as a result of injury. The physiologic response to hemorrhage into the pleura and pericardium is dramatically different. In the adult, each pleural space can accommodate as much as 3 L of blood. This large volume loss will cause rapid progression to class IV hemorrhagic shock and exsanguination (Table 65–1). In contrast, the pericardium can only acutely accommodate an additional 100 ml of blood before venous return and diastolic filling are impaired, causing cardiac tamponade and shock.

The integrity of the chest wall and the underlying pleural membrane is essential for respiratory function. Negative intrapleural pressure, the coordinated function of the thoracic musculoskeletal system, and a patent airway are all required for respiration. Airway obstruction or injury, pneumothorax, hemothorax, and a significant flail chest are life-threatening injuries unless quickly treated. An open pneumothorax related to a traumatic chest wall defect will seriously compromise spontaneous respiration. If the defect is larger than the cross-sectional area of the trachea, ventilation will preferentially occur across the defect, rather than down the trachea (Krantz et al, 1997).

PATHOPHYSIOLOGY

The pathophysiologic response to injury is related to the primary mechanism of injury. Injury can be easily classified into blunt or penetrating.

Blunt trauma is most commonly a result of vehicular accidents, followed by falls, assaults, and sports, crush, or blast injuries. The severity of a blunt injury is proportional to the force or the kinetic energy involved. Newton's second law of motion describes the relationship $F = MA$. The force (F) of a blunt injury and the resultant gross effects are directly proportional to the mass (M) and acceleration (A) of the impacting object (Pezzella et al, 1998). The most common blunt thoracic injury is a pulmonary contusion, and the extent of the alveolar hemorrhage and parenchymal injury is directly related to the magnitude of a blunt chest wall injury (Cohn, 1997). Blunt injury can be compounded by dislocated skeletal fracture, which may lacerate underlying viscera with sharp fragments.

Substantial blunt injury can also occur without direct impact. Damage from a blast pressure wave preferentially affects gas-containing organs: intestine, eardrum, and

TABLE 65–1 ■ **Estimated Blood Loss Based on Initial Vital Signs***

	Class I	*Class II*	*Class III*	*Class IV*
Blood Loss (ml)	<750	750–1500	1500–2000	>2000
Blood Loss (% blood volume)	<15%	15%–30%	30%–40%	>40%
Pulse Rate	<100	>100	>120	>140
Blood Pressure	Normal	Normal	Decreased	Decreased
Respiratory Rate	14–20	20–30	30–40	>35
Urine Output (ml/hr)	>30	20–30	5–15	Negligible
Mental Status	Anxious	Anxious	Confused	Lethargic
Fluid Replacement (3:1 rule†)	Crystalloid	Crystalloid	Crystalloid and blood	Crystalloid and blood

*70-kg man.

†An empirical resuscitation formula requiring approximately 300 ml of crystalloid solution for each 100 ml of blood loss.

Adapted from Committee on Trauma, American College of Surgeons: Advanced Trauma Life Support Program for Doctors, 6th ed. Chicago, American College of Surgeons, 1997.

lung. Shock and hypoxemia characterize the clinical response to a major blast injury. In an animal model of blast-induced circulatory shock, pulmonary hemorrhage with ventilation-perfusion mismatch and a unique type of cardiogenic shock with myocardial depression without compensatory vasoconstriction were the primary pathophysiologic processes (Irwin et al, 1997).

Additional important injury can occur as a result of torsion or rotational forces. In response to significant force or deceleration, anatomic structures, fixed in position by membranous attachments, can be avulsed at the point of mediastinal fixation. Injuries to the aortic isthmus, main bronchus, diaphragm, or atria are prototypical. Early survival is related to the integrity and strength of the mediastinal pleura.

An uncommon injury mechanism is hypothesized to occur when visceral rupture or valvular disruption occurs after blunt trauma. Coincident with blunt impact, intraluminal disruptive forces are intensified when a hollow viscus is a closed space with a fixed volume. Presumably after glottic closure, the trachea or the esophagus can burst, or during coaptation the cardiac valves and subvalvular apparatus can be avulsed (Martin de Nicholas et al, 1996; Pretre and Chilcott, 1997).

The host response to equivalent force is also variable. Immature bones are less calcified and more resilient than their adult counterparts. In comparison with adults, particularly the elderly, children have a much lower incidence of bone injury after major blunt trauma. A rib fracture in a child is usually a marker of a severe injury (Garcia et al, 1990; Nakayama et al, 1989). After motor vehicular accidents, blunt aortic rupture is associated with rib fracture in approximately 50% of adults (Lee et al, 1997). However, in children, blunt aortic rupture almost always occurs without rib fracture (Trachiotis et al, 1996). In addition, different solid organs, based on their inherent architecture, have different behavior when subject to equivalent blunt force. In the bovine model, before organ rupture occurs the heart can sustain almost twice the blunt force than can the spleen or the liver (Seki and Iwamoto, 1998).

Penetrating injury typically causes a laceration of anatomic structures in the trajectory of the weapon. Knife and bullet wounds are the most common routes of injury. Unpredictable missile ricochet can drastically alter the path of injury. However, in the thorax, large deflections in the missile trajectory are uncommon and are unlikely unless an associated fracture of the impacted bone is present (Hollerman et al, 1990). The kinetic energy of a missile is dependent on its weight and velocity. This energy disrupts cells and fragments tissues in an area around the path of the bullet. The actual size of this cavity is determined by the size, rotation, and tumbling of the missile. Close-range wounds are more destructive because less of the energy is dissipated by air friction. As the magnitude of the weapon increases from knife to low-velocity and then high-velocity bullets, the accompanying blast effect to surrounding structures rises. A high-velocity military missile (>3000 ft/sec) is 36 times more destructive than a low-velocity missile (<500 ft/sec) (Swan and Swan, 1991).

SHOCK AND RESUSCITATION

Shock is defined as a syndrome that is initiated by a global decrease in perfusion that results in inadequate delivery of oxygen to tissues and thus in organ dysfunction. Early shock after trauma generally is a result of hemorrhage and hypovolemia. After cardiac tamponade or tension pneumothorax, compressive shock can occur after mechanical compression of the heart within the confines of the pericardium or thorax. Less common is cardiogenic shock from myocardial failure and neurogenic shock secondary to loss of sympathetic tone.

The physiologic response to hemorrhagic shock is well understood. The magnitude of response is dependent on the volume of hemorrhage (see Table 65–1). A decrease in blood pressure immediately causes an increase in sympathetic activity with tachycardia and vasoconstriction. Within minutes, this is augmented by excretion of epinephrine and norepinephrine. Constriction of the microvasculature in the skin, kidneys, viscera, and the capacitance vessels in skeletal muscle and the lungs shifts blood centrally, increasing effective blood volume. This increased central blood volume, tachycardia, and increased myocardial contractility results in increased cardiac output and a state of compensated shock.

The neuroendocrine response to injury varies with the severity of injury, volume of hemorrhage, presence of shock, and preexisting medical conditions. In response to trauma, the early response results in an elevation of circulating norepinephrine and epinephrine levels. Additionally, there is an increase in circulating cortisol in response to a sudden increase in adrenocorticotropic hormone from the anterior pituitary. Cortisol levels are elevated for up to 48 hours and are responsible for tissue catabolism that provides the necessary substrates for wound healing and hepatic synthesis of glucose and acute phase proteins. The neuroendocrine response to stress also modifies salt and water excretion. Aldosterone and antidiuretic hormone both cause a decrease in urine volume and sodium reabsorption, causing fluid and sodium retention. Glucagon levels increase and insulin levels decrease, signalling hepatic gluconeogenesis. If the patient suffers no complications, this catabolic phase lasts 2 to 6 days and is followed by a prolonged period of anabolism with positive nitrogen balance with normalization of salt and water excretion (Mullins, 1996).

The cellular response to injury is a consequence of hypoperfusion and reduced oxygen delivery, below the oxygen requirements of the cellular apparatus. The hypoxemic insult initiates anaerobic metabolism and lactate production. With sustained untreated hypoperfusion, precapillary sphincters fail and cellular membrane function becomes impaired. Cellular acidosis and swelling ensue, and the patient becomes more and more resistant to resuscitation. If not rapidly corrected, this uncompensated state results in death.

As a result of resuscitation, perfusion is restored to the microvasculature of ischemic cells and a reperfusion injury is initiated. Reperfusion injury is thought to be essential to the development of systemic inflammatory syndromes and post-traumatic organ failure. The injury is amplified by an interrelated cascade of inflammatory mediators: complement cytokines, coagulation cascade proteins, kinins, and prostaglandins. In addition, free radicals, normally scavenged by healthy cells, persist in the ischemic cell long enough to degrade the lipid cellular membrane. Activated neutrophils subsequently adhere to damaged endothelial cells, resulting in microvascular thrombosis, edema, and further ischemia. Ultimately, it is endothelial cell structure and function that are the initial and final common pathways in organ dysfunction and failure seen after trauma (Calhoon and Trinkle, 1997; Mullins, 1996).

Treatment of hemorrhagic shock requires control of hemorrhage and reconstitution of circulating blood volume. After securing the airway and ensuring ventilation, the search for possible sources of hemorrhage and volume resuscitation should occur simultaneously. In hypotensive patients, 1 to 2 L of warm lactated Ringer's solution should be infused, and the response should be observed (Table 65–2). The traditional 3:1 rule suggests early resuscitation with a volume of crystalloid that is three times greater than that of the estimated blood loss (Krantz et al, 1997). If improvement in blood pressure is minimal or transient, then hemorrhage is significant and blood transfusion should be considered while additional crystalloid is infused. Transfusion is recommended if the blood loss is estimated to be greater than 25% of the total blood volume (Mullins, 1996). Crossmatched type-specific blood is ideal, but time constraints may necessitate the use of type-specific, type O–negative or autologous blood. Shed blood, particularly in an anticoagulated pleural collection system, can be autotransfused. However, blood collected from a hemothorax is deficient in platelets, fibrinogen, and the ability to form clot (Symbas, 1978).

The advantage of prompt control of active hemorrhage is undisputed. Nonetheless, the timing, volume, and extent of preoperative resuscitation and the value of massive infusion before definitive control of hemorrhage remain controversial. In a randomized prospective series of hypotensive patients with penetrating torso trauma, traditional preoperative volume resuscitation increased complications, length of hospital stay, and mortality. It is possible that aggressive administration of fluids before surgical control of bleeding causes hemodilution and relative hypertension, which disrupts thrombus, increases bleeding, and therefore decreases survival (Bickell et al, 1994). In addition, the pneumatic antishock garments, a device thought to augment autotransfusion, have been associated with an increased mortality rate, particularly in cases of cardiac or thoracic vascular injury (Mattox et al, 1989). A minimal resuscitation appears to be beneficial in patients with compensated shock who undergo expedient surgical repair, but the widespread application of this methodology to all trauma patients, particularly those with blunt trauma or with profound and persistent hypotension, remains uncertain.

The presence of a robust distal circulation, with bounding radial or pedal pulses and warm, pink extremities, almost certainly excludes hypovolemic shock. However, normalization of blood pressure, pulse rate, and urine output alone are not sensitive indicators of resolution of shock. This is particularly true for patients after class I, II, and III hemorrhage in whom vital signs are not substantially abnormal but patients remain in shock, albeit compensated shock (Porter and Ivatury, 1998). Shock may be more precisely defined as inadequate tissue perfusion and oxygenation with resultant anaerobic metabolism, and evidence of improved tissue oxygenation or tissue perfusion may provide more precise endpoints of resuscitation. Clinical markers of hypoperfusion and cellular acidosis include serum lactate and base deficit determinations. Serum lactate rises with hypovolemic shock, and increasing levels are associated with increased likelihood of death. In addition, the longer the time to normalize lactate, the worse the outcome (Abramson et al, 1993). Base deficit, calculated from the arterial blood gas, correlates with severity of injury and risk of death. It generally reflects serum lactate as well. It has the advantage that it is readily available, is inexpensive, and can provide important physiologic information about the adequacy of resuscitation (Porter and Ivatury, 1998).

HISTORY AND PHYSICAL EXAMINATION

An accurate history and physical examination are essential. Obviously, the extent of the initial evaluation may be abbreviated, owing to the severity of injury and the tempo of therapeutic intervention. Furthermore, the initial assessment may be limited by the previous paramedic intervention and it may be difficult to evaluate an intubated, restrained patient. At the minimum, an AMPLE history should be obtained: *A*llergies, *M*edications commonly used, *P*ast illnesses or *P*regnancy, *L*ast meal, and the *E*vents related to injury (Krantz et al, 1997).

Re-creation of the injury scene, from the patient's or paramedical personnel's accounts, can be rewarding. Certain types of vehicular accidents are associated with patterns of injury. A frontal impact and the pathognomonic

TABLE 65–2 ■ **Responses to Initial Fluid Resuscitation***

	Rapid Response	*Transient Response*	*No Response*
Vital Signs	Normalize	Transient improvement	Remain abnormal
Estimated Blood Loss	Minimal (<20%)	Moderate and ongoing (20%–40%)	Severe (>40%)
Need for More Crystalloid	Low	High	High
Need for Blood	Low	Moderate to high	Immediate
Need for Operative Intervention	Possibly	Likely	Highly likely

*2000 ml Ringer's lactate solution in adults; 20 ml/kg Ringer's lactate bolus in children.

Adapted from Committee on Trauma, American College of Surgeons: Advanced Trauma Life Support Program for Doctors, 6th ed. Chicago, American College of Surgeons, 1997.

bent steering wheel suggest substantial blunt trauma to the chest wall, lungs, heart, and aortic isthmus. A passenger involved in a side-impact accident as well as a pedestrian struck by an automobile both have the increased possibility of a significant injury to the solid upper abdominal organs on the side of the impact as well as blunt aortic rupture (Fabian et al, 1997; Krantz et al, 1997). Ejection from the vehicle and death of another occupant in the vehicle are both associated with a higher incidence of lethal multiple injuries (Krantz et al, 1997).

Other common blunt-injury mechanisms, which should be quantified at the time of admission, are falls from heights, crush injuries, assaults, and sports injuries. Blunt impact to the chest during sports activities, particularly baseball in children, can result in commotio cordis and sudden death (Maron et al, 1995). The history is vital because physical findings are often absent.

The specifics of a penetrating injury can also be important. The dimension of the knife, or impaling object, the position of the combatants at the time of the assault, the caliber of the weapon, and the number of shots fired are helpful. Unfortunately, this information is usually vague and unreliable, but occasionally valuable hints about the anatomic extent of injury can be obtained.

Physical examination of the trauma patient is straightforward. Vital signs must be obtained on admission to the ER and compared with those obtained in the field. The vital signs on presentation will provide an estimate of the blood loss (see Table 65–1). As a rule, profound hypotension and a depressed sensorium indicate thoracic or abdominal hemorrhage, rather than the infrequent neurologic injury and neurogenic shock. The hemodynamic responses of the heart rate and blood pressure to the ongoing resuscitation must be appraised at frequent intervals. Intact peripheral pulses and perfused extremities imply a normovolemic state. The response to early resuscitation has significant implications for the amount of hemorrhage present and the need for operative intervention (see Table 65–2).

Evaluation and Treatment of the ABCs

*A*irway, *B*reathing, and *C*irculation constitute the initial assessment (Krantz et al, 1997). Ventilation is evaluated by observing the respiratory rate and the quality of chest wall and diaphragmatic excursion. If stridor is present, a maxillofacial or tracheal injury is probable. Frank disruption of the airway can be obvious with air escaping from a cervical penetrating injury or subcutaneous emphysema (Rossbach et al, 1998). Hemoptysis is usually insignificant after trauma and suggests a parenchymal lung or tracheobronchial injury. Massive hemoptysis (>500 ml) can occasionally be seen with a major pulmonary vascular injury. A "sucking" chest wound and the concomitant open pneumothorax and impaired ventilation are equally obvious and will cause rapid ventilatory decompensation if large enough. Rarely, traumatic asphyxia can occur as a result of a massive crush injury causing temporary compression of the superior vena cava or blunt cardiac rupture and is characterized by upper body plethora, petechiae, and edema.

Both lung fields are auscultated for air entry and presence of breath sounds. The diagnosis of a pneumothorax or hemothorax is a clinical one. At the accident scene, or if the patient is unstable, chest tube decompression is often initiated before radiographic confirmation. Despite a noisy emergency department (ED), auscultation to detect hemothorax and pneumothorax is useful for both blunt and penetrating trauma patients. The absence of breath sounds has a positive predictive value of greater than 95% to detect abnormal pleural air or blood (Chen et al, 1997; Schmidt et al, 1998).

Once and if the patient is stabilized in the ED, a careful secondary survey can proceed. The entire chest wall can be palpated to evaluate for a flail segment, crepitance, soft tissue contusion, or deformity of the ribs, sternum, or clavicle. A flail chest is considered to be present if four or more ribs have fracture or dislocations in at least two places or if an obvious paradox of the chest wall occurs with inspiration. Sternal fractures or dislocations are usually indicated by point tenderness or a "step off." Fracture or dislocation of the sternoclavicular joint may cause prominence of the clavicular head in the case of the more common anterior dislocation or cause compression of the structures of the thoracic inlet along with the "hollowed-out pocket" deformity of a posterior dislocation (Mayberry and Trunkey, 1997).

Hematomas, particularly of the thoracic inlet, can be marked and measured. Peripheral pulses are documented. A pseudocoarctation syndrome can be present after blunt aortic rupture or dissection (Pretre and Chilcott, 1997). Carotid pulsations and distended neck veins are noted. The heart is auscultated, because sometimes Beck's triad (muffled heart sounds, distended neck veins, and pulsus paradoxus) is present and suggests cardiac tamponade. However, tension pneumothorax may cause similar symptoms. In addition, the axillae and the back must be carefully examined, so that a small penetrating injury is not missed. Lastly, a penetrating object impaled in the chest is left undisturbed, to be removed in the operating room (Fig. 65–2).

INITIAL EVALUATION

Bedside Procedures

The airway is secured, and respiration is maintained. If adequate ventilation is not present, the airway is usually obtained by orotracheal intubation. Extreme care must be exercised if a cervical spine fracture is suggested, and manual cervical spine alignment must be maintained during intubation. If significant maxillofacial trauma or airway obstruction is present, the airway is obtained with a cricothyroidotomy (Fig. 65–3). If there is suspicion of a blunt injury to the cervical trachea, orotracheal intubation should proceed over a flexible bronchoscope, with the ability to perform a surgical airway in reserve (Grover et al, 1979). After a major blast injury, excessive positive-pressure ventilation must be avoided to minimize alveolar disruption (Irwin et al, 1997).

Venous access is secured with large-bore (<16 gauge) peripheral catheters. If a major venous injury is suggested, access must be obtained proximal to an abdominal injury or on the contralateral side of a thoracic ve-

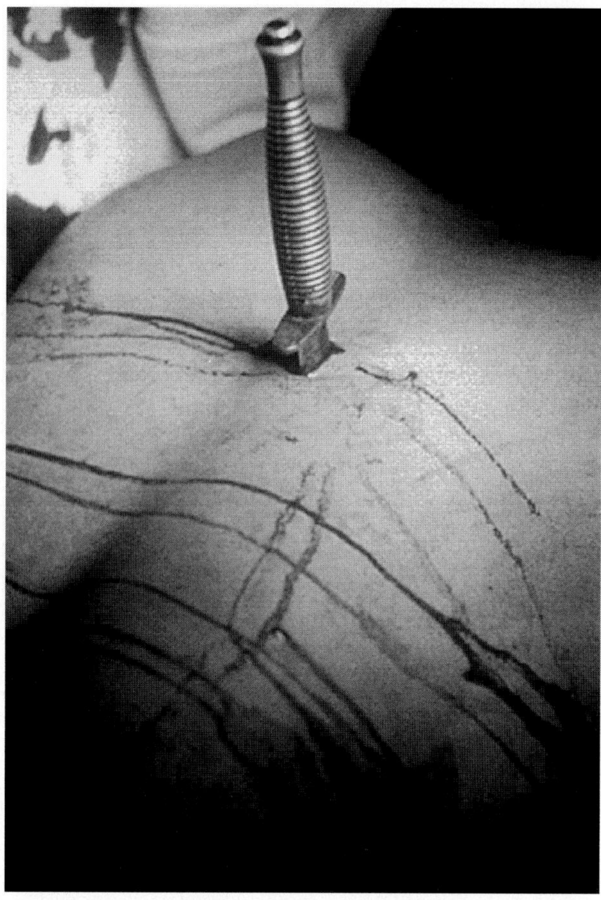

FIGURE 65–2 ■ Impaled knife in the back. A 23-year-old male who sustained a stab wound, with impalement, to the right posterior thorax. A right lateral thoracotomy identified minor pulmonary parenchymal and chest wall injuries.

nous injury to avoid extravasation of resuscitation fluid into the peritoneum or pleura. A subclavian or internal jugular central venous catheter is desirable, and in the case of a cardiac injury an elevation in the central venous pressure will suggest the diagnosis.

The heart rate and rhythm are observed with continuous electrocardiographic monitoring. In the case of penetrating cardiac trauma, normal sinus rhythm is a favorable prognostic sign (Asensio et al, 1998). Obvious electrocardiographic abnormalities, or irritability, along with creatine phosphokinase-MB isoenzyme (CPK-MB) elevation are the simplest and most accurate predictors of a significant cardiac contusion and the need for monitored observation (Maenza et al, 1996). Commotio cordis is heralded by ventricular fibrillation and cardiopulmonary arrest (Maron et al, 1995). A pulseless agonal idioventricular rhythm or asystole usually implies a prolonged arrest and irretrievable injury. Despite traumatic cardiopulmonary arrest, moribund penetrating trauma victims, but not similar blunt trauma victims, will occasionally survive (Stratton et al, 1998).

A Foley catheter is inserted and the urine output is monitored. A satisfactory urine output (>1 ml/kg/min) implies a satisfactory cardiac output and tissue perfusion (see Table 65–1). A nasogastric tube is inserted to provide gastric drainage and avoid pulmonary aspiration. A nasogastric tube may provide valuable hints about the integrity of the diaphragm or the presence of a mediastinal hematoma.

Drainage of the pleural space with a chest tube may be initiated if the diagnosis of hemothorax or pneumothorax is clinically suggested (Chen et al, 1997; Schmidt et al, 1998). Pleural drainage alone is a simple and definitive treatment in the majority of patients with thoracic trauma (Mattox and Wall, 1997; Oglesby 1971; Stewart et al, 1997; Tarantino and Bernhard, 1992). An open pneumothorax requires an occlusive dressing and subsequent chest tube decompression.

Chest tube insertion is typically performed at the level of the fifth intercostal space, on the lateral aspect of the thorax (Fig. 65–4). The skin is prepared and topical anesthetic is administered, particularly to the subdermal region, the periosteum of the rib, and the pleural membrane. A small skin incision (2 cm) is created in the anterior-axillary line, just lateral to the pectoralis muscle in males, or to the lateral mammary crease in females. With the use of a curved clamp, the intercostal space is bluntly dissected and the pleura is carefully entered over the superior aspect of the rib. A finger is placed in the pleural space to ensure that pulmonary adhesions are not present and then a large chest tube (36–40 French) is positioned posteriorly and cephalad in the pleural space. The initial amount of blood drained and the degree of air leak are noted. A massive, continuous air leak and a significant hemothorax are prime indications for a formal thoracotomy (Fig. 65–5). A second chest tube for a retained hemothorax is less desirable; rather, a video-assisted thoracoscopy and operative evacuation is preferable (Meyer et al, 1997).

Diagnostic Tests

A routine arterial blood gas analysis, complete blood cell count, and chemistry (SMA-18) values can all be obtained from a single puncture of the radial or femoral artery. An indwelling radial arterial line is desirable, particularly in patients with multiple injuries destined for a multitude of diagnostic tests or if there is significant suggestion of a blunt aortic rupture and the blood pressure must be strictly regulated (Fabian et al, 1998).

Arterial blood gas analysis will provide additional insight as to the quality of ventilation. The clinical evaluation of respiration remains paramount, but identification of significant hypoxemia or hypercarbia will support the use of mechanical ventilation. The serum pH and base deficit corresponds to the degree of shock and the quality of the resuscitative effort. A profound or persistent acidosis (pH of <7.20 or base deficit >12 mEq/L) implies decompensated shock and substantial mortality (Mullins, 1996; Porter and Ivatury, 1998).

Blood is sent for crossmatch, and routine blood analysis is performed. A complete blood cell count will provide a serum hematocrit, which has a limited role in predicting the amount of acute blood loss or the response to resuscitation. Chemistry analysis is important only to confirm electrolyte balance during volume infusion and to determine serum CPK-MB and troponin levels if blunt cardiac

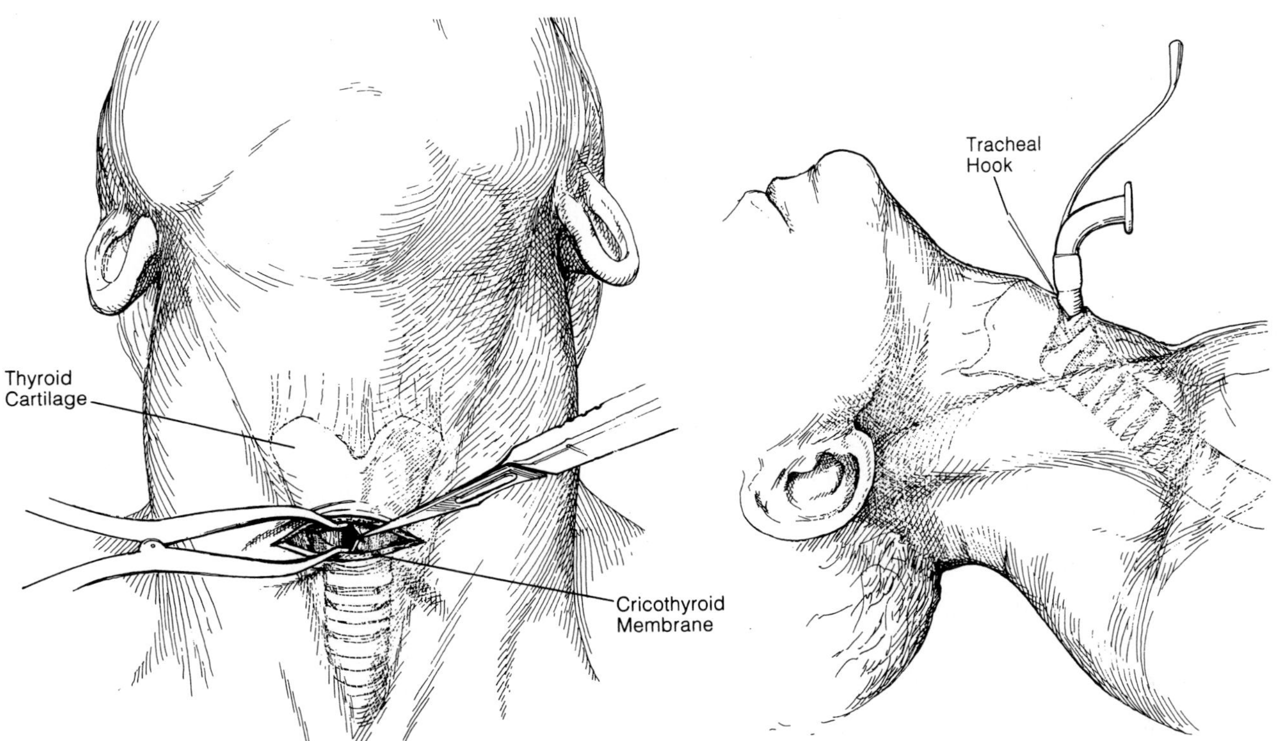

FIGURE 65–3 ■ Technique for cricothyroidotomy. A transverse skin incision is made over the cricothyroid membrane, which is then incised with a scalpel. The incision in the membrane is bluntly spread apart, and a tracheostomy tube is inserted. (From Moore FA, Moore EE: Trauma resuscitation. In Wilmore DN, Brennan MF, Harken AH et al [eds]: Care of the Surgical Patient. New York, Scientific American, 1989.)

trauma is suggested. Elevated levels of CPK-MB (>50 U/L or a fraction of >5%) or troponin T (>0.20 μg/L) are relatively nonspecific but combined with the presence of arrhythmia or electrocardiographic abnormalities confirm the diagnosis of cardiac contusion (Fulda et al, 1997; Maenza et al, 1996).

An admission chest radiograph is an essential part of the diagnostic workup (Table 65–3). The important exceptions are those moribund patients in whom immediate operative therapy is required and those patients with an obvious pneumothorax or hemothorax who require urgent chest tube decompression before radiographic confirmation. Review of the chest radiograph should be methodical and should include the pleural spaces, the diaphragm, the pulmonary parenchyma, the mediastinum, the bony structures, and indwelling tubes and catheters.

A pneumothorax can be subtle and may be apparent only when comparing inspiratory and expiratory films, or it may occur hours after the initial injury. More commonly, a traumatic pneumothorax is obvious and can progress to a tension pneumothorax with mediastinal shift (Fig. 65–6). A massive pneumothorax with complete collapse of the lung ("fallen lung sign") or abrupt cutoff of the mainstem bronchus ("bronchial cut-off sign") suggests bronchial rupture with complete distal atelectasis (Mirvis, 1992) (Fig. 65–7).

An upright chest radiograph makes the diagnosis of a hemothorax or hemopneumothorax relatively straightforward, with the loss of the costophrenic sulcus and a fluid meniscus. A supine film may be difficult to interpret, and subtle changes in pleural opacification may be missed, particularly if they are bilateral. A massive hemothorax, with retained intrapleural blood, can trap air next to the mediastinum and cause "the medial meniscus sign" or a "caked hemothorax" (Feliciano, 1992) (Fig. 65–8).

The radiographic evaluation of the diaphragm can be difficult. Persistent elevation usually suggests an intra-abdominal process, and flattening or inversion suggests a tension pneumothorax. Traumatic diaphragmatic disruption infrequently appears as an acute eventration of intra-abdominal contents into the pleural space, but it is usually suggested by a subtle loss of diaphragmatic contour or a pleural effusion in the majority of patients (Mirvis, 1992; Symbas et al, 1986).

Radiographic evaluation of the pulmonary parenchyma may reveal a spectrum of changes seen with contusion. Typically, an early contusion can appear as a fluffy, air space–occupying process located in a nonanatomic distribution ("geographic distribution") in the periphery of the lung fields and in proximity to bony fracture. However, a large pulmonary contusion, or pulmonary hematoma, can manifest with substantial opacification of the lung fields and can be confused with a hemothorax. Less common are traumatic pneumatoceles, which have an appearance similar to that of bullae or blebs.

Injury within the mediastinum produces extravasated air or blood. Pneumomediastinum is commonly a self-limited radiographic abnormality that is thought to be related to alveolar barotrauma and subsequent dissection

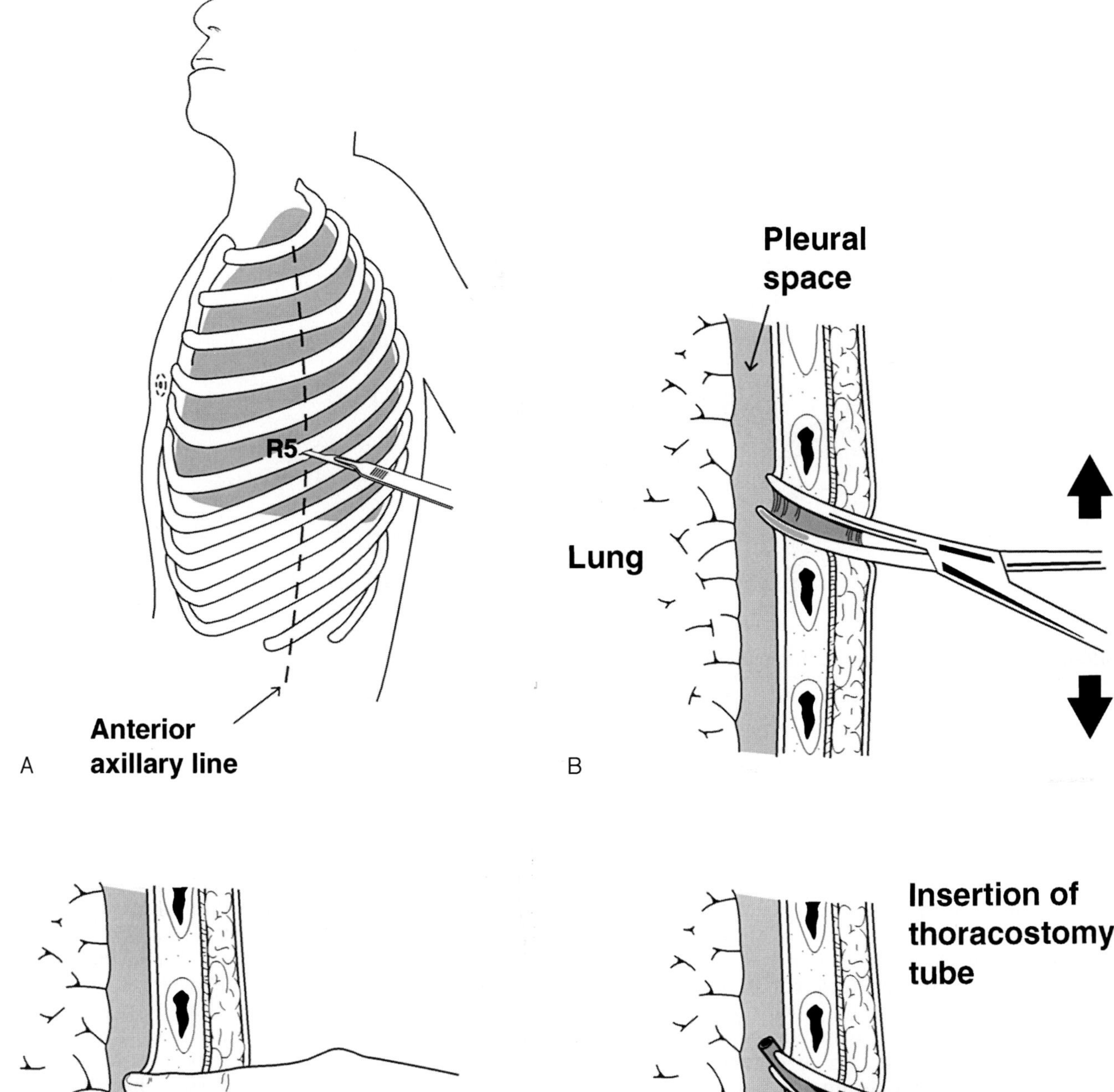

FIGURE 65–4 ■ Technique for chest tube insertion. *A*, Chest tube insertion site on the lateral thorax in the fifth intercostal space and the anterior axillary line and lateral to the pectoralis major and the breast. *B*, A skin incision has been made and a sharp, curved clamp is used to bluntly spread the intercostal muscles and enter the pleural space over the superior margin of the rib. *C*, A finger is introduced to explore the wound and to exclude significant pleural adhesions. *D*, A chest tube is inserted into the pleural space. The tube is guided with a curved clamp in a posterior and cephalad direction. The chest tube is secured to the skin and connected to a pleural drainage system.

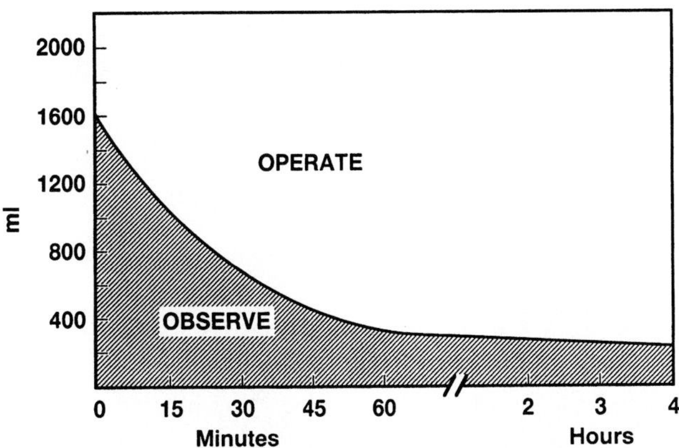

FIGURE 65–5 ■ Operation versus observation in patients with hemothorax following chest trauma. (From Mattox KL, Wall MJ: Newer diagnostic measures and emergency management. Chest Surg Clin North Am 7:213, 1997.)

of air beneath the visceral pleura into the mediastinum (Mirvis, 1992). Pneumomediastinum may also signal rupture of trachea, bronchus, or esophagus. Particularly after blunt impact, airway injury is more commonplace than esophageal injury, and endoscopic evaluation is warranted.

Mediastinal hematoma can signify blunt aortic rupture, but it is also seen after inconsequential venous injury. Widening of the mediastinum, loss of the contour of the aortic knob or aortic arch, apical pleural cap, depression of the left mainstem bronchus, and deviation of the nasogastric tube or the trachea to the right all suggest a blunt aortic rupture at the aortic isthmus. The diagnostic value of these radiographic signs is relatively low. A widened mediastinum is the most common abnormality and provides a diagnostic sensitivity and specificity of less than 50% (Fabian et al, 1997; Patel et al, 1998). The initial diagnostic efforts to screen for blunt aortic injury should be expanded to include aortobrachiocephalic injury. Blunt injury of other segments of the thoracic aorta, typically the ascending aorta or major brachiocephalic branches, can occur in up to 20% of all cases of thoracic vascular injury (Ahrar et al, 1997; Symbas et al, 1998). Major vascular injury may not be detected radiographically in up to 30% of cases (Fabian et al, 1997, 1998; Symbas et al, 1998).

The admission chest radiograph must be scrutinized for bony injury. Nondisplaced rib fractures, or costrochondral separations, can be overlooked on the initial film, and appropriate oblique views must be obtained. Despite the degree of force that is required to fracture the first rib, the injury is usually not associated with concomitant vascular injury. The incidence of isolated first rib fracture and associated major vascular injury is approximately 3%. More importantly, multiple trauma and fracture-dislocation of the first rib, along with radiographic signs of mediastinal hematoma or suggestive physical findings, are current indications for further evaluation (Gupta et al, 1997; Krantz et al, 1997).

The radiographic positions of various indwelling catheters can have important therapeutic and diagnostic implications. The endotracheal tube must be in the midtrachea, above the carina. With the nasogastric tube in the stomach, rightward displacement of the mediastinal path suggests mediastinal hematoma. If the nasogastric tube is coiled above the diaphragm, the diagnosis of blunt rupture of the left diaphragm is confirmed. The chest tube should be positioned posteriorly and superiorly, and the last side hole must be in the pleural space.

Preliminary ultrasound evaluation of the abdomen and thorax, along with formal transthoracic and transesophageal echocardiography, has become an important component of the initial evaluation of the trauma patient. Ultrasonography is advantageous because of the portability of the equipment and the rapidity of the examination. A limited FAST (Focused Assessment for the Sonographic evaluation of the Trauma patient) examination can be performed during the secondary survey by trained trauma surgeons or ED physicians. In several minutes, four standard sonographic views are obtained: the pelvis, the left and right upper quadrants and related pleural spaces, and the subxiphoid pericardial space (Rozycki et al, 1998) (Fig. 65–9).

The diagnosis of a traumatic pericardial effusion (>20 ml fluid) can be made by the visualization of an echodense region between the heart and pericardium, and the right atrial, followed by right ventricular, diastolic collapse will confirm tamponade. If a skilled sonographer is

TABLE 65–3 ■ **Diagnostic Tests**

Test	*Advantages*	*Disadvantages*	*Definitive Diagnosis*
Chest radiograph	Portable, rapid, gold standard for general screening		Pleural air or blood, lung parenchyma, fracture
FAST ultrasound	Portable, extremely rapid	Trained personnel needed	Pericardial effusion, hemoperitoneum
TTE, TEE	Portable	Trained physician needed; entire aorta and branches not seen	Pericardial effusion, valvular and wall motion abnormalities, blunt aortic rupture
CT	Already in CT scanner	Transport to suite	Mediastinal hematoma, cavity violation?
CT angiography	Already in CT scanner	Transport to suite; contrast medium needed	Vascular injury
Angiography	Anatomic detail	Transport to suite; contrast medium needed; slow	Vascular injury

CT, computed tomography; FAST, *F*ocused *A*ssessment for the *S*onographic evaluation of the *T*rauma patient; TTE, transthoracic echocardiogram; TEE, transesophageal echocardiogram.

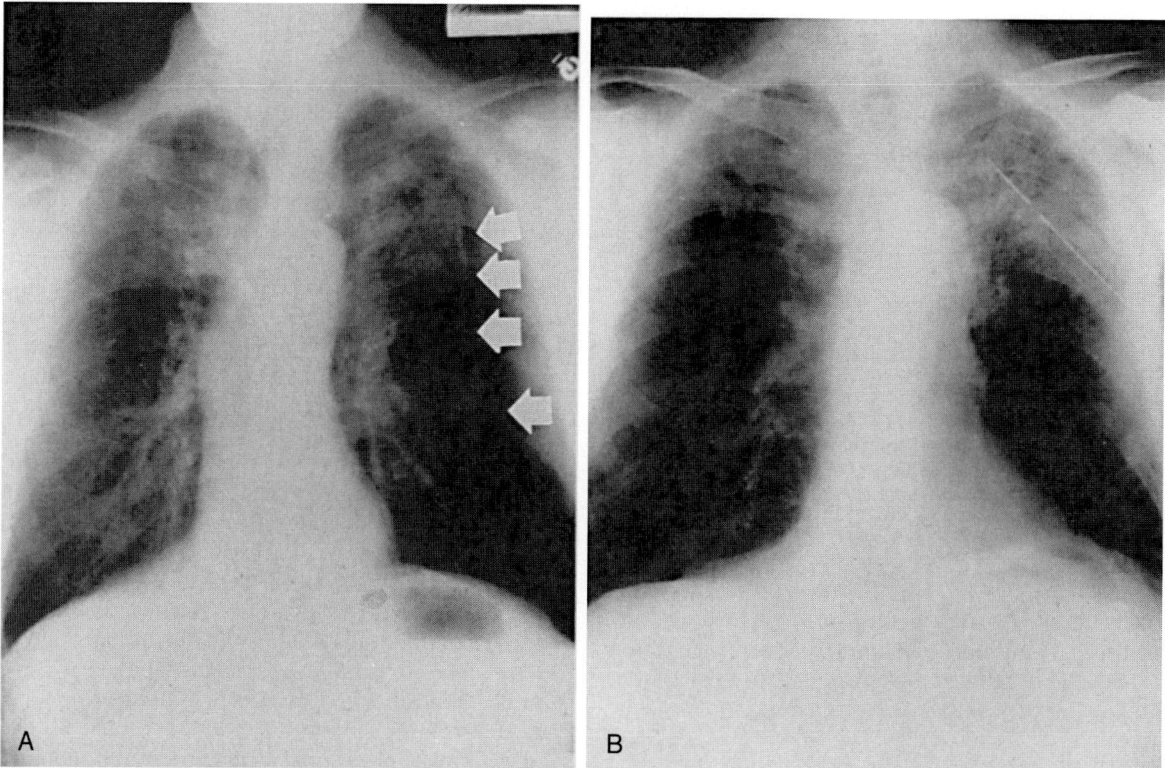

FIGURE 65–6 ■ Tension pneumothorax. *A,* Chest radiograph that shows a left-sided tension pneumothorax in a 60-year-old man who was involved in a motor vehicle accident. *B,* Complete lung re-expansion following chest tube drainage.

present, ultrasound appears as accurate as a traditional subxiphoid pericardial window in making the diagnosis of effusion, with a sensitivity and specificity above 95% (Jimenez et al, 1990; Rozycki et al, 1998). However, important false-negative results can occur if there is a clotted hemopericardium or if the pericardial effusion is completely decompressed into the pleural space through a pericardial laceration or if a hemothorax is present (Bolton et al, 1993; Meyer et al, 1995). Additionally, the presence of obesity, mechanical ventilation, hyperinflation, and subcutaneous emphysema will not permit a technically satisfactory examination in up to 30% of patients (Chan, 1998). Subxiphoid pericardial window remains an important diagnostic option for indeterminate or difficult cases.

Originally applied to stable patients with penetrating trauma in proximity to the heart, indications for FAST ultrasonography may be extended to blunt precordial

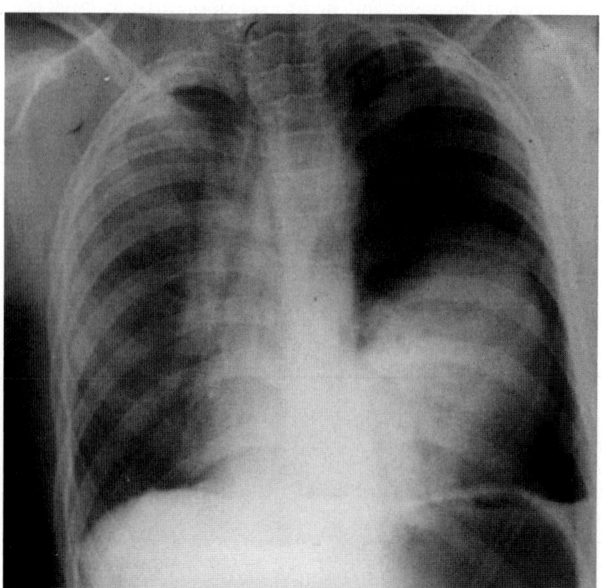

FIGURE 65–7 ■ Bronchial disruption. Chest radiograph of a 12-year-old boy who was struck by a motor vehicle. A massive left-side pneumothorax and complete atelectasis of the left lung ("fallen lung sign") are shown. A complete disruption of the proximal left mainstem bronchus was repaired primarily at thoracotomy.

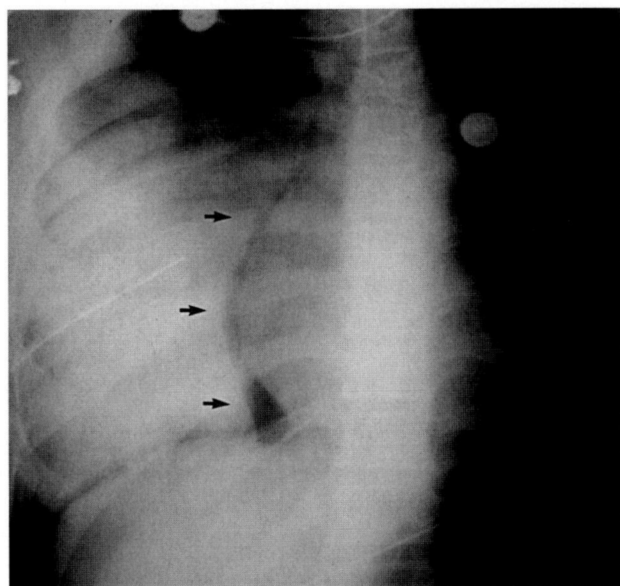

FIGURE 65–8 ■ Massive hemothorax. Chest radiograph of an 18-year-old man who sustained a close-range, single gunshot wound to the right chest. Brisk pulmonary parenchymal bleeding caused the entrapment of air between the massive hemothorax and the mediastinum ("medial meniscus sign"). A pulmonary tracheotomy and a right upper lobe wedge resection were required.

injury with signs of cardiac tamponade or thoracoabdominal injury with unexplained hypotension. The presence of a hemopericardium implying a cardiac laceration or blunt cardiac rupture can be confirmed. In the unstable patient, the choice of the initial incision can be based on the presence of hemoperitoneum or hemopericardium (Rozycki et al, 1998; Symbas et al, 1999). Additionally, in a prospective study, surgeon-sonographers were easily able to detect a traumatic pleural effusion (Sisley et al, 1998). Ultrasonography appears to have similar accuracy as a portable chest radiograph, although the breadth of information obtained is limited to the presence of pericardial or pleural fluid.

Formal echocardiography, either transthoracic or transesophageal, can be performed by a cardiologist during the trauma resuscitation. Transesophageal echocardiography can define wall motion abnormalities, valvular disruption, or septal defects (Pretre and Chilcott, 1997). The aortic isthmus can be visualized, and the rapid diagnosis of blunt aortic rupture can be confirmed. However, indeterminate signs of mediastinal hematoma or intimal hematoma can be difficult to discern from true rupture. Additionally, the entire aortic arch and brachiocephalic branches cannot be imaged because of interposition of the trachea and bronchus and other anatomic constraints. The true role of transesophageal echocardiography to diagnose blunt aortic rupture remains controversial, with accuracy reported to range between 60% and 98% (Minard et al, 1996; Smith et al, 1995). In the unstable patient, or in the patient in the midst of surgical treatment of other injuries, transesophageal echocardiography has a significant role, but angiography remains the definitive test to diagnose vascular injury (Ben-Menachem, 1997).

Computed tomography (CT) of the chest had been applied to chest trauma patients with increasing frequency, reflecting the evolving technology and the ability to reconstruct the radiographic image to produce a CT angiogram (CTA). Disadvantages include the use of an intravenous contrast agent for vascular imaging and the need to place the injured patient through the CT scanner. However, many patients, particularly patients who have sustained blunt trauma with multiple injuries, are already in the radiology suite undergoing head or abdominal CT. A standard, nonenhanced CT scan is useful to identify mediastinal hematoma and a hematoma in proximity to the great vessels with a much higher degree of accuracy than a chest radiograph provides (Mirvis et al, 1998; Trupka et al, 1997) (Fig. 65–10). It may be an ideal screening test to select those patients who require intravenous contrast to delineate a vascular injury. A CTA created by a helical CT scan with contrast angiography can visualize vascular structures, image a small intimal flap (15 mm in size), and pinpoint active extravasation into a mediastinal hematoma. The sensitivity and specificity of CTA are above 90%, and the overall accuracy approaches that of aortography (Fabian et al, 1998; Mirvis et al, 1998). A helical CT can provide both screening and the diagnostic imaging for vascular injury in the

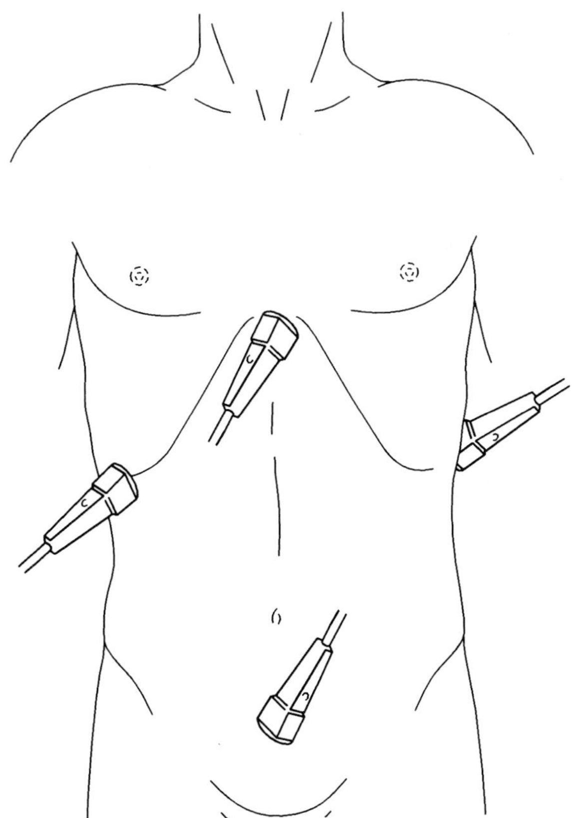

FIGURE 65–9 ■ Focused Assessment for the Sonographic evaluation of the Trauma patient (FAST) examination. Ultrasound transducer positions to examine the pelvis, subdiaphragmatic, pleural, and pericardial spaces for traumatic effusion. (From Rozycki GS, Ballard RB, Feliciano DV: Surgeon-performed ultrasound for the assessment of truncal injuries: Lessons learned from 1540 patients. Ann Surg 228:557, 1998.)

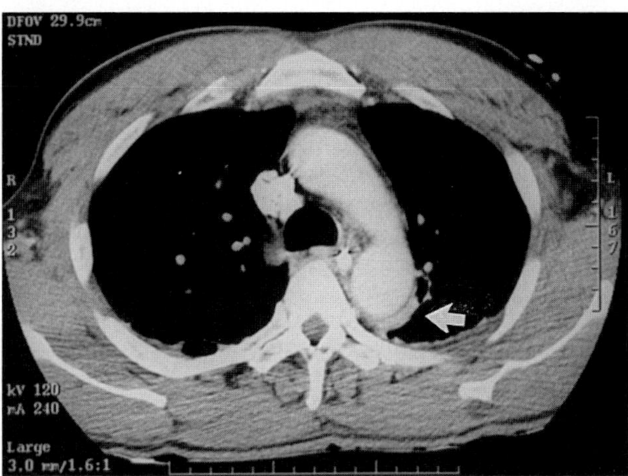

FIGURE 65–10 ■ Mediastinal hematoma. A computed tomography scan, with intravenous contrast, of a 22-year-old male who was involved in a motorcycle accident. The scan shows a small posterior mediastinal hematoma near the descending thoracic aorta. Angiography was negative for vascular injury.

majority of patients, and formal angiography may be reserved for indeterminate cases. In a recent large series of blunt trauma patients, all of whom underwent a prospective helical CT, 10% had a mediastinal hematoma. Twenty percent of those patients with hematoma had direct evidence of aortic injury. In experienced hands, with current equipment, helical CT provides a reliable means of diagnosing major vascular injury (Mirvis et al, 1998).

Widespread application of CT scans has also been suggested in the evaluation of pulmonary contusion, hemothorax, and pneumothorax, because they appear to be more accurate than portable chest radiography (Trupka et al, 1997). However, the increased time of examination and the cost of a routine CT scan may be more burdensome than the ultimate therapeutic effects of the CT diagnostics can justify. The use of the initial CT scan for all blunt chest trauma patients remains controversial (Blostein and Hodgman, 1997). In addition, in a select group of stable patients with thoracic or transmediastinal gunshot wounds, a screening CT scan can be used to define the anatomic extent and trajectory of the penetrating injury. Trivial soft tissue injuries can be differentiated from injuries with vascular proximity or those that violate the mediastinum or pleura and assist in the decision regarding further diagnostics (Grossman et al, 1998).

Angiography remains the gold standard in the evaluation of thoracic vascular injury, with accuracy rates approaching 100% (Fabian et al, 1998; Minard et al, 1996; Patel et al, 1998). However, angiography requires transport to a specialized radiology suite, the time and expertise to perform the examination, and the administration of contrast material. In the setting of blunt aortic rupture, false-positive results can be occasionally related to misinterpretation of atherosclerotic ulcers or to a prominent diverticulum of the ductus arteriosus (Mirvis, 1992). Nonetheless, angiography remains the gold standard and provides the most detailed evaluation of vascular anatomy (Fig. 65–11).

Patients with penetrating transmediastinal injury represent another diagnostic challenge. Injury traversing the mediastinum and the pleural space results in hemodynamic instability related to a thoracic vascular injury in approximately 50% of cases (Cornwell et al, 1996). Unstable patients require immediate operative intervention. Hemodynamically stable patients have been subject to the traditional algorithm of subxiphoid pericardial window, bronchoscopy, esophagoscopy, and aortography (Richardson et al, 1981). The diagnostic approach may be modified if the injury can be reasonably localized to the anterior or posterior mediastinum. Ultrasonography has replaced the subxiphoid pericardiotomy, and video-assisted fiberoptic bronchoscopy provides a superior visualization of the airway. Video-assisted fiberoptic esophagoscopy is also useful, particularly in the intubated patient, but traumatic esophageal perforation is most reliably diagnosed with contrast esophagography (Bastos and Graeber, 1997). Aortography, particularly in the stable patient with a transmediastinal gunshot injury, rarely identifies a vascular injury (Cornwell et al, 1996).

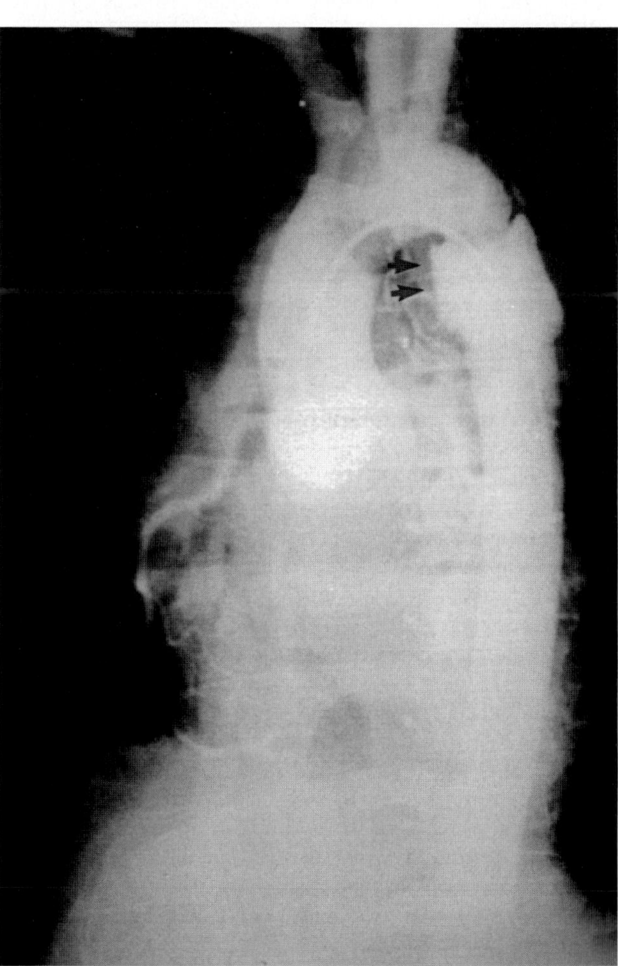

FIGURE 65–11 ■ Blunt aortic rupture. An aortogram of a 27-year-old woman who fell from the roof of a four-story building. Shown is a blunt aortic rupture with a contained mediastinal hematoma. A prosthetic interposition aortic graft was necessary at a delayed thoracotomy.

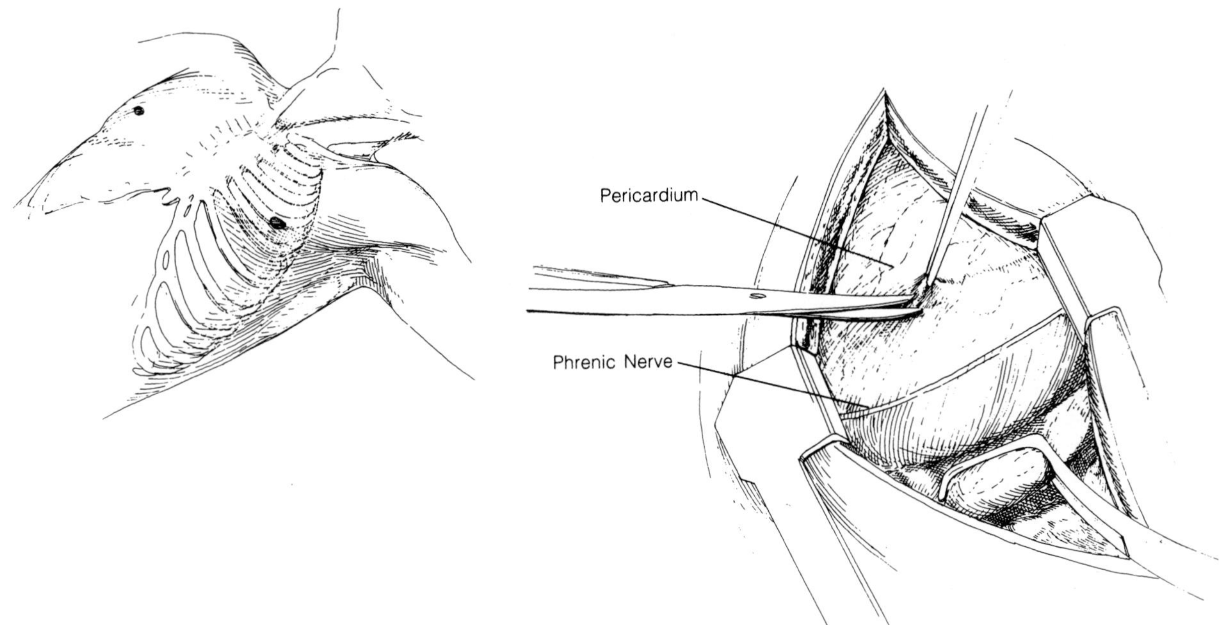

FIGURE 65–12 ■ Emergency department thoracotomy. A left anterior thoracotomy incision is made with the patient in the supine position. The fourth or fifth interspace is entered, and the descending thoracic aorta is cross-clamped. Care is taken to avoid injury to the esophagus. The pericardium is opened to initiate cardiac massage. A search for an active source of hemorrhage in the left pleural space and pericardium is performed. The sternum can be transversely divided and the right pleural space can be entered if necessary. (From Moore FA, Moore EE: Trauma resuscitation. In Wilmore DN, Brennan MF, Harken AH et al [eds]: Care of the Surgical Patient. New York, Scientific American, 1989.)

SURGICAL TREATMENT

An emergency department thoracotomy (EDT) is the final diagnostic and therapeutic option. Thoracotomy is indicated for patients in traumatic arrest or those who sustain arrest or near-arrest during the resuscitation. Obviously, exploration in the operating room is preferable if vital signs will permit rapid transfer. Adequate lighting and surgical equipment, along with anesthesia personnel and banked blood, should be available in the ED.

An EDT is a generous left anterior thoracotomy. The incision is made just below the nipple, from the sternum to the midaxillary line, and the chest is entered through the fourth or fifth intercostal space (Fig. 65–12). The descending thoracic aorta can be cross clamped just superior to the diaphragm, carefully avoiding the esophagus with its indwelling nasogastric tube. Volume resuscitation can be augmented by distal aortic occlusion, with preferential perfusion to the brain, heart, and upper extremities. A pericardial incision is made anterior to the phrenic nerve, and the heart is exposed. Open cardiac massage can proceed, and the possible site of injury in the pericardium or left pleural space can be addressed. Cardiac injuries can be managed with digital compression of ventricular injury or occlusive clamping of an atrial or great vessel injury, followed by suture repair. Significant pulmonary injuries will necessitate temporary "en masse" clamping of the pulmonary hilum to provide proximal control of hemorrhage or air leak. The right pleural space can be entered by bluntly dissecting anterior to the pericardium; and, if need be, the thoracotomy can be carried across the sternum and converted into a clamshell incision. The right atrium is available for the insertion of large intravenous catheters to facilitate transfusion.

The goal of the EDT is to rapidly diagnose the injury and perform direct repair or to temporize the injury to permit restoration of vital signs and rapid transfer to the operating room (Wall and Soltero, 1997). EDT is most successful in the treatment of penetrating cardiac injuries, particularly knife wounds, in which a reported survival of greater than 50% can be achieved (Asensio et al, 1998). Operative survival after complex penetrating thoracic injuries can occasionally occur, but survival after blunt injury or thoracoabdominal injury is almost nonexistent (Stratton et al, 1998; Wall and Soltero, 1997).

During the course of the initial resuscitation, operative decisions must be made by the trauma or thoracic surgeon. Apparent traumatic cardiac arrest and near-arrest remain the sole indications for an EDT. Indications for prompt transfer to the operating room include a confirmed or highly suspect cardiac injury, persistent hemodynamic instability despite resuscitation, massive hemothorax (>1500 ml), or a persistent hemothorax with ongoing hemorrhage (>200–300 ml/hr) (see Fig. 65–5). A major airway injury, to the cervical or thoracic trachea or main bronchus, also necessitates prompt endoscopy and operative repair (Table 65–4).

CONCLUSION

The treatment of thoracic trauma continues to evolve and improve. Careful examination and resuscitation, together with simple bedside procedures, facilitate a successful outcome in most patients. In addition, important advances in the management of hemorrhagic shock and technologic advances in diagnostic imaging, combined with prompt operative repair, continue to improve sur-

TABLE 65–4 ■ **Early Operative Indications**

Diagnosis	*Comment*
Traumatic arrest after penetrating chest trauma	ED thoracotomy
Persistent shock	Failed resuscitation
Suspect or proven cardiac injury	FAST examination if stable
Massive hemothorax (>1500 ml)	
Persistent hemothorax (>300 ml/hr)	
Retained hemothorax	Consider initial VATS
Massive air leak or airway injury suspect	Initial endoscopy in operating room

ED, emergency department; FAST, Focused Assessment for the Sonographic evaluation of the Trauma patient; VATS, video-assisted thoracic surgery.

vival in severely injured patients. In subsequent chapters in this section, the manifestations and specific treatment of injuries to the individual thoracic viscera are reviewed. In the final chapters, management of the late sequelae of chest injury is discussed.

COMMENTS AND CONTROVERSIES

Drs. Burack and Dresner provide an up-to-date review of the pathophysiology and initial management of patients suffering from thoracic trauma. Long-standing principles of management are clearly outlined. Particularly timely is the detailed discussion of FAST (Focused Assessment for the Sonographic evaluation of the Trauma patient). The technology is being increasingly used in state-of-the-art emergency departments and no doubt will improve the expeditious management of traumatized patients. Also timely is the increasing use of transesophageal echocardiography in the evaluation of blunt aortic injury. The use of this modality as opposed to contrast medium–enhanced computed tomography and standard angiography is very well covered by the authors.

G. A. P.

■ KEY REFERENCES

Bickell WH, Matthew JW, Pepe PE et al: Immediate versus delayed fluid resuscitation for hypotensive patients with penetrating torso injuries. N Engl J Med 331:1105, 1994.

Calhoon JH, Trinkle JK: Pathophysiology of chest trauma. Chest Surg Clin North Am 7:199, 1997.

Fabian TC, Richardson JD, Croce MA et al: Prospective study of blunt aortic injury: Multicenter trial of the American Association for the Surgery of Trauma. J Trauma 42:374, 1997.

Hochberg LA: Thoracic Surgery Before the 20th Century. New York, Vantage Press, 1960.

Krantz BE, Subcommittee on Trauma: Advanced Trauma Life Support Program for Doctors, 6th ed. Chicago, American College of Surgeons, 1997.

Mattox KL, Wall MJ: Newer diagnostic measures and emergency management. Chest Surg Clin North Am 7:213, 1997.

Meade RH: A History of Thoracic Surgery. Springfield, IL, Charles C Thomas, 1961.

Mullins RJ: Management of shock. In Feliciano DV, Moore EE, Mattox KL (eds): Trauma, 3rd ed. Stamford, CT, Appleton & Lange, 1996, pp 159–180.

Pezzella AT, Silva WE, Lancey RA: Cardiothoracic trauma. Curr Probl Surg 35:656, 1998.

■ REFERENCES

Abramson D, Scalea TM, Hitchcock R et al: Lactate clearance and survival following injury. J Trauma 25:584, 1993.

Acosta JA, Yang JC, Winchell RJ et al: Lethal injuries and time to death in a level 1 trauma center. J Am Coll Surg 186:528, 1998.

Ahrar K, Smith DC, Bansal RC et al: Angiography in blunt aortic injury. J Trauma 42:665, 1997.

Asensio JA, Berne JD, Demetriades D et al: One hundred five penetrating cardiac injuries: A 2-year prospective evaluation. J Trauma 44:1073, 1998.

Bastos RBN, Graeber GM: Esophageal Injuries. Chest Surg Clin North Am 7:357, 1997.

Ben-Menachem Y: Assessment of blunt aortic-brachiocephalic trauma: Should angiography be supplanted by transesophageal echocardiography? J Trauma 42:969, 1997.

Blostein PA, Hodgman CG: Computed tomography of the chest in blunt thoracic trauma: Results of a prospective study. J Trauma 43:13, 1997.

Bolton JWR, Bynoe RP, Lazar HL et al: Two-dimensional echocardiography in the evaluation of penetrating intrapericardial injuries. Ann Thorac Surg 56:506, 1993.

Chan D: Echocardiography in thoracic trauma. Emerg Med Clin North Am 16:191, 1998.

Chen SC, Markman JF, Kauder DR et al: Hemothorax missed by auscultation in penetrating chest injury. J Trauma 42:86, 1997.

Cohn SM: Pulmonary contusion: Review of a clinical entity. J Trauma 42:973, 1997.

Cornwell EE, Kennnedy F, Ayad IA et al: Transmediastinal gunshot wounds: A reconsideration of the role of aortography. Arch Surg 131:949, 1996.

Fabian TC, Davis KA, Gavant AL et al: Prospective study of blunt aortic injury: Helical CT is diagnostic and antihypertensive therapy reduces rupture. Ann Surg 227:666, 1998.

Feliciano DV: The diagnostic and therapeutic approaches to chest trauma. Semin Thorac Cardiovasc Surg 4:156, 1992.

Fulda GJ, Giberson F, Hailstone D et al: An evaluation of serum troponin t and signal-averaged electrocardiography in predicting electrocardiographic abnormalities after blunt chest trauma. J Trauma 43:304, 1997.

Garcia VF, Gotschall CS, Eichelberger MR et al: Rib fractures in children: A marker of severe trauma. J Trauma 30:695, 1990.

Grossman MD, May AK, Schwab W et al: Determining anatomic injury with computed tomography in selected torso gunshot wounds. J Trauma 45:446, 1998.

Grover FL, Ellestad C, Arom KV et al: Diagnosis and management of major tracheo-bronchial injuries. Ann Thorac Surg 28:384, 1979.

Gupta A, Jamshidi M, Rubin JR: Traumatic first rib fracture: Is angiography necessary? A review of 730 cases. Cardiovasc Surg 5:48, 1997.

Hollerman JJ, Fackler ML, Coldwell DM, Ben-Menachem Y: Radiology of gunshot wounds: II. AJR Am J Roentgenol 155:691, 1990.

Irwin RJ, Lerner MR, Bealer JF et al: Cardiopulmonary physiology of major blast injury. J Trauma 43:650, 1997.

Jimenez E, Martin M, Krukenkamp I et al: Subxiphoid pericardotomy versus echocardiography: A prospective analysis of the diagnosis of occult penetrating cardiac injury. Surgery 108:676, 1990.

Kovaric JJ, Aaby G, Hamit HF et al: Vietnam casualty statistics: February–November, 1967. Arch Surg 98:150, 1969.

Lee J, Harris JH, Duke JH et al: Noncorrelation between thoracic skeletal injuries and acute traumatic aortic tear. J Trauma 43:400, 1997.

Maenza RL, Seaberg D, D'Amico F: A meta-analysis of blunt cardiac trauma: Ending myocardial confusion. Am J Emerg Med 14:237, 1996.

Maron BJ, Poliac LC, Kaplan JA et al: Blunt impact to the chest leading to sudden death from cardiac arrest during sports activities. N Engl J Med 333:337, 1995.

Martin de Nicolas JL, Gamez AP, Cruz F et al: Long tracheobronchial and esophageal rupture after blunt chest trauma: Injury by airway bursting. Ann Thorac Surg 62:269, 1996.

Mattox KL, Bickell W, Pepe PE et al: Prospective MAST study in 911 patients. J Trauma 29:1104, 1989.
Mayberry JC, Trunkey DD: The fractured rib in chest wall trauma. Chest Surg Clin North Am 7:239, 1997.
Meyer DM, Jessen ME, Grayburn PA: Use of echocardiography to detect occult cardiac injury after penetrating thoracic trauma: A prospective study. J Trauma 39:902, 1995.
Meyer DM, Jessen ME, Wait MA et al: Early evacuation of traumatic retained hemothoraces using thoracoscopy: A prospective, randomized trial. Ann Thorac Surg 64:1396, 1997.
Minard G, Schurr MJ, Croce MA et al: A prospective analysis of transesophageal echocardiography in the diagnosis of traumatic disruption of the aorta. J Trauma 40:225, 1996.
Mirvis SE: Imaging of thoracic trauma. Semin Thorac Cardiovasc Surg 4:27, 1992.
Mirvis SE, Kathirkamuganathan S, Buell J et al: Use of spiral computed tomography for the assessment of blunt trauma patients with potential aortic injury. J Trauma 45:922, 1998.
Nakayama DK, Ramenofsky ML, Rowe MI: Chest injuries in children. Ann Surg 210:770, 1989.
Oglesby JE: Twenty-two months war surgery in Vietnam. Arch Surg 102:607, 1971.
Patel NH, Stephens KE, Mirvis SE et al: Imaging of acute thoracic aortic injury due to blunt trauma: A review. Radiology 209:335, 1998.
Porter JM, Ivatury RR: In search of the optimal end points of resuscitation in trauma patients: A review. J Trauma 44:908, 1998.
Pretre R, Chilcott M: Blunt trauma to the heart and great vessels. N Engl J Med 336:626, 1997.
Richardson JD, Adams L, Snow NJ et al: Management of transmediastinal gunshot wounds. Surgery 90:671, 1981.
Rossbach MM, Johnson SB, Gomez MA et al: Management of major tracheobronchial injuries: A 28-year experience. Ann Thorac Surg 65:182, 1998.
Rozycki GS, Ballard RB, Feliciano DV: Surgeon-performed ultrasound for the assessment of truncal injuries: Lessons learned from 1540 patients. Ann Surg 228:557, 1998.
Schmidt U, Stalp M, Gerich T et al: Chest tube decompression of blunt chest injury by physicians in the field: Effectiveness and complications. J Trauma 44:98, 1998.
Seki S, Iwamoto H: Disruptive forces for swine heart, liver and spleen: Their breaking stresses. J Trauma 45:1079, 1998.
Sisley AC, Rozycki GS, Ballard RB et al: Rapid detection of traumatic effusion using surgeon performed ultrasonography. J Trauma 44:291, 1998.
Smith MD, Cassidy MJ, Souther S et al: Transesophageal echocardiography in the diagnosis of traumatic rupture of the aorta. N Engl J Med 332:356, 1995.
Stewart KC, Urschel JD, Nakai SS et al: Pulmonary resection for lung trauma. Ann Thorac Surg 63:1587, 1997.
Stratton SJ, Brickett K, Crammer T: Prehospital pulseless, unconscious penetrating trauma victims: Field assessments associated with survival. J Trauma 45:96, 1998.
Swan KG, Swan RC: Principle of ballistics applicable to the treatment of gunshot wounds. Surg Clin North Am 71:221, 1991.
Symbas NP: Extraoperative autotransfusion from hemothorax. Surgery 84:722, 1978.
Symbas NP, Bongiorno PF, Symbas NP: Blunt cardiac rupture: The utility of emergency department ultrasound. Ann Thorac Surg 67:1274, 1999.
Symbas NP, Vaisis SE, Hatcher C: Blunt and penetrating diaphragmatic injuries with or without herniation of organs into the chest. Ann Thorac Surg 42:158, 1986.
Symbas PJ, Horsley S, Symbas NP: Rupture of the ascending aorta caused by blunt trauma. Ann Thorac Surg 66:113, 1998.
Tarantino DP, Bernhard WN: Anesthesia considerations in thoracic trauma. Semin Thorac Cardiovasc Surg 4:187, 1992.
Trachiotis GD, Sell JE, Pearson GD et al: Traumatic thoracic aortic rupture in the pediatric patient. Ann Thorac Surg 62:724, 1996.
Trupka A, Waydhas C, Hallfeldt KKJ et al: Value of thoracic computed tomography in the first assessment of severely injured patients with blunt chest trauma: Results of a prospective study. J Trauma 43:405, 1997.
Wall MJ, Soltero E: Damage control for thoracic injuries. Surg Clin North Am 77:863, 1997.

CHAPTER **66**

Laryngeal Trauma

Philippe Pasche
Florian Lang
Philippe Monnier

HISTORICAL NOTE

The first report of a true laryngeal trauma and its treatment was from Egypt and is found in Smith's papyrus; primary wound closure and dressings were recommended. Most of the patients died immediately. Although laryngotracheal anatomy was progressively discovered by the ancient Greeks and Romans (Galien, 150 BC), its physiology was not understood, and there was no change in treatment or prognosis until the extensive anatomic works of the Renaissance (da Vinci, 1452–1519; Vesalius, 1514–1580; Paré, 1509–1590; Casserius, 1545–1616; Morgagni, 1682–1771; Guerrier, 1980; Willemot, 1981). As reported for the first time in 1620 by Habicot in Paris, tracheotomy became the standard life-saving treatment in laryngeal trauma (Willemot, 1981). Morgagni was the first to make an accurate anatomic description of a laryngeal trauma, a cricoid fracture that was found in a hanged convict. Laryngeal gunshot injuries occurred later. Some of these patients were saved by direct tracheal intubation through the wound (Sabatier, 1796).

The first breakthrough in diagnosis and treatment occurred in the second half of the 19th century with a dramatic increase of surgical possibilities thanks to the development of anesthesiology (inhalation narcosis, Priestly; chloroform, Simpson; cocaine, Jelinek; laryngeal block, Braun), better hygiene (disinfection of laryngeal instruments, Pasteur), and laryngoscopy (Garcia, Czernak, Kierstein), which allowed the ultimate comprehension of laryngeal physiology and pathology. Tracheotomy became only part of the treatment, to ensure breathing (prophylactic use, Langenbeck), and the era of surgical treatments of laryngeal injuries started: laryngotomies for reduction of laryngeal fractures (Eichman, Germany, 1850; Laney, France, during the Napoleonic wars), treatment of laryngotracheal stenoses (Dobleau, 1869), tracheal resection-anastomosis (Küster, 1885), and laryngeal reconstructions with skin flaps (Schimmelbusch, 1887; Guerrier, 1980; Willemot, 1981).

In the 20th century, a tremendous increase of the incidence and the variety of laryngeal traumas that occurred during the world wars and the Korean and Vietnam conflicts forced the development of adequate diagnostic and treatment procedures (Moure, 1981; Schwab, 1963). A study of Moure and associates' extensive textbook about laryngeal war injuries, which was published in 1918, shows that all modern surgical techniques were already known at that time. To enhance the prognosis, however, took many additional developments, especially in infection control (penicillin, Fleming, 1928; sulfonamides, Domagk, 1935), in radiology (radiography for shrapnel localization, Moure, 1915; laryngeal tomography, Canuyt, 1939; computed tomographic [CT] scanning), in surgical technology (suspension laryngoscopy, Killian, 1911; surgical microscope, Albrecht, 1954; microlaryngoscopy, Kleinsasser, 1963; CO_2 laser, Strong and Jako, 1972), and in anesthesiology (jet ventilation, Carden, 1973; Willemot, 1981).

More improvements in treatment and prognosis began in the 1960s, at the same time as a change in the epidemiology occurred, with a marked increase of traumas from car and motorcycle accidents. Therefore, epidemiology, physiopathology, and laryngeal wound healing were systematically studied (Nahum and Siegel, 1967; Olson, 1979; Piquet et al, 1975). Special care was paid to blunt traumas (Ogura and Biller, 1971) and to laryngotracheal disruptions (Alonso, 1974; Couraud et al, 1974). Natural history, classification, and timing of treatment were discussed (Harris and Tobin, 1970). Hirano became interested in the phoniatric sequelae of laryngeal trauma (Hirano et al, 1985). Diagnosis was refined because of the selective application of the CT scan (Schaefer, 1991a). The specifics of laryngeal traumas in the pediatric age group were reported (Holinger, 1972) as well as surgical novelties such as the miniplate osteosynthesis of the thyroid alae (Woo, 1990). Despite all of this knowledge and the publication of individual and small group studies (Bryce, 1972; Guerrier et al, 1979; Piquet et al, 1975; Traissac, 1979), there was no general consensus about the management of such injuries.

The major advances in laryngeal trauma management are due to people such as Gussack and Schaefer, who introduced protocol approaches to this relatively rare injury. Relying on his series of 139 consecutive cases in work over 27 years, Schaefer, in 1992, published a management algorithm of great value. During the same period, major advances in the surgery of laryngotracheal trauma sequelae were achieved because of the enlargement plasties (chondroplastic, Réthi, 1956; cricoid split, Cotton, 1992); the development of resection surgery in the trachea (Grillo, 1965), the larynx (Ogura, 1971; Gerwat and Bryce, 1974; Pearson, 1975), and the pediatric larynx (Savary, 1978); and the development of laser surgery (Duncavage, 1985; Shapshay, 1987).

The fact that it took the contributions of so many eager people and of so many different sciences to understand the larynx and to be able to repair it to its greatest functional capacity illustrates well the complexity of the organ and the multiplicity of the problems that arise when it is needed to restore breathing, swallowing, and voice, problems that are by far not all solved today.

■ *HISTORICAL READINGS*

Guerrier Y, Mounier-Kuhn P: Histoire des Maladies de l'Oreille, du Nez et de la Gorge. Paris, Les Éditions Dacosta, 1980.

Moure EJ, Liébault G, Canuyt G: Pathologie de guerre du Larynx et de la Trachée. Paris, Librairie Felix Alcan, 1918.

Sabatier C: De la Médécine Opératoire ou des Opérations de Chirurgie qui se Pratiquent le Plus Fréquemment. Paris, Imprimerie de Didot le Jeune, 1796.

Schwab W, Ey W: Verletzungen und Stenosen des Kehlkopfes und der Luftröhre. In Berendes J (ed): Kehlkopf Sprachstörungen. Stuttgart, Thieme, 1963.

Willemot J, Pirsig W, Rodegra H: Naissance et développement de l'oto-rhino-laryngologie dans l'histoire de la médecine. Acta Med Belg 35(Suppl 4):1045, 1981.

BASIC SCIENCE

This chapter addresses external laryngeal trauma and does not deal with internal iatrogenic trauma that is induced by intubation, cricothyrotomy, tracheotomy, and laser. External traumas include blunt and penetrating injuries, inhalation injuries, and injuries from caustic ingestion. Various classifications have been proposed, according to site (Bryce, 1972; Ogura, 1971; Ogura and Billa, 1971), to the tissue injured (Richardson, 1981), or to the severity (Olson, 1982). In this chapter, the different injuries are discussed according to the cause of the trauma and to the structure damaged.

Anatomy

Schematically, the larynx is a tube-like structure that is formed by mobile and articulated cartilages that are connected by pliable but resistant fibrous membranes; numerous intrinsic highly differentiated muscles and nerves that may be directly injured; and an internal mucosa that can, in certain places, be easily detached and the integrity of which is critical for normal function of the larynx.

The larynx is suspended to the hyoid bone and to the tongue base and is followed by the trachea. Although it lies anteriorly directly subcutaneously on the midline (exposed to anterior penetrating trauma), the larynx enjoys a relatively well-protected position in the neck. It is shielded laterally by the bulk of the sternocleidomastoid muscles, from behind by the cervical spine and the other muscles of the neck, and from above by the overhanging mandible. When the patient is in normal position, the larynx is shielded from the front and the sides by the mandible and the shoulder girdle because the normal reflexive reaction to impending anterior trauma is to withdraw, lower the head, and raise the shoulders (Fabre et al, 1987; Tucker, 1993). Moreover, the vertical and lateral pliability of the laryngeal structures allows a certain degree of avoidance of the trauma. In children, the larynx is situated higher in the neck than is the adult larynx and its tissue elasticity is increased. Thus, it is afforded even greater protection. Finally, the nasal filter offers the larynx a certain amount of protection against inhalation injuries.

Epidemiology

Because of the protected position of the larynx in the neck and along the upper respiratory tract, external laryngeal trauma is uncommon. When it occurs, however, it has a high mortality rate, which can be as high as 40% from blunt injuries (Edwards et al, 1987) and can range from 7% to 20% with penetrating injuries (Angood et al, 1986; Jones et al, 1967). This high mortality rate is due to immediate asphyxia, hemorrhage from an associated vascular lesion, or simply laryngeal concussion. Because the larynx is a highly innervated organ, a direct blow, even without major laryngeal lesions, can induce a nociceptive reflex to the bulbus, thus provoking (Fabre et al, 1987) a laryngospasm with temporary palsy of one or both laryngeal recurrent nerves, a respiratory arrest lasting up to several minutes, or a cardiac arrest, which is usually lethal in the absence of cardiopulmonary resuscitation.

The immediate mortality rate is even higher when the thoracic trachea is involved because of the associated vascular injuries (Minard et al, 1992) and when head and neck or other sites of the body have adjacent injury (as high as 80% of the cases reported by Danic and colleagues in 1996). Therefore, external laryngeal trauma has a low overall incidence in trauma centers, accounting for only 1 in 30,000 emergency room visits (Schaefer, 1989). In their national traffic security report in 1964, Dufflot and Hoffman found craniocerebral traumas in 21.1% of patients injured in a road accident, maxillofacial traumas in 17.7%, and laryngeal traumas in 1.7%. Other data suggest that one laryngeal fracture to every 650 peacetime fractures of the facial bone (0.15%) can be expected (Haugh and Giles, 1992). The introduction of seat belts and airbags may explain a decrease of the incidence of external laryngeal trauma since the 1980s. In a hospital with a well-established emergency service and trauma center, two to five cases of laryngeal trauma are encountered each year (Yen, 1994).

External laryngeal traumas are caused by motor vehicle accidents in 60% of the cases (car 37%, motorcycle, 23%), by assault or suicide attempts in 20% (mainly knife wounds or hanging), and by blows to the neck (sport accidents, e.g., karate, soccer; or occupational accidents, e.g., from rotating blades, motor chain saws, or elevator repair) or by falls (ski, mountain bike) in the remaining 20% (Piquet et al, 1975; Yen, 1994). In peacetime, blunt injuries are more common (83%) compared with penetrating injuries (17%) (Yen, 1994). The ratio of knife injuries to gunshot injuries depends strongly on geographic factors, and the frequency of gunshot wounds is increasing, especially in the United States (Schaefer, 1998).

In penetrating traumas to the neck, the larynx, with its anterior subcutaneous position, is the most frequently injured organ (10.1% of the cases; pharynx and esophagus, 9.6%; jugular vein, 9%; carotid artery, 6.7%; spinal nerve, 3.0%) (McConnell, 1994). Supraglottic and transglottic injuries are the more frequent causes. Subglottic injuries are rare, and cricoid cartilage fractures are usually combined with fractures of the thyroid cartilages (Danic et al, 1996).

Because of its high localization in the neck, the pediatric larynx is not commonly injured, and indeed, in infants who are younger than 18 months of age, trauma is largely the result of impacted foreign bodies, intubation, or hypopharyngeal aspiration. In older children, the activities of childhood play a greater role (falls, sports accidents). Automobile-related injuries increase in older children, whereas in adolescents, they outweigh all other causes in laryngeal trauma incidence (Holinger and Schild, 1972).

Mechanisms of Injury

Blunt Trauma

The basic mechanism for blunt external injury to the laryngotracheal skeleton consists of the compression of the laryngotracheal cartilages on the cervical spine. The larynx is particularly exposed to crushing forces in a car accident when no seat belt is worn, when the belt is too loose, or when only a lap belt is used. The occupant of the car is thrust forward during rapid deceleration with the neck hyperextended (Fig. 66–1). This position removes the bony protection that is afforded by the mandible, and the steering wheel, dashboard, and back of the front seats are then ideally positioned for crushing impact (Chagnon and Mulder, 1996; Schaefer, 1998; Tucker, 1993). In motorcycle riders, the larynx is usually hit by the handlebar or the brake handle (Piquet et al, 1975).

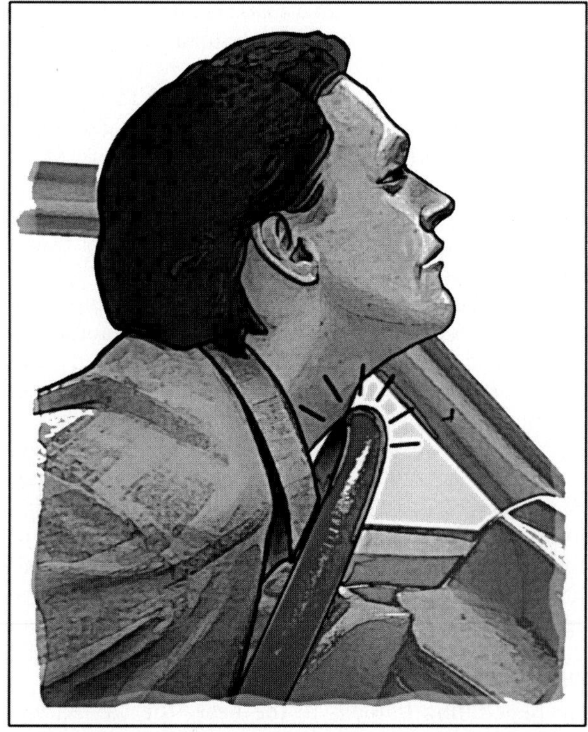

FIGURE 66–1 ■ Blunt laryngeal trauma due to a car accident. In cases of unfastened or loose seat belts, the body is thrust forward with the neck hyperextended. The unprotected larynx crashes against the steering wheel.

Young and flexible larynges may absorb the impact and spring back into position without fracturing. Only submucosal edema or submucosal hemorrhage may ensue, but these can still result in an airway compromise, especially in children because of the small cross-sectional area of the pediatric airway and because the medical personnel underestimate the situation because of a lack of fractures (Schaefer, 1998). Indeed, the flexible cartilages potentiate the mechanism of dislocation of the arytenoid cartilages and rupture of the membranous vocal folds. The anterior convex surface of the vertebral bodies acts like a wedge to force the thyroid alae apart when the thyroid cartilage is driven against it (Fig. 66–2). The posterior cricoid lamina is driven anteriorly by its impact on the spine, releasing all tension on the vocal ligaments and simultaneously displacing the arytenoid cartilages anteriorly.

If the anterior force of the trauma is then suddenly withdrawn, the larynx springs back instantaneously, massively increasing the tension on the vocal ligaments. This may result in rupture of the membranous vocal folds, typically at their insertion at the anterior commissure; dislocation of the arytenoid cartilage that is anterior to the cricoid lamina; or rupture of the thyroepiglottic ligament with posterior dislocation of the petiolus (Figs. 66–2 and 66–3).

Fractures of any or all of the cartilaginous structures occur by the same mechanism, especially in calcified larynges. The fracture pattern corresponds to the point of impact (see Figs. 66–2 and 66–3). Associated pharyngeal wounds are common and are due to the impact of the thyroid cornua of the hyoid bone, the posterior margins of the thyroid cartilage, and the cricoid lamina against the vertebral bodies, squashing the lateral and posterior pharyngeal wall between them and causing hematomas, lacerations, or perforations (see Fig. 66–2).

Striking the lower neck on a rigid wire or rope ("clothesline injury") at high speed while riding a bicycle, a motorcycle, or an all-terrain vehicle exerts a large amount of energy on a small area and results in massive trauma. The elasticity of the supporting structures of the airway tends to pull the larynx cephalad and the trachea caudad, with the point of impact acting as the dividing point (Alonso et al, 1974). Depending on the point of impact, the result is a crushed larynx, a separation of the cricoid from the larynx, or more commonly a cricotracheal disruption, which is often followed by immediate death. Two other blunt mechanisms may lead to an acute laryngotracheal disruption: (1) a sudden increase of intratracheal pressure with closed glottis can result in a linear rupture; and (2) a blow to the chest or an acceleration-deceleration injury produces a sudden movement of the trachea around its fixed points at the cricoid and carina, leading to a shearing force that sometimes results in complete transsection.

In hanging injuries, the hyoid and thyroid are uncommonly fractured, as they may be in ligature or manual strangulation. The cricoid is usually not fractured in either hanging or in strangulation. Typically, both types of injuries cause a marked laryngeal edema with loss of airway in 12 to 24 hours.

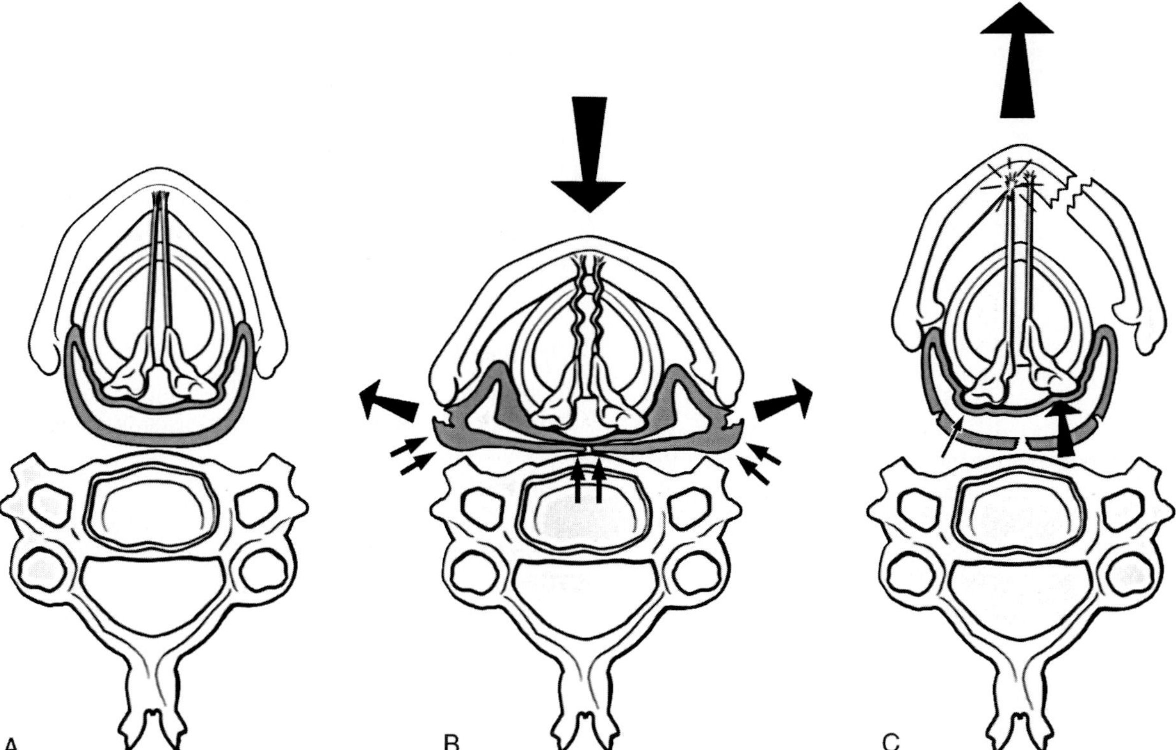

FIGURE 66–2 ■ Blunt laryngeal trauma: mechanism of injury. *A*, Larynx in normal position. *B*, Anterior force driving the cartilage against the vertebral body, spreading the thyroid alae apart. This typically causes vertical median or paramedian fractures of the thyroid cartilage. Note the places *(small double arrows)* where the thyroid alae and the cricoid lamina impact into the pharyngeal mucosa, causing lacerations. *C*, Sudden withdrawal of the anterior force, with a springing back of the larynx. The overextension of the ligaments causes disruption of the vocal folds especially at their anterior insertion (see left vocal fold, *small thin arrow*) or an anterior arytenoid dislocation (see right vocal fold, *small thick arrow*).

Penetrating Trauma

Penetrating trauma is mainly caused by razor or knife cuts, gunshots, or splinters of mines or gun shells. Associated vascular injuries are frequently the cause of death. The larynx may be displaced by knife thrusts without serious injury, and there is no tissue destruction distant to the path of injury. The course of the injury may be estimated from the entrance and exit wounds. Nevertheless, the wound may be narrow, and by its aspect one might be tempted not to suspect deep-lying, especially vascular lesions.

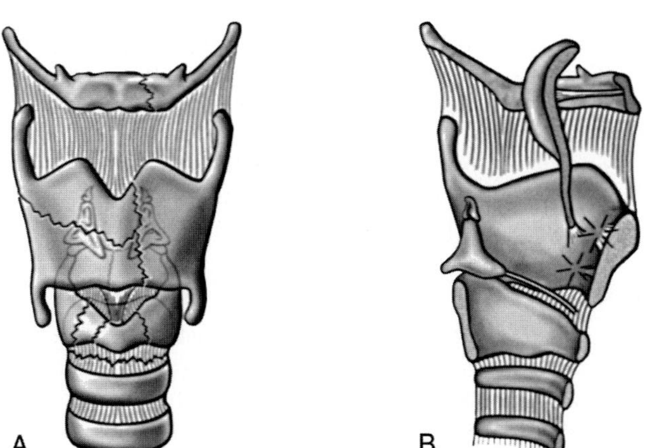

FIGURE 66–3 ■ Blunt laryngeal trauma: typical lesions. *A*, Typical hyoid, thyroid, and cricoid fracture lines. Vertical fractures are the most frequent ones. *B*, Posterior dislocation of the epiglottic petiolus and disruption of the vocal fold at the anterior commissure.

Injury from a gunshot depends on the type of weapon used and the range from which it was fired. Shots at close range cause intense energy and are usually lethal, whereas shots from a long range may cause only minimal damage. Low-velocity handguns have a moderate blast effect on soft tissues, but the bullet may be deviated by harder structures such as laryngeal cartilages and may follow an erratic course in the soft tissues. This may be misleading during the initial examination.

Military or hunting weapons and, even more so, splinters of mines and shells impart a considerable amount of kinetic energy to the tissues, occasioning necrosis that is far beyond the limits of the obviously nonviable tissues, necessitating a wide débridement of the surrounding tissues (Schaefer, 1998; Tucker, 1993).

Inhalation Injuries

Inhalation injuries can be thermal or chemical. Thermal injury is the most rare because the regulation system of the nose and oral cavity can dissipate most of the heat; however, if the air is supersaturated with steam, thermal injury may occur. With hot steam, significant laryngeal edema occurs before any pulmonary injury, whereas with smoke, necrotizing tracheitis, bronchitis, and intra-alveolar hemorrhagic edema may develop first.

When it comes in contact with the mucosa, inhaled ammonia gas forms ammonium hydroxide, a strong alkali that causes liquefaction necrosis. The supraglottis is predominantly involved, and edema, ulcerations, and slough cause laryngeal narrowing and spasm. The larynx protects the lower airway. Laryngeal edema often appears briskly but late, sometimes as long as 24 hours after the inhalation.

Injuries from caustic ingestion typically occur in children and may result from various household products. In adults, they are usually the result of a suicide attempt. The larynx is injured by direct contact during ingestion or regurgitation of the ingested caustic material. Reflex glottic closure limits these injuries to the supraglottis (Gluckman and Ajay, 1991; Schaefer, 1998; Tucker, 1993).

Sites of Traumatic Lesions to the Larynx and Trachea

Hyoid Bone

Fractures of the hyoid bone are rare and are mainly caused by strangulation or hanging (see Fig. 66–3). They usually do not induce respiratory distress but are very painful, especially during coughing and swallowing. Special care should be paid to the diagnosis of associated pharyngeal lacerations.

Epiglottis

The most common lesion of the epiglottis is a posterior avulsion of the petiolus due to the rupture of the thyroepiglottic ligament (see Fig. 66–3). It is frequently associated with fractures of the thyroid cartilage. It provokes a marked anteroposterior shortening of the supraglottic lumen. Ruptures of the hyoepiglottic ligament are rare and may be associated with a fracture of the hyoid bone. Direct lesions of the epiglottic cartilage are reported only in penetrating traumas.

Thyroid Cartilage

The damage to the thyroid cartilage depends on the degree of calcification. In children and young adults, a blunt injury usually results in a vertical, linear, median or paramedian fracture (see Fig. 66–3). This type of fracture is the most common injury encountered in the larynx. It may be unique or associated with a fracture of the cricoid cartilage. It leads in many cases to a disruption of the vocal cords. In men and in older patients, the fracture pattern is comminuted. The larynx is shortened in the anteroposterior axis, with airway restriction. The external perichondrium often remains intact, whereas the internal perichondrium is breached by fractured cartilage fragments, resulting in internal soft tissue damage, mucosal lacerations, and exposure of pieces of cartilage.

Cricoid Cartilage

An isolated fracture of the cricoid is rare. A fracture of the thyroid cartilage or, less frequently, a cricotracheal disruption is associated. The most likely site of fracture is the anterior arch, but a direct crushing blow to the cricoid generally results in a comminuted type of fracture (see Fig. 66–3). Because the cricoid is a complete ring, there is not much space for expansion of soft tissue, which may result from edema or hemorrhage, and the airway restriction is early and severe. The incidence of concomitant recurrent laryngeal nerve palsy and esophageal injuries is high because of the close anatomic relationship of these structures to the cartilage.

Arytenoids

Depending on the mechanism of injury, the arytenoids are either dislocated, subluxated, or completely avulsed.

Soft Endolaryngeal Tissues

The mucosa can show edema (peak at 12 hours, gradually subsiding within 2 to 3 days), hemorrhage, laceration, or complete avulsion of underlying structures, with displacement and contraction of the mucosal flaps and exposure of the submucosal structures. The muscle can show hemorrhage, even in cases of minor trauma, tearing, or separation, the last mainly associated with ligamentous and cricoarytenoid joint lesions. The vocal cords can lack tension and can be shorter than normal in cases of an anteroposterior shortening of the larynx due to a thyroid cartilage fracture (even without other internal signs) or in cases of an arytenoid cartilage dislocation. With the spring-back mechanism of the larynx in anterior blunt trauma, avulsion of the anterior commissure attachment of one or both vocal cords may occur. Tears of the vocal cords, the false cords, or the aryepiglottic folds result from more severe trauma.

Cricotracheal Ligament

A laryngotracheal disruption is one of the most severe laryngeal injuries. It is nearly always associated with a unilateral or bilateral recurrent laryngeal nerve injury. A comminuted fracture of the cricoid cartilage is also reported to be associated (Couraud et al, 1974). Initially, the outward signs may be few, and the respiratory distress may be surprisingly minimal. Breathing is possible for a time, but the collapse of the avulsed soft tissues surrounding the segment of the disruption always results in a sudden airway loss, which is lethal when the condition has not been recognized before. The diagnosis is often made only when the condition is suspected with regard to the mechanism of injury.

Trachea

The tracheal cartilage is extremely elastic and tolerates impact well. Severe blunt injury or injury by increase of intratracheal pressure results mainly in disruption of the intercartilaginous membranes, with varying degrees of tracheal cartilage prolapse.

Recurrent Laryngeal Nerves

Except for penetrating traumas with transsection of the nerve, an injury of the recurrent laryngeal nerve is encountered in cricoid fractures or in laryngotracheal separation. It is caused by distention, complete disruption, or a direct lesion from a displaced cartilaginous fragment. Clinical presentation depends on the type of the laryngeal trauma and the unilaterality or bilaterality of the injury.

NATURAL HISTORY AND PROGNOSIS

Death can occur immediately even after minor laryngeal traumas by reflexive respiratory or cardiorespiratory arrest. Asphyxia and hemorrhage are the next immediate causes of death in more severe traumas. The functional prognosis is proportional to the severity of the trauma, especially to the degree of dislocation of the structures or to the importance of the tissue loss. Harris and Tobin best summarized the long-term natural history in 1970: "Anything short of immediate repair will lead to infection, distortion of the cartilaginous framework, scar tissue contraction of the lacerated mucosa, and, finally, stricture of the airway." However, the life and the life quality of the patient depend not only on the restoration of the airway but also on the restoration of the other dynamic functions of the pharyngolarynx, namely swallowing and speech.

The greatest challenge to the specialist in charge, and the situation with the worst functional prognosis, is the immobile larynx, resulting either from neurologic damage or from cricoarytenoid ankylosis. The final outcome is a delicate compromise between degree of physical activity and nutrition and phonation possibilities, none of which are optimal. These situations are encountered in complex cricoid fractures, cricotracheal disruptions, and severe penetrating traumas; they also occur when diagnosis and treatment of less severe forms of laryngeal trauma intervene too late and the fibrosis has set in.

DIAGNOSIS

Clinical Presentation

The challenge in penetrating laryngeal trauma is less a diagnostic problem than the detection of the associated injuries. The situation differs with blunt trauma, in which diagnosis can be more subtle. Early diagnosis and treatment of blunt laryngeal trauma are crucial to avoid acute complication, and any delay may lead to disastrous late sequelae. The physician is confronted with two situations: a conscious patient who will provide information and will cooperate for the laryngeal examination, or an unconscious patient with either an unsecured airway or one that is already intubated or tracheostomized. In the first situation, the diagnosis of laryngeal trauma is evident most of the time, but the larynx must be carefully examined after the patient is stable to exclude an insidious delayed development of airway obstruction. In the second situation, delayed diagnosis of laryngotracheal trauma still occurs and becomes apparent at the time of failed extubation.

Although the diagnosis is evident in cases of penetrating injuries, many cases of blunt laryngeal trauma may remain asymptomatic at an early stage and can be missed by the physician. Minor symptoms may hide serious underlying injuries; therefore, an aggressive diagnostic investigation must be done, particularly in cases of multiple trauma when preoccupation with the other life-threatening injuries can hide an apparent minor pathology. Knowledge of the mechanisms of the injury may depend on the degree of the wound and the severity of the injury; therefore, witnesses can be helpful when the patient is unconscious. The following symptoms are suggestive of laryngeal trauma:

- *Change of voice.* This symptom is constant and ranges from slight dysphonia to hoarseness and aphonia. Hematoma of a vocal cord often causes hoarseness, whereas dislocation of the cricoarytenoid joint, vocal cord paralysis, or avulsion can lead to a weak and breathy voice. Aphonia may be encountered in severe trauma.
- *Dyspnea.* This is not constant but represents the most serious symptom of laryngeal trauma. Dyspnea ranges from slight stridor to acute respiratory distress. It may be absent during the early stages of a contusion or nondisplaced fracture, when edema and hematoma are not large enough to create an obstruction, and may only become significant after a few hours when the lesion has enlarged. On the other hand, immediate onset of dyspnea with dramatic acute obstruction may follow a laryngeal crush, an epiglottis avulsion, or a laryngotracheal disruption.
- *Neck pain.* This may appear spontaneously or may occur only during swallowing as a result of the mobilization of the injured larynx.
- *Dysphagia and odynodysphagia.* These can result from a contusion, a crush, or a laceration of the pharyngeal or esophageal mucosa.
- *Cough.* An irritative cough may appear as an initial symptom of a lesion of the larynx.
- *Hemoptysis.* Laceration of the pharynx or larynx or disruption of the trachea or bronchi can be followed by hemoptysis, which can be severe enough to cause respiratory distress.
- *Aspiration.* This may appear later when the patient begins to eat; it is usually caused by a unilateral or bilateral paralysis of the vocal cord.

A discordance may exist between the clinical symptoms and the underlying lesions, and major injuries may be poorly symptomatic initially and suddenly decompensate, as in a laryngotracheal disruption occurring in two stages. Therefore, all patients with suspicion of neck trauma should be carefully examined to exclude laryngeal lesions.

Signs

Blunt Laryngeal Trauma

Observation of the neck may reveal contusion, mild bruising or laceration, loss of the thyroid prominence, or edema or fleshiness of the cervical tissues. A gentle palpation of the neck is performed to discover crepitus of a subcutaneous emphysema, soft tissue swelling and tenderness, or depression of the thyroid cartilage due to a fracture. Emphysema can diffuse to the face and the thorax. Examination of the face is done to exclude an associated mandibular fracture. The cervical spine should be palpated to look for any bony step-offs.

Penetrating Trauma

Clinical findings include subcutaneous crepitus, dyspnea, shock or hemorrhage, expanding neck hematoma, hemoptysis, hematemesis, and neurologic deficit (Grewal et al, 1995; McConnell and Trunkey, 1994; Miller and Duplechain, 1991). The entrance and exit wounds are carefully examined, and the path of travel of the projectile is estimated to evaluate the potential risk for underlying injuries.

Laryngeal Examination

Conscious Patient

After the initial evaluation demonstrates a stable airway, examination of the pharynx and the larynx is attempted. Transnasal fiberoptic laryngoscopy has replaced indirect laryngoscopy and allows immediate assessment of airway integrity while maintaining cervical spine immobilization. The risk for laryngospasm during the examination is increased in cases of laryngeal lesion and may precipitate an airway obstruction. Therefore, the medical team should be ready for an emergency intubation or tracheostomy. Examination of the larynx should assess vocal cord mobility and the presence of mucosal edema, hematomas, tears, and exposed or avulsed arytenoid cartilages. Arytenoid luxation is suspected in cases of a change of the shape or an unusual position or when there is a disparity between the level of the two vocal cords. In moderate to severe injuries, a detailed examination should be performed by direct laryngoscopy under general anesthesia; in most situations, a tracheotomy is performed initially to establish a safe airway.

Intubated Patient

Patients are frequently already intubated when transferred, and transnasal flexible laryngoscopy is thus not possible to check the active mobility of the vocal cords. The larynx is examined by direct laryngoscopy that is performed with an intubation laryngoscope and a 4-mm, zero- or 30-degree telescope. Depending on the severity of the lesions, the endotracheal tube is temporarily removed or a tracheotomy is performed, permitting a precise evaluation of the endolarynx and the subglottis. Passive mobilization of the arytenoids helps differentiate between paralysis and arytenoid dislocation or fixation.

Radiologic Evaluation

Radiologic evaluation is performed only after the airway and the hemodynamic parameters are stabilized. It adds diagnostic elements in suspected laryngeal trauma, increases the precision in the topography of lesions, and assesses associated injuries of the spine, the vessels, the esophagus, and the chest. Plain radiographs of the cervical spine are taken to exclude vertebral fractures and the presence of deep cervical and prevertebral air. Pneumothorax, pneumomediastinum, pleural effusion, and subcutaneous emphysema are detected by plain chest radiography, which is performed routinely.

CT scans of the larynx have replaced tomograms, xeroradiograms, and lateral radiographs in the evaluation of the traumatized larynx (Duda et al, 1996; Schaefer, 1991a). CT scanning shows fractures or dislocations of the cricoid, the hyoid, and the thyroid cartilage and accurately reveals arytenoid luxation, hematoma, and subcutaneous emphysema, but it may fail to demonstrate some forms of cricotracheal separation (Lupetin, 1997). Three-dimensional CT scanning may provide significant additional useful information in subtle laryngeal fractures or cricoarytenoid dislocation and may be helpful in preoperative planning by increasing diagnostic accuracy (Meglin et al, 1991). Controversies are ongoing about the indications for CT examination.

According to Schaefer (1991a), CT scanning of the larynx should not be performed routinely but only when the result of the examination will influence the treatment. CT scan should be reserved for subtle abnormalities to avoid an unnecessary open surgical procedure. Thus, in cases of significant injuries, such as exposed cartilage, evident fracture, deinsertion of the vocal cord, and supraglottic or subglottic disruption, Schaefer states that the CT scan adds no valuable diagnostic element to the external and laryngoscopic examination in patients who require surgical exploration anyway. He limits his indications to two situations: (1) for making the decision of an open approach in patients with extensive edema of the laryngeal mucosa that precludes an accurate assessment in direct laryngoscopy; and (2) in patients with minimal symptoms and a history of trauma important enough to cause a fracture. In this condition, the CT scan excludes an occult thyroid fracture, which may have adverse effects on the quality of the voice. Detection of occult thyroid fractures may have therapeutic consequences. Hirano and associates (1985) reported functional disturbances in only 1-mm displacements. Other authors, however, found CT scanning valuable in anticipating injuries and planning the operative approach (Bent et al, 1993; Fuhrman et al, 1990).

Angiography or color Doppler of the cervical vessels is reserved for cases of penetrating trauma.

Associated Injuries

Facial and spinal fractures, chest trauma, and closed head injury are commonly observed in patients with blunt laryngotracheal trauma, whereas injuries to organs that are adjacent to the larynx (vessels, esophagus, spinal cord) and chest injuries are frequently associated with penetrating laryngotracheal trauma.

Pharyngeal and Esophageal Injuries

The frequency of associated pharyngeal or esophageal injuries varies from 15% in blunt trauma up to 42% in penetrating trauma (Fuhrman et al, 1990; Grewal et al, 1995; Minard et al, 1992). Pharyngeal laceration or perforation after blunt trauma is the result of impaction of the cricoid or thyroid cartilage through the mucosa (Fig. 66–4). Odynophagia, hematemesis, and subcutaneous

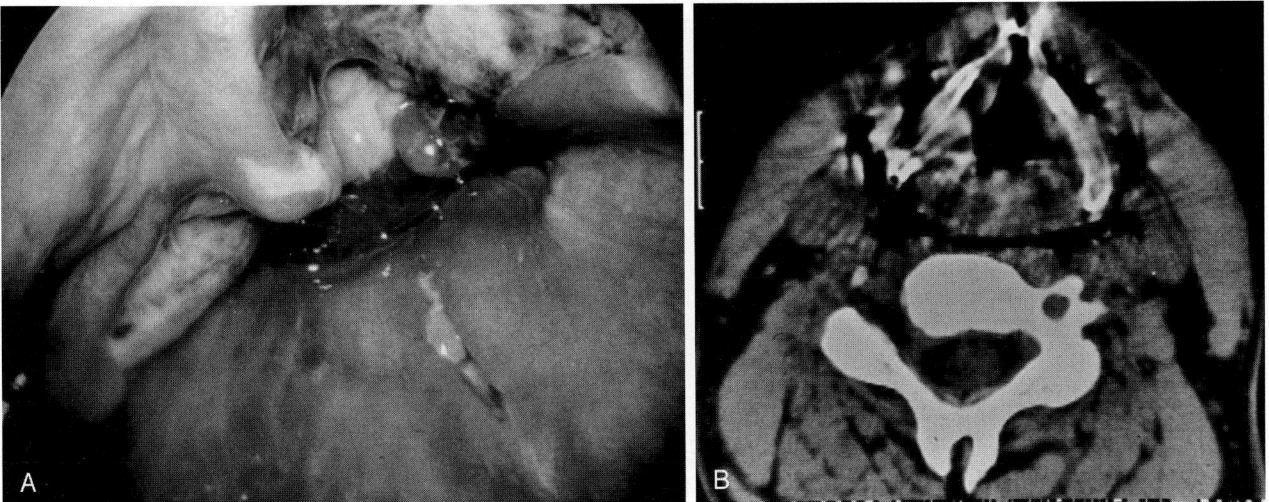

FIGURE 66–4 ■ *A*, Blunt trauma with horizontal supraglottic disruption and vertical laceration of the posterior pharyngeal wall made by impaction of the cricoid cartilage. The petiolus of the epiglottis has moved backwards at the level of the arytenoids. *B*, A computed tomography scan of the same patient showing a fracture of the right thyroid ala and cervical emphysema.

emphysema are the most reliable clinical signs that have motivated some authors to recommend investigations only in symptomatic or unconscious patients (Demetriades et al, 1996). However, it is the most commonly missed injury in the neck, and delay in diagnosis may result in severe complication. Thus, other authors recommend aggressive investigation based on the fact that the history and physical examination do not always have diagnostic value. Moreover, a primary closure within the first 24 hours drastically decreases the mortality rate, which increases to 40% if the treatment is delayed (Velmahos, 1994).

We recommend routine esophagoscopy in all unconscious patients and in patients with symptoms that require laryngeal exploration. The average false-negative rate of 21% for flexible esophagoscopy is similar to that of esophagography. A combination of the two examinations has a 100% rate of sensitivity and specificity, but this falls to 67% for hypopharyngeal perforation (White and Morris, 1992). For that reason, we strongly advise rigid esophagoscopy, which also checks the hypopharynx. It can be associated with esophagography with a water-soluble contrast agent injected through a catheter to exclude a small occult perforation. In patients at high risk for associated tracheobronchial injuries, the addition of routine tracheobronchoscopy (panendoscopy) is warranted.

Complication rates of combined esophageal and tracheal injuries reach up to 50%, and fistulas on adjacent structures such as the trachea, skin, and pleura are common. Although the trachea may be closed in one layer, esophageal lacerations are repaired with a two-layer suture and a muscle flap, usually of proximally detached sternohyoid muscle, which should be inserted between the esophagus and the trachea to prevent fistula formation (Mathisen and Grillo, 1987).

Vascular Injuries

The incidence of vascular injury is much higher in penetrating trauma (up to 38%) than it is in blunt trauma (less than 2%), and gunshots are more likely to cause vascular damage than are stab wounds (Grewal, 1995; Minard et al, 1992). Routine angiography is recommended by many authors; however, its disadvantages are its high cost and its invasive character. Demetriades and coauthors (1993) reported, in a series of 176 patients with penetrating trauma to the neck, that 19% of vascular lesions were diagnosed by routine angiography; among them, only 8% required treatment. In another study, these authors showed that the combination of physical examination and color-flow Doppler was a safe and cost-effective method to detect vascular injuries requiring treatment (Demetriades et al, 1995).

MANAGEMENT

Acute Management

Prompt initial diagnosis and management of laryngeal trauma is the key to the success of the treatment to avoid both fatal respiratory distress and catastrophic long-term sequelae. Data collected by centers over the years have permitted improvement of the diagnostic strategies and initial management through established protocols and clarification of the indications for conservative and surgical treatments (Fuhrman et al, 1990; Gussack and Jurkovich, 1988; Schaefer, 1992). Grading of the injuries has been established to standardize the reports and to define management options (Table 66–1).

Securing the airways is the most important first step in the management of a laryngeal trauma victim. Disagreement exists about the best way to establish the airway. Some authors advocate orotracheal intubation under the pretext that iatrogenic tracheal injury may result from emergency routine tracheotomy; thus, intubation should remain the primary method of airway control, but this should move quickly to tracheostomy if intubation is difficult (Gussack et al, 1986). Other authors recommend tracheotomy under local anesthesia, arguing that intubation can be hazardous and may exacerbate mucosal injur-

TABLE 66–1 ■ **Laryngotracheal Injury Classification**

Grade	*Description*
I	Minor endolaryngeal hematoma or laceration without detectable fracture
II	Edema, hematoma, minor mucosal injury without exposed cartilage; nondisplaced fractures noted on a computed tomography scan; absence of dislocation
III	Massive edema or hematoma, mucosal tears with exposed cartilage, cord immobility, displaced fractures
IV	As grade III, with multiple fractures, disruption of the anterior half of the larynx, unstable laryngeal framework
V	Complete laryngotracheal separation

Modified from Schaefer SD: Acute management of laryngeal trauma update. Ann Otol Rhinol Laryngol 98:98, 1989; and Fuhrman GM, Stieg FH, Buerk CA: Blunt laryngeal trauma: Classification and management protocol. J Trauma 30:87, 1990.

ies or complete a partial laryngotracheal separation (Fuhrman et al, 1990; Harris and Tobin, 1970; Schaefer, 1992). In agreement with Schaefer (1992), we believe that only patients without injuries involving the lumen can undergo a safe intubation. Other patients with mild to moderate lesions and those with severe injuries should undergo tracheostomy under local anesthesia. This decisional protocol highly reduces the risk for loss of or damage to the airway. Tracheotomy is performed lower than usual on the trachea, at the level of the fourth or fifth ring. Exceptionally, cricothyroidotomy may be necessary in urgent situations, but in principle should be avoided to prevent the airway from sustaining additional trauma. Therefore, it should be converted to a formal tracheotomy as soon as possible (Bent et al, 1993). Care should be taken to avoid manipulation of the neck until a cervical spine fracture has been excluded.

Timing

Timing of the surgical exploration has been a topic of controversy in the past; however, more recently, it is generally admitted that early treatment yields the best result. Delays in operative intervention lead to a higher complication rate (infection, perichondritis, stenosis), more difficult surgery, and poorer voice and airway results (Bent et al, 1993; Gussack et al, 1986; Schaefer, 1992). Open exploration should be performed within 24 hours of injury to help in the identification of specific damage before the onset of edema.

Conservative Management

Conservative management of laryngeal trauma is reserved for cases in which spontaneous healing without alteration of laryngeal function can be expected. The injuries correspond to grade I and II lesions (see Table 66–1): laryngeal edema, hematomas, and small lacerations without exposed cartilage and those not involving the anterior commissure. Single stable and nondisplaced fractures usually require no open exploration because a good functional prognosis is expected. Nevertheless, some authors advocate repair of minimally displaced fractures and asymptomatic thyroid cartilage fractures, arguing the possibility of changes in vocal dynamics (Hirano et al, 1985; Stanley et al, 1987).

Conservative management consists of close observation, elevation of the head of the bed, humidification of inspired air, prophylactic antibiotics, and daily fiberoptic laryngeal examination until the edema has decreased. H_2-blockers may be helpful, particularly in patients with gastroesophageal reflux and in the prevention of irritation of the traumatized mucosa. Corticosteroids are used inconsistently and may be useful if administered early after injury. Tracheotomy is necessary if laryngeal edema is expected to be present for several days. Functional results after conservative treatment are good; nearly 90% of grade I and II injuries have good results (Bent et al, 1993; Schaefer, 1992).

Surgical Management

Open surgical exploration is indicated for more severe laryngeal injuries corresponding to grade III to V injuries (see Table 66–1): large mucosal lacerations, exposed cartilage, multiple or displaced cartilaginous fractures, vocal cord immobility, laceration of the anterior commissure or of the free margin of the vocal cords, or arytenoid dislocation. Criteria for neck exploration include the following: progressive subcutaneous emphysema, active bleeding, hematoma of the neck, and neurologic deficit (Bent et al, 1993; Fuhrman et al, 1990; Grewal et al, 1995; Schaefer, 1989).

The larynx is exposed through a transverse incision usually at the level of the cricothyroid membrane. The strap muscles are divided in the midline and retracted laterally. The larynx is explored through a midline thyrotomy. If a vertical fracture exists within 3 mm of the midline, the larynx is explored through the fracture. The true vocal cords are the first anatomic landmark to identify. Starting posteriorly, pharyngeal mucosal lacerations are first carefully readapted with 4–0 or 5–0 absorbable sutures followed by laryngeal and tracheal repair. Dislocated arytenoids are replaced in their normal position or removed if severely damaged. All exposed cartilages are covered with local mucosal flaps (mainly harvested in the piriform fossae) to prevent scarring and perichondritis. Although skin graft and mucous graft harvested in the mouth are described in the literature, they are rarely required.

Vocal cord injuries are repaired first by the reconstitution of the anterior commissure. This is achieved by suturing the anterior margin of the true vocal cord to the outer perichondrium of the thyroid cartilage (Schaefer, 1992). A soft Silastic feeding tube is used for 1 week in case of esophageal or pharyngeal laceration. Direct laryngotracheoscopy is performed after 10 days and repeated if further treatment is necessary. After 1 week, the tracheostomy cannula is progressively occluded to stimulate phonation.

Hyoid Bone Fracture

An isolated fracture of the hyoid bone is treated conservatively. Displaced or comminuted fractures are managed

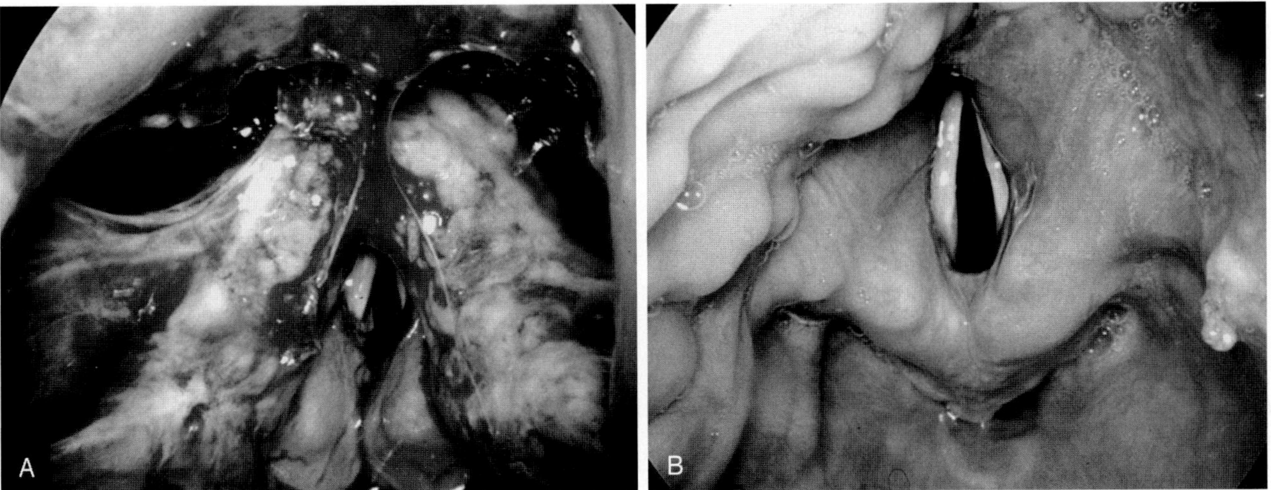

FIGURE 66–5 ■ *A*, Horizontal supraglottic disruption above the arytenoids with a large communication in the soft tissue of the neck after a blunt trauma during a car accident. *B*, Result after horizontal laryngectomy; the epiglottis was removed and the base of the tongue was sutured at the anterior commissure.

by removing the cartilaginous fragments and re-establishing the continuity between the suprahyoid and infrahyoid musculature with large sutures, to facilitate onset of swallowing.

Supraglottic Injury

Exploration of the supraglottic area is made through the thyrohyoid membrane. Disruption of the attachment of the epiglottis is treated by anterior fixation with resorbable sutures. If anterior anchorage support is not available, the lower one third of the epiglottis is resected, and the remaining cartilage is suspended to the hyoid bone. Significant injuries of the supraglottic area with extensive lacerations are managed with a supraglottic laryngectomy, as performed for oncologic purposes (Fig. 66–5).

Thyroid Cartilage Fracture

Minimally displaced or nondisplaced thyroid fractures have an excellent prognosis with conservative treatment, although changes in vocal dynamics have been reported (Hirano et al, 1985). Any single displaced thyroid fracture should be reduced and repaired with No. 24 wire. In soft cartilage, 3–0 nonabsorbable sutures are preferred over wire, which can cut through the cartilage. Simple, nondisplaced fractures are fixed by suturing only the outer perichondrium. If the cartilage is ossified, holes are made with a minidrill to facilitate suture placement. Rigid fixation with miniplates can facilitate the stabilization of multiple unstable segments and restore the exact geometry of the laryngeal framework, mainly the anterior angulation of the thyroid cartilage, and also offer the ability to bridge large defects (Woo, 1990).

Arytenoid Dislocation

Early diagnosis facilitates treatment, and reduction within 3 weeks of injury is associated with good functional results. Open reduction through laryngofissure is performed during the surgical revision of a laryngeal trauma. Avulsed arytenoids are covered with the piriform sinus mucosa or removed if the damage is too extensive (Fig. 66–6). If the arytenoid remains dislocated for an extended period, fibrotic ankylosis of the joint prevents the reposition; however, it is difficult to predict until what time reduction can be attempted. Successful late reductions have been described even after a delay of 1 year. Sataloff and colleagues (1994) reported a series of 26 cases in which patients with good results had an average time interval of 10 weeks between injury and surgical reduction, whereas the time interval for the group of patients with residual alteration was 29 weeks.

Closed reduction remains a difficult procedure. It is performed under general anesthesia in suspension laryn-

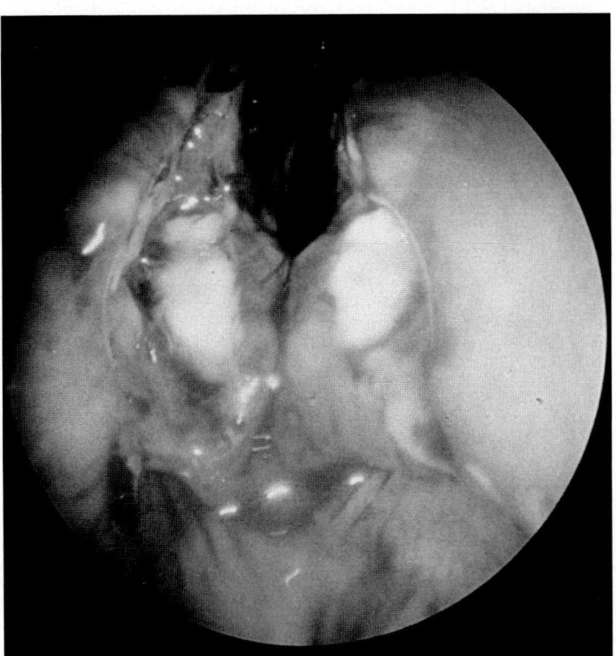

FIGURE 66–6 ■ Blunt trauma with avulsed arytenoids.

goscopy or with local anesthesia and sedation using the blade of a Miller laryngoscope (Sataloff et al, 1994). Pressure is exerted on the lateral surface of the vocal process and the body of the arytenoid to push it posteriorly or anteriorly according to the type of luxation. Delicate and thin instruments may lacerate the mucosa; therefore, large and smooth instruments are preferred. Unsuccessful reduction may necessitate delayed endoscopic procedures, such as arytenoidectomy in cases of airway compromise, or intracordal fat or collagen injection in cases of glottic incompetence. Vocal cord medialization through a thyroplasty is another option.

Laryngotracheal Disruption and Cricoid Fractures

Laryngotracheal disruption with cricoid fractures is a serious, but rare, injury and has been reported by several authors (Alonso, 1979; Alonso et al, 1974; Bryce, 1972; Couraud et al, 1974; Harris, 1972; Mathisen and Grillo, 1987; Offiah and Endres, 1997; Ogura and Biller, 1971). An immediate low tracheotomy is advocated to secure the airway. Although intubation may exacerbate the soft tissue lesions around the dehiscence, it may be the only way to save the patient's life on the site of the accident (Fig. 66–7). Many patients have no injury to the thyroid cartilage, and exploration can be adequately performed through the cricotracheal dehiscence.

Associated injuries to the pharynx and the esophagus are repaired first, and the tracheal stumps of the disruption are then mobilized and "freshened" to create a tension-free anastomosis. For this purpose, a laryngeal release may be necessary and is performed by cutting the infrahyoid muscle attachments at the hyoid bone and freeing the superior horns of the thyroid cartilage. If the integrity of the cartilages is preserved, a circumferential anastomosis is performed. Resection of damaged tracheal rings may be necessary, keeping the posterior wall of the trachea, which can serve as a local mucosal flap to cover a denuded area of the cricoid cartilage, if possible. If this flap is not available, it is replaced by an autograft of buccal mucosa, secured in place with absorbable sutures, fibrin glue, and short-term stenting. Associated cricoid fractures are reduced and fixed with wire sutures.

Internal stabilization with a Montgomery T tube may be necessary in fractures of the posterior arch. If the anterior arch of the cricoid is severely damaged, it is better to perform a partial cricotracheal resection with thyrotracheal anastomosis (see Chapter 20). Other alternatives, such as autografts of the hyoid bone, rib cartilage, or iliac crest, present a higher risk for residual cicatricial stenosis; they should be avoided (Monnier et al, 1998; Pearson et al, 1986).

Transection or severe damage to the recurrent laryngeal nerves is frequently associated with laryngotracheal disruption, and its management remains controversial. Identification of the recurrent laryngeal nerves may be difficult in swollen tissues and may lead to further damage to a potential intact nerve in an already tracheotomized patient, without having information on vocal cord mobility. For that reason, exploration of a hypothetically injured recurrent laryngeal nerve is not advocated. If there is evidence of transection, the recurrent laryngeal nerve–to–recurrent laryngeal nerve anastomosis should be avoided because it may lead to laryngeal synkinesis. The ansa cervicalis–to–recurrent laryngeal nerve anastomosis, as advocated by Crumley (1990), may be preferred.

For cases in which both recurrent laryngeal nerves are sectioned, various treatments have been proposed. Reanastomosis of the transected nerves is usually followed by poor function and increases the risk for airway compromise (Alonso, 1979; Casiano and Goodwin, 1991). Direct reimplantation of the nerve into the posterior arytenoid muscle, which acts as the main abductor muscle of the glottis, has been described with inconsistent outcomes (Snow, 1984). Couraud and associates (1974) resolved the functional stenosis with enlargement of the posterior commissure by maintaining the posterior hiatus from the fracture with a stent placed for 10 days

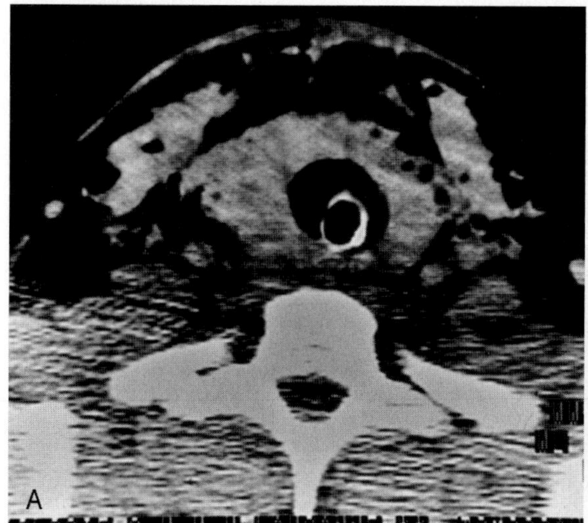

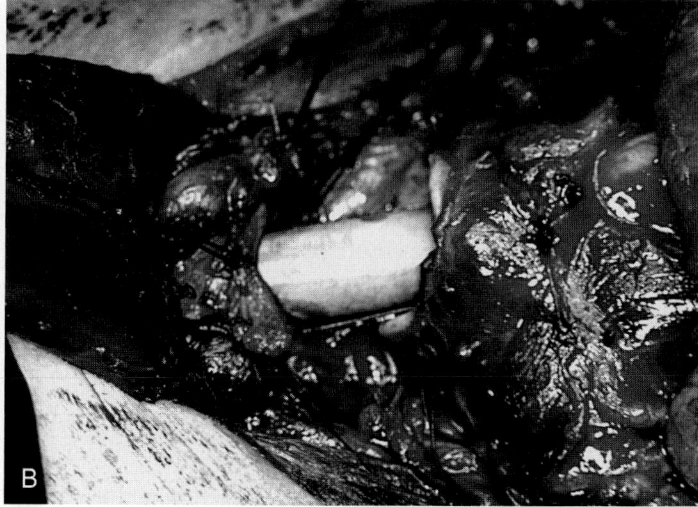

FIGURE 66–7 ■ *A*, A computed tomography scan of a total cricotracheal disruption; the endotracheal tube is surrounded by air and soft tissues without cartilages. *B*, Perioperative view of the dehiscence between the cricoid (*right*) and the trachea (*left*). The patient was successfully intubated on the site of the accident.

as described by Réthi (1956). However, unilateral laser arytenoidectomy that is performed in a second stage remains the simplest and most effective treatment for symptomatic bilateral vocal cord paralysis.

Missile Injuries to the Larynx

After an evaluation of the lesions, the treatment for penetrating injuries of the larynx follows the same general principles as those applied to the nonpenetrating traumas, with the addition of extensive infection prevention measures, especially in severe ballistic decay. Surgical exploration focuses on the search for associated injuries (present in up to half of cases) to the vessels, trachea, and particularly to the pharynx and esophagus. The extraction of the missile often requires a second incision. Surgical repair includes suturing of the mucosal lacerations with use of piriform fossa mucosal flaps and, rarely, grafts, restoration of the laryngeal architecture, and use of a stent (Danic et al, 1996). Cutaneous wounds may be left partially open if they are contaminated. Severe soft tissue damage with loss of tissue as a result of high-velocity missiles and military weapons seldom requires partial or total laryngectomy.

Indications for Stenting

The use of laryngeal stents remains controversial, and the indications, type of stent, and timing of removal are still under debate. The main functions of a stent are (1) to maintain the lumen of the larynx to prevent web formation and to promote adherence of flaps or grafts to the underlying cartilaginous structures; (2) to stabilize an unstable tracheolaryngeal framework by providing internal support as an adjunct to external fixation of cartilages; and (3) to maintain or re-create the anterior commissure by insertion of a keel when the vocal cords are seriously avulsed, which is essential to recovery of a good voice. Thus, stenting is indicated in the following situations (Bent et al, 1993; Casiano and Goodwin, 1991; Eliachar, 1996; Gussack and Jurkovich, 1988; Schaefer, 1992):

- Disruption of the anterior half of the larynx
- High instability of the cartilaginous skeleton, which cannot be maintained with fixation of the cartilaginous fractures
- Severe tracheal ring injury or loss of cricoid structural integrity
- Massive endolaryngeal laceration and avulsion with a high risk for cicatricial stenosis
- Extensive lacerations of the mucosa, preventing the restoration of a normally shaped anterior commissure

Many types of stents have been used, and many different opinions regarding the ideal material to be used remain; however, surgeons agree that the stent should have the shape of the larynx and should be made with soft material to avoid further injuries to the traumatized mucosa (Casiano and Goodwin, 1991; Eliachar, 1996). Many different stents have been described, including the finger of a surgical glove filled with a sponge, a rolled

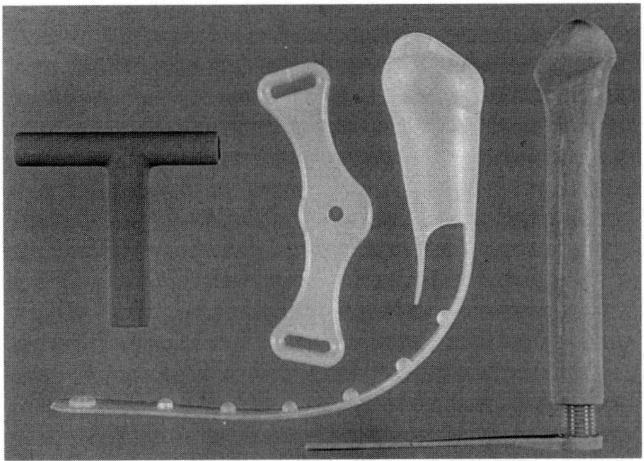

FIGURE 66–8 ■ Laryngeal stents (from the *left*): rubber silicone T tube; Eliachar laryngeal stent made in soft silicone fixed with a strap attached to the skin through the tracheostomy; Lausanne prototype stent made in rubber silicone, available in different sizes, with the same type of fixation as the Eliachar stent.

Silastic sheet, a modified endotracheal Portex tube, a silicone rubber stent, and the Montgomery T tube, without any observable difference in outcome (Fig. 66–8) (Schaefer, 1992). The stent is fixed with transcutaneous, nonabsorbable sutures, or it is fixed through the tracheotomy by a strap at the inferior extremity of the stent. Another specific stent is the Silastic keel, which may be applied to prevent anterior webbing when the anterior thirds of the true cords are avulsed.

Although experimental studies of stenting the larynx in dogs have shown a higher incidence of wound infection and granulation tissue formation (Thomas and Stevens, 1975), these complications can be avoided or reduced by short-term stenting that does not exceed 2 weeks. According to most surgeons, this appears to be enough time to promote stability of the larynx without further damage to the mucosa (Bent et al, 1993; Gussack and Jurkovich, 1988; Leopold, 1983; Schaefer, 1992). In his series, Leopold (1983) reported a duration of use for best airway results of 3.5 weeks and for best voice results of 2.1 weeks. Fixation of the stent must be handled with caution because death by airway obstruction after displacement of the stent has been reported (Gussack and Jurkovich, 1988). Broad-spectrum antibiotic coverage is advocated. The stent is removed endoscopically, and follow-up laryngotracheoscopies are performed until complete healing has occurred.

Endoscopic adjunctive procedures may be necessary to optimize the functional result. Granulations are removed with forceps, and thin webs or synechiae are treated with the CO_2 laser.

Inhalation and Caustic Injuries

Inhalation injuries of the larynx and the upper airway require endotracheal intubation as soon as slight symptoms such as hoarseness or dysphonia appear, and before the onset of edema, which can quickly lead to a glottic–subglottic obstruction. Extubation is generally possible 2 to 5 days after the laryngeal edema has resolved. Long-term intubation should be avoided, and tracheotomy is indicated after 6 days if edema is still present (Miller et al, 1988). Immediate tracheotomy is advocated by other authors to diminish the risk for subglottic stenosis (Sataloff and Sataloff, 1984).

Conservative treatment with humidification and complete voice rest is seldom complicated with cicatricial stenosis, but sequelae of intubation or tracheotomy increase up to 30% when tracheobronchial burns are associated with laryngeal burns (Nottet et al, 1997). When they occur, laryngeal sequelae consist mainly of posterior glottic stenosis, which may involve one or both cricoarytenoid joints. The consequences are a limitation or an absence of arytenoid abduction, leading to a fixed larynx. They are associated with complex multiple stenoses of the subglottis and the trachea (Eliachar et al, 1981; Flexon et al, 1989; Miller et al, 1988).

The management of laryngeal stenosis by inhalation differs from that of postintubation stenosis because of the long-standing evolution of the lesion. Stenting with a Montgomery T tube for a prolonged period of up to 28 months as soon as the stenosis appears constitutes the first stage of the treatment (Gaissert et al, 1993; Nottet et al, 1997). The second stage is accomplished later with the resection of the stenosis by an open surgical procedure when the lesion is stable (Miller et al, 1988). Nevertheless, Flexon and colleagues (1989) reported success with an earlier open surgical procedure. The surgery follows the same principles as those applied to laryngeal and subglottic stenoses of other origins, but often multiple operations are required.

Laryngeal injuries caused by caustic ingestion are mainly located in the supraglottic area and are associated with hypopharyngeal and esophageal burns. Acute management consists of securing the airway by endotracheal intubation or tracheotomy, controlling the volemia with a central venous catheter, and administering broad-spectrum antibiotics and corticosteroids to prevent fibrosis. Feeding jejunostomy or gastrostomy may be necessary in severe cases in which a nasogastric tube for feeding is contraindicated.

Cicatricial stenosis of the supraglottis and of the hypopharynx is treated in association with the esophageal stricture in a one-stage procedure. The key to success is to replace the pharyngeal fibrotic tissue with the soft mucosa of the colic transplant such as that used to replace the esophagus. The pharyngeal stenosis can be resected with the CO_2 laser, and the anastomotic zone is well delineated for immediate suture of the transplant up to the arytenoids (Fig. 66–9). Pharyngeal Z plasty, local mucosal flaps, regional chest flaps, and supraglottic laryngectomy are alternatives that are reported in the literature (Gross and Harris, 1971; Hamaker and Conley, 1979; Tran Ba Huy and Celerier, 1988).

Laryngeal Stenosis

Management of laryngeal stenosis after laryngeal trauma does not differ from the treatment of postintubation or congenital stenoses. Subglottic stenoses are best treated with partial cricoid resection and primary anastomosis (see Chapter 20). Associated glottic stenoses are treated during the same procedure through a laryngofissure. Depending on the severity of the lesion, treatment varies from endoscopic resection to enlargement laryngotracheoplasty. Anterior enlargement is performed with a laryngofissure combined with an anterior cartilage graft interposition and stenting for 4 to 6 weeks or for up to several months in severe cases. Posterior glottic stenosis requires resection of the posterior fibrosis with mobilization of the arytenoids and enlargement of the posterior commissure with the interposition of a costal cartilage graft (Réthi procedure) and stenting for several weeks (Réthi, 1956).

The development of endoscopic procedures with the CO_2 laser, dilatation, and stenting has led to overuse without thorough respect for the indications. Endoscopic treatment should not be proposed as a first attempt before an eventual open surgical procedure; but the indications and the risk of aggravating the initial condition should be rigorously considered. The indications are limited to a noncircular scar; a circular, thin diaphragm without cartilaginous collapse; an arytenoidectomy for bilateral vocal cord paralysis or a cricoarytenoid joint ankylosis; and anterior glottic synechia. A keel is often used to repair the angle of the anterior commissure. Interventional endoscopy, however, plays an important role as an adjunctive treatment after open procedures to optimize the results.

Results

The outcome of laryngeal trauma depends on the severity of the initial injuries and the timing and quality of the repair. Patients with grade I and II lesions, treated conservatively or with tracheotomy and endoscopy, most often recover normal laryngeal functions (Hirano et al, 1985; Leopold, 1983; Mathisen and Grillo, 1987). Bent and coauthors (1993) and Schaefer (1992) reported more than 90% recovery of good airway and voice. In Schaefer's series, the fair results in three patients were because of a laryngeal nerve injury and an unrepaired laceration of a vocal fold that would probably have benefited from primary closure of the laceration. Patients with grade III to V injuries have less optimal results. The same authors reported, respectively, 42% and 24% of fair voices and 1.2% and 0% of poor voices, 13% and 0% of fair airways, and 3.7% and 3.8% persistent tracheostomies. There was a higher incidence of poor results when the treatment was delayed. Suboptimal results were encountered in patients with bilateral vocal cord paralysis, displaced cricoid fracture, and arytenoid subluxation; among them, 25% of patients with complete laryngotracheal separation were still tracheostomy dependent. All patients recovered normal swallowing function.

Recent improvements in the management of laryngeal trauma, including early diagnosis and treatment, precise reconstruction of the anatomy, short-term stenting with better tolerated stents, and appropriate laryngeal stenosis treatment, have allowed a high percentage of good results to be obtained, even in severe injuries. The experience of the surgeon also plays an important role in the successful management of laryngeal trauma.

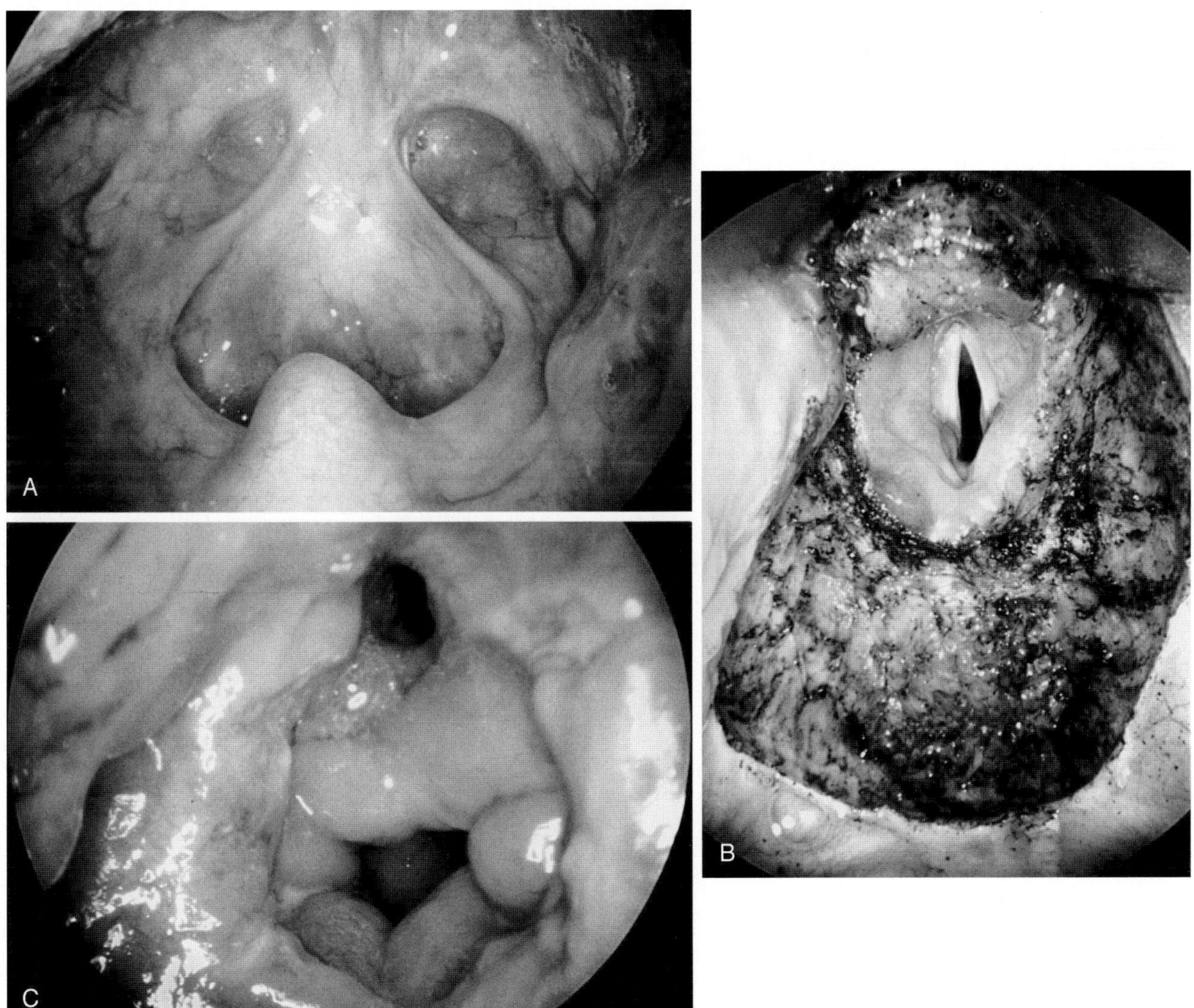

FIGURE 66–9 ■ *A*, Total pharyngolaryngeal stenosis after caustic ingestion in a 5-year-old girl. *B*, The surgery begins with the resection of the supraglottic stenosis with the CO_2 laser in suspension microlaryngoscopy. The laser cut precisely delineates the mucosal margins for the colic anastomosis during open repair. *C*, Result 1 year after the colic transplant has been sutured to the arytenoids. There is slight residual supraglottic stenosis without functional impairment.

COMMENTS AND CONTROVERSIES

Isolated laryngeal trauma is exceedingly rare. However, recognition of these injuries and their immediate management are critical because laryngeal trauma and its associated disruption of the airway often prove immediately fatal. Furthermore, proper management of these injuries is mandatory to maintain airway patency, satisfactory phonation, and avoidance of aspiration.

Dr. Monnier and his colleagues have provided an outstanding review of a very complicated subject. The complex physiology of the larynx is discussed. The mechanisms of injury, both blunt and penetrating, to various components of the larynx are covered in detail. Management strategies are thoroughly discussed with particular reference to recent major contributions to the literature. Controversial aspects of laryngeal injury are also discussed. The authors recommend early and low tracheostomy for patients who have endoluminal disruption and early exploration and anatomic repair of all laryngeal injuries to achieve optimum results. Avoidance of long-term cricothyroidotomy is stressed to minimize the likelihood of subglottic stenosis. The appropriate use of laryngeal stents in association with primary repair is covered in detail.

G.A.P.

■ KEY REFERENCES

Demetriades D, Asensio JA, Velmahos G, Thal E: Complex problems in penetrating neck trauma. Surg Clin North Am 76:661, 1996.

The authors provide an excellent review of the diagnostic strategies and management of penetrating trauma of the neck including the larynx and trachea. Investigation and therapeutic protocols are discussed in detail.

Grewal H, Rao PM, Mukerji S et al: Management of penetrating laryngotracheal injuries. Head Neck 17:494, 1995.

The authors report on a series of 57 penetrating laryngotracheal injuries, with a focus on airway management, procedure for diagnosing associated lesions, and operative management.

Pearson FG, Brito-Filomeno L, Cooper JD: Experience with partial cricoid resection and thyrotracheal anastomosis. Ann Otol Rhinol Laryngol 95:582, 1986.

The technique of partial cricoid resection for tracheal and subglottic stenosis and for laryngotracheal disruption is described extensively.

Schaefer SD: The acute management of external laryngeal trauma: A 27 year experience. Arch Otolaryngol Head Neck Surg 118:598, 1992.

The authors describe the principles of the management of laryngeal trauma, including the diagnostic strategies, criteria for surgical versus medical management, principles of surgical treatment, and indications for stenting. This article is a useful reference for the clinician interested in laryngeal trauma.

■ REFERENCES

Alonso WA: Surgical management and complications of acute laryngotracheal disruption. Otolaryngol Clin North Am 12:753, 1979.

Alonso WA, Pratt LL, Zollinger WK et al: Complications of laryngotracheal disruption. Laryngoscope 84:1276, 1974.

Angood B, Attia EL, Brown RA et al: Extrinsic civilian trauma to the larynx and cervical trachea: Important predictors of long-term morbidity. J Trauma 36:869, 1986.

Bent JP, Silver JR, Porubsky ES: Acute laryngeal trauma: A review of 77 patients. Otolaryngol Head Neck Surg 109:441, 1993.

Bryce DP: The surgical management of laryngotracheal injury. J Laryngol Otol 86:547, 1972.

Casiano RR, Goodwin WJ: Restoring function to the injured larynx. Otolaryngol Clin North Am 24:1215, 1991.

Chagnon FP, Mulder DS: Laryngotracheal trauma. Chest Surg Clin North Am 6:733, 1996.

Couraud L, Bruneteau A, Hazera JR: Désinsertion laryngo-trachéale post-traumatique avec fracture du cartilage cricoïde et arrachement bilatéral du nerf récurrent. Ann Chir Thorac Cardiovasc 13:249, 1974.

Crumley RL: Teflon versus thyroplasty versus nerve transfer: A comparison. Ann Otol Rhinol Laryngol 99:759, 1990.

Danic D, Milicic D, Progmet D et al: Acute laryngeal trauma: A comparison between peace time and war injuries. J Laryngol Otol 110:435, 1996.

Demetriades D, Asensio JA, Velmahos G, Thal E: Complex problems in penetrating neck trauma. Surg Clin North Am 76(4):661, 1996.

Demetriades D, Charalambides D, Lakhoo M: Physical examination and selective conservative management in patients with penetrating injuries of the neck. Br J Surg 80:1534, 1993.

Demetriades D, Theodorou D, Cornwell E et al: Penetrating injuries of the neck in stable patients: Physical examination, angiography, or color flow Doppler. Arch Surg 130:971, 1995.

Duda JJ, Lewin JS, Eliachar I: Evaluation of epiglottic disruption. Am J Neuroradiol 17:563, 1996.

Edwards WH, Morris JA, DeLozier JB et al: Airway injuries: The first priority in trauma. Ann Surg 95:192, 1987.

Eliachar I: Management of acute laryngeal trauma. Acta Otol Rhinol Laryngol Belg 50:151, 1996.

Eliachar I, Moscona R, Joachims HZ et al: The management of laryngotracheal stenosis in burned patients. Plast Reconstr Surg 68:11, 1981.

Fabre A, Menard M, Lacau St-Guily J et al: Traumatismes externes du larynx. Encycl Méd Chir (Paris, France) 20720:A10, 1987.

Flexon PB, Cheney ML, Montgomery WW et al: Management of patients with glottic and subglottic stenosis resulting from thermal burns. Ann Otol Rhinol Laryngol 98:27, 1989.

Fuhrman GM, Stieg FH, Buerk CA: Blunt laryngeal trauma: Classification and management protocol. J Trauma 30:87, 1990.

Gaissert HA, Lofgren RH, Grillo HC: Upper airway compromise after inhalation injury: Complex strictures of the larynx and trachea and their management. Ann Surg 218:672, 1993.

Gluckman JL, Ajay KM: Laryngeal trauma in otolaryngology. In Paparella MM, Gluckman JL, Meyerhoff WL (eds): Disorders of the Head and Neck. Philadelphia, WB Saunders, 1991, pp 2231–2244.

Grewal H, Rao PM, Mukerji S et al: Management of penetrating laryngotracheal injuries. Head Neck 17:494, 1995.

Gross CW, Harris AS: Relief of stricture in the cervical esophagus by Z-plasty technique. Laryngoscope 81:658, 1971.

Guerrier Y, Mounier-Kuhn P: Histoire des Maladies de l'Oreille, du Nez et de la Gorge. Paris, Les Éditions Dacosta, 1980.

Guerrier Y, Savary M, Meyer R et al: Les traumatismes externes du larynx. Les Cah d'O.R.L. 14:767, 1979.

Gussack GS, Jurkovich GJ: Treatment dilemmas in laryngotracheal trauma. J Trauma 28:1439, 1988.

Gussack GS, Jurkovich GJ, Luterman A et al: Laryngotracheal trauma: A protocol approach to a rare injury. Laryngoscope 96:660, 1986.

Hamaker RC, Conley J: Surgical treatment of hypopharyngeal stenosis in children. Laryngoscope 89:1593, 1979.

Harris HH: Management of injuries to the larynx and trachea. Laryngoscope 82:1924, 1972.

Harris HH, Tobin HA: Acute injuries of the larynx and trachea in 49 patients. Laryngoscope 80:1376, 1970.

Haugh RH, Giles DL: Laryngeal cartilage fracture: Report of case. J Oral Maxillofac Surg 50:528, 1992.

Hirano M, Kurita S, Terasawa R: Difficulty in high-pitched phonation by laryngeal trauma. Arch Otolaryngol 111:59, 1985.

Holinger PH, Schild JA: Pharyngeal, laryngeal and tracheal injuries in the pediatric age group. Ann J Otol 81:538, 1972.

Jones RF, Terrel JC, Salyer KE: Penetrating wounds of the neck: An analysis of 274 cases. J Trauma 7:228, 1967.

Leopold DA: Laryngeal trauma: A historical comparison of treatment methods. Otolaryngol Head Neck Surg 109:106, 1983.

Lupetin AR: Computed tomographic evaluation of laryngotracheal trauma. Curr Probl Diagn Radiol July/August:185, 1997.

Mathisen DJ, Grillo H: Laryngotracheal trauma. Ann Thorac Surg 43:254, 1987.

McConnell DB, Trunkey DD: Management of penetrating trauma to the neck. Adv Surg 27:97, 1994.

Meglin AJ, Biedlingmaier JF, Mirvis SE: Three-dimensional computerized tomography in the evaluation of laryngeal injury. Laryngoscope 101:202, 1991.

Merrit RM, Bent JP, Porubsky ES: Acute laryngeal trauma in the pediatric patient. Ann Otol Rhinol Laryngol 107:104, 1998.

Miglets AW: Functional laryngeal abduction following reimplantation of the recurrent laryngeal nerves. Laryngoscope 84:1974, 1996.

Miller RH, Duplechain JK: Penetrating wounds of the neck. Otolaryngol Clin North Am 24:15, 1991.

Miller RP, Gray SD, Cotton RT et al: Airway reconstruction following laryngotracheal thermal trauma. Laryngoscope 98:826, 1988.

Minard G, Kudsk KA, Croce MA et al: Laryngotracheal trauma. Am Surg 58:181, 1992.

Monnier P, Lang F, Savary M: Partial cricotracheal resection for severe pediatric subglottic stenosis: Update of the Lausanne experience. Ann Otol Rhinol Laryngol 107:961, 1998.

Moure EJ, Liébault G, Canuyt G: Pathologie de guerre du Larynx et de la Trachée. Paris, Librairie Felix Alcan, 1918.

Myer CM, Orobello P, Cotton RT et al: Blunt laryngeal trauma in children. Laryngoscope 97:1043, 1987.

Nahum AM, Siegel AW: Biodynamics of injury to the larynx in automobile collisions. Ann Otol Rhinol Laryngol 76:781, 1967.

Nottet JB, Duruisseau O, Herve S et al: Les brûlures par inhalation: À propos de 198 cas. Incidence de l'atteinte laryngo-trachéale. Ann Otolaryngol Cervicofac 114:220, 1997.

Offiah CJ, Endres D: Isolated laryngotracheal separation following blunt trauma to the neck. J Laryngol Otol 111:1079, 1997.

Ogura J: Management of traumatic injuries of the larynx and the trachea including stenosis. J Laryngol Otol 85:1259, 1971.

Ogura JH, Biller HF: Reconstruction of the larynx following blunt trauma. Ann Otol 80:492, 1971.

Ogura JH, Heenemann H, Spector GV: Laryngotracheal trauma: Diagnosis and treatment. Can J Otolaryngol 2:112, 1973.

Olson NR: Acute laryngeal trauma. In Gates GA (ed): Current Therapy in Otolaryngology: Head and Neck Surgery. St. Louis, CV Mosby, 1982.

Olson NR: Wound healing by primary intention in the larynx. Otolaryngol Clin North Am 12:735, 1979.

Pearson FG, Brito-Filomeno L, Cooper JD: Experience with partial cricoid resection and thyrotracheal anastomosis. Ann Otol Rhinol Laryngol 95:582, 1986.

Piller P, Herman D, Weryha JC et al: Les traumatismes externes du larynx. Notre expérience à propos de 55 cas. Rev Laryngol 112:199–204, 1991.

Piquet JJ, Desaulty A, Vaneeclo FM et al: Les traumatismes externes du larynx et de la trachée cervicale—à propos de 40 observations. Acta Otol Laryngol Belg 29:715, 1975.

Réthi A: An operation for cicatricial stenosis of the larynx. J Laryngol Otol 70:283, 1956.

Richardson MS: Laryngeal anatomy and mechanisms of trauma. Ear Nose Throat J 60:346, 1981.

Sabatier C: De la Médécine Opératoire ou des Opérations de Chirurgie qui se Pratiquent le Plus Fréquemment. Paris, Imprimerie de Didot le Jeune, 1796.

Sataloff DM, Sataloff RT: Tracheotomy and inhalation injury. Head Neck 6:1024, 1984.

Sataloff RT, Bough ID, Spiegel JR: Arythenoid dislocation: Diagnosis and treatment. Laryngoscope 104:1353, 1994.

Schaefer SD: Acute management of laryngeal trauma update. Ann Otol Rhinol Laryngol 98:98, 1989.

Schaefer SD: Use of CT scanning in the management of the acutely injured larynx. Otolaryngol Clin North Am 24:31, 1991a.

Schaefer SD: The treatment of acute external laryngeal injuries. Arch Otolaryngol 117:35, 1991b.

Schaefer SD: The acute management of external laryngeal trauma: A 27 year experience. Arch Otolaryngol 118:598, 1992.

Schaefer SD: Laryngeal and esophageal trauma. In Cummings CW (ed): Head and Neck Surgery. Philadelphia, Mosby–Year Book, 1998.

Schwab W, Ey W: Verletzungen und Stenosen des Kehlkopfes und der Luftröhre. In Berendes J (ed): Kehlkopf Sprachstörungen. Stuttgart, Thieme, 1963.

Snow JB: Diagnosis and therapy for acute laryngeal and tracheal trauma. Otolaryngol Clin North Am 17:101, 1984.

Stanley RB, Cooper DS, Florman SH: Phonatory effects of thyroid cartilage fractures. Ann Otol Rhinol Laryngol 96:493, 1987.

Thomas GK, Stevens MH: Stenting in experimental laryngeal injuries. Arch Otolaryngol 101:217, 1975.

Traissac L, Danion PH, Moure M: Les traumatismes du larynx: á propos de 21 cas. Cah Oto Rhino Laryngol 14:805, 1979.

Tran Ba Huy P, Celerier M: Management of severe caustic stenosis of the hypopharynx and esophagus by ileocolic transposition via suprahyoid or transepiglottic approach. Ann Surg April:439, 1988.

Tucker HM: The Larynx, 2nd ed. New York, Thieme, 1993.

Velhamos GC, Santer I, Degiannis E et al: Selective management in penetrating neck injuries. Can J Surg 37:487, 1994.

White RK, Morris DM: Diagnosis and management of esophageal perforations. Ann Surg 58:112, 1992.

Willemot J, Pirsig W, Rodegra H: Naissance et développement de l'oto-rhino-laryngologie dans l'histoire de la médecine. Acta Med Belg 35(Suppl 4):1045, 1981.

Woo P: Laryngeal framework reconstruction with miniplates. Ann Otol Rhinol Laryngol 99:772, 1990.

Yen PT, Lee HY, Tsai MH et al: Clinical analysis of external laryngeal trauma. J Laryngol Otol 108:221, 1994.

CHAPTER **67**

Tracheobronchial Trauma

Douglas E. Wood
Riyad Karmy-Jones
Éric Vallières

Tracheobronchial injury is uncommon but immediately life threatening. The immediate sequelae can include death from asphyxiation, whereas lack of recognition or incorrect management may result in life-threatening or disabling airway stricture. Penetrating injuries can occur with any laceration to the neck or from projectile injuries to the neck or chest. Blunt injuries can occur from a variety of direct and indirect trauma. Laryngotracheal injuries are sometimes classified together, but in this discussion they are separated from laryngeal trauma, including laryngotracheal separation, which is discussed in Chapter 66. In this chapter, we concentrate on injuries that occur between the cricoid cartilage and the right and left mainstem bronchial bifurcations. More distal injuries are covered in Chapters 68 and 70.

HISTORICAL NOTE

Paré provided the first known attempts of primary suture repair of two penetrating tracheal injuries, which he encountered while he was a young surgeon in the French army in the mid 1500s. Unfortunately, neither of these patients survived (Hamby, 1960). Blunt traumatic bronchial rupture was described by Webb in 1848, occurring in a pedestrian who was run over by a horse-drawn wagon (Webb, 1848). The first description of a surviving blunt tracheobronchial injury may be from an 1871 article by Winslow:

> The cook was preparing two of them (canvas back ducks) for baking, when she noticed something abnormal in one of them, and called my attention to it. Upon examination, it was evident that at some previous remote period the left bronchus of the duck had been ruptured upon the outer side, where it joined the trachea at the bifurcation . . . yet, in this wild bird, life and health had apparently existed with the injury for many months, and repair had made good progress until interrupted by the sportsman.

In 1927, Krinitzki provided the first report of a patient surviving a blunt bronchial disruption when he described the autopsy of a 31-year-old woman with an occluded right mainstem bronchus from a traumatic stricture due to trauma 20 years earlier (Krinitzki, 1927).

Surgical management of tracheobronchial injuries necessitated the development of endotracheal anesthesia and the techniques for pulmonary resection; therefore, the successful management of acute airway injuries is a development that is concurrent with the advent of elective airway surgery developed in the last 4 to 5 decades (Grillo, 1989). Successful repair of a penetrating bronchial injury was not reported until 1945 (Sanger, 1945), and 2 years later Kinsella and Johnsrud (1947) performed the first successful repair of a bronchial injury from blunt trauma. Late repair of a traumatic stricture was initially performed by Griffith (1949), who excised the stricture, performed a primary end-to-end anastomosis, and preserved distal pulmonary function.

ANATOMY

The trachea is a cervical and mediastinal structure that spans the inferior border of the cricoid cartilage to its bifurcation at the carina. The cervical portion of the trachea spans all of zone 1 in the neck and lies posterior to the strap muscles and thyroid gland and anterior to the esophagus and vertebral bodies. Lateral to the cervical trachea are the jugular veins, the common carotid arteries, and the vagus nerves, whereas the recurrent laryngeal nerves are closely applied to the trachea in the tracheoesophageal groove. As the trachea descends into the mediastinum through the thoracic inlet, it lies posterior to both the innominate vein and the innominate artery. Further distally, the trachea passes underneath the aortic arch and posterior and to the left of the superior vena cava. The left recurrent laryngeal nerve runs in the left tracheoesophageal groove for nearly the full length of the cervical and thoracic trachea after passing underneath the aortic arch and around the ligamentum arteriosum. The right recurrent nerve is only closely applied to the trachea in its cervical portion. The carina is located at the level of the sternal angle anteriorly and the T4-T5 intervertebral disk posteriorly and lies directly behind the posterior pericardium, the ascending aorta, and the proximal portion of the aortic arch.

The left mainstem bronchus measures 3 to 4 cm in length and passes posterior to the posterior pericardium, the aortic arch, and the left atrium and anterior to the esophagus and the proximal descending thoracic aorta. It then passes through the pleural reflection, changing from a mediastinal structure to an intrathoracic structure before bifurcating into the upper and lower lobar bronchi. The right mainstem bronchus measures 1.5 to 2 cm in length and passes medial to the azygous vein and posterior to the azygocaval junction. The right mainstem bronchus lies posterior to the right pulmonary artery as it exits the mediastinum through the pleural reflection into the right hemithorax.

On average, approximately 50% of the trachea lies within the neck and 50% within the chest. However, this can be markedly influenced by body habitus and neck position. Only 1 to 3 cm of the trachea may lie above the sternal notch in a kyphotic elderly person with a short neck. However, 7 cm or more of the trachea may lie above the sternal notch in a person with a long neck and with marked neck extension. This latter point must be kept in mind, particularly in the presence of penetrating or blunt injuries during neck hyperextension, which may result in an airway injury in an unexpectedly distal location.

The anatomic relations of the trachea within the neck and chest are fundamental in evaluating the risk of airway involvement by mechanism and location of injury, as well as in aiding in the consideration and assessment of associated injuries. These anatomic details are also critical to the appropriate choice of surgical incision and exposure for treatment of airway and associated injuries. These decisions may be particularly complex with intrathoracic tracheal or carinal injuries in which optimal airway exposure would be gained through a right posterolateral approach whereas known or suspected associated injuries may dictate an anterior approach. An intimate understanding of the relational anatomy allows a diversity of approaches to complex intrathoracic trauma that involves the airway.

INCIDENCE

The true incidence of tracheal and bronchial rupture is difficult to establish. It is estimated that only 0.5% of all patients with multiple injuries managed in modern trauma centers suffer from tracheobronchial injury (Fitz-Hugh and Powell, 1970; Gussack et al, 1986). This estimate is crude, however, because virtually all studies of airway trauma combine penetrating and blunt causes and do not publish a denominator of cervical and thoracic injuries with which to calculate the true incidence of airway involvement. It is therefore even more difficult to establish the incidence of tracheobronchial injury as a percentage of traumatic injuries overall.

Penetrating neck injuries have a 3% to 6% incidence of cervical tracheal injury (Flynn et al, 1989; Lee, 1997). Less than 1% (4/666) of patients admitted with penetrating chest trauma had tracheal injury in a series published from the Ben Taub Hospital in Houston (Graham, 1979). Because major urban trauma centers report three to four cases of penetrating tracheal trauma per year (Flynn and Thomas, 1989; Grover et al, 1979; Symbas et al, 1976, 1982), it appears that the incidence of penetrating tracheobronchial trauma constitutes 1% to 2% of thoracic trauma admissions (Lee, 1997).

A frequently quoted series by Bertelsen and Howitz (1972) provides the best information regarding tracheobronchial injuries in blunt trauma. The authors reviewed 1178 autopsy reports of patients dying of blunt trauma and found an incidence of tracheobronchial injury of 2.8%, with over 80% of these patients dying instantly of airway or associated injuries and the rest dying within 2 hours of reaching the hospital. Kemmerer and associates (1961) reported an incidence of tracheobronchial rupture of under 1% in a study of nearly 600 traffic fatalities. A review of blunt cervical trauma revealed tracheal injury in 1.6% (Shelly et al, 1974). Symbas and colleagues (1992) reviewed 20 years of English language literature, spanning from 1970 to 1990, that reported airway injury secondary to blunt trauma. In this time frame, 47 articles described 183 patients, with 6 patients added in the 20-year period from the Grady Memorial Hospital experience in Atlanta. Unfortunately, these data do not provide a meaningful denominator on which to calculate the incidence of airway injury in blunt chest trauma.

There is an apparent increase in the incidence of patients with airway injuries reaching the emergency department alive, which may occur as a result of improved prehospital care and development of specialized regional trauma units (Chagnon and Mulder, 1996). However, this is difficult to establish, given the inherent inaccuracies in the historical and current data regarding airway injuries. De La Rocha and Kayler (1985) reported an incidence of tracheobronchial injuries of 1.8% in 327 patients who were discharged from a centralized trauma unit, whereas another series reported an incidence of 0.5% in a series of 2000 patients requiring an intensive care unit admission for multiple trauma (Angood et al, 1986).

The best consolidation of these data shows an incidence of tracheobronchial injury occurring in 0.5% to 2% of individuals sustaining blunt trauma, including blunt trauma to the neck. More than 80% of tracheobronchial injuries from blunt trauma are located within 2.5 cm of the carina (Lynn and Iyengar, 1972). Most injuries related to blunt trauma involve the intrathoracic trachea and mainstem bronchi, with only 4% of these injuries reported in the cervical trachea (Symbas et al, 1992). In this review, 22% of the blunt airway injuries involved the distal thoracic trachea; 27%, the right mainstem bronchus; and 17%, the left proximal mainstem bronchus. Eight percent were complex injuries involving the trachea and mainstem bronchi, and 16% involved the lobar orifices (Symbas et al, 1992). The rate of tracheobronchial injury from penetrating thoracic trauma is also 0.5% to 2%, but, in contrast, penetrating cervical injuries involve the airway 3% to 8% of the time. Penetrating injuries predominantly involve the cervical trachea, with only 25% of the penetrating injuries involving the intrathoracic airways (Lee, 1997).

MECHANISM OF INJURY

Most tracheobronchial injuries result from blunt or penetrating trauma, although iatrogenic injuries and less common causes such as strangulation, burns, or caustic injury occasionally result in airway injury. Most penetrating trauma is due to stab wounds or gunshot wounds and only uncommonly may occur from impalement or slash injuries. Nearly all stab injuries of the trachea are cervical in origin, owing to the deep location of the intrathoracic trachea. Knife injuries produce a tearing or shearing effect, resulting in perforation, linear laceration, through and through injuries, or transsection (Lee, 1997).

Gunshot wounds are a more common cause of penetrating airway injury and can affect any portion of the cervical or intrathoracic airways. However, cervical injuries are still more common, being the site of injury in 75% to 80% of penetrating tracheal trauma overall (Lee 1997; Mulder and Ratnani, 1995). This may be, in part, because more distal penetrating injuries of the trachea may have associated fatal injuries of the heart or great vessels, and such patients never arrive at the trauma center for evaluation and management. Knowledge of the missile trajectory based on history and the entrance and exit wounds is very helpful in predicting the path of the bullet and subsequent structures at risk for injury. However, this can be unpredictable, with bullet paths frequently altered by impact with bone or other dense tissue. Therefore, a high index of suspicion for airway injury must be maintained in all cervical and upper thoracic gunshot wounds. Gunshot wounds produce a crush injury and wound cavity that varies depending on the muzzle velocity, the caliber, and the type of ammunition, with the greatest damage being produced by high-velocity rifles firing hollow-point ammunition. These injuries produce much greater cavitation and soft tissue destruction than do relatively low-velocity injuries from handguns.

Blunt injuries of the cervical trachea most commonly result from direct trauma or from sudden hyperextension. Direct cervical trauma produces a crush injury of the trachea, because it may be impinged on by the rigid vertebral bodies. This has classically been described as a "dashboard" injury because unrestrained automobile passengers may hyperextend the neck during head-on collisions, striking the neck on the steering wheel or dashboard and producing a crush injury of the larynx or cervical trachea (Lupetin, 1997). However, even the restrained passenger may incur a laryngeal or cervical tracheal injury when a high-riding shoulder harness applies a compressive and rotational force to the neck on front-impact automobile injuries (Guertler, 1988; Huelke, 1989) Clothesline injuries may produce similar direct crushing trauma but with the force concentrated across a very narrow band. Other injuries may occur with rapid hyperextension, producing a traction and distraction injury that most commonly results in laryngotracheal separation. This is discussed more thoroughly in Chapter 66. Hyperextension injuries most commonly occur in automobile accidents but can occur in any other situations in which forced rapid cervical hyperextension occurs.

The exact mechanism of intrathoracic tracheobronchial disruption from blunt trauma is unknown but, as discussed, 80% of these injuries occur within 2.5 cm of the carina (Lynn, 1972). Kirsch and associates (1976) proposed three potential mechanisms for the cause of blunt intrathoracic tracheobronchial injuries. First, they noted that sudden, forceful anteroposterior compression of the thoracic cage is the most common type of injury associated with tracheobronchial disruption. They postulated that this produces a decrease in the anteroposterior diameter with subsequent widening of the transverse diameter. Because the lung remains in contact with the chest wall because of negative intrapleural pressure, lateral motion pulls the two lungs apart, producing traction on the trachea at the carina. Airway disruption occurs if this lateral force exceeds tracheobronchial elasticity. A second mechanism may be due to airway rupture as a consequence of high airway pressures. Compression of the lung, trachea, and major bronchi between the sternum and vertebral column during blunt trauma produces a sudden increase in intratracheal airway pressure; and in a patient with a closed glottis at the moment of impact, rupture can occur when the intraluminal pressure exceeds the elasticity of the membranous trachea and bronchi. Rupture in these circumstances occurs most commonly at the junction of the membranous and cartilaginous airway or between cartilaginous rings. The third potential mechanism may be due to a rapid deceleration injury, producing shear forces at points of relative airway fixation such as the cricoid cartilage and the carina, similar to the mechanism of traumatic injuries of the thoracic aorta.

ASSOCIATED INJURIES

Because of the adjacent cervical and intrathoracic structures, penetrating airway trauma frequently is associated with other major injuries. Cervical trauma of the airway frequently involves the esophagus, the recurrent laryngeal nerves, the cervical spine and spinal cord, the larynx, and the carotid arteries and jugular veins. Intrathoracic penetrating trauma may involve the esophagus, left recurrent laryngeal nerve, and spinal cord, but it can also involve any of the great vessels, including the ascending arch and descending aorta and the pulmonary arteries, and may involve any of the four heart chambers or the lung parenchyma. Obviously, concomitant great vessel and cardiac injury from penetrating trauma is frequently fatal and may lead to exsanguination or asphyxiation on blood in the airway before presentation in a trauma unit. These associated injuries are common and frequently determine the ultimate outcome in terms of the patient's survival and morbidity (Symbas et al, 1992).

In a series of 100 penetrating tracheobronchial injuries reported by Kelly and colleagues (1985) in patients with a primary airway injury in the cervical trachea, 28% of the patients had an associated esophageal injury, 24% had a hemopneumothorax, 13% had a major vascular injury, 8% had a recurrent laryngeal nerve injury, and 3% had a spinal cord injury. In contrast, primary injuries of the intrathoracic trachea were associated with an incidence of esophageal injury of 11%; hemopneumothorax, 32%; a major vascular injury, 18%; cardiac injury, 5%; spinal cord injury, 7%; and intra-abdominal injuries, 18% (Kelly et al, 1985). Several other series have shown an overall incidence of associated major injuries with penetrating tracheobronchial trauma to be in the range of 50% to 80%, most of these being esophageal and vascular injuries, followed by spinal cord, pulmonary, and intra-abdominal injuries (Flynn and Thomas, 1989; Grover et al, 1979; Rossbach et al, 1998; Symbas et al, 1976, 1982).

Because of the magnitude of blunt trauma necessary to produce an airway injury, associated injuries are also common in this group and may be the primary determinant in patient outcome. Any other structure or organ system may be involved as in any multiple trauma patient. Head, facial, and cervical spine injuries are frequent and important predictors of mortality and morbidity.

Blunt intra-abdominal, intrathoracic, and skeletal trauma also occur frequently, as well as specific injuries to the esophagus and great vessels that are adjacent to the major airways. Major associated injuries are present in 40% to 100% of patients suffering blunt airway trauma and are dominated by orthopedic injuries in most patients, with a third to half of the patients having concomitant facial trauma, pulmonary contusions, or intra-abdominal injuries. Ten percent to 20% of the patients have major closed-head injuries, and approximately 10% have associated spinal cord injuries (Ramzy et al, 1988; Reece and Shatney, 1988; Rossbach, 1998). In one series, a very high incidence was reported of recurrent nerve injury associated with blunt airway trauma as evidenced by vocal cord dysfunction without evidence of direct laryngeal injury (Reece, 1988). In this series, 49% of patients had recurrent nerve injuries and two thirds of these had bilateral recurrent nerve palsy. In this same series, a 21% incidence of esophageal perforation was reported, clearly suggesting the need for high index of suspicion for associated esophageal injuries, even in the setting of blunt trauma. A high percentage of cervical crush injuries producing tracheal disruption may have associated laryngeal injuries that require careful assessment by an otolaryngologist during the primary assessment phase and before treatment decisions are made regarding repair of the tracheal injury.

Associated injuries are extremely common with both blunt and penetrating trauma of the airway and may be the major determinants of both short-term mortality and long-term morbidity. Knowledge of the relational anatomy, mechanism of injury, and incidence of related injuries helps define a prompt but thorough algorithm for diagnosing or excluding important injuries that require immediate or urgent management. Consideration of the known or potentially associated injuries becomes a critical factor in later choices of the surgical approach for addressing the airway injury.

DIAGNOSIS

Accurate diagnosis of tracheobronchial injury requires an understanding of the mechanism of injury and a high index of suspicion when these mechanisms or common associated injuries are present. The initial assessment of the patient with potential airway trauma involves the traditional ABCs of resuscitation outlined by the American College of Surgeons in the Advanced Trauma Life Support (ATLS) guidelines (Committee on Trauma, 1989). Airway injuries become the first priority in trauma, and because of their acuity and critical importance in stabilizing the patient, initial steps in management may precede simultaneously with the diagnosis of airway pathology and associated injuries. Dyspnea and respiratory distress are frequent symptoms, occurring in 76% to 100% of patients (Kelly et al, 1985; Reece and Shatney, 1988; Rossbach et al, 1998). The other common symptom is hoarseness or dysphonia, which occurred in 46% of the patients in a series published by Reece and Shatney (1988).

The most common signs of airway injury reported in most series were subcutaneous emphysema (35%–85%), pneumothorax (20%–50%), and hemoptysis (14%–25%) (Baumgartner et al, 1990; Flynn et al, 1989; Kelly et al, 1985; Reece and Shatney, 1988; Rossbach et al, 1998). Air escaping from a penetrating wound in the neck is a pathognomonic sign of airway laceration and occurs in approximately 60% of patients with cervical penetrating trauma to the trachea (Symbas et al, 1982).

The most useful initial diagnostic studies are those obtained routinely in the initial trauma survey (i.e., chest and cervical spine radiographs). Deep cervical emphysema and pneumomediastinum will be seen in 60% and pneumothorax occurs in 70% of patients with tracheobronchial injuries (Flynn, 1989; Stark, 1995). The cervical spine or chest radiograph may also show a disruption of the tracheal or bronchial air column on careful examination. Overdistention of the endotracheal tube balloon cuff or displacement of the endotracheal tube may give additional radiologic signs of airway injury (Stark, 1995). Complete transsection of a mainstem bronchus may result in the classic signs of atelectasis, "absent hilum," or a collapsing of the lung away from the hilus toward the diaphragm, known as the "falling lung sign of Kumpe" (Endress et al, 1991; Kumpe et al, 1970; Stark, 1995). A persistent pneumothorax with large air leak from a well-placed chest tube should increase the suspicion of intrathoracic tracheal or bronchial injury. With the chest tube on suction, the patient may experience more respiratory difficulties, and this finding is almost invariably associated with bronchial disruption (Deslauriers et al, 1982).

Although neck and upper chest computed tomography (CT) scan has become critical to the accurate diagnosis of traumatic laryngeal injuries (Lupetin, 1997), the role in more distal tracheobronchial injuries is not well established. Commonly, a chest CT may be obtained as a part of the trauma workup and is extremely valuable in detecting the presence of a mediastinal hematoma or the possibility of associated injuries of the great vessels. The CT scan may show mediastinal air, disruption of the tracheobronchial air column, deviation of the airway, or the specific site of airway disruption. Although not specifically indicated for the workup of suggested acute tracheobronchial trauma, preoperative CT can be useful in assessing associated laryngeal injuries or other unsuspected chest injuries that should be dealt with at the time of surgical exploration. CT is contraindicated in the hemodynamically unstable trauma patient or the patient with an unstable airway. A negative CT scan does not obviate the need for bronchoscopy or other diagnostic studies.

Other imaging of suspected associated injuries is performed as indicated. Because of the common association of esophageal injuries, particularly after penetrating trauma, a contrast esophagogram is often necessary. Esophageal injuries may be distant from the airway injuries because of the distortion of tissues on traumatic impact (Minard et al, 1992). Angiography of the aortic arch or cervical vessels is performed for penetrating injuries in a stable patient or in a blunt chest trauma patient when the chest radiograph or CT raises the suspicion for great vessel injury.

If the initial diagnosis of airway injury is missed, granulation tissue and stricture of the trachea or bronchus will develop within the first 1 to 4 weeks and will usually lead to symptoms, signs, and radiologic findings of pneumonia, bronchiectasis, atelectasis, and abscess. Stridor and dyspnea are the common signs of late tracheal stenosis, whereas wheezing and postobstructive pneumonia are the common presentations of bronchial stenosis. Chest radiography and CT have been useful in the delayed setting and may directly reveal the site of stenosis and the secondary consequences of airway narrowing.

Bronchoscopy provides the single definitive diagnostic study in a patient with suspected airway injury. Direct or fiberoptic laryngoscopy is an important part of the endoscopic study in patients with cervical trauma and should be performed with the assistance of an experienced otolaryngologist when laryngeal injuries are suggested. Careful examination of the tracheobronchial tree with the fiberoptic bronchoscope will allow determination of the site and extent of injury. Bronchoscopy is the only study that can reliably exclude central airway trauma, although minor lacerations may occasionally be missed. The advantages of fiberoptic bronchoscopy are that it can be performed quickly and easily, even in the setting of concomitant head and neck injuries or cervical spine trauma. If bronchoscopy is being performed for a suspected airway injury in an intubated patient, it is important to carefully withdraw the endotracheal tube during endoscopy to avoid missing proximal tracheal injuries.

Bronchoscopy may also prove critical to the initial management of the patient with an injured airway. The flexible bronchoscope can be used as a guide to help intubate across a lacerated or transsected trachea or to intubate selectively into a mainstem bronchus (Fig. 67–1). With this in mind, many major trauma units have now made the presence of a fiberoptic bronchoscope an integral part of their trauma suite equipment to help provide assistance for the establishment of an airway and quick evaluation of potential airway injuries (Mulder and Ratnani, 1995). Rigid bronchoscopy is rarely needed and, in fact, has the potential of exacerbating or extending the airway injury and is contraindicated in cervical spine trauma. However, skilled intubation with a ventilating bronchoscope may be lifesaving in cases in which tracheal transsection and displacement does not allow identification or intubation of the distal segment with the fiberoptic bronchoscope (Barmada and Gibbons, 1994). In these cases, the rigid bronchoscope may help realign the displaced airway and allow establishment of emergency ventilation before subsequent surgical repair (Fig. 67–2). In most such cases, proceeding directly to open surgical control of the airway is most expedient and appropriate, as discussed later.

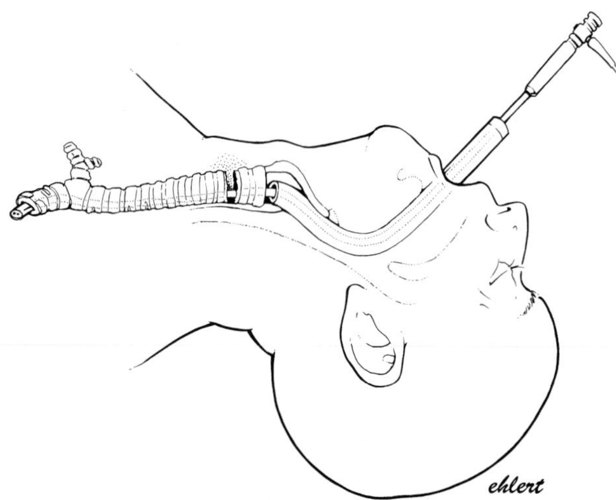

FIGURE 67–1 ■ The flexible bronchoscope can be used as a guide and obturator for passing an endotracheal tube distal to the area of injury.

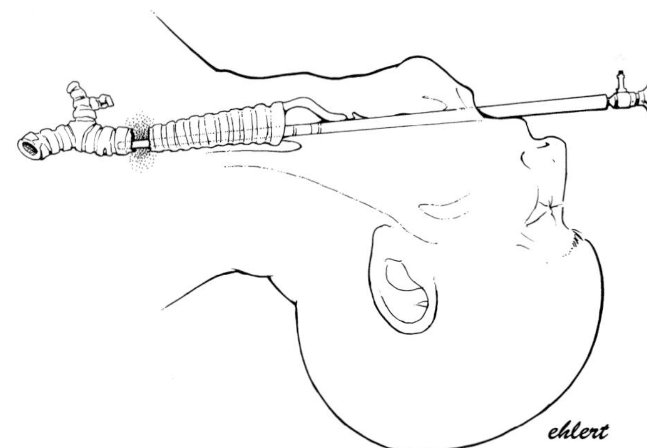

FIGURE 67–2 ■ The rigid bronchoscope may provide airway control and ventilation.

MANAGEMENT

Airway Management

The initial and most important priority in acute tracheobronchial injury is to secure a satisfactory airway. Patients with respiratory distress and the clinical suspicion of an airway injury should be intubated immediately, preferably with the guidance of a flexible bronchoscope, as described earlier (see Fig. 67–1). Fiberoptic intubation provides several advantages. First, it does not require neck extension for direct laryngoscopy and so can be performed while stabilization of the cervical spine is maintained before the exclusion of cervical spine injuries. Second, fiberoptic intubation can easily be performed in the awake, spontaneously ventilating patient. This prevents the need for sedation and paralysis, which is contraindicated in the patient with an unstable airway, until a satisfactory airway can be established. Sedation and paralysis is also contraindicated during the immediate evaluation and stabilization of an injured patient who requires several simultaneous assessments and hemodynamic stabilization. Third, flexible bronchoscopy can act as an obturator for the endotracheal tube and direct the tube past an area of injury under direct vision, allowing accurate placement into the distal trachea or either mainstem bronchus as necessary. Lastly, immediate bronchoscopy by an experienced endoscopist allows early evaluation of the location and extent of airway injury. This provides the best early information about the indications and approach for airway repair, allowing this to be calculated into the priority list of possible interventions for the multiply injured patient.

In published reports, the incidence of upper airway

obstruction or severe distress that requires immediate intubation is variable and dependent on the degree of injuries and the criteria used. Flynn and associates (1989) reported 8 of 22 patients (36%) requiring an immediate airway and 3 of these patients requiring an emergency tracheostomy or cricothyroidotomy. A series by Gussack and colleagues (1986) revealed 92% of patients requiring an emergency airway, 73% of these being successfully managed by orotracheal intubation and 3 emergently intubated through an open neck wound. Edwards and associates (1987) and Rossbach and Johnson (1998) reported that approximately 60% of their patients required prompt control of the airway. In Rossbach and Johnson's series, 74% of the patients requiring emergency intubation were successfully managed by orotracheal intubation alone, whereas 10% required intubation with fiberoptic guidance, 10% were intubated through an open neck wound, and only one patient (5%) required an emergent surgical airway through tracheostomy or cricothyroidotomy. In the series reported by Edwards and coworkers (1987), approximately 60% of the emergency airways were managed by nasotracheal or orotracheal intubation, and the other 40% required tracheostomy. Important points are raised concerning the three patients in this series who were initially stable but experienced sudden deterioration secondary to the airway injury while they were being evaluated for multiple injuries. Two patients with a transsected cervical trachea required emergency tracheostomy with intubation of the distal tracheal segment through the tracheostomy incision. In one patient, an attempted emergency cricothyroidotomy produced a significant laryngeal injury that necessitated subsequent delayed repair (Edwards et al, 1987). A high index of suspicion and prompt securing of the injured airway are paramount to both the initial resuscitation and the ultimate outcome.

Patients with air emanating from a penetrating cervical injury may be intubated through the neck injury directly into the tracheal lumen. This technique has been utilized in approximately 25% of airway trauma in reports that include penetrating cervical injuries (Edwards et al, 1987; Flynn et al, 1989; Gussack et al, 1986; Rossbach et al, 1998). However, attempts at oral intubation or blind intubation through a cervical wound may be futile and can either precipitate total obstruction or allow the progressive loss of an unstable airway if repeated attempts are unsuccessful. Although intubation guided by a flexible bronchoscope may solve most of these difficulties, delay in obtaining a bronchoscope or successfully traversing the injury may also cause complete obstruction, with the tragic loss of a salvageable patient. In cases in which airway injury is suspected, preparation for immediate tracheostomy must be made simultaneously with the attempts at intubation. In cases of severe maxillofacial trauma, immediate tracheostomy is the procedure of choice for airway control. Cricothyroidotomy is rarely useful in tracheobronchial trauma because the injury lies distal to the insertion point of the tracheostomy tube, which is placed blindly and with no additional accuracy over oral or nasotracheal intubation alone. If a tracheostomy is performed, the tracheostomy tube should be placed through the area of injury if possible to prevent extension of the tracheal injury by the tracheal stoma. A transsected cervical trachea may retract into the mediastinum; in these cases it is best found by inserting a finger into the mediastinum anterior to the esophagus, locating the distal trachea by palpation, and grasping the clamp to allow retraction into the cervical wound and distal intubation (Mathisen and Grillo, 1987).

Management of the airway for injuries of the distal trachea, the carina, and the proximal mainstem bronchi can be extremely challenging. Use of double-lumen tubes should be avoided because of their rigidity and size, which increases the possibility of injury extension. In these cases, a long endotracheal tube should be positioned beyond the injury or into the appropriate mainstem bronchus to provide single-lung ventilation. This can best be performed with the aid of the flexible bronchoscope serving as a guide and to confirm the final position. In almost all cases, standard ventilation can be initiated once distal airway control is ensured. In cases of distal injuries of the left mainstem bronchus, the bronchus intermedius, or lobar orifices, a bronchial blocker placed proximal to the injury under endoscopic guidance provides another alternative for stabilizing the airway and allowing ventilation.

Stabilization and Prioritization of Associated Injuries

Establishment of a stable airway and assurance of ventilation are the first two priorities as outlined in the ATLS guidelines of the American College of Surgeons (Committee on Trauma, 1989). Once the airway is secured, the priority shifts to circulation, with the recognition, stabilization, and resuscitation of cardiovascular injuries. Neurologic, intrathoracic and intra-abdominal, vascular, and orthopedic injuries are identified during the primary and secondary trauma surveys. A patient with multiple injuries frequently has several, simultaneous, competing priorities for the sequencing of and approach to operative procedures. Fortunately, intubation distal to the injury or into the unaffected proximal mainstem bronchus usually allows adequate oxygenation and ventilation for emergency management of associated life-threatening injuries. The sequence of operative procedures must be individualized, but establishment of effective ventilation allows the initial priority to be given to the management of life- or organ-threatening injuries. Subdural hematomas, intra-abdominal bleeding, or major cardiovascular injuries should usually be repaired before definitive repair of the tracheobronchial injury.

Anesthetic Management

Close cooperation between the anesthesiologist and surgeon is critical to the successful management of a tracheobronchial injury. In cases in which the airway has not already been established, the anesthesiologist may provide invaluable assistance in airway control and selective intubation. The choice and timing of anesthetic agents and muscle relaxants, the type of endotracheal tubes used, and the mode of intraoperative ventilation require close communication between the anesthesiologist and surgeon for planning of an efficient and effective operative strategy. If a bronchoscopy has not already been performed, it is necessary at the initiation of the procedure to define the location and extent of injury and to guide the surgeon regarding the operative approach and intended repair. This is best performed with a standard diagnostic bronchoscope through a large single-lumen endotracheal tube. In cases of mainstem bronchial or lobar injuries, a contralateral double-lumen endotracheal tube is preferred for the ease of isolated single-lung ventilation. However, in all other injuries involving the trachea or carina, a long, single-lumen tube can traverse and be seated distal to the injury and is preferred because it is less bulky and easier to guide past the torn airway without injury extension.

High-frequency jet ventilation provides an effective option for ventilation with relatively low airway pressures. Its main advantage is during airway reconstruction, because it can be delivered through a small catheter with less bulk and rigidity, allowing easier placement of sutures or approximation of the newly reconstructed airway without tension. However, in most cases, it is usually easiest to perform standard ventilation through the oral endotracheal tube or through a sterile endotracheal tube inserted through the operative field into the transsected airway. This does not require additional equipment or experience and has the added advantage of a cuffed tube preventing aspiration of blood into the distal airway and less aerosolization of blood around the surgical team (Wood et al, [in press]).

Cardiopulmonary bypass is virtually never necessary for the intraoperative management of isolated airway injuries. Associated injuries of the heart or great vessels may require cardiopulmonary bypass (CPB). In cases in which CPB is already being used, it may facilitate a concomitant tracheobronchial repair. However, CPB after major trauma can exacerbate intracerebral or intra-abdominal hemorrhage and potentiate the systemic inflammatory response that produces adult respiratory distress syndrome, with a very high subsequent mortality. In simple injuries, standard ventilation is straightforward, precluding consideration of CPB. In complex injuries, or those in which associated trauma makes ventilation difficult, the anticoagulation and added trauma of CPB probably results in exacerbation of bleeding and the systemic inflammatory response more than it helps in allowing airway repair.

Virtually all patients with isolated tracheobronchial injuries can be easily extubated at the end of the operative procedure and should be managed by the anesthesiologist with this in mind. Patients who require postoperative ventilation because of their associated injuries should finish the procedure with a large-bore, single-lumen endotracheal tube to allow good pulmonary toilet and fiberoptic bronchoscopy if necessary. If possible, this should be placed with the balloon cuff distal to the area of tracheal repair in proximal injuries or should lie proximal and away from the repair for carinal and mainstem bronchial injuries. Major laryngeal or maxillofacial injuries with the anticipated need for prolonged ventilation are indications for placement of a tracheostomy at the completion of the tracheobronchial repair. This tracheostomy should not be placed through the tracheal repair, which will lead to a contamination of the suture line with subsequent dehiscence or stenosis (Mathisen and Grillo, 1991).

Surgical Management

Definitive primary repair of major tracheobronchial injuries is almost always indicated in conjunction with other urgent operative interventions, as discussed earlier. Minor injuries may not be initially apparent or recognized, owing to a lack of clinical suspicion or concealment by prompt distal intubation for stabilization of a patient with multiple injuries. These minor injuries may heal without direct surgical repair with no negative sequelae if they involve less than one third of the circumference of the airway. However, the most reliable short- and long-term result is provided by prompt, definitive repair and should be performed whenever possible when the injury is recognized. In rare circumstances it may be appropriate to perform a delayed repair if it is not possible to perform operative correction because of the instability of the patient with multiple injuries.

Figure 67–3 shows the central airways in relation to

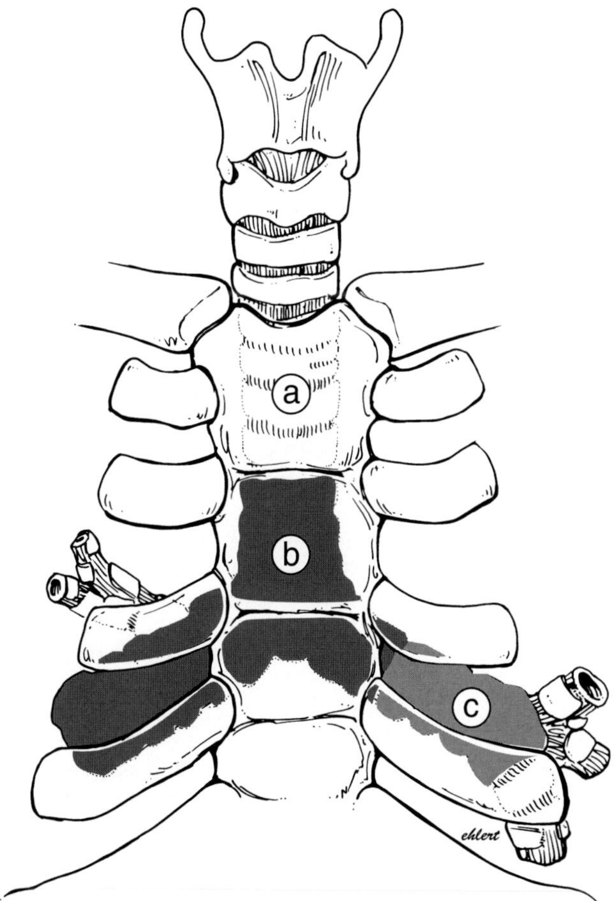

FIGURE 67–3 ■ Comparative surface anatomy and surgical approaches for repairing tracheobronchial injuries. Proximal tracheal injuries (*a*) are best approached via a cervical collar incision. The distal half of the trachea, the right main bronchus, the carina, and the proximal left main bronchus (*b*) are most easily exposed via right posterolateral thoracotomy. Most of the left main bronchus (*c*) may be exposed via a left posterolateral thoracotomy.

the anterior skeletal anatomy of the manubrium and sternum and demonstrates the preferred operative approaches for isolated tracheobronchial injuries. The proximal one half to two thirds of the trachea is best approached through a low cervical collar incision that also provides excellent exposure to vascular or esophageal injuries in the neck (see Fig. 67–3*A*). Creating a "T" incision over the manubrium and splitting the manubrium down to the second interspace opens the thoracic inlet and provides a broader exposure to the middle third of the trachea as well as proximal control of the innominate artery or veins. A full median sternotomy does not provide significant additional airway exposure except in specific circumstances, which are discussed later. The distal third of the trachea, the carina, and the right mainstem bronchus are most easily approached through a right thoracotomy, which also provides good exposure to the azygous vein, superior vena cava, and right atrium, as well as all of the intrathoracic esophagus (Fig. 67–4; see Fig. 67–3*B*). Injuries of the left mainstem bronchus are most easily approached through a left thoracotomy, which also provides good exposure to the distal portion of the aortic arch, the descending thoracic aorta, and the proximal left subclavian artery (see Fig. 67–3*C*). However, exposure to the proximal left mainstem, the carina, the distal trachea, or the right mainstem is extremely difficult through a left thoracotomy, owing to the overlying aortic arch (Fig. 67–5*A*). Adequate proximal exposure may be gained by mobilization of the arch with retraction cephalad and laterally and division of the ligamentum arteriosum (see Fig. 67–5*B*).

These approaches may not be adequate for the management of potential associated injuries. Because of the proximity of the heart and great vessels anterior to the distal trachea, the carina, and the proximal mainstem bronchi, penetrating injuries to the chest are likely to have associated life-threatening cardiovascular injuries (Fig. 67–6). A median sternotomy will often be performed to provide optimal access to the heart or great vessels but provides far less satisfactory exposure to the trachea, carina, and bronchi than did respective thoracotomies as described earlier. However, it is possible to obtain exposure to the anterior airway in the vicinity of the carina to allow anterior repair or limited primary resection and reconstruction. This requires mobilization of the superior vena cava with reflection to the right, retraction of the ascending aorta to the left, and longitudinal division of the posterior pericardium cephalad to the right pulmonary artery and caudal to the innominate vein (Fig. 67–7). Unfortunately, this does not provide any exposure to the posterior airway where blunt injuries frequently occur. It also does not provide adequate exposure for repair of concomitant esophageal injuries. A bilateral thoracosternotomy or "clamshell" incision through the fourth interspace provides good exposure to both hemithoraces and the anterior mediastinum and may be a considered as an approach because of associated injuries. However, this approach provides little additional airway exposure or airway advantages over those incisions previously described.

Simple, clean lacerations without airway devascularization can be repaired primarily with simple interrupted absorbable sutures. We prefer 4-0 Vicryl (Ethicon, Cincinnati, OH), although others have successfully utilized permanent and absorbable monofilament. In cases in which there is significant tracheobronchial damage, all devitalized tissue should be débrided, with care taken to preserve as much viable airway as possible. In these cases, a circumferential resection and end-to-end anastomosis is almost always preferable to partial wedge resections of traumatized airway with attempted primary repair. The principles of airway resection and reconstruction are similar for tracheal, carinal, or bronchial injuries, although the anatomy of reconstruction is unique to the surgical exposure, the location, and the extent of resection. This is particularly true when a portion of the carina must be resected or reconstructed, because a large variety of techniques may be necessary to achieve reconstruction in this area (Mitchell et al, 1999). Dissection of the airway is limited to the region to be resected to preserve tracheobronchial blood supply to the area of anastomosis. Precise placement of interrupted absorbable suture allows an

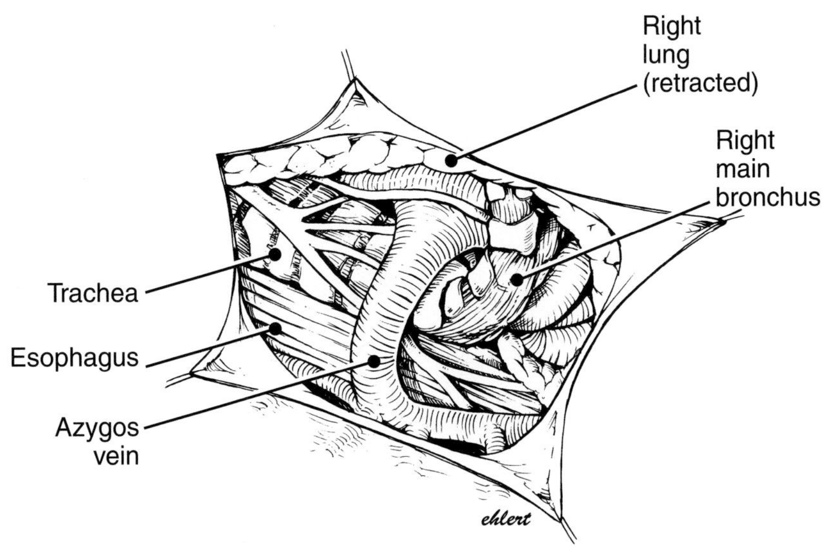

FIGURE 67–4 ■ The exposure of the trachea and right mainstem bronchus from right posterolateral thoracotomy (via either the fourth interspace or via the bed of the resected fifth rib). The lung is retracted anteriorly.

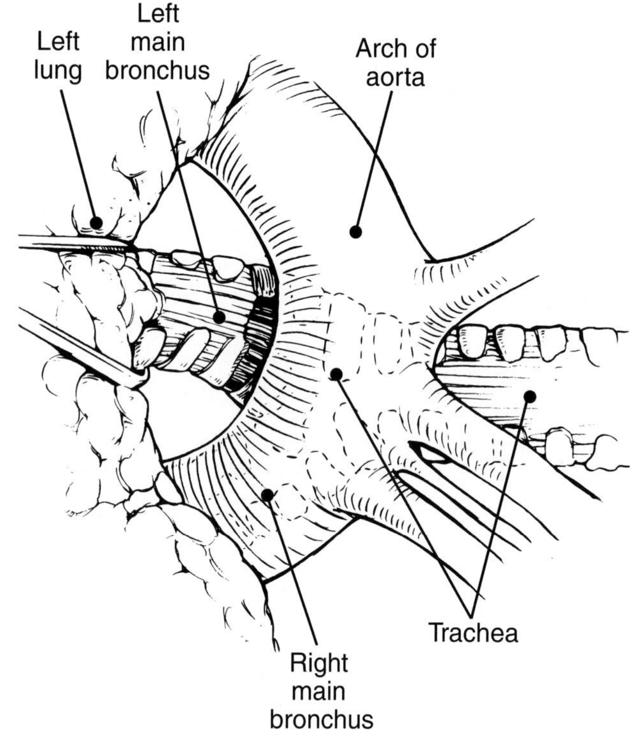

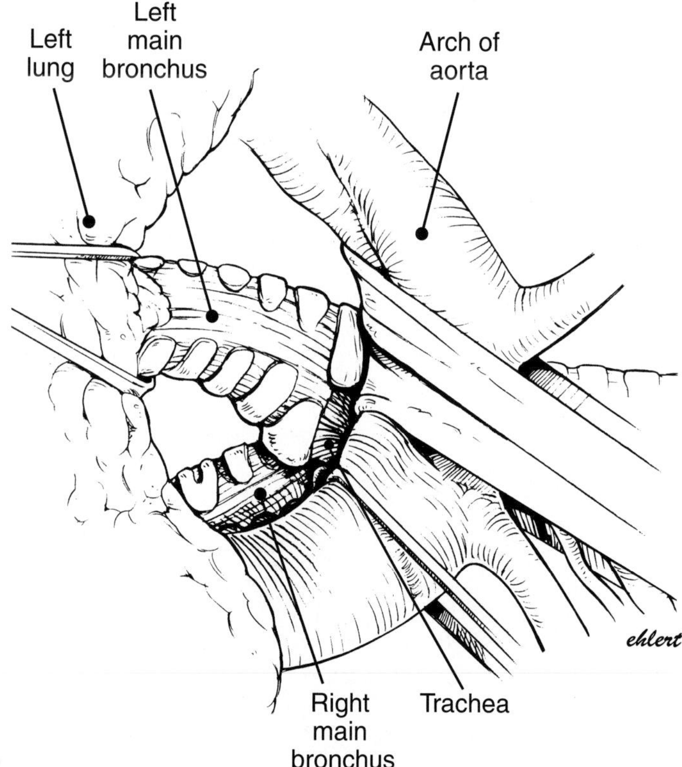

FIGURE 67–5 ■ A view of the left mainstem bronchus via the left posterolateral thoracotomy. The aortic arch overlies the proximal mainstem (*A*) and must be extensively mobilized to gain adequate proximal exposure (*B*).

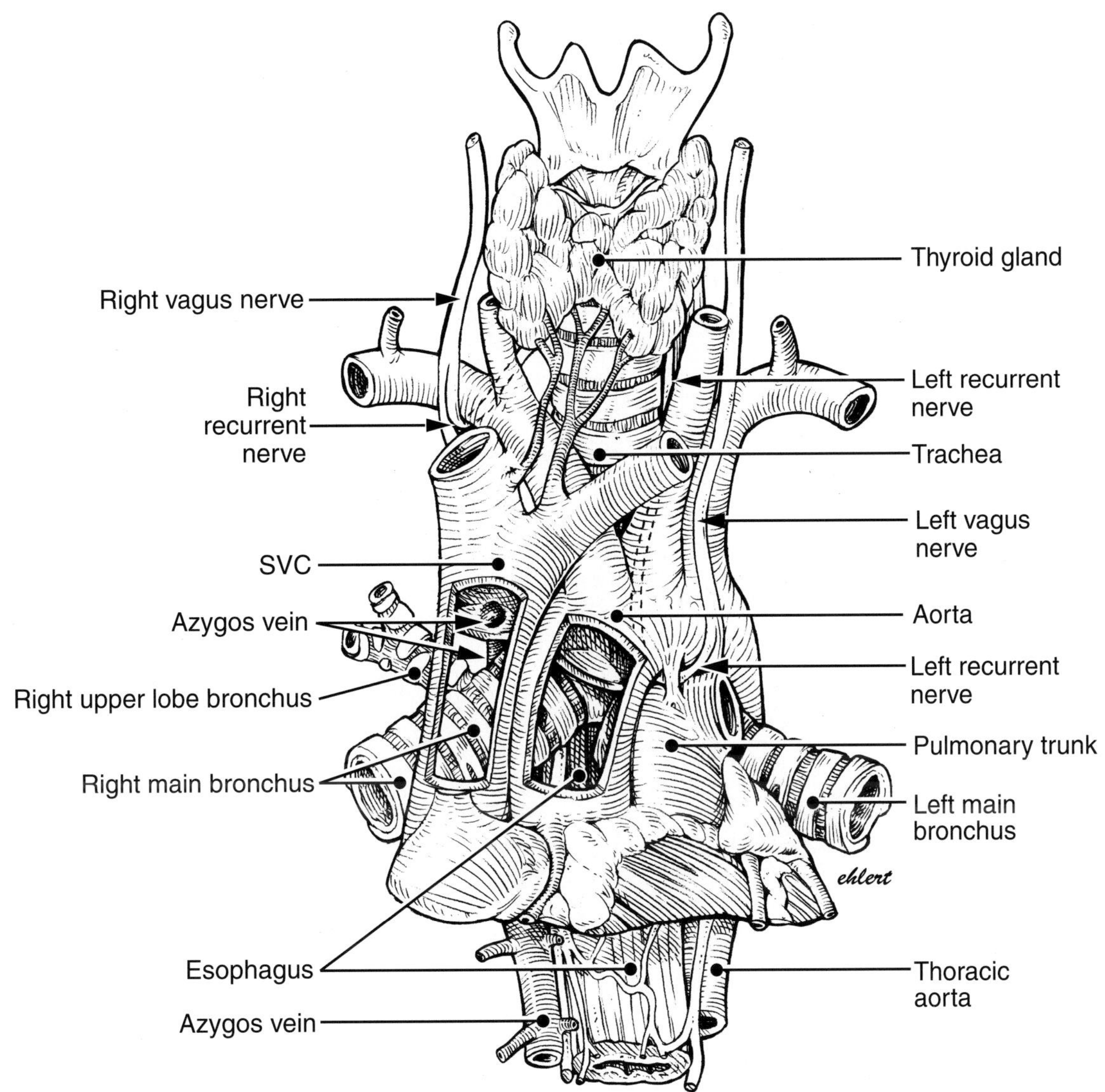

FIGURE 67–6 ■ Major structures close to the tracheobronchial tree that are at risk for simultaneous injury. SVC, superior vena cava.

airtight anastomosis, correction of size discrepancy between the distal and proximal airway, and minimal anastomotic granulations if the anastomosis is brought together without tension. These techniques of tracheobronchial reconstruction have been well described and have been fairly consistently utilized in most thoracic surgical groups who perform airway reconstruction (Grillo, 1987).

In most patients, up to half of the trachea can be resected and primarily reconstructed and so that the most significant tracheal injuries should be able to allow primary resection and reconstruction without difficulty. Both mainstem bronchi can be completely resected with primary reconstruction without tension in all cases. Extensive injuries of the carina are more problematic and should be repaired rather than resected if at all possible. Only 3 to 4 cm of airway involving the carina can be resected and allow for primary reconstruction. A variety of tracheobronchial release maneuvers have been used to allow a tension-free anastomosis. For most limited tracheal resections, blunt development of the anterior avascular pretracheal plane combined with neck flexion is all that is necessary. For more extensive proximal tracheal resections, a suprahyoid laryngeal release can provide 1 to 2 cm of additional proximal mobilization. For resections of the mainstem bronchi or carina, division of the pericardium around the inferior aspect of the hilum provides an additional 1 to 2 cm of distal airway mobilization (Heitmiller, 1996).

Associated injuries of the esophagus should be repaired in two layers. When working through an anterior cervical exposure, the esophagus may be best exposed by complete tracheal transsection through the area of planned tracheal repair. A vascularized flap of muscle or soft tissue should be interposed between the tracheal and esophageal repairs to minimize the risk of postoperative tracheoesophageal fistula. Intrathoracic tracheobronchial suture lines are also preferably wrapped with pedicled

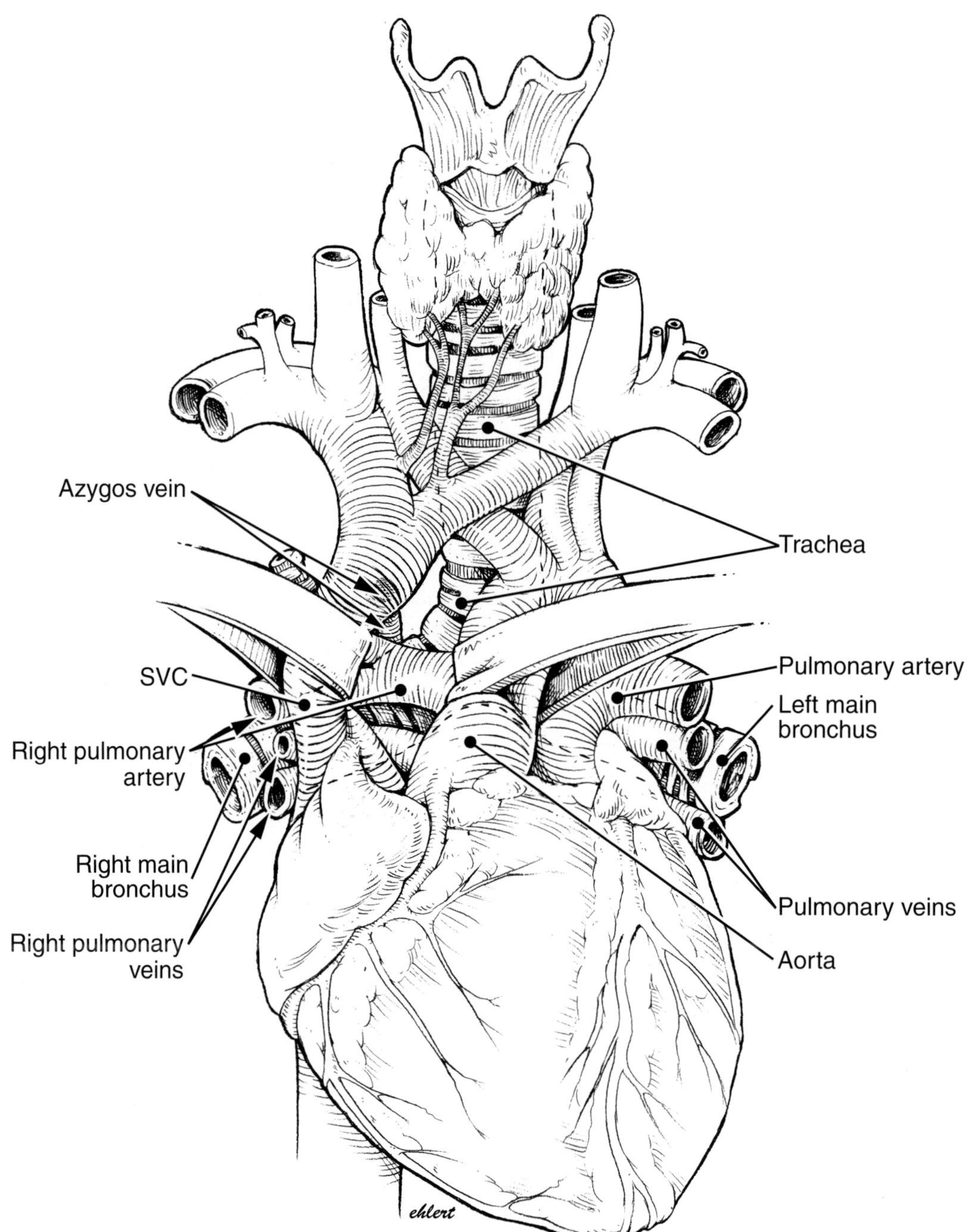

FIGURE 67–7 ■ Transpericardial exposure of the carina. The superior vena cava is retracted to the right, the ascending aorta is retracted to the left, and the pericardium is incised cephalad to the right pulmonary artery. SVC, superior vena cava.

pericardial fat, intercostal muscle, or pleura to separate the airway anastomosis from overlying blood vessels. In cases in which a portion of the trachea or carina has been resected and reconstructed, much of the airway mobility is provided by neck flexion. This position is maintained in the postoperative period by placement of a "guardian suture" between the chin and the sternum (Wood et al, 1999). As discussed earlier, patients with isolated airway injuries are routinely extubated in the operating room, even after complex reconstructions.

Postoperative Management

Careful airway observation is maintained in the early postoperative period. Aggressive pulmonary toilet, including the liberal use of bedside bronchoscopy, is important because these patients may have difficulty clearing secretions past their anastomosis or area of airway repair. Patients who have an associated vocal cord paralysis may have even more difficulty with pulmonary toilet owing to their inability to produce an effective cough.

These patients may benefit from a commercially available minitracheostomy (Minitrach II, Portex, Keene, NH), which is placed through their cricothyroid membrane to allow direct tracheal suctioning. Some patients with tracheal resection may have problems with postoperative aspiration because of difficulty in elevating the larynx during deglutition. This is more profound in the patients with associated recurrent nerve injuries or in those who have had a suprahyoid laryngeal release. The remainder of the postoperative management is similar to the routine care after other neck operations or thoracotomy for pulmonary resection. In the trauma setting, management of the associated injuries and their complications may dominate the care of the patient. For the ventilated patient, care should be taken to position the endotracheal balloon distal or proximal to the tracheal suture line and minimize airway pressures in cases where the endotracheal tube lies above the airway anastomosis by necessity. These patients should be managed at the lowest possible airway pressures that provide satisfactory oxygenation and ventilation and extubated as soon as their other injuries will allow. Bronchoscopy should usually be performed 7 to 10 days after tracheobronchial repair or before discharge to ensure satisfactory healing without granulation tissue or the early development of anastomotic stenosis.

Complications

The complications of tracheobronchial repair are similar to those of airway resection and reconstruction and consist mostly of anastomotic problems. Anastomotic dehiscence or restenosis occurs in 5% to 6% of patients after tracheal reconstruction (Grillo et al, 1986). Initial management involves securing the airway, usually with an endoluminal or tracheal T tube until healing is complete and the perioperative inflammation has subsided. Most of these patients can be managed with subsequent airway resection and reconstruction 3 to 6 months after the original repair if necessary (Donohue et al, 1997). Anastomotic dehiscence is life threatening if this results in fistula formation to the innominate artery or esophagus. Tracheal/innominate artery fistula is rare but frequently fatal and requires immediate operation for division of the innominate artery and interposition of healthy tissue between the airway and great vessels. Tracheoesophageal fistula can usually be managed initially by establishing gastric drainage, enteral nutrition, and treatment of pneumonia. When the patient is stable and no longer requires ventilatory support, the tracheoesophageal fistula can be divided, with the esophageal and tracheal defects resected or repaired and healthy soft tissue interposed between the adjacent suture lines. Associated laryngeal complications due to laryngeal injuries or vocal cord dysfunction are discussed in Chapter 66. If vocal cord paralysis is permanent, it can usually be palliated by vocal cord lateralization or medialization procedures.

Late Management

Patients may incur delayed treatment after tracheobronchial trauma for three reasons. First, the initial injury may have been subtle and initially missed in the early or intermediate trauma management. Second, severe associated injuries may have prevented early definitive management of recognized airway injury. Third, initial attempts at repair may fail, resulting in dehiscence or late stenosis.

In any of these scenarios, the sequelae are similar. Although the airway may be partially or completely disrupted at the time of initial injury, it may be held together by strong peritracheal connective tissue, allowing an airway to be established and ventilation to be maintained. However, as the primary injury or secondary dehiscence heals, granulation tissue and scar contracture result, with subsequent stricture formation that usually develops 1 to 4 weeks after injury. Taskinen and associates (1989) reported nine patients with blunt tracheobronchial rupture, five of whom had operations purposely delayed from 9 to 89 days because of complete lung expansion with suction drainage. However, in all five patients, dyspnea later developed, with bronchoscopy revealing obstruction and granulation tissue at the site of airway injury. Each of these patients required subsequent airway resection with primary reconstruction.

These patients may initially have dyspnea on exertion but may also have wheezing, stridor, cough, difficulty in clearing secretions, or recurrent respiratory infections. Any of these symptoms with a history of trauma or prolonged intubation should raise the suspicion of a late airway stenosis, which should be diagnosed or excluded by bronchoscopy. A 50% reduction in the cross-sectional area of the trachea usually results in dyspnea only with significant exertion, whereas narrowing of the lumen to less than 25% usually produces dyspnea and stridor at rest. Patients may be reasonably compensated in spite of significant stenosis but can have acute life-threatening deterioration with a minor amount of airway edema or secretions. A high index of suspicion in these patients is critical to their subsequent workup and timely diagnosis (Wood and Vallières, 1997).

Once recognized, critical airway stenosis can be evaluated and initially stabilized by bronchoscopy and dilatation (Stephens and Wood, 2000). However, the appropriate, definitive management of most of these patients is subsequent tracheal or bronchial resection with primary reconstruction as for benign airway strictures from other causes (Wood and Vallières, 1997). Except in cases of distal lung destruction by chronic infection, re-establishment of ventilation to lung parenchyma can be expected to restore significant function, even years after the injury. There may be little or no apparent function by preoperative perfusion scanning; this is likely due to reflexive pulmonary vasoconstriction and is reversible on resumption of ventilation to the lung parenchyma. Airway reconstruction should always be considered first in these instances, with pulmonary resection reserved for patients with unreconstructable lesions or those with destroyed parenchyma from chronic infection or bronchiectasis.

RESULTS

Injury to the trachea and proximal bronchi is a lethal injury, with more than 75% of patients with blunt tracheobronchial trauma dying before arrival to the emergency department (Bertelsen and Howitz, 1972). There are no known series of autopsy studies of penetrating tracheobronchial trauma to give us a similar prehospital mortality denominator. However, in both instances, death is most likely due to associated injuries rather than to the tracheobronchial injury itself.

In patients operated on for penetrating injuries, the mortality is 6% to 18% (Symbas et al, 1976, 1982). Of 17 survivors of penetrating tracheal trauma, 88% had a good result, apparently without symptoms (Symbas et al, 1976). One of 17 patients had permanent hoarseness from concomitant recurrent nerve injury and a second patient required a permanent tracheostomy because of complications and failed reconstruction of a combined tracheal and esophageal injury. In Rossbach's series of 32 patients with penetrating (59%) and blunt (41%) tracheobronchial trauma, 78% of patients required postoperative mechanical ventilation. In patients with a penetrating injury, this ranged from 1 to 3 days with a mean of 2 days, and in patients with blunt injury, intubation ranged from 3 to 9 days with a mean of 5 days. The average length of intensive care unit stay was 4 days for patients with penetrating trauma and 9 days for patients with blunt injury, whereas the mean hospitalization was 15 days and 17 days for penetrating and blunt injuries, respectively (Rossbach et al, 1998). Nineteen percent of patients in this series sustained postoperative complications but 93% of patients were ultimately asymptomatic and returned to preinjury function. Only 1 of 32 patients (3%) had a symptomatic late stenosis after repair of complex avulsion injury. The mortality rate in this series was 6% and was related to multiple injuries in the setting of blunt trauma. Results from other series show a mortality of 10% to 25% for patients undergoing repair of tracheobronchial injury in the setting of penetrating or blunt trauma with associated injuries (Edwards et al, 1987; Flynn et al, 1989; Symbas et al, 1992).

Patients with early definitive airway repair had a long-term good result in over 90% of patients, with poor airway–related outcomes generally being due to associated recurrent nerve injury or failed initial tracheobronchial repair (Gussack et al, 1986; Reece and Shatney, 1988). However, in the series by Reece and Shatney (1988), good results were only obtained in 67% of patients who had tracheal repair over a stent or with a tracheostomy, leaving the authors to conclude that primary early repair provides the best long-term outcomes. In many series, the ultimate prognosis after airway injury is dependent on the associated injuries, particularly closed-head injuries. Thirteen percent of the patients in a series published by Angood and associates (1986) were left in a vegetative state in spite of excellent functional airways after definitive tracheobronchial repair.

COMMENTS AND CONTROVERSIES

Tracheobronchial trauma represents a genuine life-threatening risk after cervical thoracic trauma. This chapter covers in great detail the steps involved in accurate diagnosis and emergent management. These cases often provoke injudicious treatment strategies such as emergency tracheostomy or ill-advised rigid bronchoscopy in an attempt to establish an airway. As Dr. Wood points out, the safest and most expeditious way to deal with such life-threatening injuries is careful examination by flexible bronchoscopy followed by a planned stepwise treatment strategy.

G. A. P.

REFERENCES

Angood B, Attia EL, Brown RA, Mulder DS: Extrinsic civilian trauma to the larynx and cervical trachea: Important predictors of long-term morbidity. J Trauma 26:869–873, 1986.

Barmada H, Gibbons JR: Tracheobronchial injury in blunt and penetrating chest trauma. Chest 106:74–78, 1994.

Baumgartner F, Sheppard B, deVirgilio C et al: Tracheal and main bronchial disruptions after blunt chest trauma: Presentation and management. Ann Thorac Surg 50:569–574, 1990.

Bertelsen S, Howitz P: Injuries of the trachea and bronchi. Thorax 27:188–194, 1972.

Chagnon FP, Mulder DS: Laryngotracheal trauma. Chest Surg Clin North Am 6:733–748, 1996.

Committee on Trauma, American College of Surgeons: Advanced Trauma Life Support Program Instructor's Manual. Chicago, American College of Surgeons, 1989.

De La Rocha AG, Kayler D: Traumatic rupture of the tracheobronchial tree. Can J Surg 28:68–71, 1985.

Deslauriers J, Beaulieu, M, Archambault G et al: Diagnosis and long-term follow-up of major bronchial disruptions due to non-penetrating trauma. Ann Thorac Surg 33:32–38, 1982.

Donahue DM, Grillo HC, Wain JC et al: Reoperative tracheal resection and reconstruction for unsuccessful repair of postintubation stenosis. J Thorac Cardiovasc Surg 114:934–939, 1997.

Edwards WH Jr, Morris JA Jr, DeLozier JB III, Adkins RB Jr: Airway injuries: The first priority in trauma. Am Surg 53:192–197, 1987.

Endress C, Guyot DR, Engels JA et al: The "fallen lung with absent hilum" signs of complete bronchial transection. Ann Emerg Med 20:317–318, 1991.

Fitz-Hugh GS, Powell JB III: Management of laryngotracheal injuries. Va Med 97:490–493, 1970.

Flynn AE, Thomas AN, Schecter WP: Acute tracheobronchial injury. J Trauma 29:1326–1330, 1989.

Graham JM, Mattox KL, Beall AC: Penetrating trauma of the lung. J Trauma 19:665, 1979.

Griffith JL: Fracture of the bronchus. Thorax 4:105, 1949.

Grillo HC, Zannini P, Michelassi F: Complications of tracheal reconstruction. J Thorac Cardiovasc Surg 91:322–328, 1986.

Grillo HC: Tracheal surgery. In Ranitch M, Steichen F (eds): Atlas of General Thoracic Surgery. Philadelphia, WB Saunders. 1987, pp 293–331.

Grillo HC: Notes on the windpipe. Ann Thorac Surg 47:9–26, 1989.

Grover FL, Ellestad C, Arom KV et al: Diagnosis and management of major tracheobronchial injuries. Ann Thorac Surg 28:384–391, 1979.

Guertler AT: Blunt laryngeal trauma associated with shoulder harness use. Am Emerg Med 17:838–839, 1988.

Gussack GS, Jurkovich GJ, Luterman A: Laryngotracheal trauma: A protocol approach to a rare injury. Laryngoscope 96:660–665, 1986.

Hamby WB (ed): The Reports and Autopsy Records of Ambrose Paré. Springfield, IL, Charles C Thomas, 1960, pp 47–49.

Heitmiller RF: Tracheal release maneuvers. Chest Surg Clin North Am 6:675–682, 1996.

Huelke DF: Shoulder belts and laryngeal trauma (Letter; Comment). Am Emerg Med 18:1257–1258, 1989.

Kelly JP, Webb WR, Moulder PV et al: Management of airway trauma: I. Tracheobronchial injuries. Ann Thorac Surg 40:551–555, 1985.

Kemmerer WT, Eckert WG, Gathright JB et al: Patterns of thoracic injuries in fatal traffic accidents. J Trauma 1:595–599, 1961.

Kinsella TJ, Johnsrud LW: Traumatic rupture of the bronchus. J Thorac Cardiovasc Surg 16:571, 1947.

Kirsch MM, Orringer MB, Behrendt DM, Sloan H: Management of

tracheobronchial disruption secondary to non-penetrating trauma. Ann Thorac Surg 22:93–101, 1976.

Krinitzki SI: Zur Kasuistik einer vollstandigen Zerreibung der rechten Luftrohrenastes. Virchows Arch A Pathol Anat Histopathol 266:815, 1927.

Kumpe DA, Oh KS, Wyman SM: A characteristic pulmonary finding in unilateral complete bronchial transection. AJR Am J Roentgenol 110:704–706, 1970.

Lee RB: Traumatic injury of the cervico-thoracic trachea and major bronchi. Chest Surg Clin North Am 7:285–304, 1997.

Lupetin AR: Computed tomographic evaluation of laryngotracheal trauma. J Curr Probl Diagn Radiol 26:185–206, 1997.

Lynn RB, Iyengar K: Traumatic rupture of the bronchus. Chest 61:81–83, 1972.

Mathisen DJ, Grillo H: Laryngotracheal trauma. Ann Thorac Surg 43:254–261, 1987.

Mathisen DJ, Grillo HC: Airway trauma: Laryngotracheal trauma. In Webb WR, Vesson A (eds): International Trends in General Thoracic Surgery, Vol 7, Thoracic Surgery: Surgical Management of Chest Injuries. St Louis, CV Mosby, 1991, pp 385–389.

Minard G, Kudsk RA, Croce MA et al: Laryngotracheal trauma. Am Surg 58:181–187, 1992.

Mitchell JD, Mathisen DJ, Wright CD et al: Clinical experience with carinal resection. J Thorac Cardiovasc Surg 117:39–52, 1999.

Mulder DS, Ratnani S: Tracheobronchial trauma. In Pearson FG, Deslauriers J, Ginsberg RJ et al (eds): Thoracic Surgery. New York, Churchill Livingstone, 1995, pp 1543–1554.

Ramzy AI, Rodriguez A, Turney SZ: Management of major tracheobronchial ruptures in patients with multiple system trauma. J Trauma 28:1353–1356, 1988.

Reece GP, Shatney CH: Blunt injuries of the cervical trachea: Review of 51 patients. South Med J 81:1542–1548, 1988.

Rossbach MM, Johnson SB, Gomez MA et al: Management of major tracheobronchial injuries: A 28-year experience. Ann Thorac Surg 65:182–186, 1998.

Sanger PW: Evacuation hospital experience with war wounds and injuries of the chest. Ann Surg 122:147, 1945.

Shelly CH, Mattox KL, Beall AC: Management of acute cervical tracheal trauma. Am J Surg 128:805–808, 1974.

Stark P: Imaging of tracheobronchial injuries. J Thorac Imaging 10:206–219, 1995.

Stephens KE Jr, Wood DE: Bronchoscopic management of central airway obstruction. J Thorac Cardiovasc Surg 119:289–296, 2000.

Symbas PN, Hatcher CR, Boehm GAW: Acute penetrating tracheal trauma. Ann Thorac Surg 22:473–477, 1976.

Symbas PN, Hatcher JCR, Vlasis SE: Bullet wounds of the trachea. J Thorac Cardiovasc Surg 83:235–238, 1982.

Symbas PN, Justicz AG, Ricketts RR: Rupture of the airways from blunt trauma: Treatment of complex injuries. Ann Thorac Surg 54:177–183, 1992.

Taskinen SO, Salo JA, Halttunen PE, Sovijärvi ARA: Tracheobronchial rupture due to blunt chest trauma: A follow-up study. Ann Thorac Surg 48:846–849, 1989.

Webb A: Pathologica Indica of the Anatomy of Indian Diseases, 2nd ed. Calcutta, Thacker, 1848.

Winslow WH: Rupture of bronchus from wild duck. Philadelphia Med Times 1:225, 1871.

Wood DE, Vallières E: Tracheobronchial resection and reconstruction. Arch Surg 132:850–856, 1997.

Wood DE, Vallières E, Karmy-Jones R: Tracheobronchial resection and reconstruction. Semin Respir Crit Care Med (in press).

CHAPTER **68**

Blunt Trauma: Chest Wall, Lung, Pleura, Heart, Great Vessels, Thoracic Duct, and Esophagus

Kamal A. Mansour

Philip F. Bongiorno

HISTORICAL NOTE

The first known description of chest trauma appeared in the Edwin Smith Papyrus written in ancient Egypt circa 1600 BC and was probably a copy of an older text originally written circa 3000 BC (Breasted, 1930). In *The Iliad*, written circa 850 BC, Homer described numerous blunt and penetrating chest injuries. In the 5th century BC, Hippocrates described hemoptysis after rib fractures. He recognized that hemoptysis indicates injury to the underlying lung and signifies a much more serious injury than does simple rib fracture (Withington, 1959). Morgagni, Pare, and Hewson each described pulmonary disruption that was secondary to blunt chest trauma and open pneumothorax in the 18th century (Meade, 1961). Thoracentesis was a widely used therapy for hemothorax during World War I. Later in that war, thoracotomy was performed to evacuate clotted hemothoraces. During World War II, decortication for clotted hemothoraces and trapped lung was standard therapy.

The modern era of treatment for thoracic trauma has evolved with the advent of positive-pressure ventilation, endotracheal intubation, cardiopulmonary bypass, intensive care units (ICUs), and a multitude of other advances. Cardiac wounds throughout history were recognized for their lethality. Aristotle wrote, "The heart among the viscera cannot withstand injury. This is to be expected because when the main source of strength is destroyed there is no aid that can be brought to the other organs which depend upon it" (Peck, 1937). In 1896, Paget wrote, "Surgery of the heart has probably reached the limits set by nature to all surgery, no new method and no new discovery can overcome all the natural difficulties that attend a wound to the heart" (Paget, 1896). One year later, in 1897, the first successful cardiorrhaphy for a traumatic cardiac injury was reported by Rehn.

Vesalius described a blunt injury to the thoracic aorta in 1557 (Glinz, 1981), but the first successful repair of a traumatic aortic injury was not reported until 1922 by Dshanelidze (Lilienthal, 1926).

The earliest reference to esophageal perforation is also in the Edwin Smith Papyrus, which describes a complication thereof—a cervical esophagocutaneous fistula. In 1676, Wiseman advised closure with sutures of an esophageal injury, and in 1695, Purmann acknowledged the difficulties that may be encountered in an effort to expose an injured esophagus and recommended to leave it alone (Hochberg, 1960). Brewer and Burford (1965) reported the successful repair of a traumatic esophageal perforation in 1947.

■ *HISTORICAL REFERENCES*

Breasted JH: The Edwin Smith Surgical Papyrus, Vol 1. Chicago, University of Chicago Press, 1930.

Brewer LA, Burford TH: Special types of thoracic wounds. In Medical Department: U.S. Army Surgery in World War II, Thoracic Surgery, 38th ed. Washington, D.C., U.S. Government Printing Office, 1965, p 269.

Hochberg LA: Thoracic Surgery Before the 20th Century. New York, Vantage, New York, 1960.

Homer (Alexander Pope, translator): Homer's Poetical Works. The Iliad: Book XVI. New York, Leavitt & Allen, pp 362–363.

Lilienthal H: Thoracic Surgery: The Surgical Treatment of Thoracic Diseases. Philadelphia, WB Saunders, 1926.

Meade RH: A History of Thoracic Surgery. Springfield, IL, Charles C Thomas, 1961.

Paget S: The Surgery of the Chest. London, John Wright, 1896.

Peck A: Aristotle: De Partisbus Animalum. Cambridge, MA, Harvard University Press, 1937.

Rehn L: Ueber penetrirende Herzwunden und Herznaht. Arch Clin Chir 55:315, 1897.

Withington ET (translator): Hippocrates, Vol 3. Cambridge MA, Harvard University Press, 1959, pp 307–313.

BLUNT TRAUMA TO THE CHEST WALL

The chest wall consists of the bony skeleton; ribs, sternum, clavicles, scapulae, and associated muscles, including the intercostal, latissimus dorsi, serratus anterior, and trapezius muscles. The two functions of the chest wall are to protect the internal thoracic organs and to serve as the "motor" of respiration. Thus, the chest wall has a central and critical role in the blunt trauma patient. Chest wall injuries have been estimated to result in 60 to 180 deaths per day in the United States (Mayberry and Trunkey, 1997). Motor vehicle accidents account for about 70% of the total number of chest wall injuries (Gaillard et al, 1990; Shorr et al, 1987; Ziegler and Agarwal, 1994). Falls from height are the next most common cause, with industrial and farm accidents, blast injuries, and assaults accounting for the remaining injuries (Gaillard et al, 1990; Shorr et al, 1987; Ziegler and Agarwal, 1994). In children younger than 3 years of age, child abuse is the most common cause of chest wall injury (63%) (Garcia et al, 1990). Chest wall injuries can occur as a direct result of impact and compression. Rapid deceleration may cause external injury but frequently results in internal injuries that are worse than might be anticipated from external signs alone. Chest wall injury occurs as an isolated injury only 16% of the time and is a marker for other severe thoracic and abdominal injuries (Shorr et al, 1987).

Chest Wall Contusion and Hematoma

The chest wall has a luxurious blood supply that is relatively exposed. The internal thoracic, lateral thoracic, and intercostal vessels are all susceptible to injury leading to significant blood loss requiring transfusion. Additionally, bleeding from rib and other skeletal fractures can produce significant hematomas.

Management

Observation alone or with transfusion is adequate therapy for most patients. Other patients have required intervention, including evacuation of the hematoma and ligation of the bleeding vessels or control of other bleeding sites. Angiographic embolization has been used to control bleeding from chest wall vessels after blunt trauma (Mayberry and Trunkey, 1997).

Rib Fracture

Simple rib fractures are common, with one series reporting a 10% incidence of rib fractures occurring in patients admitted to a level II trauma center after blunt trauma (Ziegler and Agarwal, 1994). The actual incidence is likely higher because of the difficulty in detecting rib fractures on chest radiographs. Additional studies such as rib detail films are not clinically useful for directing therapy but may be important in cases of suspected child abuse. Clearly, multiple rib fractures are a marker for severe trauma, and one group of authors has advocated that patients with three or more rib fractures are transferred to a trauma center to diagnose and treat likely associated injuries (Lee et al, 1990). The fourth through the ninth ribs are the most commonly fractured and are associated with lung, pleural, bronchial, and cardiac injuries. Fractures of ribs 9 through 12 are associated with renal, hepatic, and splenic injuries.

Management

Treatment of patients with rib fractures includes pain control, pulmonary toilet, and treatment of associated injuries. Analgesia is tailored to the individual clinical situation with two goals: pain control and maintenance of pulmonary function. Most patients can be treated with enteral or parenteral pain medications in the form of nonsteroidal analgesics or narcotics. Regional anesthetic techniques can be effective for more severe pain. Options include intercostal nerve blocks with 1% lidocaine or 0.25% bupivacaine. Ideally, ribs above and below the fractures should be blocked. The major disadvantage is a need to reblock at specific intervals. Epidural analgesia with narcotics, local anesthetics, or both is very effective in pain relief and provides minimal complications and a documented improvement in pulmonary function (Cicala et al, 1990; Wisner, 1990). These patients are best managed by a consulting pain service along with a primary surgical service.

Flail Chest

Flail chest is caused by four consecutive ribs being fractured in at least two places, which leads to paradoxic motion of the chest wall during respiration (Fig. 68–1). The diagnosis is made by careful observation of the patient's respiration and by examination of the chest radiograph for rib fractures. Pulmonary contusion is commonly associated with flail chest and is a major factor in determining the degree of respiratory compromise (Freedland et al, 1990).

Management

Patients with minimal compromise can be managed with good pain control, including use of epidural anesthesia and aggressive pulmonary toilet. Patients with more significant respiratory compromise require intubation and mechanical ventilation. Patients are weaned from the ventilator as pain is controlled and the chest wall stabilizes with fibrosis over time. Early tracheostomy is useful for both pulmonary toilet and decreasing dead space while weaning from the ventilator.

Surgical, internal fixation can be achieved by a variety of techniques, including wire sutures, intramedullary wires, Judet staples, or external metal plate (Barioni et al, 1992; Trunkey, 1994). Internal fixation has not proved to be effective in preventing the need for intubation or decreasing the time on mechanical ventilator (Trunkey, 1994). Indications for internal fixation include thoracotomy for bleeding with coexisting flail chest, failed weaning, and severe cosmetic deformity.

Sternal Fracture

Fracture most commonly occurs in the upper or middle body of the sternum as a result of striking the steering wheel in a motor vehicle accident. The injury is detected on physical examination by point tenderness, edema, and deformity. Fractures of the sternum are best seen on lateral chest radiographs. The risk for serious associated injury is probably low. The incidence of cardiac abnormality associated with sternal fracture is between 18% and 91% as assessed by various techniques (Harley and Mena, 1986; Wojcik and Morgan, 1988). The mortality rate of patients with sternal fracture is less than 1% and is 0% when sternal fracture is an isolated injury (Brookes et al, 1993).

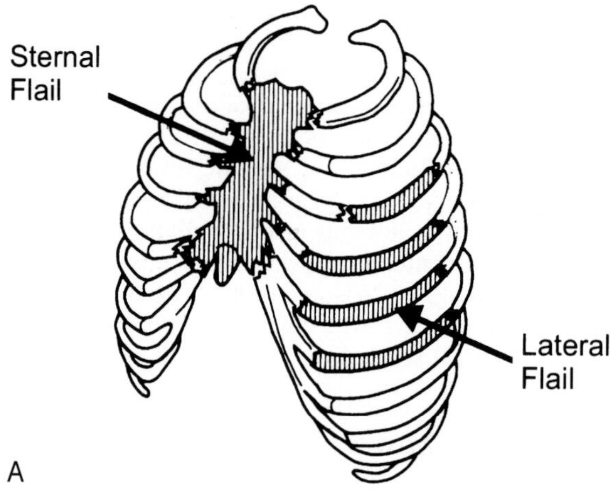

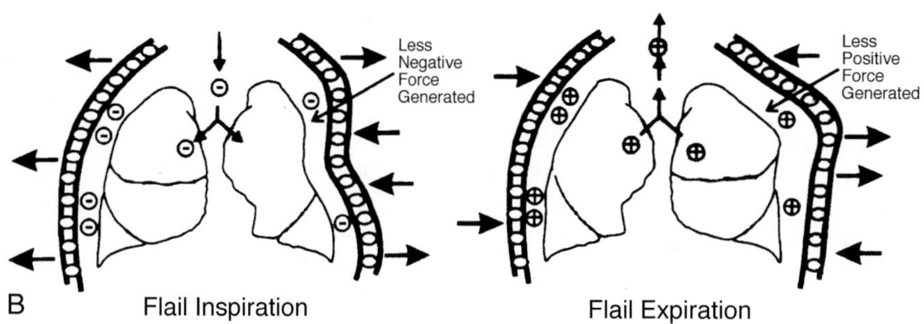

FIGURE 68–1 ■ *A,* Anatomic drawing indicating flail segments involving four ribs fractured at two locations with and without sternal flail. *B,* Drawing of the chest in *A* illustrating the paradoxical movement of the chest during respiration.

Management

Patients should undergo a 12-lead electrocardiogram (ECG) study and be placed on a cardiac monitor. Careful evaluation for associated injury should be undertaken. Repair of a sternal fracture is rarely necessary but is indicated for persistent pain or marked cosmetic deformity. Some authors have advocated external plates to achieve a more stable repair (Kitchens and Richardson, 1993).

Clavicular Fracture and Dislocation

The clavicles are exposed and thin in their midportions and are thus easily fractured. Fracture is signaled by point tenderness, deformity, and crepitus and is usually visible on chest radiograph. Careful examination for evidence of associated upper extremity neurovascular injury is important. Dislocations are rare because the sternoclavicular joint is supported by stout ligamentous attachments. Dislocation is detected by palpation as a prominent clavicular head with anterior dislocation and a depression at the sternal edge with posterior dislocation. Plain radiographs generally confirm the diagnosis.

Management

Treatment is geared toward patient comfort, and figure-eight slings are used to provide stability. Nonunion is rare, but malunion with cosmetic deformity may be an indication for operation. Rarely, neurovascular, thoracic outlet obstruction can occur as a late complication of callous formation (Connolly and Dehne, 1989).

Reduction of an anterior dislocation can be achieved with conscious sedation. The arm is abducted with lateral traction, and firm downward pressure is applied to the medial head of the clavicle. Posterior dislocations are more difficult to reduce and usually require general anesthesia. Again, the arm is placed in abduction and extension, and the head of the clavicle is then grasped with a penetrating towel clip and pulled anteriorly while applying lateral traction on the arm. Open repair is required if closed reduction fails.

Scapular Fracture and Scapulothoracic Dislocation

The scapula is a thick, well-protected bone. Thus, scapular fractures are rare and are the result of high-energy impact. These injuries are usually associated with other chest injury, including rib fracture and pulmonary contusion (Thompson et al, 1985). The diagnosis is difficult to make but is suggested by local pain, edema, and crepitus. Chest radiographs and oblique films confirm the diagnosis. Most injuries are to the neck and the body of the scapula. The less common injuries to the glenoid, acromion, and coracoid process may be associated with brachial plexus injury and long-term loss of shoulder mobility (Thompson et al, 1985). Scapulothoracic dislocation occurs with severe shoulder traction that leads to separation of the scapula from the chest wall with disruption of neurovascular, ligamentous, and muscular attachments (Sampson et al, 1993).

Management

Treatment of scapular fracture is usually immobilization with a sling; open fixation is rarely required. In patients with scapulothoracic dislocation, complex vascular repairs are not usually indicated. Distal ischemia is rarely present, even with axillary artery occlusion, because adequate collateral circulation is usually present. Brachial plexus and vascular injuries lead to long-term disability. Many patients eventually require amputation for a severely debilitated, insensate extremity.

Traumatic Asphyxia

Severe thoracic crush injuries cause a marked increase in superior vena cava pressure with reversal of flow into the veins of the face and neck leading to capillary rupture. Patients suffering traumatic asphyxia have a moribund appearance with craniofacial cyanosis, edema and petechiae, subconjuctival hemorrhage, and periorbital bruising. Patients suffer seizures, confusion, coma, and blindness.

Management

Treatment is directed toward resuscitation, supporting respiration, and detection and treatment of other injuries. Careful serial neurologic examinations should be performed with the patient monitored in an ICU. The head of the bed should be elevated to 30 degrees. Long-term results after traumatic asphyxia are good and are related to the duration of the asphyxia and associated injuries. Long-term neurologic problems are unusual (Jongewaard and Coghill, 1992).

BLUNT TRAUMA TO THE LUNG

Approximately one third of all patients admitted to trauma centers have sustained serious injuries to the chest. Lung parenchyma, which fills such a large portion of the chest cavity and which lies in close proximity to the bony thorax, is injured in many of these patients. Many lung injuries are associated with trauma to other critical structures.

Pulmonary Contusion

Pulmonary contusion is the most common injury seen in association with thoracic trauma (Wiot, 1975). It occurs in 30% to 75% of patients suffering major chest injuries (Chopra et al, 1977). Pulmonary contusion is seen with both blunt and penetrating wounds but is most common after motor vehicle accidents, such as when the chest strikes the steering wheel or a car door. It is also seen after falls from great heights and from blast injuries.

Isolated pulmonary contusions are encountered much less commonly than are contusions that are associated with other thoracic and nonthoracic injuries. Because pulmonary contusions are so commonly associated with other injuries, the pathophysiology of the associated injuries, the resuscitative and therapeutic measures that are necessary for their treatment, and the effects of aspiration, infection, and adult respiratory distress syndrome (ARDS) on the lung parenchyma have clouded the understanding of isolated pulmonary contusion (Ratliff et al, 1971).

Pathology

Wagner and colleagues (1988) have presented convincing evidence, based on computed tomography (CT) scan findings and limited pathologic material, that a pulmonary laceration with resultant hemorrhage into adjacent alveolar spaces, rather than alveolar capillary wall injury, is the basis for the development of pulmonary contusions. They have also described four types of lacerations that are associated with pulmonary contusions. Type I lacerations are the result of compression of the elastic chest wall that causes the underlying air-filled lung to rupture. Type II lacerations result from compression of the lower chest wall that causes a sudden displacement of the lower lobe across the vertebral column and produces a shearing tear in the adjacent lung. Type III lacerations are small peripheral lacerations that are close to rib fractures and are thought to be penetrating injuries caused by the ends of the fractured ribs. Type IV lacerations are tears caused by sudden chest wall compression that displaces the lung inwardly next to a thick pleuropulmonary adhesion. Type I is the most commonly encountered laceration and is almost always seen in patients who are younger than 40 years of age. Type III lacerations are the next most commonly seen and usually occur in older patients.

Diagnosis

Blunt trauma to the chest, falls, and blast injuries of the chest should all suggest the possibility that a pulmonary contusion may develop. Dyspnea, tachypnea, hemoptysis, cyanosis, and hypotension are frequently seen. Physical examination may be unrevealing; however, in the presence of a severe contusion, inspiratory rales and decreased breath sounds may be found. A chest radiograph shows either singular or multiple patchy alveolar infiltrates caused by intra-alveolar hemorrhage (Stevens and Templeton, 1965). These patchy infiltrates can coalesce into homogenous infiltrates that involve a lobe or an entire lung. CT scans of the chest have been shown to be much more sensitive in demonstrating the changes seen with pulmonary contusions than are routine chest radiographs (Wagner et al, 1988). In patients with pulmonary contusions, arterial PaO_2, alveolar-arterial oxygen gradients, and pulmonary compliance are usually abnormally low (Blair, 1976). Hyperventilation may induce hypocapnia and respiratory alkalosis (Erikson et al, 1971). If the contusion is massive or if aspiration, infection, or ARDS develops, carbon dioxide may be retained, and respiratory acidosis may ensue.

Treatment

Patients with pulmonary contusions should be hospitalized for careful monitoring because they can become critically ill rapidly. Oxygen should be administered as necessary to maintain an arterial oxygen saturation that is higher than 90%. Patient-controlled analgesia, intravenous or epidural, should be used as necessary to control pain. Vigorous chest physiotherapy is important to keep the airway clear and help prevent the development of atelectasis. If ventilation is inadequate, intubation and mechanical ventilation are indicated. If large volumes of fluid are necessary for resuscitation, a pulmonary artery catheter should be positioned so that pulmonary artery pressures and pulmonary capillary wedge pressures can be measured.

The use of steroids and antibiotics is controversial. Some authors advocate the use of high doses of steroids for a short time, whereas others feel that the use of steroids is not indicated (Svennevig et al, 1980). Prophylactic antibiotics are used in some institutions; in others, antibiotics are used only when evidence of infection is present.

Pulmonary contusions are not innocuous injuries. In one series, 11% of patients with serious isolated pulmonary contusions died, whereas the mortality rate was much higher (22%) in patients with associated injuries (DeMuth and Smith, 1965). ARDS developed in 17% of patients with isolated pulmonary contusions and in 78% of patients with two or more simultaneous associated injuries in other series (Pepe et al, 1982).

Pulmonary Parenchymal Injuries

Pulmonary Lacerations

Pulmonary parenchymal lacerations, although seen more commonly after penetrating chest trauma, are also seen after blunt trauma. Although both blood vessels and air passages may be disrupted, pneumothorax is in many cases the major problem, and bleeding is of minor consequence. If the laceration involves the visceral pleura and the communication with the pleural space remains patent, a hemothorax, pneumothorax, or hemopneumothorax results. If the visceral pleura is torn but quickly seals, blood, air, or both can accumulate within the parenchyma and result in the development of a hematoma, cyst, or a cyst containing blood.

As a result of high-speed motor vehicle crashes, extensive pulmonary lacerations, occasionally with volvulus or torsion of lung parenchyma, are being encountered with increasing frequency. Such lacerations often are centrally located, are associated with severe chest wall injuries and pulmonary contusion, and disrupt large vessels and major bronchi.

Pulmonary Hematoma

Pulmonary lacerations resulting from either blunt or penetrating injuries may fill with blood, forming a pulmonary hematoma. The reported incidence of hematomas developing in pulmonary contusions has varied from 4% (Wagner et al, 1988) to 11% (Westermark, 1941). Because hematomas are recognized infrequently in clinical situations, the true incidence is likely to be less than 4%. Despite an unimpressive radiographic appearance, the injury represents a significant collection of intraparenchymal blood. It may not become visible radiographically for 24 to 72 hours after trauma resuscitation, during which time it increases insidiously. Pulmonary hematomas generally do not interfere with gas exchange, nor do they produce significant intrapulmonary shunting. A pulmonary hematoma, however, is a major risk factor for infection and lung abscess formation (Hankins et al, 1973). The use of CT scans probably permits much more accurate evaluation of hematomas than conventional radiographs. On CT scan, hematomas have been found to shrink less than 0.5 cm in 3 weeks, whereas on conventional radiographs, they are reported to resolve within 2 to 4 weeks of injury (Wagner et al, 1988). In the absence of previous radiographs, serial films, or serial CT scans demonstrating the evolution of the hematoma, the exact nature of the nodule or lesion may be unclear, and the possibility of a neoplasm must be considered. If the nodule remains stable after 4 weeks, showing no evidence of resolution, fine-needle aspiration of the nodule or surgical excision should be performed to establish the nature of the lesion (Engelman, 1973).

Management

In most cases, pulmonary lacerations heal promptly after chest tube insertion, without any significant long-lasting ill effects. Peripheral lacerations encountered at operation can be oversewn (pneumonorrhaphy), stapled, or wedged out (Fig. 68–2). Extensive lacerations may be centrally located and disrupt major vessels and bronchi. Resultant massive bleeding, large air leaks, and, although rarely seen, bronchopulmonary venous fistulas resulting in systemic air embolization require immediate operation. The thoracotomy incision is determined by the urgency of this situation, location of the injury, and structures presumed to be involved. After thoracotomy, hilar compression with the fingers and then with a large vascular clamp, such as a Satinsky or curved DeBakey, is used to control bleeding and air leak and to stop systemic air embolization (Fig. 68–3). When the hilum is controlled, if embolization occurred, air is aspirated from the left heart, aorta, and coronary arteries. The vascular and bronchial injuries are then repaired, if possible, and the laceration is left open and drained with appropriately placed chest tubes.

Torsion or volvulus of the lung suggested by atypically oriented lobar collapse also necessitates prompt diagnosis and operation (Groskin et al, 1988). At thoracotomy, the involved lung is untwisted and observed to ensure that the lobe is viable. If there is any question about its viability, the lung should be resected. Otherwise, the involved lobe should be stapled, if possible, to an adjacent lobe to prevent retwisting.

If either pulmonary hematoma or pulmonary contusion is identified at the time of thoracotomy, the surgeon should resist the temptation to resect the involved lung. Despite the gross appearance, there is rarely an indication for the resection of an injured lung (Graham et al, 1979), unless there is associated significant injury to the airway or pulmonary vessels.

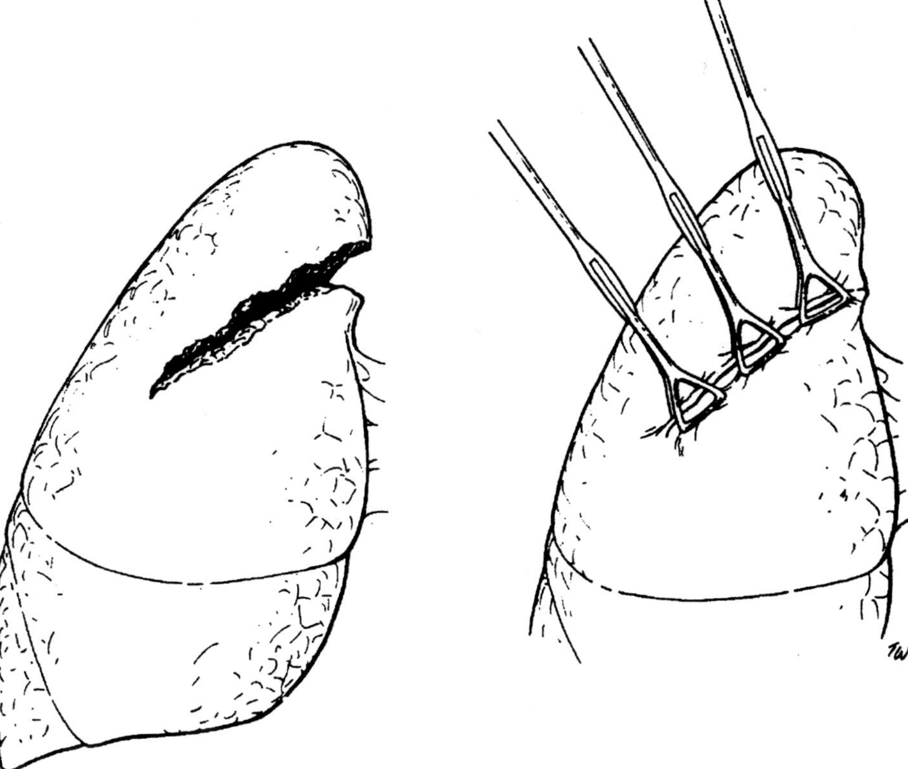

FIGURE 68–2 ■ Duvall lobe forceps used for hemostasis of a large lung laceration.

Pulmonary Vascular Injury

Vascular injury within the pulmonary parenchyma occurs within a low-pressure system compressed by the surrounding parenchyma. Such hemorrhage generally stops with complete expansion of the lung (Beall et al, 1966; Graham et al, 1979). Uncorrected injury to the main pulmonary arteries or veins or to their principal lobar branches, however, is usually lethal from rapid exsanguination because these structures bleed freely into the pleural space. Major pulmonary vascular injuries usually result from sudden deceleration. Mortality rates for pulmonary arterial or venous injuries exceed 75%. Therefore, these patients rarely survive long enough to reach a trauma center (Mattox, 1989).

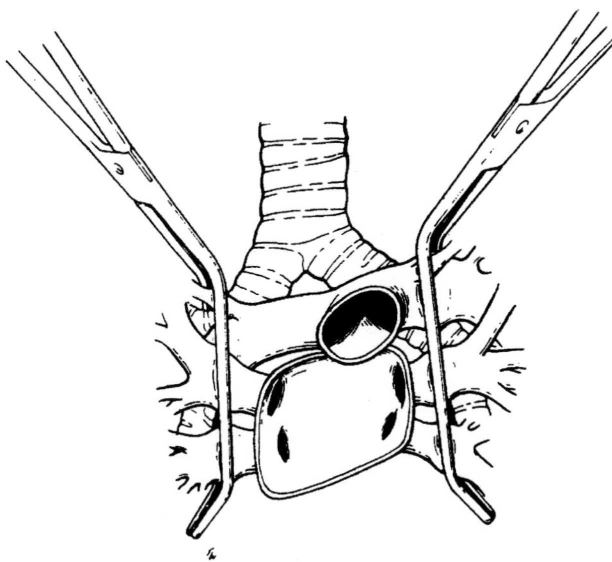

FIGURE 68–3 ■ Technique to stop major pulmonary vascular hemorrhage. The entire pulmonary hilum is grasped with one hand as a large vascular clamp is applied across the hilum with the other hand.

Management

If major pulmonary vascular injury is diagnosed or suspected, immediate thoracotomy should be performed. Temporary vascular control may be obtained at the pulmonary hilum by clamping the entire hilum. Through a thoracotomy incision, the hilum of the lung is grasped firmly with one hand as the surgeon uses the other hand to apply a long vascular clamp across the entire pulmonary hilum (see Fig. 68–3). This maneuver excludes the main pulmonary artery and veins from the circulation. This may prevent exsanguination and provide time to resuscitate the patient. If there is a significant amount of blood in the airway, a double-lumen endotracheal tube or a bronchial blocker may be used to protect the opposite lung from aspiration of blood. Next, the vascular injury should be isolated and repaired using standard vascular techniques (Carr, 1980). If a lobar pulmonary artery is irreparable, it may be ligated without fear of pulmonary necrosis. The bronchial blood supply is usually sufficient to maintain parenchymal viability (Wolfe and Sabiston, 1980). If the venous drainage to a parenchymal region must be sacrificed, the involved parenchyma should be resected to prevent infarction of the lung (Carr, 1980).

BLUNT TRAUMA TO THE PLEURA

Traumatic Pneumothorax

Blunt trauma results in pneumothorax from direct lung puncture by fractured ribs or rapid deceleration, or from an abrupt rise in the intrathoracic pressure against a closed glottis (Thal et al, 1989). In the latter mechanism, the acute rise in the airway pressure causes rupture of distal alveolar air spaces, and air tracks proximally along the bronchial tree into the mediastinum. If sufficient air collects within the mediastinum, the mediastinal pleura may rupture, producing pneumothorax.

Pneumothorax should be suspected in the initial evaluation of all traumatized patients. Signs on physical examination include dyspnea, hyper-resonance of the chest to percussion, and diminished or absent breath sounds. Tension pneumothorax is life-threatening and is a true emergency that requires immediate diagnosis and chest tube insertion. The presence of subcutaneous emphysema, absent breath sounds, mediastinal shift, and acute respiratory distress warrants chest tube insertion without waiting for the chest radiograph to be taken. The diagnosis may be confirmed radiographically before tube thoracostomy if the patient's condition allows it. While waiting for a tube insertion, a needle should be placed into the chest in the second intercostal space anteriorly. This maneuver could be diagnostic if there is a large gush of air, and it may also be life saving. Chest tube insertion can be in the fourth or fifth intercostal space in the midaxillary line and directed anteriorly and superiorly (Fig. 68–4) (Hughes, 1965). If the lung does not completely re-expand or a large or continuous air leak persists, a major airway injury should be suspected.

Thoracotomy is rarely, if ever, indicated for the control of a parenchymal air leak. If a parenchymal air leak is identified at the time of thoracotomy for another reason, it should be closed surgically during that procedure. The area of the parenchymal laceration should be repaired using fine absorbable sutures over Teflon felt pledges if necessary. Staples could also be used over strips of bovine pericardium or over Gore-Tex strips (Seamguard, WL Gore and Assoc., Flagstaff, AZ), but lung resection is almost never indicated (Graham et al, 1979; Sherman, 1966).

Traumatic Hemothorax

Hemothorax usually results from parenchymal laceration, intercostal vessel injury, chest wall injury, bronchial arterial injury, or major thoracic vascular injury (Hughes, 1965). When hemothorax is identified on the chest radiograph, a tube thoracostomy should be performed. To evacuate blood, a 36 French tube is best placed in the fifth or sixth intercostal space and directed posteriorly. Bleeding usually ceases and re-expansion of the lung occurs in more than 85% of such patients. In the acute situation, if the volume of blood obtained immediately exceeds 1000 ml or if bleeding continues in amounts that exceed 100 ml/hr for more than 4 hours, emergent thoracotomy should be performed. The recommended practice guidelines of the Ben Taub General Hospital for operation versus observation may be followed (Fig. 68–5).

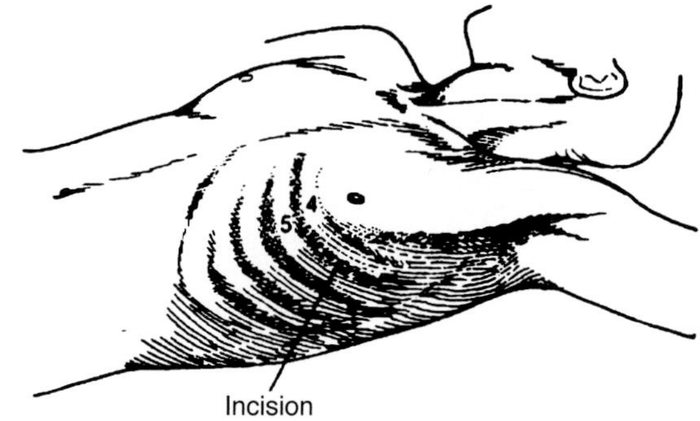

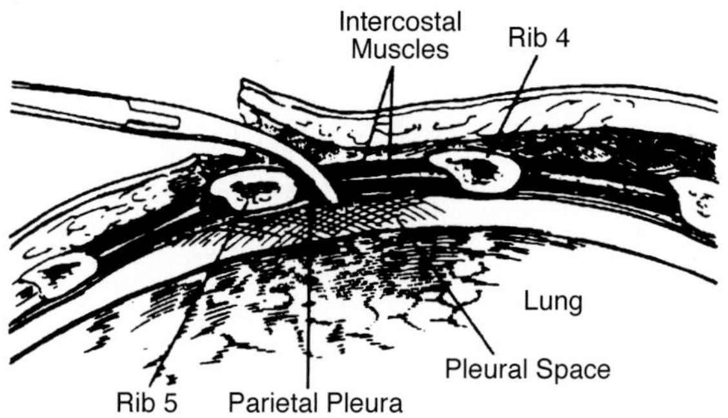

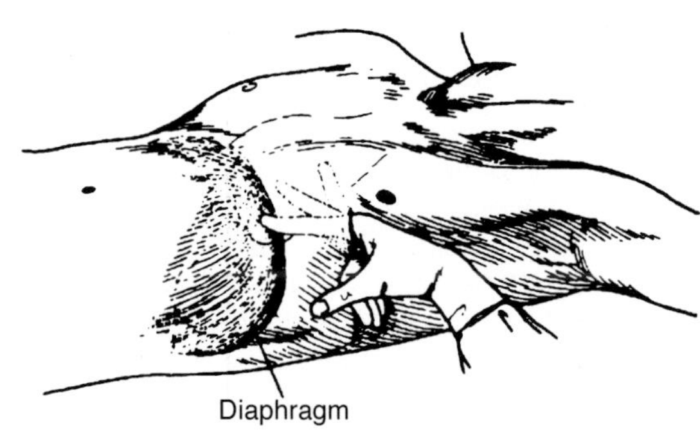

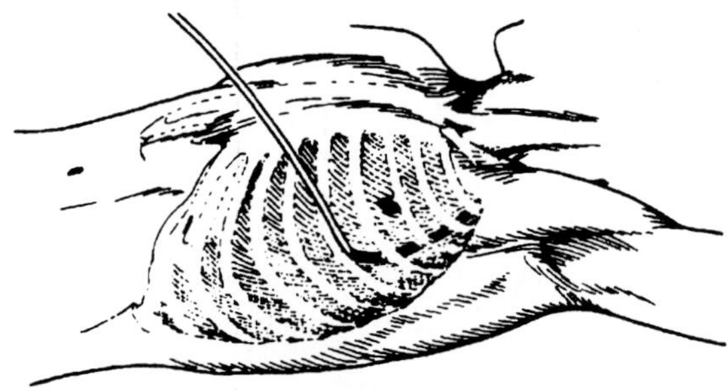

FIGURE 68–4 ■ Technique for tube thoracostomy. When the tube is placed emergently for trauma, an incision is made in the anterior axillary line. The fourth intercostal space is entered. A clamp and finger exploration is performed to be certain that the pleural space is entered. The tube is directed to the apex of the chest. (From Moore FA, Moore EE: Trauma resuscitation. In Wilmore DN, Brennan MF, Harken AH et al [eds]: Care of the Surgical Patient. New York, Scientific American, 1989.)

It is essential that all blood is evacuated. If the first chest tube does not completely evacuate the pleural space, a second or third tube should be placed. Failure to evacuation hemothorax may cause a clotted hemotho-

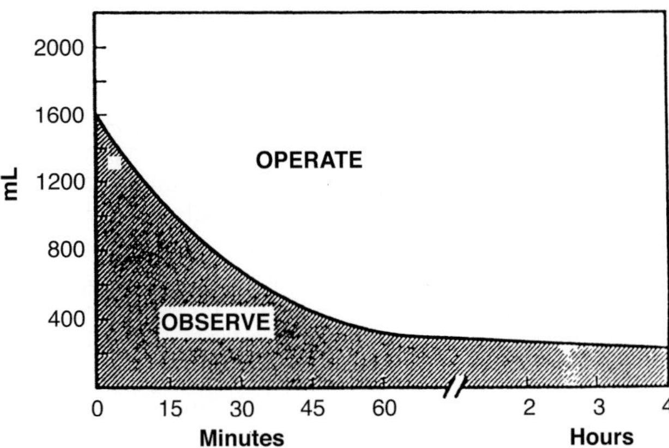

FIGURE 68–5 ■ Recommended practice guidelines for operation versus observation in patients with hemothorax following thoracic trauma.

rax and a trapped lung (Gray et al, 1960). Several studies have shown that incomplete evacuation of traumatic hemothorax is a major risk factor for the development of post-traumatic empyema (Eddy et al, 1989; Kish et al, 1976).

Controversy surrounds the management of clotted hemothorax. Some advocate limited thoracotomy and surgical evacuation of the hemothorax (Collins et al, 1978). Others recommend instillation of liquefying agents such as urokinase before considering thoracotomy. Still others acknowledge the potential risk for empyema but prefer to reserve thoracotomy for a specific indication, such as the presence of empyema evidenced by fever and leukocytosis or lung entrapment evidenced by at least a 25% reduction in the ipsilateral lung volume (Arom et al, 1977).

The management of clotted hemothorax should be individualized. In patients with a significant volume of clotted hemothorax or suspected pleural sepsis, surgical evacuation is advisable when an anesthetic and a limited thoracotomy are believed to pose minimal morbidity. In the multiple-injury patient with significant pulmonary dysfunction that necessitates high levels of support from mechanical ventilation, the risks associated with transport to the operating room, anesthesia, and potential intraoperative lung injury may outweigh the potential benefits of thoracotomy. In this situation, reserving thoracotomy for a specific indication is appropriate. If surgical evacuation of the clotted hemothorax is to be performed, it should be performed early. Within the first 7 days, the clot is relatively easy to scoop out through a limited thoracotomy (Coselli et al, 1984). Thereafter, the clot begins to organize and becomes adherent to both the parietal and visceral pleura, making extraction more difficult and traumatic. Beyond 6 weeks after injury, a fibrous peel develops, creating a fibrothorax, which may require a more difficult decortication (Collins et al, 1978).

Video-assisted thoracic surgery (VATS) may be used for early evacuation of clotted hemothorax. Experience with this approach is limited but shows promise. The thoracoscope is placed in the chest, and blood is removed by a combination of suction, irrigation, and instillation of lytic agents. The timing of thoracoscopy for residual hemothorax is important. When done immediately after the trauma, it is unlikely to succeed because of the difficulties with ongoing bleeding. Delaying thoracoscopy beyond several days may also decrease chances of success. Because it is more difficult to remove peel and organized clot from the chest thoracoscopically than with an open technique, it is important to do the procedure before the hemothorax becomes too organized. The low morbidity rate of thoracoscopy as opposed to thoracotomy permits a low threshold for the procedure and makes a strong argument for early intervention before a prolonged trial of tube thoracostomy drainage has run its course (Wisner, 1995).

Data conflict about whether patients with chest tubes placed for trauma should routinely receive antibiotics. The argument for antibiotic coverage of common skin pathogens is that it prevents empyema. The argument against routine antibiotic coverage is that it produces resistant organisms and does not prevent empyema. Although there is no consensus on this issue, some evidence indicates that prophylactic antibiotics are beneficial (Fallon and Wears, 1992; Lo Cicero and Mattox, 1989; Lo Curto et al, 1986).

BLUNT TRAUMA TO THE HEART

The most common cause of blunt cardiac injury is a high-speed motor vehicle crash in which the driver's chest impacts the steering wheel. Less common causes of cardiac injury include falls from height, blast injury, crush injury, high-speed projectiles, animal kicks, and physical assaults (Fulda et al, 1991; Kato et al, 1994). Various mechanisms for injury have been described: direct precordial impact, compression of the heart between the sternum and vertebral column, hydraulic force transmitted through the venous system from a blow to the abdomen or extremities, deceleration with displacement or twisting of the heart on its fixed attachments, and penetration from fractured ribs and sternum (Martin et al, 1984).

The spectrum of cardiac lesions related to blunt trauma ranges from myocardial contusion, which may have little clinical significance, to free-wall cardiac rupture, which is generally fatal. Most patients with cardiac injury have other significant thoracic injuries, most commonly multiple rib fractures but also flail chest, ruptured diaphragm, and rupture of the descending thoracic aorta (Calhoon et al, 1986). Simultaneous head injury occurs in more than 50% and abdominal trauma in about 40% of patients with blunt cardiac injury (Fulda et al, 1991).

When evaluating and treating blunt trauma patients, a high index of suspicion for cardiac injuries needs to be balanced by a comprehensive knowledge of the range and significance of potential injuries to diagnose and treat injuries in a cost-effective manner.

Myocardial Contusion

Myocardial contusion is a frequent event, occurring in at least 10% of blunt chest trauma victims (Baxter et al, 1989; Fabian et al, 1988). A historical autopsy series in motor vehicle crash fatalities demonstrated a 15% to 17% incidence of myocardial contusion (Kissane, 1952). The most common complaint after myocardial contusion is nonspecific chest pain. Fortunately, significant clinical cardiac events are rare in patients who are suffering myocardial contusion, and these usually manifest as benign arrhythmias (McLean et al, 1991). Arrhythmias can be of any type but most commonly are premature atrial and premature ventricular contractions (Cachecho et al, 1992; Fabian et al, 1991). The most severe manifestations of myocardial contusion are subendocardial, subepicardial, or intramyocardial hemorrhage and necrosis, which can lead to ventricular dysfunction, delayed rupture, or aneurysm formation (Symbas, 1991).

Management

Previously, many strategies were developed to detect or exclude myocardial contusion in patients suffering chest trauma, including the use of cardiac isoenzyme analysis, echocardiography, and nuclear cardiac scintigraphy. Clinical protocols were developed that mirrored the treatment of patients in whom angina and acute myocardial infarction were suspected. None of the tests designed to detect myocardial contusion was found to be especially sensitive or specific. Additionally, strategies to monitor or treat patients for myocardial contusion were not found to change patient outcome.

Because most patients manifest no dysfunction, specific attempts to diagnose and treat myocardial contusion should not be made. Instead, current recommendations are that patient management should be expectant and that patients should be treated for specific cardiac abnormalities as they are detected and given specific diagnosis other than myocardial contusion (Mattox et al, 1992). Appropriate evaluation of symptom-free patients suffering blunt chest trauma includes a 12-lead ECG upon arrival to the emergency center and then continuous telemetered cardiac monitoring and invasive hemodynamic monitoring as determined by the patient's clinical course.

Cardiac and Pericardial Rupture

Rupture of the heart occurring during blunt trauma is not rare; it has been estimated to cause 2500 motor vehicle fatalities per year in the United States and is present along with other fatal injuries in up to 15% of all motor vehicle accidental deaths (Calhoon et al, 1986). As delineated earlier, a spectrum of causes and mechanisms can lead to cardiac rupture. Most patients with blunt cardiac rupture die shortly after the injury, but a subset of patients survive 30 minutes or longer. In a series of 59 patients with blunt cardiac rupture reported by Fulda and colleagues (1991), 51% of patients who were alive at the accident scene died during transport to the emergency center, and 24% arrested in the emergency room.

The classic auscultatory sign of cardiac rupture is the "bruit de Moulin," an attempt to describe the sound of the heart beating in a pericardium that is partially filled with air and blood as analogous to the sound of a splashing millwheel. The clinical manifestations of rupture of the free cardiac wall are dependent on the presence or absence of a concomitant tear in the pericardium. Most patients with cardiac rupture have an intact pericardium and signs of cardiac tamponade, such as hypotension, distended neck veins, and pulsus paradoxus. Patients with an associated pericardial tear usually manifest with hemothorax and hemorrhagic shock.

In reported series, most cardiac injuries occur to the right-sided chambers, with the atria being more commonly injured than the ventricles (Calhoon et al, 1986; Fulda et al, 1991; Pevec et al, 1989). Injuries are only rarely multiple. Clearly, some selection bias may skew the reported incidence toward the more survivable injuries. Isolated pericardial injuries occur about half as commonly as isolated cardiac injuries, with most of these being left-sided pleuropericardial tears that are parallel to the phrenic nerve (Fulda et al, 1991). The risk for cardiac herniation through a pleuropericardial tear is real and may occur in up to one third of patients with such an injury (Fulda et al, 1991).

Diagnosis

The diagnosis of cardiac rupture should be considered in any patient suffering blunt injury with signs of cardiac tamponade or unexplained hypotension. Emergency department ultrasound is a diagnostic modality that may be immediately available and has been clinically demonstrated to be both sensitive and specific in detecting pericardial effusion in a trauma setting (Rozycki et al, 1993; Symbas et al, 1999). Rarely, the injury is detected incidentally by CT scanning or another diagnostic modality. Most injuries are detected during emergency thoracotomy in a patient who loses vital signs while being evaluated and resuscitated in the emergency room.

Pericardiocentesis should not be used to diagnose hemopericardium in a stable patient with suspected cardiac rupture; instead, the patient should be transported to the operating room to undergo pericardial window exploration. Patients who undergo exploratory laparotomy with suspected cardiac injury can easily have a pericardial exploration through a concomitant pericardial window.

Management

The operative approach to repair blunt cardiac injury is a median sternotomy. A left anterior thoracotomy should be converted to a clamshell incision by performing a transverse sternotomy and bilateral thoracotomy (Fig. 68–6). Initial control of the injury should be made by applying direct digital pressure or, in the case of atrial injuries, by judicious application of a side-biting clamp. Occasionally, occluding inflow of blood by clamping the superior and interior vena cava can aid repair by improving visualization and by decompressing the ventricle.

Injuries can be repaired with pledgeted sutures. Cardiopulmonary bypass is usually never needed to repair injuries, the exception being the patient with valvular or septal injury that requires emergent repair. Intraoperative transesophageal echocardiography can be useful in obtaining a more complete evaluation of the heart.

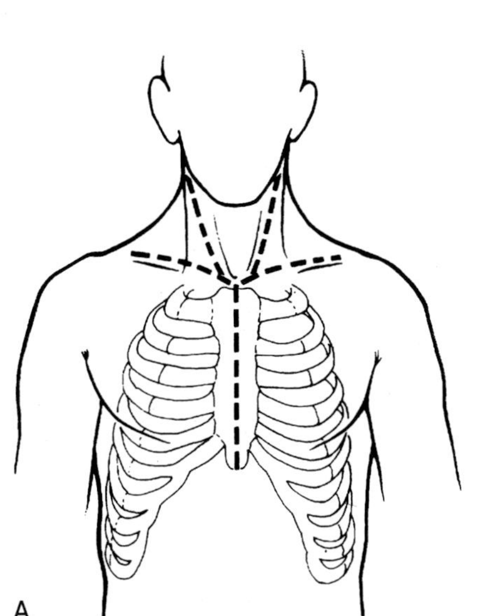

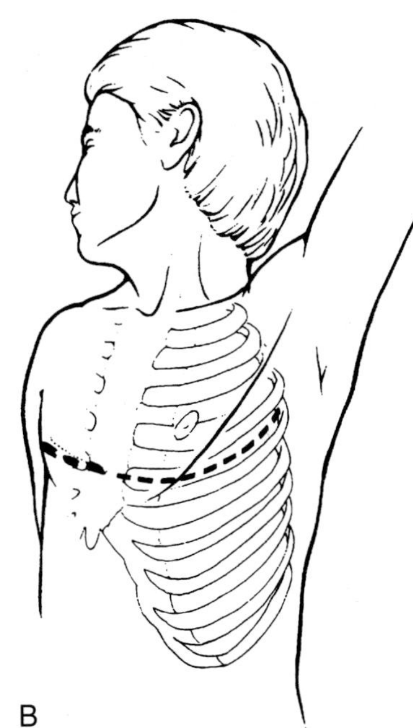

FIGURE 68–6 ■ *A*, Median sternotomy with extension to the right or left supraclavicular or cervical region. *B*, Emergent anterolateral thoracotomy with extension into a "clam shell" thoracotomy.

Other Cardiac Injuries

Coronary Artery

Blunt chest trauma can cause direct injury and occlusion of a coronary artery. The left anterior descending and right coronary arteries are the most susceptible. These injuries produce acute myocardial infarction. Successful revascularization has been reported using thrombolytic agents and coronary artery stenting (Ginzburg et al, 1998; Ledley et al, 1992).

Cardiac Valves

The most common valvular injuries produced by blunt trauma are chordal rupture with acute mitral regurgitation and aortic valve cusp rupture with acute aortic insufficiency. These injuries are usually suspected based on the presence of a murmur or signs of cardiac failure. Definitive diagnosis depends on the use of echocardiography because the clinical signs are often atypical. The timing of operation depends on the patient's condition; in patients with acute left ventricular failure, it is often prudent to operate without performing coronary angiography.

Septum

Septal defects are signaled by murmurs and are best evaluated by echocardiography. Treatment is individualized, but patients with a left-to-right shunt and a Qp:Qs ratio greater than 2:1 need operative correction (Morant et al, 1991). Initial medical therapy and elective repair are always the goal to improve long-term results.

BLUNT TRAUMA TO THE GREAT VESSELS

The thoracic great vessels consist of the aorta and its major intrathoracic branches, the pulmonary arteries and veins, the vena cava, and the azygos vein. The three mechanisms of injury that come into play are shear, compression, and intraluminal hyperextension (Pretie et al, 1997). Shear forces act when the vasculature is fixed, such as the aorta at the ligamentum arteriosum and the vena cava and pulmonary veins at the atria. Compression occurs as the great vessels are pressed against the skeleton, specifically the vertebral column and sternum. Intraluminal hyperextension occurs as large increases in intraluminal pressure act to disrupt the vasculature from inside to out.

Diagnosis

Prompt diagnosis of blunt great vessel injury rests on a high index of suspicion and an accurate history of the traumatic event. Approximately half of patients with serious blunt great vessel injury have no external signs of injury (Mattox, 1989). Important points in the history include the magnitude of deceleration, damage to the vehicles involved, other injuries or deaths at the scene, location and position of the patient at the scene, presence of hemodynamic instability, and neurologic status of the patient. Important clinical signs are indicators of severe chest trauma, such as palpable sternal fractures or flail chest, expanding hematomas, or an abnormal pulse examination and evidence of cardiac tamponade (elevated central venous pressure, hypotension, pulsus paradoxus).

Among the first diagnostic studies that should be performed on any blunt trauma patient is a standard portable chest radiograph taken with an anterior-to-posterior technique at 36 inches. Multiple findings on a portable chest radiograph have been reported to suggest great vessel injury (Table 68–1). Controversy persists regarding whether certain of these findings are truly correlated with great vessel injury, specifically first and second rib fractures and other skeletal fractures (Lee et al, 1997; Poole, 1989; Sturm et al, 1989). The chest radiograph finding that correlates most reliably with great vessel

TABLE 68–1 ■ **Radiographic Findings with Thoracic Great Vessel Injury**

FRACTURES
Sternum
Scapula
Multiple ribs
Clavicle
First rib
MEDIASTINUM
Obliteration of aortic knob contour
Widened mediastinum
Depression of left mainstem bronchus
Loss of perivertebral pleural stripe
Calcium layering of aortic knob
OTHER
Anterior displacement of trachea
Lateral displacement of trachea
Loss of aortopulmonary window
Deviation of nasogastric tube to left
Apical hemothorax
Blunt injury to the diaphragm

injury is loss of aortic knob contour, which produces an abnormal-appearing mediastinal silhouette (Miller et al, 1989; Mirvis et al, 1987). Unfortunately, chest radiographs are normal in up to 25% of patients with significant thoracic vascular injuries (Kirsch, 1976; Woodridge, 1990).

In adopting a posture of high index of suspicion, clinicians should consider arteriography in evaluating patients with significant mechanisms of injury despite the absence of external signs of injury or abnormal chest radiographs. This may be the clinical scenario in up to 2% of patients with thoracic great vessel injury (Feliciano, 1997). The other diagnostic modalities that have been used to evaluate for vascular injury include CT scanning, magnetic resonance imaging, transesophageal echocardiography, and digital subtraction arteriography (Johnson et al, 1997; Kearney et al, 1993; Mirvis et al, 1996; Nunez et al, 1998). Despite local expertise with certain of these modalities, none has the proven accuracy and long-term track record of biplane contrast aortography in detecting great vessel injury (Raptopoulos, 1994; Saletta et al, 1995; Trerotala, 1995).

Management

Thoracic great vessel injury generally warrants an urgent but not necessarily emergent surgical approach. Patients with contained aortic rupture who are appropriately managed nonoperatively or at least with delayed operation include patients with severe central nervous system injury, severe burns, hemodynamic instability from other injuries, or pulmonary contusion and respiratory failure (Akins et al, 1981; Pate et al, 1995). Additionally, stable patients who have small intimal defects, specifically those with descending aortic injuries without significant false aneurysm, can do well without operation (Fischer et al, 1990; Wigle et al, 1991) The advocates of this approach call for the patient to be placed in a well-monitored setting with careful control of blood pressure using β-blockers and serial evaluation (Fabian et al, 1998; Pate, 1998). Careful follow-up is warranted with a repeat aortogram, helical CT, or transesophageal echocardiography at some defined interval.

Descending Aorta

When the diagnosis of contained, blunt rupture of the descending aorta is made, other life-threatening injuries are evaluated and treated before proceeding with repair. Specifically, laparotomy to control intra-abdominal bleeding and treatment of bleeding from extremity injury are appropriate before thoracotomy. A complete neurologic examination before operation is imperative to assess and document any preoperative deficits. The approach to repair is through a fourth interspace left posterolateral thoracotomy. The site of injury is usually medial at the site of the ligamentum arteriosum. Multiple injuries are possible; thus, preoperative arteriography is essential in evaluating the location of injury. Distal control is obtained below the level of the hematoma, with care taken to preserve the maximal number of intercostal vessels to minimize the risk for injury to the artery of Adamkiewicz and subsequent spinal cord ischemia. Proximal control is obtained by encircling the left subclavian artery and then the aortic arch between the left carotid artery and left subclavian artery, with care taken to avoid the recurrent laryngeal and vagus nerves.

The simplest approach to repair is to "clamp and sew" (Fig. 68–7*A*) (Mattox et al, 1985). The aorta is clamped proximally and distally, the area of injury is débrided, and the aortic continuity is re-established by placing a Dacron graft or by primary anastomosis if the area of injury is limited. The advantages of this approach are simplicity and rapidity. The disadvantages are the severe increase in afterload created by the aortic cross-clamp application and the distal ischemia during the period of cross-clamp. Reported mortality rates range between 5% and 25%, with death related mostly to the severity of other injuries (von Oppell et al, 1994). The incidence of postoperative paraplegia ranges from 8% to 30% with this technique (Mauney et al, 1995; von Oppell et al, 1994).

Techniques that unload the left heart proximally and shunt blood distally include the insertion of a Gott shunt from the ascending aorta to the distal descending aorta (see Fig. 68–7*B*) and the institution of left heart bypass with a centrifugal pump and left atrial drainage and femoral arterial return (see Fig. 68–7*C*). Neither of these techniques necessitates systemic heparinization, although a small dose of heparin (5000 to 10,000 U) is frequently given. Cardiopulmonary bypass with systemic heparinization and an oxygenator can be used with femoral cannulation. Bleeding complications with heparinization can occur with either central nervous system injury or pulmonary contusion (Pate, 1998). Although good results have been reported using various techniques, left heart bypass has obvious physiologic advantages and can be used by both thoracic and trauma surgeons with facility (Feliciano, 1997; Rim et al, 1994).

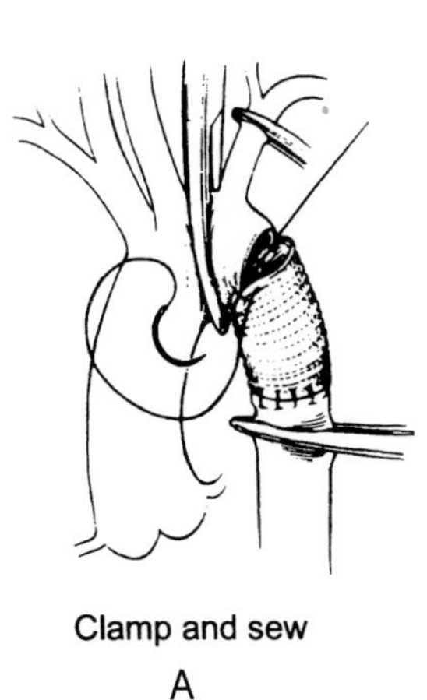

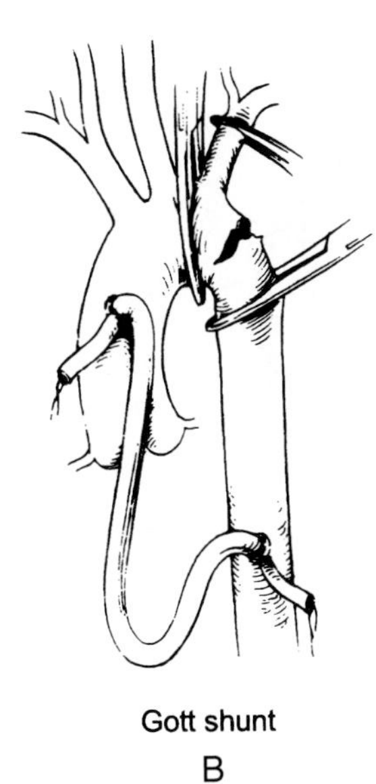

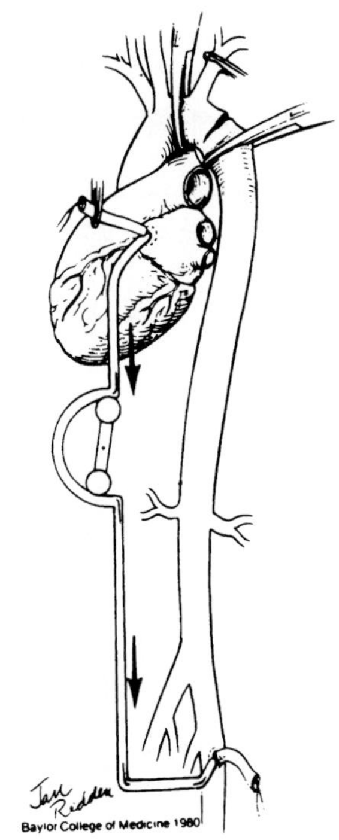

FIGURE 68–7 ■ Techniques for repair of a descending aortic rupture. *A*, Clamp and sew; *B*, Gott shunt; and *C*, Left-heart partial bypass.

The most devastating postoperative complication after aortic operation is paraplegia. The cause of paraplegia after aortic operation is related to preoperative, intraoperative, and postoperative factors (Table 68–2). The variable anatomy of the spinal cord blood supply plays a central role in the unpredictable occurrence of postoperative paraplegia (Fig. 68–8). There is no operative technique that can completely prevent the risk for paraplegia.

Ascending Aorta

These injuries are often fatal at the scene because of exsanguinating hemorrhage or cardiac tamponade. The ascending aorta is approached through a median sternotomy and requires cardiopulmonary bypass and use of a Dacron interposition graft (Mattox, 1989). When the injury extends into the arch, extension of the incision into the neck may aid in exposure. When the quality of the distal aorta is poor, performing the distal anastomosis under hypothermic circulatory arrest without applying a cross-clamp should be considered.

Innominate Artery

Blunt trauma produces proximal innominate artery injury at the level of the aortic arch. The repair is approached

TABLE 68–2 ■ **Paraplegia After Aortic Injury Repair**

INJURY FACTORS	OPERATIVE FACTORS
Anatomic location of aortic injury	Required occlusion of segmental arteries
Direct segmental artery injury	Length of aorta excluded
Direct radicular artery injury	Pharmacologic pressors required
Direct spinal artery injury	Intraoperative hypotension
Direct spinal cord injury	Required crossclamp time
Spinal canal compartment syndrome	Flow and blood pressure in aorta distal to crossclamp
PREOPERATIVE FACTORS	POSTOPERATIVE FACTORS
Anatomy of artery radicularis magna	Spinal cord swelling
Continuity of anterior spinal artery	Delayed occlusion of spinal cord arterial blood supply
Anatomy of segmental radicular arteries	Pharmacologically induced spasm of arterial blood supply to spinal cord
Caliber of spinal canal	
Perispinal collateral blood supply	
Blood alcohol levels	

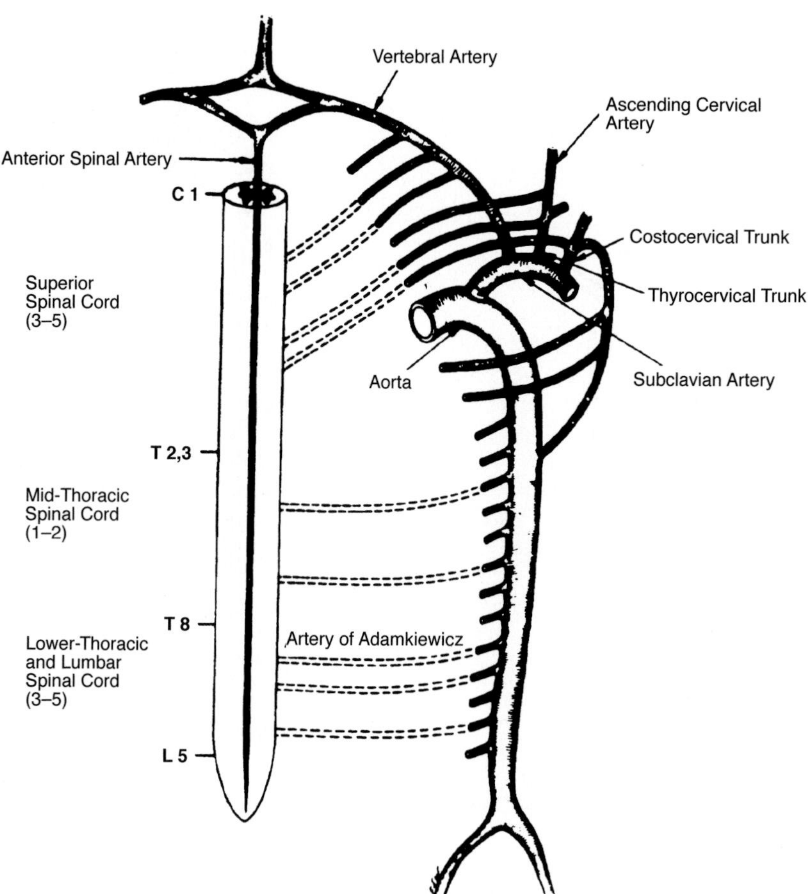

FIGURE 68–8 ■ Variable blood supply to the spinal cord.

through a median sternotomy to expose the ascending aorta. The area of injury is bypassed and then excluded. Neither cardiopulmonary bypass nor shunts are generally employed (Weinman et al, 1998). The proximal anastomosis is constructed first, by applying a side-biting clamp on the ascending aorta. A prosthetic graft of Dacron or polytetrafluoroethylene, 8 to 10 mm in diameter, is usually used (Johnston et al, 1993). The distal anastomosis is constructed by clamping the innominate artery distally, allowing retrograde flow through the bifurcation of subclavian and right carotid arteries. If necessary for exposure, the innominate vein can be ligated. The area of injury is oversewn with pledgeted sutures.

Subclavian Artery

Approach to the subclavian arteries is difficult because injury can be at the level of the aortic arch, thoracic outlet, or upper extremity. Proximal control is imperative because blood loss can be significant. The right subclavian artery is approached through a median sternotomy with cervical extension. The left subclavian artery can be approached with a left supraclavicular incision with proximal control obtained through a left fourth interspace anterior thoracotomy. Additionally, the clavicular head can be resected to gain exposure, although similar exposure may be gained with supraclavicular and infraclavicular incisions. Repair is best performed by clamping proximally and distally, débriding the injured portion, and creating an end-to-end anastomosis either primarily or with interposed, prosthetic material or saphenous vein (McCoy et al, 1997).

Left Carotid Artery

Blunt injury to the proximal left carotid artery is approached through a median sternotomy with a left cervical extension. Repair is similar to the technique that is described for the innominate artery. Cardiopulmonary bypass and shunts are generally not used. The area of injury is bypassed using an 8- to 10-mm prosthetic graft, and then the area of injury is oversewn proximally with pledgeted suture.

Pulmonary Artery and Veins

See the section Blunt Trauma to the Lung for a description of injury to the pulmonary artery and veins.

Vena Cava

Blunt injury to the superior vena cava or intrathoracic inferior vena cava is rarely an isolated injury. Superior vena cava injuries can be repaired by either primary or patch closure. Inferior vena cava injuries often necessitate the use of cardiopulmonary bypass to gain exposure. The injuries can be complex and require Dacron or bovine pericardial patch reconstruction.

Azygos Vein

Injury to the azygos vein is frequently associated with other intrathoracic injuries and is associated with a potential for significant blood loss. These injuries are managed through a right thoracotomy and vein ligation.

BLUNT TRAUMA TO THE THORACIC DUCT

Thoracic duct injury is rare after blunt trauma to the chest. It is usually overshadowed by associated life-threatening damage to other structures in the chest. Chylous leak after nonpenetrating trauma is usually attributed to hyperflexion-extension of the vertebral column with shearing of tethered lymphatics. Alternatively, sudden compression of lipemic and engorged mesenteric lymphatics, adjacent nodes, and the lower thoracic duct, aggravated by deformities associated with stretching and tearing motions, may also directly disrupt chyle-containing lymphatics. Rupture of the thoracic duct superior to the sixth thoracic vertebra generally results in a left-sided chylothorax; below that level, injury usually results in a right-sided chylothorax (Cariati et al, 1996).

Diagnosis

Traumatic injury to the thoracic duct may occur at any level along the course of the duct, making localization difficult. Skala and colleagues (1992) reported three patients who developed chylous leakage after major blunt trauma. In a patient with nonremitting right-sided chylothorax, lymphangioscintigraphy and conventional oil-contrast lymphography demonstrated disruption of the thoracic duct at the aortic hiatus, which eventually necessitated transpleural mediastinal ductal ligation. The other two patients had chylous retroperitoneum or chylous peritoneum, which was self-limited, although one patient died of multiple-organ failure from associated pulmonary contusions and cervical spine injuries.

Management

After the diagnosis is made, total parenteral nutrition or a fat-restricted diet should be started. Closed-tube thoracostomy should be performed for drainage. This nonoperative treatment should be continued for 2 to 3 weeks, and the lymphatic fistula will ideally close spontaneously. Surgical intervention is indicated if nonoperative management fails after 3 weeks or when the daily output exceeds 800 to 1000 mL. Ligation of the thoracic duct on the side of the leakage should be done. Intrathoracic identification of the leak may be aided by ingestion of a fatty meal 4 to 5 hours before thoracotomy or by instillation of olive oil through the nasogastric tube.

Graham and associates (1994) reported 10 cases of chylothorax, one of which was due to blunt trauma. VATS was used as the principal mode of therapy in these patients. Talc pleurodesis alone was used in eight patients, talc pleurodesis with clipping of the thoracic duct and application of fibrin glue was used in one patient, and in another patient, clipping of a pleural defect with application of fibrin glue was used.

Lymphatic–venous anastomoses have also been recommended (Cariati et al, 1996). Demonstration of long-term patency of these shunts, however, is rarely documented. The anatomy and management of thoracic duct injury are discussed in more detail in Chapter 44.

BLUNT TRAUMA TO THE ESOPHAGUS

Blunt injuries to the esophagus are rare, with an incidence among traumatized patients that is less than 0.1% (Kemmerer et al, 1961). In a review of 45 patients who sustained traumatic rupture of the esophagus, 75.5% of cases were due to gunshot wounds, 20% due to stab wounds, and 4.4% due to blunt trauma (Steinman et al, 1990). Although these injuries are uncommon, a high index of suspicion must be maintained. A delay in the diagnosis of thoracic esophageal perforation beyond 24 hours carries a high mortality rate. A chemical mediastinitis is incited with progression to multiple-organ failure. More than half of traumatic esophageal injuries are associated with tracheal injury (Beal et al, 1988; Nissen, 1980).

The cervical esophagus is the most commonly injured site in virtually all series. It has been diagnosed after boxing and forcible neck hyperextension (Latimer et al, 1991; Niezgoda et al, 1990). Thoracic esophageal disruption has been described with motor vehicle collisions (Micon et al, 1990). Rupture of the distal thoracic esophagus is an unusual injury after blunt abdominal trauma from a minor motor vehicle crash; an improperly positioned seat belt is presumed contributory.

Diagnosis

The diagnosis may be suggested on the initial chest radiograph by the presence of pneumomediastinum or pleural effusion. In both blunt and penetrating injuries, however, up to one third of patients have a normal initial chest radiograph (Glatterer et al, 1985).

Contrast esophagography, particularly when Gastrografin is used, is notoriously insensitive in making the diagnosis, with false-negative rates ranging from 0% to 50% (Attar et al, 1991; Symbas et al, 1980). If the diagnosis is entertained, it is best evaluated by a combination of esophageal endoscopy (Kemmerer et al, 1961) and barium esophagography when feasible. A chest CT scan with contrast studies confirms the diagnosis in certain situations. A pleural effusion containing high levels of amylase should be considered diagnostic in this setting.

Management

Although successful nonoperative management of small iatrogenic esophageal perforations has been reported, these data should not be considered applicable to the trauma patient. The extent of both penetrating and blunt esophageal injuries is much less predictable than it is in simple iatrogenic perforations. All traumatic esophageal injuries should be explored early. Cervical esophageal injuries may be débrided and closed primarily with drainage of the mediastinum. A right thoracotomy using the fourth or fifth intercostal space may be advantageous for

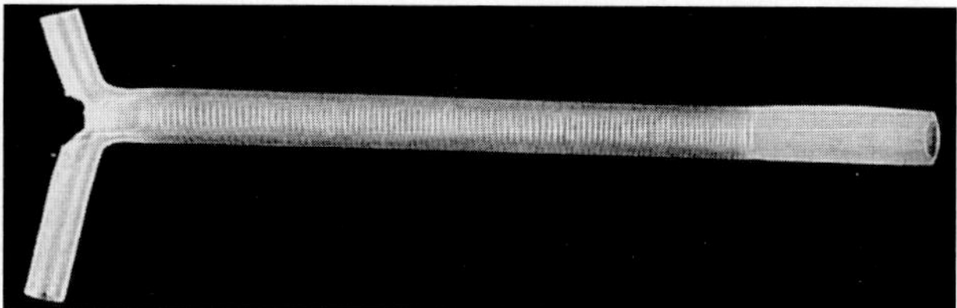

FIGURE 68–9 ■ T-tube (Research Medical, Inc., Salt Lake City, UT) for late esophageal perforations.

injuries to the upper or middle thoracic esophagus, and the sixth intercostal space on the left side is used for injuries of the distal esophagus.

When the injury involves less than half the circumference of the esophagus, suturing with ample drainage should be performed. In more extensive injuries involving more than half of the circumference of the esophagus, a total esophagectomy is the treatment of choice. In abdominal esophageal injuries, laparotomy, suture, and drainage should be done. Two-layered closure is achieved using 3–0 silk interrupted sutures for the mucosal and muscular layers. The suture line is usually reinforced using nearby structures, such as parietal pleura or gastric fundus in most instances. Occasionally, a flap fashioned from the diaphragm, pericardium, intercostal muscles, or omentum is used.

If primary esophageal closure cannot be satisfactorily attained, it may be possible to approximate the wound edges over a T-tube placed in the lumen of the esophagus through the perforation and then brought out the chest wall to convert the perforation to a controlled fistula (Fig. 68–9) (Abbott et al, 1970; Bufkin et al, 1996; Mansour and Wenger, 1992). This procedure may be combined with decompression gastrostomy and feeding jejunostomy. Nasogastric drainage combined with central hyperalimentation would be another alternative.

Placement of an esophageal T-tube in a lower-third injury should be precise (Fig. 68–10). The long arm is directed toward the stomach, with the short arm in the esophagus proximal to the site of injury. The T-tube should be brought out through a separate stab incision and secured in a lateral position away from the aorta. The tube remains in place for 2 to 3 weeks to allow development of a definite tract. There have been reports of aortic erosion from malpositioned T-tubes; hence, attention to these details is important.

Some authorities advocate exclusion and diversion for management of delayed esophageal perforations (Urschel et al, 1974). In selected circumstances, this option may be considered. Careful attention should be directed to creation of the lateral cervical esophagostomy to ensure diversion of the oropharyngeal secretions. The need for a second operation to establish cervical esophageal continuity and the creation of a distal esophageal stricture after temporary banding are undesirable consequences of exclusion and diversion. Successful exclusion with late resumption of function has been achieved by Lewis and Sisler (1985) using Rummell tourniquets and catheter drainage.

Pharyngeal esophageal perforation that is secondary to blunt neck trauma is an uncommon injury that can cause serious morbidity and mortality if not recognized and treated. Pharyngeal perforation that is secondary to blunt trauma sustained while boxing is reported. A review of the world literature revealed 10 patients with pharyngeal esophageal perforation that was secondary to blunt neck trauma (Niezgoda et al, 1990). Analysis of these patients indicates that perforations that are smaller than 2 cm and limited to the pharynx may be treated conservatively

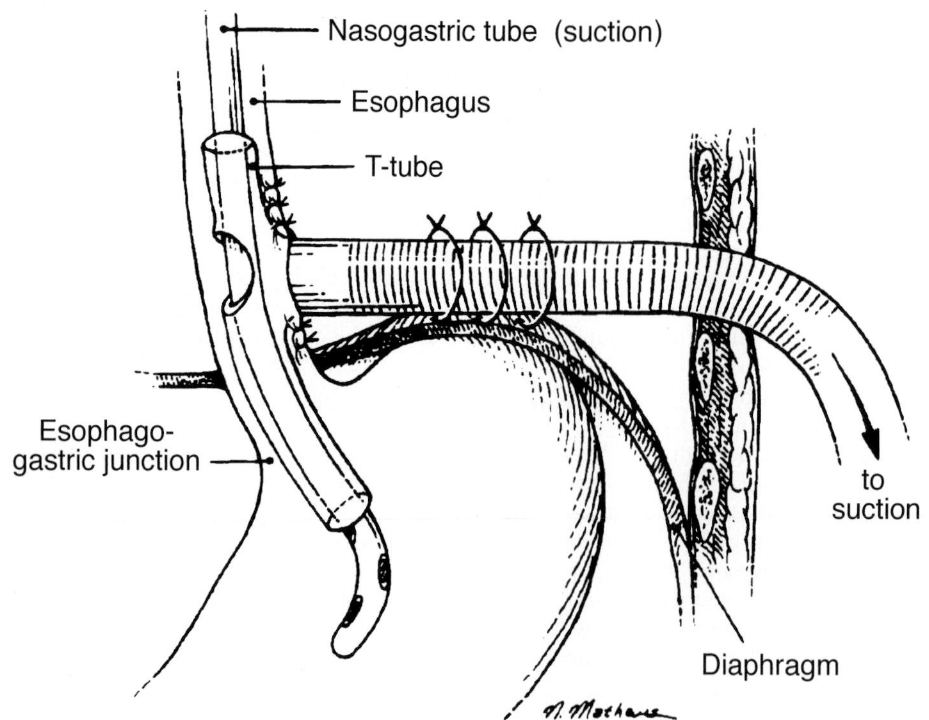

FIGURE 68–10 ■ T-tube placed within esophageal perforation, fixed to the diaphragm, and exiting the chest wall.

with close observation. Large perforations and those that extend to the esophageal inlet or involve the esophagus exclusively are best treated surgically.

Because of the association with tracheal injuries, tracheoesophageal fistula formation may result from esophageal trauma. These fistulas are found in the distal trachea. Initial presentation is usually one of subcutaneous emphysema followed by aspiration when the patient begins to take oral feedings. This repair should include débridement and primary closure of both the trachea and the esophagus, with interposition of intercostal muscle flap or pericardial flap between the two repairs.

COMMENTS AND CONTROVERSIES

The authors have thoroughly stressed the importance of adequate analgesia following blunt chest trauma. Simple rib fracture can be a major injury in the elderly with limited lung function. Local nerve blocks above and below the injury or epidural anesthesia with narcotic or local anesthetic can dramatically improve pain control and pulmonary function. Effective pain control and judicious fluid administration can often avoid the need for mechanical ventilation even in a flail chest injury. Early tracheostomy for patients with major injuries is also stressed. Early tracheostomy maximizes patient comfort and decreases the likelihood of subsequent laryngeal or subglottic stenosis from prolonged translaryngeal intubation.

In their discussion of blunt injury to the lung, the authors stress the importance of conservative therapy and lung preservation techniques if open exploration is required. The lung has a remarkable capability to heal injury of contusion and laceration resulting in functional parenchyma. Resection should also be avoided even if lobar or pulmonary arteries must be sacrificed to control bleeding.

In their discussion of cardiac and great vessel injuries, the authors thoroughly discuss current techniques of diagnosis and management. Great vessel injuries are increasingly and precisely documented by contrast computed tomography scan or magnetic resonance imaging. The discussion of descending aortic injury outlines the controversy between the no-bypass, "clamp and sew" technique and the more commonly employed techniques of left heart bypass during aortic cross clamp and repair. The authors stress the fact that there is no operative technique that can completely eliminate the risk of postoperative paraplegia. The authors correctly stress the importance of early exploration and repair of all esophageal perforations in the trauma patient. Pre-emptive repair and drainage minimizes the likelihood and consequence of subsequent cervical or mediastinal sepsis as a result of the esophageal disruption being managed conservatively.

G.A.P.

■ REFERENCES

Abbott OA, Mansour KA, Logan WD Jr et al: Atraumatic so-called "spontaneous" rupture of the esophagus: A review of 47 personal cases with comments on a new method of surgical therapy. J Thorac Cardiovasc Surg 59:67–83, 1970.

Akins C, Buckley M, Daggett W: Acute traumatic disruption of the thoracic aorta: A 10 year experience. Ann Thorac Surg 31:305, 1981.

Arom KV, Griver FL, Richardson JD, Trinkle JK: Post-traumatic empyema. Ann Thorac Surg 23:254, 1977.

Attar S, Hankins JR, Suer CM et al: Esophageal perforation: A therapeutic challenge. Ann Thorac Surg 50:45, 1991.

Barioni R, Renzo C, Actis Dato C: Surgical stabilization of the flail chest (Letter). Ann Thorac Surg 54:397–398, 1992.

Baxter B, Moore E, Moore F: A plea for sensible management of myocardial contusion. Am J Surg 158:557–562, 1989.

Beal SL, Pottmeyer EW, Pisso S: Esophageal perforation following external blunt trauma. J Trauma 28:1425, 1988.

Beall AC, Crawford HW, Debakey ME: Considerations in the management of acute traumatic hemothorax. J Thorac Cardiovasc Surg 52:351, 1966.

Blair E: Pulmonary barriers to oxygen transport in chest trauma. Am Surg 42:55, 1976.

Breasted JH: The Edwin Smith Surgical Papyrus, Vol 1. Chicago, University of Chicago Press, 1930.

Brewer LA, Burford TH: Special types of thoracic wounds. In Medical Department: U.S. Army Surgery in World War II, Thoracic Surgery, 38th ed. Washington, D.C., U.S. Government Printing Office, 1965, p 269.

Brookes J, Dunn R, Rogers I: Sternal fractures: A retrospective analysis of 272 cases. J Trauma 35:46–54, 1993.

Bufkin BR, Miller JI, Mansour KA: Esophageal perforation: Emphasis on management. Ann Thorac Surg 61:1447–52, 1996.

Cachecho R, Grindlinger G, Lee V: The clinical significance of myocardial contusion. J Trauma 33:68–73, 1992.

Calhoon J, Hoffman T, Trinkle J et al: Management of blunt rupture of the heart. J Trauma 26:495–502, 1986.

Cariati A, Taviani M, Pescio G et al: Management of thoracic duct complex lesions (chylothorax): Experience in 16 patients. Lymphology 29:83–86, 1996.

Carr RE: Injuries to the pulmonary parenchyma and vasculature. In Daughtry DC (ed): Thoracic Trauma. Boston, Little, Brown, 1980.

Chopra P, Kroncke G, Berkoff H et al: Pulmonary contusion: A problem in blunt chest trauma. Wisc Med J 76:1, 1977.

Cicala R, Voella G, Fox T: Epidural analgesia in thoracic trauma: Effects of lumbar morphine and thoracic (bupivacaine) on the pulmonary function. Crit Care Med 18:229–231, 1990.

Collins MP, Shuck JM, Wachtel TL et al: Early decortication after thoracic trauma. Arch Surg 113:44, 1978.

Connolly J, Dehne R: Nonunion of the clavicle and thoracic outlet syndrome. J Trauma 29:1127–1133, 1989.

Coselli JS, Mattox KL, Beall AC: Re-evaluation of early evacuation of clotted hemothorax. Am J Surg 148:785, 1984.

DeMuth WE Jr, Smith JM: Pulmonary contusion. Am Surg 109:819, 1965.

Eddy AC, Luna GK, Copass MK: Factors affecting the incidence of empyema thoracic in patient undergoing emergent closed tube thoracostomy for thoracic trauma. Am J Surg 157:494, 1989.

Engelman RM, Boyd AD, Blum M et al: Multiple circumscribed pulmonary hematomas masquerading as metastatic carcinoma. Ann Thorac Surg 15:291, 1973.

Erikson D, Shinozaki T, Beekman E et al: Relationship of arterial blood gases and pulmonary radiographs to the degree of pulmonary contusion. J Trauma 11:689, 1971.

Fabian T, Cicala R, Croce M et al: A prospective evaluation of myocardial contusion: Correlation of significant arrhythmias and cardiac output with CPK-MB measurements. J Trauma 32:653–657, 1991.

Fabian T, Davis K, Gavant M et al: Prospective study of blunt aortic injury: Helical CT diagnostic and antihypertensive therapy reduces rupture. Am Surg 227:666–677, 1998.

Fabian T, Mangiante E, Patterson R: Myocardial contusion in blunt trauma: Clinical characteristics, means of diagnosis, and implications for patient management. J Trauma 28:50–57, 1988.

Fallon WF Jr, Wears RL: Prophylactic antibiotics for the prevention of infectious complications including empyema following tube thoracostomy for trauma: Results of meta analysis. J Trauma 33:110, 1992.

Feliciano D: Trauma to the aorta and major vessels. Chest Surg Clin N Am 7:305–323, 1997.

Fischer R, Oria R, Mattox K: Conservative management of aortic lacerations due to blunt trauma. J Trauma 30:1562, 1990.

Freedland M, Wilson R, Bender J, Levison M: The management of flail check injury: Factors affecting outcome. J Trauma 30:1460–1468, 1990.

Fulda G, Brathwaite C, Rodriguez A et al: Blunt traumatic rupture of the heart and pericardium: A ten year experience (1979–1989). J Trauma 31:167–173, 1991.

Gaillard M, Herve C, Mandin L, Raynaud P: Mortality prognostic factors in chest injury. J Trauma 30:93–96, 1990.

Garcia V, Gatschall C, Eichelberger M, Bowman L: Rib fractures in children: A marker for severe trauma. J Trauma 30:695–700, 1990.

Ginzburg E, Dygert J, Para-Davila E et al: Coronary artery stenting for occlusive dissection after blunt chest trauma. J Trauma 45:157–161, 1998.

Glatterer MS Jr, Toon RS, Ellestad C et al: Management of blunt and penetrating external esophageal trauma. J Trauma 25:784, 1985.

Glinz W: Chest Trauma: Diagnosis and Treatment. West Berlin, Springer-Verlag, 1981.

Graham DD, McGahren ED, Tribble CG et al: Use of video-assisted thoracic surgery in the treatment of chylothorax. Ann Thorac Surg 57(6):1507–1511; discussion 1511–1512, 1994.

Graham JM, Mattox Kl, Beall AC: Penetrating trauma of the lung. J Trauma 19:655, 1979.

Gray AR, Harrison WH, Couves CM et al: Penetrating injuries to the chest: Clinical results in the management of 769 patients. Am J Surg 100:709, 1960.

Groskin S, Maresca M, Heitzman RE: Thoracic trauma. In Moore EE, Mattox KL, Feliciano DV (eds): Trauma. Norwalk, CT, Appleton & Lange, 1988.

Hankins J, Attar S, Turndy S et al: Differential diagnosis of pulmonary parenchymal changes in thoracic trauma. Am Surg 39:309, 1973.

Harley D, Mena I: Cardiac and vascular sequelae of sternal fractures. J Trauma 26:553–555, 1986.

Hochberg LA: Thoracic Surgery Before the 20th Century. New York, Vantage, New York, 1960.

Homer (Alexander Pope, translator): Homer's Poetical Works. The Iliad: Book XVI. New York, Leavitt & Allen, pp 362–363.

Hughes RK: Thoracic trauma. Ann Thorac Surg 1:778, 1965.

Johnson M, Shah H, Harris V et al: Comparison of digital subtraction and cut film arteriography in the evaluation of suspected thoracic aortic injury. J Vasc Intervent Radiol 8:799–807, 1997.

Johnston R, Wall M, Mattox K: Innominate artery trauma: A thirty year experience. J Vasc Surg 17:134–140, 1993.

Jongewaard W, Coghill T, Landercasper J: Neurologic consequences after traumatic asphyxia. J Trauma 32:28–31, 1992.

Kato K, Kushimoto S, Mashiko K et al: Blunt traumatic rupture of the heart on experience in Tokyo. J Trauma 36:859–864, 1994.

Kearney P, Smith W, Johnson S et al: Use of transesophageal echocardiography in the evaluation of traumatic aortic injury. J Trauma 24:696–701, 1993.

Kemmerer NT, Exkert WG, Gathright JB et al: Patterns of thoracic injuries in fatal accidents. J Trauma 1:595, 1961.

Kirsch M, Behredt D, Orringer M: The treatment of acute traumatic rupture of the aorta. Ann Surg 184:308, 1976.

Kish G, Kozloff L, Joseph WL et al: Indications for early thoracotomy in the management of chest trauma. Ann Thorac Surg 22:23, 1976.

Kissane R: Traumatic heart disease. Circulation 6:241, 1952.

Kitchens J, Richardson J: Open fixation of sternal fracture. Surg Gynecol Obstet 177:423–424, 1993.

Landreneay R, Hinson J, Hazelring S: Strut fixation of an extensive flail chest. Ann Thorac Surg 51:473–475, 1991.

Latimer EA, Clevenger FW, Osler TM: Tear of the cervical esophagus following hyperextension from manual traction: Case report. J Trauma 31:1448–1449, 1991.

Ledley G, Yazdanfar S, Friedman O, Kotler M: Acute thrombotic coronary occlusion secondary to chest trauma treated with intracoronary thrombolysis. Am Heart J 123:518–521, 1992.

Lee J, Harris JH, Duke JH, Williams JS: Non-correlation between thoracic skeletal injuries and acute traumatic aortic tear. J Trauma 43:400-404, 1997.

Lee R, Bass S, Morris J: Three or more rib fractures as an indicator for transfer to a level I trauma center: A population based study. J Trauma 30:689–694, 1990.

Lewis RJ, Sisler GE: Reversible total esophageal exclusion. Ann Thorac Surg 39:476, 1985.

Lilienthal H: Thoracic Surgery: The Surgical Treatment of Thoracic Diseases. Philadelphia, WB Saunders, 1926.

Lo Cicero J, Mattox KL: Epidemiology of chest trauma. Surg Clin North Am 69(1):15, 1989.

Lo Curto JH Jr, Tischler CD, Swan KG et al: Tube thoracostomy and trauma: Antibiotics or not? J Trauma 26:1067, 1986.

Mansour KA, Wenger RK: T-tube management of late esophageal perforations. Surg Gynecol Obstet 175:571–572, 1992.

Martin T, Flynn T, Rowlands B et al: Blunt cardiac rupture. J Trauma 24:287–290, 1984.

Mattox K: Approaches to trauma involving the major vessels of the thorax. Surg Clin North Am 69:77, 1989.

Mattox K, Flint L, Carrico C et al: Blunt cardiac injury (Editorial). J Trauma 33:649–650, 1992.

Mattox K, Holtzman M, Pickard L et al: Clamp/repair: A safe technique for treatment of blunt injury to descending thoracic aorta. Ann Thorac Surg 40:456–469, 1985.

Mauney M, Blackbourne L, Langenburg S et al: Prevention of spinal cord injury after repair of the thoracic or thoracoabdominal aorta. Ann Thorac Surg 59:245–252, 1995.

Mayberry J, Trunkey D: The fractured rib in chest wall trauma: Trauma of the chest. Chest Surg Clin N Am 7:239–261, 1997.

McCoy D, Weiman D, Pate J et al: Subclavian artery injuries. Am Surg 63:761–764, 1997.

McLean R, Devitt J, Dubbin J, McLellan B: Incidence of abnormal RNA studies and dysrhythmias in patients with blunt chest trauma. J Trauma 31:968–970, 1991.

Meade RH: A History of Thoracic Surgery. Springfield, IL, Charles C. Thomas, 1961.

Micon L, Geis L, Sidreys H et al: Rupture of the distal thoracic esophagus following blunt trauma: Case report. J Trauma 30:214–217, 1990.

Miller F, Richardson J, Thomas H: Role of CT in the diagnosis of major arterial injury after blunt thoracic trauma. Surgery 106:596, 1989.

Mirvis S, Bidwell J, Buddemeyer E: Value of chest radiography in excluding traumatic aortic injury. Radiology 163:487, 1987.

Mirvis S, Shanmuganathan K, Miller B et al: Traumatic aortic injury: Diagnosis with contrast enhanced thoracic CT. Five year experience at a major trauma center. Radiology 200:413–422, 1996.

Morant M, Lefrak A, Akl B: Traumatic rupture of the interventricular septum and tricuspid valve: Case report. J Trauma 31:134–136, 1991.

Niezgoda JA, McMenamin P, Graeber GM: Pharyngoesophageal perforation after blunt trauma. Ann Thorac Surg 50:615–617, 1990.

Nissen R: Total pneumonectomy. Ann Thorac Surg 29:390, 1980.

Nunez D, Rivas L, McKenney K et al: Helical CT of traumatic arterial injuries. Am J Roentgenol 170:1621–1626, 1998.

Paget S: The Surgery of the Chest. London, John Wright, 1896.

Pate J: Modern management of traumatic rupture of the aortic isthmus. Ann Thorac Surg 66:611–612, 1998.

Pate J, Fabian T, Walker W: Traumatic rupture of the aortic isthmus: An emergency? World J Surg 19:119–126, 1995.

Peck A: Aristotle: De Partisbus Animalum. Cambridge, MA, Harvard University Press, 1937.

Pepe P, Potkin R, Reus D et al: Clinical predictors of the adult respiratory distress syndrome. Am J Surg 144:124, 1982.

Pevec W, Udekwu A, Peitzman A: Blunt rupture of the myocardium. Ann Thorac Surg 48:139–142, 1989.

Poole GV: Fracture of the upper ribs and injury to the great vessels. Surg Gynecol Obstet 169:275, 1989.

Pretie R, Chilcott M: Blunt trauma to the heart and great vessels. N Engl J Med 336:626–632, 1997.

Raptopoulos V: Chest CT for aortic injury: Maybe not for everyone. Am J Roentgenol 162:1053, 1994.

Ratliff JL, Fletcher JR, Kopriva CJ et al: Pulmonary contusion: A continuing management problem. J Thorac Cardiovasc Surg 62:638, 1971.

Rehn L: Ueber penetrirende Herzwunden und Herznaht. Arch Clin Chir 55:315, 1897.

Rim F, Moore G, Moore F: Trauma surgeons can render definitive surgical care for major thoracic injuries. J Trauma 36:871–876, 1994.

Rozycki G, Ochsner M, Jaffin J, Champion H: Prospective evaluation of surgeons' use of ultrasound in the evaluation of trauma patients. J Trauma 34:516–526, 1993.

Saletta S, Lederman E, Fein S et al: Transesophageal echocardiography for the initial evaluation of the widened mediastinum in trauma patients. J Trauma 39:137–142, 1995.

Sampson L, Britton J, Eldrop-Jorgensen J: The neurovascular outcome of scapulothoracic dissociation. J Vasc Surg 17:1083–1089, 1993.

Sherman RT: Experience with 472 civilian penetrating wounds of the chest. Milit Med 131:63, 1966.

Shorr R, Crittenden M, Indeck M et al: Blunt thoracic trauma: Analysis of SIS patients. Ann Surg 206:200–205, 1987.

Skala J, Witte C, Bruna J et al: Chyle leakage after blunt trauma. Lymphology 25(2):62–8, 1992.

Steinman E, Utiyama EM, Pires PW, Birolini D: Traumatic wounds of the esophagus. Rev Hosp Clin Fac Med 45:127–131, 1990.

Stevens E, Templeton A: Traumatic nonpenetrating lung contusion. Radiology 85:247, 1965.

Sturm J, Luxenberg M, Moundy B: Does sternal fracture increase the risk for aortic rupture? Ann Thorac Surg 48:697, 1989.

Svennevig J, Bugge-Asperheim B, Birkeland S et al: Efficacy of steroids in the treatment of lung contusion. Acta Chir Scand Suppl 499:87, 1980.

Symbas N, Bongiorno P, Symbas P: Blunt cardiac rupture: The utility of emergency department ultrasound. Ann Thorac Surg 67:1274, 1999.

Symbas P: Traumatic heart disease. Curr Probl Cardiol 16:539–582, 1991.

Symbas P, Hatcher CR Jr, Vlasis SE: Esophageal gunshot injuries. Ann Surg 191:709, 1980.

Thal ER, Ramenofsky MI, Aprahamian C: Advanced Trauma Life Support Course for Physicians, Subcommittee Trauma, 1987–1988. Chicago, American College of Surgeons, 1989.

Thompson D, Flynn T, Miller P, Fischer R: The significance of scapular fractures. J Trauma 25:974–977, 1985.

Trerotala S: Can helical CT replace aortography in thoracic trauma? Radiology 197:13, 1995.

Trunkey D: Chest wall injuries. In Blaisdell F, Trunkey D (eds): Cervico Thoracic Trauma, 2nd ed. New York, Thieme Medical Publishers, 1994, pp 190–214.

Urschel HC Jr, Razzuk MA, Wood RE et al: Esophageal perforation: Exclusion and diversion in continuity. Ann Surg 179:587, 1974.

von Oppell U, Dunne T, De Groot M, Zilla P: Traumatic aortic rupture; Twenty year metaanalysis of mortality and risk of paraplegia. Ann Thorac Surg 58:585–593, 1994.

Wagner RB, Crawford WO Jr, Schimpf PP: Classification of parenchymal injuries of the lung. Radiology 167:77–82, 1988.

Weinman D, McCoy D, Haan C et al: Blunt injuries of the brachiocephalic artery. Am Surg 64:383–387, 1998.

Westermark N: A roentgenological investigation into traumatic lung changes arisen through blast violence to the thorax. Acta Radiol (Stockholm) 22:331, 1941.

Wigle R, Moran J: Spontaneous healing of a traumatic thoracic aortic tear: Case report. J Trauma 31:280, 1991.

Wiot J: The radiographic manifestations of blunt chest trauma. JAMA 231:500, 1975.

Wisner DH: A stepwise logistic regression analysis of factors affecting morbidity and mortality after thoracic trauma: Effect of epidural analgesia. J Trauma 30:799–805, 1990.

Wisner DH: Trauma to the chest. In Sabiston DC, Spencer FC (eds): Surgery of the Chest, 6th ed. Philadelphia, WB Saunders, 1995, pp 456–493.

Withington ET (translator): Hippocrates, Vol 3. Cambridge MA, Harvard University Press, 1959, pp 307–313.

Wojcik J, Morgan A: Sternal fractures: The natural history. Ann Emerg Med 17:912–914, 1988.

Wolfe WG, Sabiston DC Jr: Pulmonary embolism. Major Probl Clin Surg 25:1, 1980.

Woodridge J: The normal mediastinum in blunt traumatic rupture of the thoracic aorta and brachiocephalic arteries. J Emerg Med 8:467, 1990.

Ziegler D, Agarwal N: The morbidity and mortality of rib fractures. J Trauma 37:975–979, 1994.

CHAPTER **69**

Traumatic Diaphragmatic Rupture

Stanley C. Fell

Advances in the logistics of evacuation, triage, and resuscitation of trauma victims have increased the number of viable patients receiving hospital care. As a result, traumatic diaphragmatic rupture (TDR) is being reported with increasing frequency. Although TDR may be discovered and treated during emergency laparotomy or thoracotomy, it may not be diagnosed in cases in which urgent surgery is not required because of lack of sensitivity of the diagnostic modalities used. TDR inevitably results in traumatic diaphragmatic hernia (TDH), either immediately or over a course of time varying from days to years after the initial injury. If TDR is not recognized, the TDH that follows may have catastrophic consequences.

HISTORICAL NOTE

Reid, in 1840, reported autopsy findings of gangrenous colon in the left chest after TDH; he credited Sennertus with first reporting, in 1541, a case of TDH after a self-inflicted stab wound 7 months before death. At autopsy, gangrenous stomach was found within the left chest. Paré, in 1579 (Bowditch, 1853), reported the autopsy finding in a French artillery captain who, after surviving an abdominal gunshot wound, died 8 months later of gangrenous colon that had herniated through a fingertip-sized defect in the left hemidiaphragm. Bowditch made the antemortem diagnosis of left TDH in a man who sustained a crushing injury of the chest on the basis of displacement of the heart, absent breath sounds on auscultation, and audible bowel sounds in the chest. He found 88 previously reported cases in the literature before 1846. Riolfi, in 1886 (Hedblom, 1925), repaired a stab wound of the left hemidiaphragm in which omentum prolapsed through the chest wall. Naumann, in 1888, made a preoperative diagnosis of TDH, but the patient died after attempted repair. Walker, in 1889, reported the first successful laparotomy for TDH after a crushing injury caused by a falling log.

■ *HISTORICAL REFERENCES*

Bowditch H: Diaphragmatic hernia. Buffalo Med Surg J 9:65–94, 1853.

Hedblom C: Diaphragmatic hernia. JAMA 85:947–953, 1925.

Naumann G: Diaphragmatic hernia; laparotomy; died. Hygea 5:524–528, 1888.

Reid J: Case of diaphragmatic hernia produced by a penetrating wound. Edinburgh Med Surg J 53:104–108, 1840.

Walker E: Diaphragmatic hernia. JAMA 35:778, 1900.

INCIDENCE

TDR has been reported to occur in 0.8% to 1.6% of cases of blunt trauma and 10% to 15% of cases of penetrating trauma requiring hospital admission (Boulanger et al, 1993; Rosati, 1998; Rizoli et al, 1994). The actual incidence may be higher, because the diagnosis is missed on initial evaluation in 7% to 66% of multiple injury cases (Guth et al, 1995; Shapiro et al, 1996). Of patients undergoing laparotomy or thoracotomy for trauma, 6% have TDR (Shah et al, 1995).

ETIOLOGY

The relative frequency of blunt versus penetrating trauma causing TDR varies with the time period and the demography whence the report originates. In the pastoral era of the 19th century, excepting war wounds, falls, and crushing injuries were the common causes of TDR. In inner-city areas, where guns and knives are commonly used to settle disputes, penetrating wounds may be more common than are high-speed vehicular accidents as causes of TDR (Estrera et al, 1979). Overall, motor vehicle accidents account for 75% of cases of TDR (Shah et al, 1995). Gunshot and stab wounds account for 25% of cases. Rare causes are iatrogenic injury such as faulty placement of chest tubes, disruptions of closure of diaphragmatic incisions, and failure to adequately close these incisions after esophageal and other transdiaphragmatic surgery (Fig. 69–1).

MECHANISM OF INJURY

TDR must be considered in patients with stab wounds that traverse the fourth intercostal space anteriorly to the 12th rib posteriorly (Fig. 69–2). Gunshot wounds are entirely unpredictable and may injure the diaphragm through any point of truncal entry. In Wiencek's series (1986) of 190 cases, bilateral TDRs were present in 19 (21%) of 89 patients with gunshot wounds, 10 of which were due to a single wound and 9 to multiple wounds. Of 65 patients with stab wounds, 6 had bilateral injuries from multiple stab wounds. Almost two thirds (64%) of gunshot wounds causing diaphragm injury entered through the abdomen and similarly almost two thirds (62%) of stab wounds causing diaphragmatic injury entered the chest. Single stab wounds usually penetrate the left hemidiaphragm because most assailants are right handed. Multiple stab and gunshot wounds are associated with an increased incidence of bilateral TDR.

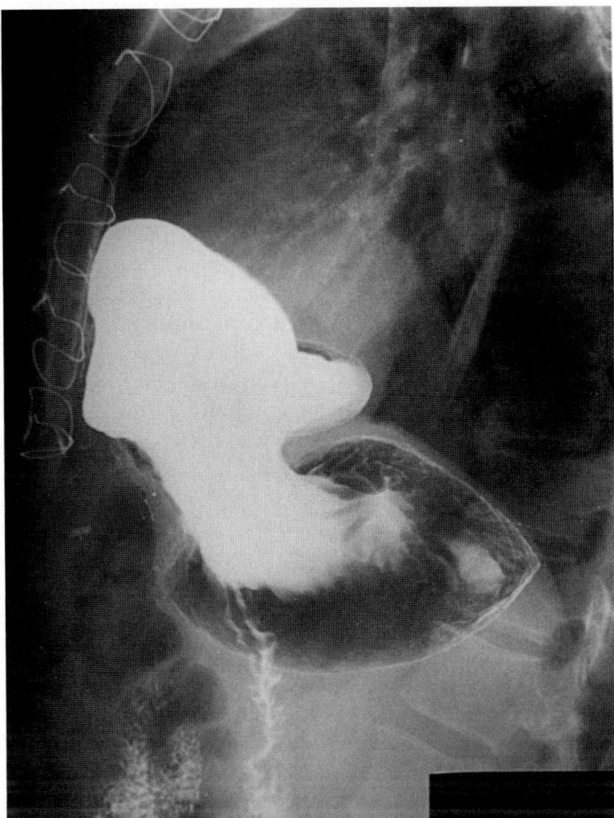

FIGURE 69–1 ■ Gastric obstruction 2 years following transdiaphragmatic placement of a gastroepiploic arterial graft to the right coronary artery. (Courtesy of Keith Naunheim, MD.)

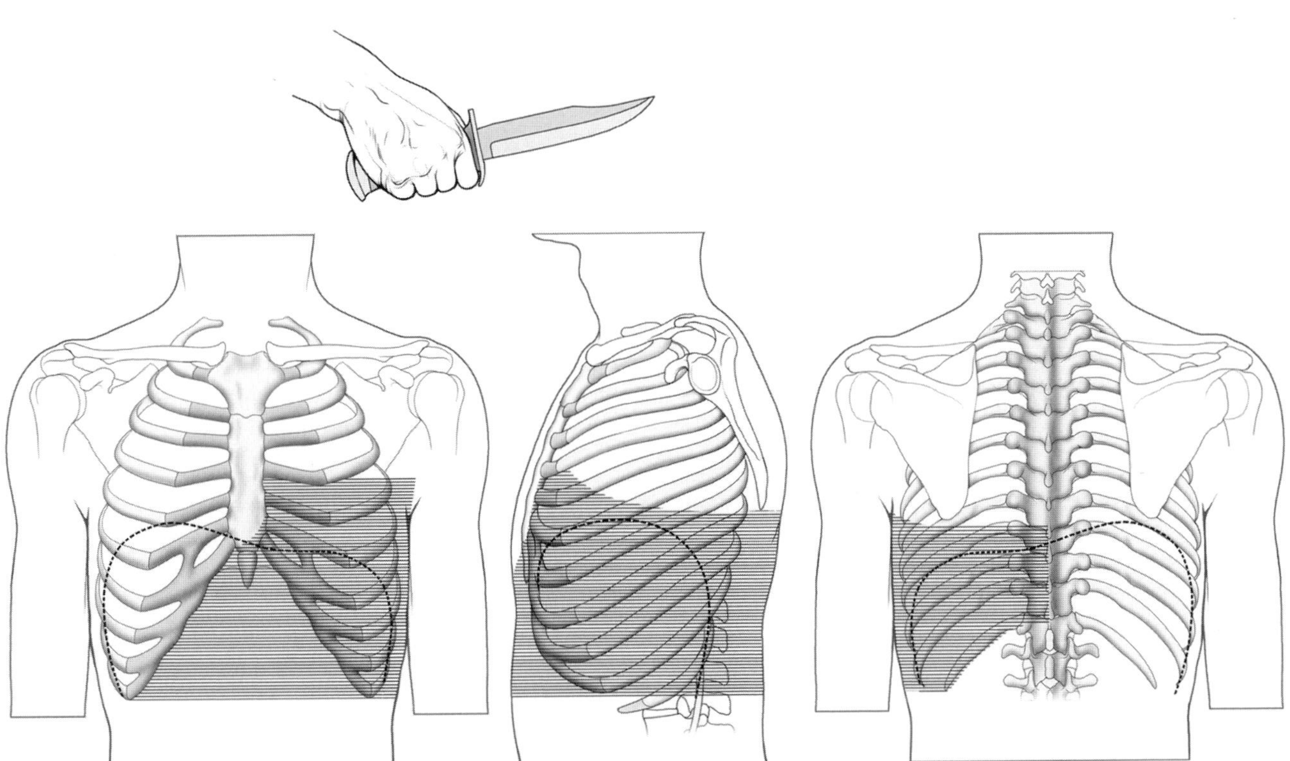

FIGURE 69–2 ■ Left diaphragm is vulnerable to stab wounds from the fourth interspace to the 12th rib. (Modified from Madden M, Paull D, Shires GT et al: Occult diaphragmatic injury from stab wounds to the lower chest and abdomen. J Trauma 29:293, 1989.)

Although the early series of Carter (1951) and Hood (1971) reported that TDR was overwhelmingly left sided (95% and 88%, respectively), Shah's review (1995) of 980 cases noted left-sided rupture in 65.5% of cases, right-sided rupture in 24.2%, bilateral rupture in 1.5%, and intrapericardial rupture in 0.9%, with 4.9% of cases unclassified.

In a review of right-sided blunt TDR in 1968, Epstein and Lempke noted that many did not survive long enough to reach a hospital for diagnosis and treatment. Because autopsy studies of trauma victims who die before reaching the hospital demonstrate an essentially equal incidence of right- and left-sided rupture, and right-sided TDRs are less common in hospital admissions, it would appear that right-sided TDR has a higher prehospital mortality rate (Boulanger et al, 1993; Estrera et al, 1979).

The mechanism of TDR caused by blunt trauma is still entirely speculative. To explain why left-sided injuries are more common, it had been theorized that the liver serves as a protective buffer for the right hemidiaphragm, diminishing the transmission of pressure from the abdomen to the thorax in cases of frontal impact (Mansour, 1997). It had also been postulated that the left hemidiaphragm is more susceptible to rupture than the right because of inherent weakness at points of embryologic fusion (Carter et al, 1951).

Kearney and colleagues (1989) studied the site of vehicular impact in motor vehicle accidents in relation to the site of TDR and concluded that victims of side-impact motor vehicle accidents were three times more likely to have TDR than those in front-impact accidents. They suggested that deformity of the chest wall and shearing force on the diaphragm are responsible for TDR in side-impact injuries.

PATHOPHYSIOLOGY

Acute Phase

In the acute phase of TDR, clinical signs may be obscured by those of associated injuries, present in almost 100% of cases. They are head, neck, and central nervous system, 10% to 40%; cardiothoracic, 20% to 60%; musculoskeletal, 30% to 40%; and intra-abdominal, 60% to 100% (Rosati, 1998). Hood (1971) noted in his collected series an average of 1.6 injuries per patient, the most common being rib fractures, skeletal fractures, and ruptured spleen.

Nevertheless, abdominal or thoracic pain, shoulder pain, respiratory insufficiency, hemopneumothorax, mediastinal shift, and scaphoid abdomen associated with diminished or absent breath sounds on chest auscultation suggest diaphragmatic injury. Severe respiratory insufficiency and hypotension may result from compression of the lung and mediastinal structures by dilated viscera in the chest. This situation has been aptly termed *tension enterothorax* (Wiencek et al, 1986).

The location of the tear in blunt TDR varies in different series; some report the highest incidence in the posterolateral portion of the left leaf of the diaphragm, whereas others note the greatest frequency of tears to be in the anterolateral portion (Mansour, 1997). Boulanger (1993), reporting on 80 cases, noted a random distribution of tears, with visceral herniation in 58% of left-sided and 19% of right-sided blunt TDR. All of the right-sided TDRs had associated intra-abdominal injury necessitating surgical repair, whereas 23% of those with the left-sided tears had no intra-abdominal injuries but did have associated skeletal fractures.

Intra-abdominal injuries are more commonly associated with right-sided than left-sided blunt TDR, thus leading to earlier laparotomy. Liver laceration and hepatic vein and inferior vena cava injuries are more prevalent in right-sided TDR. Liver and colon herniation may occur. Thoracic aortic rupture (juxtaductal) occurred in approximately 10% of cases of blunt TDR, both right- and left-sided (Rizoli et al, 1994). The mortality rate in the acute phase has been reported to be 20% to 40% and is primarily due to the associated injuries (Rosati, 1998).

Penetrating injuries of the diaphragm may not be initially associated with organ herniation. Healing is, however, unlikely because of rhythmic muscular contraction of the diaphragm with respiration and the pressure differential between the abdomen (positive pressure) and the thorax (subatmospheric pressure). Inevitably, a tag of omentum insinuates itself into the thorax, and visceral herniation subsequently occurs.

Interval Phase

If the TDR is not diagnosed and treated by laparotomy or thoracotomy during the acute phase of injury, the interval phase may be relatively asymptomatic and TDH is discovered only by serendipitous incidental radiography (Carter et al, 1951). In other cases, the patient may have symptoms that suggest peptic ulcer, biliary tract disease, angina, or subacute intestinal obstruction.

Phase of Obstruction or Strangulation

Carter and co-workers (1951) reported that 85% of patients develop signs of obstruction or strangulation within 3 years of injury; obstruction has been reported as late as 45 years after injury. The clinical picture is that of abdominal and chest pain and gastric or colonic obstruction. If the stomach has undergone organoaxial volvulus within the chest, there may be substantial pain, intractable retching without vomiting, and inability to pass a nasogastric tube because of the closed-loop gastric obstruction (Borchardt's triad).

DIAGNOSIS

Modalities for the diagnosis of TDR include the following:

- Chest radiograph
- Standard, nasogastric tube in situ, or after oral administration of contrast medium
- Computed tomography
- Ultrasonography
- Peritoneal lavage
- Peritoneography (dye, contrast, radioisotopic scintigraphy)

Liver-spleen radioisotopic scintigraphy
Magnetic resonance imaging
Thoracoscopy

The standard chest radiograph, augmented by a repeat study after passage of a nasogastric tube, and, if required, instillation of contrast material through the tube, are the most valuable studies used to diagnose TDR. Nevertheless, the reported sensitivity of chest radiography varies from 30% to 60% for left-sided TDR and approximately 17% for right-sided TDR (Shapiro et al, 1996).

Felson (cited in Carter et al, 1951) emphasized the following chest radiographic findings for TDR: (1) arch-like shadow stimulating an abnormally high hemidiaphragm; (2) amorphous densities or gas bubbles above the level of the diaphragm; (3) contralateral shift of the mediastinal structures; and (4) atelectasis at the lung bases.

Intubated patients on ventilatory support are less likely to have diagnostic chest radiographs and computed tomographic scans (Shapiro et al, 1996). Mechanical ventilation has been demonstrated to reduce hernias through experimental diaphragmatic ruptures (Ali and Qi, 1992).

Reviews of the value of abdominothoracic computed tomography for the diagnosis of TDR suggest that the sensitivity ranges from 33% to 83% (Guth et al, 1995; Murray et al, 1996). The diaphragmatic defect may not be visualized because of associated hemothorax or hemoperitoneum. This is especially true for right-sided TDR.

Ultrasonography has the advantage of being a bedside procedure, but its sensitivity varies with the experience of the observer (Somers et al, 1990). It is diagnostic when the tear appears as a flap between fluid on both the thoracic and the abdominal surfaces of the diaphragm. Peritoneal lavage has been reported to be falsely negative in 10% to 20% of cases (Guth et al, 1995). If, however, the lavage fluid is retrieved by means of a previously placed chest tube, the diagnosis of TDR is established.

Radioisotopic liver-spleen scans (Blumenthal et al, 1984) and scanning after the intraperitoneal instillation of technetium sulfur colloid have not been widely used (Halldrosson et al, 1992). Magnetic resonance imaging is unique in its ability to generate images in the axial, coronal, and sagittal planes, but its use is incompatible with patients requiring monitoring and ventilatory support (Boulanger et al, 1992). Furthermore, respiratory and cardiac motion may obscure the images. Thoracoscopy has proved reliable in the diagnosis of TDR after penetrating injury, especially in cases in which urgent laparotomy is not required (Ochsner et al, 1993). It may be useful in cases in which bilateral TDR is suggested.

Angiography may be required when injury to the inferior vena cava or aorta is suspected. If the aorta is injured, transesophageal echocardiography, a bedside procedure, may be preferable.

In TDH, the diagnosis is usually readily established by standard chest radiography, upper gastrointestinal series, barium enema, and computed tomography during the interval phase as well as the obstructive phase.

The following are examples of the cases of TDH that I treated between 1990 and 1996:

Case 1. A woman, age 36, two years after a motor vehicle accident, was admitted to the medical service with a 4-day history of cough, left-sided chest pain, and low-grade fever. Chest radiography (Fig. 69–3*A*) was thought to demonstrate left pleural effusion. After nonproductive

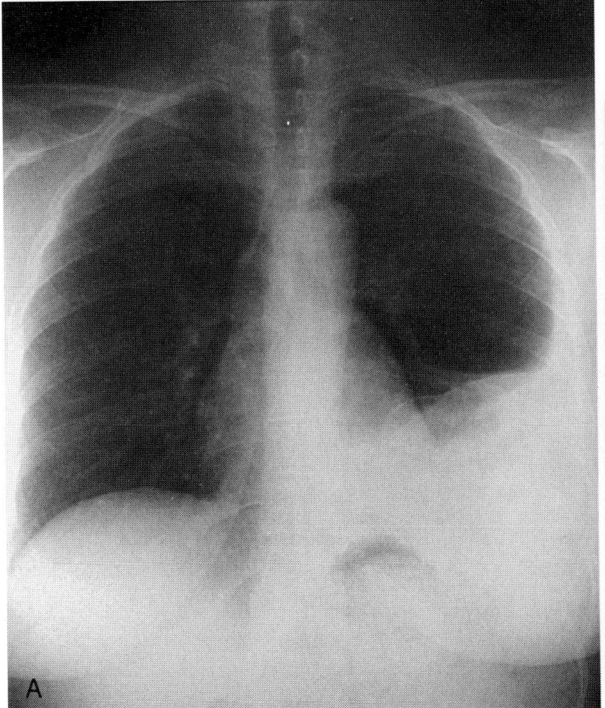

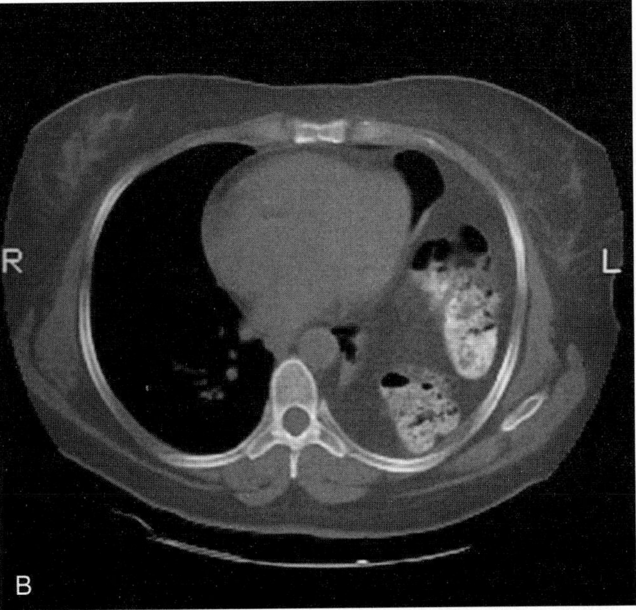

FIGURE 69–3 ■ Transdiaphragmatic hernia with symptoms of pneumonia.

thoracentesis, computed tomography demonstrated TDH (see Fig. 69–3*B*).

Case 2. A male farmer, age 39, noted postprandial dyspnea and left-sided chest pain after blunt trauma sustained when his tractor overturned 2 years previously. Breath sounds were absent over the lower left chest and scaphoid abdomen. Chest radiography and barium swallow demonstrated viscera in the left chest (Fig 69–4). At surgery, the colon, small intestine, and spleen were replaced into the abdomen.

Case 3. A 37-year-old man was admitted to the general surgery service with abdominal pain and distention. He had been in a motor vehicle accident 3 years previously (Fig. 69–5*A*). At laparotomy, appendectomy and colostomy were performed because of colonic distention. A preoperative chest radiograph was not obtained. On the second postoperative day, the patient became dysneic and febrile. Chest radiography demonstrated distended bowel in the left chest, confirmed by contrast enema (see Fig. 69–5*B*, *C*). Gangrenous colon resection was done through left thoracotomy, with complementary transverse colostomy. The patient survived following a stormy postoperative course.

Case 4. A 39-year-old man visited a chiropractor because of back pain of 4 months' duration and was referred because of a right-sided chest abnormality noted on the spine films. The patient had sustained an injury from a motor vehicle accident 6 months earlier and had been comatose, and intubated because of closed-head injury. The patient was discharged when his neurologic status improved. Chest radiography and computed tomography demonstrated the liver had herniated into the right side of the chest (Fig. 69–6*A*, *B*). Repair was easily accomplished without a prosthetic patch.

MANAGEMENT

Because TDR is almost always associated with other injuries, resuscitation, ventilatory support, blood volume restoration, and control of bleeding are required. Military antishock trousers should not be used in cases of TDR because they may cause cardiopulmonary collapse (Shah et al, 1995). Occasionally, massive intrathoracic visceral herniation that displaces the heart and impedes ventilation necessitates reduction of the hernia and repair of the diaphragm before the treatment of associated injuries. Laparotomy is usually the preferred route for repair because of the high incidence of other intra-abdominal injuries. Injury to the inferior vena cava and hepatic veins may necessitate median sternotomy in association with laparotomy. If exposure of the right-sided TDR is difficult from the abdominal approach, a short right thoracotomy will facilitate the repair.

The technique I prefer for repair is one of interrupted horizontal mattress sutures of heavy, nonabsorbable suture material such as silk, Dacron, or polypropylene followed by a continuous suture of synthetic material as a second layer.

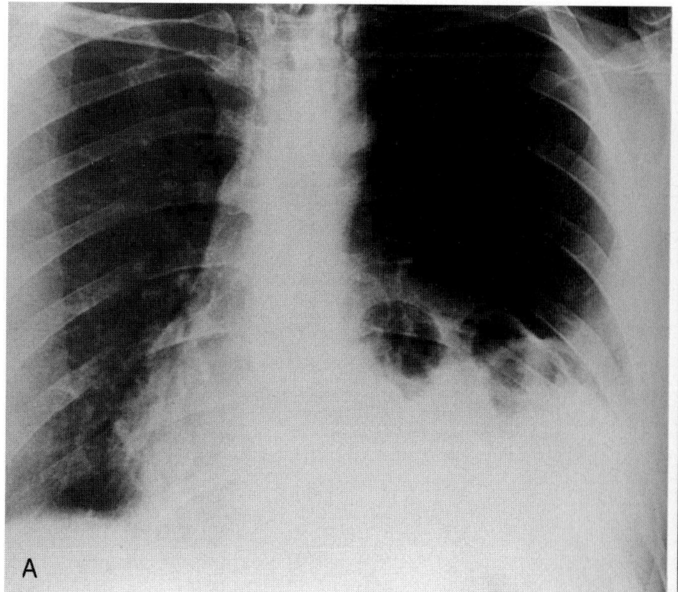

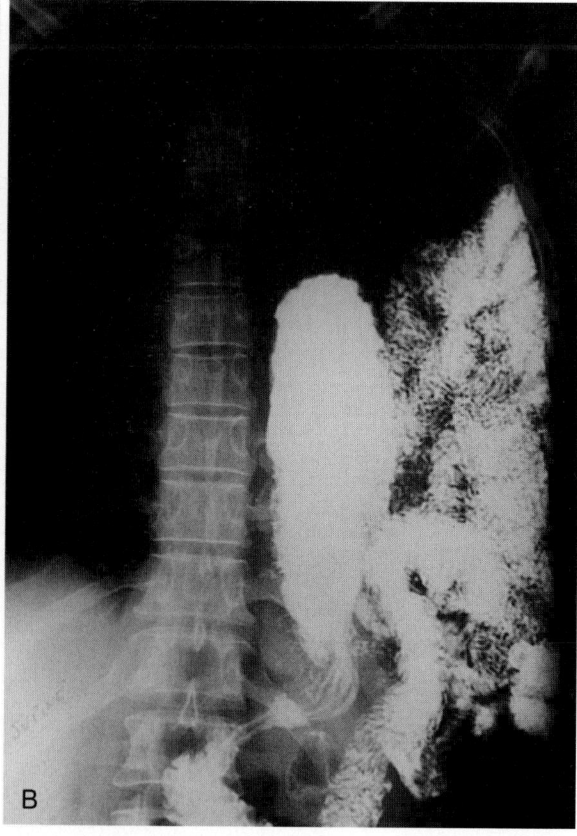

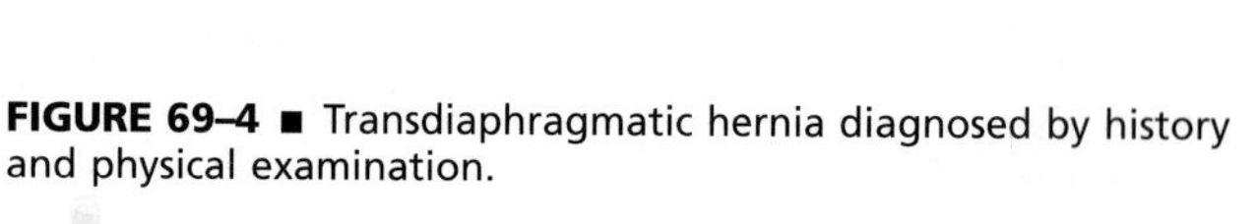

FIGURE 69–4 ■ Transdiaphragmatic hernia diagnosed by history and physical examination.

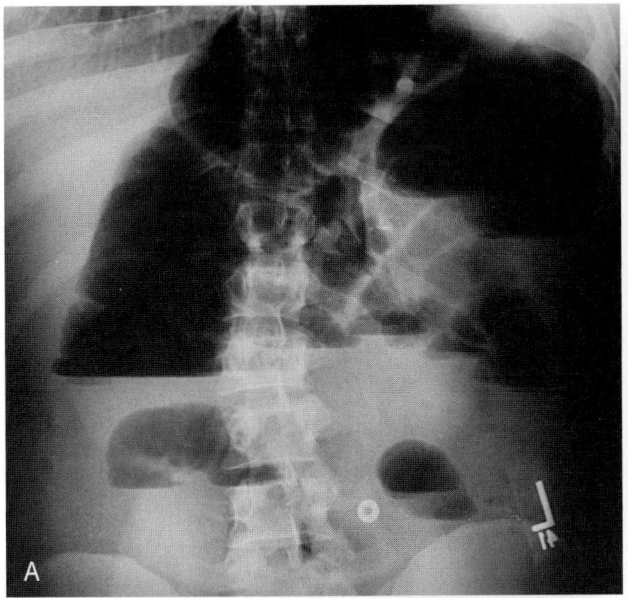

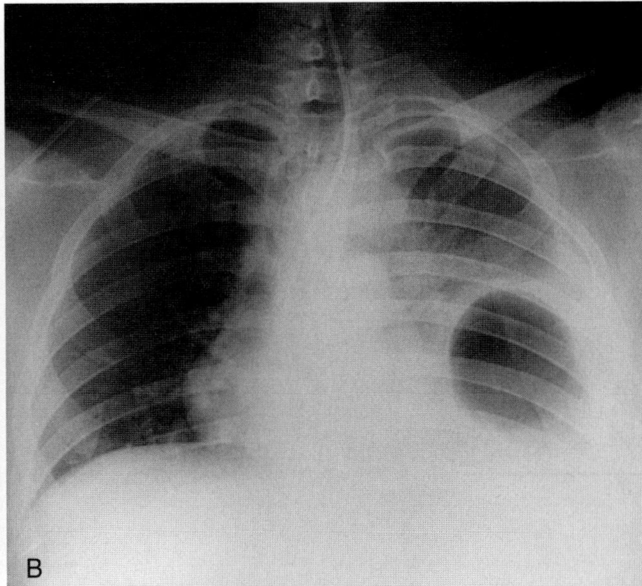

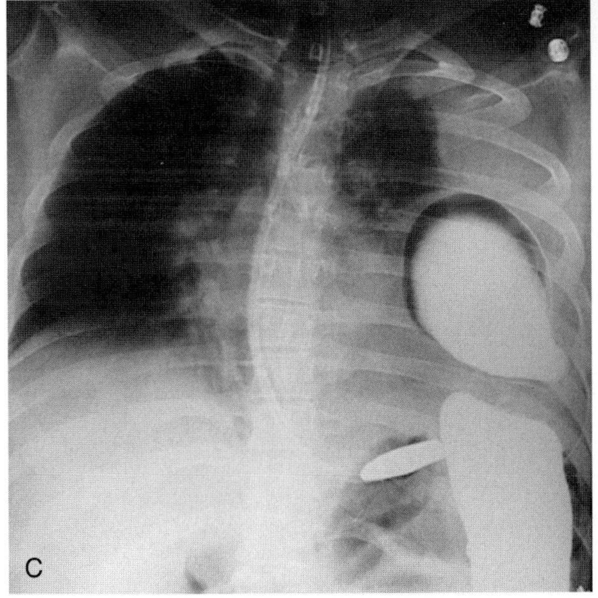

FIGURE 69–5 ■ Chest radiograph must be obtained prior to laparotomy.

In patients who undergo surgery a week or more after the injury, thoracotomy is the preferred approach because of the development of intrathoracic adhesions. In these cases, reduction of the incarcerated viscera may be facilitated by judicious enlargement of the defect in the diaphragm, avoiding branches of the phrenic nerve. Prosthetic patching of the defect is rarely required. In situations in which the diaphragm has been avulsed from its costal attachment, it may be reattached by pericostal sutures, reattaching the diaphragm either at its previous level or one level higher, if there is tension on the sutures.

The operative repair of TDR is not especially technically demanding, yet the diagnosis of this injury is often fraught with difficulty (Fig 69–7). The "gold standard" for the diagnosis of TDR is laparotomy, yet there are anecdotal reports of this injury being missed during emergency laparotomy and, even more disturbing, of recurrence of the defect because of inadequate repair (Naclerio, 1971).

COMMENTS AND CONTROVERSIES

This chapter covers in great detail the subject of diaphragmatic rupture. Dr. Fell has included a very nice historical background to introduce the subject. The pitfalls of diagnosis are reviewed in depth. Dr. Fell points out the difficulties in establishing this diagnosis by imaging studies. Diaphragmatic rupture is an often missed diagnosis that should always be considered during evaluation of a victim of major blunt trauma.

G.A.P.

Acknowledgment

This work was supported by the Feldesman Fund for Thoracic Surgery.

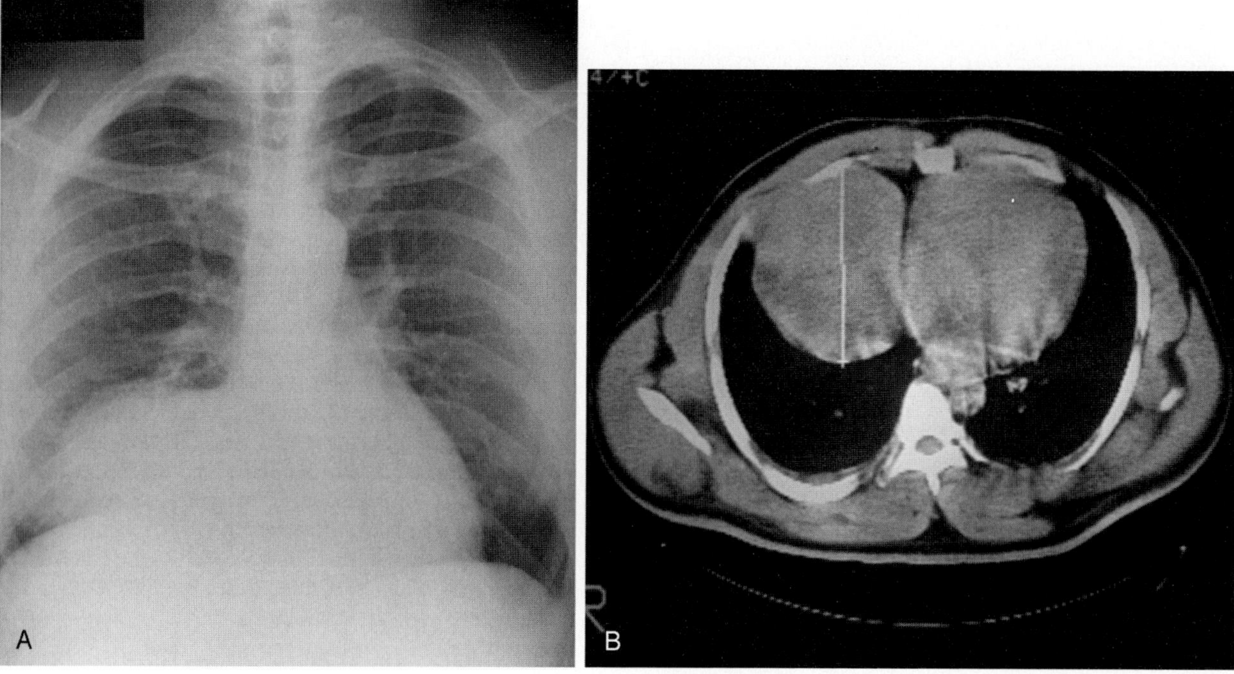

FIGURE 69–6. ■ Transdiaphragmatic hernia causing chronic backache.

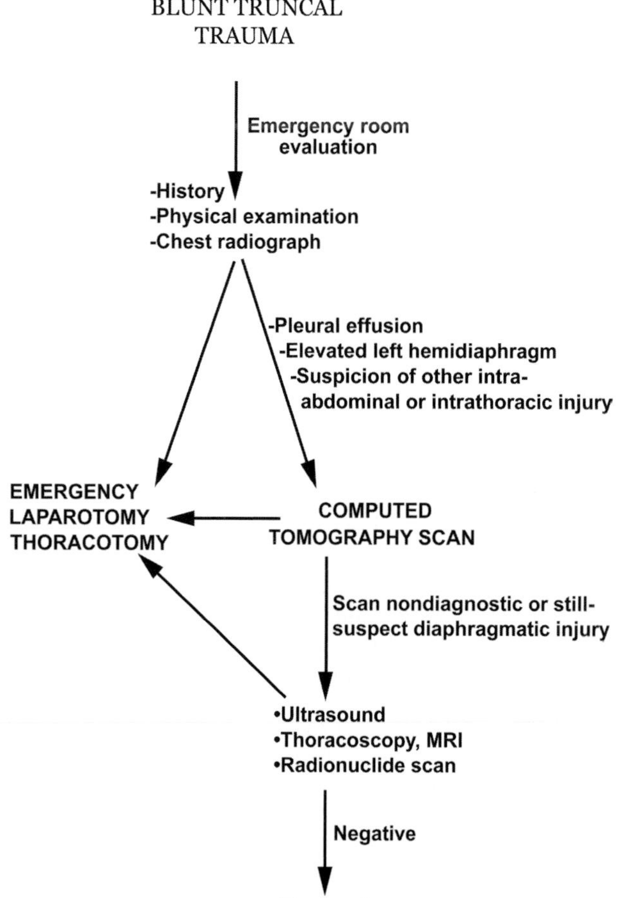

FIGURE 69–7. ■ Algorithm for the evaluation of diaphragmatic injury. MRI, magnetic resonance imaging. (Modified from Guth AA, Pachter L, Kim U et al: Pitfalls in the diagnosis of blunt diaphragmatic injury. Am J Surg 170:5–9, 1995.)

■ *REFERENCES*

Ali J, Qi W: The effect of positive airway pressure and intraabdominal pressure in diaphragmatic rupture. World J Surg 16:1120–1125, 1992.

Blumenthal DH, Raghu G, Rudd TG: Diagnosis of right hemidiaphragmatic rupture by liver scintigraphy. J Trauma 24:536, 1984.

Boulanger B, Mirvis S, Rodriguez A: Magnetic resonance imaging in traumatic diaphragmatic rupture: Case reports. J Trauma 32:89, 1992.

Boulanger B, Milzman D, Rosati C: Comparison of right and left blunt traumatic diaphragmatic rupture. J Trauma 35:255, 1993.

Bowditch H: Diaphragmatic hernia. Buffalo Med Surg J 9:65–94, 1853.

Carter BN, Giuseffi J, Felson B: Traumatic diaphragmatic hernia. AJR A J Roentgenol 65:56–82, 1951.

Epstein L, Lempke R: Rupture of the right hemidiaphragm due to blunt trauma. J Trauma 8:19, 1968.

Estrera AS, Platt MR, Mills LI: Traumatic injuries of the diaphragm. Chest 75:306–313, 1979.

Guth AA, Pachter HL, Unsup K: Pitfalls in the diagnosis of blunt diaphragmatic injury. Am J Surg 170:5–9, 1995.

Halldrosson A, Esser MJ, Rappaport W et al: A new method of diagnosing diaphragmatic injury using intraperitoneal technetium: Case report. J Trauma 33:140–143, 1992.

Hedblom C: Diaphragmatic hernia. JAMA 85:947–953, 1925.

Hood RM: Traumatic diaphragmatic hernia. Ann Thorac Surg 23:311–324, 1971.

Kearney PA, Rouhana SW, Burney RE: Blunt rupture of the diaphragm: Mechanism, diagnosis and treatment. Ann Emerg Med 18:1326–1330, 1989.

Mansour K: Trauma to the diaphragm. Chest Surg Clin North Am 7:373, 1997.

Murray JG, Caioili E, Gruden JF: Acute rupture of diaphragm due to blunt traumas: Diagnostic sensitivity and specificity of CT. AJR Am J Roentgenol 166:1035, 1996.

Naclerio E: Discussion of Carter R, Brewer LA: Strangulating diaphragmatic hernia. Ann Thorac Surg 12:281–290, 1971.

Naumann G: Diaphragmatic hernia; laparatomy; died. Hygea 5:524–528, 1888.

Ochsner MG, Rozycki GS, Lucente F: Prospective evaluation of thoracoscopy for diagnosis of diaphragmatic injury in thoracoabdominal trauma: A preliminary report. J Trauma 34:704, 1993.

Reid J: Case of diaphragmatic hernia pruduced by a penetrating wound. Edinburgh Med Surg J 53:104–108, 1840.

Rizoli S, Brenneman F, Boulanger B: Blunt diaphragmatic and thoracic aortic rupture: An emerging injury complex. Ann Thorac Surg 58:1404; 1994.

Rosati C: Acute traumatic injuries of the diaphragm. Chest Surg Clin North Am 8:371, 1998.

Shah R, Sabaratnam S, Mearns AJ et al: Traumatic rupture of diaphragm. Ann Thorac Surg 60:1444–1449, 1995.

Shapiro M, Hieberg E, Duram R: The unreliability of CT scans and initial chest radiographs in evaluating blunt trauma induced diaphragmatic rupture. Clin Radiol 51:27, 1996.

Somers JM, Gleeson FU, Flower CD: Rupture of the right hemidiaphragm following blunt trauma: The use of ultrasound in diagnosis. Clin Radiol 42:97–101, 1990.

Walker E: Diaphragmatic hernia. JAMA 35:778, 1900.

Wiencek RG, Wilson RF, Steiger Z: Acute injuries of the diaphragm: An analysis of 165 cases. J Thorac Cardiovasc Surg 92:989–993, 1986.

CHAPTER **70**

Penetrating Trauma

Matthew J. Wall, Jr.
Ernesto Soltero
Kenneth L. Mattox

Penetrating thoracic injury may be the result of stab wounds from a sharp object or weapon, low- or high-velocity missile, shotgun wounds, or iatrogenic injury. The incidence of low- and high-velocity gunshot wounds and iatrogenic injury is increasing. Most penetrating injury is secondary to social violence and is potentially preventable (LoCicero and Mattox, 1989).

Iatrogenic penetrating thoracic injury occurs during various diagnostic and therapeutic procedures. Percutaneous aspiration of lung masses can produce pneumothorax and pulmonary hemorrhage and occasionally systemic air embolism. Penetration of subclavian, cervical, and mediastinal vascular structures by percutaneously inserted trocars, catheters, pacemaker lead wires, introducers, and other instruments can result in significant hemorrhage and death. Percutaneously introduced balloon-directed catheters may cause injury to the superior vena cava, right atrium, right ventricle, or pulmonary arteries. These iatrogenic injuries may occur in environments in which no surgical personnel are available, and surgeons are frequently summoned too late to reverse an iatrogenic vascular catastrophe. In spite of the trend away from this procedure, pericardiocentesis is included in the American College of Surgeons' Advanced Life Support course. Iatrogenic injury to the heart and coronary vessels is occurring with increasing frequency from this maneuver. Careless placement of a tube thoracostomy may produce injury. Because partial pleural symphysis is present in 25% of the population, puncture of the lung with resultant pulmonary hematoma, arteriovenous fistula, and air embolism can occur.

HISTORICAL NOTE

The insulting victor with disdain bestrode
The prostrate prince, and on his bosom trod.
Then withdrew the weapon from his panting heart,
The reeking fibers clinging to the dart;
From the wide wound gush'd out a stream of blood,
And the soul issued in the purple flood.

—*The Iliad*, Homer

Penetrating wounds of the thorax have been the subject of medical writings, ancient literature, and works of art since antiquity. The Edwin Smith and Evers papyri of Egypt described the consequences of penetrating thoracic wounds.

During each period, artists in Europe have depicted thoracic penetration by knives, spears, and musket balls. The first recorded operation for penetrating chest trauma in North America occurred in Texas. Cabeza de Vaca wrote in his diary in 1535 of the extraction of an arrowhead from the sternum of an Indian (Sparkman et al, 1965). One of the early and incapacitating injuries reported with survival was William Beaumont's (1833) famous patient, Alexis Saint Martin, who sustained a traumatic lung herniation at the entrance site of a musket ball.

MORTALITY RATES FROM PENETRATING THORACIC INJURY

World War II: 4.5%
Korean Conflict: 2.5%
Vietnam Conflict: 2.0%

The mortality rate from thoracic wounds decreased with each ensuing major war. Although many patients with penetrating thoracic injury died shortly after injury, Harken (1946) was able to tabulate 134 operations for the removal of foreign bodies in and around the heart and great vessels without a single death among this group arriving at his thoracic surgery referral center in World War II. Through the 1960s, pericardiocentesis, rather than thoracotomy and cardiorrhaphy, was the preferred method of treating pericardial tamponade from penetrating injury. In the 1970s and 1980s, large series, primarily from inner-city trauma centers, reported significant numbers of patients with penetrating thoracic injury. At that time, thoracotomy and cardiorrhaphy replaced pericardiocentesis. A high-velocity gunshot wound to the chest nearly took the life of Governor Connally at the time of the assassination of President John F. Kennedy in 1963. An injury to the chest from a handgun seriously injured President Ronald Reagan. Both required thoracotomy.

■ *HISTORICAL READINGS*

Beaumont W: Experiments and Observations on the Gastric Juice and Physiology of Digestion. Pittsburgh, FP Allen, 1833.

Harken DE: Foreign bodies in, and in relation to, thoracic blood vessels and heart. I. Techniques for approaching and removing foreign bodies from chambers of the heart. Surg Gynecol Obstet 83:117, 1946.

Sparkman RS, Nixon PI, Crosthwait RW et al: The Texas Surgical Society: The First Fifty Years. Dallas, Texas Surgical Society, 1965.

INVESTIGATIVE TECHNIQUES

Penetrating injuries require a precise definition of the anatomy. Arteriography is useful in the evaluation of the hemodynamically stable trauma patient with suspected vascular injuries, whether it is a transsected aorta or innominate artery, or a cervical injury. Arteriography for these conditions is usually performed in the arteriography suite. The option of the retrograde brachial-axillary arteriogram for selected subclavian and axillary artery injuries should be considered. These arteriograms can be performed in the emergency center by surgical personnel (Itani et al, 1992). In general, the usefulness of arteriography for penetrating trauma is limited to suspected innominate, carotid, or subclavian artery injury to guide the proper choice of incision. Arteriography for penetrating thoracic aortic injury may yield false-negative results related to prior sealing of the penetration or inadequate projections. Neither computed tomography (CT) nor magnetic resonance imaging (MRI) has been shown to be as effective as arteriography for diagnosing aortic injuries (Miller et al, 1989). Transesophageal endocardiography has been reported to be useful in demonstrating internal flaps and mediastinal hematomas. However, this technique appears to be overly sensitive and often requires angiography for clarification, a duplication of effort.

INDICATIONS FOR THORACOTOMY

Following penetrating chest trauma, 85% of patients can be treated with either observation or tube thoracostomy and surgery for concomitant cervical or abdominal injury. Only 15% require thoracotomy.

Urgent thoracotomy is usually performed in the emergency center on patients who arrive in extremis or who have an arrest shortly after arrival. Emergency-center thoracotomy should be performed by surgical personnel who are familiar with this procedure. It should not be performed on unintubated patients who have undergone prehospital cardiopulmonary resuscitation (CPR) for longer than 5 minutes or intubated patients with prehospital CPR in progress longer than 10 minutes (Durham et al, 1992). Anterolateral thoracotomy is performed through a fourth interspace incision (below the inframammary crease in female patients), with transsternal extension if necessary. The descending thoracic aorta may be cross-clamped to increase cerebral and coronary flow, effective open cardiac massage may be instituted, the pericardium may be entered, and cardiorrhaphy may be performed. For such urgent procedures, the survival rate may be as high as 30% following stab wounds and 8% following gunshot wounds to the heart.

Acute indications for thoracotomy include post-traumatic cardiovascular collapse, pericardial tamponade, vascular injury to the thoracic outlet, traumatic thoracotomy, massive air leak, proven tracheobronchial injury, proven esophageal injury, suspected great vessel injury, continued hemothorax, a bullet path traversing the mediastinum, bullet embolism, and systemic air embolism. Chronic conditions requiring thoracotomy include unevacuated clotted hemothorax, chronic traumatic diaphragmatic hernia, chronic cardiac septal or valvular injuries, chronic false aneurysm of the thoracic aorta, chronic nonclosure of thoracic duct fistula, chronic empyema, infected intrapulmonary hematomas, missed tracheal bronchial lesions, and traumatic arteriovenous fistula. A small-volume hemothorax, thoracoabdominal wounding alone, a bullet in proximity to a major vessel, tension pneumothorax, and pneumomediastinum are not appropriate indications for thoracotomy following trauma (Mattox, 1989).

INDICATIONS FOR EMERGENCY-CENTER THORACOTOMY

Postinjury cardiac arrest
Profound shock as a result of pericardial tamponade
Profound shock caused by air embolization
Refractory shock (blood pressure <60 mm Hg) as a result of massive abdominal hemorrhage
Refractory shock (blood pressure <80 mm Hg) caused by thoracic bleeding

CHEST WALL PENETRATION

Penetrating injury to the chest wall from knives and low-caliber missiles rarely produces loss of chest wall substance but may require thoracotomy to control injuries to the intercostal vascular bundle or the internal mammary artery. High-velocity missiles and shotgun blasts can cause extensive loss of chest wall tissue, leaving a traumatic open thoracotomy. In such injuries, the underlying lung and other adjacent structures are likely to be severely injured. Plastic sheets, such as Saran Wrap or sterile plastic drapes, can be used to close these defects temporarily until the definitive procedure can be done. At times, such surgical procedures as acute thoracoplasty or immediate reconstruction of the chest wall with plastic surgery techniques may be required.

Injuries to the internal mammary artery or intercostal bundle are frequently found at the time of thoracotomy for continued hemothorax. The internal mammary artery can simply be suture ligated, with control of the bleeding. The intercostal bundle may require a secondary intercostal incision approached through the same skin incision or through a ligature encircling the rib proximal and distal to the area of the bleeding because suture ligature and clips may not control the hemorrhage.

Cardiac and Pericardial Penetration

Surgeons are seeing penetrating cardiac injury more frequently. At the Ben Taub General Hospital in Houston, four to five patients per month are treated for penetrating injury to the heart or pericardium. Of this group, the largest number of injuries are stab wounds, with gunshot wounds accounting for most of the remainder. The diagnosis of cardiac injury must be considered any time the chest is penetrated by a missile or knife. This is especially true when the entry is medial to the nipple anteriorly or medial to the scapula posteriorly. If this type of injury is accompanied by restlessness and hypotension, the diagnosis of pericardial tamponade must be strongly considered. The patient with these injuries most commonly presents with cardiac tamponade, in extremis, with vital signs still present, or with CPR in progress.

Patients with penetrating chest trauma have the best results from emergency-department thoracotomy. This is especially true in patients with cardiac wounds. Most patients with this injury present with cardiac tamponade, and a significant number are in extremis. Emergency-department thoracotomy allows the release of the pericardial tamponade, assessment of cardiac function, and control of the cardiac injury. If needed, open cardiac massage and cross-clamping of the descending thoracic aorta can be accomplished.

To perform the urgent thoracotomy, the patient is positioned supine on the operating table, with the left side tilted up slightly. The incision of choice is a left anterolateral thoracotomy. If the injury requires access to the right heart, this incision can be extended to the right, across the sternum, and into the right chest. Should access to the descending aorta be required, the incision can be taken posteriorly to expose the descending thoracic aorta. Rapid access to the heart can be gained through this incision. After the chest is opened, the pericardium is easily visualized. If blood is present, the pericardium will be distended and have a blue appearance. The pericardium is opened anterior to the phrenic nerve with a large incision. After this is done, the cardiac action is assessed, and the site of preparation is identified and controlled. Subxiphoid pericardiotomy is not recommended because it may convert a contained hemorrhage into an exsanguinating hemorrhage with no means of rapid control.

The most common site of penetrating injury is the right ventricle because it has greatest anterior exposure, followed by the left ventricle and then by the right atrium. Digital pressure is used to control the injury until adequate suture control can be accomplished. Metal skin staples have been used in some cases to protect the surgeon from needle sticks. The myocardium can be either penetrated or lacerated without complete cavitary penetration. These injuries may penetrate the septum, producing a traumatic ventricular septal defect, and may result in a shunt between chambers. Patients surviving penetrating cardiac injury should undergo daily evaluations of heart sounds. Special attention should be given to "new" murmurs because septal perforation may manifest itself late. Most septal injuries from penetrating trauma close spontaneously. No patient should be considered for operation acutely. Only after several months of observation should surgery be considered, and then only if a significant intracardiac shunt greater than 2:1 is confirmed by cardiac catheterization. If a coronary artery injury is found, it must be repaired because ligation of a proximal coronary artery leads to myocardial infarction and death in many patients. Valve penetration can occur but is very rare in our experience.

A significant number of patients have only pericardial injuries. Should the wound be a stab wound with the knife still in place, the weapon is left in place until the patient reaches the operating room, where operative control of the penetrating injury can be accomplished.

Some cardiac injury results in marked swelling of the heart, often secondary to excessive fluid administration. On occasion, the thoracotomy cannot be closed without adverse cardiac compression. These patients are managed by leaving the sternum and chest open and sewing sterile plastic material into the incision, allowing transfer to the intensive care unit (ICU) until swelling abates. They can be returned to the operating room later for definitive closure of the thoracotomy.

GREAT VESSEL PENETRATION

Penetrating injury to thoracic vessels is usually obvious on presentation. The prehospital phase of assessment and management includes the initial level of hypotension and fluid volume required for resuscitation and stability during transfer. Examination of all entrance and exit wounds may give some indication of the missile's trajectory, although a missile, after it enters the body, can deviate markedly from a straight line between entry and exit sites. Should the entry be medial to the nipples anteriorly or medial to the scapula posteriorly, major mediastinal vascular injury is highly probable. If the mediastinum has been traversed by a missile, exploration is required. Auscultation of the chest and an assessment of distal pulses are helpful if the blood pressure is sufficient to produce extremity pulses. The chest radiograph demonstrates an enlarging mediastinal hematoma or hemothorax if present.

If the patient is stable enough to undergo the procedure, arteriography gives significant information about the extent of injury. It demonstrates a false aneurysm, arteriovenous fistula, intimal disruption, and arterial occlusion. However, the majority of these patients are too unstable to permit this examination. Arteriography has a low diagnostic yield for penetrating aortic injury.

After the patient reaches the emergency center, injuries are rapidly assessed as are airway patency, systemic blood pressure, blood volume loss, and the presence of external hematomas, hemothorax, cardiac tamponade, or pneumothorax. Intravenous access and, frequently, endotracheal intubation are required. Resuscitation of the patient includes restoration of circulating blood volume with aggressive fluid and colloid management. A chest radiograph and an arterial blood gas evaluation are obtained. Chest-tube insertion may be required.

At this point, patients can be stratified into three categories. Patients in extremis, but with signs of life, are in the first category and require an emergency-center thoracotomy. The objective of this maneuver is to release pericardial tamponade, to control intrathoracic hemorrhage, to provide access for temporary clamping of the descending aorta to raise the central blood pressure, and to give access for open cardiac massage. Patients in the second category are those who are unstable following volume replacement or who may have an expanding hematoma. This group requires immediate thoracotomy in the operating room. The stable patient falls into the third category. In this group, the physician has time to perform aortography, endoscopy, and esophography.

After the patient reaches the operating room, the surgeon must have an idea of the pattern of injury. If the surgeon is faced with uncontrolled bleeding from an unknown site, the recommended incision is a left anterolateral thoracotomy. The chest is prepared so that an incision can cross the midline and be converted into a bilateral anterior thoracotomy by crossing the sternum. In the case of an anterior injury to the ascending aorta or great vessels, the incision should be a median sternotomy, which easily can be extended into the neck for access to the innominate or the right subclavian arteries. Should the injured vessel be the descending aorta, a posterolateral thoracotomy incision is required. One of the more difficult surgical exposures is that required to repair the proximal left subclavian artery. For proximal control, a high (third intercostal space) left anterolateral thoracotomy is used. The injury is then approached by a supraclavicular incision. On rare occasions, these incisions may need to be joined to create a "book" or "trap door" type of incision. The medial end of the clavicle can be resected for better exposure of this area.

In patients with ascending aortic injury, good exposure can be obtained through a median sternotomy. The injury is initially controlled by digital pressure, and 4–0 monofilament sutures are used to oversew the injury as the finger is withdrawn. The evaluation of other vessels for injury after the control of the initial bleeding point is imperative. Should the injury be in the aortic arch, the sternotomy incision is extended into the neck for better exposure. The brachiocephalic vein is divided, and occasionally, if digital control can not be obtained, a balloon catheter or Hegar dilator can be inserted into the defect to facilitate tamponade control of the bleeding point.

Descending thoracic aortic injury is associated with a high prehospital mortality rate of 85% (Parmely et al, 1958). If this injury is not discovered during the initial assessment of the trauma patient, the hospital mortality rate is 50% in the first 48 hours. This injury can be associated with a large hemothorax on the left. The approach to the descending aorta is through a left posterolateral thoracotomy incision. For penetrating trauma proximal and distal, control is gained, the aorta is clamped, and lateral repair is accomplished.

Penetrating injury to the innominate artery usually occurs in its distal portion; however, the injury can be located in any portion. The innominate artery can be visualized in its entirety through a median sternotomy with neck extension. If the injury is small, a primary repair can be accomplished. However, if a segment is missing or a large defect is present, then the bypass principle is used. A polytetrafluoroethylene (PTFE) graft is attached on the ascending aorta with a side-biting clamp and then anastomosed to the distal innominate artery. Complex techniques, using hypothermia, temporary shunting, or heparinization, are not required for this operation. The brachiocephalic vein can be ligated and divided with impunity for better visualization.

The subclavian arteries are the more difficult to expose, and gaining proximal control is of the utmost importance. Control of the proximal right subclavian artery is accomplished through a median sternotomy with a right neck extension. The brachiocephalic vein or the jugular vein may be divided, and then the first part of the right subclavian artery can be seen. The artery is then isolated with a tape for clamp control when needed. The proximal left subclavian artery is exposed through a left anterolateral thoracotomy incision placed in the third or fourth interspace. The left subclavian artery is easily visualized as it arises from the aorta. The middle and distal subclavian artery is exposed through a supraclavicular incision, whether injury is on the right or left side, and exposure for repair may require removal of a segment of the clavicle. The incision can be made over the course of the subclavian artery, dissecting down until both the proximal and distal ends of the artery are exposed. Injuries to the subclavian artery frequently require graft replacement. Both autogenous saphenous vein and 6-mm Gore-Tex grafts have been used for this purpose. A notable potential pitfall to this repair is injury to the brachial plexus, the vagus, the phrenic nerves, or to recurrent laryngeal nerves. On the left side, the thoracic duct should be identified and avoided, as should the jugular duct on the right.

An intrapericardial injury to the pulmonary artery or vein is usually best managed by bilateral anterior thoracotomy incision because these patients are usually in extremis on admission to the emergency center. Bleeding may be profuse, and control of the injury may be difficult. Usually, digital control can be gained and suture repair can be accomplished. A significant problem seen with this injury and injury to the pulmonary hilum is air embolization. The use of cardiopulmonary bypass has not improved the outcome for the patient with an air embolus (Graham et al, 1977).

Injury to the superior vena cava is often associated with injury to the innominate artery and jugular or brachiocephalic veins. Although the jugular or brachiocephalic vein can be ligated, the superior vena cava must be reconstructed. Previous experience with the use of prosthetic material in the superior vena cava has not yielded long-term patency (Doty, 1976). Construction of a conduit using the spiral saphenous vein technique (Doty, 1976) or substituting another vein, such as the common femoral vein, has been recommended for the repair of the superior vena cava. Shunting of the blood may be required while this repair is being accomplished in the acute setting.

Injuries of the intrapericardial inferior vena cava are associated with a very high mortality rate, especially when the injury occurs at the junction of the inferior vena cava and right atrium. Management is likely to require cardiopulmonary bypass with repair accomplished transatrially. Injury to the azygos vein is potentially fatal and is usually associated with another injury, especially to the innominate artery, the trachea, the bronchus, or the superior vena cava. Injury to the azygos vein can be difficult to control through a median sternotomy incision. A right anterolateral or a right posterolateral thoracotomy incision is preferred. The azygos vein is suture ligated for control.

Penetrating injury to the great vessels in the chest must be approached with a high index of suspicion by a surgical team ready and able to perform a definitive life-saving thoracotomy in the emergency center or the operating room. An aggressive approach to these injuries is advised. For patients presenting with signs of life and arrest secondary to pericardial tamponade, emergency-center thoracotomy has yielded a survival rate of 8% (Durham et al, 1992).

PENETRATING TRACHEOBRONCHIAL INJURIES

Penetrating injury of the vascular structures of the pulmonary hilum is usually manifested by massive hemothorax, incomplete evacuation of hemothorax, or hemothorax with continued active bleeding. Patients with these injuries can be surprisingly stable initially, but thoracotomy should not be delayed when indicated. Penetrating injury to tracheobronchial structures of the pulmonary hilum usually causes respiratory distress and an inability to ventilate the patient adequately (Ecker et al, 1971; Pate, 1989). If the injury is intrapleural, it may be a pneumothorax or a large air leak after tube thoracostomy with incomplete expansion of the lung. If the injury is extrapleural, it may be pneumomediastinum with subcutaneous and cervical emphysema.

The procedure of choice for the diagnosis of this injury is bronchoscopy. The bronchoscope may be used therapeutically to pass an endotracheal tube through the disrupted trachea. The bronchoscope can also be used to pass an uncut endotracheal tube selectively into the uninjured bronchus. A large amount of bleeding into the pulmonary parenchyma is always associated with this injury, and aggressive tracheobronchial suction is required. If the patient is stable enough to permit it, selective bronchial intubation with a double-lumen endotracheal tube is a helpful adjunct. Many of the details of the operative technique and ventilation are discussed in Chapter 67.

Positioning

For proximal tracheal injuries, the patient is positioned supine with the neck extended and the head elevated to decrease the central venous pressure. The neck and entire chest should be prepared and draped. The groin should be prepared for cannulation for cardiopulmonary bypass, although it is not commonly needed. For distal tracheal and bronchial injuries, the patient is positioned in the standard posterolateral thoracotomy position. The patient in extremis is placed in the supine position and prepared and draped from the neck to the groin so that a rapid anterolateral thoracotomy can be performed.

Incisions

The patient in extremis from hemorrhage is approached by an anterolateral thoracotomy on the appropriate side. In the stable patient with isolated proximal tracheal injuries, the repair is accomplished through a cervical collar incision at the level of the injury. Superior and inferior flaps are raised for exposure, and knowledge of the anatomy of the neck is essential. The chest is prepared so that a median sternotomy can be performed if needed. For distal tracheal or bronchial injuries, a right standard posterolateral thoracotomy is the incision of choice, allowing access to the distal trachea, the rimae, and the right mainstem bronchus. For the left mainstem bronchus beyond the carina, a left posterolateral thoracotomy incision is performed (Fig. 70–1).

Technique

The principle for tracheobronchial repair is mucosa-to-mucosa apposition. The repair of tracheal or bronchial

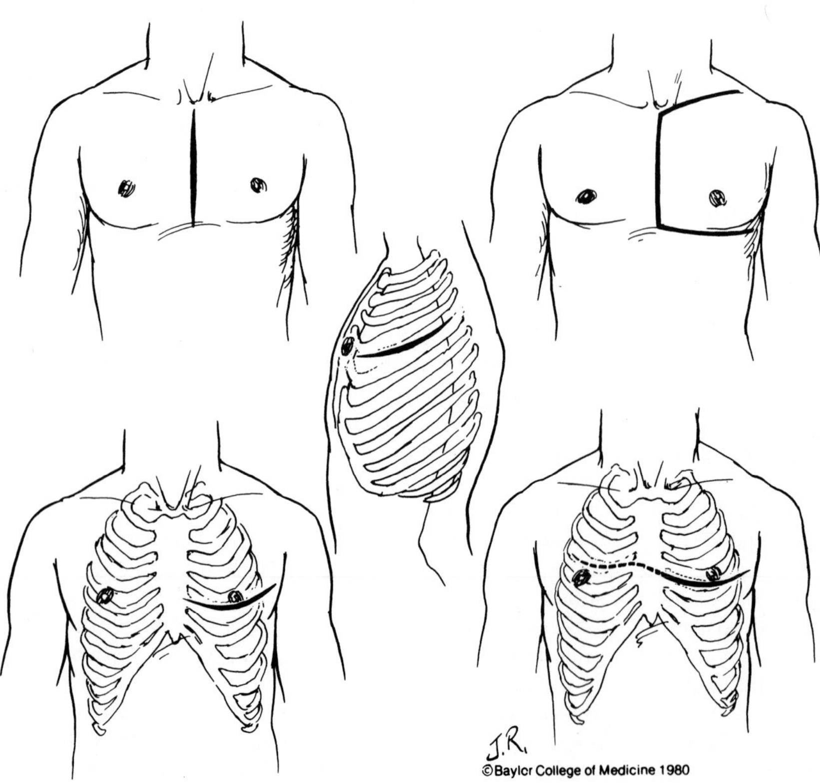

FIGURE 70–1 ■ Incision options that might be used in penetrating thoracic trauma.

transsection requires adequate débridement without interruption of the blood supply, with anastomosis performed in one layer using interrupted absorbable sutures. This can be reinforced with a pleural or intercostal muscle patch. Standard bronchoplasty techniques can be used as needed. Cardiopulmonary bypass can be used selectively in these patients; however, this adjunct has its own set of complications. Alternatives to cardiopulmonary bypass may be the intubation of each bronchus with selective ventilation during repair. Penetrating and blunt injuries to the pulmonary hilum require rapid control by digital compression followed by hilar cross-clamping. The patient's condition commonly necessitates pneumonectomy, and time should not be wasted attempting a lesser resection in a critically ill trauma patient.

Injuries to the tracheobronchial tree result in mortality rates ranging from 0% to 30%. The risk of death depends on the anatomy, initial condition of the patient, and whether the injury is secondary to blunt or penetrating injury (Burke, 1962; De La Rocha and Kayler, 1982; Deslauriers et al, 1982; Grover et al, 1979; Jones et al, 1984; Mills et al, 1982; Pate, 1989).

ESOPHAGEAL INJURY

The management of esophageal injury is discussed elsewhere. The essential step in management is alertness in looking for the injury at the time of presentation. Closure of penetrating injuries is usually readily done by using a two-layered interrupted suture technique.

BULLET EMBOLISM

Intravascular migratory missiles produce confusing clinical findings because the entrance site is often misleading. Symptoms and physical findings do not match anticipated and projected injuries. In the chest, missile emboli may lodge either in the right ventricle or the pulmonary arteries. Missiles entering the heart and aorta may embolize to distant sites, such as the carotid and iliac arteries (Fig. 70–2). In all instances, control of the entrance site is achieved first, and then the embolized missile is removed. In general, missile emboli are removed from the heart using cardiopulmonary bypass, although nonbypass and angiographic means have been used. A missile embolus in the heart should be removed to prevent complications of endocarditis, tricuspid valve dysfunction, cardiac arrhythmias, and secondary embolization to pulmonary and systemic arteries. A radiologic clue that suggests a bullet embolus to the heart is a bullet appearing out of focus (secondary to the beating heart) while the rest of the radiograph is in focus (Fig. 70–3). Bullet emboli to the pulmonary arteries should be removed with the patient in a supine position to prevent the bullet from falling into the dependent lung during lateral thoracotomy. Very small emboli, such as small pellets from a shotgun wound, can be left undisturbed.

AIR EMBOLISM

The physiology of the pulmonary vasculature and current techniques for positive pressure-assisted ventilation are

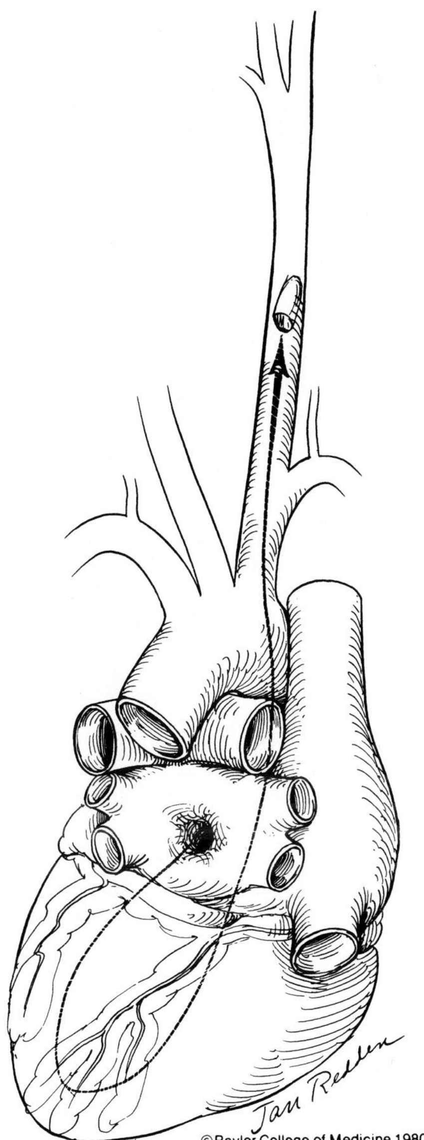

FIGURE 70–2 ■ A bullet embolizing from the heart to the carotid artery.

conducive to the formation of a systemic air embolism. The normal pressures within the pulmonary artery are 25/5 to 15/0. The pressures within the pulmonary veins are frequently 5 cm H_2O. During positive-pressure breathing, pressure at the site of the endotracheal tube normally peaks at 30 cm H_2O. During resuscitation in ambulances and emergency centers, ventilatory bags are capable of delivering pressures in excess of 120 cm H_2O (Fig. 70–4). Many manufacturers of ventilatory bags have removed the pop-off valve that prevented positive pressure ventilation in excess of 50 mm Hg. Numerous clinical and experimental studies have documented that systemic air embolism can occur when pressure in the positive pressure ventilatory circuit exceeds 60 cm H_2O. In this situation, a fistula is created between the bronchioles and adjacent pulmonary veins, with air then going to the aorta, coronary arteries, cerebral circulation, and other areas in the body (Graham et al, 1977).

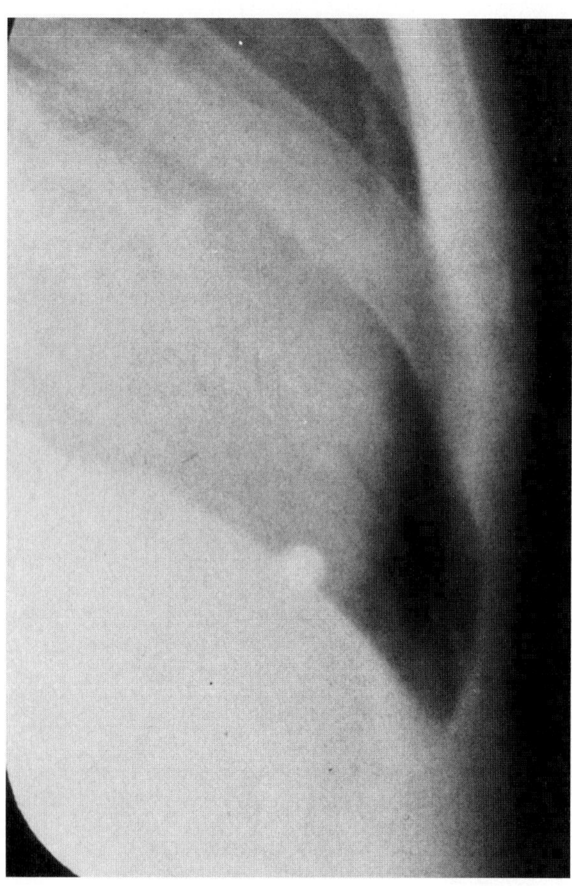

FIGURE 70–3 ■ Radiograph of the chest showing a bullet embolism to the right ventricle; note that the bullet appears to be out of focus.

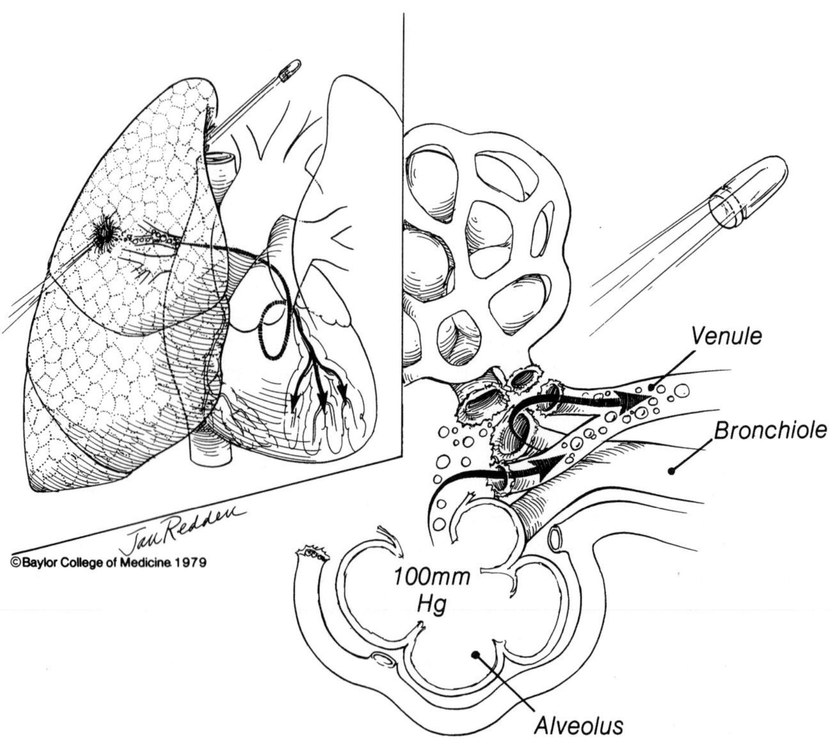

FIGURE 70–4 ■ Mechanism of systemic air embolism from a penetrating lung injury.

THORACIC DAMAGE CONTROL

One of the newer concepts in the treatment of the critically injured patient with abdominal trauma is damage control surgery. This is a different operative philosophy in that rather than a meticulous operation addressing all injuries, only the injuries that threaten the patient's life are addressed. Thus, the operation continues only long enough to achieve a survivable physiology. For example, vascular injuries would be controlled but bowel injuries may be addressed expectantly with ligation. The abdomen is then rapidly closed using varying techniques (e.g., towel-clips closure). The patient is then brought to the intensive care unit, resuscitated, and rewarmed to a survivable physiology. A planned reoperation is then undertaken to restore bowel continuity and to remove packs. This has resulted in a significant increase in the survival of patients who have near-fatal injuries. This technique has evolved from one of a bail-out to one that is proactive. An important principle is to anticipate exceeding the patient's physiologic limits and to limit the operation prior to that occurring.

Although philosophically similar to traditional methods, damage control surgery is being applied to the chest in a different manner. The extremes of the chest such as the apices, the upper mediastinum, and the diaphragmatic areas may be packed, but the mass effect can interfere with pulmonary and cardiac function. In the chest, a different approach with simpler techniques to address life-threatening injuries are used, instead of an abbreviated technique with planned reoperation. Rapid stapling of cardiac injuries to control bleeding has become common. En masse stapled lung resections are performed obviating formal resections in critical patients. One damage control technique that is used increasingly is the pulmonary tractotomy (Wall et al, 1998). In the past, a deep through-and-through injury that was addressed with simple oversewing often resulted in continued intrapulmonary bleeding. Pulmonary tractotomy was developed in parallel with hepatic tractotomy. The wound tract is opened between vascular clamps or with a stapler. Selective vascular ligation is then performed, controlling bleeding and air leaks. Although this occurs across nonanatomic planes, it is tolerated well owing to the dual blood supply of the lung. Pulmonary tractotomy has thus evolved from a technique to preserve lung tissue to one that is simple, quick, and effective in the hands of the trauma surgeon and has the advantage of avoiding a formal lobectomy.

Abbreviated closures of the chest are somewhat different from those for the laparotomy incision. The midline of the abdomen is an avascular area, and towel clips function well for closing. The lateral thoracotomies that are performed in the patient in extremis cut chest wall muscles, which continue to bleed significantly. Although towel-clip closure is used in patients who are near death, it is often more effective to use a continuous, single-layer stitch that closes all layers at once. As in the abdomen, should chest closure interfere with cardiac filling, patch closures (such as those achieved with the sterile intravenous bag) can be employed.

UNRESOLVED ISSUES

Unresolved areas for focused future research and dialogue include (1) the appropriate volume of fluid to administer to patients with penetrating chest trauma (Martin et al, 1992), (2) the development and application of techniques to prevent systemic air emboli, (3) appropriate approaches for the management of penetrating wounds of the thoracic inferior vena cava, and (4) reconstructive techniques for injuries to the superior vena cava and the innominate vein.

COMMENTS AND CONTROVERSIES

In this chapter, the practical management of an epidemic problem of injury to the chest by knives and guns, derived from the extensive experience and thoughtful analysis of Dr. Mattox and his colleagues in Houston, is reviewed. There is a difference in the opinions expressed regarding the approach to hemopericardium. Dr. Mattox recommends against subxiphoid drainage, favoring anterior thoracotomy to allow immediate placement of a pledgeted suture, which is commonly needed with penetrating wounds. Transverse sternotomy is added for the less common penetrating injury requiring cardiopulmonary bypass.

In contrast, Grover and others endorse subxiphoid pericardial drainage in the chapters on initial management of trauma and the management of blunt cardiac injury, with median sternotomy as the next step if the pericardium continues to fill (see Ch. 65). The probability of needing cardiopulmonary bypass rather than digital pressure and a pledgeted suture is probably higher with a blunt injury, which causes persistent pericardial bleeding. The ease and familiarity of the median sternotomy for this purpose is certainly advantageous. Thus, both approaches have merit and a rational basis for application.

Recently the use of externally stented Gore-Tex grafts has been associated with improvement in the patency rate when superior vena caval replacement is required (Dartevelle et al, 1991). This is an encouraging development because the spiral vein graft technique of Doty, which works well, is time-consuming and demanding.

Hyperbaric oxygen treatment should be considered in patients with air embolism following penetrating trauma. Good results have been reported in patients with systemic air embolism from other causes, and hyperbaric oxygen was responsible for recovery in a patient treated 23 hours after massive air embolism unresponsive to cardiopulmonary bypass (Lar et al, 1990).

M.F.M.

■ KEY REFERENCES

Durham LA, Richardson RJ, Wall MJ et al: Emergency center thoracotomy: Impact of prehospital resuscitation. J Trauma 32:775, 1992.

Patients with penetrating thoracic trauma requiring prehospital CPR (who are not intubated) for more than 5 minutes or more than 10 minutes (intubated) do not survive. Extensive resuscitative efforts must be carefully chosen.

LoCicero J, Mattox K: Epidemiology of chest trauma. Surg Clin North Am 69:15, 1989.

In civilian practice, penetrating thoracic trauma is on the increase. Twenty-five percent of the 150,000 annual U.S. deaths caused by trauma have thoracic injury as a cause.

Martin RR, Bickell WH, Pepe PE et al: Prospective evaluation of preoperative fluid resuscitation in hypotensive patients with penetrating trauma injury: A preliminary report. J Trauma 33:1, 1992.

Preoperative crystalloid fluid restriction (during the ambulance ride and in the emergency center) decreases the incidence of adult respiratory distress syndrome (ARDS) and the length of stay in the ICU. It increases the survival time in patients with penetrating thoracic trauma.

Mattox KL: Indications for thoracotomy: Decision to operate. Surg Clin North Am 69:53, 1989.

Only 1% of patients with penetrating thoracic trauma require a formal thoracotomy. A decision to operate follows precise and reproducible indications.

Mattox KL, Feliciano DV, Beall AC et al: Five thousand seven hundred sixty cardiovascular injuries in 4459 patients: Epidemiologic evolution 1958–1988. Ann Surg 209–698, 1989.

Although military vascular injuries occur in the extremities more than 90% of the time in civilian vascular trauma cases, penetrating injury is seen in the trunk in more than 60% of the cases. Penetrating thoracic vascular injury produces especially complex lesions.

■ REFERENCES

Beaumont W: Experiments and Observations on the Gastric Juice and Physiology of Digestion. Plattsburgh, NY, FP Allen, 1833.

Burke JK: Early diagnosis of traumatic rupture of the bronchus. JAMA 181:682, 1962.

Dartevelle P, Chapelier A, Pastorino U et al: Long-term follow-up after prosthetic replacement of the superior vena cava combined with resection of mediastinal-pulmonary malignant tumors. J Thorac Cardiovasc Surg 102:159, 1991.

DeLa Rocha AG, Kayler D: Traumatic rupture of the tracheobronchial tree. Can J Surg 28:68, 1982.

Deslauriers J, Beaulieu M, Archambault G et al: Diagnosis and long-term follow-up of major bronchial disruptions due to nonpenetrating trauma. Ann Thorac Surg 33:32, 1982.

Doty DB: Bypass of superior vena cava: Six years experience with spiral vein graft for obstruction of superior vena cava due to benign and malignant disease. Ann Thorac Surg 22:490, 1976.

Ecker RR, Libertine RV, Rea WJ et al: Injuries of the trachea and bronchi. Ann Thorac Surg 11:289, 1971.

Graham JM, Beal AC Jr, Mattox KL, Vaughn GD: Systemic air embolism following penetrating trauma to the lung. Chest 72:449, 1977.

Grover FL, Ellestad C, Arom KV et al: Diagnosis and management of major tracheobronchial injuries. Ann Thorac Surg 28:384, 1979.

Harken DE: Foreign bodies in, and in relation to, thoracic blood vessels and heart. I. Techniques for approaching and removing foreign bodies from chambers of the heart. Surg Gynecol Obstet 83:117, 1946.

Itani KMF, Burch JM, Richardson R et al: Emergency center arteriography. J Trauma 32:302, 1992.

Jones WS, Mavroudis C, Richardson JD et al: Management of tracheobronchial disruption resulting from blunt trauma. Surgery 95:319, 1984.

Lar LW, Lai LC, Ren LW: Massive arterial air embolism during cardiac operation: Successful treatment in a hyperbaric chamber under 3 ATA. J Thorac Cardiovasc Surg 100:928, 1990.

Miller FB, Richardson JD, Thomas HA: Role of CT in the diagnosis of major arterial injury after blunt thoracic trauma. Surgery 106:596, 1989.

Mills SA, Johnston FR, Hudspeth AS et al: Clinical spectrum of blunt tracheobronchial disruption illustrated by seven cases. J Thorac Cardiovasc Surg 84:4, 2982, 1982.

Parmely LF, Mattingly TW et al: Non-penetrating traumatic injury of the aorta. Circulation 17:1086, 1958.

Pate JW: Tracheobronchial and esophageal injuries. Surg Clin North Am 69:111, 1989.

Sparkman RS, Nixon PI, Crosthwait RW et al: The Texas Surgical Society: The First Fifty Years. Texas Surgical Society, Dallas, 1965.

Wall MJ, Jr. Villavicencio RT, Miller CC et al: Pulmonary tractotomy as an abbreviated thoracotomy technique. J Trauma 45:1015, 1998.

CHAPTER **71**

Adult Respiratory Distress Syndrome

Thomas R. J. Todd

Adult respiratory distress syndrome (ARDS) has become a synonym for respiratory failure of multiple etiologies. Following pulmonary resection, respiratory failure, whether as a result of ARDS or of other etiologies, carries a mortality of 36% (Todd, 1992). This is probably because respiratory reserve has already been permanently altered by the resection itself. Morbidity is also high as reflected in prolonged length of stay in intensive care for those who survive. If sepsis supervenes, the prospect of multiple-system organ failure becomes a distinct possibility, and under such circumstances, the mortality and morbidity increase sharply. In this chapter, the management of the patient in incipient and established respiratory failure is discussed, with special emphasis on ARDS.

HISTORICAL NOTE

The definition and management of ARDS has undergone many changes since its original description. It may develop via several mechanisms. In particular, the role of endothelial lung injury after trauma and sepsis was defined in the classic article by Ashbaugh and colleagues (1967) and later summarized with great clarity by Moore (1969) in his monograph. It was left to Pepe and coworkers (1982) to note the major association between sepsis and what would become known as ARDS.

The therapy of ARDS was until recently restricted to supportive measures only and in particular to the provision of mechanical ventilatory support. Alternatives to volume-cycled mechanical ventilation have occupied intensive care physicians since the 1970s in an effort to support patients for longer periods and to reduce the barotrauma that has been recorded by several authors after the inspiratory pressures increase (Tsuno et al, 1991). Particularly noteworthy are the efforts of Bartlett and colleagues (1977) in the establishment of extracorporeal membrane oxygenation (ECMO). The reader is referred to the landmark study of Zapol and associates (1979), which concluded that ECMO provided no survival benefit over conventional forms of ventilation. The latter study, although often quoted, was undertaken without a sample size calculation and has an inherently large beta error; that is, the chance that there was a positive result that was not recorded by the study because of insufficient numbers is quite high. Carlon and colleagues (1981) are credited with bringing high-frequency ventilation (HFV) to our attention. HFV plays a significant role in the management of patients with bronchopleural fistulas. These means of ventilatory support are discussed in the section on ventilatory support that follows.

HISTORICAL READINGS

Ashbaugh DG, Bigelow DB, Petty TL et al: Acute respiratory distress in adults. Lancet 2:319, 1967.

Barlett RH, Gazzamiga AB, Fong SW et al: Extracorporeal membrane oxygenat or support for cardiopulmonary failure: Experience in 28 cases. J Thorac Cardiovasc Surg 73:375, 1977.

Carlon GC, Kahn RC, Howland WS et al: Clinical experience with high frequency jet ventilation. Crit Care Med 9:1, 1981.

Moore E: Clinical pathologic ARDS. In Moore FD, Lyons JH, Pierce EC et al (eds): Post-traumatic Pulmonary Insufficiency. Philadelphia, WB Saunders, 1969.

Pepe PE, Potkin RT, Reus DH et al: Clinical predictors of the adult respiratory distress syndrome. Am J Surg 144:124, 1982.

Tsuno K, Miura K, Takeya M et al: Histopathologic pulmonary changes from mechanical ventilation at high peak airway pressures. Am Rev Respir Dis 143:1115, 1991.

Zapol WM et al: Extracorporeal membrane oxygenation in severe acute respiratory failure. JAMA 193:2193, 1979

PATHOPHYSIOLOGY OF RESPIRATORY FAILURE AND ARDS

Despite adequate perioperative evaluation and preparation, respiratory failure may develop in the postoperative period. It is useful to classify respiratory failure as in Table 71–1, because the diagnosis may be facilitated by an appreciation of the pathophysiology.

Pure ventilatory failure usually occurs in the immediate postoperative period secondary to inadequate reversal

TABLE 71–1 ■ **Achieving the Lowest Therapeutic Intervention**

Means of lowering fraction of inspired oxygen
- Positive end-expiratory pressure
- Diuresis
- Postural changes
- Ventilatory changes (e.g., high-frequency jet ventilation or inverse ratio)

Means of lowering airway pressure
- ↑ Rate and ↓ tidal volume
- Permissive hypercarbia
- Bronchoscopy
- Pleural drainage
- High-frequency jet ventilation

Means of lowering preload
- Diuresis and fluid restriction
- β-adrenergic agents (e.g., dopamine)

of anesthesia, opiate overdosage, unrecognized pneumothorax, or airway obstruction. As a result, early assessment of arterial blood gases in the recovery room is important. If the initial arterial carbon dioxide tension ($Paco_2$) is normal, further assessments of a gas exchange can usually be achieved with noninvasive oxygen saturation monitoring. However, if the $Paco_2$ is elevated, careful evaluation of the patient, further blood gas assessment, and possibly the administration of narcotic antagonists or the further reversal of muscle relaxation are indicated. The latter is particularly indicated when there is significant respiratory acidosis (pH < 7.2). Under such circumstances, pharmacologic intervention or reintubation is required.

Ventilatory failure later in the postoperative period most commonly occurs in a mixed fashion, with associated hypoxemia. The most common causes are respiratory muscle fatigue, bronchial spasm, pneumonia, and bronchopleural fistula. Often the clinician is under the impression that pure ventilatory failure is present because supplemental oxygenation has achieved a satisfactory arterial oxygen tension (Pao_2) or oxygen saturation as the $Paco_2$ is rising. In the patient with marginal preoperative pulmonary function, postoperative atelectasis, pneumonia, pulmonary edema, or poor relief of pain, respiratory muscle fatigue may eventually develop. At this point ventilatory failure, if not apparent before, quickly ensues, and the $Paco_2$ will rise abruptly.

Hypoxemic respiratory failure is fairly common and is the hallmark of ARDS. The onset of hypoxemia implies a mismatching of ventilation and perfusion (V/Q abnormality) (Fig. 71–1). The degree of V/Q imbalance will determine the severity of the venous admixture and subsequent hypoxemia. Hypoxemia may be caused by a number of clinical situations. In the first 72 hours following major thoracic procedures, atelectasis and excessive extravascular lung water are common. Both can result in mismatching of ventilation and perfusion. The former is usually secondary to secretional retention during anesthesia or the failure to adequately expand areas of the lung that were purposely collapsed during the surgical procedure. The latter is often due to excessive fluid administration, cardiac failure, or alterations in pulmonary capillary permeability from the handling of the lung. Chest physiotherapy, adequate pain relief, and diuretic therapy usually result in an improvement in alveolar arterial oxygen gradients that occur in the first 48 hours following surgery. This early hypoxemia should not be interpreted as the harbinger of ARDS. In the next few days following surgery, however, sputum retention and resultant microatelectases, the aspiration of gastric contents, or the onset of ARDS may lead to further impairment of oxygenation or the establishment of pneumonia.

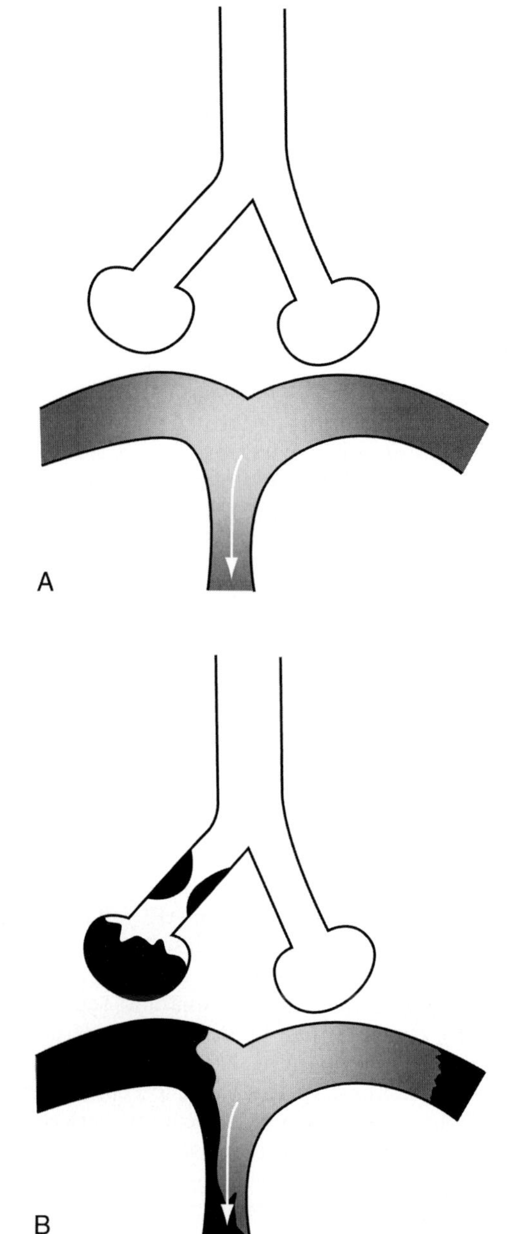

FIGURE 71–1 ■ *A*, Two-alveoli model of normal V/Q distribution. *B*, Two-alveoli model of abnormal V/Q distribution. The abnormally ventilated alveolus contributes desaturated blood to the left atrium for mixing with saturated blood from well-ventilated alveoli.

PATHOPHYSIOLOGY OF ARDS

The term *ARDS* was coined by Ashbaugh and colleagues (1967) to describe a clinicopathologic entity of acute lung injury. Moore (1969) provided a comprehensive review of the knowledge at that time. He identified several clinical stages in the disorder from an initial stage of respiratory distress, which is indistinguishable from acute pulmonary edema, to a late stage that is characterized by stiff, poorly compliant lungs and both hypercarbia and hypoxia. The pathologic descriptions of the latter stages perfectly paralleled those described in subsequent reports. The clinical situations associated with ARDS are legion and have led to considerable confusion in regard to the pathophysiology of ARDS. Shock, pancreatitis, and perfusion-reperfusion injuries (such as in transplantation), multiple blood transfusions, trauma, and, most importantly, sepsis have all been associated with the development of ARDS. Sepsis is perhaps the most frequent predisposing situation (Pepe et al, 1982).

The common clinical picture involves the rapid development of hypoxemia and diffuse pulmonary infiltrates 24 to 48 hours after the inciting event in a clinical situation where left ventricular preload is normal (Fig. 71–2). Frequently, however, the clinical picture is confused with either pulmonary edema secondary to cardiac failure or with pulmonary sepsis. Common to all the predisposing entities is the clinical and radiologic picture of pulmonary edema. The lungs become poorly compliant and filled with copious frothy pink secretions. It was initially suggested that the pulmonary edema was secondary to an increase in microvascular pressure (Kusajima et al, 1974; Webb, 1982). However, capillary pressures in both humans and experimental models of ARDS were subsequently shown to be normal or low (Brigham et al, 1974; Todd et al, 1968). Staub and coworkers (Brigham et al, 1974; Vreim and Staub, 1976) demonstrated that, in awake sheep, pulmonary capillary permeability was altered. It is now generally accepted that the basic defect is an increase in pulmonary capillary permeability. The permeability characteristics of the pulmonary capillary are altered by mechanical trauma during surgery, infection, aspiration, and sepsis. The filtration of fluid across the pulmonary capillary is described by the Starling equation, as follows:

$$FM = K[(P_C - P_{is}) - \gamma(P_C - P_{is})]$$

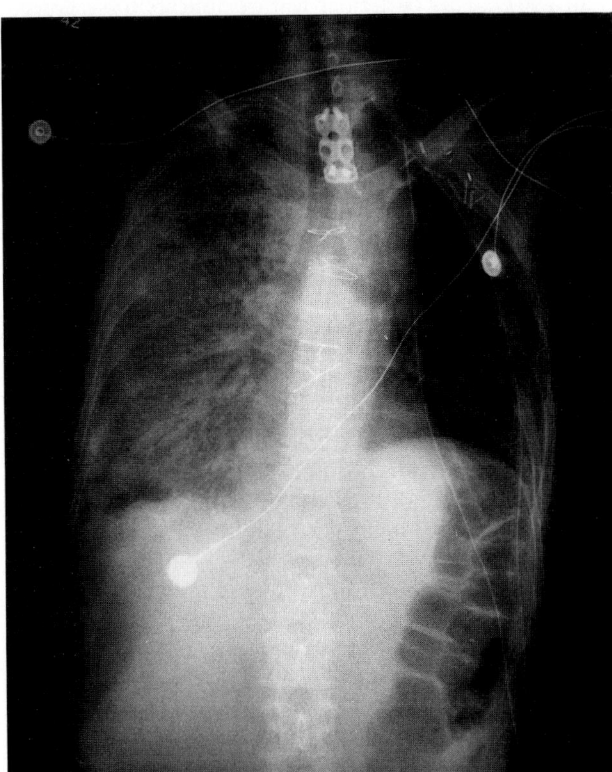

FIGURE 71–2 ■ Postoperative chest radiograph in a patient who has undergone left upper lobectomy and chest wall resection following neoadjuvant chemotherapy. Note the air-space disease in the right lung. No organisms were ever cultured, and the patient recovered without antibiotic therapy.

where FM is the fluid movement across the capillary, K is the permeability coefficient of the membrane, P_C is capillary hydrostatic pressure, and P_{is} is interstitial hydrostatic pressure. Gamma (γ) = the osmotic reflection coefficient of the membrane, P_C is the capillary osmotic pressure, and P_{is} is interstitial osmotic pressure.

When the permeability coefficient is altered, the major determinants of transcapillary fluid movement are hydrostatic capillary pressure and capillary osmotic pressure. There is no recognized therapeutic maneuver to alter osmotic pressure, other than the temporary effect of colloid administration. Hydrostatic pressure can, however, be modified by fluid restriction and diuretic therapy. Thus, diuresis is a useful therapeutic adjunct whether the extravascular fluid accumulation is secondary to fluid overload or altered permeability.

The numerous clinical predisposing factors associated with ARDS suggest that either the lung has one pathophysiologic response or that there is a common pathway of biochemical injury to the alveolar-capillary membrane that results in altered permeability. In pulmonary surgery, the incidence of ARDS has been variously reported as occurring between 5% and 15% (Parquin et al 1996; Williams et al, 1996). No doubt some of the reported cases are secondary to fluid overload or congestive heart failure rather than due to permeability changes in the pulmonary capillary. Predisposing factors were examined recently by Parquin and coworkers (1996). Following pneumonectomy, they concluded, previous radiation or chemotherapy, remaining lung perfusion less than 55%, and intraoperative fluid administration of more than 2 L were associated with pulmonary edema. The association with induction chemotherapy has also been noted and bears consideration during an era of increased interest in this therapeutic modality.

ARDS may have its onset after the development of respiratory failure that has occurred for other reasons. Patients who require ventilatory support because of sputum retention, pneumonia, or reasons that are unrelated to primary lung failure such as myocardial ischemia and congestive failure may develop an ARDS clinical picture following several days of ventilatory support. This situation is not unique to the thoracic population and has been called ventilator-associated lung injury (Dreyfuss et al, 1988; Tsuno et al, 1991). Indeed, there is speculation that the prolonged course of ARDS may not be related to the initial inciting event but rather may be the result of ventilatory support at high pressures. It has been generally accepted that regional overdistension of alveoli can occur from high ventilation volumes and pressure that is likely related to shear factors during the opening and closing of lung units. The availability of computed tomography (CT) scans in the intensive care unit population has now permitted us to recognize that the radiologic injury at least is not uniform but rather is frequently restricted to the dependent areas of the lung (Puybasset et al, 1998) (Fig. 71–3). These observations have led to proposals that the mode of ventilatory support may be the most important aspect of care after the onset of respiratory failure. This will be discussed in the section of therapy of ARDS.

The onset of ARDS is particularly devastating after

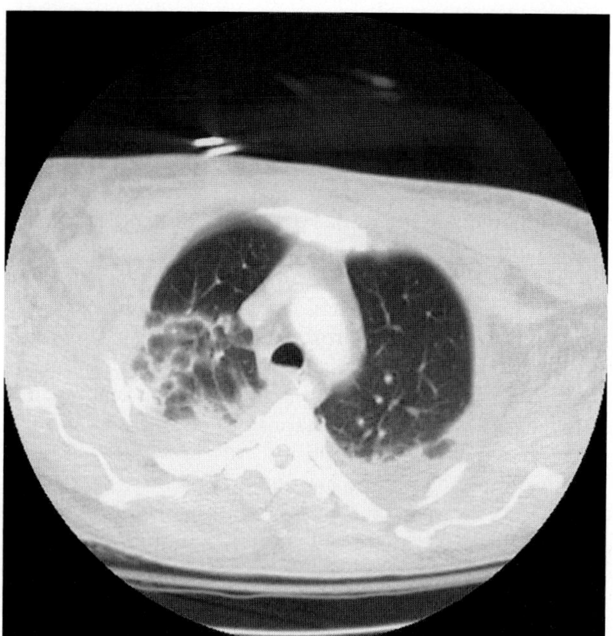

FIGURE 71–3 ■ A computed tomography scan of a patient with ARDS following Boerhaave's syndrome.

pneumonectomy. The etiology remains unclear but recent attention has focused on the fact that it may represent a form of ischemia reperfusion injury caused by the collapse of the diseased lung, which results in alterations in perfusion or endothelial function in the contralateral remaining lung (Williams et al, 1996). More likely, it may be the result of white-cell sequestration and activation in the remaining lung during the surgical procedure. Granulocyte elastase levels have been shown to increase 300% following pneumonectomy as opposed to lobectomy in which increases are modest (Martin, 1994). If this were the case, one would expect the abnormality to become clinically apparent in the first 24 hours following resection (rather than at 48 to 72 hours); however, the white-cell and inflammatory mediators were the focus of most basic research at the end of the 20th century.

A summary of the available experimental literature suggests that neutrophils and macrophages are required to produce the permeability defect. It would appear that this occurs by virtue of the inflammatory mediators that these cells produce. Almost all experimental models of ARDS record a biphasic increase in pulmonary artery pressure, the second phase also being associated with an increase in capillary permeability. The complement system has also received a great deal of attention, but its involvement is likely to be related to the stimulation of leukocytes. In addition, arachidonic acid metabolites (Fig. 71–4) appear to be responsible for many of the physiologic alterations noted in the clinical and the experimental disorder. The degradation of arachidonic acid results in the production of several compounds that have profound effects on vascular reactivity, inflammation, and capillary permeability. In particular, experimental observation has focused on the generation of thromboxane A_2 and prostacyclin. The latter has been shown to initiate platelet aggregation (Whittle et al, 1978) and dilation of both the systemic and the pulmonary vascular trees (Watkins et al, 1980). On the other hand, thromboxane A_2 is a potent vasoconstrictor and a stimulus to platelet aggregation (Oats et al, 1988; Schmeck et al, 1998). Both of these metabolites are released from the lung, probably from the vascular endothelium during the injection of endotoxin or bacteria into the circulation (Demling et al, 1981). In experimental models, the appearance of prostanoids or endothelin is temporarily correlated with pulmonary changes that mimic ARDS in humans (Schmeck et al, 1998). In addition, the inhibition of cyclooxygenase by nonsteroidal anti-inflammatory drugs (NSAIDs) has been shown to blunt the pulmonary hypertensive response (Schmeck et al, 1998) and resultant arterial hypoxemia that were noted in the early stages of all animal models of ARDS. This observation is consistently noted both pretreatment and post-treatment with these mediators (Metz and Sibbald, 1991). The degree of protection afforded by NSAIDs is variable. It is greatest with ibuprofen, which suggests that such drugs individually possess properties beyond their observed effects on cyclooxygenase. This latter point is emphasized by the relatively poor effects of corticosteroids, also cyclooxygenase inhibitors, in the early phase I stage of experimental ARDS. NSAIDs also have been shown to ameliorate the phase II arterial oxygen desaturation phase of ARDS.

An important role for leucocytes has been suggested by the observation that they are sequestered in the lung after endotoxemia, bacteremia, or the administration of compounds that activate the complement system (Smith et al, 1981). This particular feature appears to be consistent in most animal models of ARDS. Leucocytes adhere to the pulmonary endothelium, and the oxidative burst that follows their activation can certainly produce the permeability changes noted in the full-blown syndrome. Several studies in human subjects support a prominent role for leucocytes in the pathogenesis of ARDS (Nahum et al, 1991; Rivkind et al, 1981; Simms and Damico, 1991; Tagan et al, 1981). These reports have compared the expression of leucocyte antigen and the incidence of white-cell activation in patients with ARDS or at risk for ARDS with similar parameters in nonseptic control subjects. These results are consistent with the clinical observations of increases in white-cell elastase following pneumonectomy by Schmeck and colleagues (1998). In some animal models of ARDS, depletion of white cells prior to the induction of injury has prevented or attenuated the defect (Egan et al, 1985).

Recognition of an important role for tumor necrosis factor (TNF) or cachectin has focused attention on the macrophage. TNF is a 15-amino acid polypeptide that is released by macrophages in response to various stimuli. Responsible for several biologic interactions, it can mediate the adhesion of leucocytes to endothelial cells (Gamble et al, 1985), and its levels have been shown to increase dramatically during experimental sepsis (Leeper-Woodford et al, 1991). After the white blood cells adhere to the pulmonary endothelium, a superoxide release occurs that appears to be augmented by TNF and can lead to significant pulmonary destruction (Tracey et al, 1987). Of considerable interest is the fact that anti-TNF monoclonal antibodies have been shown to prevent the pulmo-

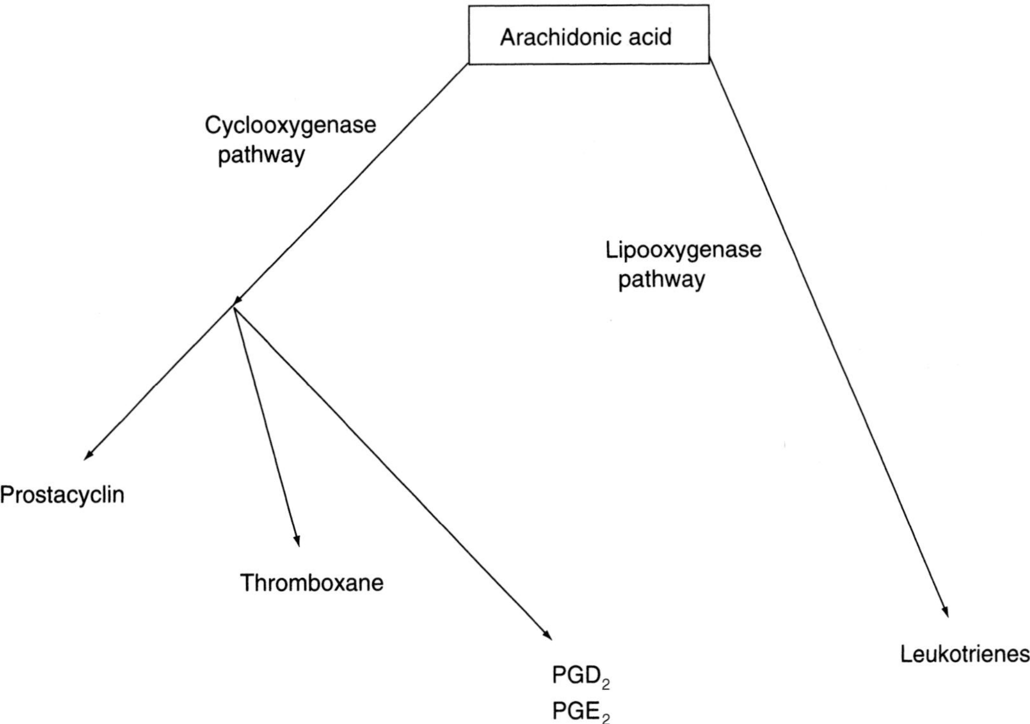

FIGURE 71–4 ■ Arachidonic acid metabolism.

nary complications and ventilatory failure that is associated with a 50% lethal-dose intravenous injection of live bacteria in baboons. Elevation of the TNF level has been observed in the bronchoalveolar lavage fluid and serum of patients with established ARDS and also in those at risk of this syndrome (Hers et al, 1991).

The interleukin family of mediators has also been implicated in ARDS. Interleukin-8 is elevated in patients with early ARDS (Goodman et al, 1998). The alveolar macrophage is also capable of generating several inflammatory mediators. In a recent experimental study, interleukin-10 was shown to significantly reduce the production of TNF and prostaglandin E_2 (PGE_2) (Lo et al, 1998).

In summary, it would appear that there are a series of interrelated events and pathways to ARDS. As noted by Metz and Sibbald (1991), the two main components are the inflammatory process (as represented by the stimulation of the complement system and leucocytes) and the generation of the products of arachidonic acid metabolism.

CLINICAL ASSESSMENT

The first signs of respiratory difficulty may be subtle. Tachypnea and sinus tachycardia often precede the radiographic changes. Although most patients undergoing pulmonary resection require supplemental oxygen, the presence of a wide alveolar-arterial oxygen gradient ($P_{AO_2} - Pa_{O_2}$) suggests that an unexpected and significant V/Q problem has developed. Thus, the high oxygen requirements should be of concern. Arterial blood gas determinations may enable the surgeon to appreciate not only the severity of the problem but also the progression of the difficulty over time. A widening of the $P_{AO_2} - Pa_{O_2}$ suggests that the V/Q abnormality is progressive. The development of hypercarbia alerts the physician to the fact that there is now either an increase in dead space or that respiratory fatigue is incipient. The rapidity of any of these changes reflects the urgency for intervention, most specifically the requirement of mechanical ventilatory support. Fatigue may be clinically manifest by the development of tachypnea, confusion, somnolence, or the use of the accessory muscles of respiration. A more specific indicator of fatigue and the need for ventilatory support is the presence of abdominal–chest wall respiratory paradox. During normal spontaneous inspiration, both the chest wall and the abdomen expand; the latter is secondary to diaphragmatic descent (Fig. 71–5). With the development of respiratory muscle fatigue, the diaphragm no longer functions properly. As a result, as the chest expands from the contraction of the chest wall muscles, the diaphragm is drawn upward as pleural pressure falls. Thus, during clinical assessment, the hand on the abdomen follows the abdomen inward as the hand on the chest expands. Although new Pa_{CO_2} elevations that occur in association with V/Q abnormalities may alert the clinician to the onset of a mixed respiratory failure pattern, the presence of chest wall–abdominal paradox indicates established respiratory fatigue and the need for intubation and ventilatory support. In determining that a particular patient requires ventilatory assistance, the three most reliable parameters are:

1. The rapidity of change in Pa_{O_2} and P_{CO_2}.
2. The observation of diaphragmatic fatigue.
3. The observation that the patient is no longer able to speak in uninterrupted sentences.

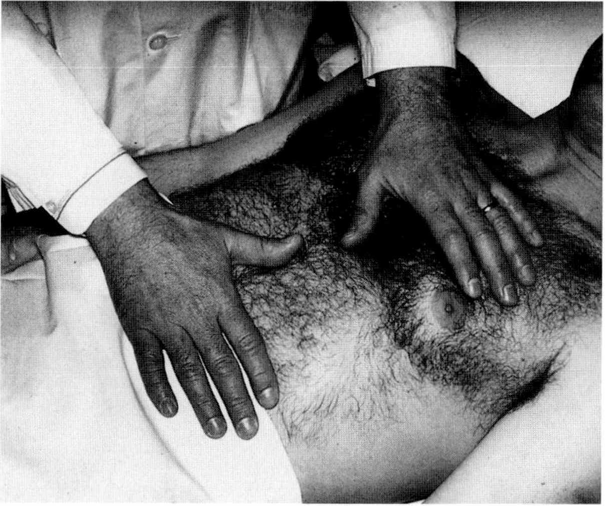

FIGURE 71–5 ■ Physical examination to detect abdominal–chest wall paradox.

In the postoperative period, the first signs of impending respiratory difficulty may be subtle radiographic changes that usually become apparent on the second day following pulmonary resection. Early airspace disease or an increase in perihilar markings suggest either fluid overload or impending ARDS. An accurate interpretation of the chest radiograph will permit the surgeon to intervene not only earlier but more appropriately. The radiographic features peculiar to ARDS, as opposed to pneumonia, are the diffuse nature of the alveolar infiltrate, the presence of interstitial edema, and the occasional appearance of peribronchial cuffing as seen in Figure 71–2 (although the latter is more commonly seen with cardiac edema). It is important to remember that pneumonia may complicate established ARDS, particularly in the ventilated patient. In the first few postoperative days, chest films are usually portable and may be of less than ideal quality and therefore difficult to interpret. The first thing to determine when one has appreciated that there is new airspace disease is whether the distribution of the alveolar infiltrate is generalized or focal. The latter suggests a pneumonic process (Fig. 71–6) whereas the former is more typical of ARDS (Fig. 71–7), congestive failure, or fluid overload. An appreciation of these differences can form the basis of an interventional algorithm as noted later.

THERAPEUTIC CONSIDERATIONS

General Measures

During the period of assessment, there are several interventions that may provide assistance to the patient and avoid the progression to ventilatory support. These include supplemental oxygen administration, chest physiotherapy, adequate analgesia, inhalation therapy, bronchoscopy, and diuretic therapy when applicable. The latter three deserve further comment. Inhalation therapy is important. These patients, most of whom have been smokers, frequently have small airways disease, and bronchospasm is exacerbated in the postoperative period from sputum retention, bronchial infection, and fluid overload. As a result, albuterol therapy through an ultrasonic nebulizer is an important adjunct. The ultrasonic nebulizer ensures adequate deposition of the bronchodilator compared with the standard hand-held inhalers that depend on the patient's performance. Acetylcysteine (Mucomyst) is an additional aid when secretions are thick and tenacious. Although acetylcysteine can cause bronchial irritation and bronchospasm, these complications are unusual if it is given with albuterol. Fiberoptic bronchoscopy can be undertaken in a step-down area or intensive care unit to aid in the elimination of secretions or to obtain specimens in the diagnosis of pulmonary sepsis. It is important to remember that, in the face of significant hypoxemia, bronchoscopy is not without risk. As a result, it should be performed under controlled circumstances with adequate local analgesia, oxygen supplementation, and oxygen saturation monitoring. If hypoxemia requires high-flow oxygen (>60%), endotracheal intubation should be considered to permit safe bronchoscopy. Diuresis is often necessary because most postoperative pulmonary bronchial disease is complicated by extravascular fluid accumulation. As noted above, there are obligate alterations in capillary permeability, and there has frequently been the administration of significant amounts of intravenous fluids. Even in the absence of radiographic

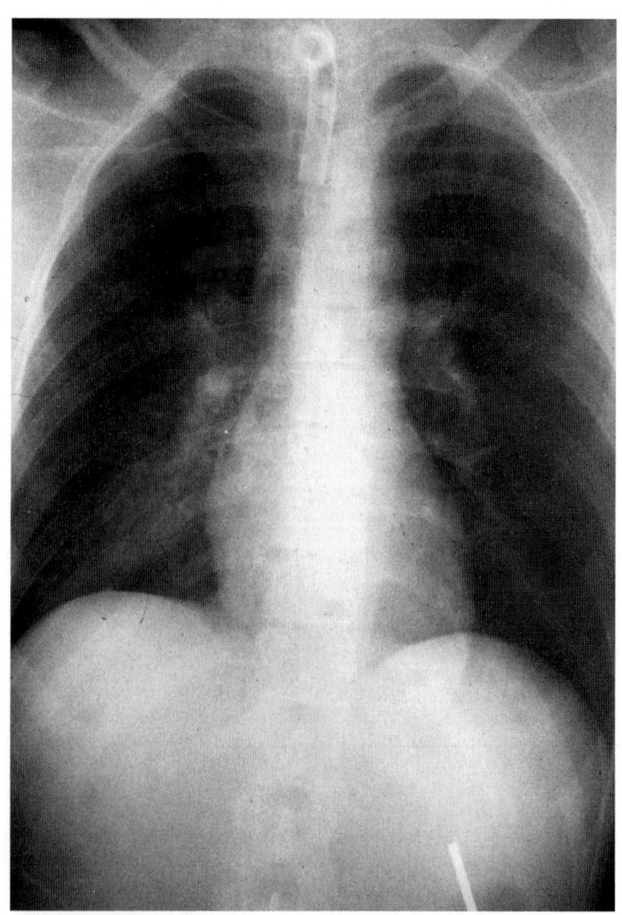

FIGURE 71–6 ■ Chest radiograph demonstrating a focal alveolar infiltrate.

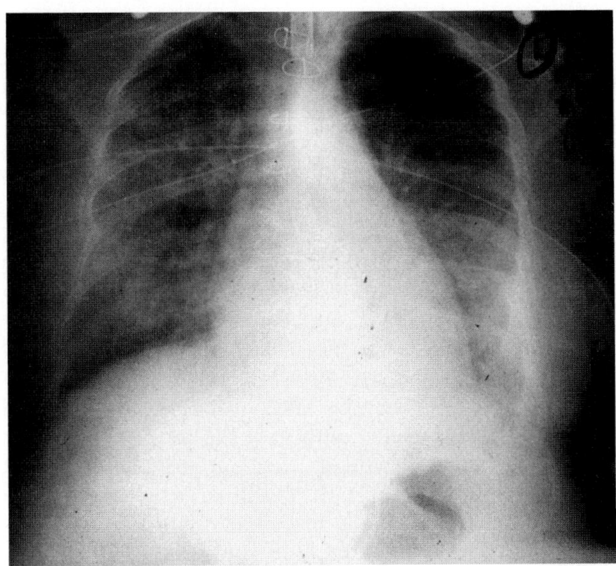

FIGURE 71–7 ■ Chest radiograph demonstrating a generalized infiltrate that proved to be ARDS.

abnormalities, there may be significant increases in extravascular lung water.

In the experience of this author, the presence of an elevated white cell count or purulent sputum is helpful in differentiating pneumonia from ARDS but is so often equivocal that a treatment algorithm proves more effective (Fig. 71–8). If the patient has a focal pulmonary infiltrate, sputum is obtained for Gram stain and culture and antibiotics are started. Diuresis is also frequently employed. An excellent guide to the requirement for diuresis is the patient's preoperative weight. If the postoperative weight is greater than that recorded at admission, diuresis is undertaken, even if the clinical diagnosis is pneumonia. If the chest film suggests a generalized alveolar infiltrate, diuresis is the mainstay of therapy until the results of sputum cultures are available. Aggressive diuresis is performed irrespective of the patient's weight under this circumstance. Assuming that a permeability abnormality is present, the only means the clinician has to decrease extravascular lung water is to lower capillary pressure. A decrease in left ventricular preload is the only means of accomplishing this. If therapy fails to achieve prompt results, re-evaluation is essential. A positive culture in the generalized radiographic case demands appropriate antimicrobial therapy.

Unfortunately, both ARDS and pneumonia may be unresponsive to therapeutic interventions, and respiratory failure may ensue (Fig. 71–9). The presence of an endotracheal tube permits the early use of bronchoscopic surveillance of airway secretions. Thus, irrespective of whether a focal or generalized infiltrate is present, bronchoscopy, bronchoalveolar lavage (BAL), and protected specimen brushing (PSB) of abnormal areas is undertaken. These are the most sensitive (BAL) and specific (PSB) means of diagnosing pneumonia (Chastre et al, 1988; Decastro et al, 1991). Gram stains are obtained. If the alveolar abnormality is generalized, antibiotic therapy is withheld until cultures return; but appropriate antibiotics are commenced on the basis of the Gram stain. Meduri and coworkers (1998) noted a positive return in just under 30% of patients with clinical ARDS who underwent bronchoscopic assessment. As a result, antibiotic therapy was frequently modified.

When respiratory failure persists and the radiographic abnormalities fail to resolve, there are two other interventions that should be considered. First, a pulmonary artery

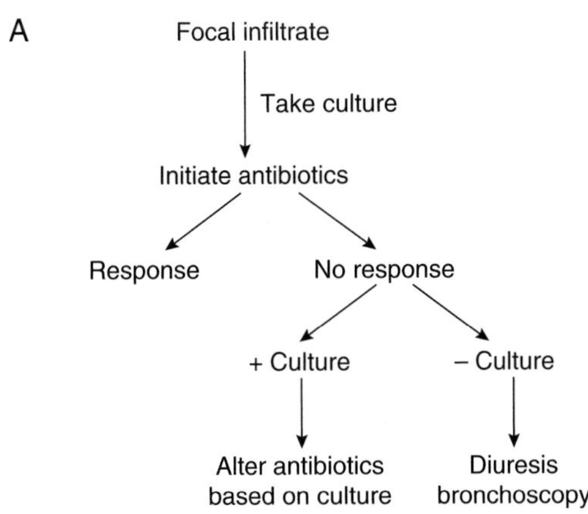

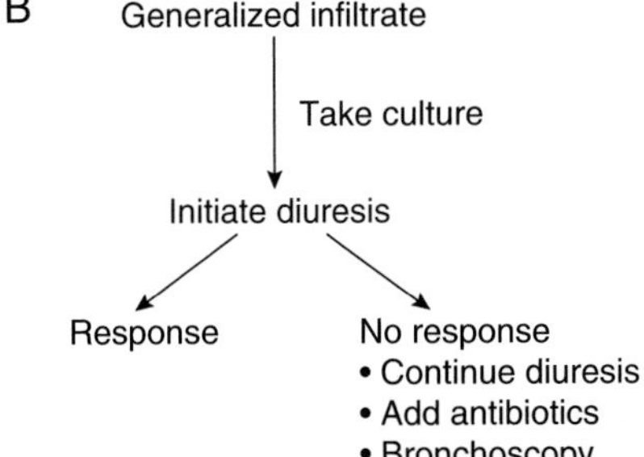

FIGURE 71–8 ■ Algorithm for therapy of parenchymal infiltrates in nonventilated patients.

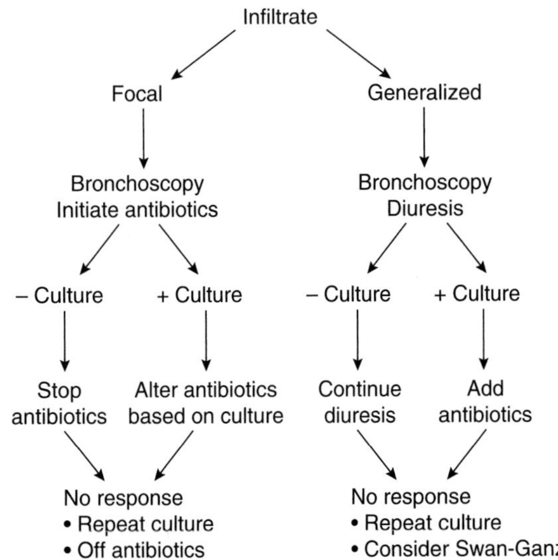

FIGURE 71–9 ■ Algorithm for therapy of parenchymal infiltrates in ventilated patients.

catheter may provide more accurate information concerning left ventricular preload and cardiac function. In addition, one should begin to consider the value of an open lung biopsy. However, in the nonimmunosuppressed patient, the latter is unlikely to yield useful information.

Pharmacologic Support

Specific pharmacologic intervention is directed at the interruption of the pathophysiologic changes. For the most part, it has been concerned with the blockade of the proposed mediators discussed earlier. Experimentation with corticosteroids in animal models, either therapeutically or prophylactically, has not produced consistent results (Begley et al, 1984; Demling et al, 1980; Modig and Bord, 1985; Traber et al, 1984). Clinical trials of methylprednisolone in patients with ARDS or at risk of acquiring it have not demonstrated a beneficial effect (Bernard et al, 1987; Bone et al, 1987; Luce et al, 1988). As a result, routine use of corticosteroid has fallen out of favor. The literature demonstrated that there was a discrepancy in therapeutic effect of corticosteroids between experimental and clinical studies. The former usually demonstrated significant benefits in experimental models of ARDS wherein the steroid was administered either prophylactically or immediately after the inciting event. This, however, was not possible in the randomized clinical trials. Recent evidence suggests that the clinical role of corticosteroid may actually be later in the course of the disease and that administration is required for a more prolonged period than was considered in any of the other clinical trials. In that regard, Meduri and colleagues (1998) undertook a double-blind, randomized clinical trial of methylprednisolone versus placebo in patients with established ARDS that showed no sign of resolving after 7 days. Corticosteroid was administered for 32 days. A significant improvement in survival was noted for the steroid group. This study had a small sample size, but the results suggest a new role for corticosteroid administration during the chronic fibroproliferative phase of the disease. This conclusion is supported by another retrospective review of clinical experience with steroid use in established ARDS 1 week after the initiation of mechanical ventilatory support (Keel et al, 1998). If steroids are used in ARDS, the state of the art would suggest that treatment be reserved for those patients who are 7 days into the process and, most importantly, who have no evidence of superimposed pneumonia.

There is a wealth of experimental literature on the use of NSAIDs as preventive therapy or post-injury therapy in ARDS. The most impressive evidence for their therapeutic role has been found with the use of ibuprofen. In experimental models, pretreatment with ibuprofen in bacteriologically induced ARDS has uniformly resulted in significant amelioration of the pulmonary vascular responses and resultant hypoxemia (Balk et al, 1984; Barke et al, 1983; Kopolovic et al, 1984). There have been two clinical reports of ibuprofen therapy in human lung injury. One showed no benefit, but the other—an anecdotal report—suggested that there was considerable improvement in both pulmonary vascular pressures and hypoxemia (Hallemans et al, 1984; Hasselstrom et al, 1985).

There have been no clinical trials of the other half of the arachidonic acid metabolic pathway, that is, the lipooxygenase pathway. Blockade of this pathway in ARDS has not been as intensively studied as has the cyclooxygenase pathway. Pretreatment has been the rule, and attenuation of the pathophysiologic changes, but no complete protection, has been observed (Cohn et al, 1991; Turner et al, 1991). Other prostanoids have been used in the therapy of ARDS, particularly prostaglandin E_1 (PGE_1). Holcroft and colleagues (1986) conducted a randomized trial of PGE_1 in ARDS and reported a significant improvement in the mortality rate. The trial involved a small group of patients in whom remarkable improvement occurred. In a large randomized trial, the results could not be duplicated, although the trial did conclude that PGE_1 had a beneficial effect on oxygen transport (Silverman et al, 1990). If PGE_1 is beneficial in this disorder, its effect is likely to be secondary to pulmonary and systemic vasodilatation, with a resultant reduction in right ventricular afterload and improvement in oxygen delivery. Prostacyclin (PGI_2) has also been reported to have beneficial effects in experimentally induced ARDS (Slotman et al, 1982). A selective pulmonary artery vasodilator, PGI_2 can also be administered as an aerosol. In doses of 7.5 ng/kg/min, PGI_2 was found to be equivalent to nitric oxide as far as improvement in oxygenation was concerned (Walmrath et al, 1996).

Interest has been generated in the use of inhaled nitric oxide. Roissant and colleagues (1993) demonstrated an improvement in gas exchange without an influence on the overall mortality rate. Since this publication, there have been several other case series (Brett et al, 1998; Iotti et al, 1998; Johannigman et al, 1997) and randomized clinical trials (Dellinger et al, 1998; Michael et al, 1998; Troncey et al, 1998) addressing the efficacy of inhaled nitric oxide. These trials have indicated an improvement in oxygenation and a decrease in pulmonary artery pressure in 40% to 65% of patients with ARDS. The improvement is not always sustained beyond 24 hours. None of the trials has demonstrated an increase in survival. When the fraction of inspired oxygen (FIO_2) requirements are high or pulmonary artery pressures are increased, inhaled nitric oxide offers acute benefits. It is certainly worth implementation in doses of 5 to 30 parts per million, although there are no known predictors of response (Brett et al, 1998).

The search continues for a therapy that is specific and can interrupt the sequence of events that leads to ARDS. Another exciting prospect is the development of a monoclonal antibody against TNF. In a rabbit model of endotoxic shock, administration of anti-TNF antibodies prevented the deposition of fibrin in the lung and the appearance of pulmonary edema (Mathison et al, 1988). Similar results were observed in baboons that were given a lethal injection of bacteria; pulmonary edema and subsequent ventilatory failure did not occur (Tracey et al, 1987).

VENTILATION

Tracheal Intubation

Despite prophylactic measures, respiratory failure may ensue, which requires the institution of mechanical ventilation. Clinical judgment rather than laboratory numbers should determine when conservative methods of support are inadequate. The increased work of breathing is signaled by accessory muscle recruitment. Progression to dis-coordinated breathing patterns in which abdominal-diaphragmatic excursion is paradoxic to chest wall movement is a certain sign of impending respiratory failure (see Fig. 71–5). Tachypnea and a rising $Pa{CO_2}$ should prompt action. The combination of hypoxemia and hypercarbia should signal the need for immediate intubation. The fatigued patient often presents the most difficult problem. When does the clinician decide that it is time for mechanical support? Often the patients are the best guide. Lucid patients who can speak in sentences and report that they are the same or better provide a reliable index for continued conservative therapy. The onset of confusion, agitation, and inability to speak in sentences indicates that intubation is essential. A combination of impending respiratory failure and hemodynamic instability can be lethal and warrants tracheal intubation and ventilatory support at an earlier stage. In general, ongoing and frequent re-evaluation of the patient and arterial blood gases provides the best guide. The rapidity of change is of prognostic importance. Under such circumstances, early intubation and ventilation before overt signs are present is preferable to a respiratory or cardiopulmonary arrest.

At the time of intubation, it is imperative that the clinician have all the equipment that might be required readily available should difficulties arise. Most hospitals have accumulated this equipment into a specific intubation tray. Intubation for ventilatory or respiratory failure is best done with the patient awake but sedated. During awake intubation, patients must be subjected to minimal trauma and stress. The act of intubation itself can activate ventricular arrhythmias, cause aspiration, and exacerbate hypoxemia. The procedure should be explained to the patient in a reassuring manner. Intravenous diazepam, at a dose of 5 to 10 mg, induces light sedation and relieves anxiety. A short-acting intravenous analgesic such as fentanyl (50 to 100 mg) may further reduce the patient's awareness. The mouth is suctioned to remove secretions, and the back of the throat is sprayed with a 1% lidocaine aerosol. The laryngoscope blade is inserted, and the vocal cords are visualized and sprayed with the local anesthetic. This takes time. The lidocaine should be applied to the pharynx and the larynx intermittently, with 100% oxygen supplied by a tandem set-up between applications. A pulse oximeter can ensure that oxygen saturation is appropriate throughout the procedure. During the application of the local anesthetic, the patient's respiration should be assisted by an Ambu bag. It is important to ensure synchrony with the patient's efforts. Under such circumstances, oxygenation can usually be maintained and reassurance of the same obtained with continuous noninvasive saturation monitoring. In addition, the patient should not be positioned supine because the diaphragm is then placed in a disadvantageous position, which further increases the work of breathing. Rather, the patient should be positioned in a high Fowler's position. Not only will it be easier to assist the patient's respiratory effort but the intubation itself will be facilitated, particularly if a pillow is placed behind the head to ensure that the oropharynx and glottis are in alignment.

An alternate approach is nasotracheal intubation. The nares and the throat must be anesthetized with lidocaine spray. A 7.5- to 8-mm tube is usually well tolerated. Successful blind intubation requires practice, although with Magill forceps and a laryngoscope, the tube can often be guided into the proper position. Again with the patient in a Fowler's position, the endotracheal tube is positioned through the nares into the oropharynx. By listening over the end of the tube, the clinician can appreciate the point at which the tube lies over the vocal cords. For nasotracheal intubation, it is imperative that the clinician ensures that the endotracheal tube has not already been cut, in which case it may be too short to reach from the anterior nares to the upper trachea.

With flexible bronchoscopes available to the thoracic surgeon, intubation should be neither blind nor difficult. Flexible bronchoscopy can be used for either oral or nasal routes. Pharmacologic management is the same as described earlier. The bronchoscope is passed through the endotracheal tube and placed into the mouth or nostril (Fig. 71–10). Gentle traction on the tongue facilitates exposure of the larynx. Once the vocal cords have been visualized, 5 ml of 1% lidocaine is flushed through the suction port to anesthetize the vocal cords. The bronchoscope is passed between the vocal cords into the upper trachea and into either mainstem bronchus. In this position, the bronchoscope acts as a stent, and the endotracheal tube is advanced into the airway. Should difficulty be encountered on advancing the endotracheal tube, rotation of the tube usually ensures that the tip does not "hang up" on the arytenoid cartilages or the vocal cords. The proper position is confirmed by withdrawal of the bronchoscope into the endotracheal tube. The tube is then fixed at a suitable distance above the tracheal carina. If flexible bronchoscopy is unavailable or is unsuccessful because of the patient's anatomy, rigid bronchoscopy may be attempted. The thoracic surgeon should be both familiar and adept at passage of a rigid bronchoscopy in the face of airway obstruction. The Noseworthy adapter cap for attachment to the ventilator tubing should be removed from the endotracheal tube

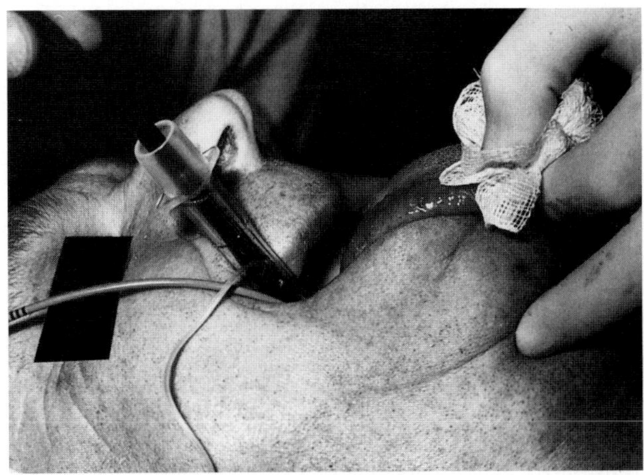

FIGURE 71–10 ■ Bronchoscopic intubation.

because it limits the internal diameter. A lubricated 7-mm rigid bronchoscope will pass through a 7.5-mm endotracheal tube. The principles of intubation are the same as those for flexible bronchoscopy. Obviously, the nasal approach cannot be used. The rigid scope, however, can be used as a laryngoscope to lever the tongue and epiglottis out of the way to view the vocal cords better. After the scope has been passed through the cords, ventilation can be initiated with the Venturi technique to relieve hypoxemia caused by the intubation attempts. Once through the vocal cords, the endotracheal tube simply slides into the airway as the rigid bronchoscope is removed.

Should all attempts at reintubation fail and a surgical airway seem necessary, apneic oxygenation may provide support until proper ventilation can be established. This can be achieved with the insertion of an Intracath catheter through the cricothyroid membrane. The catheter is then connected to wall oxygen at 6 to 10 L/min. Such endotracheal gas flow usually provides satisfactory oxygenation, which is similar to that provided during an apnea test for brain death. Although the $Pa\text{CO}_2$ level continues to rise, oxygen saturation can be restored or maintained.

Specifics of Ventilator Management

The following is designed as a pragmatic approach to ventilatory management. This information reflects the author's personal bias, and it is recognized that there are several means to achieve the same end. The objectives of ventilatory management are improvement in oxygenation, as assessed by $Pa\text{O}_2$, and the maintenance of appropriate ventilation, as assessed by both the $Pa\text{CO}_2$ and the maintenance of arterial pH in an acceptable range.

As noted earlier, mechanical ventilation itself has been implicated in the development or the persistence of ARDS through the damaging effects of high peak-airway pressures on the alveolar walls. Therefore, in determining the specifics of ventilator management it is useful to remember the rule of lowest therapeutic intervention. This involves the achievement of the lowest $F\text{IO}_2$, the lowest peak airway pressure (PAW), and the lowest left ventricular pre-load to maximize therapy and avoid the complications of therapy itself.

Oxygen has a variety of deleterious effects, particularly when the $F\text{IO}_2$ exceeds 50% (Fox et al, 1981; Sackner et al, 1976). The surgeon should, therefore attempt to achieve the lowest possible $F\text{IO}_2$ that produces an oxygen saturation of 90%. There are several avenues available. First and foremost is positive end-expiratory pressure (PEEP). There is no question that, under most circumstances, PEEP improves $P\text{AO}_2 - Pa\text{O}_2$ and hence permits a decrease in $F\text{IO}_2$. PEEP, however, can produce deleterious effects; especially a decrease in cardiac output and an increase in barotrauma. The former is unusual if PEEP is less than 10 cm H_2O. If a PEEP of more than 10 cm H_2O is required, it is advisable to place a pulmonary artery catheter that permits measurement of cardiac output by thermodilution. Barotrauma is an important complication. PEEP can adversely affect peak airway pressure and thus contribute to the development of pneumothorax, subcutaneous emphysema, or more subtle parenchymal damage. Other measures to lower the $F\text{IO}_2$ are noted below. In situations in which excessive lung water has accumulated (e.g., pulmonary edema and ARDS), diuresis improves lung compliance and ventilation perfusion equally. Parenchymal lung disease is rarely homogeneous. Some areas of the lung are more severely affected than are others. If the V/Q relationship in one lung is superior to that on the contralateral side, then nursing the patient on that side may improve oxygenation by ensuring that pulmonary arterial blood flow is favored to the side that receives the most efficient alveolar ventilation. In addition, if the patient's position is alternated between supine and prone on a circle electric or Stryker frame, V/Q mismatching can be improved mismatching (German et al, 1998; Gillart et al, 1998; Papazian et al, 1998). These reports have suggested an additive effect when nitric oxide and the prone position are used together. With time, the dependent area of the lung becomes more atelectatic because of the accumulation of secretions and the effect of the pleural hydrostatic pressure gradient, but the dependent area of the lung receives most of the pulmonary arterial blood flow. A quick change from supine to prone brings the previously nondependent but well-ventilated area into a dependent position in which the blood supply is optimal for gas exchange. The improvement is short-lived, but the maneuver can be repeated every 3 to 4 hours.

Respiratory failure that requires excessive levels of $F\text{IO}_2$ may suggest that alternative means of ventilation, such as inverse ratio or high-frequency jet ventilation (HFJV), should be used. Although each can at times lower the $F\text{IO}_2$, there is no convincing evidence that the outcome is altered. Inverse ratio ventilation involves changing inspiratory time. Under normal circumstances the ventilator is cycled to allow expiration to be longer than inspiration. When the inspiratory-expiratory ratio is reversed, more of the total time is spent on inspiration on the assumption that the inspired volume is more evenly distributed and that the pulmonary volume will be maintained by the shortening of expiration. Intrathoracic volume and pressure are increased by this maneuver. Both inverse ratio and high frequency ventilation increase mean airway pressure and thus lung volume (Yanos et al, 1998), and although this may result in improved oxygenation and decreased $Pa\text{O}_2/F\text{IO}_2$ ratios, concern remains over the increased risk of barotrauma (Zavala et al, 1998). Therefore, interest in ventilation dynamics that maintain peak airway pressures in the lowest possible range has increased.

Pressure-Limited Ventilation

High peak-airway pressures may result in pneumothoraces or, worse, the separation of bronchial anastomosis or the disruption of bronchial stumps. Tsuno and colleagues (1991) reported on the deleterious effects of modest increases in peak airway pressure on the pulmonary parenchyma. As noted earlier, Dreyfuss and colleagues (1988) have also suggested that high peak-airway pressures are deleterious. The peak pressure can be lowered by decreasing the tidal volume. To maintain the same $Pa\text{CO}_2$, the minute ventilation must be preserved by increasing the ventilatory rate. The required change is quickly calculated from the following:

$$\text{Minute ventilation} = \text{Tidal volume} \times \text{Rate}$$

Several authors have argued that $Paco_2$ is unimportant and can be allowed to increase as long as the pH is maintained at 7.2 (Darioli and Perret, 1984; Hickling, 1990). Such permissive hypercarbia or pressure-limited ventilation strategies have been utilized in ARDS. There are several forms of ventilation (e.g., permissive hypercarbia, pressure preset ventilation, and pressure-limited ventilation) that differ from each other in relatively minor ways. Common to each is the goal of limiting the peak inflation pressure or the mean airway pressure. On the basis of the work of several authors, as noted above, the advocates of these modes of ventilatory support suppose that barotrauma is perhaps responsible for additive pulmonary parenchymal damage after the initiation of ventilatory support for other reasons. As a result, an effort is made to limit the airway pressure.

Marini and coworkers (1989) introduced a concept of pressure preset ventilation, a square wave form of ventilatory drive that focuses on three parameters: a preset pressure, an inspiratory time fraction, and frequency. PEEP is usually set at 10 to 12 cm H_2O, and, hence, ventilatory pressure becomes the difference between the preset pressure and PEEP. This is a reliable means of ventilatory support that should limit or reduce barotrauma.

The inspiratory time fraction is a particularly intriguing parameter of which the benefits were largely unappreciated until they were better defined by Marini and colleagues (1992). Basically, the authors demonstrated that an extension of the inspiratory time fraction results in an improvement in arterial oxygenation unless the minute ventilation was already high. It is postulated that a slowing in inspiratory time may permit a better distribution of ventilation. This is particularly appealing in ARDS in which there may be lung units with vastly different time constants. It was previously demonstrated that increases in inspiratory time would improve alveolar ventilation (Pesanti et al, 1985). However, if the minute ventilation is already high, such a maneuver may result in an increase in auto-PEEP (auto-PEEP is defined as the increase in end-expiratory pressure that is generated unintentionally by the ventilator when the expiratory time is insufficient to allow for full expiration of the expired gas). This circumstance, rather than improving alveolar ventilation, should result in an increase in dead space.

At high frequencies, therefore, pressure preset ventilation may result in hypercarbia. Such, however, should not be considered a failure of ventilatory support as long as the metabolic compensation is sufficient to prevent respiratory acidosis below a pH of 7.2. Indeed, a ventilatory mode called "permissive hypercarbia or pressure-limited ventilation" has become increasingly popular. This involves limiting the inflation pressure irrespective of tidal volume. Initial requirements for increased ventilation can be achieved by increases in rate. However, if the $Paco_2$ is allowed to rise gradually, renal compensation should prevent a major deterioration in the acid–base balance. It seems that a pH of 7.2 is well tolerated without undue hematologic or hemodynamic sequelae. If it is done gradually, the $Paco_2$ may rise to substantial levels. Favorable results with this form of ventilatory support have been reported in asthmatic patients (Darioli and Perret, 1984) and in ARDS (Hickling, 1990).

Reports on studies of pressure limitation in a controlled fashion have been given. A retrospective study by Weg and colleagues (1998) suggested that pneumothorax was not strictly related to inspiratory distending pressures. Two subsequent randomized trials conventional ventilatory support reported conflicting results as far as lung damage and survival were concerned. The disparity in results is less real than apparent as the means of limiting pressure were different and the severity of pulmonary compliance change was also substantially different in the two groups. Stewart and colleagues (1998) reported no survival advantage with pressure-limited ventilation, but it is noteworthy that the peak inflation pressure in the control group was relatively low, suggesting that the the degree of lung damage was insufficient for a benefit from low pressure ventilation to be demonstrated. Amato and colleagues (1998) found an improved survival for patients in intensive care, but hospital survival was identical, suggesting again that mortality is greatly affected by accompanying organ dysfunction. It would seem prudent to lower tidal volumes and peak pressures to avoid pressures in excess of 35 to 40 cm of water (Hudson, 1998).

However, the clinician should remember simple measures of decreasing peak airway pressures. Bronchoscopy and drainage of pneumothoraces are obvious interventions. Bronchoscopy is warranted whenever the peak airway pressure exceeds 40 cm H_2O for a sustained period.

Measurements of preload can be obtained either through central venous pressure (CVP) or pulmonary arterial wedge pressure, measured by a Swan-Ganz catheter. As noted earlier, even if excessive water in the lung is the result of altered permeability, a reduction in preload can reduce the amount of extravascular water. Fluid restriction and diuresis are the simplest means to achieve this end. The addition of β-adrenergic doses of dopamine helps to preserve renal cortical flow and urine output. The attainment of the lowest wedge pressure that is compatible with normal renal function is desirable.

High-Frequency Ventilation

HFV offers an alternative when conventional ventilation fails and gas exchange is insufficient. The delivery of small tidal volumes at high frequencies may improve alveolar mixing and alleviate the gas exchange problem. Such is achieved with the maintenance of the mean airway pressure and a reduction of peak airway pressure. There are several forms of HFV. High-frequency positive-pressure ventilation (HFPPV) refers to conventional ventilators set to deliver small tidal volumes at rates that exceed 40 breaths/min. This technique is useful for bronchoscopy and some open chest operations, as shown by

Malina and colleagues (1981). To avoid overextension of the lungs, sufficient time for exhalation must be allowed.

High-frequency oscillation (HFO) delivers some volumes of fresh gas at rates of 900 to 3000 breaths/min. The gas flow is rapidly interrupted by a piston or ball to produce oscillations. The mechanism for gas exchange is unclear. Molecular diffusion of gas in the airways may be enhanced by the turbulence that is generated by the oscillations.

During HFJV, jets of gas at rates of 80 to 400 breaths/min are delivered through a small cannula into the distal trachea. By the Venturi principle, additional gas is drawn into the airway (the biased gas flow). Traditionally, these systems have been open; the biased gas is drawn from the atmosphere or from an oxygen source. Because the degree of mixing of jet-stream gas and biased gas remained unknown, the true FIO_2 was also uncertain. These systems have been particularly useful in the ventilatory management of patients with large bronchopleural fistulas. Table 71–2 displays the arterial blood gases that are associated with ventilation by a standard volume cycle ventilator and then by HFJV in a patient with an iatrogenically created defect in the trachea and left mainstem bronchus after complicated esophageal surgery, as reported by Panos and colleagues (1986). These systems have, however, been hampered by several difficulties. As noted, the mixing of biased gas and jet gas leads to an unknown FIO_2. In addition, humidification of the biased gas is often difficult, which results in drying of the airways. An important factor is that many of these systems lack disconnect and high-pressure alarms. It is, however, possible to use a standard volume-cycle ventilator set in an intermittent mechanical ventilation (IMV) mode (at 2 to 6 breaths/min and a tidal volume of 200 ml) as the source of the biased gas flow. Thus, a constant FIO_2, adequate humidification, and the alarm systems of a conventional ventilator are supplied. This method also allows the surgeon to use PEEP to a greater extent, should such be desired.

Although general agreement exists about the efficacy of HFJV in the management of bronchopleural fistulas, controversy concerning its role in hypoxemic respiratory failure continues. MacIntyre and associates (1986) did not demonstrate any advantage of HFJV over conventional ventilators in their patients with respiratory failure. Carlon and associates (1981) documented their experience in 17 patients with various abnormalities that caused hypoxemia that was refractory to conventional ventilation. Of these 17, 8 patients improved and survived as a result of HFJV, and none of the 17 patients experienced a deterioration when switched to HFJV. Experimental work by Lucking and coworkers (1986) demonstrated an improvement in cardiac output and systemic hemodynamic parameters with maintenance in gas exchange in dogs with induced right ventricular dysfunction. In our experience, the closed system mentioned earlier has provided improved gas exchange even in hypoxemic respiratory failure.

Table 71–2 ■ Comparison of Arterial Blood Gases Under Two Forms of Ventilation

Arterial Blood Gases	*Volume Cycle Ventilation*	*High-Frequency Jet Ventilation*
Rate	20	120
Tidal volume	1.0 L	—
Positive end-expiratory pressure	10 cm H_2O	10 cm H_2O
Fraction of inspired oxygen	0.60	0.60
Pounds per square inch	—	10
pH	7.23	7.37
Arterial carbon dioxide tension	102 mm Hg	63 mm Hg
Arterial oxygen tension	57 mm Hg	85 mm Hg

Extracorporeal Membrane Oxygenation

Occasionally, maximum ventilatory support, which includes the use of HFJV, is insufficient to reverse hypoxemia, hypercarbia, or both. ECMO may salvage a few of these patients in terminal respiratory failure. A multicenter National Institutes of Health trial reported by Zapol and colleagues (1979) concluded that ECMO provided no survival advantage over continued conventional ventilatory support. The study had a large beta error. Several authors, including Solca and colleagues (1985), Egan and associates (1988), and Bartlett and coworkers (1977), have reported their successes with varying forms of ECMO.

A technique for the rapid institution of ECMO with percutaneous catheters and a Bio-Medicus pump, the so-called mini-membrane, has been developed. Girotti and colleagues (1986) described the techniques, and Rice and associates (1986) presented the results in five patients. Rapid percutaneous cannulation of the femoral veins provided venous drainage. Blood was returned through a canula placed in the internal jugular vein. Oxygenation improved from 37 mm Hg pre-ECMO to 186 mm Hg post-ECMO. The carbon dioxide level was normalized in all cases. Three of the five patients survived their pulmonary insult and were discharged from the hospital.

A further refinement of the use of extracorporeal circuits has been formalized by Gattinoni and coworkers (1986). They extended the principle of pressure-limited ventilation by removing CO_2 through extracorporeal circuits while providing the support of oxygenation (at least to some degree) with a low-frequency positive-pressure ventilation system.

WEANING

Most patients who require mechanical assistance for respiratory failure present different challenges because varying degrees of continued parenchymal disease, increased bronchial reactivity, respiratory muscle debility, and cardiovascular compromise demand a more cautious approach to weaning. The initial problem is to identify that weaning has become possible. This is usually signaled by an FIO_2 that is less than 50%, PEEP that is less than or equal to 7 cm H_2O, and clearing of infiltrates on chest radiography. Further support for the initiation of the weaning effort can be obtained in the conscious patient who has the ability to generate a forced vital capacity of at least 7 ml/kg of body weight and a minimal negative inspiratory force of −15 cm H_2O. There are several methods of weaning. We focus on the classic method, IMV, and pressure support. Although weaning through an open airway (T-piece method) has often been quoted as a variant of a classic weaning method, it possesses no distinct advantage. On the contrary, there are potential disadvantages in that the removal of end-expiratory pressure results in a progressive fall in functional residual capacity and the potentiation of V/Q mismatching. Annest and colleagues (1980) and Quan and associates (1981) showed that this leads to increased work in breathing. The continuous positive airway pressure (CPAP) method (or classic method) places the entire ventilatory responsibility on the patient. It provides for intermittent stresses with periods of complete rest at levels of assisted ventilation. Theoretically, this maximal stress followed by rest should provide beneficial respiratory muscle exercise. When using the classic technique, it is important to recognize that patients initially tolerate CPAP for only a short time. The extension of the interval should proceed slowly; patients should not be stressed to the point of impending failure. Cohen and coworkers (1982) described the clinical signs of respiratory muscle fatigue. An increased respiratory rate is followed by an alteration between rib cage and abdominal breathing, which they called "respiratory alternans," the paradoxic abdominal–chest wall motion described earlier, and finally decreased PaO_2 accompanied by a fall in minute ventilation and hypercarbia. Electromyographic recordings from their patients revealed high- and low-frequency discharges from the intercostal muscles. A fall in the ratio of high- to low-frequency power indicated fatiguing muscle and preceded the clinical signs of failure. Clinically, a simple guide to a patient's tolerance of the weaning process can be obtained by a measurement of vital capacity and negative inspiratory force at the beginning and at the end of the CPAP weaning. The weaning period should not be extended unless the beginning and end values are comparable.

During the use of the IMV technique, a patient must work constantly and may not be able to sustain the effort. As noted, failure occurs when fatigue results in diminishing tidal volumes, which in turn reduces functional residual capacity. Gas exchange becomes increasingly impaired. In addition, the ventilator may itself impose an increased burden on the work of breathing. Marini and colleagues (1986) demonstrated higher workloads during patient-triggered ventilatory breaths than during spontaneous breathing. Part of the explanation for this phenomenon lies in the resistance threshold in the ventilator itself. The resistance within the internal circuitry of respirators varies greatly. For this reason, when CPAP is used, it is wise to use external circuits.

Pressure support ventilation and the use of pressure support during weaning has become popular. During weaning, the amount of pressure support is gradually decreased until it is eliminated or at least until 10 cm H_2O has been achieved. This is a well-tolerated form of weaning. However, as with the classic method, adequate rest with maximal pressure support is a prerequisite between weaning intervals.

Failure to wean should prompt further investigations to reveal possible causes. A finding of a dead space to tidal volume ratio (VD/VT) of greater than 0.7 suggests an inability to wean. However, this is a dynamic measurement, and patients often improve over time. It is an accurate measurement of subtle improvement in long-term patients who have severe inspiratory insults. In our experience, it may require up to 3 months of stable respiratory maintenance before VD/VT improves and the criteria for weaning are reached. Open lung biopsy sometimes reveals unsuspected and treatable disease, but this is less useful that it was in the past given the advent of protected specimen brushing and bronchoalveolar ravage. V/Q scanning may show areas of gross mismatch that contribute to the intrapulmonary shunt. Several patients are unable to be weaned because of hemodynamic instability, which is evident only during the weaning period. Insertion of a pulmonary artery catheter may uncover significant pulmonary arterial hypertension, which can be corrected with appropriate vasodilator therapy. Figure 71–11 documents the results seen in a patient with left ventricular dysfunction and mitral valve replacement. Several weaning attempts had failed in this patient over several weeks. After pulmonary artery pressures were controlled, weaning proceeded rapidly and successfully.

Aubier and colleagues (1987) showed that digoxin improved diaphragmatic strength by 19.5% in ventilated patients with chronic obstructive pulmonary disease. The mechanism of action is unclear.

OUTCOME

The recovery from ARDS may be prolonged, and in the absence of multi-system organ failure one should persist with mechanical ventilatory support as the ability of the lung to recover remains upredictable. The mortality after the first several days is rarely secondary to respiratory failure but rather due to sepsis and other organ dysfunction. Some have noted that the development of pneumothorax and bronchopleural fistulas has resulted in an increased mortality. However, recent data from a large prospective trial suggests that the presence of pneumothoraces does not confer a greater risk of mortality (Weg et al 1998). The authors of the latter report also confirm that the modern mortality of ARDS is approximately 40%, considerably less than classically reported (Ashbaugh et al, 1967). In the absence of other systems failure, this author encourages continued aggressive management, because the predictors of mortality are generally unreliable and often not applicable to the individual case. Monchi and colleagues (1998) recently undertook a thorough analysis of 259 patients with ARDS and an overall mortality of 65%. They concluded from logistical regression analysis that the prognosis of ARDS was related to the severity of the triggering event, the degree of respiratory embarrassment (which likely affects early mortality), and the onset of right ventricular dysfunction. Nonetheless, these data simply provide guidelines to management and outline clinical scenarios in which prognosis may be guarded. These data should not influence the decision to withdraw therapy because of speculation of a poor prognosis. ARDS remains an obscure clinical entity 30 years after the original description, and, therefore, it is

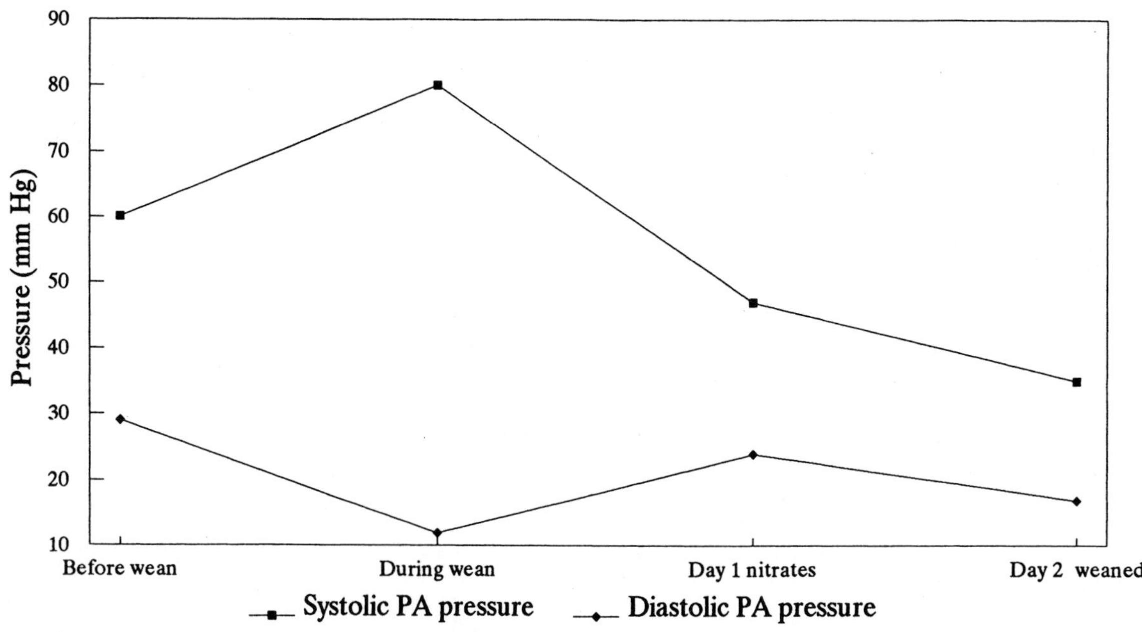

FIGURE 71–11 ■ Systolic and diastolic pulmonary artery pressures after prolonged ventilatory support. Note the increase in systolic pressure with weaning. This was accompanied by pulmonary edema. Weaning proceeded smoothly with the addition of nitrates. PA, pulmonary artery.

advised that the clinician persist with therapy and support until the support itself can no longer provide for the delivery of adequate oxygen to the tissues.

■ *REFERENCES*

Amato MB, Barbas CS, Medeiros DM et al: Effect of a protective-ventilation strategy on mortality in the acute respiratory distress syndrome. N Engl J Med 338:347, 1998.

Annest SJ, Gottlieb M, Paloski WH et al: Detrimental effects of removing end-expiratory pressure prior to extubation. Ann Surg 191:539, 1980.

Ashbaugh DG, Bigelow DB, Petty TL, Levine, BE: Acute respiratory distress in adults. Lancet 2:319, 1967.

Aubier M, Murciano D, Viires N et al: Effects of digoxin on diaphragmatic strength generation in patients with chronic obstructive pulmonary disease during acute respiratory failure. Am Rev Respir Dis 135:544, 1987.

Balk RA, Tryka AF, Bone RC: The effect of ibuprofen on endotoxin induced sheep. Am Rev Respir Dis 129(Suppl):A144, 1984.

Barke RA, Dunn RL, Dalmasso P: Effects of ibuprofen treatment versus ibuprofen pretreatment of pulmonary micro-vascular permeability and pulmonary function following *Escherichia* cold peritoneal contamination. Surg Forum 34:144, 1983.

Bartlett RH, Grzzaniga AB, Fong SW et al: Extracorporeal membrane oxygenator support for cardiopulmonary failure: Experience in 28 cases. J Cardiovasc Thorac Surg 73:375, 1977.

Begley CJ, Ogletree ML, Meyrick BO: Modification of pulmonary response to endotoxemia in awake sheep by steroidal and nonsteroidal anti-inflammatory agents. Am Rev Respir Dis 130:1140, 1984.

Bernard JR, Luce JM, Sprung CL: High-dose corticosteroids in patients with the adult respiratory distress syndrome. N Engl J Med 317:1365, 1987.

Bone RC, Hisha JR, Clemer TP: Early methylprednisolone treatment for septic syndrome in the adult respiratory distress syndrome. Chest 92:1032, 1987.

Brett SJ, Hansell DM, Evans TW: Clinical correlates in acute lung injury: Response to inhaled nitric oxide. Chest 114:1397, 1998.

Brigham KR, Wolverton WC, Blake JH: Increased sheep lung vascular permeability caused by *Pseudomonas*. J Clin Invest 54:792, 1974.

Carlon GC, Kahn RC, Howland WS et al: Clinical experience with high frequency jet ventilation. Crit Care Med 9:1, 1981.

Chastre J, Fagon JV, Soles P et al: Diagnosis of nosocomial bacterial pneumonia in intubated patients undergoing ventilation: Comparison of the usefulness of BAL and PSB. Am J Med 85:498, 1988.

Cohen CA, Zagalbaum G, Gross D et al: Clinical manifestations of inspiratory muscle fatigue. Am J Med 73:308, 1982.

Cohn SM, Cruithoff KL, Rothchild HR: Beneficial effects of LY203647, a novel leukotriene C4/D4 antagonist, on pulmonary function and mesenteric perfusion in a porcine model of endotoxin shock in ARDS. Circ Shock 33:7, 1991.

Darioli R, Perret C: Mechanical controlled hypertension in status asthmaticus. Am Rev Respir Dis 129:385, 1984.

Decastro FR, Violan JS, Capuz BL et al: Reliability of the bronchoscopic-protected catheter brush in the diagnosis of pneumonia in mechanically ventilated patients. Crit Care Med 19:171, 1991.

Dellinger RP, Zimmerman JL, Taylor RW et al: Effects of inhaled nitric oxide in patients with acute respiratory distress syndrome: Results of a randomized phase II trial. Inhaled Nitric Oxide in ARDS Study Group. Crit Care Med 26:15, 1998.

Demling RH, Smith M, Gunther R et al: Pulmonary injury and prostaglandin production during endotoxemia in conscious sheep. Am J Physiol 240:H348, 1981.

Demling RJ, Proctor R, Grossman J: Comparison of systemic and pulmonary vascular response to plasma and lung lymph lysosomal enzyme release: The effects of steroid treatment. Circ Shock 7:317, 1980.

Dreyfuss D, Soler P, Bassett G, Saumon G: High inflation pressure pulmonary edema: Respective effects of high airway pressure, high tidal volume, and positive end-expiratory pressure. Am Rev Respir Dis 137:1159, 1988.

Egan TM, Duffin J, Glynn MF et al: Ten-year experience with ECMO for severe respiratory failure. Chest 94:681, 1988.

Egan TM, Saunders NR, Dubois P: Contribution of circulating formed elements to prostanoid production in complement mediated lung injury in sheep. Surgery 98:350, 1985.

Fox RB, Shasti DM, Harada N: A novel mechanism for pulmonary oxygen toxicity-phagocyte mediated lung injury. Chest 80 (Suppl): 35, 1981.

Gamble JR, Harlan JM, Klebanoff SI: The stimulation of the adherence of neutrophils to umbilical vein endothelium by human recombinant tumor necrosis factor. Proc Natl Acad Sci USA 82:8667, 1985.

Gattinoni L, Pesenti A, Mascheroni D et al: Low-frequency positive pressure ventilation with extracorporeal CO_2 removal in severe acute respiratory failure. JAMA 256:881, 1986.

Germann P, Poschl G, Leitner C et al: Additive effect of nitric oxide inhalation on the oxygenation benefit of the prone position in the adult respiratory distress syndrome. Anesthesiology 89:1401, 1998.

Gillart T, Bazin JE, Cosserant B et al: Combined nitric oxide inhalation, prone positioning, and almitrine infusion improve oxygenation in severe ARDS. Can J Anaesth 45:402, 1998.

Girotti MJ, Pym J, Todesco J et al: Simultaneous use of membrane oxygenation and high-frequency jet ventilation in acute pulmonary failure. Crit Care Med 14:511, 1986.

Goodman ER, Kleinstein E, Fusco AM et al: Role of interleukin-8 in the genesis of acute respiratory distress syndrome through an effect on neutrophil apoptosis. Arch Surg 133:1234, 1998.

Hallemans R, Naelde R, Malot C: Do cyclo-oxygenase products mediate hypoxic pulmonary vasoconstriction in man? Am Rev Respir Dis 129(Suppl):A341, 1984.

Hasselstrom LJ, Ekkasen K, Mogensen T: Lowering pulmonary arterial pressure in a patient with severe acute respiratory failure. Intensive Care Med 11:48, 1985.

Hers TM, Tricomi SM, Dettenmeir PA: Tumor necrosis factor levels in serum and broncho-alveolar ravage fluid of patients with the adult respiratory distress syndrome. Am Rev Respir Dis 144:268, 1991.

Hickling KG: Permissive hypercarbia. Intensive Care Med 16:219, 1990.

Holcroft JW, Vassar MJ, Weber CJ: Prostaglandin F_1 and survival in patients with the adult respiratory distress syndrome: A prospective study. Ann Surg 203:371, 1986.

Hudson LD: Protective ventilation for patients with acute respiratory distress syndrome. N Engl J Med 338:385, 1998.

Iotti GA, Olivei MC, Palo A et al: Acute effects of inhaled nitric oxide in adult respiratory distress syndrome. Eur Respir J 12:1164, 1998.

Johannigman JA, Davis K, Campbell RS et al: Inhaled nitric oxide in acute respiratory distress syndrome. J Trauma 43:904, 1997.

Kopolovic R, Thraillkill KM, Martin DT et al: Effects of ibuprofen on a porcine model of acute respiratory failure. J Surg Res 36:300, 1984.

Keel JB, Hauser M, Stocker R et al: Established acute respiratory distress syndrome: Benefit of corticosteroid rescue therapy. Respiration 65:258, 1998.

Kusajima K, Waks SP, Webb WR: Effect of methylprednisolone on the pulmonary microcirculation. Surg Gynecol Obstet 139:1, 1974.

Leeper-Woodford SK, Carey PD, Byrne K et al: Tumor necrosis factor: Alpha and beta subtypes appear in circulation during onset of sepsis-induced lung injury. Am Rev Respir Dis 143:1076, 1991.

Lo CJ, Fu M, Cryer HG: Interleukin-10 inhibits alveolar macrophage production of inflammatory mediators involved in adult respiratory distress syndrome. J Surg Res 79:179, 1998.

Luce JM, Montgomery AB, Marks JD: Ineffectiveness of high dose methylprednisolone in preventing parenchymal lung injury and in improving mortality in patients with septic shock. Am Rev Respir Dis 138:62, 1988.

Lucking SE, Fields AI, Mahfood S et al: High-frequency ventilation versus conventional ventilation in dogs with right ventricular dysfunction. Crit Care Med 14:798, 1986.

MacIntyre NR, Follett JV, Dietz JL et al: Jet ventilation at 100 breaths per minute in adult respiratory failure. Am Rev Respir Dis 134:897, 1986.

Malina JR, Nordstrom SG, Sjostrand UH, Wattwil LM: Clinical evaluation of high-frequency positive-pressure ventilation (HFPPV) in patients scheduled for open-chest surgery. Anesth Analg 60:324, 1981.

Marini JJ et al: New approaches to the ventilatory management of the adult respiratory distress syndrome. J Crit Care 87:256, 1992.

Marini JJ, Crooke PS, Truwitt JD: Determinants and limits of pressure preset ventilation: A mathematical model of pressure control. J Appl Physiol 67:1081, 1989.

Marini JJ, Rodriguez M, Lamb V: The inspiratory workload of patient-initiated mechanical ventilation. Am Rev Respir Dis 134:902, 1986.

Martin P, Gebitekin C, Gupta NK et al: Effect of type of resection on plasma granulocyte elastase levels following surgery for non–small cell lung carcinoma. Eur J Cardiothorac Surg 8:517, 1994.

Mathison JC, Wolfson E, Ulevitch RJ: Participation of tumor necrosis factor in the mediation of gram negative bacterial lipopolysaccharide induced injury in rabbits. J Clin Invest 81:1925, 1988.

Meduri GU, Headley SA, Golden E, Carson SJ: Effect of prolonged methylprednisolone therapy in unresolving acute respiratory distress syndrome. JAMA 280:159, 1998.

Meduri GU, Reddy RC, Stanley T, El-Zeky F: Pneumonia in acute respiratory distress syndrome: A prospective evaluation of bilateral bronchoscopic sampling. Am J Respir Crit Care Med 158:870, 1998.

Metz C, Sibbald WJ: Anti-inflammatory therapy of acute lung injury. Chest 100:1110, 1991.

Michael JR, Barton RG, Saffle JR et al: Inhaled nitric oxide versus conventional therapy: Effect on oxygenation in ARDS. Am J Respir Crit Care Med 157:1372, 1998.

Modig J, Bord T: High-dose methylprednisolone in a porcine model of ARDS induced by endotoxemia. Acta Chir Scand 526:94, 1985.

Monchi M, Bellenfant F, Cariou A et al: Early predictive factors of survival in the acute respiratory distress syndrome: A multivariate analysis. Am J Respir Crit Care Med 158:1076, 1998.

Moore F: Clinical pathologic review ARDS. In Moore FD, Lyons JH, Perce EC et al (eds): Post-Traumatic Pulmonary Insufficiency. Philadelphia, WB Saunders, 1969.

Nahum A, Chamberlain W, Sznajder J: Differential activation of mixed venous and arterial neutrophils in patients with sepsis syndrome and acute lung injury. Am Rev Respir Dis 143:1083, 1991.

Oats JA, Fitzgerald GA, Branch RA: Clinical implications of prostaglandin and thromboxane A_2 formation. N Engl J Med 319:689, 1988.

Panos A, Demajo W, Todd TR: High frequency jet ventilation in the management of bronchopleural fistula (BPF). Chest 89 (Suppl):521S, 1986.

Papazian L, Bregeon F, Gaillat F et al: Respective and combined effects of prone position and inhaled nitric oxide in patients with acute respiratory distress syndrome. Am J Respir Crit Care Med 157:580, 1998.

Parquin F, Marchal M, Mehiri S et al: Post-pneumonectomy pulmonary edema: Analysis and risk factors. Eur J Cardiothorac Surg 10:929, 1996.

Pepe PE, Potkin RT, Reus DH: Clinical predictors of the adult respiratory distress syndrome. Am J Surg 144:124, 1982.

Pesanti A et al: Mean airway pressure versus positive end expiratory pressure during mechanical ventilation: A review of 39 cases. Crit Care Med 13:34, 1985.

Puybasset L, Cluzel P, Chao N et al: A computed tomography scan assessment of regional lung volume in acute lung injury: The CT scan ARDS study group. Am J Respir Crit Care Med 158:1644, 1998.

Quan SF, Falltrick RT, Schlobolm RM: Extubation from ambient or expiratory positive airway pressure in adults. Anesthesiology 55:53, 1981.

Rice TW: The mini-membrane: A new method of extracorporeal membrane oxygenation (ECMO) for profound acute respiratory failure. Clin Invest Med 9:A8, 1986.

Rivkind AK, Seigel GH, Littleton M: Neutrophil oxidative burst activation and the pattern of respiratory physiological abnormalities in the fulminant posttraumatic adult respiratory distress syndrome. Circ Shock 33:48, 1981.

Roissant R, Falke KJ, Lopez F: Inhaled nitric oxide for the adult respiratory distress syndrome. N Engl J Med 328:399, 1993.

Sackner MA, Landa J, Hirsh J: Pulmonary effects of oxygen breathing: A 6-hour study in normal men. Ann Intern Med 82:40, 1976.

Schmeck J, Janzen R, Munter K et al: Endothelin-1 and thromboxane A-2 increase pulmonary vascular resistance in granulocyte-mediated lung injury. Crit Care Med 26:1868, 1998.

Silverman HJ, Slotman G, Maunder R: Effects of prostaglandin E1 on oxygen delivery and consumption in patients with adult respiratory distress syndrome. Chest 98:405, 1990.

Simms HH, Damico R: Increased polymorphonuclear CDI IB/CD18 expression following post traumatic ARDS. J Surg Res 50:362, 1991.

Slotman G, Machiedo JW, Casey KF: Histological and hemodynamic effects of prostacyclin and prostaglandin E, following oleic acid infusion. Surgery 92:93, 1982.

Smith ME, Gunther R, Gee M: Leukocytes, platelets and thromboxane A2 in endotoxin induced lung injury. Surgery 90:102, 1981.

Solca M, Pesenti A, Iapichino G et al: Multidisciplinary approach to extracorporeal respiratory assist for acute pulmonary failure. Int Surg 70:9, 1985.

Stewart TE, Meade MO, Cook DJ et al: Evaluation of a ventilation strategy to prevent barotrauma in patients at high risk for acute respiratory distress syndrome: Pressure and volume limited ventilation strategy group. N Engl J Med 338:355, 1998.

Tagan MC, Maibert M, Smaller MD: Oxidative metabolism of circulating granulocytes in adult respiratory distress syndrome. Am J Med 91:72S, 1981.

Todd TRJ: Personal data: Surgical Intensive Care Unit, Toronto General Hospital, 1988–1992.

Todd TRJ, Baile EM, Hogg JC: Pulmonary arterial wedge pressure in hemorrhagic shock. Am Rev Respir Dis 118:613, 1968.

Traber DL, Adam T Jr, Sziebert L et al: Failure of a protease inhibitor to affect the cardiopulmonary response to endotoxin when combined with a cyclooxygenase inhibitor. Circ Shock 13:319, 1984.

Tracey KJ, Fong Y, Hesse DG: Anti-cachetin/TNF monoclonal antibodies prevent septic shock during lethal bacteremia. Nature 330:662, 1987.

Troncey E, Collet JP, Shapiro S et al: Inhaled nitric oxide in acute respiratory distress syndrome: A pilot randomized controlled study. Am J Respir Crit Care Med 157:1483, 1998.

Turner CR, Lackey MN, Quinlan MF: Therapeutic intervention in a rat model of adult respiratory distress syndrome. II. Lipo-oxygenase pathway inhibition. Circ Shock 34:263, 1991.

Tsuno K, Miura K, Takeya M et al: Histopathologic pulmonary changes from mechanical ventilation at high peak airway pressures. Am Rev Respir Dis 143:1115, 1991.

Vreim CE, Staub NC: Protein composition of lung fluid in acute alloxan edema in dogs. Am J Physiol 230:376, 1976.

Walmrath D, Schneider T, Schmeruly R et al: Direct comparison of inhaled nitric oxide and aerolized prostacyclin in acute respiratory distress syndrome. Am J Respir Crit Care Med 153:991, 1996.

Watkins WD, Peterson MD, Crane RK: Prostacyclin and prostaglandin E_1 for severe idiopathic pulmonary hypertension. Lancet 1:1083, 1980.

Webb WR: Adult respiratory distress syndrome. In Delarue N (ed): Clinical Facets in International Trends in Thoracic Surgery. St. Louis, Mosby–Year Book, 1982.

Weg JG, Anzueto A, Balk RA et al: The relation of pneumothorax and other air leaks to mortality in the acute respiratory distress syndrome. N Engl J Med 338:341, 1998.

Whittle BJ, Moncada S, Vane JR: Comparison of the effects of prostacyclin (PGI_2), prostaglandin E_1 and D_2 on platelet aggregation in different species. Prostaglandins 16:373, 1978.

Williams E, Evans TW, Goldstraw P: Acute lung injury following lung resection: Is one lung anaesthesia to blame? Thorax 51:114, 1996.

Williams E, Goldstraw P, Evans TW: The complications of lung resection in adults: Acute respiratory distress syndrome (ARDS). Monaldi Arch Chest Dis 51:310, 1996.

Yanos J, Watling SM, Verhey J: The physiologic effects of inverse ratio ventilation. Chest 114:834, 1998.

Zapol WM, Snider MT, Hill JD et al: Extracorporeal membrane oxygenation in severe acute respiratory failure: A randomized prospective study. JAMA 242:2193, 1979.

Zavala E, Ferrer M, Polese G et al: Effect of inverse I/E ratio on pulmonary gas exchange in acute respiratory distress syndrome. Anesthesiology 88:35, 1998.

CHAPTER **72**

Late Sequelae of Thoracic Trauma

Reza John Mehran
Jean Deslauriers
Denis Desaulniers

Although simple chest tube drainage and nonoperative care can be used to successfully manage 85% to 90% of chest trauma victims, a number of patients will present with signs and symptoms resulting from complications of the injury months to years after the initial event. Often, these are the result of undue delay in diagnosing the initial injury or of inadequate early management. This chapter reviews the pathophysiology, diagnosis, and management of some of the most common sequelae of thoracic trauma.

LATE SEQUELAE OF TRAUMA TO THE CHEST WALL

Bony Fractures

Rib fractures with or without contusion of the underlying lung are the most common type of injury to the chest. Most of the time, they occur over the third to the seventh ribs not only because at those levels ribs are more exposed to direct impact, but also because they are more solidly attached to the bony structure of the chest wall and therefore are less mobile. Indeed, fracture of the eighth to twelfth ribs is uncommon because these ribs are more mobile. Healing of rib fractures usually results in the formation of a callus, which can become palpable as its size increases. This could be misdiagnosed as a bony tumor. The callus can also impinge on the surrounding intercostal bundle, resulting in chronic pain within the dermatome supplied by the involved intercostal nerves.

Malunion fractures are not uncommon and usually result in local pain. Malunion fractures at the level of the costochondral cartilages produce local tenderness often increased by movement or cough. Sometimes the feeling of motion over the involved cartilage or rib can be felt easily. Malunion and costochondral separations are best treated by local resection. Neurapraxic pain on the other hand is best treated with local infiltration of long-lasting anesthetic agents mixed with corticosteroid preparations.

Trauma of the first rib should alert the clinician to sometimes difficult to diagnose injury to the subclavian artery and brachial plexus, thereby highlighting the necessity for long-term follow-up (Richardson et al, 1975). Traumatic disruption of the first rib, for instance, potentially narrows the interscalene triangle, which may result in mechanical compression of the brachial plexus and subclavian artery by a callus or organizing hematoma. Injuries to the clavicle can also compromise the costoclavicular space (Mulder et al, 1973). Management of these patients is the same as that of patients with thoracic outlet syndrome due to other causes, although better results are to be expected in this group when compared with surgery done for thoracic outlet syndrome due to other etiologies (Cheng et al, 1995; Toso et al, 1999).

The authors believe that first rib excision in this group of patients is best carried out through the posterior approach. This approach allows neurolysis of the brachial plexus and complete resection of the first rib, which could be deformed. It also allows proper exposure of the subclavian and axillary vessels, which could be entrapped or aneurysmal. Patients without radiologic evidence of bony lesions involving the first rib should be further evaluated by digital substraction angiography or by magnetic resonance imaging (MRI) of the thoracic inlet done with the arm in the most symptomatic position.

A number of recent reports have shown that the transaxillary or supraclavicular route may be preferred for managing post-traumatic thoracic outlet syndromes. In 1993, Dellon suggested that the symptoms commonly referred to as *post-traumatic thoracic outlet syndrome* may, in fact, be due to entrapment of the brachial plexus at sites proximal to the interval between the first rib and clavicle. His hypothesis is that trauma victims sustain stretch-type injuries with subsequent scarring in and about the brachial plexus that would be left untreated by simple first rib resection. He suggests that the term *brachial plexus compression* may be a better description of this syndrome, and that a supraclavicular approach for brachial plexus neurolysis and anterior scalenectomy without resection of the first rib is a more suitable and less invasive procedure. In his series of 14 patients treated by this technique, Dellon (1993) reports good to excellent results in 90%.

Sternal Fractures

Most sternal fractures heal primarily without sequelae; late complications, including nonunion and overriding of the fragments with thoracic deformity (Fig. 72–1), are uncommon events. Surgical correction by open reduction

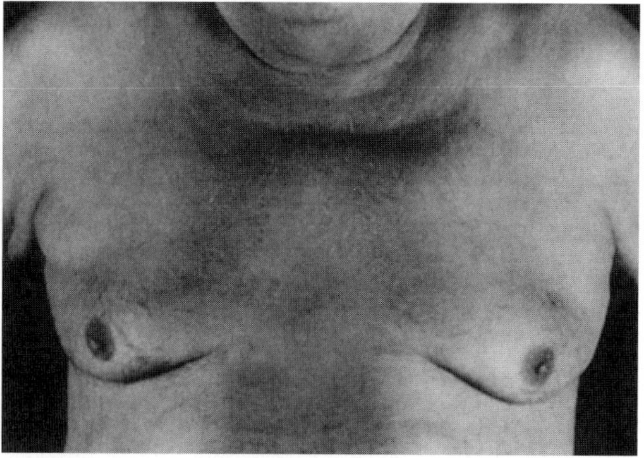

FIGURE 72–1 ■ Photograph of a patient with an anterior chest wall deformity secondary to a sternal fracture with overriding of the fragments.

and sternal wiring is indicated when the symptoms of tenderness, deformity, or abnormal motion are present and incapacitating. In the series reported by Gibson and associates (1962) of 80 sternal fracture patients, normal union of "undisplaced" fractures occurred within 6 weeks in nearly all surviving patients. There was only one patient in whom pain related to the fracture persisted for a period of 5 months. All other patients were considered to have no disability for heavy work 3 months after injury. Of the 25 patients with "displaced" fractures, 8 had pain and disability for longer than 6 weeks but only 1 for longer than 3 months. In contrast, Richardson and colleagues (1975) recommend early operation for patients with sternal fractures that have overriding defects, are unstable at the fracture site, are causing severe pain, or result in a major deformity of the sternum. Another possible indication for open fixation of sternal fractures is the presence of concomitant thoracic vertebral fracture or dislocation. In such cases, it has been shown that open fixation of the sternal fracture might increase the stability of the thoracic spine (Berg, 1993; Klaase et al, 1998).

Flail Chest

Acute flail chest associated with respiratory compromise can be treated by either mechanical ventilation or internal fixation. In some series, however, internal fixation has been shown to result in more speedy recovery, decreased complications, better cosmetic results, and better results overall (Ahmed and Mohyuddin, 1995; Mouton et al, 1997). In a group of 22 trauma victims who had sustained flail chest as their only significant injury, Beal and Oreskovich (1985) reported that 64% had long-term sequelae, the most common being persistent chest wall pain, chest wall deformity, and dyspnea on exertion. In a similar series, Mouton and co-workers (1997) showed that 95% of 21 patients who survived flail chest were able to return to full-time employment, and that 86% returned to their pre-trauma level of sports activities without complaining of chest wall or shoulder girdle pain or dysfunction. In this latter series (1997), all patients had had chest wall fixation using 3.5-mm-thick reconstruction plates. In a series of 32 patients treated by nonoperative means, Landercasper and associates (1984) showed that only 12 were able to return to full-time employment. Twenty-five percent had nonspecific chest tightness, 49% complained of thoracic cage pain, and 38% experienced moderate or severe changes in their overall level of activity. The authors also documented that 28% of patients had moderate to severe dyspnea, and spirometry was abnormal in 57% of patients, with 33% exhibiting at least a mild restrictive defect. It is the authors' opinion that patients who have had surgical stabilization of their flail chest do better overall than those who have not. We recommend the use of Judet struts for the fixation of rib fractures, although these struts may on occasion have to be removed because of chronic chest wall pain after the ribs have healed (Fig. 72–2).

Chest Wall Infection

Most post-traumatic osteomyelitis or chondritis of the chest wall is the result of penetrating injury with or without retained foreign bodies. Occasionally, they can also be due to blunt trauma with destruction of the perichondrium and necrosis of the cartilage (Brown and Trenton, 1952; Miller et al, 1978; Payne et al, 1973; Pontius et al, 1959), or they may be secondary to thermal burns (Alfie et al, 1995; Escudero-Nafs et al, 1989). Costal cartilages are particularly prone to infection because they are poorly vascularized; once they have undergone necrosis, the necrotic tissues act as foreign bodies

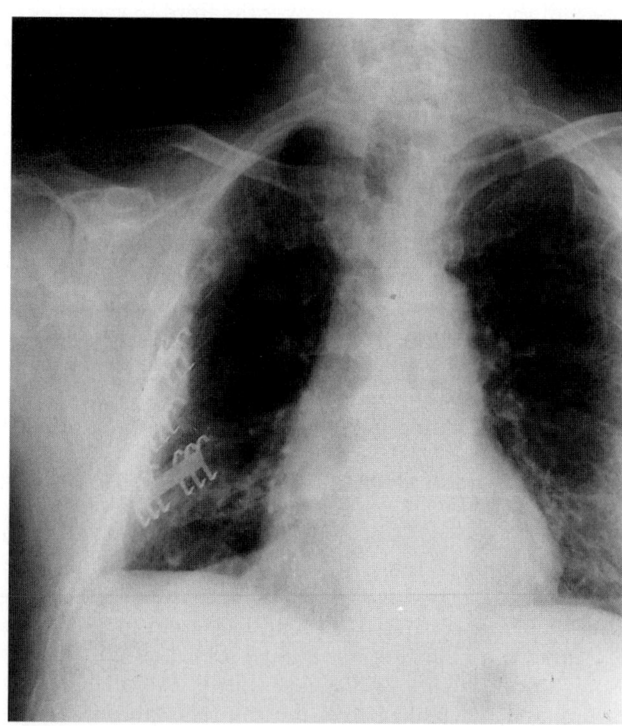

FIGURE 72–2 ■ Standard chest radiograph of a 66-year-old man who presented with continuous chest wall pain 1 year after operative stabilization of a flail chest with Judet struts.

and contribute to the chronicity of the problem. Symptoms of infection include fever, chills, local tenderness, swelling, and draining sinuses of the chest wall. Payne and colleagues (1973) noted that in several cases of posttraumatic chest wall infection, the draining sinus first appeared months or years after apparent complete healing and recovery from the initial trauma.

Management includes surgical débridement and specific antibiotic therapy. When débridement is carried out, it is most important that all infected and devitalized bone, cartilage, soft tissue, and foreign bodies be removed, as well as the full length of the involved cartilage(s). If the cartilages of the sixth to tenth ribs are involved, resection of the entire costal arch may be necessary. The wound can then be kept open until it is clean and covered with granulation tissue, at which time reconstruction is completed by transposition of well-vascularized adjacent soft tissues or distant myocutaneous flaps. With modern techniques of chest wall reconstruction, infected wounds can now be closed primarily with the use of transposed muscle flaps (Fig. 72–3) with or without cutaneous islands. Prosthetic materials such as Gore-Tex or Marlex mesh should be avoided, and indeed these prostheses are usually unnecessary because chronically infected wounds are already fibrotic and contracted.

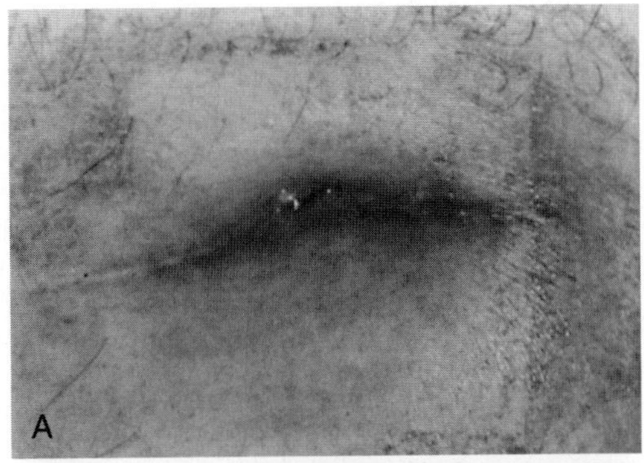

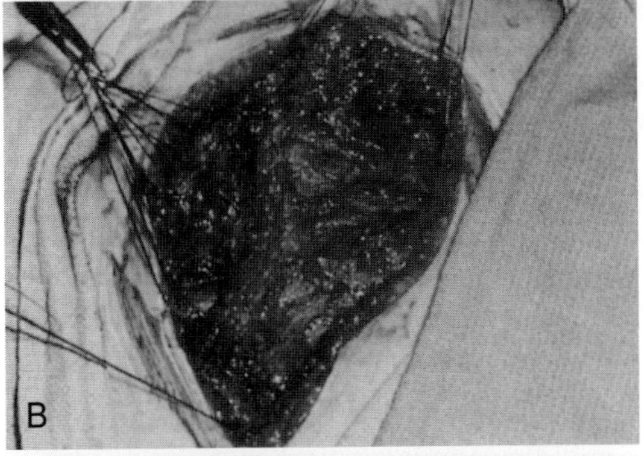

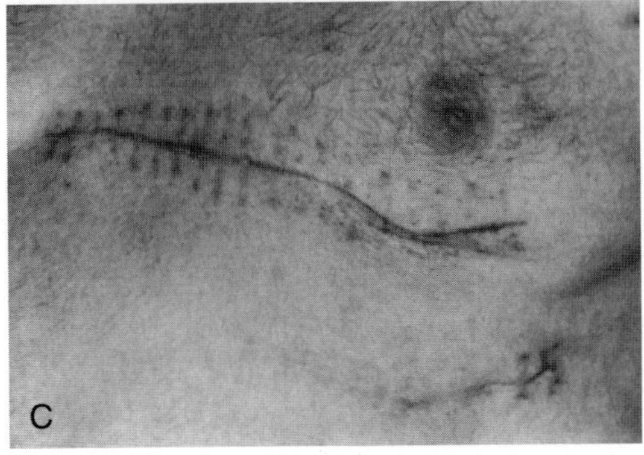

FIGURE 72–3 ■ Chest wall infection. *A*, Photograph of a chronic sinus of the anterior chest wall still draining despite previous attempts at resection. *B*, Pectoralis major muscle flap used to reconstruct the defect after wide excision of all necrotic cartilages. *C*, Complete healing of the wound.

Intercostal Hernias

Intercostal pulmonary hernias are rare (Table 72–1); most result from complications related to chest trauma. They are usually located parasternally or paravertebrally (Munnell, 1968; Salter and Hapton, 1969) (Fig. 72–4) and are small and relatively asymptomatic. Surgery, consisting of plication of the hernial sac and repair of the intercostal defect with autogenous tissue or synthetic materials, is recommended only for large and symptomatic hernias (Fig. 72–5).

Rarely, a combination of diaphragmatic and intercostal defects occurs, causing abdominal contents to herniate through the intercostal space (Fig. 72–6). Like simple lung hernias, these occur anteriorly (costochondral junction to sternum) because of the absence of external intercostal muscle, or posteriorly (costal angle to vertebra) because of the absence of internal intercostal muscle (Cole et al, 1986; Saw et al, 1976). Transdiaphragmatic intercostal hernias are repaired by closure of both the diaphragmatic and the intercostal defects (Cole et al, 1986; Francis and Barnsley, 1979).

TABLE 72–1 ■ **Etiologic Classification* of Lung Hernias with Relative Frequencies**

Type	*Frequency (%)*
Congenital	
Rib or intercostal hypoplasia or agenesis	18
Acquired	
Traumatic	52
Pathologic or spontaneous	30

*Classification based on that of Morel-Lavelle A: Hernies du poumon. Bull Soc Chir Paris 1:75, 1847.

Data from Hiscoe B, Digman J: Types and incidence of lung hernias. J Thorac Cardiovasc Surg 30:335, 1995, and Forty J, Wells FC: Traumatic intercostal pulmonary hernia. Ann Thorac Surg 49:670, 1990.

Other Late Sequelae of Trauma to the Chest Wall

Arteriovenous fistulas of the internal mammary or intercostal vessels are uncommon (Holland, 1960; Ketharanathan and Westlake, 1969; Rubino and Milnes, 1971) and have been reported following both blunt and penetrating trauma. Patients are usually asymptomatic and present with an abnormal chest radiograph taken for unrelated reasons. A continuous murmur and thrill over the fistula are the characteristic findings on physical examination. The diagnosis is confirmed by computed tomography (CT) scanning with intravenous contrast injection, or by arteriography. Therapy consists of embolization or operative ligation of the feeding vessels with excision of the fistula.

Chronic Chest Wall Pain

Post-traumatic chronic thoracic pain is a common and most challenging problem to investigate and treat. It occurs in approximately 30% of victims of thoracic trauma and can last for months or even years. Numbness or paresthesia in the cutaneous dermatomes of the involved intercostal nerves can accompany the local tenderness. Patients typically complain of tingling sensation or swelling over the anterior chest and upper abdominal wall. The swelling results from the denervation injury to the portion of abdominal wall muscles innervated by the intercostal nerves.

Therapy can be frustrating because in the majority of cases, the exact cause of pain is unknown. Initially, it should be conservative and one must take time to reassure the patient about the absence of any serious underlying problem. Mild non-narcotic analgesics can be given, but the use of narcotics should be restricted. Intercostal nerve blocks can be used, and a mixture of long-acting local anesthesia and corticosteroids is injected over the area of maximal tenderness, which often harbors a Tinel sign. Best results are usually observed after two to three injections and can be long-lasting. Other options include physical therapy consisting of heat massages and ultrasound and the administration of nonsteroidal anti-inflammatory drugs. The use of transcutaneous electrical nerve stimulation (TENS) is also recommended, especially in the presence of a myofascial pain syndrome.

If the pain persists, management benefits from a multidisciplinary approach, in which the anesthesiologist usually plays a key role in developing a plan of therapy. Intercostal neurectomy can be considered if the pain is neurogenic in origin but should be performed only in patients in whom intercostal nerve blocks have produced temporary but significant relief. Not only may neurectomy not relieve the symptoms, but it commonly results in dysesthesias that can seem worse to the patient than the original pain.

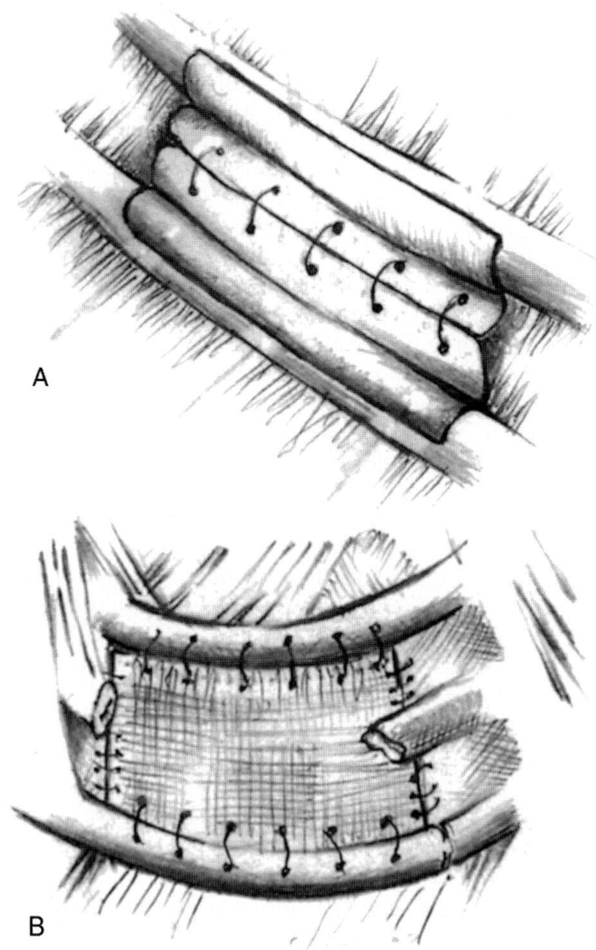

FIGURE 72–5 ■ Diagram illustrating two methods used for the repair of pulmonary hernia. *A*, Use of autologous periosteum. *B*, Use of prosthetic mesh. (Modified from Hix WR: Residua of thoracic trauma. Surg Gynecol Obstet 158:295, 1984.)

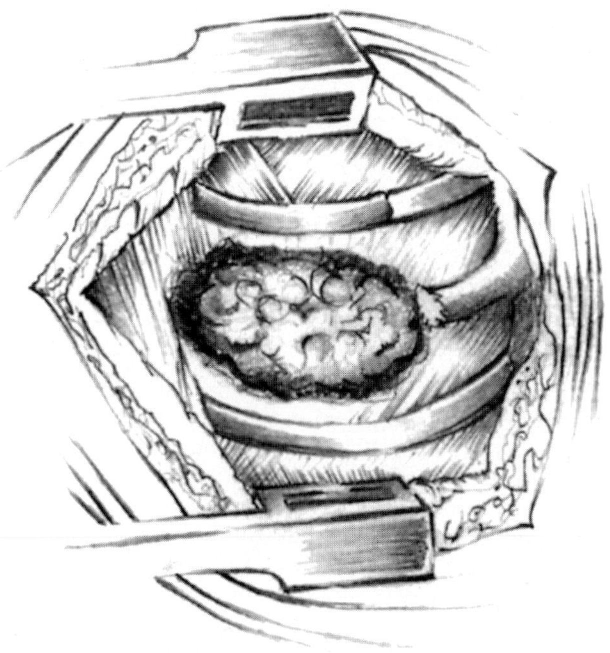

FIGURE 72–4 ■ Diagram illustrating a post-traumatic pulmonary hernia. (Modified from Hix WR: Residua of thoracic trauma. Surg Gynecol Obstet 158:295, 1984.)

LATE SEQUELAE OF TRAUMA TO MAJOR AIRWAYS

Larynx and Upper Trachea

Unrecognized injuries to the larynx and cervical trachea may result in late subglottic or tracheal stenosis with progressive airway obstruction. In most cases, an emergency tracheotomy has been performed at the time of the initial trauma, and the underlying laryngotracheal injury has been overlooked (Fig. 72–7).

The management of these chronic injuries is difficult, and the expertise of both the thoracic surgeon and the otorhinolaryngologist is required. The repair should be attempted only when the patient no longer requires mechanical ventilation and when all associated injuries have resolved. Preoperatively, the extent of injury and involvement of associated structures must be carefully evaluated

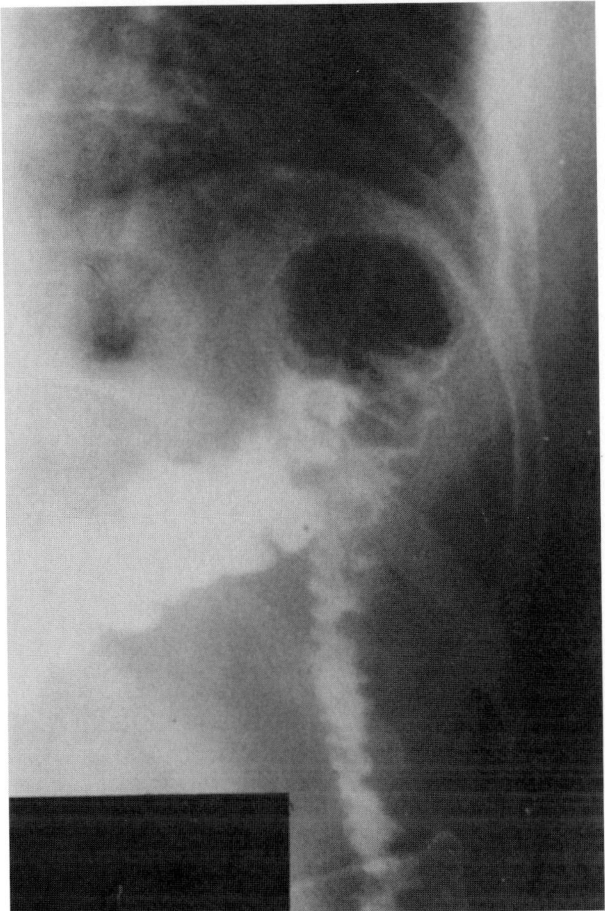

FIGURE 72–6 ■ Transdiaphragmatic intercostal hernia. Barium enema showing a left-sided diaphragmatic hernia and a defect in the anterolateral chest wall in a 33-year-old man previously involved in a car accident.

radiographically and endoscopically, and the functional status of the larynx must also be assessed. A barium swallow to rule out a tracheoesophageal fistula completes the investigation.

There are two major series reporting the results of subglottic tracheal resection for sequelae of blunt trauma. In the series of Maddaus and colleagues (1992), eight patients underwent subglottic resection for lesions resulting from blunt trauma; in all, there was complete transection of the airways at the cricotracheal junction, fracture of the cricoid, and permanent disruption of both recurrent laryngeal nerves. In addition, four of the eight patients had a vertical fracture of the posterior cricoid plate with a tracheoesophageal fistula. All of these patients were successfully managed by tracheal and subglottic resection (Fig. 72–8), with reconstruction by primary laryngeal anastomosis (Maddaus et al, 1992; Pearson et al, 1975, 1986). In Mathisen and Grillo's series (1987), 17 patients were treated for delayed traumatic laryngotracheal stenosis, and the laryngotracheal junction or upper trachea was involved in 11 patients. Results of surgery were good in 16 of the 17 patients, and the airway did not limit their activities.

Intrathoracic Trachea and Main Bronchi

Most intrathoracic tracheobronchial injuries occur within 2.5 cm of the carina. In the acute phase, the clinical presentation depends on the size and location of the rupture and, most importantly, on the presence or absence of free communication with the pleural space.

If the rupture does not communicate with the pleural space and bronchial continuity is preserved by surrounding peribronchial tissues, the clinical presentation may be subtle and the diagnosis can be missed (Deslauriers, 1987). A stricture may develop at the site of rupture, and within 4 to 6 weeks saccular bronchiectasis and irreversible parenchymal damage often develop (Fig. 72–9).

When complete rupture is missed, each of the two stumps heals separately, and this eventually causes obstruction of the airway, with distal atelectasis. These patients may be asymptomatic, or they may present with signs of arterial desaturation secondary to intrapulmonary shunting (Deslauriers, 1987; Deslauriers et al, 1991).

Management depends on the presence or absence of distal suppuration. If there is no infection, lung preservation is usually possible no matter how long the interval between the initial injury and the repair (Fig. 72–10). Pulmonary resection is usually required when there is distal suppuration. When pulmonary resection is carried out, reinforcement of the bronchial stump with well-vascularized autologous local tissues such as the intercostal muscle should be considered.

The surgical principles involved in the repair of post-traumatic bronchial strictures are the same as in any other tracheobronchial reconstruction. Proper exposure of the site of injury is essential, but extensive dissection

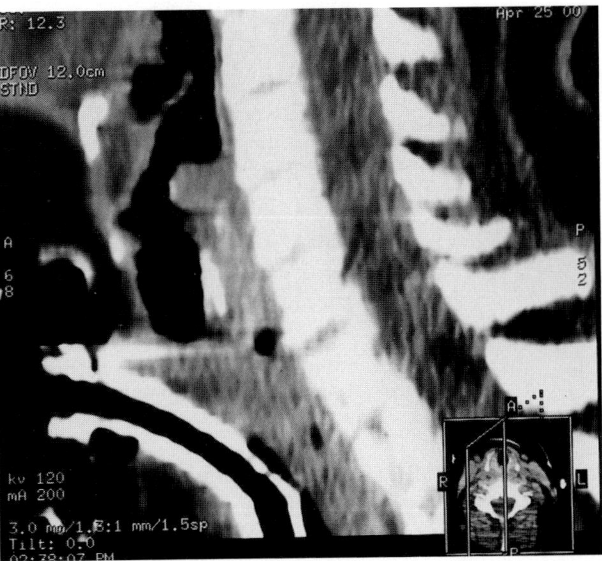

FIGURE 72–7 ■ A computed tomography reconstruction of the larynx and cervical trachea in a 60-year-old woman with complete post-traumatic obstruction of the trachea above the tracheotomy stoma. In this case, the initial unrecognized injury was likely a complete cricotracheal separation.

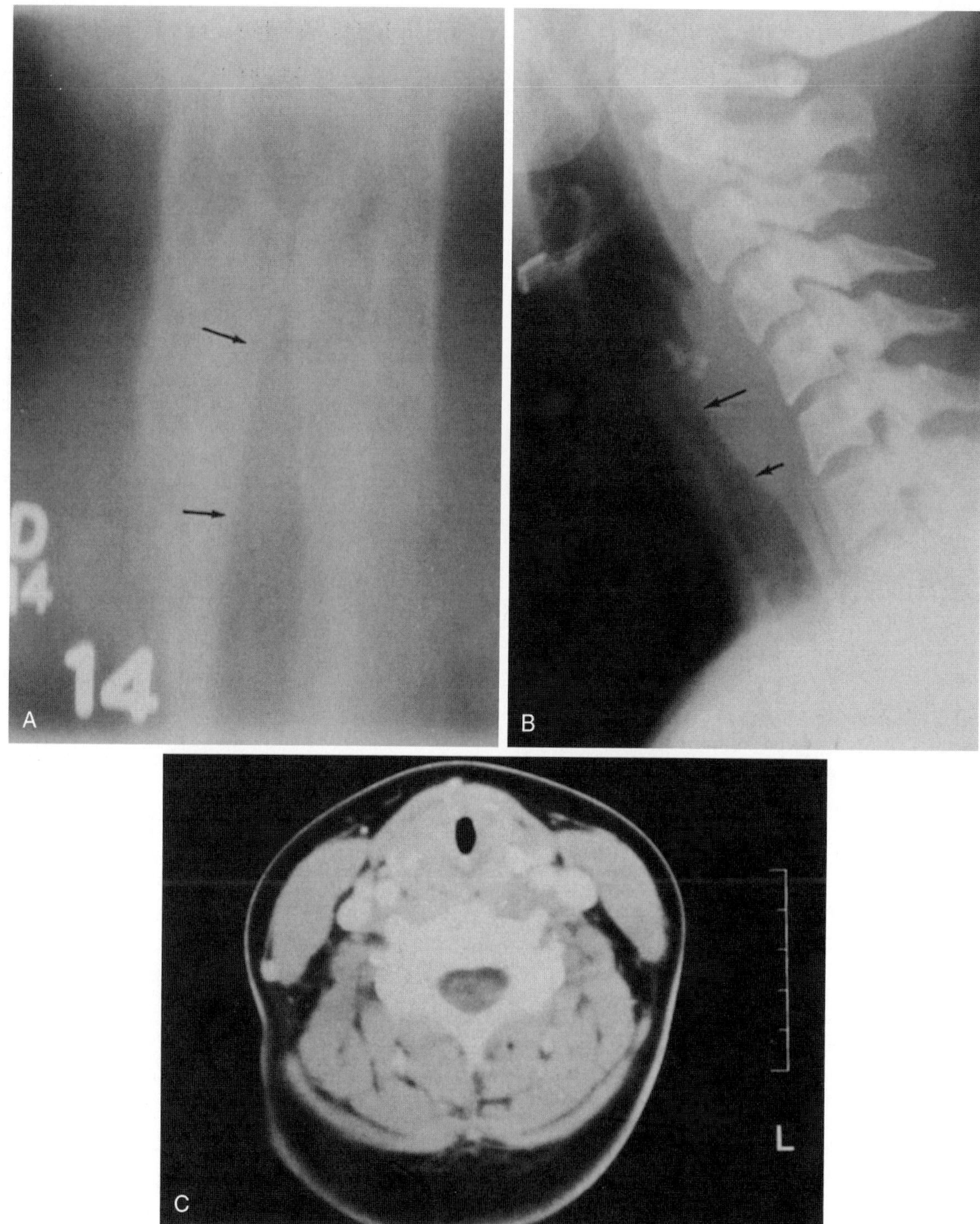

FIGURE 72–8 ■ Post-traumatic subglottic stricture. *A*, Posteroanterior and *B*, lateral tomograms. *C*, A computed tomography scan of an 18-year-old woman with a post-traumatic subglottic stricture (*arrows* in *A* and *B*). The trauma occurred at age 7, and the patient was relatively asymptomatic for over 10 years.

with bronchial devascularization should be avoided. Suturing may be more difficult than in other cases of bronchial reconstruction because of dense peribronchial scarred tissues (Deslauriers and Bussières, 1989). Occasionally, fibrosis and loss of elasticity of the lung prevent re-expansion despite adequate reconstruction. In these cases, resection may be necessary.

Lynn and Iyengar (1972) reported excellent functional results in most patients who underwent reconstruction within 6 months of injury, but they found from a literature review that early repair is best, not only to ensure more complete recovery of function but also to prevent irreversible fibrosis or pulmonary infection. In 1953, Webb and Burford reported the results of their experimental studies of the re-expanded lung after prolonged atelectasis. Dog lungs that had been atelectatic for 3, $3^1/_2$,

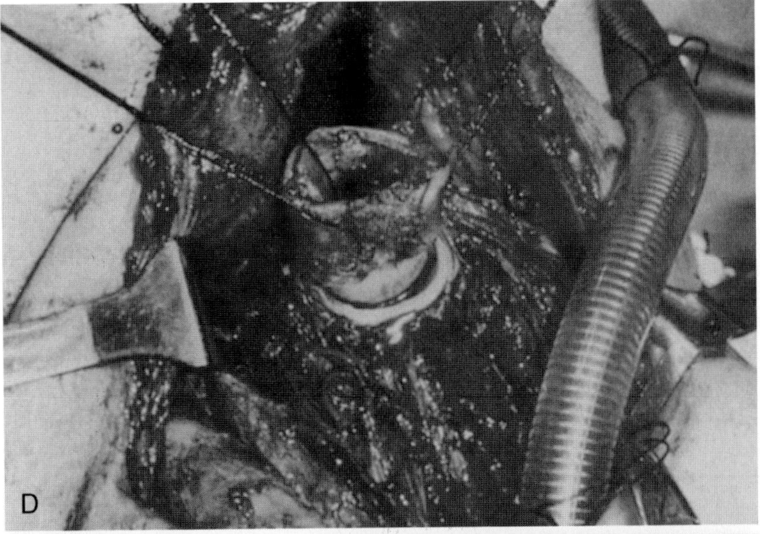

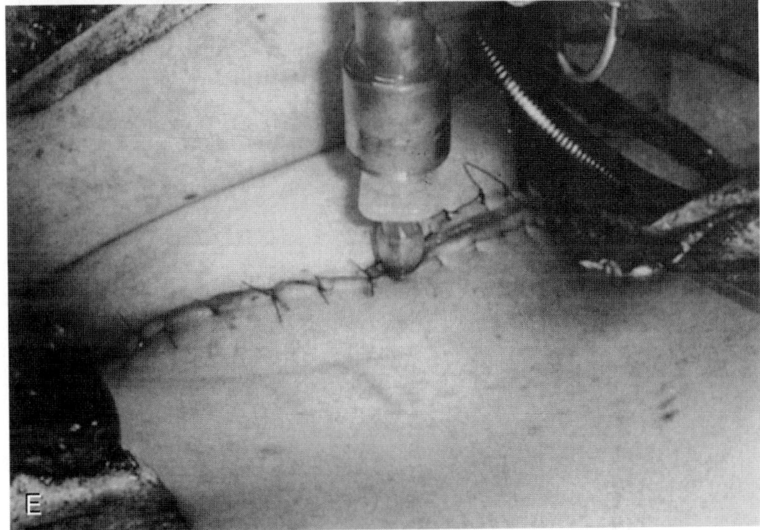

FIGURE 72–8 ■ *Continued. D*, Operative photograph showing the distal trachea, which had been transected and intubated; the proximal segment was mobilized to the inferior border of the cricoid cartilage. The lower border of the cricoid plate has been exposed subperichondrially, and a rim of white posterior cartilage is clearly seen. (Courtesy of M. A. Maddaus, MD and F. G. Pearson, MD.) *E*, Completed operation with a Montgomery T-tube.

and 7½ months re-expanded readily and completely, had a normal pattern of blood flow by angiocardiogram, and oxygenated the blood flowing through the lung.

Mahaffey and associates (1956), Logeais and colleagues (1970), and Nonoyama and co-workers (1976) reported successful reconstruction of the airway 4, 8, and 9 years, respectively, after the initial injury. The patient reported by Nonoyama and associates (1976) showed progressive improvement in pulmonary function following delayed repair 9 years after injury. Although they were slightly reduced from predicted, oxygen uptake and vital capacity in the reimplanted lung returned to almost normal 2 months after direct anastomosis. Partial return of pulmonary function should therefore be expected following resection of a post-traumatic bronchial stricture, even after prolonged intervals between injury and repair (Deslauriers et al, 1981).

Tracheoesophageal and Bronchoesophageal Fistulas

Most combined injuries to the trachea and esophagus associated with penetrating cervical trauma are recognized and repaired early (Kelly et al, 1987). Following blunt trauma, however, injuries to the trachea and esophagus may not be immediately recognized, either because of lack of symptoms or because of the extent of associated injuries.

Tracheoesophageal fistulas may develop in the upper cervical region in association with fracture of the cricoid cartilage and cricotracheal separation, or as a complication of prolonged intubation. They may also occur at or near the carina, where they are secondary to a tear of the membranous trachea, with partial disruption of the esophageal wall, necrosis, and eventually fistula formation. Layton and colleagues (1980) have shown that at the moment of impact, there is an immediate laceration of the membranous trachea, which seals rapidly, and a contusion of the anterior wall of the esophagus, which progresses to necrosis, probably accelerated by infection; within 3 to 5 days, a fistula between the trachea and esophagus is established. In a review of the literature (Layton et al, 1980), 69% of fistulas (24 of 35) were at or just above the carina, and in five cases, the fistula was located in the cervical esophagus.

A collar incision is used for a cervical fistula, and a

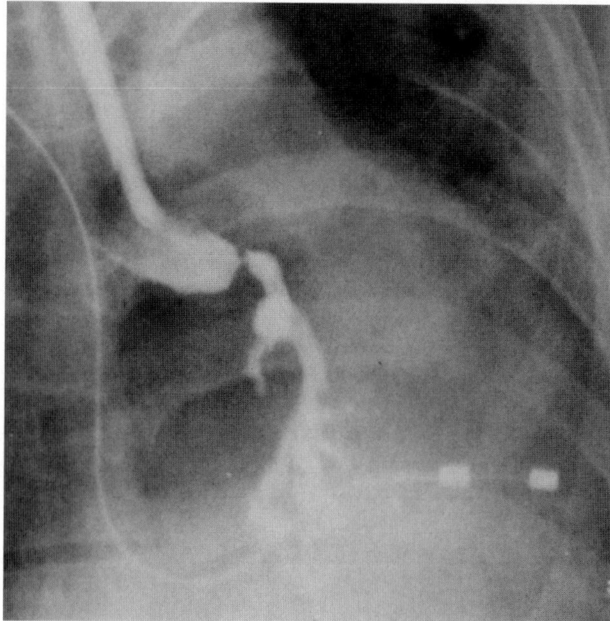

FIGURE 72–9 ■ Post-traumatic bronchial stricture; post-traumatic left main bronchial stricture with distal bronchiectasis. This patient required a left pneumonectomy.

right posterolateral thoracotomy is the best approach for a thoracic fistula. The fistula is first identified and divided; the esophageal wall is then enclosed in two layers of interrupted silk sutures. The trachea often needs to be locally resected and reconstructed (Grillo et al, 1976). Interposition of well-vascularized tissues such as pleura, pericardium, or intercostal muscle between the suture lines is highly recommended in the repair of tracheo-esophageal fistulas.

LATE SEQUELAE OF TRAUMA TO THE LUNG

Pulmonary Contusion

Although blunt thoracic trauma and missile injury often cause acute pulmonary contusion, significant late sequelae are rare, even if the contused lung becomes infected. Hanning and co-workers (1981) noted, however, that more than half of the survivors of pulmonary contusion might have increased respiratory symptoms, presenting as worsening of productive cough and wheezing. In their series, prevalence of respiratory symptoms after injury was greater than expected, with 27% claiming a persistent productive cough, 21% persistent wheezing, and 26% grade 2 dyspnea. Persistent productive cough and occasional wheezing were more common among smokers and ex-smokers than among nonsmokers. In a study of pulmonary disability after severe blunt chest trauma, Livingston and Richardson (1990) showed that pulmonary function tests were markedly abnormal soon after injury, averaging 40% to 50% of predicted values. There was, however, rapid improvement in all parameters within 4 months, and long-term respiratory disability was present in less than 5% of patients studied. By contrast, Kishikawa and associates (1991) showed that patients with pulmonary contusion had long-term respiratory dys-

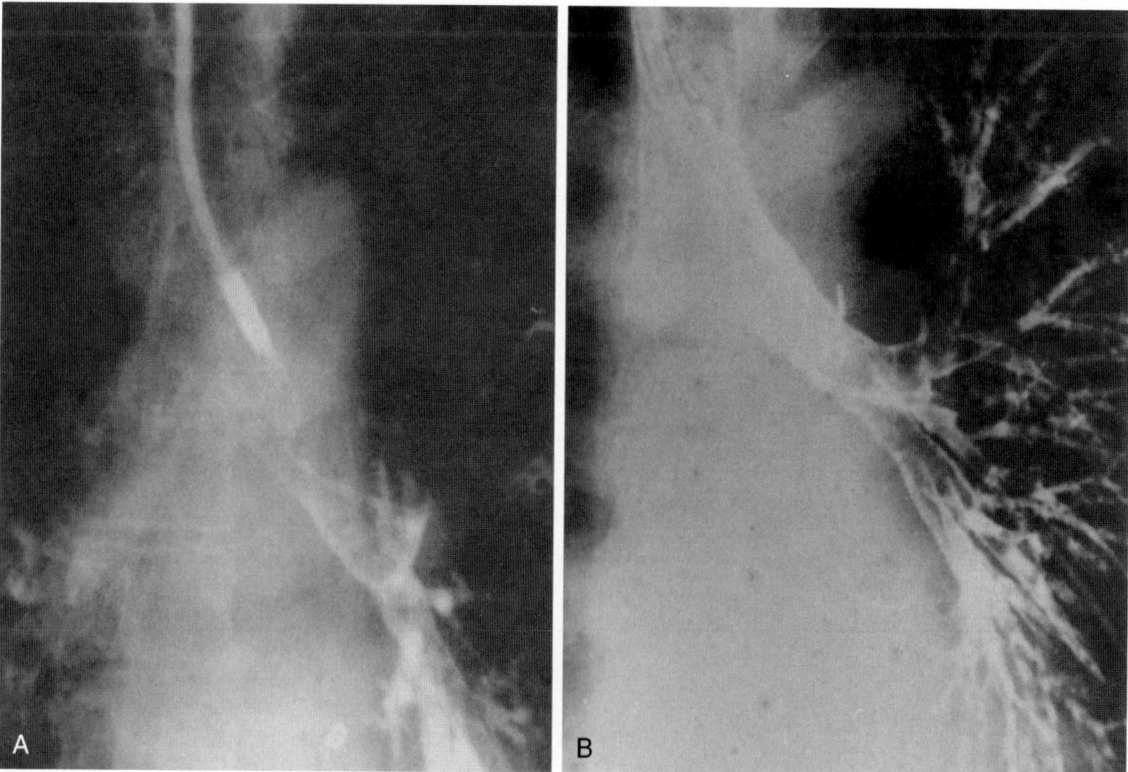

FIGURE 72–10 ■ Post-traumatic bronchial stricture. *A*, Bronchogram showing a post-traumatic stricture of the left main bronchus. *B*, Repeat bronchogram 4 years after resection and reanastomosis.

function with decreased functional residual capacity and a fall in the PaO_2 when moved from the lordotic to the supine position, even several years after injury.

Hematoma and Pneumatocele

Traumatic pulmonary hematoma and pneumatocele are related sequelae of shearing injury to the pulmonary tissue. Khan and colleagues (1974) suggested that increased intrathoracic pressure at the instant of chest compression followed by greatly increased negative intrathoracic pressure on chest rebound causes bursting lesions with pulmonary destruction. When the destruction does not result in a hemothorax and is entirely located within the lung, it may form a cavity that can fill with blood, air, or both, depending on the amount of communication with the airways. These cavities are also called *traumatic pseudocysts* because they do not contain an epithelial lining such as that seen in true bronchogenic cysts (Kato et al, 1989). Other possible mechanisms of post-traumatic pulmonary pseudocyst formation include disruption of the wall of a small bronchus in conjunction with increased intrabronchial pressure (Fagan, 1966), and increased pressure in areas distal to a traumatically occluded bronchus (Fagan and Swischuk, 1976). In a review of the literature, Santos and Mahendra (1979) noted that most reported traumatic lung pseudocysts occurred in children or young adults, probably because of the increased elastic recoil present in the lungs of this group of patients.

The clinical picture varies with the size of the cavity and the importance of the associated pulmonary contusion. About 40% of patients present with cough or hemoptysis. Unless they become infected, most pneumatoceles resolve spontaneously over a period of a few months. In the series of Kato and colleagues (1989), all 12 traumatic pulmonary pseudocysts resolved with no specific treatment, and late sequelae were only those of radiologic scarring in an area of previous lung injury. The differential diagnosis should include a localized pneumothorax, a diaphragmatic hernia, a pre-existing cystic lesion of the lung (Desrues et al, 1988), or even lung cancer. Post-traumatic pneumatoceles can involve the inferior pulmonary ligament (Ravin et al, 1976) where they can be confused with hemidiaphragmatic hernias. In 1990, Ulstad and co-workers reported a patient whose bilateral post-traumatic paramediastinal lung cysts were presumed to be bilateral hemidiaphragmatic hernias, which led to unnecessary surgery.

Secondary infection of post-traumatic cavitary lung lesions is unusual. Because these lesions may not respond to a conservative approach owing to the lack of direct anatomic communication with the main airways, percutaneous drainage or exploratory thoracotomy should be considered in the face of prolonged fever and pulmonary deterioration (Carroll et al, 1989).

Pulmonary Arteriovenous Fistula and Pulmonary Artery Aneurysm

Rarely, penetrating or blunt trauma to the thorax will cause a pulmonary arteriovenous fistula or a pulmonary artery aneurysm. These lesions should be suspected in patients with a history of trauma, signs and symptoms of pulmonary arteriovenous fistula with shunting (Arom and Lyons, 1975), and chronic residual, well-circumscribed density on chest radiograph. The diagnosis is confirmed by pulmonary arteriography (Fig. 72–11), or most commonly by CT with intravenous contrast. When these lesions are localized peripherally, embolization by coils or other foreign material can successfully obliterate the fistula (Kerr and Sauter, 1993). When the fistula is centrally located, however, embolization may not be possible, and excision of the lesion with preservation of the lung or resection of the involved lobe becomes the therapy of choice (Symbas et al, 1980).

LATE SEQUELAE OF TRAUMA TO THE PLEURAL SPACE

Chronic empyema and fibrothorax with entrapment of the lung often result from undrained or inadequately drained traumatic hemothoraces. Incomplete drainage leads to clot formation, recurrent pleural effusions due to clot lysis, loculation of the pleural space, and organization of the collection.

Hemothorax

Culiner and associates (1959), Milfeld and colleagues (1978), and Coselli and co-workers (1984) have recommended early thoracotomy for residual hemothoraces because of their significant potential for developing empyema or fibrothorax. In the series of Milfeld and associates (1978), 3.3% of 3000 patients with hemothorax or pneumohemothorax developed a clotted hemothorax or post-traumatic empyema. Among 10 patients undergoing evacuation of a clotted hemothorax within 5 days of admission, there was zero mortality and an average hospital stay of 10 days. Among 41 patients undergoing decortication more than 5 days after injury, there was one death (2.4% mortality); among 34 patients requiring decortication and drainage of empyema, 4 died (12% mortality), and the average hospital stay was 41 days. By contrast, Wilson and colleagues (1979) concluded that early thoracotomy is often unnecessary. They reviewed the management and results in 452 patients with hemothorax caused by penetrating (n = 338) or blunt trauma (n = 114). The overall incidence of empyema was 4.9%, and this incidence was not changed by thoracotomy or by the presence of residual hemothorax. Shock, pleural contamination, pneumonia, and duration of pleural catheter drainage were found to be significant variables. The authors currently recommend the use of videothoracoscopic techniques to remove residual clots that remain in the pleural space after trauma, despite proper initial chest drainage. This technique is less invasive than thoracotomy, and probably achieves the same overall result (Lang-Ladzunski et al, 1997).

Empyema

Post-traumatic empyema is defined as an empyema that develops secondary to infection of a traumatic hemotho-

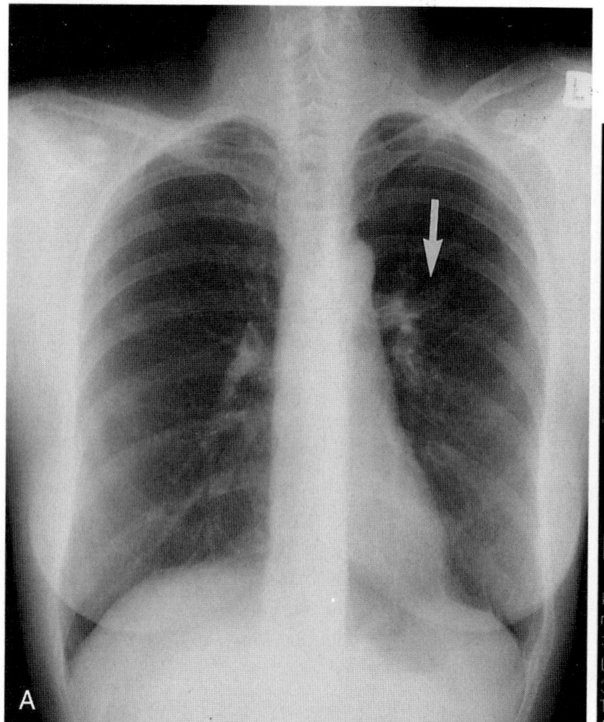

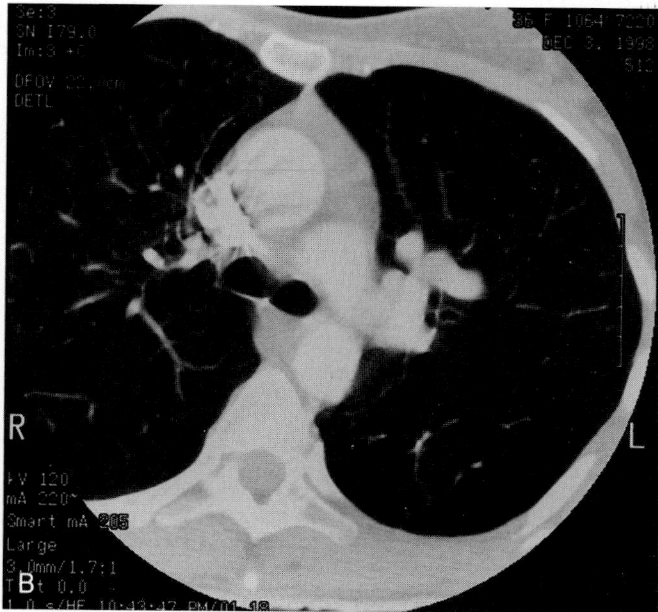

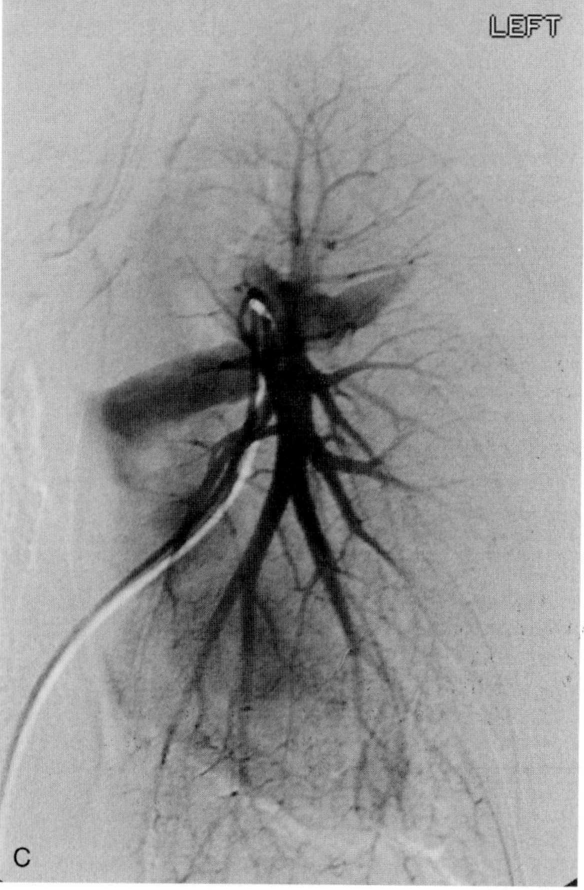

FIGURE 72–11 ■ *A*, Standard chest radiograph showing a left upper lobe density in a 32-year-old woman shot through the chest 5 years prior to consulting for dyspnea. *B*, A computed tomography scan shows a vascular mass in the left hilum. *C*, Angiography reveals the mass to be a vascular malformation connecting the pulmonary artery to the pulmonary vein. Because of hilar proximity, the lesion could not be embolized. It was successfully treated by operative ligation of the fistula without pulmonary resection.

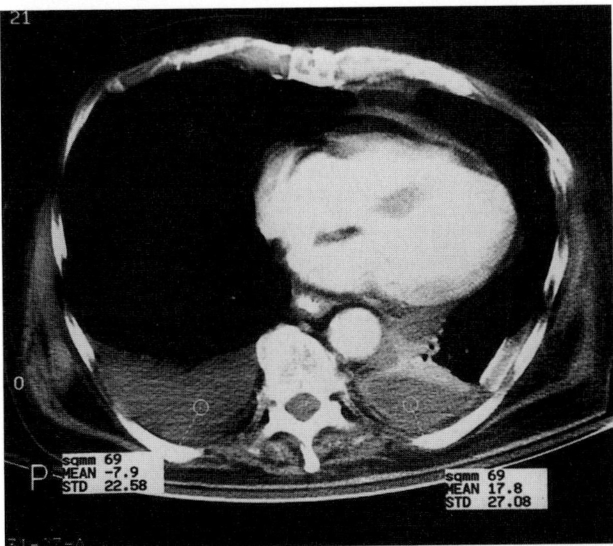

FIGURE 72–12 ■ A computed tomography scan showing a left-sided empyema in a 77-year-old male 2 weeks after blunt chest trauma. The empyema was treated by open decortication with successful result.

rax (Symbas, 1989). It is usually related to incomplete drainage of intrapleural blood, with contamination either from an open thoracic wound, from the chest tube, or from an infection in the adjacent lung (Fig. 72–12). Predisposing factors (Table 72–2) include delay in initial chest tube insertion, improper positioning or unnecessary manipulation of the tube, tube occlusion, prolonged drainage (Eddy et al, 1989), and the presence of an intrapleural foreign body. Larger hemothoraces (more than 500 ml) are more likely to become infected (Ogilvie, 1950; Young et al, 1972) (Table 72–3) than smaller ones. Residual pneumothorax (incomplete re-expansion of the lung or loculated spaces), missed diaphragmatic perforation, lung contusion, extrapleural hematomas, shock, pleural contamination, pneumonia, and duration of pleural catheter drainage are other factors considered important in the development of post-traumatic empyemas (Hix, 1984; Villalba et al, 1979).

Post-traumatic empyemas should be treated in the same way as empyemas of other etiologies. The principles of management include adequate drainage of the collection, lung re-expansion, and obliteration of the pleural space. The authors recommend early decortication as soon as pleural infection is evident and cannot be controlled by closed tube drainage. With early decortication and immediate removal of the infected peel, chronic empyema with additional weeks of disability is prevented, and the patient is spared considerable discomfort (Arom et al, 1977; Neef, 1991).

TABLE 72–2 ■ **Predisposing Factors for the Development of Post-Traumatic Empyemas**

- Delay in initial chest tube insertion
- Improper positioning of the tube
- Manipulations of the tube
- Tube occlusion
- Large hemothoraces (>500 ml)
- Pneumohemothoraces
- Foreign body driven into pleural space
- Open thoracic wounds
- Bronchopneumonia
- Diaphragmatic perforation
- Extrapleural hematomas

TABLE 72–3 ■ **Size of Hemothorax in Relation to Pleural Infection**

	Number of Hemothoraces			
Size	*Sterile*	*Infected*	*Total*	*Infected (%)*
Large	123	43	166	26
Small	57	7	64	11
Total	180	50	230	22

From Ogilvie AG: Final results in traumatic haemothorax: A report of 230 cases. Thorax 5:116, 1950, with permission.

Fibrothorax

Post-traumatic fibrothorax is the abnormal deposition of a fibrous scar over the surface of the lung and over the inner surface of the chest wall. Fibrothorax is an end-stage manifestation of an undrained or incompletely drained hemothorax, empyema, or chylothorax and causes entrapment and loss of function of the lung.

Patients present with decreased exercise tolerance and pain. Chest radiography and CT scanning often show a thick peel surrounding a cavity. The inflammatory vascular peel is better seen on CT with intravenous contrast injection. Symptomatic patients should be offered surgery to remove the fibrous tissue and to allow the lung and chest wall to re-expand. Successful surgery generally improves pulmonary function and lowers the incidence of infection in the underlying lung (Ilie, 1996; Nieminen et al, 1985; Petty et al, 1961; Siebens et al, 1956).

Chylothorax

Traumatic chylothorax is an accumulation of chyle in the pleural space secondary to an injury to the thoracic duct. Traumatic chylothorax can be encountered in association with vertebral fractures (Crnojevic et al, 1997; Ikonomidis et al, 1997) after hyperextension injuries of the spine, after a violent Valsalva maneuver while coughing or vomiting, or after compressive trauma of the chest. Often chylothoraces become apparent or symptomatic only 4 to 6 weeks after the injury. They will be right-sided if the spinal lesion is below the fifth thoracic vertebra where the thoracic duct crosses from right to left, and they will be left-sided if the lesion is above that level.

The initial management of post-traumatic chylothorax is chest drainage and intravenous hyperalimentation, but if lung expansion is not complete, surgical decortication of the lung and concomitant ligation of the thoracic duct may become necessary. It has also been shown that chylothorax fluid can be autotransfused to the patient with no apparent deterrent side effects (Montebugnoli et al, 1998). If the amount of chyle drainage does not decrease after a latency period of about 2 weeks, the thoracic duct should be ligated. In patients unfit for surgery, the use of a pleuroperitoneal shunt has been shown to be effective in relieving and sometimes preventing the reaccumulation of the effusion (Milano et al, 1994).

In 1986, Saibil and associates reported the case of a patient who developed a subcutaneous chest wall lymphocele following trauma to the thoracic duct and continued chyle leak in the mediastinum. The diagnosis was made by computed tomography and lymphangiography, and the condition was treated by ligation of the thoracic duct.

LATE SEQUELAE OF TRAUMA TO THE ESOPHAGUS

Because of its protected position, small size, and resiliency, the esophagus is rarely the site of trauma. In 1973, Andréassiam and colleagues reported 63 cases (collective review), and most were secondary to blunt thoracic trauma incurred in high-speed motor vehicle accidents. Isolated ruptures of the cervical esophagus (Niezgoda et al, 1990) or of the abdominal esophagus (Barrié et al, 1961) are extremely unusual.

Late sequelae of esophageal injuries include stricture or fistula formation. Strictures are secondary to ischemia or initial loss of tissue, and most can be treated by dilatation alone, although resection and reconstruction of the esophagus may occasionally be necessary. Fistulas between the esophagus and the pleural space, airway, aorta, and pericardium have all been described as the result of undetected perforation of the esophagus due to external trauma or to erosion of impacted foreign bodies. Chronic nasogastric intubation can result in chronic reflux and chronic distal esophagitis, which can leave injury if the patient survives the traumatic event to a distal esophageal stricture formation. In these cases, which occur often in very debilitated patients, the authors have used self-expandable metallic stents to successfully relieve the dysphagia.

Most esophagopleural fistulas present as empyemas. The diagnosis is suspected when drainage of the empyema yields food particles and yeast organisms. The diagnosis can be readily confirmed by a barium swallow. As with any other type of esophageal perforation, management of an established esophagopleural fistula depends on the location and extent of injury, the local inflammatory reaction, the degree of pleural contamination, the significance of associated injuries, and the overall condition of the patient. In debilitated patients, drainage of the empyema by either chest tube or thoracic window associated with gastrostomy for drainage of the stomach and feeding jejunostomy for caloric gavage can improve the patient until he or she is strong enough to sustain a more permanent procedure. A number of reports have shown satisfactory results with the use of decortication of the lung followed by the insertion of a T tube within the perforation to create a controlled fistulous track (Larson et al, 1991; Özcelik et al, 1994).

LATE SEQUELAE OF TRAUMA TO THE DIAPHRAGM

Like many other injuries previously considered rare, diaphragmatic rupture is being reported with increasing frequency. This relates not only to a net increase in the number of high-speed motor vehicle accidents but also to a higher index of suspicion for this type of injury. When the diagnosis of blunt diaphragmatic injury is missed, the most likely sequela is that of either a chronic herniation of abdominal contents in the pleural space or an eventration.

Diaphragmatic Hernia

Chronic post-traumatic diaphragmatic hernias are usually seen in patients previously involved in deceleration injuries. Because of the extent of associated injuries, the diagnosis is overlooked at the time of injury; often, the typical radiologic signs are obscured by the presence of atelectasis, hemopneumothorax, pulmonary contusion, or subcutaneous emphysema or mechanical ventilation, which reduces intra-abdominal contents back within the abdomen.

Patients with chronic post-traumatic diaphragmatic hernia are usually asymptomatic or may present with minor symptoms such as postprandial chest pain and dyspnea (Childress and Grimes, 1961). The time between injury and diagnosis ranges from months to years, but an average figure from the literature is 10 years after the initial trauma (Mansour et al, 1975). At this stage, the diagnosis can again be missed because the radiologic signs are falsely attributed to late pleural sequelae. However, the diagnosis should be suspected when standard chest radiographs show elevation of the diaphragmatic shadow, an abdominal viscus within the pleural space, or a contralateral mediastinal shift. Additional helpful studies are CT scanning, gastroesophageal contrast studies, and pneumoperitoneum. The latter study, in which 500 ml of air is introduced into the peritoneal cavity, is diagnostic in virtually all cases. When the diagnosis is still not made or the hernia is left unrepaired, the patient can eventually go on to incarcerate or strangulate the contents of the hernia, an event more likely to occur with left-sided hernias (Estrera et al, 1985).

Because of the high likelihood of incarceration or strangulation, surgical repair of a traumatic diaphragmatic hernia is always indicated when the diagnosis is made (Fig. 72–13). On the right side, the repair is best accomplished through a right posterolateral seventh interspace thoracotomy, whereas on the left side, controversy exists as to whether it should be done by the transthoracic or transabdominal route. Because of often dense adhesions between the contents of the hernia and the lung, the authors prefer the transthoracic approach. Unless infected or necrotic tissues exist within the hernia, the morbidity and mortality rates associated with the repair of a diaphragmatic hernia are low and the long-term results excellent.

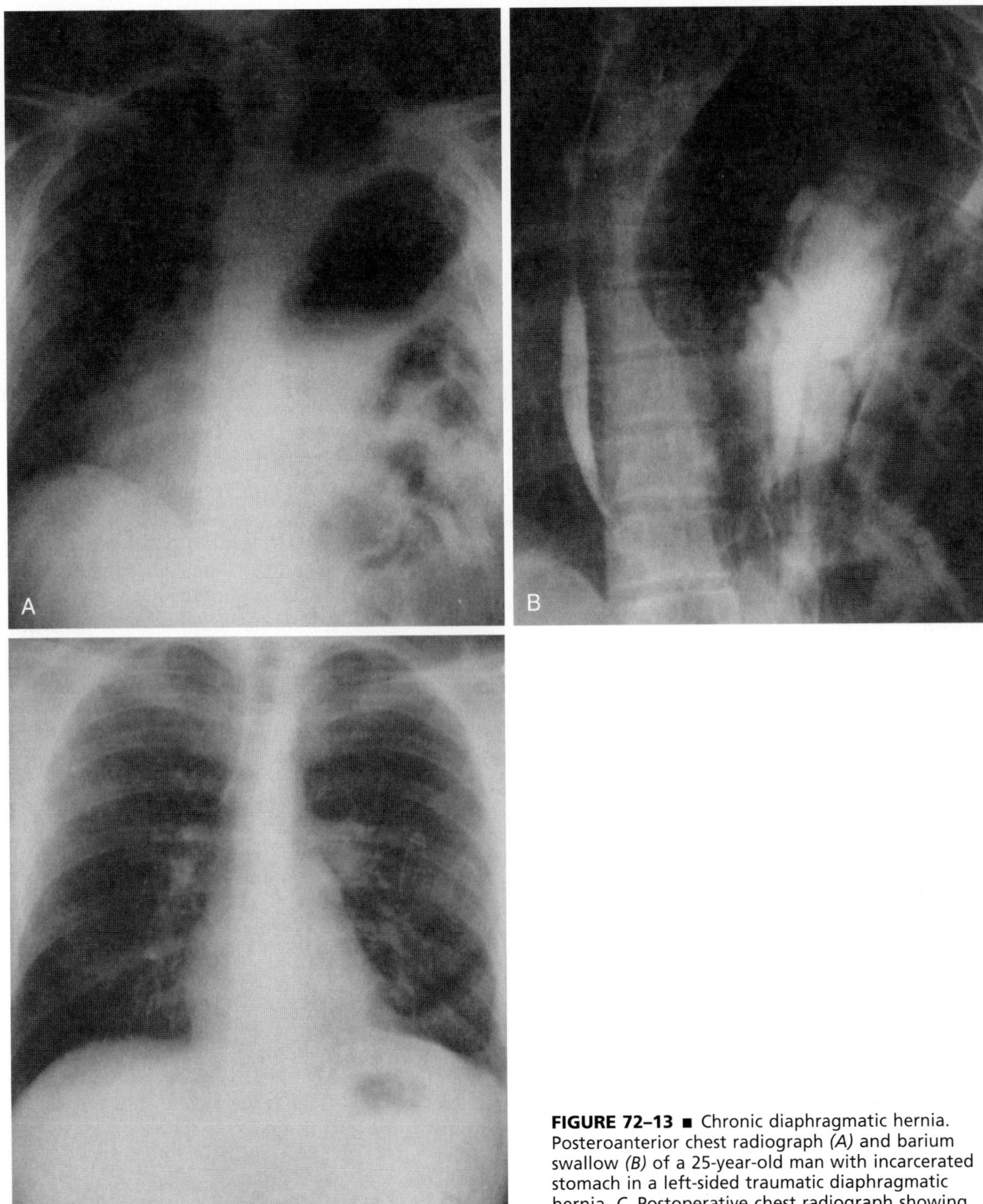

FIGURE 72–13 ■ Chronic diaphragmatic hernia. Posteroanterior chest radiograph *(A)* and barium swallow *(B)* of a 25-year-old man with incarcerated stomach in a left-sided traumatic diaphragmatic hernia. *C*, Postoperative chest radiograph showing the repaired hemidiaphragm in normal position.

Diaphragmatic Eventration

The term *eventration of the diaphragm* is used in the pediatric population to describe congenital absence of the diaphragm. When used in the setting of trauma, it indicates diaphragmatic paralysis and it is best referred to as elevation of the hemidiaphragm. Post-traumatic elevation of the diaphragm can be caused either by an injury to the phrenic nerve or by partial disruption of the diaphragmatic muscle itself (Waldschmidt and Laws, 1980). The chest radiograph shows an elevated hemidiaphragm, and paralysis of the diaphragm can be confirmed by fluoroscopy or by electromyographic studies. Occasionally, one can use pneumoperitoneum to confirm the diagnosis at bedside (Fig. 72–14).

Because most of these injuries are due to traction injuries to the phrenic nerve, regeneration is possible and the diaphragm can resume its normal position and function. Therefore, surgical correction is never indicated before 6 to 8 months have elapsed after the injury. Plica-

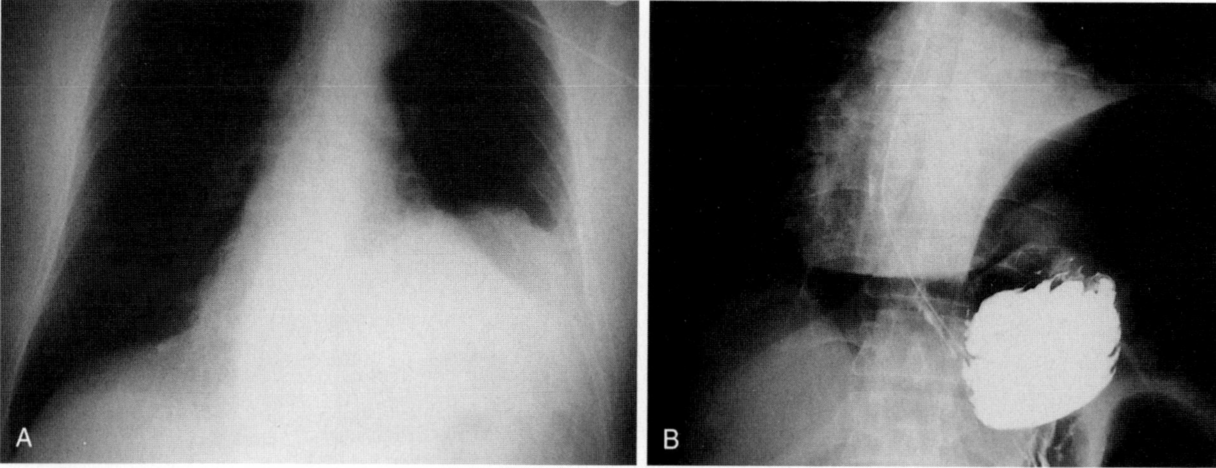

FIGURE 72–14 ■ *A*, Standard posteroanterior chest radiograph showing an elevated left hemidiaphragm in a 40-year-old patient. *B*, As determined by bedside pneumoperitoneum, the elevation was due to an eventration rather than a true hernia.

tion of the diaphragm may be indicated in patients in whom there is evidence of respiratory restriction due to lung compression during abdominal paradoxical breathing.

LATE SEQUELAE OF TRAUMA TO THE HEART AND GREAT VESSELS

Late sequelae of injuries to the heart and great vessels are rare and have generated very few reports (Antunes et al, 1988; Deslauriers et al, 1991; Hix and Aaron, 1987; Sturaitis et al, 1986). In general, less than 5% of survivors from penetrating wounds of the heart and great vessels will have symptomatic sequelae up to 10 years after the injury (Cha et al, 1993); complete recovery from myocardial contusion due to blunt chest trauma is the rule when associated complications are promptly recognized and properly managed (Sturaitis et al, 1986).

Penetrating Cardiac Trauma

Because of the initial cardiac tamponade, injuries such as intra- or even extracardiac shunts may be unrecognized at the time of trauma only to become symptomatic and functionally significant when the perforation becomes larger as a result of fibrous contraction of its edges. Although the prevalence of extracardiac shunts is unknown, Antunes and co-workers (1988) reported that 42% were late sequelae of trauma in a series of 31 patients.

Symptoms are usually those of congestive heart failure, and the shunt can be easily documented by noninvasive techniques such as Doppler echocardiography (Antunes et al, 1988; Kirklin and Barratt-Boyes, 1993; Sturaitis et al, 1986). Intracardiac shunts include ventricular septal defects and fistulas between the aorta and right atrium, the aorta and right ventricle, or the left ventricle and right atrium. The most common extracardiac shunts are fistulas between aorta and innominate vein, or between aorta and main pulmonary artery. Surgical repair is always indicated and should be carried out by standard techniques. Coronary artery fistulas can, on occasion, be the result of penetrating cardiac injuries as reported by Lowe and associates (1983). In their series, such fistulas were caused by penetrating trauma in 80% of cases and were secondary to blunt trauma in the remaining 20%. Right and left coronary arteries were equally involved; the fistula was between a coronary artery and the right ventricle in 50% of patients, and between a coronary artery and the right atrium in an additional 35% of patients.

Lacerations of cardiac valves, particularly of the tricuspid or pulmonary valves, can also be diagnosed late after thoracic trauma. These lacerations can be safely repaired (Antunes et al, 1988; Symbas, 1989), although postoperative recovery may be impaired by traumatic neurosis, a syndrome similar to that which has been reported in patients who have sustained violent and major abdominal trauma (Abbott et al, 1978).

Blunt Cardiac Trauma

Post-traumatic left ventricular aneurysms were described in 1892, but since then, very few cases have been reported (Fig. 72–15) as is shown in a recent literature review in which only 35 documented cases could be found (Grieco et al, 1989). In that review, the interval between injury and diagnosis ranged from 5 days to 18 years (with a median interval of 3 months), and in most cases, associated coronary artery disease was thought to be the cause of the aneurysm rather than myocardial contusion. The thin walls of post-traumatic ventricular aneurysms and their liability to rupture make surgical resection advisable in most patients (Kirklin and Barratt-Boyes, 1993). In 1989, Grieco and co-workers reported that 10 of 12 patients treated conservatively died from complications directly attributed to the aneurysm.

Tricuspid incompetence (Fig. 72–16) from chordal or papillary muscle rupture is rare, and progression from injury to severe disability may take as long as 5 or even 10 years (Kirklin and Barratt-Boyes, 1993). Because of the severe disability often present when patients are referred for surgery, and because of the technical difficulties

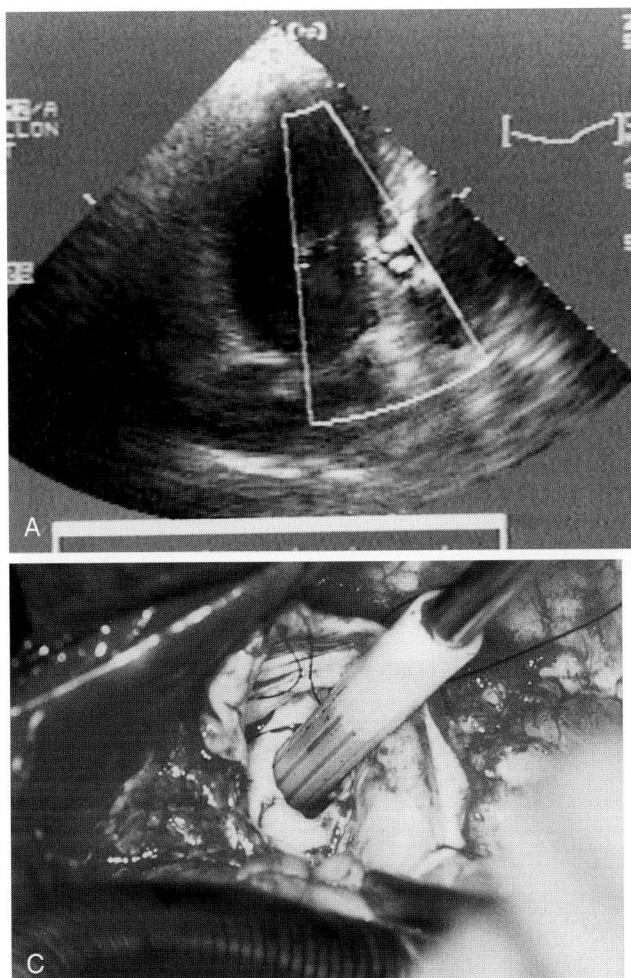

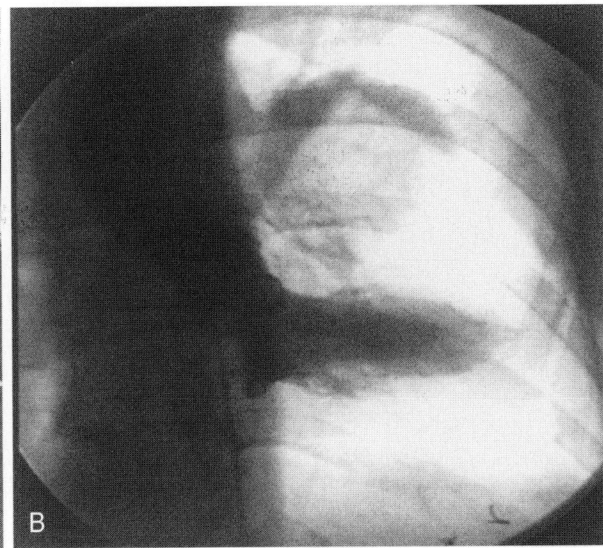

FIGURE 72–15 ■ *A*, Echocardiogram of a patient with post-traumatic left ventricular aneurysm discovered 9 years after trauma. *B*, The diagnosis was confirmed by left ventriculography. *C*, At operation, the neck of the aneurysm measured 12 mm in diameter and was simply closed with mattress sutures.

associated with the repair of tricuspid chordal or papillary muscles, tricuspid valve replacement with a bioprosthesis is the procedure of choice.

Coronary artery injuries may be the cause of angina or heart failure, especially in patients with previous arteriosclerotic coronary artery disease. In such patients, the intimal tear with secondary thrombosis and platelet aggregation and the myocardial contusion contribute to occlude the coronary artery. Blunt chest trauma may also occlude aortocoronary bypass grafts. In 1996, Masuda and associates reported the case of a traumatic coronary artery dissection that healed spontaneously in a young woman

Atrial septal rupture is rare, and it can be diagnosed long after trauma. This delay in recognition is often due to severe associated injuries, as a massive force is required to rupture the atrial septum (Jenson et al, 1993).

In children, few series have reported sequelae of blunt trauma to the heart (Dowd and Krug, 1996; Ildstad et al, 1990). As the majority of these children have multiple system injuries, the diagnosis of cardiac injury is often missed initially, and long-term follow-up is mandatory to diagnose sequelae.

Great Vessels

Traumatic rupture of the thoracic aorta is responsible for approximately 10% of all deaths associated with blunt trauma (Desaulniers and Bruneau, 1972), but because of associated injuries or lack of suspicion, the diagnosis is often overlooked or missed completely at the time of trauma. Indeed, Utley (1987) reported that the interval between trauma and diagnosis of aneurysm is greater than 10 years in about half the patients. Symptoms are usually those of compression of adjacent organs, such as the lung, esophagus, or recurrent nerve.

Post-traumatic aneurysms of the descending aorta should always be resected, even in asymptomatic patients. In contrast with arteriosclerotic aortic aneurysms, post-traumatic aneurysms are false aneurysms because the aortic wall is held in place only by the adventitia. The authors recommend that the resection of a chronic post-traumatic aneurysm be done with temporary blood shunting (Verdant et al, 1988) or with the use of partial heart-lung bypass in association with an autotransfusion system. Because this is an elective procedure, every precaution to prevent spinal cord ischemia and blood loss should be taken.

Pericardium

Post-traumatic constrictive pericarditis was first described by Goldstein and Yu (1965). It is a rare sequela that is secondary to local post-traumatic immunoreaction (Blake et al, 1983) or to the organization of large intrapericardial

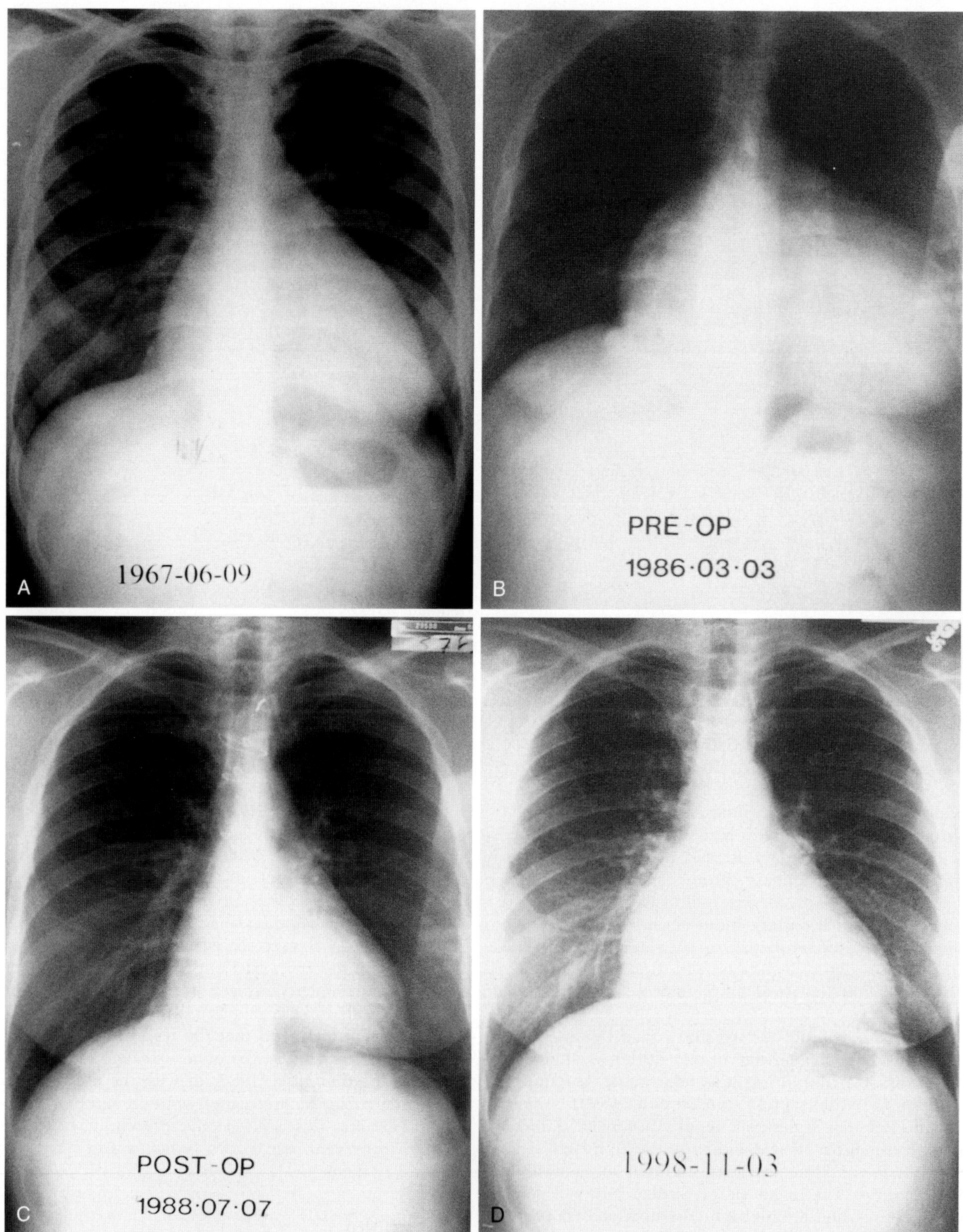

FIGURE 72–16 ■ Serial posteroanterior chest radiographs of a patient with post-traumatic tricuspid regurgitation 7 years after trauma *(A)*, 16 years after trauma *(B)*, 2 years after valve replacement *(C)*, and 12 years after valve replacement *(D)*.

hematomas (Meleca and Hoit, 1995). Indications for pericardectomy are based on clinical and hemodynamic symptoms. Results of surgery are similar to those obtained after pericardectomy for pericarditis due to other causes.

MISCELLANEOUS SEQUELAE

Retained Intrathoracic Foreign Bodies

Retained intrathoracic foreign bodies such as shrapnel fragments, bullets, knife tips, and small aspirated fragments rarely cause symptoms after the initial injury period. As part of the natural healing process, they stimulate the formation of scar capsule, which locks the particle in place. Only occasionally do they erode into surrounding structures (Bogedain, 1984; Sounders et al, 1992).

If the initial injury does not require thoracotomy, and if the patient is asymptomatic, a retained intrathoracic foreign body need not be removed (Vogt-Moykopf and Krumhar, 1966). These foreign bodies can, however, be associated with the development of serious complications, which will require surgical removal at a later date. Intrapulmonary foreign bodies, for instance, can migrate into surrounding airways to cause hemoptysis, lung abscesses, and airway obstruction years after the initial injury. The scar around the foreign body can also become the stimulus for the formation of carcinomas.

The migration and impaction of retained foreign bodies, located near major hilar vascular structures or the heart, can result in life-threatening events. In this group of patients, surgical exploration is recommended at the time of presentation not only to verify the integrity of the major vessels and heart but also to extract the foreign particle and thereby prevent future complications.

When it is decided not to remove an intrapulmonary foreign body, regular chest radiographs are probably not justified owing to the rarity of migration. The patient should, however, be warned about potential complications, and any change in the position of the foreign body should lead to the suspicion of possible migration and erosion into surrounding structures. If the change of position is associated with new symptoms such as cough, hemoptysis, chest pain, or recurrent bouts of infection, resection of the scar and foreign body should be considered.

Traumatic Asphyxia

In 1837, d'Angers described the syndrome of traumatic asphyxia on the basis of autopsy findings in 23 patients who had suffered thoracic compression as victims of a panic in Paris (Glinz, 1991). The term *traumatic asphyxia*, however, was introduced by Burrell and Crandon (1899) to designate the clinical picture of bluish-red discoloration of the head and neck caused by petechiae secondary to acute, severe compression of the chest, which produces a massive increase of intrathoracic pressure, resulting in increased central venous pressure (Glinz, 1991). Most patients survive the acute episode, and the syndrome gradually disappears. Late sequelae are rare, but lasting neurologic impairment (Sandfford and Sickler, 1974) or chronic vena cava thrombosis (Daughtry, 1980) has been reported. Because of this last potential problem, patients may benefit from long-term anticoagulation.

Thoracic Splenosis

Thoracic splenosis is a rare entity in which autotransplantation of splenic tissue occurs in the pleural cavity after combined splenic and diaphragmatic injury (Roucos et al, 1990). It was first reported by Shaw and Shafi (1937). Preoperative diagnosis of thoracic splenosis depends on a high index of suspicion in patients who have a mass or masses in the left hemithorax that on CT scan appear to be subpleural and scattered in the chest and who also have a history of thoracoabdominal trauma with splenectomy (Roucos et al, 1990). If the diagnosis of thoracic splenosis is well documented, surgery is usually unnecessary.

CONCLUSION

Late sequelae of thoracic trauma are rare, and most can be prevented by proper understanding and management of the initial injury. When they do occur, successful therapy depends on a complete evaluation of the problem before surgery is undertaken or other measures are employed that may lead to more damage. This is especially true in complicated problems related to sequelae of airway trauma, in which hurried surgery may lead to irreversible disabilities.

■ *KEY REFERENCES*

Hix WR: Residua of thoracic trauma. Surg Gynecol Obstet 158:295, 1984

Collective review summarizing all late sequelae of thoracic injuries. Good description of pathogenesis and principles of management.

Hix WR, Aaron BL: Residua of Thoracic Trauma. Mount Kisco, NY, Futura Publishing, 1987.

Excellent volume detailing all sequelae of thoracic injuries.

Maddaus MA, Toth JLR, Gullane PJ, Pearson FG: Subglottic tracheal resection and synchronous laryngeal reconstruction. J Thorac Cardiovasc Surg 104:1443, 1992.

Excellent review of indications for surgery, operative techniques, and results for patients with postintubation or post-traumatic laryngotracheal strictures.

■ *REFERENCES*

Abbott JA, Cousineau BS, Cheitlin M et al: Late sequelae of penetrating cardiac wounds. J Thorac Cardiovasc Surg 75:510, 1978.

Ahmed Z, Mohyuddin Z: Management of flail chest injury: Internal fixation versus endotracheal intubation and ventilation. J Thorac Cardiovasc Surg 110:1676, 1995.

Alfie M, Benmeir P, Caspi R et al: Costal osteomyelitis due to an electrical burn. Burns 21:147, 1995.

Andréassiam B, Lacombe M, Nussaume O et al: Ruptures de l'oesophage par traumatisme fermé. Ann Chir 12:409, 1973.

Antunes MJ, Fernandes LE, Oliveira JM: Ventricular septal defects and arteriovenous fistulas, with and without valvular lesions, resulting from penetrating injury to the heart and aorta. J Thorac Cardiovasc Surg 95:902, 1988.

Arom KV, Grover FL, Richardson JD, Trinkle JK: Post-traumatic empyema. Ann Thorac Surg 23:254, 1977.

Arom KV, Lyons GW: Traumatic pulmonary arteriovenous fistula. J Thorac Cardiovasc Surg 70:918, 1975.

Barrié J, Sarrazin R, Bonnett-Eymard J: Rupture traumatique de l'oesophage abdominal. Mem Acad 87:662, 1961.

Beal SL, Oreskovich MR: Long-term disability associated with flail chest injury. Am J Surg 150:324, 1985.

Berg EE: The sternal-rib complex. A possible fourth column in thoracic spine fractures. Spine 18:1916, 1993.

Blake S, Bonar S, O'Neill H et al: Aetiology of chronic constrictive pericarditis. Br Heart J 50:273, 1983.

Bogedain W: Migration of shrapnel from lung to bronchus. JAMA 251:1862, 1984.

Brown RB, Trenton J: Chronic abscesses and sinuses of the chest wall. Ann Surg 135:44, 1952.

Burrell HL, Crandon LRG: Traumatic apnea or asphyxia. Boston Med Surg J 51:599, 1899.

Carroll K, Cheeseman SH, Fink MP et al: Secondary infection of post-traumatic pulmonary cavitary lesions in adolescents and young adults: Role of computed tomography and operative débridement and drainage. J Trauma 29:109, 1989.

Cha EK, Mittal V, Allaben RD: Delayed sequelae of penetrating cardiac injury. Arch Surg 128:836, 1993.

Cheng SWK, Reilly LM, Nelken A et al: Neurogenic thoracic outlet decompression: Rationale for sparing the first rib. Cardiovasc Surg 3:617, 1995.

Childress ME, Grimes OF: Immediate and remote sequelae in traumatic diaphragmatic hernia. Surg Gynecol Obstet 113:573, 1961.

Cole FH, Miller MP, Jones CV: Transdiaphragmatic intercostal hernia. Ann Thorac Surg 41:565, 1986.

Coselli JS, Mattox KL, Beall AC Jr: Reevaluation of early evacuation of clotted hemothorax. Am J Surg 148:786, 1984.

Crnojevic LJ, Hogetts TJ, Chambers D, Partridge RJ: Bilateral traumatic chylothorax: A complication of a fracture of the thoracic spine. Injury 28:681, 1997.

Culiner MM, Roe BR, Grimes OF: The early elective surgical approach to the treatment of traumatic hemothorax. J Thorac Cardiovasc Surg 38:780, 1959.

d'Angers O: Relation medicale des événements survenus au Champde-Mars 14 juin 1837. Ann Hyg Publique Med Legale 18:485, 1837.

Daughtry DC: Thoracic Trauma. Boston, Little, Brown, 1980, p 198.

Dellon AL: The results of supraclavicular brachial plexus neurolysis (without first rib resection) in management of post-traumatic "thoracic outlet syndrome." J Reconstr Microsurg 9:11, 1993.

Desaulniers D, Bruneau L: Rupture traumatique de l'aorte thoracique. Union Med Can 101:1055, 1972.

Deslauriers J: Bronchial rupture. In Grillo HG, Eschapasse H (eds): Major Challenges. In International Trends in General Thoracic Surgery, Vol 2. St. Louis, CV Mosby, 1987, p 246.

Deslauriers J, Beaulieu M, Archambault G et al: Diagnosis and long-term follow-up of major bronchial disruptions due to nonpenetrating trauma. Ann Thorac Surg 33:32, 1981.

Deslauriers J, Bussières J: Bronchial rupture. In Grillo HC et al (eds): Current Therapy in Cardiothoracic Surgery. Philadelphia, BC Decker, 1989, p 42.

Deslauriers J, Desaulniers D, Pomerleau S, Sasseville N: Late sequelae of thoracic injuries. In Webb WR, Besson A (eds): Thoracic Surgery: Surgical Management of Chest Injuries, Vol 7. In International Trends in General Thoracic Surgery. St. Louis, CV Mosby, 1991, p 513.

Desrues B, Delaval P, Motreff C et al: Pneumatocèle et hémato-pneumatocèle post-traumatique du poumon. Rev Mal Resp 5:67, 1988.

Dowd MD, Krug S: Pediatric blunt cardiac injury: Epidemiology, clinical features, and diagnosis. J Trauma Injury Infect Crit Care 40:61, 1996.

Eddy AC, Luna GK, Copass M: Empyema thoracis in patients undergoing emergent closed tube thoracostomy for thoracic trauma. Am J Surg 157:494, 1989.

Escudero-Nafs FJ, Rabanal-Suarez F, Leiva-Oliva RM: Costal chondritis following very deep flame burns involving the chest wall. Burns 15:394, 1989.

Estrera AS, Landay MJ, McClelland RN: Blunt traumatic rupture of the right hemidiaphragm: Experience in 12 patients. Ann Thorac Surg 39:525, 1985.

Fagan CT: Traumatic lung cyst. AJR 97:186, 1966.

Fagan CT, Swischuk LE: Traumatic lung and paramediastinal pneumatoceles. Radiology 120:11, 1976.

Forty J, Wells FC: Traumatic intercostal pulmonary hernia. Ann Thorac Surg 49:670, 1990.

Francis DMA, Barnsley WC: Intercostal herniation of abdominal contents following a penetrating chest injury. Aust NZ J Surg 49:357, 1979.

Gibson LD, Carter R, Hinshaw DB: Surgical significance of sternal fracture. Surg Gynecol Obstet 144:443, 1962.

Glinz W: Acute thoracic compression syndrome-"traumatic asphyxia." In Webb WR, Besson A (eds): Thoracic Surgery: Surgical Management of Chest Injuries. In International Trends in General Thoracic Surgery, Vol 7. St. Louis, CV Mosby, 1991, p 344.

Goldstein S, Yu PN: Constrictive pericarditis after blunt chest trauma. Am Heart J 69:544, 1965.

Grieco JG, Montoya A, Sullivan HJ et al: Ventricular aneurysm due to blunt chest injury. Ann Thorac Surg 47:322, 1989.

Grillo HC, Moncure AC, McEnany MT: Repair of inflammatory tracheoesophageal fistula. Ann Thorac Surg 22:112, 1976.

Hanning CD, Ledingham E, Ledingham IM: Late respiratory sequelae of blunt chest injury: A preliminary report. Thorax 36:204, 1981.

Hiscoe B, Digman J: Types and incidence of lung hernias. J Thorac Cardiovasc Surg 30:335, 1955.

Hix WR: Residua of thoracic trauma. Surg Gynecol Obstet 158:295, 1984.

Hix WR, Aaron BL: Residua of Thoracic Trauma. Mount Kisco, NY, Futura Publishing, 1987.

Holland RH: Arteriovenous fistula of the left internal mammary vessels stimulating a patent ductus arteriosus. J Thorac Cardiovasc Surg 39:767, 1960.

Ikonomidis JS, Boulanger BR, Brenneman FD: Chylothorax after blunt chest trauma: A report of 2 cases. Can J Surg 40:135, 1997.

Ildstad ST, Tollerud DJ, Weiss RG et al: Cardiac contusion in pediatric patients with blunt thoracic trauma. J Pediatr Surg 25:287, 1990.

Ilie N: Functional effects of decortication after penetrating war injuries to the chest. J Thorac Cardiovasc Surg 111:967, 1996.

Jenson BP, Hoffman I, Follis FM: Surgical repair of atrial septal rupture due to blunt trauma. Ann Thorac Surg 56:1172, 1993.

Kato R, Horinouchi H, Maenaka Y: Traumatic pulmonary pseudocyst. J Thorac Cardiovasc Surg 97:309, 1989.

Kelly P, Webb WR, Moulder PV: Management of airway trauma. II: Combined injuries of the trachea and esophagus. Ann Thorac Surg 43:160, 1987.

Kerr A, Sauter D: Acquired traumatic pulmonary arteriovenous fistula: Case report. J Trauma 35:484–486, 1993.

Ketharanathan V, Westlake GW: Traumatic arteriovenous fistula between the internal thoracic artery and vein. Aust NZ J Surg 38:278, 1969.

Khan FA, Phillips W, Khan A, Seriff NS: Unusual unilateral blunt chest trauma without rib fractures leading to pulmonary laceration requiring pneumonectomy. Chest 66:211, 1974.

Kirklin JW, Barratt-Boyes BG: Cardiac Surgery. New York, Churchill Livingstone, 1993.

Kishikawa M, Yoshioka T, Shimazu T et al: Pulmonary contusion causes long-term respiratory dysfunction with decreased functional residual capacity. J Trauma 31:1203, 1991.

Klaase JM, Zimmerman KW, Veldhuis EF: Increased kyphosis by a combination of fractures of the sternum and thoracic spine. Eur Spine J 7:69, 1998.

Landercasper J, Cogbill TH, Lindesmith LA: Long-term disability after flail chest injury. J Trauma 24:410, 1984.

Lang-Lazdunski L, Mouroux J, Pons F et al: Role of videothoracoscopy in chest trauma. Ann Thorac Surg 63:327–333, 1997.

Larson S, Petterson G, Lepore V: Esophagocutaneous drainage to treat late and complicated esophageal perforation. Eur J Cardiothoracic Surg 5:579, 1991.

Layton TR, Dimarco RF, Pellegrini RV: Tracheoesophageal fistula from nonpenetrating trauma. J Trauma 20:802, 1980.

Livingston DH, Richardson JD: Pulmonary disability after severe blunt chest trauma. J Trauma 30:562, 1990.

Logeais Y, DeSaint Florent G, Danrigal A et al: Traumatic rupture of the right main bronchus in an 8 year old child successfully repaired 8 years after injury. Ann Surg 172:1039, 1970.

Lowe JE, Adams DH, Cummings RG et al: The natural history and recommended management of patients with traumatic coronary artery fistulas. Ann Thorac Surg 36:295, 1983.

Lynn RB, Iyengar R: Traumatic rupture of the bronchus. Chest 61:81, 1972.

Maddaus MA, Toth JLR, Gullane PJ, Pearson FG: Subglottic tracheal resection and synchronous laryngeal reconstruction. J Thorac Cardiovasc Surg 104:1443, 1992.

Mahaffey DE, Creech O, Boren HG, Debakey ME: Traumatic rupture of the left main bronchus successfully repaired eleven years after injury. J Thorac Surg 32:312, 1956.

Mansour KA, Clements JL, Hatcher CR et al: Diaphragmatic hernia caused by trauma: Experience with 35 cases. Am Surg 13:97, 1975.

Masuda T, Akiyama H, Kurosawa T, Ohwada T: Long-term follow-up of coronary artery dissection due to blunt chest trauma with spontaneous healing in a young woman. Intensive Care Med 22:450, 1996.

Mathisen DJ, Grillo H: Laryngotracheal trauma. Ann Thorac Surg 43:254, 1987.

Meleca MJ, Hoit BD: Previously unrecognized intrapericardial hematoma leading to refractory abdominal ascites. Chest 108:1747, 1995.

Milano S, Maroldi R, Vezzoli G et al: Chylothorax after blunt chest trauma: An unusual case with long latent period. Thorac Cardiovasc Surg 42:187, 1994.

Milfeld DJ, Mattox KL, Beall AC Jr: Early evacuation of clotted hemothorax. Am J Surg 136:686, 1978.

Miller DR, Murphy K, Cesario T: *Pseudomonas* infection of the sternum and costal cartilages. J Thorac Cardiovasc Surg 76:723, 1978.

Montebugnoli M, Borghi B, Bugamelli B: Salvage and reinfusion of chyle in closed chest injury. Int J Artif Organs 21:235, 1998.

Morel-Lavelle A: Hernies du poumon. Bull Soc Chir Paris 1:75, 1847.

Mouton W, Lardinois D, Furrer M, Regli B: Long-term follow-up of patients with operative stabilisation of a flail chest. Thorac Cardiovasc Surg 45:242, 1997.

Mulder DS, Greenwood AH, Brooks CE: Post-traumatic thoracic outlet syndrome. J Trauma 13:706, 1973.

Munnell ER: Herniation of the lung. Ann Thorac Surg 5:204, 1968.

Neef H: Post-traumatic and post-operative empyema. In Webb WR, Besson A (eds): Thoracic Surgery: Surgical Management of Chest Injuries. In International Trends in General Thoracic Surgery. St. Louis, CV Mosby, 1991, p 253.

Nieminen MM, Antila P, Markkula H, Karvonen J: Effect of decortication in fibrothorax on pulmonary function. J Respiration 48:94, 1985.

Niezgoda JA, McMenamin P, Graeber GM: Pharyngoesophageal perforation after blunt neck trauma. Ann Thorac Surg 50:615, 1990.

Nonoyama A, Masuda A, Kasahara K et al: Total rupture of the left main bronchus successfully repaired 9 years after injury. Ann Thorac Surg 21:445, 1976.

Ogilvie AG: Final results in traumatic haemothorax: A report of 230 cases. Thorax 5:116, 1950.

Özcelik C, Inci I, Özgen G, Eren N: Near-total esophageal exclusion in the treatment of late-diagnosed esophageal perforation. Scand J Cardiovasc Surg 28:91–93, 1994.

Payne WS, Cardoza F, Weed LA: Chronic draining sinuses of the chest wall. Surg Clin North Am 53:927, 1973.

Pearson FG, Brito-Filomeno L, Cooper JD: Experience with partial cricoid resection and thyrotracheal anastomosis. Ann Otol Rhinol Laryngol 95:582, 1986.

Pearson FG, Cooper JD, Nelems JM, Van Nostrand AWP: Primary tracheal anastomosis after resection of the cricoid cartilage with preservation of the recurrent laryngeal nerves. J Thorac Cardiovasc Surg 70:806, 1975.

Petty TL, Filley GF, Mitchell RS: Objective functional improvement by decortication after twenty years of artificial pneumothorax for pulmonary tuberculosis. Report of a case and review of the literature. Am Rev Respir Dis 84:572, 1961.

Pontius JG, Clagett OT, McDonald JR: Costal chondritis and perichondritis. Surgery 45:852, 1959.

Ravin CE, Walkersmith G, Lester PD et al: Post-traumatic pneumatocele on the inferior pulmonary ligament. Radiology 121:39, 1976.

Richardson JD, Grover FL, Trinkle JK: Early operative management of isolated sternal fractures. J Trauma 15:156, 1975.

Richardson JD, McElvein RB, Trinkle JK: First rib fracture: A hallmark of severe trauma. Ann Surg 181:251, 1975.

Roucos S, Tabet G, Jebara VA et al: Thoracic splenosis. Case report and literature review. J Thorac Cardiovasc Surg 99:361, 1990.

Rubino PJ, Milnes RF: Internal artery arteriovenous fistula. Int Surg 55:404, 1971.

Saibil A, Howard BA, McKee JD, Taylor G: Subcutaneous lymphocele following trauma to the thoracic duct. J Can Assoc Radiol 37:213, 1986.

Salter DG, Hapton DS: Traumatic intercostal hernia without penetrating injury in a child. Br J Surg 56:550, 1969.

Sandfford JA, Sickler D: Traumatic asphyxia with severe neurological sequelae. J Trauma 14:805, 1974.

Santos GH, Mahendra T: Traumatic pulmonary pseudocysts. Ann Thorac Surg 27:359, 1979.

Saw EC, Yokoyama T, Lee BC et al: Intercostal pulmonary hernia. Arch Surg 111:548, 1976.

Shaw AFB, Shafi A: Traumatic autoplastic transplantation of splenic tissue in man with observations on the late results of splenectomy in six cases. J Pathol 45:215, 1937.

Siebens AA, Storey CF, Newman MM et al: The physiologic effects of fibrothorax and the functional results of surgical treatment. J Thorac Cardiovasc Surg 32:53, 1956.

Sounders MS, Cropp AJ, Awad M: Spontaneous endobronchial erosion and expectoration of a retained intrathoracic bullet: Case report. J Trauma 33:909, 1992.

Sturaitis M, McCallum D, Cheung H et al: Lack of significant long-term sequelae following traumatic myocardial contusion. Arch Intern Med 146:1765, 1986.

Symbas PN: Cardiothoracic Trauma. Philadelphia, WB Saunders, 1989.

Symbas PN, Goldman M, Erbesfeld MH, Vlasis SE: Pulmonary arteriovenous fistula, pulmonary artery aneurysm and other vascular changes of the lung from penetrating trauma. Ann Surg 191:336, 1980.

Toso C, Robert J, Berney T et al: Thoracic outlet syndrome: Influence of personal history and surgical technique on long-term results. Eur J Cardiothorac Surg 16:44, 1999.

Ulstad DR, Bjelland JC, Quan SF: Bilateral para-mediastinal post-traumatic lung cysts. Chest 97:242, 1990.

Utley JR: Residua of trauma to the heart and great vessels. In Residua of Thoracic Trauma. Mount Kisco, NY, Futura Publishing, 1987, p 171.

Verdant A, Pagé A, Cossette R et al: Surgery of the descending thoracic aorta: Spinal cord protection with the Gott shunt. Ann Thorac Surg 46:147, 1988.

Villalba M, Lucas CE, Ledgerwood AM, Asfaw I: The etiology of post-traumatic empyema and the role of decortication. J Trauma 19:414, 1979.

Vogt-Moykopf I, Krumhar D: Treatment of intrapulmonary shell fragments. Surg Gynecol Obstet 123:1233, 1966.

Waldschmidt ML, Laws HL: Injuries of the diaphragm. J Trauma 20:587, 1980.

Webb WR, Burford TH: Studies of the reexpanded lung after prolonged atelectasis. Arch Surg 66:801, 1953.

Wilson JM, Boren CH, Peterson SR, Thomas AN: Traumatic hemothorax: Is decortication necessary? J Thorac Cardiovasc Surg 77:489, 1979.

Young D, Simon J, Pomerantz M: Current indications for and status of decortication for "trapped lung." Ann Thorac Surg 14:631, 1972.

INDEX

Note: Page numbers followed by f refer to figures; page numbers followed by t refer to tables; page numbers followed by b refer to text in boxes.

B

C

D

E

G

H

I

N

O

Q

R

S